OTHER EMERGENCIES

GENETIC DISEASES

NEOPLASTIC DISEASES

Harrison's

PRINCIPLES OF INTERNAL MEDICINE

EDITORS OF PREVIOUS EDITIONS

T. R. Harrison, Editor-in-Chief, Editions 1, 2, 3, 4, 5

W. R. Resnik, Editor, Editions 1, 2, 3, 4, 5

M. M. Wintrobe, Editor, Editions 1, 2, 3, 4, 5
Editor-in-Chief, Editions 6, 7

G. W. Thorn, Editor, Editions 1, 2, 3, 4, 5, 6, 7
Editor-in-Chief, Edition 8

R. D. Adams, Editor, Editions 2, 3, 4, 5, 6, 7, 8, 9

P. B. Beeson, Editor, Editions 1, 2

I. L. Bennett, Jr., Editor, Editions 3, 4, 5, 6

E. Braunwald, Editor, Editions 6, 7, 8, 9

K. J. Isselbacher, Editor, Editions 6, 7, 8
Editor-in-Chief, Edition 9

R. G. Petersdorf, Editor, Editions 6, 7, 8, 9

J. D. Wilson, Editor, Edition 9

Harrison's
PRINCIPLES OF INTERNAL MEDICINE
Tenth Edition

Editors

ROBERT G. PETERSDORF, A.B., M.D., M.A. (Hon), D.Sc. (Hon.) Professor of Medicine, Dean and Vice Chancellor, Health Sciences, University of California School of Medicine, San Diego, La Jolla

RAYMOND D. ADAMS, B.A., M.A., M.D., M.A. (Hon.), D.Sc. (Hon.), M.D. (Hon.) Bullard Professor of Neuropathology, Emeritus, Harvard Medical School; Consultant Neurologist and formerly Chief of Neurology Service, Massachusetts General Hospital; Director, Eunice K. Shriver Research Center, Boston; Médicin Adjoint, L'Hôpital Cantonale de Lausanne, Lausanne

EUGENE BRAUNWALD, M.D., M.A. (Hon.) Hersey Professor of the Theory and Practice of Physic and Hermann Ludwig Blumgart Professor of Medicine, Harvard Medical School; Chairman, Department of Medicine, Brigham and Women's and Beth Israel Hospitals, Boston

KURT J. ISSELBACHER, A.B., M.D. Mallinckrodt Professor of Medicine, Harvard Medical School; Physician and Chief, Gastrointestinal Unit, Massachusetts General Hospital, Boston

JOSEPH B. MARTIN, M.D., Ph.D., F.R.C.P.(C), M.A. (Hon.) Bullard Professor of Neurology, Harvard Medical School; Chief, Neurology Service, Massachusetts General Hospital, Boston

JEAN D. WILSON, M.D. Professor of Internal Medicine, The University of Texas Southwestern Medical School, Dallas

McGRAW-HILL BOOK COMPANY *New York St. Louis San Francisco Auckland Bogotá Guatemala Hamburg Johannesburg Lisbon London Madrid Mexico Montreal New Delhi Panama Paris San Juan São Paulo Singapore Sydney Tokyo Toronto*

NOTICE
Medicine is an ever-changing science. As new research and clinical experience broaden our knowledge, changes in treatment and drug therapy are required. The editors and the publisher of this work have made every effort to ensure that the drug dosage schedules herein are accurate and in accord with the standards accepted at the time of publication. Readers are advised, however, to check the product information sheet included in the package of each drug they plan to administer to be certain that changes have not been made in the recommended dose or in the contraindications for administration. This recommendation is of particular importance in regard to new or infrequently used drugs.

Harrison's
Principles of Internal Medicine

1234567890 DOW DOW 89876543

Foreign Editions
FRENCH (Ninth Edition)—Flammarion, © 1982
ITALIAN (Ninth Edition)—Piccin Editore, S.A.S., © 1983 (est.)
PORTUGUESE (Ninth Edition)—Editoria Guanabara Koogan, S.A., © 1983 (est.)
SPANISH (Eighth Edition)—La Prensa Medica Mexicana, © 1979
JAPANESE (Ninth Edition)—Hirokawa, © 1981
GREEK (Eighth Edition)—Parissianos, © 1979
INDONESIAN (Eighth Edition)—E.G.C., JL, © 1983 (est.)
GERMAN (Tenth Edition)—Schwabe and Company, Ltd., © 1983 (est.)

This book was set in Times Roman by Rocappi, Inc.
The editors were J. Dereck Jeffers and Moira Lerner.
The indexer was Philip James; the production supervisor was Jeanne Skahan.
R. R. Donnelley & Sons Company was printer and binder.

Library of Congress Cataloging in Publication Data
Main entry under title:

Harrison's principles of internal medicine.

Includes bibliographies and index.
1. Internal medicine. I. Petersdorf, Robert G.
II. Title: Principles of internal medicine.
RC46.H323 1983 616 82-23981
ISBN 0-07-049603-X (1-vol. ed.)
ISBN 0-07-079309-3 (2-vol. ed.)

A salute to Maxwell M. Wintrobe by the editors of Harrison's

This edition is dedicated to Professor Maxwell Wintrobe as an expression of gratitude for his contributions to *Harrison's* and to American medicine.

One of the founders of this book, along with Tinsley Harrison, George Thorn, William Resnik, and Paul Beeson, he inculcated his high standards of succinct and lucid exposition, gained through writing his own textbook, *Clinical Hematology*. More than any other of the early editors, he insisted on every chapter's being mercilessly criticized with complete objectivity and impartiality by peers of the contributor in another university department. This peer review method which he was instrumental in initiating continues to be used as a way of maintaining the standards of *Harrison's* to this day.

In the swift current of scientific progress it is easy to forget the people who make fundamental contributions. The current vogue is to cite only the most recent reference. Max Wintrobe, it will be remembered, in one of his first scientific endeavors, while still a PhD candidate, introduced a quantitative methodology for evaluating the volume, size, and hemoglobin content of red blood cells. These measurements became the basis for the classification of the anemias into macrocytic, microcytic, and hypochromic. He also standardized the measurement of the sedimentation rate by using tubes of a constant caliber, the Wintrobe tubes. Fundamental contributions to the role of trace elements in red blood cell metabolism, as well as the original studies of the effects of thiamine, pyridoxine, and pantothenic acid deficiencies, followed in rapid succession.

But the time and energy spent on these and innumerable other scientific works did not prevent or deter him from founding one of the fine medical schools and departments of medicine in the United States, at the University of Utah; guiding a generation of students to careers in scientific medicine; and giving his colleagues on *Harrison's* the benefits of his wise counsel and clinical experience over a period of nearly thirty years.

ABBREVIATED CONTENTS

CONTENTS

Functional abnormalities of the heart

Specific cardiac diseases

Section 2 Disorders of the vascular system

Section 3 Disorders of the respiratory system

Diagnostic methods

Lung disease caused by immunologic and environmental injury

Pulmonary infections

Diffuse lung disease

Vascular diseases of the lung

Other abnormalities of the respiratory tract

Section 12 Diseases of striated muscle

Section 13 Major psychiatric disorders

LIST OF CONTRIBUTORS

RAYMOND D. ADAMS, B.A., M.A., M.D., M.A. (Hon.), D.Sc. (Hon.), M.D. (Hon.)
Bullard Professor of Neuropathology, Emeritus, Harvard Medical School; Consultant Neurologist and formerly Chief of Neurology Service, Massachusetts General Hospital; Director, Eunice K. Shriver Research Center, Boston; Médicin Adjoint, L'Hôpital Cantonale de Lausanne, Lausanne

JOHN W. ADAMSON, M.D.
Professor of Medicine and Head, Division of Hematology, Department of Medicine, University of Washington School of Medicine, Seattle

RAYMOND ALEXANIAN, M.D.
Professor of Medicine, The University of Texas, M. D. Anderson Hospital and Tumor Institute, Houston

ELLIOT ALPERT, M.D.
Professor of Medicine and Chief of Gastroenterology, Baylor College of Medicine, Houston

JOSEPH S. ALPERT, M.D.
Professor of Medicine, University of Massachusetts Medical School; Director, Division of Cardiovascular Medicine, University of Massachusetts Medical Center, Worcester

RICHARD G. W. ANDERSON, Ph.D.
Professor of Cell Biology, The University of Texas Southwestern Medical School, Dallas

ROBERT J. ANDERSON, M.D.
Associate Professor of Medicine, Division of Renal Diseases, University of Colorado Medical Center, Denver

RONALD J. ANDERSON, M.D.
Assistant Professor of Medicine, Harvard Medical School; Director of Clinical Training, Division of Rheumatology and Immunology, Brigham and Women's Hospital, Boston

JACK P. ANTEL, M.D.
Associate Professor of Neurology, University of Chicago Hospitals and Clinics, Chicago

BARRY G. W. ARNASON, M.D.
Professor and Chairman, Department of Neurology, The University of Chicago and the Pritzker School of Medicine, Chicago

ARTHUR K. ASBURY, M.D.
Professor of Neurology, University of Pennsylvania School of Medicine; Chairman, Department of Neurology, Hospital of the University of Pennsylvania, Philadelphia

K. FRANK AUSTEN, M.D.
Theodore B. Bayles Professor of Medicine, Harvard Medical School; Chairman, Department of Rheumatology and Immunology, Brigham and Women's Hospital, Boston

ROBERT AUSTRIAN, M.D., D.Sc. (Hon.)
John Herr Musser Professor and Chairman, Department of Research Medicine, University of Pennsylvania School of Medicine, Philadelphia

BERNARD M. BABIOR, M.D.
Professor of Medicine, Tufts University School of Medicine, Division of Adult Hematology, New England Medical Center, Boston

JEFFREY P. BAKER, M.D., F.R.C.P. (C)
Assistant Professor of Medicine, University of Toronto; Consultant Staff Gastroenterologist, Toronto Western Hospital, Toronto

JOSEPH H. BATES, M.D.
Chief, Medical Service, Little Rock Veterans Administration Medical Center; Professor of Medicine and Microbiology, University of Arkansas College of Medicine, Little Rock

ROBERT A. BAUERNFEIND, M.D.
Assistant Professor of Medicine, University of Illinois College of Medicine; Director, Cardiac Electrophysiology Laboratory, University of Illinois Hospital, Chicago

HARRY N. BEATY, M.D.
Professor and Chairman, Department of Medicine, University of Vermont, Burlington

ARTHUR L. BEAUDET, M.D.
Professor of Pediatrics, Baylor College of Medicine, Houston

JOHN E. BENNETT, M.D.
Head, Clinical Mycology Section, LCI, National Institute of Allergy and Infectious Diseases, National Institutes of Health, Bethesda

EDWIN L. BIERMAN, M.D.
Professor of Medicine and Head, Division of Metabolism and Endocrinology, Department of Medicine, University of Washington School of Medicine, Seattle

ALAN L. BISNO, M.D.
Professor of Medicine and Chief, Division of Infectious Diseases, University of Tennessee Center for the Health Sciences, Memphis

JULIA C. BLEIER, M.N.S., R.D.
Research Nutritionist, Clinical Research Facility, Emory University School of Medicine, Atlanta

HENRY R. BOURNE, M.D.
Associate Professor of Medicine and Pharmacology and Chief, Division of Clinical Pharmacology, University of California, San Francisco

WALTER G. BRADLEY, M.D., F.R.C.P.
Professor and Chairman, Department of Neurology, University of Vermont College of Medicine and Medical Center Hospital of Vermont, Burlington

EUGENE BRAUNWALD, M.D., M.A. (Hon.)
Hersey Professor of the Theory and Practice of Physic and Hermann Ludwig Blumgart Professor of Medicine, Harvard Medical School; Chairman, Department of Medicine, Brigham and Women's and Beth Israel Hospitals, Boston

BARRY M. BRENNER, M.D., B.S., M.A. (Hon.)
Samuel A. Levine Professor of Medicine, Harvard Medical School; Senior Physician and Director, Renal Division, Brigham and Women's Hospital, Boston

MICHAEL S. BROWN, M.D.
Paul J. Thomas Professor, Department of Molecular Genetics, The University of Texas Southwestern Medical School, Dallas

THOMAS M. BUCHANAN, M.D.
Professor of Medicine and Pathobiology and Adjunct Professor of Microbiology and Immunology, University of Washington School of Medicine; Chief, Immunology Research Laboratory, Seattle Public Health Hospital, Seattle

H. FRANKLIN BUNN, M.D.
Professor of Medicine, Harvard Medical School; Senior Physician and Director, Hematology Research, Brigham and Women's Hospital; Investigator, Howard Hughes Medical Institute, Boston

GEORGE P. CANELLOS, M.D.
Associate Professor of Medicine, Harvard Medical School; Chief, Division of Medical Oncology, Sidney Farber Cancer Center; Senior Associate in Medicine, Brigham and Women's Hospital, Boston

CHARLES B. CARPENTER, M.D.
Professor of Medicine, Harvard Medical School; Physician, Brigham and Women's Hospital, Boston

CHARLES C. J. CARPENTER, M.D.
Professor and Chairman, Department of Medicine, Case Western Reserve University; Physician-in-Chief, University Hospitals of Cleveland, Cleveland

BRUCE R. CARR, M.D.
Assistant Professor, Department of Obstetrics and Gynecology and Cecil and Ida Green Center for Reproductive Biology Sciences, The University of Texas Southwestern Medical School, Dallas

WILLIAM A. CAUSEY, M.D.
Associate Professor of Medicine, University of Mississippi School of Medicine; Chief, Medical Service, Veterans Administration Medical Center, Jackson

KEITH H. CHIAPPA, M.D.
Assistant Professor of Neurology, Harvard Medical School; Director, EEG and Evoked Potentials Unit of the Clinical Neurophysiology Laboratory, Massachusetts General Hospital, Boston

BAYARD CLARKSON, M.D.
Chief of Hematology/Lymphoma Service, Memorial Sloan-Kettering Cancer Center; Professor of Medicine, Cornell University Medical College, New York

FREDRIC L. COE, M.D.
Professor of Medicine and Physiology, University of Chicago Pritzker School of Medicine; Director, Renal Division, Michael Reese Hospital and Medical Center, Chicago

ALAN S. COHEN, M.D.
Chief of Medicine and Director, Thorndike Memorial Laboratory, Boston City Hospital; Conrad Wesselhoeft Professor of Medicine, Boston University School of Medicine, Boston

PETER F. COHN, M.D.
Professor of Medicine and Chief, Cardiology Division, State University of New York, Health Sciences Center, New York

WILSON S. COLUCCI, M.D.
Assistant Professor of Medicine, Harvard Medical School; Associate Physician, Brigham and Women's Hospital, Boston

MAX D. COOPER, M.D.
Professor of Pediatrics and Microbiology, Department of Pediatrics, University of Alabama in Birmingham, The Medical Center, Birmingham

RICHARD A. COOPER, M.D.
Professor of Medicine and Chief, Hematology-Oncology Section, Hospital of the University of Pennsylvania, University of Pennsylvania School of Medicine, Philadelphia

LESTER G. CORDES, M.D.
Physician, Community Hospital of Los Gatos-Saratoga, Los Gatos, California

LAWRENCE COREY, M.D.
Associate Professor, Laboratory Medicine and Microbiology, and Adjunct Associate Professor, Medicine and Pediatrics, University of Washington School of Medicine; Head, Virology Division, Laboratory Medicine, Childrens Orthopedic Hospital, Seattle

NATHAN P. COUCH, M.D., F.A.C.S.
Associate Professor of Surgery, Harvard Medical School; Surgeon, Brigham and Women's Hospital, Boston

GEORGE W. COUNTS, M.D.
Associate Professor of Medicine, University of Washington; Chief, Infectious Diseases Division, Harborview Medical Center, Seattle

DAVID C. DALE, M.D.
Professor of Medicine and Dean, University of Washington School of Medicine, Seattle

JAMES E. DALEN, M.D.
Professor and Chairman, Department of Medicine, University of Massachusetts Medical School; Physician-in-Chief, University of Massachusetts Hospital, Worcester

JOHN R. DAVID, M.D.
John LaPorte Given Professor and Chairman, Department of Tropical Public Health, Harvard School of Public Health; Professor of Medicine, Harvard Medical School, Boston

CHANDLER R. DAWSON, M.D.
Professor of Ophthalmology and Associate Director, Francis I. Proctor Foundation for Research in Ophthalmology, University of California, San Francisco; Director, WHO Collaborating Center for Prevention of Blindness and Trachoma, San Francisco

CALVIN L. DAY, JR., M.D.
Chemosurgery Fellow, Chemosurgery Unit, New York University Medical Center, New York

G. ROBERT DELONG, M.D.
Assistant Professor of Neurology, Harvard Medical School; Associate Neurologist and Associate Pediatrician, Massachusetts General Hospital, Boston

VINCENT T. DeVITA, JR., M.D.
Director, National Cancer Institute, National Institutes of Health, Bethesda

MARC A. DICHTER, M.D., Ph.D.
Associate Professor of Neurology, Harvard Medical School; Associate Neurologist, Beth Israel Hospital and Children's Medical Center, Boston

JULES L. DIENSTAG, M.D.
Associate Professor of Medicine, Harvard Medical School; Assistant in Medicine, Gastrointestinal Unit, Massachusetts General Hospital, Boston

ROBERT G. DLUHY, M.D.
Associate Professor of Medicine, Harvard Medical School; Senior Associate in Medicine, Brigham and Women's Hospital, Boston

MURRAY J. FAVUS, M.D.
Associate Professor of Medicine, University of Chicago Pritzker School of Medicine, Michael Reese Hospital, Chicago

ALEXANDER FEFER, M.D.
Professor of Medicine, University of Washington School of Medicine; Head, Division of Oncology, University of Washington Hospital, Seattle

PHILIP J. FIALKOW, M.D.
Professor and Chairman, Department of Medicine and Professor of Genetics, University of Washington School of Medicine, Seattle

JORDAN N. FINK, M.D.
Professor of Medicine and Chief, Allergy Section, the Medical College of Wisconsin, The Medical College of Wisconsin Affiliated Hospitals, Milwaukee

ALFRED P. FISHMAN, M.D.
William Maul Measey Professor of Medicine and Director, Cardiovascular-Pulmonary Division, Hospital of the University of Pennsylvania, Philadelphia

THOMAS B. FITZPATRICK, M.D., Ph.D.
Edward Wigglesworth Professor and Chairman, Department of Dermatology, Harvard Medical School; Chief, Dermatology Service, Massachusetts General Hospital, Boston

DANIEL W. FOSTER, M.D.
Professor of Internal Medicine, The University of Texas Southwestern Medical School, Dallas

PAUL A. FRIEDMAN, M.D.
Associate Professor of Medicine and Director, Clinical Pharmacology, Harvard Medical School, Beth Israel Hospital, Boston

WILLIAM F. FRIEDMAN, M.D.
J. H. Nicholson Professor of Pediatrics and Chairman, Department of Pediatrics, University of California School of Medicine, UCLA Center for the Health Sciences, Los Angeles

PIERCE GARDNER, M.D.
Professor of Medicine and Pediatrics, Division of Biological Sciences, Department of Medicine, Pritzker School of Medicine, University of Chicago, Chicago

JAMES L. GERMAN III, M.D.
Professor (Genetics), Department of Pediatrics, Cornell University Medical College; Senior Investigator and Director, Laboratory of Human Genetics, The New York Blood Center, New York

ELOISE R. GIBLETT, M.D.
Research Professor of Medicine, University of Washington School of Medicine; Executive Director, Puget Sound Blood Center, Seattle

WILLIAM B. GILL, M.D., Ph.D.
Associate Professor of Surgery (Urology), The University of Chicago, Chicago

BRUCE C. GILLILAND, M.D.
Professor of Medicine and Laboratory Medicine and Director of Clinical Immunology Laboratory, University of Washington School of Medicine; Medical Director, Providence Medical Center, Seattle

RICHARD J. GLASSOCK, M.D.
Professor of Medicine, University of California School of Medicine, Los Angeles; Chairman, Department of Medicine, Harbor-UCLA Medical Center, Torrance

ROBERT M. GLICKMAN, M.D.
Samuel Bard Professor of Medicine, Columbia University College of Physicians and Surgeons; Director, Medical Service, Presbyterian Hospital, New York

STEPHEN E. GOLDFINGER, M.D.
Associate Professor of Medicine and Associate Dean of Continuing Education, Harvard Medical School; Physician, Gastrointestinal Unit, Massachusetts General Hospital, Boston

PAUL GOLDHABER, D.D.S.
Dean and Professor of Periodontology, Harvard School of Dental Medicine, Boston

JOSEPH L. GOLDSTEIN, M.D.
Paul J. Thomas Professor and Chairman, Department of Molecular Genetics, The University of Texas Southwestern Medical School, Dallas

HARVEY M. GOLOMB, M.D.
Associate Professor of Medicine and Chief, Section of Hematology/Oncology, Department of Medicine, Pritzker School of Medicine, University of Chicago, Chicago

RAJ K. GOYAL, M.D.
Mallinckrodt Professor of Medicine, Harvard Medical School; Chief, Division of Gastroenterology, Beth Israel Hospital, Boston

J. THOMAS GRAYSTON, M.D.
Vice President for Health Sciences and Professor of Epidemiology, School of Public Health and Community Medicine, University of Washington, Seattle

NORTON J. GREENBERGER, M.D.
Peter T. Bohan Professor and Chairman, Department of Medicine, University of Kansas School of Medicine, Kansas City

JAMES E. GRIFFIN, M.D.
Associate Professor of Internal Medicine, The University of Texas Southwestern Medical School, Dallas

RICHARD L. GUERRANT, M.D.
Professor of Medicine, Department of Medicine, University of Virginia Medical Center, Charlottesville

ELEANOR M. HACKETT
Treasurer of the Ladies Visiting Committee and Chairman of the Volunteer Patient Care Representatives Committee, Massachusetts General Hospital, Boston

THOMAS P. HACKETT, M.D.
Eben S. Draper Professor of Psychiatry, Harvard Medical School; Chief, Psychiatry Service, Massachusetts General Hospital, Boston

H. HUNTER HANDSFIELD, M.D.
Director, Sexually Transmitted Disease Control Program, Seattle-King County Department of Public Health; Associate Professor of Medicine, University of Washington School of Medicine, Seattle

JAMES P. HARNISCH, M.D.
Clinical Associate Professor, Department of Medicine, University of Washington School of Medicine, Seattle

DONALD H. HARTER, M.D.
Charles L. Mix Professor of Neurology and Chairman, Department of Neurology, Northwestern University Medical School; Chairman, Department of Neurology and Attending Neurologist, Northwestern Memorial Hospital, Chicago

HARLEY A. HAYNES, A.B., M.D.
Associate Professor of Dermatology, Harvard Medical School; Director, Dermatology Division, Brigham and Women's Hospital; Chief, Dermatology, West Roxbury Veterans Administration Hospital, Boston

WILLIAM R. HAZZARD, M.D.
Professor of Medicine, The Johns Hopkins University Medical Center; Associate Director, Department of Medicine, The Johns Hopkins Hospital, Baltimore

JANE E. HENNEY, M.D.
Deputy Director, National Cancer Institute, National Institutes of Health, Bethesda

JAN V. HIRSCHMANN, M.D.
Associate Professor of Medicine, University of Washington School of Medicine; Assistant Chief, Medical Service, Veterans Administration Medical Center, Seattle

FRED H. HOCHBERG, M.D.
Assistant Professor of Neurology, Harvard Medical School; Assistant Neurologist, Massachusetts General Hospital, Boston

PAUL D. HOEPRICH, M.D.
Professor of Medicine and Pathology, Division of Infectious and Immunologic Diseases, Department of Internal Medicine, School of Medicine, University of California, Davis

JOHN H. HOLBROOK, M.D.
Associate Professor of Medicine, Division of General Internal Medicine, Department of Medicine, University of Utah Medical Center, Salt Lake City

MICHAEL F. HOLICK, M.D., Ph.D.
Associate Professor of Medicine, Harvard Medical School; Associate Professor of Nutritional Biochemistry, Massachusetts Institute of Technology, Cambridge; Assistant in Medicine, Massachusetts General Hospital, Boston

NORMAN K. HOLLENBERG, M.D., Ph.D.
Professor and Director of Physiology Research, Department of Radiology, Harvard Medical School; Senior Associate in Medicine, Brigham and Women's Hospital, Boston

KING K. HOLMES, M.D., Ph.D.
Professor of Medicine, University of Washington School of Medicine; Head, Division of Infectious Diseases, Seattle Public Health Hospital, Seattle

EDWARD W. HOOK, M.D.
Mulholland Professor of Internal Medicine and Chairman, Department of Medicine, University of Virginia School of Medicine; Physician-in-Chief, University of Virginia Hospital, Charlottesville

EDWARD W. HOOK III, M.D.
Research Fellow in Medicine, Division of Infectious Diseases, University of Washington School of Medicine, Seattle

THOMAS H. HOSTETTER, M.D.
Assistant Professor of Medicine, University of Minnesota School of Medicine, Minneapolis

H. DAVID HUMES, M.D.
Associate Professor of Internal Medicine, University of Michigan; Chief of Nephrology, Veterans Administration Hospital, Ann Arbor

SIDNEY H. INGBAR, M.D.
William Bosworth Castle Professor of Medicine, Harvard Medical School; Director, Thorndike Laboratory, Beth Israel Hospital, Boston

ROLAND H. INGRAM, JR., M.D.
Parker B. Francis Professor of Medicine, Harvard Medical School; Director, Respiratory Division, Brigham and Women's Hospital, Beth Israel Hospital, Boston

ELI IPP, M.D.
Department of Endocrinology and Metabolism, Hadassah University Hospital, Jerusalem, Israel

KURT J. ISSELBACHER, A.B., M.D.
Mallinckrodt Professor of Medicine, Harvard Medical School; Physician and Chief, Gastrointestinal Unit, Massachusetts General Hospital, Boston

KHURSHEED N. JEEJEEBHOY, M.B.B.S., Ph.D., F.R.C.P. (Lond.), F.R.C.P. (Edin.), F.R.C.P. (C)
Professor of Medicine, University of Toronto; Director, Division of Gastroenterology, Toronto General Hospital, Toronto

JOSEPH E. JOHNSON III, M.D.
Professor and Chairman, Department of Medicine, Bowman Gray School of Medicine, Winston-Salem

ELAINE C. JONG, M.D.
Assistant Professor of Medicine, Division of Infectious Diseases, University of Washington School of Medicine, Seattle

CARLOS S. KASE, M.D.
Associate Professor of Neurology, University of South Alabama; Neurologist, South Alabama University Hospital, Mobile

SATISH KATHPALIA, M.D.
Assistant Professor of Medicine, University of Chicago Pritzker School of Medicine; Attending Physician, Renal Division, Department of Medicine, Michael Reese Hospital and Medical Center, Chicago

WILLIAM N. KELLEY, M.D.
Professor and Chairman, Department of Internal Medicine, University of Michigan Medical School, Ann Arbor

WILLIAM M. M. KIRBY, M.D.
Professor of Medicine, Division of Infectious Diseases, University of Washington School of Medicine, Seattle

VERNON KNIGHT, M.D.
Professor and Chairman, Department of Microbiology and Immunology, and Professor and Chief, Section on Infectious Diseases, Department of Medicine, Baylor College of Medicine; Senior Attending Physician, The Methodist Hospital, Houston

RAYMOND S. KOFF, M.D.
Professor of Medicine, Boston University School of Medicine; Chief, Hepatology Section, Boston University Medical Center and Veterans Administration Medical Center, Boston

PETER O. KOHLER, M.D.
Professor and Chairman, Department of Medicine, University of Arkansas Center for Medical Sciences; Chief, Medical Service, University Hospital, Little Rock

STEPHEN M. KRANE, M.D.
Professor of Medicine, Harvard Medical School; Physician and Chief, Arthritis Unit, Massachusetts General Hospital, Boston

HENRY M. KRONENBERG, M.D.
Assistant Professor of Medicine, Harvard Medical School; Chief, Endocrine Genetics Unit, Massachusetts General Hospital, Boston

J. THOMAS LaMONT, M.D.
Associate Professor of Medicine, Boston University Medical Center; Chief, Gastrointestinal Section, University Hospital, Boston

LEWIS LANDSBERG, M.D.
Associate Professor of Medicine, Harvard Medical School; Department of Medicine, Beth Israel Hospital, Boston

ALEXANDER R. LAWTON III, M.D.
Edward C. Stahlman Professor of Pediatric Physiology and Cell Metabolism, Professor of Pediatrics and Microbiology and Head, Division of Pediatric Immunology, Vanderbilt University School of Medicine, Nashville

J. MICHAEL LAZARUS, M.D.
Associate Professor of Medicine, Harvard Medical School, Brigham and Women's Hospital, Boston

A. MARTIN LERNER, M.D.
Professor of Medicine and Head, Division of Infectious Diseases, Department of Medicine, Wayne State University School of Medicine; Chief, Department of Medicine, Hutzel Hospital, Detroit

NORMAN G. LEVINSKY, M.D.
Wade Professor and Chairman, Division of Medicine, Boston University School of Medicine; Physician-in-Chief and Director, Evans Memorial Department of Clinical Research, Boston

RICHARD M. LOCKSLEY, M.D.
Senior Fellow, Department of Medicine, University of Washington School of Medicine, Seattle

WALTER C. MacDONALD, M.D.
Professor of Medicine and Head of Gastroenterology, University of British Columbia, Vancouver

HENRY J. MANKIN, M.D.
Edith M. Ashley Professor of Orthopedic Surgery, Harvard Medical School; Orthopedist-in-Chief, Massachusetts General Hospital, Boston

MART MANNIK, M.D.
Professor of Medicine, Adjunct Professor of Microbiology and Immunology and Head, Division of Rheumatology, Department of Medicine, University of Washington School of Medicine, Seattle

JOSEPH B. MARTIN, M.D., Ph.D.
Bullard Professor of Neurology, Harvard Medical School; Chief, Neurology Service, Massachusetts General Hospital, Boston

ROGER J. MAY, M.D.
Instructor of Medicine, Harvard Medical School; Clinical Assistant in Medicine, Gastrointestinal Unit, Massachusetts General Hospital, Boston

E. R. McFADDEN, JR., M.D.
Associate Professor of Medicine, Harvard Medical School; Physician, Brigham and Women's Hospital, Boston

J. DENIS McGARRY, Ph.D.
Professor of Internal Medicine and Biochemistry, The University of Texas Southwestern Medical School, Dallas

JAMES E. McGUIGAN, M.D.
Professor and Chairman, Department of Medicine, University of Florida College of Medicine, Gainesville

RIMA McLEOD, M.D.
Assistant Professor of Medicine, University of Chicago Pritzker School of Medicine; Attending Physician, Michael Reese Hospital and Medical Center, Chicago

MARK S. McPHEE, M.D.
Assistant Professor of Medicine, University of Kansas Medical Center, College of Health Sciences, Kansas City

NANCY K. MELLO, Ph.D.
Professor of Psychology, Department of Psychiatry, Harvard Medical School; Associate Director, Alcohol and Drug Abuse Research Center, McLean Hospital, Boston

JACK H. MENDELSON, M.D.
Professor of Psychiatry, Harvard Medical School; Director, Alcohol and Drug Abuse Research Center, McLean Hospital, Boston

URS A. MEYER, M.D.
Professor of Clinical Pharmacology, Department of Internal Medicine, University of Zürich Hospital, Zürich, Switzerland

JOEL D. MEYERS, M.D.
Associate Professor of Medicine, Division of Infectious Diseases, University of Washington School of Medicine; Head, Program in Infectious Diseases and Clinical Virology, Fred Hutchinson Cancer Research Center, Seattle

MARTIN C. MIHM, JR., M.D.
Associate Professor of Pathology, Harvard Medical School; Associate Pathologist and Dermatologist, Massachusetts General Hospital, Boston

EDGAR L. MILFORD, M.D.
Instructor in Medicine, Harvard Medical School; Associate Physician, Brigham and Women's Hospital, Boston

MYRON MILLER, M.D.
Professor of Medicine, State University of New York Upstate Medical Center; Chief of Medical Service, Veterans Administration Medical Center, Syracuse

JOHN D. MINNA, M.D.
Chief, NCI-Navy Medical Oncology Branch; Professor of Medicine, Uniformed Services University of the Health Sciences, National Cancer Institute, National Institutes of Health, National Medical Center, Bethesda

BEVERLY S. MITCHELL, M.D.
Associate Professor of Internal Medicine, University of Michigan Medical School, Ann Arbor

JAY P. MOHR, M.D.
Professor of Neurology, University of South Alabama; Chief, Neurology Service, South Alabama University Hospital, Mobile

KENNETH M. MOSER, M.D.
Professor of Medicine, University of California School of Medicine; Director, Pulmonary and Critical Care Division, University of California Medical Center, San Diego

ARNOLD M. MOSES, M.D.
Professor of Medicine and Director, Clinical Research Center, State University of New York Upstate Medical Center; Chief, Endocrinology, Veterans Administration Medical Center, Syracuse

DAVID B. MOSHER, M.D.
Clinical Instructor in Dermatology, Harvard Medical School; Assistant in Dermatology, Massachusetts General Hospital, Boston

JOHN F. MURRAY, M.D.
Professor of Medicine, University of California School of Medicine; Chief, The Chest Service, San Francisco General Hospital, San Francisco

ROBERT J. MYERBURG, M.D.
Professor of Medicine and Physiology and Director, Division of Cardiology, University of Miami School of Medicine, Miami

JAMES C. NIEDERMAN, M.D., D.Sc. (Hon.)
Clinical Professor of Epidemiology and Medicine, Yale University School of Medicine, New Haven

HYMIE L. NOSSEL, M.D.
Professor of Medicine, College of Physicians and Surgeons, Columbia University; Attending Physician, Presbyterian Hospital, New York

JOHN A. OATES, M.D.
The Joe and Morris Werthan Professor of Investigative Medicine, Departments of Medicine and Pharmacology, Vanderbilt University School of Medicine, Nashville

JERROLD M. OLEFSKY, M.D.
Professor of Medicine and Head, Division of Endocrinology and Metabolism, University of Colorado Medical Center, Denver

ROBERT A. O'ROURKE, M.D.
Charles Conrad and Anna Sahm Brown Professor of Medicine and Director, Cardiology Division, University of Texas Health Science Center, San Antonio

JOHN A. PARRISH, M.D.
Associate Professor of Dermatology, Harvard Medical School; Assistant Dermatologist, Massachusetts General Hospital, Boston

A. WILLIAM PASCULLE, D.Sc.
Assistant Professor of Pathology, University of Pittsburgh School of Medicine; Assistant Director of Microbiology, Presbyterian-University Hospital, Pittsburgh

MADHUKAR A. PATHAK, M.B., Ph.D.
Senior Associate in Dermatology, Harvard Medical School; Biochemist, Massachusetts General Hospital, Boston

LAWRENCE L. PELLETIER, JR., M.D.
Professor of Internal Medicine, University of Kansas School of Medicine-Wichita; Chief, Medical Service, Wichita Veterans Administration Medical Center, Wichita

PETER L. PERINE, M.D., M.P.H.
Associate Professor of Epidemiology; Adjunct Associate Professor of Pathobiology, School of Public Health and Community Medicine, University of Washington, Seattle

ROBERT G. PETERSDORF, A.B., M.D., M.A. (Hon.), D.Sc. (Hon.)
Professor of Medicine and Dean, School of Medicine; Vice Chancellor for Health Sciences, University of California School of Medicine, San Diego

KIRK L. PETERSON, M.D.
Professor of Medicine, University of California School of Medicine; Director, Cardiac Catheterization Laboratory, University of California Medical Center, San Diego

JAMES J. PLORDE, M.D.
Professor of Medicine and Laboratory Medicine, University of Washington School of Medicine; Chief, Infectious Disease Section, and Chief, Clinical Microbiology Section, Veterans Administration Medical Center, Seattle

DANIEL K. PODOLSKY, M.D.
Assistant Professor of Medicine, Harvard Medical School; Assistant in Medicine, Gastrointestinal Unit, Massachusetts General Hospital, Boston

DAVID C. POSKANZER, M.D.
Formerly Associate Professor of Neurology, Harvard Medical School; formerly Associate Neurologist, Massachusetts General Hospital, Boston

JOHN T. POTTS, JR., M.D.
Jackson Professor of Clinical Medicine, Harvard Medical School; Chief of the General Medical Service, Massachusetts General Hospital, Boston

LAWRIE W. POWELL, M.D.
Professor of Medicine, University of Queensland; Physician, Royal Brisbane Hospital, Brisbane, Queensland, Australia

PAUL G. RAMSEY, M.D.
Assistant Professor, Department of Medicine, University of Washington School of Medicine, Seattle

C. GEORGE RAY, M.D.
Professor of Pathology and Pediatrics, University of Arizona College of Medicine, Tucson

JEAN J. REBEIZ, M.D.
Professor of Neuropathology, American University of Beirut; Neurologist and Neuropathologist, American University Hospital, Beirut

PETER REICH, M.D.
Associate Professor of Psychiatry, Harvard Medical School; Chief of Psychiatry, Brigham and Women's Hospital, Boston

JACK S. REMINGTON, M.D.
Professor of Medicine, Division of Infectious Diseases, Department of Medicine, Stanford University School of Medicine; Chairman, Department of Immunology and Infectious Diseases, Research Institute, Palo Alto Medical Foundation, Palo Alto

EDWARD P. RICHARDSON, JR., M.D.
Professor of Neuropathology, Harvard Medical School; Neuropathologist, Massachusetts General Hospital, Boston

JAMES M. RICHTER, M.D.
Instructor in Medicine, Harvard Medical School; Assistant in Medicine, Massachusetts General Hospital, Boston

R. PAUL ROBERTSON, M.D.
Professor of Medicine and Director, Division of Clinical Pharmacology, University of Washington School of Medicine, Seattle

ALLAN R. RONALD, M.D.
Professor of Medicine and Medical Microbiology and Chairman, Department of Medical Microbiology, The University of Manitoba; Director, Department of Clinical Microbiology, Health Sciences Centre, Winnipeg, Manitoba

ALLAN H. ROPPER, M.D.
Assistant Professor of Neurology, Harvard Medical School; Assistant Neurologist and Director, Neurology/Neurosurgery Intensive Care Unit, Massachusetts General Hospital, Boston

KENNETH M. ROSEN, M.D. (deceased)
Chief, Cardiology Section; Professor of Medicine and Physiology, University of Illinois College of Medicine, Chicago

LEON E. ROSENBERG, M.D.
Professor of Human Genetics, Medicine and Pediatrics, and Chairman, Department of Human Genetics, Yale University School of Medicine; Attending Physician, Yale-New Haven Hospital, New Haven

JOHN ROSS, JR., M.D.
Professor of Medicine and Chief, Cardiovascular Division, Department of Medicine, University of California School of Medicine, University of California Medical Center, San Diego

ARTHUR H. RUBENSTEIN, M.D.
Professor and Chairman, Department of Medicine, Pritzker School of Medicine, The University of Chicago Medical Center, Chicago

CYRUS E. RUBIN, M.D.
Professor of Medicine, Division of Gastroenterology, University of Washington School of Medicine, Seattle

DANIEL RUDMAN, M.D.
Professor of Medicine and Surgery and Director, Clinical Research Facility, Emory University School of Medicine, Atlanta

ARTHUR I. SAGALOWSKY, M.D.
Assistant Professor of Surgery, Division of Urology, The University of Texas Southwestern Medical School, Dallas

MARIA SALAM-ADAMS, M.D.
Assistant Professor of Neurology, Harvard Medical School; Clinical and Research Fellow in Children's Neurology, Massachusetts General Hospital, Boston

MERLE A. SANDE, M.D.
Professor of Medicine and Vice Chairman, Department of Medicine, University of California, San Francisco; Chief of Medical Services, San Francisco General Hospital, San Francisco

JAY P. SANFORD, M.D.
Professor of Medicine and President, Uniformed Services University of the Health Sciences; Dean, School of Medicine, Bethesda

DENNIS SCHABERG, M.D.
Assistant Professor of Medicine, University of Michigan School of Medicine, Ann Arbor

ANDREW I. SCHAFER, M.D.
Assistant Professor of Medicine, Harvard Medical School and Brigham and Women's Hospital, Boston

I. HERBERT SCHEINBERG, M.D.
Professor of Medicine and Head, Division of Genetic Medicine, Albert Einstein College of Medicine; Attending Physician, Hospital of the Albert Einstein College of Medicine, New York

ALAN L. SCHILLER, A.B., M.D.
Associate Professor of Pathology, Harvard Medical School; Associate Pathologist and Chief, Autopsy Pathology and Bone Laboratory, Massachusetts General Hospital, Boston

R. NEIL SCHIMKE, M.D.
Professor of Internal Medicine and Director, Division of Metabolism, Endocrinology and Genetics, The University of Kansas College of Health Sciences, Kansas City

ROBERT W. SCHRIER, M.D.
Professor and Chairman, Department of Medicine, University of Colorado School of Medicine, University Hospital, Denver

CHARLES C. SHEPARD, M.D.
Chief, Leprosy Laboratory, Centers for Disease Control; Adjunct Professor of Microbiology, Emory University School of Medicine, Atlanta

LOUIS M. SHERWOOD, M.D.
Baumritter Professor and Chairman, Department of Medicine, Albert Einstein College of Medicine, New York

ELIZABETH M. SHORT, M.D.
Assistant Professor of Medicine and Associate Dean, Stanford University School of Medicine; Attending Physician, Stanford University Medical Center, Stanford

HARRY SHWACHMAN, M.D.
Professor of Pediatrics, Harvard Medical School; Senior Associate in Medicine and Chief, Clinical Nutrition Division, Children's Hospital Medical Center, Boston

WILLIAM SILEN, M.D.
Johnson and Johnson Professor of Surgery, Harvard Medical School; Surgeon-in-Chief, Beth Israel Hospital, Boston

FRED E. SILVERSTEIN, M.D.
Clinical Associate Professor of Medicine, University of Washington School of Medicine, Seattle; Senior Director, Strategic Development Squibb Medical System Group, Bellevue

DAVID H. SMITH, M.D.
Professor and Chairman, Department of Pediatrics, University of Rochester School of Medicine and Dentistry, Rochester

BURTON E. SOBEL, M.D.
Professor of Medicine, Washington University; Director, Cardiovascular Division; Cardiologist-in-Chief, Barnes Hospital, St. Louis

ARTHUR J. SOBER, M.D.
Assistant Professor of Dermatology, Harvard Medical School; Assistant Dermatologist, Massachusetts General Hospital, Boston

FRANK E. SPEIZER, M.D.
Associate Professor of Medicine, Harvard Medical School; Director, Occupational and Environmental Health Center, Brigham and Women's Hospital, Boston

WALTER E. STAMM, M.D.
Associate Professor of Medicine and Epidemiology, University of Washington, Harborview Medical Center, Seattle

WILLIAM W. STEAD, M.D.
Professor of Medicine, University of Arkansas Center for the Health Sciences; Director, Tuberculosis Program, Arkansas Department of Health, Little Rock

GENE H. STOLLERMAN, M.D.
Professor of Medicine, Boston University School of Medicine; Attending Physician, University Hospital, Boston

D. EUGENE STRANDNESS, JR., M.D.
Professor of Surgery, University of Washington School of Medicine and University Hospital, Seattle

DAVID H. P. STREETEN, M.D., D. Phil., F.R.C.P.
Professor of Medicine and Head, Section of Endocrinology, State University of New York Upstate Medical Center, Syracuse

STEVEN S. SWIRYN, M.D.
Assistant Professor of Medicine, University of Illinois College of Medicine; Director, Electrocardiography Laboratory; Attending Physician, University of Illinois Hospital, Chicago

E. DONNALL THOMAS, M.D.
Professor of Medicine and Head, Division of Oncology, University of Washington School of Medicine; Associate Director for Clinical Research, Fred Hutchinson Cancer Research Center, Seattle

GENNARO M. TISI, M.D.
Associate Professor of Medicine, University of California School of Medicine; Chief, Pulmonary Section, Veterans Administration Medical Center, San Diego

PHILLIP P. TOSKES, M.D.
Professor of Medicine and Director, Division of Gastroenterology and Nutrition, University of Florida College of Medicine and Veterans Administration Medical Center, Gainesville

MARVIN TURCK, M.D.
Professor of Medicine, University of Washington School of Medicine; Medical Director, Harborview Medical Center, Seattle

DAVID D. ULMER, M.D.
Professor and Chairman, Department of Medicine, Charles R. Drew Postgraduate Medical School; Physician, Martin Luther King Hospital, Los Angeles

JOHN E. ULTMANN, M.D.
Professor of Medicine, Section of Hematology/Oncology, Department of Medicine; Director, University of Chicago Cancer Research Center; Associate Dean for Research Programs, Biological Sciences Division, Pritzker School of Medicine, University of Chicago, Chicago

ROGER H. UNGER, M.D.
Professor of Internal Medicine, The University of Texas Southwestern Medical School; Senior Medical Investigator, Dallas Veterans Administration Medical Center, Dallas

HENRI VANDER EECKEN, H.M., M.D.
Professor of Neurology, Faculty of Medicine, University of Ghent; Head of the Department of Neurology, Akademisch Zeikenhuis, Ghent

MAURICE VICTOR, M.D.
Professor of Neurology, Case Western Reserve University School of Medicine; Director, Neurology Service, Cleveland Metropolitan General Hospital, Cleveland

JAMES F. WALLACE, M.D.
Professor of Medicine, University of Washington School of Medicine; Associate Physician-in-Chief, University of Washington Hospital, Seattle

PATRICK C. WALSH, M.D.
David Hall McConnell Professor and Director, Department of Urology, The Johns Hopkins University School of Medicine; Urologist-in-Chief, James Buchanan Brady Urological Institute, The Johns Hopkins Hospital, Baltimore

JACK R. WANDS, M.D.
Associate Professor of Medicine, Harvard Medical School; Assistant Physician, Gastrointestinal Unit, Massachusetts General Hospital, Boston

LOUIS WEINSTEIN, M.D., Ph.D., Sc.D. (Hon.)
Visiting Professor of Medicine, Harvard Medical School; Physician and Director of Clinical Services, Infectious Diseases Division, Brigham and Women's Hospital, Boston

JOHN B. WEST, M.D., Ph.D., D.Sc., F.R.A.C.P., M.R.C.P.
Professor of Medicine and Physiology, University of California School of Medicine; Physician, University of California Medical Center, San Diego

GRANT R. WILKINSON, M.D., Ph.D.
Professor of Pharmacology, Vanderbilt University School of Medicine, Nashville

GORDON H. WILLIAMS, M.D.
Associate Professor of Medicine, Harvard Medical School; Senior Associate in Medicine and Director, Endocrine Unit, Brigham and Women's Hospital, Boston

JEAN D. WILSON, M.D.
Professor of Internal Medicine, The University of Texas Southwestern Medical School, Dallas

RICHARD H. WINTERBAUER, M.D.
Head, Section of Chest and Infectious Diseases, The Mason Clinic, Seattle

KENNETH A. WOEBER, M.D.
Professor and Vice-Chairman, Department of Medicine, University of California, San Francisco; Chief of Medicine, Mount Zion Hospital and Medical Center, San Francisco

SHELDON M. WOLFF, M.D.
Endicott Professor and Chairman, Department of Medicine, Tufts University School of Medicine; Physician-in-Chief, New England Medical Center, Boston

ALASTAIR J. J. WOOD, M.D., M.B., Ch.B., M.R.C.P.
Assistant Professor of Medicine and Pharmacology, Vanderbilt University School of Medicine; Attending Physician, Vanderbilt University Hospital, Nashville

THEODORE E. WOODWARD, M.D., M.A.C.P.
Professor of Medicine, University of Maryland School of Medicine and Hospital, Baltimore

RICHARD J. WURTMAN, M.D.
Professor of Endocrinology and Metabolism and Director, Laboratory of Neuroendocrine Regulation, Massachusetts Institute of Technology; Clinical Associate in Medicine, Massachusetts General Hospital, Boston

JOSHUA WYNNE, M.D.
Assistant Professor of Medicine, Harvard Medical School; Director, Noninvasive Cardiac Laboratory, Brigham and Women's Hospital, Boston

JAMES B. YOUNG, M.D.
Assistant Professor of Medicine, Harvard Medical School; Department of Medicine, Beth Israel Hospital, Boston

ROBERT R. YOUNG, M.D.
Associate Professor of Neurology, Harvard Medical School; Neurologist and Director, Clinical Neurophysiology Laboratory, Massachusetts General Hospital, Boston

PREFACE

This is the Tenth Edition of *Harrison's Principles of Internal Medicine* to appear in the short span of thirty-three years. As has been the case with previous editions, the editors have attempted to incorporate into this edition the latest advances in pathophysiology, diagnosis, and treatment. The attempt has been made, where possible, to build a bridge between basic science and clinical medicine and to emphasize the advances in biomedicine while retaining those facts which, while not new, remain clinically useful.

In adherence to the principles of those who founded the book, the section dealing with the cardinal manifestations of disease remains a mainstay of this edition. Its 56 chapters form a comprehensive introduction to clinical medicine. The next part deals with disorders that affect multiple organs and includes genetics, clinical immunology, clinical pharmacology, neoplasia, and, in this edition for the first time, the biology and diseases of aging. These multisystem disorders are then followed by a predominantly etiologically oriented section on infections and the traditional discussion of diseases of the major organ systems.

Despite their efforts to present as much new material in this edition as possible, the amount of information that is coming to the fore exceeds the editors' abilities to keep within the confines of one volume. Therefore, following publication of the ninth edition, the editors and the publisher embarked on a new venture and have published four volumes entitled *Updates to Harrison's Principles of Internal Medicine* (Volumes I through IV). Each of these volumes contains between 15 and 18 articles, written by an expert in the field but not necessarily the author of the article in the ninth or tenth editions. The subject matter, which varies widely, was chosen to augment discussion of the same subject in the ninth edition or consists of important new topics in which there have been exciting advances since the publication of the ninth edition. These *Updates* complement the *Harrison* textbook in every sense of the word. Cognizant of the continued requirements for continuing education for licensure and relicensure, as well as the emphasis on certification and recertification, the editors and the publisher have embarked on two efforts to help the reader stay abreast of the broad field of internal medicine. The *PreTest Self-Assessment and Review* to accompany the ninth edition of *Principles of Internal Medicine* appeared shortly after the ninth edition, and a radically revised version will appear simultaneously with the tenth edition. *PreTest Self-Assessment and Review* consists of several hundred questions based upon the textbook, along with answers and explanations for the answers. A CME examination multiple-choice test which may be taken for CME credit is an optional companion to the *PreTest*. Some months after the appearance of *PreTest*, a self-assessment examination book dealing with patient management problems was published under the editorial guidance of Dr. Alfred J. Bollet. These patient management problems also refer to *Principles of Internal Medicine*.

This quadripartite effort—*Principles of Internal Medicine*, the four *Updates*, and the two examination books—represents a continuous learning system and reflects the editors' conviction that medicine is an ever-changing science and that multiple modalities of presenting new information and learning are essential if physicians want to keep up with the rapid changes in their field.

The tenth edition also pays close attention to updated and current references. Although space constraints require that references be kept to a modest number, the editors have made particular efforts to include papers that were published in 1981, 1982, and even 1983. Although this has required omission of some important older papers, these almost always appear in the bibliographies of the newer ones. The reverse is, of course, not the case and, hence, our effort to keep the references up-to-date.

Although we cannot highlight in this short preface all of the new and extensively updated parts of the tenth edition, we would like to call the reader's attention to some.

- In the section on gastroenterology, the chapters on dysphagia and diseases of the esophagus have been completely revised; there is an entirely new and comprehensive chapter on inflammatory bowel disease; the chapter dealing with diseases of the gallbladder and biliary tract is entirely new; the diagnosis, prevention, and treatment of viral hepatitis have been completely updated in line with newer advances in the field; the chapter on diseases of the pancreas has been revised to take into account the current state of imaging procedures, endoscopy, and serologic tests in the diagnosis of acute and chronic pancreatitis, as well as cancer of the pancreas; and the chapters on absorption and malabsorption have been completely revised.
- The section on metabolic pathways has been changed to emphasize the clinical relevance of the cyclic AMP system, the prostaglandins, the endorphins, and cell surface phagocytosis. In the expanded genetic section, there are new chapters on the HLA system and an essay on the implications of recombinant DNA technology for medicine. There are major new chapters on ovarian disorders, nutritional therapy, disturbances in glycogen metabolism, and pheochromocytoma. There is a totally new chapter on the autonomic nervous system, resulting from an appreciation of the importance of the autonomic nervous system in a wide variety of disease states and in understanding the responses to a variety of drugs.
- One of the spectacular advances in clinical cardiology has been the application of electrophysiologic techniques to the study of arrhythmias. Two new chapters on the brady- and tachyarrhythmias, respectively, emphasize this new approach. Cardiac surgery is playing an increasingly important role in the management of cardiac diseases and its role is emphasized in the chapters on arrhythmias, congenital heart disease, valvular heart disease, infective endocarditis, coronary heart disease, acute myocardial infarction, cardiac tumors, and pericardial disease.
- Hypersensitivity pneumonitis and environmental air pollution have been increasingly recognized in the production of interstitial lung disease, and these two topics have been emphasized in two important new chapters by new authors. Likewise, the emergence of the adult respiratory distress syndrome (ARDS) as the major cause of death in a variety of medical and surgical illnesses is now recognized, and a new chapter on this syndrome has been included.
- The section on disorders of the nervous system includes completely new chapters on coma, epilepsy, multiple sclerosis, and sleep and its abnormalities. A new chapter on commonly abused drugs has been added. New chapters on psychiatry, including the neuroses, manic-depressive psy-

choses, and schizophrenia have been included. Extensive revisions have also been made in the chapters on faintness, syncope and seizures, abnormalities in movement and posture, and traumatic diseases of the brain. The chapter on diagnostic methods has been extensively updated to include a consideration of evoked potentials and of nuclear magnetic resonance.

• The last three or four years have seen exciting developments in infectious disease. Following the discovery of *Legionella,* a number of other new as well as previously described agents were shown to cause pneumonia. These are summarized in a new chapter. The toxic-shock syndrome and the acquired immune deficiency syndrome (AIDS) in homosexuals represent two exciting developments in human biology which have been included in the tenth edition.

One of the strengths of this textbook is the close-knit character of the editors. But just as medicine progresses, the old guard must give way to the new. With the tenth edition, Dr. Raymond D. Adams, who was the editor of the section on neurology from the second through the tenth editions—giving him more seniority than any other editor who has ever been with the book—is retiring as editor. We are fortunate to welcome as a new editor Dr. Joseph B. Martin, Neurologist-in-Chief at Massachusetts General Hospital and Professor of Neurology at Harvard Medical School, as Dr. Adams's successor. In order to ensure a smooth transition, Drs. Martin and Adams worked together on the Neurology Section of the tenth edition. The editors are grateful to Ray Adams for the continuing high quality that he has given to the section on neurological medicine; more importantly, he has been a valuable critic, a wise counselor, and a warm friend. While we shall miss him as an active editor, we consider ourselves fortunate in having attracted an outstanding academic neurologist like Joseph Martin to the editorial board.

We also wish to express our appreciation to our many associates and colleagues who, as experts in their fields, have helped us with constructive and valuable criticisms of the chapters in the tenth edition. We wish to thank the following for many helpful suggestions: Drs. Elliott Antman, David W. Bilheimer, Kurt J. Bloch, Neil Breslau, H. Franklin Bunn, George Canellos, Norman Carter, Jack L. Clausen, Wayne E. Crill, J. Donald Easton, Richard W. Erbe, Clement A. Finch, Daniel W. Foster, William Franklin, Eugene Frenkel, Lawrence Friedman, Peter L. Friedman, Theodore Friedmann, Bruce Gilliland, Stephen E. Goldfinger, Joseph L. Goldstein, John L. Gollan, Mehron Goulian, Mark R. Green, Gabriel Gregoratos, James E. Griffin, Frederick G. Guggenheim, Robert I. Handin, John A. Hanson, Donald H. Harter, Lee W. Henderson, Fred Hendler, Roland H. Ingram, Jr., Jon I. Isenberg, Charles Jablecki, Robert N. Jones, Lewis L. Judd, Vern H. Kerchberger, William Kovacs, Guenther Krejs, S. Lakshminarayanan, Alexander R. Lawton, Mark Leshin, John D. Loeser, Kenneth L. Luskey, Paul C. MacDonald, Raymond J. Maciewicz, Jamie Maguire, Roger J. May, Robert J. Mayer, Donald B. McCormick, E. Regis McFadden, Alfred Merrill, Kenneth M. Moser, Robert Munford, Barbara Nath, David Nathan, Charles Y. C. Pak, Alan S. Pearlman, James E. Pennington, James Plorde, Daniel K. Podolsky, Charles E. Pope II, Samuel I. Rapaport, Joel M. Rappeport, Robert W. Rebar, Peter Reich, Herbert Y. Reynolds, James Richter, R. Paul Robertson, Russell Ross, John W. Rowe, Daniel Rudman, Martin A. Samuels, Stuart F. Schlossman, Jerry A. Schneider, William J. Schwartz, J. E. Seegmiller, Ralph Shabetai, Marc A. Shuckit, Sheldon R. Simon, Frank E. Speizer, Paul E. Strandjord, Christina M. Surawicz, Steven I. Wasserman, Henry O. Wheeler, W. C. Wiederholt, Robert R. Young, Jerome Zeldis, and Ms. Mary Ellen Collins.

This book could not be edited without the dedicated help of our coworkers in the editorial offices of the individual editors. We are especially indebted to Kristin Ahlman, Martha Conant, Rebecca Frost, Hilda Gardner, Brenda H. Hennis, Patricia Higgins, Mary Jackson, Patricia Kadlick, Kathy Kreatz, Cynthia Reid, Barbara Ann Rumson, Ruth R. Simonds, Janice Stearns, Trisha C. Walker.

Finally, we need to say a word of thanks to the senior editors at McGraw-Hill, Mr. Dereck Jeffers and Mr. Richard Laufer. They formed a most effective team who gave the editors constant encouragement and kept them on the straight and narrow.

THE EDITORS

VOLUME 1

PART ONE
INTRODUCTION TO CLINICAL MEDICINE

PART TWO
CARDINAL MANIFESTATIONS OF DISEASE: AN APPROACH TO CLINICAL PROBLEMS

PART THREE
BIOLOGICAL CONSIDERATIONS IN THE APPROACH TO CLINICAL MEDICINE

PART FOUR
DISORDERS CAUSED BY BIOLOGICAL AND ENVIRONMENTAL AGENTS

PART ONE | INTRODUCTION TO CLINICAL MEDICINE

1 THE PRACTICE OF MEDICINE

THE EDITORS

THE EVER-CHANGING FACE OF MEDICINE Nearly 35 years have passed since the first edition of this book. This period of time is approximately equivalent to a lifetime of practice. In other words, the internist who began to practice in 1950 when this book first saw the light of day will be nearing retirement when he or she opens the tenth edition. Perhaps to one engaged in the practice of medicine every day over a 33-year period, the rapid changes are not as perceptible as would become evident by comparing the first and the tenth editions.

The emphasis in the first edition was primarily on clinical diagnosis, and while this remains an important cornerstone of internal medicine, the emphasis in the tenth edition has shifted progressively to the technological advances evident in the use of sophisticated diagnostic tests that are aimed at searching for the causes of disease and to applying the many more effective treatment modalities that are now available to physicians. Most of these advances would not have been possible were it not for vastly improved understanding of pathophysiology and mechanisms of disease. Although many gaps in knowledge remain, it is remarkable how many diseases whose causes were only vaguely known 30 years ago are now sufficiently well understood to conceptualize therapeutic approaches in pathophysiological terms. Ten editions of *Harrison's Principles of Internal Medicine* have recorded a saga of unparalleled progress!

WHAT IS EXPECTED OF THE PHYSICIAN However much the knowledge base of the physician has changed in the past 35 years, the fundamental commitment of the physician to the care of the patient remains unaltered. The editors of the first edition put it so eloquently that their words bear repeating:

Tact, sympathy and understanding are expected of the physician, for the patient is no mere collection of symptoms, signs, disordered functions, damaged organs, and disturbed emotions. He is human, fearful, and hopeful, seeking relief, help and reassurance. To the physician, as to the anthropologist, nothing human is strange or repulsive. The misanthrope may become a smart diagnostician of organic disease, but he can scarcely hope to succeed as a physician. The true physician has a Shakespearean breadth of interest in the wise and the foolish, the proud and the humble, the stoic hero and the whining rogue. He cares for people.

The practice of medicine combines both science and art. The role of science in medicine is clear. Technology based on science is the foundation for the solution to many clinical problems; the dazzling advances in biochemical methodology and in biophysical imaging techniques that allow access to the remotest recesses of the body are the products of science. So too are the therapeutic maneuvers which increasingly are a major part of medical practice. Yet skill in the most sophisticated application of laboratory technology or the use of the latest therapeutic modality alone does not make a good doctor. The ability to extract from a mass of contradictory physical signs and from the crowded computer printouts of laboratory data those items that are of crucial significance, to know in a difficult case whether to "treat" or to "watch," to determine when a clinical clue is worth pursuing or when to dismiss it as a "red herring," and to estimate in any given patient whether a proposed treatment entails a greater risk than the disease are all involved in the decisions which the clinician, skilled in the practice of medicine, must make many times each day. This combination of medical knowledge, intuition, and judgment is termed the *art of medicine.* It is as necessary to the practice of medicine as a sound scientific base.

THE PHYSICIAN-PATIENT RELATIONSHIP It may be trite to emphasize that physicians need to approach patients not as "cases" or "diseases" but as individuals whose problems all too often transcend the complaints which bring them to the doctor. Most patients are anxious and frightened. Often they go to great ends to convince themselves that illness does not exist, or unconsciously they set up elaborate defenses to divert attention from the real problem that they perceive to be serious or life-threatening. Some patients use illness to gain attention or to serve as a crutch to extricate themselves from an emotionally stressful situation. Whatever the patient's attitude, the physician needs to consider the terrain in which an illness occurs—not only in terms of the patients themselves, but also their families and social backgrounds. All too often medical records fail to contain essential information about the patient's origins, schooling, job, home and family, hopes and fears. Without this knowledge it is difficult for the physician to gain rapport with the patient. Such a relationship must be based on thorough knowledge of the patient and on mutual trust and the ability to communicate with one another.

In the United States in particular, but to a progressively greater extent throughout the world, the modern hospital poses a particularly intimidating environment for most patients. Lying in a bed surrounded by air jets, buttons, and lights; invaded by tubes and wires; beset by the numerous members of the health care team—nurses, nurses' aides, physicians' assistants, social workers, technologists, physical therapists, medical students, house officers, attending and consulting physicians, and many others; transported to special laboratories and x-ray chambers replete with machines with blinking lights and emitting strange sounds, it is little wonder that patients lose their sense of reality. In fact, the patient's physician is often the only tenuous link between the patient and the real world. Only a strong personal relationship with the physician can sustain the patient in such a stressful situation.

The direct, one-to-one patient-physician relationship which traditionally has characterized the practice of medicine is changing, primarily because of the changing setting in which medicine is being practiced. Often the management of the individual patient requires the active participation of a variety of trained professional personnel in addition to physicians. In most instances, health care is a team effort. The patient can benefit greatly from such collaboration, but it is the duty of the physician to guide the patient through an illness. To carry out this increasingly difficult task, the physician must have some familiarity with the techniques, skills, and objectives of colleagues in the fields allied to medicine. In giving the patient an opportunity to receive all the benefits of the important advances of science, the physician must, in the last analysis, retain responsibility for the major decisions concerning diagnosis and treatment.

An increasing number of patients are being cared for by groups of physicians, clinics, hospitals, and health-maintenance organizations (HMOs) rather than by individual independent practitioners. There are many potential advantages in the use of such organized medical groups, but there are also potential drawbacks, the chief of which is a loss of identity of the physician who is primarily and continuously responsible for the patient. It is essential, even in the group setting, that each patient have a physician who has an overview of the patient's problems and who maintains familiarity with the patient's reaction to his or her illness, to the drugs given, and to the challenges of daily living. Moreover, because a number of physicians may, at any one time, contribute to the care of a particular patient, and because patients as well as physicians are becoming increasingly mobile, accurate and detailed medical records are essential to good patient care.

CLINICAL SKILLS **History taking** The written history of an illness should embody all the facts of medical significance in the life of the patient. If the history is recorded in chronological order, recent events should be given the most attention. Likewise, if a problem-oriented approach is used, the problems that are clinically dominant should be listed first. Ideally, the narration of symptoms or problems should be in the patient's own words. However, few patients have the power of observation or recall to give a history without some guidance from the physician, who must be careful not to suggest the answers to the questions being posed.

Often a symptom which has concerned a patient has little significance, while a seemingly minor complaint may be of considerable importance. Therefore, the physician must be constantly alert to the possibility that any event related by the patient, however trivial or apparently remote, may be the key to the solution of the medical problem.

An informative history is more than an orderly listing of symptoms. Something is always gained by listening to patients and noting the way in which they talk about their symptoms. Inflections of voice, facial expression, and attitude may betray important clues to the meaning of the symptoms to a patient. In listening to the history, the physician discovers not only something about the disease but also something about the patient.

With experience, the pitfalls of history taking become apparent. What patients relate for the most part consists of subjective phenomena colored by past experience. Patients obviously differ widely in their responses to the same stimuli. Their remarks are variably influenced by fear of disability and death, and by concern over the consequences of their illness to their families. Sometimes the accuracy of the history is affected by language or sociological barriers, by failing intellectual powers which interfere with recall, or by disorders of consciousness that make them unaware of their illness. It is not surprising, then, that even the most careful physician may at times despair of collecting factual data and be forced to proceed with evidence that represents little more than an approximation of the truth. It is in obtaining the history that the physician's skill, knowledge, and experience are most clearly in evidence. Not to be neglected is the importance of the interview in establishing a relationship between doctor and patient. Such a relationship enables the doctor to gain the patient's confidence and helps to allay apprehension and fear.

The family history serves several functions. Firstly, in rare single-gene defects a positive family history of a similarly affected individual or a history of consanguinity may have important diagnostic implications. Secondly, in diseases of multifactorial etiology that have a familial aggregation, it may be possible to identify patients at risk for disease and to intervene prior to development of overt manifestations. For example, recent weight gain is a more ominous development in a woman who has a family history of diabetes than one who does not. Finally, in certain situations the family history has major implications for preventive medicine. When a diagnosis of a hereditary condition known to predispose to cancer is made, it is the physician's obligation to survey the family and to educate them about the need for long-term follow-up.

Physical examination Physical signs are the objective and verifiable marks of disease and represent solid, indisputable facts. Their significance is enhanced when they confirm a functional or structural change already suggested by the patient's history. At times, the physical signs may be the only evidence of disease, especially when the history has been inconsistent, confused, or lacking altogether.

The physical examination should be performed methodically and thoroughly. Although attention has often been directed by the history to the diseased organ or part of the body, the examination must extend from head to toe in an objective search for abnormalities. Unless the examination procedure is systematic, important parts of it may be forgotten, an error which is common even among the most skilled clinicians. The results of the examination, like the details of the history, should be recorded at the time they are elicited, not hours later when they are subject to the distortions of memory. Many inaccuracies stem from the careless practice of writing or dictating notes long after the examination has been concluded. Skill in physical diagnosis is acquired with experience, but it is not merely technique that determines success in eliciting signs. The detection of a few scattered petechiae, a faint diastolic murmur, or a small mass in the abdomen is not a question of keener eyes and ears or more sensitive fingers but of a mind prepared to be alert to these findings. Skill in physical diagnosis reflects a way of thinking more than a way of doing. Physical findings are subject to change. Just because the examination is normal on one occasion does not guarantee that this will be the case on subsequent examinations. It is important, therefore, to repeat pertinent parts of the physical examination as long as the clinical situation warrants.

Laboratory tests The marked increase in the number and availability of laboratory tests has inevitably resulted in increasing reliance being placed on knowledge gained from these studies in the solution of clinical problems. It is essential, however, to bear in mind the limitations of such procedures, which by virtue of their impersonal quality and complexity often gain an aura of authority regardless of the fallibility of the individuals doing or interpreting them, or of their instruments. More importantly, the accumulation of laboratory data cannot relieve the physician from the responsibility of careful observation and study of the patient. Physicians also must weigh carefully the hazards and the expense involved in the laboratory procedures they order. Moreover, laboratory tests are rarely ordered and reported singly. Rather, they are produced as "batteries." A common combination is the M6, which consists of determinations of serum sodium, potassium, carbon dioxide combining power, chloride, blood urea nitrogen, and blood glucose. Even more common is the M12, which also includes serum calcium, phosphate, proteins, albumin, uric acid, cholesterol, and several enzymes. Some laboratories now perform batteries of 24 and even 40 tests! The various combinations of laboratory tests are often useful. For example, they may provide the clue to such nonspecific symptoms as generalized weakness and increased fatigability by revealing an elevated serum calcium which, in turn, would suggest the diagnosis of hyperparathyroidism.

The thoughtful use of screening tests should not be confused with indiscriminate laboratory testing. The use of screening tests is based on the fact that a group of laboratory determinations which are known to be frequent harbingers of disease can now be carried out on a single specimen of blood at relatively low cost. Biochemical measurements, together with simple laboratory examinations such as blood count, urinalysis, and sedimentation rate, often provide the major clue to the presence of a pathologic process. They are particularly helpful in identifying organic disease in a patient with evident emotional problems. At the same time the physician must learn to evaluate occasional abnormalities among the screening tests that may not necessarily connote significant disease. There is nothing more costly and unproductive than an in-depth workup following a report of an isolated laboratory abnormality in a patient who is otherwise well. Among the more than 20 tests that are performed on many patients, one is often slightly abnormal. Here it is important to distinguish a minor abnormality (less than 1 standard deviation) from a major one (more than 2 standard deviations). Even then, whether to proceed with further workup is a test of the physician's clinical judgment.

Newer imaging techniques The last decade has seen the arrival of ultrasonography, a variety of isotopic scans that employ new isotopes to visualize organs heretofore inaccessible, and computerized tomography with its varying permutations. Nuclear magnetic resonance and nuclear spin resonance, while not generally available for clinical use, are in the offing. Aside from opening up new diagnostic vistas, this new, highly sophisticated technology benefits patients because it has frequently supplanted invasive techniques which require the insertion of tubes, wires, or catheters into the body—procedures which are often painful and sometimes risky. While the enthusiasm for noninvasive technology is understandably justified, all too often the results have not been properly validated before they are disseminated as clinical dogma. Moreover, the expense entailed in performing these imaging tests is often substantial and is not always considered when ordering them. There is no question that a tool like computerized tomography has led to a reassessment of the problem of adrenal tumors, just as routine measurement of calcium caused a redefinition of hyperparathyroidism. The principles being espoused here are simply to use these examinations judiciously, preferably in lieu of, not in addition to, the invasive maneuvers they are meant to replace.

THE DIAGNOSIS OF DISEASE Accurate diagnosis requires, first of all, the collection of accurate data. But much more is required in making a diagnosis. Each datum must be interpreted in the light of what is known about the structure and function of the involved organ(s). Knowledge of anatomy, physiology, and biochemistry must be combined into a plausible pathophysiologic mechanism.

Clinical diagnosis requires both aspects of logic—analysis and synthesis—and the more difficult the clinical problem, the more important is a logical approach to it. Such an approach requires that the physician list carefully each problem suggested by the patient's symptoms and physical and laboratory findings and seek answers to each. Anatomic diagnosis should precede etiological diagnosis. The cause and mechanism of a disease can seldom be determined before ascertaining which organ is involved.

Most physicians attempt consciously or unconsciously to fit a given problem into one of a series of syndromes. *The syndrome is a group of symptoms and signs of disordered function, related to one another by means of some anatomic, physiologic, or biochemical peculiarity.* It embodies a hypothesis concerning the deranged function of an organ, organ system, or tissue. Congestive heart failure, Cushing's disease, and dementia are examples. In congestive heart failure dyspnea, orthopnea, cyanosis, dependent edema, engorged neck veins, pleural effusion, rales, and hepatomegaly are known to be connected by a single pathophysiologic mechanism—heart failure. In Cushing's disease the moon facies, hypertension, diabetes, and osteoporosis are the recognized effects of excess corticosteroids acting on many target organs. In dementia, deterioration of memory, incoherent thinking, impaired language functions, visual-spatial disorientation, and faulty judgment are related to destruction of the association areas of the cerebrum.

A syndrome does not necessarily identify the precise cause of an illness, but it greatly narrows the number of possibilities and often suggests certain special clinical and laboratory studies. The derangements of each organ system in humans are reducible to a relatively small number of syndromes. The diagnosis is greatly simplified if a clinical problem conforms neatly to a well-defined syndrome, because only a few diseases need to be considered in the differential diagnosis. In contrast, the search for the cause of an illness that does not conform to a syndrome is much more difficult because a much greater number of diseases may then have to be sought. Even here an orderly approach which proceeds from symptom to sign to laboratory findings will result in the diagnosis most of the time.

CARING FOR THE PATIENT The care of the patient begins with the development of a personal relationship between the patient and the physician. In the absence of a sense of trust and confidence on the part of the patient, the effectiveness of most therapeutic measures is diminished. In many instances, when there is confidence in the physician, reassurance is the best treatment and is all that is needed. Likewise, in those cases which do not lend themselves to easy solutions or for which no effective treatment is available, a feeling on the part of the patient that the physician is doing all that is possible is one of the most important therapeutic measures that can be provided.

Drug therapy With each succeeding year, more drugs are being released, every one with the hope and the promise that it is an improvement over its predecessor. Although the pharmaceutical industry must be given most of the credit for advances in drug therapy, it is also true that many new drugs have only a marginal advantage over the agents they are aimed to replace. The barrage of new information with which practitioners are deluged does little to help them grasp a clear picture of clinical pharmacology; on the contrary, to most physicians new drugs are confusing. There is no easy way to answer the question of when a new drug should be employed. With some exceptions, however, the approach to a new drug should be one of caution. Unless the new agent is established beyond doubt to be a real advance, it is wiser to use well-tested and well-established agents which are not only efficacious but also safe.

Iatrogenic disorders An iatrogenic disorder occurs when the deleterious effects of a procedure or drug produce pathology independent of the condition for which the drug is given. For example, the use of glucocorticoids to arrest progressive disseminated lupus erythematosus may produce Cushing's syndrome. In this instance, the benefits exceed the untoward side effects. No matter what the clinical situation, it is the responsibility of the physician to use new and powerful therapeutic measures wisely, with due regard to their action, cost, and potential dangers. Every medical procedure, whether diagnostic or therapeutic, has the potential for harm, but it would be impossible to afford the patient all the benefits of modern scientific medicine if reasonable steps in diagnosis and therapy were withheld because of possible risks. "Reasonable" implies that the physician has weighed the pros and cons of a procedure and has concluded on rational grounds that it is advisable or essential for the relief of discomfort or the cure or amelioration of disease. However, much harm can result when the deleterious effects of a procedure or a drug exceed any possible advantages that might have been anticipated. Examples include the dangerous or fatal drug reactions that occasionally follow the use of antibiotics given for trivial respiratory infections, the gastric hemorrhage or perforation caused by cortisone administered for mild arthritis, or the occurrence of fatal hepatitis B that may follow needless transfusions of blood or plasma.

But the harm that a physician can do to a patient is not limited to the imprudent use of medication. Equally important are ill-considered or unjustified remarks. Many a patient has developed a cardiac neurosis because the physician ventured a grave prognosis on the basis of a misinterpreted electrocardiogram. Not only the treatment itself but the physician's words and behavior are capable of causing injury.

The physician must never become so absorbed in the disease as to forget the patient who is its victim. As the science of medicine advances, it is all too easy to become so fascinated by the manifestations of disease that the ailing person's fears and concerns about job and family, the cost of medical care, and the specter of economic insecurity are disregarded. Treatment of a patient consists of more than the dispassionate confrontation of a disease. It embodies also the exercise of warmth, compassion, and understanding. In the now famous words of Dr. Francis Peabody,

One of the essential qualities of the clinician is interest in humanity, for the secret of the care of the patient is in caring for the patient.

Informed consent In an era of rapidly advancing technology, patients will require diagnostic and therapeutic procedures that are painful and that pose some risk. These include all surgical procedures, e.g., biopsies of tissues, radiographic maneuvers involving the insertion of catheters, endoscopy, and many others. In most American hospitals and clinics, patients undergoing such procedures are required to sign a form consenting to them. More important, however, is the notion that the patient must understand clearly the risk entailed in these procedures; this is the definition of *informed consent.* It is incumbent upon the physician to explain to the patient, in a clearly understandable fashion, the procedures which he or she faces. By doing this conscientiously much of the dread of the unknown that is inherent in hospitalization will be mitigated.

Accountability Throughout the world physicians, once licensed to practice medicine, have not had to account for their actions except to their peers. In the United States, however, during the past decade, there have been increasing demands for physicians to account for the way in which they practice medicine by meeting certain standards prescribed by federal and state governments. Hospitalized patients whose health care is reimbursed by the government (Medicare and Medicaid) have been subjected to utilization review. This means that the physician must defend the cause for and duration of a patient's hospitalization if it falls outside certain "average" standards. This concept has been extended in the form of Professional Standard Review Organizations (PSRO) under whose direction norms and standards for the care of patients have been developed. The purpose of these regulations is to improve the quality of patient care, and in some instances this has undoubtedly happened. Another important reason for implementing these regulations, however, is to contain spiraling health care costs. It is likely that this type of review will be extended to all phases of medical practice and will inevitably alter not only the practice of medicine but the traditional patient-physician relationship.

Physicians also will be expected to give account of their continuing competence by mandatory continuing education, patient record audit, recertification by examination, and relicensure. While these measures probably enhance the physician's factual knowledge, there is no evidence that they have a similar effect on the quality of practice.

Cost-effectiveness in medical care As the whole of society undertakes greater fiscal responsibility for health care, and as the cost of medical care continues to rise, it has become necessary to establish stringent priorities in the expenditure of health care dollars. In some instances, preventive measures offer the greatest return per dollar; outstanding examples include vaccination, immunization, reduction in accidents and occupational hazards, and improved environmental control. The cost of "newborn screening" for metabolic diseases is being evaluated. For example, the detection of phenylketonuria by screening of large populations may save many thousands of dollars in hospital costs.

As resources become more and more constrained, it will be necessary to weigh the justifiability of performing prohibitively costly operations that provide only a limited life expectancy against the pressing need for more primary care centers for the large segments of population who do not have adequate access to medical services. At the level of the individual patient it has become extremely important to minimize costly hospital admissions as far as possible, if total health care is to be provided at a figure which most can afford. This, of course, implies and depends upon a close cooperative effort between patients, their physicians, third-party carriers, and government, and a constant surveillance of those types of procedures which can be conducted safely and effectively on an ambulatory basis. Equally important in reducing total health care expenditures is the need for individual physicians to monitor carefully both the cost and effectiveness of the drugs they prescribe. In the last analysis the public should depend on the medical profession for leadership and guidance in matters of cost control. It is equally important, however, that consideration of these important socioeconomic aspects of the health care delivery system not be permitted to interfere with the primary humane concern of physicians for the welfare of their patients.

Incurability and death No problem is more distressing than that presented by the patient with an incurable disease, particularly when premature death is inevitable. What should the patient and family be told, what measures should be taken to maintain the patient's life, and how is death to be defined?

Although some would argue otherwise, there is no ironclad rule that the patient must be told "everything," even if the patient is an adult and may be the head of a family. How much the patient is told should depend upon the patient's ability and capacity to deal with the possibility of imminent death. This decision may take into consideration the wishes of the family and perhaps the patient's financial and business affairs and religious beliefs. First of all, the patient must be given an opportunity to speak to the physician and to ask questions. Patients may find it easier to share their feelings about death with their physician who is likely to be more objective and less emotional than their family members.

One thing is certain: it is not for you to don the black cap and, assuming the judicial function, take hope away from any patient . . . hope that comes to us all.

William Osler

Even when the patient directly inquires, "Doctor, am I dying?" the physician must attempt to determine whether this is a request for information, a demand for reassurance, or even an expression of hostility. Most would agree that only open communication between the patient and the physician can resolve these questions and guide the physician in what to say and how to say it.

The physician should provide or arrange for emotional, physical, and spiritual support, and must be compassionate, unhurried, and open. Pain should be adequately controlled, human dignity maintained, and isolation from family avoided. The last two in particular tend to be overlooked in hospitals, where the intrusion of life-sustaining apparatus can so easily detract from attention to the whole person to concentrate instead on the life-threatening disease.

The physician must also prepare to deal with guilt feelings on the part of the family when a member becomes gravely or hopelessly ill. It is important for the doctor to reassure the family that everything possible has been done.

Definition of death Traditionally, in every society, arrest of heart action has been taken as the only valid medical criterion of death. Lawbooks cite this as the only certain proof that human life has ended. But, as every modern physician knows, the heart may sometimes be restored to action, seemingly miraculously, minutes after it has stopped. On the other hand, other vital organs such as the brain may be destroyed, leaving the individual emotionally and psychologically dead.

Clinical and electroencephalographic criteria are at hand which permit the reliable diagnosis of cerebral death. According to the criteria adopted by the staff of the Massachusetts General Hospital and the Harvard Committee on Brain Death, death has occurred when, as a consequence usually of hypoxia and hypotension, all signs of receptivity and responsivity are absent, including all brainstem reflexes (pupillary reactions, ocular movement, blinking, swallowing, breathing), and the electroencephalogram is isoelectric. Occasionally, intoxications and metabolic disorders may simulate this state; hence the diagnosis requires expert medical evaluation. Under the aforementioned circumstances, to continue with heroic, highly costly, supportive measures merely for the purpose of preserving cardiac function is against the best interests of patient, family, and society. In such instances, the dilemma of continuing care could be avoided if the medical profession, in accord with social sanction, can be brought to redefine life as a state in which cerebral functions subserve awareness of the environment and the possibility of expressing intellect, awareness, and emotion, and if it can equate the opposite of this with death.

A practice which has proved acceptable in many settings is as follows:

1 The diagnosis of brain death, based on the above criteria, should be corroborated by another physician and confirmed by clinical examination and EEG, repeated one or more times.
2 The family should be informed of the irreversibility of brain function but should not be requested in any way to ratify the decision whether medical treatment should be discontinued. An exception to this limited decision-making power of the family might apply where the patient has directed the family that he or she wishes them to make the decision.
3 The physician, after consultation with a professional colleague, may withdraw supportive measures, assuming that nothing more can be offered. This interpretation is in general agreement with that of most religions.
4 The possibility that such patients may become sources of organs for grafting should not enter into the aforementioned decisions, although prior to the cessation of heart action the family may be approached and asked whether this would be their wish, or the family may suggest that organs be used for this purpose.

The issues involving death and dying are among the most difficult in medicine. In approaching them rationally and consistently, the physician must combine the art of medicine with the science.

PART TWO | CARDINAL MANIFESTATIONS OF DISEASE: AN APPROACH TO CLINICAL PROBLEMS

section 1 | Pain

2

ACUTE AND CHRONIC PAIN: PATHOPHYSIOLOGY AND MANAGEMENT

RAYMOND D. ADAMS
JOSEPH B. MARTIN

Pain, it has been said, is one of "Nature's earliest signs of morbidity." Few will deny that it stands preeminent among all the sensory experiences by which humans judge the existence of disease within themselves. There are relatively few maladies that do not have their painful phases, and in many of them pain is a characteristic without which diagnosis must always be in doubt. It seems appropriate, therefore, to begin a section on the cardinal manifestations of disease with a discussion of the more general aspects of pain.

The painful experiences of the sick pose difficult problems for practitioners of medicine. Physicians must be ready to diagnose acute disease in patients who have felt only the first rumblings of discomfort before other symptoms and signs of disease have appeared. To cope effectively with problems of this type requires a sound knowledge of the sensory supply of the body surface and of the viscera and a familiarity with the typical symptoms of many diseases. Physicians are also consulted by patients with pain symptoms that are chronic and persistent and in whom no amount of investigation will disclose evidence of either medical disease or psychiatric illness. In some, detailed inquiry may uncover possible contributing factors such as concern about compensation for an alleged injury, unsatisfactory job or marital circumstances, or anxiety and concern about the presence of a serious malady. In yet others, pain may be the presenting symptom of hidden depression, of a neurosis, or of malingering. Finally, the physician must care for patients with intractable pain, often from an established and incurable disease, who require long-term drug administration or surgical intervention to interrupt sensory pathways.

In general the concept of pain encompasses at least three components: *nociception,* the body's detection and signaling of noxious events; *pain,* the conscious perception or recognition of the nociceptive stimulus; and *suffering,* the affective, behavioral, or emotional response to the pain. In these terms, it is important to distinguish certain differences between *acute* and *chronic* pain. When acute, pain is often the crucial signal of the location and nature of the disorder. In the circumstance of chronic pain, both the quality of the discomfort and its neurologic basis seem to differ and its management then becomes much more complex.

ANATOMY OF PAIN PATHWAYS Pain is a sensation which has its own sensory apparatus. The receptors in the skin and deep structures are fine, freely branching nerve endings which form an intricate network throughout the body. A single primary pain neuron with its cell body in the posterior root ganglion subdivides into many small peripheral branches to supply an area of skin of several square millimeters. The cutaneous area of each neuron overlaps with those of other neurons, so that every spot of skin lies within the domain of two to four neurons. These freely branching nerve endings are also found in many of the other specialized sensory receptors in the skin, such as Krause's end bulbs, the ruffinian plumes, and the pacinian corpuscles, which may explain why the extremes of hot, cold, and pressure sensation become painful. Free nerve endings may also serve as receptors for other types of sensation. They are the only end organ in the cornea, where touch and temperature as well as pain are felt.

The sensory nerve fibers for pain, as they course through somatic and visceral nerves, are mixed with other sensory and motor fibers. Most sensory fibers enter the spinal cord through the spinal posterior roots. A few enter the anterior (motor) root, but these also terminate in the dorsal horn. Fibers from the head enter the brainstem through certain of the cranial nerves. The pain fibers are of two sizes, one very small and unmyelinated (2 to 4 μm in diameter), called the *C fiber,* with a slow conducting velocity, the other larger (6 to 8 μm), called the *A-delta fiber,* with more rapid transmission. As the posterior root enters the spinal cord, it separates into two divisions, medial and lateral. The medial division, heavily myelinated, synapses either with large secondary sensory neurons in the posterior horn or with anterior horn cells (serving segmental reflexes), or it passes upward in the posterior columns, with some fibers reaching the medulla. The lateral division, of thinly myelinated and nonmyelinated fibers, travels in the tract of Lissauer to reach the substantia gelatinosa, where it synapses with (1) many small neurons whose axons pass into the posterior and anterior horns of the same and adjacent segments of the spinal cord, also effecting reflex connections and (2) large secondary sensory neurons, some of which form the lateral spinothalamic tract and some of which ascend for varying distances near the gray matter as a polysynaptic pathway. The neurons on which the afferent root fibers terminate tend to lie in the first and fifth laminae of the posterior horn. It is postulated that their reactivity is influenced by large afferent myelinated fibers or by other inhibitory neurons within the spinal gray matter. Through a mechanism still rather obscure, two secondary ascending pathways for pain are activated. One is the lateral *neospinothalamic tract,* the cell bodies of which lie in the posterior horns, with axons crossing through the anterior commissure of the spinal cord within one to two segments of the level of entry. This pathway is believed to make one aware of the intensity and localization of pain. The other, the *paleospinothalamic tract,* lies more anterior in the lateral cord. This pathway is believed to subserve the arousal and emotional components of pain. The neospinothalamic tract, joined in the brainstem by the trigeminothalamic tract, courses through the lateral part of the medulla, pons, and midbrain, giving off many collaterals before terminating in the nucleus ventralis posterolateralis and the posterior nuclear group of the thalamus (Fig. 2-1). The paleospinothalamic tract extends cephalad and makes connections with the reticular formation of the brainstem and with the intralaminar and parafascicular nuclei of the thalamus which connect to limbic portions of the cerebrum (Bonica). Through a mechanism still rather obscure a pain stimulus activates both secondary ascending pathways for pain.

The secondary spinothalamic and trigeminothalamic tracts synapse with the tertiary sensory neurons of the thalamus whose axons extend to the cortex of the parietal lobe. Physiologists are not agreed as to the cortical terminus for the pain fibers, for electrical stimulation of the cortex in the conscious human seldom produces a painful sensation, and parietal lobe lesions seldom cause central pain. Presumably their cortical termination is rather diffuse and occurs in both parietal and frontal regions. Only a few end in the primary somatosensory cortex. The secondary somatosensory cortex receives more fibers than the primary. Most of the pain fibers from the periphery cross to the opposite side of the brain; only a small contingent remains ipsilateral. (See Adams and Victor for more detailed descriptions of pain neurons and tracts.)

FIGURE 2-1

Diagram of central nervous system pathway for pain. Small-diameter afferent fibers (A-delta and C) enter dorsal horn. [●, substance P (SP)—containing bipolar sensory neuron; ◆ , enkephalin (ENK)—containing interneuron in dorsal horn of spinal cord.] Crossed ascending pathways include the neospinothalamic (NSTT) tract with principal terminations in the ventral posterolateral (VPL) nucleus of the thalamus, and the paleospinothalamic (PSTT) tract with terminations in the brainstem nuclei. Sensory relay to cerebral cortex occurs primarily from VPL. Descending pathways for pain regulation arise from the periaqueductal gray (PAG) and the raphe magnus (RM) nucleus of the brainstem. (Courtesy of Dr. Ray Maciewicz.)

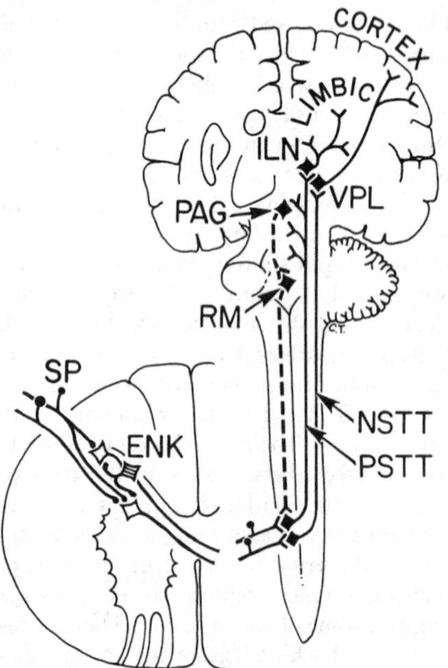

Segmental innervation As a means of quick orientation to the anatomy of the peripheral pain pathways it should be remembered that the facial structures and anterior cranium lie in the field of the trigeminal nerves; the back of the head, second cervical; the neck, third cervical; epaulet area, fourth cervical; deltoid area, fifth cervical, radial forearm and thumb, sixth cervical; index finger, seventh cervical; middle finger, eighth cervical; little finger and inner forearm, first thoracic; nipple segment, fifth thoracic; umbilical, tenth thoracic; groin, first lumbar; medial side of knee, third lumbar; great toe, fifth lumbar; little toe, first sacral; back of thigh, second sacral; genitosacral areas, third, fourth, and fifth sacral. The first to fourth thoracic nerve roots are the important sensory pathways for the intrathoracic viscera; the sixth to eighth thoracic, for the upper abdominal organs.

PHYSIOLOGY AND PHARMACOLOGY OF PAIN The stimuli that arouse pain vary for each tissue. Generally the adequate stimuli for skin are those which injure tissue, i.e., pricking, cutting, crushing, burning, and freezing. Interestingly, these same forms of stimulation have little effect when applied to the stomach and intestine. Pain in the gastrointestinal tract is produced instead by local trauma of an engorged or inflamed mucosa, distention or spasm of smooth muscle, and traction on the mesenteric attachment. Pain is induced in skeletal muscles by ischemia (the basis for the condition known as intermittent claudication), as well as by tears of connective tissue sheaths, necrosis, hemorrhage, or the injection of irritating solutions. Prolonged contraction of muscles evokes an aching type of pain. Ischemia, the only proved source of pain in the heart muscle, is responsible for angina pectoris and for the pain of myocardial infarction. Joints are insensitive to pricking, cutting, and cautery, but pain is induced in the synovial membrane by hypertonic saline solution and inflammation. Arteries give rise to pain when pierced with a needle, when induced to pulsate excessively (as in migraine), and in certain diseases of their walls such as exemplified by atherosclerotic thrombosis and arteritis of cranial arteries. Traction and displacement of intracranial vessels and the meningeal structures by which they are supported may cause headache.

Stimuli that elicit pain are thought to do so by causing release of chemical substances into the tissues. Histamine, bradykinin, prostaglandins, and potassium ions cause pain when injected into the skin or when administered intraarterially. These agents, which are present in all tissues, may be released or activated by stimuli that are potentially damaging. Excitation of nerve endings in the area of release causes depolarization of afferent pain fibers which relay the signal to the central nervous system. Strong pressure may also directly stimulate free nerve endings.

The sensory experiences resulting from these several modes of stimulation in the skin and in deep skeletomuscular and visceral structures differ in quality. Integumentary stimuli, at the lowest levels of intensity, evoke sensations of touch, pressure, warmth, cold, or tickle. When increased to the point approaching tissue destruction, pain is added, and the resulting experience is thereafter a mixed one. The painful experience itself is one of pricking or burning. The threshold for burning pain from a thermal stimulus is approximately 2000 times the threshold for warmth. This relationship of pain to tissue destruction is the basis of a biologic principle—that pain has a protective, or self-preserving, value to the organism.

There is a wide range of responses to pain to which attention is drawn. Strong, acute pain causes a startle reaction. Intense, persistent pain is usually accompanied by segmental flexion reflexes (e.g., spasm of a segment of the abdominal wall with visceral disease, flexion of knees and hips with peritoneal irritation, extension of neck with meningitis), autonomic responses, postural adjustments, avoidance movements, and vocalization. The obvious biologic function of segmental reflexes is to splint the diseased part and to facilitate healing. The altered state of receptivity of the spinal gray matter accounts for stimuli of nonreceptive type evoking pain, e.g., for subcutaneous pressure being painful.

Acute pain sensation may be induced by stimulation of the receptors or by irritation of peripheral nerves or roots; it may also be abolished by diseases which affect the peripheral or central nervous system, or by a surgical procedure which accomplishes the same result. Pain in a circumscribed region may be terminated by section of the nerve which supplies that region (neurotomy) or by section of the spinal roots (posterior rhizotomy); pain in a limb or one side of the trunk may be abolished by section of the anterolateral spinothalamic tracts (lateral spinal tractotomy in the spinal cord or tractotomy in the lateral medulla or mesencephalon). However, such lesions may fail to influence pain perception in chronic pain states.

Recent discoveries have added new information concerning the pharmacology and neurophysiology of nociception. Salicylates and other nonsteroidal anti-inflammatory drugs are peripherally acting analgesics, which exert inhibitory effects on the synthesis of prostaglandins, known to be potent stimulators of nociceptive endings. Salicylates fail to antagonize effects of other nociceptive substances such as bradykinin and histamine.

Pain transmission in the dorsal horn is believed to occur by release of substance P, an 11-amino acid peptide, present in cell bodies in the dorsal root ganglia that give rise to the C and A-delta fibers (Fig. 2-1). Electron-microscopic studies show that substance P is localized in dense core granules in the synaptic terminals of primary afferents in the dorsal horn. Peripheral nociceptive stimulation causes the release of substance P, and application of the peptide to neurons in the dorsal horn causes excitation. These observations support the idea that substance P functions as a sensory neurotransmitter for relay of pain signals to second-order neurons of the spinothalamic system. Opioid substances act centrally at several sites to modify pain transmission. Enkephalin, an endogenous opioid peptide, is found in neurons of lamina II of the spinal cord dorsal horn and in the trigeminal nuclei of the brainstem. Opiate receptors are abundant in these regions. Electron-microscopic studies show termination of substance-P neurons upon enkephalin-containing cells. There is electrophysiologic and pharmacologic evidence to indicate that the enkephalins (and perhaps β-endorphin) inhibit substance-P release and may act at the level of the spinal cord or brainstem to block pain transmission. Intrathecal administration of β-endorphin or of morphine produces potent analgesic effects that persist for several hours. Descending pathways from large neurons of the brainstem reticular formation also modulate pain transmission at the level of the dorsal horn. These descending fiber systems contain enkephalin, serotonin, and dopamine and terminate in laminae I and V of the dorsal horn.

These observations have provided support to the "gate control theory of pain" first proposed by Melzack and Wall some 15 years ago and also emphasize the importance of discrete, descending pathways from brainstem nuclei that may be important modulators of afferent nociceptive inflow at the level of the dorsal horn. According to their hypothesis, increased activity in large-fiber afferents can attenuate or block pain transmission in small fibers. Although still unproven in its full detail, there is considerable evidence that pain modulation does occur at the level of the spinal cord.

High densities of opiate receptors are also found in the periaqueductal gray matter of the brainstem and in the medial thalamus, amygdaloid nuclei, caudate nuclei, and frontotemporal cortex. This interesting distribution may account for both the antinociceptive and affective aspects of opioid compounds. Central electrical stimulation of the periaqueductal region can inhibit pain transmission by both ascending and descending effects. Such stimulation has also been shown to cause release of endorphins into the cerebrospinal fluid. The descending effects are believed to be mediated through serotonin neurons of the reticular formation relayed to the dorsal horn of the spinal cord. Other peptides, including angiotensin II and somatostatin, and the inhibitory neurotransmitters γ-aminobutyric acid (GABA) and glycine, are also found in sensory neurons of the dorsal root ganglia and substantia gelatinosa and may be involved in pain transmission.

The threshold for the perception of pain, i.e., the lowest intensity of stimulus recognized as pain, is approximately the same in all persons. It is lowered by inflammation and raised by local anesthetics (e.g., procaine), lesions of the nervous system, and certain centrally acting analgesic drugs. Distraction and suggestion by turning attention away from the painful part reduce the awareness of and the response to pain. Strong emotion (fear or rage) suppresses pain. Neurotic patients in general have the same pain threshold as normal subjects, but their reaction may be excessive or abnormal. The pain thresholds of frontal lobotomized subjects are also unchanged, but they react briefly if at all to pain. The degree of emotional reaction and the verbalization (complaint) also vary with the personality and character of the patient.

One important aspect of pain perception is the well-known "placebo effect." Up to 35 percent of patients suffering from a variety of painful conditions obtain benefit when given therapeutically inert substances. The nature of this response, although clearly substantiated, remains uncertain; recent investigations have given evidence that the placebo response is reversed by naloxone, an opioid antagonist, giving support to the contention that it is mediated by release of endogenous opioid substances. There is also evidence that analgesia induced by electroacupuncture may be mediated by activation of endogenous opioid release, perhaps through a "gating" mechanism described above.

Superficial pain Sensory impulses subserving pricking pain, being transmitted by larger pain fibers, have a more rapid rate of conductivity to the nervous system than burning pain. A hot needle applied to the toe, for example, produces a quick, pricking pain and, only 1 to 2 s later, a burning pain. Together they constitute the "double response" of Lewis. Ischemia of nerve by the application of a tourniquet to a limb abolishes pricking pain before burning pain. Both types of dermal pain are localized with precision (local sign), made possible by the overlap of sensory neurons. Analgesia means the interruption of all pain neurons to an area, and hypalgesia, the interruption of only part of them.

Visceral pain Deep pain (including that of visceral and skeletal structures) has basically the quality of aching, but if intense may be sharp and penetrating (knifelike). Occasionally there is a burning type of pain, as in the heartburn of esophageal irritation and rarely in angina pectoris. The pain is felt as being deep to the body surface. The double response is absent, localization is poor, and the margins of the pain are not well delineated, presumably because of the paucity of nerve endings in viscera.

Actually, the pain originating in deep skeletomuscular and visceral structures cannot be localized closer than two to three sensory segments. For example, pain from myocardial disease is felt to arise within the first to fourth or possibly fifth thoracic segments. Unfortunately, from the standpoint of diagnosis, these spinal segments also receive sensory fibers from other structures—the esophagus, mediastinal contents, bones, muscles, etc.—and diseases of these structures may cause pain that is difficult to distinguish from cardiac pain.

Deep musculoskeletal pain Since deep skeletal pain and visceral pain are mediated through a common deep sensory system, it is not surprising that their characteristics (type, localization, and referral) should be similar. The topography of muscle and tendinous pain has been mapped by injecting a few milliliters of normal saline solution into the various muscles and noting the location of induced pain. The ache is usually segmental and may spread one to two segments above (less often below) the site injected. A tear or injury in a lumbar muscle may give rise to a pain which, in quality and localization, including radiation into the groin and scrotum, is indistinguishable from the pain of renal colic. A hemorrhage into the right upper rectus muscle mimics the pain of gallbladder colic; and a lesion in a muscle or ligament deep in the chest wall causes pain referred to the left arm, like that of angina. The differentiation of these pains must be made on grounds other than location and reference.

Referred pain Deep visceral and somatic pains tend always to be referred superficially to those structures within a given spinal segment that have the most extensive nerve ramifications and therefore the widest cerebral representation (e.g., there are more sensory nerves in the integument than in the viscera, hence the pain in the latter is projected to the body surface). In the case of myocardial pain, sensory impulses entering the first to fourth thoracic nerves activate a pool of sensory neurons, the largest number of which also receive afferents from the skin of the inner side of the arm (T_1 and T_2) and the anterior precordium (T_3 and T_4). More of the sensory neurons from the heart enter the left side of the spinal cord than the right. These anatomic and physiologic data explain why cardiac pain is referred predominantly to the substernal, left precordial, and inner brachial zones.

Aberrant reference of pain occurs not infrequently and is explained in terms of the physiologic status of the spinal pool of sensory neurons. As was stated, a single sensory neuron entering one spinal root depolarizes to a varying degree a pool of spinal neurons over four or five spinal segments. Pain then should spread to segments adjacent to the painful lesion, where it also causes cutaneous hyperesthesia and, by activating motor neurons, involuntary muscle contraction. If some preexistent disease in *adjacent* somatic segments has already partially depolarized the spinal pool of sensory neurons, a new painful disease which will further depolarize them causes the pain to spread to them. For example, if gallbladder disease which activated sensory fibers entering at the sixth to eighth thoracic nerve root, or cervical arthritis (at the second to eighth cervical nerve root) were present before a myocardial infarct, the cardiac pain might then be referred to the upper part of the abdomen or neck, respectively. Generally these aberrant referrals occur in segments that are cephalad to the normal segmental distribution of pain because their inhibitory connections are more abundant than those of caudal ones.

Hyperesthesia, hyperalgesia, hyperpathia, involuntary spasms, and other responses It has been customary but inaccurate to use the first two of these terms to designate a lowering of the threshold to touch and pain stimuli and the third for a state of pain with a normal or raised threshold but overreaction. Hyperpathia may even occur with anesthesia, as in *anesthesia dolorosa.* Any real distinction between these states is ephemeral. Probably only with inflammation of the skin is the pain threshold consistently lowered. What is most characteristic of all chronically painful states, and these frequently implicate nerves or central nervous structures, is that the part is unusually sensitive to all stimuli, even those which normally do not evoke pain; and the elicited pain is unnatural, radiant, outlasts the initiating stimulus, and is unusually modifiable by fatigue, emotion, etc. These are the characteristics of many chronic pain states, including causalgia, spinal cord pain, phantom pain, herpes zoster neuralgia, thalamic pain, etc. Explanations offered for these states remain unsatisfactory. It is useful, in an attempt to define such chronic painful states, to distinguish between nonneuronal tissue injury (somatic pain as in metastatic cancer) and the sensations that arise from peripheral nerve or central neural injury, often referred to as *deafferentation* or *dysesthetic* pain (see Tasker for a more complete discussion). In the former, there is generally a satisfactory response to analgesic agents, particularly narcotics, and relief can be obtained in severe cases by stereotaxic lesions in the pain pathways (spinal cord tractotomy, for example), or by stimulation of the periaqueductal gray matter. In deafferentation pain, narcotic analgesics are only partially effective; the pain can be elicited or reproduced by electrical stimulation of central regions of the midbrain, thalamus, thalamocortical radiation, or even the somatosensory cortex; and the pain is not relieved by periaqueductal stimulation. These observations, made by neurosurgeons attempting to treat chronic pain states, imply separate mechanisms for somatic and dysesthetic pain. The dysesthesia of the deafferentation lesion, it is speculated, arises from the formation of functionally aberrant central neuronal pathways that subserve or give rise to the burning quality of the pain. Although only rarely indicated, such patients may show favorable responses to lesions made in certain brain regions not classically associated with the neospinothalamic system, such as the posteromedial and pulvinar regions of the thalamus, the amygdala, or the cingulate cortex, i.e., all components of the paleospinothalamic system. Thus, the pain felt in the offending extremity or in the face in such cases may be uninfluenced by central lesions placed in primary pain pathways such as the spinothalamic tract or the posterior ventrolateral nucleus of the thalamus. These observations suggest that regions of the spinoreticular and limbic systems become involved in such chronic pain states. Such lesions may not alter the threshold for pain sensation but rather change the affective component of the pain response.

Perception of pain Only upon the arrival of pain impulses at the thalamocortical level of the nervous system is there conscious awareness of the pain stimulus. Clinical study has not informed us of the exact localization of the nervous apparatus for this mental process. It is not entirely abolished by a total hemispherectomy, including the thalamus on one side. A significant fraction of the lateral spinothalamic tract arises in sacral neurons *ipsilateral* to the thalamus terminations. It is often said that impulses reaching the thalamus create awareness of the attributes of sensation and that the parietal cortex is necessary for the appreciation of the intensity and localization of the sensation. This seems to be an oversimplification. Probably a close and harmonious relationship between thalamus and cortex must exist in order for a sensory experience to be complete. The traditional separation of sensation (in this instance awareness of pain) and perception (awareness of the nature of the painful stimulus) has been abandoned in favor of the view that sensation, perception, and the various conscious and unconscious responses to a pain stimulus comprise an indivisible process.

Although similar to other sensory or perceptive phenomena in certain respects, such as predictable response to given intensity of stimulus, pain differs in other ways. One of its most remarkable characteristics is the strong feeling tone, or affect, with which it is endowed, nearly always one of unpleasantness. Furthermore, pain does not appear to be subject to negative adaptation. Most stimuli, if applied continuously, soon cease to be effective, whereas pain may persist as long as the stimulus is operative; and, by establishing a central excitatory state, may even outlast the stimulus.

Psychologic aspects of pain A discussion of this problem could hardly be complete without some reference to the influence of emotional states or to the importance of racial, cultural, and religious factors on the pain response, especially its overt expressions. It is common knowledge that some individuals, by virtue of training, habit, or phlegmatic character, are relatively stoical, and that others are excessively responsive to pain. And there are rare individuals who are totally incapable of experiencing pain throughout their lifetime, either from a lack of sensory endings or peripheral sensory apparatus, or from some peculiarity of central reception.

CLINICAL APPROACH TO THE PATIENT WITH ACUTE PAIN

One of the first points to keep in mind is that not all pain is the consequence of serious disease. Otherwise healthy individuals have thousands of pains which are part of their daily sensory experience. To mention but a few, there is the momentary, hard pain over an eye, in the temporal region, or in the ear or jaw, which strikes with alarming suddenness; the more persistent ache which arises in some fleshy part, such as the shoulder, neck, thigh, or calf; the darting pain in an arm or leg; the fleeting precordial discomfort that arouses momentarily the thought of heart disease; the breathtaking catch in the side from diaphragmatic cramp; the cluster of abdominal pains with their associated intestinal rumblings; and the brief discomfort upon movement of a joint. These *normal pains,* as they should be called, occur at all ages, tend to be brief, and depart as obscurely as they come. They acquire medical significance only when elicited by an inquiring physician, or when presented as a complaint by a worried patient; and, of course, they must always be distinguished from the *abnormal pains* of disease.

When pain, by its intensity, duration, and the circumstance of its occurrence, appears to be abnormal or constitutes one of the principal symptoms of disease, an attempt should be made to reach a tentative decision as to its cause and the mechanism of its production. This can usually be accomplished by thoroughly questioning and encouraging the patient to relate as accurately as possible the main characteristics of the pain and the circumstances under which it occurs. The physical examination is directed toward a search for evidences of suspected disease and the reproduction of the pain.

Location of pain When the pain is caused by a superficial lesion, the cause and effect are usually so obvious that no problem is posed. It is the deep lesion, whether involving somatic or visceral structures, that causes trouble, and here exact localization becomes especially important. We have already seen that the pain originating from such tissues is no longer sensed as coming from them, but is instead only roughly segmental, i.e., within the territory of the cord segments innervating the structure. The identification of the segments involved is of value, for it sets the limit on the diagnostic possibilities that must be considered, i.e., they are limited to those structures having a

corresponding innervation. Thus an epigastric or subxiphoid pain, or one in the opposite region in the back, obliges one to search for its cause in all those structures innervated by the sixth through eighth thoracic cord segments, i.e., the esophagus, stomach, duodenum, pancreas, biliary tract, the upper retroperitoneal structures, as well as the deep somatic tissues in this region. Also, one must consider the possibility that a lesion in a viscus innervated by spinal segments above or below the sixth through eighth thoracic cord segments may at times be the source of pain that has spread outside its normal boundaries and involved the epigastrium.

Provoking and relieving factors These factors are of greater value than quality of pain in providing important data concerning its mechanism. Pain related to breathing, swallowing, and defecation focuses attention on the respiratory apparatus, the esophagus, and the lower part of the intestinal tract, respectively. A pain coming on a few minutes after the beginning of general bodily movement and relieved almost at once by rest indicates ischemia or a neural mechanism as the probable cause (see Chaps. 6 and 7). Pain occurring several hours after meals and relieved by food or alkali suggests the irritative effect of acid on the mucosa of the stomach or duodenum. Pain that is brought on or relieved by certain movements or postures of parts of the body is usually due to diseased skeletal structures (bones, muscles, ligaments). Pain that is enhanced by cough, sneeze, and strain is usually radicular in origin or arises in ligamentous structures.

Quality and time-intensity characteristics of pain Much reliance is put on the patient's choice of words and account of the intensity of pain. Unfortunately this will depend, in part at least, on the patient's intelligence, vocabulary, and concept of what is taking place. "Crushing" and "squeezing" are commonly employed to describe an anginal pain, and this implication of pressure has some significance since the pain may depend on an associated involuntary contraction of the pectoral muscles. Another patient with the same disease, however, may describe the pain as "exploding" or "burning." Far more important than the adjective used for pain is the information that it is steady and does not fluctuate. Similarly, the pain of peptic ulcer is frequently designated as "gnawing," but again, the deep, steady quality is more important than the word used to denote it. Gallbladder colic and renal colic are misnomers, if by *colic* is meant a "paroxysmal abdominal pain due to spasm, obstruction, or distention of any of the hollow viscera." *In both these disorders, the pain tends to be steady.* The aching quality of all deep pains is usually characteristic, but there are also several other informative attributes. A true colicky pain, one that is rhythmic and cramping, suggests an obstructive lesion in a hollow viscus. A pain that is steady and varies little or not at all from moment to moment means that the stimulus to pain is steady and unwavering, as in angina pectoris and peptic ulcer. Thus, a pain in the anterior midsternal region whose intensity fluctuates appreciably within the space of a minute or two is not due to angina, even though the history may appear to suggest a relation to exertion. Similarly, a high epigastric pain appearing several hours after a meal and even apparently relieved by food is not caused by an ulcer if the pain fluctuates perceptibly within seconds or a few minutes. The stimulus to ulcer pain does not quickly vary in intensity. A throbbing pain indicates that an arterial pulsation is giving rise to painful stimuli. Sharp, recurrent stabs of pain are caused by disease of nerve roots or sensory ganglions, as exemplified by tic douloureux or tabes, or a single episode may be due to a tear of a muscle or ligament. Once started, in each instance there may be a background of dull, aching pain. Particularly noteworthy here is the abrupt intensification of the dull ache of root pain by cough, sneeze, or strain which momentarily stretches or alters the position of the root.

Mode of onset of pain This factor is also important. A pain reaching its full intensity almost immediately after its appearance suggests a rupture of tissue. The pain of a dissecting aortic aneurysm often develops in this manner. In fact, the suddenness and the severity of the pain, reaching a peak of intensity within seconds or minutes, sometimes provides the first clue in differentiating this type of chest pain from that caused by myocardial infarction. A similarly rapid accession of pain may occur with the rupture of a peptic ulcer.

Duration of pain This is another useful diagnostic attribute. Anginal pain, for example, rarely lasts less than 2 or 3 min or more than 10 to 15 min. Ulcer pain may continue for an hour or more, unless terminated by the ingestion of food or alkali or a tumbler of water.

Severity of pain In any given disease, the severity of pain is subject to wide variation, and patients differ in their tolerance to it. Therefore, one cannot judge the gravity of an illness solely by the patient's report of the intensity of pain. As a rule, pains that completely interrupt work or pleasurable activity, require opiates for relief, enforce bed rest, or awaken the patient from sound sleep are to be taken more seriously than those which have the opposite characteristics.

Time of occurrence An accurate determination must be made of the temporal aspects of the pain. The relationship of ulcer pain to the preceding meal has already been mentioned. Postural aches come after prolonged activity and disappear with rest; arthritic pains are usually most severe during the first movements after prolonged inactivity. The mechanisms for this latter phenomenon are not known, nor do we understand why painful lesions of the bone, such as those caused by metastatic cancer, are likely to be most disturbing during the night. It is possible that the occurrence or aggravation of the latter types of pain is due to enhanced awareness of painful stimuli at a time when the mind is not distracted by other stimuli, or it may be that the pains are now more easily evoked by unconscious movements made during sleep when protective reflexes are in abeyance.

It should be obvious from these remarks that the full significance of a pain is usually not revealed by any one single characteristic. It is only by combining all these data that one can determine its anatomic site and its mechanism. In general, *the most important and revealing clues are obtained from the answers to the questions: What brings on the pain? What relieves it?* Pain is a subjective manifestation, not a state to be observed or measured. The accuracy of our data depends on the skill with which we frame our questions and on the powers of observation and memory of the person answering them.

Finally, the diagnostic value of measures which *reproduce* and *relieve the pain* should be stressed. Not only are they important for diagnosis, but they convince the patient that the physician understands and can control pain and the illness behind it. Climbing several flights of stairs under the physician's supervision may settle the question of the presence or absence of angina pectoris. An injection of procaine into the tender area in the chest wall or some other skeletal structure, with complete disappearance of the pain, may establish its skeletal origin and exclude the possibility of visceral disease. Reproducing the distress sometimes caused by aerophagia merely by distending the esophagus or stomach with air, or reproducing the vague but sometimes alarming sensation of pressure in the chest caused by unconscious hyperventilation by having the patient deliberately hyperventilate are other examples of how the principle of the reproduction of pain may be usefully employed.

A systematic interrogation of the patient will not lead to accurate diagnosis in every instance, but the habit of searching for the identifying characteristics of pain will enable physicians to increase their skill in this difficult field. Furthermore, after becoming familiar with the customary responses to these questions, one becomes more alert to the anxious, the hysterical, or the depressed patient who while complaining of pain seems incapable of describing any of its details, or is unwilling to do so. Instead, there is preoccupation with theories of what is wrong or with the treatments or mistreatments already given.

MANAGEMENT OF ACUTE PAIN Acute pain arising in skin, bone, muscles, and joints is effectively treated with nonnarcotic analgesic agents, which decrease pain without causing alteration in the level of consciousness (Table 2-1). Aspirin, 300 to 600 mg, or acetaminophen (Tylenol), 650 mg orally every 4 to 6 h, is often effective. Other nonsteroidal anti-inflammatory agents, including phenacetin, 600 mg every 3 to 4 h; zomepirac (Zomax), 50 to 100 mg every 4 to 6 h; sulindac (Clinoril), 150 to 200 mg 2 to 3 times daily; or ibuprofen (Motrin), 200 to 600 mg every 6 h, may be used, but these agents have not been shown unequivocally to be better than their less-expensive counterparts aspirin and acetaminophen. Commercial proprietary combinations of aspirin, phenacetin, and acetaminophen often also containing caffeine (Empirin Compound, Excedrin, ASA Compound) are widely self-administered. All nonsteroidal anti-inflammatory drugs have potential side effects of gastrointestinal irritation and may cause allergic reactions. The side effects of aspirin, particularly dyspepsia, gastrointestinal bleeding, and inhibition of platelet aggregation, are not observed with acetaminophen and make the latter the safer and in many circumstances the more useful agent. Aspirin and acetaminophen in combination are not more effective than either one alone, but either in combination with codeine is more effective than codeine alone.

Unresponsiveness of pain in integumentary or musculoskeletal tissues may require the acute administration (for 5 to 7 days) of mild narcotic agents such as codeine, propoxyphene, or oxycodone (marketed in combination with aspirin and caffeine as Percodan, or with acetaminophen as Percocet). These agents provide additional analgesic effects with little risk of causing addiction with short-term administration. The more severe acute pain of myocardial infarction, pulmonary embolism, and renal and biliary colic usually requires administration of high-potency narcotic agents.

CLINICAL APPROACH TO THE PATIENT WITH CHRONIC PAIN The occurrence of acute pain most often signals a medical problem, the nature of which can be accurately divulged by a careful history and physical examination. Appropriate treatment is given (e.g., steroids for polymyositis, rest and splinting for joint or tendon injury), and the condition subsides. In many patients, however, a relatively minor injury, an obscure or indeterminate source of pain (low back pain), or a structural lesion (postoperative pain, metastatic tumor) results in a chronic pain condition. As Ambroise Paré remarked, "There is nothing that abateth so much the strength as paine." Continuous pain can be observed to have multiple adverse effects, including increased irritability, fatigue, insomnia, anorexia, and depression. Courageous individuals may be reduced to a whimpering, pitiable state that may arouse only the scorn of a healthy person. They may become irrational about illness and make unreasonable demands on the family and physician. Demand for and dependence on narcotic drugs often complicate the picture.

The management of such patients is one of the most difficult in all of medicine and requires great patience and objectivity. Specific treatment in such cases often is not applicable and the approach used may require a combination of drugs, behavioral modification, and occasionally invasive neurosurgical procedures.

MANAGEMENT OF CHRONIC PAIN The management of *chronic pain,* which may be defined as persistent pain of more than 6 months' duration, is a more difficult problem. There are five discernible categories of such patients: (1) those with pain of medical or surgical diseases yet undiagnosable, (2) those with a primary psychiatric disorder, (3) those with pain due to a neurologic lesion, (4) those with pain due to an identified somatic lesion such as metastatic tumor, and (5) those with pain of indeterminate type, commonly present for many years, in whom there is no evidence of medical, psychiatric, or neurologic abnormality.

Pain of undiagnosed medical or surgical disease Repeated, painstaking evaluation eventually reveals the commonest types of disease in this category: neoplasms in the retropharyngeal,

TABLE 2-1
Analgesic agents

		Dose		
Type	*Generic (proprietary)*	*Oral, mg*	*Parenteral, mg*	*Comment*
Nonnarcotic (nonsteroidal anti-inflammatory agents)	Aspirin Acetaminophen (Tylenol) Phenacetin (Acetophenatidin) Ibuprofen (Motrin) Naproxen (Naprosyn) Sulindac (Clinoril)	600 q 3–4 h 650 q 3–4 h 600 q 3–4 h 200–600 q 4 h 250 q 12 h 150–200 tid		Effects due to inhibition of prostaglandin biosynthesis. Side effects include gastrointestinal irritation, possible hepatic and renal toxicity, allergic reactions, and interference with platelet aggregation (aspirin). Acetaminophen is the major metabolite of phenacetin.
	Zomepirac sodium (Zomax) Indomethacin (Indocin) Phenylbutazone (Butazolidin)	100 tid 25–50 q 12 h 100 qd		May cause bone marrow suppression.
Narcotic agents (intermediate potency for moderate pain)	Codeine	15–60 q 4–6 h	60–120 q 4–6 h	Absorbed well after oral use.
	Oxycodone with aspirin, phenacetin, and caffeine (Percodan)	5–10 q 4–6 h		Short-acting, high PO/IM potency ratio, weak narcotic, high addiction potential.
	Oxycodone with acetaminophen (Percocet)	5–10 q 4–6 h		
	Propoxyphene (Darvon)	65 q 3–4 h		Structurally related to methadone, addictive potential.
	Pentazocine (Talwin)	50–100 q 4–6 h	30–60 q 4 h	Mixed narcotic agonist/antagonist: produces withdrawal in patients with physical dependence to narcotics. Low addiction potential.
Narcotic agents (high potency for severe pain)	Morphine		10 q 3–4 h	Standard narcotic, binds to opiate receptors, poor oral efficacy.
	Meperidine (Demerol, Pethidine)	50–100 q 3–4 h	50–100 q 2–4 h	Low PO/IM ratio, 75% of oral dose excreted in feces.
	Levorphanol (Levo-Dromoran)	2 q 6–8 h	2 q 6–8 h	Synthetic, long-acting oral narcotic; high PO/IM ratio.
	Methadone (Dolophine)	10–20 q 3–4 h	2.5–10 q 3–4 h	Long-acting oral narcotic, widely used in maintenance treatment of addicts.
	Hydromorphone (Dilaudid)	1–2 q 3–4 h	2 q 4–6 h	Short-acting narcotic.
Adjuvant drugs	Methotrimeprazine (Levoprome)		10–20 q 4–6 h	Nonnarcotic phenothiazine derivative, pain-relieving effects demonstrated, but mechanism unknown; available only for parenteral use.
	Dextroamphetamine	10 q 6 h		Increases narcotic effects, decreases somnolence.
	Benzodiazepine derivatives: Diazepam (Valium)	5 qid	10–20 q 2–4 h	Useful with mild analgesics for acute pain from muscle spasm or anxiety.
	Antidepressants: Amitriptyline (Elavil) Imipramine (Tofranil) Desipramine (Norpramin)	75–200 qhs 50–150 qhs 50–150 qhs		Useful in depression and painful states with insomnia. All have sedative and anticholinergic effects.
	Phenelzine (Nardil)	15 tid		Postural hypotension; may potentiate effects of narcotics.
	Phenothiazines (see text)			Reported useful in some cases of postherpetic or thalamic pain.
	Anticonvulsants: Carbamazepine (Tegretol) Phenytoin (Dilantin)	200 qid 300–400 qd		Useful in some forms of deafferentation pain, postherpetic neuralgia, diabetic neuropathy.

posterior mediastinal, retroperitoneal regions, and the spine. Other symptoms of systemic illness such as weight loss, fever, and laboratory findings of elevation in erythrocyte sedimentation rate or anemia often clue the physician to the serious nature of the illness.

Pain in psychiatric illness The diagnosis of a psychiatric disorder must be made on the basis of positive evidence and not as a diagnosis of exclusion. Since pain is a subjective experience, without a clinical or laboratory method to assess either its quality or severity, the physician must in general believe and accept the patient's account. The patient's response to the experience of chronic pain will invariably alter the physician's response to the symptom and make it tempting for the physician to ascribe the pain inappropriately to a primary psychiatric disorder. Chronic pain may occur in depression, in "compensation neurosis," in hysteria, and in malingering.

Pain in neurologic disease Among the most difficult pain-management problems are those that follow demonstrated structural lesions of the peripheral or central nervous system. Examples are minor peripheral nerve injury occurring with deep lacerations or bone fractures that give rise to *causalgia;* spinal cord lesions that evolve into a syndrome of burning, dysesthetic pain of the entire body below the level of the lesion; vascular lesions in the thalamus or adjacent internal capsule (thalamic syndrome of Déjerine-Roussy); and postherpetic neuralgia. The chronic pain evoked by these lesions does not ordinarily respond to nonnarcotic analgesics and responds only partially to the potent narcotic drugs; addiction to oral or parenterally administered drugs is common, and the patient is often rendered incapable of working or of normal function. In addition to administration of narcotic drugs, which such patients nearly always demand and usually succeed in obtaining, it is often helpful to treat the depression and anxiety states that result. Tricyclic antidepressants should be given in adequate doses; amitriptyline, 150 to 200 mg daily, or imipramine or desipramine (which have fewer anticholinergic side effects), 100 to 200 mg daily. In addition to their antidepressant actions, the effectiveness of the tricyclics in pain management may relate to their action on blockade of serotonin reuptake, thus facilitating serotonin-mediated suppression of pain transmission. These drugs can be given at bedtime where benefit of the commonly associated insomnia may also be obtained. Benzodiazepine drugs are commonly given together with antidepressants but are in general not very effective in alleviating the anxiety that is commonly present except in doses that cause sedation. The pain of *anesthesia dolorosa* or of *postherpetic neuralgia* has been shown to respond in some cases to carbamazepine (Tegretol), 200 mg given 4 or 5 times daily, or to phenytoin (Dilantin), 300 to 500 mg daily. An occasional patient appears to respond to a combination of the two drugs. Finally, administration of a major tranquilizer, such as chlorpromazine, 50 to 200 mg daily; thioridazine (Mellaril), 30 to 100 mg bid; or fluphenazine (Prolixin), 1 to 3 mg daily, should be considered. The phenothiazine methotrimeprazine (Levoprome), 20 mg every 4 to 6 h subcutaneously or intramuscularly, is reported to have analgesic actions as potent as those of morphine in postoperative pain and in cancer pain without evidence (thus far) of addiction potential. Sedation, postural hypotension, and extrapyramidal side effects may limit its usefulness in a given patient; concomitant administration of trihexyphenidyl (Artane), 2 mg tid, or benztropine (Cogentin), 1 to 2 mg daily, minimize the neurologic side effects. A combination of an antidepressant (amitriptyline) and phenothiazine (fluphenazine) is reported to be effective in postherpetic neuralgia and may be used in other pain conditions if care is given to the detection of undesirable side effects.

Physical and surgical treatments of neurologic conditions associated with pain have in general been unsatisfactory, with less than one-third of patients receiving noticeable benefit from nerve block, transcutaneous stimulation, dorsal column stimulation, rhizotomy, spinothalamic tractotomy, or thalamotomy. In the most severe cases substantial relief of pain, including the withdrawal from narcotic drugs, has been achieved with stereotaxic lesions placed in the amygdala or in the cingulum. It is common for surgical lesions to afford relief of pain for a period of weeks or months only to have the symptoms return with full force.

Pain of metastatic disease The physician's attempt to manage the chronic pain of metastatic disease can range from palliation in a dying patient to the management of bony metastases where survival may extend for many years, as in carcinoma of the prostate. In general, the principles of management follow a strategy similar to that present for neurologic lesions, except that there is less fear about addiction, particularly in terminal cases, and neurosurgical procedures have been shown to be more beneficial. Fifty to sixty percent of patients with cancer have pain, those with tumors of the bone having the highest incidence (85 percent) and those with leukemia the lowest (5 percent). The pain may be due to direct invasion of pain-sensitive structures (about 80 percent of patients), be associated with the treatment (surgery, chemotherapy, radiation—about 20 percent), or be unrelated to the tumor (less than 5 percent). With current techniques of management more than 90 percent of patients with cancer pain can be satisfactorily treated.

Narcotic analgesics are the mainstay of therapy in malignant disease. Pain relief can be achieved in over 95 percent of patients, but narcotic use must be balanced against the undesirable side effects of sedation, constipation, tolerance, physical dependence, and addiction. *Tolerance* is defined as the need to increase the dosage of the drug to achieve the desired analgesic effect. *Physical dependence* is observed when withdrawal of the drug causes symptoms of tremulousness, sweating, anxiety, insomnia, chills, and nausea and vomiting. *Addiction* should be distinguished from tolerance and physical dependence as a concomitant behavioral pattern of drug abuse in which the drug is sought by the patient for effects other than its pain-relieving benefit and which leads to aberrant behavior in the acquisition and use of the drug. Narcotic drugs are divided into two major groups, *agonists,* including morphine, methadone, meperidine, and codeine, and drugs with mixed agonist and *antagonist* properties, the most commonly used being pentazocine (Talwin). *Administration of pentazocine to a patient chronically taking narcotic agonist drugs will precipitate withdrawal symptoms.* In practical terms, the administration of narcotic agents should be given at regular intervals around the clock; intravenous administration is currently under investigation as a potentially more efficacious mode of administration for the most severe kinds of pain. Oral administration of methadone or Dilaudid is efficacious in many cases; the low oral/intramuscular ratio of meperidine (75 percent is excreted in feces) makes it less useful. Combinations of narcotic with nonnarcotic drugs should be used, particularly acetaminophen, antidepressants, and phenothiazines. The development of tolerance usually first becomes apparent by the reduced duration of effect of the narcotic. Amphetamines may be used to counter sedation caused by narcotic agents and may further potentiate analgesic effects. Chronic narcotic administration may cause inappropriate ADH secretion and, with meperidine, myoclonus and seizures.

Pain of undetermined cause This group includes the cases that are left when the first four are excluded. They defy solution. The physician can proceed only by repeatedly reexamining the patient, explaining the need for continued observation, and enlisting the patient's aid and forbearance during this trying period. Asking the patient to tolerate a certain amount of pain without the use of powerful analgesics is usually effective, particularly when the possibility of drug addiction is explained.

Physical methods of pain relief Peripheral nerve blocks or intrathecal administration of phenol or narcotic agents may be effective in regional pain due to metastatic disease. Intrathecal drugs, used widely in England, have not been extensively applied in the United States.

ELECTROANALGESIA The use of electroanalgesia for pain relief, although first used in the nineteenth century, was revived in the 1960s by the popularization of the gate-control hypothesis. Two forms are currently in use. (1) *Transcutaneous nerve stimulation:* This technique uses low-intensity, high-frequency electrical stimulation of the painful area or of its segmental nerve. Initial reports of pain relief were highly favorable, but more recent larger series with longer follow-up show less convincing efficacy. The problem of placebo effect has made accurate assessment of the effects difficult. It has been applied to postoperative pain, to malignancy, to the pain of postherpetic neuralgia, and to the pain of central nervous system lesions. Transcutaneous nerve stimulation should be considered when expert neurosurgical assistance is available, when the pain is anatomically regionalized, and when the pain is unresponsive to other modalities of treatment and the patient is willing to learn the technique. (2) *Acupuncture analgesia:* There is unequivocal evidence that acupuncture, either performed by electrical stimulation or by manual twirling, produces acute analgesia of a degree sufficient to reduce markedly acute operative pain (in some but not all patients). There is no evidence that acupuncture is an effective modality for the treatment of the chronic pains of metastatic disease. The system of meridians initially used has no established basis and segmental stimulation is the most effective in alleviating acute pain. Low-frequency, high-intensity stimulation, most often used in acupuncture, may act via endogenous opioid systems, as analgesic effects are reported to be blocked by naloxone and stimulation causes a rise in endorphin levels in the cerebrospinal fluid. In contrast, analgesia induced by high-frequency, low-intensity stimulation, commonly used with transcutaneous stimulation, is unaffected by naloxone, implying a non-opioid-mediated mechanism.

SURGERY INVOLVING THE CENTRAL NERVOUS SYSTEM Neurosurgical procedures for treatment of pain fall into two categories: (1) an ablative lesion that interrupts pain pathways within the central nervous system, and (2) electrical stimulation of central regions that induce analgesia, presumably by interference with central pain transmission. It is beyond the scope of this text to review the indications, efficacy, and complications of these procedures. Spinal cord tractotomy has been widely used and can bring great benefit to selected patients with metastatic pain. Central electrical stimulation of the thalamus or periaqueductal gray matter, and ablation of limbic system structures (amygdalotomy, cingulotomy) is available only in a few major medical centers and must at this time still be considered an investigational rather than an accepted mode of treatment.

Multidisciplinary pain clinics During the past decade a number of medical centers have established effective units for the interdisciplinary management of complex pain problems. Neurologists, neurosurgeons, anesthetists, psychiatrists, and appropriate paramedical support staff have provided a means to address the many facets of patient care.

REFERENCES

ADAMS RD, VICTOR M: *Principles of Neurology,* 2d ed. New York, McGraw-Hill, 1981

BASBAUM AJ, FIELDS HL: Endogenous pain control mechanisms: Review and hypothesis. Ann Neurol 4:451, 1978

BONICA JJ (ed): *Pain.* Assoc Res Nerv Ment Dis, New York, Raven Press, 1980, vol 58

DYKES RW: Nociception. Brain Res 99:229, 1975

FIELDS HL: Pain II: New approaches to management. Ann Neurol 9:101, 1981

FOLEY KM: The management of pain of malignant origin, in *Current Neurology,* HR Tyler, DM Dawson (eds). Boston, Houghton Mifflin, 1979, vol 2

HARDY JD et al: Pain sensations and reactions. Baltimore, Williams & Wilkins, 1952

HOSOBUCHI Y et al: Pain relief by electrical stimulation of the central gray matter in humans and its reversal by naloxone. Science 197:183, 1977

KRIEGER DT, MARTIN JB: Brain peptides. N Engl J Med 304:876, 944, 1981

LEWIS T: *Pain.* New York, Macmillan, 1942

MELZACK R, WALL PD: Interaction of fast and slow conducting fiber systems involved in pain and analgesia, in *Pharmacology of Pain,* RKS Lim et al (eds). London, Pergamon, 1968

SYNDER SH: Brain peptides as neurotransmitters. Science 209:976, 1980

TASKER R et al: Deafferentation and causalgia, in *Pain,* JJ Bonica (ed). Assoc Res Nerv Ment Dis, New York, Raven Press, 1980, vol 28

WHITE JC, SWEET WH: *Pain and the Neurosurgeon—A Forty Years Experience.* Springfield, Ill., Charles C Thomas, 1969

3
HEADACHE

RAYMOND D. ADAMS

The term *headache* should encompass all aches and pains located in the head, but in common language its application is restricted to unpleasant sensations in the region of the cranial vault. Facial, pharyngeal, laryngeal, and cervical pain will be described in Chaps. 6 and 367. (See also Table 3-1.)

Headache, along with fatigue, hunger, and thirst, represents the most frequent human discomforts. Medically speaking, its significance is often abstruse, for it may stand as a symptomatic expression of disease or of some minor tension or fatigue, incident to the affairs of the day. Fortunately, in most instances it reflects the latter, and only exceptionally does it warn of serious disease seated in intracranial structures. But it is this dual significance, the benign and the potentially malignant, that keeps the physician on the alert. Systematic approach to the headache problem necessitates a broad knowledge of the medical and surgical diseases of which it is a symptom and a clinical methodology which leaves none of the common and treatable causes unexplored.

GENERAL CONSIDERATIONS In the introductory chapter on pain, reference was made to the necessity, when dealing with any painful state, of determining its quality, location, duration, and time course, and conditions which produce, exacerbate, or relieve it. When headache is considered in these terms, a certain amount of useful information is obtained by careful history, but perhaps less than one might expect. Unfortunately, physical examination of the head itself is seldom useful.

As to quality of cephalic pain, the patient is rarely helpful in describing it. In fact persistent questioning on that point occasions surprise, for the patient usually assumes that the word *headache* should have conveyed enough information to the examiner about the nature of the discomfort. Most headaches are dull, deeply located, and of aching character, a pain recognizable as of the type that usually arises from structures deep to the skin. Seldom is there reported the superficial burning, smarting, or stinging type of pain localized to the skin. When asked to analogize the sensation to another sensory experience, the patient may make some allusion to tightness, pressure, or bursting feeling, terms which then give clue to a muscular tension or a psychologic state.

Queries about the intensity of the pain are seldom of much value since they reflect more the patient's attitude toward the condition and a customary way of reporting things that happen than the true severity. As usual the bluff, hearty person tends to minimize discomfort, whereas the neurotic dramatizes it. Degree of incapacity is a better index. A severe migraine attack seldom allows performance of the day's work. The pain which awakens the patient from sleep at night, or prevents sleep, is also more likely to have a demonstrable organic basis. As a rule, the most intense cranial pains are those that accompany subarachnoid hemorrhage and meningitis, which have grave implications, or migraine and paroxysmal nocturnal orbitotemporal (cluster) headaches, which are benign.

Data regarding *location* of the headache are apt to be more informative. If the source is in deep structures (extracranial, i.e., subdermal, or muscular), as is usually the case, the correspondence with the site of the pain is fairly precise. Inflammation of an extracranial artery causes pain well localized to the site of the vessel. Lesions of paranasal sinuses, teeth, eyes, and upper cervical vertebrae induce less sharply localized pain but one that is still referred in a regional distribution that is fairly constant. Intracranial lesions in the posterior fossa cause pain in the occipital-nuchal region, homolateral if the lesion is one-sided. Supratentorial lesions induce frontotemporal pains, again homolateral to the lesion if it is on one side. But localization can also be very uninformative or misleading. Ear pain, for example, although it may mean disease in the ear, more often is referred from other regions, and eye pain may be referred from parts as remote as the occiput or cervical spine.

Duration and *time-intensity curve* of headaches in both the attack itself and their life profile are most useful. Of course the headache of bacterial meningitis or subarachnoid hemorrhage occurs usually in single attacks over a period of days. Single, brief, momentary (1 to 2 s) pains in the cranium are presently uninterpretable and are significant only because they indicate no serious underlying disease. Migraine of the classic type has its onset in the early morning hours or daytime, reaches its peak of severity in a half hour or so, lasts, unless treated, for several hours up to 1 to 2 days, and is often terminated by sleep. In the life history a frequency of more than a single attack every few weeks is exceptional. A migraine patient having several attacks per week usually proves to have a combination of migraine and tension headaches. In contrast to this is the nightly occurrence (2 to 3 h after onset of sleep) over a period of several weeks to months of the rapidly peaking, nonthrobbing orbital or supraorbital pain of cluster headache, which tends to dissipate within an hour. The headache of intracranial tumor characteristically can occur at any time of day or night, can interrupt sleep, varies in intensity, and lasts a few minutes to hours. The life profile is one of increasing frequency and intensity over a period of months. Tension headache, once commenced, may persist continuously for weeks or months, though waxing and waning from hour to hour.

Headache that bears a more or less constant relationship to certain biologic events and also to physical environmental changes may prove to be informative. Premenstrual headaches most typically relate to premenstrual tension during the period of oliguria and edema formation; they usually vanish after the first day of vaginal bleeding. The headaches of cervical arthritis are most typically intense after a period of inactivity, and the first movements in the morning are both difficult and painful. Hypertensive headaches, like those of cerebral tumor, tend to occur on waking in the morning, but, as with all vascular headaches, excitement and tension may provoke them. Headache from infection of nasal sinuses may appear, with clocklike regularity, upon awakening and in midmorning, and is characteristically worsened by stooping and jarring of the head. Eyestrain headaches naturally follow prolonged use of the eyes, as in reading, peering for a long time against glaring headlights in traffic, or watching the cinema. Atmospheric cold may evoke pain in the so-called fibrositic or nodular headache or when the underlying condition is arthritic or neuralgic. Anger, excitement, or irritation may initiate common migraine in certain disposed persons; this is more typical of common migraine than of the classic type. Change of position, stooping, straining, cough, and sexual intercourse are each known to produce a special type of headache, to be described further on. Exertional headaches, another well-known type, are usually benign (only 1 in 10 will have an intracranial lesion) and disappear within weeks to months.

PAIN-SENSITIVE STRUCTURES AND MECHANISMS OF HEADACHE Understanding of headache has been greatly augmented by the observations of surgeons during operations. They inform us that the following cranial structures are sensitive to mechanical stimulation: (1) skin, subcutaneous tissue, muscles, arteries, and periosteum of skull; (2) delicate structures of eye, ear, and nasal cavity; (3) intracranial venous sinuses and their tributary veins; (4) parts of the dura at the base of the brain and the arteries within the dura mater and pia-rachnoid; and (5) the trigeminal, glossopharyngeal, vagus, and first three cervical nerves. The bony skull, much of the pia-arachnoid and dura, and the parenchyma of the brain lack sensitivity. Interestingly, pain is practically the only sensation produced by stimulation of the listed structures.

The pathways whereby sensory stimuli, whatever their source, are conveyed to the central nervous system are the trigeminal nerves for structures above the tentorium in the anterior and middle fossae of the skull, and the first three cervical nerves for those in the posterior fossa and infradural structures. The ninth and tenth cranial nerves supply part of the posterior fossa and refer the pain to the ear and throat. The tentorium is the border zone between the trigeminal and cervical innervation. The central connections through spinal cord and brainstem to thalamus have already been described in Chap. 2 and will be depicted in Chap. 18.

The pain of intracranial disease is referred, by a mechanism already discussed, to some part of the cranium lying within the areas supplied by the aforementioned nerves (the fifth, ninth, and tenth cranial nerves and the first three cervicals). There may be an associated local tenderness of the scalp at the site of reference. Dental or jaw pain may also have cranial reference. The pain of disease in other parts of the body is not referred to the head, although it may initiate headache by other means.

By analysis of several types of headache, Wolff and his colleagues have demonstrated that most "spontaneous" cranial pains can be traced to the operation of one or more of the following mechanisms:

1 Distention, traction, and dilatation of the intracranial or extracranial arteries
2 Traction or displacement of large intracranial veins or the dural envelope in which they lie
3 Compression, traction, or intrinsic disease of cranial and spinal nerves
4 Voluntary or involuntary spasm and possibly interstitial inflammation and trauma of cranial and cervical muscles
5 Meningeal irritation and raised intracranial pressure

Appenzeller would add to the list hysteria and some "psychogenic" disorders.

More specifically, intracranial mass lesions cause headache only if in a position to deform, displace, or exert traction on vessels and dural structures at the base of the brain, and this may happen long before intracranial pressure rises. In fact, the artificial induction of high intraspinal and intracranial pressure by the subarachnoid or intraventricular injection of sterile saline solution does not result in headache. Some have interpreted this to mean raised intracranial pressure does not cause headache, a conclusion which is called into question by the demonstrable relief of headache by lumbar puncture and lowering the cerebrospinal fluid (CSF) pressure in some patients. Actually, most patients with high intracranial pressure complain of recurrent bioccipital and bifrontal headache, probably due to traction on vessels or dura. As to localization, the pains follow the patterns mentioned above; those lesions deflecting the falx or pressing on superior longitudinal or straight sinuses induce pain behind or above the eye; if the lateral part of the lateral sinus is involved, the pain is felt in the ear. Displacement of tentorium elicits pain felt in the supraorbital region.

Dilatation of the extracranial, temporal, and intracranial arteries with stretching of surrounding sensitive structures is believed to be the mechanism of most of the pain of migraine. Extracranial, temporal, and occipital arteries, when involved in giant-cell arteritis (cranial or "temporal" arteritis), a disease which usually afflicts individuals over 50 years of age, give rise to headache of dull aching and throbbing type, at first localized and then more diffuse. Characteristically it is severe and persistent over a period of weeks or months. The offending artery, strangely, is not always tender to pressure, yet section of it, as in biopsy, may relieve the pain (Chap. 69). Evolving atherosclerotic thrombosis of internal carotid, anterior, and middle cerebral arteries is sometimes accompanied by pain in the forehead or temple; with vertebral artery thrombosis the pain is postauricular, and basilar artery thrombosis causes pain to be projected to the occiput and sometimes the forehead.

In *infection or blockage* of *paranasal sinuses,* accompanied usually by pain over the antrum or in the forehead (from the ethmoid and sphenoid sinuses the pain localizes around the eyes on one or both sides or in the vertex or other part of the cranium, especially in disease of the sphenoid sinuses), the mechanism involves changes in pressure and irritation of pain-sensitive sinus walls. Usually it is associated with tenderness of the skin in the same distribution. The pain may have two remarkable properties: (1) When throbbing, it may be abolished by compressing the carotid artery on the same side. (2) It tends to recur and subside at the same hours, i.e., on awakening, with gradual disappearance when the person is upright, and coming again in the late morning hours. The time relations are believed to yield information concerning the mechanism; morning pain is ascribed to the sinuses filling at night, and its relief on arising to emptying after the erect posture has been assumed. Stooping intensifies the pain by pressure change, as do blowing the nose and jarring the head sometimes; and inhalant sympathomimetic drugs such as Neo-Synephrine, which reduce swelling and congestion, tend to relieve the pain. Some believe that the highly sensitive orifice of the sinus is the source, but more probably the pain arises in the sensitive mucous membrane of the sinus. However, it may persist after all purulent secretions have disappeared, probably because of mechanism of blockage of the orifice by boggy membranes and a vacuum or suction effect on the sinus wall (*vacuum sinus headaches*). The condition is relieved when aeration is restored. During air flights both earache and sinus headache tend to occur on descent, when the relative pressure in the blocked viscus falls.

Headache of ocular origin, located as a rule in the orbit, forehead, or temple, is of steady, aching type and tends to follow prolonged use of the eyes in close work. Ocular muscle imbalance is believed to be the mechanism. The main faults are hypermetropia and astigmatism (not myopia), which result in sustained contraction of extraocular as well as frontal, temporal, and even occipital muscles. Convergence insufficiency is another common disorder. Correction of the refractive error abolishes the headache. Traction on the extraocular muscles during eye surgery, particularly on the iris, will evoke pain. Another mechanism is involved in the raised intraocular pressure seen in acute glaucoma or iridocyclitis, which causes steady, aching pain in the region of the eye. When intense, it may radiate throughout the distribution of the ophthalmic division of the trigeminal nerve. As for ocular pain in general, it is important that the eyes should always be refracted, but eyestrain is probably not as frequent as one would expect from the wholesale dispensing of spectacles. The pain of diabetic third nerve palsy, intracranial aneurysm, cavernous sinus thrombosis, and Raeder's paratrigeminal syndrome may also be referred to the eye.

The mechanism of *headaches accompanying disease of ligaments, muscles, and apophyseal joints* in the upper part of the spine, which are referred to occiput and nape of neck on the same side, can be in part reproduced by the injection of hypertonic saline solution into these structures. Such referred pains are especially frequent in middle and late adult life in patients with rheumatoid and hypertrophic arthritis and tend also to occur after whiplash injuries to the neck. If the pain is articular or synovial in origin, the first movements after being still for some hours are both stiff and painful. In fact, evocation of pain by active and passive motion of the spine should indicate traumatic or other disease of movable parts. The pain of myofibrositis, evidenced by tender nodules near the cranial insertion of cervical and other muscles, is more obscure. There are no pathologic data as to the nature of these vaguely palpable lesions, and it is uncertain whether the pain actually arises in them. They may represent only the deep tenderness felt in the region of referred pain or the involuntary secondary protective spasm of muscles. Characteristically, the pain is steady (nonthrobbing) and spreads from one to both sides of the head. Exposure to cold or draft may precipitate it. Though severe at times, it seldom prevents sleep. Massage of muscles and heat have unpredictable effects but relieve the pain in some cases.

The *headache of meningeal irritation* (infection or hemorrhage), which is of acute onset, severe, generalized, deep-seated, constant, especially intense at the base of the skull, and associated with stiffness of neck on bending forward, has been ascribed by some authorities to increased intracranial pressure. Indeed the withdrawal of CSF may afford some relief. But dilatation and congestion of inflamed meningeal vessels must also be a factor. It seems more probable, therefore, that the pain is due to the chemical irritation of nerve endings in the meninges.

Lumbar puncture headache, which is characterized by a steady occipital-nuchal pain and also by frontal pain coming on a few minutes after arising from a recumbent position and relieved within a few minutes by lying down, has as its cause a persistent leakage of CSF into the lumbar tissues through the needle site. The CSF pressure is low (often 0 in the lateral decubitus position), and the injection of sterile isotonic saline solution intrathecally relieves it. The headache is usually increased by compression of the jugular veins and is unaffected by digital obliteration of one carotid artery. It seems probable that in the upright position a low intraspinal and negative intracranial pressure exerts traction on dural attachments and dural sinuses by caudal displacement of the brain. Understandably, then, headache following cisternal puncture is rare. As soon as the leakage of CSF stops and CSF pressure is gradually restored (usually from a few days up to a week or so), the headache disappears. "Spontaneous" low-pressure headache may also follow a sneeze or strain, presumably because of rupture of the spinal arachnoid along a nerve root.

The mechanism of the throbbing or steady headache which accompanies febrile illnesses, located in frontal or occipital regions or generalized, is probably vascular. It is much like histamine headache in being relieved on one side by carotid artery compression and on both sides by jugular vein compression or the subarachnoid injection of saline solution. It is increased by shaking the head. It seems probable that the meningeal vessels pulsate unduly and stretch pain-sensitive structures around the base of the brain. In certain cases, however, the pain may be lessened by compression of temporal arteries, and in these cases a component of the headache seems to be derived from the walls of extracranial arteries, as in migraine.

The claims of insufferable headaches by the hysteric are undecipherable. The so-called tension headaches of patients with anxiety states and depression are allegedly due to chronic spasm of cranial and cervical muscles. Combinations of the tension and vascular headaches give rise to the "mixed headaches" of many psychiatric patients.

PRINCIPAL CLINICAL VARIETIES OF HEADACHE Usually there is no difficulty in diagnosing the headache of glaucoma, purulent sinusitis, bacterial meningitis, and brain tumor, and a fuller account of these special headaches will be found where these diseases are described in later sections of the book. It is when headache is chronic, recurrent, and unattended by other important signs of disease that the physician faces one of the most difficult medical problems.

The following types of headache should then be considered.

Migraine The term *migraine* refers to periodic, hemicranial throbbing headaches which usually begin in childhood, adolescence, or early adult life and recur in diminishing number and intensity during advancing years. Migraine is frequent, found in an estimated 5 percent of the population. Women are slightly more susceptible than men. There is a tendency for the headaches to occur during the period of premenstrual tension and fluid retention and to cease during pregnancy.

Two closely related syndromes have been identified. The first is called *classic* or *neurologic migraine,* the second *common migraine.* The classic type is ushered in by prominent neurologic symptoms such as visual scintillations and spreading scotomata, hemisensory disorder, aphasic difficulty, and hemiparesis. These neurologic symptoms last for 15 to 30 min and cease or merge into a hemicranial or generalized throbbing headache with nausea and sometimes vomiting, all of which last for several hours up to 1 to 2 days. In the common type there is an unheralded onset of headache, nausea, and vomiting, following the same temporal pattern but without the antecedent neurologic symptoms. Both headache syndromes respond to ergot preparations, if administered early in the attack. Their genetic nature is evidenced by concurrence in near relatives in 60 to 80 percent of cases, but inheritance is somewhat less clear in the common than the classic variety, perhaps because diagnosis is less accurate.

Neurologic migraine presents such a dramatic and at times confusing sequence of events that it merits further description. On awakening in the morning, or at any time of day, the patient may have a premonition of an attack in the form of a feeling of elation, excessive energy, thirst, a craving for sweet foods, or drowsiness. Or there may be no warning whatsoever. In either instance abruptly there is a disturbance of vision consisting of bright spots or dazzling zigzag lines (fortification spectra) which gives way within minutes to scotomatous or homonymous hemianopic field defects; sometimes they are bilateral and even total blindness may rarely occur. Soon thereafter numbness and tingling of the lips, face, hand, and leg on one side occurs, sometimes in combination with an aphasic disorder. The arm and leg may become weak or paralyzed on one side, raising the specter of a stroke. Only one or a few of these symptoms may be present in any given patient and they tend to occur in the same combination in each attack. If the numbness or weakness spreads from one part of the body to another, it does so slowly over a period of minutes. The symptoms last for 5 to 30 min and then recede with complete recovery of function. Within a few minutes they are followed by the unilateral headache, usually on the side of the cerebral dysfunction, which gradually increases in intensity. At its peak in an hour or so or earlier, nausea and vomiting may occur. The headache is usually the most unpleasant feature of the illness.

A number of special neurologic syndromes have been delineated and certain clusterings of symptoms implicate particular cerebral arteries. The neurologic syndrome described above is explainable by involvement of a middle cerebral artery, though a purely hemianopic defect could be due to spasm of a posterior cerebral artery. Bickerstaff first called attention to *basilar migraine* in which the visual disorder and paresthesias are bilateral and are accompanied by confusion, stupor, rarely coma, aggressive outbursts, vertigo, diplopia, and dysarthria. While the full syndrome is infrequent, partial basilar syndromes are found in some 30 percent of children with migraine (Hockaday). Alternating hemiplegias in children have also been attributed to basilar migraine but could as well be due to alternating involvement of the middle cerebral arteries. An attack of confusion may be the presenting syndrome in basilar migraine, as was noted in the cases of Gascon and Barlow, and it may be difficult to diagnose, especially if preceded by cranial trauma. Ophthalmoplegic migraine, usually with involvement of the third nerve on one side, can be due to spasm of carotid or posterior cerebral artery.

Much variation occurs in the main clinical components of the migraine attack, and since there is no reliable laboratory test for confirmation of the diagnosis, one never knows the acceptable limits of neurologic migraine. The neurologic syndromes may occur and not be followed by any headache whatsoever. The first neurologic syndrome may not occur until late adult life in a person not known to have migraine. According to Fisher this state accounts for many of the transitory strokes in young and middle-aged adults. Instead of the neurologic symptoms preceding the headache they may occur simultaneously. And they may not be completely reversible; a residual visual field defect or hemisensory defect or mental backwardness (in a few of the malignant hemiplegic migraines of children) may be permanent. In general the headache part of the syndrome tends to lessen with age. In children abdominal pain and vomiting, sometimes cyclical, may accompany the headache or be the sole expression of migraine; and the same is true of paroxysmal vertigo of children. Without the headache it would be called the benign vertigo syndrome of childhood or labyrinthitis.

There are also wide variations in the intensity of headache in the common migraine. When the "sick headache" comes on in the daytime the patient is usually forced to lie down and shun light and noise. Milder forms, especially if partially controlled by medication, do not force withdrawal from accustomed activities. The headache, though typically hemicranial (the word *migraine* is said to be derived from *megrim,* meaning hemicranial), may always be bifrontal or generalized. Some patients vomit frequently and are pale and deathly ill; others experience only anorexia or minimal nausea.

Between attacks the migrainous patient is essentially normal. For a time years ago, when psychosomatic medicine was much in vogue, there was insistence on a migrainous personality characterized by rigidity of thinking, meticulousness, and perfectionism. The migrainous attack was said to occur during the let-down period after many hours and days of hard work under stressful conditions. But personality analyses on a larger population have not borne out these ideas, and the temporal relationship between headache and the day's activities have not been consistent. Moreover, the genetic factor and the beginning of the headaches in infancy and early childhood, when the personality is relatively amorphous, would argue against the importance of a personality type.

MECHANISM A complete theory of pathogenesis has eluded clinical investigators. All agree that the migraine attack consists of a neurovascular disorder of the intracranial as well as extracranial vessels. Sequential studies of cerebral blood flow, the most recent being those of Oleson, Larson, and Lauritzen, show a reduction, either in the territory of the affected artery or generalized, and an increased perfusion of 35 to 50 percent during the later headache period. In some recordings a period of hyperemia also preceded the oligemia.

The cause of the circulatory changes is disputed. Histamine, serotonin, and norepinephrine levels are increased in the blood during attacks. Couch and Hassanein found an increase in platelet aggregability in migraine patients during an attack and they suggest that it may be responsible for the stroke that complicates migraine. Clover and his associates have measured a transitory decrease in platelet monoamine oxidase activity during attacks. Also, the platelets are increased in number and are depleted of their serotonin content. Increased amounts of the catabolites of the biogenic amines, especially 5-hydroxyindoleacetic acid (5-HIAA) derived from serotonin, and of vanillylmandelic acid (VMA), a product of norepinephrine and epinephrine, are excreted in the urine during the attack. Lance interprets the premonitory hypothalamic symptoms (thirst, hunger, etc.) as being under dopaminergic control.

The headache part of the syndrome has been attributed to excessive pulsation of extracranial arteries (and possibly intracranial ones) since the time of the original observations of it by Graham and Wolff. Liberation of pain-producing substances such as kallikrein and bradykinin (neurokinin) from the extracranial vessels into the perivascular edematous tissue has been found and may account for the tenderness of scalp in some cases. Their algogenic action is potentiated by serotonin.

There is some evidence that the cranial vessels of the migraine patient are hypersensitive. In headache-free intervals they are abnormally responsive to intravenous histamine and to inhalation of CO_2.

But what triggers the attack? Some patients describe exposure to sunlight, exercise, tension, alcohol, and the eating of certain foods (the use of oral contraceptives increases the frequency and severity of migraine in some women), but these are exceptional. Onset may occur during sleep. Plainly, we cannot answer this question.

DIAGNOSIS Classic migraine should occasion no difficulty in diagnosis if the above facts are kept in mind and if a good history is obtained. That is possible, as a rule, for migraine patients tend to be intelligent.

The real difficulties come from three sources: (1) ignorance of the fact that a progressively unfolding neurologic syndrome may be migrainous in origin; (2) lack of appreciation that the neurologic disorder may occur without headache; (3) lack of awareness that recurrent headaches, which may be an isolated phenomenon, may take many forms, some of which may prove difficult to distinguish from the other common types of headache described in this chapter.

Some of these problems merit further elaboration because of their practical importance, as follows:

The neurologic part of the migraine syndrome may resemble focal epilepsy, the clinical picture of a vascular malformation such as an angioma or aneurysm, or some other vascular disease such as a thrombotic or embolic stroke. Here it is the pace of the neurologic symptoms of migraine more than their character that reliably distinguishes the condition from epilepsy. The clinical profile of the aura of epilepsy is measured in seconds, for it depends on spreading neural excitation, in contrast to the slow progression of migraine, which is based on spreading vascular spasm. Nevertheless, there are instances where episodes of coma with EEG abnormality could be either migraine or epilepsy. A seizure is often followed by a generalized headache.

Ophthalmoplegic migraine will always suggest a carotid aneurysm, but in relatively few cases has carotid arteriography revealed such an abnormality. Despite many claims that the question of a vascular malformation should be raised in cases of hemicranial painful attacks occurring invariably on the same side of the head (unlike migraine), in a large series of cases this has only rarely been confirmed by arteriography. Of course, focal epilepsy, protracted headache, stiff neck and bloody cerebrospinal fluid, a persistent neurologic deficit, and cranial bruit would be indicative of a vascular type of headache associated with angioma or aneurysm. Only in the earlier stages, when periodic throbbing headache is the sole symptom, might it be confused with true migraine.

Attacks indistinguishable from migraine may also appear in association with the hypertensive and cerebral arteriosclerotic vascular diseases of late life. Here one is aided by late age of onset, more persistent and frequent headaches, and the evidence of vascular disease of heart, lower extremities, and brain.

A special problem relates to paroxysms of throbbing headache, not hemicranial in distribution, not preceded by a neurologic aura, and not accounted for by other known cause. Are they examples of common migraine? Unfortunately, since diagnosis depends on the interpretation of the patient's description of symptoms, the controversy as to where migraine begins and ends is of the armchair type. Favoring the diagnosis of migraine are lifelong history, childhood onset, positive family history, and response of the headache to ergot derivatives.

A variety of episodic attacks have been described as migraine equivalents: attacks of abdominal pain with nausea, vomiting, and diarrhea; pain localized in the thorax, pelvis, and extremities; bouts of fever; paroxysmal vertigo; transient disturbances in mood (psychic equivalents); recurrent nocturnal orbital (cluster) headache, or migrainous neuralgia. Watson and Steele attribute these associated conditions to a paroxysmal disequilibrium which they find in approximately one-third of migrainous children. The only advantage of considering such attacks as migrainous is that this view protects some patients from unnecessary diagnostic procedures and surgical intervention—but it may also prevent necessary surgery.

From all this discussion the reader should be left with the

idea that the migraine syndromes are more numerous and more protean than the rigid stereotyped descriptions we have given would suggest. In these days of complicated diagnostic procedures it is tempting to take x-rays or do computerized tomography (CT scan) of the skull and perform arteriography and electroencephalography on every patient. A conservative approach would lead to temporization, reserving CT scan or EEG for the exceptional case.

Cluster headache This headache is also called *paroxysmal nocturnal cephalalgia, migrainous neuralgia, histamine headache,* and Horton's syndrome. It is characterized by a fourfold higher incidence in men than in women, constant, unilateral orbital localization, and onset usually within 2 or 3 h after falling asleep, during the phase of rapid eye movement (REM) sleep (it may occur, but is infrequent, during the waking hours). The pain is intense and steady (nonthrobbing) with lacrimation, blocked nostril, then rhinorrhea, and sometimes miosis, ptosis, flush, and edema of cheek, all lasting approximately an hour or two. It tends to recur nightly for several weeks or a few months (hence the term *cluster*), followed by complete freedom for years. The pain of a given attack may leave as rapidly as it began. Clusters may recur over the years, being possibly more likely in times of stress, prolonged strain, overwork, and with upsetting emotional experiences. Occasionally alcohol, nitroglycerine, or tyramine-containing foods precipitate an attack. Rarely, the condition may occur in daytime and may not cluster but continue for years.

The picture is so characteristic that it cannot be confused with any other disease, though to those unfamiliar with it the possibility of a carotid aneurysm, hemangioma, brain tumor, or sinusitis may be suggested. Appropriate roentgenograms and carotid arteriography will always exclude such conditions but usually are unnecessary. In the differential diagnosis orbital, nasociliary, supraorbital, Sluder's sphenopalatine, and neuralgias must also be considered (see Chap. 367).

In the life history profile the clusters of headache may last for weeks. The clusters may be single or recur two, three, or more times, with years of freedom in between, during which such precipitating factors as alcohol are no longer effective. Often the pain involves the same orbit in each cluster. Examples are seen in which the same type of headache may last a year or more or even for a period of 10 to 20 years.

The relationship of the cluster headache to migraine remains conjectural. A portion of the cases have a background of migraine, which led to the earlier postulation of migrainous neuralgia, but the majority do not. The face of the patient with cluster headache turns red (by infrared photography), whereas that of the migraine patient is pale. Several investigators (Henry et al.) found no change in cerebral blood flow. Doppler studies of supraorbital and frontal extracranial arteries evidenced a reduced blood flow at the onset of an attack of headache and an increased pulsation later. In migraine there is hyperperfusion during the headache period. Some investigators have found a drop in the blood pressure of migraine patients; none occurs with cluster headaches.

Tension headache and various other cranial pains with psychiatric disease The headache is usually bilateral, often with diffuse extension over the top of the cranium. Occipital-nuchal localization is also common. Although the sensation may be described as pain, close questioning may uncover other sensations, viz., fullness, tightness, or pressure (as if the head is surrounded by a band or in a vise), on which waves of aching pain are superimposed. The onset of a given attack is more gradual than in migraine and not infrequently a throbbing "vascular" type of headache is added intermittently to a pressure ache. Tension headache may occur acutely under conditions of emotional excitement or intense worry and lasts for hours or a day or two. More often it persists unremittingly for weeks or months. In fact, this is the only type of headache that exhibits the peculiarity of being absolutely continuous day and night for long periods of time. Although sleep may be possible, whenever the patient awakens, the headache is present; the common analgesic remedies have no beneficial effect unless the pain is intense and of aching type.

As to mechanism, the ascription of it to sustained muscle activity, shown by the electromyogram, can at best be only a partial explanation. Indeed, several recent investigations have revealed no consistent changes in the EMG of forehead or neck muscles. The continuous pressing quality of milder cephalic sensations at times when the patient is relaxed hardly seems to be attributable to physiologic stimulation and suggests instead that the condition is maintained by focused attention on the head (occasioned sometimes by worry and fear of intracranial disease). Moreover, it must be remembered that all types of headache in their late stages may give rise to muscle tension, and that this is of an aching rather than a pressure type. In contrast to migraine, in which pain is periodic and lifelong, with tendency to lessen in late adult years, tension headache occurs more often in middle age and usually coincides with anxiety and depression in the trying times of life. Many premenstrual headaches are of this type, and there is an increased incidence of this type of tension headache at menopause. Worried medical students may have it.

Psychologic studies of groups of patients with tension headaches have revealed prominent symptoms of depression, anxiety, and to a lesser extent hypochondriasis. Kudrow records that 65 percent of depressed patients have this type of headache and that over 60 percent of his patients with tension headaches were depressed. When psychiatric syndromes are searched for in headache patients, it is evident that the majority of those with anxiety neurosis, hysteria, obsessive-compulsive neurosis, and schizophrenia, in which anxiety is a prominent symptom, exhibit this type of headache. Migraine and traumatic headaches may be complicated by tension headache.

Other odd cephalic pains, e.g., boring pains, "clavus hystericus," may occur in hysteria and raise perplexing problems in diagnosis. Their bizarre character, persistence in the face of every known therapy, absence of other signs of disease, and the presence of the stigmata of the hysterical personality provide the basis for correct diagnosis (see Chap. 375).

Headache of angioma and aneurysm The temporal profile of any given attack shows the onset to be sudden or very acute, with the pain reaching a peak within minutes. Neurologic disturbances such as defects in vision, unilateral numbness, weakness, or aphasia may precede or occur after the onset of headache and outlast it. Should hemorrhage occur the headache is often extremely severe and localizes more toward the occiput and neck, lasting many days in association with stiff neck. A cranial or cervical bruit and, of course, blood in the cerebrospinal fluid establish the diagnosis, but it may require verification by arteriography. The claim that vascular malformations may give rise to migraine is probably untenable. Statistical data show migraine to be no more frequent in this group of patients than in the general population. There are, however, a few notable exceptions to this statement. Of course, vascular lesions may exist for long periods of time without headache, or the latter may develop many years after other manifestations, such as epilepsy and hemiplegia (see Chap. 356).

Traumatic headaches Severe, chronic, continuous, or intermittent headaches appear as the cardinal symptom of four posttraumatic syndromes, separable in each instance from the headache that immediately follows head injury (i.e., that of scalp laceration, contusion with sanguineous cerebrospinal fluid and increased intracranial pressure, the syndrome of posttraumatic nervous instability, and posttraumatic dysautonomic cephalagia). The latter term was given by Vijayan and Dreyfus to severe, episodic, throbbing, unilateral headaches accompanied by ipsilateral mydriasis and excessive facial sweating. The condition followed injury to the neck in the region of the carotid sheath. It was postulated that the sympathetic nervous supply of the cranium had been disinhibited, and there was clinical and pharmacologic evidence of sympathetic dysfunction (see Chap. 357).

Headache of chronic subdural hematoma Headache and dizziness of fluctuating severity, followed by drowsiness, stupor, coma, and hemiparesis, are the usual manifestations of chronic subdural hematoma. The head injury may have been minor and forgotten by patient and family. The headaches are deep-seated, steady, unilateral or generalized, and respond to the usual analgesic drugs. The typical attack profile of the headache and other symptoms is one of increasing frequency and severity over several weeks or months. Diagnosis is now established by CT scan and arteriography (see Chap. 357).

Headaches of brain tumor Headache is the outstanding symptom of cerebral tumor. Unfortunately, the quality of the pain has no specific feature. It tends to be deep-seated, nonthrobbing (or throbbing), and aching or bursting. Attacks last a few minutes to an hour or more and occur once or many times during the day. Activity and frequently change in the position of the head may provoke pain, while rest in bed diminishes its frequency. Nocturnal awakening because of pain, although typical, is by no means diagnostic. Unexpected forceful (projectile) vomiting may punctuate the illness in its later stages. As the tumor grows the pain becomes more frequent and severe; it sometimes is nearly continuous terminally. But there are exceptions: some headaches are mild and tolerable, others as agonizing as that of the headache of bacterial meningitis and subarachnoid hemorrhage. If unilateral, the headache is homolateral to the tumor in 9 out of 10 patients. Supratentorial tumors are felt anterior to the interauricular circumference of the skull; posterior fossa tumors behind this line. Bifrontal and bioccipital headache, coming on after unilateral headache, signifies the development of increased intracranial pressure.

HEADACHES RELATED TO MEDICAL DISORDERS Experienced physicians are aware of many conditions in which headache figures as a dominant symptom. These include fevers of any cause, carbon monoxide exposure, chronic lung disease with hypercapnia (headaches often nocturnal), hypothyroidism, Cushing's disease, withdrawal of corticosteroid medication, chronic nitrite or ergot exposure, occasionally Addison's disease, aldosterone-producing adrenal tumors, use of "the pill" in some instances, acute rises in blood pressure, e.g., from pheochromocytoma, and acute anemia with hemoglobin below 10 g.

With reference to chronic hypertension the relation to headache is less clear. Approximately 50 percent of patients with hypertension complain of headaches. Wolff and colleagues state that except with hypertensive encephalopathy where the intracranial pressure may be increased, the mechanism of the headache is similar to that of migraine, i.e., it is vascular. Perhaps the headache is due to the release of vasodilating prostaglandins. The headaches of renal dialysis tend to increase as the blood pressure falls and sodium and osmolality decrease.

An erythromelalgic syndrome (flushing, red hands, numb fingers, blotchy skin) with severe headaches has been described in association with serotonin-secreting tumors, carcinoid tumors, and mastocytosis. In one type reported by Streeter and associates there were high levels of circulating bradykinin.

HEADACHE AND FACIAL PAIN The facial neuralgias discussed in Chap. 367 overlap headache syndromes. For comparison see Table 3-2.

APPROACH TO THE PATIENT WITH HEADACHE Obviously very different possibilities are raised by a patient who presents for the first time with severe headache and a patient who has had recurrent headache over a period of years. The chances of uncovering the cause in the first instance are much greater than in the latter, and some of the potential underlying conditions (meningitis, subarachnoid hemorrhage, epidural or subdural hematoma, glaucoma, and purulent sinusitis) are more serious. The simple rules to follow are that severe, persistent headache with stiff neck and fever always means meningitis and the same combination without fever, subarachnoid hemorrhage. A lumbar puncture is mandatory. Acute persistent headache over a period of hours or days may occur in systemic infections such as influenza (febrile) or as a manifestation of an acute tension state. If there is a diagnosable febrile disease and no stiffness of the neck, lumbar puncture may be deferred. The first attack of migraine may also present in this way, but of course there is no fever.

In searching for the cause of recurrent headache one should investigate the status of cardiovascular and renal systems by blood pressure and urine examination, eyes by fundoscopic, intraocular pressure, and refraction, the sinuses by transillumination and x-rays, the cranial arteries by palpation (and biopsy?), the cervical spine by effect of passive movement of the head and x-rays, the nervous system by neurologic examination, and psychic function by mental status.

Hypertension is, of course, frequent in the general population and when present is always difficult to prove as a cause of recurrent headaches. Minor elevations of blood pressure may be a result rather than the cause of nervous tension. No doubt severe hypertension with diastolic blood pressures of over 110 mmHg is more regularly associated with headache than is moderate hypertension. If headache is severe and frequent, one should always consider the possibilities of underlying anxiety or tension state, or a common migraine syndrome exacerbated by blood vessel disease. The mechanism of the puzzling hypertensive phenomenon of occipital pain, present on awakening in the morning and wearing off during the first hour of the day, is uncertain.

The adolescent with daily frontal headaches represents a special type of problem. Often their relationship to eyestrain is unclear, and refraction of the eyes and new eyeglasses do not relieve the condition. Anxiety or tension is probably a factor in such cases, but it is difficult to be certain of a causal relationship. Some of the most persistent and inexplicable headaches, which have led to a survey by a battery of diagnostic procedures for tumor, have proved in the end to be caused by endogenous depression.

Equally puzzling is the somber, tense adult whose primary complaint is headache, or the migrainous person who in late life or at menopause begins to have daily headaches. Here it becomes important to assess mental status along the lines suggested in Chaps. 11 and 24, looking for evidences of anxiety, depression, and hypochondriasis. The quality and persistence of the headache are suggestive of the possibility of psychiatric illness. Sometimes a direct question as to the patient's idea of what is the matter may elicit suspicion and fear of brain tumor. Antidepressant drugs given as an empirical test may relieve the headache, thus clarifying the diagnosis.

The most worrisome type of patient is the one who has

headache of increasing frequency and severity over a period of months or a year or so. Since an intracranial mass lesion (tumor, abscess, subdural hematoma) is a leading possibility, it becomes necessary to resort to a complete neurologic survey, including careful inspection of optic disks, CT and radioactive isotope scans, and electroencephalogram.

Every elderly person (over 50 to 55 years) with severe headache of some few days or weeks duration should be considered as possibly having cranial arteritis. In this disease women are more often affected than men (4:1) and there is an associated polymyalgia in 25 percent of cases. Conversely, in 50 percent of polymyalgia rheumatica patients there is a cranial arteritis. Increased sedimentation rate, fever, and anemia may be conjoined, but only in a minority of cases, unfortunately. The finding of a thickened temporal artery is important, and arterial biopsy and response to corticosteroids establish the diagnosis; treatment with corticosteroids often relieves the pain (see Chap. 69).

TREATMENT The most important steps in the treatment of headache are those measures which uncover and remove the underlying disease or functional disturbance.

For the common everyday headache due to fatigue, stuffy atmosphere, or excessive use of alcohol and tobacco, it is simply enough to advise avoidance of the offending activity or agent, and symptomatic therapy in the form of aspirin, 0.6 g (some brand such as Anacin), or acetaminophen (Tylenol), 0.6 g, will suffice. Some patients who invariably have headache when constipated and hypochondriacs who not infrequently suffer incapacitating headache, fatigue, and depression whenever bowel elimination does not meet their expectations are not easily helped. Certainly, simple explanation, an anticonstipation regimen, and drugs which counteract depression (see Chap. 11) are preferable to the continuous use of analgesics. Premenstrual headache, if troublesome, can usually be helped by the use of a diuretic compound for the week preceding the menstrual period and a mixture of mild analgesic and tranquilizing medications (aspirin or acetaminophen, 0.6 g, and phenobarbital, 30 mg). If the headaches are severe and incapacitating, they should be treated as common migraine.

Migraine may require no treatment at all, other than an explanation of its nature to the patient and a reassurance that it will do no harm. Some patients know, or allege to know, that certain acts induce attacks, and it is obvious enough that they should be urged to avoid these acts, if possible. In certain instances alcoholic drinks, particularly red wine, are invariably

TABLE 3-1
Common types of headache

Type	*Site*	*Age and sex*	*Clinical characteristics*	*Diurnal pattern*	*Life profile*
Common migraine	Frontotemporal Uni- or bilateral	Children, young to middle-aged adults, both sexes	Throbbing and/or dull ache; worse behind one eye or ear Becomes generalized	Upon awakening or later in day Duration: hours to 1–2 days	Irregular interval, weeks to months Tends to disappear in middle age and during pregnancy
"Neurologic" migraine	Same as above	Same as above	Same as above	Same as above	Same as above
Cluster, histamine headache, or migrainous neuralgia	Orbital Temporal Unilateral	Adolescent and adult males (80–90%)	Intense, nonthrobbing pain	Usually nocturnal; occurs one or more hours after falling asleep Rarely diurnal	Nightly for several weeks to months (cluster) Recurrence: years later
Tension headaches	Generalized	Adolescents and adults, both sexes	Pressure (nonthrobbing); tightness Aching	Continuous, variable intensity, for weeks and months	One or more periods of months to years
Meningeal irritation (meningitis subarachnoid hemorrhage)	Generalized	Any age, both sexes	Intense, steady deep pain, may be worse in neck	Duration: days to a week or more	Single episode
Brain tumor	(See text)	Any age, both sexes	Variable in intensity May awaken patient Steady pain	Lasts minutes to hours; increasing severity	Once in a lifetime: weeks to months
Temporal arteritis	Unilateral, temporal, or occipital	Over 50 years, either sex	Persistent burning, aching	Continuous or intermittent	Persists for weeks to a few months

SOURCE: *After J Patten, Neurological Differential Diagnosis, London, Harold Starke, Springer-Verlag, 1977.*

followed by a migraine. Others claim reduction of attacks of headache by an elimination diet, correction of refractive error, or by psychotherapy. There has been a recent claim that biofeedback reduced the number of migraine attacks by one-third (Lake, Rainey, and Papsdorf), and Lance believes that practiced relaxation is beneficial. However, the author's efforts along the latter lines have seldom been successful.

Treatment of the neurologic aura of migraine is rarely required or possible because of its brevity. If the deficits are lasting, inhalation of an ampul of amyl nitrate should be tried as a preventive measure; it should be used at the first premonition of the attack. The time to initiate treatment of the oncoming headache is during the neurologic disorder. If many of the headaches are mild, the patient may already have learned that 0.6 g aspirin and possibly 5 mg dextroamphetamine sulfate (Dexedrine) will suffice to control the pain. A combination of analgesic and suporific medicine (small dose of phenobarbital) are also helpful. If severe disabling attacks are expected, they, too, respond to simple analgesic medication and rest in a quiet, darkened room. Success has been claimed with ergot preparations, and indeed ergotamine tartrate, 0.25 mg by intravenous injection or 1 to 3 mg held under the tongue until dissolved, will interrupt a headache in 80 to 90 percent of cases if given near the onset of the headache. Sometimes the combination of caffeine, 100 mg with 1 mg ergotamine (Cafergot), is preferred. It may be taken in the form of a tablet (two at the onset of headache and a third in half an hour) or as a rectal suppository (2 mg ergotamine and 100 mg caffeine) if vomiting prevents oral administration.

Because of the danger of prolonged vascular spasm in patients who have vascular disease or are pregnant, ergot preparations must be used cautiously, if at all. Even in healthy individuals more than 10 to 15 mg ergotamine per week is risky, for it may in itself produce headache. Hakkareinen et al. report that tolfenamic acid, an anti-inflammatory agent that blocks prostaglandin receptors in oral doses of 200 mg, was found to be as effective as ergotamine tartrate. For the frequent atypical migraine headaches, some of which respond poorly to ergot, one should prescribe a preparation containing 150 mg aspirin, 160 mg acetophenetidin, and dextroamphetamine sulfate, 5 mg, with phenobarbital, 30 mg. This can be repeated once or twice in a severe attack. Once the headache has become intense (after 30 min), ergot is of little help, and one must resort to codeine sulfate, 30 mg, or meperidine (Demerol), 50 mg, as the only means of terminating the pain. If sleep customarily terminates headache, 50 mg of promethazine (Phenergan) orally is helpful; it also relieves vomiting.

In individuals with frequent migrainous attacks (more than one to three times a month), efforts at prevention are worthwhile. Some success has been obtained with preparations of ergot, 0.5 mg, atropine, 0.3 mg, and phenobarbital (Bellergal), 15 mg, two or three times a day for a few weeks. Propranolol (Inderal), 40 mg tid, has been effective in reducing the frequency and intensity of attacks in approximately one-third of cases. For the most severe forms of the disease, methysergide (Sansert) in a dose of 6 to 8 mg per day given for several weeks or months has proved to be most promising in reducing the frequency of or abolishing attacks. The main contraindication has been retroperitoneal fibrosis; this complication has been reported in several dozen cases when the patient has been treated continuously for more than 4 to 5 months. Discontinuing treatment for 1 month out of every 6 has greatly reduced the incidence of this complication. Recently, claims have been made for pizotifen (a histamine- and serotonin-blocking agent), for amitriptyline, apart from its antidepressant action, and for phenelzine, a monoamine oxidase inhibitor.

All experienced physicians appreciate the importance of helping patients rearrange their schedules so as to control tensions and hard-driving ways of living, so often a feature of many migrainous patients. There is no one way of accomplishing this, but in general, long and costly psychotherapy has not been helpful, or at least one can say there are no substantial data as to its value.

Cluster headaches have proved to be most resistant to treatment. One capsule of Cafergot or 1.0 mg of ergotamine tartrate at bedtime is most widely recommended. However, if the headaches are frequent, severe, and diurnal as well as nocturnal, the intake of ergot may reach dangerous levels. Success has also been claimed for amitriptyline (Elavil), 25 to 100 mg tid, and methysergide, 6 to 8 mg per day, as means of interrupting a cluster. Lance recommends prednisone, 40 mg daily for 5 days then reduced to an amount necessary to control headaches. Lithium carbonate in an initial dose of 250 mg tid is said to give relief in 80 to 90 percent of cases. Histamine desensitization, originally proposed by Horton, has been little used in recent years because of inconsistent results. In rare cases of persistent cluster headaches lasting for 10 to 20 years spectacular success has been obtained by indomethacin (Indocin).

Hypertensive headaches respond to agents which lower

Provoking factors	*Associated features*	*Treatment*
Bright light, noise, tension, alcohol Dark room and sleep relieve Scalp sensitive Pressure helps	Nausea in some cases	Ergot preparation at onset Phenergen in established phase Inderal and Bellargol Methysergide (Sansert) for prevention
Same as above	Blindness and scintillating lights Unilateral numbness Disturbed speech Vertigo Confusion	Same as above
Alcohol in some	Lacrimation, congested eye	Ergot preparation at bedtime Amytryptaline (Elavil) and lithium carbonate for prevention
Fatigue and nervous strain	Depression, nervousness, anxiety, insomnia	Antianxiety and antidepressant drugs
None	Neck stiff on forward bending Kernig and Brudzinski signs	For meningitis or bleeding (see text)
None Sometimes position	Papilledema Vomiting Slow mentation	Corticosteroids Mannitol Glycerol Treatment of tumor
Scalp sensitive Tender arteries	Intermittent or permanent loss of sight Rheumatic myalgia Fever	Corticosteroid therapy

blood pressure and relieve muscle tension. Chlorothiazide (Diuril), 250 to 500 mg twice a day, and methyldopa (Aldomet), 250 to 500 mg per day, when combined with a small amount of phenobarbital, 15 mg tid, or propranolol (Inderal) 40 mg tid, have given the best results. Meprobamate, 200 mg tid, or chlordiazepoxide hydrochloride (Librium), 5 mg tid, may be administered in place of phenobarbital. For the morning occipital ache a capsule containing sodium nitrite, 30 mg, caffeine sodium benzoate, 0.5 g, and acetophenetidin, 0.6 g, has been useful. A simplified method of treating this kind of headache is to supply the caffeine in a cup of strong black coffee and to give aspirin with it. Blocks under the head of the bed may be helpful.

The muscle tension headaches respond best to massage, relaxation, and a combination of drugs which relieve depression [e.g., amitriptyline (Elavil) or imipramine (Tofranil)] and anxiety (e.g., phenobarbital, amobarbital, meprobamate, and chlordiazepoxide hydrochloride). Pain-relieving medicine of non-habit-forming type [e.g., aspirin and propoxyphene hydrochloride (Darvon)], should be added when throbbing headache is present. Stronger analgesic medication (codeine or meperidine hydrochloride) should be avoided. Psychotherapy may be helpful in this group of patients.

The headache of the syndrome of posttraumatic nervous instability requires supportive psychotherapy in the form of reassurance and frequent explanation of its benign and transient nature, a program of increasing physical activity, and drugs which allay anxiety and depression. However, the tricyclic antidepressants are generally less effective than in the mixed tension and throbbing headaches of anxious depressions. Tender scars from scalp laceration may be novocainized repeatedly (subcutaneous injection of 5 ml of 1% procaine) with some degree of success. Settlement of litigation as soon as possible works to the patient's advantage.

Heat, massage, salicylates, and indomethacin or phenylbutazone (Butazolidin) usually effect some improvement in those arthritic diseases of the cervical spine which are associated with cervicocranial pain (see Chaps. 346 and 351).

Corticosteroid therapy is indicated in cranial arteritis to prevent disastrous blindness by occlusion of the ophthalmic arteries, which occurs in 50 percent of untreated patients. Prednisone should be given in full doses (40 mg per day) for at least a month and continued until all symptoms and laboratory abnormalities have disappeared. The headaches of cranial

TABLE 3-2
Types of facial pain

Types	*Site*	*Clinical characteristics*	*Aggravating-relieving factors*	*Diseases*	*Treatment*
Trigeminal neuralgia (tic douloureux)	Second to third division of trigeminal nerve, unilateral	Men : women = 1:3 Over 50 years Paroxysms (10–30 s) of stabbing, burning pain Trigger points, intermittent ache No sensory or motor paralysis	Touching face, chewing, smiling, talking, blowing nose	Idiopathic If in young adults unilateral or bilateral, multiple sclerosis Vascular anomaly Tumor of fifth cranial nerve	Carbamazepine (Tegretol) Phenytoin Surgical section of nerve
Atypical facial neuralgia	Unilateral or bilateral	Predominantly female 30–50 years Continuous intolerable pain Mainly maxillary areas	None	Depressive and anxiety states Hysteria Idiopathic	Antidepressant and antianxiety medication
Supraorbital ciliary, infraorbital, sphenopalatine neuralgias	Unilateral in eye, cheek, ear, neck	Persistent, aching pain	Occasional nasal obstruction	Idiopathic Paranasal sinus disease	Decongestant nasal medication ?Nerve section and injection
Postzoster neuralgia	Unilateral Any one of trigeminal divisions	History of zoster Aching, burning pain; jabs of pain Paresthesia, slight sensory loss Dermal scars	Contact, movement	Herpes zoster	Carbamazepine and phenytoin and antidepressants
Costen's syndrome	Unilateral, near temporomandibular joints	Elderly females Severe aching pain, intensified by chewing Tenderness over joints Malocclusion	Chewing, pressure over temporomandibular joint	Loss of teeth, rheumatoid arthritis	Bite correction and surgery
Tolosa-Hunt syndrome	Unilateral, mainly orbital	Intense sharp, aching pain; associated ophthalmoplegias of varying degree Pupil inequality, sensory loss	None	?Arteritis and granulomatous lesions	Corticosteroids Nerve section (trigeminal)
Raeder's paratrigeminal syndrome	Unilateral, frontotemporal and maxilla	Intense sharp, aching pain Pupil inequality, sensory loss	None	Tumors, granulomatous lesions, injuries	Depends on type of lesion
Migrainous neuralgia	Orbitofrontal	See cluster headache, Table 3-1	None		Ergot

SOURCE: *After J Patten, Neurological Differential Diagnosis, London, Harold Starke, Springer-Verlag, 1977.*

tumor often respond surprisingly well to large doses of methylprednisolone acetate and like compounds.

In conclusion, it is well to mention the importance of general hygienic measures. Young physicians in particular are apt to seek a specific therapy for each headache syndrome and give little thought to the general health of the patient. We have observed that most of the recurrent and chronic headaches are likely to be more severe and disabling whenever the patient becomes nervous, sick, and tired. A well-rounded diet, adequate rest, a reasonable amount of physical exercise, and a balanced view of the sources of daily anxieties and how to cope with them should be the goal of all therapeutic programs.

REFERENCES

Appenzeller O: *Pathogenesis and Treatment of Headache.* New York, Spectrum, 1976

Bickerstaff ER: Basilar artery migraine. Lancet 1:15, 1961

Clover V et al: Transitory decrease in platelet monoamine oxidase activity during migraine attacks. Lancet 1:391, 1977

Couch JR, Hassaneim RS: Platelet aggregability in migraine. Neurology 27:843, 1977

Fisher CM: Personal communication

Gascon G, Barlow C: Juvenile migraine presenting as an acute confusional state. Pediatrics 45:628, 1970

Hakkareinen H et al: Tolfenamic acid is as effective as ergotamine during migraine attacks. Lancet 2:326, 1979

Henry PY et al: Cerebral blood flow in migraine and cluster headache. Res Clin Studies, Headache 6:81, 1978

Hockaday JM: Basilar migraine in childhood. Dev Med Child Neurol 21:455, 1979

Lake A, Rainey J, Papsdorf JD: Biofeedback and rational-emotive therapy in the management of migraine headache. Appl Behav Anal 12:127, 1979

Lance JW: Headache. Ann Neurol 10:1, 1981

Lance JW, Hintzenberger H: The control of cranial arteries by humoral mechanisms and its relation to the migraine syndrome. Headache 7:93, 1967

Oleson J et al: Focal hyperemia followed by spreading oligemia in classic migraine. Ann Neurol 9:344, 1981

Vijayan N, Dreyfus PM: Posttraumatic dysautonomic cephalalgia: Clinical observations and treatment. Arch Neurol 32:649, 1976

Vinken PJ, Bruyn GW: *Handbook of Clinical Neurology*, vol 5: *Headache and Cranial Neuralgias.* Amsterdam, North-Holland, 1968

Watson P, Steele JC: Paroxysmal dysequilibrium in the migraine syndrome of childhood. Arch Otolaryngol 99:177, 1974

4
CHEST PAIN AND PALPITATION

EUGENE BRAUNWALD

CHEST PAIN

There is little parallelism between the severity of chest pain and the gravity of its cause. Therefore, a frequent problem in patients who complain of chest pain is distinguishing trivial disorders from coronary artery disease and other serious disorders. An incorrect positive diagnosis of a hazardous condition such as angina pectoris is likely to have harmful psychologic and economic consequences, and may lead to unnecessary complex procedures, such as coronary arteriography, while failure to recognize a serious disorder, such as coronary artery disease or mediastinal tumor, may result in the dangerous delay of much-needed treatment.

The apparently bizarre radiation of pain arising in the thoracic viscera can usually be explained in terms of the known facts concerning nerve supply (Chap. 2). One occasionally sees a patient with extension of pain to a location which cannot be logically explained. In most instances, such a person will be found to have more than one disorder capable of causing pain in the chest. The presence of one condition may affect the radiation of the pain produced by the other disorder. For example, when the pain of transient myocardial ischemia, i.e., angina pectoris, extends to the back or abdomen, the patient may be found to have also a significant degree of spinal arthritis or an upper abdominal disorder, such as hiatus hernia, disease of the gallbladder, pancreatitis, or peptic ulcer. Pain impulses which enter one cord segment may spill over and excite nearby cord segments. In this manner, the pain of myocardial ischemia may be referred to the epigastrium in a patient with chronic cholecystitis.

The common tendency to assume that the presence of an objective abnormality, such as a hiatus hernia or an electrocardiographic abnormality, necessarily means that an atypical chest pain arises in the stomach or the heart is to be strongly condemned. Such an assumption is justified only if a careful history indicates that the behavior of the pain is compatible with the site of origin suggested by the objective finding.

THE LEFT-ARM MYTH There is a long tradition, widely accepted by physicians and nonphysicians, alike, that pain in the left arm, especially when appearing in conjunction with chest pain, has a unique and ominous significance as being almost certain evidence of the presence of ischemic heart disease. This is a myth that has neither theoretic nor clinical foundation. Impulses from somatic structures, such as the skin, and visceral structures, such as the esophagus and heart, converge on a common pool of neurons in the posterior horn of the spinal cord. Their origin may be confused by the cortex. Also, stimulation of one of the thoracic nerves that also innervates the heart by, for example, protrusion of an intervertebral disk, may be misinterpreted as pain originating from the heart.

From a theoretic standpoint, *any* disorder involving the deep afferent fibers of the left upper thoracic region should be capable of causing pain in the chest, the left arm, or both areas. Hence a pain of trivial significance arising in skeletal tissues innervated by upper (first to fourth) thoracic nerves may produce left-arm-area pain; almost any condition capable of causing pain in the chest may induce radiation to the left arm. Such localization is common not only in patients with coronary disease but also in those with numerous other types of chest pain. Although pain due to myocardial ischemia most frequently is substernal, radiates down the ulnar aspect of the left arm (Chap. 260), and is pressing and constricting in nature, the location, radiation, and quality of pain are of less diagnostic significance than the behavior of the pain, in terms of the conditions which induce it and relieve it.

Most persons also believe that cardiac pain is situated in the region of the left breast, and therefore left inframammary pain is one of the common symptoms that brings the patient to seek medical advice. It differs radically from the pain due to myocardial hypoxia, i.e., angina pectoris, in that it is either momentary, sharp and lancinating, or a long-lasting, dull ache, occasionally accentuated by sharp stabs. Relief is often sudden, or occurs slowly and after prolonged rest, and may not be temporally related to nitroglycerin administration. In contrast to angina pectoris, such precordial pain has no relationship to exertion and may be accompanied by tenderness over the precordium and is frequently observed in patients who are tense, easily fatigued, unusually anxious, or psychoneurotic, or who have neurocirculatory asthenia.

PAIN DUE TO OXYGEN DEFICIENCY OF THE MYOCARDIUM

Physiologic considerations of the coronary circulation Pain due to myocardial ischemia occurs when the oxygen supply to the heart is deficient in relation to the oxygen need. The oxygen consumption of this organ is closely related to the physiologic effort made during contraction. It is dependent primarily on three factors: (1) the tension developed by the myocardium, (2) the contractile (inotropic) state of the myocardium, and (3) the heart rate. When these three factors remain constant, or almost so, an elevation of stroke volume produces an efficient type of response because it leads to an increase in the external work of the heart (i.e., in the product of cardiac output and arterial pressure) with little accompanying augmentation of myocardial oxygen requirements. Thus, a rise in flow load causes less increment in myocardial oxygen consumption than does a comparable increase in cardiac work brought about by elevation either of pressure or of heart rate. However, the net effects of these hemodynamic variables depend not on oxygen need alone, but rather on the balance between the demand and the supply of oxygen. The heart is always active, and the coronary venous blood is normally much more desaturated than that draining other areas of the body. Thus the removal of more oxygen from each unit of blood, which is one of the adjustments commonly utilized by exercising skeletal muscle, is already employed in the heart in the basal state. Therefore, the heart must rely primarily on an increase in the coronary blood flow for obtaining additional oxygen.

The blood flow through the coronary arteries is directly proportional to the pressure gradient between the aorta and the ventricular myocardium during systole and the ventricular cavity during diastole, but is also proportional to the fourth power of the radius of the coronary arteries. Thus a relatively slight alteration in coronary diameter will produce a large change in coronary flow, provided that other factors remain constant. In the normal heart, coronary blood flow occurs primarily during diastole, when it is unopposed by myocardial compression of the coronary vessels. Coronary flow is regulated primarily by myocardial oxygen needs, probably through the release of vasodilator metabolites, such as adenosine, and through variations in myocardial P_{O_2}. Control of the lumen of the coronary arterial bed through autonomic nerves constitutes a second mechanism of regulation of coronary blood flow.

The coronary dilatation which normally occurs during exercise and emotion results from the increased myocardial metabolism during these conditions and is impaired in patients with fixed coronary narrowing due to coronary arteriosclerosis. Thus, any condition in which increased heart rate, arterial pressure, or myocardial contractility occurs tends, particularly in the presence of coronary obstruction, to precipitate anginal attacks by increasing myocardial oxygen needs. Bradycardia, when not severe, usually has the opposite effects, and this apparently explains the rarity of angina in patients with complete heart block, even when this disorder is associated with coronary disease.

Causes of myocardial hypoxia By far the most frequent underlying cause is organic narrowing of the coronary arteries secondary to coronary atherosclerosis. Less frequently, narrowing of the coronary orifices due to syphilitic aortitis or to distortion by an aortic dissection may be responsible. There is no evidence that systemic arterial constriction or increased cardiac contractile activity (rise in heart rate or blood pressure, or increase in contractility due to liberation of catecholamines or adrenergic activity) due to emotion can precipitate angina unless there is also structural narrowing of the coronary vessels. While this is usually on an organic basis and secondary to arteriosclerosis, recently it has become clear that coronary artery spasm, with or without accompanying atherosclerosis, can also precipitate angina.

Aside from conditions which narrow the lumen of the coronary arteries, the only other frequent causes of myocardial hypoxia are disorders, such as aortic stenosis and/or regurgitation (Chap. 258), which cause a marked disproportion between the perfusion pressure and the heart's oxygen requirements. Under such conditions the rise in left ventricular systolic pressure is not, as in hypertensive states, balanced by a corresponding elevation of aortic perfusion pressure.

An increase in heart rate is especially harmful in patients with coronary atherosclerosis and with aortic stenosis, because on the one hand it increases myocardial oxygen needs, and on the other it shortens diastole more than systole and thereby decreases the total available perfusion time per minute.

Patients with marked *right ventricular hypertension* may have exertional pain which is, in most respects, identical with that of the common type of angina. It is likely that this discomfort results from relative ischemia of the right ventricle brought about by the increased oxygen needs and by the elevated intramural resistance, with sharp reduction of the normally large systolic pressure gradient which perfuses this chamber. Angina is common in patients with *syphilitic aortitis*, in whom the relative roles of aortic regurgitation and of coronary ostial narrowing are difficult to assess. The importance of tachycardia, decline in arterial pressure, thyrotoxicosis, or diminution in arterial oxygen content (such as occurs in anemia or arterial hypoxia) in the production of myocardial hypoxia will be apparent from the above discussion. However, these are precipitating and aggravating factors rather than the underlying cause of angina; as already noted, the latter is, in almost all instances, coronary atherosclerosis.

Effects of myocardial hypoxia The most common of these is *anginal pain*, considered in some detail in Chap. 260. Usually it is described as a heavy pressure or squeezing, a sensation of strangling or constriction in the chest, a "burning" or "heavy feeling," or difficulty in breathing, and it occurs particularly on walking, especially after meals, on cold days, against a wind or uphill. It is not a stabbing pain. Typically it occurs during exertion, after heavy meals, and with anger, excitement, and other emotional states; it is not precipitated by coughing or respiratory movements or other motion. When anginal pain is induced by walking, it forces the patient to stop or to reduce his speed; it is characteristically relieved by rest and nitroglycerin. The exact mechanism of the pain stimulus is still unknown, but it is probably related to an accumulation of metabolites within the heart muscle. Anginal pain occurs most typically in the substernal region, anteriorly across the midthorax; it may radiate to or rarely occur alone in the interscapular region, in the arms, shoulders, and teeth. The more severe the attack, the greater the radiation from the substernal areas to the left arm, especially its ulnar aspect.

Myocardial infarction is usually associated with a pain similar in quality and distribution to that of angina but of greater intensity and longer duration. In contrast to angina, the pain of myocardial infarction is not relieved by rest or by coronary dilator drugs and may require large doses of narcotics. It may be accompanied by diaphoresis, nausea, and hypotension (Chap. 261).

A second effect of myocardial ischemia consists of *electrocardiographic changes* (Chaps. 249, 260, and 261). Many patients with angina have normal tracings between attacks, and the record may even remain normal during the episode of pain. However, often depression of the ST segments appears during exertion. The finding of flat or downsloping ST-segment depressions of 0.1 mV or greater during an attack of pain, with a return to normal after the pain subsides, strongly suggests that the pain is anginal in origin. The value and limitation of electrocardiographic changes occurring after exercise in the diagnosis of angina pectoris are discussed in Chap. 260.

A third effect of myocardial hypoxia is depression of *myocardial contraction.* The left ventricular end-diastolic and pulmonary vascular pressures may rise during anginal attacks, particularly if they are prolonged and are caused, presumably, by the decreased contractility and reduced distensibility of the ischemic areas. A fourth heart sound is also frequently heard during the anginal episode; paradoxic pulsations may be evident on palpation of the precordium and can be recorded by apex cardiography.

Another characteristic effect of myocardial hypoxia is liability to sudden death (Chap. 30). This may never occur, despite thousands of anginal episodes. However, it may supervene early in the disease and even in the first attack. The usual mechanism is probably ventricular fibrillation, but occasionally sudden death may be due to ventricular standsill in patients with impaired atrioventricular conduction.

PAIN DUE TO IRRITATION OF SEROUS MEMBRANES OR JOINTS **Pericarditis** The visceral surface of the pericardium is ordinarily insensitive to pain, as is the parietal surface, except in its lower portion, which has a relatively small number of pain fibers carried in the phrenic nerves. The pain associated with pericarditis is believed to be due to inflammation of the adjacent parietal pleura. These observations explain why noninfectious pericarditis (that associated with uremia and with myocardial infarction) and cardiac tamponade with relatively mild inflammation are usually painless or accompanied by mild pain, whereas infectious pericarditis, being nearly always more intense and spreading to the neighboring pleura, is usually associated with pain having some pleuritic features, i.e., it is aggravated by breathing, coughing, etc. Since the central part of the diaphragm receives its sensory supply from the phrenic nerve (which arises from the third to fifth cervical segments of the spinal cord), pain arising from the lower parietal pericardium and central tendon of the diaphragm is felt characteristically at the tip of the shoulder, the adjoining trapezius ridge, and the neck. Involvement of the more lateral part of the diaphragmatic pleura, supplied by branches from the sixth to ninth intercostal nerves, causes pain not only in the anterior part of the chest but also in the upper part of the abdomen or corresponding region of the back, thus sometimes simulating the pain of acute cholecystitis or pancreatitis.

Pericarditis causes two distinct types of pain (Chap. 265). The commonest is pleuritic pain, related to respiratory movements and aggravated by cough or deep inspiration. It is sometimes brought on by swallowing, because the esophagus lies just beyond the posterior portion of the heart and is often altered by a change of bodily position, becoming sharper and more left-sided in the supine position and reduced when the patient sits upright, leaning forward. It is frequently referred to the neck and lasts longer than the pain of angina pectoris. This type of pain is due to the pleuritic component of the pleuropericarditis so commonly present in the infectious forms.

The second form of pericardial pain is the steady, crushing substernal pain which mimics that of acute myocardial infarction. The mechanism of this steady substernal pain is not certain, but it may arise from marked inflammation of the relatively insensitive inner parietal surface of the pericardium, or from irritated afferent cardiac nerve fibers lying in the periadventitial layers of the superficial coronary arteries. Occasionally both types of pain may be present simultaneously.

The painful syndromes which may follow trauma to or operations on the heart (i.e., the postcardiotomy syndrome) or myocardial infarction are discussed in later chapters (Chaps. 261 and 265). Such pains often but not always arise in the pericardium.

Pleural pain is very common; it generally results from stretching of inflamed parietal pleura and may be identical with that of pericarditis. It occurs in fibrinous pleurisy, as well as when pneumonic processes reach the periphery of the lung. Pneumothorax and tumors involving the pleural space may also irritate the parietal pleura and cause pleural pain; the latter is sharp, knifelike, superficial in quality, and its aggravation by each breath and by coughing distinguishes it from the deep, dull, steady unwavering pain of myocardial ischemia.

The pain resulting from *pulmonary embolism* may resemble that of acute myocardial infarction, and in massive embolism it is located substernally. In patients with smaller emboli the pain is located more laterally, is pleuritic in nature, and may be associated with hemoptysis (Chap. 282). Massive pulmonary emboli and other causes of acute pulmonary hypertension may cause severe, persistent substernal pain, presumably due to distention of the pulmonary artery. The pain of *mediastinal emphysema* (Chap. 285) may be intense and sharp and may radiate from the substernal region to the shoulders; often a distinct crepitus is heard. The pain associated with *mediastinitis* and *mediastinal tumors* usually resembles that of pleuritis but is more likely to be maximal in the substernal region, and the associated feeling of constriction or oppression may cause confusion with myocardial infarction. The pain due to *acute dissection of the aorta* or to an expanding aortic aneurysm results from stimulation of the adventitia; it is usually extremely severe, is localized to the center of the chest, lasts for hours, and requires unusually large amounts of analgesics for relief. It often radiates into the back but is not aggravated by changes in position or respiration (Chap. 268).

The *costochondral and chondrosternal articulations* are the commonest sites of anterior chest pain. Objective signs in the form of swelling (Tietze's syndrome), redness, and heat are rare, but sharply localized tenderness is common. The pain may be darting and lasting for only a few seconds, or a dull ache enduring for hours or days. An associated feeling of tightness due to muscle spasm (see below) is frequent. When the discomfort persists for a few days only, a story of minor trauma or of some unaccustomed physical effort can often be obtained. This variety of discomfort is common in persons with arthritis of the spine and also in patients with ischemic heart disease, but in many instances no associated disorder is found. It should be emphasized that *pressure on the chondrosternal and costochondral junctions is an essential part of the examination of every patient with chest pain.* A large percentage of patients with costochondral pain, especially those who also have minor and innocent T-wave alterations, are erroneously labeled as having coronary disease. The dire consequences of such a mistake have already been emphasized.

Pain secondary to *subacromial bursitis* and *arthritis of the shoulder and spine* may be precipitated by exercise of the local area but not by general exertion. It may be brought about by passive movement of the involved area as well as by coughing.

PAIN DUE TO TISSUE DISRUPTION Rupture or tear of a structure may give rise to pain that sets in abruptly and reaches its peak of intensity almost instantly. Such a story should arouse the suspicion of aortic dissection, pneumothorax, mediastinal emphysema, a cervical disk syndrome, or rupture of the esophagus. However, the patient may be too ill to recall the precise circumstances, or the pain may be atypical and increase gradually in severity. Likewise, other and more benign conditions, such as a slipped costal cartilage or an intercostal muscle cramp, may also produce pain with an abrupt onset.

CLINICAL ASPECTS OF THE COMMONER CAUSES OF CHEST PAIN The more serious causes of chest pain such as myocardial ischemia (angina pectoris and infarction), aortic dissection, pericarditis, and disorders of the pleura, esophagus, stomach, duodenum, and pancreas are considered in the appropriate chapters dealing with these problems. Here, we are concerned with the discussion of those causes which are not considered in more detail elsewhere.

Pain arising in the chest wall or upper extremity This may develop as a result of muscle or ligament strains brought on by unaccustomed exercise and felt in the costochondral or chondrosternal junctions or in the chest wall muscles. Other causes are *osteoarthritis* of the dorsal or thoracic spine and *ruptured cervical disks.* Pain in the left upper extremity and precordium may be due to compression of portions of the brachial plexus by a cervical rib or by spasm and shortening of the scalenus anticus muscle secondary to high fixation of the ribs and sternum. Finally, pains in the upper extremity (shoulder-hand syndrome) and in the pectoral muscles may, through unknown mechanisms, occur in patients following myocardial infarction.

Pains in the chest wall or shoulder girdles or arms are usually recognized by the presence of localized tenderness of the affected area and the clear relation between pain and motion. Thus deep breathing, turning or twisting of the chest, and movements of the shoulder girdle and arm will elicit and duplicate the pain of which the patient complains. The pain may be very brief, lasting only a few seconds, or full and aching and enduring for hours. The duration is, therefore, likely to be either longer or shorter than untreated anginal pain, which usually lasts for only a few minutes.

These skeletal pains often have a sharp or sticking quality. In addition, there is frequently a feeling of tightness, which is probably due to associated spasm of intercostal or pectoral muscles. This may produce the "morning stiffness" seen in so many skeletal disorders. The discomfort is unaffected by nitroglycerin but often is abolished by infiltration of the painful areas with procaine. When chest wall pain is of recent origin and follows trauma, strain, or some unusual activity involving the pectoral muscles, it presents no problem in diagnosis. However, since both disorders are very common, long-standing skeletal pain is frequent in persons who also have angina pectoris. This coexistence of the two different types of chest pain in the same patient is a frequent cause of a confusing history, because in the patient's mind the anginal needle may be hidden in the skeletal haystack. Thus every middle-aged or elderly patient who has long-standing anterior chest wall pain merits careful study for the presence of ischemic heart disease.

The confusion created by the presence of innocent skeletal pain impairs the reliability of the history and is probably the commonest cause of errors—both positive and negative—in the diagnosis of angina pectoris. It may be necessary also to learn by direct observation whether exercise alone or postprandial exertion is capable of producing the pain. Repeated tests may be required, comparing the relative effects of preceding placebos and nitroglycerin on the amount of exertion required to induce the pain. When the history is inconclusive, the exercise electrocardiogram, or in patients with equivocal or nondiagnostic tests, the exercise stress test with thallium scintigraphy (Chap. 250), may furnish useful information concerning the existence of myocardial ischemia. In rare instances coronary arteriography may be required.

Esophageal pain This usually presents as deep thoracic pain; it results from chemical (acid) irritation of the esophageal mucosa or from spasm of the esophageal muscle and characteristically follows deglutition. Accompanying dysphagia, regurgitation of undigested food, and weight loss direct attention to the esophagus (see Chaps. 32 and 305). The Bernstein acid perfusion test, in which an attempt is made to reproduce the pain by infusing 0.1 *M* HCl into the esophagus, is helpful in establishing acid gastric reflux into the esophagus as the cause of pain. Esophageal manometry and measurement of lower esophageal sphincter pressure, sometimes with ergonovine stimulation, are useful in identifying esophageal spasm as the origin of the pain.

Emotional disorders These are also common causes of chest pain. Usually, the discomfort is experienced as a sense of "tightness," sometimes called "aching," and occasionally it may be sufficiently severe as to be designated a pain of considerable magnitude. Since the discomfort has almost always the additional quality of tightness or constriction, and since it is often localized at least in part beneath the sternum, it is not surprising that this type of pain is frequently confused with that of myocardial ischemia. Ordinarily, it lasts for a half hour or more and may persist for a day or less with slow fluctuation of intensity. The association with fatigue or emotional strain is usually clear, although this may not be recognized by the patient until called to his or her attention. The pain probably develops through unconscious and prolonged increase of muscle tone, often enhanced by an accompanying hyperventilation (by causing a contraction of the chest wall muscles similar to the painful tetany of the extremities). When the hyperventilation and/or the associated adrenergic effect due to anxiety also causes innocent changes in the T waves and ST segments, the confusion with coronary disease is strengthened. However, the long duration of the pain, the lack of any relation to exertion but association rather with fatigue or tension, and the usually periodic occurrence on successive days without any limitation of capacity for exercise usually make the differentiation from ischemic pain quite clear.

As compared with these two causes (the chest wall muscle and ligament strains and the contraction of the pectoral muscles due to reflex influences, fatigue, or tension), the various other conditions that may cause skeletal discomfort are uncommon and readily recognized after appropriate observation. These include spinal arthritis, herpes zoster, anterior scalene and hyperabduction syndromes, malignant disease of the ribs, etc.

Other causes of chest pain The several *abdominal disorders* which may at times mimic anginal pain may usually be suspected from the history, which, as in esophageal pain, ordinarily indicates some relationship to swallowing, eating, belching, etc. Pain resulting from gastric or duodenal ulcer (Chap. 306) is epigastric or substernal, commences about 1 to $1\frac{1}{2}$ h after meals, and is usually promptly relieved by antacids or milk. The gastrointestinal roentgenogram is of crucial significance, and roentgenographic examination is also often helpful in differentiating biliary, gastrointestinal, aortic, pulmonary, and skeletal disease pain from angina pectoris. It should be emphasized again that the demonstration of the presence of a coexistent abdominal disorder such as a hiatus hernia does not constitute proof that the chest pain of which the patient complains is due to this. Such disorders are frequently asymptomatic and are not at all uncommon in patients who also have angina pectoris.

Substernal discomfort also frequently occurs in the presence of *tracheobronchitis;* it is described as a burning sensation accentuated by coughing. A variety of *disorders involving the breast,* including inflammatory breast disease, benign and malignant tumors, as well as mastodynia, are common causes of thoracic pain. The localization and superficial swelling and tenderness are of diagnostic importance.

APPROACH TO THE PATIENT WITH PAIN IN THE CHEST

Most persons with this complaint will fall into one of two general groups. The first consists of persons with prolonged and often severe pain without obvious initiating factors. Such persons will frequently be gravely ill. The problem is that of differentiating such serious conditions as myocardial infarction, aortic dissection, and pulmonary embolism from each other and from less grave causes. In some such instances, a careful history will provide significant clues, while objective evidence of crucial importance will appear within the subsequent 2 or 3 days. Thus, when the initial examinations are not decisive, a watch-and-wait policy, with repeated electrocardiograms coupled with measurements of serum enzymes, pulmonary scintigraphy, and chest roentgenograms, will commonly provide the correct answer.

The second group of patients comprises those who have brief episodes of pain and are otherwise in apparently excellent health. Here, the resting electrocardiogram will rarely supply decisive information, but records taken during or immediately after exercise or pain will often reveal characteristic changes (Chap. 260). However, in many instances it is the study of the subjective phenomenon, i.e., of the pain itself, that will lead to the diagnosis. Of the several methods of investigation which are available for such patients, three are of cardinal importance.

A detailed and *meticulous history* of the behavior of the pain is the most important method. The location, radiation, quality, intensity, and, especially, duration of the episodes are important. Even more so is the story of the aggravating and alleviating factors. Thus a history of sharp aggravation by breathing, coughing, or other respiratory movements will usually point toward the pleura and pericardium or mediastinum as the site, although chest wall pain is likewise affected by respiratory motions. Similarly, a pain which regularly appears on rapid walking and vanishes within a few minutes upon standing still suggests the diagnosis of angina pectoris, although here, once again, a similar story will rarely be obtained from patients with skeletal disorders.

When the history is inconclusive, the *study of the patient at the time of the spontaneous episode* will often supply crucial information. Thus the electrocardiogram, which may be normal both at rest and even during or after exercise in the absence of pain, will occasionally demonstrate striking changes when recorded during an anginal episode. Similarly, radiographic study of the esophagus or of the stomach may show no evidence of cardiospasm or of hiatal hernia except when the observation is made during the pain.

The third method of study represents the *attempt to produce and alleviate the pain at will.* This procedure is necessary only when doubt exists following the history or when needed for psychotherapeutic purposes. Thus the demonstration that a localized pain, which can be reproduced by pressure on the chest, is completely relieved by local infiltration with procaine will often be of conclusive importance in convincing the patient that the heart is not the site. When the pain is precipitated by intravenous injections of ergonovine and this is accompanied by electrocardiographic ST-segment elevations and coronary spasm on arteriography, the diagnosis of Prinzmetal's angina can be made.

When, as is often the case, the history is atypical, the correct diagnosis of angina pectoris may be aided by noting the response to nitroglycerin. Relief of pain after its sublingual administration does not necessarily prove that there is a cause-and-effect relationship. It is necessary to be certain that the pain vanishes more rapidly (usually within 5 min) and more completely when the drug is used than when it is not employed. A false-negative impression concerning the effect of nitroglycerin may be the result of the use of a deteriorated preparation which has been exposed to light. In doubtful instances, repeated exercise tests, with and without preceding administration of nitroglycerin, are necessary. The demonstration that the time required for a given exercise to produce pain is consistently and considerably longer when it is undertaken within a few minutes after a sublingual nitroglycerin pill than after a placebo may, in some instances, represent the sole method for accurate recognition of angina pectoris. A completely negative response to such repeated tests constitutes almost conclusive evidence against angina.

In patients in whom the question of whether there is coronary disease cannot be resolved despite the aforementioned clinical and laboratory tests, including exercise electrocardiography (Chap. 260), cardiac catheterization and coronary arteriography may be required. A useful stress test that can be carried out at the time of catheterization is to elevate the heart rate in stepwise fashion by electrical pacing; the development of ST-segment depressions on the electrocardiogram and the reproduction of the pain support the diagnosis of myocardial ischemia. Coronary arteriography will show severe (more than 75 percent) reduction of the lumen in patients with obstructive coronary artery disease (Chaps. 251 and 260).

PALPITATION

Palpitation is a common, disagreeable symptom which may be defined as an awareness of the beating of the heart, an awareness most commonly brought about by a change in the heart's rhythm or rate or by an augmentation of its contractility. Palpitation is not pathognomonic of any particular group of disorders; indeed, often it signifies not a primary physical disorder but rather a psychologic disturbance. Even when it occurs as a more or less prominent complaint, the diagnosis of the underlying disease is made largely on the basis of other associated symptoms and data. Nevertheless, palpitation is frequently of considerable importance in the minds of patients, who fear that it may indicate heart disease. Concern is all the more pronounced in patients who have been told that they may have heart disease; to them palpitation may seem to be an omen of impending disaster. Since the resulting anxiety may be associated with increased activity of the autonomic nervous system, with consequent increases of the cardiac rate and rhythm and the vigor of contraction, the patient's awareness of these changes may then lead to a vicious cycle, which may ultimately be responsible for his or her incapacitation.

Palpitation may be described by the patient in various terms, such as "pounding," "fluttering," "flopping," and "skipping," and in most cases it will be obvious that the complaint is of a sensation of disturbed heartbeat. The wide variability in the sensitivity to alterations in cardiac activity among different individuals must be appreciated. Some patients seem to be unaware of the most serious and chaotic dysrhythmias; others are seriously troubled by an occasional extrasystole. Patients with anxiety states often exhibit a lowered threshold at which disorders of rate and rhythm result in palpitation. The awareness of the heartbeat also tends to be more common at night and during introspective moments, but is less marked during activity. Patients with organic heart disease and chronic disorders of cardiac rate, rhythm, or stroke volume tend to accommodate to these abnormalities and are often less sensitive than normal persons to such events. Persistent tachycardia and/or atrial fibrillation may not be accompanied by continual palpitation, in contrast to a sudden, brief alteration in cardiac rate or rhythm which often causes considerable subjective discomfort. Thus, palpitation is particularly prominent when the precipitating cause for increased heart rate or contractility or arrhythmia is recent, transient, and episodic. Conversely, in emotionally well-adjusted individuals palpitation becomes progressively less disconcerting as the cause (e.g., anemia, frequent extrasystoles, complete atrioventricular block) persists.

PATHOGENESIS OF PALPITATION Under ordinary circumstances the rhythmic heartbeat is imperceptible to the healthy individual of average or placid temperament. Palpitation may be experienced by normal persons who have engaged in strenuous physical effort or have been aroused emotionally or sexually. This type of palpitation is physiologic and represents the normal awareness of an overactive heart—i.e., a heart that is beating at a rapid rate and with an increased contractility. Palpitation due to overactivity of the heart may also occur in certain pathologic states, e.g., high fever, severe anemia, or thyrotoxicosis.

When palpitation is heavy and regular, it is usually caused by an augmented stroke volume, and it should raise the question of aortic or mitral regurgitation, ventricular septal defect, or of a variety of hyperkinetic circulatory states (anemia, arteriovenous fistula, thyrotoxicosis, and the so-called idiopathic hyperkinetic heart syndrome). It may also occur immediately after the onset of cardiac slowing, as with the sudden development of heart block, or upon the conversion of sinus rhythm from atrial fibrillation. But unusual movements of the heart within the thorax are also frequently the mechanism of palpitation. Thus, the ectopic beat and/or the compensatory pause may be appreciated, since both are associated with alterations in cardiac motion.

IMPORTANT CAUSES OF PALPITATION See also Chap. 255.

Extrasystoles In most cases the diagnosis will be suggested by the patient's story. The premature contraction and postpremature beat are often described as a "flopping," or the patient may say that it feels as if "the heart were turning over." The pause following the premature contraction may be felt as an actual cessation of the heartbeat. The first ventricular contraction succeeding the pause may be felt as an unusually vigorous beat and will be described as "pounding" or "thudding."

When extrasystoles are numerous, clinical differentiation from atrial fibrillation can be made by any procedure that will bring about a definite increase in the ventricular rate; at increasingly rapid heart rates, the extrasystoles usually diminish in frequency and then disappear, whereas the ventricular irregularity of atrial fibrillation increases.

Ectopic tachycardias These conditions, which are considered in some detail in Chap. 255, are common and medically important causes of palpitation. Ventricular tachycardia, one of the most serious arrhythmias, rarely is manifested as palpitation; this may be related to the abnormal sequence, and hence impaired coordination and vigor, of ventricular contraction. If the patient is seen between attacks, the diagnosis of ectopic tachycardia and its type will have to depend on the history, but of course the precise diagnosis can be made only when an electrocardiogram and observations on the effect of carotid sinus pressure are made during the episode. The mode of onset and offset gives the most important lead in distinguishing sinus from one of the various forms of ectopic tachycardias; sinus tachycardia commences and ceases over the course of minutes or seconds, but not instantaneously as is characteristic of ectopic rhythms. Monitoring of the electrocardiogram with a portable tape recording system and asking the patient to record the time of onset and cessation of the palpitations are extremely helpful in determining their cause (Chap. 255).

Other causes Other causes include thyrotoxicosis (Chap. 111), hypoglycemia (Chap. 116), pheochromocytoma (Chap. 113), fever (Chap. 9), and drugs. The relationship between the development of palpitation and the use of tobacco, coffee, tea, alcohol, epinephrine, ephedrine, aminophylline, atropine, or thyroid extract is usually obvious.

Palpitation as a manifestation of the anxiety state Persons who are healthy physically and well adjusted emotionally may have palpitation under certain circumstances. Thus, during or immediately after vigorous physical exertion or during sudden emotional tension, palpitation is common and is usually associated with sinus tachycardia. In poorly conditioned persons without organic heart disease, the sinus tachycardia of exercise may be excessive and associated with palpitation.

In some patients, palpitation may be one of the outstanding manifestations of an episode of acute anxiety. In other persons the palpitation may, with other symptoms, represent prolonged anxiety neurosis or a lifelong disorder characterized by volatile autonomic function. The latter condition has been called *neurocirculatory asthenia.* Whether these illnesses are simply an expression of a chronic, deep-seated anxiety state superimposed on a normal autonomic nervous system or whether they depend on instability of the autonomic nervous system is not clear. At any rate, the clinical significance of the differentiation between the transitory and the enduring forms is that the former is often dissipated by firm reassurance from the physician, whereas the latter is usually resistant even to the most thorough and expert psychiatric care. In the latter case, the patient must be treated with most carefully planned psychologic support and tranquilizing medications. This chronic form of palpitation is known by various names such as *Da Costa's syndrome, soldier's heart, effort syndrome, irritable heart, neurocirculatory asthenia,* and *functional cardiovascular disease.* Aside from palpitation, the chief symptoms are those of an anxiety state.

Physical examination usually reveals the typical findings of the hyperkinetic syndrome. These include a left parasternal lift, a precordial or apical systolic murmur, a wide pulse pressure, rapidly rising pulse, and excessive perspiration. The electrocardiogram may display minor depressions of the ST junction and inversion of T waves and so occasionally lead to a mistaken diagnosis of coronary disease; this is particularly likely to occur when these findings are associated with complaints by the patients of an aching feeling of substernal tightness, commonly present in emotional stress. The presence of any kind of organic disease is one of the commonest causes of the underlying anxiety which frequently precipitates this functional syndrome.

Even when a patient presents undoubted objective evidence of structural cardiac disease, the possibility that a superimposed anxiety responsible for the symptoms when the clinical picture is that which has been described should be considered. Palpitation associated with organic cardiac disease is nearly always accompanied by arrhythmia or by marked tachycardia, whereas the symptom may exist with regular rhythm and with a heart rate of 80 beats per minute or less in patients with the

TABLE 4-1
Items to be covered in history

Does the palpitation occur:	*If so, suspect:*
As isolated "jumps" or "skips"?	Extrasystoles
In attacks, known to be of abrupt beginning, with a heart rate of 120 beats per minute or over, with regular or irregular rhythm?	Paroxysmal rapid heart action
Independent of exercise or excitement adequate to account for the symptom?	Atrial fibrillation, atrial flutter, thyrotoxicosis, anemia, febrile states, hypoglycemia, anxiety state
In attacks developing rapidly though not absolutely abruptly, unrelated to exertion or excitement?	Hemorrhage, hypoglycemia, tumor of the adrenal medulla
In conjunction with the taking of drugs?	Tobacco, coffee, tea, alcohol, epinephrine, ephedrine, aminophylline, atropine, thyroid extract, monoamine oxidase inhibitors
On standing?	Postural hypotension
In middle-aged women, in conjunction with flushes and sweats?	Menopausal syndrome
When the rate is known to be normal and the rhythm regular?	Anxiety state

anxiety state. It is noteworthy that an anxiety state, in contrast to heart disease, causes a sighing type of dyspnea. Also pain localized to the apex, either brief and lancinating in character or lasting for hours or days and accompanied by hyperesthesia, is due usually to an anxiety state, not to structural cardiac disease. Giddiness due to this syndrome can usually be reproduced by hyperventilation (Chap. 12) or by change from the recumbent to the erect posture.

The *treatment* of the anxiety state with palpitation is difficult and depends on removal of the cause. In many instances a thorough examination of the heart and a statement that it is normal will suffice. Instructions to take more rather than less physical exercise will reinforce these statements. When the anxiety state is a manifestation of chronic anxiety neurosis or depressive psychosis, the symptoms are more likely to persist.

Table 4-1 summarizes the main points of information to be ascertained in the history in elucidating the significance of palpitation. The recording of the electrocardiogram using a portable tape recorder in an ambulatory subject, and the precise temporal correlation of the cardiac rate and rhythm with the presence of palpitation are extremely useful in the identification or exclusion of a rhythmic disturbance. The effectiveness of antiarrhythmia treatment can also be assessed objectively in this manner, without the necessity of relying only on the patient's subjective symptoms. Beta-adrenergic blockade with propranolol, beginning with 40 mg per day in divided doses, and ranging as high as 400 mg per day, can be extremely effective in patients with palpitation and sinus rhythm or sinus tachycardia.

One point merits special emphasis. *As a rule palpitation produces anxiety and fear out of all proportion to its seriousness.* When the cause has been accurately determined and its significance explained to patients, their concern is often ameliorated and may disappear entirely.

REFERENCES

ARESKOG NH, TIBBLING L (eds): Differential diagnostic aspects of chest pain. Acta Med Scand (suppl):644, 1980

BRAUNWALD E: Control of myocardial oxygen consumption: Physiologic and clinical considerations. Am J Cardiol 27:416, 1971

———: Coronary artery spasm as a cause of myocardial ischemia. J Lab Clin Med 97:299, 1981

BURCH GE et al: Cardiac causalgia. Am Heart J 76:725, 1968

CHRISTIE LG et al: Systematic approach to evaluation of angina-like chest pain: Pathophysiology and clinical testing with emphasis on objective documentation of myocardial ischemia. Am Heart J 102:897, 1981

COHEN S: Diagnosis and management of gastroesophageal reflux disease, in *Update I: Harrison's Principles of Internal Medicine*, KJ Isselbacher et al (eds). New York, McGraw-Hill, 1981, p 23

COHN PF, BRAUNWALD E: Coronary artery disease, in *Heart Disease*, E Braunwald (ed). Philadelphia, Saunders, 1980, chap 38

DRESSLER W: *Clinical Aids in Cardiac Diagnosis.* New York, Grune & Stratton, 1970

HILLIS DF, BRAUNWALD E: Myocardial ischemia. N Engl J Med 296:971, 1034, 1093, 1977

LEVENE DL: *Chest Pain.* Philadelphia, Lea & Febiger, 1977, p 203

LOWN B, PODRID PJ: Ventricular premature beats: Why, when, and how to treat, in *Update II: Harrison's Principles of Internal Medicine*, KJ Isselbacher et al (eds). New York, McGraw-Hill, 1982, p 131

5 ABDOMINAL PAIN

WILLIAM SILEN

The correct interpretation of acute abdominal pain is one of the most challenging demands made of any physician. Since proper therapy often requires urgent action, the luxury of the leisurely approach suitable for the study of other conditions is frequently denied. Few other clinical situations demand greater experience and judgment, because the most catastrophic of events may be forecast by the subtlest of symptoms and signs. Nowhere in medicine is a meticulously executed detailed history and physical examination of greater importance. The etiologic classification in Table 5-1, although not complete, forms a useful frame of reference for the evaluation of patients with abdominal pain.

The diagnosis of "acute or surgical abdomen" so often heard in emergency wards is not an acceptable one because of its often misleading and erroneous connotation. The most obvious of "acute abdomens" may not require operative intervention, and the mildest of abdominal pains may herald the onset of an urgently correctable lesion. Any patient with abdominal pain of recent onset requires early and thorough evaluation with specific attempts at accurate diagnosis.

SOME MECHANISMS OF PAIN ORIGINATING IN THE ABDOMEN **Inflammation of the parietal peritoneum** The pain of parietal peritoneal inflammation is steady and aching in character and is located directly over the inflamed area, its exact reference being possible because it is transmitted by overlapping somatic nerves supplying the parietal peritoneum. The intensity of the pain is dependent upon the type and amount of foreign substance to which the peritoneal surfaces are exposed in a given period of time. For example, the sudden release into the peritoneal cavity of a small quantity of *sterile* acid gastric juice causes much more pain than the same amount of grossly contaminated neutral fecal material. Enzymatically active pancreatic juice incites more pain and inflammation than does the same amount of sterile bile containing no potent enzymes. Blood and urine are often so bland as to go undetected if exposure of the peritoneum has not been sudden and massive. In the case of bacterial contamination, such as in pelvic inflammatory disease, the pain is frequently of low intensity early in the illness until bacterial multiplication has caused the elaboration of irritating substances.

So important is the rate at which the irritating material is applied to the peritoneum that cases of perforated peptic ulcer may be associated with entirely different clinical pictures dependent only upon the rapidity with which the gastric juice enters the peritoneal cavity.

The pain of peritoneal inflammation is invariably accentuated by pressure or changes in tension of the peritoneum, whether produced by palpation or by movement, as in coughing or sneezing. Consequently, the patient with peritonitis lies quietly in bed, preferring to avoid motion, in contrast to the patient with colic, who may writhe incessantly.

Another of the characteristic features of peritoneal irritation is tonic reflex spasm of the abdominal musculature, localized to the involved body segment. The intensity of the tonic muscle spasm accompanying peritoneal inflammation is dependent upon the location of the inflammatory process, the rate at which it develops, and the integrity of the nervous system. Spasm over a perforated retrocecal appendix or perforated ulcer into the lesser peritoneal sac may be minimal or absent because of the protective effect of overlying viscera. As in pain of peritoneal inflammation, a slowly developing process often greatly attenuates the degree of muscle spasm. Catastrophic abdominal emergencies such as a perforated ulcer have been repeatedly associated with minimal or occasionally no detectable pain or muscle spasm in obtunded, seriously ill, debilitated elderly patients or in psychotic patients.

TABLE 5-1
Some important causes of abdominal pain

- *I* Pain originating in the abdomen
  - *A* Parietal peritoneal inflammation
    - *1* Bacterial contamination, e.g., perforated appendix, pelvic inflammatory disease
    - *2* Chemical irritation, e.g., perforated ulcer, pancreatitis, mittelschmerz
  - *B* Mechanical obstruction of hollow viscera
    - *1* Obstruction of the small or large intestine
    - *2* Obstruction of the biliary tree
    - *3* Obstruction of the ureter
  - *C* Vascular disturbances
    - *1* Embolism or thrombosis
    - *2* Vascular rupture
    - *3* Pressure or torsional occlusion
    - *4* Sickle cell anemia
  - *D* Abdominal wall
    - *1* Distortion or traction of mesentery
    - *2* Trauma or infection of muscles
    - *3* Distention of visceral surfaces, e.g., hepatic or renal capsules
- *II* Pain referred from extraabdominal sources
  - *A* Thorax—e.g., pneumonia, referred pain from coronary occlusion
  - *B* Spine—e.g., radiculitis from arthritis
  - *C* Genitalia—e.g., torsion of the testicle
- *III* Metabolic causes
  - *A* Exogenous
    - *1* Black widow spider bite
    - *2* Lead poisoning and others
  - *B* Endogenous
    - *1* Uremia
    - *2* Diabetic coma
    - *3* Porphyria
    - *4* Allergic factors (C'1 esterase inhibitor deficiency)
- *IV* Neurogenic causes
  - *A* Organic
    - *1* Tabes dorsalis
    - *2* Herpes zoster
    - *3* Causalgia and others
  - *B* Functional

Obstruction of hollow viscera The pain of obstruction of hollow abdominal viscera is classically described as intermittent, or colicky. Yet the lack of a truly cramping character should not be misleading, because distention of a hollow viscus may produce steady pain with only very occasional exacerbations. Although not nearly as well localized as the pain of parietal peritoneal inflammation, some useful generalities can be made concerning its distribution.

The colicky pain of obstruction of small intestine is usually periumbilical or supraumbilical and is poorly localized. As the intestine becomes progressively dilated with loss of muscular tone, the colicky nature of the pain may become less apparent. With superimposed strangulating obstruction, pain may spread in the lower lumbar region if there is traction on the root of the mesentery. The colicky pain of colonic obstruction is of lesser intensity than that of the small intestine and is often located in the infraumbilical area. Lumbar radiation of pain is common in colonic obstruction.

Sudden distention of the biliary tree produces a steady rather than colicky type of pain; hence the term *biliary colic* is misleading. Acute distention of the gallbladder usually causes pain in the right upper quadrant with radiation to the right posterior region of the thorax or to the tip of the right scapula, and distention of the common bile duct is often associated with pain in the epigastrium radiating to the upper part of the lumbar region. Considerable variation is common, however, so that differentiation between these may be impossible. The typical subscapular pain or lumbar radiation is frequently absent. Gradual dilatation of the biliary tree as in carcinoma of the head of the pancreas may cause no pain or only a mild aching sensation in the epigastrium or right upper quadrant. The pain of distention of the pancreatic ducts is similar to that described for distention of the common bile duct but in addition is very frequently accentuated by recumbency and relieved by the upright position.

Obstruction of the urinary bladder results in dull suprapubic pain, usually low in intensity. Restlessness without specific complaint of pain may be the only sign of a distended bladder in an obtunded patient. In contrast, acute obstruction of the intravesicular portion of the ureter is characterized by severe suprapubic and flank pain which radiates to the penis, scrotum, or inner aspect of the upper region of the thigh. Obstruction of the ureteropelvic junction is felt as pain in the costovertebral angle, whereas obstruction of the remainder of the ureter is associated with flank pain, which often extends into the corresponding side of the abdomen.

Vascular disturbances A frequent misconception, despite abundant experience to the contrary, is that pain associated with intraabdominal vascular disturbances is sudden and catastrophic in nature. The pain of embolism or thrombosis of the superior mesenteric artery or that of impending rupture of an abdominal aortic aneurysm certainly may be severe and diffuse. Yet just as frequently, the patient with occlusion of the superior mesenteric artery has only mild continuous diffuse pain for 2 or 3 days before vascular collapse or findings of peritoneal inflammation appear. The early, seemingly insignificant discomfort is caused by hyperperistalsis rather than peritoneal inflammation. Indeed, absence of tenderness and rigidity in the presence of continuous diffuse pain in a patient likely to have vascular disease is quite characteristic of occlusion of the superior mesenteric artery. Abdominal pain with radiation to the sacral region, flank, or genitalia should always signal the possible presence of a rupturing abdominal aortic aneurysm. This pain may persist over a period of several days before rupture and collapse occur.

Abdominal wall Pain arising from the abdominal wall is usually constant and aching. Movement and pressure accentuate the discomfort and muscle spasm. In the case of hematoma of the rectus sheath, now most frequently encountered in association with anticoagulant therapy, a mass may be present in the lower quadrants of the abdomen. Simultaneous involvement of muscles in other parts of the body usually serves to differentiate myositis of the abdominal wall from an intraabdominal process which might cause pain in the same region.

REFERRED PAIN IN ABDOMINAL DISEASES Pain referred to the abdomen from the thorax, spine, or genitalia may prove a vexing problem in differential diagnosis, because diseases of the upper part of the abdominal cavity such as acute cholecystitis, perforated ulcer, or subphrenic abscesses are frequently associated with intrathoracic complications. A most important, yet often forgotten, dictum is that the possibility of intrathoracic disease must be considered in every patient with abdominal pain, especially if the pain is in the upper part of the abdomen. Systematic questioning and examination directed toward detecting the presence or absence of myocardial or pulmonary infarction, pneumonia, pericarditis, or esophageal disease (the intrathoracic diseases which most often masquerade as abdominal emergencies) will often provide sufficient clues to establish the proper diagnosis. Diaphragmatic pleuritis resulting from pneumonia or pulmonary infarction may cause pain in the right upper quadrant and pain in the supraclavicular area, the latter radiation to be sharply distinguished from the referred subscapular pain caused by acute distention of the extrahepatic biliary tree. The ultimate decision as to the origin of abdominal pain may require deliberate and planned observation over a period of several hours, during which time repeated questioning and examination will provide the proper explanation.

Referred pain of thoracic origin is often accompanied by splinting of the involved hemithorax with respiratory lag and decrease in excursion more marked than that seen in the presence of intraabdominal disease. In addition, apparent abdominal muscle spasm caused by referred pain will diminish during the inspiratory phase of respiration, whereas it is persistent throughout both respiratory phases if it is of abdominal origin. Palpation over the area of referred pain in the abdomen also does not usually accentuate the pain and in many instances actually seems to relieve it. The frequent coexistence of thoracic and abdominal disease may be misleading and confusing, so that differentiation might be difficult or impossible. For example, the patient with known biliary tract disease often has epigastric pain during myocardial infarction, or biliary colic may be referred to the precordium or left shoulder in a patient who has suffered previously from angina pectoris. For the explanation of the radiation of pain to a previously diseased area, see Chap. 2.

Referred pain from the spine, which usually involves compression or irritation of nerve roots, is characteristically intensified by certain motions such as cough, sneeze, or strain and is associated with hyperesthesia over the involved dermatomes. Pain referred to the abdomen from the testicles or seminal vesicles is generally accentuated by the slightest pressure on either of these organs. The abdominal discomfort is of dull aching character and is poorly localized.

METABOLIC ABDOMINAL CRISES Pain of metabolic origin may simulate almost any other type of intraabdominal disease. Here several mechanisms may be at work. In certain instances, such as hyperparathyroidism, the metabolic disease itself may produce an intraabdominal process such as pancreatitis. Primary hyperlipemia may also be accompanied by severe pancreatitis, which can lead to unnecessary laparotomy unless recognized. C'1 esterase deficiency associated with angioneurotic edema is also often associated with episodes of severe abdominal pain. Whenever the cause of abdominal pain is obscure, a metabolic origin must always be considered. Abdominal pain is also the hallmark of familial Mediterranean fever (Chap. 236).

The problem of differential diagnosis is often not readily resolved. The pain of porphyria and of lead colic usually is difficult to distinguish from that of intestinal obstruction, because severe hyperperistalsis is a prominent feature of both. The pain of uremia or diabetes is nonspecific, and the pain and tenderness frequently shift in location and intensity. Diabetic acidosis may be precipitated by acute appendicitis or intestinal obstruction, so that if prompt resolution of the abdominal pain does not result from correction of the metabolic abnormalities, an underlying organic problem should be suspected. Black widow spider bites produce intense pain and rigidity of the abdominal muscles and of the back, an area infrequently involved in disease of intraabdominal origin.

NEUROGENIC CAUSES Causalgic pain may occur in diseases which injure nerves of sensory type. It has a burning character and is usually limited to the distribution of a given peripheral nerve. Normal stimuli such as touch or change in temperature may be transformed into this type of pain, which is also frequently present in a patient at rest. A helpful finding is the demonstration that cutaneous pain spots are now irregularly spaced, and this may be the only indication of an old nerve lesion underlying causalgic pain. Even though the pain may be precipitated by gentle palpation, rigidity of the abdominal muscles is absent, and the respirations are not disturbed. Distention of the abdomen is uncommon, and the pain has no relationship to the intake of food.

Pain arising from spinal nerves or roots comes and goes suddenly and is of a lancinating type (see Chap. 6). It may be caused by herpes zoster, impingement by arthritis, tumors, herniated nucleus pulposus, diabetes, or syphilis. Again it is not associated with food intake, abdominal distention, or changes in respiration. Severe muscle spasm, as in the gastric crises of tabes dorsalis, is common but is either relieved or is not accentuated by abdominal palpation. The pain is made worse by movement of the spine and is usually confined to a few dermatome segments. Hyperesthesia is very common.

Psychogenic pain conforms to none of the aforementioned patterns of disease. Here the mechanism is hard to define. The most common problem is the hysterical adolescent or young woman who develops abdominal pain; she frequently loses an appendix and other organs because of it. Ovulation or some other natural event that causes brief mild abdominal discomfort may be maximized as an abdominal catastrophe.

Psychogenic pain varies enormously in type and location but usually has no relation to meals. It is often at its onset markedly accentuated during the night. Nausea and vomiting are rarely observed, although occasionally the patient reports these symptoms. Spasm is seldom induced in the abdominal musculature and if present does not persist, especially if the attention of the patient can be distracted. Persistent localized tenderness is rare, and if found, the muscle spasm in the area is inconsistent and often absent. Restriction of the depth of respiration is the most common respiratory abnormality, but this is in the nature of a smothering or choking sensation and is part of an anxiety state (see Chap. 11). It occurs in the absence of thoracic splinting or change in the respiratory rate.

APPROACH TO THE PATIENT WITH ABDOMINAL PAIN There are few abdominal conditions which require such urgent operative intervention that an orderly approach need be abandoned, no matter how ill the patient. Only those patients with exsanguinating hemorrhage must be rushed to the operating room immediately, but in such instances only a few minutes are required to assess the critical nature of the problem. Under these circumstances, all obstacles must be swept aside, adequate access for intravenous fluid replacement obtained, and the operation begun. Many patients of this type have died in the radiology department or the emergency room while awaiting such unnecessary examinations as electrocardiograms or films of the abdomen. *There are no contraindications to operation when massive hemorrhage is present.* Although exceedingly important, this situation fortunately is relatively rare.

Nothing will supplant an orderly painstakingly *detailed history,* which is far more valuable than any laboratory or roentgenologic examination. This kind of history is laborious and time-consuming, making it not especially popular even though a reasonably accurate diagnosis can be made on the basis of the history alone in the majority of cases. The *chronological sequence of events* in the patient's history is often more important than emphasis on the location of pain. If the examiner is sufficiently open-minded and unhurried, asks the proper questions, and listens, the patient will often provide the diagnosis. Careful attention should be paid to the extraabdominal regions which may be responsible for abdominal pain. An accurate menstrual history in a female patient is essential. Narcotics or analgesics should be withheld until a definitive diagnosis or a definitive plan has been formulated, because these agents often make it more difficult to secure and to interpret the history and physical findings.

In the examination, simple critical inspection of the patient, e.g., of facies, position in bed, and respiratory activity, may provide valuable clues. The amount of information to be gleaned is directly proportional to the *gentleness* and thoroughness of the examiner. Once a patient with peritoneal inflammation has been examined in a brusque manner, accurate assessment by the next examiner becomes almost impossible. For example, eliciting rebound tenderness by sudden release of a deeply palpating hand in a patient with suspected peritonitis is cruel and unnecessary. The same information can be obtained by gentle percussion of the abdomen (rebound tenderness on a miniature scale), a maneuver which can be far more precise and localizing. Asking the patient to cough will elicit true rebound tenderness without the need for placing a hand on the abdomen. Furthermore, the brusque demonstration of rebound tenderness will startle and induce protective spasm in a nervous or worried patient in whom true rebound tenderness is not present. A palpable gallbladder will be missed if palpation is so brusque that voluntary muscle spasm becomes superimposed upon involuntary muscular rigidity.

As in history taking, there is no substitute for sufficient time spent in the examination. It is important to remember that abdominal signs may be minimal but nevertheless, if accompanied by consistent symptoms, may be exceptionally meaningful when carefully assessed. Signs may be virtually or actually totally absent in cases of pelvic peritonitis, so that careful *pelvic and rectal examinations are mandatory in every patient with abdominal pain.* The presence of tenderness on pelvic or rectal examination in the absence of other abdominal signs must not lead the examiner to exclude such important operative indications as perforated appendicitis, diverticulitis, twisted ovarian cyst, and many others.

Much attention has been paid to the presence or absence of peristaltic sounds, their quality, and their frequency. Auscultation of the abdomen is probably one of the least rewarding aspects of the physical examination of a patient with abdominal pain. Severe catastrophes, such as strangulating small-intestinal obstruction or perforated appendicitis, may occur in the presence of normal peristalsis. Conversely, when the proximal part of the intestine above an obstruction becomes markedly distended and edematous, peristaltic sounds may lose the characteristics of borborygmi and become weak or absent even when peritonitis is not present. It is usually the severe chemical peritonitis of sudden onset which is associated with the truly silent abdomen. Assessment of the patient's state of hydration is important. The hematocrit and urinalysis permit an accurate estimate of the severity of dehydration, so that adequate replacement can be carried out.

Laboratory examinations may be of enormous value in the assessment of the patient with abdominal pain, yet with but a few exceptions they rarely establish a diagnosis. Leukocytosis should never be the single deciding factor as to whether or not operation is indicated. A white blood cell count greater than 20,000 per cubic millimeter may be observed with perforation of a viscus, but pancreatitis, acute cholecystitis, pelvic inflammatory disease, and intestinal infarction may be associated with marked leukocytosis. A normal white blood cell count is by no means rare in cases of perforation of abdominal viscera. The diagnosis of anemia may be more helpful than the white blood cell count, especially when combined with the history.

The urinalysis is also of great value in indicating to some degree the state of hydration or to rule out severe renal disease, diabetes, or porphyria. Determination of the blood urea nitrogen, blood sugar, and serum bilirubin levels may also be helpful. The serum amylase determination is overrated, since in carefully controlled series of patients with proved pancreatitis where the determination has been done within the first 72 h, amylase was less than 200 Somogyi units in one-third of the cases, between 200 and 500 in another one-third of the cases, and greater than 500 in one-third. Since many diseases other than pancreatitis, e.g., perforated ulcer, strangulating intestinal obstruction, and acute cholecystitis, may be associated with very marked increase in the serum amylase, great care must be exercised in denying an operation to a patient solely on the basis of an elevated serum amylase level. The determination of the amylase-to-creatinine clearance ratio is of somewhat greater accuracy than either serum amylase or lipase determinations in the diagnosis of pancreatitis but has not proved to be specific.

Abdominal paracentesis is a safe and effective diagnostic maneuver in patients with acute abdominal pain. It is of special value in patients with blunt trauma to the abdomen where evaluation of the abdomen may be difficult because of other multiple injuries to the spine, pelvis, or ribs and where blood in the peritoneal cavity produces only a very mild peritoneal reaction. The gallbladder is the only organ which may continue to seep fluid following accidental perforation, so that the region of this organ must be assiduously avoided. Determination of the pH of the aspirated fluid to ascertain the site of a perforation is misleading, because even highly acid gastric juice is rapidly buffered by peritoneal exudate.

Plain and upright or lateral decubitus roentgenograms of the abdomen may be of the greatest value. They are usually unnecessary in patients with acute appendicitis or strangulated external hernias. However, in cases of intestinal obstruction, perforated ulcer, and a variety of other conditions, films may be diagnostic. During a search for free air, the patient should be kept in the decubitus or upright position for at least 10 min before the appropriate film is taken lest a small pneumoperitoneum be missed. In rare instances, barium or water-soluble medium examination of the upper part of the gastrointestinal tract may demonstrate partial intestinal obstruction which may elude diagnosis by other means. If there is any question of obstruction of the colon, oral administration of barium sulfate should be avoided. On the other hand, barium enema is of inestimable value in cases of colonic obstruction and should be used with greater frequency where the possibility of perforation does not exist. Ultrasound recently has proved to be useful in detecting an enlarged gallbladder or pancreas, the presence of gallstones, or a localized collection of fluid or pus.

Sometimes, even under the best of circumstances with all available auxiliary aids and with the greatest of clinical skill, a definitive diagnosis cannot be established at the time of the initial examination. Nevertheless, despite lack of a clear anatomic diagnosis it may be abundantly clear to an experienced and thoughtful physician and surgeon on clinical grounds alone that operation is indicated. Should that decision be questionable, watchful waiting with repeated questioning and examination will often elucidate the true nature of the illness and indicate the proper course of action.

REFERENCES

Bonica JJ: Neurophysiologic and pathologic aspects of acute and chronic pain. Arch Surg 112:750, 1977

Lasser RB et al: The role of intestinal gas in functional abdominal pain. N Engl J Med 293:524, 1975

Leek BF: Abdominal and pelvic visceral receptors. Br Med Bull 33:163, 1977

Silen W: *Cope's Early Diagnosis of the Acute Abdomen*, 15th ed. London, Oxford Press, 1979

Staniland JR et al: Clinical presentation of acute abdomen: Study of 600 patients. Br Med J 2:393, 1972

Swarbick ET et al: Site of pain from the irritable bowel. Lancet 2:443, 1980

6 PAIN IN THE BACK AND NECK

HENRY J. MANKIN
RAYMOND D. ADAMS

The remarks in the first part of this chapter concern mainly the lower part of the back, since it is most frequently the site of disabling pain. The lower portions of the spine and pelvis, with their many muscular and tendinous attachments, are relatively inaccessible to palpation and inspection. Although certain physical signs and radiographs are helpful, it is often necessary to depend on the patient's description of a pain (which may not be altogether accurate) and behavior during the execution of certain maneuvers to fully assess the nature of the problem. Seasoned clinicians, for these reasons, come to appreciate the need of a systematic clinical approach, the description of which is one of the main purposes of this chapter.

ANATOMY AND PHYSIOLOGY OF THE LOWER PART OF THE BACK

The bony spine is a complex structure, anatomically divisible into two parts. The anterior part consists of a series of cylindrical vertebral bodies articulated by the intervertebral disks and held together by the anterior and posterior longitudinal ligaments. The posterior part consists of more delicate elements that extend from the vertebral body as pedicles and laminae, fused by ligaments to form the vertebral canal. Stout transverse and spinous bony processes project laterally and posteriorly and serve as the attachments of muscles which support and protect the vertebral column. The stability of the spine depends on two types of support: that provided by the bony articulations (principally the posterior elements) and a second type provided by the ligamentous (passive) and muscular (active) supporting structures. The ligamentous structures are quite strong, but because neither they nor the vertebral body-disk complexes have sufficient integral strength to resist the

enormous forces acting on the column during even simple movements, voluntary and reflex contractions of the sacrospinalis, abdominal, gluteal, psoas, and hamstring muscles afford most of the stability.

The vertebral and paravertebral structures derive their innervation from the recurrent branches of the spinal nerves. Pain endings and fibers have been demonstrated in the ligaments, muscles, periosteum of bone, outer layers of annulus fibrosus, and synovium of the articular facets. The sensory fibers from these structures and the sacroiliac and lumbosacral joints join to form the sinovertebral nerves which pass via the recurrent branches of the spinal nerves of the first sacral and the fifth to first lumbar vertebrae into the gray matter of the corresponding segments of the spinal cord. Efferent fibers emerge from these segments and extend to the muscles through the same nerves. The sympathetic nerves contribute only to the innervation of blood vessels and appear to play no part in voluntary and reflex movement, though they do contain sensory fibers.

The parts of the back that possess the greatest freedom of movement, and hence are most frequently subject to injury, are the lumbar and cervical. In addition to the voluntary motions required for bending, twisting, and other movements, many actions of the spine are reflex in nature and are the basis of posture.

GENERAL CLINICAL CONSIDERATIONS

TYPES OF LOW BACK PAIN Of the several symptoms of disease of the spine (pain, stiffness or limitation of movement, and deformity), pain is of foremost importance by virtue of its frequency and its disabling effects. Four types of pain may be differentiated: local, referred, radicular, and that arising from secondary (protective) muscular spasm. One must identify these several types of pain by the patient's description, and here reliance is placed mainly on the character, location, and the conditions which modify them. The mechanism of the several types of pain has already been described in Chap. 2.

Local pain is caused by any pathologic process which impinges upon or irritates sensory endings. Involvement of structures which contain no sensory endings is painless. The central, medullary portion of the vertebral body may be destroyed by tumor, for example, without evocation of pain, whereas cortical fractures, or tears and distortions of the periosteum, synovial membranes, muscles, annulus fibrosus, and ligaments are often exquisitely painful. Although painful states are often accompanied by swelling of the affected tissues, this may not be apparent if a deep structure of the back is the site of disease. Local pain is often described as steady but may be intermittent, varying considerably with position or activity. The pain may be sharp or dull and although often diffuse is always felt in or near the affected part of the spine. Reflex splinting of the spine segments by paravertebral muscles is frequently noted, and certain movements or postures that alter the position of the injured tissues aggravate the pain. Firm pressure or percussion upon superficial structures in the region involved usually evokes tenderness, which is of aid in identifying the site of the abnormality.

Referred pain is of two types, that projected from the spine into regions lying within the area of the lumbar and upper sacral dermatomes and that projected from the pelvic and abdominal viscera to the spine. Pain due to diseases of the upper part of the lumbar spine is usually referred to the anterior aspects of the thighs and legs; that from the lower lumbar and sacral segments is referred to the gluteal regions, posterior thighs, and calves. Pain of this type, although of deep, aching quality and rather diffuse, tends at times to be superficially projected. In general the referred pain parallels in intensity the local pain in the back. In other words, maneuvers which alter local pain have a similar effect on referred pain, though not with such precision and immediacy as in radicular, or "root," pain. Referred pain may be confused with pain from visceral disease, but the latter is usually described as "deep" and tends to radiate from the abdomen through to the back. Also, visceral pain is usually unaffected by movement of the spine, does not improve with recumbency, and may be modified by the activity of the involved viscus.

Radicular, or "root," *pain* has some of the characteristics of referred pain but differs in its greater intensity, distal radiation, circumscription to the territory of a root, and the factors which excite it. The mechanism is distortion, stretching, irritation, or compression of a spinal root, most often central to the intervertebral foramen. Although the pain itself is often dull or aching, various maneuvers which increase the irritation of the root may greatly intensify the pain. Nearly always the radiation of pain is from a central position near the spine to some part of the lower extremity. Cough, sneeze, and strain are characteristically evocative maneuvers; but since they may also jar or move the spine, they may aggravate local pain as well. Any motion which stretches the nerve, e.g., forward bending with the knees extended or "straight-leg raising," in disease of the lower part of the lumbar spine excites radicular pain; jugular vein compression, which raises intraspinal pressure and may cause a shift in the position of the root, may have a similar effect. The fourth and fifth lumbar and first sacral roots, which form the sciatic nerve, cause pain which extends mainly down the posterior aspects of thigh, the postero- and anterolateral aspects of the leg, and into the foot, in the distribution of this nerve—so called sciatica. Tingling, paresthesias, and numbness or sensory impairment of the skin, soreness of the skin, and tenderness along the nerve usually accompany radicular pain. Also reflex loss, weakness, atrophy, fascicular twitching, and often stasis edema may occur if motor fibers of the anterior root are involved.

Pain resulting from muscular spasm is usually mentioned in relation to local pain. Muscle spasm may be associated with many disorders of the spine and can produce significant distortions of the normal posture. Chronic tension in muscles may give rise to a dull and sometimes cramping ache. One can in this instance feel the tautness of the sacrospinalis and gluteal muscles and demonstrate by palpation that the pain is localized to them.

Other pains often of undetermined origin are sometimes described by patients with chronic disease of the lower part of the back. In the legs, drawing, pulling, cramping sensations (without involuntary muscle spasm), tearing, throbbing, or jabbing pains, or feelings of burning or coldness are difficult to interpret and, like paresthesias and numbness, should always suggest the possibility of nerve or root disease.

Since it is often difficult to secure physical or laboratory confirmation of painful disease of the lower region of the spine, it is extremely important to obtain an accurate history. In addition to assessing the character and location of the pain, one should determine the factors which aggravate and relieve it, its constancy, and its relationship to recumbency and such stereotypical movements and maneuvers as forward bending, cough, sneeze, and strain. Frequently the most important lead comes from the knowledge of the mode of onset and circumstances which initiated the pain. Inasmuch as many painful afflictions of the back are the result of injury incurred during work or in an accident, the possibility of exaggeration or prolongation of pain for purposes of compensation or other personal reasons, or because of hysteria or malingering, must always be kept in mind.

EXAMINATION OF THE LOWER PART OF THE BACK

Much information may be gained by "inspection" of the back, buttocks, and lower extremities in various positions and movements. The normal spine shows a dorsal kyphosis and lumbar lordosis in the saggital plane, which in some individuals may be somewhat exaggerated (swayback). Normally the spine is relatively straight in the coronal plane, although slight curvature is frequent, particularly in females. In spinal disorders, one should observe the spine closely for excessive curvature, list, flattening of the normal lumbar arch, presence of a gibbus (a short, sharp, kyphotic angulation usually indicative of a fracture), pelvic tilt or obliquity, or asymmetry of the paravertebral or gluteal musculature. In severe sciatica, one may observe abnormalities of posture of the affected leg, presumably to reduce tension on the irritated part.

The next step in the examination is observation of the spine, hips, and legs during certain motions. During the procedure it is well to remember that no advantage accrues from trying to find out how much the patient can be hurt. Instead, it is much more important to determine when and under what conditions the pain commences. One looks for limitation of the natural motions of the patient while he or she is disrobing, standing, and reclining. When standing, the motion of forward bending normally produces flattening and reversal of the lumbar lordotic curve and exaggeration of the dorsal curve. With lesions of the lumbosacral region which involve the posterior ligaments, articular facets, or sacrospinalis muscle and with ruptured lumbar disks, protective reflexes prevent stretching of these structures. As a consequence, the sacrospinalis muscles remain taut and limit motion in the lumbar part of the spine. Forward bending then occurs at the hips and at the lumbar-thoracic junction. With disease of the lumbosacral joints and spinal roots, the patient bends in such a way as to avoid tensing the hamstring muscles and putting undue leverage upon the pelvis. In unilateral "sciatica," with its increased curvature toward the side of the lesion, lumbar and lumbosacral motions are splinted, and bending is mainly at the hips; at a certain point the knee on the affected side is flexed to relieve hamstring spasm and tilting of the pelvis occurs to slacken the lumbosacral roots and sciatic nerve.

It is sometimes of value to record the degree of flexion achieved either by measuring the distance between the fingertips and the floor or by estimating the degree of bending of the spine. Lateral bending is usually less instructive than forward bending. However, in unilateral ligamentous or muscular strain, bending to the opposite side aggravates the pain by stretching the damaged tissues. Moreover, in lateral disk lesions, bending of the spine toward the side from which the trunk lists is restricted. In diseases of the lower part of the spine, flexion while sitting with the hips and knees flexed can normally be performed easily, even to the point of bringing the knees in contact with the chest. The reason is that knee flexion relaxes the tightened hamstring muscles and also relieves stretch of the sciatic nerve.

The study of motions in the supine position yields the same information as study of motions in the standing and sitting positions, with the difference that there is less intradiskal pressure. With lumbosacral lesions and sciatica, passive lumbar flexion causes little pain and is not limited as long as the hamstrings are relaxed and there is no stretching of the sciatic nerve. With lumbosacral and lumbar spine disease (e.g., arthritis), passive flexion of the hips is free, whereas flexion of the lumbar spine may be impeded and painful. Passive straight-leg raising (possible in most normal individuals up to 90° except in those who have unusually tight hamstrings), like forward bending in the standing posture with the legs straight, places the sciatic nerve and its roots under tension, thereby producing pain. It may also cause an anterior rotation of the pelvis around a transverse axis, increasing stress on the lumbosacral joint, and thus causing pain if this segment is arthritic or otherwise impaired. Consequently, in diseases of the lumbosacral joints and lumbosacral roots, this movement is limited on the affected side and to a lesser extent on the opposite side. Lasègue's sign (pain and limitation of movement during elevation of the leg when the knee is extended) is a useful test of this condition. Straight-leg raising of the opposite leg may also cause contralateral pain but of lesser degree and is believed by some to be a sign of a more extensive lesion, such as an extruded disk fragment, rather than a simple prolapse or protrusion. It is important to remember, however, that the evoked pain is always referred to the diseased side, no matter which leg is flexed.

The motion of hyperextension is best performed with the patient standing or lying prone. If the condition causing back pain is acute, it may be difficult to extend the spine in the standing position. A patient with lumbosacral strain or disk disease can usually extend or hyperextend the spine without aggravation of pain. If there is an active inflammatory process or fracture of the vertebral body or posterior elements, hyperextension may be markedly limited.

Palpation and percussion of the spine are the last steps in the examination. The approach must always be gentle since rough percussion of the designated area of pain may antagonize the patient and only serve to confuse the physician. It is preferable to palpate first those regions which are the least likely to evoke pain. At all times the examiner should know what structures are being palpated (see Fig. 6-1). Localized tenderness is seldom pronounced in disease of the spine because the involved structures are so deep that they rarely give rise to surface tenderness. Mild superficial and poorly localized tenderness signifies only a disease process within the affected segment of the body, i.e., dermatome.

Tenderness over the costovertebral angle often indicates genitourinary disease, adrenal disease (Rogoff's sign), or an injury to the transverse processes of the first or second lumbar vertebra [Fig. 6-1 (1)]. Hypersensitivity on palpation of the transverse processes of the other lumbar vertebrae as well as the overlying sacrospinalis muscles may signify fracture of the transverse process or a strain of muscle attachments. Tenderness of a spinous process or aggravation of pain by the jarring of gentle percussion may be nonspecific but frequently indicates the presence of a disk lesion at the site deep to it, inflammation (as in disk space infection), or pathologic fracture.

In palpation of the spinous processes, it is important to note any deviation in the lateral plane (this may be indicative of fracture or arthritis) or in the anteroposterior plane. A "step-off" forward displacement of the spinous process may be an important clue to a spondylolisthesis, one segment below the displaced level.

Tenderness in the region of the articular facets between the fifth lumbar and first sacral vertebrae is consistent with disease of a lumbosacral disk [Fig. 6-1 (3)]. It is also frequent in rheumatoid arthritis.

Abdominal, rectal, and pelvic examination and assessment of the status of the peripheral vascular system are important parts of the examination of the patient with complaints in the lower back and should not be omitted. They may provide evidence for vascular, visceral, neoplastic, or inflammatory disorders which may extend to the spine or cause pain to be referred to this region.

Finally, a careful neurologic examination should be performed, with special attention given to motor, reflex, and sensory changes (see "Protrusion of Lumbar Intervertebral Disks," below), particularly in the lower extremities.

SPECIAL LABORATORY PROCEDURES Useful laboratory tests, depending on the nature of the problem and the circumstances, include a complete blood count, erythrocyte sedimentation rate (especially helpful in screening for infection or myeloma), measurement of serum calcium, phosphorus, alkaline phosphatase, acid phosphatase (the last mentioned is of importance if one suspects metastatic carcinoma from the prostate), protein electrophoresis, immunoglobulin electrophoresis, tuberculin test, and tests for febrile agglutinins and rheumatoid factor. Roentgenograms of the lumbar part of the spine should be taken in every case of low back pain and sciatica (preferably with the patient standing) in the anteroposterior, lateral, and oblique planes. Special spot views or stereoscopic or laminographic films may provide further information in certain cases. Bone scans are of aid in revealing some fractures and neoplastic and inflammatory lesions.

Examination of the spinal canal with a contrast medium (air or other contrast myelogram) is often of great value, especially if a spinal cord tumor is suspected or if a patient is thought to have a disk herniation and fails to improve on a conservative regimen. Myelography can be combined with

FIGURE 6-1

(1) Costovertebral angle. (2) Spinous process and interspinous ligament. (3) Region of the articular fifth lumbar to the first sacral facet. (4) Dorsum of sacrum. (5) Region of iliac crest. (6) Iliolumbar angle. (7) Spinous processes of fifth lumbar to first sacral vertebrae (tenderness = faulty posture or occasionally spina bifida occulta). (8) Region between posterior superior and posterior inferior spines. Sacroiliac ligaments (tenderness = sacroiliac sprain, often tender with fifth lumbar to first sacral disk). (9) Sacrococcygeal junction (tenderness = sacrococcygeal injury, i.e., sprain or fracture). (10) Region of sacrosciatic notch (tenderness = fourth to fifth lumbar disk rupture and sacroiliac sprain). (11) Sciatic nerve trunk (tenderness = ruptured lumbar disk or sciatic nerve lesion).

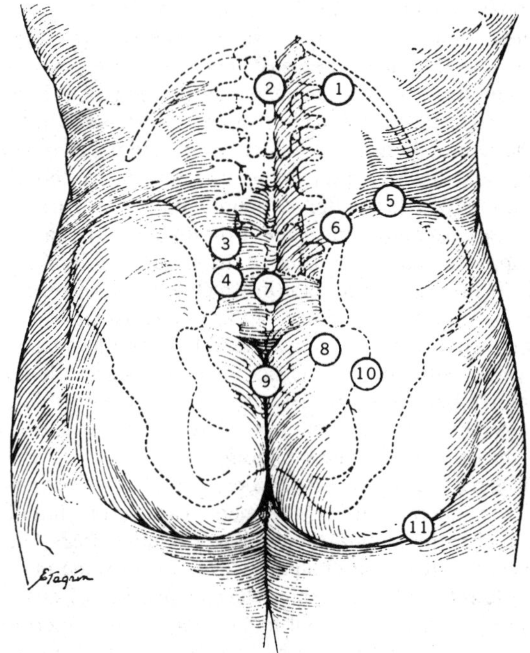

tests of dynamics of the cerebrospinal fluid, and a sample of the fluid should always be removed for cytologic and chemical examination prior to the instillation of the contrast medium (Pantopaque, Myodil, air, or some of the newer contrast media which are resorbed). Injection and removal of Pantopaque require special skill and should not be attempted without previous experience with the procedure. If done properly, the procedure has a very low incidence of significant complications. Injection of contrast medium directly into the intervertebral disk (diskograms) has waxed and waned in popularity over the years but remains controversial. The technique of this procedure is more complicated than that of myelographic examination, and the risk of damage to the disk or nerve roots and the possibility of introduction of infection is not inconsiderable. In the authors' opinion, such a procedure is indicated only under very special circumstances.

In recent years, computerized tomography (CT) has become a very valuable instrument for study of the spinal canal, bony segments, and adjacent soft tissues. The newest equipment, particularly if combined with instillation of water-soluble contrast media, will not only provide excellent definition of the narrow canal, destructive lesions of the vertebral bodies in posterior elements, or presence of a paravertebral soft tissue mass, but by appropriate computerized reconstruction techniques can also identify disk herniations with what appears to be even greater accuracy than the myelogram. Even without radiopaque material in the canal, the reconstructed CT scans have a high resolution and provide a noninvasive method of study of disk disease with a relatively low level of radiation.

PRINCIPAL CONDITIONS WHICH GIVE RISE TO DISABLING PAIN IN THE LOWER PART OF THE BACK

CONGENITAL ANOMALIES OF THE LUMBAR SPINE Anatomic variations of the spine are not at all infrequent, and although rarely of themselves the source of pain and functional derangement, they may predispose an individual to excessive stress because of the altered mechanics or alignment of the spine.

One of the most common disorders is a failure of fusion of the laminae of the neural arch (spina bifida) of one or several of the lumbar vertebrae or of the sacrum. Hypertrichosis or hyperpigmentation in the sacral area may betray the condition, but in most patients the spine defect remains entirely occult until disclosed by x-ray. The anomaly has greater potentiality for pain if accompanied by malformation of vertebral joints. Usually the pain is induced by injury. There are many other congenital anomalies which affect the lower lumbar vertebrae such as asymmetrical facetal joints, abnormalities of the transverse processes, sacralization of the fifth lumbar vertebra (in which L5 appears to be firmly fixed to the sacrum), or lumbarization of the first sacral vertebra (in which the first sacral resembles a sixth lumbar). Any one of these is occasionally observed in patients with symptoms referable to the low back, but they occur with equal frequency in individuals with no evidence of low back problem. Their role in the genesis of low back derangement is unclear, but in the authors' opinion, they are rarely the cause of specific symptomatology.

Spondylolysis consists of a bony defect, probably congenital, in the pars interarticularis (a segment near the junction of the pedicle with the lamina) of the lower lumbar area. The defect is best visualized on oblique projections. In some individuals the defect is bilateral. Under the circumstance of single or multiple injuries, the vertebral body, pedicle, and superior articular facet move anteriorly, leaving the posterior elements behind. This latter abnormality, known as *spondylolisthesis*, usually results in symptoms. The patient complains of pain in the low back radiating into the thighs, and there is limitation of motion. Often tenderness is elicited near the segment which has "slipped" forward (most often L5 or occasionally L4), and one can feel a "step" on deep palpation of the posterior elements. The pelvis is sometimes rotated and hip flexion limited by hamstring spasm; a variety of neurologic deficits indicative of radiculopathy complete the clincial syndrome. In exceptionally severe cases, the trunk may be shortened and the abdomen protuberant, both the result of the forward shift of L5 on S1.

TRAUMATIC AFFLICTIONS OF THE LOWER PART OF THE BACK Trauma constitutes the most frequent cause of low back pain.

In severe acute injuries, the examining physician must be careful to avoid further damage. In tests of mobility, all movements must be kept to a minimum until a diagnosis has been made and adequate measures have been instituted for the proper care of the patient. A patient complaining of back pain and inability to move the legs may have a fractured spine. The neck should not be flexed, nor should the patient be allowed to sit up. (See Chap. 366 for further discussion of spinal cord injury.)

Sprains, strains, and derangements The terms lumbosacral *sprain* and *strain* are used loosely by most physicians, and it is probably impossible to distinguish between them. The authors prefer the term *low back derangement* or *strain* for minor, self-limited injuries usually associated with lifting a heavy object, a fall, or a sudden deceleration as may occur in an automobile accident. Occasionally, these syndromes are more chronic in nature, suggesting that postural, muscular, or arthritic factors may play a role. The patients with low back derangement or strain are often acutely discomfited and may assume unusual postures related to spasm of the sacrospinalis muscles. The pain is usually confined to the lower back and is almost invariably relieved by rest. What formerly was regarded as sacroiliac strain or sprain is now known to be due to disk disease in most instances. This is caused by lifting heavy objects with the spine in a position of imperfect mechanical balance, as when lifting and turning at the same time. Sudden, unexpected motion is particularly likely to cause this injury.

The diagnosis of lumbosacral and sacroiliac strains with injury of the various structures of the lower part of the back depends upon the description of the injury, the localization of the pain by the patient, the finding of localized tenderness, and the augmentation of pain when tension is exerted on the involved structures by the appropriate maneuvers. The prompt alleviation of the pain by rest and relaxation indicates the existence of a strain. The rate of recovery depends on the degree of damage, preexisting disk disease, etc. Pain may be immediately relieved by local infiltration of an anesthetic agent, a finding which is also helpful in diagnosis.

Vertebral fractures Most fractures of the lumbar vertebral body are the result of flexion injuries and consist of anterior wedging or compression. With more severe trauma the patient may sustain a fracture dislocation, "bursting" fracture, or asymmetrical fracture involving not only the body but the posterior elements. The initiating trauma which causes fractures of the vertebrae is usually a fall from a height (in which case the calcanei may also be fractured) or may result from an automobile accident or other violence. When fractures occur with minimal trauma (or spontaneously), the bone is presumed to have been previously weakened by some pathologic process. Most of the time, particularly in older individuals, the cause of such an event is idiopathic osteoporosis, but there are many other underlying systemic disorders such as osteomalacia, hyperparathyroidism, hyperthyroidism, multiple myeloma, metastatic carcinoma, and a large number of local conditions that may play a role in weakening the vertebral body. Spasm of the lower lumbar muscles, limitation of motion of the lumbar section of the spine, and the roentgenographic appearance of the damaged lumbar portion (with or without neurologic abnormalities) are the basis of clinical diagnosis. The pain is usually immediate, though occasionally it may be delayed in onset for a few days. The patient may develop a mild paralytic ileus or urinary retention during the acute period.

Fractures of the transverse processes are almost always associated with tearing of the paravertebral muscles, principally the psoas. They may cause significant retroperitoneal hemorrhage resulting in a marked depression in hematocrit and, in extensive fractures, hypovolemic shock. Such injuries may be diagnosed by the finding of deep tenderness at the site of the injury, local muscle spasm on one side, and limitation of all movements which stretch the lumbar muscles. Radiologic evidence including body CT scan provides the final confirmation. Fractures of multiple transverse processes, although seemingly trivial, should be the object of considerable concern, and the patient should be carefully watched over the initial period for internal hemorrhage.

Protrusion of lumbar intervertebral disks This condition is now recognized as the major cause of severe and chronic or recurrent low back and leg pain. It is most likely to occur between the fifth lumbar and first sacral vertebrae, and, with lessening frequency, between the fourth and fifth lumbar, the third and fourth lumbar, the second and third lumbar, and the first and second lumbar vertebrae. Rare in the thoracic portion of the spine, it is next most frequent between the sixth and seventh and fifth and sixth cervical vertebrae. The cause is usually a flexion injury, but in a considerable proportion of cases no trauma is recalled. Degeneration of the posterior longitudinal ligaments and the annulus fibrosus, which occurs in most adults of middle and advanced years, may have taken place silently or have been manifested by mild, recurrent lumbar ache. A sneeze, lurch, or other trivial movement may then cause the nucleus pulposus to prolapse, pushing the frayed and weakened annulus posteriorly. In more severe cases of disk disease, the nucleus may protrude through the annulus or become extruded to lie as a free fragment in the vertebral canal.

The fully developed syndrome of ruptured lumbar intervertebral disk consists of backache, abnormal posture, and limitation of motion of the spine (particularly flexion). Nerve root involvement is indicated by radicular pain, sensory disturbances (paresthesias, hyper- and hyposensitivity in dermatome pattern), coarse twitching and fasciculation, muscle spasms, and impairment of a tendon reflex. Motor abnormalities (weakness and muscle atrophy) may also occur but are usually less prominent than the pain and sensory disorder. Since herniation of the intervertebral lumbar disks most often occurs between the fourth and fifth lumbar vertebrae and the fifth lumbar and first sacral vertebrae with irritation and compression of the fifth lumbar and first sacral roots, respectively, it is important to recognize the clinical characteristics of lesions of these two roots. *Lesions of the fifth lumbar root* produce pain in the region of the hip, groin, posterolateral thigh, lateral calf to the external malleolus, dorsal surface of the foot, and the first or second and third toes. Paresthesias may be in the entire territory or only in the distal parts of these territories. The tenderness is in the lateral gluteal region and near the head of the fibula. Weakness, if present, involves the extensors of the great toe and of the foot. The knee and ankle reflexes are seldom altered, although occasionally the ankle jerk is moderately depressed. Walking on the heels may be more difficult, because of weakness of dorsiflexion of the foot, and more uncomfortable than walking on the toes. In *lesions of the first sacral root* the pain is felt in the midgluteal region, posterior part of the thigh, posterior region of the calf to the heel, and the plantar surface of the foot and fourth and fifth toes. Tenderness is most pronounced over the midgluteal region (sacroiliac joint), posterior thigh area, and calf. Rarely it may be referred to the rectum, testicles, or labia. Paresthesias and sensory loss are mainly in the lower leg and outer toes, and weakness, if present, involves the flexor muscles of the foot and toes, abductors of the toes, and hamstring muscles. The ankle reflex is diminished to absent in the majority of cases. Walking on the toes is more difficult, because of weakness of plantar flexors, and more uncomfortable than walking on the heel. With lesions of either root there may be limitation of straight-leg raising during the acute, painful stages.

Degeneration of the intervertebral disk without frank extrusion of a fragment of disk tissue may give rise to low back pain, or the disk may herniate into the adjacent vertebral body, giving rise to a Schmorl's node (seen on x-ray). Such cases often show no signs of nerve root involvement though the back pain may be referred to the thigh and leg.

The rarer *lesions of the fourth and third lumbar roots* give rise to pain in the anterior part of the thigh and knee, with corresponding sensory loss. The knee jerk is diminished or abolished. An inverted Lasègue sign (pain with hypertension of the limb in relation to the trunk, best elicited with the patient in the prone position) is positive when the third lumbar root is affected.

The lumbar disk syndromes are usually unilateral. Only with massive derangements of the disk or the extrusion of a large, free fragment into the canal do bilateral symptoms and signs occur, and these may sometimes be associated with paralysis of the sphincters. The pain may be mild or severe. All or part of the above syndrome may be present. There may be back pain with little or no leg pain; rarely only leg pain may be experienced. The rupture of multiple lumbar or lumbar and cervical disks is not infrequent, suggesting a diffuse disorder of the connective tissue of the disks, including both the annulus fibrosus and the nucleus pulposus.

When all components of the syndrome are present, the diagnosis is easy; when only one part is present (particularly backache), it may be difficult, especially if there has been a clearly remembered initiating traumatic event. Since similar symptoms may occur without demonstrable disk rupture, other diagnostic procedures are required. Plain roentgenograms usually show no abnormality or at most a narrowing of the intervertebral space, sometimes more on the side of the rupture. Traction spurs, which are indicative of disk degeneration, may be present; in extreme cases, there may be a "vacuum" disk sign, in which a gas-density shadow is present in the intervertebral space, usually on lateral roentgenogram. Frequently, however, one must resort to Pantopaque or air myelography, which in most cases will reveal an indentation of the lumbar subarachnoid space or deformity of the root sleeve. Occasionally, with large lesions there is a complete interruption of the flow of contrast material. In some patients, CT with or without contrast material may show the disk herniation clearly even when it is small or laterally placed. A small ruptured disk may not show any abnormality in the CT scan or myelogram, especially at the fifth lumbar to first sacral level where there is a large space between the spinal canal and dura. Some clinics use diskograms (opaque material is injected directly into the disk) to reveal any evidence of extrusion, but the procedure is risky, and the results are difficult to interpret. The electromyogram is helpful in showing denervation of leg muscles (see Chap. 369). The protein level of the cerebrospinal fluid may be elevated in some instances.

Tumor of the spinal canal, epidural or intradural, may produce a syndrome similar to that of ruptured disk (see Chap. 366).

ARTHRITIS Arthritis of the spine is a major cause of backache, cervical pain, and occipital headache.

Osteoarthritis This more frequent type of osteoarthritic spinal disease occurs usually in later life and may involve any part of the spine. It is most prevalent in the cervical and lumbar regions, however, and the exact location determines the localization of the symptoms. Patients often complain of pain centered in the spine, which is increased by motion and is almost invariably associated with complaints of stiffness and limitation of motion. There is a notable absence of systemic symptoms such as fatigue, malaise, and fever, and the pain usually can be relieved by rest. The severity of the symptoms often bears little relation to the radiologic findings; pain may be present when there are minimal findings on an x-ray, and, conversely, marked osteophytic overgrowth with spur formation, ridging, and bridging of vertebrae can be seen in asymptomatic patients in middle and later life. Osteoarthropathic changes in the cervical spine and to a lesser extent in the lumbar spine may by their location compress roots or even the cauda equina or spinal cord, giving rise to the spondylitic form of myelopathy (see Chaps. 366 and 368).

Spondylitic caudal radiculopathy (SCR) is another variant of hypertrophic arthritis. A congenital smallness of the lumbar canal, especially at the L4 to L5 level, renders the individual susceptible to either a rupture of an intervertebral disk or arthrosis. The latter condition further narrows the anteroposterior diameter of the canal and leads to compression of lumbosacral roots and even to a block of the spinal canal. The roots are actually caught between the posterior surface of the vertebral body and the ligamentum flavum posterolaterally. Lumbosacral pains are followed by weakening of the lower legs, impairment of ankle and knee reflexes, and numbness and paresthesia in the feet and legs. Extension of the lumbar spine during walking and standing produces or aggravates the neurologic symptoms, and flexion relieves them. The clinical picture and its intermittency correspond to the so-called intermittent claudication of the spinal cord. The diagnosis may be suspected on the basis of history and radiographic findings but may be confirmed by myelography or CT scan, both of which will demonstrate the narrowed lumbar canal. Decompression of the spinal canal relieves the symptoms in a considerable proportion of the cases but should be approached with caution since it may lead to instability, necessitating an arthrodesis. SCR is the lumbar equivalent of spondylitic cervical myelopathy (SCM), described below. SCR is a cauda equina syndrome, and its differential diagnosis is discussed in Chap. 366, "Diseases of the Spinal Cord."

Rheumatoid arthritis and ankylosing spondylitis Arthritic disease of the spine takes two distinct forms, ankylosing spondylitis (the more common) and rheumatoid arthritis.

Patients with *ankylosing spondylitis* (also called Marie-Strümpell arthritis) are usually young men who complain of mild to moderate pain, which early in the course of the disease is centered in the back, and on occasion radiates to the back of the thighs. The symptoms may be vague at first (tired back, "catches" up and down the back, sore back) and the diagnosis may be overlooked for a considerable period. Although the pain is often intermittent, the finding of limitation of movement is constant and progressive and over a period of time tends to dominate the picture. Early in the course, this finding is described as "morning stiffness" or increasing stiffness after periods of inactivity, and may be present long before radiologic changes are manifest. Limitation of chest expansion, tenderness over the sternum, and decreased motion and flexion contractures of the hips may also be present early in the course. The radiologic hallmarks of the disease are destruction and subsequent obliteration of the sacroiliac joints, development of syndesmophytes on the margins of the vertebral bodies, followed by bridging by bone to produce the characteristic "bamboo spine." The entire spine becomes immobilized, often in a flexed position, and usually the pain then subsides. Patterns of restricted movement, indistinguishable from those of ankylosing spondylitis, may accompany Reiter's syndrome, psoriatic arthritis, and inflammatory diseases of the intestine. Patients with these disorders rarely show the joint manifestations of peripheral rheumatoid arthritis, and seldom do they display involvement of the hips or knees. The rheumatoid factor is usually absent, but the sedimentation rate is often rapid, and many of the patients are found to have a HLA-B27 antigen.

Occasionally ankylosing spondylitis is complicated by progressively destructive vertebral lesions. This complication should be suspected whenever the pain returns, after a period of quiescence, or becomes localized. The etiology of these lesions is not known, but they may represent an exaggerated healing response to fracture or excessive production of fibrous inflammatory tissues. Rarely they may result in collapse of a segment of the spine and compression of the spinal cord. Another complication of severe ankylosing spondylitis is bilateral ankylosis of the ribs to the spine, which, coupled with a decrease in the height of axial thoracic structures, causes marked impairment of respiratory function.

Spinal rheumatoid arthritis tends to be localized to the cervical apophyseal joints and atlantoaxial articulation; the pain, stiffness, and limitation of motion are then in the neck and back of the head. Unlike ankylosing spondylitis, rheumatoid arthritis is rarely confined to the spine, and it does not lead to significant degrees of intervertebral bridging. Because of major affection of other joints, the diagnosis is relatively easy to make, but significant involvement of the neck may be overlooked. In the advanced stages of the disease, one or several of the vertebrae may be displaced anteriorly, or a synovitis of the atlantoaxial joint may damage the transverse ligament of the atlas, resulting in forward displacement of the atlas on the axis, i.e., atlantoaxial subluxation. In either instance serious and even life-threatening compression of the spinal cord may occur gradually or suddenly (see Chaps. 346 and 366). Lateral roentgenograms in flexion and extension, performed cautiously, are necessary to visualize dislocation or subluxation.

OTHER DESTRUCTIVE DISEASES Neoplastic, infectious, and metabolic diseases Metastatic carcinoma (breast, lung, prostate, thyroid, kidney, gastrointestinal tract), multiple myeloma, and non-Hodgkin's and Hodgkin's lymphomas are the malignant tumors which most frequently involve the spine. Since the primary site may be overlooked or asymptomatic, the presenting complaint in such patients may be pain in the back. The pain tends to be constant and dull, and is often unrelieved by rest. Indeed, it may be worse at night. Radiographic changes may be absent early in the disease, but when they appear, usually are manifest as destructive lesions in one or several vertebral bodies with little or limited involvement of the disk space, even in the face of a compression fracture. A ^{99m}Tc diphosphonate bone scan is helpful in lighting up "hot spots," indicating areas of increased blood flow and reactive bone formation associated with destructive inflammatory or arthritic lesions. It should be noted, however, that myeloma and sometimes metastatic thyroid carcinoma may fail to show increased activity on a bone scan.

Infection of the vertebral column is usually the result of pyogenic organisms (staphylococci or coliform bacilli) or tubercule bacilli and is often diffcult to distinguish on the basis of clinical findings. Patients complain of pain in the back of subacute or chronic nature that is exacerbated by motion but not materially relieved by rest. There is limitation of motion, tenderness over the spine of the involved segments, and pain with jarring of the spine, such as occurs with walking on the heels. Usually, these patients are afebrile and often do not have a leukocytosis although the erythrocyte sedimentation rate is almost invariably elevated. Radiographs may demonstrate narrowing of a disk space with erosion and destruction of the two adjacent vertebrae. A paravertebral soft tissue mass may be present, indicating an abscess, which may in the case of tuberculosis drain spontaneously, at sites quite remote from the vertebral column. In addition to a bone scan, a gallium scan is somtimes helpful in identifying a soft tissue inflammatory or infectious lesion even when overt bone destruction is not visible in x-rays.

Special mention should be made of the spinal *epidural abscess* (usually staphylococcal), which necessitates urgent surgical treatment. The symptoms are a localized pain, occurring spontaneously, aggravated by percussion and palpation. The patient is febrile and usually has severe radicular complaints, often bilaterial, progressing rapidly to a flaccid paraplegia (see Chaps. 359 and 366).

In so-called metabolic bone diseases (osteoporosis or osteomalacia) a considerable degree of loss of bone substance may occur without any symptoms whatsoever. Many patients with such conditions do, however, complain of aching in the lumbar or thoracic area. This is most likly to occur following an injury, sometimes of trivial degree, which leads to collapse or wedging of a vertebra. Certain movements greatly enhance the pain, and certain positions relieve it. One or more spinal roots may be involved. Paget's disease of the spine is nearly always painless but may lead to compression of the spinal cord or roots because of encroachment on the canal or foramina by the pagetoid bone. The recognition of these bone disorders is discussed in some detail elsewhere (Chaps. 341 and 342).

In general, patients thought to have neoplastic, infectious, or metabolic disease of the spine should be thoroughly evaluated by means of radiographs, bone scans, CT scans, and appropriate laboratory studies (see above).

REFERRED PAIN FROM VISCERAL DISEASE The pain of disease of the pelvic, abdominal, or thoracic viscera is often felt in the region of the spine; i.e., it is referred to the more posterior parts of the spinal segment which innervates the diseased organ. Occasionally back pain may be the first and only sign. The general rule is that pelvic diseases are referred to the sacral region, lower abdominal diseases to the lumbar region (centering around the second to fourth lumbar vertebrae), and upper abdominal diseases to the lower thoracic spine (eighth thoracic to the first and second lumbar vertebrae). Characteristically there are no local signs or stiffness of the back, and motion is of full range without augmentation of the pain. However, some positions, e.g., flexion of the lumbar area of the spine in the lateral recumbent position, may be more comfortable than others.

Low thoracic and upper lumbar pain in abdominal disease Peptic ulceration or tumor of the wall of the stomach and of the duodenum most typically induces pain in the epigastrium (see Chaps. 306 and 325); but if the posterior wall is involved, and particularly if there is retroperitoneal extension, the pain may be felt in the region of the spine. The pain may be central in location or more intense on one side, or it may be felt in both locations. If very intense, it may seem to encircle the body. It tends to retain the characteristics of pain from the affected organ; e.g., if due to peptic ulceration, it appears about 2 h after a meal and is relieved by food and antacids.

Diseases of the pancreas (peptic ulceration with extension to the pancreas, cholecystitis with pancreatitis, cyst, or tumor) are apt to cause pain in the back, being more to the right of the spine if the head of the pancreas is involved and to the left if the body and tail are implicated.

Diseases of retroperitoneal structures, e.g., lymphomas, sarcomas, and carcinomas, may evoke pain in this part of the spine with some tendency toward radiation to the lower part of the abdomen, groin, and anterior thighs. A secondary tumor of the iliopsoas region on one side often produces a unilateral lumbar ache with radiation toward the groin and labia or testicle; there may also be signs of involvement of the upper lumbar spinal roots. An aneurysm of the abdominal aorta may induce pain which is localized to this region of the spine but may be felt higher or lower, depending on the location of the lesion.

The sudden appearance of obscure lumbar pain in a patient receiving anticoagulants should arouse the suspicion of retroperitoneal bleeding.

Lumbar pain with lower abdominal diseases Inflammatory diseases of segments of the colon (colitis, diverticulitis) or tumor of the colon cause pain which may be felt in the lower part of the abdomen between the umbilicus and pubis, in the midlumbar region, or in both places. If very intense, the pain may have a beltlike distribution around the body. A lesion in the transverse colon or first part of the descending colon may be central or left-sided, and its level of reference to the back is to the second to third lumbar vertebrae. If the sigmoid colon is implicated, the pain is lower, in the upper sacral region and anteriorly in the midline suprapubic region or left lower quadrant of the abdomen.

Sacral pain in pelvic (urologic and gynecologic) diseases Although gynecologic disorders may manifest themselves by back pain, the pelvis is seldom the site of a disease which causes obscure low back pain. The diagnosis of painful pelvic lesions may prove to be difficult. Less than a third of such cases are due to inflammatory disease; and other more hypothetical entities, such as traumatism of uterine supports, retroversion of uterus, pelvic varicosities, and adnexal edema, have been largely discredited. Recently, diagnostic laparoscopy has been recommended as a valuable supplement to rectal and pelvic examinations, sigmoidoscopy, and intravenous pyelography. The importance of psychiatric illness in the majority of undiagnosed cases has been stressed in a recent editorial in *Lancet*.

Menstrual pain itself may be felt in the sacral region. It is rather poorly localized, tends to radiate down the legs, and is of a crampy nature. The most important source of chronic back pain from the pelvic organs, however, is the uterosacral ligaments. Endometriosis or carcinoma of the uterus (body or cervix) may invade these structures, while malposition of the uterus may pull on them. The pain is localized centrally in the sacrum below the lumbosacral joint but may be more on one side. In endometriosis the pain begins during the premenstrual phase and often continues until it merges with menstrual pain. Malposition of the uterus (retroversion, descensus, and prolapse) is thought by some to lead to sacral pain, especially after the patient has been standing for several hours. One may observe the effect of postural influences here as when a fibroma of the uterus pulls on the uterosacral ligaments. Carcinomatous pain due to involvement of nerve plexuses is continuous and becomes progressively more severe; it tends to be more intense at night. The primary lesion may be inconspicuous, being overlooked upon pelvic examination. Papanicolaou smears, pyelogram, and CT scan are the most useful diagnostic procedures. X-ray therapy of these tumors may produce sacral pain consequent to necrosis of tissue and injury to nerve roots. Low back pain with radiation into one or both thighs is a common phenomenon during the last weeks of pregnancy.

Chronic prostatitis, evidenced by prostatic discharge, burning and frequency of urination, and slight reduction in sexual potency, may be attended by a nagging sacral ache; it may be mainly on one side, with radiation into one leg if the seminal vesicle is involved on that side. Carcinoma of the prostate with metastases to the lower part of the spine is another more common cause of sacral or lumbar pain. It may be present without urinary frequency or burning. Spinal nerves may be infiltrated by tumor cells, or the spinal cord itself may be compressed if the epidural space is invaded. The diagnosis is established by rectal examination, roentgenograms and bone scans of the spine, and measurement of acid phosphatase (particularly the prostatic phosphatase fraction). Lesions of the bladder and testes are usually not accompanied by back pain. When the kidney is the site of disease, the pain is ipsilateral, being felt in the flank or lumbar region.

Visceral derangements of whatever type may intensify the pain of arthritis, and the presence of arthritis may alter the distribution of visceral pain. With disease of the spine in the lumbosacral region, for example, distention of the ampulla of the sigmoid by feces or a bout of colitis may aggravate the arthritic pain. In patients with arthritis of the cervical or thoracic spine the pain of myocardial ischemia may radiate to the back.

OBSCURE TYPES OF LOW BACK PAIN AND THE QUESTION OF PSYCHIATRIC DISEASE The practitioner is frequently consulted by persons who complain of low back pain of obscure origin. Usually the disorder is benign in nature and results from some minor derangement, muscular strain, or diskal prolapse. This is particularly true for those lesions which are of acute onset, aggravated by motion, and relieved by rest. Considerably more difficult are patients with chronic pain, especially those who have had prior back surgery or chronic visceral disease, or those who have severe and progressive pain in which neoplasia or infection is considered.

Even when exhaustive studies have been performed, there remains a group of patients in whom no anatomic or pathologic lesion can be found. These patients generally fall into two categories: those with postural back pain and those with psychiatric illness.

Postural back pain Many slender asthenic individuals and some obese middle-aged individuals have discomfort in the back. Their backs ache much of the time, and the pain interferes with effective work. The physical examination is negative except for slack musculature and poor posture. The pain is diffuse in the mid or low region of the back and characteristically is relieved by bed rest and induced by the maintenance of a particular posture over a period of time. Pain in the neck and between the shoulder blades is a common complaint among thin, tense, active women and seems to be related to taut trapezius muscles.

Psychiatric illness Low back pain may be encountered in compensation hysteria and malingering, in anxiety or neurocirculatory asthenia (formerly called neurasthenia), in depression and hypochondriasis, and in many nervous persons whose symptoms and complaints do not fall within any category of psychiatric illness. It is probably correct to assume that pain in the back in such patients usually signifies diseases of the spine and adjacent structures, and one should always search for a specific cause. However, even when organic factors are found, the pain may be exaggerated, prolonged, or woven into a pattern of invalidism or disability because of coexistent psychological factors. This is especially true when there is the possibility of secondary gain (notably compensation). Patients seeking compensation for protracted low back pain without obvious structural disease, tend, after a time, to become suspicious, uncooperative, and hostile toward the medical profession or anyone who might question the authenticity of their illness. One notes in them a tendency to describe their pain poorly and to prefer, instead, to discuss the degree of their disability and their mistreatment at the hands of the medical profession. These features and a negative examination of the back should lead one to suspect a psychological factor. A few patients, usually frank malingerers, adopt the most bizarre attitudes, such as being unable to straighten up or walking with the trunk flexed at almost a right angle (camptocormia) (see Chap. 11).

The depressed and hypochondriacal patient represents a troublesome problem, and a common error is to minimize the importance of anxiety and depression or to ascribe them to worry over the illness and its social effects. The more common and minor back ailments, e.g., those due to osteoarthritis and postural ache, are enhanced and rendered intolerable by irritable moodiness and self-concern. Such patients are often subjected to surgical procedures which prove ineffective. The disability seems excessive for the degree of spinal malfunction, and misery and despair are the prevailing features of the syndrome. One of the more reliable diagnostic measures is the favorable response to drugs that alleviate the depression (see Chaps. 11 and 24).

PAIN IN THE NECK AND SHOULDER

This topic is discussed to some extent in Chap. 4, and further references are found in Chap. 7.

It is useful to distinguish here three major categories of painful disease—of the spine, brachial plexus (thoracic outlet), and shoulder. Although pain in these three regions of the body may overlap, the patient usually can indicate the site of origin. Pain arising from the cervical spine is felt in the neck and back of the head (though it may be projected to the shoulder and arm), is evoked or enhanced by certain movements or positions of the neck, and is accompanied by tenderness and limitation of motions of the neck. Similarly, pain resulting from abnormalities of the thoracic outlet is experienced in and around the shoulder in the supraclavicular region, or between the shoulders; is induced by the performance of certain tasks and by certain positions; and is associated with tenderness of structures above the clavicle. There may be a palpable abnormality above the clavicle (aneurysms of the subclavian artery, tumor, cervical rib). The combination of circulatory symptoms and signs referable to the lower part of the brachial plexus, manifested in the hand by obliteration of pulse when the patient holds a full breath with the head tilted back or turned (Adson's test), unilateral Raynaud's phenomenon, trophic changes in the fingers, and sensory loss over the ulnar side of the hand with or without interosseous atrophy complete the clinical picture. Roentgenograms showing a cervical rib, deformed thoracic outlet, or superior sulcus tumor of the lung (Pancoast's syndrome) corroborate disease in this location. Electromyography and conduction studies along the plexus from points stimulated above and below the clavicle, and studies of arterial and venous circulation (venograms, noninvasive Doppler techniques) are especially helpful in evaluating this problem.

Pain localized to the shoulder region, often worse at night, associated with tenderness and aggravated by abduction, internal rotation, and extension points toward a lesion of the tendinous structures about the shoulder. Most often these are in the form of a calcific tendonitis or bursitis usually affecting the supraspinatus tendon and the adjacent subdeltoid bursa; occasionally the lesion is more extensive and consists of a rupture of the rotator cuff, in which case the patient may have weakness on abduction and forward flexion. In some such patients there is an adhesive capsulitis, leading to profound limitation of motion, designated as a "frozen shoulder." Shoulder pain may radiate into the arm or hand, but the sensory, motor, and reflex changes which indicate disease of nerve roots, plexus, or peripheral nerves are absent.

Osteoarthritis of the cervical part of the spine may cause pains which radiate into the back of the head, shoulders, and arms on one or both sides of the thorax. Coincident involvement of nerve roots is manifested by paresthesias, sensory loss, weakness, or deep tendon reflex change. Should bony ridges form in the spinal canal (spondylosis) the spinal cord may be compressed (see Chap. 366). A myelogram or CT scan may reveal the degree of encroachment on the spinal canal (narrowing of the canal to less than 11 mm in the anteroposterior diameter) at the level at which the spinal cord is affected. The authors have experienced difficulty in distinguishing spondylosis with or without disk rupture and spinal cord compression from primary neurologic diseases (syringomyelia, amyotrophic lateral sclerosis, or tumor) with an unrelated osteoarthritis of the cervical portion of the spine, particularly at the fifth to sixth and sixth to seventh cervical vertebrae, where the disk spaces are often narrowed in the adult. A combination of nervous tension with osteoarthritis of the cervical part of the spine or a painful injury to ligaments and muscles after an accident in which the neck is forcibly extended and flexed (e.g., whiplash injury to spine) raises extremely vexatious clinical syndromes. If the pain is persistent and limited to the neck, the problem will sometimes prove to have been due to disruption of a disk, but it is often complicated by psychological factors.

RUPTURED CERVICAL DISKS One of the commonest causes of neck, shoulder, and arm pain is disk herniation in the lower cervical region. As with rupture of the lumbar disks, the complete syndrome includes the disorder of spinal function and evidence of neural involvement. It may develop after trauma either major or minor (sudden hyperextension of the neck, diving, forceful manipulations, etc.). Virtually every patient exhibits an abnormality in range of motion of the neck (limitation and pain). Hyperextension is the movement that most consistently aggravates the pain, although one occasionally sees patients whose principal limitation is in flexion. With laterally situated disk lesions between the fifth and sixth cervical vertebrae, the symptoms and signs are referred to the sixth cervical roots. The full syndrome is characterized by pain felt at the trapezius ridge, tip of the shoulder, anterior upper part of the arm, radial forearm, and often in the thumb; paresthesias and sensory impairment or hypersensitivity in the same regions; tenderness in the area above the spine of the scapula and in the supraclavicular and biceps regions; weakness in flexion of the forearm; diminished to absent biceps and supinator reflexes (triceps retained or exaggerated). When the protruded disk lies between the sixth and seventh cervical vertebrae, the seventh cervical root is involved. Under these circumstances, in the patient with the complete syndrome, the pain is in the region of the shoulder blade, pectoral region and medial axilla, posterolateral upper arm, elbow and dorsal forearm, index and middle fingers, or all the fingers; tenderness is most pronounced over the medial aspect of the shoulder blade opposite the third to fourth thoracic spinous processes, in the supraclavicular area and triceps region; paresthesias and sensory loss are most pronounced in the second and third fingers or tips of all the fingers; weakness is seen in extension of the forearm, in the extension of the wrist, and in the hand grip; the triceps reflex is diminished to absent, and the biceps and supinator reflexes are preserved. Either of these syndromes may be incomplete in that only one of several of the typical findings (e.g., pain) is present. Usually the patient states that cough, sneeze, and downward pressure on the head in the hyperextension position exacerbate pain and traction (even manual) tends to relieve it.

Unlike lumbar disks, the cervical ones, if large and centrally situated, may result in compression of the spinal cord (central disk, all the cord; paracentral disk, part of the cord). The central disk is often nearly painless, and the cord syndrome may simulate a degenerative disease (amyotrophic lateral sclerosis, combined system disease). A common error is to fail to think of a ruptured disk in the cervical region in patients with obscure symptoms in the legs. The diagnosis of ruptured cervical disk should be confirmed by the same laboratory procedures that were mentioned under "Spondylosis," above.

OTHER CONDITIONS Metastases to the cervical spine are fortunately less common than to other parts of the vertebral column. They are frequently painful and the cause of disordered root function. Compression fractures or extension of the tumor posteriorly may lead to rapid development of quadriplegia.

Shoulder injuries (rotator cuff), subacromial or subdeltoid bursitis, the frozen shoulder (periarthritis or capsulitis), tendonitis, and arthritis may develop in patients who are otherwise well, but these conditions are also frequent in hemiplegics or in individuals suffering from coronary heart disease. The pain is often severe and extends toward the neck and down the arm into the hand. The dorsum of the latter may tingle without other signs of nerve involvement. Vasomotor changes also may occur in the hand (shoulder-hand syndrome), and after a time, osteoporosis and atrophy of cutaneous and subcutaneous structures occur (Sudeck's atrophy or Sudeck-Leriche syndrome). These conditions fall more within the province of orthopaedics than of medicine and are not discussed here in detail. The physician, however, must know that they can often be prevented by proper exercises (Chap. 269).

The *carpal tunnel syndrome,* with paresthesias and numbness in palmar distribution of the median nerve and aching pain which extends up into the forearm, may be mistaken for disease of the shoulder or neck. Similarly, other less common forms of nerve entrapment may involve the ulnar, radial, or median nerves and lead to a mistaken diagnosis of brachial plexus lesion or cervical syndrome. Electromyography and conduction studies are especially helpful in such conditions (Chap. 368).

MANAGEMENT OF BACK PAIN

Without doubt the preventive aspects of back pain are important. There would be far fewer back problems if adults kept their trunk muscles in optimal condition by regular exercise such as swimming, bicycle riding, walking briskly, running, or calisthenic programs. Morning is the ideal time since the back of the older adult tends to stiffen during the night because of inactivity. This happens regardless of whether a bed board or a stiff mattress is used. Sleeping with back hyperextended and sitting for long times in an overstuffed chair or a badly designed auto seat are particularly risky. It is estimated that pressures between disks are increased 200 percent by changing from a recumbent to a standing position and by 400 percent by sitting slumped in an easy chair. Correct sitting posture lessens this. Long trips in a car or plane without change in position put maximal strain on disk and ligamentous structures in the spine. Lifting from a position of flexed trunk, as in removing a suitcase from the trunk of a car, is dangerous (always lift with the object close to the body). Sudden strenuous activity without conditioning and warm-up also is likely to cause trouble to disks and their ligamentous envelopes (the commonest sources of back pain); certain families seem disposed.

The diagrams in Figs. 6-2 to 6-6 are useful guides in strengthening trunk muscles.

Muscular and ligamentous strains and minor disk prolapses are usually self-limited, responding to simple measures in a relatively short period of time. The basic principle of therapy is rest in a recumbent position for several days to weeks. When weight bearing is resumed, a light lumbosacral support is usually helpful in continuing the immobilization until the patient is restored to full health. Physical measures such as heat, cold, diathermy, or massage are of limited value; of considerably greater importance are active exercises to both reduce the spasm and improve muscle tone. Analgesic medication should be given liberally during the first few days: codeine, 30 mg, and aspirin, 0.6 g, or pentazocine (Talwin), 50 mg, propoxyphene (Darvon), 65 mg, or meperidine (Demerol), 50 mg. Muscle relaxants are often a valuable adjunct, particularly in that such drugs as Valium, 8 to 40 mg in divided doses, and carisoprodol (Soma), 350 mg, twice daily, make bed rest more tolerable. If an inflammatory component is suspected, indomethacin, 75 mg per day (in divided doses), or ibuprofen (Motrin), 400 mg 3 or 4 times daily, may be helpful.

In the treatment of an acute or chronic rupture of a lumbar or cervical disk, complete bed rest is essential, and strong analgesic medication may be required. Traction is of little value in lumbar disk disease, and it is best to permit the patient to find the most comfortable position. Cervical traction with a halter may be of considerable benefit to patients with cervical disk syndrome. It can be administered with the patient in recumbency, or after sufficient improvement to allow ambulation, can be performed intermittently in the erect position using special equipment. During the recumbent phase of treatment of lumbar disk disease, exercises to reduce spasm, muscle relaxants, and anti-inflammatory agents as described above may be of considerable value. After 2 to 3 weeks in bed, the patient can be allowed to slowly resume activities, usually with the protection of a brace or light spinal support. Exercise programs designed to increase the strength of the abdominal and gluteal muscles are helpful at this point. The patient may suffer some minor recurrence of the pain but be able to carry on his or her usual activities, and eventually most individuals will recover. If the pain and neurologic findings do not disappear on prolonged, conservative management, or if the patient suffers frequently recurring acute episodes, surgical management may

FIGURE 6-2
A. With knees bent, feet flat on floor, and hands clasped behind head, pinch buttocks together, pull in abdomen, and flatten back against floor. At first, hold position for a count of 5, relax for 5, then gradually increase to counts of 20. B. Next do this same exercise with legs extended and arms raised straight overhead. (From U.S. News & World Report. Copyright 1975, U.S. News & World Report).

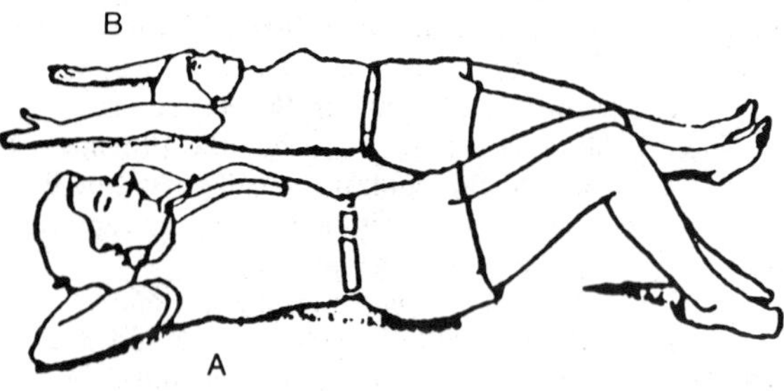

FIGURE 6-3
A. Keeping shoulders flat on floor, draw knees toward chest, clasp hands around knees, and pull knees tightly against chest. B. Next bring forehead up to knees. (From U.S. News & World Report. Copyright 1975, U.S. News & World Report.)

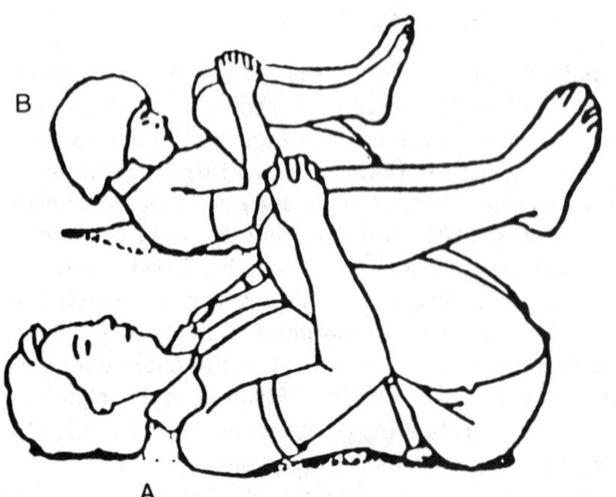

FIGURE 6-4
A. With knees bent, keep feet flat on floor and held or hooked under a heavy piece of furniture to provide leverage. B. Cross arms on chest, raise head and shoulders, and curl up to a sitting position. Keep back round and pull with abdominal muscles. Lower self slowly. (From U.S. News & World Report. Copyright 1975, U.S. News & World Report.)

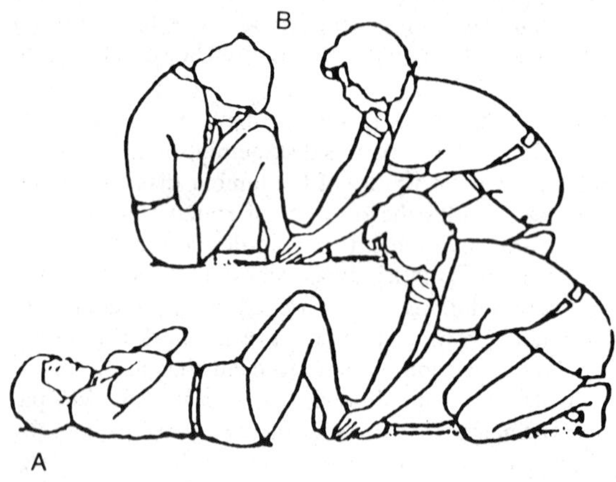

FIGURE 6-5
A. Bend knees, keeping feet flat on floor and arms straight forward. Raise up and touch head to knees. B. Lower self, then pull knees up tightly against chest and bring forehead up to knees. (From U.S. News & World Report. Copyright 1975, U.S. News & World Report.)

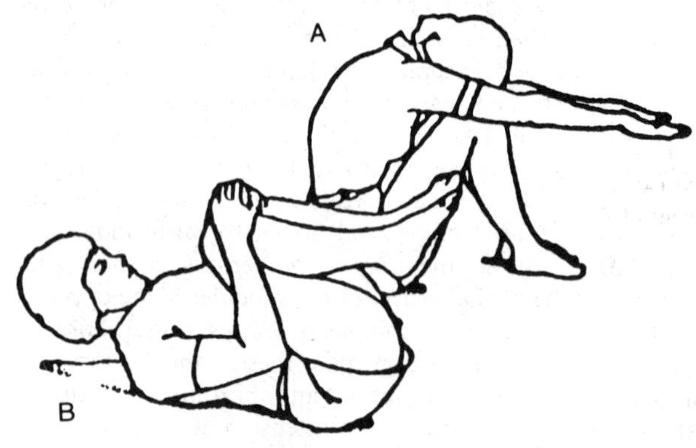

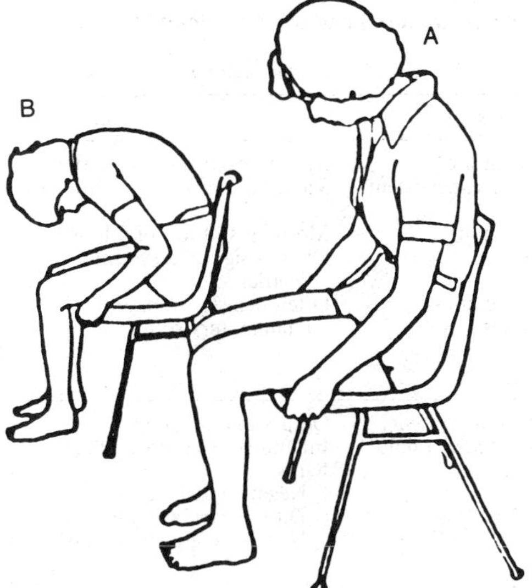

FIGURE 6-6
A. Place hands at edge of chair. B. Bend forward to bring head to knees, pulling in abdomen as you curl forward. Keep weight well back on hips. Release abdominal muscles slowly as you come up. (From U.S. News & World Report. Copyright 1975, U.S. News & World Report.)

be indicated. This should always be preceded by a myelogram or a computerized reconstructed body scan to localize the lesion (and rule out the presence of intra- or extradural tumors). The surgical procedure most often indicated is a hemilaminectomy with excision of the disk involved. Arthrodesis of the involved segments is indicated only in cases in which there is extraordinary instability usually related to an anatomic abnormality (such as spondylolysis) or in the cervical region when an extensive laminectomy has rendered the spine unstable. The results of conservative management of so-called sciatica cases in the controlled study of Coxhead et al. was approximately 80 percent improved at the end of 4 weeks, regardless of whether traction, exercises, manipulation, or corset, or some combination thereof, was used.

Spondylosis of the cervical part of the spine, if painful, is helped by bed rest and traction; if signs of spinal cord involvement are present, a collar to limit movement may halt the progression and even lead to improvement. Decompressive laminectomy or anterior fusion is reserved for severe instances of the disease with advancing neurologic symptoms. The shoulder-hand syndrome may benefit from stellate ganglion blocks or ganglionectomy, but the basic treatment is physiotherapy, with or without prednisone, and surgical procedures are used only as measures of last resort.

REFERENCES

Armstrong JR: *Lumbar Disc Lesions,* 3d ed. Baltimore, Williams & Wilkins, 1965

Brady LP et al: An evaluation of the electromyogram in the diagnosis of lumbar disk lesion. J Bone Joint Surg 51A:539, 1969

Coxhead CE et al: Multicenter trial of physiotherapy in the management of sciatic symptoms. Lancet 1:1065, 1981

Edeiken J, Pitt MJ: The radiologic diagnoses of disk disease. Orthop Clin North Am 2:405, 1971

Editorial: Pelvic pain, Lancet 2:617, 1981

Friedenberg AB, Miller WT: Degenerative disk disease of the cervical spine. J Bone Joint Surg 45A:1171, 1963

Golub B et al: Cervical and lumbar disk disease: A review. Bull Rheum Dis 21:635, 1971

Grabias SL, Mankin HJ: Pain in lower back. Bull Rheum Dis 30:1040, 1980

Murphy RW: Nerve roots and spinal nerves in degenerative disk disease. Clin Orthop 129:46, 1977

Naylor A: The changes in the human intervertebral disk in degeneration and nuclear prolapse. Orthop Clin North Am 2:343, 1971

Rothman RC, Simeone F: *Lumbar Disc Disease.* Philadelphia, Saunders, 1975, pp 443–458

Williams AL et al: Computed tomography in the diagnosis of herniated nucleus pulposus. Radiology 135:95, 1980

Wilson ES, Brill RF: Spinal stenosis: The narrow lumbar canal syndrome. Clin Orthop 122:244, 1977

7
PAIN IN THE EXTREMITIES

RONALD ANDERSON
NATHAN P. COUCH

There are inherent functional and anatomic differences between the upper and lower extremities. Because of this, the two sets of extremities differ not only in their pattern of symptoms but also in the pathological states which they are prone to develop. The basic distinctions to consider are as follows:

1 The essential functions are locomotion in the lower extremity and manipulation in the upper extremity.
2 The lower extremity is more subject to traumatic injury due to its weight-bearing function.
3 The effects of gravity upon the circulatory system are accentuated in the lower extremity.
4 The increased muscle mass with its concomitant increased oxygen requirements during work make the lower extremity more sensitive to ischemia.
5 Lower extremity function is dependent upon bilateral integrated activity. An isolated lesion, therefore, usually is associated with a gait disturbance.
6 The upper extremity is not dependent upon bilaterality and can better adapt to an isolated dysfunction of one of its parts.

The basic approach to extremity pain initially concerns the diagnosis of the organ system involved and an understanding of its anatomy and physiology. Because these structures are readily accessible by physical examination, identification of the character of the lesion can usually be made by history and physical examination alone.

ARTICULAR PAIN Joints consist of cartilage covering the articular surface of bone, an encompassing synovial membrane, and, peripherally, the periarticular supporting structures consisting of ligaments, tendons, and muscles. Bursae and tendon sheaths, which histologically resemble synovial membrane, often provide the interface upon which these supporting structures move. Articular cartilage is an elastic substance with a low coefficient of friction. Cartilage loss is an irreversible process which is due either to mechanical stress as in degenerative joint disease or to erosive synovitis in conditions such as rheumatoid arthritis. Synovitis, if arrested prior to the development of cartilage loss, is potentially reversible. The cause of articular pain involves either reversible synovitis, irreversible structural damage, or a mixture of the two. The initial step in approaching articular pain is to determine whether the problem is primarily structural or consists primarily of synovitis.

The pain associated with cartilage loss is due to the friction created by two imperfect surfaces grinding against each other. For this reason structural pain is usually experienced only with activity and the patient is free of pain at rest. Although physical stress increases joint pain in either condition, synovitis is invariably associated with symptoms at rest and, in acute inflammatory forms of arthritis such as gout or septic arthritis, pain sufficient to awaken the patient at night is common.

Because the process or cartilage wear is gradual and irreversible, the symptoms of structural disorders are slowly progressive and the rate of deterioration is measured in terms of years. In synovitis the sudden, rapid development of joint pain is common and, because of the inherent variability of inflammatory activity, flare-ups alternate with periods of quiescence. Because synovitis plays a minimal role in a purely structural condition such as osteoarthritis, anti-inflammatory therapy does little to alter its symptoms. However, these medications often significantly reduce the symptoms of synovitis. Moreover, while mechanical damage to a joint is a localized process, many of the conditions which produce synovitis are systemic disorders and the patient, in addition to joint pain, has generalized symptoms such as malaise and fatigue.

Most patients with systemic rheumatic diseases have an accentuation of their symptoms, accompanied by clear-cut changes in the physical examination, after a period of sleep. The duration of morning stiffness is in the range of 2 to 4 h, in contradistinction to "gelling," a 5- to 15-min accentuation of stiffness associated with other articular disorders.

Degenerative joint disease, in the absence of a unique repetitive trauma or injury, occurs only in those joints subjected to mechanical stress. These consist of the metacarpal-carpal joint of the thumb, hip, and knees and the metatarsal-phalangeal joint of the great toe. The appearance of a deformity in a non-weight-bearing joint such as the elbow or a metacarpal-phalangeal joint implies synovitis rather than structural abnormality.

A definitive diagnosis of synovitis can be made by demonstrating leukocytosis in the synovial fluid (white blood cell count > 2000) or by the presence of a swollen, inflamed joint. Joints such as the hips or spinal articulations are so deep that visual or palpable findings of inflammation are obscured. The shoulder and ankle are incorporated into their supporting structures so that the distinction between periarticular and articular disease is often difficult. In structural conditions, joint effusions are rare, the joint is seldom warm or tense, and synovial fluid leukocytosis does not occur.

The extent of cartilage loss can only be estimated on radiography by the degree of approximation of the opposing articular surfaces. In synovial inflammation, joint films tend to show no abnormalities in the early preerosive phase. While some cartilaginous erosion may occur in long-standing synovitis, new bone formation, represented by osteophytes, is not seen in persistent erosive synovitis, whereas osteophytes are common when cartilage loss results from mechanical wear and tear. Moreover, because mechanical stress varies in different regions of the cartilage surface, localized cartilage loss occurs in degenerative joint disease, as opposed to synovitis where diffuse cartilage loss is the rule. By the time that a structural lesion has progressed far enough to cause symptoms, radiographic evidence of cartilage loss is almost always present.

The differentiation between structural lesions due to mechanical factors and synovitis governs the management of the patient. The former is an irreversible process alterable only by surgical reconstruction. Synovitis, on the other hand, is potentially reversible and can often be altered by medical therapy.

TABLE 7-1
Differences between structural and synovitic joint lesions

Structural lesions	*Synovitic lesions*
SUBJECTIVE FEATURES	
Symptoms only with use	Symptoms at rest and with use
Gradually progressive, persistent course	Variable course, often with flare-up
"Gelling" phenomenon	Morning stiffness of 2 h or more
Localized process	Often a sign of a systemic disorder
Minimal response to anti-inflammatory drugs	Often benefits from anti-inflammatory drugs
OBJECTIVE FEATURES	
Occurs in weight-bearing joints	Occurs in any joint
Noninflammatory synovial fluid	Inflammatory synovial fluid
X-ray	X-ray
Usually abnormal	Negative early in course
Localized cartilage loss	Diffuse cartilage loss
Osteophytes seen	New bone growth absent
MANAGEMENT	
Surgical	Medical

The differences between these two conditions are summarized in Table 7-1.

PERIARTICULAR PAIN Symptoms referable to periarticular tissues arise from either an injury or inflammation of the periarticular supporting structures—the joint capsule, tendons, ligaments, and bursae. The differentiation from articular pain is predicated on finding localized tenderness and on reproducing the pain by maneuvers designed to stress the structure but not the joint. For example, the symptoms of *tennis elbow* are reproduced by dorsiflexion of the wrist, against resistance, with the elbow immobilized. The diagnosis can be confirmed by alleviating the pain with an injection of lidocaine (Xylocaine) into the structure felt to be responsible for the symptoms. Periarticular pain is frequently nocturnal as pressure is applied to the injured structure during sleep. The most common sites involved are the subdeltoid, trochanteric, and anserine bursae, and the bicipital and de Quervain's tendons. Contracture of the joint capsule as a cause of pain most frequently occurs in the shoulder following an attack of bursitis or tendonitis which leads to immobilization and secondary contracture of the shoulder capsule. The resulting "frozen shoulder syndrome" is painful when the joint capsule is stretched to its full range of motion. This most commonly occurs at night when the shoulder, unconsciously immobilized during the day, is stressed by its contact with the pillow during sleep. Arthrography may be employed to document the decreased volume of the capsule. Therapy for this condition requires full-range-of-motion exercises.

MUSCLE PAIN Myalgias occur after severe exertion, are limited in duration, and seldom come to the attention of a physician. They are also seen in metabolic abnormalities such as phosphorylase deficiency, toxic myopathies due to alcohol or "brown heroin," tetanus, and severe electrolyte disturbances. Although sometimes a component of polymyositis, muscle pain is seldom observed in this condition unless there is marked inflammation accompanied by muscle weakness, elevation of muscle enzymes, and, frequently, palpable tender edema of the muscles. A major component of the pain of chronic arterial insufficiency arises from muscle ischemia. Polymyalgia rheumatica (see Chap. 69) presents in an abrupt fashion with proximal myalgias which increase with exercise. The syndrome of masseter claudication is virtually specific for this condition. The pattern of proximal myalgias in the absence of articular abnormalities tends to distinguish polymyalgia from arterial insufficiency or arthritis.

A common clinical problem is presented by the "achey" patient with a normal physical examination. The causes of this clinical picture run the gamut from metastatic carcinoma to malingering. The term *fibrositis* (see Chap. 353) is applied to many of these patients who seem to react to stress and other noxious stimuli with musculoskeletal symptoms. Because of the high rate of false-negative and false-positive tests in the laboratory evaluation of rheumatic diseases, the distinction between the "walking wounded" and the "worried well" is best made by history and physical examination. Three features seem to be diagnostic of "benign aches and pains":

1 *An intermittent pattern of symptoms with asymptomatic intervals.* The occurrence of an asymptomatic interval in the recent past permits exclusion of a structural lesion of the joint and also places into perspective radiographic findings in the bones which obviously don't fluctuate with the symptoms.
2 *Lack of specific functional loss.* Any condition which alters the anatomy of a joint will be associated with a highly specific functional defect. For example, patients with hip disease cannot get out of bathtubs. Patients with the fibrositis syndrome either do not lose specific function or describe their complaints in vague terms such as "I've slowed down." When those presenting with vague complaints are questioned carefully, it is found that they have not lost a specific function.
3 *Negative physical examination.* This finding confirms that none of the symptoms which have occurred in the past have brought about any anatomic change. Patients who are asymptomatic on the day of the examination should be reexamined at the time they have symptoms to exclude an intermittent synovitis. Patients with persistent complaints should be reexamined after an appropriate time interval to determine whether their symptoms have brought about any alteration in the physical examination or have resulted in measurable functional loss.

BONE PAIN The cardinal features of bone pain are localized tenderness on palpation of the bone and accentuation with weight bearing. The etiologies include fractures, tumors, osteomyelitis and periostitis, and Paget's disease. All these conditions have characteristic radiographic abnormalities. In fact, almost any condition causing bone pain will be accompanied by an abnormal x-ray. Historical features, such as the abrupt onset associated with trauma characteristic of fractures or a progressive course in tumors and infections, are helpful in the diagnosis.

THE PAIN OF VASCULAR DISEASE (Table 7-2) Pain is the most common symptom of vascular disease in the extremities. In taking the history, attention should be given to the rapidity of onset, duration, progression, distribution, association with exercise, dependency, weight bearing, use of tobacco, and the presence of generalized systemic disease, such as heart disease or diabetes mellitus.

Chronic extremity pain which is not accompanied by skin ulceration, such as occurs in chronic arterial occlusive disease or lumbosacral nerve root compression, may be defined by determining its association with exercise. Typically, claudication (from the Latin *claudicare*, "to limp"), a symptom characteristic of chronic arteriosclerosis obliterans in the leg, is produced by walking or climbing and its discomfort may be described in a variety of ways as "pain," "cramping," "fatigue," "tiredness," or "weakness." (Nocturnal leg cramps must be distin-

TABLE 7-2
Primary vascular disorders producing pain

	Historical setting predominant			*Character of pain*				
Diagnosis	*Age group*	*Sex*	*Pain-inciting activity*	*Location*	*Rate of onset*	*Duration*	*Key physical findings*	*Laboratory findings*
Acute major arterial:								
Embolism	> 45	M>F	Rest or exercise	Distal extremity	S	H–D	Pallor, cool or cold hand or foot, absent pulses	ECG abnormal, low ankle or wrist pressure (by Doppler flowmeter)
Thrombosis	> 45	M>F	Rest or exercise	Distal extremity	S	H–D	Same	Low ankle or wrist pressure (by Doppler flowmeter)
Chronic arterial occlusion	> 45	M>F	Exercise	Distal extremity	G	W–M–Y	Pallor, atrophy, skin ulcer in severe cases	Same as for arterial thrombosis
Acute deep venous thrombosis	All ages	M=F	Dependency	Usually calf; thigh; occlusion arm	G S	H–D	None in 50% of cases, calf or ankle swelling, tenderness	Phlebogram positive
Chronic postphlebitic syndrome	> 35	M=F	Dependency	Leg, arm	G	Y	Swelling, stasis, pigmentation, ulcer	Not helpful
Acute superficial thrombophlebitis	None	M=F	Dependency	Leg, arm	S–G	H–D	Firm, red, tender venous cord	Not helpful (except in blood diseases)
Varicose veins	Affects all ages equally	F	Prolonged dependency	Thighs, calves	S	Y	Varicosities, swelling	Not useful
AV fistula	Affects all ages equally	M=F	Rest	Variable	S	H	Thrill, bruit, ↑pulse pressure	Proved by arteriogram

NOTE: *For rate of onset and duration, S = sudden, G = gradual, H = hours, D = days, W = weeks, M = months, Y = years.*

guished from those of claudication because they are not the product of vascular disease.) Claudication of the calf can occur with any level of arterial occlusion from the abdominal aorta to the tibial arteries. In patients who can walk on a flat surface for more than 50 yards, the more advanced symptoms of rest pain or necrosis are rare. As the required muscle energy expenditure increases, as in climbing stairs or carrying luggage, exercise tolerance decreases. A more accurate evaluation of exercise tolerance or disability may be gained by asking the question, "Does your leg pain prevent you from doing things you have to do?" Other useful information can be gained by walking or climbing stairs with the patient. If severe ischemia is present, the patient will describe rest pain, numbness, or paresthesias in the foot, most frequently in the toes. This is most likely to occur when lying down or elevating the leg, i.e., in circumstances wherein the marginal arterial flow is not augmented by gravity. The patient will describe sleeping in a sitting position or with the affected leg dependent. These symptoms indicate that peripheral nerve injury has begun, because even the arterial flow at rest is inadequate. This is referred to as a *pregangrenous* state. If the flow deficiency is not corrected, skin necrosis, sometimes resulting from very minor trauma, will begin. The symptoms of *acute arterial embolism or thrombosis* are qualitatively similar, but accelerated, when compared with the symptoms of chronic arterial occlusion. The patient will usually complain of sudden onset of pain, coldness, and numbness in the part, symptoms that may wane prior to seeing the physician. The severity of such symptoms is directly related to the size of the blocked artery, the degree of cross-sectional occlusion, the length of the clot, and the adequacy of the collaterals. The more severe the occlusion, the worse the symptoms, and the shorter the interval from onset to the visit with a physician. Patients with this complaint may have as the source of embolism an endocardium injured by myocardial infarction, a left ventricular aneurysm, or a fibrillating left atrium. Less common sources for emboli small enough to lodge in 1- or 2-mm arteries include valvular vegetations, such as those occurring in subacute bacterial endocarditis, and atheromas. Although the symptoms of arterial embolism sometimes relent after a few hours, such improvement is more frequent in association with arterial thrombosis because it occurs at the site of a stenotic arterial plaque, a situation that will have already promoted development of arterial collaterals.

Traumatic interruption of arterial flow should always be suspected in severely injured extremities, especially in fractures or dislocations at the shoulder, elbow, wrist, knee, and ankle. In the acute stage the complaint of pain may be too diffuse to raise suspicion of ischemic injury to the distal limb. Physical examination often holds the key to diagnosis. Venous injury with laceration or thrombosis can often accompany arterial injury, and pain owing to venous malfunction may be impossible to distinguish from that due to the arterial lesion or the trauma.

Regardless of the type of arterial occlusion, the physical findings of greatest importance include the pulse, the heart rate and rhythm, presence and width of the abdominal aortic pulse, and presence of femoral arterial bruits. In traumatized extremities, large hematomas, local bruits or thrills, and unstable fractures or dislocations are common. The most important indicator of arterial occlusive disease is the absence of a palpable pulse below the obstruction, while the level of temperature demarcation (which can be in two gradations), skin color changes, atrophy, necrosis, and hyperesthesia add important information to determining the severity of ischemia and provide a good estimate of the urgency with which the disorder should be corrected. (The Doppler ultrasonic flowmeter is a most valuable device in determining specific arterial patency and pressure.) Chronic occlusions (treated by bypass grafts or endarterectomy) rarely require urgent correction, while acute occlusions nearly always demand acute relief, either by thromboembolectomy (often feasible with local anesthesia) or arterial repair.

Venous disease The pain of venous thrombosis is rarely severe but may, like arterial occlusion, occur acutely. The degree of thrombosis may vary from a few centimeters of saphenous or saphenous branch vein to the entire iliofemoral popliteal system. In the lesser degrees of either superficial or deep phlebitis, swelling is usually absent. But the more extensive the clot, especially where the proximal vein is affected, the greater the likelihood of swelling. In the most extreme cases of iliofemoral phlebothrombosis, in which the venous outflow is critically compromised, the entire leg is swollen, cyanotic, and painful and the foot pulses may be absent. Elevation of the part almost always relieves the pain of venous thrombosis, in contrast to arterial occlusion. If the pain is not relieved by elevation, an arterial occlusion should be suspected.

With the conservative measures of continuous intravenous heparin and elevation, the extremity pain usually subsides in 2 to 4 days and both the pain and swelling are mitigated for a longer period by elastic support. However, postphlebitic limbs are subject to late recurrences of moderate pain and swelling which are not usually due to acute phlebitis but to venous distension and soft-tissue edema. Postphlebitic symptoms are most likely to occur when the patient has not been using elastic supports. In the most severe cases of postphlebitic syndrome, there is pigmentation of the lower leg and medial or lateral, painful ankle ulcers.

Most varicose veins do not cause severe pain, but the small fraction of patients who suffer discomfort describe a low-grade aching, burning, heaviness, cramping, or itching, especially after prolonged dependency. Relief after elevation or after use of elastic supports is diagnostically helpful. The degree of pain does not correlate with the size of the varicosity.

Occasionally varicose veins may be the site of superficial thrombophlebitis, which typically appears as a tender, firm, easily defined rubbery cord with a red blush. This form of thrombophlebitis may extend either proximally or distally, but usually begins to subside in less than 5 days.

The least common form of extremity thrombosis involves the subclavian-axillo-brachial vein, so-called effort thrombosis. This usually has a sudden onset which occurs in the wake of unusually vigorous, awkward arm activity. The patient complains of pain, heaviness, and even weakness of the arm and both swelling and cyanosis are apparent. Heparin, elevation, and, in certain cases, fibrinolysis bring prompt relief.

Pain caused by small-vessel insufficiency (Table 7-3) The pain of *vasculitis* is encountered infrequently (see Chap. 69). In its early stages, it is most likely to single out one or a few finger- or toe tips or some other focal area of the extremity. The historical setting commonly includes a prior diagnosis of rheumatic disease, i.e., rheumatoid arthritis, lupus erythematosus, scleroderma, or polyarteritis nodosa, or the kind of angiitis seen in especially sensitive smokers, sometimes referred to as thromboangiitis obliterans (Buerger's disease). The initial site of focal pain and pallor or cyanosis may evolve to ulceration of the digital tip, in the presence of good wrist or pedal pulses. When such complaints occur in patients with no known rheumatic disease, the careful history should include questions about joint pain or swelling, fever, rashes, smoking, pleuritic pain, symptoms of phlebothrombosis, or dysphagia.

In contrast to vasculitis, but sometimes confused with it, *Raynaud's disease* does not usually entail loss of digital skin

TABLE 7-3
Disorders of small-vessel insufficiency

	Historical setting predominant			Character of pain				
Diagnosis	*Age group*	*Sex*	*Pain-inciting activity*	*Location*	*Rate of onset*	*Duration*	*Key physical findings*	*Laboratory findings*
Vasospastic disorders (e.g., Raynaud's disease)	< 50	F	Cold, anxiety	Hands, feet	S	H	Pallor, cold, cyanosis	Normal digital arteries in Raynaud's disease; absent D.A.'s in other types
Sympathetic dystrophy, causalgia	< 50	M=F	Cold, mechanical stimulus	Variable	S	Y	Clamminess, swelling, tenderness, cyanosis	Not helpful
Erythromelalgia	< 60	M=F	Walking, warmth or cold	Legs and feet	S	M–H	Swelling; heat (during attack)	Occasional polycythemia
Frostbite, immersion injury	May affect all ages	M=F	Cold	Hands and feet	S	D–W	Pallor, cold (early); cyanosis, occasional gangrene (late)	Not useful
Pernio	< 60	F	Cold	Legs and feet	S	H–D	Cyanosis, swelling, occasional blebs	Not useful

NOTE: *See Table 7-2 for abbreviations.*

but can nevertheless result in severe pain. Typically this follows exposure to cold and is accompanied first by numbness and pallor of the digits, then cyanosis, and finally severe reactive hyperemia when the pain is particularly severe. The wrist and pedal pulses remain normal. Raynaud's disease is much more common in females, does not result in permanent disability, and usually "burns out" after several years. Alternatively, these symptoms may be the first signs of a systemic rheumatic disease.

Pernio (*chilblains*) is a vasospastic disorder that may occur both acutely and chronically and chiefly affects children and women whose feet and legs have been exposed to excessive cold and dampness. The result is a patchy vasoconstriction of the skin, cyanosis, slight edema, blistering, and intense itching. The acute symptoms may persist for several days. The chronic form may occur if exposure to cold is recurrent leading to red, hemorrhagic, ulcerated skin lesions.

Other conditions related to vasoconstriction include frostbite (see Chap. 8) (usually resulting from freezing of soft tissue) and trench or immersion foot (resulting from severe cooling without freezing). The history almost always makes the diagnosis obvious, but because the resulting injury includes similar findings for both conditions it is not always possible, or even useful, to distinguish the freezing injury from the immersion injury. Both conditions begin with a vasospastic phase (cold, pale, or cyanotic skin), continue with an edematous phase followed by a hyperemic phase (red, hot blistered skin), and end, in the more severe injuries, with a necrotic stage. It is in the latter stage, which may last 2 or 3 weeks, that the patient is most likely to see a physician.

TABLE 7-4
Nonvascular diseases that mimic vascular disease

	Historical setting predominant			Character of pain				
Diagnosis	*Age group*	*Sex*	*Pain-inciting activity*	*Location*	*Rate of onset*	*Duration*	*Key physical findings*	*Laboratory findings*
Carpal tunnel syndrome	> 40	F> M	Motion, flexion of wrist	Wrist, hand	G	D–M	Occasionally thenar atrophy	Delayed nerve conduction
Herniated lumbar nucleus pulposus	> 20	M=F	Lumbar flexion, standing	Lumbo-sacral, leg	S or G	H–D–M	Lumbar spasm, ↓muscle power, ↓reflexes, ↓sensation	Protrusion of disk (myelogram), narrow disk space, spondylolisthesis
Cervical radiculitis	> 30	M=F	Neck motion	Neck, shoulder, arm	S or G	H–D–M	Limited neck motion	Narrow disk spaces, spurring of vertebral bodies
Nocturnal muscle cramps	> 30	F	Sleeping	Calves, occasionally thighs	S	M	Tight muscle "knot"	Not useful
Thoracic outlet syndromes	None	M=F	Variable shoulder motion	Compressed nerve root distribution	S	M–Y	Supraclavicular bruit (occasional)	Cervical rib, compression of subclavian artery in arteriogram

NOTE: *See Table 7-2 for abbreviations.*

OTHER CAUSES OF EXTREMITY PAIN (Table 7-4) *Bacterial infections* may be a cause of pain in the extremities and most often result from invasion at wound sites, such as areas of interdigital fungus infection ("athlete's foot"), or areas of ischemic or postphlebitic ulceration. The diffuse tenderness, heat, and erythema found on examination make the diagnosis obvious. If swelling is also present, and circumferential, the erroneous diagnosis of thrombophlebitis may be made. Patients who are otherwise healthy will usually have fever, tachycardia, and malaise, but those who are immunosuppressed or aged may be unable to respond with the usual manifestations of inflammation.

Erythema nodosum (see Chap. 50), wherein subcutaneous red tender nodules appear along with fever and arthralgia, may also mimic infection. It is occasionally associated with chronic inflammatory conditions, such as tuberculosis, coccidioidomycosis, ulcerative colitis, and sarcoidosis.

Pain from *thermal injury* is present in first- and second-degree burns, but not in those which are third-degree or deeper. The diagnosis is generally obvious because the history is available.

Neuropathic pain is discussed in Chap. 2. In addition to sensory and motor abnormalities its characteristic feature is constancy, because it is not altered by motion or weight bearing. Most patients describe neuropathic pain as being worse at night, and the most plausible explanation for this is that the stimuli which normally distract the patient during the waking hours are eliminated so that the pain is perceived more clearly.

Referred pain is simply pain appearing in a site other than its real origin. In the extremities, it is usually the result of nerve root or peripheral nerve stimulation by compression or other local trauma. It is discussed in Chap. 2. The commonest causes of referred pain include cervical osteoarthritis with radiculopathy, herpes zoster, herniated lumbosacral nucleus pulposus, and the thoracic outlet syndromes. Of the lesions that are not primarily neurologic, psoas muscle spasm, due to an adjacent infection such as appendicitis or lymphadenitis (where pain sometimes appears to originate in the hip joint), and osteoarthritis of the hip (in which pain may be referred to the knee) are common.

REFERENCES

Juergens JL et al (eds): *Peripheral Vascular Diseases,* 5th ed. Philadelphia, Saunders, 1980

Kelley WN et al: *Textbook of Rheumatology.* Philadelphia, Saunders, 1981

section 2 | Alterations in body temperature

8 DISTURBANCES OF HEAT REGULATION

ROBERT G. PETERSDORF

CONTROL OF BODY TEMPERATURE In health, the body temperature of human beings is maintained within a narrow range despite extremes in environmental conditions and physical activity. This is also true for most birds and mammals, and such animals are termed *homeothermic,* or warm-blooded. An almost invariable accompaniment of systemic illness is a disturbance in temperature regulation, usually an abnormal elevation, or *fever.* In fact, fever is such a sensitive and reliable indicator of the presence of disease that thermometry is probably the commonest clinical procedure in use. Even in the absence of a frank febrile response, interference with heat regulation by disease is evident. This may take the form of flushing, pallor, sweating, shivering, and abnormal sensations of cold or warmth, or it may consist of erratic fluctuations of body temperature within normal limits when a patient is at bed rest.

Heat production The major source of basal heat production is through thyroid thermogenesis and the action of adenosine triphosphatase (ATPase) on the sodium pump of all membranes. The muscles are most important in promoting increased heat production through increased shivering. Heat production by muscle is of particular importance because the quantity can be varied according to the need. In most circumstances this variation consists of small increases and decreases in the number of nerve impulses to the muscles, causing inapparent tensing or relaxing. When, however, there is a strong stimulus for heat production, muscle activity may increase to the point of shivering, or even to a generalized rigor.

Heat loss Heat is lost from the body in several ways. Small amounts are used in warming food or drink and in the evaporation of moisture from the respiratory tract. Most heat is lost from the surface of the body, by *convection,* i.e., the transfer of heat to a fluid medium. Heat loss by convection depends on the existence of a temperature gradient between the body surface and the ambient air. A second mechanism for heat loss is *radiation,* which may be defined as an exchange of electromagnetic energy between the body and the radiant environment. *Evaporation* is the third major mechanism for dissipating heat and is particularly important when the ambient temperature exceeds that of the body.

The principal method of regulating heat loss is by varying the volume of blood flowing to the surface of the body. A rich circulation in the skin and subcutaneous tissues carries heat to the surface, where it can escape. In addition, sweating increases heat loss by providing water to be vaporized. The sweat, or eccrine, glands are under the control of the sympathetic nerves which, in this instance, mediate cholinergic stimuli. Heat loss by sweating may be tremendous, and as much as 1 liter per hour of sweat may be evaporated. The amount of heat loss through sweating is also dependent upon the humidity in the air. The greater the humidity, the less the ability to lose heat through sweat.

When there is need for conservation of heat, adrenergic autonomic stimuli cause a sharp reduction in the blood flow to the surface. This causes vasoconstriction and transforms the skin and subcutaneous tissue into layers of insulation.

Heat transfer within the body This depends upon *conduction,* i.e., the transfer of heat between adjacent organs, and upon *circulatory convection,* which is governed by bulk movement of body fluids and which is responsible for the transfer of heat between the cells and the bloodstream. It is useful, although oversimplified, to visualize the body as a central core at uniform temperatures surrounded by an insulating shell. The role of the shell as a mediator for heat conservation and heat loss is determined in part by its blood supply and by vasoconstriction or vasodilatation. Although insulation is relatively uniform throughout the body, some parts, such as the digits, are particularly susceptible to cold because of the increased surface-to-volume ratio. Moreover, blood that reaches the digits has already been cooled on the way. Insulation may be enhanced by the addition of clothing.

Neural control of temperature The control of body temperature, integrating the various physical and chemical processes for heat production or heat loss, is a function of cerebral centers located in the hypothalamus. A high-decerebrate animal has a normal temperature if the hypothalamus is left intact. On the other hand, an animal whose brainstem has been sectioned loses ability to control body temperature, which consequently tends to vary with the environment, a condition referred to as *poikilothermia.* Animal experiments suggest that the preoptic anterior hypothalamus and some centers in the spinal cord have neurons which respond directly to local temperature and act as a sensor for internal temperature. This function is distinct from the integrative function which responds to temperature-sensitive structures all over the body.

FACTORS AFFECTING NEURAL CONTROL OF TEMPERATURE The temperature-regulating system is a negative feedback control system, and possesses three elements essential to such a system: (1) receptors which sense the existing central temperatures; (2) effector mechanisms, consisting of the vasomotor, sudomotor, and metabolic effectors, and (3) integrative structures which determine whether the existing temperature is too high or too low and which activate the appropriate motor response. It is a negative feedback system because a rise in central temperature initiates mechanisms for losing heat while a fall in central temperature activates mechanisms for heat production and heat conservation. The activation of these effector responses is governed by a central integrative mechanism which may be compared with a thermostat and which responds to a variety of stimuli, such as the sensory impulses engendered in flushing or sweating, behavioral impulses, exercise, endocrine influences, and probably the temperature of the blood circulating through the hypothalamic centers. In a sense all these stimuli reset the thermostat.

A classic example of the endocrine influence on temperature is the effect of menstruation. The mean body temperature of women is higher during the second half of the menstrual cycle than it is between the onset of menstruation and the time of ovulation. The sensations of intense heat followed by diaphoresis that characterize the vasomotor instability experienced by some women at the menopause are undoubtedly the result of endocrine imbalance. The activation of the adrenal medulla in response to cold is another example of the relationship between the endocrine system and the thermoregulatory apparatus.

Normal body temperature It is not practical to designate an exact upper level of normal body temperature because there are small differences among normal persons. There are rare individuals whose temperatures are always elevated slightly above accepted "normal" levels, and there is considerable variation in temperature in a given individual. In general, however, it is safe to regard an oral temperature above 99°F (37.2°C) in a person at bed rest as probable indication of disease. The temperature may be as low as 96.5°F (35.8°C) in healthy persons. Rectal temperature is usually 0.5 to 1.0°F higher than oral temperature. In very hot weather the body temperature may be elevated by 0.5 or even 1.0°F.

There is a distinct diurnal variation in body temperature in healthy human beings. Oral readings of 97°F (36.1°C) are relatively common on arising in the morning. Body temperature rises steadily through the day, reaches a peak of 99°F (37.2°C) or greater between 6 P.M. and 10 P.M., and then drops slowly to reach a minimum at 2 A.M. to 4 A.M. Although it has been postulated that this diurnal variation is dependent upon increasing activity during the day and rest at night, the pattern is not reversed in individuals who work at night and sleep during the day for long periods of time. The febrile patterns of most human diseases also tend to follow this normal diurnal pattern. Fevers tend to be higher, to "spike," in the evening, and many patients with febrile disease have relatively normal temperatures in the early morning hours.

Body temperature is more labile in young children, and transient elevations after relatively slight exertion in warm weather are frequently observed in them.

Severe or prolonged exercise can produce considerable elevation in body temperature. For example, marathon runners often have temperatures between 103.2 and 105.8°F (39 and 41°C). Although this marked increase in temperature with exercise tends to be balanced by compensatory cutaneous vasodilatation, resulting in loss of heat, and hyperventilation, these compensatory mechanisms may fail, leading to hyperpyrexia and, if uncontrolled, to heat stroke. Many of the adverse effects of long-distance running can be prevented by holding races only if the ambient temperature is below 82°F (27.8°C), preferably in the early morning or early evening, and by assuring ample fluid intake both before and during a race.

Disordered thermoregulation In exercise, there is a temporary imbalance between heat production and heat loss with prompt reestablishment of normal temperatures at rest due to continuing activation of heat loss mechanisms. In fact, in prolonged exercise, cutaneous vasodilatation in response to an increase in central body temperature stops in order to preserve central temperature. Less adaptation occurs in fever because once a stable body temperature is reached, heat production equals heat loss, but both are greater than in the basal state. Cutaneous blood flow plays a greater role in controlling heat production and heat loss in fever than does sweating. At the beginning of fever, the body temperature as sensed by the thermoreceptors is low and the individual responds physiologically as if he or she were cold. *Heat production* is increased by shivering, and *heat loss* is decreased by vasoconstriction. These events explain the sensation of cold or chills that characterizes the beginning of fever. Conversely, when the cause of fever is removed, the temperature returns to normal, and the individual responds as if warm. Cutaneous vasodilatation, sweating, and inhibition of shivering are the compensatory responses.

Deviations of 5°F (approximately 3.5°C) from the normal body temperature do not interfere appreciably with most bodily functions. Convulsions are common at temperatures higher than 106°F (41.1°C) in children, and irreversible brain damage, presumably due to protein denaturation (impairment of normal enzymic functions), is common when temperatures of 108°F (42.2°C) are reached. Fortunately, when hyperthermia reaches dangerous levels, the mechanisms for heat loss are suddenly activated; consequently, oral temperatures above 106°F (41.1°C) are relatively rare in humans. Conversely, when temperatures are lowered to 91°F (32.8°C), loss of consciousness occurs; at 86°F (30°C) poikilothermia sets in, and between 83 and 84°F (28.5°C) slow atrial fibrillation supervenes. Ventricular fibrillation occurs at extremely hypothermic temperatures.

The systemic symptoms accompanying deviations in temperature are poorly understood. For example at temperatures of 102°F (39°C) many patients have malaise, drowsiness, weakness, and generalized aches and pains. Many others, however, feel entirely well. Why some individuals are able to tolerate fever so well while others become markedly ill remains an enigma. Perhaps the inciting stimulus rather than fever per se is the major determinant of systemic complaints.

DISEASES OF THE NERVOUS SYSTEM Disease of the regulatory centers in the hypothalamus may affect body temperature. Cases have been observed in which there was destruction of the centers controlling heat-conserving mechanisms, with resulting hypothermia. More commonly, cerebral lesions are manifested by hyperthermia; this may occur with tumors, degenerative diseases, vascular accidents, particularly cerebral hemorrhage, or infections involving the hypothalamus, such as encephalitis. All these may result in loss of neurons and gliosis. Central fever is accompanied by lack of a diurnal variation, absence of sweating, resistance to antipyretic drugs, excessive response to external cooling, and loss of consciousness.

There are several diseases, of which heat stroke is the cardinal example, in which the central mechanisms for cooling suddenly fail and the patient ceases to sweat, despite the fact that his temperature is rising. Some of the highest temperatures ever observed in human beings [112 to 113°F (44.4°C)] have been in cases of heat stroke. A temperature higher than 114°F (45.6°C) is probably not compatible with life.

INCREASED HEAT PRODUCTION Patients with thyrotoxicosis show exaggerated heat production, and their temperature is often 1 to 2°F above the normal range.

IMPAIRMENT OF HEAT LOSS Patients with *congestive heart failure* often have an elevation of body temperature between 0.5 and 1.5°F. Perhaps this elevation is caused by impairment of heat dissipation as a result of diminished cardiac output, decline in cutaneous blood flow (with increasing insulation of the central temperature core), the insulating effect of edema, and the increased heat production incident to the muscular activity of dyspnea. On the other hand, patients with congestive heart failure are likely to have other causes of fever, such as venous thrombosis, pulmonary embolism and infarction, myocardial infarction, pneumonia, and urinary tract infection. However, since slight fever is so regularly present even in the absence of such complications, the circulatory disturbance may be responsible.

Patients with skin disorders such as *ichthyosis* and *congenital absence of sweat glands* may have fever in a warm environment because of inability to lose heat from the surface of the body. Individuals with congenitally absent sweat glands lack the ability of active cutaneous vasodilatation and hence are unable to dissipate heat by at least two mechanisms. Drugs which impair sweating, such as atropine, scopolamine, phenothiazines, monoamine oxidase inhibitors, glutethimide, lysergic acid diethylamide (LSD), amphetamines, and inhalation anesthetics may result in elevated temperatures.

Patients with severe burns tend to be hyperthermic, probably because occlusive dressings interfere with heat loss despite large areas of denuded skin.

PATHOGENESIS OF FEVER Fever is a consequence of many stimuli, including bacteria and their endotoxins; viruses; yeasts; spirochetes; antigen-antibody reactions; hormonal substances, exemplified by progesterone; drugs; and synthetic polynucleotides like poly I:poly C. These substances, which have been termed collectively *exogenous pyrogens,* are both diverse and complex. It has been postulated that they act through an intermediary substance termed *endogenous pyrogen* (EP). Most of the knowledge concerning EP has come from work in experimental animals.

EP is a basic protein of low molecular weight that is derived primarily from blood monocytes and from tissue macrophages. EP has not been isolated from lymphocytes, but these cells may react with antigens and, through the action of lymphokines, may stimulate macrophages to release EP.

Production of EP [henceforth called leukocytic pyrogen (LP)] requires synthesis of new messenger ribonucleic acid (mRNA) from a DNA genome coded for LP. LP is present in very small amounts and has been difficult to detect in human serum or exudates. LP is similar to other inducible proteins. The resting leukocyte is repressed and LP synthesis does not occur. During activation by the stimulators mentioned above, the genome is derepressed, new mRNA is transcribed with subsequent translation into new LP.

Once released, LP probably acts on the thermosensitive neurons in the preoptic region of the hypothalamus. These neurons control the constancy of body temperature and are the point where fever is initiated.

The action of LP on the hypothalamus is by no means simple. It appears as if LP induces hypothalamic prostaglandin synthesis by the following mechanisms:

1 LP releases arachidonic acid with subsequent release of prostaglandin and prostaglandin-like molecules.
2 These products of arachidonic acid synthesis most likely modulate the hypothalamic regulatory mechanism resulting in an increased set point from normothermic to fever levels. The precise mechanism for upward resetting is not known.
3 Antipyretics that inhibit prostaglandin synthetase decrease fever by preventing the synthesis of prostaglandins E_1 and E_2 from arachidonic acid.

ROLE OF THE THERMOSTAT During fever the thermostat in the hypothalamus shifts upward (for example, from 37°C to 39°C). This results in signals from the posterior hypothalamus to increase heat production (by muscular contractions such as shivering) and to decrease heat loss by peripheral vasoconstriction. These processes continue until the temperature of the blood supplying the hypothalamus matches the higher thermostat setting. In contrast to fever, in hyperthermia the thermostat setting remains unchanged at its normothermic level, while the body's mechanisms for heat loss fail.

DISORDERS ASSOCIATED WITH HIGH TEMPERATURES Heat syndromes Four clinical syndromes are associated with high environmental temperature: *heat cramps, heat exhaustion, exertional heat injury,* and *heat stroke.* Although each of these entities may be separated from the other on clinical grounds, there is considerable overlap between them, and they may be considered as a series of syndromes along a single spectrum. The incidence of heat syndromes is unknown, but during an ordinary summer about 200 cases of heat stroke are reported. During the heat wave of July 1980, 1265 deaths from heat stroke were reported—784 from Kansas City and St. Louis alone. Heat syndromes occur primarily at elevated temperatures (>90°F) and at high humidities (>60%); and elderly individuals, those with mental illness or alcoholism or who receive antipsychotic drugs, diuretics, and anticholinergics, or those who reside in poorly ventilated places without air conditioning are most susceptible. Heat syndromes are especially prevalent during the first days of a heat wave before effective acclimatization can occur. Prophylaxis by augmenting fluid intake prior to exposure and by ensuring that susceptible individuals, particularly the elderly or the very young, wear light clothing, take frequent cool baths, remain in a cool environment, and avoid strenuous physical activity can help prevent the full-blown syndrome, especially heat stroke.

ACCLIMATIZATION The basic mechanism by which humans accommodate to excessive temperatures is unknown. Acclimatization does not increase the threshold for sweating. However, sweating is the most effective natural means of combating heat stress and can occur with little or no change in the core temperature of the body. As long as sweating continues, humans can withstand remarkably high temperatures, provided water and sodium chloride, the most important physiologic constituents of sweat, are replaced. The concentration of sodium chloride varies between that of interstitial fluid and very low concentrations, and the ability to secrete sweat with low sodium chloride content, as well as to increase the quantity of sweat, is a major mechanism for the conservation of salt in hot weather. Dilatation of the peripheral blood vessels in an attempt to dissipate heat is another major way for the body to acclimatize to hot temperatures. Other alterations include a decrease in total circulating blood volume, a decrease in renal blood flow, an increase of antidiuretic hormones (ADH) as well as aldosterone, a decrease in urine sodium, and an increase in respiratory and pulse rates. Ordinarily, acclimatization takes from 4 to 7 days. The hyperaldosteronism may result in potassium loss, which may be aggravated by replacement of sodium without concomitant repletion of potassium. Initially there is an increase in cardiac output but as heat stress persists, venous return diminishes and heart failure may occur. If environmental temperatures in excess of the body's temperature persist, heat is retained and hyperpyrexia develops.

HEAT CRAMPS Heat cramps, called "miner's cramps" and "stoker's cramps," are the most benign heat syndrome. Cramps are characterized by painful spasms of the voluntary muscles and usually follow strenuous exercise. In general, only individuals in good physical condition develop this syndrome. External temperatures need not exceed the body temperature, and direct exposure to the sun is not necessary. The body temperature is usually not elevated. Muscle cramps usually occur after excessive sweating and may even be precipitated by strenuous exercise in cold environments in untrained persons heavily clothed. Muscles of the extremities bear the brunt of physical activity and hence show the highest incidence of cramps. Physical examination of the patient is normal between the paroxysms. Examination of the blood reveals a concentration of the formed elements and a decreased sodium and chloride concentration. Excretion of these ions in the urine is characteristically low. Treatment consists of sodium chloride; cessation of cramps with replacement of sodium chloride and water is striking and supports the hypothesis that the cause of heat cramps is depletion of these essential electrolytes. Occasionally cramps involve the abdominal musculature, mimicking an intraabdominal emergency. Such patients have had mistaken exploratory surgery performed, often with disastrous results. Replacement of saline prior to surgery would have obviated such operations.

HEAT EXHAUSTION Heat prostration, or heat collapse, is probably the most common heat syndrome. It represents a failure of the cardiovascular responses to high external temperatures and is particularly common in elderly individuals who are receiving diuretics. Weakness, vertigo, headache, anorexia, nausea, vomiting, the urge to defecate, and faintness may precede collapse. Heat collapse occurs in both physically active and sedentary individuals. The onset is usually sudden and the duration of collapse brief. During the acute stage, the patient looks ashen-gray. The skin is cold and clammy. The pupils are dilated. The blood pressure may be low and the pulse pressure elevated. Since prostration develops before exposure to heat is prolonged, body temperature is subnormal or normal. The duration of exposure and the extent to which sweat is lost determine the degree of hemoconcentration. Treatment consists of removal of the patient to a cool area and placing him or her in the recumbent position. Spontaneous recovery then usually takes place. Intravenous administration of saline solution or whole blood is necessary only rarely. Although the pathogenetic mechanism of heat prostration is not primarily a depletion of water and salt, it is likely that maintenance of these electrolytes will prevent heat prostration in individuals exposed to high temperatures.

EXERTIONAL HEAT INJURY This syndrome occurs in individuals who are exerting themselves in hot ambient temperatures (about 80°F) when the humidity is high. It is particularly common in runners who enter races with insufficient acclimatization, inadequate conditioning, or improper hydration (before and during the race). Obesity, age, and previous heat stroke are contributing predisposing factors. In contrast to classic heat stroke, individuals with exertional heat injury usually sweat freely, and their temperatures are lower (102°F to 104°F as opposed to 106°F and higher in heat stroke). Symptoms consist of headache, piloerection (gooseflesh) on the chest and upper arms, chills, overbreathing, nausea, vomiting, muscle cramps, ataxia, unsteady gait, and incoherent speech. In some individuals, loss of consciousness occurs. Physical examination shows tachycardia, hypotension, and evidence of low peripheral resistance. Laboratory data show hemoconcentration, hypernatremia, abnormal liver and muscle enzymes, hypocalcemia, hypophosphatemia, and, in some instances, hypoglycemia. An occasional patient has thrombocytopenia, hemolysis, disseminated intravascular coagulation, rhabdomyolysis, myoglobinuria, and acute tubular necrosis. These severe complications can be avoided by prompt treatment, which consists of placing the victim under wet cold sheets to lower core temperature to 38°C as quickly as possible, massaging the extremities to improve blood flow from the core to the periphery, and infusing fluids consisting primarily of hypotonic glucose-saline. Patients should be hospitalized for 36 h of observation.

Exertional heat injury can be prevented by (1) running races early in the morning (before 8 A.M.) when the temperature and humidity are likely to be low, (2) educating runners to enter a race well hydrated by drinking 300 ml of water 10 min before a race and 250 ml every 3 to 4 km (salt and glucose solutions should be avoided), (3) placing aid stations at 5-km intervals, (4) instructing runners not to increase their pace after most of the race has been run, and (5) avoiding alcohol before a race.

HEAT STROKE Heat hyperpyrexia, heat stroke, or sunstroke is most common in elderly individuals with preexisting chronic disease. Among these are arteriosclerosis and congestive heart failure, particularly when patients receive diurectics. Other predisposing factors include diabetes mellitus, alcoholism, the use of anticholinergic drugs, and skin disorders in which it may be difficult to lose heat such as ectodermal dysplasia, congenital absence of the sweat glands, or severe scleroderma. Heat stroke is also common in military recruits undergoing basic training, and in an occasional long-distance runner. The mechanism for heat stroke is not known. Although most patients with heat stroke cease sweating, in some sweating is preserved. The vasoconstriction that accompanies heat stroke prevents dissipation of heat from the core, but whether this vasoconstriction is cause or effect is not clear. Direct exposure to the sun is not a necessary prerequisite.

There may be few premonitory symptoms of heat stroke, and loss of consciousness may be the first sign. Other patients may complain of headache, vertigo, faintness, abdominal distress, confusion, or hyperpnea. Delirium may develop in more severe cases.

Pyrexia and prostration are the significant findings on physical examination. A rectal temperature greater than 106°F (41.1°C) is common and internal body temperatures as high as 112 to 113°F (44.4°C) have been recorded. The skin is hot and dry, and, in most cases, sweating is absent. The pulse rate is increased, and respirations are rapid and weak. The blood pressure is usually low. The muscles are flaccid, and tendon reflexes may be diminished. Lethargy, stupor, or coma, depending on the severity, is present. Shock is common in fatal cases.

Examination of the blood and urine may show few abnormalities. Hemoconcentration is common. Leukocytosis is characteristic as are proteinuria, cylinduria, and an elevation in BUN. There is usually a respiratory alkalosis which is followed by a metabolic acidosis. Lactic acidemia is common. Serum potassium is normal or low and there are usually hypocalcemia and hypophosphatemia. The electrocardiogram may show, in addition to tachycardia and sinus arrhythmia, flattening and subsequent inversion of the T wave and depression of the ST segment. Diffuse myocardial necrosis with ECG evidence of myocardial infarction has been reported. Other major laboratory abnormalities include thrombocytopenia; prolonged bleeding, clotting, and prothrombin times; afibrinogenemia and fibrinolysis; and disseminated intravascular coagulation. All these may be responsible for diffuse bleeding. Liver damage is common; it appears 24 to 36 h after admission and is characterized by clinically apparent jaundice and, often, by abnormalities in hepatocellular enzymes. Renal failure is a common complication of heat stroke.

Patients with heat stroke may die within a few hours after being discovered, or may die of complications such as acute renal failure. However, a number of patients will die several weeks after the acute episode, usually of myocardial infarction, heart failure, renal failure, bronchopneumonia, or complicating bacteremia. In them autopsy may show extensive parenchymal damage to various organs, either from hyperpyrexia per se or from petechial hemorrhages in the brain, heart, kidneys, or liver.

Heat stroke requires heroic emergency measures. Time is most important. The patient should be placed in a cool place with adequate circulation of fresh air and with most of the clothing removed. Because the pathogenesis of heat stroke involves failure of the heat-regulating mechanism with cessation of sweating, external means of heat dissipation must be employed. The most effective measure is to immerse the patient in an ice-water bath, and there is no effective substitute for this seemingly drastic treatment. An ice-water bath does not induce shock or stimulate significant cutaneous vasoconstriction. The bath should be given with a minimum of delay. The patient should be watched constantly by a nurse or physician and the rectal temperature monitored. The bath may be discontinued when the rectal temperature falls below 101°F (38.3°C), but treatment should be resumed if there is a febrile rebound. Compared with immersion in ice water, other forms of therapy are less effective, but covering the patient with cold wet towels under a fan may be satisfactory if a bath is not available. After the bath the patient should be placed in a cool, well-ventilated room. Massage of the skin should be employed along with cooling because it stimulates return of the cool peripheral blood to the overheated brain and viscera and aids acceleration of heat loss. The patient should be well hydrated with hypotonic crystalloid solutions. Phenothiazine may be helpful in reducing shivering. Stimulants such as epinephrine and narcotics are contraindicated. Central venous pressure and urinary output need to be monitored. Prompt ice-bath cooling, massage of the limbs, and vigorous hydration, along with establishment of a proper airway, avoidance of aspiration, treating coma and convulsions, and watching for arrhythmia, will lead to survival of most patients, particularly if they are young and were previously well. Unfortunately, the poor, ill, and elderly who are often not discovered until heat hyperpyrexia has been present for some hours have a much less favorable outcome. Both dehydration and heart failure must be avoided. Fresh blood should be given in case of bleeding, and clear-cut evidence of disseminated intravascular coagulation calls for heparin (7500 units per hour). Persistent oliguria is an indication for early dialysis.

Malignant hyperthermia ETIOLOGY Malignant hyperthermia (MH) consists of a group of inherited disorders that are characterized by a rapid increase in temperature to 102.2 to 107.6°F (39 to 42°C) in response to inhalational anesthetics such as halothane, methoxyflurane, cyclopropane, and ethyl ether or muscle relaxants, notably succinylcholine. In one form of the disease where the mechanism of inheritance is autosomal dominant, the individuals are normal between attacks although about 50 percent have an elevation in creatine phosphokinase (CPK), and in 90 percent, muscle from susceptible individuals contracts on exposure to concentrations of caffeine, halothane, or hexamethonium that causes only minimal changes in normal muscle. A second recessive form occurs in young boys and, less commonly, girls, with a number of congenital abnormalities including short stature, undescended testes, lumbar lordosis, thoracic kyphosis, pectus carinatum, webbed neck, winged scapulae, small chin, low-set ears, and an antimongoloid obliquity of the palpebral fissures. This form is called the *King syndrome.* MH has also been described in several other myopathies including myotonia congenita, central core disease, and Duchenne muscular dystrophy. The incidence of the autosomal dominant form is 1:50,000 to 1:100,000.

PATHOGENESIS The triggering anesthetic releases calcium from the membrane of the muscle cell's sarcoplasmic reticulum, which is defective in storing this ion. The result is a sudden increase in myoplasmic calcium. The calcium activates myosin ATPase, which converts adenosine triphosphate (ATP) to adenosine diphosphate, phosphate, and heat. There are also inhibition of tropanin, uncoupling of oxidative phosphorylation, activation of phosphorylase kinase, and increased glycolysis. Muscular contraction occurs and it, as well as the chemical events, leads to production of heat.

MANIFESTATIONS Existence of malignant hyperthermia can be suspected if less relaxation is noted during induction of anesthesia and muscle fasciculations become evident when succinyl choline is given. In some patients trismus during intubation is the first sign of a muscle disorder. Although the elevation in temperature is the result of muscular contraction, it may rise very rapidly, and if the temperature is not monitored, the first signs may be a hot skin and tachycardia or a cardiac arrhythmia. In addition to the high fever, there is muscle rigidity, hypotension, and mottled cyanosis.

Early laboratory abnormalities include respiratory and metabolic acidosis, hyperkalemia and hypermagnesemia, and elevation in blood lactate and pyruvate. Late complications include massive skeletal muscle swelling, pulmonary edema, disseminated intravascular coagulation, and acute renal failure.

TREATMENT Malignant hyperthermia is a medical emergency. Surgery must be interrupted and the patient cooled with ice. One hundred percent oxygen should be given, along with sodium bicarbonate, to combat the severe metabolic acidosis. A diuresis should be induced with fluids and diuretics to reduce myoglobinemia and hyperkalemia. Specific treatment consists of dantrolene sodium, 1 mg/kg, by rapid intravenous infusion. The drug should be continued until symptoms have begun to subside or up to a maximum single dose of 10 mg/kg. The regimen can be repeated if symptoms recur. Procainamide to combat arrhythmias, in dosage of 0.5 to 1 (mg/kg)/min with ECG monitoring should be administered as well.

PREVENTION Because of the tendency of this syndrome to run in families, its detection is essential. This can be achieved by monitoring the temperature of all patients under anesthesia; the best way to avert it altogether is to take a thorough family history. Examining patients preoperatively is often not helpful because, between attacks, persons susceptible to malignant hyperthermia may be entirely normal. Some have increased muscle bulk, some have localized areas of muscle weakness, some have spontaneous muscle cramps, and a few have generalized muscle weakness. In some of these patients, the CPK is elevated, but in many this test is entirely normal. Prophylactic dantrolene orally has not been successful in preventing MH. In susceptible patients, surgery should be performed under spinal, epidural, or regional anesthesia. If this is not possible, a combination of pentothal and diazepam is probably safest. Phosphorylase A and adenylate cyclase are elevated in muscles of MH patients and along with their increased contractility provide useful biochemical markers of MH.

Neuroleptic malignant syndrome (NMS) This syndrome is characterized by muscular rigidity, hyperthermia, altered consciousness, and autonomic dysfunction. Rigidity and akinesia develop concomitantly with fever as high as 41°C. Consciousness fluctuates from alertness to coma. Autonomic dysfunction is manifested by tachycardia, labile blood pressure, profuse sweating, dyspnea, and incontinence. Laboratory abnormalities consist of leukocytosis (15,000 to 30,000) and elevation in CPK. The syndrome occurs after use of potent neuroleptics in therapeutic doses. Most cases have been reported after haloperidol, thiothixene, or piperazine phenothiazine. Young adult males predominate. The NMS lasts 5 to 10 days after administration of oral neuroleptics is discontinued, and longer after depot injection. The overall mortality is 20 percent and fatalities have occurred as late as 30 days after onset and have been due to renal failure or arrhythmias. Although the etiology of NMS is unknown, its similarity to malignant hyperthermia is striking, and the fact that MH has occurred in the wake of neuroleptic drugs strengthens the hypothesis that NMS may be a variant of MH. No specific treatment for NMS has been described, although dantrolene sodium may be worth trying if supportive measures, cooling, and drug withdrawal do not result in improvement.

DISORDERS ASSOCIATED WITH LOW TEMPERATURES

Cold acclimatization The state of increased resistance to cold injury is the result of exposure to a cold but tolerable environment. Adaptive responses consist of circulatory adjustments protecting the temperatures of exposed portions of the body, metabolic adaptation providing greater heat production to compensate for increased heat loss, and behavioral and neural adaptations minimizing either the actual cold stress or the discomfort resulting from physiologically tolerable hypothermia. In contrast with heat acclimatization, it is not possible to delineate adaptive physiologic changes to cold. Nevertheless, primitive people live at zero temperatures wearing little or no clothing; pain perception is less in persons, such as fishermen, who work periodically with their hands in ice water; and military personnel shiver less during cold exposure after training in the Arctic. Adaptation may take place either by shivering, with production of excess heat, or, as is the case with Australian aborigines, by a drop of internal temperature with only minimal shivering.

Hypothermia Although far less common than is elevation in temperature, hypothermia is of considerable importance because it represents a medical emergency which lends itself to treatment.

ACCIDENTAL HYPOTHERMIA This is a well-known complication of exposure and has been reported frequently during the winter months. It usually occurs in elderly or inebriated individuals after prolonged exposure, not necessarily to excessively low external temperatures. It is true, however, that both of these groups detect low temperatures less well than normal. The diagnosis of hypothermia has proved elusive largely because *clinical thermometers do not record temperatures below 95°F (35°C). Whenever a patient presents with a temperature below this level, the true temperature should be determined with an incubator thermometer or a thermocouple.* Accidental hypothermia has been found in association with myxedema, pituitary insufficiency, Addison's disease, hypoglycemia, cerebrovascular disease, Wernicke's encephalopathy, myocardial infarction, cirrhosis, pancreatitis, and ingestion of drugs or alcohol. For example, it is not uncommon to find a derelict in a railroad yard or under a bridge following an alcoholic debauch with a temperature between 85 and 90°F (28.5 and 32.3°C) or lower. These patients usually appear cold and pale and, when their temperatures are very low, give the appearance of having rigor mortis, so stiff is their musculature. Patients with temperatures less than 80°F (26.7°C) are usually unconscious. The pupils are usually miotic, respirations tend to be shallow and slow, there is bradycardia, and most patients are hypotensive. Generalized edema is often present. When the temperature falls below 25°C, coma, areflexia, and lack of pupillary response are present. Laboratory data tend to show hemoconcentration, mild azotemia, and metabolic acidosis. The acidosis is due to lactic acidemia which is, in part, a result of hypoxemia in peripheral tissues. At cold temperatures, the hemoglobin dissociation curve is shifted to the left, and there is decreased unloading of oxygen in the peripheral tissues. Some patients have hypoglycemia while others show evidence of diabetes mellitus. Thyroid function tests may give results typical of myxedema. Some patients have elevations in serum amylase, and a few show pancreatitis at autopsy. The electrocardiogram is distorted by muscular tremors and may show bradycardia or slow atrial fibrillation and a characteristic J wave (occurring at the junction of the QRS complex and ST segment). Other arrythmias are common; ventricular fibrillation is usually a terminal event. The mortality is five times higher in people over 75.

Hypothermia is a medical emergency, and therapy should be instituted at once. The following steps are indicated:

1. An airway must be established and maintained, and the patient should be well oxygenated. Warmed oxygen may be helpful.
2. Blood gases should be monitored; they should be corrected for temperature.

3 Blood volume should be expanded with glucose and saline, low-molecular-weight dextran, or albumin. Maintenance of blood volume is necessary to prevent the infarctions which have been a hallmark in fatal cases and to avert "rewarming shock."

4 Because of the tendency to arrythmias, serum potassium should be monitored carefully; a transvenous pacemaker may be indicated.

5 Sodium bicarbonate should be given if pH $\leq$ 7.25.

6 Although external rewarming with blankets or placing the patient in a warm room is appropriate in patients with mild hypothermia, patients who are moderately hypothermic require reestablishment of core temperature. This can be done effectively by placing the patient in a warm bath or a Hubbard tank at 40 to 42°C. External warming tends to dilate the constricted peripheral blood vessels and to divert blood from the visceral organs. In severely hypothermic patients, this may result in rewarming shock and does not lead to sufficient restoration of the core temperature to warm the myocardium sufficiently to make it responsive to antiarrhythmic agents. In this situation hemodialysis, during which the blood is warmed externally, or peritoneal dialysis, during which the dialysate is warmed to 98.6°F (37°C), is the method of choice. It is particularly important to rewarm the myocardium because, in cases of ventricular fibrillation, defibrillation will not be successful until myocardial temperature is raised to near normal levels.

7 There is a tendency for these patients to develop pneumonia which should be treated promptly with antibiotics.

8 Finally, resuscitative efforts should be vigorous and prolonged despite the poor prognosis which is related primarily to the advanced age and associated debilitating disease of these patients. In younger individuals, some remarkable rescues have been recorded; one young woman was resuscitated even after her temperature had dropped to 69°F (20.6°C). *Authorities agree that hypothermia victims without vital signs (prolonged asystole) should not be pronounced dead until they have been rewarmed to 36°C and remain unresponsive to CPR at that temperature.*

HYPOTHERMIA SECONDARY TO ACUTE ILLNESS There is a group of patients who develop moderate hypothermia in association with acute diseases including congestive heart failure, uremia, diabetes mellitus, drug overdose, acute respiratory failure, and hypoglycemia. These patients are generally elderly and upon admission to the hospital are found to have temperatures of 92 to 93.9°F (33.3 to 34.4°C). They also have a severe metabolic acidosis, due to increased production of lactic acid, and cardiac arrhythmias. Most of these patients are comatose. This entity differs from accidental hypothermia only in the absence of exposure; these cases have all occurred at normal ambient temperatures. The mechanism appears to be an acute failure of thermoregulation; shivering did not occur in any of these patients. Usually these patients have been rewarmed within a few hours by means of an alcohol-circulating blanket. Upon return to normal temperature, cardiac arrythmias, which were present in most of these patients, responded to treatment, and the sensorium returned to normal. With the exception that core rewarming was established by external means, other facets of therapy should follow the steps outlined above. In addition, treatment of the underlying disease such as diabetes with insulin, uremia with dialysis, or congestive heart failure with appropriate cardiac drugs and diuretics is essential. The prognosis is good provided the syndrome is recognized early and treatment is instituted at once.

IMMERSION HYPOTHERMIA Responses to cold-water immersion may be classified as (1) stimulatory, with deep body temperature normal to 95°F (35°C); (2) depressant, with deep body temperature 95 to 86°F (35 to 30°C); and (3) critical, with deep body temperature 86 to 77°F (30 to 25°C).

The long-distance swimmer is able to maintain a normal body temperature for periods of 15 to 25 h or more in water that may plunge skin temperature to 59°F (15°C) or lower, which is some 28°F below deep body temperature, lending support to the concept of a body core insulated by a body shell. The vasoconstriction operative in cold water greatly reduces heat loss. However, there is great individual variability in heat loss in cold water. The relatively obese swimmer may maintain a normal rectal temperature for 2 h without shivering in 61°F (16°C) water. A lean person under the same conditions, despite violent shivering, may experience a fall in rectal temperature of several degrees and become incapacitated from the rigor. In hypersensitive persons, immersion in cold water may be followed by vascular spasm, vomiting, and syncope.

Other compensatory responses include bradycardia, a slight rise in blood pressure, and an early rise in rectal temperature followed by a fall. At 86°F (30°C), atrial fibrillation is common.

Rewarming in warm water has been recommended as the treatment of immersion hypothermia. In severe cases, hemodialysis or peritoneal dialysis should be instituted.

Local cold injuries MECHANISMS OF FREEZING INJURY These can be divided into phenomena which affect cells and extracellular fluids (direct effects) and those which disrupt the function of organized tissues and the integrity of the circulation (indirect effects).

When tissue freezes, ice crystals form and, concomitantly, solutes in the residual liquid become concentrated. The physical dislocation during slow freezing is extreme. Ice crystals many times the size of individual cells form but only in the extracellular spaces. Large ice crystals can develop between cells in soft tissue without producing irreversible injury as long as the percentage of water frozen does not exceed a critical amount. A major source of damage to living cells during freezing and thawing appears to be the strong salt solutions which develop during formation and dissolution of ice; changes in the proportions of lipids and phospholipids in the cell membrane are also of great importance.

The fulminating vascular reaction and stasis which supervene are associated with production of histamine-like substances which increase the permeability of the capillary bed. Within blood vessels, cellular elements aggregate. Irreversible occlusion of small blood vessels by cell masses has been demonstrated in thawed tissue following freezing injury. The damaged frozen tissue simulates tissue damage produced by burns.

MANIFESTATIONS The mildest form of cold injury is called *frostnip* and tends to occur in organs farthest removed from the core of the body such as the earlobes, nose, cheeks, fingers and toes, and hands and feet. It can be prevented by warm clothing and treated with simple rewarming. More consequential local cold injuries may be divided into freezing (frostbite) and nonfreezing (immersion-foot) injuries. The two types may be observed in the same extremity or in different extremities in the same individual.The diagnosis of freezing versus nonfreezing injury generally can be made on the basis of history and clinical manifestations.

Immersion foot is an entity observed in shipwreck survivors or in soldiers (trench foot) whose feet have been wet but not freezing cold for prolonged periods. There is primarily injury to nerve and muscle tissue, but no gross or irreparable pathologic changes occur in blood vessels and skin. The clinical picture reflects primary hypoxic trauma giving rise to three clearly recognizable conditions: (1) *ischemia*, denoted by a pale, pulseless extremity; (2) *hyperemia*, characterized by a bounding pulsatile circulation in red, swollen, painful feet; and (3) the *posthyperemic* or recovery period. The initial cold-induced vasoconstriction, increased blood viscosity, and impaired oxygen transport in the ischemic state are aggravated by such factors as malnutrition, general hypothermia, dehydration, and trauma from relatively fixed, pendant extremities. The problem of rewarming is critical in these patients during the stage of ischemia, when overheating of tissue may lead to gangrene. In the state of hyperemia, the red, swollen feet require judicious cooling. Severe cases may show muscular weakness, atrophy, ulceration, and gangrene of superficial areas. Sensitivity to cold and pain on weight bearing, which may cause discomfort for many years, are sequelae even of milder injuries.

Frostbite stands in contrast with immersion foot because the blood vessels may be severely and irreparably injured, the circulation of blood ceases, and the vascular bed of the frozen tissue is occluded by agglutinated cell aggregates and thrombi. The cutaneous injury consists in part of separation of the epidermal-dermal interface. Early, the intravascular clumping is reversible. However, with the passage of time, clumped red blood cells within vessels in injured tissue lose their morphologic identity and take on the appearance of a homogenous, hyalinaceous plug. It has been shown in some, but not all, experimental studies that much of the intravascular aggregation following freezing injury can be reversed and microcirculatory perfusion improved if low-molecular-weight dextran is given intravenously shortly after injury but the data in humans are less convincing. Frostbitten tissues unfortunately are often neglected and with thawing become macerated; if this is the situation, the method of rewarming is not important. The method of rewarming has been a matter of controversy. It seems most rational to warm the core of the body before treating the local area of frostbite. Following restoration of the core temperature to normal, warming of a frostbitten limb should begin in water at 50 to 59°F (10 to 15°C), which is then increased 9°F (5°C) every 5 min to a maximum of 104°F (40°C).

Once the frost-bitten limb has been rewarmed, treatment should be conservative and consists of bed rest, elevation of the injured part, tetanus toxoid administration, and use of antibiotics if infection is present; early drainage of blebs and bullae; daily washes with chlorhexidine or an iodophor; and early institution of physiotherapy. Alcohol and cigarettes are strongly contraindicated. Surgical amputation and reconstruction is usually not necessary. Regional sympathectomy performed 24 to 48 h after thawing has not been of value in acute frostbite although it has prevented some late complications, and recurrent episodes of cold injury in individuals who have been reexposed. The effect of regional sympathectomy is probably due to ablation of persistent vasospasm and to restoration of cold perception. Intraarterial reserpine has effects similar to sympathectomy.

Some patients with frostbite have residua consisting of excessive sweating, pain, cold feet, numbness, abnormal color, and pain in the joints. The symptoms are generally worse in the winter and following exposure to cold. These patients also often show abnormal nails, discoloration and pigmentation, hyperhydrosis, and, by x-ray, osteoporosis and cystic defects near the joints. These abnormalities tend to be milder in patients who have had sympathetic blockade. Most cold injuries are preventable by graded exposure to cold, as well as appropriate clothing in freezing temperatures.

REFERENCES

Temperature regulation

BERNHEIM HA et al: Fever: pathogenesis, pathophysiology and purpose. Ann Int Med 91:261, 1979

BRENGELMAN G: Temperature regulation, in *Physiology and Biophysics*, TC Ruch, HD Patton (eds). Philadelphia, Saunders, 1973

DINARELLO CA, WOLFF SM: Molecular basis of fever in humans. Am J Med 72:799, 1982

EDELMAN IS: Thyroid thermogenesis. N Engl J Med 290:1303, 1974

Heat injury

BRITT BA: Etiology and pathophysiology of malignant hyperthermia. Fed Proc 38:44, 1979

CLOWES GHA JR, O'DONNEL TF JR: Current concepts: Heat stroke. N Engl J Med 291:564, 1974

CAROFF SN: The neuroleptic malignant syndrome. J Clin Psych 41:79, 1980

COSTRINI AM et al: Cardiovascular and metabolic manifestations of heat stroke and severe heat exhaustion. Am J Med 66:296, 1979

GRONERT GA: Malignant hyperthermia. Anesthesiology 53:395, 1980

HANSON PG, ZIMMERMAN SW: Exertional heat stroke in novice runners. JAMA 242:159, 1979

MCPHERSON EW, TAYLOR CA JR: The King syndrome: Malignant hyperthermia, myopathy and multiple anomalies. Am J Med Genet 8:159, 1981

SHIBOLET S et al: Heat stroke: A review. Aviat Space Environ Med 47:280, 1976

SPRUNG CL et al: The metabolic and respiratory alterations of heat stroke. Arch Intern Med 140:665, 1980

WILLNER JH et al: Increased myophosphorylase A in malignant hyperthermia. N Engl J Med 303:138, 1980

——— et al: High skeletal muscle adenylate cyclase in malignant hyperthermia. J Clin Invest 68:1119, 1981

WYNDHAM CH: Heat stroke and hyperthermia in marathon runners. Ann NY Acad Sci 301:128, 1977

Cold injury

BOUWMAN DL et al: Early sympathetic blockade for frostbite—Is it of value? J Trauma 20:744, 1980

GAGE AM: Frostbite. Trauma and Emergency Med 7:25, 1981

MACLEAN D et al: Metabolic aspects of spontaneous recovery in accidental hypothermia and hypothermic myxedema. Q J Med (n.s.) 43:371, 1974.

SOUTHWICK FS, DALGLISH PH JR: Recovery after prolonged asystolic cardiac arrest in profound hypothermia. JAMA 243:1250, 1980

VAUGHN PB: Local cold injury—Menace to military operations: A review. Military Med 143:305, 1980

WHITTLE JL, BATES JH: Thermoregulatory failure secondary to acute illness: Complications and treatment. Arch Intern Med 139:418, 1979

WICKSTROM P et al: Accidental hypothermia. Am J Surg 131:622, 1976

9 CHILLS AND FEVER

ROBERT G. PETERSDORF

Omitting disorders which may involve cerebral thermoregulatory centers directly, such as brain tumors, intracranial hemorrhage or thrombosis, or heat stroke, the following disease states may be accompanied by fever:

1 All *infections,* whether caused by bacteria, rickettsias, chlamydia, viruses, or parasites, cause fever.
2 *Mechanical trauma,* e.g., a crushing injury, frequently gives rise to fever lasting 1 or 2 days. Not infrequently, however, complicating infection sets in.
3 Many *neoplastic diseases* are associated with fever. In most patients, fever in patients with cancer is related to obstruction or infection produced by the tumor. In some solid tumors, however, fever may be due to the tumor per se, particularly following metastasis to the liver. Tumors which are associated with fever include hypernephroma, carcinoma of the pancreas, lung, or bone, and hepatoma. In tumors of the reticuloendothelial system, including Hodgkin's disease, non-Hodgkin's lymphoma, acute leukemias, and malignant histiocytosis, fever may be one of the prominent early manifestations.
4 *Hematopoietic disorders,* e.g., acute hemolytic episodes, may be characterized by pyrexia.
5 *Vascular accidents* of any magnitude, e.g., myocardial, pulmonary, and cerebral infarctions, nearly always cause fever.
6 *Diseases due to immune mechanisms* are almost always febrile. These include the connective tissue diseases, drug fevers, and fever due to other immunologic abnormalities.
7 Certain *acute metabolic disorders,* such as gout, porphyria, hypertriglyceridemia, Fabry's disease, and Addisonian or thyroid crises, sometimes are associated with fever.

ACCOMPANIMENTS OF FEVER **Systemic symptoms** The perception of fever by patients varies enormously. Some persons can tell with considerable accuracy whether their body temperatures are elevated; others, especially patients with tuberculosis, may be wholly unaware of body temperature as high as 103°F (39.4°C). Often, patients may pay no attention to fever because of other unpleasant symptoms such as headache and pleuritic pain. Pain in the back, generalized myalgias, and arthralgia without arthritis are commonly associated with fever. Whether these symptoms reflect the presence of an infectious agent or are merely a nonspecific accompaniment of pyrexia is not clear.

Chills Abrupt onset of fever with a *chill* or *rigor* is characteristic of some diseases and, in the absence of antipyretic drugs, rare in others. Although repeated rigors are typical of pyogenic infection with bacteremia, a similar pattern of fever may occur in noninfectious diseases such as lymphoma. It is important to differentiate a true chill, which is accompanied by teeth chattering and bed shaking, from the chilly sensation which occurs in almost all fevers, particularly those in viral infections. In some instances, however, a true rigor occurs in viremia. Chills may be evoked or perpetuated by the intermittent administration of aspirin or other antipyretics. These agents may cause a sharp depression in temperature, which is followed by compensatory involuntary muscular contractions, i.e., a chill. This unpleasant side effect of antipyretic drugs can be averted by administering these agents no less frequently than every 3 h, around the clock, rather than by prescribing them only for elevations in temperature above a certain level.

Herpes labialis So-called fever blisters result from activation of latent herpes simplex virus infection by elevations in temperature. For reasons which are obscure, fever blisters are common in pneumococcal infections, streptococcosis, malaria, meningococcemia, and rickettsioses but are rare in mycoplasma pneumonia, tuberculosis, brucellosis, smallpox, and typhoid.

Delirium This may result from elevation of body temperature and is particularly common in patients with alcoholism, cerebral arteriosclerosis, or senility.

Convulsions These are frequent in febrile children, especially those with a family history of epilepsy, although febrile convulsions do not, in general, reflect serious cerebral disease.

CLINICAL IMPORTANCE OF FEVER The temperature is a simple, objective, and accurate indicator of a physiologic state and is much less subject to external and psychogenic stimuli than the other vital signs, such as pulse, respiratory rate, and blood pressure. For these reasons, determination of the body temperature assists in estimating the severity of an illness, its course and duration, and the effect of therapy, or even in deciding whether a person has an organic illness.

Benefit of fever There are a few infections of humans in which pyrexia appears definitely to be beneficial to the host, such as neurosyphilis, some forms of chronic arthritis, and widespread cancer. Certain other diseases, such as uveitis and rheumatoid arthritis, sometimes improve after fever therapy. There is some experimental evidence that fever, associated with release of endogenous pyrogen, leads to activation of T cells and presumably enhanced host defenses. Aged and debilitated patients with infection may have little or no fever, and this is generally interpreted as a bad prognostic sign. In the great majority of infectious diseases, however, there is no reason to believe that pyrexia accelerates phagocytosis, antibody formation, or other defense mechanisms.

Detrimental aspects of fever Fever accelerates many metabolic processes and accentuates weight loss and nitrogen wastage. The work and the rate of the heart are increased. Sweating aggravates loss of salt and water. There may be discomfort due to headache, photophobia, general malaise, or unpleasant sensation of warmth. Fever may precipitate seizures in epileptic patients. The rigors and profuse sweats of hectic fevers are particularly unpleasant for the patient. In elderly individuals with overt or potential cardiac or cerebral vascular disease, fever may be particularly deleterious.

MANAGEMENT OF FEVER Since fever ordinarily does little harm and imposes no great discomfort, antipyretic drugs are rarely essential to patient welfare and may obfuscate the effect of a specific therapeutic agent or of the natural course of the disease. There are situations, however, in which lowering of the body temperature is of vital importance; e.g., heat stroke, postoperative hyperthermia, delirium due to hyperpyrexia, epileptic seizures, or shock associated with fever and heart failure. Under these circumstances lowering the temperature is indicated. Cooling blankets which can be set at hypothermic temperatures are a highly effective means for external cooling. Alternatively, sponging the body surface with cool saline solution or the application of cool compresses to the skin and forehead may be employed. There is no advantage in sponging with alcohol, which, because of its pungent odor, makes some patients ill. When high internal temperature is combined with cutaneous vasoconstriction, as in heat stroke or postoperative hyperthermia, the cooling measures should be combined with massage of the skin in order to bring blood to the surface, where it may be cooled. Immediate immersion in a tub of ice water should be considered a lifesaving emergency procedure in patients with heat stroke if the internal body temperature is in excess of 108°F (42.2°C). If cooling blankets are available, they are preferable to immersion in ice in most instances.

Antipyretic drugs, such as aspirin (0.3 to 0.6 g) or acetaminophen (0.5 g), are often employed in lowering temperature, particularly if patients are uncomfortable or if fever poses a high risk to them, as is the case in patients with heart failure, febrile seizures (usually children), head injury, mental disorders, or pregnancy. Antipyretics are sometimes associated with unpleasant diaphoresis, an alarming fall in blood pressure, and the subsequent return of fever occasionally accompanied by a chill. These can be mitigated by enforcing a liberal fluid intake and by administering the drugs regularly and frequently at 2- to 3-h intervals. Although adrenal steroids are also potent antipyretics, they must be used with caution because of their tendency to precipitate abrupt falls in temperature accompanied by hypotension. The capacity of these drugs to mask other manifestations of infection also constitutes a relative contraindication to their use.

The discomfort of a rigor can be alleviated in many patients by the intravenous injection of calcium salts. This procedure will stop the shivering and chilliness but has no influence on the ultimate height of the fever. Severe disruptive rigors sometimes need to be abolished with morphine sulfate (10 to 15 mg subcutaneously) or with parenteral chlorpromazine.

DIAGNOSTIC CONSIDERATIONS IN FEVER In many illnesses fever is the most prominent and often the only manifestation of disease. It is not an indication of any particular type of disease; rather it should be considered a reaction to injury comparable with an elevated leukocyte count or a rapid erythrocyte sedimentation rate.

Definitions of fever Fever is classically described as intermittent, remittent, sustained, and relapsing. In *intermittent fever* the temperature falls to normal each day. When the variation between the peak and the nadir is very large, the fever is called *hectic* or *septic.* Intermittent fevers are characteristic in pyogenic infections, particularly abscesses, lymphomas, and miliary tuberculosis. In *remittent fever* the temperature falls each day but does not return to normal. Most fevers are remittent, and this type of febrile response is not characteristic of any disease. A *sustained fever* is characterized by persistent elevation without significant diurnal variation. It is exemplified by the fever of untreated typhoid or typhus. With *relapsing fever* short febrile periods occur between one or several days of normal temperature. Examples of relapsing fever are:

Malaria (see Chap. 218) had vanished from the United States almost completely, but for several years Vietnam war veterans constituted an important and sizable reservoir of this infection, as do other persons recently arrived from foreign countries. It is most unusual, however, for malaria to recur after a symptom-free interval of 1 year or more. Febrile bouts recur at 2- or 3-day intervals, or more irregularly in falciparum infections, depending on the maturation cycle of the parasite. The diagnosis depends on demonstration of the parasites in the blood.

Relapsing fever (see Chap. 180) occurs in the southwest part of the United States, as far east as Texas, and in many other parts of the world. The recurrences are related to the cyclic development of parasites. Diagnosis is by demonstration of the spirochetal organisms in stained films of the blood.

Rat-bite fever (see Chap. 161) is brought about by two agents—*Spirillum minus* and *Streptobacillus moniliformis,* both transmitted by the bite of a rat. Both may cause an illness characterized by periodic exacerbations of fever. The clue to the diagnosis depends on obtaining a history of rat bite 1 to 10 weeks prior to the onset of symptoms. The cause can be established by appropriate laboratory procedures.

Localized *pyogenic infections* in rare instances give rise to periodic bouts of fever separated by afebrile and relatively symptom-free intervals. The so-called Charcot's intermittent biliary fever, i.e., cholangitis with biliary obstruction due to stones, is an example. *Urinary tract infection,* with episodes of ureteral obstruction due to small stones or inspissated pus, can also cause recurrent fever.

A few patients with Hodgkin's disease at some time have so-called Pel-Ebstein fever—bouts of fever lasting 3 to 10 days, separated by afebrile and asymptomatic periods of 3 to 10 days. These cycles may be repeated regularly over a period of several months. In rare instances this periodicity of the fever has been sufficiently striking to suggest the correct diagnosis before lymphadenopathy or splenomegaly became evident. However, relapsing fevers indistinguishable from Pel-Ebstein fever usually have causes other than Hodgkin's disease.

Epidemiology of fever The diagnosis of febrile illnesses must take into consideration the context of the epidemiologic setting. For example, an acute febrile illness in southeast Asia or Africa is probably due to one of the arboviruses (see Chap. 208) or malaria (see Chap. 218); in a college student in the United States it may result from infectious mononucleosis or some other viral infection; and in an octogenarian following prostatectomy it is probably an indication of urinary tract infection, wound infection, pulmonary infarction, or aspiration pneumonia. In children, infections are more likely to be responsible for prolonged fevers than in adults. Likewise, travelers returning from short trips to foreign countries are much more likely to have febrile illnesses indigenous to their home than to the foreign country they have visited.

Rare versus common diseases Most of the time fever is a manifestation of a common disease, and fever associated with a pulmonary infiltrate is much more likely to be due to pneumococcal than to pneumocystis pneumonia. Failure to appreciate this cardinal principle has led to many prolonged and futile diagnostic workups.

Febrile illnesses of short duration Acute febrile illnesses of less than 2 weeks' duration are common in medical practice. In many instances they run their course, progressing to complete recovery, and a precise diagnosis is not made. In most instances, however, it is safe to assume that the illness is of infectious origin. Although short febrile illnesses may be noninfectious (e.g., allergic fevers due to drugs, thromboembolic disease, hemolytic crises, or gout), they are decidedly in the minority.

Most undiagnosed acute febrile infectious diseases are probably viral and remain undiagnosed because diagnostic methods are unavailable, cumbersome, or not cost-effective. It is not practical to carry out tests needed to identify all the known viruses, and, furthermore, there must be a considerable number of still unidentified viruses pathogenic for humans. In bacterial infections, on the other hand, laboratory diagnosis is simpler, and these infections are often rapidly controlled with chemotherapy.

The following characteristics, though not restricted solely to acute infections, are highly suggestive that infection is present:

1 Abrupt onset
2 High fever, i.e., 102 to 105°F (38.9 to 40.6°C), with or without chills
3 Respiratory symptoms—sore throat, coryza, cough
4 Severe malaise, with muscle or joint pain, photophobia, pain on movement of the eyes, headache
5 Nausea, vomiting, or diarrhea
6 Acute enlargement of lymph nodes or spleen

7 Meningeal signs, with or without spinal fluid pleocytosis
8 Leukocyte count above 12,000 or below 5000 per cubic millimeter
9 Dysuria, frequency, and flank pain

None of the symptoms or signs listed is encountered only in infection. Many of these features could be seen in acute leukemia or in disseminated lupus erythematosus. Nevertheless, in a given instance of acute febrile illness with some of or all the manifestations listed, the probabilities strongly favor infection, and the patient may be given reasonable reassurance that he or she will probably recover in a week or two, regardless of a precise diagnosis.

It is desirable, of course, to establish an accurate diagnosis, and whatever steps are practicable in the circumstances to establish the cause should be taken. Cultures of the throat, blood, urine, or feces should be obtained before institution of antibacterial chemotherapy. Skin and/or serologic tests should be carried out when indicated.

There is a tendency to rely immediately and excessively on the laboratory in ascertaining the cause of fever. In many instances, a thorough history and a complete and, if necessary, repeated physical examination, along with a complete blood count (CBC), urinalysis, and sedimentation rate will provide the answer. Often a little patience, in the form of watchful waiting, before plunging into an expensive and extensive laboratory workup, will lead to the diagnosis.

Prolonged febrile illnesses Some of the knottiest problems in the field of internal medicine are found in cases of prolonged fever in which the diagnosis remains obscure for weeks or even months. Eventually, however, the true nature of the illness usually reveals itself, since a disease which causes injury sufficient to evoke temperature elevations to 101°F (38.3°C) or higher for several weeks does not often subside without leaving some clue as to its nature. The elucidation of problems of this sort calls for skillful application of all diagnostic methods—careful history, thorough physical examination, and the carefully considered use of laboratory examinations and imaging techniques.

FEVER OF UNKNOWN ORIGIN In some patients fever becomes the dominant sign or symptom in a patient's illness, and when its cause escapes detection it is defined as fever of unknown origin (FUO). It is appropriate to use this term only in patients who have elevations in temperature [>101°F (38.3°C)] for a prolonged period (at least 2, and preferably 3, weeks) and in whom the diagnosis cannot be made during at least 1 week of intensive study. These rigid criteria eliminate from this diagnostic category patients with common bacterial or viral infections, those in whom the diagnosis is obvious, and those whose fever is due to a sequential occurrence of etiologically unrelated diseases. An example is a patient who is febrile following a myocardial infarction, who then develops thrombophlebitis that is associated with fever, and in whom this is followed by multiple pulmonary emboli, also a febrile disease. Much of the confusion in the literature concerning causes of FUO is due to failure to define the criteria employed in classifying patients who have had fever of unknown origin.

DISEASES CAUSING PROLONGED FEVERS Table 9-1 lists some of the diseases responsible for prolonged fever. Some of these disorders must initially be considered to be FUO; in others the diagnosis comes to mind readily.

Infections Infections occupy a less prominent position among causes of prolonged fever now than formerly because of the common practice of administering antibiotics to any patient in whom fever persists for more than a few days. Consequently, many infections are eradicated by more or less "blind" therapy without accurate determination of their nature or location. In the 1950s, patients with infections comprised about 40 percent of patients with FUO, but in a comparable series collected in the 1970s this figure had fallen to 32 percent, while neoplasms had risen from 20 to 33 percent.

ABSCESSES Abscesses are the most common form of infection presenting as FUO and are important because they can be cured with early diagnosis and treatment, while failure to make the diagnosis may eventuate fatally. These abscesses usually arise in the abdomen or pelvis including the subphrenic space, the liver or spleen, or a ruptured diverticulum or appendix. Ultrasonography, liver-spleen scan, or CT scan, should provide the diagnosis in most instances. Laparotomy is usually necessary to confirm the diagnosis and to achieve cure.

MYCOBACTERIAL INFECTIONS Although less common than formerly, mycobacterial infections, such as tuberculosis (see Chap. 174) and, less commonly, atypical mycobacterial infections (see Chap. 176), cause FUO. These infections are more common among blacks, native Americans, southeast Asians, and individuals from outside the United States. Most of these infections are extrapulmonary and involve the bones, lymph nodes, genital or urinary organs, peritoneum, or liver. Extrapulmonary or miliary tuberculosis may not be detectable by x-ray until late in the course. Many of these patients are debilitated and have overwhelming disease. Despite this, the diagnosis, which is usually made by biopsy of lymph nodes or involved tissue, is essential because these patients respond well to treatment, particularly with bactericidal drugs such as isoniazid and rifampin.

RENAL INFECTIONS Ordinary pyelonephritis is rarely accompanied by prolonged fever; if pyrexia occurs in these patients, intrarenal or extrarenal obstruction should be considered. Ureteral obstruction by either a mass of leukocytes or renal epithelium, as in papillary necrosis, may be accompanied by prolonged fever. Prostatic abscess should be considered in males. These patients may not have dysuria or rectal pain.

OTHER BACTERIAL INFECTIONS These include sinusitis, vertebral osteomyelitis (usually occurring in association with chronic bacteruria, and more easily diagnosed by bone scan), infected intravenous or intraarterial catheters, and retroperitoneal infection such as aneurysms that have become filled with organizing clot and debris that have become secondarily infected. Enteric pathogens (including *Escherichia coli*, bacteroides, and *Salmonella*), have been isolated frequently from patients with such infections. Surgery is mandatory for both diagnosis and therapy. In addition, some patients with dissecting aneurysms have fever without superimposed infections.

BACTERIAL ENDOCARDITIS Perhaps because of a high index of suspicion, the ubiquitous use of blood cultures, and the indiscriminate use of antibiotics, which must cure some patients, bacterial endocarditis has become a rare cause of FUO. Similarly, bacteremia due to *Neisseria, Salmonella,* and *Brucella* rarely cause FUO.

IATROGENIC INFECTIONS These include catheter infections, infected arteriovenous fistulas, and sometimes ordinary wound infections in obscure locations. Usually, their cure requires removal of a foreign body in addition to antimicrobial therapy.

VIRAL, RICKETTSIAL, AND CHLAMYDIAL INFECTIONS These are rarely the cause of prolonged fevers, but occasionally patients with Epstein-Barr or cytomegalovirus infections may have febrile illnesses, which are often characterized by spontaneous remissions and exacerbations. Cytomegalovirus (with or without *Pneumocystis*) is becoming a progressively more common cause of prolonged fever in immunocompromised hosts. In them, it should not pose a diagnostic problem, but an infectious mononucleosis-like syndrome or postperfusion fever in otherwise healthy patients may be difficult diagnostic dilemmas. Since these patients are generally not very ill and improve spontaneously, they should not be subjected to prolonged, expensive FUO workups. *Psittacosis* may look much like typhoid fever, and *Q-fever endocarditis* has been a particularly puzzling and lethal illness that must be treated both with antibiotics and valve replacement.

PARASITIC DISEASES Amebiasis presents as an FUO, either in the form of diffuse hepatitis or liver abscess. The diagnosis of malaria demands a history of recent exposure.

Neoplasms HODGKIN'S DISEASE Fever may be the principal symptom and only objective finding early in the course of Hodgkin's disease, especially because patients with this disease who present with FUO usually have intraabdominal or retroperitoneal disease. The diagnosis is usually made by biopsy or staging laparotomy. It is important to arrive at the diagnosis early because, with proper chemotherapy, prolonged remissions may be achieved.

LYMPHOMA-LIKE SYNDROMES Several disease entities have been described which are clinically and histologically similar to non-Hodgkin's lymphoma but which may have a better prognosis or respond differently to steroids and antitumor agents. Among these entities, all of which may present as FUOs, are immunoblastic lymphadenopathy, lymphadenoid granulomatosis, acute megakaryocytic myelosis, and, in children, the mucocutaneous lymph node syndrome (Kawasaki's disease). These diseases are discussed more fully in Chap. 56.

NON-HODGKIN'S LYMPHOMA These illnesses usually present with fever, nonspecific symptoms, and lymphadenopathy which the patient recognizes. Hepatosplenomegaly and bone pain and tenderness are common. The laboratory findings usu-

TABLE 9-1
Common disease entities in the United States causing prolonged fever

- *I* Infections
  - *A* Granulomatous infections
    - *1* Tuberculosis
    - *2* Deep-seated fungus infections
    - *3* Atypical mycobacterial infections
  - *B* Pyogenic infections
    - *1* Upper abdominal infections
      - *a* Cholecystitis (stone), empyema of gallbladder
      - *b* Cholangitis
      - *c* Liver abscess
      - *d* Lesser sac abscess
      - *e* Subphrenic abscess
      - *f* Splenic abscess
    - *2* Lower abdominal infections
      - *a* Diverticulitis (± abscess)
      - *b* Appendicitis
    - *3* Pelvic inflammatory disease
    - *4* Urinary tract infections
      - *a* Pyelonephritis (rare)
      - *b* Intrarenal abscess
      - *c* Perinephric abscess
      - *d* Ureteral obstruction
      - *e* Prostatic abscess
    - *5* Sinusitis
    - *6* Osteomyelitis
  - *C* Intravascular infections
    - *1* Bacterial endocarditis (acute and subacute)
    - *2* Intravascular catheter infections
  - *D* Bacteremias without overt primary focus
    - *1* Meningococcemia
    - *2* Gonococcemia
    - *3* Vibriosis
    - *4* Listeriosis
    - *5* Brucellosis
    - *6* Coliform bacteremia in patients with cirrhosis
  - *E* Viral, rickettsial, and chlamydial infections
    - *1* Infectious mononucleosis
    - *2* Cytomegalovirus
    - *3* Hepatitis
    - *4* Group B coxsackievirus diseases
    - *5* Q fever (including endocarditis)
    - *6* Psittacosis
  - *F* Parasitic diseases
    - *1* Amebiasis
    - *2* Malaria
    - *3* Trichinosis
  - *G* Spirochetal infections
    - *1* Leptospirosis
    - *2* Relapsing fever
- *II* Neoplasms
  - *A* Solid (localized)
    - *1* Kidney
    - *2* Lung
    - *3* Pancreas
    - *4* Liver
    - *5* Large bowel
    - *6* Atrial myxoma
  - *B* Metastatic
    - *1* From gastrointestinal tract
    - *2* From lung, kidneys, bone, cervix, ovary
    - *3* Melanoma
    - *4* Sarcoma
  - *C* Tumors of the reticuloendothelial system
    - *1* Hodgkin's disease
    - *2* Non-Hodgkin's lymphoma
    - *3* Malignant histiocytosis
    - *4* Immunoblastic lymphadenopathy
    - *5* Lymphomatoid granulomatosis
    - *6* Mucocutaneous lymph node syndrome (children)
- *III* Connective tissue disease
  - *A* Rheumatic fever
  - *B* Systemic lupus erythematosus
  - *C* Rheumatoid arthritis (particularly Still's disease)
  - *D* Giant-cell arteritis (polymyalgia rheumatica)
  - *E* Hypersensitivity vasculitis
  - *F* Periarteritis nodosa
  - *G* Wegener's granulomatosis
  - *H* Panaortitis
- *IV* Granulomatus diseases
  - *A* Crohn's disease (regional enteritis)
  - *B* Granulomatous hepatitis
  - *C* Sarcoidosis
  - *D* Erythema nodosum
- *V* Miscellaneous
  - *A* Drug fever
  - *B* Pulmonary emboli
  - *C* Thyroiditis
  - *D* Hemolytic states
  - *E* Cryptic trauma with bleeding into enclosed spaces (hematomas)
  - *F* Dissecting aneurysm (with or without infection)
  - *G* Whipple's disease
- *VI* Metabolic and inherited diseases
  - *A* Familial Mediterranean fever
  - *B* Hypertriglyceridemia and hypercholesterolemia
  - *C* Fabry's disease
- *VII* Psychogenic fevers
  - *A* Habitual hyperthermia
  - *B* Factitious fever
- *VIII* Periodic fevers (e.g., cyclic neutropenia)
- *IX* Thermoregulatory disorders
- *X* Undiagnosed
  - *A* Resolved
    - *1* Without treatment
    - *2* With antibiotics
    - *3* With anti-inflammatory drugs
  - *B* Recurrent
    - *1* Suppressed with steroids

ally consist of anemia, leukocytosis, and atypical lymphocytosis. The diagnosis is usually made by lymph node biopsy, but biopsies are often mistaken for reactive hyperplasia or atypical lymphocytic infiltrates, at least initially. Survival after the diagnosis is made is disappointingly short, despite transient improvement following radiation and chemotherapy.

MALIGNANT HISTIOCYTOSIS This is a rare infiltrative disease, with a poor prognosis that presents with fever, wasting, generalized lymphadenopathy, and hepatosplenomegaly. The bone marrow, lung, and skin may also be involved by this rapidly progressing illness. There tends to be anemia, leukopenia, and thrombocytopenia, or a combination of the three. Biopsied tissue is often difficult to diagnose definitively but a rapidly progressive febrile illness, and the presence of large, malignant, primitive reticuloendothelial cells with histiocytic predominance and erythrophagocytosis should yield the answer.

LEUKEMIAS It is not uncommon for acute leukemia to be mistaken for acute infection at the onset. The acute leukemias are nearly always accompanied by fever, sometimes as high as 105°F (40.6°C). The diagnosis is characteristically delayed by the absence of blast cells in the blood or bone marrow. However, the patients are usually anemic and leukopenic and often have been labeled as having preleukemia. Chronic lymphatic or granulocytic leukemia may be characterized by fever, but such fever is usually due to concomitant infection. Because of the typical changes in circulating leukocytes, fever does not often cause a diagnostic problem. Before it is assumed that fever in a patient with leukemia is due to the blood dyscrasia, infection must be ruled out by appropriate tests and cultures, and attempts to treat the "most likely" pathogen must be made.

SOLID TUMORS An invariable feature of solid tumors causing FUO is the presence of tumor in the abdomen. These patients are usually older; the diagnosis is characteristically made by laparotomy which is directed to the proper location on the basis of history, physical examination, and noninvasive studies. The sites of the primary vary widely and include the kidney, liver, pancreas, stomach, pleura, lung, and bowel. Not surprisingly, survival is short.

ATRIAL MYXOMA Patients with changing heart murmurs, peripheral embolic phenomena, and joint pains are usually suspected of having bacterial endocarditis, rheumatic fever, or occasionally some other connective tissue disease. In the face of persistence of these symptoms and signs without a positive diagnosis, two-dimensional echocardiography and, if the echocardiogram is positive, angiography should be performed with the possibility that an atrial myxoma may be responsible.

Connective tissue disease RHEUMATIC FEVER Perhaps because of the common use of immunologic diagnostic tests, connective tissue diseases now form a smaller part of FUO series. For example, both rheumatic fever and disseminated lupus erythematosus are notorious by their absence.

RHEUMATOID ARTHRITIS In its classic form, this disease is not difficult to recognize, but in certain patients who initially have FUO, arthritis is absent early in the course of the illness; these patients have primarily fever, hepatosplenomegaly, lymphadenopathy, evanescent rashes, anemia, and leukocytosis. Joint changes do not appear until late in the disease. This disease usually occurs in young adults and may be considered the adult counterpart of juvenile rheumatoid disease. The diagnosis is made usually only after prolonged observation, in part because serologic tests for rheumatoid disease are characteristically negative. The prognosis is generally good, and patients respond well to aspirin, nonsteroidal anti-inflammatory drugs, or steroids. Lyme arthritis has sometimes caused confusion in the diagnosis (see Chap. 353).

GIANT-CELL ARTERITIS (POLYMYALGIA RHEUMATICA) This is a disease of elderly persons who complain of fever, headache, and pain in the muscles and joints. Overt arthritis is unusual. At times, fever is the only symptom, and there are no abnormal physical findings. The sedimentation rate tends to be very rapid, and there may be anemia, leukocytosis, or eosinophilia. Occasionally, the temporal or occipital arteries are inflamed and tender, but usually they are normal. In either instance, the diagnosis must be made by temporal artery biopsy. There may be accompanying visual defects or blindness because of involvement of the retinal artery. This disease responds extremely well to steroids, which may be used as a therapeutic trial.

OTHER CONNECTIVE TISSUE DISEASES These include classical periarteritis nodosa, with or without hepatitis B infection, a disease that classically involves small and medium-sized arteries as well as large vessel disease of the aorta and its main branches (see Chap. 69).

Granulomatous diseases SARCOIDOSIS Ordinarily, fever is not characteristic of sarcoidosis, but it is prominent in a minority of cases, especially those characterized by arthralgia, hilar lymphadenopathy, and cutaneous lesions resembling erythema nodosum, or in those with extensive hepatic lesions. The diagnosis is suggested by lymphoid enlargement, ocular lesions, and hyperglobulinemia and is clinched by biopsy of skin, lymph nodes, muscle, and liver. The diagnosis may be obfuscated by the presence of erythema nodosum or other vascular rashes long before granulomas are found.

REGIONAL ENTERITIS Inflammatory lesions of the large and small intestine rarely present as FUO, but an occasional patient who has only fever, abdominal pain, recurrent bouts of diarrhea, or subtle changes in bowel habits which may indicate low-grade obstruction will be found to have regional enteritis. Likewise, Whipple's disease may make itself known by fever, without arthritis or malabsorption.

GRANULOMATOUS HEPATITIS This disease of unknown etiology is a relatively common cause of FUO. It is probably a manifestation of hypersensitivity, perhaps to penicillin. Liver biopsy shows only nonspecific granulomas. The fever generally subsides spontaneously over a period of weeks or months. Sometimes defervescence can be achieved with anti-inflammatory drugs or steroids, but because the diagnosis of tuberculosis cannot be ruled out completely, patients in whom steroid therapy is given should also be given antituberculous medication.

Miscellaneous causes of fever DRUG FEVER This is an important cause of cryptic fever; a careful history of drug intake should be taken in every patient with unexplained fever. Fever due to allergy to one of the antibiotics may become superimposed on the fever of the infection for which the drug was given, resulting in a very confused picture. Often, fever is due to common drugs, including sulfonamides, bromides, arsenicals, iodides, thiouracils, barbiturates, and laxatives, especially those containing phenolphthalein. Any questions of drug fever can be resolved rapidly by discontinuing all medications. The diagnosis can be further substantiated by giving a test dose of the drug after fever has subsided, but this may result in a very unpleasant or even dangerous reaction.

MULTIPLE PULMONARY EMBOLI Multiple pulmonary emboli are decreasing as a cause of FUO; in fact, in one series, they were overdiagnosed. Nevertheless, symptomless thrombosis of deep calf or pelvic veins may cause prolonged febrile illness either because of the thrombophlebitis or as a result of repeated small pulmonary emboli. These emboli may not be manifested by pleuritic pain or hemoptysis, but cough, dyspnea, and vague thoracic discomfort are likely to be present. Lung scans and venography should reveal the diagnosis. Sometimes these patients present with a nephrotic syndrome due to renal vein thrombosis. Pelvic thrombophlebitis with or without pulmonary emboli is an important cause of FUO in postpartum patients.

HEMOLYTIC EPISODES Most hemolytic diseases are characterized by bouts of fever, and acute hemolytic crises may give rise to shaking chills and marked elevations of temperature. The difficulty sometimes encountered in differentiating sickle cell disease from acute rheumatic fever is well known. The presence of these hemolytic disorders is suggested by the more rapid development of anemia than occurs in other febrile illnesses and by the usual accompaniment of reticulocytosis and jaundice. Fever is not characteristic of severe anemia due to external blood loss or of the anemia of uremia.

CRYPTIC HEMATOMAS Blood in closed spaces such as sites of remote trauma, particularly in the perisplenic area, in the pericardium, or in the retroperitoneal area, particularly in patients receiving anticoagulants, are among the sites in which accumulated old blood has resulted in prolonged fever. The diagnosis is important because evacuation of the clot is often curative.

NONSPECIFIC PERICARDITIS Occasionally, this entity escapes diagnosis and presents as an FUO.

FAMILIAL MEDITERRANEAN FEVER (see Chap. 236) Either the disease is decreasing in incidence, or it is being recognized more readily.

THERMOREGULATORY DISORDERS Rare patients have fever due to an abnormality in their temperature-regulating mechanism. They may be febrile without any other cause or may have exaggerated responses in temperature during the course of other fever-producing diseases. The diagnosis is made by exclusion. Some patients have responded to chlorpromazine.

Psychogenic fever HABITUAL HYPERTHERMIA Not infrequently, a patient, while not appearing acutely ill, has been subject to elevation of body temperature above the "normal" range level, i.e., temperatures in the range of 99.0 to 100.5°F (37.2 to 38°C). Prolonged low-grade fever may be a manifestation of serious illness, or it may be a matter of no real consequence. Possibly there are some persons whose "normal" temperatures are in this range. However, there is no certain way of identifying such individuals. The possibilities to be considered in such cases vary considerably according to the age groups concerned. A special problem termed *habitual hyperthermia* is encountered in young females. The patient may have temperatures ranging from 99.0 to 100.5°F (37.2 to 38.0°C) regularly or intermittently for years and also usually has a variety of complaints characteristic of psychoneurosis, such as fatigability, insomnia, bowel distress, vague aches, and headache. Prolonged careful study and observation fail to reveal evidence of organic disease. Unfortunately, many of these people go from physician to physician and are subjected to a variety of unpleasant, expensive, and even harmful tests, treatments, and operations. The diagnosis of this syndrome can be made with reasonable certainty after a suitable period of observation and study, and if the patient can be convinced of its validity, a real service will have been rendered.

In a patient past middle age, even low-grade fever should always be regarded as a probable indication of organic disease. The possibilities to be considered in this age group are the same as those discussed earlier under "Prolonged Febrile Illness."

FACTITIOUS FEVER Occasionally, patients will produce purposeful false elevations in temperature. Usually these patients are young women, many of whom are allied health professionals. They fall into two groups—one infects itself with bacteria or other contaminated materials and the second finds a way to cause the thermometer to register higher than the true temperature. If malingering is suspected, all that is necessary to prove it is to repeat the temperature determination immediately after a high reading has been obtained, with someone remaining at the bedside while the thermometer is in place. Other clues to false elevations in the temperature are a dissociation between pulse and temperature, and excessively high fevers [greater than 106°F (41.1°C) in adults] and the absence of chills, sweats, or tachycardia. These patients fall into the psychiatric diagnostic category of "borderline syndrome," a state between neurosis and psychosis, in which the prognosis is guarded. Others, mostly young girls, falsify their temperatures as a means of asking for psychiatric help and do well with psychotherapy.

Patients with FUO who remain undiagnosed These patients divide themselves into several groups. Some have a self-limited, prolonged viral infection that resembles infectious mononucleosis, cytomegalovirus, hepatitis virus or adenovirus infection, but in which these agents are never isolated. They recover spontaneously. Others appear to have responded to antibiotics and can be presumed to have had a cryptic bacterial infection. A third group has a steroid-responsive fever which resembles, but is not diagnostic of, immunologically mediated diseases. Some of these patients eventually no longer require steroids for suppression of fever, but some do not stay free of pyrexia or other inflammatory symptoms without steroids. An occasional elderly patient looks like an example of a superannuated juvenile rheumatoid arthritis (Still's disease).

DIAGNOSTIC PROCEDURES IN FEVER OF UNKNOWN ORIGIN

With so large a number of possibilities, it is obvious that no single plan can be outlined for the systematic study of every problem in unexplained fever. In any given patient, the history, physical examination, and, most importantly, epidemiologic setting must determine the diagnostic approach. If the features suggest infectious disease, the main dependence will be upon bacteriologic methods, whereas when a person in the "cancer age group" has an obscure febrile disorder, the best chance of early diagnosis may lie in x-ray studies, scans, and biopsy.

History Careful attention to the patient's past history and the chronologic development of symptoms may provide important leads. Places of recent residence, contact with domestic or wild animals and birds, preceding acute infectious diseases such as diarrheal illness or boils, and contact with persons with tuberculosis may provide clues to infection. Localizing symptoms may provide a lead to the affected organ system. It is important to query the patient repeatedly. All too often facts of historical importance do not come to light until several interviews have been held.

Physical examination Careful search should be made for skin lesions and for petechial hemorrhages in the ocular fundi, conjunctivas, nail beds, and skin. The lymph nodes should be carefully palpated, with special attention given to the supraclavicular, axillary, and epitrochlear areas. The finding of a heart murmur may be important, particularly if it occurs in diastole. Detection of an abdominal mass may be the first lead to the diagnosis of neoplastic disease. Palpable enlargement of the spleen suggests infection, leukemia, or lymphoma and points away from a diagnosis of solid tumors. Enlargement of the liver and spleen suggests lymphoma, leukemia, chronic infection, or cirrhosis. A large liver without a palpable spleen points to liver abscess or metastatic cancer. The rectum and the female pelvic organs may reveal masses or abscesses; the testicles may reveal tumor or tuberculosis.

Laboratory tests Patients with FUO are subjected to a large number of laboratory tests, often repeatedly and to excess. The following may be useful guidelines in the use of these tests.

HEMATOLOGY These are often abnormal, showing anemia, leukopenia, thrombocytopenia or thrombocytosis, and elevation in the sedimentation rate. They are rarely specific. Blood smears for morphology show many abnormalities but, by virtue of the type of patient who presents with FUO, are rarely diagnostic.

CHEMISTRY These are rarely useful. Even serum enzymes indicating hepatic infiltrative disease such as the alkaline phosphatase or 5′-nucleotidase are often normal even in the presence of liver disease.

IMMUNOLOGIC TESTS These are almost never helpful in the diagnosis of FUO, perhaps because they eliminate patients with immunologic diseases from FUO series.

BACTERIOLOGY Blood cultures rarely contribute to the diagnosis of FUO, and in no instance should more than six blood cultures (which are expensive) be performed on any one patient. Smears and cultures of pus are useful but in sick patients should not delay institution of therapy. Anaerobic cultures should be performed in all abscesses. Mycobacterial cultures continue to be the mainstay in the diagnosis of acid-fast bacilli.

SEROLOGY Serologic testing is useful in cytomegalovirus (CMV) infections and in amebiasis. Routine febrile agglutinins are rarely helpful.

SKIN TESTS These are rarely helpful. Many patients with far-advanced neoplasia had negative skin tests. Patients with disseminated tuberculosis usually have positive tuberculin tests.

Imaging techniques ROENTGENOGRAMS Chest x-rays and intravenous urograms are the most valuable films in the diagnosis of FUO. Review of earlier films, including those performed at other institutions, often turns up important clues when viewed by a fresh observer. Conversely, there is nothing to be gained by repeating earlier films that are technically satisfactory, provided such films were obtained within a reasonable period of time. Sinus and bone films are also often useful. In contrast, gastrointestinal x-rays; oral, intravenous, transhepatic, or retrograde endoscopic cholangiograms; aortograms; and lymphangiograms are helpful only if there are clues that clearly indicate the likelihood of an abnormality in the organ or organ system to be imaged.

ULTRASONOGRAPHY This technique has come into vogue to detect abdominal, renal, retroperitoneal, or pelvic mass lesions. While both false-positive and false-negative results are common, the techniques are still evolving and with further improvement will provide relatively inexpensive, noninvasive screening for masses. It may be the method of choice for imaging the gallbladder and biliary tree.

RADIONUCLIDE SCANS Of all nuclide scans, the technetrium sulfocolloid liver-spleen scan remains the most useful. Gallium scanning, on the other hand, is subject to many false-positive and false-negative tests and has been overrated. Indium 111 leukocyte scanning may be more reliable in the diagnosis of intraabdominal abscesses. Lung scans may reveal pulmonary emboli, and simultaneous liver and lung scans are useful in delineating subphrenic abscess. Bone scans may detect osseous metastases or osteomyelitis more readily than x-rays. Renal scans are helpful in the diagnosis of hypernephroma.

COMPUTERIZED TOMOGRAPHY (CT) SCANS CT scans are likely to be useful in the detection of subphrenic, abdominal, and pelvic abscesses and are the most effective method for imaging the retroperitoneum, which is often the site of the cause of FUO in the form of retroperitoneal lymph nodes, tumors, abscesses, or hematomas. CT scanning is excellent for detecting space-occupying lesions in the liver, although some feel that ultrasound is more effective for visualizing the gallbladder and biliary tree.

Biopsies Often the best means of definitive diagnosis is a biopsy.

Bone marrow biopsy may be helpful not only in clarifying the histologic nature of the marrow but also for occasional demonstration of other disease processes such as metastatic carcinoma or granulomas, and for culture. It is one location where blind sampling is productive.

Needle biopsy of the liver, while often abnormal, has a low diagnostic yield. It is useless in the diagnosis of reticuloendothelial malignancy but is helpful in granulomatous diseases. It rarely yields the diagnosis if there are no abnormalities in liver function tests.

Biopsy of other tissues. Biopsies of tissues that appear abnormal on physical examination or by noninvasive imaging tests are more likely to be helpful in the diagnosis than tissues that are biopsied blindly. These include biopsies of the lung, muscle, skin, gastrointestinal mucosa, bone, and arteries. Occasionally, "blind biopsies" of muscle or temporal artery will yield abnormalities, but even here tenderness of the affected part makes finding an abnormality much more likely.

Lymph node biopsy is helpful in the diagnosis of many diseases, including the lymphomas, metastatic cancer, tuberculosis, and mycotic infections. Inguinal nodes are notoriously unsatisfactory for biopsy and are too frequently chosen because of their easy accessibility. Axillary, cervical, and supraclavicular nodes are much more likely to yield helpful information, and the node excised need not necessarily be large.

Exploratory laparotomy Exploratory laparotomy has been advocated as the most definitive diagnostic maneuver in FUO but is valuable only when other investigations, including history, physical examination, noninvasive imaging techniques, and laboratory data point to the abdomen as a possible source of disease. Laparotomies are most helpful in patients with solid tumors or intraabdominal abscesses. The clues to intraabdominal disease are often subtle, but they are present nonetheless. Blind exploration of the abdomen simply because the diagnosis is obscure is poor practice.

Therapeutic trials It is common practice to give a trial of antibiotics to patients with unidentified febrile disorders. Occasionally, this kind of marksmanship is effective, but in general, blind therapy does more harm than good. Undesirable features include drug toxicity, superinfection due to resistant pathogenic bacteria, and interference with accurate diagnosis by cultural methods. Furthermore, a coincidental fall in temperature not due to therapy is likely to be interpreted as response to treatment, with the conclusion that an infectious disease is present. If therapeutic trials are instituted, they should be as specific as possible. Examples are *isoniazid* or *ethambutol* for tuberculosis; *aspirin* for rheumatic fever; *metronidazole* for hepatic amebiasis; *penicillin* and *gentamicin* for enterococcal endocarditis; and *chloramphenicol* for *Salmonella* bacteremia. Relatively few trials with antibiotics will be successful; those with aspirin, nonsteroidal anti-inflammatory agents, and steroids are more likely to be effective but these drugs should be used with caution and only in patients in whom the likelihood of connective tissue disease is high and in whom granulomas, infection, and cancer have been ruled out as definitively as possible.

Prognosis in FUO The intelligent application of appropriate diagnostic maneuvers should provide the answer in approximately 90 percent of patients with prolonged obscure febrile illness. The mortality rate in patients with FUO is high among elderly patients, particularly since cancer is the most likely cause of the fever in this age group. Fortunately, most of the remaining patients respond to medical or surgical treatment or recover spontaneously. Of those who do come to autopsy (about 10 percent), fewer than half have had potentially curable disease.

A brief philosophy about patients with FUO Many patients are placed in the FUO category because attending physicians overlook, disregard, or reject an obvious clue. This statement implies no malice; it simply means that physicians, being human instruments, are far from perfect. No algorithms or computers are likely to reverse this trend; moreover, even the new technology is not sufficiently sophisticated to sort out the causes of fever in these patients who often present in very atypical fashion.

In order to mitigate these human errors, clinicians have to work harder. This requires repeated histories and physical examinations, frequent chart reviews to look for the "clue" that is there but has not been appreciated, extensive discussion of the problem with colleagues, and last but not least, time spent in quiet contemplation of the clinical enigma. It does not mean yet another barrage of tests, some of which might be painful

and all of which are likely to be expensive, or dousing the patient with more drugs, or, in the absence of corroborating data and as a last resort, subjecting the patient to exploratory surgery. Physicians who care for patients with FUO need to observe them, to talk to them, and to think about them. There are no substitutes for these simple clinical principles.

REFERENCES

ADUAN RP et al: Factitious fever and self-induced infection. Ann Intern Med 90:230, 1979

BUJAK JS et al: Juvenile rheumatoid arthritis present in the adult as fever of unknown origin. Medicine 52:431, 1973

DINARELLO CA, WOLFF SM: *Fever. Current Concepts.* The Upjohn Company, 1980, pp 3–38

FAUCI AS et al: The spectrum of vasculitis: Clinical pathologic, immunologic and therapeutic considerations. Ann Intern Med 89:660, 1978

GHOSE MK et al: Arteritis of the aged (giant cell arteritis) and fever of unexplained origin. Am J Med 60:429, 1976

JACOBY GA, SWARTZ MN: Fever of undetermined origin. N Engl J Med 289:1407, 1973

KLATSKIN G: Hepatic granulomata: Problems in interpretation. Mt Sinai J Med 44:798, 1977

LARSON EB et al: Fever of undetermined origin: The second hundred cases. Medicine, 1982 (in press)

MALMVALL BE et al: The clinical pictures of giant cell arteritis: Temporal arteritis, polymyalgia rheumatica and fever of unknown origin. Postgrad Med 67:141, 1980

McDOUGALL IR et al: Evaluation of 111_{In} leukocyte whole body scanning. Am J Roentgenol 133:849, 1979

McNEIL BJ et al: A prospective study of computed tomography, ultrasound and gallium imaging in patients with fever. Radiology 139:647, 1981

MITCHELL DP et al: Fever of unknown origin: Assessment of the value of percutaneous liver biopsy. Arch Intern Med 137:1001, 1977

PETERSDORF RG, BEESON PB: Fever of unexplained origin: Report of 100 cases. Medicine 40:1, 1961

QUINN MJ et al: Computed tomography of the abdomen in evaluation of patients with fever of unknown origin. Radiology 136:407, 1980

SIMON HB, WOLFF SM: Granulomatous hepatitis and prolonged fever of unknown origin: A study of 13 patients. Medicine 52:1, 1973

WOLFF SM et al: Unusual etiologies of fever and their evaluation. Ann Rev Med 26:277, 1975

section 3 | Alterations in nervous system function

10

APPROACH TO THE PATIENT WITH NERVOUS SYSTEM DISEASE

RAYMOND D. ADAMS

The symptoms and signs of disordered nervous system function, to be described in the following chapters, are probably the most frequent and complicated in all of medicine. A lucid exposition of them is difficult because the more complex phenomena may be viewed from either a *neurologic* or *psychologic* standpoint. The neurologist is inclined to assume that all are manifestations of diseases of the nervous system. The psychiatrist thinks of many of them in terms of abnormal psychologic reactions. Naturally the bias of the author is more toward the neurologic, for it draws on all the principles of medicine and biological science. But each extreme can be criticized. The aim, therefore, in these introductory chapters is lucid description of each of the major symptoms and signs of disordered nervous system function. The most generally accepted explanations in terms of anatomy, physiology, pharmacology, and chemistry will be offered. In discussing some of the most complex and abstruse cerebral derangements, a particular effort will be made to present both the neurologic and psychologic conceptions, for the latter have received much attention in recent years.

A few additional comments concerning the broad field of neuropsychiatry and the overlap between the disciplines of neurology and psychiatry are required. The neurologist has defined disease of the nervous system as any condition that produces a visible lesion. However, it is now recognized that many neurologic disorders which present with severe clinical manifestations lack any demonstrable neuropathologic abnormality, even when scrutinized by the most modern techniques of electron microscopy or neurochemistry (examples are dystonia musculorum deformans, spasmodic torticollis, tardive dyskinesia, Gilles de la Tourette's syndrome). The likelihood that a disorder of neurotransmitter release or of receptor function occurs in these conditions is strong in view of their partial response to newer neuropharmacologic drugs, yet their basic abnormality remains elusive. In several disorders traditionally treated by the psychiatrist, in particular the major psychoses of schizophrenia and of manic-depressive disease, accumulated evidence based on genetic analysis, responses to neuropharmacologic drugs, and documented neuroendocrine-biochemical abnormalities suggest that these, too, are *primary* disorders of nervous system function. This conclusion is supported further by observations that similar psychotic symptomatology can be observed in patients with readily identifiable lesions of the nervous system (neurosyphilis, chronic temporal lobe seizures, brain tumor). Although the major psychoses may one day fall within the general purview of the neurologist, they are at present, because of their psychologic expressions and chronicity, of interest to the psychiatrist. They are discussed in this book in the section on psychiatry (Chaps. 376 and 377).

More difficult conceptual problems for both the neurologist and the psychiatrist are the disorders presumed to be based upon *abnormal psychologic reactions,* defined as a disorder of mental function or of behavior (or manifest as a somatic disease) occasioned by, or associated with, abnormal life experiences, environmental stresses, or social maladjustments; examples include unusually protracted grief, obsessional fear of disease, anxiety over family illness, and persistent neurotic disorders. The latter are discussed in detail in Chap. 375.

There are two areas of neuropsychiatry which are particularly controversial: psychosomatic disorders and the sociopathies. Included under psychosomatic diseases are such conditions as peptic ulcer, Raynaud's disease, ulcerative colitis, asthma, hypertension, hyperthyroidism, "neurodermatitis," rheumatoid arthritis, migraine, and paroxysmal tachycardia. These diseases have been set apart from others on the basis of three lines of evidence: (1) a large series of observations which have revealed that the malfunctioning organ is susceptible to changes in function by influences mediated via the autonomic nervous system, (2) the discovery in the biographies of some patients of an inordinately high incidence of resentment, hostility, and suppressed emotionality, (3) a demonstrable relationship between onset and successive exacerbations of disease and the presence of disturbing and frustrating incidents in the patient's life.

These psychosomatic diseases differ from the neuroses described in Chap. 375 in that the symptoms are different, are of longer duration, have a known pathologic basis, and often a known cause (e.g., allergy in asthma, hay fever, and atopic dermatitis). Finally, the incidence of frank neuroses in this group of patients is no greater than in the population at large, and neurotics are not more liable to psychosomatic diseases than are normal individuals. For many reasons, not the least of which is that a psychogenesis has never been proved in any one of these diseases, we have chosen to present the relevant psychologic data in the discussions of these diseases within the organ systems involved.

The sociopathies, which include the large number of people who from childhood exhibit abnormal degrees of impulsivity, aggressiveness, and various antisocial behaviors (truancy, running away, repeated thefts, drug abuse, etc.), involve so many sociologic, educational, economic, and political factors that they almost fall outside the orbit of medicine. While a medical position is often of value, particularly if there are questions of a psychiatric nature, there is no clear evidence that a medical opinion contributes significantly to the understanding and management of these problems. The same may be said of the large group of patients with deviant sexual behaviors (homosexuality, voyeurism, exhibitionism, etc.). While neurologic opinion is inclined to view them as having a biological basis, so few facts are available that we have not thought it advisable to include them in a textbook of medicine.

NEUROLOGIC ASSESSMENT OF THE PATIENT: THE NEUROLOGIC METHOD In neurologic diagnosis several problems emerge that are not encountered in other branches of internal medicine. *First,* there is the bewildering array of clinical abnormalities that require documentation and interpretation. These may range from simple muscle paresis to a disorder of memory. The analysis and interpretation become difficult because similar symptoms (for example, headache or dizziness) may be the presenting complaint in a patient with any of several disorders. A careful assessment of the character and pattern of the symptoms and of their temporal profile, and a recognition of associated complaints, together with a well-constructed neurologic examination, permit a conclusion to be reached among the various alternatives. *Second,* the anatomic localization of the lesion assumes special significance in neurology, as certain diseases are known to affect certain regions of the nervous system and not to involve others. Thus recognition of a constellation of symptoms and signs (a syndrome) points to the possible existence of certain diseases and to the exclusion of others. *Third,* the physician must acquire skill in coping with two orders of clinical phenomena—one known only to the patient (introspective data) and reported by him or her under conditions of mental clarity; the other, obvious to an outside observer, the extrospective data of behavioral change. *Lastly,* in all diseases of the cerebrum an outside source of information about disease (someone who knows the patient well, usually a member of the family) is needed if the patient's capacity for self-examination and reporting is impaired.

Since the physician must first determine by the elicitation of symptoms whether the nervous system has been affected, and, if so, what part of it, anatomic diagnosis takes precedence over etiologic diagnosis. The clinical neurologic method thus proceeds in a series of steps, as follows:

1 The essential clinical data are collected by history from the patient and family and by a systematic physical examination that encompasses a survey of all functions from the cerebrum to peripheral nerve and muscle, i.e., from the mental to the simplest reflexes.
2 The clinical data relevant to the current problems are assembled into one of the known syndromes and are interpreted and translated in terms of neuroanatomy and neurophysiology.
3 From the syndrome the physician should be able to determine the anatomic localization(s) that best explain the clinical findings.
4 The anatomic localization, mode of onset and course of illness, other medical data, and laboratory findings are then integrated.
5 Finally, the etiologic diagnosis is reached, and therapy appropriate for the causative agent is proposed.

The neurologic history It is obvious that in this logical step-by-step analysis great premium attaches to the accuracy of the clinical data. Imprecise and unreliable historical data concerning the disordered functioning of the nervous system in the course of illness (when the examiner was not present) will often result in erroneous diagnosis. Often when there is uncertainty or disagreement about neurologic diagnosis it will be found that the source of the difficulty lies in an inadequate or incomplete history, incomplete usually in the sense that the temporal profile of each symptom is not known.

The neurologic examination The neurologic examination requires the performance of a series of physical tests aimed at eliciting the functional capacities of different parts of the nervous system. The examiner must acquire skills that come only from the repeated use of the same techniques and instruments on a large number of normal and abnormal individuals. Errors and serious omissions are avoided if the examination procedure is orderly and systematic, beginning always with mental (cerebral) functions and continuing with cranial nerves, then with motor, reflex, and sensory functions of the arms, trunk, and legs, and finishing or starting with an analysis of gait.

The mental status may be tested while the history is being taken. One looks for faults of memory, incoherence of thought, dominating ideas, peculiarities of mood and outlook, aphasic errors, and loss of insight and judgment. If abnormalities are noted a more formal analysis of these functions is undertaken along the lines suggested in Chaps. 5, 20, 21, 22, and 23. The function of each cranial nerve is then examined in order, beginning with olfaction (see Chaps. 17 and 367). Examination of the motor system should include estimates of power of each of the major muscle groups (as outlined in Chaps. 14 and 369); the tone of the musculature during passive manipulations, looking for signs of spasticity, rigidity, hypotonia (as outlined in Chaps. 14 and 15), and speed and coordination of the limbs are assessed. Next, prevailing postures and the stance and gait are examined (Chap. 16). The tendon reflexes are next assessed for evidence of increased or decreased (or absent) response or of asymmetry between right and left sides or between arms and legs. The superficial cutaneous reflexes, abdominal and plantar, are then evaluated. Touch, pain, vibration, and joint-position sense are tested as the final part of the examination (see Chap. 18 for details).

This detailed neurologic examination is undertaken only if there are symptoms of disturbed nervous system functioning. If none are present it suffices to do an abbreviated examination which includes evaluation only of pupils, ocular movements, optic fundi, facial movements, speech, strength of arm and leg muscles, tendon and plantar reflexes, and pain and vibratory sensation in hands and feet. All of this can be completed in 2 to 3 min. The findings, even in the short examination, should be recorded in the patient's record for future reference.

Experience teaches that the neurologic examination may be normal even in patients with a serious neurologic disease, such as one which causes seizures or syncope, and the physician then proceeds along lines indicated in Chaps. 11 through 13. Or the patient may arrive in coma with no available history, in which case the clinical study should follow the plan described in Chap. 20. An inadequate history may to some extent be replaced by a succession of examinations from which the course of the illness may be plotted.

The formulation of the problem and establishment of an etiologic diagnosis The interpretations of symptoms and signs from which anatomic diagnosis is deduced may be aided by the discussions of applied anatomy and physiology which have been appended to each of the chapters on cardinal manifestations (Chaps. 10 to 23).

The proper selection of laboratory tests which will assist in arriving at anatomic but more particularly at etiologic diagnosis poses another set of problems for the student. The tests and the interpretation of results require an experience which the student often lacks. In Chaps. 354 and 369 we have tried to describe the principal tests and when they should be used. Of course in some neurologic and in all psychiatric disease, there are no available laboratory tests so one must rely entirely on the history and physical examination.

Once it is decided from the syndrome and the course of the illness that the problem is of neuropathic, muscular, vascular, traumatic, neoplastic, or psychiatric type, a fairly complete discussion of each of these categories of disease and the ways in which they can be distinguished will be found in Chaps. 354 to 377. For an account of the rare diseases which could not be included for lack of space, the physician is advised to turn to the references at the end of the chapters.

The assiduous application of the neurologic method described above offers an assured and rational approach to the majority of neuropsychiatric diseases and conditions. But of course there are some problems seen daily in a general hospital which defy solution. This is not surprising when one considers the many hundreds of diseases to which the human nervous system is subject. Sometimes, one reaches an anatomic diagnosis without being able to determine etiologic diagnosis, and one must wait patiently for further developments. Clinical responsibility begins and ends with the diagnosis of diseases for which we have a treatment. In view of the irreversibility of lesions which destroy neurons, the major objective is diagnosis and treatment in the earliest stage of disease or, even better, prevention. For the clinical investigator the diagnosis of untreatable disease is equally important, for the identification of a disease entity is the first step in the scientific study of it.

11
ANXIETY, DEPRESSION, ASTHENIA, AND PERSONALITY DISORDERS

RAYMOND D. ADAMS

In this chapter and the following one, the main phenomena discussed are complaints for which there are relatively few or at most ambiguous physical findings and no reliable corroborative laboratory tests. Yet as symptoms they are no less real and important than are others such as cough or paralysis. Their elicitation requires a careful history and reports of family members, and demands of the physician the same attention to detail and objectivity as other dysfunctions of the nervous system and viscera. When any one of the symptoms appearing in the titles of this chapter and Chap. 12 are presented by the patient, their cause(s) should be pursued along the lines described in the following pages, and the patient should be scrutinized for subtle behavioral accompaniments. Recurrent patterns of behavioral abnormality should also be sought, for they portend reactions to illness and disease that are predictable and helpful in the care of the patient.

Clinical experience teaches that the majority of patients who enter a physician's office or hospital will admit to being or having been nervous, anxious, or depressed. The stress of contemporary life or the prospect of real or imaginary illness is thought to induce these reactions. If they stand in clear relationship to a stressful event or situation, such as worry over economic reverses or grief over the death of a loved one, such states can be accepted as normal. Only when excessively intense and uncontrollable or when accompanied by obscure derangements of visceral function do they become the basis for medical consultation.

Such problems become more abstruse when similar symptoms occur in persons who are not being subjected to immediately stressful or unhappy experiences, and awareness of such threatening situations, if it exists at all, lies buried in the subconscious mind of the patient. One may assume that these causal events either have been suppressed from consciousness or are part of an elaborate subjective interpretation of which the patient is unaware. The relationship between social stimulus and prevailing anxiety or nervousness, if there is any such association, can then be discovered only by the gentle probings of a psychologically sophisticated physician. But once the connection is established and the problem dealt with realistically, the symptoms allegedly become understandable and disappear. One recognizes here all the elements of a *psychoneurotic reaction.* The line of separation between the latter and normal emotional reactions is admittedly ambiguous.

There is still another category of nervousness, anxiety, and depression wherein the emotional states are intense and prolonged, and may occur in cycles, but again without obvious explanation. Such states may overwhelm the individual and cause derangement of all that individual's activities. Delving into the unconscious mind or studying lifelong reaction patterns fails to reveal a plausible psychogenesis. One recognizes here all the elements of a more complete, pervasive *psychotic reaction.* In many such instances a genetic factor appears to operate, and the features of the illness are so stereotyped as to indicate a disease of the parts of the nervous system which control the affective, emotional life. Yet a consistent biochemical change in the blood or brain tissue has not been found, and no lesion has been discerned. Treatment must proceed empirically, along nonpsychologic lines.

The problem confronting every physician is to recognize all these nuances of reaction, personality disorder, and disease, which obviously shade into one another, and to determine to what extent they figure in the medical condition of the patient. Some type of therapeutic maneuver must then be initiated, varying from simple reassurance and realistic management of existing personal difficulties, to suppression of symptoms by drugs. Often, referral to a psychiatrist is necessary for more expert management, including, in severe cases, electroconvulsive therapy.

In this chapter we shall first consider the cardinal features of these common reactive states and then the personality and character disorders from which they are believed to arise, together with currently accepted views of their origins. The major neuroses of which they may be a part are discussed in Chap. 375 and the psychoses in Chaps. 376 and 377. See also the citation of Nicholi in the references.

NERVOUSNESS By this vague term the lay person usually refers to a state of restlessness, tension, uneasy apprehension, irritability, or hyperexcitability. But it may connote other states, such as thoughts of suicide, fear of killing one's child or spouse, a distressing hallucination, a paranoid idea, or a frankly hysterical outburst. Careful inquiry as to what the patient means when complaining of nervousness is always a necessary first step.

In its most common presentation, a period of nervousness may represent no more than a psychic and behavioral state in which an organism is maximally challenged by difficult personal problems, and there are periods in normal life when this is more likely to happen. For example, adolescence rarely passes without its period of turmoil as the person attempts emancipation from parental dominance or adjustment to demands of a scholastic or social nature. The menses are regularly accompanied by increased tension and moodiness, and, of course, the menarche and menopause are other critical periods. Some persons, because of early patterning or character formation, claim to have been nervous in all their social relationships throughout life; one should then suspect a psychoneurosis or unstable character formation or an oncoming psychosis, even though performance within the family unit, at school, and at work are said to be adequate. When nervousness is a recent development, one must consider such conditions as an upheaval in personal affairs, the first attack or exacerbation of a psychoneurosis, an endogenous depression, an endocrine disease (hyperthyroidism, adrenal hypersecretion, or corticosteroid therapy), or withdrawal from a sedative drug (alcohol, barbiturate). Some patients complain of a nervousness that attends or follows the onset of a medical or neurologic disease; and it would then appear to be secondary, occasioned by fear of disability, dependency, or death.

Nervousness, even in its simplest form, is reflected in many important activities of the human organism. There are often a mild somberness of mood and an increased tendency to tears and anger (irritability). Fatigue that bears no proper relationship to activity and rest is frequent, and sleep is often disturbed, as are eating and drinking habits. Headaches may increase in number and intensity. There is a tendency to sweat, tremble, be aware of heart action, feel a bit "queer in the head" or giddy, have an upset stomach, and urinate more often, though these recognized autonomic accompaniments of anxiety are seldom as conspicuous as in anxiety neurosis. Thus, it would appear that nervousness and anxiety constitute a graded series of reactions, the latter in many instances being only a more intense and protracted form of nervousness.

ANXIETY Anxiety is "the fundamental phenomenon and central problem of the neurosis . . . a nodal point, linking up all kinds of most important questions, a riddle of which the solution must cast a flood of light upon our whole mental life" (Freud). From the viewpoint of the social historian, anxiety is said to be "the most prominent mental characteristic of Occidental civilization" (Willoughby). These comments should inform the reader of the broad implications of this reaction.

The more strictly medical meaning of the term *anxiety,* and the one used in this chapter, is a state characterized by a subjective feeling of fear and uneasy anticipation (apprehension), usually with a definite topical content and associated with the physiologic accompaniments of strong emotion, i.e., breathlessness, choking sensation, palpitation, restlessness, increased muscular tension, tightness in the chest, giddiness, trembling, sweating, and flushing. By *topical content* is meant the idea, person, or object about which the person is anxious. The several vasomotor and visceral alterations that underlie the symptoms are mediated through the autonomic nervous system, particularly the sympathetic part of it, and involve also the thyroid and adrenal glands. One would expect such autonomic discharges to alter the levels of epinephrine or norepinephrine or their metabolites in the blood or urine, but efforts to measure them have not yielded consistent results. Aldosterone excretion is said to be raised to two or three times the normal level during an anxiety attack.

Forms of anxiety Anxiety is manifested in acute episodes, each lasting a few minutes and clearly related to a disturbing event in the patient's life; or it may represent an inexplicable protracted state that may last for weeks, months, or years. There may be a succession of acute *attacks,* or *panics* as they are called; the patient is plunged into an inexplicable mental state and fears death, loss of reason or self-control, and insanity, or feels that he or she may commit some horrible crime. The patient is breathless, has a racing heart, chokes, sweats, trembles, and feels gastric distress and anorexia. In a persistent, protracted form there are lesser and fluctuating degrees of nervousness, restlessness, irritability, fatigue, insomnia, intolerance of physical exertion, and pressure or tension headaches. Discrete anxiety attacks and chronic states of anxiety merge into one another.

Episodic anxiety without disorder of mood (i.e., depression) is usually classified as *anxiety neurosis.* The chronic form with prominent exercise intolerance is called *neurocirculatory asthenia.* Anxiety may, however, be combined with other somatic symptoms in hysteria and may be the restraining factor in *phobic neurosis.* Persistent anxiety with insomnia, lassitude, and fatigue, regardless of mood, should always raise suspicion of a *depressive psychosis,* especially if it begins late in life. Panic attacks are said to occur at the beginning of a schizophrenic illness, but this is rare in our experience. Both anxiety and depression are prominent features of the posttraumatic syndrome of nervous instability (see Chap. 357).

Thus, the differential diagnosis of an anxiety state requires that the physician consider all the major syndromes in psychiatry. Often it is but one component of a far more serious condition, one which may result in suicide or some other antisocial act. Also, without the psychic counterparts of fear and apprehension, the visceral symptoms alone should arouse suspicion of thyrotoxicosis, epilepsy, corticosteroid overdosage, pheochromocytoma, hypoglycemia, or menopause.

Physiologic and psychologic basis The question to be asked is, What is the source and mechanism of this intense emotional state? Answers to this question have taken two forms, one mainly psychologic, the other based on anatomic and psychopharmacologic evidence.

PSYCHOLOGIC Anxiety is interpreted as a fear, perhaps somewhat muted, that is aroused under conditions not overtly threatening. In terms of psychoanalytic theory it is a reaction to a situation that undermines the security of the individual, and its purpose is self-protection. The topical content of the anxiety, i.e., what one is fearful of, lies hidden in the unconscious mind. The postulated danger is internal rather than external. A primitive drive has been aroused that is not compatible with current social practices, and it can be satisfied only at risk of harm to the person. In other words, the anxiety prevents the execution of the unacceptable action. The reader readily appreciates that such hypotheses, even when accepted as an explanation of a neurotic reaction, are essentially teleological and would not necessarily explain the mechanism of a cycle of unprovoked anxiety in an endogenous hereditary anxious depression.

PSYCHOPHARMACOLOGIC BASIS Drugs such as the barbiturates and particularly the benzodiazepines, which have long been known to assuage anxiety, have recently been found by Costa et al. to interact with γ-aminobutyric acid (GABA) receptors in the brain. Binding sites for benzodiazepines have been found in several parts of the brain which correspond closely to the distribution of GABA receptors. The neuronal systems subserving anxiety are believed to be located in the limbic regions, including the amygdala and hippocampus. Destruction of these latter structures renders the individual placid and fearless. Pharmacologic analysis shows them to be rich in benzodiazepine receptors. The existence must be assumed, therefore, of naturally occurring substances (endogenous ligands) that are involved in neurotransmission at these receptor sites and which control anxiety in the same way as opioid peptides are related to opioid receptors in the control of pain. Although a number of leads for the isolation of such endogenous substances have been forthcoming, including the finding of an acidic protein that interacts with GABA and β-carbolines which inhibit the action of benzodiazepines by binding to the receptors, the endogenous ligand has yet to be identified. But one can see in these findings the making of a theory for an endogenous mechanism of anxiety. And of course it need not be incompatible with a psychologic hypothesis such as that of Gray (see reference).

DEPRESSION (UNHAPPINESS, GLOOM, AND GRIEF) There are few persons who do not experience periods of discouragement and despair, and these periods become manifestly more frequent in modern society where individual freedom is constrained and one's impulses must be inhibited. As with nervousness and anxiety, depression of mood that is appropriate to a given situation in life is a natural, healthy reaction and seldom is the basis of medical complaint. The depression is of reactive type and this probably includes most depressions secondary to medical or neurologic disease and probably the neurotic depressions. The patient tends to seek help only when grief or unhappiness becomes uncontrollable. But there are numerous instances in which the patient is miserable, unhappy, and hopeless for reasons which are not apparent. The depression is endogenous. Many of the symptoms are interpreted as ill health, being so similar to those of many disease states as to bring the patient first to the internist. Sometimes another disease is found (such as chronic hepatitis, brucellosis, or postinfluenzal asthenia or other infections) in which chronic fatigue is confused with depression, but often an endogenous depression is itself the essential problem. Since the risk of suicide is not inconsiderable, if the illness is mistaken for another or overlooked as a complication, an error in diagnosis may be life-threatening.

Information about depression, like that about all psychiatric syndromes, is gained from three sources: the history obtained from the patient, the history obtained from the family or close friend, and the findings on examination.

From the patient and family it is learned that the patient has been "feeling unwell," "low in spirits," "blue," "glum," "unhappy," or "morbid." There has been a change in emotional reactions of which the patient may not be fully aware. Activities that were formerly pleasurable are no longer so. Often, however, change in mood is less conspicuous than reduction in psychic and physical energy. Fatigue is almost invariable; not uncommonly, it is worse in the morning after a night of restless sleep. The words "loss of pep," "weak," "tired," "no energy to work," "my job seems more trying and difficult" appear in the language of the patient. The outlook is pessimistic. The patient is preoccupied with uncontrollable worry over trivialities. With excessive worry the ability to think with accustomed efficiency is reduced; there is complaint that the mind does not function properly, of being forgetful and unable to concentrate. If the patient is naturally of suspicious nature, paranoid tendencies may assert themselves.

Particularly troublesome in medical diagnosis is the patient's tendency to become hypochondriacal about associated diseases. Indeed, most cases formerly diagnosed as hypochondriasis are now regarded as depression. Pain from whatever cause—a stiff joint, a toothache, fleeting abdominal pains, or other troubles such as constipation, frequency of urination, insomnia, pruritus, burning tongue, weight loss—may become an obsessive focus of complaint. The patient passes from doctor to doctor seeking relief from symptoms that would not trouble the average person, and no amount of reassurance relieves this state of mind. The nervousness and anxiety felt by many of these persons may be obscured by their preoccupation with visceral functions.

When examined, the patient's facial expression is often plaintive, troubled, pained, or anguished. The attitude and manner betray a prevailing mood of depression, discouragement, and despondency. In other words, the affective response, which is the outward expression of feeling, is consistent with the depressed mood. During the interview the patient's eyes may be tearful, or he or she may cry openly. In some there is a kind of immobility of the face that mimics parkinsonism, though others are restless and agitated (pacing the floor, wringing their hands, etc.). Occasionally the patient will smile, but the smile impresses one as more of a social gesture than an expression of feeling.

The stream of speech, from which the ideational content is determined, is slow. At times the patient is mute and speaks neither spontaneously nor in response to questions. Again there may be a long pause between questions and answers. The latter are brief and may be monosyllabic. There is a paucity of ideas. The retardation extends to all topics of conversation and affects movement of limbs as well. The most extreme forms of decreased motor activity, rarely seen in the medical clinic, border on stupor.

Content of speech is found to be abnormal if examined carefully. Conversation is replete with pessimistic thoughts, fears, expressions of unworthiness, inadequacy, inferiority, and sometimes guilt. In severe depressions bizarre ideas, delusions about the body ("blood drying up," "bowels are blocked with cement," "I am half dead") may be expressed.

Etiology and mechanism (see Chap. 376) Like anxiety, depression is a state which may stand as a simple reaction to an environmental circumstance, a form of neurosis, or a major psychosis. It is the writer's belief that depression is one of the most commonly overlooked diagnoses in clinical medicine. Part of the trouble is with the word itself, which implies being unhappy about something. The persistent or recurrent endogenous depression or involutional depression should be suspected in all chronic states of ill health, hypochondriasis, multiple complaints involving many organ systems, chronic pain, disability that exceeds manifest signs of a medical disease, neurasthenia, and suicide attempts. Inasmuch as recovery is the rule, the suicide is a tragedy for which the medical profession must often share responsibility.

For endogenous depressions there seems to be little doubt that a causative genetic factor is operative. The prevalence of depression in the first-degree relatives of patients ranges from 10 to 25 percent, in comparison to a 1 to 2 percent incidence in the general population. In identical twins the concordance rate is approximately 70 percent and for nonidentical twins 25 percent.

Biochemical theories are receiving increased support. Tricyclic antidepressant drugs and monoamine oxidase (MAO) inhibitors, the major therapeutic agents now in use, are believed to exert their effect by increasing one or another of the biogenic amines at adrenergic receptor sites in the hypothalamus and limbic regions of the cerebrum. It would follow logically enough that an increase or a deficiency of biogenic amines might result in the mood and energy changes. Levels of methoxy-4-hydroxyphenylglycol (MHPG), a metabolite of norepinephrine, were found to be reduced in the cerebrospinal fluid (CSF) of depressed patients and increased in manic patients. Also 5-hydroxyindoleacetic acid (5-HIAA), a deaminated metabolite of serotonin, was reduced in the CSF of depressed patients. However, the findings are not consistent, which some investigators have interpreted to mean that all depressions are not the same. Maas identifies two groups of depressive patients, one with normal and the other with low levels of MHPG. The first group responded to amitriptyline and the second to imipramine.

Other observations, by Schlesser et al., suggest a basic derangement of the hypothalamic-pituitary-adrenal axis. In cases of monopolar and bipolar depression the oral administration of 1 to 2 mg of dexamethasone failed to suppress cortisol levels while the patient was ill, but did so after recovery. In a comparable group of reactive depressions cortisol levels were suppressed. This test is believed to separate the two large groups of depressed patients and to predict their therapeutic response (see Chap. 376).

LASSITUDE AND ASTHENIA The terms *weakness* and *fatigue* are used by patients to describe a variety of subjective complaints which vary in their import and prognostic significance. The different meanings can usually be fitted into the following classification:

1 Lassitude, fatigue, lack of energy, listlessness, and languor.

These terms, though not synonymous, shade into one another. All refer to a weariness and a loss of that sense of well-being typically found in persons healthy of body and mind.

2 Weakness, loss of strength, paresis, paralysis. These may be persistent or episodic.
   a Persistent weakness: This may be (1) restricted to certain muscles or groups of muscles (see Chap. 14) or (2) more or less generalized, i.e., involving the entire musculature (see Chaps. 372 and 373).
   b Episodic, often recurrent: Attacks of weakness may occur in the periodic paralyses. [Many patients confuse "attacks of weakness" with a diminished sense of alertness, lightheadedness, feeling of faintness. These usually turn out to be episodes of partial or threatening syncope, attacks of anxiety or vertigo, or seizures (see Chaps. 12 and 13).]

Of all the symptoms in this group, lassitude and fatigue are among the most frequent and abstruse. More than half of all patients entering a general hospital register direct complaint of fatigability or admit to it when questioned. During the Second World War fatigue was so prominent as to be given a separate place in medical nosology, viz., "combat fatigue," which came to refer to all acute psychiatric illnesses that happened on the battlefield. The common clinical antecedents and accompaniments of fatigue, its significance, and its physiologic and psychologic bases should, therefore, be matters of common medical knowledge.

Patients who complain of weariness and tiredness have a more or less characteristic way of describing their condition. They say that they "are all in," "have lost pep," "have no ambition" or "no interest," are "turned off" or "fed up." They manifest their condition by showing an indifference to the tasks at hand, by talking much about how hard they are working; they are inclined to sit around or lie down, occupying themselves with trivial tasks. On closer analysis one observes that they have a difficulty in initiating activity and also in sustaining it.

This condition is the familiar aftermath of prolonged labor or great physical exertion, and under such circumstances it is accepted as a normal physiologic reaction. When, however, the same symptoms or similar ones appear in no relation to such antecedents, they are suspected of being the manifestations of disease.

The physician's task begins, then, with an attempt to determine whether the patient is merely suffering from the physical and mental effects of overwork without realizing it. Overworked, overwrought people are everywhere observable in our society. Their actions are both instructive and pathetic. They seem to be impelled by notions of duty and refuse to think of themselves. Or, as is often the case, some personal inadequacy seems to prevent them from deriving pleasure from any activity except their work, in which they indulge themselves as a kind of defense mechanism. Such persons show their fatigue by other symptoms, such as irritability, restlessness, and sleeplessness. Their symptoms and behavior are best understood by referring to psychologic studies of the effect of fatigue on the normal individual.

Effects of fatigue on the normal person According to several authoritative sources, fatigue has both explicit and implicit effects, logically grouped under (1) a series of biochemical and physiologic changes in many organs of the body, (2) an overt disorder in behavior, a reduced output of work, known as *work decrement,* and (3) an expressed dissatisfaction and a subjective feeling of tiredness.

As to the biochemical and physiologic changes, continuous muscular work leads to depletion of muscle glycogen and an accumulation of lactic acid and other metabolites, which in themselves reduce the power of contraction and delay recovery. Extreme degrees of muscle work, in which activity exceeds provision of substrate, result in necrosis of fibers and rise in serum levels of creatine phosphokinase and aldolase even in normal persons. The muscles are slightly swollen and sore for several days. It is said that the injection of blood from a fatigued animal into a rested one will produce overt manifestations of fatigue in the latter. During repeated contractions of muscle, its action is observed to become tremulous, movements are less adept, and the coordination of agonist, antagonist, and synergic muscles is less perfect. The rate of breathing increases, the pulse quickens, the blood pressure rises and pulse pressure widens, and the white blood cell count and metabolic rate are increased. These alterations bear out the hypothesis that fatigue is in part a manifestation of altered metabolism.

The decreased capacity for work or productivity which is a direct consequence of fatigue has been investigated by industrial psychologists. Their findings show clearly the importance of the motivational factor on work output, whether it be in manual or clerical tasks. Individual differences in energy potential appear also to be important, as are differences in physique, intelligence, and temperament.

The subjective feelings of fatigue have been carefully recorded. Aside from feeling weary tired persons are unable to deal effectively with complex problems and tend to be unreasonable, often about trivialities. The number and quality of their associations in psychologic tests are reduced. The ability to deliberate and to reach judgments is impaired; decisions made late at night may appear unsound the next day. The worker after a long, hard day is unable to perform adequately his or her duties as head of a household; the example of the tired business person who becomes the proverbial tyrant of the family circle is well known. A disinclination to try and the appearance of ideas of inferiority are other characteristics of the fatigued mind.

Instances of fatigue and lassitude resulting from overwork are not difficult to recognize. Descriptions of patients' daily routines and talks with associates and family will usually suffice. Moreover if they can be persuaded to live at a more reasonable pace and allow time for outside pleasurable activities, their symptoms will promptly subside. A common error in diagnosis, however, is the ascription of fatigue to overwork when actually it is a manifestation of a psychoneurosis or depression.

Fatigue as a manifestation of psychiatric disorder The great majority of patients who enter a hospital because of unexplained chronic fatigue and lassitude have been found to have some type of psychiatric illness. Formerly this state was called *neurasthenia;* but since fatigue rarely exists as an isolated phenomenon, the current practice is to label such cases according to the total clinical picture. The usual associated symptoms are nervousness, irritability, anxiety, depression, insomnia, headaches, difficulty in concentrating, sexual disorders, and loss of bodily appetites. In one series in a general hospital 75 percent of persons admitted because of chronic fatigue and nervousness were diagnosed, finally, as having *anxiety neurosis* and *tension states.* Depression accounted for another 10 percent, and the remainder of the patients had a miscellany of medical and psychiatric illnesses.

Several features are common to the psychiatric group. The fatigue may be worse in the morning. There is an inclination to lie down and rest, but sleep does not come. The fatigue relates more to some activities than to others. Inquiry as to what was happening when the fatigue was first experienced may reveal an unpleasant event, a grief reaction, a surgical operation, or a medical illness. The feeling of fatigue interferes with mental as well as physical activities. The psychic aspects are manifested as difficulty in concentrating on the solution of a problem or in carrying on an involved conversation.

Depressing emotion, as was remarked above, has its characteristic effect on impulse life and energy. Also, it impairs sleep, with a tendency to early-morning waking. Such persons are at their worst in the morning, both in spirit and in energy output. Their tendency is to improve as the day wears on, and they may even feel fairly normal by evening. It is often difficult in them to decide whether the fatigue is a primary manifestation of the depression or is secondary to a lack of interest.

Many physicians question whether all chronically fatigued individuals deviate enough from normal to justify the diagnosis of psychoneurosis or depression. Many people in society, because of circumstances beyond their control, have no purpose in life and much idle time. They are bored with the monotony of their routine. Such circumstances are conducive to fatigue, just as the opposite is also true—that a new enterprise that excites optimism and enthusiasm will dispel fatigue. Other individuals seem normal until some adversity is encountered, arousing worry or fear, and then it becomes apparent that their adjustment is unstable. Such reactions are understandable to anyone who has ever had stage fright or "buck fever" and who remembers the sense of physical weakness, the utter incapacity to act, the intellectual chaos that overwhelms the previously well-ordered mind, and the exhaustion which follows.

Psychologic theories The enervating effect of a strong emotion such as anxiety is well known, and it might be supposed that the simple prolongation of the emotional experience would provide a rational explanation for a chronic fatigue of anxiety. But even if true, however, this explanation does not account for the occurrence of emotion at a time when there is no reason for it.

The dynamic schools of psychiatry, particularly the psychoanalytic, have postulated that chronic fatigue, in the broadest sense, is like the anxiety from which it derives; it is a danger signal that something is wrong—that some attitude or activity has been too intense or too persistent. The fatigue is self-preservative, serving not merely as a protection against physical injury but also as a protection of the individual's self-esteem and confidence in self. As to mechanism, it is claimed that the fatigue is the result of exhaustion of the store of psychic energy required to maintain repression of unacceptable ideas. Others, however, claim to have evidence that fatigue is not a negative symptom, a lack or depletion of energy, but an unconscious desire for inactivity. A reciprocal relationship is said to exist between fatigue and anxiety. Both are protective, but anxiety is the more imperative. It calls for the individual to take some positive action to extricate him- or herself from a predicament, whereas fatigue calls for inactivity. Both operate blindly, however, for the person cannot perceive what it is that must be done or not done. All this happens at the unconscious level.

It is also observed that some persons are low in impulse and energy throughout life, being more so at times of stress. Some psychiatrists believe that they have a constitutional inadequacy. Kahn classifies such individuals as "psychopaths weak in impulse," and points out in his description their inability throughout life to play games vigorously, to compete successfully, to work hard without exhaustion, to withstand or recover quickly from illness, or to assume a dominant role in a social group. The physician caring for them expects greater disability and more prolonged convalescence from every illness.

It is obvious that these several psychologic hypotheses could not all be correct, nor could they be applicable to all situations in which chronic fatigue is the complaint. Undoubtedly there are persons who are underactive and weak because of genetic factors or early life experiences. It is equally clear that psychic and physical energy are closely linked to mood. The more chronic varieties of acquired fatigue, without a basis in medical disease, have in nearly all instances a psychologic basis.

Lassitude and fatigue in chronic infection and in endocrine and other medical diseases Infection is another cause of chronic fatigue, though a much less frequent one. Everyone has at some time or other sensed the abrupt onset of extreme exhaustion, the tired ache in the muscles, an inexplicable listlessness, only to discover later that one is "coming down with the flu." In chronic infections such as hepatitis, tuberculosis, brucellosis, infectious mononucleosis, the infection may not be at once evident. But it should always be suspected when the fatigue is out of proportion to other symptoms such as mood change, nervousness, and anxiety. Often this syndrome will begin with an obvious infection but will persist for several weeks after it should have terminated, and it may then be difficult to decide whether there is still a lingering infection or the infection has been complicated by psychiatric illness during convalescence. In many diseases such as infectious hepatitis, brucellosis, infectious mononucleosis, and a host of other systemic viral infections, long-standing neurotic symptoms appear to have been uncovered. Nevertheless it is difficult to dismiss an obscure secondary metabolic disorder consequent to the infection.

Metabolic and endocrine diseases (see Chaps. 362 and 110) of various types may cause inordinate degrees of lassitude and fatigue. Sometimes there is in addition a true muscular weakness (see Chaps. 12 and 373). In Addison's disease and Simmonds' disease fatigue may dominate the clinical picture. Aldosterone deficiency is another established cause of fatigue (see Chap. 112). In persons with hypothyroidism, with or without frank myxedema, lassitude and sluggishness are frequent complaints. These same symptoms may also be present in patients with hyperthyroidism but are usually less troublesome than nervousness. Uncontrolled diabetes mellitus may be accompanied by excessive fatigability, as are hyperparathyroidism, hypogonadism, and Cushing's disease.

Anemia, when moderate or severe (hematocrit less than 25) should be considered as a possible cause of unexplained lassitude. Mild grades of anemia are usually asymptomatic; lassitude is far too often ascribed to it.

Any type of nutritional deficiency may, when severe, cause lassitude, and in its earlier stages this may be the chief complaint. Weight loss and the history of dietary inadequacy may provide the only other clues to the nature of the illness. Many patients feel weak and tired after a myocardial infarct, but usually there is an accompanying depression.

Among neurologic diseases in which fatigability is a prominent symptom should be mentioned the posttraumatic nervous instability syndrome, Parkinson's disease, and multiple sclerosis. The fatigue of Parkinson's disease may precede the recognition of neurologic signs by months or even years. It is probably a reaction to the increasing disability occasioned by subjective awareness of the akinesia. The majority of patients who recover from a stroke complain of being weak and tired. Hot temperatures worsen the fatigue and other symptoms of the multiple sclerotic patient.

Differential diagnosis If one looks critically at the patients who enter a hospital because of lassitude and fatigability (sometimes incorrectly called weakness), it is clear that the most commonly overlooked diagnoses are psychoneurosis and depression. The correct conclusion can usually be reached by keeping these illnesses in mind as one elicits the principal symptoms of these psychiatric illnesses from patient and family. Difficulty arises when such symptoms are so inconspicuous as not to be appreciated; one comes then to suspect the psychiatric diagnosis only by having eliminated the common medical causes. Observations in the hospital may bear out the existence of a tension state or gloomy mood, as the patient resists attempts to be mobilized. Strong reassurance in combination with a therapeutic trial of 2.5 to 5.0 mg dextroamphetamine morning and noon and, if there are prominent features of anxiety and depression, 100 to 200 mg sodium amobarbital three times a day may suppress symptoms of which the patient was barely aware and may clarify diagnosis. The danger of mistaking a depression for a neurosis has already been mentioned. Of course, asthenic psychopaths are recognized by their actions as revealed in biographies.

Obscure infections such as pulmonary tuberculosis, brucellosis, subclinical hepatitis, subacute bacterial endocarditis, malaria, hookworm, and parasitic infections should be recognizable by the characteristic symptoms and signs described elsewhere in the book. An endocrine survey, particularly for adrenal insufficiency and thyroid disease, is in order in all obscure cases. There should also be a search for occult tumors. It should be remembered that chronic intoxications with barbiturates, alcohol, or bromides, some of which are given to suppress nervousness, may contribute to fatigability.

Finally, when onset of fatigue is rapid and recent, the cause is likely to be an infection, a disturbance in fluid balance, or rapidly developing circulatory failure of either peripheral or cardiac origin.

GENERALIZED WEAKNESS AND ASTHENIA As can be judged from the foregoing remarks, weakness must be distinguished from lassitude and fatigue. The demonstration of reduced muscular power sets the case analysis along rather different lines, for it raises consideration more particularly of diseases of the nervous system or of the musculature.

True neural or myopathic weakness is probably never due to psychologic factors, though the hysteric or malingering patient may claim weakness. Usually this can be detected by the criteria outlined here and in Chap. 375. In anemia, chronic infection, malignancy, and nutritional depletion (except when polyneuropathy is present), the thin muscles are always stronger during tests of peak contraction than one would expect, though of course strength falls short of that of a healthy individual (see Chap. 369 for description of tests of peak power and endurance of muscles).

The proper ascertainment of muscular weakness depends on two lines of inquiry: (1) a history of reduced efficiency; and (2) demonstrable failure in ability to contract the muscles forcefully one or more times. If one proceeds to test each of the major groups of muscles from head to foot, comparing the patient's performance with one's idea of normalcy for man or woman, one may ascertain whether all or certain groups fall below standard. Quantitative and qualitative changes (myasthenia, inverse myasthenia, myotonia, paramyotonia, pathologic cramping) may also be detected by the methods outlined in Chap. 369. The topography of weakness and associated neurologic findings permit distinction between the various types of spinal, peripheral nerve, and myopathic pareses. Rare diseases, difficult to diagnose, that cause inexplicable muscle weakness are masked hyperthyroidism, hyperparathyroidism, ossifying hemangiomas with hypophosphatemia, some of the kalemic periodic paralyses, and hyperinsulinism.

PERSONALITY DISORDERS When the above nervous states occur repeatedly and without explanation, there is likelihood that they derive from chronic lifelong patterns of maladaptation and peculiarities of character. Psychiatrists speak of such states as *borderline character disorders,* implying that they account for the ways different individuals cope with life.

The origins of these peculiarities of character are obscure. To avoid the dispute as to whether they are conditioned by early life experiences or are the product of genetic factors, the adjective *constitutional* is sometimes used in reference to them. The formal types of neuroses are believed to originate in these personality disorders.

If one examines Table 11-1, the specific personality types clearly shade into particular neuroses, and one wonders if they are not merely milder forms of neurosis, differing from the latter in that they less frequently present as medical problems. Personality disturbances are important to recognize, however, for the perceptive physician must take account of them as well as of the related neuroses in the diagnosis of disease and the management of patients with medical illnesses. Such patients may sabotage a needed diagnostic test or therapy. Actually, it is the physician's knowledge of human nature and skill in the care of these difficult and often exasperating patients that enable him or her to be the leader of a therapeutic team.

NEUROSES When nervousness, anxiety, and depression are persistently or episodically joined with various combinations

TABLE 11-1
Personality disorders

Type of disorder	*Characteristics*
1 Paranoid	Chronic wariness, suspiciousness, litigiousness; lack of insight or humor; tendency to blame others; sense of self-importance and entitlement
2 Cyclothymic	Recurring periods of depression and elation not readily explained by circumstances; severe moodiness
3 Schizoid	Isolation, seclusiveness, secretiveness; discomfort in relationships; often eccentric and lacking in energy; few friends
4 Explosive	Outbursts of rage and aggression not in keeping with usual personality, often in response to minor provocation; sense of loss of control followed by regret
5 Obsessive-compulsive	Chronic worries about standards; excessive concern about self-image; tension in relationships, leading to isolation; inability to relax and excessive inhibitions; predisposition to depression
6 Hysterical	Immaturity, histrionic behavior, sexualization of relationships, low frustration tolerance, and shallow interpersonal ties; dependency
7 Asthenic	Chronic weakness, easy fatigability, sense of vulnerability, poor response to stress, little ambition or aggression
8 Passive-aggressive	Obstructive behavior, stubbornness, intentional errors or omissions; intolerance of authority with struggles over control, often creating difficulties in medical settings; externalization of conflicts and blaming others for untoward events
9 Inadequate	Chronic inability to meet ordinary life demands in the absence of mental retardation; severe dependency on others; tendency to become institutionalized or to become dependent on institutions
10 Antisocial	Unsocialized or antisocial behavior in conflict with society; selfishness, callousness, impulsiveness, lack of loyalty, and little guilt; frustration tolerance is low; tendency to blame others and have a long history of interpersonal and social difficulties and arrests

of irrational fears, obsessive thoughts, compulsions, lassitude and fatigue, insomnia, preoccupation with trivial symptoms, and a number of different somatic disturbances for which no cause can be found, the condition is properly called *neurosis* or *psychoneurosis.*

The neuroses represent a specific group of mental disorders appearing in adolescence and early to middle adulthood in individuals who have already achieved relatively adequate mental function. Since these disorders have no demonstrable organic basis, they are often called "functional," a term that is incorrect, for all functional disorders must have a physical basis. In all instances the neurotic patients are normally alert and correctly oriented, have considerable insight into their troubles, and manifest *unimpaired reality testing,* meaning that they do not confuse their subjective experiences and fantasies with external reality, more explicitly that they are not deluded and do not suffer hallucinations. The personality remains organized, and conduct is within socially acceptable limits. Neurotic patients can usually study, work, and function in the family and social circle even though assailed by doubts, loss of self-confidence, and despondency. They know that the troublesome symptoms originate within the mind, but are incapable of overcoming them by force of will, and hence they feel ashamed and inadequate. In these several ways neuroses are to be distinguished from the more pervasive and disorganizing psychoses.

Within this multitude of symptoms certain natural clusterings occur, and these are the basis of the classification in Table 11-2, which has been sanctioned by an international committee of psychiatrists.

In general medicine we have frequently encountered types 1 to 4, whereas type 6 (neurasthenia) and type 8 (hypochondriasis) will usually prove to be manifestations of a depressive state. Type 5 (depressive neurosis) will be difficult to distinguish from the nonpsychotic depression. Type 7 (depersonalization neurosis), a relatively rare condition in the author's experience, probably is a form of depression or pseudoneurotic schizophrenia.

For clarity of concept the term neurosis should be reserved for these particular groupings of symptoms and signs, and not loosely applied to individuals who are transiently upset by some circumstance or are emotional or eccentric. Each type may occur in relatively pure form, but often there are overlappings of symptoms. Anxiety, for example, may occur in pure form with a depressive reaction, in hysteria, and with phobic states. These combinations of neuroses are called "mixed neuroses."

The diagnosis of a neurosis depends largely on a thorough history that covers much of the medical biography of the patient. The physical examination seldom yields abnormal findings. Moreover, there is no laboratory test to which one can turn for final confirmation of diagnosis, which is true also of manic-depressive psychosis and schizophrenia. Subjective impressions supersede objective data, reducing accuracy of diagnosis.

Most psychiatrists hold the opinion that the neuroses have their genesis in the early life experiences that mold character and personality; that is, the neurosis stems from a neurotic character (hysterical, hypochondriacal, etc.). Reich and Kelly, who wrote the chapter on neuroses in the eighth edition of this textbook, regard them as psychologic decompensations of a neurotic personality that are basically maladaptive and inappropriate to the level of stress. The form of the neurotic episode is believed to be determined by the personality structure of the patient. But such explanations do not seem relevant to the most frequent of all the neuroses, the anxiety neurosis, which may strike a well-balanced person at any time during life. Furthermore, the stress of urban living conditions seems not to be a factor in the development of neurosis, for surveys of urban and rural populations show approximately the same incidence of neurotic behavior. The lifetime prevalence, regardless of social environment, is approximately 15 percent.

Neuroses vary in severity from mild periods of uneasiness that may not come to medical attention to episodes of severe, incapacitating illnesses that may require hospitalization. Since neuroses are frequent and may masquerade as medical illnesses with which the internist must contend, or complicate certain disease states, these descriptive data and the material in Chap. 375 should be fixed in mind.

Treatment In the management of acute anxiety states, it is important to explain to patients that they suffer from a real medical illness and not just "nerves," or an imaginary condition. They should be allowed to express their feelings, doubts, and fears. Superficial psychotherapy, involving support, insight, and reeducation proves to be the most practical. Often, as the patient is mobilized and returned to usual activities, the symptoms subside. If the anxiety is persistent and severe, one should be alert to the risk of suicide and be prepared to send the patient to a psychiatric hospital for treatment of depression. If mild, antianxiety drugs such as meprobamate, 400 mg tid; chlordiazepoxide, 10 to 20 mg tid; diazepam, 5 to 10 mg tid; propranolol, 40 mg tid; or sodium amytal, 100 to 200 mg tid, prescribed in the lowest possible dose, may suffice to bring the symptoms under control.

In the management of patients with prominent somatic complaints and a hysterical type of personality, prolonged psychotherapy has seldom produced successful results. Often, any suggestion that the illness is psychiatric arouses a hostile reaction, and the patient may refuse to see a psychiatrist. The author has obtained the best results by explaining to the patient and the family that the illness is really a chronic constitutional

TABLE 11-2
The neuroses

Type of neurosis	*Characteristics*
1 Anxiety neurosis	Episodic diffuse anxiety in attacks or waves; somatic complaints such as palpitations, paresthesias, weakness, dizziness; pessimism and irritability
2 Hysterical neurosis:	
a Conversion type	Physical symptoms involving voluntary musculature and sensory system, such as paradoxic paralyses, seizures, sensory deficits, and pain; attitude of indifference
b Dissociative type	Alterations in consciousness and sense of identity, such as fugue states, amnesias, somnambulism; anxiety not evident
3 Phobic neurosis	Intense irrational fears of objects or situations; anxiety attacks may occur with corresponding physical symptoms
4 Obsessive-compulsive neurosis	Persistent or intrusive thoughts, often distressing in content, and uncontrollable minor acts, often to expiate, cleanse, or counteract evil; depression and guilt are prominent; preoccupations with disease may occur
5 Depressive neurosis	Episodic excessive self-criticism, low self-esteem, and lowered vitality, often accompanied by physical complaints
6 Neurasthenic neurosis	Weakness, fatigability, exhaustion, with low self-esteem but little self-criticism
7 Depersonalization neurosis	Feelings of unreality and estrangement from self, body, and surroundings; panic may occur
8 Hypochondriacal neurosis	Morbid preoccupations with bodily processes and diseases, accompanied by multiple physical complaints; anxiety and agitation may occur; depression is common

nervous weakness which is now abating. After all tests for other physical ailments are concluded, the patient is urged to begin walking and resuming normal activities. Sometimes this positive approach can overcome a paralysis within a few minutes, but if it has been present a long time, a vigorous physical program will be needed to restore lost function. Subjective complaints are disregarded, and if the patient continues to emphasize them, reassurance is offered that they will soon recede. Hypnosis, electric stimulation, and dramatic curative methods (Lourdes, acupuncture, etc.) have no advantage. Once rid of the pressing complaint, the patient is best managed by a kindly, understanding physician, sensitive to the nuances of this psychologic disorder, who will analyze each new illness to make sure it is hysterical and not some new intervening disease. Hysterical symptoms should be treated symptomatically, with simple non-habit-forming drugs.

The treatment of compensation problems requires a thorough medical survey, reassurance, symptomatic therapy, and early settlement of the compensation claims. The results in the older worker are far from satisfactory.

It is best to assume that most patients with hypochondriacal reactions have a depression. A few express frankly delusional ideas about their viscera. Severe hypochondriasis in a young person should always suggest schizophrenia. But there are many individuals who have no other mental illness. They go through life being concerned and worried about disease in themselves and their families. Often, one finds that they have been raised in a family atmosphere of overconcern about health. It has become part of their character.

After the proper physical examination procedure and laboratory tests have eliminated serious disease, the physician should tell hypochondriacal patients that they have a neurosis and need help. Symptomatic therapy, a regulated program of daily activities, frequent visits with an understanding physician for explanation and reeducation, and group psychotherapy are all beneficial. But whenever there is suspicion of despondency and depression, a psychiatric opinion should be sought and antidepressive measures as outlined in Chap. 376 should be initiated.

Many patients with depressive states may feel trapped, hopeless, and gloomy—a natural reaction to the symptomatology over which they have no control. Unlike the endogenous and involutional depressions, the mood change may be transitory and variable from day to day, and vegetative symptoms such as loss of appetite, weight loss, constipation, loss of libido, and impotence do not occur. Many psychiatrists distinguish this neurotic type of depression and the reactive depression from the endogenous or organic types, and they caution that the drugs and electroconvulsive therapy used in the endogenous and organic types are usually unsuccessful in neurotic depressions. The line between the two types is thin, however, and the physician is well advised to let a psychiatric consultant stand responsible for separating them and making sure the patient is not suicidal.

COMMON PROBLEMS IN DIAGNOSIS OF PSYCHIATRIC ILLNESSES THAT PRODUCE PHYSICAL SYMPTOMS The physician's greatest concern is misdiagnosis, and physicians rightly appreciate the difficulty of deciding when mental symptoms appear to accompany, mask, or mimic physical disease. There is often the impression that diagnosis is reduced to inspired guesswork. Shulman, in a discussion of psychogenic illness with physical manifestations, states that the common problems are relatively few and not difficult to recognize. He believes the most frequent source of error to be the too strict application of the law of parsimony, which tries to subsume all symptoms under one diagnosis. At least one-fourth to one-half of all adult medical problems represent a cluster or complex of functional-organic or physical-psychosocial illnesses. Most astute physicians can separate the effects of diseases from the associated psychologic reactions.

Probably the largest and most serious diagnostic error may be committed when there are recurrent symptoms in many organ systems for which no obvious cause can be found. Here one must suspect the *masked depression,* i.e., the form of endogenous illness in which the leading complaint is pain (headache, precordial pain, backache, etc.) or exhaustion, and it is a mistake to consider the despondency a secondary reaction (see Woods). A safe rule to follow is that whenever an unexplained syndrome is accompanied by complaints in two or three other organ systems, a serious psychiatric illness with anxiety and depression should be suspected. Complications of pharmacologic therapy and chronic liver or pancreatic disease may rarely give rise to a similar picture.

Another perplexing problem is the anxiety state that is misdiagnosed as menopause, thyrotoxicosis, hypoglycemia, pheochromocytoma, carcinoid tumor, left-sided heart failure, or temporal lobe epilepsy. Each of these diseases causes visceral derangements not unlike those of anxiety. But the latter differs descriptively in that there is always a prominent psychic component of fear and apprehension. It is the combination of mental and autonomic symptoms that should always lead to the suspicion of an anxiety state or anxious depression.

And finally there is the problem of misdiagnosing a neurologic disease (e.g., multiple sclerosis) in a patient who has the conversion form of hysteria or a compensation problem. The lifelong history, the context of the illness, and discrepancy between symptoms and signs should direct thinking along the right path.

In all these problems, a good history is the cornerstone of diagnosis, especially if it includes a kind of life chart of key personal events, medical illnesses, and psychologic derangements. The history is more important than the physical examination and laboratory tests. Incongruities between complaints and between symptoms and physical findings and disabilities are the most important leads. It is "the old crock" with a long history of ill health that is most subject to misdiagnosis.

REFERENCES

ADAMS, RD: *Pathology of Muscle Diseases,* 3d ed. New York, Harper & Row, 1976

COSTA E et al: New concepts on the mechanism of action of benzodiazepines. Life Sci 17:167, 1975

EASTON D, SHERMAN DG: Somatic anxiety attacks and propranolol. Arch Neurol 33:689, 1976

GRAY JA: Anxiety as a paradigm case of emotion. Br Med Bull 37:193, 1981

KAHN E: *Psychopathic Personalities.* New Haven, Yale University Press, 1931

MAAS JW: The clinical and biochemical heterogeneity of the depressive disorders. Ann Intern Med 88:556, 1962

MAYER-GROSS W et al: *Clinical Psychiatry,* 3d ed. Baltimore, Williams & Wilkins, 1969

NICHOLI AM (ed): *The Harvard Guide to Modern Psychiatry.* Cambridge, Mass., Harvard University Press, 1978

OLSEN RW: GABA, benzodiazepine-barbiturate receptor interactions. J Neurochem 37:1, 1981

SCHLESSER MA et al: Hypothalamic-pituitary-adrenal axis activity in depressive illness. Arch Gen Psychiat 37:737, 1980

SHULMAN R: Psychogenic illness with physical manifestations: A practical approach. Lancet 1:524, 1977

WALTON JN (ed): *Diseases of Voluntary Muscle,* 4th ed. London, Churchill, 1981

Woods B: The medical and neurological aspects of depression. *Update III: Harrison's Principles of Internal Medicine,* KJ Isselbacher et al (eds). New York, McGraw-Hill, 1981

12
FAINTNESS, SYNCOPE, AND SEIZURES

RAYMOND D. ADAMS
JOSEPH B. MARTIN

Episodic faintness, light-headedness or giddiness, and reduced alertness are frequently difficult to distinguish, tending to shade into one another. The difference between faintness and frank syncope is only quantitative. Types of episodic weakness, such as myasthenia gravis, cataplexy, and familial periodic paralysis, which cause striking reduction of muscular strength but no impairment of consciousness, should be set apart (see Chaps. 372 and 373). Seizures, an important cause of altered consciousness, usually differ from syncope, but in some instances the distinction may be difficult. The features that distinguish seizures from syncope are discussed at the end of this chapter and in Chap. 355.

SYNCOPE AND FAINTNESS

Syncope comprises a generalized weakness of muscles, with inability to stand upright, and a loss of consciousness. The term *faintness,* in contrast, refers to lack of strength, with sensation of impending loss of consciousness. At the beginning of a syncopal attack the patient is nearly always in the upright position, either sitting or standing [the Stokes-Adams attack (see Chap. 254) is exceptional in this respect]. Usually an individual is warned of the impending faint by a sense of "feeling bad." The patient is assailed by giddiness, the floor seems to move, and surrounding objects begin to sway. The senses become confused; the patient yawns or gapes, there are spots before the eyes, vision may dim, and the ears may ring. Nausea and sometimes vomiting accompany these symptoms. There is a striking pallor or ashen gray color of the face, and very often the face and body are bathed in cold perspiration. The deliberate onset may often allow the patient time for protection against injury; a hurtful fall is exceptional. If the patient can lie down promptly, the attack may be averted without complete loss of consciousness.

The depth and duration of unconsciousness vary. Sometimes the patient is not completely oblivious of the surroundings, or there may be profound coma with complete lack of awareness and of capacity to respond. The patient may remain in this state for seconds to minutes or even as long as half an hour. Usually the patient lies motionless with skeletal muscles relaxed, but a few clonic jerks of the limbs and face may occur shortly after the beginning of the unconsciousness. Sphincter control is usually maintained. The pulse is feeble or cannot be felt; the blood pressure may be low and breathing may be almost imperceptible. Once the patient is in a horizontal position, perhaps from having fallen, gravitation no longer hinders the flow of blood to the brain. The strength of the pulse then improves, color begins to return to the face, breathing becomes quicker and deeper, and consciousness is regained. There is from this moment onward a correct perception of the environment. The patient is, nevertheless, keenly aware of physical weakness, and rising too soon may precipitate another faint. Headache and drowsiness, which, with mental confusion, are the usual sequelae of a convulsion, do not follow a syncopal attack.

ETIOLOGY The list of causes in Table 12-1 is based on established or assumed physiologic mechanisms. The commoner types of faint are reducible to a few simple mechanisms. Syncope results from a sudden impairment of brain metabolism usually brought about by a hypotensive reduction of cerebral blood flow.

Nature has provided humans with several mechanisms by which circulation adjusts to the upright posture. Approximately three-fourths of the systemic blood volume is contained in the venous bed, and any interference with venous return may lead to a reduction in cardiac output. Cerebral blood flow may still be maintained, as long as systemic arterial vasoconstriction occurs; but when this adjustment fails, serious hypotension with resultant cerebral underperfusion to less than half of normal results in syncope. Normally, the pooling of blood in the lower parts of the body is prevented by (1) pressor reflexes which induce constriction of peripheral arterioles and venules, (2) reflex acceleration of the heart by means of aortic and ca-

TABLE 12-1
Causes of recurrent weakness, faintness, and disturbances of consciousness

- *I* Circulatory (deficient quantity of blood to the brain)
  - *A* Inadequate vasoconstrictor mechanisms
    - *1* Vasovagal (vasodepressor)
    - *2* Postural hypotension
    - *3* Primary autonomic insufficiency
    - *4* Sympathectomy (pharmacologic due to antihypertensive medications such as Aldomet and hydralazine, or surgical)
    - *5* Diseases of central and peripheral nervous systems, including autonomic nerves (Chap. 368)
    - *6* Carotid sinus syncope (see also "Bradyarrhythmias," below)
    - *7* Hyperbradykininemia
  - *B* Hypovolemia
  - *C* Mechanical reduction of venous return
    - *1* Valsalva maneuver
    - *2* Cough
    - *3* Micturition
    - *4* Atrial myxoma, ball valve thrombus
  - *D* Reduced cardiac output
    - *1* Obstruction to left ventricular outflow: aortic stenosis, hypertrophic subaortic stenosis
    - *2* Obstruction to pulmonary flow: pulmonic stenosis, primary pulmonary hypertension, pulmonary embolism
    - *3* Myocardial: massive myocardial infarction with pump failure
    - *4* Pericardial: cardiac tamponade
  - *E* Arrhythmias (Chap. 254)
    - *1* Bradyarrhythmias
      - *a* Atrioventricular (AV) block (II° and III°), with Stokes-Adams attacks
      - *b* Ventricular asystole
      - *c* Sinus bradycardia, sinoatrial block, sinus arrest
      - *d* Carotid sinus syncope (see also inadequate vasoconstrictor mechanisms, above)
      - *e* Glossopharyngeal neuralgia (and other painful states)
    - *2* Tachyarrhythmias
      - *a* Episodic ventricular fibrillation with or without associated bradyarrhythmias
      - *b* Ventricular tachycardia
      - *c* Supraventricular tachycardia without AV block
- *II* Other causes of weakness and episodic disturbances of consciousness
  - *A* Altered state of blood to the brain
    - *1* Hypoxia
    - *2* Anemia
    - *3* Diminished carbon dioxide due to hyperventilation (faintness common, syncope seldom occurs)
    - *4* Hypoglycemia (episodic weakness common, faintness occasional, syncope rare)
  - *B* Cerebral
    - *1* Cerebrovascular disturbances (cerebral ischemic attacks, see Chap. 356)
      - *a* Extracranial vascular insufficiency (vertebral-basilar, carotid)
      - *b* Diffuse spasm of cerebral arterioles (hypertensive encephalopathy)
    - *2* Emotional disturbances, anxiety attacks, and hysterical seizures (see Chaps. 11 and 24)

rotid reflexes, and (3) improvement of venous return to the heart by activity of the muscles of the limbs. Placing a normal person on a tilt table to relax the muscles and tilting upright slightly diminishes cardiac output, and allows the blood to accumulate in the legs to a slight degree. This may then be followed by a slight transitory fall in systolic arterial pressure and, in patients with defective vasomotor reflexes, may be a means of producing faints.

TYPES OF SYNCOPE **Vasovagal (vasodepressor) syncope** This is the common faint that may be experienced by normal persons; it is frequently recurrent and tends to take place during emotional stress (especially in a warm, crowded room), after an injurious, shocking accident, and during pain. Mild blood loss, poor physical condition, prolonged bed rest, anemia, fever, organic heart disease, and fasting are other factors which increase the possibility of fainting in susceptible individuals. A short premonitory phase is characterized by nausea, perspiration, yawning, epigastric distress, hyperpnea, tachypnea, weakness, confusion, tachycardia, and pupillary dilatation. Physiologically, there is first a marked fall in arterial pressure and systemic vascular resistance which is most notable in the skeletal muscular beds. Cardiac output may be within normal limits but fails to exhibit the expected increase which normally occurs with hypotension. Output declines when vagal activity leads to marked bradycardia, replacing tachycardia, resulting in further lowering of arterial pressure and reduction of cerebral perfusion. Assumption of the supine posture with elevation of the legs and removal of the offending stimulus will rapidly restore consciousness.

Postural hypotension with syncope This type of syncope affects persons who have a chronic defect in, or variable instability of, vasomotor reflexes. The fall in blood pressure on assumption of upright posture is due to a loss of vasoconstriction reflexes in resistance and capacitance vessels of the lower extremities. Though the character of the syncopal attack differs little from that of the vasovagal or vasodepressor type, the effect of posture is its cardinal feature; sudden arising from a recumbent position or standing still are the circumstances under which it is most likely to happen.

Postural syncope tends to occur under the following conditions:

1 In otherwise normal persons who for some unknown reason have defective postural reflexes (this may be familial). In such individuals fainting may occur when tilted on a table. Under such circumstances it has been found that at first the blood pressure diminishes slightly and then stabilizes at a lower level. Shortly thereafter, the compensatory reflexes suddenly fail and the arterial pressure falls precipitously.

2 In *primary autonomic insufficiency* and in the *dysautonomias.* At least three syndromes have been delineated.

a *Acute or subacute dysautonomia.* In this disease an otherwise healthy adult or child is afflicted over a period of a few days or weeks with a partial or complete paralysis of the parasympathetic and sympathetic nervous systems. Pupillary reflexes are lost, as are lacrimation, salivation, and sweating, and there is impotence, paresis of bladder and bowel musculature, and orthostatic hypotension. The CSF protein is increased. Sensory and motor nerve fibers are demonstrably intact, but nonmedullated autonomic ones have degenerated. Recovery occurs within a few months, possibly hastened by prednisone therapy. The disease is believed to represent a variant of acute idiopathic polyneuritis, akin to Landry-Guillain-Barré syndrome.

b *Chronic postganglionic autonomic insufficiency.* This is a disease of middle-aged and elderly individuals who gradually develop chronic orthostatic hypotension, sometimes in conjunction with impotence, and sphincter disturbances. Upon standing for 5 to 10 min, the blood pressure decreases at least 35 torr and the pulse pressure narrows, both without increase in pulse rate, pallor, or nausea. Men are more often affected than women. The condition is relatively benign and seemingly irreversible.

c *Chronic preganglionic autonomic insufficiency.* In this condition orthostatic hypotension with variable anhidrosis, impotence, and sphincter disturbances is combined with any one of three or more disorders of the central nervous system. These include (1) tremor, extrapyramidal rigidity, and akinesia (Shy-Drager syndrome); (2) progressive cerebellar degeneration, some instances of which are familial; and (3) a more variable extrapyramidal and cerebellar disorder (strionigral degeneration). These syndromes lead to disability and often death within a few years.

The differentiation of the chronic peripheral postganglionic and central preganglionic insufficiency is based on pathologic and pharmacologic evidence. In the postganglionic type, neurons of the sympathetic ganglia degenerate, whereas in the central type, the lateral horn cells of the thoracic spinal cord degenerate. In the postganglionic peripheral type, the resting levels of norepinephrine are subnormal because of failure to release norepinephrine from postganglionic endings, and there is hypersensitivity to injected norepinephrine. In the central type, resting levels of norepinephrine are normal. On standing, unlike the normal individual, there is little if any rise in norepinephrine levels in either type. And in both types, the levels of plasma dopamine β-hydroxylase (the enzyme that converts dopamine to norepinephrine) are subnormal.

The distinction between the various types of orthostatic hypotension has therapeutic significance. In the peripheral postganglionic type, the most effective treatment is 9α-fluorohydrocortisone (oral dose 0.1 to 0.2 mg per day) and salt loading to increase blood volume, supplemented by mechanical devices to prevent pooling of blood in the legs and lower trunk (g suit). However, salt together with mineralocorticoids may induce serious supine hypertension and the dose of the drug must be adjusted for this. For the central preganglionic type, there has been greater success with use of a sympathomimetic amine such as tyramine (which releases norepinephrine from intact postganglionic endings) supplemented by a monoamine oxidase inhibitor (to prevent destruction of the amine), and possibly propranolol (Inderal). Levodopa has been effective in some cases. In the postganglionic type, judicious use of phenylephrine or ephedrine may be beneficial. Initial reports of the effectiveness of indomethacin in chronic orthostatic hypotension have not been substantiated.

3 After physical deconditioning, e.g., after prolonged illness with recumbency, especially in elderly individuals with reduced muscle tone.

4 After a sympathectomy that has abolished vasopressor reflexes.

5 In diabetic, alcoholic, and other neuropathies; tabes dorsalis; syringomyelia; subacute combined sclerosis; and diseases of the nervous system which cause muscular atrophy and paralysis of vasopressor reflexes. The most common form of neurogenic orthostatic hypotension is that which accompanies diseases of the peripheral nervous system. Diabetic polyneuropathy, beriberi, amyloid polyneuropathy, and the Adie syndrome are examples. Usually the orthostatic hypotension is associated with disturbances in sweating, impotence, and sphincter difficulties. Presumably the lesion involves postganglionic, nonmedullated fibers in peripheral nerves.

6 In patients receiving antihypertensive and vasodilator drugs as well as those who may be hypovolemic because of diuretics, excessive sweating, or adrenal insufficiency.

Micturition syncope, a condition usually seen in the elderly during or after urination, particularly after arising from the recumbent position, is probably a special type of postural syncope. It has been suggested that release of intravesicular pressure causes sudden vasodilatation, augmented by standing, and that vagally mediated bradycardia is a contributory factor.

Hyperbradykininemia Deficient kinin-inactivating enzymes with apparently normal sympathetic function may result in symptoms of faintness or syncope on assumption of upright posture. Hyperbradykininemia causes arteriolar and venular dilatation giving rise to postural hypotension and syncope with tachycardia. The pathophysiology of this condition remains uncertain. Treatment with beta-receptor antagonists has been beneficial.

Syncope of cardiac origin (cardiac syncope) Cardiac syncope results from a sudden reduction in cardiac output, caused most commonly by a cardiac arrhythmia. In normal individuals slow ventricular rates, but above 35 to 40 beats per minute, and fast ones not exceeding 180 beats per minute do not reduce cerebral blood flow, especially if the person is in the supine position, but changes in pulse rate outside these limits may impair cerebral circulation and function. The upright posture, cerebrovascular disease, anemia, and coronary, myocardial, or valvular disease all reduce the tolerance to alterations in rate.

Complete atrioventricular block is the commonest arrhythmia that leads to fainting, and syncopal episodes associated with this arrhythmia are known as the Stokes-Adams-Morgagni syndrome. The etiology of disturbances in atrioventricular conduction is considered elsewhere (Chap. 254), but in patients with these attacks the block may be persistent or intermittent; it is often preceded or followed by disturbed conduction in one or two of the three fascicles through which the ventricles are normally activated, by second-degree atrioventricular block (Mobitz type II), or bifascicular or trifascicular block. When the block is complete and the pacemaker below the block fails to function, syncope occurs. A brief bout of ventricular tachycardia or fibrillation may also be responsible for the syncopal episode. Recurrent syncope due to ventricular fibrillation, characterized by a prolonged QT interval (sometimes associated with congenital deafness), has been reported; this condition may be familial or sporadic.

Stokes-Adams attacks occur usually without more than a momentary sense of weakness, the patient suddenly losing consciousness. After cardiac standstill of more than several seconds, the patient turns pale, falls unconscious, and, as in other types of fainting, may exhibit a few clonic jerks. With longer periods of asystole, the ashen gray pallor gives way to cyanosis, stertorous breathing, fixed pupils, incontinence, and bilateral Babinski signs. Prolonged confusion and neurologic signs due to cerebral ischemia may occur in some patients, and permanent impairment of mental function may result, although focal neurologic signs are rare. Cardiac faints of this type may recur several times a day. Occasionally the heart block is transitory, and the electrocardiogram taken later may not show any arrhythmia.

Less commonly, a decreased rate of discharge of the sinoatrial node leads to syncope. Recurrent attacks of tachyarrhythmias—including atrial flutter and paroxysmal atrial and ventricular tachycardia with normal AV conduction—may also suddenly reduce cardiac output to a degree sufficient to cause syncope.

In another form of cardiac syncope the heart block is reflexive and is due to irritation of the vagus nerves. Examples of this phenomenon have been observed in patients with esophageal diverticula, mediastinal tumors, gallbladder disease, carotid sinus disease, glossopharyngeal neuralgia, and pleural and pulmonary irritation. However, in these conditions reflex bradycardia is more commonly of the sinoatrial than the atrioventricular type.

Cardiac syncope may also result from *acute massive myocardial infarction,* particularly when associated with cardiogenic shock. *Aortic stenosis* often sets the stage for exertional syncope, most commonly by limiting cardiac output in the face of peripheral vasodilatation, but sometimes during exertion, with resultant myocardial and cerebral ischemia and occasionally arrhythmias. *Idiopathic hypertrophic subaortic stenosis* may also lead to exertional syncope, because of intensified obstruction and/or ventricular arrhythmias (Chap. 254). In *primary pulmonary hypertension* a relatively fixed cardiac output and bouts of acute right ventricular failure may be associated with syncope (Chap. 281). However, vagal reflexes may be involved in this condition as well as in the syncope that occurs with *pulmonary embolism.* Ball valve thrombus in the left atrium, left atrial myxoma, or thrombosis or malfunction of a prosthetic valve may produce sudden mechanical obstruction of the circulation and syncope. *Tetralogy of Fallot* is the congenital cardiac malformation most commonly responsible for syncope. In this condition systemic vasodilatation, perhaps associated with infundibular spasm, greatly increases the right-to-left shunt and produces arterial hypoxia, which leads to syncope (Chap. 256).

Carotid sinus syncope The carotid sinus is normally sensitive to stretch and gives rise to sensory impulses carried via the nerve of Hering, a branch of the glossopharyngeal nerve, to the medulla oblongata. Massage of one or both of the carotid sinuses, particularly in elderly persons, causes (1) a reflex cardiac slowing (sinus bradycardia, sinus arrest, or even atrioventricular block), the so-called vagal type of response and (2) a fall of arterial pressure without cardiac slowing, the so-called depressor type of response. Both types of carotid sinus response may coexist.

Syncope due to carotid sinus sensitivity may be initiated by turning of the head to one side, by a tight collar, or, as in a few reported cases, by shaving over the region of the sinus. But the absence of such stimuli is of no aid in diagnosis, since spontaneous attacks may occur. The attack nearly always begins when the patient is in an upright position, usually when standing. The period of unconsciousness seldom lasts longer than a few minutes. The sensorium is immediately clear when consciousness is regained. The majority of the reported cases have been in men. In a patient displaying faintness on compression of one carotid sinus, it is important to distinguish between the benign disorder (hypersensitivity of one carotid sinus) and a much more serious condition—atheromatous narrowing of the opposite carotid or of the basilar artery (see Chap. 356).

Other forms of vasovagal syncope have been described. Exceptionally intense pain of visceral origin may inhibit cardiac action through vagal stimulation, e.g., cardiac standstill during an attack of gallbladder colic, a lesion of the esophagus or mediastinum, bronchoscopy, pleural or peritoneal taps, intense vertigo from labyrinthine or vestibular disease, and needling of body cavities.

Vagal and glossopharyngeal neuralgia Occasionally this induces a reflex type of fainting. Again the sequence is always pain, then syncope; in this instance the pain is localized to the base of the tongue, pharynx or larynx, tonsillar area, and ear. It may be triggered by pressure at these sites. Section of the appropriate branches of the ninth or tenth cranial nerve relieves the condition. The cardiovascular effects are attributable to excitation of the dorsal motor nucleus of the vagus via collateral fibers from the nucleus of the tractus solitarius.

Tussive syncope (laryngeal vertigo) This is a rare condition that results from a paroxysm of coughing, usually in men with chronic bronchitis. After hard coughing the patient suddenly becomes weak and loses consciousness momentarily. The intrathoracic pressure becomes elevated and interferes with the venous return to the heart, as does the Valsalva maneuver (exhaling against a closed glottis).

Syncope associated with cerebrovascular disease This is usually caused by partial or complete occlusion of the large arteries in the neck. Physical activity may then critically reduce blood flow to the upper part of the brainstem, causing abrupt loss of consciousness (see Chap. 356).

PATHOPHYSIOLOGY OF SYNCOPE The loss of consciousness in each type of syncope is caused by reduction of oxygenation to those parts of the brain which subserve consciousness. During syncopal attacks, there are demonstrable reductions in cerebral blood flow, cerebral oxygen utilization, and cerebrovascular resistance. The electroencephalogram reveals high-voltage slow waves, two to five per second, coincident with the loss of consciousness. If the ischemia lasts only a few minutes, there are no lasting effects on the brain. If it persists for a longer time, it may result in necrosis of brain tissue in the border zones of perfusion between the vascular territories of the major cerebral and cerebellar arteries.

DIFFERENTIAL DIAGNOSIS OF CONDITIONS INVOLVING EPISODIC WEAKNESS AND FAINTNESS BUT NOT SYNCOPE

Anxiety attacks and the hyperventilation syndrome These are discussed in detail in Chaps. 11 and 376. The giddiness of anxiety is frequently interpreted as a feeling of faintness without actual loss of consciousness. Such symptoms are not accompanied by facial pallor and are not relieved by recumbency. The diagnosis is made on the basis of the associated symptoms, and part of the attack can be reproduced by hyperventilation. Two of the mechanisms known to be involved in the attacks are reduction in carbon dioxide as the result of hyperventilation and the release of epinephrine. Hyperventilation results in hypocapnia, alkalosis, increased cerebrovascular resistance, and decreased cerebral blood flow.

Hypoglycemia When severe, hypoglycemia is usually traceable to a serious disease, such as a tumor of the islets of Langerhans or advanced adrenal, pituitary, or hepatic disease, or to excessive administration of insulin. The clinical picture is one of confusion or even a loss of consciousness. When mild, as is usually the case, hypoglycemia is often of the reactive type (Chap. 116), occurring 2 to 5 h after eating, and is not usually associated with a disturbance of consciousness. The diagnosis depends on the history and the documentation of reduced blood sugar during an attack.

Acute hemorrhage Acute blood loss, usually within the gastrointestinal tract, is an occasional cause of syncope. In the absence of pain and hematemesis the cause of the weakness, faintness, or even unconsciousness may remain obscure until the passage of a black stool.

Cerebral ischemic attacks These occur in some patients with arteriosclerotic narrowings or occlusion of the major arteries of the brain. The main symptoms vary from patient to patient

and include dim vision, hemiparesis, numbness of one side of the body, dizziness, and thick speech, and to these may be added an impairment of consciousness. In any one patient all attacks are of identical type and indicate a temporary deficit of function in a certain region of the brain due to inadequate circulation.

Hysterical fainting Hysterical fainting is rather frequent and usually occurs under dramatic circumstances (Chap. 375). The attack is unattended by any outward display of anxiety. The evident lack of change in pulse and blood pressure or color of the skin and mucous membranes distinguishes it from the vasodepressor faint. The diagnosis is based on the bizarre nature of the attack in a person who exhibits the general personality and behavioral characteristics of the hysteric.

Different types of syncope Differentiation of the several conditions that diminish cerebral blood flow is discussed in greater detail in Chap. 29.

When faintness is related to reduced cerebral blood flow resulting directly from a disorder of cardiac function, there is likely to be a combination of pallor and cyanosis. When, on the other hand, the peripheral circulation is at fault, pallor is usually striking but is not accompanied by cyanosis or respiratory disturbances. When the primary disturbance lies in the cerebral circulation, the face is likely to be florid and the breathing slow and stertorous. During the attack a heart rate faster than 150 beats per minute indicates an ectopic cardiac rhythm, while a striking bradycardia (rate of less than 40 beats per minute) suggests complete heart block. In a patient with faintness or syncope attended by bradycardia, one has to distinguish that due to failure of neurogenic reflexes from that due to a cardiogenic (Stokes-Adams) attack. The electrocardiogram is decisive, but even without it, the Stokes-Adams seizures can be recognized clinically by their longer duration, by the greater constancy of the slow heart rate, by the presence of audible sounds synchronous with atrial contractions, by atrial contraction (A) waves in the jugular venous pulse, and by marked variation in intensity of the first sound, despite the regular rhythm (Chap. 254).

In cases of recurrent syncope of unknown cause, the use of intracardiac electrophysiologic techniques with programmed stimulation can be helpful in determining cardiac abnormalities and in establishing effective treatment. During stimulation, up to two-thirds of such patients can be shown to have rapid ventricular tachycardia, His bundle conduction delays, atrial flutter, sick-sinus syndrome, or hypervagotonia.

Type of onset When the attack begins over the period of a few seconds, carotid sinus syncope, postural hypotension, sudden atrioventricular block, ventricular standstill, or fibrillation is likely. When the symptoms develop gradually during a period of several minutes, hyperventilation or hypoglycemia should be considered. Onset of syncope during or immediately after exertion suggests aortic stenosis or idiopathic hypertrophic subaortic stenosis and, in elderly subjects, postural hypotension. Exertional syncope is seen occasionally in persons with aortic insufficiency and with severe occlusive disease of cerebral arteries. In patients with ventricular standstill or ventricular fibrillation, loss of consciousness occurs several seconds later, followed rapidly by cessation of electroencephalographic activity and then often by brief clonic contractions.

Position at onset of attack Epilepsy and syncopal attacks due to hypoglycemia, hyperventilation, or heart block are likely to be independent of posture. Faintness associated with a decline in blood pressure (including carotid sinus attacks) and with ectopic tachycardia usually occurs only in the sitting or standing position, whereas faintness resulting from orthostatic hypotension is apt to set in shortly after change from the recumbent to the standing position.

Associated symptoms Palpitation is likely to be present when the attack is due to anxiety or hyperventilation, to ectopic tachycardia, or to hypoglycemia. Numbness and tingling in the hands and face are frequent accompaniments of hyperventilation. Genuine convulsions during the attack may occasionally occur with heart block, ventricular standstill, or fibrillation.

Duration of attack When the duration is very brief, i.e., a few seconds to a few minutes, carotid sinus syncope or one of the several forms of postural hypotension is most likely. A duration of more than a few minutes but less than an hour suggests hypoglycemia or hyperventilation.

SPECIAL METHODS OF EXAMINATION In many patients who complain of recurrent weakness or syncope but do not have a spontaneous attack while under observation, an attempt to reproduce attacks is of great assistance in diagnosis.

When hyperventilation is accompanied by faintness, the pattern of symptoms can be reproduced readily by having the subject breathe rapidly and deeply for 2 to 3 min. This test is often of therapeutic value also, because the underlying anxiety tends to be lessened when the patient learns that the symptoms can be produced and alleviated at will simply by controlling breathing.

Among other conditions in which the diagnosis is commonly clarified by reproducing the attacks are carotid sinus hypersensitivity (massage of one or the other carotid sinus), orthostatic hypotension and orthostatic tachycardia (observations of pulse rate, blood pressure, and symptoms in the recumbent and standing positions), and tussive syncope (by inducing the Valsalva maneuver). In all these instances the crucial point is not whether symptoms are produced (the procedures mentioned frequently induce symptoms in healthy persons) but whether the exact pattern of symptoms that occurs in the spontaneous attacks is reproduced in the artificial ones. Careful, continuous Holter monitoring of the electrocardiogram in the hospital or the recording of the electrocardiogram over 1 or 2 days using a portable lightweight tape recorder in an ambulatory patient may be extremely useful in identifying an arrhythmia responsible for the syncopal episode. Monitoring is most helpful if it shows that the syncopal episode is characterized by a bout of cardiac standstill, extreme bradycardia, or tachyarrhythmia.

The electroencephalogram may be helpful in differentiating syncope from seizures. In the interval between epileptic seizures it may show some degree of abnormality in 40 to 80 percent of cases. In the interval between syncopal attacks it should be normal.

TREATMENT In most instances fainting is relatively benign. In dealing with patients who have fainted, the physician should think first of those causes of fainting that constitute a therapeutic emergency. Among them are massive internal hemorrhage and myocardial infarction, which may be painless, and cardiac arrhythmias. In elderly persons a sudden faint, without obvious cause, should arouse the suspicion of complete heart block, even though all findings are negative when the patient is seen.

Patients seen during the preliminary stages of fainting or after they have lost consciousness should be placed in a position which permits maximal cerebral blood flow, i.e., with head lowered between the knees, if sitting, or in the supine position. All tight clothing and other constrictions should be loosened and the head turned so that the tongue does not fall back into the throat, blocking the airway. Peripheral irritation, such as sprinkling or dashing cold water on the face and neck or the application of cold moist towels, is helpful. If the temperature is subnormal, the body should be covered with a warm blanket. Since emesis is frequent, aspiration should be prevented. The head should be turned to the side and nothing should be given by mouth until the patient has regained consciousness. Patients should not be permitted to rise until the sense of physical weakness has passed, and they should be watched carefully for a few minutes after rising.

The *prevention* of fainting depends on the mechanisms involved. In the usual vasovagal faint of adolescents, which tends to occur in periods of emotional excitement, fatigue, hunger, etc., it is enough to advise the patient to avoid such circumstances. In postural hypotension, patients should be cautioned against arising suddenly from bed. Instead, they should first exercise their legs for a few seconds, then sit on the edge of the bed and make sure they are not lightheaded or dizzy before starting to walk. Sleeping with the headposts of the bed elevated on wooden blocks 8 to 12 in high and wearing snug elastic abdominal binder and elastic stockings are often helpful. Drugs of the ephedrine group may be useful if they do not cause insomnia. If there are no contraindications, a high intake of sodium chloride, which expands the extracellular fluid volume, may be beneficial.

In the syndrome of chronic orthostatic hypotension, special corticosteroid preparations (Florinef Acetate tablets, 0.1 to 0.2 mg per day in divided doses) have given relief in some cases. Binding of the legs (g suit) and sleeping with head and shoulders elevated are helpful.

The treatment of carotid sinus syncope involves first of all instructing the patient in measures that minimize the hazards of a fall (see below). Loose collars should be worn, and the patient should learn to turn the whole body, rather than the head alone, when looking to one side. Atropine or the ephedrine group of drugs should be used, respectively, in patients with pronounced bradycardia or hypotension during attacks. If atropine is not successful, a demand pacemaker should be inserted into the right ventricle. Radiation or surgical denervation of the carotid sinus has apparently yielded favorable results in some patients, but it is rarely necessary. Once it has been concluded that the attacks are due to a narrowing of major cerebral arteries, some of the surgical measures discussed in Chap. 356 must be considered.

The treatment of the various cardiac arrhythmias which may induce syncope is discussed in Chap. 254. The treatment of hypoglycemia will be found in Chap. 116 and of the hyperventilation syndrome and hysterical fainting in Chap. 11.

The chief hazard of a faint in most elderly persons is not the underlying disease but fracture or other trauma due to the fall. Therefore, patients subject to recurrent syncope should cover the bathroom floor and bathtub with rubber mats and should have as much of their home carpeted as is feasible. Especially important is the floor space between the bed and the bathroom, because faints are common in elderly persons when walking from bed to toilet. Outdoor walking should be on soft ground rather than hard surfaces, and the patient should avoid standing still, which is more likely than walking to induce an attack.

SEIZURES

A cerebral seizure or convulsion is defined as an abrupt alteration in cortical electrical activity manifested clinically by a change in consciousness or by a motor, sensory, or behavioral symptom. Seizures, which may be due to a variety of causes, become important in the differential diagnosis of syncope when the episode occurs with minimal or no warning and results in only a brief loss of consciousness. *Epilepsy* (discussed in Chap. 355) is the term used to describe recurrent seizures present over months or years, often with a stereotyped clinical pattern.

CLINICAL CHARACTERISTICS OF SEIZURES A detailed account of the types of seizures, of their pathophysiology, and of their treatment is found in Chap. 355. The purpose here is to recount briefly the varieties of seizures that occur (Table 12-2), and to outline their clinical presentation, particularly with respect to their distinction from syncope. A single seizure may occur during the course of many medical illnesses; its importance derives from the fact that it signifies involvement of the central nervous system by the disease process.

Partial seizures (focal seizures) The appearance of focal motor or sensory manifestations provide clinical documentation of the localization of the cerebral lesion. Deviation of the eyes and head to one side (adversive seizure) points to an irritative focus in the opposite prefrontal region. A Jacksonian seizure begins as a clonic movement in one portion of the body, often the thumb, the corner of the mouth, or the great toe, and spreads to adjacent muscular groups over a few seconds or minutes. The order of the march corresponds to the spread of the electrical discharge in the motor cortex and has precise localizing value. The seizure may progress to involve the entire side or become generalized with attendant loss of consciousness. Jacksonian seizures almost always are accompanied by an abnormal interictal EEG. *Epilepsia partialis continua* is a persistently focal motor seizure which may involve only a small excursion of a finger or toe. The seizure can recur intermittently over weeks or months and has great value in localizing intrinsic central nervous system disease.

Complex partial seizures (temporal lobe or psychomotor seizures) These differ from generalized motor seizures by (1) subjective presence of an aura that arises from discharges in the autonomic, visceral, and olfactory portions of the temporal lobe and limbic system; and (2) objective manifestation of behavioral and often complex motor movements for which the patient is amnesic after the attack. Subjective experiences of the aura include hallucinations (olfactory, gustatory, visual, or auditory), illusions (spatial distortions, shrinkage, or angulation), aberrations in cognition (déjà vu, a sense of familiarity; jamais vu, a sense of unfamiliarity; or recurrent memory), and affective changes (anxiety, fear, and, very rarely, rage). The seizure may terminate with only the subjective component or may progress to the motor phase which is often evident by repetitive motor acts like smacking the lips, swallowing, undressing, and incoherent or dysphasic speech.

TABLE 12-2
Classification of seizures

I Partial or focal seizures
- *A* Simple partial seizures—usually without loss of consciousness
  - *1* Motor—Jacksonian
  - *2* Sensory—somatosensory, visual, auditory, olfactory
- *B* Complex partial seizures
  - *1* Temporal lobe or "psychomotor" seizures (usually accompanied by loss of consciousness)

II Primary generalized seizures—bilaterally symmetric, without focal onset, associated with loss of consciousness
- *A* Tonic-clonic (grand mal)
- *B* Absence (petit mal)
- *C* Atypical absence—myoclonic, akinetic

III Partial seizure with secondary bilateral generalization associated with warning (vertiginous, autonomic, olfactory, etc.) followed by loss of consciousness

The abrupt onset of complex partial seizures indicates a disorder of the temporal lobe and its connection to the limbic system. Complete investigation in search of the cause is indicated.

Tonic-clonic (grand mal) seizure The abrupt presentation, without warning, of a generalized motor seizure is one of the commonest indications of involvement of the cerebral cortex by a disease process. Grand mal seizures usually begin with opening of the eyes and mouth, flexion and abduction of the arms, and extension of the legs. The *tonic* phase of the seizure is often heralded by contraction of the respiratory muscles resulting in a vocalization. These motor signs are followed by closure of the jaw, often with laceration of the tongue, respiratory arrest with plethora and cyanosis, and urinary, or less commonly, fecal incontinence. The tonic phase of the seizure, which usually persists for only 15 to 30 s, is followed immediately by the *clonic* phase, characterized by violent rhythmic muscular contractions affecting the whole body including the muscles of respiration. Eye movements, facial grimacing, and persistence of respiratory apnea are evident. The clonic movements subside in amplitude and frequency and the seizure terminates, usually within 1 to 2 min. Normal respiration resumes and the patient falls asleep; arousal may occur in a few minutes but lethargy, fatigue, and postseizure (postictal) confusion are common and may persist for several hours. Postictal headache is common.

The generalized seizure occurring in the course of a major medical illness signifies involvement of the central nervous system by the disorder and requires careful assessment and investigation. Such a seizure may accompany high fever, hyponatremia, metabolic acidosis, alcohol or drug withdrawal, and renal or liver failure, indicating the presence of a *metabolic encephalopathy*, without requiring the postulation of another separate neurologic illness. The determination that a metabolic encephalopathy may be responsible is dependent upon documentation of the systemic illness and careful attention to the exclusion of an additional infectious, vascular, or neoplastic lesion in the nervous system. Central nervous system evaluation should include a careful history, a detailed neurologic examination searching for focal neurologic deficit, and, in many cases, electroencephalography and CT scan. If infection is suspected, an examination of the cerebrospinal fluid is mandatory. Recurrent seizures (status epilepticus) indicate a serious compromise of cerebral cortical function and require vigorous treatment to prevent hypoxic damage to the brain and, following termination of the seizures, a thorough investigation of the cause.

An isolated generalized seizure occurring in an otherwise healthy, asymptomatic patient when observed by family or other bystanders is not difficult to distinguish from syncope. More difficult to assess is the circumstance of sudden loss of consciousness occurring without warning and unwitnessed by an observer or an akinetic "drop-seizure" (atypical petit mal). The latter may be indistinguishable from syncope. Postictal confusion or drowsiness, injury such as laceration of the tongue, urinary or fecal incontinence, or muscle soreness suggests that a convulsion has occurred. One common clinical presentation is the sudden occurrence of a brief clonic seizure during a minor surgical or dental procedure. The patient is usually in a seated position and the episode is considered to be due to cerebral ischemia associated with systemic hypotension and bradycardia accompanying vasovagal syncope. There are usually only two or three clonic movements, without a prior tonic phase, and recovery is rapid without postictal symptoms.

Such patients should have a neurologic examination and an EEG and, if these are normal, be treated with reassurance and not given anticonvulsants. There is no evidence to indicate an underlying cerebral lesion in such patients.

Generalized seizures may be preceded by a specific warning or *aura* and attention to these symptoms may be important in aiding in the localization of the seizure focus and assist in distinguishing the episode from syncope. Tingling or numbness points to involvement of the parietal lobe and visual or auditory sensations suggest occipitotemporal localization. More complex psychologic and cognitive sensations may accompany temporal lobe seizures. Such symptoms may also accompany transient cerebral ischemic attacks (see Chap. 356), but in this case the symptoms usually persist for many minutes or hours.

Absence (petit mal) seizures Absence seizures, in contrast to grand mal, are noted for their brevity and for the degree of loss of consciousness accompanied by minimal motor manifestations. They are abrupt in onset and are often evident only by a stare or cessation of ongoing behavior; they may be accompanied by fluttering of the eyelids or by a few facial twitches. Full recovery occurs in 5 to 10 s, and the episode may go unnoticed by the patient, the family, or the teacher. Loss of postural tone (atonic or akinetic seizure) with falling is uncommon but when present requires distinction from syncope. The EEG is diagnostic in such cases, consisting of three-per-second spike and wave discharges. This condition, which indicates a specific generalized disorder of cerebral electrical activity, is responsive to specific drug treatments (see Chap. 355).

DIFFERENTIAL DIAGNOSIS OF SEIZURES AND SYNCOPE
Syncope must be distinguished from other disturbances of cerebral function, the most frequent of which is an atonic or some other form of seizure. A seizure may occur day or night, regardless of the position of the patient; syncope rarely appears when the patient is recumbent, the only common exception being the Stokes-Adams attack. The patient's color may not change in seizures, though there may be cyanosis; pallor is an early and invariable finding in all types of syncope, except chronic orthostatic hypotension and hysteria, and it precedes unconsciousness. Seizures are more sudden in onset and if an aura is present, it rarely lasts longer than a few seconds before consciousness is lost. The onset of syncope is usually more deliberate and without aura. Injury from falling is frequent in a seizure and rare in syncope, for the reason that only in seizures are protective reflexes abolished instantaneously. Tonic-convulsive movements with upturning eyes are a feature of seizures and not syncope. The period of unconsciousness tends to be longer in seizures than in syncope. Urinary incontinence is frequent in seizures and rare in syncope. The return of consciousness is prompt in syncope, slow after a seizure. Mental confusion, headache, and drowsiness are common sequelae of seizures; physical weakness with a clear sensorium characterizes the postsyncopal state. Repeated spells of unconsciousness in a young person at a rate of several per day or month are more suggestive of epilepsy than of syncope. No one of these points will absolutely differentiate a seizure from syncope, but taken as a group and supplemented by electroencephalograms, they provide a means of distinguishing the two conditions.

TREATMENT See Chap. 355.

REFERENCES

CRILL WE: Neuronal mechanisms of seizure initiation, in *Antiepileptic Drugs: Mechanisms of Action,* GH Glaser et al (eds). New York, Raven Press, 1980, p 169

DIMARCO JP et al: Intracardiac electrophysiologic techniques in recurrent syncope of unknown cause. Ann Intern Med 95:542, 1981

EWING DJ et al: The natural history of diabetic autonomic neuropathy. Q J Med 49:95, 1980

GLAZER GH: Epilepsy, in *Recent Advances in Clinical Neurology,* WB Mathews (ed). Edinburgh, Churchill Livingstone, 1975, pp 23–68

HAUSER WA, KURLAND LT: The epidemiology of epilepsy in Rochester, Minnesota. Epilepsia 16:1, 1975

HICKLER R: Fainting, in *Signs and Symptoms,* 6th ed, RS Blacklow (ed). Philadelphia, Lippincott, 1977, chap 33

JASPER HH et al (eds): *Basic Mechanisms of the Epilepsies.* Boston, Little Brown, 1969

JOHNSON RH, SPAULDING JMK: *Disorders of the Autonomic Nervous System.* Philadelphia, Davis, 1974

LEE JE et al: Episodic unconsciousness, in *Diagnostic Approaches to Presenting Syndromes,* JA Barondess (ed). Baltimore, Williams & Wilkins, 1971, pp 133–167

LENNOX W, LENNOX M: *Epilepsy and Related Disorders.* Boston, Little, Brown, 1960

POLINSKY RJ et al: Pharmacologic distinction of different orthostatic hypotension syndromes. Neurology 31:1, 1981

SCHMIDT RP, WILDER BJ: Epilepsy, in *Contemporary Neurology Series,* F Plum, FH McDowell (eds). Philadelphia, Davis, 1968

STREETER DHP et al: Hyperbradykininism: A new orthostatic syndrome. Lancet ii:1048, 1972

SUTHERLAND JM, EADIE MJ: *The Epilepsies,* 3d ed. Edinburgh, Churchill Livingstone, 1980

WEISSLER AM, WARREN, JV: Syncope and shock, in *The Heart,* 4th ed, JW Hurst et al (eds). New York, McGraw-Hill, 1978, p 705

WRIGHT KE JR, MCINTOSH MD: Syncope: Review of pathophysiological mechanisms. Prog Cardiovasc Dis 13:580, 1971

YOUNG RR et al: Pure pandysautonomia with recovery. Description and discussion of diagnostic criteria. Brain 98:613, 1975

13

DIZZINESS AND VERTIGO

MAURICE VICTOR
RAYMOND D. ADAMS

Dizziness and other similar sensations are remarkably common symptoms, the significance of which varies greatly. Most often they are benign, but in many instances a correct analysis of the complaint provides the clue to an important medical disorder.

The patient uses the term to describe a number of different sensory experiences—a feeling of whirling or rotation (true vertigo), as well as nonrotatory swaying, weakness, faintness, and lightheadedness. Blurring of vision, feelings of unreality, syncope, and even petit mal may be incorrectly called dizzy spells; hence close questioning as to how the patient is using the term becomes a necessary first step in clinical study. A distinction is sometimes drawn between subjective vertigo, meaning a sense of turning of one's body, and objective vertigo, an illusion of movement of objects in the environment, but its validity is doubtful.

In this chapter the term *vertigo* is used to refer to all subjective and objective illusions of rotation. Other nonrotatory forms of dizziness are referred to as *giddiness,* or *pseudovertigo.* The distinction between these two groups of symptoms is elaborated below. Equilibrium, the state of equipoise whereby the posture of the body is maintained against the forces of gravity, is deranged in vertigo but is also affected by other disorders—e.g., loss of joint or muscle sense (sensory ataxia), cerebellar disease (cerebellar ataxia), and motor abnormalities (spasticity and rigidity, myotonia, and the pseudomyotonia of hypothyroidism).

ANATOMIC, PHYSIOLOGIC, AND PSYCHOLOGICAL CONSIDERATIONS The labyrinthine-vestibular sensory system is the main apparatus for the maintenance of equilibrium and awareness of the body's position in relation to its environment. It serves to transduce forces associated with linear and angular movements of the head into nerve impulses that reflexly control movement and posture. Five sensory organs are included: the two saccular and utricular macules sense linear movements of the head; the three semicircular canals sense angular accelerations of the head. Each macule supports otoliths (calcareous material embedded in a gelatinous matrix), the position of which is altered by linear motion and (statically) by the effects of gravity. The cristae (the sensory receptors of the semicircular canals) are attached to their walls and are activated by motions of the fluid within the canals. Currents can also be induced in this fluid by warming and cooling the tympanic membrane (as in the caloric test). The otoliths and cristae deform hair cells of the sensory membranes, which induce nerve impulses. The latter are transmitted by ganglion cells (Scarpa's ganglion located in the internal auditory canal) and reach the brainstem via the vestibular nerve (a division of the eighth cranial nerve). The central termination of the vestibular nerve is the vestibular nuclei, which in turn connect by way of the vestibulo- and reticulo-spinal tracts and the medial longitudinal fasciculus with spinal motor nerve cells, the cerebellum, and oculomotor nuclei. These motor neurons are responsible for the reflex postural movements and the tonic influences on ocular muscles manifested in lateral pulsions and nystagmus. Vestibular impulses also ascend to the contralateral ventroposterolateral nucleus of the thalamus and then to the parietal lobe for the perception of vertigo. Impulses also pass to the dorsal motor nucleus of the vagus and nucleus solitarius, accounting for attendant nausea, vomiting, salivation, and sweating, of which seasickness is an example.

Nonlabyrinthine mechanisms are also important. These are:

1 Impulses from the retinas which are coordinated by ocular motor mechanisms to supply information about the position and movement of the body and its surroundings.
2 Impulses from the proprioceptors of joints and muscles—essential to all reflex, postural, and volitional movements. Those of the neck are of special importance in relating the position of the head to that of the rest of the body.

The cerebellum and certain ganglionic centers in the brainstem (particularly the vestibular nuclei, oculomotor nuclei, and red nuclei) and the basal ganglia are the important coordinators of these sensory data and provide for postural adjustment, i.e., upright stance and locomotion.

Important psychophysiologic mechanisms are also involved in the maintenance of equilibrium and the proper relationship of our bodies to the external world. Early in life we come to coordinate the parts of our body in relation to one another and to perceive that portion of space occupied by our bodies. The construct of these integrated sensory data has been designated by Russell Brain as the *body schema.* The space around our body is said to be represented by another set of data, the *environmental schema.* These two schemata are dynamic and interdependent, since both are changed simultaneously in every activity. For example, we learn to see objects as being stationary when we are moving. Thus, the motion of ourselves and of objects in space is always relative. At times, when sensory information is incomplete, we mistake movement of our surroundings for those of our own body, as in the illusion caused by motion of a neighboring train. A disturbance in the awareness of one's own body schema is postulated by some psychiatrists as the basis of neurotic disorientation and psychotic feelings of unreality.

CLINICAL CHARACTERISTICS OF VERTIGO AND GIDDINESS The clinical recognition of *vertigo* proves to be relatively easy when the patient states that objects in the environment turn or move in one direction or that the head and body whirl. Often, however, the patient is not so explicit. The feeling may be described as oscillation, or veering or being pulled to one side or to the ground, as though drawn by a magnet (impulsion). Again, the floor or walls may seem to tilt, sink, or rise up. Such feelings are notable features of a labyrinthine disorder, as is the sensation of being pulled or tilted. Past pointing to one side when the eyes are closed is part of the same mechanism.

All but the mildest forms of vertigo are accompanied by perspiration, pallor, nausea, and vomiting. The nystagmus which is invariably present causes objects in the field of vision to move rhythmically. As a rule the patient can walk only with difficulty, or not at all if the vertigo is intense. A sudden attack may even catapult the patient to the ground, and only then is vertigo experienced. Forced to lie down, the patient realizes that one position, usually on one side with eyes closed, reduces the vertigo and nausea, and that the slightest motion of the head aggravates them. One form of vertigo, the *benign positional vertigo of Bárány,* occurs only for a few seconds after lying down and sitting up. If the vertigo is less severe, the patient can walk unsteadily but may veer to one side. With the mildest form, the patient is conscious only of a disequilibrium on walking. The source of the ataxia of gait with vertigo (vertiginous ataxia) is recognized as being in the head, and not primarily in the control of the legs and trunk. It is noteworthy that in these circumstances the coordination of the individual movements of the limbs is not impaired—another point of difference from cerebellar disease. There may be headache or a sensation of pressure, especially in the region of the affected ear. Loss of consciousness as part of a vertiginous attack nearly always signifies another type of disorder (seizure or faint).

Giddiness and other types of pseudovertigo are usually described as feelings of swaying; lightheadedness; a swimming sensation, and, more rarely, a sensation of walking on air; "queer in the head"; uncertain; about to fall or "pass out." These sensory experiences are particularly common in psychiatric illnesses characterized by anxiety attacks. They may be reproduced by hyperventilation, and then it is appreciated that panic and apprehensiveness, palpitation, breathlessness, trembling, and sweating occur concurrently.

Other pseudovertiginous symptoms are less definitive. In severe anemic states weakness and languor may be attended by lightheadedness related to postural change and exertion. In the emphysematous patient physical effort may be associated with weakness and peculiar cephalic sensations, and coughing may lead to giddiness and even fainting (tussive syncope) because of impaired return of venous blood to the heart. The dizziness that so often accompanies hypertension is even more difficult to evaluate. Sometimes it is an expression of anxiety, or it may be due to unstable adjustment of cerebral blood flow. *Postural dizziness* is another example of unstable vasomotor reflexes preventing a constancy of cerebral circulation and is notably frequent in persons recently bedfast, in the weak and ill, and in the elderly. Abrupt arising from a recumbent or sitting position is followed immediately by a swaying type of dizziness, dimming of vision, and spots before the eyes which last a few seconds. The patient is forced to stand still and hold onto a nearby object until steady. A syncopal attack may occur at this time (see Chap. 12).

In practice it is not difficult to separate these types of pseudovertigo from true vertigo, for there is none of the feeling of rotation or impulsion so characteristic of the latter. Lacking also are the ancillary symptoms of true vertigo, namely nausea, vomiting, nystagmus, and staggering and sometimes tinnitus and deafness.

NEUROLOGIC AND OTOLOGIC CAUSES OF VERTIGO Vertigo may constitute the aura of an epileptic seizure, but this event is rare. The lesion is then on the posterolateral aspects of the temporal lobe or the inferior parietal lobule near the sylvian fissure. A sensation of movement, either of the body away from the side of the lesion or of the environment in the opposite direction, lasts for a few seconds before being submerged in other seizure activity. Rarely, vertiginous sensations provide the stimulus for *reflex epilepsy* (see Chap. 355), and rotational or caloric tests for this form of vertigo may provoke the seizure.

Oculomotor disorders are a source of a spatial disorientation simulating vertigo. This is maximal when the patient looks in the direction of action of the paralyzed muscle; it is attributable to the patient's receiving two conflicting visual images. In fact some normal individuals even experience dizziness for a time when adjusting to bifocal glasses or when looking down from a height.

Whether lesions of the cerebellum can produce vertigo seems to depend on the part involved. Large destructive processes in the cerebellar hemispheres and vermis may cause no vertigo whatsoever, unless they extend to the central vestibulocerebellar connections. However, Duncan et al. have described intense vertigo in two patients with verified lesions of the flocculonodular lobe on one side due to occlusion of the cerebellar branch of the posterior inferior cerebellar artery.

Labyrinthine (aural) lesions are the usual causes of paroxysmal vertigo. In the classic variety, that of *Ménière's disease,* the onset is abrupt, the vertigo is clearly of the rotary type, and it lasts a few minutes to hours. Concomitant tinnitus, first low then high, pressure or pain in the ear, pure tone deafness with auditory recruitment (see Chap. 17), nystagmus, nausea, vomiting, and staggering constitute the full syndrome. The patient preferentially lies with the faulty ear uppermost and is disinclined to look toward the normal side because it exaggerates the nystagmus and dizziness. The nystagmus is fine, rotatory, and most pronounced when the eyes are turned away from the offending ear. Vertiginous attacks of this type may recur frequently and give rise to mild, chronic states of disequilibrium which may persist for days. Seldom is the vertigo long-lasting, however, for central mechanisms compensate for permanent deficits of one labyrinth. Frequently, recurring attacks of vertigo may be complicated by the giddiness of a secondary anxiety state. *Vestibular neuronitis* (neuropathy) is a term that refers to severe vertigo, often of several days' duration and recurrent, without tinnitus or deafness. Its pathologic basis is uncertain, but Schuknecht has reported a degeneration of the vestibular nerve (possibly viral). Most cases of benign positional vertigo are of unknown etiology. Schuknecht and Kitamura offer evidence of cupolithiasis (dislocation of otoliths) as the mechanism of the postural effects. Viral infection and trauma are responsible for the symptoms in a few cases. Other causes of labyrinthine vertigo are: viral infections (respiratory and others), occlusive vascular lesions of the vestibular artery, reaction to aminoglycosides (particularly streptomycin and gentamicin), temporal bone fractures, and labyrinthine concussion. These conditions and Ménière's disease are described in Chap. 367.

Vertigo of acoustic nerve origin, the commonest cause of which is an acoustic neuroma, tends usually to be mild and intermittent (lasting weeks or months). Seldom does it come in discrete attacks separated by free intervals. Vertigo has rarely been observed as the initial symptom of eighth nerve tumors, but the usual sequence is deafness of high-frequency type (without recruitment), followed some time later by a sense of imbalance and impaired caloric responses, then cranial nerve palsies (involving the eighth, fifth, and tenth nerves), ipsilateral ataxia of limbs, and headache, the other common signs of a cerebellopontine angle tumor (see Chap. 358).

Vertigo of brainstem origin implicates the vestibular nuclei and their connections. In these cases auditory function is nearly always spared, since the vestibular and cochlear fibers separate upon entering the medulla and pons. The nystagmus which accompanies such central lesions tends to be coarse, protracted, and variable; it is more marked on lateral gaze to one side than the other and may be disjunctive (not the same in the two eyes). There may also be a nonrotary vertical component. The central localization is evidenced further by the attendant signs of involvement of other structures within the brainstem (cranial nerves, sensory and motor tracts, etc.). Mode of onset, duration, and other features of the clinical picture depend upon the nature of the causative disease, usually vascular (occlusion of branches of the basilar or vertebral arteries), traumatic, neoplastic, or demyelinative (see Table 13-1).

Electronystagmography is often helpful in the diagnosis of vertigo of brainstem origin. It will reveal vertical nystagmus with eyes closed, types I and II positional nystagmus, lack of nystagmus on caloric stimulation, and other ocular deviations with eyes closed.

APPROACH TO THE PATIENT WITH DIZZINESS As already stated, a careful history and physical examination of the dizzy patient usually afford a basis for separating true vertigo from the swaying dizziness of the hyperventilating, anxious patient and from the other types of pseudovertigo (such as partial syncope and feelings of unreality). If the patient is unobservant or imprecise in his or her descriptions, a helpful tactic is to provoke a number of dissimilar sensations by rotating the patient, irrigating the ears with warm or cold water, asking the patient to stoop for a minute and straighten up and to hyperventilate for 3 min, and by measuring the blood pressure as the patient changes from a recumbent to a standing position and remains upright for 3 to 4 min. Should the patient be unable to distinguish among these several types of induced sensation or to ascertain the similarity of one of the types to his or her own condition, the history is probably too inaccurate for purposes of diagnosis.

When vertigo is mild or difficult for the patient to describe, small items of the history, such as a disinclination to walk during an attack, a tendency to list to one side, aggravation by riding in a vehicle, or a preference for one position, are helpful in distinguishing vertigo from giddiness.

In some patients an attack of vertigo is so abrupt and intense that they are virtually flung to the ground, sometimes sustaining a serious injury. Such an attack has been called an "otolithic catastrophe of Tumarken," but without proof of involvement of the utricle or saccule. The diagnosis is usually substantiated by the occurrence of vertigo, nausea, and vomiting once the patient is on the ground, distinguishing the event from a seizure, faint, or cataplexy. Probably this attack differs from other forms of labyrinthine vertigo only in its severity.

In the differentiation of types of labyrinthine and vestibular nerve disease, inspection of eardrums, x-rays of mastoids, middle ears, and inner ears, and auditory and caloric tests are useful, especially in excluding labyrinthitis. In caloric testing, with the patient supine the head is tilted forward 30° from the horizontal (bringing the horizontal semicircular canal into a vertical plane), which is the position of maximal sensitivity to thermal stimuli. The external auditory meati are irrigated in turn

TABLE 13-1
Vertiginous syndromes with lesions of different parts of the vestibular system*

	Findings on ear exam	*Other neurologic findings*	*Disorders of equilibrium*	*Pathologic type of nystagmus*	*Hearing*	*Laboratory exam*
Labyrinths (postural vertigo, trauma, Ménière's disease, aminoglycosides, labyrinthitis)	Abnormalities of eardrum Positive fistula test	None	Ipsilateral past pointing and lateral propulsion	Rotatory to side of lesion, paroxysmal, positional	*Normal* or conduction or neurosensory deafness with recruitment	Vestibular paresis by caloric testing, directional proponderance X-ray and CT scan may be abnormal
Vestibular nerve and ganglia (vestibular neuropathy, herpes zoster)	Zoster vesicles in external auditory canal and palate	Seventh and auditory eighth nerve, and other cranial nerves	Ipsilateral past pointing and lateral propulsion to side of lesion	Vestibular, positional	Usually sensorineural deafness present No recruitment Speech discrimination diminished	X-ray and CT scan may be normal or abnormal Vestibular paresis on caloric test Directional preponderance
Cerebellopontine angle (acoustic neuroma, glomus, and other tumors)	Negative	Ipsilateral fifth, seventh, ninth, tenth cranial nerves, cerebellar ataxia Increased intracranial pressure (late)	Ataxia and falling ipsilaterally	Gaze paretic, positional, coarser to side of lesion	Sensorineural deafness without recruitment	X-ray and CT scan abnormal Vestibular paresis on caloric test Directional preponderance
Brainstem and cerebellum (infarcts, tumors, viral infections)	Negative	Multiple cranial nerves, brainstem tracts, cerebellar ataxia	Ataxia present with eyes open	Coarse lateral and vertical gaze, paretic	None	Hyperactive labyrinths or directional preponderance on caloric testing CT scan abnormal in some cases
Higher central (cortical) connections	Negative	Aphasia visual field, hemimotor, hemisensory, other cerebral abnormalities, seizures	No change	Usually absent	None	No change in caloric responses CT scan and EEG may be abnormal

* *See Chap. 17 for description of types of nystagmus.*

for 40 s with ice water. The nystagmus persists 90 to 120 s. Comparison of the two labyrinths reveals which one is paretic or hypersensitive. Special rotational chairs and electronystagmography are other more refined means of assessing disordered labyrinthine function. The diagnosis of benign positional vertigo is settled at the bedside by reproducing brief vertigo and nystagmus (lasting for 15 s or less) by moving the patient from the sitting position to recumbency, with the head to one side in one trial and to the other in the second. Going from a recumbent to a sitting position reverses the direction of vertigo and nystagmus. This specific pattern and its reversibility are not observed in the more malignant positional vertigo of posterior fossa tumors and other lesions. The application of some of the maneuvers designed to elicit weakness and syncope (see Chap. 12) will distinguish these forms of pseudovertigo.

The association of vertigo with auditory signs and symptoms always signifies a disease process of end organ or eighth cranial nerve. Labyrinthine and auditory tests and the presence or absence of neurologic signs referable to structures adjacent to the eighth cranial nerve nuclei are useful as a means of differentiation.

Pure vertigo as a manifestation of disease of the brainstem is rare, and a trustworthy rule is that unless other symptoms and signs appear within 1 to 2 weeks, one can nearly always postulate an aural origin and exclude vascular or other disease of the brainstem. This is also true of multiple sclerosis, which may be the explanation of persistent vertigo and nystagmus in some adolescents or young adults.

MANAGEMENT OF THE VERTIGINOUS PATIENT Only the severe and persistent forms compel admission to the hospital. Recumbency in one position and closure of the eyes are chosen almost automatically by the patient. Meclizine or dimenhydrinate (Dramamine) in oral doses of 25 mg reduces the irritability of the labyrinths. Nausea and vomiting are controllable by antiemetic medication such as trimethobenzamide (Tigan) in 200-mg suppositories every 6 h. One proceeds with diagnostic tests only after the acute attack has subsided. For the patient with giddiness, one employs the measures outlined in Chaps. 375 and 376.

REFERENCES

Adams RD, Victor M: *Principles of Neurology,* 2d ed. New York, McGraw-Hill, 1981

Altmann F: Diagnostic significance of vertigo, in *The Vestibular System and Its Diseases,* RF Wolfson (ed). Philadelphia, University of Pennsylvania Press, 1966, p 353

Baloh RW, Honrubia V: *Clinical Neurophysiology of the Vestibular System,* Philadelphia, FA Davis, 1979

Dix MR: Modern tests of vestibular function, with special reference to their value in clinical practice. Br Med J 3:317, 1969

DUNCAN GW et al: Acute cerebellar infarction in the PICA territory. Arch Neurol 32:364, 1975

FISHER CM: Vertigo in cerebrovascular disease. Arch Otolaryngol 85:529, 1967

SCHUKNECHT HF, KITAMURA K: Vestibular neuritis. Ann Otol Rhinol Laryngol 90:1, 1981

14
MOTOR PARALYSIS

RAYMOND D. ADAMS
HENRI VANDER EECKEN

Impairments of motor function may be subdivided into (1) paralysis due to affection of lower motor neurons, (2) paralysis due to disorder of upper motor (corticospinal and corticobrainstem) neurons, (3) abnormalities of coordination (ataxia) due to lesions in the cerebellum, (4) abnormalities of movement and posture due to disease of the extrapyramidal motor system, and (5) apraxic or nonparalytic disturbances of purposive movement due to involvement of the cerebrum. The first two types of motor disorder and the cerebral disorders of movement are discussed briefly in the following pages; purely muscular weakness and paralysis will be discussed in Chap. 369; cerebellar ataxia and extrapyramidal motor abnormalities are considered in Chap. 15.

A logical approach to the problem of muscular weakness, paralysis, and motor ineptitude is presented at the end of this chapter.

DEFINITIONS When applied to voluntary muscles, *paralysis* means loss of contraction due to interruption of one of the motor pathways from the cerebrum to the muscle fiber. Lesser degrees of paralysis are sometimes spoken of as *paresis,* but in everyday medical parlance motor paralysis usually stands for either partial or complete loss of function. The word *plegia* comes from the Greek word meaning stroke; and the word *palsy,* from an old French word, has the same meaning as paralysis. It is preferable to use *paresis* for slight and *paralysis* or *plegia* for severe loss of motor function.

PARALYSIS DUE TO DISEASE OF THE LOWER MOTOR NEURONS Each motor nerve cell, through the extensive arborization of the terminal part of its fiber, comes into contact with 100 to 200 or more muscle fibers; altogether they constitute "the motor unit." All the variations in force, range, and type of movement are determined by differences in the number and size of motor units called into activity and the frequency of their action. Feeble movements recruit few units, stronger ones many more units of increasing size. Histochemical methods show that motor units involved in slow, tonic contractions (type I) have muscle fibers rich in oxidative enzymes and mitochondria, and those involved in fast, phasic contractions (type II), more phosphorylase. When a motor neuron becomes diseased, as in progressive muscular atrophy, it may manifest increased irritability, and all the muscle fibers that it controls may discharge sporadically, in isolation from other units. The result of the contraction of one or several such units is a visible twitch, or *fasciculation,* which can be seen and recorded in the electromyogram as a large diphasic or multiphasic action potential. If the motor neuron is destroyed, all the muscle fibers to which it is attached undergo a profound atrophy, namely, denervation atrophy. For some unknown reason the individual denervated muscle fibers now begin to be hypersensitive and to contract spontaneously, though they can no longer do so in response to a nerve impulse as a part of the motor unit. This isolated activity of individual muscle fibers is called *fibrillation* and is so fine that it cannot be seen through the intact skin and can be recorded only as a repetitive short-duration spike potential in the electromyogram. The motor nerve fibers of each anterior root intermingle with adjacent roots as they join to form plexuses, and although the innervation of the muscles is roughly according to segments of the spinal cord, each large muscle comes to be supplied by two or more roots. In contrast, a single peripheral nerve usually provides the complete motor innervation of a muscle or group of muscles. For this reason the distribution of paralysis due to disease of the anterior horn cells or anterior roots differs from that which follows a lesion of a peripheral nerve.

All motor activity, even the most elementary reflex type, requires the cooperation of several muscles. The analysis of a relatively simple movement, such as clenching the fist, affords some idea of the complexity of the underlying neural arrangements. In this act the primary movement is a contraction of the flexor muscles of the fingers, the flexor digitorum sublimis and profundus, the flexor pollicis longus and brevis, and the abductor pollicis brevis. These muscles act as *agonists,* or *prime movers,* in this act. In order for flexion to be smooth and forceful, the extensor muscles (antagonists) must relax at the same rate at which the flexors contract. The muscles which flex the fingers also flex the wrist; and since it is desired that only the fingers flex, the muscles which extend the wrist must be brought into play to prevent its flexion. The action of the wrist extensors is *synergic,* and these muscles are called synergists in this particular act. Lastly the wrist, elbow, and shoulder must be stabilized by appropriate flexor and extensor muscles, which serve as *fixators.* The coordination of agonists, antagonists, synergists, and fixators involves reciprocal innervation and is managed entirely by segmental spinal reflexes under the guidance of proprioceptive sensory stimuli. Only the agonist movement in a voluntary act is believed to be initiated at a cortical level.

In addition, there are many basic motor activities, such as the maintenance of certain postures and stepping movements, which do not involve reciprocal innervation. For these activities agonists and antagonists contract simultaneously. The alternating movements of spinal stepping represent an even more elaborate type of coordination. Also in the support of the body in an upright posture, when the limb must be as rigid as a pillar, and in shivering, the agonists and antagonists must act together. In general, the more delicate the movement, the more precise the coordination between agonist and antagonist muscles.

If all or practically all peripheral motor nerves supplying a muscle are destroyed, all voluntary, postural, and reflex movements are abolished. The muscle becomes soft and yields excessively to passive stretching, a condition known as flaccidity. Muscle tone—the slight resistance that normal relaxed muscle offers to passive movement—is reduced (hypotonia or atonia). The denervated muscles undergo extreme atrophy, usually being reduced to 20 to 30 percent of their original bulk within 4 months. The reaction of the muscle to sudden stretch, as by tapping its tendon, is lost. If only a part of the motor units in the muscles is affected, partial paralysis will ensue. Quantitative testing by determination of strength-duration curves is a means of showing partial denervation, and electromyographic evidence of fibrillations may also be obtained.

The tonus of muscle and the tendon reflexes are known to depend on the muscle spindles and the afferent fibers to which they give origin and on the small anterior horn cells whose axons terminate on the small muscle fibers within the spindles. These small spinal motor neurons are called *gamma neurons,* in contrast to the large *alpha neurons.* Two different gamma neurons are now recognized, one, connected with nuclear bag spindle muscle fibers for phasic actions; the other, with nuclear chain spindle fibers for tonic actions. A tap on a tendon, by stretching the spindle muscle fibers, activates afferent neurons which transmit impulses to alpha motor neurons. The result is the familiar brief muscle contraction or tendon reflex. The spindle muscle fibers are then relaxed (unloaded), which terminates the reflex. Thus the setting of the spindle fibers and the state of excitability of the gamma neurons (normally inhibited by the corticospinal fibers and other supranuclear neurons) determine the level of activity of the tendon reflexes and the responsiveness of muscle to stretch. Other mechanisms of an inhibitory nature, involving Golgi tendon organs, are brought into play in more powerful stretching of muscle.

The neurotransmitters for excitation and inhibition of alpha and gamma spinal neurons by the corticospinal, rubrospinal, vestibulospinal, and reticulospinal tracts, or by peripheral sensory afferents, have not been fully elucidated. At least five neurotransmitters—acetylcholine (ACh), noradrenaline, serotonin, glycine, and γ-aminobutyric acid (GABA) have been identified. Some, such as ACh, are excitatory; others, like glycine and GABA, are inhibitory. But their localization (for example, that of the inhibitory transmitters in the presynaptic endings of the corticospinal and rubrospinal tracts which normally inhibit the intermediate neurons and anterior horn cells of extensor muscles of the arm and leg) has not been established. Even in spasticity, where the neurons responsible for excitation of the extensor muscles of the leg and flexors of the arm are overactive, it is not known whether there is a functional excess of excitatory neurotransmitter or a deficiency of inhibitory transmitter. Current evidence indicates that drugs that decrease spasticity act at the spinal cord level to alter neurotransmitter function. Baclofen (Lioresal) interferes with release of excitatory neurotransmitters and diazepam (Valium) facilitates GABA-mediated presynaptic inhibition (cf. Young and Delwaide).

Lower motor neuron paralysis is the direct result of physiologic arrest or destruction of anterior horn cells or their axons in anterior roots and nerves. The signs and symptoms vary according to the location of the lesion. Probably the most important question for clinical purposes is whether sensory changes coexist. The combination of flaccid, areflexic paralysis and sensory changes usually indicates involvement of mixed motor and sensory nerves or affection of both anterior and posterior roots. If sensory changes are absent, the lesion must be situated in the gray matter of the spinal cord, in the anterior roots, in a purely motor branch of a peripheral nerve, or in motor axons alone. The distinction between nuclear (spinal) and anterior root (radicular) lesions may at times be impossible to make. Retention of reflexes and spasticity in muscles weakened by a spinal lesion point to a lesion of the corticospinal tracts and integrity of the segments below the level of the lesion.

PARALYSIS DUE TO DISEASE OF THE CORTICOSPINAL AND CORTICO-BRAINSTEM NEURONS It was formerly believed that the corticospinal tract originated from the large motor cell of Betz in the fifth layer of the precentral convolution. However, there are only about 25,000 to 30,000 Betz cells, whereas the corticospinal tract at the level of the medulla contains approximately 1 million axons. This tract must, therefore, contain many fibers that arise not from the giant Betz cells of the motor cortex (area 4 of Brodmann) but rather from the smaller Betz cells of area 4, the cells of the adjacent precentral cortex (area 6), as well as those of the secondary motor cortex in the superior frontal convolution and postcentral cortex (areas 1, 2, 3, 5, 7). The most critical degeneration studies of van Crevel have shown that when areas 4, 6, 1, 2, 3, 5, and 7 are removed in the cat, if one waits several months, all of the pyramidal fibers will be found to have degenerated. The corticospinal tract is the only long-fiber connection between the cerebrum and the spinal cord. At the level of the internal capsule these corticospinal fibers are intermingled with many others destined to end in the striatum, globus pallidus, substantia nigra, red nucleus, and reticular substance and with others ascending from the thalamus. The fibers to the cranial nerve nuclei become separated at about the level of the midbrain and cross the midline to the contralateral cranial nerve nuclei (Fig. 14-1). These fibers form the corticomesencephalic, corticopontine, and corticobulbar tracts, and since they have functions similar to those of the corticospinal tract, they may be included in the pyramidal system of motor neurons. The decussation of the corticospinal tract at the lower end of the medulla is variable in different persons. Most of the crossing fibers come to occupy a position in the posterolateral part of the lateral funiculus; a few cross to form an anterior fasciculus. A small number of fibers, 10 to 20 percent, do not cross but descend ipsilaterally as the uncrossed corticospinal tract. Exceptionally, all of them cross; rarely, none. The termination of the corticospinal tract is in relation to nerve cells in the intermediate zone of gray matter, and not more than 10 to 15 percent establish direct synaptic connection with anterior horn cells. These facts, derived from degeneration studies, must of necessity modify current views of the anatomy of the corticospinal tract and suggest new interpretations.

The motor area of the cerebral cortex is difficult to define. It includes that part of the precentral convolution which contains Betz cells (area 4), but, as already mentioned, it probably extends anteriorly into area 6 and the secondary motor area of the superior frontal convolution and posteriorly into the anterior parietal lobe, where it overlaps the sensory areas. Physiologically it is defined as the region of electrically excitable cortex from which isolated movements can be evoked by stimuli of minimal intensity. The muscle groups of the contralateral

FIGURE 14-1
Diagram of the corticospinal and corticobulbar tracts. Lesion at A produces ipsilateral oculomotor palsy and contralateral paralysis involving face, arm, and leg. Lesion at B causes ipsilateral facial paralysis of peripheral type and contralateral paralysis of arm and leg. Lesion at b results in ipsilateral facial weakness of upper motor neuron of central type and contralateral paralysis of arm and leg. (Courtesy of Bergmann and Staehln, Krankheiten des Nervensystems, Berlin, Springer-Verlag, 1939.)

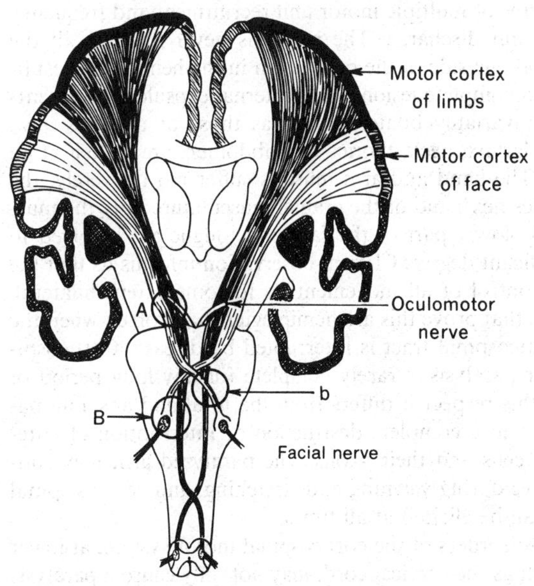

face, arm, trunk, and leg are represented in the motor cortex, those of the face being at the lower end of the precentral convolution and those of the leg in the paracentral lobule on the medial surface of the cerebral hemisphere. The parts of the body capable of the most delicate movements have, in general, the largest cortical representation. Very strong stimuli elicit movements from a wide area of premotor frontal and parietal cortex, and the same movements may be obtained from several points. From this it may be assumed that one of the functions of the motor cortex is to synthesize simple movements into an infinite variety of finely graded, highly differentiated patterns.

Corticospinal motor neuron paralysis may be due to lesions in the cerebral cortex, subcortical white matter, internal capsule, brainstem, or spinal cord. Usually much more is involved than the corticospinal, or pyramidal, tract. There has been a dispute as to the effects of a pure lesion of the corticospinal system. A lesion which severs the corticospinal system at midbrain level is said to cause only hemiparesis. Moreover in 12 autopsied cases where the pyramid of the medulla was destroyed on one side, there was a remarkable degree of recovery of motor function in the contralateral arm and leg, leaving only a variable degree of spasticity (usually slight), an increase in phasic myotatic or tendon reflexes, and an inverted plantar reflex (Babinski's sign). One of our patients, reported by Ropper and Fisher, recovered sufficiently after 6 months to finger the strings of a cello with her left (affected) hand and had only a slight limp. This recovery may be due to preservation of a few fibers of the pyramid (Trelles et al.), but the more important idea revealed by such cases is that complete spastic hemiplegias in humans involve interruption not only of the corticospinal tract but of other descending fibers from the cerebral cortex (corticorubral, corticostriatal, corticopallidal, corticopontine, and corticoreticular) and from the brainstem (reticulospinal, vestibulospinal, and rubrospinal). The influence of these nonpyramidal fibers not only is reflected in the degree of paralysis but also in the status of the disconnected segmental motor neurons subserving reflex, postural, and locomotory functions. From such observations our concept of the pyramidal lesion has had to be modified (see Brodal).

In general it may be said that with corticospinal lesions in humans the distribution of the paralysis varies with the locale of the lesion, but there are certain common features. Paralysis due to a lesion of these supranuclear motor neurons always involves a group of muscles, never individual muscles. If any volitional movement is possible, the maximum effort is attained more slowly than in the normal limb, and there is a lesser degree of multiple motor unit recruitment and frequency of single-unit discharge. The paralysis never involves all the muscles on one side of the body, even in the hemiplegia resulting from a complete lesion of the internal capsule. Movements that are invariably bilateral, such as those of the eyes, jaw, pharynx, larynx, neck, thorax, and abdomen, are little if at all affected. The hand and arm muscles suffer most severely, the leg muscles next, and of the cranial musculature only the muscles of the lower part of the face and tongue are involved to any significant degree. Clinical observation informs us that the cortical control of all movements is to some extent bilateral. Examples that prove this are hemiplegias that worsen when the other corticospinal tract is interrupted by disease. Corticospinal motor paralysis is rarely complete for any long period of time; in this respect it differs from the total and absolute paralysis due to a complete destruction or interruption of anterior horn cells and their axons. The paralyzed arm may suddenly move during yawning and stretching, and various spinal reflexes can be elicited at all times.

Acute disorders of the corticospinal motor system, at lower levels such as the cervical cord, may not only cause a paralysis of voluntary movement but may also abolish temporarily the spinal reflexes subserved by segments below the lesion. This condition is known as *spinal shock*. After a few days to weeks the shock disappears and gives way to a phenomenon known as *hypertonicity*. The latter is a feature of all acute and chronic lesions of the pyramidal system at cerebral, capsular, midbrain, and pontine levels. In cerebral and brainstem lesions it does not usually appear immediately, and in exceptional cases the paralyzed limbs remain flaccid but with lively reflexes. Spasticity is related to the excessive activity of the released or disinhibited spinal motor neurons. The tendon reflexes are hyperactive, and clonus may appear. The posture of the arm and leg inform us that certain spinal neurons are more active than others. The arm, for example, is maintained in a pronated, flexed position and the leg in an adducted, extended position. Any attempts to extend the arm or flex the leg passively will encounter, after a brief free interval, a resistance which quickly yields (clasp-knife phenomenon). When the limb is left in the new position, the resistance reappears (lengthening and shortening reactions). Actually the clasp-knife type of spasticity is infrequent. It is more usual for combined lesions of corticospinal and other suprasegmental tracts (see further on) to produce a sustained resistance to movement, as pointed out by Calne. But the tendon reflexes are hyperactive and the muscles weakened. The nocifensive spinal flexion reflexes, of which Babinski's sign is a part, are also released, and the cutaneomuscular abdominal and cremasteric reflexes abolished. The flexion reflexes are not actually a component of spasticity. In the hemiplegic patient they are less prominent than in the spinal paraplegic or quadriplegic patient. With cerebral lesions exaggerated stretch and cutaneous cranial reflexes can also be elicited in cranial as well as limb and trunk muscles, and when the corticospinal disorder is bilateral, there is pseudobulbar paralysis (dysarthria, dysphonia, and dysphagia with bifacial paralysis). Prolonged flexor and extensor spasms may occur with lesions of the spinal cord; they are due to a release of tonic myotatic reflexes.

Spasticity may be present when the limbs are not paralyzed but only paretic, and it then produces interesting effects on voluntary movements. In general all attempts by the patient to move the hemiparetic extremities appear to be hampered. Discrete movements of individual fingers and finely coordinated movements of the hand are lost. Proximal muscles are under better voluntary control. Synergies of movements eventually appear. For example, in the upper extremity a flexion synergy consisting of finger flexion, wrist flexion and pronation, elbow flexion, and shoulder elevation and abduction is produced in a slow, massive, stereotyped fashion upon attempted grasp of an object. Attempts to push with the hand result in a weaker pronation of the hand, extension or flexion of the fingers, extension of the wrist and elbow, adduction of the upper arm, and lowering of the shoulder. In the lower extremity the extensor synergy (thigh adduction, thigh and knee extension, and plantar flexion of the toes and foot) is more powerful than the flexor synergy of hip abduction, hip and knee flexion, and dorsiflexion and inversion of toes and foot. The latter part of this flexion synergy is called Strumpell's tibialis sign, which appears during attempts to elevate the leg. This bias toward extensor synergy facilitates weight-bearing and walking, which are eventually achieved by nearly all hemiplegic patients. These synergies indicate that there is not only a diminution in anterior horn cell activation (the negative effect of a corticospinal lesion), but a "deficit in the dynamic range and degree of reciprocal motor neuron control" (Sohrman and Norton). Strong-willed effort to move the paretic limb may also evoke symmetric associated (mirror) movements in the normal limb. The anatomic basis of all these synergic movements is not known. One possibility is the activation of anterior horn cells via the uncrossed ipsilateral corticospinal fibers.

OTHER DESCENDING SUPRASEGMENTAL TRACTS One cannot think about spasticity and spinal reflexes without considering the rubrospinal, vestibulospinal, and reticulospinal tracts, which also terminate on internuncial spinal neurons and possibly anterior horn cells. Of these tracts only the rubrospinal, which arises from the red nucleus, and reticulospinal receive cortical fibers. The vestibulospinal, which arises in Deiter's lateral vestibular nuclei, and the medullary reticulospinal arise in nuclei that are essentially under cerebellar control. Interestingly the rubrospinal, like the corticospinal, tract inhibits extensor and facilitates flexor mechanisms, whereas the vestibulospinal has the opposite effect. The release of the vestibulospinal and the interruption of the rubrospinal in upper brainstem lesions accounts for the exaggerated extensor postures and hyperactive tendon reflexes of decerebrate rigidity. The lower pontine reticular nuclei give rise to a tract whose principal effect on anterior horn cells is facilitatory, and the more lateral medullary reticular nuclei to a tract whose main influence is inhibitory. The rubrospinal and the lateral reticulospinal tracts are situated close to the lateral corticospinal tract and they are often simultaneously involved by spinal cord lesions. And, as was already remarked, lesions at higher levels, e.g., internal capsule, interrupt a number of tracts other than the corticospinal (cf. Young and Delwaide concerning pharmacotherapy of spasticity).

Table 14-1 shows the main differences between corticospinal and lower motor neuron syndrome.

Not all hemiplegias of cerebral origin are spastic.

APRAXIC OR NONPARALYTIC DISORDERS OF MOTOR FUNCTION Aside from upper and lower motor neuron paralysis with cerebral lesions, there may be loss of learned purposive movement that may simulate paresis of a limb. This is called *apraxia* and may be explained as follows. Many simple actions are acquired by learning or practice. These depend on the formation of movement patterns, particularly those which involve the use of tools and instruments as well as gestures. Once established, they are remembered and may be reproduced under the proper circumstances. Any purposive act of these types may be conceived as occurring in several stages. First, the idea of an act must be aroused in the mind of the subject by an appropriate stimulus situation, perhaps by a spoken command to do something. This idea is then translated into action by excitation of patterns of premotor or motor cortical neurons in proper sequence, which are transmitted to lower centers by the corticospinal tracts. These initiate particular movements of individual muscle groups but also modify or suppress the subcortical mechanisms that control the basic attitudes and postures of the body. In right-handed and most left-handed persons the neural mechanisms for the formulation of an idea of an act (motor schema or image) in response to a spoken command or a verbal stimulus and its reproduction are believed to be centered in the posterior and inferior parts of the left parietal lobe; these areas, near the language mechanism, are connected with the left premotor regions for the control of the right hand and thence with the motor areas of the right cerebral hemisphere through the corpus callosum for the control of the left side.

A failure to execute certain acts in the correct context while retaining the ability to carry out the individual movements upon which such acts depend is the main feature of *apraxia.* The most adequate clinical test of motor deficits of this type is to observe a series of self-initiated actions such as using a comb, a razor, a toothbrush, or a common tool, or gesturing, e.g., waving goodbye, saluting, shaking the fist as though angry, or blowing a kiss. These actions may be called forth by a command or a request to imitate the examiner. Of course, failure to follow a spoken or written request may be due to an aphasia that prevents understanding of what is asked, or an agnosia may prevent recognition of the tool or object to be used. But when these difficulties are excluded, there remains a peculiar motor deficit in which the patient appears to understand but has lost the memory of how to perform a given act, especially if it is called for in an unnatural setting. The patient may have the idea of what to do, but cannot translate the idea of the sequence of movements into a precise, well-executed act. This is sometimes called *ideomotor apraxia.* The failure may be evident both after a spoken command and in requests to imitate the gestures of the examiner. Sometimes these two conditions may be dissociated; the patient, while not aphasic, cannot execute a spoken command but can still imitate the act if it is called forth by gesture. Also if merely given the tool, the patient may use it properly in an automatic fashion. There is also another level of motor ineptitude. The performance may be executed, but in a clumsy manner. The motor cortex seemingly has either not coordinated parts of the action, or a magnetic grasp reaction, avoidance reaction, or perseveration interferes with the act. This state has been called innervatory apraxia by Kleist, and kinetic apraxia by Denny-Brown.

Apraxia may be limited to one group of muscles, such as tongue or lips, as in Broca's aphasia (Chap. 23), or the loss of commanded actions of the left arm and leg in right-sided hemiplegics (sympathetic apraxia). (See Chap. 24.)

If this motor disorder can be singled out, it reflects a specific loss of certain learned patterns of movement (a "specific amnesia," so to speak, analogous to the amnesia of words in aphasia). The added element of mental confusion or dementia tends often to obscure the disorder (cf. Ajuriaguerra and Tissot). Dressing apraxia and constructional apraxia are other types which will be discussed with the entire subject of apraxia in Chap. 24.

DIFFERENTIAL DIAGNOSIS OF PARALYSIS The diagnostic consideration of paralysis may be simplified by the following subdivisions, which relate to the location and distribution of weakness.

Monoplegia The examination of patients who complain of weakness of one extremity often discloses an unnoticed weak-

TABLE 14-1
Differences between paralysis of corticospinal and lower motor neurons

Upper, corticospinal motor paralysis	*Lower, spinomuscular, or nuclear-infranuclear paralysis*
Muscle groups affected diffusely, never individual muscles	Individual muscles may be affected
Atrophy slight and due to disuse	Atrophy pronounced, 70 to 80 percent of total bulk
Spasticity with hyperactivity of the tendon reflexes	Flaccidity and hypotonia of affected muscles with loss of tendon reflexes
Extensor plantar reflex, Babinski's sign	Plantar reflex, if present, is of normal flexor type
Fascicular twitches not produced	Fascicular twitches may be present
Normal electromyogram	Electromyogram reveals reduced numbers of motor units and fibrillations

ness in another limb, and the condition is actually hemiplegia or paraplegia. Or instead of weakness of all the muscles in a limb, only isolated groups are found to be affected. Ataxia, sensory disturbances, or pain in an extremity will often be interpreted by the patient as weakness, as will the mechanical limitation resulting from arthritis or the rigidity of parkinsonism.

In general, the presence or absence of atrophy of muscles in a monoplegic limb can be of diagnostic help.

PARALYSIS WITH LITTLE OR NO ATROPHY Long-continued disuse of a limb may lead to atrophy, but this is usually not so marked as in diseases that denervate muscles; the tendon reflexes are normal, and the response of the muscles to electric stimulation and the electromyogram are unaltered.

The most frequent cause of monoplegia without muscular wasting is a lesion of the cerebral cortex. Only occasionally does it occur in diseases which interrupt the corticospinal tract at the level of the internal capsule, brainstem, or spinal cord. A vascular lesion (thrombosis or embolus) is the commonest cause, and, of course, a tumor or abscess may have the same effect. Multiple sclerosis and spinal cord tumor, early in their course, may cause weakness of one extremity, usually the leg. Weakness due to damage to the corticospinal system is usually accompanied by spasticity, increased reflexes, and an extensor plantar reflex (Babinski's sign), and the electromyogram is normal. However, acute diseases that destroy the motor tracts in the spinal cord may at first (for several days) reduce the tendon reflexes and cause hypotonia (*spinal shock*). This does not occur in partial or slowly evolving lesions and occurs only to minimal degree, if at all, in lesions of brainstem and cerebrum. In acute diseases affecting the lower motor neurons the tendon reflexes are always reduced or abolished, but atrophy may not appear for several weeks. Hence one must take into account the mode of onset and the duration of the disease in evaluating the tendon reflexes, muscle tone, and degree of atrophy before reaching an anatomic diagnosis.

PARALYSIS WITH MUSCULAR ATROPHY This is more frequent than paralysis without muscular atrophy. In addition to the paralysis and reduced or abolished tendon reflexes, there may be visible fasciculations. If completely paralyzed, the muscles exhibit an electric reaction of degeneration, and the electromyogram shows reduced numbers of motor units (often of large size), fasciculations at rest, and fibrillations. The lesion may be in the spinal cord, spinal roots, or peripheral nerves. Its location can usually be decided by the distribution of the palsied muscles (whether the pattern is one of nerve, spinal root, or spinal cord involvement), by the associated neurologic symptoms and signs, and by special tests (cerebrospinal fluid examination, roentgenogram of spine, and myelogram).

Brachial atrophic monoplegia is relatively rare, and when present, it should suggest in an infant a brachial plexus trauma, in a child poliomyelitis, in an adult poliomyelitis, syringomyelia, amyotrophic lateral sclerosis, or other brachial plexus lesions. Crural monoplegia is more frequent and may be caused by any lesion of thoracic or lumbar cord, i.e., trauma, tumor, myelitis, multiple sclerosis, etc. Multiple sclerosis almost never causes atrophy, and ruptured intervertebral disk and the many varieties of neuritis rarely paralyze all or most of the muscles of a limb. Muscle dystrophy may begin in one limb, but by the time the patient is seen the typical more or less symmetric pattern of proximal limb and trunk involvement is evident. A unilateral retroperitoneal tumor may paralyze the leg by implicating the lumbosacral plexus.

Hemiplegia Loss of strength in arm, leg, and sometimes face on one side of the body is the most frequent distribution of paralysis in humans. With rare exceptions (a few unusual cases of poliomyelitis or motor system disease) this pattern of paralysis is due to involvement of the corticospinal tract.

LOCATION OF LESION-PRODUCING HEMIPLEGIA The site or level of the lesion can usually be deduced from the associated neurologic findings. Diseases localized in the cerebral cortex, cerebral white matter (corona radiata), and internal capsule usually evoke weakness or paralysis of the face, arm, and leg on the opposite side. The occurrence of convulsive seizures or the presence of a defect in speech (aphasia), a cortical type of sensory loss (astereognosis, loss of two-point discrimination, etc.), anosognosia, or defects in the visual fields suggest a cortical or subcortical location. A pure, isolated hemiplegia affecting simultaneously the face, arm, and leg indicates a lesion in the posterior limb of the internal capsule, often a vascular lacuna.

Damage to the corticospinal and cortico-brainstem tracts in the upper portion of the brainstem (see Fig. 14-1) may cause paralysis of the face, arm, and leg on the opposite side. The lesion in such cases is localized by the presence of a paralysis of the muscles supplied by the oculomotor nerve on the same side as the lesion (Weber's syndrome) or other neurologic findings. With low pontine lesions a unilateral abducens or facial palsy is combined with a contralateral weakness or paralysis of the arm and leg (Millard-Gubler syndrome). Lesions of the lowermost part of the brainstem, i.e., in the medulla, affect the tongue and sometimes the pharynx and larynx on one side and arm and leg on the other side. These "crossed paralyses," so common in brainstem diseases, are described in Chap. 367. Ataxic hemiplegia with or without dysarthria also indicates a lesion in the contralateral basis pons. Here Fisher has traced the involvement to the uncrossed corticospinal, corticobulbar, and corticopontocerebellar tracts.

Rarely, a homolateral hemiplegia (sparing cranial muscles) may be caused by a lesion in the lateral column of the cervical spinal cord. At this level, however, the pathologic process often induces bilateral signs, with resulting quadriparesis or quadriplegia. Homolateral paralysis, if combined with a loss of vibratory and position sense on the same side and a contralateral loss of pain and temperature (Brown-Séquard syndrome), signifies disease of the spinal cord on one side (Chaps. 18 and 366).

Muscle atrophy of minor degree often follows lesions of the corticospinal system but never reaches the proportions seen in diseases of the lower motor neurons. The atrophy is due to disuse. When the motor cortex and adjacent parts of the parietal lobe are damaged in infancy or childhood, the normal development of the muscles and the skeletal system in the affected limbs is retarded. The palsied limbs and even the trunk on one side are small. This does not occur if the paralysis begins after the greater part of skeletal growth is attained (after puberty). In the hemiplegia due to spinal cord injury, muscles at the level of the lesion may undergo atrophy if there is associated damage to anterior horn cells or ventral roots.

CAUSES OF HEMIPLEGIA In this condition vascular diseases of the cerebrum and brainstem exceed all others in frequency. Trauma (brain contusion, epidural and subdural hemorrhage) ranks second, and other diseases such as brain tumor, brain abscess and encephalitis, demyelinative diseases, complications of meningitis, tuberculosis, and syphilis are of decreasing order of importance.

Paraplegia Paralysis of both lower extremities may occur in diseases of the spinal cord and the spinal roots or of the peripheral nerves. If the onset is acute, it may be difficult to distinguish spinal from neural paralysis, for in any acute myelopathy spinal shock may result in abolition of reflexes and flaccidity. As a rule in acute spinal cord diseases with involvement of corticospinal tracts, the paralysis affects all muscles below a given level; and often, if the white matter is extensively damaged, sensory loss below a particular level (loss of pain and temperature sense with lateral spinothalamic tracts and loss of vibratory and position sense with posterior columns) is conjoined. Also, in bilateral disease of the spinal cord, the bladder and bowel sphincters are paralyzed. Alterations of cerebrospinal fluid (dynamic block, increase in protein or cells) are frequent. In peripheral nerve diseases both sensory loss and motor loss tend to involve the distal muscles of the legs more than the proximal ones (an exception is acute idiopathic polyneuritis), and the sphincters are spared or only briefly deranged in function. Sensory loss, if present, is more likely to consist of distal impairment of touch, vibration, and position sense, with pain and temperature sense spared in many instances. The cerebrospinal fluid protein level may be normal or elevated.

Acute paraplegia beginning at any age is relatively infrequent. Rarely it may be due to a medial pontine lesion affecting the leg fibers which are near to the midline (as in pontine infarction or central pontine myolinolysis). Fracture dislocation of the spine with traumatic necrosis of the spinal cord, spontaneous hematomyelia with bleeding from a vascular malformation (angioma, telangiectasis), thrombosis of a spinal artery with infarction (myelomalacia), and dissecting aortic aneurysm or atherosclerotic occlusion of nutrient spinal arteries arising from the aorta with resulting infarction (myelomalacia) are the commonest varieties of sudden paraplegia (or quadriplegia, if the cervical cord is involved). Postinfectious or postvaccinal myelitis, acute demyelinative myelitis (Devic's disease if the optic nerves are affected), necrotizing myelitis, and epidural abscess or hemorrhage with spinal cord compression tend to develop somewhat more slowly, over a period of hours or days, or they may have an acute onset. Poliomyelitis, a purely motor disorder with meningitis, must be distinguished from the other acute myelopathies.

In adult life multiple sclerosis, subacute combined degeneration, spinal cord tumor, ruptured cervical disk and cervical spondylosis, syphilitic meningomyelitis, chronic epidural infections (fungous and other granulomatous diseases), Erb's spastic paraplegia and motor system disease, familial spastic paraplegia, and syringomyelia represent the most frequently encountered forms of spinal paraplegia. (See Chap. 366 for discussion of these spinal cord diseases). The several varieties of polyneuritis and polymyositis must be considered in their differential diagnosis, for they, too, may cause paraparesis. Friedreich's ataxia and familial paraplegia, progressive muscular dystrophy, and the chronic varieties of polyneuritis tend to appear during late childhood and adolescence and are slowly progressive.

Theoretically paraplegia may be due to a lesion of the leg areas of the motor cortex. Arterial (anterior cerebral arteries) or venous (superior sagittal sinus and tributary cerebral veins) infarction with an anterior communicating aneurysm are causes of acute paraplegia, and a parasagittal meningioma of asymmetrical chronic paraplegia. Usually other signs such as confusion, stupor, or seizures indicate the cerebral localization, hence differential diagnosis is not a problem.

Quadriplegia All that has been written about the common causes of paraplegia applies to quadriplegia. The lesion is usually in the cervical rather than the thoracic or lumbar segments of the spinal cord. If it is situated in the low cervical segments and involves the anterior half of the spinal cord, as in occlusion of the anterior spinal artery, the arm paralysis may be flaccid and areflexic and the leg paralysis spastic (anterior spinal syndrome). There are only a few points of difference between the common paraplegic and quadriplegic syndromes. Repeated cerebral vascular accidents may lead to bilateral hemiplegia, usually accompanied by pseudobulbar palsy.

Isolated paralysis Paralysis of isolated muscle groups usually indicates a lesion of one or more peripheral nerves. The diagnosis of a lesion of an individual peripheral nerve is made on the presence of weakness or paralysis of the muscle or group of muscles and impairment or loss of sensation in the distribution of the nerve in question (Chap. 368). Complete transection or severe injury to a peripheral nerve is usually followed by atrophy of the muscles it innervates and by loss of their tendon reflexes. Trophic changes in the skin, nails, and subcutaneous tissue may also occur. It is of considerable importance to decide whether the lesion is a temporary one of conduction only (neuropraxia) or whether there has been a pathologic dissolution of continuity, requiring nerve regeneration for recovery. Electromyography is of value here.

EXAMINATION SCHEME FOR MOTOR PARALYSIS AND APRAXIA The first step is to inspect the paralyzed limb, taking note first of its posture and of the presence or absence of muscle atrophy, hypertrophy, and fascicular twitchings. The patient is then called upon to move each muscle group, and the power and facility of movement are graded and recorded. The range of passive movement is then determined by moving all the joints. This provides information concerning alterations of muscle tone, i.e., hypotonia, spasticity, and rigidity. Dislocations, diseased joints, and ankyloses may also be revealed by these same maneuvers. Muscle bulk is then inspected. Slight atrophy may be due to disuse from any cause, i.e., pain, fixation as the result of a cast, or any type of paralysis. Pronounced atrophy usually occurs only with denervation of several weeks' or months' standing.

The tendon reflexes are then tested. The usual routine is to try to elicit the jaw jerk (increased in pseudobulbar palsy) and the supinator, biceps, triceps, quadriceps, and Achilles tendon reflexes. Two cutaneous reflexes are then tested, the abdominal and plantar reflexes.

If there is no evidence of upper or lower motor neuron disease, but certain acts are nonetheless imperfectly performed, one should look for a disorder of postural sensibility or of cerebellar coordination or rigidity with abnormality of posture and movement due to disease of the basal ganglia (Chap. 15). In the absence of these disorders, the possibility of an apraxic disorder may be investigated by watching the patient's own movements and those called forth by specific command and gesture.

Hysterical paralysis may pose problems. Usually it is easily distinguished from chronic lower motor neuron disease by absence of areflexia and severe atrophy. Diagnostic difficulty arises only in certain acute cases of upper motor neuron disease that lack all the usual changes in reflexes and muscle tone. In hysterical paralysis one arm or one leg or all one side of the body may be affected. The hysterical gait is sometimes diagnostic (Chap. 16). Often there is loss of all forms of sensation (touch, pain, smell, vision, and hearing) in the paralyzed side, a group of sensory changes that is never seen in organic brain disease. The patient should be asked to move the affected limbs; the movement is seen to be slow and jerky, often with contraction of both agonist and antagonist muscles simultaneously or intermittently. Hoover's sign and Babinski's combined leg flexion test are helpful in distinguishing hysterical from organic hemiplegia. To elicit Hoover's sign, the patient, lying on the back, is asked to raise one leg from the bed against resistance; in a normal individual the back of the heel of the contralateral leg is pressed firmly down, and the same is true when the patient with organic hemiplegia attempts to lift the paralyzed leg. The hysteric will contract the good leg more strongly under these circumstances than as a primary willed action. To carry out Babinski's combined leg flexion test, a patient with an organic hemiplegia is asked to sit up without using the arms; in doing this, the paralyzed or weak leg flexes at the hip, and the heel is lifted from the bed while the heel of the sound leg is pressed into the bed. This sign is absent in hysterical hemiplegia.

MUSCULAR PARALYSIS AND SPASM UNATTENDED BY VISIBLE CHANGE IN NERVE OR MUSCLE A group of diseases appears to have no basis in visible structural light microscopic change in motor nerve cells, nerve fibers, motor end plates, and muscular fibers. This group is composed of myasthenia gravis, myotonia congenita (Thomsen's disease), familial periodic paralysis, disorders of potassium, sodium, calcium, and magnesium metabolism, tetany, tetanus, botulinus poisoning, black widow spider bite, and the thyroid myopathies. In these diseases, each of which possesses a fairly distinctive clinical picture, the abnormality is purely biochemical, and even if the patient survives for a long time, no visible microscopic changes develop. An understanding of these diseases requires knowledge of the processes involved in nerve and muscle excitation and the contraction of muscle. They are discussed in Chaps. 369 and 374.

REFERENCES

AJURIAGUERRA J, TISSOT R: The apraxias, in *Handbook of Clinical Neurology,* PJ Vinken, GW Bruyn (eds). Amsterdam, North-Holland, 1969, chap 3

BRODAL A: *Neurological Anatomy in Relation to Clinical Medicine.* 3d ed. New York, Oxford, 1981

CALNE DB: Drug treatment of spasticity and rigidity, in *Modern Trends in Neurology,* D Williams (ed). London, Butterworths, 1975, chap 11

FISHER CM: Ataxic hemiparesis—a pathological study. Arch Neurol 2:126, 1978

LANCE JW, MCLEOD JG: *A Physiological Approach to Clinical Neurology,* 3d ed. London, Butterworths, 1981

ROPPER AH et al: Pyramidal infarction in the medulla. Neurology, 29:41, 1979

SOHRMAN SA, NORTON BJ: The relationship of voluntary movement to spasticity in the upper motor neuron syndrome. Ann Neurol 2:460, 1977

TRELLES JO et al: Spasticity in hemiplegia due to lesion of anterior pyramid. Rev Neurol 129:105, 1973

YOUNG RR, DELWAIDE PJ: Drug therapy: Spasticity. N Engl J Med 304:28, 1981

15
ABNORMALITIES OF MOVEMENT AND POSTURE

RAYMOND D. ADAMS
JOSEPH B. MARTIN

The preceding chapter described the functions, in the control of movement, of the corticospinal system and of the lower motor neuron. Disorders of these pathways were shown to affect power, speed, and precision of muscular movements. This chapter presents an overview of two other central nervous system pathways, namely those of the *basal ganglia,* commonly called the *extrapyramidal system,* and of the *cerebellum,* both of which are important for the organization of facile, coordinated movements of the axial (trunk) and extremity musculature. Disorders of these systems will be seen to affect walking, posture, balance, and the trajectory of movements of the limbs.

The organization of coordinated movements depends upon the integration of neural activity at all levels of the nervous system. Sensory inputs from joint and tendon proprioceptors and muscle spindles influence local spinal cord reflexes and provide afferent information to the brainstem, cerebellum, basal ganglia, and cerebral cortex, which function to align the output of the motor pathways. The *corticospinal* system is essential for the fine movements of dexterity that are characteristic of the fingers and hands and is responsible for rapid (ballistic) movements. A number of other descending systems, arising principally in the brainstem (*bulbospinal*), including the *vestibulospinal, reticulospinal, rubrospinal,* and *tectospinal* pathways, are involved in the integration of the automatic and static axial postures required for upright stance and locomotion. The corticospinal and the bulbospinal pathways are influenced by the two other major neuronal loop systems, one comprising the basal ganglia and the other the cerebellum. In this chapter these two systems are considered, and the clinical symptoms that arise from dysfunction within them, namely, tremor, bradykinesia, rigidity, ataxia, chorea, athetosis, and myoclonus, are described.

THE BASAL GANGLIA

ANATOMIC CONSIDERATIONS As an anatomic entity the basal ganglia have no precise definition. In addition to the recognized nuclear structures of the *caudate nucleus* and *putamen* (together commonly called the *neostriatum* or the striatum), the *globus pallidus* (which together with the putamen is called the lentiform nucleus), the *substantia nigra,* and the *subthalamic nucleus of Luys,* it is common to include portions of the red nucleus, the superior colliculus (tectum), the brainstem reticular formation, and the amygdala. The principal anatomic components of the basal ganglia are shown in Fig. 15-1.

It is useful first to summarize the major anatomic pathways involved in this system and then to consider them in more detail. Multiple inputs to the basal ganglia converge upon the neostriatum, which projects to the globus pallidus and the substantia nigra. The striatal-pallidal inputs are joined by the loop afferents from the substantia nigra and project to the thalamus, which in turn projects to the motor cortex to complete the basal ganglia loop. It is important to recognize that the major cerebellar output involved in motor control, which exits from the cerebellum through the superior cerebellar peduncle, terminates with the pallidal-thalamic fibers in the ventroanterior and ventrolateral thalamic nuclei. This region of the thalamus forms an essential link in the ascending fiber systems from both the basal ganglia and the cerebellum to the motor cortex. Indeed, it would seem that most of the basal ganglionic and

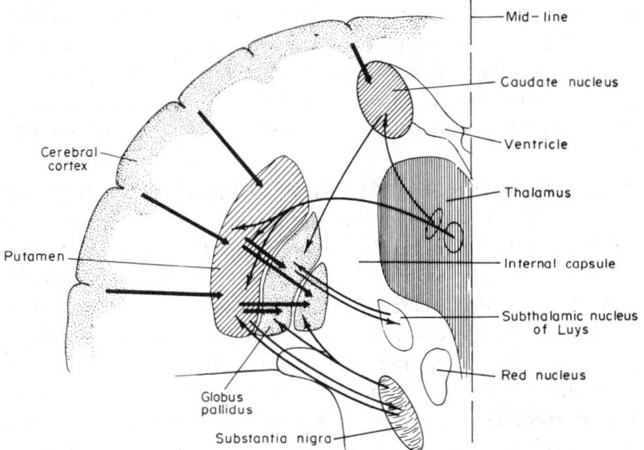

FIGURE 15-1
Basal ganglia in the coronal plane, illustrating major connections between the nuclear groups. (From RD Adams and M Victor, Principles of Neurology, New York, McGraw-Hill, 1977.)

cerebellar influences on the motor system are funneled through this ventral plane of the thalamic nuclei. Lesions in the ventral thalamus can both abolish the tremor of Parkinson's disease and attenuate, in some circumstances, the limb dyskinesia or ataxia associated with cerebellar disorders. The ascending thalamocortical fibers pass through the internal capsule and cerebral white matter; hence lesions in these parts may simultaneously affect both corticospinal and extrapyramidal systems.

As to the details of the anatomy of the basal ganglia, there are four main afferent connections to the neostriatum: (1) the corticostriatal, which projects from all regions of the neocortex to the caudate and putamen; (2) the nigrostriatal system, a dopaminergic projection from the pars compacta of the substantia nigra; (3) a raphé-striatal system, arising in the brainstem raphé nuclei and providing a serotoninergic input; and (4) the thalamostriatal system, projecting principally from the intralaminar and fascicular nuclei of the thalamus.

The neostriatum contains a large and a small cell population, and both project within and beyond the caudate and putamen, principally to the two segments (inner and outer) of the globus pallidus and to the pars reticulata of the substantia nigra. The substantia nigra projects back to the striatum and the two segments of the globus pallidus, but also connects with the tectum of the brainstem and directly with the thalamus. The segments of the globus pallidus project to the ventroanterior and ventrolateral nuclei of the thalamus; these fibers are divided into two separate fascicles as they leave the pallidum, the *ansa lenticularis,* which loops posteriorly around the internal capsule, and the *fasciculus lenticularis,* which traverses the internal capsule. One additional loop consists of the subthalamic nucleus of Luys, which receives input from the pallidum and projects back to it. The importance of this link is demonstrated by the observation that vascular lesions of the subthalamic nucleus result in a motor disorder called *hemiballismus* in which the arm and leg of the opposite side are thrown about in a violent fashion.

The basal ganglia do not project directly to the spinal cord or in any major way to the brainstem. The influences on movement are effected principally via the cerebral cortex. Taken as a whole, the basal ganglia form a *cortico-striatal-pallidal-thalamic-cortical* loop.

PHYSIOLOGICAL CONSIDERATIONS Although experimental studies and clinicopathologic correlations have provided data upon which concepts of basal ganglia physiology have been built, the picture has been little clarified by physiologic studies. Electrophysiologic recordings in the caudate and putamen in awake monkeys and humans show little spontaneous activity, suggesting tonic inhibition; the activity of the neurons in the globus pallidus is considerably greater. An increase in neuronal firing in the striatum and in the pallidum has been found to occur *before* the initiation of movement. Over 50 percent of neurons in the pallidum show an increase in firing with slow (ramp) movements, whereas only about 10 percent respond in this way with fast (ballistic) movements. The basal ganglia are considered essential for the initiation of movements, particularly those of a slow, postural kind. However, ballistic (fast) movements may persist in patients with the bradykinesia and rigidity of Parkinson's disease, as, for example, when the patient observed to be immobile can suddenly reach out to catch an object thrown to him or her.

NEUROPHARMACOLOGY The neuronal pathways of the basal ganglia contain certain specific neurotransmitters believed to be important for normal function. The corticostriatal pathway contains glutamate, an excitatory neurotransmitter; the nigrostriatal system contains dopamine (DA), which is believed to be inhibitory, and the raphé-striatal system serotonin (function unknown). The projections of the caudate and putamen to the pallidum and substantia nigra contain γ-aminobutyric acid (GABA) and also the neuropeptides, substance P and leucine- and methionine-enkephalin. Interneurons in the striatum contain acetylcholine (ACh) and the enkephalins. The concentration of opiate receptors in the striatum is very high. The neurotransmitters involved in the pallidothalamic and the pallidosubthalamic nuclear pathways have not been identified.

The biogenic amines [DA, norepinephrine (NE); and serotonin] are inactivated by reuptake into the presynaptic nerve terminals; acetylcholine is inactivated by hydrolysis within the synaptic cleft. Specific receptors for these neurotransmitters are found both on the postsynaptic membrane and also on the

FIGURE 15-2
Neurotransmitters that are identified in the principal pathways of the basal ganglia. Excitatory (+) and inhibitory (−) effects are indicated. ACh = acetylcholine; DA = dopamine; ENK = enkephalin; 5-HT = serotonin; GABA = γ-aminobutyric acid; Glu = glutamate; p.c. = pars compacta; p.r. = pars reticulata; SUB. P = substance P. (From Growdon and Scheife, with permission.)

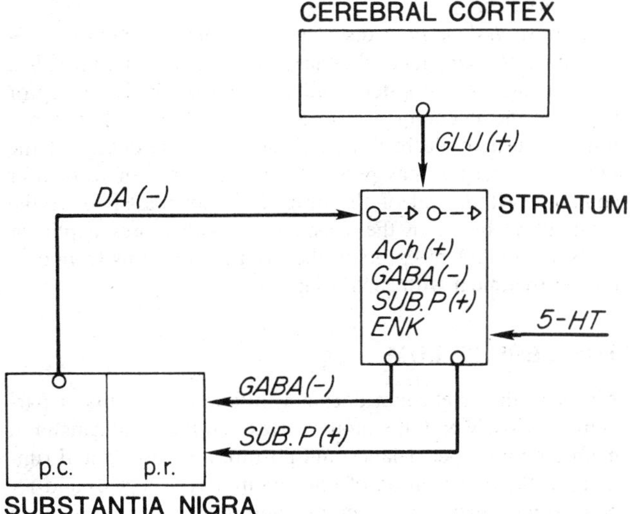

presynaptic terminal; the latter are called autoreceptors, and their stimulation causes a decrease in synthesis and release of the transmitter, a mechanism which serves an autoregulatory function. The affinity of the neurotransmitter for the autoreceptor is often much greater than that of the postsynaptic receptor. Thus, drugs that stimulate DA autoreceptors decrease DA transmission. Two separate populations of DA receptors have been described; stimulation of D_1 sites activates adenylate cyclase, whereas D_2-receptor stimulation does not.

Neuropharmacological analysis of neurotransmitter content, together with anatomic studies and neuropathological correlations, provides the basis for an understanding of certain disorders involving the basal ganglia and for their treatment. In *Parkinson's disease,* which is manifested by a combination of akinesia, tremor, rigidity, and flexed posture, the DA content of the striatum is depleted owing to a loss of neurons in the substantia nigra and degeneration of the nigrostriatal tract to which they give rise. The loss of DA in the striatum, which is believed to have a predominant inhibitory control on the intrinsic striatal cholinergic neurons, results in an overactivity of the cholinergic component of the striatum. Restoration of this equilibrium, by giving L-dopa (often in combination with anticholinergic medication) is the basis of the main therapeutic rationale for the disorder. On the other hand, administration of DA-receptor blockers (phenothiazines, butyrophenones) or depletion of DA with reserpine or tetrabenzine, may cause a more or less typical parkinsonian syndrome in an otherwise normal patient.

An excess of L-dopa in the patient with Parkinson's disease, probably by the stimulation of DA receptors in the striatum, may induce a wide variety of abnormal movements that seem to be dose-related. The most frequent of these is craniofacial athetosis, but a more generalized choreoathetosis, facial and cervical spasms, tremors, and myoclonic jerks (see below) may also occur. Presumably, certain striatal neurons other than the ones causing the Parkinson's syndrome have been rendered hypersensitive, for L-dopa appears not to have this effect on normal individuals.

In contrast, in *Huntington's disease* there is loss of neurons in the caudate and putamen, accompanied by depletion of GABA and of ACh, but with preservation of DA content. The symptoms of chorea, which form so prominent a part of the disorder, are believed due to the dopaminergic excess; they can be effectively treated, albeit transiently, with DA blockers like haloperidol. L-Dopa increases and physostigmine, which enhances cholinergic activity, is said to lessen the chorea. Isoniazid, which increases GABA concentrations, also lessens chorea in some cases. Other attempts at GABA replacement have not been successful.

Tardive dyskinesia, a disorder consisting of repetitive, stereotypical movements of the face, tongue, and extremities, is a complication of long-term administration of DA-receptor blockers and is commonly seen in schizophrenia. The symptoms are usually decreased by reduction in the dosage of the DA antagonist but may persist for months or even years after complete withdrawal of the drug. It is postulated to be the result of a change in the sensitivity of either presynaptic or postsynaptic DA receptors in the striatum, resulting from prolonged treatment with such drugs.

THE CEREBELLUM

Although the cerebellum does not initiate movements, it participates closely with the motor cortex and the basal ganglia in maintaining proper balance and posture for walking and running, in the organization of fine voluntary (projected) and repetitive movements of the cranial and limb musculature (such as those used in hammering, turning a screwdriver, or tapping a foot), and in the coordination of smooth pursuit movements of the eyes, as in following a moving target. The cerebellum provides the ability to locate accurately an object in space by analyzing the correct trajectory and velocity of the movement.

ANATOMIC AND PHYSIOLOGICAL CONSIDERATIONS The cerebellum straddles the pons and medulla and is connected to the brainstem on each side by three fiber bundles, the inferior (restiform body), middle, and superior cerebellar peduncles. The massive middle cerebellar peduncle is estimated to contain 20 million fibers (compared with 1 million in the medullary pyramid). The anatomic subdivisions of the cerebellum are best understood by a consideration of its afferent inputs. Vestibulocerebellar inputs go principally to the flocculonodular lobe (also called the archicerebellum), spinocerebellar afferents distribute to the vermis and the anterior lobe (paleocerebellum), and medullo- and pontocerebellar fibers distribute to the lateral hemispheres (neocerebellum). Anatomic studies indicate that there is more overlap between these various afferent inputs than had previously been thought. The restiform body carries afferents from the spinal cord (dorsal spinocerebellar tract), from the vestibular nuclei (vestibulocerebellar), and olivocerebellar and reticulocerebellar fibers from the medulla and pons. The middle cerebellar peduncle contains the pontocerebellar fibers, which carry the primary input from the cerebral cortex. The superior cerebellar peduncle contains both afferents (the ventral spinocerebellar tract) and efferents, including the fibers that reach the red nucleus and the thalamus, the latter to complete the cerebello-thalamo-cortico-ponto-cerebellar loop, important for the integration of motor functions with the corticospinal and extrapyramidal systems. Recent studies have documented that the cerebellum also receives sensory inputs from the visual, auditory, and somatosensory cortex.

Histologically, three types of afferent fibers to the cerebellum can be differentiated: (1) mossy fibers that terminate in the granule cell layer of the cortex, and which arise from all inputs except those of the olivary nucleus; (2) climbing fibers that terminate on the dendrites of the Purkinje cells, and which are derived exclusively from the olivary nucleus in the medulla; and (3) monoaminergic fibers containing either norepinephrine or serotonin that terminate diffusely in the granular and molecular layers. The output of the cerebellum originates in the Purkinje cells and is relayed through the deep cerebellar nuclei, the principal one of which is the dentate nucleus. GABA is the main neurotransmitter in the cerebellar efferent system, both within the Purkinje cells and in the efferents from the deep cerebellar nuclei.

CLINICAL MANIFESTATIONS OF LESIONS OF THE BASAL GANGLIA

The symptoms that lend themselves best to clinical analysis are akinesia, rigidity, chorea, athetosis, dystonia, myoclonus, and tremor. Table 15-1 presents clinicopathologic correlations accepted by most neurologists.

AKINESIA When extrapyramidal disease is analyzed along classic neurologic lines into primary functional deficits and secondary release effects, akinesia stands as the principal negative or deficit symptom. The term *akinesia* refers to the disinclination of the patient to use an affected part of the body, to engage it freely in all the natural actions of the body. In contrast to paralysis, the negative symptom of corticospinal lesions, strength is relatively undiminished in the part, and it can be used effectively in the desired movement under conditions of maximal attention and motivation. In this respect, too, it is unlike apraxia, where movements are lost because of a lesion

TABLE 15-1
Clinicopathologic correlations

Symptoms	*Principal location of morbid anatomy*
Unilateral plastic rigidity with static tremor and regular slowness of movement (Parkinson's syndrome)	Contralateral substantia nigra plus (?) other structures
Unilateral hemiballismus and hemichorea	Contralateral subthalamic nucleus of Luys, prerubral area, and Forel's fields
Chronic chorea of Huntington's type	Caudate nucleus, putamen
Athetosis and dystonia	Contralateral putamen or thalamus
Cerebellar ataxia, i.e., intention tremor; irregular slowness in starting and stopping alternating voluntary movements; hypotonia; rebound phenomenon	Homolateral cerebellar hemisphere or middle and inferior cerebellar peduncles, superior brachium conjunctivum (ipsilateral if below the decussation, contralateral if above)
Decerebrate rigidity, i.e., opisthotonos, extension of arms and legs	Lesion usually bilateral in tegmentum, involving upper brainstem, particularly red nucleus or structures between red nucleus and vestibular nuclei
Palatal and facial myoclonus (rhythmic)	Lesion in the central tegmental tract, inferior olivary nucleus, and olivodentate connections
Diffuse myoclonus	Cerebellar cortex (?), thalami (?)

which erases the "memory" of the motor schema that directs the sequence of movements for intended action. Parkinsonian patients exhibit the phenomenon of akinesia most clearly in their extreme underactivity. They sit motionless for long times. In looking to the side they move the eyes, not the head. In arising from a chair they fail to make all the little adjustments needed (pulling feet back, putting hands on arms of chair, etc.). They neglect the affected arm. Yet they are not weak (paretic) or apraxic. Formerly, akinesia was attributed to rigidity, which could reasonably hamper all movements, but now that stereotaxic surgery has been shown to abolish both tremor and rigidity, it becomes clear that the motor deficit, or akinesia, is still there. Strictly interpreted, it would appear that apart from their contribution to the maintenance of postures, the substantia nigra and other pigmented neurons must provide something essential to the performance of the large variety of semiautomatic actions that make up the full repertoire of natural human motility.

ALTERATIONS OF MUSCLE TONE (SPASTICITY, RIGIDITY, HYPOTONIA) Muscle tone (the small resistance to muscle stretch offered by healthy muscle) is enhanced in the many conditions that cause a paralysis of voluntary movement by interrupting the corticospinal tract. The special distribution of the increased tone (i.e., greater in antigravity muscles—leg extensors and arm flexors in humans), the sudden augmentation of tone with gradual yielding upon quick movement, the clasp-knife phenomenon, the absence of resistance upon slow movement and its disappearance in relaxed muscle with "electromyographic silence when relaxed," and exaggerated tendon (phasic myotatic) reflexes are the identifying characteristics of spasticity. This type of hypertonus is believed to be due in some instances to hyperactivity of the small gamma motor neurons, resulting in increase in the sensitivity of the spindle muscle fibers to stretch. In other instances especially when a voluntary movement evokes a persistent, diffuse resistance to active and passive movement (tonic myotatic reflex activity), it seems clearly related to excessive activity (or disinhibition) of the larger alpha motor neurons. The "gamma spasticity" is abolished by procaine injection of the motor nerve, which paralyzes the small gamma motor and sensory fibers, leaving the larger ones intact, without weakening the willed contractions of the muscle; the "alpha spasticity" is not affected by procaine.

In the state known as *rigidity* the muscles are continuously or intermittently firm, tense, and prominent; and the resistance to passive movement is intense and even, like that noted in bending a lead pipe or in stretching a strand of toffee. Although rigidity is present in all muscle groups, both flexor and extensor, on the whole it tends to be more prominent in those which maintain a flexed posture, i.e., the flexor muscles of trunk and limbs. It appears to be somewhat greater in the large muscle groups, but this may be merely a question of muscle mass. Certainly the smaller muscles of the face and tongue and even those of the larynx are often affected. Nevertheless, like gamma spasticity, this rigidity is said to be abolished by procaine, and it is eradicated by posterior root section. In the electromyographic tracing, motor unit activity tends to be more continuous than in spasticity, persisting even after relaxation (Table 15-2).

A special type of rigidity is the *cogwheel phenomenon*. When the hypertonic muscle is passively stretched, the resistance may be rhythmically jerky, as though the resistance of the limb were controlled by a ratchet. A number of different explanations of this phenomenon have been suggested. Wilson postulated that it might be due to a minor form of the lengthening-shortening reaction, but a more likely explanation is an associated static tremor that is masked by rigidity during an attitude of repose but emerges faintly during manipulation.

Rigidity is prominent in extrapyramidal diseases such as paralysis agitans, postencephalitic Parkinson's syndrome, and dystonia musculorum deformans.

The *tension hypertonus of athetosis* differs from both spasticity and rigidity. Strictly speaking, it takes two forms, one which occurs during the involuntary athetotic movement, and another which appears in the absence of any involuntary motion. Clinically these forms of hypertonus are variable from one moment to the next and are paradoxical in that they sometimes disappear during a rapid passive movement or when the limb is passively shaken. The tendon reflexes may be normal or brisk. The lengthening and shortening reactions are absent. This form of variable hypertonus is found in double athetosis and choreoathetosis and in some cases of dystonia musculorum deformans.

Hypotonia refers to slackness of the muscles. It is most striking in diseases of spinal motor neurons and peripheral nerve diseases. With reference to basal ganglia and cerebellar diseases hypotonia is most evident in acute cerebellar lesions, in Sydenham's chorea, and in Huntington's chorea.

INVOLUNTARY MOVEMENTS Chorea Derived from the Greek word meaning "dance," *chorea* refers to widespread arrhythmic movements of a forcible, rapid, jerky type. These movements are involuntary and are noted for their irregularity, variability, relative speed, and relatively brief duration. They may be simple or quite elaborate and of variable distribution. In some respects they resemble a voluntary movement in their complexity, yet they are never combined into a coordinated act. The patient may, however, incorporate them into a deliberate movement, as if to make them less noticeable. When superimposed on voluntary movements, these may take on a grotesque and exaggerated character. Grimacing and peculiar respiratory sounds may be other expressions of the movement disorder. Usually the movements are discrete, but if very numerous, they may flow into one another; the resultant picture then resembles athetosis. They may be limited to a limb or one side of the body (hemichorea), or they may involve all parts of the body. Normal volitional movements are, of course, possible, for there is no paralysis, but they too may be excessively quick and poorly sustained. The limbs are often unusually slack, or hypotonic. A choreic movement may be superimposed on a tendon reflex, giving rise to the "hung-up reflex." The tendon reflexes tend to be pendular because of the associated hypotonia; when the knee jerk is elicited with the patient sitting, the leg swings back and forth four or five times, like a pendulum, rather than one or two times as in a normal person. (See Table 15-2 for list of common pathologies.)

A special variety of chorea (sometimes choreoathetosis or dystonia) is clearly paroxysmal and sometimes familial (dominant inheritance). Paroxysms lasting minutes to hours appear during childhood or adolescence and continue throughout life. In one special subtype the chorea is kinesogenic, meaning that it is initiated by a sudden voluntary movement. Alcohol, hypernatremia, and phenytoin (especially in patients who have had Sydenham's chorea in childhood) may precipitate paroxysmal chorea. In some cases anticonvulsive drugs (clonazepam, phenobarbital) have prevented attacks, and in others L-dopa has been effective.

Athetosis This term is from a Greek word meaning "unfixed" or "changeable." The condition is characterized by an inability to sustain the fingers and toes, tongue, or any other group of muscles in one position. The maintained posture is interrupted by continuous, slow, sinuous, purposeless movements. These are most pronounced in the digits and the hands but often involve the tongue, throat, and face. One can detect as basic patterns of movement an extension and pronation and flexion and supination of the arm, and alternating flexion and extension of the fingers. Athetosis may be unilateral, especially in children who have suffered a hemiplegia at some previous date (posthemiplegic athetosis). The movements are slower than those associated with chorea, but in many cases gradations between the two (choreoathetosis) are seen. Most athetotic patients exhibit variable degrees of motor deficit due in some

TABLE 15-2
Nontremorous extrapyramidal movement disorders

Type	*Physiologic characteristics*	*Pathologic anatomy*	*Common diseases*	*Treatment*
Plastic rigidity, static tremor, slowness of movement (Parkinson's syndrome)	Present during rest and activity Worsened by excitement No change in tendon or cutaneous reflexes unilateral or bilateral See Table 15-3	Substantia nigra- and nigrostriatal pathway Contralateral if one-sided	Paralysis agitans (Parkinson's disease) Postencephalitic parkinsonism Wilson's disease Hallevorden-Spatz disease Dopamine receptor-antagonist drugs (phenothiazines, butyrophenones)	Anticholinergic drugs L-Dopa Amantadine Stereotaxic thalamic surgery
Chorea and choreoathetosis:				
Generalized	Moderately fast, arrhythmic, usually with hypotonia but without change in reflexes or ataxia	Striatum, caudate nucleus, and putamen	Rheumatic (Sydenham's chorea) Huntington's chorea Senile chorea Tardive dyskinesia Rarely thyrotoxicosis, "the pill," lupus erythematosus, polycythemia vera, hypernatremia	Prednisone Haloperidol Diazepam
Unilateral or localized	Same	Contralateral striatum	Infarct or hemorrhage in thalamus or striatum (contralateral)	Rest, quiet, sedatives Stereotaxic thalamic surgery
Athetosis and dystonia:				
Generalized	Present at rest, worse on willed movement Aggravated by excitement Reflexes normal or abnormal	Anterior thalamus or ventricular nuclei with intact pyramidal tracts	Cerebral palsy Wilson's disease Rigid form of Huntington's chorea Overdose of L-dopa Postanoxic sequela Other degenerative diseases Dystonia musculorum deformans	Stereotaxic thalamic surgery Penicillamine
Unilateral (restricted dystonias, see text)	Same	Same	Posthemiplegic states	As above Surgical denervation of affected muscles
Hemiballismus	Arrhythmic; large excursion; usually unilateral; no weakness or pyramidal signs	Contralateral subthalamic nucleus	Vascular lesions (hemorrhage or infarct) Posttraumatic (rare)	Stereotaxic thalamic surgery Diazepam and other sedatives
Myoclonus:				
Arrhythmic	Movements quicker than chorea Associated ataxia (often) or dementia and seizures	Cerebellum, ?cortex, ?dentate nuclei, ?thalamus	Postanoxic Lipidoses Jakob-Creutzfeldt disease Subacute sclerosing encephalitis Familial myoclonic epilepsy and other degenerative diseases	5-Hydroxytryptophan Anticonvulsant and sedative medications
Rhythmic (restricted, palatal myoclonus)	Continuous, awake and asleep; other brainstem signs	Central segmental tracts of pons, medulla, and inferior olivary nuclei	Vascular lesions, gliomas	None known

instances to associated corticospinal tract disease. Discrete individual movements of the tongue, lips, and hand are often impossible, and attempts to perform such voluntary movements result in a contraction of all the muscles in the limb and other parts of the body (*intention spasm*). Variable degrees of rigidity are generally associated, and these may account for the slower quality of movement in athetosis, in contrast to chorea. It must be admitted, however, that in some cases it is almost impossible to distinguish between chorea and athetosis.

Torsion spasm, or dystonia Torsion spasm is closely allied to athetosis, differing only in that the larger axial muscles (those of the trunk and limb girdles) rather than appendicular muscles are involved. It results in bizarre, grotesque movements and positions of the body. The word *dystonia* has been given to these movements but, unfortunately, is also applied to any fixed posture which may be the end result of a disease of the motor system. Thus Denny-Brown speaks of hemiplegic dystonia, the flexion dystonia of parkinsonism, and extensor dystonia with retraction of the head and arching or twisting of the back. If the latter meaning is given, it would be better to speak of athetosis of the trunk as torsion spasms or phasic dystonia, in contrast to fixed dystonia. The former, like athetosis, may show remarkable fluctuations; sometimes the whole musculature of the body may be thrown into spasm by an effort to move an arm or to speak. If mild, the torsion spasm may be limited to the lumbar or cervical muscles or those of one limb and may cease when the body is at rest (see below).

Torsion spasm may be seen in the condition of double athetosis after hypoxic damage to the brain, in kernicterus, in chronic manganese intoxication, rarely in Wilson's hepatolenticular degeneration, in postphenothiazine dyskinesias, and in Hallevorden-Spatz disease (Chap. 364). But it is most characteristic of the syndrome designated as *dystonia musculorum deformans*.

Chorea, athetosis, and torsion spasm are all closely related. The movements are elaborate and depend for their expression on cortical mechanisms. Paralytic lesions involving the corticospinal tract abolish these involuntary movements. The hypotonia in chorea and some cases of athetosis, the pendular reflexes, and some degree of interference with natural movements are also reminiscent of the syndrome that follows disease of the cerebellum. Lacking, however, are intention tremor and true incoordination, or ataxia.

Myoclonus This term refers to several different motor disorders, some localized, others diffuse. As in chorea, the myoclonic movement is involuntary and arrhythmic, but it is much faster than chorea, being concluded in a few hundred milliseconds or less. Variations in degree are noteworthy; it may consist of no more than a flick of a single muscle or part of a muscle simulating a fasciculation, but the larger movements always betray its nature, involving as they do a group of muscles. Sensory relationships are another prominent attribute. Flickering light, a series of loud sounds, or abrupt contact with some part of the body in some instances may regularly initiate a jerk, sometimes as a direct sensorimotor effect, again through the mechanism of startle. One special variety is evoked by willed movement, presumably through a proprioceptive mechanism. Hence, one may speak of action or intention myoclonus, auditory or visual myoclonus. A series of intense stimuli may recruit a series of myoclonic jerks that progress to a full-blown seizure, as happens often in the familial myoclonic epilepsy syndrome of Unverricht-Lundborg. The pathologic disturbance in the latter is usually a lipid storage disease or an amyloid Lafora body inclusion disease (Chap. 364). See Table 15-2 for list of common disorders associated with myoclonus.

The term *myoclonus* unfortunately has also been assigned to a rather different motor phenomenon—that of repetitious, rhythmic clonus of some part of the "branchial cleft" or craniocervical musculature. Examples are "nystagmus of the palate" (rhythmic contractions at the rate of 10 to 50 or more per minute of the soft palate) and rhythmic contractions of the pharyngeal muscles, vocal cords, facial muscles, and diaphragm. The lesions producing this state, which we would prefer to designate as a form of continuous *bulbar, facial,* or *diaphragmatic clonus,* have been situated in all instances in the central tegmental tract, inferior olivary nucleus, or olivocerebellar tract. The causative lesions have been infarcts, tumors, and encephalitic processes.

The main fault with our concept of myoclonus is that it covers too many motor disorders. When movements are grouped according to their brevity or involuntary nature, one must include the normal dormescent start or jerk of a limb as one falls asleep, and the motor components of a natural startle reaction. The obligatory Moro response also falls within the group, as well as the form of epilepsy known as infantile or salaam spasms and the falling spells of the petit mal triad. Pentylenetetrazol (Metrazol) injections cause myoclonus of the limbs, which has been shown to depend on a lower brainstem (medullary reticular) mechanism. Another problem arises on the clinical side in distinguishing diffuse myoclonus from other abrupt involuntary movements such as tremors, chorea, and restricted forms of epilepsy (epilepsia partialis continua). Speed of movement, lack of rhythmicity, and relationships to sensory stimulation prove to be the most reliable identifying features of the larger group of myoclonic disorders. There is an advantage in separating the arrhythmic diffuse form from the rhythmic restricted form in that each stands as a diagnostic attribute of a separate category of nervous diseases.

Tremor This consists of a more or less regular rhythmic oscillation of a part of the body around a fixed point. The rate varies from three to eight oscillations per second; in a particular person the rate is fairly constant in all affected parts, regardless of the size of the muscle or of the part of the body. Tremors usually involve the distal part of the limbs, the head, tongue, or jaw, and rarely the trunk.

There are many different types of tremor, and only a few are recognized as bearing any meaningful relationship to disease of the extrapyramidal motor system; but since tremors have not been discussed elsewhere, all the different types will be considered here.

Tremors may be subdivided according to their distribution, amplitude, regularity, and relationship to volitional movement. The tremors described in the following paragraphs should be familiar to every physician (Table 15-3).

STATIC (PARKINSONIAN) TREMOR This is a coarse, rhythmic tremor, with an average rate of four to five beats per second, most often localized in one or both hands, and, occasionally, in the jaw or tongue. Its most characteristic feature is that it occurs when the limb is in an attitude of repose, and willed movement at least temporarily suppresses it. If the tremulous limb is completely relaxed, the tremor usually disappears, but the average patient rarely achieves this state. In some cases the tremor is constant; in others it varies from time to time and with the progress of the disease extends from one group of muscles to another. In paralysis agitans the tremor tends to be rather gentle and more or less limited to the distal muscles, whereas in postencephalitic parkinsonism and hepatolenticular degeneration it often has a wider range and involves proximal muscles. In many cases there is a variable degree of rigidity of a plastic type in the tremulous limb or elsewhere. The tremor interferes with voluntary movements surprisingly little; it is not uncommon to see a patient who has been trembling violently raise a full glass of water to the lips and drain the contents without spilling a drop. The handwriting of these patients is often small and cramped (micrographia). The gait may be of festinating type (see Chap. 16). It is the combination of static tremor, slowness of movement, rigidity, and flexed postures without true paralysis that constitutes Parkinson's syndrome (also called *amyostatic* syndrome).

The exact pathologic anatomy of static tremor is unknown. In paralysis agitans and postencephalitic Parkinson's syndrome, the visible lesions are predominantly in the substantia nigra. In hepatocerebral degeneration, where this syndrome is mixed with cerebellar ataxia, the lesions are more diffuse. A similar tremor, without rigidity, slowness of movement, flexed postures, or masked facies, is seen in senile persons. Unlike Parkinson's disease, it does not progress to motor disability and usually does not respond to antiparkinsonian drugs. In any given case one cannot always predict whether it is the initial sign of Parkinson's disease.

ACTION TREMOR This term refers to a tremor present when the limbs are actively maintained in a certain position, as when outstretched, and throughout voluntary movement. It may increase slightly as the action of the limbs becomes more precise, but it never approaches the degree of augmentation in fine movement seen in intention tremor. It is easily made to disappear when the limbs are relaxed. Probably some of the *action tremors* are but an exaggeration of normal or physiologic tremor, which ranges from eight to ten per second, being slower in childhood and old age. In adults the tremor is of small excursion, has a frequency of seven to eight per second, and is somewhat irregular. The tremor involves the outstretched hand, head, and, less often, the lips and tongue, and usually it interferes little with voluntary movements such as handwriting and speech. This type of tremor is seen in numerous medical, neurologic, and psychiatric diseases and is therefore more difficult to interpret than static tremor.

There is another, somewhat slower frequency type of action tremor, and instead of rather irregular potentials in both agonist and antagonist muscles (as in the aforementioned type), their activity alternates. These two types respond differently to drugs. Either form, when occurring as the only neurologic abnormality in several members of a family, is known as *familial* or *hereditary tremor.* Familial tremor may begin in childhood, but usually comes on later and persists throughout adult life. Being worse when the patient is under observation, it becomes a source of embarrassment because it suggests to the onlooker that the patient is nervous. A curious fact about familial tremors is that one or two drinks of an alcoholic beverage may abolish them, and they may become worse after the effects of the alcohol have worn off. The fast-frequency type of action tremor is seen in delirious states, such as delirium tremens, in chronic alcoholism as an isolated symptom (the morning shakes), and in general paresis. An action tremor, usually more rapid than the above, is also characteristic of hyperthyroidism and other toxic states, and a similar tremor is frequently observed in patients suffering intense anxiety. In fact it can be reproduced by injections of epinephrine. Severe action tremor may also accompany certain diseases of the basal ganglia, in-

TABLE 15-3
Tremors

Types	*Physiologic characteristics*	*Anatomic pathology*	*Common diseases*	*Treatment*
Fast frequency (7–10 per second), slightly arrhythmic action tremor	Generalized (usually) Present during activity; increased in precise movement and excitement; ceases during full relaxation Increased by epinephrine	Unknown ?Peripheral or spinal	One of hereditary types Hyperthyroidism Intense fright Corticosteroid and lithium therapy Pheochromocytoma and carcinoid Alcoholic withdrawal	Reduced by propranolol (Inderal) and beta-blocking agents Reduced by alcohol Sometimes helped by diazepam or primidone
Medium frequency (5–7 per second), rhythmic action tremor	Same as above except for rhythmic alternations of agonists and antagonists	Unknown ?Central (spinal or higher centers)	One of hereditary types General paresis (syphilis) Rare in other diseases Some cases of corticosteroid therapy	Variably reduced by propranolol and alcohol Reduced by diazepam or primidone
Ataxic intention tremor (4–6 per second)	Present in terminal phase of projected (willed) movement; absent during relaxation May be unilateral Associated with cerebellar ataxia	Cerebellum—especially dentatothalamic tracts (superior cerebellar peduncle and brachium conjunctivum)	Multiple sclerosis Cerebellar and brainstem tumors Vascular lesions	Drugs ineffective Light weights on limbs occasionally help
Combined rest and intention tremor (4–6 per second, erroneously called "rubral tremor")	Wide range and rhythmic; worse during willed movement, but present at rest Associated with cerebellar ataxia and/or parkinsonism May be unilateral	Tegmentum of midbrain and subthalamus ?Brachium conjunctivum	Multiple sclerosis Wilson's disease Vascular lesions and traumatism	Stereotaxic surgery of ventromedial nucleus may help Drugs ineffective
Tremor at rest (4–5 per second, static tremor or "parkinsonian tremor")	Rhythmic alternation of agonist-antagonist muscles Present in attitude of repose; temporarily abolished by willed movement May be combined with fast-frequency tremor Usually associated with rigidity and slowness of movement	Lesions in substantia nigra and nigrolenticular pathway	Paralysis agitans (Parkinson's disease) Postencephalitic parkinsonism Wilson's disease Senile syndromes Postphenothiazine (tardive) dyskinesia	Reduced by anticholinergic drugs and L-dopa Reduced by stereotaxic surgery (ventral thalamus and pallidum)

cluding parkinsonism. Some of the fast-frequency action tremors are suppressed by beta-adrenergic blocking agents such as propranolol (Inderal, 40 mg tid). The slower type may respond to isoniazid (300 mg tid) but not consistently to propranolol.

INTENTION TREMOR The word *intention* is ambiguous in this context because the tremor itself is not intentional. The term means, instead, that the tremor requires for its full expression the performance of an exacting, precise, willed movement. The term *ataxic* or *kinetic tremor* has been suggested because it is always combined with and adds to cerebellar ataxia. The tremor is absent when the limbs are inactive and during the first part of a voluntary movement, but as the action continues and greater precision is demanded (e.g., in touching a target such as the patient's nose or the examiner's finger), a jerky, more or less rhythmic interruption of forward progression, with side-to-side oscillation, appears. It continues for a fraction of a second or so after the act is completed. The tremor may seriously interfere with the patient's performance of skilled acts. Sometimes the head is involved (titubation). This type of tremor invariably indicates disease of the cerebellum and of its connections. When the disease is very severe, every movement, even the lifting of a limb, results in a wide-ranging tremor of such violence as to throw the patient off balance. This latter state is occasionally seen in multiple sclerosis, Wilson's disease, and vascular, traumatic, and other lesions of the tegmentum of the midbrain and subthalamus but not of the cerebellum.

Other involuntary movements There are other abnormalities of movement, about which only a few words can be said. They vary from simple irritative phenomena to complex psychologically related disorders, such as compulsions, mannerisms, etc.

The first group are the isolated or restricted dystonias (dyskinesias) of adult life. These include idiopathic spasmodic torticollis, oromandibular dystonia, blepharospasm, spastic dysphonia, and dystonic writer's cramp.

SPASMODIC TORTICOLLIS This is an intermittent or continuous spasm of sternomastoid, trapezius, and other neck muscles, usually more pronounced on one side, with turning or tipping of the head. It is involuntary and cannot be inhibited and thereby differs from habit spasm or tic. This condition should be considered a form of dystonia. It is worse when the patient sits, stands, or walks, and usually contactual stimulation of the chin or of the back of the head partially alleviates the muscle imbalance.

Women are affected twice as often as men and the average age of onset is 40 years. Rarely it appears in early adult life or adolescence. Extranuchal dystonia, tremor, and facial masking are associated findings in some cases.

Various modes of therapy have been tried with inconsistent results. L-Dopa (1 g per day) with carbidopa, carbamazepine (Tegretol, 200 to 1200 mg per day), haloperidol (2 to 12 mg per day) and biofeedback therapy have each been beneficial in certain cases. Psychiatric treatment is ineffectual. In severe cases muscle sectioning, neurectomy, or section of the anterior cervical roots has given favorable results in over 75 percent of patients.

OTHER CRANIOCERVICAL SPASMS Blepharoclonus (inability to keep the eyes open), lingual spasms, "spastic" dysphonia, facial spasms, cervicothoracic spasms, and writer's cramp are all special varieties of involuntary movement, appearing usually in late middle life and the senium. Such facial, cervical, and thoracic spasms have occurred with striking frequency during phenothiazine medication, but they also appear de novo. Marsden refers to them as restricted dystonias. Nonprogressivity, unresponsiveness to psychotherapy, and uncertain amelioration by all pharmacologic agents characterize most of them. Exceptionally, when these disorders are induced by drugs of the phenothiazine class, they persist after discontinuance of the drug (tardive or postphenothiazine dyskinesias). The only therapy of value in severe spasmodic torticollis has been surgical denervation of the affected muscles (C1 to C3 and unilateral C4 roots).

TICS AND HABIT SPASMS Many persons throughout life are given to habitual movements, such as sniffing, clearing the throat, protruding the chin, or blinking, whenever they become tense. The patient admits that the movements are voluntary and that he or she feels compelled to make them in order to relieve tension; they can be inhibited for a time by an effort of will but reappear when attention is diverted. Children between 5 and 10 years of age are especially likely to have habit spasms. The movements are often purposive coordinated acts which normally serve the organism; it is only their incessant repetition when uncalled for that constitutes a habit. In certain cases they become so ingrained that the person is unaware of them and unable to control them. Stereotypy, purposelessness, and repetitiveness at irregular intervals are their main identifying features. Multiple convulsive tics with coprolalia (compulsive utterance of vile words; *Gilles de la Tourette's disease*) constitute a more severe and often unremitting form of the same condition. In children with transitory habit spasms it is best to ignore the habit spasm and at the same time to arrange for more rest and calmer environment. In adults, relief of nervous tension by tranquilizing drugs (chlorpromazine, 25 to 75 mg tid) and psychotherapy is helpful, but the disposition to tic formation persists. In the chronic tic or Tourette's syndrome large doses of haloperidol (10 to 20 mg per day orally) or administration of clonidine have been beneficial in some cases.

Mentally retarded children and adults often display, when idle, a wide variety of rhythmic body-rocking, head-bobbing, arm-and-finger movements. These are of the nature of mannerisms and have no known basal ganglion pathology.

It would be a mistake to assume that each of the above disorders of movement occurs separately in specific relationships to certain diseases. This may happen, as in paralysis agitans, but there is sometimes much overlap in the degenerative diseases and birth injuries.

MOTOR DISTURBANCES DUE PRIMARILY TO DISEASES OF THE CEREBELLUM Isolated lesions in the midline flocculonodular lobe result in grave disturbances of equilibrium. Often the symptoms are exhibited only when the patient attempts to stand and walk. Then he or she sways, staggers, titubates, and reels (see "Disturbance of Movement and Posture," below). There may be no disturbance in coordination and no intention tremor of the limbs. A midline tumor (such as medulloblastoma), hemorrhage, or other lesion in the same locale produces this syndrome.

Extensive lesions of one cerebellar hemisphere, especially the anterior lobe, cause disturbances in coordination of volitional movements of the ipsilateral arm and leg. This is known as *ataxia.* The movements are characterized by an inappropriate range, rate, and strength of each of the various components of a motor act and by an improper combination of those components. Electromyographic analysis has shown that ataxia is manifested as a decomposition of movement consisting of abnormal duration and timing of bursts of contraction and relaxation of agonists and antagonists of a joint, usually a large one. This incoordination is also called *asynergia.* The defects are particularly noticeable in acts that require rapid alternation of movements. Irregular slowness in acceleration and deceleration, which is almost invariably present, impedes the performance. Babinski called this dysdiadochokinesis. The direction of projected (purposive) movement is frequently inaccurate. Owing to delay in arresting a movement, the patient may overshoot the mark. The antagonist muscles do not come into play at the proper time, possibly because of the hypotonia that is almost always present. This may be demonstrated by having the patient flex the arm against a resistance that is suddenly released. The patient with cerebellar disease will sometimes strike the face because of failure to check the flexion movement. In movements requiring accurate direction, as the limb approaches its destination it may stop short and then advance by a more or less rhythmic series of jerks and oscillations (intention tremor). In addition to hypotonia, there may be, in acute cerebellar lesions, some slight weakness.

A similar ataxia, asynergia, and dysmetria, usually with hypotonia and only a little intention tremor, may accompany lesions of the lateral and inferior parts of the cerebellar hemisphere. Bilateral lesions of the cerebellar hemispheres and midline flocculonodular lobe lead to such a severe disturbance in all movements that the patient may be unable to stand or walk or use the limbs effectively. In addition, there are ocular and speech disturbances, namely, nystagmus, dysmetria and skew deviation of the eyes, and an uneven dysarthria. Lesions of the cerebellar peduncles have the same effect as extensive hemispheral lesions. This syndrome, due to involvement of one cerebellar hemisphere, may be observed in a tumor or abscess or in vascular lesions of the brainstem and cerebellar peduncles. The ataxia tends to be bilateral and symmetric in primary atrophy or degeneration of the cerebellum.

There have been numerous attempts to explain in physiologic terms the hypotonia, mild degrees of weakness and fatigability, and abnormalities in the rate and regularity of projected movement that accompany cerebellar lesions in humans. It has been found that depression of fusimotor (spindle) efferent activity in the spinal cord leads to decreased spindle afferent discharge and lessened tonic facilitation of alpha motor neuron activity. The cerebellar facilitation that is lost with acute lesions is normally mediated through two systems of fibers—the fastigioreticulospinal and the dentatorubrothalamocortical. The latter, acting specifically on cortical areas 4 and 6, is the more important in humans. The corticospinal tract is probably essential for expression of cerebellar deficits in humans. Tremor, ataxia, and hypotonia seem to be separable, independent entities, but all are believed related to the disturbed fusimotor activity.

A kind of pseudoataxia, especially of gait, may be caused by the improper timing of the components of complex actions, e.g., with defects in postural sense (sensory ataxia), with defects in afferents entering the spinocerebellar system, and with slow relaxation of muscles in hypothyroidism (myxedema with ataxia).

SOME GENERAL FEATURES OF ALL EXTRAPYRAMIDAL MOTOR DISTURBANCES

Motor disorder seldom appears in pure form. Various combinations occur in diseases. For example, Wilson's disease usually presents with a Parkinson-like picture of tremor, rigidity, slowness of movement, and flexion dystonia of trunk, but exceptionally there is athetosis, tonic innervation (inability to relax a voluntary movement), phasic dystonia, and intention tremor. Hallevorden-Spatz disease may take the form of universal rigidity and flexion dystonia or choreoathetosis. Occasionally the degeneration of Huntington's chorea leads to rigidity rather than choreoathetosis. Corticospinal and various of these extrapyramidal disorders may be associated in patients with cerebral diplegia. Nonetheless certain combinations tend to occur with greater or lesser frequency in certain diseases, as discussed in Chaps. 364 and 365.

In broad terms all the extrapyramidal disorders should be viewed in terms of the primary deficit (negative symptom) and of the new phenomena (movements, abnormal postures, tremors, etc.) which have appeared. These latter positive symptoms are presently ascribed to release from or disequilibrium of undamaged motor parts of the nervous system. The clearest negative effect is usually evidenced as an akinesia, or disinclination to use the affected muscles. The difficulty in rapid alternating sequences of movement stands as another negative effect in diseases of both the basal ganglia and the cerebellum. In fact this latter symptom, presenting as a clumsiness, may be the only fault manifest in certain congenitally maladroit children. Stress and nervous tension characteristically worsen both the motor deficiency and the abnormal movements in all these extrapyramidal syndromes, just as relaxation helps the motor performance. All the movement disorders are abolished in sleep.

Tremors, rigidity, and involuntary movements of the limbs have been abolished by a surgical lesion in the medial segment of the globus pallidus or the ventrolateral nucleus of the thalamus. The effects are contralateral. Usually the lesion has been made first by the injection of procaine (Novocain) and then by use of alcohol, cooling and freezing, or electrocoagulation. The operation has been successful in temporarily alleviating tremor or rigidity (or both) on one side. The procedure is successful in approximately 80 percent of cases of paralysis agitans, and the postural abnormality in dystonia musculorum deformans and double athetosis has responded somewhat less consistently. The operations have been perfected to the point at which the mortality rate is less than 1 percent, and the risk of hemiplegia or some other sequel is less than 10 percent. Of course, as the disease progresses, the beneficial effects are lost. The therapeutic procedure indicates that the pallidum and ventrolateral nucleus, probably through their connections with the cerebral cortex (motor cortex and its corticospinal pathway), are essential for the expression of these extrapyramidal syndromes. The indications for these surgical procedures are discussed in Chap. 364.

DISTURBANCE OF MOVEMENT AND POSTURE: EXAMINATION AND DIFFERENTIAL DIAGNOSIS

In Chap. 14 the methods of examining the motor system are described at some length, so only a few additional remarks concerning extrapyramidal disorders need be made here. These abnormalities are best demonstrated by seeing the patient in action. Patients who complain of a limp after walking a distance or of difficulty in climbing stairs should be observed under these conditions. Tests of rate, regularity, and coordination of voluntary movement must be sufficiently varied and demanding of the patient's motor coordination to bring out the defect. The physician must cultivate the habit of accurately observing and describing abnormalities of movement and must not be content merely to give the condition a name or to force it into some category such as chorea, tic, or myoclonus. The main postures of the body in all common acts should be noted. Aside from the assessment of muscle power and of gait, the usual test applied to the upper limb is to ask the patient to touch the examiner's fingertip and then the tip of his or her own nose repeatedly (*finger-to-nose test*). To test the leg, the patient is asked to place a heel on one knee and then to run it down the shin and back to the knee (*heel-to-knee-to-shin test*). Finer movements of the hand may be tested by having the patient successively touch each finger to the thumb, pat a thigh rapidly, or use tools or handle objects. Rapidly alternating movements such as repeatedly touching the index finger with the thumb, pronation and supination of wrist, or opening and closing the hands are valuable tests.

The fully developed extrapyramidal motor syndromes can be recognized without difficulty once the physician has become familiar with the typical pictures. The mental picture of Parkinson's syndrome, with its slowness of movement, poverty of facial expression, and static tremor and rigidity should be fixed in mind. Similarly, the gross distortions and postural abnormalities of dystonia, whether widespread in trunk muscles or involving only neck muscles, as in spasmodic torticollis, once seen should thereafter be familiar. Athetosis, with its instability of postures, ceaseless movements of fingers and hands, and intention spasm; chorea, with its more rapid and complicated movements; and the abrupt movements of myoclonus that flit over the body are other standard syndromes. Characteristic of all is a mild defect in the voluntary use of the affected parts.

The clinical differences between corticospinal and extrapyramidal disorders are summarized in Table 15-2.

Early or mild forms of these conditions, like all medical diseases, may offer special difficulties in diagnosis. Cases of paralysis agitans, seen before the appearance of tremor, are often overlooked. The patient may complain of being nervous and restless or may have experienced an indescribable stiffness and aching in certain parts of the body. Because there is no weakness or reflex changes, the disorder may be considered psychogenic or rheumatic. Parkinson's syndrome often begins in a hemiplegic distribution, and for this reason the illness may be misdiagnosed as cerebral thrombosis. A slight masking of the face, a suggestion of a limp, blepharoclonus (uninhibited blinking of eyes when the bridge of the nose is tapped), a mild rigidity, failure of an arm to swing naturally in walking, or loss of certain movements of cooperation will help in diagnosis at this time. Every case presenting the syndrome of Parkinson or other abnormality of movement and posture in adolescence or early adult life should be surveyed for hepatolenticular degeneration (Wilson's disease) by tests of liver function and slit-lamp examination for corneal pigmentation (Kayser-Fleischer ring); measurement of plasma ceruloplasmin (lowered) and urinary copper excretion (increased) confirm the diagnosis.

Mild or early chorea is often mistaken for simple nervousness. If one sits for a time and watches the patient, the diagnosis will often become evident. There are cases, nonetheless, in which it is impossible to distinguish simple fidgits from early Sydenham's chorea, especially in children, and there is no laboratory test upon which one can depend. The first postural manifestation of dystonia may suggest hysteria, and it is only later, when the fixity of the postural abnormality, the lack of the usual psychological picture of hysteria, and the relentlessly progressive character of the illness become evident, that accurate diagnosis is reached. Another common error is to assume that a bedfast patient who has complained of dizziness, staggering, and headaches and exhibits no other neurologic abnormality is suffering from hysteria. The flocculonodular cerebellar syndrome is demonstrable only when the patient attempts to stand and walk.

The uncertainty of balance and short-stepped gait (*marche à petit pas*) in the elderly is often incorrectly attributed to loss of confidence and fear of falling.

REFERENCES

BIRD ED: Chemical pathology of Huntington's disease. Annu Rev Pharmacol Toxicol 20:533, 1980

CARPENTER M: Anatomy of the basal ganglia and related nuclei: A review, in *Advances in Neurology,* vol 14: *Dystonia,* D Williams (ed). London, Butterworths, 1975

COOPER IS: *Involuntary Movement Disorders.* New York, Hoeber, 1969

CUMINGS JN: Biochemistry of the basal ganglia, in *Handbook of Clinical Neurology,* PJ Vinken, GW Bruyn (eds). Amsterdam, North-Holland, 1968, vol 6, p 116

DENNY-BROWN D: Clinical symptomatology of disease of the basal ganglia, in *Handbook of Clinical Neurology,* PJ Vinken, GW Bruyn (eds). Amsterdam, North-Holland, 1968, vol 6, p 133

GILMAN S et al: *Disorders of the Cerebellum.* Philadelphia, FA Davis, 1981

GROWDON J, SCHEIFE RT: Medical treatment of extrapyramidal diseases, in *Update III: Harrison's Principles of Internal Medicine,* KJ Isselbacher et al (eds). New York, McGraw-Hill, 1982, p 185.

LANCE JW: Familial paroxysmal dystonic choreoathetosis and its differentiation from related syndromes. Ann Neurol 2:285, 1977

MARSDEN CD: The neuropharmacology of abnormal involuntary movement disorders (the dyskinesias), in *Modern Trends in Neurology,* D Williams (ed). London, Butterworths, 1975

YAHR MD (ed): *The Basal Ganglia, Assoc Res Nerv Ment Dis,* vol 55. New York, Raven Press, 1976

YOUNG RR, SHAHANI BT: Pharmacology of tremor, in *Clinical Neuropharmacology,* HL Klawans (ed). New York, Raven Press, 1979, vol 4

16
DISTURBANCES OF EQUILIBRIUM AND OF GAIT

MAURICE VICTOR
RAYMOND D. ADAMS

In Chap. 13, "Dizziness and Vertigo," it was pointed out that vertigo, of whatever cause, is associated with a disturbance of equilibrium, predicated, in this instance, upon a disorientation in space. However, there are other forms of neurologic abnormality with a prominent disequilibrium of the body but no vertigo whatsoever. Since these are manifested most clearly as an impairment of upright stance and locomotion, their evaluation depends on a knowledge of the nervous mechanisms underlying these peculiarly human functions.

The maintenance of normal body posture and locomotion requires appropriate visual information, labyrinthine function, and proprioception, and it is of interest to note the effect of deficits in these senses on stance and gait. Blind persons or normal persons who are blindfolded may walk quite well. They move cautiously to avoid collision with objects, and on smooth pavement shorten their step slightly; with the shortening there is less rocking of the body, and they seem unnaturally stiff. A person deprived of labyrinthine function shows a slight unsteadiness in walking and an inability to descend stairs without holding onto a banister. Running is also difficult. Characteristically, there is great difficulty in focusing on a stationary object when the individual is moving, so that he or she has difficulty in driving a car. Proof of dependence on visual cues comes from blindfolded performance, when unsteadiness and staggering increase to a varying extent, sometimes to the point of falling. A loss of proprioception, as in a complete lesion in the posterior columns of the spinal cord in the high cervical region, abolishes for a long time the capacity for independent locomotion. After years of training, the patients will still have difficulty in starting to walk and in propelling themselves forward. As Purdon Martin has illustrated, they hold the hands in front of the body, bend the body and head forward, walk with a wide base and irregular uneven steps, but they do rock the body. If they lose their balance, they do not react appropriately to the altered posture. If they fall, they cannot arise without help, and they cannot get up from a chair. They are unable to crawl or to get into an all-fours posture. When standing, if blindfolded, they immediately fall. In these latter patients, postural reactions are demonstrably more dependent on proprioceptive than on visual or labyrinthine information.

CLINICAL APPROACH TO GAIT DISORDERS When confronted with a disorder of gait, the examiner must observe the patient's natural stance and the attitude and dominant positions of the legs, trunk, and arms. Questions about coexistent vertigo and giddiness should be asked. If present, one proceeds as outlined in Chap. 13. It is a good practice to watch patients as they walk into the examining room, because they are apt to walk more naturally then than during special tests. They should be asked to stand with the feet together, head erect, with eyes first open and then closed. Swaying due to nervousness may be overcome by diverting the patient's attention by asking him or her to touch the tip of the nose with the finger of first one hand and then the other. Next the patient should be asked to walk forward and backward, with the eyes first open and then closed. Any tendency to veer to one side, as in cerebellar disease, can be checked by having the patient walk around a chair. When the affected side is toward the chair, the patient tends to walk into it; when it is away from the chair, the patient veers outward in ever-widening circles. More delicate tests of gait are walking a straight line heel to toe or having the patient arise quickly from a chair, walk briskly, and then stop or turn suddenly. If all these tests are successfully executed, it may be assumed that any difficulty in locomotion is not due to disease of the proprioceptive mechanisms or cerebellum. Detailed neurologic examination is then necessary in order to determine the presence of other mechanisms that derange stance and gait and to determine which of the many other possible diseases is responsible for the disorder.

The following abnormal gaits are so distinctive that with a little practice they can be recognized at a glance.

Cerebellar gait The main features of this gait are *wide base* (separation of legs), *unsteadiness, irregularity,* and *lateral reeling.* Steps are uncertain, some are shorter and others longer than intended, and the patient may lurch to one side or the other. The unsteadiness is more prominent on quickly arising from a chair and walking, on stopping suddenly while walking, or on turning abruptly. If the ataxia is severe, the patient cannot stand without assistance. If it is less severe, standing with feet together and head erect, with eyes either open or closed, may be difficult. In its mildest form the ataxia is best demonstrated by having the patient walk a line heel to toe. After two or three steps there is loss of balance and the patient must place one foot to the side to avoid falling. Romberg's sign, i.e., marked swaying or falling with the eyes closed but not with the eyes open, is not a feature of cerebellar disease. Compensation may be effected by shortening the step and shuffling, i.e., keeping both feet simultaneously on the ground. The defect in cerebellar gait is not in antigravity support, steppage, or propulsion but in the coordination of proprioceptive, labyrinthine, and visual information in the reflex coordination of movements. The abnormality of gait may or may not be accompanied by other signs of cerebellar incoordination and intention tremor of the arms and legs. The presence of the latter signs depends on involvement of the cerebellar hemispheres as distinct from the superior midline structures. If the lesion is unilateral, the signs are always on the same side.

Cerebellar gait is the major symptom in some instances of multiple sclerosis, in cerebellar tumors, particularly medulloblastoma of the cerebellar vermis, and in paraneoplastic and other forms of cerebellar degeneration. In certain forms of cerebellar degeneration (e.g., the type associated with chronic alcoholism) the disease process reaches a plateau and then remains stable for many years, and the gait disorder, in these circumstances, becomes altered to some extent. The base is wide and the steps are still short, but more regular; the trunk is inclined slightly forward, the arms are held away from the sides, and the gait assumes a somewhat mechanical, rhythmic quality. In this way the patient can walk for long distances but lacks the capacity to make the necessary postural adjustments in response to sudden changes in position.

A slowness in muscle relaxation as in myxedema may give rise to a gait disorder that may simulate a cerebellar defect.

Gait of sensory ataxia This gait is due to an impairment of proprioception resulting from interruption of afferent nerve fibers in the peripheral nerves, posterior roots, posterior columns of the spinal cords, or medial lemnisci; it may also be produced occasionally by a lesion of both parietal lobes. Whatever the location of the lesion, the patient is deprived of knowledge of the position of his or her limbs. The principal features of the resulting gait disorder are *uncertainty, irregularity,* and the *stamp* of the feet. Ramsay Hunt aptly characterized this type of gait when he said that the ataxic patient is recognized by "his stamp and stick." More explicitly, there are varying degrees of difficulty in standing and walking, and in advanced cases a complete failure of locomotion, even though muscular power is retained. The legs are kept far apart to correct the instability, and the patient carefully watches the ground and the feet. As the patient steps out, the legs are flung abruptly forward and outward, often lifted higher than necessary. The steps are of variable length, and many are attended by an audible stamp as the foot is brought down forcibly on the floor. The body is held in a slightly flexed posture, and the weight may be supported on the cane that the severely ataxic patient usually carries. The incoordination is greatly exaggerated when the patient is deprived of visual cues, as in walking in the dark. Most patients, when asked to stand with feet together and eyes closed, show greatly increased swaying or actual falling (Romberg's sign). It has been said that a lame person whose shoes are not worn in any one place is probably suffering from sensory ataxia. There is invariably a loss of vibratory and position sense in the feet and legs. A disordered gait of this type is observed in tabes dorsalis, Friedreich's ataxia, subacute combined degeneration, syphilitic meningomyelitis, chronic polyneuritis, and those cases of multiple sclerosis in which posterior column disease predominates.

Hemiplegic and paraplegic (spastic) gait In walking, the hemiplegic leg is held stiffly and does not flex freely and gracefully at the knee and hip. It tends to rotate outward and describes a semicircle, first away from and then toward the trunk (circumduction). The foot scrapes along the floor, and the toe and outer side of the sole of the shoe are worn. One can diagnose the hemiplegic gait by the sound of the slow, rhythmic scuff of the foot along the floor. The other muscles of the body on the affected side are weak and stiff to a variable degree, particularly the arm, which is carried in a flexed position and does not swing naturally. This type of gait disorder is most frequently a sequela of cerebral infarction or trauma.

The spastic paraplegic gait is entirely different from the gait of sensory ataxia, though the two may be combined. Each leg is advanced slowly and stiffly with restricted motion at the knee and hip. The patient looks as though he or she is wading waist-deep in water. The legs are extended or slightly bent at the knees and may be strongly adducted at the hips, tending almost to cross ("scissors" gait). The steps are regular and short. Movements of the legs are slow, and the patient may be able to advance only with great effort. An easy way to remember the main features of the hemiplegic and paraplegic gait is by the letter S, which begins each of its descriptive adjectives—spastic, slow, scuffing. The defect is in the stepping mechanism and in propulsion, not in support or equilibrium. Cerebral spastic diplegia, multiple sclerosis, syringomyelia, spinal syphilis, combined system disease, spinal cord compression, and familial spinal spastic ataxia are the common causes of spastic paraparesis.

Festinating gait The term *festinating* comes from the Latin *festinare,* to hasten, and appropriately describes the involuntary increase or hastening of the gait that characterizes both paralysis agitans and postencephalitic Parkinson's syndrome (see Chap. 364). *Rigidity* and *shuffling,* in addition to *festination,* are the cardinal features of this gait. When they are joined to the typical tremors, rigidity, and slowness of movement, there can be little doubt as to the diagnosis.

The general attitude of the patient is one of flexion; rigidity and immobility of the body are other conspicuous features. There is a paucity of the automatic movements made in sitting, standing, and walking; the head does not turn in looking to one side, the arms are seldom folded, and the legs are rarely crossed. The arms are held stiffly as though in preparation for writing, and the facial expression is unblinking and masklike. This slight, generalized stiffness is also common in psychiatric patients treated with phenothiazine drugs.

In walking, the trunk is bent forward and the arms are carried slightly flexed and ahead of the body and do not swing. The legs are stiff and bent at the knees and hips. The steps are short, and the feet barely clear the ground as the patient shuffles along. Once forward or backward locomotion is started, the upper part of the body advances ahead of the lower part, as though the patient were chasing his or her center of gravity. Steps become more and more rapid, and the patient may fall if not assisted. This is the festination, and it may occur when the patient is walking forward or backward, taking the form of either propulsion or retropulsion. The defect is in rocking the body from side to side so that the legs clear the floor and in moving the legs quickly enough to catch the center of gravity in forward propulsion. Other unusual gaits are sometimes observed in postencephalitic patients. For example, they may be unable to take the first step forward because they cannot lift one foot, or they may be unable to step forward until they hop or take one step backward; walking may be initiated by a series of short steps that give way to a more normal gait; occasionally such a patient may run better than walk or walk backward better than forward. Choreoathetotic movements may be added to the festinating gait in the L-dopa-treated patient with Parkinson's disease.

Athetotic, dystonic, and choreic gaits Extrapyramidal motor diseases that are characterized by involuntary movements and abnormal postures seriously affect gait. In fact, a disturbance of gait may be the initial and dominant manifestation of these diseases, and the testing of gait often serves to provoke abnormalities of movement and posture that are otherwise not conspicuous. The *athetotic* patient often assumes the most grotesque postures. One arm may be held aloft and the other one behind the body with wrist and fingers alternately undergoing slow flexion, extension, and rotation. The head may be inclined first in one direction, then in another; the lips alternately retract and purse as part of a grimace; and the tongue intermittently protrudes. The legs advance slowly and awkwardly, the result of superimposed involuntary movements and postures. Sometimes the foot is plantarflexed at the ankle, and the weight is carried on the toes; or it may be dorsiflexed or inverted or flung to one side. This type of gait is typical of congenital athetosis and Huntington's chorea.

In *dystonia musculorum deformans* the first symptom may be a limp due to inversion or plantar flexion of the foot or a distortion of the pelvis. The patient stands with one leg rigidly extended or one shoulder elevated. The trunk may be in a position of exaggerated lordosis, and the hips partly flexed, with a tilting forward of the pelvis. Because of the muscle spasms that deform the body in this manner, the patient may have to walk with knees flexed. The gait may seem normal as the first steps are taken, but as the patient walks, the lumbar lordosis becomes exaggerated and one or both legs become flexed, giving rise to the "dromedary gait." In the more advanced stages walking becomes impossible, owing to torsion of the trunk or continuous flexion of the leg(s).

In *Sydenham's chorea* the gait is often bizarre (see Chap. 364). As the patient stands or walks, there is a continuous play of irregular "choreic" movements affecting the face, neck, hands, and, in the advanced stages, the large proximal joints and trunk. The positions of the trunk and upper parts of the body vary with each step. There are jerks of the head, grimacing, squirming, twisting movements of the trunk and limbs, and peculiar respiratory noises.

Steppage, or equine, gait This is caused by paralysis of the pretibial and peroneal muscles, with resultant foot drop and the need to lift the legs abnormally high in order for the feet to clear the ground. There is a slapping noise as the foot strikes the floor. The anterior and lateral borders of the sole of the shoe become worn. The steps are regular and even; otherwise, walking is not remarkable. Foot drop may be unilateral or bilateral and occurs in diseases that affect the peripheral nerves of the legs or motor neurons in the spinal cord, such as poliomyelitis, progressive spinal muscular atrophy, and Charcot-Marie-Tooth disease (peroneal muscular atrophy). It may also be observed in patients with peripheral types of muscular dystrophy. The most common cause of unilateral foot drop is compression of the anterior tibial nerve, where it crosses the head of the fibula (see Chap. 368).

Waddling gait This gait is characteristic of progressive muscular dystrophy. The attitude of the body may be straight, but more often the lumbar lordosis is accentuated. The steps are regular but a little uncertain. With each step there is an exaggerated elevation of one hip and depression of the other. Normally, as weight is placed on one leg, the corresponding hip is fixated by the gluteus medius, allowing the opposite hip to rise slightly and the trunk to tilt to the weight-bearing side. With weakness of these muscles, there is a failure to stabilize the weight-bearing hip, causing the opposite side of the pelvis to drop and the trunk to incline to that side. With the next step there is an overinclination of the trunk to the opposite side. This alternation of lateral trunk movements results in the rolling gait, or *waddle,* a term suggested by Oppenheim. The gluteal musculature is weak and inefficient, although leg muscles may appear well developed. Muscular contractures leading to a position of the foot as in equinovarus may complicate childhood cases, so that the waddle is combined with circumduction of the legs and "walking on the toes."

Staggering or drunken gait This is characteristic of alcoholic and barbiturate intoxication. The drunken patient totters, reels, tips forward and then backward, threatening each moment to lose balance and fall. Control over trunk and legs is greatly impaired. The steps are irregular and uncertain. The patient appears stupefied and indifferent to the quality of performance, but under certain circumstances can momentarily correct the defect.

The frequently used adjectives *drunken* and *reeling* do not describe aptly the gait of cerebellar disease, except, perhaps, the most acute and severe cases. The intoxicated patient reels in many different directions, unlike the patient with cerebellar disease, and no effort is made to correct the staggering by watching the legs or the ground, as in cerebellar or sensory ataxia. In the drunken patient, despite a wide diversity of excursions of all parts of the body, the base may be narrow and balance may be exquisitely maintained. In contrast, patients with cerebellar disease have great difficulty in maintaining balance if they sway or lurch too far to one side.

Toppling gait Toppling, meaning abrupt tottering and falling, may occur with brainstem lesions, especially in older persons and in those with lateral medullary infarction. Also, this type of gait disorder is an early and prominent feature of progressive supranuclear palsy, in which case it is combined with paralysis of vertical gaze and dystonia of the neck (see Chap. 364). In addition to sudden lurches and frequent falls, the gait is hesitant and uncertain, features that are enhanced by the hazard of falling unpredictably. The exact cause of toppling is not known; it cannot be attributed to weakness, ataxia, or deep sensory loss.

Hysterical gait This may take one of several forms—monoplegic, paraplegic, or hemiplegic. The monoplegic or hemiplegic patient does not lift the foot from the floor while walking; instead, it is dragged as a useless member or pushed ahead as though it were a skate. The characteristic circumduction is absent in hysterical hemiplegia, and the typical hemiplegic posture, hyperactive tendon reflexes, and Babinski sign are missing. The hysterical paraplegic cannot very well drag both legs, and usually depends on a crutch or remains helpless in bed; the muscles may be rigid with pseudocontractures or flaccid. The gait may be quite dramatic. Some patients look as though they were walking on stilts, and others lurch wildly in all directions, actually demonstrating by their gyrations a remarkable ability to make rapid postural adjustments.

Astasia-abasia, in which the patient, though unable to either stand or walk, retains normal use of the legs while in bed, is nearly always hysterical. When such patients are placed on their feet, they take a few normal steps and then become unable to advance the feet; they lurch wildly and crumple to the floor if not assisted.

Frontal lobe disorder of gait Equilibrium and the capacity to stand and walk may be severely disturbed by diseases that affect the frontal lobes, particularly their medial parts. Although this disorder of gait is sometimes spoken of as an *ataxia* or as an *apraxia,* since the difficulty in walking cannot be accounted for by weakness or loss of sensation, it is probably neither. It most likely represents a loss of integration at the cortical and basal ganglionic level of the essential elements of stance and locomotion which were acquired in infancy and are often lost in senility.

These patients assume a posture of slight flexion, with the feet placed farther apart than normal. They advance slowly, with small, shuffling, hesitant steps. At times they halt, unable to advance without great effort, although they do much better with a little assistance. Turning is accomplished by a series of tiny, uncertain steps which are made with one foot, the other being planted on the floor as a pivot. The initiation of walking becomes progressively more difficult, and in advanced cases patients may be unable to take a step, as though the feet were glued to the floor. Finally they become unable to stand or even to sit, and without support fall backward or to one side.

Some patients are able to make complex movements with their legs, such as drawing imaginary figures, at a time when their gait is seriously impaired. Eventually, however, all movements of the legs become slow and awkward, and the limbs, when passively moved, offer variable resistance (gegenhalten). An inability to turn and sit in a chair or to lie down or turn over in bed is highly characteristic, and may eventually become complete. These motor disabilities are usually associated with dementia, but there need be no parallelism in their evolution. Grasping, groping, hyperactive tendon reflexes, and Babinski signs may or may not be present. The end result in some cases is a "cerebral paraplegia in flexion" (Yakovlev), in which the patient lies curled up in bed, immobile and mute, the limbs fixed by contractures in an attitude of flexion.

Senile gait Elderly persons often complain of difficulty in walking, and examination may disclose no abnormality other than the slightly flexed posture of the senile and short uncertain steps, *marche à petit pas.* Speed, balance, and all the graceful, adaptive movements are lost. The exact nature of this gait disorder is not understood. Probably it is a combination frontal lobe and basal ganglionic defect and represents a mild degree of the frontal lobe disorder described above. It should be noted, however, that a short-stepped, cautious gait lacks specificity, being a general defensive reaction to all forms of defective locomotion.

Disorders of gait due to blindness and loss of labyrinthine function These have been described in the introduction to this chapter. Loss of labyrinthine function is attributable most often to the prolonged administration of streptomycin, kanamycin, or neomycin, which destroy the hair cells of the specialized sensory epithelium of the semicircular canals, saccule, and utricle.

REFERENCES

ADAMS RD, VICTOR M: *Principles of Neurology,* 2d ed. New York, McGraw-Hill, 1981

MARTIN JP: The basal ganglia and locomotion. Ann R Coll Surg Engl 32:219, 1963

YAKOVLEV PI: Paraplegia in flexion of cerebral origin. J Neuropathol Exp Neurol 13:267, 1954

17
COMMON DISTURBANCES OF VISION, OCULAR MOVEMENT, AND HEARING

MAURICE VICTOR
RAYMOND D. ADAMS

Diseases of the eyes and ears, by virtue of their frequency, unusual nature, and serious consequences, make up separate medical specialties and, therefore, fall outside the field of internal medicine. Yet disturbances of visual and auditory function may be the initial or leading manifestations of many systemic diseases. Of more general interest is the fact that these two special senses represent the most finely developed parts of the entire sensory nervous system; hence the study of their disorders may yield important information about neurologic diseases.

THE EYE AND DISORDERS OF VISION

The eye, with its diverse epithelial, vascular, collagenous, neural, and pigmentary components, is a medical microcosm, susceptible to manifold diseases. Moreover, its transparency makes it accessible to direct inspection by the ophthalmoscope, and affords an opportunity to observe many of the specific lesions of medical diseases.

Since the eye is the organ of vision, it is obvious that impairment of visual acuity of varying degree should stand as the most frequent symptom of eye disease. Strabismus and diplopia, ocular pain, irritation, redness and photophobia, inability to read or recognize objects and people, and drooping or closure of the eyelids are also important. The impairment of eyesight may be unilateral or bilateral, sudden or gradual, episodic or enduring. The common causes vary with age. In late childhood and adolescence, nearsightedness, or myopia, is the usual cause, though an optic nerve tumor or suprasellar tumor must be excluded. In middle age, farsightedness, or presbyopia, is almost invariable and requires refraction and eyeglasses. Still later in life, cataracts, glaucoma, and retinal hemorrhages and detachments are the most frequent causes of visual disturbance. Episodic blindness (amaurosis fugax) in early life is usually due to migraine; later, stenosis of the carotid artery or embolism of the retinal arterioles are the common causes. Cerebrovascular disease deranges vision with increasing frequency in late life.

Some of the terms used to describe a loss of vision are *amaurosis,* which refers to blindness from any cause, *amblyopia,* which refers to visual loss which is not due to an error of refraction or to other disease of the eye, and *nyctalopia,* which means poor twilight or night vision. The latter is associated with either vitamin A deficiency or pigmentary degenerations of the retina.

Thus failing eyesight may be due to an abnormality of the refractive media of the eye or to a lesion of the retina or optic nerve or the parts of the brain with which they are connected. In approaching this problem one begins always by inquiring as to precisely what patients mean when they say they cannot see properly, for they may be referring to symptoms as varied as excessive tearing, diplopia, partial syncope, or even giddiness or dizziness. Fortunately these statements can be checked by the measurement of visual acuity, a technique which is the single most important part of the ocular examination. If visual acuity is less than 20/20 and cannot be improved by refraction and if the media of the eye are transparent, there is some sensory defect, the nature of which must be ascertained.

In the measurement of visual acuity the *Snellen chart,* which contains rows of letters of diminishing size (those of each row subtending 5 min of an arc when held at various distances from the eye), is utilized. The letters at the top of the chart subtend 5 min of an arc at a distance of 200 ft; those at the bottom subtend an arc of 5 min at 20 ft. Thus if the patient can see only the top letters at 20 ft, rather than 200 ft, vision is 20/200; if those letters at the bottom are seen at this distance, the acuity is 20/20. The patient with a corrected refractive error should wear eyeglasses for the test; if the visual acuity is then less than 20/20, either the refractive error has not been properly corrected or there is some other reason for it. The former possibility can be ruled out if the patient sees clearly while looking through a pinhole in a cardboard with the glasses still on. The pinhole permits a narrow shaft of light to fall on the fovea without being refracted.

Light entering the eye is focused on the outer layer of the retina (the rods and cones). Consequently the media (tissues and fluids) through which the light passes must be transparent. These media are the cornea, the aqueous humor of the anterior chamber, the lens, the vitreous humor of the vitreous cavity, and the retina itself. The clarity of these media can be determined ophthalmoscopically, but this examination requires that the pupil be dilated to at least 6 mm in diameter. This is best accomplished by instilling a few drops of 10% phenylephrine (Neo-Synephrine) in each eye after the visual acuity is measured, the pupillary response recorded, and the intraocular pressure estimated. *Rarely an attack of angle-closure glaucoma may be precipitated by pupillary dilatation;* this should be treated by the intravenous administration of mannitol (50 g of a 20% solution) and oral administration of the carbonic anhydrase inhibitor, acetazolamide (Diamox, 250 mg qid), followed by the topical instillation of 4% pilocarpine. The cycloplegic action of phenylephrine lasts only an hour or two. Looking through a +6 ophthalmoscopic lens from a distance of 15 to 20 cm permits the visualization of any opacity in refractive media against the diffuse bright red of reflected light from the retina. By adjusting the lens of the ophthalmoscope from a high plus to zero or a minus setting, one can "depth-focus" from the cornea to the retina. Clarity of all media means that reduced vision uncorrected by glasses must be due to a lesion in the macula, optic nerve, or structures further back in the visual system.

More specifically, alterations in the refractile media that affect vision have certain medical implications, as follows.

CORNEAS In hypercalcemia secondary to sarcoid (Chap. 235), hyperparathyroidism (Chap. 339), and vitamin D intoxication (Chap. 340), calcium phosphates and carbonates precipitate, primarily beneath the corneal epithelium in a plane corresponding to the interpalpebral tissue—so-called *band keratopathy* (see Plate 7-8); cystine crystals are deposited in cystinosis (Chap. 93), cholesterol esters in hypercholesterolemia (*arcus senilis*) (Chap. 103), chloroquine crystals in treatment of discoid lupus by this drug, polysaccharides in Hurler's disease (Chap. 104), and copper in hepatolenticular degeneration [Kayser-Fleischer ring (Plate 8-8 and Chap. 98)]. Opacification of the cornea (keratitis) may also occur after herpes simplex and herpes zoster infections (Chaps. 210 and 204), or it may be combined with uveitis and iritis in Behçet's disease, Reiter's disease (Chap. 348), Stevens-Johnson disease (Chap. 69), and idiopathic infections. Keratitis may be a manifestation also of congenital syphilis (Chap. 177), and of more innocent states such as drying and injury during coma.

AQUEOUS HUMOR The common problem is one of high pressure due to an impediment to the outflow of the aqueous fluid. This is termed *glaucoma.* In 90 percent of cases (of the wide-angle type) the cause is unknown; in 5 percent the angle between pupil and lateral cornea is narrow and blocked when the pupil is dilated; and in the remaining 5 percent the condition is secondary to some disease process that blocks the outflow channels (inflammatory debris of uveitis, or red blood cells from hemorrhage in the anterior chamber, i.e., hyphema). Glaucoma occurs in about 2 percent of all patients over the age of 40; it may be asymptomatic and go unrecognized for years before it progresses to rapid loss of vision. Therefore, the intraocular pressure should be measured routinely, using a Schiotz tonometer. This is a simple procedure which should be practiced by every physician. With the patient supine, a drop of local anesthetic is put into each eye and the tonometer is then placed on the cornea so that the instrument is perfectly vertical. When the tonometer is pressed against the eye, the scale is read and the units are converted into millimeters of mercury from the chart in the tonometer case. The normal pressure is about 15 mmHg. Pressures of 20 to 30 mmHg may damage the optic nerve, leading first to a nasal quadrant defect and finally to blindness. With the ophthalmoscope one can see also that the optic disc is excavated and, in some instances, atrophic (Plate 7-2).

THE LENS Here the common abnormality is one of cataract formation. Opacities form in diabetes mellitus (Chap. 114) ("sugar cataracts") from sustained high levels of blood glucose, which is changed to sorbitol (the accumulation of which leads to a high osmotic gradient within the lens fibers, see Chap. 339); in galactosemia, a much rarer disease, a similar mechanism is operative, namely, disruption of lens fibers due to the accumulation of dulcitol (Chap. 101); in hypoparathyroidism the lowering of the concentration of calcium in the aqueous humor opacifies newly formed lens fibers; prolonged high doses of chlorpromazine and corticosteroids in some cases result in lenticular opacities and in myotonic dystrophy (Chap. 371); and Wilson's disease is also associated with a special type (Chap. 98) of cataract. Weakening of the zonular ligaments of the lens allows a dislocation (iridodonesis) in Marfan's syndrome and homocystinuria (Plate 8-7 and Chap. 58).

VITREOUS HUMOR Hemorrhage may occur from rupture of a ciliary or retinal vessel. The common causes are trauma; diabetes mellitus, in which the bleeding occurs from newly formed retinal vessels, i.e., retinitis proliferans; or after a retinal tear which may progress to retinal detachment. The vitreous humor may also be affected by deposition of calcium soaps (seen as small white opacities with the ophthalmoscope)—so-called asteroid hyalosis of diabetes mellitus. The commonest vitreous opacities are benign "floaters," which appear to patients as gray or black spots when they move their eyes.

RETINA The search for neurologic explanations of reduced vision begins with an ophthalmoscopic examination of the retina. This thin (350 μm) sheet of transparent tissue and the optic nerve head (optic disc) into which the visual information is channeled are the only parts of the central nervous system that can be inspected during life.

Light entering the eye passes through the full thickness of the retina to reach the receptor layer of rods and cones. Impulses arising in these photoreceptors are transmitted via secondary neurons, the bipolar cells, to the innermost ganglion cell layer, the axons of which in turn travel through the optic nerve head, optic nerve, chiasm, and optic tracts to the lateral geniculate bodies. These retinal neurons normally acquire a myelin sheath only after piercing the lamina cribrosa. The macular region, which lies two disc diameters or 3 mm lateral to the optic disc, is the most sensitive part of the retina. The vascular supply (of the retina) comes from the ophthalmic branch of the internal carotid artery, which in turn gives origin to the central retinal artery. The latter, upon issuing from the optic disc, divides into four arterioles, which supply the four quadrants of the retina (Plate 7-1). The ganglion cells and bipolar cells receive their blood supply from these arterioles and their capillaries, whereas photoreceptor elements receive nourishment from the underlying choroidal vascular bed. The posterior ciliary arteries, which also arise from the ophthalmic artery, supply the optic nerve head.

In disease states the retinal vessels react like vessels of corresponding size in the brain. Since the walls of the retinal arterioles are transparent to the ophthalmoscope, what is seen is a column of blood. In arteriosclerosis (usually coexistent with hypertension), the lumina of the vessels are narrowed because of fibrous tissue replacement of the media and thickening of the basement membrane. The light reflection from the vessel then has a different refractive index than the adjacent retinal tissue. Tortuosity of vessels, arteriolar-venular compressions, and narrowed segments are other signs of hypertension and arteriolosclerosis. In malignant hypertension there are also so-called soft exudates or cotton-wool patches (actually infarcts of the nerve fiber layer), splinter hemorrhages and papilledema, changes that may be present in and around the intracerebral arterioles. Atheromatous deposits, which form in larger arteries, are observed in the retina only with extreme degrees of hyperlipemia because of the small size of the vessels. Occasionally atheromatous and other emboli from the carotid artery and aorta may lodge in them. Capillary-venular aneurysms may develop, most often in diabetes mellitus (Plate 8-3). Since the central retinal vein and artery share a common adventitial sheath, atheromatous plaques in the artery may result in thrombosis of the vein. Round or oval hemorrhages always lie in the outer plexiform layer and linear or flame-shaped ones in the superficial layer of the retina, their shape being determined by the arrangement of the nerve fibers in these particular zones. Rupture of arterioles on the inner surface of the retina, as occurs with ruptured aneurysms and other conditions causing extremely high intracranial pressure, permits the accumulation of a lake of blood between the retina and vitreous body (subhyaloid or preretinal hemorrhage).

The systemic coagulopathies (thrombotic thrombocytopenia and disseminated intravascular coagulopathy) may cause clotting, preferentially in the submacular choriocapillaries. Sometimes this is associated with choroidal hemorrhage and detachment of the retina. The patient will complain of blurred vision because of a scotoma.

Aside from visible vascular lesions, other more specific alterations of the retina may impair vision. The most important of these are tears and detachments. Important also are several types of retinal degeneration:

1 *Degeneration of the outer receptor layer and subjacent pigment epithelium* occurs as a hereditary trait in *retinitis pigmentosa* (Plate 7-7), and also in Laurence-Moon-Biedl syndrome, progressive ophthalmoplegia, Bassen-Kornzweig disease (Chap. 103), Refsum's disease (Chap. 368), Kearns-Sayre syndrome (Chap. 371), Batten-Mayou juvenile lipid storage disease, and idiopathic senile macular degeneration (Chaps. 103 and 364).
2 *Degeneration of Bruch's membrane* (which supports the layer of pigment epithelium next to the rods and cones) and its repair by fibrosis give rise to angioid streaks (Plate 7-4) typical of pseudoxanthoma elasticum (Chap. 353), Paget's disease (Chap. 342), hyperphosphatemia, and acromegaly.
3 *Phenothiazine derivatives may conjugate with the melanin* of the pigment layer and result in degeneration of the outer retinal layers. When these drugs are used, the doses should be kept low and the central visual fields tested with small colored test objects.

Sarcoidosis, toxoplasmosis, and *histoplasmosis* involve both the retina and the choroid. The latter is the site of noninfective inflammatory reactions, often in association with iridocyclitis.

THE OPTIC DISC The optic nerves, chiasm, and tracts which constitute the third visual neuron can be inspected only in part, from the foveal or macular region to the optic disc. The latter reflects raised intracranial pressure (papilledema or choked disc), papillitis (disease of the optic nerve close to the disc), optic nerve atrophy, and glaucoma (Plates 7-2, 7-5, and 7-6).

Papilledema (choked disc) refers to venous congestion and edema and elevation of disc margins. The depression of the optic disc is obliterated. The elevation ranges from 1 to 4 mm and when extreme may be surrounded by hemorrhages. Visual acuity is little affected until late, except for constriction of visual fields and enlargement of blind spots, which is in contrast to papillitis where visual loss occurs early. The cause is raised intracranial pressure (tumors, abscesses, hemorrhages) which is transmitted to the subarachnoid space around optic nerves. This leads, after some days, to obstruction of venous outflow from the retinas, usually more so on the side of the lesion (see Plates 7-3 and 8-6).

Minor degrees of disc swelling are difficult to distinguish from the disc of the normal hyperopic eye. Lack of vein pulsation suggests increased pressure. Fluorescein retinography reveals early papilledema by the leakage of the dye into the disc and surrounding retina. Myelination of optic nerve fibers and drusen must not be confused with papilledema.

With most diseases of the optic nerve, the nerve head will eventually become pale (optic atrophy). This may require several weeks or months, as illustrated by the delay between the sudden blindness of a traumatic severance of one optic nerve and the pallor. If the optic nerve degenerates [e.g., in multiple sclerosis, Leber's hereditary optic atrophy (Chap. 364), or syphilitic optic atrophy], the disc becomes chalk-white, with sharp, clean margins. If the atrophy is secondary to papillitis or papilledema, the margins are obscure and irregular, with pigment deposits in the adjacent retina. Since the optic nerve also contains the afferent fibers for the pupillary light reflex, lesions of the nerve will cause pupillary disturbances (see further on).

THE CENTRAL VISUAL PATHWAY *Central visual disturbances* (caused by defects in the retina, optic nerves and tracts, lateral geniculate bodies, geniculocalcarine path, and striate cortex of occipital lobes) are evidenced by changes in the visual fields. In good light, if one of the patient's eyes is covered and the other aligned with the corresponding eye of the examiner and a cotton pledget or white object on a stick is brought from the outside toward the center, the periphery of the patient's visual field can be compared with that of the examiner. The types of visual field defect resulting from lesions in different parts of the visual pathways are shown in Fig. 17-1. A prechiasmal lesion causes either a scotoma (an island of impaired vision within the visual field) or a cut in the peripheral part of the visual field. A small scotoma in the macular part of the visual field may seriously impair visual acuity, giving rise to a central scotoma; patients may complain of distortion of vision, particularly for straight lines (metamorphopsia). One may test for this at the bedside by asking the patient to look at the center of a checkerboard or a jigsaw puzzle. The straight lines in the center appear curved or kinked. Metamorphopsia is diagnostic of retinal disease and aids in the distinction between a macular lesion and one in the optic nerve or occipital lobe. Demyelinative, toxic (methyl alcohol, quinine, and certain of the phenothiazine tranquilizing drugs), nutritional (so-called tobacco-alcohol amblyopia), and vascular diseases are the usual causes of scotomas. The toxic states are characterized by symmetric bilateral scotomas, and the nutritional disorders by more or less symmetric central scotomas (involving the fixation point) or centrocecal scotomas (involving both the fixation point and the blind spot). These latter scotomas are predominantly in the distribution of the papillomacular bundle, but their presence does not establish whether the primary effect is in the nerve fibers or the ganglion cells. Demyelinative diseases are characterized by unilateral or asymmetric bilateral scotomas. As indicated above, if the lesion is near the optic disc, there may be swelling of the optic nerve head, i.e., *papillitis,* which can usually be distinguished from papilledema by the marked impairment of vision it produces. Vascular lesions as a rule give rise to unilateral scotomas. The lesions take the form of retinal hemorrhages, hard exudates, or cotton-wool patches (occluded

vessels which cause infarction of the retina). Large zones of retinal infarction may follow occlusion of a branch of the central retinal artery (Plates 8-1 through 8-5).

Ischemic optic neuropathy is another well-recognized entity. The onset is abrupt, usually in an elderly person. It may be painful. Vision may be abolished completely, or there may be an altitudinal or segmental defect in one eye. Examination of the fundus may show no abnormality, but later the optic disc may become pale; rarely there is congestion, hemorrhage, and swelling of the disc. The pathologic basis of this disturbance is thrombosis or embolism of the posterior ciliary artery. If preceded by headache, pain on chewing, and arthralgia, the diagnosis is usually temporal arteritis. Both eyes may be affected simultaneously or in succession. Prognosis for recovery of vision is poor. Fluorescein retinography (see below) is a valuable method for revealing retinal vascular abnormalities.

Another common defect encountered on visual field examination is concentric constriction. This may be due to papilledema, in which case it is usually accompanied by an enlargement of the blind spot. A concentric constriction of the visual field, at first unilateral and later bilateral, and pallor of the optic disc (optic atrophy) should suggest chronic syphilitic meningooptic neuritis. Glaucoma is another cause of this type of field defect. Tubular vision, i.e., constriction of the visual field

FIGURE 17-1

Diagram showing the effects on the fields of vision produced by lesions at various points along the optic pathway. A. Complete blindness in left eye. B. Bitemporal hemianopia. C. Nasal hemianopia of left eye. D. Right homonymous hemianopia. E and F. Right upper and lower quadrant hemianopia. G. Right homonymous hemianopia with preservation of central vision. (From Homans, A Textbook of Surgery, Springfield, Ill., Charles C Thomas, 1945.)

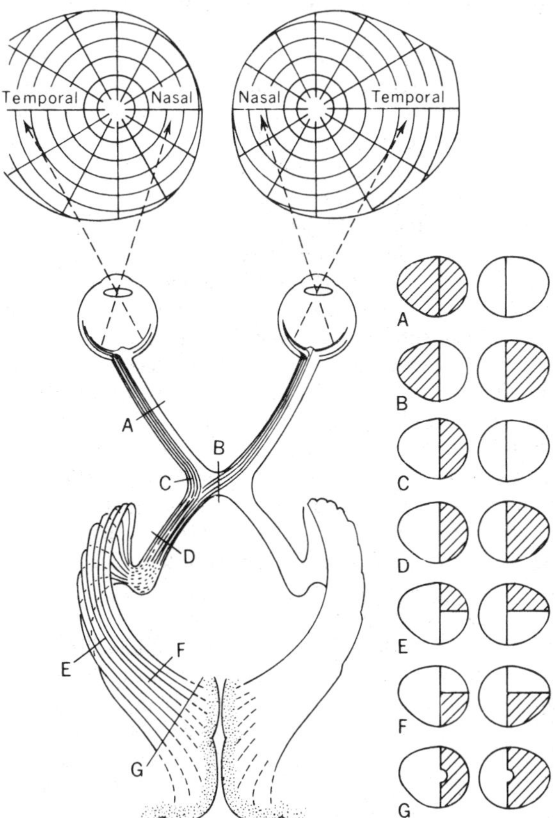

to the same degree regardless of the distance of the visual test stimulus from the eye, is a sign of hysteria. In organic disease, for example, chorioretinitis, the area of the constricted visual field naturally enlarges as the distance between the patient and the stimulus increases.

Hemianopia means blindness in one-half of the visual field. *Bitemporal hemianopia* indicates a lesion of the decussating nasal retinal fibers of the optic chiasm and is due usually to a tumor of the pituitary gland, infundibulum, or third ventricle, to meningioma of the diaphragm of the sella, or occasionally to a large suprasellar aneurysm of the circle of Willis. *Homonymous hemianopia* (a loss of vision in corresponding halves of the visual fields) signifies a lesion of the visual pathway behind the chiasm and, if *complete*, gives no more information than that. *Incomplete homonymous hemianopia* has more localizing value: if the field defects in the two eyes are identical (*congruous*), the lesion is likely to be in the calcarine cortex; if *incongruous*, the visual fibers in the parietal or temporal lobe are more likely to be implicated. Since the fibers from the peripheral lower quadrants of the retina extend for a variable distance into the temporal lobe, lesions of this lobe may be accompanied by a homonymous upper quadrantic field defect. Parietal lobe lesions may affect the lower quadrants more than the upper.

If the entire optic tract or calcarine cortex on one side is destroyed, there is a complete homonymous hemianopia, including that part of the field supplied by the macula. Incomplete lesions of the optic tract and radiation usually spare central (macular) vision. Apparent macular sparing is frequently due to imperfect fixation of gaze. A lesion of the tip of one occipital lobe produces central homonymous hemianopia because half the macular fibers of both eyes terminate there. Lesions of both occipital poles (as in embolization of the posterior cerebral arteries) result in bilateral central scotomas; if all the calcarine cortex on both sides is completely destroyed, there is "cortical" blindness. Altitudinal or horizontal hemianopias are more often due to lesions of the occipital lobes below or above the calcarine sulcus than to lesions of the optic chiasm.

In addition to blindness, i.e., "visual anesthesia," there is another category of visual impairment, which consists of a defect of visual perception, i.e., *visual agnosia*. With this disorder patients can see but cannot recognize objects unless they hear, smell, taste, or palpate them. The failure of visual recognition of words alone is called *alexia*. The ability to recognize visually presented objects and words depends upon the integrity not only of the visual pathways and primary areas of the cerebral cortex but also of those secondary and tertiary visual cortical areas which lie just anterior to them and the angular gyrus of the dominant hemisphere. Visual-object agnosia and alexia result from lesions of these latter areas or from a lesion of the left calcarine cortex combined with one which interrupts the fibers crossing from the right occipital lobe. These subjects are discussed further in Chaps. 18 and 24.

Other disturbances of vision include various types of distortion in which the perceived objects appear too small (micropsia), too large (macropsia), or askew. If this disturbance is in only one eye, a local retinal lesion should be suspected. When bilateral, such phenomena suggest disease of the temporal lobes, in which case the visual disturbances tend to occur in attacks and are accompanied by complex visual hallucinations and other manifestations of temporal lobe seizures (Chap. 12).

In the analysis of retinal, optic nerve and tract, and geniculocalcarine lesions, two other techniques are especially valuable—the electroretinogram (ERG) and the patterned stimulus visual-evoked responses (VER). The human ERG is a mass response that is reduced only in diseases of the retina. The VER provides evidence of the speed of visual impulse conduction between the retina and occipital lobe. With diseases of the optic nerve, even with normal visual acuity and a normal appearance of the retina, it may be abnormal.

DIPLOPIA, STRABISMUS, AND DISORDERS OF THE THIRD, FOURTH, AND SIXTH NERVES *Strabismus* (squint) refers to a muscle imbalance that results in improper alignment of the two eyes. It may be due to paralysis of an eye muscle or to inequality of tone in the muscles that yoke the two eyes together in a central position. The former is called *paralytic strabismus* and is primarily a neurologic problem; the latter is *nonparalytic strabismus* (referred to as comitant strabismus if the angle between the visual axes is the same in all fields of gaze) and is an ophthalmologic problem. Once binocular fusion is established, any type of ocular muscle imbalance causes diplopia, for the reason that images then fall on disparate or noncorresponding parts of the two retinas. After a time, however, the patient learns to suppress the image of one eye. This almost invariably happens early in comitant strabismus of congenital nature, and the person may then have a diminished visual acuity in that eye (*amblyopia ex anopsia*). The vision may remain normal in both eyes when each eye is used alternately for fixation; this is *alternating strabismus*.

The oculomotor, trochlear, and abducens nerves innervate the extrinsic musculature of the eye. A knowledge of their origin and anatomic relationships is essential to an understanding of the various paralytic ocular syndromes. The oculomotor nucleus consists of several groups of nerve cells ventral to the aqueduct of Sylvius, at the level of the superior colliculi. All nuclear neurons send fibers to the ipsilateral eye except those innervating the superior rectus muscle, which are contralateral like those of the trochlear nucleus. The nerve cells that innervate the iris and ciliary body are situated dorsally in the so-called Edinger-Westphal nucleus. Ventral to this nucleus are the cells for the levator of the lid, superior and inferior recti, inferior oblique, and medial rectus muscles, in this dorsoventral order. Convergence is under the control of an unpaired medial group of cells. The cells of origin of the trochlear nerves are just inferior to those of the oculomotor nerves. The sixth nerve arises at a considerably lower level, from a paired group of cells in the floor of the fourth ventricle at the level of the lower pons. The intrapontine portion of the facial nerve loops around the sixth nerve nucleus before it turns anterolaterally to make its exit; a lesion in this locality usually causes a homolateral paralysis of both the lateral rectus and facial muscles.

All three nerves, after leaving the brainstem, course anteriorly and pass through the cavernous sinus, where they come into close proximity with the ophthalmic division of the fifth nerve, and together they enter the orbit through the superior orbital fissure. The oculomotor nerve supplies all the extrinsic ocular muscles except two—the superior oblique and the external rectus—which are innervated by the trochlear and the abducens nerves, respectively. The levator palpebrae muscle is also supplied by the oculomotor nerve, the involuntary part being under the control of autonomic fibers. Parasympathetic fibers of the oculomotor nerve supply the sphincter pupillae and the ciliary muscles (muscles of accommodation).

Although all the extraocular muscles probably participate in every movement of the eyes, particular muscles move the eyes in certain fields. The lateral rectus deviates the eye outward; the medial rectus, inward. The function of the vertical recti and the oblique muscles varies according to the position of the eye. When the eye is turned outward, the elevators and depressors of the eye are the superior and inferior recti; when the eye is turned inward, they are the inferior and superior oblique muscles, respectively. In contrast, torsion of the eyeball is effected by the oblique muscles when the eye is turned outward.

Accurate binocular vision is achieved by the associated action of the ocular muscles, which allows a visual stimulus to fall on exactly corresponding parts of the two retinas. Conjugate movement of the eyes is controlled by centers in the cerebral cortex and brainstem. Area 8 in the frontal lobe is the center for voluntary conjugate movements of the eyes to the opposite side. In addition, there is a center in the occipital lobe concerned with contralateral following movements. Fibers from these centers pass to the opposite sides of the brainstem, where they connect with lower centers for conjugate movements: those for right lateral gaze are thought to be in the proximity of the right abducens nucleus; those for left lateral gaze are near the left abducens. Simultaneous innervation of one internal rectus and the other external rectus during lateral gaze is mediated through the medial longitudinal fasciculus which connects one abducens nucleus with the opposite oculomotor nucleus. The arrangements of nerve cells and fibers for vertical gaze and convergence are situated in the pretectal areas and paramedian zones of the midbrain tegmentum.

The coordination of eye movement by these cerebral and brainstem structures involves the interaction of several physiologic systems: (1) voluntary conjugate movements, which are characteristically rapid and jerky (saccadic) and whose purpose is to quickly change ocular fixation (saccadic movements can also be elicited reflexly); (2) largely involuntary pursuit or following movements, the function of which is to stabilize the image of a moving object on the fovea or to track a fixated object ("smooth tracking"); (3) vergence movements; and (4) vestibuloocular reflex movements, by means of which the vestibular system stabilizes ocular fixation during body movement (the clinical importance of this subdivision relates to the fact that each system may be affected independently by disease).

OCULAR MUSCLE AND GAZE PALSIES There are three types of paralysis of extraocular muscles: (1) paralysis of isolated ocular muscles, (2) paralysis of conjugate movements (gaze), and (3) mixed gaze and ocular muscle paralysis.

Characteristic clinical disturbances result from single lesions of the third, fourth, or sixth cranial nerves. A complete *third nerve lesion* causes ptosis (since the levator palpebrae is supplied mainly by the third nerve), an inability to turn the eye upward, downward, or inward; a divergent strabismus due to unopposed action of the lateral rectus muscle; a dilated nonreactive pupil (iridoplegia); and paralysis of accommodation (cycloplegia). When only the muscles of the iris and ciliary body are paralyzed, the condition is termed *internal ophthalmoplegia. Fourth nerve lesions* result in extorsion of the eye and a weakness of downward gaze most marked when the eye is turned inward, so that patients commonly complain of special difficulty in going downstairs. Head tilting, to the opposite shoulder, is especially characteristic of a fourth nerve lesion; this causes a compensatory intorsion of the unaffected eye and ablates the diplopia. Such patients may also have difficulty in reading with their bifocal glasses. Lesions of the *sixth nerve* result in paralysis of abduction and a convergent strabismus, owing to the unopposed action of the internal rectus muscles. With incomplete sixth nerve palsies, turning the head toward the side of the paretic muscle may overcome diplopia by relaxing the affected lateral rectus muscle. (The foregoing signs may occur with various degrees of completeness, depending on the severity and site of the lesion or lesions.)

Ocular palsies may be central, i.e., due to a lesion of the nucleus or the intramedullary portion of the cranial nerve, or peripheral. Ophthalmoplegia due to a lesion in the brainstem is usually accompanied by involvement of other cranial nerves or long tracts. Peripheral lesions, which may or may not be solitary, have a great variety of causes; the most common are aneurysm of the circle of Willis, tumors of the base of the brain, carcinomatosis of the meninges, herpes zoster, syphilitic and other chronic forms of meningitis. A practical rule is that any nontraumatic oculomotor palsy with a dilated, unreactive pupil will usually be traced to a tumor or aneurysm. The third nerve palsy that occurs with diabetes is most often due to infarction of the third nerve, and the prognosis for recovery in such cases, as with other nonprogressive diseases of the peripheral nerve, is usually excellent. The points of difference between lesions within and outside the brainstem are tabulated in Table 17-1, and the various intramedullary and extramedullary cranial nerve syndromes are described in Tables 367-1 and 367-2. See also the diagrams in Chap. 367.

Paralysis of conjugate movement (gaze) The term *conjugate gaze,* or *conjugate movement,* refers to the simultaneous movement of the two eyes in the same direction. An acute lesion, such as an infarct, in one frontal lobe may cause paralysis of contralateral gaze, and the eyes will turn toward the side of the lesion. The ocular disorder in this circumstance is temporary (several days' duration). In bilateral frontal lesions the patient may be unable to turn the eyes voluntarily in any direction—up, down, or to the side—but retains fixation and following movements, which are believed to be occipital lobe functions. Gaze paralysis of cerebral origin is not attended by strabismus or diplopia. The usual causes are vascular occlusion with infarction, hemorrhage, and abscess or tumor of the frontal lobe. With certain extrapyramidal disorders, e.g., postencephalitic parkinsonism, Huntington's chorea, and progressive supranuclear palsy, ocular movements may be limited in all directions, especially upward. Lesions of the high midbrain tegmentum, ventral to the superior colliculi and near the posterior commissure, interfere with voluntary upward gaze, and often movements of convergence as well as the pupillary light reflex are abolished (Parinaud's syndrome). There also exists a pontine center for conjugate lateral gaze, probably in the vicinity of the abducens nucleus. A lesion here causes ipsilateral gaze palsy, with the eyes turning to the opposite side. Vertical and lateral gaze palsies are combined in progressive supranuclear palsy. The palsy is persistent, unlike that of cerebral lesions, and is frequently accompanied by other signs of midbrain disease. Fully developed forms of gaze paralysis are readily discerned, but lesser degrees may be overlooked unless one pays special attention to the predominant position of the eyes at rest and the ability to sustain conjugate movement.

TABLE 17-1
Comparison of lesions within and outside the brainstem

Effect	*Lesions within the brainstem*	*Lesions external to the brainstem*
Involvement of multiple contiguous nerves	±	+
Involvement of sensorimotor tracts	+, often "alternating" or crossed sensory motor palsies	±
Disturbance of consciousness	+	0 (+ late)
Evidence of other segmental disturbances of the brainstem such as decerebrate rigidity, tonic neck reflexes, pseudobulbar palsy	+	0 (+ late)
X-ray evidence of erosion of cranial bones or enlargement of foramens	0	+

Ocular apraxia is another special gaze disorder. Normally, on looking to the side, the eyes and head turn together, but in this condition the head turns and the eyes actually go in the opposite direction. The head is flung too far, in order not to lose sight of the target, and then the eyes "catch up." This may be a solitary congenital abnormality (Cogan), the anatomy of which is unknown, or it may be acquired as in ataxia telangiectasia (see Chap. 365).

In skew deviation, a poorly understood disorder of gaze, the eyes diverge, one looking down, the other up, and the patient complains of vertical diplopia. The deviation may be constant in all fields of gaze or it may be variable. It may occur with any lesion of the posterior fossa but particularly with one in the brainstem. The lesion is on the side of the lower eye.

Mixed gaze and ocular paralyses These are always a sign of intrapontine or mesencephalic disease. A lesion of the lower pons in or near the sixth nerve nucleus causes a homolateral paralysis of the lateral rectus muscle and a failure of adduction of the opposite eye, i.e., a combined paralysis of the sixth nerve and of conjugate lateral gaze. Lesions of the medial longitudinal fasciculi interfere with lateral conjugate gaze in another way. When the patient looks to the right, the left eye fails to adduct; when looking to the left, the right eye fails to adduct. Nystagmus is more prominent in or limited to the abducting eye. This condition is referred to as *internuclear ophthalmoplegia* and should always be suspected when only adduction of the eyes is affected. It may be unilateral or bilateral. If unilateral, the lesion is always on the side of the weak adducting eye. If the lesion is in the higher (midbrain) part of the medial longitudinal fasciculus, convergence may be lost in addition to paralysis of the medial recti on attempted lateral gaze (anterior internuclear ophthalmoplegia); if the lesion is in the lower (pontine) part, convergence is normal, but there may be some degree of associated limitation of conjugate lateral gaze or sixth nerve palsy (posterior internuclear ophthalmoplegia).

NYSTAGMUS AND OTHER INVOLUNTARY EYE MOVEMENTS

The term *nystagmus* refers to involuntary rhythmic movements of the eyes. It may be a normal physiologic phenomenon, as when one is riding in a train and watching the landscape, or a rotating drum with vertical stripes. Then the eyes drift to one side because of visual fixation in following the moving object and are repeatedly repositioned by a quick compensatory jerk. This is called optokinetic nystagmus. Rotation of the body also induces nystagmus, as does caloric irrigation of one external auditory meatus (cold water induces nystagmus to the opposite side). And in many normal individuals on extreme lateral gaze one observes a few irregular "nystagmoid" jerks; this is called end-point nystagmus. It is probably similar to the tremulousness of a muscle that is maximally contracted.

Pathologic nystagmus is subdivided into two types, oscillating (pendular) and rhythmic (jerk). Although practical, this classification is an oversimplification. The cause of pendular nystagmus is in some instances due to a fault in vision, e.g., amblyopic nystagmus where the wandering eye movements occur irregularly in every possible direction. Nevertheless similar eye movements are present in congenital nystagmus where visual acuity is normal. And in the latter on lateral gaze the pendular nystagmus changes to rhythmic jerk nystagmus. The anatomic and physiologic basis of congenital nystagmus is unknown.

All other types of pathologic nystagmus are of the rhythmic jerk type of which the following are the most important:

1 *Labyrinthine—vestibular type.* Here a disease of one semicircular canal which decreases the flow of action potentials causes a slow deviation of the eye to the side of the lesion and quick corrective movements to the opposite side. The abnormality is the slow drift to one side, but by convention the side of the nystagmus is designated by the direction of the fast phase. Since more than one canal is nearly always affected the nystagmus is usually rotatory but more horizontal than vertical. It is accompanied by the usual effects of canal paresis—disequilibrium, lateral pulsion and past pointing to the side of the affected ear, nausea, and in some instances vomiting. Fixation of the eyes tends to suppress it.

2 *Positional nystagmus.* This is characteristically induced by change of position. Reclining the patient from a sitting position with the affected ear down is followed within a few seconds by nystagmus and vertigo, lasting 10 to 15 s. Sitting up from the reclining position reproduces the nystagmus and vertigo but usually in the opposite direction. This is the benign form, shown by Schuchnecht to be due to cuprolithiasis (see Chap. 13). A malignant form with less consistent pattern and lack of reversibility occurs with tumors of the posterior fossa.

3 *Fixation and gaze-paretic nystagmus.* This is usually a coarse horizontal or vertical, upward or downward, nystagmus which is elicited by having the patient turn the eyes in the direction of the fast phase of the nystagmus and fixate on a target. In its most extreme degree there is difficulty in maintaining the eyes in the deviated position. Loss of fixation arrests the nystagmus; increasing the effort of lateral gaze increases its amplitude. Usually there is no vertigo or disequilibrium. Lateral and vertical fixation nystagmus are commonly observed in states of intoxication [alcohol, barbiturates, phenytoin (Dilantin)]. Lesions involving the vestibular connections of the brainstem, such as Wernicke's disease, multiple sclerosis, pontine gliomas, cause this type of nystagmus. Acoustic neuromas, by involving the vestibular nerve and compressing the brainstem, induce an asymmetrical gaze-paretic and vestibular nystagmus, coarser to the side of the lesion. Lesions of the lower brainstem such as the Arnold-Chiari malformation are associated with a vertical downward nystagmus; vertical upward nystagmus is usually related to lesions in the pons.

4 *Dissociated nystagmus (monocular nystagmus).* Usually this type is observed with lesions that implicate the medial longitudinal fasciculus. On lateral gaze there is nystagmus only in the abducting eye. Multiple sclerosis and other lesions of the pontine tegmentum are the usual cause.

5 *Convergence and retraction nystagmus.* With a variety of lesions of the midbrain which interfere with upward gaze (Parinaud's syndrome) when the patient attempts to look up the eyes converge in a series of rhythmic synchronous movements and may retract at the same time.

6 *Periodic alternating nystagmus.* Here there is horizontal nystagmus on straight-ahead gaze in one direction for 1 to 2 min, and then nystagmus in the reversed direction occurs. This has been observed with lesions in the fastigial nuclei an flocculonodular lobes of the cerebellum.

7 *See-saw nystagmus.* In this type of dissociated nystagmus, in which one eye rhythmically rises and intorts and the other descends and extorts, there has usually been a lesion in or near the optic chiasm. A congenital form also is known. See-saw nystagmus has been observed with craniopharyngiomas, optic gliomas, and upper brainstem infarcts.

In testing for nystagmus the eyes should first be examined in the central position and then during upward, downward, and lateral gaze. If nystagmus is monocular, each eye should be tested separately, with the other one covered. Labyrinthine nystagmus is most obvious when visual fixation is prevented by shielding the eyes; and brainstem and cerebellar nystagmus are brought out by having the patient fixate on the examiner's finger. Labyrinthine nystagmus may vary with the position of the head, hence these various tests should be performed with the head in several different positions, including the head-hanging position (neck retroflexed in recumbency), i.e., during the so-called Barany maneuvers. Optokinetic nystagmus is elicited by having the patient fixate on the vertical stripes of a moving piece of cloth or rotating drum. In most large clinics it is possible to do quantitative caloric testing and electronystagmography.

OTHER ABNORMALITIES OF OCULAR MOVEMENT *Oscillopsia* refers to illusory movement of the environment, in which objects seem to move back and forth, up or down, or side to side. It may or may not occur with turning of the eyes and consequent displacement of the image on the retina. Such movement of all objects in the environment is usually associated with coarse nystagmus due to lesion of the brainstem but may also accompany vestibular (labyrinthine) nystagmus. Movement of distortion of position of single visualized objects may be part of a metamorphopsia from cerebral lesions.

Opsoclonus is the term applied to sustained, irregular, conjugate "dancing" movements of the eyes in a horizontal, rotary, and vertical direction. The neurologic basis for these movements is not clear, but in most cases they are associated with signs of cerebellar disease due to a viral infection or occult neuroblastoma. In some viral infections causing stupor or coma, the eye movements are constant and chaotic.

Ocular dysmetria consists of an overshoot of the eyes on attempted fixation, followed by several cycles of oscillations of diminishing amplitude until precise fixation is attained. The overshoot may occur on eccentric fixation or on refixation in the primary position of gaze. This sign occurs in disease of the cerebellum or its pathways and is analogous to cerebellar dysmetria of the limbs. *Ocular flutter* further refers to quick, multiphasic, usually horizontal oscillations around the point of fixation; this abnormality is also associated with cerebellar disease. A fast downward movement of both eyes followed by a slow drift back to the midposition (called *ocular bobbing* by Fisher) is characteristic of pontine lesions such as hypertensive hemorrhage.

ALTERATIONS OF PUPILS Pupil size is determined by the balance of innervation between the dilator and constrictor fibers. The pupillodilator (sympathetic) fibers arise in the posterior part of the hypothalamus and descend in the lateral tegmentum of the midbrain, pons, medulla, and cervical spinal cord to the eighth cervical and first thoracic segments, where they synapse with the lateral horn cells. These give rise to preganglionic fibers that synapse in the superior cervical ganglion; the postganglionic fibers course along the internal carotid artery and traverse the cavernous sinus to join the first division of the trigeminal nerve, finally reaching the eyes as the long ciliary nerves. The pupilloconstrictor (parasympathetic) fibers arise in the nucleus of Edinger-Westphal, join the oculomotor nerve, and synapse in the ciliary ganglion with the postganglionic neurons that innervate the iris and ciliary body.

The afferent fibers for the pupillary light reflexes run in the optic nerve, chiasm, and optic tract. These fibers leave the optic tract and synapse in the pretectal nucleus of the midbrain, and thence, via intercalated neurons with the ipsilateral and contralateral Edinger-Westphal nuclei.

The sympathetic fibers dilate the pupil and the parasympathetic ones constrict it. A lesion of the optic nerve or tracts may abolish the pupillary light reflex; the pupil is dilated and unreactive. Cerebral lesions, on the other hand, leave the pupillary light reflex unaltered. The lack of a direct reflex in the blind eye and of a consensual reflex in the sound one means that the afferent limb of the reflex arc is the site of the lesion. A lack of direct light reflex with retention of the consensual reflex places the lesion in the efferent limb of the reflex (the homolateral oculomotor nucleus or nerve).

Interruption of the sympathetic fibers either centrally, between the hypothalamus and their point of exit from the spinal cord (first thoracic segment), or peripherally (superior or cervical ganglion in the neck or along the carotid artery) results in miosis and ptosis (because of paralysis of Müller's muscle), with loss of sweating of the face, and occasionally enophthalmos (Bernard-Horner syndrome). Irritation of the pupillodilator fibers has the opposite effect, i.e., lid retraction, slight proptosis, and dilatation of the pupil. The ciliospinal pupillary reflex, evoked by pinching the neck, is effected through these efferent sympathetic fibers. Abnormal dilatation of the pupils (mydriasis), often with loss of pupillary light reflexes, may result from midbrain lesions and is a frequent finding in cases of deep coma. Extreme constriction of the pupils (miosis) is commonly observed with pontine lesions, presumably because of bilateral interruption of the pupillodilator fibers.

The functional integrity of the sympathetic and parasympathetic nerve endings in the iris may be determined by the use of certain drugs. Atropine and homatropine dilate the pupils by paralyzing the parasympathetic nerve endings; physostigmine and pilocarpine constrict them, the former by inhibiting cholinesterase activity at the neuromuscular junction, and the latter by direct stimulation of the sphincter muscle of the iris. Epinephrine and phenylephrine cause mydriasis by stimulating the dilator muscle directly. Cocaine dilates the pupils by preventing the reuptake of norepinephrine into the nerve endings. Morphine acts centrally to constrict the pupils. Sensitivity to extremely low doses of these drugs (2.5% methadroline, 1/1000 dilution of epinephrine) indicate parasympathetic and sympathetic denervation, respectively (Pallis).

In chronic syphilitic meningitis and other forms of late syphilis, particularly tabes dorsalis, the pupils are usually small, irregular, and unequal; they do not dilate properly in response to mydriatic drugs and fail to react to light, although they do constrict on accommodation. In some cases there is an associated atrophy of the iris. This is known as the *Argyll Robertson pupil.* The exact locality of the lesion is not certain; it is generally believed to be in the tectum of the midbrain proximal to the oculomotor nuclei, where the descending pupillodilator fibers are in close proximity to the light-reflex fibers. A dissociation of the light reflex from the accommodation-convergence reaction is sometimes observed with other midbrain lesions, e.g., pinealoma, multiple sclerosis, and diabetes mellitus; in these diseases miosis, irregularity of pupils, and failure to respond to a mydriatic are not constantly present. Therefore, in the usual Argyll Robertson pupillary abnormality of tabes and of diabetic and amyloid polyneuropathy the lesion is probably peripheral, in the oculomotor nerve or ciliary ganglion. Another interesting pupillary abnormality is the myotonic reaction, sometimes referred to as *Adie's pupil.* The patient may complain of blurring of vision or may have suddenly noticed that one pupil is larger than the other. The reaction to light and convergence are absent if tested in the customary manner, although the size of the pupil will change slowly on prolonged stimulation. Once contracted or dilated, the pupils remain in that state for some minutes. The affected pupil reacts promptly to the usual mydriatic and miotic drugs but is unusually sensitive to a 0.125% solution of pilocarpine, a strength that will not affect a normal pupil. The myotonic pupil usually appears during the third or fourth decade of life; it may be associated with absence of knee or ankle jerks and hence be mistaken for tabes dorsalis.

Ocular movement, pupillary contraction, and visual acuity may be affected by diseases which alter the contents of the orbit. Usually this is accompanied by bilateral exophthalmos, as in thyroid or pituitary disease (Chap. 111). Unilateral exophthalmos may occur with orbital tumors (dermoids, adenoma of lacrimal gland, optic nerve glioma, neurofibroma, metastatic carcinoma, meningioma, or granuloma), or cavernous sinus thrombosis (Chap. 359). Sometimes thyroid disease will have an asymmetric effect with more exophthalmos and/or limitation of motion on one side than the other. Progressive paralysis of the eyelids, which may obstruct vision, occurs separately or as part of an external ophthalmoplegia, as in ocular dystrophy or in oculopharyngeal dystrophy.

DISTURBANCES OF HEARING

Tinnitus and *deafness* are frequent symptoms and always indicate disease of the ear or of the auditory nerve and its central connections.

Tinnitus, or ringing in the ears, is a purely subjective phenomenon and may also be reported as a buzzing, whistling, hissing, or roaring sound. It is a very common symptom in adults and always indicates a primary dysfunction of the auditory neural mechanism (cochlea and eighth nerve). Low-frequency vibratory clicks, pops, roarings, etc., are mechanical in nature and are due to contraction of muscles of the eustachian tube, middle ear, palate, or pharynx. Severe and prolonged tinnitus in the presence of normal hearing is very rare. If tinnitus is localized to one ear and is described as having a tonal character, such as ringing or a bell-like or high, steady musical tone, it is probably cochlear in origin. In Ménière's disease, the tinnitus usually has a low-pitched buzzing or roaring sound and is associated with reduced hearing and the recruitment phenomenon (see below). A pulsating tinnitus synchronous with the pulse may be related to an intracranial vascular malformation; however, this symptom must be carefully judged, since introspective persons often report hearing their pulse when lying with one ear on a pillow. Certain drugs such as salicylates and quinine produce tinnitus and transient deafness. Nervous persons are less tolerant of tinnitus than more stable ones; depressed or anxious patients may demand relief from tinnitus that has existed for years.

Examination of hearing should always begin with inspection of the external auditory canal and the tympanic membrane. A ticking watch or whispered words are suitable means of testing hearing at the bedside, the opposite ear being closed by the finger. If there is any suspicion of deafness or a complaint of tinnitus or vertigo, or if the patient is a child with a speech defect, then hearing must be tested further. This can be done with the use of tuning forks of different frequencies, but the most accurate results are obtained by the use of an electric audiometer and the construction of an audiogram which reveals the entire range of hearing at a glance.

Deafness is frequent. In the United States it is estimated that there are more than 6 million persons with hearing loss; in one-third to one-half of these persons the loss is hereditary. Deafness is of two general types: (1) nerve deafness (also called perceptive or sensorineural), due to disease of the cochlea or of the cochlear division of the eighth cranial nerve, and (2) conductive deafness, due to disease of the middle ear, such as otosclerosis or chronic otitis, or to occlusion of the external auditory canal or eustachian tube. In differentiating these two types, the tuning fork tests are of value. When a tuning fork vibrating at 256 Hz is held about 25 mm from the ear (the test for air conduction), sound waves can be appreciated only as they are transmitted through the middle ear and are reduced with disease in this location. When the fork is applied to the skull (test for bone conduction), the sound waves are conveyed directly to the cochlea, without the intervention of the middle ear apparatus, and are therefore not reduced with middle ear disease. Normally air conduction is better than bone conduction. These principles form the basis for several tests of auditory function.

In *Weber's test,* the vibrating fork is applied to the forehead in the midline. In middle ear deafness the sound is localized in the affected ear; in nerve deafness, in the normal ear. In *Rinne's test,* the vibrating fork is applied to the mastoid process, the other ear being closed by the observer's finger. At the moment the sound ceases, the fork is held at the auditory meatus. In middle ear deafness the sound cannot be heard by air conduction after bone conduction has ceased (abnormal or negative Rinne's test). In nerve deafness the reverse is true (normal or positive Rinne's test), although both air and bone conduction may be quantitatively decreased. In *Schwabach's test,* the patient's bone conduction is compared with that of a normal observer. In general, high-pitched tones are lost in nerve deafness and low-pitched ones in middle ear deafness, but there are frequent exceptions to this rule.

The following audiologic tests, taken together, help distinguish between cochlear and retrocochlear (nerve) lesions:

1 *Auditory recruitment.* The difference in hearing between the two ears is estimated, and the loudness of the stimulus delivered to each ear is then increased by regular increments. In nonrecruiting deafness (characteristic of nerve trunk lesion) the original difference in hearing persists in all comparisons of loudness above threshold. In recruiting deafness (as occurs in Ménière's disease) the more defective ear gains in loudness and finally is equal to the better one.
2 *Speech discrimination.* Retrocochlear lesions are indicated by a failure to recognize more than 30 percent of phonetically balanced monosyllabic words (e.g., *thin and sin*) at suprathreshold levels.
3 *Short-increment sensitivity index* (SISI). The patient responds to a series of twenty 1-decibel (dB) increments in amplitude superimposed on a steady tone of the same frequency presented at a sensation level of 20 dB. The patient's score is the percentage of these 20-dB increments which he or she is able to detect at a given frequency. Low SISI scores, below 60 percent, point to an end-organ lesion.
4 *Threshold sensitivity recorded via Békésy audiometry for both continuous and interrupted tonal stimuli.* Four types of tracing may be obtained; the type II tracing is obtained in patients with end-organ lesions, and type III or IV, usually the former, characterizes retrocochlear lesions.
5 *Threshold tone decay.* This test quantifies auditory adaptation and requires only a conventional pure tone audiometer. With retrocochlear lesions a continuous tone seems to decrease gradually in loudness, in contrast to cochlear lesions.

The common causes of middle ear deafness are otitis media, otosclerosis, and rupture of the eardrum. Nerve deafness has many causes. The internal ear may be aplastic from birth (hereditary deaf-mutism), or it may be damaged by rubella in the pregnant mother. Acute purulent meningitis or chronic infection spreading from the middle ear may cause nerve deafness in childhood. The auditory nerve may be involved by tumors of the cerebellopontine angle or by syphilis. Deafness may also result from a demyelinative plaque or infarct in the brainstem. A large series of genetically determined syndromes which feature a neural type of deafness, some congenital, others with onset in childhood or early adult life, has come to light (see article by Konigsmark). Most of these are inherited as an autosomal dominant trait, some as autosomal recessive or sex-linked traits. Konigsmark has classified these hereditary forms of deafness on the basis of associated defects caused by the same gene: hereditary deafness with malformations of external ears, face, and neck (Treacher-Collins disease and Engelmann's diaphyseal dysplasia); with various combinations of mental retardation, retinitis pigmentosa, and polyneuropathy (as in Hallgren's disease, Alstrom's disease, Refsum's disease); with skin abnormalities such as albinism, lentigines, piebaldness, white forelock (Waardenburg's disease), onchydystrophy and pegged teeth, atopic dermatitis, and anhydrosis; and with renal, thyroid, and cardiac abnormalities.

Of the types of progressive conduction deafness, hereditary otosclerosis is the most frequent (cause of 50 percent of deafness in adulthood). Hysterical deafness may be difficult to distinguish from organic disease. In the case of bilateral deafness, the distinction can be made by observing a blink (cochleoorbicular reflex) or an alteration in skin sweating (psychogalvanic skin reflex) in response to a loud sound. Unilateral hysterical deafness may be detected by an audiometer, with both ears connected, or by whispering into the bell of a stethoscope attached to the patient's ears, closing first one tube and then the other without the patient's knowledge.

In otosclerosis and hereditary sensorineural deafness, vestibular function is usually retained (caloric responses are normal).

REFERENCES

Ashworth B: Neuro-ophthalmology, in *Recent Advances in Clinical Neurology,* WB Mathews (ed). Edinburgh, Churchill-Livingstone, 1975

Bach-y-Rita P, Collins CC: *The Control of Eye Movements.* New York, Academic, 1971

Cogan DG: *Neurology of the Ocular Muscles,* 2d ed. Springfield, Ill., Charles C Thomas, 1956

———: *Neurology of the Visual System.* Springfield, Ill., Charles C Thomas, 1966

Daroff RB: Ocular oscillations. Ann Otol Rhin Laryng 86:102, 1977

Glaser JM: *Neuro-ophthalmology.* New York, Harper & Row, 1978

Konigsmark BW: Medical progress. Hereditary deafness in man. N Engl J Med 281:713, 774, 827, 1969

———: Hereditary diseases of the nervous system with hearing loss, in *Handbook of Clinical Neurology,* PJ Vinken, GW Bruyn (eds). Amsterdam, North Holland, 1975, vol 22, chap 23, pp 499–526

Pallis C: The pupil as an indicator of denervation hypersensitivity in the autonomic nervous system, in *Neurotransmitter Systems and Their Clinical Disorders,* NJ Legg (ed). London, Academic Press, 1978

Rucker CW: The causes of paralysis of the third, fourth and sixth cranial nerves. Am J Ophthalmol 61:1293, 1966

Tillman TW: Special hearing tests in otoneurologic diagnosis. Arch Otolaryngol 89:25 1969

Zee DS et al: Ocular motor abnormalities in hereditary cerebellar ataxia. Brain 99:207, 1976

18 DISORDERS OF SENSATION

MAURICE VICTOR
RAYMOND D. ADAMS

Loss or perversion of somatic sensation is not infrequently the principal manifestation of disease of the nervous system. The reason for this is clear enough, since the major anatomic pathways of the sensory system are distinct from those of the motor system and may be selectively disrupted by disease. An understanding of these sensory pathways and their functional derangements may provide important leads to neurologic diagnosis.

GENERAL CONSIDERATIONS Unfortunately, space does not permit a detailed review of the anatomy of the sensory system or of its physiology. The interested reader may turn to the references at the end of the chapter. One form of somatic sensation—pain—has already been considered in Chap. 2. The cutaneous distribution of sensory spinal roots is depicted in Fig. 18-1 (see also Chap. 2).

Disorders of the somatic sensory apparatus pose special problems. Patients are confronted with derangements of sensation which may be unlike anything they have previously experienced, and they have few words in their vocabulary to describe what they feel. They may say that a limb feels "numb" and "dead" when in fact they mean it is weak. Observant individuals may occasionally discover a loss of sensation, for example, inability to feel discomfort on touching an object hot enough to blister the skin or unawareness of articles of clothing and other objects in contact with the skin. But more often disease has induced a new and unnatural series of sensory experiences. If nerves, spinal roots, or spinal tracts are only partially interrupted, a tactile stimulus may arouse a tingling or pricking sensation, meaning presumably that at least some of the remaining touch and pain fibers are functioning but are conducting impulses abnormally. Tightness and drawing and pulling sensations, a feeling of a band or girdle around the limb or trunk, are common complaints with partial involvement of deep sensory fibers. Similarly, burning and pain (cau-

FIGURE 18-1
Distribution of the sensory spinal roots on the surface of the body. (From Holmes.)

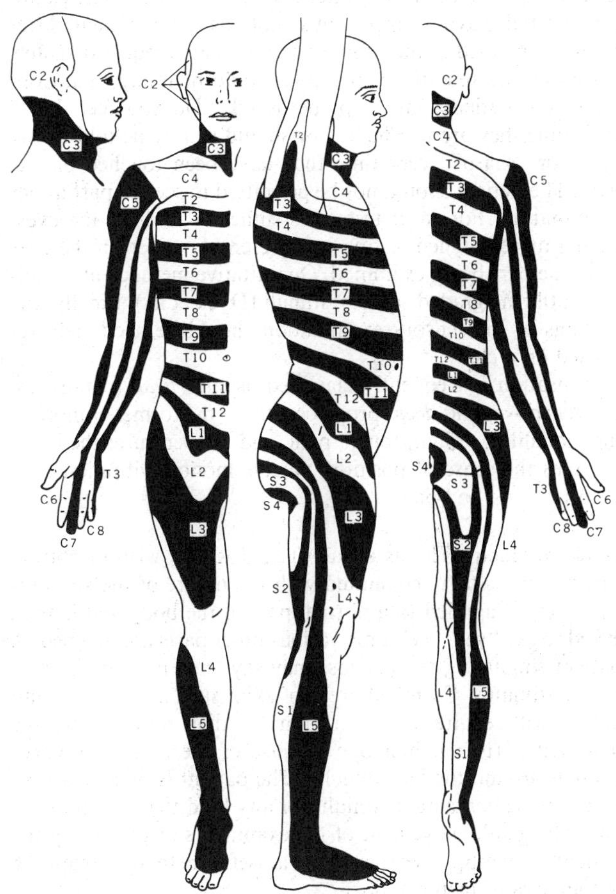

salgia) may represent overactivity of surviving thermal and pain fibers. The responsible lesion may be in the peripheral nerve, in the gray matter or sensory tracts in the spinal cord or brainstem, or in the thalamus. Also, hyperesthesia and hyperpathia are frequent. All of these abnormal sensations are called *paresthesias,* or *dysesthesias,* if they are unpleasant; and their character and distribution inform us of the anatomy of the lesion involving the sensory system.

EXAMINATION OF SENSATION The examination of sensation is the most difficult part of the neurologic examination. For one thing, test procedures are relatively crude and inadequate. And, embarrassingly often, no objective sensory loss can be demonstrated despite symptoms that clearly indicate the presence of such a deficit. Also, a response to a sensory stimulus is difficult to evaluate objectively, since the examiner's conclusions depend on the patient's interpretations of sensory experiences. This presupposes a general responsiveness, alertness, and desire to cooperate, as well as intelligence and a certain level of education. Hypersuggestibility and fatigue may interfere with the obtaining of accurate test data.

The detail in which sensation is tested will be determined by the clinical situation. If the patient has no sensory complaints, it is sufficient to examine vibration and position sense in the fingers and toes, to test the perception of pain over the face, trunk, and extremities, and to determine whether the sensory findings are the same in symmetric parts of the body. A rough survey of this sort may detect sensory defects of which the patient is unaware. On the other hand, more thorough testing is in order if the patient has complaints referable to the sensory system or if there is localized atrophy or weakness, ataxia, trophic changes of joints, or painless ulcers.

A few other general principles should be mentioned. One should not press the sensory examination in the presence of fatigue, for an inattentive patient is a poor witness. The examiner must also avoid suggesting symptoms to the patient. After having explained in the simplest terms what is required, as few questions and remarks as possible should be interposed. Consequently, patients must not be asked, "Do you feel that?" each time they are touched; they should simply be told to say "yes" or "sharp" every time they have been touched or feel pain. The patient should not be permitted to see the part under examination. For short tests it is sufficient to close the eyes; during more detailed testing it is preferable to screen the eyes from the part being examined. Quantitative methods are available, utilizing graded sensory stimuli (Dyck et al.). Finally, the findings of the sensory examination should be accurately recorded on a chart.

Sensation is frequently classified as *superficial* (cutaneous, exteroceptive) and *deep* (proprioceptive); the former comprises the modalities of light touch, pain, and temperature; the latter includes the sense of position, passive motion, vibration, and deep pressure and pain.

Sense of touch This is usually tested with a wisp of cotton. The patient is first acquainted with the nature of the stimulus by feeling it applied to a normal part of the body and is then asked to say "yes" each time various other parts are touched. A patient simulating sensory loss may say "no" in response to a tactile stimulus. Cornified areas of skin, such as the soles and palms, will require a heavier stimulus than normal, and the hair-clad parts a lighter one because of the numerous nerve endings around the hair follicles. The patient is more sensitive to a moving contactual stimulus of any kind than a stationary one. The gentle movement of the examiner's or preferably the patient's fingertip over the skin is a useful method of mapping out an area of tactile loss.

Sense of pain This is most efficiently estimated by pinprick, although it may be evoked by a diversity of noxious stimuli. The patient must understand that he or she is to report the degree of sharpness of the pin, not simply the feeling of contact or pressure of the point. If the pinpricks are applied rapidly, their effects may be summated and excessive pain may result; therefore, they should be delivered not too rapidly, about one per second, and not over the same spot.

If an area of diminished or absent touch or pain sensation is encountered, its boundaries should be demarcated to determine whether it has a segmental or peripheral nerve distribution or whether sensation is lost below a certain level. Such areas are best delineated by proceeding from the region of impaired sensation toward the normal, and the changes may be confirmed by dragging a pin lightly over the skin.

Thermal sense The following procedure for testing thermal sensation is suggested. The areas of skin to be tested should be exposed for some time before the examination. The test objects should be large, preferably Erlenmeyer flasks containing hot and cold water. Thermometers which extend into the water through the flask stoppers indicate the temperature of the water at the moment of testing. At first, extreme degrees of heat and cold (e.g., 10 and 45°C) may be employed to delineate roughly an area of thermal sensory disturbance; the patient will report that the flask feels "less hot" or "less cold" over such an area than over a normal part. If areas of impaired sensation are found, the borders may be accurately determined by moving the flask along the skin from the insensitive to the normal region. The qualitative change should then be quantitated as far as possible by estimating the *differences in temperature* which the patient is able to recognize. The patient is asked to report whether one stimulus is *warmer or colder* than another, not whether a given stimulus is warm or cold, since the cooler of the two may be interpreted as warm. The range of temperature difference between the two flasks is gradually narrowed by mixing their contents. A normal person is capable of detecting a difference of 1°C when the temperature of the flasks is in the range of 28 to 32°C. In the warm range one should readily recognize differences between 35 and 40°C, and in the cold range, between 10 and 20°C. In many normal older persons and in others with poor peripheral circulation (especially in cold weather), the responses may be modified.

The sensation of heat or cold depends not only on the temperature of the stimulus but also on the duration of the stimulus and the area over which it is applied. This principle may be employed to detect slight degrees of impaired thermal sensation; the patient may be able to distinguish small differences in temperature when the bottom of the flask is applied for 3 s but unable to do so if only the side of the flask is applied for 1 s. Throughout the test procedure, especially when small temperature differences are involved, the area of sensory disturbance should be continually checked against perception in normal parts.

Postural sense and the appreciation of passive movement These modalities are usually lost together, although in any particular case one may be disproportionately affected.

Abnormalities of postural sensation may be revealed in several ways. When the patient extends the arms forward and closes the eyes, the affected arm will wander from its original position; if the fingers are spread apart, they may undergo a series of slow-changing postures ("piano-playing" movements, or *pseudoathetosis*). In attempting to touch the tip of the nose with the index finger, the patient may miss the target repeatedly.

The lack of position sense in the legs may be demonstrated by displacing the limb from its original position and asking the patient to point to the large toe. If postural sensation is defective in both legs, the patient will be unable to maintain balance with feet together and eyes closed (Romberg's sign). This sign should be interpreted with caution. Even a normal person in the Romberg position will sway slightly more with the eyes closed than open. A patient with lack of balance due to motor disorders or cerebellar disease will also sway more if visual cues are removed. Only if there is a marked discrepancy between the state of balance with eyes open and closed can one confidently state that the patient shows Romberg's sign, i.e., loss of joint-position (kinesthetic) sense. Mild degrees of unsteadiness in nervous or suggestible patients may be overcome by diverting their attention, e.g., by having them alternately touch the index finger of each hand to their nose while standing with their eyes closed.

The appreciation of passive movement is first tested in the fingers and toes, and the defect, when present, is reflected maximally in these parts. It is important to grasp the digit firmly at the sides opposite the plane of movement; otherwise the pressure applied by the examiner in displacing the digit may allow the patient to identify the direction of movement. This applies to the testing of the more proximal segments of the limb as well. The patient should be instructed to report each movement as "up" or "down" in relation to the previous stationary position. It is useful to demonstrate the test with a large and easily identified movement, but once the idea is clear to the patient, the smallest detectable changes in position should be tested. The range of movement normally appreciated in the digits is said to be as little as 1°. Clinically, however, defective appreciation of passive movement is judged by comparison with a normal limb or, if bilaterally defective, on the basis of what the examiner has through experience learned to regard as normal. Slight impairment may be disclosed by a slow response or, if the digit is displaced very slowly, by a relative unawareness that movements have occurred; or after the digit has been displaced in the same direction several times, the patient may misjudge the first movement in the opposite direction; or after the examiner has moved the toe, the patient may make a number of small voluntary movements of the toe, in an apparent attempt to determine its position or the direction of the movement.

The sense of vibration This is a composite sensation comprising touch and rapid alterations of deep pressure sense, the end organ of which is the pacinian corpuscle. Its conduction depends on both cutaneous and deep afferent fibers which ascend in the dorsal columns of the cord. It is therefore rarely affected by lesions of single nerves but will be disturbed in cases of polyneuritis and disease of the dorsal columns, medial lemniscus, and thalamus. For this reason, vibration and position sense are usually lost together, although one of them (usually vibration sense) may be affected disproportionately. With advancing age, vibration sense may be diminished at the toes and ankles.

Vibration sense is tested by placing a tuning fork with a low rate (and long duration) of vibration (128 Hz) over the bony prominences. The examiner must make sure that the patient responds to the vibration, not simply to the pressure of the fork. Although there are mechanical devices to quantitate vibration sense, it is sufficient for clinical purposes to compare the point tested with a normal part of the patient or the examiner. Thus, if the fork is allowed to run down until vibration is no longer appreciated but is still felt at an analogous point on the opposite limb, and if this finding is consistent, one can be certain of a significant impairment of vibration sense. In a similar way, the appreciation of vibration at the tibial tuberosity after it has disappeared in the ankle, or at the anterior iliac spine after it has disappeared at the tibial tuberosity, is an indication of a peripheral nerve lesion. The level of vibration sense loss due to spinal cord lesions may be estimated by placing the fork over successive vertebral spines.

Sense of deep pressure and pain This can be estimated simply by gently pinching or pressing deeply on the tendons and muscles. Pain can often be elicited by heavy pressure even when superficial pain is diminished; conversely, in some diseases, such as tabetic neurosyphilis, the loss of deep pressure and pain may be more prominent.

DISCRIMINATIVE SENSORY FUNCTIONS Damage to the sensory cortex or to the thalamocortical projections results in a special type of disturbance that affects mainly the patient's ability to make sensory discriminations. Lesions in these structures usually disturb postural sense but leave the so-called primary modalities (touch, pain, temperature, and vibration sense) relatively little affected. In such a situation, or if a cerebral lesion is suspected on other grounds, discriminative function should be tested further in the following ways:

Two-point discrimination The ability to distinguish two points from one is tested by using a compass, the points of which should be blunt and applied simultaneously and painlessly. The distance at which such stimuli can be recognized as double varies greatly; 1 mm at the tip of the tongue, 2 to 3 mm on the lips, 3 to 5 mm on the dorsa of the hands and feet, and 4 to 7 cm on the body surface. It is characteristic of the patient with a lesion of the sensory cortex to mistake two points for one, although occasionally the opposite occurs.

Cutaneous localization and number writing The ability to localize cutaneous stimuli is tested by touching or pricking various parts of the patient's body and asking the patient to point to the part touched or pricked, or to the corresponding part on the examiner's limb. Recognition of numbers or letters (these should be larger than 4 cm) or of the direction of lines drawn on the skin also depends on localization of tactile stimuli.

Appreciation of texture, size, and shape Appreciation of texture depends mainly on cutaneous impressions, but the recognition of shape and size of objects is based on impressions from deeper receptors as well. The lack of recognition of shape and form, therefore, though frequently found with cerebral cortical lesions, may also be present with lesions of the spinal cord and brainstem because of interruption of tracts transmitting postural and tactile sensation. The latter type of sensory defect, called *stereoanesthesia,* should be distinguished from *astereognosis,* which connotes an inability to identify an object by palpation, the primary sense data (touch, pain, temperature, and vibration) being intact. In practice, a pure astereognosis is rarely encountered, and the term is employed where the impairment of superficial and vibratory sensation in the hands seems to be of insufficient severity to account for the defect. Defined in this way, astereognosis is either right- or left-sided and the product of a lesion in the opposite hemisphere, involving the postcentral gyrus or the thalamoparietal projections. Astereognosis should not be confused with *tactile agnosia.* The latter disorder is due to a lesion lying posterior to the postcentral gyrus of the *dominant* parietal lobe, and causes an inability to recognize an object by touch or handling in both hands.

Extinction of sensory stimuli and sensory inattention In response to bilateral simultaneous testing of symmetric parts, the patient may acknowledge only the stimulus on the sound side or may improperly localize the stimulus on the affected side, whereas stimuli applied to each side separately are properly appreciated. This phenomenon of extinction, or cortical inattention, is characteristic of parietal lobe lesions, the symptoms of which are considered in Chap. 24.

A few other terms require definition, since they may be encountered in descriptions of sensation. *Anesthesia* refers to a loss of all forms of sensation, and *hypesthesia* to a diminution of all sensation. Loss or impairment of specific cutaneous sensations is indicated by an appropriate prefix or suffix, e.g., thermoanesthesia or thermohypesthesia, analgesia (loss of pain) or hypalgesia, tactile anesthesia (loss of sense of touch), and pallanesthesia (loss of vibratory sense). The term *hyperesthesia* requires special mention; although it implies a heightened receptiveness of the nervous system, careful testing will usually demonstrate an underlying sensory defect, i.e., an elevated threshold to tactile, painful, or thermal stimuli; once the stimulus is perceived, however, it may have a severely painful or unpleasant quality (hyperpathia).

Laboratory methods for demonstration of sensory loss As described in Chap. 354 a lack of or slowing of sensory nerve fiber conduction from one point in a peripheral nerve to another is clearly an indication of disease of sensory nerve fibers. Techniques of somatosensory-evoked potential also permit the measurement of the transmission of the impulse from a peripheral stimulus to a proximal part of the nerve. Also revealed is its speed of conduction in the posterior columns of the spinal cord to the nucleus of Goll or Burdach, and then through the medial lemniscus to the posterolateral nucleus of the thalamus and to the parietal lobe cortex. Delay at any one of these points is indicated by the wave forms recorded in the neck and at the cranial surface (see Desmedt).

SYNDROMES OF SENSORY ABNORMALITY **Sensory changes due to single nerve involvement** Sensory changes may be due to interruption of a single peripheral nerve. These changes will vary with the composition of the nerve involved, depending on whether it is predominantly muscular, cutaneous, or mixed. In lesions of cutaneous nerves, the area of tactile anesthesia is more extensive than the one for pain, because of greater overlapping of pain fibers. Also, because of overlap from adjacent nerves, the area of sensory loss following division of a cutaneous nerve is always less than its anatomic distribution. If a large area of skin is involved, the sensory defect characteristically consists of a central portion, in which all forms of cutaneous sensation are lost, surrounded by a zone of partial loss, which becomes less marked as one proceeds from the center to the periphery. The perception of deep pressure and passive movement is intact because these modalities are carried by special nerve fibers from subcutaneous structures and joints. Along the margin of the hypesthetic zone the skin becomes excessively sensitive. According to Weddell, this is because of collateral regeneration from surrounding healthy nerves into the denervated region (see Chap. 2).

Particular types of lesions differentially affect the fibers in a sensory nerve. Compression paralyzes large touch and pressure fibers more than the small pain, thermal, and autonomic motor fibers; procaine and cocaine have opposite effects.

In lesions involving the brachial and lumbosacral plexuses, the sensory disturbance is no longer confined to the territory of a single nerve and is almost invariably accompanied by muscle weakness and reflex changes.

Sensory changes due to multiple nerve involvement (polyneuropathy) In most instances of polyneuropathy the sensory changes are accompanied by varying degrees of motor and reflex loss. Usually the sensory impairment is symmetric, with notable exceptions in some instances of diabetic and periarteritic neuropathy. Since the longest and largest fibers tend to be the most affected, the sensory loss is most severe over the feet and legs and less severe over the hands and arms. The abdomen, thorax, and face are spared except in the most severe cases. The sensory loss usually involves all the modalities, and although it is manifestly difficult to equate the impairment of pain, touch, temperature, vibration, and position sense, one of these may seemingly be impaired out of proportion to the others. One cannot accurately predict from the patient's symptoms which mode of sensation will be disproportionately affected. The term *glove-and-stocking anesthesia* is frequently employed to describe the sensory loss of polyneuropathy and draws attention to the predominantly distal pattern of involvement. It is a less accurate term insofar as the change from normal to impaired sensation is not sharp, but gradual. In hysteria, by contrast, the border between normal and absent sensation is usually sharp. (See Chap. 368 for description of special varieties of sensory changes in polyneuropathies.)

Sensory changes due to involvement of single or multiple spinal nerve roots Because of considerable overlap from adjacent roots, division of a single sensory root does not produce complete loss of sensation in any area of skin. Compression of a single sensory cervical or lumbar root (e.g., in herniated intervertebral disks) causes varying degrees of impairment of cutaneous sensation in a segmental pattern, however. When two or more roots have been completely divided, a zone of sensory loss can be found which is greater for pain than for touch. Surrounding the area of complete loss is a narrow zone of partial loss, in which a raised threshold accompanied by overreaction (*hyperpathia*) may or may not be demonstrated. The presence of muscle paralysis and atrophy indicates involvement of ventral roots as well.

Tabetic syndrome This, too, is a radicular syndrome, resulting from damage to the large proprioceptive and other fibers of the posterior lumbosacral roots. It is usually caused by neurosyphilis, less often by diabetes mellitus, cauda equina tumors, etc. Numbness or paresthesias and lightning pains are frequent complaints, and areflexia, atonicity of the bladder, abnormalities of gait (Chap. 16), and hypotonia without muscle weakness are found on examination. The sensory loss may consist only of loss of vibration and position sense in the lower extremities, but in severe cases, loss or impairment of superficial or deep pain sense or of touch may be added. The feet and legs are most affected, much less often the arms and trunk.

Complete spinal sensory syndromes In a complete transverse lesion of the spinal cord, all forms of sensation are abolished below a level that corresponds to the lesion. There may be a narrow zone of "hyperesthesia" at the upper margin of the anesthetic zone. During the evolution of such a lesion there may be a discrepancy between the level of the lesion and that of the sensory loss, the latter ascending as the lesion progresses. This can be understood if one conceives of a lesion evolving from the periphery to the center of the cord, affecting first the outermost fibers of the spinothalamic tract, carrying pain and temperature sensation from the legs. Conversely, a lesion advancing from the center of the cord may affect these modalities in the reverse order. (See Chap. 366 for a more complete discussion.)

Partial spinal sensory syndromes (hemisection of the spinal cord, Brown-Séquard's syndrome) In rare instances disease is confined to one side of the spinal cord; pain and thermal sensation are affected on the opposite side, and proprioceptive sensation is affected on the same side as the lesion. The loss of pain and temperature sensation begins two or three segments below the lesion. An associated motor paralysis on the side of the lesion completes the syndrome. Tactile sensation is not involved, since the fibers from one side of the body are distributed in tracts on both sides of the cord.

Lesions of the central gray matter (syringomyelic syndrome) Since fibers conducting pain and temperature cross the cord in the anterior commissure, a lesion in this location will characteristically abolish these modalities on one or both sides but will spare tactile sensation. The commonest cause of such a lesion is syringomyelia, less often, tumor and hemorrhage. This type of dissociated sensory loss usually occurs in a segmental distribution (sensation is normal above and below the affected segments), and since the lesion frequently involves other parts of the gray matter, varying degrees of segmental amyotrophy and reflex loss may be added. If the lesion has spread to the white matter, signs of involvement of corticospinal and spinothalamic tracts and posterior columns will be present as well.

Posterior column syndrome There is loss of vibratory and position sense below the lesion, but the senses of pain, temperature, and touch are affected relatively little or not at all. This condition may be difficult to distinguish from an affection of large fibers in sensory roots (tabetic syndrome). In some diseases vibratory sensation may be involved predominantly, whereas in others position sense is more affected. An interruption of proprioceptive fibers may interfere with discriminative sensory function, such as two-point discrimination and recognition of size, shape, and weight; and impairment of these functions may occur with posterior column disease alone. Paresthesias in the form of tingling and "pins-and-needles" sensations or girdle sensations are a common complaint with diseases of posterior columns, and pinprick may produce a diffuse, burning, unpleasant sensation.

The "anterior spinal artery syndrome" With occlusion of the anterior spinal artery or other destructive lesions that predominantly affect the ventral portion of the cord, there is a relative or absolute sparing of the posterior column functions and only a loss of pain and temperature sensation below the level of the lesion. Since the corticospinal tracts and the ventral gray matter also fall within the area of distribution of the anterior spinal artery, paralysis of motor function forms a prominent part of this syndrome.

Disturbances of sensation due to lesions of the brainstem A characteristic feature of lesions of the medulla and lower pons is crossed sensory disturbance, i.e., loss of pain and temperature sensation of one side of the face and of the opposite side of the body. This is accounted for by involvement of the trigeminal tract or nucleus and the lateral spinothalamic tract on one side of the brainstem. This is nearly always due to a lateral medullary infarction (Wallenberg's syndrome). In the upper midbrain, where the spinothalamic tract and the medial lemniscus become confluent, an appropriately placed lesion may cause a loss of all superficial and deep sensation over the contralateral side of the body. Cranial nerve palsies, cerebellar ataxia, or motor paralysis are often associated (see Chap. 367).

Sensory loss due to a lesion of the thalamus (syndrome of Déjerine-Roussy) Involvement of the nucleus ventralis posterolateralis of the thalamus, usually due to a vascular lesion and less often to a tumor, causes loss or diminution of all forms of sensation on the opposite side of the body. Position sense is affected more frequently than any other sensory function, and deep sensory loss is usually, but not always, more profound than cutaneous loss. Sooner or later, often as sensation improves, spontaneous pain or discomfort ("thalamic pain"), sometimes of the most distressing and disabling type, appears on the affected side of the body; and any form of stimulus may acquire a diffuse, unpleasant, lingering quality. Emotional disturbance also aggravates the painful state. The thalamic pain syndrome may occasionally accompany lesions of the white matter of the parietal lobe (Chap. 24).

Sensory loss due to a lesion of the parietal lobe There is a unique disturbance mainly of discriminative sensory functions on the opposite side of the body, particularly the face, arm, and leg. Loss of position sense, impaired ability to localize touch and pain stimuli, elevation of two-point threshold, a general inattentiveness to sensory stimuli or sensory extinction on one side of the body, and astereognosis are the most prominent findings. With cortical lesions, the patient's reports are variable; one examination may disclose no sensory abnormalities, whereas another does. This type of response may be incorrectly attributed to hysteria. As to the anatomic localization of lesions that impair tactile discrimination, they have been found consistently in the postcentral gyrus of the contralateral parietal lobe (Roland). More frequent with lesions of the parietal lobe is a global reduction of all forms of somatic sensation on the opposite side of the body. Other features of parietal lobe symptomatology and the differences between dominant and nondominant parietal lobe syndromes are considered in Chap. 24

Sensory loss due to suggestion and hysteria Hysterical patients almost never complain spontaneously of cutaneous sensory loss, although they may use the term *numbness* to indicate a paralysis of a limb. Complete hemianesthesia, often with reduced hearing, sight, smell, and taste, as well as impaired vibration sense over only half the skull, is a common finding in hysteria. Anesthesia of one entire limb or a sharply defined sensory loss over part of a limb, not conforming to the distribution of root or cutaneous nerve, may also be observed. Postural sensation is rarely affected. The diagnosis of hysterical hemianesthesia is best made by eliciting the other relevant symptoms of hysteria or, if this is not possible, by noting the discrepancies between this type of sensory loss and that which occurs as part of the usual sensory syndromes.

REFERENCES

Adams RD, Victor M: *Principles of Neurology,* 2d ed. New York, McGraw-Hill, 1981

Brodal A: The somatic afferent pathways, in *Neurological Anatomy,* 3d ed. New York, Oxford, 1981, pp 46–147

Desmedt JE (ed): *Progress in Clinical Neurophysiology,* vol 7: *Clinical Uses of Cerebral, Brainstem and Spinal Evoked Potentials.* Basel, Karger, 1980

Dyck PJ et al: Clinical vs. quantitative evaluation of cutaneous sensation. Arch Neurol 33:651, 1976

Holmes GM: *Introduction to Clinical Neurology,* 2d ed. Baltimore, Williams & Wilkins, 1952, chaps 8, 9

Mayo Clinic: *Clinical Examinations in Neurology,* 5th ed. Philadelphia, Saunders, 1981

Mountcastle VB: Central nervous mechanisms in sensation, in *Medical Physiology,* 13th ed, VB Mountcastle (ed). St. Louis, Mosby, 1974, vol I, chaps 9–11

Roland PE: Astereognosis: Tactile discrimination after localized hemispheric lesions in man. Arch Neurol 33:543, 1976

Semmes J et al: *Somatosensory Changes after Penetrating Brain Wounds in Man.* Cambridge, Mass, Harvard University Press, 1960

19
THE SLEEP-WAKE CYCLE AND DISORDERS OF SLEEP

JOSEPH B. MARTIN

All organisms show daily rhythmic changes in physiologic functions and behavior. Such rhythms are commonly *circadian* (*circa*, "approximately"; *dian*, "day"), because in the absence of a time cue such as a regular daily time of awakening, they emerge as "free-running" with a periodicity of about 1 day. In humans, the most important of these rhythms is the sleep-wake cycle.

Sleep is a complex biological function with marked individual variations in depth and length. The average total sleep period is 7.5 h but ranges in healthy adult individuals from 4 to 10 h. Short-duration sleepers often tend to be more active and productive during the waking hours, whereas long-duration sleepers are frequently underachievers and have low-key personalities. Increased mortality rates are reported for men and women who sleep less than 4 h or more than 10 h per night. Total sleep time is highest in infancy, decreases to adult levels after completion of body growth, and declines with old age.

STAGES OF SLEEP The use of continuous recordings of brain waves (electroencephalogram, EEG), muscle electrical activity (electromyogram, EMG), and eye movements (electro-oculogram, EOG), together with measurements of the respiratory rate, blood pressure, and heart rate, has provided important information about normal patterns of sleep and given clues to the nature of sleep disorders. For such studies, EEG electrodes are attached to the scalp, EOG electrodes to the skin at the outer canthus of both eyes, and EMG electrodes to the skin overlying the chin (mentalis) muscle.

The characteristic EEG pattern during wakefulness, with the eyes closed, is a sinusoidal posterior alpha rhythm of 8 to 12 Hz combined with low-voltage fast (beta) activity of mixed frequency (13 to 22 Hz). The EMG shows high-amplitude tonic discharge activity. There are two distinct phases of sleep, *nonrapid eye movement* (NREM) sleep, and *rapid eye movement* (REM) sleep. NREM sleep consists of four stages. Stage I sleep is characterized by low-voltage, mixed-frequency EEG activity, accompanied by slow, rolling eye movements recorded on the EOG. The EMG shows moderately high amplitude discharges, which are decreased in size from that of the waking stage. Stage II sleep is represented by a moderately low voltage EEG, interspersed with brief (0.2 to 0.75 s) high-voltage discharges (K complexes) and vertex waves, interspersed with low- to moderate-amplitude discharges (sleep spindles) recorded at 12 to 15 Hz. Stage III sleep consists of high-amplitude background activity of theta (5 to 7 Hz) and delta (1 to 3 Hz) waves, as well as K complexes and sleep spindles. Such high-voltage, slow-wave activity is present for 20 to 50 percent of the record. Stage IV sleep consists of high-voltage (75 μV or greater) delta waves. Spindles are rare. Delta activity is present for 50 percent or more of the record. Low-voltage muscle potentials persist during each NREM sleep stage. Eye movements are infrequent or absent in stages III and IV.

The transition to REM sleep occurs abruptly and consists of a change in the EEG to low-voltage, fast-frequency (8 to 22 Hz) activity which resembles closely that seen during waking or stage I sleep; however, sawtooth waves consisting of moderately high amplitude, 3- to 5-Hz triangular-shaped waveforms are also commonly observed. The EOG shows clusters of conjugate eye movements occurring in all directions of gaze (REM activity). EMG activity becomes either totally absent or markedly suppressed, an effect due to descending inhibition of motor unit discharges from the brainstem reticular formation. The deep tendon reflexes are also absent. Upon awakening from REM sleep, subjects commonly report dreams.

REM sleep alternates with NREM sleep approximately every 90 to 100 min, the first REM period usually occurring about 90 to 100 min after the onset of sleep. The full sequence of transition through stages I, II, III, and IV of NREM typically occurs after first going to sleep (Fig. 19-1). The sequence is then reversed through stages IV, III, and II, and REM sleep ensues. Normal night sleep consists of three to five such alternating cycles, characterized as the night progresses by an increasing duration and percentage of the REM-sleep period. Stages III and IV occur predominantly during the first one-third of the sleep period. Stage I sleep normally occupies approximately 5 to 10 percent of total sleep, stage II about 50 percent, stage III approximately 15 percent, stage IV about 10 percent, and REM sleep approximately 20 percent.

Cyclic autonomic and endocrine changes also occur during normal sleep. Blood pressure and heart and respiratory rates decrease during progressive stages of NREM sleep. Abrupt fluctuations in blood pressure, heart rate, respiratory rate, and penile erection occur during REM sleep. In terms of endocrine functions, there is a major surge of growth hormone secretion during the first 2 h of sleep that is commonly, but not exclusively, associated with stages III and IV sleep. ACTH-cortisol secretion occurs as a series of individual surges during the latter half of night sleep, the accumulation of which produces the high concentrations on awakening that are characteristic of the circadian pituitary-adrenal rhythm. Prolactin secretion in both men and women also increases during the night, with highest plasma concentrations found immediately after sleep onset. Increased sleep-associated luteinizing hormone (LH) secretion has been shown to occur during puberty in boys and girls.

PHYSIOLOGIC MECHANISMS OF SLEEP Experimental studies indicate that the oscillator(s) controlling the sleep cycle is located in the pontine reticular formation of the brainstem. The sleep cycle appears to be influenced by the two biogenic

FIGURE 19-1
The states of wake, NREM sleep, and REM sleep. Polygraph recordings define stages of sleep. Associated sensation and perception, thought, and movements are characteristic of each state. The neuronal model is based on fluctuations in aminergic and cholinergic tone in brainstem centers. (Modified from Sleep: Order and Disorder by permission of J.A. Hobson.)

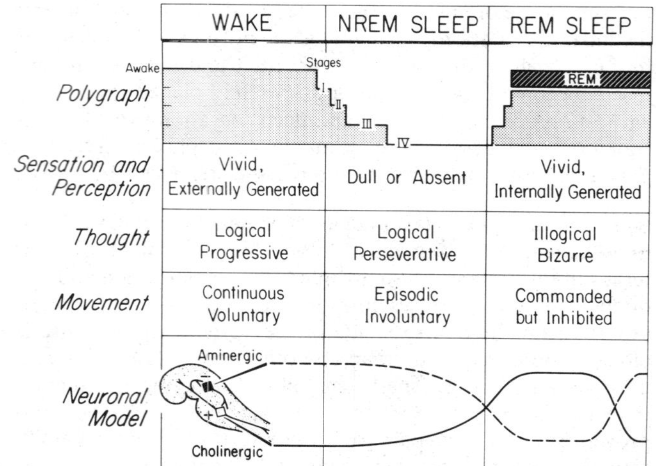

amines, 5-hydroxytryptamine (serotonin) and norepinephrine, and by acetylcholine. The serotonergic neurons are located in the dorsal raphé nuclei of the medial tegmentum of the medulla, pons, and lower midbrain. The noradrenergic neurons are clustered in the locus ceruleus.

Two general hypotheses of the neurotransmitter control of sleep have been advanced. In the 1960s, on the basis of experimental work, Jouvet proposed a major role of serotonin in the induction of NREM sleep and provided evidence that norepinephrine was involved in the transition from NREM to REM sleep. More recently, Hobson and colleagues have invoked a shift in brainstem cholinergic and bioaminergic tonic activity to explain sleep cycles (Fig. 19-1). Single-unit recordings of brainstem neurons suggest that the pontine clock is composed of these two reciprocally interconnected neuronal populations. During wakefulness the integrated activity in the aminergic nuclei of the brainstem (serotonergic and noradrenergic) is high. The resting activity level of cholinergic neurons in the reticular formation is low as a consequence of aminergic inhibition. During NREM sleep aminergic inhibition declines; simultaneously, cholinergic excitation gradually increases so that at midcycle the balance between aminergic inhibition and cholinergic excitation shifts. The REM period occurs when aminergic inhibition has fallen to its lowest point and cholinergic excitation becomes maximal.

As predicted by this model, microinjection of either cholinergic agonists or aminergic antagonists into the pontine brainstem can convert an animal's state from awake to REM sleep. This hypothesis is attractive because it provides a basis for understanding the efficacy of certain drugs in the treatment of sleep disorders.

There is also evidence that peptides may be important in the regulation of sleep. The plasma of drowsy or sleeping animals was shown by Monnier to contain a peptide substance that induces somnolence and increases NREM sleep in alert animals. A factor has been isolated from the cerebrospinal fluid and urine of animals and humans that when injected into rats and rabbits induces slow-wave sleep lasting 4 to 6 h. Its molecular weight is about 350 to 700 daltons and it is destroyed by peptidases, suggesting that it is a peptide.

EFFECTS OF SLEEP LOSS Human beings deprived of NREM and REM sleep for periods of 60 to 200 h experience increasing fatigue and irritability and find it difficult to concentrate. Illusions and hallucinations intrude into consciousness, primarily in the visual and tactile sensory fields, becoming more intense as the period of sleeplessness is prolonged. Performance of motor tasks deteriorates. Motivation declines and actions are interrupted by lapses of attention. Neurologic signs include mild and fleeting nystagmus, a slight tremor of the hands, ptosis of the eyelids, and thickness of speech, with mispronunciation and incorrect choice of words. A decrement of alpha waves appears in the EEG, and closing of the eyes no longer generates alpha activity.

Recovery after prolonged sleep deprivation shows that the amount of sleep required to recuperate is never equal to the amount lost. During the first recovery sleep period the subject rapidly falls into stage IV of NREM sleep, often with "supernormal" slow waves in the EEG, and remains there at the expense of stage II sleep; REM sleep is decreased. By the second night, there is REM sleep "rebound" which exceeds that of the predeprivation period.

The effects of partial and differential deprivation are difficult to test. Total REM sleep deprivation cannot be sustained for more than a few days. Episodes of REM sleep begin to intrude rapidly into the waking state, making it impossible to maintain total deprivation. There is no convincing evidence that selective REM sleep deprivation leads to psychological instability or psychosis.

SLEEP DISORDERS Sleep disorders can occur at any period of life. Some are peculiar to specific age groups, such as nocturnal enuresis, night terrors, and somnambulism in children and adolescents, and insomnia and hypersomnia in middle and old age. Others, such as the narcolepsy-cataplexy syndrome, may begin in childhood and persist throughout life.

Data on the prevalence of sleep disorders are fragmentary, but it appears that between 8 and 15 percent of the adult population in the United States has frequent and chronic complaints about the quality and the amount of their sleep. From 3 to 11 percent of adults use sedative-hypnotic drugs and the percentage increases with age. Sleep disorders are a major problem both in terms of the frequency of complaint and the tendency to excessive drug usage, but also because there is evidence for an increased risk of mortality in persons with chronic sleep disorders.

The classification of sleep disorders is still evolving. Recently, a committee of the Association of Sleep Disorders Centers proposed a classification based principally on clinical symptomatology (see Table 19-1 and reference by Weitzman).

Insomnia Insomnia, defined as want of sleep, is used popularly to indicate any impairment in duration, depth, or restorative properties of sleep. Sleep depth and duration are so variable and complaints of insomnia so common as to raise difficult questions about when complaints of too little sleep are to be regarded as abnormal. Insomnia may occur as a primary disorder or be associated with other disorders of sleep such as sleep apnea and the hypoventilation syndromes. Insomnia may also be a secondary manifestation of the affective disorders, of psychoneurosis, and of anxiety, or occur with the use of drugs or alcohol.

The term *primary insomnia* is applied when individuals throughout life have a persistent disorder of restful, restorative sleep. There may be symptoms of difficulty falling asleep, of frequent awakening, or of persistent early morning arousal, each contributing to feelings of chronic fatigue and irritability. Such individuals may show no evidence of a neurosis or a psychosomatic disorder. Sleep recordings may confirm that such individuals sleep for shorter periods than normal persons, awaken more often, spend less time in stages III and IV of NREM sleep, and have decreased REM sleep. As data on sleep disorders accumulate it becomes apparent that many such individuals are better classified in other categories, such as sleep apnea.

INSOMNIA ASSOCIATED WITH THE AFFECTIVE PSYCHIATRIC DISORDERS The sleep abnormalities found in the affective disorders consist of chronic or recurrent inability to maintain sleep through the expected sleep period. Patients complain of persistent restlessness at night and of a tired, "washed-out" feeling during the day. More frequent arousal throughout the night, failure to "sleep deeply," and early morning awakening complete the clinical picture.

The affective disorders have been divided into major depressive and bipolar (manic-depressive) disorders (see Chap. 376). Patients with unipolar depression have different sleep patterns from those with bipolar depression. The sleep disorder in unipolar depression is characterized by repeated awakenings with a shortened REM latency (time from sleep onset to first episode of REM sleep) and decreased stages III and IV NREM sleep. By contrast, patients with bipolar depression often have excessive daytime sleepiness (take naps) and have extended sleep periods at night. Despite documented polygraph recordings showing "normal" sleep periods of 5 to 6 h, patients with bipolar depression awaken feeling unrefreshed. During periods of hypomania, partial or total sleeplessness may occur lasting for several days.

INSOMNIAS ASSOCIATED WITH THE USE OF DRUGS AND ALCOHOL The widespread use and abuse of central nervous system depressants (hypnotic and sedative drugs, tranquilizers, or bedtime use of alcohol) is well documented. Psychopathology is present in many insomniac patients, and most fail to respond to hypnotics for more than a short period of time. The effectiveness of long-term use (greater than 30 days) of any hypnotic drug has not been established. Flurazepam (Dalmane) is now the most frequently used "sleeping pill" in the United States.

Tolerance to or withdrawal from central nervous system depressants may produce drug-dependency insomnia. The short-term sleep-inducing and sleep-maintaining effects of such drugs are lost, and the patient and the physician often increase the dosage or combine it with other drugs. Specific sleep-disturbing symptoms caused by partial withdrawal can develop, even though administration of the drug is continued. The symptoms are often misinterpreted as evidence of persistence of the underlying insomniac syndrome. Sleep studies in patients who regularly and chronically use hypnotic agents demonstrate that sleep is interrupted by frequent awakenings lasting more than 5 min, especially during the second half of the night. As the drug's effectiveness decreases, partial withdrawal occurs each night and contributes to the early morning arousal. Stages III and IV and REM sleep are decreased, and sleep-stage demarcations are less clear. These observations point to a considerable degree of sleep disorganization.

The sleep pattern is very disrupted following rapid or acute withdrawal from hypnotic agents that have been used chronically in high daily doses. A high percentage of REM sleep appears, presumably due to a compensatory REM rebound. Sleep-related periodic movements (nocturnal myoclonus) may also occur during the withdrawal period. In addition, daytime symptoms appear, including restlessness, nervousness, generalized muscle aches, and, in severe cases, drug withdrawal symptoms, including confusion, hallucinations, and grand mal convulsions. These complications are most common after barbiturate and glutethimide (Doriden) withdrawal. In patients who are chronic high-dose and multiple hypnotic drug users, withdrawal should be gradual and direct patient supervision should be continued after withdrawal. Many patients show remarkable improvement in both objective and subjective sleep patterns, although they may not return immediately to a fully normal sleep.

With heavy and sustained ingestion of alcohol, sleep-stage organization is severely disrupted. REM sleep periods are abbreviated and associated intrusive awakenings occur. Acute withdrawal from alcohol in the chronic alcoholic leads to a lengthening of the sleep onset time, a decrease in total sleep, and an increase in REM sleep. The REM latency shortens. If severe, acute toxic withdrawal syndrome (delirium tremens) may develop. In the chronic "dried out" alcoholic, an abnormal sleep pattern may persist for many weeks, although most show a return to normal sleep within 2 weeks.

TABLE 19-1
Classification of sleep disorders

I Insomnias: Disorders of initiating and maintaining sleep
- *A* Psychophysiological—transient or persistent
- *B* Associated with psychiatric disorders, particularly affective disorders
- *C* Associated with drugs and alcohol
  - *1* Sustained use of or withdrawal from drugs
  - *2* Chronic alcoholism
  - *3* Tolerance to or withdrawal from CNS depressants
  - *4* Sustained use of CNS stimulants
- *D* Associated with sleep-induced respiratory impairment
  - *1* Sleep apnea syndrome
  - *2* Alveolar hypoventilation syndrome
- *E* Associated with sleep-related (nocturnal) myoclonus or "restless legs"
- *F* Miscellaneous—other medical, toxic, or environmental conditions

II Hypersomnias: Disorders of excessive somnolence
- *A* Psychophysiological—transient or persistent
- *B* Associated with psychiatric disorders, particularly affective disorders
- *C* Associated with use of drugs or alcohol
- *D* Associated with sleep-induced respiratory impairment (as in D above)
- *E* Narcolepsy-cataplexy
- *F* Miscellaneous and idiopathic
  - *1* Kleine-Levin syndrome

III Disorders of the sleep-wake schedule
- *A* Transient—jet lag, work shift
- *B* Persistent
  - *1* Delayed sleep phase syndrome
  - *2* Advanced sleep phase syndrome
  - *3* Non-24-h sleep-wake syndrome

IV Dysfunctions associated with sleep, sleep stages, or partial arousal (parasomnias)
- *A* Sleepwalking
- *B* Sleep terrors
- *C* Enuresis
- *D* Other sleep-related events
  - *1* Seizures
  - *2* Cluster headaches
  - *3* Gastroesophageal reflux
  - *4* Sleep palsies

OTHER CAUSES OF INSOMNIA Recurrent pain due to spinal cord or nerve root involvement or to abdominal discomfort secondary to gastrointestinal disorders may also cause insomnia. Tired, aching, restless legs, an obscure benign state known as the "restless legs syndrome," may regularly delay the onset of sleep. Paresthesia of the fingers secondary to carpal tunnel syndrome may awaken the patient at night. Patients who complain of frequent awakenings and restless, unrefreshing sleep may have sleep apnea or hypoventilation (see below).

In some patients with primary insomnia and in many with other forms of insomnia, *periodic movements of sleep* (PMS) occur, usually during NREM sleep. The movements consist of stereotyped, repetitive dorsiflexion of the foot and toes and sometimes flexion of the knee and hip. They are to be distinguished from the common and benign "night starts" which occur at the onset of sleep. Sleep recordings indicate that PMS occur in a wide variety of sleep disorders. In one study, 53 of 409 patients (13 percent) showed the disorder, including patients with narcolepsy-cataplexy, sleep apnea, drug-dependency insomnia, and the restless legs syndrome. The symptoms appear to be secondary to a chronic sleep-wake disturbance rather than representing a primary disorder.

Movements similar to PMS have been observed in patients with *Parkinson's disease* receiving high dosages of L-dopa, and in patients with narcolepsy on high doses of chlorimipramine for the treatment of cataplexy. Although a wide variety of drugs have been tried in clinical and experimental treatment trials, none has been clearly effective in eliminating PMS. The neurophysiological mechanisms responsible for PMS are unknown.

Restless legs syndrome is a disorder in which the afflicted individual feels an irresistible urge to move the legs, generally when sitting or lying down, and especially in bed, at night, just prior to getting to sleep. The patient has an extremely unpleasant deep discomfort inside the calves, which, although not truly painful, is perceived as a "dysease," requiring that the legs be moved. This interferes with sleep onset but may also recur during the night. Usually by morning the restless legs symptoms have either disappeared or become considerably attenuated, and the patient is able to fall asleep more easily. PMS is present in all cases of restless legs syndrome studied polygraphically.

APPROACH TO THE PATIENT WITH INSOMNIA In order to understand the nature of the sleep disturbances causing insomnia, it is important to document the sleep-wake rhythm of the patient. A sleep log provided by the patient (and the bed partner) may be helpful to the physician. Observations of snoring, grinding of teeth (bruxism), or kicking may point to a more specific diagnosis.

For best management of insomnia, treatment should be based on the symptoms exhibited by the patient. There are three types of complaints. The first is the inability to fall asleep. For these patients, if the condition is chronic, a short trial (not longer than 2 to 3 weeks) of flurazepam, 15 to 60 mg; chloral hydrate (Noctec), 500 to 1000 mg; glutethimide, 500 mg; or methaqualone (Sopor), 150 to 300 mg, may be given 15 to 30 min before going to bed. Flurazepam has less REM sleep–suppressing effects than the others.

The second type of insomnia is exhibited by patients who are able to go to sleep but who awaken in 2 or 3 h and are alternately awake and asleep the rest of the night. Sometimes these are persons with a debilitating or painful illness which generates more pain and restlessness as muscles relax to leave painful areas unsplinted. Medical illness such as paroxysmal nocturnal dyspnea, nocturnal asthma, and discomforts associated with rheumatic or gastrointestinal disorders may cause insomnia. These conditions should receive appropriate attention and treatment. For patients with midsleep insomnia, administration of flurazepam, 30 to 60 mg, at bedtime may be beneficial. Recurrent pain causing wakefulness after an initial period of sleep may be treated with aspirin, 0.3 to 0.6 g, together with a sedative. Occasionally, codeine phosphate, 30 mg; meperidine (Demerol), 50 mg; or morphine sulfate, 10 to 15 mg, may be required when pain is severe.

The third type of insomnia is seen in patients who go to sleep promptly and sleep well most of the night, only to awaken too early in the morning. Some of these individuals are older persons who turn night into day. They go to bed and get up earlier and earlier and are soon sleeping during the day and are alert during the night. Into this category commonly fall individuals with depression and anxiety who are overworked and exhausted. They face sleep easily through sheer exhaustion, but awaken around 4 or 5 A.M. with worry and discouragement, unable to get back to sleep.

Changes in working patterns and establishment of a regular exercise regimen may be of more benefit in the treatment of such individuals than prescription of sedative drugs, which are largely ineffective. Patients with serious psychiatric illness or dementia require appropriate attention. For frankly delirious or psychotic patients, the administration of potent antipsychotic drugs is required; chlorpromazine (Thorazine), 25 to 50 mg tid, and haloperidol (Haldol), 1 to 5 mg tid, are sometimes effective. Depression is treated by nighttime administration of antidepressant drugs such as amitriptyline (Elavil), 100 to 150 mg; desipramine (Norpramin), 100 to 150 mg; or phenelzine (Nardil), a monoamine oxidase inhibitor, 45 to 60 mg. Several new non-drug-related treatments for depression are currently under study, including manipulation of the timing of sleep within the circadian rhythm. Progressive *phase advance* of the onset of sleep has been reported to reverse acutely the depressive phase in bipolar depression.

The widespread use of the benzodiazepines as nighttime sedatives is now complicated by recognition of certain undesirable properties. First, they are mildly addictive; second, rebound insomnia following intermediate-term use may occur; and, third, there is buildup of active metabolites which may have a biological effect for 36 to 48 h.

DISORDERS OF EXCESSIVE SOMNOLENCE These disorders are typified by inappropriate and undesirable sleepiness leading to sleep during a time when the patient wishes to be awake. The patient complains of an irresistible urge to sleep during the day, decreased concentration, excessive yawning, and an increase in total sleep time over a 24-h period. The complaint of excessive sleep need should be distinguished from other symptoms of lethargy, fatigue, and lack of motivation that commonly accompany anxiety or depression.

A classification of disorders of excessive daytime somnolence is given in Table 19-1. In clinical practice two major disorders, sleep-induced respiratory impairment and the narcolepsy-cataplexy syndrome, account for about 80 percent of patients with complaints of hypersomnia.

Sleep-induced respiratory impairment (the sleep apnea–hypersomnia syndrome) Excessive daytime somnolence is the primary complaint. In addition, disturbing nighttime symptoms occur in almost all patients. They are observed to have periods of sleep apnea and inspiratory snoring. The snoring tends to increase in prominence over a period of 20 to 60 s, culminating in a series of loud, partially obstructive gasps. Brief arousal followed by a variable period of apnea ensues. Episodes recur in a cyclic pattern. The patient often talks during sleep (somniloquy) and awakens in the morning unrefreshed, tired, and sleepy, often with a generalized headache.

In adults, the ratio of men to women with the sleep apnea–hypersomnia syndrome is 15:1 to 25:1, and the age range is the fourth to sixth decade. Approximately two-thirds of the patients are obese (Pickwickian syndrome). A rapid weight gain may precipitate or increase the severity of the symptoms.

Hypertension, often severe, may be associated. Direct endoscopic observations of the airway during the apneic episode show that the site of obstruction is in the oral pharynx at the level of the velopharyngeal sphincter. Obstruction is caused by apposition of the lateral pharyngeal walls and by posterior movement of the base of the tongue (obstructive apnea). Apnea may also result in such patients from cessation of respiratory movements (central or nonobstructive sleep apnea—Ondine's curse) or from partial obstruction (subobstructive apnea). Each of these patterns of apnea may be present in an individual patient.

The period of apnea may result in oxygen desaturation (often below 50 percent), bradycardia alternating with tachycardia, and transient episodes of cardiac arrhythmias or brief asystole. The cause of the respiratory abnormality is unknown. It may occur with central failure of respiratory regulation in association with obesity, or with narrowing of the upper airway secondary to enlarged tonsils or adenoids, mandibular shortening, or pharyngeal soft tissue masses. Disorders of the respiratory neuromuscular apparatus (chronic poliomyelitis, myotonic dystrophy) may also lead to symptoms. The common lack of identifiable otolaryngologic abnormalities during wakefulness suggests a role of airway incoordination in the pathogenesis of sleep apnea.

The most effective treatment is the establishment of an adequate airway, which in severe cases may require tracheotomy. Other treatments for milder forms have included tricyclic antidepressants, progesterone (in children), and weight loss. Improvement in night sleep is followed by reduction in daytime sleepiness.

Narcolepsy and cataplexy The narcolepsy-cataplexy syndrome is a distinct clinical entity characterized by recurrent attacks of uncontrollable daytime sleepiness (*narcolepsy*) and sudden decreases in muscle tone (*cataplexy*). It is estimated that the disorder occurs with a prevalence of 40 per 100,000 population. It affects men and women equally, usually begins in adolescence or early childhood, and is a lifelong illness. The daytime sleepiness occurs episodically and irresistibly, especially when the patient is physically inactive. The impulse to sleep is so insistent that it may be impossible to sit through a single class in school or drive a car. The subject appears to enter a natural sleep; the eyes close, breathing slows, and the head falls forward. The period of sleep usually lasts 10 to 20 min and the subject may awaken refreshed. In about 80 percent of cases, there is also a history of *cataplexy*, characterized by sudden, brief episodes of loss of muscle tone without loss of consciousness. Cataplexy is commonly triggered by an emotional event such as laughter, anger, fear, or surprise. In its most severe form, the cataplectic attack results in total flaccid paralysis (with sparing of diaphragmatic and extraocular eye muscle movements), resulting in collapse to the floor. Less severe symptoms may consist of sagging of the jaw or head, speechlessness, or a feeling of weakening of the knees. Full recovery occurs within a minute or two. Two other symptoms complete the clinical tetrad of the narcolepsy-cataplexy syndrome. *Sleep paralysis* is a frightening sensation of inability to move the voluntary muscles, occurring at the transition of sleep onset or at awakening. *Vivid hallucinations* (usually visual) may occur either at sleep onset (hypnagogic) or on awakening (hypnopompic). Narcoleptics frequently complain that despite troublesome daytime sleepiness night sleep is also disturbed and unrestful.

PATHOPHYSIOLOGY Narcolepsy may occur as a familial genetic disorder; animal models with autosomal recessive transmission are described in dogs and horses. The central nervous system localization of the defect in narcolepsy is unknown. Lesions in the pontomesencephalic reticular formation of the brainstem have been described in a few cases. Narcolepsy is best understood as a disorder of the REM sleep process due to increased activity of the pontine REM sleep generator. The sleep attacks that occur suddenly during the waking state are often sleep-onset REM attacks, and cataplexy, with loss of muscle tone, resembles the quiescent state of the EMG during REM sleep. Hypnagogic hallucinations and sleep paralysis are the subjective equivalent of dreaming and muscle paralysis, respectively, which occur at the waking-sleeping interphase as manifestations of the activated REM state. The hypothesis proposed by Hobson of diminished aminergic and increased cholinergic tone resulting in an enhanced REM state is supported by the evidence obtained from the effectiveness of the drugs used in treatment of the disorder.

TREATMENT The treatment of narcolepsy is symptomatic. Two separate classes of drugs are effective in the management of narcolepsy and cataplexy, respectively. Narcoleptics may show improvement with strategically timed naps (during lunch hour or after meals), but most require administration of central adrenergic stimulant drugs. Methylphenidate (Ritalin), 10 mg two to three times daily, or amphetamine sulfate (Benzedrine), 5 to 10 mg three to four times daily, are given to sustain the patient through the most difficult periods of the day. Late afternoon or evening administration should be avoided since it may interfere with night sleep. Cataplexy responds best to imipramine (Tofranil) or desipramine, in doses ranging from 75 to 200 mg daily. These drugs suppress REM sleep by facilitation of adrenergic transmission and inhibition of cholinergic systems. Each class of drugs should be titrated separately to achieve best results for the symptoms of narcolepsy and cataplexy, respectively.

Other conditions associated with excessive daytime somnolence The Kleine-Levin syndrome (periodic hypersomnia) is a rare disorder that first presents between the ages of 12 and 20. It is more common in men but is also described in women. Recurrent periods of hypersomnolence lasting from a few days to several weeks alternate with asymptomatic intervals of months or years.

During a bout of hypersomnolence, the patient develops a voracious appetite and may exhibit disturbances in mood, show sexual hyperactivity and exhibitionism, and have hallucinations, disorientation, and memory deficits. The condition is usually self-limited, rarely occurring beyond the fourth or fifth decade. The cause is unknown and no specific neuropathology has been reported, although the disorder has been postulated to be a dysfunction of limbic and hypothalamic rhythms. Rarely, cerebrospinal fluid pleocytosis has been found, which suggests that an episode of encephalitis may underlie the disorder in some cases.

Excessive somnolence is a feature of many endocrine and metabolic disorders, including uremia, liver failure, hypothyroidism (severe, with myxedema), chronic pulmonary disease (with hypercapnia), and diabetes mellitus with incipient coma or with severe hypoglycemia. In addition, hypersomnolence may occur in other central nervous system disorders, such as a tumor in the area of the third ventricle (glioma, pinealoma, dysgerminoma, craniopharyngioma, pituitary adenoma), obstructive hydrocephalus, viral encephalitis, and other infections of the brain and its surrounding membranes. Although uncommon, excessive daytime somnolence also can occur in various degenerative diseases of the brain, including dementia of the Alzheimer type, multiple sclerosis, and cerebrovascular disease. The postconcussion syndrome has been associated with increased sleepiness. In all the above conditions, it is important to distinguish complaints of tiredness, fatigue, depression, lack of interest, malaise, and lethargy secondary to metabolic, endocrine, neurologic, and psychiatric disease from sleepiness per se.

DISORDERS OF THE SLEEP-WAKE SCHEDULE Recent observations of the physiology of human sleep and its disorders have revealed the importance of circadian timekeeping systems. Normal humans studied in controlled laboratory conditions have demonstrated that the preferred length of the "free-running" period for humans is approximately 25 h. Measurements of body temperature and sleep duration and sleep-stage organization have shown that consistent changes of timing relationships between body temperature and the sleep-wake cycle occur and that different physiologic rhythms develop independent cycle lengths under such time-isolated conditions. This has led to the hypothesis that multiple oscillators exist that are normally synchronized with each other but which can become desynchronized in certain sleep disorders.

Disorders of the circadian sleep-wake cycle are classified under two major categories, transient and persistent. In the transient category, the dyssomnia of a rapid time-zone change ("jet lag") is very familiar, as is that found in an acute work-shift change. The sleep disturbance that results is due to both sleep deprivation and the circadian phase-shift change. The symptoms vary considerably from subject to subject, but generally consist of a deficiency in the sustained sleep period, with frequent arousals primarily at the end of the sleep episode associated with excessive daytime sleepiness and falling asleep at inappropriate times. For varying periods of time (usually several days to 2 weeks), the person affected is intermittently sleepy, fatigued, and inattentive during the waking period, with partial insomnia during the sleep period.

The persistent category of the sleep-wake cycle disorders is divided into three subcategories: (1) delayed sleep phase syndrome, (2) advanced sleep phase syndrome, and (3) non-24-h sleep-wake syndrome. The delayed sleep phase syndrome is a sleep disorder that can be differentiated from other forms of insomnia. The patient reports a chronic inability to fall asleep at a desired clock time required to meet work or study schedules, typically being unable to fall asleep until 2 to 6 A.M. However, when not required to maintain a strict schedule (e.g., weekends, holidays, and vacation periods), the patient will sleep without difficulty and after a sleep period of normal length will awaken spontaneously, feeling refreshed. Such patients have been successfully treated by a progressive phase delay of the sleep time (chronotherapy). By delaying the time of going to sleep by 3 h each day (i.e., a 27-h sleep-wake cycle) the patient's sleep timing can be "reset" to occur at the clock time preferred by the patient.

It has been suggested that individuals who have chronic sleep-onset and wake times that are undesirably early but who have no disturbance of the sleep process itself might fall into the category of an *advanced sleep phase syndrome.* Since the "early to bed—early to rise" rhythm conforms very well with our socioeconomic and solar-day timing systems, these individuals rarely seek medical or psychological help. The process of aging leads to a characteristic change in the timing of sleep such that older individuals spontaneously awaken earlier in the morning and become sleepy and go to sleep earlier in the evening.

The non-24-h sleep-wake (hypernyctohemeral) syndrome is characterized by an inability to be entrained to society's 24-h day. These individuals develop a 25- to 27-h biological day length in spite of all attempts to do otherwise. Blindness or a personality disorder may predispose to this condition.

DYSFUNCTIONS ASSOCIATED WITH SLEEP, SLEEP STAGES, OR PARTIAL AROUSALS (PARASOMNIAS) There is a group of conditions in which undesirable behavioral and physiologic events occur in association with or during sleep but in which the sleep and waking process per se is not abnormal. In the present state of our knowledge, it seems best to use clinical descriptions, although an attempt has been made to organize several of these around the concept of "disorders of the state of partial arousal."

Sleepwalking (somnambulism) This condition consists of a sudden behavioral sequence that interrupts the quiet state of sleep by a motor performance that consists of either sitting up in bed or leaving the bed and walking about. Full consciousness does not occur. Somnambulism characteristically occurs during stage III or IV of NREM sleep. The complex behavior includes repetitive automatic and semipurposeful motor acts such as dressing, walking, opening and closing doors, and climbing stairs. On occasion patients will carry out an act that may be harmful to themselves, such as climbing out a window. Patients are not easily arousable during the episode and typically will strongly resist being aroused. The episode generally lasts no more than 15 min and is terminated by either a spontaneous arousal, returning to the bed, or going to sleep in another place. There is no evidence of seizure activity either preceding or during the episode, although clinically it must be distinguished from a nocturnal seizure disorder originating in the temporal lobes.

Somnambulism occurs normally in children and adolescents; 15 percent of all children have one or more episodes. A small percent of children (1 to 6 percent) have frequent attacks (at times, nightly). If the episodes persist into adulthood or begin in adulthood, there is a high association with serious psychopathology.

Nightmares and night terrors (pavor nocturnus) Awakening in a state of terror is an occasional occurrence familiar to nearly everyone. Such attacks are most common in children and are best understood as a state of partial arousal from stage III or IV NREM sleep. Almost without exception, the attacks occur during the first 1 to 2 h of sleep and are characterized by a frightened vocalization and sitting up in bed, with agitated and panicked behavior. Autonomic changes appear, including sweating, tachycardia, hyperventilation, and pupillary dilatation. It may be difficult to arouse the child fully and the attack may persist for several minutes. There is no report of dream imagery after the attack, which differentiates the episode from a nightmare. Typically, the child falls asleep again and has no memory for the event the following morning. Night terrors are almost always benign and time-limited so that reassurance is both adequate and sufficient. Differentiation between night terrors and nightmares (which occur during REM sleep) is important because the latter are more likely to reflect underlying psychological conflicts, particularly if they are recurrent.

Sleep-related enuresis Bed-wetting occurs during stage III and IV of NREM sleep, usually during the first third of the night. Primary enuresis is the persistence of bed-wetting from infancy to childhood, whereas secondary enuresis occurs after a period of successful toilet training. Both need to be distinguished from symptomatic enuresis, which is caused by a known organic lesion affecting bladder regulation. All forms need to be separated from nocturnal seizures associated with incontinence.

Nocturnal seizures Paroxysmal abnormalities of brain electrical activity of the type seen in seizure disorders sometimes occur in epileptic patients during or shortly after the onset of sleep. An individual subject to grand mal attacks may have them only at night during sleep. They are often accompanied by tongue biting and incontinence and by muscle soreness the following day.

Sleep-related cluster headaches Many patients with cluster headaches or migraine have attacks during sleep. A cluster headache awakens the patient with severe pain either directly out of REM sleep or in the immediate post-REM period. Cluster headaches are characterized by the rapid development of severe unilateral eye and upper facial pain in association with tearing, rhinorrhea, and conjunctival redness. An ipsilateral Horner's syndrome may be present. Nausea may also occur. The attack may last from 30 min to several hours.

Sleep-related gastroesophageal reflux The clinical symptoms of sleep-related gastroesophageal reflux are recurrent awakening from sleep with a burning substernal pain (heartburn) associated with a sour taste, coughing, choking, and respiratory discomfort. These symptoms are often associated with postprandial regurgitation, dysphagia, esophagitis, laryngopharyngitis, and heartburn during the waking state. Recent studies have demonstrated that gastric acid refluxes into the lower esophagus during sleep and that a decreased clearing mechanism is present.

Sleep palsies Curious and at times distressing paresthetic disturbances develop during sleep. Everyone is familiar with the phenomenon of an arm or leg "falling asleep." The ulnar, radial, and peroneal nerves are most often affected. If pressure is continued for half an hour or longer, a sensory or motor paralysis, sometimes referred to as "sleep palsy," may develop. This condition usually lasts only a few minutes or hours, but if the compression is prolonged, the nerve may be severely damaged so that functional recovery must await remyelination or regeneration. Unusually deep sleep, as in alcoholic intoxication, renders the patient especially liable to sleep palsies merely because the patient does not heed the discomfort of an unnatural posture (Saturday night palsy).

REFERENCES

COLEMAN R et al: Periodic movements in sleep (nocturnal myoclonus): Relation to sleep disorders. Ann Neurol 8:416, 1980

CZEISLER CA et al: Human sleep: Its duration and organization depend on its circadian phase. Science 210:1264, 1980

GUILLEMINAULT C, DEMENT WC: Two hundred thirty-five cases of excessive daytime sleepiness: Diagnosis and tentative classification. J Chron Dis 29:733, 1976

GUILLEMINAULT C et al: The sleep apnea syndromes. Ann Rev Med 27:465, 1976

HOBSON JA, BRAZIER MAB (eds): *The Reticular Formation Revisited.* New York, Raven Press, 1980

JOUVET M: Neurophysiology of the states of sleep. Physiol Rev 47:117, 1967

KALES A, KALES JD: Recent findings in the diagnosis and treatment of disturbed sleep. N Engl J Med 290:487, 1974

PAPPENHEIMER JR et al: Peptides in cerebrospinal fluid and their relation to sleep and activity, in *Brain Dysfunction in Metabolic Disorders,* F Plum (ed). *Res Publ Assoc Nerv Ment Dis,* New York, Raven Press, 1974, vol 53, p 201

WEITZMAN E: Disorders of sleep and the sleep-wake cycle, in *Update I: Harrison's Principles of Internal Medicine.* New York, McGraw-Hill, 1981, p 245

20
COMA AND OTHER DISORDERS OF CONSCIOUSNESS

ALLAN H. ROPPER
JOSEPH B. MARTIN

Coma is a common problem in general medicine, and a systematic approach to its diagnosis and management is essential. It is estimated that up to 3 percent of total admissions to the emergency ward of large municipal hospitals is due to diseases that cause a disorder of consciousness. Such data serve to emphasize the importance of this class of neurologic disorders and point to the necessity to acquire a theoretic as well as a practical knowledge of coma.

The increased availability of computerized tomography (CT) has resulted in an artificial orientation to the diagnosis of coma by focusing attention on lesions that are detectable by CT (e.g., hemorrhages, tumors, or hydrocephalus). This approach, although at times expedient, is often imprudent. The physician confronted with an unresponsive patient should formulate a differential diagnosis based on the history and the clinical signs before leaving the bedside. Certain signs observed during general and neurologic examination allow the physician to decide which of several generic diseases is responsible for coma, thus limiting the diagnostic possibilities. A rational approach to the precise diagnosis and subsequent management can then be planned and clinical changes anticipated. The clinical approach to diagnosis must also be coupled with knowledge of the pathologic entities that cause coma. This chapter describes a practical approach to coma based on the anatomy and physiology of consciousness and a consideration of the general and neurologic examination and CT.

Coma is epitomized by unresponsiveness and as such is easily recognized. The interesting and sometimes subtle distinctions made between coma, stupor, and drowsiness are largely semantic because there is no anatomical or physiological basis for distinguishing them except as relative degrees of unresponsiveness. A narrative description of the clinical state of the patient and of responses evoked by various stimuli, precisely as they are observed at the bedside, remains the optimal way to characterize coma and related disturbances of consciousness. Such a description is preferable to summary terms such as *stupor, semicoma,* or *obtundation,* which are often ambiguous and commonly differ between observers.

Although the definition of consciousness is a psychological and philosophical matter, the distinction between *level* of consciousness, or wakefulness, and *content* of consciousness, or awareness, has physiological significance. The neurologist views awareness as composed of integrated and organized material thoughts, subjective experience, emotions, and mental processes, each of which resides to some extent in anatomically defined regions of the brain. The inability to maintain a coherent sequence of thoughts and actions is called *confusion* and is a disorder of content of consciousness. In contrast, wakefulness is maintained by a diffuse system of upper brainstem and thalamic neurons, the reticular activating system (RAS), and its connections to the cerebral hemispheres as a whole. Therefore, depression of either hemispheral or RAS activity may cause reduced wakefulness. Reduced wakefulness often precludes evaluation of content of consciousness, but content of consciousness can be severely impaired, as in confusion, without affecting arousal. Because drowsy or stuporous patients are often also confused, diagnostic considerations should address the primary problem as an alteration in the level of consciousness.

ANATOMICAL CORRELATES OF CONSCIOUSNESS A normal level of consciousness (wakefulness) depends upon activation of the cerebral hemispheres by groups of neurons located in the brainstem RAS. Both of the cerebral hemispheres, the RAS, and the connections between them must be preserved for normal consciousness. The principal causes of coma are, therefore, (1) bilateral hemispheral damage and (2) a brainstem lesion that damages the RAS. There is some evidence that large, purely unilateral hemispheral lesions may cause drowsiness (though not coma), even in the absence of damage to the opposite hemisphere or RAS.

Reticular activating system The RAS is best defined as a physiological system, not an anatomical one. It is contained within the reticular formation, which consists of loosely grouped neurons located bilaterally in the medial tegmental gray matter of the brainstem extending from the medulla to the posterior diencephalon. These neurons have been shown in neuroanatomical studies to span long rostrocaudal distances within the reticular formation. Animal experiments and human clinical-neuropathological observations have established that the *neurons located in the region extending from the rostral pons* *to the caudal diencephalon are of primary importance for maintaining wakefulness.* Lesions here produce coma by damaging the RAS. Such lesions also commonly affect adjacent brainstem structures concerned with control of pupillary constriction and mechanisms for eye movements (Fig. 20-1). Abnormalities in these systems on physical examination provide signposts of brainstem damage. Lesions confined to the cerebral hemispheres do not directly affect the brainstem RAS, though secondary damage may result from transtentorial herniation of a cerebral hemisphere.

Brainstem RAS neurons project rostrally to the cortex, primarily via "nonspecific" thalamic relay nuclei. The relay nuclei exert a tonic influence on the cerebral cortex and are considered a part of the RAS. Experimental work suggests that the brainstem RAS indirectly affects the level of consciousness by suppressing the activity of the nonspecific nuclei. Electrical stimulation of the pontine and midbrain RAS desynchronizes the electroencephalogram (EEG), a pattern associated with behavioral arousal. Stimulation of the thalamic relay nuclei opposes this activity, resulting in synchronization and slowing of the EEG. Consciousness can be disturbed by lesions of the upper pontine, midbrain, or diencephalic components of the RAS. Conversely, the basis of behavioral arousal by environmental stimuli (somesthetic, auditory, and visual) depends on the rich innervation of the RAS by each sensory system.

The relay between the RAS and thalamic and cortical areas is accomplished by neurotransmitters. Of these, the influence of acetylcholine on arousal is the best established. Cholinergic fibers connect the midbrain to other areas of the upper brainstem, thalamus, and cortex. These pathways are thought to mediate the clinical and EEG arousal observed after administration of cholinergic drugs such as physostigmine. Specialized groups of biogenic amine-containing neurons in the midbrain and pons are also known to project diffusely to the cortex. Serotoninergic and noradrenergic fibers subserve important functions in the regulation of the sleep-wake cycle (see Chap. 19). Their roles in arousal and coma have not been clearly established, although the alerting effects of amphetamines are thought to be mediated by catecholamine release.

Cerebral hemispheres and consciousness The specialized functions of the cerebral cortex in language, control of movement, and perception are regionalized. In contrast, wakefulness is related in a semiquantitative way to the total mass of functioning cortex (and RAS connections) and is not focally represented in the hemispheres. Hemispheral lesions may cause coma in one of three ways: (1) bilateral, generalized hemispheral lesions or metabolic derangements such as occur in encephalitis, generalized epilepsy, drug ingestion, ischemia, and hypoglycemia interfere with awareness in a graded fashion as more cortical territory is damaged or rendered functionally inactive; (2) enlarging masses or secondary brain swelling initially confined to one side of the brain may compress the contralateral hemisphere, effectively creating bilateral hemispheral lesions; and (3) large lesions in one or both hemispheres may compress the brainstem and diencephalon causing coma indirectly by damaging the RAS. The degree of decrease in alertness is often related to the acuteness of onset of the cortical dysfunction.

PATHOPHYSIOLOGY OF COMA The pathophysiological basis of coma is either mechanical destruction of crucial areas of the brainstem or cerebral cortex (anatomical coma) or global disruption of brain metabolic processes (metabolic coma). Coma of metabolic origin may be produced by interruption of energy substrate delivery (hypoxia, ischemia, hypoglycemia) or by alteration of the neurophysiological responses of neuronal membranes (drug or alcohol intoxication, epilepsy, or acute head injury).

The brain is markedly dependent on continuous blood flow and delivery of oxygen and glucose. They are consumed at rates of 3.5 ml per 100 g per minute and 5 mg per 100 g per minute, respectively. Brain stores of glucose provide energy for approximately 2 min after blood flow is interrupted, although consciousness is lost within 8 to 10 s. When hypoxia occurs simultaneously with ischemia, available glucose is exhausted more rapidly. Normal resting cerebral blood flow (CBF) is approximately 75 ml per 100 g per minute in gray matter and 30 ml per 100 g per minute in white matter (mean = 55 ml per 100 g per minute). This provides for adequate metabolic supplies with a modest safety factor to accommodate most physiologic changes. When mean CBF diminishes to 25 ml per 100 g per minute the EEG becomes diffusely slowed (typical of metabolic encephalopathies), and at 15 ml per 100 g per minute brain electrical activity ceases. If all other conditions such as temperature and arterial oxygenation remain normal, CBF less than 10 ml per 100 g per minute causes irrevocable brain damage.

Coma due to hyponatremia, hyperosmolarity, hypercapnia, and the encephalopathies of hepatic and renal failure are associated with a variety of metabolic derangements of neurons and astrocytes. The toxic effects of these conditions on the brain are frequently multifactorial, producing impaired energy supplies, changes in resting membrane potentials, neurotransmitter abnormalities, and in some instances morphological changes. For example, hepatic coma may be related in part to a high brain ammonia concentration which interferes with cerebral energy metabolism and the Na-K-ATPase pump. The increased number and size of astrocytes seen in the brains of patients who die as a result of hepatic encephalopathy may contribute to neurologic symptoms. This change may be due to the need to detoxify ammonia. In addition, abnormalities of neurotransmitters have been found in experimental hepatic coma, including possible "false" neurotransmitters, which may act competitively at monoaminergic receptor sites.

The exact cause of the encephalopathy of renal failure is also poorly understood. Urea itself does not produce nervous system toxicity. A multifactorial cause is likely, including increased permeability of the blood-brain barrier to toxic substances such as organic acids and an increase in brain calcium or cerebrospinal fluid (CSF) phosphate content. Cellular membrane potentials change in uremia due to brain potassium shifts, but the magnitude of this effect is small and unlikely to account for neurologic symptoms. Parathyroid hormone excess may also play a part in uremic encephalopathy.

Abnormalities of osmolarity are involved in the coma and seizures caused by several medical disorders including diabetic ketoacidosis, the nonketotic hyperosmolar state, and hyponatremia. In hyperosmolarity, brain volume is reduced while hypoosmolarity leads to brain swelling. Brain water volume correlates best with level of consciousness in hyponatremic-hypoosmolar states but other factors probably also play a role. Sodium levels below 115 meq per liter are associated with coma and convulsions, depending to some extent on the rapidity with which the hyponatremia develops. Serum osmolarity is generally above 350 mosmol per liter in hyperosmolar coma.

Hypercapnia produces a diminished level of consciousness proportional to the P_{CO_2} tension in the blood and to acuteness of onset. A relationship between CSF acidosis and severity of symptoms has been established. The pathophysiology of other metabolic encephalopathies such as hypercalcemia, hypothyroidism, vitamin B_{12} deficiency, and hypothermia are incompletely understood but probably reflect multifaceted derangements of cerebral biochemistry.

Central nervous system (CNS) depressant drugs and some endogenous toxins probably produce coma by suppression of metabolic and membrane electrical activities in both the RAS and cerebral cortex. For this reason combinations of cortical and brainstem signs occur in drug overdose and other metabolic comas which may lead to a specious diagnosis of structural brainstem damage. Certain anesthetic agents have a predilection for affecting the brainstem RAS neurons out of proportion to the cortex.

Although all metabolic derangements alter neuronal electrophysiology, the disturbance of brain electrical activity most commonly encountered in clinical practice is epilepsy. Continuous, generalized electrical discharges of the cortex may be associated with coma even in the absence of epileptic motor activity. Coma following seizures (postictal state) may be due to exhaustion of energy metabolites or be secondary to locally toxic molecules produced during the seizures. Recovery from postictal unresponsiveness occurs when neuronal metabolic balance is restored. The postictal state produces a pattern of continuous, generalized slowing of the background EEG activity similar to that of metabolic encephalopathy.

PRACTICAL APPROACH TO THE COMATOSE PATIENT The diagnosis and acute management of coma depend on understanding the pitfalls of examining the comatose patient, an interpretation of brainstem reflexes, and on the wise use of selected diagnostic tests. Respiratory and cardiovascular problems should be attended to prior to neurologic diagnosis. The general medical evaluation, except for the vital signs and examination for nuchal rigidity, should be deferred until the neurologic evaluation has established the severity and nature of coma.

History In many cases the cause of coma is immediately evident (e.g., trauma, cardiac arrest, and known drug ingestion). However, in the remainder, historical information about the onset of coma is often sparse. The most useful historical points, when obtainable, are (1) the circumstances and temporal profile of the onset of neurologic symptoms, (2) the precise details of preceding neurologic symptoms (weakness, headaches, seizures, dizziness, diplopia, or vomiting), (3) the use of drugs or alcohol, (4) history of liver, kidney, lung, heart, or other medical disease. Telephone calls to family and observers on the scene are an important part of the initial evaluation of coma.

PHYSICAL EXAMINATION AND GENERAL OBSERVATIONS The temperature, pulse, respiratory rate and pattern, and blood pressure should be measured. Fever suggests systemic infection, bacterial meningitis, or a brain lesion that has disturbed the temperature-regulating centers. High body temperature, 42 to 44°C, associated with dry skin should arouse the suspicion of heat stroke. Hypothermia is observed with bodily exposure; alcoholic, barbiturate, or phenothiazine intoxication; hypoglycemia; peripheral circulatory failure; or myxedema. Hypothermia causes coma directly only when the temperature is below 31°C. Aberrant respiratory patterns commonly reflect brainstem disorders and are discussed below. A change of pulse rate combined with hyperventilation and hypertension may signal an increase in intracranial pressure. Marked hypertension occurs in patients with hypertensive encephalopathy, cerebral hemorrhage, and, at times, in those with other causes of increased intracranial pressure. Hypotension may occur in the coma of alcohol or barbiturate intoxication, internal hemorrhage, myocardial infarction, gram-negative bacillary septicemia, and Addisonian crisis. The funduscopic examination is useful in detecting subarachnoid hemorrhage (subhyaloid hemorrhages), hypertensive encephalopathy (exudates, hemorrhages, vessel-crossing changes), and increased intracranial pressure (papilledema).

General neurologic assessment An exact description of spontaneous and elicited movements in coma is of great value in establishing the level of neurologic dysfunction. The patient's state is observed first without examiner intervention. Likeness to sleep and the nature of respirations and spontaneous movements are the most helpful features. Patients who toss about, reach up toward the face, cross the midline with an arm, cross their legs, yawn, swallow, cough, or moan are closest to being awake. Adventitious movements or postures may be subtle and must be specifically sought. For example, the only sign of seizures may be small excursion twitching of a foot, finger, or facial muscle. An outturned leg at rest or lack of restless movements on one side suggests a hemiparesis.

The terms *decorticate* and *decerebrate rigidity* or "posturing" have been adapted from animal experiments to describe stereotyped tonic flexor and extensor arm movements, respectively, with extension of the legs. Spontaneous flexion of the elbows and wrists and arm supination (decortication) suggest severe bilateral damage in the hemispheres above the midbrain, while extension of the elbows and wrists with pronation (decerebration) suggests damage in the midbrain or diencephalon. Arm extension with weak leg flexion or flaccid legs has been associated with lesions in the low pons. Acute lesions, however, frequently cause limb extension regardless of location, and almost all extensor posturing becomes flexor in nature as time passes. Metabolic coma, especially after acute hypoxia, may produce vigorous spontaneous extensor (decerebrate) rigidity. Posturing may alternate or coexist with purposeful limb movements, usually reflecting subtotal damage to the motor system.

Elicited movements and level of arousal A sequence of increasingly intense stimuli is used to determine the patient's best level of arousal and the optimal motor response of each limb. If the patient is not aroused by conversational voice, shouting should be tried. Shaking the patient is attempted next, then painful pressure on the limbs. Nasal tickle with a cotton wisp is a strong arousal stimulus. Deep pressure on the knuckles or bony prominences is the preferred and humane form of noxious stimulus. Pinching the skin over the face or chest may cause unsightly ecchymoses and is rarely necessary.

Responses to painful stimuli should be appraised critically. Abduction avoidance of a limb is a purposeful, cortically derived movement and denotes an intact corticospinal system to that limb. If abduction is present in all limbs it is a reliable sign of only minimal motor dysfunction. Stereotyped posturing following stimulation of a limb indicates severe dysfunction of the corticospinal system. Adduction and flexion of the stimulated limbs may occur as reflex movements and do not imply an intact corticospinal system. Brief oscillatory limb movements frequently occur at the end of elicited extensor posturing excursions and should not be mistaken for seizures.

Brainstem reflexes Brainstem signs are the key to the localization of the causative lesion in coma (Fig. 20-1). As a rule, coma associated with normal brainstem function indicates widespread and bilateral hemispheral disease. The brainstem contains several intrinsic reflexes that are convenient to examine. Normal pupillary symmetry, size, shape, and reaction to light indicate intact functioning of the midbrain and efferent parasympathetic fibers of the third cranial nerve responsible for pupillary constriction. The afferent component of the light reflex utilizes the optic nerve. Pupillary reaction should be examined with a bright diffuse light and, if absent, confirmed with a magnifying lens. Excessive room lighting mutes pupillary reactivity. Equal and reactive round pupils (2.5 to 5 mm in diameter) usually exclude midbrain damage as the cause of coma. An enlarged (greater than 5 mm) and unreactive or poorly reactive pupil can result either from an intrinsic midbrain lesion (on the same side) or be secondary to compression of the midbrain and/or third nerve as occurs in transtentorial herniation. Unilateral pupillary enlargement usually denotes an ipsilateral mass but rarely can occur contralaterally by compression of the cerebral peduncle of the midbrain against the opposite tentorial margin. Oval and slightly eccentric pupils (corectopia) often accompany early midbrain–third nerve compression. Bilaterally dilated and unreactive pupils indicate severe midbrain damage, usually from secondary compression by transtentorial herniation or metabolically by ingestion of drugs with anticholinergic activity. The unannounced use of mydriatic eye drops by a previous examiner or direct ocular trauma may cause misleading pupillary enlargement. Reactive and bilaterally small but not pinpoint pupils (1 to 2.5 mm) are most commonly seen in metabolic encephalopathy or after deep bilateral hemispheral lesions such as hydrocephalus or thalamic hemorrhage. This has been attributed to dysfunction of sympathetic nervous system efferents emerging from the posterior hypothalamus. Profound barbiturate-induced coma may produce similar-sized pupils. Very small but reactive pupils (less than 1 mm) denote narcotic overdose but may also occur with acute, extensive bilateral pontine damage. The response to naloxone and the presence of reflex eye movements (see below) will distinguish between these causes. The unilaterally small pupil of a Horner's syndrome is rare in coma but may occur ipsilateral to a large cerebral hemorrhage.

Eye movements are the foundation of physical diagnosis in coma because their examination permits exploration of a large portion of the rostrocaudal extent of the brainstem. The eyes are first observed by elevating the lids and noting the resting position and spontaneous movements of the globes. Horizontal divergence of the eyes at rest is normally observed in drowsiness. As patients either awaken or as coma deepens, the ocular axes become parallel again. An adducted eye at rest indicates lateral rectus paresis (weakness) due to a sixth nerve lesion and may indicate damage to the pons. However, sixth nerve paresis, often bilateral, occurs with increased intracranial pressure and is not a localizing sign. An abducted eye at rest indicates medial rectus paresis due to third nerve paresis. With few exceptions, vertical separation of the ocular axes, or "skew," results from pontine or cerebellar lesions.

When spontaneous eye movements are present in coma they generally take the form of conjugate horizontal roving. This motion exonerates the midbrain and pons and has the same meaning as normal reflex eye movements (see below). Cyclic vertical downward movements are seen in specific circumstances. "Ocular bobbing" describes a brisk conjugate downward and slow upward movement of the globes in situations where horizontal eye movement mechanisms have been disrupted and is diagnostic of bilateral pontine damage. "Ocular dipping" is a slow downward movement followed by fast upward movement in patients with normal reflex horizontal gaze. Dipping occurs particularly in patients with diffuse anoxic damage to the cerebral cortex and may be preceded by sustained up or down gaze. The eyes may turn down and inward in thalamic and upper midbrain lesions. Conjugate ocular deviation at rest is discussed below.

Doll's-eye, or *oculocephalic,* movements are tested by moving the head from side to side or vertically, first slowly then briskly. Reflex eye movements are evoked in the opposite direction to head turning (Fig. 20-1). These responses are mediated by brainstem mechanisms originating in the labyrinths and vestibular nuclei and cervical proprioceptors. They are normally suppressed by visual fixation mediated by the cerebral hemispheres in awake patients. The neuronal pathways for reflex horizontal eye movements require integrity of the region surrounding the sixth nerve nucleus and are yoked to the contralateral third nerve via the medial longitudinal fasciculus (MLF) (Fig. 20-1). Two disparate pieces of information can be obtained from the reflex eye movements. *First,* in coma result-

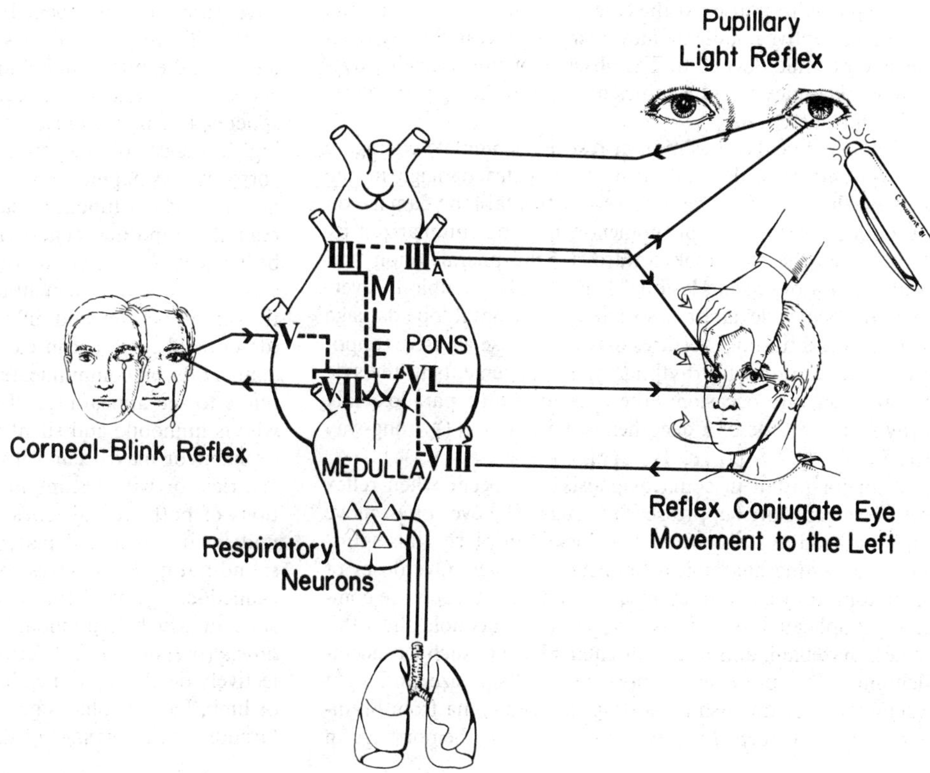

FIGURE 20-1
Brainstem reflexes in the coma examination. Midbrain and third nerve function are tested by pupillary reaction to light, pontine function by spontaneous and reflex eye movements and corneal responses, and medullary function by respiratory and pharyngeal responses.

Reflex conjugate, horizontal eye movements are dependent upon the medial longitudinal fasciculus (MLF) interconnecting the sixth and contralateral third nerve nuclei. Eye movements are elicited by head rotation (oculocephalic reflex) or caloric stimulation of the labyrinths (oculovestibular or vestibuloocular reflex).

ing from bihemispheral disease, the eyes move easily or "loosely" from side to side in a direction opposite to the direction of head turning. The ease with which the globes move toward the opposite side is a reflection of disinhibition of brainstem reflexes by damaged cerebral hemispheres. In drowsy patients, the first two or three head rotations cause opposite conjugate eye movements following which the maneuver itself usually causes arousal and the reflex movements stop. *Second,* full conjugate oculocephalic movements require integrity of the brainstem pathways extending from the high cervical spinal cord and medulla, where vestibular and proprioceptive input from head turning originates, to the midbrain where the third nerve originates, and the MLF running between these regions. Thus, the oculocephalic maneuver is a convenient way to demonstrate the functional integrity of a large segment of brainstem tegmental pathways and the cranial nerves involved in eye movements. Faulty abduction of an eye suggests a sixth nerve lesion, due either to ipsilateral pontine damage or the distant effects of increased intracranial pressure. Lack of complete adduction indicates an ipsilateral midbrain (third nerve) lesion or, alternatively, damage to the pathways mediating reflex eye movements in the MLF (i.e., internuclear ophthalmoplegia). Third nerve damage is usually associated with an enlarged pupil and horizontal ocular divergence at rest, whereas MLF destruction shows neither. Adduction of the globes is by nature more difficult to obtain with head turning than abduction, and subtle symmetric abnormalities in the doll's-eye maneuver should be interpreted with caution.

Caloric stimulation of the vestibular apparatus (*oculovestibular* or *vestibuloocular response*) is a useful adjunct to the oculocephalic test and acts as a stronger stimulus to reflex eye movements. Irrigation of the external auditory canal with ice-cold water causes convection currents in the endolymph of the labyrinths of the inner ear. With the head placed at 30° elevation from the supine position, endolymph movement is induced primarily in the horizontal semicircular canals. An intact brainstem response is indicated by tonic deviation of both eyes (lasting 30 to 120 s) to the side of cold-water irrigation. Bilateral conjugate eye movements have the same significance as full oculocephalic responses. If the cerebral hemispheres are intact, a rapid corrective conjugate movement is generated away from the side of tonic deviation. The absence of this saccadic, nystagmus-like quick phase signifies damage to the opposite cerebral hemisphere.

Conjugate ocular deviation at rest or incomplete conjugate eye movements with head turning indicates damage in the pons on the side of the gaze paresis or frontal lobe damage on the opposite side. This phenomenon may be summarized by the phrase "the eyes look toward a hemispheral lesion and away from a brainstem lesion." It is usually possible to overcome the ocular deviation associated with frontal lobe damage by brisk head turning. Seizures may also cause aversive (opposite) eye deviation with rhythmic, jerky movements to the side of gaze. On rare occasions, the eyes may turn paradoxically away from the side of a deep hemispheral lesion ("wrong-way eyes").

A major pitfall in coma diagnosis may occur when reflex eye movements are suppressed by drugs. The eyes often move with the head as it is turned as if locked in place, thus spuriously suggesting anatomical brainstem damage. Overdoses of phenytoin, tricyclic antidepressants, and barbiturates are commonly implicated as well as, on occasion, alcohol, phenothiazines, diazepam, and neuromuscular blockers such as succinylcholine. The presence of normal pupillary size and light reaction will distinguish most drug-induced coma from brainstem damage (except for pontine infarction or hemorrhage in which the pupils remain small). Both absent oculocephalic responses and dilated, fixed pupils may occur with glutethimide intoxication. Small to midposition, nonreactive pupils may also occur with very high serum levels of barbiturates.

Although the *corneal reflexes* are rarely useful alone, they may corroborate eye movement abnormalities because they also depend on the integrity of pontine pathways. By touching the cornea with a wisp of cotton, a response consisting of brief bilateral lid closure may be observed. The corneal response may be lost when the afferent fifth nerve, the efferent seventh nerve, or their reflex connections within the pons are damaged. The normal efferent response is bilateral, with closure of both eyelids. Nervous system depressant drugs diminish or eliminate the corneal responses soon after the reflex eye movements become paralyzed but before the pupils become unreactive to light.

Respiration Respiratory patterns have received much attention in coma diagnosis but are of inconsistent localizing value. Shallow, slow, but well-timed regular breathing suggests metabolic or drug depression. Rapid, deep (Kussmaul) breathing usually implies metabolic acidosis but may also occur with pontomesencephalic lesions. Cheyne-Stokes respiration in its classic cyclic form, ending with a brief apneic period, signifies mild bihemispheral damage or metabolic suppression and commonly accompanies light coma. Gasps, held-in inspiration, reflect bilateral lower brainstem damage and are well known as the terminal respiratory pattern of severe brain damage. In brain-dead patients, shallow respiratory-like movements with irregular, nonrepetitive back arching may be stimulated by hypercapnia or hypoxia and are probably generated by the surviving cervical spinal cord and lower medulla. Other cyclic breathing variations are not usually diagnostic of specific local lesions.

COMALIKE SYNDROMES AND RELATED STATES The simple observation of inability to arouse a patient characterizes most comatose states. Several syndromes, however, appear to render patients unresponsive or insensate but are considered separately because of their unusual features. The *vegetative state* occurs in patients who were earlier comatose but whose eyes have subsequently opened giving the appearance of being awake. There may be yawning, grunting, picking with the hands, and random limb and head movements. These are associated with signs of extensive damage to both cerebral hemispheres, i.e., Babinski signs, decerebrate or decorticate posturing, absence of response to visual stimuli, and absent corrective nystagmus on vestibuloocular testing. Autonomic nervous system functions such as cardiovascular and thermoregulatory and neuroendocrine control are preserved and may be subject to periods of overactivity. The syndrome is best viewed as a severe dementia resulting from global damage to the cerebral cortex and differs somewhat from akinetic mutism (described below) because of a complete inability to respond to commands or communicate. *Akinetic mutism,* or coma vigil, refers to the appearance of a partially or fully awake patient who is immobile and silent. The state may result from hydrocephalus or may occur with masses in the region of the third ventricle or with lesions in the cingulate gyrus or other portions of both frontal lobes. *Abulia* is a mild form of akinetic mutism in which the patient is hypokinetic and slow to respond but generally gives correct answers. Lesions in the periacqueductal, low diencephalic regions may cause a similar state in which hypophonia is prominent. The *locked-in syndrome* (pseudocoma) describes patients who are awake but selectively deefferented, i.e., have no means of producing speech or limb, face, or pharyngeal movements. This results from infarction or hemorrhage of the ventral pons which transects all descending corticospinal and corticobulbar pathways but spares the RAS arousal system. Vertical eye movements and blinking are generally normal because these midbrain functions are outside the field of infarction in basilar artery thrombosis. Such movements can be used by the patient to signal to the examiner. A similar awake state simulating unresponsiveness may occur in severe cases of acute polyneuritis or myasthenia gravis as a result of total paralysis of limb and bulbar musculature. Unlike basilar artery stroke, vertical eye movements are not selectively spared in these nerve and muscle diseases.

Certain psychiatric states mimic coma because they produce apparent unresponsiveness. *Catatonia* is a generic term for peculiar motor activities associated with major psychosis. In the typical hypomobile form catatonic patients appear awake with eyes open but make no voluntary or responsive movements, though they blink spontaneously and may not appear distressed. There may be associated "waxy flexibility" in which limbs maintain their posture when lifted by the examiner. Upon recovery, such patients have full memory of events that occurred during their catatonic stupor. Patients with *pseudocoma conversion* states (trance) have signs which indicate voluntary attempts to appear comatose. They may resist eyelid elevation, blink to threat when the lids are held open, and move the eyes concomitantly with head rotation, all signs belying brain damage.

LABORATORY EXAMINATION IN COMA Four laboratory tests are used most frequently in the diagnosis of coma: CT, EEG, CSF examination, and chemical-toxicologic analysis of blood. CT depends on computer reconstruction of the differential radiologic densities of brain, blood, ischemic areas, edema, cerebrospinal fluid, tumor, and iodinated dye. With the current generation of scanners, single lesions of approximately 0.5 cm are visible as well as normal brain and ventricular architecture. The notion that a normal CT scan excludes anatomical lesions as the cause of coma is erroneous. Early infarction, small brainstem lesions, encephalitis, mechanical shearing of axons as a result of closed head trauma, absent cerebral perfusion associated with brain death, cortical vein thrombosis, and subdural hematomas which are isodense to adjacent brain are some of the lesions which may be overlooked by CT. Nevertheless, in coma of unknown etiology, a CT scan should be obtained early in the evaluation. In those cases where the etiology is clinically apparent the CT provides verification and defines the extent of the lesion.

The EEG is rarely diagnostic in coma, with the occasional exceptions of coma due to ongoing clinically unrecognized seizures, herpes virus encephalitis, and Creutzfeldt-Jakob disease. Examination of the EEG does, however, provide important information about the general electrophysiologic state of the cortex, and asymmetries may point to unilateral lesions not visualized on the CT scan. The amount of background slowing of the EEG is useful for gauging and following the severity of any diffuse encephalopathy. The EEG pattern of "alpha coma" deserves separate mention. It is defined by widespread, invariant 8- to 12-Hz activity superficially resembling the normal alpha rhythm of waking, but which is unresponsive to environmental stimuli. Alpha coma results from either high pontine or diffuse cortical damage and is associated with a poor prognosis. Coma due to persistent epileptic discharges that are not clinically manifested may be revealed by EEG recordings. Normal alpha activity on the EEG may also alert the clinician to the "locked-in" syndrome. Evoked potential recordings (auditory and somatosensory) are currently under investigation as additional methods of coma diagnosis and monitoring.

Lumbar puncture is now used more judiciously than previously because the CT scan excludes intracerebral hemorrhages and most subarachnoid hemorrhages. The use of lumbar puncture in coma is limited to diagnosis of meningitis-encephalitis, occasional cases of subarachnoid hemorrhage, and cases with normal CT where the origin of coma is obscure. If the CT is normal or unavailable and suspicion of meningeal infection or subarachnoid hemorrhage remains, then the CSF should be examined for white cells, microorganisms, and blood. Xanthochromia is documented by spinning the CSF in a large tube and comparing the supernatant to water. Yellow coloration indicates preexisting blood in the CSF and permits exclusion of a traumatic puncture. In addition, initial and final tubes should be inspected for a decrement in the number of erythrocytes, indicating traumatic puncture.

Chemical blood determinations are routinely made to investigate metabolic, toxic, or drug-induced encephalopathies. The major metabolic aberrations encountered in clinical practice are those of electrolytes, calcium, BUN, glucose, and hepatic dysfunction. Toxicologic analysis is of great value in any case of coma where the diagnosis is not immediately clear. However, the presence of exogenous drugs or toxins, especially alcohol, does not assure that other factors, particularly head trauma, may not also contribute to the clinical state.

DIFFERENTIAL DIAGNOSIS OF COMA In most instances, coma is part of an obvious medical problem such as known drug ingestion, hypoxia, stroke, trauma, or liver or kidney failure. Attention is appropriately focused on the primary illness. A complete listing of all diseases which cause coma would serve little purpose since it would not aid diagnosis. Some general rules, however, are helpful. Illnesses which cause sudden or acute coma are due to drug ingestion or to one of the catastrophic brain lesions—hemorrhage, trauma, or hypoxia. Coma which appears subacutely is usually related to preceding medical or neurologic problems, including the secondary brain swelling which surrounds a preexisting lesion. Coma diagnosis, therefore, requires familiarity with the common intracerebral catastrophies. These are described in more detail in Chap. 356, but may be summarized as follows: (1) basal ganglia and thalamic hemorrhage (acute but not instantaneous onset, vomiting, headache, hemiplegia, and characteristic eye signs); (2) subarachnoid hemorrhage (instantaneous onset, severe headache, neck stiffness, vomiting, third or sixth nerve lesions, transient loss of consciousness, or sudden coma with vigorous extensor posturing); (3) pontine hemorrhage (sudden onset, pinpoint pupils, loss of reflex eye movements and corneal responses, ocular bobbing, posturing, hyperventilation, and sweating); (4) cerebellar hemorrhage (occipital headache, vomiting, gaze paresis, and inability to stand); (5) basilar artery thrombosis (neurologic prodrome or warning spells, diplopia, dysarthria, vomiting, eye movement and corneal response abnormalities, and asymmetric limb paresis). The commonest stroke, namely, infarction in the territory of the middle cerebral artery, does not cause coma acutely.

If the history and examination are not typical for any neurologic diagnosis, then information obtained from CT, guided by the findings on physical examination, may be used as outlined in Table 20-1. The neurologic examination remains preeminent because it allows localization of lesions to one or both hemispheres or to the brainstem (with the exceptions noted above.) The CT scan is then utilized to focus the differential diagnosis, and because of its accuracy and general availability the diagnoses which it facilitates are listed in the table. The majority of causes of coma are established without a CT or with the study being normal. The authors repeat the admonition that CT is most useful in the context of a properly conducted neurologic examination.

COMA AFTER HEAD TRAUMA Concussion is a common form of transient coma which probably results from torsion of the hemispheres about the midbrain-diencephalic junction with brief interruption of RAS function. Persistent coma after head trauma presents a more complex and serious problem. Bilateral hemispheral mass lesions such as subdural or intracerebral hematomas or brain contusions account for most cases. Large unilateral lesions, particularly epidural hematomas, may secondarily compress the opposite hemisphere and/or RAS and cause coma with asymmetric eye and motor signs. All these lesions are associated with elevated intracranial pressure and an abnormal CT scan. Direct brainstem contusion–hemorrhage with signs of midbrain damage is occasionally invoked as the cause of coma when intracranial pressure is normal but is, in fact, extremely rare. Severe closed head trauma is commonly associated with a unique injury consisting of microscopic shearing of axonal fibers in the corpus callosum, central hemispheral white matter, and dorsolateral pons. Intracranial pressure is usually normal, and coma with vigorous extensor posturing is probably due to the bilateral hemispheral shearing lesions rather than brainstem injury. The CT scan may be unremarkable or show small hemorrhagic areas, particularly in the anterior corpus callosum.

TABLE 20-1
Approach to the differential diagnosis of coma

I Normal brainstem reflexes, no lateralizing signs
- *A* Diagnosis facilitated by CT
  - *1* Hydrocephalus
  - *2* Bilateral subdural hematomas
  - *3* Bilateral contusions, edema, or axonal shearing of hemispheres due to closed head trauma
  - *4* Subarachnoid hemorrhage
- *B* Diagnosed without CT (CT normal or unhelpful)
  - *1* Drug-toxin ingestion (toxicologic analysis)
  - *2* Endogenous metabolic encephalopathy (glucose, ammonia, calcium, osmolarity, P_{O_2}, P_{CO_2}, urea, sodium)
  - *3* Shock, hypertensive encephalopathy
  - *4* Meningitis (CSF analysis)
  - *5* Nonherpetic viral encephalitis (CSF analysis)
  - *6* Epilepsy (EEG)
  - *7* Reye's syndrome (ammonia, increased intracranial pressure)
  - *8* Conversion reaction, catatonia
  - *9* Subarachnoid hemorrhage with normal CT (CSF analysis)
  - *10* Acute disseminated encephalomyelitis (CSF analysis)
  - *11* Acute hemorrhagic leukoencephalitis
  - *12* Advanced Alzheimer's and Creutzfeldt-Jakob disease

II Normal brainstem reflexes (with or without unilateral compressive third nerve palsy), lateralizing motor signs
- *A* Diagnosis facilitated by CT
  - *1* Cerebral hemorrhage (basal ganglia, thalamus)
  - *2* Large infarction with surrounding brain edema
  - *3* Herpes virus encephalitis
  - *4* Subdural or epidural hematoma
  - *5* Tumor with edema
  - *6* Brain abscess with edema
  - *7* Vasculitis with multiple infarctions
  - *8* Metabolic encephalopathy superimposed on preexisting focal lesions (i.e., stroke)
  - *9* Pituitary apoplexy
- *B* Diagnosed without CT (CT normal or unhelpful)
  - *1* Metabolic encephalopathies with asymmetrical signs (blood chemical determinations)
  - *2* Isodense subdural hematoma (brain scan, angiogram)
  - *3* TTP (blood smear, platelet count)
  - *4* Epilepsy with focal seizures or postictal state (EEG)

III Multiple brainstem reflex abnormalities
- *A* Diagnosis facilitated by CT
  - *1* Pontine, midbrain hemorrhage
  - *2* Cerebellar hemorrhage, tumor, abscess
  - *3* Cerebellar infarction with brainstem compression
  - *4* Mass in hemisphere causing advanced bilateral brainstem compression
  - *5* Brainstem tumor or demyelination
- *B* Diagnosed without CT (CT normal or unhelpful)
  - *1* Basilar artery thrombosis causing brainstem stroke (clinical signs, angiogram)
  - *2* Severe drug overdose (toxicologic analysis)
  - *3* Traumatic brainstem contusion–hemorrhage (clinical signs, auditory-evoked potentials)
  - *4* Basilar artery migraine
  - *5* Brain death

EMERGENCY TREATMENT OF THE COMATOSE PATIENT The immediate goal in acute coma is prevention of further nervous system damage. Hypotension, hypoglycemia, hypoxia, hypercapnia, and hyperthermia should be rapidly and assiduously corrected. An oropharyngeal airway is adequate to keep the pharynx open in drowsy patients who are breathing normally. Tracheal intubation is indicated if there is obvious apnea, hypoventilation, or emesis, or if the patient is liable to aspirate. Mechanical ventilation is required if the patient is apneic or hypoventilating or if there is an intracranial mass and hypocapnia is therapeutically necessary. An intravenous access is established and naloxone and dextrose administered if narcotic overdose or hypoglycemia are even remote possibilities. Thiamine is generally administered with glucose in order to prevent an exacerbation of Wernicke's encephalopathy. The veins of intravenous drug abusers may be difficult to cannulate; in such cases, naloxone can be injected sublingually through a small-gauge needle. In cases of suspected basilar thrombosis with brainstem ischemia, intravenous heparin is administered after obtaining a CT scan, keeping in mind that cerebellar and pontine hemorrhages bear some resemblance to the syndrome of basilar occlusion. Physostigmine, when used by experienced physicians with careful monitoring, may awaken patients with anticholinergic-type drug overdose, but many physicians believe that this is justified only if cardiac arrhythmias are a problem. Intravenous fluid administration should be carefully monitored in any serious acute nervous system illness because of the potential for exacerbating brain swelling. Neck injuries must not be overlooked, particularly prior to attempting the oculocephalic maneuver.

Enlargement of one pupil usually indicates secondary midbrain compression by a hemispheral mass and demands immediate reduction of intracranial pressure. Intravenous fluids are slowed to the minimum necessary to support blood pressure. Therapeutic hyperventilation is then used to achieve an arterial P_{CO_2} of 28 to 32 mmHg. This acts rapidly to reduce intracranial pressure but the beneficial effect rarely lasts more than 2 h. Hyperosmolar therapy with mannitol may be used simultaneously with hyperventilation in critical cases, but its effects are not apparent for several minutes. The effective duration of mannitol is only a few hours or less. A ventricular puncture may be necessary to decompress the intracranial compartment by removing CSF if medical measures fail. Virtually all patients who survive to arrive in an emergency room can be protected from further brain damage by these means until definitive therapy is possible. In some patients, high-dose barbiturates may reduce intracranial pressure beyond that obtained by the conventional means listed above. Their use has a good rationale in intractable intracranial hypertension but they are not without risk and should be confined to units experienced in intracranial pressure monitoring. The use of barbiturates remains investigative until evidence demonstrates a clear improvement in outcome.

BRAIN DEATH Brain death is defined as resulting from total cessation of cerebral blood flow and global infarction of the brain at a time when cardiovascular and respiratory functions remain preserved, the latter requiring artificial support. It is the only type of irrevocable loss of brain function recognized by law as death. Many sets of roughly equivalent criteria have been advanced for the diagnosis of brain death, and it is essential to adhere to those approved locally and recognized as standard practice. Ideal criteria are ones that are simple and conducted at the bedside and which allow no chance of diagnostic error. Cortical death is usually shown by an isoelectric EEG and unresponsiveness to the environment, midbrain death by absent pupillary light reaction, pontine death by absent oculovestibular and corneal reflexes, and medullary death by apnea. Some period of observation, usually 6 to 24 h, is desirable during which this state is shown to be sustained. The pupils need not be fully dilated but should not be constricted. The absence of spinal reflexes is not required since the spinal cord remains functional in many cases of brain death. The possibility of profound drug-induced or hypothermic nervous system depression should always be excluded.

The demonstration of apnea generally requires that the P_{CO_2} be high enough to stimulate respiration. This can be safely accomplished in most patients by removing the respirator and using diffusion oxygenation sustained by a tracheal cannula connected to an oxygen supply. In brain-dead patients, CO_2 tension increases approximately 2.5 mmHg/min during apnea. At the end of an appropriate interval, arterial P_{CO_2} should be at least above 45 mmHg (higher limits have been suggested) for the test to be valid. Large posterior fossa lesions which compress the brainstem, nervous system depressant drugs, and profound hypothermia can simulate brain death, but adherence to recognized protocols for diagnosis will avoid these errors. Radionuclide brain scanning or cerebral angiography may be used to demonstrate the absence of cerebral blood flow in brain death. These techniques have the virtue of rapidity but are often unfeasible and expensive and have not been extensively correlated with pathological study or conventional criteria of brain death.

There is no implicit pressure to make the diagnosis of brain death except when organ transplantation or difficult resource allocation (intensive care) issues are involved. Although it is eminently reasonable to disconnect the respirator from a brain-dead patient after proper explanations to the family, there is no obligation to do so and some physicians prefer to await the inevitable cardiovascular failure that follows brain death, usually within a week.

PROGNOSIS OF COMA Interest in predicting the outcome of coma is oriented toward allocating medical resources and limiting the support of hopeless cases. To date, no collection of clinical signs except those of brain death assuredly predicts coma outcome. Children and young adults may have ominous, early clinical findings such as abnormal brainstem reflexes and yet recover normally. All schemes for prognosis should, therefore, be taken as only approximate indicators, and medical judgments must be conservatively tempered by other factors such as age, underlying disease, general medical condition, and the previously expressed wishes of the patient. In an attempt to collect prognostic information from large numbers of patients with head injury, a "coma scale" scoring system has been devised which empirically has predictive value in cases of brain trauma. Major points include a 95 percent death rate in patients whose pupillary reaction or reflex eye movements were absent 6 h after onset of coma, and a 91 percent death rate if the pupils were unreactive at 24 h (though 4 percent made a good recovery).

Prognostication of nontraumatic coma is more difficult because of the heterogeneity of contributing diseases. Unfavorable signs in the first hours after admission have been reported to be the absence of any two signs of pupillary reaction, corneal reflex, or the oculovestibular response. One day after the onset of coma, the above signs, in addition to absence of eye opening and muscle tone, predicted death or severe disability and the same signs at 3 days strengthened the prediction of a poor outcome. Favorable signs at 1 and 3 days included any verbal output, normal oculovestibular response, localization of stimuli by appropriate limb movements, and normal muscle tone. In approximately 50 percent of patients precise combinations of predictive signs do not occur and coma scales lose their prognostic value. It may be wisest to fully support all but those patients whose extreme signs convincingly suggest a poor outcome. Medical practitioners are becoming less reluctant to withdraw support from brain-dead patients as predictions become more reliable and resources more limited.

REFERENCES

FINKLESTEIN S, ROPPER A: The diagnosis of coma: Its pitfalls and limitations. Heart Lung 8:1059, 1979

FISHER CM: The neurological examination of the comatose patient. Acta Neurol Scand 45 (suppl 6):1, 1969

JENNET B et al: Prognosis of patients with severe head injury. Neurosurgery 4:283, 1979

LEVY D et al: Prognosis in non-traumatic coma. Ann Intern Med 94:229, 1981

PLUM F, POSNER J: *The Diagnosis of Stupor and Coma,* 3d ed. Philadelphia, Davis, 1980

21 DELIRIUM AND OTHER ACUTE CONFUSIONAL STATES

RAYMOND D. ADAMS
MAURICE VICTOR

All physicians sooner or later discover through clinical experience the need for special competence in assessing the mental faculties of their patients. They must be able to observe with detachment and complete objectivity the patient's character, intelligence, mood, memory, judgment, and other attributes of personality, in much the same fashion as they observe the nutritional state and the color of the mucous membranes. The systematic examination of these affective and cognitive functions permits the physician to reach certain conclusions regarding patients' mental status. Without such data, errors will be made in evaluating the reliability of the patient's history in diagnosing the neurologic or psychiatric disease from which he or she suffers, and in conducting an appropriate therapeutic program.

DEFINITION OF TERMS

The definition of normal and abnormal states of mind is difficult because the terms used to describe these states have been given so many different meanings in both medical and nonmedical writings. Compounding the difficulty is the fact that the pathophysiology of the confusional states, delirium and dementia, is not fully understood, and the definitions depend on their clinical relationships, with all the lack of precision which this entails. The following nomenclature, though tentative, has been found useful by the authors, and is employed throughout this textbook.

Confusion is a general term denoting an incapacity of the patient to think with customary speed and clarity. This abnormality may depend on any one of several factors. In delirium, for example, inattention, impairment of perception, and the intrusion of illusory and hallucinatory experiences are mainly responsible. At certain stages in the evolution or devolution of stupor and coma, as indicated in Chap. 20, confusion is aligned with a disorder of conscious awareness and perception. In patients with dementia, confusion is related to a derangement of intellectual function, i.e., an inability to learn, remember, calculate, make appropriate deductions from given premises, reason abstractly, etc. Also, intense emotional experiences may interfere with coherence of thinking.

The term *delirium* is used here to denote a special type of confusional state, acute in onset and transient in nature, and characterized by gross disorientation in the presence of heightened alertness, i.e., an increased readiness to respond to stimuli, a disorder of perception in which illusions and vivid hallucinations are prominent, and overactivity of psychomotor and autonomic nervous functions. Implicit in the definition are certain nonmedical connotations of the term—agitation, excitement, vivid dreams, and creations of the imagination. Most stuporous and demented patients, in contrast to those with delirium, show a *reduced* state of arousal, alertness, and attentiveness, *decreased* psychomotor activity, and a *relatively slight* tendency to hallucinate. For these reasons, and also because of the particular clinical settings in which they occur, it seems worthwhile to set the delirious states apart from those of depressed consciousness on the one hand and of dementia and amnesia on the other. Such a concept is far from new. To a greater or lesser extent, the terms *exogenous reaction type, symptomatic psychosis, toxic psychosis, infective-exhaustive psychosis,* and *drug, traumatic,* or *febrile delirium* all have reference to the syndrome of delirium. All these terms convey the idea of an acute and transient (reversible) confusional state, occurring in a particular clinical setting and carrying a serious prognosis, by virtue of adding its burden to an already serious medical illness.

It should be pointed out that not all psychiatrists agree with our distinction between delirium and other confusional states. Some, such as Engel and Romano, and Lipowski, use the term *delirium* in reference to confusional states of all types. Our insistence on their separation is based on their different clinical manifestations and the clinical settings in which they occur.

The term *amnesia* refers to a loss of past memories coupled with an inability to form new memories, i.e., to learn. It presupposes an alert state of mind, an ability to grasp the problem, to use language normally, and to maintain adequate motivation. The failure is mainly one of retention, recall, and reproduction, and it should be distinguished from the loss of memory that accompanies states of drowsiness and acute confusion, in which information seems never to have been adequately registered in the first place or assimilated.

Dementia literally means an undoing of the mind or, more particularly, a deterioration of all intellectual and cognitive functions, without disturbance of consciousness or perception. Implied in the word is a gradual and in most instances irreversible enfeeblement of mental powers in a person who formerly possessed a normal mind. *Amentia,* by contrast, indicates a congenital feeblemindedness.

OBSERVABLE ASPECTS OF BEHAVIOR AND THEIR RELATION TO CONFUSION, DELIRIUM, AMNESIA, AND DEMENTIA

The components of mentation and behavior that lend themselves to bedside examination are (1) the processes of sensation and perception; (2) the capacity for memorizing; (3) the ability to think and reason; (4) temperament, mood, and emotion; (5) initiative, impulse, and drive; (6) insight. Of these number 1 is sensorial, 2 and 3 are cognitive, 4 is affective, and 5 is conative or volitional. Insight includes all introspective observations made by patients concerning their own normal or disordered functioning. Each component of behavior and intellection has its objective side, expressed in behavioral responses that are produced by certain stimuli, and its subjective side, expressed in what patients think and feel in relation to the stimuli.

DISTURBANCES OF PERCEPTION Perception, i.e., the processes utilized in acquiring through the senses a knowledge of the "world about" or of one's own body, involves many things aside from the simple sensory phenomenon of being aware of the attributes of a stimulus. It includes the maintenance of attention, the selective focusing on a stimulus, the elimination of all extraneous stimuli, and the identification of the stimulus by recognizing its relationship to personal remembered experience. The perception of a stimulus undergoes predictable types of derangement in disease. Most often there is a reduction in the number of perceptions in a given unit of time and failure to synthesize them properly and relate them to the ongoing activities of the mind. There may be inattention or fluctuations of attention, distraction (pertinent and irrelevant stimuli now having equal value), and inability to persist in an assigned task. Qualitative changes also appear, mainly in the form of sensory distortions, causing misinterpretation and misidentification of objects and persons (illusions). These changes, at least in part, form the basis of hallucinatory experience in which the patient reports and reacts to stimuli not present in the environment. There is also an inability to perceive simultaneously all elements of a large complex of stimuli, which is referred to by some as a "failure of subjective reorganization." These major disturbances in the perceptual sphere, sometimes called "clouding of the sensorium," occur most often in deliria and other acute confusional states, but quantitative deficiency may also become evident in the advanced stages of amentia and dementia.

DISTURBANCES OF MEMORY Memory, i.e., the retention of learned experiences, is involved in all mental activities. It may be arbitrarily subdivided into several parts, namely, (1) registration, which includes all that was mentioned under perception; (2) mnemonic integration and retention; (3) recall; and (4) reproduction. In disturbances of perception and attention there may be a complete failure of learning and consequently of memory for the reason that the material to be learned was never registered and assimilated. In Korsakoff's amnesic syndrome, newly presented material appears to be temporarily registered but cannot be retained for more than a few minutes, and there is always an associated defect in the recall and reproduction of memories that had been formed some days, weeks, or even years before the onset of the illness (retrograde amnesia). The fabrication of stories, *confabulation,* constitutes a third, but not invariable, feature of the syndrome. Sound retention with failure of recall is at times a normal state; when it is severe and extends to all events of past life, it is usually due to hysteria or malingering. Proof that the processes of registration and retention are intact under these circumstances comes from hypnosis and suggestion, and questioning under amobarbital (Amytal) or thiopental sodium (Pentothal) narcosis, whereby the lost items are fully recalled and reproduced. In Korsakoff's amnesic state the patient fails on all tests of learning and recent memory, and behavior accords with the deficiencies of information. Since some aspect of memory is involved to some extent in all mental processes, it becomes the most testable component of mentation and behavior.

DISTURBANCES OF THINKING Thinking, which is central to so many important intellectual activities, remains one of the most elusive of all mental operations. If by thinking we mean selective ordering of symbols for problem solving and capacity to reason and form sound judgments (the usual definition), obviously the working units of most mental activity of this type are words and numbers. The substitution of words and numbers for the objects for which they stand (symbolization) is a fundamental part of the process. These symbols are formed into ideas or concepts, and the arrangement of new and remembered ideas into certain orders or relationships according to the rules of logic constitutes another intricate part of thought. One test is problem solving—the capacity to formulate a problem into several hypotheses, to analyze critically the evidence for and against each hypothesis, and to make a correct choice. In a general way one may examine thinking for speed and efficiency, ideational content, coherence and logical relationships of ideas, quantity and quality of associations to a given idea, and the propriety of the feeling and behavior engendered by an idea.

Information concerning the thought processes and associative functions is best obtained by analyzing the patient's spontaneous verbal productions and by engaging him or her in conversation. If the patient is taciturn or mute, one may then have to depend on the responses to direct questions or upon written material, i.e., letters, etc. One notes the prevailing trends of the patient's thoughts; whether the ideas are reasonable, precise, and coherent or vague, circumstantial, tangential, and irrelevant; and whether the thought processes are shallow and fragmented. Disorders of thinking are frequent in deliria and other confusional states and in dementia and schizophrenia. The organization of thought may be disrupted with fragmentation, repetition, and perseveration. This is spoken of as *incoherence of thinking* and characterizes many confusional states of all types. The patient may be excessively critical, rationalizing, and hairsplitting; this type of thinking is often manifest in depressive psychoses. Derangements of thinking may also take the form of a flight of ideas; the patient moves nimbly from one idea to another, and associations are numerous and loosely linked. This is a common feature of hypomanic or manic states. The opposite condition, poverty of ideas, is characteristic both of depression, where it is combined with gloomy thoughts, and of dementing diseases, where it is part of a general reduction in intellectual activity. Thinking may be distorted in such a way that the patient fails to check his or her ideas against reality. When a false belief is maintained in spite of normally convincing contradictory evidence, the patient is said to have a *delusion.* Delusions are common to many illnesses, particularly manic-depressive and schizophrenic states. Ideas may seem to the patient to have been implanted in his or her mind by some outside agent such as radio, television, or atomic energy. These reflect the "passivity feelings" characteristic of schizophrenic psychoses. Other distortions of thinking, such as gaps or condensations of logical associations, are also typical of schizophrenia, of which they constitute a diagnostic feature.

DISTURBANCES OF EMOTION, MOOD, AND AFFECT The emotional life of the patient is expressed in a variety of ways. In the first place, rather marked individual differences in basic temperament are to be observed in the normal population; some persons are throughout their life cheerful, gregarious, optimistic, and free from worry, whereas others are just the opposite. The unusually volatile, cyclothymic person is believed to be liable to manic-depressive psychosis, and the suspicious, withdrawn, introverted person to schizophrenia and paranoia. Strong, persistent emotional states such as fear and anxiety may occur as reactions to life situations and may be accompanied by derangements of visceral function. If disproportionate to the stimulus and persistent, they are usually manifestations of an anxiety neurosis, depression, or schizophrenia. Variations in the degree of responsiveness to emotional stimuli are also frequent and, when excessive and persistent, assume importance. In depression all stimuli tend to enhance the somber mood of unhappiness. Emotional responses that are excessively labile and poorly controlled or uninhibited are a common manifestation of many diseases of the cerebrum, particularly those involving the corticopontine and corticobulbar pathways. Such responses constitute a part of the syndrome of pseudobulbar palsy. All emotional expression may be lacking, as in apathetic states or severe depressions, or the patient may be a victim of every trivial problem in daily life; i.e., cannot control worries. Finally, the emotional response may be inappropriate to the stimulus, e.g., a depressing or morbid thought may seem amusing and be attended by a smile or arouse no emotional reaction, as appears to be the case in schizophrenia.

Temperament, mood, and other emotional experiences described above are evaluated by the appearance of the patient and by verbalized accounts of his or her feelings. For these purposes it is convenient to divide emotionality into mood and feeling (affect). By *mood* is meant the prevailing emotional state of the individual without reference to the impinging stimuli. It may be pleasant and cheerful or melancholic. The language, e.g., the adjectives used, and the facial expressions, attitudes, postures, and speed of movement most reliably betray the patient's mood. By contrast, *feelings* (or *affect*) are said to be emotional experiences evoked by particular stimuli.

DISTURBANCES IN IMPULSE Impulse, that basic biologic urge, driving force, or purpose by which every organism is directed to reach its full potentialities, is another important and observable, though somewhat neglected, dimension of behavior. Again, one notes wide normal variations from one person to another in strength of impulse to action and thought, and these individual differences are present throughout life. One of the most conspicuous pathologic deviations is an apparent constitutional weakness in impulse in certain neurotic persons. Moreover, with many types of cerebral disease (particularly those which involve the upper and medial parts of the frontal lobes), a reduction in impulse is coupled with an indifference or lack of concern about the consequences of actions. In such cases all other measurable aspects of psychic function may be normal. Extreme degrees of lack of impulse, or *abulia,* may take the form of mutism and immobility, a state sometimes called *akinetic mutism.* Psychomotor retardation is a lesser degree of the same state and is a feature of both cerebral disease and depression. In the latter instance mood alteration and extreme fatigability are conjoined.

LOSS OF INSIGHT Insight, the state of being fully aware of the nature and degree of one's deficits, becomes manifestly impaired or abolished in relation to all types of cerebral disease that cause complex disorders of behavior. Rarely does the patient with any of these disorders seek advice or help for the illness. Instead, the family usually brings the individual to the physician. Thus, it appears that the diseases which produce many of the high-order or complex mental abnormalities not only evoke observable changes in mentation and behavior but also alter or reduce the patient's capacity for self-observation.

DELIRIUM

CLINICAL FEATURES These are most perfectly depicted in the alcoholic patient. The symptoms usually develop over a period of 2 or 3 days. The first indications of the approaching attack are difficulty in concentrating, restless irritability, tremulousness, insomnia, and poor appetite. One or several generalized convulsions are the initial major symptom in almost 30 percent of the cases. The patient's rest becomes troubled by unpleasant and terrifying dreams or by hallucinations. There may be momentary disorientation or an occasional inappropriate remark.

These initial symptoms rapidly give way to a clinical picture that, in severe cases, is one of the most colorful and dramatic in medicine. The state of consciousness becomes altered (sensorium is "clouded") in that the patient is inattentive and unable to perceive all elements of the situation. The patient may talk incessantly and incoherently and look distressed and perplexed; the facial expression is in keeping with vague notions of being annoyed or pursued by some threatening person. From the patient's manner and speech content it is evident that the patient misinterprets the meaning of ordinary objects and ambient sounds and has vivid visual, auditory, and tactile hallucinations, often of a most unpleasant type. At first the patient can be brought momentarily into touch with reality and may in fact answer questions correctly; but almost at once there is a relapse into the preoccupied, confused state; the patient gives wrong answers, is unable to think coherently, and is incapable of proper self-orientation. Before long the patient is unable to shake off the hallucinations even for a second and does not recognize family or physician. Tremor and restless movements are usually present and may be violent. Sleep is impossible or occurs only in brief naps. The countenance is flushed, the pupils are dilated, and the conjunctivas are injected; the pulse is rapid, and the temperature may be raised. There is much sweating, and the urine is scanty and of high specific gravity. The signs of overactivity of the autonomic nervous system, more than any others, distinguish delirium from all other confusional states.

The symptoms abate, either suddenly or gradually, after 2 or 3 days, although in exceptional cases they may persist for several weeks. The most certain indication of the end of the attack is the occurrence of sound sleep and of lucid intervals of increasing length. Recovery is usually complete.

Delirium is subject to all degrees of variability, not only from patient to patient but in the same patient from day to day and hour to hour. The entire syndrome may be observed in one patient and only one or two components in another. In its mildest form, as so often occurs in febrile diseases, it consists of an occasional wandering of the mind and incoherence of verbal expression, interrupted by periods of lucidity. This form, lacking motor and autonomic overactivity, is sometimes referred to as a *quiet delirium* (or *hypokinetic delirium*) and is difficult to distinguish from other confusional states. The most severe form, best exemplified by delirium tremens, ends fatally in 3 to 5 percent of patients.

MORBID ANATOMY AND PATHOPHYSIOLOGY The brains of patients who have died in delirium tremens usually show no pathologic changes of significance. A number of diseases, however, may cause delirium and also give rise to focal lesions in the brain, such as focal embolic encephalitis, viral encephalitis, or trauma. The topography of these lesions is of particular interest. They tend to be localized in the high midbrain and subthalamus and in the temporal lobes, where they involve the reticular activating and limbic systems.

Penfield's studies of the human cortex during surgical exploration clearly indicate the importance of the temporal lobe in producing visual, auditory, and olfactory hallucinations. With subthalamic and midbrain lesions there may be visual hallucinations that are pleasant, animated, and accompanied by good insight (the peduncular hallucinosis of Lhermitte).

The electroencephalogram in delirium may show nonfocal slow activity in the 5- to 7-per-second range, a state that rapidly returns to normal as the delirium clears. In other cases only low-voltage, fast activity in the fast beta frequency range is seen, and in milder degrees of delirium there is usually no abnormality at all.

An analysis of the several conditions conducive to delirium suggests at least three different physiologic mechanisms. The withdrawal of alcohol, barbiturates, or other sedative hypnotic drugs, following a period of chronic intoxication, is the most common cause of delirium (Chaps. 242 and 243). These drugs are known to have a strong depressant effect on certain areas of the central nervous system; presumably the release and overactivity of these parts, after withdrawal of the drug, are the basis of delirium. In the case of bacterial infections and poisoning by certain drugs, such as atropine and scopolamine, the delirious state probably results from the direct action of the toxin or chemical agent on these same parts of the brain. Thirdly, destructive lesions, such as those of the temporal lobes in herpes simplex encephalitis, may cause delirium by disturbing the function of these particular areas.

ACUTE CONFUSIONAL STATES ASSOCIATED WITH REDUCED ALERTNESS AND PSYCHOMOTOR ACTIVITY

In the most typical examples, all mental functions are reduced to some degree, but alertness, attentiveness, and the ability to grasp all elements of the immediate situation suffer most. In the mildest form the patient may pass for normal, and only failure to recollect and reproduce happenings of the past few hours or days reveals the inadequacy of mental function. The more obviously confused patient spends much time in idleness, and what is done may be inappropriate and annoying to others. Only the more automatic acts and verbal responses are properly performed, but these may permit the examiner to obtain from the patient a number of relevant and accurate replies to questions about age, occupation, and residence. Reactions are slow and indecisive, and it is difficult for the patient to sustain a conversation. The patient may fall asleep during the interview and if left alone sleeps more hours each day than is natural. Responses tend to be rather abrupt, brief, and mechanical. Disturbances of perception are frequent, causing misinterpretation of voices, common objects, and the actions of other persons. Often one cannot discern whether the patient hears voices and sees things that do not exist, i.e., whether he or she is hallucinating, or is merely misinterpreting stimuli in the environment. Inadequate perception and forgetfulness result in a constant state of bewilderment. Failing to recognize the surroundings and having lost all sense of time, the patient repeats the same question and makes the same remarks over and over again. Irritability may or may not be present. Some patients are extremely suspicious, demanding, and aggressive; in fact, a paranoid trend may be the most pronounced and troublesome feature of the illness.

As the confusion deepens, conversation becomes more difficult, and at a certain stage the patient no longer notices or responds to much of what is occurring. Questions may be answered with a single word or a short phrase spoken in a soft tremulous voice or whisper, or the patient may be mute. In its most advanced stages confusion gives way to stupor and finally to coma. As the patient improves, there may again be a stage of stupor and confusion, occurring in the reverse order. All this informs us that at least one category of confusion is but a manifestation of the same disease processes that in their severest form cause coma.

In the most typical cases, this type of confusional state is readily distinguished from delirium; in others with more than the usual degree of irritability and restlessness, one cannot fail to notice the resemblance of one to the other. Similarly, when a delirium is complicated by an illness that superimposes stupor (e.g., delirium tremens with pneumonia or meningitis), it may be difficult to distinguish from other confusional states.

When clouding of consciousness is minimal and the confusion is of insidious onset and several weeks' duration, it may mimic dementia. Lipowski has called it "reversible dementia," claiming it to be an intermediate state between delirium and dementia and still potentially reversible. We would classify it as a protracted confusional state.

MORBID ANATOMY AND PATHOPHYSIOLOGY Confusional states are so diverse and are associated with such a wide variety of diseases that one would hardly expect a common anatomy or pathophysiologic basis. In general there is a more frequent occurrence with lesions of the right nondominant hemisphere, especially the posterior parts of it. As will be remarked upon in Chap. 24, large vascular and other acute lesions of the right parietal lobe tend to render the patient underactive, apathetic, and unaware of his or her neurologic disabilities. With this there may be disorientation and inattentiveness. Only if the lesion is large enough to cause a hemiplegia, hemisensory disorder, or homonymous hemianopia will the focal nature of the lesion be appreciated. The same may be said of left temporooccipital lesions.

More frequently the basis of the confusional state is an acute metabolic disease, and the pathologic changes, if detectable (many are not visible by light microscopy), are bilateral and diffuse. Hypoxia, hyperglycemia, uremia, metabolic acidosis or alkalosis, hepatic stupor, hyponatremia, and certain drug intoxications are some of the recognized causes, readily corroborated by appropriate biochemical analyses of blood, urine, and cerebrospinal fluid. Clues to these biochemical derangements are often provided by observations of respiration, presence of asterixis, myoclonus, tremor, and preserved pupillary reflexes. Correction of the biochemical derangements may result in rapid improvements in the patient's condition. (See Chap. 20.)

SENILE DEMENTIA AND OTHER CEREBRAL DISEASES COMPLICATED BY MEDICAL OR SURGICAL ILLNESS (BECLOUDED DEMENTIA)

Many elderly patients who enter the hospital with a medical or surgical illness are mentally confused. Presumably the liability to this state is determined by preexisting brain disease, in most instances senile dementia, which may or may not have been obvious to the family before the onset of the complicating illness. Other cerebral diseases (vascular, neoplastic, demyelinative) may have the same effect.

All the clinical features that one observes in the acute confusional states may be present. The severity may vary greatly. The confusion may be reflected only in the patient's inability to relate sequentially the history of the illness, or it may be so severe that the patient is virtually *non compos mentis.*

Although almost any complicating illness may bring out the confusion, it is particularly frequent with infectious disease; with posttraumatic and postoperative states, notably after concussive brain injuries and the removal of cataracts (in which case the confusion is probably related to being temporarily deprived of vision); and with congestive heart failure, chronic respiratory disease, and severe anemia, especially pernicious anemia. Often it is difficult to determine which of several possible factors is responsible for the confusion, and there may be more than one. In a cardiac patient with a confusional psychosis, for example, there may be fever, a marginally reduced cerebral blood flow, intoxication with one or more drugs, and electrolyte imbalance.

When these patients recover from their medical or surgical illness, they usually return to their premorbid state, though their shortcomings, now drawn to the attention of the family and physician, may be more obvious than before.

CLASSIFICATION AND DIAGNOSIS (See Table 21-1)

The first step in *diagnosis* is to recognize that the patient is confused. This is obvious in most cases, but, as pointed out above, the mildest forms of confusion, particularly when some other acute alteration of personality is prominent, may be overlooked. In these mild forms a careful analysis of the patient's thought patterns as the history of the illness and the details of personal life are recited will usually reveal an incoherence. Digit span and serial subtraction of 3s and 7s from 100 are useful bedside tests of the patient's capacity for sustained mental activity. Memory of recent events is one of the most delicate tests of adequate mental function and may be accomplished by having the patient relate all the details of entry into the hospital, laboratory tests, etc.

A certain proportion of psychoses of the schizophrenic or manic-depressive type first become manifest during an acute

TABLE 21-1
Classification of delirium and acute confusional states

I Delirium
- *A* In a medical or surgical illness (no focal or lateralizing neurologic signs; cerebrospinal fluid usually clear)
  - *1* Typhoid fever
  - *2* Pneumonia
  - *3* Septicemia, particularly erysipelas and other streptococcal infections
  - *4* Rheumatic fever
  - *5* Thyrotoxicosis and ACTH intoxication (rare)
  - *6* Postoperative and postconcussive states
- *B* In neurologic disease that causes focal or lateralizing signs or changes in the cerebrospinal fluid
  - *1* Vascular, neoplastic, or other diseases, particularly those involving the temporal lobes and upper part of the brainstem
  - *2* Cerebral contusion and laceration (traumatic delirium)
  - *3* Acute bacterial and tuberculous meningitis
  - *4* Subarachnoid hemorrhage
  - *5* Viral encephalitis
- *C* The abstinence states, exogenous intoxications, and postconvulsive states; signs of other medical, surgical, and neurologic illnesses absent or coincidental
  - *1* Withdrawal of alcohol (delirium tremens), barbiturates, and nonbarbiturate sedative drugs, following chronic intoxication (Chaps. 242 and 243)
  - *2* Drug intoxications: camphor, caffeine, ergot, bromides, scopolamine, atropine, amphetamine
  - *3* Postconvulsive delirium

II Acute confusional states associated with psychomotor underactivity
- *A* Associated with a medical or surgical disease (no focal lateralizing neurologic signs; cerebrospinal fluid clear)
  - *1* Metabolic disorders: hepatic stupor, uremia, hypoxia, hypercapnea, hypoglycemia, porphyria
  - *2* Infective fevers
  - *3* Congestive heart failure
  - *4* Postoperative and posttraumatic psychoses
- *B* Associated with drug intoxication (no focal or lateralizing signs; cerebrospinal fluid clear): opiates, barbiturates, bromides, trihexyphenidyl (Artane), etc.
- *C* Associated with diseases of the nervous system (the focal or lateralizing neurologic signs and cerebrospinal fluid changes of these conditions are commoner than in delirium)
  - *1* Cerebral vascular disease, tumor, abscess
  - *2* Subdural hematoma
  - *3* Meningitis
  - *4* Encephalitis
- *D* Beclouded dementia, i.e., senile or other brain disease in combination with infective fevers, drug reactions, heart failure, or other medical or surgical disease

medical illness or following an operation or parturition. A causal relationship between the two is sought but cannot be established. Usually the psychosis began long before but was not recognized. The diagnostic studies of the psychiatric illness must proceed along the lines suggested below. Close observation will usually reveal a clear sensorium and relatively intact memory, which permits differentiation from the acute confusional states.

Once it is established that the patient is confused, the differential diagnosis must be made between delirium, acute confusional states associated with psychomotor underactivity, and a beclouded dementia. This may be difficult at times but can usually be accomplished by careful attention to the patient's degree of wakefulness, alertness and responsiveness, capacity to solve new problems, memory, accuracy of perception, mode of onset, degree of reversibility, and so forth.

CARE OF THE DELIRIOUS AND CONFUSED PATIENT

The physician must be secure in his or her ability to manage the delirious and confused patient because such illnesses are observed almost daily on the medical and surgical wards of a general hospital. Occurring as they do during an infective fever, in the course of another illness such as cardiac failure, or following an injury, operation, or withdrawal from alcohol, they never fail to create grave problems. The physician's program of treatment may constantly be threatened by the patient's agitation, sleeplessness, and uncooperative attitude. The nursing personnel are often sorely taxed by the necessity of providing a satisfactory environment for the convalescence of the patient and, at the same time, maintaining a tranquil atmosphere for the other patients. And the family is appalled by the sudden specter of insanity and all that it entails.

The primary therapeutic effort is directed to the control of the underlying medical disease. Other important objectives are to quiet the patient and protect him or her against injury. A private nurse, an attendant, or a member of the family should be with the patient at all times, if this can be arranged. Depending on how active and vigorous the patient is, a locked room, screened windows that cannot be opened by the patient, and a low bed should be arranged. It is often better to allow the patient to walk about the room rather than to be tied into bed, which may excite or frighten him or her into struggling to the point of complete exhaustion and collapse. If less active, the patient can be kept in bed by leather wrist restraints, a restraining sheet, or a net thrown over the bed. Unless it is contraindicated by the primary disease, the patient should be permitted to sit up or walk about the room part of the day.

All drugs that could possibly be responsible for the acute confusional state or delirium—particularly opioids, barbiturates, bromides, atropine, hyoscine, cortisone, adrenocorticotropic hormone (ACTH), and salicylates in large doses—should be discontinued (unless withdrawal effects are believed to underlie the illness). Paraldehyde and choral hydrate are trustworthy sedatives under these circumstances. Paraldehyde, which is preferred, may be given orally or rectally in doses of 10 to 12 ml. For oral administration, mixing it with fruit juices makes it more palatable. Chlordiazepoxide and diazepam are equally effective if given in full doses, and should be continued until natural sleep is restored. One must be cautious in attempting to suppress agitation completely. To accomplish this may require very large doses of drugs, and vital functions may then be dangerously impaired. The purpose of sedation is to blunt the agitation so that the patient does not become exhausted and nursing care is facilitated.

Confusional states related to antidepressant drugs, e.g., amitriptyline, are said to be reversed by a 2-mg dose of physostigmine.

A fluid intake and output chart should be kept, and any fluid and electrolyte deficit should be corrected. The pulse and blood pressure should be recorded at frequent intervals in anticipation of circulatory collapse. Transfusions of whole blood and vasopressor drugs may be lifesaving if shock develops.

Finally, the physician should be aware of many small therapeutic measures that may allay fear and suspicion and reduce the tendency to hallucinations. The room should be kept dimly lighted at night, and if possible the patient should not be moved from one room to another. Every procedure should be explained in detail, even such simple ones as the taking of blood pressure or temperature. The presence of a member of the family may enable the patient to maintain contact with reality.

Most delirious patients tend to recover if they receive competent medical and nursing care. The family should be reassured on this point and must also understand that the abnormal behavior and irrational actions of the patient are not willful but rather are symptomatic of a brain disease. Once recovered, the patient will be at least partly amnesic for the period of confusion, a gap which must be filled by information provided by physician and family.

REFERENCES

Adams RD, Victor M: *Principles of Neurology,* 2d ed. New York, McGraw-Hill, 1981

Benson FD, Blumer D: *Psychiatric Aspects of Neurologic Disease.* New York, Grune & Stratton, 1975, chap 2

Engel GL, Romano J: Delirium, a syndrome of cerebral insufficiency. J Chronic Dis 9:260, 1959

Lipowski ZJ: *Delirium: Acute Brain Failure in Man.* Springfield, Ill., Thomas, 1980

Lishman WA: *Organic Psychiatry: The Psychological Consequences of Cerebral Disorders.* Oxford, Blackwell, 1978

22
DERANGEMENTS OF INTELLECT, MOOD, AND BEHAVIOR

RAYMOND D. ADAMS
MAURICE VICTOR

As mental, emotional, and behavioral disorders are increasingly recognized as manifestations of disease, the internist is likely to be consulted because an otherwise healthy person begins to lose his or her mental capability of functioning as a student, a worker, or as head of a family. Changes of these types may have any one of several pathologic bases—the beginning of a brain tumor, the formation of a subdural hematoma, a chronic drug intoxication, a degenerative cerebral disease (sometimes hereditary), or a schizophrenic or depressive psychosis, to mention only a few. In former times, when there was little that could be done about any of these clinical states, no great premium was attached to diagnosis; the matter was more or less academic. But modern medicine now offers a means of treating several of the underlying diseases, and in some instances of restoring the patient to normal health and effectiveness. Early recognition of the causative pathologic process improves the chances of recovery.

In this chapter we shall consider first the global deterioration of mental functions subsumed under the heading of dementia and then certain special impairments such as Korsakoff's amnesic state, the schizophrenic syndrome, and affective or mood disorders. A discussion of other special types of intellectual failure will be described in Chaps. 23 and 24, which the student should read in conjunction with this chapter.

THE CLINICAL SYNDROME OF DEMENTIA

The term *dementia* denotes a clinical state in which there is loss of retentive memory and other of the intellectual (cognitive) functions due to a chronic progressive degenerative disease of the brain. It may be associated with signs of disease in one or more of the motor, sensory, visual, or language areas of the cerebrum or may occur in relatively pure form. The chronicity of the process is ordinarily emphasized, but the illogic of setting apart one constellation of cerebral symptoms on the basis of speed of onset, rate of development, or duration is obvious. We would insist that the state of dementia is a generic syndrome of variable type and multiple causation and mechanism, and that a diffuse degeneration of neurons is only one of the underlying diseases.

To be more explicit we find reason for criticizing the concept of dementia as a global loss of all intellectual functions. When the latter are carefully analyzed they are found to include several separable though related functions, such as memory, verbal facility, ability to deal with mathematical symbols, to perceive visuospatial relationships, and to think abstractly and solve problems. Each of these functions (except thinking) has a definable anatomy in the cerebrum and can be affected individually by a disease. For example, retentive memory involves neural mechanisms located bilaterally in the medial parts of the temporal lobes, and the language mechanisms lie in the central part of the left (dominant) hemisphere. It comes as no surprise, therefore, that the dementing illnesses may affect various ones or combinations and sequences of these intellectual deficits. Preferably one should speak not of dementia in the singular but in the plural, i.e., the dementias.

Another point of some importance is that the majority of dementing diseases appear during the senium, and many others during late adult life. It is estimated that 2 to 5 percent of all individuals over 70 years of age show a degree of intellectual decline that threatens their independence. Since the elderly population in the western world is increasing both in percentage of the population and in absolute numbers, the magnitude of the medical problems they will present reaches an alarming dimension. In 1978 the percentage of the population over 65 years was 11 percent; in the United States the number comes to approximately 22 million persons, and by the year 2000 it will be 17 to 20 percent, or approximately 50 million. The dementias of the elderly are not to be regarded as merely the ineluctable consequences of growing old but as age-linked diseases, some 15 percent of which are treatable (Wells). Their prevention is a challenge to the ingenuity of the neuroscientists.

Clinical findings Here we shall first describe the syndrome of progressive global dementia, as most regularly manifested by Alzheimer and Pick forms of senile dementia.

The earliest signs of dementia may be so subtle as to escape the notice of even the most discerning physician. Often an observant relative of the patient or an employer is the first to become aware of certain lack of initiative, irritability, loss of interest, forgetfulness, and inability to perform up to the usual standard. Later there is distractibility of attention; inability to think with accustomed clarity; reduced general comprehension; perseveration in speech, action, and thought; and defective memory, especially for recent events. Frequently a change in mood becomes apparent, deviating more often toward apathy than depression or elation. The direction of this deviation is said to depend on the previous personality of the patient rather than upon the character of the disease, but this is open to question. Excessive lability of mood may be observed, i.e., easy fluctuation from laughter to tears on slight provocation. Lapses in social graces and conduct occur, and judgment becomes impaired, early in some cases and late in others. Paranoid ideas and delusions may develop. As a rule, the patient has little or no realization of these changes in behavior and lacks insight into their meaning. However, in some cases the patient is so painfully aware of the decline that he or she is obviously depressed.

As the condition progresses, particularly in the degenerative diseases, there is loss of almost all intellectual faculties. Dysarthria, aphasia, and sphincteric incontinence, reduced responsivity, and finally mutism may be added to the clinical picture. In a late stage a secondary physical deterioration also takes place. Food intake, which may be increased in the beginning of the illness, is in the end usually limited, with resulting emaciation. Locomotion fails; voluntary movements become poorly coordinated. Any febrile illness or metabolic upset induces a marked increase in confusion and even stupor or coma, indicating the precarious state of cerebral compensation. Finally, the patient remains in bed most of the time and dies of pneumonia or some other intercurrent infection. This whole process may evolve over a period of months or years, usually the latter.

Many of the alterations of behavior are the direct result of disease of the nervous system; expressed in another way, the symptoms are the primary manifestations of neurologic disease. Others are secondary; i.e., they are reactions to the catastrophe of losing one's mind. For example, the dement is said to seek solitude to hide the affliction and may thus appear asocial or apathetic. Again, excessive orderliness may be an attempt to compensate for failing memory; apprehension, gloom, or irritability may reflect general dissatisfaction with a necessarily restricted life. It would appear that even in a state of fairly advanced deterioration the patient is still capable of reacting to the illness and to the persons who care for him or her.

Degenerative diseases may terminate in virtually complete decortication. The patient is unaware of what is happening but lies with eyes open. He or she no longer responds to spoken commands or speaks. There is no interest in food or drink, though they are swallowed if placed in the mouth. The facial and limb muscles are stiff with increased tendon reflexes and Babinski signs. Grasping and sucking are prominent. The sphincters are incontinent.

Morbid anatomy and pathologic physiology of dementia Dementia is related usually to obvious structural disease of the cerebrum and the diencephalon. In some, such as the Alzheimer–senile dementia complex and Pick's disease, the main process appears to be a degeneration and loss of nerve cells in the association areas of the cerebral cortex, with secondary changes in the cerebral white matter. A degeneration of neurons confined to the thalamus may also cause dementia. In others, such as Huntington's chorea and certain of the spinocerebellar and cerebral-basal ganglionic degenerations, loss of neurons in the cerebral cortex is accompanied by a similar degeneration of neurons in the putamen and caudate nuclei. Arteriosclerotic vascular disease may result in multiple foci of infarction throughout the thalami, basal ganglia, brainstem, and cerebrum with dementia. Cerebral involvement may include the motor, sensory, or visual projection areas as well as the association areas. This condition, which takes many forms, is called *multi-infarct dementia,* where mental deterioration dominates the clinical picture. Severe trauma may cause contusions of cerebral convolutions and white matter as well as necroses and hemorrhages in the midbrain, lesions which are responsible for protracted stupor, coma, or dementia. Most diseases that produce dementia are quite extensive, and the frontal lobes are affected more often than other parts of the cerebrum.

Mechanisms other than the destruction of brain tissue may be operative in some cases. Chronic increased intracranial pressure or chronic hydrocephalus (with large ventricles the pressure may not exceed 180 torr), regardless of cause, is often associated with a general impairment of mental function. Compression of cerebral white matter is the main factor. The compression of one or both of the cerebral hemispheres by chronic subdural hematomas may cause a widespread disturbance of cortical function. A diffuse inflammatory process is at least in part the basis for dementia in syphilis and in certain virus infections such as "inclusion body encephalitis"; presumably there is loss of some neurons as well as inflammatory derangement of the function of other neurons. Lastly, several of the toxic and metabolic diseases discussed in Chaps. 242, 361, and 362 may interfere with nervous function over a period of time and create a clinical picture similar to, if not identical with, that of dementia. One must suppose that the altered biochemical environment has affected the excitability of the neurons.

Bedside classification of dementia

I Diseases in which dementia is usually the only evidence of neurologic or medical disease
- *A* Alzheimer's disease and senile dementia
- *B* Pick's disease

II Diseases in which dementia is associated with other neurologic signs but not with other obvious medical disease
- *A* Invariably associated with other neurologic signs
  - *1* Huntington's chorea (choreoathetosis)
  - *2* Leukodystrophies (Schilder's disease, adrenoleukodystrophy)
  - *3* Metachromatic leukodystrophy, and related demyelinative diseases (spastic weakness, pseudobulbar palsy, blindness, deafness)
  - *4* Lipofuscinosis and other lipid-storage diseases (myoclonic seizures, blindness, spasticity, cerebellar ataxia)
  - *5* Myoclonic epilepsy (diffuse myoclonus, generalized seizures, cerebellar ataxia)
  - *6* Jakob-Creutzfeldt disease (diffuse myoclonus and cerebellar ataxia)
  - *7* Cerebrocerebellar degeneration (cerebellar ataxia of olivopontocerebellar type and others)
  - *8* Cerebral-basal ganglionic degenerations (apraxia-rigidity) and supranuclear palsy (paralysis of vertical gaze, neck dystonia)
  - *9* Dementia with spastic paraplegia
  - *10* Basal ganglia calcification (idiopathic and hypoparathyroidism)
  - *11* Hallervorden-Spatz disease
  - *12* Dementia with Parkinson's disease (tremor, rigidity, bradykinesia)
- *B* Often associated with other neurologic signs
  - *1* Cerebral arteriosclerosis
  - *2* Brain tumor
  - *3* Brain trauma, such as cerebral contusion, midbrain hemorrhage, chronic subdural hematoma
  - *4* Marchiafava-Bignami disease (often with apraxia and other frontal lobe signs)
  - *5* Low-pressure hydrocephalus (always with ataxia of gait and often with sphincteric incontinence)

III Diseases in which dementia is usually associated with clinical and laboratory signs of other medical disease
- *A* Hypothyroidism
- *B* Cushing's disease
- *C* Nutritional deficiency states such as pellagra, the Wernicke-Korsakoff syndrome, and subacute combined degeneration of spinal cord and brain (vitamin B_{12} deficiency)
- *D* Neurosyphilis: general paresis and meningovascular syphilis
- *E* Hepatolenticular degeneration, familial and acquired
- *F* Chronic drug intoxication (bromidism, chronic barbiturate intoxication)

Not all of these diseases are of equal importance as causes of dementia. Some are rare. In a series of 84 cases of established presenile dementia (< 65 years of age) admitted to a British Neurological Center, 58 percent had brain atrophy, probably of the Alzheimer type, and 10 percent had multi-infarct dementia. Being a primary neurologic referral hospital, the incidence of tumors was high, nearly 10 percent. Normal-pressure hydrocephalus, alcoholic dementia, Creutzfeldt-Jakob disease, Huntington's chorea, posttraumatic sequelae, and alcoholism accounted for the remaining 30 percent. In an older population (> 65 years) the incidence of brain atrophy was found in approximately 80 percent and multi-infarct dementia 15 percent (Tomlinson). Probably the statistics amassed by Wells from a survey of patients with dementia entering a university hospital are the most representative. These are presented in Table 22-1.

The degenerative diseases that cause dementia are discussed in Chap. 364. The special features of the dementia that accompanies arteriosclerotic, senile, syphilitic, traumatic, nutritional, and degenerative diseases are discussed in the appropriate chapters.

Differential diagnosis The first task in dealing with this class of patients is to make sure that the central problem is one of progressive general deterioration of intellect and personality change. It may be necessary to examine the patient several times before one is confident of the clinical findings.

An easy mistake is to assume that mental function is normal if there is complaint only of nervousness, fatigue, insomnia, or vague somatic symptoms, and to label such patients as psychoneurotic. *This will be avoided if one keeps in mind that*

TABLE 22-1
Frequency of dementing cerebral diseases (417 patients)

	Number	*Percent*
Dementia of unknown cause	199	47.7
Alcoholic dementia (Korsakoff's syndrome)	42	10.0
Multi-infarct dementia	39	9.4
Normal-pressure hydrocephalus	25	6.0
Intracranial masses	20	4.8
Huntington's chorea	12	2.9
Drug toxicity	10	2.4
Posttraumatic	7	1.7
Other identified cerebral diseases (subarachnoid hemorrhage, hypo- and hyperthyroidism, encephalitis, hypoxia, pernicious anemia, etc.)	28	6.7
Pseudodementias:		
Schizophrenia	5	
Depression	16	
Mania	2	
	23	5.5
No diagnosis	7	
No dementia	4	
	11	2.6

SOURCE: *Wells.*

psychoneuroses rarely begin in middle or late adult life. A practical rule is to assume that all mental illnesses beginning during this period are due either to structural disease of the brain or to a depressive psychosis.

A mild dysphasia must not be mistaken for dementia. Aphasic patients appear uncertain of themselves, and their speech may be incoherent. Furthermore, they may be anxious and depressed over this ineptitude. Careful attention to the language performance of these patients, which reveals misuse of words, mispronunciation of words, and impaired comprehension of spoken and written words, will lead to the correct diagnosis in most instances. Further observation will disclose that their behavior, except that which is related to the language disorder, is within normal limits.

Depressed patients present another type of problem. They may remark that their mental function is poor or that they are forgetful and cannot concentrate. Scrutiny of these remarks will show, however, that they actually remember the details of their illness and that no qualitative change in mental ability has taken place. The difficulty is either a lack of energy and interest or an anxiety that prevents the focusing of attention on anything except their own problems. Even during mental tests their performance may be impaired by their emotions in much the same way as the performance of worried students is impaired during examinations. This condition of emotional blocking is called *experiential confusion.* When patients are calmed by reassurance and given more time in the performance of tests, mental function improves, indicating that intellectual deterioration has not occurred. Hypomanic patients fail in tests of intellectual function because of restlessness and distractibility. It is helpful to remember that demented patients, except in the early phases of their illness, rarely have sufficient insight to complain of mental deterioration and those who admit to poor memory seldom realize the degree of their disability. The physician must never rely on patients' statements of the efficiency of mental function and must always evaluate a poor performance on tests in the light of the emotional state and motivation at the time the test is given. Especially difficult is the mildly demented patient who is also depressed and whose computerized tomography (CT) scan shows some degree of ventricular enlargement and sulcal widening, raising the question of normal-pressure hydrocephalus. Sometimes the contribution of depression can only be ascertained by an empirical trial of antidepressant drugs.

The neurologic syndromes associated with metabolic or endocrine disorders, i.e., ACTH therapy, hypothyroidism, Cushing's disease, Addison's disease, or the postpartum state may be difficult to separate from that of dementia because of the wide variety of clinical pictures by which they manifest themselves. Some such patients appear to be suffering from a dementia, others from an acute confusional psychosis; or if mood change or delusions predominate, a manic-depressive psychosis or schizophrenia is suggested. In these conditions some degree of clouding of sensorium and impairment of intellectual function can usually be recognized, and these findings alone should be enough to exclude schizophrenia and manic-depressive psychosis. It is well to remember that acute onset of mental symptoms always suggests confusional psychosis or delirium. Inasmuch as many of these conditions are completely reversible, they must be distinguished from the dementia of degenerative diseases (see Chap. 21).

Once it is decided that the patient suffers from a dementing disease, the next step is to determine by careful physical examination whether there are other neurologic signs or indications of a particular medical disease. This enables the physician to place the case in one of the three categories in the bedside classification. X-rays of the skull, electroencephalogram, lumbar puncture, and CT scans should be carried out in most cases. Usually these procedures necessitate admission to a hospital. The final step is to determine by the total clinical picture which disease within any one category the patient has.

ONE SPECIAL TYPE OF INTELLECTUAL IMPAIRMENT—AMNESIC DEMENTIA (Also Korsakoff's psychosis, amnesic confabulatory psychosis)

Clinical findings These terms are used interchangeably to designate a unique but common disorder of cognitive function, in which memory is deranged out of all proportion to other components of mentation and behavior. It possesses two salient features which may vary in severity but are always conjoined: (1) an impaired ability to recall events and other information that has been recorded in the mind before the onset of the illness (retrograde amnesia); and (2) an impaired ability to acquire new information, i.e., to learn or to form new memories (anterograde amnesia). Other cognitive functions (particularly the capacity for concentration, spatial organization, visual and verbal abstraction), which depend little or not at all on memory, may also be impaired but to a relatively minor degree. The patient tends to be lacking in initiative and spontaneity and is usually complacent. Ability to repeat a series of numbers or a spoken sentence (immediate memory) is intact. Recent memories are affected much more than remote ones (Ribot's law) but the extent of this varies with the disease. In Wernicke's disease early or remote memories are retained better than in Huntington's chorea. Performance on a general intelligence test may be relatively unimpaired. *Confabulation,* meaning false or fabricated accounts of recent events, is present in most cases, especially in the acute phase of the illness.

The definition of Korsakoff's psychosis demands also that certain aspects of behavior and mental function be intact. The patient should be alert, attentive, responsive, and capable of understanding the written and spoken word, of making appropriate deductions from given premises, and of solving such problems as can be concluded within his or her forward memory span. These "negative" features are of particular importance because they help to distinguish Korsakoff's psychosis from a number of other disorders in which the basic defect is not necessarily in retentive memory but in some other psychologic mechanism, e.g., in attention and perception (as in the delirious, confused, or stuporous patient), in recall (as in the hysterical patient), or in volition (as in the patient with frontal lobe disease).

Pathologic anatomy The anatomic structures of particular importance in memory function are the diencephalon (specifically the medial portions of the medial dorsal nuclei of the thalamus) and the inferomedial portions of the temporal lobes, particularly the hippocampal formations and underlying white matter. Bilaterally placed lesions in either of these regions derange memory and learning out of all proportion to other cognitive functions, and even unilateral lesions in the dominant hemispheres produce a lesser degree of the same effect. It would appear that the aforementioned anatomic structures are involved in all forms of learning and integration of newly formed memories and that they form a tenuous but vital link between the high brainstem reticular formation (the integrity of which is necessary to maintain an alert state of mind, a prerequisite for any learning) and the cerebral cortex, which is the locus for special memories such as words, geometric figures, and numbers.

Classification of diseases characterized by an amnesic syndrome

I Amnesic syndrome of sudden onset—usually with gradual but incomplete recovery
  A Bilateral hippocampal infarction due to atherosclerotic-thrombotic or embolic occlusion of the posterior cerebral arteries or their inferior temporal branches
  B Trauma to the diencephalic or inferomedial temporal regions
  C Spontaneous subarachnoid hemorrhage
  D Carbon monoxide poisoning and other hypoxic states (rare)

II Amnesia of sudden onset and brief duration with full recovery
  A Temporal lobe seizures
  B Postconcussive states
  C "Transient global amnesia"

III Amnesic syndrome of subacute onset with varying degrees of recovery, usually leaving permanent residue
  A Wernicke-Korsakoff disease
  B Inclusion body (herpes simplex) encephalitis
  C Tuberculous and other forms of meningitis characterized by a granulomatous exudate at the base of the brain

IV Slowly progressive amnesic states
  A Tumors involving the walls of the third ventricle and temporal lobes
  B Alzheimer's disease and other degenerative disorders (early stage only)

Some of these amnesic syndromes are unique. For example, in *episodic global amnesia,* described originally by Adams and Fisher, an elderly person (usually over 50 years) will suddenly reveal uncertainty as to whereabouts, the time of day, and what he or she is doing by asking questions. If told, the person quickly forgets and asks the same questions repeatedly. In contrast to the patient having a seizure, the patient with global episodic amnesia is in contact with the environment and can reply to complex questions, read, calculate, and perform routine tasks. There is also a loss of memories of events that happened hours or days before the attack began. There is no evidence at the time of pallor, twitching, or altered consciousness. Within a few hours the patient makes a complete recovery but is left with a gap in memory that covers the period of the attack and a short period before its onset. Minor changes in the temporal regions during the attack are disclosed in an EEG. An ischemic attack due to obstructive disease of the temporal branches of the posterior cerebral arteries is one postulated cause. The patient usually has only a single attack and no treatment is necessary. Second, third, or several attacks may occur, however, and nothing is known about how to prevent them.

Acute inclusion-body encephalitis is the viral infection that is recognized as the cause of an amnesic state, because of its tendency to localize in the medial parts of the temporal lobes (see Chap. 360). Evidence of herpes simplex virus has been obtained in the majority of such cases. In some patients with carcinomatosis, a limbic encephalitis of unknown etiology has been found (see Chap. 358). Some gliomas infiltrate the temporal lobes, fornices, and thalamus over a period of weeks to months, resulting in an almost specific amnesic syndrome.

In many of these diseases other components of intellectual function are impaired and other neurologic disorders are conjoined. Lack of impulse—a psychomotor retardation—is the most frequent.

The differentiation of the diseases that give rise to the amnesic syndrome proceeds along the lines indicated in Chaps. 357, 358, 360, and 364.

The abulic-hypokinetic-mute syndrome In varying degree this mental state is the most common in all of neuropsychiatry and will be referred to in the description of a variety of cerebral diseases. The change is one which touches all aspects of the psychic life of the individual and is best regarded as a quantitative reduction in activity. In its mildest degree, often undetected in a clinical setting, the patient has fewer thoughts, fewer words, and fewer movements per unit of time. Idleness, which is poorly tolerated by the healthy person, is accepted with seeming indifference. An intelligent person whose life is largely verbal no longer reads or watches television; he or she is content to sit or lie in bed. Tasks which require a series of ideational associations or serial steps are finished after long pauses or left uncompleted. Every type of assignment, whether involving words, numbers, a sequence of movements, or memorization of events, reflects the slowness and impersistence. There is every gradation from this mild form of the syndrome to complete mutism and akinesia.

In respect to mechanism, attention is clearly reduced while consciousness is maintained. One must suppose that cortico-thalamic interaction is impeded, and it seems not to make much difference which part(s) of the cerebrum is affected, nor by what type of disease process, though some of the most striking examples of vigilance with total akinesia have been bifrontal-thalamic.

Psychologic tests may be performed without error and fail to reveal the abnormality, unless timed.

Delusional-hallucinatory (schizophreniform) syndrome and related mental states (psychoses) From the neurologist's standpoint this syndrome is basically a subtle disorder in attention and thinking associated in its most flagrant form with self-preoccupation, hallucinatory experiences and delusions, and inability to separate subjective experience from reality. Often conjoined are disturbances in affect, verbal expression, and social behavior.

Originally Kraepelin, one of the pioneers in German psychiatry, referred to this syndrome as *dementia praecox,* but it soon became evident that it bore little resemblance to the general deterioration described above under "The Clinical Syndrome of Dementia." Indeed, memory function, lost early in the latter syndrome, is usually preserved, except in the most advanced stages. Even then the sensorium tends to remain clear, and language functions, arithmetic ability, and all gnosic and praxic functions of the brain are preserved. Bleuler decided that the term *schizophrenia,* meaning a splitting of the mind (or dissociation of content of thought and affect) was more appropriate. He emphasized disturbances in the association of ideas, an inclination to withdraw from reality, and a preference for rumination and fantasy (autism) as the primary derangements.

Discerning analyses of the abnormal mentation, mood, and behavior inform us that this unique syndrome has multiple causes. While characteristic of a genetic disease, known in the medical world as schizophrenia, the syndrome may also be the clinical expression of manic-depressive psychosis, alcoholic auditory hallucinosis, amphetamine psychosis, temporal lobe epilepsy, some cases of puerperal metabolic and endocrine psychoses, and rarely of focal cerebral disease of other types.

CLINICAL ASPECTS OF THE SYNDROME The clinical state is the most abstruse of any in the realm of neuropsychiatry. Thinking and behavioral abnormalities are both present. In some instances they may be so obvious that diagnosis offers no difficulty whatsoever, but in many others the symptoms may be subtle, vague, and difficult to elicit. The clinician must always depend for diagnosis on the verbal expressions and actions of the patient. If the patient is mute, taciturn, or incapable of freely expressing his or her thoughts, or reluctant to talk because of hostility and suspicion toward the examiner, the primary disorder of thought may not be discovered or may be only inferred from his or her actions. A detailed account of the patient's speech and behavior by an observant member of the family then is particularly helpful.

The most striking feature of the syndrome is a curious alteration of awareness of what is going on. Such patients are seemingly preoccupied with their own thoughts so that their responses to questions are neither constant nor prompt. In their replies to questions and in their spontaneous remarks, one finds that orientation to time, place, and person is intact, and usually the names of doctors, nurses, medications, etc., can be given accurately. In other words, the general aspects of formal intelligence are preserved. However, during the most intense phases of the syndrome, in which mental disorganization is profound, there may be inattentiveness to ambient surroundings.

The thoughts of these patients are often interrupted by the intrusion of distressing ideas and by hallucinations (usually auditory) and unreal dreamlike experiences. Sometimes the hallucinations consist of voices coming from outside the body, but often no clear distinction is drawn between a hallucination and an idea that has been planted in the mind. In the struggle to retain sanity, patients try vainly to separate their own thoughts and perceptual experiences from those of others who are ostensibly trying to control them. Communication of this melange of confusing experiences is difficult. Even when obviously preoccupied with voices, the patients may be reluctant or unable to admit that they are hallucinating.

The patients may feel that their thoughts are being read by others or that they are under outside control. When extraneous ideas are forced upon them they may feel powerless, as though they are passive recipients of the ideas of others (passivity feelings). They may believe these ideas have been transmitted to them by wireless electronic devices, laser beams, or whatever is culturally in vogue. Sometimes they may believe that their own thoughts are made known to others by similar devices. Trying to cope with this confusion of strange and disturbing ideas, patients become so self-absorbed that simple questions may evoke no reply or only one that seems tangential, inappropriate, and incomplete.

Psychologists have attempted for decades to categorize this thought disorder and to educe its essential character. They have remarked on the apparent "disregard for the logical limits of time and space," the "confusion of parts for wholes," "the lumping and condensation of separate items," the acceptance of "the identity of opposites," and the inability to think abstractly. None of these attributes appear to be inclusively descriptive.

Associated with this thought disorder are delusions. These are expressed at some time in the majority of cases. Patients may come to believe they have a disease, that their lives are in danger, that they have been singled out or are threatened for some obscure reason, or that they have suddenly gained remarkable insight into world events. The delusions, based as they are on accusatory or controlling hallucinatory and imagined experiences, cannot be eradicated by logical argument. Such thoughts may be acted upon and occasionally lead to suicide or homicide.

This disorder of thought may vary in intensity from time to time. If it is severe and persistent, patients appear overwhelmed; they may lie mute and frozen in a state of suspended activity (catatonia), or they may be found wandering aimlessly, perplexed, and fearful or excited. The mental state then may resemble a confusion or delirium but without the characteristic clouding of consciousness. If the thought disorder is mild, there are periods when patients appear relatively normal and only withdrawal, disregard of social customs, and preoccupations prevent adequate school or work performance. However, at any time the thought disorder may break through, and seemingly well persons may for no obvious reason once again become vague, preoccupied, and deluded.

The typical and allegedly characteristic affect of the delusional-hallucinatory syndrome is difficult to interpret. Often it seems to be a reflection of the patients' mental state and content of thought. When they are preoccupied, they appear to be detached and indifferent to surroundings. Irritability and undue sensitivity are prominent in some patients and are expressed as resentment toward the therapist and sometimes as unreasonable hostility. If voices and ideas threaten, they first excite patients, but later, if the threats continue, patients become more or less inured to them. While some of the emotional reactions seem inappropriate to the immediate situation, it is usually discovered that they are not inappropriate to the patients' thoughts and mental preoccupations. If one can probe the content of thought, one may then find that the emotions are not at all incongruous, but in some instances the incongruity of thought and feeling is obvious and impossible to understand.

In summary, it is the combination of a subtle *alteration of clear awareness and the intrusion of hallucinatory and dreamlike experiences,* occurring all during the waking hours and making separation of fantasy and reality impossible, and *the delusional systems of ideas* that identifies this psychotic syndrome. Semiologically it falls between delirium on one side and a vague personality and character disorder on the other.

This syndrome, beginning in childhood, adolescence, or early adult life in a patient whose family is known to include other members who are schizophrenic, and causing persistent school failure and continuously inadequate social and occupational adjustment is called *schizophrenia.* This disease will be described in Chap. 377.

PSYCHOTIC FORM OF MANIC-DEPRESSIVE DISEASE Descriptions of manic-depressive disease and dementia praecox, from the earliest ones by Kraepelin, cannot fail to impress the readers with the similarities between these disease states. Contemporary psychiatrists attest to the difficulty in distinguishing some cases of these two diseases by positing a category of *schizoaffective* or *schizothymic* states in which are combined attributes of both. Pope and Lipinski, after a review of the literature and a 4-year personal experience with admissions to the McLean Hospital, and Robins and Guze and their associates, observe that the full delusional-hallucinatory psychotic syndrome of schizophrenia occurs frequently in the manic phase of manic-depressive disease. They insist that this psychotic syndrome when viewed in "cross section" is not diagnostic of either schizophrenia or manic-depressive disease; i.e., it is nonspecific. If it occurs acutely in association with a prominent affective or mood disorder in a previously well-adjusted individual, especially if it is preceded by euphoria, hyperactivity, flight of ideas, pressure of speech, grandiosity, hostility, and sleeplessness (the usual symptoms and signs of mania), the diagnosis will usually turn out to be manic-depressive disease. The hypomanic patient often will have a family history of manic-depressive disease, and over 70 percent will respond to lithium therapy and make a full recovery within a few weeks to months. Schizophrenia differs in the lack of manic-depressive disease in the family, lack of affective symptoms and an emotional state incongruent with thought content, a more gradual onset, incomplete recovery, and little or no response to lithium. Some psychiatrists (Goodwin and Guze) divide schizophrenic illnesses into poor-prognosis and good-prognosis types. The majority of the latter are forms of manic-depressive disease. Depressive states of nonpsychotic type are more fully discussed below.

ALCOHOLIC AUDITORY HALLUCINOSIS This disease begins as a withdrawal or abstinence syndrome in the chronic alcoholic. Usually it subsides in 1 to 2 weeks, but in some the hallucinosis persists indefinitely. The illness comes in time to resemble schizophrenia (see Chap. 240). Affected individuals do not have a premorbid schizoid personality and have no family history of schizophrenia. Such cases reinforce the authors' argument that a slightly altered consciousness, delusions, and hallucinatory experiences stand as the primary abnormalities in the schizophrenic syndrome and are not of themselves diagnostic of the disease schizophrenia.

SCHIZOPHRENIC PSYCHOSIS IN PATIENTS WITH TEMPORAL LOBE EPILEPSY Quite apart from the psychomotor seizures, which in themselves induce curious behavioral abnormalities, such patients may develop an acute psychosis with prominent thought disorder, hallucinations and delusions, ideas of reference, remoteness, and a disorganization of behavior and social relations that simulates schizophrenia. The psychosis appears not to be due to continuous subclinical firing of a seizure focus, for the EEG contains no paroxysmal discharge. The patients respond to antipsychotic drugs and recover within a few weeks.

AMPHETAMINE PSYCHOSIS High dosage and prolonged usage of amphetamines can induce a typical paranoid psychosis with characteristic autistic thought disorder, delusions, and hallucinations. Once started it may continue for several weeks and is said to respond to antipsychotic drugs. A similar syndrome is occasionally observed in a metabolic disease, and after marijuana and lysergic acid overdosage. The authors have had little experience with these states and cannot document the similarity of such syndromes to the one under consideration.

PUERPERAL PSYCHOSIS Brief psychologic disturbances are not infrequent in the puerperium. The most typical reaction is a depression which may last for days, weeks, or months, and may recur after the next pregnancy. There is another type of psychosis featured by variable degrees of confusion and autistic thought disorder. The deluded mother may claim the baby not to be her own, and there are tragic instances where she has killed the infant. Recovery occurs over many weeks or months, and opinion is divided as to whether this is a confusional psychosis or delirium or is a delusional-hallucinatory psychosis of either schizophrenic or manic type.

ENDOCRINE PSYCHOSIS In patients receiving high-dose corticosteroid or ACTH therapy and occasionally in a person suffering from hyperthyroidism, there may occur poor sleep, hallucinations, delusions, disordered thought, and frenzied excitement in varying combinations. Discontinuation of the steroid or treatment of the thyrotoxicosis usually restores the patient to normalcy within a few weeks. Here once again is an example of an illness that overlaps the acute confusional and delirious state where there is clouding of consciousness on the one hand and the more protracted delusional-hallucinatory syndrome with relatively clear consciousness on the other.

DIFFERENTIAL DIAGNOSIS At times a schizophrenic illness that never explodes into an overt psychosis but leads to persistent inability to function in school, at work, or as a member of a family unit may be difficult to distinguish from one in which there is adolescent turmoil, maladjustment, preoccupation with philosophical ideas and eastern religions, and involvement in the activist affairs of the counterculture. Abuse of drugs adds to the problem. Suspiciousness, dramatic behavior, unreasonable attitudes, and indifference to conventional practices are common to both conditions. Only by identification of the basic cognitive disorders of the schizophrenic syndrome with the added stipulation that it persist for many months will the diagnosis of schizophrenia be established, and this may require a period of observation in the neutral environment of a hospital. It is said that some social derelicts, vagrants, chronic drug abusers, and sociopathic individuals are actually suffering from simple schizophrenia.

The elderly patient who becomes paranoid while still mentally intact and who is not depressed presents another difficult clinical problem. Such cases need to be studied over a period of time before one can eliminate the possibility of a dementing illness or a depressive psychosis. Only if the latter are excluded is one justified in the conclusion that they have the rare and special psychiatric illness known as pure *paranoia*.

SYNDROMES OF EMOTIONAL (AFFECT AND MOOD) DISTURBANCE The term *emotion* is used in medical practice in so many ways that it virtually loses all meaning. It refers indiscriminately to the nervous, the neurotic, the unhappy and maladjusted, and to the patient with obscure medical disease. The neurologist assigns to it a more precise definition—a complex state of the organism comprised of a mental component of fear, anger, love, or hate in association with certain visceral changes that are mainly under the control of the autonomic nervous system and lead to a certain pattern of motor expression. Intense emotion may disturb rational thought, and the resulting behavior, while apparently degraded and stereotyped, is nonetheless protective of the organism. Mild emotion may take the form of anxiety, depression, or elation with only the most subtle visceral accompaniments and somatic manifestations.

Human emotion upon strict analysis consists of a stimulus, the accurate perception of which requires the memory of specific associations drawn from previous experience. The psychic state aroused by the perception includes a *feeling* or *affect* known only to the experiencing individual and manifested through verbal expressions and behavior. Thus, on the one side, an emotion includes the same perceptive-cognitive processes as does any induced sensory experience, but it differs with respect to its affective component with the associated visceral reactions and with respect to certain specific patterns of behavior.

Cannon and Bard and their associates studied the ways in which the two parts of the autonomic nervous system participate in the emotional state—the parasympathetic mediating trophotropic, restorative, and reproductive functions, viz., the general homeostatic functions; and the sympathetic (including the adrenal glands) mediating self-protective or ergotropic functions. Hess and Bard localized the central control mechanisms in the hypothalamus which are ideally situated to send impulses via descending tracts to the parasympathetic and sympathetic segmental apparatus and via releasing factors to the pituitary-adrenal-thyroid system. This entire complex of emotional activities, including visceral, glandular, and motor reactions, could be elicited from decerebrate animals as long as the hypothalamus remained intact. Papez postulated that the limbic parts of medial temporal and orbital parts of the frontal lobes, which have rich connections with the hypothalamus, could sustain and modulate the long-acting emotional states. His ideas have been corroborated by the experiments of Bard.

Clinical observations The affective and emotional apparatus is known to be disordered in a number of ways by diseases of the brain. There may be an unnatural *apathy* and *placidity*, wherein the usual stimuli of fear, anger, love, and anxious concern have little or no effect on the patient. Bilateral temporal lesions may result in this condition, along with a remarkable failure of visual recognition, a tendency to examine every object by touch or oral exploration, and either hyper- or hyposexuality. This entire complex is known as the *Kluver-Bucy syndrome.* The right parietal (nondominant) lobe seemed very important in emotional experience, and large lesions here result in an unusual blunting of all emotional reactions. In contrast, a focal lesion in the dominant temporoparietal region rarely may plunge the patient into a state of frenzied excitement, rage, and fear; every stimulus, even innocuous ones, excite the individual, who may lash out blindly at everyone who approaches. One may imagine that the dominant cerebral lesion has disinhibited the intact right parietal lobe. Inferior bifrontal lesions may cause either apathy along with abulia or, rarely, excitement and aggressive behavior, depending on their anatomy. Complete disinhibition of the facial-respiratory apparatus for laughter and crying (syndrome of forced or pathologic laughter and crying) is a frequent accompaniment of pseudobulbar palsy. Here it is the apparatus for emotional expression and not the mental state that is out of control. Lesser degrees of this, in the forms of emotional lability, occur in many cerebral diseases.

The emotional disorders that are the most subtle and difficult to comprehend are *acute* and *chronic anxiety, depression,* and *mania.* They stand as separate syndromes that may appear as the dominant features of certain mental disturbances. They bear no clear relationship to the circumstances which may have occurred in the patient's life. In some instances the prevailing emotional state, on close examination, has been induced by a hallucination or delusion. In a delirium or the schizophreniform syndrome, for example, voices which threaten the patient's life naturally excite fear. In other mental illnesses, the patient experiences an overwhelming anxiety or depression. Unlike the normal person, in whom anxiety, depression, and elation are the natural reactions to life situations such as loss of livelihood or grief over the death of a loved one, or the winning of a coveted treasure, these patients have no conscious awareness of any provocative stimulus. In this sense their emotional state is endogenous. Manic-depressive psychosis, involutional melancholia, and anxiety neurosis (actually a form of depression in most instances) are the most familiar examples, and in the opinion of most neurologists and many psychiatrists they represent diseases of the brain.

Manic-depressive disease Manic-depressive psychosis is a hereditary disease characterized by a cyclic disorder of mood. There may be episodes of depression or of mania, appearing once or many times during the lifetime of the patient. Depression is more frequent than mania, and some patients have only depressions. Thus, the mood disorder may be subdivided into monopolar or bipolar type; but in some individuals, there may be features of both within a given episode, i.e., mixed manic-depressive. For further description see Chap. 376.

OTHER BEHAVIORAL DISORDERS ASSOCIATED WITH CEREBRAL DISEASE

When one attempts to categorize all the patients with relatively acute or subacute disorders of mentation and behavior under the section headings above and under those listed in Chap. 24, there are still a considerable number that remain difficult to classify. They present themselves as an almost infinite variety of syndromes in which the following abnormalities of function may occur: reduced or increased levels of speech, thought, and action; disorientation as to time and place; idleness and lack of interest; loss of spontaneity and sense of humor; muteness and hypokinesia, resistiveness and negativism; hostility, lack of observance of social customs, use of abusive and vulgar language; inexplicable fright, euphoria, and lack of proper concern; complaint of visual distortion, of excess sensitivity to sounds; distortions of smell and taste; inability to find the names of objects, to follow a conversation, to think coherently; sexual indiscretion, lack of modesty, and other signs of disinhibition; seizures; disturbances of sleep. Obviously these many symptoms do not all have the same basic significance, and the majority possess only relative localizing value. They may be associated with definite hemiparesis, hemihypesthesia, frank aphasia, or homonymous hemianopia, but even without these lateralizing signs they point to the existence of cerebral disease.

Syndromes comprising these elements may be observed in subacute sclerosing panencephalitis, listeriosis with meningoencephalitis, Behçet's meningoencephalitis, adult toxoplasmosis, infectious mononucleosis, acute or subacute demyelinative diseases (acute or subacute recurrent multiple sclerosis), granulomatous and other forms of angiitis, gliomatosis cerebri, carcinomatosis with encephalopathy of multifocal type, multiple tumor metastases, acute and subacute bacterial endocarditis, and thrombopenia with multiple-platelet thromboses in small vessels (Moschkowitz's disease). A fuller account of some of the cerebral symptoms enumerated above is found in chapters dealing with these diseases.

APPROACH TO THE PATIENT

The physician presented with a patient suffering from delirium, confusional states, dementia and psychoses of manic-depressive or schizophrenic type must adopt an examination technique designed to expose fully the intellectual defect. Abnormalities of posture, movement, sensation, and reflexes cannot be relied upon for the full demonstration of the neurologic deficit, for it must be remembered that the association and limbic areas of the brain may be severely damaged without demonstrable neurologic signs of this type.

Three sources of data are required for the recognition and differential diagnosis of these mental disorders:

1 A reliable history of the illness
2 Findings on mental examination, i.e., so-called mental status, as well as on the rest of the neurologic examination
3 Special laboratory procedures, CT and radionuclide scanning of the brain, lumbar puncture, x-rays of the skull, electroencephalogram, arteriography, and sometimes pneumoencephalogram

The history should always be supplemented by information obtained from a person other than the patient. Through lack of insight, patients are often unaware of their illness; indeed, they may be ignorant even of their chief complaint. Special inquiry should be made about the patient's general behavior, social adjustment, capacity for work, personal habits, etc., and family history.

The examination of the mental status must be systematic. At a minimum it should provide answers to the questions listed below.

1 Insight (patients' replies to questions about their chief symptoms): What is your difficulty? Are you ill? When did your illness begin?
2 Orientation (knowledge of personal identity and present situation): What is your name? What is your occupation? Where do you live? Are you married? Where are you now?
   a Place: What is the name of the place where you are now? How did you get here? What floor is it on? Where is the bathroom? What are you doing now?
   b Time: What is the date today? What time of day is it? What meals have you had? When was the last holiday?
3 Memory
   a Remote: Tell me the names of your children and their birth dates. When were you married? What was your mother's maiden name? What was the name of your first school teacher? What jobs have you held?
   b Recent past: Tell me about your recent illness (compare with previous statements). What did you have for breakfast today? What is my name or the nurse's name? When did you see me for the first time? What tests were done yesterday? What were the headlines in the newspaper today? Give patients a simple story, oral or written, and ask him to recall it after 3 to 5 min.
   c Immediate recall (short-term memory): Repeat these numbers after me (give a series of 3, 4, 5, 6, 7, and then 8 digits at the speed of one per second). Now when I give a series of numbers, repeat them in reverse order.
   d Visual span: Show patients a picture of several objects, ask them to name what they have seen and note any inaccuracies.
4 General information: Ask about names of presidents, well-known historic dates, the names of large rivers or cities, etc.
5 Capacity for sustained mental activity
   a Calculation: Test ability to add, subtract, multiply, and divide. Serial subtraction of 7s or 3s from 100 is a good test of calculation as well as of concentration.
   b Abstract thinking: See if patients can detect similarities and differences between classes of objects, or explain a proverb or a fable.
6 General behavior: Attitudes, general bearing, attentiveness, manner of dress, etc.
   a Content of thought: What ideas occupy the thoughts of patients? Do they believe that their thoughts and actions are controlled or are being broadcast to others? Are there hallucinations and/or delusions? Is there a press of speech or lack of speech?
   b Mood: Do patients appear gay or sad? How do they feel? Are they nervous and worried or apprehensive? What feeling is revealed through speech, attitude, facial expression?
7 Special tests of localized cerebral functions: Grasping, sucking, aphasia battery, praxis with both hands, cortical sensory function, drawing of clock face, map of United States or Europe, floor plan of patient's house, etc.

Another simple bedside test for dementia is what Isaacs and coworkers call the "set test." The patient is asked to name as many items as he or she can recall in each of four categories or sets—colors, animals, fruits, and towns. The maximum score is 10 for each set. A total score of over 25 usually excludes a global type of dementia.

In order to enlist the full cooperation of patients, physicians must prepare them for questions of this type. Otherwise, their first reaction will be one of embarrassment or anger because of the implication that their mind is not sound. It should be pointed out to patients that some individuals are rather forgetful and that it is necessary to ask specific questions in order to form some impression about their degree of nervousness when being examined. Reassurance that these are not tests of intelligence or of sanity is helpful. A more formal and reliable method of examining the mental capacity of adults is the Wechsler-Bellevue test. The Wechsler Memory Test is a reliable method for quantitating the degree of impairment of retentive memory.

Correct diagnosis of treatable forms of mental disease (e.g., general paresis, subdural hematoma, brain tumor, bromide or other chronic drug intoxication, normal-pressure hydrocephalus, pellagra and other deficiency states, and hypothyroidism) is of greater practical importance than the diagnosis of the untreatable ones.

The separation of the Korsakoff amnesic syndrome and dementia depends on the relative integrity of all cognitive functions except retentive memory. The two major so-called functional psychoses, schizophrenia and manic-depressive disease, are distinguished from the amnesic state and dementia on the basis of the retention of an alert state of mind, relative retention of all cognitive functions including retentive memory, and the identification of disordered thinking with prominent hallucinations, delusions, and/or alteration of mood. The separation of these two latter types of mental illness, both of which are chronic, is based on the presence or absence of premorbid psychic peculiarity, age of patient, mode of onset, duration of illness, recovery, recurrence, etc. (Chaps. 375 and 376). If of recent onset while using drugs and alcohol, or associated with temporal lobe seizures or an endocrine disease, a period of observation may be required before the diagnosis can be settled. Information concerning the bizarre thinking disorder in these psychotic states is often revealed by the Rorschach and thematic apperception tests.

MANAGEMENT OF THE PATIENT

These major mental derangements and psychoses are clinical states of the most serious nature, and usually it is worthwhile to admit the patient to the hospital for a period of observation. The physician then has an opportunity to see the patient several times in a neutral and fairly constant hospital environment, and certain special procedures such as x-rays of the skull, lumbar puncture, analysis of blood for drugs, basal metabolic rate, an EEG, CT scan, and sometimes a pneumoencephalogram can be carried out at this time. The management of the demented patient in the hospital may be relatively simple if the person is quiet and cooperative. If the disorder of mental function is severe, i.e., the patient is psychotic, a nurse, attendant, or member of the family must stay with the patient at all times. Provision must be made for adequate food and fluid intake and control of infection, using the same measures outlined for the delirious patient (see Chap. 21).

Once it is established that the patient has an untreatable dementing, amnesic, schizophrenic, or manic-depressive brain disease, a responsible member of the family should be apprised of the medical facts. The patient should be told that he or she has a nervous condition for which rest and treatment has been prescribed. Nothing is accomplished by telling the individual more. The family should be given diagnosis and prognosis if the diagnosis is sufficiently certain for this to be done. If the psychic or mood abnormalities are slight and circumstances are suitable, the patient should remain at home, continue customary activities, and receive appropriate medication. If depressed and suicidal, the patient should remain in a psychiatric hospital. He or she should be spared responsibility and guarded against injury that might result from imprudent action. If the patient becomes demented while still at work, plans for occupational retirement should be carried out. In more advanced stages of disease, mental and physical enfeeblement become pronounced and institutional care should be advised. Seizures should be treated symptomatically. Nerve tonics, vitamins, and hormones are of no value in checking the course of dementia or in regenerating decayed tissue. They may, however, offer some support to the patient and family. Sometimes, stimulants in the form of dextroamphetamine, caffeine, and nicotinic acid cause transitory improvement in mental function. Undesirable restlessness, nocturnal wandering, belligerency, or anxiety may be reduced by some of the "minor" tranquilizing drugs (see Chap. 241).

REFERENCES

ADAMS RD, VICTOR M: *Principles of Neurology,* 2d ed. New York, McGraw-Hill, 1981

BENSON L, BLUMER D: *Psychiatric Aspects of Neurologic Disease.* New York, Grune & Stratton, 1975

FISHER CM, ADAMS RD: Episodic global amnesia. Acta Neurol Scand, vol 40, suppl 9, 1964

GOODWIN DW, GUZE SB: *Psychiatric Diagnosis,* 2d ed. New York, Oxford University Press, 1979

HOREL JA: The neuroanatomy of amnesia. A critique of the hippocampal memory hypothesis. Brain 101:403, 1978.

ISAACS B, KENNIE AT: The set test as an aid to the detection of dementia in old people. Br J Psych 123:467, 1973

LURIA AR: *Higher Cortical Functions in Man.* New York, Basic Books, 1966

POPE HG, LIPINSKI JF: Diagnosis in schizophrenia and manic depressive illness. Arch Gen Psychiatry 35:811, 1978

ROBINS E et al: Diagnostic criteria for use in psychiatric research. Arch Gen Psychiatry 26:57, 1972

TOMLINSON, BE: Dementia, in *Contemporary Neurology Series,* CE Wells (ed). Philadelphia, Davis, 1977

WELLS CW: Treatable forms of dementia, in *Update II: Harrison's Principles of Internal Medicine,* KJ Isselbacher et al (eds). New York, McGraw-Hill, 1981

23
AFFECTIONS OF SPEECH

JAY P. MOHR
RAYMOND D. ADAMS

Language and speech are of fundamental significance to humanity both in social intercourse and private intellectual life. When disordered as a consequence of disease of the brain, the loss exceeds in gravity even blindness, deafness, and paralysis.

GENERAL CONSIDERATIONS

The terms *speech* and *language* refer to some of the most complex and poorly understood activities of the cerebrum. The terms are not synonymous.

Speech involves the execution of acquired skills of the vocal, manual, auditory, and visual systems in the conveyance of interpersonal communication. These skills include pronunciation of words; variations in stress, intonation, and melody; the production of graphic marks in the accepted spatial orientation; the auditory discrimination of spoken speech and its classification as to speaker; the visual discrimination of handwritten or printed speech; the visual search patterns involved in scanning a text; and the use of other, less specifiable behaviors. Deficiencies in these skills impede interpersonal communication apart from any separate impairment in language usage; when intact, these skills do not suffice for any but elemental communication, such as that between two individuals who speak languages unfamiliar to each other.

Language has a wider connotation and refers to the selection and serial ordering of individual words according to accepted rules that permit a person using the speech modalities to modify the behavior of another and to externalize that poorly understood cerebral activity referred to as *thinking.* A disturbance of language usage, usually accompanied by a disturbance in speech from cerebral dysfunction, is referred to as *aphasia,* or more properly as *dysphasia* (see below).

CEREBRAL DOMINANCE AND ITS RELATIONSHIP TO SPEECH AND HANDEDNESS

Of the general population approximately 90 to 95 percent are right-handed. A person who chooses the right hand for intricate, complex acts and is more skillful with it is said to be right-handed. The preference is more complete in some persons than in others. Most individuals are neither right-handed nor completely left-handed but favor one hand for more complicated tasks.

Left-handedness may result from disease of the left cerebral hemisphere in early life; this fact probably accounts for its higher incidence among the feebleminded and brain-injured. Presumably the neural mechanisms for language then become centered in the right cerebral hemisphere. Handedness and cerebral dominance may fail to develop in some individuals; this is particularly true in certain families.

The reason for hand preference is still controversial. There is strong evidence of a hereditary factor, but learning is also a factor; many children are shifted at an early age from left to right (shifted sinistrals) because it is a handicap to be left-handed in a right-handed world. Anatomic differences between the dominant and the minor cerebral hemispheres have recently attracted attention. The left planum temporale, part of Wernicke's language zone, in the left hemisphere, is larger in right-handed individuals.

Unilateral brain damage that produces a disturbance in language affects the left hemisphere in over 95 percent of right-handed individuals. Furthermore, in left-handed individuals who suffer cerebral derangements of speech, approximately 75 percent also have lesions in the left cerebral hemisphere. Further, in those extremely rare cases of aphasia due to right cerebral lesions, the patient is nearly always left-handed, and the speech disorder tends to be less severe and enduring. The functional capacities of the minor hemisphere in language are not fully understood.

The anatomic substrate for improvement in language function after unilateral brain lesions is also poorly understood, whether it is due to recovery of parts of its language zones or to the activity solely of the minor hemisphere.

TYPES OF LANGUAGE DISORDERS ENCOUNTERED IN MEDICAL PRACTICE

These may be divided into four categories:

1. *Cerebral disturbances* in which there is a loss more or less exclusively of the production and/or comprehension of speech and language. Such a condition is called *aphasia,* or, in milder degrees, *dysphasia.*
2. *Defects in articulation* with intact mental functions. These are pure motor disorders of the muscles of articulation and may be due to flaccid or spastic paralysis, rigidity, repetitive spasms (stuttering), or ataxia. The term *dysarthria* refers to these conditions.

3 *Loss of voice* due to a disease of the larynx or its innervation, designated as *aphonia* or *dysphonia.*
4 *Disturbances of language* that occur with diseases that produce delirium and dementia (see Chaps. 21 and 24). Speech is seldom lost in these conditions but its language content is deranged as part of a general impairment of all elements of higher cerebral functions.

APHASIA OR DYSPHASIA No experimental models exist to test hypotheses of speech and language function. The only reliable source materials are humans with cerebral disease, and the study of such cases is hampered by a number of uncontrollable variables such as the difficulty in the precise delineation of the basic functional deficit and the changes in symptomatology at different periods in the time-course of the disease. The anatomic site of the lesion is now more easily characterized with the advent of computerized tomography (CT scan) but difficulties are still encountered in clinicopathologic correlation. And, finally, of theoretical importance is the problem of ascribing normal function to a part of the cerebrum by a study of the abnormal diseased brain.

As a general orientation, most of the lesions that lead to aphasia occur in the perisylvian or *opercular* regions (frontal, temporal, and parietal) that cover the insula of the dominant cerebral hemisphere, i.e., the left in right-handed individuals.

The clinical deficit is most easily demonstrated in the acute phase of a lesion. The changes that occur with time make estimation of lesion site and size more difficult later on, especially with the smaller lesions. Lesions one or more centimeters in diameter are usually associated with an evanescent deficit that fades to functional insignificance within weeks or months. Diseases affecting the cerebral surface gray matter produce a more significant deficit than those more confined to the white matter; tumors, confined as they are largely to the white matter, usually reach discouragingly large size before speech or language deficit is evident.

The site is more significant than the size of the lesion, for the former determines the qualitative features of the deficit; but the size determines the quantitative features and, in the larger lesions, appears to produce additional qualitative features not present in the smaller lesions. In particular, deficits in speech function are more evident in smaller lesions, while in the larger lesions deficits in language occur as well.

The study of the types of disturbance in speech modalities observed in diseases affecting the sylvian territory show that those that lie anteriorly produce deficits in the acts of speaking. These disorders include mutism, impaired articulation, disordered transitions from syllable to syllable, and defective stress, intonation, and melody. Those located more posteriorly produce malpositioning of the oral cavity and some anticipatory errors out of sequence that result in gross mispronunciations of the intended syllables and words, more evident when the expected utterance is lengthy. Lesions grouped around the posterior sylvian fissure including the superior temporal lobe and its auditory gyri are manifested by disordered discrimination of spoken words, resulting in poor repetition of speech sounds and faulty understanding of spoken language.

Language deficits are well understood and less well correlated with anatomic pathology. Traditional formulations of aphasia envision only one "true" language deficit, the detection of which by any method of testing suffices to label the patient as aphasic. But formulations based more on pathoanatomic correlations are leaning more toward separation of two large categories of language disorder. Large anterior lesions involving the bulk of the frontal operculum and insula result in *agrammatism,* which features sharply contracted sentence structure, lack of most small grammatic words, often with faulty use of grammar in the words remaining, the surviving words serving mainly a predicative or substantive function. Large posterior sylvian lesions show almost the opposite, with substantive elements missing or substituted by errors in which the desired response is only approximated (paraphasias). These latter may consist of faulty pronunciations (literal paraphasias) or faulty word selections (verbal paraphasias). Disturbances in understanding language, both the auditory and visual speech forms, occur in both types of major paraphasias.

Lesions in other parts of the cerebrum either cause no disturbance of human communicative skills or alter them only secondarily. An example of the latter is the lesion of the *anterior frontal lobes,* especially the medial and orbital parts, which impairs all motor activities, and often results in abulia, verging on akinetic mutism. The speech is laconic with long pauses between utterances, and there is an inability to sustain monologue and narrative. Extensive *occipital lesions* impair reading and reduce the utilization of all visual, lexic stimuli. Thalamic and deep *cerebral lesions* impair alertness and cause fluctuating states of inattention and disorientation, thereby inducing fragmentation of words (neologisms) and phrases, and protracted uncontrollable talking (logorrhea). Strong stimulation which momentarily stabilizes behavior and speech informs us of the essential integrity of language mechanisms.

The following functions are not disturbed in lesions of the hemisphere dominant for language: motor responses of mimicry, social anticipation (smiling, handshaking, modesty reactions) and self-care (washing and feeding), avoidance behavior to noxious stimuli, and capability of training in performances of cross-matching visually presented simple words with pictures.

In the initial formulations of cerebral function in the last century, a working hypothesis was developed that lesions of the frontal (motor) regions produced syndromes independent from those of the posterior (sensory) regions, that the dysphasias could be classified as motor (Broca's) or sensory (Wernicke's), and could be further specified as subcortical, cortical, or transcortical in location. Subcortical lesions were believed to cut off the main efferent or afferent projections of the cortical "center." Cortical lesions involved the centers themselves. Transcortical lesions isolated the centers from one another, i.e., a kind of "conduction" aphasia, or from other regions of the brain related to speech. In modern times, the difficulties in attempting to understand the disorders of language that usually accompany the disorders of speech in focal brain disease, the improvements in techniques to document the extent of the lesion, and data available in longitudinal studies have led to a greater awareness of the complexity of these relationships.

TYPES OF APHASIA The examination of patients with disturbances of speech and language discloses a number of different abnormalities. Attempts have been made to classify them in terms of their predominant form, their presumed physiologic or psychologic bases, or the anatomy of the underlying diseases. No one of the many schemes has been accepted, and the leading students of language have railed against the premature acceptance of incomplete simplistic theories of language.

The syndromes of aphasia described below have fairly specific anatomic localizing value and can be diagnosed from their clinical presentation without much difficulty. Since the middle cerebral artery nourishes all the speech areas, nearly all aphasic syndromes due to vascular occlusion are caused by involvement of this artery or its branches. The prognoses attached to several syndromes are helpful in management and in the use of different corrective measures in therapy.

Complete (global) aphasia This major syndrome is due to a lesion that destroys a large part of the speech and language areas of the major cerebral hemisphere. As such, it represents the maximal aphasic deficit possible and shows the least improvement of all aphasic syndromes. Occlusion of the left internal carotid or the middle cerebral artery at its origin is usually responsible. Less often, the syndrome may be caused by a large hemorrhage, tumor, or other lesions. Rapid improvement frequently occurs when the main cause is edema, postconvulsive paralysis, or transient hyperthermic and metabolic derangements such as infection, or hyponatremia, which worsen aphasia due to old lesions.

Most patients with total aphasia can say at most a few words; they cannot read or write, and they understand only a few words and phrases of the speech of others. Related signs include right hemiplegia, hemianesthesia, and homonymous hemianopia. The state of consciousness may vary from full alertness to semicoma. The alert patient may participate in common gestures of greeting, may show modesty and avoidance reactions, and is able to engage in self-help activities. Early appearance of clearly vocalized stereotyped words, such as "hi," are often falsely encouraging signs and may reflect the uninhibited function of the right hemisphere. With the passage of time some degree of understanding of spoken speech may be evident, and a few spoken words may emerge.

Broca's aphasia (major motor aphasia) This term is used to designate a complex syndrome, predominantly a failure of motor aspects of speaking and writing, with an accompanying *agrammatism* and a variable impairment in language comprehension. Although commonly thought due to a circumscribed lesion in the inferior frontal convolution (Broca's area), this major syndrome is usually the result of a larger lesion which involves cortical and subcortical structures along the frontal and superior sylvian fissure and the insula, in the territory of supply of the upper division of the left middle cerebral artery.

The lesion of Broca's aphasia is most often an infarction of frontal, anterior parietal, and anterior insular parts of the cerebrum due to embolic occlusion of the upper division of the left middle cerebral artery. Major putaminal hypertensive hemorrhage is also a common cause. A huge frontal lobe tumor or abscess is occasionally responsible; metastatic lesions, subdural hematoma, and encephalitis only rarely cause the syndrome.

Although smaller than the lesion causing complete aphasia, the large lesion involves the sensorimotor rolandic region, with a more or less dense right hemiparetic and hemisensory syndrome that usually persists. Initially, a transient right hemianopia and an ipsilateral deviation of the eyes are observed.

In the acute phase of the syndrome, the entire language mechanism appears inactivated, and the helplessly mute, noncommunicative, and uncomprehending patient presents the syndrome of *complete or global aphasia,* indistinguishable by present methods from that resulting from infarction of the whole left middle cerebral artery territory. Within weeks to years, the disorder of comprehension abates somewhat but remains forever easily detected by formal testing. This improvement in comprehension exceeds that in speaking and writing, allowing the traditional label of *motor aphasia.*

For a time, despite satisfactory comprehension of spoken words and ability to read simple commands, an *apraxia* of the linguooropharyngeal apparatus is manifested in faulty efforts to make purposeful or commanded movements of these parts. In these circumstances imitation of the examiner's actions are better performed than execution of acts on command. Self-initiated actions, by contrast, are often normal. The patient who speaks at all may repeat his or her few remaining words over and over, as if compelled to do so. Certain stereotyped phrases tend to be uttered more easily, such as "hi," "good morning," "how are you," and the words of popular songs when sung. When angered or excited, the patient may curse. The patient's efforts and facial expressions suggest an awareness of his or her own ineptitudes and mistakes. Repeated failures cause exasperation and despair.

As improvement occurs, and in the milder forms of motor aphasia, the patient is able to speak aloud to some degree. Words are enunciated slowly and laboriously. Articulation and the melody of speech (prosody) are impaired. This dysfluency takes the form of improper accent or stress on certain syllables, incorrect phrasing of words in a series, pacing of the speed of word sequences, and even a stammering quality to the uttered phrases. Speech is sparse and consists mainly of nouns, transitive verbs, and important adjectives; many of the small words (articles, prepositions, conjunctions) are omitted, giving the speech an *agrammatic* and telegraphic character. The substantive content allows the patient to communicate to some extent despite the gross mechanical and language difficulties. Once fully established, these speech impediments persist and improve only slightly despite years of speech therapy.

Most patients with Broca's aphasia have a correspondingly severe impairment in writing. Should their right hand be paralyzed, they cannot print with their left one; if manual mobility is spared, they fail as completely in writing out their commands or replies to questions as in speaking them. Writing from dictation is severely impaired, though letters and words can still be copied. On careful testing, however, communication by writing can be shown superior to that of speaking, suggesting a certain independence between these two acts as vehicles of language.

Minor motor aphasia More circumscribed focal lesions along the anterior and superior sylvian operculum and insula produce remarkably discrete effects on the mechanical elaboration of speech which can be observed alone or in combinations, depending on the site and extent of the lesion. The important point with all these minor motor aphasias is that at first they may resemble major motor aphasia except for the satisfactory understanding of spoken and written words. The prognosis for nearly full recovery is excellent. However, *none of these focal lesions produces significant or lasting deficits in language usage;* the experienced listener can easily detect the error patterns in speech and, through them, discern the nature of the communicative difficulties of the sufferer, who is acutely aware of and discouraged by the deficit. The effects on speech of focal opercular lesions take several forms. *Broca's area infarction* involves the lower premotor cortex adjacent to the motor cortex for the oropharynx, larynx, and respiratory apparatus; the infarct interrupts skilled movements of these muscle groups, and the resultant dyspraxia in speech takes the form of impaired transitions between syllables and words, and disruption of the melodic intonation of phrases (dysprosody). Involvement of this region appears insufficient to produce the major syndrome referred to as Broca's aphasia. *Rolandic infarction* involves the sensorimotor cortex itself; poor articulation, lowered volume and pitch of speech, and a nasal quality to the voice reveal the pareses of the involved musculature. *Postcentral, anterior parietal infarction* appears to be associated with errors in the positioning of the oral cavity for individual sounds, syllables, and whole words; the acoustic features of the utterance are often distorted by these malpositions of the oral cavity and strike the listener's ear as literal paraphasias. Since they are easily produced in tests of repeating and reading aloud and occur in conversation, the patient could be labeled as having "conduction" aphasia.

Most such focal lesions are embolic in nature. The sequential branching of the upper division of the middle cerebral artery provides a series of separate sites for emboli to lodge.

Deeper, larger lesions, or larger emboli involving the stem of the upper division, encompass several deficit types in a single patient, making these individual distinctions less clear, and blend with the major syndromes of Broca's aphasia. Facial, lingual, and sometimes brachial paresis and ideomotor dyspraxia of the face and *left, nondominant limbs* commonly accompany the speech disorder. Most of these syndromes fade in clinical significance within weeks or months.

Wernicke's aphasia (major central or sensory aphasia) This term encompasses a wide range of syndromes that arise from lesions from the posterior perisylvian structures to the posterior parietooccipital regions supplied by the lower division of the middle cerebral artery. There is disruption of the whole array of language behavior. When more restricted to the temporal lobe, the main disturbance is most evident in language tasks involving words heard; when more parietooccipital, words seen.

Spoken and written efforts in communication as well as in auditory and visual comprehension are affected, a combination which justifies the term *central aphasia.* The older term, *sensory aphasia,* was formerly used to accentuate the contrast with motor (Broca's) aphasia. Instead of the difficult articulation, faulty transitions, dysmelodic speaking, and disproportionate condensation of grammatical forms that characterize Broca's aphasia, the speech of Wernicke's aphasia is fluent, hence the name *fluent aphasia.* We prefer the eponym *Wernicke's aphasia,* for it serves to encompass all the syndromes while avoiding the many sharp controversies that still surround unsuccessful attempts to characterize these aphasias by a single functional term.

In severe cases, the patient utters a series of incomprehensible syllables, makes illegible marks on a page in attempts at writing, cannot be made to repeat aloud or copy correctly at sight, and treats the examiner's attempts at written and verbal communication as if they were in a wholly unfamiliar foreign language. In less severe cases, the patient can be made to repeat aloud and copy, but in so doing frequently echoes the words heard with faulty pronunciation, or copies the words seen in a slavish manner, imitating even the examiner's handwriting style, as though the test words were unfamiliar. The disturbance in language does not simply reflect a disturbance in hearing or in vision. In the mildest cases, the deficits are reflected in errors in word comprehension and usage that show some approximation to the desired response, the words often belonging to the same functional class [i.e., *cow* for *pig,* but not *cow* for *yellow* (such errors are labeled *verbal paraphasias*)]; errors in word structure, with improper tenses, prefixes, suffixes (i.e., *beautifuling*); and other errors that resemble performances by normal people unfamiliar with the language in question. Some such patients pass for normal in casual conversation. Their speech resembles the performance of people tired or distracted, and their abnormality is detected only on tests of complex language function. This milder state is often the residual of a more severe initial deficit.

As a rule, the syndrome is due to an embolic occlusion of the lower division of the left middle cerebral artery. A "slit hemorrhage" in the subcortex of the temporoparietal region or involvement of the temporal isthmus and adjacent white matter by tumor, abscess, or extension of a small putaminal or thalamic hemorrhage may have similar effects.

The posterior sylvian region, comprising posterosuperior temporal, opercular supramarginal, and posterior insular gyri, appears to encompass a variety of language functions, since seemingly minor changes in size and locale of the lesion are associated with important variations in the elements of Wernicke's aphasia detailed below.

Minor central aphasia syndromes In time the patient with Wernicke's aphasia improves, and a number of lesser syndromes appear. These latter, however, may be present in comparatively pure form from the beginning, when only a small, restricted lesion involves some part of the territory of the lower division of the middle cerebral artery. Depending on the exact locale of lesion, language behavior dependent on auditory function (hearing spoken words, echoing sounds and speech, relating the spoken to the written word, and finally repeating and writing it) may be deranged partially or in its entirety. The same is true of language behavior dependent upon visual function, when the left posterior parietal lobe is involved.

These partial syndromes have been traditionally labeled as conduction aphasia, pure word deafness, and pure word blindness.

Attempts to correlate complete and partial posterior sylvian syndromes with arteriographic findings during life frequently fail. Since most partial vascular aphasias are due to cerebral embolism, the latter may have lodged in the artery long enough to cause infarction and then disintegrated. The arteriogram done after this happens is normal. Or a fragment of the disintegrating embolus may drift distally and permanently block only a more distal branch, sometimes permitting part of the ischemic tissue to recover. Computerized tomography has proved a helpful addition to attempts to delineate the areas involved.

CONDUCTION APHASIA: SEPARATION OF WERNICKE'S AND BROCA'S LANGUAGE AREAS Here the principal abnormality resembles Wernicke's aphasia in certain respects. There is the same degree of paraphasia in self-initiated speech, in repeating what is heard, and in reading aloud. However, no difficulty is encountered in comprehending words that are heard or seen. Because the motor regions are unaffected, no element of dysarthria or dysprosody occurs. The patient is alert and aware of the deficit. The mistakes take the form of literal paraphasia, i.e., errors in oropharyngeal positioning produce detectably different sounds from those intended. The disorder in repeating from dictation becomes more apparent when the rate of presentation of auditory material is increased, the uttered words are more polysyllabic, or when they are unfamiliar, e.g., sets of nonsense syllables. Since nouns are the longest words in the sentence, one may gain an impression that they are specifically affected.

The lesion in autopsied cases is located in the cortex and subcortical white matter in the upper bank of the sylvian fissure, involving the supramarginal gyrus of the inferior parietal lobule. The posterior part of the superior temporal region is the other site occasionally affected. The usual cause is an embolus in the ascending parietal or posterior temporal branch of the middle cerebral artery. Deeper, larger lesions in position to interrupt the arcuate fasciculus connecting the temporal and frontal lobes may produce the syndrome, but usually involve other pathways as well, giving rise to a more extensive speech deficit (Wernicke's aphasia or amnestic aphasia). However, these latter types of aphasia, as they regress, may resolve into conduction aphasia. More anterior insular lesions usually include some degree of Broca's aphasia.

"PURE" WORD DEAFNESS Instead of a disturbance confined to auditory comprehension, this syndrome is more inclusive, being the auditory form of Wernicke's aphasia. The most obvious findings are an impaired auditory comprehension and inability to repeat what is said or to write to dictation. Spoken language is far better performed but is rarely normal, and occasionally the patient is initially diagnosed as having Wernicke's aphasia. By audiometric testing no hearing defect is found, or minor abnormalities appear which may well reveal the underlying deficit in individual cases. Ordinary sounds can be distinguished. The patient is forced to depend heavily on visual cues in understanding the remarks of others and frequently uses these cues well enough to obviate much of the difficulty. But tests which prevent the use of visual cues readily uncover the deficit. Comprehension of visually presented material, for example, printed matter such as newspapers, while not normal, is far better than auditory comprehension. It occasionally approaches normal and justifies use of the traditional term, *pure word deafness.*

In most recorded autopsy studies the lesion has been embolic, bilateral in the superior temporal gyrus, in position to damage the primary auditory cortex in the transverse gyrus of Heschl and its relations to the association areas of the superior, posterior part of the temporal lobe. The few unilateral lesions are localized in this part of the major (dominant) temporal lobe and encroach on those regions whose involvement precipitates the larger syndrome of Wernicke's aphasia.

DYSLEXIA WITH DYSGRAPHIA This syndrome features a language disturbance most evident in reading and writing. The errors in response to lexical stimuli take a form typical of those encountered in the larger syndrome of Wernicke's aphasia. Yet auditory comprehension, while not normal, is superior to visual comprehension. The syndrome should be considered the visual form of Wernicke's aphasia. Since conversational testing frequently is the extent of many casual clinical evaluations of such patients, satisfactory auditory comprehension, ability to repeat aloud, and only mild paraphasic errors in spontaneous speech frequently lead to a misdiagnosis of very mild Wernicke's aphasia. Detailed testing of reading aloud and for comprehension, and tests of spontaneous writing and writing in response to dictated and visually presented material, will reveal a far greater disturbance on these tasks and expose the syndrome. This type of aphasia is often another of the late sequelae of the larger syndrome of Wernicke's aphasia.

The parietooccipital region is the anatomic site of this deficit. A lesion here is unusual in embolism, which more often affects structures more proximal in the territory of the lower division of the middle cerebral artery. However, a small embolus may pass through the more proximal territory and lodge distally in a branch. Tumors, abscess, and the like disrupt other structures as well, and this syndrome is often a less conspicuous part of a larger clinical picture. Systemic hypotension and hypoxia may leave dyslexia with dysgraphia as a residual; but more often they have produced a more severe defect described below under "Isolation of speech areas."

Pure word blindness In this state literate persons lose their ability to read and often to name colors. They can no longer name or point on dictated command to visual letter stimuli or the words of which they are composed. However, understanding spoken language, repetition of what is heard, writing to dictation, and conversation are all intact. Often the patient is unaware of the difficulty and registers no complaint; it is discovered almost by accident. In lesser degrees of the affection, reading aloud is possible, but the patient manages only a single letter at a time (this may be seen in otherwise normal patients who have bilateral hemianopia with only central vision remaining); commonly letter or name responses that seem to have little connection with the presented ones are expressed. The response may be corrected and the defect obscured if other visual cues are available, such as the bottle on which the words *Coca-Cola* appear. The naming of common colors presented singly and of objects is also impaired. The right homonymous hemianopia, an amnesic defect (see Chap. 24), and a hemisensory defect on the right reflect the involvement of the left occipital lobe, the left fornix and its decussation, and the left thalamus, respectively, a combination which nearly always signifies thrombosis or embolism of the left posterior cerebral artery, placing the origin of this syndrome rather remote from the main language zone supplied by the middle cerebral artery territory.

The autopsy of such lesions has usually demonstrated a lesion that destroys the left visual striate cortex (area 17) and visual association areas (18 and 19), as well as the connections of the right visual cortex and association areas with the temporoparietal region. This latter "disconnection" usually is due to interruption of the fibers passing through the posterior part (splenium) of the corpus callosum, which connect the visual association areas of the two hemispheres. A lesion deep in the left parietooccipital region may also prevent visual information from both occipital lobes reaching the left angular gyrus. In this case the right homonymous hemianopia may be absent. With purely left cerebral lesions, aside from vascular lesions there may be a primary or secondary tumor, or, rarely, multifocal leukoencephalopathy may be the underlying disease.

Isolation of speech areas Following prolonged hypotension or carbon monoxide poisoning, widespread cerebral ischemia affects the vascular anatomic border zones linking the major cerebral arteries and their distal branches on the cerebral surfaces, and spreads centripetally into their adjacent territories. The central fields of supply of these arteries are spared. In the middle cerebral artery territory, this sparing leaves largely intact the sylvian region and its speech areas. With much of the rest of the brain out of action in patients who have survived such hypoxic-hypotensive accidents, the speech mechanism is preserved and can be activated by spoken words. There is parrot-like repetition of words and sounds (echolalia) and similar findings which indicate that the auditory-vocal loop remains functional. Scant evidence of comprehension or self-initiated conversation has been observed, findings that are thought to reflect the widespread injury outside the speech regions. The syndrome is common in patients surviving cardiac arrest.

Amnesic-dysnomic aphasia This may be a relatively early or an isolated manifestation of disease of the nervous system. The patient loses only the ability to produce names on demand, including nouns, adjectives, and other descriptive parts of speech. There are typical pauses in speech, groping for words, and substitution of another word or phrase that conveys the meaning (circumlocution). When shown a series of common objects, the patient may tell of their use instead of giving their names. The difficulty applies not only to objects seen but to the names of things heard or felt. By contrast, other verbal tasks, including recall of the names for letters, digits, reading, writing, spelling, etc., are almost invariably preserved. That the deficit is principally one of naming is shown by the patient's correct use of the object and, usually, by an ability to point to the correct object on hearing or seeing the name. There is a tendency among patients to attribute their failure to forgetfulness, or to give some other lame excuse for the disability, suggesting that they are not completely aware of the nature of their difficulty.

The causative lesion is usually deep in the temporal lobe, in position, probably, to interrupt connections of sensory speech areas with the hippocampal-parahippocampal regions concerned with learning and memory. Mass lesions, such as a tumor or an otogenic abscess, are the most frequent, and as they enlarge, an upper contralateral quadrantic visual field defect or Wernicke's aphasia is added. Occasionally, dysnomia appears with diseases which occlude the temporal branches of the posterior cerebral artery. Alzheimer's disease and senile dementia may begin with a dysnomic or amnesic type of aphasia. By the time the patient's difficulty is fully recognized, other disorders of speech and indifference, apathy, and abulia are conjoined. This deficit may also be discovered in testing patients with a confusional state caused by metabolic, infectious, intoxicative, or other acute medical illnesses, but then it has no certain localizing value.

DISORDERS OF ARTICULATION AND PHONATION In simple dysarthria there is no abnormality of the cortical centers. Dysarthric patients are able to understand perfectly what they hear, and if literate, read and have no difficulty in writing, even though they are unable to utter a single intelligible word.

The act of speaking is a highly coordinated sequence of contractions of the larynx, pharynx, palate, tongue, lips, and respiratory musculature. These are innervated by the hypoglossal, vagal, facial, and phrenic nerves. The nuclei of these nerves are controlled through the corticobulbar tracts by both motor cortices. As with all movements, there are also extrapyramidal influences from the cerebellum and basal ganglia. A current of air is produced by expiration, and the force of it is finely regulated by the activity of the various muscles engaged in speech. *Phonation,* or the production of vocal sounds, is a function of the larynx. Changes in the size and shape of the glottis and in the length and tension of the vocal cords are controlled by the action of the laryngeal muscles. Vibrations are set up and transmitted to the column of air passing over the vocal cords. Sounds thus formed are modified as they pass through the nasopharynx and mouth, which act as resonators. Articulation consists of contractions of the tongue, lips, pharynx, and palate, which interrupt or alter the vocal sounds. Vowels are of laryngeal origin, as are some consonants, but the latter are formed for the most part during articulation. For instance, the consonants *m, b,* and *p* are labial, *l* and *t* are lingual, and *nk* and *ng* are nasoguttural.

Defective articulation and phonation are recognized at once by listening to patients during ordinary conversation or while they are reading aloud from a newspaper or book. Test phrases or attempts at rapid repetition of lingual, labial, and guttural consonants (e.g., la-la-la-la or me-me-me-me) bring out the particular abnormality. Disorders of phonation call for a precise analysis of the voice and its apparatus. The movements of the vocal cords should be inspected with the aid of a hand mirror, or, even better, a laryngoscope, and those of the tongue, palate, and pharynx by direct observation.

Defects in articulation may be subdivided into several types; paretic dysarthria, spastic and rigid dysarthria, choreic, myoclonic, and ataxic dysarthria.

Paretic dysarthria This is due to a neural or bulbar (medullary) weakness or paralysis of the articulatory muscles (lower motor neuron paralysis). In the latter condition the shriveled tongue lies inert on the floor of the mouth, and the lips are relaxed and tremulous. Saliva constantly collects in the mouth because of dysphagia, and spills over the lips causing drooling. Speech becomes less and less distinct. There is a special difficulty in the correct utterance of vibratives, such as *r;* as the paralysis becomes more complete, lingual and labial consonants are finally not pronounced at all. Degrees of this abnormality are observed in myasthenia gravis. Bilateral paralysis of the palate may occur with diphtheria, poliomyelitis, and progressive bulbar palsy. Bilateral paralysis of the lips, as in the facial diplegia of idiopathic polyneuritis, interferes with enunciation of labial consonants; *p* and *b* are slurred and sound more like *f* and *v*.

Spastic and rigid dysarthria These are more frequent than the paralytic variety. Diseases that involve the corticobulbar tracts, usually vascular disease or motor system disease bilaterally, either simultaneously or in stages, result in the syndrome of pseudobulbar palsy. The patient may have had a minor stroke some time in the past affecting the corticobulbar fibers on one side; but since the bulbar muscles are probably represented in both motor cortices, there is no impairment in speech or swallowing from a unilateral lesion. Should another stroke then occur, involving the other corticobulbar tract and possibly the corticospinal tract at the pontine, midbrain, or capsular level, the patient immediately becomes anarthric or dysarthric and dysphagic. Often the muscles of facial expression on both sides are weakened as well. Unlike bulbar paralysis due to lower motor neuron involvement, this condition entails no atrophy or fasciculation of the paralyzed muscles; the jaw jerk and other facial reflexes soon become exaggerated; the palatal reflexes are retained; emotional control is poor (pathologic laughter and crying); and sometimes breathing becomes periodic (Cheyne-Stokes). When the frontal operculum alone is involved, the speech deficit may be a pure dysarthria but usually without the impairment in emotional control. In the beginning, the patient may be totally anarthric and aphonic, but as improvement occurs or in mild degrees of the same condition, speech is notably slow, thick, and indistinct, much like that of partial bulbar paralysis.

In Parkinson's syndrome, one observes an extrapyramidal disturbance of articulation. The patient speaks hastily and articulates poorly, slurring over many syllables and trailing off the end of sentences. The words are pronounced hastily. The voice is low-pitched, monotonous, and lacking in inflection; voice volume diminishes. In advanced cases speech is almost unintelligible; only whispering is possible.

Pyramidal and extrapyramidal disturbances of speech may be combined in generalized cerebral diseases such as general paresis, in which slurred speech is one of the cardinal signs.

In many cases of capsular hemiplegia or partially recovered Broca's aphasia the patient is left with a dysarthria that may be difficult to distinguish from a pure articulatory defect.

Choreic and myoclonic dysarthria In chorea and myoclonus, speech may also be affected in a highly characteristic way. Unlike the defect of pseudobulbar palsy or parkinsonism, chorea and myoclonus abruptly interrupt the pronunciation of words by the abnormal movements. Grimacing and other characteristic motor signs must be depended upon for diagnosis.

Ataxic dysarthria This is characteristic of acute and chronic cerebellar lesions. It may be observed in multiple sclerosis, Friedreich's ataxia, cerebellar atrophy, and heat stroke. The principal speech abnormality is slowness; imprecise enunciation, monotony, and unnatural, irregular separation of the syllables of words (scanning) are other features. Coordination of speech and respiration are poor. There may not be enough breath to utter certain words, and others may be ejaculated explosively. *Scanning dysarthria* is distinctive, but in some cases, especially if there is a possibility of spastic weakness of the tongue from corticobulbar tract involvement, it is impossible to predict the anatomy of disease from analysis of speech alone. Myoclonic jerks involving the speech musculature may be superimposed on cerebellar ataxia in a number of diseases.

APHONIA AND DYSPHONIA Finally, a few points should be made concerning the group of speech disorders involving disturbances of voice.

Paresis of the respiratory movements, as in poliomyelitis and acute infectious polyneuritis, or incoordination as part of extrapyramidal disease, may affect voice because insufficient air is provided for phonation and speech. Reduced volume of speech due to limited excursion of the breathing muscles is another common feature; the patient is unable to speak above a whisper or to shout. Whispering speech is also a feature of stupor, but strong stimulation may make the voice audible.

Paresis of both vocal cords causes complete aphonia. There is no voice, and the patient can speak only in whispers. Since the vocal cords normally separate during inspiration, their failure to do so when paralyzed may result in an inspiratory stridor. If one vocal cord is paralyzed, the voice becomes hoarse, low-pitched, and rasping. Involvement of one of the tenth cranial nerves by tumor, for example, may also cause a certain nasality of voice because the posterior nares do not close during phonation. Certain consonants such as *b, p, n,* and *k* are followed by escape of air into the nasal passages. The abnormality is sometimes less pronounced in recumbency and increases when the head is thrown forward. Hoarseness may also be due to structural changes in the vocal cords caused by cigarette smoking, chronic inflammation, polyps, etc.

Another curious condition about which little is known is *spastic dysphonia.* The authors have seen many patients, middle-aged or elderly men and women, otherwise healthy, who gradually lose the ability to speak quietly and fluently. Any effort to speak results in contraction of all the speech musculature so the patient's voice is strained and phonation is labored. This is apparently a neurologic disorder similar to writer's cramp, i.e., a kind of restricted dystonia. The patients are not neurotic, and psychotherapy and speech therapy have been ineffective. This condition differs from the stridor caused by spasm of the laryngeal muscles in tetany. It is nonprogressive but in some instances is combined with other of the restricted extrapyramidal disorders such as blepharospasm and spasmodic torticollis.

CLINICAL APPROACH TO LANGUAGE DISORDERS **Aphasia** In investigating a case of aphasia, it is first necessary to inquire into the patient's native language, handedness, and previous education. Many naturally left-handed children are trained to use their right hand for writing; therefore, in determining this point we must ask which hand is used for throwing a ball, threading a needle, or using a spoon and common tools such as a hammer, saw, or bread knife. It is important before the beginning of the examination to determine whether the patient is alert and can be made to participate reliably in testing, as accurate assessment of language depends on these factors. One should quickly ascertain whether the patient has other signs of a gross cerebral lesion such as hemiplegia, facial weakness, homonymous hemianopia, or cortical sensory loss. When hemiplegia, hemianesthesia, and homonymous hemianopia coexist, the aphasic disorder is usually complete or global. Such a constellation of major neurologic signs is seldom associated with the less complete forms of language disorder, the posterior sylvian syndromes, or one of the dissociative syndromes, though one defect may exceed others. Dyspraxia of limbs and speech musculature, in response to spoken commands or to visual mimicry, is generally associated with Broca's aphasia and sometimes with Wernicke's aphasia. Bilateral or unilateral homonymous hemianopia without motor weakness tends often to be linked to "pure" word blindness (alexia or dyslexia) or to amnesic-dysnomic aphasia. Bilateral hemiplegias due to extensive frontal lesions are accompanied not infrequently by "pure" word muteness. The special types of aphasia—alexia, "pure" word deafness, etc.—are often associated with evidence of embolism to other parts of the brain or other organs.

Conversational testing permits quick assessment of the motor aspects of speech (praxis and prosody) and apparent language formulation and auditory comprehension.

Disabilities in the purely motor aspects of speech suggest a motor aphasia, and this possibility can be pursued further by tests of repeating from dictation and by special tests of praxis of the oropharyngeal and respiratory apparatus. Disabilities in language formulation in the form of literal paraphasias with impaired comprehension are indicative of Wernicke's aphasia. Disorders confined to naming, generally without paraphasias, when other language functions (reading, writing, spelling, etc.) are found adequate, are diagnostic of amnesic dysnomia.

When conversation shows virtually no disabilities, other tests may still be revealing. Reading aloud single letters, words, and text may reveal the dissociative syndrome of pure word blindness, while tests of writing in this syndrome will show little abnormality. Literal and verbal paraphasic errors may appear in milder cases of Wernicke's aphasia as the patient reads aloud from text or from words in the examiner's handwriting. Similar errors appear even more frequently when the patient is asked to explain the text, read aloud, or give explanations in writing. Adequacy of response channels is next determined by presenting the patient with tasks that permit a response physically identical with the test stimulus. Copying visual stimuli and repeating aloud from auditory stimuli are examples of this kind of testing. Inadequacy of receptive or response channels will then preclude further analysis of the deficit involving that channel in more complex types of tests, except in the unlikely instance that the more complex test is better performed. If reception and response channels are found adequate in these initial tests, they may then be used in tests requiring all types of language function, such as writing from dictation, vocal naming of visual stimuli, matching physically dissimilar stimuli having a name in common (e.g., the word *cow* and a picture of a cow). By utilizing the same test material used in the earlier tests, direct comparison of performances in spoken naming, written naming, and matching can be compared from visual, auditory, and palpated stimuli. A performance profile can be constructed separately for each type of stimulus material tested (objects, pictures, words, letters, numbers, colors, etc.). The resultant profile can then be used to determine whether the main deficits fall across one or more input or response channels. These data then provide a base line against which later changes may be compared.

Articulatory-phonation disorders Disturbances of articulation point to involvement of a different set of neural structures, such as the motor cortices, the corticobulbar pathways, the seventh, ninth, and tenth nuclei, the brainstem, and extrapyramidal nuclei and tracts. Often it is necessary to use other neurologic findings to decide which of these are implicated in any given case. The important distinction between the pseudobulbar or supranuclear palsies and the bulbar palsies is grasped only with difficulty by the average student. The information obtained by localizing these two major types of dysarthria is extremely helpful in differential diagnosis.

Dysphonia should lead to an investigation of laryngeal disease, either primary or secondary to an abnormality of innervation. Inspection of vocal cords is a necessary step in the clinical study.

TREATMENT The sudden loss of speech would be expected to cause great apprehension, but except for almost pure motor defects, most patients show remarkably little concern. It appears that the very lesion that deprives them of speech also causes a partial loss of insight into their own disability. This reaches almost a ludicrous extreme in some cases of Wernicke's aphasia, in which patients become indignant when others cannot understand their jargon. Nonetheless, as improvement occurs, many patients do become discouraged.

Reassurance and a positive program of speech rehabilitation are the best ways of helping the patient at this stage.

Most aphasic difficulties are due to vascular disease of the brain, and nearly always this is accompanied by some degree of spontaneous improvement in the days, weeks, and months that follow the stroke. Sometimes recovery is complete within hours or days; at times not more than a few words are regained after a year or two of assiduous speech training. Nevertheless, it is the opinion of many experts in the field that speech training is worthwhile.

One must decide for each patient whether speech training is needed and when it should be started. As a rule, therapy is not advisable in the first few days of an aphasic illness, because one does not know how lasting it will be. Also, if the patient suffers a severe global aphasia and can neither speak nor understand spoken and written words, the speech therapist is helpless. Under such circumstances, one does well to wait a few weeks until some one of the language functions has begun to return. Then the physician may begin to encourage and help the patient to use the function to a maximal degree. In milder aphasic disorders the patient may be sent to the speech therapist as soon as the illness has stabilized.

The methods of speech training are specialized, and it is advisable to call in a person who has been trained in this field.

There is no special treatment for the dysarthric disturbance of speech.

PROGNOSIS The outcome of aphasia depends on the nature of the underlying disease and the magnitude of the lesion within the speech areas. Global aphasias lasting more than a week or two usually have a bad outcome. Seldom is there enough recovery of communicative speech to permit resumption of occupation or profession. Partial aphasias frequently improve, sometimes to a gratifying degree, if of vascular or encephalitic origin. Aphasias due to embolism, whether global or restricted, may disappear in hours to days, like all cerebral embolic deficits, or persist.

REFERENCES

Brain R: Aphasia, apraxia, agnosia, in *Neurology*, 2d ed, SAK Wilson, N Bruce (eds). Baltimore, Williams & Wilkins, 1955, vol 3, chap 83

Geschwind N: Disconnection syndromes in animals and man. Brain 88:237, 585, 1965

Mohr JP: Broca's area and Broca's aphasia, in *Studies in Neurolinguistics*, H Whitaker (ed). New York, Academic, 1975, chap 6

———, Sidman M: Aphasia: Behavioral aspects, in *American Handbook of Psychiatry*, vol 4, M Reiser (ed). New York, Basic Books, 1975, pp 279–298

Nielsen JM: *Agnosia, Apraxia, Aphasia: Their Value in Cerebral Localization*, 2d ed. New York, Hafner, 1962

24
SYNDROMES DUE TO FOCAL CEREBRAL LESIONS

RAYMOND D. ADAMS
MAURICE VICTOR

Apart from the general syndromes described in Chap. 22, there are many others which relate to anatomic lesions of particular parts of the cerebrum. Their recognition constitutes irrefutable evidence that all parts of the cerebrum are not functionally equivalent. Some of the symptoms and signs of which these syndromes are comprised have the same diagnostic value as a hemiplegia, and, once identified, require the same type of clinical analysis as to cause and pathophysiologic mechanism.

These focal syndromes will be described in terms of the conventional anatomic divisions of the cerebrum, but it will be obvious that most diseases do not respect these boundaries. Hence the syndromes may overlap or occur in a number of combinations.

FRONTAL LOBE SYNDROMES In Fig. 24-1, it is seen that the frontal lobes lie anterior to the central, or rolandic, sulcus and superior to the sylvian fissure. They consist of several functionally different parts, which are conventionally designated in the neurologic literature by numbers (according to a scheme devised by Brodmann) and by letters (according to a scheme of von Economo and Koskinas).

The posterior parts, areas 4 and 6 of Brodmann, are specifically related to motor function. There is also a secondary motor area in the posterior part of the superior frontal convolution. Voluntary movement in humans depends on the integrity of these areas, and lesions in them produce spastic paralysis of the contralateral face, arm, and leg. This is discussed in Chap. 14. Lesions limited more or less to the premotor areas (area 6) are accompanied by prominent grasp and sucking reflexes. Lesions in area 8 of Brodmann interfere with the mechanism concerned with turning the head and eyes contralaterally. Lesions in area 44 (Broca's area) of the dominant cerebral hemisphere, usually the left one, result in at least a temporary loss of verbal expression. Lesions in the medial limbic or piriform cortex

FIGURE 24-1
Diagram to show cortical areas, numbered according to the scheme of Brodmann. The speech areas are in black, the three main ones of which are 39, 41, and 45. The zone marked by vertical stripes in the superior frontal convolution is the secondary motor area which, like Broca's area 45, if stimulated, causes vocal arrest. (After Handbuch der Inneren Medizin, Berlin, Springer-Verlag, 1939.)

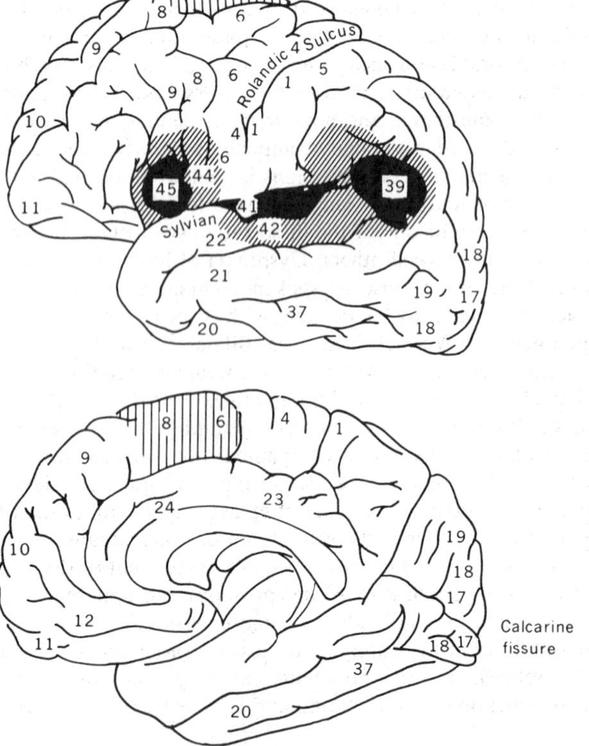

(areas 23 and 24), wherein are bilaterally organized the mechanisms controlling respiration, circulation, and micturition, have relatively unclear clinical effects.

The remaining parts of the frontal lobes (areas 9 to 13 of Brodmann), sometimes called the *prefrontal areas,* have less specific and measurable functions. In contrast to the motor areas of the frontal lobes and other areas of the brain, stimulation of the prefrontal areas in humans has yielded a paucity of findings. Many patients with gunshot wounds of these areas have shown only mild and inconsistent abnormalities of behavior. Nevertheless, the following groups of symptoms have been observed in patients with large lesions of one or both of the frontal lobes and of the central white matter and the anterior part of the corpus callosum by which they are joined:

1 Lack of initiative and spontaneity in conjunction with diminished speech and motor inactivity (apathetic-akinetic-abulic state). Necessary daily activities are neglected. Interpersonal social reactions are reduced and shallow.
2 Change of personality, usually expressed as lack of concern over the consequences of any action, which may take the form of a childish excitement, an inappropriate joking and punning, a thoughtless impulsivity, an instability and superficiality of emotion, or irritability. This puerility and euphoria may at times assume a pseudopsychopathic form.
3 Slight impairment of intelligence, usually described as lack of concentration, vacillation of attention, inability to carry out planned activity, difficulty in changing from one activity to another, or slight loss of recent memory. Goldstein reduces the difficulty to a loss of the capacity for abstract thinking. According to Luria, who views the frontal lobe as a regulating mechanism of the organism's activities, planned action is deficient with respect to steady control and goal orientation.
4 Motor abnormalities such as decomposition of gait and upright stance, wide base, flexed posture, and small shuffling steps, culminating in an inability to stand (truncal ataxia of Bruns), abnormal postures, reflex grasping or sucking, and incontinence of sphincters.

Some differences have been noted between the dominant (left) and right frontal lobes. In psychologic tests left frontal lesions impair verbal fluency and cause perseveration, and right frontal lesions impair the learning of visual spatial patterns and cause impersistence (see Hecaen and Albert, and Luria for further details).

TEMPORAL LOBES The boundaries of the temporal lobes may be seen in Fig. 24-1. The sylvian fissure separates the superior surface of each temporal lobe from the frontal and anterior parts of the parietal lobes. There is no definite anatomic boundary between the temporal and occipital lobes or the posterior temporal and parietal lobes. The temporal lobe includes the superior, middle, and inferior temporal, fusiform, and hippocampal convolutions and the transverse convolutions of Heschl, which are the auditory receptive area present on the superior surface within the sylvian fissure. The hippocampal convolution was once believed to be related indirectly to the olfactory bulb, but now it is known that lesions here do not cause anosmia. Only the medial and anterior parts of the temporal lobes (uncal regions) are related to smell. The lower fibers of the geniculocalcarine pathway (from the inferior retina) swing in a wide arc over the temporal horn of the ventricle into the white matter of the temporal lobe en route to the occipital lobes, and lesions that interrupt them characteristically produce a contralateral homonymous upper quadrant defect of visual fields. Hearing, also localized in the temporal lobes, is bilaterally represented, which accounts for the fact that unless both temporal lobes are affected, there is little or no demonstrable loss of hearing. Loss of equilibrium has not been observed with temporal lobe lesions. Extensive disease in the superior and middle convolutions of the left temporal lobe in right-handed individuals results in Wernicke's aphasia. This syndrome, discussed in Chap. 23, consists of jargon aphasia and inability to read, to write, or to understand the meaning of spoken words.

Between the auditory and olfactory projection areas there is a large expanse of temporal lobe which has no assignable function. This is the temporal association area. Dysnomia has been the most frequent symptom in lesions of the dominant hemisphere. The most careful psychologic studies have shown a difference between cases involving loss of the dominant and nondominant temporal lobe. With lesions of the dominant side there is impairment in learning auditorially presented material; with nondominant lesions there is a similar failure in tests with visually presented material. In addition, about 20 percent of both right and left lobectomy patients have shown a syndrome similar to that described for the prefrontal parts of the brain; but more significant is the fact that the other cases exhibited little or no alteration of personality. The study of cases of uncinate epilepsy, with the characteristic dreamy state, olfactory or gustatory hallucinations, and masticatory movements, suggests that all these functions are organized through the temporal lobes. Similarly, stimulation of the posterior parts of the temporal lobes of fully conscious epileptic patients during surgical procedures has brought to light the interesting fact that complex memories and visual and auditory images, some with strong emotional content, can be aroused. Studies of the effect of stimulation of the amygdaloid nucleus, which is in the anterior and medial part of the temporal lobe, have shed additional light on this subject. Symptoms not unlike some of those of schizophrenic and manic patients may be evoked. Complex emotional experiences that have occurred previously may be revived. There are remarkable autonomic effects: blood pressure rises, pulse increases, respirations increase in frequency and depth, and the patient looks frightened. In temporal lobe epilepsy, reviewed by Geschwind, there may be an intensification of the patient's emotional reactions, an intense concern about moral and religious issues, a tendency to write excessively, and sometimes aggressiveness. Ablation of the amygdaloid nuclei has eliminated uncontrollable rage reactions in psychotic patients. Hippocampal and adjacent convolutions have been excised bilaterally, with a disastrous loss of ability to learn or to establish new memories (Korsakoff's psychosis). Bilateral destruction of the temporal lobes in both humans and monkeys results in placidity, loss of visual recognition, tendency to examine objects by touch and mouthing, and hypersexuality (Kluver-Bucy syndrome). All this indicates an important role of the temporal lobes in auditory and visual perception and imagery, in learning and memory, and in the emotional life of the individual.

1 Effects of unilateral disease of the dominant temporal lobe
  a Homonymous quadrantanopia
  b Wernicke's aphasia
  c Impairment in verbal tests of material presented through the auditory sense
  d Dysnomia or amnesic aphasia
2 Effects of unilateral disease of nondominant temporal lobe
  a Homonymous quadrantanopia
  b Impairment of mental function with inability to judge spatial relationships in some cases
  c Impairment in nonverbal tests of visually presented material

3 Effects of bilateral disease
  a Korsakoff's amnesic defect
  b Apathy and placidity
  c Loss of sexual capacity
  d Loss of other of the unilateral functions
  e Kluver-Bucy syndrome

PARIETAL LOBES The postcentral convolution is the terminus of somatic sensory pathways from the opposite half of the body. However, destructive lesions here do not abolish cutaneous sensation but instead cause mainly a defect in sensory discrimination with variable impairment of primary sensation. In other words, the perception of painful, tactile, thermal, and vibratory stimuli is more or less normal, whereas stereognosis, sense of position, distinction between single and double contacts (two-point threshold), and the localization of sensory stimuli are impaired or lost. There is also the phenomenon of extinction; i.e., if both sides of the body are touched simultaneously, only the stimulus on the normal side is perceived. This type of sensory disturbance, sometimes called *cortical sensory defect,* is discussed in Chap. 18. Extensive lesions deep in the white matter of the parietal lobes produce an impairment of all forms of sensation contralaterally as well as a contralateral homonymous hemianopia, often incongruous and greater in the inferior quadrants. Lesions in the angular gyrus of the dominant hemisphere result in an inability to read.

More recent investigations have centered on the function of the parietal lobes in the perception of one's position in space and of the relationship of the various parts of the body to one another. Since the time of Babinski it has been known that patients with a large lesion of the minor parietal lobe are often unaware of their hemiplegia and hemianesthesia. Babinski called this condition *anosognosia.* Related psychologic disorders are lack of recognition of the left arm and leg, neglect of the left side of the body (as in dressing) and of external space on the left side, and constructional apraxia (an inability to perform the movements of constructing simple figures). All these disorders of parietal lobe function may occur with left-sided lesions as well but are observed only infrequently, since aphasic difficulties with lesions of the left hemisphere make it difficult to adequately test these functions.

Another frequent constellation of symptoms, usually referred to as *Gerstmann's syndrome,* occurs only with lesions of the dominant parietal lobe. This consists of inability to write (agraphia), inability to calculate (acalculia), failure to distinguish right from left, and inability to indicate the fingers and toes when asked. This is a true *agnosia,* since it represents a defect in the formulation and use of symbolic concepts, including the significance of numbers and letters and the names of parts of the body. An ideomotor apraxia may or may not be associated. *Apraxia* and *agnosia* are discussed in Chaps. 14 and 18.

The effects of disease of the parietal lobes may be organized into three major categories:

1 Effects of unilateral disease of the parietal lobe, right or left
  a Cortical sensory syndrome and sensory extinction (or total hemianesthesia with large acute lesions of white matter)
  b Mild hemiparesis, unilateral hemiatrophy of the body in children
  c Homonymous hemianopia or visual inattention, and sometimes anosognosia, neglect of one-half of the body and of extrapersonal space
  d Abolition of opticokinetic nystagmus to one side
2 Effects of unilateral disease of the dominant parietal lobe (left hemisphere in right-handed patients), additional phenomena
  a Disorders of language (especially alexia)
  b Gerstmann's syndrome
  c Bimanual astereognosis (tactile agnosia)
  d Bilateral apraxia of the ideomotor type
3 Effects of nondominant parietal lobe (additional phenomena)
  a Dressing apraxia
  b Constructional apraxia
  c Misidentification of left arm and leg
  d Bland mood, indifference to illness, or neurologic defects

In all these lesions, if the disease is sufficiently extensive, there may be a reduction in the capacity to think clearly, inattentiveness, and impaired memory.

OCCIPITAL LOBES The occipital lobes are the terminus of the geniculocalcarine pathways and are essential for visual sensation and perception. Lesions in one occipital lobe result in homonymous defects in the contralateral visual fields. Most often the defect takes the form of loss of vision in part or all of the homonymous fields. Occasionally patients complain of changes in the form and contour of visually perceived objects (metamorphopsia), as well as illusory displacement of images from one side of the visual field to another (visual allesthesia), or of abnormal persistence of the visual image after the object has been removed (palinopsia). Bilateral lesions cause "cortical" blindness, a state of blindness without change in optic fundi or pupillary reflexes. Visual illusions, hallucinations, and metamorphopsias (distortion of form, size, movement, and color) may also occur.

Lesions in Brodmann's areas 18 and 19 of the dominant hemisphere (Fig. 24-1) cause a loss of visual recognition with retention of some degree of visual acuity, a state termed *visual agnosia.* In the classic form of this blindness individuals with intact mental powers are unable to recognize objects, even though by tests of visual acuity and perimetry they appear to see sufficiently well to do so; they are able to recognize objects by tactile or other extravisual sense. In these terms, *alexia,* or inability to read, represents a visual verbal agnosia or "word blindness." Patients can see letters and words but cannot recognize their meaning, although they can still recognize them through tactile or auditory senses. Other types of agnosia for recognition of faces (prosopagnosia), for a complex of objects the elements of which are perceived but not the whole (simultanagnosia), color agnosia, and Balint's syndrome (inability to look at and grasp an object and inattention) are observed with unilateral and bilateral occipital lesions (see Adams and Victor).

The details of these syndromes of the different lobes of the cerebrum are well presented in the monograph by Walsh.

CORPUS CALLOSUM AND THE DISCONNECTION SYNDROMES Considerable attention has been devoted to the study of each of the two cerebral hemispheres in isolation. This is possible only when the corpus callosum which forms a bridge between the two hemispheres is congenitally defective, surgically sectioned (for epilepsy), or destroyed by infarction or tumors. From these studies emerges the well-known fact that the left hemisphere is dominant in all language functions and auditory perception and the right hemisphere is superior in spatial and visual perception. Partial lesions of the corpus callosum or of the long tracts in the cerebral white matter are found to be associated with a number of interesting syndromes (commissural and intrahemispheric) which will be described below. (See reference to disconnection syndromes by Dimond.)

When the entire corpus callosum is missing because of a

congenital defect or destroyed by a surgical procedure or anterior cerebral artery occlusion (anterior four-fifths), the speech and perceptual areas of the left hemisphere are isolated from those of the right hemisphere. These patients, if blindfolded, are unable to match an object held in one hand with that in the other hand. Further, they cannot match an object seen in the right half of the visual field with one in the left half. If given verbal commands to execute, they perform correctly with the right hand but not with the left. Without vision, objects placed in the right hand are named correctly, but not those in the left. In lesions confined to the posterior fifth of the corpus callosum (splenium), only the visual part of the disconnection syndrome occurs. Occlusion of the left posterior cerebral artery provides the best examples of the latter. Since infarction of the left occipital lobe causes a right homonymous hemianopia, thereafter all visual information needed for activating the speech areas of the left hemisphere must come from the right occipital lobe and cross the splenium of the corpus callosum. If there is a lesion in the corpus callosum, the patient cannot read or name colors because the visual information cannot reach the left angular gyrus. There is no difficulty in copying words, though the patient cannot read what he or she has written; matching colors without naming them is done without error. Apparently the visual information for activating the left motor area crosses the corpus callosum more anteriorly. A disconnection in the anterior third of the corpus callosum, where fiber systems between the right and left premotor areas must pass, results only in failure of the left hand to obey commands, the right one performing perfectly (left-sided apraxia). The left hand can still imitate the examiner's movements or carry out the patient's intention.

There are also intrahemispheric disconnections, of which the most important are the following:

1 Conduction (also called *central*) aphasia. The patient has fluent but paraphasic speech and writing with nearly perfect comprehension of spoken or written language. Repetition of

what is heard or read is, however, severely impaired. The lesion is presumably in the arcuate fasciculus, which connects Wernicke's area with Broca's area.

2 Pure word deafness. Although the patient is able to hear and identify nonverbal sounds, there is loss of ability to comprehend spoken language. The patient's speech remains normal. The defect has been attributed to a subcortical lesion near to but sparing Wernicke's area.

The reader is referred to Adams and Victor and to Dimond for further details on the disconnection syndromes.

DIAGNOSTIC MEASURES FOR THE IDENTIFICATION OF FOCAL CEREBRAL LESIONS These involve the same principles as were described in Chap. 22. Special tests, mostly of psychologic type, are available for each of the focal cerebral syndromes (Walsh).

MANAGEMENT OF PATIENTS See Chap. 22.

REFERENCES

Adams RD, Victor M: *Principles of Neurology*, 2d ed. New York, McGraw-Hill, 1981

Dimond SJ: The disconnection syndromes, in *Modern Trends in Neurology*, D Williams (ed). London, Butterworth, 1975

Hecaen H, Albert ML: Disorders of mental functioning related to the frontal lobes, in *Modern Trends in Neurology*, D Williams (ed). London, Butterworth, 1975

Luria AR: *The Working Brain. An Introduction to Neuropsychology.* New York, Basic Books (translation Penguin Books Ltd), 1973

Walsh KW: *Neuropsychology. A Clinical Approach.* London, Churchill Livingstone, 1978

section 4 | Alterations in circulatory and respiratory function

25
COUGH AND HEMOPTYSIS

GENNARO M. TISI
EUGENE BRAUNWALD

COUGH

Cough, one of the most frequent cardiorespiratory symptoms, is an explosive expiration which provides a means of clearing the tracheobronchial tree of secretions and foreign bodies.

MECHANISM Coughing may be initiated either voluntarily or reflexly. As a defensive reflex it has both afferent and efferent pathways. The *afferent limb* includes cough receptors within the sensory distribution of the trigeminal, glossopharyngeal, superior laryngeal, and vagus nerves. The *efferent limb* includes the recurrent laryngeal nerve (which causes glottic closure) and the spinal nerves (which cause contraction of the thoracic and abdominal musculature). The *sequence of a cough* includes an appropriate stimulus which initiates a deep inspiration. This is followed by glottic closure, relaxation of the diaphragm, and muscle contraction against a closed glottis so as to produce maximally positive intrathoracic and intraairway pressures. These positive intrathoracic pressures result in a narrowing of the trachea, produced by an infolding of its more compliant posterior membrane. Once the glottis opens, the combination of a large pressure differential between the airways and the atmosphere coupled with this tracheal narrowing produces flow rates through the trachea close to the speed of sound. The shearing forces which are developed aid in the elimination of mucus and foreign materials. A tracheostomy short-circuits glottic closure and therefore decreases the effectiveness of the cough mechanism.

ETIOLOGY Cough is produced by inflammatory, mechanical, chemical, and thermal stimulation of the cough receptors. *Inflammatory* stimuli are initiated by edema and hyperemia of the respiratory mucous membranes, and by irritation from exudative processes. Such stimuli may arise either in the airways (as in laryngitis, tracheitis, bronchitis, and bronchiolitis) or in the alveoli (as in pneumonitis and lung abscess). *Mechanical* stimuli are produced by inhalation of particulate matter, such as dust particles, and by compression of the air passages and pressure or tension upon these structures. Lesions associated with airway compression may be either extramural or intramural in type. The former include aortic aneurysms, granulomas, pulmonary neoplasms, and mediastinal tumors; intramural lesions include bronchogenic carcinoma, bronchial adenoma, foreign bodies, granulomatous endobronchial involvement, and contraction of airway smooth muscle (bronchial asthma). Pressure or tension upon the air passages is usually produced by lesions associated with a decrease in pulmonary compliance. Examples of specific causes include acute and chronic interstitial fibrosis (Chap. 280), pulmonary edema, and atelectasis. *Chemical* stimuli may result from inhalation of irritant gases, including cigarette smoke and chemical fumes. Finally, *thermal* stimuli may be produced by inhalation of either very hot or cold air.

Cough is commonly associated with episodic wheezing secondary to bronchoconstriction in symptomatic patients with bronchial asthma (Chap. 273). Recent reports have drawn attention to patients with chronic, persistent cough as the *sole* presenting manifestation of bronchial asthma. Such patients are characterized by (1) absence of a history of episodic wheezing and (2) no evidence of expiratory airflow obstruction by spirometry, but (3) hyperreactive airways (characteristic of asthma) when challenged with a cholinergic agent, methacholine.

DIAGNOSTIC EVALUATION When one is considering the above list of causes, answers to the following general questions will significantly narrow the diagnostic possibilities: Is the cough acute or chronic? Is it productive of sputum or nonproductive? A chronic productive cough may be caused by diseases such as chronic bronchitis, pulmonary tuberculosis, and pulmonary neoplasms. Are the findings on physical examination of the chest normal or abnormal? Is the chest roentgenogram normal or abnormal?

Features of the history, physical examination, chest roentgenogram, screening pulmonary function studies (static lung volumes and dynamic flow rates), and sputum examination may indicate a specific cause. The *history* may indicate specific diagnoses. Acute episodes of cough may be associated with such viral infections as acute tracheobronchitis or pneumonitis or with bacterial bronchopneumonia. Cough associated with an acute febrile episode and associated with hoarseness is usually produced by viral laryngotracheobronchitis. The character of the cough may suggest the anatomic site of involvement: the patient with a "barking" type of cough may have epiglottal involvement, while the cough associated with tracheal or major airway involvement is often loud and "brassy." Cough associated with generalized wheezing may be produced by acute bronchospasm. The time of occurrence of a cough may indicate a specific cause: a cough which occurs selectively at night suggests congestive heart failure; one related to meals suggests a tracheoesophageal fistula, a hiatal hernia, or an esophageal diverticulum; a cough precipitated by a change in position suggests a lung abscess or a localized area of bronchiectasis. The description of sputum or secretions produced in conjunction with the cough may also be helpful: putrid sputum suggests a lung abscess; bloody sputum, bleeding (see "Hemoptysis," below); frothy and pink-tinged sputum, pulmonary edema; mucoid and massive sputum, alveolar cell carcinoma; purulent and/or large amounts of sputum, lung abscess and bronchiectasis.

On *physical examination* the character of the auscultatory findings may suggest the site of disease: inspiratory stridor and wheezing may be present in laryngeal disease, inspiratory and expiratory rhonchi favor tracheal and major airway involvement, coarse subcrepitant inspiratory rales may indicate interstitial fibrosis and/or edema, fine crepitant rales may indicate a process such as pneumonitis or pulmonary edema, which fills the alveoli with fluid. The *chest roentgenogram* may reveal the cause of the cough; it may show an intrapulmonary mass lesion which may be either central or peripheral (Chap. 284), an alveolar filling process which may be pneumonic or nonpneumonic, an area of honeycombing and cyst formation which may indicate an area of localized bronchiectasis, or bilateral hilar adenopathy which may indicate sarcoidosis or a lymphoma.

Screening pulmonary function studies (Chap. 271) may also indicate specific diagnoses. Significant expiratory obstruction to airflow (as determined from a forced expiratory flow maneuver), coupled with a history of cough and significant sputum production, suggests that irrespective of other lesions the patient has significant bronchitis. Decreased lung volume (as determined from the static lung volumes) indicates that a restrictive type of lung disease is present—reduction of lung volumes produced by thoracic, pleural, alveolar, or interstitial disease. Finally, a careful *sputum examination* may be more enlightening than a patient's description of the character of the sputum. Examination shows whether the sputum is thin or viscid, purulent or not, foul-smelling or not, blood-tinged or not, scant or copious. Gram stain and culture of the deep-cough specimen may reveal a specific bacterial, fungal, or mycoplasmal causation, while sputum cytology may result in a positive diagnosis of a pulmonary neoplasm.

Two features of cough should be highlighted: (1) A cough is often so common in the cigarette smoker as to be ignored or minimized. *Any change in the nature or character of a chronic cigarette cough should initiate immediate diagnostic evaluation, with particular attention directed to detection of bronchogenic carcinoma.* (2) Female patients are inclined to swallow sputum and not to expectorate as male patients do. This tendency may lead to the incorrect conclusion that a cough in a female patient is irritative and nonproductive.

COMPLICATIONS Three complications may be produced by the coughing mechanism: paroxysms of coughing may precipitate syncope (cough syncope, Chap. 12), and strenuous coughing may produce rupture of an emphysematous bleb and rib fractures. A potential mechanism for cough syncope includes the development of markedly positive intrathoracic and alveolar pressures which decrease venous return, producing a decrease in cardiac output and resultant syncope. Although cough fractures of the ribs may occur in otherwise normal patients, their occurrence should at least raise the possibility of pathologic fractures, which are seen in multiple myeloma, osteoporosis, and osteolytic metastases.

THERAPY Definitive treatment of cough depends on determining its precise cause and then initiating specific therapy for the underlying cause. Symptomatic therapy should be considered when the cause of the cough is idiopathic and the cough performs no useful function or represents a potential hazard to the patient. An irritative, nonproductive cough may be suppressed by an antitussive agent, such as codeine or dextromethorphan, 15 mg qid. These drugs are particularly useful in interrupting prolonged, self-perpetuating paroxysms. However, a cough productive of significant quantities of sputum should not be suppressed, since retention of sputum in the tracheobronchial tree may interfere with the distribution of ventilation, alveolar aeration, and the ability of the lung to resist infection. When secretions are tenacious and thick, adequate hydration, expectorants, and humidification of the air with an ultrasonic nebulizer may be helpful.

HEMOPTYSIS

For purposes of definition hemoptysis includes both blood-streaked sputum and gross hemoptysis. It is apparent that any patient with gross hemoptysis should be given appropriate diagnostic tests so that a specific cause may be found. The patient with blood-streaked sputum should also be studied unless one can be certain that this type of hemoptysis is due to a benign condition. A major pitfall in dealing with hemoptysis is to ascribe recurrent episodes of hemoptysis to a previously established diagnosis, such as chronic bronchiectasis or bronchitis. Such an approach may result in missing a serious but potentially treatable lesion. The safest approach to a recurrent episode of hemoptysis is to treat it as if it were the initial episode and proceed with a complete diagnostic evaluation.

ETIOLOGY AND INCIDENCE Prior to embarking upon an extensive diagnostic workup of hemoptysis, it is essential to determine that the blood is in fact coming from the respiratory tract, not from the nasopharynx or gastrointestinal tract. Once this point is established, the diagnostic tests for hemoptysis may proceed. Although there are numerous single case reports of diseases which have been associated with hemoptysis, Table 25-1 presents the more common disorders.

The incidence of the diagnoses listed in Table 25-1 depends upon the nature of the series reported and whether one includes both gross bleeding and blood streaking of the sputum. If both types of bleeding are included, then the major causes (approximately 60 to 70 percent) are chronic bronchitis and bronchiectasis. If the definition is restricted to gross bleeding (greater than several tablespoons) then the incidence depends upon the type of series reported. Surgical series favor the incidence of mass lesions and operable lesions (carcinoma, 20 percent; localized, segmental, or lobar bronchiectasis, 30 percent). Those from centers with a large tuberculosis population favor this condition (incidence varying between 2 and 40 percent). Combined medical-surgical series include a wider representation of those lesions which present with hemoptysis (carcinoma, 20 percent; bronchiectasis, 30 percent; bronchitis, 15 percent; other inflammatory lesions including tuberculosis, 10 to 20 percent; other lesions including the vascular, traumatic, and hemorrhagic etiologies listed in Table 25-1, 10 percent).

TABLE 25-1
Causes of hemoptysis

1 Inflammatory
- *a* Bronchitis
- *b* Bronchiectasis
- *c* Tuberculosis
- *d* Lung abscess
- *e* Pneumonia, particularly *Klebsiella*

2 Neoplastic
- *a* Lung cancer: squamous cell, adenocarcinoma, oat cell
- *b* Bronchial adenoma

3 Other
- *a* Pulmonary thromboembolism
- *b* Left ventricular failure
- *c* Mitral stenosis
- *d* Traumatic, including foreign body and lung contusion
- *e* Primary pulmonary hypertension; arteriovenous malformation; Eisenmenger's syndrome; pulmonary vasculitis including Wegener's granulomatosis and Goodpasture's syndrome; idiopathic pulmonary hemosiderosis; and amyloid
- *f* Hemorrhagic diathesis including anticoagulant therapy

Despite the most extensive of evaluations, 5 to 15 percent of cases entailing gross hemoptysis remain undiagnosed.

Two points should be highlighted with reference to diseases associated with hemoptysis: (1) *hemoptysis is rare in metastatic carcinoma to the lung;* (2) *although hemoptysis may occur at some time during the course of a viral or pneumococcal pneumonia, it is usually scanty and its occurrence should always raise the question of a more serious underlying process.*

DIAGNOSIS The *history* may suggest specific diagnoses: recurrent, chronic hemoptysis in a young, otherwise asymptomatic female favors the diagnosis of a bronchial adenoma; recurrent hemoptysis with chronic, marked sputum production associated with ring shadows, tram lines (abnormal air bronchograms), and cyst formation on the roentgenogram suggests a diagnosis of bronchiectasis; putrid sputum production suggests a lung abscess; weight loss and anorexia in a male smoker over the age of 40 raises the possibility of a bronchogenic carcinoma; a recent history of blunt trauma to the chest suggests a lung contusion; and acute pleuritic chest pain raises the possibility of pulmonary embolism with infarction or some other pleurally based lesion (lung abscess, coccidioidomycosis cavity, and vasculitis). Several findings on the *physical examination* may also suggest a specific diagnosis: a pleural friction rub suggests those diagnoses just mentioned in connection with pleuritic pain; the findings of pulmonary hypertension raise the diagnostic possibilities of primary pulmonary hypertension, mitral stenosis, recurrent or chronic thromboembolism, and Eisenmenger's syndrome; a localized wheeze over a major lobar airway suggests an intramural lesion such as a bronchogenic carcinoma or a foreign body; systemic arteriovenous communications or the presence of a murmur over the lung fields suggest the diagnosis of Osler-Weber-Rendu disease with pulmonary ateriovenous malformation; evidence of significant expiratory obstruction to airflow coupled with sputum production suggests that whatever other lesion may be present, the patient has significant bronchitis. Finally, the *chest roentgenogram* is critical to diagnosis. The presence of ring shadows favors a diagnosis of bronchiectasis; an air-fluid level, the diagnosis of a lung abscess; and a mass lesion, the diagnosis of a central or peripheral pulmonary neoplasm. A mass lesion which may cause hemoptysis should be distinguished from an area of blood pneumonitis caused by aspiration of blood into contiguous areas.

One of the most demanding diagnostic problems is the identification of the side of bleeding in a patient with normal findings on physical examination and a normal roentgenogram of the chest. A patient with hemoptysis tends to keep the bleeding side dependent. Otherwise, gravitational drainage would cause aspiration into the noninvolved dependent lung. The patient may also be able to give a history of a burning or deep pain which may localize the side of bleeding; bronchoscopy may then be useful. This procedure generally is most helpful when the bleeding is scant, and of least help when the bleeding is massive, since blood may be aspirated into contiguous airways.

Following the history and physical examination, the diagnostic approach to a patient with hemoptysis includes whatever specialized studies and procedures are required to make a specific diagnosis. The first step is to obtain a roentgenogram. Usually bronchoscopy is the procedure employed next. Fiberoptic bronchoscopy (Chap. 272) includes within the range of visualization airways as small as several millimeters in diameter. This endoscopic technique may provide definitive visual, biopsy, or cytologic information. Since direct visualization of more peripheral portions of the airway system is now possible, the indications for bronchography in the evaluation of hemoptysis are being modified. The principal indications for bronchography in such patients are (1) to establish the presence of localized bronchiectasis (including a sequestered lobe) and (2) to rule out the presence of more generalized bronchiectasis in a patient with localized disease who is regarded as a surgical candidate because of either repetitive hemoptysis or recurrent infections. The majority of patients with bronchiectasis have a normal chest roentgenogram. If bronchoscopy in such patients is also negative, bronchography is the only means of establishing an anatomic diagnosis of bronchiectasis. If the chest roentgenogram is abnormal, revealing either ring shadows or tram lines, a diagnosis of bronchiectasis may be made without the need for bronchography.

THERAPY Since hemoptysis is such an alarming symptom, there is a tendency to overtreat the patient. Usually hemoptysis is scant and will stop spontaneously without specific therapy. If the hemoptysis is substantial, the mainstays of therapy include keeping the patient calm, instituting complete bed rest, excluding unnecessary diagnostic procedures until the hemoptysis has begun to subside, and suppressing cough if it is present and an aggravating feature of the hemoptysis. The emergency care of such a patient demands that intubation and suctioning equipment be at the bedside. In patients in danger of asphyxiation by flooding of the lung contralateral to the site of hemorrhage, intubation by a technique which isolates the hemorrhaging lung and prevents contralateral aspiration of blood should be carried out. This can be accomplished by strategic location of a balloon catheter whose introduction into the bronchus in question is facilitated by direct visualization through a fiberoptic bronchoscope.

The management of potentially lethal massive hemoptysis remains controversial. The choice between a medical approach and surgical intervention hinges on the words *potentially lethal.* Massive hemoptysis, usually defined as greater than 1000 ml in 24 h, is an alarming clinical situation in which asphyxiation due to aspiration of blood represents the principal threat to life. The choice between surgical and medical management relates most often to the anatomic basis for the massive hemoptysis. In patients with cavitary tuberculosis, anaerobic lung abscess, and lung cancer, the risk of mortality is far greater than when the cause of the hemoptysis is bronchitis or bronchiectasis. Operation may occasionally be necessary in the former, but virtually never in the latter group. In either case the initial management should include the conservative measures suggested above. With such management, spontaneous cessation of bleeding usually occurs. Surgical intervention should be considered in that small group of patients with a definable lesion on chest roentgenogram (i.e., cavitary disease, lung abscess, lung cancer) who have evidence of uncontrollable respiratory or hemodynamic compromise. If a patient is a surgical candidate, bronchoscopy should be performed to identify the specific site of bleeding. Otherwise bronchoscopy should be deferred for several days because of the tendency of this procedure to aggravate cough and thereby perpetuate the hemoptysis. Bronchial arterial catheterization and embolization are new modalities of treatment currently under evaluation for the nonsurgical control of massive hemoptysis, especially in patients with nonresectable lung cancer.

REFERENCES

Chai H et al: Standardization of bronchial inhalation challenge procedures. J Allergy Clin Immunol 56:323, 1975

Committee on Etiology of Chronic Bronchitis, Medical Research Council: Definition and classification of chronic bronchitis. Lancet 1:775, 1965

Committee on Therapy, American Thoracic Society: The management of hemoptysis. Am Rev Resp Dis 93:471, 1966

Corrao WMC et al: Chronic cough as the sole presenting manifestation of bronchial asthma. N Engl J Med 300:633, 1979

Fishman AP: Manifestations of respiratory disorders, in *Pulmonary Diseases and Disorders,* AP Fishman (ed). New York, McGraw-Hill, 1980, pp 44–83

Irwin RS et al: Cough: A comprehensive review. Arch Intern Med 137:1186, 1977

Loudon RG, Shaw GB: Mechanics of cough in normal subjects and in patients with obstructive respiratory disease. Am Rev Resp Dis 96:666, 1967

Wolfe JD, Simmons DH: Hemoptysis: Diagnosis and management (medical progress). West J Med 127:383, 1977

26 DYSPNEA AND PULMONARY EDEMA

ROLAND H. INGRAM, JR.
EUGENE BRAUNWALD

DYSPNEA

The breathing pattern is controlled by a series of higher central and peripheral mechanisms which can increase ventilation in excess of metabolic demands in conditions such as anxiety and fear, and can increase ventilation appropriate to increased metabolic demands during physical activity. A normal resting person is unaware of the act of breathing, and while he or she may become conscious of breathing during mild to moderate exertion, no discomfort is experienced. However, during and following exhausting exertion an individual may become unpleasantly aware of breathing, yet feel reasonably assured that the sensation will be transitory and is appropriate to the level of exercise. Therefore, as a cardinal symptom of diseases affecting the cardiorespiratory system, dyspnea is defined as an *abnormally uncomfortable awareness of breathing.*

Although dyspnea is not painful in the usual sense of the word, it is, like pain, involved with both the perception of a sensation and the reaction to that perception. Patients experience a number of uncomfortable sensations related to breathing and use an even larger number of verbal expressions to describe these sensations, such as "cannot get enough air," "air does not go all the way down," "smothering feeling in the chest," "tightness in the chest," "fatigue in the chest," and a "choking sensation." It may be necessary, therefore, to review meticulously the patient's history in order to ascertain whether the more abstruse descriptions do, in fact, represent dyspnea. Once it is established that a patient does have dyspnea, it is of paramount importance to define the circumstances in which it occurs and to assess associated symptoms. There are situations in which breathing appears labored but in which dyspnea does not occur. For example, the hyperventilation in association with metabolic acidemia is rarely accompanied by dyspnea. On the other hand, patients with apparently normal breathing patterns may complain of shortness of breath.

QUANTITATION OF DYSPNEA The gradation of dyspnea may usefully be based upon the amount of physical exertion required to produce the sensation. In actual practice the major functional classifications of patients with heart or lung disease are based largely on dyspnea in relation to degree of exertion. However, in assessing the severity of dyspnea, it is important to obtain a clear understanding of the patient's general physical condition, work history, and recreational habits. For example, the development of dyspnea in a trained runner upon running 2 mi may signify a more serious disturbance than a similar degree of breathlessness in a sedentary person upon running a fraction of this distance. Some patients with lung or heart disease may have such reduced capabilities due to other disease that exertional dyspnea is precluded despite serious impairment of pulmonary or cardiac function.

Some patterns of dyspnea are not directly related to physical exertion. Sudden and unexpected dyspneic episodes at rest can be associated with pulmonary emboli, spontaneous pneumothorax, or anxiety. Nocturnal episodes of severe paroxysmal dyspnea are characteristic of left ventricular failure. Dyspnea upon assuming the supine posture, *orthopnea* (see below), thought to be mainly characteristic of congestive heart failure, may also occur in some patients with asthma and chronic obstruction of the airways and is a regular finding in the rare occurrence of bilateral diaphragmatic paralysis. *Trepopnea* is used to describe the unusual circumstance in which dyspnea occurs only in the left or right lateral decubitus position, most often in patients with heart disease, while *platypnea* is dyspnea which occurs only in the upright position. Both of these patterns remain to be fully explained but may be related to positional alterations in ventilation-perfusion relations (Chap. 271).

MECHANISMS OF DYSPNEA Physicians usually relate the symptom of dyspnea to a process such as obstruction of the airways or congestive heart failure and generally proceed with further diagnostic and/or therapeutic attempts, having satisfied themselves that they understand the mechanism of the dyspnea. In fact, elucidation of the *actual* mechanism(s) of dyspnea has eluded clinical investigators.

Dyspnea occurs whenever the work of breathing is excessive. Increased force generation is required of the respiratory muscles to produce a given volume change if the chest wall or lungs are less compliant or if resistance to airflow is increased. Increased work of breathing also occurs when the ventilation is excessive for the level of activity. Although an individual is more apt to become dyspneic when the work of breathing is increased, the work theory does not account for the perceptual difference between a deep breath with a normal mechanical load and a normal-sized breath with an increased mechanical load. The work might be the same with both breaths, but the normal one with the increased load will be associated with discomfort. In fact, with respiratory loading, such as adding a resistance at the mouth, there is an increase in respiratory center output, as gauged by newer indexes, that is disproportionate to the increase in work of breathing. Hence, a more appealing theory is one that links inappropriate length to tension in the respiratory muscles. Campbell has proposed that a sense of discomfort arises when there is misalignment of the nerve spindles, which are sensing tension, in relation to muscle length. This misalignment would lead to the sensation that a person is getting an insufficient breath for the tension generated by the respiratory muscles. Such a theory is difficult to test and, if tested and proved in some circumstances, would still not explain why patients who are completely paralyzed, either by cord transections or neuromuscular blockade, experience dyspnea although aided by a mechanical ventilator. It is probable, in these circumstances, that signals from the lungs and/or airways travel via the vagus nerve to the central nervous system to account for the sensation.

In all likelihood a number of different mechanisms operate to different degrees in the various clinical situations in which dyspnea occurs. Perhaps, in some circumstances, dyspnea is evoked by stimulation of receptors in the upper respiratory tract; in others it may originate from receptors in the lungs, airways, respiratory muscles, or some combination of those structures. In any event, dyspnea is characterized by an excessive or abnormal activation of the respiratory centers in the brainstem. This activation comes about from stimuli transmitted from or through a variety of structures and pathways including (1) intrathoracic receptors via the vagi; (2) afferent somatic nerves, particularly from the respiratory muscles and chest wall, but also from other skeletal muscles and joints; (3) chemoreceptors in the brain, aortic and carotid bodies, and elsewhere in the circulation; (4) higher (cortical) centers; and perhaps (5) afferent fibers in the phrenic nerves. In general, there is a reasonably good correlation between the severity of dyspnea and the disturbances of pulmonary or cardiac function which are responsible.

DIFFERENTIAL DIAGNOSIS **Obstructive disease of airways** (see also Chaps. 273 and 279) Obstruction to airflow can be present anywhere from the extrathoracic airways out to the small airways in the periphery of the lung. Large extrathoracic airway obstruction can occur acutely, as with aspiration of food or a foreign body or with angioneurotic edema of the glottis. Circumstantial evidence or testimony from witnesses should cause the physician to suspect aspiration, and an allergic history together with a few scattered hives should raise the possibility of glottic edema. The acute form of upper airway obstruction is a medical emergency. More chronic forms can occur with tumors or with fibrotic stenosis following tracheostomy or prolonged endotracheal intubation. Whether acute or chronic, the cardinal symptom is dyspnea, and the characteristic signs are stridor and retraction of the supraclavicular fossae with inspiration.

Obstruction of intrathoracic airways can occur acutely and intermittently or can be present chronically with worsening during respiratory infections. Acute intermittent obstruction with wheezing is typical of *asthma*. Chronic cough with expectoration is typical of *chronic bronchitis* and *bronchiectasis*. Most often there is a prolongation of expiration and coarse rhonchi which are generalized in chronic bronchitis and may be localized in the case of bronchiectasis. Intercurrent infection results in worsening of the cough, increased expectoration of purulent sputum, and more severe dyspnea. During such episodes the patient may complain of nocturnal paroxysms of dyspnea with wheezing relieved by cough and expectoration of sputum.

Many years of exertional dyspnea progressing to dyspnea at rest characterize the patient with predominant *emphysema* (Chap. 279). Although a parenchymal disease by definition, emphysema is invariably accompanied by obstruction of airways.

Diffuse parenchymal lung diseases (see also Chap. 280) This category includes a large number of diseases ranging from acute pneumonia to chronic disorders such as sarcoidosis and the various forms of *pneumoconiosis*. History, physical findings, and radiographic abnormalities often provide clues to the diagnosis. The patients are often tachypneic with arterial P_{CO_2} and P_{O_2} values below normal. Exertion often further reduces the arterial P_{O_2}. Lung volumes are decreased and the lungs are stiffer, i.e., less compliant.

Pulmonary vascular occlusive diseases (see also Chap. 282) Repeated episodes of dyspnea at rest often occur with repeated emboli. A source for emboli, such as phlebitis of a lower extremity or the pelvis, is quite helpful in leading the physician to suspect the diagnosis. Arterial blood gases are almost invariably abnormal, but lung volumes are frequently normal or only minimally abnormal.

Diseases of the chest wall or respiratory muscles (see also Chap. 286) The physical examination establishes the presence of a chest wall disease such as severe kyphoscoliosis, pectus excavatum, or spondylitis. Although all three of these deformities may be associated with dyspnea, only severe kyphoscoliosis regularly interferes with ventilation sufficiently to produce chronic cor pulmonale and respiratory failure. Even though vital capacity, lung volumes, and airflow rates are normal with pectus excavatum, there is some evidence that cardiac compression from the posteriorly displaced sternum interferes with diastolic filling of the ventricle during the increased demands of exercise. Hence a cardiogenic component to the dyspnea may be present in this condition.

Both weakness and paralysis of respiratory muscles can lead to respiratory failure and dyspnea (Chap. 286), but most often the signs and symptoms of the neurologic or muscular disorder are more prominently manifested in other systems.

Heart disease In patients with cardiac disease exertional dyspnea occurs most commonly as a consequence of an elevated pulmonary capillary pressure; aside from uncommon causes such as obstructive disease of the pulmonary veins (Chap. 256), pulmonary capillary hypertension is a consequence of left atrial hypertension, which in turn may be due to left ventricular dysfunction (Chaps. 252 and 253), reduced left ventricular compliance, and mitral stenosis. The elevation of hydrostatic pressure in the pulmonary vascular bed tends to upset the Starling equilibrium (see "Pulmonary Edema," below) with resulting transudation of liquid into the interstitial space, reducing the compliance of the lungs and stimulating J (juxtacapillary) receptors in the alveolar interstitial space. When prolonged, pulmonary venous hypertension results in thickening of pulmonary vessels and an increase in perivascular cells and fibrous tissue, causing a further reduction in compliance. The competition for space between vessels, airways, and increased liquid within the interstitial space compromises the lumina of small airways, increasing the airways' resistance. Diminution in compliance and an increase in airways' resistance increase the work of breathing which, to some degree, is minimized by both an increase in frequency of respiration and a reduction in tidal volume. In severe heart disease, usually involving elevation of both pulmonary and systemic venous pressures, hydrothorax may develop, further interfering with pulmonary function and intensifying dyspnea. In patients with heart failure and a severely diminished cardiac output, dyspnea may also be related to fatigue of the respiratory muscles as a consequence of their reduced perfusion. The metabolic acidosis characteristic of severe heart failure may play a contributory role. Dyspnea may also be associated with severe systemic and cerebral anoxia, as occurs during exertion in patients with congenital heart disease and right-to-left shunts.

Cardiac dyspnea usually begins as breathlessness on strenuous exertion and, over the course of months or years, progresses until the patient is dyspneic at rest. Occasionally, a nonproductive cough developing in the recumbent position, particularly at night, may be the first complaint.

Orthopnea, i.e., dyspnea in the recumbent position and *paroxysmal nocturnal dyspnea*, i.e., attacks of shortness of breath which generally occur at night and awaken the patient from sleep, are characteristic of more advanced forms of heart failure associated with elevations of pulmonary venous and capillary pressures and are discussed in Chap. 253. Orthopnea is the result of the alteration of gravitational forces when the recumbent position is assumed. This augmentation of intrathoracic blood volume elevates pulmonary venous and capillary pressures which increases the pulmonary closing volume (Chap. 271) and reduces the vital capacity. An additional factor associated with recumbency is the elevation of the diaphragm, which results in a lower end-expiratory lung volume. This combination of lower end-expiratory lung volume and increase in closing volume results in a significant alteration of alveolar-capillary gas exchange.

PAROXYSMAL (NOCTURNAL) DYSPNEA Also known as *cardiac asthma,* this condition is characterized by attacks of severe shortness of breath which generally occur at night and usually awaken the patient from sleep. The attack is precipitated by stimuli which aggravate the previously existing pulmonary congestion; frequently the total blood volume is augmented at night because of the reabsorption of edema from dependent portions of the body during recumbency; the redistribution of blood volume which takes place results in an increase in intrathoracic blood volume and therefore produces pulmonary congestion. A sleeping patient can tolerate relatively severe pulmonary engorgement and may awaken only when actual pulmonary edema and bronchospasm have developed, with the feeling of suffocation and with wheezing respirations.

CHEYNE-STOKES RESPIRATION See Chap. 253.

DIAGNOSIS The diagnosis of cardiac dyspnea depends on the recognition of heart disease on the basis of the history and physical examination. There may be a history of antecedent myocardial infarction, third and fourth heart sounds may be audible, and/or there may be evidence of left ventricular enlargement, jugular neck vein distention, and/or peripheral edema. Often there are radiographic signs of heart failure, with evidence of interstitial edema, pulmonary vascular redistribution, and accumulation of liquid in the septal planes and pleural cavity. Cardiomegaly is often present, but the overall heart size may be normal, particularly in patients with dyspnea due to acute myocardial infarction or mitral stenosis; an enlarged left atrium is usually evident in the latter condition. The electrocardiogram (Chap. 249) is rarely specific for heart disease and cannot specifically indicate whether a patient's dyspnea is caused by heart disease; however, it is rarely normal in patients with cardiac dyspnea.

Differentiation between cardiac and pulmonary dyspnea In most patients with dyspnea there is obvious clinical evidence of disease of either heart or lungs. The dyspnea of chronic obstructive lung disease tends to develop more gradually than that of heart diseases; exceptions, of course, occur in patients with obstructive lung disease who develop an episode of infectious bronchitis, pneumonia, or pneumothorax, or an exacerbation of asthma. Like patients with cardiac dyspnea, patients with chronic obstructive lung disease may also waken at night with dyspnea, but this is usually associated with sputum production; the dyspnea is relieved after these patients rid themselves of secretions.

The difficulty in the distinction between cardiac and pulmonary dyspnea may be compounded by the coexistence of diseases involving both organ systems. Patients with a history of chronic bronchitis or asthma who develop left ventricular failure tend to develop recurrences of bronchoconstriction and wheezing in association with bouts of paroxysmal nocturnal dyspnea and pulmonary edema. This condition, i.e., cardiac asthma, usually occurs in patients with overt clinical evidence of heart disease. Acute cardiac asthma is further differentiated from acute attacks of bronchial asthma by the presence of diaphoresis, more bubbly airway sounds, and the more common occurrence of cyanosis.

It is desirable to carry out pulmonary function testing in patients in whom the etiology of dyspnea is not clear, for these tests should be helpful in determining whether dyspnea is produced by heart disease, lung disease, abnormalities of the chest wall, or anxiety. In addition to the usual means of assessing patients for heart disease (Chap. 247), determination of the ejection fraction at rest and during exercise by radionuclide ventriculography (Chap. 250), is helpful in the differential diagnosis of dyspnea; the left ventricular ejection fraction is depressed in left ventricular failure while the right ventricular ejection fraction may be low at rest or may decline during exercise in patients with severe lung disease; both ejection fractions are normal both at rest and during exercise in dyspnea due to anxiety or malingering. Careful observation during the performance of an exercise treadmill test will often help in the identification of the patient who is malingering or whose dyspnea is secondary to anxiety. Under these circumstances the patient usually complains of severe shortness of breath but appears to be breathing either effortlessly or totally irregularly.

Anxiety neurosis Dyspnea experienced by someone with an anxiety neurosis is a difficult symptom to evaluate. The signs and symptoms of acute and chronic hyperventilation do not serve to distinguish between anxiety neurosis and other processes, such as recurrent pulmonary emboli. Another potentially confusing situation is seen when chest pain and electrocardiographic changes accompany the hyperventilation syndrome. When present and attributable to this condition, often referred to as *neurocirculatory asthenia* (Chap. 4), the chest pain is often sharp, fleeting, and in various loci, and the electrocardiographic changes are most often seen during repolarization; yet occasional ventricular ectopic activity can be seen as well. A rather extensive series of pulmonary and cardiac function tests, carried out both at rest and during exercise, may be needed to be certain that anxiety is, in fact, the cause of the dyspnea. Certain clues are helpful in leading one to suspect a psychogenic origin. Frequent sighing respirations and a bizarre, irregular breathing pattern are helpful. Often the breathing pattern returns to normal during sleep.

PULMONARY EDEMA

CARDIOGENIC PULMONARY EDEMA An increase in pulmonary venous pressure, which results initially in the engorgement of the pulmonary vasculature, is common in most instances of dyspnea in association with congestive heart failure. The lungs become less compliant, the resistance of small airways increases, and there is an increase in lymphatic flow which apparently serves to maintain a constant pulmonary extravascular liquid volume. At this early stage there is usually mild tachypnea, and if arterial blood gases are measured, the arterial P_{O_2} and P_{CO_2} are both lowered with an increase in the alveolar-to-arterial oxygen difference. Tachypnea itself, which might result from stimulation of receptors in the pulmonary interstitium, apparently increases lymphatic flow by augmenting ventilatory pumping of lymphatic vessels. The changes described are seen well in advance of auscultatory findings or radiographic signs pointing to congestive heart failure. If sufficient both in magnitude and duration, the increase in intravascular pressure results in a net gain of liquid in the extravascular space despite further increases in lymphatic flow. It is at this point that symptoms worsen, tachypnea increases, gas exchange deteriorates further, and radiographic changes, such as Kerley B lines and loss of distinct vascular margins, are seen. Even at this intermediate stage, the capillary endothelial intercellular junctions have been shown to widen and allow passage of macromolecules into the interstices. Up to and including this stage, the edema is purely *interstitial.* Sufficient further elevations in intravascular pressure result in disruption of the tighter junctions between alveolar lining cells, and alveolar edema ensues with outpouring of liquid, which contains both red blood cells and macromolecules. At this point *alveolar edema* is present. Although originally considered an early and subtle radiographic sign of interstitial edema, recent evidence suggests that an antigravity redistribution of pulmonary blood flow occurs only after the onset of alveolar edema. With yet more severe disruption of the alveolar-capillary membrane, edematous liquid floods the alveoli and airways. At this point, full-blown clinical pulmonary edema with bilateral wet rales and rhonchi will occur, and the chest radiograph may show diffuse haziness of the lung fields with greater density in the more proximal hilar regions. Typically, the patient is anxious and perspires freely, and the sputum is frothy and blood-tinged. Gas exchange is more severely compromised with worsening hypoxia and possibly hypercapnia. Without effective treatment (Chap. 253) progressive acidemia, hypoxia, and respiratory arrest ensue.

The earlier sequence of fluid accumulation described above follows the Starling law of capillary–interstitial fluid exchange:

$$\text{Fluid accumulation} = K[(P_c - P_{IF}) - \sigma(\pi_{pl} - \pi_{IF})] - Q_{lymph}$$

where K = permeability coefficient
P_c = mean intracapillary pressure
π_{IF} = oncotic pressure of interstitial fluid
σ = reflection coefficient of macromolecules
P_{IF} = mean interstitial liquid pressure
π_{pl} = oncotic pressure of the plasma
Q_{lymph} = lymphatic flow

The pressures tending to move liquid out of the vessel are P_c and π_{IF}, which are normally more than offset by pressures tending to move liquid back into the vasculature, i.e., the algebraic sum of P_{IF} and π_{pl}. Implicit in the above equation is that lymphatic flow can increase in the case of imbalance of forces and result in no net accumulation of interstitial fluid. However, in later sequences, with opening of first the endothelial and then the alveolar intercellular junctions, the permeability and reflection coefficients change strikingly. Thus, the initial process of hemodynamic pulmonary edema is one of liquid filtration and clearance. With further increasing pressures, disruption of both the structure and the function of the alveolar-capillary membrane occurs.

NONCARDIOGENIC PULMONARY EDEMA There are several clinical conditions which are associated with pulmonary edema based upon an imbalance of Starling forces other than through primary elevations of pulmonary capillary pressure. Although diminished plasma oncotic pressure in hypoalbuminemic states (e.g., severe liver disease, nephrotic syndrome, protein-losing enteropathy) might be expected to lead to pulmonary edema, the balance of forces normally so strongly favors resorption that even under these conditions some elevation of capillary pressure is necessary before interstitial edema develops. Increased negativity of interstitial pressure has been implicated in the genesis of unilateral pulmonary edema following rapid evacuation of a large pneumothorax. In this situation the findings are apparent only by radiography. It has been recently proposed that large negative intrapleural pressures during acute severe asthma may be associated with the development of interstitial edema. If this proposal can be supported by sufficient clinical data, then asthma would represent an additional example of edema due to increased negativity of interstitial pressure. Lymphatic blockade secondary to fibrotic and inflammatory diseases or lymphangitic carcinomatosis may lead to interstitial edema. In such instances both clinical and radiographic manifestations are dominated by the underlying disease process.

There are other conditions characterized by increases in the interstitial liquid content of the lungs which begin neither with an imbalance between intravascular and interstitial forces nor with alterations in lymphatics, but rather appear to be associated primarily with disruption of the alveolar-capillary membranes. Experimentally the prototype for such conditions is the pulmonary edema following alloxan administration. Any number of spontaneously occurring or environmental toxic insults, including diffuse pulmonary infections, aspiration, shock (particularly due to gram-negative septicemia and hemorrhagic pancreatitis, and following cardiopulmonary bypass), are associated with diffuse pulmonary edema which clearly does not have a hemodynamic origin. These conditions, which may lead to the adult respiratory distress syndrome, are discussed in Chap. 287.

Other forms of pulmonary edema There are three forms of pulmonary edema which have not been clearly related to increased permeability, inadequate lymphatic flow, or an imbalance of Starling forces; hence their precise mechanism remains unexplained. *Narcotic overdose* is a well-recognized antecedent to pulmonary edema. Although illicit use of parenteral heroin has been the most frequent cause, parenteral and oral overdoses of legitimate preparations of morphine, methadone, and dextropropoxyphene have also been associated with pulmonary edema. Thus the earlier idea that injected impurities lead to the disorder is untenable. Available evidence suggests that there are alterations in the permeability of alveolar and capillary membranes rather than elevation of pulmonary capillary pressure. *Exposure to high altitude* in association with severe physical exertion is a well-recognized setting for pulmonary edema in unacclimatized, yet otherwise healthy, persons. Recent data show that acclimatized high-altitude natives also develop this syndrome upon return to high altitude after a relatively brief sojourn at low altitudes. The mechanism for high-altitude pulmonary edema remains obscure, and studies have been conflicting, some suggesting pulmonary venous constriction and others indicating pulmonary arteriolar constriction as the prime mechanisms. The hypoxia at altitude appears to play no role. *Neurogenic* pulmonary edema has been suspected in patients with central nervous system disorders and without apparent preexisting left ventricular dysfunction. Although most experimental equivalents have implicated sympathetic nervous system activity, the mechanism whereby sympathetic efferent activity leads to pulmonary edema is a matter of speculation. It is known that a massive adrenergic discharge leads to peripheral vasoconstriction with elevation of blood pressure and shifts of blood to the central circulation. In addition, it is probable that a decrease in left ventricular compliance also occurs, and both factors serve to increase left atrial pressures sufficiently to induce pulmonary edema on a hemodynamic basis. Recent experimental evidence suggests that stimulation of adrenergic receptors increases capillary permeability directly, but this effect is relatively minor as compared to the imbalance of Starling forces.

TREATMENT OF PULMONARY EDEMA See Chap. 253.

REFERENCES

AYRES SM: Mechanism and consequences of pulmonary edema: Cardiac lung, shock lung, and principles of ventilatory therapy in adult respiratory distress syndrome. Am Heart J 103:97, 1982

CAMPBELL EJM et al: *Breathlessness.* Oxford, Blackwell, 1966

——— et al: *The Respiratory Muscles: Mechanisms and Neural Control.* Philadelphia, Saunders, 1970

FISHMAN AP, RENKIN EM (eds): *Pulmonary Edema.* Washington, DC, American Physiological Society, 1979

INGRAM RH JR, BRAUNWALD E: Pulmonary edema: Cardiogenic and noncardiogenic, in *Heart Disease*, E. Braunwald (ed). Philadelphia, Saunders, 1980, chap 17, pp 571–589

MCFADDEN ER, INGRAM RH JR: Relationship between diseases of the heart and lungs, in *Heart Disease,* E Braunwald (ed). Philadelphia, Saunders, 1980, chap 53, p 1893

ROUSSOS C, MACKLEM PT: Disorders of the respiratory muscle function, in *Update III: Harrison's Principles of Internal Medicine,* KJ Isselbacher et al (eds). New York, McGraw-Hill, 1982, p 83

SCOGGIN CH et al: High altitude pulmonary edema in the children and young adults of Leadville, Colorado. N Engl J Med 297:1269, 1977

SPRUNG, CL et al: The spectrum of pulmonary edema: Differentiation of cardiogenic, intermediate, and noncardiogenic forms of pulmonary edema: Am Rev Respir Dis 124:718, 1981

STAUB NC: The pathogenesis of pulmonary edema. Prog Cardiovasc Dis 23:53, 1980

———: Pulmonary edema due to increased microvascular permeability. Ann Rev Med 32:291, 1981

27 CYANOSIS, HYPOXIA, AND POLYCYTHEMIA

EUGENE BRAUNWALD

CYANOSIS

Cyanosis refers to a bluish color of the skin and mucous membranes resulting from an increased amount of reduced hemoglobin, or of hemoglobin derivatives, in the small blood vessels of those areas. It is usually most marked in the lips, nail beds, ears, and malar eminences. The "red cyanosis" of polycythemia vera (Chap. 336) must be distinguished from the true cyanosis discussed here. A cherry-colored flush, rather than cyanosis, is caused by carboxyhemoglobin (Chap. 238). In *argyria,* the skin is bluish because of the deposition of silver salts, and the discoloration persists despite pressure, unlike cyanotic skin which blanches. The degree of cyanosis is modified by the quality of cutaneous pigment, the color of the blood plasma, and the thickness of the skin, as well as by the state of the cutaneous capillaries. The accurate clinical detection of the presence and degree of cyanosis is difficult, as proved by oximetric studies. In some instances central cyanosis can be reliably detected when the arterial saturation has fallen to 85 percent; in others it may not be detected until the saturation has reached 75 percent.

The increase in the amount of reduced hemoglobin in the cutaneous vessels, which produces cyanosis, may be brought about either by an increase in the quantity of venous blood in the skin as the result of dilatation of the venules and venous ends of the capillaries, or by a decrease in the oxygen saturation in the capillary blood. In general, cyanosis becomes apparent when the mean capillary concentration of reduced hemoglobin exceeds 5 g/dl. It is the *absolute* rather than the *relative* amount of reduced hemoglobin which is important in producing cyanosis. Thus, in a patient with severe anemia the relative amount of reduced hemoglobin in the venous blood may be very large when considered in relation to the total amount of hemoglobin. However, since the latter is markedly lowered, the absolute amount of reduced hemoglobin may still be small, and therefore patients with severe anemia and marked arterial desaturation do not display cyanosis. Conversely, the higher the total hemoglobin content, the greater the tendency toward cyanosis; thus, patients with marked polycythemia tend to be cyanotic at higher levels of arterial oxygen saturation than patients with normal hematocrit values. Likewise, local passive congestion, which causes an increase in the total amount of reduced hemoglobin in the vessels in a given area, may cause cyanosis. Cyanosis also is observed when nonfunctional hemoglobin is present in the blood; as little as 1.5 g/dl methemoglobin or 0.5 g sulfhemoglobin is sufficient to produce cyanosis (Chap. 330).

True cyanosis may be subdivided into *central* and *peripheral* categories. In the *central* type, there is arterial blood unsaturation or an abnormal hemoglobin derivative, and the mucous membranes and skin are both affected. *Peripheral* cyanosis is due to a slowing of blood flow to an area and abnormally great extraction of oxygen from normally saturated arterial blood. It results from vasoconstriction and diminished peripheral blood flow, such as occurs in cold exposure, shock, congestive failure, and peripheral vascular disease. Often, in these conditions, the mucous membranes of the oral cavity or those beneath the tongue may be spared. Clinical differentiation between central and peripheral cyanosis may not always be simple, and in conditions such as cardiogenic shock with pulmonary edema there may be a mixture of both types.

DIFFERENTIAL DIAGNOSIS (See Table 27-1) **Central cyanosis** Decreased arterial oxygen saturation results from a marked reduction in the oxygen tension in the arterial blood. This may be brought about by a decline in the tension of oxygen in the inspired air without sufficient compensatory alveolar hyperventilation to maintain alveolar oxygen tension. Cyanosis does not occur in a significant degree in an ascent to an altitude of 8000 ft but is marked in a further ascent to 16,000 ft. The reason for this becomes clear on studying the S shape of the oxygen dissociation curve (Fig. 54-4). At 8000 ft the tension of oxygen in the inspired air is about 120 mmHg, the alveolar tension is approximately 80 mmHg, and the hemoglobin is nearly completely saturated. However, at 16,000 ft the oxygen tensions in atmospheric air and alveolar air are about 85 and 50 mmHg, respectively, and the oxygen dissociation curve shows that the arterial blood is only about 75 percent saturated. This leaves 25 percent of the hemoglobin in the reduced form, an amount likely to be associated with cyanosis in the absence of anemia. Similarly, a mutant hemoglobin with a low affinity for oxygen (Hb Kansas) causes lowered arterial oxygen saturation and resultant central cyanosis (Chap. 330).

Seriously *impaired pulmonary function,* through alveolar hypoventilation or perfusion of unventilated or poorly ventilated areas of the lung, is a common cause of central cyanosis (Chap. 271). This may occur acutely, as in extensive pneumonia or in pulmonary edema, or with chronic pulmonary diseases (e.g., emphysema). In the last situation clubbing of the fingers and polycythemia are generally present. However, in many types of chronic pulmonary disease with fibrosis and obliteration of the capillary vascular bed, cyanosis does not occur because there is relatively little perfusion of underventilated areas.

TABLE 27-1
Causes of cyanosis

- *I* Central cyanosis
  - *A* Decreased arterial oxygen saturation
    - *1* Decreased atmospheric pressure—high altitude
    - *2* Impaired pulmonary function
      - *a* Alveolar hypoventilation
      - *b* Uneven relationships between pulmonary ventilation and perfusion
      - *c* Impaired oxygen diffusion
    - *3* Anatomic shunts
      - *a* Certain types of congenital heart disease
      - *b* Pulmonary arteriovenous fistulas
      - *c* Multiple small intrapulmonary shunts
    - *4* Hemoglobin with low affinity for oxygen
  - *B* Hemoglobin abnormalities
    - *1* Methemoglobinemia—hereditary, acquired
    - *2* Sulfhemoglobinema—acquired
    - *3* Carboxyhemoglobinemia (not true cyanosis)
- *II* Peripheral cyanosis
  - *A* Reduced cardiac output
  - *B* Cold exposure
  - *C* Redistribution of blood flow from extremities
  - *D* Arterial obstruction
  - *E* Venous obstruction

Another cause of decreased arterial oxygen saturation is *shunting of systemic venous blood into the arterial circuit.* Certain forms of congenital heart disease are associated with cyanosis (Chap. 256). Since blood normally flows from a high-pressure to a low-pressure region, in order for a cardiac defect to result in a right-to-left shunt, it must ordinarily be combined with an obstructive lesion distal to the defect or with elevated pulmonary vascular resistance. The commonest congenital cardiac lesion associated with cyanosis is the combination of ventricular septal defect and pulmonary outflow tract obstruction (tetralogy of Fallot). The more severe the obstruction, the greater the degree of right-to-left shunting and resultant cyanosis. The mechanisms for the elevated pulmonary vascular resistance which may produce cyanosis in the presence of intra- and extracardiac communications without pulmonic stenosis are discussed elsewhere (Chap. 256). In patients with patent ductus arteriosus, pulmonary hypertension, and right-to-left shunt, *differential cyanosis* results; i.e., cyanosis occurs in the lower extremities but not in the upper extremities.

Pulmonary arteriovenous fistulas may be congenital or acquired, solitary or multiple, microscopic or massive. The degree of cyanosis produced by these fistulas depends upon their size and number. They occur with some frequency in hereditary hemorrhagic telangiectasia (Chap. 333). Arterial oxygen unsaturation also occurs in some patients with cirrhosis, presumably as a consequence of pulmonary arteriovenous fistulas or portal vein–pulmonary vein anastomoses.

In patients with cardiac or pulmonary right-to-left shunts, the presence and severity of cyanosis depend on the size of the shunt relative to the systemic flow as well as on the oxyhemoglobin saturation of the venous blood. In patients with central cyanosis due to arterial oxygen unsaturation, the severity of cyanosis increases with exercise. With increased extraction of oxygen from the blood by the exercising muscles, the venous blood returning to the right side of the heart is more unsaturated than at rest, and shunting of this blood or its passage through lungs incapable of normal oxygenation intensifies the cyanosis. Also, since the systemic vascular resistance normally decreases with exercise, the right-to-left shunt is augmented by exercise in patients with congenital heart disease and communications between the two sides of the heart. Secondary polycythemia occurs frequently in patients with arterial unsaturation and contributes to the cyanosis.

Cyanosis can be caused by small amounts of circulating methemoglobin and by even smaller amounts of sulfhemoglobin (Chap. 330). Although they are uncommon causes of cyanosis, these abnormal hemoglobin pigments should be sought by spectroscopy when cyanosis is not readily explained by malfunction of the circulatory or respiratory systems. Generally, clubbing does not occur with them. The diagnosis of methemoglobinemia can be suspected, if, on mixing the patient's blood in a test tube, it remains brown.

Peripheral cyanosis Probably the most common cause of peripheral cyanosis is generalized vasoconstriction resulting from exposure to cold air or water. This is clearly a normal response to the stimulus and is transient. When cardiac output is low, as in severe congestive heart failure or shock, cutaneous vasoconstriction occurs as a compensatory mechanism, so that blood is diverted to more vital areas [central nervous system, heart (Chap. 253)], and intense cyanosis associated with cool extremities may result. Even though the arterial blood is normally saturated, the reduced volume flow through the skin and the reduced oxygen tension at the venous end of the capillary result in cyanosis.

Arterial obstruction to an extremity, as with an embolus, or arteriolar constriction, as in cold-induced vasospasm (Raynaud's phenomenon, Chap. 269), generally results in pallor and coldness, but there may be associated slight cyanosis. If there is venous obstruction, the extremity is usually congested and also cyanotic, and there is true stagnation of blood flow. Venous hypertension, which may be local (as in thrombophlebitis) or generalized (as in tricuspid valve disease or constrictive pericarditis), dilates the subpapillary venous plexuses and intensifies cyanosis.

APPROACH TO THE PATIENT WITH CYANOSIS Certain features are important in arriving at the proper cause of cyanosis:

1 The history, particularly the duration (cyanosis present since birth is usually due to congenital heart disease); possible exposure to drugs or chemicals which may produce abnormal types of hemoglobin.
2 Clinical differentiation of central as opposed to peripheral cyanosis. Objective evidence by physical or radiographic examination of disorders of the respiratory or cardiovascular systems. Massage or gentle warming of a cyanotic extremity will increase peripheral blood flow and abolish peripheral but not central cyanosis.
3 The presence or absence of clubbing of the fingers. Clubbing without cyanosis is frequent in patients with infective endocarditis and in association with ulcerative colitis, it may occasionally occur in healthy persons, and in some instances it may be occupational, e.g., in jackhammer operators. Slight cyanosis of the lips and cheeks, without clubbing of the fingers, is common in patients with well-compensated mitral stenosis and is probably due to minimal arterial hypoxia resulting from fibrotic changes in the lungs secondary to longstanding congestion combined with reduction of cardiac output (Chap. 258). The combination of cyanosis and clubbing is frequent in many patients with certain types of congenital cardiac disease and is seen occasionally in persons with pulmonary disease such as lung abscess or pulmonary arteriovenous shunts. On the other hand, peripheral cyanosis or acutely developing central cyanosis is not associated with clubbed fingers.
4 Determination of arterial blood oxygen tension or oxygen saturation, spectroscopic and other examinations of the blood for abnormal types of hemoglobin.

CLUBBING Clubbing is the selective bullous enlargement of the distal segment of a digit due to an increase in soft tissue. It may be hereditary or idiopathic, or acquired and associated with a variety of disorders, including cyanotic heart disease, infective endocarditis, and a variety of pulmonary conditions (among them, primary and metastatic lung cancer, bronchiectasis, lung abscess, and mesothelioma), as well as with some gastrointestinal diseases (including regional enteritis, chronic ulcerative colitis, and hepatic cirrhosis). Primary lung cancer, mesothelioma, neurogenic diaphragmatic tumors, and rarely cyanotic congenital heart disease may be associated with hypertrophic osteoarthropathy, the subperiosteal formation of new bone in the distal diaphyses of the long bones of the extremities. Although the mechanism of clubbing is unclear, it appears to be secondary to a (presumably humoral) substance, which causes dilation of the vessels of the fingertip.

HYPOXIA

The fundamental purpose of the cardiorespiratory system is to deliver oxygen (and substrates) to the cells and to remove carbon dioxide (and other metabolic products) from them. Proper maintenance of this function depends on intact cardiovascular and respiratory systems and a supply of inspired gas containing adequate oxygen. Changes in oxygen and in carbon dioxide tension as well as changes in the intraerythrocytic concentration of certain *organic phosphate compounds,* especially 2,3-diphosphoglyceric acid (2,3-DPG), cause shifts in the oxygen dissociation curve. These are discussed in detail in Chap. 54 and are illustrated in Fig. 54-4. When hypoxia results as a consequence of respiratory failure, arterial P_{CO_2} usually rises (Chaps. 279 and 287), and the oxygen dissociation curve tends to be displaced to the right. Under these conditions the percentage saturation of the hemoglobin in the arterial blood at a given level of alveolar oxygen tension declines. Thus arterial hypoxia and cyanosis are likely to be more marked in proportion to the degree of depression of alveolar oxygen tension when such depression results from pulmonary disease than when the depression occurs as the result of a decline in the partial pressure of oxygen in the inspired air, in which case arterial P_{CO_2} falls and the oxygen dissociation curve is displaced to the left.

DIFFERENTIAL DIAGNOSIS **Anemic hypoxia** Any decrease in hemoglobin concentration is attended by a corresponding decline in the oxygen-carrying power. The P_{O_2} in the arterial blood remains normal, but the absolute amount of oxygen transported per unit volume of blood is diminished. As the anemic blood passes through the capillaries, and the usual amount of oxygen is removed from it, the P_{O_2} in the venous blood declines to a greater degree than would normally be the case.

Carbon monoxide intoxication (Chap. 238) This condition is accompanied by the equivalent of anemic hypoxia in that the hemoglobin which is combined with the carbon monoxide (carboxyhemoglobin) is unavailable for oxygen transport. In addition, the presence of carboxyhemoglobin shifts the lower portion of the dissociation curve of hemoglobin to the left, so that the oxygen can be unloaded only at lower tensions. By such formation of carboxyhemoglobin a given degree of reduction in oxygen-carrying power produces a far greater degree of tissue hypoxia than the equivalent reduction in hemoglobin due to simple anemia.

Circulatory hypoxia As in anemic hypoxia, arterial P_{O_2} is normal but venous and tissue P_{O_2} are reduced as a consequence of reduced tissue perfusion in the face of normal tissue oxygen consumption. For this reason the term *stagnant hypoxia* may be used for this condition. Generalized circulatory hypoxia occurs in heart failure, as discussed in Chap. 253.

Specific organ hypoxia Decreased circulation to a specific organ resulting in localized stagnant hypoxia may be due to organic arterial or venous obstruction or may occur as a reflex phenomenon. The latter may occur when vasoconstriction of, for instance, the limbs results from an attempt to maintain adequate perfusion to more vital organs, as in severe congestive heart failure. When organic arterial obliterative disease develops, ischemic hypoxia results, with accompanying pallor. Localized hypoxia may also result from venous obstruction which results in congestion. Edema, which increases the distance through which oxygen diffuses before it reaches the cells, can also cause localized hypoxia.

Increased oxygen requirements Even if oxygen diffusion into blood perfusing the pulmonary capillary bed is unhampered and the hemoglobin is qualitatively and quantitatively normal, the P_{O_2} in venous blood (hence, capillary and tissue P_{O_2}) may be reduced if the oxygen consumption of the tissues is elevated without a corresponding increase in volume flow per unit of time. Such a situation may be encountered in febrile states and in thyrotoxicosis. Under such conditions the circulation may be considered deficient relative to the metabolic requirements.

Ordinarily, the clinical picture of patients with hypoxia due to an elevated basal metabolic rate is quite different from that in other types of hypoxia; the skin is warm and flushed, owing to increased cutaneous blood flow which dissipates the excessive heat produced, and cyanosis is absent in these patients.

Exercise is a classic example of increased tissue oxygen requirements. The increased demands are normally met by several mechanisms: (1) increasing the cardiac output and thus oxygen delivery to the tissues; (2) preferentially directing the blood to the exercising muscles and away from resting muscles (by changing vascular resistances in various circulatory beds, directly and/or reflexly); (3) increasing oxygen extraction from the delivered blood and widening the arteriovenous oxygen differences. If the capacity of these mechanisms is exceeded, then hypoxia, especially of the exercising muscles, will result.

Improper oxygen utilization Cyanide (Chap. 238) and several other similarly acting poisons cause a paradoxic state in which the tissues are unable to utilize oxygen and as a consequence the venous blood tends to have a high oxygen tension. This condition has been termed *histotoxic hypoxia.* Cyanide produces cellular hypoxia by paralyzing the electron-transfer function of cytochrome oxidase so that it cannot pass electrons to oxygen, whereas diphtheria toxin is believed to inhibit the synthesis of one of the cytochromes and thus interfere with oxygen consumption and energy production by the cells involved.

EFFECTS OF HYPOXIA Changes in the central nervous system, particularly the higher centers, are especially important. Acute hypoxia produces impaired judgment, motor incoordination, and a clinical picture closely resembling that of acute alcoholism. When hypoxia is long-standing, the symptoms consist of fatigue, drowsiness, apathy, inattentiveness, delayed reaction time, severe fatigue, and reduced work capacity. As hypoxia becomes more severe, the centers of the brainstem are affected, and death usually results from respiratory failure. With reduction of arterial oxygen tension, cerebrovascular resistance decreases and cerebral blood flow increases, which tends to minimize the cerebral hypoxia. On the other hand when the reduction of arterial P_{O_2} is accompanied by hyperventilation and diminution of P_{CO_2}, cerebrovascular resistance rises, blood flow falls, and hypoxia is enhanced. Compared with the brain, the phylogenetically older spinal cord and peripheral nerves are relatively insensitive to hypoxia. Hypoxia also causes pulmonary arterial constriction, which serves the useful function of shunting blood away from poorly ventilated areas toward better-ventilated portions of the lung. However, it has the disadvantage of causing increased pulmonary vascular resistance and an increased burden on the right ventricle.

A complex disturbance of cellular functions results from the metabolic effects of severe acute hypoxia. In liver and muscles the breakdown of the primary foodstuff, carbohydrate, normally proceeds anaerobically (i.e., without oxidation) to the stage of formation of pyruvic acid. The breakdown of pyruvate requires oxygen, and when this is deficient, increasing proportions of pyruvate are reduced to lactic acid, which cannot be broken down further (Chap. 85). Hence, there is an increase in the blood lactate, with decrease in bicarbonate and a corresponding acidosis. Under these circumstances the total energy obtained from foodstuff breakdown is greatly reduced, and the amount of energy available for continuing resynthesis of energy-rich phosphate compounds becomes inadequate, leading to a complex disturbance of cellular function.

Most of the useful respiratory response to hypoxia originates in special chemosensitive cells in the carotid and aortic bodies, although the respiratory center is also stimulated directly by oxygen lack. The resultant increase in ventilation, with loss of carbon dioxide, leads to respiratory alkalosis. On the other hand, the diffusion of additional quantities of lactic acid from the tissues into the blood tends to produce metabolic acidosis. In either case the total amount of bicarbonate, and hence the carbon dioxide–combining power, tends to be diminished.

Diminished oxygen tension in any tissue results in local vasodilatation, and the diffuse vasodilatation which occurs in generalized hypoxia results in an elevation of total cardiac output (Fig. 54-5). In patients with preexisting heart disease, particularly coronary artery disease, the combination of hypoxia and the requirements of the peripheral tissues for an increase of cardiac output may precipitate congestive heart failure. Prolonged or severe hypoxia may also impair hepatic and renal function.

One of the important mechanisms of compensation for prolonged hypoxia is an increase in the amount of hemoglobin in the blood (Fig. 54-5). This is due not to direct stimulation of the bone marrow but to the effect of an erythropoiesis-stimulating factor (erythropoietin) which originates primarily in the kidneys. Assayable levels of erythropoietin are increased by hypoxia, and its production has been found to be regulated by the balance between tissue oxygen supply and demand.

POLYCYTHEMIA (See also Chap. 336)

The term *polycythemia* signifies an increase above the normal in the number of red corpuscles in the circulating blood. This increase is usually, though not always, accompanied by a corresponding increase in the quantity of hemoglobin and in the volume of packed red corpuscles. The increase may or may not be associated with an increase in the total quantity of red blood cells in the body. It is important to distinguish between *absolute* polycythemia (an increase in the total red corpuscle mass) and *relative* polycythemia, which occurs when, through loss of blood plasma, the concentration of the red corpuscles becomes greater than normal in the circulating blood. This may be the consequence of abnormally lowered fluid intake, of the loss of plasma into the interstitial fluid, or of the marked loss of body fluids, such as occurs in persistent vomiting, severe diarrhea, copious sweating, or acidosis (Chap. 44).

Because the term polycythemia is used loosely to refer to all varieties of increase in the number of red corpuscles, the terms *erythrocytosis* and *erythremia* are preferred in referring to two forms of absolute polycythemia. Erythrocytosis denotes absolute polycythemia which occurs in response to some known stimulus (secondary polycythemia); erythremia (polycythemia rubra vera) refers to the disease of unknown etiology (Chap. 336). An approach to the differential diagnosis of erythrocytosis should begin with a consideration of its mechanisms (Table 27-2). Erythrocytosis develops as a consequence of a variety of factors and represents a physiologic response to conditions of hypoxia. Sojourn at high altitudes leads to defective saturation of arterial blood with oxygen and stimulates the production of more red corpuscles. The oxygen saturation, rather than oxygen tension, appears to be the more important determinant of the erythropoietic response to chronic hypoxia (Fig. 27-1). A disorder may set in insidiously after several years of continued residence at high altitudes, leading to the development of a condition known as *chronic mountain sickness* or *seroche* (Monge's disease). Prominent manifestations are a florid color which turns to cyanosis on mild exertion, mental torpor, fatigue, and headache. Those affected are usually in the fourth to sixth decades. Return to sea level promptly relieves the symptoms. Living at high altitudes also evokes a number of compensatory reactions which act to increase oxygen delivery to the tissues. These include hyperventilation, which reduces the oxygen gradient between ambient and alveolar air, an augmentation of pulmonary capillary blood volume, a reduction of diffusing capacity, and an increase in cardiac output.

Any chronic pulmonary disease which produces chronic hypoxia may lead to erythrocytosis. The increased blood viscosity secondary to the polycythemia elevates pulmonary arterial pressure and, combined with the elevation of pulmonary vascular resistance resulting from hypoxia, further elevates right ventricular pressure, contributing to the development or intensification of cor pulmonale (Chap. 262).

The *abnormal ventilatory conditions* present in very obese individuals may cause alveolar hypoventilation and result in arterial unsaturation, erythrocytosis, hypercapnia, and somnolence (the Pickwickian syndrome, Chap. 286). This syndrome is observed less commonly in nonobese persons (sleep-apnea syndrome), in whom decreased sensitivity of the respiratory center to CO_2 may play a role (Chap. 286).

The partial shunting of blood from the pulmonary circuit, such as occurs in *congenital heart disease,* causes the most striking erythrocytosis resulting from abnormalities in the heart or lungs. Erythrocyte counts as high as 13 million per cubic millimeter, which are possible only when the red corpuscles are smaller than normal, have been observed in such cases, with volumes of packed red blood cells even as high as 86 ml/dl of blood. As the polycythemia develops, there is a progressive rise in blood viscosity, the sharpest increase beginning when the volume of packed red blood cells reaches 65 to 70 percent. The commonest defect producing such polycythemia is tetralogy of Fallot (obstruction to right ventricular outflow and ventricular septal defect). Other conditions include transposition of the great arteries, tricuspid atresia, and persistent truncus arteriosus (Chap. 256). The polycythemia of cyanotic congenital heart disease may lead to spontaneous thrombosis at any site, including the central nervous system. It may also be accompanied by a variety of blood coagulation defects, including reduced fibrinogen and prothrombin concentrations, as well as thrombocytopenia. Reduction in red blood cell volume (phlebotomy with reinfusion of the plasma) is sometimes performed in severely symptomatic patients with extremely high hematocrit levels, but it must be carried out slowly and with great caution. It results in a reduction of the elevated blood viscosity which improves blood flow.

FIGURE 27-1

Relationship between mean arterial oxygen saturation (percent) and the mean hemoglobin content (grams per deciliter) in healthy male residents at various altitudes. (From Hurtado, by permission of Annals of Internal Medicine.)

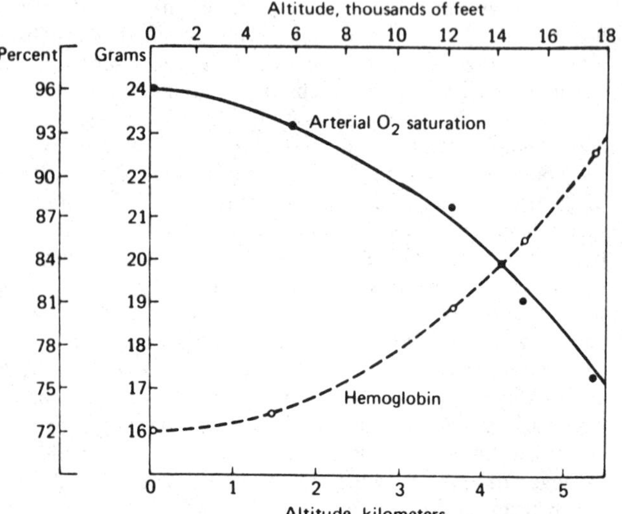

TABLE 27-2
Differential diagnosis of erythrocytosis

I Autonomous erythroid proliferation (↓ EP*); polycythemia vera
II Secondary erythroid proliferation
- *A* Autonomous or inappropriate increase in EP
  - *1* Neoplasm
  - *2* Renal lesions
  - *3* Familial erythrocytosis (autosomal recessive inheritance)
- *B* Secondary increase in EP
  - *1* Hypoxemia (↓ arterial P_{O_2})
    - *a* High altitude
    - *b* Alveolar hypoventilation
    - *c* Pulmonary disease
    - *d* Cardiac right-to-left shunt
  - *2* Abnormal hemoglobin function (normal arterial P_{O_2})
    - *a* High-affinity variants (autosomal dominant inheritance)
    - *b* Congenital methemoglobinemia
    - *c* Carboxyhemoglobin (smokers)
- *C* Hormonal stimulus to erythropoeisis
  - *1* Cushing's syndrome

* *Erythropoietin.*
SOURCE: *HF Bunn et al, Human Hemoglobins, Philadelphia, Saunders, 1977.*

The excessive use of coal-tar derivatives and other forms of chronic poisoning, by producing abnormal hemoglobin pigments such as *methemoglobin* and *sulfhemoglobin* (Chap. 330), also may cause erythrocytosis. Carriers of certain abnormal hemoglobins which displace the oxygen dissociation curve to the left and interfere with oxygen unloading in the tissues stimulate the production of erythropoietin and a secondary erythrocytosis unassociated with leukocytosis or thrombocytosis (Chap. 330).

Erythrocytosis is found in *Cushing's syndrome* (Chap. 112) and can be produced by the administration of large amounts of adrenocortical steroids. Especially intriguing are the instances of polycythemia observed in association with various *tumors.* These have been chiefly of two varieties, *infratentorial* and *renal.* The tumors in the posterior fossa of the skull have usually been vascular (hemangioblastomas). The renal tumors have included hypernephroma, adenoma, and sarcoma. Other tumors that have been associated with polycythemia include uterine myoma and hepatic carcinoma. Polycythemia also has been reported in association with polycystic disease of the kidneys and hydronephrosis. However, only a small proportion (0.3 to 2.6 percent) of the various renal disorders mentioned above have been associated with polycythemia. Plasma erythropoietin levels have been found to be elevated in a number of these patients. Erythropoiesis-stimulating activity has been demonstrated in tumor extracts and in renal cyst fluid, and polycythemia has disappeared after the associated tumor was removed.

The term *stress erythrocytosis* has been applied to the polycythemia seen occasionally in very active, hard-working persons in a state of anxiety, who appear florid but who have none of the characteristic signs of erythremia—no splenomegaly or leukocytosis with immature cells in the blood. In such persons the total red blood cell mass is normal, and the plasma volume is below normal.

The differential diagnosis of polycythemia is discussed in Chap. 336. However, it should be pointed out that in secondary polycythemia with hypoxia, arterial P_{O_2} is reduced, erythropoietin levels are elevated, while levels of leukocyte alkaline phosphatase, serum vitamin B_{12}, platelet, total white blood cell, and differential counts are all normal, and the liver and spleen are not enlarged; the bone marrow shows only erythroid hyperplasia. In polycythemia vera, erythropoietin levels are normal or decreased and leukocyte alkaline phosphatase and vitamin B_{12} levels and platelet and total white blood cells are normal, and hepatosplenomegaly is common; the bone marrow shows hyperplasia of all elements.

REFERENCES

Golde DW et al: Polycythemia: Mechanisms and management. Ann Intern Med 95:71, 1981

Harkness DR: The regulation of hemoglobin oxygenation, in *Advances in Internal Medicine,* GH Stollerman (ed). Chicago, Year Book, 1971, p 189

Hurtado A: Some clinical aspects of life at high altitudes. Ann Intern Med 53:247, 1960

Jepson JH, Frankl W: *Haematological Complications in Cardiac Practice.* Philadelphia, Saunders, 1975

Lanken PN, Fishman AP: Clubbing and hypertrophic osteoarthropathy, in *Pulmonary Diseases and Disorders,* AP Fishman (ed). New York, McGraw-Hill, 1980, chap 4, pp 84–91

Rosenthal A, Tyler DC: Effect of red cell volume reduction or pulmonary blood flow in polycythemia of cyanotic congenital heart disease. Am J Cardiol 33:410, 1974

Smith JR, Landaw SA: Smokers' polycythemia. N Engl J Med 298:6, 1978

28 EDEMA

EUGENE BRAUNWALD

Edema is defined as an increase in the extravascular (interstitial) component of the extracellular fluid volume, which may increase by several liters before the abnormality is recognized. Therefore, a weight gain of several kilograms usually precedes overt manifestations of edema, and a similar weight loss resulting from diuresis can be induced in a slightly edematous patient before "dry weight" is achieved. *Ascites* (Chap. 39) and *hydrothorax* refer to accumulation of excess fluid in the peritoneal and pleural cavities, respectively, and are considered to be special forms of edema. *Anasarca,* or "dropsy," refers to gross, generalized edema. Depending on its etiology and mechanism, edema may be localized or have a generalized distribution; it is recognized in its generalized form by puffiness of the face, which is most readily apparent in the periorbital areas, and by the persistence of an indentation of the skin following pressure; this is known as "pitting" edema. In its more subtle form, it may be detected by the fact that the rim of the bell of the stethoscope leaves an indentation on the skin of the chest that lasts a few minutes. One of the early symptoms a patient may note is the ring on a finger fitting more snugly than in the past, or difficulty in putting on shoes, particularly in the evening.

PATHOGENESIS (See also Chap. 43) About one-third of the total body water is confined to the extracellular space. This compartment, in turn, is composed of the plasma volume and the interstitial space. Under ordinary circumstances the plasma volume represents about 25 percent of the extracellular space, and the remainder is interstitial fluid. The forces that regulate the disposition of fluid between these two components of the extracellular compartment are frequently referred to as the Starling forces (page 161). In general terms, the hydrostatic pressure within the vascular system and the colloid oncotic pressure in the interstitial fluid, tend to promote movement of fluid from the vascular to the extravascular space. In contrast, the colloid oncotic pressure contributed by the plasma proteins, and the hydrostatic pressure within the interstitial fluid, referred to as the *tissue tension,* promote a movement of fluid into the vascular compartment. As a consequence of these forces there is a movement of water and diffusible solutes from the vascular space at the arteriolar end of the microcirculation. Fluid is returned from the interstitial space into the vascular system by way of the lymphatics, and unless these channels are obstructed, lymph flow tends to increase if there is a tendency toward a net movement of fluid from the vascular compartment to the interstitium. All these forces are usually balanced so that a steady state exists in the size of the intravascular and interstitial compartments, and yet a large exchange between them is permitted. However, should any one of these forces be altered significantly, a net movement of fluid from one component of the extracellular space to the other will occur.

An increase in capillary pressure may result from an increase in venous pressure due to local obstruction in venous drainage, to congestive heart failure, or rarely to the simple expansion of the vascular volume by the administration of large volumes of fluid at a rate in excess of the ability of the kidneys to excrete these excesses. The colloid oncotic pressure of the plasma may be reduced, owing to any of the factors that may induce hypoalbuminemia, such as malnutrition, liver disease, and loss of protein into the urine or into the gastrointestinal tract, or to a severe catabolic state.

Edema may also result from damage to the capillary endothelium, which increases the permeability of these vessels, permitting the transfer to the interstitial compartment of a fluid containing more protein than usual. Injury to the capillary walls may be the result of chemical, bacterial, thermal, or mechanical agents. Increased capillary permeability may also be a consequence of a hypersensitivity reaction and is characteristic of immune injury. Damage to the capillary endothelium is presumably responsible for inflammatory edema, which is nonpitting, usually localized, and readily recognized by the presence of other signs of inflammation—redness, heat, and tenderness.

In an attempt to formulate a hypothesis about the pathophysiology involved in edematous states, it is important to discriminate between the *primary* events, such as venous or lymphatic obstruction, reduction of cardiac output, hypoalbuminemia, or trapping of fluid in spaces such as the peritoneal cavity, and the predictable *secondary* consequences, which include the renal retention of salt and water. There are instances in which an abnormal positive balance of salt and water may, in fact, be the primary disturbance. In these circumstances the edema is a secondary manifestation of the generalized increase in extracellular fluid volume. These special instances are usually related to conditions characterized by an acute reduction in renal function, such as acute tubular necrosis or acute glomerulonephritis (Fig. 28-1).

These circumstances aside, a hypothesis can be advanced, which, although admittedly incomplete, leads to improved understanding of the events in a variety of edematous states and enhances the perception of their pathophysiology. The basic premise is that the primary disorder concerns one or more alterations in the Starling forces so that there is a net movement of fluid from the vascular system into the interstitium or into a "third space," or from the arterial compartment of the vascular space into the chambers of the heart or into the venous circulation itself. The *effective arterial blood volume,* an as yet poorly defined parameter of the filling of the arterial tree, is reduced, and a series of physiologic responses which are designed to restore it to normal are set into motion. A key element of these responses is the retention of an increment of salt and water, and in many instances this repairs the deficit of the effective arterial blood volume; often this occurs without the development of overt edema. If, however, the retention of salt and water is insufficient to restore and maintain the effective arterial blood volume, the stimuli are not dissipated, the retention of salt and water continues, and edema develops. The sequence of events described above is operative in a variety of circumstances, including dehydration and hemorrhage. Although there is a reduction of effective arterial blood volume and activation of the entire sequence shown on the right side of Fig. 28-1, including the retention of salt and water, edema does not occur because the total extravascular fluid volume is reduced.

Certain data suggest that the increase in volume of some component(s) of the extracellular space normally promotes the secretion of natriuretic hormone(s), also referred to as "third factor." The unambiguous demonstration of such a hormone, its site(s) of secretion, and its characterization is yet to be presented. The retention of sodium is accompanied by an increased reabsorption of water. This is attested to by (1) the usual failure to accumulate edema if sodium is not available in the diet, and (2) the successful use of pharmacologic agents and other measures that promote the excretion of sodium chloride in the urine. In most circumstances the mechanisms responsible for maintaining a normal effective osmolality in the body fluids continue to operate efficiently so that sodium retention promotes thirst and secretion of the antidiuretic hormone, which, in turn, lead to the ingestion and retention of approximately 1 liter of water for each 140 mmol sodium retained. Similarly, measures which promote the loss of sodium into the urine are accompanied by the net loss of an equivalent volume of water from the body.

Obstruction of venous and lymphatic drainage of a limb In this condition the hydrostatic pressure in the capillary bed increases so that more fluid than normal is transferred from the vascular to the interstitial space; since the alternate route (i.e., the lymphatic channels) is obstructed as well, this event must of necessity cause an increased volume of interstitial fluid in the limb, i.e., a trapping of fluid in the extremity, at the expense of the blood volume in the remainder of the body, thereby reducing effective arterial blood volume and leading to the consequences shown in Fig. 28-1.

As fluid accumulates in the interstitium of the limb, in which venous and lymphatic drainage are obstructed, tissue tension rises until it is great enough to counterbalance the primary alterations in the Starling forces, at which time no further fluid will accumulate in that limb. At this point the additional accumulation of fluid will repair the deficit in plasma volume, and the stimuli to retain more salt and water are dissipated. The net effect is an increase in the volume of interstitial fluid in a local area, and the secondary responses repair the plasma volume deficit incurred by the primary event. This same sequence may be translated to many other edematous states.

Congestive heart failure (see also Chap. 253) In this disorder it is postulated that the defective systolic emptying of the chambers of the heart promotes an accumulation of blood in the heart and venous circulation at the expense of the arterial volume, and the aforementioned sequence of events (Fig. 28-1) is initiated. In many instances of mild heart failure a small increment of volume may be achieved, which repairs the volume deficit and establishes a new steady state because through the operation of Starling's law of the heart, up to a point an increase in the volume of blood within the chambers of the heart promotes a more forceful contraction and may thereby increase the volume ejected in systole (Fig. 252-4). However, if the cardiac disorder is more severe, retention of fluid cannot repair the deficit in effective arterial blood volume. The increment accumulates in the venous circulation, and the increase in hydrostatic pressure therein promotes the formation of edema. The formation of edema in the lungs (Chap. 26) impairs gas exchange and may induce hypoxia, which embarrasses cardiac function still further.

In addition to the sequence shown on the right-hand side of Fig. 28-1, incomplete ventricular emptying leads to an elevation of ventricular end-diastolic pressure. If the impairment of cardiac function involves the right ventricle primarily, then incomplete ventricular emptying leads to an elevation of right ventricular end-diastolic volume and pressure; as a consequence pressures in the systemic veins and capillaries also rise, thereby augmenting transudation of fluid into the interstitial space and enhancing the likelihood of peripheral edema. The elevated systemic venous pressure is transmitted to the thoracic duct with consequent reduction of lymph drainage, fur-

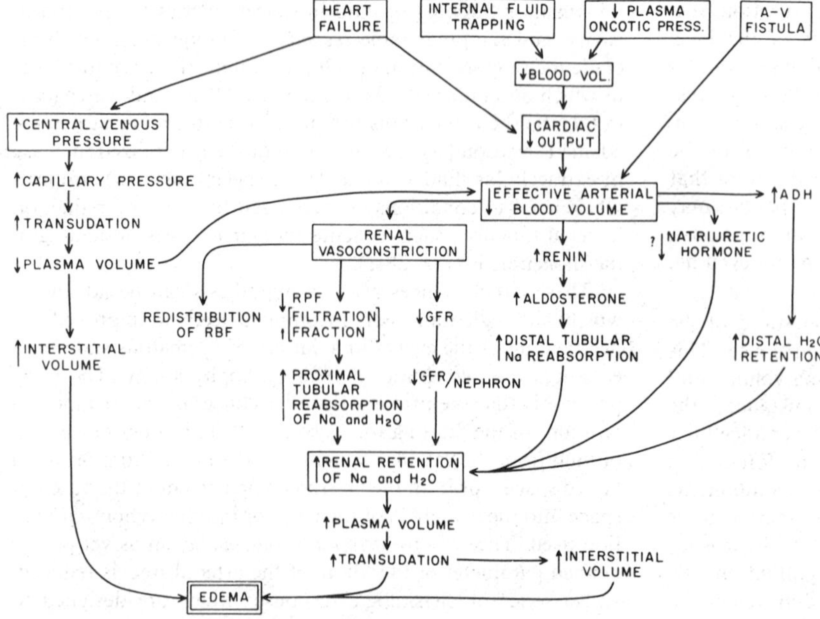

FIGURE 28-1
Sequence of events leading to the formation and retention of salt and water and the development of edema.

ther increasing edema formation. If the impairment of cardiac function involves the left ventricle, then pulmonary venous and capillary pressures rise [leading in some instances to pulmonary edema (Chap. 26)], as does pulmonary artery pressure; this in turn interferes with the systolic emptying of the right ventricle, leading to an elevation of right ventricular end-diastolic and central and systemic venous pressures, enhancing the likelihood of edema formation.

A reduction of cardiac output is associated with a reduction of the effective arterial blood volume as well as of renal blood flow and an elevation of the filtration fraction, i.e., the ratio of glomerular filtration rate to renal plasma flow. In severe heart failure the blood flow to the outer renal cortex, in particular, is significantly reduced with less depression in the more central regions of the kidney, and there is a reduction in the glomerular filtration rate. This constriction of renal cortical vessels appears to play an important role in the retention of salt and water and the formation of edema in heart failure. Indirect evidence suggests that at different stages of heart failure, activation of the sympathetic nervous system and of the renin-angiotensin systems is responsible for renal vasoconstriction. Activation of the former can be counteracted by the administration of alpha-adrenergic blocking agents, a finding which indicates that the elevated renal vascular resistance in heart failure is mediated, at least in part, by sympathetic stimuli. The augmented renal blood flow and profound diuresis induced by treatment with angiotensin converting enzyme inhibitors points to the involvement of the renin-angiotensin system in the retention of salt and water in heart failure.

It is generally agreed that an increase in the tubular reabsorption of glomerular filtrate plays a principal role in the salt and water retention of heart failure. However, the precise site(s) in the system composed of the renal tubules, loops of Henle, and collective ducts which is involved is not clear, nor have the responsible mechanism(s) been identified. Alterations in intrarenal hemodynamics appear to play a significant role. Heart failure, by augmenting renal arteriolar constriction, reduces the hydrostatic pressure and raises the colloid osmotic pressure in the peritubular capillaries, thus enhancing salt and water reabsorption in the proximal tubule. The aforementioned distribution of intrarenal blood flow characteristic of heart failure may be responsible for augmentation of sodium reabsorption in the ascending limb of the loop of Henle.

In addition, the diminished renal blood flow characteristic of all states in which the effective arterial blood volume is reduced is translated by the renal juxtaglomerular cells into a signal for increased renin release (Chap. 112). The specific nature of the signal is complex. One factor involves a baroreceptor mechanism, in which reduced renal perfusion results in incomplete filling of the renal arterioles and diminished stretch of the juxtaglomerular cells, a signal that provides for the elaboration or release, or both, of renin. A second mechanism involves the macula densa; as a result of reduced glomerular filtration the sodium load reaching the distal renal tubules is reduced. This is sensed by the macula densa, which in an as yet undefined manner signals the neighboring juxtaglomerular cells to secrete renin. A third mechanism involves the sympathetic nervous system and circulating catecholamines. Activation of the beta-adrenergic receptors in the juxtaglomerular cells stimulates them to release renin. These three mechanisms generally act in concert.

Renin, an enzyme that has a molecular weight of about 40,000, acts on its substrate, angiotensinogen, an alpha$_2$ globulin synthesized by the liver, resulting in the elaboration of angiotensin II, an octapeptide with vasoconstrictor properties. The intrarenal production of angiotensin II may also contribute to renal vasoconstriction in heart failure and to the salt and water retention in this state. Angiotensin II also passes through the circulation and stimulates the production of aldosterone by the zona glomerulosa region of the adrenal cortex. In patients with heart failure, not only is aldosterone secretion elevated, but the biologic half-life of aldosterone is prolonged, indicating a reduced catabolic rate and further increasing the plasma level of the hormone. A depression of hepatic blood flow, particularly during exercise, secondary to a reduction in cardiac output, is responsible for the reduced hepatic catabolism of aldosterone.

Although increased quantities of aldosterone have been demonstrated to be secreted during heart failure and other edematous states, and blockade of the action of aldosterone by spironolactone often induces a moderate diuresis in edematous states, augmented levels of aldosterone (or other mineralocorticoids) alone do not always promote accumulation of edema, as witnessed by the lack of striking fluid retention in most instances of primary aldosteronism. Furthermore, although normal subjects will retain some salt and water under the influence of a potent mineralocorticoid, such as deoxycorticosterone acetate or 9α-fluorohydrocortisone, the accumulation appears to be self-limiting, despite continued exposure to the steroid and to salt and water. It is probable that the failure of normal subjects to accumulate large quantities of fluid is a consequence of an increase in glomerular filtration rate, other hemodynamic influences, and most importantly the increase in volume which promotes an increased excretion of salt independent of the filtered load of sodium, i.e., through the action of natriuretic substance(s). The role of aldosterone in the accumulation of fluid in edematous states may be more important because these patients are unable to repair the crucial deficit in volume.

Nephrotic syndrome and other hypoalbuminic states (see also Chap. 294) The primary alteration in this disorder is a diminished colloid oncotic pressure due to massive losses of protein into the urine. This promotes a net movement of fluid into the interstitium, causes hypovolemia, and initiates the sequence of events described above. As long as the hypoalbuminemia is severe, the salt and water retained cannot be restrained within the vascular compartment, and hence the stimuli to retain salt and water are not abated. A similar sequence of events occurs in other conditions which lead to severe hypoalbuminemia, including severe nutritional deficiency states, protein-losing enteropathy, congenital hypoalbuminemia, and severe, chronic liver disease.

Cirrhosis (see also Chaps. 39 and 320) The total blood volume in cirrhosis of the liver is commonly increased when the disorder is accompanied by a system of dilated venous radicles and multiple small arteriovenous fistulas. Effective systemic perfusion, the effective arterial blood volume, and the intrathoracic blood volume appear to be diminished, probably as a consequence of the passage of blood through these fistulas, as well as from the portal venous obstruction and the obstruction of the lymphatic drainage of the liver. These alterations are frequently complicated by the reduced serum albumin characteristic of cirrhosis, which reduces the effective arterial blood volume even further, leading to activation of the renin-angiotensin-aldosterone system and other salt and water–retaining mechanisms. Initially, the excess interstitial fluid is localized preferentially behind the congested portal venous system and obstructed hepatic lymphatics, i.e., in the peritoneal cavity. In late stages of the disease, particularly when there is hypoalbuminemia, peripheral edema may also be noted.

Idiopathic cyclic edema This syndrome, which occurs predominantly in women, particularly those with psychosocial difficulties, is characterized by periodic episodes of edema, frequently accompanied by abdominal distention. Fairly large, diurnal alterations in weight occur, so that the patient may well weigh several pounds more in the evening than in the morning after having been in the upright posture most of the day. Such large diurnal weight changes suggest an increase in capillary permeability which appears to fluctuate in severity. The fact that it occurs most commonly in women and appears to have some temporal relation to the menstrual cycle suggests that there may be some hormonal influence in the permeability of the vessels which permits the loss of plasma volume into the interstitial space and the sequence of events secondary to a contraction in plasma volume.

The treatment of idiopathic cyclic edema includes a reduction in salt intake, education in the use of rest in the supine position for several hours each day, the wearing of elastic stockings which are put on before arising in the morning, and an attempt to understand the underlying emotional problems. Diuretics are initially effective but may lose their effectiveness with continuous administration; accordingly, they should be employed sparingly. It has been reported that the plasma concentration of cyclic adenosine monophosphate (AMP) is high in patients with idiopathic edema in both the recumbent and upright positions, and its renal clearance, unlike that of creatinine, is low. If a relationship between extracellular cyclic AMP and the action of hormones on beta-adrenergic receptors could be established, the favorable therapeutic effect of propranolol in cases where diuretics alone did not satisfactorily control the disease could be explained.

DIFFERENTIAL DIAGNOSIS As a rule, localized edema can be readily differentiated from generalized edema. The great majority of patients with noninflammatory generalized edema of significant degree suffer from advanced cardiac, renal, hepatic, or nutritional disorders. Consequently, the differential diagnosis of generalized edema should be directed toward implicating or excluding these several conditions.

Localized edema Edema originating from inflammation or hypersensitivity is usually readily identified. Localized edema due to venous or lymphatic obstruction may be caused by thrombophlebitis, chronic lymphangitis, resection of regional lymph nodes, filariasis, etc. Lymphedema is particularly intractable because restriction of lymphatic flow results in increased protein concentration in the interstitial fluid, a circumstance which severely impedes removal of retained fluid.

Edema of heart failure Evidence of heart disease, as manifested by cardiac enlargement and gallop rhythm together with evidence of cardiac failure, such as dyspnea, basilar rales, venous distention, and hepatomegaly, usually provides an indication on clinical examination of the pathogenesis of edema resulting from heart failure. Rarely, echocardiography, radionuclide angiography, or even cardiac catheterization are required to establish the diagnosis of heart failure (see also Chap. 253).

Edema of the nephrotic syndrome Massive proteinuria, severe hypoproteinemia, and in some instances hypercholesterolemia are present. This syndrome may occur during the course of a variety of kidney diseases, which include glomerulonephritis, diabetic glomerulosclerosis, and hypersensitivity reactions. A history of previous renal disease may or may not be elicited (see also Chap. 294).

Edema of acute glomerulonephritis The edema occurring during the acute phases of glomerulonephritis is characteristically associated with hematuria, proteinuria, and hypertension. Although some evidence supports the view that the fluid retention is due to increased capillary permeability, in most instances the edema in this disease results from primary retention of sodium and water by the kidneys owing to renal insufficiency. This state differs from congestive heart failure in that it is characterized by a normal or increased cardiac output, normal or diminished circulation time, a reduction in the packed cell volume, and a normal arteriomixed venous oxygen difference. Patients commonly have evidence of pulmonary congestion on chest roentgenograms before cardiac enlargement is significant and do not develop orthopnea.

Edema of cirrhosis Ascites and evidence of hepatic disease (collateral venous channels, jaundice, and spider angiomas) characterize edema of hepatic origin. The ascites is frequently refractory to treatment because it collects as a result of a combination of obstruction of hepatic lymphatic drainage, portal hypertension, and hypoalbuminemia. Edema may also occur in other parts of the body in these patients as a result of hypoalbuminemia. Furthermore, the sizable accumulation of ascitic fluid may be expected to increase intraabdominal pressure and impede venous return from the lower extremities; hence, it tends to promote accumulation of edema in this region as well (see also Chap. 320).

Edema of nutritional origin An inadequate diet over a prolonged period may produce hypoproteinemia and edema, which may be intensified by beriberi heart disease, in which multiple peripheral arteriovenous fistulas result in reduced effective systemic perfusion and effective arterial blood volume, thereby enhancing edema formation. More striking edema is commonly observed when these famished subjects are provided with an adequate diet. The ingestion of more food may increase the quantity of salt ingested, which is then retained along with water.

Distribution The distribution of edema is an important guide to the cause. Thus, edema of one leg or of one or both arms is usually the result of venous and/or lymphatic obstruction. Edema resulting from hypoproteinemia characteristically is generalized, but it is especially evident in the very soft tissues of the eyelids and face and tends to be most pronounced in the morning because of the recumbent posture assumed during the night. Edema associated with heart failure, on the other hand, tends to be more extensive in the legs and to be accentuated in the evening, a feature also determined largely by posture. In the rare types of cardiac disease, such as tricuspid stenosis and constrictive pericarditis, in which orthopnea may be absent and the patient actually prefers the recumbent posture, the factor of gravity may be equalized and facial edema observed. Less common causes of facial edema include trichinosis, allergic reactions, and myxedema. Unilateral edema occasionally results from lesions in the central nervous system affecting the vasomotor fibers on one side of the body; paralysis also reduces lymphatic and venous drainage on the affected side.

Additional factors in diagnosis The color, thickness, and sensitivity of the skin are significant. Local tenderness and increase in temperature suggest inflammation. Local cyanosis may signify a venous obstruction. In individuals who have had repeated episodes of prolonged edema, the skin over the involved areas may be thickened, hard, and often red.

Measurement of the venous pressure is also of great importance in evaluating edema. Elevation in an isolated part of the body usually reflects localized venous obstruction. Generalized elevation of systemic venous pressure suggests the presence of congestive heart failure, although it may be present in the congested state that accompanies acute renal insufficiency. Ordinarily, significant increase in venous pressure can be recognized by the level at which cervical veins collapse; in doubtful cases and for accurate recording, the central venous pressure should be measured. In patients with obstruction of the superior vena cava, edema is confined to the face, neck, and upper extremities, where the venous pressure is elevated compared with that in the lower extremities. Measurement of venous pressure in the upper extremities is also useful in patients with massive edema of the lower extremities and ascites; it is elevated when the edema is on a cardiac basis (e.g., constrictive pericarditis or tricuspid stenosis), but is normal when it is secondary to cirrhosis.

Determination of the concentration of serum proteins, and especially of serum albumin, clearly differentiates those patients in whom edema is due, at least in part, to diminished intravascular colloid osmotic pressure. The presence of proteinuria affords useful clues. The complete absence of protein in the urine is evidence against, but does not exclude, either cardiac or renal disease as a cause of edema. Slight to moderate proteinuria is the rule in patients with heart failure, whereas persistent massive proteinuria usually reflects the presence of the nephrotic syndrome.

APPROACH TO THE PATIENT WITH EDEMA A significant question to ask is whether the edema is localized or generalized. If it is localized, those phenomena alluded to above that may be responsible should be concentrated upon. In this context, localized edema may include hydrothorax, ascites, or both, in the absence of congestive heart failure or hypoalbuminemia. Either of these collections may be a consequence of local venous or lymphatic obstruction, as in inflammatory disease or carcinoma. In instances of either hydrothorax (Chap. 285) or ascites (Chap. 39), an examination of the characteristics of the fluid is extremely important. This should include bacterial culture, smear with stains for ordinary and less common infectious agents, determination of protein concentration, cell count, and the presence or absence of blood; the cells should be concentrated by centrifugation and preparation for histologic examination for evidences of malignancy and other characteristics.

If the edema is generalized, it should be determined, first, if there is hypoalbuminemia of significant degree, e.g., serum albumin concentration less than 2.5 g/dl. If there is, a history, physical examination, and other laboratory data will help evaluate the question of cirrhosis, severe malnutrition, protein-losing gastroenteropathy, or the nephrotic syndrome as the underlying disorder. If hypoalbuminemia is not present, it should be determined if there is evidence of congestive heart failure of a severity to promote generalized edema. Finally, it should be ascertained whether the patient has an adequate urine output, or if there is significant oliguria or even anuria. These abnormalities are discussed in Chaps. 40, 290, and 291. The major differential diagnosis in these instances is frequently the discrimination between overload with fluid and a congested state as opposed to congestive heart failure.

REFERENCES

Brenner BM, Stein JH (eds): *Sodium and Water Homeostasis.* New York, Churchill Livingstone, 1978

De Wardener HE: The control of sodium excretion, in *Handbook of Physiology,* vol 8: *Renal Physiology,* J Orloff et al (eds). Washington, The American Physiological Society, 1973, chap 21, p 677

Guyton AC: Edema, in *Textbook of Medical Physiology,* 5th ed. Philadelphia, Saunders, 1976, p 403

Levy M, Seely J: Pathophysiology of edema formation, in *The Kidney,* 2d ed, BM Brenner, FC Rector Jr (eds). Philadelphia, Saunders, 1980, chap 15

Skorecki KL, Brenner BM: Body fluid homeostasis in man. Am J Med 70:77, 1981

———, ———: Body fluid homeostasis in congestive heart failure cirrhosis with ascites. Am J Med 72:325, 1982

29 ALTERATIONS IN ARTERIAL PRESSURE AND THE SHOCK SYNDROME

EUGENE BRAUNWALD
GORDON H. WILLIAMS

CONTROL AND MEASUREMENT OF ARTERIAL PRESSURE

Arterial pressure must be maintained at levels sufficient to permit adequate perfusion of the capillary networks in the systemic vascular bed. The pressure in the central arterial bed is dependent on the product of two factors—the volume of blood ejected by the left ventricle per unit of time, i.e., the cardiac output, and the resistance to blood flow offered by the vessels in the peripheral vascular bed. The resistance of a blood vessel, in turn, varies inversely as the fourth power of its radius, and at any given level of cardiac output arterial pressure is therefore largely dependent upon the degree of constriction of the smooth muscle in the walls of the arterioles. Though resistance to flow also varies with the viscosity of the fluid and the length of the vessels, alterations in these factors are ordinarily of only secondary importance.

Cardiac output is controlled largely by factors which regulate ventricular end-diastolic volume (preload), the level of myocardial contractility, the impedance against which the left ventricle ejects (afterload), and heart rate (Chap. 252). The autonomic nervous system (Chap. 73) plays a major role in the maintenance of arterial pressure by its influences on all four determinants of cardiac output through activation of adrenergic receptors in the sinoatrial node, myocardium, smooth muscle in the walls of the arterioles, venules, and veins. The afferent limbs of the autonomic reflex arcs regulating arterial pressure acutely arise in stretch receptors in the carotid sinuses, the aortic arch, the chambers of the heart, and the lungs. Impulses are transmitted along afferent fibers in the glossopharyngeal and vagus nerves to extensive central autonomic connections in the medulla. Synapses connect not only the sympathetic and parasympathetic nuclei and efferent arcs, but also the cerebral cortex and hypothalamic nuclei which control hormonal secretion via the pituitary gland.

A rapid reduction of arterial pressure diminishes the stimulation of pressoreceptors, which in turn activates sympathetic outflow and inhibits parasympathetic activity. As a result, the vascular smooth muscle in arterioles and veins constricts, while heart rate and myocardial contractility are augmented. In addition, as arterial pressure falls, adrenal medullary secretion increases, along with the output of antidiuretic hormone (ADH), adrenocorticotropic hormone (ACTH), renin, and aldosterone; all these effects act to restore the arterial pressure to control levels. Opposite changes occur if arterial pressure is raised acutely. Thus, the operation of the pressoreceptor and a number of humoral systems normally serve to buffer the body from a variety of influences which would otherwise produce marked alterations in arterial pressure.

MEASUREMENT OF ARTERIAL PRESSURE Arterial pressure is determined clinically with a pneumatic cuff; ordinarily, this indirect method provides slight underestimation of the true arterial pressure. However, considerable error may be introduced if proper precautions are not taken in determining blood pressure by this method. The arterial pressure may be significantly underestimated if the air in the cuff is released too rapidly, especially in the presence of bradycardia or an irregular rhythm, or if inadequate inflation of the cuff does not result in complete vascular occlusion. This indirect method is most accurate when, in normal-sized adults, cuffs 12 to 14 cm in width are employed. However, when a cuff of this size is used on children or adults with unusually thin arms, blood pressure may be seriously underestimated, or conversely, it may be overestimated when employed on an arm or thigh greater than 20 cm in girth. Marked vasoconstriction resulting in severely attenuated limb blood flow and/or marked reductions in pulse pressure may also result in serious underestimation of arterial pressure by the auscultatory method. Direct intraarterial recordings may reveal a normal or even an elevated pressure, while the absence of Korotkoff sounds makes the pressure unobtainable by the indirect methods. Diastolic pressure usually corresponds closely to the disappearance (phase V) of the Korotkoff sounds, but in severe aortic regurgitation it corresponds with the muffling (phase IV) of the sounds.

THE "NORMAL" BLOOD PRESSURE The "normal" blood pressure is difficult to define. Traditional statistical approaches define normality on the basis of values included within two standard deviations of the mean of pressures obtained in a large population of presumably healthy individuals. However, a better definition of abnormality would be based on demonstrated deleterious effects of blood pressure levels exceeding certain limits. If such criteria are used, chronic *hypotension* would seem to occur very rarely. However, the incidence of hypertension based on casual blood pressure levels exceeding 140/90 (widely accepted as hazardous because it is associated with increased risk of vascular disease which can be reduced by therapy) is estimated to be approximately 20 percent in the adult population of the United States, the incidence in the black population exceeding that in the nonblacks by 50 to 100 percent. Even these statistics may understate the prevalence of hypertension if one accepts the validity of actuarial data indicating that longevity is shortened progressively in adults whose blood pressures exceed 100/60.

ACUTE HYPOTENSION AND SHOCK

Hypotension or shock are not synonymous; although shock is usually associated with hypotension, a previously hypertensive patient may be in shock despite an arterial pressure within normal limits, and hypotension may occur in the absence of shock. *Shock* may be defined as a state in which there is widespread, serious reduction of tissue perfusion, which, if prolonged, leads to generalized impairment of cellular function.

CAUSES The most common clinical causes of shock are listed in Table 29-1. Since arterial pressure is dependent on cardiac output and peripheral vasomotor tone, marked reductions in either of these variables without a compensatory elevation of the other results in systemic hypotension. Reduction of cardiac output may be due to (1) hypovolemia, with volume loss being external (e.g., hemorrhage) or endogenous (e.g., anaphylaxis); (2) myocardial failure (e.g., cardiogenic shock); (3) circulatory obstruction (e.g., pulmonary embolism); (4) redistribution of blood into the venous capacitance bed ("distributive shock," e.g., septic shock); and (5) failure of neurogenic vasoconstriction (e.g., spinal cord injury). In many patients, particularly in the late stages of shock, multiple factors are involved in the development of circulatory failure.

Hypovolemia has been studied much more extensively than any other cause of shock; the mechanism of development is usually readily evident and well understood, and therapy, i.e., restoration of blood volume, is both simple and effective if applied before irreversible tissue damage occurs. Whether the primary insult is the external loss of blood, plasma, or water and salt or the internal sequestration of these fluids in a hollow viscus or body cavity, the general effect is similar, i.e., reduced venous return and decreased cardiac output. This leads to a set of reflex responses designed to maintain the supply of oxygen to critical organs, such as the brain and heart. However, these responses may so limit perfusion of other organs, such as the gut, as to produce necrosis. For purposes of a general discussion of shock, hemorrhagic hypovolemia will be used as the model, but the consequences of general reduced tissue perfusion are similar in other forms of shock.

Stages of hypovolemic shock Depending upon the severity and rate of development of hypovolemia, the shock syndrome

TABLE 29-1
Etiologic factors in shock

- *I* Hypovolemia
  - *A* External fluid losses
    - *1* Hemorrhage
    - *2* Gastrointestinal
      - *a* Vomiting (pyloric stenosis, intestinal obstruction)
      - *b* Diarrhea
    - *3* Renal
      - *a* Diabetes mellitus
      - *b* Diabetes insipidus
      - *c* Excessive use of diuretics
    - *4* Cutaneous
      - *a* Burns
      - *b* Exudative lesions
      - *c* Perspiration and insensible water loss without replacement
  - *B* Internal sequestration
    - *1* Fractures
    - *2* Ascites (peritonitis, pancreatitis, cirrhosis)
    - *3* Intestinal obstruction
    - *4* Hemothorax
    - *5* Hemoperitoneum
- *II* Cardiogenic
  - *A* Myocardial infarction
  - *B* Arrhythmia (paroxysmal tachycardia or fibrillation, severe bradycardia)
  - *C* Severe congestive heart failure with low cardiac output
  - *D* Cardiac mechanical factors
    - *1* Acute mitral or aortic regurgitation
    - *2* Rupture of interventricular septum
- *III* Obstruction to blood flow
  - *A* Pulmonary embolus
  - *B* Tension pneumothorax
  - *C* Cardiac tamponade
  - *D* Dissecting aortic aneurysm
  - *E* Intracardiac (ball valve thrombus, atrial myxoma)
- *IV* Neuropathic
  - *A* Drug induced
    - *1* Anesthesia
    - *2* Ganglion-blocking or other antihypertensive drugs
    - *3* "Ingestion" (barbiturates, glutethimide, phenothiazines)
  - *B* Spinal cord injury
  - *C* Orthostatic hypotension (primary autonomic insufficiency, peripheral neuropathies)
- *V* Other
  - *A* Infection
    - *1* Gram-negative septicemia (endotoxin)
    - *2* Other septicemias
  - *B* Anaphylaxis
  - *C* Endocrine failure (Addison's disease, myxedema)
  - *D* Anoxia

may develop abruptly or evolve gradually. If the precipitating factors progress unabated, the endogenous defense mechanisms, while initially competent to maintain adequate circulation, eventually are extended beyond their capacity for compensation. The development of the shock syndrome may be thought to evolve through several stages which merge with one another. The first is the period in which the blood volume deficit is relatively minor and in which the patient may be asymptomatic. In a previously healthy individual compensation for an acute blood loss of as much as 10 percent of the normal blood volume (as with venesection of 500 ml blood from a donor) is achieved acutely by constriction of the arteriolar bed and an augmentation of heart rate, effects mediated by reflex increases in sympathetic neural discharge of norepinephrine from sympathetic nerve endings and of both norepinephrine and epinephrine from the adrenal medulla. Other responses with more gradual effects include the increased secretion of antidiuretic hormone and the activation of the renin-angiotensin-aldosterone axis (Chap. 112). Arterial pressure is maintained and cardiac output is normal, or only slightly reduced, primarily as a consequence of selective reductions of blood flow to the skin and muscle beds. Heart rate may rise and arterial pressure decline modestly when the patient assumes the erect posture. Hemorrhage may be associated with thrombocytosis, increased platelet adhesiveness, and resultant stasis in blood flow in some capillary beds.

During the second stage, with a reduction in blood volume of 15 to 25 percent, cardiac output falls markedly, even in the recumbent position, and despite intense arteriolar constriction in most vascular beds, arterial pressure declines, although proportionately less than cardiac output. Generalized venoconstriction occurs, increasing the fraction of the total blood volume in the central circulation and tending to sustain venous return. Accompanying this massive reflex adrenergic discharge are tachycardia, tachypnea, intense cutaneous vasoconstriction, pallor, diaphoresis, piloerection, oliguria, apprehension, and restlessness. The latter mental signs relate to a reduction in cerebral circulation due to decreased perfusion pressure rather than to local vasoconstriction. Angina may occur in patients who have intrinsic coronary vascular disease. Reduced availability of oxygen to tissues activates anaerobic glycolysis, and plasma lactate levels rise.

Once the patient has achieved this state of maximal mobilization of compensatory mechanisms, small additional losses of blood result in the third stage characterized by rapid deterioration of the circulation, with life-threatening reductions of cardiac output, blood pressure, and tissue perfusion. The duration of this shock state, the severity of tissue anoxia, and the age and underlying physical state of the patient are of primary importance in determining the ultimate outcome. If tissue perfusion is restored rapidly, recovery may be expected. However, if shock persists, the severe vasoconstriction, a compensatory mechanism which aids in the maintenance of arterial pressure, may itself become a complicating factor, and by reducing tissue perfusion even further may initiate a vicious cycle leading to an irreversible state due to widespread cellular injury. Blood flow to the brain, heart, and kidneys is further reduced, and severe ischemia of these vital organs leads to irreversible tissue damage which may result in impaired function of the organ and, eventually, death. Impaired coronary perfusion depresses cardiac function, particularly in patients with some coronary vascular obstruction, and this may lead to further lowering of cardiac output, thus perpetuating a vicious cycle. Cardiac function may also be depressed by the release of myocardial *depressant factor(s)* from other hypoperfused organs. Reduced flow to the medullary vasomotor center late in the stage of shock depresses the activity of compensatory reflexes. Anoxia, hypercapnia, and lactic acidosis result from hypoperfusion of tissues and anaerobic metabolism. These metabolic derangements ultimately result in failure of the energy-requiring active transport systems of cell membranes. The cellular high-energy phosphate reserves are depleted. The integrity of the cells is compromised, and potassium ions, intracellular lysosomal enzymes, peptides, and other vasoactive compounds are released into the circulation. The integrity of capillary membranes is disrupted, and fluid, proteins, and cellular constituents of the blood seep into the extravascular space of tissues.

In profound shock from any cause an additional important factor which may exacerbate the status of the microcirculation is widespread disseminated intravascular coagulation (DIC, Chap. 334) in the bowel, kidney, and other organs. The resultant ischemia produced in the bowel may further complicate the circulatory compensation as a result of breakdown of the mucosal barrier, leading to entry of bacteria and toxic bacterial products into the circulation. Similar changes in the capillary network of the lungs result in interstitial and alveolar edema (noncardiogenic pulmonary edema), impaired respiratory gas transfer, and ultimately development of the adult respiratory distress syndrome (ARDS, Chap. 287), a common lethal complication of shock. Acute tubular necrosis, caused by prolonged renal hypoperfusion, may result in prolonged postshock renal insufficiency (Chap. 290). Because many bacterial substances are potent vasodilators, vasoconstrictor mechanisms may be inhibited, with a further decrease in blood pressure despite intense sympathetic activity.

Just as tissue perfusion may fall to dangerous or even fatal levels because of actual fluid losses or sequestration with diminished venous return, cardiac failure or intrathoracic obstruction to blood flow may have similar effects. Furthermore, even in the presence of a normal blood volume and cardiac function, "vasomotor collapse" due to drug-induced or neuropathic failure of sympathetic vasomotor activity can result in shock because of reduction of peripheral resistance, the pooling of blood in the venous bed, and reduction of cardiac output.

Other forms of shock A complex form of shock may result from infection, especially gram-negative bacteremia with endotoxin release (Chap. 139). This form of shock is associated with vascular pooling, diminished venous return, and reduced cardiac output. Sometimes there is inadequate vasoconstriction with a decline in perfusion pressures. When cutaneous vasodilatation is present, the skin is warm and dry and cardiac output may be increased, even though perfusion of critical organs is reduced. At other stages there is intense vasoconstriction with tissue damage secondary to reduced perfusion. In anaphylactic shock, release of histamine or a histamine-like substance causes venous dilatation and an attendant reduction in venous return and cardiac output. Also, it results in arteriolar dilatation and a reduction of perfusion pressure, as well as increased capillary permeability with loss of intravascular volume.

TREATMENT This should be directed toward the rapid restoration of cardiac output and tissue perfusion. General supportive measures must be undertaken immediately, sometimes even before the cause of the shock state has been identified. Whether shock results from decreased cardiac output due to a primary reduction in intravascular volume or from a reduction of "effective blood volume" with pooling of blood in certain vascular beds, the most effective means of restoring adequate circulation is by the rapid infusion of volume-expanding fluids (whole blood, plasma, plasma substitutes, or isotonic electrolyte solutions). However, when shock is secondary to, or is accompanied by, cardiac failure with increased pulmonary vascular and central venous pressures, the infusion of volume-expanding fluids may result in pulmonary edema. Here attention must be directed toward restoring cardiac function with cardiotonic drugs such as digitalis glycosides and isoproterenol (Chap. 253), and an attempt should be made to support arterial pressure at levels sufficient to maintain the coronary perfusion pressure (Chap. 261). Intraaortic balloon counterpulsation, together with augmentation of contractility with a sympathomimetic amine, and adjustment of preload to an optimal level of left ventricular filling pressure (18 to 20 mmHg) may be used to treat this state. Arrhythmias, which may also contribute to the low cardiac output, should be corrected (Chaps. 254 and 255).

The appearance of the external jugular veins may be helpful in differentiating between shock with high or low central venous pressure. However, catheters inserted into the superior vena cava and, if possible, into the pulmonary artery (a Swan-Ganz balloon-tipped catheter) are the best means for continuously monitoring ventricular filling pressure and of considerable value in guiding therapy; such catheters should be inserted in patients with shock whenever possible. Serial measurements of central venous pressure, urine flow rate, heart rate, and the clinical and mental state of the patient often provide more important indexes of the efficacy of therapy than arterial pressure changes do. In patients with shock and impaired left ventricular function, e.g., cardiogenic shock due to massive acute myocardial infarction, the balloon-tipped catheter "floated" into the pulmonary artery at the bedside without the aid of fluoroscopy is essential in guiding treatment (Chap. 261). Shock secondary to cardiac tamponade may be recognized by the presence of a paradoxical pulse, jugular venous distention, and, if time permits, fluid in the pericardial space recognized by echocardiography (Chap. 265). Pericardiocentesis may be life-saving.

There is considerable debate concerning the efficacy of va-
There is considerable debate concerning the efficacy of va-
soconstrictor drugs in shock. In patients with severe peripheral constriction these agents are often ineffective and may actually reduce the already lowered tissue perfusion. However, these drugs may be helpful in patients with inadequate vasoconstrictor responses who are not in heart failure. The use of alpha-adrenergic blocking agents or massive doses of adrenal glucocorticoids in shock secondary to gram-negative septicemia with endotoxin release is also a matter of considerable controversy and cannot yet be considered a routine procedure. The release of the endogenous opiate β-endorphin in many forms of stress has led to trials with the specific opiate antagonist naloxone, with favorable responses having been reported in patients with septic shock. Following immediate attention to improvement of perfusion, attention should be directed to treating the underlying etiologic factor, such as diabetic acidosis, pneumothorax, or septicemia (Table 29-1).

CHRONIC HYPOTENSION

Although many patients have been treated for chronic "low blood pressure," most of them, with systolic pressures in the range of 90 to 110 mmHg, are normal and may actually have a greater life expectancy than those with "normal" pressures. Patients with true chronic hypotension may complain of lethargy, weakness, easy fatigability, and dizziness or faintness, especially if arterial pressure is lowered further when the erect position is assumed. These symptoms are presumably due to a decrease in perfusion of the brain, heart, skeletal muscle, and other organs.

Chronic hypotension occasionally results from severe reductions of the cardiac output. The major endocrine causes of chronic hypotension are associated with deficient gluco- and mineralocorticoid secretion and resultant reductions of the intravascular and interstitial fluid volume. Hypotension is usually more pronounced in patients with primary adrenocortical insufficiency than in those with hypopituitarism because secretion of the salt-retaining adrenocortical hormone, aldosterone, is partially preserved in pituitary insufficiency (Chap. 112).

Malnutrition, cachexia, chronic bed rest, and a variety of neurologic disorders may result in chronic hypotension, especially in the standing position. Interference with the neural pathways anywhere between the vasomotor center and the efferent sympathetic nerve endings on the blood vessels or heart may prevent the vasoconstriction and increase in cardiac output which occur as a normal response to a reduction in arterial pressure. Multiple sclerosis, amyotrophic lateral sclerosis, syringomyelia, syphilitic or diabetic tabes dorsalis, peripheral neuropathies, spinal cord section, diabetic neuropathy, extensive lumbodorsal sympathectomy, and the administration of drugs interfering with nerve transmission in the sympathetic nervous system are all associated with orthostatic hypotension.

IDIOPATHIC ORTHOSTATIC HYPOTENSION (PRIMARY AUTONOMIC INSUFFICIENCY) This is a rare condition occurring mostly in older men in which there is degeneration of central and/or peripheral autonomic nervous structures, may result in such severe orthostatic hypotension that syncope or seizures occur when the patient arises from recumbency. This condition is progressive and characterized by ascending anhydrosis and loss of hair, decreased basal metabolic rate (BMR), reduced norepinephrine production, deficient secretion of lacrimal and salivary glands, ileus, bladder atony, and absence of tachycardia on standing despite the marked reduction of blood pressure.

Those patients with orthostatic hypotension and central nervous system disease (*Shy-Drager syndrome*) have prominent degeneration of the extrapyramidal tracts, the basal ganglia, and the dorsal nucleus of the vagus and have normal resting plasma norepinephrine levels, while those with only peripheral autonomic disease have depressed levels at rest. Both groups fail to increase their circulating concentrations of the neurotransmitter during standing and exercise. Thus, it appears that patients with orthostatic hypotension and central nervous system disease have an intact peripheral sympathetic nervous system, but are unable to activate it, while those without central disease have true insufficiency of the peripheral autonomic nervous system.

Specific therapy is not available for most of the neurologic causes of orthostatic hypotension, and treatment with sympathomimetic drugs has not proved effective over prolonged periods. However, the expansion of extracellular volume, which may be achieved with a high-salt diet (10 to 20 g per day), and/or the potent synthetic salt-retaining steroid, 9α-fluorohydrocortisone (0.1 to 0.5 mg per day) may be useful. Tight, full-length elastic supportive hose to reduce orthostatic pooling of blood in the legs may also be helpful in sustaining arterial pressure, and in the most severe cases pressurized aviator suits may be necessary to permit ambulation. Occasionally, favorable results may be achieved with sympathomimetic amines such as ephedrine, particularly in combination with a monoamine oxidase inhibitor, such as tranylcypromine.

HYPERTENSION (See also Chap. 267)

DIAGNOSIS Patients with elevations of arterial pressure are usually asymptomatic, and the blood pressure abnormality often arouses attention only incidentally during military, life insurance, or other periodic physical examinations. Because hypertension results in secondary organ damage and a reduced life span, it should be evaluated fully and, when appropriate, treated.

Often, however, the first question is whether patients with a moderately elevated routine blood pressure recording are truly hypertensive. It is well established that anxiety, discomfort, physical activity, or other stress can acutely and transiently raise arterial pressure. Most persons have a higher pressure when initially examined than after several measurements made in the course of a single visit; in order to establish the diagnosis of hypertension, it is necessary to document in the course of several examinations that arterial pressure remains elevated. This precaution need not be taken in patients with markedly elevated blood pressure and/or in those in whom significant target organ damage is already manifest. Patients with transient or "labile" hypertension may not require immediate treatment but should be reexamined periodically, since over the course of time they often develop sustained hypertension.

MECHANISM Regardless of the primary cause, the hemodynamic abnormality in most patients with increased systolic, mean, and diastolic arterial pressures is increased vascular resistance, especially at the level of the smaller muscular arteries and arterioles, though a small number of patients may have an increased cardiac output, particularly in the early stages of the illness. In some patients in whom hypertension is associated with an increase of cardiac output, hypervolemia is present.

Peripheral resistance is determined by the intrinsic physical characteristics of the resistance vessels, i.e., the ratio of lumen to wall thickness, as well as the neurohumoral influences that act on vascular smooth muscle; the latter include the neurotransmitters norepinephrine, a vasoconstrictor, and in some vessels, acetylcholine, a vasodilator. Humoral and locally acting substances include angiotensin II (a vasoconstrictor) and prostaglandins and kinins (vasodilators). Hypoxia and products of metabolism, such as H^+, lactic acid, and perhaps most important, adenosine, also exert potent *local* vasodilating influences.

Systolic hypertension is most commonly seen in elderly patients with decreased compliance of the aortic wall and, like diastolic hypertension, is a risk factor for the development of atherosclerosis. When systolic hypertension is due to an elevated stroke volume, as in patients with severe bradycardia, thyrotoxicosis, severe anemia, aortic valvular regurgitation, arteriovenous shunts or fistulas, patent ductus arteriosus, or the hyperkinetic heart syndrome, it is usually accompanied by a reduced diastolic pressure and a normal mean pressure, and under these circumstances it does not appear to be a risk factor for atherosclerosis.

In 1963, Borst and Borst de Geus proposed that "hypertension is part of a homeostatic reaction to deficient renal sodium output." The proposed abnormality in renal function, i.e., reduced sodium excretion at normal arterial pressure, might be secondary to (1) a primary (perhaps genetic) tubular defect, (2) mild increases in mineralocorticoid activity, (3) decreased renal kallikrein-kinin or prostaglandin activity, or (4) *local* increases in vasoconstrictor activity (angiotensin II or sympathetic nervous system), reducing renal blood flow and secondarily sodium excretion. Regardless of the mechanism of salt retention, according to this concept, blood volume rises because of the decreased sodium excretion, raising central venous pressure and preload, and thereby, cardiac output, i.e., systemic blood flow. However, tissues have the intrinsic capacity to regulate this overperfusion down to appropriate levels by increasing local vascular resistance. When resistance is increased in many vascular beds, arterial pressure rises and serves as negative feedback by increasing cardiac afterload, thereby depressing stroke volume and cardiac output (Fig. 252-6). As has been shown by Guyton, and others, the elevated arterial (renal perfusion) pressure also increases the urinary excretion of sodium, thereby serving as a source of negative feedback and reducing blood volume, central venous pressure, preload, and ultimately cardiac output. Thus, the end result of this process would be increased peripheral resistance and arterial pressure, with all other parameters, including blood volume, cardiac output, and renal sodium excretion, remaining normal. Indeed, this sequence has been documented in experimental human (desoxycorticosterone) and animal (renal artery stenosis) hypertension. However, in patients with essential hypertension, most investigations have reported only a normal cardiac output and elevated peripheral resistance, suggesting either that the studies have not been performed early enough in the course of the disease or that this theory is incorrect in that a change in peripheral resistance is actually a *primary* rather than secondary event.

Such a primary elevation in peripheral resistance can occur either because of an increase in factors tending to produce vasoconstriction, a reduction in factors producing vasodilation, or a change in the arterial smooth muscle—i.e., an increase in muscle mass or an increase in its responsiveness and/or sensitivity to vasoconstrictor stimuli. Each theory has it advocates. Thus, the hypertension associated with emotional stress, some neurologic disorders, and perhaps early essential hypertension is accompanied by increased plasma or urine levels of norepinephrine. Presumably, this reflects augmented neural releases of the vasoconstrictive adrenergic neurotransmitter which is responsible for the increased arterial pressure. Secondly, there is an increased vascular response to vasoconstrictor agents (e.g., angiotensin II, norepinephrine) in many patients with essential hypertension. Finally, since the early 1930s, hypertensive patients have been noted to exhibit a decrease in the urinary excretion of kinins, and thus it is possible that reduced vasodilator activity could also result in increased peripheral resistance and arterial pressure.

The "primary increase in peripheral resistance" hypothesis and the "deficient renal sodium output" theory are not necessarily mutually exclusive. For example, an increased retention of sodium enhances vascular reactivity, at least to angiotensin II, even in normotensive subjects. Thus, a primary defect of sodium excretion could simultaneously increase both cardiac output and peripheral resistance. It appears that all the factors mentioned above play some role in the development of essential hypertension; individual patients may differ in the relative importance of each. Thus, essential hypertension might be best regarded as a multifactorial disease related to abnormalities of the regulatory mechanisms normally concerned with the control of systemic vascular resistance, sodium excretion, blood volume, cardiac output, and ultimately arterial pressure. The specific parameter which is improperly regulated may differ from patient to patient.

ETIOLOGY A specific cause for the elevated arterial pressure cannot be defined for most patients with hypertension. The percentage of patients with so-called idiopathic, essential, or primary hypertension is high, varying from 80 to 95 percent depending on both the patient population and how extensive the "routine" evaluation is.

More specific etiologic relationships have been established for a smaller group of patients with systemic hypertension (Table 267-1). Primary renal diseases associated with the development of serious hypertension (as distinguished from renal damage secondary to hypertension) have been recognized for years, although in many cases the exact mechanism of blood pressure elevation is unknown. In some instances it is due to activation of the renin-angiotensin-aldosterone axis; in others, perhaps it is related to a reduced ability to excrete sodium and the sequence already described.

The most clearly defined etiologic relationships in the development of hypertension are found among the endocrine disorders. Adrenocortical hormones have also been implicated in the hypertensive syndromes associated with tumors or hyperplasia of the anterior pituitary (Cushing's syndrome, primary hyperaldosteronism, Chap. 112), as well as with various congenital or hereditary enzyme defects (hypertensive adrenogenital syndromes). Secretion of excessive quantities of the pressor catecholamines, norepinephrine and epinephrine, associated with pheochromocytomas, i.e., chromaffin cell tumors arising from the adrenal medulla or sympathetic ganglia, is also commonly associated with hypertension (Chap. 113). Up to 50 percent of patients with acromegaly (Chap. 109) may have hypertension, but the mechanism of their blood pressure elevation is less clear.

EFFECTS OF HYPERTENSION Patients with untreated hypertension die prematurely, most commonly due to heart disease (Chaps. 253 and 267), with strokes (Chap. 356) and renal failure (Chap. 298) also frequently occurring.

APPROACH TO THE PATIENT WITH HYPERTENSION The physician's first task is to determine whether or not a patient with a given level of arterial pressure has hypertension. Then, determinations of the extent of pretreatment evaluation, whether or not to treat, how to treat, and how frequently to reevaluate are necessary. In general, it is preferable to measure arterial pressure on several occasions prior to starting therapy using a mercury sphygmomanometer with the patient seated.

Initial history, physical examination, and laboratory evaluation should be directed at uncovering correctable secondary forms of hypertension (Table 267-1).

An assessment of the following areas in the medical history is particularly important: family or personal history of hypertension; drugs or dietary factors which may aggravate the hypertension, e.g., high salt intake, oral contraceptives, and hormones; cardiovascular risk factors including diabetes mellitus, smoking, lipid abnormalities, or strokes; cardiac or renal disease; and symptoms suggestive of secondary forms of hypertension, e.g., muscle cramps and weakness associated with primary aldosteronism (Chap. 112) or episodic headaches, palpitations, and sweating associated with pheochromocytoma (Chap. 113).

The *physical examination* should include a standing blood pressure, height, weight, funduscopic examination, assessment of thyroid size, bruits in neck or abdomen, peripheral pulses including determination of synchrony between upper and lower extremities, examination of the heart for size, rate, murmurs, gallops, auscultation of the lungs, examination of the abdomen for masses, and particularly kidney size, and a neurologic examination to assess the presence of deficits associated with a stroke.

The basic *laboratory evaluation* should consist of hematocrit, urinalysis, blood urea nitrogen or creatinine, serum potassium, ECG, and chest x-ray. Often blood glucose, uric acid, and cholesterol determinations and a blood count are also useful, particularly since they may be part of a battery of automated blood tests that as a group are about the same price as the individual tests listed above. Other studies to identify secondary forms of hypertension may be indicated on the basis of the initial therapy or physical examination.

If the diastolic pressure is consistently higher than 90 mmHg, therapy is almost always indicated unless contraindications exist.

Therapy should be directed at reducing the arterial pressure to or near normal levels, since studies have documented that morbidity and mortality are reduced. In order to minimize drug side effects in achieving this goal, a "step-care approach" has been advocated. The principle involves initiating therapy with a small dose of a single drug, usually a thiazide diuretic, increasing the dose of that drug, and then adding a beta-adrenergic blocker and, if necessary, other drugs one at a time (Chap. 267). The therapeutic regimen should be revised as dictated by the arterial pressure measured at periodic intervals. The frequency of reevaluation should be as often as weekly while blood pressure is being lowered in patients with initial diastolic pressures greater than 115 mmHg, and approximately every 4 months in symptom-free patients on stable treatment programs.

The specific drugs are discussed elsewhere (Chap. 267). However, it is important to emphasize here that control of arterial pressure is a lifelong endeavor the success of which is often dependent on the physician's ability to motivate the patient to adhere to the therapeutic program and to recognize the pharmacologic interactions and adverse reactions of antihypertensive agents.

REFERENCES

ABBRUZZESE JL et al: Postural hypotension. Johns Hopkins Med J 148:127, 1981

BORST JGG, BORST DE GEUS A: Hypertension explained by Starling's theory of circulatory homeostasis. Lancet 1:677, 1963

GENEST J (ed): *Hypertension: Physiopathology and Treatment.* New York, McGraw-Hill, 1977

GUYTON AC: Circulatory shock and physiology of its treatment, in *Textbook of Medical Physiology,* 6th ed. Philadelphia, Saunders, 1981, chap 28, p 332

———: Regulation of arterial pressure, in *Textbook of Medical Physiology,* 6th ed. Philadelphia, Saunders, 1981, pp 246–273

HYPERTENSION DETECTION AND FOLLOW-UP PROGRAM COOPERATIVE GROUP: Five year findings. JAMA 242:2562, 1979

KAPLAN NM (ed): *Clinical Hypertension,* 2d ed. Baltimore, Williams & Wilkins, 1978

———: Systemic hypertension, in *Heart Disease,* E Braunwald (ed). Philadelphia, Saunders, 1980, pp 852–951

LEDINGHAM IM et al: Prognosis in severe shock. Brit Heart J 284:443, 1982

MACLEAN LD: Shock: Causes and management of circulatory collapse, in *Davis-Christopher Textbook of Surgery,* 12th ed, DC Sabiston Jr (ed). Philadelphia, Saunders, 1981, pp 58–90

PETERS WP et al: Pressor affect of naloxone in septic shock. Lancet 1:529, 1981

SHINE KI et al: Aspects of the management of shock. Ann Intern Med 93:723, 1980

SOBEL BE: Shock, in *Heart Disease,* E Braunwald (ed). Philadelphia, Saunders, 1980, chap 18, pp 590–629

———, Roberts R: Hypotension and syncope, in *Heart Disease,* E Braunwald (ed). Philadelphia, Saunders, 1980, chap 27, pp 952–966

WEIL MH et al: Treatment of circulatory shock. JAMA 231:1280, 1975

ZIEGLER MG et al: The sympathetic nervous system defect in primary orthostatic hypotension. N Engl J Med 296:293, 1977

30
SUDDEN CARDIOVASCULAR COLLAPSE AND DEATH

BURTON E. SOBEL
EUGENE BRAUNWALD

Sudden cardiac death claims more than 400,000 lives annually in the United States alone, a frequency on the order of one death per minute. Definitions vary, but most include death occurring unexpectedly and instantaneously or within 1 h of the onset of symptoms or signs. Usually only several minutes elapse between sudden cardiovascular collapse (without effective cardiac output) and irreversible ischemic changes in the central nervous system. Nevertheless, prolonged survival without functional impairment may result from prompt treatment of certain forms of cardiovascular collapse.

MECHANISMS Sudden cardiovascular collapse may be due to (1) dysrhythmia (Chaps. 254 and 255)—(*a*) most commonly, ventricular tachycardia or fibrillation, sometimes occurring following a bradyarrhythmia, or (*b*) in as many as 25 percent of cases, ventricular asystole or severe bradycardia, factors generally presaging failure of resuscitative efforts; (2) a marked, abrupt reduction in cardiac output, such as occurs with mechanical blockade of the circulation; massive pulmonary thromboembolism (Chap. 282) and cardiac tamponade are two examples of this form; (3) sudden ventricular (pump) failure, which may occur in the presence of critical aortic stenosis (Chap. 258) or acute myocardial infarction ("nonarrhythmic cardiac death") with or without ventricular rupture (Chap. 261); (4) activation of vasodepressor reflexes, which may contribute to sudden reductions in arterial pressure and heart rate, and which are activated in diverse conditions, including primary pulmonary hypertension (Chap. 281), pulmonary thromboembolism, and the hypersensitive carotid sinus syndrome (Chap. 12).

Sudden death and coronary atherosclerosis Sudden death is primarily a complication of severe, multivessel coronary atherosclerosis. However, in contrast to the high prevalence of complete coronary occlusion in patients dying with transmural myocardial infarction, complete occlusion is evident in only 20 to 30 percent of autopsied cases of sudden death; nonetheless, acute myocardial ischemia appears to be the precipitating event. A form of injury resembling that induced by stress or by catecholamines (myocytolysis) is common. In victims of sudden death less than 45 years of age, platelet thrombi in the coronary microcirculation are often seen. Approximately 60 percent of patients who die because of coronary artery disease succumb before they reach the hospital. In fact, in 25 percent of patients with coronary artery disease, death is the first indication of the presence of the disorder (Chap. 261). By extrapolation from experience in coronary care units, in which control of electrical activity of the heart has affected the mortality rate favorably, it would appear that the incidence of sudden death in the community might be reduced substantially by prophylactic therapy in populations at particularly high risk, if such therapy could be demonstrated to be effective, of low toxicity, and convenient to the patient. However, sudden death may be but one mode of expression of coronary artery disease, and effective prevention of sudden death will almost certainly require reduction in the incidence and severity of atherosclerosis.

Factors associated with increased risk of sudden death in nonhospitalized persons When electrocardiograms are recorded for 24 h during the course of normal activities, supraventricular premature contractions are found to occur in most American men over 50 years of age, and ventricular premature contractions occur in almost two-thirds. Simple ventricular premature beats are not associated with increased risk of sudden death, but conduction abnormalities and couplets or high-grade ventricular ectopic beats (repetitive, or R-on-T complexes) are associated with an increased risk. Among patients with acute myocardial infarction, late ventricular ectopic beats are particularly prone to be associated with malignant ventricular dysrhythmia.

Ventricular premature beats may trigger ventricular fibrillation, particularly with concomitant myocardial ischemia. On the other hand, they may be manifestations of common fundamental electrophysiologic disturbances predisposing to both ventricular premature beats and ventricular fibrillation or totally independent phenomena associated with electrophysiologic mechanisms different from those responsible for fibrillation. Thus, it is not surprising that in many patients who develop ventricular fibrillation, no premonitory warning dysrhythmias have occurred.

In general, ventricular dysrhythmias are of greater significance and more ominous in the presence of acute ischemia and of severe left ventricular dysfunction secondary to ischemic heart disease or cardiomyopathy than in their absence.

Severe coronary artery disease, not necessarily accompanied by morphological evidence of an acute infarction, hypertension, or diabetes mellitus, is present in more than 75 percent of persons dying suddenly, and perhaps more significantly, the incidence of sudden death in persons with at least one of the three abnormalities is substantially increased. More than 75 percent of men without known prior coronary artery disease who die suddenly exhibit at least two of the following four risk factors: hypercholesterolemia, hypertension, hyperglycemia, and cigarette smoking. Obesity and electrocardiographic criteria of left ventricular hypertrophy are also associated with an increased incidence. The incidence of sudden death is higher in cigarette smokers than in nonsmokers, perhaps because of the elevation of circulating catecholamines and fatty acids and the production of increased circulating carboxyhemoglobin with consequently diminished oxygen-carrying capacity by the blood. The proclivity of cigarette smoking to cause sudden death is not cumulative and appears to be reversible when smoking is discontinued.

Cardiovascular collapse on exertion occurs only rarely in patients with ischemic heart disease undergoing exercise testing, and with appropriate personnel and facilities these episodes respond promptly to electrical defibrillation. Acute emotional stress may precipitate acute myocardial infarction and sudden death, findings which are in keeping with recent clinical observations of their association with type A personality, and experimental observations of increased susceptibility to ventricular tachycardia and ventricular fibrillation after coronary occlusion in emotionally stressed animals or those with augmented sympathetic activity, and protection of experimental animals with selected central nervous system neurotransmitter precursors.

Two major clinical syndromes may be recognized in patients who die suddenly and unexpectedly; both are generally associated with ischemic heart disease. In the larger group, the dysrhythmia occurs totally unexpectedly and without preceding symptoms or prodromata. This form is *not* associated with acute myocardial infarction; following resuscitation, there is a propensity for early recurrence, probably reflecting the myocardial electrical instability responsible for the intitial episode, and a relatively high 2-year mortality rate (approximately 50 percent). Clearly, these patients can be salvaged only by a rapidly responsive system, and pharmacologic prophylaxis is required to enhance survival. The second, smaller group consists of patients who, following resuscitation, exhibit evidence of acute myocardial infarction. These patients often exhibit prodromal symptoms—chest pain, dyspnea, and syncope—and show a much lower recurrence and 2-year mortality rate (15 percent). Survival in this subgroup is similar to that following resuscitation from ventricular fibrillation complicating acute myocardial infarction in the coronary care unit. Although the propensity for developing ventricular fibrillation at the time of acute infarction is of short duration, in contrast to the prolonged interval of high risk among patients in whom fibrillation occurs without infarction, the risk of sudden death remains particularly high among some survivors of infarction. Risk factors include extensive infarction; severe impairment of ventricular function; persistent, complex ventricular ectopic activity; QT prolongation after the acute episode; loss of the normal hypertensive response to exercise after convalescence; and persistently positive myocardial infarct scintigrams.

Other causes of sudden death Sudden cardiovascular collapse may result from a number of disorders other than coronary atherosclerosis (Table 30-1). Severe aortic stenosis (congenital or acquired) with sudden dysrhythmias or pump failure, hypertrophic cardiomyopathy, and myocarditis or cardiomyopathy associated with dysrhythmia may be responsible. Massive pulmonary embolism leads to circulatory collapse and death within minutes in approximately 10 percent of patients; some of the remainder succumb gradually with progressive right ventricular failure. Acute circulatory collapse may be presaged by smaller emboli occurring at variable intervals before the lethal attack. Accordingly, implementation of therapy during the premonitory sublethal phase, including anticoagulant administration, may be lifesaving (Chap. 282).

Cardiovascular collapse and sudden death are rare but always potential complications of infective endocarditis (Chap. 259). Sudden, unexpected death in infants, so-called crib death, is responsible for approximately 10,000 deaths per year in the United States. A defect in the regulation of ventilation may be responsible.

A number of less common causes of sudden death have been recognized increasingly in recent years. Sudden cardiac death has been associated with liquid-protein, modified-fast diet programs. Distinguishing features include QT prolongation as well as the less specific morphological cardiac lesions typical of cachexia seen in autopsied cases. Primary degeneration of the atrioventricular conduction system, with or without deposition of calcium or cartilage, may lead to sudden death in the absence of severe coronary atherosclerosis. Trifascicular atrioventricular (AV) block is often seen in these conditions, which account for more than two-thirds of the cases of chronic AV block in adults (Chap. 254). However, the risk of sudden death is substantially greater with impaired conduction associated with ischemic heart disease than that due to primary conduction system disease itself. Electrocardiographic QT-interval prolongation, nerve deafness, and autosomal recessive inheritance (the Jervell-Lange-Nielsen syndrome) is associated with a high proportion of cases of ventricular fibrillation. The same electrocardiographic abnormality and electrophysiologic instability without nerve deafness (the Romano-Ward syndrome) appears to be inherited in an autosomal dominant mode. Electrocardiographic changes in these disorders may be manifest only after exercise, and so they may be more important causes of sudden death than has been generally recognized. Other conditions with QT prolongation and increased temporal dispersion of repolarization, such as hypothermia and phenothiazine, emetine, or quinidine toxicity, have been associated with sudden death, particularly when accompanied by episodes of torsades de pointes, a form of rapid ventricular tachycardia with distinctive electrocardiographic and pathophysiologic features (Chap. 255). Sinoatrial arrest or block with depression of lower pacemakers or the sick sinus syndrome, usually accompanied by conduction system dysfunction as well, may also lead to asystole. Rarely, fibromas or inflammatory processes in the region of the sinus or AV nodes and conduction system elements (ganglionitis and neuritis) may precipitate sudden death in subjects without prior manifestations of heart disease. Sudden rupture of a papillary muscle, the ventricular septum, or free wall, usually occurring within the first few days following acute myocardial infarction, occasionally causes sudden death (Chap. 261). Sudden cardiovascular collapse is also a major, and frequently the terminal, event in patients with major cerebrovascular accidents, sudden alterations of intracranial pressure, or lesions affecting the brainstem. It may also occur with asphyxia, and the toxicity of cardioactive drugs such as digitalis and quinidine may result in life-threatening arrhythmias, leading to sudden cardiovascular collapse and, if treatment is not immediate, to death (Chap. 255).

TABLE 30-1
Conditions associated with cardiovascular collapse and sudden death in adults

Ischemic heart disease secondary to coronary atherosclerosis (including acute myocardial infarction)
Prinzmetal's variant angina; coronary artery spasm
Congenital coronary artery disease (including anomalous origins, coronary arteriovenous fistula)
Coronary embolism
Acquired, nonatherosclerotic coronary disease (including aneurysms occurring with Kawasaki's disease)
Myocardial bridges that demonstrably impair perfusion
Wolff-Parkinson-White syndrome
Hereditary QT-interval prolongation (with or without congenital deafness)
Sinoatrial node disease
Atrioventricular block (Stokes-Adams syndrome)
Secondary disease of the conduction system (e.g., amyloid, sarcoid, hemochromatosis, thrombotic thrombocytopenic purpura, myotonia dystrophica)
Drug toxicity or idiosyncrasy (e.g., digitalis, quinidine)
Electrolyte derangements (with myocardial magnesium and potassium deficiencies having been implicated)
Valvular heart disease, especially aortic stenosis
Infective endocarditis
Myocarditis
Cardiomyopathies, particularly idiopathic hypertrophic subaortic stenosis
Liquid-protein, modified-fast diet programs
Pericardial tamponade
Mitral valve prolapse (despite the benignity of most cases)
Cardiac tumor
Ruptured or dissecting aortic aneurysm
Pulmonary thromboembolism
Cerebrovascular accident, particularly hemorrhage

Electrophysiologic mechanisms underlying ventricular fibrillation Potentially lethal ventricular dysrhythmias in patients with acute myocardial infarction may result from reentry, enhanced automaticity, or both. It would appear that reentry plays a dominant role in early dysrhythmia, for example, within the first hour, and that increased automaticity is an important contributing factor later.

Several factors appear to set the stage for ventricular fibrillation and other rhythms dependent upon reentry early after the onset of ischemia (see also Chap. 255). Local accumulation of hydrogen ions, an increased ratio of extra- to intracellular potassium, and regional adrenergic stimulation tend to shift diastolic transmembrane potentials toward zero and elicit anomalous depolarizations possibly mediated by calcium currents or indicative of depressed, fast sodium-mediated depolarizations. This type of depolarization appears to contribute to slowed conduction required for the development of reentry early after the onset of ischemia.

Another mechanism implicated in reentry early after ischemia is focal reexcitation. Anoxia results in marked abbreviation of the duration of the action potential. Accordingly, during electrical systole, cells within an ischemic zone may be repolarized before cells in adjacent nonischemic tissue. The consequent disparity between prevailing transmembrane potentials may give rise to an uneven depolarization of adjacent cells and hence contribute to dysrhythmia dependent upon reentry. Concomitant pharmacologic or metabolic factors may predispose toward reentry. For example, quinidine may depress conduction velocity, thereby facilitating dysrhythmias dependent upon reentry early after the onset of ischemia.

The so-called vulnerable period, corresponding to the ascending limb of the T wave, represents that portion of the cardiac cycle when temporal dispersion of ventricular refractoriness is maximum and, accordingly, when reentrant rhythms leading to sustained, repetitive activity can be initiated most readily. In patients with severe myocardial ischemia, the vulnerable period is prolonged and the intensity of stimulus required to evoke repetitive tachycardia or ventricular fibrillation is reduced, so that a single ventricular premature contraction may initiate the rhythm.

Temporal dispersion of refractoriness may be increased in nonischemic tissue in the presence of a slow heart rate. Accordingly, profound bradycardia due to decreased automaticity of the sinus node or AV block may also be particularly dangerous in patients with acute myocardial infarction since it may potentiate reentry.

Malignant ventricular dysrhythmia occurring later after the onset of ischemia appears to be dependent in part on enhanced automaticity of Purkinje fibers and possibly of myocardial cells as well. Reduction of diastolic transmembrane potential in response to regional biochemical alterations induced by ischemia may contribute to the enhanced automaticity by facilitating repetitive depolarizations of Purkinje fibers triggered by a single depolarization. Since catecholamines facilitate propagation of such slow-current responses, enhanced regional adrenergic stimulation may be an important contributing factor. The apparent efficacy of beta-adrenergic blockade in suppressing some ventricular dysrhythmias and the relative inefficacy of conventional antiarrhythmic agents such as lidocaine in patients with sympathetic hyperactivity may be reflections of the importance of regional adrenergic stimulation to enhanced automaticity.

Asystole and/or profound bradycardia are less common electrophysiologic mechanisms underlying sudden death due to coronary atherosclerosis. They may be manifestations of complete right coronary artery occlusion and usually presage failure of resuscitative efforts. They often result from failure of impulse formation in the sinus node, AV block, and failure of subsidiary pacemakers to function effectively.

PREVENTION OF SUDDEN DEATH The difficulties entailed in ambulatory electrocardiographic monitoring or other procedures for mass screening to detect candidates at risk for sudden death are formidable, since the population at risk comprises more than one-third of all men 35 to 74 years of age, and since ventricular ectopic activity occurs so commonly and is so variable from day to day in the same subject. At greatest risk are patients who have previously experienced primary ventricular fibrillation without associated acute myocardial infarction. Also, patients with ischemic heart disease who exhibit bouts of rapid ventricular tachycardia as well as those within 6 months after recovery from acute myocardial infarction with frequent, early, and/or multifocal ventricular premature contractions at rest, during physical activity, or during psychologic stress are particularly susceptible to sudden death. Patients with prolonged QT intervals and frequent premature contractions, particularly those who present with a history of syncope, represent another vulnerable group. Although identification of patients at high risk is particularly important, selection of an effective prophylactic regimen remains difficult, and none has clearly demonstrated effectiveness in reducing the risk. Induction of ventricular tachycardia or ventricular fibrillation by ventricular stimulation techniques with catheter electrodes and selection of a regimen based on abolition of subsequent induction of the dysrhythmia at a defined blood level suffers from the demanding and invasive nature of the procedure. In addition, inducibility is much less common among patients with prior primary ventricular fibrillation as opposed to those with recurrent ventricular tachycardia. Nevertheless, information acquired with this approach appears to be predictive of the prophylactic efficacy of specific pharmacologic regimens or pacemaker modalities for preventing or interrupting recurrent malignant dysrhythmia, particularly ventricular tachycardia.

In carefully selected survivors of sudden cardiac death with recurrent malignant dysrhythmia, surgical approaches may be indicated. Endocardial mapping with catheter electrodes has permitted localization of the origin of the spontaneous or inducible dysrhythmia, facilitating effective treatment by endocardial excision or encircling ventriculotomy rather than simple resection of a detectable aneurysm which may fail if the reentrant pathway or automatic focus involves its border, the intraventricular septum, or other regions of the heart.

Treatment with antiarrhythmic drugs in doses sufficient to maintain "therapeutic" drug levels has been claimed to be effective in reducing recurrent ventricular fibrillation in survivors of sudden death, if during acute drug testing, advanced grades of ventricular premature contraction (early or repetitive forms) can be eliminated or reduced, although the number of patients evaluated prospectively is small. It is reasonable to propose prophylactic treatment, on an individual basis, for patients with known or suspected coronary artery disease with recurrent or complex dysrhythmias or in survivors of sudden cardiac death. Conventional doses of procainamide (50 mg/kg per day by mouth in divided doses every 4 h), quinidine gluconate (15 mg/kg per day by mouth in divided doses every 6 h), or disopyramide (10 mg/kg per day by mouth in divided doses every 6 h) may be effective in suppressing these dysrhythmias. Dosage of quinidine may be increased up to 3 g per day if found necessary, unless gastrointestinal disturbances or electrocardiographic evidence of toxicity occurs. Some patients benefit from long-acting preparations of procainamide in somewhat reduced total daily dosage administered at 6-h intervals. Another agent, amiodarone (investigational only in the United States at this time) has striking antifibrillatory actions but a very slow rate of onset with peak effects seen only after several days or weeks of administration.

Ambulatory electrocardiographic monitoring with or without exercise stress may be particularly helpful in documenting the efficacy of treatment, since the incomplete knowledge regarding the pathogenesis of sudden death makes rational prophylactic drug selection and dosage difficult, and a stereotyped regimen for all patients impractical. However, marked reduction of ventricular ectopic activity (at least 80 percent) must be documented before attributing efficacy to a specific regimen. Some patients require concomitant administration of multiple drugs. Since the fundamental electrophysiologic derangements underlying ventricular fibrillation and premature beats may not be the same, even documented suppression of premature beats, while desirable, provides no reassurance of prevention of sudden death.

Decreased incidence of sudden death in a random selection of patients surviving acute myocardial infarction has been documented in several prospective double-blind studies utilizing beta-adrenergic blocking agents, although the effect of treatment on dysrhythmia was not quantified and the mechanism of apparent protection has not yet been identified. The reinfarction rate, overall mortality, and incidence of sudden cardiac death were all significantly decreased during a follow-up interval of 12 to 33 months among 1884 survivors of myocardial infarction by treatment with Timolol initiated within 7 to 28 days after the infarct.

Delays by the patient, physician, and transportation system and in the emergency room after the occurrence of acute myocardial infarction are significant impediments to prevention of sudden death. The median elapsed time between onset of symptoms and hospitalization averages 5 to 8 h in most areas of the United States. Denial by the patient of the seriousness of the condition and indecision by both the patient and physician contribute most to total delay.

Experience gained in Seattle, Washington, has shown that in order to deal effectively on a communitywide basis with the problem of sudden cardiovascular collapse and death, it is necessary to develop a system that provides rapid and effective response for these emergencies. Important elements of the system include a citywide emergency call number through which the system can be activated, a well-trained group of paramedical personnel such as fire fighters to respond, a short average time of response (under 4 min), and a large number of lay people trained in techniques of resuscitation. Clearly, the success in immediate resuscitation and for long-term survival is directly related to how soon following collapse resuscitation efforts are initiated. The availability of special ambulances (mobile coronary care units) equipped and staffed to handle acute cardiac emergencies appears to reduce delay by increasing community and physician awareness of the urgency of prompt medical attention. Such a system can be effective in resuscitating more than 40 percent of patients who have undergone cardiovascular collapse, and more than 25 percent of such patients are discharged from the hospital.

Therefore, providing instructions to susceptible persons on how to seek medical care on an emergency basis upon the development of symptoms of myocardial infarction is of great importance in the prevention of sudden cardiac death. This strategy includes instructing the patient that prompt entry into an effective emergency care system is not only urgent but also what the physician expects of the patient, regardless of whether symptoms suggestive of myocardial infarction occur during the day or night (Chap. 261); this concept also means instructing the patient to bypass the physician and to contact the emergency care system directly. Unsupervised physical stress, such as jogging, should be discouraged in patients with known ischemic heart disease and prohibited in those at high risk of sudden death, as defined above.

APPROACH TO THE PATIENT WITH SUDDEN CARDIOVASCULAR COLLAPSE Sudden death can often be averted even when cardiovascular collapse has occurred. When a patient under close medical observation develops sudden collapse from a dysrhythmia, the immediate goal must be restoration of effective cardiac rhythm. Circulatory collapse must be recognized and confirmed immediately. Its cardinal features are (1) loss of consciousness, syncope, and seizures; (2) absent peripheral arterial pulses; and (3) absent heart sounds. Since external cardiac massage provides only limited cardiac output, presently no more than 30 percent of the lower limit of normal, definitive restoration of effective rhythm should be the immediate goal, and in the absence of evidence to the contrary, abrupt circulatory collapse should be assumed to be due to ventricular fibrillation. If the physician sees the patient within 1 min of the collapse, time should not be wasted by attempting to achieve oxygenation. An immediate blow to the precordium ("thump version") may be attempted, since this is occasionally effective and takes only seconds. Rarely, when circulatory collapse is due to ventricular tachycardia and the patient is still conscious when first seen, a vigorous cough may terminate the dysrhythmia. In the absence of immediate restoration of the circulation, electrical defibrillation (Chap. 255) should be attempted immediately thereafter, without necessarily even pausing first to record an electrocardiogram on separate equipment, although use of portable defibrillators capable of electrocardiographic recording directly from the defibrillating electrodes may be helpful. Maximum electrical output of conventionally available equipment (400 W · s) is generally adequate, even for obese patients, and should be used. Efficacy is potentiated by application of the electrode paddles with firm pressure, application of the shock during the expiratory phase of the respiratory cycle when transthoracic impedance is lowest, and delivery of the electrical discharge promptly and before the energy requirements for defibrillation increase with the duration of ventricular fibrillation. If these immediate attempts are unsuccessful, external cardiac massage and complete cardiopulmonary resuscitation should be implemented.

If collapse is due to unequivocal asystole, transthoracic or transvenous electrical pacing should be implemented immediately. Intracardiac epinephrine, 1 ml of 1:1000 solution diluted 1:10 with intracavitary blood, may facilitate the heart's response to artificial pacing or be helpful when a slow ventricular focus is present but ineffective. If these initial definitive measures fail despite adequate technical performance, prompt restitution of a favorable metabolic milieu and monitoring are necessary. This is best accomplished by these three procedures: (1) External cardiac massage. (2) Correction of acid-base balance, often requiring intravenous sodium bicarbonate administration in an initial dose of 1 mg/kg repeated once within 5 to 10 min. Administration of subsequent doses of bicarbonate should be guided by frequent determinations of arterial pH, particularly since intracellular pH may paradoxically decrease, despite a rise in extracellular pH, because permeability to carbon dioxide is so much greater than to bicarbonate. (3) Assessment and correction of electrolyte imbalance. Definitive efforts to restore an effective cardiac rhythm should be attempted again as soon as possible, certainly within minutes. When effective cardiac rhythm is restored but rapidly degenerates again into ventricular tachycardia or fibrillation, lidocaine should be administered as a bolus, 1 mg/kg intravenously, then continued by intravenous infusion at a rate up to 1 to 5 (mg/kg)/h, and countershock repeated.

Cardiac massage External cardiac massage is designed to lead to the ejection of blood from the heart by manual compression of the ventricles between the sternum and the spine, and cyclic passive ventricular filling. Adherence to several aspects of technique is essential (Fig. 30-1). (1) The patient should be placed supine on a firm surface (a wooden board serves well). (2) Compression of the chest should be performed with the heel of one hand on the lower third of the sternum cephalad to the xiphoid process (to avoid lacerations of the liver) and the other hand applied on top of the first. (3) The frequency of external massage should approximate one per second to permit adequate time for ventricular filling. (4) The resuscitator's waist must be higher than the patient's chest in order to permit the resuscitator to administer the approximately 100-lb force required to depress the anterior chest wall of an adult male the necessary 5 cm per beat. (5) Depression and release of the chest wall should be smooth, with each occupying 50 percent of the cycle, since sudden compression may elicit a pressure wave palpable at the femoral or carotid artery but able to eject little blood. (6) Massage should not be interrupted, even momentarily, since cardiac output increases cumulatively during the first 8 to 10 compressions and even brief interruptions are detrimental. (7) Effective ventilation must be carried out. To accomplish this, the chin must be retracted and the neck fully extended. Mouth-to-mouth or mouth-to-nose technique must be continued throughout the resuscitative effort at a frequency of about 12 per minute and monitored by arterial blood gas analyses. If the latter are clearly abnormal, endotracheal intubation should be carried out expeditiously.

Each external cardiac compression limits venous return, and the optimal anticipated cardiac index during external massage approximates only 40 percent of the lower limit of normal, well below that seen in most patients after spontaneous ventricular contractions have returned. Therefore, prompt restoration of effective cardiac rhythm is essential.

Recently, the mechanisms involved in external cardiac massage have been clarified. The antegrade propulsion of blood has been found to result largely from compression of the aorta and left heart (which act as a conduit) by the augmented intrathoracic pressure achieved by compression of the lungs. Thus, the lungs serve as the compression pump. Maneuvers such as binding the abdomen to preclude downward excursion of the diaphragm or maintenance or positive airway pressure during compression, both of which augment intrathoracic pressure, increase the cardiac output achieved by compression. The equal pressures during compression in the pulmonary veins, left atrium, left ventricle, and intrathoracic aorta—all of which reflect the augmented intrathoracic pressure—exceed systemic arterial pressure thereby providing a gradient for antegrade flow. Systemic venous pressure is increased because of closure of venous valves at the thoracic inlet as well as venous collapse due to the increased intrathoracic pressure, both of which preclude retrograde transmission of the augmented intrathoracic pressure into the jugular venous system.

FIGURE 30-1
Cardiopulmonary resuscitation (CPR) and external chest compression. A diagrammatic representation of the steps required for resuscitation by a single rescuer. [Modified from Standards and guidelines for cardiopulmonary resuscitation (CPR) and emergency cardiac care (ECC). JAMA 244:453, 1980.]

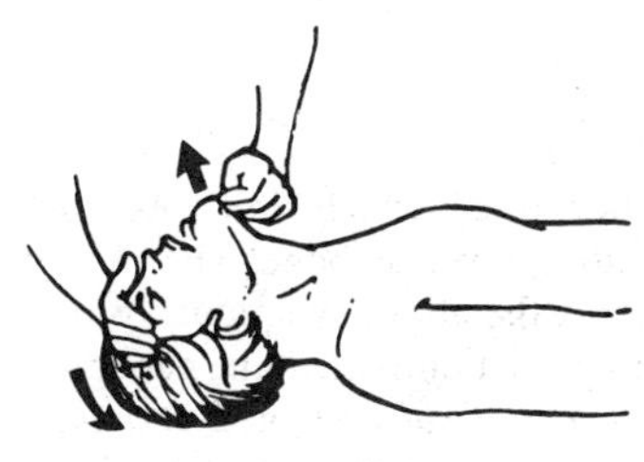

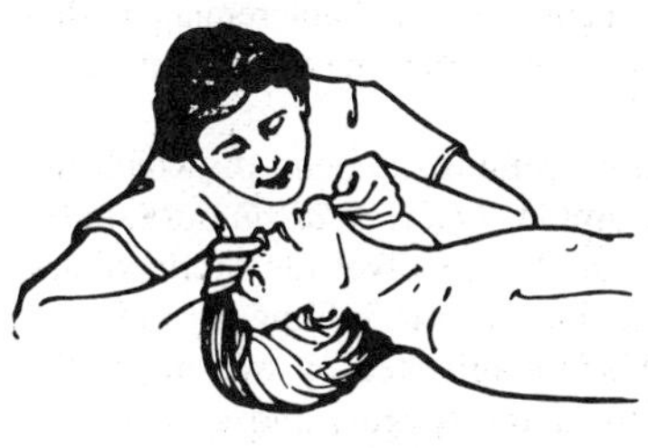

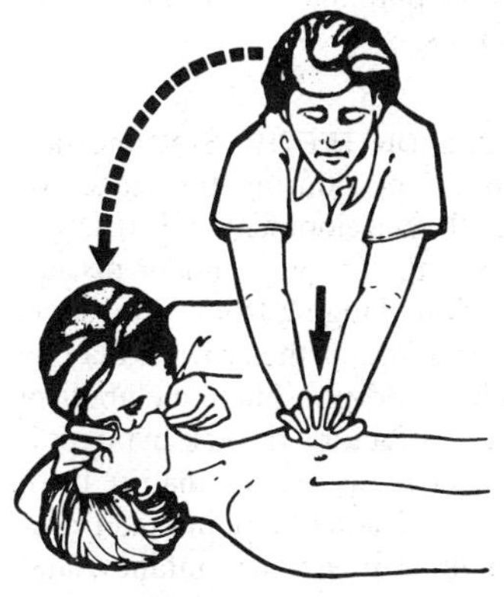

During the relaxation phase of cardiopulmonary resuscitation, when the chest is allowed to expand the right heart acts as a conduit and the decreased intrathoracic pressure potentiates flow of blood from the systemic veins into the pulmonary arterial circulation. During this phase negative airway pressure potentiates venous return and augments cardiac output elicited by subsequent compression.

It is likely that some modifications of the classical technique will become established in the near future aimed at (1) augmenting intrathoracic pressure during compression (positive airway pressure, abdominal binding, initiating compression at end-inspiration), (2) reducing intrathoracic pressure during relaxation (negative airway pressure during this phase), and (3) reducing intrathoracic aortic and systemic arterial collapse during compression (augmentation of vascular volume). One application of these concepts that has already been employed is "cough CPR," a technique with which a still-conscious patient can maintain cardiac output despite ventricular fibrillation, at least for brief intervals, by repetitive, rhythmic coughing which phasically augments intrathoracic pressure simulating the changes induced by conventional chest compression.

Rarely, organized electrocardiographic activity unaccompanied by effective cardiac contraction (electromechanical dissociation) may occur and respond to intracardiac epinephrine (1 ml of 1:1000 solution diluted 1:10 with blood) or calcium gluconate (1 g). Refractory or repetitively recurrent ventricular fibrillation may respond to intravenous administration of bretylium tosylate, 5 to 12 mg/kg over several minutes, although the antifibrillatory effect may not develop for 20 min or more. Cardiac massage should be terminated as soon as effective cardiac contractions serve to produce a detectable pulse and systemic arterial blood pressure.

The therapeutic approach outlined above is based on several considerations: (1) irreversible brain damage often occurs after a few (approximately 4) minutes of circulatory collapse; (2) the likelihood of restoring effective cardiac rhythm and successfully resuscitating the patient diminishes rapidly with time; (3) 80 to 90 percent survival can be anticipated in patients developing primary ventricular fibrillation, as when undergoing cardiac catheterization or exercise testing, in whom definitive treatment is prompt; (4) survival rates in the general hospital setting are much lower, approximately 20 percent, depending in part on the coexisting or underlying disease process; (5) survival rates in the community approach zero, unless special emergency care systems have been perfected, probably because of unavoidable delays in initiating definitive therapy and limitations of equipment and available personnel; and (6) external cardiac massage can provide only a limited cardiac output. When ventricular fibrillation occurs, the earliest application of electrical countershock is the one most likely to succeed. Thus, when circulatory collapse is a primary event, therapy must be directed toward prompt restoration of effective cardiac rhythm.

Complications External cardiac massage is not free from significant complications, including rib fracture, hemopericardium and tamponade, hemothorax, pneumothorax, liver laceration, fat embolus, and ruptured spleen with late, occult blood loss. However, these complications can be minimized by proper technique and, if appropriately considered, can be readily recognized and often managed effectively. The decision to terminate unsuccessful cardiopulmonary resuscitation is always difficult. In general, if effective cardiac rhythm has not been restored and if the patient's pupils are fixed and dilated despite 30 min or more of cardiac massage, a successful resuscitation cannot be expected.

REFERENCES

BAROLDI G et al: Sudden coronary death: A postmortem study in 208 selected cases compared to 97 "control" subjects. Am Heart J 98:20, 1979

COBB LA et al: Sudden cardiac death 1. A decade's experience with out-of-hospital resuscitation. Mod Concepts Cardiovasc Dis 49:31, 1980

EL-MARAGHI N et al: The relevance of platelet and fibrin thromboembolism of the coronary microcirculation, with special reference to sudden cardiac death. Circulation 62:936, 1980

GELTMAN EM et al: The influence of location and extent of myocardial infarction on long-term ventricular dysrhythmia and mortality. Circulation 60:805, 1979

ISERI LT et al: Prehospital brady-asystolic cardiac arrest. Ann Intern Med 88:741, 1978

ISNER JM et al: Sudden, unexpected death in avid dieters using the liquid-protein-modified-fast diet. Circulation 60:1401, 1979

LEWIS RP et al: Reduction of mortality from prehospital myocardial infarction by prudent patient activation of mobile coronary care system. Am Heart J 103:123, 1982

LOWN B: Cardiovascular collapse and sudden cardiac death, in *Heart Disease: A Textbook of Cardiovascular Disease,* E Braunwald (ed). Philadelphia, Saunders, 1980, chap 22, pp 778–817

———, PODRID PT: Ventricular beats: Why, when, and how to treat, in *Update II: Harrison's Principles of Internal Medicine,* KJ Isselbacher et al (eds). New York, McGraw-Hill, 1982

MCINTYRE KM, LEWIS AJ: *Textbook of Advanced Cardiac Life Support.* Dallas, 1981

THE NORWEGIAN MULTICENTER STUDY GROUP: Timolol-induced reduction in mortality and reinfarction in patients surviving acute myocardial infarction. N Engl J Med 304:801, 1981

RUDIKOFF MT et al: Mechanisms of blood flow during cardiopulmonary resuscitation. Circulation 61:345, 1980

section 5 | Alterations in gastrointestinal function

31 ORAL MANIFESTATIONS OF DISEASE

PAUL GOLDHABER

DISTURBANCES OF THE TEETH AND DENTAL TISSUES

DENTAL CARIES, PULPAL AND PERIAPICAL INFECTION, AND SEQUELAE Dental caries, the principal cause of tooth loss up to the fourth decade of life, is characterized by a bacteria-induced progressive destruction of the mineral and organic components of the outer enamel and underlying dentin. Numerous long-term studies have clearly shown that the artificial fluoridation of drinking water supplies to a level of 1 part per million leads to a 50 to 75 percent reduction in the occurrence of dental caries in permanent teeth of children, presumably because of an alteration of the developing enamel crystals during tooth formation which makes them more resistant to acid dissolution.

If the carious lesion progresses unchecked, there is eventual infection of the dental pulp, giving rise to an *acute pulpitis.* During the early stages of pulpitis moderately severe pain may result from thermal changes, particularly with cold drinks. As more of the pulp becomes involved because of advanced caries, heat or reclining may stimulate the onset of even more severe and continuous pain. At this stage, damage to the pulp is irreversible, and treatment consists of either extraction or thorough removal of the remaining contents of the pulp chamber and root canals followed by sterilization and filling with an inert material (root canal therapy).

If the pulpitis is not treated, infection may spread beyond the apex of the tooth into the periodontal ligament, giving rise to pain on chewing or percussion. The most common manifestation of periapical disease is the *periapical granuloma,* a localized mass of chronic granulation tissue which slowly expands at the expense of the surrounding alveolar bone. The *chronic periapical granuloma* may present the above symptoms or may be asymptomatic. If allowed to persist untreated, the periapical granuloma may give rise to a *periapical cyst* or a *periapical abscess*—all three lesions appearing as radiolucent areas on roentgenograms. The acute periapical abscess may extend into the surrounding bone marrow, resulting in an *osteomyelitis.* More frequently, the abscess perforates the cortical plate and, following the path of least resistance, spreads through various tissue spaces, giving rise to cellulitis and bacteremia, or discharges into the oral cavity, into the maxillary sinus, or through the skin.

The symptoms produced by cellulitis depend on which tissue space is affected. For example, *Ludwig's angina* originates from an infected mandibular molar, involves the submaxillary space, and subsequently extends into the sublingual and submental spaces. Clinically, this is manifested by swelling of the floor of the mouth, elevation of the tongue, and difficulty in swallowing and breathing. With continued swelling, there may be edema of the glottis, necessitating an emergency tracheotomy. Spread of the infection to the parapharyngeal spaces may lead to cavernous sinus thrombosis.

EFFECT OF SYSTEMIC FACTORS ON TEETH Systemic factors, occurring in utero or in infancy during the stages of crown formation, may influence the development and structure of the teeth. *Enamel hypoplasia* of the primary and/or permanent teeth, manifested by alterations ranging from white spots to gross defects in the surface structure of the crowns, may be caused by disturbances of calcium and phosphate metabolism such as are found in vitamin D–refractory rickets, hypoparathyroidism, gastroenteritis, and celiac disease. Premature birth or high fevers may also give rise to enamel hypoplasia. Tetracycline, given during the last half of pregnancy, infancy, and childhood up to 8 years of age, causes both a permanent discoloration of the teeth as well as enamel hypoplasia. Daily ingestion of more than 1.5 mg fluoride can result in enamel discoloration (mottling). Prenatal factors appear to influence crown size. Larger teeth are associated with maternal diabetes, maternal hypothyroidism, and large birth size. Tooth size is reduced in *Down's syndrome.* Premature loss of the deciduous dentition is frequently the first symptom in *juvenile hypophosphatasia.* Systemic disease may give rise to pain that simulates pulpal disease. *Maxillary sinusitis* is frequently manifested by pain in the maxillary teeth, including sensitivity to thermal changes and percussion. *Cardiac disease* with *angina pectoris* may result in referred pain to the lower jaw.

PERIODONTAL DISEASE

After the third decade chronic destructive periodontal disease *(periodontitis)* is responsible for the loss of more teeth than dental caries. It begins as a marginal inflammation of the gingivae (gingivitis), which slowly spreads to involve the underlying alveolar bone and periodontal ligament. As the disease progresses, the alveolar bone is resorbed, resulting in loss of periodontal ligament fiber attachment from the tooth to the bone. The separation of the soft tissue from the tooth surface results in "pocket" formation, the inner aspect of which bleeds readily on probing or spontaneously during chewing. Frank pus sometimes exudes from under the gingival margin, accounting for the use of the now outmoded term "pyorrhea." With continued loss of alveolar bone the involved teeth become mobile. As the periodontal pockets deepen, the pocket orifice may become occluded, leading to the formation of a *periodontal abscess.* The prognosis for teeth with advanced bone loss, extreme mobility, and recurrent abscess formation is usually poor or hopeless, and the usual treatment is extraction.

The most important local etiologic factors associated with this disease are thought to be *poor oral hygiene,* resulting in the accumulation of grossly visible adherent masses of bacteria *(bacterial plaque),* calculus (mineralized bacterial plaque), and food impaction. The margins of overextended fillings also play a role as local irritating factors. Occlusal trauma, particularly trauma due to grinding and clenching habits, may be involved. Therapy is aimed at elimination of these factors and the development of a local environment which can be maintained in health by good oral hygiene. It appears that specific groups of organisms found subgingivally correlate with the different types and severity of periodontal disease. In advanced periodontitis, the flora is dominated by motile rods and spirochetes.

Systemic factors are thought to modify the response of the host to the local factors, but their nature is more obscure. Reduced neutrophil functions, such as chemotaxis and phagocytosis, appear to predispose to *juvenile periodontitis,* a form of periodontitis characterized by early and severe alveolar bone loss and a familial pattern of occurrence. Of possible etiologic importance is the finding that a sonic extract of *Actinobacillus actinomycetemcomitans,* a microorganism consistently isolated from patients with juvenile periodontitis, contains a leukotoxin which specifically kills human polymorphonuclear leukocytes and monocytes. *Capnocytophaga,* another organism implicated in periodontal disease, has also been reported to be associated with morphologic and functional abnormalities of neutrophils. On the other hand, patients with IgA deficiency and agammaglobulinemia have less periodontal disease and dental caries than matched immunocompetent controls. Individuals with *Down's syndrome* seem to be particularly susceptible to periodontal disease and may demonstrate advanced alveolar bone loss around the permanent mandibular incisors and maxillary first molars. Severe chronic periodontal disease may be present in uncontrolled *diabetes mellitus.* In some instances, however,

there are characteristic alterations in the gingiva in response to a number of specific systemic conditions. For example, during *pregnancy* the gingiva may become edematous and friable, with a raspberry-like appearance of the interdental papillae. Occasionally, a tumorlike mass may develop in an interdental area; this usually regresses following parturition. Oral contraceptives may lead to an increase in gingival inflammation. The use of the anticonvulsant drug *phenytoin* (Dilantin) frequently results in fibrous hyperplasia of the gingiva, which may actually cover the teeth, interfere with mastication, and cause a serious aesthetic problem. A similar clinical picture, although usually more generalized and extensive, occurs in *idiopathic familial fibromatosis.* The latter condition appears to be hereditary.

A relatively common gingival disease, found predominantly in young adults, is *acute necrotizing ulcerative gingivitis* (Vincent's infection, trench mouth). This disease is characterized by tender or painful gingivae, bleeding on pressure, and the pathognomonic sign of papillary or marginal gingival necrosis and ulceration. Clinical evidence suggests that the cause of this disease has a psychosomatic component. Vincent's infection differs from *acute herpetic gingivostomatitis,* with which it is most frequently confused, in that fever or malaise rarely develops, and patients respond rapidly to penicillin or broad-spectrum antibiotics.

It should be noted that both infected periapical lesions and periodontal disease provide potential sources of infection which may spread to other sites. Transient bacteremias have been demonstrated after simple massage of inflamed gingivae or use of an oral irrigative device, as well as during tooth extraction. The frequent association of tooth extraction with the subsequent occurrence of subacute bacterial endocarditis has led to the prophylactic use of antibiotics in dental patients with a history of rheumatic fever or other evidence of valvular disease. Similar precautions should be taken with dental patients having heart valve or joint prostheses. Prophylactic extraction of healthy teeth in leukemic patients is not justified.

DISEASES OF THE ORAL MUCOSA AND TONGUE

HEMATOLOGIC DISTURBANCES Oral manifestations are common in both the acute and chronic forms of all types of leukemia, particularly *monocytic leukemia.* They consist of local gingival bleeding, enlargement, and necrosis. Petechiae and ulceration of the oral mucosa may also be evident. Extensive ulcerations of the gingivae, buccal mucosa, lips, soft palate, pharynx, and tonsils may also occur in *agranulocytosis.* In thrombocytopenic states multiple petechiae, ecchymoses, and bleeding gingivae may be observed. The mucous membranes of the oral cavity, including the papillae of the tongue, are atrophic in the *Plummer-Vinson syndrome* (see Chaps. 32 and 305). As a result, the tongue is red, smooth, and sore, and there is difficulty in swallowing. Of interest is the finding that the atrophic mucous membranes have a predisposition toward the development of oral carcinoma. The oral symptoms in *pernicious anemia* are similar (see Chap. 327). Ulceration, mucositis, xerostomia, and infection (bacterial or fungal) are relatively common oral complications among patients receiving chemotherapy and/or radiotherapy for malignancies not involving the head or neck.

VITAMIN DEFICIENCIES *The oral effects of deficiency of the B group of vitamins* involve the soft tissues primarily, giving rise to reddening and ulceration of the oral mucosa and tongue, swelling and burning of the tongue, and fissuring at the corners of the lips (*angular cheilosis*). Severe vitamin C deficiency (*scurvy*) is manifested by petechiae in the oral mucosa; swollen, ulcerated, bleeding gingivae; and loosening of teeth.

PIGMENTATIONS (See Table 31-1) The spread of irregular spots or blotches or brown pigment throughout the oral mucosa, primarily the buccal mucosa, may be the first sign of *Addison's disease.* The pigmentation associated with the *Peutz-Jeghers syndrome* is readily differentiated because of its characteristic distribution around the lips, eyes, and nostrils, as well as its intraoral distribution. Both *lead poisoning* and *bismuth poisoning* may be manifested by a dark line along the gingival margin, particularly in individuals who have poor oral hygiene. Bismuth poisoning may also demonstrate pigmented patches elsewhere in the oral mucosa.

INFECTIONS See Tables 31-2 and 31-3.

DERMATOLOGIC DISEASES See Tables 31-2 and 31-3 and Chaps. 49 to 53.

TONGUE ALTERATIONS See Table 31-4.

MALODOROUS BREATH A distinctly unpleasant odor of the breath (halitosis) may emanate from any patient with *infections of the upper part of the respiratory tract,* especially in bronchiectasis and lung abscess. Halitosis may occur with oral sepsis as in *stomatitis, gingivitis,* or extensive *caries.* Some persons who smoke excessively may have halitosis. Occasionally otherwise normal persons will have halitosis without obvious cause. The primary oral sources of bad breath are inflamed periodontal pockets and the coating on the dorsoposterior surface of the tongue. A *fishy odor* of the breath is found in patients with hepatic failure, an *ammoniacal* or *urinary odor* is found in azotemia, and a *sweet, fruity odor* is typical of diabetic acidosis.

DISEASES OF THE SALIVARY GLANDS

Conditions affecting the salivary glands include mumps parotitis (Chap. 206), Mikulicz's disease, Sjögren's syndrome (Chap. 346), and sarcoidosis. Inflammation of the salivary glands (*sialadenitis*) is usually associated with the presence of a salivary stone (*sialolithiasis*) in the duct of one of the major salivary glands. The classic history of pain and swelling of the gland at mealtimes is due to the partial blockage of salivary flow by the stone. Localization of the stone may be accomplished by palpation or by roentgenograms with or without the use of an intraductal injection of radiopaque material (*sialography*). Acute or recurrent parotitis, with or without a defined microorganism, may occur in children and is marked by sudden onset of swelling of the whole gland or side of the face, accompanied by suppuration from Stensen's duct.

Xerostomia, or dryness of the mouth, is due to salivary gland dysfunction and may be temporary or permanent. Among the factors which cause temporary dryness are emotional factors (such as fear), infection of the glands, and administration of drugs such as atropine, antihistamines, or tricyclic antidepressants and phenothiazines. Radiation of the area may produce a more permanent xerostomia because of atrophy of the glands. A similar dryness may occur in Sjögren's syndrome. The dry mouth may give rise to rampant caries, particularly if sugar-containing candies are sucked in an attempt to stimulate salivary flow. Other symptoms may include disturbances in taste, difficulty in speech or swallowing, and inflammation of the oral mucosa. Extensive dental caries, especially around the gum margins of the teeth, may be seen in drug addicts and alcoholics, presumably due to xerostomia and lack of oral hygiene and dental care. Xerostomia-induced caries may be prevented or arrested by the daily topical application of a 1% sodium fluoride gel. The soft tissue complications may be relieved by the utilization of an artificial saliva.

Benign or malignant tumors may arise in the major or minor salivary glands. The benign *mixed tumor* accounts for the vast majority of all salivary gland tumors and has a relatively high recurrence rate. Malignant tumors of the parotid gland may affect the facial nerve.

ORAL CANCER

Oral cancer constitutes more than 5 percent of all human cancers. *Squamous cell carcinoma* is the most common malignant oral tumor, accounting for approximately 90 to 95 percent of

TABLE 31-1
Pigmented lesions of the oral mucosa

Condition	*Usual location*	*Clinical features*	*Course*
Black, hairy tongue	Dorsum of tongue	Elongation of filiform papillae of tongue, which take on a brown to black coloration	Long-lasting but may disappear spontaneously
Heavy metal pigmentation (bismuth, mercury, lead)	Gingival margin	Thin blue-black pigmented line along gingival margin due to prior treatment for syphilis with bismuth or mercury or from accidental absorption of lead	Long-lasting
Drug ingestion (tranquilizers, oral contraceptives, antimalarials)	Any area in mouth	Brown, black, or gray areas of pigmentation	Disappears following cessation of drug
Amalgam tattoo	Gingiva and mucobuccal fold	Small blue-black pigmented areas associated with embedded amalgam particles in soft tissues; these will show up on radiographs as radiopaque particles	Remains indefinitely
Fordyce's disease	Buccal and labial mucosa	Aggregation of numerous, small yellowish spots just beneath mucosal surface; no subjective symptoms	Remains without apparent change indefinitely
Addison's disease	Any area in mouth but mostly on buccal mucosa	Blotches or spots of bluish-black to dark-brown pigmentation occurring early in the disease, accompanied by diffuse pigmentation of skin; other symptoms of adrenal insufficiency	Condition controlled by steroid therapy
Peutz-Jeghers syndrome	Any area in mouth	Dark brown spots on lips, buccal mucosa, and palate with characteristic distribution of pigment around lips, nose, eyes, and on hands; concomitant intestinal polyposis	Lesions remaining indefinitely
Malignant melanoma	Any area in mouth	May appear as a raised, painless, brown-black lesion or may be amelanotic; may be ulcerated and infected	Early metastasis leading to death

TABLE 31-2
Vesicular, bullous, or ulcerative lesions of the oral mucosa

Condition	*Usual location*	*Clinical features*	*Course*
VIRAL DISEASES			
Acute herpetic gingivostomatitis (herpes simplex, type 1)	Lip and oral mucosa	Labial vesicles which rupture and crust, and intraoral vesicles which quickly ulcerate; extremely painful to pressure; acute gingivitis, fever, malaise, foul odor, and cervical lymphadenopathy; occurs primarily in infants and children	Heals spontaneously in 10–14 days unless secondarily infected
Recurrent herpes labialis	Mucocutaneous junction of lip	Eruption of groups of vesicles which may coalesce, then rupture and crust; painful to pressure or spicy foods	Lasts about 1 week, but condition may be prolonged if secondary infection occurs
Primary herpes, type 2	Mouth, oral pharynx, and genitalia	Large, painful, discrete vesicles on zone of erythema; anterior cervical glands enlarged	Lasts several weeks; may recur
Herpangina (coxsackievirus A; also possibly coxsackievirus B and echovirus)	Oral mucosa, pharynx, tongue	Sudden onset of fever, sore throat, and oropharyngeal vesicles usually in children under 4 years, during summer months; diffuse pharyngeal injection and vesicles (1–2 mm), grayish white surrounded by red areola; vesicles enlarge and ulcerate	Incubation period 2–9 days; fever for 1–4 days; recovery uneventful
Hand, foot, and mouth disease (type A coxsackieviruses)	Oral mucosa, pharynx, palms, and soles	Fever, malaise, headache with oropharyngeal vesicles which become painful, shallow ulcers	Incubation period 2–18 days; lesions heal spontaneously in 2–4 weeks
Chickenpox	Gingiva and oral mucosa	Skin lesions may be accompanied by small vesicles on oral mucosa that rupture to form shallow ulcers; may coalesce to form large bullous lesions that ulcerate; mucosa may have generalized erythema	Lesions heal spontaneously within 2 weeks
Herpes zoster	Cheek, tongue, gingiva, or palate	Unilateral vesicular eruption and ulceration in linear pattern following sensory distribution of trigeminal nerve	Gradual healing without scarring
Infectious mononucleosis	Oral mucosa	Fatigue, sore throat, malaise, low-grade fever, and enlarged cervical lymph nodes; numerous small ulcers usually appear several days before lymphadenopathy; gingival bleeding and multiple petechiae at junction of hard and soft palates	Oral lesions disappear during convalescence
Warts	Any place on skin and oral mucosa, primarily lips and vestibule	Single or multiple papillary lesions, with thick, white, keratinized surfaces containing many pointed projections	Lesions grow rapidly and spread
BACTERIAL OR FUNGAL DISEASES			
Acute necrotizing ulcerative gingivitis ("trench mouth," Vincent's infection)	Gingiva	Painful, bleeding gingiva characterized by necrosis and ulceration of gingival papillae and margins plus lymphadenopathy and foul odor	Continued destruction of tissue followed by remission, but may recur
Prenatal (congenital) syphilis	Palate, jaws, tongue, and teeth	Gummatous involvement of palate, jaws, and facial bones; Hutchinson's incisors, mulberry molars, glossitis, mucous patches, and fissures of corners of mouth	Tooth deformities in permanent dentition irreversible
Primary syphilis (chancre)	Lesion appears where organism enters body; may occur on lips, tongue, or tonsillar area	Small papule developing rapidly into a large, painless ulcer with indurated border; unilateral lymphadenopathy; chancre and lymph nodes containing spirochetes; serologic tests positive by third to fourth weeks	Healing of chancre in 1–2 months, followed by secondary syphilis in 6–8 weeks
Secondary syphilis	Oral mucosa frequently involved with mucous patches, primarily on palate but also at commissures of mouth	Maculopapular lesions of oral mucosa, about 5–10 mm in diameter with central ulceration covered by grayish membrane; eruptions occurring on various mucosal surfaces and skin accompanied by fever, malaise, and sore throat	Lesions may persist from several weeks to a year
Tertiary syphilis	Palate and tongue	Gummatous infiltration of palate or tongue followed by ulceration and fibrosis; atrophy of tongue papillae may produce characteristic bald tongue and glossitis	Gumma may destroy palate, causing complete perforation
Gonorrhea	Lesions may occur in mouth at site of inoculation or secondarily by hematogenous spread from a primary focus elsewhere	Earliest symptoms are burning or itching sensation, dryness, or heat in mouth followed by acute pain on eating or speaking; tonsils and oropharynx most frequently involved; oral tissues may be diffusely inflamed or ulcerated; saliva develops increased viscosity and fetid odor; submaxillary lymphadenopathy with fever in severe cases	Lesions resolve with appropriate antibiotic therapy
Tuberculosis	Tongue, tonsillar area, soft palate	A solitary, irregular ulcer covered by a persistent exudate; ulcer has an undermined, indurated border	Lesion may persist
Cervicofacial actinomycosis	Swellings in region of face, neck, and floor of mouth	Infection may be associated with an extraction, jaw fracture, or eruption of molar tooth; in acute form resembles an acute pyogenic abscess, but contains yellow "sulfur granules" (gram-positive mycelia and their hyphae)	Acute form may last a few weeks; chronic form lasts months or years; prognosis excellent; actinomycetes respond to antibiotics (tetracyclines or penicillin) but not to antifungal drugs
Histoplasmosis	Any area in mouth, particularly tongue, gingiva, or palate	Numerous small nodules which may ulcerate; hoarseness and dysphagia may occur because of lesions in larynx, usually associated with fever and malaise	May be fatal

TABLE 31-2 (*Continued*)

Vesicular, bullous, or ulcerative lesions of the oral mucosa

Condition	*Usual location*	*Clinical features*	*Course*
DERMATOLOGIC DISEASES			
Mucous membrane pemphigoid	Primarily mucous membranes of the oral cavity, but may also involve the eyes, urethra, vagina, and rectum	Painful, grayish white collapsed vesicles or bullae with peripheral erythematous zone; gingival lesions desquamate, leaving ulcerated area	Protracted course with remissions and exacerbations; involvement of different sites occurs slowly; corticosteroids may control severe cases
Erythema multiforme (Stevens-Johnson syndrome)	Primarily the oral mucosa and skin of hands and feet	Intraoral ruptured bullae surrounded by an inflammatory area; lips may show hemorrhagic crusts; the "iris," or "target" lesion, on the skin is pathognomonic; patient may have severe signs of toxicity	Onset very rapid; condition may last 1–2 weeks; may be fatal
Pemphigus vulgaris	Oral mucosa and skin	Ruptured bullae and ulcerated oral areas; mostly in older adults	With repeated recurrence of bullae, toxicity may lead to cachexia, infection, and death within 2 years
NEOPLASTIC DISEASES			
Squamous cell carcinoma	Any area in mouth, most commonly on lower lip, tongue, and floor of mouth	Ulcer with elevated, indurated border; failure to heal, pain not prominent; lesions tend to arise in areas of leukoplakia or in smooth or atrophic tongue	Invades and destroys underlying tissues or may metastasize to regional lymph nodes
Acute leukemia	Gingiva	Gingival swelling and superficial ulcerations followed by hyperplasia of gingiva with extensive necrosis and hemorrhage; deep ulcers may occur elsewhere on the mucosa complicated by secondary infection	Fatal
Lymphosarcoma	Gingiva, palate, tongue, and tonsillar area	Elevated, ulcerated area which may proliferate rapidly, giving the appearance of a traumatic inflammatory lesion; swelling of regional lymph nodes	Fatal
OTHER CONDITIONS			
Recurrent aphthous stomatitis	Any place on oral mucosa	Single or clusters of painful ulcers with surrounding erythematous border, found anywhere on mucosa; lesions may be 1–15 mm in diameter	Lesions heal in 1–2 weeks but may recur monthly or several times a year. Topical corticosteroid ointments give symptomatic relief in mild cases. Systemic corticosteroids are used in severe cases. A tetracycline oral suspension may decrease ulcer severity.
Behçet's syndrome	Oral mucosa, eyes, and genitalia	Multiple aphthouslike ulcers in mouth; inflammatory ocular changes and ulcerative lesions on genitalia	Ulcers may persist for several weeks and heal without scarring
Traumatic ulcers	Any place on oral mucosa; dentures frequently responsible for ulcers in vestibule	Localized, discrete ulcerated lesion with red border; produced by accidental biting of mucosa, penetration by a foreign object, or chronic irritation by a denture	Lesion usually heals in 7–10 days when irritant is removed, unless secondarily infected

TABLE 31-3

White lesions of oral mucosa

Condition	*Usual location*	*Clinical features*	*Course*
Pachyderma oralis	Any area in mouth	Elevated white lesion due to hyperkeratosis and thickening of the oral epithelium secondary to chronic irritation	Removal of irritant leads to healing in 2–3 weeks
Leukoplakia	Any area in mouth	White patch or raised plaque with sharply defined borders; in more severe cases the lesion is indurated and rough, and may be fissured and eroded; pain not present in early lesions	Carcinoma frequently arises in the more severe type of lesion
Lichen planus	Any area in mouth but most often on buccal mucosa	Varied appearance of lesion due to arrangement of grayish-white papules which coalesce to make up the pattern; a reticular network is most common; oral lesions may precede skin lesions	May disappear spontaneously
Moniliasis (thrush)	Any area in mouth	Creamy white curdlike patches which reveal a raw, bleeding surface when scraped; found in sick infants, debilitated elderly patients, or patients receiving high doses of corticosteroids or broad-spectrum antibiotics	Responds favorably to antifungal therapy after correction of predisposing causes
Chemical burns	Any area in mouth	White slough due to necrosis of epithelium and underlying connective tissue caused by contact with agents (e.g., aspirin) applied locally or the use of undiluted sodium perborate or hydrogen peroxide as a mouthwash; removal of slough leaves a raw, painful surface	Lesion heals in several weeks if not secondarily infected

TABLE 31-4
Alterations of the tongue

Type of change	*Clinical features*
SIZE OR MORPHOLOGY CHANGES	
Macroglossia	Enlarged tongue which may be part of a syndrome found in developmental conditions such as Down's syndrome; may be due to tumor (hemangioma or lymphangioma), metabolic disease (such as primary amyloidosis), or endocrine disturbance (such as acromegaly or cretinism)
Fissured ("scrotal") tongue	Dorsal surface and sides of tongue covered by painless shallow or deep fissures which may collect debris and become irritated
Median rhomboid glossitis	Congenital abnormality of tongue with ovoid, denuded area in the median posterior portion of the tongue
COLOR CHANGES	
"Geographic" tongue ("wandering rash")	Asymptomatic inflammatory condition of the tongue, with rapid loss and regrowth of filiform papillae, leading to appearance of denuded red patches "wandering" across the surface of the tongue
Hairy tongue	Elongation of filiform papillae of the medial dorsal surface area due to failure of keratin layer of the papillae to desquamate normally; brownish-black coloration may be due to staining by tobacco, food, or chromogenic organisms
"Strawberry" and "raspberry" tongue	Appearance of tongue during scarlet fever due to the hypertrophy of fungiform papillae plus changes in the filiform papillae
"Bald" tongue	Complete atrophy of papillae which may occur in pernicious anemia, severe iron-deficiency anemia, pellagra, or syphilis; may be accompanied by painful, burning sensations

all oral malignant tumors. Most of these tumors occur on the lips, primarily the lower lip, rather than intraorally. About half the intraoral tumors involve the tongue, primarily the posterior two-thirds and the lateral borders. The major etiologic factor in lip cancer appears to be exposure to intense sunlight. Predisposing factors for intraoral carcinoma include tobacco (usually in the form of cigar or pipe smoking, or snuff placed in the mucobuccal fold), excessive consumption of alcohol, syphilitic glossitis, and the atrophic mucosa of the Plummer-Vinson syndrome. Although numerous instances of carcinoma of the tongue adjacent to a sharp tooth or dental appliance have been reported, animal studies with chronic irritation per se, as well as epidemiologic studies, cast doubt on this apparent relationship. The most common *precancerous lesion* in the oral cavity is *leukoplakia,* a whitish patch on the mucosa that histologically shows hyperkeratosis, acanthosis, and dyskeratosis. Nodular leukoplakias have a much higher potential for malignant transformation than homogeneous leukoplakias. Recent evidence suggests that the asymptomatic, red velvety (erythroplastic) lesion of the floor of the mouth, ventrolateral aspect of the tongue, or soft palate–anterior pillar complex is more likely to be carcinoma in situ or invasive carcinoma than is the white lesion. *All chronic ulcerative lesions which fail to heal within 1 to 2 weeks should be considered potentially malignant* and must be biopsied in order to make the definitive diagnosis. It is noteworthy that in their early stages intraoral epidermoid carcinomas are rarely painful, in contrast to similar-appearing inflammatory lesions.

The prognosis for patients with carcinoma of the lip is usually good, since these malignant tumors are noted sooner and apparently metastasize later. Patients with carcinoma of the tongue have a poorer prognosis, particularly as the tumor occurs more posteriorly on the tongue. Intraoral carcinomas may spread by direct invasion to the underlying bone. Depending on the site of origin of the intraoral carcinoma, metastases usually spread to the submaxillary or cervical lymph nodes. Death may result from recurrent or uncontrollable disease above the clavicles; metastatic disease beyond the neck; treatment complications; or a second primary cancer, usually in the oral cavity or the upper parts of the gastrointestinal or respiratory tract.

NEUROLOGIC DISTURBANCES

A number of neurologic disturbances have a direct effect on oral and paraoral structures. *Trigeminal neuralgia* (tic douloureux) is an example of a syndrome involving the trigeminal nerve. It is characterized by extremely severe, unilateral, lancinating pain of the face occurring spontaneously or set off by pressure on a "trigger zone" on the face (see Chap. 367). In some cases of idiopathic trigeminal neuralgia, dental and oral pathoses, primarily in the form of jawbone cavities at sites of previous extractions, may be major etiologic factors. Facial palsy is a unilateral disturbance of the motor branch of the facial nerve due to either trauma, surgical sectioning, or tumor involvement. When it is of acute onset and unknown cause, possibly a localized infection in the nerve, it is called *Bell's palsy.* It may be due to cranial herpes zoster in some instances. The condition is manifested by drooping of the corner of the mouth, inability to close the eye on the same side, and difficulty in speech and eating. In mild cases the symptoms may disappear spontaneously within a month. Alteration in taste sensation in the anterior two-thirds of the tongue due to disturbance of the sensory component of the facial nerve occurs in some cases and indicates a more central location of the lesion in the nerve (see Chap. 367). Taste acuity declines with age for salty and bitter, but not for sour and sweet. This change may be associated in part with the number of missing teeth and the size of any artificial prosthesis used, thereby influencing food preferences, palatability, intake, and nutritional status of the elderly.

The pain associated with the *glossopharyngeal neuralgia syndrome* is similar in type and intensity to that found in trigeminal neuralgia, being set off by a trigger zone in the pharynx and affecting the posterior region of the tongue, pharynx, soft palate, and ear. Disturbance of the hypoglossal nerve leads to dysfunction of the tongue musculature and atrophy. Bilateral nerve involvement prevents protrusion of the tongue; unilateral involvement leads to deviation of the protruded tongue toward the affected side.

DISTURBANCES OF THE TEMPOROMANDIBULAR JOINT

Pain in the area of the temporomandibular joint frequently causes the patient to seek therapy. It may be due to posterior displacement of the condyle in the fossa leading to displacement of the meniscus and chronic trauma. *Dislocation of the condyle anteriorly* beyond the articular eminence due to sudden stretching or tearing of the capsular ligament may result in a locking of the mandible in an open position. In *osteoarthritis* the clinical signs and symptoms may be minimal despite extensive changes in the condyle. Temporomandibular joint involvement occurs less frequently in *rheumatoid arthritis.* When affected, the joints are swollen and painful, leading to limitation of movement, particularly on arising in the morning. In children the disease may lead to malocclusion. *Ankylosis* of the joint may occur eventually, necessitating a condylectomy (see Chap. 346).

The myofascial pain syndrome, the most common disorder of the temporomandibular joint, is characterized by facial pain and mandibular dysfunction in the absence of clinical or radiologic evidence of organic disease. The pain is often localized in the ear or jaw and may extend to the neck and shoulder. The mandibular dysfunction is manifested by limitation of movement, particularly an inability to open the jaw to the fullest extent. It is thought that such patients have increased musculature tension and hyperexcitable reflexes related to emotional tension. The precipitating factor appears to be the stretching of an abnormal focus of pain which initiates a self-sustaining pain-spasm-pain cycle. Treatment of the pain-dysfunction syndrome involves the use of drugs to relieve the pain, lessen cortical excitability, and relax the muscles. Local heat therapy, elimination of gross occlusal discrepancies, and jaw-opening exercises are also used. Local anesthetics are used intramuscularly in the region of the trigger zone or as superficial sprays in an attempt to break the pain-spasm-pain cycle.

REFERENCES

BAEHNI PC et al: Leukotoxic activity in different strains of the bacterium *Actinobacillus actinomycetemcomitans* isolated from juvenile periodontitis in man. Arch Oral Biol 26:671, 1981

BEITMAN RG: Oral manifestations of gastrointestinal disease. Dig Dis Sc 26:741, 1981

GOLDMAN HM, COHEN DW (eds): *Periodontal Therapy*, 6th ed. St Louis, Mosby, 1978

GOLDMAN HS, MARDER MZ: *Physician's Guide to Diseases of the Oral Cavity*. Oradell, NJ, Medical Economics, 1982

MASHBERG A: Erythroplasia: The earliest sign of asymptomatic oral cancer. J Am Dent Assoc 96:615, 1978

MCCARTHY PL, SHKLAR G: *Diseases of the Oral Mucosa*, 2d ed. Philadelphia, Lea & Febiger, 1980

SHAW JH et al: *Textbook of Oral Biology*. Philadelphia, Saunders, 1978

32 DYSPHAGIA

RAJ K. GOYAL

Dysphagia is defined as a sensation of "sticking" or obstruction of the passage of food through the mouth, pharynx, or the esophagus.

Dysphagia should be distinguished from other symptoms related to swallowing. *Aphagia* signifies complete esophageal obstruction which is usually due to bolus impaction and represents a medical emergency. *Difficulty in initiating a swallow* occurs in disorders of the voluntary phase of swallowing. Once initiated, however, swallowing is completed normally. *Odynophagia* means painful swallowing. Frequently, odynophagia and dysphagia occur together. *Globus hystericus* is the sensation of a lump lodged in the throat. No difficulty, however, is encountered when actual swallowing is performed. *Refusal to swallow* and *fear of swallowing* may occur in hysteria, rabies, tetanus, and pharyngeal paralysis due to fear of aspiration. Painful inflammatory lesions that cause odynophagia may also cause refusal to swallow. Some patients may feel the food as it goes down the esophagus. This esophageal sensitivity is not associated with sticking of the food or obstruction, however. Similarly, the *feeling of fullness in the epigastrium* that occurs after a meal or after swallowing air should not be confused with dysphagia.

PHYSIOLOGY OF SWALLOWING The process of swallowing begins with a voluntary (oral) phase during which a bolus of food is pushed backward into the pharynx. The bolus activates oropharyngeal sensory receptors which initiate the involuntary (pharyngeal and esophageal) phase or deglutition reflex. The deglutition reflex is a complex series of events which serves both to propel food through the pharynx and the esophagus and to prevent its entry into the airway. At the same time as the bolus is propelled backward by the tongue, the larynx moves forward and the upper esophageal sphincter opens. As the bolus moves into the pharynx, contraction of the superior pharyngeal constrictor against the contracted soft palate initiates a peristaltic contraction that proceeds rapidly downward to move the bolus through the pharynx and the esophagus. The lower esophageal sphincter opens as the food enters the esophagus and remains open until the peristaltic contraction has swept the bolus into the stomach. Peristaltic contraction in response to a swallow involves the entire swallowing passages and is called *primary peristalsis*. Local distention of the esophagus due to food activates intramural reflexes in the smooth muscle which result in *secondary peristalsis*, limited to the lower esophagus. *Tertiary contractions* are nonperistaltic as they occur simultaneously over a long segment of the esophagus. Tertiary contractions may occur in response to a swallow or esophageal distention, or they may occur spontaneously.

PATHOPHYSIOLOGY OF DYSPHAGIA The normal transport of an ingested bolus through the swallowing passage depends on (1) the size of the ingested bolus, (2) the luminal diameter of the swallowing passage, (3) the peristaltic contraction, and (4) deglutitive inhibition, which includes normal relaxation of upper and lower esophageal sphincters during swallowing and inhibition of persisting contractions in the esophageal body, for example, due to an immediately preceding swallow. Dysphagia caused by a large bolus or luminal narrowing is called *mechanical dysphagia*, while dysphagia due to incoordination or weakness of peristaltic contractions or to impaired deglutitive inhibition is called *motor dysphagia*.

Mechanical dysphagia Mechanical dysphagia could be caused by luminal factors, intrinsic narrowing or extrinsic compression of the lumen. In an adult, the esophageal lumen can distend to a diameter of well over 4 cm because of the elasticity of the esophageal wall. When the esophagus cannot dilate to more than 2.5 cm in diameter, dysphagia can occur, but it is always present when it cannot distend beyond 1.3 cm. Circumferential lesions produce dysphagia more consistently than eccentric lesions. Eccentric benign tumors and lesions causing extrinsic compression cause dysphagia infrequently. The causes of mechanical dysphagia are listed in Table 32-1. Common causes are carcinoma, peptic and other benign strictures, and lower esophageal ring.

Motor dysphagia Motor dysphagia may result from difficulty in initiating a swallow or abnormalities in peristalsis and deglutitive inhibition due to diseases of the esophageal skeletal or smooth muscle.

Diseases of the skeletal muscle involve the pharynx, upper esophageal sphincter, and the upper part of the esophagus. The striated muscle is innervated by a somatic component of the vagus with cell bodies of the lower motor neurons located in the nucleus ambiguus. These neurons are cholinergic and excitatory and are the sole determinant of the muscle activity. Peristalsis in the skeletal muscle segment is due to sequential central activation of neurons innervating muscles at different levels. Motor dysphagia of the pharynx results from neuromus-

TABLE 32-1
Causes of mechanical dysphagia

- *I* Luminal
  - *A* Large bolus
  - *B* Foreign body
- *II* Intrinsic narrowing
  - *A* Inflammatory condition causing edema and swelling
    - *1* Stomatitis
    - *2* Pharyngitis, epiglottitis
    - *3* Esophagitis (e.g., viral, monilial)
  - *B* Webs
    - *1* Pharyngeal (Plummer-Vinson syndrome)
    - *2* Esophageal
  - *C* Lower esophageal ring
    - *1* Mucosal ring (Schatzki ring)
  - *D* Benign strictures
    - *1* Peptic
    - *2* Caustic
    - *3* Inflammatory (Crohn's disease, moniliasis, epidermolysis bullosa)
    - *4* Ischemic
    - *5* Postoperative, postirradiation
    - *6* Congenital
  - *E* Malignant tumors
    - *1* Primary carcinoma
    - *2* Squamous-cell carcinoma
    - *3* Adenocarcinoma
    - *4* Carcinosarcoma
    - *5* Pseudosarcoma
    - *6* Lymphoma
    - *7* Melanoma
    - *8* Metastatic carcinoma
  - *F* Benign tumors
    - *1* Leiomyoma
    - *2* Lipoma
    - *3* Angioma
    - *4* Inflammatory fibroid polyp
    - *5* Epithelial papilloma
- *III* Extrinsic compression
  - *A* Cervical spondylitis
  - *B* Vertebral osteophytes
  - *C* Retropharyngeal abscess and masses
  - *D* Enlarged thyroid gland
  - *E* Zenker's diverticulum
  - *F* Vascular compression
    - *1* Aberrant right subclavian artery
    - *2* Right-sided aorta
    - *3* Left atrial enlargement
    - *4* Aortic aneurysm
  - *G* Posterior mediastinal masses
  - *H* Pancreatic tumor, pancreatitis
  - *I* Postvagotomy hematoma and fibrosis

NOTE: *Some lesions can occur anywhere along the swallowing passages while others occur in a specific location.*

cular disorders causing muscle paralysis, simultaneous nonperistaltic contraction, or loss of opening of the upper esophageal sphincter. Loss of opening of the upper sphincter is caused by paralysis of geniohyoid and other suprahyoid muscles or loss of deglutitive inhibition of the cricopharyngeus muscle. Because each side of the pharynx is innervated by ipsilateral nerves, a lesion of motor neurons occurring only on one side leads to unilateral pharyngeal paralysis. Although lesions of skeletal muscle also involve the upper part of the esophagus, the clinical manifestations of pharyngeal dysfunction usually overshadow the manifestations due to esophageal involvement.

Diseases of the smooth-muscle segment involve the lower part of the esophagus and the lower esophageal sphincter. This smooth muscle is innervated by the parasympathetic component of the vagal preganglionic fibers and postganglionic noncholinergic neurons in the myenteric ganglia. These nerves exert a predominantly inhibitory influence on the lower esophageal sphincter and cause inhibition followed by contraction in the esophageal body. Peristalsis in this segment is due to neuromuscular mechanisms in the wall of the esophagus itself. Dysphagia results when the peristaltic contractions are weak or nonperistaltic or when the lower sphincter fails to open normally. Loss of contractile power occurs due to muscle weakness, as in scleroderma, or to loss of myenteric neurons, as in achalasia. The cause of simultaneous onset of contractions, typically seen in diffuse esophageal spasm, is not understood. Impairment of deglutitive inhibition of the lower esophageal sphincter is associated with a defect in inhibitory nerves to the sphincter and is the major cause of dysphagia in achalasia.

The causes of motor dysphagia are listed in Table 32-2. The important causes are achalasia, diffuse esophageal spasm and related motor disorders, pharyngeal paralysis, cricopharyngeal achalasia, and scleroderma of the esophagus.

APPROACH TO THE PATIENT WITH DYSPHAGIA History The history can provide a correct presumptive diagnosis in over 80 percent of patients. The type of food causing dysphagia provides useful information. Difficulty only with solids implies mechanical dysphagia with a lumen that is not severely narrowed. The impacted bolus may be forced through the narrowed area by drinking liquids. In advanced obstruction dys-

TABLE 32-2
Causes of motor (neuromuscular) dysphagia

- *I* Difficulty in initiating swallowing reflex
  - *A* Oral lesions and paralysis of tongue
  - *B* Oropharyngeal anesthesia
  - *C* Lack of saliva
  - *D* Lesions of sensory components of vagus and glossopharyngeal nerves
  - *E* Lesions of swallowing center
- *II* Disorders of esophageal skeletal muscle
  - *A* Muscle weakness
    - *1* Lower motor neuron lesion (bulbar paralysis)
      - *a* Cerebrovascular accident
      - *b* Motor neuron disease
      - *c* Poliomyelitis
      - *d* Polyneuritis
      - *e* Amyotrophic lateral sclerosis
      - *f* Familial dysautonomia
    - *2* Neuromuscular
      - *a* Myasthenia gravis
    - *3* Muscle disorders
      - *a* Polymyositis
      - *b* Dermatomyositis
      - *c* Myopathies (myotonic dystrophy, oculopharyngeal myopathy)
  - *B* Simultaneous onset contractions or impaired deglutitive inhibition
    - *1* Pharynx and upper esophagus
      - *a* Rabies
      - *b* Stiff-man syndrome
      - *c* Extrapyramidal tract disease
      - *d* Upper motor neuron lesions (pseudobulbar paralysis)
    - *2* Upper esophageal sphincter (UES)
      - *a* Paralysis of suprahyoid muscles (causes same as paralysis of pharyngeal musculature)
      - *b* Cricopharyngeal achalasia
- *III* Disorders of esophageal smooth muscle
  - *A* Paralysis of esophageal body causing weak contractions
    - *1* Scleroderma and related collagen vascular diseases
    - *2* Myotonic dystrophy
    - *3* Metabolic neuromyopathy (amyloid, alcohol?, diabetes?)
    - *4* Achalasia (classical)
  - *B* Simultaneous-onset contractions or impaired deglutitive inhibition
    - *1* Esophageal body
      - *a* Diffuse esophageal spasm
      - *b* Achalasia (vigorous)
      - *c* Variants of diffuse esophageal spasm
    - *2* Lower esophageal sphincter (LES)
      - *a* Achalasia
        - *(1)* Primary
        - *(2)* Secondary
          - *(a)* Chagas' disease
          - *(b)* Carcinoma
          - *(c)* Lymphoma
          - *(d)* Intestinal pseudoobstruction syndrome
          - *(e)* Toxins and drugs
          - *(f)* Irradiation
      - *b* Lower esophageal muscular (contractile) ring

phagia occurs to liquids as well as solids. In contrast, motor dysphagia due to achalasia and diffuse esophageal spasm is equally affected by solids and liquids from the very onset. Patients with scleroderma have dysphagia to solids that is unrelated to posture and to liquids in the recumbent but not in the upright posture. When peptic stricture develops in these patients dysphagia becomes more persistent.

The duration and course of dysphagia are helpful in diagnosis. Transient dysphagia of short duration may be due to an inflammatory process. Progressive dysphagia of a few weeks to a few months duration is suggestive of carcinoma of the esophagus. Episodic dysphagia to solids of several years' duration indicates a benign disease and is characteristic of a lower esophageal ring.

The localization of dysphagia is helpful when it is described in the chest, where the site of dysphagia generally correlates with the site of esophageal obstruction. However, localization of dysphagia to the neck is of no diagnostic value because lesions of the pharynx, cervical esophagus, and even lower esophagus may cause dysphagia to be perceived in the neck.

Associated symptoms provide important diagnostic clues. Nasal regurgitation and tracheobronchial aspiration with swallowing are hallmarks of pharyngeal paralysis or a tracheoesophageal fistula. Tracheobronchial aspiration unrelated to swallowing may be secondary to achalasia, a Zenker's diverticulum, or gastroesophageal reflux. Severe weight loss out of proportion to the degree of dysphagia is highly suggestive of carcinoma. When hoarseness precedes dysphagia the primary lesion is usually in the larynx. Hoarseness following dysphagia may suggest involvement of the recurrent laryngeal nerve by extension of esophageal carcinoma beyond the walls of the esophagus. Sometimes hoarseness may be due to laryngitis secondary to gastroesophageal reflux. Association of laryngeal symptoms and dysphagia also occurs in various neuromuscular disorders. Hiccups suggest a lesion in the distal portion of the esophagus. Unilateral wheezing with dysphagia indicates a mediastinal mass involving the esophagus and a large bronchus. Chest pain with dysphagia occurs in diffuse esophageal spasm and in related motor disorders. Chest pain resembling diffuse esophageal spasms also may occur in acute aphagia due to a large bolus. A prolonged history of heartburn and reflux preceding dysphagia indicates peptic stricture. Similarly, a history of prolonged nasogastric intubation, ingestion of caustic agents, previous radiation therapy, or associated mucocutaneous diseases may provide the cause of esophageal stricture. If odynophagia is present, monilial or herpes esophagitis should be suspected, particularly in debilitated patients with carcinoma or those receiving immunosuppressive therapy.

Physical examination Physical examination is important in motor dysphagia due to skeletal muscle, neurologic, and oropharyngeal diseases. Signs of bulbar or pseudobulbar palsy, including dysarthria, dysphonia, ptosis, tongue atrophy, and hyperactive jaw jerk, in addition to evidence of generalized neuromuscular disease, should be carefully searched for. The neck should be examined for thyromegaly or a spinal abnormality. A careful inspection of the mouth and pharynx should disclose lesions that may cause interference with passage of food from the mouth or esophagus because of pain or obstruction. Changes in the skin and extremities may suggest a diagnosis of scleroderma and other collagen vascular diseases, or mucocutaneous diseases such as pemphigoid or epidermolysis bullosa which may involve the esophagus. Metastatic diseases to lymph nodes and liver may be evident. Pulmonary complications of acute aspiration pneumonia or chronic aspiration may be present.

Diagnostic procedures Dysphagia is one of the major symptoms of esophageal disease, and a cause for this symptom can invariably be determined. Therefore, all patients with dysphagia must be thoroughly investigated until a specific cause is determined. This is particularly important because the treatment depends upon the underlying cause of dysphagia. Barium swallow with cineradiography, esophagogastroscopy with biopsy and exfoliative cytology, and esophageal motility are the main diagnostic procedures (see Chap. 305).

REFERENCES

EDWARDS DAW: Discriminatory value of symptoms in the differential diagnosis of dysphagia. Clin Gastroenterol 5(1):49, 1976

GERSHON MD, ERDE SM: The nervous system of the gut. Gastroenterology 80:1571, 1981

GOYAL RK, COBB BW: Motility of pharynx, esophagus and esophageal sphincter, in *Physiology of the Gastrointestinal Tract*, LR Johnson (ed). New York, Raven Press, 1981, pp 359–391

HURWITZ AL et al: *Disorders of Esophageal Motility*. Philadelphia, Saunders, 1979

33
INDIGESTION

KURT J. ISSELBACHER

Indigestion is a term frequently used by patients to describe a multitude of symptoms generally appreciated as distress associated with the intake of food. The term is thus nonspecific and may not have the same meaning for the patient and the physician. In approaching the patient with indigestion, it is important for the physician first to elicit a good description of this complaint. To some patients indigestion refers to a feeling that digestion has not proceeded naturally. They may describe a sense of abdominal fullness, pressure, or actual pain. Others may use the term to describe heartburn, belching, distention, or flatulence. These complaints are considered in this chapter. Discussed elsewhere are the closely related symptoms of dysphagia, nausea and vomiting, and anorexia (Chaps. 32 and 34).

Indigestion may occur as a result of disease of the gastrointestinal tract or in association with pathologic states in other organ systems. As a result of systematic clinical and laboratory tests, a definable pathophysiologic process often can be shown to be responsible for the symptoms in a given case of indigestion. Frequently, however, clear etiologic explanation for the patient's complaints of indigestion are not established. Such cases are often designated as "functional indigestion," with a strong implication that psychosomatic factors underlie the complaints. Although it is clear that psychic factors may lead to symptoms of indigestion, the designation of "functional indigestion" is rarely, if ever, a satisfactory explanation, serving only to rephrase the patient's description of the symptoms. A psychogenic cause should not be assumed until organic causes of indigestion have been thoroughly excluded.

After having ascertained the patient's definition of indigestion, it is also important to determine (1) the location and duration of the discomfort, (2) the temporal relation of the symptoms to the ingestion of food, and (3) the possible relation of the symptoms to the ingestion of specific types of food (e.g., fatty foods, milk, and drugs).

PAIN PATTERNS True visceral abdominal pain as seen in indigestion is mediated over visceral afferent nerves which accompany the abdominal sympathetic pathways (see Chap. 5).

Visceral pain is generally described as dull and aching in nature (with a diffuse midline localization) or as fullness or pressure. The location of the discomfort corresponds generally to the segmental level of the affected organ. Abdominal visceral pain can be produced experimentally by artificially increasing pressure in a hollow viscus. Usually this pain is the result of distention or exaggerated muscular contraction of a viscus. Inflammation generally lowers the threshold to such stimuli.

The visceral pain of indigestion should be distinguished from the sharp, lateralized, and localized pain patterns seen in many acute abdominal processes involving the peritoneum. In contrast to true visceral pain, this pain is mediated over cerebrospinal afferent nerves. Again it is of a dull, aching type, whether from inflammation of the viscera or of peritoneal surfaces.

In view of the diffuse nature of true visceral abdominal pain, the main clue comes from the segmental level of the viscus; in any given segmental region there is no way of determining which of several viscera are the source of it (Table 33-1). The following rules, already given in Chap. 5, are useful: *Substernal pain* of gastrointestinal origin usually arises from disorders in the esophagus or cardia of the stomach. Because pain in this area is frequently of cardiac origin, heart disease must be considered carefully and excluded. *Epigastric pain* is generally of gastric, duodenal, biliary, or pancreatic origin. As the pathologic process in the biliary tract and pancreas becomes more intense, it tends to lateralize and localize, e.g., biliary pain to the right upper quadrant and tip of the right scapula and pancreatic pain to the epigastrium, left upper quadrant, and back. *Periumbilical pain* is generally associated with small-intestinal disease. *Pain below the umbilicus* is often of appendiceal, large-intestinal, or pelvic origin.

TEMPORAL RELATIONSHIPS OF PAIN AND INDIGESTION The unraveling of the temporal relationships of the patient's symptoms often provides the most significant diagnostic information. It is important to ascertain whether the symptoms are *constant* (continually present over extended periods of time), as may occur, for example, with an infiltrating gastric carcinoma, or *intermittent,* as in acute gastritis following an alcoholic binge or in association with the use of certain drugs. The symptoms may have a *diurnal* pattern; e.g., pain occurring *nocturnally* and with *recumbency* is seen in esophagitis and hiatus hernia.

TABLE 33-1
Distribution of visceral pain and examples of disorders frequently involving the specific organ

Organ	*Location of referred pain*	*Frequent disorders*
Esophagus	Substernum, epigastrium	Peptic esophagitis, hiatus hernia, stricture, carcinoma
Stomach	Epigastrium	Gastritis, peptic ulcer, carcinoma
Duodenum (first and second portions)	Epigastrium	Peptic ulcer
Duodenum (third portion, jejunum, and ileum)	Periumbilical	Regional enteritis, lymphoma, gastroenteritis (infectious), intestinal obstruction
Gallbladder	Epigastrium, right upper quadrant, right side of back	Cholelithiasis, cholecystitis
Pancreas	Epigastrium, left side of back	Pancreatitis, pancreatic carcinoma
Liver	Right upper quadrant	Passive congestion of liver, hepatitis, cirrhosis
Colon	Below umbilicus	Ulcerative colitis, carcinoma, partial obstruction

Symptoms are occasionally *seasonal;* this may occur in peptic ulcer disease, in which some patients experience more discomfort in the spring and autumn.

Another important and often diagnostic feature is the relation of pain or indigestion to ingestion of food. This relationship is especially significant or helpful if symptoms occur either during or minutes after the meal or if they occur several hours (4 or more) after eating. *Early postprandial symptoms* may reflect esophageal disease, because they may be associated with disordered swallowing function. In such instances, the distress or other symptoms of indigestion often are experienced substernally. Early postprandial complaints occur also in gastric disorders such as acute gastritis or carcinoma. *Late postprandial indigestion,* i.e., that occurring several hours after eating, may reflect failure of the stomach to empty adequately, as in pyloric stenosis or gastric atony. It may also be a symptom of duodenal ulcer, in which case it classically occurs several hours after the meal, when the ulcerated mucosa is exposed to acid secretions of the stomach unbuffered by food. Conversely, the relief of pain following food ingestion is also seen in patients with peptic ulcer and is presumably due to the neutralization of the acid by the ingested food. Such pain also is typically alleviated quickly by oral antacids. Late postprandial indigestion also may result from impaired digestive and absorptive processes, as in pancreatic insufficiency.

FOOD INTOLERANCE In a number of situations specific foods or types of foods appear to be related to indigestion. Careful documentation of this relationship is sometimes of great help in arriving at an etiologic diagnosis.

Some foods may be poorly tolerated because of their consistency. Patients with esophageal stricture or carcinoma may tolerate liquids well, but the ingestion of solids may be associated with discomfort, especially substernal distress (see Chap. 305). Certain foods may be tolerated poorly because the intestinal tract cannot assimilate them adequately. This may occur following the ingestion of fatty foods in patients with pancreatic or biliary tract disease. Citrus fruits, with their relatively low pH, often provoke symptoms in patients with peptic ulcer disease.

Individuals may lack a specific enzyme required for assimilation of a certain nutrient. Patients may have a deficiency of the mucosal enzyme lactase, which catalyzes the hydrolysis of lactose. When lactase deficiency exists on a hereditary or acquired basis (e.g., in sprue, ulcerative colitis) (Chap. 308), the ingestion of milk (which contains lactose) results in abdominal cramps, distention, flatulence, and diarrhea.

There are a number of other conditions or disorders in which specific foods are poorly tolerated. Foods may be poorly tolerated because they initiate *allergic reactions* or exert a deleterious or *toxic effect* on the intestinal tract of susceptible persons (e.g., gluten in patients with nontropical sprue). Finally, certain substances may lead to systemic effects because of biochemical defects in the patient which render the substances particularly hazardous. An example of the latter is galactose intolerance in galactosemia (Chap. 101).

The above mechanisms do not explain the majority of clinical situations in which indigestion is associated with the eating of specific foods. For example, a history of fatty-food intolerance or an inability to eat cabbage, cucumbers, or spicy foods is commonly obtained from patients with indigestion. However, the mechanisms underlying the production of symptoms in these circumstances are still unclear.

ADDITIONAL SYNDROMES COMMONLY DESCRIBED AS INDIGESTION **Gaseousness, flatulence, aerophagia** A number of common clinical syndromes which may be described by the patient as "indigestion" appear to be related to increased quantities of gas in the intestinal tract. About 20 to 60 percent of intraluminal gas represents swallowed air. A degree of air swallowing, or *aerophagia,* occurs in normal persons, and the swallowed air can be observed at fluoroscopy. Under certain circumstances, such as chronic anxiety, poor eating habits, or actual intestinal disease itself, aerophagia may increase in magnitude and lead to symptoms in its own right.

The combination of early postprandial fullness and pressure, relieved by eructation and accompanied by a large amount of air seen in the gastric fundus on roentgenogram, is often referred to as the *magenblase* (i.e., gastric bubble) *syndrome.* Acute gastric distention by swallowed air can occasionally produce sharp pains which may mimic angina pectoris. This sequence of events may be especially perplexing in older patients with coronary artery disease, because it is well recognized that true angina pectoris may itself be precipitated by the ingestion of a large meal. Fatty meals delay gastric emptying and hence the passage of swallowed air in the intestine. This relationship may explain, in part, the prolonged sense of fullness and eructations experienced by many individuals after a fatty meal.

Swallowed air that is not eructated passes on in the intestinal tract and may either produce diffuse abdominal distention or become trapped in the splenic flexure of the colon. Distention of this segment of the colon produces a sensation of left upper quadrant fullness and pressure with radiation to the left side of the chest. This is known as the *splenic flexure syndrome.* Patients will often describe relief of pain with defecation or with the expulsion of flatus. Diagnosis may be made by demonstrating, on physical examination, a note of increased tympany in the extreme left lateral portion of the upper part of the abdomen or by the visualization of large amounts of air in the splenic flexure of the colon by radiography.

A second major source of intestinal gas is the fermentative action of bacteria on carbohydrates and proteins within the lumen. Increased amounts of intraluminal gas production due to this mechanism have been demonstrated in conditions associated with abnormal bacterial colonization of the small intestine and in patients with carbohydrate malabsorption.

Increased gas production may occur following the ingestion of certain foods (e.g., the legumes) which contain significant quantities of nonabsorbable sugars. As in the case of swallowed air, increased amounts of intraluminally produced gas can produce symptoms by causing distention, pain, increased motility (with diarrhea), or flatulence.

Heartburn Heartburn, or pyrosis, is a sensation of warmth or burning located substernally or high in the epigastrium. Experimental studies in human beings have shown that esophageal distention or increased motor activity is associated in most subjects with a feeling of fullness and burning in this area.

Heartburn may occur with organic disease of the intestinal tract and is usually associated with gastroesophageal reflux. This is frequently the case in hiatus hernia. In this setting, heartburn occurs after a large meal or with stooping or bending. Esophageal reflux of acid contents at these times leads to symptoms by either the production of abnormal motor activity or direct mucosal irritation (i.e., esophagitis). Heartburn may arise following the ingestion of certain foods or drugs (e.g., alcohol and aspirin). It may also be seen in the absence of a demonstrable anatomic or motor pathologic condition, in which case it is frequently accompanied by aerophagia and for lack of other explanation is often attributed to psychological factors.

INDIGESTION DUE TO DISEASE OUTSIDE THE INTESTINAL TRACT A multitude of extraintestinal disease processes may result in indigestion by mechanisms which are poorly understood. Indigestion may be the presenting complaint, for example, in congestive heart failure, uremia, pulmonary tuberculosis, and neoplastic disease. Under these circumstances the symptoms of indigestion may present with no unique features to suggest that they are in fact due to some other systemic disease process. Drugs such as aspirin, corticosteroids, indomethacin, and phenylbutazone affect gastric secretion and are ulcerogenic; thus they may lead to symptoms of indigestion.

DIAGNOSTIC APPROACH TO THE PATIENT WITH INDIGESTION Indigestion represents a challenging and difficult diagnostic problem because of the nonspecific nature of its manifestations. The evaluation of indigestion must include initially a thorough medical workup, with ultimate confirmation or exclusion of pathophysiologic derangements by the appropriate diagnostic procedures.

A careful history should include an assessment of the patient's general medical health, including the possibility of diseases in extraintestinal organ systems which may produce indigestion. Careful evaluation of psychological factors is crucial, because they often play an etiologic or contributory role in the patient's problem. Of particular importance are anxiety, depressive reactions, and hysteria (Chap. 11). Evaluation of the patient's intestinal problem must include an assessment of nutritional status, changes in weight, and appetite.

A clear and detailed description of the specific symptoms should be obtained, particularly the patient's definition of the term "indigestion." The nature of the pain, its frequency and time of occurrence, its relationship to meals, and the special circumstances which lead to its exacerbation or relief should be elicited. Associated intestinal symptoms such as nausea and vomiting, abnormal bowel habits, steatorrhea, diarrhea, and melena should also be sought. Physical examination rarely establishes the specific diagnosis, but it may be useful in detecting disease in other organ systems (e.g., congestive heart failure) which can affect intestinal physiology.

X-ray examination of the alimentary tract is crucial to the evaluation of indigestion. This may involve examination of the esophagus, stomach, small intestine, colon, and biliary tract. Esophagoscopy, gastroscopy, colonoscopy, or sigmoidoscopy also may be helpful or necessary. Stools should be examined for appearance, occult blood, fat, and muscle fibers. As stated above, careful attempts must be made to exclude nonintestinal disease, especially cardiac disease.

Unfortunately, even after completion of careful diagnostic studies, many cases of indigestion will turn out to have no clear explanation. Some of these are psychogenic and may respond to appropriate psychiatric measures. Others represent physiologic derangements which are undetectable by currently available diagnostic methods. Still others represent actual disease processes in early stages which may be diagnosable by conventional methods at a later date. The ultimate evaluation of indigestion requires, therefore, the utmost in sensitivity, diligence, and patience on the part of the examining physician.

REFERENCES

BOND JH, LEVITT MD: A rational approach to intestinal gas problems. Viewpoints Digestive Dis, vol 9, no 2, 1977

COGHILL NF: Dyspepsia. Br Med J 4:97, 1967

LASSER RB et al: The role of intestinal gas in functional abdominal pain. N Engl J Med 293:524, 1975

LEVITT MD: Methane production in the gut. N Engl J Med 291:528, 1974

34 ANOREXIA, NAUSEA, AND VOMITING

KURT J. ISSELBACHER

ANOREXIA Anorexia, or loss of the desire to eat, is a prominent symptom in a wide variety of intestinal and extraintestinal disorders. It must be clearly differentiated from satiety and from specific food intolerance. Anorexia occurs in many disorders and as a result *by itself is of little specific diagnostic value.* The mechanisms whereby hunger and appetite are modified in various disease states are poorly understood. Normally food intake is regulated by two hypothalamic centers—a lateral "feeding center" and a ventromedial "satiety center." The latter inhibits the feeding center following a meal, leading to the sensation of satiety. There is increasing evidence to suggest that the brain-gut peptide cholecystokinin (CCK) has a satiety effect and is involved in the regulation of feeding behavior.

Anorexia is commonly seen in diseases of the gastrointestinal tract and liver. For example, it may precede the appearance of jaundice in hepatitis, or it may be a prominent symptom in gastric carcinoma. In the setting of intestinal disease, anorexia should be clearly differentiated from *sitophobia,* or fear of eating because of subsequent or associated discomfort. In such circumstances, appetite may persist, but the ingestion of food is curtailed nonetheless. Sitophobia may be seen, for example, in regional enteritis (especially with partial obstruction) or in patients with gastric ulcer following partial or total gastrectomy.

Anorexia may also be a prominent feature of severe extraintestinal diseases. For example, anorexia may be profound in severe congestive heart failure and is often associated with cardiac glycoside intoxication. It may be a major symptom in patients with uremia, pulmonary failure, and various endocrinopathies (e.g., hyperparathyroidism, Addison's disease, and panhypopituitarism). Anorexia also often accompanies psychogenic disturbances, such as anxiety or depression. For a discussion of anorexia nervosa, see Chap. 80.

NAUSEA AND VOMITING Nausea and vomiting may occur independently of each other, but generally they are so closely allied that they may conveniently be considered together. *Nausea* denotes the feeling of the imminent desire to vomit, usually referred to the throat or epigastrium. *Vomiting* refers to the forceful oral expulsion of gastric contents; *retching* denotes the labored rhythmic respiratory activity that frequently precedes emesis. Extremely forceful *projectile vomiting* is a special form of vomiting which has significance because it connotes the presence of increased intracranial pressure.

Nausea often precedes or accompanies vomiting. It is usually associated with diminished functional activity of the stomach and alterations of the motility of the duodenum and small intestine. Accompanying severe nausea there is often evidence of altered autonomic (especially parasympathetic) activity: pallor of the skin, increased perspiration, salivation, and the occasional association of hypotension and bradycardia (vasovagal syndrome). Anorexia is also often present.

Following a period of nausea and a brief interval of retching, a sequence of involuntary visceral and somatic motor events occurs, resulting in emesis. The stomach plays a relatively passive role in the vomiting process, the major ejection force being provided by the abdominal musculature. With relaxation of the gastric fundus and gastroesophageal sphincter, a sharp increase in intraabdominal pressure is brought about by forceful contraction of the diaphragm and abdominal wall. This, together with concomitant annular contraction of the gastric pylorus, results in the expulsion of gastric contents into the esophagus. Increased intrathoracic pressure results in the further movement of esophageal contents into the mouth. Reversal of the normal direction of esophageal peristalsis may play a role in this process. Reflex elevation of the soft palate during the vomiting act prevents the entry of the material into the nasopharynx, whereas reflex closure of the glottis and inhibition of respiration help to prevent pulmonary aspiration.

Repeated emesis may have deleterious effects in a number of different ways. The process of vomiting itself may lead to traumatic rupture or tearing in the region of the cardioesophageal junction, resulting in massive hematemesis, the Mallory-Weiss syndrome. Prolonged vomiting may lead to dehydration and the loss of gastric secretions (especially hydrochloric acid), resulting in metabolic alkalosis with hypokalemia. Finally, in states of central nervous system depression (coma, etc.), gastric contents may be aspirated into the lungs, with a resulting aspiration pneumonitis.

Vomiting mechanism The act of vomiting is under the control of two functionally distinct medullary centers: the *vomiting center* and the *chemoreceptor trigger zone.* They lie close to each other near other brainstem centers regulating vasomotor and autonomic functions. The vomiting center controls and integrates the actual act of emesis. It receives afferent stimuli from the intestinal tract and other parts of the body, from higher cortical centers, especially the labyrinthine apparatus, and from the chemoreceptor trigger zone. The important efferent pathways in vomiting are the phrenic nerves (to the diaphragm), the spinal nerves (to the abdominal musculature), and visceral efferent nerves (to the stomach and esophagus).

The chemoreceptor trigger zone is also located in the medulla but by itself is incapable of mediating the act of vomiting. Activation of this zone results in efferent impulses to the medullary vomiting center, which in turn initiates the act of emesis. Dopamine receptors in the chemoreceptor trigger zone can be activated by many stimuli, including drugs such as apomorphine and levodopa, after decarboxylation to dopamine.

Phenothiazine derivatives such as prochlorperazine and metoclopramide inhibit cerebral dopamine receptors and can be effective against both nausea and vomiting. Metoclopramide is the prototype of selective dopamine antagonists called *substituted benzamides.* In contrast to the phenothiazines, which have anticholinergic effects, metoclopramide has powerful cholinergic effects. The latter, together with its dopamine antagonism, have made metoclopramide a useful agent equal or superior to drugs such as prochlorperazine in the treatment of nausea and vomiting. The usual oral dosage is 10 mg four times daily; it can be used intravenously in doses up to 1 to 3 mg/kg. Metoclopramide is also effective in hastening esophageal clearance, accelerating gastric emptying, and shortening small-bowel transit.

Clinical classification Nausea and vomiting are common manifestations of organic and functional disorders. The precise mechanisms triggering vomiting in the various clinical states are poorly understood, making classification of mechanisms difficult. The categories mentioned below serve to illustrate some of the many disorders which may be accompanied by nausea and vomiting.

Many *acute abdominal emergencies* which lead to the "surgical abdomen" are associated with nausea and vomiting. Notably, vomiting may be seen with inflammation of a viscus as in acute appendicitis or acute cholecystitis, obstruction of the intestine, or acute peritonitis (see Chap. 5).

In many of the disorders involving *chronic indigestion* (see Chap. 33) nausea and vomiting may be prominent. Emesis may be either spontaneous or self-induced and may lead to relief of symptoms, as, for example, in uncomplicated peptic ulcer. Nausea and vomiting may accompany the distention and pain seen in the aerophagic syndromes. Often in patients with chronic indigestion, nausea and vomiting may be provoked by specific foods (e.g., fatty foods), for reasons that are poorly understood.

Acute systemic infections with fever, especially in young children, are frequently accompanied by vomiting and often by severe diarrhea. The mechanism whereby infections remote from the gastrointestinal tract produce these manifestations is unclear. Viral, bacterial, and parasitic infections of the intestinal tract may be associated with severe nausea and vomiting, often with diarrhea. Severe nausea and vomiting may be prominent in viral hepatitis, even before the appearance of jaundice.

Central nervous system disorders which lead to increased intracranial pressure may be accompanied by vomiting, often projectile. Brain swelling due to inflammation, anoxemia, acute hydrocephalus, neoplasms, etc., may thus be complicated by vomiting. Disorders of the labyrinthine apparatus and its central connections which underlie vertigo may be accompanied by vomiting with nausea and retching. Acute labyrinthitis and Ménière's disease are examples of such disturbances. Migraine headaches, tabetic crises, and acute meningitis are additional examples of disorders of the nervous system which may lead to vomiting. In the reactive phase of hypotension with syncope, there may also be nausea and vomiting.

Severe nausea and vomiting may be present in *acute myocardial infarction,* especially of the posterior wall of the heart. Nausea and vomiting may also be seen in *congestive heart failure,* perhaps in relation to congestion of the liver. The possibility that these symptoms may be due to drugs (e.g., opiates or digitalis) should always be borne in mind in patients with cardiac disease.

Nausea and vomiting commonly accompany several *endocrinologic disorders,* including diabetic acidosis and adrenal insufficiency, especially adrenal crises. The morning sickness of early pregnancy is another instance of nausea and vomiting possibly related to hormonal changes.

The *side effects of many drugs and chemicals* include nausea and vomiting. In some instances this is because of gastric irritation which stimulates the medullary vomiting center.

Psychogenic vomiting means vomiting which may occur as part of any emotional upset on a transitory basis or more persistently as part of a psychic disturbance. Close observation will usually disclose the condition to be one of regurgitation rather than of vomiting, and weight loss may not correspond at all to the patient's description of the frequency and severity of vomiting. As discussed in Chap. 80, anorexia nervosa is an emotional disturbance which may be associated not only with anorexia but also with vomiting. Often patients with emotional disorders and vomiting maintain a relatively normal state of nutrition because a relatively small amount of the ingested food is vomited.

Differential diagnosis Vomiting should be distinguished from *regurgitation,* which refers to the expulsion of food in the absence of nausea and without abdominal diaphragmatic muscular contraction which is part of vomiting. Regurgitation of esophageal contents may occur with esophageal stricture or diverticula. Regurgitation of gastric contents is generally seen with gastroesophageal sphincter incompetence, especially with hiatus hernia or in association with peptic ulcer, usually when pylorospasm supervenes.

The temporal relationships of vomiting to eating may be of help diagnostically. Vomiting which occurs predominantly in the morning is often seen early in pregnancy and uremia. Alcoholic gastritis is commonly accompanied by early-morning emesis, the so-called dry heaves. Vomiting which occurs shortly after eating may suggest pylorospasm or gastritis. On the other hand, vomiting which occurs 4 to 6 h or longer after eating and involves the elimination of large quantities of undigested food often indicates gastric retention (e.g., diabetic gastric atony or pyloric obstruction).

The character of the vomitus offers clues to the diagnosis. If the vomitus contains free hydrochloric acid, the obstruction may be due to an ulcer; absence of free hydrochloric acid is more compatible with gastric malignancy. A feculent or putrid odor reflects the results of bacterial action on the intestinal contents. Such vomiting may be seen with low-intestinal obstruction, peritonitis, or gastrocolic fistula. Bile is commonly present in gastric contents whenever vomiting is prolonged. It has no significance unless constantly present in large quantities, when it may signify an obstructive lesion below the ampulla of Vater. The presence of blood in the gastric contents usually denotes bleeding from the esophagus, stomach, or duodenum.

REFERENCES

HALL RJC: Normal and abnormal food intake. Gut 16:744, 1975

LUMSDEN K, HOLDEN SW: The act of vomiting in man. Gut 10:173, 1969

SCHULZE-DELRIEU K: Metoclopramide. N Engl J Med 305:28, 1981

SMITH GP: Satiety effect of gastrointestinl hormones, in *Polypeptide Hormones*, RF Beers, EG Bassett (eds). New York, Raven Press, 1980, pp 413–420

35

GAIN AND LOSS IN WEIGHT

DANIEL W. FOSTER

GENERAL PRINCIPLES

In normal persons weight is stable because caloric intake is matched to caloric expenditure by the coordinated activities of the feeding and satiety centers in the brainstem. Energy costs fall into three categories: (1) calories needed for maintenance of basal metabolism, (2) calories necessary for food absorption (specific dynamic action), and (3) calories required for physical activity. *Basal metabolism* is defined as the total caloric requirement when the body is in the supine position, motionless except for quiet respiration. It can be translated as the energy required to maintain structural and functional integrity of the organism in the absence of physical activity. About half the total daily caloric intake is normally consumed by basal processes. In nonobese, nonsedentary subjects another 10 percent of intake is used for food absorption. The remainder is spent in physical activity. In active persons this represents about 40 percent of daily intake, though athletes may use greater than 50 percent of calories for physical activity.

Gain or loss in tissue mass is determined by the net balance between caloric intake and caloric expenditure. Change in body weight as a consequence of voluntary alteration in diet or exercise is never worrisome; change in weight that is not deliberately sought, on the other hand, is a frequent reason for consultation with the physician and often indicates the presence of disease. Changes in weight may reflect alteration in either tissue mass or body fluid content. Rapid swings almost always indicate the latter. Even when tissue mass is changing, fluid loss or gain plays a major role in the measured change in weight, particularly over the short run. This point is well illustrated by the data of Table 35-1, where the composition of weight loss was estimated during a 24-day period of semistarvation in 13 normal soldiers (daily intake 1010 cal). During the first 3 days 70 percent of the weight loss was due to water, while in subsequent stages protein and fat accounted for essentially all the decreased mass. This varying contribution of fluid accounts for the fact that one cannot use a fixed formula for predicting weight loss or gain. It is frequently stated that a net change of 7700 cal will be accompanied by a 1-kg change in body mass (3500 cal/lb). While this figure is reasonable as an estimate for long-term changes in caloric intake, the apparent caloric cost per kilogram of weight lost or gained varies with the accompanying fluid shifts. In the experiment summarized in Table 35-1, for example, a negative balance of only 2596 cal resulted in the loss of a kilogram of weight between days 1 and 3, while between days 22 and 24, loss of a kilogram required a deficit of 8700 cal. In general if weight loss or gain has occurred over a period of weeks or months, it is safe to assume that change in tissue mass has occurred; weight loss or gain limited to a several-day period may be due to fluid shifts alone. Occasionally true loss of tissue mass is obscured by fluid retention as in the case of the cirrhotic patient who develops ascites or the patient with anorexia nervosa and edema.

WEIGHT GAIN

While obesity is a major public health concern (see Chap. 79), its diagnosis is usually uncomplicated. Obese subjects often deny overeating, but the true situation can usually be assessed either by tabulating actual food intake and determining its caloric content from standard tables or by interviewing the patient's family and friends. Regardless of history, excess caloric intake is the cause of obesity in the overwhelming majority of cases. Pathological causes of obesity are rare. In the adult, Cushing's syndrome can result in acquired obesity in a previously nonobese patient, but usually the diagnosis suggests itself by the pattern of fat distribution and the clinical picture. Other endocrine diseases such as hypothyroidism, hypogonadism, and insulin-secreting tumors are frequently listed in the differential diagnosis of obesity but do not represent significant diagnostic problems. Congenital diseases that cause obesity such as the Prader-Willi and Laurence-Moon-Biedl syndromes are usually readily recognizable and appear early in life. Rarely neoplastic disease involving the hypothalamus, particularly craniopharyngioma, may be a cause of acquired obesity. Extensive workup of the central nervous system in obesity is not indicated, however, in the absence of suspicious symptoms (headache, visual difficulties, vomiting, or endocrine changes).

WEIGHT LOSS

Weight loss in the absence of deliberate dieting is a more serious problem than weight gain because there is a high chance that organic disease is present. Mechanisms include decreased appetite, accelerated metabolism, and loss of calories in urine or stool, acting singly or in combination. No attempt will be made to list all diseases capable of causing weight loss. The majority of cases fall into one of seven categories, but in one large prospective series 35 percent of patients had no identifiable physical illness.

TABLE 35-1
Percentage composition of mean daily weight loss in 13 young men during caloric restriction for 24 days

Days	*Mean weight loss, kg/day*	*Water, %*	*Fat, %*	*Protein, %*	*Calorie equivalents of weight loss, cal/kg*
1–3	0.80	70	25	5	2596
11–13	0.23	19	69	12	7043
22–24	0.17	0	85	15	8700

SOURCE: *After Brožek et al.*

DIABETES MELLITUS Initial weight loss with the onset of diabetes is largely fluid and is due to the osmotic diuresis induced by hyperglycemia. Subsequently loss of tissue mass occurs in the insulin-dependent form of the disease due both to caloric wastage (the consequence of glycosuria) and to the hormonal abnormalities that characterize the illness. Insulin deficiency and glucagon excess result in impaired synthesis of protein and fat and simultaneously cause accelerated proteolysis and lipolysis such that the net energy state is catabolic. Weight loss in diabetes is frequently associated with increased food intake.

ENDOCRINE DISEASE The most important endocrine disease causing weight loss is thyrotoxicosis. While weight loss is not inevitable (indeed, thyrotoxicosis may rarely be found in a patient who has gained weight), it is common. Increased appetite and food intake are the rule, and patients often consume a high-carbohydrate diet. Caloric expenditure is enormous, primarily because of an increased metabolic rate, but increased motor activity also plays a role. The molecular mechanism whereby thyrotoxicosis causes weight loss is not settled, but thyroid hormone is thought to increase sodium-potassium adenosine triphosphatase (ATPase) activity in many tissues, suggesting that the diminished efficiency of ingested calories is due to a futile cycle of adenosine triphosphate (ATP) synthesis and breakdown with energy lost as heat. Another cause of weight loss due to hypermetabolism is pheochromocytoma, the inducing agent being catecholamine release. Panhypopituitarism and adrenal insufficiency may also be associated with weight loss, largely as a consequence of diminished appetite secondary to cortisol deficiency.

GASTROINTESTINAL DISEASE A variety of gastrointestinal diseases may cause weight loss. Overt or occult steatorrhea due to sprue, chronic pancreatitis, or cystic fibrosis may produce wasting despite major increases in food intake. Chronic diarrhea due to inflammatory bowel disease (with or without fistulas) or parasites, esophageal disease with reflux or vomiting, even ordinary peptic ulcer have to be considered in the differential diagnosis. The mechanism of weight loss in alimentary tract disease is generally either decreased food intake or malabsorption, though inflammation per se probably plays a major role in ulcerative colitis and regional enteritis.

INFECTION Hidden infection must always be sought in patients with unexplained weight loss. Tuberculosis, fungal diseases, amebic abscess, and subacute bacterial endocarditis should be high on the list of suspects. The mechanism probably involves both anorexia and inflammation-induced acceleration of cellular metabolic demands. It has been suggested that glucagon plays a major role in the induction of negative nitrogen balance and tissue wastage in inflammation, but it is likely that the catabolic state also requires changes in a number of other hormones.

MALIGNANCY Occult malignancy is probably the most common cause of weight loss in the absence of major signs and symptoms. In the search for malignancy particular emphasis must be placed on the gastrointestinal tract, pancreas, and liver. Lymphoma and leukemia should also be considered. While silent (except for weight loss) malignancy can occur in any organ, the gastrointestinal tract is the most common site.

PSYCHIATRIC DISEASE The classic psychiatric illness associated with profound weight loss is anorexia nervosa (Chap. 80). However, anorexia may also occur in depressive states and schizophrenia. The presence of anorexia is usually clear from the history. While organic disease causing both anorexia and depression has to be ruled out, ordinarily the psychiatric nature of the problem will be clear.

RENAL DISEASE One of the earliest manifestations of uremia is anorexia. As a consequence all patients with unexplained weight loss should be given screening renal function tests.

SUMMARY

Weight loss is more often a diagnostic problem than weight gain and more often a sign of serious organic illness. If the weight loss is associated with increased food intake, the diagnosis will likely be diabetes, thyrotoxicosis, or malabsorption. If food intake is normal or decreased, malignancy, infection, renal disease, psychiatric syndromes, or endocrine deficiency are more common.

REFERENCES

Brožek J et al: Changes in body weight and body dimensions in men performing work on a low calorie carbohydrate diet. J Appl Physiol 10:412, 1957

Konishi F: Food energy equivalents of various activities. J Am Diet Assoc 46:186, 1965

Marton KI et al: Involuntary weight loss: Diagnostic and prognostic significance. Ann Intern Med 95:568, 1981

Runcie J, Hilditch TE: Energy provision, tissue utilization and weight loss in prolonged starvation. Br Med J 2:352, 1974

Yang M-U, Van Itallie TB: Composition of weight loss during short-term weight reduction. Metabolic responses of obese subjects to starvation and low calorie ketogenic and non-ketogenic diets. J Clin Invest 58:722, 1976

36 CONSTIPATION, DIARRHEA, AND DISTURBANCES OF ANORECTAL FUNCTION

STEPHEN E. GOLDFINGER

NORMAL COLONIC FUNCTION Each day approximately 9 liters of fluid enters the digestive tract; 2 liters represents ingested fluids and the remainder comes from salivary, gastric, biliary, pancreatic, and intestinal secretions that are needed to provide an appropriate milieu for food digestion. Most of this fluid is absorbed in the upper bowel. A residual of approximately 1 liter containing undigested dietary residue and cellular debris passes across the ileocecal valve to the colon. Little of nutritional value remains following the extensive digestive processing and absorption that occurs in the small intestine. The colon's principal function is to convert this liquid ileal effluent to solid feces before it is advanced to the rectum and evacuated. Several important physiologic processes underlie normal colonic function; among these are *absorption* of fluid and electrolytes; *peristaltic contractions* that facilitate mixing, dessication, and passage of feces to the rectum; and, finally, *defecation*.

Absorption of fluid and electrolytes (see also Chap. 308) In western societies where dietary fiber content is relatively low, the average daily stool weight is less than 200 g, of which 60 to 80 percent is water. Thus, the colon normally absorbs approximately 80 to 90 percent of the fluid it receives, and this occurs well within its absorptive capacity of 6 liters water and 800 meq sodium per day. Fluid and electrolyte absorption occurs primarily in the ascending and transverse colon. Water absorption occurs passively, osmotically following the active transport of sodium and chloride ions. In addition, bicarbonate is secreted in exchange for chloride, and sodium is reabsorbed in exchange for potassium. The secreted bicarbonate is converted, in part, to carbon dioxide by reacting with acids produced by colonic bacteria. Analysis of fecal electrolyte concentration in normal subjects reveals considerable variation, but average values for sodium, potassium, chloride, and bicarbonate are 32, 75, 16, and 40 meq per liter, respectively. The hyperosmolality of normal stool, which averages 375 mosmol, is largely due to osmotically active organic compounds produced by bacteria.

The term *diarrhea* generally connotes *frequent* or *loose* stools. Based on physiologic events described above, diarrhea may be defined more quantitatively as a fecal output exceeding 200 g per day when dietary fiber content is low. Diarrhea can be further classified on the basis of underlying mechanisms (see Table 36-1). In *secretory diarrhea*, fecal fluid rich in sodium and potassium is lost as a consequence of impaired absorption and/or excessive secretion of electrolytes by the bowel. In *osmotic diarrhea*, absorption of water is decreased by the osmotic effect of nonabsorbable, intraluminal molecules. *Exudative diarrhea* is caused by an outpouring of necrotic mucosa, colloid, fluid, and electrolytes from an inflamed colon which, in addition, is less able to carry out its normal absorp-

TABLE 36-1
Classification of diarrhea

Type	*Mechanism*	*Stool characteristics*	*Examples*
Secretory	↓ absorption of electrolytes; ↑ secretion of electrolyte	Clear $Na^+ + K^+ \simeq 2 \times$ osmolality No polymorphs	Cholera Toxigenic *E. coli* enteritis Diarrheogenic islet cell tumors Bile salt enteropathy
Osmotic	Nonabsorbable intraluminal molecules	Clear $Na^+ + K^+ < 2 \times$ osmolality No polymorphs	Lactase deficiency Mg^{2+} containing cathartics Unabsorbed carbohydrates in malabsorption states
Exudative	Impaired colonic absorption; outpouring of cells and colloid; mucosal sloughing	Purulent Polymorphs present Gross or occult blood	Ulcerative colitis Shigellosis Amebiasis Pseudomembranous colitis
Anatomical derangement	Decreased absorption surface	Variable	Subtotal colectomy Major small bowel resection Inadvertent gastroileostomy

tive function. *Anatomical derangements* of the bowel that reduce absorptive surface area may also cause diarrhea.

Motility (contraction) patterns of the colon The colon and rectum are innervated by fibers that release norepinephrine, acetylcholine, and a variety of other neurotransmitters, which may include bioactive amines, peptides, and nucleotides. Signals transmitted by autonomic nervous system fibers originating centrally, local reflex arcs confined to the autonomous "enteric nervous system," and intrinsic contractile responses of smooth muscle all play a part in the coordination of colonic motility. Parasympathetic nerves, which stimulate peristaltic contraction, dominate the neurogenic regulation of colonic motor activity; adrenergic tone inhibits cholinergic stimulation. The precise integration of all neural and nonneural mediators of colonic motility remains poorly understood.

Basal colonic motor activity relates to the function of the various colonic segments. In the ascending colon, where most fluid absorption occurs, rhythmic, retrograde contractions occur to promote prolonged fecal retention. In the midcolon, segmental contractions continue the process of absorption while feces are gradually advanced to the left colon. The most distal portion of the colon, which is under the greatest neurogenic control, propels feces caudally in preparation for defecation. In addition, massive peristalsis occurs several times per day, with resulting rectal distention stimulating the defecatory urge.

Since colonic motility plays an important role in both absorption and movement of contents to the rectum, alterations of bowel tone occurring as a result of disease, stress, or various drugs tend to have an important influence on bowel movements. In view of the number of pharmacologic agents that may influence smooth-muscle contractility, it is essential to take a careful drug history when evaluating patients with constipation or diarrhea of recent onset.

Defecation The defecatory reflex is initiated by acute distention of the rectum. When it is allowed to progress by supraspinal centers, sigmoidal and rectal contractions heighten the pressure within the rectum and also obliterate the rectosigmoidal angle. Concomitant relaxation of the internal and external anal sphincters then permits the evacuation of feces. This can be augmented by an increase in intraabdominal pressure created by the Valsalva maneuver (i.e., voluntary closure of the glottis, diaphragmatic fixation, and abdominal-wall contraction). Conversely, defecation may be consciously prevented by the voluntary contraction of the striated muscles of the pelvic diaphragm and external anal sphincter. The functional value of voluntary control of defecation requires little elaboration, but the opportunity for individuals to resist the defecatory urge, when abused, may lead to chronic rectal distention, reduced afferent signals, lax motor tone, and chronic constipation.

DIARRHEA AND CONSTIPATION The bowel habits of apparently healthy persons vary widely. For this reason, the terms *diarrhea* and *constipation* have most meaning when viewed as a change from an individual's customary pattern. Reasonably detailed information is important in evaluating either abnormality. When patients complain of diarrhea, it is important to obtain an estimate of the volume as well as frequency of fecal output and, in addition, to examine directly a stool sample for consistency, blood, oiliness, and malodor. For example, the repeated elimination of small quantities of solid material admixed with gas, so typical in the irritable bowel syndrome, has a far different connotation than the same number of movements of liquid, blood-tinged feces. The term *constipation* may be used by the patient to refer to a variety of changes including reduction in frequency of defecation, a constant sensation of rectal fullness with incomplete evacuation of feces, and some-

times painful defecation due to hard stools or perianal pathology. Excessively hard stools are usually due to increased absorption of fluid as a result of prolonged contact of the luminal contents with the colonic mucosa consequent to delayed transit. In some instances ingested material such as calcium carbonate can explain "rocklike" feces. In an assessment of complaints of diarrhea or constipation, it is important to consider the patient's emotional state since in many instances the recent onset of psychological stress is the major reason for altered bowel habits. However, it can be hazardous to assume this to be the case, even when the relationship seems convincing. For this reason, the judicious use of laboratory, proctoscopic, and radiologic procedures is recommended to make certain that organic disease will not be overlooked.

Acute diarrhea Diarrhea of abrupt onset occurring in otherwise healthy persons is most often related to an infectious process. A variety of accompanying symptoms are often observed, including fever, headache, anorexia, vomiting, malaise, and myalgia, but they cannot be used to distinguish with certainty among viral, bacterial, and protozoal causes. Because bacterial and protozoal pathogens are usually not recovered from the feces, so-called nonspecific diarrhea is often considered to be of viral etiology. However, the demonstration of enterotoxins produced by strains of *Escherichia coli*, which are not distinguishable from "normal flora" on routine culture, suggests that these bacteria may account for a number of cases that are usually ascribed to viral infection.

Acute diarrhea presumed to be of viral etiology typically persists for a period of 1 to 3 days; death is extremely rare except in previously debilitated individuals who become severely dehydrated. When human volunteers have been infected with the Norwalk virus, which is believed to account for approximately one-third of epidemics of acute viral diarrhea in adults, transient malabsorption of fat and xylose has been described. Changes in the small intestine include abnormalities of intestinal cell morphology such as villous shortening, an increase in the number of crypt cells, and increased cellularity of the lamina propria. The colonic mucosa is unaffected in viral diarrhea; this is consistent with the absence of polymorphonuclear leukocytes when fresh stool is examined microscopically after preparation with Loeffler's methylene blue.

Bacterial diarrhea may be suspected if there is a history of a similar and simultaneous illness in individuals who have shared contaminated food with the patient. Diarrhea developing within 12 h of the meal is most likely due to ingestion of a preformed toxin (e.g., staphylococcal exotoxin). A lag period of up to 3 days after consumption of contaminated food can occur with salmonellosis. The pathogenesis of bacterial diarrhea is due to two principal mechanisms, *mucosal invasion* and *enterotoxin-induced hypersecretion*. Bacterial invasion of the colonic wall leads to mucosal hyperemia, edema, leukocytic infiltration, and frank ulceration. Lower abdominal cramps and tenderness are prominent, as are tenesmus and rectal urgency. In severe cases the stool is grossly bloody. At other times, microscopic examination of the stool will reveal erythrocytes along with pus cells. In *shigellosis*, diarrhea is mainly due to mucosal destruction by the invading microorganisms, but small-intestinal hypersecretion may also occur in the early stage of enteritis caused by some enterotoxin-producing strains of *Shigella*. The prototype of hypersecretory bacterial diarrhea is *cholera*, in which the organism *Vibrio cholerae* adheres to, but does not invade, the surface epithelial cells and releases an enterotoxin which stimulates massive secretion of fluid and electrolytes by the small intestine. This may be produced experimentally in animals by placing the enterotoxin, free of the organism itself, into isolated intestinal loops. Hypersecretion reaches a peak at 4 to 6 h and is mediated by the stimulation of mucosal adenylate cyclase by the toxin. It should be emphasized that in cholera, mucosal morphology is essentially normal and intestinal absorptive capacity is preserved. This provides the basis for oral rehydration therapy with solutions containing glucose and sodium chloride, the former stimulating absorption of the latter. Because other species of bacteria, such as *E. coli, Clostridium,* and *Salmonella*, have been shown to produce enterotoxins, the finding of an exudate-free stool does not preclude bacterial infection as the cause of diarrhea.

Protozoal infections may also be responsible for acute diarrhea. *Entamoeba histolytica*, prevalent in some areas of the United States and in the homosexual male population, produces an inflammatory colitis which can closely mimic idiopathic ulcerative colitis. Giardiasis is a cause of prolonged, watery diarrhea that often afflicts travelers returning from endemic areas where the water supply has been contaminated. Careful examination of fresh stools by experienced technicians is required for the diagnosis of protozoal infection. Duodenal samples in the form of aspirate and biopsy touch preparations may be necessary to make the diagnosis of giardiasis.

Travelers' diarrhea may result from any one or several of the pathogens described above. When no specific agent is identified, the etiology is usually assumed to be due to enterotoxin-producing coliform organisms or viruses; both Norwalk virus and rotavirus have been implicated. Not infrequently prolonged bowel irregularity will occur following the acute illness.

Ulcerative colitis and *regional enteritis* (Crohn's disease) may begin as acute diarrhea (Chap. 309). Bloody stools and generalized abdominal cramping and tenderness are more apt to occur in the patients with ulcerative colitis; in regional enteritis the diarrhea tends to be milder, is often nonbloody, and is associated with right lower quadrant pain and tenderness. Diarrhea may be caused by a variety of *drugs*, including cholinergic agents, magnesium-containing antacids, antimetabolites used in cancer chemotherapy, and many antibiotics. A necrolytic toxin produced by *Clostridium difficile* has been shown to be the cause of pseudomembranous colitis occurring during or after antibiotic use. Diarrhea due to *diverticulitis* is usually accompanied by fever, tenesmus, and rectal urgency, together with cramps and tenderness in the left lower quadrant (Chap. 310). When there is no evidence of acute inflammation, diarrhea in the presence of colonic diverticula is probably due to a spastic (irritable) colon, a disorder which may set the stage for the development of diverticula. In elderly and debilitated individuals with *fecal impaction,* the presenting symptom may be the frequent expulsion of small amounts of liquid stool overflowing from colonic distention behind the impaction. Fecal incontinence due to anal sphincter impairment is a problem that may be encountered in certain neurologic disorders or following local surgical procedures (e.g., hemorrhoidectomy, episiotomy). Acute *psychological stress* can cause diarrhea at any age.

DIAGNOSTIC APPROACH The appropriate tempo and approach in the evaluation of acute diarrhea depend so heavily on the clinical setting in which it occurs that only very general guidelines can be offered. It is entirely reasonable to withhold studies in mild, self-limited cases such as are seen as part of an epidemic viral illness. When dealing with sporadic severe diarrhea or when a suggestive epidemiologic history is obtained, bacterial cultures and microscopic examination of the stool for parasites and inflammatory cells are appropriate. Proctoscopy is generally reserved for patients with bloody diarrhea, or those who do not show improvement within 5 days. Likewise, radiologic studies should usually be deferred until the initial course of the illness has been observed. In cases of massive fluid loss, measurement of serum electrolytes is useful to aid in determining replacement therapy.

TREATMENT General and nonspecific treatment of acute diarrhea includes rest, encouragement of fluid intake, and prescription of opiate-containing agents by mouth. Intravenous fluid and electrolyte replacement may be desirable and necessary in infants and the elderly. As a result of success achieved with cholera patients, the use of oral glucose-electrolyte solutions is being extended to the treatment of patients with acute diarrhea considered to be due to other enterotoxin-producing bacteria.

Chronic diarrhea Diarrhea persisting for weeks or months, whether constant or intermittent, may be a functional symptom or a manifestation of serious illness. For this reason, it is incumbent upon the physician to search carefully for evidence of organic disease, such as fever, weight loss, malnutrition, or anemia. Abdominal tenderness and fever suggest the presence of inflammation. When there is involvement of the large bowel, the major diseases to be considered include ulcerative colitis, Crohn's disease of the colon, amebiasis, and diverticulitis. Crohn's disease of the small intestine may involve one or more of its segments. The ileum is most frequently affected. Other diarrheal conditions which may resemble Crohn's disease radiographically include tuberculous and fungal enteritis, lymphosarcoma, amyloidosis, and argentaffin (carcinoid) tumors of the small bowel.

Prolonged diarrhea without evidence of inflammation may reflect impairments of absorption, secretion, or digestion. Selective derangements, such as those due to *bile salt enteropathy* and *lactase deficiency,* are usually not accompanied by weight loss or malnutrition. *Mucosal disorders,* best exemplified by sprue, are frequently associated with weight loss, malodorous stools, abdominal distention, and anemia, and, when more severe, with osteomalacia, hypoprothrombinemia, avitaminotic neuropathies, and tetany. *Pancreatic insufficiency* resulting from chronic pancreatitis, carcinoma, or resection produces steatorrhea and weight loss of varying severity. A number of mechanisms may be responsible for *postgastrectomy diarrhea* (see Chap. 306). These include the dumping syndrome, postvagotomy motility derangements, inadequate stimulation of pancreatic digestive enzymes, and incomplete mixing of these enzymes with food. On rare occasions severe postgastrectomy diarrhea and malnutrition are due to the inadvertent creation by the surgeon of a gastroileostomy instead of a gastrojejunostomy. *Bacterial overgrowth* in the small intestine, as may occur with extensive diverticulosis and prolonged bowel stasis secondary to disorders of peristalsis (e.g., scleroderma, diabetic visceral neuropathy), can also lead to chronic diarrhea and weight loss. This has been attributed to bacterial deconjugation of bile salts and hydroxylation of long-chain fatty acids, to consumption of nutrients by the organisms, and to mucosal abnormalities believed to be caused by bacteria or their metabolites (see Chap. 308). At times, diarrhea may accompany stasis in the absence of bacterial overgrowth.

Endocrine disorders that may be accompanied by chronic diarrhea include thyrotoxicosis, diabetes mellitus, adrenal insufficiency, and hypoparathyroidism. The release of potent secretagogues from neoplastic tissue in the Zollinger-Ellison syndrome (gastrin), medullary carcinoma of the thyroid (calcitonin, prostaglandins), and pancreatic cholera syndrome (vasoactive intestinal peptide) makes diarrhea a prominent feature of these disorders. The passage of excessive amounts of clear liquid, at times sufficient to cause dehydration, occurs in some patients with large villous adenomas of the rectum.

Habitual *cathartic abuse* must be suspected when the cause of prolonged diarrhea remains perplexing. Even if this is denied by the patient, a stool sample should be alkalinized with sodium hydroxide; this will produce a red color if phenolphthalein-containing laxatives have been surreptitiously ingested. The observation of melanosis coli by sigmoidoscopy indicates chronic usage of anthraquinone laxatives.

Constipation Constipation is a common complaint often resulting from the inordinate expectation of "regularity" in bowel-conscious individuals. Stools are described as infrequent, incomplete, or unduly hard; unusual straining may be required to achieve defecation. A review of the patient's habits often reveals contributory and correctable causes, such as insufficient dietary roughage, lack of exercise, suppression of defecatory urges arising at inconvenient moments, inadequate allotment of time for full defecation, and prolonged travel. Appropriate adjustments of these patterns and reassurance are preferable to the prescription of laxatives and may be all that is required for improvement. When the patient also has symptoms such as fatigue, malaise, headaches, or anorexia, the possibility should be considered that such symptoms reflect an underlying depression of which constipation is but one component. Decreased colonic motility is responsible for the constipation associated with the use of parasympatholytic drugs, spinal cord injury, scleroderma, and Hirschsprung's disease.

Hemorrhoids, anal fissures, perineal abscesses, and rectal strictures often prevent easy and adequate stool evacuation. When constipation and tenesmus of recent onset are reported, the possibility of carcinoma of the rectum or descending colon must be seriously considered. In such instances sigmoidoscopic and barium enema examinations should be obtained early and are virtually obligatory if fecal blood has been observed or if occult blood is detected on any of three successive stool specimens. Stools of abnormally thin caliber occur in patients with rectal or sigmoid colon carcinoma but are even more commonly due to an irritable colon. Other mechanical causes of constipation include volvulus of the sigmoid colon, diverticulitis, intussusception, and hernias. A variety of metabolic abnormalities, such as hypothyroidism, hypercalcemia, hypokalemia, porphyria, lead poisoning, and dehydration are often associated with constipation. Tremendous fecal retention and impaction may occur in certain neurologic disorders (e.g., spinal cord injury, multiple sclerosis, cerebral palsy, senility), and in these instances, when autonomous regulation of evacuation is unachievable, vigorous and sustained enema programs are often necessary.

IRRITABLE BOWEL The irritable bowel syndrome (also referred to as *spastic colon* and *mucous colitis*) is one of the most frequent gastrointestinal disorders (see Chap. 310). This condition is characterized by periodic or chronic bowel symptoms which include diarrhea, constipation, and abdominal pain. These symptoms are often associated with psychiatric illness, but the anxiety produced by the bowel disturbance is sometimes regarded by the patient as the fundamental cause of the emotional upset. During periods of discomfort, stools are apt to become thin, fragmented, or pelletlike, and accompanied by excessive mucus and gas. Efforts to ameliorate symptoms with mild cathartics or antispasmodic drugs may yield adverse and exaggerated responses. A variety of therapeutic approaches, including the avoidance of foods which tend to upset the patient, addition of bulk-forming agents, judicious use of antispasmodics and tranquilizers, and psychotherapy may provide some relief. If the patient's life goals can be shifted away from the quixotic search for the perfect stool, much can be accomplished. At the same time, it must be remembered that such individuals are not exempt from developing bowel cancer, and any worrisome deviation from their general pattern of derangement must be seriously evaluated.

FLATULENCE A significant amount of flatus is passed each day by normal persons, and the complaint of flatulence often reflects a heightened and embarrassing awareness of this natural occurrence. Excessive quantities of flatus may be caused by aerophagia or the formation of increased amounts of gas by intestinal bacteria. The latter process can be associated with malabsorption syndromes but is more frequently a consequence of eating foods such as beans, broccoli, and cabbage which have a high content of nondigestible polysaccharides. The oligosaccharides stachyose and raffinose, isolated from beans, are particularly effective substrates for fermentation to carbon dioxide, hydrogen, and methane by colonic flora. Chromatographic analysis of a sample of flatus will show these gases to predominate, in contrast to the high nitrogen levels that occur when excessive flatus is caused by aerophagia. The treatment of flatulence is generally undertaken to reduce embarrassment and consists of measures to decrease aerophagia along with avoidance of foods that cause excessive gas.

REFERENCES

Blacklow NR, Cukor GC: Viral gastroenteritis. N Engl J Med 304:397, 1981

Christensen J: Motility of the colon, in *Physiology of the Gastrointestinal Tract,* LR Johnson et al (eds). New York, Raven Press, 1981, vol 1, chap 14

Debongnie JC, Phillips SF: Capacity of the human colon to absorb fluid. Gastroenterology 74:698, 1978

Drossman DA et al: The irritable bowel syndrome. Gastroenterology 73:811, 1977

Field M, Fordtran S, Schultz SG (eds): *Secretory Diarrhea,* Clinical Physiology Series. Bethesda, Md., American Physiological Society, 1980

Gershon MD, Erde SM: The nervous system of the gut. Gastroenterology 80:1571, 1981

Plotkin GR et al: Gastroenteritis: Etiology, pathophysiology and clinical manifestations. Medicine 58:95, 1979

Read NW et al: Chronic diarrhea of unknown origin. Gastroenterology 78:2644, 1980

Schultz SG: Ion transport by mammalian large intestine, in *Physiology of the Gastrointestinal Tract,* LR Johnson et al (eds). New York, Raven Press, 1981, vol 2, chap 38

37
HEMATEMESIS, MELENA, AND HEMATOCHEZIA

KURT J. ISSELBACHER
JAMES M. RICHTER

Hematemesis is defined as the vomiting of blood, and *melena* as the passage of stools rendered black and tarry by the presence of altered blood. These symptoms of gastrointestinal hemorrhage should bring the patient to medical attention and, within certain limits, suggest the anatomic site of bleeding. Exsanguinating gastrointestinal hemorrhage will rarely occur without the appearance of altered or gross blood passed by mouth or rectum. The color of vomited blood will vary depending on the concentration of hydrochloric acid in the stomach and its admixture with the blood. Thus, if vomiting occurs shortly after the onset of bleeding, the vomitus appears red; if there is a delay in vomiting, the appearance will be dark red, brown, or black. Precipitated blood clots in the vomitus will produce a characteristic "coffee grounds" appearance. Hematemesis usually indicates bleeding proximal to the ligament of Treitz, since blood entering the gastrointestinal tract below the duodenum rarely reenters the stomach.

While bleeding sufficient to produce hematemesis usually results in melena, less than half of patients with melena have hematemesis. *Melena* usually denotes bleeding from the esophagus, stomach, or duodenum, but lesions in the jejunum, ileum, and even ascending colon may cause melena provided the gastrointestinal transit time is sufficiently prolonged. Approximately 60 ml of blood is required to produce a single black stool; acute blood loss greater than this may produce melena for up to 3 days. After the stool color returns to normal, tests for occult blood may remain positive for up to a week or longer.

The black color of stools secondary to intestinal bleeding results from contact of the blood with hydrochloric acid to produce hematin. Characteristically, such stools are tarry ("sticky"). This tarry consistency is in contrast to black or dark stools occurring after the ingestion of iron, bismuth, or licorice. Similarly, red stools may result from the ingestion of beets or intravenous administration of sulfobromophthalein. Gastrointestinal bleeding, even if detected only by positive tests for occult blood, indicates potentially serious disease and must be further investigated.

Hematochezia, the passage of bright red blood per rectum, generally signifies bleeding from a source distal to the ligament of Treitz. However, since blood must remain in the gut for approximately 8 h to produce melena, rapid hemorrhage into the esophagus, stomach, or duodenum may also result in hematochezia.

The clinical manifestations of gastrointestinal bleeding depend upon the extent and rate of hemorrhage, and the presence of coincidental diseases. Blood loss of less than 500 ml is rarely associated with systemic signs; exceptions include bleeding in the elderly or in the anemic patient in whom smaller amounts of blood loss may produce hemodynamic alterations. Rapid hemorrhage of greater volume results in decreased venous return to the heart, decreased cardiac output, and increased peripheral resistance due to reflex vasoconstriction. Orthostatic hypotension greater than 10 mmHg usually indicates a 20 percent or greater reduction in blood volume. Concomitant symptoms include syncope, lightheadedness, nausea, sweating, and thirst. When blood loss approaches 40 percent of blood volume, shock frequently ensues with pronounced tachycardia and hypotension. Pallor is prominent, and the skin is cool.

It is important to recognize that the hematocrit, when determined immediately after the onset of bleeding, may not accurately reflect blood loss, since equilibration with extravascular fluid and hemodilution require several hours. Common laboratory findings include mild leukocytosis and thrombocytosis which develop within 6 h after the onset of bleeding. The blood urea nitrogen may be mildly elevated, particularly in upper gastrointestinal bleeding, due to breakdown of blood proteins to urea by intestinal bacteria as well as from a mild reduction in the glomerular filtration rate.

ETIOLOGY OF UPPER GASTROINTESTINAL BLEEDING A careful history and physical examination of the oropharynx should serve to exclude swallowed blood as a source of hematemesis or melena.

The three most common causes of upper gastrointestinal hemorrhage are (1) peptic ulceration, (2) erosive gastritis, and (3) variceal bleeding. These entities account for up to 90 percent of all cases of upper gastrointestinal hemorrhage in which a definite lesion can be found.

Peptic ulcer Peptic ulcer is probably the most common cause of upper gastrointestinal bleeding; the majority of such ulcers are found in the duodenum. Approximately 20 to 30 percent of patients with documented ulcers will have significant bleeding sometime during the course of their disease. Since hemorrhage may be the initial manifestation of a peptic ulcer, this lesion should be seriously considered even when a history characteristic of ulcer disease is not obtained.

Gastritis Gastritis may be associated with recent alcohol ingestion or with the use of anti-inflammatory drugs, such as aspirin or indomethacin. Gastric erosions also frequently develop in patients with major trauma, surgery, and severe systemic disease, particularly burn victims and patients with increased intracranial pressure. Since there are no characteristic physical findings, the diagnosis of gastritis must be suspected when the appropriate clinical setting is encountered. Gastroscopy is usually needed to confirm the diagnosis since radiologic examination generally lacks the sensitivity required to detect gastritis.

Variceal bleeding Variceal bleeding is characteristically abrupt and massive; chronic gastrointestinal blood loss is unusual. Bleeding from esophageal or gastric varices is usually the result of portal hypertension, secondary to hepatic cirrhosis. Although alcoholic cirrhosis is the most prevalent cause of esophageal varices in the United States, any condition producing portal hypertension, even in the absence of hepatic disease (i.e., portal vein thrombosis or idiopathic portal hypertension), may result in variceal bleeding. Further, while the presence of varices usually connotes long-standing portal hypertension, acute hepatitis or severe fatty infiltration of the liver may occasionally produce varices which disappear once the hepatic abnormality resolves. It should be emphasized that although upper gastrointestinal bleeding in a patient with cirrhosis suggests a variceal source, approximately half those patients will be bleeding from other lesions (e.g., gastritis, ulcers). Consequently, it is essential to exclude nonvariceal causes of bleeding so that the appropriate treatment can be instituted. Finally, since varices may occur at any site in the gastrointestinal tract, angiography may be required to identify hemorrhage from varices distal to the duodenum.

Other lesions With the advent of esophagogastroduodenoscopy, the Mallory-Weiss syndrome has been demonstrated with increasing frequency as a cause of acute upper gastrointestinal hemorrhage. This syndrome refers to laceration in the region of the esophagogastric junction characterized historically by retching or nonbloody vomiting followed by hematemesis. Less common bleeding esophageal lesions include esophagitis (with or without hiatus hernia) and carcinoma; these generally cause chronic blood loss and rarely produce massive bleeding.

Gastric carcinoma may result in chronic gastrointestinal bleeding. Lymphoma, polyps, and other tumors of the stomach and small bowel are uncommon and, consequently, are infrequent causes of hemorrhage. Leiomyoma and leiomyosarcoma are likewise rare, but they can lead to massive hemorrhage. Bleeding from duodenal and jejunal diverticula is relatively unusual. Vascular insufficiency of the mesenteric vessels, including occlusive and nonocclusive disease, may lead to bloody diarrhea.

Arteriosclerotic aortic aneurysms may rupture into the small intestine; such an event is almost always fatal. Rupture may also occur following arterial reconstructive surgery with fistula formation between synthetic graft and bowel lumen. Sudden bleeding may also occur after trauma resulting in hepatic laceration; this may result in blood loss into the bile ducts (i.e., hemobilia).

Primary blood dyscrasias, including leukemia, thrombocytopenic states, the hemophilias, and disseminated intravascular coagulation may result in significant gastrointestinal bleeding. Polycythemia vera, although associated with an increased incidence of peptic ulceration, may also result in gastrointestinal bleeding due to mesenteric or portal vein thrombosis. Periarteritis nodosa, Henoch-Schönlein purpura, and other forms of vasculitis may lead to gastrointestinal blood loss.

Mild gastrointestinal bleeding may be seen with amyloidosis, Osler-Weber-Rendu disease, pseudoxanthoma elasticum, Turner's syndrome, intestinal hemangiomas, neurofibromatosis, Kaposi's sarcoma, and Peutz-Jeghers syndrome. Uremia may produce gastrointestinal blood loss; the most common presentation is chronic, occult bleeding from diffuse involvement of the mucosa of the stomach and small bowel.

ETIOLOGY OF LOWER GASTROINTESTINAL BLEEDING Anal and rectal lesions Small amounts of bright red blood on the surface of the stool and toilet tissue are often caused by hemorrhoids; such bleeding is generally precipitated by the strained passage of a hard stool. Anal fissures and fistulas may present in a similar fashion. Proctitis is another source of rectal bleeding; it is frequently seen in young adults, especially in male homosexuals. In the latter situation, proctitis may be nonspecific or due to gonorrheal infection. Rectal trauma is a cause of hematochezia, and the placement of foreign objects in the rectal vault may precipitate perforation as well as acute rectal hemorrhage. It must be emphasized that anal pathology does not preclude other sources of blood loss, and these must be sought and excluded.

Colonic lesions Carcinoma of the colon, as well as colonic polyps, may produce chronic blood loss. Frankly bloody diarrhea is common and may be the presenting symptom in patients with ulcerative colitis; it is less frequent in granulomatous colitis, but occult blood may be present in the stool. Bleeding may also accompany diarrhea due to infections such as shigellosis, amebiasis, campylobacterosis, and rarely, salmonellosis. In the elderly patient, ischemic colitis may be a cause of bloody diarrhea; this lesion may also be seen in the younger age group associated with the use of oral contraceptive agents. Angiodysplastic lesions, usually involving the ascending colon, can be a major source of bleeding in elderly patients; such vascular lesions can be identified by angiography or colonoscopy.

Diverticula Colonic diverticula are most often located in the sigmoid colon; however, most episodes of diverticular bleeding originate in the ascending colon. Bleeding from colonic diverticula is one of the most common causes of massive lower gastrointestinal hemorrhage. The usual presentation of a diverticular hemorrhage is that of painless passage of a maroon-colored stool. Mild blood loss is more often associated with diverticulitis. Meckel's diverticulum, a congenital anomaly of the distal ileum, is present in about 2 percent of the population and may cause bleeding. Although only about 15 percent of these diverticula contain gastric mucosa, the lesions which cause acute bleeding contain gastric mucosa half the time. This anomaly is an important cause of acute hemorrhage in children and young adults.

APPROACH TO THE PATIENT WITH GASTROINTESTINAL BLEEDING The approach to the bleeding patient depends upon the site, extent, and rate of bleeding. Patients with hematemesis have usually bled greater amounts (often greater than 1000 ml) than those who have melena alone (usually 500 ml or less), and mortality with the former is about twice that of the latter. When first seen, the patient may be in shock. Prior to taking a history and performing a thorough physical examination, vital signs should be noted, blood sent for typing and cross-matching, and a large-bore intravenous line placed for infusion of saline or other plasma expanders. The physician initiating the evaluation of the bleeding patient must be aware that the primary consideration is the necessity of maintaining adequate intravascular volume and hemodynamic stability during the diagnostic workup.

History A history of prior ulcer disease or symptoms suggestive thereof may provide a useful clue. Similarly, recent abuse of alcohol or ingestion of anti-inflammatory drugs should make erosive gastritis more suspect. If alcohol abuse has been long-standing, esophageal varices may be a more likely source of hemorrhage. Aspirin use may also cause bleeding by aggravating a preexisting lesion (e.g., peptic ulceration). Prior history of gastrointestinal bleeding may be helpful, as may a family history of intestinal disease or hemorrhagic diathesis. Recent retching followed by hematemesis should suggest the possibility of the Mallory-Weiss syndrome. The acute onset of bloody diarrhea may indicate the presence of inflammatory bowel disease or infectious involvement of the colon. It is also important to exclude associated systemic illnesses or recent trauma, since bleeding from erosive gastritis is frequently seen under such conditions.

Physical examination Following evaluation for orthostatic changes in pulse and blood pressure and institution of volume repletion, the patient should be examined for clues to the underlying illness. A nonintestinal bleeding source should be excluded by careful examination of the nasopharynx. Dermatologic examination may disclose the characteristic telangiectasia of Osler-Weber-Rendu disease (although these will not be visible if severe anemia is present), the perioral pigmentation of Peutz-Jeghers syndrome, the dermal fibromas of neurofibromatosis, the sebaceous cysts and bony tumors of Gardner's syndrome, the palpable purpura frequently seen with vasculitis, or the diffuse pigmentation seen in hemochromatosis. Stigmata of chronic liver disease such as spider angiomata, gynecomastia, testicular atrophy, jaundice, ascites, and hepatosplenomegaly should suggest portal hypertension resulting in bleeding from esophageal or gastric varices. Significant lymph node enlargement or abdominal masses may reflect underlying intraabdominal malignancy. Careful rectal examination is important to exclude local pathology as well as to observe the color of the stool.

Laboratory studies Initial studies should include the hematocrit, hemoglobin, careful assessment of red blood cell morphologic features (hypochromic, microcytic red blood cells suggest that blood loss is chronic), white blood cell count, differential, and platelet count. Prothrombin time, partial thromboplastin time, and other coagulation studies may be in order to exclude primary or secondary clotting defects. A radiograph of the abdomen is rarely helpful in establishing a diagnosis unless a perforated viscus is suspected. Though the initial studies are valuable and essential, repeated evaluation of the laboratory data is important as one follows the clinical course of the bleeding.

Diagnostic and therapeutic approach The diagnostic approach to the patient with gastrointestinal hemorrhage must be individualized. The initial management of gastrointestinal bleeding may be under the direction of the internist, but it is prudent to consult a surgeon in the event that the bleeding cannot be controlled by medical means.

When there is a history of melena or hematemesis or the suspicion of bleeding from the upper part of the gastrointestinal tract, the patient should have a nasogastric tube passed to empty the stomach and to determine whether the bleeding is in the upper part of the gastrointestinal tract. If the initial nasogastric aspirate is clear, the tube should be left in place until bile-stained material appears, since active duodenal bleeding may occur with a clear nasogastric aspirate. The latter situation is due to failure of duodenal contents to reflux into the stomach secondary to pyloric irritability and spasm. If the aspirate is bile-stained and negative for occult blood, one can assume that active bleeding is not occurring in the gastroduodenal region, and the nasogastric tube can be removed.

If red blood or "coffee grounds" material is aspirated from the nasogastric tube, saline irrigation of the stomach should be initiated. Irrigation serves two purposes: it provides the clinician with an assessment of the rapidity of the bleeding, and clears the stomach of old blood prior to possible gastroscopy. Subsequent diagnostic maneuvers will depend on whether bleeding continues; this can be assessed by vital signs, transfusion requirements, and the number and consistency of stools. Most medical centers now have available experienced endoscopists as well as radiologists with facilities for selective arteriography so that it is possible to have emergency endoscopic, angiographic, and barium studies performed within hours of the patient's admission to the hospital. It must be emphasized that demonstration of a lesion in a patient with gastrointestinal bleeding should also be accompanied by evidence that this lesion is the site of bleeding.

If the nasogastric aspirate suggests that bleeding has stopped, one may proceed with either esophagogastroduodenoscopy or upper gastrointestinal barium studies. Although *endoscopy* provides a higher diagnostic yield, it has not been proved conclusively that survival is increased by early endoscopy. *Barium examination* often identifies a potential source of hemorrhage, but there are important limitations to such x-rays. First, lesions such as erosive gastritis and Mallory-Weiss lacerations are not visualized by x-ray. Second, if the patient rebleeds following a barium exam, the retained contrast material will make endoscopy difficult and angiography impossible. Clearly the approach in this setting must be individualized. The decision to employ esophagogastroduodenoscopy or barium studies will depend on several variables, including the availability of an experienced endoscopist and the condition of the patient. Some studies have shown that emergency endoscopy and a vigorous diagnostic approach do not generally decrease patient morbidity or mortality. However, emergency endoscopy may be important in planning therapy in certain patients with cirrhosis or previous gastric surgery. Newer techniques for coagulation of bleeding ulcers or sclerosis of varices via the endoscope may broaden the indications for and utility of early endoscopy in the future.

Persistent upper gastrointestinal hemorrhage must be viewed differently, and most clinicians would proceed immediately to esophagogastroduodenoscopy. Determination of the site and cause of bleeding is essential for appropriate therapy, particularly if varices are responsible. Such information is beneficial both to the surgeon, who may be asked to intervene, and to the angiographer, should injection of vasoconstricting agents into the artery supplying the lesion be deemed appropriate. Thus, anticipation of surgery, angiography, or the suspicion of bleeding varices are strong indications for esophagogastroduodenoscopy in the evaluation of the patient with persistent upper gastrointestinal bleeding.

In contrast, esophagogastroduodenoscopy is less vital in the evaluation of *massive* hemorrhage, since large amounts of blood obscure visualization of mucosal pathology. In such a setting, selective arteriography or surgery is more appropriate. Should bleeding continue and gastric aspiration fail to reveal fresh blood, the site of hemorrhage may be beyond the ligament of Treitz. In this situation angiography is frequently valuable in establishing a diagnosis. Angiographic demonstration of the bleeding site requires blood loss at a rate of at least 0.5 ml/min. Clinical correlates reflecting this degree of blood loss include postural hypotension and the necessity for blood transfusion to maintain stable vital signs. Emergency angiography may localize the site of bleeding; however, the cause of the

FIGURE 37-1
Angiographic findings on a patient with massive upper gastrointestinal bleeding. Angiographic studies revealed the bleeding to be secondary to hemorrhagic gastritis; it was controlled by the selective left gastric arterial infusion of vasopressin. A. Selective left gastric arteriography demonstrates massive extravasation of contrast material (arrow) from a branch of the left gastric artery. B. Selective left gastric arteriography during the infusion of 0.1 unit of vasopressin per minute demonstrates a marked decrease in the caliber of the left gastric artery and cessation of hemorrhage.

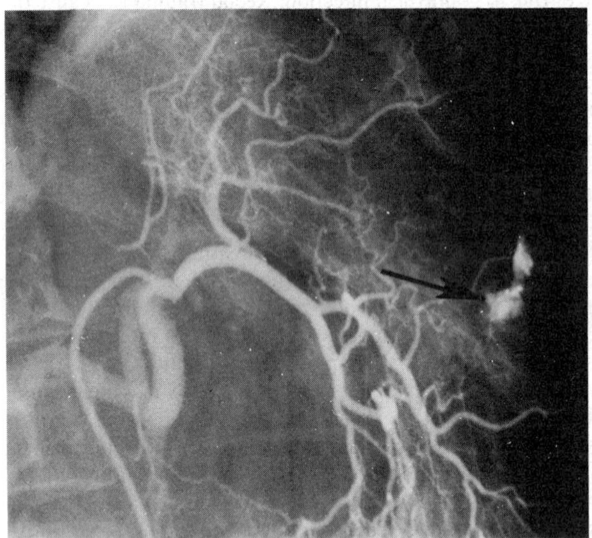
A

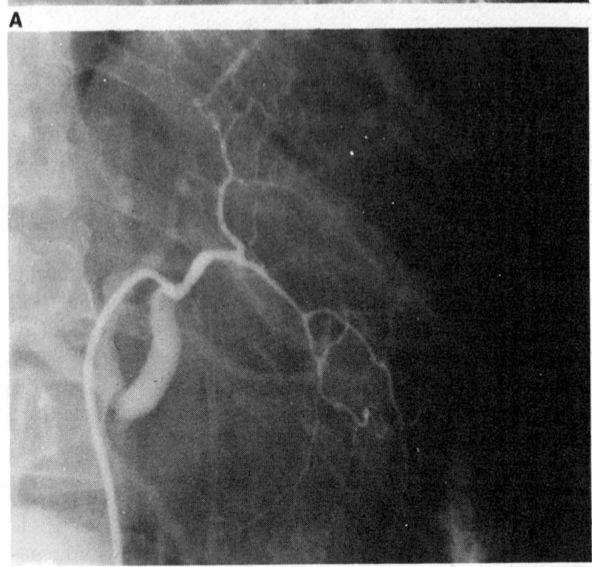
B

bleeding may not be determined unless varices, vascular malformations, or aneurysms are present.

Therapeutic angiography is a promising approach to the control of persistent hemorrhage. Continuous intraarterial infusion of vasoconstrictor agents, such as vasopressin, is often successful in controlling hemorrhage (Fig. 37-1) due to gastric ulcer or Mallory-Weiss tear. Additionally, embolic material may be injected directly into the artery perfusing the bleeding site. Intravenous infusions of vasopressin and endoscopic sclerosis for control of variceal bleeding appear more valuable than angiographic techniques.

If bleeding esophageal varices are identified on upper endoscopy, peripheral infusions of vasopressin (Pitressin) may control the bleeding. The response to such therapy depends upon the general condition of the patient as assessed by certain clinical and laboratory parameters (Child's criteria). It has been shown that intraarterial vasopressin is no more effective than intravenous administration in the control of variceal bleeding. Varices may also be controlled by balloon tamponade with a Sengstaken-Blakemore tube. Unlike vasopressin, this technique is generally used as a stabilizing preoperative measure which should be followed by surgical decompression of the portal system within 48 h whenever possible.

In the evaluation of lower gastrointestinal bleeding the most important procedures are the digital examination, anoscopy, and sigmoidoscopy. The last of these may identify a bleeding site or document bleeding coming from above the range of the instrument. If brisk bleeding continues, arteriography may serve to localize the bleeding site and allow local infusion of vasoconstrictor agents to control bleeding. Since arteriography detects actively bleeding lesions only when blood loss exceeds 0.5 ml/min and gastrointestinal bleeding tends to be intermittent, arteriography is often nondiagnostic. Radiolabeled erythrocyte scanning is more sensitive than arteriography in detecting blood loss of 0.1 ml/min and may be used to investigate less severe bleeding. However, bleeding scans are less specific than arteriography, generally localizing the lesion and seldom making a discrete diagnosis. Bleeding scans are most helpful in detecting active, low-grade, or intermittent bleeding in order to better time arteriography and obtain the maximal diagnostic yield. Several investigations are currently being conducted to assess the efficacy of colonoscopy in identifying bleeding lesions proximal to the sigmoid colon. As with esophagogastroduodenoscopy, massive hemorrhage precludes effective use of colonoscopy, and in such instances it should not be attempted. Finally, a barium enema has a limited role in the evaluation of acute rectal bleeding. A barium-filled colon may localize potential bleeding sources, but will not necessarily define the bleeding site. Furthermore, if brisk bleeding recurs, subsequent colonoscopy or angiography will be difficult to interpret due to retained contrast material. Therefore, it is advisable to withhold barium studies of both the upper and lower bowel for at least 24 h after the cessation of active bleeding.

REFERENCES

ATHANASOULIS CA: Angiography. Its contribution to the emergency management of gastrointestinal hemorrhage. Radiol Clin North Am 14:265, 1976

BAUM S et al: Angiodysplasia of the right colon: A cause of gastrointestinal hemorrhage. Am J Roentgenol 129:789, 1977

CHOJKIER M et al: A controlled comparison of continuous intra-arterial and intravenous infusions of vasopressin in hemorrhage from esophageal varices. Gastroenterology 77:540, 1979

LEBREC D et al: Propranolol for prevention of recurrent bleeding in patients with cirrhosis: A controlled study. N Engl J Med 305:1371, 1981

LICHTENSTEIN JL: Accuracy and reliability of endoscopy and x-ray in upper gastrointestinal bleeding. Dig Dis Sc 26:70s, 1981

MACDOUGALL BRD et al: Increased long term survival in variceal hemorrhage using injection sclerotherapy. Lancet 1:124, 1982

PETERSON WL et al: Routine early endoscopy in upper gastrointestinal tract bleeding: A randomized, controlled trial. N Engl J Med 304:925, 1981

PRIEBE HJ et al: Antacid versus cimetidine in preventing acute gastrointestinal bleeding. A randomized trial in 75 critically ill patients. N Engl J Med 302:426, 1980

TERES J et al: Upper gastrointestinal bleeding in cirrhosis: Clinical and endoscopic correlations. Gut 17:37, 1976

38
JAUNDICE AND HEPATOMEGALY

KURT J. ISSELBACHER

JAUNDICE

Jaundice, or *icterus,* refers to the yellow pigmentation of the skin or scleras by bilirubin. This in turn is a result of elevated levels of bilirubin in the bloodstream. Jaundice may be brought to clinical attention by a darkening of the urine or a yellow discoloration of the skin or sclera; the latter often is the site where clinical icterus may first be detected. Scleral pigmentation is attributed to richness of this tissue in elastin, which has a special affinity for bilirubin. Jaundice must be distinguished from other causes of yellow pigmentation such as carotenemia (see Chaps. 52 and 111), which is due to carotenoid pigments in the bloodstream and is associated with a yellowish discoloration of the skin but not of the sclera. Atabrine treatment (see Chap. 218) may produce a yellow color of the skin and urine, but the scleras are usually only minimally discolored, and when pigment is present, it is seen only in the regions of the scleras exposed to light.

Normal serum bilirubin concentrations range from 0.5 to 1.0 mg/dl, and normally most of this is unconjugated (see Fig. 38-1). The precise level at which jaundice becomes clinically evident varies, but usually it can be recognized when the total serum bilirubin exceeds 2 to 2.5 mg/dl. Not infrequently in deep jaundice the skin may take on a greenish hue because of the conversion of bilirubin to biliverdin, an oxidation product of bilirubin. Oxidation occurs more readily with conjugated bilirubin, and hence a greenish hue is seen more frequently in conditions with pronounced conjugated hyperbilirubinemia. When bilirubin is exposed to visible blue light (430 to 470 nm), metastable isomers of bilirubin are produced. These photoisomers are polar (because they permit no intramolecular hydrogen bonding) and can be excreted by the liver into bile without having to be conjugated (see below and Fig. 38-2).

PRODUCTION AND METABOLISM OF BILIRUBIN Normal sources of bilirubin (Fig. 38-2) The greater part of the bilirubin is derived from the catabolism of hemoglobin present in senescent red blood cells. This normally accounts for about 80 to 85 percent of the daily bilirubin production. When a circulating red blood cell reaches the end of its normal life span of approximately 120 days, it is destroyed in the reticuloendothelial system. In the catabolism of hemoglobin, globin is first dissociated from heme, after which the heme moiety (ferroprotoporphyrin IX) is oxidatively cleaved and converted to biliverdin by a microsomal heme oxygenase. This enzyme system requires oxygen and a cofactor, reduced nicotinamide adenine dinucleotide phosphate (NADPH). Bilirubin (in the chemical form of bilirubin IXα) is then formed from biliverdin by biliverdin reductase.

About 15 to 20 percent of the bilirubin is derived from sources other than senescent erythrocytes. One source is the *destruction of maturing erythroid cells in the bone marrow,* or so-called ineffective erythropoiesis (see Chap. 329). The other is *nonerythroid components,* especially in the liver, and involves the turnover of heme and heme proteins (such as cytochrome, myoglobin, and heme-containing enzymes). These two sources of bilirubin are collectively referred to as the *early labeled fraction,* a term derived from experiments with labeled glycine and Δ-aminolevulinic acid (ALA). Thus when labeled glycine is administered to a normal subject, approximately 15 percent of the label appears in stool urobilinogens in the first 3 to 5 days; 85 percent of the label appears over a broad range with the peak at about 120 days and reflects the bilirubin produced from the normal destruction of senescent red blood cells.

Transport of bilirubin Following liberation of bilirubin into the plasma, virtually all the pigment is tightly *bound to albumin.* The maximum binding capacity is 2 mol bilirubin per mole of albumin. Because in a normal adult this corresponds to plasma unconjugated bilirubin concentrations of 60 to 80 mg/ml, saturation of the binding capacity of the plasma almost never occurs. It is clinically relevant that certain organic anions, such as sulfonamides and salicylates, compete with bilirubin for common binding sites on albumin and may displace bilirubin from albumin, permitting it to enter tissues such as the central nervous system. Most of the evidence for albumin binding has been obtained from studies using unconjugated bilirubin. The conjugated pigment also appears to be bound primarily to albumin, although the binding to albumin is much weaker than with unconjugated bilirubin. This may account for the fact that conjugated, but not unconjugated, bilirubin may be filtered by the renal glomeruli.

Bilirubin is found in body fluids (cerebrospinal fluid, joint effusions, cysts, etc.) in proportion to the albumin content of the fluids and is absent from true secretions such as tears, saliva, and pancreatic juice. Scar tissue is rarely bilirubin-stained. The appearance of jaundice is also influenced by blood flow and edema. Paralyzed extremities and edematous areas tend to remain uncolored, and "unilateral" jaundice in patients with hemiplegia and edema may be seen if jaundice develops.

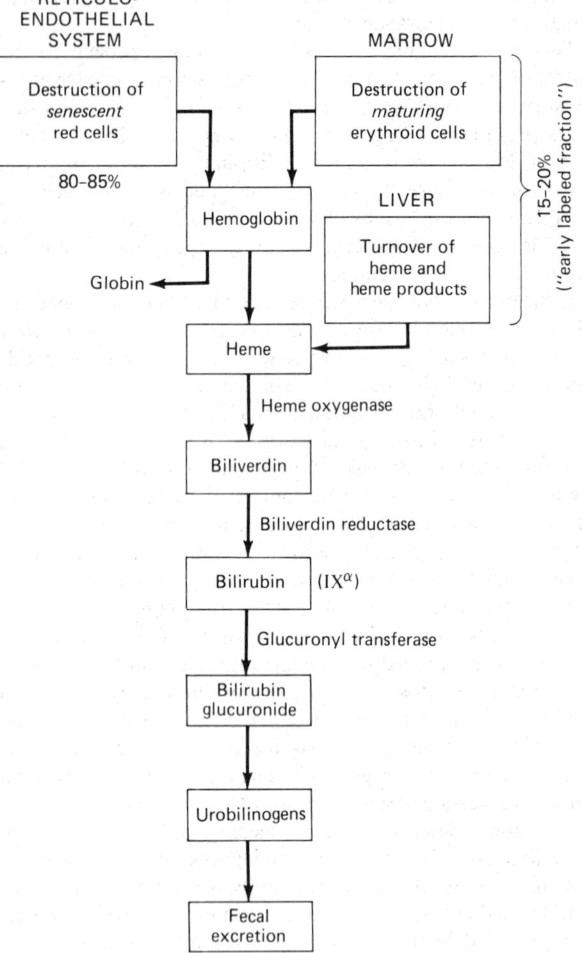

FIGURE 38-1
The sources and precursors of bilirubin and steps in its subsequent metabolism and excretion.

Hepatic metabolism of bilirubin (Fig. 38-3) The liver occupies a central role in the metabolism of the bile pigments. Three distinct phases are recognized: (1) *hepatic uptake,* (2) *conjugation,* and (3) *excretion* into bile. Of these three steps, excretion appears to be the rate-limiting step and the one most susceptible to impairment when the liver cell is damaged.

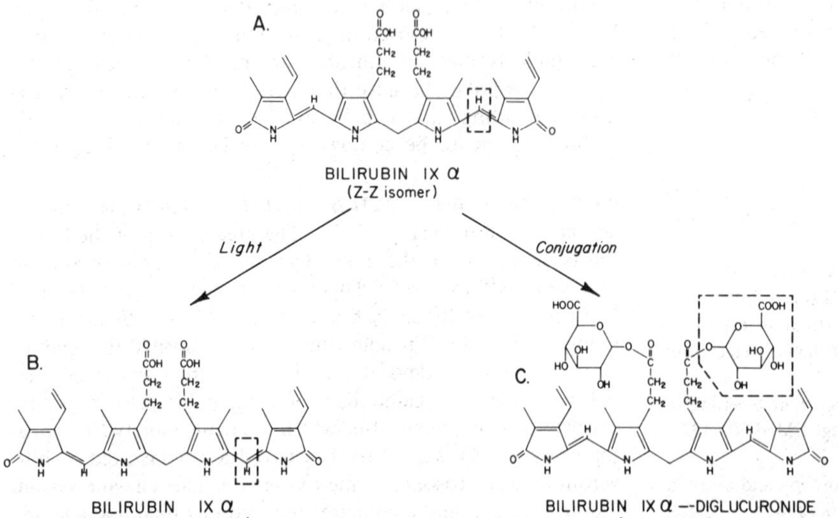

FIGURE 38-2
Scheme showing the conversion of bilirubin IXα to water-soluble derivatives by photoisomerization or conjugation. In A the normal, unconjugated pigment Z-Z isomer is shown; the dashed line shows the upright *position of the hydrogen at the methene bridges linking the pyrrole molecules. B shows the effect of light leading to the formation of the water-soluble E-E isomer; the dashed-line box serves to emphasize the inversion of the hydrogens at the methene bridges between the pyrrole molecules. C shows the formation of water-soluble bilirubin diglucuronide formation; the dashed-line box encloses one of the two glucuronic acid moieties.*

UPTAKE Unconjugated bilirubin bound to albumin is presented to the liver cell, and upon entry the pigment and albumin become dissociated. The uptake phase is believed to involve the binding of bilirubin to certain cytoplasmic anionic binding proteins (ligandins). Hepatic uptake appears to be reversible.

CONJUGATION Unconjugated bilirubin is water-insoluble and must be converted to a *water-soluble derivative* in order to be excreted by the liver cell into bile. This is accomplished by conjugation whereby bilirubin is predominantly converted to bilirubin glucuronide. The reaction occurs in the endoplasmic reticulum of the hepatocytes by action of bilirubin glucuronyl transferase. As shown in Fig. 38-3, this appears to be a two-step reaction, resulting first in the formation of the monoglucuronide followed by the production of the diglucuronide. Although there is general agreement that the conversion of the monoglucuronide to the diglucuronide is also mediated by glucuronyl transferase, some have suggested that a separate plasma membrane enzyme (transglucuronidase) may be involved. Normally, bile contains 85 percent of bilirubin diconjugates and 15 percent monoconjugates. Unconjugated bilirubin usually is *not* excreted by the liver into the bile (except following photooxidation, see below). Bile also contains small amounts of bilirubin conjugated with other sugars (e.g., with xylose and aldobiuronic acid). The physiologic significance of these nonglucuronide conjugates is not known.

EXCRETION OR SECRETION INTO BILE Normally, for bilirubin to be excreted into bile, *the pigment must be in the conjugated form.* Although the overall process is not well understood, the excretion of conjugated bilirubin into bile appears to be an energy-dependent process and the *rate-limiting* step in the hepatic metabolism of bilirubin. When this step is compromised, two consequences occur: (1) decreased excretion of bilirubin into the bile, and (2) "regurgitation," or reentry of conjugated bilirubin from the liver cells into the bloodstream.

As indicated above, bilirubin IXα can exist as four geometric isomers. The naturally occurring isomer is of Z-Z form (see Fig. 38-2) which permits intramolecular hydrogen bonding making the molecule hydrophobic. The other isomers (Z-E, E-Z, and E-E, depending on the position of the hydrogens at the two bridge double bonds) can be formed upon exposure to blue light and are unstable. They are water-soluble because their geometric configuration prevents intramolecular hydrogen bonding. Thus, these isomers (photoisomers) can be excreted into bile without having to be conjugated. The natural Z-Z isomer is also rendered water-soluble by conjugation with glucuronic acid. Bilirubin glucuronide formation prevents intramolecular hydrogen bonding, makes the molecule polar, and permits excretion of the pigment into bile (Fig. 38-2).

Intestinal phase of bilirubin metabolism After its appearance in the intestinal lumen, bilirubin glucuronide may be excreted in the stool or metabolized to urobilinogen and related products. Because of its polarity, *conjugated bilirubin is not reabsorbed* by the intestinal mucosa, a mechanism which may serve to rid the body of this pigment. The formation of urobilinogen from conjugated bilirubin requires the action of bacteria and occurs in the lower part of the small intestine and colon.

In contrast to conjugated bilirubin, *urobilinogen is reabsorbed* from the small intestine into the portal blood and is thus subject to enterohepatic circulation. Some urobilinogen is reexcreted by the liver into the bile; the rest is excreted in the urine in an amount usually not exceeding 4 mg daily. When the hepatic excretory mechanism is impaired (e.g., in hepatocellular disease) or the production of bilirubin is greatly increased (e.g., in hemolytic anemia), the urinary urobilinogen may increase significantly.

The normal output of fecal urobilinogen ranges from 50 to 280 mg per day. Under conditions of decreased excretion of conjugated bilirubin into the intestine (e.g., liver disease, bile duct obstruction) or suppression of intestinal flora by antibiotics, fecal output will be diminished. In hemolytic anemia, urinary and fecal urobilinogen excretion is greatly increased.

In a normal person with a blood volume of 5 liters and a hemoglobin concentration of 15 g/dl, the total circulating hemoglobin is 750 g. Because approximately 0.8 percent of the red blood cells are destroyed daily, 6.3 g hemoglobin is released for catabolism.

Renal excretion of bilirubin Normally the urine contains no bilirubin that can be detected by the methods usually employed, although traces may be detectable by sensitive spectrophotometric procedures. Unconjugated bilirubin, being tightly bound to albumin, is not filtered by the renal glomeruli, and because there is no tubular secretory process for bilirubin, *unconjugated bilirubin (as the IXα, Z-Z isomer) is not excreted in urine.* On the other hand, conjugated bilirubin is less tightly bound to albumin, and a small fraction (about 5 percent) is unbound. The unbound fraction is dialyzable and is filtered by the renal glomeruli. Thus, in contrast to the unconjugated pigment, a fraction of plasma *conjugated bilirubin appears in the urine.* Bile salts enhance the dialyzability of conjugated bilirubin, and in obstructive jaundice, the elevated level of plasma bile acids may account for an increased renal excretion of conjugated bilirubin. This may also explain why in biliary tract obstruction, serum conjugated bilirubin levels tend to plateau

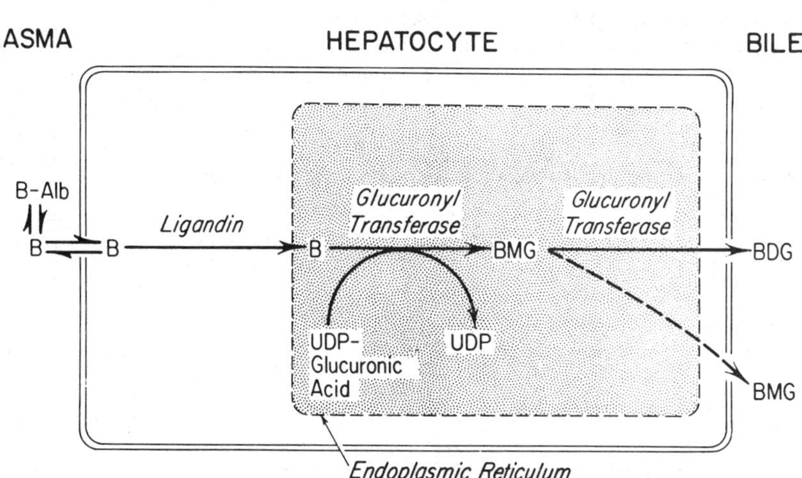

FIGURE 38-3
Scheme of bilirubin uptake, conjugation, and excretion by the liver cell. Although the conversion of BMG to BDG appears to be catalyzed by glucuronyl transferase, some have also postulated its formation by a plasma membrane transglucuronidase. B = bilirubin; BMG = bilirubin monoglucuronide; BDG = bilirubin diglucuronide; UDP = uridine diphosphate.

and not to exceed 30 to 40 mg/dl, while with severe hepatocellular injury bilirubin levels higher than this may occur.

CHEMICAL TESTS FOR BILE PIGMENTS The most widely employed chemical test for the bile pigments in serum is the van den Bergh reaction. In this reaction the bilirubin pigments are diazotized with sulfanilic acid, and the chromogenic products are measured colorimetrically. The van den Bergh reaction can be used to distinguish between unconjugated and conjugated bilirubin because of the different solubility properties of the pigments. When the reaction is carried out in an *aqueous* medium, the water-soluble conjugated bilirubin reacts to give the so-called direct van den Bergh reaction. When the reaction is carried out in *methanol,* the intramolecular hydrogen bonds of unconjugated bilirubin are broken; thus both conjugated and unconjugated pigments react, giving a measure of the *total* bilirubin level. The total minus the direct-reacting bilirubin give the *indirect* value, which is a measure of the unconjugated bilirubin level.

In the direct van den Bergh reaction, the most accurate measurements are those carried out at 1 min. If the reaction is allowed to proceed longer, a small amount of the unconjugated pigment may begin to react in the aqueous medium. As a result, if the reaction is carried out at 30 min in a patient with unconjugated hyperbilirubinemia, falsely low values for the indirect-reacting bilirubin may be obtained. This serves to emphasize that the direct and indirect van den Bergh reactions represent *approximations* (not absolute measurements) of the conjugated and unconjugated pigments.

The most accurate method for measuring bilirubin in biologic fluids involves the formation of bilirubin methyl esters (by alkaline methanolysis) and measuring the products by high-performance liquid chromatography (HPLC). Studies with this procedure show that *normal serum contains only unconjugated bilirubin.* This confirms the long-held suspicion that the small amount of conjugated bilirubin measured in normal serum by the diazo method (0.1 to 0.3 mg/ml) is most likely an artifact of the van den Bergh method. The HPLC method also shows that in patients with liver disease and conjugated hyperbilirubinemia, the serum contains significant amounts of *monoconjugates as well as diconjugates.* A summary of the key differences in the properties and reactions of the bilirubin pigments is presented in Table 38-1.

The qualitative measurement of bilirubin in the urine may be carried out with Ictotest tablets or the dipstick method. The foam test is also a simple and qualitatively valid procedure. When normal urine is vigorously shaken in a test tube, the foam is absolutely white. In urine containing bilirubin, the foam will be yellow. This difference may be subtle and may become evident only by comparing a normal urine specimen and one containing bilirubin side by side.

Except for concentrated urine, the most common cause of a deep yellow-brown or dark urine is bilirubinuria. However, other mechanisms and diseases associated with a dark urine need to be considered. These include yellow urine due to drugs (e.g., sulfasalazine); red urine due to porphyria, hemoglobinuria, myoglobinuria, or drugs (e.g., pyridium); and dark brown or black urine due to homogentisic acid (in ochronosis) or melanin (with melanoma).

APPROACH TO THE PATIENT WITH JAUNDICE Once jaundice is recognized clinically or chemically, it is important to determine whether it is predominantly due to unconjugated or conjugated hyperbilirubinemia. *A simple clue in this regard is to determine whether bilirubin is present in the urine.* Its absence in the urine suggests unconjugated hyperbilirubinemia (since this pigment is not filtered by the glomerulus); its presence indicates conjugated hyperbilirubinemia. One can then proceed to the chemical measurement of the bilirubin pigments in the serum. In predominantly unconjugated hyperbilirubinemia, 80 to 85 percent of the total serum bilirubin is unconjugated (i.e., less than 15 to 20 percent is conjugated). The patient is considered to have predominantly conjugated hyperbilirubinemia when more than 50 percent of the serum bilirubin is of the conjugated type. The serum of such patients will contain both mono- and diconjugates.

An approach to the classification of jaundice based on this important distinction is presented in Table 38-2. Derangements of bilirubin metabolism may occur through any of four mechanisms: (1) overproduction, (2) decreased hepatic uptake, (3) decreased hepatic conjugation, and (4) decreased excretion of bilirubin into bile (due to both intrahepatic and extrahepatic factors). Jaundice may also be described on the basis of the pathogenetic mechanisms or disease processes leading to increased bilirubin levels. Thus, the terms *hemolytic jaundice, hepatocellular jaundice,* and *obstructive* (or cholestatic) *jaundice* are often used.

Though these classifications and terms are helpful, in any one patient more than a single derangement or more than one

TABLE 38-1
Comparison of the major differences between conjugated and unconjugated bilirubin

Properties and reactions	*Unconjugated**	*Conjugated*
Water solubility	0	+
Affinity for lipids	+	0
Bound to serum albumin	+++	+
Renal excretion	0	+
Van den Bergh reaction	Indirect (total minus direct)	Direct
Lipid membrane permeability	+	0

* *These properties apply to the naturally occurring bilirubin IXα. Other geometric and photoisomers behave like conjugated bilirubin. See text for details.*

TABLE 38-2
Classification of jaundice based on underlying derangement of bilirubin metabolism

I Predominantly *unconjugated* hyperbilirubinemia
- *A* Overproduction
  - *1* Hemolysis (intra- and extravascular)
  - *2* Ineffective erythropoiesis
- *B* Decreased hepatic uptake
  - *1* Drugs (e.g., flavaspidic acid)
  - *2* Prolonged fasting (< 300 cal per day)
  - *3* Sepsis
- *C* Decreased bilirubin conjugation (decreased glucuronyl transferase activity)
  - *1* Gilbert's syndrome (*mild* decrease in transferase)
  - *2* Crigler-Najjar type II (*moderate* decrease in transferase)
  - *3* Crigler-Najjar type I (absent transferase)
  - *4* Neonatal jaundice
  - *5* Acquired transferase deficiency
    - *a* Drug inhibition (e.g., pregnanediol, chloramphenicol)
    - *b* Hepatocellular disease (hepatitis, cirrhosis)*
  - *6* Sepsis

II Predominantly *conjugated* hyperbilirubinemia
- *A* Impaired hepatic excretion (intrahepatic defects)
  - *1* Familial or hereditary disorders
    - *a* Dubin-Johnson syndrome; Rotor syndrome
    - *b* Recurrent (benign) intrahepatic cholestasis
    - *c* Cholestatic jaundice of pregnancy
  - *2* Acquired disorders
    - *a* Hepatocellular disease* (e.g., viral or drug-induced hepatitis)
    - *b* Drug-induced cholestasis (e.g., oral contraceptives, methyltestosterone)
    - *c* Sepsis
- *B* Extrahepatic biliary obstruction (mechanical obstruction, e.g., stones, stricture, tumor of bile duct)

* *In hepatocellular disease (hepatitis and cirrhosis) there is usually interference in the three major steps of bilirubin metabolism—uptake, conjugation, and excretion. However, excretion is the rate-limiting step and is usually impaired to the greatest extent. As a result, conjugated hyperbilirubinemia predominates.*

"type" of jaundice may be present. For example, a patient with cirrhosis may have not only impaired liver cell function (and hence hepatocellular jaundice) but also hemolysis. Furthermore, obstructive jaundice may be due to either *mechanical* obstruction of the biliary radicles or *functional* factors causing impaired hepatic excretion of bilirubin into bile.

In the present chapter a brief description of the major types of jaundice is given. A more detailed discussion of the individual disease entities is found in Chap. 317.

Jaundice with predominantly unconjugated bilirubin in the serum OVERPRODUCTION OF BILIRUBIN When an increased amount of hemoglobin is released from red blood cells into either the bloodstream or tissues, increased bilirubin production occurs. Hyperbilirubinemia develops when the capacity of the liver to remove the pigment from the circulation is exceeded. In most cases of hemolysis, the total serum bilirubin concentration ranges from 3 to 5 mg/dl. A slight increase in direct-reacting pigment may also be found, but this usually constitutes less than 15 percent of the total serum bilirubin. This finding is probably analogous to the slight elevations of direct-reacting bilirubin which occur when normal subjects are infused with unconjugated bilirubin. Both instances appear to be a reflection of the fact that the rate-limiting step in hepatic bilirubin metabolism is excretion and that when the excretory capacity of the liver is exceeded, some reentry of conjugated bilirubin into the bloodstream occurs. However, as indicated above, future measurements using alkaline methanolysis and HPLC may show that much of the diazo reacting material is an artifact of the van den Bergh reaction and is largely unconjugated bilirubin. For a detailed description of the causes of increased bilirubin production, see Chap. 317.

IMPAIRED HEPATIC UPTAKE OF BILIRUBIN As indicated previously, the uptake of bilirubin by the liver cell involves dissociation of the pigment from albumin, and presumably binding to certain cytoplasmic proteins (i.e., ligandins). In some cases of drug-induced jaundice (e.g., due to flavaspidic acid) and possibly in some patients with Gilbert's syndrome, there may be a derangement in this phase of bilirubin metabolism (see Chap. 317).

IMPAIRED GLUCURONIDE CONJUGATION Both acquired and genetic derangements in hepatic glucuronyl transferase occur. In the fetus and at birth, glucuronyl transferase activity is low and appears to account in part for the *neonatal jaundice* normally found between the second and the fifth days of life. *Mild* decreases in glucuronyl transferases occur in Gilbert's syndrome, *moderate* decreases are found in Crigler-Najjar syndrome type II, and the enzyme is totally absent in the rare Crigler-Najjar syndrome type I (see Chap. 317).

Acquired defects in bilirubin glucuronyl transferase activity may be produced by drugs (i.e., enzyme inhibition) or intrinsic liver disease. However, with liver cell damage, the excretory capacity of the liver is impaired to a greater extent than is the conjugating capacity. Therefore in most hepatocellular diseases, the hyperbilirubinemia is predominantly of the conjugated type (see Chap. 317).

Jaundice with predominantly conjugated bilirubin in the serum IMPAIRED EXCRETION OF BILIRUBIN BY THE LIVER The impaired excretion of bilirubin into the biliary canaliculi, whether due to functional or mechanical factors, results in predominantly conjugated hyperbilirubinemia and bilirubinuria. The presence of *bilirubin in the urine is evidence of conjugated hyperbilirubinemia* and is a most important point in the differential diagnosis of jaundice. Such findings are identical to those occurring in complete obstruction of the bile duct, emphasizing that *jaundice due to hepatocellular disease can seldom be differentiated from that due to extrahepatic obstruction solely on the basis of changes in bile pigment metabolism.* Indeed there are often instances when the two conditions are not distinguishable by any biochemical criteria, and liver biopsy or other diagnostic procedures are needed for the definitive diagnosis.

When there is interference in the excretion of conjugated bilirubin into bile, by what mechanism does this pigment enter the systemic circulation? Several postulates have been proposed for this "reentry": (1) rupture of the bile canaliculi secondary to the necrosis of the hepatic cells that constitute their walls; (2) occlusion of the canaliculi by inspissated bile or their compression by swollen hepatic cells; (3) obstruction of the terminal intrahepatic bile ducts (cholangioles) by inflammatory cells; (4) altered hepatic cell permeability; and (5) as a result of impaired excretion, accumulation of conjugated bilirubin in the hepatocytes and secondary diffusion into the plasma. Although some of these postulates are speculative, it is likely that several of these mechanisms occur. For example, occasionally in histologic sections, escape of bile through rents in the walls of canaliculi in areas of necrosis is apparent. Also, microscopic studies of the liver of rats injected with fluorescent dyes have shown reflux of bile from canaliculi into sinusoids. However, no anatomic damage needs to be invoked, because when unconjugated bilirubin is infused into normal subjects at high rates, conjugated hyperbilirubinemia occurs; this is explained most logically by passive diffusion.

EXTRAHEPATIC BILIARY OBSTRUCTION Complete obstruction of the extrahepatic bile ducts leads to jaundice with predominantly conjugated hyperbilirubinemia, bilirubinuria, and clay-colored stools. Failure of bile to reach the intestine results in virtual disappearance of urobilinogen from the stool and urine. The concentration of bilirubin rises progressively but then usually plateaus at a level of 30 to 40 mg/dl. To some extent this plateau may be explained by a balance between renal excretion and diversion of bilirubin to other metabolites. In hepatocellular jaundice, such a plateau tends not to occur, and bilirubin levels in excess of 50 mg/dl may be found, in part due to concomitant hemolysis and renal insufficiency.

Partial obstruction of the extrahepatic bile ducts can also give rise to jaundice but only if the intrabiliary pressure is increased, because the excretion of bilirubin does not diminish until the intraductile pressure approaches the maximal secretory pressure of approximately 250 mmHg bile. Jaundice may occur at much lower pressures if the obstruction is complicated by infection of the ducts or hepatocellular injury. Therefore, jaundice, bilirubinuria, and clay-colored stools are inconstant findings in partial biliary obstruction, and the amount of urobilinogen in urine and stool varies with the degree of occlusion.

The functional reserve of the liver is so great that *occlusion of the intrahepatic bile ducts* does not give rise to jaundice unless the drainage of bile from a large segment of the parenchyma is interrupted. Either of the two major hepatic ducts or a large number of secondary radicles may be occluded without production of jaundice. In experimental animals the ducts draining at least 75 percent of the parenchyma must be occluded before jaundice appears.

Additional points of terminology In clinical practice, a patient may be described as having *obstructive*, or *cholestatic*, jaundice. By this is meant that clinically, and especially biochemically, there is little to suggest hepatocellular damage and that the main features point to interference with, or obstruction in, the flow of bile. Typically one would expect such a patient to show (1) predominantly conjugated hyperbilirubinemia, (2) minimal biochemical changes of parenchymal liver damage, and (3) a moderate to a marked increase in the serum alkaline phosphatase level [usually three or four times normal (or greater than 250 IU per liter)]. As emphasized in Chaps. 315 and 316, an *elevated alkaline phosphatase level* in a patient with jaundice or liver disease, in the absence of other disorders such as bone disease, is most suggestive of interference with bile secretion or an infiltrative process in the liver. However, *laboratory tests alone may not permit differentiation of intrahepatic from extrahepatic cholestasis.*

Some clinicians reserve the term obstructive jaundice for those situations in which anatomic obstruction can be demonstrated and use the term cholestatic jaundice for cases of parenchymal liver disease in which the obstructive phase is on a junctional basis. Nevertheless, because these two entities frequently are indistinguishable by clinical and biochemical criteria, the terms obstructive jaundice and cholestatic jaundice are often used interchangeably.

Hepatocellular disorders in which jaundice associated with an obstructive, or cholestatic, phase occurs include (1) occasional cases of viral hepatitis, (2) drug reactions, especially those due to chlorpromazine and methyltestosterone, (3) some cases of alcoholic hepatitis or alcohol-induced fatty liver, (4) jaundice in the last trimester of pregnancy, (5) most cases of Dubin-Johnson or Rotor syndrome, (6) benign recurrent intrahepatic cholestasis, and (7) certain types of postoperative jaundice. These and other conditions are discussed in Chaps. 317 and 318.

In summary, all forms of conjugated hyperbilirubinemia have by definition an impairment in the excretion of bilirubin into bile. In most cases of parenchymal liver disease, a broad derangement is shown by the biochemical tests of liver function. However, when the major detectable alterations of liver function tests include (1) conjugated hyperbilirubinemia and (2) moderate to marked elevation of the serum alkaline phosphatase level, the terms obstructive or cholestatic jaundice may be appropriate. Additional procedures, including operation, are often needed to determine the cause of the cholestasis (see Chaps. 314 and 316).

HEPATOMEGALY

In the supine position, the major part of the liver lies beneath the right rib cage. In some normal persons the liver edge may be palpable 1 to 2 cm below the right costal margin, and a palpable liver edge by itself does not necessarily indicate hepatomegaly. In evaluating liver size by physical examination, two factors other than ability to palpate the liver edge need to be considered, namely, (1) the location of the upper border of liver dullness by percussion, and (2) the body habitus.

Normally, the upper edge of liver dullness on the right side in the midclavicular line is at the level of the fifth rib, but in asthenic habitus it may be lower. The liver edge normally descends 1 to 3 cm with deep inspiration. In hypersthenic subjects, the liver may extend over to the left side of the abdominal wall, with the lower edge high and not palpable; in hyposthenic subjects with a very acute costal angle, the liver may lie in the right half of the abdomen, the edge being palpable by as much as 6 to 8 cm below the right costal margin lateral to the right rectus abdominis muscle. Thus, palpability does not necessarily imply hepatomegaly.

In determining liver enlargement by palpation, one should be certain that the liver is being palpated rather than other right upper quadrant masses such as gallbladder, colonic neoplasm, or fecal material in the colon. Liver enlargement is often confirmed by radiologic studies, including hepatic scintiscans, celiac axis angiography, and echography.

TABLE 38-3
Causes of a palpable liver and hepatomegaly

I Palpable liver without hepatomegaly
- *A* Right diaphragm displaced downward (e.g., emphysema, asthma)
- *B* Subdiaphragmatic lesion (e.g., abscess)
- *C* Aberrant lobe of liver (Riedel's lobe)
- *D* Extremely thin or relaxed abdominal muscles
- *E* Occasionally present in normal persons

II Hepatomegaly
- *A* Vascular congestion (e.g., congestive heart failure, hepatic vein thrombosis)
- *B* Bile duct obstruction (e.g., lesion in common duct leading to hepatomegaly and subsequently biliary cirrhosis)
- *C* Infiltrative disorders
  - *1* Bone marrow and reticuloendothelial cells
    - *a* Extramedullary hematopoiesis
    - *b* Leukemia
    - *c* Lymphoma
  - *2* Fat
    - *a* Fatty liver (e.g., secondary to alcohol, diabetes, or toxins)
    - *b* Gaucher's disease and some other lipidoses
  - *3* Glycogen (e.g., diabetes, especially after insulin excess)
  - *4* Amyloid
  - *5* Iron (hemochromatosis and hemosiderosis)
  - *6* Granuloma (tuberculosis, sarcoid)
- *D* Inflammatory disorders
  - *1* Hepatitis—due to drugs or infectious agents
  - *2* Cirrhosis—except in late stages when prolonged scarring may lead to a *small*, shrunken liver
- *E* Tumors—primary or metastatic
- *F* Cysts—polycystic disease, congenital hepatic fibrosis

In many cases of generalized liver enlargement, the left lobe will be felt in the epigastrium between the xiphoid and umbilicus. The liver should be carefully palpated during deep inspiration to determine whether the edge is tender, regular or irregular, firm or soft, rounded and thickened, or sharp. The edge is tender and often rounded with hepatic inflammation, as in hepatitis, or when the liver is acutely congested, as in cardiac decompensation. Pulsation of the liver may be found with tricuspid valvular incompetence. A carcinomatous liver may be rocklike in hardness; the cirrhotic liver is very firm in consistency. The largest livers are often found with carcinoma (primary or metastatic), marked fatty infiltration, congestive cardiac decompensation, Hodgkin's disease, and amyloidosis. Rapid decrease in liver size may occur with improvement of congestive failure, mobilization of fat from the liver, or massive hepatic necrosis.

In a patient with hepatomegaly, auscultation is sometimes helpful. A friction rub may be audible (and palpable) in the right upper quadrant; it is usually due to a recent biopsy, tumor, or perihepatitis. In portal hypertension a venous hum may be audible between the umbilicus and the xiphoid. An arterial murmur or bruit over the liver may indicate tumor, usually hepatoma.

Some of the causes of a palpable liver and hepatomegaly are given in Table 38-3.

REFERENCES

BERTHELOT P, DHUMEAUX D: New insights into the classification and mechanisms of hereditary, chronic non-hemolytic hyperbilirubinemias. Gut 19:474, 1978

BILLING BH: Twenty-five years of progress in bilirubin metabolism. Gut 19:481, 1978

BLANKAERT N et al: Measurement of bilirubin and its monoconjugates and diconjugates in human serum by alkaline methanolysis and high performance liquid chromatography. J Lab Clin Med 96:1980

FEVERY J et al: Unconjugated bilirubin and an increased proportion of bilirubin monoconjugates in the bile of patients with Gilbert's syndrome and Crigler-Najjar disease. J Clin Invest 60:970, 1977

GOLLAN J, SCHMID R: Bilirubin update: Formation, transport and metabolism, in *Progress in Liver Diseases,* H Popper et al (eds). New York, Grune & Stratton, 1982, vol VII

McDONAGH AF et al: Blue light and bilirubin excretion. Science 208:145, 1980

39 ABDOMINAL SWELLING AND ASCITES

ROBERT M. GLICKMAN
KURT J. ISSELBACHER

ABDOMINAL SWELLING Abdominal swelling or distention is a common problem in clinical medicine and may be the initial manifestation of a systemic disease or of otherwise unsuspected abdominal disease. *Subjective* abdominal enlargement, often described as a sensation of fullness or bloating, is usually transient and is often related to a functional gastrointestinal disorder when it is not accompanied by objective physical findings of increased abdominal girth or local swelling. *Obesity* and lumbar lordosis, which may be associated with prominence of the abdomen, may usually be distinguished from true increases in the volume of the peritoneal cavity by history and careful physical examination.

Clinical history Abdominal swelling may first be noticed by the patient because of a progressive increase in belt or clothing size, the appearance of abdominal or inguinal hernias, or the development of a localized swelling. Often, considerable abdominal enlargement has gone unnoticed for weeks or months, either because of coexistent obesity or because the ascites formation has been insidious, without pain or localizing symptoms. Progressive abdominal distention may be associated with a sensation of "pulling" or "stretching" of the flanks or groins and vague low back pain. Localized *pain* usually results from involvement of an abdominal organ (e.g., a passively congested liver, large spleen, or colonic tumor). Pain is uncommon in cirrhosis with ascites and when it is present pancreatitis, hepatoma, or peritonitis should be considered. Tense ascites or abdominal tumors may produce increased intraabdominal pressure, resulting in *indigestion* and *heartburn* due to gastroesophageal reflux or *dyspnea, orthopnea,* and *tachypnea* from elevation of the diaphragm. A coexistent pleural effusion, more commonly on the right, presumably due to leakage of ascitic fluid through lymphatic channels in the diaphragm, may also contribute to respiratory embarrassment. The patient with diffuse abdominal swelling should be questioned about increased alcoholic intake, a prior episode of jaundice or hematuria, a change in bowel habits, or a past history of rheumatic heart disease. Such historic information may provide the clues that will lead one to suspect an occult cirrhosis, a colonic tumor with peritoneal seeding, congestive heart failure, or nephrosis.

Physical examination A carefully executed *general physical examination* can yield valuable clues concerning the etiology of abdominal swelling. Thus palmar erythema and spider angiomas suggest an underlying cirrhosis, while supraclavicular adenopathy (Virchow's node) should raise the question of an underlying gastrointestinal malignancy. *Inspection* of the abdomen is an important but often cursorily performed aspect of the abdominal examination. By noting the abdominal contour, one may be able to distinguish localized from generalized swelling. The tensely distended abdomen with tightly stretched skin, bulging flanks, and everted umbilicus is characteristic of ascites. A prominent abdominal venous pattern with the direction of flow away from the umbilicus often is a reflection of portal hypertension; venous collaterals with flow from the lower part of the abdomen toward the umbilicus suggest obstruction of the inferior vena cava; flow downward toward the umbilicus suggests superior vena cava obstruction. "Doming" of the abdomen with visible ridges from underlying intestinal loops is usually due to intestinal obstruction or distention. An epigastric mass, with evident peristalsis proceeding from left to right, usually indicates underlying pyloric obstruction. A liver with metastatic deposits may be visible as a nodular right upper quadrant mass moving with respiration.

Auscultation may reveal the high-pitched, rushing sounds of early intestinal obstruction or a succussion sound due to increased fluid and gas in a dilated hollow viscus. Careful auscultation over an enlarged liver occasionally reveals the harsh bruit of a vascular tumor, especially a hepatoma, or the leathery friction rub of a surface nodule. A venous hum at the umbilicus may signify portal hypertension and an increased collateral blood flow around the liver. A fluid wave and flank dullness which shifts with change in position of the patient are important signs that indicate the presence of peritoneal fluid. In obese patients, small amounts of fluid may be difficult to demonstrate; on occasion the fluid may be detected by abdominal percussion with patients on their hands and knees. Doubt about the presence of peritoneal fluid may be resolved by careful paracentesis with a small-gauge (no. 19 or 20) needle. Careful percussion should serve to distinguish generalized abdominal enlargement from localized swelling due to an enlarged uterus, ovarian cyst, or distended bladder. Percussion can also outline an abnormally small or large liver. Loss of normal liver dullness may result from massive hepatic necrosis; it may also be a clue to free gas in the peritoneal cavity, as from perforation of a hollow viscus.

Palpation is often difficult with massive ascites, and ballottement of overlying fluid may be the only method of palpating the liver or spleen. A slightly enlarged spleen in association with ascites may be the only evidence of an occult cirrhosis. When there is evidence of portal hypertension, a soft liver suggests that obstruction to portal flow is extrahepatic; a firm liver suggests cirrhosis as the likely cause of the portal hypertension. A very hard or nodular liver is a clue that the liver is infiltrated with tumor, and when accompanied by ascites, it suggests that the latter is due to peritoneal seeding. The presence of a hard periumbilical lymph node (Sister Marie Joseph's nodule) suggests metastatic disease from a pelvic or gastrointestinal primary tumor. A pulsatile liver and ascites may be found in tricuspid insufficiency.

An attempt should be made to determine whether a mass is solid or cystic, smooth or irregular, and whether it moves with respiration. The liver, spleen, and gallbladder should descend with respiration unless they are fixed by adhesions or extension of tumor beyond the organ. A fixed mass not descending with respiration may indicate that it is retroperitoneal. Tenderness, especially if localized, may indicate an inflammatory process such as an abscess; it may also be due to stretching of the visceral peritoneum or tumor necrosis. Rectal and pelvic examinations are mandatory; they may reveal otherwise undetected masses due to tumor or infection.

Radiographic and laboratory examinations are essential for confirming or extending the impressions gained on physical examination. Upright and recumbent films of the abdomen may demonstrate the dilated loops of intestine with fluid levels characteristic of intestinal obstruction or the diffuse abdominal haziness and loss of psoas margins suggestive of ascites. Ultrasonography is often of value in detecting ascites, determining the presence of a mass, or evaluating the size of the liver and spleen. Computerized axial tomography (CT scanning) provides similar information. A plain film of the abdomen may reveal the distended colon of otherwise unsuspected ulcerative colitis and give valuable information as to the size of the liver and spleen. An irregular and elevated right side of the diaphragm may be a clue to a liver abscess or hepatoma. Studies of the gastrointestinal tract with barium or other contrast media are usually necessary in the search for a primary tumor.

ASCITES In most cases the clinical and laboratory evaluation of the patient with ascites is sufficient to reveal the cause of the fluid accumulation. Often the ascites is a component or complication of cirrhosis, congestive heart failure, nephrosis, or disseminated carcinomatosis. However, even when the cause of ascites seems obvious, it is often important to determine whether another separate or related disease process has supervened. For example, when the patient with compensated cirrhosis and minimal ascites develops progressive ascites that is increasingly difficult to control with sodium restriction or diuretics, the obvious temptation is to attribute the worsening of the clinical picture to progressive liver disease. However, an occult hepatoma, portal vein thrombosis, spontaneous bacterial peritonitis, or even tuberculosis may be responsible for the decompensation. The disappointingly low success of diagnosing tuberculous peritonitis or hepatoma in the patient with cirrhosis and ascites reflects the too-low index of suspicion for the development of such superimposed conditions. Similarly, the patient with congestive heart failure may develop ascites from a disseminated carcinoma with peritoneal seeding. The thorough evaluation of each patient with ascites, even in the presence of an "obvious" cause, will help avoid these errors.

Diagnostic paracentesis (50 to 100 ml) should be part of the routine evaluation of the patient with ascites. The fluid should be examined for its gross appearance, protein content, cell count, and differential cell count, as well as Gram's and acid-fast stains and culture. Cytologic and cell-block examination may disclose an otherwise unsuspected carcinoma. Table 39-1 presents some of the features of ascitic fluid typically found in various disease states. In some disorders, such as cirrhosis, the fluid has the characteristics of a transudate (less than 2.5 g protein per deciliter and a specific gravity less than 1.016); in others, such as peritonitis, the features are those of an exudate. Although there is variability of the ascitic fluid in any given disease state, some features are sufficiently characteristic to suggest certain diagnostic possibilities. For example, blood-stained fluid with more than 2.5 g protein per deciliter is unusual in uncomplicated cirrhosis but is consistent with tuberculous peritonitis or neoplasm. Cloudy fluid with a predominance of polymorphonuclear cells and a positive Gram stain are characteristic of bacterial peritonitis; if most cells are lymphocytes, tuberculosis should be suspected. The complete examination of each fluid is most important, for occasionally only *one* finding may be abnormal. For example, if the fluid is a typical transudate but contains more than 250 white blood cells per cubic millimeter, the finding should be recognized as atypical for cirrhosis, nephrosis, or congestive heart failure and should warrant a search for tumor or infection. This is especially true in the evaluation of cirrhotic ascites where occult peritoneal infection may be present with only minor elevations in the white blood cell count of the peritoneal fluid (300 to 500 cells per cubic millimeter). Since Gram's stain of the fluid may be negative in a high proportion of such cases, careful culture of the peritoneal fluid is mandatory. Direct visualization of the peritoneum (peritoneoscopy) may disclose peritoneal deposits of tumor, tuberculosis, or metastatic disease of the liver. Biopsies are taken under direct vision often adding to the diagnostic accuracy of the procedure.

Chylous ascites refers to a turbid, milky, or creamy peritoneal fluid due to the presence of thoracic or intestinal lymph. Such a fluid shows Sudan-staining fat globules microscopically and an increased triglyceride content by chemical examination. A turbid fluid due to leukocytes or tumor cells may be confused with chylous fluid, and it is often helpful to carry out alkalinization and ether extraction of the specimen. Alkali will tend to dissolve cellular proteins and thereby reduce turbidity; ether extraction will lead to clearing if the turbidity of the fluid is due to lipid. Chylous ascites is most often the result of lymphatic obstruction from trauma, tumor, tuberculosis, filariasis (see Chap. 227), or congenital abnormalities. It may also be seen in the nephrotic syndrome.

Rarely, ascitic fluid may be *mucinous* in character, suggest-

TABLE 39-1
Ascitic fluid characteristics in various disease states

Condition	*Gross appearance*	*Specific gravity*	*Protein, g/100 ml*	*Cell count: Red blood cells, >10,000/mm³*	*Cell count: White blood cells, per mm³*	*Other tests*
Cirrhosis	Straw-colored or bile-stained	<1.016 (95%)*	<2.5 (95%)	1%	<250 (90%);* predominantly endothelial	
Neoplasm	Straw-colored, hemorrhagic, mucinous, or chylous	Variable, >1.016 (45%)	>2.5 (75%)	20%	>1000 (50%); variable cell types	Cytology, cell block, peritoneal biopsy
Tuberculous peritonitis	Clear, turbid, hemorrhagic, chylous	Variable, >1.016 (50%)	>2.5 (50%)	7%	>1000 (70%); usually >70% lymphocytes	Peritoneal biopsy, stain and culture for acid-fast bacilli
Pyogenic peritonitis	Turbid or purulent	If purulent, >1.016	If purulent, >2.5	Unusual	Predominantly polymorphonuclear leukocytes	+Gram's stain, culture
Congestive heart failure	Straw-colored	Variable, <1.016 (60%)	Variable, 1.5–5.3	10%	<1000 (90%); usually mesothelial, mononuclear	
Nephrosis	Straw-colored or chylous	<1.016	<2.5 (100%)	Unusual	<250; mesothelial, mononuclear	If chylous, ether extraction, Sudan staining
Pancreatic ascites (pancreatitis, pseudocyst)	Turbid, hemorrhagic, or chylous	Variable, often >1.016	Variable, often >2.5	Variable, may be blood-stained	Variable	Increased amylase in ascitic fluid and serum

* *Since the conditions of examining fluid and selecting patients were not identical in each series, the percentage figures (in the parentheses) should be taken as an indication of the order of magnitude rather than as the precise incidence of any abnormal finding.*
SOURCES: *Borhanmanesh et al; Coder and Olander; Malagelada et al.*

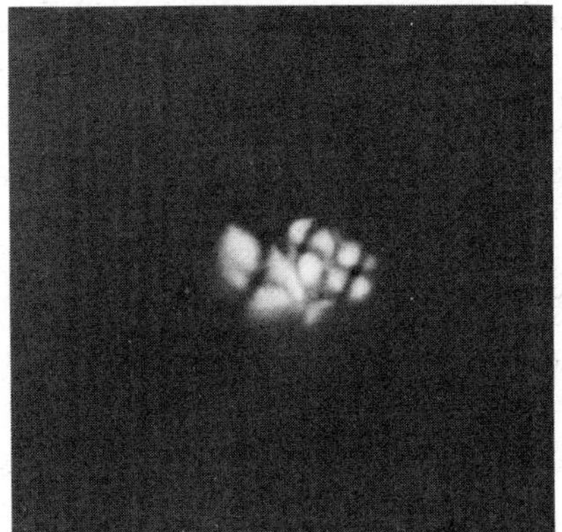

FIGURE 39-1
Starch peritonitis. Examination of ascitic fluid under polarized light reveals doubly refractile starch granules.

ing either pseudomyxoma peritonei (Chap. 313) or rarely a colloid carcinoma of the stomach or colon with peritoneal implants.

On rare occasions a syndrome may be seen of fever and ascites, without infection, occurring several weeks after abdominal surgery. This seems to result from starch (from surgical gloves) introduced into the peritoneum at the time of surgery, with a subsequent foreign-body reaction and ascites formation. Given the proper index of suspicion, diagnosis can be made by paracentesis and finding double refractile particles (i.e., starch) when polarized light is used (Fig. 39-1).

The etiology of ascites may remain uncertain even after the usual diagnostic procedures have been carried out. Under those circumstances a high proportion of the cases will be due to (1) cirrhosis of the liver, (2) carcinomatosis with peritoneal involvement, (3) tuberculous peritonitis, or (4) hepatoma. In all these conditions pronounced weight loss, wasting, anorexia, and fever may be found, and hepatomegaly, splenomegaly, and deranged liver function tests may be present. Procedures such as peritoneal biopsy, peritoneoscopy, liver biopsy, splenoportography, or laparotomy may be necessary to provide the diagnosis. Other less common causes of ascites include constrictive pericarditis, hepatic vein obstruction, myxedema and benign tumors of the ovary, particularly fibroma (Meigs's syndrome, with ascites and hydrothorax). The physiologic and metabolic factors involved in the production of ascites are described in Chap. 320.

REFERENCES

BAR-MEIR S: Analysis of ascitic fluid in cirrhosis. Dig Dis Sc 24:136, 1979

BORHANMANESH F et al: Tuberculous peritonitis: Prospective study of 32 cases in Iran. Ann Intern Med 76:567, 1972

CATTAN EL JR et al: The accuracy of the physical examination in the diagnosis of suspected ascites. JAMA 247:1146, 1982

CONN HO: Spontaneous bacterial peritonitis: Multiple revisitations. Gastroenterology 70:455, 1976

———, FESSEL JH: Spontaneous bacterial peritonitis in cirrhosis: Variations on a theme. Medicine 50:161, 1971

GRAKE TMS et al: Peritoneoscopy in the diagnosis of tuberculous peritonitis. Gastrointest Endosc 27:66, 1981

MALAGELADA JR et al: Origin of fat in chylous ascites of patients with liver cirrhosis. Gastroenterology 67:878, 1974

WARSHAW AL: Diagnosis of starch peritonitis by paracentesis. Lancet 2:1054, 1972

section 6 | Alterations in urinary function

40 PROTEINURIA, HEMATURIA, AZOTEMIA, AND OLIGURIA

FREDRIC L. COE

PROTEINURIA

Normal adults may excrete up to 150 mg protein daily. Of this, only 10 to 15 mg is albumin; the rest is composed of over 30 different plasma proteins and of glycoproteins that derive from the renal cells. Tamm-Horsfall mucoprotein, the most prevalent of the urine proteins that do not arise from plasma, is produced by the cells of the ascending limb of the loop of Henle and is excreted at the rate of 25 mg per day. Daily excretion of more than 150 mg protein is properly termed *pathological proteinuria,* but in common usage the word *proteinuria* suffices. Protein excretion above 3.5 g per 24 h is termed *massive* proteinuria and usually occurs when glomeruli have been damaged enough to allow plasma proteins, especially albumin, to enter the urine. Urinary albumin loss lowers serum albumin concentration, and the consequent fall in intracapillary oncotic pressure fosters the accumulation of tissue edema (Chap. 28); serum lipids rise. The combination of *massive proteinuria, hypoalbuminemia, edema,* and *hyperlipidemia* is often called the *nephrotic syndrome,* but this term is becoming synonymous with massive urinary protein loss alone. Hypoalbuminemia, elevated blood lipids, and edema are pathophysiologic consequences of massive proteinuria and occur only when hepatic albumin synthesis, though normal or even increased, fails to compensate for urine albumin losses; they are not a direct result of renal disease.

DETECTION OF PROTEINURIA Detection of proteinuria is usually by urine "dipsticks" that register a trace result in response to as little as 50 mg protein per liter, and a distinct color change of the 1+ level at about 300 mg per liter. Since proteinuria can be missed if the urine is very dilute, fasting morning samples that tend to be concentrated are usually studied. Dipsticks respond best to albumin, so that a negative result can occur when large amounts of other protein, or protein fragments such as light chains, are being excreted. Dipstick proteinuria requires additional evaluation by the measurement of 24-h excretion rate. If total protein excretion is abnormal, it is helpful to characterize the proportions of albumin and globulins in the urine by cellulose acetate electrophoresis or other methods. Immunoelectrophoresis is required to identify immunoglobulin fragments, kappa or lambda light chains, when their presence is suggested by a monoclonal peak on routine urine electrophoresis.

MECHANISMS OF PROTEINURIA **Tubular proteinuria** Normal low-molecular-weight serum proteins below 40,000 daltons, such as beta$_2$ microglobulin (11,600 mol wt), lysozyme (14,000 mol wt), or light chains (22,000 mol wt) are readily filtered by the glomeruli but are normally present in urine in only trace amounts because tubular reabsorption of them is very efficient. Diseases that selectively damage the tubules more than glomeruli (Chap. 297) cause excessive excretion of these small proteins with little or no increase in albumin excretion. The resulting proteinuria is usually between 1 and 3 g per 24 h, and edema and lipid disorders do not occur because albumin losses are small. Bence-Jones protein, which is probably a dimer of two light chains, light chains themselves, and myoglobin are examples of proteins whose plasma concentrations may increase as a consequence of disease. If their filtered load rises enough to exceed tubular reabsorptive capacity, "overflow" proteinuria may occur.

Glomerular proteinuria When glomerular damage is present, albumin and even larger globulin molecules may be filtered excessively because normal selective filtration is lost. The glomerular capillary endothelial cells form a barrier penetrated by pores of about 1000 Å diameter that holds back cells and other particles but offers no impediment to most proteins. The glomerular basement membrane traps molecules above 50 Å in effective radius. These usually have a molecular weight above 100,000 daltons. The *foot processes (podocytes)* of the visceral epithelial cells (Fig. 40-1) cover the urinary aspect of the glomerular basement membrane and produce a series of narrow channels through which molecules that traverse the basement membrane must pass. Anionic molecules, like albumin, are filtered less freely than are neutral or positively charged molecules of the same size, so little albumin enters the filtrate. This charge selectivity appears to be due to anionic glycoproteins that cover the surfaces of the foot processes and contribute to the matrix structure of the basement membrane (Chap. 289). The glycoproteins are anionic because they contain the dicarboxylic amino acids, glutamic and aspartic acid, and sialic acid. At the pH of blood (7.4) or urine (4.5 to 7.5) carboxylic and sialic acid residues are dissociated and, therefore, have a negative charge. Albumin also carries an overall negative charge. The negatively charged portions of the glycoproteins repel those of albumin and retard filtration.

Glomerular disease can disrupt any of these filtration barriers. Injury limited to the polyanion glycoproteins would tend to produce selective losses of anionic proteins, such as albumin, that would be filtered more completely by the normal

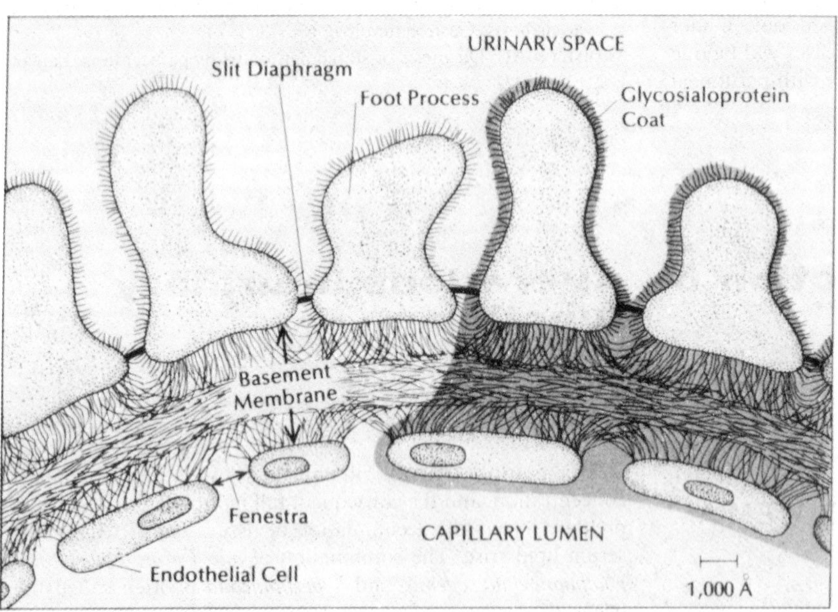

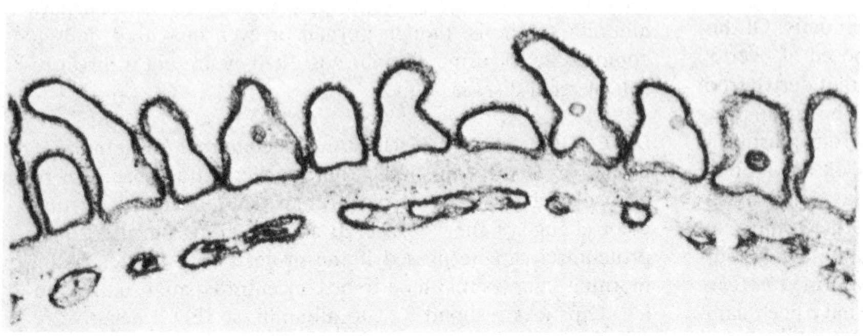

FIGURE 40-1
Top. Diagram showing normal structures separating the capillary lumen and urinary space in the glomerulus. In the process of glomerular filtration, an ultrafiltrate of plasma traverses the glomerular capillary wall through endothelial fenestrae, basement membrane, and slit diaphragms. Macromolecules in the plasma are believed to be restricted from entry into glomerular urine by each of these wall structures. In addition, circulating polyanions (e.g., albumin) are thought to be retarded by negatively charged glycosialoproteins, which, as shown by the shaded area in the upper panel, are distributed throughout the glomerular wall. Bottom. A corresponding electron micrograph of the same structures. (Drawing by NL Gahan from BM Brenner, R Beeuwkes, Hosp Prac, vol 13, no 7, 1978. Reproduced with permission.)

glomerulus but for their charge. Extensive injury that involves the entire basement membrane, not only its polyanion components, may increase losses of very large proteins, as well as albumin.

The selectivity of proteinuria varies with the extent of glomerular injury. However, the clinical value of measuring selectivity has not been fully defined. The basis of such measurements is to express the excretion rate of a protein as a fraction of its theoretical maximum filtered load, which is the product of its serum concentration and the glomerular filtration rate (GFR). This fraction must reflect the relative filtration efficiency of the protein to that of a completely filtered GFR marker, usually inulin or creatinine, provided that tubular reabsorption and renal production or catabolism are negligible. The slope of a plot of such a clearance ratio against molecular weight for a variety of serum proteins is one index of filtration selectivity. A more practical version of this test is based upon the ratio of the clearance fractions of two proteins of different molecular weight. For example, the IgG/transferrin clearance fraction ratio is below 0.1 in most children with lipoid nephrosis, a proteinuric disorder in which fusion of foot processes is the only detectable glomerular abnormality (Chap. 294) and progressive renal failure is very uncommon. In chronic membranous glomerulopathy (Chap. 294) the basement membrane is filled with immune complex deposits, and progressive loss of renal function is not uncommon. Here, the clearance ratio usually is between 0.1 and 0.2. The ratio usually is above 0.2 in membranoproliferative glomerulonephritis, a severe renal disease that can progress rapidly to renal failure and in which glomerular architecture is severely disturbed (Chap. 294). These and other aspects of the relationship between glomerular pathology and proteinuria are considered in greater detail in Chaps. 293 to 295.

APPROACH TO THE PATIENT WITH PROTEINURIA Given dipstick proteinuria of the 1+ level or more, 24-h urine protein excretion should be measured. If it is above 150 mg, electrophoresis should be carried out to determine the proportions of albumin and other proteins. Excretion mainly of albumin signifies a glomerular lesion. When the total daily protein excretion exceeds 3.5 g, by definition the nephrotic syndrome is considered to be present; milder albuminuria is called an *asymptomatic urinary abnormality*. The initial steps in evaluating proteinuria are outlined in Chap. 288. Subsequent details of differential diagnosis are in Chaps. 294 and 295. Tubular proteinuria usually reflects a hereditary or acquired tubular disorder or tubulointerstitial nephropathy (Chap. 297). The presence of large amounts of Bence-Jones protein suggests that multiple myeloma may be present (Chap. 65).

HEMATURIA

ISOLATED HEMATURIA Urinary tract bleeding from the urethra to the renal pelvis produces isolated hematuria, without significant proteinuria, cells, or urinary casts. Total hematuria, which occurs evenly throughout voiding, means that blood has had the opportunity to mix fully with the bladder urine. When bleeding occurs mainly at the beginning or end of micturition, a prostatic or urethral origin is more likely.

Common causes of *isolated* hematuria are urinary tract stones, benign and malignant neoplasms of the urinary tract, tuberculosis, trauma, and prostatitis; few primary renal diseases cause it. As discussed in Chaps. 288 and 294, *focal glomerulitis*, in the syndrome of benign recurrent hematuria or in Berger's disease, i.e., IgA nephropathy, is usually associated with red blood cell casts. Analgesic nephropathy and sickling states cause isolated hematuria, but modest proteinuria, papillary necrosis, or azotemia often is present and suggests a renal origin. Hemoglobin electrophoresis is appropriate whenever a sickling disorder is suspected.

Prostatic and external urethral examination is the basic first step in the evaluation of isolated hematuria. Intravenous pyelography is the next. If no lesion is found, cystoscopy and retrograde pyelography may become necessary. At cystoscopy, blood may be found to issue from only one ureter, a helpful clue which indicates a localized lesion rather than a primary renal disease. Disorders of coagulation, and thrombocytopenia, as well as urinary infection, must be excluded. Because infection with tuberculosis and fungi may be difficult to detect, multiple urine samples must be cultured and examined by microscopy. Renal arteriography may be needed to disclose anatomic lesions such as cysts or tumors.

HEMATURIA ASSOCIATED WITH URINARY TRACT INFECTION Bacterial infection of the lower urinary tract or of the kidneys occasionally causes hematuria. The presence of associated pyuria suggests the diagnosis of infection and the demonstration of pathogenic bacteria in concentrations above 10^5 colonies per milliliter of urine establishes it. Acute cystitis or urethritis in women is an especially common cause of gross hematuria. Urinary tuberculosis can produce isolated hematuria, but pyuria often is present as well.

HEMATURIA WITH EVIDENCE OF RENAL DISEASE **Nephronal hematuria** Blood may enter the tubular fluid anywhere along the nephron, from the glomerulus to the end of the collecting duct. Tamm-Horsfall protein tends to gel when concentrated at a low pH, as occurs during dehydration, or when exposed to myoglobin, hemoglobin, albumin, Bence-Jones protein, and pyelographic contrast media. Red blood cells in the tubule lumens can be trapped in a cylindrical mold of the gelled protein to produce red blood cell casts, which provide conclusive evidence of bleeding into the nephron. Degenerated red blood cells and clumps of hemoglobin can produce deeply pigmented casts that have the same significance as red blood cell casts.

Bleeding from the nephron itself, like glomerular proteinuria, always connotes significant renal disease such as glomerulonephritis, tubulointerstitial injury, or a vasculitis that has damaged the circulation of the nephron. Glomerular or tubular proteinuria often accompanies renal bleeding, as a consequence of nephron injury. In general, nephronal hematuria or proteinuria alone arises from primary renal diseases that have a better prognosis than those in which proteinuria and hematuria occur in combination.

Hematuria with proteinuria or casts Frequently, hematuria is accompanied by proteinuria, but red blood cell and deeply pigmented granular casts are absent. The presumption then is that bleeding is of nephronal origin, but a coincident independent lesion of the urinary tract must always be considered, because common renal diseases, such as diabetic glomerulosclerosis and arteriolar nephrosclerosis associated with hypertension, produce mainly proteinuria.

Heavy albuminuria or dehydration can cause showers of transparent, refractile "hyaline" casts. During heavy proteinuria tubule cells fill with cholesterol-rich lipid droplets that display a Maltese-cross appearance in polarized light. Casts that incorporate these cells are called *fatty casts* because the lipid droplets are prominent. The same lipid-rich cells free in urine are called *oval fat bodies*.

White blood cell and *epithelial cell casts* can occur in any inflammatory state that involves the nephrons. White blood cell casts are particularly common in pyelonephritis, nephritis associated with systemic lupus erythematosus, and during transplant rejection. When white blood or epithelial cells degenerate, they form granular nonpigmented casts that contain cellular debris and aggregated proteins. So-called *waxy* casts, with few granules and very distinct margins, arise when cell debris has broken down to a fine dispersion so that granules are no longer visible.

Broad casts, of unusual width, are thought to arise in the dilated tubules of enlarged nephrons that have undergone compensatory hypertrophy in response to a reduction of functioning renal mass. A urine sample that contains a combination of broad and waxy casts as well as cellular or granular casts or red blood cells indicates a chronic smouldering process and has been termed a *telescoped* urine. This abnormality, first described in polyarteritis nodosa and systemic lupus erythematosus, can also be found in many chronic forms of glomerulonephritis with active glomerulitis.

APPROACH TO THE PATIENT WITH HEMATURIA The most important step is to determine whether the hematuria is isolated or associated with other features of primary renal disease, i.e., cells, casts, or proteinuria. Many urinalyses may be needed to define the casts, cells, and proteins which accompany the hematuria, and the magnitude and type of associated proteinuria should be determined. As a general rule intravenous pyelography should be performed, if it can be done safely, even when the hematuria is of definite nephronal origin. Not only lesions of the urinary tract, but renal tumors or cysts, discrete areas of papillary necrosis, or signs of renal venous obstruction may be present. The source of isolated hematuria must always be ascertained, and this means a progressively detailed examination of the urinary tract by cystoscopy, retrograde pyelography, and arteriography to disclose tumor, stone, cysts, or other cause. Renal ultrasonography and computer-assisted tomography are particularly helpful in detecting and evaluating renal cysts and tumors and should precede cystoscopy and arteriography. If all the studies disclose normal structures, a nephronal origin of hematuria is likely even if no red blood cell casts are present. Hematuria with infection or overt renal disease usually requires no steps beyond intravenous pyelography. Evaluation of hematuria is detailed further in Chap. 288.

AZOTEMIA, OLIGURIA, AND ANURIA

AZOTEMIA Measurements of urea and creatinine concentrations in serum are often obtained to assess the GFR. Both substances are produced at a reasonably constant rate, by the liver and muscles, respectively. As discussed in Chap. 289, they undergo complete glomerular filtration and are not reabsorbed extensively by the renal tubules; hence their clearances tend to reflect the GFR. An increase in their serum concentrations, termed *azotemia* (*azo*, "containing nitrogen"), occurs as the GFR falls. Renal failure is reflected by a high blood nitrogen level. Of the two substances, creatinine is a more reliable index of GFR because of its lower back diffusion from tubule lumen to peritubular blood. Although azotemia is a laboratory finding, rather than a symptom, it is an almost universal clue to the presence of abnormal renal function and often of renal disease, now that multiple-test biochemical screening of blood has become a common practice.

Glomerular filtration rate may be reduced by a fall in the filtration rates of individual functioning nephrons, or by a reduction in the total number of functioning nephrons. (See Table 40-1.)

TABLE 40-1
Pathophysiologic mechanisms of azotemia

		Laboratory findings					
Mechanism of reduced GFR	*Clinical examples*	*Oliguria*	*Urine osm, mosmol/kg*	*Urine $[Na^+]$, meq/L*	$\left(\frac{U}{P}\right)_{creat}$	$\left(\frac{U}{P}\right)_{urea}$	*BUN / Serum creat*
REDUCED SNGFR							
Tubules normal (prerenal azotemia)	Severe dehydration, edema-forming states, diuretic agents, systemic hypotension, acute glomerular disease, acute urinary obstruction, incomplete renal vascular obstruction	Nearly always present	>500	<20	>40	>8	>10
Tubules damaged (acute renal failure)	Acute tubular necrosis, nephrotoxic agents, glomerulonephritis with tubule injury	Common	<350	>40	<20	<2	10
REDUCED NEPHRON NUMBER							
Elevated SNGFR	Chronic tubulointerstitial/renal disease Surgical loss of renal tissue	Rare*	290	>40	3–10	3–10	10
Normal SNGFR	Diffuse chronic glomerulonephritis Diabetic nephropathy	Rare†	100–350‡	10–100‡	>10	>3	>10
Reduced SNGFR	Any of the factors that can reduce SNGFR (listed above) may lower SNGFR in a patient who has a reduced number of functioning nephrons	Common	290	>20	>10	<3	>10

* *Occurs only when total GFR is below 5% normal.*
† *Rare as long as GFR is above 5% normal.*
‡ *Varies with diet and with the level of GFR. When GFR is below 20% normal, osmotic concentration of the urine is usually impossible.*
NOTE: *osm = osmolality; creat = creatinine concentration; U = urine; P = plasma.*

Reduced single-nephron glomerular filtration rate TUBULAR FUNCTION NORMAL The physiological response of the normal kidney to a sodium-conserving stimulus is reduction of the single-nephron glomerular filtration rate (SNGFR) and subsequent reabsorption of an increased fraction of the reduced amounts of NaCl and water that enter the tubules. Depletion of extracellular fluid volume is a most instructive example of such a stimulus. Azotemia occurs and urine Na concentration falls below 20 (often below 1 meq per liter). Secretion of vasopressin is stimulated by depletion of extracellular fluid volume, and as a consequence, the distal tubules and collecting ducts become fully permeable to water. The concentrating mechanisms in the inner medulla (Chap. 289) are very efficient when flow rates through the loops of Henle and the collecting ducts are low. As a result, the filtrate that escapes reabsorption in the proximal tubule undergoes maximal osmotic concentration, the urine volume becomes small, and it has a high osmolality, above 500 mosmol per kilogram of water. Most of the filtered creatinine escapes tubular reabsorption, and so the ratio of the urine-to-plasma (U/P) creatinine concentrations is very high, 40 or more. Because urea can back-diffuse more completely than creatinine, the urea U/P ratio is less elevated, above 8, and the blood urea nitrogen (BUN) level rises more than the serum creatinine concentration. Normally, the ratio of BUN to serum creatinine concentration is 10:1; with depletion of the extracellular fluid volume the ratio rises. An elevated ratio can also be produced by unrelated factors such as tetracycline administration, adrenocortical steroid therapy, and the presence of blood in the gastrointestinal tract.

The pattern of renal response to extracellular fluid volume depletion appears in any edema-forming condition during the phase of NaCl and water accumulation. Typical examples include the nephrotic syndrome and hepatic cirrhosis with ascites (Chaps. 28 and 294). When a diuretic is being administered to inhibit the tubular reabsorption of NaCl, urine volume and sodium concentration may be normal or elevated, even though SNGFR falls in response to the combination of the underlying edema-forming stimulus and further extracellular fluid volume depletion from the drug. Severe oliguria may appear upon withdrawal of the drug as the renal tubules resume intense reabsorption of NaCl and water. The pattern of low SNGFR with well-preserved tubule function may also be seen when renal blood flow is reduced, by systemic hypotension, incomplete renal arterial or venous occlusion, or other cause (Chap. 298). Acute incomplete obstruction of the ureter and acute glomerular injury may also reduce SNGFR and leave tubule function relatively intact, but whenever chronic obstruction or glomerulonephritis damages nephrons extensively, the high urinary osmolality, U/P ratios for creatinine or urea, and low urinary sodium concentrations disappear.

TUBULAR FUNCTION IMPAIRED Certain acute renal diseases which produce azotemia lower SNGFR and at the same time damage the tubules sufficiently to reduce or even abolish their reabsorptive functions. Acute tubular necrosis, exposure to nephrotoxic agents, and all forms of acute tubulointerstitial disease are excellent examples. Azotemia and oliguria appear, but the urine sodium concentration is above 20 meq per liter and usually above 40 meq per liter, the U/P ratios for urea and creatinine are below 2 and 20, respectively, and urine osmolality is below 350 mosmol per kilogram of water. The ratio of BUN to serum creatinine is not elevated.

Reduced nephron number INCREASED SNGFR If one kidney is removed, the other grows larger, its nephrons enlarge, and the SNGFR increases until the total GFR becomes nearly normal for two kidneys. The tubules are overperfused with filtrate, but they appear to cope well with their increased reabsorptive burdens, perhaps in part because they are longer and wider and possess more cells. If more kidney tissue is removed, the remnant nephrons enlarge further, and their SNGFR rises. Extreme overperfusion of the tubules interferes with sodium conservation. At the same time, total GFR comes to depend more and more upon expansion of the extracellular fluid volume largely because the increase in SNGFR is due not only to anatomic growth of the glomeruli but also to a relatively high rate of blood flow per glomerulus.

Azotemia occurs because the total GFR, the product of the elevated SNGFR and the markedly reduced nephron number, is low. The ratio of BUN to serum creatinine concentration is approximately 10. Urine-to-plasma ratios for creatinine and urea are usually between 3 and 10, urine sodium concentration is above 40 meq per liter, and urine osmolality approaches that of plasma. Tubule conservation of filtered water and sodium conservation are poor, so fluid and salt intake must be liberal. Clinical states that produce this picture include surgical loss of renal substance because of trauma, neoplasm, stone, and destruction of kidneys by bacterial infection or tuberculosis, polycystic and medullary cystic renal diseases, and all the chronic tubulointerstitial nephropathies (Chaps. 297 and 299). In each of these disorders, the nephrons that remain viable are either fully intact or behave as though the SNGFR is better preserved than tubule function.

SNGFR NORMAL The SNGFR does not appear to increase despite a reduction of nephron number in diseases such as glomerulonephritis and diabetic glomerulosclerosis, where the glomerulus is the primary site of damage. In these diseases total GFR falls directly with nephron number and is not supported by elevated SNGFR. Since the tubules are not confronted with an excessive reabsorptive burden, sodium conservation is adequate. In these disorders, superimposed conditions that lower SNGFR, such as depletion of extracellular fluid volume, can cause oliguria with low urine sodium concentration and U/P ratios for creatinine and urea above 20 and 3, respectively. The serum urea to creatinine ratio will rise distinctly.

SNGFR REDUCED In patients with chronic renal disease in whom total GFR has been sufficient to support life only because of a very high SNGFR, inadvertent dehydration or any other factor that lowers the SNGFR can provoke oliguria and severe azotemia. Under these circumstances, urine sodium concentration will fall, but not below 20 meq per liter, as in the normal person, because SNGFR, though reduced from a previously elevated level, may still be above normal. The U/P ratios for creatinine and urea will be low, usually below 10 and 3, respectively, despite oliguria, and urine osmolality will not rise above the plasma level. The serum urea to creatinine ratio may rise, but not above 20. In less extreme situations, reduction of SNGFR will worsen azotemia and alter urine chemistry in the same directions but to a lesser extent.

OLIGURIA In this condition urine volume is insufficient to sustain life in a steady state; it is usually less than 400 ml per 24 h (16.6 ml/h) in an adult of average size. Daily urine volume is difficult to measure when flow rate is low, because small absolute errors of volume measurement, in the range of 50 to 100 ml of urine each day, or of timing of collection, may represent large percentage errors.

APPROACH TO THE PATIENT WITH AZOTEMIA OR OLIGURIA Clinical history, physical examination, and urinalysis often disclose an obvious reason for azotemia or oliguria. The most discriminating additional measurements include serum urea and creatinine concentrations, and the sodium, urea, and creatinine concentrations and osmolality of a concurrent urine sample. Reduction of SNGFR with well-preserved tubular function is usually present when urine osmolality exceeds 500 mosmol per kilogram of water, sodium is below 20 meq per liter, the U/P ratios for urea and creatinine exceed 8 and 40, respectively, and the BUN is more than 10 times the serum creatinine concentration. The prognosis for recovery of adequate GFR is good, if the cause of reduced SNGFR can be reversed. When urine osmolality is below 350 mosmol per kilogram of water, sodium is above 40 meq, the U/P values for urea and creatinine are below 2 and 20, respectively, and the BUN exceeds the serum creatinine by only tenfold, tubule function has been lost, and some form of acute or chronic renal failure usually is present.

ANURIA This extreme condition is uncommon. Urinary obstruction is the main cause and must be excluded as a first step (Chap. 301). Complete renal arterial and venous occlusion are other important causes. Few severe renal diseases produce anuria in the adult, and anuria should never be ascribed to a primary renal disease until patency of the urinary tract and major renal blood vessels has been established.

REFERENCES

BRENNER BM et al: Molecular basis of proteinuria of glomerular origin. N Engl J Med 298:826, 1978

CARRIE BJ et al: Minimal change nephropathy: An electrochemical disorder of the glomerular membrane. Am J Med 70:262, 1981

COHEN JJ et al (eds): Nephrology forum: Isolated proteinuria in asymptomatic patients. Kidney Int 18:395, 1980

GLASSOCK RJ, BENNETT CM: The glomerulopathies, in *The Kidney*, 2d ed, BM Brenner, FC Rector Jr (eds). Philadelphia, Saunders, 1981

KURTZMAN NA (ed): *Seminars in Nephrology: Acute Renal Failure*, JP Knochel (guest ed). New York, Grune & Stratton, 1981

——— (ed): *Seminars in Nephrology: Chronic Renal Failure*, G Eknoyan (guest ed). New York, Grune & Stratton, 1981

OKEN DE: On the differential diagnosis of acute renal failure. Am J Med 71:916, 1981

PARDO V et al: Benign primary hematuria: Clinicopathologic study of 65 patients. Am J Med 67:817, 1979

41 POLYURIA AND NOCTURIA

FREDRIC L. COE

Though considered together in this chapter because they bear superficial clinical similarities to one another, polyuria and nocturia have little in common pathophysiologically. True polyuria that is not due to a deliberate, habitual high fluid intake always points to an important defect of renal water handling or of the secretion of vasopressin. Nocturia is less specific. It can arise from defective renal water conservation, excretion of an abnormal fraction of the daily salt load at night, low bladder capacity, irritable bladder, or partial bladder obstruction.

POLYURIA

Patients cannot always distinguish urinary frequency from polyuria. Voiding of small volumes is typical of frequency, whereas large volumes characterize the polyuric states. Since voiding volumes may not be clear from the history, polyuria must be substantiated by 24-h urine collection before one begins an investigation of causes. A reasonable definition of polyuria is a urine volume above 3 liters per day, but should be qualified to exclude normal individuals who desire a large fluid intake and therefore form large volumes of urine. The presence of nocturia is best established by the history alone.

CAUSES Polyuria can arise from inadequate secretion of vasopressin, failure of the renal tubules to respond to vasopressin, solute diuresis, or natriuresis (Table 41-1). It may also occur as a physiological adaptation to deliberate excessive water drinking. The normal physiology of urine formation and mechanisms responsible for renal water conservation are discussed in Chap. 289.

Diabetes insipidus (see also Chap. 110) The term *diabetes insipidus* is applied to situations in which renal water conservation is so inadequate that polyuria occurs. Either vasopressin insufficiency (central diabetes insipidus) or renal unresponsiveness to vasopressin (nephrogenic diabetes insipidus) produces severe polyuria and secondary thirst. In both, water reabsorption is reduced all along the distal nephron, because passive water movement from tubules into the hypertonic outer and inner medullary interstitium is slow. But even though the rate of water movement out of the collecting ducts is low for a given osmotic difference between the tubule lumen and interstitial fluid, the fluid that enters the collecting ducts is so abnormally dilute and copious in volume that more water enters the inner medulla than under normal circumstances and medullary solutes are washed out into the vasa recta. Washout is incomplete and vasopressin administration can lead to formation of an osmotically concentrated urine, but the maximum urine osmolality that can be attained is below normal.

Vasopressin-sensitive (central) diabetes insipidus may be idiopathic or secondary to hypophysectomy or trauma or to neoplastic, inflammatory, vascular, or infectious causes (Table 41-1). Idiopathic diabetes insipidus can be familial, and then it is usually inherited as an autosomal dominant trait; but more commonly it is sporadic and appears in childhood. In both

TABLE 41-1
Causes of polyuria

I Inadequate renal water conservation
- *A* Diabetes insipidus
  - *1* Vasopressin-sensitive (posthypophysectomy; posttrauma; postpituitary ablation; idiopathic, supra- or intrasellar tumors or cysts; histiocystosis or granuloma; encroachment by aneurysm; Sheehan's syndrome, meningoencephalitis; Guillain-Barré's syndrome; fat embolus; empty sella)
  - *2* Nephrogenic
    - *a* Acquired tubulointerstitial renal disease (pyelonephritis, analgesic nephropathy, multiple myeloma, amyloidosis, obstructive uropathy, sarcoidosis, hypercalcemic or hypokalemic nephropathy, Sjögren's syndrome, sickle cell anemia, renal transplantation)
    - *b* Drugs or toxins (lithium, demeclocycline, methyoxyflurane, ethanol, diphenylhydantoin, propoxyphene, amphotericin)
    - *c* Congenital (hereditary nephrogenic diabetes insipidus, polycystic or medullary cystic disease)
- *B* Solute diuresis (glucosuria, high-protein tube feedings, urea or mannitol infusion, radiographic contrast media, chronic renal failure)
- *C* Natriuretic syndromes (salt-losing nephritis, diuretic phase of acute tubular necrosis, diuretic agents)

II Primary polydipsia

forms there is selective destruction of the neurons that produce vasopressin in the supraoptic nucleus.

Failure of the kidney to respond to vasopressin, i.e., nephrogenic diabetes insipidus, may be acquired or congenital. Nephrogenic diabetes insipidus acquired from renal disease (Table 41-1) probably is the most common form; the familial form is rare. Hypercalcemia and hypokalemic nephropathy are important reversible causes of nephrogenic diabetes insipidus. Lithium carbonate, methoxyflurane (1,1-difluoro-2,2-dichloroethyl methyl ether) anesthetic, and demeclocycline, a tetracycline derivative, can also produce nephrogenic diabetes insipidus.

Solute diuresis Excessive filtration of a poorly resorbed solute such as glucose, mannitol, or urea can depress reabsorption of NaCl and water in the proximal tubule and cause their loss in the urine, producing polyuria. Urine sodium concentration is below that of blood, so that more water than salt is lost from the body and serum hypertonicity can be produced. Glucosuria in diabetes mellitus is a common cause of solute diuresis. Iatrogenic solute diuresis may arise from mannitol infusion, angiographic contrast media, and high-protein gavage feedings, which produce excessive excretion of urea.

Natriuretic syndromes Excessive chronic sodium loss may occur during the course of tubulointerstitial or cystic renal diseases. Polyuria and polydipsia are accompanied by an unusually large daily sodium requirement. Examples of this phenomenon include medullary cystic disease, Bartter's syndrome, and the diuretic phase of acute tubular necrosis, in which sodium and water losses are very large.

Primary polydipsia Whether because of habit, predilection, psychiatric disorder, or a specific lesion in the brain, some people drink enough water every day to produce polyuria. The body and the kidneys rarely if ever are injured by chronic polydipsia, but the condition can be confused with diabetes insipidus, which it resembles closely. During deliberate polydipsia, extracellular fluid volume is normal or high, and vasopressin secretion is reduced to a basal level because serum osmolality tends to be near the lower limits of normal. Reabsorption of water from the end distal convoluted tubule and collecting ducts is reduced so that all the surplus water can be excreted into the urine. The inner medulla loses its urea and NaCl gradients because of washout, as in diabetes insipidus. Washout may be more severe than in diabetes insipidus because primary polydipsia tends to cause expansion of the extracellular fluid volume, whereas primary renal water loss does the opposite. Volume expansion raises total delivery of NaCl and water to the thick ascending limb of Henle's loop and therefore to the inner medulla, all things being equal. It also raises renal blood flow, and increased flow through the vasa rectae reduces their ability to trap solutes in the medulla.

APPROACH TO THE PATIENT Solute diuresis and natriuretic syndromes usually are apparent from the history, physical examination, urinalysis, clinical setting, blood count, and serum creatinine or the BUN. Diagnostic problems occur mainly when stable, chronic polyuria and polydipsia of uncertain origin are present. Here, one must try to distinguish between vasopressin-sensitive diabetes insipidus, nephrogenic diabetes insipidus, and primary polydipsia; and the best-established way to do this is by measuring the response of urine osmolality to water deprivation and the administration of vasopressin.

The patient should have free access to water and receive a normal diet that provides approximately 100 mmol NaCl per day for 3 days; then a total fast is instituted. During the fast, pulse and blood pressure should be measured every 30 min and body weight every hour, using an accurate balance. When 3 percent of the initial body weight has been lost or 14 h have elapsed, urine and serum osmolality are measured. A normal subject will lower urine volume below 0.5 ml/min and raise urine osmolality to above 700 mosmol per kilogram of water. In complete diabetes insipidus, nephrogenic or vasopressin-sensitive, the urine osmolality will remain below 200 mosmol/kg and urine flow will remain above 0.5 ml/min, but some rise in osmolality and fall in flow will occur given incomplete diabetes insipidus. If urine osmolality is below 700 mosmol/kg, by the end of the fasting period, 5 mU/min of aqueous vasopressin is administered by intravenous drip. Patients with complete or partial vasopressin-sensitive diabetes insipidus will raise their urine osmolality above the level achieved by fasting alone. No increase will occur given complete nephrogenic diabetes insipidus, although incomplete forms of nephrogenic diabetes insipidus will permit some response to vasopressin.

The response of patients with primary polydipsia is quite different. During fluid restriction the secretion of vasopressin increases, and at the completion of the test the flow rate and osmolality of the urine will reflect a physiological level of vasopressin acting upon normal tubules that traverse a medullary interstitium whose urea and NaCl concentrations have been reduced by chronic washout. In other words, the washout will set the upper limit on urine osmolality, and patients with primary polydipsia thus demonstrate a submaximal concentrating ability in spite of intact vasopressin secretion. Exogenous vasopressin can increase urine osmolality very little, if at all, because medullary washout, not vasopressin insensitivity, is the main limiting factor. Usually the urine osmolality will be above 400 mosmol/kg by the end of the fluid deprivation test, in contrast to the lower values of approximately 200 mosmol/kg encountered in patients with nephrogenic diabetes insipidus; but it may be impossible to distinguish incomplete nephrogenic diabetes insipidus from primary polydipsia, in some cases, by using the fluid deprivation test alone. However, measurement of serum antidiuretic hormone levels by radioimmunoassay may increase diagnostic accuracy.

NOCTURIA

Whether an individual sleeps through the night without urinating depends upon a diurnal rhythm in which the volume of urine formed during sleep does not exceed bladder capacity. Nocturia results when nocturnal urine volume exceeds bladder capacity, because of reduced renal osmotic concentration, high sodium excretion, solute diuresis, or low bladder capacity.

All the polyuric states may cause nocturia. Urinary concentrating ability falls in most renal diseases (Chap. 289), often at an early stage. Even though overt polyuria may be absent, overnight urine volume frequently exceeds bladder capacity. Nocturia also occurs in edema-forming states. In congestive heart failure, nephrotic syndrome, and hepatic cirrhosis with ascites, fluid accumulates preferentially in dependent portions of the body during the day. At night, with recumbency, tissue capillary forces change and some edema fluid is mobilized, producing the effect of an intravenous saline infusion. Venous insufficiency may produce dependent edema of the legs that is often also mobilized at night, causing nocturia.

Reduced bladder capacity is present when infection, tumor, or stone causes inflammation or increased irritability. Chronic partial bladder-outflow obstruction, from prostatic hypertrophy, urethral stricture, or benign or malignant neoplasm or stone, causes a frequent stimulus to void and also a thickening of the muscular wall that reduces its compliance. Frequent small voidings may be a clue to this lower urinary tract cause of nocturia, but in its earlier phases chronic obstruction may lead to only one nocturnal voiding of reasonable volume.

REFERENCES

HAYS RM, LEVINE SD: Pathophysiology of water metabolism, in *The Kidney*, 2d ed, BM Brenner, FC Rector Jr (eds). Philadelphia, Saunders, 1981

SCHRIER RW, BICHET DG: Osmotic and nonosmotic control of vasopressin release and the pathogenesis of impaired water excretion in adrenal, thyroid, and edematous disorders. J Lab Clin Med 98:1, 1981

WEITZMAN R, KLEEMAN CR: Water metabolism and the neurohypophyseal hormones, in *Clinical Disorders of Fluid and Electrolyte Metabolism*, MH Maxwell, CR Kleeman (eds). New York, McGraw-Hill, 1980, p 531

ZERBE RL, ROBERTSON GL: A comparison of plasma vasopressin measurements with a standard indirect test in the differential diagnosis of polyuria. N Engl J Med 305:1539, 1981

42
DYSURIA, INCONTINENCE, AND ENURESIS

WILLIAM GILL
FREDRIC L. COE

NORMAL BLADDER FUNCTION

The detrusor muscle, which provides the propulsive force for emptying the bladder, consists of interlacing fibers of smooth muscle that are under parasympathetic autonomic control through the pelvic nerves from sacral spinal cord segments S2, S3, and S4. The smooth muscle of the trigonal portion of the bladder, between the ureteral orifices and the posterior area of the bladder outlet, is innervated by motor fibers from thoracolumbar segments (T11 to L2) of the sympathetic nervous system, in which alpha receptor sites predominate. This layer of muscle extends into the posterior urethra and acts as an involuntary internal sphincter that helps maintain urinary continence even in the absence of voluntary control. The external urethral sphincter and perineal muscles are under voluntary control via the pudendal nerves.

Sensory tracts for pain, temperature, and distention pass from the bladder via the pelvic nerves to sacral spinal levels S2, S3, and S4, creating a simple spinal voiding reflex between the bladder and the sacral spinal cord. The sensory tracts from the bladder further ascend through sacrobulbar pathways to the medulla of the brain and ultimately to cortical centers (superomedial portion of the frontal lobes), from which impulses arise, pass back down the lateral and ventral reticulospinal tracts, and normally suppress the sacral spinal reflex arc controlling bladder emptying.

The normal adult bladder can accommodate as much as approximately 400 ml fluid without a significant increase in intravesical pressure (< 20 cmH_2O). Above this point, sensations of fullness are transmitted to the sacral cord. If not suppressed by cortical control, the sacral cord reflexly discharges motor impulses that cause powerful sustained detrusor contraction. Urination can be prevented by cortical suppression of the reflex arc or by voluntary contraction of the external sphincter and perineal muscles. Infants, and adults with spinal cord damage above S2, urinate spontaneously when the bladder fills sufficiently.

Normal micturition is initiated by voluntary suppression of cortical inhibition of the reflex arc and by relaxation of the muscles of the pelvic floor and the external sphincter. The base of the bladder falls; then the trigone contracts, an action that occludes the ureters as they pass through the bladder wall and helps to prevent vesicoureteral reflux of urine during voiding. Finally, the detrusor contracts and voiding occurs.

DYSURIA

Dysuria refers to anything abnormal having to do with urination, such as urinary frequency, nocturia, hesitancy in starting urination, straining to urinate, burning upon urination, urgency, decreased size of urinary stream, dribbling at the end of urination, and combinations of these symptoms. Some clinicians restrict the use of the term *dysuria* to burning or pain upon urination, but the broader definition is preferable.

MECHANISMS OF DYSURIA **Reduced bladder compliance** When the bladder has a decreased ability to expand, frequency, nocturia, and urgency usually result. When decreased expansion is due to inflammation of the mucosa (cystitis) from infection, radiation, chemicals, or foreign bodies (catheters, stones), burning usually is more prominent than when it is due to infiltration of the muscle by tumors of the bladder or from adjacent organs (prostate, rectum, uterus). Any upper motor neuron lesion that interferes with cortical inhibition of the voiding reflex produces a spastic hypertonic bladder, and incontinence is then a frequent manifestation.

Impaired bladder emptying Increased outflow resistance because of obstruction of the bladder neck or urethra causes hesitancy, reduced caliber of the stream, and dribbling. Damage to the sacral nerves involved in vesical emptying can produce a completely autonomous bladder, or a sensory paralytic or motor paralytic neurogenic bladder. Thus, the individual whose bladder has lost all sensory and motor innervation must rely for emptying upon distention of the organ leading to muscle stretching and automatic contraction, because the sacral voiding reflex is absent. Hesitancy, incomplete emptying, and even gross retention of urine can result. Symptoms of bladder fullness will depend upon whether the sensory tracts are intact. Since the bladder cannot empty itself properly in the worst cases of deficient innervation, gross overflow incontinence occurs.

CAUSES OF DYSURIA **Infection** *Acute bacterial cystitis*, which occurs more frequently in women, usually causes great frequency day and night, burning on urination, and, not infrequently, gross hematuria. *Prostatitis* or *prostatocystitis* in men can cause a picture similar to acute cystitis in women. When only the prostate is involved, milder symptoms such as vague pain or discomfort in the lower abdomen, groin, perineum, rectum, testes, or penis occur. The symptoms may be associated with urination, but more frequently are noticed at times other than during micturition or ejaculation.

Benign prostatic hypertrophy This condition afflicts upwards of 75 percent of older men. It is manifested by nocturia, reduced size and force of the urinary stream, straining to urinate, and terminal dribbling, all due to outflow obstruction.

Neurological disorders Any lesion that disrupts the lateral and vertical reticulospinal tracts can reduce or abolish descending inhibiting impulses to the sacral spine reflex and can result in a loss of bladder compliance due to increased detrusor tone. Frequency will result, because intravesical pressure will be abnormally elevated even at low bladder volumes. If the descending tracts are completely destroyed, the bladder will empty automatically, producing incontinence. Sacral motor damage produces incomplete emptying and, in the extreme case, overflow incontinence.

Psychosomatic cystitis The functional bladder syndrome and chronic glandular urethrotrigonitis are synonyms for a very common but poorly understood affliction of middle-aged and older women, in which pain is usually vague, aching in nature, and in the lower abdomen or vagina. There is daytime frequency without nocturia; pyuria is absent. A complete urologic evaluation usually becomes necessary because symptoms are chronic and hard to eradicate. The functional bladder syndrome must be distinguished from the effects of a cystocele, which can be repaired surgically. (See also Chap. 296.)

APPROACH TO THE PATIENT The medical history should focus on past as well as present urinary problems. A pelvic examination in women and prostatic examination in men are necessary components of the physical examination. Microscopic examination of a two-glass urinary sediment in all patients and of the prostatic fluid in men, obtained by prostatic massage, is also necessary. The first 20 ml of a voiding, if collected separately, may contain a higher concentration of leukocytes and bacteria than the remainder of the voided urine, when the urethra is the principal site of inflammation or infection. Normal prostatic fluid, not subjected to centrifugation, contains less than 10 leukocytes per high-power field; excessive leukocytes in the prostatic fluid are an important clue to prostatitis and may, when prostatitis is chronic, be the only detectable abnormality. Further diagnostic studies will depend upon such positive findings as a history of chronic or recurrent episodes or associated fever, which are rare in lower urinary tract infections except in acute prostatitis, or an abnormality on physical examination such as a pelvic or rectal mass or tenderness, hematuria or pyuria, or excessive leukocytes and macrophages in the prostatic fluid. Serum acid phosphatase may be elevated when carcinoma of the prostate has extended beyond the boundary of the prostatic capsule.

Additional evaluation of dysuria, when the cause is not evident from clinical examination, may include cultures of urine and prostatic fluid for aerobic and anaerobic bacteria, tubercle bacilli, and mycoplasma, excretory urography and voiding cystourethrography. If these examinations do not reveal the diagnosis, but the symptoms are sufficiently troublesome, urologic consultation should be sought. The urologist may carry out cystoscopy and urethroscopy with endoscopic biopsies where abnormalities are found. Functional urodynamic studies, gas cystometry, sphincter electromyography, urethral pressure profile, uroflometry, and urine spectrometry may be needed in special cases.

INCONTINENCE

Incontinence refers to the inability to retain urine in the bladder. The diagnostic approach to the evaluation of the patient should be the same as that used for dysuria.

Stress incontinence This condition is common in postmenopausal parous women. The structures of the female urethra atrophy when deprived of estrogen and many become unable to resist the passage of urine under the stress of increased intraabdominal pressure during coughing, sneezing, climbing stairs, and other physical activity. Parturition may damage the pelvic support of the bladder so that the bladder and urethra can slip downward from their normal position above the pelvic diaphragm. As they do, the urethra shortens, and the normal urethrovesical angle, important in closing the urethral sphincter, is lost. In men, stress incontinence usually is secondary to prostatic surgery for benign prostatic hypertrophy or prostatic carcinoma. If the external sphincter has also been damaged during operation, total, complete incontinence may result.

Inflammatory lesions of the bladder mucosa, especially in the trigone area, can cause uncontrollable detrusor contractions and unwanted passage of urine, often called *urgency incontinence.* Common inflammatory lesions include infection, stones in the intravesical ureter, bladder tumors, and catheters in the bladder. Upper motor neuron lesions of the spinal cord or brain may produce a hypertonic, spastic, neurogenic bladder with frequent, uncontrollable, urgency incontinence.

Overflow or paradoxical incontinence This form of incontinence arises from large residual volumes of urine secondary to obstruction at the bladder neck or along the urethra (urethral stricture) or from neurological damage. Hypotonic neurogenic bladders may occur in diseases which produce autonomic peripheral neuropathy, such as diabetes mellitus, uremia, hypothyroidism, chronic alcoholism, Guillain-Barré syndrome, collagen vascular diseases, and toxic neuropathies associated with some carcinomas (especially lung and kidney). It may also occur because of prolonged overdistention of the bladder. Hydronephrosis and impaired renal function can occur in patients with chronic overflow incontinence.

Some congenital anomalies, extrophy of the bladder, patent urachus, and ectopic ureteral openings distal to the vesical neck cause *mechanical incontinence.* Acquired mechanical incontinence can follow transurethral resection of the prostate in which damage has occurred to both the internal and external sphincter mechanisms. Pelvic surgery or irradiation of the uterus or rectum may cause incontinence because of vesicovaginal, ureterovaginal, vesicoperineal, or ureteroperineal fistulae.

Children, and even some young adults, draw attention to themselves by feigning incontinence and thereby derive some secondary emotional satisfaction. A complete diagnostic evaluation usually is necessary to rule out organic disease even when *psychogenic incontinence* is strongly suspected.

ENURESIS

Enuresis refers to the involuntary passage of urine at night or during sleep—hence, the synonym *bed-wetting.* Some clinicians reserve the term enuresis for those bed wetters who have no gross urologic abnormalities, but it should be used for bed-wetting in general.

The sacral spinal reflex arc alone controls urination in the infant; therefore, enuretic incontinence is normal under the age of 2 years. As the nervous system matures, cortical control over the spinal reflex arc results in the voluntary control over urination and defecation by the age of $2\frac{1}{2}$ years. Even so, enuresis beyond the age of 3 years occurs to some degree in approximately 10 percent of all otherwise normal children and probably is due to a delay in maturation of bladder control, which may be familial.

Although the majority of bed wetters will be dry by the age of puberty, organic diseases, especially infections of the urinary tract, obstructive lesions with overflow incontinence, neurovesical dysfunction, and polyuric conditions that overload the bladder must be suspected in any child who is enuretic beyond the age of 3 years. Patients with organic disease usually, but not always, are incontinent during the day as well as at night. The approach to the patient with enuresis is the same as that used for dysuria or incontinence.

REFERENCES

BRADLEY WE: Autonomic neuropathy and the genitourinary system. J Urol 119:299, 1978

———: Diagnosis of urinary bladder dysfunction in diabetes mellitus. Ann Intern Med 92:323, 1980

———, SCOTT FB: Physiology of the urinary bladder, in *Urology*, 4th ed, JH Harrison et al (eds). Philadelphia, Saunders, 1978, vol 1, chap 4, p 87

DEGROAT WC, BOOTH AM: Physiology of the urinary bladder and urethra. Ann Intern Med 92:312, 1980

HARRISON JH et al (eds): Infections and inflammations of the genitourinary tract, in *Urology*, 4th ed. Philadelphia, Saunders, 1978, vol 1, sec IV, p 451

HINDMARSH HR, BYRNE PO: Adult enuresis: A symptomatic and urodynamic assessment. Br J Urol 52:88, 1980

MEARES EM Jr: Prostatitis syndromes: New perspectives about old woes. J Urol 123:141, 1980

MIKKELSEN EJ, RAPOPORT JL: Enuresis: Psychopathology, sleep stage, and drug response. Urol Clin N Am 7:361, 1980

TURNER-WARWICK R, WHITESIDE CG (eds): *Symposium on Clinical Urodynamics: The Urologic Clinics of North America.* Philadelphia, Saunders, 1979, vol 6

43
FLUIDS AND ELECTROLYTES

NORMAN G. LEVINSKY

SODIUM AND WATER

PHYSIOLOGIC CONSIDERATIONS (See also Chap. 289) Both physiologically and clinically, sodium and water metabolism are closely interrelated. The sodium content of the body depends on the balance between dietary intake and renal excretion of sodium. In health, extrarenal losses of sodium are negligible. Renal sodium excretion is closely regulated to match dietary content. Within 2 to 4 days after sodium intake stops, urinary excretion decreases to 5 meq per day or less. If dietary sodium is abruptly increased, sodium excretion promptly rises. About one-half of the surfeit is excreted within the first 24 h and the remainder over the next few days. Thus, in normal persons the sodium content of the body remains quite constant despite wide variations in sodium intake; over the range of 0 to 400 meq per day, total body sodium varies only by about 10 percent.

Although detailed knowledge of the mechanism of this renal response is limited, certain general points deserve emphasis because of their clinical relevance. Sodium loads tend to increase glomerular filtration and to depress proximal tubular reabsorption of sodium, while sodium deficits have the opposite effects. Thus, delivery of sodium to the distal segments of the nephron tends to vary in parallel with extracellular sodium. Reabsorption in the loop of Henle and distal convolutions appears to change proportionately with the rate of sodium delivery. This modulates variations in the amount of sodium entering the collecting ducts, where final adjustments are made. Multiple regulatory factors control these tubular adjustments. Of these, only the role of aldosterone is well established; its principal action is to stimulate sodium transport in distal nephron segments, especially the cortical collecting ducts. There is some evidence for a "natriuretic hormone" which inhibits sodium reabsorption, perhaps at a distal tubular site such as the collecting duct. Prostaglandins may have a similar action. Changes in proximal tubular reabsorption in response to altered sodium balance appear to be mediated, at least in part, by changes in hemodynamic factors in the peritubular microcirculation. Undoubtedly, other regulatory mechanisms remain to be defined. The multiplicity of control mechanisms prevents abnormalities of any single mechanism from grossly distorting the regulation of sodium excretion. For example, increased aldosterone secretion leads only to limited and transient sodium retention, because the initial accumulation of sodium stimulates opposing natriuretic factors such as increased glomerular filtration and decreased proximal tubular reabsorption.

All but 2 to 5 percent of the sodium in the body is located in the extracellular fluids. (Approximately 40 percent of total body sodium is located in bone, but this fraction does not participate significantly in most physiologic processes and will not be considered further.) Except for minor differences in concentration due to the Gibbs-Donnan effect of plasma proteins, the electrolyte compositions of plasma and interstitial fluid are essentially equal. For practical purposes, plasma composition can be considered representative of the entire extracellular compartment. Total extracellular volume approximates 20 percent of body weight. Of this, 5 percent represents plasma volume and 15 percent the volume of interstitial fluids. Thus, in a 70-kg individual with plasma sodium concentration of 140 meq per liter, extracellular sodium content will approximate 2000 meq. The volume of intracellular fluid is approximately twice as great as that of extracellular fluid, i.e., about 40 percent of body weight. However, since intracellular sodium concentration is less than 5 meq per liter, total intracellular sodium content is only about 100 to 150 meq. The asymmetric distribution of sodium across cell membranes is maintained by expenditure of a large fraction of the energy derived from cell metabolism, which is required constantly to pump sodium out of cells against its electrochemical gradient. All the principal electrolytes are asymmetrically distributed across cell membranes. The principal electrolytes of the extracellular fluids are sodium, chloride, and bicarbonate. The major electrolytes of the intracellular fluids are potassium, magnesium, calcium, and organic anions, including proteins.

Since sodium salts account for more than 90 percent of the total osmolality of the extracellular fluid, variations in plasma sodium concentration are almost always reflected in equivalent changes in plasma osmolality. Exceptions due to accumulation of other solutes in plasma are discussed later. Although the electrolyte compositions of intracellular and extracellular fluids differ markedly, they are always in osmotic equilibrium, since water moves rapidly across cellular membranes to dissipate osmotic gradients. Therefore, although sodium is largely confined to extracellular fluids, plasma sodium concentration is an index of not only the relative proportions of sodium and water in those fluids but also the relation between total body solute and total body water. An example is the effect of shift of sodium from extracellular to intracellular fluid without a change in total body solute. Movement of sodium into cells would not cause hyponatremia, since water would shift into cells with the sodium. On the other hand, a primary decrease in the concentration of osmotically active solute within cells would decrease total body solute; although there would be no change in total body sodium or water, hyponatremia would result from the shift of intracellular water into the extracellular compartment.

A very effective mechanism involving the hypothalamus, the neurohypophysis, and the kidney regulates plasma osmolality. Changes of 2 percent or less in plasma osmolality can be detected by osmoreceptors in the hypothalamus. Small increases in osmolality stimulate the secretion of antidiuretic hormone (ADH) from the neurohypophysis, while small decreases suppress secretion of the hormone. Normal plasma osmolality is approximately 280 to 300 mosmol per kilogram of water; the exact level is determined by the "set" of the hypothalamic osmoreceptors in a given individual. When ADH secretion is maximal, urine volume will be about 500 ml per day, and urine osmolality will be 800 to 1400 mosmol/kg. In the absence of ADH, minimal urine osmolality is 40 to 80 mosmol/kg, and maximum water diuresis can reach 15 to 20 liters per day or more. The capacity of this receptor-effector system is sufficient to maintain plasma osmolality within narrow limits despite large variations in the volume and concentration of dietary fluids.

The total sodium *content* of the body is determined by the renal sodium regulatory mechanisms described earlier. However, the principal determinant of plasma sodium *concentration* is water metabolism rather than total body sodium content. If excess sodium were to be ingested and retained, hypernatremia would be only transient. Water intake would increase because of thirst, and the fluid ingested would be retained because hypernatremia (hyperosmolality) would stimulate ADH secretion. Expanded extracellular volume, not hypernatremia, would be the end result. Conversely, if the osmoregulatory system is functioning normally, loss of sodium without water would not result in permanent reduction of plasma sodium concentration. The initial reduction would shut off secretion of ADH, and a water diuresis would ensue. The final outcome would be contraction of extracellular volume, while plasma sodium concentration would be restored to normal. It should be apparent that changes in total sodium content tend to cause changes in extracellular volume. In this sense, the sodium content of the extracellular fluid determines extracellular volume. On the other hand, changes in plasma sodium concentration reflect altered regulation of water excretion, not changes in total body sodium content alone. Clinically, plasma sodium concentration per se gives no information about the amount of sodium present in the body. Total body sodium content is determined by the volume of extracellular fluids as well as by the concentration of sodium in these fluids. Extracellular volume is usually the dominant factor since changes in volume tend to be greater than changes in sodium concentration. Plasma sodium concentration reflects merely the relative proportions of sodium and water (or, more exactly, of total body solute and water), not the absolute amount of sodium in the body. Either hyponatremia or hypernatremia may occur when total body sodium content is decreased, normal, or increased.

CLINICAL DISORDERS Deficits and excesses of sodium and water occur in a great variety of clinical circumstances. The manifestations of the underlying illness may overshadow the clinical features of the fluid and electrolyte disorder. Theoretically, disturbances of sodium and water metabolism can be classified into four categories, reflecting a primary excess or deficit of water or sodium. Practically, such isolated disturbances are uncommon. A primary excess of sodium leads to edema; it is not ordinarily considered as an electrolyte disorder but as a feature of underlying disease, such as congestive heart failure, hepatic cirrhosis, or nephrotic syndrome. Primary sodium deficits are nearly always accompanied by water depletion, leading to the clinical syndrome of extracellular volume depletion. Pure or disproportionate water excess leads to hyponatremia, relative or absolute water depletion to hypernatremia. A practical clinical classification of disorders of sodium and water metabolism is given in Table 43-1.

VOLUME DEPLETION Combined sodium and water deficits are far more frequent than isolated deficits of either constituent. Although the term *dehydration* is often used for combined deficits, this usage is confusing. Dehydration should be used to describe relatively pure water depletion leading to hypernatremia; *volume depletion* or some similar term should be used for combined deficits.

Pathogenesis As noted earlier, elimination of sodium from the diet will not by itself lead to sodium depletion, since urinary sodium excretion will quickly fall to very low levels. Therefore, sodium depletion is always due either to extrarenal losses or to abnormal renal losses.

GASTROINTESTINAL The most common cause of volume depletion is loss of a significant fraction of the 8 to 10 liters of gastrointestinal fluids normally secreted daily. Since the principal secretions contain potassium and hydrogen ion or bicarbonate in large amounts, volume depletion due to gastrointestinal losses is often combined with potassium depletion and acidosis or alkalosis.

Significant volume depletion may be caused by sequestration of secretions within an obstructed gastrointestinal tract or within the peritoneal cavity in peritonitis. Rapid reaccumulation of ascites after paracentesis may cause contraction of the effective circulating blood volume.

SKIN The sodium concentration of sweat varies from 5 to 50 meq per liter; sodium concentration increases with higher rates of sweating and in adrenal insufficiency. Because sweat is always a hypotonic solution, sweating leads to water deficits out of proportion to sodium losses. In burns, capillary damage may lead to sequestration of large amounts of sodium and water in the injured skin.

RENAL Abnormal losses of sodium in the urine may occur in both acute and chronic renal diseases. Early in the recovery

TABLE 43-1
Disorders of sodium and water metabolism

I Combined sodium and water depletion (volume depletion)
- *A* Extrarenal losses
  - *1* Gastrointestinal (vomiting, diarrhea, gastrointestinal suction, fistulas)
  - *2* Abdominal sequestration (peritonitis, rapid reaccumulation of ascites)
  - *3* Skin (sweating, burns)
- *B* Renal losses
  - *1* Renal disease (chronic renal failure, salt-wasting tubular disease, diuretic phase of acute renal failure)
  - *2* Diuretic excess
  - *3* Osmotic diuresis (diabetic glycosuria)
  - *4* Adrenal insufficiency

II Hyponatremia
- *A* Associated with extracellular volume depletion (see list of causes above)
- *B* Associated with extracellular volume excess and edema
- *C* Associated with normal or modestly expanded extracellular volume (no edema)
  - *1* Acute and chronic renal failure
  - *2* Temporary impairment of water diuresis (pain, drugs, emotion)
  - *3* Syndrome of inappropriate secretion of antidiuretic hormone (SIADH)
  - *4* Severe polydipsia
  - *5* Essential ("sick-cell syndrome")
- *D* Without plasma hypoosmolality
  - *1* Osmotic (hyperglycemia, mannitol)
  - *2* Artifactual (hyperlipemia, hyperproteinemia, laboratory error)

III Hypernatremia
- *A* Extrarenal water loss
  - *1* Skin (insensible losses, burns, sweat)
  - *2* Lungs (insensible)
- *B* Renal water loss
  - *1* Diabetes insipidus (pituitary, nephrogenic)
  - *2* Osmotic diuresis (glycosuria, urea diuresis)
- *C* Primary excess of sodium (excessive salt administration without access to water)
- *D* Adrenal hyperfunction (Cushing's disease, primary hyperaldosteronism)

(diuretic) phase of *acute renal failure*, urinary sodium concentration tends to be high (50 to 100 meq per liter), and substantial deficits may ensue. With rare exceptions, severe sodium wasting does not persist beyond the first few days. It is important to discriminate between increased sodium excretion which represents elimination of excess salt retained during the oliguric period and true tubular sodium wasting which depletes normal extracellular sodium. Only the latter requires replacement. Acute salt wasting due to tubular damage may also occur immediately after relief of prolonged *obstruction* of the urinary tract. Although such a postobstructive diuresis may be severe, it rarely persists for more than several days as a clinically important phenomenon.

Patients with *chronic renal failure* have limited ability to decrease sodium excretion in response to decreased intake. They will become progressively volume-depleted if their intake is restricted by the anorexia, nausea, and vomiting characteristic of uremia or because of their physician's instructions. Large deficits may develop insidiously over many days or weeks. A "vicious circle" may result, in that volume depletion will tend further to compromise renal function. Sodium-wasting renal disease, i.e., negative sodium balance when dietary sodium is normal, is very rare. It occurs in occasional patients with tubulointerstitial diseases of the kidney, especially medullary cystic disease.

Renal sodium wasting in the presence of normal intrinsic renal function occurs in three clinical circumstances. Perhaps the most common is sodium depletion due to continued administration of potent *diuretics* after edema has been relieved or to patients whose edema is sequestered and cannot be mobilized. For example, attempted treatment of cirrhotics with ascites may result in depletion of overall extracellular volume rather than mobilization of ascitic fluid. An obligatory *osmotic diuresis* may also cause renal sodium wasting despite normal renal function. Marked glycosuria in uncontrolled diabetes mellitus is the most frequent clinical example. Administration of osmotic diuretics such as mannitol and urea is a common iatrogenic cause. Volume depletion in patients receiving high-protein tube feedings may be due to an osmotic diuresis of urea formed by protein metabolism. Finally, renal sodium wasting despite normal intrinsic function occurs in *adrenal insufficiency* due to a deficiency of mineralocorticoids.

Clinical features and diagnosis The cause of volume depletion can usually be suspected from a history of inadequate salt and water intake together with vomiting, diarrhea, or excessive sweating; the symptoms of poorly controlled diabetes mellitus or of renal or adrenal disease may be elicited. The key findings on physical examination are those of plasma and extracellular volume depletion. Decreased skin turgor is usually present in patients with significant volume contraction but may be difficult to evaluate in the elderly. It can be estimated clinically by noting the slow rate of return of skin to its original position when it is raised between the examiner's fingers. An area of skin normally free of wrinkles and not subject to wide variations in the thickness of subcutaneous tissue, such as that over the sternum, should be selected for this maneuver. Oral mucous membranes may be dry and axillary sweating decreased; these are less reliable diagnostic features than decreased skin turgor. With moderate volume depletion, blood pressure is usually normal when the patient is recumbent, although resting tachycardia may be present. Postural hypotension, i.e., a drop of at least 5 to 10 mmHg in the sitting or standing position, is often present. With greater degrees of volume depletion, even recumbent blood pressure is reduced, and frank shock may occur. The patient with moderate or severe degrees of volume contraction is often lethargic, weak, confused, or obtunded. Such patients are usually oliguric, even when recumbent blood pressure is normal. However, an osmotic diuresis, as occurs in hyperglycemia, will tend to prevent oliguria despite volume contraction.

LABORATORY FINDINGS The hematocrit and plasma protein concentration are increased, but values within the normal range are interpretable only if prior values are known. Plasma sodium concentration may be decreased, normal, or increased, depending upon the proportion between deficits of sodium and of water. Plasma creatinine and urea nitrogen are usually increased, since the glomerular filtration rate is decreased ("prerenal azotemia"). Urinary sodium concentration may be of value in differentiating extrarenal and renal sources of sodium loss if the probable cause is not clear from the history. With extrarenal losses, urinary sodium concentration will be less than 10 meq per liter; the concentration will usually exceed 20 meq per liter if renal or adrenal disorders are at fault. However urinary sodium may ultimately fall below this level even in patients with renal salt wasting if sodium depletion becomes very severe.

Treatment The principal clinical manifestations of extracellular volume depletion are due to reduction of plasma and interstitial fluid volume. Since there is no convenient clinical method for assessing these volumes, the effect of treatment must be determined by following the clinical response through evaluation of changes in parameters such as blood pressure, urine output, and skin turgor. Modest deficits of sodium and water can often be corrected by increased oral intake in patients not suffering from gastrointestinal disorders. Severe depletion requires therapy with intravenous solutions. Isotonic saline (0.85%) is the infusion of choice in patients whose serum sodium concentration is approximately normal. The amount to be infused can be estimated from the history of prior losses and from the severity of the physical findings of extracellular volume contraction. Patients with clinically moderate volume contraction usually require replacement with 2 to 3 liters of saline, while patients with severe depletion may require much larger volumes. The need for correction of other concurrent electrolyte abnormalities may alter the composition of the required infusion; e.g., some of the sodium may be given as bicarbonate to patients with volume contraction and metabolic acidosis, or potassium may be added in patients with concurrent potassium depletion. In estimating the total amount to be infused, allowance for ongoing losses must be included. Since the amount to be infused cannot be calculated precisely, patients should be monitored carefully to avoid fluid overload and congestive failure.

HYPONATREMIA Pathophysiology Hyponatremia indicates that the body fluids are diluted by an excess of water relative to total solute. Hyponatremia is not equivalent to sodium depletion, which is only one of a number of clinical states in which it may occur (see Table 43-1). Most types of hyponatremia can be considered to result from defective urinary dilution. The normal response to dilution of body fluids is a water diuresis, which corrects the hypoosmotic state. Normal water diuresis requires three factors: (1) Secretion of ADH must be suppressed. (2) Sufficient sodium and water must reach the diluting sites of the nephron, in the ascending limb of Henle's loop and the distal convoluted tubule. (3) These nephron segments must function normally, reabsorbing sodium while remaining impermeable to water.

Correspondingly, three general types of mechanisms may cause defective water diuresis in patients with hyponatremia. (1) Secretion of ADH may continue "inappropriately" despite hypotonicity of extracellular fluid, which normally shuts off secretion of the hormone. Nonosmotic stimuli to ADH secretion include volume depletion and neural factors such as pain and emotion. (2) Insufficient sodium may reach the diluting segments to permit the formation of an adequate amount of dilute urine. Inadequate delivery of tubular fluid to distal sites may be due to reduced glomerular filtration and/or enhanced proximal tubular reabsorption. Even in the absence of ADH, distal tubular segments are not absolutely impermeable to water; small amounts of water continue to leak from the hypotonic tubular fluid into the isotonic cortical and slightly hypertonic medullary interstitial fluid. The amount of water leaking back in this manner becomes an increasingly larger fraction of the volume of dilute urine formed, as the diluting process is progressively limited by decreasing delivery. Hence, urine osmolality rises progressively. In some instances, this mechanism may even result in excretion of a urine hypertonic to plasma, despite the absence of ADH. (3) Sodium transport in the diluting segments may be defective or water permeability may be excessive at these sites even in the absence of ADH. One of these three factors can account for most types of hyponatremia.

Paradoxically, hyponatremia in *volume depletion* and in some edematous states appears to result from similar mechanisms. Delivery of sodium and water to the diluting segments of the nephron is reduced because of decreased gomerular filtration, increased proximal tubular reabsorption, or both. Volume-mediated secretion of ADH also occurs in these conditions. Contraction of plasma or extracellular volume is the stimulus to these changes in renal function and hormone secretion during salt depletion. These volumes appear to be normal or increased in most edematous patients. However, it is believed that the "effective" volume is reduced by decreased cardiac output or sequestration of fluid beyond the central circulation. Essential hyponatremia may be an additional mechanism in some edematous patients (see below).

In a number of clinical disorders, hyponatremia results from excess body water not associated with a substantial deficit or excess of salt. In these disorders, extracellular volume is only modestly expanded. Since excess water is distributed throughout both intracellular and extracellular fluids in proportion to their volumes, only one-third of a water excess will be retained in the extracellular compartment. *Oliguric* patients will develop dilutional hyponatremia if the volume of oral and intravenous fluids is not restricted appropriately. The ability to excrete a normal volume of dilute urine is progressively limited in advancing *chronic renal failure.* Regulation of water intake by thirst usually prevents dilutional hyponatremia. However, hyponatremia may be precipitated by increased fluid intake (for example, if the patient is instructed to force fluids). Since the ability to regulate salt excretion is also limited in chronic renal failure, in many patients hyponatremia is associated with edema or salt depletion.

Water diuresis may be limited temporarily by ADH secretion induced by various neural stimuli such as pain and narcotics. In the postoperative state, these factors, together with administration of large volumes of hypotonic fluids, may cause hyponatremia. Hyponatremia in patients with the *syndrome* of chronic *inappropriate* secretion of *antidiuretic hormone* (SIADH) is principally due to water retention, but continued urinary losses of sodium also contribute to producing a mild negative sodium balance. Renal sodium wasting is related to modest volume expansion, since it can be eliminated by restricting fluid intake. The mechanisms by which extracellular expansion may increase sodium excretion have been discussed above.

The normal kidney can excrete 15 to 20 liters of dilute urine per day. Normal water intake, regulated by thirst and habit, is a small fraction of this maximum excretory capacity. Very rarely, psychogenic polydipsia may be so severe that the rapid ingestion of huge quantities of fluids may overwhelm normal excretory capacity and produce symptomatic dilutional hyponatremia despite normal renal diluting mechanisms.

A limited number of observations suggest that some patients may be hyponatremic in the absence of a defect in water diuresis. The terms *essential hyponatremia* and *sick-cell syndrome* have been applied to this category. Osmoreceptor cells in the hypothalamus are thought to be "reset" to maintain a decreased level of body fluid osmolality as though it were normal. Urine becomes dilute or concentrated, respectively, if plasma sodium falls or increases slightly from the new "normal" level for the particular patient. The genesis of such a syndrome is speculative. It has been suggested that changes in cellular metabolism might lead to a primary reduction in cellular osmolality. Another possibility is that essential hyponatremia is a variant of SIADH in which there is a nonosmotic stimulus to ADH secretion. When plasma osmolality is reduced sufficiently, osmotic suppression of ADH secretion overcomes the nonosmotic stimulus.

Multiple factors appear to play a role in limiting water diuresis in patients with *adrenal insufficiency.* Deficient secretion of mineralocorticoid hormones may lead to sodium depletion, with consequent reduction of glomerular filtration and enhancement of proximal tubular sodium reabsorption. Moreover, glucocorticoid deficiency directly reduces filtration. Therefore, adrenal insufficiency will tend to decrease delivery of sodium to diluting sites. In addition, glucocorticoid deficiency prevents the maintenance of normal water impermeability in distal diluting segments of the nephron. This appears to be due to inappropriate secretion of ADH, although some evidence suggests a direct effect of glucocorticoid deficiency on water permeability of distal tubular epithelium.

Multiple factors also contribute to hyponatremia caused by *diuretics.* Salt loss may cause volume depletion, which limits water diuresis by mechanisms already described. Furosemide, ethacrynic acid, and thiazides inhibit salt reabsorption in the diluting segments of the nephron and thereby directly limit water diuresis. In addition, potassium depletion caused by many diuretics contributes to hyponatremia through uncertain mechanisms.

Hyponatremia due to *accumulation* of *osmotically active solutes* in the plasma is the sole exception to the rule that hyponatremia means decreased plasma osmolality. In this type of hyponatremia, plasma osmolality is increased. Plasma sodium is diluted by movement of water out of cells along the osmotic gradient created by addition to the plasma of a solute such as glucose or mannitol. (High plasma urea levels in patients with renal failure do not cause hyponatremia because urea concentration is equal across cell membranes.)

Clinical features and diagnosis In *sodium* (volume) *depletion,* hyponatremia per se is usually of little clinical significance. The major features are those of extracellular volume contraction, described above. Reduction of plasma sodium concentration by more than 10 to 15 meq per liter is rare in the absence of obvious decreases in skin turgor, postural or recumbent hypotension, and some degree of azotemia.

In *edematous states* such as congestive heart failure, cirrhosis, and the nephrotic syndrome, the severity and frequency of hyponatremia correlates to some extent with the magnitude of the edema and the seriousness of the underlying condition. Hyponatremia is usually present in patients with advanced disease unless water intake is restricted. The hyponatremia itself is often of little clinical significance. The principal features are those of the underlying disease. However, symptomatic hyponatremia may occur, most often in connection with vigorous diuretic therapy or excessive oral or parenteral intake of dilute fluids.

The diagnosis of *dilutional hyponatremia* is usually evident from the history. This diagnosis should be considered in postoperative patients and in patients with acute or chronic renal failure. Since extracellular fluid volume is normal or modestly expanded by water retention, blood pressure and skin turgor are normal. Plasma creatinine and urea are normal unless preexisting renal disease is present.

SIADH is defined by a unique group of clinical features. (1) Urine osmolality is not maximally dilute even when marked hyponatremia is induced by water loading. In most cases, urine osmolality exceeds plasma osmolality. (The elaboration of hypertonic urine is presumptive evidence of ADH secretion if the glomerular filtration rate is normal.) (2) Plasma creatinine and urea are normal or low, indicating that the glomerular filtration rate is normal or increased. (3) During fluid loading, hyponatremia increases due to water retention and urinary sodium wasting. During restriction of fluid intake, hyponatremia and urinary sodium wasting are corrected. It should be noted that sodium wasting during volume expansion may be minimal or even absent in patients with extreme degrees of hyponatremia. In clinical testing to demonstrate these features, patients with symptomatic hyponatremia or plasma sodium concentrations below 125 meq per liter should first have their fluid intake restricted to 800 to 1000 ml per day or less. Infusion of small volumes of hypertonic saline may be appropriate in symptomatic patients. During restriction of fluid intake, hyponatremia should disappear promptly, and urinary sodium excretion should not exceed intake. Thereafter, plasma and urinary parameters should be evaluated during daily administration of 2 to 3 liters of fluids by mouth or intravenously. Urine osmolality will always exceed 100 mosmol per liter (urine specific gravity greater than 1.003); in the great majority of instances, it will exceed plasma osmolality, despite progressive dilution of body fluids. Urinary sodium excretion will usually exceed sodium intake during this phase of fluid loading. Two to three days of this regimen are ordinarily sufficient to demonstrate the requisite clinical pattern for SIADH without inducing symptomatic hyponatremia.

SIADH has been found frequently in patients with oat-cell carcinoma of the lung but has also been described in patients with a variety of other *neoplasms*. In some of these patients there is evidence that the tumor is secreting ADH or a substance with analogous biological activity (see also Chap. 110). The syndrome has also been reported in patients with various disorders which affect the *central nervous system*, including meningitis, encephalitis, tumors, trauma, stroke, and porphyria. It is assumed that ADH in these patients is secreted in response to direct stimulation of the hypothalamic osmoreceptors. *Pulmonary* diseases associated with SIADH, in addition to tumors, include a wide variety of infections.

An ever-increasing list of pharmacological agents has been reported to induce SIADH. The list includes (1) the oral hypoglycemic agents chlorpropamide and tolbutamide; (2) the antineoplastic and immunosuppressive agents vincristine and cyclophosphamide; (3) psychoactive drugs, such as carbamazepine (Tegretol) and amitriptyline (Elavil); and (4) clofibrate. These agents exert their antidiuretic effects either by potentiating the tubular action of small amounts of ADH or by stimulating inappropriate secretion of ADH.

Since patients with *adrenal insufficiency* may have the combination of defective dilution of the urine and sodium wasting, hyponatremia due to Addison's disease can occasionally be confused with SIADH. Usually, other clinical features of adrenal insufficiency such as hyperkalemia, pigmentation, and hypoglycemia will suggest the correct diagnosis. However, specific tests of adrenal cortical function are indicated whenever the diagnosis is in doubt.

Essential hyponatremia (sick-cell syndrome) may occur in a variety of chronic illnesses, such as pulmonary tuberculosis, congestive heart failure, and hepatic cirrhosis. This type of hyponatremia is asymptomatic; skin turgor, blood pressure, and renal function are normal, unless altered by the primary disease. Definitive diagnosis of essential hyponatremia requires the demonstration of normal urinary dilution in response to water loading, normal urinary concentration during dehydration, and normal renal sodium excretory responses to sodium loading and restriction.

The diagnosis of hyponatremia due to *increased plasma concentrations* of *osmotically active solute* is usually apparent from the history and clinical features of uncontrolled diabetes. Plasma sodium concentration will decrease by about 1.6 meq per liter with every elevation of 100 mg/dl in plasma glucose above normal. This type of hyponatremia should also be considered whenever there is a history of recent administration of mannitol, especially to oliguric patients unable to excrete it promptly. Since plasma osmolality is increased, clinical manifestations of hypotonicity are absent in this type of hyponatremia.

In patients with severe hyperlipemia or, very rarely, with extreme hyperproteinemia, hyponatremia which is clinically *artifactual* may be reported by the laboratory. In severe hyperlipemia part of any unit volume of plasma taken for analysis will be lipid, which is sodium-free. This type of hyponatremia is rarely reported unless the plasma is grossly milky. In patients with extreme hyperproteinemia, proteins occupy more than the normal 7 percent of plasma volume, thereby reducing the proportion of aqueous sodium-containing fluid per unit of plasma taken for analysis. In both cases, hyponatremia will be reported by the laboratory because the sodium concentration will be low in milliequivalents per liter of plasma. However, sodium concentration per liter of plasma water and plasma osmolality are normal; hence, this type of hyponatremia has no clinical significance.

DIFFERENTIAL DIAGNOSIS Although the type of hyponatremia can be defined easily in most patients, precise diagnosis may be very difficult in some cases. More than one type of hyponatremia may occur in a specific disease entity. For example, hyponatremia in patients with hepatic cirrhosis is usually associated with edema or is due to excessive administration of diuretics, but essential hyponatremia may also occur in this condition. Moreover, current categories may prove artificial or inaccurate when the pathophysiology of hyponatremia is more completely understood and specific diagnostic tests such as a sensitive assay for ADH are readily available. Despite these limitations, the classification outlined above is a useful framework for diagnosis and treatment.

The history is often the most important factor in differential diagnosis. For example, prolonged vomiting, diarrhea, or nasogastric suction will suggest volume depletion, or the history of a lung tumor will suggest SIADH. Critical information to be derived from the physical examination includes the presence or absence of edema or signs of volume depletion. The history and physical examination are usually sufficient to determine whether the hyponatremia is associated with a decreased, increased, or normal extracellular volume. Laboratory studies may help to confirm and refine the diagnosis. The plasma creatinine will tend to be increased when hyponatremia is associated with volume depletion, normal or decreased when associated with normal or slightly expanded extracellular volume, as in SIADH. Urine sodium concentration will be low (under 10 meq per liter) if hyponatremia is associated with edema or with volume depletion due to extrarenal causes. Urine sodium concentration will usually exceed 20 meq per liter if the hyponatremia is due to renal salt losses or to renal failure with water retention. In SIADH, urine sodium concentration will usually exceed 20 meq per liter, unless the patient is salt-restricted. Since impaired water diuresis is the mechanism of most types of hyponatremia, urinary osmolality is not usually of differential diagnostic value. A maximally dilute urine would be expected only in essential hyponatremia and hyponatremia due to extreme polydipsia. With other causes, urinary osmolality will at least exceed 150 mosmol per kilogram of water; usually the urine will be hypertonic to plasma.

CLINICAL MANIFESTATIONS Neurologic dysfunction is the principal clinical feature of hyponatremia. The severity of symptoms is related to the degree of hyponatremia and the rapidity with which it develops. Patients may be lethargic, confused, stuporous, or comatose. If hyponatremia develops rapidly, signs of hyperexcitability such as muscular twitches, irritability, and convulsions may occur. These are believed due to intracellular movement of water, leading to swelling of brain cells. Hyponatremia rarely causes clinical symptoms when plasma sodium is above 125 meq per liter, although symptoms may occur occasionally at higher levels if the decrease in concentration has been rapid.

Treatment Hyponatremia itself is often of little clinical significance and requires no specific treatment. When hyponatremia is associated with volume depletion, treatment is directed to correction of the volume deficits. In the occasional symptomatic patient with sodium depletion whose plasma sodium concentration is less than 125 meq per liter, some of the intravenous sodium replacement fluids should be administered as hypertonic saline. Hyponatremia associated with edema responds to effective treatment of the underlying disease. Moderate, nonprogressive hyponatremia in edematous patients usually does not cause symptoms. Attempts to correct such hyponatremia by restriction of fluid intake induce thirst and discomfort without improving the clinical picture or longevity. Patients with severe or progressive hyponatremia may require some restriction of water intake, especially during vigorous treatment with diuretics. However, moderate limitations to the range of 1000 to 1500 ml per day will often suffice to avoid symptoms or progressive hyponatremia. More severe restriction should be instituted only if specific clinical or laboratory observations warrant. Since edematous subjects have excess total extracellular sodium, hypertonic saline solution should not be administered, except in rare instances in which clinical manifestations of extreme hyponatremia, such as coma or convulsions, justify emergency measures. Dilutional hyponatremia is treated by water restriction. Only if severe symptoms occur is hypertonic saline infusion required. Hyponatremia due to SIADH responds to limitation of fluid intake; restriction to the range of 1000 to 1200 ml per day is ordinarily adequate. Occasional patients with marked hyponatremia due to this syndrome may be symptomatic and require initial therapy with hypertonic saline infusions.

If severe hyponatremia of any type is to be treated intravenously, the amount of sodium to be given should be calculated by multiplying the deficit in plasma sodium concentration (milliequivalents per liter) by total body water (approximately 50 to 60 percent of body weight). Although the administered sodium will remain in the extracellular compartment, the osmotic effect of the hypertonic saline will cause water to shift out of cells. The amount needed to raise plasma sodium concentration to the range of 125 to 130 meq per liter should be calculated and infused over several hours. The patient's symptoms and clinical status, especially with respect to circulatory congestion, should be carefully assessed throughout the infusion. Furosemide may be given if fluid overload is present initially or develops during the infusion. Complete correction of hyponatremia, if clinically indicated, is usually best carried out more slowly, by water restriction or oral sodium supplementation if possible.

HYPERNATREMIA Pathophysiology Hypernatremia is due to a deficit of body water relative to total body solute or sodium content. Without exception, hypernatremia indicates that the body fluids are hypertonic. Normally, minimal increases in tonicity stimulate both thirst and release of ADH. Although renal water retention induced by ADH helps to correct hypernatremia, thirst appears to be the principal defense mechanism. Hypernatremia is usually modest in patients with diabetes insipidus, who lack ADH and may excrete 15 liters or more of urine per day. Thirst stimulates water intake enough to balance even such large water losses. Severe persistent hypernatremia occurs only in patients who cannot respond to thirst by voluntary ingestion of fluid, e.g., infants or mentally obtunded patients. In such individuals, loss of dilute body fluids will progressively elevate body fluid osmolality. Initial losses of water are from the extracellular compartment, but water deficits are rapidly equilibrated throughout total body water. The rise in extracellular fluid tonicity causes intracellular water to shift into the extracellular compartment. In effect, approximately two-thirds of pure water deficits are derived from intracellular fluid. Hence, the clinical findings of extracellular volume depletion occur in patients with relatively pure deficits of water only when such deficits are large. The principal clinical features are attributable to decreased intracellular volume, especially dehydration of cells in the central nervous system. Brain cells appear to adapt to chronic hyperosmolality by accumulating increased intracellular solute. When hyperosmolality is rapidly corrected, the increase in total intracellular solute may promote brain swelling even at normal or slightly elevated plasma osmolality. These mechanisms may account for the clinical observation that rapid correction of hypertonicity sometimes causes deterioration of central nervous function. The identity of the excess brain solute is uncertain; experimental data suggest that electrolyte accumulation accounts only for part of the excess in chronic hypernatremia.

Minimal persistent hypernatremia may be seen in some patients with Cushing's disease and hyperaldosteronism. Presumably stimulation of renal tubular reabsorption by adrenal steroids initiates the hypernatremia. It is not known why the thirst mechanism fails to maintain normal body fluid osmolality.

Pathogenesis The principal causes of hypernatremia are listed in Table 43-1. The most frequent is unreplaced loss of hypotonic fluid from the skin and lungs. Insensible losses of water from these sources may reach several liters per day, especially in patients with fever or increased respirations. Since sweat is hypotonic fluid, hypernatremia will develop if sweating patients are unable to drink. Major losses of insensible water may occur in patients with extensive burns. Renal losses may lead to hypernatremia in two clinical circumstances, diabetes insipidus and solute diuresis. Alert patients with diabetes insipidus ordinarily maintain normal or only slightly hypertonic body fluids despite massive renal water wasting by increasing fluid intake appropriately. However, diabetes insipidus may develop acutely in patients who suffer cerebral trauma or undergo neurosurgical procedures. In such patients, careful attention to replacement of urinary losses is mandatory to avoid severe hypernatremia. In an osmotic diuresis, urinary sodium concentration is less than plasma concentration; therefore, hypernatremia tends to occur. Hypernatremia due to a urea diuresis may develop when patients unable to complain of thirst are placed on a high-protein tube feeding. Examples include patients with severe cerebrovascular accidents who are unable to swallow and postoperative neurosurgical patients. In the syndrome of hyperosmolar nonketotic diabetic coma, severe hyperosmolality of the body fluids is due to a combination of hyperglycemia and relative or absolute hypernatremia. The hypernatremia is a consequence of an intense glucose osmotic diuresis in patients who are unable to ingest fluids. Since hyperglycemia itself causes hyponatremia by inducing a shift of water from cells, the presence of hypernatremia in the face of extreme hyperglycemia indicates that total body water is severely depleted. Hypernatremia due to an osmotic diuresis is usually accompanied by significant extracellular volume depletion, since both sodium and water are lost.

In rare instances, hypernatremia may result from an absolute excess of sodium rather than from water depletion. Examples are hypernatremia caused by accidental substitution of salt for sugar in infant feeding formulas and administration of excessive amounts of hypertonic saline to comatose adults.

Clinical features and diagnosis The principal clinical manifestations of hypernatremia are observed in the central nervous system. Confusion and other evidence of altered mental state; increased neuromuscular irritability, such as twitching and seizures; and obtundation, stupor, or coma may all occur. The magnitude of symptoms depends on the severity of the hyperosmolality. The clinical symptoms are similar whether hyperosmolality is due to hypernatremia or extreme hyperglycemia. The neurologic symptoms appear to be due to dehydration of brain cells. The clinical manifestations of acute hypernatremia are more marked than those of hypernatremia which develops more slowly. Severe hyperosmolality may cause irreversible neurologic sequelae, apparently due to vascular abnormalities such as venous sinus thrombosis and hemorrhage from vessels which rupture when the brain shrinks. High mortality rates are associated with extreme hyperosmolality, especially in children and in the elderly.

In patients with pure water deficits, manifestations of extracellular volume depletion are minimal because only one-third of the deficit is derived from extracellular fluid. As already noted, combined deficits are common, especially in patients who are sweating or undergoing an osmotic diuresis; in such individuals, the signs and symptoms of volume depletion may overshadow those due to hypernatremia.

The cause of hypernatremia can usually be inferred from the history when it is due to extrarenal water loss, an osmotic diuresis, or sodium excess. In these cases, the urine is hypertonic to plasma. The differential diagnosis of the various forms of pituitary and nephrogenic diabetes insipidus, in which urine concentrating ability is impaired, is discussed in Chap. 110.

Treatment Water by mouth or intravenous administration of a dilute solution (5% dextrose or 0.45% saline) is the treatment of hypernatremia. Calculation of water requirements must be based on total body water, since water deficits are drawn from both intracellular and extracellular fluid and both must be repleted. Hypernatremia should be corrected slowly; no more than half the water deficit should be replaced in the first few hours. Excessively rapid correction of hypernatremia may cause clinical deterioration of central nervous function.

POTASSIUM

PHYSIOLOGIC CONSIDERATIONS Potassium is the principal intracellular cation. Active transport mediated by Na-K–stimulated adenosine triphosphatase (ATPase) in cell membranes maintains a cellular concentration of approximately 160 meq per liter, 40 times that in extracellular fluid. All but 2 percent of the 2500 to 3000 meq potassium in the body is within cells. Since potassium is a large fraction of total cellular solute, it is a major determinant of the volume of the cell and the osmolality of the body fluids. Moreover, potassium is an important cofactor in a number of metabolic processes. Extracellular potassium, while a small fraction of the total, greatly influences neuromuscular function. The ratio of intracellular to extracellular potassium concentration is the principal determinant of membrane potential in excitable tissues. Since extracellular potassium concentration is low, small deviations in absolute concentration will produce large variations in this ratio; conversely, only large changes in intracellular potassium will influence the ratio significantly. These relationships have practical consequences. For example, toxic effects of hyperkalemia can be mitigated by inducing movement of potassium from extracellular fluid into cells.

The relation between plasma and cellular potassium is complex and influenced by a number of factors, prominent among them being acid-base balance. Acidosis tends to shift potassium out of cells, and alkalosis favors movement of potassium from extracellular fluid into cells. The exact relation between blood pH and plasma potassium is complex. Experimental evidence indicates that the magnitude of potassium shifts is influenced by a number of factors, including the type of acidosis, the duration of the altered acid-base state, and the change in plasma bicarbonate per se. In general, plasma potassium changes less with respiratory acidosis than with metabolic acidosis and less with alkalosis than with acidosis. While the exact magnitude of the change in plasma potassium cannot be predicted from changes in blood pH alone, a patient with normal total body potassium will tend to be hyperkalemic if acidotic and hypokalemic if alkalotic. Hormones also influence the distribution of potassium between extracellular fluid and cells. Insulin, beta-adrenergic catecholamines, and possibly aldosterone promote movement of potassium into cells. These hormones appear to be important parts of the mechanism for moving potassium loads out of plasma. During potassium depletion, plasma potassium initially decreases about 1 meq per liter for each 100 to 200 meq lost. However, plasma potassium falls much more slowly after it reaches 2 meq per liter. Thus, a plasma potassium in the range of 2 to 3.5 meq per liter is a reasonably accurate guide to the magnitude of depletion, but plasma potassium concentrations less than 2 meq per liter may reflect a wide range of deficits, from moderate to very severe. Plasma concentration increases about 1 meq per liter after acute administration of 100 to 200 meq potassium. Assuming an extracellular volume of 15 liters, 150 meq would be expected to raise plasma potassium by about 10 meq per liter. Thus, it is evident that the largest fraction of administered potassium rapidly enters cells. Renal excretion also increases promptly. Chronic exposure to high-potassium diets enhances both tissue uptake and renal excretion of the ion; the mechanism of these adaptations is uncertain. Sustained hyperkalemia rarely is caused by excess intake, because these mechanisms normally function so efficiently. Impaired renal excretion and cellular transfer are the usual causes of hyperkalemia.

Of the usual potassium intake of 50 to 150 meq per day, all but a few milliequivalents are excreted in the urine. Normally, stool and sweat contain only about 5 meq per day. As already noted, the kidneys respond to acute and chronic changes in potassium intake by corresponding changes in excretion. Excess potassium is excreted promptly; about half of an acute load appears in the urine within 12 h. The renal response to potassium depletion is more sluggish. Excretion does not fall to minimal levels for 7 to 14 days. During this period, a deficit of 200 meq or more may develop in an individual on a potassium-deficient diet. Renal excretory mechanisms for potassium are complex. Potassium in the urine is secreted in the distal convoluted tubule and collecting duct; filtered potassium is nearly quantitatively reabsorbed in more proximal segments. Potassium secretion appears to be determined by the potassium concentration of tubular cells and by an electrochemical gradient favoring diffusion of the ion into tubular fluid. Net excretion is the resultant of secretion and concurrent reabsorption in the distal segments. Among the key influences on this complex system are aldosterone, distal tubular fluid flow rate, and acid-base balance. Aldosterone stimulates potassium secretion. Thus, hyperkalemia increases potassium excretion by two mechanisms: it stimulates adrenal secretion of aldosterone, and it directly enhances renal secretion, presumably via increased tubular cell potassium. Potassium secretion in the distal tubule is flow-dependent; increased distal delivery of tubular fluid will favor potassium excretion. For example, loop diuretics, which enhance distal volume delivery, will increase potassium excretion, especially in patients with edema and secondary aldosteronism. Alkalosis enhances and acidosis depresses renal potassium secretion, probably by inducing corresponding changes in tubular cell potassium.

POTASSIUM DEPLETION AND HYPOKALEMIA **Pathogenesis** The principal causes of potassium depletion are listed in Table 43-2. As noted earlier, renal excretion of potassium falls slowly in persons on potassium-deficient diets. During the 10 to 14 days before balance is achieved, significant deficits may occur. Thus, in contrast to sodium, moderate potassium depletion may result from *poor intake* alone. Potassium deficiency is frequent in various *gastrointestinal disorders* in which vomiting, diarrhea, or loss of gastrointestinal secretions is prominent. Diarrhea may cause large potassium deficits, since the potassium concentration of liquid stool is 40 to 60 meq per liter. *Loss* of *gastric secretions* through vomiting or vasogastric suction is also a common cause of potassium depletion. The potassium concentration of gastric fluid is 5 to 10 meq per liter; direct losses of potassium contribute only modestly to negative potassium balance. The potassium deficit is primarily due to increased renal excretion. Potassium excretion appears to be stimulated by three mechanisms. Loss of gastric acid leads to *metabolic alkalosis,* which increases tubular cell potassium concentration. The elevated plasma bicarbonate concentration also increases delivery of bicarbonate and fluid to the distal nephron. Finally, secondary hyperaldosteronism due to associated extracellular volume contraction may play a role in maintaining potassium excretion at high levels despite potassium depletion.

All *diuretics* in common use except spironolactone, triamterene, and amiloride promote potassium excretion. In edematous patients with secondary aldosteronism, these agents often cause significant hypokalemia and potassium depletion. Although hypokalemia also occurs in patients receiving diuretics for treatment of hypertension, significant potassium depletion appears to be infrequent if dietary potassium is normal and there are no other factors which stimulate potassium excretion. Therefore, dietary potassium supplements or potassium-sparing diuretics need not routinely be administered to all patients receiving diuretic therapy but often are required by patients with aldosteronism or inadequate diets, especially if they are on digitalis preparations.

Potassium excretion is increased during an *osmotic diuresis.* This mechanism regularly leads to potassium depletion in patients with diabetic ketoacidosis, in whom the osmotic diuresis is due to glycosuria and to increased excretion of keto acid anions. However, potassium depletion may be masked by the shift of potassium out of tissues caused by the diabetic acidosis. Failure to recognize potassium depletion may lead to serious cardiotoxicity from sudden hypokalemia when the acidosis is corrected with insulin or alkali. A normal plasma potassium concentration in an acidotic patient strongly suggests potassium depletion.

Urinary potassium loss is often due to *excessive mineralocorticoid activity.* Hypokalemia is characteristic of *primary aldosteronism,* but may be minimal in patients with restricted sodium intake. *Secondary aldosteronism* causes renal potassium wasting and hypokalemia in patients with malignant hypertension, Bartter's syndrome, and renin-secreting renal tumors. *Licorice* contains a compound with mineralocorticoid activity; patients who consume huge amounts may become hypokalemic. Excessive levels of *glucocorticoids* stimulate secretion of renal potassium (and hydrogen), leading to hypokalemia and alkalosis in patients with *Cushing's syndrome* and those receiving *therapeutic steroids.*

Renal tubular potassium wasting is a feature of *renal tubular acidosis* (Chap. 299). Some patients with monocytic or myelomonocytic *leukemia* have developed hypokalemia. The mechanism is uncertain. Renal potassium wasting in some patients appears to correlate with lysozymuria, and it has been suggested that the enzyme may interfere with tubular function. In *Liddle's syndrome,* a rare familial disorder (Chap. 299), renal potassium wasting is an intrinsic tubular abnormality.

Clinical features and diagnosis The most prominent features of hypokalemia and potassium depletion are neuromuscular. Moderate degrees of depletion may be asymptomatic, especially if they develop slowly. Some patients, however, may complain of muscle weakness. With more severe or acute degrees of hypokalemia and potassium deficiency, marked and generalized weakness of skeletal muscles is prominent. Very severe or abrupt development of hypokalemia may lead to virtually total paralysis, including the respiratory muscles. Rhabdomyolysis may occur in patients with potassium depletion. On physical examination, in addition to decreased motor power, the patient may demonstrate decreased or absent tendon reflexes.

Abnormalities in the electrocardiogram are common in patients with hypokalemia and potassium depletion (Chap. 249). The characteristic changes include flattening and inversion of the T wave, increased prominence of the U wave, and sagging of the ST segment. These alterations are not well correlated with the severity of the disturbance in potassium metabolism and cannot be relied on as indexes of the clinical significance of a potassium deficit. Although moderate potassium depletion

TABLE 43-2
Causes of potassium depletion and hypokalemia

I Gastrointestinal
- *A* Deficient dietary intake
- *B* Gastrointestinal disorders (vomiting, diarrhea, villous adenoma, fistulas, ureterosigmoidostomy)

II Renal
- *A* Metabolic alkalosis
- *B* Diuretics, osmotic diuresis
- *C* Excessive mineralocorticoid effects
  - *1* Primary aldosteronism
  - *2* Secondary aldosteronism (including malignant hypertension, Bartter's syndrome, juxtaglomerular cell tumor)
  - *3* Licorice ingestion
  - *4* Glucocorticoid excess (Cushing's syndrome, exogenous steroids, ectopic ACTH production)
- *D* Renal tubular diseases
  - *1* Renal tubular acidosis
  - *2* Leukemia
  - *3* Liddle's syndrome

III Hypokalemia due to shift into cells (no depletion)
- *A* Hypokalemic periodic paralysis
- *B* Insulin effect
- *C* Alkalosis

rarely affects cardiac action, severe or rapid reduction in serum potassium may cause cardiac arrest. Potassium deficiency enhances the cardiac toxicity of digitalis preparations.

Renal tubular function is markedly impaired by potassium depletion (Chap. 297). The most prominent abnormality is decreased concentrating ability, which may cause polyuria and polydipsia. Glomerular filtration rate is normal or only slightly reduced; moderate reductions may occur in occasional patients with chronic potassium depletion nephropathy. Renal regulation of potassium excretion remains normal. The urinalysis is benign: protein excretion is normal or minimally increased, and the urinary sediment is normal or demonstrates only a slight increase in hyaline or granular casts.

DIAGNOSIS The cause of hypokalemia and potassium depletion is usually evident from the history. However, patients whose potassium deficiency is caused by chronic abuse of laxatives; psychogenic, self-induced vomiting; or surreptitious use of diuretics will rarely volunteer an accurate history. Patients with villous adenomas of the rectum sometimes report that their feces are formed; careful questioning will reveal the elimination of the characteristic mucous secretion of the tumor.

When the history is obscure, evaluation of urinary potassium excretion may be helpful in determining the origin of the potassium deficit. If gastrointestinal losses have occurred, urinary excretion will usually be less than 20 to 25 meq per liter. Although renal conservation of potassium is slow, excretion will have fallen to these levels by the time that clinically significant deficits of potassium have accumulated. On the other hand, when renal potassium wasting is the cause, urinary concentration will usually exceed 20 meq per liter. However, lower concentrations may be found in severely depleted patients, in those with excessive mineralocorticoid activity while on low sodium intake, and in patients where diuretics have been stopped at the time of examination. Measurement of blood pH also may help in differential diagnosis. A normal pH or alkalosis is present in most patients who are potassium-depleted. Hypokalemia is associated with acidosis in renal tubular acidosis, diarrhea, and diabetic ketoacidosis, and in patients treated with carbonic anhydrase inhibitors. A third clue to diagnosis is the presence of hypertension, which suggests the various causes of hyperaldosteronism (except Bartter's syndrome) and glucocorticoid excess. Blood pressure is normal in patients whose potassium depletion is due to the other causes listed in Table 43-2.

Treatment When possible, potassium depletion should be corrected by increased dietary intake or supplementation with potassium salts. Potassium chloride is the salt of choice, especially in alkalotic patients. It may be given in the form of an elixir or in tablets in which potassium chloride crystals are imbedded in a wax (Slow-K). Enteric-coated potassium chloride tablets have been responsible for ulceration of the small bowel, due to release of high concentrations of potassium salts. Organic salts such as gluconate or citrate are adequate in patients who are not severely alkalotic.

Intravenous treatment is required for patients with gastrointestinal disorders or when the potassium deficiency is severe. It must be emphasized that the potassium *concentration* in commonly available intravenous solutions of potassium chloride is 2000 meq per liter. Concentrations in intravenous infusions should not exceed 40 or at the most 60 meq per liter. The rate of infusion should not exceed 20 meq/h or approximately 200 to 250 meq per day, unless the need for more rapid infusion has been demonstrated in the individual patient by evidence of continuing losses large enough to justify more intensive therapy. The results of treatment are best monitored by repeated determinations of plasma potassium and evaluation of clinical symptoms such as muscular weakness or paralysis. Disappearance of electrocardiographic abnormalities correlates only roughly with improvement in total body potassium content. However, during rapid intravenous administration of potassium, the electrocardiogram should be monitored to avoid cardiac toxicity from inadvertent hyperkalemia.

Hypokalemia and hypocalcemia may occur together, for example, in patients with malabsorption syndrome. The neuromuscular effect of each electrolyte abnormality is masked by the other. Treatment of either disorder alone may precipitate symptoms. Thus, treatment of hypokalemia alone may precipitate tetany, and conversely, treatment of hypocalcemia without correcting the hypokalemia may exacerbate the manifestations of potassium deficiency.

HYPERKALEMIA Pathogenesis The causes of hyperkalemia are shown in Table 43-3. *Inadequate renal excretion* is the most frequent cause (see also Chaps. 291 and 292). When oliguria or anuria is present, as in acute renal failure, progressive hyperkalemia is the rule. Plasma potassium will rise by about 0.5 meq per liter per day if there are no abnormal loads. Chronic renal failure does not cause severe or progressive hyperkalemia unless oliguria supervenes. Adaptive changes of unknown etiology increase potassium excretion per residual nephron as chronic renal failure progresses. However, patients with chronic renal failure are functioning at the limits of their excretory capacity. Hence, hyperkalemia may develop rapidly if the potassium load is increased or excretory capacity is limited, e.g., by administration of spironolactone. Selective renal *tubular potassium secretory defects* have been described in a few patients with nonazotemic renal disease caused by lupus erythematosus, sickle cell disease, or rejection of a transplanted kidney.

Hyperkalemia is a cardinal feature of adrenal insufficiency (Addison's disease) and of selective *hypoaldosteronism.* The common form of the latter disorder in adults is *hyporeninemic hypoaldosteronism* (Chap. 112).

A kilogram of tissue such as muscle or erythrocytes contains about 80 meq potassium, and damaged cells release potassium into the plasma. Hence hyperkalemia may be seen when there is *muscle-crushing injury, hemolysis,* or *internal hemorrhage.* Acidosis drives potassium out of cells and leads to hyperkalemia. Severe progressive hyperkalemia is not ordinarily a consequence of increased release of potassium from damaged or acidotic tissues alone. However, acidosis and tissue damage often occur together with acute renal insufficiency; under these circumstances, severe hyperkalemia may develop

TABLE 43-3
Causes of hyperkalemia

I Inadequate excretion
- *A* Renal failure
  - *1* Acute renal failure
  - *2* Severe chronic renal failure
  - *3* Tubular disorders
- *B* Adrenal insufficiency
  - *1* Hypoaldosteronism
  - *2* Addison's disease
- *C* Diuretics which inhibit potassium secretion (spironolactone, triamterene, amiloride)

II Shift of potassium from tissues
- *A* Tissue damage (muscle crush, hemolysis, internal bleeding)
- *B* Drugs: succinylcholine, arginine, digitalis poisoning
- *C* Acidosis
- *D* Hyperkalemic periodic paralysis

III Excessive intake

IV Pseudohyperkalemia
- *A* Thrombocytosis
- *B* Leukocytosis
- *C* Poor venipuncture technique
- *D* In vitro hemolysis

quickly. In contrast to the increase of 0.5 meq per liter per day typical of uncomplicated anuria, plasma potassium in anuric patients with tissue damage may increase 2 to 4 meq per liter per day. Such rapidly progressive hyperkalemia may be an important cause of death in military casualties. In patients with trauma, burns, or neuromuscular diseases such as paraplegia and multiple sclerosis, the muscle relaxant succinylcholine may cause dangerous hyperkalemia. This agent apparently releases potassium from muscle by depolarizing cell membranes. *Arginine hydrochloride*, used to treat metabolic alkalosis, drives potassium out of cells. If potassium excretion is impaired, clinically significant hyperkalemia may occur during arginine infusions. Extreme digitalis poisoning may cause severe hyperkalemia; potassium leaks out of cells because Na-K-ATPase is inhibited by the drug. *Metabolic acidosis* causes hyperkalemia by shifting potassium out of cells. Respiratory acidosis has less striking effects. In *hyperkalemic periodic paralysis*, the hyperkalemia is associated with repeated attacks of muscular paralysis. The mechanism of this syndrome is not understood. Ingestion of increased amounts of potassium may precipitate attacks.

The severity of hyperkalemia caused by potassium loads is influenced by the various factors which modulate tissue uptake and renal excretion of potassium. For example, insulin deficiency and treatment with beta-adrenergic blockers will tend to augment hyperkalemia by limiting tissue uptake of potassium loads. Volume depletion will enhance hyperkalemia by limiting the rate at which the kidney excretes endogenous or exogenous loads.

Patients with extreme thrombocytosis or, more rarely, extreme leukocytosis in leukemia may demonstrate the phenomenon of pseudohyperkalemia. Platelets or white blood cells release potassium during blood clotting in vitro. While serum potassium may be grossly abnormal, plasma potassium is not increased. Artifactual elevation of plasma potassium may occur if blood is drawn after repeated fist clenching to make veins more prominent during application of a tourniquet. Artifactual hyperkalemia may be suspected when electrocardiographic abnormalities are absent despite apparently marked elevation of serum potassium.

Clinical features and diagnosis The most important toxic effects of hyperkalemia are cardiac arrhythmias. The characteristic sequence of electrocardiographic changes is shown in Fig. 43-1. The earliest manifestation is the development of high-peaked T waves, especially prominent in precordial leads. Hyperkalemia does not prolong the QT interval, unlike other disorders which induce peaking of the T waves. Later changes include prolongation of the PR interval, complete heart block, and atrial asystole. As plasma potassium rises further, ventricular complexes may deteriorate. The QRS complex becomes progressively prolonged and finally tends to merge with the T wave in a sine wave configuration. Terminally, ventricular fibrillation and standstill may occur (see also Chap. 249).

Occasionally moderate or severe hyperkalemia may have striking effects on peripheral muscles. Ascending muscular weakness can occur, progressing to flaccid quadriplegia and respiratory paralysis. Cerebral and cranial nerve function are normal, as is sensation.

Treatment In considering appropriate therapy, it is helpful to classify hyperkalemia according to degree of severity. The seriousness of hyperkalemia is best estimated by considering both the plasma potassium and the electrocardiogram. When the plasma potassium is less than 6.5 meq per liter and electrocardiographic changes are limited to peaking of T waves, hyperkalemia can be considered to be mild. When the plasma potassium is 6.5 to 8 meq per liter and T-wave peaking is the only electrocardiographic abnormality, hyperkalemia may be considered moderate. Severe hyperkalemia is present if the plasma potassium exceeds 8 meq per liter or if electrocardiographic abnormalities include absent P waves, widened QRS complexes, or ventricular arrhythmias. Minimal hyperkalemia can usually be treated by elimination of a cause, such as potassium-sparing diuretics, or by treatment of accompanying acidosis. More severe or progressive hyperkalemia requires vigorous therapy. Severe cardiac toxicity responds most rapidly to infusion of calcium; 10 to 30 ml of 10% calcium gluconate may be infused intravenously within a period of 1 to 5 min under constant electrocardiographic monitoring. While calcium infusions do not alter plasma potassium, they counteract the adverse effects of potassium on neuromuscular membranes. The effect of calcium infusions, while almost immediate, is relatively transient if the hyperkalemia is not treated directly.

In moderately severe hyperkalemia, infusion of hypertonic glucose solutions will decrease toxicity by shifting potassium into cells. In the first 30 min, 200 to 500 ml of 10% glucose may be given. An additional 500 to 1000 ml may be infused over the next several hours. Ten units of regular insulin may be given subcutaneously, although this is probably necessary only in insulin-deficient diabetic patients. This treatment may reduce serum potassium by 1 to 2 meq per liter, and effects persist for a number of hours. The infusion of sodium bicarbonate will also help lower serum potassium rapidly by causing potassium to shift into cells; 44 to 132 meq alkali (two to three ampuls) may be added to a liter of glucose. Although this agent is most valuable in acidotic patients, it also is effective in individuals with normal acid-base status. The effect occurs within 1 h and persists for a number of hours thereafter. The infusion of hypertonic sodium solutions may also be effective in reversing cardiac toxicity, especially in hyponatremic or volume-depleted patients. In part the effect depends simply on dilution of plasma potassium, but there may be a direct effect of elevated plasma sodium to antagonize hyperkalemic neuromuscular toxicity as well. Glucose, bicarbonate, and sodium may be

FIGURE 43-1

Electrocardiographic changes in hyperkalemia. A. Early toxicity in a patient with plasma potassium of 6.8 meq per liter. Note symmetrical peaking of T waves. B. Advanced toxicity in a patient with plasma potassium of 8.6 meq per liter. QRS complexes are abnormally widened, P waves have disappeared, and ventricular rhythm is irregular. (From NG Levinsky, Clinician, 1973.)

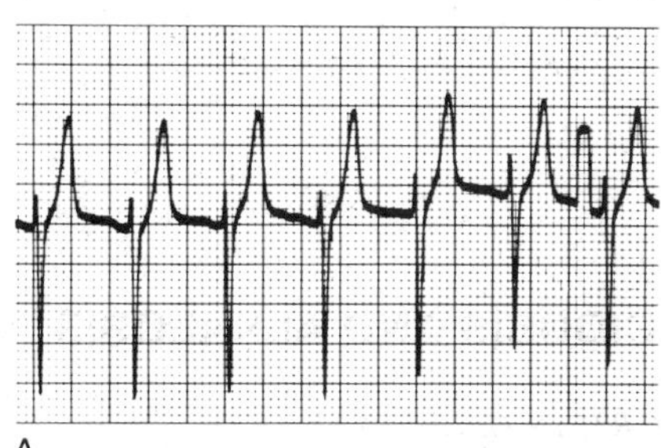
A

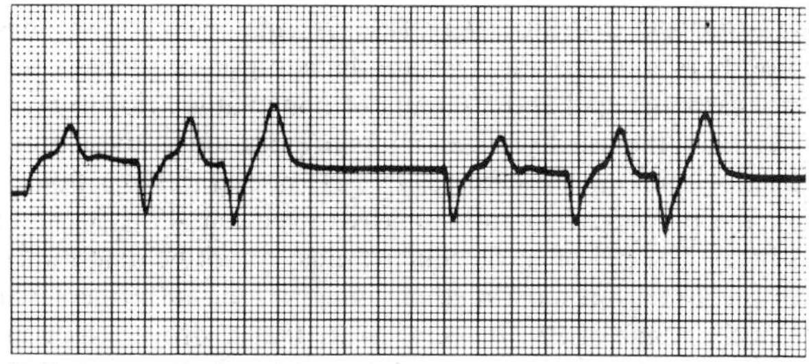
B

combined in a "therapeutic cocktail," formulated by adding an ampul or two of sodium bicarbonate to a liter of 5% dextrose in 0.9% saline.

None of the measures just described removes potassium from the body. Cation exchange resins such as sodium polystyrene sulfonate may be given by retention enema in the treatment of moderate or severe hyperkalemia. Enough potassium may be removed by a single enema to reduce potassium by 0.5 to 2 meq per liter within an hour, and repeated enemas can be given. These resins can also be given repeatedly by mouth to maintain low plasma potassium concentration. Twenty grams is given three or four times a day together with 20 ml of a 70% sorbitol solution, as required to ensure the passage of several loose stools daily. In patients with renal failure, hemodialysis and peritoneal dialysis will effectively control hyperkalemia. However, they are relatively slow techniques, and patients with severe hyperkalemia should be treated first with one of the methods previously discussed.

REFERENCES

Sodium and water

BARTTER FC: The syndrome of inappropriate secretion of antidiuretic hormone (SIADH). Dis Month Nov 1973

BERL T et al: Clinical disorders of water metabolism. Kidney Int 10:117, 1976

GABOW PA et al: Diagnostic importance of an increased serum anion gap. N Engl J Med 303:854, 1980

MILLER M, MOSES AM: Drug-induced states of impaired water excretion. Kidney Int 10:96, 1976

NARINS RG et al: Diagnostic strategies in disorders of fluid, electrolyte and acid-base homeostasis. Am J Med 72:496, 1982

WEINER M, EPSTEIN FH: Signs and symptoms of electrolyte disorders. Yale J Biol Med 43:76, 1970

ZERBE R et al: Vasopressin function in the syndrome of inappropriate diuresis. Ann Rev Med 31:315, 1980

Potassium

BIA MJ, DEFRONZO RA: Extrarenal potassium homeostasis. Am J Physiol 240:F257, 1981

KNOCHEL JP: The syndrome of hyporeninemic hypoaldosteronism. Ann Rev Med 30:145, 1979

SCHWARTZ WB, RELMAN AS: Effects of electrolyte disorders on renal structure and function. N Engl J Med 276:283, 1967

SURAWICZ B: Relationship between the ECG and electrolytes. Am Heart J 73:814, 1967

WRIGHT FS: Sites and mechanisms of potassium transport along the renal tubule. Kidney Int 11:415, 1977

44
ACIDOSIS AND ALKALOSIS

NORMAN G. LEVINSKY

PHYSIOLOGIC CONSIDERATIONS Normal metabolism continuously produces acids. Despite the addition of some 20,000 mmol carbonic acid and 80 mmol of nonvolatile acids to body fluids daily, the free hydrogen ion concentration of these fluids is fixed within a narrow range. The pH of extracellular fluid is normally between 7.35 and 7.45 (hydrogen ion, 45 to 35 nmol per liter). The pH of intracellular fluids cannot be determined with precision, but most methods suggest a mean intracellular pH in the range of 6.9. It seems likely that hydrogen ion concentration varies among intracellular organelles and cytoplasm even within individual cells. Although the free hydrogen ion concentration of body fluids is exceedingly low, protons are so reactive that even minute changes in concentration significantly influence enzymatic reactions and physiologic processes. Immediate defense against untoward changes in pH is provided by body buffers which can take up or release protons instantaneously in response to changes in acidity of body fluids. Regulation of pH ultimately depends on the lungs and the kidneys.

The principal acid product of metabolism is carbon dioxide, equivalent to potential carbonic acid. The normal concentration of carbon dioxide in body fluids is fixed at 1.2 mmol per liter (P_{CO_2} = 40 mmHg) by the lungs; at this concentration, pulmonary excretion equals metabolic production. Although carbon dioxide reacts with water and body buffers during transport from cells to pulmonary alveoli, no net change in body fluid composition results, since the CO_2 excreted by the lungs is directly equivalent to the CO_2 produced by cells. When a nonvolatile acid is produced by metabolism, the protons are removed instantaneously from body fluids by reaction with buffers. In extracellular fluid, bicarbonate is converted to water and carbon dioxide, which is excreted by the lungs. Although this mechanism effectively minimizes changes in acidity, it destroys bicarbonate and uses up cell buffer capacity. The total buffer capacity of the body fluids is about 15 meq per kilogram of body weight. Thus, the normal rate of production of nonvolatile acids would be sufficient to deplete the body buffers completely in 10 to 20 days, were it not for the unique ability of the kidney to eliminate protons from the body by secretion into the urine, thereby regenerating bicarbonate and cell buffer capacity.

The principal source of nonvolatile acid appears to be metabolism of methionine and cystine in dietary proteins, which produces sulfuric acid. Additional sources include the incomplete combustion of carbohydrates and fats, which produces organic acids; the metabolism of nucleoproteins, which produces uric acid; and the metabolism of organic phosphorus compounds, which releases protons and inorganic phosphates. The diet does not normally contain significant amounts of preformed acids or alkalis, but significant amounts of potential acid (e.g., an excess of cationic acids, such as lysine) or alkali (e.g., citrate) may be present.

The principal functions of the kidney in acid-base metabolism can be viewed as retention of existing bicarbonate and generation of new bicarbonate to replace that used to buffer nonvolatile acids. Bicarbonate is reabsorbed in both proximal and distal segments by secretion of protons into tubular fluid. New bicarbonate is generated by secretion of protons onto urinary buffers. Normally, one-third is titrated onto phosphate, converting HPO_4^{2-} to $H_2PO_4^-$, the remainder onto ammonia. The amount of free acid which can be excreted in the urine is negligible, even at the minimum urine pH of 4.8. However, acidification of the urine is essential for titration of acid onto phosphate and ammonia. Changes in the pH of body fluids lead to regulatory responses by the kidney. Acidosis stimulates renal hydrogen ion secretion. Ammonia production increases, and more protons can be excreted as ammonium. In extreme acidosis, ammonia production may increase tenfold or more above the normal rate of 40 to 50 meq per day. The bicarbonate concentration of extracellular fluid is, in effect, set by the renal rate of proton secretion (bicarbonate reabsorption and generation). If plasma bicarbonate rises without an increase in renal reabsorptive capacity, bicarbonate will be excreted rapidly and normal plasma bicarbonate will be restored promptly. For example, chronic ingestion of even large amounts of sodium bicarbonate will normally produce only minimal sustained elevation of plasma bicarbonate. The rate of proton secretion is influenced by a number of factors, important among them carbon dioxide tension of body fluids, extracellular volume, aldosterone, and body potassium stores. Bicarbonate reabsorption is directly related to carbon dioxide concentration; hypercapnia tends to stimulate and hypocapnia to inhibit renal bicarbonate retention. Contraction of extracellular volume tends to enhance tubular bicarbonate reabsorption, while volume expansion has the opposite effect. Aldosterone stimulates renal proton secretion; by this effect, hyperaldosteronism promotes metabolic alkalosis, while hypoaldosteronism tends to cause acidosis. In experimental animals, renal bicarbonate reabsorption is inversely related to body potassium stores. In humans, the relation is less clear, but severe potassium depletion has been associated with increased bicarbonate reabsorption and metabolic alkalosis.

The respiratory response to changes in blood pH is almost instantaneous. Acidosis stimulates and alkalosis depresses ventilation. The respiratory center in the medulla appears to respond to a pH intermediate between those of blood and cerebrospinal fluid.

EVALUATION OF ACID-BASE BALANCE In practice, classification of acid-base disorders is based on measurements of changes in the bicarbonate–carbonic acid system, the principal buffer of extracellular fluid. Because intracellular and extracellular buffers are functionally linked, measurement of the plasma bicarbonate system provides useful information about total body buffers. The relationship among the elements of the bicarbonate system is usually described in terms of the Henderson-Hasselbalch equation:

$$\text{pH} = \text{p}K + \log \frac{[\text{HCO}_3^-]}{[\text{H}_2\text{CO}_3]}$$

(The pK of carbonic acid is 6.1. $[H_2CO_3]$ is calculated as αP_{CO_2}; α, the solubility factor for carbon dioxide in body fluids, is 0.031 mmol per liter per mmHg P_{CO_2}. For a normal P_{CO_2} of 40 mmHg, $[H_2CO_3]$ is calculated to be $40 \times 0.031 = 1.2$ mmol per liter.)

Acidosis is defined as a physiologic disturbance which tends to add acid or remove alkali from body fluids, while *alkalosis* is any physiologic disturbance which tends to remove acid or add base. Since compensatory processes may minimize or prevent a change in the hydrogen ion concentration of the plasma, some authors prefer to use the terms *acidemia* and *alkalemia* to indicate those situations in which the pH of the plasma is measurably altered. *Respiratory* disorders are those in which the primary change is in the concentration of carbon dioxide (carbonic acid). As can be seen from the Henderson-Hasselbalch equation, a fall in carbon dioxide concentration will tend to cause alkalemia, while an increase in carbon dioxide concentration will cause acidemia. *Metabolic* disorders are those in which the primary disturbance is in the concentration of bicarbonate. Since bicarbonate appears in the numerator of the buffer salt/acid ratio in the Henderson-Hasselbalch equation, increased bicarbonate concentration causes alkalemia while a decrease in bicarbonate causes acidemia.

A major problem in the clinical assessment of acid-base disorders results from the compensatory responses of the lungs and the kidney. A primary change in carbon dioxide concentration induces a compensatory renal response which alters plasma bicarbonate in the same direction. Conversely, a primary alteration of plasma bicarbonate will induce compensatory changes in plasma carbon dioxide. Consider a patient with chronic respiratory insufficiency who has the following set of acid-base parameters: $P_{CO_2} = 70$ mmHg, $[HCO_3^-] = 31$ mmol per liter, pH = 7.25. The clinician needs to know whether the elevation of plasma bicarbonate is merely the appropriate renal response to the primary hypercapnia or a metabolic acid-base disorder is superimposed. No calculations or a priori reasoning will provide the answer to this key question. Such information can be derived only from in vivo observations in which the usual compensatory response to a given degree of chronic hypercapnia is determined.

Appropriate clinical and experimental observations in humans (and animals) have been made in all common primary acid-base disturbances. They are most readily visualized and used for analysis of clinical acid-base disorders by the "confidence band" technique, as shown in Fig. 44-1. Each band represents the mean ±2 SD, that is, 95 percent of observations, for the compensatory response to each primary disturbance. In the example under discussion, inspection of the confidence band marked *chronic respiratory acidosis* indicates that 95 percent of individuals with chronic elevation of P_{CO_2} to 70 mmHg would have $[HCO_3^-]$ between 34 and 44 meq per liter, due to renal compensation. Thus, the $[HCO_3^-]$ of 31 meq per liter in the example cannot be interpreted as solely the result of an appropriate compensatory response to chronic hypercapnia. A second acid-base disorder, presumably metabolic acidosis, must be superimposed. Obviously, the use of this figure is no panacea nor does it obviate the need for commonsense clinical evaluation of alternative possibilities. For example, if the patient under discussion had only recently developed hypercapnia, the $[HCO_3^-]$ of 31 meq per liter would be too high for a purely compensatory response to acute respiratory acidosis and would be interpreted as superimposed metabolic alkalosis. The difference between these two interpretations depends entirely on the clinical recognition of the chronicity of the primary respiratory disorder. The use of Fig. 44-1 in each type of acid-base disturbance is described in the appropriate section of this chapter.[1]

[1] *Although the confidence band method does not permit automatic identification of simple or complicated acid-base disorders, it is much preferable to other techniques such as "buffer base" or "base excess-deficit" for reasons discussed in detail by Schwartz and Relman, N Engl J Med 268:1382, 1963. These terms are not used in this chapter.*

FIGURE 44-1

In vivo nomogram, showing bands for uncomplicated respiratory or metabolic acid-base disturbances. Each "confidence" band represents the mean ± 2 SD for the compensatory response of normal subjects or patients to a given primary disorder. (Modified from Arbus.)

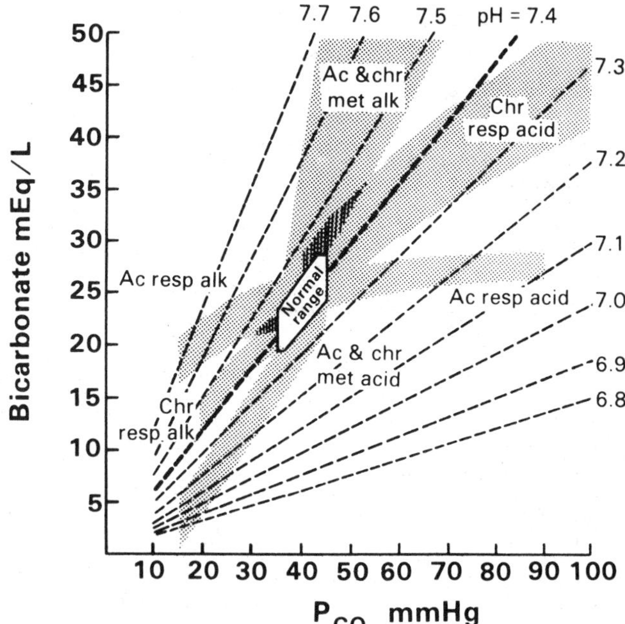

METABOLIC ACIDOSIS

PATHOPHYSIOLOGY Metabolic acidosis is caused by one of three mechanisms: (1) increased production of nonvolatile acids, (2) decreased acid excretion by the kidney, (3) loss of alkali. In intracellular fluid excess protons replace potassium, which shifts out of cells, tending to elevate plasma levels. Extracellular bicarbonate is reduced by reaction with hydrogen ions or, in patients wasting alkali, by loss of bicarbonate in urine or stool. The decrease in pH stimulates respiration, and P_{CO_2} is lowered. Inspection of the confidence band for metabolic acidosis (Fig. 44-1) indicates that a decrease in P_{CO_2} of roughly 1 mmHg can be expected for each decrement of 1 mmol per liter in plasma bicarbonate. Complete respiratory compensation for primary metabolic acidosis does not occur. Respiratory compensation for acute acidosis tends to be somewhat greater than for chronic metabolic acidosis. The minimum level of P_{CO_2} which can be attained is approximately 10 mmHg; levels below 15 to 20 mmHg are rarely maintained in chronic metabolic acidosis. When kidney function is normal, net acid excretion increases promptly in response to metabolic acidosis. Most of the initial rise is due to increased titration of urinary phosphate as urine pH falls below 5.2. Over several days, ammonia production by the kidney increases and becomes quantitatively by far the most important mechanism for excreting excess protons. Net acid excretion may increase 5 to 10 times above normal, reaching a maximum of several hundred milliequivalents per day.

The most common cause of *acute* metabolic acidosis is increased production of nonvolatile acids. In *diabetic ketoacidosis,* acetoacetic and β-hydroxybutyric acids are produced more rapidly than they can be metabolized (Chap. 114). Severe ketoacidosis may occur in *association* with *acute* and *chronic alcoholism.* Typically patients have given a history of prolonged abstention from food, protracted vomiting, and appreciable alcohol intake just before development of the ketoacidosis. β-Hydroxybutyrate, acetoacetate, and lactate accumulate in the plasma. The ketosis may be overlooked because the ratio of β-hydroxybutyrate to acetoacetate tends to be unusually high; the nitroprusside test used for clinical detection of plasma ketones responds only to the latter. Blood sugar is usually normal or mildly elevated in these patients. The mechanism of the syndrome is uncertain. *Starvation* may cause mild ketoacidosis because of increased fat metabolism.

TABLE 44-1
Causes of metabolic acidosis

Increased anion gap
- *I* Increased acid production
  - *A* Ketoacidosis
    - *1* Diabetic
    - *2* Alcoholic
    - *3* Starvation
  - *B* Lactic acidosis
    - *1* Secondary to circulatory or respiratory failure
    - *2* Associated with various disorders (see text)
    - *3* Drugs and toxins
    - *4* Enzyme defects
  - *C* Poisoning (salicylates, ethylene glycol, methanol)
- *II* Renal failure

Normal anion gap (hyperchloremic)
- *III* Renal tubular dysfunction
  - *A* Renal tubular acidosis
  - *B* Hypoaldosteronism
- *IV* Loss of alkali
  - *A* Diarrhea
  - *B* Ureterosigmoidostomy
  - *C* Carbonic anhydrase inhibitors
- *V* Ammonium chloride, cationic amino acids (excess intake)

Several types of *lactic acidosis* have been recognized. The most common is *secondary* to severe acute circulatory or respiratory failure, with poor tissue perfusion or arterial oxygen desaturation. The clinical features of shock are usually present. In these patients, lactic acidosis probably is due both to increased production of lactate by hypoxic tissues and to decreased utilization by the liver. Lactic acidosis (Chap. 115) may also be *associated* with *various disorders* such as acute hepatic necrosis, leukemia, and infections. The biguanide oral hypoglycemic agents, such as phenformin, were the drugs most often responsible for *drug-induced* lactic acidosis; they have been removed from general use. Certain sugars used for parenteral alimentation, such as fructose, may cause lactic acidosis. Increased lactic acid production contributes to acidosis in *poisoning* by methanol and salicylates. In infants and children, a variety of congenital defects in enzymes of carbohydrate metabolism have been identified as causes of lactic acidosis. Primary lactic acidosis in patients without an underlying disease has been reported but the existence of such a spontaneous disorder is uncertain.

Poisoning and drug toxicity are causes of acute metabolic acidosis. Among the more common agents are salicylates, ethylene glycol, and methyl alcohol (Chap. 238). Salicylates create a metabolic block, which leads to production of a mixture of endogenous organic acids. Methanol and ethylene glycol are converted to acid metabolites, methanol to formic acid and ethylene glycol to glyoxylic and oxalic acids. In addition, these intoxicants create metabolic blocks, which may lead to increased production of a mixture of endogenous organic acids. Salicylates have the additional effect of stimulating the respiratory center directly. Respiratory alkalosis is the earliest derangement in salicylate intoxication and may be the only acid-base disorder in some patients.

Renal disease is the most common cause of chronic metabolic acidosis. In *chronic renal failure* (Chap. 291), the principal defect is decreased ability to excrete ammonium, but some patients also waste bicarbonate, especially at plasma levels of 18 mmol per liter or above. Acidification of the urine and formation of titratable acidity are usually normal. Plasma bicarbonate tends to fall progressively as renal insufficiency becomes increasingly severe, but plasma bicarbonate usually stabilizes at levels of 12 to 18 mmol per liter; it rarely falls below 10 mmol per liter, even in advanced uremia. The mechanisms of stabilization are thought to be (1) stimulation of acid excretion by advancing acidosis, which occurs to some extent even in the diseased kidney; and (2) buffering of the daily metabolic acid load by carbonate and phosphate in bone. In *acute renal failure* (Chap. 290), plasma bicarbonate decreases by only 1 to 2 mmol per liter per day if reduced renal acid excretion is the only cause of metabolic acidosis. Greater rates of fall suggest the presence, in addition, of some cause of increased acid production.

Chronic metabolic acidosis is the hallmark of *renal tubular acidosis* (Chap. 299), which may be an isolated disorder of tubular acid excretion; part of a Fanconi syndrome, in which other tubular functions are also abnormal; or associated with a number of nonrenal primary disorders (Chap. 92). The acidosis is due to defective renal tubular acidification mechanisms, which limit renal conservation and regeneration of bicarbonate.

Aldosterone stimulates distal tubular acid and potassium secretion. In *hypoaldosteronism,* loss of this effect leads to metabolic acidosis and hyperkalemia. The acidosis is due not only to loss of the direct effect of aldosterone on acid excretion but also to the hyperkalemia, which decreases renal ammonia production.

Loss of alkali may be the cause of acute or chronic metabolic acidosis. Severe *diarrhea* or intestinal malabsorption usually causes mild to moderate acidosis due to the loss of bicarbonate in liquid stool, in which concentrations of 40 to 60 mmol per liter may be present. Ureterosigmoidostomy, i.e., transplantation of the ureters into the sigmoid colon, leads to metabolic acidosis both because of exchange of chloride for bicarbonate by intestinal epithelium and because renal disease (obstructive uropathy and pyelonephritis) often develops. However, acidosis has virtually been eliminated as a problem by the more modern technique for urinary diversion, in which a bladder is formed from a small isolated loop of ileum. Carbonic anhydrase inhibitors, such as acetazolamide, cause mild to moderate acidosis by increasing bicarbonate loss in the urine.

Acidosis can be caused by administration of ammonium chloride and lysine or arginine hydrochloride, which form HCl during metabolism. This type of acidosis also may occur during parenteral alimentation with amino acid infusates which contain an excess of the cationic amino acids arginine, lysine, and histidine.

CLINICAL FEATURES AND DIAGNOSIS There are few specific symptoms or signs of metabolic acidosis; diagnosis depends on recognition of the clinical setting and appropriate laboratory studies. In acute metabolic acidosis, hyperventilation is usually evident and may be extremely intense (Kussmaul respiration). However, it is ordinarily impossible to detect increased respiration by physical examination in patients with chronic metabolic acidosis, despite substantial reduction of P_{CO_2}. Acute, severe acidosis produces a variety of nonspecific symptoms ranging from fatigue through confusion, stupor, and coma. Cardiovascular effects include decreased cardiac contractility and vasodilatation, which may lead to heart failure or hypotension. Chronic metabolic acidosis may produce no symptoms or may be associated with fatigue and anorexia, although it is usually difficult to determine whether these symptoms reflect the acidosis per se or are related to the underlying disease.

The characteristic laboratory features are reduction of plasma bicarbonate and blood pH, together with a compensatory reduction in P_{CO_2} (see Fig. 44-1). Hyperkalemia is often present, due to shift of potassium out of cells. This phenomenon may mask significant potassium depletion (see Chap. 43). Hypokalemia is a clue to conditions in which concomitant potassium depletion is severe, for example, diarrhea or diabetic ketoacidosis, or in which renal potassium-regulating mechanisms are affected, such as renal tubular acidosis or administration of carbonic anhydrase inhibitors.

In those instances in which the cause of metabolic acidosis is not evident from the history or clinical setting, calculation of unmeasured anions (anion gap) may help in differential diagnosis. Unmeasured anions are calculated by subtracting the sum of plasma bicarbonate and chloride from plasma sodium concentration; the normal value is 8 to 16 mmol per liter. The negative charges on plasma proteins, principally albumin, make up most of the anion gap. Phosphate, sulfate, and various organic acid anions normally contribute to unmeasured anions to a lesser degree. When metabolic acidosis is due to increased acid production or renal insufficiency (categories I and II, Table 44-1), the anion gap will usually be increased. In acidosis resulting from increased acid production, the increased anion gap is due to accumulation in plasma of the anions of the various acids such as acetoacetate or lactate, which are produced faster than they can be metabolized or excreted. In renal failure, the anion gap increases because sulfate, phosphate, and organic acid anions are not excreted efficiently. In all other types of metabolic acidosis (categories III, IV, V, Table 44-1), the anion gap will be normal since there is neither increased production or decreased excretion of organic acids, sulfate, and phosphate. Plasma chloride concentration is increased approximately as much as plasma bicarbonate is decreased (hyperchloremic acidosis).

TREATMENT The treatment of metabolic acidosis depends on its cause and severity. In *chronic renal failure,* mild or moderate metabolic acidosis does not require treatment. When plasma bicarbonate falls below 15 mmol per liter, it is reasonable to treat patients with oral alkali, such as sodium bicarbonate or sodium citrate. The dose is gradually increased until plasma bicarbonate concentration rises to about 18 to 20 mmol per liter. Some patients appear to benefit symptomatically from elevation of bicarbonate to this level, and fatigue, anorexia, and malaise tend to be alleviated. Caution must be exerted to avoid excessively rapid alkalination of the plasma, which may precipitate tetany; excess sodium given with alkali may aggravate hypertension or edema. Acidosis should be corrected as completely as possible in patients with *renal tubular acidosis;* this will avoid hypercalciuria, osteomalacia, nephrocalcinosis, and lithiasis. Patients with *acute renal failure* do not ordinarily require specific therapy for acidosis. Dialysis instituted for management of the renal failure should maintain an adequate plasma bicarbonate.

Diabetic *ketoacidosis* responds to insulin, and most patients do not require treatment with alkali. However, when acidosis is extreme (pH less than 7.1 or $[HCO_3^-]$ less than 6 to 8 meq per liter), intravenous bicarbonate therapy is justified. The ketoacidosis associated with alcoholism responds rapidly to infusions of glucose and saline. Insulin is not required, nor should alkali be given unless acidosis is extreme. The ketoacidosis of starvation is mild and requires no specific treatment.

Lactic acidosis secondary to acute circulatory or respiratory failure is corrected if treatment of the underlying disorder is successful. Since this type of lactic acidosis is usually associated with severe acute circulatory or respiratory failure, the mortality rate is high. Lactic acidosis occurring in other disorders is usually resistant to treatment. Rapid administration of several hundred milliequivalents of alkali may raise plasma bicarbonate in some patients, but in others net production of lactic acid may be so rapid that correction of acidosis is difficult. Since vigorous administration of alkali may lead to circulatory overloading, dialysis may be a useful therapeutic measure. Despite rapid administration of alkali, the mortality rate in these patients is high.

The acidosis associated with *diarrhea* or loss of alkaline upper intestinal secretions is usually associated with other electrolyte abnormalities, including volume depletion and potassium deficiency. Treatment with intravenous infusions appropriate for all these abnormalities may be required.

Some general points about therapy with alkali are worth emphasis. Oral treatment with sodium bicarbonate should usually begin with 1 g three times daily and be increased to maintain the desired plasma bicarbonate level. Some patients find that sodium bicarbonate leads to upper gastrointestinal discomfort; a 10% sodium citrate solution may be more palatable. In treatment of acute metabolic acidosis by intravenous administration of alkali, sodium bicarbonate is the agent of choice. The concentration of bicarbonate to be given depends upon the severity of the acidosis and any associated disorders of serum sodium concentration. Typically, concentrations of bicarbonate between 44 and 132 meq per liter are achieved by adding one to three ampuls of sodium bicarbonate to a liter of dextrose in water. The concentration of bicarbonate in these ampuls is 880 meq per liter (44 meq in 50 ml); they should never be given undiluted in the treatment of acidosis, since rapid infusion may induce serious or even fatal cardiac arrhythmias, especially if given as a bolus through a central venous catheter. The total amount of alkali needed to raise plasma bicarbonate can be estimated from the effects of administration of acid loads. In experiments, approximately equal amounts of acid appear to be buffered by extracellular bicarbonate and by intracellular buffers. (In extremely severe acidosis, a greater fraction of the acid load may be buffered within cells.) Therefore, it is appropriate to calculate the amount of alkali needed by assuming that approximately half will accept protons from intracellular buffers and be destroyed; the other half will elevate plasma bicarbonate concentration. Thus, the calculation would be: millimoles of bicarbonate required equals desired increment in plasma concentration (millimoles per liter) times 40 percent of body weight. The 40 percent figure represents twice the extracellular volume. It is rarely desirable to infuse enough alkali to elevate plasma bicarbonate to normal. Possible untoward effects include hypokalemic cardiac toxicity in patients who are substantially potassium-depleted; tetany in patients with renal failure or hypocalcemia; and congestive failure due to excess sodium. Moreover, alkalosis may supervene. Cerebrospinal fluid bicarbonate does not equilibrate rapidly with plasma. Hence the respiratory center, which responds to acidity both of blood and cerebrospinal fluid, maintains some degree of hyperventilation as plasma bicarbonate is increasing. This type of respiratory alkalosis may sometimes persist for several days after correction of metabolic acidosis. In acute acidosis due to overproduction of metabolic acids, successful treatment of the primary disorder will cause rapid metabolic conversion of lactate and ketone bodies to bicarbonate. Thus, excessive administration of bicarbonate early in therapy also may lead to metabolic alkalosis at a later stage of treatment, when endogenous bicarbonate has been reconstituted by improvement in metabolism.

METABOLIC ALKALOSIS

PATHOPHYSIOLOGY Metabolic alkalosis is usually initiated by increased loss of acid from the stomach or the kidney. However, excretion of bicarbonate at high plasma concentrations is normally so rapid that alkalosis will not be sustained unless bicarbonate reabsorption is enhanced or alkali is continuously generated at a great rate. Clinically, maintenance of metabolic alkalosis is most often due to stimulation of bicarbonate reabsorption by a volume (chloride) deficit. During volume depletion, renal conservation of sodium takes precedence over other homeostatic mechanisms, such as correction of alkalosis. Since in alkalosis a large fraction of plasma sodium is paired with bicarbonate, complete reabsorption of filtered sodium requires reabsorption of bicarbonate as well. Alkalosis is sustained until volume depletion is corrected by administration of sodium chloride. This diminishes tubular avidity for sodium and provides chloride as an alternative anion for reabsorption with sodium; excess bicarbonate can then be excreted with sodium.

The other major mechanism which can maintain metabolic alkalosis is hypermineralocorticoidism. Mineralocorticoids stimulate renal hydrogen ion secretion. In patients with excess mineralocorticoid activity, elevation of plasma bicarbonate is initiated by increased urinary loss of protons as ammonium and titratable acidity. Stimulation of tubular acid secretion also enhances bicarbonate reabsorption, thereby sustaining the metabolic alkalosis. Patients with excess mineralocorticoid activity are not volume or chloride-deficient. Hence, this type of metabolic alkalosis does not respond to sodium chloride administration.

The relation between metabolic alkalosis and potassium is complex and incompletely understood. Alkalosis and hypokalemia often occur together. Alkalosis may cause hypokalemia and potassium depletion through mechanisms discussed in Chap. 43. Conversely, potassium depletion may help to sustain metabolic alkalosis because distal tubular acid secretion, and hence bicarbonate reabsorption, is stimulated. Whether potassium depletion alone can generate metabolic alkalosis is uncertain; if so, severe potassium depletion is required.

Respiratory compensation for metabolic alkalosis is limited. Alveolar ventilation decreases, and P_{CO_2} is elevated. However, since this response is limited by hypoxia, P_{CO_2} rarely rises above 50 to 55 mmHg.

PATHOGENESIS The principal causes of metabolic alkalosis are outlined in Table 44-2. *Vomiting* and *gastric drainage* usually induce only minimal or moderate alkalosis, but occasional patients, especially those with increased gastric acid secretion, e.g., with acid-peptic disease or the Zollinger-Ellison syndrome, may develop very severe alkalosis.

Alkalosis may be present in patients treated with any *diuretic* except those which specifically inhibit bicarbonate reabsorption, such as acetazolamide, or those which inhibit distal cation secretion, such as spironolactone and triamterene. Alkalosis due to oral treatment with diuretics is usually mild. Acute administration of very potent intravenous diuretics such as ethacrynic acid to patients on low-sodium diets may induce more severe alkalosis due to rapid loss of sodium chloride in the urine. Sudden contraction of extracellular volume elevates plasma bicarbonate; renal excretion of excess bicarbonate is prevented by the mechanism discussed above.

Patients with chronic hypercapnia due to respiratory insufficiency maintain high plasma bicarbonate concentrations (see "Respiratory Acidosis," below). If respiration improves, P_{CO_2} will fall promptly. However, urinary excretion of excess bicarbonate previously generated by renal compensatory mechanisms will take a number of days. In patients on low-salt diets or diuretics who have a volume (chloride) deficiency, *posthypercapnic* alkalosis of this type may persist indefinitely unless sodium or potassium chloride is added to the diet. The mechanism in this condition is the same as that which causes persistent alkalosis in vomiting, described earlier.

Alkalosis is variable in patients with excess mineralocorticoid activity. Minimal or moderate alkalosis is usually present in patients with *Cushing's syndrome* or *primary aldosteronism.* More marked alkalosis may be seen in patients with extreme adrenal hyperfunction associated with ACTH-secreting tumors, such as bronchogenic carcinoma. Moderate alkalosis is typical of patients with *Bartter's syndrome.*

Although alkalosis and *potassium depletion* are often associated, mild or moderate potassium depletion does not cause sustained metabolic alkalosis. However, extreme degrees of potassium depletion (serum potassium usually 2 meq per liter or less) may cause metabolic alkalosis. This type of alkalosis is

TABLE 44-2
Causes of metabolic alkalosis

I Associated with volume (chloride) depletion
- *A* Vomiting or gastric drainage
- *B* Diuretic therapy
- *C* Posthypercapnic alkalosis

II Associated with hyperadrenocorticism
- *A* Cushing's syndrome
- *B* Primary aldosteronism
- *C* Bartter's syndrome

III Severe potassium depletion

IV Excessive alkali intake
- *A* Acute
- *B* Milk-alkali syndrome

not corrected by administration of sodium chloride but does respond to administration of potassium.

For reasons noted earlier, alkalosis due to administration of alkali cannot be sustained unless large amounts are given. When renal function is compromised, alkalosis may be sustained by small exogenous loads. This is apparently the mechanism of alkalosis in the milk-alkali syndrome, in which hypercalcemic nephropathy and alkalosis develop in response to excessive intake of absorbable alkali. The nephropathy limits bicarbonate excretion, thus maintaining the alkalosis.

CLINICAL FEATURES AND DIAGNOSIS There are no specific clinical signs or symptoms. Severe alkalosis may cause apathy, confusion, and stupor. If serum calcium is borderline or low, rapid development of alkalosis may lead to tetany. The diagnosis of metabolic alkalosis depends on recognition of the clinical setting and appropriate laboratory studies. Plasma bicarbonate is increased, and elevation of P_{CO_2} is insufficient to prevent alkalemia (see Fig. 44-1). Plasma potassium concentration is often reduced, and the electrocardiogram may reveal changes in T and U waves typical of hypokalemia (Chap. 249); it is uncertain whether these changes are due to alkalosis itself or to associated alterations in potassium metabolism. Despite elevation of plasma bicarbonate, the urine pH is usually less than 7 in patients with sustained metabolic alkalosis. This "paradoxical aciduria" reflects the fact that bicarbonate reabsorption must be increased if metabolic alkalosis is to be sustained.

Differential diagnosis is usually made from clinical features, such as a history of vomiting or the manifestations of Cushing's syndrome. The urinary chloride concentration may be a helpful clue if the diagnosis is not evident. When the alkalosis is associated with volume contraction (category I, Table 44-2), urinary chloride will be low, usually less than 10 meq per liter. When the alkalosis is caused by hyperadrenocorticism or severe potassium depletion (categories II and III), urinary chloride will be higher, usually 20 meq per liter or more.

TREATMENT Mild or moderate metabolic alkalosis rarely requires specific treatment. In patients with gastric alkalosis, infusion of saline solutions is usually sufficient to enhance renal bicarbonate excretion and to correct alkalosis by mechanisms discussed above. Administration of potassium chloride is also helpful in treating or preventing alkalosis in these patients and in treating those with diuretic-induced alkalosis. In patients with adrenal hyperfunction, alkalosis is corrected by specific treatment of the underlying disease. In Bartter's syndrome hypokalemia and potassium wasting may be partly corrected by treatment with prostaglandin synthetase inhibitors such as indomethacin. Whenever alkalosis and potassium depletion occur together, potassium depletion should be treated with potassium chloride, not with an organic salt of potassium.

Rarely, metabolic alkalosis in patients with prolonged gastric losses may be severe enough to require intravenous therapy with acidifying agents. Ammonium chloride or arginine hydrochloride may be given slowly under such circumstances. In most patients the use of potentially toxic acidifying agents can be avoided by appropriate treatment with saline and potassium chloride. In patients who are volume-expanded or in whom volume loading is inadvisable, therapy with acetazolamide, which enhances renal bicarbonate excretion, may be helpful.

RESPIRATORY ACIDOSIS

PATHOPHYSIOLOGY Failure of ventilation promptly increases P_{CO_2} (carbonic acid) because metabolic production of carbon dioxide is so rapid. Acute respiratory acidosis is modulated to a limited degree by tissue buffers. As can be seen from the curve labeled *acute respiratory acidosis* in Fig. 44-1, immediate tissue buffering is insufficient to elevate plasma bicarbonate more than a few milliequivalents per liter. If hypercapnia is sustained, renal acid excretion is enhanced, and bicarbonate reabsorption stimulated. Over a period of several days, plasma bicarbonate rises approximately 3 meq per liter for each increase of 10 mmHg in P_{CO_2}, thereby minimizing the degree of acidemia. The increment in plasma bicarbonate attributable to renal activity is represented by the difference between the curves marked *chronic respiratory acidosis* and *acute respiratory acidosis*.

PATHOGENESIS *Acute* respiratory acidosis occurs whenever there is a sudden failure of ventilation. Common causes include depression of the respiratory center by cerebral disease or drugs, neuromuscular disorders, and cardiopulmonary arrest. *Chronic* respiratory acidosis occurs in pulmonary diseases such as chronic emphysema and bronchitis, in which ventilation and perfusion are mismatched and effective alveolar ventilation is decreased. Chronic hypercapnia may also result from primary alveolar hypoventilation or from alveolar hypoventilation related to extreme obesity (Pickwickian syndrome). Acute and chronic diseases characterized principally by interference with alveolar gas exchange, such as chronic pulmonary fibrosis, pneumonia, and pulmonary edema, usually cause hypocapnia rather than hypercapnia. In these conditions, hypoxia stimulates increased ventilation; since carbon dioxide is much more diffusible than oxygen, excretion of carbon dioxide is enhanced despite the barrier to gas exchange. Hypercapnia occurs only with respiratory fatigue or extremely severe disease.

CLINICAL FEATURES AND DIAGNOSIS It is often difficult to separate the manifestations of respiratory acidosis from those of associated hypoxia. Moderate hypercapnia, especially if it develops slowly, probably has no specific clinical features. When P_{CO_2} exceeds 70 mmHg, patients progressively become confused and obtunded. Asterixis may be noted. Papilledema may occur, apparently because intracranial pressure is increased by the cerebral vasodilation characteristic of hypercapnia. Dilatation of conjunctival and superficial facial blood vessels may be noted.

The diagnosis of acute respiratory acidosis is usually evident from the clinical situation, especially if respiration is obviously depressed. Proof requires laboratory confirmation that P_{CO_2} is elevated. Acidemia is always present in patients with *acute* hypercapnia. Acidosis in acute cardiopulmonary arrest is usually a combination of a metabolic lactic acidosis and acute respiratory acidosis. Patients with chronic hypercapnia are usually acidemic. However, some individuals with minimal or moderate chronic hypercapnia may have normal or even slightly elevated plasma pH, as may be seen from Fig. 44-1. The mechanism of full compensation or of "overcompensation" in such individuals is unknown. However, significant elevation of pH in patients with chronic hypercapnia is almost always due to complicating metabolic alkalosis. Diuretics, low-sodium diets, and posthypercapnic alkalosis are frequent causes of this type of superimposed acid-base disorder.

Because of the differences between plasma bicarbonate in acute hypercapnia and in chronic hypercapnia, proper interpretation of acid-base parameters in respiratory acidosis depends on clinical information.

TREATMENT The only worthwhile approach to treatment of respiratory acidosis is correction of the underlying disorder. Rapid infusion of alkali is justified in cardiopulmonary arrest. In other circumstances, attempted treatment of respiratory acidosis with infusions of alkali or with buffers such as THAM is of transient benefit and has no role in practical management.

RESPIRATORY ALKALOSIS

PATHOPHYSIOLOGY Acute reduction in carbon dioxide concentration releases hydrogen ion from tissue buffers, which minimize alkalemia by reducing plasma bicarbonate. Acute alkalosis also enhances glycolysis; increased production of lactic and pyruvic acids lowers serum bicarbonate and raises plasma concentrations of the corresponding anions by a millimole or two. In chronic hypocapnia, plasma bicarbonate is further reduced because the decreased P_{CO_2} inhibits tubular reabsorption and generation of bicarbonate. Figure 44-1 shows that, as for respiratory acidosis, compensation for the chronic state is much more complete than for the acute. In acute hypocapnia, plasma bicarbonate falls only about 2 mmole per liter for each 10 mm reduction in P_{CO_2}. In chronic hypocapnia, plasma bicarbonate is reduced by 4 to 5 mmol per liter for each 10 mm decrease in P_{CO_2}. The decrement in plasma bicarbonate attributable to renal compensatory activity is shown by the difference between the curves labeled acute and chronic respiratory alkalosis in Fig. 44-1.

PATHOGENESIS Respiratory alkalosis is due to acute or chronic hyperventilation, which lowers P_{CO_2}. The causes of respiratory alkalosis are shown in Table 44-3.

TABLE 44-3
Causes of respiratory alkalosis

I Hypoxia
- *A* Acute (e.g., pneumonia, asthma, pulmonary edema)
- *B* Chronic (e.g., pulmonary fibrosis, cyanotic heart disease, high altitudes)

II Respiratory center stimulation
- *A* Anxiety
- *B* Fever
- *C* Salicylate intoxication
- *D* Cerebral disease (tumor, encephalitis, etc.)

III Exercise
IV Gram-negative sepsis
V Hepatic cirrhosis
VI Pregnancy
VII Excessive mechanical ventilation

CLINICAL FEATURES AND DIAGNOSIS Depending on its severity and acuteness, hyperventilation may or may not be clinically apparent. In acute respiratory alkalosis, the clinical picture is rather characteristic: patients complain of paresthesias, numbness, and tingling; of light-headedness; and, if alkalosis is sufficiently severe, of manifestations of tetany. Alkalosis directly enhances neuromuscular excitability; this effect, rather than the modest decrease in ionized plasma calcium induced by alkalosis, is probably the major cause of tetany. Severe respiratory alkalosis may cause confusion or loss of consciousness, perhaps due to cerebral vasospasm induced by hypocapnia.

The diagnosis may be suspected from the clinical setting but must be confirmed by analysis of the plasma bicarbonate system. Hypocapnia together with a variable degree of alkalemia is found; plasma bicarbonate is decreased but is rarely below 15 mmol per liter.

TREATMENT The only successful treatment for respiratory alkalosis is elimination of the underlying disorder. In the acute hyperventilation syndrome, sedation, reassurance, and if symptoms are sufficiently severe, rebreathing into a bag will usually terminate the attack.

REFERENCES

ARBUS GS: An in vivo acid-base nomogram for clinical use. Can Med Assoc J 109:291, 1973

BATTLE DC et al: Clinical and pathophysiologic spectrum of acquired distal renal tubular acidosis. Kidney Int 20:289, 1981

EMMETT M, NARINS RG: Clinical use of the anion gap. Medicine 56:38, 1977

KASSIRER JP, MADIAS NE: Respiratory acid-base disorders. Hosp Practice 15:57, 1980

LEVY LH et al: Ketoacidosis associated with alcoholism in non-diabetic subjects. Ann Intern Med 78:213, 1973

NARINS RG, EMMETT M: Simple and mixed acid-base disorders: A practical approach. Medicine 59:161, 1980

NARINS RG et al: Diagnostic strategies in disorders of fluid, electrolyte and acid-base homeostasis. Am J Med 72:496, 1982

SCHWARTZ WB, RELMAN AS: A critique of the parameters used in the evaluation of acid-base disorders. N Engl J Med 268:1382, 1963

SELDIN DW, RECTOR FC: The generation and maintenance of metabolic alkalosis. Kidney Int 1:306, 1972

STINEBAUGH BJ et al: Pathogenesis of distal renal tubular acidosis. Kidney Int 19:1, 1981

TANNEN RL: Control of acid excretion by the kidney. Ann Rev Med 31:35, 1980

section 7 | Alterations in reproductive and sexual function

45
DISTURBANCES OF THE REPRODUCTIVE TRACT IN WOMEN

BRUCE R. CARR
JEAN D. WILSON

Complaints related to the female reproductive tract can usually be categorized as either disorders of menstruation, pelvic pain, disturbances in sexual function, or infertility. However any disorder, for example leiomyoma of the uterus, can present with symptoms referable to any one or more of these categories. Furthermore, sexual dysfunction can interdigitate with other complaints in several ways. On the one hand, in women who present with complaints related to other reproductive tract functions, the underlying problem may actually be severe sexual dysfunction or marital conflict. Alternatively, women who have severe organic diseases of the pelvis, for example pelvic inflammatory disease, may present with a problem of sexual function such as dyspareunia, which in fact is only a minor manifestation of the underlying disease.

Since normal reproductive function depends on the integrated action of the central nervous system, the endocrine glands, and the reproductive organs, it is to be expected that menstrual cycle abnormalities, sexual dysfunction, and infertility may be the result of a variety of systemic and psychological disorders as well as of primary disorders in the endocrine and reproductive organs. The endocrine and physiological changes—normal and abnormal—associated with puberty, reproductive life, and menopause are discussed in Chap. 118. The focus of this chapter is on the initial evaluation of women with disturbances of the reproductive tract.

DISTURBANCES IN MENSTRUATION Disorders of menstruation can be divided into abnormal uterine bleeding and amenorrhea.

Abnormal uterine bleeding The length of a menstrual cycle is defined as the interval between the onset of one bleeding episode and the onset of the next. In normal women of reproductive age the cycle averages 28 $\pm$ 3 days, the mean duration of menstrual flow is 4 $\pm$ 2 days, and the average blood loss is 40 to 100 ml. Between the menarche and the menopause almost every woman experiences one or more episodes of abnormal uterine bleeding, here defined as any bleeding pattern outside the parameters of frequency, duration, and/or amount of blood loss described above. The decision to evaluate a patient with an abnormal bleeding pattern is based on the severity and frequency of the abnormal bleeding episodes.

In every woman whose complaints suggest abnormal uterine bleeding it is essential to establish first that the blood observed by the patient is derived from the uterine endometrium. Rectal, bladder, cervical, or vaginal sources of bleeding must be excluded. Once the bleeding is documented to be uterine in origin, a pregnancy-related disorder (such as threatened or incomplete abortion or ectopic pregnancy) must be excluded by physical examination and appropriate laboratory tests. It must also be kept in mind that abnormal uterine bleeding may be the initial or principal manifestation of a generalized bleeding diathesis. The remaining causes of abnormal uterine bleeding fall into one of two general categories: those associated with ovulatory cycles and those associated with anovulatory cycles.

OVULATORY CYCLES Menstrual bleeding that occurs with ovulatory cycles is spontaneous, regular in onset, predictable in duration and amount of flow, and frequently associated with discomfort. Uterine bleeding in women with ovulatory cycles is due to progesterone withdrawal at the end of the luteal phase and requires prior estrogen priming of the endometrium during the follicular phase of the cycle. When deviations from an established pattern of menstrual flow occur but the cycles are still regular, the usual cause is organic disease of the outflow tract. For example, regular but prolonged and excessive bleeding episodes unassociated with a bleeding diathesis are commonly due to abnormalities of the uterus such as submucous leiomyomas, adenomyosis, or endometrial polyps. On the other hand, cyclic, predictable menstruation characterized by spotting or light bleeding is often due to obstruction of the outflow tract as occurs with uterine synechiae or scarring of the cervix. Intermittent bleeding between cyclic ovulatory menses is often due to cervical or endometrial lesions.

ANOVULATORY CYCLES Uterine bleeding that is irregular in occurrence and unpredictable with respect to amount and duration of flow is called dysfunctional uterine bleeding. Such bleeding is usually painless. Dysfunctional uterine bleeding is the result of a failure of normal follicular maturation with consequent anovulation and may be either transient or chronic. Transient disruption of the synchronous hypothalamic-pituitary-ovarian hormonal secretory patterns necessary for ovulatory cycles occurs most often in the early menarcheal years, during the perimenopausal period, or as the secondary consequence of a variety of stresses and intercurrent illnesses. Persistent dysfunctional uterine bleeding during the reproductive years is the result of any of several organic diseases that affect ovarian function directly and is most often due to estrogen breakthrough bleeding. Estrogen breakthrough bleeding occurs when there is prolonged continuous estrogen stimulation of the endometrium that is not interrupted by cyclic progesterone withdrawal. It is the result of chronic acyclic estrogen production that is not associated with ovulation, as occurs in patients with polycystic ovarian disease.

Amenorrhea Amenorrhea is defined as failure of menarche by age 16, regardless of the presence or absence of secondary sexual characteristics, or the absence of menstruation for 6 months in a woman with previous periodic menses. Amenorrhea in a woman who has never menstruated is termed primary; absence of menses in a woman who previously menstruated is termed secondary amenorrhea. Because some disorders can cause both primary and secondary amenorrhea, we prefer a functional classification based upon the nature of the underlying defect, namely anatomical defects of the outflow tract (uterus, cervix, or vagina), ovarian failure, and chronic anovulation.

Anatomical defects of the outflow tract include congenital defects of the vagina, imperforate hymen, transverse vaginal septae, cervical stenosis, and intrauterine adhesions (synechiae). The diagnosis of an anatomical defect is usually made by physical examination and can be confirmed by demonstrating failure of bleeding following administration of estrogen plus a progestin for 21 days.

Causes of *ovarian failure* include gonadal dysgenesis, 17α-hydroxylase deficiency, premature ovarian failure, and resistant ovary syndrome. Ovarian failure encompasses those disorders in which the ovary is deficient in germ cells and those in which the germ cells are resistant to FSH (follicle-stimulating hormone). The diagnosis of ovarian failure as the cause of amenorrhea is confirmed by a plasma FSH greater than 40 mIU/ml.

Women with *chronic anovulation* fail to ovulate spontaneously but have the capability of ovulating with appropriate therapy. Estrogen production is adequate in some patients with chronic anovulation but is not secreted in a cyclic fashion. In others estrogen production is deficient.

Women who have adequate amounts of estrogen production and therefore demonstrate withdrawal bleeding after progesterone challenge usually have the syndrome of polycystic ovarian disease (see Fig. 118-7). Unusual causes of chronic anovulation associated with estrogen production include hormone-secreting ovarian and adrenal tumors. Women with deficient or absent estrogen production, and therefore with absence of withdrawal bleeding after progesterone treatment, usually have hypogonadotropic hypogonadism due either to organic or functional disorders of the pituitary or central nervous system such as brain tumors, pituitary tumors (especially prolactin-secreting adenomas), primary hypopituitarism, or the Sheehan syndrome.

PELVIC PAIN Pelvic pain may originate in the pelvis or be referred from some other region of the body. A pelvic source as the cause of such pain is often suggested by the history (for example, dysmenorrhea and dyspareunia) and physical findings, but a high index of suspicion must be entertained for extrapelvic disorders that refer to the pelvis, such as appendicitis, cholecystitis, intestinal obstruction, and urinary tract infections (see Chap. 5).

"Physiological" pelvic pain PAIN ASSOCIATED WITH OVULATION ("MITTELSCHMERZ") Many women experience low abdominal discomfort associated with ovulation, typically a dull aching pain at midcycle in one lower quadrant lasting from a few minutes to hours in length. It is rarely severe or incapacitating. The relationship of the pain to the mechanisms of ovulation is unknown. It may result from peritoneal irritation by follicular fluid released into the peritoneal cavity at the time of ovulation. The onset at midcycle and a short duration of pain are often diagnostic.

PREMENSTRUAL OR MENSTRUAL PAIN In normal ovulatory women somatic symptoms during the few days prior to menses may be insignificant in some and disabling in others. These symptoms include edema, breast engorgement, and abdominal bloating or discomfort. A functional symptom complex consisting of cyclic irritability, depression, and lethargy is known as the *premenstrual syndrome.* The cause of this syndrome is unknown, but it is thought to be prostaglandin-mediated.

Cramping of varying degrees of severity usually accompanies ovulatory menses in the absence of demonstrable disorders of the pelvis and if severe or incapacitating is termed *primary dysmenorrhea.*

Pelvic pain due to organic causes Severe dysmenorrhea associated with organic disease of the pelvis is termed *secondary dysmenorrhea.* Organic causes of pelvic pain can be classified as (1) uterine, (2) adnexal, (3) vulvar or vaginal, and (4) pregnancy-associated.

UTERINE PAIN Pain of uterine etiology is often chronic and continuous and is increased in intensity during menstruation and intercourse. Causes include leiomyomas of the uterus (particularly submucous and degenerating leiomyomas), adenomyosis, and cervical stenosis. Infections of the uterus associated with intrauterine manipulation following dilatation and curettage or intrauterine devices can also cause significant pelvic pain (see Chap. 118). Pelvic pain due to endometrial or cervical cancer is usually a late manifestation of disseminated disease (see Chap. 118).

ADNEXAL PAIN The most common cause of pain in the adnexae (fallopian tubes and ovaries) is infection (see Chap. 114). Acute salpingo-oophoritis presents as low abdominal pain, fever, and chills, beginning a few days after a menstrual period, and is most often a consequence of gonococcal disease with or without a superimposed nongonococcal pyogenic infection. Chronic pelvic inflammatory disease results from either a single episode or multiple episodes of infection and often presents as infertility associated with chronic pelvic pain that increases in intensity with menses and intercourse. On physical examination the adnexae are tender, and adnexal thickening with or without masses may be present. Pelvic inflammatory disease may become a surgical emergency if associated with peritonitis due to rupture of a tuboovarian abscess. Ovarian cysts or neoplasms may be sources of pelvic pain that becomes more severe with torsion or rupture of the mass, and ectopic pregnancy must also be considered in the differential diagnosis (see below). Endometriosis involving fallopian tubes, ovaries, or peritoneum may cause both chronic low abdominal pain and infertility, although the magnitude of tissue involvement does not always correlate with the severity of clinical symptoms. Pain associated with endometriosis typically increases with menstruation and, if the posterior ligaments of the uterus are involved, with intercourse.

VULVAR OR VAGINAL PAIN This is most often due to infectious vaginitis caused by organisms such as *Monilia, Trichomonas,* or *Hemophilus* and is often associated with vaginal discharge and pruritus. Herpetic vulvitis, condyloma acuminata, and cysts or abscesses of Bartholin's glands may also cause vulvar pain.

PREGNANCY-ASSOCIATED DISORDERS Pregnancy must be considered in the differential diagnosis of pelvic pain in all women during the reproductive years. Threatened abortion or incomplete abortion often presents with uterine cramping, bleeding, or passage of tissue following a period of amenorrhea. Ectopic pregnancy may be insidious in its presentation and can result in severe intraperitoneal hemorrhage and maternal death.

The evaluation of pelvic pain includes a careful history and pelvic examination. This often leads to the correct diagnosis and institution of appropriate treatment. If the pain is severe and the diagnosis is unclear, the workup should follow that outlined for the acute abdomen (Chap. 5). A culdocentesis is indicated if the diagnosis of ruptured ectopic pregnancy is suspected. If there is a question of an adnexal mass such as a tubal pregnancy or if the patient is so obese as to preclude a thorough pelvic examination, sonography may be helpful in the evaluation. Finally, diagnostic laparoscopy and laparotomy may be indicated in patients with severe or prolonged pain of undetermined etiologies.

SEXUAL DYSFUNCTION Many women consult physicians because of disturbances in sexual function. Some describe minor complaints related to the reproductive tract as a means of bringing sexual problems to the attention of the physician. On the other hand, sexual dysfunction may be attributed as the cause of low abdominal discomfort or dyspareunia when the actual etiology is some organic lesion. However, more and more women seek medical advice because of sexual problems that interface in their provenance between medicine and sociology.

The normal sexual response begins with sexual arousal which causes genital vasocongestion that results in vaginal lubrication in preparation for intromission. The lubrication is due to the formation of a transudate in the vagina and in conjunction with genital congestion produces the so-called orgasmic platform prior to orgasm. Sexual stimuli (visual, tactile, auditory, and olfactory) as well as healthy vaginal tissue are prerequisites for genital vasocongestion and vaginal lubrication. During the second stage of the sexual response a series of involuntary contractions of the pelvic skeletal muscles under control of the autonomic nervous system results in a pleasurable cortical sensory phenomenon known as orgasm. Direct or indirect stimulation of the clitoris is important in the production of the female orgasm.

In simple terms, sexual dysfunction can be due to interference with the arousal or orgasmic phases of the normal sexual response. Either type of disorder can be due to organic or functional disorder or both.

Illnesses that impair neurological function such as diabetes mellitus or multiple sclerosis may prevent normal sexual arousal. Local pelvic diseases such as vaginitis, endometriosis, and salpingo-oophoritis may preclude normal sexual response because of the resulting dyspareunia. Debilitating systemic diseases such as cancer and cardiovascular diseases may impair normal sexual response indirectly.

More commonly, failure of a normal sexual response is due to psychological problems that impair sexual arousal. Such problems include misinformation, for example, the perception of sexual satisfaction as bad or feelings of guilt about previous psychologically traumatic events such as incest, rape, or unwanted pregnancy. In addition, women who have had previous hysterectomy or mastectomy may perceive themselves as "incomplete." Many such stresses, for example, anxiety, depression, fatigue, and marital or interpersonal conflicts, may lead to failure of the vasocongestive response and prevent normal vaginal lubrication. Women with such experiences may be unable to achieve normal sexual response unless they receive professional counseling. These problems are approached by attempting to identify and reduce such stresses with the assistance of a physician, psychologist, psychiatrist, or sex therapist.

Failure to achieve orgasm is a specific form of sexual dysfunction. Many women enjoy sexual encounters to variable degrees without experiencing orgasm, particularly with a loving partner, because of the pleasure derived from closeness in a cherished relationship. However, for most women sexual relations with rare or absent orgasms are frustrating and unsatisfying. In many instances, failure of orgasm is due to insufficient clitoral stimulation and may be rectified by appropriate counseling and patient education.

A specific entity, "vaginismus," painful, involuntary con-

tractions of the musculature surrounding the entrance to the vagina, is a rare cause of dyspareunia. It is a conditioned response to a previous real or imagined frightening or traumatic sexual experience. Treatment is directed to elimination of the conditioned response by progressive vaginal dilation by the patient in conjunction with marital therapy.

REPRODUCTION Problems of infertility are discussed in detail in Chap. 118. The approach to infertile couples always involves evaluation of both the man and woman. The initial evaluation includes a thorough history and physical examination. The history should elicit information as to the frequency of intercourse, the sexual responses of both, the use of contraceptives or lubricants, previous or past medical illnesses, and all medications taken.

Male-associated factors account for half of all infertility problems. Therefore, one of the first procedures in the workup of infertile couples should be a semen analysis (see Chap. 117). The initial evaluation of the female includes documentation of normal ovulatory cycles. A history of regular, cyclic, predictable, spontaneous menses usually indicates ovulatory cycles. This may be confirmed by basal body temperature graphs, properly timed endometrial biopsies, or plasma progesterone levels during the luteal phase of the cycle. Also, the diagnosis of luteal-phase dysfunction can be determined by these methods. If the woman is anovulatory, attempts to induce ovulation can be undertaken by a variety of methods including clomiphene citrate, human menopausal gonadotropins, bromocryptine mesylate, or wedge resection of the ovaries (Chap. 118).

The most common cause of infertility in the female is tubal disease most often due to infection (pelvic inflammatory disease) or endometriosis. Tubal disease can be evaluated by obtaining a hysterosalpingogram or by diagnostic laparoscopy. The treatment of tubal causes of infertility is primarily surgical.

A cervical factor as a cause of infertility is evaluated by a properly timed postcoital examination. During this examination the sperm motility in cervical mucus is observed. Also, immunological etiologies for infertility may be present and can be tested for by a variety of laboratory tests. We are unable to account for a cause of infertility in 10 percent of couples.

The desire for fertility control or contraception is also a frequent cause for women to seek medical treatment or evaluation. The most widely used methods for fertility control include (1) rhythm and withdrawal techniques, (2) barrier methods, (3) intrauterine devices, (4) oral steroid contraceptives, (5) sterilization, and (6) abortion. A discussion of these methods and the possible complications of each is found in Chap. 118.

REFERENCES

FORDNEY DS: Dyspareunia and vaginismus. Clin Obstet Gynecol 21:205, 1978

HAMMOND MG, TALBERT LM: *Infertility.* Chapel Hill, Health Sciences Consortium Inc, 1981

HATCHER RA et al: *Contraceptive Technology 1980–1981.* New York, Irvington, 1980

MASTERS W, JOHNSON V: *Human Sexual Response.* Boston, Little, Brown, 1966

———: *Human Sexual Inadequacy.* Boston, Little, Brown, 1970

ROMNEY SL et al: *Gynecology and Obstetrics: The Health Care of Women.* New York, McGraw-Hill, 1980

SPEROFF L et al: *Clinical Gynecologic Endocrinology and Infertility,* 2d ed. Baltimore, Williams & Wilkins, 1978

46
DISTURBANCES OF SEXUAL AND REPRODUCTIVE FUNCTION IN MEN

PATRICK C. WALSH
JEAN D. WILSON

A coordinated sequence of physiological events (psychic, endocrine, vascular, and neurologic) controls normal sexual and reproductive function in men. In this chapter, the discussion is focused on the clinical presentation of sexual disorders in men. (Also see Chaps. 47, "Approach to the Patient with Sexual Complaints," and 117, "Diseases of the Testis.")

SEXUAL FUNCTION

NORMAL SEXUAL FUNCTION Simply stated, normal male sexual function can be divided into five events, each of which is under diverse regulation: libido, erection, ejaculation, orgasm, and detumescence.

The first, sexual desire or libido, is regulated by poorly understood psychic factors and by testicular androgens. Castration produces a decline in libido that can be restored by treatment with testosterone.

The second phase, erection, is primarily a neurologic event that results in modification of the vascular supply to the penis, causing it to become engorged with blood. The neurologic aspect of erection is controlled by both reflex and psychic stimuli. The sensory portion begins with fibers that originate in pacinian corpuscles of the penis and pass via the pudendal nerve to the S2–S4 dorsal root ganglia. The efferent limb begins with parasympathetic preganglionic fibers from S2–S4 which synapse in the perivesicular, prostatic, and cavernous plexuses. From there, postganglionic fibers pass to blood vessels of the corpora cavernosa. Efferent fibers from S3–S4 also travel in the pudendal nerve to the ischiocavernosus and bulbocavernosus muscles. Sympathetic innervation of the male genitalia originates in fibers from the lateral columns of T12 and L1, the so-called thoracolumbar erection center, that synapse in the pelvic and perivesicular plexuses. Postganglionic fibers innervate the smooth muscle of the vas deferens, seminal vesicle, and internal sphincter of the bladder. Sympathetic innervation can act synergistically with the sacral parasympathetics to mediate erection initiated by psychic stimuli but is not mandatory for erection, because most patients have normal potency after bilateral complete sympathectomy. The central nervous system modulates erectile response via pathways thought to descend in the lateral columns of the spinal cord. The effect of the central nervous system on erection can either be stimulatory or inhibitory, thus the importance of psychic factors for erection.

While erection is primarily controlled by the parasympathetic nervous system, the transformation of the penis from a flaccid to an erect state is a vascular phenomenon. Blood reaches the penis via terminal branches of the right and left internal pudendal arteries. The erectile tissue of the penis consists of two corpora cavernosa lying side by side on the dorsal aspect of the penis and the corpus spongiosum that surrounds the urethra. This erectile tissue consists of an irregular spongelike system of vascular spaces interspersed between arteries and veins. Erection is produced by the shunting of arterial blood into the cavernous spaces through arteriovenous anastomoses. The mechanisms responsible (e.g., increased arterial inflow, opening of arteriovenous connections, etc.) are uncertain. Furthermore, it is not clear whether venous valves impede flow and thus further promote erection. Passive venous obstruction undoubtedly occurs.

The third phase, ejaculation, is under control of the sympathetic nervous system and consists of two processes, seminal emission and true ejaculation. Emission results from the contraction of the vas deferens, prostate, and seminal vesicles which causes seminal fluid to enter the urethra. True ejaculation results from contraction of the muscles of the pelvic floor including the bulbocavernosus and ischiocavernosus muscles. Retrograde ejaculation into the bladder is prevented by partial bladder neck closure mediated by the sympathetic nerves.

The fourth phase, orgasm, is a cortical sensory phenomenon in which the rhythmic contraction of the bulbocavernosus and ischiocavernosus muscles is perceived as pleasurable. It is purely psychic. The fact that orgasm can occur without either erection, ejaculation, or bladder neck closure explains why some drugs that prevent erection or ejaculation do not interfere with orgasm.

Detumescence after orgasm and ejaculation may be the result of vasoconstriction of the arterioles supplying blood to the erectile tissue, thus allowing venous drainage to empty the sinuses and the penis to become flaccid. Following orgasm, there is a refractory period that varies with age, physical condition, and psychic factors during which erection and ejaculation are inhibited.

IMPOTENCE Male sexual dysfunction, often termed *impotence,* may be manifested in various ways: loss of desire, inability to obtain or maintain an erection, premature ejaculation, absence of emission, inability to achieve orgasm. Many subjects complain of more than one abnormality simultaneously. These complaints can be secondary to other chronic or debilitating diseases, the consequence of specific disorders of the urogenital or endocrine systems, or the result of psychiatric disturbance. It is mandatory in all instances to exclude organic (and in some instances potentially correctable or treatable) causes.

Loss of desire Because androgens have a major influence on sexual desire in men, a decrease in libido may indicate androgen deficiency arising from either pituitary or testicular disease. This possibility can be tested by the measurement of plasma testosterone and gonadotropins. However, since the testosterone required to maintain libido is usually less than the amount necessary for full stimulation of the prostate and seminal vesicles, absence of emission also occurs when the loss of libido is due to hypogonadism. Conversely, if the semen volume is normal, it is unlikely that endocrine factors are responsible for their sexual dysfunction.

Loss of erection The organic causes of erectile impotence can be grouped into endocrine, drug, local, neurologic, and vascular causes (Table 46-1).

Endocrine causes of testicular failure that result in impotence usually cause such profound changes that the disorders are not difficult to recognize (Chap. 117). However, hyperprolactinemia may cause impotence in some patients with pituitary tumors and may not be obvious on physical examination (see Chaps. 109 and 119); hyperprolactinemia suppresses LHRH (luteinizing hormone–releasing hormone) production, resulting in plasma gonadotropins and testosterone values in the low normal range. Bromocriptine mesylate, a dopamine agonist, may lower prolactin levels and reverse impotence in such patients.

Many drugs cause impotence including antihistamines, antihypertensives, anticholinergics, psychogenic agents, and drugs of habituation or addiction. The usual explanation is neurologic blockade, and this may well be the case for those drugs with peripheral parasympatholytic actions such as the tricyclic antidepressants. Others may act by enhancing prolactin secretion. It is not clear whether impotence caused by drugs of addiction such as alcohol, methadone, and heroin is due to reduced testosterone levels or the general condition of the patient.

Penile diseases that cause impotence can almost always be diagnosed by history and physical examination and include previous priapism, penile trauma, and Peyronie's disease.

Many types of neurologic disorders can cause impotence including lesions in the anterior temporal lobe, spinal cord disorders, insufficiency of sensory input as can occur in diabetic neuropathy and tabes dorsalis, or damage to parasympathetic nerves, for example, following surgical procedures such as total prostatectomy. (Transurethral prostatectomy, in contrast, probably does not cause organic impotence.) If spinal cord injury is above the thoracolumbar region, reflex erections may occur. Diffuse injury of the spinal cord results in total impotence. Diabetes mellitus deserves special comment. As many as half of diabetic men develop impotence within 6 years of the onset of diabetes, and impotence may be the first clinical manifestation of diabetic neuropathy. However, when a careful neurologic examination is performed including measurement of the cystometrogram, other evidences of neurologic disturbance are usually uncovered. Many of the other polyneuropathies described in Chap. 368 have similar effects.

Vascular insufficiency causes impotence because blood flow into the vascular network of the penis is insufficient to obtain (or maintain) the erect state. The prototype of impaired penile blood supply is the Leriche syndrome. Here impedance to the

TABLE 46-1
Some organic causes of erectile impotence in men

I Endocrine causes
- *A* Testicular failure (primary or secondary)
- *B* Hyperprolactinemia

II Drugs
- *A* Antihistamines
  - *1* Cimetidine
  - *2* Diphenhydramine
  - *3* Hydroxyzine
- *B* Antihypertensives
  - *1* Clonidine
  - *2* Methyldopa
  - *3* Propranolol
  - *4* Reserpine
  - *5* Spironolactone
  - *6* Thiazides
- *C* Anticholinergics
- *D* Antidepressants
  - *1* Amitriptyline
  - *2* Doxepin
  - *3* Isocarboxazid
- *E* Antipsychotics
  - *1* Chlorpromazine
  - *2* Haloperidol
  - *3* Thioridazine
- *F* Tranquilizers
  - *1* Diazepam
  - *2* Barbiturates
  - *3* Chlordiazepoxide
- *G* Drugs of habituation or addiction
  - *1* Alcohol
  - *2* Methadone
  - *3* Heroin

III Penile diseases
- *A* Previous priapism
- *B* Penile trauma
- *C* Peyronie's disease

IV Neurologic diseases
- *A* Anterior temporal lobe lesions
- *B* Diseases of the spinal cord
- *C* Loss of sensory input
  - *1* Diabetes mellitus and various polyneuropathies
  - *2* Tabes dorsalis
  - *3* Disease of dorsal root ganglia
- *D* Disease of nervi erigentes
  - *1* Complete prostatectomy
  - *2* Rectosigmoid operations
  - *3* Aortic bypass surgery

V Vascular disease
- *A* Leriche syndrome

blood flow into the penis occurs as the result of obstruction of the distal aorta at the bifurcation of the common iliacs. This usually presents as claudication and impotence; either can occur separately. Likewise, occlusion in smaller vessels supplying the penis can also lead to impotence. Decreased blood flow to the penis may be detected using the Doppler technique. By dividing the penile systolic blood pressure by the simultaneously determined supine brachial systolic pressure, the penile/brachial index is obtained. An index of over 0.75 is normal, and one of less than 0.6 is suggestive of vasculogenic impotence. An index of 0.6 to 0.75 is indeterminate. Due to overlap of such abnormal results with those in older potent men it is not possible to be certain that arterial insufficiency is the cause of impotence in a given individual. Normal values exclude arterial insufficiency; abnormal values require confirmatory arteriography.

Premature ejaculation This disorder seldom has an organic cause. It is usually related to anxiety in the sexual situation, unreasonable expectations about performance, or an emotional disorder. A variety of successful therapeutic modalities have been described by Levine.

Absence of emission This symptom may be produced by (1) retrograde ejaculation, (2) sympathetic denervation, (3) androgen deficiency, or (4) drugs. Retrograde ejaculation may occur following surgery on the bladder neck or may develop spontaneously in diabetic men. Demonstration of sperm in a postcoital urine specimen will establish the diagnosis. Following sympathectomy or occasionally after extensive retroperitoneal surgery, the autonomic innervation of the prostate and seminal vesicles is lost, resulting in absence of smooth-muscle contraction at the time of ejaculation. Androgen deficiency results in a decrease in secretions of the prostate and seminal vesicles and results in a diminution of the volume of ejaculate. Finally, drugs such as guanethidine, phenoxybenzamine, and phentolamine primarily impair ejaculation rather than erection or libido.

Absence of orgasm If libido and erectile function are normal, the absence of orgasm is almost always due to a psychiatric disorder.

Failure of detumescence Priapism is a persistent painful erection, often totally unrelated to sexual activity. The etiology of priapism is usually idiopathic, but the disorder can be associated with sickle cell anemia, chronic granulocytic leukemia, or spinal cord injury. The disorder is thought to be secondary to clotting within the penile vascular network. The persistent erection disrupts the network and can lead to fibrosis and subsequent erectile impotence.

Evaluation of impotence The commonest cause of prolonged impotence is an anxiety or depression state. These closely related conditions can be diagnosed by the criteria enunciated in Chap. 11. Other psychologic factors such as disinterest in the sexual partner, fear of sexual incompetence, marital discord, deviant sexual attitudes, worry, fatigue, and ill health often operate in various combinations to reduce sexual impulse. The central issue in the evaluation of impotence is to separate those instances due to psychologic factors from those due to organic causes (Table 46-1). Usually, the separation can be made on the basis of history. From early childhood through the eighth decade, erections occur during normal sleep. This phenomenon, termed *nocturnal penile tumescence* (NPT), occurs during rapid eye movement sleep, and the total time of NPT averages 100 min per night. Consequently, if the impotent man gives a history of turgid erections under any circumstances (often when awakening in the early morning), the psychic, efferent neurologic, and circulatory systems that mediate erection are intact, and dysfunction is probably due to a psychiatric disorder. In these patients the physical and laboratory examinations should be limited. (Occasional patients with sensory neuropathy may have nocturnal erections.)

If the history of nocturnal erections is questionable, measurements of NPT can be made with the use of a strain gauge attached to a recorder. Alternatively, the penis can be wrapped with gummed, perforated paper; failure to break the perforations on three successive nights indicates absence of nocturnal erections. Although false-negatives due to REM sleep deprivation are possible, these procedures usually differentiate psychogenic and organic impotence. Interestingly, psychogenically impotent men may experience longer and more frequent nocturnal erections than do normal men. Other factors in favor of organic impotence include a similar degree of erectile dysfunction under all circumstances, onset not associated with any particular psychiatric symptomatology, a previous uninterrupted period of normal erectile function, and persistent sexual desire.

Having deduced an organic cause, the fundamental problem is the differential diagnosis of the etiology (Table 46-1). The patient's history should be probed for symptoms of diabetes, symptoms of peripheral neuropathy of bladder dysfunction, symptoms referable to the vascular system such as intermittent claudication, and symptoms of local disease such as a history of priapism. A thorough drug history should be obtained, and inquiry concerning past operations that may have produced neurologic damage should be made.

Physical examination should include a thorough genital examination to identify abnormalities of the penis. The testes should be palpated for size and abnormal masses; if the length is less than 4 cm, hypogonadism should be considered. Evidence of feminization such as gynecomastia and abnormal body hair distribution should be sought. All pulses should be palpated, including the penile pulse, which can be felt by pressing both corpora between the thumb and forefinger and palpating to either side of the midline. However, because only a portion of the superficial dorsal arteries reach the corpus cavernosum, normal dorsal pulse pressures do not exclude the presence of deep cavernous arterial occlusion. If there is an indication from either history or physical examination of a vascular etiology, a Doppler procedure or arteriography may be indicated.

The neurologic exam should measure anal sphincter tone, perineal sensation, and the bulbocavernosus reflex. This reflex is obtained by squeezing the glans penis and noting the degree of anal sphincter constriction. An examination for peripheral neuropathy, including distal muscle weakness, loss of tendon reflexes in the legs, and tests for impairment of vibratory, position, tactile, and pain sensation should also be performed (see Chap. 368). In the absence of a concomitant neurogenic bladder, electromyographic sacral signal tracing of the bulbocavernosus reflex may be a useful ancillary procedure for detection of localized peripheral neuropathy; the methodology involves measurement of bulbocavernosus response latencies following electrical stimulation of the glans. Although this procedure has not been studied exhaustively, improvement by revascularization surgery is unlikely if the test is abnormal.

Laboratory evaluation is probably of minimal value. Measurement of serum testosterone in the absence of evidence of feminization or hypogonadism is seldom helpful.

Treatment of impotence Medical therapy with androgens offers little more than placebo benefit except in hypogonadal men. If a prolactin-secreting pituitary tumor is present, however, either surgical removal or treatment with bromocriptine mesylate usually results in return of potency. Surgical therapy may be useful in the treatment of decreased potency related to aortic obstruction; however, potency can be lost rather than improved after aortic operation if the autonomic nerve supply to the penis is damaged. This complication is minimized if an endarterectomy is done or, in a grafting procedure, if the reconstruction of the distal end is performed above the origin of the external iliac arteries. Early surgical relief of priapism by shunting procedures, such as corpora spongiosum shunting, might prevent subsequent impotence.

In some centers a useful surgical technique for improvement of potency in refractory patients such as individuals with diabetic neuropathy is the implantation of a penile prosthesis, namely the insertion within the corpora of a small, blunt silastic rod. The patient must be made aware that full erection is not produced and that the device only prevents buckling during intercourse. Furthermore, the complication rate is high in some series. Alternatively, an inflatable prosthetic device has been devised for implantation on either side of the corpora. A connecting reservoir of material is placed in the perivesicular space and pumps are located in the scrotum. By means of these pumps the penis can be made to become nearly fully erect at the appropriate time and to relax after intercourse.

In the larger group of anxiety states and depressive illnesses measures directed at their alleviation may restore sexual potency, and sexual counseling, education, and psychotherapy are beneficial in alleviating psychogenic factors.

REPRODUCTION

Approximately a tenth of marriages in the United States are barren, and another tenth result in fewer children than desired. The husband is the cause of the infertility in about a third of these marriages.

Infertility can either be due to disorders of the hypothalamic-pituitary system, disorders of the testes, or abnormalities of the ejaculatory system (Table 117-1). When obtaining a history, the physician should collect information about the duration of infertility, fertility in prior marriages of both the husband and wife, the presence of acquired or congenital disease that may lead to infertility, technique and frequency of intercourse, and family history of infertility. To exclude the presence of gross abnormalities of the endocrine system the physical examination should evaluate the distribution of body hair, the presence of gynecomastia, the development of the scrotum and penis, the location of the urethral meatus, and the presence of normal vasa deferentia and epididymides. The size of each testis should be estimated with care. Because the seminiferous tubules account for more than 75 percent of the testicular mass, a reduction in testicular size (less than 4 cm in length) indicates a severe deficiency in the spermatogenic function of the testis. Finally, with the patient standing in the upright position, the Valsalva maneuver should be utilized to test for the presence of a varicocele.

The next step in the evaluation of the male partner is the semen analysis. This provides a semiquantitative estimation of the severity of the dysfunction. The findings are usually considered normal if the semen coagulates and then liquefies, the volume is 2 to 5 ml, the sperm count is greater than 20 million per milliliter, more than 60 percent of the sperm are actively motile, and more than 60 percent have normal morphology. If no sperm are present, the term *azoospermia* is used; if sperm are present but the count is less than 20 million per milliliter, the patient is considered to have *oligospermia.* In the azoospermic man with normal-sized testes, the differential diagnosis includes hyalinization of the seminiferous tubules, Sertoli cell-only syndrome, gonadotropin deficiency, ductal obstruction, and maturation arrest. Plasma testosterone and serum LH (luteinizing hormone) and FSH (follicle-stimulating hormone) measurements are helpful in separating these conditions. In patients with hyalinization of the seminiferous tubules LH and FSH are elevated and plasma testosterone is low or borderline normal. Patients with Sertoli cell-only syndrome usually have normal LH and testosterone levels, but FSH levels are characteristically elevated. In gonadotropin deficiency LH, FSH, and testosterone are low, and in ductal obstruction or maturation arrest all studies are normal. To differentiate between the last two disorders, a testicular biopsy is necessary. In oligospermic patients, if the history and physical examination are normal, it is unlikely that any further laboratory investigation will be useful in defining the etiology. These patients are usually classified in the large group termed *idiopathic oligospermia.*

REFERENCES

Impotence

BARRY JM et al: Nocturnal penile tumescence monitoring with stamps. Urology 15:171, 1980

BENSON GS: Mechanisms of penile erection. Invest Urol 19:65, 1981

——— et al: Neuromorphology and neuropharmacology of the human penis. An *in vitro* study. J Clin Invest 65:506, 1980

COLE NJ: Drugs that influence sexual expression. Consultant 20:3281, 1980

DAVIDSON JM et al: Effects of androgen on sexual behavior in hypogonadal men. J Clin Endocrinol 48:955, 1979

FURLOW WL: Surgical management of impotence using the inflatable penile prosthesis: Experience with 103 patients. Br J Urol 50:114, 1977

——— (ed): Male sexual dysfunction. Urol Clin N Am 8:1, 1981

GERSTENBERGER DL: Inflatable penile prosthesis. Followup study of patient-partner satisfaction. Urology 14:583, 1979

LEVINE SB: Marital sexual dysfunction: Ejaculation disturbances. Ann Intern Med 84:575, 1976

NATH RL et al: The multidisciplinary approach to vasculogenic impotence. Surgery 89:124, 1981

NEWMAN HF et al: Mechanism of human penile erection: An overview. Urology 17:399, 1981

SPARK RF et al: Impotence is not always psychogenic. JAMA 243:750, 1980

WINTER CC: Priapism. Urol Surv 28:163, 1978

Infertility

AMELAR RD et al: *Male Infertility.* Philadelphia, Saunders, 1977, p 153

GREENBERG SH et al: Experience with 425 subfertile male patients. J Urol 119:507, 1970

SHERINS RJ et al: Male infertility, in *Campbell's Urology,* 4th ed, JH Harrison et al (eds). Philadelphia, Saunders, 1978, vol 1, chap 21, p 715

47 APPROACH TO THE PATIENT WITH SEXUAL COMPLAINTS

PETER REICH

The part of the medical evaluation concerned with the assessment of sexual function is frequently handled awkwardly by the patient and by the physician. The patient may be inhibited from describing important sexual complaints by shyness, embarrassment, guilt, shame, anxiety, or feelings of inadequacy; the physician in turn may inadvertently discourage the patient from bringing up sexual concerns by subtle indications of discomfort, disapproval, or embarrassment or by failing to ask appropriate questions.

An objective approach to sexual issues reduces tensions and enables both patient and physician to deal with sensitive material. A physician does not need to be a psychotherapist or an expert on sexual behavior to be helpful. Patients who seek sexual advice from physicians are likely to be concerned about medical issues. Often sexual problems reflect fears and misconceptions, and the objective evaluation of the symptoms may lead to relief without further treatment. Alternatively, sexual symptoms may be the first manifestations of organic disorders, and a change in sexual function at any time of life is an indication for a thorough medical evaluation. The responsibility of the physician is to establish an accurate and complete diagnosis including both physiologic and psychologic factors, to evaluate the significance of the problem in the context of the patient's background and life-style, and to be familiar with the various modes of therapy available.

Despite its importance to the overall sense of well-being, physicians frequently fail to ask patients about sexual function, even as part of a general medical evaluation or when medical problems relate directly or indirectly to the sex life. Physicians avoid the subject because of concerns over their own competency to deal with sexual problems, concerns about embarrassing or disturbing the patients, and fears of starting an emotionally charged discussion with insufficient time to resolve it. In truth most physicians are competent to make an initial assessment of sexual symptoms. One study of a primary care clinic population showed that most patients felt that questions about their sexuality were appropriate to a medical workup and indicated that the physician was thorough and humane in asking such questions. Even when sexual complaints were revealed, it rarely took more than a few minutes to discuss them.

The present day openness about sexuality in the media does not necessarily mean, however, that individual patients are better educated on sexual matters or more willing to initiate discussions of sexual complaints. Physicians who inquire about sexuality routinely find that as many as a third of patients have sexual concerns and problems, many of which arise from misconceptions and respond to an educational approach.

Most medical schools now include courses on sexuality in the undergraduate curricula, and postgraduate courses and journal articles on the medical aspects of sexuality are now widely available. In addition to a basic knowledge of sexual anatomy, urogenital physiology, and sexual behavior, the physician needs to know the effects of illnesses, operative procedures, and medications upon sexual function.

THE GENERAL APPROACH TO THE PATIENT More often than in other areas of medicine, the physician needs to take an active role in initiating the discussion of sexual matters. The inclusion of routine screening questions in the review of systems is one way to ensure that the area is not overlooked. Sexuality can be brought up comfortably after questions about menstrual function in women or questions about urinary function in men. Some clinicians prefer linking questions about sexual function to inquiries about relationships and personal satisfactions. To be effective, screening questions should be nonspecific, should not assume that the patient is heterosexual, and should project a nonjudgmental attitude. One approach is to ask, "Are you sexually active?" The next question can be whether there are any physical problems associated with sexual activity and whether the sexual activities are satisfying or disappointing. The physician can also simply ask whether the patient has problems with sexual function. Even when patients respond with a hurried negative, follow-up questions about specific problems such as pain, difficulty in maintaining an erection, or inability to reach orgasm may elicit a sexual complaint nevertheless. Screening questions vary with the age and the circumstances of the patient, but such questions should be routine. Otherwise, the physician may overlook problems, may return to the subject as an afterthought, or may experience tension or show embarrassment when trying to think of a screening question during the history.

When a sexual complaint is elicited or volunteered, a detailed history of the manifestations and associated symptoms should be obtained. The assessment of a sexual problem is similar to the assessment of a problem involving any other system. The history of a sexual complaint necessarily includes information about relationships with partners; tensions, anxieties, preconceptions, attitudes, and interpersonal factors must be taken into account. A complete history that includes careful attention to multiple determinants, a thorough evaluation of the patient as a person, and a consideration of the context of the symptoms usually yields a working diagnosis that enables the physician either to treat the patient or to make an appropriate referral. A detailed guide to the assessment of sexual function has been published by the Group for Advancement of Psychiatry. Similar guides can be found in standard texts of psychiatry and of obstetrics and gynecology. It is useful to have such a framework in mind when obtaining a sexual history.

The physician has the special responsibility of initiating a discussion of sexuality when coexisting medical problems are likely to affect sexual function. Patients may fear sexual activity after myocardial infarction or episodes of cardiac arrhythmia or may anticipate loss of sexual function after transurethral prostatectomy, hysterectomy, or other procedures or conditions involving the urogenital tract. Other disorders affect sexuality directly or indirectly through loss of libido or changes in body image (Chaps. 45 and 46). By anticipating sexual problems the physician can help the patient make adjustments and can sometimes prevent disorders that are secondary to fears or misconceptions. Even when the patient initiates the discussion, an active inquiry by the physician enables the patient to discuss specific and intimate details.

Reassurances about confidentiality may be necessary during the discussion of sexual matters even though such confidentiality is ordinarily assumed in the doctor-patient relationship. The assurance of confidentiality is especially important when the physician also treats other members of the family or when the patient needs to discuss extramarital, deviant, or extralegal behavior.

The dignity of the patient should be kept in mind as the history is taken by observing such simple practices as using scientific words for sexual parts and sexual activities. Vernacular or slang expressions, which are sometimes used in a mistaken effort to put the patient at ease, and jokes or other informal remarks should be avoided even with a patient who uses them. Comments that may seem casual to the physician tend to live on in the patient's mind.

While inquiry into sexual matters requires tact and timing, the need to protect the patient from embarrassment should not be overemphasized. Anticipation of discomfort may lead physicians to choose an evasive route of inquiry while patients might appreciate a direct question. Alternatively, some patients allude to sexual problems indirectly with idiomatic phrases, such as "changing nature" or "problems in relationships"; unless the physician is sensitive to feelings and language the reference may be missed, and the patient may assume that the physician is not interested in further information. Sometimes sexual problems appear indirectly through other complaints relating to the urogenital system.

Two types of patients—the elderly and the homosexual—present special problems in regard to the evaluation of sexual function. The sexual problems of elderly patients are not well understood by most physicians. Physicians may refrain from asking questions because they incorrectly assume that sexual satisfactions can no longer be achieved because of the aging process. Alternatively, patients silently accept a loss of sexual function because of misconceptions about the effects of illness or of aging. Depression may be a factor in such instances. Here the questions of the physician, coupled with some reassuring statements about the tendencies of many persons to assume mistakenly they will never be able to enjoy sexual relations again, bring the issue into the open and awaken new hopes in the patient.

Homosexual patients with disorders of sexual function often do not receive sympathetic medical care from heterosexual physicians. Indeed, physicians share with the public at large serious misconceptions about homosexual behavior. In one study of gynecologic care for lesbians a major hindrance in communication was the assumption by physicians that all patients are heterosexual; this unwarranted assumption caused a reluctance on the part of the women to ask questions related to sexuality, and 40 percent of the women believed their health care would be affected adversely if the physicians knew they were lesbians. Homosexual men have similar problems in relating to heterosexual physicians. Some homosexual patients prefer going to homosexual physicians or to clinics run by homophile organizations.

EVALUATION Once a sexual complaint has been elicited, it is important to obtain a detailed history of specific behavior. Terms for sexual disorders may be misused, exaggerated, or misunderstood by patients. Other sexual complaints reflect misconceptions, ignorance, or fears, and the problems prove to be nonexistent when the behavior is explored in detail. Patients may overestimate or underestimate the extent of a problem, depending upon their psychologic orientation. For example, one woman believed herself to be frigid because her sexual partner, for neurotic reasons of his own, compared her in a disparaging way to his previous partners. Much can be learned from the first instance of a sexual problem, from the pattern of behavior after the onset of symptoms, and from inquiring whether the problem is present consistently or varies with the circumstances or nature of the sexual practice.

In every disorder there is a complex interaction between the physical and the emotional, and every sexual symptom needs to be evaluated in the context of the relationships between the patient and the sexual partners and in the context of the sexual practices and attitudes of the patient. A past history, including early experiences, attitudes of parents, and attitudes toward childhood sexuality, development, marriage, and pregnancy may be relevant. Establishing the relationship of sexual function to general health is of fundamental importance, and it is essential to take a complete drug history on every patient, both in regard to drug abuse and to use of prescribed drugs.

An understanding of the daily habits of a patient may provide important clues to diagnosis. Fatigue, anxiety, and stress, as well as the timing of the use of alcohol, drugs, and medications, can provide insight into the underlying cause. In addition, traumatic events, such as automobile accidents, surgical procedures, or the illness or death of another person, may exert acute or chronic effects on sexual behavior.

A general physical examination with special attention to an examination of the genitalia is essential in the evaluation. At times patients conceal or are unaware of abnormalities of the genitalia. On the other hand, otherwise sophisticated patients may harbor irrational misconceptions or feelings of shame about their bodies and may require concrete reassurance about the adequacy of the genital apparatus. Even if the diagnosis is that of a psychogenic basis for the sexual dysfunction, the patient may disregard assurances that there is no organic basis unless the workup for possible medical causes of the complaint has been thorough.

Appropriate laboratory tests to screen for systemic illnesses together with the specific test for various endocrinopathies, neurologic conditions, and other systemic disorders that may present with sexual problems may be indicated (see Chaps. 45 and 46). Attention to the mental status, including assessment of mood, affect, thought content, judgment, and reality testing, enables the physician to determine whether the sexual symptom is an aspect of a mental disorder. Rarely, sexual problems, especially loss of libido, may be the presenting sign of a disorder of the central nervous system; an examination of mental status can reveal early signs of dementia or other manifestations of organic brain conditions.

DIAGNOSTIC CONSIDERATIONS Specific disorders of sexual function are discussed in Chaps. 45 and 46. All of them can vary in severity, from complete loss of function under all circumstances to relatively minor disturbances in specific circumstances or with specific partners. Patients also may vary in their reactions to sexual symptoms, some ignoring or concealing severe disability, others reacting with panic about minor disturbances.

The first consideration is whether the condition is primarily organic or psychogenic. In clinics devoted to sexual counseling, the complaints of 10 to 20 percent of the patients are manifestations of organic problems, while the complaints of the remaining 80 to 90 percent are psychogenic in origin. When significant organic factors are present, a useful distinction can be made between sexual symptoms that arise *directly* from organic disorders, such as structural disorders of the urogenital system, neurologic disorders affecting the innervation of the sexual organs, and endocrinopathies that influence sexual physiology, and those that are *secondary* to changes in general health, such as sexual disturbances associated with rheumatoid arthritis, malignancies, renal failure, and other chronic diseases, or those that occur with acute debilitating conditions, such as myocardial infarction, major surgery, and hepatitis. Patients with primary organic disorders may need counseling to help them adjust to permanent losses of sexual function if medical measures cannot reverse the process. When sexual disturbances are secondary to changes in health, the effects of organic factors are often overemphasized by both the patient and the physician. Although libido may be affected adversely by a general loss of vitality and by toxic and metabolic factors, the sexual disturbances associated with physical illnesses are often the expression of hopelessness, depression, or anxiety and may be perpetuated by psychologic factors long after the organic problems have disappeared.

The physician can also make useful diagnostic distinctions as to the cause of psychogenic sexual disturbances. *Primary* psychogenic disturbances, those that have been present since puberty, can be distinguished from *secondary* disturbances, those that represent decompensations from previous adequate levels of function. The former often reflect chronic and deep-seated sexual conflicts. When a patient seeks help for a chronic disturbance, the key diagnostic issue may be why help has been sought at this particular time. A secondary decompensation may be the presenting symptom of a psychologic defeat or a disturbance in a relationship. Some sexual problems occur in connection with life stresses or transitions, such as retirement, pregnancy, work crises, or bereavement. The prognosis is good providing that the underlying issues are recognized and acknowledged. A disproportionate focus on sexual symptoms can actually perpetuate the problem by reinforcing anxiety about sexual performance.

Some sexual disorders are manifestations of major mental disorders and respond only to treatment directed at the mental disorders themselves. Diminished sexual responsiveness, impotence, or ejaculatory disturbances may be indications of depression. Bizarre sexual complaints with increased or diminished sexual activity can indicate incipient psychosis. The strange qualities of the symptoms or the intensity of the associated feelings may be the best diagnostic clue to the presence of a psychosis. Hypersexuality can also occur with the onset of mania or as a manifestation of depression, especially in postmenopausal women. Neuroses are often associated with sexual inhibitions.

Alcohol may play a significant role in impairment of potency. Often the first episode of secondary impotence is associated with the use of alcohol, and the midlife depressive syndrome that is often related to secondary impotence may be further complicated by alcohol abuse. Barbiturates and opiates also can cause reduced libido and impotence. Antihypertensive agents, tranquilizers, hypnotics, analgesics, and sedatives may also impair sexual function, particularly in the male.

Sexual disturbances may develop after traumatic incidents. For example, impotence can develop after cystoscopic examination or after vasectomy, even though neither procedure has any direct physiologic effect upon sexual function. An automobile accident, pregnancy, contraceptive difficulties, casual but disturbing sexual encounters, and a host of other emotionally significant episodes may cause sudden changes in sexual functioning. The patient may not be aware of the importance of such episodes or may be reluctant to discuss them. The diligent physician may inadvertently overdiagnose sexual disturbances. Most patients have self-doubts and sexual dissatisfactions even though they are functioning adequately. It is well to have in mind the concept of a threshold of disturbance to separate the normal vicissitudes from problems that require treatment.

TREATMENT Some sexual problems resolve spontaneously during the evaluation process, especially during an extensive workup. With those problems that persist, the physician must decide whether to treat the patients or to refer them elsewhere. The management of sexual dysfunction due to organic causes is described in Chaps. 45, 46, 117, and 118; sexual problems related to such physical illnesses are appropriately handled by the same physician who treats the physical disorder. A decision as to the best means of managing that large group in which the primary cause is psychogenic requires careful thought. Often a brief attempt at office counseling enables the physician to make this decision. Generally, the secondary or reactive psychogenic disorders are most amenable to brief counseling, especially when they occur in response to stress. Patients with more deep-seated problems may best be handled by psychiatrists.

The technique for counseling by the family physician cannot be mapped in a formal way. Sufficient time, a relaxed atmosphere, and genuine interest by the physician are necessary. The patient should be encouraged to tell the full story with careful attention to the circumstances surrounding the onset of symptoms, to the attitudes of the patient and partner, to the nature of the patient's relationships, and to factors that might lead to anxiety or depression. Although it may be necessary to review the physical details of the sexual practices, resolution of symptoms may occur with only indirect reference to sexual techniques. Sexual inadequacies often produce anxiety, which in turn leads to further defeats and to inhibition of libido. Without reduction of anxiety and lifting of depression, the process cannot be reversed.

Some physicians choose not to attempt sexual counseling, while others find it a satisfying aspect of medical practice. In either case, it is important for physicians to be familiar with the resources in their communities and to understand the capabilities and limitations of various treatment approaches. Physicians who do not undertake sexual counseling themselves usually have referral relationships with gynecologists, urologists, and psychiatrists. In addition, many communities now have family services and counseling services. Referral should be tailored to the nature of the problems and to the life-style and personality of the patient. Some patients prefer to discuss the intimate details of a sexual problem only with a gynecologist or urologist. Others should be directed to a reputable clinic where direct behavioral approaches to the treatment of sexual dysfunctions are available.

Referral is often a difficult transition for a patient because it implies turning to a stranger after having confided in a physician who has understood the problem. A previously eager patient may lose motivation when referred elsewhere. Some physicians have counselors associated with them in their offices. This system has the advantage of maintaining the personal relationship between counselors and physicians but has the disadvantage of encouraging physicians to rely on counselors for the evaluation of emotional problems rather than carrying through the diagnostic phase themselves. If physicians keep in touch with patients through the process of therapy, it enables them to evaluate the efficacy of the treatment program and to provide support and reassurance.

A few examples will illustrate some of the principles involved in the treatment of patients with sexual disorders.

A.R., a 56-year-old attorney who had recently suffered a myocardial infarct, complained to his physician of loss of libido. He was an energetic, competitive, aggressive self-made man, who enjoyed athletics and was "top man" in his firm. The physician asked him about the details of his daily life and found that the loss of libido was only one of many inhibitions. He avoided arguments, stopped playing handball, reduced his work load, lost weight, and developed insomnia and anorexia. Further questioning revealed fears of sudden death and the fatalistic belief that his days were numbered. He assumed that strict reduction of activity was mandatory. His wife shared his fears and urged him to avoid stress. Together they had decided not to have sexual relations during the period immediately after his heart attack, and he had no desire to resume. In the course of several sessions of counseling the physician reassured him that his fears were exaggerated and that many patients with heart trouble experienced similar feelings, clarified the extent of his disability, and helped him and his wife to plan realistic resumption of many of his previous activities, including sexual relations.

L.D., a 26-year-old woman, consulted a physician because of frigidity. She had left her husband after 6 years of an unfulfilling marriage and had sought satisfaction in a series of brief affairs. The interview revealed her to be a restless, competitive, chronically dissatisfied person who was unhappy in her career and who experienced disappointment in close relationships. After careful evaluation of the physical aspects of her sexual difficulties and experiences, the physician decided that her problem reflected long-standing psychologic conflicts and referred her to a psychiatrist.

M.B., a 34-year-old salesman, complained to his physician of impotence. He was a nervous, insecure, ineffectual man who worked for his older brother. His wife, an active real estate broker, had become withdrawn and bitter, and his two adolescent children were involved in minor delinquency. The impotence was confined to his relationship with his wife; in a recent extramarital affair he had performed adequately. He said he was unable to satisfy his wife in any way; she was either withdrawn or overly demanding. The physician determined that the impotency had no organic basis and because of the nature of the family conflicts referred the patient to a service agency where the family could be worked with as a unit. Here the wife was found to be depressed and received psychiatric treatment. Later the patient reported that when her depression improved, his potency returned.

C.W., a woman with breast cancer, was asked about her marriage. She reported that her husband had stopped having sexual relations with her when it was discovered that she had metastatic disease. The physician then saw the husband, who confessed to an extramarital affair and the wish to leave his wife. He also described irrational anger directed to his wife and feelings of shame and worthlessness. It emerged that the marriage had been an unusually close one and that he could not bear the anticipation of his wife's death. Sexual contact with her reminded him of his impending loss. His anger and the extramarital affair were responses to grief. The physician met with him for several sessions. By avoiding a moralistic position and by indicating that many spouses of patients with serious diseases have similar feelings and may even find solace in extramarital relationships, the physician helped him to overcome his shame and to share his grief. The process brought dramatic relief, and with occasional contact with the physician he was able to remain with his wife and be helpful to her throughout her terminal illness.

MARITAL COUNSELING BY THE PHYSICIAN The evaluation of sexual problems almost invariably requires some attention to marital or other sexual relationships. Counseling that focuses primarily on these relationships has been designated *marital counseling.* Instead of the usual medical relationship, which emphasizes the individual patient, marital counseling involves both partners, although each may be seen separately at times.

The specific nature of the marital counseling depends upon the complaints or upon the time of life of the couple. The main requisite is a willingness for physicians to set aside time for this kind of undertaking and to develop an interest in the functional health of patients beyond the specific issues raised by disease. The stresses and transitions in the early years of a marriage should be appreciated as well as the pressures exerted by children. In later years, job problems and conflicts over roles may emerge, followed by development of the "empty nest" syndrome, menopausal and midlife issues, and the male-depressive syndrome as horizons close in and the realities of aging appear.

Most marital problems are not due to sexual difficulties, although sexual problems may be the leading edge, especially in the modern climate where sexual adjustment is so widely publicized. Sexual satisfaction is dependent on the broader aspects of the relationship between partners and on mental and physical health. The alert physician should probe to these deeper levels during marriage counseling. In this sense, counseling about sexual problems is dependent upon the successful outcome of marriage counseling. Early in the approach the motivation of both partners should be assessed. If one partner is determined to break up the marriage, the counseling may consist of communicating this information to the other partner and perhaps advising legal assistance. On the other hand, apparent determination to seek divorce by either partner needs to be evaluated because it may mask depression, a paranoid reaction, or a hidden problem that is being avoided by flight, such as shame over an affair, fear, illness, or personal failure.

In marital counseling, as with other medical counseling, it is well to avoid giving direct advice about interpersonal relationships. By defining the problem, the physician may enable the patient to arrive at a decision on a course of action. By taking sides in family conflicts or by espousing an ethical position, physicians can inadvertently introduce their own biases or allow themselves to be manipulated by one of the marital partners.

The internist or family physician is in a strategic position to provide effective marital counseling. As preventive medicine gains importance, marital counseling can provide physicians with great professional satisfaction.

REFERENCES

BELL AP, WEINBERG MS: *Homosexualities: A Study of Diversity among Men and Women.* New York, Simon & Schuster, 1978

GROUP FOR THE ADVANCEMENT OF PSYCHIATRY, COMMITTEE ON MEDICAL EDUCATION: *Assessment of Sexual Function.* New York, Jason Aronson, 1974

JOHNSON SA et al: Factors influencing lesbian gynecological care: A preliminary study. Am J Obstet Gynecol 140:20, 1981

KOLODNY RC et al: *Textbook of Sexual Medicine.* Boston, Little, Brown, 1979

LIEF HI et al (eds): *Sexual Problems in Medical Practice.* American Medical Association, 1981

MUNJACK DJ, OZIEL LJ (eds): *Sexual Medicine and Counseling in Office Practice: A Comprehensive Treatment Guide.* Boston, Little, Brown, 1980

SAGHIR MT, ROBINS E: *Male and Female Homosexuality.* Baltimore, Williams & Wilkins, 1973

48
HIRSUTISM AND VIRILIZATION

JEAN D. WILSON

Hirsutism, the growth of hair in women in a pattern characteristic of men, is a common and perplexing problem in medicine. Numerous factors—genetic, endocrine, and unknown—influence the growth and distribution of hair so that there is considerable overlap in the patterns in normal men and women. As a consequence, abnormal hair growth is difficult to define; an unbearable burden to one woman may be an unnoticed amount of hair in another. However, if the patient thinks that hair growth is excessive, no amount of reassurance, persuasion, or argument will convince her otherwise. The central issue in dealing with such patients is the separation of those infrequent instances in which hirsutism is one manifestation of an underlying virilizing or defeminizing syndrome from the vast majority of individuals in which it is fundamentally a cosmetic problem.

CONTROL OF NORMAL HAIR GROWTH AND DISTRIBUTION

Endocrinology Androgens are the major determinants of hair distribution in both sexes. There are three principal circulating androgens in women—dehydroepiandrosterone, derived from the adrenal; androstenedione, derived equally from adrenal and ovary; and testosterone, which is both secreted from the ovary and formed by peripheral conversion from circulating dehydroepiandrosterone and androstenedione. The production of adrenal androgen is regulated primarily by ACTH, while ovarian androgen secretion is regulated by the gonadotropins. These various androgens must be converted to testosterone (or dihydrotestosterone) before they can bind to the cytoplasmic androgen receptor of target cells and induce an androgenic response. Thus, adrenal androgens virilize only insofar as they serve as precursors for testosterone formation; hence plasma testosterone correlates better with abnormal hair growth or virilization than do other plasma hormones.

In simple terms four types of relation between hair growth and androgens can be defined: (1) no androgen dependence, lanugo, eyebrows, eyelashes; (2) dependence upon adrenal androgen and hence equal growth in men and women, axillary and lower pubic hair; (3) dependence upon testicular androgen, upper pubic, facial, ear, extremity, and truncal hair; and (4) inhibition by testicular androgen, scalp hair. The reason different body regions respond differently to the same or similar androgen is unknown. Theoretically, the metabolism of androgens might differ in the various sites, or hormone receptors might vary. The hair follicle, like some other androgen-responsive cells, requires conversion of testosterone to dihydrotestosterone for expression of testicular androgen action, and hair follicles from all regions of the body perform this conversion equally well. Moreover, the same cytoplasmic receptor that is essential for androgen action in other cells (Chap. 117) is necessary for the action of dihydrotestosterone in the hair follicle. Genetic disorders with normal testosterone production but absent receptor have deficient or absent axillary, pubic, facial, truncal, and limb hair (Chap. 120). Regional differences in androgen responsiveness of hair in normal individuals are probably the consequence of regional differences in the amount of androgen receptor in hair follicles or in the postreceptor events in androgen action.

Genetic factors Despite similar hormone levels, there is considerable diversity in the distribution of hair among individuals and between different racial groups in regard to facial, truncal, and pubic hair. It is generally agreed that dark-haired, darkly pigmented whites of either sex tend to be more hirsute than blonde or fair-skinned persons. Orientals, American Indians, and blacks are less hirsute than whites. Orientals rarely have facial or body hair except in the pubic and axillary regions, and American Indians, in addition, rarely develop baldness in either sex. There is also considerable heterogeneity of hair patterns within family groups. The inheritance of hair patterns is complex and probably polygenic in nature.

Other factors Aging is a prerequisite for the expression of some types of hair development, whether mediated by androgens or otherwise. For example, in men hair on the trunk and extremities frequently increases for several years after maximal levels of plasma androgens have been reached. Conversely, loss of androgens rarely results in diminution of normal hair or reverses hirsutism. The appearance of pubic hair is frequently the heralding event of puberty in females. Women in the first trimester of pregnancy commonly observe increased hairiness of the face, extremities, and breasts. Menopause is often associated with the loss of hair in the pubic area, axillae, and extremities, whereas growth of hair on the face increases in postmenopausal women. The physiologic basis for these changes is unclear and cannot be explained entirely by changes in androgen levels.

PATHOLOGICAL HAIR GROWTH OR DISTRIBUTION **Drugs** Drug-induced hirsutism is a frequent complication of modern therapy. It may be an isolated symptom or part of a virilizing syndrome. If the onset is subtle it may go unrecognized by the physician. Drugs that produce hirsutism without actual virilization include diphenylhydantoin, minoxidil, diazoxide, hexachlorobenzene, and ACTH. Steroidal drugs that are capable of inducing virilization as well as hirsutism include progestins (which may also cause virilization of infants born to mothers given them) and androgens.

Virilizing syndromes In evaluating patients for hirsutism the most important feature is whether virilization or defeminization is also present (Table 48-1). In patients with androgen overproduction defeminizing signs are more consistent than are the signs of virilization, although the latter, if present, are valuable, since they indicate either ovarian or adrenal pathology. It is of particular interest that other evidences of virilization are common in women above the age of 20 who present with acne. Two reservations should be kept in mind in interpreting the presence or absence of virilization. First, certain signs of virilization (clitoromegaly, balding, coarsening of the hair, hirsutism) indicate androgen excess at some time in the patient's life but do not necessarily mean that active disease is present at the time of evaluation. This can be ascertained by measurement of plasma androgen levels and/or production rates. Second, severe overandrogenization may exist in the absence of marked virilization; i.e., at the same level of androgen production clitoromegaly may be present in one patient and not another.

Two types of virilizing syndromes can occur—ovarian and adrenal, recognizing that these disorders account for only a small fraction of patients who complain of hirsutism.

Ovarian androgenization Polycystic ovarian disease (PCOD) is the commonest cause of ovarian hyperandrogenism (see Chap. 118). The disorder has a wide clinical spectrum that varies from apparently normal menses and mild hirsutism to complete amenorrhea and virilization; hyperthecosis of the ovary characterized by the presence of luteinized theca-like cells in the ovarian stroma is a variant of the disorder. Luteinizing hormone (LH) is almost invariably elevated, and there is considerable overproduction of androgens by the ovary. Other causes of ovarian virilization include stromal hyperplasia, luteomas, hilar cell hyperplasia, and a variety of androgen-secreting tumors including arrhenoblastoma and Krukenberg tumor. In these disorders plasma testosterone levels are elevated, frequently to the male range; the tumors may be so small as to be undetected by pelvic examination or laparoscopy.

TABLE 48-1
Clinical signs of defeminization and virilization

Signs of defeminization	*Signs of virilization*
Amenorrhea	Frontal balding
Decrease in breast size	Increase in size of shoulder girdle muscles
Loss of female body contours	Clitoromegaly
	Coarsening of the voice
	Acne

SOURCE: *After Karp and Herrmann.*

Adrenal androgenization Adrenal androgen-secreting tumors (adenoma or carcinoma) are generally accompanied by elevated urinary 17-ketosteroid excretion. Plasma testosterone levels are usually not as high as in ovarian virilization. Hirsutism can also occur in congenital adrenal hyperplasia and Cushing's disease.

Idiopathic or simple hirsutism This term applies to those hirsute women in whom a specific etiological diagnosis cannot be made. The diagnosis should be restricted to instances in which menstruation is normal, the urinary 17-ketosteroid level is not elevated, the ovaries are not enlarged, adrenal function is normal, and there is no evidence of an adrenal or ovarian tumor. Slight elevations of plasma androstenedione and/or testosterone are common in idiopathic hirsutism, and testosterone secretion rates may be increased above the mean. The fact that the experimental antiandrogen cyproterone acetate causes improvement in the hirsutism indicates that the hirsutism is due to the elevated testosterone values. In the majority of such women the increased plasma testosterone is derived from the ovaries. However, it is unclear whether these abnormalities represent the extreme end of a normal continuum or a distinct pathological group. In some the underlying diagnosis may be mild or early polycystic ovarian disease, but in most the mild androgen excess is not accompanied or followed by signs of ovarian dysfunction. Thus, it is possible that these patients are variants of normal. Since androgens are a major determinant of hair distribution and growth it is to be expected that within the normal range higher testosterone levels would be associated on average with greater androgen-mediated hair growth. Therefore, the belief of many endocrinologists that the majority of hirsute women have no associated endocrinopathy may still be valid.

TREATMENT In the case of drugs and tumors of the ovaries or adrenal glands, treatment is straightforward—stop the drugs or remove the tumors. In polycystic ovarian disease and idiopathic hirsutism, effective therapy is ovarian suppression using a combination-type oral contraceptive; improvement in hirsutism can frequently be documented in 6 months to a year. If fertility is desired, other forms of therapy are indicated and indeed whether the risks of contraceptive therapy are justified in simple hirsutism is an individual judgment. Several series have now been reported in which treatment with spironolactone caused a decrease in testosterone production (spironolactone also blocks the androgen receptor) and an improvement in hirsutism after a few months. Favorable results have also been reported with cimetidine, which also acts as an antiandrogen. Since coarsened hairs usually do not return completely to normal, local therapy is often required for hirsutism, including depilatory agents, shaving, tweezing, or electrolysis. Other evidences of virilization such as balding, clitoromegaly, and coarsening of the voice rarely improve following cure of overandrogenization.

REFERENCES

CASEY JH: Hirsutism: Pathogenesis and treatment. Aust NZ J Med 10:240, 1980

Frolich M et al: The influence of long-term treatment with cyproterone acetate or a cyproterone acetate–ethinyl oestradiol combination on androgen levels in blood of hirsute women. J Steroid Biochem 12:499, 1980

Givens JR: Hirsutism and hyperandrogenism. Adv Int Med 21:221, 1976

Kirschner MA, Bardin CW: Androgen production and metabolism in normal and virilized women. Metabolism 21:667, 1972

Mathur RS et al: Plasma androgens and sex hormone–binding globulin in the evaluation of hirsute females. Fertil Steril 35:29, 1981

Medical Letter on Drugs and Therapeutics: Treatment of hirsutism. 23:15, 1981

Muller SA: Hirsutism. Am J Med 46:803, 1969

Rook A: Aspects of cutaneous androgen-dependent syndromes. Int J Dermatol 19:357, 1980

Shapiro G, Evron S: A novel use of spironolactone: Treatment of hirsutism. J Clin Endocrinol Metab 51:429, 1980

Steinberger E et al: The menstrual cycle and plasma testosterone levels in women with acne. J Am Acad Dermatol 4:54, 1981

section 8 | Alterations in the skin

49
INTERPRETATION OF ALTERATIONS IN THE SKIN

THOMAS B. FITZPATRICK
HARLEY A. HAYNES

CLINICAL EXAMINATION OF THE SKIN

The identification of skin lesions, or alterations, is a problem similar to the recognition of cells in a blood smear: the minute details are of the greatest importance. The individual type of skin lesion (e.g., papule, nodule) can be considered as a letter in the alphabet, forming the basic element for the identification of the pathologic change and often leading to the clinical diagnosis. Lesions may be the presenting complaint of the patient or may be incidental findings during the routine physical examination; or they may be incidental to some major presenting complaint such as fever, cough, arthralgia, and the like. The recognition of the important and nonimportant skin lesions commonly encountered during the routine physical examination of the skin is a requisite part of the physician's task (Plates 1 to 6).

Inasmuch as the identification of skin lesions is the *sine qua non* of dermatologic diagnosis, the examiner's eye is undoubtedly the most valuable instrument at his or her disposal. Adequate illumination, preferably with natural light, is necessary. The observation of the skin should begin with an overall, "low-power" general assessment of the completely disrobed patient. The systematic approach to the examination of skin should be as follows: first the fingernails and then the anterior and posterior aspects of the arm; then, in sequence, the scalp, the face, the trunk, the lower extremities and the skin between the toes; and then the mucous membranes, including the mouth and anogenital areas. The examiner of dermatologic lesions should consider (1) the specific *type* of lesion, (2) the *shape* of the lesion, and (3) the *arrangement* of the groups of lesions, such as linear, arciform, annular, polycyclic, herpetiform, zosteriform, and serpiginous.

Types of skin lesions can be classified by determining the topographic level of the lesions in relation to the normal skin (Table 49-1). For example, it is possible to distinguish lesions that are in or that protrude from or are superimposed above or below the level of the normal skin. The lesions that are encompassed within the scope of dermatology are listed in Fig. 49-1 and Table 49-1, and the histologic aspects are illustrated in Figs. 49-2 through 49-13.

The *shape* of the individual lesion and the *arrangement* of two or more lesions in relation to each other sometimes constitute important diagnostic clues. A *linear* arrangement of lesions often is indicative of an exogenous cause; also, linear lesions may occur because the pathologic process involves a vein, a lymphatic component, or an arteriole. Linearity can often be seen in various types of cutaneous hamartoma involving epidermal cells or melanocytes or even dermal connective tissue. In contrast, *annular* and *arciform* lesions and annular and arciform arrangements are relatively common and therefore only rarely lead to a specific diagnosis. The *iris* lesion, however, a special and important type of annular lesion, is an erythematous annular macule or papule with either a purplish papule or vesicle in the center. Iris lesions are characteristic of the erythema-multiforme syndrome. Annular macules may be

TABLE 49-1
Types of skin lesion

Flat lesions (in plane of skin)	*Elevated lesions (above plane of skin)*	*Depressed lesions (below plane of skin)*
Macule	Vesicle and bulla	Atrophy§
Infarct*	Pustule	Sclerosis§†
Sclerosis*†	Abscess‡	Erosion
Telangiectasia†	Cyst†	Excoriation
	Papule	Scar†
	Wheal	Ulcer
	Plaque	Sinus‡
	Nodule‡	Gangrene§
	Vegetation	
	Keratosis	
	Desquamation (scales)	
	Exudate* (crusts)	
	Lichenification	

* *May also be below the plane of the skin.*
† *May also be above the plane of the skin.*
‡ *May also be in or below the plane of the skin.*
§ *May also be in the plane of the skin.*
SOURCE: *TB Fitzpatrick, in Dermatology in General Medicine, 2d ed, TB Fitzpatrick et al (eds), New York, McGraw-Hill, 1979.*

observed in drug eruptions, secondary syphilis, and lupus erythematosus. Annular lesions with scale often suggest dermatophytosis or pityriasis rosea or psoriasis. The wheals that occur in creeping eruptions as well as the nodules in late syphilis are arranged in a *serpiginous* (snake-like) pattern.

Lesions that are contiguous are described as *grouped,* and are of relatively little diagnostic value except in the special pattern, *herpetiform,* which is pathognomonic for herpes simplex or herpes zoster. Similarly, the special arrangement, *zosteriform,* follows a dermatome in a bandlike pattern and is characteristically seen in herpes zoster; a zosteriform arrangement of skin nodules is occasionally seen in metastatic carcinoma of the breast. A *reticular* arrangement often results from vascular dilatation and is observed in cutis marmorata and livedo reticularis.

The *distribution* of sites of localization of skin eruptions has been greatly overemphasized in dermatologic diagnosis; of far more importance are the type, shape, and arrangement of the lesions. The distribution of eruptions can be classified as *isolated, regional,* or *generalized;* the term *total* (universal) denotes an involvement of all the skin, including the hair and the nails. When the eruption occurs in a bilateral and symmetric distribution, the pathologic stimulus is usually endogenous or is hematogenously disseminated. Bilateral symmetry is characteristic of hypersensitivity and is a common response to a drug. In photosensitivity eruptions, lesions are localized to the parts of the body that are exposed to sunlight. The exposed areas of the face that are usually spared include the fold of skin in the upper eyelids, the skin of the hair-covered scalp, and the region below the chin.

LABORATORY AND OTHER AIDS IN EXAMINATION OF THE SKIN

There are certain technical, clinical, and laboratory aids and procedures that are indispensable in the clinical examination and interpretation of skin conditions.

VISUAL AIDS **Magnification** Certain diagnostic signs can be revealed only by magnification of the skin lesions, e.g., the follicular plugging indicative of lupus erythematosus, the fine telangiectasia and raised border indicative of basal cell carcinoma, and, if present, the bluish color indicative of early primary malignant melanoma. A pocket magnifier (2 to 7×) is necessary for proper identification.

Transillumination Transillumination, or oblique lighting, of skin lesions, which is done in a darkened room, is often required to detect slight degrees of elevation or depression, and is also sometimes useful in estimating the extent of the eruption.

Diascopy Diascopy is an essential technique for the examination of skin because it permits the differentiation of purpura from erythematous macules. Diascopy consists of firmly pressing a microscope slide or a piece of clear plastic over the skin lesion; if the lesion is erythematous, the pressure will reveal capillary dilatation rather than an extravasation of blood. Sarcoidosis, lymphoma, and tuberculosis of the skin are suggested if diascopy of the nodules shows either a characteristic hyaline, yellowish-brown, or an "apple-jelly" appearance.

Long-wave ultraviolet light, or Wood's lamp Long-wave ultraviolet light (360 nm), or Wood's lamp, is a necessary source of illumination for examination of the skin. Wood's lamp consists of a high-pressure mercury arc lamp with a specially compounded glass filter made of nickel oxide and silica (Wood's filter). This filter permits the passage of a band of radiation of

FIGURE 49-1

Common lesions, shown on anterior and posterior views of the patient, encountered during the physical examination of the skin. See also Plates 1 to 6. [From TB Fitzpatrick, DP Johnson, in Dermatology in General Medicine, TB Fitzpatrick et al (eds), New York, McGraw-Hill, 1979.]

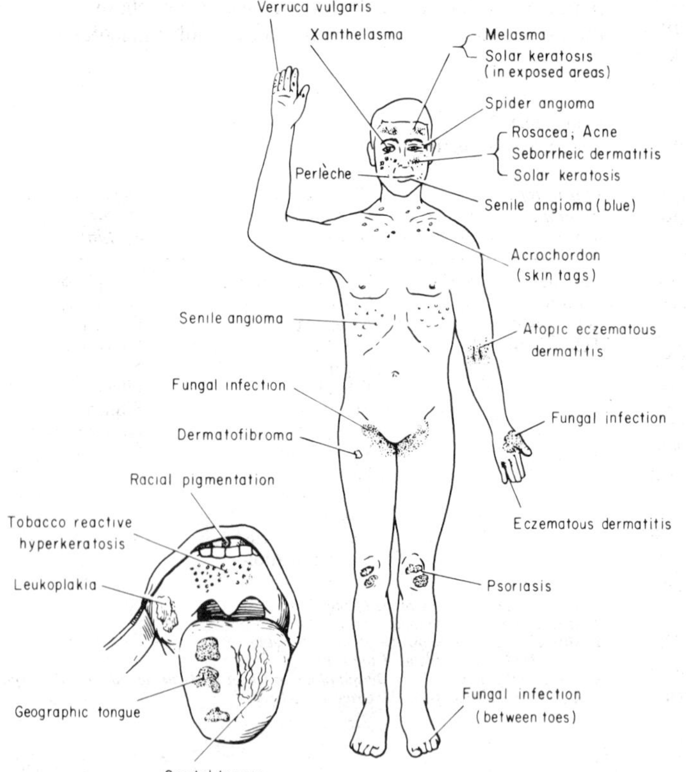

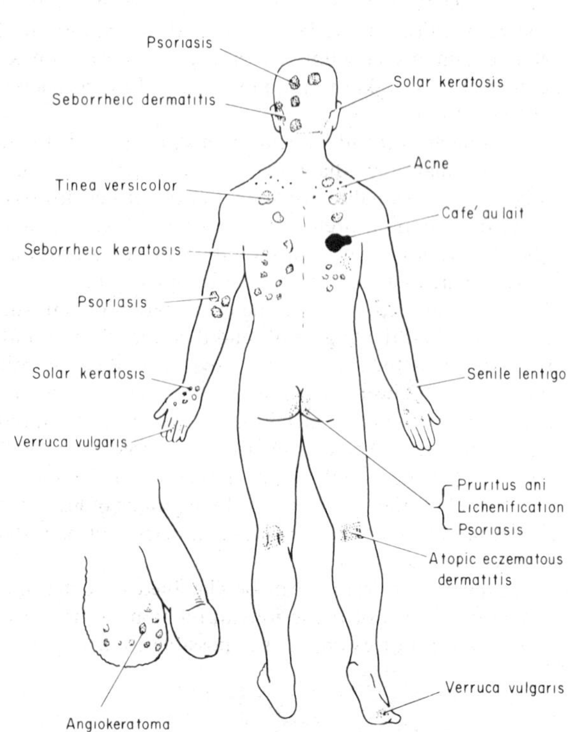

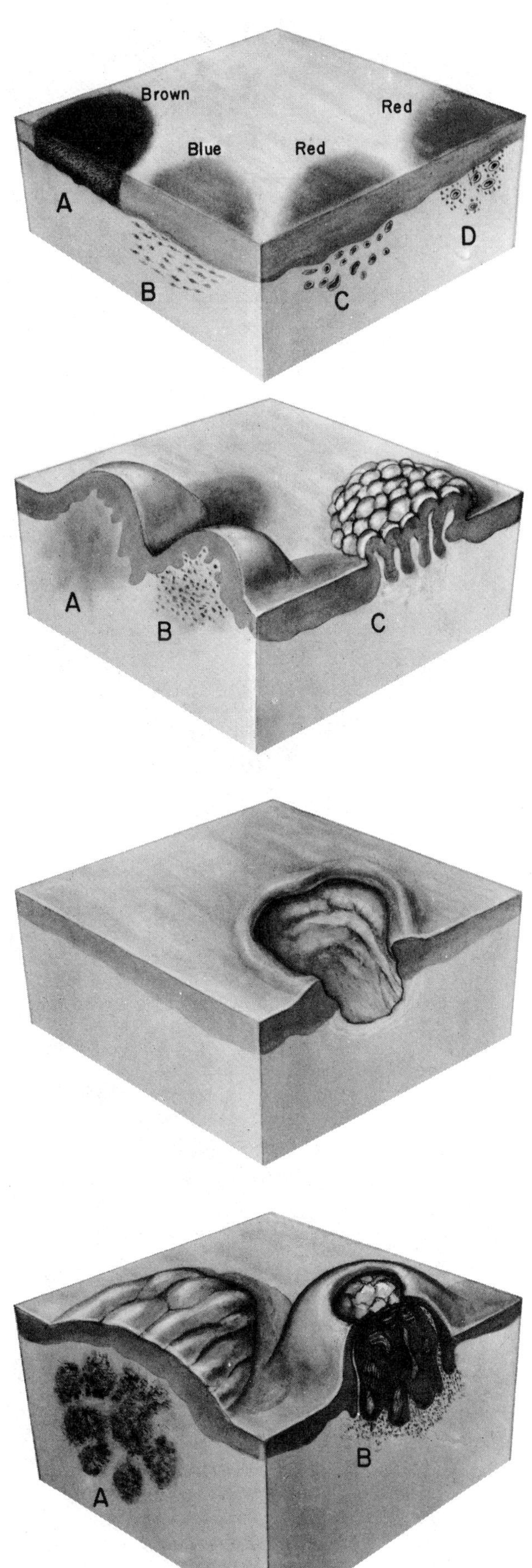

MACULE

FIGURE 49-2
A macule *is a circumscribed area of change in normal skin color without elevation or depression of the surface relative to the surrounding skin. The macules may be of any size and are the result of hypopigmentation (e.g., vitiligo) or hyperpigmentation—melanin (A) or hemosiderin (D)—such as café au lait spots and Mongolian spots (B), or permanent vascular abnormalities of the skin, as in a capillary hemangioma or transient capillary dilation (erythema) (C). Pressure of a glass slide (diascopy) on the border of a red lesion is a simple and reliable method for detecting the extravasation of red blood cells. If the redness remains under the pressure of the slide, the lesion may be purpuric (D); if the redness disappears, the lesion is erythematous and is due to vascular dilation (C).*

PAPULE

FIGURE 49-3
A papule *is a solid lesion, generally considered as less than 1 cm in diameter. Most of it is elevated above, rather than deep within, the plane of the surrounding skin. The elevation is caused by metabolic deposits (A) in the dermis or by localized infiltrates (B) in the dermis or by localized hyperplasia of cellular elements (C) in the dermis or epidermis. Superficial papules with distinct borders are seen when the lesion is the result of an increase in the number of epidermal cells (C) or melanocytes. Deeper dermal papules resulting from cellular infiltrates have indistinct borders. The topography of a papule or plaque may consist of multiple, small, closely packed, projected elevations that are known as a vegetation (C).*

ULCERS

FIGURE 49-4
An ulcer *is a lesion in which there has been destruction of the epidermis and the upper papillary layer of the dermis. Certain features that are helpful in determining the cause of ulcers include location, borders, base, discharge, and any associated topographic features of the lesions, such as nodules, excoriations, varicosities, hair distribution, presence or absence of sweating, and adjacent pulses.*

NODULE

FIGURE 49-5
A nodule *is a palpable solid, round, or ellipsoidal lesion deeper than a papule and is in the dermis or subcutaneous tissue (A) or in the epidermis (B). The depth of involvement rather than the diameter primarily differentiates a nodule from a papule. Nodules result from infiltrates (A), neoplasms (B), or metabolic deposits in the dermis or subcutaneous tissue and often indicate systemic disease. Late syphilis, tuberculosis, the deep mycoses, lymphoma, and metastatic neoplasms, for example, can present as cutaneous nodules. Therefore, biopsy should be performed on unidentified persistent nodules, and a portion of excised tissue should be ground in a sterile mortar and cultured for fungi. Nodules can develop as a result of a benign or malignant proliferation of keratinocytes, as in keratoacanthoma (B), verruca vulgaris, and squamous cell and basal cell carcinoma.*

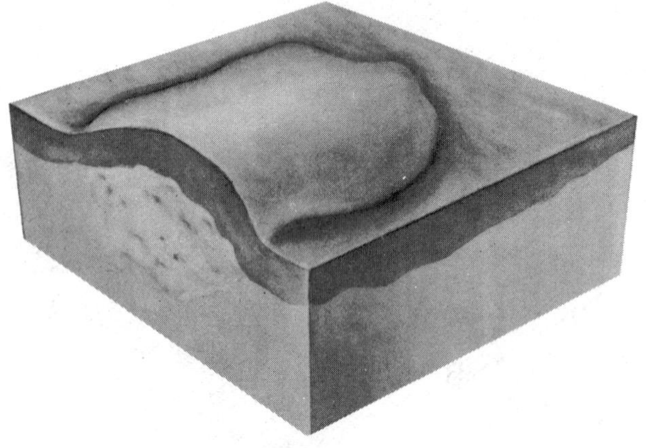

WHEAL

FIGURE 49-6
A wheal *is a rounded or flat-topped, pale-red elevation in the skin that is characteristically evanescent, disappearing within hours. Observation of the borders of wheals that have been traced with a skin-marking pencil reveals that the wheals shift relatively rapidly from the involved to the uninvolved adjacent areas. Wheals are the result of edema in the upper layer of the dermis.*

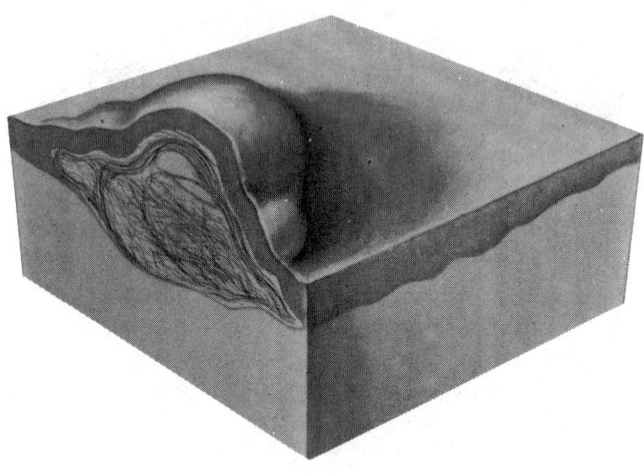

VESICLE

FIGURE 49-7
A vesicle *(less than 0.5 cm) or a* bulla *(more than 0.5 cm) is a circumscribed elevated lesion containing fluid. Often the walls are so thin that they are translucent, and the serum, lymph fluid, blood, or extracellular fluid can be seen. Vesicles and bullae arise from a cleavage at various levels of the skin; the cleavage may be within the epidermis (i.e., intraepidermal vesication), or at the epidermal-dermal interface (i.e., subepidermal).*

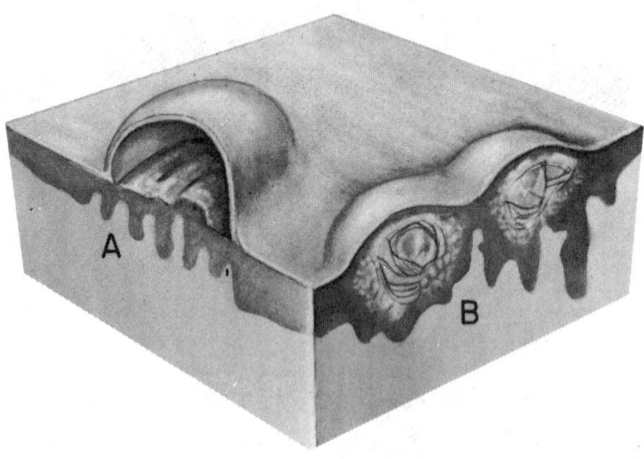

BULLA (A, subcorneal; B, spongiotic)

FIGURE 49-8
When the cleavage is just beneath the stratum corneum, a subcorneal vesicle *or* bulla *results (A), as seen in impetigo and subcorneal pustular dermatosis. Intraepidermal vesication may result from intercellular edema, or spongiosis (B), as characteristically seen in delayed hypersensitivity reactions of the epidermis (e.g., in contact eczematous dermatitis), and in dyshidrotic eczema (B).* Spongiotic vesicles *may or may not be seen clinically as vesicles.*

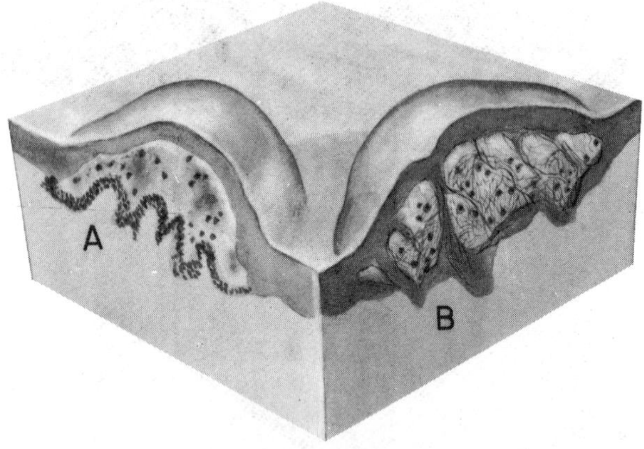

VESICLE (A, acantholytic; B, viral)

FIGURE 49-9
Loss of intercellular bridges, or desmosomes, is known as acantholysis (A), and this type of intraepidermal vesication is seen in the vesicles or bullae of pemphigus vulgaris; the cleavage is usually just above the basal layer, as in pemphigus vulgaris, but may occur just below the subcorneal layer, as in pemphigus foliaceus. Viruses cause a curious "ballooning degeneration" of epidermal cells (B), as in herpes zoster, herpes simplex, variola, and varicella. Viral bullae often have a depressed ("umbilicated") center.

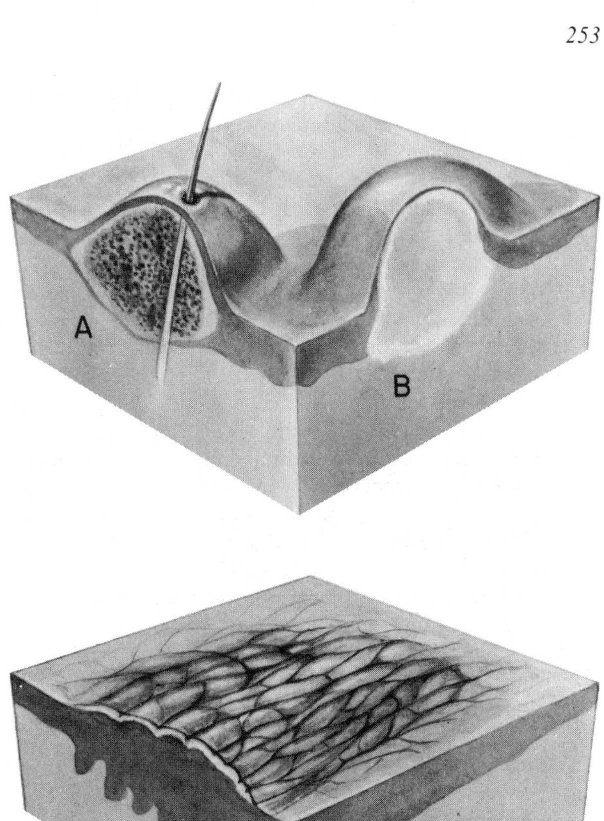

PUSTULE

FIGURE 49-10
A pustule *is a circumscribed elevation of the skin that contains a purulent exudate that may be white, yellow, or greenish yellow. This process may arise in a hair follicle (A) or independently (B). Pustules may vary in size and shape; follicular pustules, however, are always conical and usually contain a hair in the center. The vesicular lesions of the viral diseases (varicella, variola, vaccinia, herpes simplex, and herpes zoster) may secondarily become pustular. A Gram's stain and culture should be done on all pustules.*

PLAQUE

FIGURE 49-11
A plaque *is an elevation above the skin surface that occupies a relatively large suface area in comparison with its height above the skin. Frequently, it is formed by a confluence of papules, as in psoriasis and mycosis fungoides. Lichenification is a proliferation of keratinocytes and stratum corneum forming a plaquelike structure. The skin appears thickened, and the skin markings are accentuated. The process results from repeated rubbing, and frequently develops in persons with atopy. Lichenification occurs in eczematous dermatitis.*

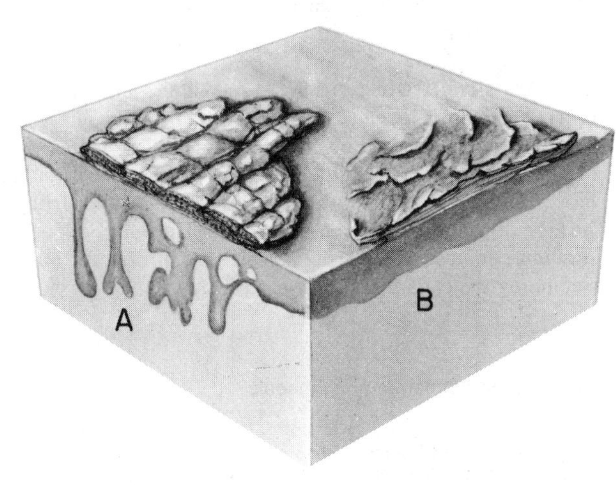

SCALES

FIGURE 49-12
Epidermal cells are completely replaced every 27 days. The end product of this holocrine process is the stratum corneum. This outermost layer of skin, the stratum corneum, normally does not contain nuclei and is imperceptibly lost. With an increased rate of proliferation of epidermal cells, as in psoriasis, the stratum corneum is not formed normally, and the outermost layers of the skin retain the nuclei. These desquamating layers of skin are seen clinically as scales. *Densely adherent scales that have a gritty feel (like sandpaper) result from a localized increase in the stratum corneum and are typically seen in solar keratosis (B).*

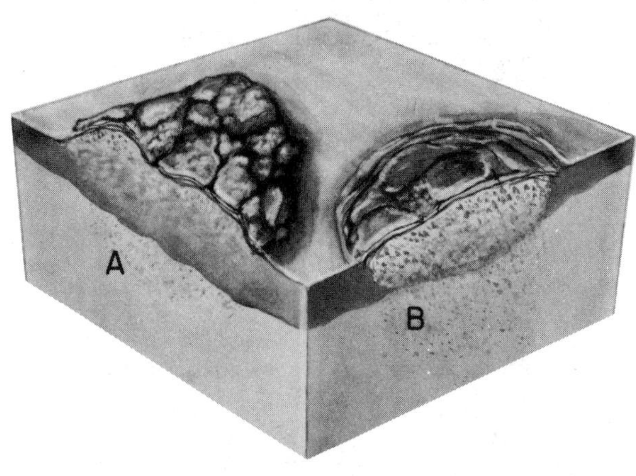

CRUSTS

FIGURE 49-13
Crusts, *resulting when serum, blood, or purulent exudate dries on the skin surface, are the hallmark of pyogenic infection. Crusts may be thin, delicate, and friable (A) or thick and adherent (B). Crusts are yellow when formed from dried serum, green or yellow-green when formed from purulent exudate, or brown or dark red when formed from blood. Superficial crusts occur as honey-colored, delicate, glistening particulates on the surface (A) and are typically seen in impetigo. When the exudate involves the entire epidermis, the crusts may be thick and adherent, and this condition is known as ecthyma (B).*

360 nm, which will reveal fluorescence when light passed through the filter impinges upon certain structures.

Wood's lamp is important for the detection of the pinkish-red fluorescence of the urine of patients with porphyria cutanea tarda; the addition of 5% hydrochloric acid greatly intensifies the fluorescence, owing to the oxidation of porphyrin precursors to porphyrins.

Wood's lamp is also a great help in estimating variation in the pigmentation of the skin; it reveals both increased and decreased pigmentation. Inasmuch as melanin is a universal absorber of ultraviolet light, areas of increased melanin will show an increased intensity under Wood's lamp; conversely, areas of decreased melanin will show a decrease in intensity (or an increased reflection) because the ultraviolet light is not absorbed. In this respect, Wood's lamp may be the only means of recognizing the sometimes indistinguishable hypomelanotic macules in tuberous sclerosis, a dominantly inherited trait associated with mental retardation and seizures. The white spots are present at birth and remain throughout life, and therefore represent important markers of this serious genetic disorder. Wood's lamp can be used in mass screening for detection of the fluorescence of dermatophytosis *in the hair shaft* in ringworm of the scalp.

CLINICAL TESTS Patch testing Patch testing is primarily used by dermatologists to detect contact sensitivity. The contactants are listed in Fisher's 1973 monograph on the subject.

Darier's sign One very useful clinical response of the skin, Darier's sign, is used as a test for urticaria pigmentosa, and is evoked by the vigorous rubbing of a pigmented macule with the blunt end of a pen. In urticaria pigmentosa (mastocytosis), a palpable red wheal occurs within a few minutes after the physical trauma, owing to the release of histamine by the mast cells in the skin.

LABORATORY PROCEDURES Examination for bacteria in crusts and biopsy specimens Gram's stains and bacterial cultures of exudates should be performed on all lesions consisting of crusts and purulent exudates. Ulcers and nodules should be biopsied by removal of a wedge of tissue that extends from the surface down to the subcutaneous fat. The biopsy specimen should be minced in a sterile mortar and cultured for bacteria (including typical and atypical mycobacteria) and fungi.

TABLE 49-2
Approach to dermatologic diagnosis

I History
- *A* Duration of lesions: days, weeks, months, years
- *B* Relationship of skin lesions to season, heat, cold, previous treatment, drug ingestion
- *C* Skin symptoms: pruritus, pain, paresthesia
- *D* Constitutional symptoms
  - *1* "Acute illness" syndrome: headache, chills, feverishness, weakness
  - *2* "Chronic illness" syndrome: fatigue, weakness, anorexia, weight loss, malaise
- *E* System review

II Physical examination
- *A* Appearance of patient: uncomfortable, "toxic," well
- *B* Changes in body temperature: elevated
- *C* Normal skin color: white, brown, black
- *D* Skin—four major skin signs: (1) type, (2) shape, (3) arrangement, (4) distribution of lesions
  - *1* Type of lesion

Basic lesions	*Sequential lesions*
Macule	Scale
Papule-plaque	Exudation: dry (crust)
Wheal	wet (weeping)
Nodule	Erosion
Cyst	Scar
Vesicle-bulla	Lichenification
Pustule	
Ulcer (also sequential)	
Hyperkeratosis (also sequential)	
Sclerosis	
Atrophy (also sequential)	
Telangiectasis	
Infarct	
Purpura	

Color of lesions or of skin (if diffuse involvement): "skin color," white, leukoderma, hypomelanosis; red, erythema, pink, violaceous; brown, hypermelanosis, black, blue, gray, orange, yellow. Red purpuric lesions do not blanch with pressure (diascopy).

Palpation
Consistency (soft, firm, hard, fluctuant, boardlike)
Deviation in temperature (hot, cold)
Mobility of lesion or of skin
Presence of tenderness
Estimate of the depth of lesion (i.e., dermal or subcutaneous)

  - *2 Shape* of individual lesions: round, oval, polygonal, polycyclic, annular (ring-shaped), iris, serpiginous (snake-like), umbilicated
  - *3 Arrangement* of multiple lesions
    Grouped: herpetiform, zosteriform, arciform, annular, reticulated (netlike), linear, serpiginous (snake-like)
    Disseminated: scattered discrete lesions or diffuse involvement, i.e., without identifiable borders
  - *4 Distribution* of lesions
    Extent: isolated (single lesion), localized, regional generalized, universal
    Pattern: symmetrical, exposed areas, sites of pressure, intertriginous areas, follicular localization, random
    Characteristic patterns: scabies, secondary syphilis, psoriasis, seborrheic dermatitis, lichen planus, pityriasis rosea, dermatitis herpetiformis, atopic dermatitis, vitiligo, acne, erythema multiforme, candidiasis, contact dermatitis, lupus erythematosus, erythrasma, ichthyosis, pemphigus, pemphigoid, porphyria cutanea tarda, xanthoma, necrotizing angiitis (vasculitis)
- *E* Hair and nails
- *F* Mucous membranes
- *G* Miscellaneous physical findings: lymphadenopathy, hepatosplenomegaly, cardiac findings, neurologic findings, ophthalmologic findings

III Laboratory and special examinations
- *A* Dermatopathology
  - *1* Light microscopy: site, process, cell types
  - *2* Immunofluorescence
  - *3* Special techniques: stains, electron microscopy, etc.
- *B* Microbiologic examination of skin material: scales, crusts, or exudate
  - *1* Direct microscopic examination of skin

For yeast and fungus:	10% potassium hydroxide preparation
For bacteria:	Gram stain
For virus:	Tzanck smear
For spirochetes:	Dark-field examination
For parasites:	Scabies mite from a burrow

  - *2* Culture
    Bacterial: for granulomas, culture
    Mycologic: minced tissue
- *C* General laboratory examinations: blood

Bacteriologic: culture
Serologic: ANA, STS
Hematologic: hematocrit or hemoglobin, cells, differential smear, erythrocyte sedimentation rate
Chemistry: Fasting blood sugar, blood urea nitrogen, creatinine

- *D* Wood's light examination

Urine: pink-orange fluorescence in porphyria cutanea tarda (add 5.0% hydrochloric acid)
Hair: (in vivo) green fluorescence in tinea capitis (hair shaft)
Skin (in vivo):

Compared to visible light examination	Erythrasma	Coral red fluorescence
	Hypomelanosis	Decrease in intensity
	Brown hypermelanosis	Increase in intensity
	Blue hypermelanosis	No change in intensity

- *E* Radiographic studies

Atlas of common lesions encountered during the physical examination of the skin

The skin and mucous membrane may frequently contain a variety of lesions that are rarely a major complaint (see Fig. 48-1). They are, therefore, incidental findings in the general physical examination. The recognition of "bumps and blemishes" is a necessary first step for physicians inasmuch as they will be required to distinguish the trivial from the serious and important skin changes. For example, such a serious lesion as a malignant melanoma may be incidentally discovered during a routine physical examination (see Plates 6-1 to 6-4 and the discussion in Chap. 330).

The common disorders of the skin that every physician should be able to recognize are presented in this series of color photographs (Plates 1 to 4).

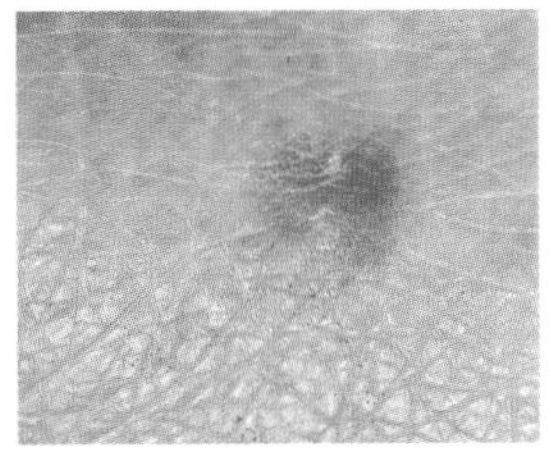

A

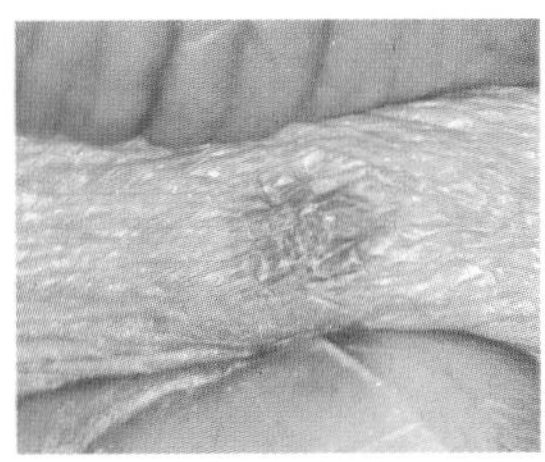

B

1-1 **Dermatofibroma** is especially common in middle life and in women. The lesions, when pigmented, are occasionally confused with malignant melanoma. They appear as isolated, slightly elevated, hard, button-like nodules *(A)*. In fair-skinned persons, the lesions are not usually skin color, but are pink or dark red, yellowish brown, or gray-black. They are usually less than 1 cm in diameter. A diagnostic sign is that a dermatofibroma dimples or becomes depressed *(B)* when it is laterally compressed; melanocytic nevus and melanoma, however, with which dermatofibroma may be easily confused, become elevated with lateral compression.

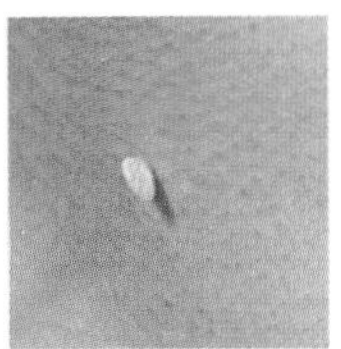

1-2 **Acrochordon** (skin tag) is very common after middle life and appears on the neck, especially in women, in the axillae, and on the upper part of the trunk. The lesions are small (1 to 5 mm), soft, pedunculated papules, usually of normal skin color.

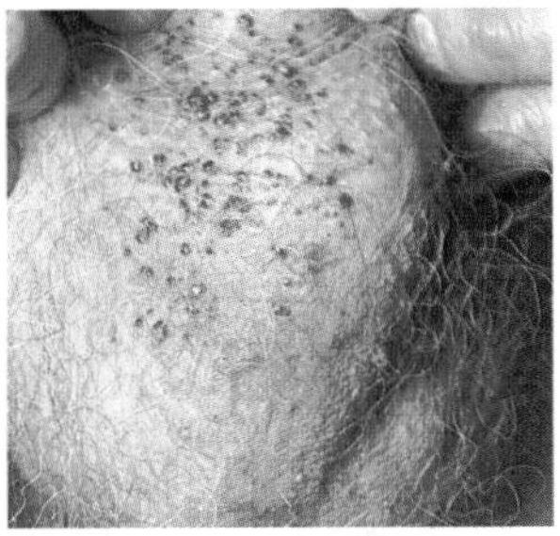

1-3 **Angiokeratomas** are bizarre vascular dilatations that occur under the tongue and on the scrotum and consist of myriads of 2- to 3-mm purplish red papules. They are of no known significance. When they occur on the trunk and extremities, a biopsy is indicated to rule out glycolipid lipidosis or Fabry's disease.

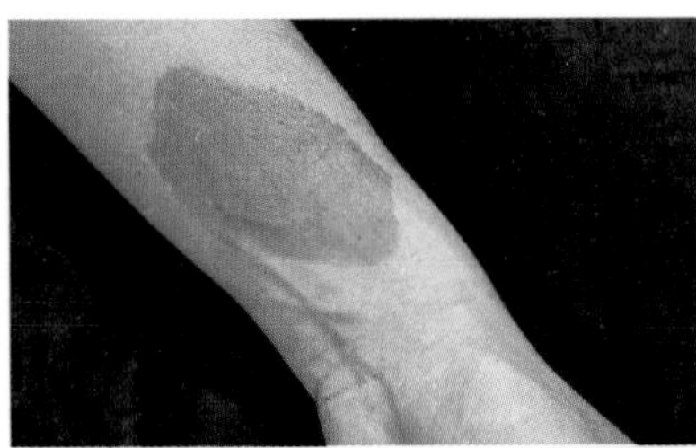

1-4 **Café au lait macules** are found in about 10 percent of the normal population and, in fair-skinned persons, are light yellowish brown macules, which may also be markers of neurofibromatosis and polyostotic fibrous dysplasia (Albright's syndrome). The presence of six or more café au lait macules with a diameter of 1.5 cm or greater is diagnostic of neurofibromatosis.

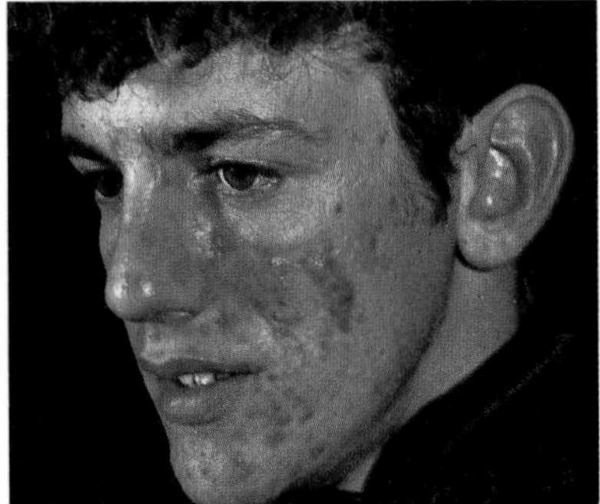

1-5 **Acne** is a condition in which the most characteristic lesion is the comedo, or "blackhead," that later becomes a conical erythematous papule or pustule. A third type of lesion is the "blind boil," which is a dermal cyst without an orifice. This lesion is often associated with atrophic or hypertrophic scarring. Cystic acne may appear with only a very few comedones; also, comedo-like acne may occur with few cysts or erythematous papules.

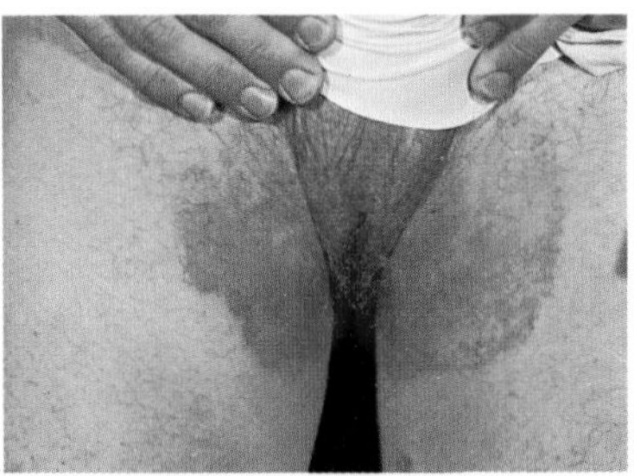

2-1 **Dermatophytosis** is identified by the striking polycyclic, annular shape of the scaling, especially on the feet and hands, where there is often a scalloped pattern. A positive diagnosis of dermatophytosis is quickly established by direct examination of scales from the advancing border; the mycelia are revealed when the scales are immersed in 10% potassium hydroxide or Swartz stain.

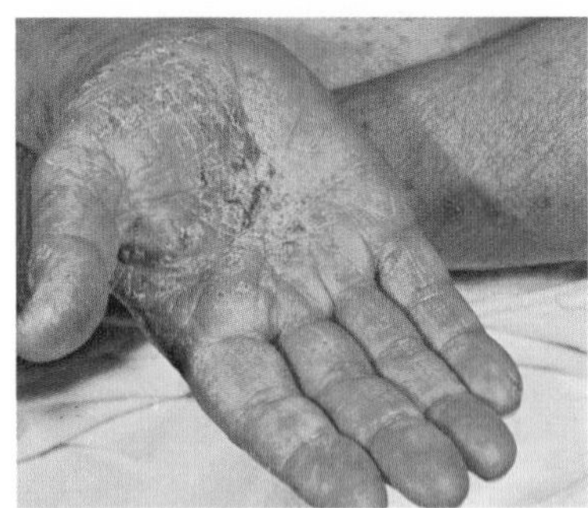

2-2 **Eczematous dermatitis** is a very common cutaneous reaction that is localized to the hands of housewives, to the legs in patients with chronic venous insufficiency, and behind the ears in patients with seborrheic dermatitis. In subacute eczematous dermatitis, there are mild erythema, dry scales, and often small red papules, many of which are excoriated. In chronic eczematous dermatitis, lichenification is the most prominent feature.

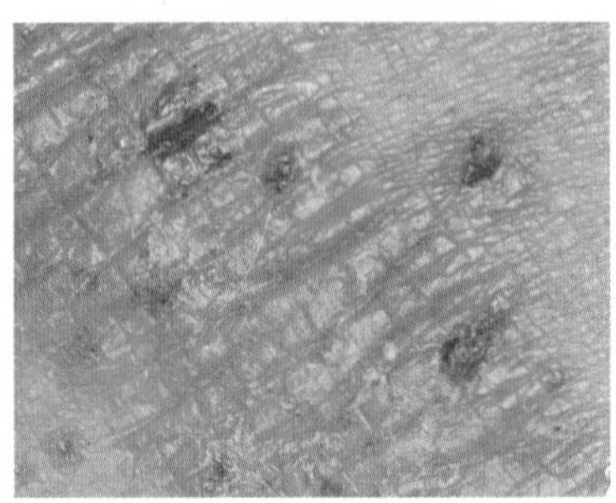

2-3 **Localized lichenification** results from repeated rubbing of the skin and consists of isolated, circumscribed plaques. These single lesions vary in size from 2 to 10 cm and occur most often on the extensor aspect of the forearm and in the scrotal, nuchal, inguinal, and anogenital areas. The perianal and vulvar areas may become diffusely lichenified. Lichenification is thought to be more frequent in persons with an atopic background.

2-4 **Melasma (chloasma)** is the so-called "mask" of pregnancy, but it also occurs in men and in women taking progestational agents. The pigmentation is uniform and is limited to the exposed areas of the face. There is no scaling or epidermal change. In fair-skinned persons, the pigment may be any shade from light tan to a very dark brown. It is most often seen on the cheeks and upper lip, as here, and on the forehead.

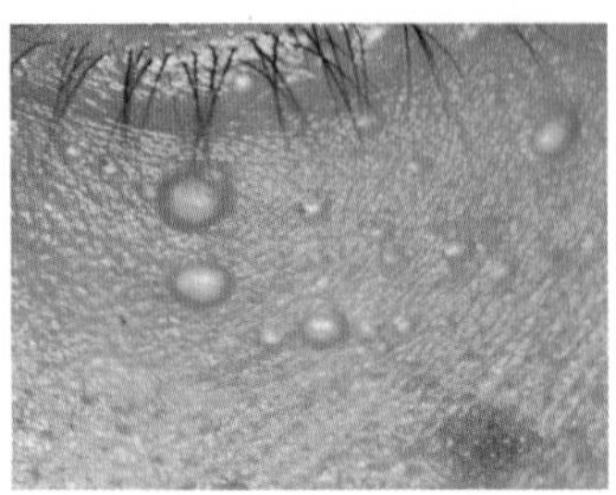

2-5 **Milia** are a collection of lesions, occurring most commonly on the face, and consist of tiny (1 to 2 mm), white, hard, rounded, superficial papules. There is no orifice, and the keratinous contents are easily expressed by lateral compression after the making of a tiny incision in the dome of the lesion.

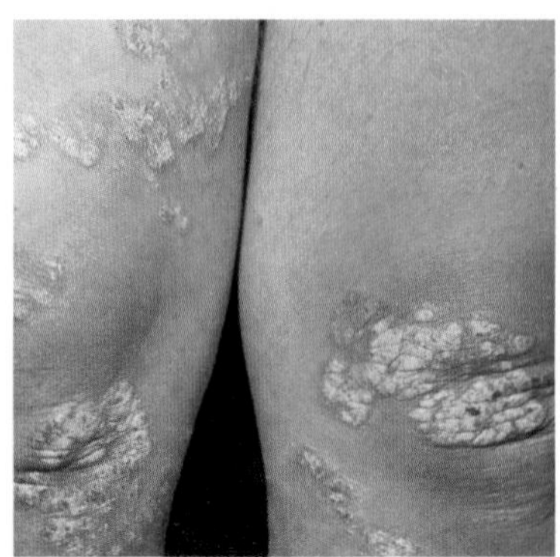

2-6 **Psoriasis,** affecting more than 2 percent of the population, consists of isolated scaling papules or plaques and is quite commonly observed in the routine physical examination. The lesions occur most frequently on the scalp, elbows, and knees. The color and type of scales are the identifying features of the lesions. The scales are either dense and lamellated with peripherally detached edges or loose and branny. The plaques are pink to deep red, and the borders are distinct.

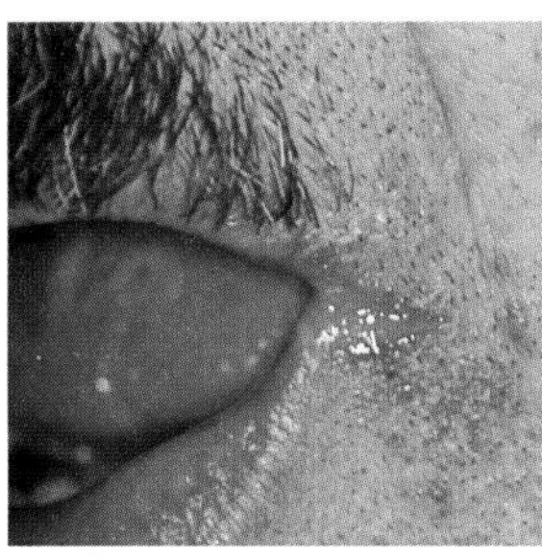

3-1 **Perlèche** consists of painful small fissures at the angles of the mouth, often covered with yellow crusts. Perlèche most often occurs with poorly fitting dentures and in moniliasis and secondary syphilis.

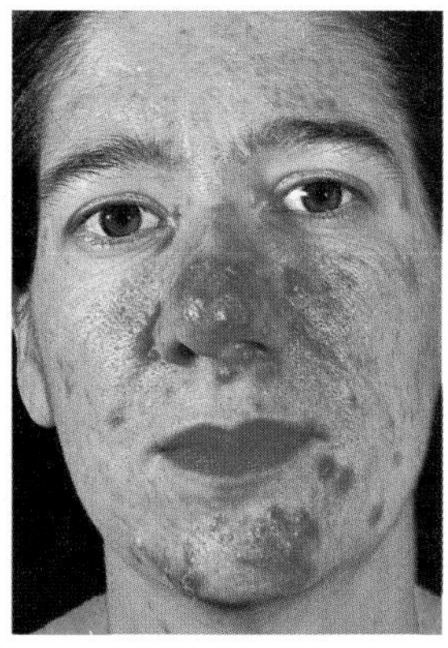

3-2 **Rosacea,** usually limited to the face, consists of tiny, erythematous papules and pustules 1 to 5 mm in size. The pustules, often tiny and sometimes hardly visible, sit on the dome of the papules. The diffuse redness of the face is due to vasodilatation, as well as to myriad telangiectases. In men, rhinophyma, a disfiguring enlargement of the nose, may occur.

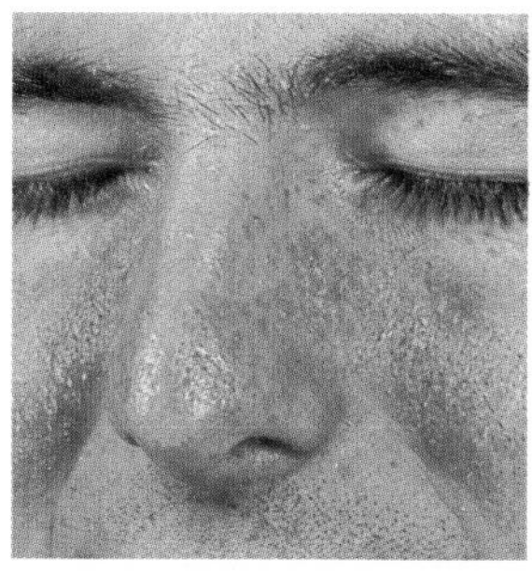

3-3 **Seborrheic dermatitis,** a common disorder found in all age groups, occurs most frequently on the scalp, eyebrows, and nasolabial folds and behind the ears. Scaling is the prominent feature and is loose and branny; it may be yellow and oily or dry and white. The lesion may become exudative and crusted or eczematous.

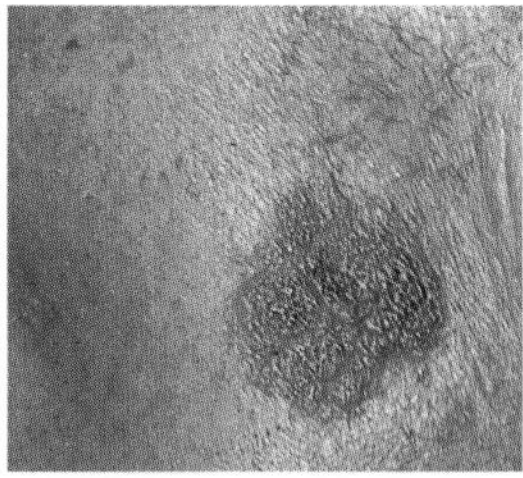

3-4 **Seborrheic keratosis** appears in middle life and may occur on exposed or unexposed areas but is especially common on the trunk. The lesions are irregularly round or oval flat-topped papules or plaques that seem "stuck" on the skin. The margins are distinct, and the surface is often warty or consists of multiple tiny projections (vegetation). In fair-skinned persons, the lesions are light brown at first but, enlarging, become more heavily pigmented and may be confused with malignant melanoma.

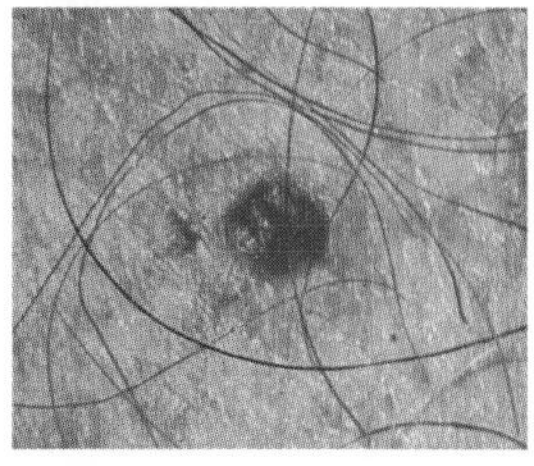

3-5 **Senile angioma ("cherry red spot")** appears in the third decade. On the lip, the lesion is usually singular and consists of a bluish red round nodule. On the trunk, the lesions are small (2 to 3 mm), bright red, globular papules.

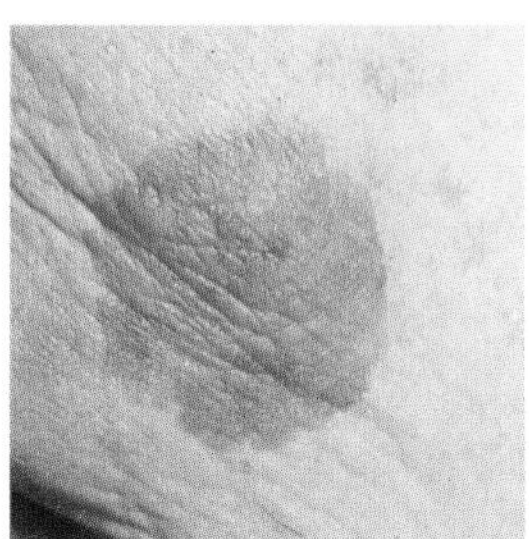

3-6 **Senile lentigo** occurs as a single macule or as a group of isolated, sharply circumscribed macules on the exposed areas, especially on the dorsal surfaces of the hands and arms and on the forehead and cheeks. The macules are usually light yellowish brown, but may be dark brown; the color is somewhat variegated, rather than uniform as it is in a café au lait macule. Rarely, dark brown *papules* develop in these lesions, and then the condition is called *lentigo maligna,* which may slowly develop, over a period of years, into a melanoma *(lentigo maligna melanoma).*

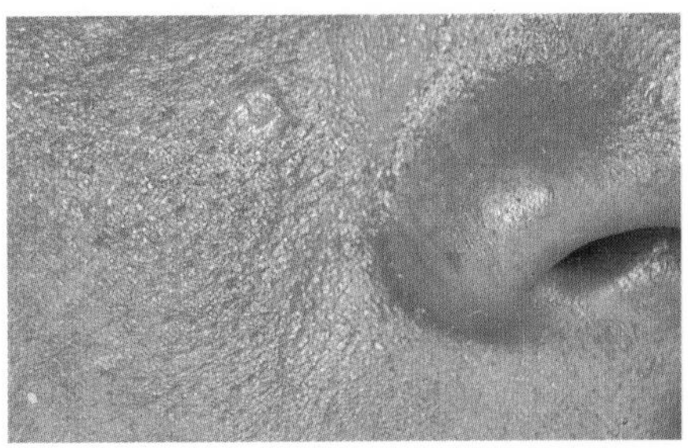

4-1 **Senile sebaceous adenoma** occurs on the face in patients over 40 and is often diagnosed as basal-cell carcinoma. The lesions are soft, small, flat-topped papules, varying in size from 1 to 8 mm, and are characterized by a minute central depression from which sebaceous material can be exuded by lateral compression.

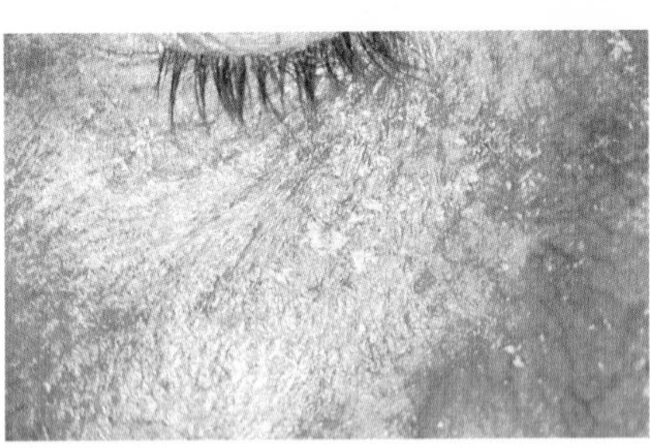

4-2 **Solar keratosis** (1) occurs usually in persons with light skin prone to sunburn or with darker skin after chronic excessive exposure; (2) is strictly limited to exposed skin, especially on the face and dorsal surfaces of the hands; (3) is more easily felt than seen (gritty and sandpaperish); (4) in fair-skinned persons, consists of skin-colored or light brown macules or slightly raised papules with superficial adherent scales not easily removed; and (5) is associated with marked wrinkling, telangiectasia, and often diffuse, tiny, pale yellow papules indicating solar degeneration of connective tissue ("turkey skin").

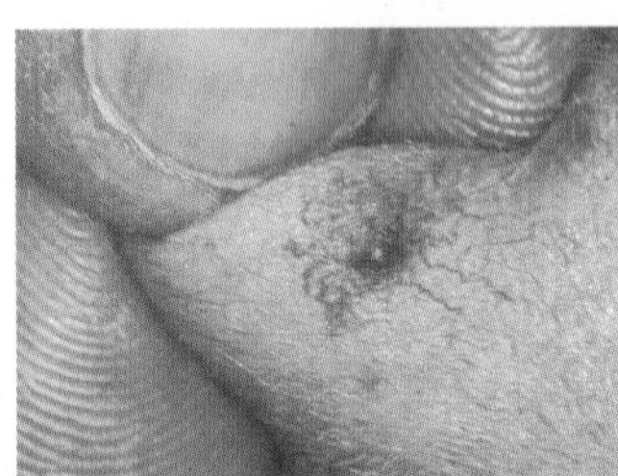

4-3 **Spider nevus** consists of a central, punctate, bright red macule or papule (the body) from which fine red lines radiate like spider legs. There is often a red flare between the radiating vessels. On diascopy, the central body pulsates.

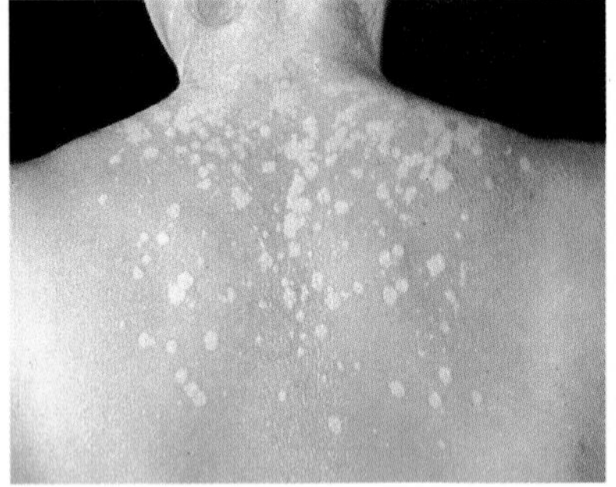

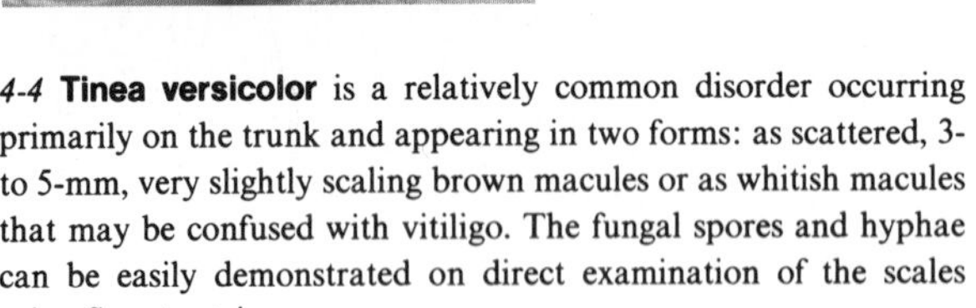

4-4 **Tinea versicolor** is a relatively common disorder occurring primarily on the trunk and appearing in two forms: as scattered, 3- to 5-mm, very slightly scaling brown macules or as whitish macules that may be confused with vitiligo. The fungal spores and hyphae can be easily demonstrated on direct examination of the scales using Swartz stain.

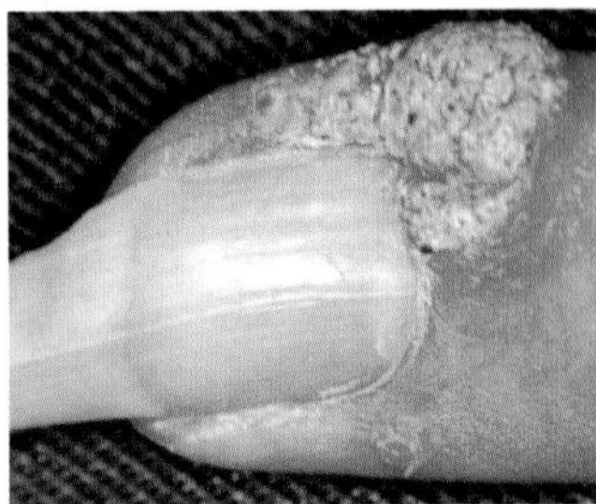

4-5 **Verruca vulgaris** may occur at any age, but it is most common in children. The lesions, which vary in size from 0.5 to 2.0 cm, are round or oval, firm, skin-colored papules with multiple tiny keratotic, rounded or filiform projections covering the surface (vegetation). They occur most frequently on the hands and soles.

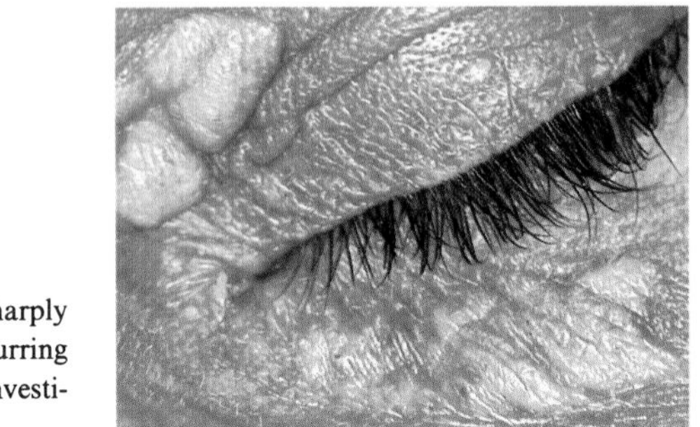

4-6 **Xanthelasma** consists of one or more bright yellow, sharply marginated plaques with no epidermal change, usually occurring on the eyelids, All patients with xanthelasma should be investigated for evidence of plasma lipid abnormalities.

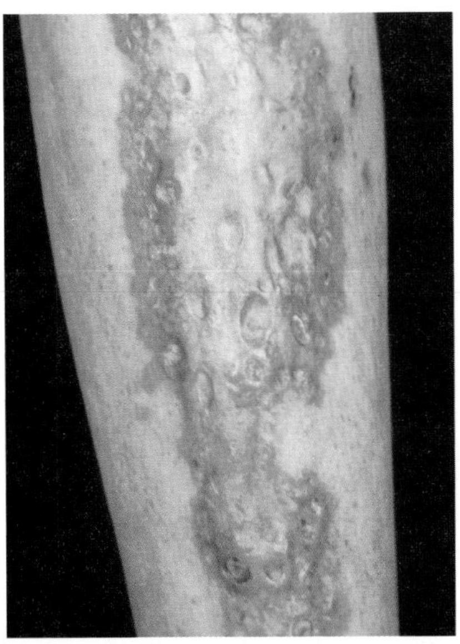

5-1 **Necrobiosis lipoidica diabeticorum.** Note the vivid colors (brown and yellow) and fine, arborizing blood vessels traversing the atrophic skin.

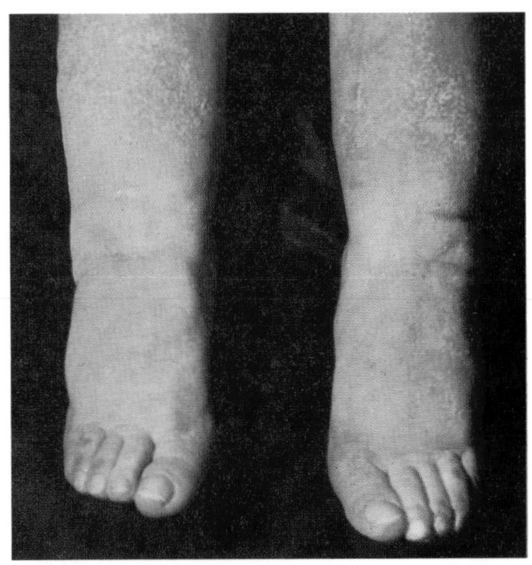

5-2 **Pretibial myxedema.**

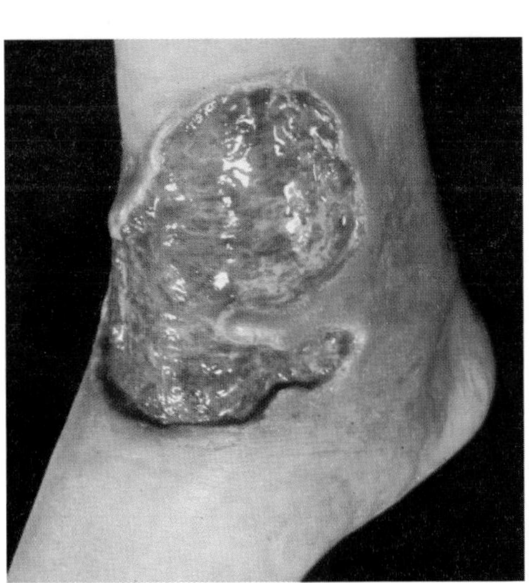

5-3 **Pyoderma gangrenosum** in a patient with ulcerative colitis.

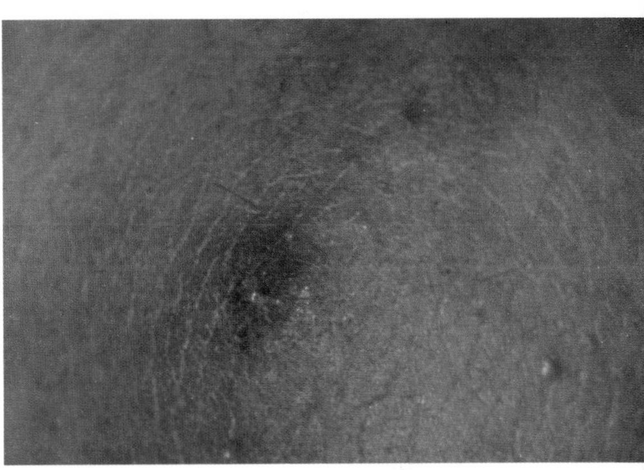

5-4 **"Palpable" purpura with inflammation occurring in gonococcemia.** An identical lesion may be seen in meningococcemia, staphylococcemia, and systemic vasculitis.

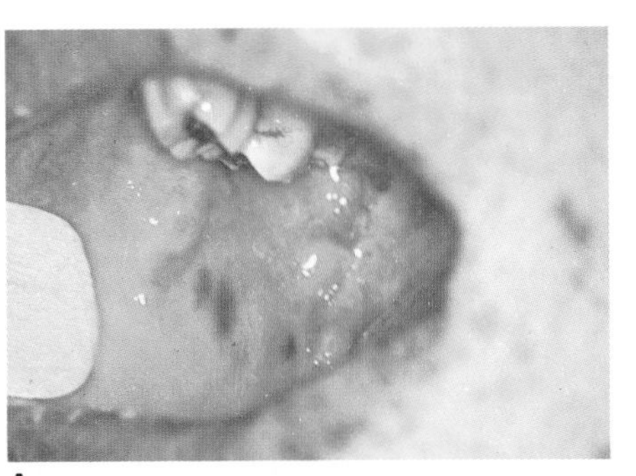

A B

5-5 **Peutz-Jeghers syndrome.** *A.* Macules on the buccal mucosae that are blue or blue-black and are pathogonomonic. *B.* Punctate dark brown macules that typically occur on the lips, around the mouth, and on the fingers. The pigmented macules may disappear on the lips but not on the buccal mucosa.

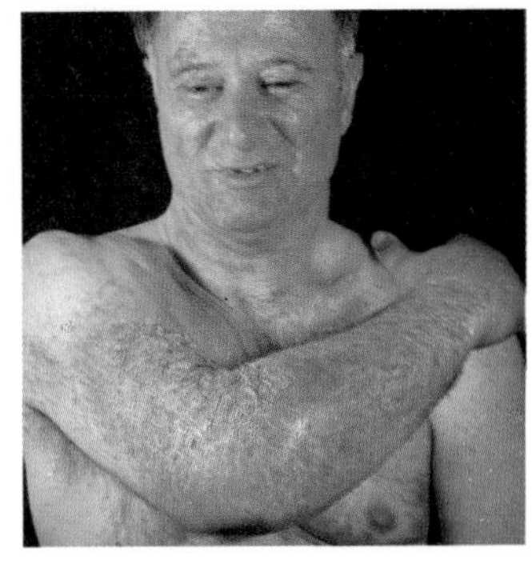

5-6 **Contact eczematous dermatitis.** The diagnosis is made by detailed history in the manner of a detective and also by the periodicity of the attacks. The artificial configuration (sharp borders, etc.) indicates an "outside job."

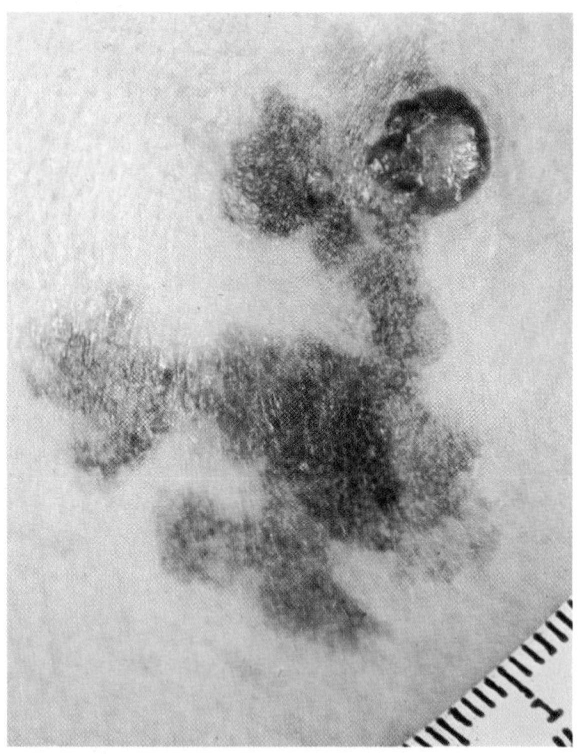

6-1 In **lentigo maligna melanoma,** the lesion is predominantly flat, but there may be a few nodules or papules. The color consists mainly of shades of brown and black, admixed with whitish gray and, occasionally, with reddish brown, bluish gray, and bluish black.

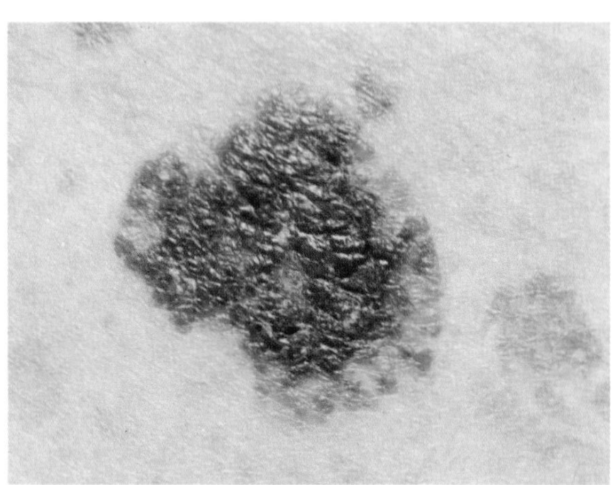

6-2 In **superficial spreading melanoma,** the lesion is usually slightly raised in its entirety and is punctuated with papules and, sometimes, nodules. The color consists mainly of brown and black, admixed with bluish red (violaceous), bluish gray, bluish black, reddish brown, and often whitish pink. The presence of a notched border is distinctive.

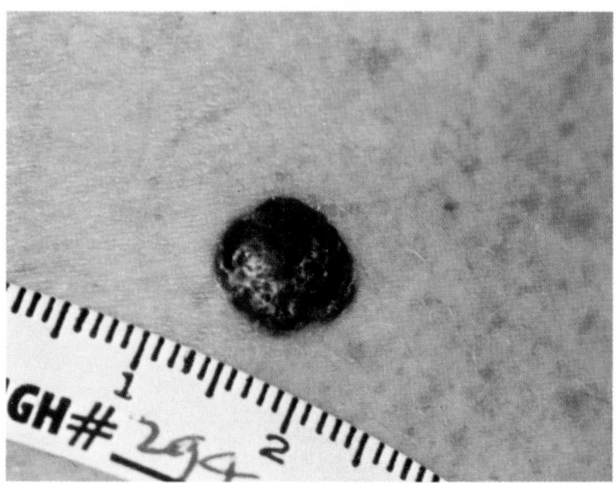

6-3 In **nodular melanoma,** the lesion is always raised and may be dome-shaped or polypoid. The color is usually uniform bluish black, but there may rarely be shades of reddish blue (purple) or an admixture of bluish black with brown or black.

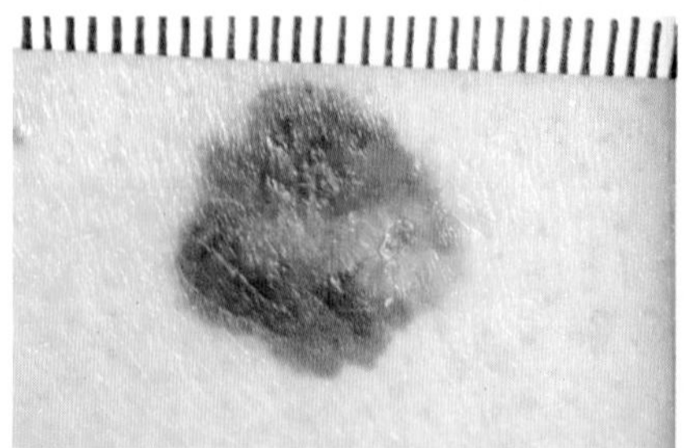

6-4 **Superficial spreading melanoma, superficially invasive.** At this very early stage in the evolution of this tumor, the variegation of color is the clue to the diagnosis.

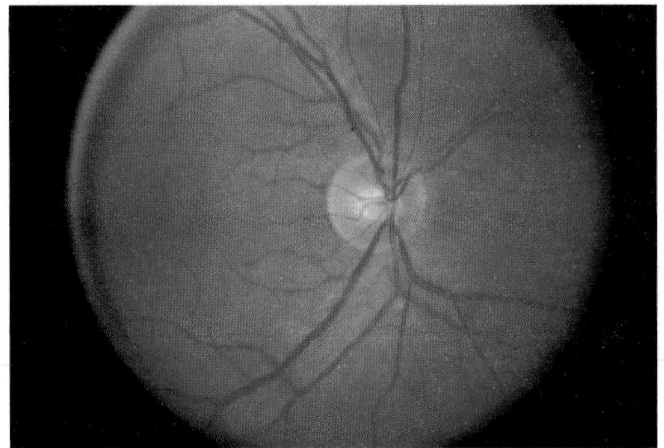

7-1 **Normal optic nerve and retina.**

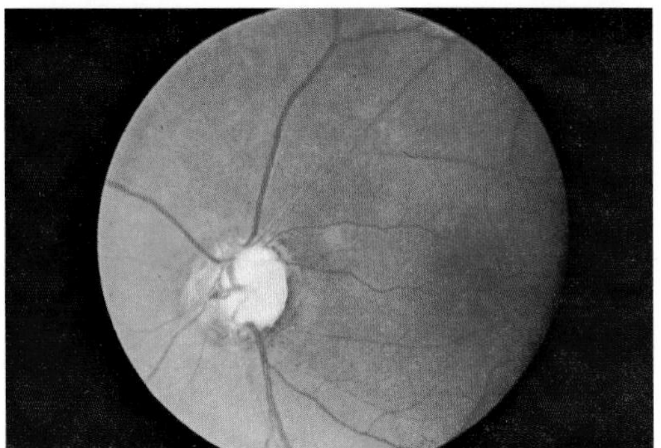

7-2 **Glaucomatous optic disk with secondary atrophy.**

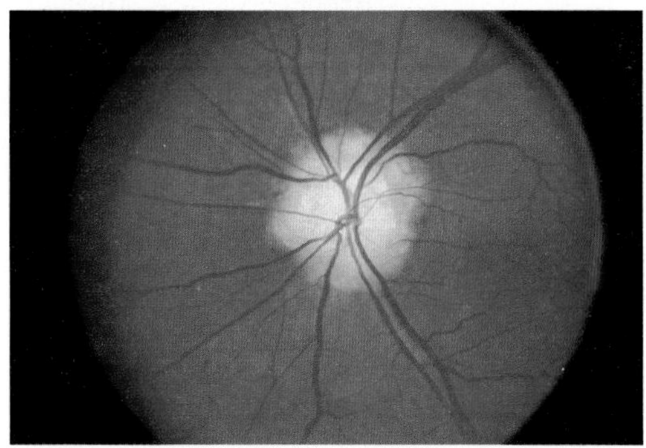

7-3 **Drusen of the optic nerve head.**

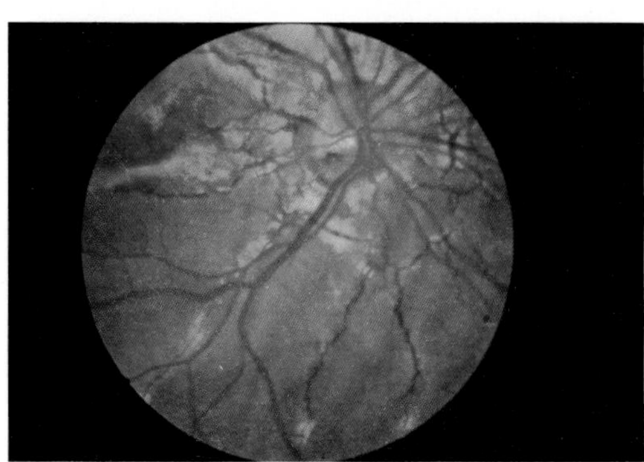

7-4 **Angioid streaks.**

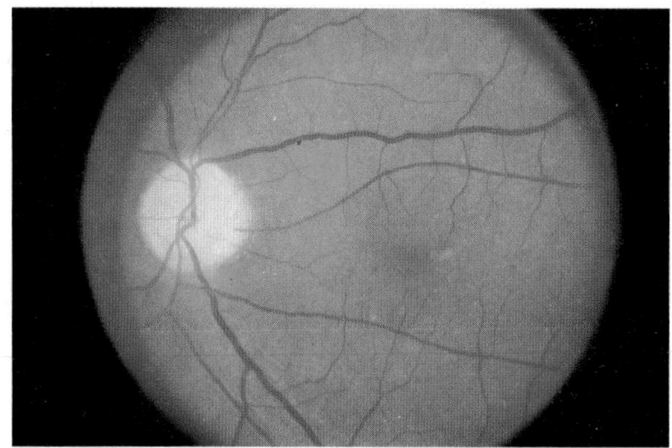

7-5 **Primary optic atrophy.**

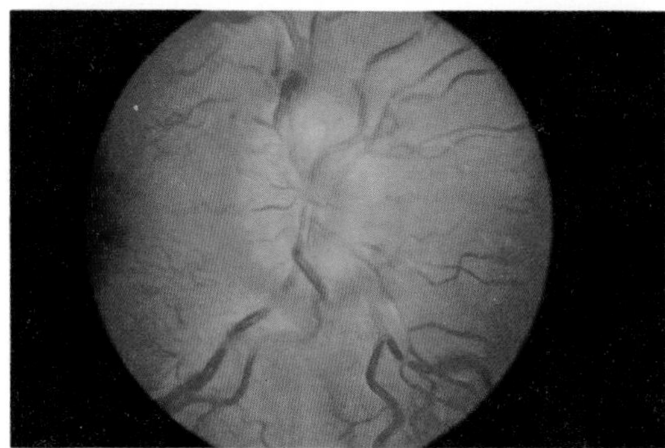

7-6 **Early papilledema.**

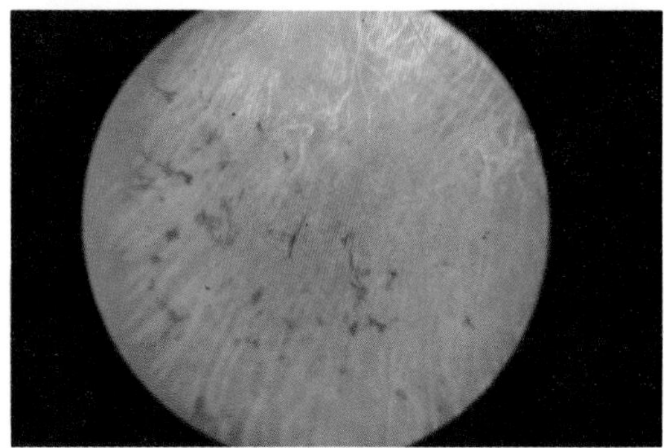

7-7 **Retinitis pigmentosa.**

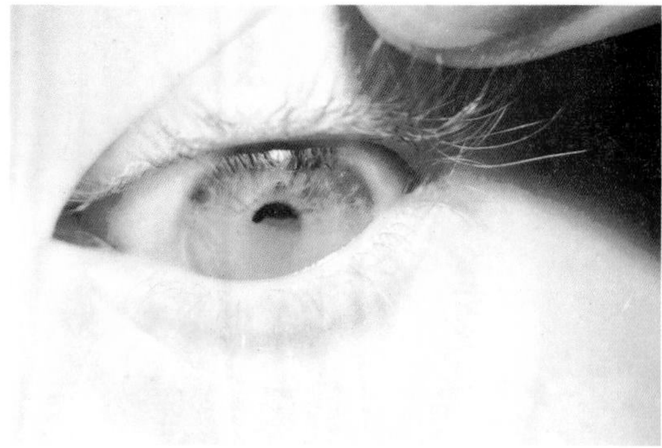

7-8 **Band keratopathy.**

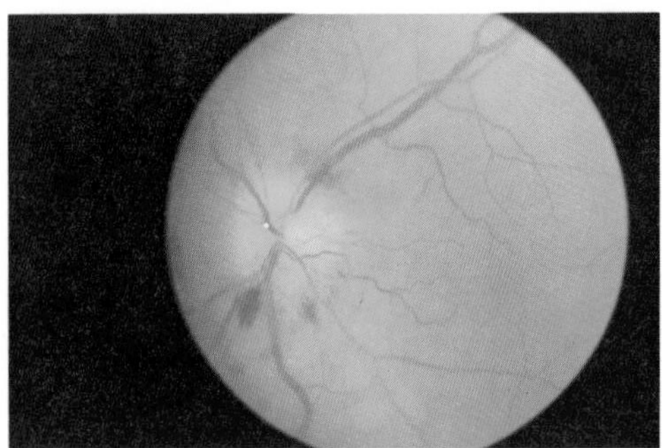

8-1 **Ischemic optic neuropathy.**

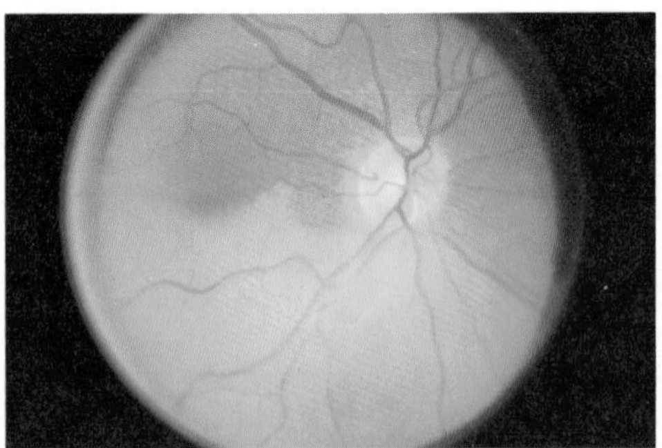

8-2 **Embolic branch artery occlusion with retinal infarction.**

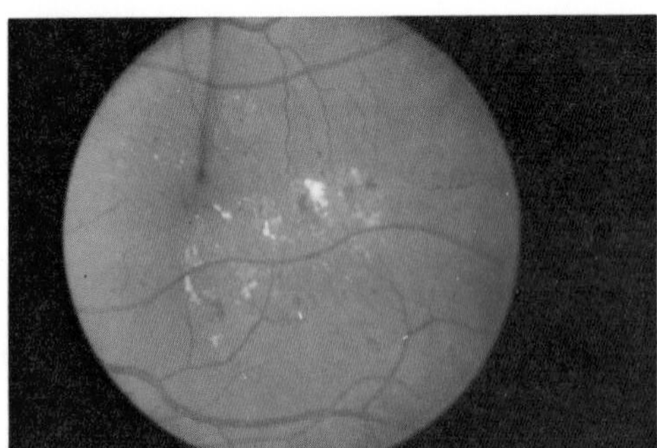

8-3 **Diabetic retinopathy with microaneurysms.**

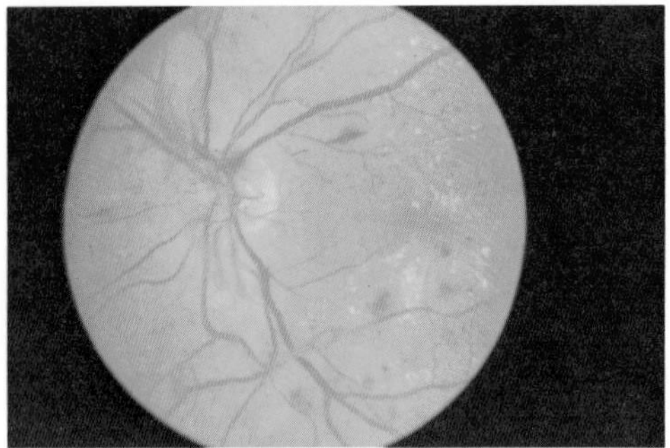

8-4 **Proliferative diabetic retinopathy.**

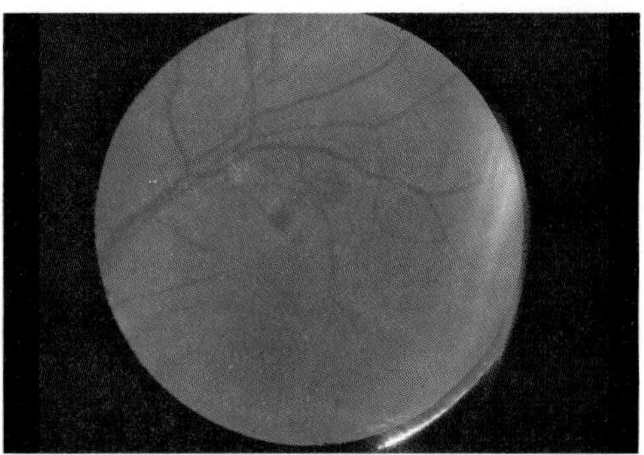

8-5 **Roth spot with subacute bacterial endocarditis.**

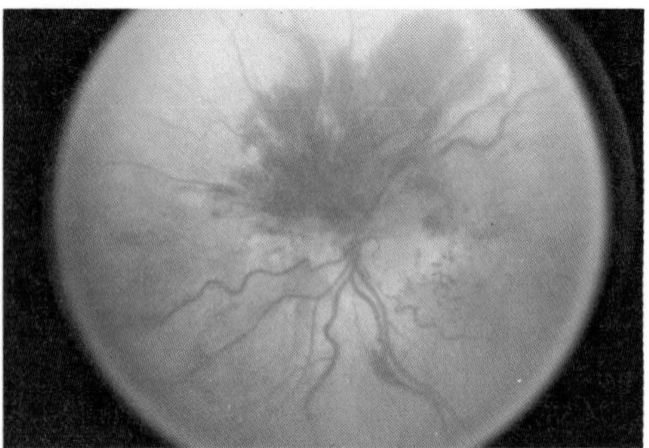

8-6 **Central retinal vein thrombosis.**

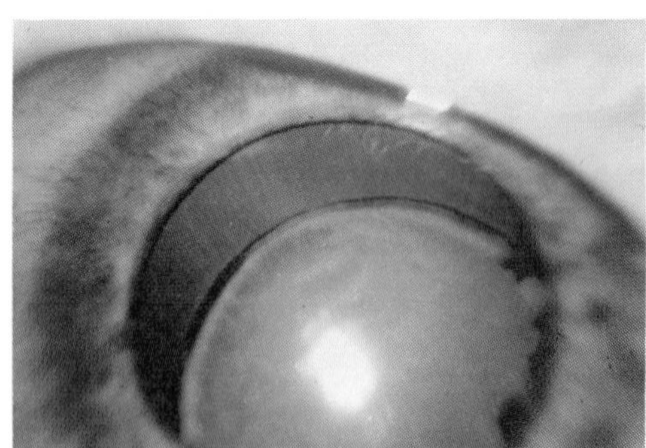

8-7 **Dislocated lens in Marfan's disease.**

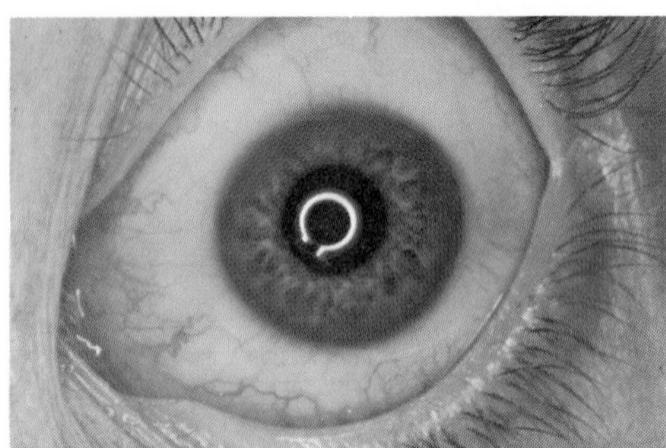

8-8 **Kayser-Fleischer ring in Wilson's disease.** (*Note:* The ring is the golden brown pigment at the periphery of the cornea and is characteristically broader superiorly and inferiorly than it is medially and laterally.)

Examination for mycelia The presence of mycelia may be ascertained by the application of 10% potassium hydroxide to a single tiny portion of scale, which is then gently heated. For fungi and yeasts, scales and hair should be cultured on Sabouraud's medium.

Tzanck test The Tzanck test, or the microscopic examination of cells from the base of vesicles, determines the presence of giant epithelial cells and multinucleated giant cells that occur in herpes simplex, herpes zoster, and varicella. Material taken from the base of a vesicle by gentle curettage with a scalpel is spread gently on a glass slide and prepared with Giemsa's or Wright's stain for the examination.

Dark-field examination of serum for *Treponema pallidum* Dark-field examination of serum from ulcers and erosions on the male and female genitalia is essential for the detection of *Treponema pallidum.* Dark-field examination of material obtained from the oral cavity is not diagnostic because of the presence of nonpathogenic treponemas that are indistinguishable from *T. pallidum.*

BIOPSY Microscopic examination of tissue is particularly applicable in dermatology because biopsies of the lesions can be easily obtained. Although the classic method is an elliptical incision followed by suturing, a satisfactory method for diagnostic purposes is "punch" biopsy. Biopsy of the skin enables correlation of gross and microscopic pathology. For punch biopsy, a small, 3.0- to 4.0-nm, disposable tubular blade is rotated between the thumb and index finger to cut through the entire thickness of the abnormal skin; the resulting cylinder of skin is then lifted out with forceps, and the skin is cut off at its base with a pointed scissors. This simple operation is done under local anesthesia, and the bleeding can be stopped by the use of pressure or absorbable foam; suturing is not usually necessary. This technique is as harmless and simple as a venipuncture, and supplies enough tissue to permit a definitive histologic diagnosis in most cases.

APPROACH TO DIAGNOSIS In Tables 49-2 and 49-3 an orderly sequence is suggested as a method of establishing a diagnosis in a patient presenting with skin lesions.

TABLE 49-3
Clinical classification of skin lesions and syndromes according to the component of the skin primarily involved

I Epidermis (keratinocytes and melanocytes)
- *A* Keratinocytes
  - *1* Scaling macules, papules, or plaques
  - *2* Vesicles and bullae
  - *3* Pustules
  - *4* Exudative (impetiginized) lesions
  - *5* Eczematous dermatitis
  - *6* Erythroderma syndrome (exfoliative dermatitis)*
  - *7* Atrophy, diffuse* or circumscribed
- *B* Melanocytes
  - *1* Hypomelanotic macules
  - *2* Diffuse hypomelanosis*
  - *3* Hypermelanotic (brown) macules
  - *4* Diffuse brown hypermelanosis*

II Dermis (connective tissue and blood vessels)
- *A* Connective tissue component
  - *1* Papules and nodules (with and without inflammation)
  - *2* Ulcers
  - *3* Sclerosis, diffuse* or circumscribed
  - *4* Edema*
  - *5* Atrophy, diffuse* or circumscribed
- *B* Blood vessels
  - *1* Morbilliform and scarlatiniform eruptions
  - *2* Urticarial syndromes
  - *3* Erythema multiforme syndrome
  - *4* Purpura (with and without inflammation)
  - *5* Infarcts
  - *6* Telangiectasia

III Panniculus adiposus (connective tissue and blood vessels)
- *A* Connective tissue component
  - *1* Nodules, noninflammatory, usually nontender
  - *2* Atrophy
- *B* Blood vessels
  - *1* Nodules, inflammatory, usually tender and red
    - *a* Erythema nodosum syndrome

* *Pathologic changes affect large areas of skin, and there are no discrete, circumscribed lesions.*

SOURCE: *TB Fitzpatrick, in Dermatology in General Medicine, 2d ed, TB Fitzpatrick et al (eds), New York, McGraw-Hill, 1979.*

REFERENCES

FISHER AA: *Contact Dermatitis,* 2d ed. Philadelphia, Lea & Febiger, 1973

FITZPATRICK TB et al (eds): *Dermatology in General Medicine,* 2d ed. New York, McGraw-Hill, 1979

LAZARUS GS, GOLDSMITH LA: Diagnosis of Skin Disease. Philadelphia, Davis, 1980, p 506

ROOK A, WILKINSON DS: The principles of diagnosis, in *Textbook of Dermatology,* A Rook et al (eds). Oxford, Blackwell Scientific Publications, 1979, p 37

50 SKIN LESIONS OF GENERAL MEDICAL SIGNIFICANCE

THOMAS B. FITZPATRICK
HARLEY A. HAYNES

The skin is one of the best indicators of serious disease; even an untrained eye can recognize the ashen pallor of shock, or cyanosis, or jaundice. The competent physician must be able to detect the subtle skin signs of life-threatening diseases and the skin clues to diseases in other organs. Skin lesions are frequently critical in the final resolution of puzzling diagnostic medical problems.

The skin (Fig. 50-1) is composed of three layers: (1) the *epidermis,* the outermost part, which consists of two main cell types, keratinocytes and melanocytes; (2) the *dermis,* upon which the epidermis rests, which is composed of a mélange of connective tissue elements, nerves, blood and lymph vessels, glands, appendages, and a few cells (mast cells, histiocytes); and (3) the *panniculus adiposus* (subcutaneous tissue), which acts as a cushion between the epidermis and dermis and the underlying bone. The specialized cells of the epidermis, the keratinocytes, produce and retain in their cytoplasm the scleroprotein keratin. They are constantly turning over, about 27 days being required to complete differentiation and maturation. Maturation of keratinocytes consists of loss of the nucleus, leaving only the cytoplasm. The latter is made up of a highly ordered, two-phase system of keratin filaments embedded in an amorphous matrix, much like the cellulose-lignin system of wood fiber, which is known to be well adapted to withstand shearing and compression forces. The anucleate outermost portion of the epidermis is the *stratum corneum,* which acts as a tough, keratinous membrane. The stratum corneum functions structurally as a "waterproof" wall between the internal fluid milieu and the environment, and is the major barrier of the skin, protecting the body against loss of fluids and entrance of toxic agents. It also serves as a passive membrane—substances move across the skin by passive diffusion in the direction of the concentration gradient.

The skin has a relatively limited number of pathologic responses. If the letters of the alphabet are taken to represent individual skin lesions (see Table 49-1), then words or phrases can be said to represent groups of lesions. The lesions in the majority of patients seen by the general physician can be classified in one of the groups of clinical reactions (see Table 49-3) or types of skin lesions listed in Table 49-1. These skin lesions or clinical reactions may consist of one type of lesion, such as a vesicle or a nodule, or aggregates of various types of lesions, such as papules or vesicles, as in erythema multiforme. Just one lesion or several solitary lesions or one or more groups of lesions may be distributed any place on the body. A pathologic process may involve the skin in the form of isolated lesions, as just mentioned, or the pathologic process may involve all the skin so that the borders of the lesions may not be defined; this latter type of diffuse involvement occurs in systemic sclerosis and in pigmentation disorders.

In the physician's attempts to identify the specific types of lesions, it is therefore essential to try to estimate the component of the skin that is *primarily* affected, as the epidermis, the dermis, the blood vessels, or the panniculus adiposus. Inasmuch as there are a finite number of disorders that produce pathologic changes in the various individual components, this method of approach will improve the physician's diagnostic acumen. For example, even though erythema multiforme involves the dermis and the epidermis, the *primary component* affected is the blood vessel, and it is this involvement that explains the erythematous macules; the inflammatory process leads subsequently to the development of the cellular infiltrates seen clinically as papules and to destruction of the basement membrane and the development of bullae.

FIGURE 50-1

Anatomy of the skin. (Copyright 1967 CIBA Pharmaceutical Company, division of CIBA-Geigy Corporation. Reproduced, with permission from the Clinical Symposia, illustrated by Frank H Netter, MD. All rights reserved.)

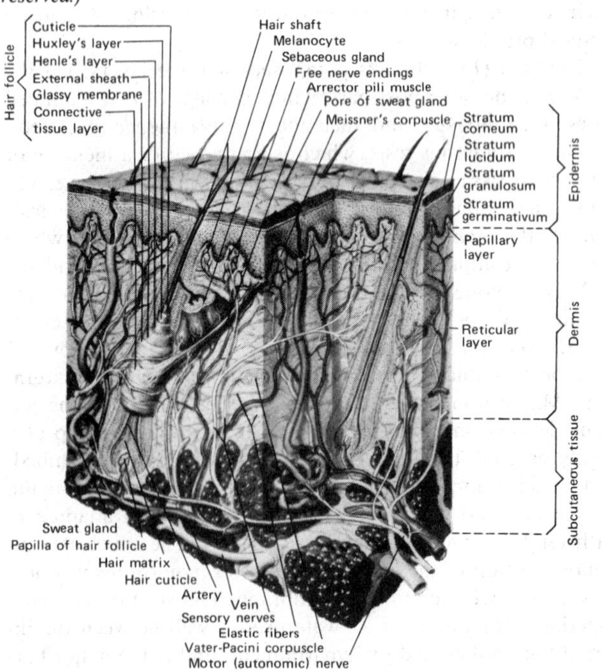

CLASSIFICATION OF LESIONS ACCORDING TO THE COMPONENT OF THE SKIN PRIMARILY AFFECTED

EPIDERMIS Scaling macules, papules, or plaques Generalized scaling macules, papules, or plaques are frequent and important diagnostic problems and are usually a presenting complaint of the patient (see Figs. 49-2, 49-3, and 49-11).

Sudden onset of symmetrical, scaling, erythematous macules or papules should suggest that drugs are the etiologic agents. Scaling erythematous papules on the scalp and extensor aspects of the arms and legs are suggestive of *psoriasis;* psoriatic lesions often are accentuated on the sites of repeated trauma, such as the elbows and knees. The papules or plaques of psoriasis often contain a silvery white micaceous scale that is relatively easily removed in layers (see Plate 2-6). In psoriasis, there is a severalfold increase in the normal number of the basal cells of the epidermis. This increase in the basal cell population reduces the turnover time of the epidermis from the normal 27 days to 3 to 4 days. With this shortened interval of epidermal cell migration from the basal layer to the skin surface, the normal events of cell maturation and keratinization do not occur (see A in Fig. 49-12); this failure of maturation is reflected by an array of abnormal morphologic and biochemical changes. In association with the basal cell hyperplasia, there is enhanced metabolism and accelerated synthesis and degradation of nucleoproteins, resulting in an elevated urinary excretion of nucleic acid metabolites such as uric acid. In addition, there is a proliferation of the subepidermal vasculature that is necessary to support the increased rate of cell division. These numerous cytologic, histologic, histochemical, and biochemical alterations are now known to be the result, rather than the cause, of the disease process. The only main fact known at this time about the fundamental cause of psoriasis is that the predisposition to its development is genetically transmitted. An erosive joint disease, *psoriatic arthritis,* is discussed in Chap. 348.

The treatment of psoriasis still remains the province of the dermatologist. The most effective treatment in the control of *localized psoriasis,* for most patients, is the use of topical corticosteroids with plastic wrap, topical coal-tar preparations, and ultraviolet light or sunlight exposures. Corticosteroids can also be injected directly into small, resistant plaques. Systemic corticosteroids not only are ineffective in psoriasis but may cause generalization of the process and are absolutely contraindicated. With certain patients who have generalized psoriasis, it has been necessary to use a variety of systemic chemotherapeutic agents, especially methotrexate; the latter has the capacity to inhibit cell replication without a proportionate inhibition of cell function, i.e., keratinization.

In 1974, a new form of photochemotherapy was introduced which uses oral methoxsalen and a high-intensity, long-wave ultraviolet light source. This approach may replace many of the other forms of therapy. In this so-called PUVA treatment, psoralen (P) is administered by mouth 2 h before total-body irradiation with a special light system that emits predominantly long-wave (320- to 400-nm) ultraviolet light (UV-A). The light alone is ineffective in producing erythema or remission of psoriatic lesions; however, in the presence of one of the psoralens (methoxsalen) the UV-A becomes a potent photoactive agent and produces a remission of psoriatic lesions after several exposures. The mechanism of action is probably related in part to the binding of psoralen to DNA by the action of UV-A. Multicenter clinical trials in the United States and Europe involving over 5000 patients have shown that oral methoxsalen photochemotherapy is highly effective in the control of severe psoriasis; in over 80 percent of such patients the psoriasis completely cleared in 3 to 4 weeks of treatment using two or four exposures per week. After clearing, the patients were given maintenance exposures once per week or less frequently. While methoxsalen photochemotherapy is effective, it requires specialized knowledge and lighting systems, delivering precisely measured amounts of UV-A. PUVA treatment is recommended only for patients with disabling psoriasis because long-term sequelae will not be known for a decade; such adverse effects could include skin cancers in certain susceptible patients (i.e., with history of previous exposure to arsenic or ionizing radiation) and cataracts.

The general physician does not always appreciate the impact of psoriasis as a major cause of disability and of disfigurement. Psoriasis affects between 2 and 8 million persons in the United States; about 100,000 are severely affected.

Psoriasiform lesions occurring on the face, lower abdomen, buttocks, groin, perineum, and legs occur in *glucagonoma syndrome.* The lesions may be almost indistinguishable from subacute psoriasis, but often they have necrosis in the center of the plaques; also stomatitis, anemia, and marked weight loss are present. Hyperglycemia may or may not be present. The eruption disappears rapidly on removal of the glucagon-secreting tumor of the pancreas.

Symmetrical scaling macules or papules localized on the palms and soles often are presenting signs of *secondary syphilis;* very frequently there is generalized lymphadenopathy and there may be mouth lesions occurring as erosions.

A relatively common and often baffling generalized scaling eruption is seen in *pityriasis rosea.* In this condition, the scale at the periphery of the lesion is very thin and forms a collarette; the center of the lesion may or may not be scaly. Pityriasis rosea typically has a "fir-tree" type of distribution, especially evident on the back. Very often, but not always, a preceding, single, isolated scaling lesion is present for several days before generalization of the lesions.

Scaling macules and papules are seen in *dermatophytosis* (Plate 2-1) and *candidiasis,* and it is therefore necessary that some of the scales be examined for the presence of mycelia (see "Laboratory Procedures," in Chap. 49).

From the clinician's point of view, *mycotic infections of the skin* may be separated into two major categories, each of which has a different etiology, associated systemic disease, and response to treatment, with only one category responding to the oral antifungal, griseofulvin.

The various types of *dermatophytosis* (so-called ringworm infections) constitute one category, and all (except tinea versicolor) respond to oral griseofulvin and are confined to the epidermis, hair, toenails, and fingernails. Dermatophytosis is due to three types of fungus: *Microsporum, Epidermophyton,* and *Trichophyton. Microsporum audouini,* a parasite of humans, is the principal pathogen causing epidemic urban fungous infection of the scalp. *Microsporum canis,* which affects the scalp and also the face, where it causes boggy nodules, is a parasite of animals and originates largely from young (usually) farm animals and pets (kittens, puppies, and calves). *Trichophyton rubrum, T. mentagrophytes,* and *E. floccosum,* which also are parasites of humans, are the agents usually causing dermatophytosis of the feet, the most common site of mycotic infection. The type of fungus infecting upper extremities, face, and trunk can be *Trichophyton* or *Microsporum* or *Epidermophyton.*

Inasmuch as *Trichophyton, Microsporum,* and *Epidermophyton* are parasites in humans, factors other than mere contact might be implicated. Variation in the host response, for instance, based on hereditary factors and mediated, possibly, through increased susceptibility or related to immune factors, has yet to be clearly defined.

The response of these three types of fungus to oral griseofulvin varies. Griseofulvin is effective, even in short courses, in fungous infection of the scalp, trunk, and groin, but even prolonged therapy rarely controls infection of the hands, fingernails, or toenails. Topical treatment with any of the antifungals is quite effective in infection of the feet, trunk, and groin, but is ineffective for infections of the fingernails or toenails.

The other major category of mycotic infections is represented by candidiasis (monilial infections). These infections do not respond at all to oral griseofulvin and are caused chiefly by *Candida albicans,* although occasionally by *C. tropicalis, C. krusei,* and *C. stellatoidea. C. albicans* can exist as a harmless saprophyte in the gastrointestinal tract and in the vagina. It is more common in females, and is most often present in those who are pregnant or who are taking oral contraceptives or broad-spectrum antibiotics. The association with diabetes mellitus, however, is so common that all patients (regardless of sex) with candidiasis should be screened for this disease.

Despite the fact that *C. albicans* is a normal saprophytic fungus in the vagina and gastrointestinal tract, it is rarely isolated from the exposed surface of the normal skin. *C. albicans* can invade the epidermis when the skin is exposed to high humidity and when the skin becomes macerated; therefore, candidiasis commonly occurs in the intertriginous areas (under the breasts and in the umbilicus, groin, and axillae) and in the oral, as well as the vaginal, mucous membranes. Chronic paronychia is usually caused by *C. albicans.* Candidiasis also may involve the lungs, urinary tract, and heart (see Chap. 184).

The treatment of candidiasis of the skin and mucous membranes depends on the site of the infection and the type of lesion. Maceration of the skin should be treated by air-drying of the area. Lotions and dusting powders containing nystatin are also very useful for intertriginous areas. Oral administration of nystatin is not of value in cutaneous moniliasis. Unless the sexual partner is treated when candidiasis is present, there will be constant retransfer of the infection. For monilial paronychia, 2% alcohol solutions of gentian violet are still the best treatment.

Differentiation between dermatophytosis caused by any of the three types of fungus already mentioned and candidiasis may be difficult, if not impossible, without cultures of the fungus. Direct examination of the scales from a scaling eruption in the intertriginous area is not diagnostic because it may reveal mycelia in both dermatophytosis and candidiasis; spores, however, are seen only in candidiasis. Too often, the general physician starts treatment with topical antifungal agents or with griseofulvin without establishing whether the eruption is a type of dermatophytosis or candidiasis. Inasmuch as candidiasis does not respond to systemic griseofulvin or to most of the topical antifungal agents, prescribing these agents for an eruption that is actually candidiasis results in prolonged disability for the patient. Newer agents such as haloprogin and miconazole are effective against both dermatophytosis and candidiasis.

In the past few years, fungous diseases have assumed a new significance in medicine because of the increased number of patients under treatment with chemotherapeutic agents for leukemia and other neoplasms. Almost all of the saprophytic fungi are now known to invade the tissues of patients who are being treated with chemotherapeutic agents or who have had kidney transplants.

Vesicles and bullae Some diseases may occasionally be associated with vesicles or bullae, such as erythema multiforme or porphyria cutanea tarda, but blisters (vesicles and bullae) are the major feature of a number of disorders: certain bacterial and viral infections; allergic contact dermatitis (such as poison ivy); trauma from mechanical, thermal, or chemical agents; and most important, the bullous diseases of unknown cause (such as pemphigus and pemphigoid).

Grouped vesicles occur in herpes zoster and herpes simplex, whereas scattered, discrete vesicles occur in varicella. A helpful sign in determining the nature of the vesicles is the Tzanck test (see "Laboratory Procedures," in Chap. 49). In herpes simplex, herpes zoster, and varicella, there will be clusters of epithelial giant cells, which are absent in vaccinia and variola. Skin biopsy will also establish the nature of the vesicle or bulla; that is, whether it is an intraepidermal (as seen in virus infections and pemphigus) or a subepidermal bulla (as seen in bullous pemphigoid) (see Figs. 49-7 to 49-9).

Vesicles arranged in linear streaks are characteristic of poison ivy dermatitis. The most reliable clue to the diagnosis of both allergic and primary-irritant contact dermatitis is the localization of vesicles to the skin areas likely to have been exposed to the agent in question. Isolated vesicles and bullae on the pressure areas of the dorsa of the hands and the face may be the only sign of porphyria cutanea tarda; the diagnosis is immediately confirmed by examination of the urine, using the Wood's lamp. These patients do not present with photosensitivity.

Scattered, isolated bullae in adults represent a special and serious problem in diagnosis and treatment. *Bullous pemphigoid* and *pemphigus* are chronic and occur primarily in adults; one of them, pemphigus, has serious consequences for the patient. These two disorders need to be distinguished by biopsy of the skin and by the newly available immunofluorescence techniques. It is impossible on the basis of clinical diagnosis alone to distinguish between bullous pemphigoid, which is a chronic and relatively benign disorder and often of limited duration, and *pemphigus vulgaris,* which is a serious disease leading in a relentless course to death, unless treatment with immunosuppressive agents or steroids is instituted. Pemphigus has been divided into four separate entities, but pemphigus vulgaris is the most important for the general physician to recognize. Pemphigus vulgaris may begin in the nasal or oral mucous membrane, and the patient may consult the dentist or otolaryngologist first for persistent erosions of the larynx (hoarseness), the mouth, or a bloody nasal discharge. The lesions tend to involve in an unpredictable fashion other parts of the body, but localize chiefly on the umbilicus, scalp, and trunk, although there is no specific distribution pattern. Pemphigus vulgaris affects primarily the middle-aged, particularly between the ages of 40 and 60. It rarely occurs before the age of 17 or after the age of 75. The clinical lesions appear as flaccid bullae from the beginning; they break easily and rarely become very large. The denuded areas that form at the site of the ruptured bullae increase in size as the epidermis detaches itself. Occasionally, almost the entire surface may be involved by large, denuded areas; this involvement represents a serious problem in the management of secondary infection and in maintenance of fluid balance—more or less the same problems that occur in a severely burned patient. Oral or nasal mucosal lesions occur in nearly all the patients, and more than half have lesions in the mucous membrane of the mouth as the first manifestation of the disease. The disease often starts with only a few lesions in the mouth and may remain limited in extent for several weeks; it then gradually spreads to other parts of the body.

The diagnosis of pemphigus is made on the basis of the light-microscopic examination of the biopsy of an early vesicle and direct immunofluorescence. The earliest change in pemphigus vulgaris consists of intercellular edema followed by disappearance of intercellular bridges in the lower epidermis (see A in Fig. 49-9). This results in loss of cohesion between the epidermal cells (acantholysis) and leads to the formation of clefts and then bullae that are predominantly in the suprabasal locations; in other words, the basal cells, although separated from one another, remain attached to the dermis much like a "row of tombstones."

Immunofluorescence allows detection of IgG antibodies specific for an intercellular substance of the skin and mucosa in the serum of patients with pemphigus, and makes possible a differentiation of pemphigus and pemphigoid by the localization of the antibody. The antibodies react with a specific intercellular antigen. The fluorescence is localized precisely to the site of acantholysis in pemphigus; IgG is confined to the glycocalyx of epidermal cells. In bullous pemphigoid, however, the antibodies react with the basement membrane, and the fluorescence is localized there.

Treatment of pemphigus with systemic corticosteroids, sometimes in combination with azathioprine, is quite successful. Azathioprine alone can control the disease in some patients.

Pustules This skin reaction (see Fig. 49-10) may result from infections or from sterile inflammation. Pustules may arise from preexisting vesicles of any etiology. Infection by pyogenic bacteria, especially staphylococci, as well as by certain fungi and mycobacteria, can produce pustules without a preceding vesicular stage. Noninfectious causes of pustules include acne, pustular psoriasis, and hypersensitivity to drugs, particularly sulfonamides, iodides, or bromides.

Exudative (impetiginized) lesions Acute infection with gram-positive cocci can occur as a primary process or may be superimposed on eczematous dermatitis or occasionally on any of the vesicular bullous diseases, and is characterized by the presence of crusts (see Fig. 49-13). Such infection on the skin has the same implications as a streptococcal pharyngitis, inasmuch as acute glomerular nephritis develops in a significant percentage of patients with impetiginized dermatitis. Patients with impetiginized dermatitis must be treated with full courses of systemic antibiotics.

Eczematous dermatitis Eczematous dermatitis (Plates 2-2 and 5-6) is not a specific disease entity but a characteristic inflammatory response of the skin due to both endogenous and exogenous agents that cause a delayed hypersensitivity reaction. Eczematous dermatitis therefore requires a qualifying etiologic term, e.g., *atopic eczematous dermatitis.* Eczematous dermatitis is sufficiently serious to account for the highest incidence of skin disease, being responsible for incalculable losses of time and productivity in industry; approximately one-third of all patients in the United States seen by dermatologists have eczema. In Tables 50-1 and 50-2 some of the types of eczematous dermatitis are summarized (see also B in Fig. 49-8 and Fig. 49-11). For the general physician, atopic eczematous dermatitis is the most important disease of this group of disorders. Over 30 percent of patients develop respiratory allergic manifestations. Furthermore, the disease may persist for 15 to 20 years. Cataracts develop in 15 percent of young patients. Finally, patients with atopic eczematous dermatitis are susceptible to infections with herpes simplex and vaccinia. The majority of patients with severe atopic eczematous dermatitis have elevated serum levels of IgE. The control of the intractable pruritus in this disease is difficult, and best results are obtained by judicious use of topical corticosteroids, tar gels, oil baths, lubrication with emollients, and limitation of emotional stress.

Erythroderma syndrome (exfoliative dermatitis) The erythroderma syndrome is an important dermatologic complication that may occur as the result of an extension of a drug reaction, as a generalized spreading of a preexisting dermatitis, such as psoriasis or atopic dermatitis, or in association with lymphoma and leukemia. This syndrome consists of a generalized, erythematous, scaling eruption involving all of the skin surface, and has important implications in general medicine because of the systemic effects occasioned by the massive and continuous exfoliation of the skin. The severity of the metabolic response to exfoliation depends on the duration and severity of the process itself. Patients with extensive exfoliative dermatitis may have negative nitrogen balance, edema, hypoalbuminemia, and loss of muscle mass. Another salient feature in these patients is the large extrarenal water loss, due to the defective cutaneous barrier that leads to markedly increased transepidermal water loss. Serious metabolic effects of chronic exfoliative dermatitis occur when the rate of scaling reaches 17 g/m^2 per 24 h. The etiology of exfoliative dermatitis determines its course: the disease eventually clears in patients with psoriasis or atopic dermatitis, whereas the prognosis is relatively poor in patients with lymphoma and leukemia. Approximately 60 percent of patients with exfoliative dermatitis recover within 8 to 10 months, 30 percent die, and 10 percent have a persistent problem unresponsive to therapy.

Atrophy, diffuse or circumscribed Epidermal atrophy is manifested by an almost transparent epidermis and is associated with a decrease in the number of epidermal cells. An atrophic epidermis may or may not retain the normal skin markings. Circumscribed epidermal atrophy occurs in discoid lupus erythematosus, in necrobiosis lipoidica diabeticorum, and in striae cutis distensae; diffuse epidermal atrophy occurs with aging and in scleroderma.

The most important atrophic-type disorder is *necrobiosis lipoidica diabeticorum* (NLD) (Plate 5-1). These lesions, which are usually asymptomatic, occur more frequently in women and *on the areas subject to trauma* such as the anterior and lateral surfaces of the lower legs. Lesions may also occur on the arms and even on the face. The lesion begins as a small, reddish, elevated nodule with a sharply circumscribed border, gradually enlarges, and becomes flattened and depressed as the skin becomes atrophic. The brownish-yellow color is prominent, and blood vessels are readily seen because of the atrophic epidermis that is smooth and loses its skin markings entirely. The lesions of NLD are extremely indolent, and shallow ulcerations that are very slow to heal may develop. NLD may apparently occur when diabetes mellitus cannot be detected, but in these patients full tests of glucose tolerance, such as the cortisone-glucose tolerance test, have not been done. It is characterized by focal changes in the dermis that present as acellular and intense eosinophilic areas of necrosis bordered by inflammation. The inflammatory cells are granulomatous and include epithelioid cells, histiocytes, and multinucleated giant cells. The blood vessels are always involved, with endothelial proliferation and sometimes even occlusion of the arterioles and arteries deep within the dermis; the capillary walls are thickened with focal deposits of PAS-positive material. NLD can be controlled with intralesional injections of suspensions of triamcinolone acetonide in some patients.

Hypomelanotic macules See Chap. 52.

Diffuse hypomelanosis See Chap. 52.

Hypermelanotic macules See Chap. 52.

Diffuse brown hypermelanosis syndrome See Chap. 52.

DERMIS Papules and nodules (with and without inflammation) Papules and nodules without epidermal change (i.e., scaling) may be either skin color, erythematous, or even slightly pigmented (yellow or brown). Dermal papules and all nodules require a biopsy for definitive diagnosis because they often

TABLE 50-1
Various types of eczematous dermatitis* of uncertain etiology

Clinical type	*Suspected pathogenesis*	*Diagnostic considerations*
Atopic eczematous dermatitis	Hereditary predisposition plus precipitating factors	Eczematous dermatitis, especially localized to the antecubital and popliteal fossae and to the face
Lichen simplex chronicus	Hereditary predisposition plus repeated local trauma	One or more lichenified plaques (see Fig. 49-11), especially on neck
Prurigo nodularis	Repeated local trauma	One or more nodules, especially on extremities
"Neurodermatitis"	Hereditary predisposition plus repeated scratching	Generalized or localized eczematous eruption at sites of repeated trauma
Stasis dermatitis	Chronic venous insufficiency	Signs of venous insufficiency
Nummular eczematous dermatitis	Various precipitating factors (contact irritants, xerosis, emotional stress, etc.)	Discrete coin-shaped patches, usually on extremities and trunk
"Dyshidrotic" eczematous dermatitis	Emotional stress plus other factors‡	Vesicles and bullae on palms and soles
Seborrheic dermatitis	Constitutional diathesis	Greasy scaling patches on scalp, eyebrows, and nasolabial area
Various patterns of eczematous dermatitis	Association with gastrointestinal malabsorption	Eczematous eruption in patient with steatorrhea and abnormal biopsy specimens of the jejunal mucosa
"Eczematous-like eruptions"† with systemic disease: Wiskott-Aldrich syndrome; X-linked agammaglobulinemia; Phenylketonuria; Ahistidinemia; Hurler's syndrome; Hartnup disease; Acrodermatitis enteropathica	Metabolic and immunologic disorders	Related features of clinical syndrome plus immunologic deficiency or biochemical abnormality

* *This term is used by many clinicians for at least four types of eczematous dermatitis that may be exclusively localized to the hands (atopic eczematous dermatitis, allergic contact eczematous dermatitis, nummular eczematous dermatitis, and "dyshidrotic" eczematous dermatitis). Possibly, contact irritants to which the hands are frequently exposed may precipitate or aggravate one of the above-mentioned basic types of eczematous dermatitis.*

† *These eruptions are reported in the literature as eczematous dermatitis, but clear, careful clinical descriptions with cutaneous biopsy specimens are frequently lacking.*

‡ *Such as constitutional diathesis and contact dermatitis.*

represent either processes that have general medical significance, such as sarcoidosis or histiocytosis X, or tuberculosis or lymphoma. Inasmuch as dermal nodules may be present in deep mycotic infections such as coccidioidomycosis, it is necessary to obtain a biopsy, not only to rule out malignancy but to culture a portion of the excised tissue for fungi. Cultures of nodules must be made from minced tissue. The histologic specimen should be carefully studied for the presence of acid-fast bacilli, since nodules are the presenting feature of leprosy or tuberculosis; nodules removed from the common areas of localization for leishmaniasis (face and arms) should be carefully examined for the presence of parasites.

Papules and nodules with and without inflammation can occur in disorders of the sebaceous glands. Sebaceous glands are distributed largely on the face and scalp, although they can also occur in the labia minora and on the scrotal skin, trunk, nipples, and eyelids. The sebaceous gland is a holocrine gland in which the entire cell is cast off into the excretory stream. Sebum is a complex lipid mixture of squalene (a major product of the steroid pathway), triglycerides, and wax ester. Sebaceous glands are controlled by direct hormonal stimulation with androgens, derived largely from the gonads in both sexes; in the female, but not in the male, adrenal androgens may be important factors in maintaining sebum production. The major disease of the sebaceous gland in humans is *acne vulgaris* (Plate 1-5), which occurs predominantly on the face and, to a lesser degree, on the back, chest, and shoulders. It is characterized by a variety of clinical lesions. These lesions may be either noninflammatory or inflammatory papules and nodules. The noninflammatory papules are called comedones, and these may be either open (blackheads) or closed (whiteheads). The closed comedones are the precursors of large inflammatory nodules and of papules and pustules. In addition, cysts and scars of various sizes may occur, the typical acne scar being a sharply punched-out pit. In the pustular and cystic lesions, despite a large amount of purulent exudate that may be recovered following incision, the lesions are usually sterile but may contain *Propionibacterium acnes.* It is believed that acne develops as a result of a primary inflammation in the follicle wall, and that the follicle partly ruptures, leading to a spilling out of its components and the development of a perifollicular inflammatory process. The inflammatory infiltrate is lymphocytic, but later, as a result of the presence of keratinous material, gram-positive diphtheroids, and sebum, the infiltrate consists essentially of a foreign-body giant-cell reaction.

The initial stimulus to the formation of comedones (both the closed and open types) is not precisely known at this time, but the initial histologic event in comedone formation is excessive keratinization within the follicular canal. It is currently believed that *Propionibacterium acnes* is responsible for lipolysis with a release of fatty acids; it is thought that these fatty acids are capable of producing an inflammatory process in the follicle wall. Acne vulgaris is a serious problem, especially common during adolescence, and its therapy is complex and prolonged. Moderate to severe acne vulgaris is best treated by a dermatologist who has a number of modalities: topical agents, incision and drainage of the cystic lesions, ultraviolet light therapy, and judicious use of systemic antibiotics; x-ray therapy has no place in the treatment of acne vulgaris.

The mechanism of action of antibiotics such as tetracycline is not completely understood, but these drugs are known to suppress the number of propionibacteria and to cause a reduction of free fatty acids recoverable from the skin. Because the organisms have been shown to have lipolytic activity in vitro, it is presumed that the antibiotic causes this reduction of free fatty acids. Benzoyl peroxide lotions and gels probably act as antibacterial agents and decrease the bacterial population; these agents are very effective and are widely used by dermatologists.

Estrogens combined with progestins (oral contraceptives) were initially considered to be effective in controlling acne; however, they have been of only limited value in the treatment of acne in females and cannot be given to males. There is no evidence suggesting that diet has any effect on the course or severity of acne vulgaris. Acne vulgaris may begin as early as the eighth year or may not appear until the twentieth. It lasts for several years and then subsides spontaneously, usually when the patients are in their early twenties. In some patients, however, acne vulgaris may continue into the third and fourth decades. Topical antibiotic solutions such as clindamycin or erythromycin are effective new agents for treatment of acne vulgaris. The most dramatically effective new treatment for severe cystic acne is orally administered 13-*cis*-retinoic acid. This drug acts rapidly and is very effective.

Pretibial myxedema (PM) also may cause nodules on the legs and dorsa of the feet (Plate 5-2). The lesions are usually bilateral and consist of elevated, firm, dermal nodules and plaques that are not easily movable. They may be skin color, pink, or, rarely, brown, and, when diascoped, appear yellow and waxy. The epidermis over the nodules may appear normal or may have a marked verrucous (warty) surface. The pathogenesis of pretibial myxedema is not clear. Pretibial myxedema may occur with or without hyperthyroidism (Graves' disease) or before or after treatment of hyperthyroidism, and its development does not parallel the ocular changes (if present). The nodules in pretibial myxedema are accumulations of mucopolysaccharides, which can be demonstrated by special staining of the histopathologic material. LATS (long-acting

TABLE 50-2
Various types of eczematous dermatitis* of known etiology

Clinical type	*Pathogenesis*	*Diagnostic considerations*
Allergic contact eczematous dermatitis	Chemical allergens (plants, medicaments, cosmetics, metals, fabrics, etc.)	Site and configuration are clues to causal agent; patch tests may confirm diagnosis; avoidance of cause cures eruption
Photoallergic contact eczematous dermatitis	Ultraviolet radiation plus topical chemicals (in soaps, perfumes, citrus fruits, etc.), which then become allergens	Occurs on exposed skin; photopatch tests confirm diagnosis
Polymorphous light-induced eruption—eczematous type	Ultraviolet radiation; sometimes visible light	Occurs on exposed skin; diagnosis implies that all known causes of light-induced eruptions have been eliminated
"Infectious eczematoid dermatitis"	Bacterial products from draining focus (e.g., ear infection)	Occurs near site of infection; responds to treatment of primary infection
Eczematous dermatophytosis	Fungus	Fungi demonstrated in scales or exudate

* *This term is used by many clinicians for at least four types of eczematous dermatitis that may be exclusively localized to the hands (atopic eczematous dermatitis, allergic contact eczematous dermatitis, nummular eczematous dermatitis, and "dyshidrotic" eczematous dermatitis). Possibly, contact irritants to which the hands are frequently exposed may precipitate or aggravate one of the above-mentioned basic types of eczematous dermatitis.*

thyroid stimulator), which is associated in the plasma with immunoglobulin G (7 S gamma globulin), has been implicated in the pathogenesis of pretibial myxedema, exophthalmos, and acropachy; the role of LATS in the pathogenesis of pretibial myxedema has not been established.

Ulcers Ulcers occur as a result of destruction of the epidermis and, at least, the papillary layer of the dermis (see Fig. 49-4). All ulcers of the skin that do not heal within a period of a month must be assumed to be carcinoma until proved otherwise, and it is essential that a biopsy be obtained to rule out malignancy. Ulcers can be divided into two categories: lesions that occur on the legs and feet, and lesions that occur elsewhere on the body. Ulcers not occurring on the legs are rather rare except in primary cancer of the skin or in malignant metastases to the skin. Ulcers arising in nodules with inflammation should be approached in the manner suggested previously for nodules—that is, a biopsy should be obtained, and the tissue examined for bacterial, mycotic, and parasitic diseases. Chancre-like ulcerations and noduloulcerative lesions with regional lymphadenopathy may occur in primary syphilis and primary tuberculosis and in tularemia, anthrax, glanders, and bubonic plague. Isolated noduloulcerative lesions may be seen in sporotrichosis, coccidioidomycosis, leishmaniasis, cryptococcosis, and tertiary syphilis. Serologic studies are necessary in the diagnosis of syphilis.

The most prominent etiologic factors in ulceration on the legs and feet are disturbances of circulation. Chronic venous insufficiency leads to ulceration, especially on the medial aspect of the ankle or lower leg, and the ulcers develop in areas of skin with brownish hemosiderin pigmentation and occasionally where there is edema or sclerosis of the area. Hypertensive or ischemic ulcerations tend to start on the lateral aspect of the ankle. Ulceration can also occur as a result of tissue infarction in areas supplied by either large or small blood vessels (arteries, arterioles); this infarction may occur as the result of occlusion or constriction due to a variety of etiologic factors, in addition to those already mentioned: emboli, thrombosis, cryoagglutinins, macroglobulinemia, cryoglobulinemia, thrombotic thrombocytopenic purpura, polycythemia, systemic lupus erythematosus, Raynaud's phenomenon, arteriosclerosis obliterans, and thromboangiitis obliterans. Ulceration of the lower extremities also occurs in hemolytic anemia, including sickle cell anemia, thalassemia, and hereditary spherocytosis.

Some ulcers show extensive necrosis of the edges, such as those in *pyoderma gangrenosum* (Plate 5-3), an indolent ulcer usually on the lower extremities and often associated with ulcerative colitis or regional ileitis. The ulcers in pyoderma gangrenosum have ragged bluish-red overhanging edges and a necrotic base. These lesions often start as pustules or tender red nodules at the site of trauma, and then gradually increase in size until liquefaction necrosis occurs and an irregular ulcer develops. The ulcers are often multiple and may cover large areas of the leg. The histopathologic findings are not specific. The healing of the ulcers usually parallels the activity of the ulcerative colitis, and, inasmuch as the ulceration extends into and involves the reticular layer of the dermis and the subcutis, scarring occurs.

The term *"tropical" ulcer,* in addition to cutaneous leishmaniasis, now also includes ulceration due to cutaneous diphtheria, treponemal disorders (syphilis, yaws, and bejel), and phagedenic ulcer, a chronic ulcer of the feet and legs caused by mixed bacteria that occurs in persons suffering from starvation and neglect.

Ulcers can be associated with peripheral neuropathy ("neuropathic" ulcer, or malum perforans) seen in diabetes mellitus, tabes dorsalis, polyneuritis, leprosy, congenital anesthesia, or hereditary sensory radicular neuropathy.

Anal and perianal ulcers are seen in histiocytosis X and in amebiasis. A hanging-drop preparation is necessary to detect *Entamoeba histolytica.*

Ulcers with artificial and bizarre shapes must be suspected of being self-induced by means of destructive agents such as acid and lighted cigarettes. Factitial ulcers are overstudied and, unfortunately, underdiagnosed by most physicians.

Stony-hard, noduloulcerative lesions, particularly around joints (elbows, knees, and fingers) are suggestive of calcinosis cutis or gout; roentgenographic examination enables the detection of calcinosis cutis but shows no opaque bodies in gout.

Sclerosis, diffuse or circumscribed Diffuse sclerosis of the skin is most often seen on the upper extremities, chest, and face in systemic scleroderma (sometimes called progressive systemic sclerosis). Initially, the skin appears yellowish and shows slight nonpitting edema; later, however, it becomes indurated, bound down, and may be markedly hyperpigmented. Calcinosis cutis and Raynaud's phenomenon commonly occur.

Circumscribed sclerosis occurs in *morphea,* which consists of one or more round or oval, firm, reddish plaques up to several centimeters in diameter that become white or yellow centrally, often with a lilac-colored, telangiectatic border. This disorder is not associated with any other organ involvement and is a localized cutaneous form of scleroderma. Another type of localized scleroderma is *linear scleroderma,* in which the morphologic change is the same as that seen in morphea except that the process occurs in bands extending parallel to the long axis of the extremity or along the paramedian line of the forehead and scalp. This form of scleroderma has no relationship to progressive systemic sclerosis.

Edema In addition to the various causes of localized edema and generalized edema, there is a type of edema of the lower extremities that is not often recognized by the physician. This is a bilateral pedal edema which is common in patients with subacute or chronic dermatitis of the lower extremities. This type of edema is most often seen with chronic eczematous dermatitis and psoriasis, but is unrelated to cardiac failure or lymphatic obstruction. It is most probably due to an increased permeability as a result of local capillary damage, which is part of the inflammatory process in the skin. The increased capillary permeability leads to an increased transfer of fluid from the intravascular to the extravascular component of the extracellular fluid space. This type of pitting edema disappears completely when the dermatitis has resolved.

Atrophy, diffuse or circumscribed Dermal atrophy results from a decrease of the papillary or reticular connective tissue and is manifested in the skin as a depression. Circumscribed dermal atrophy may follow trauma, or may occur in association with epidermal atrophy, as in the striae of pregnancy or in Cushing's disease.

PANNICULUS ADIPOSUS (SUBCUTIS) Nodules (inflammatory, usually tender, red) Nodules in the subcutis may be recognized by the fact that the skin is usually movable over the nodule; occasionally, however, in inflammatory processes, the nodule may involve both the dermis and panniculus adiposus, and the skin will then not be movable over the nodule. Acute, tender, red nodules on the leg are characteristically found in two disorders: *erythema nodosum syndrome* and *nodular subcutaneous fat necrosis* associated with pancreatitis.

The erythema nodosum syndrome refers to the occurrence of multiple bilateral tender nodules appearing principally on the anterior aspect of the lower extremities and occasionally on the upper extremities and face. The erythema nodosum syndrome is associated with a number of disorders that are unrelated to each other.

The nodules in erythema nodosum are only slightly elevated, edematous, and sometimes exquisitely tender. Bruising is a characteristic feature of the disease and is due to hemorrhage, leading to the formation of contusions. The lesions never ulcerate or become indurated and very seldom leave any scarring or atrophy. Erythema nodosum is associated with primary tuberculosis and primary coccidioidomycosis, histoplasmosis, *Yersinia* infection, beta-hemolytic streptococcal infections, lymphogranuloma venereum, leprosy, sarcoidosis, ulcerative colitis, Crohn's disease, regional enteritis, drugs (penicillin, sulfonamides, bromides, iodides), and oral contraceptives containing ethynylestradiol and norethynodrel.

Tender, red subcutaneous nodules may also appear on the legs in association with acute pancreatitis and with pancreatic neoplasms and are often erroneously called erythema nodosum. This disorder has been termed *nodular liquefying panniculitis* (NLP). These lesions are distinctive. Their morphologic features are different from those of classic erythema nodosum. The lesions in NLP vary in size from a few millimeters to several centimeters, and, in contrast to the lesions of erythema nodosum, are movable. The lesions of NLP involute in 2 to 3 weeks and may leave a hyperpigmented scar that is slightly depressed. The nodules are often associated with abdominal pain and may also be accompanied by fever and arthralgia. Rarely, lesions may be present on other parts of the body besides the legs. Some of the larger nodules may undergo an abscess-like change, becoming fluctuant, and may rupture, exuding a whitish, creamy, or oily viscous material; abscess formation with drainage rarely, if ever, occurs in erythema nodosum. The most common pancreatic neoplasm associated with NLP is an acinous adenocarcinoma of the pancreas. In *Weber-Christian panniculitis,* the subcutaneous nodules, which at first are slightly mobile, become adherent to the overlying skin; then, as the edema subsides in the area of induration, a central depression occurs.

In addition to the above-mentioned entities, various types of vasculitis may also produce tender subcutaneous nodules. Therefore, diagnosis of these lesions often requires an excisional or incisional biopsy.

Nodules (noninflammatory, usually nontender, nonerythematous) Movable, painless, noninflammatory-appearing nodules occur around joints in rheumatic fever, rheumatoid arthritis, and in certain metabolic diseases such as xanthoma, gout, and calcinosis. Metastatic carcinoma or metastatic malignant melanoma may appear as movable, nontender subcutaneous nodules. Sarcoidosis may be manifested in the skin solely as subcutaneous nodules on the lower extremities. Subcutaneous nodules also occur in onchocerciasis and loiasis. *Lipomas,* relatively common causes of subcutaneous nodules, are benign tumors composed of adipose tissue and may be single or multiple and are frequently lobulated; they are often rubbery or compressible and occur most often on the trunk and back of the neck and forearms. Occasionally, subcutaneous lipoma may be painful and associated with marked obesity; this condition, known as *Dercum's disease,* is most common in middle-aged females.

Atrophy, diffuse or circumscribed Atrophy of the panniculus adiposus produces depressions in the skin; these depressions are seen in progressive lipodystrophy, in liquefying panniculitis, and in the localized fat atrophy that occurs at the site of injections of insulin. About 25 percent of diabetics who receive insulin (most often females under the age of 20) have this type of atrophy. The depressed areas of localized fat atrophy show a complete absence of the panniculus, and there is no inflammation. In lipodystrophy, diffuse atrophy of the skin may involve large portions of the body.

BLOOD VESSELS Morbilliform and scarlatiniform eruptions Morbilliform (measle-like) and scarlatiniform eruptions are macular and papular exanthems and can be due to drug hypersensitivities, measles, German measles, erythema infectiosum, viral exanthems, rickettsial diseases including endemic murine typhus and Rocky Mountain spotted fever, scarlet fever, and secondary syphilis. Many of the diseases manifested by macules or papules and occurring in acutely ill patients with a fever are listed in Table 50-3.

Urticaria Urticaria is characterized by wheals, of which the outstanding feature is their persistence for only a few hours (see Fig. 49-6). This short duration differentiates urticarial wheals from the otherwise almost identical papules of erythema multiforme, which persist for more than 1 or 2 days rather than for a few hours. An acute onset of urticaria is usually related to ingestion of drugs or certain types of foods (shellfish, fresh berries).

Chronic recurrent urticaria is a special problem, and its causes are not easily established. Most patients with this disorder require a careful examination for cryptic diseases such as lymphoma, systemic lupus erythematosus, primary or meta-

TABLE 50-3
Rash and fever in the acutely ill patient: Diagnosis according to type of lesion

DISEASES MANIFESTED BY MACULES OR PAPULES	
Drug hypersensitivities	Rocky Mountain spotted fever (early lesions)*
Scarlet fever	Pityriasis rosea
Erythema infectiosum (fifth disease)	Erythema multiforme
Measles (rubeola)	Erythema marginatum
German measles (rubella)*	Systemic lupus erythematosus*
Enterovirus (echo- and coxsackievirus) infections	Dermatomyositis
Adenovirus infections	"Serum sickness"* (manifested only as wheals)
Typhoid fever	Urticaria, acute (viral hepatitis)
Secondary syphilis	Urticaria, persistent (necrotizing angiitis)
Typhus, murine (endemic)	

DISEASES MANIFESTED BY VESICLES, BULLAE, OR PUSTULES	
Drug hypersensitivities	Variola†
Dermatitis from plants	Enterovirus (echo- and coxsackievirus) infections, including hand-foot-mouth disease
Rickettsialpox	Toxic epidermal necrolysis
Varicella (chickenpox)†	Staphylococcal scaled-skin syndrome
Generalized herpes zoster†	Erythema multiforme bullosum
Disseminated herpes simplex†	
Eczema herpeticum†	
Disseminated vaccinia†	
Eczema vaccinatum†	

DISEASES MANIFESTED BY PURPURIC MACULES, PURPURIC PAPULES, OR PURPURIC VESICLES	
Drug hypersensitivities	Enterovirus (echo- and coxsackievirus) infections
Bacteremia:‡	Rickettsial diseases:
Meningococcemia (acute or chronic)*	Rocky Mountain spotted fever*
Gonococcemia*	Typhus, louse-borne (epidemic)
Staphylococcemia	"Allergic" vasculitis*,‡
Pseudomonas bacteremia	Purpura fulminans‡
Subacute bacterial endocarditis	

* *May have arthralgia or musculoskeletal pain.*
† *One characteristic lesion of these exanthems is an umbilicated papule or vesicle.*
‡ *Often present as infarcts.*
SOURCE: *TB Fitzpatrick, RA Johnson, in Dermatology in General Medicine, 2d ed, TB Fitzpatrick et al (eds), New York, McGraw-Hill, 1979.*

static carcinoma, intestinal parasites, acute hepatitis, systemic vasculitis, or dermatomyositis. It is especially important, even in chronic urticarias, to carry out a painstaking interrogation of the patient in search of a history of drugs. Aspirin is one of the most common causes of chronic urticaria and can often be missed even in a careful drug history because many patients do not consider aspirin a drug. It is probably true that some patients with chronic urticaria can relate their problem to emotional stress, but this should be considered only after excluding all possible organic causes.

Erythema multiforme syndrome Erythema multiforme syndrome is a characteristic response of the skin and mucous membranes that is related to a number of possible etiologies, including infectious agents (herpesvirus hominis, *Mycoplasma pneumoniae*) and drugs (especially penicillin, antipyretics, barbiturates, hydantoins, and sulfonamides). In 50 percent of patients no etiology is ascertained. The major pathologic change is an acute lymphohistiocytic inflammatory infiltrate around blood vessels and may include degenerative changes in the endothelial cells of the capillaries and marked papillary dermal edema. There is some evidence for an immune-complex etiology with hypocomplementemic vasculitis.

The lesions occur in a characteristic symmetrical distribution and favor the extensor areas of the distal parts of the limbs, the backs of the hands, and the dorsa of the feet; the palms and soles are often involved, even to the exclusion of the dorsal surfaces. Oral lesions, first as blisters and then erosions, occur on the buccal mucous membrane, gums, and tongue, and there is often swelling and crusting of the lips. The syndrome may also include severe toxemia and prostration, high fever, cough, and "patchy" inflammation of the lungs. The skin lesions are often characterized by a vivid redness that gradually becomes duller, and they become more indurated, with the development of centers that are pale or may have bullae; these "target" or "iris" lesions, which are characteristic of erythema multiforme but do not invariably occur, are identified by the clear red area at the periphery that surrounds a pale pink zone and a central livid area, which may contain a bulla. The efficacy of systemic corticosteroids has not been proved, but this therapy is commonly used.

Purpura (with and without inflammation) A purpuric eruption demands immediate exploration for its etiology. Purpura arises in the skin of the vascularized dermis and is almost always confined to the dermis. The purpuric macules gradually disappear after days or weeks, depending on their size. Punctate or tiny purpuric spots are termed *petchiae,* larger (>2.0 cm) macules are spoken of as *suggillations,* and extensive purpuric macules are called *ecchymoses* (see D in Fig. 49-2).

Purpura with inflammation is usually "palpable," i.e., papular, and is seen in systemic vasculitis and in bacteremias such as staphylococcemia, gonococcemia (Plate 5-4), and meningococcemia. In these bacteremias and in vasculitis, the examination of biopsied skin may establish a diagnosis within 8 h (the time required for processing the tissue). Gentle scraping of the purpuric lesions will produce enough material for a Gram's stain; intracellular gram-negative diplococci are occasionally found in the lesions in acute, but not in chronic, meningococcemia, and are rarely found in acute gonococcemia. The differential diagnosis of papable purpuric lesions and infarcts occurring in *systemic vasculitis* (necrotizing vasculitis) as compared with those in chronic meningococcemia is not easy. The skin lesions in systemic vasculitis are usually bilateral, and almost symmetrical, in their distribution. They tend to be concentrated on the lower extremities, especially on the lower portion and around the ankles and the dorsa of the feet. The lesions in chronic meningococcemia are more randomly distributed, with occurrence on the trunk, lower and upper extremities, and face. Nevertheless, in meningococcemia, lesions can occur in a bilateral distribution, which makes the distinction between chronic meningococcemia and systemic vasculitis difficult, if not impossible, at times. The individual lesions in both chronic meningococcemia and systemic vasculitis may be identical, consisting of a mixture of palpable purpura and urticarial-type papules without purpura. Unfortunately, the histologic findings in biopsy specimens of the lesions in both diseases do not permit a distinction. Therefore, a patient with bilaterally distributed palpable purpuric lesions and fever is best treated with antibiotics before the results of blood cultures are available.

Purpura without inflammation is completely macular, and examination of a blood smear can quickly establish the presence of platelets; if platelets are seen in the smear, thrombocytopenic purpura can be safely ruled out as a possibility.

On the lower legs of older people, a great variety of inflammatory skin diseases, including various types of contact dermatitis, may be associated with purpura; under these circumstances, the purpura does not have the same importance as it does when present on the trunk or upper extremities. Perifollicular purpura, however, on the lower extremities (usually accompanied by a follicular hyperkeratosis) is almost pathognomonic of scurvy.

Purpura frequently develops in amyloidosis when the lesions (waxy macules and papules) are pinched. This "pinch" purpura, however, may also occur in the normal skin of patients with thrombocytopenic purpura or in the skin of apparently normal elderly persons. (For a full discussion of the classification and differential diagnosis of purpura, see Chaps. 55 and 332.)

Infarcts Infarcts in the skin are usually not pale like those that occur in the kidney but have a variegated dusky red, grayish hue. They are irregularly shaped macules, sometimes slightly depressed below the plane of the skin, and often surrounded by a pink zone of hyperemia. Infarcts are usually slightly tender.

Cutaneous infarctions are important and often diagnostic signs of serious multisystem disease, including both acute and chronic meningococcemia, streptococcal and staphylococcal septicemia, gonococcemia, pseudomonas septicemia, systemic vasculitis, purpura fulminans, systemic lupus erythematosus, and, rarely, dermatomyositis.

Telangiectasia Redness of the skin is most freqently caused by transient dilatation of blood vessels (erythema). In contrast to the color produced by fixed blood pigments, as in purpura, the erythema will disappear under the pressure of a glass or plastic slide (see "Diascopy," in Chap. 49). Telangiectasia is the condition in which the redness of the skin is the result of a permanent enlargement in the caliber of the blood vessels (which will be revealed by examination with a hand lens) and an increase in the number of the vessels. Telangiectasia may be composed of fine linear branches of blood vessels appearing distinctly red (i.e., not blue), which are often seen on the nose and face, or of confluent macular areas that appear as a permanent erythema. Telangiectasia is the cause of the erythema in discoid and systemic lupus erythematosus, dermatomyositis, and psoriasis.

Telangiectasia may also occur in a scattered, discrete fashion on the upper trunk or on the extremities and is seen characteristically in progressive systemic sclerosis (systemic scleroderma). Telangiectasia occurring around the nail beds, i.e., periungual telangiectasia, is an important diagnostic sign in lupus erythematosus (both discoid and systemic) and in dermatomyositis; these lesions are seen rarely, if at all, in systemic scleroderma or rheumatoid arthritis.

Sharply outlined, red macules or papules 1 to 2 mm in diameter, with an area of radiating telangiectasia, are seen in *hereditary hemorrhagic telangiectasia* (Chap. 334). These occur on the lips, tongue, nasal mucosa, face, and hands.

Generalized telangiectasia occurring in the form of red macules over most of the body surface may be the presenting sign of mastocytosis or urticaria pigmentosa.

Telangiectasia is a prominent and diagnostic feature of *ataxia-telangiectasia,* or Louis-Bar syndrome. Telangiectasia may be present as early as the second year of life but usually develops by the fifth year; it appears first on the bulbar conjunctiva and subsequently involves the ears, the eyelids, the butterfly area of the face, the upper aspect of the chest, and the extremities.

Telangiectasia may occur in a characteristic form known as the *arterial spider,* or spider nevus, spider angioma, or naevus araneus. The main vessel of the spider is an arteriole, and it is usually faintly pulsating, which will show under the diascope. A less common skin lesion usually found with vascular spiders in liver disorders is the telangiectatic *mat* or net, a small red patch composed of intermeshed fine vessels that blanch on pressure. Spider angiomas, usually three or fewer, occur not infrequently in normal children and adults. Numerous spider angiomas often develop during pregnancy or after the ingestion of progestational agents or in rheumatoid arthritis or thyrotoxicosis. Most patients with numerous and prominent vascular spiders, however, have some form of underlying diffuse liver disease, e.g., alcoholic cirrhosis. The progression of subacute hepatitis is often paralleled by the appearance of crops of spiders, and in alcoholic and postnecrotic cirrhosis, almost half the patients have multiple vascular spiders. The mechanism responsible for the development of spider angiomas in liver disease is not known, nor has it been firmly established that the lesions result from disordered metabolism of estrogens by the liver.

REFERENCES

FARBER EM, COX AJ (eds): *Psoriasis: Proceedings of the Third International Symposium.* New York, Yorke Medical Books, 1981

FITZPATRICK TB: Fundamentals of dermatologic diagnosis, in *Dermatology in General Medicine,* 2d ed, TB Fitzpatrick et al (eds). New York, McGraw-Hill, 1979

———, JOHNSON RA: Atlas of differential diagnosis of rashes in the acutely ill febrile patient and in life-threatening diseases, in *Dermatology in General Medicine,* 2d ed, TB Fitzpatrick et al (eds). New York, McGraw-Hill, 1979

HENSELER T et al: Oral 8-methoxypsoralen photochemotherapy of psoriasis. Lancet 1:853, 1981

PARRISH JA et al: Photochemotherapy of psoriasis with oral methoxsalen and longwave ultraviolet light. N Engl J Med 291:1207, 1974

PECK GL et al: Prolonged remissions of cystic acne with 13-*cis*-retinoic acid. N Engl J Med 300:329, 1979

WOLFF K, HÖNIGSMANN H: Clinical aspects of photochemotherapy. Pharmac Ther, vol 12, p 381, Pergamon Press, 1981

51 GENERALIZED PRURITUS

THOMAS B. FITZPATRICK
HARLEY A. HAYNES

Generalized pruritus is a frequent and important problem in differential diagnosis for the general physician. In many patients, intense generalized pruritus is the only symptom. Unfortunately, there are no good studies that have described in detail the special qualities of pruritus that permit a specific diagnosis; in other words, it is not really known what type of pruritus is seen, for example, in obstructive biliary disease as opposed to lymphoma. In the absence of these data, the clinician must rely on the history, physical examination, and laboratory studies to establish the nature of the pruritus. The receptors for the itch stimuli reside in the papillary layer of the dermis but there are no specific end organs for itching. Itching is a sensation carried principally by unmyelinated slowly conducting fibers of the C group to central neuronal pools in the spinal cord. The stimuli are then carried by the posterior roots of the spinal nerves, enter the thalamus from the anterolateral spinothalamic tracts, and then proceed to the sensory area of the gyrus postcentralis of the cortex. Intracutaneous histamine, trypsin, proteases, and bile salts all cause pruritus when introduced intracutaneously. Prostaglandin E lowers the threshold to itching evoked by both histamine and papain. Since prostaglandins are known to be increased in inflamed skin, perhaps they potentiate pruritus in inflammatory dermatoses. The opiate antagonist naloxone hydrochloride lowers the threshold to itching evoked by histamine. This may indicate a role of central nervous system opiate receptors in the perception of pruritus and might explain how opiates relieve pain but exacerbate pruritus.

Patients with pruritus associated with obvious skin lesions, such as vesicles and papules, usually have a primary cutaneous cause for their pruritus. Some of the dermatologic disorders in which pruritus is a common symptom include scabies, dermatitis herpetiformis, lichen planus, urticaria, mycosis fungoides, insect bites, psoriasis, and eczematous dermatitis, including atopic dermatitis. Many of these disorders require specialized dermatologic approaches, particularly biopsy of the skin, in order to establish the diagnosis.

The itching patient without an apparent skin eruption and with or without the sequelae of chronic scratching (linear excoriations) and rubbing (lichenification, polished nails), poses a diagnostic challenge. Initially, a search should be undertaken for the subtle evidence of a cutaneous disorder.

Thorough evaluation of the patient with generalized pruritus in an attempt to discover an underlying systemic disease should include, in addition to history and physical examination, the following basic laboratory screening tests: complete blood count; sedimentation rate, urinalysis; blood glucose, liver, thyroid, and renal function tests; chest x-ray; Papanicolaou smear; and stool exam for ova, parasites, and occult blood. Additional tests such as serum protein electrophoresis, serum calcium, and radiologic surveys should be performed when indicated. A psychological assessment is helpful. Attributing generalized pruritus of uncertain etiology to a psychological disturbance is unwise.

An important cause of pruritus is psychogenic, that is, a reaction to stress and strain. This type of pruritus often affects the skin of the scalp, and may be associated with other sensory complaints such as a bitter taste in the mouth or burning of the tongue. Some patients with psychogenic pruritus are convinced that the itching is caused by some sort of parasite in their skin that cannot be seen by themselves or the physician. Such patients may scratch their skin until the lesions become excoriated, and then assert that the itching has disappeared, owing, they believe, to removal of the parasite or "germ" by the appearance of bleeding.

Older persons in whom dry skin is a common occurrence may have generalized pruritus unrelated to multisystem disease. Some other older persons, however, usually more than 60 years of age, who do not have obvious dry skin may also have generalized ("senile") pruritus that is intense and does not seem to be caused by emotional stress. This pruritus is usually most severe when the patients disrobe to go to bed, and usually begins in one area, particularly the back, and spreads to involve the entire body. Neither psychogenic nor senile pruritus leads to a loss of sleep.

A subtle and important cause of pruritus without a visible rash may be a reaction to drugs, such as aspirin and, especially, opiates and their derivatives, and quinidine.

The itching that is associated with pediculosis corporis may be so intense that it will interfere with the patient's sleep. This type of eruption is usually relatively easy to diagnose by the linear excoriations that occur along the back and often the insect can be found in the clothing, particularly along the seams.

For a list of conditions in which generalized pruritus occurs without any evidence of primary skin disease, see Table 51-1.

The pruritus in hepatic disease has no special qualities. Generalized pruritus may frequently be the first sign of biliary cirrhosis and may occur many months before the onset of jaundice. It may be the first sign also of lymphoma, and, rarely, of carcinoma. The pruritus may be of sudden onset and may be very severe from the beginning.

The treatment of generalized pruritus is unsatisfactory if the primary cause cannot be corrected or eliminated. Exceptions are the excellent response of uremic pruritus to ultraviolet radiation therapy (UV-B) of all or part of the skin surface and the response of patients with various forms of cholestasis to the ion-exchange resin cholestyramine. Not one of the systemic medications has been shown to be effective in generalized pruritus. A topical preparation containing 0.5% menthol and 1% phenol in Nivea oil is somewhat helpful in relieving pruritus temporarily. The topical anesthetics containing benzocaine should be avoided because of the high risk of allergic sensitization. When the patient with pruritus also has insomnia, a hypnotic or a sedative should be prescribed. Antihistamines are of little value except in pruritus due to urticaria. It is a general clinical impression that aspirin is helpful in pruritus of any origin, but this has not been proved. The development of drugs that control pruritus remains one of the great challenges of medical research, and it is paradoxical that, at this juncture, severe pain can be immediately controlled with a variety of agents but there is not one single agent that is so effective for generalized pruritus.

TABLE 51-1
Conditions with generalized pruritus without diagnostic skin lesions

Psychogenic states:
- Transitory: periods of emotional stress
- Persistent: delusions of parasitosis

Metabolic and endocrine conditions:
- Hyperthyroidism
- Diabetes mellitus*
- Carcinoid syndrome

Malignant neoplasms:
- Lymphoma and leukemia
- Abdominal cancer*
- CNS tumors*
- Multiple myeloma*

Drug ingestion:
- Opium derivatives
- Subclinical drug sensitivities

Infestations:
- Pediculosis corporis
- Scabies†
- Hookworm (ancylostomiasis)
- Onchocerciasis

Renal disease:
- Chronic renal failure

Hematologic disease:
- Polycythemia vera‡
- Iron deficiency
- Mastocytosis

Hepatic disease:
- Obstructive biliary disease
- Pregnancy (intrahepatic cholestasis)

Miscellaneous conditions:
- Dry skin§
- "Senile" pruritus§

* *Not definitely proven.*
† *Diagnostic lesions may be present.*
‡ *Especially after a bath.*
§ *Unexplained intense pruritus in patients over 65 years old without obvious "dry skin" and with no apparent emotional stress.*
SOURCE: *TB Fitzpatrick, in Dermatology in General Medicine, 2d ed, TB Fitzpatrick et al (eds), New York, McGraw-Hill, 1979.*

REFERENCES

ARNDT KA, CLARK RAF: Principles of topical therapy, in *Dermatology in General Medicine,* 2d ed, TB Fitzpatrick et al (eds). New York, McGraw-Hill, 1979, pp 1753–1758

BERNSTEIN JE et al: Antipruritic effect of an opiate antagonist, naloxone hydrochloride. J Invest Dermatol 78:82, 1982

BOSS M, BURTON JL: Lack of effect of the antihistamine drug clemastine on the potentiation of itch by prostaglandin E_1. Arch Dermatol 117:208, 1981

BOTERO F: Pruritus as a manifestation of systemic disorders, in *Cutaneous Aspects of Internal Disease,* JP Callen (ed), Chicago, Year Book, 1981, pp 627–633

CAIRNS RJ: The skin and the nervous system, in *Textbook of Dermatology,* A Rook et al (eds). Oxford, Blackwell Scientific Publications, 1972, p 1791

CUNLIFFE WJ: The skin and the nervous system, in *Textbook of Dermatology,* 3d ed, A Rook et al (eds). Oxford, Blackwell, 1979

FREEDMAN MR et al: Pruritus in cholestasis: No direct causative role for bile acid retention. Am J Med 70:1011, 1981

GILCHREST BA et al: Ultraviolet phototherapy of uremic pruritus. Ann Intern Med 91:17, 1979

HERNDON, JH, JR: Itching: The pathophysiology of pruritus. Int J Dermatol 14:465, 1975

52
PIGMENTATION OF THE SKIN AND DISORDERS OF MELANIN METABOLISM

THOMAS B. FITZPATRICK
DAVID B. MOSHER

THE MELANOCYTE SYSTEM

DEFINITION OF MELANIN The presence of melanin, oxyhemoglobin, reduced hemoglobin, and carotene accounts for the kaleidoscope of normal human skin colors, but melanin is the principal pigment responsible for the color of human skin, hair, and eyes. Melanin is also a filter that decreases the harmful effects of ultraviolet light on the dermis and thereby provides protection against acute sunburn reaction and chronic actinic damage, including skin cancer.

Derived from the Greek word *melas,* "black," melanin is a protein-bound polymer formed by the oxidation of tyrosine by tyrosinase to dihydroxyphenylalanine (dopa) within melanocytes, which are specialized epidermal dendritic cells of neural crest origin. The structure of melanin is unknown because it is so insoluble that all attempts to degrade it into identifiable fragments have failed. However, all animal melanins are known to contain indoles and are composed basically of indole 5,6-quinone units, in contrast to plant melanins which contain catechols. Radioactive dopa studies have shown that melanin is a copolymer of dopa quinone, indole 5,6-quinone, and indole 5,6-quinone 23-carboxylic acid in a ratio of 3:2:1. Recently, sulfur-containing pigments present in hair and known as trichochromes have been isolated and characterized; these are benzothiazylolamines and are the subunit structures of pheomelanins, the yellow-red pigments present in humans and mammals exclusively in the hair.

Skin color is derived from the presence of melanin within the keratinocytes, which are receptor cells for melanocyte-formed melanin-containing organelles called *melanosomes.* Normal skin color is "constitutive"—that of habitually unexposed skin, as the buttocks—and "facultative"—that resulting from the sun-induced tanning reaction or from increased pigmentation by pituitary melanocyte-stimulating hormones (MSH).

BIOSYNTHESIS OF MELANIN The melanocyte system is composed of melanocytes found at the dermoepidermal interface, in the hair bulb, uveal tract, retinal pigment epithelium, inner ear, and leptomeninges (Fig. 52-1). The melanocyte system is analogous to, but not known to be related to, the chromaffin system, the cells of which are also derived from the neural crest and which possess biochemical mechanisms for the hydroxylation of tyrosine to dopa. However, in the latter system the enzyme is not tyrosinase, but tyrosine hydroxylase, and dopa is converted to adrenochrome and not to tyrosine melanin.

FIGURE 52-1
Diagram showing the embryonic origin, dispersal, and developmental fate of melanocytes in humans. [By permission from JB Stanbury et al (eds), The Metabolic Basis of Inherited Disease, 2d ed, New York, McGraw-Hill, 1966.]

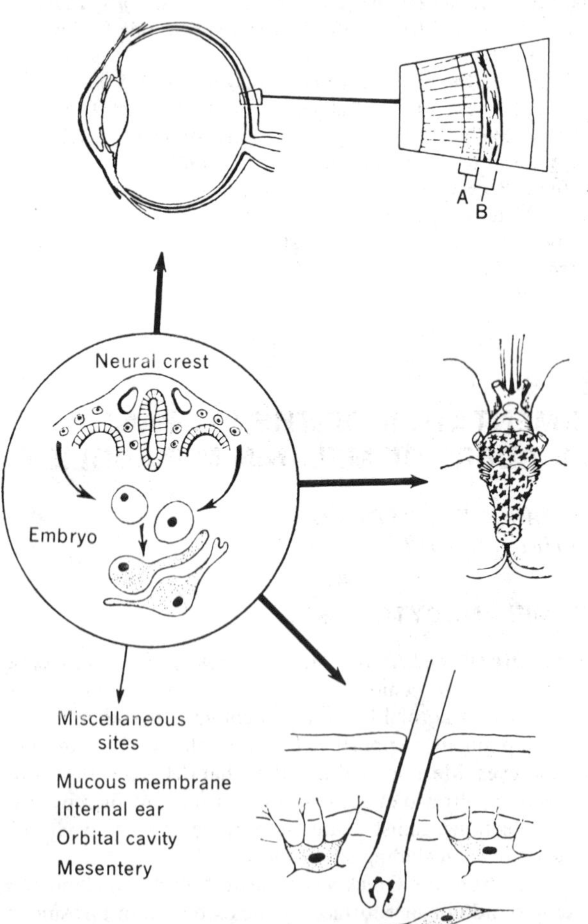

FIGURE 52-2
Epidermal melanin unit. Four biologic processes in melanin pigmentation underscore the differences in melanosome formation and packaging between Negroes and Caucasians: (1) Formation of melanosomes in melanocytes; (2) melanization of melanosomes in melanocytes; (3) secretion of melanocytes by keratinocytes; and (4) transport of melanocytes by keratinocytes, either with degradation of melanosomes within lysosome-like organelles (in Caucasoids) or without apparent degradation of melanosomes (in Negroids). Note the difference in size between the melanosomes in the Negroid and Caucasoid epidermal keratinocytes. In the Negroid keratinocytes, the melanosomes are nonaggregated. In the Caucasoid keratinocytes, groups of several melanosomes are aggregated within membrane-limited lysosome-like organelles, and the melanosomes often appear fragmented (G, Golgi apparatus; N, nucleus; I to IV, the four stages in the development of the melanosome). The epidermal melanin unit is shown at the top. The melanocyte supplies melanosomes to a group of keratinocytes.

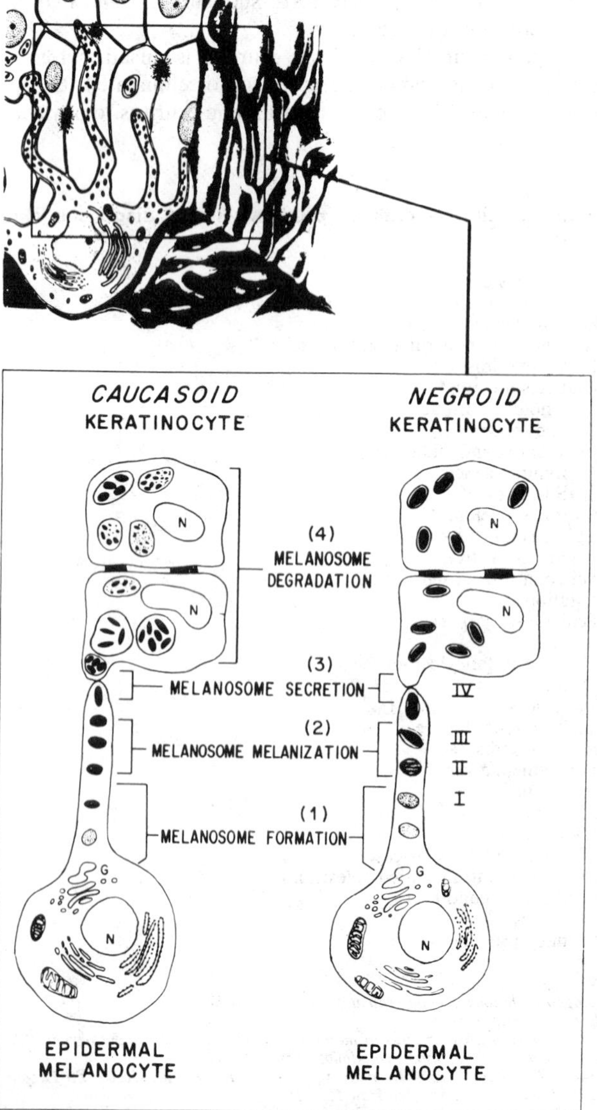

Melanocytes within the epidermis at the dermoepidermal interface are dendritic cells that are functionally linked to a number of keratinocytes; each melanocyte and its corresponding associated 36 keratinocytes compose an epidermal melanin unit (Fig. 52-2). This functional unit permits organized transfer of specialized tyrosinase-containing, melanin-producing organelles, or melanosomes, to associated keratinocytes. Melanosomes are ellipsoidal organelles which are thought to arise in the area of the endoplasmic reticulum and Golgi apparatus; they are formed as unmelanized spherical structures that darken and become more dense and oval in shape with increasing melanization.

Tyrosinase, the only enzyme in the pathway of melanin production, is one of a large group of copper-containing aerobic oxidases that catalyze the oxidation of both monohydroxy and *o*-dihydroxy phenols to orthoquinones. There are at least three isozymes of tyrosinase. In humans and other mammals, this oxidase catalyzes the hydroxylation of the melanin precursor, tyrosine, to dopa and dopa quinone (Fig. 52-3). Tyrosinase is required only for the first step in the biosynthesis of tyrosine melanin, i.e., the orthohydroxylation of tyrosine. It is noteworthy that zinc ions catalyze the conversion of dopachrome to 5,6-dihydroxyindole and that melanosomes have been shown to contain high concentrations of zinc. Recently some new factors have been shown to augment or block the synthesis of melanin *after* the action of tyrosinase.

BIOLOGY OF MELANIN PIGMENTATION Melanin pigmentation (Fig. 52-4), from the clinical point of view, results from the melanin present in the keratinocytes and also in the melanocytes. Inasmuch as the ratio of keratinocytes to melanocytes in the epidermis is 36:1, it is apparent that the amount of melanin present in the keratinocytes must be the predominant factor in the determination of skin color. The relationship of skin color to the location of melanin in the epidermis was studied with the light microscope in Negro Americans of various hues of brown coloration. In lightly pigmented skin, there was a great variation in both the number and location of melanin particles within the epidermis; only scanty melanin deposits were in the malpighian layer, and no deposits were in the stratum corneum. In fact, in the most lightly pigmented skin, the only melanin particles were in the keratinocytes of the basal layer. In the most heavily pigmented skin, there were melanin particles in the keratinocytes of the basal layer, throughout the malpighian cells, and in the stratum corneum.

It is apparent from studies of normal skin and of pigmentary disorders, that the intensity of pigmentation, as viewed clinically, depends not only on the rate of melanosome production but also on the number of melanosomes that are transferred to the keratinocytes (Fig. 52-2). Another factor that determines normal and abnormal melanin pigmentation is the degree of melanization of the individual melanosomes. Until recently, three factors—melanosome formation, melanosome melanization, and melanosome secretion—were considered to be the major variables in normal and abnormal melanin pigmentation. In the past few years, however, a fourth variable has been implicated in melanin pigmentation, i.e., the phenomenon of aggregation and degradation of melanosomes that occurs during their transport in the keratinocytes.

Melanosomes are present in melanocytes mainly as nonaggregated (single), membrane-delimited, discrete organelles. In keratinocytes, however, melanosomes occur either as single, or nonaggregated, particles or as aggregates of three or more within a membrane-delimited organelle. These melanosome-

FIGURE 52-3
Biosynthesis of tyrosine melanin.

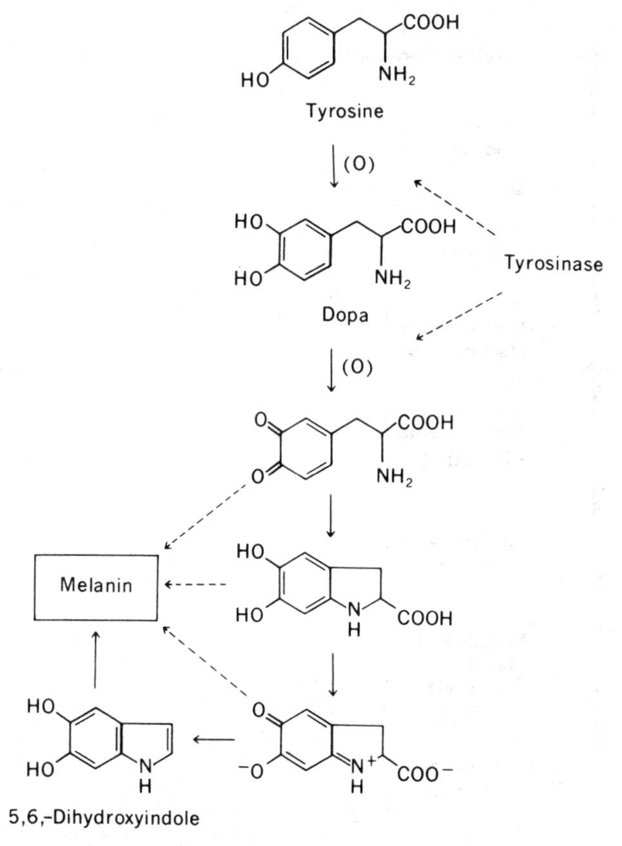

FIGURE 52-4
Melanogenesis in human skin, as seen in the light and the electron microscopes and at the molecular level.

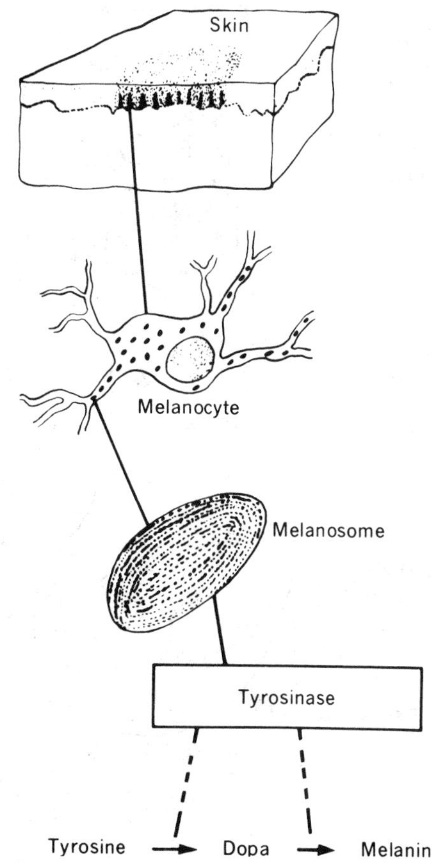

containing organelles resemble the melanosome-containing organelles within macrophages that have been identified as lysosomes. In the epidermal keratinocyte, melanosomes appear to undergo a gradual degradation. In heavily pigmented skin, however, intact melanosomes remain in the stratum corneum, indicating that some melanosomes are apparently not degraded with the lysosomes in the epidermis. Numerous studies in recent years have shown that there appears to be a considerable variation in the arrangement of melanosomes in the nonfollicular keratinocytes in different racial groups. In the keratinocytes of the hair follicle in all racial groups, there are, in the growing phase of the hair growth cycle, single, or nonaggregated, melanosomes. In Negroids and Australian aborigines, however, melanosomes are found, in the epidermal keratinocytes, to be nonaggregated (single), whereas in Caucasoids, Mongoloids, and American Indians, melanosomes are found, in the keratinocytes, to be mostly aggregated, and there is often a suggestion of fragmentation of the melanosomes within these lysosome-like organelles. Some recent observations have shown that the size of the melanosome determines whether a melanosome becomes aggregated in the keratinocytes. Melanosomes that are smaller than 1 mm can aggregate in the form of a phagosome and undergo degradation—a process that could gradually decrease the intensity of skin color.

Melanin pigmentation of the skin is related to 10 biologic processes as shown in Fig. 52-5. Aggregation[1] and dispersion of melanosomes probably play little part in the pigmentary anomalies of humans. Such movement has thus far been observed only in specialized effector cells, *melanophores,* present only in vertebrates below mammals in the phylogenetic scale; this movement of melanosomes is under neural and hormonal control in these animals.

[1] *Aggregation in this sense refers to the clustering of melanosomes around the nucleus of the melanocyte, e.g., the phenomenon that occurs when a frog is placed on a white background; when the frog is placed on a dark background, however, there is movement, or dispersion, of the melanosomes into the dendrites.*

DISORDERS OF THE MELANOCYTE SYSTEM; HYPOMELANOSES AND HYPERMELANOSES

Disorders of melanin pigmentation have been increasingly found to be markers for diseases of other organ systems (Tables 52-1 and 52-2) and may be classified as hypomelanoses (decreased or absent epidermal melanin) or hypermelanoses (increased epidermal or dermal melanin). Hypomelanoses, in general, result from the absence of melanocytes, failure of formation of normal melanosomes, or failure of transfer of melanosomes to keratinocytes. The hypermelanoses are further classified as epidermal disorders which present as brown, or as dermal disorders which are blue, blue-gray, or gray. Brown hypermelanoses arise from increased melanin in the epidermis, resulting from increased melanocyte activity, increased numbers of secretory melanocytes, increased numbers of melanosomes, or increased size of melanosomes. The blue-gray hypermelanoses represent a virtual "melanin tattoo"—the presence of melanin in the dermis in ectopic dermal melanocytes or in dermal macrophages which, because of the Tyndall effect, imparts a characteristic slate, blue, or gray color to the skin. Blue or slate-gray coloration of the skin may also arise from nonmelanin sources—ochronosis, tattoos, and deposition of other foreign materials in the dermis.

Clinical recognition of hypomelanosis and of gray or slate or blue hypermelanosis is usually not difficult. When the degree of hypomelanosis is very slight, when the patient's normal skin color is very light, or when the patient's skin is untanned, the lesions may be inapparent, and the diagnosis may be facilitated by the use of black light (Wood's lamp; see Chap. 49), which will heighten the contrast between abnormal epidermal

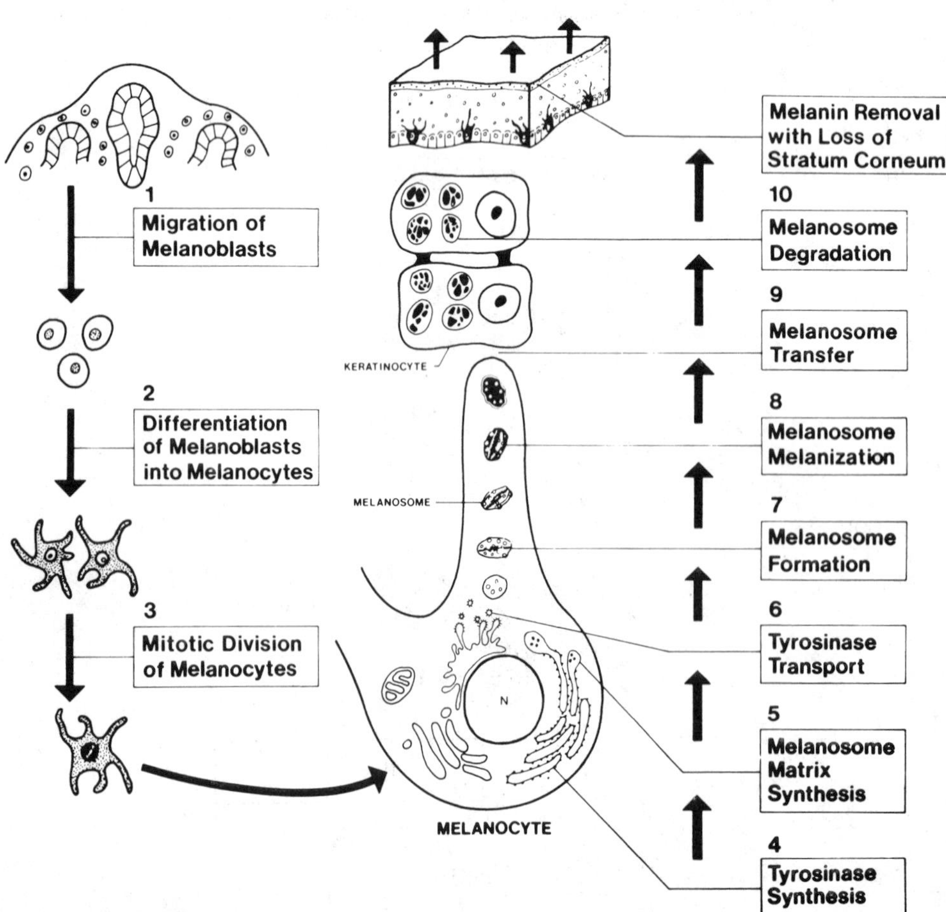

FIGURE 52-5
Morphological and metabolic pathway of epidermal melanin pigmentation.

pigmentation and normal skin but will not increase the contrast between increased dermal pigmentation and normal skin. Differentiation between abnormal diffuse brown hyperpigmentation and normal pigmentation frequently poses a problem because there is such a wide range of skin coloration in normal individuals. Diffuse color changes may be insidious; often patients themselves have been unaware of an unusual or unexplained progressive or gradual deepening of their skin color, such as a summer tan which is not fading. The degree of hypermelanosis that develops appears to be related to the basic skin color of the patient involved. With the onset of primary Addison's disease, a patient of Mediterranean extraction (such as Italian, French, or Spanish) may become intensely pigmented, whereas a light-skinned individual may have only a minimal degree of hypermelanosis that may or may not be apparent. Localized pigmentation that develops in mucous membranes and in specific areas, such as axillae and palmar creases, is usually easier to identify as an abnormality than is generalized brown hyperpigmentation.

GENETIC MELANIN DISORDERS *Oculocutaneous albinism* is an autosomal recessive trait characterized by congenital, decreased, uniform hypomelanosis of skin and hair; albinism involving the skin alone has not been reported, but ocular albinism with minimal or no cutaneous involvement has been observed. The classic constellation of findings in oculocutaneous albinism includes marked hypomelanosis or amelanosis of skin, white or faintly blondish hair, photophobia, nystagmus, hypopigmented fundus oculi, and translucent irides. Oculocutaneous albinism may be classified according to the presence or absence of tyrosinase in plucked hair follicles of the scalp (the hair bulb incubation test). In normal individuals hair bulbs darken when incubated with tyrosine; in some persons with oculocutaneous albinism the hair follicles darken when incubated in tyrosine, i.e., *tyrosinase-positive,* while in others no

TABLE 52-1
Pigmentary Changes as Diagnostic Signs in General Medicine

Chief complaint or presenting problem	*Pigmentary change*	*Diseases*	*Systems involved*
ADDISONIAN BROWN HYPERPIGMENTATION			
"Getting dark"	Generalized diffuse brown hypermelanosis	Addison's disease	Adrenal insufficiency
		Hemochromatosis	Cirrhosis of liver, diabetes
		ACTH-producing tumors	Pituitary tumor, primary; metastatic cancer
		Systemic scleroderma	Dysphagia; pulmonary insufficiency
		Porphyria cutanea tarda	Liver: increased iron stores Diabetes mellitus (25%)
CIRCUMSCRIBED BROWN MACULES			
"Abdominal pain, brown spots on lips, fingers"	Circumscribed, mostly small dark-brown macules (many)	Peutz-Jegher syndrome	Polyposis of small intestine
"Brown spots all over"	Circumscribed small dark-brown macules	Progressive lentiginosis	Abnormal ECG Pulmonary stenosis
"Birth mark"; hypertension; precocious puberty	Circumscribed, uniformly brown macules, small or large (café au lait) (few or many)	Neurofibromatosis	Neurofibromatosis of skin and peripheral nervous system; pheochromocytoma
		Albright's syndrome	Polyostotic fibrous dysplasia Precocious puberty
		Watson's syndrome	Pulmonary stenosis
"Funny moles"	Circumscribed dark-brown macules or slightly raised papules with irregular borders and variegation of color (few or many)	Dysplastic nevus syndrome	
CIRCUMSCRIBED WHITE MACULES			
"White spots"	Circumscribed, mostly large white macules (few or many)	"Vitiligo"	Hypothyroidism Thyrotoxicosis Pernicious anemia Adrenal insufficiency Diabetes mellitus
"Convulsions"; mental retardation	Congenital circumscribed small (1–3 cm) white macules (more than 3)	Tuberous sclerosis	Mental retardation, abnormal EEG Abnormal CT scan Rhabdomyoma of heart
"Eye trouble"; deafness	Circumscribed white macules, poliosis	Vogt-Koyanagi-Harada disease	Uveitis, dysacousia
"Deafness"	White forelock, congenital circumscribed large white macules	Waardenburg's syndrome	Nerve deafness, heterochromia
UNIVERSAL HYPOMELANOSIS			
"Sun sensitivity"; decreased vision	Universal hypomelanosis of skin, hair, and uveal tract	Oculocutaneous albinism, recessive	Decreased visual acuity, iris translucency, nystagmus
"Sun sensitivity"; "Poor tanner"	Type I or type II skin	Oculocutaneous albinoidism, dominant	Iris translucency, normal vision, nystagmus (rare)

such darkening occurs, i.e., *tyrosinase-negative.* These two types of albinism are known to have separate gene loci. In oculocutaneous albinism melanocytes are present, but formation of melanosomes is interrupted in the early stages so that few mature melanosomes are present in albino skin or hair. Whatever tyrosinase is present must be functionally defective and unable to convert enzymatically tyrosine to dopa. Other variants of oculocutaneous albinism include yellow mutant, Cross-McKusick-Green syndrome (oculocerebral-hypopigmentation syndrome), Hermansky-Pudlak syndrome (hemorrhagic diathesis secondary to storage pool platelet defect), and Chédiak-Higashi syndrome (recurrent infections, hematologic and neurologic abnormalities, and early death from lymphoma). The deficiency of melanin in oculocutaneous albinism has two disturbing consequences for humans: decreased visual acuity and an abnormal degree of intolerance to sunlight. The sensitivity of human albinos to ultraviolet light often leads to the development of carcinoma in exposed areas of the skin. Nearly all

TABLE 52-2
Disturbances of human melanin pigmentation

Hypomelanosis[a] *White*	*Hypermelanosis*[a] *Brown, gray, slate, or blue*[b]
GENETIC FACTORS	
Piebaldism[c] Waardenburg's syndrome[c] Vitiligo[c,d] Hypomelanotic macules in tuberous sclerosis[c,e] Albinism, oculocutaneous:[f,g] Tyrosinase-negative Tyrosinase-positive Yellow mutant Hermansky-Pudlak syndrome Chédiak-Higashi syndrome Cross-McKusick-Green syndrome Albinism, ocular[c,g,h] Albinoidism, oculocutaneous[f,g,h] Phenylketonuria[f,g,h] Fanconi's syndrome[h] Homocystinuria[f,h] Histidinemia[f] Menkes' kinky hair syndrome[h] Canities, premature[h]	Café au lait and freckle-like macules in neurofibromatosis[c] Melanotic macules in polyostotic fibrous dysplasia (Albright's syndrome)[c] Ephelides (freckles)[c] Lentigines[c] Lentigines with cardiac arrhythmias[c] Melanocytic nevus[c] Neurocutaneous melanosis[c] Xeroderma pigmentosum[c] Acanthosis nigricans Fanconi's syndrome[c] Dermal melanocytosis (Mongolian spot)[b,c] Blue melanocytic nevus[b,c] Incontinentia pigmenti[b,c]
METABOLIC FACTORS	
	Hemochromatosis[f] Hepatolenticular disease (Wilson's disease)[f] Porphyria (congenital erythropoietic, variegata and cutanea tarda)[f] Gaucher's disease[i] Niemann-Pick disease[i] Hemochromatosis[f]
ENDOCRINE FACTORS	
Hypopituitarism[f] Addison's disease[c] Hyperthyroidism[c]	ACTH-producing and MSH-producing pituitary and other tumors[f] ACTH therapy[f] Pregnancy[i] Addison's disease[f] Melasma[c,k]
NUTRITIONAL FACTORS	
Chronic protein deficiency or loss:[h,l] Kwashiorkor Nephrosis Ulcerative colitis Malabsorption Vitamin B_{12} deficiency[h]	Pellagra[i] Sprue[i] Vitamin B_{12} deficiency[i] Chronic nutritional insufficiency[c]
CHEMICAL AND PHARMACOLOGIC AGENTS	
Hydroquinone, monobenzylether[c] Hydroquinone[c,e] Miscellaneous catechol and phenol compounds[f] Chloroquine and hydroxychloroquine[h] Arsenical ingestion[c] Corticosteroids, topical and intradermal[c,e]	Arsenical intoxication[f] Busulfan administration[f] Photochemical agents (topical or systemic drugs)[c] 5-Fluorouracil, systemic[f] Cyclophosphamide[f] Nitrogen mustard, topical[c] Bleomycin[c] Fixed (drug) eruption[b,c]
PHYSICAL AGENTS	
Burns: Thermal, ultraviolet, ionizing radiation[c,m] Trauma[c,m]	Ultraviolet light (suntanning)[c] Thermal radiation[c] Alpha, beta, and gamma ionizing radiation[c] Trauma (e.g., chronic pruritus)[c]
INFLAMMATION AND INFECTION	
Sarcoidosis[c,e] Pinta[c] Yaws[c] Leprosy[c,e] Tinea versicolor[c,e] Post–kala azar[c] Eczematous dermatitis[c,e] Psoriasis[c] Discoid lupus erythematosus[c] Vagabond's leukoderma[c] Miscellaneous postinflammatory hypomelanoses[c,e]	Postinflammation melanoses (exanthems, drug eruptions)[c] Lichen planus[c] Lupus erythematosus, discoid[c] Lichen simplex chronicus[c] Atopic dermatitis[i] Psoriasis[c] Tinea versicolor[c] Pinta in exposed areas[b,c]
NEOPLASMS	
Leukoderma acquisitum centrifugum (including halo nevus)[c] Malignant melanoma around primary neoplasms[c] Vitiligo-like hypomelanosis[c,e] around nevi and metastatic melanoma[c]	Malignant melanoma[c,h] Mastocytosis (urticaria pigmentosa)[c] Acanthosis nigricans, with adenocarcinoma and lymphoma[c] Slate-gray dermal pigmentation with metastatic melanoma and melanogenuria[f]
MISCELLANEOUS FACTORS	
Vogt-Koyanagi-Harada syndrome[c] Scleroderma, circumscribed or systemic[c] Canities[h] Alopecia areata[o] Horner's syndrome, congenital and acquired[g] Idiopathic, guttate hypomelanosis[c]	Scleroderma, systemic[f] Chronic hepatic insufficiency[f] Whipple's syndrome[f] Lentigo, senile ("liver spots")[c] Cronkhite-Canada syndrome[c]

[a] *Listing includes the pigmentation disorder itself or the condition with which it is associated.*
[b] *Gray, slate, or blue color results from the presence of dermal melanocytes or phagocytized melanin in the dermis.*
[c] *Pigment change is circumscribed.*
[d] *Total loss of pigment in the skin and hair may occur.*
[e] *Loss of pigmentation is usually partial (hypomelanosis); viewed with Wood's lamp, the lesions are not completely devoid of pigment (amelanosis), as in vitiligo.*
[f] *Pigment change is diffuse, not circumscribed, and there are no identifiable borders.*
[g] *Pigment is decreased in the iris.*
[h] *Pigment is decreased in the hair.*
[i] *Pigment change may be diffuse or circumscribed.*
[j] *Nipples are affected.*
[k] *Idiopathic or due to progestational agents.*
[l] *Hair is gray or reddish.*
[m] *There is a loss of melanocytes.*
[n] *Areas of brown may be admixed with the slate-gray and blue discoloration.*
[o] *Regrown hair is white.*

SOURCE: *DB Mosher et al, in Dermatology in General Medicine, 2d ed, TB Fitzpatrick et al (eds), New York, McGraw-Hill, 1979.*

albinos in the tropics are said to have actinic keratoses or skin cancers by the third decade. Daily use of effective topical sunscreens and avoidance of unnecessary sun exposure are indicated for all albinos (see Chap. 53).

Phenylketonuria is an autosomal recessive disorder of phenylalanine metabolism in which there is a single metabolic block in the conversion of phenylalanine to tyrosine. There is pigmentary dilution of the skin, hair, and irides. The lightening of hair, which is characteristically light blond to dark brown, may be appraised only by comparison with uninvolved siblings. The melanocytes are normal but lack a full complement of melanosomes. Decreased melanin formation results from the fact that excess phenylalanine and its metabolites, present in serum and extracellular fluid, act as competitive inhibitors of tyrosinase and block melanin synthesis.

Vitiligo is an idiopathic, acquired, circumscribed hypomelanosis which is familial in about 30 percent of cases and is characterized by progressively enlarging amelanotic macules (Table 52-3). Vitiligo may be localized, segmental (one or more dermatomes), or generalized. On occasion, vitiligo may become so extensive that all or nearly all the skin becomes white. Characteristic distribution patterns of vitiligo involve extensor surfaces and bony prominences (elbows, knees), the small joints in the hands, and the area around the eyes and mouth. The low back, axillae, and flexor wrists may also be involved. Genitalia, palms and soles, and mucous membranes are often affected. Typically, the vitiligo macules gradually enlarge centrifugally, and new macules appear. In up to 30 percent of cases some minimal spontaneous repigmentation occurs, particularly in sun-exposed areas of skin. White hairs are common in macules of vitiligo, but may also be normally pigmented. Most vitiligo patients are generally healthy, although thyroid disease, diabetes mellitus, Addison's disease, and pernicious anemia occur with increased frequency. Thyroid disease—hyperthyroidism, thyroiditis, hypothyroidism, and nontoxic goiter—may, in fact, be a common coexisting disorder with vitiligo in patients over the age of 50. Syndromes with multiple endocrinopathies and with hyperthyroidism, hypoparathyroidism, Addison's disease, chronic mucocutaneous candidiasis, and alopecia areata have been described. Circulating complement-binding antimelanocyte antibodies have been found in two such patients.

Electron microscope studies show a total absence of melanocytes in the white vitiligo macules and decreased numbers of melanocytes in "trichrome" areas (macules or margins of vitiligo patches in which a color intermediate between the normal skin color and the vitiligo white is present).

In over half the patients treated with psoralens and ultraviolet A [UV-A (sunlight or an artificial UV-A light system; see Chap. 53)] significant repigmentation occurs, particularly on the face and neck, and usually on the trunk, upper arms, and legs. Up to 200 or more treatments may be required, however. In some older patients with extensive areas of depigmentation, irreversible depigmention with topical monobenzylether of hydroquinone cream is a more practical and feasible approach. These persons look essentially normal but need to use sun-protective lotions.

Piebaldism is a congenital, autosomal dominant, stable, circumscribed hypomelanosis which resembles vitiligo except that it has a characteristic distribution pattern different from vitiligo and does not usually progress or resolve over time. The hypomelanosis in piebaldism occurs in circumscribed areas on the extremities and anterior surface of the thorax. A white forelock is typical. The eyes are normal, and the patients are otherwise healthy.

Tuberous sclerosis is an autosomal dominant disease which manifests itself by the presence of congenital, circumscribed, white macules in up to 98 percent of cases, and classically by the development (by the fourth year) of seizures, mental retardation, and adenoma sebaceum. The white macules are characteristically on the trunk or buttocks, hypomelanotic, number from 3 to 100, and of typical shape—oval, lance-ovate, or polygonal, like a "thumbprint." The most characteristic, though not the most frequent, is the lance-ovate or American mountain "ash-leaf" macule, which is usually less than 3 cm in its longest dimension and off-white, not pure white, in color. The macules are usually oriented transversely on the trunk and axially on the extremities. The size and color of these lesions do not change over time. The presence of three or more circumscribed macules in a patient is strongly suggestive of tuberous sclerosis. Examination with Wood's lamp is often necessary to visualize the lesions. Histologically, these macules contain melanocytes which have decreased numbers of small melanosomes.

All persons with unexplained seizures or mental retardation should be screened with a Wood's lamp examination for the presence of white spots to exclude tuberous sclerosis. In addition, examination of parents and siblings with CT scans is necessary.

Neurofibromatosis (von Recklinghausen's disease) is an autosomal dominant trait characterized by the appearance, usually by the age of 3 and primarily on the trunk and the extremities, of numerous pale yellow-brown macules (Plate 1-4), or café au lait spots, that vary in diameter from less than 1 cm to more than 15 cm. Spotty generalized pigmentation and axillary freckling may also be present. Often, a few or many soft, rounded, cone-shaped, or pendulous cutaneous tumors covered by normal skin appear by the first or second decade.

The presence of six or more café au lait spots—which are uniformly hypermelanotic, circumscribed, oval macules with a

TABLE 52-3
Disorders associated with circumscribed vitiligo-type hypomelanosis

Associated disorder
GENETIC
Vitiligio, with or without:
Hyper/hypothyroidism
Diabetes mellitus
Addison's disease
Pernicious anemia
Hypoparathyroidism
Addison's disease
Chronic mucocutaneous candidiasis syndrome
Piebaldism
Waardenburg's syndrome
Tuberous sclerosis
Ataxia-telangiectasia
CHEMICAL EXPOSURE
Phenolic germicides (O-Syl, Phebocide, etc.)
Hydroquinone, monobenzylether of
Hydroquinone, monomethylether of
NEOPLASTIC
Malignant melanoma (in sites of regression)
Melanocytic nevi (halo nevi)
INFECTIOUS
Leprosy
Pinta
Tinea versicolor
IDIOPATHIC
Vogt-Koyanagi-Harada syndrome
Postinflammation: atopic dermatitis, psoriasis
Sarcoidosis
Scleroderma

diameter greater than 1.5 cm—is characteristic of neurofibromatosis even in the absence of a positive family history. In *Albright's disease* (polyostotic fibrous dysplasia), however, there are rarely more than three or four such macules, which are usually unilaterally distributed on the buttocks or cervical areas. A single, large, isolated café au lait spot of neurofibromatosis resembles the macule of Albright's disease. It is possible, however, using light microscopy, to detect large pigmented globules in whole amounts of epidermis prepared from café au lait macules of neurofibromatosis; these pigmented globules, or macromelanosomes, are usually not found in the macular pigmented areas present in Albright's disease or in the café au lait macules observed in 10 percent of the normal population. Café au lait spots have also been associated with pulmonic stenosis (Watson's syndrome).

Generalized lentigines may be a feature of *Moynahan's syndrome,* or the "leopard" syndrome, which is an autosomal dominant trait in which the diffuse presence of multiple, small, dark-brown, circumscribed hypermelanotic macules has been associated with ECG abnormalities and, in its fully expressed form, with other findings (*lentigines, ECG abnormalities, ocular hypertelorism, pulmonary stenosis, abnormal genitalia, retardation of growth,* and *deafness).*

Peutz-Jeghers syndrome is an autosomal dominant disorder in which hyperpigmented, brown to blue macules on the lips and buccal mucosa are associated with similar cutaneous lesions and gastrointestinal polyps. The cutaneous macules, but not the buccal pigmented lesions may fade, by adulthood. Chronic gastrointestinal blood loss may occur.

METABOLIC FACTORS Generalized brown hypermelanosis of the skin is a characteristic manifestation of hemochromatosis and of porphyria cutanea tarda. The hyperpigmentation observed in hemochromatosis may be grayish brown or brown and indistinguishable from that of Addison's disease. The diagnosis of hemochromatosis may be established from a skin biopsy which shows hemosiderin deposition in the sweat glands. Porphyria cutanea tarda may be diagnosed by the clinical presence of vesicles, bullae, atrophic macules, sclerodermoid changes, and milia on the skin of the dorsal hands and face, and in the laboratory by red fluorescence of acidified urine, or the presence of increased urinary uroporphyrin (uroporphyrin to coproporphyrin ratio usually is greater than 3:1). Similar changes may be seen in patients with *variegate porphyria,* which has a distinctive porphyrin profile, especially high fecal protoporphyrin. The lesions in variegate porphyria are identical to porphyria cutanea tarda and the diseases must be differentiated as they have different responses to treatment and very different associated medical problems (see Chaps. 53 and 99).

NUTRITIONAL FACTORS In chronic nutritional deficiency, in general, splotches of dirty-brown hyperpigmentation appear, especially on the trunk. In selective deficiencies, such as protein deficiency in kwashiorkor, or when there is protein loss as in chronic nephrosis, ulcerative colitis, and malabsorption syndrome, there is sometimes dilution of hair color so that the hair becomes a reddish-brown and eventually gray. In other selective deficiencies, such as sprue, there may be a brown hypermelanosis over any area of the body. In pellagra, however, the pigmentation is limited to areas of skin exposed to light or to trauma. In vitamin B_{12} deficiency, there is premature graying of hair and a hypermelanosis most apparent overlying the small joints of the hands.

ENDOCRINE FACTORS Diffuse brown hypermelanosis is a striking feature of primary adrenocortical insufficiency (Addison's disease). There is a marked hyperpigmentation over certain areas, namely, the pressure points (vertebrae, knuckles, elbows, and knees), and in body folds, palmar creases, and gingival mucous membrane. An identifiable type of diffuse hyperpigmentation has also been reported to follow adrenalectomy in patients with Cushing disease. In these patients, there usually are signs and symptoms of pituitary tumors; all tumors recorded have been chromophobe adenomas. A third example of the Addisonian type of melanosis has also been observed in patients with pancreatic and lung tumors. The generalized brown hypermelanosis found in all these conditions results from overproduction of melanocyte-stimulating hormone (MSH) and adrenocorticotropic hormone (ACTH), which share common amino acid sequences. It appears that an excess of α-MSH plays a dominant role in the abnormal pigmentation that occurs in Addison's disease. Both MSH and ACTH are increased in adrenal insufficiency as a result of decreased output of cortisol by the adrenals. Hypermelanosis of the Addisonian type can be produced in adrenalectomized human subjects by the administration of large amounts of homogeneous ACTH and α-MSH. α-MSH is a single-polypeptide chain of 13 amino acid residues and is identical in sequence to the terminal portion of ACTH except for the acetylation of the terminal serine residue. Recent evidence has shown that the polypeptide hormones themselves are produced by cleavage of the larger polypeptides. In mammals, MSH causes a significant darkening of skin as early as 24 h after administration. Mammalian melanocytes have been shown to be uniquely sensitive to α-MSH. Melanocytes appear to possess a unique membrane-bound receptor molecule that is present in the G_2 phase of the cell cycle. Following interaction of this receptor with α-MSH, an enzyme also found within the membrane, adenylate cyclase, is stimulated, leading to an increase in the formation and level of intracellular cyclic AMP. Eight hours following treatment with MSH, tyrosinase activity begins to increase. This effect is followed at 16 h by an increase in melanin formation. Current information suggests that cyclic AMP is the mediator of the MSH effect; this evidence includes the fact that cyclic AMP levels rise soon after exposure to MSH.

Melasma, or the "mask of pregnancy," is found in pregnant women, women on oral contraceptives, and in some otherwise normal women and men. This is a circumscribed hypermelanosis of the epidermis, usually of the forehead, cheeks, upper lip, and chin, probably secondary to progestational effects. MSH levels are normal in these patients. Melasma-like hyperpigmentation has also been observed in patients taking phenytoin or mesantoin.

CHEMICAL FACTORS Use of various chemicals, particularly phenol derivatives may cause depigmentation. Topical use of hydroquinone induces a temporary lightening which may be useful in some patients with melasma; monobenzylether of hydroquinone, however, causes a permanent vitiligo-like leukoderma, even remote from the site of application, and is used only to depigment completely the normal skin in patients with extensive vitiligo. Addisonian-like hypermelanosis of the skin follows busulfan therapy, and hypermelanosis may also be seen after use of cyclophosphamide and nitrogen mustard. Inorganic trivalent arsenicals may also produce generalized Addisonian-like hypermelanosis as well as scattered macular hypomelanosis and punctate keratosis of the palms and soles. Blue-gray pigmentation has been observed due to chlorpromazine, minocycline, and other drugs.

PHYSICAL FACTORS Mechanical trauma, as well as burns caused by heat, ultraviolet light, or alpha, beta, and gamma radiation, can lead to hypomelanosis or hypermelanosis. The effects of these physical agents on pigmentation are determined by the intensity and duration of exposure and are limited to the site of injury. Hypomelanosis results from destruction of melanocytes.

INFLAMMATORY AND INFECTIOUS FACTORS Many epidermal proliferative processes resolve and leave aberrations of pigmentation at the sites of involvement; both postinflammatory hypermelanosis (blue-gray, brown, or both) and hypomelanosis may occur following resolution of eczema, psoriasis, lichen planus, drug reactions, pemphigus, viral exanthems, etc. Usually these hypermelanoses disappear spontaneously within several months. White halos surrounding psoriatic plaques are a result of abnormal prostaglandin synthesis and are not an abnormality of melanin biology.

Tinea versicolor, a hypomelanotic, not amelanotic, scaling, circumscribed eruption of the upper anterior and posterior chest in young people, results from the presence in the skin of *Pityrosporum orbiculare* which contains an enzyme that forms azelaic acid, a tyrosinase inhibitor, and results in decreased melanin pigmentation. Repigmentation with sun exposure follows appropriate topical therapy.

Tuberculoid and *lepromatous leprosy* have hypomelanotic macules that are anesthetic. The color, unlike vitiligo, is not pure white, rather, off-white, and the margins of these macules are characteristically indiscrete.

NEOPLASTIC FACTORS Disorders of melanin pigmentation are uncommon features of skin neoplasms. Hypomelanosis has been found around benign nevi (halo nevi) in healthy patients but may also be found in or around malignant melanoma (primaries or metastases); vitiligo-like hypomelanotic macules remote from the melanoma may also occur. A Vogt-Koyanagi-Harada syndrome has been reported following bacillus Calmette-Guérin (BCG) therapy of melanoma. During terminal stages of malignant melanoma, striking development of blue hypermelanosis may be observed, associated with large amounts of a conjugated derivative of 5,6-dihydroxyindole excreted in the urine (melanogenuria). This intermediate in the metabolic pathway from tyrosine to melanin can be oxidized to melanin in the absence of tyrosinase; therefore, melanin can be synthesized at almost any site in which oxidation can take place. Consequently, diffuse black pigmentation may develop in peritoneum, liver, heart, muscle, and dermis of patients during the late stages of malignant melanoma. The brown melanin in the dermal phagocytes appears clinically as blue in the skin because of the Tyndall light-scattering phenomenon. Velvety textured hypermelanotic (brown) macules, representing *acanthosis nigricans,* may be found in the axillae and other areas in patients with various carcinomas, particularly adenocarcinomas of the gastrointestinal tract. Acanthosis nigricans may also be congenital or benign and associated with diabetes mellitus, Cushing's disease, Addison's disease, pituitary adenoma, and other disorders.

The multiple, irregular, round or oval, yellowish brown to reddish brown macules and papules characteristic of *urticaria pigmentosa* are related to the presence of melanin in the epidermis overlying clusters of mast cells. Vigorous rubbing of such lesions results in the development of urticarial wheals (Darier's sign). Systemic mastocytosis, in which mast cells infiltrate diffusely into the liver, spleen, gastrointestinal system, and bones, is a rare condition. Mast-cell leukemia occasionally develops. In children, the skin lesions usually appear in infancy and often spontaneously disappear in several years. The usual course is quite benign, but symptoms of flushing, itching, and urticaria occur in about 30 percent of patients; less than 15 percent experience vomiting, syncope, or shock. The symptoms are presumed to be due to histamine release from mast cells and often coincide with increased urinary excretion of free histamines and metabolites. Urinary levels of 5-hydroxyindoleacetic acid are normal. Antihistamines are of little value.

UNKNOWN CAUSES Generalized brown hypermelanosis of the type seen in Addison's disease may be associated with systemic scleroderma early in the course of the disorder. Generalized hyperpigmentation occasionally develops in patients with chronic hepatic insufficiency, especially that due to portal cirrhosis. The pathogenesis of the pigmentation in both conditions is unknown; MSH levels are not elevated. Hypomelanotic macules may also be found in a small percentage of patients with sarcoidosis. These macules are characteristically not pure white and are circumscribed with indiscrete margins. They may overlie dermal nodules, particularly on the extremities but also at times on the trunk.

REFERENCES

Fitzpatrick TB et al: Biology of the melanin pigmentary system, in *Dermatology in General Medicine,* 2d ed, TB Fitzpatrick et al (eds). New York, McGraw-Hill, 1979

Jimbow K et al: Congenital circumscribed hypomelanosis: A characterization based on electron microscopic study of tuberous sclerosis, nevus depigmentosis, and piebaldism. J Invest Dermatol 64:50, 1975

Mosher DB et al: Abnormalities of pigmentation, in *Dermatology in General Medicine,* 2d ed, TB Fitzpatrick et al (eds). New York, McGraw-Hill, 1979

Pawelek JM: Factors regulating growth in pigmentation of melanoma cells. J Invest Dermatol 66:201, 1976

Prota G, Thompson RH: Melanin pigmentation in mammals. Endeavour 35:32, 1976

Riley PA: Melanins and melanogenesis, in *Pathobiology Annual,* HL Ioachim (ed). New York, Raven Press, 1980, vol 10

Witkop CV et al: Albinism, in *The Metabolic Basis of Inherited Diseases,* 5th ed, JB Stanbury et al (eds). New York, McGraw-Hill, 1982

53 PHOTOSENSITIVITY AND OTHER REACTIONS TO LIGHT

MADHUKAR A. PATHAK
THOMAS B. FITZPATRICK
JOHN A. PARRISH

Humans have evolved in sunlight and depend upon it for much more than an indirect source of food and maintenance of the earth's temperature. The natural light has always been recognized for, and endowed with, health-giving powers. Our skin, eyes, blood vessels, and certain endocrine gland functions respond to radiation from the electromagnetic spectrum of the sun. The formation of vitamin D from sterol precursors in the skin by solar ultraviolet radiation (UVR) exposure has long been recognized in the management of rickets. Certain of our daily biorhythms are dependent upon the cycles of sunlight. Yet, sunlight can be harmful and damage or kill living cells. Sunlight causes sunburn, damage to deoxyribonucleic acid (DNA), skin cancer, wrinkling and aging of the skin, eye inflammation, and possibly cataracts. During the last decade, interest in the reaction of human skin to light has been renewed as a result of:

1 The public's obsession with sunbathing, resulting in premature "aging" of the skin (solar elastosis).
2 Demographic data indicating that exposure to sunlight is an important cause of basal-cell and squamous-cell carcinoma and even melanoma of the sun-exposed parts of the body.

3 The widespread use of certain drugs such as phenothiazines, thiazides and related sulfonamide diuretics, and antibiotics (demethylchlortetracycline), which alter the cutaneous responses to sunlight and cause undesirable photosensitivity reactions.

4 Increased awareness that sunlight is a major cause of discomfort and photosensitivity reactions in patients with certain types of porphyria, especially for those with erythropoietic protoporphyria.

5 The emergence of a new science of photomedicine and photochemotherapy based on the recent advances in molecular photobiology and the availability of high-intensity ultraviolet irradiation systems; this has enabled both researchers and practicing physicians to use UVR and visible radiation with or without the systemic administration of the drug to achieve a striking, therapeutic response in diseases such as psoriasis, polymorphous photodermatitis, mycosis fungoides, lichen planus, vitiligo, uremic pruritus, etc. Visible radiation also has been successfully used in newborn infants in the treatment of neonatal jaundice to prevent bilirubin encephalopathy. Light emitted by certain types of lasers is being increasingly used in the treatment of port-wine stains, telangiectasia, and other vascular lesions.

6 The increased recognition that the exposure of UVR can alter the function and viability of cellular components of the immune system; normal and abnormal immune responses can be altered and can result in local alterations of immune function at the site of exposure or some specific systemic alterations at distant nonexposed sites.

There are more than 25 human disorders that are either caused by or aggravated by exposure of the skin to sunlight. These range from degenerative and neoplastic changes to disability and discomfort associated with chemically induced photosensitivity reactions. These abnormal reactions to light in humans are briefly presented in Table 53-1.

TABLE 53-1
Diseases induced or exacerbated by light

I By light alone
- *A* Genetic: ephelides (freckles)
- *B* Idiopathic
  - *1* Acute solar skin damage (sunburn)
  - *2* Connective tissue degeneration (wrinkling)
  - *3* Telangiectasia
  - *4* Solar keratoses and solar lentigo
  - *5* Basal-cell carcinoma
  - *6* Squamous-cell carcinoma
  - *7* Malignant melanoma
  - *8* Polymorphous photodermatosis
  - *9* Solar urticaria
  - *10* Actinic reticuloid

II By light plus exogenous agents
- *A* Chemical or drug
  - *1* Phototoxic reactions
  - *2* Phytophotodermatitis
  - *3* Lupus erythematosus (with hydralazine, procainamide)
- *B* Chemical and immunologic: photoallergic reactions

III By light plus metabolite(s)
- *A* Porphyrias
- *B* Porphyria cutanea tarda associated with hexachlorobenzene, estrogens, alcohol

IV By light plus preexisting disease
- *A* Genetic
  - *1* Xeroderma pigmentosum
  - *2* Oculocutaneous albinism
  - *3* Vitiligo
  - *4* Hartnup syndrome
- *B* Nutritional or metabolic
  - *1* Pellagra
  - *2* Malignant carcinoid
- *C* Viral: herpes simplex
- *D* Unknown: lupus erythematosus (cutaneous, systemic)

This chapter will be concerned with (1) common conditions such as sunburn, the degenerative and neoplastic conditions associated with solar radiation [basal-cell carcinoma, squamous-cell carcinoma, malignant melanoma, solar keratoses (Plate 4-2)] and chronic sun-induced degeneration; (2) photosensitivity related to drugs and to increased blood or plasma levels of photosensitizing porphyrins in patients with all types of porphyria (except acute intermittent porphyria); (3) certain idiopathic forms of commonly occurring photodermatoses; (4) photochemotherapy; and (5) photoprotection.

The unit of wavelength most commonly used to measure and express nonionizing UVR or visible light is the nanometer (1 nm $= 10^{-9}$ m $=$ 10 Å).

Electromagnetic emanations from the sun comprise a wide range of radiation and include electric waves, radio waves, infrared rays, visible light, UVR, roentgen rays (x-rays), gamma rays, and cosmic rays. The shortest wavelengths that reach the surface of the earth through the atmosphere are about 286 to 290 nm. Wavelengths shorter than 286 nm are principally absorbed by ozone in the stratosphere. In terrestrial sunlight, the UV region extends from 290 to 400 nm, the visible spectrum from 400 to 760 nm, and the infrared spectrum from wavelengths longer than 760 nm.

The solar spectrum that can affect human skin includes wavelengths of 290 to 760 nm; however, infrared radiation (1.5 to 1000 μm) can produce thermal effects (including burn) and potentiate the photochemical and biologic reactions initiated by UVR or visible radiation. For practical reasons, UVR is often arbitrarily subdivided into three bands designated as (1) UV-A (320 to 400 nm, or long-wave ultraviolet), (2) UV-B (290 to 320 nm, or sunburn spectrum), and (3) UV-C (shorter than 290 nm, or germicidal radiation).

The amount and type of solar radiation that may reach a given part of the earth at any given time are determined by a great variety of factors, including latitude, time of day, season, altitude, local atmospheric conditions (smog, cloudiness, haze, smoke, dust, fog, humidity, aerosol particles), variations in the thickness of the ozone layer, and height of the sun above the horizon.

Approximately 50 percent of the sun's radiant energy is in the visible portion of the spectrum (400 to 760 nm), about 40 percent in the infrared region, and about 10 percent in the UV region. The damage to skin (sunburn, skin cancer) is evoked by 3 percent of the ultraviolet radiation wavelengths, namely, from 290 to 320 nm.

The transmission of radiant energy varies with wavelength and different areas of the human skin; it may range from 0 to 70 percent. Shorter wavelengths ($<$ 285 nm) are mostly absorbed by the dead-cell layer of the stratum corneum; wavelengths that produce sunburn (290 to 315 nm) are also mostly absorbed in the epidermis. Longer wavelengths (320 to 760 nm) penetrate more deeply into the dermis. Transmission of different wavelengths depends upon (1) the regional thickness of the epidermis, (2) the degree of hydration, (3) the concentration of UV and visible light-absorbing components such as melanin, proteins (keratin, elastin, collagen), nucleic acid, urocanic acid, carotenoids, and hemoglobin, and (4) the number and spatial arrangement of melanosomes and of blood vessels. In fair-skinned individuals, about 85 to 90 percent of 290- to 315-nm radiation is absorbed by the epidermis and only about 10 to 15 percent can penetrate through the epidermis to reach the dermis. In dark-skinned individuals, nearly 90 to 95 percent of 290- to 315-nm radiation is absorbed by the epidermis. The transmission through the epidermis of long-wave UV radiation (320 to 400 nm) and visible radiation (400 to 760 nm) may range from 20 to 70 percent. The optical properties of hypopigmented epidermis of fair-skinned individuals are such that approximately 2 percent of 250-nm (germicidal) radiation, about 12 to 15 percent of 300 nm radiation, and about 50 percent of 360-nm radiation can be transmitted to the dermis. Since cutaneous blood flow is about 500 ml/min, the equivalent entire blood volume of an adult person at rest can circulate through the skin every 11 min. Thus, UVR penetrating through the epidermis and impinging on the network of capillaries and small vessels can affect lymphocytes circulating through the skin, and prolonged exposure (over 90 min) may damage a significant portion of the circulating cells. It is now known that UVR induces loss of mononuclear cell viability; they are most sensitive to UV-C (< 290 nm) and less sensitive to UV-B and UV-A radiation (sensitivity ratios of 10^4:10:1). UV-induced alterations in immune function appear to be involved in the pathogenesis of experimental photocarcinogenesis in mice. The significance of the alteration of lymphocyte function following exposure to UVR is not well understood, but it is possible that such alterations may play a role in the pathogenesis of UV-induced skin cancer, lupus erythematosus, and some photosensitivity disorders. The alteration of lymphocyte function and immune responses may explain the beneficial effects of phototherapy and photochemotherapy in certain skin diseases.

The most detrimental effect of UVR is cell death. Other effects include mutagenesis, carcinogenesis, interference or inhibition in the synthesis of DNA, RNA, and protein, and also in immune functions. The mutagenic and carcinogenic effects appear to be mediated largely through the action of UV-B radiation on DNA. The most common reactions, such as sunburn, tanning or melanin pigmentation, synthesis of vitamin D, keratosis, and skin aging are also caused by UV-B radiation. Although the longer wavelengths (320 to 400 nm or 400 to 760 nm) penetrate more deeply into the skin, they are much less effective at causing these types of photobiologic phenomena. However, in the presence of certain chemical agents (e.g., drugs that are given orally or endogenous porphyrins in certain porphyrias), these wavelengths become highly damaging and can cause severe skin photosensitization.

Protection against this damage to the "normal" skin has been the subject of much investigation, and many commercially available sunscreens can be recommended in the prevention of sunburn, skin cancer, aging of skin, and in various types of photosensitivity disorders.

SUNBURN AND TANNING

CLINICAL CHANGES Erythema, or sunburn reaction Erythema is caused principally by 290- to 320-nm radiation, maximum solar effectiveness being 300 to 307 nm. UVR emitted by artificial light sources produces erythema maximally at 297 and 254 nm. Light greater than 320 nm (320 to 760 nm) is generally considered to be nonerythemogenic, although prolonged exposure to 320- to 400-nm radiation (2 h of midday summer sun in northern latitudes) can produce mild sunburn in normal subjects. The minimal erythema dose (MED) is defined as the lowest UVR dose which produces perceptible redness up to 24 h following exposure to a defined spectral band (either UV-B or UV-A). In fair-skinned individuals, the MED of UV-B is approximately 20 to 50 mJ/cm². UV doses larger than 3, 6, or 9 times the MED have a short latent period, and the subsequent erythema reaction is more severe; marked erythema, edema, and even bullae may occur. If the total dose is large, pain and systemic symptoms such as fever may occur. The MED of 320 to 400 nm (UV-A) is approximately 25 to 100 J/cm² or about 800 to 1000 times greater than that of UV-B.

Sunburn, suntan, and peeling are experiences familiar to almost the entire fair-skinned population. Individuals vary in their susceptibility to sunburn and suntan. Personal history of sunburning (e.g., easy, moderate, severe, or difficult), peeling, and the ability to acquire tan (minimal, moderate, profuse, etc.) is very helpful to classify people of different ethnic backgrounds into six sun-reactive types as described in Table 53-2.

The sunburn reaction is a complex inflammatory process. The observed histologic changes include the appearance of dyskeratotic cells (containing pyknotic nuclei), spongiosis, vacuolation of keratinocytes, and edema. The dermal changes include an inflammatory infiltrate (mostly lymphocytes), endothelial swelling, and capillary leakage manifested by extravasation of red blood cells. The severity of these changes and the rate at which they evolve depend on the exposure dose, the incident wavelength, and degree of skin pigmentation. Hypopigmented, fair-skinned individuals (e.g., red-haired, freckled individuals such as the Irish or Scottish) are more susceptible to sunburn than pigmented individuals who tan well. The nature of the chromophore that absorbs the light energy which initiates the primary photochemical responses is not well established, although the bulk of evidence suggests that nucleic acids (DNA) are primary targets for the absorption of the 290- to 320-nm radiation. Vasodilatation which accompanies the sunburn reaction appears to result from the activation and release of one or more chemical mediators (e.g., kinins, serotonin, histamine).

There has been considerable focus on the role of prostaglandins (PG) and related derivatives of arachidonic acid as mediators of the delayed erythema reaction induced by UV-B. Prostaglandins of the PGE and PGF series are low-molecular-weight, oxygenated fatty acid structures synthesized by microsomal enzymes (PG synthase, lipoxygenase, and cyclooxygenase) present in all mammalian cells, including epidermal cells. Increased levels of prostaglandins (PGE series) have been observed in widely different types of cutaneous inflammation reaction, including the UV-induced sunburn reaction. Indomethacin, a nonsteroidal anti-inflammatory agent, when applied topically or given intradermally, can decrease a delayed sunburn response of human skin produced by UV-B radiation. Since indomethacin is known to inhibit prostaglandin synthesis, these findings support the possible role of prostaglandins as mediators of the delayed erythemal response to UV-B radiation. It is of interest to note that prostaglandin levels are increased in skin exposed to an erythemogenic dose of UV-C (germicidal) radiation. However, a PUVA (psoralen + UV-A)–induced phototoxic reaction does not seem to generate elevated levels of prostaglandins, and indomethacin, applied topically or given intradermally, has no effect in decreasing the intensity of the erythema reaction, suggesting that the mechanism of photosensitization reaction evoked by PUVA is not mediated by PGs. Other mediators including histamine are also believed to be involved in UV-B–induced delayed erythema reaction. Ultraviolet radiation may also have a direct effect on the blood vessels of the upper layer of the dermis (capillaries, venules, and arterioles). The formation of peroxides, superoxide anions, or free radicals may play an important role in the damage to lysosomal membranes associated with lipid peroxidation. In fair skin 290- to 320-nm spectrum is

TABLE 53-2
Classification of sun-reactive skin types

Skin type	*History of sunburning and tanning*
I	Always burn, never tan, often peel (Celtics)
II	Always burn, tan slightly
III	Always burn, tan moderately (average Caucasians)
IV	Sometimes burn (minimally), always tan (olive skin)
V	Rarely burn, tan easily and substantially (brown skin)
VI	Never burn, tan profusely (Blacks)

known to produce damaging free radicals (molecules with unpaired electrons).

Melanin pigmentation, or tanning Tanning (increase in melanin pigment) that follows exposure of the skin to solar radiation involves two distinct photobiologic processes. The first, *immediate pigment darkening* (IPD), or darkening of preformed pigment in the epidermis, is elicited by wavelengths of 320 to 720 nm. The second, *melanogenesis,* or delayed tanning reaction, is an intricate process that consists of the *erythema response (sunburn)* followed usually in 3 to 4 days by formation of new pigment. Immediate pigment darkening results from oxidation of melanin through the production of semiquinone-like free radicals in the melanin polymer; transfer of melanosomes from melanocytes and redistribution of already existing melanosomes within the keratinocytes also may occur.

Melanogenesis involves (1) an increase in the number of functional melanocytes, resulting from increased proliferation of melanocytes, and activation of dormant melanocytes; (2) increased arborization of melanocytic dendrites; (3) an increase in the number of melanosomes in proliferating melanocytes; (4) an increase in tyrosinase activity; and (5) an increase in the transfer of melanosomes from melanocytes to keratinocytes. The degree of melanin pigmentation, however, that can be achieved in an individual by exposure to solar radiation is genetically predetermined. People with fair skin who burn easily but do not tan or tan poorly (skin types I and II) cannot with repeated sun exposures achieve that degree of tanning which can be easily achieved by someone genetically able to tan profusely with minimal exposure. Delayed tanning reaction appears to have a protective effect on the skin against subsequent exposures.

CELLULAR AND MOLECULAR CHANGES Hyperplasia Within 72 h after exposure, there is an increase in the number of epidermal cells with a high rate of mitotic activity. The rate of cell proliferation decreases after 7 to 10 days, and the thickness of the epidermis gradually returns to normal within the next 30 to 60 days. In UV-induced hyperplasia the activities of polyamine biosynthetic enzymes, ornithine-decarboxylase (ODC) and *S*-adenosyl-methionine decarboxylase are increased in UV-B irradiated skin, resulting in the elevation of putrescine and spermidine. PUVA and UV-C also induce increased epidermal ODC activity, reflecting the potential role of polyamines in cell growth and hyperplasia.

DNA and RNA changes Damage to DNA by sunburn-producing UV light (290 to 320 nm) may result in mutation or cell death. The principal epidermal DNA photoproducts are pyrimidine dimers (e.g., thymine dimers); these are of the cyclobutane type and are formed between adjacent pyrimidine bases. Cell membranes, DNA, RNA, protein, and other molecules may be altered, and the synthesis of DNA, RNA, and protein may be temporarily inhibited immediately after irradiation. New synthesis is evident by 24 h and is maximal by 60 to 70 h.

Mitosis Inhibition of epidermal mitosis and retardation of basal-cell turnover occur within 1 h after irradiation. The epidermal cell cycle is interruped at the S phase of DNA synthesis. Inhibition of mitosis can persist for 7 to 24 h; it is followed by an acceleration of mitotic rate and basal-cell turnover that reaches a peak by 48 to 72 h and is associated with epidermal hyperplasia. The mitotic cycle appears to be interrupted in the G_2 stage, in the prophase stage, or in both. The increased mitotic activity and the associated hyperplasia may last for 30 to 60 days. This hyperplasia appears to be due to a combination of the removal of the epidermal mitotic inhibitors (chalones) and stimulation of growth by the action of cyclic adenosine monophosphate (AMP) and guanosine 5′-monophosphate (GMP).

Formation of vitamin D The skin has long been recognized as the site for sun-induced photosynthesis of vitamin D. The photochemical mechanisms involved have been recently elucidated and are described in Chap. 351.

SUN-INDUCED CARCINOMA

The malignancies and premalignancies unequivocally associated with sun exposure include solar or actinic keratoses, basal-cell epitheliomas, squamous-cell carcinomas, and keratoacanthomas. Some studies have established that carcinoma of the skin occurs more frequently on the parts of the body habitually exposed to sunlight; thus, the lesions of the head and hands are concentrated on the nose, central portions of the cheeks, eyelids, and dorsum of the hands. In fair-skinned Caucasoids who sunburn easily, these cancers are limited almost exclusively to the exposed portions of the face, head, neck, arms, and hands. Negroid skin, on the other hand, is remarkably resistant to the development of skin cancer on the exposed surfaces, and a similar resistance is seen among the pigmented Caucasoids (e.g., East Indians), American Indians, and Asiatics.

Carcinoma of the exposed skin is more prevalent among persons who are outdoors a great deal and is the common cause of cancer in Caucasoids in Australia, South Africa, and the southern parts of the United States. The action spectrum for photocarcinogenesis is similar to that of sunburn reaction.

Several studies based on the distribution of local populations in the United States, Australia, and Ireland have emphasized that skin cancer develops earlier and more frequently in people who have light skin and freckles, who burn easily and do not tan on exposure to the sun, and who are of mostly Celtic ancestry (people with skin types I and II). *Australia, with the highest reported incidence of skin cancer* in the world, has a population largely descended from British stock, with about 25 percent claiming Celtic (i.e., Irish, Scottish, and Welsh) extraction. In all three countries surveyed, persons of Celtic ancestry were found to have a disproportionately high incidence of skin cancer. Dark-pigmented races and people who tan well (skin types IV to VI) are least susceptible to skin cancer. Chronically exposed areas of many fair-skinned individuals may develop small hyperkeratotic lesions commonly referred to as *solar keratoses.* These may progress to squamous-cell or basal-cell carcinomas and may be seen as early as the third decade. Susceptible individuals may exhibit more than one lesion. These can be readily recognized by the use of topical 5-fluorouracil.

All varieties of skin cancer develop in patients with *xeroderma pigmentosum,* an autosomal recessive disorder. This rare defect represents, in the extreme, the basic problem of solar radiation and skin cancer. Patients with this disease have a greatly increased susceptibility to malignant tumors of the skin in the light-exposed areas. The characteristic skin manifestations are atrophy, telangiectasia, hyperpigmented macules, keratoses, and ulcerations, all occurring in sun-exposed areas. Within the first few years of life, basal-cell or squamous-cell carcinomas or sarcomas or malignant melanomas develop. An inherited enzyme defect may be responsible, at least in part, for the cancer-forming potential in patients with xeroderma pigmentosum. Cultured fibroblasts from patients with xeroderma pigmentosum are incapable of releasing thymine dimers from DNA and, in consequence, are deficient in their ability to repair their UV-damaged DNA. Xeroderma pigmentosum is the most notable human disease in which there is a defect in the excision repair process involving the removal of UV-induced dimers followed by the synthesis and re-forming of new segments of DNA. This enzymatic deficiency may result in a high somatic mutation rate of skin cells after sun exposure and, eventually, in cancer formation. The fact that mutagenesis is largely the result of errors made during the repair of photo-damaged DNA and that UVR is known to be mutagenic suggests that the first step toward UV-induced carcinogenesis may be the result of an error made during the repair and replication of the damaged DNA.

DEGENERATIVE CHANGES OF THE SKIN

Degenerative skin changes (wrinkling, telangiectasia, keratoses) are more frequent in white-skinned people living in areas where the intensity of UVR is great (e.g., southwestern United States, Australia, South Africa). The term *solar degeneration* or *dermatoheliosis* implies a group of changes in the exposed areas of the skin, including wrinkling, atrophy, hypermelanotic and hypomelanotic macules, telangiectasia, yellow papules and plaques, and keratoses. The furrowed and leathery condition of the skin is seen particularly in persons who have fair skin and poor tanning ability and are constantly exposed to the sun. The most conspicuous and characteristic change may result from biochemical and structural alterations of connective tissue (elastin as well as collagen). The generative changes are caused by sunburn-producing (290 to 320 nm) and UV-A (320 to 400 nm) radiation that can penetrate deeply into the dermis. Heat (infrared radiation) may accelerate actinic degeneration.

Chronically light-damaged human epidermis shows shortening or flattening of the rete ridges, thinning of the epidermis (decrease in malpighian cells), and many abnormal cells in disorderly arrangement. There is a progressive degeneration in the papillary and subpapillary zones of the dermis. Other changes include (1) the development of vascular ectasia, (2) accumulation of acid mucopolysaccharides, (3) appearance of abnormal fibrocytes, (4) loss of collagen, (5) degeneration of elastic tissue ("actinic elastosis") and disorganization of the connective tissue into amorphous masses. In actinically damaged skin the concentration of elastin may be increased and collagen decreased. These changes are mostly irreversible but can be minimized by daily topical application of effective sunscreens.

PHOTOTOXICITY AND PHOTOALLERGY

Sensitivity to sunlight is a common clinical problem. Continuous daily exposure to sun alone may be the major factor responsible for irreversible skin changes (e.g., freckles, telangiectasia, wrinkling, keratoses, atrophy, hypermelanotic and hypomelanotic macules, and carcinomas in the sun-exposed regions). Apart from these chronic changes, human skin can also become hypersensitive to UVR and visible light. The interface between humans and their environment is the skin, and the physical (light) and chemical agents acting directly on it are important etiologic or precipitating factors in photosensitivity disorders.

EFFECT OF DRUGS AND OTHER CHEMICALS IN ASSOCIATION WITH LIGHT EXPOSURE Some chemicals and drugs by themselves may not act as contact irritants and are generally innocuous to skin in the absence of light exposure. However, when the skin is challenged with proper concentrations of

TABLE 53-3
Contact photosensitizers: Chemicals that induce photosensitivity reactions in humans

Name	*Use*	*Reported clinical observations*
Halogenated salicylanilides; 3,3′,4′,5-tetrachlorosalicylanilide; 3,4′,5- and 3,3′,5-trichlorosalicylanilide; 3,4′,5- and 3,3′,5-tribromosalicylanilide; 3,5- and 4,5′-dibromosalicylanilide	Deodorant, bacteriostatic agents in soaps	Phototoxic and eczematous photoallergic reactions, burning, itching, cross-photosensitivity reactions
Hexachlorophene	Antimicrobial, antiseptic	Phototoxic reactions
Bithionol or bis(2-hydroxy-3,5-dichlorophenyl) sulfide	Antimicrobial, antiseptic	Photoallergic reactions
Fentichlor (2,2′-dihydroxy-5,5′-dichlorodiphenyl sulfide); multifungin (bromochlorosalicylanilide); Jadit (4-chloro-2-hydroxybenzoic acid *N*-*n*-butylamide)	Antifungal	Phototoxic and photoallergic reactions
5-Flurouracil	Antineoplastic	Acceleration of inflammatory process
p-Aminobenzoic acid (PABA) and esters of PABA	Sunscreen	Photoallergic reactions
4,4′-Bis(3-phenylureido)-2,2′-stilbenedisulfonic acid or blankophor	Fluorescent brightening agent for cellulose, nylon, or wool fibers	Phototoxic and photoallergic reactions
Cadmium sulfide	In tattoos	Erythema
Furocoumarins: psoralen, 8-methoxypsoralen, 5-methoxypsoralen, 4,5′,8-trimethylpsoralen	In vitiligo for increased pigment formation and sun tolerance	Marked erythema, vesicles, bullae, hyperpigmentation
Essential oils: oil of bergamot, oil of lime, oil of cedar, oil of lavender, oil of citron, oil of sandalwood	Cosmetics and beauty aids	Phototoxic reactions and postinflammatory hyperpigmentation
Plants: Umbelliferae, Rutaceae	Used in perfumes or flavorings or as spices	Phytophotodermatitis, hyperpigmentation, vesicles, bullae
6-Methylcoumarin	Used in cosmetics	Photoallergic reactions
Musk ambrette	Used in cosmetics	Photoallergic reactions
Dyes: fluorescein, rose bengal, eosin, erythrocine, trypaflavin, orange red, paraphenylenediamine, methylene blue, toluidine blue, trypan blue, anthraquinone	Cosmetics and dye industry	Erythema, edema, vesicles, pigmentation, phototoxic reaction
Coal tar and coal tar derivatives containing anthracene, phenanthrene, naphthalene, thiophene, and many phenolic agents; pitch, acridine	In therapy for psoriasis and chronic eczema; in hair shampoos	Smarting, exaggerated sunburn, urticarial wheals, tar melanosis

SOURCE: *TB Fitzpatrick et al, in Sunlight and Man: Normal and Abnormal Photobiologic Responses, MA Pathak et al (eds), Tokyo, University of Tokyo Press, 1974.*

the agent and the appropriate light wavelengths, these agents can induce undesirable skin reactions.

Cutaneous photosensitivity is a general term used to refer to the abnormal reaction of the human skin to the stimulus of light. Chemical or drug photosensitivity reactions may be defined clinically as adverse skin responses resulting from the combination of exposure to certain therapeutic or chemical agents and UVR. In most of the drug or chemical photosensitivity reactions, the wavelengths that evoke abnormal reactions are usually but not always in the 320 to 400-nm region. Adverse cutaneous reactions can occur in some individuals who either have ingested certain drugs or have been in contact with certain chemicals (Tables 53-3 and 53-4). These reactions may include an acute, abnormal sunburn response, namely, edema, papules, macules, vesicles, bullae, or acute eczematous or urticarial reactions. There may be desquamation and hyperpigmentation or hypopigmentation. These adverse photosensitivity reactions are classified into two broad categories: (1) phototoxic reactions and (2) photoallergic reactions.

Phototoxic reactions are those reactions exaggerated by UVR in which there is no evidence of participation of the immune system; these reactions usually can be elicited in almost everyone with enough light energy of the appropriate wavelengths and when appropriate concentrations of the agent are either applied topically or given orally. Light plus the offending agent leads to an exaggerated sunburn reaction, with or without painful edema. The reaction can occur within 5 to 18 h after exposure to the sun and is usually maximum at 36 to 72 h. Hyperpigmentation and desquamation can also occur. The reaction is usually confined to the site of exposure. If the applied concentration of the implicated agent is high, bullae or small vesicles may develop. The most common chemicals that induce phototoxicity reactions in humans are (1) anthraquinone dyes; (2) chorothiazides; (3) chlorpromazines and phenothiazines; (4) coal tars containing anthracene, acridine, phenanthrene, etc.; (5) nalidixic acid; (6) protriptyline; (7) psoralens (8-methoxypsoralen and 4,5',8-trimethylpsoralen); (8) sulfonamides; and (9) tetracycline (demethylchlortetracycline, etc.) (see Table 53-4).

Certain *phototoxic reactions* require the presence of molecular oxygen (e.g., hematoporphyrin, several dyes). The oxygen-dependent reactions are referred to as *photodynamic reactions.* On the other hand, many phototoxic reactions can occur in the absence of oxygen (e.g., psoralen photosensitization). Most reactions have been reported to require UV-A (320 to 400 nm) radiation; however, certain phototoxic reactions can be initiated by the UV-B (290 to 320 nm) as well as by the visible (400 to 700 nm) spectra. The phototoxic reactions in general should

TABLE 53-4
Systemic photosensitizers: Chemicals that induce photosensitivity reactions in humans

Name	*Uses*	*Clinical observations*	*Action spectrum, nm*
SULFONAMIDES			
Sulfanilamide, sulfathiazole, sulfapyridine, sulfamethazine, sulfaguanidine, sulfisoxazole, monochlorphenamide	Chemotherapy, antibacterial agents	Phototoxic and photoallergic reactions	290–320
SULFONYLUREA			
Carbutamide, tolbutamide (Orinase), chlorpropamide (Diabinese)	Hypoglycemic or antidiabetic drugs	Phototoxic reactions	290–360
CHLORTHIAZIDES			
6-Chloro-7-sulfamyl-3,4-dihydro-1,2,4-thiodiazine 1,1-dioxide (HydroDiuril)	Diuretics, antihypertensive	Papular and edematous eruption, plaques	290–320
Quinethazone (Diuril)	Antihypertensive	Phototoxic and photoallergic reactions	320–400
PHENOTHIAZINES			
Chlorpromazine (Thorazine), promethazine (Phenergan), mepazine, Stelazine, trimeprazine, Compazine, promazine (Sparine)	Tranquilizer, nematode infestation agent, urinary antiseptic, antihistamine	Exaggerated sunburn, maculopapular and urticarial eruptions, gray-blue hyperpigmentation	290–400
ANTIBIOTICS			
Demethylchlortetracycline (Declomycin), chlortetracycline, oxytetracycline, doxycycline	Broad-spectrum antibiotic	Exaggerated sunburn, phototoxic reaction	320–400
Griseofulvin	Antimycotic	Exaggerated sunburn, phototoxic and photoallergic reactions	320–400
Nalidixic acid (NegGram)	Antibacterial	Erythema, bullae	320–400
FUROCOUMARINS			
4,5′,8-Trimethylpsoralen (trioxsalen), 8-methoxypsoralen (methoxsalen), psoralen	In photochemotherapy of psoriasis and vitiligo; for sun tolerance and increased pigment formation	Erythema, bullae, hyperpigmentation	320–400
ESTROGENS AND PROGESTERONES			
Mestranol and norethynodrel, diethylstilbestrol	Oral contraceptives	Melasma, phototoxic reactions	?290–320
Chlordiazepoxide (Librium)	Tranquilizer, psychotropic	Eczematous eruption	290–360
Triacetyldiphenolisatin	Laxative	Eczematous photoallergic reaction	290–320
Cyclamates, calcium cyclamate, sodium cyclohexylsulfamate	Artificial sweeteners	Phototoxic and photoallergic reactions	290–360

SOURCE: *TB Fitzpatrick et al, in Sunlight and Man: Normal and Abnormal Photobiologic Responses, MA Pathak et al (eds), Tokyo, University of Tokyo Press, 1974.*

be regarded as the undesirable sequelae of augmentation of the primary photochemical reactions that underlie the inflammatory response of skin evoked by UVR. It is believed that a deleterious amount of radiant energy is absorbed by the skin and the photosensitizing agents. This absorbed energy can directly cause cell damage by creating a covalent linking of the sensitizing molecule to the pyrimidines (e.g., thymine) in the cellular DNA. This linkage (the formation of cyclobutane photoadducts of the sensitizer and the pyrimidines) can be lethal to the cell. Photosensitizers like the psoralens selectively intercalate between two base pairs and produce interstrand cross-links with epidermal DNA. In addition, the photosensitizing molecule can transfer the absorbed energy and promote formation of free radicals (molecules with unpaired electrons that are highly reactive) and cause damage to the cell membranes and lysosomes. In the presence of certain porphyrins (e.g., hematoporphyrin, protoporphyrin), a reactive singlet form of oxygen can be generated by these photosensitizing molecules. Drug-induced phototoxic reactions may thus involve damage to the DNA, RNA, lysosomes, cell membranes, and other organelles.

Photoallergy to drugs is an acquired and altered capacity of the skin to respond to light in the presence of a photosensitizer, and involves the immune system. The absorbed light energy may promote a photochemical reaction between the drug and the skin proteins. The drug may act to form a haptenic group and either combines directly with the protein to form a photoantigen or is altered by the absorbed energy; this altered haptenic group then reacts with the proteins to form an antigen. The photoantigen is then processed by macrophages and is believed to come in contact with T-cells to manifest any ordinary type of delayed hypersensitivity immunologic response. The complete photoantigen is recognized on subsequent exposure to sensitized T-cells in the form of a papulovesicular or an eczematous response.

The clinical manifestations in drug-induced photoallergic reactions may range from acute urticarial lesions, developing within a few minutes after exposure, to eczematous or papular lesions appearing within 24 h or later. The eruption may extend beyond the exposed areas. In recurrent cases, flare-ups of distant, previously uninvolved sites may also occur. Some edema and vasodilatation are common in most of these eruptions. The action spectrum is generally in the long-wave range (320 to 400 nm), and less energy is required than is necessary for the production of phototoxic reactions. In general, photoallergy is much less common than phototoxic reaction, and the light-microscopic examination of a lesional biopsy reveals a characteristic, though not diagnostic, dense perivascular round-cell infiltrate.

The various systemic therapeutic agents and their effects on the skin in the presence of light (whether phototoxic or pho-

TABLE 53-5
Topical sunscreens

Formulation ingredient	Concentration	Commercial name	SPF*	Recommended for skin type nos.†
PABA SUNSCREENS				
Aminobenzoic acid in 50–70% ethyl alcohol	5%, clear lotion	PreSun Pabanol	>10–15 >6–8	I and II III and IV
ESTERS AND DERIVATIVES OF PABA				
1-Hydroxy-4-methoxybenzophenone, + octyldimethyl PABA (Padimate O)	3% + 7%, creamy lotion	Coppertone Supershade	10	I and II
Isoamyl-*p*-*N*,*N*-dimethyl aminobenzoate (Escalol 506, Padimate A)	2.5% or 3.3%, clear lotion	Block Out PABA Film Spectraban	6 6 6	III and IV III and IV III and IV
Glyceryl PABA + octyldimethyl PABA or 2-ethylhexyl ester of dimethylaminobenzoate (Escalol 507)	2.5% + 2.5%, milky lotion	Eclipse, total	>8–10	I and II
Escalol 507 + dioxybenzone	2.5% + 3%, clear lotion	Sungard	6	III and IV
Escalol 507 (octyldimethyl PABA) in ammonium acrylate–acrylate polymer	3.3%, milky lotion	Sundown	6–8	III and IV
Homomenthyl salicylate + *p*-dimethylaminobenzoate	5%, clear lotion	Aztec	6	III and IV
NON-PABA CHEMICAL SUNSCREENS				
2-Hydroxy-4-methoxybenzophenone 5-sulfonic acid	10%, milky lotion	UVAL	7	III and IV
Ethylhexyl-*p*-methoxycinnamate + 2-hydroxy-4-methoxybenzophenone + 2-phenylbenzamidazole sulfonic acid (G6)	5% + 3% + 4%, cream	Piz Buin Exclusiv Extrem Cream, Tisol	>10–15	I and II
Ethylhexyl-*p*-methoxycinnamate	4%–4.5% cream or lotion	Piz Buin-4	>6	III and IV
Ethylhexyl-*p*-methoxycinnamate + 2-hydroxy-4-methoxybenzophenone	5% + 3% milky lotion	Piz Buin-6, Tisol	>8 8–10	I and II I and II
PHYSICAL SUNSCREENS				
Titanium dioxide, zinc oxide, kaolin, talc, iron oxide, etc.	Heavy cream or paste	A-fil RVPaque Shadow Reflecta Covermark	>4–8	All skin types—for protection against UV-A, UV-B, and visible light.

* *SPF = Sun protection factor; it is the ratio of MED of sunscreen-protected skin to MED of protected skin.*
† *See Table 53-2 for skin types.*
NOTE: *Eyes should be always protected with ultraviolet-opaque goggles or sunglasses while sunbathing or skiing.*

toallergic reactions) are listed in Table 53-4. The biologic action spectra that induce either the phototoxic or photoallergic reactions are also given.

EFFECT OF PLANTS PLUS LIGHT *Phytophotodermatitis* (phototoxic reactions) can develop as the result of contact with many plants (belonging principally to the families Rutaceae and Umbelliferae, e.g., certain limes, parsley, celery, bishop's weed, figs) and subsequent exposure of the skin to sunlight. The photodermatitis involves a mild-to-severe erythematous reaction with or without vesicles or bullae. Dense postinflammatory hyperpigmentation is visible within 3 to 5 days. Perfumes and colognes containing oil of bergamot are also known to induce hyperpigmentation with or without erythema. The pigmentation in berloque dermatitis occurs in configurations that seem bizarre but actually represent the areas to which the scent was applied; sometimes the hyperpigmentation may be droplike or pendant-like, and has therefore been named accordingly (*berloque* or *berlock,* meaning trinket or pendant). This phytophotodermatitis, as well as that which follows contact with various other plants, is thought to be caused by furocoumarins (e.g., 5-methoxypsoralen, 8-methoxypsoralen, and other psoralens) characteristically present in these plants. The combination of exposure to long-wave UVR (320 to 400 nm) and furocoumarins greatly enhances the erythema and the pigmentation response.

Treatment Therapy of acute phototoxic reactions induced by topical or systemic agents is best achieved by removal of the offending agent and avoidance of exposure to the sun, or both. If necessary, the usual dermatologic procedures for minimizing the discomforts of the inflammatory response should be undertaken. However, in instances in which continued systemic use of the drug is vital, cutaneous photoreactions may be prevented by instructing the patient to remain indoors or by avoiding exposure to sunlight between 10 A.M. and 4 P.M. Generally the problem subsides within a week after discontinuation of the stress (sun and the drug). Sunscreens listed in Table 53-5 also should be prescribed.

EFFECT OF LIGHT PLUS ENDOGENOUS PHOTOSENSITIZERS This category includes several photosensitivity reactions in patients with various types of porphyria (see Chap. 99). The photosensitivity reactions are related to the overproduction in vivo of either photo-, uro-, or coproporphyrins and their precursors. In the porphyrias, endogenously synthesized porphyrin molecules, when exposed to light, cause burning, itching, urticaria, edema, crusting and scarring, vesiculation, atrophy, and many other disabling cutaneous changes. The light-absorbing molecules involved in evoking the cutaneous reactions are a complex of oxidized porphyrins present in abnormal amounts in red blood cells, plasma, skin, liver, stool, and urine. The photodermatitis is optimally produced by a narrow band of light in the region of 400 to 410 nm, which corresponds to one of the absorption peaks of porphyrins. Patients, however, are sensitive to wavelengths from 380 to 600 nm. The most disabling types of photosensitivity reactions are encountered in erythropoietic (congenital) porphyria and in erythropoietic protoporphyria (Chap. 99). Symptoms and signs of sensitivity to sunlight occur in early childhood.

The adverse cutaneous responses to sunlight in patients with erythropoietic protoporphyria (EPP) have been found to be ameliorated by oral ingestion of β-carotene (Chap. 99). Patients who take β-carotene are able to withstand prolonged exposures to sunlight and experience relief from their usual photosensitivity reactions. A recommended treatment is the daily oral ingestion of β-carotene (Solatene) sufficient to maintain blood levels of 600 to 800 μg/dl (usually adults receive a dose of 120 to 180 mg per day; children under 12 years receive 30 to 90 mg per day). Photoprotective effect of β-carotene is observed after 4 to 6 weeks, and the therapy is generally continued throughout the year. In vitro, β-carotene has been found to be an effective quencher for the "singlet" oxygen generated in certain photosensitivity reactions. During porphyrin-mediated photosensitivity reactions, peroxides are generated which damage the lipid membranes. It is presumed that β-carotene is preferentially oxidized and that by quenching the "singlet" oxygen, it inhibits lipid peroxide formation.

POLYMORPHOUS LIGHT ERUPTIONS

Polymorphous light eruption (PMLE) is an idiopathic, acquired syndrome characterized by a delayed abnormal response to light and varied morphology. The clinical patterns are pleomorphic or polymorphic in nature. The most common pattern consists of multiple small papules, or papules and vesicles that may become confluent and present at times an eczematous clinical picture. Lichenification due to scratching of the pruritic lesions is not common but certainly occurs. Less frequently, the primary lesion is a large papule that may present an erythema multiforme–like pattern or become confluent to form plaques. This variety is usually, but not exclusively, confined to the face and neck. The only consistent histologic feature in all cases is a dense perivascular infiltrate in the upper and middle dermis. Typically the lesions appear in early spring and after each exposure. The latent period between exposure and the appearance of rash may range from a few hours to 2 days, with the most common interval being 24 to 36 h. Itching is frequent and may occur during sun exposure and even preceding the eruption. Irritating papules may coalesce into plaques, and frequently excoriate and subside within 2 to 5 days if sun exposure is avoided. In the majority of patients, the PMLE condition is seasonal, occurring in the early spring and summer months. Patients tend to improve as the summer progresses.

The sunburn-producing spectrum (UV-B, or 290 to 320 nm) is the most effective waveband for eliciting abnormal PMLE responses. However, in many instances, the action spectrum may extend into the UV-A (320 to 400 nm) region; in some instances it may extend into the visible region. Even alpha particles, x-rays, and germicidal radiation (290 nm) may produce PMLE. Although the mechanisms underlying these reactions are not known, the evidence suggests a delayed hypersensitivity reaction to an antigen induced by radiation.

TREATMENT Photoprotection, either through avoidance or with the use of highly effective sunscreens (Table 53-5), may be adequate to control symptoms and appearance of new lesions. The synthetic antimalarials are effective in PMLE, but they must be used with great caution to prevent retinopathy and optic nerve atrophy. The lesions of PMLE are often responsive to topical corticosteroids; systemic steroids are rarely indicated. Desensitization by repeated graduated exposure to sunlight or to artificial radiation (UV-A) in combination with psoralens (methoxsalen) has been successful in a limited number of cases. Oral administration of β-carotene (Solatene) has been found to be of limited value.

Several other idiopathic forms of photodermatoses are seen that constitute a rare but large group of light-induced abnormal reactions. *Solar urticaria* following brief exposure to sunlight or artificial radiation is a rare but distinctive condition. The exposed skin reddens, scattered wheals appear and coalesce, and an erythematous flare develops around the wheals with or without urticaria; the cause is unknown. In some patients exposure to UV-B, UV-A, or visible radiation has been followed by the elevation of histamine and chemotactic factors into the circulation, suggesting that mast cells may play a role. Although antihistamines may benefit some patients, topical broad-spectrum sunscreens and gradual induction of tolerance to natural or artificial radiation by repeated and graded exposures to radiation of appropriate wavelengths have been found to diminish the urticarial reaction.

Actinic reticuloid is another form of chronic, persistent photodermatitis occurring mainly in males who are middle-aged or elderly. It is a most distressing form of persistent photosensitivity characterized by erythematous papular and eczematous eruption; pruritus is generally severe. Lymphomatoid infiltrate is observed histologically with microscopic features implied by the term reticuloid. The patients are severely sensitive to UV-B, UV-A, and even visible radiation. There is a frequent history of eczema present for many years; in some, photosensitivity starts with photocontact dermatitis to a chemical agent. Oral psoralen photochemotherapy appears to help the clearance of photodermatoses.

PHOTOTHERAPY AND PHOTOCHEMOTHERAPY

Phototherapy refers to the therapeutic effectiveness of UVR (usually 290 to 320 nm) or visible radiation without the systemic use of a drug. Photochemotherapy, on the other hand, involves the combination of nonionizing electromagnetic radiation and a systemically administered, photochemically reactive agent. Generally in the doses used, neither the drug alone nor the radiation alone has any therapeutic response; only the combination of the photoactive drug and the radiation, administered at the appropriate time, is therapeutic. Indications for phototherapy include various dermatoses, uremic pruritus, and neonatal hyperbilirubinemia. Phototherapy with blue visible light (430 to 500 nm) causes the photoisomerization of bilirubin, and the bilirubin photoproducts are readily excreted in bile and urine. Psoriasis, eczema, and pityriasis rosea may improve with controlled sun exposures. UV-B radiation (290 to 320 nm) is, therefore, a part of the therapeutic regimen for these dermatoses.

The treatment of psoriasis and other proliferative diseases of the skin has involved attempts to inhibit cellular proliferation and DNA synthesis.

The topical application of crude coal-tar products followed by subsequent UV exposure has been a standard treatment for severe generalized psoriasis and was first described by W. H. Goeckerman, M.D., of the Mayo Clinic more than 50 years ago. Although tar-induced phototoxicity affecting DNA synthesis is believed to be responsible for therapeutic effects, it is not yet clear whether the beneficial effects are due to the chemical ingredients of tar alone or the photosensitizing action of UV-A (320 to 400 nm) or UV-B.

ORAL PSORALEN PHOTOCHEMOTHERAPY Psoralens are naturally occurring furocoumarins that are tricyclic compounds, many of which are photochemically reactive [e.g., 8-methoxypsoralen (methoxsalen) and 4,5′,8-trimethylpsoralen (trioxsalen)]. It has been shown that in the presence of psoralens irradiation with UV-A (320 to 400 nm) can result in covalent binding of psoralens to pyrimidine bases in DNA. This photoconjugation may lead to interstrand cross-linking of psoralen between base paired strands of DNA, inhibition of DNA synthesis, and cell death. Methoxsalen in combination with UV-A (PUVA) is now widely used in treating psoriasis, vitiligo, eczema, and mycosis fungoides. Two hours after ingestion of methoxsalen (0.6 to 0.9 mg/kg), patients are exposed to a measured dose of UV-A radiation. The initial dose depends on the patient's skin reactivity to UVR (sunburn history) and degree of melanin pigmentation of skin. Repeated psoralen plus UV-A treatments cause disappearance of psoriatic lesions; a

total of 10 to 20 treatments given two or three times weekly will usually result in clearance of psoriasis. Maintenance treatments are recommended, and it appears that gradually tapering the frequency of treatments is most effective. The scalp and areas to which UV-A does not penetrate do not respond to therapy. Data verifying the efficacy of PUVA have come from several carefully designed, prospective clinical trials involving over 4000 patients at university medical centers throughout the United States and western Europe.

In vitiligo, a disease characterized by amelanotic macules of varying sizes and absence of melanocytes, methoxsalen plus UV-A treatment can be used in restoring the normal skin color to pigmentless areas of vitiligo macules. Over 70 percent of repigmentation in vitiliginous areas can be achieved. Over 100 to 200 treatments are needed, and this long duration of treatment can often be frustrating, especially when the pigment response is slow, unpredictable, and subject to the presence of functional melanocytes.

The potential long-term concerns of photochemotherapy include premature aging (irreversible changes in connective tissue, blood vessels, and keratinocytes), cataract, and skin cancer. Oral methoxsalen photochemotherapy using long-wave UVR sources is a new approach. Although over 30,000 patients with psoriasis and thousands of patients with vitiligo have been treated, well-documented examples of actinic keratoses or early squamous-cell carcinoma have been infrequently observed with patients receiving over 80 treatments. Prior skin cancer, the exposure to ionizing radiation, and arsenic ingestion appear to be predisposing factors for increased incidence of squamous-cell carcinoma. However, there is no evidence of cataractogenesis in humans treated with psoralens and sunlight or high-intensity UVR over the past 25 years, and adequate eye protection with appropriate UV-A–opaque lenses would largely obviate this risk. Photochemotherapy is an effective treatment which, when compared with other available treatments for generalized psoriasis or vitiligo, appears to have the most acceptable risk/benefit ratio.

Another type of photochemotherapy that appears to be promising is the treatment of tumors with a photosensitizer and visible light. A hematoporphyrin derivative in combination with visible radiation is now being increasingly used for the local treatment of a wide variety of malignant lesions (e.g., metastatic breast carcinoma), including those involving skin. The therapy is based upon the ability of hematoporphyrin to localize in the tumor mass, and its photodynamic efficiency in killing of malignant cells by the photoactivated hepatoporphyrins through the generation of reactive singlet oxygen and subsequent damage to the DNA and other cellular components.

TOPICAL SUNSCREENS IN HEALTH AND DISEASES

Since exposure of skin to UVR is the major cause of skin cancer and actinic aging, the risk can be significantly reduced by decreasing the quantity of harmful radiation reaching the skin with topical application of effective sunscreens. Sunscreens protect viable cells of the skin by absorbing and reflecting the radiation impinging on the skin (see Table 53-5). The majority of sunscreens are designed to protect the user against UV-B (290 to 320 nm). Sunscreens that contain two or more UVR-absorbing chemicals [e.g., benzophenones + cinnamic acid derivatives or benzophenones + PABA ester (padimate O)] appear to filter out both UV-B and UV-A radiation, and at times are referred to as broad-spectrum sunscreens. The effectiveness of a sunscreen is rated on the basis of the sun protection factor

(SPF), a term that designates a ratio of MED of the sunscreen-protected skin to the MED of the nonprotected skin; the higher the SPF, the better the skin protection. In counseling people in the prevention of sunburn, skin cancer, aging of the skin, actinic elastosis, and various forms of sun sensitivity, the choice and recommendations of sunscreen depend upon several factors. The most important consideration should be the individual's reactivity to sunlight. People with fair skin, blue eyes, with or without freckles, who burn easily and tan poorly (skin types I and II, Table 53-2) should be given those sunscreens that have an SPF of 10 or greater (Table 53-5). Individuals with skin types III and IV, who burn moderately or minimally but tan well, may be recommended sunscreens with an SPF of 6 to 8.

For the greatest protection patients should apply sunscreens with SPF of 10 or more or 5.0 percent *p*-aminobenzoic acid (PABA) lotions in 50 to 70 percent ethyl alcohol 1 h before exposure. PABA esters in 2.5 percent concentration in ethanol are less effective than PABA. Most sunscreens should be reapplied after swimming or during prolonged sunbathing. In many instances patients may be exquisitely sensitive, irrespective of skin type, and they may require combination therapy with two or more sunscreens (preferably an opaque sunscreen). The drug-induced photosensitization reactions can be minimized or prevented by prescribing topical sunscreens containing benzophenones (Table 53-5). Sunscreens containing PABA or its derivatives should *not* be prescribed for individuals who are photosensitive to certain drugs and manifest phototoxic or cell-mediated delayed hypersensitivity reactions. In patients receiving antihypertensive thiazide diuretics or sulfonamides there may be a cross-reaction with PABA leading to eczematous dermatitis. These patients should be prescribed sunscreens containing benzophenones (e.g., Piz Buin Exclusive Extrem Cream or Tisol) or opaque sunscreens containing zinc oxide, titanium oxide, and other light-scattering agents such as kaolin.

Individuals with acute sunburn reaction manifesting severe erythema, edema, and painful blistering reaction may be treated with systemic corticosteroids. Oral prednisone, beginning with 40 to 60 mg and tapering over 4 to 8 days, will help to control the severe sunburn reaction.

REFERENCES

MAGNUS IA: *Dermatological Photobiology.* Oxford, Blackwell, 1976

MORISON WL: Photoimmunology. J Invest Dermatol 77:71, 1981

PARRISH JA: Phototherapy and photochemotherapy of skin diseases. J Invest Dermatol 77:167, 1981

——— et al: Photomedicine, in *Dermatology in General Medicine,* 2d ed, TB Fitzpatrick et al (eds). New York, McGraw-Hill, 1979

PATHAK MA et al (eds): *Sunlight and Man: Normal and Abnormal Photobiologic Responses.* Tokyo, University of Tokyo Press, 1974

———, EPSTEIN JH: Normal and abnormal reactions of man to light, in *Dermatology in General Medicine,* TB Fitzpatrick et al (eds). New York, McGraw-Hill, 1971

——— et al: Evaluation of topical agents that prevent sunburn. N Engl J Med 280:1459, 1969

——— et al: Topical and systemic approaches of protection in human skin against harmful effects of solar radiation, in *The Sciences of Photomedicine,* JD Reagan, JA Parrish (eds). New York, Plenum Press, 1981

section 9 | Hematologic alterations

54
ANEMIA

H. FRANKLIN BUNN

By definition patients with anemia have a significant reduction in red cell mass and a corresponding decrease in the oxygen-carrying capacity of the blood. Normally, blood volume is maintained at a nearly constant level. Therefore, anemia entails a decrease in the concentration of red cells or hemoglobin in peripheral blood. Normal values for individuals of various ages are shown in the Appendix. In women in the childbearing age group the normal blood values are 10 percent lower than in men. At high altitudes, higher values are found, roughly in proportion to the elevation above sea level. Anemia may be defined as a reduction of more than 10 percent below the mean values for the sex. However, since the variations in normal hemoglobin values approach this limit, the documentation of mild anemia may be uncertain.

RED BLOOD CELL PRODUCTION Red cells are derived from an undifferentiated progenitor cell in the bone marrow called the *pluripotent stem cell* (Fig. 54-1). A stem cell is one which is capable of both self-renewal and differentiation. *Pluripotent* implies that granulocytes, monocytes, and platelets also evolve from this ancestor cell. The pluripotent stem cell probably has the morphological characteristics of a mature lymphocyte. The control of proliferation into differentiated cell lines is poorly understood. Experiments have been hampered by difficulty in isolating early red cell precursors from the bone marrow. However, in the past 5 years, considerable advances have been made in culturing erythroid progenitor cells in vitro. As Fig. 54-1 shows, the most primitive erythroid progenitor which has been cultured from both bone marrow and peripheral blood is called the *erythroid burst-forming unit* (BFU_e). After 10 to 15 days in tissue culture it produces a large colony of recognizable red cell precursors. The BFU_e is responsive only to high doses of the erythroid-promoting hormone, erythropoietin. A more mature cell, the *erythroid colony-forming unit* (CFU_e), produces a smaller clone of erythroid cells after 4 to 7 days in culture and is very sensitive to erythropoietin. Various other factors such as catecholamines, steroids, thyroid hormone, growth hormone, and cyclic nucleotides may influence erythroid cell differentiation. In addition, macrophages and lymphocytes may also play a role. Well-designed experiments involving erythroid cells in culture should provide considerably more information about the mechanism underlying the differentiation and maturation of erythroid cells, as well as insights into certain disorders involving erythroid precursor cells.

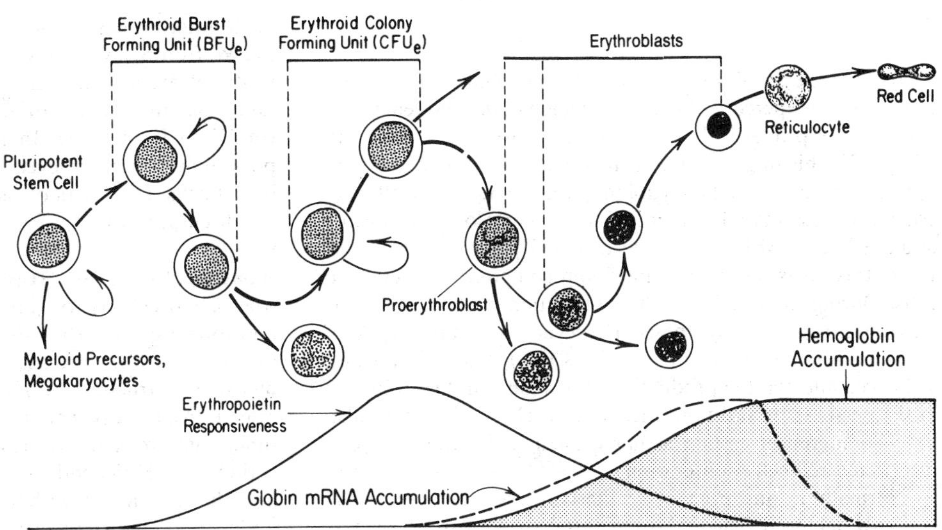

FIGURE 54-1
Differentiation and morphological maturation of erythroid cells. Erythroid cells are derived from pluripotent stem cells shown on left. Under the influence of erythropoietin, erythroid stem cells ($BFU_e \rightarrow CFU_e$) differentiate into proerythroblasts, the earliest recognizable red blood cell precursor in the bone marrow. During further maturation, globin mRNA accumulates, directing the cell to synthesize hemoglobin. (After Nienhuis and Benz.)

Erythropoietin, a glycoprotein having a molecular weight of about 32,000, has been purified nearly to homogeneity. Original experiments indicated that this hormone is produced primarily by the kidneys. Alternatively, the kidneys may produce a substance, renal erythropoietic factor, which converts a biologically inactive plasma protein into erythropoietin, analogous to the formation of angiotensin II. Erythropoietin production is stimulated by hypoxia. The recent purification of erythropoietin has permitted the development of a radioimmunoassay which is more accurate and sensitive than conventional bioassays. Reliable measurements of erythropoietin will have a number of diagnostic applications and also provide new information about the pathogenesis of several types of anemias.

Erythropoietin probably interacts with specific receptors on the surfaces of committed erythroid stem cells, inducing them to differentiate into pronormoblasts, the earliest red cell precursor that can be recognized on examination of the bone marrow. In addition, erythropoietin acts on later red cell precursors, stimulating hemoglobin synthesis. Normally the transition from the proerythroblast to the most mature normoblast involves three or four cell divisions over a 4-day period (Fig. 54-1). During this time, the nucleus becomes smaller, and an increasing amount of hemoglobin is produced in the cytoplasm. Following the last division, the pyknotic nucleus is removed from the normoblast, forming the reticulocyte which stays in the bone marrow for 2.5 to 3 days. The reticulocyte is then released into the general circulation, where it remains for another 24 h before it loses its mitochondria and ribosomes and assumes the morphological appearance of a mature red cell.

Erythroid precursor cells ranging from the pronormoblast to the reticulocyte possess a specific surface receptor for the iron-transferrin complex, enabling them to incorporate sufficient iron for hemoglobin production (Fig. 54-2). The use of a radioactive iron label such as ^{59}Fe permits a quantitative assessment of erythropoiesis. From the rate at which injected ^{59}Fe-labeled transferrin disappears from the plasma, plasma iron turnover can be calculated. This parameter is generally proportional to the total developing erythroid cell mass. Normally, about 80 percent of ^{59}Fe bound to plasma transferrin goes to erythroid cells in the marrow. After 4 to 6 days the labeled iron reappears in circulating erythrocytes. The extent to which circulating red cells acquire the label provides an index of the efficiency or effectiveness of erythropoiesis.

The normal marrow is capable of increasing its red cell production about three to five times normal within a week or two following maximal stimulation. In chronic hemolytic anemias, erythropoiesis may increase five- to sevenfold. As the erythroid marrow expands, fat is replaced by erythroid cells, and formerly inactive or "yellow" marrow becomes active or "red."

HEMOGLOBIN BIOSYNTHESIS Erythroid cell development involves the production of hemoglobin-containing cells. About 98 percent of the protein in the cytoplasm of circulating red cells is hemoglobin. This protein is a tetramer composed of two pairs of polypeptide chains designated α, β, γ, and δ, each of which is covalently linked to a heme group. The synthesis of a particular globin subunit is directed by a corresponding gene inherited from each parent. As shown in Fig. 54-1, there is a marked amplification in the transcription of globin chain mRNA during the development of proerythroblasts.

FIGURE 54-2
Erythrocyte production, circulation, and destruction. Circulating iron-bound transferrin (TF) is bound to specific receptors on the surface of red blood cell precursors in the marrow. Most of this iron is incorporated into hemoglobin; the remainder is stored as ferritin. Following maturation of the erythroid precursor, the nucleus is shed and the red blood cell emerges from the marrow into the plasma where it circulates for approximately 120 days. The senescent red blood cell is taken up by the mononuclear-macrophage system and is destroyed. The heme-iron is initially incorporated into ferritin. This storage iron is available for transport to the marrow via transferrin.

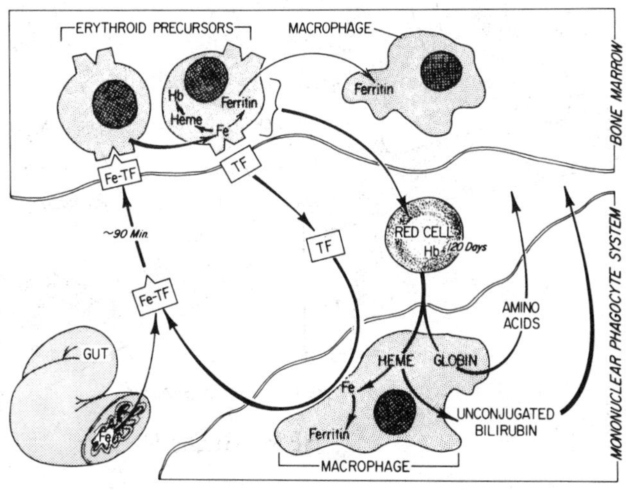

In the red cells of normal adults, hemoglobin A ($\alpha_2\beta_2$) composes about 97 percent of the total hemoglobin. The remaining 3 percent is primarily hemoglobin A_2 ($\alpha_2\delta_2$). As discussed in Chap. 330, this minor component is increased in patients with β thalassemia. Fetal hemoglobin (HbF or $\alpha_2\gamma_2$) usually accounts for less than 1 percent of total hemoglobin in normal adult red cells. HbF is localized to 1 to 7 percent of red cells. In contrast, it is the main hemoglobin component of fetal red cells. During the last 3 months of gestation, γ-chain synthesis switches to β-chain synthesis. However, in certain types of congenital hemolytic anemias such as the β thalassemias and sickle cell anemia, the production of γ chains (and therefore of HbF) persists. In addition, increased levels of HbF may also be encountered in certain acquired anemias in which there is disordered red cell proliferation.

Normally α- and β-chain synthesis in erythroid precursors is evenly balanced. The thalassemias (Chap. 330) are characterized by imbalance in globin chain synthesis.

The synthesis of *heme* in red cell precursors is closely matched to globin chain production. As shown in Fig. 54-3 the initial and rate-limiting step is the condensation of succinyl CoA and glycine to form δ-aminolevulinic acid. This reaction which takes place in mitochondria requires that glycine be activated by pyridoxal phosphate. Accordingly, patients with sideroblastic anemia in whom heme synthesis is usually defective may sometimes respond to pyridoxine therapy (Chap. 326). The next steps of heme synthesis take place in the cytosol. Two molecules of δ-aminolevulinic acid condense to form a ring structure, porphobilinogen. This colorless pyrrole is elevated in acute intermittent porphyria and can be detected in urine by the Watson-Schwartz test. The subsequent steps in porphyrin synthesis are also shown in Fig. 54-3. The last three reactions take place in mitochondria. Iron is inserted into protoporphyrin IX to form heme. In iron deficiency, as well as in lead poisoning, increased levels of protoporphyrin can be detected in red cells. Disorders of porphyrin synthesis and metabolism are discussed in Chap. 99.

HEMOGLOBIN STRUCTURE AND FUNCTION The primary role of red cells is to transport oxygen from lungs to tissues and to transport carbon dioxide in the reverse direction. Both of these functions are assumed by hemoglobin. The three-dimensional structure of human hemoglobin has been determined from x-ray crystallographic analysis. The important functional properties of hemoglobin such as heme-heme interaction, the pH dependency of oxygen affinity (the Bohr effect), and the interaction with 2,3-diphosphoglycerate can now be understood on a stereochemical basis. This structural information has also been useful in explaining the abnormal functional properties of a number of human hemoglobin variants which are associated with clinical and hematologic manifestations (see Chap. 330).

During the circulation through the lungs, hemoglobin becomes almost fully saturated with oxygen (1.34 ml O_2 per gram of hemoglobin). As red cells perfuse the capillary beds, oxygen is extracted. Efficient unloading of oxygen at relatively high oxygen tensions is possible because of the sigmoid shape of the oxygen dissociation curve (heme-heme interaction) (see Fig. 54-4). The affinity of hemoglobin for oxygen is modified by three intracellular cofactors: hydrogen ion, carbon dioxide,

FIGURE 54-3
The biosynthesis of heme. The following abbreviations are used: CoA, coenzyme A; GTP, guanosine triphosphate; GDP, guanosine diphosphate; Pi, inorganic phosphorus; GSH, glutathione; Δ-ALA-DH, Δ-aminolevulinate dehydrase; UIS, uroporphyrinogen I synthetase; UIII CoS, uroporphyrinogen III cosynthetase; UD, uroporphyrinogen decarboxylase; CO, coproporphyrinogen oxidase; HS, heme synthetase. Enzymatic steps that occur in mitochondria are shown.

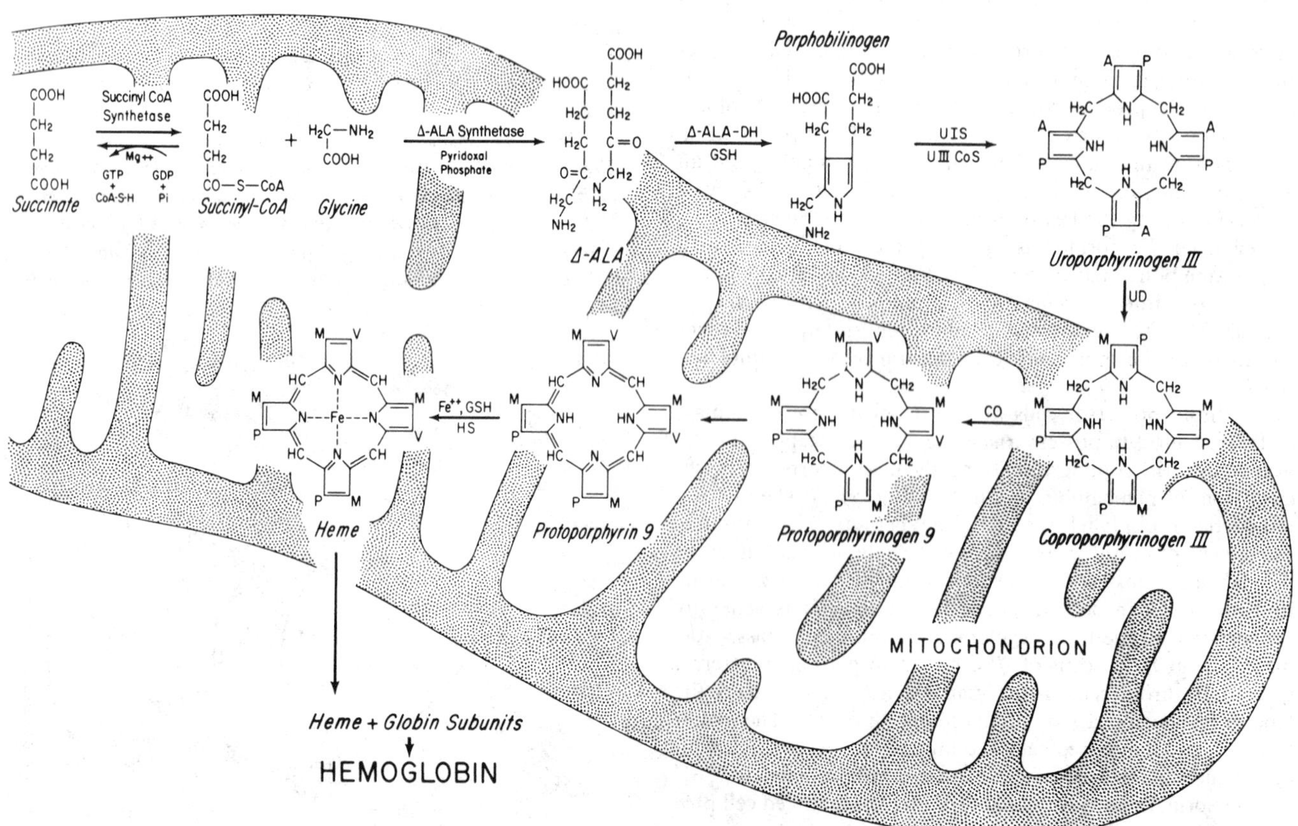

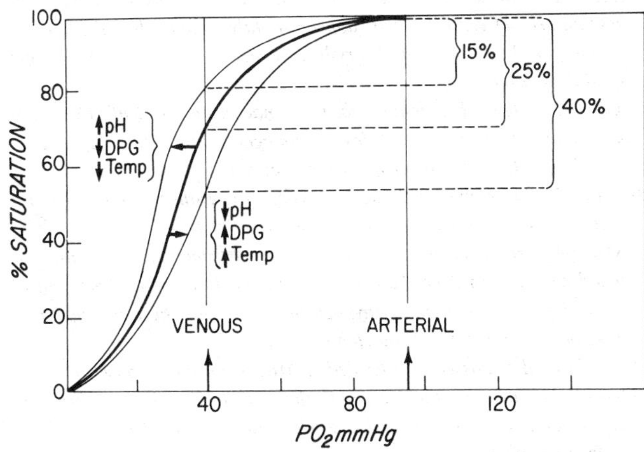

FIGURE 54-4

The oxyhemoglobin dissociation curve of normal blood. The major factors influencing the position of the curve are pH, temperature, and the intracellular concentration of 2,3-DPG. An increase in plasma pH or a decrease in temperature and 2,3-DPG causes an increase in oxygen affinity (shift to the left) and a relative decrease in oxygen unloading when going from an arterial P_{O_2} *of 95 mmHg to a venous* P_{O_2} *of 40 mmHg. Conversely, a decrease in pH or an increase in temperature and 2,3-DPG causes a decrease in oxygen affinity (shift to the right) and a relative increase in oxygen unloading.*

and 2,3-diphosphoglycerate (2,3-DPG). Increasing concentrations of each of these three effectors results in a "shift to the right" in the oxygen dissociation curve. In human red cells, 2,3-DPG appears to be an important regulator of hemoglobin function. One molecule of 2,3-DPG binds to the β chains of deoxyhemoglobin, thereby decreasing oxygen affinity. Elevated levels of 2,3-DPG have been noted in various states of hypoxia. The resulting decrease in oxygen affinity permits enhanced oxygen release. The oxygenation of a particular organ or tissue depends on three main factors (depicted in Fig. 54-5): blood flow, oxygen-carrying capacity of the blood (hemoglobin concentration), and the affinity of the hemoglobin for oxygen. Patients with a primary abnormality of one of these three factors depend on adjustments in one or both of the other two in order to maintain optimal tissue oxygenation. For example, patients with anemia have two available modes of compensation: enhanced blood flow and decreased oxygen affinity, mediated by increased levels of 2,3-DPG. Conversely, individuals with a hemoglobin variant having increased oxygen affinity have a primary defect in oxygen unloading. As discussed in Chap. 330, such patients compensate by developing secondary erythrocytosis.

FIGURE 54-5

Oxygen delivered to an organ or tissue is directly proportional to (1) blood flow, (2) hemoglobin concentration, and (3) the difference in oxygen saturation of the arterial and venous blood. Patients with various types of hypoxia may compensate in the following ways: (1) The distribution of blood flow is altered to maintain oxygenation of vital organs; total cardiac output increases when hypoxia is severe. (2) Increased erythropoietin production stimulates erythropoiesis. (3) Oxygen unloading is enhanced by a shift to the right in the oxygen dissociation curve, mediated by an increase in red cell 2,3-DPG.

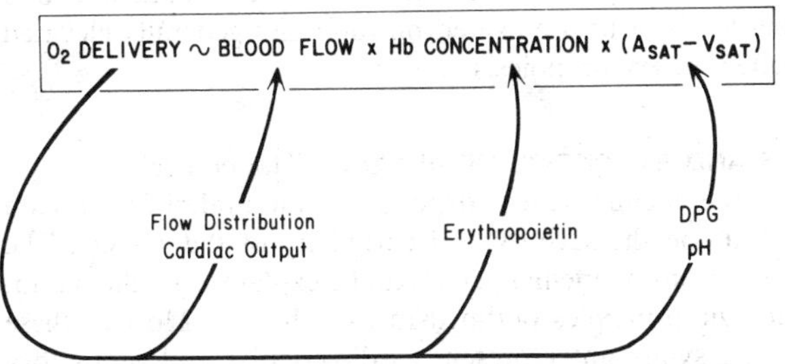

RED BLOOD CELL METABOLISM As the red cell emerges from the bone marrow, it loses its nucleus, ribosomes, and mitochondria and therefore all capability for cell division, protein synthesis, and oxidative phosphorylation. Compared with other cells, the erythrocyte has a rather simple scheme of intermediary metabolism. Glucose is virtually the only fuel utilized by the red cell. It readily enters the red cell by facilitated diffusion and is then converted to glucose 6-phosphate. There are two major pathways available for glucose 6-phosphate (Fig. 329-2). About 80 to 90 percent of this intermediate is converted to lactate by means of the glycolytic (or Embden-Meyerhof) pathway. Two moles of adenosine triphosphate (ATP) are generated for every mole of glucose that is metabolized. The intracellular mediator of hemoglobin function, 2,3-diphosphoglycerate, is synthesized in a side reaction shown in Fig. 329-2. About 10 percent of intracellular glucose 6-phosphate may undergo oxidation by means of the hexose-monophosphate shunt. This pathway maintains glutathione in the reduced form, thereby protecting sulfhydryl groups in hemoglobin and the red cell membrane from oxidation by peroxides and superoxide as well as by certain drugs and toxins. Such oxidant stress can compromise red cell function and viability in patients with a deficiency in glucose 6-phosphate dehydrogenase, the first enzymatic step in the hexose monophosphate shunt (see Chap. 329). Less commonly, individuals may have a deficiency in one of the enzymes of the glycolytic pathway or in one of the other enzymes of the hexose monophosphate shunt.

The red cell has rather modest metabolic obligations in keeping with its simplified structure. A significant portion of the ATP generated by glycolysis is spent in operating the so-

FIGURE 54-6

Diagram of a cross section of the red blood cell membrane. Spectrin and actin form a meshwork which laminates the inner surface of the membrane. Several other proteins of varying sizes including the enzyme glyceraldehyde 3-phosphate dehydrogenase (G3PD) also bind to the inner surface. In contrast, other proteins such as the glycophorins A and B (GP-A and GP-B) and the anion transport protein traverse the lipid bilayer. Long polysaccharide chains are covalently attached to these proteins on the outer surface of the cell and also to glycolipid. Phospholipids include phosphatidyl choline (PC) and sphingomyelin (SM), which are located primarily on the outer surface of the membrane, and phosphatidyl serine (PS) and phosphatidyl ethanolamine (PE), which are located primarily on the inner surface of the membrane. (This figure was prepared by Dr. Samuel Lux IV.)

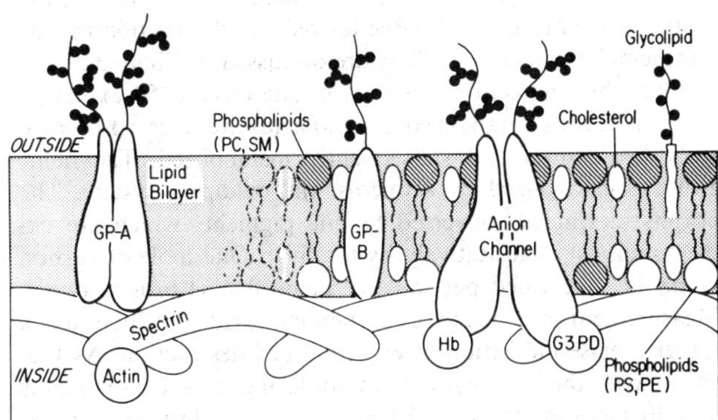

dium-potassium pump, necessary to preserve the ionic milieu in the cytoplasm and prevent colloid osmotic lysis. In addition, some metabolic energy is expended on maintenance and repair of the red cell membrane. Certain proteins in the membrane become phosphorylated by means of ATP and protein kinases, but the physiologic significance of this process is not yet understood. Finally, a small amount of metabolic currency is spent on maintaining hemoglobin iron atoms in the reduced form (Fe^{2+}).

The 120-day survival of the circulating red cell is dependent on preservation of the pliability of its membrane. The red cell membrane is composed of 50 percent protein, 40 percent lipid, and 10 percent carbohydrate. According to the most widely accepted model, it is a bilayer consisting of molecules of phospholipid and cholesterol in a 1.2:1 molar ratio oriented in a stacked array so that the hydrophobic portions of the molecules are oriented toward the interior while the polar side groups are either on the external surface of the cell (the plasma membrane) or on the inner cytoplasmic surface (see Fig. 54-6). The distribution of phospholipids differs significantly in the two portions of the bilayer. The outer surface is relatively rich in lecithin and sphingomyelin while the inner surface has relatively more phosphatidyl serine and phosphatidyl ethanolamine. The lipids on the outer surface exchange freely with plasma lipids.

The red cell membrane contains about eight major proteins (depicted in Fig. 54-6) and a large number of minor components. These proteins can be divided into two groups. A few span the lipid bilayer so that one end of the polypeptide is on the external cell surface and the other is on the inner surface. Examples include glycophorin which contains a number of polysaccharide blood group antigens and band 3, which serves as a channel for the passage of anions in and out of the red cell. Other proteins bind only to the inner surface of the red cell membrane. These include several enzymes as well as structural proteins such as spectrin and actin, which interact to form a meshwork that laminates the cytoplasmic surface of the membrane.

It is likely that the physiologic demise of 120-day-old red cells is due to a loss of membrane flexibility preventing them from negotiating the narrow-bore channels of the microcirculation including the sinusoids of the spleen. The factors responsible for red cell senescence are poorly understood. Experimental evidence indicates that deterioration of the red cell's metabolic machinery, sufficient to deplete it of ATP, can cause the cell to become spiculated (ecchinocytic) and lose its normal pliability. Depletion of ATP disrupts the spectrin and actin meshwork lining the inner membrane surface, resulting in aggregation of these proteins. Other factors such as enhanced rigidity due to accumulation of calcium and, perhaps, alterations in charge on the external surface of the membrane may also contribute to the recognition of the senescent red cell by the mononuclear-phagocyte system. In contrast to normal red cells, there is a large and well-documented body of information on the mechanisms responsible for red cell destruction in various hemolytic anemias. These are discussed in Chap. 329.

Once the senescent red cell is sequestered (Fig. 54-2), hemoglobin is readily catabolized. Amino acids are released by proteolytic digestion and subsequently metabolized. The heme group is catabolized by a microsomal oxidizing system. The porphyrin ring is converted to bile pigments which are excreted almost quantitatively by the liver. One mole of carbon monoxide is formed per mole of heme that is broken down. Measurement of endogenous carbon monoxide production is a rather precise indication of erythroid cell destruction. As Fig. 54-2 shows, the iron that is released during heme catabolism is initially incorporated into the storage protein, ferritin, but it is

PLATE 9-1 *Normal blood smear. Normal red blood cells are round, possess an area of central pallor, appear slightly smaller than the nucleus of a mature lymphocyte, and vary little in size (anisocytosis) or in shape (poikilocytosis).*

PLATE 9-2 *Megaloblastic anemia. Oval macrocytes, well filled with hemoglobin, are admixed with lesser numbers of small teardrop-shaped red blood cells. Note also hypersegmented granulocyte.*

PLATE 9-3 *Liver disease. Round macrocytes of rather uniform size are seen. Many of the macrocytes are also target cells.*

PLATE 9-4 *Iron-deficiency anemia. In severe iron deficiency, the red blood cells are smaller than normal (microcytosis), and their central area of pallor is expanded (hypochromia) so that the cells appear to have only a thin rim of hemoglobin.*

PLATE 9-5 *β thalassemia intermedia. Microcytic and hypochromic red blood cells are seen that resemble the red blood cells of severe iron deficiency anemia shown in Plate 9-4. Many elliptical and teardrop-shaped red blood cells are noted.*

PLATE 9-6 *Sickle cell anemia. The elongated and crescent-shaped red blood cells seen on this smear represent circulating irreversibly sickled cells. Target cells and a nucleated red blood cell are also seen.*

PLATE 9-7 *Traumatic hemolysis. The helmet-shaped red blood cell and the small triangular-shaped red blood cells seen on this smear represent morphologic evidence of mechanical damage to red blood cells within the circulatory tree.*

PLATE 9-8 *Spur cell anemia. Spur cells are recognized as distorted red blood cells containing several irregularly distributed thornlike projections. Cells with this morphologic abnormality are also called acanthocytes.*

PLATE 9-9 *Uremia. The red blood cells in uremia may acquire numerous, regularly spaced, small spiny projections. Such cells, called burr cells or echinocytes, are readily distinguishable from the irregularly spiculated acanothocytes shown in Plate 9-8.*

PLATE 9-10 *Hereditary spherocytosis. Small, densely staining red blood cells are seen that have lost their central area of pallor (microspherocytes). Microspherocytes may also be found in other hemolytic disorders (Plate 9-11).*

PLATE 9-11 *Immunohemolytic anemia. Microspherocytes are seen on this blood smear along with several macrocytes with a slight purple tinge (polychromasia). The latter represent new red blood cells released early from the bone marrow. The microspherocytes seen in immunohemolytic anemia may be indistinguishable from the microspherocytes seen in hereditary spherocytosis (Plate 9-10).*

PLATE 9-12 *Myeloid metaplasia. Teardrop-shaped red blood cells, a nucleated red blood cell, and immature myeloid cells are seen on this blood smear.*

---

eventually transported to marrow erythroid precursors by transferrin, the plasma-iron-binding protein.

If red cell production is disordered, there may be significant destruction of erythroid cells within the bone marrow. A number of anemias are characterized by *ineffective erythropoiesis*, particularly those in which erythroid maturation is morphologically abnormal and the circulating red cells are abnormal in size. Examples discussed in detail elsewhere include megaloblastic anemias, sideroblastic anemias, and β thalassemia major. Such disorders are characterized by erythroid hyperplasia in the bone marrow and rapid uptake of labeled iron into the marrow but a low recovery of the labeled iron in circulating red cells. Endogenous carbon monoxide production and plasma levels of unconjugated bilirubin are generally elevated in ineffective erythropoiesis.

SIGNS AND SYMPTOMS OF ANEMIA The clinical presentation of the anemic patient depends on the underlying disease as well as on the severity and chronicity of the anemia. The manifestations of anemia per se can be explained by the pathophysiologic principles outlined in this chapter. Most of these signs and symptoms represent cardiovascular and ventilatory

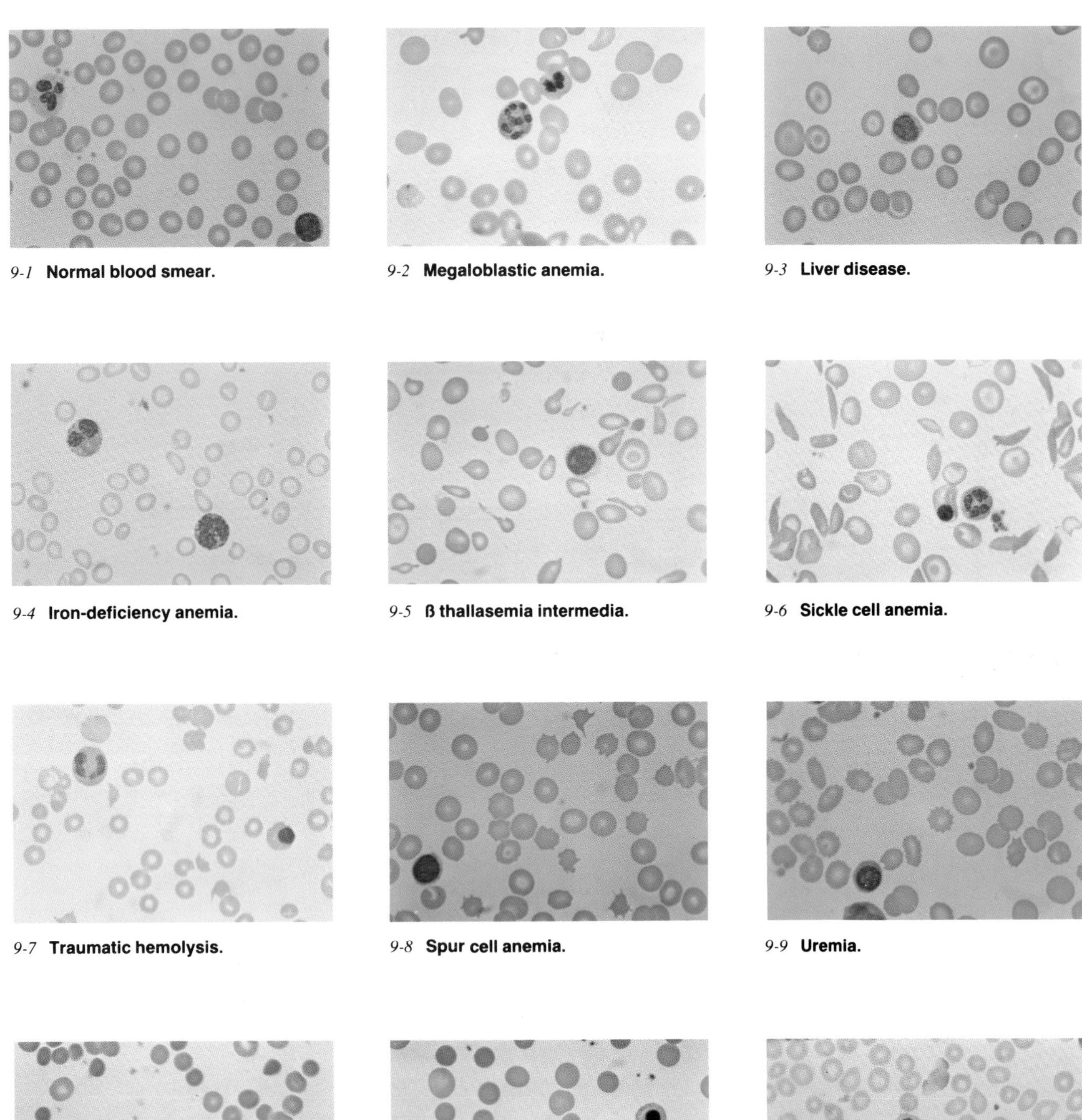

9-1 **Normal blood smear.**

9-2 **Megaloblastic anemia.**

9-3 **Liver disease.**

9-4 **Iron-deficiency anemia.**

9-5 **ß thallasemia intermedia.**

9-6 **Sickle cell anemia.**

9-7 **Traumatic hemolysis.**

9-8 **Spur cell anemia.**

9-9 **Uremia.**

9-10 **Hereditary spherocytosis.**

9-11 **Immunohemolytic anemia.**

9-12 **Myeloid metaplasia.**

PLATE 9

Peripheral blood smears illustrating abnormalities of red blood cell morphology. Smears were stained with Wright's stain. 760X (reproduced at 150 percent of original slide). (Courtesy of C. von Kapff and H. Franklin Bunn.)

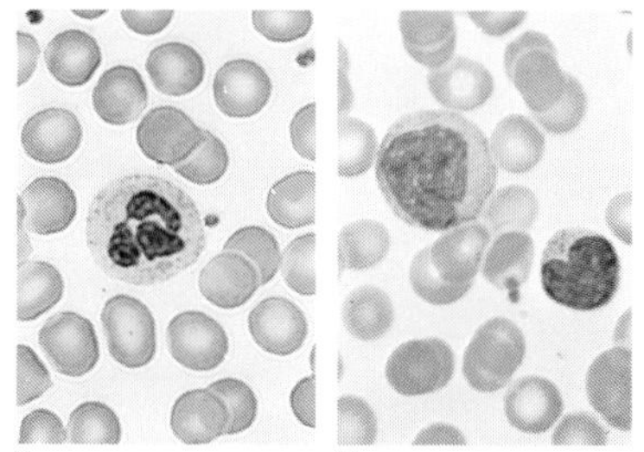

10-1 *A.* **Normal granulocyte.** *B.* **Normal monocyte and lymphocyte.**

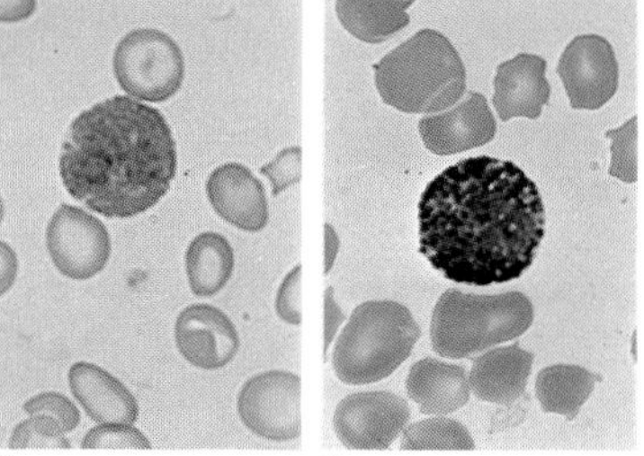

10-2 *A.* **Normal eosinophil.** *B.* **Normal basophil.**

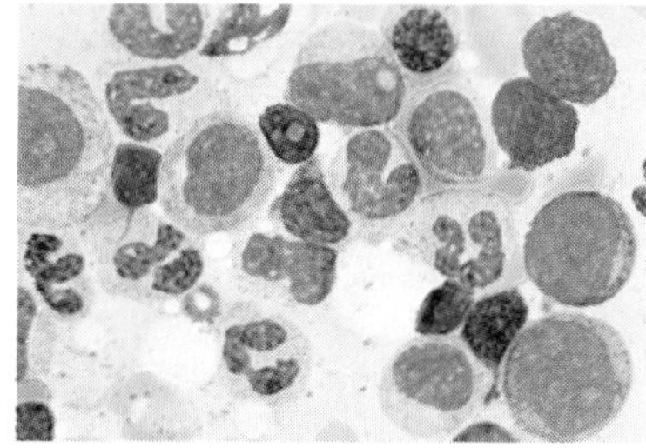

10-3 **Normal granulocyte precursors in marrow.**

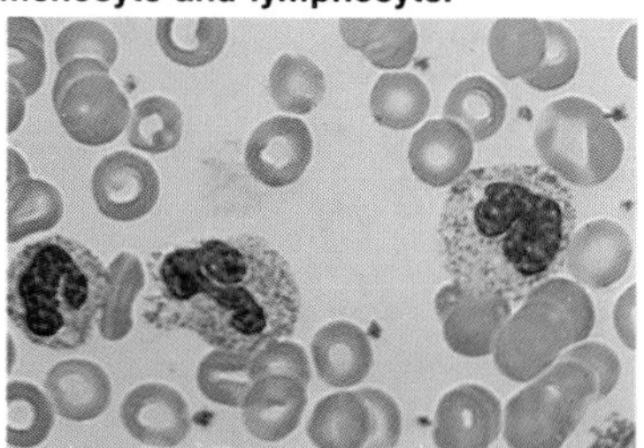

10-4 **Neutrophils with toxic granulation.**

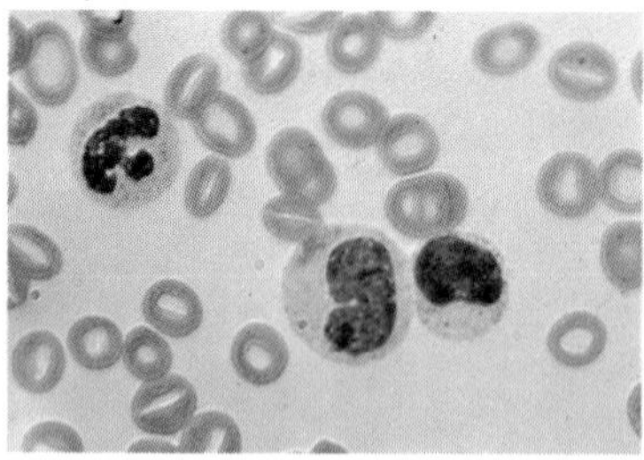

10-5 **Band with Döhle body** (center).

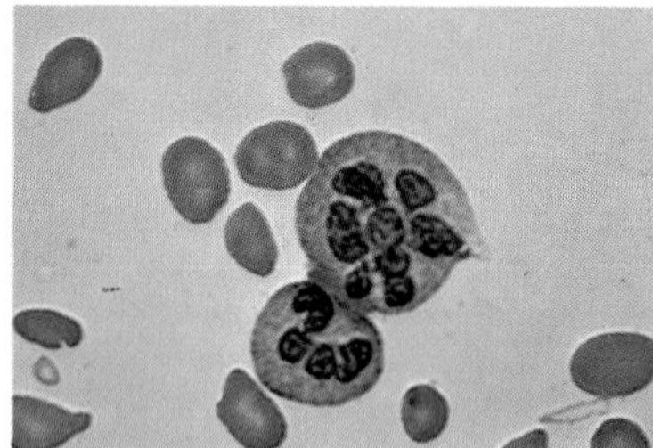

10-6 **Hypersegmentation.**

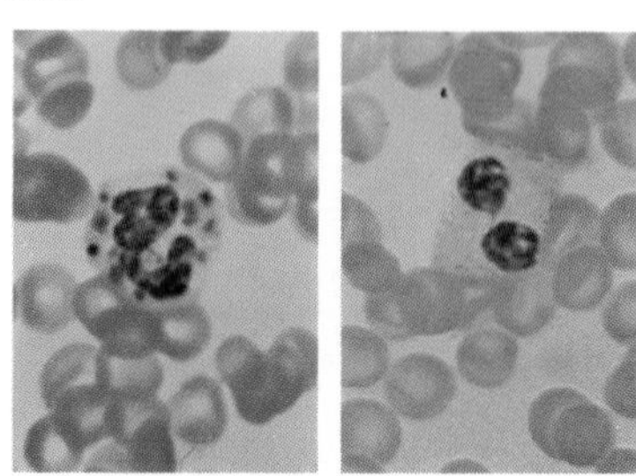

10-7 *A.* **Chédiak-Higashi anomaly.** *B.* **Pelger-Hüet anomaly.**

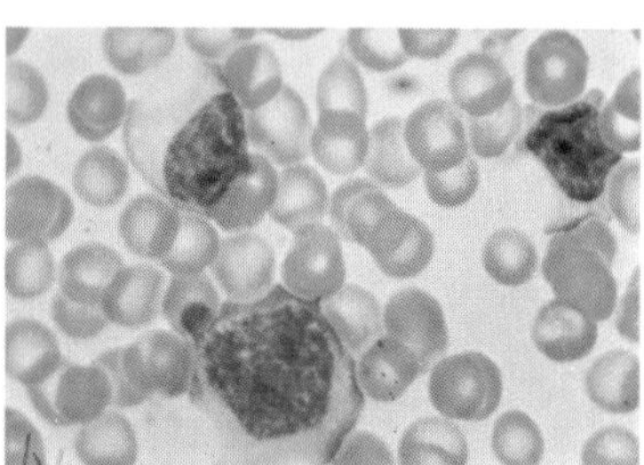

10-8 **Reactive lymphocytes** (infectious mononucleosis).

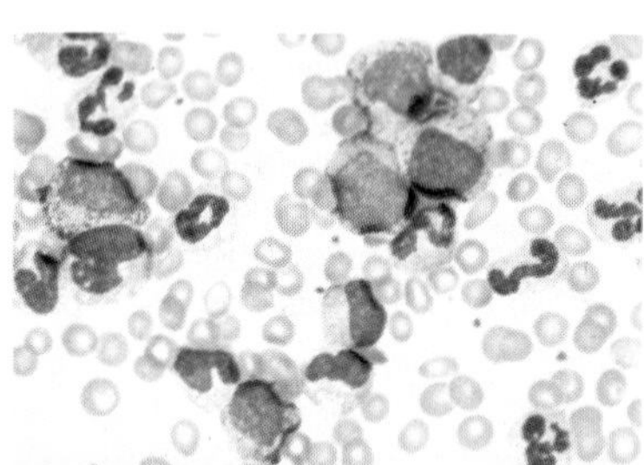

10-9 **Chronic granulocytic leukemia.**

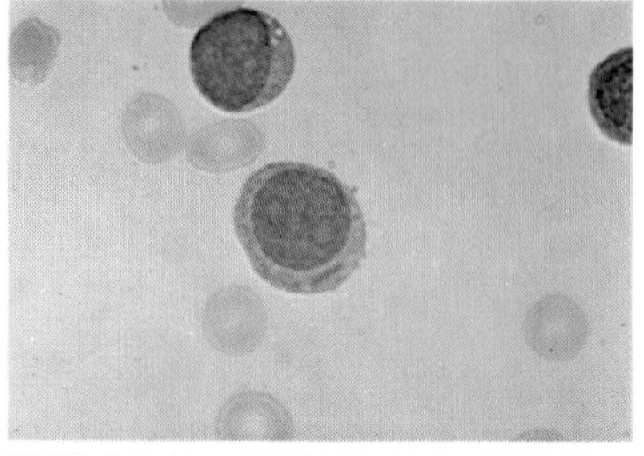

10-10 **Acute myelogenous leukemia:** myeloblast with Auer rod (center).

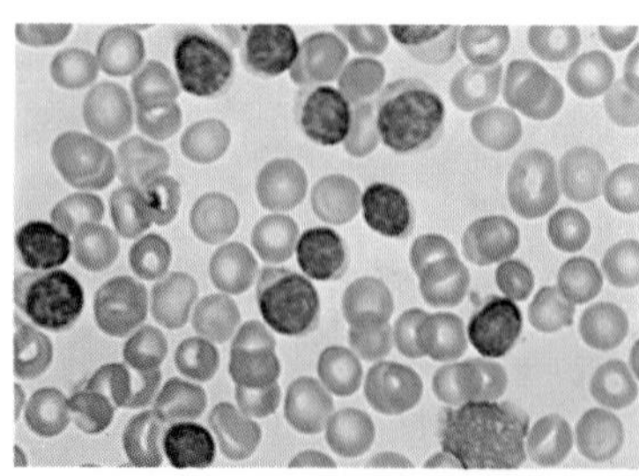

10-11 **Chronic lymphocytic leukemia.**

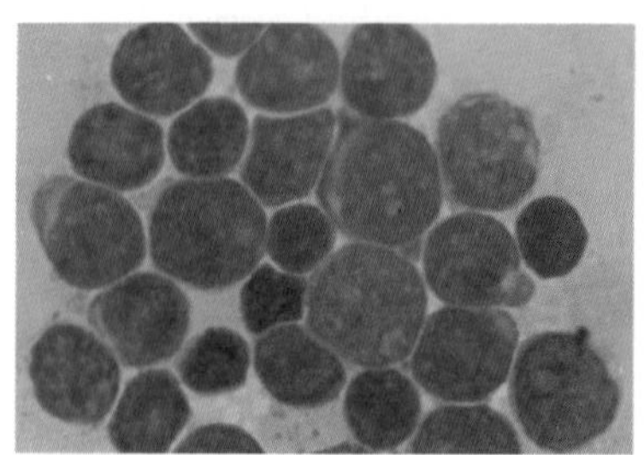

10-12 **Acute lymphoblastic leukemia** (marrow).

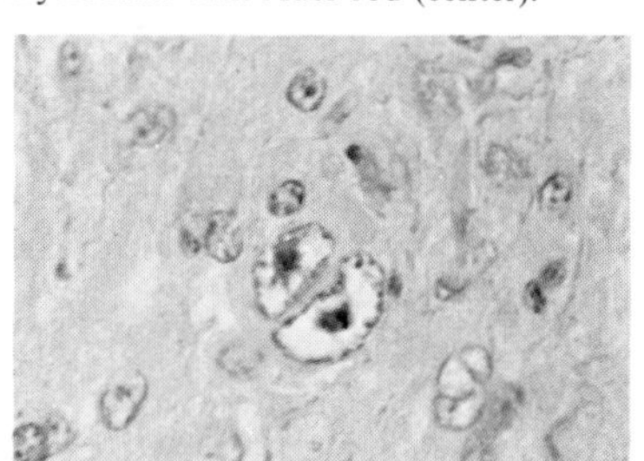

10-13 **Hodgkin's disease:** Reed-Sternberg cell in marrow (center).

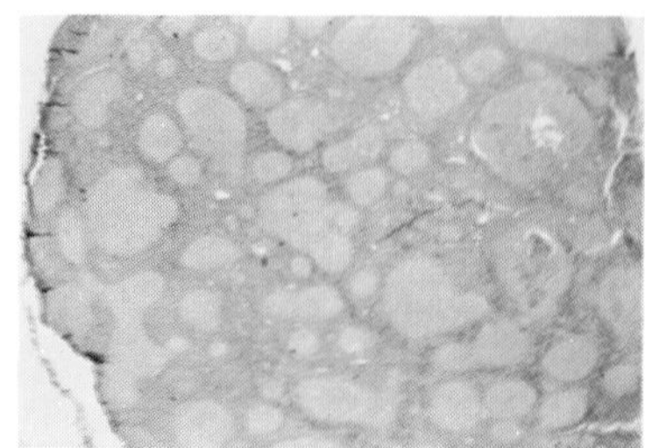

10-14 **Non-Hodgkin's nodular lymphoma** (lymph node).

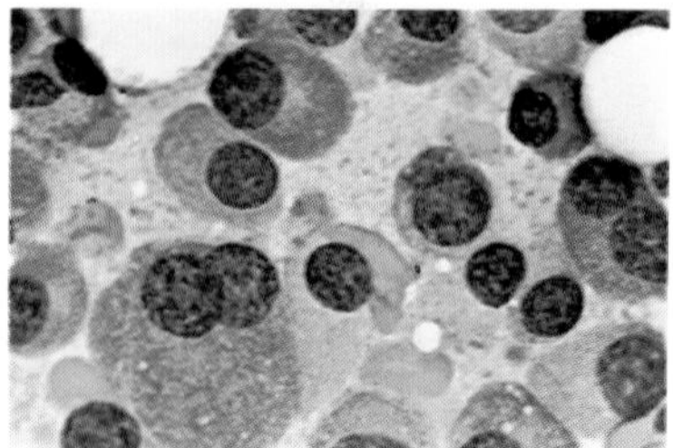

10-15 **Multiple myeloma** (marrow).

PLATE 10

Normal and abnormal leukocytes. (From American Society of Hematology Slide Bank, 2d ed, 1977. Used with permission.)

PLATE 10-1 *A. Normal granulocyte. The normal granulocyte has a segmented nucleus with heavy, clumped chromatin; fine neutrophilic granules are dispersed throughout its cytoplasm. B. Normal monocyte and lymphocyte. The normal monocyte is a large cell with an indented or folded nucleus containing loose, strandlike chromatin; the cytoplasm is a blue-gray color and usually contains fine azurophilic granules. The normal lymphocyte is a smaller cell. Its nucleus is usually round but may be indented, as in the cell shown in this plate. The nuclear chromatin has a smudgy appearance; the cytoplasm is a blue color.*

PLATE 10-2 *A. Normal eosinophil. The eosinophil contains large, bright-orange granules; the nucleus is bilobed. B. Basophil. The basophil contains large purple-black granules which fill the cell and obscure the nucleus.*

PLATE 10-3 *Normal granulocyte precursors in marrow. The earliest granulocytic precursor (myeloblast) possesses a round nucleus with fine, punctate chromatin and one or more nucleoli; the cytoplasm is blue. As nuclear differentiation proceeds, the nucleoli disappear, the chromatin coarsens, and the nucleus becomes increasingly indented and finally segmented. As cytoplasmic differentiation proceeds, azurophilic granules appear and the cytoplasm changes color from blue to the yellow-pink-gray hue of the mature granulocyte, and as this occurs the azurophilic granules become obscured by fine neutrophilic granules.*

PLATE 10-4 *Neutrophils with toxic granulation. In infection and other toxic states, azurophilic granules may become visible in mature granulocytes as coarse, dark-staining cytoplasmic granules.*

PLATE 10-5 *Band with Döhle body (center). Döhle bodies are discrete, blue-staining, nongranular areas found in the periphery of the cytoplasm of the neutrophil in infections and other toxic states. They represent aggregates of rough endoplasmic reticulum.*

PLATE 10-6 *Hypersegmentation. Frequent five-lobed granulocytes on a blood smear or granulocytes with more than five lobes are evidence of hypersegmentation, an important clue to the diagnosis of megaloblastic anemia.*

PLATE 10-7 *A. Chédiak-Higashi anomaly. In this ultimately fatal disorder, the granulocytes contain huge cytoplasmic granules, formed from aggregation and fusion of azurophilic and specific granules. Large, abnormal granules are found in other granule-containing cells throughout the body. B. Pelger-Hüet anomaly. In this benign disorder, the majority of granulocytes are bilobed. The nucleus frequently has a spectacle-like or "pince-nez" configuration.*

PLATE 10-8 *Reactive lymphocytes (infectious mononucleosis). Reactive lymphocytes are usually large, cytoplasmic lymphocytes. The nucleus may be eccentrically placed and may have irregular borders and indentations (not seen on this plate). The cytoplasm contains areas that stain a darker blue due to their increased content of RNA. The cytoplasm may be indented where it abuts against a red blood cell.*

PLATE 10-9 *Chronic granulocytic leukemia. The peripheral blood WBC count is high due to increased numbers of granulocytes and their precursors. The majority of the WBCs are segmented granulocytes or band forms, but as seen on this plate, myelocytes and promyelocytes are also present in substantial numbers. Smaller numbers of myeloblasts (not seen on this plate) may also be found on review of the blood smear.*

PLATE 10-10 *Acute myelogenous leukemia: myeloblast with Auer rod (center). The center cell is recognized as a blast because of its fine nuclear chromatin and prominent nucleoli. A thin, red, rodlike structure, an Auer rod, is readily visible in its cytoplasm. Auer rods are not found in normal blasts or in leukemic lymphoblasts. Their discovery permits an unequivocal diagnosis to be made of acute nonlymphocytic leukemia (acute myelogenous leukemia, acute monocytic leukemia).*

PLATE 10-11 *Chronic lymphocytic leukemia. The peripheral blood WBC count is high due to increased numbers of small, well-differentiated lymphocytes that do not differ in appearance from normal small lymphocytes. However, the leukemic lymphocytes are fragile, and substantial numbers of broken, smudged cells are usually also present on the blood smear.*

PLATE 10-12 *Acute lymphoblastic leukemia (marrow). A monomorphous infiltrate of leukemic lymphoblasts is seen. The erythroid and granulocytic precursors found in normal marrow are not present.*

PLATE 10-13 *Hodgkin's disease: Reed-Sternberg cell in marrow (center). The Reed-Sternberg cell is recognized by its bilobed, mirror-image nucleus, which contains in each lobe a giant, inclusion body–like nucleolus. The cytoplasmic borders of the cell cannot be identified on this plate.*

PLATE 10-14 *Non-Hodgkin's nodular lymphoma (lymph node). This low-power view illustrates that a proliferative process has caused the normal architecture of the lymph node to be replaced by multiple nodules of varying size that extend throughout the entire lymph node.*

PLATE 10-15 *Multiple myeloma (marrow). A cluster of plasma cells is seen. A plasma cell is recognized by its small, round, eccentrically placed nucleus with nuclear chromatin distributed in a clock-face pattern, and by its deep-blue cytoplasm, which frequently contains a perinuclear clear area. Bilobed plasma cells are also seen on this plate.*

---

adjustments which compensate for the decrease in red cell mass.

The degree to which symptoms occur in an anemic patient depends on several contributing factors. If the anemia has developed rapidly, there may not be adequate time for compensatory adjustments to take place, and the patient may have more marked symptoms than if an anemia of equivalent severity had developed insidiously. Furthermore, the patient's complaints may depend on the presence of local vascular disease. For example, angina pectoris, intermittent claudication, or transient cerebral ischemia may be unmasked by the development of anemia.

Individuals with mild anemia are often asymptomatic. They may complain of fatigue as well as dyspnea and palpitation, particularly following exercise. Severely anemic patients will often be symptomatic at rest and unable to tolerate significant exertion. When the hemoglobin concentration falls below 7.5 g/dl, resting cardiac output rises significantly with an increase in both heart rate and stroke volume. The patient may be aware of this hyperdynamic state and complain of palpitation or a pounding pulse. Symptoms of cardiac failure may develop if the patient's myocardial reserve is reduced.

The clinical manifestations of severe anemia extend to other organ systems. Patients often complain of dizziness and headache and may experience syncope, tinnitus, or vertigo. Many patients are irritable and have difficulty sleeping or concentrating. Because of decreased blood flow to the skin, patients may become hypersensitive to cold. Gastrointestinal symptoms such as anorexia, indigestion, and even nausea or bowel irregularity are attributable to shunting of blood away from the splanchnic bed. Females commonly develop abnormal menstruation, both amenorrhea and increased bleeding. Males may complain of impotence or loss of libido.

Physical findings *Pallor* is the physical finding most commonly associated with anemia. However, the usefulness of this sign is limited by other factors that affect the color of the skin. The thickness and texture of the skin vary widely among individuals. Furthermore, the blood flow to the skin can undergo wide fluctuations. Normal individuals will appear sallow when blood is shunted away from the skin, whereas anemic patients may appear flushed when overheated or during periods of excitement. The concentration of melanin in the epidermis is another important determinant of skin color. Individuals with a fair complexion may look pale even though they are not anemic. Conversely, pallor is difficult to detect in deeply pigmented individuals. Furthermore, acquired disorders of melanin pigmentation (e.g., Addison's disease, hemochromatosis)

TABLE 54-1
Laboratory evaluation of anemias

	Reticulocytes	*Peripheral smear*	*Marrow*	*Additional lab tests*	*Diagnosis*
↓ Hematocrit	Normal, decreased	Hypochromic: Microcytic	0 Iron	↓ Fe, ↑ TIBC	Iron deficiency
			+ Iron	↑ Hb A_2, ↑ Hb F	β thalassemia
			Ring sideroblasts	↓ Hb A_2	Sideroblastic anemia
		Macrocytic	Megaloblastic	↓ Serum B_{12} achlorhydria	Vitamin B_{12} deficiency, pernicious anemia
				↓ Serum folate	Folic acid deficiency
		Normochromic: Normocytic	Normal	↓ Fe, ↓ TIBC	Anemia of chronic inflammation
				↑ Creatinine	Anemia of uremia
				Abnormal LFT	Anemia of liver disease
				↓ T_4	Anemia of myxedema
			Aplastic		Aplastic anemia
		Normoblasts, teardrops	Infiltrated: Tumor, lymphoma, etc.		Myelophthisic
			Fibrosis	↑ LAP	Myeloid metaplasia
	Increased	Polychromatophilia +	Erythroid hyperplasia ↓	+ Sucrose lysis	Paroxysmal nocturnal hemoglobinuria
		Schistocytes, helmet cells			Traumatic hemolytic anemia
		Spherocytes		+ Coombs' test	Immunohemolytic anemia
				↑ Osmotic fragility	Hereditary spherocytosis
		Spur cells		Abnormal LFT	Spur cell anemia
		Sickle cells		Positive sickle prep	Sickle cell syndromes
		Target cells		Abnormal Hb electrophoresis	Hb C, D, etc.
		Heinz bodies		Abnormal Hb electrophoresis	Congenital Heinz body hemolytic anemia
				↓ G6PD	G6PD deficiency
				Blood in stomach, stool	Blood loss anemia

NOTE: *Fe, iron; TIBC, total iron-binding capacity; Hb, hemoglobin; LAP, leukocyte alkaline phosphatase; G6PD, glucose 6-phosphate dehydrogenase, LFT, liver function tests.*

or jaundice may interfere with detection of pallor. Nevertheless, even in blacks, the presence of anemia may be suspected by the color of the palms or of noncutaneous tissues such as oral mucous membranes, nail beds, and palpebral conjunctivas. The color of the creases of the palm is a useful sign. When they are as pale as the surrounding skin, the patient usually has a hemoglobin of less than 7 g/dl.

Two factors contribute to the development of pallor in patients with anemia. There is, of course, a decrease in the hemoglobin concentration of blood perfusing the skin and mucous membranes. Also, blood is shunted away from the skin and other peripheral tissues, permitting enhanced blood flow to vital organs. Redistribution of blood flow is an important mode of compensation in anemia (see Fig. 54-5).

Other physical findings associated with anemia include tachycardia, wide pulse pressure, and a hyperdynamic precordium. A systolic ejection murmur is often heard over the precordium, particularly at the pulmonic area. In addition, a venous hum may be detected over the neck vessels. These cardiac findings disappear when the anemia is corrected. Patients with hemolytic anemia often have icterus and splenomegaly and occasionally develop superficial skin ulceration over the ankle bones.

APPROACH TO THE PATIENT WITH ANEMIA In evaluating the anemic patient, the physician should proceed in an orderly fashion so that the correct diagnosis can be established with a minimum of laboratory tests and procedures. As in other clinical disciplines, a comprehensive history and meticulous physical examination are of paramount importance in the initial workup of the anemic patient. For example, a family history which reveals a dominant inheritance pattern provides strong support for the diagnosis of hereditary spherocytosis. The discovery of a heart murmur and splenomegaly raises the possibility that the anemic patient may have subacute bacterial endocarditis.

The evaluation of the anemic patient should be based on a firm understanding of the pathophysiologic principles outlined earlier in this chapter. Table 54-1 shows an overview of the laboratory tests that are useful in the diagnosis of anemias. The clinician must first ask whether the anemia is due to a decreased production of red cells or enhanced destruction. In addition, the possibility of blood loss either as the sole etiology or as a contributing factor must always be considered. At this crossroad, laboratory information can be gathered which will establish whether the patient is failing to produce an adequate number of circulating red cells or is undergoing hemolysis.

The *reticulocyte count* is the most useful laboratory test for answering this question. When an appropriate supravital stain is applied to a sample of peripheral blood, the 1- to 2-day-old red cells exhibit a network of purple strands, which are aggregates of ribosomes. Reticulocytosis is a reflection of the release of an increased number of young cells from the bone marrow. The degree of increased erythropoiesis can be assessed more quantitatively by determining the reticulocyte index, which uses the hematocrit or packed cell volume (PCV) and is calculated as follows:

$$\text{Reticulocyte index} = \text{reticulocyte \%} \times \frac{\text{patient's PCV}}{\text{normal PCV}}$$

This measure fails to consider the distribution of reticulocytes between the bone marrow and the peripheral blood. When the marrow is greatly stimulated, marrow reticulocytes enter the circulation prematurely. Since the circulation of these "shift reticulocytes" in the peripheral blood is prolonged, the reticulocyte index should be divided by about 2. This factor varies from 1.5 to 3 depending upon the severity of the anemia and the degree of erythropoietin stimulation. This correction should always be made if normoblasts are encountered in the peripheral blood since this finding indicates the premature release of red cell precursors into the circulation. On a routinely prepared smear, "shift reticulocytes" appear larger than average and have a lavender hue, so-called polychromatophilia.

A failure to produce red cells is reflected in an inappropriately low reticulocyte count. In contrast, a significant elevation of reticulocytes is suggestive of hemolysis. Exceptions include (1) the brisk reticulocyte response that is seen in a patient with hemorrhage, (2) reticulocytosis encountered in patients recovering from impaired erythropoiesis (e.g., an individual with pernicious anemia who received an injection of vitamin B_{12} 1 week earlier), and (3) mild to moderate elevations in reticulocytes (3 to 7 percent) encountered in myelophthisic anemia in which the orderly release of cells is affected by alterations of the marrow stroma owing to tumor, fibrosis, or granulomata. These exceptions are often readily appreciated in the initial evaluation of the patient. Furthermore, a number of ancillary laboratory tests described below are useful in determining to what extent hemolysis is occurring. The measurement of unconjugated bilirubin in the serum is a particularly useful guide to the presence of accelerated red blood cell breakdown. Once this information is obtained, the workup can be directed toward the establishment of a specific etiology.

Four additional base-line studies are of critical importance in the initial workup of the patient with anemia: *measurement of red cell indexes, examination of the peripheral blood smear, testing the stool for occult blood,* and, in many patients, *bone marrow examination.*

Red cell indexes Red cell indexes can be calculated from determinants of hematocrit, hemoglobin concentration, and red blood count. Measuring the hematocrit or PCV is the simplest and one of the most precise ways to ascertain the concentration of red cells in the blood. Generally, a small sample of anticoagulated blood is drawn into a capillary tube which is sealed at one end and centrifuged. The PCV is the ratio of the volume of packed red cells to the total volume. Alternatively, the concentration of hemoglobin can be determined spectrophotometrically from the absorbance of the cyanmethemoglobin form at a specific wavelength. With the advent of automated red blood cell counting technology, very precise measurements of red blood cell indexes are now readily available in nearly all hospitals and clinical laboratories. The electronic counter makes a direct measurement of the red cell count (RBC/μl) and the mean red cell volume (MCV):

TABLE 54-2
Anemias due to decreased red cell production

I Microcytic anemias
- *A* Iron deficiency (Chap. 326)
- *B* Sideroblastic anemias (Chap. 326)
- *C* Thalassemias (Chap. 329)

II Macrocytic (megaloblastic) anemias (Chap. 327)
- *A* Vitamin B_{12} deficiency, including pernicious anemia
- *B* Folic acid deficiency
- *C* Others: drug-induced, orotic aciduria, some refractory anemias, erythroleukemia

III Normocytic anemias
- *A* Primary bone marrow failure (Chap. 331)
  - *1* Aplastic anemia (rare: pure red cell anemia)
  - *2* Myelophthisic anemias: leukemia and lymphoma, other neoplasms, myelofibrosis, granulomas
- *B* Secondary anemias (Chap. 328)
  - *1* Anemias of chronic inflammation (infections, connective tissue disorders, etc.)
  - *2* Anemia of uremia
  - *3* Anemias associated with endocrinopathies
  - *4* Anemia of chronic liver disease

$$\text{MCV (fl)} = \frac{\text{PCV (liters/liters)}}{(\text{RBC}/\mu\text{l}) \times 10^{-9}}$$

This instrument calculates the PCV from the direct measurement of MCV and RBC/μl. In addition, hemoglobin concentration is measured directly on a separate channel. The mean corpuscular hemoglobin concentration (MCHC) is then computed as follows:

$$\text{MCHC (g/dl)} = \frac{\text{Hb (g/dl)}}{\text{PCV (liters/liters)}}$$

A third red blood cell index, the mean corpuscular hemoglobin (MCH), is determined as follows:

$$\text{MCH (pg)} = \frac{\text{Hb (g/dl)}}{(\text{RBC}/\mu\text{l}) \times 10^{-7}}$$

When calculated by an electronic counter, the MCHC is not reliable and is of little use to the clinician. Generally, an automated system provides a printout which includes hemoglobin concentration, red cell count, packed cell volume, and the three red cell indexes (MCV, MCHC, and MCH).

As Table 54-2 shows, the MCV is particularly useful in classifying the anemias due to decreased red cell production. Microcytic anemias have low values for MCV. On microscopic examination, the red cells appear small and often pale. In contrast, in the macrocytic anemias the MCV is elevated and large oval cells (macroovalocytes) are seen on microscopic examination. Unlike the anemias of underproduction, nearly all the hemolytic anemias are normocytic. Exceptions include the severe forms of thalassemias in which microcytic red cells are accompanied by brisk hemolysis.

Examination of the blood smear In the evaluation of patients with anemia, the physician should take the time to examine a well-stained peripheral blood film. Plate 9 shows examples of abnormalities in red cell morphology encountered in various types of anemia. Many subtleties escape the attention of the technologist whose primary purpose in examining the slide is to obtain a white cell differential count. Furthermore, the clinician can approach the specimen with a prepared mind and can scrutinize it for specific abnormalities. As suggested above, the examination can confirm the size and color of red cells as estimated by RBC indexes. Furthermore, while these indexes provide mean statistical values, the microscopic examination can reveal variation in red cell size (anisocytosis) or shape (poikilocytosis), changes which are helpful in the diagnosis of specific anemias. Examination of the blood smear is particularly important in evaluating a patient with hemolysis. Most hemolytic anemias have characteristic morphological abnormalities. Finally, this practice may yield unexpected dividends. The finding of rouleaux suggests the presence of dysproteinemia as occurs in multiple myeloma. The examination may provide the initial clue that the patient has significant thrombocytopenia.

Bone marrow examination A microscopic examination of the bone marrow is generally indicated in the workup of any *unexplained* anemia. The more severe the anemia, the more likely that the procedure will be informative. An assessment of the quantity and quality of red cell precursors may determine whether there is a primary defect in cell production. A marrow biopsy is particularly useful in estimating overall cellularity. The normal differential of nucleated cells in the marrow is shown in the Appendix. The ratio of myeloid (M) to erythroid (E) precursors is normally about 2:1 but may be artifactually increased by the inclusion of circulating leukocytes. The ratio is increased in patients with infection, a leukemoid reaction, or neoplastic proliferation of myeloid cells. Rarely, a high M:E ratio is due to selective aplasia of the red cell precursors. A decreased M:E ratio indicates erythroid hyperplasia (seen in hemolysis or hemorrhage) or ineffective erythropoiesis (megaloblastic and sideroblastic anemias). The morphology of the precursors may reveal a maturation deficit such as megaloblastic anemia. The bone marrow examination is also important in demonstrating the presence of cellular infiltrates such as those found in leukemia, lymphoma, or multiple myeloma. The demonstration of tumor, fibrosis, or granulomata usually requires a biopsy. A portion of the marrow specimen should be stained with Prussian blue. In addition to providing an assessment of iron stores, the iron stain is required for the identification of sideroblasts.

ANEMIA DUE TO BLOOD LOSS This form of anemia varies considerably in its clinical presentation depending upon the site, severity, and rapidity of the hemorrhage. At opposite extremes are acute fulminant bleeding producing hypovolemic shock and chronic occult blood loss leading to iron-deficiency anemia.

Patients who have sustained an acute hemorrhage generally present with signs and symptoms secondary to hypoxia and hypovolemia. Depending on the severity of the process, the patient will have weakness, fatigue, light-headedness, stupor, or coma and will often appear pale, diaphoretic, and irritable. Vital signs are a reflection of cardiovascular compensation to the acute blood loss (Chap. 29). The patient will have hypotension and tachycardia in proportion to the degree of hemorrhage. Elicitation of postural signs is useful in the initial evaluation of patients with acute blood loss. If the pulse rises 25 percent or more, or the systolic blood pressure falls 20 torr or more upon going from a supine to sitting position, the patient is likely to have significant hypovolemia (blood loss $>$ 1000 ml) and requires prompt replacement. Acute blood loss in excess of 1500 ml usually leads to cardiovascular collapse.

If the blood loss has been acute and recent, the peripheral blood may not reveal a significant decrease in packed cell volume or hemoglobin, since the red cell mass and plasma volume are contracted in parallel. There often is a moderate leukocytosis and a "shift to the left" in the white cell differential count. Thrombocytosis may be encountered in both acute and chronic blood loss, particularly when the patient is iron-deficient. During the first few days following an acute hemorrhage there is usually an increase in reticulocytes. Occasionally nucleated red cells may appear in the peripheral blood. Since young red cells are larger than old ones, the patient may develop slightly macrocytic red cell indexes (MCV = 100 to 105 fl). As mentioned above, sustained reticulocytosis will be seen if significant blood loss continues, until iron stores have been exhausted. Internal bleeding may be accompanied by an increase in unconjugated bilirubin. This abnormality is a reflection of an increase in catabolism of heme from extravasated red cells. Patients with acute gastrointestinal blood loss will often have an elevation of blood urea nitrogen owing to impaired renal blood flow and perhaps to the absorption of digested blood protein.

It is of critical importance to assess these patients promptly and institute treatment without delay. A large-bore intravenous line should be placed. While blood is being typed and cross matched, saline, Ringer's lactate, or, preferably, a colloid such as 5% albumin should be infused to correct hypovolemia. Whole blood is then administered as soon as it is available. Monitoring of vital signs and central venous pressure is useful in determining the appropriate amount of volume replacement. During and following these emergency measures, diagnostic studies may reveal the site or sites of bleeding. If there appears to be generalized hemorrhage from skin, mucous membranes, urine, etc., an emergency coagulation profile should be obtained. Demonstration of bleeding from the gastrointestinal tract may require the insertion of a nasogastric tube. Appropriate radiologic studies may be indicated to determine sites of internal bleeding such as retroperitoneal hemorrhage.

Chronic blood loss is usually due to lesions in the gastrointestinal tract or the uterus. The testing of stool specimens for occult blood is an essential, though frequently overlooked, part of the evaluation of anemia. It may be necessary to examine serial specimens over a prolonged period of time since gastrointestinal bleeding is often intermittent. The hematologic manifestations of chronic blood loss are those of iron-deficiency anemia, discussed in detail in Chap. 326.

ANEMIAS DUE TO DECREASED RBC PRODUCTION As shown in Table 54-2, red cell indexes are useful in classifying the anemias due to underproduction of red cells. They can be conveniently grouped into three major categories: microcytic, macrocytic, and normocytic.

The *microcytic* anemias include iron-deficiency anemia (Chap. 326), some sideroblastic anemias (Chap. 326), and the thalassemias (Chap. 330). Collectively, they represent a decrease in the availability or synthesis of one of the three major constituents of the hemoglobin molecule: iron, porphyrin, and globin. Since hemoglobin composes over 90 percent of the protein within the erythrocyte, it is not surprising that these defects in hemoglobin synthesis result in the formation of small, pale red cells. As mentioned above, these disorders involve a variable degree of ineffective erythropoiesis. In addition, the anemias of chronic inflammation and malignancy may be slightly microcytic (Chap. 328). This phenomenon may be due to a poorly understood defect in the availability of iron. However, these disorders are more often normocytic and have been so classified in Table 54-2. As shown in Table 54-1, measurement of serum iron and iron-binding capacity and evaluation of marrow iron stores are particularly useful in distinguishing between these anemias.

The *macrocytic* anemias generally are associated with megaloblastic morphology in the bone marrow. In most cases, a deficiency of either vitamin B_{12} or folic acid results in an impairment of the replication of DNA, particularly in cells having a high turnover rate. Because nuclear maturation lags behind cytoplasmic development, large red cells tend to be produced in the bone marrow. Megaloblastic anemias are discussed in detail in Chap. 327. Like the microcytic anemias, these disorders are maturation defects associated with ineffective erythropoiesis. Macrocytosis, generally of a lesser degree, may also be encountered in patients with liver disease, hypothyroidism, hemolytic anemia, aplastic anemia, and alcoholism. However, in these conditions, the red cell precursors in the bone marrow do not appear megaloblastic. The macrocytes in liver disease and hypothyroidism may be related to an increased deposition of lipid in the red cell membrane.

The *normocytic* anemias of underproduction[1] comprise a diverse group of disorders. As shown in Table 54-2, this group can be conveniently subdivided into two categories: those due to intrinsic pathology within the bone marrow and those secondary to some other underlying disease.

The primary disorders of the bone marrow are best approached by microscopic examination of a marrow aspirate and biopsy. This group of anemias is often accompanied by leukopenia and thrombocytopenia. Pancytopenia, usually to a lesser degree, can also be seen in hypersplenism and in the megaloblastic anemias. Aplastic anemia and the myelophthisic anemias are discussed in Chap. 331.

[1] *As mentioned above, the hemolytic anemias are also normocytic.*

The diagnosis of anemia secondary to some underlying disease is usually quite straightforward. Conversely, the presence of an unexplained normocytic anemia should prompt the search for an underlying disorder such as chronic renal failure, infection, or myxedema. If the presence of such an illness is established, the physician is obliged to investigate whether other factors such as blood loss or a nutritional deficiency contribute to the patient's anemia. Generally, the anemias due to liver disease, chronic inflammation, or an endocrinopathy are of only moderate severity, unlike the other "secondary" anemias that due to chronic renal failure can be severe. All these anemias are discussed in more detail in Chap. 328.

HEMOLYTIC ANEMIAS Hemolytic anemias are encountered much less frequently than the anemias due to decreased red cell production. Although they are a diverse group, the hemolytic anemias have a number of clinical features in common. Signs and symptoms of patients with hemolysis are briefly mentioned above.

A number of laboratory tests are available to establish the presence of accelerated breakdown of red cells. The reticulocyte count is the single most useful test. Patients with hemolysis nearly always have an elevated reticulocyte count. A variety of serum and urine tests are useful in confirming the presence of hemolysis and assessing its magnitude. These are described in detail in Chap. 329 and are summarized in Table 329-2.

Classification of hemolytic anemias Once the presence of hemolysis is established, a large battery of laboratory tests is available for determining the specific diagnosis. Some of these tests are listed in Table 54-1. No other area of internal medicine is better suited to detailed and fruitful diagnostic probing. In the interest of time and money, the clinician should use the available tests in an orderly fashion. This complex group of disorders is easier to approach diagnostically if a concise and workable classification is used. The hemolytic anemias can be grouped in several ways: congenital versus acquired, intracorpuscular versus extracorpuscular, or by anatomic site of the erythrocyte defect. The various kinds of hemolytic anemia are discussed in Chap. 329.

THERAPEUTIC CONSIDERATIONS The effective treatment of anemia, like other disorders, is predicated upon a thorough diagnostic evaluation. There is no reason to administer hematinics such as iron, vitamin B_{12}, or folic acid unless a specific deficiency of these substances has been demonstrated or is anticipated. Although the indiscriminate administration of vitamin B_{12} is not deleterious per se, it lulls both the patient and the physician into false security. In contrast, the inappropriate use of iron preparations over a prolonged period of time can be directly harmful, leading to a state of iron overload. Pyridoxine is indicated only in the treatment of sideroblastic anemias.

Many kinds of anemias can be corrected if a precipitating cause can be uncovered and reversed. If a drug or toxin can be incriminated, its withdrawal may allow full recovery. The outcome of the "secondary" anemias is dependent on whether the underlying condition can be corrected. Anemias due to an endocrinopathy or infection should respond favorably to appropriate treatment. Occasionally, the anemia of malignancy is corrected by the removal of the primary tumor. One of the most dramatic sequelae of a successful renal transplant is the prompt correction of the "anemia of uremia." In chronic disorders such as hepatic cirrhosis or rheumatoid arthritis, the anemia is likely to persist, along with the underlying disease.

Primary disorders of the bone marrow such as aplastic anemia or myelophthisic anemia are often irreversible and are treated with supportive measures. *Androgens* are sometimes employed in this group of anemias, but their efficacy is marginal. Many of these patients require transfusions of red cells and platelets. Because prognosis is so bleak in these disorders, a radical approach to treatment seems justified. As described in Chap. 331, bone marrow transplantation is now a reasonable therapeutic alternative in selected cases of severe aplastic anemia and acute leukemia.

Several factors should be weighed in determining whether an anemic patient should be transfused. The risks and complications of the administration of blood products are discussed in Chap. 335. Patients with chronic or long-standing anemias are able to compensate in several ways, discussed earlier in this chapter. A considerable reduction in red cell mass can be surprisingly well tolerated, especially if the patient is young or sedentary. Transfusion is seldom indicated in a patient with a chronic anemia whose hemoglobin is 9 g/dl or greater. Those who are expected to respond to the administration of a specific agent such as iron, folic acid, or vitamin B_{12} can usually be spared transfusions. If the anemia has precipitated an episode of congestive heart failure or myocardial ischemia, prompt but cautious administration of packed red cells is indicated. In general, whole blood should be given only if the patient is hypovolemic.

Corticosteroids have only a limited role in the treatment of anemia. These agents are not effective in stimulating erythropoiesis. High doses of a glucocorticoid are indicated in the treatment of immunohemolytic anemia, thrombotic thrombocytopenic purpura, and pure red cell anemia. Otherwise, steroids should be prescribed sparingly unless some coexisting condition dictates their use.

Splenectomy is indicated in the treatment of certain hemolytic anemias. The efficacy of splenectomy correlates with the degree to which the abnormal or defective red cells are sequestered. Splenectomy is virtually curative in hereditary spherocytosis. The operation may be beneficial in selected patients with immunohemolytic anemia, congestive splenomegaly, spur cell anemia, and certain hemoglobinopathies and enzymopathies. Splenectomy has also been recommended early in the treatment of thrombotic thrombocytopenic purpura. The operative morbidity and mortality from elective splenectomy is very low. Occasional patients develop a left subphrenic abscess. Following splenectomy, young children are at risk of developing overwhelming septicemia. This complication is much rarer in adults. Thrombocytosis generally develops promptly following splenectomy. However, in most cases, it is transient. In patients with continued hemolysis, the thrombocytosis usually persists and may occasionally be associated with thromboembolic phenomena.

REFERENCES

BECK WS (ed): *Hematology.* Boston, MIT Press, 1981

BUNN HF, FORGET BG: *Human Hemoglobins,* 2d ed. Philadelphia, Saunders, 1983

CROSBY WH: Red cell mass: Its precursors and perturbations. Hosp Prac 15:2, 71, 1980

ERSLEV AJ, GABUZDA TG: *Pathophysiology of Blood.* Philadelphia, Saunders, 1979

HILLMAN RS, FINCH CA: *Red Cell Manual.* Philadelphia, Davis, 1974

LICHTMAN MA (ed): *Hematology for Practitioners.* Boston, Little, Brown, 1978

NIENHUIS AW, BENZ EJ: Regulation of hemoglobin synthesis during the development of the red cell. N Engl J Med 297:1318, 1371, 1430, 1977

WILLIAMS WJ et al (ed): *Hematology*. New York, McGraw-Hill, 1977
WINTROBE MM (ed): Blood, pure and eloquent. New York, McGraw-Hill, 1980

55
BLEEDING

HYMIE L. NOSSEL

Bleeding is one of the most serious and significant of the cardinal manifestations of disease. It may occur from a local site or may be generalized. Bleeding associated with a local lesion may be superimposed on either a normal or a defective hemostatic mechanism; in contrast, general bleeding is usually associated with a hemorrhagic diathesis. Spontaneous bleeding also suggests defective hemostasis.

LOCAL BLEEDING

In the evaluation of local bleeding, the site, appearance of the blood, signs of blood loss, and evidence for disordered hemostasis should be considered. The sites and common causes of bleeding are listed in Table 55-1. The appearance of the blood may provide a clue as to the cause of the bleeding. Bleeding from the lungs and bronchi is influenced by the degree of aeration and the presence of mucus and pus. In pneumococcal pneumonia the sputum is characteristically rusty. In tuberculosis it is usually bright red. Pus is usually mixed with the blood when infection is present. Massive hemorrhage occasionally occurs in mitral stenosis when a bronchial varicosity ruptures or in tuberculosis when a vessel is eroded. In pulmonary infarction the blood is usually dark red. Blood derived from the gastrointestinal tract may be darkened because of conversion of hemoglobin to brown hematin by gastric acid. Blood vomited from the stomach may be dark ("coffee ground") or bright red if the vomiting is sufficiently rapid. When it appears in the stool, it may be pitch black (melena). Blood derived from the colon is red or brown, and, if inflammation is the cause, mucus or pus is mixed with it (see Chap. 37). If bleeding from the urinary tract is profuse, clots or bright blood may be present in the urine. Small amounts of blood impart a smoky appearance to urine, whereas lesser degrees of hematuria may be detected only by microscopy.

The signs and symptoms of blood loss depend on the amount and rate of bleeding. If very acute, syncope occurs rapidly; with a slower rate of loss, signs and symptoms of peripheral circulatory collapse occur. Shock may occur without external blood loss if a large amount of blood is lost into a serous cavity. Slow and prolonged blood loss will gradually result in symptoms of iron-deficiency anemia.

Local bleeding which is out of proportion to the injury suggests a hemostatic defect. For example, when a patient suffers bleeding sufficient to require blood transfusion following dental extraction, a defect of the coagulation or platelet systems can almost always be defined.

HEMOSTASIS AND ITS DISORDERS

The successful management of patients with a disorder of the hemostatic mechanism depends on accurate diagnosis. Correct diagnosis and rational therapy depend on an understanding of the normal mechanisms for preserving hemostasis.

Normal hemostasis comprises mechanisms operative immediately following an injury and those acting over a longer period to maintain hemostasis. The immediate mechanism consists principally of two components: *vasoconstriction* due to active contraction of the smooth muscle of the vessel wall, and *plug formation* by masses of aggregated platelets. The maintenance mechanism consists of the *fibrin clot* produced by the coagulation system.

Platelet plug formation is especially important in capillary hemostasis, while vasoconstriction and fibrin clot formation seem to be more important in larger vessel hemostasis. These several mechanisms involved in achieving normal hemostasis are interconnected at several points, but for the sake of clarity they will be described as separate entities.

PLATELETS The normal platelet count is 150,000 to 400,000 per cubic millimeter and is accurately measured by electronic particle counting or by phase-contrast microscopy. An estimate of platelet number may be made by examination of the stained peripheral blood smear. When the red cells are almost touching one another and the platelets are evenly distributed, 1 platelet per oil immersion field is equivalent to about 20,000 per microliter; 10 platelets, to about 200,000 per microliter; and so on.

Structure Normal platelets are anucleate bodies 2 to 3 μm in diameter which appear light blue and contain small purple-red granules when stained with Giemsa's solution. With the electron microscope, three distinct structural zones may be identified in the platelet, each related to specific platelet functions. The *peripheral* zone is involved in adhesion, the *cytoplasm* (sol-gel zone) in contraction, and the *organelle* zone in secretion.

The peripheral zone comprises a surface coat of acid mucopolysaccharides (the glycocalyx), the trilaminar plasma membrane, which contains specific glycoproteins oriented toward the exterior surface of the membrane, and a submembranous area. The surface coat is involved in adhesion, and the membrane provides a trigger mechanism whereby stimuli are transmitted from the exterior into the interior. The unique quality

TABLE 55-1
Causes of localized bleeding

Locations	*Commonest causes*
Skin (petechiae, purpura, ecchymoses)	Thrombocytopenia
Limbs:	
Joints	Hemophilia
Intramuscular and subcutaneous hematomas	Hemophilia
Central nervous system	Trauma, hypertension, congenital vascular malformations
Head and neck:	
Nose and sinuses	Trauma, inflammation, hypertension, polyps and tumors, hereditary telangiectasia
Ears	Trauma
Optic fundi	Hypertension, nephritis, diabetes, thrombocytopenia, trauma
Chest:	
Respiratory tract	Tumors, infections, bronchiectasis, pulmonary embolism, mitral stenosis
Serous cavity	Tumors, tuberculosis, pulmonary infarction
Nipples	Fissure, tumor
Gastrointestinal tract	Esophageal varices, hiatal hernia, peptic ulcer, gastritis, tumors, colitis, hemorrhoids, hereditary telangiectasia
Abdominal cavity	Trauma, splenic rupture, ectopic gestation
Urinary tract	Calculi, infections, glomerulonephritis, tumors, cystitis, prostatic hypertrophy
Vagina	Obstetric and endocrine disorders, tumors

of the platelet is its ability to adhere to foreign surfaces and form aggregates in response to a variety of stimuli including thrombin, adenosine diphosphate (ADP), and catecholamines. Specific binding sites are present for thrombin, ADP, fibrinogen, the von Willebrand protein, and catecholamines.

The submembranous area and cytoplasmic zone contain microfilaments composed of actin and myosin which form the contractile protein actomyosin (also termed *thrombosthenin*). The microfilaments are responsible for the centripetal movement and coalescence of granules occurring during platelet aggregation, the contraction of pseudopods, and clot retraction. Also present in the submembranous area are bundles of microtubules which encircle the platelet, forming a cytoskeleton that stabilizes the cell, permitting it to circulate as a flattened disk. The microtubules are composed of polymers of tubulin, a protein distinct from actin and myosin.

Distinct components in the organelle zone include granules, mitochondria, glycogen-containing particles, and, in an occasional platelet, stacks of flattened saccules resembling a Golgi apparatus. Three types of membrane-enclosed granules can be distinguished: (1) alpha granules which contain proteins specific to the platelet such as platelet factor 4 (which has heparin-neutralizing activity), beta thromboglobulin, the platelet-derived growth factor (which stimulates smooth-muscle and fibroblast mitosis), and those present in plasma such as fibrinogen, von Willebrand protein, and fibronectin; (2) dense granules in which calcium, ADP, serotonin, and catecholamines are localized; and (3) lysosomal granules with enzymes such as phosphatase, β-glucuronidase, and cathepsin. The three granule populations constitute the secretory organelles of the platelet and release their contents in response to stimuli such as thrombin, collagen, ADP, and epinephrine. The threshold for release for each type of granule is different; the sequence in order of increasing threshold is alpha granules, dense granules, and lysosomal granules. Active intermediary metabolism occurs in the mitochondria. ATP is generated from both glycolysis and the tricarboxylic acid cycle. Glycogen and lipid are also synthesized.

FIGURE 55-1
Platelet plug formation.

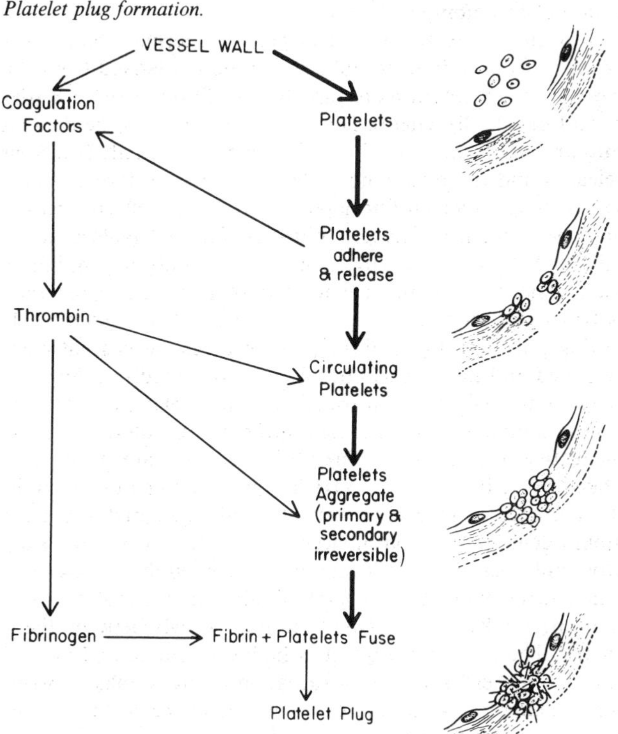

Distribution and fate Platelets are formed in the marrow and released into the circulation. At any moment, about 80 percent of the platelets are in the circulation and 20 percent are in the spleen; free movement occurs between these two pools. If the spleen enlarges markedly, the distribution shifts and up to 80 percent of the platelets may be pooled in the spleen. Survival curves of ^{51}Cr-labeled platelets are linear and suggest that most platelets become senescent and die after a life span of about 10 days.

Some platelets appear to be consumed in repairing the minor vascular injuries of daily life. There is evidence that younger platelets are physiologically more active and have higher enzyme concentrations than old platelets. This distinction is most apparent when thrombopoiesis is accelerated in response to increased platelet destruction. Senescent platelets are probably removed by the reticuloendothelial system. In thrombocytopenia due to increased platelet destruction, the destruction is random. Damaged platelets may be removed primarily in the spleen or in both the spleen and the liver. The bone marrow does not contain a reserve of platelets, and if circulating platelets are rapidly destroyed or lost, thrombocytopenia persists for several days until enough new platelets are formed. Governing normal platelet production are one or more thrombopoietic factors which have not yet been isolated and characterized.

Function in hemostasis The platelets contribute to hemostasis by forming platelet plugs and by promoting thrombin production. Platelet plug formation may be divided into a number of stages (Fig. 55-1).

ADHESION Platelets adhere to subendothelial structures exposed by trauma. Such structures include collagen fibers and basement membranes. Regularly spaced free amino groups on the collagen molecule are required for platelet adhesion. In addition von Willebrand factor is required for normal platelet adherence (see Chap. 334).

RELEASE REACTION Following adherence to collagen, platelets extrude the contents of their granules—a process termed the *release reaction.* This reaction is also induced by thrombin, and in physiologic hemostasis very likely both collagen and thrombin initiate release. Epinephrine and ADP also promote platelet aggregation and release.

Detailed understanding of the mechanism of release is incomplete, but certain facts are clear. The reaction has an absolute requirement for energy derived from glycolysis and the Krebs cycle. A major control mechanism for both aggregation and release is the platelet concentration of cyclic adenosine 3′, 5′-monophosphate (AMP) which is produced from ATP by adenylate cyclase and degraded by phosphodiesterase. Release is inhibited by substances which increase the platelet concentration of cyclic AMP. These agents include prostacyclin (PGI_2, a potent prostaglandin produced only in endothelial cells and not in platelets), which stimulates adenylate cyclase, and theophylline, which inhibits phosphodiesterase. Epinephrine and thromboxane A_2 (a prostaglandin produced in platelets) lower platelet cyclic AMP levels and promote release.

It has been shown that an intermediate of platelet prostaglandin synthesis plays a major role in mediating the release reaction (Fig. 55-2). When platelets are stimulated by a release-inducer, such as thrombin or ADP, phospholipases A_2 and C cleave platelet phospholipids, resulting in the release of free arachidonic acid. Arachidonic acid is converted to the cyclic endoperoxide PGG_2 by a cyclooxygenase. PGG_2 is spontaneously converted to PGH_2, which is converted to thromboxane A_2 by thromboxane synthetase. Thromboxane A_2 directly induces the release reaction but is unstable and is rapidly transformed to thromboxane B_2, which is inactive. Aspirin irreversibly acetylates cyclooxygenase, rendering it inactive, thus inhibiting formation of endoperoxide and thromboxane A_2. Inhibition of cyclooxygenase prevents platelet release resulting from weak or moderate stimulation. High concentrations of collagen or thrombin will overcome the inhibitory effect of aspirin and produce full release, indicating the presence of an alternative release mechanism. Calcium ionophores, which allow movements of calcium ions between subcellular compartments, may induce release independent of prostaglandin metabolism. Platelets contain the calcium-binding protein calmodulin, and when the calcium concentration increases, calcium-calmodulin complexes are formed which activate a myosin kinase. The active myosin kinase phosphorylates myosin, which then reacts with actin to produce contraction and the "release" reaction. It is an attractive but unproven hypothesis that these calcium-dependent reactions form the mechanism whereby all release inducers act.

AGGREGATION The released ADP causes additional platelets to aggregate and is thus a key component for amplifying the extent of platelet aggregation. Exposure of platelets to ADP results in binding of fibrinogen to the platelet surface. The bound fibrinogen, derived either from the plasma or from platelet alpha granules, mediates ADP-induced aggregation. Low concentrations of ADP ($\sim 10^{-6}$ M) cause only primary platelet aggregation, which is reversible, whereas two- to threefold higher concentrations of ADP produce irreversible aggregation. Low concentrations of thrombin or collagen, in addition to causing primary aggregation, stimulate the release of ADP, which promotes secondary irreversible aggregation.

Platelets participate in coagulation factor reactions leading to thrombin formation by providing a lipoprotein surface ("platelet factor 3") on which coagulation enzymes and substrates interact. Factor X_a is bound via factor V_a to the platelet membrane lipoprotein and there activates prothrombin. "Activation" of the platelet is necessary for factor X_a binding and consequent promotion of coagulation (Fig. 55-5). Hence, a defect in platelet activation will be detected as a defect in the activity of "platelet factor 3" coagulant activity.

FUSION The action of thrombin produced by the coagulation mechanism leads to coalescence. Fibrin (also a product of thrombin action) and fused platelets form a stable hemostatic plug.

FIGURE 55-2
Generation of thromboxane A_2 in platelets and prostacyclin PGI_2 in endothelial cells.

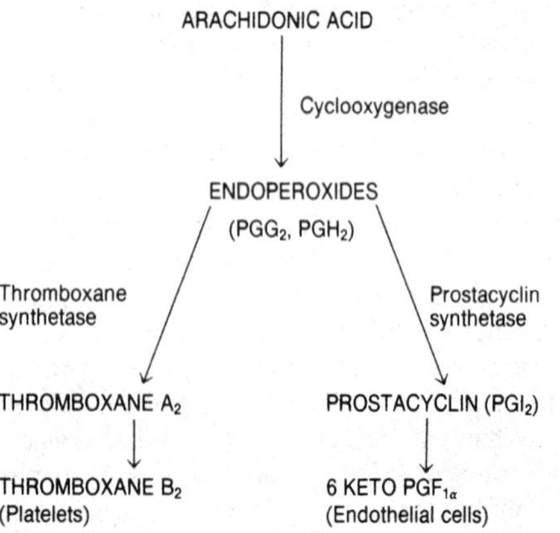

Tests of platelet function Platelet plugs rapidly stop bleeding from ruptured capillaries and small vessels. The integrity of the platelet plug-forming mechanism is tested by measuring the *bleeding time.* This is most commonly determined by the Ivy bleeding time technique, in which the time is measured for bleeding to cease from three incisions 1 cm long and 1 mm deep in an avascular area of the forearm. Venous return is obstructed by a blood pressure cuff set at 40 mmHg pressure over the upper forearm. The bleeding time is normal in disorders of the coagulation system but is abnormal in the presence of severe thrombocytopenia, defects of platelet function, deficiency of the von Willebrand plasma protein, or total absence of blood fibrinogen. Generally, clinically significant defects in platelet function are found only if the bleeding time is prolonged. Platelet aggregation, a measure of platelet function, may be studied by recording the increase in light transmitted through a cuvette containing continuously stirred platelet-rich plasma when aggregating agents are added to the plasma. The aggregating agents usually tested are collagen, epinephrine, adenosine diphosphate, thrombin, and ristocetin.

BLOOD COAGULATION: MECHANISM AND FUNCTION The two main functions of the blood coagulation mechanism are as follows:

1 Production of thrombin which stabilizes the platelet plug
2 Formation of fibrin which, by rendering the platelet plug permanent, mechanically blocks the flow of blood through ruptured vessels

A number of discrete proenzymes and proteins (termed *coagulation factors*), platelets, and calcium participate in the coagulation process. The process consists of several stages and ends with fibrin formation.

Fibrin formation Fibrinogen is a 340,000-dalton dimeric protein, each half of which contains three polypeptide chains termed $A\alpha$, $B\beta$, and γ. Fibrinogen is converted to fibrin by the action of thrombin (Fig. 55-3).

Thrombin releases two small peptides, termed the *fibrinopeptides,* from fibrinogen. Fibrinopeptide A (derived from the $A\alpha$ chain) is released more rapidly than fibrinopeptide B (derived from the $B\beta$ chain). Hence, the reaction may be divided into an *initial stage* in which fibrinopeptide A only has been released and the remaining molecule is termed fibrin I and a *second stage* in which fibrinopeptide B has also been released and the residual molecule is fibrin II. Fibrin I molecules are initially held in solution by complexing with fibrinogen, but as their concentration relative to that of fibrinogen rises they polymerize with one another to form a visible coagulum. Following polymerization, fibrinopeptide B release is greatly accelerated and the fibrin I coagulum is converted to a fibrin II coagulum in which polymerization is more extensive. This fibrin is soluble in acid and concentrated urea solutions and is ineffective in hemostasis. The fibrin polymers are then cross-linked by activated factor XIII (a transglutaminase) which, in the presence of calcium, covalently links glutamyl and lysyl amino acid residues on adjacent fibrin molecules. Two such cross-links per molecule form rapidly between the carboxy-terminal segments of the γ chains of adjacent molecules; up to four cross-links per molecule form more slowly between the α chains. The resulting product is highly insoluble and is very effective in hemostasis. The formation of cross-links between the α chains markedly increases the resistance of the clot to proteolysis by plasmin.

FIGURE 55-3

Schematic diagram of the fibrinogen molecule and its proteolysis by thrombin and plasmin. The molecule is elongated and has three nodules. The E region, containing the amino terminus, is the central nodule and the D regions are at the ends of the molecule. The molecule is a dimer, each half of which has three chains (α, β, and γ). Thrombin releases fibrinopeptide A and the residual molecule is fibrin I which polymerizes with other fibrin I molecules so that the D and E regions of adjacent molecules are juxtaposed. Thrombin releases fibrinopeptide B from fibrin I to form fibrin II. Plasmin first releases Bβ 1–42 and COOH-terminal Aα chains from fibrinogen, the residual molecule being termed fragment X. Fragment X is degraded to form fragments Y and D; fragment Y is then converted to fragments D and E.

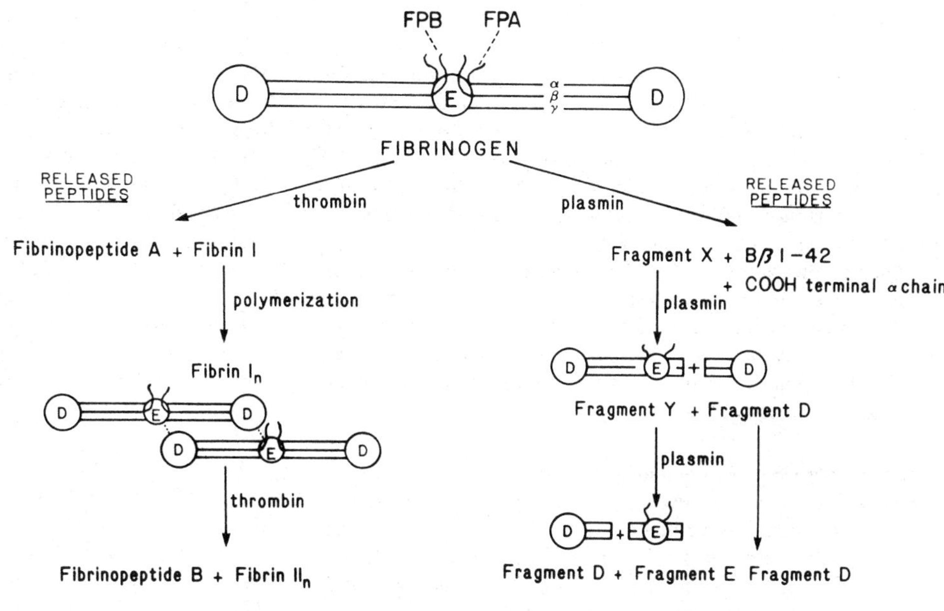

Prothrombin activation Thrombin is formed by the proteolytic cleavage of a proenzyme, prothrombin. Proteolysis is produced by activated factor X (X_a) which binds to the surface of activated platelets via factor V_a and cleaves prothrombin in the presence of calcium. Activation of factor X may occur by either of two separate pathways, the extrinsic or the intrinsic. Clinical experience suggests that effective hemostasis requires the participation of both. In the *extrinsic pathway,* a tissue factor (tissue thromboplastin), released from damaged cells, activates factor X in the presence of factor VII and calcium (Fig. 55-4). In the *intrinsic* or *cascade pathway* (Fig. 55-5), the contact of blood with a "foreign" surface, such as collagen or skin, activates factor XII. Activated factor XII, in the presence of prekallikrein and high-molecular-weight kininogen, activates factor XI which, in the presence of calcium, cleaves a peptide from factor IX producing activated factor IX. Activated factor IX proteolytically converts factor X into the activated form (X_a) in the presence of platelet membrane lipoprotein, factor VIII, and calcium. The scheme shown in Fig. 55-6 is useful in understanding how defects in specific coagulation factors affect the clotting time of blood or plasma. This scheme, however, does not explain (1) why deficiency of factors VIII or IX causes a *severe* bleeding syndrome, (2) why deficiency of factor XI causes a *mild* bleeding syndrome, and (3) why deficiency of factor XII, prekallikrein, or high-molecular-weight kininogen produces no defect in hemostasis. These clinical observations suggest that physiologically activation does not occur exclusively in sequence, suggesting the existence of bypass mechanisms. Such physiologic bypass mechanisms have not been identified, but it has been shown that tissue factor (factor VII) can cleave and activate factor IX.

Tests of the coagulation mechanism The intrinsic pathway of blood coagulation including fibrin polymerization is tested by measuring the *whole-blood clotting time* and *partial thromboplastin time* (Fig. 55-6). The whole-blood clotting time is the time taken for 1 ml of whole blood to clot at 37°C with control of both temperature and exposure of the blood to the glass surface of the test tube. The test is influenced by gross defects in the intrinsic clotting system. The partial thromboplastin time (celite or kaolin cephalin time) is the time required for recalcified citrated plasma to clot. A standardized platelet substitute (cephalin or "partial thromboplastin") and standard surface activation (provided by celite or kaolin) are used to eliminate variability due to the platelet count and surface factors. The test is influenced by moderate defects in the intrinsic clotting system.

The activity of any of the coagulation factors involved in the intrinsic pathway (i.e., factors XII, XI, IX, and VIII) may be measured by comparing the ability of control and test plasma samples to shorten the partial thromboplastin time of a plasma sample known to be deficient in the specific factor.

The extrinsic clotting system is tested by the *one-stage prothrombin time.* In this test, the time taken for recalcified ci-

FIGURE 55-4

Activation of factor X by steps in the intrinsic coagulation pathway.

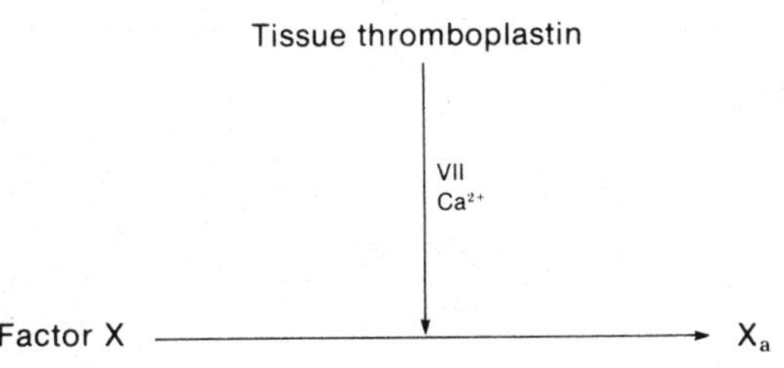

FIGURE 55-5

Activation of factor X by the steps in the extrinsic coagulation pathway.

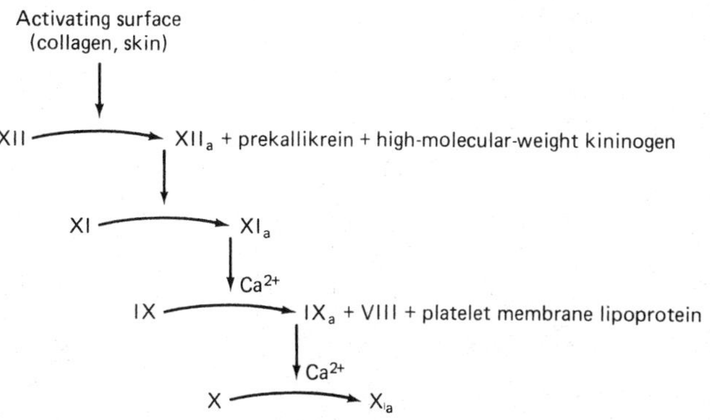

trated plasma to clot in the presence of tissue thromboplastin is measured. The test is sensitive to defects in the extrinsic clotting system (Figs. 55-4 and 55-6). The activity of factor VII and the common pathway coagulation factors (factors II, V, and X) may be measured by comparing the ability of control and test plasma samples to shorten the prothrombin time of plasma deficient in the specific factor.

The polymerization of fibrinogen is tested by measuring the *thrombin clotting time.* This test measures the time for citrated plasma to clot in the presence of added thrombin. The test is abnormal in the presence of heparin or of congenital or acquired abnormalities of the fibrinogen molecule such as occur in disseminated intravascular coagulation.

Blood fluidity system (regulator mechanisms) In addition to the coagulation factors, several mechanisms exist in the circulation for maintaining the blood in a fluid state. In the absence of this system, sufficient thrombin would be generated by the clotting of only 1 ml blood to coagulate all the fibrinogen in 3 liters of blood. The fluidity-maintaining system consists of both cellular and humoral components.

The cellular component consists of macrophages in the reticuloendothelial system and the liver, which specifically remove activated clotting factors and fibrin without affecting precursor (unactivated) coagulation factors. The humoral component consists of several proteins which specifically inactivate the activated coagulation factors. These proteins include antithrombin III and alpha$_2$ macroglobulin. Antithrombin III inactivates thrombin and each of the activated intermediates of the clotting mechanism which are serine proteases—i.e., not including VIII$_a$ or V$_a$.

The humoral system also includes the fibrinolytic mechanism for dissolving fibrin. Fibrinolysis is produced by the action of an enzyme, plasmin, which is formed from a precursor, plasminogen. Plasminogen is proteolytically converted to plasmin by an extrinsic system in which a tissue activator is supplied by endothelial cells present in the blood vessel wall or by an intrinsic system in which the components are all present in the blood. The intrinsic plasmin system is initiated by the contact of plasma with a foreign surface which leads to conversion of factor XII to factor XII$_a$. In turn, factor XII$_a$ in the presence of a high-molecular-weight kininogen converts prekallikrein to kallikrein. Kallikrein then converts plasminogen to plasmin.

Plasmin sequentially digests the fibrinogen molecule (see Fig. 55-3). Initially polypeptides from the *C*-terminal part of the Aα chain and from the *N*-terminal part of the Bβ chain (Bβ 1–42) are released and the residual molecule, which is still clottable by thrombin, is termed *fragment X.* Clots formed from fragment X have little tensile strength, cannot form α chain cross-links, and are readily dissolved by plasmin. Fragment X is further degraded to fragment Y, which is then converted to the final products D and E. These products of plasmin action are termed *fibrinogen-fibrin degradation products* and exert a variety of effects by competitively interfering with the normal functions of fibrinogen. They delay the polymerization of fibrin, thus prolonging the thrombin clotting time. In addition to fibrin, factors V and VIII are also digested by plasmin. These powerful effects of plasmin are controlled by a number of effective inhibitors, the most important being a 63,000-dalton alpha$_2$ globulin which rapidly and irreversiby inactivates plasmin.

As fibrin is deposited it adsorbs tissue plasminogen activator and enhances the conversion of plasminogen to plasmin. The plasmin adsorbed to the fibrin digests it, producing discrete local lysis of the fibrin. Plasmin escaping into the ambient plasma is rapidly neutralized by the alpha$_2$ inhibitor so that circulating fibrinogen is not proteolyzed.

Production, distribution, and life span of coagulation factors Because the concentrations of all plasma clotting factors, except factor VIII, are decreased in patients with massive liver necrosis, it is thought that hepatic parenchymal cells synthesize all factors except factor VIII. There is evidence that von Willebrand protein, which is closely related to factor VIII, is synthesized by endothelial cells. It is not known where factor VIII coagulant activity is synthesized. It does not appear to be made in endothelial cells. Levels of factor VIII rise sharply after a burst of muscular exercise or an infusion of epinephrine. The rise apparently reflects the release of stores of factor VIII into the circulation. Stress, fever, and infection elevate fibrinogen and factor VIII levels by an unknown mechanism. Gram-negative bacterial endotoxin also stimulates fibrinogen production. Levels of factors VII, VIII, and X and fibrinogen are elevated in pregnancy and in patients using oral contraceptives.

The plasma clotting factors have short intravascular half-lives compared with other plasma proteins. These can be grouped (in order of decreasing intravascular half-life) as follows (see also Table 55-2):

1 Fibrinogen, factor XIII: 4 to 5 days
2 Prothrombin, factors V, IX, X, XI, and XII: 1 to 3 days
3 Factor VIII: 12 h
4 Factor VII: 5 h

Because of these relatively short half-lives, postoperative prophylaxis or control of bleeding following trauma in a patient with a severe clotting-factor deficiency usually requires repeated replacement therapy during the period of healing.

FIGURE 55-6
Coagulation tests.

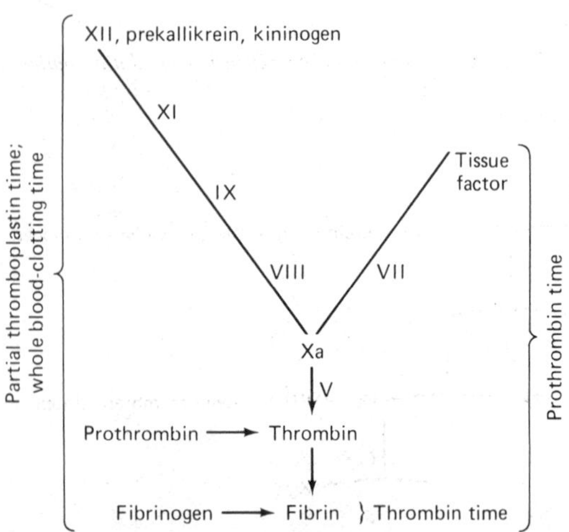

TABLE 55-2
Properties of coagulation factors

Factor	*Plasma concentration, μg/ml*	*Hemostatic level, % of normal*	*In vivo recovery, % of infused material*	$t_{\frac{1}{2}}$, *h*
Fibrinogen	3000	100 mg/dl	50	100
Prothrombin	150	?40	50	72
V	10	25	?50–100	16
VII	0.5	10	?100	6
VIII (antihemophilic)	?	30	80	12
IX	3	25	50	24
X	15	20	50–100	48
XI	6	?25	90	60
XII	29	—	—	60
XIII	20	3	50–100	120

TABLE 55-3
Clinical distinction between blood coagulation defects and capillary and platelet defects

	Coagulation defects	*Capillary and platelet defects*
Family history	Usually positive	Usually negative
Sex predominance	Males	Females
Type of bleeding	Visceral and intramuscular deep hematomas; usually after trauma	Skin and mucosal surfaces; petechiae and ecchymoses; spontaneous
Duration	Delayed after trauma and persistent	Immediate after trauma; short-lived
Local pressure	Not effective	May stop bleeding

Vessel wall The endothelial cells which line the vasculature form an important component of the hemostatic system. Endothelial cells have tissue thromboplastic activity in an inactive or sequestered form. Following injury the material is activated or released by still unknown mechanisms and is then available to initiate the extrinsic pathway of blood coagulation. Endothelial cells synthesize and secrete plasminogen activator, and this function may be important in preventing venous thrombosis. At least two functions of endothelial cells relate importantly to platelet function. These are synthesis of von Willebrand protein, which is necessary for normal platelet function in vivo, and synthesis of prostacyclin.

Since prostacyclin is derived from arachidonic acid via cyclic endoperoxides, aspirin, which inhibits endoperoxide generation, also inhibits prostacyclin formation. It is hypothesized that platelet reaction with the vessel wall is regulated by the balance between the production of thromboxane A_2 by the platelet and of prostacyclin by the endothelial cell.

Subendothelial collagen fibers cause platelet adherence, release, and aggregation and thereby initiate the formation of platelet plugs when vessels are severed. Collagen and other unidentified subendothelial constituents also initiate the intrinsic pathway of blood coagulation by activating factor XII.

Smooth-muscle cells are an important constituent of arterial and arteriolar walls. Attention has been focused on these cells following recognition that the fibrous plaques, characteristic of the advancing lesions of atherosclerosis, consist of an intimal accumulation of proliferated smooth-muscle cells, surrounded by a cap of connective tissue that covers a deeper accumulation of lipids. A factor (or factors) that promotes the proliferation of smooth-muscle and other cells is present in the alpha granules of platelets, the platelet-derived growth factor, and is extruded to the exterior by the platelet-release reaction.

DIAGNOSTIC APPROACH TO DISORDERS OF HEMOSTASIS

The diagnosis of coagulation disorders is based on both clinical and laboratory evidence. A careful and knowledgeably collected history is essential if the results obtained from laboratory studies are to be properly interpreted.

CLINICAL HISTORY (Table 55-3) A history taken to evaluate hemostasis should answer these questions: (1) Has *abnormal bleeding* or *bruising* occurred either spontaneously or after injury, dental extraction, or surgery? Was there *delayed* or *prolonged* bleeding, suggesting a coagulation disorder, or immediate and transient bleeding, suggesting a platelet disorder? (2) Was there bleeding from the umbilical stump or after circumcision? (3) Is there a history of *prolonged nose bleeds?* Brief epistaxis, stopping within minutes, even if frequent, is usually associated with normal tests of hemostasis.

One should try to determine the degree and frequency of the following:

1 *Bruising.* Spontaneous bruises larger than the palm of the hand are generally significant; a history of hematomas and bruises at the sites of injections or immunizations may likewise be suggestive of a hemostatic disorder.
2 *Excessive bleeding from small cuts.* Specific details as to the size of laceration and duration of bleeding should be elicited.

One should question the patient for (1) evidence of an underlying *systemic disorder* that may be accompanied by defective hemostasis, such as liver disease, systemic lupus erythematosus, uremia, or a hematologic malignancy; (2) a *family history* of bleeding and, if present, the hereditary pattern of transmission; and (3) *drug ingestion.* Drugs that interfere with hemostasis fall into two categories: (1) drugs that impair formation of the hemostatic plug by inhibiting platelet function or causing thrombocytopenia and (2) drugs that interfere with blood coagulation.

Drugs that impair plug formation include aspirin in ordinary doses, but such prolongation in bleeding time usually remains within the normal range unless platelet function is al-

TABLE 55-4
Diagnosis of bleeding disorders involving coagulation

	Tests					
Disorders	*Prothrombin time*	*Partial thromboplastin time*	*Thrombin time*	*Fibrinogen concentration*	*Fibrinogen proteolysis*	*Factor assays*
Congenital deficiency of factor VII	Abnormal	Normal	Normal	Normal	Normal	Specific factor abnormal
Congenital deficiency of factors VIII, IX, XI, XII, high-molecular-weight kininogen or prekallikrein	Normal	Abnormal	Normal	Normal	Normal	Specific factors abnormal
Deficiency of prothrombin, factor V, factor X, or vitamin K; or coumarin or warfarin effect	Abnormal	Abnormal	Normal	Normal	Normal	Specific factor abnormal
Dysfibrinogenemia, heparin effect	Abnormal	Abnormal	Abnormal	Normal	Normal	Normal
Disseminated intravascular coagulation, liver failure, congenital hypofibrinogenemia	Abnormal	Abnormal	Abnormal	Decreased	Abnormal	Abnormal

TABLE 55-5
Diagnosis of bleeding disorders involving platelets

	Tests			
			Platelet function	
Disorders	*Bleeding time*	*Platelet count*	*PF 3**	*Platelet aggregation*
Thrombocytopenia	Prolonged	Decreased		
Thrombasthenia	Prolonged	Normal	Abnormal	Abnormal with ADP and other aggregating agents
Release defects	Prolonged	Normal	Abnormal	Primary normal, secondary abnormal
Von Willebrand's disease (usually has low factor VIII coagulant activity and antigenic activity)	Prolonged	Normal	Normal	Usually abnormal with ristocetin, normal with ADP, epinephrine, thrombin, and collagen

* *Activity of "platelet factor 3."*

ready abnormal; aspirin should be discontinued several days before surgery. Other drugs which interfere with platelet function are dipyridamole, sulfinpyrazone, carbenicillin, penicillin, clofibrate, phenylbutazone, antihistamines, and tranquilizers. These drugs do not generally produce a bleeding tendency.

Drugs that interfere with blood coagulation include heparin and the oral coumarin drugs. Although preoperative patients are rarely receiving parenteral heparin, patients on long-term oral anticoagulant therapy are frequently encountered.

PHYSICAL FINDINGS The patient should be examined for the following.

1 *Abnormal bleeding in the skin.* Ecchymoses suggest abnormal bleeding from relatively large vessels due to a defect in blood clotting. Petechiae, which may be small, require a careful search, particularly around the ankles. Petechiae suggest increased vascular fragility secondary to thrombocytopenia.
2 *Mucosal bleeding.* Look for purpura of the buccal mucosa and the conjunctival surfaces of the eyelids. Hemorrhagic bullae in the mouth are found only in the presence of thrombocytopenia. Hemorrhages in the optic fundi, however, may reflect local eye disease, hypertension, diabetes, severe anemia, or thrombocytopenia. The presence of telangiectasia on or under the tongue should be noted.
3 *Hemarthrosis and ankylosis.* These suggest a deficiency of factor VIII or IX.
4 *Hereditary connective tissue disorder.* Abnormal elasticity of the skin and hyperextensibility of the joints (Ehlers-Danlos syndrome) may be associated with vascular bleeding.
5 *Chronic liver disease,* including jaundice, spider angiomas, palmar erythema, dilated abdominal veins, hepatomegaly, or splenomegaly.

LABORATORY STUDIES **Screening tests** A careful history is the best screening test. Nevertheless, laboratory tests for the integrity of the coagulation and platelet components of the hemostatic mechanism are indicated under a number of circumstances, including (1) historical or physical evidence of abnormal hemostasis; (2) family history of abnormal hemostasis; (3) presence of a disorder which may be associated with abnormal hemostasis, e.g., liver disease, systemic lupus erythematosus; and (4) prior surgical procedures known to be associated with a high incidence of hemorrhage.

Coagulation system tests (Table 55-4) A commonly used set of screening tests for coagulation defects include (1) *prothrombin time,* (2) *partial thromboplastin time,* (3) *thrombin clotting time,* and (4) *fibrinogen concentration* (most tests of fibrinogen depend on measuring the concentration of thrombin-clottable protein in the plasma). If one or more of these tests are abnormal, an assessment is made, based on the history as well as the test results, as to the most likely defect. The factor(s) most likely to be abnormal should be specifically assayed, including factor XIII. If all the coagulation system screening tests are normal, no further tests are necessary unless the history strongly suggests abnormal hemostasis.

Platelet system tests (Table 55-5) Basic screening tests include (1) the *bleeding time* and (2) the *platelet count.*

Tests which screen for defects of platelet function include (1) activity of "platelet factor 3" and (2) platelet aggregation.

If the bleeding time is prolonged and thrombocytopenia is detected, the etiology of the thrombocytopenia should be pursued by a careful history of drug or toxin exposure, physical examination for splenomegaly and systemic disease, a complete blood count, examination of the bone marrow, and tests for systemic lupus erythematosus and platelet antibodies. If the bleeding time is prolonged and the platelet count is normal, tests for von Willebrand's disease and for platelet function should be undertaken (see Chaps. 332 and 334).

REFERENCES

BIGGS R (ed): *Human Blood Coagulation, Haemostasis and Thrombosis,* 2d ed. Oxford, Blackwell, 1976

BLOOM AL, THOMAS DP: *Haemostasis and Thrombosis.* London, Churchill Livingstone, 1981

COLMAN RW et al: *Textbook of Hemostasis and Thrombosis,* Philadelphia, Lippincott, 1982

Haemostasis. Br Med Bull, vol 33, no 3, 1977

MONCADA S, VANE JR: Arachidonic acid metabolites and the interactions between platelets and blood vessel walls. N Engl J Med 300:1142, 1979

WILLIAMS WJ et al (eds): *Hematology,* 2d ed. New York, McGraw-Hill, 1977, chaps 128–162

56
ENLARGEMENT OF LYMPH NODES AND SPLEEN

ALEXANDER FEFER

LYMPH NODES **Structure and function** The principal cells in lymph nodes are the B lymphocytes, located in the lymphoid follicles, the T lymphocytes, in the paracortical areas, and the reticuloendothelial cells, or macrophages, which line nodal sinuses. The chief function of lymphocytes is to respond to antigens presented to the node from the structures being drained. The cells either differentiate into plasma cells and produce antibody (B cells) or enlarge, proliferate, and generate a T-cell-mediated response. Histiocytes or macrophages, which can also proliferate, participate in immunity but function chiefly in the phagocytosis of cellular debris and microorganisms which may have gained access to the node from the area being drained by it.

Mechanisms of lymph node enlargement Lymphadenopathy may be due to an increase in the number and size of lymphoid follicles with proliferation of lymphocytes or reticuloendothelial cells or to infiltration of the node by cells normally not present in it. Nodal cells proliferate in response to antigens, to stimuli which evoke greater phagocytic activity, and to unknown stimuli which cause nodal cells to become transformed to lymphoma cells and to proliferate autonomously. Nodes can be infiltrated by leukemia or metastatic carcinoma cells, by polymorphonuclear cells in lymphadenitis, or by metabolite-laden macrophages in the lipid storage diseases.

Significance of lymphadenopathy In normal persons nodes are not palpable or barely palpable. Whether a palpable node is clinically significant depends partly on its location and on the age and occupation of the patient. The number and size of nodes are greater at puberty. Children are more likely than adults to respond with lymphoid hyperplasia and generalized adenopathy even to minor stimuli, such as mild infections of the upper respiratory tract or skin, and develop appendicitis, mesenteric adenitis, and tonsillitis more often than do adults.

Lymphadenopathy reflects significant disease more often in adults than in children. However, palpable nodes do not always connote serious disease. They may reflect minor trauma and infections of the structures being drained, such as the hands of a manual laborer (epitrochlear nodes), the upper extremities (axillary), upper respiratory tract and teeth (cervical), and, most frequently, the lower extremities (inguinal). Although usually benign, enlargement of the inguinal nodes may reflect significant disease, and enlarged posterior auricular, supraclavicular, epitrochlear (not in a manual laborer), popliteal, mediastinal, and abdominal nodes must always be considered pathological.

Diseases associated with lymphadenopathy Enlarged nodes may reflect no significant disease, a benign disease, or a severe or even fatal one. Table 56-1 lists some of the conditions associated with enlarged nodes. The likelihood of each diagnosis varies with age, sex, and geography. Although most patients with significant adenopathy will have either a malignancy, an infection, or a connective tissue disease, the likelihood of each of those conditions is greatest, respectively, in the old, the young, and the female.

TABLE 56-1
Conditions associated with lymph node enlargement

1 Neoplastic
- *a* Hematologic: lymphomas, acute leukemia, chronic lymphocytic leukemia, myeloproliferative syndromes, histiocytoses
- *b* Nonhematologic: carcinomas of head and neck, lung, breast, kidney

2 Immunologic or inflammatory
- *a* Infections: pyogenic streptococcal, staphylococcal, and salmonella infections, brucellosis, tuberculosis, syphilis, infectious mononucleosis, cytomegalovirus, infectious hepatitis, rubella, lymphogranuloma venereum, toxoplasmosis, histoplasmosis, coccidioidomycosis, malaria
- *b* Connective tissue diseases: rheumatoid arthritis, systemic lupus erythematosus, dermatomyositis
- *c* Serum sickness
- *d* Reaction to hydantoins
- *e* Sarcoidosis
- *f* Miscellaneous: giant (angiofollicular) lymph node hyperplasia, sinus histiocytosis, dermatopathic lymphadenitis, immunoblastic lymphadenopathy

3 Endocrine: hyperthyroidism, Addison's disease

4 Lipid storage diseases: Gaucher's and Niemann-Pick disease

Physical characteristics of enlarged nodes Some nodal characteristics provide clues to the diagnosis. Nodes involved by lymphomas tend to be large, symmetric, rubbery, firm, movable, discrete, and nontender, whereas nodes in acute leukemia are often tender because of rapid enlargement. Nodes containing metastatic carcinoma are stony-hard, nontender, well-localized, bound to surrounding tissues, and nonmovable. In acute infections nodes are firm, tender, asymmetric, and matted, and the overlying skin may be red and edematous, whereas in chronic infections the nodes are nontender and there is no edema. Such nodal characteristics are only helpful clues, not pathognomonic signs.

Location of enlarged nodes The location of enlarged nodes also provides diagnostic clues. Generalized adenopathy, i.e., involving more than two separate node groups, is common in non-Hodgkin's lymphomas, chronic lymphocytic leukemia, the histiocytoses, and immunoblastic lymphadenopathy but not with nonhematologic malignancies. Generalized adenopathy is uncommon in adults with infections except in infectious mononucleosis, brucellosis, cytomegalovirus, tuberculosis, infectious hepatitis, secondary syphilis, toxoplasmosis, and histoplasmosis.

Enlargement of specific lymph node groups can be helpful diagnostically. Posterior auricular adenopathy suggests rubella. Unilateral anterior auricular adenopathy is associated with lesions of the conjunctiva and eyelids with a resultant oculoglandular syndrome as is seen with trachoma, tularemia, cat-scratch fever, tuberculosis, syphilis, epidemic keratoconjunctivitis, and swimming pool outbreaks of adenovirus type III pharyngoconjunctival fever. Oropharyngeal or dental infections can cause cervical adenopathy. Bilateral cervical adenopathy is prominent in tuberculosis, coccidioidomycosis, infectious mononucleosis, toxoplasmosis, sarcoidosis, lymphomas, and leukemias. However, a unilateral cervical mass often represents a metastasis from an undetected asymptomatic nasopharyngeal tumor. In one study of 1600 patients admitted to surgery with a nonthyroid neck mass, 88 percent of the patients had a malignancy, most often a metastatic tumor or a lymphoma. Therefore, a nonthyroid neck mass in adults, but not children, should be considered neoplastic until proved otherwise and requires an examination of the mouth, pharynx, nasopharynx, and larynx in search of a malignancy.

Palpable supraclavicular nodes are always abnormal and, in the absence of generalized adenopathy, reflect neoplastic disease in the abdomen or chest. The right node drains parts of the lungs and mediastinum and is involved by intrathoracic lesions especially of the lung and esophagus, whereas the left (Virchow's) node is close to the thoracic duct and is involved by intraabdominal tumor, especially from the stomach, ovary, testis, and kidney. Axillary nodes drain part of the breast and are favorite sites for metastatic breast carcinoma. Epitrochlear nodes often are chronically enlarged bilaterally in secondary lues. Inguinal adenopathy is especially common in lymphogranuloma venereum, chancroid, and syphilis.

Enlarged nodes in certain areas cannot be palpated but are suspected in the presence of clinical problems. For example, enlarged mediastinal or hilar nodes detectable on chest x-ray may be asymptomatic or may cause tracheobronchial compression with cough and wheezing, recurrent laryngeal nerve compression with hoarseness and stridor, paralysis of the left leaf of the diaphragm, esophageal compression with dysphagia, superior vena caval compression with swelling of the neck and face, and subclavian vein compression with swelling of the arm. Hilar nodes are often asymmetrically involved by lung carcinoma. Bilateral asymmetric mediastinal adenopathy is common with non-Hodgkin's lymphomas and is characteristic of nodular sclerosing Hodgkin's lymphoma. Hilar adenopathy is rarely associated with bacterial or viral pneumonias. It is seen, however, in tuberculosis (usually unilateral) and in coccidioidomycosis (usually bilateral). Bilateral hilar adenopathy is characteristic of sarcoidosis. One study of 100 patients with bilateral hilar adenopathy documented its strong association with sarcoidosis and revealed that such adenopathy in patients without symptoms or only with erythema nodosum or uveitis was nearly diagnostic for sarcoidosis. Unlike lymphomatous nodes, hilar nodes in sarcoidosis, coccidioidomycosis, and tuberculosis often show roentgenographically detectable calcification.

Abdominal nodes can enlarge in any disorder which causes generalized adenopathy. However, the cause of intraabdominal or retroperitoneal adenopathy in adults is most often neoplastic, especially lymphomatous. The nodes may cause abdominal pain, nausea, constipation, intestinal obstruction, urinary complaints, backache, fever, ascites, or peripheral edema. If sufficiently large, they can be detected by abdominal or pelvic examination, but they are most often detected by lymphangiography, ultrasonography, and computerized tomography (CT) scanning.

Approach to the patient with enlarged nodes In most patients, a diagnosis can be made by a careful history and physical examination, hematologic and other laboratory tests, skin tests, and routine x-rays. The association of some diagnoses with age and sex is helpful, e.g., systemic lupus erythematosus in the young female, breast carcinoma in the older female, infectious mononucleosis in the young adult, and chronic lymphocytic leukemia in the old. A history of exposure to potential sources of infection, and of constitutional complaints such as fever, malaise, fatigue, and weight loss, which accompany hematologic malignancies and systemic infections, is important. The duration of symptoms and signs is suggestive. Patients whose nodes are neoplastic tend to present with a longer history—often months—of adenopathy, whereas patients with painful infectious or inflammatory adenopathy often present within days after the nodes appear.

Physical examination should include a search for associated findings of special significance, e.g., splenomegaly for its myriad implications (see below), hepatomegaly for hepatitis and malignancies, skin rashes for viral infections, heart murmurs as in subacute bacterial endocarditis, and evidence of local infection such as chancre. An oral and nasopharyngeal examination for tumor is essential in any patient with a neck mass.

Routine hematologic studies may be diagnostic. The immature cells of leukemia or the atypical lymphocytes of infectious mononucleosis and other viral infections may be detected. A chest x-ray might reveal mediastinal nodes with or without pulmonary nodules or infiltrates. A liver and spleen scan might reveal increased size and defects associated with neoplasia. Cultures of blood, throat, sputum, urine, bone marrow, and other possible infectious sites should be obtained when appropriate, as should special serologic tests such as a test for syphilis, antibody titers for toxoplasmosis and cytomegalovirus, and a heterophil test for infectious mononucleosis. A marrow aspiration is indicated for anemia, thrombocytopenia, or leukopenia and may reveal leukemia or metastatic carcinoma or, when cultured, tuberculosis or other infections. A marrow biopsy is more likely than an aspirate to reveal a lymphoma.

If the above workup is not diagnostic and a neoplasm or infection for which treatment should not be delayed is suspected, then a lymph node should be biopsied, examined, and cultured. It is best to biopsy cervical or supraclavicular nodes and to avoid axillary or inguinal nodes, which are subject to local trauma and infections. Excision biopsy of an entire node provides a look at the nodal architecture. A node biopsy can be diagnostic in lymphoma, carcinoma, immunoblastic lymphadenopathy, infections such as tuberculosis or histoplasmosis, or a granuloma without caseation suggestive of sarcoidosis.

However, in 40 percent of patients the node biopsy will not yield a specific diagnosis. This failure has been attributed to inability to differentiate histologically conditions such as hydantoin-induced hyperplasia from a true lymphoma, to noninvolvement of the node obtained, or to distortion of the involved node by other processes. If another node is palpable or detectable on chest x-ray, an open biopsy or biopsy via mediastinoscopy should be obtained. If no nodes are evident and lung carcinoma, sarcoidosis, or tuberculosis is considered likely, a biopsy of the scalene node and fat pad in the supraclavicular area should be obtained. However, if despite a nondiagnostic biopsy lymphoma remains a strong possibility, no other nodes are accessible, and progressive disease is apparent, a lymphangiogram and CT scan are indicated. If abnormal abdominal or retroperitoneal nodes are detected, abdominal laparotomy may be necessary for diagnostic biopsies. However, if the patient with the nondiagnostic biopsy is otherwise well or improving and has no other accessible nodes, watchful waiting is acceptable. Adenopathy secondary to infections will almost always regress within 2 to 3 weeks. However, in long-term follow-up studies, 25 to 60 percent of patients with nondiagnostic lymph node biopsies were found within a few months largely to have lymphomas and, less often, carcinomas, connective tissue disease, or infection. The need for careful and frequent follow-up evaluations of such patients and for a node biopsy as nodes become available is obvious.

Lymph node syndromes In addition to the diagnostic entities cited, several new diseases of lymph nodes, with or without involvement of other organs, have been discovered. These include the combination of fever, rash, and lymphadenopathy, also termed the *mucocutaneous lymph node syndrome* (*Kawasaki's disease*), in children (see Chap. 199) and a lymphoproliferative and granulomatous disease involving predominantly the lungs called *lymphomatoid granulomatosis*. This process usually spares the lymph nodes, spleen, and bone marrow, although sometimes generalized atypical lymphoid hyperplasia may antedate the pulmonary lesions.

IMMUNOBLASTIC LYMPHADENOPATHY This is a disease characterized by the morphological triad of (1) predominant infiltration of immunoblasts, (2) proliferation of arborizing small blood vessels, and (3) deposition of acidophilic material in the lymph nodes, liver, spleen, and other organs. Clinically, the disease is characterized by weakness, fever, sweats, weight loss, generalized lymphadenopathy, and often hepatosplenomegaly. Rashes, which vary from maculopapular to urticarial, are common. An autoimmune hemolytic anemia is a commonly associated finding as is polyclonal hypergammaglobulinemia, involving at one time or another gamma-G, gamma-M, and gamma-A immunoglobulins. Most of the patients are elderly; most die with progressive disease within 18 months, but a few have a benign course on modest doses of steroids. Aggressive chemotherapy is not indicated in these patients.

Because many cases have followed drug ingestion, an immunologic basis has been suggested for this disease. Although it is not considered a neoplastic disease, 30 percent of the patients develop lymphoma.

ENLARGEMENT OF THE SPLEEN

Structure of the spleen Splenic function reflects the specialized cells and unique circulation of this organ. The spleen has a capsule and trabeculae which enclose the white and red pulp. The white pulp consists of periarterial sheaths of lymphocytes with follicles containing germinal centers in which there are plasma cells and macrophages. The red pulp consists of cords of reticulum containing phagocytic macrophages separated from sinuses by a basement membrane. The narrow, tortuous splenic circulation sequesters blood within the pulp and exposes the traversing blood cells to phagocytic cells and to metabolic and immunologic hazards, as well as to barriers which make it necessary for the cells to change their size and shape in order to squeeze through the cords and sinuses and return into the circulation.

Function of the spleen The spleen functions as the largest lymph node. It responds to antigens with proliferation of T lymphocytes in the lymphatic sheath and of the antibody-forming B cells in the germinal centers, as well as with proliferation of phagocytic cells. The spleen functions to clear bacteria. Its phagocytic function also includes "culling" and "pitting," which occur mostly in the tortuous red pulp. Culling refers to phagocytosis of red blood cells which have been damaged physically or immunologically and of cells containing nuclei or Howell-Jolly bodies, reticulocytes, siderocytes, target cells, and spherocytes. Pitting refers to the removal of inclusions, e.g., red blood cell nuclei, Heinz bodies, and malarial parasites from red blood cells without destroying the cells. The spleen serves as a reservoir of platelets but not of red blood cells or leukocytes. It normally sequesters 30 to 40 percent of the blood platelets. The spleen is normally the site of blood formation through the fifth fetal month, but not after birth—except in some abnormal conditions.

Hyposplenism Hyposplenism occurs when the spleen is absent or nonfunctional. The spleen may be absent congenitally, often in association with congenital heart disease. Splenic atrophy and decreased function occur in patients with multiple splenic infarcts (as in sickle cell disease), and in celiac disease or dermatitis herpetiformis associated with an enteropathy. Splenic atrophy is documented by splenic scan and by decreased clearance of ^{51}Cr-labeled heat-damaged red blood cells.

Hyposplenism usually causes no significant disease. However, splenectomy in young children and in patients with immunologic or hematologic diseases is associated with increased susceptibility to fulminant infection by *Streptococcus pneumoniae* and *Hemophilus influenzae.* Hyposplenism with decreased culling and pitting also causes laboratory abnormalities. The peripheral blood shows an increase in nucleated red blood cells, red blood cells with Howell-Jolly bodies, target cells, acanthocytes, and siderocytes, as well as cells containing Heinz bodies. After splenectomy, a leukocytosis of up to 20,000 cells per cubic millimeter and a thrombocytosis of up to 1 million cells per cubic millimeter occur within 1 to 2 weeks, but the white blood cell count and blood platelet count usually return to normal within a month. Since thrombosis may be more likely above 1 million platelets per cubic millimeter, anticoagulants or salicylates have been suggested by some if the platelet count does not fall. If an accessory spleen exists, it may undergo hyperplasia and assume normal splenic function and prevent hyposplenism.

Mechanisms of splenic enlargement Like other lymph nodes, the spleen enlarges with reactive hyperplasia in infection and inflammation and with proliferation of lymphoma cells or with infiltration by other neoplastic cells, mostly in chronic leukemias, or by lipid-laden macrophages. It also enlarges with extramedullary hemopoiesis, with proliferation of phagocytic cells in response to increased destruction of blood cells, and, uniquely, by vascular congestion in the presence of portal hypertension.

Diseases associated with splenomegaly Table 56-2 lists the principal conditions associated with splenomegaly. Any condition which causes generalized lymphadenopathy can cause splenomegaly. Splenomegaly is frequent in the infections listed. It occurs in 10 to 20 percent of patients with systemic lupus erythematosus and in rheumatoid arthritis which, when associated with splenomegaly and anemia, thrombocytopenia, or, most often, leukopenia, is designated *Felty's syndrome.* The cytopenia often responds to splenectomy. Splenomegaly also occurs in most patients with immunoblastic lymphadenopathy.

Lymphomas often involve the spleen even when it is not palpable, and laparotomy to determine the extent of Hodgkin's disease always includes splenectomy. The spleen is often massively enlarged in myeloproliferative syndromes. Splenomegaly may also be prominent in chronic lymphocytic leukemia and may be associated with autoimmune hemolytic anemia. Splenomegaly associated with increased destruction of red blood cells occurs with many hemolytic anemias, some of which, such as hereditary spherocytosis, respond dramatically to splenectomy.

Chronic congestive splenomegaly due to portal hypertension is associated with gastrointestinal bleeding and pancytopenia. It is most often secondary to cirrhosis of the liver. Many splenomegalic conditions are accompanied by the syndrome of hypersplenism, with anemia, leukopenia or thrombocytopenia, and a hyperactive marrow.

Approach to the patient with an enlarged spleen A palpable spleen in an adult is almost always clinically significant. In one study, the spleen was palpable in only 3 percent of students entering an American college and persisted in only a third of them. The spleen is even less likely to be palpable in normal persons beyond college age. Therefore, patients with a palpable spleen but without other signs or symptoms should have at least a spleen scan and complete blood count. Colloid tagged with technetium 99 injected intravenously is taken up by reticuloendothelial cells and visualizes splenic size, shape, and defects suggestive of tumor or abscess. The scan will detect an enlarged spleen and rule out a nonsplenic mass, e.g., cyst or metastatic tumor, which might cause splenic displacement rather than enlargement. A complete blood count and smear are often helpful or even diagnostic in asymptomatic splenomegalic patients with chronic myelogenous or lymphocytic leukemia.

TABLE 56-2
Conditions associated with splenomegaly

1 Immunologic-inflammatory
- *a* Infections: subacute bacterial endocarditis, brucellosis, tuberculosis, infectious mononucleosis, cytomegalovirus, syphilis, histoplasmosis, malaria, kala azar, schistosomiasis
- *b* Connective tissue diseases: rheumatoid arthritis, Felty's syndrome, systemic lupus erythematosus
- *c* Sarcoidosis

2 Hematologic disorders
- *a* Neoplastic: lymphomas, histiocytoses, myeloproliferative syndromes (chronic myelocytic leukemia, polycythemia vera, myelofibrosis, and myeloid metaplasia), chronic lymphocytic leukemia, acute leukemia
- *b* Nonneoplastic: hemolytic anemias, e.g., hereditary spherocytosis, autoimmune hemolytic anemia, hemoglobinopathies, immunoblastic lymphadenopathy

3 Congestive splenomegaly due to portal hypertension: hepatic cirrhosis, portal or splenic vein thrombosis or stenosis, myeloid metaplasia, vinyl chloride

4 Metabolic-infiltrative: Gaucher's and Niemann-Pick diseases, amyloidosis

5 Miscellaneous: cyst, splenic abscess, aneurysm of splenic artery, cavernous hemangioma

Since most conditions which cause splenomegaly also cause lymphadenopathy, the approach to diagnosis is that presented in the section on adenopathy. The cause of splenomegaly should be determined not by tests on the spleen itself but by tests—possibly including a lymph node biopsy—for diseases known to cause splenomegaly and lymphadenopathy. Splenomegaly in acute leukemia is usually a minor clinical feature—the diagnosis is made by blood count and marrow examinations. Splenomegaly in lymphomas is almost always associated with adenopathy, and the diagnosis made by node biopsy or at laparotomy.

Most conditions which cause splenomegaly without adenopathy can also be suspected and diagnosed by history and physical and laboratory examination. For example, a hemolytic anemia is detectable by routine laboratory tests for anemia and for hemolysis, including reticulocyte counts and serum bilirubin. Specific causes for hemolysis can then be determined by other studies such as Coombs' test, osmotic fragility, and hemoglobin electrophoresis. Similarly, splenomegaly and hypersplenism secondary to portal hypertension caused by cirrhosis of the liver are readily diagnosed by a history of alcoholism or previous liver disease, physical signs of liver dysfunction and portal hypertension, laboratory abnormalities consistent with liver dysfunction and hypersplenism, and evidence of esophageal varices. The diagnosis of the rare vascular causes of portal hypertension requires angiography.

Some patients with splenomegaly may have systemic symptoms but no nodes available for biopsy. If an underlying lymphoma or serious infection is considered likely but is not detected by the usual examinations, including lymphangiograms and CT scans, a laparotomy with biopsy of the liver and abdominal nodes, and splenectomy, may be necessary. Appropriate cultures and pathological examinations are essential. Such laparotomies on patients with splenomegaly of unknown cause have revealed lymphoma in one-third, congestive splenomegaly in one-fourth, and inflammatory disease in one-fifth of patients.

DISEASES OF THE SPLEEN AND RETICULOENDOTHELIAL SYSTEM **Splenic rupture** Rupture is usually due to trauma or to palpation of spleens enlarged by infection, especially infectious mononucleosis and sepsis, or, rarely, by leukemia. The spleen can also be ruptured by dissection by pancreatic pseudocysts into it. If the trauma causes a subcapsular hemorrhage, rupture may not occur for several hours. The patient with a ruptured spleen presents with severe acute left upper quadrant pain which may be referred to the left scapular region, with abdominal guarding and rigidity, and with rapidly developing evidence of internal hemorrhage, shock, and anemia. Surgery must be immediate.

Splenic infarct Splenic infarcts occur in patients with massive spleens due to a myeloproliferative syndrome or with vascular occlusive phenomena associated with hemoglobinopathies (SS, SA, S Thal, SC). The infarcts may be "silent" (asymptomatic) or may cause severe left upper quadrant pain often radiating to the left shoulder with splinting of the left diaphragm, abdominal guarding, and, at times, a friction rub in the splenic area. Sedation and bed rest are sufficient except rarely when a septic infarct causes an abscess and necessitates splenectomy.

Splenic artery aneurysm An aneurysm may be asymptomatic or may cause cramping left upper abdominal pain or vague nonspecific gastrointestinal complaints. The diagnosis may be suspected in unexplained splenomegaly with, at times, a calcified ring and adjacent mottled densities seen on x-ray. The aneurysm, most often seen in women beyond middle age, may be palpable, and a bruit may be audible. Rupture with sudden pain and, later, abdominal hemorrhage and shock is most likely to occur during pregnancy. If rupture occurs, transfusions should be given, and the ruptured aneurysm as well as the spleen must be removed.

Splenic tumors The only tumor which involves the spleen frequently is a lymphoma. Tumors arising in the vascular or sinus endothelium, i.e., lymphangioma or hemangioma, or in the capsular or trabecular framework, i.e., fibrosarcomas or leiomyosarcomas, are rare. They may cause local problems, e.g., rupture, or systemic complaints and may be diagnosed by spleen scan and angiography. Carcinomatous metastases to the spleen do not cause splenomegaly, are not clinically significant in life, and are usually detected at autopsy.

Splenic cyst Cysts cause only vague gastrointestinal symptoms. Parasitic cysts are mostly due to *Echinococcus* and are associated with peripheral eosinophilia and roentgenographically detectable calcification of the cyst wall. Nonparasitic cysts are quite rare. They consist of true cysts formed from embryonal rests and include dermoids and mesenchymal inclusion cysts, or false cysts secondary to trauma and containing serous or hemorrhagic fluid. CT scans can distinguish cysts from tumors.

Hypersplenism The syndrome consists of splenomegaly, pancytopenia (anemia, leukopenia, or thrombocytopenia) in the presence of a normal or hyperactive marrow, and reversibility by splenectomy. Hypersplenism is *primary* when no underlying disease is identified. It can also be *secondary* to other splenomegalic states (Table 56-2), especially congestive splenomegaly, connective tissue diseases, myeloproliferative disorders, subacute bacterial endocarditis, kala azar, and lymphomas.

MANIFESTATIONS The clinical manifestations of hypersplenism reflect the severity of the pancytopenia. Signs and symptoms of anemia may be predominent. If neutropenia is severe (less than 1000 cells per cubic millimeter), bacterial infections may be frequent. If the platelet count is under 50,000 per cubic millimeter, there may be easy bruising, and if it is under 20,000 per cubic millimeter, spontaneous hemorrhage from mucous membranes, from gastrointestinal and genitourinary tracts, and from cerebral vessels may occur. The manifestations of secondary hypersplenism reflect the underlying disease as well as the pancytopenia.

DIAGNOSIS The diagnosis of hypersplenism is aided by documentation of red blood cell or platelet destruction by or in the spleen. ^{51}Cr-labeled red blood cells or platelets are infused intravenously, and the relative accumulation of label in the spleen, liver, and precordium is determined. A decrease in the $t_{\frac{1}{2}}$ of infused red blood cells, e.g., to 15 days, coupled with a high (above 2) spleen/liver ratio of radioactivity at $t_{\frac{1}{2}}$ indicates significant sequestration and destruction. The mechanism of the anemia in hypersplenism is complex and may reflect increased pooling and sequestration, or actual destruction of red blood cells in the spleen. The anemia may appear to be more severe due to an increase in the total plasma volume.

Similar studies can be performed with labeled blood platelets. Usually 20 to 40 percent of the blood platelets are sequestered in a normal spleen, whereas up to 90 percent of the platelet pool may be sequestered in hypersplenism. The mechanism for leukopenia in hypersplenism is not clear, but increased sequestration and destruction are postulated. The severity of hypersplenism does not correlate with the degree of splenomegaly. Moreover, splenomegaly does not always cause hypersplenism.

TREATMENT In addition to treating the underlying disease, the treatment for hypersplenism is splenectomy. The usual indication for splenectomy is granulocytopenia of under 500 cells per cubic millimeter or thrombocytopenia of under 20,000 cells per cubic millimeter, although splenectomy may be justified for less severe cytopenias. The response to splenectomy in some patients is dramatic. The laboratory data on sequestration often fail to predict a response to splenectomy. Although strong laboratory evidence for sequestration and destruction of cells in the spleen often predicts a response to splenectomy, some patients will respond even when data fail to document sequestration.

Chronic congestive splenomegaly (Banti's syndrome) DEFINITION The syndrome is characterized by splenomegaly, pancytopenia, portal hypertension, and gastrointestinal bleeding.

ETIOLOGY The syndrome is caused by portal hypertension due, in turn, to an intrahepatic or extrahepatic pathological condition. Intrahepatic obstruction is seen with Laennec's cirrhosis or schistosomiasis; extrahepatic obstruction occurs with thrombosis of the portal or splenic vein, cavernous transformation of the portal vein, or compression of the splenic vein by pancreatic tumor or fibrosis. Portal vein thrombosis also may be associated with abdominal trauma, pregnancy, or intravascular coagulation. The hematologic changes are those of hypersplenism.

PATHOLOGY The spleen is congested, weighs 4 to 10 times normal, and has a thickened capsule, distended veins, and venous collaterals. There are distention of the sinuses, periarteriolar hemorrhage and siderotic nodules, an increase in the reticulum, and hyperplasia of the pulp. Progressive fibrosis of the reticulum, trabeculae, and capsule is seen. The bone marrow is normocellular or somewhat hypercellular with myeloid or erythroid hyperplasia.

CLINICAL MANIFESTATIONS These reflect the pancytopenia of hypersplenism (see above) and the condition underlying the congestive splenomegaly. Splenomegaly may be massive and may be accompanied by gastrointestinal complaints such as flatulence, indigestion, or pain. Evidence of gastrointestinal bleeding, especially hematemesis due to rupture of gastric or esophageal varices, is often present but is not necessary for the diagnosis of Banti's syndrome.

DIAGNOSIS The diagnosis requires detectable splenomegaly, changes consistent with portal hypertension, and the pancytopenia of hypersplenism. The anemia is normocytic-normochromic unless bleeding has induced a microcytic-hypochromic iron-deficiency anemia. The chief diagnoses to be ruled out are other causes of hypersplenism. A history of alcoholism is helpful. The liver should be evaluated by laboratory tests, liver scan, and, if necessary, liver biopsy. The detection of esophageal varices requires barium examinations and endoscopy. If no liver disease is detected, portal or splenic vein thrombosis should be suspected, and splenoportal venography should be performed in a setting in which a laparotomy may follow immediately. Congestive splenomegaly due to extrahepatic causes is more likely in patients under 18 than in older patients.

PROGNOSIS AND TREATMENT The prognosis is determined largely by the underlying cause of the chronic congestive splenomegaly. The pancytopenia can be tolerated for years. Hepatic failure or variceal bleeding represents the most unfavorable prognostic indicator. Intrahepatic obstruction requires not only splenectomy but also a shunting procedure, most often a portacaval shunt, to relieve the portal pressure. Congestive splenomegaly secondary to extrahepatic obstruction responds well to splenectomy.

Histiocytoses Due to a shared pathological lesion, eosinophilic granuloma, Hand-Schüller-Christian disease, and Letterer-Siwe disease have traditionally been considered as a single group of neoplastic diseases designated "histiocytosis X." This relationship has been questioned; Letterer-Siwe disease is regarded as a lymphomatous proliferation of poorly differentiated histiocytes, whereas eosinophilic granuloma and Hand-Schüller-Christian disease are thought to represent a nonneoplastic reaction of well-differentiated histiocytes to an unknown stimulus and should be referred to as *unifocal* and *multifocal eosinophilic granuloma,* respectively.

UNIFOCAL EOSINOPHILIC GRANULOMA This benign disease occurs in children and young adults, especially males. It presents as a solitary osteolytic lesion in the femur, skull, ribs, pelvis, or vertebrae. The lesion may be asymptomatic or may cause bone pain, tenderness, swelling, and pathological fracture. There are usually no systemic manifestations, no involvement of viscera or blood, and no eosinophilia. If no other lesion appears within 6 months, subsequent lesions are very unlikely.

The diagnosis requires biopsy. The lesion consists of well differentiated benign histiocytes and mature eosinophils and, at times, some necrosis. If the lesion is healing, fibrosis may be seen. The disease is not fatal. The treatment of choice is curettage or excision. The rare lesion which is inaccessible to surgery can be eradicated by moderate doses of x-ray. Lesions in hazardous sites such as weight-bearing bones or cervical vertebrae should be irradiated with a total of 300 to 600 R. Higher doses should be avoided. Supportive therapy should include rest and a cast to prevent collapse and compression fractures of vertebrae. Physical examinations should be performed monthly and a skeletal survey obtained every 6 months for 3 years.

MULTIFOCAL EOSINOPHILIC GRANULOMA The disease usually occurs before the age of 5. The patient presents with an osteolytic lesion and, within 6 months, with additional lesions. Alternatively, the patient will present with multiple lesions, especially in the flat bones. Nonspecific complaints such as malaise, anorexia, fever, and irritability are frequent, as is mastoiditis with recurrent bouts of otitis media and upper respiratory infections. Skin lesions in the form of seborrheic dermatitis are seen. Adenopathy and hepatosplenomegaly occur in 25 to 50 percent of the patients. The classic triad of skull lesions, exophthalmos, and diabetes insipidus occurs in 25 percent of the patients, but any one element of the triad occurs in up to one-half the patients. Diabetes insipidus is manifested by polydipsia and polyuria. Pneumonitis with diffuse pulmonary infiltrates chiefly in central and perihilar areas may represent eosinophilic granulomas, and may be accompanied by bacterial infection or, rarely, by interstitial fibrosis. The blood is usually not involved.

The diagnosis is made by biopsy of the lesion, and the pathology is described above. The prognosis is good. In half the patients the lesions spontaneously resolve over many years. Almost all patients ultimately recover, although some will have persistent orthopedic problems or diabetes insipidus.

Treatment for multifocal granuloma is similar to that for unifocal eosinophilic granuloma, but chemotherapy may be required to decrease the morbidity. However, this should not be as vigorous as the therapy for malignant disease. Modest doses of vinblastine, prednisone, or cyclophosphamide will benefit most patients.

LETTERER-SIWE DISEASE This disease, which occurs in children under the age of 3, is characterized by hepatosplenomegaly, lymphadenopathy, bleeding diathesis, bony lesions, skin involvement, and a rapidly fatal course. The skin lesions are diffuse. The patient usually has fever, recurrent infections, and pancytopenia due to marrow replacement by histiocytes.

Diagnosis is made by biopsy of bone, liver, or lymph nodes, which are replaced by moderately immature histiocytes. Treatment involves supportive care, including transfusions and antibiotics, and chemotherapy, which is, unfortunately, not very effective.

REFERENCES

BELL DM et al: Kawasaki syndrome: Description of two outbreaks in the United States. N Engl J Med 304:1568, 1981

BLUMFELDER TM et al: Felty's syndrome: Effects of splenectomy upon granulocyte count and granulocyte-associated IgG. Ann Intern Med 94:623, 1981

CHRISTENSEN BE: Pathophysiology of "hypersplenism syndrome." Scand J Haematol 11:5, 1973

GOPAL V, BISNO AL: Fulminant pneumococcal infections in "normal" asplenic hosts. Arch Intern Med 137:1526, 1977

GROOPMAN JE, GOLDE DW: The histiocytic disorders: A pathophysiologic analysis. Ann Intern Med 94:95, 1981

NATHWANI BN et al: Malignant lymphoma arising in angioimmunoblastic lymphadenopathy. Cancer 41:578, 1978

SCHROER KR, FRANSSILA KO: Atypical hyperplasia of lymph nodes: A follow-up study. Cancer 44:115, 1979

WEINSTEIN IM: Lymph node enlargement and splenomegaly, in *Hematology,* WJ Williams et al (eds). New York, McGraw-Hill, 1977, chap 106, p 950

WINTERBAUER RH et al: A clinical interpretation of bilateral hilar adenopathy. Ann Intern Med 78:65, 1973

WINTROBE MM et al (eds): *Clinical Hematology,* 7th ed. Philadelphia, Lea & Febiger, 1974

ZUERLZER WW, KAPLAN J: The child with lymphadenopathy. Semin Hematol 12:323, 1975

57
ABNORMALITIES OF LEUKOCYTES

DAVID C. DALE

Alterations of leukocyte counts and functions occur in a wide variety of hematologic, infectious, inflammatory, metabolic, and neoplastic diseases. Because leukocytes are affected by so many diseases, the routine laboratory evaluation of many patients begins with determination of the leukocyte count and the examination of a stained blood smear. From the clinical examination and these blood studies, certain diagnoses can be made or strongly suspected, e.g., leukemia, agranulocytosis, infectious mononucleosis, systemic mastocytosis, and the Chédiak-Higashi syndrome. In patients with infectious and inflammatory diseases, the leukocyte count usually serves as a useful guide to the severity of the disease process. The leukocyte count and blood smear examination plus special studies of leukocyte function also will identify certain patients with heightened susceptibility to infections.

Five types of circulating leukocytes can be identified by their morphology on blood smears: neutrophils, lymphocytes, monocytes, eosinophils, and basophils. It is generally accepted that all these leukocyte types, along with erythrocytes and platelets, derive from a common pluripotent stem cell. However, beyond this common origin, independent regulatory mechanisms govern the production, distribution, and function of each type of leukocyte. For simplicity, inferences are often made about the presence or severity of illness from the total leukocyte count and the differential leukocyte count expressed as a percentage. It is more precise to express the counts of each type of leukocyte in terms of the concentration, or absolute count per cubic millimeter of blood. This is usually determined simply by multiplying the total leukocyte count by the percent value. Normal values for blood leukocyte counts are shown in Table 57-1.

NEUTROPHILS

NORMAL PHYSIOLOGY The primary function of neutrophils is phagocytosis, killing, and digestion of microorganisms. The cells develop the capacity to perform these special functions in the bone marrow. Early neutrophil precursors, myeloblasts and promyelocytes, differentiate from hematopoietic stem cells by developing an active Golgi apparatus and endoplasmic reticulum and beginning the formation of cytoplasmic granules. The initial or *primary granules* stain reddish purple with azure dyes; hence they are also called *azurophilic granules.* They contain myeloperoxidase, acid hydrolases, lysozyme, and cationic antibacterial proteins. With further development the cells become myelocytes. At this stage the cytoplasm becomes packed with characteristic secondary or *specific granules* which stain faintly pink with the usual blood stains. These granules contain alkaline phosphatase, collagenase, lactoferrin, lysozyme, and aminopeptidase. Beyond the myelocyte stage, neutrophilic cells do not divide; instead their nuclear chromatin becomes condensed, the cell diminishes modestly in size, and cytoplasmic glycogen accumulates. Normally neutrophils are not released to the blood until the nucleus is segmented, that is, the cells have matured beyond the metamyelocyte and "band" stages.

Approximately 8 to 14 days are required for a cell to move through the sequence of four to six cell divisions and complete maturation, that is, from the myeloblast stage to a mature blood neutrophil. Measurement of the time required for the early developmental stages is difficult, but it is clear that there are normally 3 to 4 days of neutrophil maturation after cell division is finished. During this time the maturing cells can be released from the bone marrow to the blood under sufficient stress, and therefore they are described as being in the marrow neutrophil reserves. Morphologic and radioisotopic studies on bone marrow indicate that there are normally about 10 times as many nearly mature neutrophils in the marrow as in the blood. The size of the marrow neutrophil reserves can be estimated by administration of endotoxin, etiocholanolone, or glucocorticosteroids and measuring the increase in the neutrophil counts. In normal individuals, these agents roughly double the

TABLE 57-1
Normal values for concentration of blood leukocytes*

Cell type	*Mean, cells/mm³*	*95% confidence limits, cells/mm³*
Neutrophil	3650	1830–7250
Lymphocyte	2500	1500–4000
Monocyte	430	200–950
Eosinophil	150	0–700
Basophil	30	0–150

* *Total leukocyte counts from venous blood samples were done in a Coulter counter, and 200 leukocytes were differentiated on Wright-stained blood smears made on cover glass.*

count or increase blood neutrophils by a minimum of 2000 cells per cubic millimeter.

The regulation of neutrophil production and release remains poorly understood. Normal individuals maintain their own characteristic neutrophil count, but this is subject to substantial day-to-day variation and is greatly affected by activity and many other factors. A humoral substance has been identified which will stimulate neutrophil release from the bone marrow (neutrophilia-inducing factor). Colony-stimulating factor, a substance present in serum and urine which will stimulate neutrophilic bone marrow cells to grow in tissue culture systems, is another possible neutrophil regulator. The precise physiologic role of these substances is not clear.

The blood serves to transport neutrophils to areas of acute inflammation as well as to the mucosal surfaces of the body where these cells serve to maintain the normal defensive barrier to microbial invasion. Normally only about half of the neutrophils in the vascular system are circulating freely and are described as being in the circulating neutrophil pool. Only these cells are counted in routine blood samples. The other half of the blood neutrophils are loosely adherent to the walls of blood vessels throughout the body in the marginal neutrophil pool. In response to inflammation, neutrophils are shifted to the marginal pool. Certain drugs, i.e., epinephrine, glucocorticosteroids, and other anti-inflammatory agents, may reduce margination.

The neutrophil blood half-disappearance time (blood half-life) is only about 6 to 7 h. Neutrophils leave the vascular compartment by passing between endothelial cells presumably because they are attracted to sites of inflammation by chemotactic factors. Bacteria can release low-molecular-weight chemotactic substances. A well-characterized chemotactic factor, C5a, is generated from the complement system when plasma reacts with endotoxin, antigen-antibody complexes, and other foreign substances. Kallikrein, plasminogen activator, transfer factor, and other substances will also attract neutrophils.

At the inflammatory site, phagocytosis is facilitated by humoral substances, opsonins, which have coated the surface of the foreign material to be ingested. Immunoglobulins (IgG) and complement (C3) are the best-characterized opsonins. Phagocytosis stimulates numerous intracellular events including increased oxygen consumption, glycogenolysis, glucose oxidation via the hexose monophosphate shunt, and hydrogen peroxide production. Within the cell, the phagocytized particle is held in a vacuole, and the contents of the secondary and then the primary granules are sequentially emptied into this vacuole. The vacuolar pH is dramatically lowered, and the granule enzymes are activated. The neutrophil possesses a variety of bactericidal mechanisms giving it an "overkill" capacity. The best characterized bactericidal mechanism involves myeloperoxidase, hydrogen peroxide, and a halide such as iodide or chloride. The highly reactive oxygen derivatives, superoxide anion ($O_2^{\bar{}}$), hydroxyl radical ($OH\cdot$), and perhaps singlet oxygen ($'O_2$) also participate in the microbicidal systems of the cell. An interesting result of the cell's respiratory burst and the generation of these oxygen derivatives is the emission of light, or chemiluminescence. The neutrophil usually degenerates after it digests the phagocytized material. Neutrophils, cellular debris, and digested foreign matter become the pus which characterizes acute inflammation, and to which the residual myeloperoxidase imparts the slightly greenish color.

NEUTROPHIL DISORDERS

NEUTROPHILIA An absolute neutrophil count of greater than 10,000 per cubic millimeter should be regarded as elevated in most patients, although for a few individuals neutrophil counts of 10,000 to 15,000 per cubic millimeter are normal. The causes of neutrophilia are listed in Table 57-2. Exercise, excitement, epinephrine administration, or stress of any sort will increase the count up to twice the resting level within a few minutes. The duration of this neutrophilia is brief. It is largely due to a shift of cells from the marginal to circulating pool and is not accompanied by an increase in the number of nonsegmented blood neutrophils. Most acute bacterial infections are associated with neutrophilia, especially those that are accompanied by bacteremia, involve substantial amounts of tissue, or are localized in a closed space. This neutrophilia initially occurs because of accelerated release of cells from the bone marrow reserves and is often accompanied by an increase in the number of nonsegmented neutrophils in the blood, i.e., a "shift to the left." With prolonged inflammation from any cause, neutrophil production is stimulated and the bone marrow shows granulocytic hyperplasia. Toxic granulation, due to increased staining of the primary granules, and cytoplasmic vacuolization also occur under these circumstances. In all the usual conditions causing neutrophilia, the counts are generally between 10,000 and 25,000 per cubic millimeter. Persisting neutrophilia with counts greater than 30,000 to 50,000 per cubic millimeter is called a *leukemoid reaction*. This term is sometimes used to describe any persisting high leukocyte count because this degree of leukocytosis suggests leukemia. Characteristically in a leukemoid reaction the raised count is due predominantly to an increase in mature neutrophils with some increase of band neutrophils and metamyelocytes. Blood myelocytes are rare. The leukocyte alkaline phosphatase is generally high, and the cells do not contain Auer rods. The erythrocyte and platelet counts also are usually not strikingly abnormal. The differentiation between leukemoid reactions, leukemia, and myeloproliferative diseases is discussed further in Chaps. 129 and 337.

NEUTROPENIA Neutrophil counts of less than 2000 per cubic millimeter are relatively uncommon in normal individuals although some healthy resting adults, particularly black persons and Yemenite Jews, may have counts as low as 1000 per cubic millimeter with no apparent disease. Neutropenia occurs in a wide variety of clinical circumstances (Table 57-3). In general, as the count declines below about 1000 per cubic millimeter, the risk of infection increases. However, the risk of infection is related to both the nature of the primary disease process and the cell count. For instance, many patients with chronic idiopathic neutropenia have counts of less than 500 per cubic millimeter for years without infections, whereas few patients with leukemia or aplastic anemia will survive for even a few weeks at these levels without developing an infection.

Neutropenia occurs by several mechanisms: reduced precursor cell proliferation, cell loss in the maturation process, increased margination in the circulation, and accelerated utili-

TABLE 57-2
Causes of neutrophilia

Physiologic: Exercise, excitement, stress, epinephrine
Infections: Chiefly bacterial, also fungal, parasitic, and some viral diseases
Inflammation: Burns, tissue necrosis as in myocardial and pulmonary infarction, collagen vascular diseases, hypersensitivity states, other inflammatory diseases
Metabolic disorders: Ketoacidosis, acute renal failure, eclampsia, acute poisoning
Myeloproliferative diseases: Myelocytic leukemia, myeloid metaplasia, polycythemia vera
Other: Metastatic carcinoma, acute hemorrhage or hemolysis, glu[illegible] corticosteroids, lithium therapy, idiopathic

zation at sites of inflammation. In the individual patient, precise delineation of the mechanism of neutropenia is very difficult without refined methods for clinical investigation. For clinical purposes, most patients will fit into one of the following general categories.

Chronic neutropenia without splenomegaly (Chronic idiopathic neutropenia or granulocytopenia, familial benign neutropenia, chronic hypoplastic neutropenia, and chronic benign neutropenia of childhood) Isolated individuals and families are occasionally observed with neutropenia as their sole hematologic abnormality. Characteristically, the spleen is not enlarged. Onset may occur at any age; frequently, the syndrome is recognized on an incidental blood count. In adults, there is a striking female predominance, whereas in children both males and females are affected. Neutrophil counts may be as low as 50 to 200 per cubic millimeter with only infrequent infections, usually involving the upper respiratory tract. Bacteremia is rare. The blood usually contains normal-appearing mature neutrophils in reduced numbers; blood monocytes are often increased, and hypergammaglobulinemia may be present. The marrow is normocellular and shows few or no mature neutrophils. In a few cases, not readily distinguished from the rest of these patients on clinical grounds, leukoagglutinating antibodies to normal neutrophils have been detected and may be of etiologic significance (chronic idiopathic immunoneutropenia). The disease mechanisms remain largely unknown. Kinetic studies suggest that most cases occur because of reduced proliferation or cell loss during maturation. In periods of observation up to 25 years, evolution to leukemia has been reported only extremely rarely. A few children with this disorder have had spontaneous remissions. In a few patients with frequent infections and extremely low counts, alternate-day glucocorticosteroids have elevated the neutrophil counts and reduced infections.

Several other groups of patients with chronic neutropenia without splenomegaly can be recognized which have distinctly different clinical characteristics. *Infantile genetic agranulocytosis* is usually a rapidly fatal disorder associated with anemia and atypical, vacuolated marrow precursor cells. *Neutropenia associated with hypogammaglobulinemia* leads to fatal infections at an early age. Other patients are occasionally encountered with episodic severe neutropenia associated with febrile illnesses. Many other unusual neutropenic disorders have been observed; undoubtedly these neutropenias will be categorized further as their etiologies are better understood.

Cyclic neutropenia This disorder is characterized by the periodic absence of neutrophils from the blood and bone marrow associated with fever, malaise, mouth ulcers, and cervical adenopathy. These findings recur regularly at approximately 21-day intervals. Between episodes the patients are usually well. Symptoms characteristically begin in early childhood, although adult onset has been described. Cyclic fluctuations of other blood leukocytes, platelets, and reticulocytes occur, and bone marrow investigations indicate that the disease is due to a defect in the regulation of hematopoietic cell proliferation. Treatment with glucocorticosteroids, androgens, or splenectomy is not of predictable benefit, although cases improving with each of these treatments have been reported. Early recognition and prompt treatment of infectious complications are very important.

TABLE 57-3
Clinical conditions characterized by neutropenia

…atologic diseases: Chronic idiopathic neutropenia; cyclic neutro- … Chédiak-Higashi syndrome; leukemia; aplastic anemia
…ed conditions: Agranulocytosis; myelotoxic drugs
…eficiencies: Vitamin B_{12}; folate, especially in alcoholics;

…ıer diseases: Infections including typhoid fever, infec- …ıcleosis, malaria, overwhelming sepsis; diseases with …y, Felty's syndrome, congestive splenomegaly, Gaucher's …coidosis; malignancies with marrow infiltration

Neutropenia in the leukemias and aplastic anemia In leukemia, particularly the acute leukemias, neutropenia is frequently present at the time the disease is recognized. The predisposition to infection is severe, in part because the neutrophils which are present may not be functionally normal. The number of neutrophils and other host defenses are further suppressed by chemotherapy. When the neutrophil count is less than 500 per cubic millimeter, especially in patients in relapse, fever and infection should be expected (see Chap. 137).

In aplastic anemia, the infection risk is probably roughly proportional to the neutrophil count, with the chance of a severe and possibly fatal infection being substantially increased with neutrophil counts below 500 per cubic millimeter. The monocytopenia observed in these patients coupled with their neutropenia contributes substantially to the predisposition to infection.

Agranulocytosis (Schultz syndrome) Severe neutropenia occurs as an occasional or rare reaction to a great variety of drugs (Table 57-4). In most instances the patient is seen by the physician several weeks or months after beginning the offending agent and presents acutely ill with fever, sore throat, and oral or perianal ulceration. The total leukocyte count is often 1000 to 2000 per cubic millimeter, and neutrophils are absent from the blood and bone marrow. Marrow examination generally will exclude leukemia as the cause. Marrow recovery is the rule if the patient can be sustained long enough after the drug is discontinued. The pathophysiologic mechanisms for these reactions remain poorly understood. Both toxic effects of drugs on neutrophil formation and immunologic mechanisms causing accelerated cell destruction have been proposed and demonstrated in a few instances.

With some drugs, e.g., chloramphenicol, phenothiazines, carbamazepine (Tegretol), and propylthiouracil, patients may have a gradually declining neutrophil count, probably due to suppressed neutrophil production. It is not absolutely certain that these patients will develop agranulocytosis if the drug is not discontinued. However, as a rule, the presumed offending agent should be discontinued if the neutrophil count falls below 3000 per cubic millimeter.

Neutropenia and hematotoxic drugs In sufficient doses, a great number of therapeutic agents predictably cause leukopenia and neutropenia. This is particularly true for the agents used in cancer chemotherapy and for immunosuppressive ther-

TABLE 57-4
Drugs producing neutropenia

INFREQUENTLY CAUSE NEUTROPENIA

Analgesics: Aminopyrine, dipyrone, salicylates
Anticonvulsants: Phenytoin (Dilantin), carbamazepine
Anti-inflammatory drugs: Phenylbutazone
Antimicrobial agents: Chloramphenicol, penicillins, sulfonamides, organic arsenicals
Antithyroid agents: Propylthiouracil, methimazole
Phenothiazine: Chlorpromazine, promazine
Tranquilizers: Meprobamate

REGULARLY CAUSE NEUTROPENIA

Alkylating agents: Nitrogen mustard, busulfan, chlorambucil, cyclophosphamide
Antibiotics: Daunomycin
Antimetabolites: Methotrexate, 6-mercaptopurine, 5-fluorocytosine

apy of nonmalignant inflammatory diseases (see Chap. 125). These drugs reduce neutrophil production. If the neutrophil count is not allowed to drop below 1000 to 2000 cells per cubic millimeter or if the period of neutropenia is brief, infectious complications are infrequent.

Neutropenia and nutritional deficiencies Vitamin B_{12} and folic acid deficiencies are sometimes accompanied by neutropenia as well as neutrophil hypersegmentation, particularly when folate deficiency is coupled with alcoholism. Copper deficiency, which may occur with chronic hyperalimentation, also reduces blood neutrophils.

Neutropenia with infections Certain infections may be accompanied by neutropenia. These include typhoid and paratyphoid fevers (see Chap. 154), brucellosis (see Chap. 158), tularemia (see Chap. 159), infectious mononucleosis (see Chap. 212), infectious hepatitis (see Chap. 318), yellow fever (see Chap. 208), measles (see Chap. 200) and many other viral infections, malaria (see Chap. 218), kala azar (see Chap. 219), and rickettsial diseases (see Chap. 189). For the most part, these neutropenias are mild and their precise mechanisms are not known. It is postulated that they are largely due to redistribution of cells out of the circulating pool into an enlarged marginal pool. In certain overwhelming infections, for example, gram-negative bacteremia, pneumococcal pneumonia, and miliary tuberculosis, the occurrence of neutropenia portends a poor prognosis. This is particularly true in alcoholics, malnourished individuals, and patients with preexisting hematopoietic diseases.

Neutropenia with splenomegaly Neutropenia occurs in Felty's syndrome (see Chap. 56), congestive splenomegaly (see Chap. 56), Gaucher's disease (see Chap. 105), and sarcoidosis (see Chap. 235) as well as in infectious diseases with splenomegaly. There are often an associated mild thrombocytopenia and anemia. Splenic sequestration, as well as increased peripheral utilization, are proposed mechanisms. The predisposition to infection with these disorders is quite variable. Splenectomy to attempt to alter the neutropenia should be reserved for patients with repeated severe infections.

NEUTROPHIL DYSFUNCTION The normal functions of mature neutrophils are chemotaxis, phagocytosis, microbicidal action, and digestion of foreign material. There are a few specific diseases and syndromes in which these functions are abnormal. More commonly, defects in neutrophil function are observed which are secondary to other diseases such as alcoholism, diabetes mellitus, uremia, rheumatoid arthritis, and lupus erythematosus. Other defects occur secondary to abnormalities of complement and immunoglobulin metabolism.

Chemotaxis Accumulation of neutrophils in response to inflammation is most often deficient because of neutropenia. The tissue neutrophil response is also reduced by drugs, such as alcohol and glucocorticosteroids, which impair neutrophil adherence to the vascular endothelium. Chemotactic defects due to complement abnormalities have been observed chiefly in patients with either C3 or C5 deficiency. In general, defects permitting complement activation and C3 generation by the alternate complement pathway, for example, C1r, C2, and C4 deficiency, are associated with only a temporary delay in generation of chemotactic factor, and these patients have comparatively few infections. Defects in chemotaxis also may occur because of complement depletion in essential C3 hypercatabolism and possibly in acute glomerulonephritis and systemic lupus erythematosus. Chemotactic factor inactivators and inhibitors have been described in Hodgkin's disease, cirrhosis, uremia, and a few other circumstances. In patients with these complement-related disorders, the cells are usually normal when tested with normal serum. Cellular defects in chemotaxis have been described in the Chédiak-Higashi syndrome, Kartagener's syndrome, newborn infants, and some patients with congenital ichthyosis, diabetes mellitus, rheumatoid arthritis, burns, hypogammaglobulinemia, and acute infections. In *Job's syndrome,* characterized by recurrent staphylococcal abscesses, eczema, and high IgE levels, a cellular defect in chemotaxis is also observed. Abnormal chemotaxis and defective phagocytosis have been recognized with hypophosphatemia and consequently diminished intracellular ATP. Specific chemotactic defects have been described also with abnormal actin polymerization and abnormal microtubule assembly; both of these defects prevent normal cell movement.

Phagocytosis Reduced serum opsonic activity is the best-known cause for abnormal phagocytosis. This occurs in hypo- and agammaglobulinemia and certain complement disorders, including most of those with reduced chemotaxis, especially if activated C3 is not generated normally. Defective opsonic activity has been documented in premature infants, sickle cell anemia, lupus erythematosus, and cirrhosis.

Microbicidal defects A number of patients have been described with abnormalities of neutrophil primary and secondary granules and abnormalities in oxidative metabolism of these cells. Patients with a deficiency of myeloperoxidase, a primary granule enzyme, are easily recognized by histochemical staining of blood smears. Their neutrophils have a detectable abnormality in the killing of bacteria, but overall these patients are not necessarily prone to developing infections. Patients lacking neutrophil alkaline phosphatase and lactoferrin, constituents of the secondary granules, as well as patients totally lacking secondary granules, also have been reported. The best-characterized disorders of neutrophil microbicidal function are chronic granulomatous disease and the Chédiak-Higashi syndrome.

CHRONIC GRANULOMATOUS DISEASE (CGD) This inherited disorder is characterized by severe recurrent infections of the skin, lymph nodes, lungs, liver, and bones. The infections are caused chiefly by staphylococci and certain gram-negative bacteria (particularly *Escherichia coli, Serratia marcescens,* and *Salmonella*). Histologically the tissues usually show a granulomatous reaction, lipid-filled macrophages, and multiple small abscesses. The neutrophils are morphologically normal. Neutrophil production, blood counts, and chemotaxis are also normal. Other measures of host defenses, including delayed hypersensitivity and lymphocyte functions, are normal, but immunoglobulins may be increased. The neutrophils, as well as the monocytes, have a greatly impaired ability to kill the types of microorganisms with which these patients usually become infected. Phagocytosis of bacteria is normal, but the metabolic burst which follows ingestion is markedly blunted. Superoxide and H_2O_2 are not generated normally, and chemiluminescence is not observed. When CGD neutrophils phagocytize streptococci or pneumococci, these bacteria are killed normally because the bacteria contribute reactive oxygen derivatives from their own metabolism to the intracellular environment. This observation emphasizes the key role of oxygen and its derivatives in the intracellular bactericidal mechanism. Chronic granulomatous disease is most easily diagnosed by determining the amount of nitroblue tetrazolium (NBT) reduction which occurs when the patient's cells are incubated with this dye. Normally NBT is reduced intracellularly to a blue-black substance, blue formazan, which precipitates in the cell and can be seen as black intracellular particles. In CGD cells this reaction does not occur. The diagnosis is confirmed by observing that postphagocytic O_2 consumption, glucose C-1 oxidation, or the iodination reaction is reduced.

NADPH oxidase is probably the critically deficient enzyme in CGD. However, deficiencies of NADH oxidase and glutathione peroxidase have been described in patients having typical CGD. The genetic heterogeneity indicated by family studies and the variable clinical presentations of CGD suggest that several different molecular lesions may result in this clinical picture. In *familial lipochrome histiocytosis* the neutrophils have a similar defect, but this disorder is described only in women, has a late onset, and presents very striking lipid-laden histiocytes in many tissues. Severe *deficiency of leukocyte glucose 6-phosphate dehydrogenase* with G6PD levels less than 5 percent of normal is also accompanied by neutrophil dysfunction similar to CGD. The management of CGD and its variants depends upon careful observation and detection of infections as early as possible. Cultures of affected tissues are critical for the correct diagnosis and selection of the appropriate antibiotic. Prophylactic antibiotics have probably been useful for some cases but may be accompanied by the usual problems of superinfections and emergence of resistant organisms (see Chap. 145).

CHÉDIAK-HIGASHI SYNDROME This rare autosomal recessive disease is characterized by partial albinism, giant lysosomal granules in most granule-containing cells (neutrophils, monocytes, hepatocytes, renal tubular cells), and increased susceptibility to infections. The abnormal blood cells are readily seen on routine blood smears. The disease is usually recognized in children. There are several neutrophil abnormalities including moderately severe neutropenia, reduced marrow neutrophil reserves, and reduced neutrophil chemotaxis. In addition, in microbicidal studies, the giant primary granules are observed to degranulate slowly and thereby delay the killing of phagocytized bacteria. The disease is also accompanied by an accelerated phase with lymphohistiocytic infiltration in the liver, spleen, nerves, and other tissues, with accompanying dysfunctions. Treatment is limited to prompt antimicrobial therapy of infections, which usually resolve slowly. In the accelerated phase, vincristine and prednisone have been used to retard organ infiltration.

Other neutrophil abnormalities Unusual morphologic abnormalities of neutrophils include hereditary hyposegmentation (Pelger-Huët anomaly); hereditary hypersegmentation; retained remnants of endoplasmic reticulum, chiefly composed of RNA (May-Hegglin anomaly and Doehle bodies); and abnormally large azurophilic granules (Alder-Reilly anomaly). These abnormalities apparently do not interfere with neutrophil function.

OTHER LEUKOCYTIC CELLS

LYMPHOCYTES In blood smears, lymphocytes are recognized as a reasonably homogenous population of mononuclear cells with a small amount of blue cytoplasm containing a few granules. Through the analysis of antigens and receptors on the surface of these cells and their responses to culture with various antigenic and mitogenic stimuli in vitro, it has been learned that there are two main types of circulating lymphocytes, T and B cells. Characteristically T cells form rosettes when incubated with sheep erythrocytes, whereas B cells do not; this is the principal way these populations have been distinguished in most clinical studies (see Table 57-5 and Chap. 63). Approximately 80 percent of blood lymphocytes are T cells and 12 to 15 percent are B cells in normal individuals; these percentages and the absolute numbers of T and B cells are altered by many disease states. The remaining small percentage of lymphocytes lack the characteristic surface receptors of T and B cells and are called "null" cells.

Both T and B cells originate from stem cells of hematopoietic tissues. Their maturation involves the acquisition of distinctive surface properties. Pre-T cells, or prothymocytes, derived from the hematopoietic stem cells, emigrate to the thymus, where they proliferate and differentiate into three major populations which can be detected by monoclonal antibodies to surface antigens. These three groups of cells are early thymocytes, expressing the antigenic determinants T-9 and T-10; common thymocytes, expressing T-10, T-6, T-4, and T-5; and mature thymocytes, expressing either T-10, T-1, T-3, and T-4, or T-10, T-1, T-3, and T-5. The presence of the T-4 or the T-5 antigen on the cell surface reflects a major difference in functional capacities of the T cells (see below). When the thymocytes mature, they lose the T-10 antigen, leave the thymus, and enter the circulation as T cells. They migrate to the various lymphoid organs, i.e., the lymph nodes, spleen, and bone marrow. In lymph nodes they populate the perifollicular and deep cortical areas. B cells also originate from hematopoietic stem cells. They migrate through the blood to the lymphoid organs, where they populate the germinal centers and function chiefly to produce immunoglobulins. Labeling studies indicate that there is a huge overproduction of lymphocytes, but that a substantial portion of the cells which reach the blood may live for years. These are principally long-lived T cells, which recirculate repeatedly through the spleen, lymph nodes, thoracic duct, bone marrow, and blood.

T lymphocytes of the T-1, T-3, T-4 subpopulation proliferate in response to phytohemagglutinin (PHA), concanavalin A (ConA), and certain soluble antigens. They also serve to induce and enhance T-cell–T-cell and T-cell–B-cell interactions, i.e., they increase the proliferative response of purified lymphocytes in certain in vitro culture systems. These cells are called "helper" T cells. In contrast, the T-1, T-3, and T-5 cells have proliferative responses to PHA and ConA, but suppress T-cell–T-cell and T-cell–B-cell interactions. They are called "suppressor" T cells. The recognition of these specific subpop-

TABLE 57-5
Characteristics of T and B cells

	T cells	*B cells*
Origin	Hematopoietic stem cells	Hematopoietic stem cells
Development	In thymus	In bone marrow, lymph nodes, and spleen
Life span	Generally long (months to years)	Short (probably days or weeks)
Circulation pattern	Chiefly recirculating	Chiefly non-circulating
Major location in lymph nodes	Deep cortical, perifollicular	Germinal centers
Identification	Sheep RBC rosettes Surface antigens	Surface immunoglobulin Surface Fc and complement receptors Surface antigens
Functions	Mediate delayed hypersensitivity Lymphokine production Modulate function of other cells (helper/inducer cells or suppressor cells)	Antibody synthesis

ulations and their interaction has greatly improved our understanding of basic immunology and the mechanism of immunologically mediated diseases such as infectious mononucleosis (see Chap. 212), systemic lupus erythematosus (see Chap. 70), and agammaglobulinemia (see Chap. 64). The failure of lymphoid cells to develop normal surface antigens and receptors is also useful for diagnosing malignancies of these cell lines (see Chaps. 128 and 130).

Lymphocytosis An increase in the absolute lymphocyte count occurs in certain infections: infectious mononucleosis, infectious hepatitis, infectious lymphocytosis, pertussis, tuberculosis, brucellosis, syphilis, thyrotoxicosis, and adrenal insufficiency. A lymphocyte count of greater than 10,000 per cubic millimeter usually indicates chronic lymphocytic leukemia, especially in older patients. The term *relative lymphocytosis* is sometimes used to describe situations where neutrophils are decreased with an increase in the percentage, but not absolute number, of lymphocytes. This term is misleading and should not be used.

Lymphocytopenia An absolute lymphocyte count of less than 1000 per cubic millimeter is observed in less than 5 percent of normal individuals but commonly occurs with acute, stressful illnesses such as myocardial infarction, pneumonia, or sepsis. A transient lymphocytopenia regularly occurs even with very small doses of glucocorticosteroids. Chronic lymphocytopenia occurs in a variety of malignancies, uremia, congestive heart failure, lymphomas (especially Hodgkin's disease), aplastic anemia, lupus erythematosus, intestinal lymphangiectasia, and other immunologic deficiency syndromes (Wiskott-Aldrich syndrome, ataxia-telangiectasia, Di George's syndrome, Swiss-type agammaglobulinemia, and thymic alymphoplasia) (see Chap. 64). It also occurs following treatment with antilymphocyte globulin and certain chemotherapeutic agents.

MONOCYTES Monocytes are phagocytic cells with bactericidal capacities similar to neutrophils but with distinctive physiologic characteristics. They form in the bone marrow from promonocytes and have lysosomal granules containing myeloperoxidase, lysozyme, and acid phosphatases. They spend less time in the marrow than neutrophils and enter the blood with mitochondria and protein synthetic capacity intact, able to complete their differentiation as the circumstances demand. Monocytes leave the blood more slowly than neutrophils, with a half-disappearance time estimated to be 12 to 24 h. They accumulate after neutrophils in acute inflammation in response to monocyte chemotactic factors.

In response to pinocytosis of serum proteins or ingestion of foreign material, monocytes enlarge and synthesize increased amounts of lysosomal enzymes and thereby are transformed to more active phagocytes called *macrophages*. Blood monocytes are the precursors of the pulmonary alveolar macrophages, spleen macrophages, and fixed macrophages of the *monocyte-macrophage system* (sometimes less precisely called the *reticuloendothelial system*). This system serves chiefly to remove foreign matter from the blood, e.g., bacteria, fungi, injected colloidal substances, and damaged or effete blood cells. During differentiation in each tissue site, monocytes acquire unique characteristics for that particular site. For instance, alveolar macrophages utilize chiefly oxidative phosphorylation to meet energy requirements, whereas peritoneal macrophages may chiefly utilize glycolysis. Generally, in all tissue sites these cells maintain the capacity to divide.

Monocytes have surface receptors for IgG, IgM, and complement; form rosettes with antibody-coated (IgG) erythrocytes; and are capable of synthesizing components of the complement system, transferrin, interferon, endogenous pyrogen, and colony-stimulating factor. In chronic inflammatory states, such as tuberculosis, sarcoidosis, and regional enteritis, they are probably responsible for the high serum and urine lysozyme concentrations. Monocytes serve a critical role in processing of antigen essential for both cellular and humoral immunity. They respond to lymphocyte-derived chemotactic and immobilizing factors (migration inhibitory factor, MIF). The incompletely catabolized endogenous materials generated in Gaucher's, Niemann-Pick, and Fabry's diseases also accumulate in monocytes.

Monocytosis Increases in blood monocytes are observed in certain infections: tuberculosis, subacute bacterial endocarditis, brucellosis, Rocky Mountain spotted fever, malaria, and kala azar; in granulomatous diseases: sarcoidosis, regional enteritis; in some collagen vascular diseases; and in malignancies. Monocytosis may occur in leukemia and preleukemia, lymphomas, myeloproliferative syndromes, hemolytic anemias, and chronic idiopathic neutropenia.

Monocytopenia Reduced blood monocyte counts are seen acutely with stress and following glucocorticosteroid administration. Monocytopenia is observed in many acute infections, with aplastic anemia and acute leukemia, and as a direct effect of myelotoxic and immunosuppressive drugs.

EOSINOPHILS Many diseases are encountered where blood or tissue eosinophils are increased (Table 57-6). Eosinophils develop in the bone marrow similar to neutrophils. Their characteristic red-staining granules contain a unique peroxidase. Eosinophils have microbicidal capacities similar to neutrophils and monocytes, although they are somewhat less efficient than these cells in killing bacteria. By secreting the contents of their cytoplasmic granules in the vicinity of large parasites such as *Schistosoma mansoni*, they can inflict damage to the cell wall of these organisms. Eosinophils are selectively attracted by an eosinophilic chemotactic factor elaborated by lymphocytes in response to certain stimuli. Eosinophils also accumulate in the skin in response to the topical application of allergens in allergic individuals. Animal studies indicate that the blood pool of eosinophils is relatively small compared with the number of these cells in various tissues. Significant tissue eosinophilia may occur in many inflammatory states, not necessarily accompanied by marked blood eosinophilia.

Eosinophilia More than 500 eosinophils per cubic millimeter of blood is infrequent in normal individuals. The most common cause for mild eosinophilia in hospitalized patients is probably some form of drug allergy. Parasitic infections, principally helminthic infections, cause eosinophilia, especially during the invasive phase. Some parasites may be difficult to recognize, e.g., *Strongyloides* (see Chap. 229), *Trichinella* (see

TABLE 57-6
Causes of blood eosinophilia

Drug reactions: Iodides, aspirin, sulfonamides, nitrofurantoin
Parasitic infections: Hookworm disease, strongyloidiasis, toxocariasis, trichuriasis, trichinosis, filariasis, schistosomiasis, echinococcosis, cysticercosis
Allergic diseases: Hay fever, asthma, angioedema, serum sickness, allergic vasculitis, eczema, pemphigus
Collagen vascular diseases: Rheumatoid arthritis, dermatomyositis, periarteritis nodosa
Malignancy: Hodgkin's disease, carcinomatosis, mycosis fungoides, chronic myelogenous leukemia
Hypereosinophilic syndromes: Loeffler's syndrome, Loeffler's endocarditis, eosinophilic leukemia

Chap. 226), *Toxocara* (see Chap. 229), and filariae (see Chap. 227). In these diseases the eosinophil count is rarely greater than 25,000 per cubic millimeter with the highest counts probably occurring in trichinosis. Protozoan infections generally do not cause eosinophilia. Eosinophilia is usually mild and irregularly present in allergic and collagen vascular diseases and malignancies and is not necessarily a clear guide to disease activity. The hypereosinophilic syndromes cause the highest eosinophil counts, occasionally in the 50,000 to 100,000 per cubic millimeter range or higher. Many tissues become infiltrated by eosinophils, a condition leading to organ dysfunction, particularly congestive heart failure.

Eosinopenia A reduction in eosinophils occurs with any stress or following corticosteroid administration. No known adverse effects result.

BASOPHILS These are the least common blood leukocytes; usually none are seen in the routine examination of a blood smear. The distinctive deep blue granules, characteristically obscuring the cell nucleus, are rich in histamine. These cells are thought to be involved in certain acute allergic responses. Basophils are increased in chronic myelogenous leukemia, myelofibrosis, and polycythemia vera. This finding helps to distinguish these diseases from leukemoid reactions. Basophilia may also be observed occasionally in some chronic inflammatory conditions.

REFERENCES

Butterworth AE, David JR: Current concepts: Eosinophil function. N Engl J Med 203:154, 1981

Chusid MJ, Dale DC: The hypereosinophilic syndrome. Medicine 54:1, 1975

Cooper MD et al: Effects of anti Ig antibodies on the development and differentiation of B-cells. Immunol Rev 52:29, 1981

Dale DC et al: Chronic neutropenia. Medicine 58:128, 1979

Gallin JI et al: Disorders of phagocyte chemotaxis. Ann Intern Med 92:520, 1980

Klebanoff SJ: Oxygen metabolism and the toxic properties of phagocytes. Ann Intern Med 93:480, 1980

Mills EL, Quie PG: Congenital disorders of the functions of polymorphonuclear neutrophils. Rev Infect Dis 2:505, 1980

Parry MF et al: Myeloperoxidase deficiency: Prevalence and clinical significance. Ann Intern Med 95:293, 1981

Price TP, Dale DC: The selective neutropenias. Clin Hematol 7:501, 1978

Reinherz EL, Schlossman SF: Current concepts in immunology: Regulation of immune response—Inducer and suppressor T-lymphocyte subsets in human beings. N Engl J Med 303:370, 1980

Walker RI, Willemze R: Neutrophil kinetics and the regulation of granulopoiesis. Rev Infect Dis 2:282, 1980

Wright DG et al: Human cyclic neutropenia: Clinical review and long-term follow-up of patients. Medicine 60:1, 1981

PART THREE | BIOLOGICAL CONSIDERATIONS IN THE APPROACH TO CLINICAL MEDICINE

section 1 | Genetics and human disease

58
GENETIC ASPECTS OF DISEASE

JOSEPH L. GOLDSTEIN
MICHAEL S. BROWN

GENETIC PRINCIPLES

More than one-fifth of the proteins (and hence genes) in each human being exist in a form that differs from the one present in the majority of the population. This remarkable genetic variability, or polymorphism, among "normal" people accounts for much of the naturally occurring variation in body traits such as height, intelligence, and blood pressure. Moreover, these genetic differences cause variability in the ability of individuals to handle every environmental challenge, including those that produce disease. Thus, human disease can be considered to occur as a result of an interaction between an individual's genetic makeup and the environment. In certain diseases, however, the genetic component is so overwhelming that it expresses itself in a predictable manner without a requirement for extraordinary environmental challenges. Such diseases are termed *genetic disorders.*

MOLECULAR BASIS OF GENE EXPRESSION All hereditary information is transmitted from parent to offspring through the inheritance of specific molecules of deoxyribonucleic acid (DNA). DNA is a linear polymer composed of purine and pyrimidine bases whose sequence ultimately determines the sequence of amino acids in every protein molecule made by the body. The four types of bases in DNA are arranged in groups of three, each group forming a code word, or codon, that signifies a particular amino acid. A *gene* represents the total sequence of bases in DNA that specifies the amino acid sequence of a single polypeptide chain of a protein molecule.

Genetic information encoded in the DNA of the chromosomes is first transcribed into a *ribonucleic acid* (RNA) copy. During transcription the ribose nucleotides align themselves along the DNA according to base-pairing rules. Thus, adenine of DNA pairs with uridine of RNA, cytosine pairs with guanine, thymine pairs with adenine, and guanine pairs with cytosine. The ribose bases are joined together by RNA polymerase. The resulting *RNA transcript* forms the template for translation into the amino acid sequence of a protein. Figure 58-1 shows the DNA and mRNA code words for each of the amino acids in protein.

Figure 58-2 illustrates a schematic diagram of the genetic control of protein synthesis in higher organisms, including humans. The DNA of many genes is fragmented into discrete coding regions (exons) separated by noncoding regions (introns or intervening sequences). The *coding regions* contain the information specifying the sequence of amino acids in the polypeptide chain. The *intervening sequences* are composed of sequences of bases that act as spacers between the coding regions; they are not translated into protein. The transcription of DNA produces a faithful copy of the entire gene sequence; thus, the RNA transcript contains a mosaic of coding and intervening sequences. The RNA transcript is edited in the nucleus before it passes into the cytoplasm. In the editing process, the intervening sequences are excised and the coding regions are spliced together to form one continuous gene (Fig. 58-2).

After processing, the edited RNA, which is called *messenger RNA* (mRNA) leaves the nucleus and enters the cytoplasm where it becomes associated with *ribosomes* and thereby serves as a template for the ribosomal synthesis of proteins. Each of the 20 precursor amino acids for protein synthesis is attached in the cell cytoplasm to specific molecules called *transfer RNA* (tRNA). Each tRNA contains a sequence of purine and pyrimidine bases that is "complementary" to a specific codon in the mRNA. These tRNA molecules with their attached amino acids line up along the mRNA molecule in the precise order dictated by the mRNA code. Under the action of a variety of cytoplasmic enzymes (initiation factors, elongation factors, and termination factors), peptide bonds are formed between the various amino acids, and the completed protein is released from the ribosome.

MAINTENANCE OF GENETIC DIVERSITY THROUGH TRANSMISSION AND SEGREGATION OF GENES It is estimated that the amount of DNA in the nucleus of each human cell is sufficient to code for more than 100,000 genes and hence to specify more than 100,000 polypeptide chains. The genes are arranged in a linear sequence of DNA that together with certain histone proteins form rod-shaped bodies called *chromosomes.* Each somatic cell contains 46 chromosomes, arranged in 23 pairs, one of each pair derived from each of the individual's parents. Thus, each individual inherits two copies of each chromosome and hence two copies of each gene. The chromosomal location of the two copies of each gene is termed the *genetic locus.*

First nucleotide	Second nucleotide: A or *U*			G or *C*			T or *A*			C or *G*			Third nucleotide
A or *U*	**AAA**	*UUU*	Phe	**AGA**	*UCU*	Ser	**ATA**	*UAU*	Tyr	**ACA**	*UGU*	Cys	**A** or *U*
	AAG	*UUC*		**AGG**	*UCC*		**ATG**	*UAC*		**ACG**	*UGC*		**G** or *C*
	AAT	*UUA*	Leu	**AGT**	*UCA*		**ATT**	*UAA*	Stop	**ACT**	*UGA*	Stop	**T** or *A*
	AAC	*UUG*		**AGC**	*UCG*		**ATC**	*UAG*		**ACC**	*UGG*	Trp	**C** or *G*
G or *C*	**GAA**	*CUU*	Leu	**GGA**	*CCU*	Pro	**GTA**	*CAU*	His	**GCA**	*CGU*	Arg	**A** or *U*
	GAG	*CUC*		**GGG**	*CCC*		**GTG**	*CAC*		**GCG**	*CGC*		**G** or *C*
	GAT	*CUA*		**GGT**	*CCA*		**GTT**	*CAA*	Gln	**GCT**	*CGA*		**T** or *A*
	GAC	*CUG*		**GGC**	*CCG*		**GTC**	*CAG*		**GCC**	*CGG*		**C** or *G*
T or *A*	**TAA**	*AUU*	Ile	**TGA**	*ACU*	Thr	**TTA**	*AAU*	Asn	**TCA**	*AGU*	Ser	**A** or *U*
	TAG	*AUC*		**TGG**	*ACC*		**TTG**	*AAC*		**TCG**	*AGC*		**G** or *C*
	TAT	*AUA*		**TGT**	*ACA*		**TTT**	*AAA*	Lys	**TCT**	*AGA*	Arg	**T** or *A*
	TAC	*AUG*	Met	**TGC**	*ACG*		**TTC**	*AAG*		**TCC**	*AGG*		**C** or *G*
C or *G*	**CAA**	*GUU*	Val	**CGA**	*GCU*	Ala	**CTA**	*GAU*	Asp	**CCA**	*GGU*	Gly	**A** or *U*
	CAG	*GUC*		**CGG**	*GCC*		**CTG**	*GAC*		**CCG**	*GGC*		**G** or *C*
	CAT	*GUA*		**CGT**	*GCA*		**CTT**	*GAA*	Glu	**CCT**	*GGA*		**T** or *A*
	CAC	*GUG*		**CGC**	*GCG*		**CTC**	*GAG*		**CCC**	*GGG*		**C** or *G*

Note: The DNA codons appear in boldface type; the complementary RNA codons are in italics. A = adenine, C = cytosine, G = guanine, T = thymine, U = uridine (replaces thymine in RNA). In RNA, adenine is complementary to thymine of DNA; uridine is complementary to adenine of DNA; cytosine is complementary to guanine, and vice versa. "Stop" = termination. The amino acids are abbreviated as follows:

Ala = alanine; Arg = arginine; Asn = asparagine; Asp = aspartic acid; Cys = cysteine; Gln = glutamine; Glu = glutamic acid; Gly = glycine; His = histidine; Ile = isoleucine; Leu = leucine; Lys = lysine; Met = methionine; Phe = phenylalanine; Pro = proline; Ser = serine; Thr = threonine; Trp = tryptophan; Tyr = tyrosine; Val = valine

FIGURE 58-1
The genetic code.

When a gene occupying a genetic locus exists in two or more different forms, these alternate forms of the gene are referred to as *alleles.*

In humans, a given gene always resides at a specified genetic locus on one particular chromosome. For example, the genetic locus for the Rh blood group is on the short arm of chromosome 1; at this chromosomal site there are two Rh genes, one on chromosome 1 derived from the mother and the other on chromosome 1 derived from the father. When two genes at the same genetic locus are identical, the individual is a *homozygote.* When the two genes differ (i.e., two alleles are present at the locus), the individual is a *heterozygote.* Each normal human is heterozygous at approximately 20 percent of genetic loci and homozygous at 80 percent. Figure 58-3 shows a map of human chromosome 1, illustrating the location of those genes that have been assigned loci on this chromosome.

The genetic information carried on chromosomes is transmitted to daughter cells under two different sets of circumstances. One of these occurs whenever a somatic cell (i.e., a nongerm cell) divides. This process, called *mitosis,* functions to transmit identical copies of each gene to each daughter cell, thus maintaining a uniform genetic makeup in all cells of a single individual. The other set of circumstances prevails when genetic information is to be transmitted from one individual to an offspring. This process, called *meiosis,* functions to produce germ cells (i.e., ova or spermatozoa) that possess only one copy of each parental chromosome, thus allowing for new combinations of chromosomes to occur when ovum and sperm cell fuse during fertilization.

During the process of meiosis, the 46 chromosomes of an immature germ cell arrange themselves in 23 pairs at the center of the nucleus, each pair being composed of one chromosome derived from the mother and its homologous chromosome derived from the father. At a specified point in the meiotic process, the two partner chromosomes separate, only one of each pair going into each daughter cell, or gamete. Thus, meiosis produces gametes with a reduction in the number of chromosomes from 46 to 23, each gamete having received one chromosome from each of the 23 pairs. The assortment of the chromosomes within each pair is random so that each germ cell

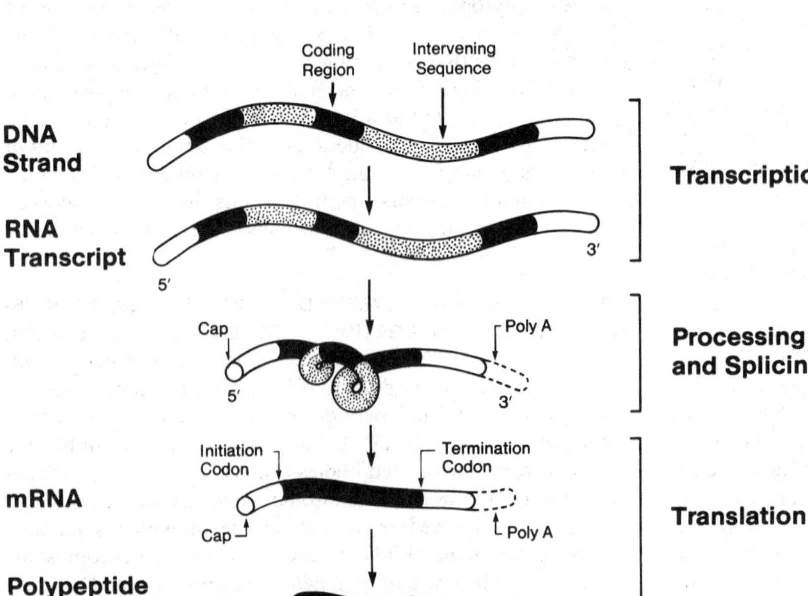

FIGURE 58-2
A schematic diagram of the genetic control of protein synthesis, illustrating the flow of genetic information from the base sequence of DNA to the RNA transcript (transcription) to mRNA (processing) to the polypeptide chain of a protein molecule (translation). Although DNA exists in a double-stranded form, only one of the two strands is used as a template for transcribing the RNA transcript. Solid sections represent coding regions in DNA, RNA transcript, mRNA, and amino acid sequence in polypeptide chain; dotted sections represent intervening sequences in DNA and RNA transcript.

receives a different combination of maternal and paternal chromosomes. During the process of fertilization, the fusion of ovum and sperm cell, each of which has 23 chromosomes, results ultimately in an individual with 46 chromosomes.

The independent assortment of chromosomes into gametes during meiosis produces an enormous diversity among the possible genotypes of the progeny. For each 23 pairs of chromosomes, there are 2^{23} different combinations of chromosomes that could occur in a gamete, and the likelihood that one set of parents will produce two offspring with the identical complement of chromosomes is one in 2^{23} or one in 8.4 million (assuming no monozygotic or identical twins).

RECOMBINATION Adding to the genetic diversity in humans is the phenomenon of *genetic recombination.* During meiosis, when homologous chromosomes are paired, bridges frequently form between corresponding regions of the chromosome pair. These bridges, or *chiasmata,* are regions in which the two chromosomes break at identical points along their length and subsequently rejoin, the distal segments having been switched from one homologous chromosome to another. This process is designated *crossing over.* Although no net change in the amount of genetic material occurs during crossing over, a recombination of genes does occur. For example, consider a chromosome with two loci, A and B, located at opposite ends of the same chromosome. On this particular chromosome, the A locus has a rare allele x and the B locus also has a rare allele y. Without the phenomenon of recombination every offspring that inherited the x allele at the A locus would also inherit the y allele at the B locus. However, if recombination occurs, the A locus with the x allele would then be on the opposite chromosome from the B locus with the y allele. In this case any offspring that inherited the x allele at the A locus could not inherit the y allele at the B locus.

FIGURE 58-3
Gene map of human chromosome 1. The black bands represent those genetic regions of the chromosome that stain brightly by a fluorescent dye such as quinacrine; the white bands are the negatively staining regions; the hatched area is a variable region that stains differently (i.e., either brightly or negatively) in the chromosomes of different individuals. Each gene that has been localized to this chromosome is listed opposite its genetic locus on the right. (Data provided by FH Ruddle and VA McKusick.)

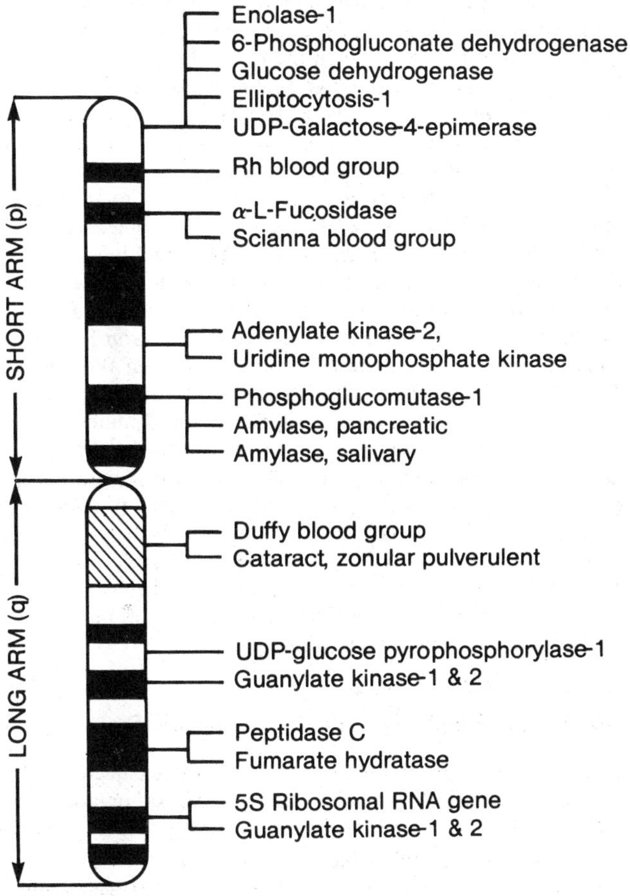

Crossing over occurs with great frequency in every meiosis in humans, and the resultant recombination of genes may occur at any point on a chromosome. The farther apart two genes are on the same chromosome, the greater is the likelihood that a crossing over will occur in the space between them. When two genes are on the opposite ends of a long chromosome, the probability of recombination is so great that their respective alleles are transmitted to offspring almost independently of one another, just as if the two gene loci were on different chromosomes. On the other hand, gene loci that are close together on the same chromosome are said to be *linked* so that there is a great likelihood that offspring will inherit the same combination of alleles that are present on the parental chromosome.

Several examples of *gene linkage* can be seen from the map of human chromosome 1 (Fig. 58-3). For example, the locus for the gene specifying the Rh blood group factor and the locus for the gene producing one form of the dominant trait, hereditary elliptocytosis, occur in close proximity on this chromosome. Thus, if a subject with hereditary elliptocytosis transmits the disease to an offspring, the offspring will usually inherit the allele that is present at the Rh locus on this chromosome. If the Rh allele happens to be a rare one in the population (such as r'), one can assume that whichever offspring inherits the r' allele at the Rh locus will also inherit the abnormal allele at the elliptocytosis locus. On the other hand, if an offspring does not exhibit the r' allele, he or she will not usually have elliptocytosis. The concept of linkage does not imply an association between any particular set of Rh alleles and the disease state elliptocytosis, rather between the two genetic loci. Thus, in different families the abnormal elliptocytosis allele may be linked to the R^1, R^0, r_2, or any other allele at the Rh locus, depending on the allele that happened to be at that locus when the elliptocytosis mutation occurred. Stated another way, the elliptocytosis locus is linked to the Rh locus in every family, but the particular Rh allele with which it is associated will differ from family to family.

MUTATION Broadly defined, a *mutation* is a stable, heritable alteration in DNA. Although the causes of mutation in humans are largely unknown, a variety of environmental agents, such as radiation, viruses, and chemicals, are among the factors that are implicated.

Mutations can involve a visible alteration in the structure of a chromosome, such as a deletion or translocation of a portion of a chromosome, or they can involve a minute change in one of the purine or pyrimidine bases of a single gene. Most commonly, such "point" mutations consist of the substitution of one base for another, changing the meaning of the codon containing that base, hence their designation as *missense mutations.* For example, in the gene coding for the β chain of hemoglobin, the sixth position normally contains the nucleotide triplet CTC, which codes for the amino acid glutamic acid (Fig. 58-1). The mutation that gives rise to hemoglobin C produces a change of the first base of this triplet from cytosine to thymine, changing the triplet to TTC, which codes for lysine. On the other hand, the mutation that gives rise to hemoglobin S produces a change in the second base of the same triplet (from thymine to adenine), producing CAC, which codes for valine. Thus, in the sixth position of the β chain of hemoglobin, the normally occurring glutamic acid may be replaced with either lysine (producing hemoglobin C) or valine (producing hemoglobin S). More than 84 such single-base mutations in the hemoglobin β chain have been identified in different population groups, and many of these mutations produce distinct clinical syndromes. Of all the mutations so far elucidated in humans, the vast majority involve such single-base changes.

Besides producing an amino acid substitution, a single-base substitution can also cause another abnormality in protein synthesis—premature chain termination. Three mRNA code words (UAA, UAG, and UGA) normally do not specify an amino acid but constitute the signal that the message has ended and that the protein chain should be released from the ribosome (Fig. 58-1). If a change occurs in DNA that produces one of these mRNA code words [for example, a switch in an mRNA triplet from UAU (tyrosine) to UAA (termination)], the polypeptide chain would be terminated prematurely when translation had reached that point. Such mutations, called *nonsense mutations,* produce short fragments of proteins that have reduced function.

CELLULAR MECHANISM BY WHICH MUTANT GENES PRODUCE DISEASES Critical to the modern understanding of heredity is the concept that the only information transmitted from generation to generation is the sequence of bases in DNA and that these sequences in turn specify only the primary structure of RNA and protein molecules. All other chemical reactions within a cell—such as the synthesis of complex lipids and carbohydrates, the formation of membranes and other cellular organelles, and the accumulation and partitioning of inorganic ions—occur as a secondary consequence of the action of specific proteins. Many of these proteins are enzymes that catalyze the biochemical conversion of one molecule into another. Others are structural proteins such as collagen and elastin, and still others are regulatory proteins that dictate how much of each enzyme and each structural protein is to be made.

Since proteins are the cellular molecules whose structures are encoded by genes, mutations in genes exert their deleterious effects by altering the structure of enzymes, structural proteins, or regulatory proteins. For example, in a disease such as glycogen storage disease, type I (von Gierke's disease), massive accumulation of glycogen in the liver is due not to a primary structural abnormality in the polysaccharide glycogen but to a structural abnormality in a protein, glucose 6-phosphatase, an enzyme that is required to liberate glucose so as to permit glycogen breakdown. Other examples of the biochemical mechanisms by which mutant genes alter cellular metabolism are discussed below in "Simply Inherited Disorders."

GENETIC HETEROGENEITY When two or more mutations can produce a similar clinical syndrome, genetic heterogeneity is said to exist. Hemophilia is one example of a genetically heterogeneous syndrome. A clinically similar bleeding disorder can be caused by mutations at either of two loci on the X chromosome, one leading to a deficiency of factor VIII (classic hemophilia) and the other causing a deficiency of factor IX (Christmas disease). It is now generally believed that most, if not all, hereditary diseases, when carefully analyzed, will be shown to be genetically heterogeneous.

Genetic heterogeneity may result from the existence of a series of different mutations at a single genetic locus (allelic mutations) or from mutations at different genetic loci (nonallelic mutations). For example, drug-induced hemolysis of red blood cells can occur in patients with several different types of allelic mutations at the glucose 6-phosphate dehydrogenase locus. On the other hand, hemophilia is an example of a syndrome in which nonallelic mutations can produce a similar clinical picture (see above).

In some cases of heterogeneity, both the genetic locus and the mode of inheritance differ, depending on the mutation. Diseases such as spastic paraplegia, Charcot-Marie-Tooth peroneal muscular atrophy, and retinitis pigmentosa are inherited as autosomal dominant traits in some families, as autosomal recessives in others, and as X-linked recessives in still others. The identification of such genetic heterogeneity in these disorders is of obvious importance for correct genetic counseling.

TAKING THE FAMILY HISTORY

The investigation of a patient with a possible genetic disorder begins with the *family history.* The first step is to obtain certain information on the *proband* or *index case* (i.e., the clinically affected person who has brought the family to attention) and on each of the *first-degree relatives* (i.e., the parents, siblings, and offspring of the proband). This information includes the given name, surname, maiden name, birth date or current age, age at death, cause of death, and name or description of any disease or defect.

The second step is to ask questions designed to survey the family for the presence of disease or defect. (1) Has any relative an identical or similar trait? (2) Has any relative a trait that is absent in the proband but is known to occur in some patients with the same disease? This question requires that the physician have some knowledge about the manifestations of the disease in question. For example, when obtaining the family history from a proband with dissecting aneurysm caused possibly by Marfan's syndrome, one should ask about the occurrence of eye abnormalities, cardiac abnormalities, and skeletal abnormalities in the relatives. (3) Has any relative a trait that is recognized to be genetically determined? The purpose of this question is to ascertain the occurrence of hereditary disease in the family even though the particular patient may not be involved. (4) Has any relative an unusual disease, or has any relative died of a rare condition? The purpose of this question is to identify a condition that might be genetically determined though not recognized as such by the informant. In addition, this question may help to identify conditions in relatives that might be etiologically related to the patient's problem. For example, a patient with pheochromocytoma should be suspected of having von Recklinghausen's disease if he or she has a brother with scoliosis and mental retardation, both of which can be manifestations of the neurofibromatosis (von Recklinghausen's) gene. (5) Is there any consanguinity in the family? This inquiry should be made directly. In addition, one should ask whether common last names appear in the families of husband-wife pairs. Consanguineous marriage may be the source of a rare autosomal recessive syndrome, and sometimes its presence in the family may not be known by the proband. (6) What is the ethnic origin of the family? Persons of various ethnic origins, such as blacks, Jews, and Greeks, have increased chances of specific genetic diseases. Table 58-1 lists examples of simply inherited disorders that are found with increased frequency in various ethnic groups.

CATEGORIES OF GENETIC DISORDERS

Genetic diseases generally fall into one of three categories: (1) *Chromosomal disorders* involve the lack, excess, or abnormal arrangement of one or more chromosomes, producing excessive or deficient genetic material. (2) *Mendelian or simply inherited disorders* are determined primarily by a single mutant gene. These disorders display inheritance patterns which can be classified into autosomal dominant, autosomal recessive, or X-linked types. (3) *Mulifactorial disorders* are caused by an interaction of multiple genes and multiple exogenous or environmental factors. Although many of these multifactorial disorders, such as essential hypertension and cleft lip and palate, are said to run in families, the inheritance pattern is complex and the risk to relatives is less than in the single-gene (mendelian) disorders. Each of these categories presents different problems with respect to causation, prevention, diagnosis, genetic counseling, and treatment.

CHROMOSOMAL DISORDERS The karyotype of an individual (i.e., the number and structure of the chromosomes) can be ascertained from readily accessible body tissues, such as peripheral blood lymphocytes or skin, by growing them in tissue culture until active cell proliferation occurs and then preparing single cells for examination of chromosomes by microscopy. Recent developments have made it possible to identify accurately each individual chromosome by special staining of DNA sequences, by the affinity of fluorescent dyes (such as quinacrine hydrochloride) for certain chromosomal segments that can be visualized by fluorescence microscopy, and by treatment with special dyes (Giemsa) and proteolytic enzymes (trypsin). These techniques produce characteristic *banding patterns* for each chromosome (Fig. 58-4).

TABLE 58-1
Examples of simply inherited disorders that occur with increased frequency in specific ethnic groups

Ethnic group	*Simply inherited disorder*
African blacks	Hemoglobinopathies, especially Hb S, Hb C, persistent Hb F, α and β thalassemias Glucose 6-phosphate dehydrogenase deficiency
Armenians	Familial Mediterranean fever
Ashkenazi Jews	Abetalipoproteinemia Bloom's syndrome Dystonia musculorum deformans (recessive form) Factor XI (PTA) deficiency Familial dysautonomia (Riley-Day syndrome) Gaucher's disease (adult form) Neimann-Pick disease Pentosuria Tay-Sachs disease
Chinese	α thalassemia Glucose 6-phosphate dehydrogenase deficiency Adult lactase deficiency
Eskimos	Pseudocholinesterase deficiency Adrenogenital syndrome
Finns	Congenital nephrosis Mulibrey nanism
French Canadians	Tyrosinemia
Japanese	Acatalasemia
Lebanese	Homozygous familial hypercholesterolemia
Mediterranean peoples (Italians, Greeks, Sephardic Jews)	β thalassemia Glucose 6-phosphate dehydrogenase deficiency Familial Mediterranean fever Glycogen storage disease, type III
Northern Europeans	Cystic fibrosis
Scandinavians	α_1-Antitrypsin deficiency LCAT (lecithin:cholesterol acyltransferase) deficiency
South African whites	Porphyria variegata Homozygous familial hypercholesterolemia

The number of chromosomes in normal individuals is 46, of which 44 are the 22 pairs of *autosomes* and the other two are the *sex chromosomes.* Females have two X chromosomes (XX), and males have one X chromosome and one Y chromosome (XY). Each of the 22 pairs of autosomes and the two sex chromosomes can be distinguished on the basis of size, location of the centromere (which divides the chromosome into arms of equal or unequal length), and the unique banding pattern (Fig. 58-4). The relative length of the arms and the position of the centromere are used as further criteria to divide the human chromosomes into seven groups (designated A to G) (Fig. 58-4).

For a complete discussion of the etiology and clinical features of chromosomal abnormalities affecting humans, the reader is referred to Chap. 61.

SIMPLY INHERITED DISORDERS Disorders caused by the transmission of a single mutant gene show one of three simple (or mendelian) patterns of inheritance: (1) autosomal dominant, (2) autosomal recessive, or (3) X-linked. The distinction between "dominant" and "recessive" is one of convenience in pedigree analysis and does not imply a fundamental difference in genetic mechanism. The term *dominant* implies that a mutation will be clinically manifest when an individual has a single dose of this mutation (or is *heterozygous* for it), while *recessive* implies that a double dose (or *homozygosity*) is required for clinical detection. Genes are never dominant or recessive; their effects, however, produce clinical patterns that are classified as dominant or recessive. Despite their overall clinical "normality," individuals who are heterozygous for "recessive" genes often have biochemical abnormalities that are demonstrable in the laboratory; on the other hand, those who are homozygous for "dominant" genes are usually more severely affected than are the heterozygotes.

With few exceptions, each of the approximately 1200 mendelian diseases is rare. However, as a group these disorders

FIGURE 58-4
The karyotype of a normal male showing the chromosomes of a single somatic cell in the metaphase stage of cell division. The photographic images of the chromosomes have been cut out and arranged according to descending length and varying arm ratio. The chromosomes have been stained by the Giemsa technique, which allows each chromosome pair to be identified by its unique banding pattern. Chromosomes 1 to 22 are the autosomes. The sex chromosomes in this normal male are an X and a Y. The normal female has an identical karyotype except for the absence of the Y chromosome and the presence instead of a second X chromosome. (Courtesy of K Hirschhorn.)

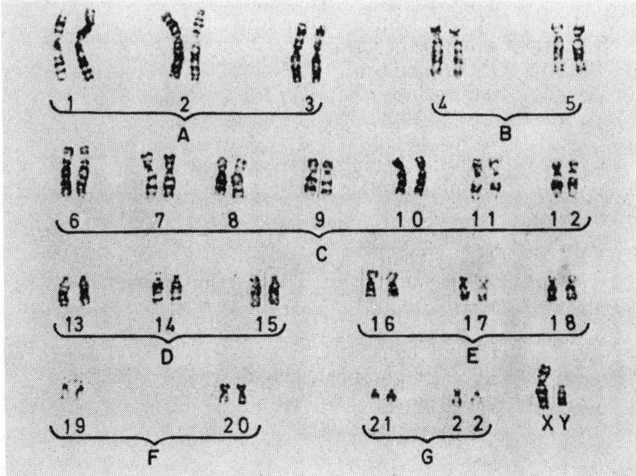

constitute an important cause of morbidity and death, accounting directly for more than 5 percent of all hospital admissions.

As of 1982, the genes for about 60 simply inherited diseases have been assigned to specific chromosomes, 45 to the 22 autosomes and 15 to the X chromosome. Disease-producing genes assigned to the X chromosome outnumber those so far assigned to any single autosome. This is because assignment to the X chromosome requires only pedigree studies showing X-linked inheritance (see below). Assignment to an autosome is more complicated, requiring sophisticated techniques of somatic cell hybridization or pedigree studies showing linkage between a disease-producing gene and a "marker" gene that is known to be on a certain chromosome. Table 58-2 lists those human genetic diseases that have been mapped to specific chromosomes.

TABLE 58-2
Human genetic diseases that have been mapped to specific chromosomes

Chromosome	*Disease*
1	Elliptocytosis
	Galactose epimerase deficiency
	Fucosidosis
2	? Aniridia
3	Generalized gangliosidosis
4	Atypical phenylketonuria
	Sclerotylosis
5	Sandhoff's disease
	Maroteaux-Lamy syndrome (mucopolysaccharidosis VI)
6	Asymmetric septal hypertrophy
	Complement C2 deficiency
	Complement C4 deficiency
	Hemochromatosis
	Congenital adrenal hyperplasia (21-hydroxylase deficiency)
	Olivopontocerebellar atrophy I
7	Argininosuccinicaciduria
	β-Glucuronidase deficiency (mucopolysaccharidosis VII)
9	Citrullinemia
	Galactosemia
	Nail-patella syndrome
10	Hexokinase deficiency (hemolytic anemia)
	Cholesteryl ester storage disease, Wolman's syndrome
11	Acatalasemia
	Syndrome of Wilms' tumor, aniridia, gonadoblastoma, retardation
	β thalassemia, sickle cell anemia
	Acute intermittent porphyria
12	Triosephosphate isomerase deficiency (hemolytic anemia)
13	Retinoblastoma
14	Nucleoside phosphorylase deficiency (immunodeficiency)
15	Prader-Willi syndrome
	Tay-Sachs disease
16	α thalassemia
	Gout due to adenine phosphoribosyltransferase deficiency
	LCAT deficiency
17	Galactokinase deficiency
	Glycogen storage disease II (acid maltase deficiency)
19	Glucosephosphate isomerase deficiency (hemolytic anemia)
	Mannosidosis
20	Adenosine deaminase deficiency (immunodeficiency)
22	Metachromatic leukodystrophy
X	X-linked ichthyosis due to placental steroid sulfatase deficiency
	Ocular albinism
	Retinoschisis
	Chronic granulomatous disease
	Duchenne muscular dystrophy
	Testicular feminization syndrome
	Phosphoglycerate kinase deficiency (hemolytic anemia)
	Fabry's disease
	Lesch-Nyhan syndrome
	Fragile site associated with X-linked mental retardation
	Color blindness
	Hemophilia A
	Glucose 6-phosphate dehydrogenase (G6PD) deficiency
	Adrenoleukodystrophy

SOURCE: *McKusick.*

The demonstration that a particular disease or syndrome shows one of the three mendelian patterns of inheritance implies that its pathogenesis, no matter how complex, is due to an abnormality in a single protein molecule. For example, in sickle cell anemia, the entire clinical syndrome, including such seemingly unrelated disturbances as anemia, pain crises, nephropathy, and predisposition to pneumococcal infections, are all the physiologic consequences of having thymine instead of adenine at a specific site in the gene that codes for the β chain of hemoglobin, producing a substitution of a valine for a glutamic acid in the sixth amino acid position in the protein sequence.

In many mendelian disorders, especially in those with dominant inheritance, it is not possible to demonstrate directly the protein that is primarily altered by the mutation. In such cases (e.g., adult polycystic kidney disease and tuberous sclerosis) only the distal physiologic effects of the mutation are recognizable. Nevertheless, it is safe to assume that a single primary defect exists whenever a disease is transmitted by a single gene mechanism and that the various manifestations of the disease all can be related to the mutational event by a more or less complicated "pedigree of causes." Table 58-3 lists the most commonly encountered mendelian disorders affecting adults.

TABLE 58-3
Some relatively frequent mendelian disorders affecting adults

AUTOSOMAL DOMINANT DISORDERS
Familial hypercholesterolemia
Hereditary hemorrhagic telangiectasia
Marfan's syndrome
Hereditary spherocytosis
Adult polycystic kidney disease
Huntington's chorea
Acute intermittent porphyria
Osteogenesis imperfecta tarda
von Willebrand's disease
Myotonic dystrophy
Idiopathic hypertrophic subaortic stenosis (IHSS)
Noonan's syndrome
Neurofibromatosis
Tuberous sclerosis
AUTOSOMAL RECESSIVE DISORDERS
Deafness
Albinism
Wilson's disease
Hemochromatosis
Sickle cell anemia
β thalassemia
Cystic fibrosis
Hereditary emphysema (α_1-antitrypsin deficiency)
Homocystinuria
Familial Mediterranean fever
Friedreich's ataxia
Phenylketonuria
X-LINKED DISORDERS
Hemophilia A
Glucose 6-phosphate dehydrogenase deficiency
Fabry's disease
Ocular albinism
Testicular feminization
Chronic granulomatous disease
Hypophosphatemic rickets
Color blindness

Autosomal dominant disorders Dominant diseases are those manifest in the heterozygous state, that is, when only one abnormal gene (*mutant allele*) is present and the corresponding partner allele on the homologous chromosome is normal. The gene responsible for an autosomal dominant disorder is located on one of the 22 autosomes, and both males and females can be affected. Since alleles segregate independently at meiosis, there is a 1 in 2 chance that the offspring of an affected heterozygote will inherit the mutant allele and, similarly, a 1 in 2 chance of the offspring inheriting the normal allele.

Figure 58-5 shows a typical pedigree involving an autosomal dominant trait. The following features are characteristic: (1) Each affected individual has an affected parent (unless the condition arose by a new mutation or is mildly expressed in the affected parent); (2) an affected individual will bear, on the average, both normal and affected offspring in equal proportions; (3) normal children of an affected individual will have only normal offspring; (4) males and females are affected in equal proportions; (5) each sex is equally likely to transmit the condition to male and female offspring, with male-to-male transmission occurring; and (6) vertical transmission of the condition through successive generations occurs, especially when the trait does not impair reproductive capacity.

While half of the offspring of an individual with an autosomal dominant condition will inherit the disease, it is not necessarily true that each affected person must have an affected parent. In every autosomal dominant disease a certain proportion of affected persons owe their disorder to a new mutation rather than to an inherited mutation. Since the estimated frequency of mutation is 5×10^{-6} mutations per gene per generation and since a dominant trait, by definition, requires a mutation in only one of a pair of alleles, one would expect that about 1 in 100,000 newborn persons would possess a new mutation at any given genetic locus. Many of these mutations either do not impair the function of the gene product or involve a recessive function so that the mutation is clinically silent. Others, however, cause a defective gene product that gives rise to a dominant trait. The parent in whose germ cells the mutation arose will be clinically normal. Likewise, the siblings of the affected individual are normal since the mutation will affect only a single germ cell. However, the affected individual will be able to transmit the disease, and half of his or her children will be affected.

The proportion of patients with dominant disorders who represent new mutations is inversely proportional to the effect of the disease in question on biologic fitness. The term *biologic fitness* refers to the ability of an affected individual to produce children who survive to adult life and reproduce. In the extreme case, if a dominant mutation produced absolute infertility, then all observed cases would of necessity represent new mutations, and it would be impossible to prove the genetic transmission of the trait. In less severe disorders, as in tuberous sclerosis, the severe mental retardation reduces biologic fitness to about 20 percent of normal, and the proportion of cases due to new mutations is about 80 percent. Other examples of the relation between biologic fitness and the proportion of new mutations in dominant disorders are shown in Table 58-4.

Many new mutations appear to occur in the germ cells of fathers who are of relatively advanced age. Such a "paternal age effect" is seen, for example, in Marfan's syndrome in which the average age of fathers of sporadic or "new mutation" cases (37 years) is in excess of the mean age of fathers generally (30 years) and also in excess of the age of fathers who transmit Marfan's disease due to an inherited mutation (30 years).

Before one concludes that a dominant disorder in a given patient with unaffected parents is the result of a new mutation, it is important to consider two other possibilities: (1) that the gene may be carried by one parent in whom the disease is of low expressivity (discussed below), and (2) that extramarital paternity may have occurred, since such is found in about 3 to 5 percent of randomly studied children in the United States.

Most autosomal dominant disorders show two characteristic features that are not usually seen in recessive syndromes: (1) *delayed age of onset* and (2) *variability in clinical expression.* Delayed age of onset is seen in disorders such as Huntington's chorea and adult polycystic kidney disease. These disorders do not manifest clinically until adult life, even though the mutant gene is present from the time of conception. Variability in clinical expression is illustrated dramatically by the multiple endocrine adenoma–peptic ulcer syndrome. Patients in the same family inheriting the same abnormal gene may have hyperplasia or neoplasia of one or all of a wide variety of endocrine tissues such as the pancreas, parathyroid glands, pituitary gland, or adipose tissue. The resulting clinical manifestations are diverse; different members of the same family may develop peptic ulcers, hypoglycemia, kidney stones, multiple lipomas of

FIGURE 58-5
Pedigree pattern of an autosomal dominant trait. Note the vertical *pattern of inheritance.*

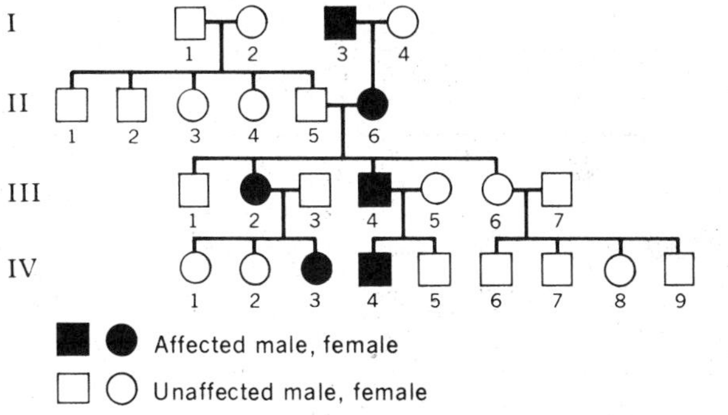

FIGURE 58-6
Pedigree of a family affected with the multiple endocrine adenoma–peptic ulcer syndrome, a disorder inherited as an autosomal dominant trait. Circles denote females; squares, males. Open circles and squares denote unaffected relatives; closed circles and squares denote affected relatives. Deceased relatives are indicated by the oblique line. The age of each relative is indicated above his or her symbol. Note the marked variation in clinical expression among living affected heterozygotes.

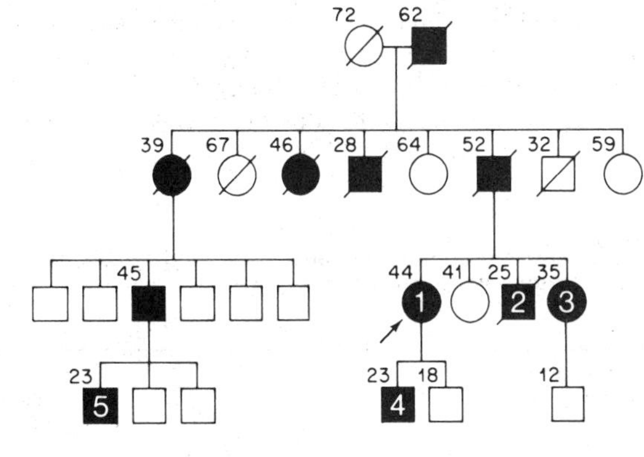

the skin, or bitemporal hemianopsia. The recognition that each family member suffers from the same genetic abnormality can be difficult, as illustrated by the family pedigree in Fig. 58-6.

Since dominant mutations involve a type of gene product that in a 50 percent abnormality is capable of producing clinical symptoms in heterozygotes, the responsible mutations are likely to involve abnormalities in two classes of proteins: (1) those that regulate complex metabolic pathways, such as membrane receptors and rate-limiting enzymes in pathways under feedback control, and (2) key structural proteins, such as hemoglobin or collagen.

The basic biochemical defects have been identified in only a handful of the approximately 600 autosomal dominant disorders. These include familial hypercholesterolemia (abnormal cell surface receptor that binds plasma low-density lipoprotein and thereby regulates cholesterol metabolism); hereditary methemoglobinemia and several hemolytic anemias due to unstable forms of hemoglobin (abnormal hemoglobin molecule); hereditary angioneurotic edema (abnormal protein inhibitor of an enzyme involved in the serum complement system); acute intermittent porphyria (abnormal enzyme that catalyzes a rate-limiting step in the heme biosynthetic pathway); and pseudohypoparathyroidism, type 1 (abnormal guanine nucleotide-binding regulatory component or *N*-protein of the adenylate cyclase system).

Autosomal recessive disorders Autosomal recessive conditions are clinically apparent only in the homozygous state, that is, when both alleles at a particular genetic locus are mutant. By definition, the gene responsible for an autosomal recessive disorder must be on one of the 22 autosomes; thus, both males and females can be affected.

Figure 58-7 shows a pedigree in which an autosomal recessive trait is present in the family. The following features are characteristic: (1) the parents are clinically normal; (2) only siblings are affected, and vertical transmission does not occur; and (3) males and females are affected in equal proportions.

The relative infrequency of recessive genes in the population and the requirement for two abnormal genes for clinical expression combine to create special conditions for autosomal recessive inheritance: (1) the more infrequent the mutant gene in the population, the stronger the likelihood that affected individuals are the product of consanguineous matings (see below); (2) if a husband and a wife are both carriers for the same autosomal recessive gene, 25 percent of the children will be normal, 50 percent will be heterozygous carriers, and 25 percent will be homozygous and affected with the disease; (3) if an affected individual marries a heterozygote (as may occur with consanguineous marriage), half the children will be affected, and a pedigree simulating dominant inheritance will result; and (4) if two individuals with the same recessive disease marry, all their children will be affected.

The clinical picture in autosomal recessive disorders tends to be more uniform than that of dominant diseases, and the age of onset is often early in life. As a general rule, recessive disorders are more commonly diagnosed in children, while dominant diseases are more frequently encountered in adults.

Since with recessive inheritance only one of four children in a sibship is expected to be affected, multiple cases in a family may not occur. This is especially true in a society in which small families are common. Consider, for example, 16 families in which both parents are heterozygous for the same recessive disorder. If each family has two children, 9 of the families will have no affected children, 6 will have one affected and one normal child, and only 1 of the 16 families will have two affected children. In the United States physicians usually see sporadic or isolated cases of a recessive disorder without an affected sibling to alert them to the possibility of a genetic disorder. Fortunately, because of the relatively uniform clinical picture of recessive disorders and because most can be diagnosed directly by biochemical tests, the correct diagnosis can usually be made even when no other members of a family are clinically affected.

The basic biochemical lesions underlying many autosomal recessive disorders have been identified. Of the three types of proteins in which mutations could occur (i.e., enzymes, structural proteins, and regulatory proteins), the one most easy to study has been the enzymes. A mutation that destroys the catalytic activity of an enzyme generally does not impair the health of a heterozygote (i.e., an individual who has one mutant allele specifying a functionless enzyme and one normal allele on the partner chromosome specifying a normal enzyme). In this situation each cell in the body usually produces about 50 percent of the normal number of active enzyme molecules. However, normal regulatory mechanisms function to avert any clinical consequences of this 50 percent deficiency, and so heterozygotes usually are clinically normal. On the other hand, when an individual inherits functionless alleles at both loci specifying an enzyme, the reduction in enzyme activity is too great for a compensatory mechanism to overcome, and a disease results. For example, heterozygotes for phenylketonuria who have half the normal activity of phenylalanine hydroxylase are clinically asymptomatic because the body compensates for the half-normal level of the enzyme by raising the substrate concentration approximately twofold. Under these conditions a normal amount of phenylalanine can be metabolized with no symptoms. On the other hand, the homozygote for phenylketonuria has such a severe reduction in phenylalanine hydroxylase activity that enormous levels of phenylalanine and its derivatives accumulate, causing detrimental brain development. As in the case of phenylketonuria, the majority of enzyme deficiency states produce *simultaneously* both a simple accumulation of

TABLE 58-4
Approximate proportion of patients affected by new mutations in some autosomal dominant disorders

Disorder	*Percentage*
Achondroplasia	80
Tuberous sclerosis	80
Neurofibromatosis	40
Marfan's syndrome	30
Myotonic dystrophy	25
Huntington's chorea	4
Adult polycystic kidney disease	1
Familial hypercholesterolemia	Very low

FIGURE 58-7
Pedigree pattern of an autosomal recessive trait. Note the horizontal *pattern of inheritance.*

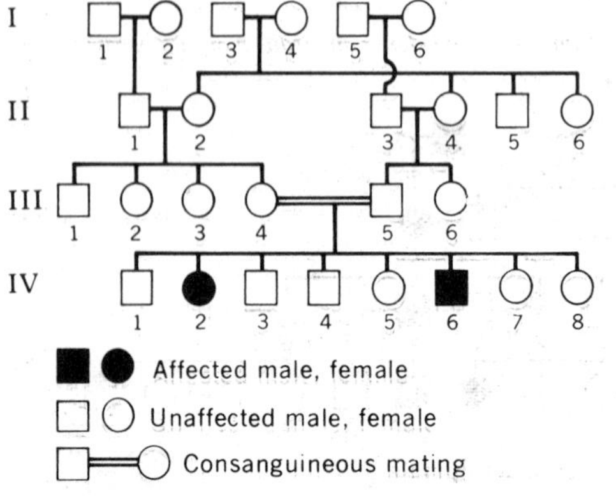

one or more metabolites preceding the enzymatic block and a deficient production of other metabolites distal to the block in the metabolic pathway.

Most of the genetic enzyme deficiencies that have been elucidated are not only inherited as recessive traits but also tend to involve enzymes that participate in catabolic pathways. Frequently these enzymes degrade organic molecules that are ingested in the diet, such as galactose (galactosemia), phenylalanine (phenylketonuria), and phytanic acid (Refsum's syndrome). A special class of such catabolic diseases is that in which the deficiency affects an acid hydrolase that occurs within lysosomes. In these *lysosomal storage disorders* the substrate, usually a complex lipid or polysaccharide, accumulates within swollen lysosomes in specific organs, giving the cells a foamy appearance. Examples of such lysosomal diseases include the mucopolysaccharidoses such as Hurler's syndrome (α-iduronidase deficiency) and the lipid storage diseases such as Gaucher's disease (glucocerebrosidase deficiency).

In general, recessive diseases are rare because the reduced biologic fitness of homozygotes acts to remove the mutant gene from the population. However, a few recessive disorders, such as cystic fibrosis and sickle cell anemia, are common. To explain this paradox, it has been postulated that the biologic fitness of heterozygotes is greater than that of noncarriers for these genes. In such a case the frequency of the gene in the population depends on the balance between the increased fitness of the relatively numerous heterozygotes and the reduced fitness of the less common homozygotes. A small selective advantage of the heterozygote over the normal results in a high gene frequency and hence a high birth frequency of homozygotes even when the disease is lethal. Thus, about 1 in 22 Caucasians is a heterozygous carrier for the genetically lethal disease cystic fibrosis, and the disease occurs in about 1 in 2000 Caucasian births. To maintain such a high gene frequency, heterozygotes for cystic fibrosis must have a definite reproductive advantage over noncarriers, but the nature of this advantage is unknown. In sickle cell anemia, another recessive disorder with high frequency among certain populations, heterozygotes appear to have increased resistance to malaria.

Inasmuch as recessive diseases require the inheritance of a mutation at the same genetic locus from each parent, when the genes are rare, the likelihood of any two parents being carriers for the same defect becomes small. However, if the parents have a common ancestor and if that ancestor was a carrier for the recessive gene, then the likelihood that two of the descendants have inherited the gene becomes relatively great. The rarer the recessive gene, the stronger becomes the likelihood that an affected individual will have resulted from such a consanguineous mating. On the other hand, certain recessive genes are so common in the population that the likelihood of two random parents being carriers is great enough to eliminate the need for consanguinity. For common traits such as sickle cell anemia, phenylketonuria, cystic fibrosis, and Tay-Sachs disease, all of which have a high carrier frequency in certain populations, consanguinity is usually not present in the parents.

In general, consanguinity is an infrequent finding clinically in families with recessive diseases in the United States. This is because the background rate of consanguinity in the general population is low. In most of the United States (as opposed to areas with relative geographic isolation such as northern Norway and Switzerland), a disorder must indeed be rare before it is associated with an important frequency of consanguinity. For example, consanguinity is expected in a large proportion of families having children with very rare disorders such as the Laurence-Moon-Biedl syndrome and abetalipoproteinemia.

Genetic compounds represent a special type of recessively inherited disorder in which the affected individual's two mutant genes, although derived from the same genetic locus, are not identical. The mutations in the paternal and maternal alleles presumably involve different alterations in the DNA of the same gene. SC hemoglobinopathy is an example of such a *heteroallelic* compound state in which individuals have a gene for sickle cell hemoglobin on one chromosome and a gene for hemoglobin C on the homologous chromosome.

X-linked disorders The genes responsible for X-linked disorders are located on the X chromosome; therefore, the clinical risk and severity of the disease are different for the two sexes. Since a female has two X chromosomes, she may be either heterozygous or homozygous for a mutant gene, and the trait may therefore demonstrate either recessive or dominant expression. Males, on the other hand, have only one X chromosome, so they can be expected to display the full syndrome whenever they inherit the gene regardless of whether the gene behaves as a recessive or as a dominant trait in the female. Thus, the terms *X-linked dominant* or *X-linked recessive* refer only to the expression of the gene in women.

An important feature of all X-linked inheritance is the absence of male-to-male (i.e., father-to-son) transmission of the trait. This follows because a male must always contribute his Y chromosome to his sons; hence, he can never contribute his X chromosome. On the other hand, a male contributes his one X chromosome to all his daughters.

The pedigree in Fig. 58-8 illustrates the characteristic features of X-linked recessive inheritance. (1) In contrast to the vertical transmission in dominant traits (parents and children affected) and the horizontal transmission in autosomal recessive traits (siblings affected), the pedigree pattern in X-linked recessive traits tends to be oblique because of the occurrence of the trait in the sons of normal carrier sisters of affected males (uncles and nephews affected) (Fig. 58-8*A*); (2) male offspring of carrier women have a 50 percent chance of being affected; (3) all female offspring of affected males are carriers, and affected males do not transmit the disease to their sons (Fig. 58-8*C*); (4) unaffected males do not transmit the trait to any offspring; and (5) affected homozygous females occur only when an affected male fathers the child of a carrier female (Fig. 58-8*B*).

Examples of X-linked recessive disorders in humans include hemophilia A, nephrogenic diabetes insipidus, the Lesch-Nyhan syndrome, Duchenne form of muscular dystrophy, glucose 6-phosphate dehydrogenase deficiency, testicular feminization, and Fabry's disease. Color blindness is also inherited as an X-linked recessive trait, but it is sufficiently frequent (occurring in about 8 percent of white males) that the occurrence of homozygous color-blind females is no rarity.

X-linked dominant inheritance is illustrated by the pedigree in Fig. 58-9. Its characteristic features are as follows: (1) Females are affected about twice as often as males; (2) an affected female transmits the disorder to half of her sons and half of her daughters; (3) an affected male transmits the disorder to all his daughters and to none of his sons; and (4) the syndrome is more variable and less severe in heterozygous affected females than in hemizygous affected males. One common trait, the Xg(a+) blood group, is inherited as an X-linked dominant trait, as is vitamin D–resistant rickets (hypophosphatemic rickets).

Some rare conditions may be inherited as X-linked dominant traits in which there is lethality in the hemizygous male. The characteristics of this form of inheritance are illustrated by the pedigree in Fig. 58-10: (1) The disorder occurs only in females who are heterozygous for the mutant gene, (2) an af-

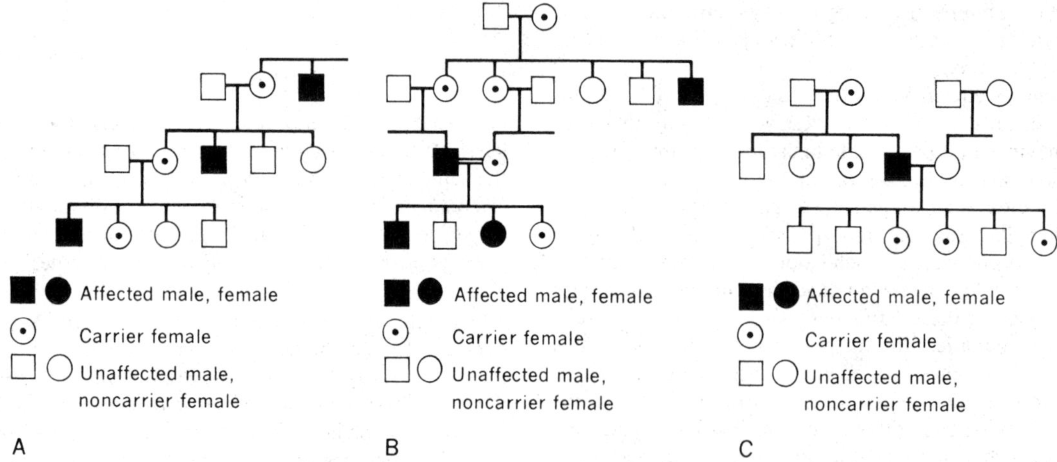

FIGURE 58-8
Pedigree patterns of an X-linked recessive trait. A. Note the oblique pattern of inheritance. B. An affected female can result from the mating of an affected male and a carrier female, as in the consanguineous marriage shown here. C. An affected male mating with a normal noncarrier female has all normal sons and all carrier daughters.

fected mother transmits the trait to half of her daughters, (3) an increased frequency of abortions occurs in affected women, the abortions representing affected male fetuses. Conditions that appear to be transmitted by this mode of inheritance include incontinentia pigmenti, focal dermal hypoplasia, orofaciodigital syndrome, and hyperammonemia due to ornithine transcarbamylase deficiency.

Expression of X-linked traits in females tends to be variable because of the phenomenon of X-chromosome inactivation. Early in embryonic development one of the two X chromosomes in each somatic cell of a female is inactivated. The inactivation process is random, so that for each cell there is an equal probability that the paternally or maternally derived X chromosome will be inactivated. The inactivated X chromosome is rendered permanently nonfunctional, so that all progeny of the initial cell inherit the same active and inactive X chromosomes. Thus, each female is a mosaic; on the average, half of her cells express the X chromosome of the father, and half express the X chromosome of the mother. If a mutation in a gene is carried on one of her X chromosomes, about one-half of the cells in each tissue will be normal and the other half will manifest the mutant phenotype. However, chance or selection of one or the other set of clones of cells may disturb these proportions in any given individual. Depending on the proportions of mutant and normal X chromosomes in each tissue, a genetically heterozygous female may either be clinically normal or have mild or severe manifestations of the disease. To illustrate, mothers of boys with the X-linked recessive Duchenne form of muscular dystrophy may occasionally show mild manifestations of the disease, such as limb girdle weakness or hypertrophied calves.

In each female cell the nonfunctional X chromosome can be visualized by several techniques. By ordinary staining, the inactivated X chromosome in metaphase appears heteropyknotic (condensed in appearance), and it replicates late in the mitotic cycle ("late-labeling" with tritiated thymidine). In nondividing cells the inactivated X chromosome can be observed as a clump of chromatin at the periphery of the nucleus—the so-called X chromatin or Barr body. In abnormal states with more than two X chromosomes such as 47 XXX, all but one of the X chromosomes are inactivated, so female cells may have multiple X chromatin bodies (see Chap. 61).

Since a single mutant allele is sufficient for the expression of X-linked recessive disorders, consanguinity does not increase the likelihood of expression in males, unlike the case in the rare autosomal recessive disorders. On the other hand, just as in the dominantly inherited disorders, new mutations can be a factor. In general, if an X-linked recessive condition reduces biologic fitness to zero, one-third of affected males will be a result of new mutations, and an additional one-third will be born to mothers who themselves are carriers as a result of a new mutation. Thus, only one-third will come from a classic pedigree

FIGURE 58-9
Pedigree pattern of an X-linked dominant trait.

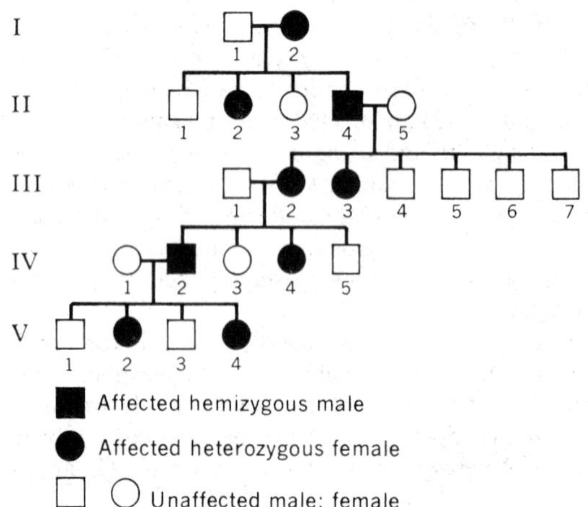

FIGURE 58-10
Pedigree pattern of an X-linked dominant trait lethal in the hemizygous male.

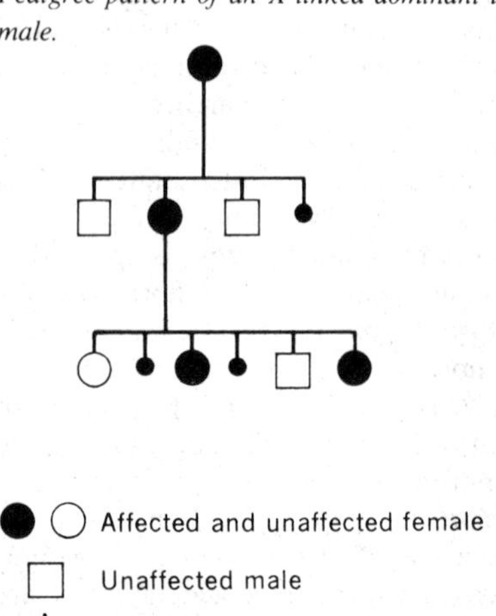

manifesting oblique transmission. An example of such a disease is the Duchenne form of muscular dystrophy in which affected hemizygous males are so severely disabled that they never reproduce. In hemophilia A, in which the biologic fitness is greater than zero, about 20 percent of affected males represent new mutations.

In families in which only one male is affected with an X-linked recessive disease and there is no other family history of the trait, it is essential for proper genetic counseling that the mother undergo biochemical tests or other relevant studies to determine whether she is a carrier. If she is a carrier, half of her daughters will be carriers and half of her sons will be affected. On the other hand, if her affected son represents a new mutation, only his daughters will inherit the gene. At present, biochemical tests can identify female carriers for several X-linked diseases including the Lesch-Nyhan syndrome, Fabry's disease, Hunter's syndrome, hemophilia, and the Duchenne form of muscular dystrophy.

The distinction between X-linked inheritance and *sex-influenced autosomal dominant inheritance* is important. Baldness is probably inherited as an autosomal dominant trait, yet it is manifested mainly in men and rarely in women. Heterozygous females express the baldness gene only when a source of testosterone becomes available as occurs with a masculinizing tumor of the ovary.

MULTIFACTORIAL GENETIC DISEASES The common chronic diseases of adults (such as essential hypertension, coronary heart disease, diabetes mellitus, peptic ulcer disease, and schizophrenia) as well as the common birth defects (such as cleft lip and palate, spina bifida, and congenital heart disease) have been long known to "run in families." They fit best into the category of *multifactorial genetic diseases.* The genetic element in these disorders rarely manifests itself in an all-or-none fashion as it does in the simply inherited (mendelian) disorders and in chromosomal aberrations. Instead, it is the interaction of multiple genes with multiple environmental factors that produces the familial aggregation.

In the multifactorial genetic diseases, there is a *polygenic component* consisting of a series of genes that interact in a cumulative fashion. An individual who inherits just the right combination of these genes passes beyond a "threshold of risk," at which point an *environmental component* determines whether and to what extent that person is clinically affected. In order for another individual in the same family to express the same syndrome, the same or similar combination of genes must be inherited. Since the first-degree relatives of an affected individual (i.e., parents, siblings, and offspring) each share half of that person's genes, they are all at increased risk of exhibiting the same polygenic syndrome. Second-degree relatives (uncles, aunts, and grandparents) share on the average one-fourth of an individual's genes $(\frac{1}{2})^2$, and third-degree relatives (cousins) share one-eighth $(\frac{1}{2})^3$. Thus, as the degree of relation becomes more distant, the likelihood of a relative inheriting the same combination of genes becomes less. Moreover, the chances of any relative inheriting the right combination of risk genes decrease as the number of genes required for the expression of a given trait increases.

Since the precise number of genes responsible for polygenic traits is unknown, the risk of inheritance for a relative of an affected individual is difficult to calculate, and the standard is based on empiric risk figures (i.e., a direct tally of the proportion of affected relatives in previously reported families). In contrast to the simply inherited disorders in which 25 or 50 percent of the first-degree relatives of an affected proband are at genetic risk, multifactorial genetic disorders are generally observed empirically to affect no more than 5 to 10 percent of first-degree relatives. Moreover, in contrast to mendelian traits, the recurrence risk of multifactorial conditions varies from family to family, and its estimation is significantly influenced by two factors: (1) the number of affected persons already present in the family, and (2) the severity of the disorder in the index case. The greater the number of affected relatives and the more severe their disease, the higher the risk to other relatives. For example, the risk of cleft lip in the siblings of a child with unilateral cleft lip is about 2.5 percent, but if the lesion in the index case is bilateral, the risk in the siblings rises to 6 percent. Table 58-5 lists the empirical risk figures for the familial recurrence of a number of multifactorial genetic diseases.

The hypothesis of a polygenic component in the inheritance of multifactorial diseases has been given a sound basis in recent years by the demonstration that at least one-third of all gene loci harbor polymorphic alleles that vary among individuals. Such a large degree of variation in normal genes undoubtedly provides the substrate for variations in genetic predisposition with which environmental factors can interact. So far, the genetic loci most strikingly associated with predisposition to specific diseases are those that constitute the HLA system (also called the *major histocompatibility gene complex*) (see Chap. 60). The HLA gene complex is located on the short arm of chromosome 6. It consists of four closely linked but distinct loci (A, B, C, and D). The products of these genes are proteins that are found on the surface of body cells and that enable an individual's immune system to distinguish its own cells from those of someone else. Each HLA locus in the population consists of multiple alleles, each of which produces an immunologically distinct protein. For example, an individual may inherit any 2 of 20 alleles at the HLA-B locus.

An important observation of recent years has been the finding that certain alleles at the HLA loci predispose individuals to certain specific diseases. For example, if the B27 allele at the HLA-B locus is inherited by an individual, that person has a 121-fold greater chance of developing ankylosing spondylitis than an individual who lacks this allele (Table 58-6). Ankylosing spondylitis remains a multifactorial disease, however, because its development clearly requires one or more other factors in addition to the B27 allele. Thus, less than 15 percent of people who inherit this allele develop this disease. Table 58-6 lists some of the diseases associated with alleles at the HLA loci. Several of them in the past have been suspected to be of viral etiology, suggesting that the HLA loci may dictate the mode of expression of certain viral diseases. A more detailed discussion of the HLA system is presented in Chap. 60.

Multifactorial disorders are heterogeneous in the sense that

TABLE 58-5
Empiric risks for some common multifactorial genetic diseases affecting adults

Disorder in index case	*Estimated absolute risk for first-degree relatives, %*
Cleft lip and/or palate	3
Congenital heart disease	4
Coronary heart disease	8 for male relatives 3 for female relatives
Diabetes mellitus	5–10
Epilepsy	5–10
Hypertension	10
Manic-depressive psychosis	10–15
Psoriasis	10–15
Schizophrenia	15
Thyroid disease (autoimmune disorders including hyperthyroidism, thyroiditis, primary myxedema, simple goiter)	10

TABLE 58-6

Alleles at the HLA loci associated with multifactorial genetic diseases

Disease	*HLA locus*	*Specific allele*	*Relative risk**
Ankylosing spondylitis	B	B27	121
Reiter's syndrome	B	B27	40
Psoriasis with arthritis	B	B27	5
Celiac disease	B	B8	10
Chronic active hepatitis	B	B8	4
Myasthenia gravis	B	B8	4
Diabetes mellitus	B	B8, B15	3
(insulin-dependent)	D	D3	3
Hyperthyroidism	D	D3	4
Addison's disease	B	B8	7
	D	D4	10
Multiple sclerosis	D	D2	7

* Relative risk *is the probability of the disease developing in an individual with the specific allele, divided by the probability of its development in an individual who does not possess this specific allele.*

the relative contribution of the polygenic factors ("risk genes") and environmental factors to the etiology vary greatly from patient to patient. However, it is important to remember that among common phenotypes which are largely multifactorial, often a small proportion will be created by major mutant genes. For example, although coronary heart disease is usually of multifactorial etiology, about 5 percent of subjects with premature myocardial infarctions are heterozygotes for familial hypercholesterolemia, a single-gene disorder that produces atherosclerosis in the absence of any other predisposing factor. Similarly, in a small proportion of patients with other common diseases such as peptic ulcer disease or "essential" hypertension, the condition is not multifactorial but determined by a single gene, as in the multiple endocrine adenoma–peptic ulcer syndrome or the medullary thyroid carcinoma–pheochromocytoma syndrome, respectively.

INTERACTION BETWEEN SINGLE GENETIC AND ENVIRONMENTAL FACTORS

Many diseases result from an interaction between a specific genotype and a specific environmental factor. In particular, inherited single-gene mutations may produce clinically significant and often life-threatening idiosyncratic responses to certain drugs.

Table 58-7 lists the most important of these *pharmacogenetic disorders,* which encompass all the mendelian modes of inheritance. Perhaps the most common is glucose 6-phosphate dehydrogenase deficiency, an X-linked recessive trait in which a variety of drugs may precipitate a hemolytic anemia. Plasma pseudocholinesterase deficiency and hepatic transacetylase deficiency are examples of autosomal recessive traits which alter drug catabolism so that when the muscle relaxant suxamethonium or the antituberculous drug isoniazid is administered, apnea or peripheral neuropathy, respectively, may ensue. Malignant hyperthermia is an autosomal dominant trait in which acute hyperpyrexia, muscle rigidity, and hyperkalemic cardiac arrest may be induced by administration of any one of several anesthetic agents. Acute intermittent porphyria is another ex-

TABLE 58-7

Examples of inherited disorders involving an abnormal response to drugs

Disorder	*Molecular abnormality*	*Mode of inheritance*	*Frequency*	*Clinical effect*	*Drugs producing abnormal response*
Slow inactivation of isoniazid	Isoniazid acetylase in liver	Autosomal recessive	~50% of U.S. population	Polyneuritis	Isoniazid, sulfamethazine, sulfamaprine, phenelzine, dapsone, hydralazine
Suxamethonium sensitivity	Pseudocholinesterase in plasma	Autosomal recessive	Several mutant alleles; most common affects 1 in 2500	Apnea	Suxamethonium, succinylcholine
Coumadin	? Altered receptor or enzyme in liver with increased affinity for vitamin K	Autosomal dominant	Rare	Inability to achieve anticoagulation with usual doses of drug	Coumadin
Glaucoma	Unknown	? Autosomal dominant	Common	Increased intraocular pressure	Corticosteroids
Malignant hyperthermia	Unknown	Autosomal dominant	~1 in 20,000 anesthesized patients	Severe hyperpyrexia, muscle rigidity, death	Such anesthetics as halothane, succinylcholine, methoxyflurane, ether, cyclopropane
Unstable hemoglobins:					
Hemoglobin Zurich	Arginine substitution for histidine at sixty-third position of β chain of hemoglobin	Autosomal dominant	Rare	Hemolysis	Sulfonamides
Hemoglobin H	Hemoglobin composed of four β chains	Autosomal dominant	Rare	Hemolysis	Sulfisoxazole
Glucose 6-phosphate dehydrogenase deficiency	Glucose 6-phosphate dehydrogenase in erythrocytes	X-linked recessive	~ 1×10^8 affected persons in world; common in persons of African, Mediterranean, Asiatic origin; multiple mutant alleles	Hemolysis	Analgesics, sulfonamides, antimalarials, nitrofurantoin, other drugs

SOURCE: *ES Vesell, N Engl J Med 287:904, 1972.*

ample of a genetic disorder that is exacerbated by drugs, such as barbiturates.

Misinterpretation of adverse drug reactions may result in serious harm to patients. In general, all unusual idiosyncratic reactions should be considered to be genetically determined until proved otherwise. Fortunately, the pharmacogenetic disorders are a group of diseases for which therapy is straightforward: avoidance of the noxious drug by patient and relatives.

In addition to drugs, other factors in the environment may aggravate specific genetic traits. Cigarette smoke may have deleterious effects on persons homozygous and possibly heterozygous for alpha_1-antitrypsin deficiency, who are predisposed to the development of emphysema. Patients with xeroderma pigmentosa and anhydrotic ectodermal dysplasia are unusually sensitive to sunlight and high temperatures, respectively. Avoidance of milk at an early age prevents many of the complications ordinarily seen in persons with galactosemia.

Genetic-environmental interactions are particularly important in pregnancy. Women who are affected with phenylketonuria may develop high plasma phenylalanine levels during pregnancy, and thus their offspring may suffer from a variety of phenylalanine-induced birth defects even though the offspring may not themselves have phenylketonuria. Other examples of diseases resulting from an adverse genetic relation between the mother and fetus include erythroblastosis caused by Rh incompatibility and diabetic embryopathy, a term that refers to a series of major birth defects occurring in about 5 percent of the offspring of women who are clinically diabetic during pregnancy.

REFERENCES

HARRIS H: *The Principles of Human Biochemical Genetics,* 3d ed. New York, American Elsevier, 1981

JACKSON LG, SCHIMKE RN: *Clinical Genetics: A Source Book for Physicians.* New York, Wiley, 1979

LEWIN B: *Gene Expression 2,* 2d ed. New York, Wiley, 1980

MCKUSICK VA: *Mendelian Inheritance in Man: Catalogs of Autosomal Dominant, Autosomal Recessive and X-Linked Phenotypes,* 5th ed. Baltimore, Johns Hopkins, 1978

———: The anatomy of the human genome. Am J Med 69:267, 1980

STANBURY JB et al: *The Metabolic Basis of Inherited Disease,* 5th ed. New York, McGraw-Hill, 1983

VOGEL F, MOTULSKY AG: *Human Genetics: Problems and Approaches.* Berlin, Springer-Verlag, 1979

59 RECOMBINANT DNA GENETICS AND MEDICINE

HENRY M. KRONENBERG

Development of recombinant DNA technology has made it possible to isolate DNA sequences or genes from mammalian cells and to replicate these genes in bacteria. At an operational level the technological advances that have permitted this capacity are straightforward and sensitive. At the clinical level they have led to remarkable advances that affect many aspects of medicine, including the identification of mutations, the diagnosis of affected and carrier states for hereditable diseases, the mapping of human genes on the chromosomes, the isolation and alteration of genes, the transfer of genes from one organism to another, and the production of hormones, vaccines, and other biological agents of pharmacological impor-

tance. In this chapter the principles of recombinant DNA technology will be reviewed, and the uses of the technology for medicine will be discussed.

THE STRUCTURE OF GENES DNA is a polymer of nucleotides (Fig. 59-1). Each nucleotide contains one of four nitrogenous bases [adenine (A), cytosine (C), guanine (G), or thymine (T)], the sugar deoxyribose, and phosphate that is linked to the 5′-hydroxyl group of the deoxyribose. The phosphate group of one nucleotide is covalently bonded to the 3′-hydroxyl group of the adjacent nucleotide, thus creating a backbone of alternating sugar and phosphate, from which the nitrogenous bases extend. The fact that the 5′-hydroxyl of one sugar is linked to the 3′-hydroxyl of the adjacent sugar gives each DNA molecule polarity—one end with a free 5′-phosphate and the other with a free 3′-hydroxyl group. In nature, DNA is usually double stranded—the familiar double helix. As a result of base pairing, the sequence of bases in each strand is related to each other in that A in one strand always bonds with T in the other; similarly, G and C are always paired. Such related DNA sequences are called complementary sequences. Since appropriate A-T and G-C pairing stabilizes the DNA helix, single-stranded DNA binds (hybridizes) to its complementary strand with high affinity and specificity.

Human DNA differs from bacterial DNA in several respects. Genes that are transcribed into messenger RNA are often interrupted by sequences not found in messenger RNA (Fig. 58-1). These intervening sequences (introns) are transcribed along with the messenger RNA sequences (exons) to form a large, short-lived precursor of messenger RNA. The transcription of DNA produces a faithful RNA copy of the entire gene sequence (exons plus introns). This RNA transcript is edited in the nucleus before it passes into the cytoplasm; in this process RNA corresponding to intervening sequences is excised, and the coding sequences are spliced together to form a functionally active messenger RNA (mRNA) molecule (Fig. 58-2). Biochemical characterization of human genes was made even more difficult by the fact that the various genes are covalently linked into 46 larger molecules, the chromosomes, and by the size of the human genome—some 9×10^8 nucleotides in the haploid state. For example, a gene of typical size represents only a millionth of the total DNA. As in bacteria certain DNA sequences regulate the transcription of genes. Human regulatory sequences, however, can be located hundreds of nucleotides away from the genes they regulate or in the middle of

FIGURE 59-1
DNA molecule (see text for details).

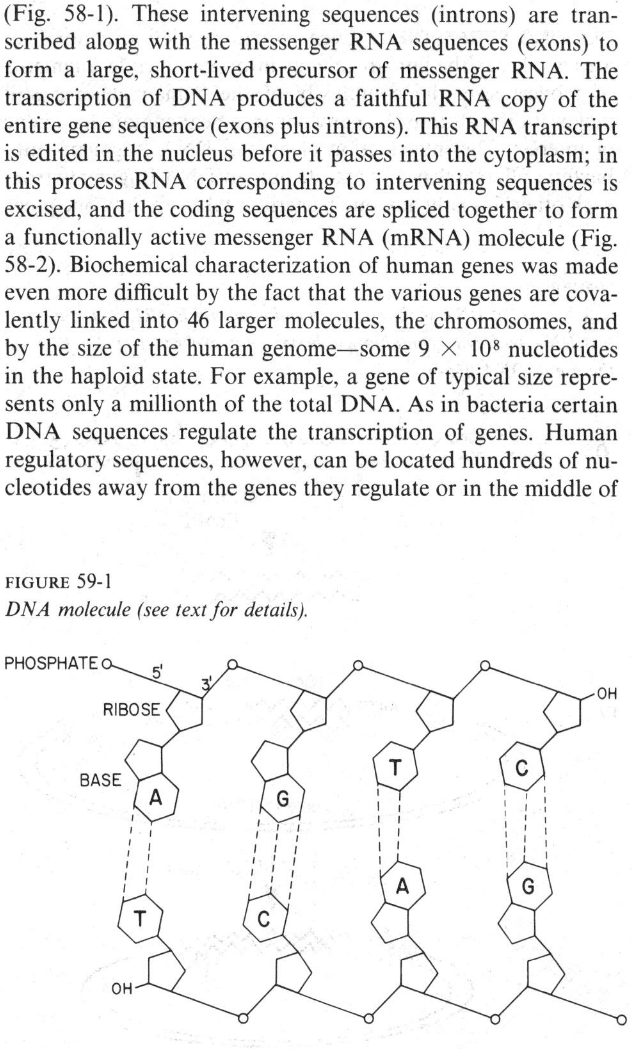

transcribed genes. The mechanisms by which these sequences regulate gene transcription are under investigation.

RESTRICTION ENDONUCLEASES Discovery of restriction endonucleases has made it possible to fragment the huge DNA molecules that comprise the 46 human chromosomes into smaller fragments and consequently to isolate genes from these large molecules. These restriction enzymes, isolated from bacteria, cleave DNA only at specific DNA sequences. The enzyme EcoRI, for example, recognizes the sequence 5′GAATTC3′ (Fig. 59-2*A*). The enzyme cleaves each strand of the double-stranded DNA between the first nucleotide, G, and the second nucleotide, A, creating two free ends, each with a short single-stranded DNA extension (AATT or TTAA). Thus, EcoRI cleaves DNA only when the sequence GAATTC appears, generating fragments of characteristic size for each type of DNA substrate. In this way restriction endonucleases allow the reproducible fragmentation of DNA, analogous to the reproducible fragmentation of proteins by proteases such as trypsin. Note that each single-stranded end generated by EcoRI cleavage can hybridize to the complementary sequence extending from the terminus of the other newly created end. In similar fashion this so-called cohesive end can hybridize to the complementary strand from any EcoRI-cut piece of DNA. Thus a piece of human DNA cleaved with EcoRI can bind to a piece of bacterial DNA cleaved with the same enzyme, and the two nicks in the resulting single molecule of DNA can be repaired by the enzyme DNA ligase to form an intact, new, and hence *recombinant DNA* molecule (Fig. 59-2*B*).

CLONING STRATEGIES Even though restriction endonucleases can break the human genome into reproducible fragments of modest size, the complexity of the human genome still makes it difficult to isolate any one fragment containing a gene of interest. The introduction of human DNA fragments into bacteria offers a way to separate human DNA fragments from each other. Usually any one bacterium takes up only one piece

FIGURE 59-2
A. Cleavage of DNA with restriction endonuclease EcoRI. B. Ligation of two DNA molecules containing cohesive ends generated by EcoRI with the use of DNA ligase.

A. human DNA 5′ GAATTC GAATTC 3′
3′ CTTAAG CTTAAG 5′
cleave with EcoRI
AATTC G
G CTTAA

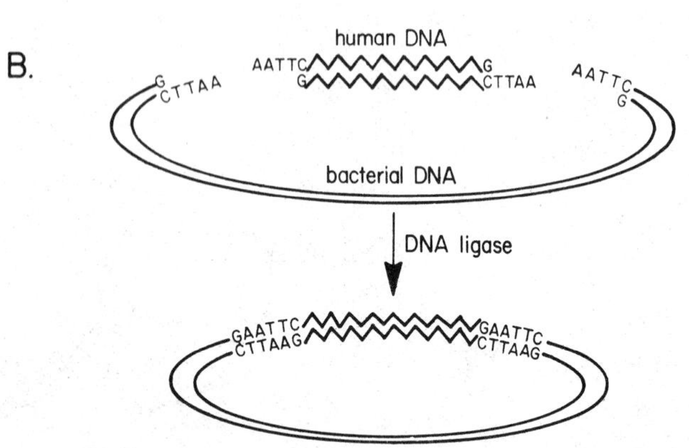

of exogenous DNA. After these bacteria are spread on agar dishes and incubated, each resultant colony represents the progeny of only one bacterium. Consequently, any one colony (clone) contains the sequence of only one fragment of exogenous human DNA. The cloning procedure thus separates individual human DNA fragments and makes it possible to isolate large amounts of this DNA, since bacteria are easy to grow.

To replicate in bacteria the human DNA must be linked to specific DNA sequences that direct bacterial DNA replication. Since bacterial plasmids and DNA viruses (phage) contain such replication sequences, human DNA must be ligated either to plasmid DNA or to phage DNA before it is introduced into the bacteria. These plasmids or phage are called *vectors* and can be designed with features that make them useful cloning vehicles. The use of plasmids containing genes encoding antibiotic resistance allows the selection of the few bacteria that take up and replicate the plasmid DNA. If the plasmid encodes penicillinase, for example, growth of bacteria in ampicillin allows replication only of the bacteria that took up the exogenous plasmid.

The introduction of a human gene into a bacterial plasmid allows the human DNA to replicate in bacteria but does not necessarily allow the gene to be expressed. To transcribe the gene into RNA a specific sequence directing bacterial RNA polymerase to initiate transcription (a so-called promoter sequence) must be adjacent to the human gene. Further, for the newly transcribed mRNA to be translated, specific sequences directing the mRNA to bind to bacterial ribosomes must also be present near the beginning of the sequence encoding the human protein. With the use of appropriately constructed plasmid or phage vectors, human gene products can become quantitatively major proteins in the bacterial cell.

In addition to bacteria (and yeasts), other host cells can be used to purify, amplify, and express sequences of human DNA. Mammalian cells, with their large genomes, slow doubling times, and demanding growth conditions are more difficult to use as hosts for purification and amplification of human genes, but they do have certain properties that make them attractive hosts for recombinant DNA vectors. For example, mammalian cells recognize specific regulatory signals in human DNA such as binding sites for RNA polymerase, and they contain the appropriate machinery for removing intervening sequences that interrupt the sequences coding for many human mRNAs. (Bacteria cannot remove intervening sequences from precursors of mammalian mRNA.) Mammalian cells also recognize peptide signals that trigger posttranslational modification of protein (such as cleavage or glycosylation) and that direct proteins to specific cellular compartments. Finally, mammalian cells are large enough to allow direct injection of DNA into nuclei. These cells can also be induced to take up naked DNA from culture medium. Thus, bacteria, yeast, and mammalian cells can all be hosts for recombinant DNA vectors; the choice depends on the particular goals of the experiment.

SOURCES OF DNA FOR CLONING Native DNA is the most straightforward source of DNA for cloning, but so many genes are present in every cell that it is difficult to isolate individual specific fragments. Consequently, DNA for cloning is often made enzymatically by copying mRNA into DNA with the enzyme reverse transcriptase (copy DNA, or cDNA). mRNA is a preferred starting material, because tissues that make particular proteins are enriched for the mRNAs that code for these proteins. In contrast, all tissues contain the same DNA. Generally, specific mRNAs of interest make up 0.01 to 1 percent of the mRNA in appropriate cells, in contrast to individual genes, which usually make up about 0.0001 percent of DNA. A third source of DNA for cloning is chemically synthesized DNA. If a desired protein's amino acid sequence is known, the genetic code can be used to predict possible DNA sequences that can encode the protein. These sequences can then be synthesized and cloned using plasmid vectors. In each of the latter instances the DNA sequence does not contain any intervening sequences that would be present in the native gene. The source of DNA used depends on the particular objectives of the cloning and the feasibility of obtaining DNA from alternative sources.

CLINICAL IMPLICATIONS One contribution of recombinant DNA technology to clinical medicine is a new understanding of gene expression. Human genes can now be isolated and analyzed, and their RNA and protein derivatives can be produced in vitro and in vivo. The ability to clone and sequence the human alpha- and beta-globin genes, for example, made it possible to define multiple causes of the thalassemia syndromes. Beta thalassemia occurs, for example, when little or no beta globin is made in red cell precursors. By cloning the beta-globin genes from patients, a variety of causes of the beta-thalassemia phenotype have been discovered. One gene is missing part of the beta-globin sequence. Others contain single base changes that instruct the cell to stop protein synthesis prematurely. An unanticipated group of mutants causes abnormal removal of intervening DNA sequences, thereby decreasing the amount of normal, functional mRNA in the cell. One abnormal gene results from a single base change in the region that is thought important for regulation of gene transcription. These analyses are helping us understand the heterogeneity of beta thalassemia, suggesting methods of prenatal diagnosis (see below), and broadening our understanding of gene regulation (see Chap. 330).

Detection of specific genes In theory, any disease caused by the alteration of a particular gene can now be diagnosed in utero through the analysis of genes from amniotic fluid cells. Sickle cell anemia is an example of the importance of this phenomenon. To detect sickle cell hemoglobin itself it is necessary to analyze relatively inaccessible fetal erythrocytes. In contrast, to identify sickle cell hemoglobin genes, any fetal cells, including amniotic fluid cells, can be utilized. The simplest way to detect the sickle cell gene is illustrated in Fig. 59-3. DNA from amniotic fluid cells is cleaved with a restriction endonuclease, and the resultant DNA fragments are separated by size using gel electrophoresis. The DNA is then transferred to a sheet of nitrocellulose and hybridized with a radioactive copy of previously cloned human beta globin. The radioactive beta-globin DNA binds only to the DNA fragments containing beta-globin sequences, and this binding is detected by autoradiography.

The normal beta-globin gene has the nucleotide sequence CCTGAGGAG corresponding to the amino acids proline–glutamic acid–glutamic acid at one specific region of the gene. In contrast, the sickle beta-globin gene has the sequence CCTGTGGAG corresponding to the amino acids proline–valine–glutamic acid at the corresponding positions. One restriction endonuclease cleaves DNA at the sequence CCTGAGG but not at CCTGTGG and therefore cleaves the normal but not the sickle cell gene. The cleaved (normal) DNA has a different electrophoretic mobility than does the uncleaved (sickle) DNA, and the two can be distinguished as shown in Fig. 59-3. Of course, not all abnormal genes are associated conveniently with an alteration in a restriction endonuclease cleavage site. Nevertheless, the blot hybridization technique is likely to find increasing applicability in prenatal diagnosis and gene mapping. Even though mutations usually do not themselves change digestion patterns, mutations are often found linked closely to other DNA sequences that vary from person to person and that alter restriction enzyme digestion patterns. Consequently, digestion patterns generated by particular enzymes differ so often in the population that it is frequently possible to associate a mutant gene with a nearby restriction enzyme site. Family studies then make it possible to associate specific restriction enzyme patterns with particular paternal and maternal chromosomes. The use of these so-called restriction site polymorphisms has already aided in the prenatal diagnosis of beta thalassemia and sickle cell anemia and is likely to have widespread applicability.

The same sort of analysis used to detect abnormal human genes can be used to detect viral DNA genes in cells and tissues. Hepatitis viral DNA, for example, has been detected in liver biopsy samples from patients with chronic active hepatitis and hepatomas. The diagnosis of illness caused by other DNA viruses such as cytomegalovirus will be facilitated by similar sensitive hybridization assays using cloned DNA.

Synthesis of human proteins in bacteria Since a number of diseases are caused by deficiency of specific proteins, replacement therapy with proteins is an attractive strategy. Proteins can also be used as drugs, not to replace a deficiency but simply as bioactive agents; for example, calcitonin is used to inhibit bone resorption in Paget's disease. The current sources of natural proteins are limited, and as a consequence the ability to use polypeptides as drugs is also limited. Only small proteins can be synthesized chemically. Animal proteins are unsatisfactory in many instances because their antigenicity is unacceptable or because the animal protein is inactive in humans. Human proteins can be isolated from urine, blood, and pla-

FIGURE 59-3

A. Mst II restriction endonuclease cutting sites adjacent to human beta-globin gene. Starred Mst II site is missing in sickle beta-globin gene. B. Schematic depiction of autoradiographic analysis of DNA from normals (AA), homozygous sickle cell patients (SS), and patients with sickle cell trait (AS). DNA is digested with Mst II, fragments are separated according to size using agarose gel electrophoresis, transferred to nitrocellulose, hybridized with radioactive human beta-globin DNA, and exposed to x-ray film.

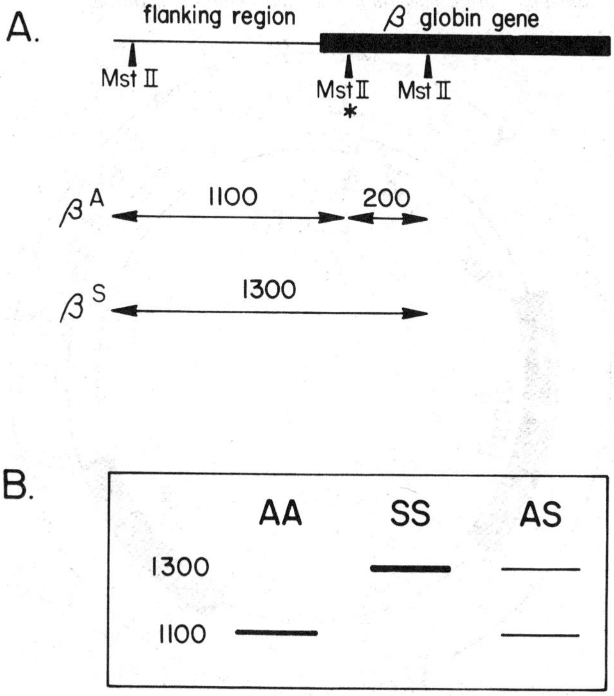

centa, but these are obviously in short supply. Moreover, a number of important proteins have never been purified from any source because they are present in such small amounts. The ability to synthesize human proteins in microorganisms may solve the problem of availability of human protein and the problem of the antigenicity of animal proteins and promises rapid advances in therapeutics.

For human DNA to direct protein synthesis in bacteria, the human DNA must be linked to DNA sequences instructing RNA polymerase to initiate RNA synthesis and to DNA sequences that encourage binding of mRNA to ribosomes. Such sequences can be synthesized chemically or isolated from bacterial sources. The optimal distance between the ribosomal binding site and the first triplet encoding a human protein varies from sequence to sequence and must be determined empirically. Figure 59-4 illustrates, for example, the plasmid first used to make human growth hormone in bacteria. Fragments of DNA from four different sources were attached, using restriction endonucleases to generate cohesive ends and DNA ligase to reattach the ends of the fragments together. Fragment A from the *Escherichia coli* genome provides a promoter sequence and a ribosomal binding sequence. Fragment B was synthesized chemically. It was designed to have an EcoRI recognition sequence to provide a cohesive end for binding to fragment A, followed by a nucleotide sequence coding for the first 24 amino acids of human growth hormone. Fragment C contains the rest of the human growth hormone nucleotide sequence. This fragment was obtained by prior cloning of a cDNA copy of part of the mRNA for human growth hormone. Fragment D comes from a bacterial plasmid and contains a sequence that allows the recombinant plasmid to replicate the *E. coli* and a sequence that encodes β-lactamase (penicillinase). The presence of the penicillinase gene, as described above, guarantees that all the bacteria that grow in the presence of ampicillin contain the recombinant plasmid.

Technical problems make the synthesis of some proteins a challenge. When mRNA is used as the source of cloned DNA, the nucleotide sequence often contains codons of amino acids found in precursor proteins rather than simply the codons of

FIGURE 59-4
Plasmid that directs bacteria to make human growth hormone.

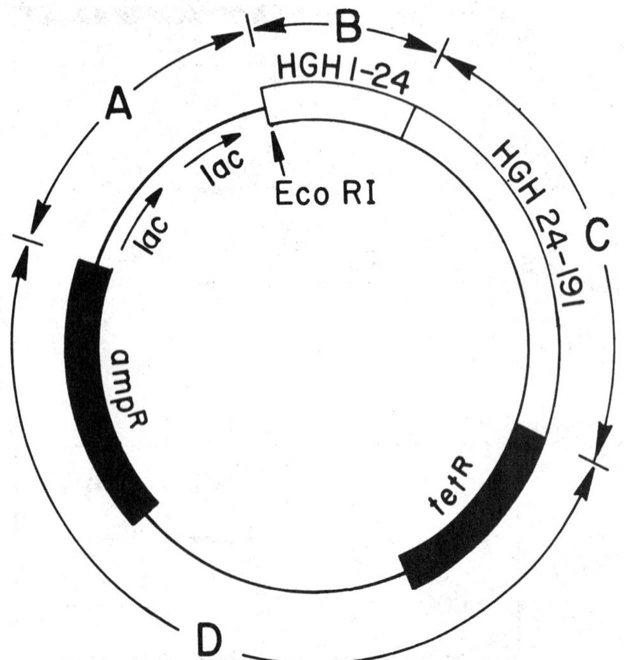

the desired mature protein, and sometimes the bacteria do not remove the precursor sequences from the synthesized proteins. Worse still, the bacteria degrade some foreign proteins rapidly, making it impossible to accumulate large amounts of the protein of interest. Proteins containing more than one polypeptide chain or requiring posttranslational modifications such as glycosylation and acetylation for activity, may be impossible to make in active form in bacteria or may need further processing after isolation from the bacteria. Finally, the most challenging constraint limiting the synthesis of a protein in bacteria can be the initial isolation of DNA encoding the protein. Even if the protein's amino acid sequence is known, synthesis of large DNA molecules is difficult. If the protein's amino acid sequence is unknown, then the corresponding DNA must be isolated from the genome or synthesized from mRNA using reverse transcriptase. Human genomic DNA often cannot be used because it is interrupted by intervening DNA sequences that microorganisms cannot remove. mRNA can be difficult to isolate if the tissue that makes the protein of interest is unknown or if the methods for assaying the protein's presence are insensitive. Despite these difficulties human insulin, interferon, and growth hormone synthesized in bacteria have already been used in clinical trials, and hepatitis B antigen has been synthesized for use in vaccines.

Gene replacement therapy It is theoretically possible to cure genetic disorders and manipulate the human genome by the introduction of recombinant DNA into cells. One approach would be the introduction of individual, well-defined genes into individual cells in vitro and the subsequent readministration of these cells into patients. For example, to restore beta-globin production in thalassemia the goal is to place normal beta-globin genes into the erythroblasts of affected individuals in a way that allows the normal expression of the gene. However, the problems of regulating gene expression in human cells are different from those of regulating gene expression in bacteria. Gene regulation in bacteria was understood prior to the development of recombinant DNA technology, and as a consequence recombinant DNA technology was exploited rapidly in bacteria. In contrast, the regulation of gene expression in mammalian cells was poorly understood prior to the development of the new technology. Remarkable progress has been made in this problem. Sequences analogous to bacterial promoters that signal the start of transcription have been identified. Other regulatory sequences, like those required for modulation of gene transcription by glucocorticoids and progestins have also been identified. Most important has been the discovery of sequences that allow the regulated transcription of the mouse beta-globin gene in a tissue culture model of erythrocyte differentiation. In the less differentiated tissue culture cell, the inserted mouse beta-globin gene is inactive, but the gene is activated by procedures that trigger the differentiation of the cell. These experiments suggest that DNA sequences adjacent to mammalian genes may contain information necessary for their regulated expression, even when the genes are inserted into cells in vitro.

An even more difficult problem in gene therapy is devising a means of reintroducing the treated cells in sufficient numbers into the affected subject in such a way that these cells will compete successfully with the mutant cells. Modifications of the strategies employed by transplantation teams might be suitable for use in life-threatening disorders. Less hazardous ways of promoting the growth of altered cells in recipients will be required before gene therapy can be more widely applied to a broad range of genetic disorders.

It is theoretically possible to introduce genes into fertilized eggs or early embryos in a way that will allow the genes to function only in the appropriate differentiated cells. In some experimental systems genes introduced into embryos are expressed in the adult animals, and the expression occurs only in the appropriate differentiated tissues. In these instances, then, DNA sequences immediately adjacent to a gene of interest contain sufficient information to allow normal expression of the gene during differentiation. On the other hand, some genes may have to be located in particular chromosomal regions or must participate in all of the stages of gametogenesis to function normally. The simple introduction of these genes into fertilized eggs would not be enough to guarantee normal regulation of differentiated expression of the genes.

Safety considerations Because of concern that the introduction of genes into cells never before containing those genes might be dangerous, recombinant DNA work in the United States has been practiced under guidelines promulgated by the National Institutes of Health. As data concerning the safety of recombinant DNA procedures have accumulated, the guidelines have been modified. In fact, recombinant DNA techniques may provide the safest way of handling dangerous genomes, such as those of pathogenic viruses. Antigens suitable for use in vaccines can be synthesized without the use of live virus. Complete viral genomes can be packaged inside bacterial cells ill-suited for survival in higher organisms. Not only have the potential dangers of recombinant DNA work failed to materialize, but the practical benefits of research using recombinant DNA techniques are appearing faster than even the most optimistic originally dared to predict.

REFERENCES

BRINSTER RL et al: Somatic expression of herpes thymidine kinase in mice following injection of a fusion gene into eggs. Cell 27:233, 1981

GOEDDEL DV et al: Direct expression in *Escherichia coli* of a DNA sequence coding for human growth hormone. Nature 281:544, 1979

ORKIN SH et al: Improved detection of the sickle mutation by DNA analysis and its application to prenatal diagnosis. N Engl J Med 307:32, 1982

60
THE MAJOR HISTOCOMPATIBILITY GENE COMPLEX

CHARLES B. CARPENTER

Antigenic differences between members of a species are called *alloantigens,* and when these play a determining role in the rejection of allogenic tissue grafts they are called *histocompatibility antigens.* Evolution has conserved a single closely linked region of histocompatibility genes, the products of which are prominently displayed on cell surfaces and provide a strong barrier to allotransplantation. The terms *major histocompatibility antigens* and *major histocompatibility gene complex* (MHC) refer to the gene products and genes of this single chromosomal region. Minor histocompatibility antigens, in contrast, are multiple and are encoded throughout the genome. They represent weaker allotypic differences on molecules that subserve a variety of functions. Structures bearing MHC antigens play a major role in immunity and possibly also in processes of self-recognition in the differentiation of cells and tissues. Much of the evidence for MHC control of the immune response comes from work in animal models in which immune-response genes have been mapped within the mouse (H-2), rat (RT1), or guinea pig (GPLA) MHC. In humans the MHC is called *HLA.* The individual letters of HLA have various meanings, and by international agreement HLA is the logo for the human MHC.

There are several generalities to be made about the MHCs of humans and other species. *First,* there are three classes of gene products encoded within the small [<2 cM (centimorgans)] region of the MHC: class I molecules, expressed on virtually all cell surfaces, consist of one heavy and one light polypeptide chain and are the products of three or more reduplicated loci (e.g. HLA-A, B, C, and H-2D, K, L). Class II molecules, restricted in expression to B lymphocytes, some monocytes, activated T lymphocytes, and sperm, consist of two polypeptide chains (α and β) of unequal length and are the products of the HLA-D and H-2I regions in human and mouse, respectively. Class III molecules are the C4, C2, and Bf complement proteins. *Second,* class I and class II molecules either form complexes with nominal antigens or the histocompatibility antigens are conjointly recognized by T lymphocytes having appropriate antigen receptors. Self versus nonself discrimination in the initiation and effector phase of the immune response is thereby intimately directed by class I and II molecules. *Third,* genes for cell-to-cell interactions involving suppressor T lymphocytes are part of the mouse H-2I region, though not yet clearly defined in humans. *Fourth,* genes for enzyme systems having no apparent relationship to immunity are located in the region of the MHC, as are genes of impor-

FIGURE 60-1
Human chromosome 6, showing the location of the HLA region in the 21 region of the short arm. The HLA-A, B, C loci encode class I heavy chains (44,000 daltons), while the beta$_2$ microglobulin light chain (11,500 daltons) of the class I molecule is encoded by genes of chromosome 15. The relative distance between loci is shown in recombination units (cM = centimorgans). HLA-D/DR (class II) is centromeric to the A, B, C loci, with genes for closely linked complement components C4A, C4B, Bf, and C2 in the B-D region. Genes for diseases clearly linked to HLA, 21-hydroxylase deficiency (21-OH^0) and idiopathic hemochromatosis, have been mapped as shown. Enzyme polymorphisms useful in mapping studies are glyoxylase (GLO) and phosphoglucomutase isomer 3 (PGM$_3$). Mapping of immunoglobulin Gm genes is uncertain, with some evidence for weak linkage to PGM$_3$.

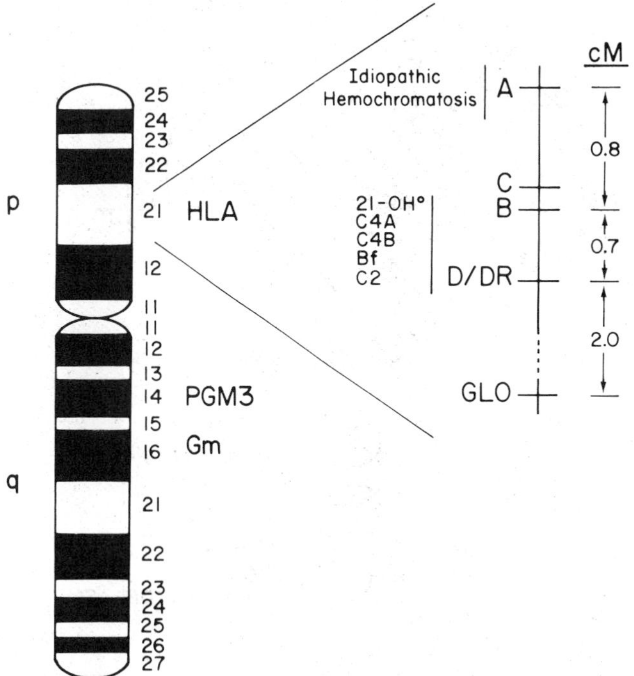

tance in skeletal growth and development. The known loci of the HLA region on the short arm of chromosome 6 are shown in Fig. 60-1.

LOCI OF THE HLA SYSTEM **Class I antigens** HLA antigens are defined serologically by human sera, principally from multiparous females, and are present in varying densities in most body tissues, including B cells, T cells, and platelets but not in mature red blood cells. The number of serologically defined specificities is large, and the HLA system is at present the most polymorphic genetic system known in humans. There are three clearly defined loci within the HLA complex for class I, serologically defined (SD), HLA antigens. Each class I antigen consists of an 11,500-dalton beta$_2$ microglobulin subunit and a 44,000-dalton heavy chain which carries the antigenic specificity (Fig. 60-2). The A and B loci were recognized as such in 1970, and the C locus was identified shortly thereafter. There are over 60 clearly defined A and B specificities, while eight C-locus specificities are known. Antigens of the major complex are all prefixed by HLA, but this may be omitted when the context is clear. Antigens tentatively accepted by the World Health Organization as a result of the series of International Histocompatibility Workshops have a *w* after the locus designation. The number following the locus designation is the name of the antigen. The HLA antigens of African, Asian, and Oceanic peoples are not as well defined at present, although they include some of the antigens commonly found in Caucasians. The distribution of HLA antigens is distinctive for certain racial groups and can serve as anthropologic markers in the study of migration patterns.

Since chromosomes are paired, each individual has six serologically defined HLA-A, HLA-B, and HLA-C antigens, three from each parent. Each of these chromosomal sets is termed a *haplotype*, and by simple mendelian inheritance 25 percent of siblings will have identical haplotypes, 50 percent will share a haplotype, and the remaining 25 percent will be completely incompatible (Fig. 60-3). Evidence that this gene complex plays the major role in the transplantation response comes from the fact that haplotype-matched sibling donor-recipient combinations show excellent results in kidney transplantation, in the vicinity of 85 to 90 percent long-term survival.

Class II antigens Linked to the serologically defined antigens, but distinct from them, is another locus which determines the in vitro proliferative response of lymphocytes to mismatched haplotypes. Because haplotype-matched identical siblings for class I antigens have negative mixed lymphocyte culture responses, it was first assumed that the A and B antigens were responsible for the proliferative response of lymphocytes mixed in tissue culture. However, a number of recombinants in families have shown clearly that a distinct locus, called *D*, exists for the mixed lymphocyte response (MLR) and is responsible for a vigorous mixed lymphocyte culture (MLC) proliferative response, even in the presence of identical HLA-A, HLA-B, and HLA-C antigens (Fig. 60-3). The recombinant rate in families is less than 1 percent between B and D loci and less than 1 percent between the A and B loci (Fig. 60-1). HLA-D antigens are defined by reference-stimulating lymphocytes which are homozygous for HLA-D and inactivated by x-irradiation or mitomycin C to make the reaction unidirectional. Serologically defined specificities closely related to the D locus have been defined. They have the special property of not being expressed on platelets or unstimulated T lymphocytes. These specificities are termed *class II*, having two glyco-

FIGURE 60-2
Schematic representation of an HLA-B7 (class I) molecule in the plasma membrane. Class I molecules are composed of two chains. The 44,000-dalton heavy chain passes through the plasma membrane. Its external portion consists of three regions (α1, α2, α3), has a small carbohydrate moiety, and bears the alloantigenic determinants. The beta$_2$-microglobulin light chain (11,500 daltons), encoded by chromosome 15, is noncovalently bound to the heavy chain. The amino acid sequences of the B7 and A2 heavy chains are known, and the sequence homology is in the range of 80 to 85 percent, falling to 50 percent or less in portions of α1 and α2 which most likely represent the alloantigenic sites. Of interest is a significant sequence homology in portions of α3 to immunoglobulin C region domains. Beta$_2$ microglobulin is also homologous to immunoglobulin C region domains. (From Strominger.)

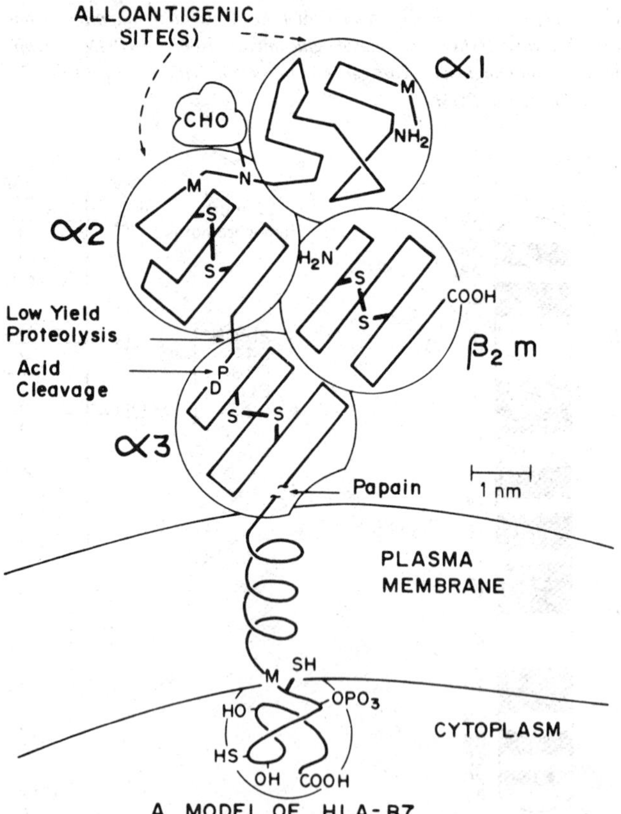

FIGURE 60-3
HLA region, chromosome 6: inheritance of HLA haplotypes. Each chromosomal segment of linked genes is termed a haplotype, and each individual inherits one haplotype from each parent. The A, B, C, and D antigens of haplotypes a and b are shown for this hypothetical individual in chromosomal order on the diagram, and also below as they would be written in text. If individual ab were to marry cd, their offspring would be of four types only, as far as HLA is concerned. Occasionally (dotted cross) recombination occurs in the germ line (meiosis) of a parent, resulting in an altered haplotype. The frequency of recombinant children is a measure of the map distance (1 percent recombination frequency = 1 cM; see Fig. 60-1). (From CB Carpenter, Kidney International, 14:283, 1978.)

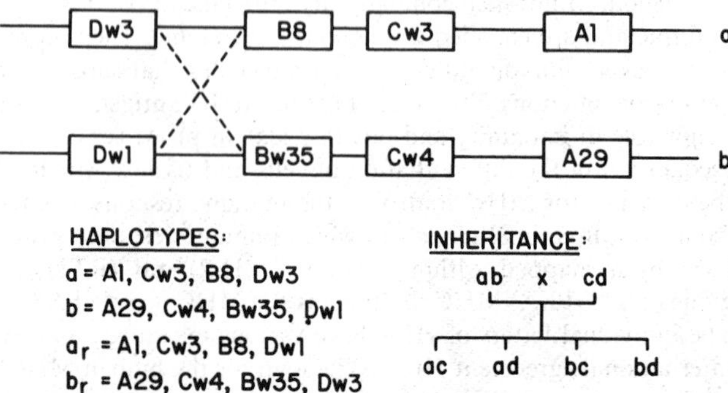

protein chains of 29,000 (β) and 34,000 (α) daltons, and lacking $beta_2$ microglobulin (Fig. 60-4). They are termed *HLA-DR* (D-related) and are markers for closely linked D-locus determinants and putative immune response (Ir) genes. The precise relationship between HLA-D and class II serologically defined antigens (HLA-DR) has yet to be established. They could be determinants on the same molecule or the products of closely linked genes. In addition, preliminary evidence exists for class II antigens unrelated to HLA-D type, which may represent a second set of class II molecules.

Other HLA antigens Two additional methods are under investigation for defining histocompatibility antigens. In the primed lymphocyte test (PLT), responder cells which have completed a proliferative response in MLC are restimulated with the same or different stimulating cells. The secondary response of primed lymphocytes is rapid (24 to 36 h instead of 5 to 6 days), and the specificity of restimulation is a test for antigenic similarity between priming and restimulating cells. Data thus far indicate that PLT antigens are more closely related to class II HLA-DR than to HLA-D. In addition, a new series of HLA-linked antigens called *SB* has been defined by PLT and not as yet by serological techniques. In the cell-mediated lympholysis (CML) test the specificity of killer T cells, which arise as a result of proliferation in MLC, is determined upon target cells from donors other than those providing the MLC-stimulating cells. Antigen systems defined by this method show a close but imperfect correlation with class I antigens. It is unknown whether antigenic determinants recognized by T cells are on

FIGURE 60-4

Schematic representation of an HLA-DR (class II) molecule in the plasma membrane. Two polypeptide chains (p29 = 29,000-dalton β chain; p34 = 34,000-dalton α chain) are noncovalently linked, and both traverse the plasma membrane. The light (β) chain is most polymorphic and is the likely site of the HLA-encoded alloantigenic determinants. Sugar complexes are shown as dark symbols. (From Strominger.)

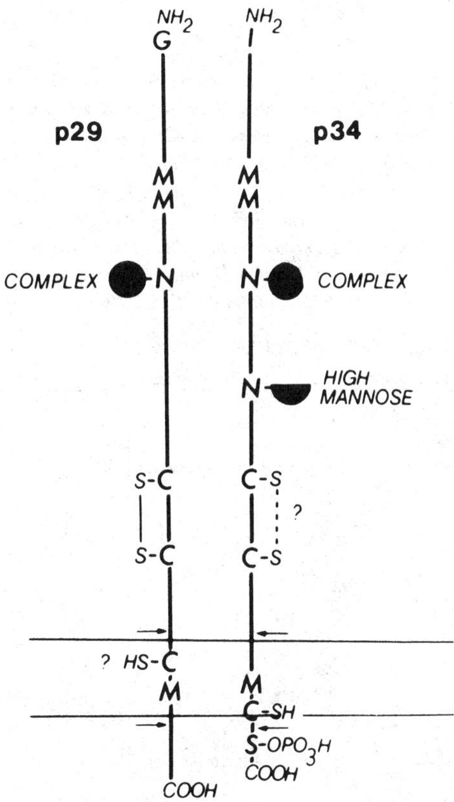

the same molecules as those determinants defined by antibodies. It is clear, however, that multiple serologically defined determinants are present on class I and class II molecules. Some of these are the specific private determinants of the HLA-A, B, C, DR loci, while others are more public (sometimes called *supertypic*) because they are found in association with several private determinants. One such system of public HLA-B antigens has two components, Bw4 and Bw6. Most HLA-B private antigens are associated with either Bw4 or Bw6. Other systems are more restricted to certain HLA-B antigen groups. For example, HLA-B-bearing heavy chains carry other sites which are shared among antigen groups, such as B7, B27, Bw22, and B40 or B5, B15, B18, and Bw35. Other types of shared antigenic determinants exist, as exemplified by a monoclonal antibody which reacts with a site shared between HLA-A and B heavy chains. A similar situation is found with HLA-DR, where two public systems, MB and MT, are supertypic to the DR antigens and represent distinct antigenic sites on the class II polypeptide chains. Precise localization of DR, MB, and MT determinants to the α and β chains of the class II molecule(s) has not been accomplished.

Complement (class III) Structural genes for three complement components, C4, C2, and Bf, have been mapped to the HLA-B-D region (Fig. 60-1). In addition, deficiency states for C4 and C2 have been shown to be linked to HLA. These deficiencies represent defects in the structural genes and are recognized by electrophoretic polymorphisms of the gene products. There are two loci for C4, coding for C4A and C4B, formerly recognized as the Rodgers and Chido red blood cell antigens, respectively. These antigens are, in fact, absorbed plasma C4 molecules.

No crossovers have been found between C4A and C4B, nor between the C2, Bf, and C4 loci. Other complement components are not closely linked to HLA. There are four alleles of C2, four of Bf, six of C4A, and two of C4B. The extensive polymorphism of complement types will make them useful for genetic studies. The close linkage of C2, C4, and Bf in the area of HLA-B-D will allow better definition of the fine structure of this region.

Other sixth-chromosome genes Deficiency of steroid 21-hydroxylase, an autosomal recessive trait, results in the syndrome of congenital adrenal hyperplasia (Chaps. 112 and 120). Extensive family studies have linked the mutant gene to HLA, and observed recombinants localize it to the HLA-B-D region. A late-onset variant of 21-hydroxylase deficiency is also linked to HLA, although congenital adrenal hyperplasia due to 11β-hydroxylase deficiency is not HLA-linked. Idiopathic hemochromatosis, an autosomal recessive disorder, is linked to HLA, as has been shown in several family studies (see Chap. 97). Although the pathogenesis of this disease is unknown, the gene that modulates gastrointestinal iron absorption is near HLA-A (Table 60-1).

Immune response genes Several studies indicate that HLA-D is analogous to the mouse H-2I region. These studies included measurement of in vitro responses to synthetic polypeptide antigens, keyhole limpet hemocyanin, and tetanus toxoid. Presentation of antigenic fragments on the surfaces of macrophages or dendritic or other cells bearing class II molecules seems to require conjoint recognition of a class II (DR or Ia) + antigen complex by T lymphocytes bearing the appropriate receptor(s). The crux of this "self + X" or "altered self" hypothesis is that in the T-dependent immune response, help from the T helper/

inducer cell (T_H) ocurs only if the appropriate class II determinant can be synthesized. The genes for the latter are Ir genes. Since allogenic class II determinants are perceived as already altered, the allogenic MLC response represents a model for the immune system in which additional nominal antigen does not need to be added (Fig. 60-5). In the effector phases of immunity there is again a demonstrated requirement for recognition of nominal antigen together with a self structure. The latter in humans, as in mice, is the molecule bearing class I histocompatibility antigens. Human cell lines infected with influenza virus are lysed by immune cytotoxic T lymphocytes (Tc) only if an HLA-A- or B-locus antigen is shared between the attacking and target cells. Again, the allogenic MLC provides a model for class I directed cytotoxic T lymphocytes (Fig. 60-5). Although predicted by work with suppressor cells in mice, no human HLA-linked suppressor T-cell locus has yet been discerned.

DISEASE ASSOCIATIONS If the major histocompatibility complex serves a critical natural biological function, what might that be? Hypotheses have been put forth relating to immune surveillance against neoplastic cells which develop in the course of an individual's lifetime. The system could also play an important role in pregnancy because of the histoincompatibility that always exists between the mother and the fetus. Work in inbred mouse models indicates the importance of some of the gene products of this locus during the phase of antigen recognition of cell-to-cell cooperation in initiating an immune response. It is possible also that the high degree of polymorphism ensures the survival of the species in relation to the large numbers of microbiological agents present in the environment. Self-tolerance which happens to cross react with microbiological agents would produce a high degree of susceptibility, resulting in lethal infection, whereas the high degree of polymorphism present in the HLA system provides assurance that segments of the population will recognize the offending agent as foreign and initiate the appropriate response. All these hypotheses relate to the survival value of the system under selective evolutionary pressures, and there is some evidence for each of them.

The most striking circumstantial evidence for the role of the HLA complex in immunobiology comes from the finding that a number of disease processes are positively associated with certain HLA antigens within the population. The search for such associations has been stimulated by the discovery of immune response genes linked to the H-2 complex in the mouse and also by the H-2 complex–linked susceptibility to murine oncogenic viruses. Although surveys of human malignancies, including leukemias and lymphoproliferative disorders, have not shown consistent associations with serologically defined HLA phenotypes, some striking correlations exist between HLA antigens and a number of diseases in which the pathogenesis is unclear. Table 60-2 summarizes the most significant HLA and disease associations.

TABLE 60-1
Linkage of genetic defects to HLA

	Gene location	*Common haplotype found*
C2 deficiency	HLA-B-D	Aw25, B18, BfS, DR2
21-OH deficiency	HLA-B-D	A3, Bw47, BfF, DR7
21-OH deficiency (late onset)	HLA-B-D,	B14, BfS, DR1
Idiopathic hemochromatosis	HLA-A	A3, B14
Paget's disease	HLA-A-D	
Spinocerebellar ataxia	HLA-A-D	

Most striking is the increased frequency of HLA-B27 in certain rheumatic diseases, particularly ankylosing spondylitis, a condition with a strong familial tendency. B27 is present in about 7 percent of the Caucasian population, while it appears in 80 to 90 percent of over 2000 patients with ankylosing spondylitis. Expressed as a relative risk, the antigen B27 confers a susceptibility to the development of ankylosing spondylitis which is 87 times that in the general population. Similarly, acute anterior uveitis, Reiter's syndrome, and reactive arthritis to at least three bacterial infections (yersinia, salmonella, and gonococcus) show a high degree of association with B27. Since it is well known that significant overlap exists among these conditions (spondylitis, Reiter's syndrome, and uveitis), it seems likely that B27 is a marker for a clustering of connective tissue responses to a number of infectious agents or unknown environmental factors. Although the ordinary form of juvenile rheumatoid arthritis (JRA) also shows a similar association with B27, the pauciarticular form of JRA with iritis is DR5-associated. The increased incidence of B27 in psoriatic arthritis is also highly significant for the central type of the disorder, while Bw38 is associated with both the central and peripheral types. Psoriasis is most significantly associated with Cw6. Patients with degenerative arthritis or gout show no alteration in antigen frequencies. Rheumatoid arthritis patients show an association with Dw4 and DR4, and Sjögren's syndrome is associated with Dw3.

Gluten-sensitive enteropathy (celiac disease, nontropical sprue) in both children and adults is associated with DR3 and less significantly with HLA-B8. The actual percentage of such patients having this antigen ranges from 63 to 96 percent compared to 22 to 27 percent of controls. The same antigen is also present in increased frequency in patients with chronic active hepatitis and in patients with dermatitis herpetiformis who also have gluten-sensitive enteropathy.

Initially reported to have associations with B8 and B15, juvenile-onset insulin-dependent diabetes mellitus (type I) is most significantly associated with DR4 and DR3 and is negatively associated with DR2. Maturity-onset diabetes is not HLA-associated. A rare allele of Bf (F1) is also found in 17 to 25 percent of cases of type I diabetes. Graves' disease in Cau-

FIGURE 60-5
Schema of the relative roles of HLA-A, HLA-B, HLA-C, and HLA-D antigens in initiation of the alloimmune response and in the development of effector cells and antibodies. Two main classes of T lymphocytes recognize antigens: T_c, the precursors to the cytotoxic "killer" cells, and T_H, the helper cells for amplification of the cytotoxic response. T_H also provide help to B lymphocytes for production of a fully mature IgG response. Note that T_c generally recognize class I antigens, while the T_H signal is provided principally by HLA-D, which has class II antigens closely associated. (From CB Carpenter, Kidney International, 14:283, 1978.)

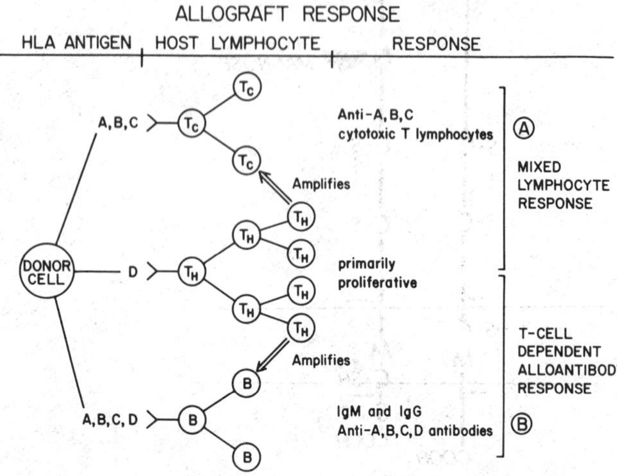

casians is B8, Dw3-associated, while in Japanese populations the association is with Bw35. More extensive studies of healthy and diseased members of various races will help in clarification of which HLA markers are universal. For example, B27 is rare in healthy Japanese but is common in subjects with ankylosing spondylitis. Also, DR4 seems to be the common marker for type I diabetes in all races, whereas B8 and B15 are secondary markers only in Caucasians. Sometimes an HLA marker is clearly associated only with a subgroup within a syndrome. For example, myasthenia gravis without thymoma is B8-associated, and the association of DR2 with multiple sclerosis is particularly strong in patients having rapidly progressive deterioration. Goodpasture's syndrome due to autoimmunity to glomerular basement membrane and idiopathic membranous glomerulonephritis, which is now viewed as possibly an autoimmune process involving antibodies to an antigen of the glomerulus, are HLA-DR-associated.

Most of the known associations are with HLA-B-D locus antigens. Psoriasis vulgaris and the response to vaccinia immunization are Cw6-associated, and the tuberculoid form of leprosy in Asians and paralytic polio are HLA-B-associated. However, most of the conditions having HLA-B or -C associations are not as yet adequately studied for HLA-D/DR. Infectious diseases are more difficult to study because only the survivors are typable. Discrepancies exist for HLA associations in diseases such as IgA nephropathy and systemic lupus erythematosus. Such differences most likely are a reflection of heterogeneity within the disease or possibly in the ethnic backgrounds of patients and control populations being compared.

LINKAGE DISEQUILIBRIUM Although the distribution of HLA alleles varies in racial and ethnic populations, the most salient feature of population genetics of HLA antigens is the presence of linkage disequilibria among certain antigens of the A and B, B and C, and B and D loci. Linkage disequilibrium means that antigens of closely linked loci appear together more frequently than predicted by random association. The classic example is the linkage disequilibrium present between the A-locus antigen, HLA-A1, and B-locus antigen, HLA-B8, in Caucasian populations of western Europe and America. The coincidence of A1 and B8 should be the product of their individual gene frequencies, or 0.17 times 0.11 equals approximately 0.02. The observed frequency of A1 and B8 in Caucasians is 0.08, four times that expected, an increase of 0.06. The latter value is termed Δ (delta), and is a measure of the disequilibrium. Other A- and B-locus haplotype disequilibria have been recognized and include (A3, B7), (A2, B12), (A29, B12), and (A11, Bw35). Furthermore, some D-locus determinants are in linkage disequilibrium with B-locus antigens (for example, Dw3 and B8), as are some B-locus and C-locus antigens. Just as the serologically defined HLA antigens can serve as markers for the genes of an entire haplotype within a family, they may also serve as markers for specific genes within a population, but only where a linkage disequilibrium exists.

Linkage disequilibrium is a matter of some importance because such gene associations may have some bearing on their function. For example, selective pressures during the course of evolution may have been the major factor in the survival of certain gene combinations in a haplotype. Such a theory would suggest, for example, that A1 and B8, along with certain D-locus and other determinants, conferred a selective advantage in the face of epidemics such as the plague or smallpox. It

TABLE 60-2
HLA antigens and disease, showing the most highly associated antigens in white populations

Disease	*Antigen*	*Relative risk**
RHEUMATIC		
Ankylosing spondylitis	B27	87
Reiter's syndrome	B27	37
Acute anterior uveitis	B27	10.3
Reactive arthritis (yersinia, salmonella, gonococcus)	B27	18
Psoriatic arthritis, central	B27	10.7
	Bw38	9.1
Psoriatic arthritis, peripheral	B27	2.0
	Bw38	6.5
Juvenile rheumatoid arthritis	B27	4.5
Juvenile arthritis pauciarticular	DR5	5.2
Rheumatoid arthritis	Dw4/ DR4	6.0
Sjögren syndrome	Dw3	9.7
GASTROINTESTINAL		
Gluten-sensitive enteropathy	DR3	21
Chronic active hepatitis	DR3	6.8
Ulcerative colitis	B5	3.8
HEMATOLOGIC		
Idiopathic hemochromatosis	A3	8.2
	B14	26.7
	A3,B14	90
Pernicious anemia	DR5	5.4
SKIN		
Dermatitis herpetiformis	Dw3	13.5
Psoriasis vulgaris	Cw6	4.8
Psoriasis vulgaris (Japanese)	Cw6	10.7
Pemphigus vulgaris (Jews)	DR4	32
	A10	5.9
Behçet's disease	B5	6.3
		12.7

Disease	*Antigen*	*Relative risk**
ENDOCRINE		
Juvenile diabetes mellitus	DR4	5.3
	DR3	2.8
	DR2	0.2
	BfF1	15.0
Graves' disease	B8	3.6
	Dw3	3.7
Graves' disease (Japanese)	Bw35	3.9
Addison's disease	Dw3	10.5
Subacute thyroiditis (de Quervain)	Bw35	13.7
Hashimoto's thyroiditis	DR5	3.2
NEUROLOGIC		
Myasthenia gravis (without thymoma)	B8	4.4
Multiple sclerosis	DR2	3.9
Manic-depressive disorder	Bw16	2.3
Schizophrenia	A28	2.3
RENAL		
Idiopathic membranous glomerulonephritis	DR3	5.7
Goodpasture's syndrome (anti-GBM)	DR2	15.9
Minimal change disease (steroid response)	B12	3.5
Polycystic kidney disease	B5	2.6
INFECTIOUS		
Tuberculoid leprosy (Asians)	B8	6.8
Paralytic polio	Bw16	4.3
Low vs. high response to vaccinia virus	Cw3	12.7

$$\text{* Relative risk} = \frac{(\%\ \text{antigen-positive patients})(\%\ \text{antigen-negative controls})}{(\%\ \text{antigen-negative patients})(\%\ \text{antigen-positive controls})}$$

would also follow that the descendants of the survivors now display susceptibility to certain diseases because their unique gene complex happens to confer an abnormal response to other environmental agents. The major difficulty with this hypothesis is the assumption that selection would have to work on several genes simultaneously to account for the observed Δ's; however, the need for complex interactions among the products of the several loci of the major histocompatibility complex is only beginning to be appreciated, and it is possible that selection could force multiple linkage disequilibria.

On the other hand, the selection hypothesis is not necessary to explain linkage disequilibrium. When a population lacking certain antigens is crossed with one having a high frequency of antigens in equilibrium, a Δ can develop within a very small number of generations. For example, the increasing Δ value for A1, B8, found in populations from east to west, from India to western Europe, can be explained on the basis of migration and fusion. In smaller groups, consanguinity, founder effects, and gene drift may account for disequilibria. Finally, certain linkage disequilibria could occur as a result of nonrandom crossing over during gametic meiosis, because of chromosomal segments which are either more or less likely to break. Unless there are selective pressures or restrictions in crossing over, linkage disequilibria will disappear over a period of several generations. A large number of nonrandom associations currently exist throughout the HLA gene complex, and elucidation of the reasons for their existence may provide insight into the mechanism underlying certain disease susceptibilities.

LINKAGE AND ASSOCIATION The diseases listed in Table 60-1 are examples of HLA linkage wherein the inherited conditions are closely marked within families by the relevant HLA haplotypes. For C2 deficiency, 21-hydroxylase deficiency, and idiopathic hemochromatosis the mode of inheritance is recessive, with heterozygotes showing partial deficiencies when tested appropriately. These genetic defects are also HLA-associated, with an excess of certain HLA alleles in affected unrelated individuals. C2 deficiency is commonly linked to the HLA-Aw25, B18, BS5, D/DR2 haplotype, and both are found in the heterozygous state in 6 percent of systemic lupus erythematosus (SLE) patients as compared to 2 percent of controls. It is apparent that SLE is not inherited as a simple mendelian trait, although C2 deficiency is HLA-linked, being present in individuals with and without SLE. SLE, in turn, is a disease process showing some association with HLA but determined by other genetic factors. 21-Hydroxylase deficiency is characterized by the inability to synthesize cortisol and consists of two clinical types, each showing strong HLA associations to Bw47 or B14 in unrelated populations. Secondary associations with alleles of linked genes (linkage disequilibrium) occur with Bf and DR, as exists with C2 deficiency. Preliminary data on C4A and C4B polymorphisms also show unique alleles for the 21-hydroxylase-deficient haplotype. Idiopathic hemochromatosis shows both linkage and strong association with HLA-A3 and B14. The simplest explanation for the high degree of linkage disequilibria in these HLA-linked diseases is that they result from mutations in a single founder and that there have not been enough subsequent generations to bring the gene pool back into equilibrium. In this view, the HLA antigens are simple markers for the linked gene. Alternatively, expression of the defect may require interaction with specific HLA alleles. This hypothesis would require a higher mutation rate, with defective gene expression occurring only when linked with certain HLA genes.

Paget's disease and spinocerebellar ataxia are HLA-linked autosomal dominant traits in families having multiple affected members. No HLA associations have been discerned, suggesting that there were multiple founders with mutations in linkage with different HLA alleles.

HLA linkage is readily recognized when simple mendelian recessive or dominant inheritance patterns are present, i.e., when expressivity is high and the process is mostly, if not entirely, determined by a single gene defect. HLA-D-associated juvenile-onset (type I) diabetes mellitus illustrates a more complex situation, suggestive of an HLA-linked recessive disorder, but analysis is hampered by the variable expressivity. Whereas the concordance of maturity-onset (type II) diabetes mellitus in identical twins approaches 100 percent, it is only 30 to 40 percent in type I diabetes. When families having both affected and nonaffected type I diabetic sibs are HLA-typed, there *is* a high degree of concordance in HLA identicals, but it is not complete since 4 to 6 percent of affected sib pairs differ for *both* HLA haplotypes. Environmental and polygenic factors are likely to be of critical importance. In fact, most of the associations between HLA and disease are in a similar category, with HLA markers representing risk factors involving the operation and modulation of the immune response in many instances. An example of the polygenic nature of a disease is atopic allergy, in which the association to HLA may be evident only in individuals whose genetically controlled (non-HLA) levels of IgE production are low. HLA associations may indicate only that the relevant gene is in linkage disequilibrium with the HLA marker and not necessarily that a particular HLA molecule is contributing to an altered immune response.

CLINICAL APPLICATIONS The clinical value of HLA typing for diagnosis of disease is limited to B27 and ankylosing spondylitis, where 10 percent false-positive and false-negative rates still exist. HLA studies are also of value in genetic counseling and preventive therapy in families with idiopathic hemochromatosis or congenital adrenal hyperplasia, particularly as HLA typing can be performed upon cells obtained by amniocentesis. The high degree of polymorphism of the HLA system also makes it a powerful tool for paternity testing and other medicolegal applications. Finally, the implications for diseases such as juvenile-onset (type I) diabetes mellitus and the dozens of other diseases showing HLA associations will require further study of the components of the HLA system and their role in the pathogenesis of disease.

REFERENCES

ALPER CA: Complement and the MHC, in *The Role of the Major Histocompatibility Complex in Immunobiology*, ME Dorf (ed). New York, Garland STPM Press, 1981, pp 173–220

BODMER WF (ed): The HLA system. Br Med Bull 34:213, 1978

DEGOS L, DAUSSET J: Human migrations and linkage disequilibrium of HLA system. Immunogenetics 3:195, 1974

RYDER LP et al (eds): *HLA and Disease Registry. Third Report.* Copenhagen, Munksgaard, 1979

SCHALLER JG, HANSEN JA: HLA relationship to disease. Hosp Prac 16:41, 1981

STROMINGER J: Structure of products of the major histocompatibility complex in man and mouse, in *Immunology 80, Progress in Immunology IV*, M Fougereau, J Dausset (eds). London, Academic, 1980, pp 541–554

VAN ROOD, JJ et al: Genetics and biology of the HLA system, in *The Role of the Major Histocompatibility Complex in Immunobiology*, ME Dorf (ed). New York, Garland STPM Press, 1981, pp 59–113

61 CYTOGENETIC ASPECTS OF HUMAN DISEASE

JAMES GERMAN

The chromosome complement of humans, like that of other species, is guarded carefully against change; most chromosome mutations, either structural or numerical, are deleterious. Only rarely is a balanced structural rearrangement (one that results in neither deficiency nor duplication of significant chromosome segments) introduced into the population and transmitted from generation to generation. (Figure 61-1 shows the normal human chromosome complement. In the legend of the figure several terms used in human cytogenetics are defined.) As a rule an abnormal number of autosomes results in early death, except for trisomy of the shortest chromosome. In contrast, an abnormal number of sex chromosomes is often tolerated reasonably well, although infertility or subfertility usually is present. Nevertheless, among human embryos abnormalities in chromosome structure and number are common and are, in fact, the major known cause of embryonic and early fetal wastage. However, not every fetus with an abnormal chromosome complement is aborted, and those that survive constitute the material of medical cytogenetics.

Clinical disorders resulting from chromosome imbalance present varying features including abnormal anatomic development, mental deficiency, behavioral disorders, and disturbances in growth and sexual development. Sometimes infertility, repeated abortion, or the birth of malformed children is the presenting complaint of persons with abnormal chromosome complements whose own general development is normal.

The disorders just referred to are due to chromosome imbalance that affects tissues throughout the body. In addition, change can occur in the chromosome complement in a single cell of some somatic tissue. Such a mutant cell may have a proliferative advantage over normal cells, in which case a clone bearing the abnormal chromosome complement can develop amid otherwise normal cells. Although such mutant clones are in many cases clinically insignificant, much evidence suggests that they are also important in the etiology of cancer.

This chapter is addressed to those aspects of normal chromosome structure and function that constitute the basis for an understanding of the chromosome alterations in human disease. In addition, the classes of alterations important in adult medicine and their consequences are summarized.

CHROMOSOME STRUCTURE AND FUNCTION The human autosomes are numbered 1 through 22, and the sex chromosomes are denoted X and Y (Fig. 61-1). Each is recognizable microscopically by morphological features such as relative length and position of the centromere and by staining characteristics (banding pattern). Each mammalian chromosome is believed to be composed of one double-stranded chain of deoxyribonucleic acid (DNA) that extends from one end through the centromere to the other end.

Cell-division cycle Chromosomes must duplicate before cell division can occur. This duplication occurs over a period of several hours prior to the onset of mitosis or meiosis in a phase of the cell cycle termed S, for synthesis of DNA (Fig. 61-2). Thus, from the completion of S to the completion of metaphase, each chromosome contains two identical double-stranded chains of DNA, and the nucleus contains four times as much DNA as a spermatozoon or ovum. During mitosis chromosomes are condensed, and the two sister chromatids can be visualized by late prophase or early metaphase (Fig. 61-1). (Metaphase is the stage in the cell-division cycle ordinarily employed for cytogenetic analysis.)

At the onset of anaphase the centromeric regions of each chromosome separate, and the two chromatids move quickly to opposite poles of the mitotic spindle. As soon as each pole receives one full complement of chromatids (chromosomes), a nuclear membrane (disassembled late in prophase) is reassembled about each cluster to complete formation of the nuclei of the two sister cells that emerge at telophase. The sister cells emerge in what is usually called the G_1 phase of the cell cycle, in which they remain unreplicated unless another division is to be prepared for, whereupon they enter the S phase. Cells engaged in some differentiated function ordinarily remain unreplicated.

Most normal cells in the human body are diploid; i.e., they have twice the haploid number (the number in a gamete) of chromosomes (haploid = 23, diploid = 46). In the germ-cell line, which is devoted to gamete formation, cells destined eventually to differentiate into spermatozoa or ova undergo mitotic cell cycles until they enter the two specialized divisions termed *meiosis*. In meiosis, pairing of homologous chromosomes occurs (the paternally derived chromosome 1 with the maternally derived chromosome 1, and so on), and genetic recombination takes place (see Chap. 58). At the first meiotic division homologous chromosomes are segregated, and the diploid chromosome number is reduced to the haploid; i.e., each cell then contains one of each of the 22 (duplicated) autosomes plus one (duplicated) sex chromosome. No S phase takes place between the first and second meiotic divisions (depicted in Fig. 61-2, right) so that at the second division, in which sister chromatids separate, emerging cells maintain the haploid number of chromosomes but are reduced in their content of DNA to half the amount of diploid G_1 cells of somatic tissues. With fertilization of an ovum by a spermatozoon, both the chromosome constitution and the DNA content of the zygote are restored to that of a G_1 somatic cell. An S period in the zygote then permits reinstitution of regular cell-division cycles characteristic of the somatic cells.

Chromosome differentiation A chromosome is differentiated along its length, and some aspects of this differentiation are resolvable in the light microscope. The DNA is complexed with a number of proteins in a highly specific way. The DNA-protein complex together with some associated ribonucleic acid (RNA) is referred to as *chromatin*. The fine structure and the manner in which the DNA is compacted and interacted with proteins are thought to pertain to the control of RNA production and DNA replication, perhaps to cellular differentiation itself.

The sequences of nucleotide bases in DNA that constitute the genes and that can be transcribed into messenger RNA are distributed throughout the length of the various chromosomes. (These sequences are too short to be resolved microscopically.) Over 200 genes have been mapped to specific chromosomes, in many cases to specific regions of a chromosome; for example, the Rh blood group locus has been assigned to the short arm of chromosome 1, and the ABO blood group locus has been assigned to a band near the end of the long arm of chromosome 9.

Certain segments of at least 12 chromosomes vary in length

among individuals. These segments can be delineated by their staining characteristics (Fig. 61-3). The variable segments consist of nontranscribed, highly repetitive nucleotide sequences of DNA and are transmitted from parent to child in a straightforward mendelian fashion. Variations in these segments are unassociated with detectable phenotypic effect. (They can serve as useful cell markers in determination of zygosity of twins, paternity, and survival of transplants.)

Other microscopically recognizable segments in the short arms of the acrocentric autosomes are devoted to the production of ribosomal RNA and nucleoli. As mitosis progresses, these nucleolus-organizer regions tend to remain relatively uncondensed later than other regions. Consequently, at metaphase they appear understained and thereby demarcate condensed segments of chromatin distal to them on the chromosome arms—*satellites.* (Satellites are examples of the polymorphic segments just mentioned.) Other examples of segmental specialization along the chromosome include regions

FIGURE 61-1

Normal human lymphocyte chromosomes arrested in metaphase and stained for G bands (G standing for Giemsa). The inset shows the arrangement of chromosomes in an intact cell, and the remainder of the figure shows their ordered arrangement into a karyotype. By the time mitosis begins, each chromosome consists of two identical parts called sister chromatids and is identified by the relative length, the location of the centromere, and a distinctive sequence of bands of varying lengths and depth of staining. The number of bands visible microscopically varies from cell to cell, depending on the degree of chromosome condensation. The 300 to 400 bands seen in this particular cell can be increased to several times that number if cells with longer chromosomes are chosen for analysis, i.e., many of the bands seen here will resolve into subbands. Normally, the G-band patterns of the two chromosomes of a pair are alike, with the exception of certain polymorphic regions, examples of which are shown in Fig. 61-3.

The centromere of a chromosome divides it into a short arm (p) and a long arm (q). Numbers 13 to 15, 21, 22, and Y are called acrocentric because of the nearly terminal positions of their centromeres; the minute p of each acrocentric autosome bears a nucleolus-organizing region which often causes a secondary constriction in the metaphase chromosome (the constriction at the centromere being the primary constriction). Telomeres are the nonvisible, somewhat theoretical, "structures" at the ends of each chromosome.

By standard nomenclature, this karyotype is described as 46,XY, indicating that its chromosome number is 46, its sex chromosomes are an X and a Y, and the autosomes (those besides the X and Y) number 44. The following examples show the general use of this nomenclature: A normal female karyotype is described as 46,XX. A female cell with an extra chromosome 18 (trisomic for 18) would be described as 47,XX,+18. A cell with only one sex chromosome, an X, and with deletion in the short arm of chromosome 5 would be described as 45,X,5p−. A male cell with a translocation between the long arm of chromosome 2 and the short arm of chromosome 3 would be described as 46,XY,t(2q;3p); exact breakpoints could be indicated by additional characters and symbols.

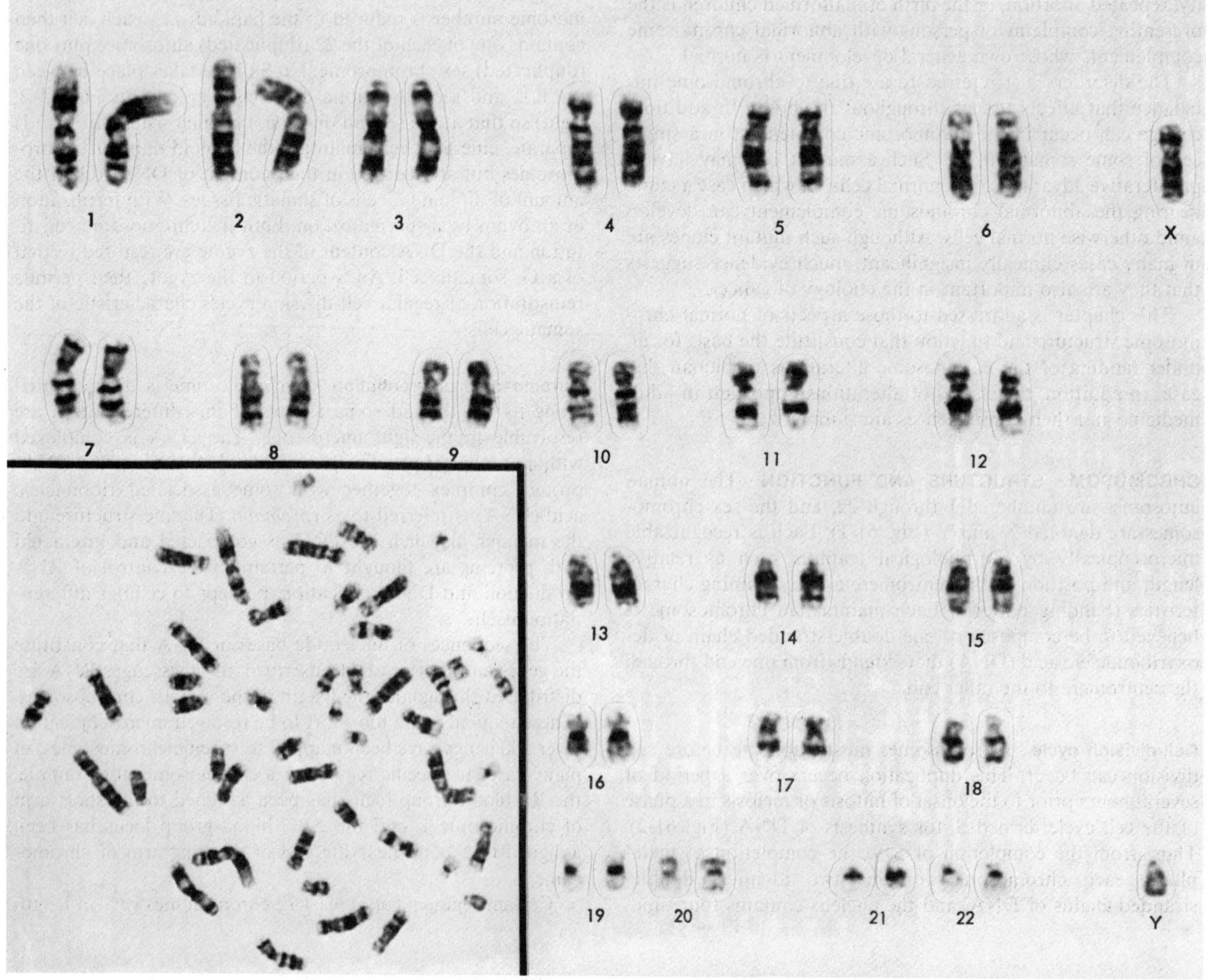

known as *telomeres* and *centromeres.* Telomeres, the distal termini of each arm, have some relationship to the nuclear membrane and probably are important in the maintenance of order in the interphase nucleus; centromeric regions are sites of microtubule attachment at metaphase.

A further example of chromosome differentiation is the established sequence by which various segments replicate during S; certain segments replicate early, others late. In general, late replication of a chromosome segment correlates with genetic inertness. This correlation is exemplified by one of the two X chromosomes in female cells; the chromosome inactivated by the Lyon effect is almost entirely late-replicating (see Chap. 58 for an explanation of the Lyon hypothesis).

A little-understood type of chromatin is that which has long been referred to as *heterochromatin.* It is tightly condensed, not just at metaphase but throughout interphase. Such condensation of chromatin correlates positively with genetic inactivity and also with late replication. Some regions are condensed and inactive in all cells (constitutive heterochromatin), while others, for example, the X chromosome, may be either condensed and inactive or decondensed and active (facultative heterochromatin). Many chromosome imbalances that permit viability beyond intrauterine life involve chromosome segments that are rich in this apparently inactive, or inactivatable, type of chromatin, e.g., chromosomes that can be trisomic in live-born individuals or, in the case of X, monosomic. The activity of genes can sometimes be affected, even inactivated, if they are positioned near regions of heterochromatin.

Therefore, in chromosomal imbalance both the specific genetic loci and the particular types of chromatin deleted or duplicated are important. Also, the significance of a structural rearrangement probably depends on the new and abnormal positioning of structural and regulatory genes in relation to each other and to heterochromatin.

Fortunately for the cytologist, several differentiated features of the chromosome correlate with cytological artifacts that can be produced and visualized in the laboratory. A number of techniques are now in use to display a pattern of bands of various lengths and staining characteristics (Figs. 61-1 and 61-3). These patterns are identical in each chromosome 1, each chromosome 2, etc., varying only in the inert polymorphic regions mentioned above, so that they can be used in clinical cytogenetics to identify chromosomes and to detect and define structural rearrangements.

Sources of error Every aspect of the cell-division cycle is complicated. Doubtless a large number of genetic loci must be active to produce the numerous enzymes and structural proteins required to initiate and complete a cycle. Remarkable precision and accuracy are demanded over and over in matters such as the passage of a cell from G_1 into S, orderly progression of replication, assembly of the mitotic spindle, and spindle function in segregating chromatids during mitosis. An additional battery of loci is activated to permit a cell of the germ line to pass successfully through the complicated stages of meiotic prophase, including pairing of homologous chromosomes, genetic recombination, and then disjoining of chromosomes. Probably all these mechanisms and processes are subject to errors, some spontaneous, others promoted by some unfavorable environmental influence (e.g., Fig. 61-4) or by the presence of deleterious mutations involving one of the many steps just mentioned. Furthermore, the genetic material itself is subject to damage, and certain types of unrepaired or erroneously repaired lesions in DNA theoretically may predispose to chromosome rearrangement. Errors at many of these steps lie behind chromosome imbalance. Errors that occur in germ cells, during fertilization, and in early postfertilization divisions are important in relation to embryonic maldevelopment and infertility; errors in somatic cells may be important in relation to neoplasia.

CHROMOSOME ABNORMALITIES Mutations of a single base in a gene and chromosome deletions and duplications involving even hundreds of base pairs are not visible to the cytogeneticist. In fact, for the normal chromosome banding pattern to be detectably disturbed, a lengthy segment of DNA must be

FIGURE 61-2
Schematic representation of the mitotic and meiotic cell-division cycles, as described in the text. G_1 and G_2 = time gaps before and after S, the period in which DNA replicates. Each of these intervals is several hours in duration; together they constitute interphase. M=mitosis; I and II = the two divisions of meiosis. The DNA content of the cycling cells is indicated on the vertical axis: 1c= the content in a gamete; 2c = that in either an egg immediately postfertilization or a somatic cell emerging from mitosis; 4c = the amount in a cell which has completed chromosome duplication and is ready to enter mitosis or meiosis.

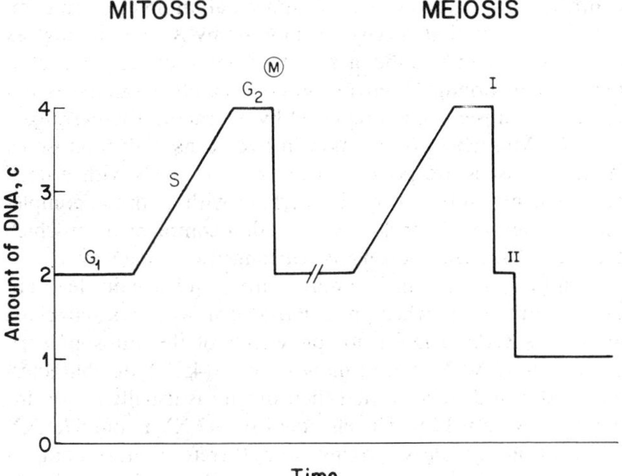

FIGURE 61-3
Metaphase chromosomes stained for C bands (C standing for centromeric or constitutive heterochromatin), showing inherited variation in lengths of C bands in chromosome 1 (arrows).

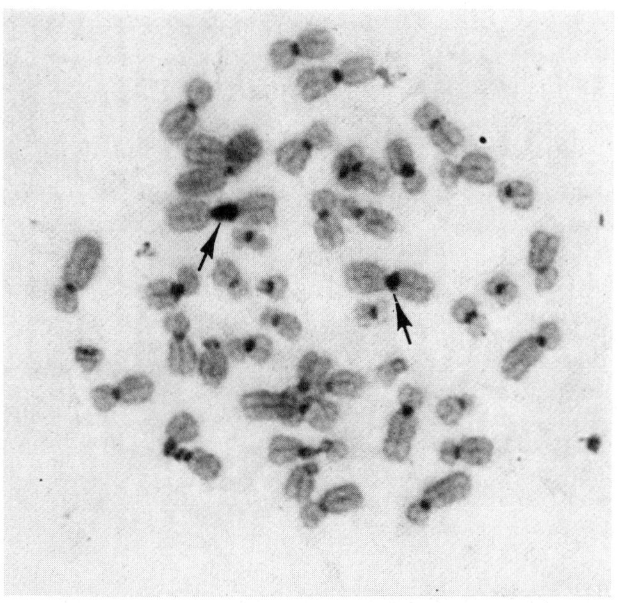

deleted, duplicated, or transposed. This means that a microscopically detectable chromosome mutation must involve relatively huge amounts of DNA. It is noteworthy, however, that the same environmental agents known to produce point mutations (mutagens in the usual sense) are in general also chromosome-breaking agents, and vice versa. Thus, it seems safe to assume the existence of a spectrum extending from mutations visible to the cytogeneticist to those that must be defined by nucleotide sequencing. Mutations visible to the cytogeneticist ordinarily exert a more widespread effect on development than do point mutations; ordinary genes—often many of them—as well as other specialized types of chromatin whose function usually is unknown, are involved in cytologically visible mutations.

If an entire chromosome is affected in an imbalance, the genome is said to be either trisomic or monosomic for the chromosome (thus, trisomy 13, monosomy X). Genes and chromatin carried on the affected chromosome then are present in triple or single dose, respectively, rather than the normal double dose. Abnormal dosage affecting less than an entire chromosome, the result of chromosome breakage and rearrangement, is often termed *partial trisomy* or *partial monosomy,* to indicate that segments rather than entire chromosomes are involved (thus, partial trisomy 13q, partial monosomy 4p).

Incidence The frequency with which chromosomal imbalance is detectable depends on the population investigated. It is estimated that a minimum of 1 in 10 recognized conceptions has a chromosome abnormality. In human embryos and fetuses aborted spontaneously, the incidence of chromosome imbalance is higher the earlier in pregnancy the sampling is made. The contribution of imbalance to late abortion and stillbirth, though not well studied, probably also is significant. In the more than 50,000 consecutive or random live-born babies that have now been examined in different laboratories, approximately 1 in 200 has a significant chromosome abnormality, either numerical or structural. In such studies, at least 1 in 700 newborns is trisomic for one of the autosomes 21, 18, or 13; about 1 in 350 newborn males has the complement 47,XXY or 47,XYY. One in every several thousand newborns has monosomy X. One in five hundred has some structural rearrangement, most of which are genetically balanced. Samplings of the general adult population reveal an occasional inherited balanced structural rearrangement as well as the expected number of XXY, XYY, and XXX complements; the inherited, apparently innocuous segmental polymorphisms (e.g., Fig. 61-3) and minor structural rearrangements demonstrable by banding techniques are found in abundance.

FIGURE 61-4

Breaks and rearrangements (arrows) in metaphase chromosomes of a blood lymphocyte that received ionizing irradiation before being stimulated by phytohemagglutinin to enter S and divide.

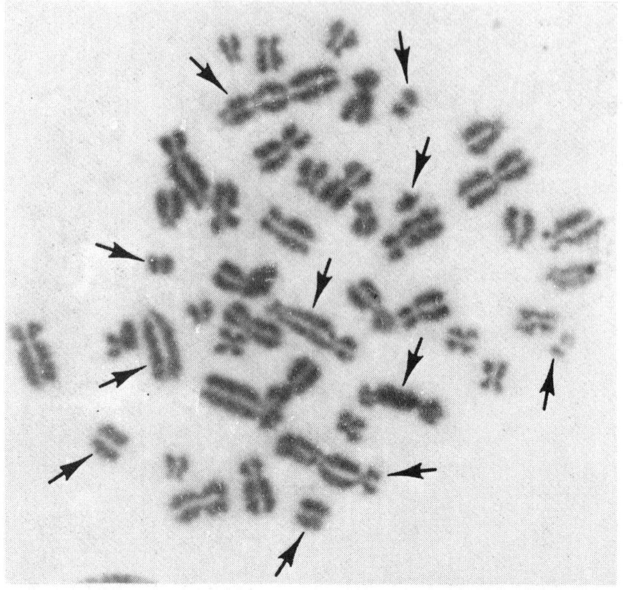

In populations of individuals with mental deficiency, 10 to 15 percent have a chromosome abnormality, the proportion being greater if the individuals also have anatomic malformations. In some groups of male criminals and in all infertile men an increased incidence of individuals with an extra sex chromosome, an X or a Y, is found. Infertile women also include many individuals with extra or missing sex chromosomes and an appreciable number with structural chromosome rearrangement; approximately one-fourth of women with primary amenorrhea have some abnormality of the X chromosome. Among infertile men and women, individuals with genes that interfere with meiosis, so-called meiotic mutants, are also found occasionally.

Numerical abnormalities Trisomy (47 chromosomes) is the most common chromosome imbalance in early spontaneous abortuses, followed by monosomy (45 chromosomes) and triploidy (69 chromosomes). The extra or missing chromosomes can be either paternal or maternal in origin, and the error in segregation of chromosomes can occur in the germ line, fertilized egg (zygote), or early embryo. Trisomy of every chromosome has been observed in spontaneous abortions, trisomy 16 most frequently.

Sex chromosomal trisomy (XXY, XYY, and XXX) is compatible with intrauterine survival; in contrast, autosomal trisomy rarely permits survival to term. However, a small proportion of autosomal trisomics is live-born. For practical purposes these are only trisomy 21, 18, and 13, in decreasing frequency. Trisomies 18 and 13 cause death during infancy. Trisomies of significance in adults are trisomy 21, XXY, XXX, and XYY. A few other autosomal trisomies, such as trisomy 8, have occasionally been reported, usually in mosaicism with a normal cellular component. (Mosaicism is the coexistence of multiple, genetically different populations of cells, derived originally from a single zygote.)

Autosomal monosomy is rare even among abortion material. In contrast, monosomy X (45,X) occurs in approximately 1.5 percent of recognized conceptions. It is common (approximately 10 percent) among spontaneously aborted human embryos and is present in one in every several thousand live-born babies. The reason for the death of 45,X embryos and fetuses is unknown, although developmental abnormalities doubtless contribute to it; cardiovascular and renal anomalies are common in the few that survive. In monosomy X, the missing sex chromosome can be either a Y or an X and is either paternal or maternal in origin. Often the second sex chromosome is not completely absent but is replaced by a structurally rearranged Y or X. Mosaicism is common in live-borns with monosomy X; here, tissues are populated not only by cells with a 45,X complement but by other cells, perhaps with a normal complement, either 46,XY or 46,XX, or with a complement in which the second sex chromosome is rearranged in some way.

Triploidy is rare in live-born babies and usually leads to early death, even when in a mosaicism with normal cells: 46,XY/69,XXY. The phenotypic effects of the autosomal trisomies, of 47,XXY, and of monosomy X (45,X) are characteristic and well defined so that their diagnosis usually is not difficult (see Chap. 120). The effects of the 47,XYY and 47,XXX constitutions are less striking, and therefore these complements are underdiagnosed. Mosaicism with coexistence of abnormal and normal populations of cells can cause an abnormal phenotype to approach the normal.

The mechanisms responsible for the numerical abnormalities are undefined and may be multiple. A striking but unexplained maternal age effect exists in trisomies 21, 18, 13, XXY, and XXX. Over one-third of babies with trisomy 21 are born to women over 35, whereas only one-tenth of all births occur in this group. The frequency of trisomy 21 rises from 0.5 to 0.7 per 1000 live births between ages 21 and 23 to 3.1 per 1000 at age 35, 10.5 per 1000 at age 40, and 33.6 per 1000 at age 45. (A paternal age effect may also exist in trisomy 21.) Maternal x-ray irradiation in low dosage is also associated with an increased incidence of trisomy 21. After a child with trisomy 21 is born, the risk to the parents of recurrence in future pregnancies is increased to approximately 1 percent. As to the etiology of monosomy X, the frequent association of the 45,X complement in mosaicism with normal complements and with structural rearrangements of the X and Y suggests that the zygote or early embryo may often be the target of a chromosome-breaking event.

Structural abnormalities Some structural chromosome rearrangements are inherited, and others represent new mutations. The etiology of the new rearrangements is unknown although they are assumed to be partly spontaneous and partly the effect of environmental agents such as mutagenic chemicals or ionizing radiation acting on the germ line, zygote, or early embryo (Fig. 61-4). The majority of de novo rearrangements are paternal in origin.

Many of the known chromosome rearrangements have been detected only once or a few times. Others are detected repeatedly, the same one occurring in unrelated individuals and families. For example, the commonest translocation, one that can occur either as result of de novo mutation or by inheritance, affects one chromosome 13 and one 14 at or near their centromeres. In this translocation, only inert chromatin is lost from the tiny short arms. A similar translocation affecting chromosomes 14 and 21 is also common.

Chromosome complements bearing rearrangements can be genetically balanced or effectively so, thus imparting no unfavorable phenotypic effect to their bearers; about two-thirds of rearrangements detected during surveys of consecutive live-born babies are balanced. Or, the complement can be unbalanced and affect development unfavorably, the usual case when rearrangements are detected during surveys of spontaneous abortuses or of individuals with multiple anomalies and mental deficiency.

Some balanced rearrangements are transmitted from generation to generation without producing clinical effects. In other cases, however, they are profoundly important to members of the kindred transmitting them, by being responsible for the conception of embryos with unbalanced genomes. For example, bearers of some 13;14 translocations are at risk of having children with the trisomy 13 syndrome, and inherited translocations involving chromosome 21 predispose to the trisomy 21 syndrome. Approximately 5 percent of live-borns with the trisomy 21 syndrome have a translocation, and in about a fifth of those it is detectable in one of the parents. Because most babies with the trisomy 21 syndrome due to translocation are born to women under 30, a search for a translocation is important when a child with this clinical syndrome is born to young parents.

Different translocations bestow on their carriers different risks of having offspring with unbalanced rearrangements. These risks cannot be predicted on the theoretical basis of the way the translocation might be expected to behave during meiosis. Useful empiric risk figures have been accumulated for common translocations; e.g., the 14;21 translocation bestows a 2 percent risk on a balanced male carrier and more than a 10 percent risk on a female carrier of having a child with the trisomy 21 syndrome. In contrast, the balanced carrier of a 21;21 translocation can expect only unbalanced offspring. Information of this type is indispensable to those undertaking genetic counseling in relation to chromosome disorders.

Although the phenotypic effects of many of the different segmental chromosome imbalances which can occur are varied and nonspecific, the resulting anomalies sometimes compose a recognizable clinical syndrome. Two examples are the following: (1) If a rearrangement causes partial trisomy of just the distal band of the long arm of 21, the clinical features composing the full syndrome associated with an extra chromosome 21 develop. (A triple dose of other segments of the long arm of chromosome 21 also produces adverse effects but not the trisomy 21 syndrome.) (2) Partial monosomy of a short segment within the short arm of chromosome 5 causes mental deficiency, a characteristic facies, and a characteristic cry during infancy. This group of signs is known as the *5p−* (five-p-minus) or *cri-du-chat syndrome.*

Because of the large number of karyotype-phenotype correlations made in recent years, additional specific syndromes produced by imbalance of many different segments now are known, e.g., the 4p−,9p partial trisomy, 13q−, and 18q− syndromes, to name a few. Rearrangements not previously described and their corresponding clinical syndromes are still being recognized. Any of these syndromes may appear as result either of de novo chromosome rearrangement or through formation of a genetically unbalanced gamete in a person carrying in balanced state a rearrangement affecting the segment involved.

In most individuals with chromosome imbalance, regardless of which segments are affected, a degree of phenotypic similarity is present. These recurring and nonspecific features include mental deficiency, growth deficiency, dysmorphic ears, nose, and mouth, cardiac malformations of standard types, abnormalities of dermal ridges and creases, and dysmorphic digits. (As a rule, autosomal imbalance need not be considered in the etiology of anatomic defects unaccompanied by mental deficiency.) Why similar abnormalities occur with so many different segmental imbalances is unknown, but when several such features are observed in a single individual, they can be a valuable clinical indication for cytogenetic analysis. Imbalance affecting certain segments also causes specific phenotypic changes; an example is the anomalous cry in the 5p− syndrome mentioned above. Other examples of specificity are retinoblastoma, which may develop when one particular band of chromosome 13 is present in single dose and the Prader-Willi syndrome, which is often associated with a disturbance of a band near the centromere of chromosome 15. Whereas the nonspecific changes serve to call the clinician's attention to the possibility of some chromosome imbalance, the specific features can suggest the exact segment of the genome affected.

DISEASE ASSOCIATIONS Various combinations of abnormalities in malformed and defective individuals have been correlated with variations in the chromosome complement. In this way, clinical syndromes due to specific chromosome imbalances have been defined. (Many of the pediatric conditions are of little significance in adult medicine because of their lethality in infancy or early childhood.)

Autosome imbalance Of the three autosomal trisomies found in live-born babies, only trisomy 21 is compatible with survival past infancy. The phenotype produced by the presence of an extra chromosome 21, formerly known as *mongolism* but now termed the *Down syndrome* or *trisomy 21 syndrome*, is characteristic and easily diagnosed from birth: mental deficiency, short stature, muscular hypotonia, brachycephaly, short neck, typical facies (oblique orbital fissures, flat nasal bridge, small simple or folded ears, nystagmus, mouth hanging open), narrow palate, short broad hands with incurving fifth fingers, gaps between the first and second toes, and characteristic dermatoglyphics. Additional findings may include congenital heart disease, blepharitis, and conjunctivitis, Brushfield's spots of the iris, straight pubic hair, abnormal teeth, a protruding furrowed tongue, a high-arched palate, loose skin of the neck, transverse palmar creases, and hyperflexibility of the joints. Cardiac malformations lead to death in infancy in a third of individuals with trisomy 21, and other malformations and infections may also cause early death. However, subjects who survive infancy often reach adulthood, and some even old age. The proneness to develop leukemia in affected infants is not maintained in later life. Females occasionally become pregnant, and, as expected, approximately half their children have trisomy 21.

Mosaicism of trisomy 21 with normal cells (46/47,+21) may occur in individuals with modified features of the trisomy 21 syndrome, and it is probable that many individuals with this mosaicism go undiagnosed. The risk of such persons having trisomic children is increased, but unfortunately their mosaicism is usually detected only after they have had an affected child. Partial trisomy, partial monosomy, or a combination of the two explains many of the instances in both children and adults of multiple developmental defects combined with mental deficiency. Sometimes a balanced autosomal translocation is detected in normally developed adults who have repeated spontaneous abortion or subnormal fertility, with or without abnormal live-born children.

Sex chromosome imbalance (see also Chap. 120) In contrast to autosome imbalance, sex chromosome imbalance has relatively mild phenotypic effects. This is because X chromosomes beyond one in the complement of somatic cells are usually almost totally inactivated and because the Y chromosome bears few if any genes other than the testis determinants. X-linked loci (in contrast to autosomal loci) function normally in single dose: the male is hemizygous for X-linked genes, having only one X chromosome (with the possible exception of a few loci on the Y that may be homologous to a segment on the X); the female is functionally hemizygous through the Lyon effect. The addition of an extra sex chromosome to the normal male or female complement has a phenotypic effect but insufficient to interfere with intrauterine survival. Since major anatomic defects are usually absent, individuals with the complements 47,XXY and 47,XYY, both of whom are males, and 47,XXX, who are females, ordinarily go unrecognized till adolescence or later, often never to be diagnosed at all.

The *Klinefelter syndrome* (Chap. 120), which in classic form consists of small testes, infertility, gynecomastia, and variable degrees of underandrogenization, sometimes with mild mental deficiency, antisocial behavior, or both, is the consequence of the addition of an extra X to the male complement: 47,XXY. The extra X interferes in some way with the survival of germ cells, and atrophy of the spermatogenic tubules and azoospermia are the consequence. Sometimes the phenotypic effects are surprisingly mild, the testicular atrophy being the only noteworthy feature in otherwise healthy and socially well-adjusted men. The mosaicism 46,XY/47,XXY sometimes occurs and may ameliorate the phenotypic effect of the extra X. More extreme phenotypic effects and mental deficiency result when more than one extra sex chromosome is added to the normal male complement: 48,XXXY or 49,XXXXY.

The phenotypic effect of 47,XYY is less well defined; although increased height, behavioral difficulties, and infertility are common, the extra Y is sometimes found in otherwise normal men. The rare complement 48,XXYY results in infertility, probably because of the extra X, as in the 47,XXY Klinefelter's syndrome. The phenotype associated with 47,XXX is also poorly defined, but women with mild mental deficiency, psychosis, and menstrual abnormalities are increased in frequency; this complement is sometimes detected in normal, healthy women. Further clarification is needed concerning the effects on personality and behavior of all three complements: 47,XXY, 47,XYY, and 47,XXX.

Loss of the Y or of the second X has drastic effects on development. If it does not cause abortion, it may or may not be recognizable at birth. Loose nuchal skin folds and edema of the hands and feet in a newborn girl, with or without renal or cardiovascular anomalies, may point to the diagnosis of the 45,X complement. The *Turner syndrome* (gonadal dysgenesis) is the manifestation in subsequent life (Chap. 120): short stature resistant to all treatment, infantilism of otherwise normal female external and internal genitalia, germ-cell-free gonads referred to as *gonadal streaks*, and variable renal, cardiovascular, skeletal, and ectodermal anomalies. Without estrogen administration breast development remains infantile and menstruation does not occur. Although mental deficiency is not a feature, a poorly defined emotional immaturity is common.

The Turner syndrome may be the developmental consequence of several chromosome constitutions besides 45,X. Mosaicism as well as structural abnormalities of a second sex chromosome, either a Y or an X, cause a spectrum of disorders at both the clinical and cytogenetic levels. A normal male or normal female cellular component may be present along with the 45,X cellular component, or one component may bear a structurally abnormal chromosome. Common abnormalities of the Y and X are isochromosome formation (one arm deleted and the other duplicated) or deletion of part of or all one arm. In some affected individuals, all cells have 46 chromosomes, with one normal X plus an abnormal Y or X, for example, 46,XXp−, deletion from the short arm of one of the X chromosomes. In others, a second or third cellular component may be present as well, for example, 45,X/46,XX/46,XXp−. Clinically pure Turner syndrome may be found in association with various combinations of these karyotypes if one of them is either monosomic or partially monosomic for X. However, when Y-bearing cells coexist with the 45,X cells, for example, 45,X/46,XY, genital ambiguity often develops, and gonads may vary from streaks to functional testes (the syndrome of *mixed gonadal dysgenesis*); here the risk of malignant gonadal neoplasia is significant. When 46,XX cells coexist with 45,X, varying degrees of ovarian function may be maintained, including ovulation. Although the phenotype may approach a normal male or female pattern when normal and abnormal cells coexist, the effects of mosaicism are unpredictable. Thus, the clinical syndrome associated with monosomy X and structurally abnormal Ys or Xs ranges from a predominantly male phenotype through Turner syndrome to an almost normal female phenotype.

Two other rare conditions deserve mention—*true hermaphroditism* and the *46,XX male* (see also Chap. 120). *True hermaphroditism* is present when both testicular and ova- and follicle-containing ovarian tissue exist in the same individual. In most cases 46,XX is the chromosome complement, and it appears normal by banding; here the most plausible explanation is that an occult translocation of the testis-determining segment of the Y to an X or autosome has occurred. Sometimes true hermaphrodites have the complement 46,XY; rarely the chimerism 46,XY/46,XX is found, the two cellular components having been derived from two zygotes.

Males occasionally have the complement 46,XX. As in 47,XXY men, the second X interferes with meiosis, and azoospermia results. In both the 46,XX true hermaphrodite and the 46,XX male the rule that a Y is required for testicular differentiation appears to break down. However, the two conditions may have the same etiologic basis, undetected translocation of Y material onto another chromosome.

X-linked mental deficiency Generally more males than females are mentally deficient, and mental deficiency when familial affects males preferentially. In some such kindreds, severe mental deficiency segregates as an X-linked trait, and in a proportion of those the X in the affected males and that same X in their mothers can be made recognizable cytologically. Near the end of its long arm (Xp) is a "fragile site" at which point gaps and breaks tend to occur. Mothers of the affected males may exhibit a degree of mental deficiency. In some families macroorchia may accompany the mental deficiency. The "fragile X" is not demonstrable in all families with X-linked mental deficiency.

Chromosome change in cancer The theory that an alteration in the chromosomal complement may be the cause of cancer was advanced almost seven decades ago, but the matter is still unsettled. Chromosome changes are plentiful in cancer, but this very fact—too many changes—has been a major reason many have rejected them as of etiologic significance. However, support for the idea that chromosome alteration is significant in the etiology of human cancer has come from two observations: (1) the known environmental "causes" of human cancer (carcinogenic chemicals and ionizing radiation) are also chromosome-breaking agents (Fig. 61-4); and (2) three recessively inherited disorders result in increased chromosome breakage and rearrangement in cells in culture, and in each the risk of cancer is increased—the Bloom syndrome, Fanconi's anemia, and ataxia-telangiectasia. Thus, the known environmental and the known genetic causes of increased chromosome mutation all predispose to cancer.

Most human cancers have altered chromosome complements. In the leukemias, lymphomas, and certain myeloproliferative disorders, the alterations, although detectable with refined technique, are less extensive than in solid tumors and, therefore, easier to define. In certain lymphomas, chromosome 14 is often found to have undergone structural rearrangement. In over 80 percent of chronic granulocytic leukemias, a translocation affecting chromosome 22 (usually chromosome 9 is the other chromosome affected) is detected, the so-called Ph^1 chromosome; if the disease progresses into a "blastic" phase, the karyotype often evolves, certain additional chromosome changes being added stepwise in a nonrandom sequence. In this and certain other leukemias, the various chromosome changes appear to have some value in prognosis and choice of therapy.

Solid tumors, which generally are studied later in their course than conditions affecting the bone marrow, show extensive karyotypic changes, both structural and numerical. Different cells from a single tumor have similar numerical changes and structural rearrangements, but in the same type tumor from another person the changes usually seen are different. This apparent lack of specificity is partly due to the complexity of the changes, however, and a few examples of chromosome alterations specific for a solid tumor are known; for example, meningiomas are associated with a deletion of chromosome 22 in almost every case. The findings in both solid tumors and leukemias demonstrate the clonal nature of human cancer.

TECHNICAL CONSIDERATIONS Human metaphase chromosomes can be examined in any tissue in which sufficient cells are cycling. Preparations can therefore be made directly from almost any embryonic tissue and from adult bone marrow, lymphoid tissue, and selected malignant tissues. In searches for mosaicism, the study of multiple tissues is often required. Some tissues unlikely to yield cells in metaphase can be placed in culture, and chromosome preparations can be made after many cells have been brought into mitosis. Blood lymphocytes stimulated to enter cell-division cycles by phytohemagglutinin are the standard material for diagnosing constitutional chromosome imbalance. In some myeloproliferative disorders and leukemias, unstimulated circulating blood cells divide spontaneously after a few hours in culture. Long-term cultures of fibroblasts can be derived from minute skin biopsies or from most any tissue, although more elaborate laboratory facilities and a longer period of time are required before cytogenetic preparations can be made. Amniotic fluid is among the sources of cells suitable for culture, and these embryonic cells are widely used in the diagnosis of fetal chromosome imbalance.

Nucleated cells in interphase can be used for the study of sex chromatin. Cells from buccal mucosa and hair follicles are perhaps the most readily obtained, but surgical and autopsy specimens or cells in culture are at times useful also. X chromatin (formerly called the Barr body), a condensed body of chromatin characteristically apposed to the nuclear membrane, is present in normal female cells. The X responsible for X chromatin in any particular cell is the one genetically inactivated and late-replicating. The number of X-chromatin masses is an indication of the number of X chromosomes in excess of 1. Y chromatin, a condensed segment of the Y demonstrated by quinacrine staining and fluorescence microscopy, is present in interphase nuclei of Y-bearing cells (for example, 48,XXYY cells contain one X-chromatin plus two Y-chromatin masses).

Meiotic chromosome preparations from testicular biopsies are sometimes useful in obscure cases of infertility. Here translocations and genetically determined disturbances in meiotic pairing may be identified.

REFERENCES

BERG K et al (eds): *Cytogenetics and Cell Genetics,* vol 32: *Human Gene Mapping 6 (1981). Sixth International Workshop.* Basel, Karger, 1982

DE GROUCHY J: *Clinical Atlas of Human Chromosomes.* New York, Wiley, 1977

GERMAN JL: Studying human chromosomes today. Am Sci 58:182, 1970

SCHWARZACHER HG: *Methods in Human Cytogenetics.* New York, Springer-Verlag, 1974

SIMPSON JL: *Disorders of Sexual Differentiation.* New York, Academic, 1976

62
PREVENTION AND TREATMENT OF GENETIC DISORDERS

JOSEPH L. GOLDSTEIN
MICHAEL S. BROWN

APPROACHES TO PREVENTION

In view of the present trend for couples to have smaller families, there is increasing concern that children should be healthy and free of genetic diseases, and primary-care physicians are called upon to play a more active role in the prevention and treatment of hereditary diseases. In most clinical situations, genetic advice can be given by the primary physician once the relatively simple principles of medical genetics (Chap. 58) and genetic counseling (discussed below) have been mastered.

RETROSPECTIVE GENETIC COUNSELING The prevention of genetic diseases requires the identification of matings that are capable of producing defective genotypes. These may involve matings in which one of the two individuals is carrying a dominant or X-linked gene mutation or a balanced translocation, or matings in which both individuals are carriers of a deleterious recessive gene. Such individuals are usually identified through an affected child or near relative, in which case retrospective genetic counseling can be provided.

When advising family members about the risk of transmit-

TABLE 62-1
Methods for detection of asymptomatic heterozygotes in frequently encountered dominantly inherited disorders

	Method of heterozygote detection		
Disorder	*Physical findings*	*Laboratory tests*	*Therapeutic advantage of early diagnosis*
GASTROINTESTINAL, LIVER, AND PANCREAS			
Gilbert's disease		Serum bilirubin	Avoid confusion with more serious forms of liver disease
Peutz-Jeghers syndrome	Melanin spots on lips, buccal mucosa, and digits	X-ray of small intestine	Clarify cause of gastrointestinal bleeding
Familial polyposis		X-ray of colon; colonoscopy	Prevent colon carcinoma
Gardner's syndrome	Multiple sebaceous cysts; lipomas; fibromas; osteomas; dental abnormalities; desmoid tumors	X-ray of colon and small intestine; colonoscopy	Prevent colon carcinoma
METABOLIC AND ENDOCRINE			
Medullary thyroid carcinoma-pheochromocytoma syndrome		Serum calcitonin; measurement of blood pressure	Prevent thyroid carcinoma and complications of hypertension
Multiple endocrine adenomatosis	Multiple lipomas	Serum calcium, gastrin, blood sugar; x-rays of sella turcica, stomach, and small intestine	Prevent complication of hyperparathyroidism, hypoglycemia, peptic ulcer, metastatic cancer
Familial hyperparathyroidism		Serum calcium, parathyroid hormone	Prevent renal damage and other complications of hypercalcemia
Familial hypercholesterolemia	Tendon xanthomas, xanthelasma, arcus corneae	Serum cholesterol; low-density lipoprotein receptor activity of cultured fibroblasts	Prevent premature coronary heart disease
HEART AND VASCULAR			
Holt-Oram syndrome	Abnormality of thumb and carpals; murmur of atrial septal defect	X-ray of hands; cardiac evaluation	Prevent complications of atrial septal defect
Noonan's syndrome	Hypertelorism; small chin; low-set ears; ptosis; pectus deformity; cryptorchidism; murmur of pulmonic stenosis	Cardiac evaluation; x-ray of skeleton; intravenous pyelogram (renal anomalies)	Prevent heart failure
Idiopathic hypertropic subaortic stenosis (asymmetric septal hypertrophy)	Presystolic gallop; characteristic carotid arterial pulse	ECG; echocardiogram	Prevent sudden death, syncope, angina, heart failure
Dominantly inherited form of atrial septal defect	Heart murmur	ECG showing first degree heart block, right bundle branch block, right axis deviation	Prevent complications of atrial septal defect
HEMATOLOGIC			
Hereditary spherocytosis	Splenomegaly; jaundice	Blood smear; reticulocyte count; hemoglobin; osmotic fragility test	Prevent anemia, cholelithiasis
Hereditary hemorrhagic telangiectasia	Telangiectasia of tongue, lips, conjunctiva, ears, fingers; pulmonary AV fistula	X-ray of lungs	Clarify cause of nosebleeds and gastrointestinal bleeding
Von Willebrand's disease		Immunologic and functional assays of plasma antihemophilic globulin levels; bleeding time	Prevent gastrointestinal and urinary bleeding
CONNECTIVE TISSUE AND BONE			
Ehler-Danlos syndromes (types I, II, III)	Loose-jointedness; fragile, stretchable, bruisable skin; subcutaneous calcified spherules		
Marfan's syndrome	Ectopic lens; mitral and aortic murmurs; excessive length of extremities	Slit-lamp examination; metacarpal index by x-ray	Reduce risk of aortic dissection; prevent blindness
Osteogenesis imperfecta	Multiple fractures; loose-jointedness; blue scleras; deafness; aortic regurgitation	X-ray of bones	

ting a disorder that has already affected someone in the family, the counselor's first step is to be certain of the *correct diagnosis*—in particular, to make certain that the problem in question is really of genetic origin. This is especially important in disorders that may have either a genetic or a nongenetic etiology, such as deafness or mental retardation. Second, if the disease has a hereditary element, the possibility of *genetic heterogeneity,* i.e., a situation in which clinically similar genetic disorders show varying patterns of inheritance, must be considered. For example, there are two types of hereditary methemoglobinemia that resemble each other quite closely, but one shows autosomal recessive and the other autosomal dominant inheritance.

To estimate the *recurrence risk,* one must initially determine what is known of the genetic mechanisms controlling the rel-

TABLE 62-1 *(continued)*
Methods for detection of asymptomatic heterozygotes in frequently encountered dominantly inherited disorders

	Method of heterozygote detection		
Disorder	*Physical findings*	*Laboratory tests*	*Therapeutic advantage of early diagnosis*
RENAL			
Alport's syndrome	Nerve deafness; cataracts, lenticonus, spherophakia	Urinalysis, slit-lamp examination	Prevent uremia
Nail-patella syndrome	Dysplastic nails; absent patellas	X-ray of pelvis (iliac horns); urinalysis	Clarify cause of hematuria and azotemia
Polycystic kidney disease		Urinalysis; intravenous pyelogram; renal arteriogram; measurement of blood pressure	Prevent uremia and complications of hypertension
Renal tubular acidosis		X-ray of kidneys (nephrocalcinosis); urine pH, calcium; serum electrolytes, calcium	Prevent acidosis, osteoporosis, kidney stones
RESPIRATORY			
Hereditary angioneurotic edema		Serum level of Cl esterase inhibitor of complement	Reduce risk of sudden death caused by laryngeal edema and clarify cause of acute abdominal pain
DERMATOLOGIC			
Neurofibromatosis	Café au lait spots; neurofibromas; scoliosis		Prevent malignant degeneration of neurofibromas
Waardenburg syndrome	Wide bridge of nose; frontal white blaze of hair; heterochromia iridis; white eyelashes; deafness		Clarify cause of deafness
Basal-cell nevus syndrome	Multiple basal-cell carcinomas; jaw cysts; pits on palms and soles; skeletal defects (ribs, spina bifida, scoliosis)	X-rays of skull (calcification of falx cerebri) and skeleton	Removal of cutaneous cancers; provide cosmetic surgery
NEUROLOGIC			
Charcot-Marie-Tooth disease	Pes cavus; atrophy of anterior tibial and calf muscles ("stork legs"); absence of deep tendon reflexes	Biopsy of muscle and of sural cutaneous nerve	Improve walking by corrective shoes and orthopedic measures
Myotonic dystrophy	Myotonia; muscle wasting of temporal and sternocleidomastoid muscles; cataracts; frontal baldness; signs of hypogonadism	Slit-lamp examination; electromyography; measurement of serum immunoglobulins; electrocardiogram	Anticipate complete heart block
Acute intermittent porphyria		Measurement of uroporphyrinogen synthetase activity in red blood cells	Reduce risk of neuropathic attacks by avoidance of aggravating drugs such as barbiturates
Tuberous sclerosis	Adenoma sebaceium; cutaneous white macules; shagreen patch; periungual fibromas		Prevent seizures
Huntington's chorea	Paranoia, other personality changes; choreic movements; dementia		
Periodic paralysis syndromes (hypo-, hyper-, and normokalemic types)	Cold-induced myotonia	Electromyogram; serum potassium	Reduce frequency of attacks by avoidance of aggravating agents such as high-carbohydrate diet and exposure to cold
PHARMACOGENETIC			
Malignant hyperthermia		Serum creatine phosphokinase	Prevent fatal episode of hyperthermia induced by general anesthesia

evant disorder. When more than one genetic mechanism exists, or when environmental factors can cause clinically indistinguishable traits, the *relative probabilities* of the different mechanisms operating in the particular family are computed. For conditions determined by simple mendelian inheritance, there is no difficulty in predicting the probability of an offspring being affected, provided that the genotypes of the parents can be recognized. Identification of the parental genotype is easiest for autosomal recessive and X-linked disorders since the basic lesions in these two forms of mendelian inheritance frequently involve simple enzyme deficiencies for which biochemical tests are now available.

For autosomal dominant disorders, identification of the parental genotype is more difficult since the basic defect is known for only a few of these disorders, and the diagnosis of the heterozygote for a dominant disorder depends almost exclusively on the clinical evaluation and a careful pedigree analysis. In counseling a family in which one relative is affected with a dominant disorder, it is important that appropriate clinical examination of all first-degree relatives and selected distant relatives be carried out. If relatives appear unaffected, the clinical symptoms may be masked by *delayed age of onset* and *variability in expression,* or the possibility of a new dominant mutation must be entertained. Table 62-1 lists the most commonly encountered dominant disorders affecting adults and the methods available for detection of the heterozygote.

When advising families about multifactorial genetic diseases, such as diabetes mellitus, in which the inheritance pattern is not clear-cut, the physician must resort to empiric risk estimates that have been derived from retrospectively assembled data (Table 58-5).

Once the parental genotypes are determined, the genetic prognosis is usually presented in terms of probability that a given couple will produce an affected offspring. The physician must make certain that the couple understands not only the meaning of such risk figures, but also the severity of the disease and the variability in clinical expression. In other words, in dealing with a disorder such as neurofibromatosis, it is important for the parents to realize not only that they have a 50 percent risk of producing a child with this disorder but also that a certain proportion of patients with the disorder have severe disease, a certain proportion have mild disease, etc. They should also have an understanding of the potential impact of the disease on their family; a disease that is lethal at birth might be classified as more "severe" than one that is lethal at age 16, but the latter is likely to have a more profound impact on the family.

Although different families react in different ways to the same risk, most couples who seek genetic advice take a responsible course of action that is based on the information quoted. Generally, the physician should avoid giving direct advice as to whether a couple "should" or "should not" have children. For serious genetic disease, with a recurrence risk equal to or greater than 1 in 10, most parents are deterred from planning further children. When the risk is less than 1 in 10, most parents continue with additional pregnancies.

PROSPECTIVE GENETIC COUNSELING In contrast to retrospective genetic counseling in which advice is given after the birth of at least one affected family member, in prospective genetic counseling advice is provided to possible carriers of recessive genes before an affected individual is born. As a first step, this requires the identification of heterozygous individuals by a population-screening procedure. Second, unmarried heterozygotes are instructed about the risk of their having af-

TABLE 62-2
Inborn errors of metabolism for which prenatal diagnosis is feasible

DISORDERS OF CARBOHYDRATE METABOLISM
Glycogen storage diseases—Types II, III, and IV
Galactosemia
Galactokinase deficiency
Pyruvate decarboxylase deficiency
DISORDERS OF AMINO ACID METABOLISM
Argininosuccinicaciduria
Citrullinemia
Homocystinuria
Maple syrup urine disease
Methylmalonic aciduria
Isovaleric acidemia
Ketotic hyperglycinemia
DISORDERS OF LIPOPROTEIN AND LIPID METABOLISM
Homozygous familial hypercholesterolemia (receptor-negative type)
Refsum's syndrome
DISORDERS OF LYSOSOMAL ENZYMES
Mucopolysaccharidosis, type I (Hurler's syndrome)
Mucopolysaccharidosis, type II (Hunter's syndrome)
Mucopolysaccharidosis, type III (Sanfillipo's syndrome, types A and B)
Mucopolysaccharidosis, type VI (Maroteaux-Lamy syndrome)
Mucopolysaccharidosis, type VII (β-glucuronidase deficiency)
I-cell disease
Lysosomal acid phosphatase deficiency
Wolman's syndrome and cholesteryl ester storage disease
Fabry's disease
Gaucher's disease
Krabbe's disease (globoid cell leukodystrophy)
Metachromatic leukodystrophy
Niemann-Pick disease
Tay-Sachs disease
Sandhoff's disease
Generalized gangliosidosis
Juvenile gangliosidosis
Fucosidosis
Mannosidosis
Farber's disease (lipogranulomatosis)
DISORDERS OF STEROID METABOLISM
21-Hydroxylase deficiency—congenital adrenal hyperplasia
Steroid sulfatase deficiency (X-linked ichythosis)
DISORDERS OF PURINE AND PYRIMIDINE METABOLISM
Lesch-Nyhan syndrome
Hereditary orotic aciduria
Xeroderma pigmentosum
Adenosine deaminase deficiency (combined immunodeficiency)
DISORDERS OF METAL METABOLISM
Menkes' syndrome
DISORDERS OF PORPHYRIN AND HEME METABOLISM
Acute intermittent poryphyria
DISORDERS INVOLVING CONNECTIVE TISSUE, MUSCLE, AND BONE
Hypophosphatasia (some types)
DISORDERS OF THE BLOOD AND BLOOD-FORMING TISSUES
Sickle cell anemia
α Thalassemias
β Thalassemias
Glucose 6-phosphate dehydrogenase deficiency
DISORDERS OF TRANSPORT
Cystinosis

fected children if they marry another heterozygote for the same gene. Finally, if two heterozygotes are already married, there is the possibility of interrupting the birth of affected infants if the disease can be diagnosed in utero by amniocentesis.

Population screening for heterozygote detection is possible for several autosomal recessive disorders (such as sickle cell anemia, thalassemia major, and Tay-Sachs disease) that occur in certain populations with high frequency. For example, 8 percent of the American black population carries the sickling gene, and 4 percent of Ashkenazi Jews are carriers of the Tay-Sachs gene.

Screening programs raise many ethical and social problems. Informing a healthy person that he or she is carrying a specific mutant gene that may cause disease in the children if a certain type of mate is chosen differs from counseling parents who have already had an affected child. Little is known about the social and psychologic effects as well as occupational discrimination that may result from discovering that a person carries a "bad" gene.

PRENATAL DIAGNOSIS The use of transabdominal amniocentesis permits diagnosis of certain genetic diseases at a stage early enough to terminate a pregnancy and to prevent the birth of a defective child. This procedure gives high-risk couples the opportunity to have unaffected children provided they are willing for the pregnancy to be terminated in the event that an abnormal fetus is detected. Amniocentesis consists of the transabdominal aspiration of amniotic fluid from the uterus. The procedure is preferably performed between the fourteenth and sixteenth weeks of pregnancy. When performed by a trained gynecologist, the technique is relatively safe for both mother and fetus.

Direct examination of the amniotic fluid itself may be diagnostic. For example, an elevated level of α-fetoprotein is a relatively good indicator of the presence of spina bifida or another neural tube abnormality. More frequently, prenatal diagnosis requires culture of the fetal cells in vitro, a process which usually takes 3 weeks. By this means the karyotype of the fetus can be determined to ascertain fetal sex and to detect chromosomal aberrations. Moreover, many inborn errors of metabolism can be detected by assays of specific enzyme activities in the cultured fetal cells. Table 62-2 lists those enzyme deficiency states for which prenatal diagnosis is currently feasible. More disorders are constantly being added to this list.

Prenatal diagnosis by amniocentesis is currently indicated in the following high-risk situations: (1) couples having a previous child with spina bifida or anencephaly, (2) couples having a previous child with a chromosomal aberration such as the

TABLE 62-3
Major indications for prenatal diagnosis

Clinical situation	*Estimated risk to fetus, %*	*Method of detection of abnormal fetus*
Couples having a previous child with spina bifida or anencephaly	5	Measurement of α-fetoprotein in amniotic fluid
Couples having a previous child with a chromosomal disorder such as the trisomy 21 form of Down's syndrome	2	Chromosomal analysis of cultured amniotic fluid cells
Couples in whom either the husband or wife carries a balanced translocation for Down's syndrome	5–20	Chromosomal analysis of cultured amniotic cells
Pregnant women 38 years of age and older whose risk of having a child with Down's syndrome is increased	1–2	Chromosomal analysis of cultured amniotic fluid cells
Couples at risk for having a child with a detectable inborn error of metabolism (see Table 62-2)	25 or 50	Biochemical analysis of cultured amniotic fluid cells

TABLE 62-4
Some treatable hereditary disorders affecting adults

Method of Treatment	*Disorder*
DIETARY RESTRICTION OF SUBSTRATE	
Lactose	Lactase deficiency
Galactose	Galactosemia and galactokinase deficiency
Fructose	Fructose intolerance
Neutral fats	Familial lipoprotein lipase deficiency
Phytanic acid	Refsum's syndrome
Phenylalanine	Phenylketonuria
REPLACEMENT OF DEFICIENT END PRODUCT	
Vitamin D and phosphate	Hypophosphatemic rickets
Cortisol	Adrenogenital syndromes
Thyroxine	Familial goiters
Uridine	Orotic aciduria
DEPLETION OF STORAGE SUBSTANCE	
Sterol removal by bile-acid binding resins	Familial hypercholesterolemia
Cystine removal by D-penicillamine	Cystinuria
Copper removal by D-penicillamine	Wilson's disease
Iron removal by phlebotomy	Hemochromatosis
Uric acid removal by uricosuric agents	Gout
AMPLIFICATION OF ENZYME ACTIVITY	
Pyridoxine (vitamin B_6)	Homocystinuria
Vitamin B_{12}	Methylmalonic aciduria
Phenobarbital	Crigler-Najjar variant and other forms of unconjugated hyperbilirubinemia
REPLACEMENT OF MUTANT PROTEIN	
Gamma globulin	Agammaglobulinemia
Factor VIII (AHG)	Hemophilia
Infusion of irradiated erythrocytes containing adenosine deaminase	Severe combined immunodeficiency disease
ORGAN TRANSPLANTATION	
Kidney	Fabry's disease, cystinosis, Alport's syndrome, polycystic kidney disease (adult form)
Allogeneic bone marrow	Lymphopenic hypogammaglobulinemia (Swiss type), Wiscott-Aldrich syndrome, severe combined immunodeficiency disease
SURGICAL REMOVAL	
Splenectomy	Hereditary spherocytosis
Portacaval shunt	Glycogen storage disease (type I) and homozygous familial hypercholesterolemia
Colectomy	Familial polyposis of the colon
Thyroidectomy	Medullary thyroid carcinoma syndrome

trisomy 21 form of Down's syndrome, (3) couples in whom either the husband or wife carries a balanced translocation chromosome for Down's syndrome, (4) couples at high risk for having a child with a detectable inborn error of metabolism, and (5) pregnant women 38 years of age and older. Table 62-3 lists the major indications for prenatal diagnosis, the risks involved, and methods by which the abnormal fetus can be detected.

APPROACHES TO TREATMENT

The goal of treatment for genetic diseases is to modify the natural history of the genetic trait so that an affected person may live a comfortable and healthy life despite a mutant genotype. Such treatment can be achieved for a number of inherited diseases using a variety of approaches, including (1) the exclusion or restriction of toxic foods, (2) metabolic supplementation, (3) removal of toxic products, (4) surgery, and (5) organ transplantation. Table 62-4 lists examples of hereditary diseases affecting adults that can be successfully treated at the present time.

REFERENCES

EPSTEIN CJ: Prenatal diagnosis of genetic disorders. Adv Intern Med 20:325, 1975

GALJAARD H: *Genetic Metabolic Diseases: Early Diagnosis and Prenatal Analysis.* Amsterdam, Elsevier/North-Holland, 1980

STANBURY JB et al: *The Metabolic Basis of Inherited Disease,* 5th ed. New York, McGraw-Hill, 1983

WORLD HEALTH ORGANIZATION: *Genetic Disorders: Prevention, Treatment, and Rehabilitation.* WHO Tech Rep 497, 1972

section 2 | Clinical immunology

63 INTRODUCTION TO CLINICAL IMMUNOLOGY

BRUCE C. GILLILAND

Clinical immunology is a rapidly expanding field with increasing practical application to medicine. The scope of immunology covers defense against infections, prevention of diseases by immunization, organ transplantation, blood banking, deficiencies of the immune system, and a variety of disorders that are mediated by immunologic mechanisms. Besides the clinical relevance of immunology, immunologic techniques are frequently used in the clinical laboratory, as in the measurement of hormones and drugs.

The intent of this chapter is to provide the reader with a review of the essential fundamentals of immunology. The cellular components of the immune system, lymphocytes, plasma cells, and macrophages, along with their role in antibody-mediated or humoral immunity and in cell-mediated or cellular immunity, will be discussed first. This will be followed by a review of the immunoglobulins, cellular immunity, the interrelationship of the B and T lymphocytes and macrophages in the immune response, tolerance, and autoimmunity. The last sections cover the complement system and types of immunologically mediated inflammation and tissue damage.

CELLS OF THE IMMUNE SYSTEM The principal cells of the immune system are lymphocytes, plasma cells, and macrophages which are collectively organized into lymphoid tissue. The thymus, lymph nodes, and spleen are examples of highly developed lymphoid tissues. Other lymphoid tissue is found along the gastrointestinal tract (tonsils, Peyer's patches, appendix) and also may accumulate at sites of inflammation.

A large body of experimental evidence has affirmed the existence of two populations of lymphocytes. These two populations were first demonstrated in chickens by removal of the thymus or by removal of the bursa of Fabricius (a lymphoid organ near the cloaca) during the neonatal period. Excision of the bursa resulted in low immunoglobulin levels and impaired antibody synthesis. Lymphoid nodules did not develop in lymph nodes and spleen, and only a few plasma cells were present. Cell-mediated immunity, however, remained intact as demonstrated by delayed hypersensitivity and allograft rejection. Evidence for two populations of immunocompetent cells in humans has largely come from study of congenital and acquired defects of immunity (see Chap. 64) and from development of techniques for identification of populations of lymphocytes. These observations clearly indicate the existence of two separate systems for the differentiation of lymphoid cells involved in humoral and cellular immunity (Fig. 63-1). The two populations of immunocompetent lymphocytes are referred to as B cells and T cells (Table 63-1). The designation *B*

FIGURE 63-1
Schematic representation of the development of the immune system and the immune response. Upon exposure to immunogen, T cells proliferate and become sensitized lymphocytes that form the basis of cell-mediated immunity. The B cells proliferate and evolve to antibody-synthesizing plasma cells that constitute the basis of humoral immunity. Macrophages process and present immunogen to T and B cells. Subsets of T cells function as helper T cells which stimulate B-cell activity, or as suppressor T cells which suppress humoral and cell-mediated immune responses.

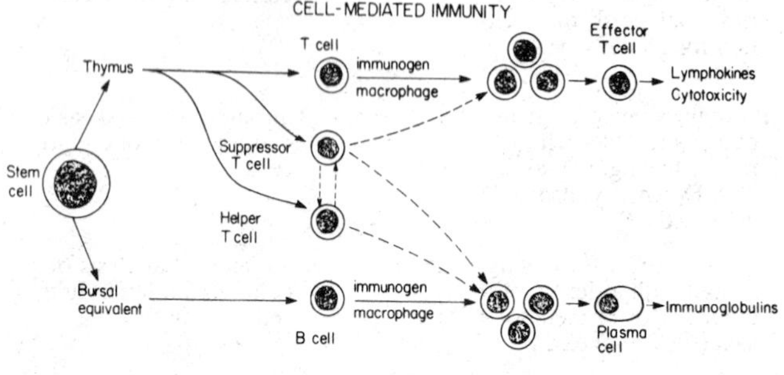

cell was used originally because these cells depend for their development on the presence of the bursa in birds or its equivalent in humans. The equivalent of the bursa in humans remains unknown but might be the fetal liver, spleen, or bone marrow. The designation *T cell* connotes the role of the thymus in the development of these cells.

B cells B cells represent approximately 12 to 15 percent of the normal peripheral blood lymphocytes, 50 percent of the splenic lymphocytes, and 75 percent of the lymphocytes in the bone marrow in normal individuals. They are the principal cells in the cortical germinal centers and medullary cords of lymph nodes. Their chief role is the production of antibodies.

The B cells carry membrane-bound immunoglobulins as demonstrated by immunofluorescence staining with anti-immunoglobulin antiserum. The main immunoglobulin classes on the surface of peripheral blood B cells are IgM, present in the low-molecular-weight (7-S subunit) monomeric form, and IgD. Approximately three-quarters of the peripheral blood B cells carry these two immunoglobulins; the remaining cells stain mostly for IgG, while about 1 percent stain for IgA. The membrane-bound immunoglobulin molecule is attached by its crystallizable fragment (Fc) portion to the plasma membrane, leaving the antigen-binding sites freely available. Upon contact with specific antigen and with modulatory signals from other cells, B cells bearing the complementary antigen-binding site will evolve through a series of events leading to clonal expansion and differentiation into antibody-synthesizing plasma cells.

The most widely accepted theory of antibody formation is clonal selection, which suggests that there are large numbers of precommitted lymphocytes, each with its specific membrane receptor capable of reacting with specific immunogen. The selective binding of immunogens is followed by clonal expansion and antibody production.

Most of the B cells have a membrane receptor for the Fc portion of IgG in the form of either antigen-antibody complexes or aggregated IgG. Approximately one-half of the B cells also carry membrane receptors for the activated third component of complement (C3b). Receptors for other complement components (C3d, C4, and Clq) have also been identified on B cells. These various membrane receptors and membrane-bound immunoglobulins have membrane mobility and can undergo redistribution and capping. For example, when membrane-bound immunoglobulin binds with specific antigen, the immunoglobulin molecules reorganize into patches on the membrane and then these molecules localize at one pole of the cell (capping). The polar cap of molecules is interiorized by endocytosis. As this process is occurring, the B cell is synthesizing new immunoglobulins for insertion into its membrane.

TABLE 63-1
Characteristics of T and B lymphocytes

	T cells	*B cells*
Function	Delayed hypersensitivity	Humoral immunity
Product	Lymphokines	Immunoglobulins
Identification	Sheep RBC rosettes	Surface Ig Fc and activated complement receptors
Assessment	Proliferative response to PHA, Con A Delayed skin test	Immunoglobulin levels Antibody response to immunization Blastogenic response to PWM

NOTE: *Ig, immunoglobulin; PHA, phytohemagglutinin; Con A, concanavalin A; PWM, pokeweed mitogen.*

These events may be important in the initiation of cell proliferation and antibody production. It has also been suggested that the capping process may serve only to remove excess antigen from the cell surface.

T cells Approximately 70 to 80 percent of normal peripheral blood lymphocytes and 90 percent of lymphocytes in thoracic duct fluid are T cells. They circulate primarily as long-lived small lymphocytes. These cells are the principal lymphocytes in the deep cortical areas of lymph nodes and in the periarteriolar areas of the splenic white pulp. The T cells are the main effectors of cell-mediated immunity and also are involved as helper or suppressor cells in modulating the immune response.

T cells possess cell surface antigens that are identified by a panel of monoclonal antibodies to surface antigens. Differentiation of T cells from precursor cells to immunologically competent cells requires a thymic microenvironment and is characterized by acquisition and loss of cell surface antigens (see Chaps. 57, 64). Precursor bone marrow cells (prothymocytes) migrate to the thymus where they undergo stages of development. The early thymocytes express $T9^+$ and $T10^+$, and with further development they lose $T9^+$, retain $T10^+$, and acquire $T6^+$, $T4^+$, $T5^+$. The thymocytes then lose $T6^+$, gain $T1^+$ and $T3^+$, and segregate into two populations of mature cells having differences in cell surface antigens and future function. The two subsets are $T10^+$, $T1^+$, $T3^+$, $T4^+$, and $T10^+$, $T1^+$, $T3^+$, $T5^+$. The mature thymocytes lose $T10^+$ on entering the circulation and become fully immunologically competent cells. T cells with surface antigens $T1^+$, $T3^+$, $T4^+$ function as helper-inducer cells and those with $T1^+$, $T3^+$, $T5^+$ as cytotoxic-suppressor cells. These cells migrate to various lymphoid tissues such as spleen, lymph nodes, and bone marrow. Once the T cell has left the thymus, this gland may continue to exert an effect on T cells by secretion of thymic hormones.

The T cells in humans are usually identified by the presence of membrane receptors for sheep red blood cells which form rosettes around T cells when they are incubated together. Several subpopulations of T cells are recognized on the basis of differences in function, surface antigens, and membrane receptors for immunoglobulins. The various subsets of T cells function as helper-inducer cells, suppressor cells, or cytotoxic effector cells (see "Immune Response" below). The nature of the antigen-binding receptor on T cells is uncertain. One candidate for antigen receptor is a monomeric IgM-like molecule which has been identified on the T-cell membrane by some investigators. Other candidates include the cell membrane product of histocompatibility genes and the membrane product (Ia antigen) of immune response genes (Ir genes).

A small number of lymphocytes in blood (2 to 10 percent) do not have the usual surface membrane markers for B or T cells and are referred to as *null cells.* Some of these cells may represent incompletely differentiated B or T cells. Others have an Fc receptor for IgG and are referred to as *K* or *killer cells,* since they are the effector cell in antibody-dependent cell-mediated cytotoxicity (see "Immune Mechanisms of Tissue Injury" below).

Macrophages Macrophages originate from promonocytes in the bone marrow and are released into the circulation as monocytes. Monocytes comprise 3 to 8 percent of the circulating leukocyte population. An even greater number of monocytes, estimated to be approximately three times the circulating population, exists in a marginal pool consisting of monocytes adhering to endothelial surfaces. Upon entering tissue, monocytes develop into macrophages. Tissue sites where macrophages are commonly found include the liver (where they are called *Kupffer cells*), peritoneum, lung, spleen, and lymph nodes. Macrophages have surface receptors for IgG1 and IgG3, and also a receptor for C3b. Through these receptors, macrophages can effectively bind and interiorize antigen-antibody complexes consisting of IgG antibodies or immune complexes which contain activated C3. Macrophages kill bacteria, fungi, and tumor cells. They also function in the induction of the immune response by processing and presenting immunogenic material to lymphocytes (see "Immune Response" below).

IMMUNOGLOBULINS Immunoglobulins are synthesized by the B-cell series and have common structural features and structural units. Immunoglobulin molecules are composed of two kinds of polypeptide chains (Fig. 63-2); each molecule consists of larger identical polypeptide chains referred to as *heavy chains* (H chains) and two identical smaller ones referred to as *light chains* (L chains). These polypeptide chains are held together by disulfide bonds and by noncovalent bonds, which are primarily hydrophobic. The heavy and light polypeptide chains are synthesized on separate ribosomes, assembled in the cell, and secreted as an intact molecule. A slight to moderate excess of light chains is synthesized and secreted as free light chains.

The understanding of the structure and function of immunoglobulins was facilitated by studies of fragments produced by enzymatic cleavage of the antibody molecule (Fig. 63-3). For example, treatment of antibody molecules with papain results in two Fab fragments, which are the antigen-binding fragments of the molecule, and one Fc fragment, which is responsible for the biological activities discussed below. The amino-terminal half of the light chains and the amino-terminal quarter of the heavy chains of the immunoglobulin molecules vary in their amino acid sequence and are termed the *variable region* (V region) of the polypeptide chains. Portions of the V region of one heavy and one light polypeptide chain contribute the site for antigen binding. Considerable variation of the amino acid sequence must exist in this portion of the immunoglobulin molecule in order to explain the estimated 1 million antibody specificities. The constant region of H chains allows their differentiation into a class or subclass and confers to the immunoglobulins certain biological properties such as the ability to activate complement, to cross the placenta, and to bind to polymorphonuclear leukocytes or macrophages.

Five immunoglobulin classes (IgG, IgA, IgM, IgD, and IgE) are recognized on the basis of structural differences of their heavy chains including the amino acid sequence and length of the polypeptide chain. The antigenic determinants on the heavy chains also permit the identification and quantitation of the immunoglobulin classes by immunochemical techniques. On protein electrophoresis at a pH of 8.6, the immunoglobulins migrate mainly in the gamma region. Significant amounts of immunoglobulins also may be found in the beta region. The bulk of the gamma globulin consists of IgG immunoglobulin. The wide range in which immunoglobulins can migrate on protein electrophoresis is due to amino acid differences in the variable region of the molecules. A narrow band of protein staining in the gamma to beta region usually indicates the presence of a monoclonal population of immunoglobulins, the product of a single clone of cells as in multiple myeloma or macroglobulinemia (see Chap. 65). Antibodies to a given antigen may be detected in all or several classes of immunoglobulins or may be restricted to a single class or subclass of immunoglobulin. Autoantibodies likewise may belong to one or several classes of immunoglobulins. For example, rheumatoid factors (antibodies to IgG) are most often recognized as an IgM immunoglobulin, but can also consist of IgG or IgA. The physical and biological properties of immunoglobulins are listed in Table 63-2.

IgG The most abundant immunoglobulin is IgG; approximately 50 percent of its distribution is in the intravascular compartment. It has a molecular weight of 150,000 daltons. IgG is the only immunoglobulin that crosses the placenta and thereby provides maternal antibodies to the neonate. The structural features that mediate the transport across the placenta reside in the Fc fragment of IgG molecules. Four subclasses of IgG have been defined. While each has a common antigenic determinant for IgG, some differences in their amino acid sequences provide antigens that permit separation into subclasses. IgG1 and IgG3 are able to activate the complement system upon formation of immune complexes and to react with

FIGURE 63-2
Schematic model of the variable and constant regions of an antibody molecule. The blackened areas represent the variable regions in the amino terminal half of each L chain and the amino terminal quarter of each H chain. The remainder of the molecules constitutes the constant regions. Amino acid sequences in the variable regions provide the basis for antibody specificity.

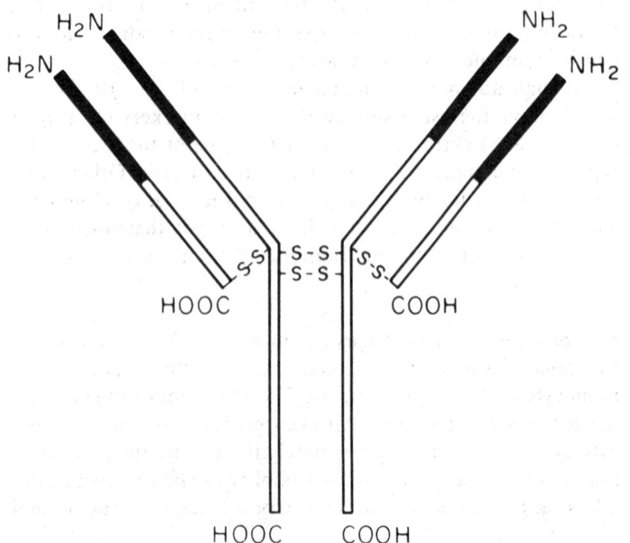

FIGURE 63-3
Schematic representation of enzyme cleavage of immunoglobulin molecules. Papain cleaves the molecule into three parts, two Fab fragments with antigen-binding sites and one Fc fragment. Pepsin produces a bivalent F(ab')$_2$ fragment, and the Fc portion is cleaved into small peptides.

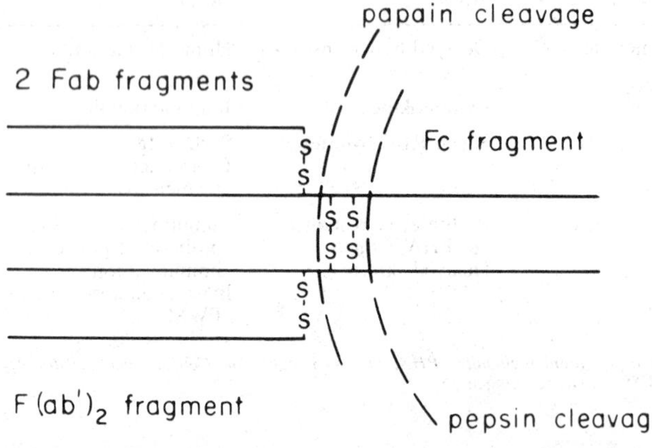

IgG receptors on monocytes and polymorphonuclear leukocytes. Both of these properties of IgG reside in the Fc portion of the molecule. Approximately 70 percent of the total IgG is IgG1, 18 percent is IgG2, 8 percent is IgG3, and 4 percent is IgG4.

IgA The predominant immunoglobulin in external secretions of the respiratory tree, gastrointestinal tract, and genitourinary system, and in tears, saliva, and colostrum is IgA. The IgA-producing plasma cells are the predominant plasma cells in the submucosa. For example, in the lamina propria of the intestine, approximately 20 IgA-producing plasma cells exist for each IgG-producing cell, compared with a 1:3 ratio in the peripheral lymph nodes and spleen. Secretory IgA is composed of two IgA molecules bound to a secretory piece by disulfide bonds. The secretory piece is a polypeptide chain with a molecular weight of 70,000 daltons that is synthesized by epithelial cells. The dimeric IgA is held together by a single J chain which is also synthesized by submucosal plasma cells and has a molecular weight of 15,000 daltons. Once the dimeric IgA leaves the plasma cell, it enters the epithelial cell and becomes covalently bound to a secretory piece. It is then secreted into the lumen. Secretory IgA has a molecular weight of approximately 400,000 daltons. Low concentrations of secretory IgA sometimes are found in the normal serum. Secretory IgA is more resistant to digestion by most proteolytic enzymes than monomeric IgA. An IgA protease that specifically cleaves human IgA1 has been discovered. This protease occurs in certain microorganisms such as *Neisseria gonorrhoeae* and *Streptococcus sanguis,* both of which are known to invade mucosal membranes in spite of prior immunity. Secretory IgA can have antibody activity to bacterial and viral antigens, toxins, and dietary macromolecules. Secretory antibodies bind microorganisms and prevent their attachment to epithelial cells, and administration of antigens by either the gastrointestinal or respiratory route results in enhanced production of secretory IgA in these organ systems.

In the serum, IgA exists as a monomer with a molecular weight of 160,000 daltons, and to a lesser extent in polymeric forms. Two subclasses of IgA have been identified; approximately 75 percent of the total IgA is IgA1, and 25 percent IgA2. No biological differences are known to exist between IgA1 and IgA2 except that IgA2 appears to be resistant to cleavage by the specific IgA proteases.

IgM Approximately 10 percent of the serum immunoglobulins are IgM, which is a pentamer of the usual four polypeptide chain structure of immunoglobulins, having a molecular weight of 900,000 daltons. The five IgM subunits are linked by disulfide bonds in association with a single J chain to constitute the IgM molecule. While the J chain apparently assists in the polymerization of IgM, polymers form in the absence of the J chain. Even though the pentameric IgM has 10 antigen-binding sites, these antibodies have a functional valence of 5 with large antigenic molecules. The distribution of IgM is predominantly intravascular. Activation of the complement system requires only one molecule of IgM antibody to react with antigen. IgM antibody is prominent in the early immune response and is the major class of antibodies to blood group substances A and B. Autoantibodies, such as rheumatoid factor (anti-IgG) and cold agglutinins, are also predominantly IgM immunoglobulins. A natural subunit of IgM is called *low-molecular-weight IgM* and has a molecular weight of 180,000 daltons. It is found on the surface of B cells, in fetal blood, and in certain diseases such as rheumatoid vasculitis, systemic lupus erythematosus, ataxia-telangiectasia, progressive muscular atrophy and idiopathic chronic neuropathy, Waldenström's macroglobulinemia, and lymphoma. The biological significance of this molecule in the circulation is not known.

IgD IgD has a molecular weight of 180,000 daltons and is found mainly in the intravascular space and on resting B cells as a cell surface immunoglobulin. IgD is easily degraded by proteolytic enzymes and by heat. The function of free IgD in blood is not known, but the IgD on B cells may, in association with monomeric IgM, play an important role in the binding of antigen to B cells.

IgE The distinctive biological feature of IgE is its role in the immediate allergic or hypersensitivity reaction (reaginic property) (see Chap. 67). IgE has a molecular weight of 190,000 daltons and binds to basophils and mast cells through its Fc region. When a specific antigen combines with the antigen-binding sites on IgE, histamine, serotinin, and the slow-reacting substance of anaphylaxis are released from these cells. The allergen must bind to two or more adjacent molecules of IgE to evoke the release of histamine. These pharmacological mediators lead to the characteristic wheal and flare reaction in the skin. In the lung, the same sequence of events leads to bronchospasm and asthma. The bulk of the body's pool of IgE is bound to basophils and mast cells, and the serum concentration of this immunoglobulin is extremely low, in the order of 0.1 to 0.2 μg/ml.

TABLE 63-2
Properties of immunoglobulins

	IgG	*IgA*	*IgM*	*IgD*	*IgE*
Molecular weight, daltons	150,000	160,000	900,000	180,000	190,000
Average serum concentration, mg/dl	1200	280	100	3	0.025*
Percent of total body pool in intravascular compartment	50	40	75	75	
Half-life, days	23	5.5	5.1	2.8	2.3
Complement fixation by classic pathway	Yes†	No‡	Yes	No	No
Reagenic properties	No	No	No	No	Yes
Selective secretion by mucous membranes	No	Yes	No	No	No
Placental transfer	Yes	No	No	No	No
Macrophage binding	Yes¶	No	No	No	No

* *Serum concentration in normal nonatopic individuals is less than 0.025 mg/dl.*
† *IgG4 does not activate complement and IgG2 only weakly.*
‡ *IgA activates complement system only by the alternative pathway.*
¶ *Only IgG1 and IgG3.*

CELL-MEDIATED IMMUNITY (DELAYED TYPE OF HYPERSENSITIVITY) The principal effectors of cell-mediated immunity are T cells that have become sensitized to foreign substances. These specifically sensitized T cells, along with macrophages, play a very important role in the defense of the host against a variety of infectious microorganisms including *Mycobacterium tuberculosis,* fungi, viruses, and protozoa. Cell-mediated immunity is most prominent in infections due to intracellular organisms. The killing of tumor cells and rejection of allografts such as kidney transplants are also expressions of cell-mediated immunity.

Cell-mediated immunity is exemplified by the delayed type of hypersensitivity reaction in skin. The intradermal or subcutaneous injection of antigen into an individual previously sensitized to that antigen results in a reaction that consists of erythema followed by induration and reaches a peak in approximately 2 days. Lymphocytes and macrophages are the predominant cells in the lesion. If the inflammation is intense, necrosis of the skin may occur. Cell-mediated immunity can be transferred to a previously unimmunized individual with T cells but not with serum. In addition, cell-mediated immunity can also be transferred to a normal recipient with *transfer factor,* a low-molecular-weight material derived from disrupted sensitized lymphocytes or from the supernatant of a stimulated lymphocyte culture.

The events of cell-mediated immunity are initiated as the result of interaction of antigen with a few specifically sensitized T cells. The sensitized T cells, activated by antigen, elaborate soluble products referred to as *lymphokines,* which have several biological activities. Lymphokines mediate and amplify cell-mediated immune reactions by affecting the activities of macrophages, polymorphonuclear leukocytes, B cells, and other T cells. Several of the products of activated lymphocytes are listed in Table 63-3. While the T cell is considered the principal cell in cell-mediated immunity, the concept of cell-mediated immunity has taken on a broader connotation with the observation that B cells also release lymphokines, including macrophage chemotactic factor, macrophage-activating factor, and macrophage inhibitory factor.

The development of the cell-mediated immune reaction in vivo may occur as follows: Antigen activates specifically sensitized T cells resulting in the elaboration of lymphokines. One of these factors, macrophage chemotactic factor, attracts macrophages to the site of immunologically induced inflammation where they are activated by macrophage-activating factor which is either identical or similar to macrophage migration inhibitory factor (MIF). Properties of the activated macrophages include an increase in their size and number of lysosomes, greater phagocytic ability, and enhanced killing of bacteria or tumor cells. The biological property of MIF is most likely to reduce the random migration of macrophages, thereby keeping them at the site of inflammation. Mitogenic factors amplify the response by increasing the number of activated lymphocytes. The sensitized T cells kill antigen-specific target cells, such as tumor cells, either by direct cell-to-cell contact or by the elaboration of lymphotoxin. Bacteria or tumor cells are also killed by macrophages, and polymorphonuclear leukocytes attracted to the site of inflammation by chemotactic factor secreted by T cells.

TABLE 63-3
Products of activated lymphocytes

1 Affecting macrophages
 a Migration inhibitory factor (MIF)
 b Macrophage-activating factor (identical to MIF?)
 c Chemotactic factor for macrophages
2 Affecting lymphocytes
 a Mitogenic factor
 b Transfer factor
3 Affecting polymorphonuclear leukocytes
 a Chemotactic factors for neutrophils, eosinophils, and basophils
 b Migration-inhibiting factor
4 Affecting other cell types
 a Cytotoxic factors (lymphotoxin)
 b Interferon
 c Growth inhibitory factors (inhibits proliferation of target cells)
 d Osteoclast activation factor

For the clinical assessment of cell-mediated immunity, skin tests continue to be useful. The diagnosis of several infectious diseases is aided by the finding of a positive skin test which indicates prior exposure and T-cell sensitization to the particular organisms but not necessarily active disease. Since at least 80 percent of the population have been sensitized to *Candida, Trichophyton,* streptokinase-streptodornase, or purified protein derivative (PPD), these antigens are suitable for determining the general status of cell-mediated immunity. The absence of a response to a battery of antigens that previously elicited a cell-mediated immune response is termed *anergy* and may signify an underlying disorder such as lymphoma or sarcoidosis. Several drugs, diseases, and other conditions may suppress skin tests of the delayed type. These include glucocorticosteroids, malignant diseases such as Hodgkin's disease or lymphoma, sarcoidosis, infections (measles, infectious mononucleosis, miliary tuberculosis), old age, malnutrition, acquired and congenital immunodeficiency disorders, and, in some instances, fever.

The ability of an individual to develop cell-mediated immunity de novo can be determined by applying directly to the skin a chemical such as dinitrochlorobenzene (DNCB) to which the individual has not been previously exposed. The chemical combines with skin proteins to form an immunogenic substance that stimulates the sensitization of T cells to DNCB. Ten to fourteen days following this initial exposure to DNCB, the reapplication of DNCB on the skin will result in a positive skin test if cell-mediated immunity is intact. In suspected anergic patients, a negative test with DNCB confirms a cutaneous anergic state.

Cell-mediated immunity can be assessed in vitro by stimulating lymphocytes with specific antigens, unrelated lymphocytes, or nonspecific substances such as the plant lectins, phytohemagglutinin or concanavalin A. The functional capacity of T cells is determined by culturing lymphocytes with phytohemagglutinin or concanavalin A. These lectins bind to the carbohydrate moieties of cell membrane receptors and stimulate transformation or blastogenesis of lymphocytes which is measured by the incorporation of radioactive precursors (tritiated thymidine) into DNA. These two lectins are primarily T-cell mitogens; however, they stimulate different subsets of T cells (see "Cell Cooperation" below).

T cells previously sensitized to an antigen will also undergo blastogenesis when cultured with the specific antigen. The blastogenic response of T cells on exposure to antigen in vitro corresponds fairly well with the in vivo skin tests of delayed hypersensitivity. The response of T cells to specific antigens can also be determined by measuring the biological activity of the various soluble mediators or lymphokines released from the activated T cells (e.g., quantitating the amount of inhibition of macrophage migration resulting from the release of MIF). The release of soluble mediators from T cells may occur without the cells undergoing blastogenesis.

The mixed lymphocyte culture (MLC) is an assay widely used in the field of transplantation for the typing of histocompatibility antigens (see Chap. 60). The test is usually performed in unidirectional method by treating the stimulating lymphocyte population with either radiation or mitomycin C which prevents these cells from responding without affecting their stimulatory properties. When the lymphocytes from a normal individual are cultured with these treated lymphocytes, the individual's T cells will undergo blastic transformation if the antigens on the stimulatory cells are sufficiently different. The cell antigens recognized in the MLC reaction are the products of genes at the HLA-D locus. The absence of a response indicates the presence of identical antigens in the two cell populations. The MLC reaction can also be used to assess the functional capacity of T cells.

IMMUNE RESPONSE Upon exposure to a foreign substance, an individual can respond by producing specific antibodies, by developing cell-mediated immunity (delayed hypersensitivity), or by becoming immunologically unresponsive. The substances that elicit an immune response are termed *immunogens,* and their ability to evoke this response is called *immunogenicity.* Antigens are substances that will react specifically with available antibodies or sensitized lymphocytes. Certain small molecules with molecular weights of less than 1000 daltons usually are not capable of inducing an immune response but can interact as antigens with available antibodies and are called *haptens.* However, an immune response can be elicited with haptens if they are coupled to a larger carrier molecule which is immunogenic in the host.

The route of administration, the dose of the immunogen, and the response of the host are all factors determining the immune response. For example, the oral administration of poliomyelitis virus leads to effective immunization by stimulating the production of IgA antibodies in the gastrointestinal tract. Skin contact with chemicals (e.g., resins of poison ivy) evokes primarily a cell-mediated or delayed hypersensitivity reaction involving the skin. The dose of immunogen also affects the immune response. Both very high doses and low doses of immunogen may produce tolerance. The failure to detect an immune response, therefore, is not conclusive, since a substance may be immunogenic at a different dose or by a different route of administration.

One of the most exciting areas in immunology is the role of genetic factors in the immune response. Evidence for a genetic influence on the immune response to a given immunogen is based on studies in inbred strains of mice and other laboratory animals. Genetic differences within a species are associated with an immune response to a given immunogen in one strain and with no response in another. These differences may also lead to a high level of antibody production in one strain and to low levels in another strain. In several species including humans, the ability of an individual to respond to a specific immunogen is under the control of immune response genes that are located in the chromosomal region referred to as *major histocompatibility gene complex.* Genes within this region code for molecules that are involved in the initiation, stimulation, and suppression of the immune response (see Chap. 60).

Cell cooperation Many immunogens require an interaction of B and T cells to generate a humoral immune response. These immunogens are referred to as being *thymus dependent.* Examples of some thymus-dependent antigens are glycoproteins, natural proteins, heterologous serum proteins, and erythrocytes. The interaction of T cells with B cells is termed *cooperation,* and the T cells that function in this context are called *helper T cells.* Other immunogens, referred to as being *thymus independent,* are able to initiate B-cell proliferation and antibody production without the help of T cells. The biochemical characteristics that differentiate thymus-independent from thymus-dependent immunogens have not been fully identified, but some differentiating features are the repeating linear polymeric structure of the thymus-independent immunogens and the slow degradation of these molecules in the host. Examples of thymus-independent immunogens include pneumococcal polysaccharides, polymerized *Salmonella* flagellin, dextran, and lipopolysaccharides.

T cells play a central role in the induction and regulation of the immune response. Various subsets of mature peripheral T cells are genetically programmed to be helper-inducer cells or cytotoxic-suppressor cells. Subsets of T cells with these functions are identified by cell surface antigens detected by using a panel of monoclonal antibodies. Helper-inducer T cells express the surface antigens $T1^+$, $T3^+$, $T4^+$ ($T4^+$) and represent approximately 65 percent of peripheral T cells. The $T4^+$ cells provide helper-inducer function in T cell–T cell, T cell–B cell, and T cell–macrophage interactions. The proliferation and differentiation of B cells into antibody-containing plasma cells is induced by $T4^+$ cells. Antigen-stimulated $T4^+$ elaborate lymphocyte mitogenic factor which induces stimulation of all major lymphocyte subclasses. $T4^+$ cells after antigen stimulation express Ia surface antigens (I-region–associated antigens) which may act as recognition sites or signals for the interaction of T cells, B cells, and macrophages involved in the immune response. Cytotoxic-suppressor T cells express $T1^+$, $T3^+$, $T5^+$ ($T5^+$) cell surface antigens and when stimulated suppress B-cell immunoglobulin production. Approximately 25 percent of peripheral T cells are $T5^+$. This subset also contains cells with cytotoxic function. The presence of $T4^+$ cells, however, is required for the optimal development of cytotoxic-effector T cells. A small number of peripheral T cells that are $T4^-$ $T5^-$ also play a role in immunoregulation. These cells and the $T5^+$ population express $T8^+$ on their cell surface. A subpopulation of T cells that carries receptors for the Fc portion of IgM and that may represent helper T cells has been recognized. Another group has membrane receptors for the Fc portion of IgG and may represent suppressor T cells. The interaction of these subsets of T cell provides a mechanism for self-regulation and homeostasis of the immune response. In a clinical context, hyperactivity of the suppressor T-cell system in patients with common variable hypogammaglobulinemia may induce low levels of immunoglobulins by suppressing B-cell proliferation and antibody production (see Chap. 64). Hypergammaglobulinemia, on the other hand, may represent too much helper T-cell activity owing to loss of suppressor T-cell function.

Macrophages are also critical cells in the immune response and especially involve thymus-dependent antigens. An important function of the macrophage is the presentation of immunogenic material to B and T cells. In this setting, immunogens may interact directly with the surface of macrophages. Macrophages also express Ia antigens on their surface which may function as antigen recognition sites. Macromolecules or particulate substances, however, require digestion by macrophages to become immunogenic. A few immunogenic molecules of the digested material are retained on the surface of the macrophages. Macrophages also elaborate soluble biologic substances that stimulate both T and B cells.

Models of antibody production Several models of antibody production involving T- and B-cell cooperation have emerged from studies in animals. In one such model, immunogenic material may be initially processed by macrophages or may directly bind with a specific antigen receptor on T cells. As mentioned above, the nature of the antigen receptor on T cells may be an IgM-like molecule or Ia antigen. This T-cell-antigen receptor and the antigen dissociate as a complex from the T cell and bind to the macrophage, perhaps through the Fc receptor on the macrophage. As a result of this binding, the necessary density and frequency of antigenic determinants are created for the interaction with antigen receptors on B cells and subsequent stimulation of antibody production. The antigen-activated T cells may also elaborate nonspecific helper factors that stimulate antibody production.

Other models for antibody production take into greater consideration the genetic control of the immune response. The antigen receptor on T cells in one such model is referred to as the *T-cell recognition factor* and is coded for by an immune response gene. The T cell, through its recognition factor, can directly bind immunogen or can interact with immunogen presented on the surface of a macrophage. The recognition factor is associated with an interaction factor which is coded for by an I-region gene. I-region genes are located within the major histocompatibility complex and control immune responsiveness. The complex of antigen, recognition factor, and interaction factor dissociates from the T cell and binds to B cells carrying the specific immunoglobulin receptor for antigen and the complementary receptor site for interaction factor. The receptor site for interaction factor on these B cells is also coded for by the same I-region gene. Antigen-stimulated T cells may also react directly with the B cells carrying the complementary antigen receptor and site for interaction factor. The interactions between T cells, B cells, and macrophages may depend on the sharing of common histocompatibility antigens.

Primary and secondary immune responses On a first exposure to a new immunogen, several days are required before humoral and cell-mediated immunity are detected. This initial response to a new immunogen is termed the *primary* immune response. When the immunogen is thymus-dependent, IgM and IgG classes of antibody are initially secreted by the B cells, and IgM appears first. As the titer of IgG rises during the second week following immunogenic stimulation, the IgM titer falls. The antibody titer reaches a peak in approximately 2 weeks and then falls gradually. However, low levels of antibody can be demonstrated for months and even years. The switch from IgM synthesis to predominantly IgG synthesis in B cells requires T-cell cooperation. The synthesis of IgA and IgE also is dependent on T-cell cooperation. In the absence of T-cell cooperation, the B cells stimulated by thymus-dependent antigens produce low levels of antibody belonging to the IgM classes. The thymus-independent immunogens such as pneumococcal polysaccharides and *Salmonella* O stimulate the production of antibodies belonging to the IgM class even after repeated injections.

Following a second exposure to the same immunogen, heightened cell-mediated or humoral responses are observed. This is termed a *secondary* or *anamnestic* response. These responses occur sooner than the primary response, usually in 4 to 5 days in humans, and depend on a marked proliferation of antibody-producing cells or effector T cells of cell-mediated immunity. The antibody produced is of the IgG class and has a greater affinity for antigen than the antibody synthesized initially during the primary immune response. The secondary response depends on immunologic memory that must be demonstrated by both T and B cells.

Tolerance A state of specific immunologic unresponsiveness to substances that would normally evoke an immune response is termed *tolerance*. It is an active physiologic process and not merely the lack of an immune response. Humoral immunity, cell-mediated immunity, or both may be suppressed. Tolerance provides the essential mechanism for the prevention of immunologically induced self-injury. The impairment of self-tolerance is considered the basic pathogenic mechanism in autoimmune diseases.

Tolerance can be induced in several ways. The physical form and dose of an antigen are important factors determining whether tolerance or an immune response develops. In experimental models, the administration of soluble antigen in monomeric form produces tolerance, while the same antigen in aggregated or polymeric form leads to an immune response. High doses of antigen lead to tolerance of both B and T cells. In comparison with B cells, tolerance in T cells is induced with lower doses of antigen and persists longer. Tolerance is more readily achieved in the neonate than in the adult. The maintenance of tolerance requires repeated or chronic exposure to the tolerogenic antigen. Tolerance may also be induced and maintained by the stimulation of suppressor T-cell activity which can suppress both humoral and cell-mediated immunity.

Immunologic unresponsiveness also can be caused by antibody. Antibody binding to antigen may produce conformational changes in the antigen, preventing its interaction with lymphocytes. Antibody in the form of an immune complex can also suppress the immune response by interacting with suppressor T cells enhancing suppressor activity.

Autoimmunity The development of immunologic responsiveness to self is called *autoimmunity* and reflects the impairment of self-tolerance. Immunologic, environmental, and genetic factors are closely interrelated in the pathogenesis of autoimmunity. Clinical disorders in which autoimmune responses play a role in the pathogenesis of the illness are referred to as *autoimmune diseases*. Autoantibodies, however, are found in some normal persons without evidence of autoimmune disease. The frequency of autoantibodies in the general population increases with age, suggesting a breakdown of self-tolerance with aging. Autoantibodies also may develop as an aftermath of tissue damage. The spectrum of autoimmune disorders ranges from thyroiditis, which is organ specific, to systemic lupus erythematosus, which is characterized by an array of autoantibodies to cell and tissue antigens.

The development of autoimmunity usually involves the breakdown or circumvention of self-tolerance. The potential for the development of autoantibodies probably exists in most individuals. For example, normal human B cells are capable of reacting with several self-antigens (e.g., thyroglobulin) but are suppressed from producing autoantibodies by one or more mechanisms of tolerance. Precommitted B cells in tolerant individuals can be stimulated in several ways. Tolerance involving only T cells, induced by persistent low levels of circulating self-antigens, may be circumvented by substances such as endotoxin. Such substances would stimulate the B cells directly to produce autoantibodies, thus obviating the need for helper T cells. A decrease in suppressor T cell activity could also lead to production of autoantibodies (see below).

Autoimmunity may develop to antigens that were sequestered or anatomically separated from the immune system during embryonic development. For example, in the absence of low levels of circulating antigen, both B and T cells are immunocompetent. In later life, exposure to such antigens through trauma or infection results in autoimmune responses (e.g., release of myelin in experimental allergic encephalomyelitis).

Viruses also play an important role in the pathogenesis of autoimmunity. Several animal models of autoimmunity such as F_1 hybrids of the New Zealand black (NZB) and white (NZW) mice have persistent viral infections from birth (Chap. 70). It is difficult to determine whether the viral infection interferes with the immune system or if preexisting abnormal immunity permits chronic viral infection. In any event, these animals develop circulating immune complexes, composed of antibodies to nuclear antigens and to viral antigens, which deposit in the glomerular basement membrane and other tissue sites, leading to the manifestations of immune complex disease. The expression of viral antigens on the surfaces of the host's cells may elicit autoantibodies to cell membrane antigens. Furthermore, autoantibodies may develop from exposure to exogenous viral antigens that cross-react with autoantigens. Bacteria or other foreign substances may also act as cross-reacting antigens.

It has been proposed that autoimmunity is a disorder of abnormal immunologic regulation resulting in excessive B-cell activity and diminished T-cell activity. A decrease in suppressor T-cell activity or an increase in helper T-cell activity would result in uncontrolled excessive production of autoantibodies. The strongest support for this concept of autoimmunity comes from studies in animal models and human autoimmune disorders in which the loss of suppressor T-cell function and excessive B-cell antibody production can be demonstrated.

A role for genetic factors in the pathogenesis of autoimmunity has been clearly demonstrated in animal models and clinical autoimmune disorders. New Zealand black mice manifest autoimmune hemolytic anemia, whereas the NZB/NZW F_1 hybrids develop a disease analogous to systemic lupus erythematosus (SLE). The relatives of patients with SLE may have clinical and serologic abnormalities of SLE: a high concordance of SLE is also found in monozygotic twins. Associations with histocompatibility antigens are noted in several clinical autoimmune disorders. Chronic active hepatitis, Graves' disease, and Addison's disease occur more often in individuals who are HLA-B8 positive. An association with genes located at the HLA-D locus has been noted in adult rheumatoid arthritis, Sjögren's syndrome, and multiple sclerosis. These associations may be significant because of the close relationship between genes determining histocompatibility antigens and genes controlling the type and magnitude of the immune response.

Complement system The complement system consists of a group of at least 15 plasma proteins which interact sequentially, producing substances that mediate several functions of inflammation and serve a role in host defense (Table 63-4). The activated complement components and the enzymatically cleaved fragments of components exert many of their biological activities by interaction with cell membranes. The actions of the complement system include cell lysis, release of histamine from mast cells and basophils, vascular permeability, contraction of smooth muscle, chemotaxis of leukocytes, stimulation of polymorphonuclear leukocyte oxidative metabolism, release of lysosomal enzymes from phagocytic cells, and neutralization of certain viruses. The complement system also is interrelated with the coagulation, fibrinolytic, and kinin systems. Complement is involved in the pathogenesis of tissue injury observed in many immunologically mediated diseases which include SLE, rheumatoid arthritis, glomerulonephritis, and immune-hemolytic anemia.

The activation of complement is initiated either by the classic pathway or by the alternative (properdin) pathway (Fig. 63-4). Both pathways lead to activation of a common terminal sequence of complement components. The complement components of the classic pathway are C1, C4, and C2. C1 is composed of three subunits, C1q, C1r, and C1s, which are held together by calcium. The classic pathway is activated by the interaction of antibody and antigen. The antigen can either be soluble or a constituent of a cell membrane or extracellular surface such as the basement membrane of the renal glomerulus. Immunoglobulin classes of antibody which activate the classic pathway are IgM and IgG. The subclasses of IgG with this property are IgG1, IgG2, and IgG3 but not IgG4. When antibody unites with antigen, the antibody undergoes conformational change which permits binding of C1q with the Fc portion of the antibody molecule. The binding of C1q activates C1r, which in turn activates C1s, which is an esterase. The esterase cleaves C4 into a small fragment, C4a, and a large fragment, C4b, which binds to the immune complex or cell membrane. Activated C1s and C4b act together to split C2 into a small fragment, C2b, which has kinin-like properties, and a larger fragment. The larger fragment, C2a, combines with C4b to form C3 convertase (C4b2a), a magnesium-dependent enzyme that acts on C3.

The alternative (properdin) complement pathway produces activation of C3 by a series of reactions that bypass C1, C4, and C2. The components of the alternative complement system include factor D, which is an esterase similar to C1s, factor B, properdin, and C3. This pathway is activated by lipopolysaccharides (e.g., bacterial endotoxin), complex polysaccharides (e.g., inulin), immune complexes containing IgA or IgD, or nephritic factors. The latter are most likely IgG immunoglobulins which function by binding to the alternative pathway C3 convertase (factor $\overline{B}$ C3b), and may be autoantibodies to this enzyme complex. Nephritic factors are present in the serum of some patients with membranoproliferative glomerulonephritis or with partial lipodystrophy. Certain bacteria and fungi (e.g., *Staphylococcus epidermidis, Candida albicans*) can activate the alternative pathway. The C3 convertase of the alternative pathway is formed by the interaction of factor D, factor B, and C3b and requires divalent Mg^{2+} ions. In the normal catabolism of C3, small amounts of C3b are present which are protected from further degradation when bound to factor B. The C3 convertase is stabilized by properdin and nephritic factor when

TABLE 63-4
Biological functions of complement

Biological function	*Complement components*
Chemotaxis	C5a, $\overline{C567}$
Histamine release (anaphylatoxin)	C3a, C5a
Opsonization	C3b
Cytolytic	C5 to C9
Kinin-like activity	C2 fragment
Viral neutralization	C1, C4

FIGURE 63-4
Diagram of the classic and alternative complement pathways. These two pathways converge at C3 to form a common terminal pathway that results in cell lysis. Cleavage of complement components produces biologically active fragments. (See text for details.)

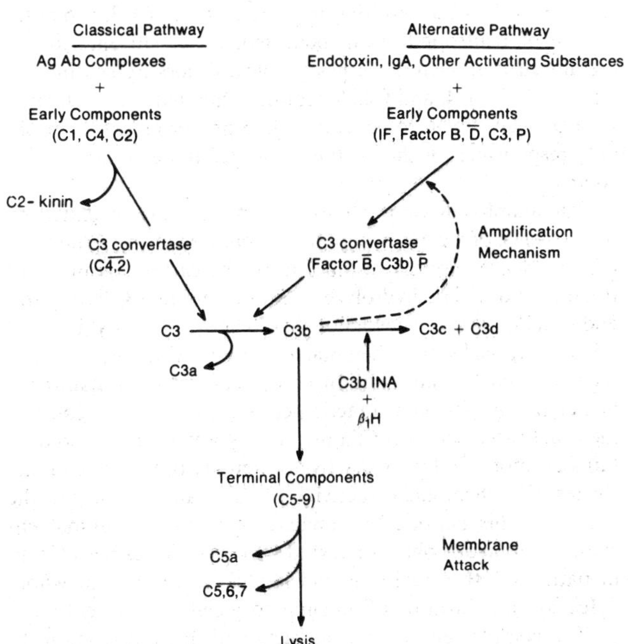

present. Cleavage of C3 by either pathway results in a small peptide, C3a, and a large molecule, C3b. The latter interacts with factor B as previously described, resulting in C3 activation with formation of C3b which leads to more activation of C3, and amplification of complement activity. Regulators of this pathway are C3b inactivator and its cofactor, β1H.

The two complement pathways converge at C3. Activation of the terminal complement components (C5 to C9) is initiated by C5 convertase, which consists of C3b in association with C3 convertase from either pathway. The C5 convertase cleaves a small fragment C5a from C5, and the remaining larger fragment C5b along with C6 to C9 self-assemble on the cell membrane. The insertion of these components into the membrane results in hydrophobic characteristics and reorientation of the lipid bilayer leading to the formation of a transmembrane channel permitting bidirectional flow of ions and eventually macromolecules. Membrane injury and disruption of the cell result.

The regulation of the complement system is through the rapid decay of C2 to C5 once they have been activated. C4-binding protein binds to C4b to regulate this step. There is also decay of C3 convertase of both the classic and alternative pathways. C1 inhibitor (C1 INH) inhibits activated C1r and C1s by combining with these enzymes. The inactivation of C3b by C3b inactivator and its cofactor β1H is important in preventing the continued formation of C3b which interacts with factor B of the alternative pathway to produce a functional C3 convertase and thus more cleavage of C3 to C3b. In the inactivation of C3b, β1H binds first with C3b to render it susceptible to proteolytic cleavage by C3b inactivator.

The peptides C3a and C5a are referred to as *anaphylatoxins.* C5a and the trimolecular complex of fluid phase $\overline{C567}$ are chemotactic for neutrophils, eosinophils, and monocytes. C3b on cell membranes coated with IgG antibodies enhances phagocytosis by interaction of these coated cells with phagocytic cells possessing receptors for C3b. The interaction of C5a with neutrophils stimulates release of lysosomal enzymes, increases oxidative metabolism, and causes these cells to become adherent and to aggregate. In renal dialysis, the cellophane dialysis membrane activates the alternative complement pathway leading to coating of neutrophils with C5a. The neutrophils marginate and aggregate in the pulmonary vasculature, producing transient neutropenia and hypoxemia. Another small peptide, C3a, resulting from activation of C3, promotes release of neutrophils from bone marrow. Neutralization of certain viruses, such as herpes simplex, occurs by coating the virus with C1, C4, and C2. A peptide generated from activated C3 has been shown to have kinin-like properties and is probably responsible for the swelling observed in hereditary angioedema.

The anaphylatoxin peptides C3a and C5a are regulated by the presence of a carboxypeptidase B enzyme in the serum that rapidly cleaves arginyl residues from the carboxyterminus of these peptides. The hydrolyzed peptides, termed C3a des Arg and C5a des Arg, are devoid of anaphylatoxin activity. Purified C5 des Arg lacks also chemotactic activity which is, however, reconstituted by the addition of normal serum containing a helper factor. The chemotactic peptide, therefore, in complement-activated serum is C5a des Arg. Normal serum also contains chemotactic factor inactivator activity (CFI) which inactivates the chemotactic activity of C5a and abrogates the ability of this peptide to stimulate release of lysosomal enzymes from neutrophils. Increased CFI activity has been found in patients with sarcoidosis and Hodgkin's disease, in whom defects in mobilization of inflammatory cells are present.

The complement system interacts with the coagulation, fibrinolytic, and kinin-generating systems. The activation of Hageman factor (factor XII) not only leads to clotting but also to the formation of plasmin, a fibrinolysin. Plasmin also activates C1 and cleaves C3 to produce C3a (anaphylatoxin). Plasmin also cleaves Hageman factor to produce Hageman factor fragments which convert prekallikrein to kallikrein. Kallikrein cleaves kininogen to bradykinin. Lysosomal enzymes can activate C1 and cleave C5 to form C5a.

Measurement of complement may be useful in diagnosis, assessment of disease activity, and evaluation of treatment. The serum level of complement depends on the balance of synthesis, catabolism, and consumption of the various complement components. Evidence for complement activation may be reflected in a low hemolytic complement level, decreased levels of individual components, or the finding of cleavage fragments of complement components. Low complement levels, however, may be the result of decreased synthesis or an inherited deficiency of a complement component. Normal or elevated complement levels do not exclude the participation of complement since synthesis of complement may equal or exceed consumption. Serum complement levels do not necessarily reflect intense local consumption of complement as might occur in synovial and pleural fluid. Further evidence of complement activation in disease can be adduced by the demonstration of complement components in lesions by immunofluorescence microscopy.

Complement is measured by its hemolytic activity expressed in CH_{50} units. Normal hemolytic activity depends on optimum concentrations of all the major components, C1 through C9. If any one component is markedly reduced or absent, little or no hemolytic activity is measured. The C3 and C4 components are readily measured immunochemically. In most instances, the measurements of C3 and C4 and hemolytic complement activity provide sufficient clinical information. Measurements of C1q and factor B may also be useful. For example, low levels of C1q, C4, C3, and CH_{50} indicate activation of complement primarily through the classic pathway. Immune complex disease such as systemic lupus erythematosus may show this complement profile. Reduced C3, CH_{50}, and factor B with a normal C4 reflect activation of complement by the alternative complement pathway, and may be seen in patients with membranoproliferative glomerulonephritis and in patients with bacterial endotoxin shock. The absence of CH_{50} may signify a hereditary deficiency of a complement component.

Hereditary deficiencies of complement The most common hereditary deficiency of complement is C2 deficiency which is inherited as an autosomal recessive trait (Table 63-5). Homozygous C2 deficiency has been recognized in normal individuals and in patients with SLE and other syndromes with a

TABLE 63-5
Clinical disorders associated with hereditary complement deficiencies

Complement component	*Clinical disorders*
Clq, Clr, Cls	SLE-like syndrome
C2	SLE-like syndrome, dermatomyositis, vasculitis, glomerulonephritis, normal persons
C3	Recurrent bacterial infections
C4	SLE-like syndrome
C5	SLE-like syndrome
C5 dysfunction	Recurrent infections with gram-negative bacteria and eczema (Leiner's syndrome)
C6	Neisserial infections
C7	Raynaud's phenomenon, neisserial infections, normal persons
C8	Neisserial infections, SLE-like syndrome
Cl inhibitor	Hereditary angioedema, SLE-like syndrome
C3b inactivator	Recurrent bacterial infections

NOTE: *SLE, systemic lupus erythematosus; neisserial infections,* Neisseria gonorrhoeae *and* N. meningitidis.

comparable clinical picture. Heterozygous C2 deficiency may also be associated with rheumatic disorders. Inherited as well as acquired deficiencies of the early components (C1, C4, C2) appear to be more common in diseases resembling SLE. Lupus-like illness has also been noted in persons with hereditary angioedema who lack C1 inhibitor. Serum levels of C4 and C2 are often low in these individuals. Systemic lupus erythematosus has been observed in patients with the homozygous deficiency of C5 or C8. Severe recurrent bacterial infections occur in patients with homozygous C3 deficiency and in those patients with low levels of C3 secondary to the continued activation of C3 in the absence of C3b inactivator. In addition, acquired or hereditary deficiencies of early complement components may predispose individuals to infection because of inefficient activation of C3. The homozygous deficiency of a terminal complement component (C6, C7, or C8) has been noted in patients with disseminated *Neisseria* infections, including both *N. gonorrhoeae* and *N. meningitidis.* These persons may be more susceptible to infection with bacteria which are normally killed by complement-mediated cell lysis, a function which depends on the terminal complement components.

Hereditary deficiencies of C2 and C4 are linked to histocompatibility antigens (HLA). The genes determining immune responses are located near the genes for the HLA system. This has raised the possibility that relationships exist between inherited deficiencies of the complement system, HLA, the immune response, and the development of SLE or lupus-like illnesses. In view of the current hypothesis of a viral etiology for SLE, it has been suggested that the inherited deficiencies of early complement components predispose these individuals to viral infections. The development of lupus-related illnesses in patients with acquired deficiencies of early complement components also supports this notion and makes the possibility less likely that a direct causative relationship exists between HLA and SLE. Another explanation is that inherited deficiency of C2 or C4 is more closely associated with a particular type of immune response that predisposes these individuals to autoimmune disease. Further work is needed to elucidate the meaning of the associations between complement synthesis and SLE or lupus-like illnesses.

Hereditary angioedema is characterized by acute episodes of circumscribed edema involving skin, gastrointestinal tract, and upper respiratory tract and an imminent danger of life-threatening laryngeal edema. The basic abnormality is the absence of C1 inhibitor. The disorder has an autosomal dominant pattern of inheritance, and the affected heterozygote has low levels of C1 inhibitor. In approximately 10 to 15 percent of these individuals, normal amounts of C1 inhibitor can be measured immunochemically, but the protein does not possess C1 inhibitor activity (see Chap. 67).

IMMUNE MECHANISMS OF TISSUE INJURY The immune system protects the individual from the attacks of microorganisms by preventing their entry or facilitating their removal. The same immunologic mechanisms that protect the individual, however, may cause damage to normal tissue, especially if the immune response is excessive or prolonged. Moreover, damage to normal cells and tissue occurs in autoimmune disorders because immune responses are directed against autoantigens. The mechanisms of immune injury have been divided into four types: anaphylactic (type I), cytotoxic (type II), immune-complex-mediated (type III), and cell-mediated reactions (type IV). An additional mechanism interferes with the function of biologically active substances and is referred to as type V. Clinical manifestations of disease may be the consequence of one or any combination of these five mechanisms of tissue injury.

Anaphylactic reaction (type I) This reaction is characterized by the release of pharmacologically active substances from mast cells or basophils as a result of the binding of antigen to IgE antibody attached to the surface of these cells. Histamine, slow-reacting substances of anaphylaxis, and eosinophil chemotactic factor of anaphylaxis are the major substances released from the mast cells in this reaction. The anaphylactic reaction is also referred to as *immediate hypersensitivity.* Clinical features of the anaphylactic reaction include generalized anaphylaxis, urticaria, angioedema, and atopic disorders (allergic rhinitis or hay fever, bronchial asthma, atopic dermatitis) (see Chap. 67).

Cytotoxic reactions (type II) In the cytotoxic mechanism of injury, antibodies belonging to either IgG or IgM class react with antigenic determinants on cell membranes or tissue. The antigens may be intrinsic or result from the firm binding of free antigens to cell membranes or tissues. The ensuing tissue damage from antigen-antibody reactions occurs through the activation of the complement system when the antibody belongs to the IgM class. Receptors for IgM are not present on phagocytic cells, and complement activation is necessary for generation of inflammation. Antigen-antibody reactions involving IgG antibodies, however, can lead to tissue damage with or without the activation of complement. Since macrophages and neutrophils have receptors for IgG, these phagocytic cells will bind to the IgG antibodies that are attached to cell membranes or tissue. Examples of type II reactions include immune hemolytic anemia, transfusion reactions, erythroblastosis fetalis, immune thrombocytopenia, and Goodpasture's syndrome. In immune hemolytic anemia of the warm antibody type, IgG-antibody-coated red blood cells become bound to macrophages mainly in the spleen and in other reticuloendothelial tissues. A portion of the red blood cell membrane is removed by the macrophage. The red blood cell with its decreased membrane returns to the circulation as a spherocyte which has both increased mechanical and osmotic fragility. Penicillin-induced hemolytic anemia is an example of a cytotoxic reaction in which free antigen (penicillin) becomes firmly bound to the red blood cell membrane. If patients on high doses of penicillin form anti-penicillin antibodies of the IgG class, these antibodies will react with the penicillin antigens bound to the red blood cell membrane and lead to increased red blood cell destruction by the process of erythrophagocytosis. In Goodpasture's syndrome, antibodies develop that are specific for antigens intrinsic to the glomerular basement membrane and for antigens in the walls of pulmonary blood vessels. The inflammation generated by these antigen-antibody reactions leads to glomerulonephritis and pulmonary vasculitis, and these patients often present with hemoptysis as their initial complaint.

Antigen-antibody complex-mediated reactions (type III) The deposition of circulating antigen-antibody complexes in tissue leads to inflammation (Chap. 68). An understanding of immune complex disease has come largely from studies of experimental serum sickness. Many human diseases in which immune complexes play a pathogenetic role are now recognized. Circulating immune complexes have been identified in SLE, bacterial endocarditis, and malignancies, to name only a few. Immune complex disease may develop locally at a tissue site such as in the rheumatoid joint or in the lung in patients with hypersensitivity pneumonitis. The systemic form of immune complex disorders such as SLE is characterized by deposition of circulating immune complexes in various sites such as the glomerular basement membrane, pleura, pericardium, synovium, and in cutaneous blood vessels. The process by which immune complexes generate inflammation involves the following steps: (1) antigen-antibody complexes deposit at tissue sites, (2) complement activation provides chemotactic factors and vasoactive peptides which dilate blood vessels and attract neutrophils, and (3) interaction of phagocytic cells with immune complexes leads to release of lysosomal enzymes which damage surrounding tissue.

Cell-mediated reactions (type IV) This form of immune injury, also referred to as *delayed type of hypersensitivity,* centers on the role of the cytotoxic effector T cell (see "Cell-mediated Immunity" above). Sensitized T cells activated by antigen become cytotoxic cells capable of killing bacteria, tumor cells, or other target cells. They also release lymphokines, which stimulate macrophages, neutrophils, and other lymphocytes. Macrophages attracted to the site of immunologically mediated inflammation by T cells also cause tissue damage. Cell-mediated reactions play a significant role in the development of immunity and/or formation of lesions in tuberculosis, mycotic infections, and certain viral infections such as mumps, hepatitis, vaccinia, and herpes. Cell-mediated reactions are also involved in the pathogenesis of rheumatoid synovitis, Hashimoto's thyroiditis, and contact dermatitis resulting from exposure to oily resins of plants (e.g., poison oak) or to a variety of simple chemicals in the home or work environment. Renal allograft rejection and the graft versus host reaction observed in bone marrow transplantation are also in part a consequence of cell-mediated reactions (see Chap. 67).

Another form of cell-mediated tissue injury is antibody-dependent cell-mediated cytotoxicity (ADCC). First, antibodies of the IgG class react with antigens on target cells such as tumor cells. Effector lymphocytes or macrophages through their receptors for the Fc portion of IgG then bind to IgG antibodies on the target cells without involving immunologic specificity. This interaction of lymphocytes or macrophages with target cells results in the killing of target cells. Only small amounts of antibody are required to initiate this form of immune injury. The type of lymphocyte participating in ADCC is not clear. While these cells have receptors for the Fc fragment of IgG, other markers that would distinguish them as B or T cells are absent. As noted in the description of T cells (above), these lymphocytes are referred to as *K* or *killer cells* and may be the same as the null cell which lacks T- and B-cell markers.

Interference with function of biologically active substances (type V) The interaction of antibodies with biologically active substances can interfere with their function. Antibodies to clotting factors, in particular factor VIII, may lead to serious bleeding abnormalities. Antibodies to intrinsic factors in patients with pernicious anemia may interfere with the absorption of vitamin B_{12}. In patients with myasthenia gravis, antibodies to acetylcholine neural receptors may be responsible for the block of neural transmission. In most diabetic patients receiving foreign insulin, antibodies to insulin develop. Anti-insulin antibodies are responsible for the insulin resistance observed in some patients. In other patients, antibodies to cell membrane receptors for insulin produce severe insulin resistance. These examples illustrate the potential clinical importance of recognizing this form of immune reaction.

REFERENCES

Agnello V: Complement deficiency states. Medicine 57:1, 1978

——— Assessment of the new immune complex assay technology, in *Update IV: Harrison's Principles of Internal Medicine,* KJ Isselbacher et al (eds). New York, McGraw-Hill, 1982

Bellanti JA (ed): *Immunology II.* Philadelphia, Saunders, 1978

Cooper NR: The complement system, in *Basic and Clinical Immunology,* HH Fudenberg et al (eds). Los Altos, Lange, 1980, chap 8, p 83

Reinherz EL, Schlossman SF: The differentiation and function of human T lymphocytes. Cell 19:821, 1980

Samter M (ed): *Immunological Diseases.* Boston, Little, Brown, 1979

Talal N: Autoimmunity, in *Basic and Clinical Immunology,* HH Fudenberg et al (eds). Los Altos, Lange, 1980, chap 18, p 220

Unanue ER: The regulatory role of macrophages in antigenic stimulation: Part two. Symbiotic relationship between lymphocytes and macrophages. Adv Immunol 31:1, 1981

Diseases of under- and overproduction of immune globulins

64
IMMUNE DEFICIENCY DISEASES

ALEXANDER R. LAWTON III
MAX D. COOPER

INTRODUCTION Immunologic functions are mediated by two developmentally independent, but functionally interacting, families of lymphocytes. The activities of B and T lymphocytes, and their products, in host defense are closely integrated with the functions of other cells of the reticuloendothelial system. Fixed and wandering macrophages play an important role in the trapping and processing of antigens and become effector cells, especially when activated by products of lymphocytes. The scavenger activity of polymorphonuclear leukocytes is directed and made specific by antibodies in concert with products of the complement system (see Chap. 63). The interaction of basophils and tissue mast cells with IgE antibodies in causation of immediate hypersensitivity is discussed in Chap. 67. Consideration of these interrelationships is an important part of the analysis of patients with suspected immune deficiency.

CLINICAL DISEASE FEATURES COMMON TO IMMUNE DEFICIENCY Immunodeficiency syndromes, whether congenital, spontaneously acquired, or iatrogenic, are characterized by unusual susceptibility to infection and, sometimes, to autoimmune disease and lymphoreticular malignancies. The types of infection often provide the first clue to the nature of the immunologic defect.

Patients with defects in humoral immunity have recurrent

or chronic sinopulmonary infection, meningitis, and bacteremia, most commonly caused by pyogenic bacteria such as *Hemophilus influenzae, Streptococcus pneumoniae,* and staphylococci. The same pathogens tend to infect patients with normal immune responses, but with either neutropenia or a deficiency of the pivotal third component of complement (C3), suggesting that a tripartite collaboration involving antibody, complement, and phagocytes exists as the chief mechanism of host defense against pyogenic organisms. Binding of antibody to the bacterial surface causes activation of the complement system. One cleavage product of activated C3 serves as a chemotactic factor for polymorphonuclear leukocytes. Activated C3b fixed to bacterial surfaces facilitates phagocytosis by interaction with C3b receptors on neutrophils.

Agammaglobulinemic patients in whom cell-mediated immunity is intact have an interesting response to viral infections. The clinical course of primary infection with viruses such as varicella zoster or rubeola, unless complicated by bacterial infection, does not differ significantly from that of the normal host. However, long-lasting immunity may not develop, and as a result multiple bouts of chickenpox and measles may occur. Such observations suggest that intact T cells may be sufficient for control of established viral infections, while antibodies play an important role in limiting the initial dissemination of virus and in providing long-lasting protection. Exceptions to this generalization are becoming more widely recognized. Agammaglobulinemic patients fail to clear hepatitis B virus from their circulation and have a progressive, and often fatal, course. Poliomyelitis has occurred following live-virus vaccination in some patients. Chronic encephalitis, which may progress over a period of months to years, is being observed with apparently increasing frequency. Echoviruses and adenoviruses have been isolated from brain, spinal fluid, or other sites in such patients; in others no agent has been detected. Immunologic injury resulting from a partial and ineffective immune response may contribute as much to the pathogenesis of these diseases as the direct effects of the viruses.

The occurrence of unusual serious infection, for example, *H. influenzae* meningitis in an older child or adult, warrants consideration of humoral immune deficiency. Bacterial infections in certain sites may also suggest this possibility. Chronic otitis media occurs frequently in patients with hypogammaglobulinemia, and is significant because of its relative rarity in normal adults. Pansinusitis, although almost invariably present in immunoglobulin deficiency, is a less helpful finding because it is not rare in apparently normal people. Bacterial infections of the skin or urinary tract are less frequent problems in hypogammaglobulinemic patients.

Infestation with the intestinal parasite *Giardia lamblia* is a frequent enough cause of diarrhea in antibody-deficient patients to warrant diagnostic duodenal aspiration and intestinal biopsy when the organism cannot be demonstrated in the stool.

Abnormalities of cell-mediated immunity predispose to *disseminated virus infections,* particularly with latent viruses such as herpes simplex (see Chap. 210), varicella zoster (see Chap. 204), and cytomegalovirus (see Chap. 211). Patients so affected also almost invariably develop mucocutaneous candidiasis and frequently acquire widely disseminated fungal infections.

Pneumonia caused by the protozoan *Pneumocystis carinii* is also common (see Chap. 222).

T-cell deficiency is probably always accompanied by some abnormality of antibody responses, although this may not be reflected by hypogammaglobulinemia. This may explain in part why patients with primary T-cell defects are also subject to overwhelming bacterial infection.

The most severe form of immune deficiency occurs in individuals, usually infants, who lack both cell-mediated and humoral immune functions. They are susceptible to the whole range of infectious agents including organisms not ordinarily considered pathogenic. Multiple infections with viruses, bacteria, and fungi occur, often simultaneously. Because donor lymphocytes cannot be rejected by the recipients, blood transfusions can produce fatal graft-versus-host disease.

DIFFERENTIATION OF T AND B CELLS The functional deficits which occur in both congenital and acquired immunodeficiencies are most usefully viewed as being caused by defects at various points along the differentiation pathways of immunocompetent cells. For this reason certain features of the development and differentiation of T and B cells that are especially relevant to the analysis of immunodeficiency are briefly presented here; Chap. 63 provides a general account of their roles in cellular and humoral immunity.

A subpopulation of hematopoietic stem cells may become restricted to lymphoid differentiation prior to migration to the thymus, where T cells are generated, or to the fetal liver and adult bone marrow, where B-cell development occurs (Fig. 64-1). A major function of central lymphoid tissues is to generate the clonal diversity characteristic of the immune system. Each T or B lymphocyte is induced to express surface receptor molecules of a unique specificity for antigen. The receptors of B lymphocytes are immunoglobulins. The nature of T-cell receptors is not yet precisely defined. Generation of clonal diversity requires cellular proliferation, such that each of the different receptor specificities encoded in the genome comes to be uniquely expressed by individual cells. A clone consists of all cells that express the identical antigen-binding receptors. Estimates for the total number of B-cell clones usually vary between 10 and 100 million. The process of clonal development is independent of antigen and reflects a genetically programmed sequence of differentiation analogous to that of primary erythropoiesis or myelopoiesis. This phase, termed *primary differentiation,* begins early in human fetal development but probably continues into adult life.

The most primitive morphologically identifiable cell in the B lineage is called a pre-B cell. These cells express cytoplasmic μ chains (the heavy chain of IgM) but not light chains, and lack the membrane-bound immunoglobulin receptors which characterize B lymphocytes. Pre-B cells are first generated in fetal liver but are produced exclusively in bone marrow of adults. Pre-B cells proliferate rapidly and spawn immature B lymphocytes which express surface IgM receptors and divide rarely. Young B lymphocytes differ from their more mature counterparts in an important physiologic characteristic; they are highly susceptible to inactivation when their receptors bind antigen. This phenomenon almost certainly is one important mechanism for the development of tolerance to self-antigens.

The developmental sequence for expression of diverse immunoglobulin classes by human B lymphocytes begins with expression of IgM. The expression of IgD on IgM-bearing cells occurs later. Lymphocytes committed to synthesis of IgG, IgA, and IgE are all derived from IgM-bearing precursors through a genetic switch mechanism.

The expression of a group of differentiation antigens, defined by their reactivity with monoclonal antibodies, has become a powerful tool in elucidating developmental relationships of both T and B lymphocytes (Fig. 64-1). Of major clinical importance is the demarcation of two independent sets of T lymphocytes. T cells bearing the T4 or Leu 3 markers constitute approximately 70 percent of total T cells and function as helper-inducer cells, necessary for expression of effector functions of both T and B cells. $T8^+$ (or Leu 2^+) lymphocytes, constituting 20 to 30 percent of circulating T cells, are responsible for suppression of immune responses and mediate cytotoxic reactions. Developmental arrests or failure of function of one or the other of these T-cell subsets may be responsible for immunodeficiency or autoimmune diseases.

In addition to generating T cells, the thymus apparently secretes hormonal products which regulate cellular maturation in peripheral lymphoid tissues. These hormones have been called *thymosin* or *thymopoetin;* deficiencies of these factors have been implicated in some immunodeficiencies.

The events designated *secondary differentiation* (Fig. 64-1) follow stimulation of specific clones of lymphocytes by antigen. These processes are synonymous with the immune response (see Chap. 63). Particularly important in consideration of immunodeficiencies are the collaborative interactions among macrophages, T cells, and B cells. B lymphocytes can proliferate in response to thymus-dependent antigens without the help of T cells, and may differentiate to IgM-secreting plasma cells when stimulated by thymus-independent antigens such as polysaccharides. However, production of normal quantities of antibodies, particularly those of the IgA and IgG classes, requires the collaboration of T cells.

Differentiation of T or B cells may be arrested at either the primary or secondary stage (Fig. 64-1). Reflecting the complex cellular interactions involved in immune responses and the pivotal role played by T lymphocytes, immune deficiencies primarily involving T cells are usually also associated with abnormal B-cell function. Conversely, immunodeficiencies manifested primarily by inability to produce antibodies may be caused by T-cell defects not associated with abnormal cell-mediated immunity.

EVALUATION OF IMMUNODEFICIENT PATIENTS Many of the laboratory assays used for precise evaluation of immunologic functions in humans are available only in specialized centers; nevertheless, most immunodeficiencies may be diagnosed by thoughtful use of tests available in most clinical laboratories. Table 64-1 presents a résumé of laboratory investigations roughly in order of increasing complexity.

A careful history will usually indicate whether the major problem involves the antibody-complement-phagocyte system or cell-mediated immunity. A history of a normal response to smallpox vaccination or of contact dermatitis due to poison ivy suggests intact cellular immunity. Lymphopenia and the absence of palpable lymph nodes may be important findings. However, patients with profound immunodeficiency may have diffuse lymphoid hyperplasia.

Humoral immunity With rare exceptions, deficiency of humoral immunity is accompanied by diminished serum concentration of one or more classes of immunoglobulin. Normal values vary with age, and adult concentrations of IgM (100 mg/dl) are reached at about 1 year, of IgG (1000 mg/dl) at 5 to 6 years, and of IgA (200 mg/dl) at puberty (see Chap. 63). Also, the wide range of values among normal adults creates difficulty in defining the lower limits of normal. Reasonable estimates for low normal values are 40 mg/dl for IgM, 500 mg/dl for IgG, and 50 mg/dl for IgA. In the presence of borderline hypogammaglobulinemia, assessing the patient's capacity to pro-

FIGURE 64-1

Differentiation of lymphoid cells is accompanied by acquisition and loss of specific cell-surface antigens as well as morphological and functional changes. Some antigens first expressed as stem cells differentiate within the thymus and are shared by all mature T cells; commercially available monoclonal antibodies to such pan-T-cell antigens include T1, T3, and Leu 1. T6, the human counterpart to the mouse thymic leukemia (TL) antigen, is expressed only by thymocytes. Within the thymus, cells acquiring helper-inducer functions selectively lose the T8 (Leu 2) antigen, while T4 (Leu 3) antigen is lost by cells destined to serve cytotoxic and suppressor functions. HLA-DR antigens are expressed by all cells of the B lineage, up to and including some plasma cells. T cells, in contrast, express HLA-DR only when they have been activated. These differentiation antigens serve as useful markers for evaluation of disorders of development and function of T and B cells. Failure to develop T and B cells may result from defective stem cells or from inborn metabolic errors affecting both cell types. Rarely, other hematopoietic cell lines are also absent. Absence of either T or B cells suggests malfunction of central lymphoid tissues, including the thymus and the fetal liver–bone marrow complex. B-cell deficiency may result from failure to generate pre-B cells from their stem-cell precursors or from failure of pre-B cells to give rise to their B-lymphocyte progeny. Similarly, differentiation may be arrested at several levels within the T-cell lineage; arrests at the thymocyte level and failure to develop the helper-inducer subset have been observed in immunodeficient patients. Agammaglobulinemia and deficiencies of some T-cell functions may occur despite the presence of normal numbers of B or T cells in the circulation. Failure of B lymphocytes to differentiate to plasma cells can be due to intrinsic cellular abnormalities or to faulty T-cell regulation.

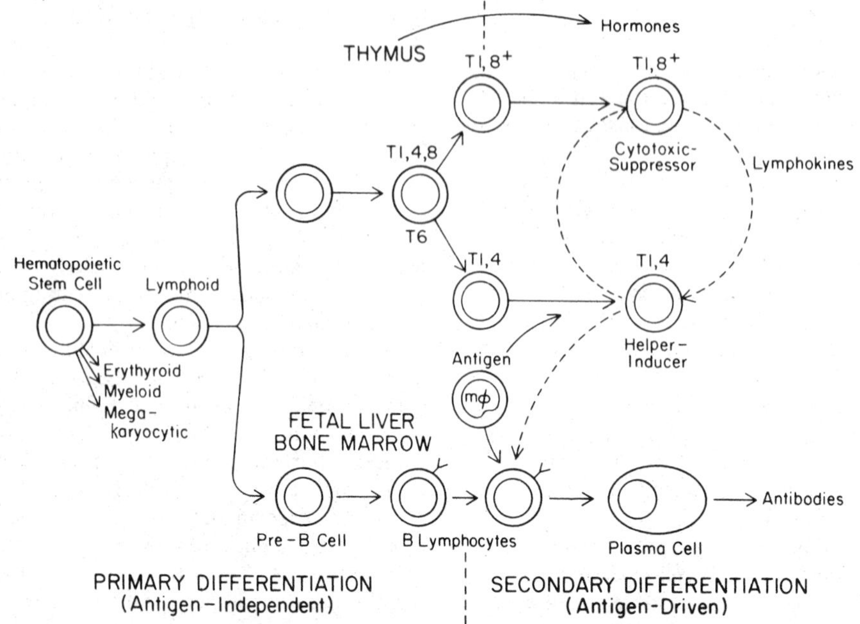

duce specific antibodies becomes particularly important. Most hospital laboratories can measure isohemagglutinins, antistreptolysin O, and "febrile agglutinins." Typhoid H and O agglutinins can be measured before and after immunization with standard typhoid vaccine. Many state public health laboratories can perform titrations for antibodies to common viral agents.

Since antibody deficiency may be mimicked clinically by deficiency of complement components, measurement of total hemolytic complement (CH_{50}) should be a part of the evaluation of host defense. Measurement of C3 alone is inadequate for screening, since deficiencies of both early and late complement components may predispose to bacterial infection (see Chap. 63). Estimation of numbers of circulating B lymphocytes has been of great value in determining the pathogenesis of certain types of immune deficiency. B lymphocytes are identified by the presence of membrane-bound immunoglobulins; additional markers include HLA-DR antigens, receptors for aggregated IgG (Fc receptor), receptors for the third component of complement (C3 receptor), and receptors which specifically bind the Epstein-Barr virus. Fc receptors and C3 receptors are also found on circulating monocytes. Moreover, not all B lymphocytes bear the C3 receptor. The Epstein-Barr virus receptor appears to be highly specific for B lymphocytes. They can also be identified and enumerated by specific heterologous antiserums or monoclonal antibodies.

TABLE 64-1
Laboratory evaluation of host defense defects

- *I* Preliminary screen*
  - *A* Complete blood count with differential smear
  - *B* Quantitative immunoglobulin levels
- *II* Readily available studies†
  - *A* B-cell function
    - *1* Natural or commonly acquired antibodies: isohemagglutinins, "febrile" agglutinins, antibodies to common viruses (rubella, rubeola, influenza), and toxins (diphtheria, tetanus)
    - *2* Response to immunization (typhoid, polio, diphtheria-tetanus vaccines)
  - *B* T-cell function
    - *1* Skin tests (PPD, *Candida, Trichophyton,* histoplasmin), tetanus toxoid (1:100 dilution)
    - *2* Contact sensitization with dinitrochlorobenzene
    - *3* Chest x-ray (thymus shadow in infants, thymoma in adults)
  - *C* Complement
    - *1* C3
    - *2* CH_{50} (total hemolytic complement)
  - *D* Phagocyte function
    - *1* Reduction of nitroblue tetrazolium
    - *2* Inflammatory skin window (Rebuck)
- *III* In-depth investigation
  - *A* B cell
    - *1* Pre-B cell examination in bone marrow samples
    - *2* B-lymphocyte membrane markers: IgM, IgD, IgG, IgA; receptors for aggregated IgG (Fc receptor), C3, Epstein-Barr virus; antigens detected by anti-B antibodies
    - *3* Induction of B-lymphocyte differentiation in vitro stimulated by pokeweed mitogen, Epstein-Barr virus, or other polyclonal B-cell activators
    - *4* Kinetics and immunoglobulin class of antibody produced in response to specific primary and secondary immunization
    - *5* Measurement of IgG subclasses and κ/λ ratio
    - *6* Histologic and immunofluorescent examination of biopsy specimens (intestinal mucosa, lymph node, bone marrow)
  - *B* T cell
    - *1* Surface markers: binding of sheep erythrocytes (E rosettes), reactivity with monoclonal antibodies recognizing all T cells and the helper and suppressor subsets
    - *2* In vitro correlates of delayed hypersensitivity
      - *a* Proliferative response to mitogens: phytohemagglutinin, concanavalin A–specific antigens (PPD, *Candida*); allogeneic cells (one-way mixed lymphocyte response)
      - *b* Quantification of lymphokines (migration inhibitory factor, etc.)
      - *c* Induction of killer cells by stimulation with allogeneic lymphocytes
    - *3* Measurement of thymus hormones
    - *4* Assays for T-cell "helper" function using supernatants of antigen-activated T cells or T cells plus PWM or antigens to trigger B-lymphocyte differentiation
    - *5* Skin graft rejection
  - *C* Phagocytes and complement
    - *1* Chemotactic response in vitro
    - *2* Bactericidal function
    - *3* Classic and alternative complement components
  - *D* Natural killer cells
    - *1* Enumeration with monoclonal antibodies
    - *2* Functional assay using appropriate target cells
  - *E* Miscellaneous
    - *1* Lymphocytotoxic antibodies
    - *2* Measurement of adenosine deaminase and purine nucleoside phosphorylase enzyme activities

* *Together with a history and physical examination, these tests will identify more than 95 percent of patients with primary immunodeficiencies.*

† *These assays are generally available in either hospitals or state public health laboratories. With rare exceptions, information gained from tests in categories I and II is sufficient to diagnose and treat those immunodeficiencies amenable to conventional treatment with gamma globulin or plasma.*

Pokeweed mitogen (PWM), an extract of the plant *Phytolacca americana,* has the capacity to induce B lymphocytes in culture to proliferate and differentiate to plasma cells. This activity requires the presence of T lymphocytes, which also proliferate in response to PWM. Thus, this assay can measure not only the capacity of B lymphocytes to differentiate, but can also assess the "helper" or "suppressor" function of patients' T lymphocytes.

Cellular immunity Human T lymphocytes may be enumerated by their capacity to bind sheep erythrocytes in the cold, forming what are called *E rosettes.* The nature and function of these receptors are unknown, but they are not related to the antigen-specificity of T cells. Monoclonal antibodies which recognize all peripheral T cells (T3 and Leu 1) and distinguish the helper-inducer subset ($T4^+$, Leu 3^+) from cytotoxic-suppressor T cells ($T8^+$, Leu 2^+) are commercially available and may soon supplant the E rosette test.

T-lymphocyte function can be measured in vivo by delayed hypersensitivity skin testing, using a variety of antigens to which the majority of older children and adults have been sensitized. The most generally useful skin test antigen is a 1:100 dilution of tetanus toxoid injected intradermally, since almost all individuals will have been sensitized. Purified protein derivative (PPD), histoplasmin, mumps antigen, and extracts of *Candida* or *Trichophyton* may also be used. The capacity to become sensitized to a new antigen may be tested by application of dinitrochlorobenzene to the skin, followed 2 weeks later by patch testing at a different site.

T-lymphocyte function may be estimated in vitro by the capacity of cells to proliferate in response to antigens to which the patient has been sensitized, to lymphocytes from an unrelated donor, or to the T-cell mitogens, which include phytohemagglutinin, concanavalin A, and pokeweed mitogen. The response is usually quantified by measurement of incorporation of radioactive thymidine into newly synthesized DNA. It is also possible to measure the production of lymphokines by activated T cells. Finally, the ability of T cells activated in mixed lymphocyte culture to lyse target cells sensitized by phytohemagglutinin can be measured.

The capacity of T lymphocytes from immunologically normal persons to be activated in vitro with antigens or mitogens may be abolished or markedly diminished by acute febrile illness, treatment with corticosteroids, or stress. Caution should be exercised in interpreting abnormal results in these circumstances.

CLASSIFICATION Primary immunodeficiencies may be either congenital or acquired, and are currently classified according to mode of inheritance and whether the defect involves T cells,

B cells, or both. Unfortunately, the best current classification, established by an expert committee of the World Health Organization, still places the majority of immunodeficiency diseases in an ill-defined category called *common varied immunodeficiency*. In general, this classification will be followed in the following discussion, which emphasizes three related concepts; first, that immunodeficiencies are most logically viewed as defects of cellular differentiation; second, that these defects may involve either primary development of T or B cells or the antigen-dependent phase of their differentiation; and third, that defects of secondary B-cell differentiation may in some instances reflect T-cell abnormalities resulting from faulty T-B collaboration.

Secondary immunodeficiencies are those not caused by intrinsic abnormalities in development or function of T and B cells. Examples are immune deficiency associated with malnutrition, protein-losing enteropathy, and intestinal lymphangiectasia. Also considered secondary are immunodeficiencies resulting from hypercatabolic states such as occur in myotonic dystrophy, immunodeficiency associated with lymphoreticular malignancy, and immunodeficiency resulting from treatment with x-rays, antilymphocyte serum, or cytotoxic drugs.

Incidence As a group, the immunodeficiency syndromes discussed in this chapter are relatively common. Isolated IgA deficiency occurs in approximately 1 in 600 individuals; no other specific category approaches this frequency, but the cumulative total is not insignificant. The incidence of diagnosed immunodeficiency diseases is clearly a function of the awareness of physicians in a community. An epidemic of immunodeficiency diseases commonly follows the addition of a clinical immunologist to a medical center staff.

The more severe forms of primary immunodeficiency have their onset early in life and all too frequently result in death during childhood. Immunodeficiencies may be acquired at any age, however, and a substantial number of patients with congenital hypogammaglobulinemia survive to middle age or beyond. In a referral center for patients with immunodeficiency diseases, approximately two-thirds of the immunodeficient patients under care are adults. Improved methods of diagnosis and treatment can be expected to increase this ratio in the future.

Severe combined immunodeficiency (SCID) This syndrome is characterized by gross functional impairment of both humoral and cell-mediated immunity. It is usually congenital, may be inherited either as an X-linked or autosomal recessive defect, or may occur sporadically. Affected infants rarely survive beyond 1 year. This syndrome has been associated with a diversity of defects in development of immunocompetent cells, some of which may be related to specific enzymatic abnormalities.

The classic example of SCID, *Swiss-type agammaglobulinemia*, is characterized by severe lymphopenia involving both T and B cells, and is inherited with an autosomal recessive pattern. Rarely, other hematopoietic cell lines fail to develop. The cellular defect in these forms of SCID logically rests with the precursor common to both T and B cells. The immunologic defects in a few of these patients have been repaired following transplantation of fetal liver as a source of stem cells, confirming the hypothesis that they have a thymus and bursa equivalent capable of supporting differentiation of normal stem cells. About half of patients with autosomal recessive SCID are deficient in an enzyme involved in purine metabolism, adenosine deaminase (ADA). These patients have varying degrees of lymphopenia, T cells usually being more deficient than B cells. The pathophysiologic relationship of ADA deficiency to lymphoid differentiation is slowly being unraveled. The best current evidence suggests that intracellular accumulation of deoxy-ATP, by inhibiting ribonucleotide reductase enzymes, interferes with synthesis of DNA precursors, particularly deoxycytidine. Improvement of both clinical status and immunologic function has occurred in some but not all patients treated with a source of exogenous ADA; therapy with deoxynucleosides is currently being investigated.

SCID may also occur with an X-linked inheritance pattern. Affected boys may not have severe lymphopenia; some have had normal numbers of B lymphocytes with few or no circulating T lymphocytes. This developmental pattern (which may also occur with autosomal recessive inheritance) suggests the possibility of a faulty thymus epithelium. Mononuclear cells from bone marrow of such patients have been induced to express T-cell characteristics by coculture on normal thymus epithelium or by treatment with thymus hormones.

The SCID syndrome may occur as a consequence of more subtle defects of T-cell maturation. In one patient, circulating T cells present in normal numbers had the phenotypic markers of cortical thymocytes (Fig. 64-1) and lacked functions of mature T cells. Another patient had a selective deficiency of $T4^+$ Leu 3^+ helper T cells.

Patients with SCID have been successfully treated by transplantation of histocompatible bone marrow from sibling donors. The same treatment has been used in children and adults with leukemia or aplastic anemia (see Chap. 331) following purposeful destruction of the immune system by irradiation and cytotoxic drugs. Other modes of treatment, including fetal liver and thymus transplants, have been successful in restoring immunocompetence, but as yet there are only short-term survivors. Treatment of these patients should probably be attempted only in centers with a strong research interest in this problem. It is crucial that these patients be recognized early and not be given blood transfusions which may cause fatal graft-versus-host disease.

T-cell immunodeficiency Reflecting the diversity of T-cell functions, abnormalities of T-cell development may be responsible for a wide spectrum of immune deficiencies including severe combined immunodeficiency, apparently isolated defects in cell-mediated immunity, and syndromes presenting as antibody deficiency with apparently normal cell-mediated immunity. These defects may be acquired as well as congenital. Until recently, laboratory assays of T-lymphocyte function were limited to correlates of cell-mediated immunity; no means were available for studying T-cell regulatory functions. Quantification of T-cell subsets using monoclonal antibodies, accompanied by functional measurements of helper, suppressor, and cytotoxic activity, are expanding the spectrum of immunodeficiencies primarily related to T-cell abnormalities.

DI GEORGE'S SYNDROME This is the classic example of isolated T-cell deficiency and results from maldevelopment of organs derived embryologically from the third and fourth pharyngeal pouches. Affected infants usually present with congenital cardiac defects, particularly those involving the great vessels, hypocalcemic tetany due to failure of parathyroid development, and absence of the thymus. Associated abnormalities may include abnormal ears, shortened philtrum, and hypertelorism. Serum immunoglobulin concentrations are frequently normal. Lymphocyte counts may be normal, but virtually all the lymphocytes are B cells. Carefully performed autopsies have often revealed a tiny, histologically normal thymus, usually in an ectopic location. With time, a few patients developed functional T cells. Several patients with Di George's syndrome transplanted with fetal thymus have developed immunocompetent T cells of host origin. However, it is difficult to be certain whether long-term improvement is the result of a small thymus gland in an ectopic location or due to grafted thymus epithelium.

Children lacking the congenital anomalies associated with Di George's syndrome may present with severe impairment of cell-mediated immunity. Some have normal or even increased immunoglobulin levels, while others have selective deficiencies of one or more immunoglobulin classes. Specific antibody responses are usually impaired even in patients with normal concentrations of immunoglobulins. This ill-defined entity has been called the *Nezelof's syndrome.*

Inherited deficiency of the enzyme purine nucleoside phosphorylase (PNP) is associated with an often severe and selective deficiency of T-lymphocyte function. This enzyme functions in the same purine salvage pathway as ADA; toxic effects of its deficiency may be related to intracellular accumulation of deoxy-GTP.

A few patients with isolated T-cell deficiency have been treated with fetal thymus grafts. Some have shown improvement in numbers of circulating T cells, in vitro reactivity to mitogens, and clinical condition, while others have had no change in status.

ATAXIA-TELANGIECTASIA This is an autosomal recessive genetic disorder characterized by cerebellar ataxia, oculocutaneous telangiectasia, and immunodeficiency. Onset of truncal ataxia usually occurs in infancy and is progressive. Immunodeficiency is clinically manifest by recurrent and chronic sinopulmonary infection leading to bronchiectasis. However, not all patients have immunodeficiency. The two most frequent causes of death are chronic pulmonary disease and malignancy. Lymphomas are most common, although carcinomas have also occurred.

The immunologic abnormalities seem to be related to maldevelopment of the thymus. If found at all, the thymus in autopsied patients has been markedly hypoplastic and similar in appearance to an embryonic thymus. Patients' lymphocytes frequently respond poorly to T-cell mitogens in vitro. Cutaneous anergy and delayed rejection of skin grafts are common. Although the number and class distribution of B lymphocytes are usually normal, most patients are deficient in serum IgE and IgA, and a smaller number have reduced serum levels of IgG. IgM and IgD are usually normal.

There is circumstantial evidence that ataxia-telangiectasia may involve a generalized defect in cellular differentiation. Ovarian agenesis occurs frequently. Persistence of very high levels of oncofetal proteins, including α-fetoprotein and carcinoembryonic antigen, are found in patients' serum. Cultured cells from these patients are highly susceptible to radiation-induced chromosomal damage. Evidence for a defect in DNA repair mechanisms has been obtained. This defect may account for the high incidence of malignancies in these patients.

Only symptomatic treatment is available. Unless severe deficiency of IgG is present, therapy with gamma globulin is not indicated. Unusual sensitivity to x-irradiation should be kept in mind in planning therapy for patients who develop cancer.

Immunoglobulin deficiency syndromes X-LINKED AGAMMAGLOBULINEMIA This syndrome was long thought to represent a central failure of development of all elements of the B-cell lineage. Recent evidence has modified this concept. Affected males have very few immunoglobulin-bearing B lymphocytes in their circulation and lack primary and secondary lymphoid follicles. However, pre-B cells are found in normal frequency in their bone marrow. This developmental block contrasts with earlier and later arrests in B-cell differentiation characterizing other immunodeficiencies (see below and Fig. 64-1). Patients usually have a substantial number of small mononuclear cells bearing receptors for aggregated immunoglobulin and C3. Although resembling B lymphocytes, these cells have been shown to have markers characteristic of the monocyte line and to lack the B-lymphocyte specific surface antigen(s) and receptors for Epstein-Barr virus. A few patients with well-documented X-linked agammaglobulinemia have had a normal number of B lymphocytes, suggesting that there may be two distinct forms of this disease.

Agammaglobulinemia is a misnomer, as most patients with this and other forms of severe panhypogammaglobulinemia synthesize some immunoglobulins, primarily of the IgG class. Within the same family some affected males have had substantial levels of IgM, IgG, and IgA, while others have been nearly agammaglobulinemic. All these patients were markedly deficient in circulating B lymphocytes. This observation suggests that the few B lymphocytes which are generated are fully capable of differentiating to plasma cells and secreting immunoglobulins. A form of arthritis with some of the features of rheumatoid disease occurs in some of these patients and may remit following treatment with gamma globulin. Chronic encephalitis, of proven or presumed viral etiology, appears to be an increasingly frequent terminal complication. Some of these patients have also had an associated dermatomyositis.

TRANSIENT HYPOGAMMAGLOBULINEMIA OF INFANCY This is a reversible syndrome in which normal physiologic hypogammaglobulinemia of infancy is unusually prolonged and severe. IgG levels of normal-term infants commonly drop to levels of 300 to 400 mg/dl between 3 and 6 months of age as maternally derived IgG is catabolized; levels subsequently rise reflecting the infants' increased synthetic capacity. In transient hypogammaglobulinemia, the rate of synthesis of IgM, IgG, and IgA remains low for long periods. Reduced numbers of $T4^+$ helper T cells have recently been reported in infants with this condition.

ISOLATED DEFICIENCY OF IgA This is by far the most commonly encountered immunodeficiency, occurring with a frequency of approximately 1 in 600 individuals of European origin. With rare exceptions, both serum and secretory IgA are involved. Many adults with isolated IgA deficiency do not seem to have unusual problems with infection. Nevertheless, this condition is not benign. A substantial proportion of IgA-deficient individuals develop precipitating antibodies to IgA. These patients may have severe anaphylactic reactions when transfused with normal blood from a blood bank.

As a group, individuals with IgA deficiency have an increased number of respiratory infections of varying severity, and a few have had severe pulmonary disease such as bronchiectasis. Chronic diarrheal disease also occurs. The incidence of asthma and other atopic diseases among IgA-deficient patients is high, and, conversely, the incidence of IgA deficiency among atopic children has been found to be 20 to 40 times that in the normal population. In one study it was found that combined deficiency of IgE and IgA (or IgE deficiency alone) did not predispose to recurrent respiratory infections, while IgA-deficient patients with normal or elevated IgE had recurrent sinopulmonary disease. Selective reductions in the IgG_2 and IgG_4 subclasses have also been associated with increased infections in IgA-deficient individuals. IgA deficiency is also significantly associated with autoimmune diseases such as rheumatoid arthritis and systemic lupus erythematosus.

IgA deficiency may be familial, but no single pattern of inheritance has been encountered consistently. It has occurred in association with congenital intrauterine infections, such as toxoplasmosis, rubella, and cytomegalovirus infection. Several patients with abnormalities of chromosome 18 have had isolated IgA deficiency. Most commonly, the syndrome appears as a sporadic defect. It may be transient or acquired late in life.

The pathogenesis of IgA deficiency, whether genetic or caused by environmental insult, involves a block in terminal differentiation of B lymphocytes. Virtually all patients have detectable IgA-bearing B lymphocytes, although their numbers may be reduced. In normal children and adults, B lymphocytes bearing IgA have only that immunoglobulin class on their surface, while in IgA-deficient patients and normal neonates, IgA-bearing lymphocytes also bear surface IgM. This immature phenotype is associated in many patients with failure of their cultured lymphocytes to secrete IgA when stimulated by pokeweed mitogen. Selective T-cell suppression of IgA responses has been described in some patients, and a variety of other, usually mild, defects of T-cell function in others. While there is as yet no generally accepted pathogenetic mechanism, suspicion remains high that many of these patients have a primary defect in regulatory T-cell function.

Treatment of IgA deficiency is symptomatic. IgA cannot be effectively replaced by exogenous gamma globulin or plasma, and use of either would greatly increase the risk of development of antibodies to IgA. IgA-deficient patients in need of transfusion should be screened for the presence of antibodies to IgA, and ideally should be given blood only from IgA-deficient donors. All patients known to be IgA-deficient should be warned of the risk of severe transfusion reactions which may occur following infusion of only a few milliliters of blood.

X-LINKED IMMUNODEFICIENCY WITH INCREASED LEVELS OF IgM This is a specific syndrome only because of its inheritance pattern. IgG levels are usually very low, and IgA low or undetectable, while IgD levels may be high. The clinical patterns of infection are similar to those occurring with other hypogammaglobulinemic states. The number and distribution of B lymphocytes bearing IgM, IgG, and IgA have been normal, suggesting that this type of immunodeficiency may also involve a block in terminal differentiation of B lymphocytes. Neutropenia often occurs in affected males and can increase their vulnerability to infections.

ISOLATED DEFICIENCY OF IgM This syndrome has been reported rarely in this country but was detected frequently in a British population. Approximately 20 percent of these patients were asymptomatic while 60 percent had severe recurrent infections, often with bacteremia. Pneumococcal pneumonia and meningitis have often been noted in IgM-deficient patients. Other associated conditions included gastrointestinal disease, atopy, splenomegaly, and development of malignancy. The condition was frequently familial, and was four times more common in males than females. The number of circulating B lymphocytes has varied from very low to normal.

COMMON VARIED IMMUNODEFICIENCY This represents a heterogeneous group of syndromes which may be congenital or acquired, sporadic or familial, and which occur in both males and females. These patients have in common the clinical manifestations of antibody deficiency associated with panhypogammaglobulinemia, with deficiency of IgG and IgA, or rarely, with selective IgG deficiency.

Less than one-third of these patients have few or no circulating B lymphocytes, suggesting a central failure of development of this cell line. The remainder have B lymphocytes, and more than half have a normal number and class distribution. In the few patients studied, B lymphocytes capable of binding specific antigens were present and increased in frequency following immunization. Consistent with the evidence that B lymphocytes in these patients are able to recognize antigens and proliferate, but fail to differentiate to plasma cells, is the fairly common finding of lymphoid hyperplasia, including splenomegaly and nodular lymphoid hyperplasia of the gut.

In agammaglobulinemic patients having B lymphocytes, the pathogenesis of immune deficiency must involve the failure of these cells to differentiate to plasma cells. By use of assays capable of measuring B-lymphocyte differentiation to plasma cells in vitro, three major types of defect have been tentatively identified. First, and most common, is an intrinsic abnormality of B lymphocytes. B lymphocytes from these patients cannot differentiate into immunoglobulin-secreting plasma cells even when provided with help from normal T cells. In other instances, plasma cells containing intracytoplasmic immunoglobulin develop but fail to secrete this product. Second, there is evidence that in some patients the T cells, or their products, may actively suppress terminal differentiation of autologous or normal B lymphocytes. The increase in suppressor activity could be either a primary or secondary abnormality; the latter could explain the increase in T-cell suppressor activity in patients with abnormal B lymphocytes and others in whom B lymphocytes are congenitally absent. Third, quantitative deficiency of helper T-cell function has been observed in some patients, usually also in association with defective B-cell function. This functional defect may or may not be associated with reduced numbers of $T4^+$ cells.

Patients with common varied immunodeficiency may present with signs and symptoms highly suggestive of lymphoid malignancy, including fever, weight loss, splenomegaly, generalized lymphadenopathy, and lymphocytosis. Routine histologic examination of lymphoid tissues usually reveals germinal center hyperplasia which may be extremely difficult to distinguish from nodular lymphoma (see Chap. 130). Demonstration of a normal distribution of immunoglobulin isotypes and light chain classes on circulating and tissue B lymphocytes can serve to distinguish these patients from those having a monoclonal B-cell malignancy with secondary hypogammaglobulinemia. Treatment of several patients with gamma globulin has resulted in relief of symptoms and reversal of lymphoid hyperplasia.

IMMUNODEFICIENCY WITH THYMOMA Recognition of the association of hypogammaglobulinemia with spindle-cell thymoma provided one of the early clues as to the role of the thymus in immunobiology. Although T-cell numbers and cell-mediated immunity are frequently intact, several T-cell abnormalities have been identified. Patients' T cells suppress differentiation of normal B lymphocytes in the pokeweed mitogen assay and may also suppress development of erythroid precursors. Suppressor T-cell activity is mediated by the subset of T cells bearing receptors for IgG, which are found in increased numbers. These patients are very deficient in circulating B lymphocytes, frequently have eosinopenia, and may develop erythroid aplasia. Failure to produce B lymphocytes has been traced to the stem-cell level, since pre-B cells could not be found in their bone marrow. The relationship between the thymoma, T-cell dysfunction, and apparent abnormalities of hematopoietic stem cells remains conjectural.

WISKOTT-ALDRICH SYNDROME This is an X-linked genetic disease characterized by eczema, thrombocytopenia, and repeated infections. Affected boys often present with bleeding in infancy. Most do not survive childhood, dying of complications of bleeding, infection, or lymphoreticular malignancy. The immunologic defects in this disease are well characterized but poorly understood. Serum concentrations of IgM are usually decreased, while IgA and IgG are normal and IgE is frequently increased. However, synthetic rates for all three classes may be elevated, indicating a significant element of hypercatabolism. The number and class distribution of B lymphocytes usually have been normal. Some patients acquire a diminished number of T cells as evaluated by the E rosette test and appraisal of lymph node biopsies. Functionally, these boys are unable to make antibodies to polysaccharide antigens normally; responses to protein antigens are often not impaired. They are frequently anergic, and their T cells do not respond normally to challenge with ubiquitous antigens. However, responses to T-cell mitogens, such as phytohemagglutinin, are generally normal. Serial appraisal of affected males suggests that the defects in T-cell function are secondary. It is possible that the Wiskott-Aldrich syndrome reflects a primary defect in the B lymphocyte.

Transplantation of histocompatible bone marrow from a sibling donor has corrected both hematologic and immunologic abnormalities in several patients. In patients lacking a suitable donor, splenectomy may improve platelet counts and reduce the risk of serious hemorrhage. Because of the increased risk of pneumococcal bacteremia, splenectomized patients should probably receive prophylactic penicillin. Treatment with transfer factor was once held to benefit these patients, but this has not been substantiated in controlled studies.

Miscellaneous immunodeficiency syndromes Infection with *Candida albicans* is the almost universal accompaniment of severe deficiencies in cell-mediated immunity. The syndrome of *chronic mucocutaneous candidiasis* is different because superficial candidiasis is usually the only major manifestation of immunodeficiency. These patients rarely develop systemic infection with *Candida* or other fungal agents and are not unusually susceptible to virus or bacterial disease. The syndrome is often congenital and may be associated with single or multiple endocrinopathies as well as iron deficiency. Treatment of associated conditions may lead to improvement or even cure of *Candida* infection.

No uniformity of immunologic defects has been identified in these patients, although defects of antibody formation have been detected occasionally. Humoral immunity, including ability to make specific anti-*Candida* antibodies, is usually normal. Many patients are anergic, some to a variety of antigens and some only to *Candida;* anergy in some patients has been related to inability of their lymphocytes to produce migration inhibition factor.

Results of treatment with antifungal agents, such as amphotericin B, have been variable but generally not encouraging. In some patients, intensive treatment with amphotericin B coupled with surgical removal of infected nails has led to sustained improvement. Ketoconazole, an oral antifungal agent, is reported to be quite effective.

IMMUNODEFICIENCY ASSOCIATED WITH SERUM LYMPHOCYTOTOXINS This syndrome has been reported in a few patients with recurrent bacterial and fungal infections. Most have had fluctuating lymphopenia. Both cellular immunity and specific antibody responses were impaired, although immunoglobulin levels were usually normal. Antibodies specific for B-cell antigens have also been reported as a cause of selective elimination of B cells and resultant hypogammaglobulinemia.

IMBALANCES OF IgG SUBCLASSES Some patients with repeated infections and only moderately decreased serum IgG levels may have an imbalance of IgG subclasses. A few such patients appeared to benefit from administration of gamma globulin. *Kappa light chain deficiency* has also been reported in association with recurrent infections, and doubtless many more subtle gaps in antibody diversity, which may be clinically significant, will be elucidated.

X-LINKED LYMPHOPROLIFERATIVE SYNDROME This is an X-linked recessive disease in which there appears to be a selective impairment in immune elimination of Epstein-Barr virus (EBV). Infectious mononucleosis in affected males may have a fulminant and fatal outcome, may be associated with development of B-cell malignancies, or may result in acquired hypogammaglobulinemia, aplastic anemia, or agranulocytosis. Antibodies to EBV have been detected in some patients but are often absent in the face of infection. Generation of cytotoxic T cells appears to be the primary mechanism of control of EBV infection in normal persons and natural killer cells may also play a role in eliminating EBV-infected B cells. While a reduction of natural killer-cell activity has been noted, the nature of the defect which prevents a normal response to EBV in patients with the X-linked lymphoproliferative syndrome has not been defined.

Acquired deficiency of cell-mediated immunity in young homosexual men *Pneumocystis carinii* pneumonia is a disease classically associated with either congenital or acquired immunodeficiency, usually as a consequence of treatment with immunosuppressive drugs. A recent epidemic of *Pneumocystis* pneumonia and other opportunistic infections in previously healthy young men has led to the description of a new syndrome of acquired deficiency of cell-mediated immunity.

The patients, mostly males, are homosexual or drug abusers or both. Malaise, fever, anorexia, weight loss, and generalized lymphadenopathy preceded the onset of respiratory signs and symptoms by several months. Oral and anal mucosal lesions from which *Candida albicans,* herpes simplex virus type 2, and cytomegalovirus have been isolated alone or in combination occur commonly. A variety of other opportunistic infections with viral, bacterial, protozoal, or fungal agents have occurred in individual patients (see Chap. 137). Kaposi's sarcoma has appeared during the course of the disease in several patients. The mortality has been very high, despite intensive and repeated treatment with appropriate antimicrobials.

The affected men are uniformly severely lymphopenic and anergic. Isolated lymphocytes have diminished proliferative responses to mitogens and specific antigens. Although absolute numbers of both T and B cells are reduced, T cells are affected to a greater degree. Phenotyping with monoclonal antibodies has revealed distinctive abnormalities in some but not all patients. The frequency of Leu 2^+ $T8^+$ suppressor T cells was relatively increased, while the proportion of Leu 3^+ $T4^+$ helper T cells was greatly diminished. The T10 antigen, normally a marker for thymocytes, was present on a high proportion of circulating T cells. Humoral immune function, as measured by the antibody response to specific immunization, is normal in most patients. Serum concentrations of IgM and IgG are generally normal, while IgA levels are increased in more than half the reported patients. Increased concentrations of circulating immune complexes are present in many patients, but complement levels are not reduced. Decreased natural killer-cell function has been described in some patients.

The pathogenesis of the acquired immunodeficiency is not known. Because of its high frequency among homosexual men, persistence in semen, and propensity to cause immunosuppression, cytomegalovirus infection has been suspected of playing a role. However, the apparent absence of the syndrome in women and its emergence among homosexual men argue that other factors must be involved.

The high case fatality rate warrants aggressive diagnostic procedures, including open lung biopsy, in patients suspected of having this syndrome. The defect in cell-mediated immunity is apparently unremitting. Since *Pneumocystis* pneumonia may recur, prophylactic treatment with trimethoprim-sulfamethoxazole has been recommended.

Metabolic abnormalities associated with immunodeficiency The relation of deficiencies of the purine salvage enzymes, adenosine deaminase and purine nucleoside phosphorylase, to immunodeficiency was discussed earlier. Other inherited metabolic defects should be briefly mentioned because of their potential importance in understanding the molecular basis of immunologic function. Inherited *deficiency of transcobalamin II*, the serum carrier molecule responsible for transport of vitamin B_{12} to tissues, was associated with failure of immunoglobulin production as well as megaloblastic anemia, leukopenia, thrombocytopenia, and severe malabsorption. All abnormalities were reversed by administration of pharmacologic doses of vitamin B_{12}. The syndrome of *acrodermatitis enteropathica* includes severe desquamating skin lesions, intractable diarrhea, bizarre neurologic symptoms, variable combined immunodeficiency, and an often fatal outcome. This disease is apparently caused by an inborn error of metabolism resulting in malabsorption of dietary zinc, and can be effectively treated by parenteral or large oral doses of zinc. Similar disease manifestations have occurred in mice and cattle with different inherited defects leading to zinc malabsorption. Zinc deficiency might in part account for the immunodeficiency which accompanies severe malnutrition.

TREATMENT OF IMMUNODEFICIENCIES Treatment of immunodeficiency diseases involving severe abnormalities of T-cell function, with or without hypogammaglobulinemia, is currently limited in effectiveness and extremely complicated. Experimental approaches, including transplantation of bone marrow, fetal liver, and thymus, were mentioned in preceding sections. Also under investigation is the use of thymic hormones and of pharmacologic agents which may correct defects in lymphoid function caused by inherited metabolic disorders.

Replacement therapy with human gamma globulin should be used in patients who have recurrent bacterial infections and are deficient in IgG. Maintenance of serum IgG levels between 100 and 300 mg/dl is sufficient to prevent most overwhelming infections, although chronic sinusitis, otitis media, and bronchitis often persist. These serum levels usually can be achieved by intramuscular injection of IgG, 100 mg/kg, at monthly intervals, following a loading dose of twice this amount given over a period of several days. Forty milliliters of 16% gamma globulin, given in two or more sites at one time, is about the maximum tolerable in adults. If more is needed, it is preferable to increase the frequency of injections. Many hypogammaglobulinemic patients and their physicians normally prefer division of the monthly doses into bimonthly injections. In patients with mild to moderate IgG deficiency (300 to 400 mg/dl), the decision to treat must be based on clinical symptoms and on failure to respond to antigenic challenge, because injection of gamma globulin at the recommended doses will not significantly elevate serum IgG levels. Gamma globulin treatment is of no value in patients with deficiencies of immunoglobulins other than IgG. This form of treatment is not benign. Many patients become intolerant, having symptoms of diaphoresis, tachycardia, and hypotension immediately following injections. This reaction is thought to be mediated by aggregates of IgG in the gamma globulin preparation, but why it develops after years of treatment in some patients, and never in others has not been adequately explained. Most patients intolerant of gamma globulin injections can be treated successfully with plasma.

Infusion of fresh plasma, 10 to 20 ml/kg at intervals of 3 to 4 weeks, has the advantages of being less painful and of replacing IgM and IgA as well as IgG; however, both IgM and IgA have a half-life of only a few days. The major disadvantage of plasma is the risk of transmitting hepatitis, which is particularly devastating in immunodeficient patients. This risk can be minimized by use of selected donors, usually family members, carefully screened for the absence of Australia antigen or antibody.

A preparation of IgG suitable for intravenous administration has recently been approved by the Food and Drug Administration. Reports from this country and more extensive experience in Europe indicate that this preparation may be more effective and better tolerated than standard intramuscular gamma globulin.

Use of plasma or gamma globulin selected on the basis of a high titer of antibodies to a particular agent may be indicated in certain situations. For example, antibodies to the causative echovirus may dramatically improve encephalitis in immunodeficient patients.

Therapy with exogenous IgG usually does not prevent chronic sinopulmonary infection and its all too frequent progression to pulmonary fibrosis and bronchiectasis. Therefore, maintenance of good pulmonary toilet with regular postural drainage is an especially important part of patient management. The principles of antibiotic therapy are not different in these than other patients, except that the index of suspicion of bacterial infection should remain very high.

REFERENCES

Aiuti F et al: Identification, enumeration, and isolation of B and T lymphocytes from human peripheral blood. Scand J Immunol 3:521, 1974

Bergsma D et al (eds): *Immunodeficiency in Man and Animals, Birth Defects*, Original Article Series, vol XI, no 1. The National Foundation–March of Dimes, Sunderland, Mass., Sinauer Associates, 1975

Chandra RK et al: Immunodeficiency: Report of a WHO scientific group. WHO Tech Rep 630, 1978

Gottlieb MS et al: *Pneumocystis carinii* pneumonia and mucosal candidiasis in previously healthy homosexual men. N Engl J Med 305:1426, 1981

Japan Medical Research Foundation (eds): *Immunodeficiency: Its Nature and Etiological Significance in Human Disease.* Tokyo, University of Tokyo Press, 1978

Meischer PA, Müller-Eberhard HJ (eds): *Seminars in Immunopathology*, vol 1: *Immunodeficiency Diseases.* Berlin, Springer-Verlag, 1978

Reinherz EL et al: Abnormalities of T cell maturation and regulation in human beings with immunodeficiency disorders. J Clin Invest 68:699, 1981

Siegal FP et al: Severe acquired immunodeficiency in male homosexuals, manifested by chronic perianal ulcerative herpes simplex lesions. N Engl J Med 305:1439, 1981

Stiehm ER, Fulginiti VA (eds): *Immunologic Disorders in Infants and Children*, 2d ed. Philadelphia, Saunders, 1979

Update on Immune Deficiency Syndrome (AIDS)—United States. Morb Mort Week Rep 31:507, 1982

65 PLASMA CELL NEOPLASMS AND RELATED DISORDERS

RAYMOND ALEXANIAN

Plasma cell diseases represent a group of related disorders in which a clone of cells proliferates abnormally. The clone usually has the capability of synthesizing and secreting immunoglobulins or their components, which may be recognized as a peak on protein or urine protein electrophoresis. The most important of these diseases is multiple myeloma; other related conditions include Waldenström's macroglobulinemia, benign monoclonal gammopathy, primary amyloidosis, and the heavy chain diseases. A combination of clinical and immunologic laboratory studies is necessary to distinguish these entities, to stage the extent of disease, and to evaluate change in tumor mass with or without therapy.

The understanding of these disorders requires an understanding of immunoglobulin structure, synthesis, secretion, catabolism, and excretion. Immunoglobulins are synthesized by the B-cell series, with the mature plasma cell representing the end stage of differentiation. The heavy and light chains are synthesized on separate ribosomes and assembled and secreted as an intact molecule consisting of two heavy and two light chains linked together by disulfide bonds. A slight to moderate excess of light chain synthesis by the plasma cell leads to secretion of free light chains which are rapidly filtered through the glomeruli and catabolized by renal tubular cells. Normal persons excrete up to 10 mg of light chains in 24 h since not all of the filtered light chains are degraded in the kidney. Immunoglobulin molecules in normal persons are products of a multiplicity of clones resulting in diversity of classes, subclasses, light chain composition, electrophoretic mobility, and other immunologic characteristics. Serum protein electrophoresis shows a wide range of electrophoretic mobility for immunoglobulins, producing a broad band of gamma globulin. Likewise, polyclonal light chains in the urine produce a broad band of gamma globulin on protein electrophoresis (Fig. 65-1). In plasma cell disorders, one clone or a limited number of clones proliferates disproportionately, resulting in the appearance of a homogeneous population of an immunoglobulin or its component, which is seen as a narrow band or peak in the gamma or beta region on protein electrophoresis, since all the molecules from the clone will have an identical charge. Further evidence that the protein in the peak represents the product of a single clone is the demonstration of a single immunoglobulin class, subclass, and light chain composition.

The most common immunoglobulin class associated with monoclonal gammopathies is IgG, followed by IgA, IgM, IgD, and IgE. The frequency of the immunoglobulin type of monoclonal gammopathy correlates with the serum concentration of the immunoglobulin class. Monoclonal gammopathies of IgG type are more common than those of IgA or IgM classes. A monoclonal gammopathy is usually recognized on electrophoresis when about 10^{11} cells of a single clone are present, as in benign gammopathy or primary amyloidosis. When tumor growth approaches 10^{12} cells, clinical disease in the form of multiple myeloma, macroglobulinemia, or heavy chain disease is recognized. In addition to the increased production of intact monoclonal immunoglobulin, the clone also synthesizes and secretes an excess number of free light chains which appear in the urine as monoclonal light chains (Bence Jones protein). In approximately 20 percent of patients with multiple myeloma, the clone secretes only monoclonal light chains. In heavy chain disease, only the Fc fragment of the immunoglobulin molecule is secreted. Rarely, patients may have manifestations of multiple myeloma in which no monoclonal immunoglobulin can be demonstrated in serum or urine. Immunofluorescence studies of bone marrow plasma cells in these patients may show immunoglobulins within the cytoplasm, indicating a defect in their release from the cell.

In addition to the markedly increased production of a monoclonal protein, the quality of immunoglobulin synthesis may also be defective. For example, there may be a markedly excessive rate of monoclonal light chain production, and some patients excrete up to 40 g protein (Bence Jones protein) a day in the urine. In fact, about 20 percent of the patients with multiple myeloma show only light chain production, although immunofluorescent studies of the involved cells indicate that a low level of heavy chain synthesis also may occur. Some patients produce only the Fc fragments of heavy chains, and have heavy chain disease. Others with myeloma or macroglobulinemia have smaller deletions of segments of their heavy or light chains. The autonomously proliferating cells in these malignant disorders are capable of producing immunoglobulins that are structurally normal in some patients, and a few even demonstrate immunologic reactivity. In contrast, still other patients produce a distorted proportion of heavy and light chains, or an excessive quantity of defective globulins.

FIGURE 65-1
Electrophoresis of normal serum (top) and serum from a patient with diffuse hypergammaglobulinemia. In this condition, an increased number of plasma cells produce larger quantities of different globulins so that a broad elevation is apparent. Normal urine electrophoresis shows a broad band of gamma globulin (middle panel).

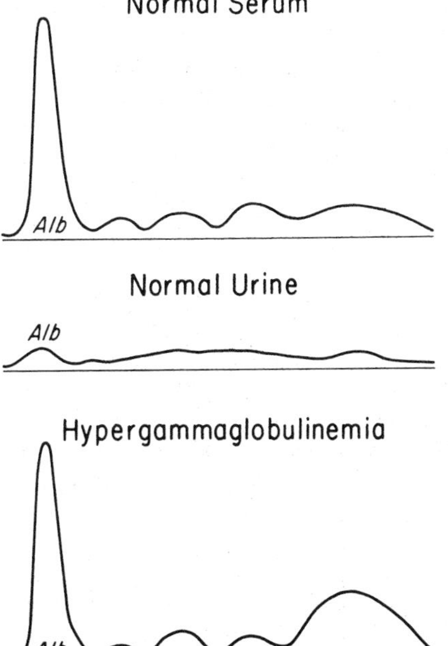

MULTIPLE MYELOMA Multiple myeloma is a disseminated malignancy of plasma cells that may be associated with bone destruction, bone marrow failure, hypercalcemia, renal failure, and recurrent infections. The disease is most common in the middle-aged and elderly; the median age of onset is 60 years. Males are affected slightly more frequently than females. The annual incidence of the disease is about 3 per 100,000 population.

Clinical and laboratory findings The clinical manifestations of multiple myeloma result primarily from the damage produced by plasma cell tumors in the bone marrow and from the effects of monoclonal proteins. There is a wide spectrum of pathologic features, and the complications of the disease as well as the modes of therapy required vary markedly among patients.

Bone pain from pathologic fractures constitutes the most common symptom and usually is due to compression fractures of the thoracic or lumbar spine. Typically, the pain is well localized, sometimes radicular, and is usually aggravated by movement, as on arising. In about 5 percent of patients, extradural plasmacytomas arising from a vertebra may produce spinal cord compression, paraplegia, and bladder dysfunction. Pathologic fractures of the ribs and proximal bones of the extremities are common. In about two-thirds of the patients, skeletal radiographs demonstrate punched-out lesions that are best seen on lateral skull films, but demineralization without focal destruction may be present. Isotopic bone scans are less useful than x-rays in demonstrating most bone lesions that may be superior in confirming pathologic rib fractures. Multiple vertebral compression fractures frequently result in a painless kyphosis of the dorsal spine and a diminution in height that may be as much as 6 in. Osteolysis appears to result from the increased production by the malignant plasma cells of a factor (osteoelastic activating factor) that stimulates osteoclast proliferation. Rarely, a diffuse osteoblastic bone reaction may occur. In about 15 percent of patients, firm plasmacytomas grow from areas of underlying bone destruction; these lesions usually develop over the skull, sternum, and clavicles and may be evident on physical examination because of their proximity to the skin.

In about 90 percent of patients, the bone marrow infiltration by plasma cells produces a normochromic, normocytic anemia at the time of diagnosis, and the anemia becomes more severe as the number of malignant cells increases. Other factors that contribute to anemia include the hypoferremia of chronic disease, renal failure, chemotherapy, and radiotherapy. The monoclonal immunoglobulins may coat the red blood cells, causing rouleaux formation and a markedly increased erythrocyte sedimentation rate. When there is marked hyperglobulinemia the plasma volume may be increased to an extent to reduce the hematocrit by as much as 6 volume percent lower than the value expected for the red blood cell volume. Occasionally, plasma cells may be present in the peripheral blood, but plasma cell leukemia with more than 1000 cells per cubic millimeter is unusual. Granulocytopenia or thrombocytopenia occurs in less than 10 percent of untreated patients. Some monoclonal immunoglobulins may produce an increased bleeding tendency by interfering with platelet function or by interactions with specific coagulation factors. When present in high concentrations and polymerized, monoclonal IgG or IgA may result in a symptomatic hyperviscosity syndrome.

Bone marrow aspirates usually contain prominent focal collections of immature plasma cells. The cells are usually large, ovoid, and basophilic, and contain an eccentric nucleus with finely clumped chromatin. Multinucleated cells, prominent nucleoli, and intracytoplasmic deposits of protein may be present. Electron microscopy always reveals a highly developed endoplasmic reticulum characteristic of cells elaborating extracellular protein, even in those few patients without apparent evidence of a monoclonal IgG or its component. Yet, there are no pathognomonic cytologic features that will always distinguish malignant from normal plasma cells.

A variety of chemical abnormalities may result from bone or kidney damage. Hypercalcemia with levels in excess of 11.5 mg/dl is found in about one-fourth of the patients at the time of diagnosis and is due to increased bone resorption. Symptoms due to hypercalcemia, such as nausea, mental confusion, and constipation, may constitute the patient's major complaint. Mild or severe renal failure with elevations of blood urea nitrogen to more than 40 mg/dl is a serious complication that occurs in about 20 percent of the patients. Although tubular damage from large quantities of filtered monoclonal light chains is considered the major factor, other important causes include hypercalcemia, uric acid nephropathy, and amyloidosis. Renal failure may be precipitated by dehydration, induced by preparation for some radiographic procedures. In rare patients, an adult Fanconi syndrome may result from derangement of specific tubular functions. An elevated serum uric acid level may occur as a consequence of an increased plasma cell turnover, increased cell destruction from chemotherapy, and/or decreased uric acid clearance from renal impairment. A symmetrical peripheral neuropathy that most frequently involves the lower extremities has been described in some patients. An increased susceptibility to bacterial infection results primarily because the levels of normal immunoglobulins are decreased in about 85 percent of the patients. This has been attributed to an increased number of monocytes that suppress the growth of normal plasma cells. Previously untreated patients are not more anergic to a battery of skin tests than normal persons of similar age. Pneumonia, urinary tract infection, and bacteremia may develop, particularly when the myeloma has not been controlled by chemotherapy. Herpes zoster occurs in about 10 percent of the patients.

One of the major features of the disease that is seen in about 97 percent of patients is a homogeneous globulin peak on electrophoresis of the serum, urine, or both (Fig. 65-2). This is present in the serum of about 80 percent of patients and is usually an intact monoclonal immunoglobulin [e.g., IgGK (kappa) or IgAL (lambda)]. The most common monoclonal protein associated with multiple myeloma is IgG, which is three times more frequent than IgA. Monoclonal IgD or IgE is rare. Bence Jones or monoclonal light chains may be demonstrated in the serum when renal failure is present. Since 20 percent of patients with multiple myeloma secrete only monoclonal light chains, which because of their small size (20,000 daltons) are rapidly filtered, they will not be detected by serum protein electrophoresis. In these patients, a urine protein electrophoresis will reveal a peak of monoclonal light chain, either kappa or lambda (Bence Jones protein). Patients suspected of having multiple myeloma or one of its variants, should have electrophoretic studies of both serum and urine. In about 3 percent of patients a monoclonal protein cannot be detected in either serum or urine, but immunofluorescence studies of bone marrow plasma cells will usually show the presence of a monoclonal protein in the cytoplasm. These cells apparently are unable to release their synthesized proteins.

Diagnosis The diagnosis should be suspected when one or more of the following abnormalities is present: bone pain from pathologic fractures of the spine or ribs, anemia, proteinuria, azotemia, hypercalcemia, recurrent infection, or spinal cord compression. In patients with severe bone pain and anemia who demonstrate bone marrow plasmacytosis, the presence of lytic bone lesions and a peak on serum or urine electrophoresis is diagnostic. Both serum and urine protein electrophoresis

FIGURE 65-2

Serum and urine electrophoresis in upper and lower panels from two patients with multiple myeloma. On the left, increased production of a complete monoclonal globulin is reflected in a serum peak; excessive light chains are excreted and produce a urine peak of different mobility. A second patient on the right has a normal serum electrophoresis with evidence only of light chain excretion in the urine.

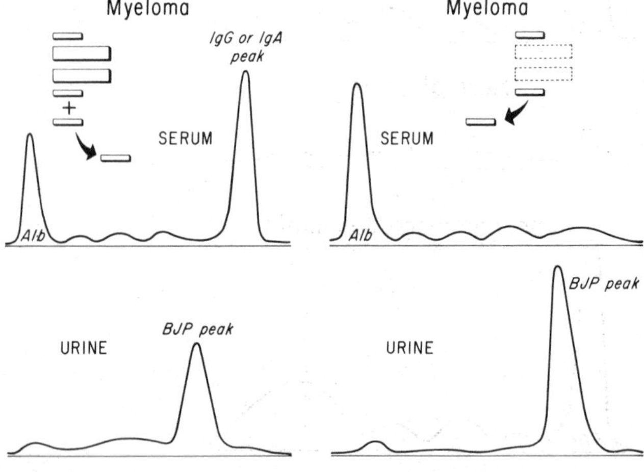

must be evaluated in patients suspected of having myeloma, and electrophoresis of concentrated urine may be necessary for the detection of small amounts of light chains. Examination of the marrow alone may not distinguish the plasma cell infiltration of multiple myeloma from the reactive plasmacytosis found in chronic infection, chronic liver disease, or collagen diseases. In these disorders, the generalized plasma cell reaction will usually produce a diffuse hypergammaglobulinemia on electrophoresis (Fig. 65-1). The occurrence of hypercalcemia or azotemia is also not specific, but the finding of markedly depressed normal immunoglobulins helps to distinguish myeloma from other nonmalignant plasma cell dyscrasias. In patients with equivocal findings, the presence of large IgG or IgA peaks in the serum (>3.0 g/dl), depressed values of normal serum immunoglobulins, or more than 100 mg per day of Bence Jones protein in the urine supports the diagnosis of myeloma. The excretion of monoclonal light chains of either kappa or lambda type usually signifies myeloma, macroglobulinemia, or primary amyloidosis, but the patient may not be clinically symptomatic for a long time when this is the only abnormality. Diseases that must be distinguished from myeloma include benign monoclonal gammopathy, primary amyloidosis, Waldenström's macroglobulinemia, the heavy chain diseases, and metastatic bone tumors. In addition, patients with localized plasmacytoma or indolent multiple myeloma need to be identified because in them chemotherapy is not indicated.

Treatment and prognosis The best treatment for multiple myeloma requires the prevention and control of the complications of this disease, as well as simultaneous efforts to reduce the number of malignant plasma cells. In disabled patients, increased physical activity should be encouraged by the rational use of analgesics, corsets, and walkers. Radiation therapy is useful for disabling bone pain from pathologic fractures, particularly when there is little improvement after the first course of chemotherapy. Immediate radiotherapy to areas of spinal cord compression may prevent the need for decompressive laminectomy after tumor masses are identified by prompt myelography or CT scan. Adequate hydration is essential in order to prevent and control renal complications from the precipitation of Bence Jones protein in the renal tubules; dehydration must be avoided in preparing patients for radiologic procedures. For patients with severe renal failure, hemodialysis may maintain life for the period required to reduce Bence Jones protein production with chemotherapy. Hypercalcemia in previously untreated patients is almost always reversible with fluids, increased activity, and chemotherapy with drug combinations that include prednisone. If a bacterial infection develops, prompt and rational use of antibiotics is essential. Prophylactic gamma globulin has no value, and vaccinations with live organisms must be avoided in these immunosuppressed patients.

For symptomatic patients with multiple myeloma and asymptomatic patients with rising myeloma proteins or progressive lytic bone lesions, chemotherapy is required in order to reduce the number of plasma cells. Serial assessments of myeloma protein levels in serum and/or urine are essential for evaluating changes in tumor mass. Before each course of drug therapy, blood counts must be monitored to ensure adequate recovery of granulocytes to a level of 2000 per cubic millimeter and platelets to a level of 100,000 per cubic millimeter. Intermittent courses of a vincristine (1.0 mg intravenously)–cyclophosphamide (100 mg/m^2 per day for 4 days)–prednisone (60 mg/m^2 per day for 4 days) combination repeated at 3- to 4-week intervals will produce tumor reductions of greater than 75 percent in about two-thirds of previously untreated patients. Recalcification of lytic bone lesions and an elevation of low immunoglobulin levels occur in 15 percent of patients who respond. Intermittent treatment should be continued for at least 12 months because many patients respond slowly. After a year, patients who have responded and whose abnormal monoclonal protein has disappeared from the serum can be followed without chemotherapy. Serial electrophoretic measurements must continue to be made because tumor recurrence, recognized by the reappearance of myeloma proteins, can usually be controlled with chemotherapy. Patients who respond but who have persistently elevated serum levels of monoclonal protein should be maintained on intermittent courses of melphalan (7 mg/m^2 per day for 4 days) and prednisone (60 mg/m^2 per day for 4 days) until relapse occurs, when the doxorubicin combination should be resumed.

The median survival time for patients who receive combination chemotherapy is about 30 months. But there is a wide variation in prognosis that depends on the extent of tumor mass at the time of diagnosis and the maximum degree of tumor reduction following chemotherapy. The pretreatment tumor mass can be estimated from such laboratory data as the degree of anemia, hypercalcemia, and bone lesions; the degree of tumor mass reduction can be assessed by the degree of reduction in myeloma proteins. The median survival is less than 1 year for patients with a high cell mass and no response, about 4 years for those with a low tumor mass and a marked response, and various intermediate responses depending on the residual number of plasma cells. When irreversible renal failure is present, the median survival is short regardless of the tumor mass and the degree of remission. About 2 percent of all patients and about 6 percent of responding patients who live longer than 2 years will develop acute myelogenous and monocytic leukemia; the long-term treatment with alkylating agents is probably the major cause. The incidence of second solid tumors is not increased.

INDOLENT MYELOMA An increasing number of asymptomatic patients with multiple myeloma in an indolent phase have been recognized. In many patients, the diagnosis was first suspected after routine biochemical studies revealed an elevated total protein level which on serum electrophoresis was found to be due to a monoclonal gammopathy. Further studies usually confirm bone marrow plasmacytosis and depressed normal immunoglobulins; mild anemia and other evidence of disease characterized by a low tumor mass may also be present. Chemotherapy should be withheld in patients unlikely to experience major morbidity, but changes in the level of myeloma protein, hemoglobin, and bone lesions must be monitored to evaluate progression. Patients with Bence Jones proteinuria, compression fractures of the vertebrae, numerous lytic bone lesions, recurrent infection, or rising myeloma proteins should receive chemotherapy without delay.

LOCALIZED MYELOMA In occasional patients considered to have a localized plasmacytoma, only one plasma cell tumor can be identified without other areas of bone destruction or bone marrow plasmacytosis. All the major disease complications usually associated with myeloma, such as severe anemia and hypercalcemia, are absent. About one-half of the patients do not show a monoclonal globulin peak in the serum or urine; even when present, the level is always low. Normal serum immunoglobulins are usually not depressed. Local radiotherapy in a dose of about 40,000 mGy (4000 rads) is recommended for treatment, but prophylactic chemotherapy is not indicated. Periodic evaluation of serum and urine globulins and of skeletal radiographs in those without abnormal globulins is necessary to detect the presence of multiple myeloma.

WALDENSTRÖM'S MACROGLOBULINEMIA Waldenström's macroglobulinemia is a chronic lymphoproliferative disorder with a wide range of manifestations. This disease affects the middle-aged and elderly and has a slightly higher frequency in men than women. The presence of a peak on electrophoresis consisting of monoclonal IgM is a prerequisite for the diagnosis (Fig. 65-3). Aside from uncommon patients with idiopathic IgM peaks, most patients have evidence of an underlying lymphoma which is characterized by bone marrow infiltration, enlargement of lymph nodes and/or spleen, chronic lymphocytic leukemia, or a combination of these features. Conversely, in about 80 percent of patients with chronic lymphocytic leukemia or lymphocytic lymphoma, the affected cells show evidence of monoclonal IgM synthesis by immunofluorescent studies; about 5 percent of patients with these diseases also have an IgM peak on serum electrophoresis.

Clinical and laboratory features The most common clinical features are anemia, lymphadenopathy, chronic lymphocytic leukemia, and the hyperviscosity syndrome. The anemia usually results from a marked bone marrow infiltration by lymphocytes, plasma cells, and lymphocytes that resemble plasma cells. Histologically, the nodes are infiltrated diffusely in a pattern that usually resembles a lymphocytic lymphoma, although the picture may be closer to that of a histiocytic lymphoma. Because of the large molecular weight of the pentameric IgM molecule (Fig. 65-3) and the propensity to polymerize, increased serum concentrations of monoclonal IgM may produce marked hyperviscosity of the blood. The symptoms of the hyperviscosity syndrome are most commonly lassitude and confusion, segmental dilatation of retinal veins with retinal hemorrhages, and an increased bleeding tendency due to an interaction of the monoclonal IgM with coagulation factors and interference with platelet function. Some monoclonal macroglobulins may have antibody activity such as rheumatoid factor (anti-IgG) and cold agglutinins. Monoclonal cold agglutinins may produce hemolytic anemia by binding complement to the red cell membrane. Renal failure is rare in macroglobulinemia, probably because Bence Jones proteinuria is absent or minimal. About 2 percent of patients show lytic bone destruction, as in myeloma. IgG and IgA are usually not reduced to the degree found in multiple myeloma. The monoclonal proteins observed in both macroglobulinemia and multiple myeloma may have the properties of a cryoglobulin. This type of cryoglobulin should be differentiated from the mixed cryoglobulins (e.g., IgG-IgM or IgG-IgA), in which the IgM or IgA component may be a monoclonal antibody to IgG. The mixed cryoglobulins are seen in a variety of infectious and collagen vascular disorders. The presence of a monoclonal immunoglobulin in mixed cryoglobulins does not signify that these patients have a plasma cell neoplasia. Raynaud's phenomenon, acrocyanosis, and ulcers of the fingers and toes may develop. In the workup of a patient suspected to have cryoglobulins, blood should be collected into prewarmed syringes, with subsequent separation at 37°C. Serum is then allowed to precipitate at 4°C, followed by quantitation and characterization of the cryoprecipitates.

FIGURE 65-3
In macroglobulinemia, the excessive production of a single pentameric globulin is demonstrated as a peak and requires immunoelectrophoretic studies for identification. With heavy chain disease, IgG heavy chains are present in serum and urine without monoclonal kappa or lambda light chains.

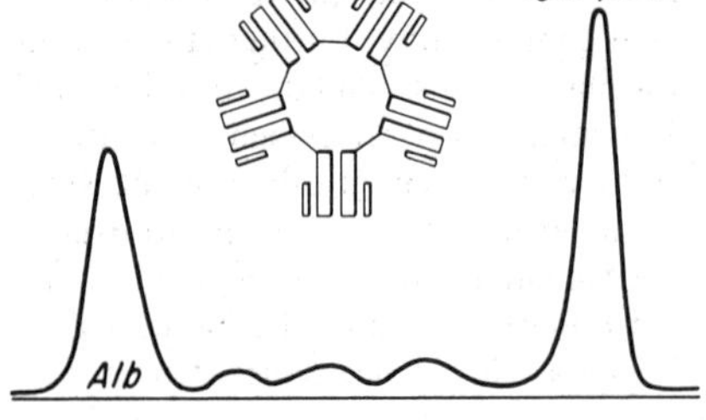

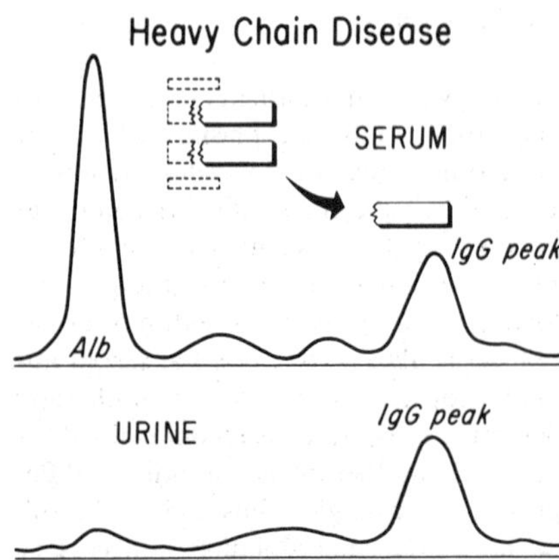

Treatment For most patients, the best management includes the reduction of the tumor mass with chemotherapy and the simultaneous control of complications. Transfusion of either whole blood or packed red cells should be instituted with caution in patients with high levels of macroglobulins because the addition of red cells will increase both the plasma volume and blood viscosity. For patients with symptoms due to cryoglobulinemia, protection of the extremities from the cold is necessary. When fatigue or neurologic changes occur, and whole blood viscosity measurements are abnormal, plasmapheresis is indicated. This procedure is carried out most expeditiously with an automatic blood cell separator. Because about 80 percent of the macroglobulin is located within the intravascular bed, efficient removal of IgM molecules is possible.

Intermittent courses of a chlorambucil (8 mg/m^2 per day for 10 days) and prednisone (25 mg/m^2 per day for 10 days) combination, repeated at 6-week intervals, are effective in reducing the tumor mass by at least 50 percent in approximately three-fourths of the patients. As in myeloma, periodic monitoring by serum electrophoresis is necessary because changes in the monoclonal IgM concentration are helpful in assessing the change in tumor mass. Irradiation may be necessary for aggregates of large lymph nodes. After 18 months, chemotherapy can be withheld from selected patients who achieve a marked reduction in tumor mass and can be resumed should relapse occur. When there is progressive tumor growth despite repeated courses of alkylating agents and prednisone or when the histologic features of a histiocytic lymphoma are present, other drug combinations that include doxorubicin (Adriamycin) and bleomycin may be helpful. The prognosis is better than for multiple myeloma; the median survival is about 4 years.

BENIGN MONOCLONAL GAMMOPATHY About 0.5 percent of normal individuals over the age of 40 years show a small monoclonal peak on serum electrophoresis. The incidence increases with advancing age so that about 3 percent of individuals over the age of 70 show this abnormality. Usually, monoclonal gammopathy is not suspected when the electrophoresis is ordered, and none of the laboratory or radiographic abnormalities associated with myeloma are present. The concentration of the monoclonal protein is almost always less than 3.0 g/dl, and Bence Jones proteinuria is rarely present. The monoclonal protein is IgG in about 85 percent of patients, and IgA and IgM account for the remainder. In contrast to myeloma, immunoglobulin levels other than the monoclonal protein are usually normal.

When a peak is detected, appropriate studies should rule out the presence of myeloma, macroglobulinemia, or amyloidosis. Most authorities agree that any relationship between monoclonal peaks and other specific underlying diseases, such as an occult solid tumor, is probably coincidental. Periodic long-term follow-up usually shows no changes in the level of the monoclonal protein for the remainder of the patient's life. Less than 20 percent of these individuals have developed multiple myeloma, lymphoma, or amyloidosis after many years of evaluation. Prophylactic chemotherapy, as is used in myeloma, is unjustified. Some benign peaks are transient, particularly those associated with acute hepatitis and other viral infections.

PRIMARY AMYLOIDOSIS (See Chap. 66) Amyloidosis is a disease in which major organs are damaged by the depositing of monoclonal light chains in the vascular endothelium. The organs most commonly affected are the kidneys (nephrotic syndrome), heart (congestive failure), joints (carpal tunnel syndrome and arthritis), tongue (macroglossia), nerves (peripheral neuropathy), and gastrointestinal tract (malabsorption syndrome). "Secondary" amyloidosis occurs in association with familial Mediterranean fever or prolonged chronic infection or inflammation, such as rheumatoid arthritis and is usually associated with the deposition of AA protein in the tissue. "Primary" amyloidosis with the organ involvement described above has no apparent inflammatory basis and occurs in about 15 percent of patients with overt myeloma or macroglobulinemia; usually it is recognized in these patients only on postmortem examination. In addition, about 80 percent of patients with primary amyloidosis and without evidence of myeloma have a small monoclonal peak on serum or urine electrophoresis. Fragments of light chains are present in amyloid fibrils both in myeloma-associated and in primary amyloidosis without myeloma. Therefore, primary amyloidosis must be considered a monoclonal gammopathy. The disease apparently results from a single clone of plasma cells that has expanded to a stable size of about 10^{11} cells, as in idiopathic monoclonal gammopathy, but with an excess secretion of free light chains that produces tissue damage in the form of amyloidosis. Biopsies of skin lesions, gums, and rectum provide the best histologic evidence for the disease. All histologic material should be stained with Congo red, and the presence of green birefringence should be sought by polarized microscopy. Because of the risks of hemorrhage, liver and renal biopsies should be employed only when biopsies of other sites are negative. Chemotherapy as for myeloma is ineffective in resolving amyloid infiltration, but a 6- to 12-month program may slow the rate of amyloid production by reducing the size of the plasma cell clone.

HEAVY CHAIN DISEASES These rare malignant disorders are characterized by an excessive production of heavy chain fragment, related mainly to the Fc portion of the gamma-globulin molecule. Each of the three described types (gamma, alpha, and mu) has different clinical features and requires immunoelectrophoretic and other special studies for diagnosis.

Patients with *gamma heavy chain disease* are elderly and have easy fatigability, recurrent infections, lymphadenopathy, and splenomegaly. The clinical picture resembles a diffuse lymphoma. Palatal edema may be present because the nodes of Waldeyer's ring are frequently enlarged. Anemia, thrombocytopenia, and eosinophilia are often present, and the bone marrow and lymph nodes are replaced by plasma cells or lymphocytes that resemble plasma cells. The diagnosis is made by finding a monoclonal peak of identical electrophoretic mobility in both serum and urine. The heavy chain molecule represents the Fc fragment or deleted portions of the fragment. Because of its small size (~60,000 daltons), studies on blood and urine will show precipitation with anti-IgG, but no reactivity with antibodies to light chains. The finding of a monoclonal peak in the serum, with a monoclonal peak in the urine that does not react to antibodies to kappa or lambda light chains, strongly suggests the diagnosis of gamma heavy chain disease (Fig. 65-3). Chemotherapy has usually been ineffective and the prognosis is poor; most patients die of infection within a year of the diagnosis.

Alpha chain disease is the most common of the heavy chain diseases, and afflicted patients have an extensive plasmacytic infiltrate throughout the small intestinal mucosa. The result is a severe malabsorption syndrome with all its attendant complications. Chronic diarrhea, abdominal pain, nausea, and weight loss are common. Young adults between 20 and 30 years of age who live in the Mediterranean region are affected most commonly. There is no sexual preponderance. The diagnosis requires the demonstration of a monoclonal gammopathy in serum or urine that consists only of alpha heavy chains and that is devoid of light chains. Because serum electrophoresis may appear normal, sensitive immunoelectrophoretic procedures and other special studies are often necessary to establish the diagnosis. The disease is progressive in most patients, although spontaneous remissions in some patients have suggested that the disease may represent an unusual reaction to infection.

Very few patients with *mu chain disease* have been described. Most have had a chronic lymphocytic leukemia with a small monoclonal component that is usually difficult to detect on serum electrophoresis. The diagnosis requires the demonstration by serum immunoelectrophoresis of an IgM monoclonal globulin that is devoid of light chains, although free light chains may be present in the urine. Insufficient data are available to determine whether the natural history of this disease differs from that of chronic lymphocytic leukemia.

REFERENCES

ALEXANIAN R et al: Prognostic factors in multiple myeloma. Cancer 36:1192, 1975

———: Chemoimmunotherapy for multiple myeloma. Cancer 47(8):1923, 1981

FRANGIONE B, FRANKLIN EC: Heavy chain diseases: Clinical features and molecular significance of the disorder immunoglobulin structure. Semin Hematol 10:53, 1973

GLENNER GG: Amyloid deposits and amyloidosis. N Engl J Med 302:1283, 1333, 1980

ISOBE T, OSSERMAN EF: Patterns of amyloidosis and their associations with plasma cell dyscrasia, monoclonal immunoglobulins and Bence Jones proteins. N Engl J Med 290:473, 1974

KYLE RA: Monoclonal gammopathy of undetermined significance. Natural history in 241 cases. Am J Med 64:814, 1978

———, Bayrd ED: *The Monoclonal Gammopathies.* Springfield, Ill., Charles C Thomas, 1977

66
AMYLOIDOSIS

ALAN S. COHEN

DEFINITION AND CLASSIFICATION Amyloidosis may be defined as the extracellular deposition of the fibrous protein amyloid in one or more sites of the body. This protein has unique ultrastructural, x-ray diffraction, and biochemical characteristics. It can be deposited locally where it has no clinical consequences or may involve virtually any organ system of the body leading to severe pathophysiologic changes, or the disease may fall between these two extremes. The natural history of amyloidosis is poorly understood, and the clinical diagnosis is often not made until the disease is far advanced. The following classification is clinically the most useful: (1) primary (AL type) amyloidosis (no evidence for preexisting or coexisting disease); (2) amyloid associated with multiple myeloma; (3) secondary (AA type) amyloidosis associated with chronic infectious diseases (e.g., osteomyelitis, tuberculosis, leprosy) or chronic inflammatory diseases (e.g., rheumatoid arthritis and ankylosing spondylitis); (4) heredofamilial amyloidosis, the amyloidosis associated with familial Mediterranean fever and a variety of neuropathic, renal, cardiovascular, and other syndromes; (5) local amyloidosis (local, often tumor-like, deposits occur in isolated organs without evidence of systemic involvement); and (6) amyloidosis associated with aging.

PATHOLOGY AND STRUCTURE Amyloid is amorphous, eosinophilic, hyalin, extracellular, and ubiquitous in distribution. The involved organs may have a rubbery, firm consistency and a waxy, pink or gray appearance. Organ enlargement, especially of the liver, kidney, spleen, and heart, may be prominent.

Microscopically, amyloid stains pink with the hematoxylin-eosin stain and shows metachromasia with crystal violet or methyl violet. The Congo red stain imparts a unique green birefringence when sections are viewed in the polarizing microscope. This is the single most useful procedure for establishing the presence of amyloid. Amyloid deposits may be focal in almost any area of the body but are most often perivascular.

The heart may show focal or diffuse interstitial deposits in the myocardium, endocardium, or pericardium. In the aged heart, the atrium is usually focally involved or there may occur more diffuse lesions of the atria and ventricles. In the kidney, the glomerulus is primarily affected, although interstitial, peritubular, and vascular amyloid occur. In early lesions, small nodular or diffuse deposits appear near the basement membrane and, as the disease progresses, the glomerulus may be massively laden with amyloid, and its capillary bed will be occluded. In the gastrointestinal tract, there may be perivascular deposits only, or irregular or diffuse deposits may be found in the submucosa, in the muscularis mucosa, or subserosa. The amyloid may appear at any level or portion of the gastrointestinal tract including the gallbladder and pancreas. In the nervous system, amyloid has been described along peripheral nerves, in autonomic ganglia, and in senile plaques, in neurofibrillary tangles, as well as blood vessels ("congophilic angiopathy") of the central nervous system. It may be found in any portion of the orbit including the vitreous humor and cornea. In summary, there is virtually no area of the body that is spared. This ubiquitous distribution elicits a wide variety of clinical symptoms and signs.

All types of human amyloid consist of fine, nonbranching rigid fibrils that in tissue sections measure approximately 100 Å in diameter. The amyloid fibrils are usually seen earliest in the mesangial cell in the kidney and Kupffer cell in the liver. Isolated amyloid fibrils have a delicate, thin, nonbranching fibrous character. The individual fibril (or filament) has a diameter of about 70 Å and tends to aggregate laterally. Each fibril (filament) has subunit protofibrils of 30 to 35 Å diameter.

A second component, the plasma component or pentagonal unit (P component) with a different ultrastructure, x-ray diffraction pattern, and chemical characteristics, has also been isolated from amyloid and is identical with a serum alpha globulin. It has many similarities to C-reactive protein, but it does not behave as a classic acute phase protein. It is not responsible for the characteristic tinctorial properties or ultrastructure of amyloid.

BIOCHEMISTRY OF AMYLOID FIBRILS The bulk of amyloid deposits consists of fibrils. The homology of the fibril of primary and myeloma amyloid to the *N*-terminal region of the variable fragment of an immunoglobulin light chain and subsequently, in a limited number of cases, to a homogeneous light polypeptide chain, has been demonstrated. These light chain–related proteins range in size from about 5000 to 25,000 daltons and are now termed amyloid light chain (AL) or A_κ or A_λ (Table 66-1). Amino acid sequence analysis indicates that most primary amyloid proteins contain the *N*-terminal amino acid residue identical to the variable regions of the light chain (Asp-Ile-Gln-Ser-Pro-Ser-Ser-Leu- . . .).

Another protein that is unrelated to any known immunoglobulin has been described in the secondary amyloid deposits. This protein, amyloid A (AA) protein, can be isolated from the amyloid of patients with secondary amyloidosis and from that associated with familial Mediterranean fever. It is a unique protein with a molecular weight of about 8500 daltons made up of 76 amino acid residues arranged in a single chain, and an amino acid sequence beginning with Arg-Ser-Phe. . . . Some heterogeneity has been demonstrated (i.e., AAs of different molecular weights).

Antiserums to alkali-degraded amyloid fibrils of the AA protein have detected an antigenically related serum component, SAA. Amino acid analysis, peptide maps, and sequence studies suggest that AA protein is an amino terminal fragment of SAA and is derived from it by proteolysis. SAA appears to behave as an acute phase reactant and is elevated in infection and inflammation, and with aging. In addition, SAA is elevated in amyloid-resistant animals suggesting that the appearance of amyloid is not solely determined by the level of SAA. An SAA inducing factor (which seems to be identical to interleukin I) has been shown to be released from stimulated macrophages and to cause the release of SAA from hepatocytes, the site of SAA synthesis. SAA appears to suppress antibody response, suggesting that it might act as an immune regulator. Heterogeneity of SAAs has also been recognized.

TABLE 66-1
Preliminary nomenclature for amyloid fibril proteins

Current amyloid clinical or organ or fibril frame of reference	*Preliminary terminology*	*Chemical description*
A protein	AA	AA (prototype)(7) AA^{Trp53} (variant)(8)
Light chain protein	AL	A_{λ_1}, etc
Familial	AF	
Portuguese	AF_P	A protein name
Japanese	AF_J	A protein name
Endocrine organ–related	AE	
Thyroid	AE_t	A protein name
Senile amyloid	AS	
Cardiac	AS_{c_1}, AS_{c_2}*	A protein name
Brain	AS_{b_1}	A protein name
Dermal (cutaneous)	AD^1	A protein name

* *These are included in this fashion since preliminary reports suggest that two types of senile cardiac amyloid may exist.*
SOURCES: *AS Cohen, O Wegelius, Arthritis Rheuma 23:644, 1980; GG Glenner et al, 1980.*

A third form of amyloid protein that has been biochemically identified is that of familial amyloid polyneuropathy. These deposits have the primary structure of prealbumin molecules. Finally, the amyloid associated with certain endocrine organs appears to be made up of local hormone precursors.

P component of amyloid In addition to the characteristic fibrils described above, a second component, the P component, has been noted in most amyloid deposits. P component (AP) has been recognized by electron microscopy as a pentagonal-shaped structured unit having an outside diameter of about 90 Å and an inside diameter of about 40 Å. On immunoelectrophoresis it migrates as an alpha globulin, and it possesses antigenic identity with a constituent of normal human plasma (SAP). The amino acid sequence is distinct from that of the amyloid fibrils. Its pentagonal ultrastructure is similar to C-reactive protein (CRP), but the latter is one-half the molecular weight of AP and has other well-defined differences despite a 50 to 60 percent homology on amino acid sequence. AP binds to amyloid fibrils in a calcium-dependent fashion.

IMMUNOBIOLOGY OF AMYLOID The etiology and pathogenesis of amyloidosis are unknown. Electron-microscopic autoradiographic studies have revealed high concentrations of fibrils adjacent to reticuloendothelial cells.

Endotoxin stimulation of macrophages has been shown to produce a mediator (SAA inducer) that stimulates hepatic cells, now recognized as a major source of SAA synthesis, to produce SAA. Other studies suggest that SAA is partially degraded by monocyte or leukocyte surface enzymes to form tissue AA. The other form of amyloid (AL) is probably produced by the partial degradation of immunoglobulins by macrophages.

An excess antigenic stimulus has been shown to induce amyloid in animals. However, the basic conditions for the experimental induction of amyloidosis have not been clearly defined. Marked depression of T cells with maintenance of normal or hyperactive B-cell function has been described. These findings suggest that disturbances in immunoregulatory mechanisms may be an important step in the pathogenesis of amyloid disease. A transferable amyloid enhancing factor (AEF) that can be isolated from the spleens of experimental animals has also been identified.

CLINICAL MANIFESTATIONS The clinical manifestations of amyloidosis are varied and depend entirely on the area of the body which is involved.

Kidney Renal involvement may consist of mild proteinuria or frank nephrosis. In some cases, the urinary sediment may show only a few red blood cells. The renal lesion is usually not reversible and in time leads to progressive azotemia and death. The prognosis does not appear to be related to the degree of the proteinuria; when azotemia finally develops, the prognosis is grave. In one series the mean survival of patients with renal amyloid from the time of biopsy was 29 months, but in a few cases there was presumptive evidence of regression of the renal amyloid. Hypertension is rare except in long-standing amyloidosis. Renal tubular acidosis or renal vein thrombosis may occur. Localized accumulation of amyloid may be noted in the ureter, bladder, or other parts of the genitourinary tract.

Liver While hepatic involvement is common, liver function abnormalities are minimal and occur late in the disease. The two tests most useful in indicating hepatic amyloid are the Bromsulphalein (BSP) extraction and serum alkaline phosphatase activity. Liver scans produce variable and nonspecific results. Portal hypertension occurs but is uncommon. Intrahepatic cholestasis has been noted in about 5 percent of patients with AL (primary) amyloidosis. In a series of 54 patients in which liver tissue was available for examination, all 54 had some amyloid present either in the parenchyma or blood vessels, irrespective of the type of amyloidosis (primary or secondary). Amyloidosis of the spleen characteristically is not associated with leukopenia and anemia.

Heart Cardiac manifestations consist primarily of congestive failure and cardiomegaly (with or without murmurs) and a variety of arrhythmias. Although the cardiac manifestations reflect predominantly diffuse myocardial amyloid, the endocardium, the valves, and the pericardium may be involved as well. Pericarditis with effusion is rare, although the differential diagnosis of constrictive pericarditis versus restrictive cardiomyopathy frequently arises. Echocardiography has demonstrated symmetrical thickening of the left ventricular wall, hypokinesia and decreased systolic thickening of the interventricular septum and left ventricular posterior wall, and left ventricular cavities of small to normal size. Two-dimensional echocardiography is said to produce the characteristic findings of thickened right and left ventricles, a normal left ventricular cavity, and especially a diffuse hyperrefractile "granular sparkling" appearance. Hearts which are heavily infiltrated with amyloid may or may not show an enlarged silhouette. Fluoroscopy usually shows decreased mobility of the ventricular wall; angiographic studies usually demonstrate thickened ventricular wall, decreased ventricular mobility, and absence of rapid ventricular filling in early diastole. Cardiac amyloidosis can present as intractable heart failure. Electrocardiographic abnormalities include a low-voltage QRS complex and abnormalities in atrioventricular and intraventricular conduction, often resulting in varying degrees of heart block. Owing to their propensity to develop conduction defects and arrhythmias, patients with cardiac amyloidosis appear to be especially sensitive to digitalis, and this drug should be used with caution.

Skin Involvement of the skin is one of the most characteristic manifestations of so-called primary amyloidosis. The lesions may consist of slightly raised, waxy papules or plaques which usually are clustered in the folds of the axillae, anal, or inguinal regions, the face and neck, or mucosal areas such as ear or tongue. The lesions are seldom pruritic. Involvement of the skin or mucosa may not be apparent clinically but may be disclosed by biopsy. Gentle rubbing of the skin may induce bleeding into the skin, leading to purpura. Cutaneous involvement also can occur in secondary amyloidosis; in one series it was found in 42 percent of such patients, in 55 percent of a group of patients with primary disease, and in all 11 patients with hereditary amyloid neuropathy.

Gastrointestinal tract Gastrointestinal symptoms are common in amyloidosis. They may result from direct involvement of the gastrointestinal tract at any level or from infiltration of the autonomic nervous system with amyloid. The symptoms include those of obstruction, ulceration, malabsorption, hemorrhage, protein loss, and diarrhea. Infiltration of the tongue occasionally leads to macroglossia. When not enlarged, the tongue may become stiffened and firm to palpation. While infiltration of the tongue is characteristic of primary amyloidosis or amyloidosis accompanying multiple myeloma, it is occasionally seen in the secondary form of the disease.

Gastrointestinal bleeding may occur from any of a number of sites, notably the esophagus, stomach, or large intestine, and may be severe. Amyloid infiltration of the esophagus may lead to an incompetent or nonrelaxing lower esophageal sphincter, nonspecific motility disorders of the esophageal body, or rarely achalasia. Small-bowel lesions may lead to clinical and x-ray changes of obstruction. A malabsorption syndrome is seen at times. Amyloidosis may develop in association with other entities involving the gastrointestinal tract, especially tuberculosis, granulomatous enteritis, lymphoma, and Whipple's disease; differentiation of these conditions, which give rise to secondary amyloidosis, from diffuse primary amyloidosis of the small bowel may be difficult. Similarly, amyloidosis of the stomach may closely mimic gastric carcinoma, with obstruction, achlorhydria, and the radiologic appearance of tumor masses.

Nervous system Neurologic manifestations may include peripheral neuropathy, postural hypotension, inability to sweat, Adie pupil, hoarseness, and sphincter incompetence. These manifestations are especially prominent in the heredofamilial amyloidoses. The cranial nerves are generally spared except for those involving the pupillary reflexes. Amyloid occurs in the central nervous system as a component of senile plaques, possibly neurofibrillary tangles, and in blood vessels ("congophilic angiopathy"). The protein concentration in the cerebral spinal fluid may be increased. Infiltrates of the cornea or vitreous body may be present in hereditary amyloid syndromes. Certain of these syndromes are characterized by a bilateral scalloping appearance of the pupil. Amyloid may infiltrate the thyroid or other endocrine glands but rarely causes endocrine dysfunction. Local amyloid deposits almost invariably accompany medullary carcinoma of the thyroid. Amyloid infiltration of muscle may lead to a pseudomyopathy.

Joints Amyloid can directly involve articular structures by its presence in the synovial membrane and synovial fluid or in the articular cartilage. Amyloid arthritis can mimic a number of rheumatic diseases because it can present as a symmetrical arthritis of small joints, including nodules, morning stiffness, and fatigue. Most patients with amyloid arthropathy eventually are found to have multiple myeloma. The synovial fluid usually has a low white blood cell count, a good to fair mucin clot, a predominance of mononuclear cells, and no crystals. Studies of surgical specimens suggest a significant incidence of amyloid in cartilage, capsule, and synovium in osteoarthritis.

Respiratory system The nasal sinuses, larynx, and trachea may be involved by accumulations of amyloid which block the ducts, in the case of the sinuses, or the air passages. Amyloidosis of the lung involves the bronchi and alveolar septa diffusely. The lower respiratory tract is affected most frequently in primary amyloidosis and in the disease associated with dysproteinemia. Pulmonary symptoms attributable to amyloid are present in about 30 percent of these patients and in some are the most serious manifestations of the disease. In secondary amyloidosis, pulmonary disease is a frequent histopathologic accompaniment but seldom gives rise to clinically significant symptoms. Amyloid may also be localized in the bronchi or pulmonary parenchyma and may resemble a neoplasm. In these cases, local excision should be attempted and, when successful, may be followed by prolonged remissions.

Hematopoietic system Hematologic changes may include fibrinogenopenia, increased fibrinolysis, and selective deficiency of clotting factors. Deficient factor X seems to be due to nonspecific calcium-dependent binding to the polyanionic amyloid fibrils. Splenectomy in the patient with such a factor-X deficiency can relieve the deficiency and the associated bleeding disorder.

HEREDOFAMILIAL AMYLOIDOSIS There is no generally accepted nosology for the heredofamilial amyloid syndromes. Some reports emphasize the site of predominant organ involvement as neuropathic, nephropathic, or cardiopathic amyloidosis, while others stress the genetic aspects. To date, virtually all analyses of pedigrees have shown that, with one major exception, the mode of inheritance is autosomal dominant. The exception is amyloidosis of familial Mediterranean fever which is inherited as an autosomal recessive disorder (Chap. 236). Since there are no specific biochemical, hematologic, or immunologic tests that enable the differentiation of one type of amyloid from another, the specific and recognizable clinical patterns form the basis for classification. Table 66-2 proposes a tentative classification and is based largely on the major site of organ involvement, in addition to genetic data and ethnic background.

The heredofamilial amyloidoses include a group primarily involving the nervous system. Among these are lower limb neuropathy, first described in Portugal, which has a poor prognosis and is characterized by progressively severe neuropathy including marked autonomic nervous system involvement. This variety also has been described in Japan, Sweden, and in families of Greek and of Swedish origin in the United States. In some of these individuals, bilateral "scalloped" pupils are pathognomonic of the disease. The second type of neuropathy has been found in families of Swiss origin in Indiana and of German origin in Maryland. It is a milder disease and is often associated with a carpal tunnel syndrome and vitreous opacities. A more severe variety of generalized neuropathy associated with renal amyloidosis has been described in Iowa in a family of English-Irish-Scottish ancestry.

Several types of severe familial renal disease in association with amyloid have been described. Possibly the most remarkable is familial Mediterranean fever (FMF), a disorder subdivided into phenotype I, with irregularly occurring fever and abdominal, chest, or joint pain, preceding or accompanying renal amyloid, and phenotype II, in which amyloidosis is the first or only manifestation of the disease (Chap. 236). Colchicine treatment prevents attacks of FMF and appears to prevent subsequent deposition of amyloid as well. Sporadically, other hereditary forms of renal amyloidosis have been described, including the curious association of urticaria, deafness, and renal amyloid.

Severe familial amyloid heart disease has been described in a Danish family, and familial persistent atrial standstill with amyloid in a family of Mexican-American origin. Miscellaneous hereditary amyloid syndromes include hereditary multiple endocrine neoplasms type II (including medullary carcinoma of the thyroid with amyloid) as well as others listed in Table 66-2.

TABLE 66-2
Heredofamilial amyloidoses

1 Neuropathy
- *a* Lower limb (Portuguese, Japanese, Swedish, other)
- *b* Upper limb (Swiss-Indiana, German-Maryland)

2 Nephropathy
- *a* Familial Mediterranean fever
- *b* Fever and abdominal pain (Swedish, Sicilian)
- *c* Urticaria, deafness, and renal disease
- *d* Renal disease and hypertension

3 Cardiopathy
- *a* Progressive heart failure (Danish)
- *b* Persistent atrial standstill (Mexican-American)

4 Miscellaneous
- *a* Medullary carcinoma of the thyroid
- *b* Lattice corneal dystrophy and cranial neuropathy (Finland)
- *c* Cerebral hemorrhage (Iceland)

SOURCE: *Cohen AS, Rheumatology-Immunology: The Scientific Basis of Clinical Medicine, New York, Grune & Stratton, 1979, with permission.*

DIAGNOSIS The specific diagnosis of amyloidosis depends upon obtaining a tissue specimen by biopsy and the demonstration of amyloid with appropriate stains. First, of course, the disease must be suspected. When a patient with a chronic disorder predisposing to amyloid such as rheumatoid arthritis, tuberculosis, paraplegia, multiple myeloma, bronchiectasis, or leprosy develops hepatomegaly, splenomegaly, malabsorption, cardiac disease, or, most importantly, proteinuria, amyloid should come to mind. In addition, in any heredofamilial syndromes, especially those which have a dominant autosomal mode of inheritance and are characterized by peripheral neuropathy, nephropathy, or cardiopathy, the diagnosis of amyloid should be considered. Finally, primary systemic amyloid should be considered in any individual with a diffuse noninflammatory infiltrative disease involving either mesenchymal tissues—blood vessels, heart, gastrointestinal tract—or parenchymal tissues—kidney, liver, spleen, adrenal.

When the diagnosis is suspected, it is good practice to perform a rectal biopsy. If there is a specific reason for not carrying out this procedure, other sites including skin, gums, or the suspected organ—kidney, liver—may be biopsied. Aspiration of the abdominal subcutaneous fat pad has recently been shown to be a very high yield procedure. All tissues obtained must be stained with Congo red and examined in the polarizing microscope for green birefringence.

In order to establish the relationship of immunoglobulin-related amyloid to multiple myeloma, electrophoretic and immunoelectrophoretic studies on serum or urine should be performed when the biopsy reveals amyloid deposition. Most of these patients will have only relatively small paraprotein components and only a few will have frank multiple myeloma. The therapeutic implications of these findings are discussed in greater detail in Chap. 65.

PROGNOSIS AND TREATMENT The course of amyloidosis is difficult to document since dating the time of origin of the disease is rarely possible. When amyloidosis develops in patients with rheumatoid arthritis, it seldom becomes evident when the arthritis is less than 2 years in duration. The mean duration of arthritis before amyloidosis was detected was 16 years in one series. When amyloidosis develops in patients with multiple myeloma, manifestations leading to initial hospitalization are more apt to be related to amyloid disease than to myeloma. In these cases prognosis is very poor, and life expectancy is usually less than 6 months.

Instances have been reported of amyloidosis accompanying treatable infections, such as osteomyelitis, in which at least partial remission has occurred following treatment of the primary disease. There have been similar experiences following successful treatment of tuberculosis or drainage of chronic empyema. However, many such reports are not substantiated by biopsy proof of resorption.

Generalized amyloidosis is usually a slowly progressive disease and leads to death in several years, but it may have a better prognosis than was suspected in the past. The average survival in most large series is 1 to 4 years, but a number of individuals with amyloid have been followed 5 to 10 years and longer.

The major cause of death is renal failure. Sudden death, presumably due to arrhythmias, is also quite common. Occasionally, gastrointestinal hemorrhage, respiratory failure, intractable heart failure, and superimposed infections are the terminal events.

There is no specific therapy for any variety of amyloidosis. Rational therapy should be directed at (1) decreasing chronic antigenic stimuli that produce amyloid, (2) inhibition of the synthesis and extracellular deposition of amyloid fibrils, and (3) promoting lysis or mobilization of existing amyloid deposits.

A variety of agents have been used to treat amyloidosis. Proof of their efficacy is not available. The finding that a portion of the immunoglobulin light chain is incorporated in the amyloid of patients with primary amyloidosis and its presumed synthesis by plasma cells has led to the use of alkylating agents. However, these agents cause bone marrow depression, and there are reports of acute leukemia developing in patients receiving melphalan. Moreover, there is experimental evidence that immunosuppressive agents may enhance the deposition of preexisting amyloid. Hence, conservative and supportive measures provide the mainstay of management. It is important to provide these patients with a more optimistic outlook.

Two patients with severe renal amyloidosis and azotemia were subjected to bilateral nephrectomy and renal transplantation followed by immune therapy. One patient died of infection 5 months after surgery. The donor kidney showed no evidence of amyloidosis. The second patient is in clinical remission 7 years after receiving a transplanted kidney. Notwithstanding the hazards of operating upon patients with systemic amyloidosis who may have cardiac involvement, carefully selected azotemic patients could benefit from transplantation.

Colchicine has been shown to be effective in preventing acute attacks in patients with familial Mediterranean fever, and two groups of investigators independently have reported the inhibition of amyloid deposition in the mouse model by colchicine. It is conceivable, therefore, that colchicine is effective in blocking amyloid deposition. One large preliminary study has shown it to be effective in prolonging life in primary (AL) amyloidosis using a life-table survivorship analysis. However, the exact mechanism of its action is unknown, and no controlled human clinical study has been reported. The role of dimethylsulfoxide (DMSO) in the treatment of amyloid is also under investigation.

REFERENCES

COHEN AS: Amyloidosis. N Engl J Med 277:522, 1967

———: Diagnosis of amyloidosis, in *Laboratory Diagnostic Procedures in the Rheumatic Diseases*, 2d ed, AS Cohen (ed). Boston, Little, Brown, 1975, p 395

——— et al: Amyloidosis: Current trends in its investigation. Arthritis Rheum 21:153, 1978

FRANKLIN EC, ZUCKER-FRANKLIN D: Current concepts of amyloid. Adv Immunol 15:249, 1972

GLENNER GG et al: Amyloid fibril proteins: Proof of homology with immunoglobulin light chains. Science 172:1150, 1971

——— et al: *Amyloid and Amyloidosis*. Excerpta Medica, 1980

Diseases of immune-mediated injury

67 DISEASES OF IMMEDIATE TYPE HYPERSENSITIVITY

K. FRANK AUSTEN

The term *atopic allergy* implies a familial tendency to manifest alone or in combination such conditions as asthma, rhinitis, urticaria, and eczematous dermatitis (atopic dermatitis). However, individuals without an atopic background may also develop hypersensitivity reactions, particularly urticaria and anaphylaxis, associated with the same class of antibody found in atopic individuals. The designation *diseases of immediate type hypersensitivity* presents a more suitable framework than the broad term *allergy* or the restrictive definition of atopy.

The passively transferred activity in human serum belongs to a unique immunoglobulin class, IgE; a myeloma protein with skin-fixing capacity was independently recognized and shown to be of the same class. The fixation of IgE to human basophils has been demonstrated by radioautography and electron microscopy and to intraepithelial and perivenular mast cells in tonsils, adenoids, and nasal polyps of humans by immunofluorescence. IgE-dependent mediator generation and release also occur in the mast cells of human lung slices, nasal polyps, or skin and have been observed in those tissues most involved in diseases of immediate type hypersensitivity.

Studies with purified rat peritoneal mast cells have indicated that the IgE receptor is transmembrane-linked to adenylate cyclase and that stereospecific receptor perturbation generates second messenger cyclic 3′,5′-adenosine monophosphate (cyclic AMP). Cyclic AMP then activates cytoplasmic cyclic AMP–dependent protein kinase, which presumably acts to phosphorylate cell proteins, thereby continuing the biochemical sequence of the coupled activation-secretion response. A parallel membrane response to stereospecific IgE receptor perturbation involves the transmethylation of phospholipids, the formation of calcium ion channels with augmented ion influx, and the activation of phospholipases. Phospholipases then cleave membrane phospholipids to generate lysophospholipids or diacylglycerol which, being fusogenic, may facilitate the fusion of the secretory granule perigranular membrane with the cell membrane, a step which releases the membrane-free granule containing the preformed or primary mediators of mast cell effects. The arachidonic acid, generated simultaneously by phospholipase action, is processed oxidatively into secondary mediators of the prostaglandin and leukotriene classes. The secretory granule of the human mast cell has a crystalline structure, unlike mast cells of lower species, and IgE-dependent cell activation can be characterized morphologically by solubilization and swelling of the granule contents within the first minute of receptor perturbation; this reaction is followed by the ordering of intermediate filaments about the swollen granule, movement toward the cell surface, and fusion of the perigranular membrane with that of other granules and with the plasmalemma to form extracellular channels for mediator release while maintaining cell viability.

Because there is significant species variation in the nature and concentration of primary chemical mediators, the tabulation presented in Chap. 273 is limited to the human cell. The secretory granules of human and rat mast cells contain histamine; eosinophilactic acidic peptides; acid hydrolases such as β-hexosaminidase, β-glucuronidase, and arylsulfatase; neutral protease; and heparin proteoglycan. The heparin proteoglycan apparently serves to store, concentrate, and "transport" the solubilized granule complex so that primary mediators can dissociate into the extracellular channels by ion exchange. Mast cells appear to be the major source of tissue neutral protease with the rat supplying about 35 μg of chymase and carboxypeptidase A per 1 million cells and the human about 15 μg of tryptase per 1 million cells; in both cases the neutral proteases represent the major proteins not only of the secretory granules, but of the entire cell. The human mast cell differs from the rat's in having about one-tenth the histamine and heparin content, in lacking serotonin, and in containing a physicochemically and functionally different neutral protease.

Human mast cells that have been enzymatically dispersed from lung fragments and concentrated by differential centrifugation and purified rat peritoneal mast cells both respond to receptor perturbation by generation of prostaglandin D_2 (PGD_2) in preference to any other oxidative product of arachidonate. However, the remarkable vasoactive and spasmogenic potency of the leukotriene products in human skin and airways in vivo, compared to histamine, prostaglandins, and other mediators, indicates that this class of compounds represents an additional important group of mediators in immediate hypersensitivity reactions. The mast cell, bearing a specific recognition unit in the form of IgE, and positioned in tissues, has the capacity to respond to a foreign substance by eliciting a local increase in venular permeability and by initiating the influx of certain cell types from the marginated cell pool; this response allows plasma proteins such as antibody and complement and various phagocytic cells to be recruited to the reaction site without the necessity for extensive local tissue injury. On the other hand, an uncontrolled response could proceed from a physiologic local reaction to a self-perpetuating inflammatory state.

Consideration of the mechanism of immediate type hypersensitivity diseases in the human has focused largely on the IgE-dependent recognition of otherwise nontoxic substances. Support for this thesis has come from the finding that clinical atopic allergy is associated with elevated total levels of IgE and in some instances with an immune response that is specifically linked to the histocompatibility locus. Populations of allergic Caucasians have a significantly higher total serum level of IgE than nonallergic individuals, and highly atopic persons with asthma have significantly higher serum levels of IgE than those with fewer allergic manifestations. Further, IgE distribution in families is consistent with the dominant inheritance of the low IgE phenotype. As a result of the action of a single IgE regulator gene the majority of family members would have elevated IgE levels as a possible basis for their atopic state. The association between HLA histocompatibility type and the immediate hypersensitivity response has been noted in persons of the low IgE phenotype who were studied with highly purified allergens, generally of small size. Such presumptive evidence of immune response (Ir) genes by linkage disequilibrium, that is, the association of the hypersensitivity response with a particular histocompatibility haplotype, represents an additional element in the polygenic atopic allergic state. Nonetheless, all the studies taken together, both of families and of populations, seem to indicate that the genetically determined elevated IgE levels found in about three-fourths of atopic allergic subjects exert the predominant influence on most specific IgE responses. It is also likely that diseases of immediate type hypersensitivity may occur because of deficient intracellular controls of mediator generation or release, or both, or that the extracellular controls directed against mediator inactivation may be impaired.

ANAPHYLAXIS **Definition** The life-threatening anaphylactic response of a sensitized human appears within minutes after administration of specific antigen and is manifested by respiratory distress often followed by vascular collapse, or shock without antecedent respiratory difficulty. Cutaneous manifestations exemplified by pruritus and urticaria with or without angioedema are characteristic of such systemic anaphylactic reactions.

Predisposing factors and etiology There is no convincing evidence that age, sex, race, occupation, or geographic location predisposes a human to anaphylaxis except through exposure to some immunogen. According to some studies, but not others, atopy predisposes individuals to penicillin anaphylaxis.

The materials capable of eliciting the systemic anaphylactic reaction in the human include the following: heterologous proteins in the form of antiserum, hormones, enzymes, Hymenoptera venom, pollen extracts, and foods; polysaccharides such as iron dextran; and most commonly diagnostic agents and drugs such as antibiotics and even vitamins. The diagnostic and therapeutic agents are generally of low molecular weight and are considered to function as haptens which form immunogenic conjugates with host proteins. The conjugating hapten may be the parent compound, a nonenzymatically derived storage product, or a metabolite formed in the host.

Pathophysiology and manifestations Individuals differ in the time of appearance of perception of symptoms and signs, but the hallmark of the anaphylactic reaction is the onset of some manifestation within seconds to minutes after introduction of the antigen, generally by injection or less commonly by ingestion. There may be upper or lower airway obstruction or both. Laryngeal edema may be experienced as a "lump" in the throat, hoarseness, or stridor, while bronchial obstruction is associated with a feeling of tightness in the chest or audible wheezing. A particularly characteristic feature is the eruption of well-circumscribed, discrete cutaneous wheals with erythematous, raised, serpiginous borders and blanched centers. These urticarial eruptions are intensely pruritic and may be localized or distributed. They may coalesce to form giant hives, and seldom persist beyond 48 h. A localized, nonpitting, deeper edematous cutaneous process, angioedema, may also be present. It may be asymptomatic or cause a burning or stinging sensation.

In fatal cases with clinical bronchial obstruction, the lungs show marked hyperinflation on gross and microscopic examination. The microscopic findings in the bronchi, however, are limited to luminal secretions, peribronchial congestion, submucosal edema, and eosinophilic infiltration, and the acute emphysema is attributed to intractable bronchospasm which subsides with death. The angioedema resulting in death by mechanical obstruction occurs in the epiglottis and larynx, but the process is also evident in the hypopharynx and to some extent the trachea; on microscopic examination there is wide separation of the collagen fibers and the glandular elements; vascular congestion and eosinophilic infiltration are also present. Patients dying of vascular collapse without antecedent hypoxia from respiratory insufficiency have visceral congestion but no major shift in the distribution of blood volume. Whether the associated electrocardiographic abnormalities, with or without infarction, noted in such patients reflect a primary cardiac event or are secondary to a critical reduction in plasma volume has not been established.

The angioedematous and urticarial manifestations of the anaphylactic syndrome have been attributed to release of endogenous histamine. The role of leukotrienes in altering pulmonary mechanics by causing marked bronchiolar constriction awaits further definition. Vascular collapse without respiratory distress in response to experimental challenge with the sting of a hymenopteran was associated not only with marked and prolonged elevations in blood histamine but also with evidence of intravascular coagulation and kinin generation. Based upon the findings that patients with systemic mastocytosis and episodic hypotension, proceeding to vascular collapse in some instances, excrete large amounts of PGD_2 in addition to histamine, it may be that PGD_2 is also of importance in the hypotensive anaphylactic reactions.

Diagnosis The diagnosis of an anaphylactic reaction depends largely upon an accurate history revealing the onset of the appropriate symptoms and signs within minutes after the responsible material is encountered. When only a portion of the full syndrome is present, such as isolated urticaria, sudden bronchospasm in an asthmatic patient, or vascular collapse after intravenous administration of an agent it is difficult to exclude a nonimmunologic, toxicologic or idiosyncratic, response. For example, intravenous administration of a chemical mast-cell–degranulating agent may elicit generalized urticaria, angioedema, and a sensation of retrosternal oppression with or without clinically detectable bronchoconstriction or hypotension. Furthermore, nonsteroidal anti-inflammatory agents such as indomethacin, aminopyrine, mefenamic acid, and aspirin may precipitate a life-threatening episode of obstruction of upper or lower airways in asthmatic subjects which is clinically reminiscent of anaphylaxis but is not associated with a detectable IgE response. This syndrome may reflect a unique reactivity to an imbalance in the ratio of prostaglandin to leukotriene products when cyclooxygenase is inhibited.

The presence of a labile reagin (IgE) in the heart blood of a patient dying of systemic anaphylaxis has been demonstrated at postmortem by passive transfer of the serum intradermally into a normal recipient, followed in 24 h by antigen challenge into the same site, with subsequent development of a wheal and flare, the Prausnitz-Küstner reaction. Indeed, such a reagin can be transiently identified in the serum of most patients who develop systemic anaphylaxis to a variety of different agents. In order to avoid the hazards of transferring hepatitis to the recipient in the Prausnitz-Küstner reaction, it is preferable to employ the less sensitive monkey recipient or a human leukocyte suspension enriched with basophils for subsequent antigen challenge. It is presumed that the activity responsible for most cases of systemic anaphylaxis resides with the IgE class, since the Prausnitz-Küstner activity in the serums of patients with systemic reactions to Hymenoptera venom or human seminal plasma protein can be removed by IgE immunosorbent columns. Furthermore, radioimmunoassays have demonstrated specific IgE antibodies in patients with anaphylactic reactions to insulin and to parathormone, but such approaches require purified antigens. In the transfusion anaphylactic reaction which occurs in patients with IgA deficiency, the responsible specificity resides in IgG anti-IgA rather than in IgE; the mechanism of the reaction is presumed to be complement activation with secondary mast cell participation.

Treatment and prevention Early recognition of an anaphylactic reaction is mandatory, since death occurs within minutes to hours after the first symptoms. Mild symptoms such as pruritus and urticaria can be controlled by administration of 0.2 to 0.5 ml of 1:1000 epinephrine subcutaneously, with repeated doses as required at 3-min intervals for a severe reaction. If the antigenic material was injected into an extremity, the rate of absorption may be reduced by prompt application of a tourniquet proximal to the reaction site, administration of 0.2 ml of 1:1000 epinephrine into the site, and removal without compression of an insect stinger, if present. An intravenous infusion should be initiated to provide a route for administration of epinephrine, diluted 1:50,000, volume expanders, and vasopressive agents if intractable hypotension occurs. Epinephrine most likely acts to reverse the action of mediators on target tissues, and its early administration appears critical. When epinephrine fails to control the situation, hypoxia due to airway obstruction or related to a cardiac arrhythmia, or both, must be considered. Oxygen via a nasal catheter or intermittent positive pressure breathing of oxygen with 0.5 ml isoproterenol diluted 1:200 in saline may be helpful, but either endotracheal intubation or a tracheostomy is mandatory if progressive hypoxia exists. Ancillary agents such as the antihistamine diphenhydramine, 50 to 80 mg intramuscularly or intravenously, and aminophylline, 0.25 to 0.5 g intravenously, are appropriate for urticaria-angioedema and bronchospasm, respectively. Intravenous corticosteroids are not effective for the acute event but may be considered for persistent bronchospasm and hypotension.

Prevention of anaphylaxis must take into account the sensitivity of the recipient, the dose and character of the diagnostic or therapeutic agent, and the effect of the route of administration on the rate of absorption. If there is a definite history of a past anaphylactic reaction, even though mild, it is advisable to select another agent or procedure. A skin test should be performed before the administration of certain materials producing a high incidence of anaphylactic reactions, such as horse serum or allergenic extracts, or when the nature of the past adverse reaction is unknown. Since even a skin or conjunctival test can produce a serious reaction, a scratch test should precede these tests in a high-risk situation. With regard to penicillin, two-thirds of patients with a positive reaction history and positive intradermal skin tests to benzylpenicilloyl-polylysine (BPL) and/or the minor determinant mixture (MDM) of benzylpenicillin products experience allergic reactions with treatment, and these are almost uniformly of the anaphylactic type in those patients with minor determinant reactivity. Even patients without a history of previous clinical reactions have a 6 percent incidence of positive skin tests to the two test materials, and about 3 per 1000 with a negative history experience anaphylaxis with therapy with a mortality of about 1 per 100,000. The value of skin testing is both to permit therapy with the agent in question when the risk does not exist and to emphasize the hazards where the sensitivity is confirmed. In the event that an agent must be used despite a positive history, a positive skin test, or both, the following precautionary measures should be taken. An intravenous infusion should be started, with intubation equipment and a tracheostomy set at hand; the material should be given intradermally, then subcutaneously, and then intramuscularly in increasing doses at 20- to 30-min intervals so that the initial dose by the next route does not exceed the final dose by the previous route. It is difficult to be certain that the mediator-containing cells have been exhausted, and therapeutic use of the agent may be accompanied by untoward consequences. It may be critical to give the therapeutic agent at regular intervals to prevent the reestablishment of a sensitized cell pool of large size. A different form of protection involves the development of blocking antibody of the IgG class which is protective against Hymenoptera venom–induced anaphylaxis by interacting with antigen so that less reaches the sensitized tissue mast cells; to be effective this immunotherapy requires the use of specific or cross reacting Hymenoptera venom rather than whole insect body extracts.

URTICARIA AND ANGIOEDEMA Definition Urticaria and angioedema may appear separately or together as cutaneous manifestations of localized nonpitting edema; a similar process may occur at mucosal surfaces of the upper respiratory or gastrointestinal tract. *Urticaria* involves only the superficial portion of the dermis presenting as well-circumscribed wheals with erythematous raised serpiginous borders with blanched centers which may coalesce to become giant wheals. *Angioedema* is a well-demarcated localized edema involving the deeper layers of the skin including the subcutaneous tissue. Recurrent episodes of urticaria and/or angioedema of less than 6 weeks duration are considered acute, while attacks persisting beyond this period are designated chronic.

Predisposing factors and etiology The occurrence of urticaria and angioedema is probably more frequent than usually described because of the evanescent, self-limited nature of such eruptions, which seldom require medical attention when limited to the skin. Although persons in any age group may experience acute or chronic urticaria and/or angioedema, these lesions increase in frequency after adolescence, with the highest incidence occurring in persons in the third decade of life; indeed, one survey of college students indicated that some 15 to 20 percent had experienced a pruritic wheal reaction.

The classification of urticaria/angioedema presented in Table 67-1 focuses on the different mechanisms for eliciting clinical disease. Only the IgE-dependent and the IgG-mediated reactions in IgA-deficient persons should be considered immediate hypersensitivity. However, the other mechanisms are important for differential diagnosis, and most cases of chronic urticaria are idiopathic. The appearance of urticaria and angioedema in atopic persons in the absence of a specific exposure is attributed to the atopic diathesis and implies an IgE mechanism. Urticaria and/or angioedema occurring during the appropriate season in patients with seasonal respiratory allergy or as a result of exposure to animals or molds is attributed to inhalation of pollens, animal dander, and mold spores, respectively. However, urticaria and angioedema secondary to inhalation are relatively uncommon compared with ingestion

TABLE 67-1
Classification of urticaria with angioedema

1 IgE-dependent
- *a* Atopic diathesis
- *b* Specific antigen sensitivity (pollens, foods, drugs, fungi, molds, Hymenoptera venom, helminths)
- *c* Physical: dermographism; cold; light; cholinergic; vibratory

2 Complement-mediated urticaria
- *a* Hereditary angioedema
- *b* Acquired angioedema with lymphoproliferative disorders
- *c* Necrotizing vasculitis
- *d* Serum sickness
- *e* Reactions to blood products

3 Nonimmunologic urticaria
- *a* Direct mast-cell–releasing agents: opiates; antibiotics; curare, D-tubocurarine; radiocontrast media
- *b* Agents which presumably alter arachidonic acid metabolism: aspirin and nonsteroidal anti-inflammatory agents; azo dyes and benzoates

4 Idiopathic urticaria

of fresh fruits, shellfish, chocolate, nuts, tomatoes, and various drugs, including penicillin-contaminated milk products, which may elicit not only the anaphylactic syndrome with prominent gastrointestinal complaints but also chronic urticaria. Additional etiologies include physical stimuli such as cold, solar rays, exercise, and mechanical irritation (dermographism). Angioedema without urticaria occurs with $C\bar{1}$ inhibitor ($C\bar{1}$INH) deficiency that can be inborn as an autosomal dominant characteristic or can be acquired in association with lymphoproliferative disorders. The urticaria and angioedema associated with classical serum sickness or with idiopathic cutaneous necrotizing angiitis is believed to be an immune-complex disease when hypocomplementemia is a concomitant. The idiosyncratic drug reactions to mast cell granule-releasing agents and to nonsteroidal anti-inflammatory drugs can be systemic, resembling anaphylaxis, or limited to cutaneous sites.

Pathophysiology and manifestations Urticarial eruptions are distinctly pruritic, involve any area of the body from the scalp to the soles of the feet, and appear in crops of 24- to 72-h duration with old lesions fading as new ones appear. The most common sites are the extremities, external genitalia, and face, particularly the region of the eyes and lips. Although self-limited in duration, angioedema of the upper respiratory tract may be life-threatening due to laryngeal obstruction, while gastrointestinal involvement may present with abdominal colic, with or without nausea and vomiting, and may precipitate unnecessary surgical intervention. No residual discoloration occurs with either urticaria or angioedema unless there is an underlying process leading to superimposed extravasation of erythrocytes.

The pathology of urticaria and angioedema is usually characterized by massive edema of the dermis in urticaria, and the subcutaneous tissue as well as dermis in angioedema. Collagen bundles in affected areas are widely separated, and the venules are sometimes dilated. The perivenular infiltrate may consist of lymphocytes, eosinophils, and neutrophils that are present in varying combination and number throughout the dermis. Allergen-induced wheal and flare reactions are characterized by mast-cell degranulation and an accumulation of eosinophils over hours to days. The elicitation of a wheal and flare response upon injection of the relevant allergen into a patient with urticaria and/or angioedema, or into a site in a normal recipient prepared with serum from the patient, the Prausnitz-Küstner reaction, indicates an IgE-dependent, mast-cell–mediated reaction.

Perhaps the best-studied example of mast-cell–mediated urticaria and angioedema is *cold urticaria.* Acquired cold urticaria is a disorder in which patients exposed to cold experience an urticarial eruption that may evolve into angioedema and be associated with syncope. Cryoglobulins, cryofibrinogens, cold agglutinins, or hemolysins may be recognized, but not in the majority of patients. The finding in a number of patients of a serum factor, characterized as being of the IgE class, that is capable of transferring the cold urticaria reaction to a skin site of a normal recipient has focused attention upon the mast cell in this condition. Immersion of an extremity in an ice bath precipitates angioedema of the distal portion with urticaria at the air interface within minutes of the challenge. Histologic studies reveal marked mast-cell degranulation with associated edema of the dermis and subcutaneous tissues. The venous effluent of the cold-challenged and angioedematous extremity reveals a marked rise in plasma content of histamine, low-molecular-weight eosinophilotactic activity, and high-molecular-weight neutrophil chemotactic activity which are presumably of mast-cell origin, whereas the venous effluent of the contralateral normal extremity contains none of these mediators.

Diagnosis The rapid onset and self-limited nature of urticarial and angioedematous eruptions are distinguishing features. Additional characteristics are the occurrence of the urticarial crops in various stages of evolution and the asymmetric distribution of the angioedema. Urticarial and/or angioedema involving IgE-dependent mechanisms are often appreciated by historical considerations implicating specific allergens, by seasonal incidence, by exposure to certain environments, or by physical stimuli such as cold, exercise, sunlight (solar urticaria), or trauma (dermographism). Direct reproduction of the lesion with physical stimuli is particularly valuable because it so often establishes the cause of the lesion. The diagnosis can be confirmed by careful testing with the putative foreign substance to determine if a local wheal and flare results, and by passive transfer of such a reaction with serum of the patient to a skin site in a normal recipient, the Prausnitz-Küstner phenomenon. Passive transfer to the skin of a nonhuman primate or in vitro to human basophils may also be attempted. IgE-mediated urticaria and/or angioedema may or may not be associated with an elevation of total IgE or with peripheral eosinophilia. Fever, leukocytosis, or an elevated sedimentation rate are characteristically absent.

The classification of urticarial and angioedematous states noted in Table 67-1 in terms of possible mechanisms necessarily includes some differential diagnostic points. Hypocomplementemia is not observed in IgE-mediated mast-cell disease and can reflect either an acquired abnormality generally attributed to the formation of immune complexes or a genetic deficiency of $C\bar{1}$INH. Chronic recurrent urticaria, generally in females, associated with arthralgias, an elevated sedimentation rate, and normo- or hypocomplementemia suggests an underlying cutaneous necrotizing angiitis. Confirmation depends upon a biopsy which reveals cellular infiltration, nuclear debris, and fibrinoid necrosis of the venules.

Hereditary angioedema is an autosomal dominant state associated with the absence of functional $C\bar{1}$INH. The diagnosis is suggested not only by family history but also by the lack of urticarial lesions, the prominence of recurrent gastrointestinal attacks of colic, and episodes of laryngeal edema. Laboratory diagnosis depends upon demonstrating the antigenic lack of $C\bar{1}$INH in most kindreds, but some kindreds have an antigenically intact nonfunctional protein and require a functional assay to establish the diagnosis. The natural substrates of uninhibited $C\bar{1}$, C4, and C2 are chronically depleted but fall further during attacks due to the activation of additional C1 to $C\bar{1}$. The pathogenetic peptide is cleaved from the C2 substrate and then fully activated by the additional proteolysis of plasmin. An acquired form of $C\bar{1}$INH deficiency, associated with lymphoproliferative disorders, has the same clinical manifestations and differs only in the lack of a familial element and in the reduction of C1/C1 as well as $C\bar{1}$INH, C4, and C2.

Urticaria and angioedema must be differentiated from contact sensitivity, an acute vesicular eruption that progresses to chronic thickening of the skin with continued allergenic exposure. They must also be differentiated from atopic dermatitis, a condition that may present as erythema, edema, papules, vesiculation, and oozing proceeding to a subacute and chronic stage in which vesiculation is less marked or absent, and in which scaling, fissuring, and lichenification predominate in a distribution that characteristically involves the flexor surfaces.

Prevention and treatment Identification of the etiologic factor(s) and their elimination provide the most satisfactory therapeutic program; this approach is feasible to varying degrees with IgE-mediated reactions to allergens or physical stimuli. Topically applied steroids are of no benefit in the management of urticaria and/or angioedema, and while systemic steroids have no general value, they are helpful in an occasional patient with necrotizing cutaneous angiitis, pressure urticaria, or even ordinary urticaria and angioedema. Antihistamines and sympathomimetic agents often provide symptomatic relief; cyproheptadine, hydroxyzine, and similar drugs are held to be even more beneficial. The therapy of $C\bar{1}INH$ deficiency has been simplified by the finding that attenuated androgens correct the biochemical defect and afford prophylactic protection. Since the affected individuals are heterozygous, with the depletion of $C\bar{1}INH$ being due to a combination of deficient synthesis and excessive utilization of the normal gene product, the efficacy of the attenuated androgens is attributed to production by the normal gene of an amount of functional $C\bar{1}INH$ sufficient to contain the spontaneous activation of C1 to $C\bar{1}$. Since the use of such agents for children and pregnant women is not yet accepted, the antifibrinolytic agent ε-aminocaproic acid may be used occasionally to control spontaneous attacks or for preoperative prophylaxis in some patients.

ALLERGIC RHINITIS

Definition Allergic rhinitis is characterized by sneezing, rhinorrhea, obstruction of the nasal passages, conjunctival and pharyngeal itching, and lacrimation. Although commonly seasonal because of its relation to airborne pollens, other patterns and etiologies occur. The use of the term "hay fever" to describe seasonal allergic rhinitis is a common convention but is literally inappropriate because the symptom complex is neither produced by hay nor associated with fever.

Predisposing factors and etiology Allergic rhinitis generally presents in atopic individuals, that is, in persons with a family history of a similar or related symptom complex and a personal history of collateral allergy expressed as eczematous dermatitis, urticaria, and/or asthma (see Chap. 273). Symptoms generally appear before the fourth decade of life and tend to diminish gradually with aging, although complete spontaneous remissions are uncommon. A relatively small number of weeds which depend upon wind rather than insects for cross-pollination, as well as certain grasses and trees, produce sufficient quantities of pollen suitable for wide distribution by air currents to elicit seasonal allergic rhinitis. The dates of pollination of these species generally vary little from year to year in a particular locale but may be quite different in another climate. Molds, which are widespread in nature because they occur in soil or decaying organic matter, may propagate spores in a pattern dependent upon climatic conditions. Perennial allergic rhinitis occurs in response to allergens that are present throughout the year such as in desquamating epithelium in animal dander, the processed materials or chemicals utilized in an industrial setting, or the dust accumulating at work or at home. Dust has a diverse content including mites, and many patients with perennial rhinitis are sensitive only to house dust. Moreover, in many patients with perennial rhinitis, no clear-cut allergen can be demonstrated. The ability of allergens to cause rhinitis rather than lower respiratory symptoms may be attributed to their size, 10 to 100 μm, and retention within the nose. However, even when the allergen penetrates to the lower respiratory tract, whether it elicits a bronchoconstrictor response resulting in mediator release depends on the presence of chronically hyperirritable airways.

Pathophysiology and manifestations Episodic rhinorrhea, sneezing, and obstruction of the nasal passages with lacrimation and pruritus of the conjunctiva, nasal mucosa, and oropharynx are the hallmarks of allergic rhinitis. The nasal mucosa is pale and boggy, but the nares are not reddened or excoriated. The conjunctiva may be congested and edematous; the pharynx is generally unremarkable but may appear injected. Swelling of the turbinates and mucous membranes with obstruction of the sinus ostia and eustachian tubes precipitates secondary infections of the sinuses and middle ear, respectively, commonly in perennial but rarely in seasonal disease. Nasal polyps often arise concurrently with edema and/or infection within the sinuses and increase obstructive symptoms.

The nose presents a large mucosal surface area through the folds of the turbinates and serves to adjust the temperature and moisture content of inhaled air and to filter out particulate materials. The convoluted nasal passages readily filter out particles above 10 μm in size by impingement in a mucous blanket at bends in their course; ciliary action then moves the entrapped particles toward the pharynx. Entrapment of pollen and digestion of the outer coat by mucosal enzymes such as lysozymes release protein allergens generally of 10,000 to 40,000 molecular weight. Although the initial interaction occurs between the allergen and intraepithelial mast cells sensitized with specific IgE, the bulk of the mast cells are located beneath the mucosal surface and are recruited secondarily. During the symptomatic season when the mucosa are already swollen and hyperemic, there is enhanced adverse reactivity to the seasonal pollen as well as to antigenically unrelated pollens for which there is underlying hypersensitivity. This priming effect is attributed to improved penetration of the allergens to the deeper perivenular mast cells. Biopsy specimens of nasal mucosa during an episodic allergic reaction show profound submucosal edema with infiltration predominantly by eosinophils, although some neutrophil polymorphonuclear leukocytes are present. Polyps, a feature in perennial rhinitis, are mucosal protrusions containing chiefly edema fluid with variable degrees of eosinophilic infiltration.

The mucosal surface fluid contains not only IgA that is present preferentially because of its secretory piece, but also IgE, which apparently arrives by diffusion from plasma cells distributed in proximity to mucosal surfaces. IgE fixes to mucosal and submucosal mast cells, and the intensity of the clinical response to inhaled allergens is quantitatively related to the naturally occurring or experimentally defined pollen dose. Specific IgE is distributed not only to tissue mast cells but also to circulating basophilic leukocytes; patients with more severe clinical disease have basophils which release histamine in response to lesser concentrations of allergen in vitro than do cells from patients with milder disease. Human nasal polyps from ragweed-sensitive patients release histamine, eosinophilotactic peptides, and spasmogenic leukotrienes upon challenge with ragweed allergen in vitro. Polyps from nonallergic patients with cystic fibrosis or chronic sinusitis, passively sensitized by interaction with serum of a ragweed-sensitive patient, release the same mediators upon challenge with the allergen. Thus, the mast cells of nasal polyp tissue, and presumably of the nasal mucosa and submucosa, generate and release mediators through IgE-dependent reactions which are capable of producing tissue edema and eosinophilic infiltration.

Diagnosis The diagnosis of seasonal allergic rhinitis depends largely upon an accurate history of occurrence coincident with the pollination of the offending weeds, grasses, or trees. The continuous character of perennial allergic rhinitis due to contamination of the home or place of work makes historical analysis difficult, but there may be a variability in symptoms that can be related to animal exposure or work habits. Patients with perennial rhinitis commonly develop the problem in adult life, are more often women than men, and manifest nasal polyps and thickening of the sinus membranes by x-ray. The term *vasomotor rhinitis* designates a symptom complex resembling perennial allergic rhinitis without an established allergic basis. Other entities to be excluded are exposure to irritants, upper respiratory infection, pregnancy with prominent nasal mucosal edema, prolonged topical use of alpha-adrenergic agents in the form of nose drops, and the use of certain therapeutic agents such as rauwolfia. Nasal polyps are a characteristic of perennial allergic rhinitis and are often associated with sinus infection.

The nasal secretions of allergic patients are rich in eosinophils, and peripheral eosinophilia with elevations in relation to clinical exacerbations is a common feature. Local or systemic neutrophilia implies infection. Total serum IgE is frequently elevated, but the demonstration of immunologic specificity for IgE is critical to an etiologic diagnosis. Some normal individuals will exhibit a wheal and flare skin response to intracutaneous inoculation of high concentrations of common airborne allergens. The diagnosis rests not only on the skin test alone, but also on the correlation of the clinical history with skin reactivity to concentrations of allergen selected by controlled testing. This provides the best balance of selectivity with specificity. Scratch tests with food allergens are unreliable, while intracutaneous testing may be dangerous, and elimination diets are the best approach to the diagnosis. Regardless of method of testing, food allergy is uncommon as a significant cause of allergic rhinitis.

Although standard radioimmunodiffusion techniques can be used to screen for patients with markedly elevated levels of IgE, their sensitivity of less than 1000 ng/ml is insufficient to detect the elevations in most atopic allergic patients. A commonly employed technique, sensitive to about 50 ng/ml, is known as the competitive radioimmunosorbent test (RIST). In this procedure, the IgE of the serum competes with radiolabeled IgE for solid-phase-bound anti-IgE; the displacement of radiolabeled IgE is compared to a standard curve to yield the IgE concentration of the serum. Other assays, such as the noncompetitive RIST, in which the anti-IgE immunosorbent is exposed to a series of standard IgE preparations before introducing the unknown, and double antibody radioimmunoprecipitin test (RIP), have greater sensitivity and reproducibility, respectively, and, like the competitive RIST, establish a normal geometric mean serum IgE for nonallergic Caucasians of less than 120 ng/ml. Even more useful is the measurement of specific anti-IgE in serum by its binding to a solid-phase allergen and quantitation by the subsequent uptake of radiolabeled anti-IgE. This radioallergosorbent technique (RAST) correlates satisfactorily with the bioassay of specific IgE by skin test or histamine release from peripheral blood leukocytes and is convenient for the patients; however, it requires defined allergens and full standardization. Further, neither the immunochemical nor bioassay detection of a previous immune response to a foreign material mandates a therapeutic intervention, unless there is relevant concomitant evidence of a significant clinical problem.

Prevention and treatment Avoidance of exposure to the offending allergen is the most effective means of controlling allergic diseases; removal of pets from the home to avoid animal danders, utilization of air filtration devices to minimize the concentrations of airborne pollens, travel to nonpollinating areas during the critical periods, and even a change of domicile to eliminate a mold spore problem may be necessary. *Immunotherapy,* often termed *hyposensitization,* consists of repeated subcutaneous injections of gradually increasing concentrations of the allergen(s) considered to be specifically responsible for the symptom complex. Controlled studies in ragweed and grass allergic rhinitis have established that patients are partially relieved of their symptoms by such treatments applied over a period of years. Improvement appears to be dose-related, and the end point is based either on severe adverse local or systemic reactions to the allergen injection or on satisfactory relief of symptoms. The immunologic characteristics of a response include a rise in antibodies of the IgG class, a small increase in specific IgE early in the treatment course followed by a plateau or decline, and a decline in the percentage of histamine released from peripheral blood basophilic leukocytes challenged with a fixed concentration of the allergen. The antibodies of the IgG class might well reduce or neutralize the quantity of allergen available for interaction with the tissue mast cells but, more importantly, could modify the seasonal booster response in specific IgE synthesis. None of the individual parameters of the response to immunotherapy correlates well with the assessments of clinical efficacy, suggesting that benefit is derived from a complex of effects. Immunotherapy should be reserved for clearly documented seasonal diseases that cannot be managed with drugs because of their side effects.

Management with pharmacologic agents offers a diverse approach. Antihistamines are the only specific end-organ antagonists available for control of a mast-cell–derived reaction and are limited to competition with but one mediator. Nonetheless, antihistamines are very effective for some patients, and the side effects such as drowsiness and gastrointestinal distress, which limit the dosage of a particular preparation, can sometimes be circumvented by use of an agent of different structure. An orally active agent with alpha-adrenergic activity is often employed for its decongestant effects and to partially counteract the drowsiness produced by antihistamines. Topical administration of alpha-adrenergic agents may be helpful but has the immediate disadvantage of rebound vasodilatation and prolonged usage may produce a chronic rhinitis. The topically active steroids of the beclamethasone class ameliorate symptoms of both seasonal and perennial rhinitis without detectable adrenal suppression and represent a major advance in therapy. Cromolyn sodium inhaled nasally has also given encouraging prophylactic results and is of particular merit because it acts to prevent mast-cell activation.

REFERENCES

AUSTEN KF: Biologic implications of the structural and functional characteristics of the chemical mediators of immediate-type hypersensitivity. The Harvey Lectures, Series 73, 1977–1978, p 93

CAULFIELD JP et al: Secretion in dissociated human pulmonary mast cells. Evidence for solubilization of granule contents before discharge. J Cell Biol 85:299, 1980

GREEN GR et al: Evaluation of penicillin hypersensitivity: Value of clinical history and skin testing with penicilloyl-polylysine and penicillin G. J Allerg Clin Immunol 60:339, 1977

KALINER M et al: Immunologic release of chemical mediators from human nasal polyps. N Engl J Med 289:277, 1973

LEWIS RA, AUSTEN KF: Mediation of local homeostasis and inflammation by leukotrienes and other mast cell–dependent compounds. Nature 292:103, 1981

LICHTENSTEIN LM, NORMAN PS: Allergic rhinitis, in *Immunological Diseases,* 3d ed, M Samter (ed). Boston, Little, Brown, 1978, p 832

MARSH DG et al: Genetics of the human immune response to allergens. J Allerg Clin Immunol 65:322, 1980

MARX JL: The leukotrienes in allergy and inflammation. Science 215:1380, 1982

SOTER NA et al: Urticaria and arthralgias as manifestations of necrotizing angiitis (vasculitis). J Invest Dermatol 63:485, 1974

———: Release of mast cell mediators and alterations in lung function in patients with cholinergic urticaria. N Engl J Med 302:604, 1980

68
IMMUNE-COMPLEX DISEASES

BRUCE C. GILLILAND
MART MANNIK

DEFINITION Immune-complex diseases are characterized by the presence of antigen-antibody complexes in vascular and glomerular basement membranes in the circulation and in other body fluid compartments. Immune complexes in tissues initiate immunologically mediated inflammation with resultant tissue damage. Immune-complex diseases have a common pathogenic mechanism, but the etiology is variable since the sources of antigens differ from disease to disease. The immune-complex diseases constitute a clinical syndrome which includes glomerulonephritis, arthritis, skin eruptions, pericarditis, pleuritis, and vasculitis at diverse sites.

The presence of immune-complex deposits in tissues can result by two mechanisms. The pathogenetic immune complexes are either deposited from the circulation or they are formed locally. In local formation of immune complexes the antigen or antigens are part of the involved organ, or unrelated antigens are selectively deposited in the organ. Subsequently, antibodies from the circulation react with these antigens to form immune complexes. Characteristically, in this mechanism one organ system is involved that contains the structural or selectively deposited antigen, and immune complexes are not present in circulation. In contrast, when immune complexes are present in circulation, usually more than one organ is involved because these materials are deposited from the circulation.

PATHOGENESIS Upon the first exposure to a foreign substance, the host develops an antibody response after a week or 10 days. The synthesized antibodies result in formation of antigen-antibody complexes, which facilitate removal of the antigen. Normally, the majority of circulating immune complexes are removed by cells in the reticuloendothelial system (also called the mononuclear phagocyte system). However, when complexes are deposited at other sites, such as along vascular and glomerular basement membranes, inflammation may develop at these sites, leading to the signs and symptoms of immune-complex disease.

The concepts of immune-complex disease in humans have evolved largely through the study of animal models, including both spontaneous and experimentally induced disease. Acute serum sickness can be induced in experimental animals by injection of a foreign protein such as bovine serum albumin. Antigen disappears from the circulation in three phases: the first represents equilibration of the antigen between the intra- and extravascular compartments; the second is produced by catabolism of the antigen; the third involves the immune clearance of the antigen due to newly made specific antibodies. During the initial part of the immune-clearance phase, small circulating immune complexes are formed. As more antibody is synthesized, the lattice structure of the immune complexes increases until the complexes reach a critical lattice structure. Then the complexes are rapidly removed from the circulation by the reticuloendothelial system in the liver and elsewhere. Once the circulating immune complexes reach a critical size, the complement system is activated. This is manifested by a decrease in total hemolytic complement or individual complement components. This event does not ensue if the complexes are formed by antibodies incapable of complement activation. The overwhelming bulk of the antigen in the form of immune complexes is removed from the circulation by the reticuloendothelial system. For example, in experimental animals less than 1 percent of the circulating immune complexes becomes entrapped in the kidneys as determined in chronic serum sickness models or by intravenous injection of preformed immune complexes. Yet these small quantities of immune complexes suffice to cause glomerulonephritis. In rabbits, the release of vasoactive amines facilitates the deposition of immune complexes in the glomeruli, but in humans this mechanism has not been demonstrated. Coincident with circulating immune complexes and complement utilization, clinical abnormalities develop in experimental animals (Fig. 68-1). These abnormalities include glomerulonephritis, vasculitis, arthritis, skin eruptions, pleuritis, and pericarditis. Once the antigen is completely cleared, the complement levels return to normal, and gradually the lesions in target organs subside. Acute serum sickness is a limited disease and progresses only as long as antigen persists in the recipient.

In experimental animals the acute serum sickness model can be converted to a chronic serum sickness or immune-complex disease model by repeated administration of antigen. The development of clinical abnormalities in such models can be achieved by frequent (daily or several times a week) administration of an appropriate dose of antigen. In such a model, renal failure due to chronic proliferative glomerulonephritis can be achieved. These animals also develop vasculitis in other locations, and extensive antigen, antibody, and C3 deposits are identifiable.

A chronic immune-complex disease can develop spontaneously in animals with viral or other microbial infection that provides a continued source of antigen for immune-complex formation. Glomerulonephritis develops in mice with persistent lymphocytic choriomeningitis virus, Maloney sarcoma virus, or lactic dehydrogenase virus infection and in Aleutian disease of mink. Immune complexes consisting of antivirus antibody, virus antigen, and complement components (mainly C3) can be identified in the kidney and serum of these animals. Immune-complex nephritis resembling closely that of systemic lupus erythematosus occurs in the female F_1 hybrid of New Zealand black and New Zealand white mice and in certain other strains of mice (see Chap. 70).

Immune-complex–induced glomerulonephritis in experimental animals has immune deposits in the subendothelial

FIGURE 68-1
Schematic presentation of events in experimental acute serum sickness. In this experimental animal, antibody production began on the eighth day with the appearance of circulating immune complexes and subsequent decrease in serum complement (C). Vasculitis, glomerulonephritis, and arthritis develop after deposition of immune complexes. With the clearance of immune complexes by the reticuloendothelial system, the pathogenic process ceases, free antibody can be detected, and the inflammatory events run their course and gradually abate.

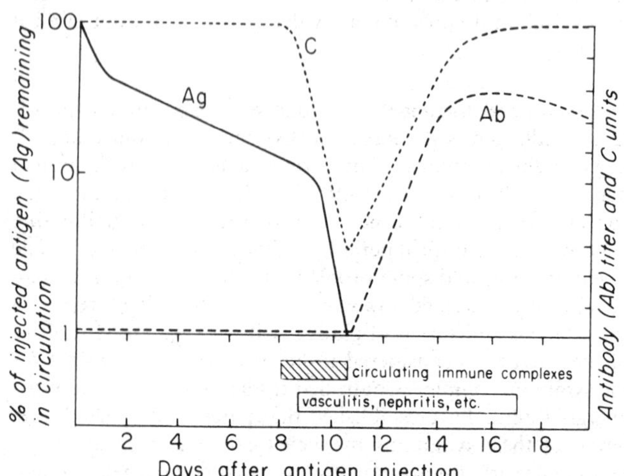

area, mesangial matrix, or subepithelial area. These immune complexes were thought to be deposited from the circulation. Recent studies, however, have indicated that circulating immune complexes are deposited in the subendothelial and mesangial areas and do not penetrate the glomerular basement membrane. Furthermore, only large-latticed immune complexes, containing more than two antibody molecules of the immunoglobulin G class, are deposited in these areas and immune complexes with smaller lattices are not deposited in glomeruli. The subepithelial deposits, as seen in membranous glomerulonephritis, are thought to develop by local immune-complex formation. The involved antigens first pass through the glomerular basement membrane and are then followed by antibodies. The sequential presence of free antigen and free antibody may contribute to this process. In addition, certain antigens may bind to the glomerular basement membrane or be deposited in the mesangial matrix, and if antibodies are present in the circulation, immune complexes are formed locally. These observations indicate that all glomerular immune complexes in human diseases may not be derived from the circulation. Similar possibilities in other organs have not been adequately investigated in experimental animals.

A localized experimental immune-complex disease can be generated by repeated injection of a foreign substance into the same location of an immunized animal. For example, rabbits immunized with a foreign protein, such as bovine serum albumin, develop arthritis when the same protein is injected into the joint cavity. Intense inflammation can be induced in a similar manner in the pericardial and pleural cavities. Again, the local immunologically induced inflammation progresses as long as antigen is present. The synovitis of rheumatoid arthritis appears to be a local immune-complex disease of joints.

Immune complexes activate complement components, leading to formation of vasoactive peptides and chemotactic factors. Neutrophils accumulate in the involved area and phagocytize the immune complexes, resulting in release of lysosomal enzymes and subsequent damage to structural components of tissue. Later in the course of the lesions monocytes, T cells, and B cells accumulate because of specific chemotactic factors. Newly arrived B cells evolve to plasma cells that synthesize antibodies to the antigen present at the site. For example, if bovine serum albumin is used to induce arthritis in the rabbit, the bulk of plasma cells in the synovium of this animal will synthesize antibodies to bovine serum albumin.

PATHOLOGY Light microscopy of the renal lesion of acute serum sickness or immune-complex disease reveals swelling of endothelial cells and the presence of a few leukocytes. In the chronic form, thickening of the basement membrane is accompanied by proliferation and swelling of endothelial cells. Epithelial cells proliferate to form crescents with eventual obliteration of Bowman's space. The renal lesions may be classified as showing mesangioproliferative, focal proliferative, diffuse proliferative, or membranous glomerular involvement, depending on the extent of the disease and the characteristics of the inflammatory response. Immunofluorescence studies of the kidney in both the acute and chronic forms of disease reveal granular deposits of immunoglobulin and complement (C3) in the mesangial matrix or along the glomerular basement membrane. Transmission electron microscopy shows electron-dense deposits in the mesangial matrix, the subendothelial space, the subepithelial space, and the glomerular basement membrane.

This history of the vascular lesion initially shows accumulation of neutrophils and proliferation of endothelial cells. This is followed by disruption of the internal elastic lamina and fibrinoid necrosis of the vessel wall. Mononuclear cells appear later. The vasculitis may vary from an intense inflammatory lesion consisting mainly of polymorphonuclear cells to one in which only perivascular cuffing with mononuclear cells is seen at the time of biopsy. If the examination is made early in the course, granular deposits of immunoglobulin and complement may be identified by immunofluorescence. However, within hours, these immune deposits are removed by the inflammatory response.

ETIOLOGY For any given immune-complex disease the etiology depends on the nature and source of the antigens that form immune complexes as well as the immunogens that incite the immune response. In most immune-complex diseases the antigen and immunogen are the same substance, but in certain autoimmune diseases they may differ. Thus, in immune complex diseases the etiologic factors may be drugs, microorganisms, tumors, or the host's own tissues. If strict criteria are employed, the etiology of an immune-complex disease is defined when the specific antigens and antibodies causing the tissue inflammation are identified. This has been achieved largely by elution of antigens and antibodies from the target tissues or by immunofluorescent microscopy using specific antigens and antibodies. The list of established immune-complex diseases has grown steadily (Table 68-1). A number of diseases, particularly glomerulonephritis and vasculitis, have all the hallmarks of immune-complex diseases in terms of the clinical pattern of the disorder and the deposition of immunoglobulins at sites of inflammation, but the involved antigens are not defined—therefore, these disorders are often listed as "probable" immune-complex diseases.

Drugs produce immune-complex disease either by acting as immunogens or by inducing synthesis of autoantibodies by an unknown mechanism. Numerous drugs and foreign proteins (e.g., penicillins, sulfonamides, horse antitoxin to tetanus, and horse antihuman lymphocyte serum) are potentially immunogenic and cause immune-complex disease. Binding of a drug or its metabolite to a serum protein may be necessary for its immunogenicity.

A form of immune-complex disease restricted to the destruction of platelets or red blood cells is occasionally observed after administration of stibophen, phenacetin, quinine, or quinidine. Antibodies made in response to one of these drugs combine with the drug to form immune complexes. These complexes are absorbed to the blood cell surface and activate complement, leading to either hemolytic anemia or thrombocytopenia. Some drug-induced neutropenias may also develop by this mechanism.

TABLE 68-1
Immune-complex diseases in humans

1 Administered (exogenous) antigens
- *a* Serum sickness (animal antitoxins, antiserums, hormones, drugs)
- *b* Drug-induced hemolytic anemia and thrombocytopenia (stibophen, quinine, quinidine, phenacetin)
- *c* Hypersensitivity pneumonitis (e.g., farmer's lung)

2 Microbial antigens
- *a* Poststreptococcal glomerulonephritis
- *b* Glomerulonephritis of bacterial endocarditis, infected ventriculoatrial shunts, syphilis, typhoid fever, toxoplasmosis, quartan malaria, schistosomiasis, infectious mononucleosis
- *c* Arthritis, polyarteritis, glomerulonephritis of hepatitis B infection

3 Autologous antigens
- *a* Systemic lupus erythematosus
- *b* Rheumatoid arthritis
- *c* Essential (mixed) cryoglobulinemia
- *d* Thyroiditis
- *e* Glomerulonephritis due to renal tubular antigen

4 Tumor antigens
- *a* Glomerulonephritis with colonic carcinoma, bronchogenic carcinoma, clear-cell renal carcinoma

Other drugs do not act as immunogens but instead stimulate the synthesis of autoantibodies, especially those with specificity to nuclear antigens. Patients receiving drugs such as procainamide, hydralazine, or hydantoins may form antibodies to nuclear antigens and manifest features of systemic lupus erythematosus (see Chap. 70). Several months of drug administration may be required before the onset of symptoms. The autoantibodies persist for months after administration of the drug has been discontinued.

Several types of infections are accompanied by immune-complex disease, and many have glomerulonephritis as a common feature. Antigens derived from the responsible microorganisms are presumed to be released at the site of their growth and then are deposited as immune complexes in glomeruli. Examples include poststreptococcal glomerulonephritis, the glomerulonephritis of bacterial endocarditis, infected ventriculoatrial shunt, osteomyelitis, quartan malaria, and hepatitis B infection.

Manifestations of immune-complex disease may accompany viral infections. For example, the preicteric phase of hepatitis B infection can be recognized by the appearance of fever, arthritis, and skin eruptions along with low serum complement and circulating hepatitis-associated antigen. As the arthritis and rash subside and complement levels return to normal, the hepatitis-associated antigen disappears from the circulation, and antibodies to the antigen can then be demonstrated. In this disorder the immune complexes consist of viral surface antigens (HBsAg) and the specific antibody.

Fungal diseases such as coccidioidomycosis may be accompanied by erythema nodosum and arthritis, most likely due to immune-complex deposition.

Patients with malignancies may develop arthritis, arthralgia, and skin eruptions. Renal biopsies in some patients with nephrotic syndrome associated with adenocarcinoma of the colon have shown IgG, complement components, and carcinoembryonic antigen in the glomerular basement membrane. As methods are developed for identifying other tumor antigens, examples of immune-complex disease will increase.

The autoimmune group of disorders is characterized by immune complexes composed of autologous antigens and their specific antibodies. The prototype of this group is systemic lupus erythematosus characterized by formation of antibodies to nuclear antigens (see Chap. 70). In particular, deposition of immune complexes consisting of native DNA, and antibodies to native DNA, in the glomerular basement membrane and other tissue leads to inflammation at these sites. Another example is essential (mixed) cryoglobulinemia in which immune complexes composed of IgG–anti-IgG can be identified in the cryoprecipitate. The antibody in these immune complexes consists of IgG, IgA, or IgM, and the antibody specificity is directed to IgG. The antibody in some instances may be monoclonal. These complexes are soluble at body temperature and show progressive insolubility as the temperature is lowered. Upon deposition, they produce glomerulonephritis, arthritis, and vasculitis. Cutaneous lesions may also develop owing to precipitation of complexes at reduced temperatures in the extremities. Immune complexes of IgG–anti-IgG are also found in rheumatoid arthritis and in hypergammaglobulinemic purpura of Waldenström, in which joint inflammation, pleuritis, pericarditis, and vasculitis are not uncommon.

Autologous antigens may be released by prior tissue damage to serve first as immunogens and later as antigens in the generation of immune-complex disease. For example, in sickle cell disease, renal tubular cell antigens are released from damaged tubular cells, antibodies to these antigens are synthesized, and the resultant immune complexes are deposited in the glomerular basement membrane.

Many forms of vasculitis, especially small-vessel vasculitis, are caused by deposition of immune complexes (see Chap. 69). Biopsy of an involved site may reveal immunoglobulins along with complement components. The absence of these substances, however, does not exclude an immune-complex pathogenesis because immune complexes may be destroyed by the inflammatory process within hours of their deposition. The nature and source of antigens that lead to immune-complex–induced vasculitis are largely unknown. In some patients with periarteritis nodosa, hepatitis-associated antigen is found in the serum. Furthermore, the antigen, antibodies, and complement components are present in the involved vessel wall, suggesting a pathogenetic role for these specific immune complexes.

A localized form of immune-complex disease occurs when antibodies come in contact with their antigens at or near the site where antigen is being released or where it is being absorbed. The gingivitis of periodontal disease is thought to be generated by complexes composed of bacterial antigens from the plaque and the specific antibodies. Studies of experimental thyroiditis indicate that antibodies specific to thyroglobulin react with this antigen as it is released from the follicular cells. Immune complexes are formed between the follicular basement membrane and the follicular cells, leading to interstitial inflammation. Thyroiditis in humans may be produced by a similar mechanism. The synovitis of rheumatoid arthritis also represents a localized immune-complex disease, in part attributed to antibodies to IgG (rheumatoid factors) that are produced in the synovium. Hypersensitivity pneumonitis, such as pigeon breeder's lung and farmer's lung, results from antibodies uniting with the respective inhaled antigen in the alveolar wall (see Chap. 274).

CLINICAL MANIFESTATIONS Since immune-complex diseases have a common pathogenetic mechanism, many of the clinical manifestations are similar even though the responsible antigens may be quite different. Glomerulonephritis, arthritis, and skin lesions are frequently observed, either individually or in various combinations. The characteristics of skin lesions can be indicative of the size of involved blood vessels. The involvement of small vessels causes palpable purpura, urticaria, morbilliform eruptions, and maculopapular eruptions. The inflammation of arterioles and small arteries leads to small infarcts, ulcerations, and bullous lesions. The involvement of even larger vessels leads to digital gangrene. Evidence for renal involvement includes proteinuria, red cells, and red cell casts. Renal infarction from immune-complex involvement of larger vessels leads to hypertension. Renal involvement may not be apparent clinically or by urinalysis; however, biopsy may show immune deposits in the mesangium or in the glomerular capillary loop. Pleuritis, pericarditis, and small-vessel vasculitis also occur. The number and severity of clinical manifestations vary among patients, even when the disorder is produced by a single etiologic agent. The reasons for this variability are not apparent.

The clinical manifestations and course of the acute, self-limited form of immune-complex disease are best exemplified by serum sickness following injection of a foreign protein such as horse antitoxin to diphtheria or tetanus. In the person who has not been previously exposed to the antitoxin, the first manifestation is reddening and swelling at the site of injection, occurring 1 to 2 weeks after antitoxin administration. This is followed within a few days by fever, myalgia, skin lesions, arthralgias or arthritis, gastrointestinal symptoms, and lymphadenopathy including nausea, vomiting, and abdominal pain. The skin lesions are most commonly urticarial; but petechial, erythematous, macular, or morbilliform lesions may be seen. Arthritis usually begins in one or two joints and rapidly progresses to include many joints. The wrists, ankles, knees, and small joints of the hand are most commonly involved. Acute glomerulonephritis with red blood cell casts, proteinuria, and decreasing renal function may develop. Vasculitis of the vasa nervorum produces peripheral neuropathy. Rarely meningoencephalitis may develop. In a person with previous exposure to the antitoxin, the above manifestations may appear 3 to 4 days following exposure. The same syndrome may occur after administration of a drug or in association with infection.

An anaphylactoid reaction may follow administration of a drug or foreign protein in a previously immunized patient who has preformed circulating antibodies to the specific antigen (see Chap. 67). This reaction begins minutes after exposure and is characterized by urticaria, bronchospasm, dyspnea, diarrhea, hypotension, and shock. This reaction may be fatal. It is caused by the release of large amounts of vasoactive peptides.

Chronic forms of immune-complex disease occur in patients who have prolonged or repeated availability of the antigen. Such conditions are seen when the antigen is released from a persisting microorganism, or when the antigen is a normal constituent of the host. Examples include infective endocarditis, adenocarcinoma of the colon, and systemic lupus erythematosus.

DIAGNOSIS Immune-complex disease should be suspected in a patient presenting with arthritis, skin eruptions, and glomerulonephritis. It should also be considered in patients with pericarditis, pleuritis, vasculitis, and/or neuropathy. When the presence of an immune-complex disease is suspected, the offending antigen must be identified by historical or laboratory inquiry. A detailed history of drug exposure is extremely important. The presence of chronic bacterial or viral infections must be sought by history and by physical and laboratory examinations.

Several diseases with diffuse vascular involvement in many organ systems may mimic immune-complex disease. Patients with a left atrial myxoma may have showers of skin lesions due to small emboli of myxomatous tissue. Similarly, patients with nonbacterial thrombotic endocarditis have peripheral embolization to small blood vessels. These patients may also have arthralgias. Patients with thrombotic thrombocytopenic purpura develop skin lesions, arthralgias, or arthritis, central nervous system abnormalities, and renal failure. The severity of the thrombocytopenia and absence of an inflammatory component in the purpuric skin lesions help to distinguish this entity from immune-complex disease. Showers of emboli from atheromatous plaques in older patients also may mimic immune-complex disease by producing multiple skin lesions. These may be unilateral or more diffuse depending on the site of the atheromatous plaques.

LABORATORY FINDINGS The laboratory abnormalities in patients with immune-complex disease include an elevated erythrocyte sedimentation rate, anemia, mild leukocytosis, and occasionally eosinophilia. The urine may contain protein, red blood cells, and red blood cell casts. Serum complement may be low. Conduction abnormalities may be present on the electrocardiogram.

In the patient suspected of having immune-complex disease, the search for antigen should include blood cultures for detection of bacteria that may release the antigens and serologic tests for viral antigens, such as the hepatitis B surface antigen. Serologic tests for detection of antibody to microbial antigens may be useful in detecting the underlying etiology. These include heterophil, anti-streptolysin O, and fluorescent treponemal antibody absorption tests, to mention just some. Tumor antigens, such as the carcinoembryonic antigen, should be sought. Antibodies to nuclear antigens and antibodies to IgG (rheumatoid factor) may suggest an underlying rheumatic disorder or infection such as infective endocarditis. Tests for cryoglobulins should be performed; if they are found, specific antigens and antibodies may be characterized in the cryoprecipitates. Measurements of serum complement can be helpful in supporting the diagnosis initially and in following the course of immune-complex diseases. Since immune complexes primarily activate the classic complement pathway, both the early and late components of complement will be consumed. A normal complement level does not exclude the presence of immune-complex disease because the rate of synthesis may compensate for the degree of complement consumption.

The biopsy and routine histologic examination of suspected vasculitic skin lesions are relatively innocuous and useful in the diagnosis of immune-complex diseases (see Chap. 69). Examination of tissue by immunofluorescence may show immunoglobulins and complement components in the wall of the involved blood vessels if the skin lesions are examined within 24 h of their development.

Immunofluorescence and electron-microscopy studies of tissue from renal biopsy are helpful in establishing the diagnosis of immune-complex–mediated renal disease. The finding of immunoglobulins, often in conjunction with complement components, by immunofluorescence indicates deposition of immune complexes. They stain in a discontinuous granular or "lumpy" pattern. In contrast, a linear pattern of staining is seen when antibody is directed to antigens of the glomerular basement membrane (e.g., in Goodpasture's syndrome). Electron microscopy reveals electron-dense deposits in the glomeruli (see Chap. 293).

The finding of decreased total hemolytic complement, decreased complement components, immunoglobulin and complement tissue deposits, or elevated titers of specific antibodies provides only inferential evidence for the presence of circulating immune complexes.

The detection and quantification of circulating immune complexes is possible with specialized techniques. Immune complexes can be identified by analytical ultracentrifugation, but this technique is insensitive. Immune complexes are precipitated by polyethylene glycol, a water-soluble polysaccharide which precipitates proteins according to size. Concentrations of polyethylene glycol below 5 percent will precipitate high-molecular-weight proteins and most immune complexes. The precipitated protein can then be quantified. This assay is not specific for immune complexes because normal macromolecules may also be precipitated. Immune complexes may also be detected by cryoglobulin assays since some immune complexes have decreased solubility at 4°C. Analysis of the cryoprecipitate may reveal the specific antigens or antibodies. Cryoglobulin assays are a reasonable, inexpensive initial screening test for detection of immune complexes but lack sensitivity. Certain monoclonal rheumatoid factors (anti-IgG antibodies) are effective in combining and precipitating with immune complexes containing IgG. Also, the first component of complement (C1q) can be used to detect complexes containing IgG or IgM in large-latticed immune complexes (C1q binding assay). It is also possible to detect circulating immune complexes by the use of a human lymphoblastoid cell line (called the Raji cell line). Complement-fixing immune complexes bind to these cells through complement (C3b, C3d, and C1q) receptors. These techniques are limited by the requirement to form an immune-complex lattice of a critical size, in order to facilitate binding of complement or interaction with cell receptors, and by the subclass of antibody. The presence of antibodies to lymphocytes may cause false-positive tests for immune complexes in the Raji cell assay. The presence of circulating DNA or endotoxin may cause false-positive tests for immune complexes in the assay with C1q. Immune complexes are detected by one or more of the above-mentioned assays in the serum of patients with a variety of clinical disorders. In many diseases the detection of immune complexes as an aid for diagnosis or a guide for management has not been adequately substantiated.

TREATMENT The principles of therapy for immune-complex diseases are to remove the offending antigen and to reduce the inflammation when it threatens to compromise organ function. When a drug is suspected of causing immune-complex disease, its administration should be stopped immediately. In patients with immune-complex disease associated with an infection, such as infective endocarditis, adequate doses of the appropriate antibiotic should be given.

The treatment of anaphylactic reactions is considered in Chap. 67.

In acute or subacute immune-complex disease, anti-inflammatory drugs such as salicylates will usually reduce joint pain. Antihistamines or small doses of epinephrine will relieve urticaria. In some patients the severity of disease warrants the use of corticosteroids which help to minimize clinical manifestations. Prednisone, 40 to 60 mg per day, can be given over a 2-week period with gradual tapering. Tissue damage may be slowed in chronic immune-complex disease by the use of corticosteroids alone or in combination with immunosuppressive drugs. Treatment of the chronic forms of immune-complex disease is discussed in detail in the chapters dealing with the specific disorders.

REFERENCES

AGNELLO V: Immune complex diseases: Assessment of the new immune complex assay technology, in *Update IV: Harrison's Principles of Internal Medicine,* KJ Isselbacher et al (eds). New York, McGraw-Hill, 1981

BEAUFILS M et al: Glomerulonephritis in severe bacterial infections with and without endocarditis. Adv Nephrol 7:217, 1978

COUSER WG, SALANT DJ: *In situ* immune complex formation and glomerular injury. Kidney Int 17:1, 1980

HAAKENSTAD AO, MANNIK M: The biology of immune complexes, in *Autoimmunity,* N Talal (ed). New York, Academic, 1977

KENNETH SR et al: Application of the solid phase C1q and Raji cell radioimmune assay for the detection of circulating immune complexes in glomerulonephritis. J Clin Invest 62:61, 1978

LAMBERT PH et al: A WHO collaborative study for the evaluation of eighteen methods for detecting immune complexes in serum. J Clin Lab Immunol 1:1, 1978

THEOFILOPOULOS AN, DIXON FJ: The biology and detection of immune complexes. Adv Immunol 28:89, 1979

WILLIAMS RC JR: Immune complexes, in *Clinical and Experimental Medicine.* Cambridge, Mass., Harvard University Press, 1980

ZUBLER RH, LAMBERT PH: Detection of immune complexes in human diseases. Prog Allergy 24:1, 1978

69 VASCULITIS

MART MANNIK
BRUCE C. GILLILAND

INTRODUCTION Many clinical syndromes of inflammation of blood vessels exist. In most of these conditions the etiology is not known, but several descriptive classifications have been offered, depending on the size of the involved blood vessels, the anatomic sites, and the histologic characteristics of the lesions. In these conditions cellular infiltration, necrosis, and fibrinoid deposits are present in the walls of blood vessels, along with perivascular cellular infiltration. The cellular infiltrates are composed of polymorphonuclear leukocytes in acute stages; with progression of the lesion, monocytes, lymphocytes, and plasma cells appear. Giant cells are encountered in some types of vasculitis. Endothelial edema and proliferation, together with hemorrhage, contribute to diminution or occlusion of the vascular lumen and subsequent ischemic symptoms and signs.

Most forms of vasculitis are thought to be caused by immunologic phenomena. Multiple reasons exist for this belief. Necrotizing inflammation of blood vessels is a common finding in experimentally induced immune-complex diseases (see Chap. 68). Vasculitis is a known manifestation of human serum sickness and occurs frequently in several known immune-complex diseases. For example, in systemic lupus erythematosus, DNA, antibodies to DNA, and complement components have been identified in vascular lesions. In essential cryoglobulinemia, IgG, antibodies to IgG, and complement components have been seen in involved vessels. Furthermore, in some patients with polyarteritis the hepatitis-associated antigen has been implicated as the causative agent with the finding of antigen, immunoglobulins, and complement in the lesions. In other types of inflammation, immunoglobulins and complement components have been visualized with immunofluorescence microscopy, but antigens have not been identified. Future work should identify the etiologic factors in many forms of vasculitis. Until then, however, the histologic and clinical features of the vasculitides serve to classify them.

Periarteritis nodosa was delineated by Kussmaul and Maier in the last century. In the early 1950s Zeek's careful descriptive work laid the foundation for most of the classifications of vasculitides. The descriptive classifications of vasculitides have been helpful in predicting the prognosis and response to therapy of individual patients. Upon microscopic examination of the lesions, in conjunction with clinical information, the vasculitides can usually be placed in one of the five categories indicated in Table 69-1. In some patients the clinical manifestations and histologic findings defy classification. Furthermore, in individual patients several sizes of blood vessels may be involved. For these reasons many classifications of vasculitides have been attempted, but none has received uniform acceptance. Finally, a single etiologic agent may cause clinically and histologically different forms of vasculitis. As an example, hepatitis B surface antigen has been identified in patients with polyarteritis, in patients with small-vessel vasculitis, and in patients with necrotizing small- and medium-vessel involvement. The nature of the antigen, the type of antibodies produced, the size of immune complexes formed, and cellular immunity are factors that may play a role in the pleomorphism of the clinical picture in the various vasculitides.

PERIARTERITIS NODOSA

PATHOLOGY In periarteritis nodosa (polyarteritis nodosa) the necrotizing inflammation involves medium and small arteries, adjacent veins, occasionally arterioles and venules, but not capillaries. The lesions involve segments of vessels, at times affecting only part of the circumference, and there is a predilection for the bifurcation of arteries. These areas may form small aneurysms, which may rupture. During the active disease each patient has acute lesions that show predominantly polymorphonuclear leukocytic infiltration of the vessel walls and perivascular areas, as well as chronic lesions with mononuclear cell infiltration and partial healing. These observations suggest that the disease process is continuous, with repeated insults, and if it is caused by immune mechanisms, there must be repeated or continuous availability of antigen(s).

The lesions of periarteritis nodosa are widespread throughout the body; they are commonly found in such places as the coronary arteries, mesenteric arteries, kidneys, muscles, and vasa nervorum. The extent and location of lesions dictate the severity of clinical symptoms. Central nervous system involvement is unusual. The lungs are usually not involved, but this question has caused controversy and confusion. Necrotizing inflammation and granuloma formation in blood vessels accompanied by lung involvement and eosinophilia should be classified as allergic granulomatosis.

CLINICAL MANIFESTATIONS Periarteritis nodosa is usually a disease of adulthood, but it occurs at any age. It affects two to three men for every woman. The onset of the disease is extremely variable. Often an antecedent history of upper respiratory tract infection or reaction to drugs is recorded.

The early complaints of patients with polyarteritis nodosa include fever, weakness, anorexia, weight loss, myalgias, and arthralgias. With the progression of the disease several organs may show involvement. Small, 5- to 10-mm nodules as a result of aneurysm formation may become palpable along the course of arteries in the extremities. Involvement of vessel walls leads to occlusion, ecchymoses, ulceration (often secondarily infected), and gangrene of fingers or toes. Muscle weakness may evolve. Arthralgias are common, but severe and persistent arthritis is uncommon. Mononeuritis multiplex develops because of involvement of the vasa nervorum. Asymmetric and multiple nerve trunks may be involved. Retinal exudates and hemorrhages may occur.

Pericarditis and pleuritis, with or without effusions, are common. Involvement of coronary arteries may lead to myocardial ischemia or infarction. Electrocardiographic abnormalities may be recorded in the absence of symptoms.

Abdominal complaints are frequent (in 60 to 70 percent of patients) and include abdominal pain, nausea, vomiting, diarrhea, and gastrointestinal bleeding. All these symptoms are related to the involvement of the mesenteric arteries. The mesenteric vasculitis may lead to mucosal ulceration with bleeding; infarction and perforation may ensue. The acute abdominal symptoms early in the disease may suggest a surgical abdomen, often resulting in unavoidable but unnecessary laparotomy. The liver may be involved, and massive hepatic infarction has been reported. Periarteritis of the gallbladder may cause cholecystitis and perforation.

Renal involvement occurs in over half the patients, and affects predominantly arteries and arterioles. Glomerulosclerosis occurs with severe involvement. Hypertension may occur early in the disease when renal function is normal. It is due to arterial occlusion. Hypertension may also accompany renal failure. Rupture of intrarenal aneurysms may cause renal infarcts or perinephric hematomas (see Chap. 298).

The causes of death in polyarteritis nodosa include renal failure, myocardial infarction, infections, congestive heart failure, and gastrointestinal bleeding.

LABORATORY FINDINGS AND DIAGNOSIS No specific chemical or serologic tests exist for periarteritis nodosa. The leukocyte count is elevated in about 80 percent of patients, principally because of neutrophilia. Anemia may be present because of inflammatory block, blood loss, or both. The erythrocyte sedimentation rate is often elevated. Other abnormalities depend on organ involvement, e.g., hematuria, proteinuria, and decreased renal function due to kidney involvement or abnormal electrocardiogram (ECG) due to coronary artery vasculitis.

Angiography has become useful in documenting the diagnosis of periarteritis nodosa. The characteristic aneurysms at branching points of arteries occur in the kidneys, mesentery, liver, pancreas, and elsewhere during the acute phase of the disease. In late stages of the disease narrowing and thrombosis of arteries predominate in the same areas. In a number of reports the finding of arterial aneurysms on angiography has been employed to support the diagnosis of periarteritis nodosa.

The diagnosis of periarteritis nodosa often causes difficulties. This disease should be suspected in patients with involvement in several of the organs mentioned above. Infections, systemic lupus erythematosus, trichinosis, heart failure, Hodgkin's disease, and most other syndromes can be ruled out. Histologic examination of tissue is essential for proper diagnosis and for distinction from other vasculitides. Clinically involved

TABLE 69-1
Classification of vasculitis

*Periarteritis nodosa**	*Allergic granulomatosis**	*Wegener's granulomatosis*	*Hypersensitivity vasculitis*	*Giant-cell arteritis*
SIZE OF INVOLVED BLOOD VESSELS				
Medium and small arteries, adjacent veins	Medium and small arteries, adjacent veins, arterioles, capillaries	Small arteries, arterioles, venules, some capillaries	Arterioles, venules, capillaries	Large and medium arteries
HISTOLOGY AND STAGE OF LESIONS				
Necrotizing inflammation, coexistence of acute and healing lesions, no giant cells	Necrotizing inflammation with extravascular granulomas, coexistence of acute and healing lesions, giant cells in granulomas, abundant eosinophils	Necrotizing inflammation with granulomas, coexistence of acute and healing lesions, giant cells in granulomas	Necrotizing inflammation, all lesions in same stage, no giant cells	Inflammation without necrosis, giant cells are present, no neutrophils
ANATOMIC PREDILECTIONS				
Widespread, common to branching points of arteries; lungs rarely involved	Widespread, but lungs frequently involved	Upper and lower respiratory tract involved; necrotizing glomerulitis	Widespread but common to skin, serosal surfaces, glomeruli	All large arteries, including aorta, coronary, vertebral, carotid, temporal, mesenteric

* *Some patients have clinical features and histologic findings of periarteritis nodosa and allergic granulomatosis. For this reason the term* systemic necrotizing vasculitis of the polyarteritis nodosa group *has been suggested to cover the spectrum of these disorders.*

tissue is best for histologic examinations, and tender subcutaneous nodules, tender muscles, tender testes, and skin infarcts are suitable. Each tissue should be examined thoroughly because of the segmental nature of the lesions. In the absence of lesions accessible for biopsy, mesenteric or renal angiography may show the presence of aneurysms. These findings, however, are not unique to periarteritis nodosa and have been observed in other types of vasculitides.

Hepatitis B surface antigen has been found in serum of 30 to 40 percent of patients with periarteritis nodosa. The same antigen has been identified in vascular lesions along with immunoglobulins and complement, suggesting that in these patients the vasculitis is caused by immune complexes containing the hepatitis antigen. The liver involvement in these patients may be mild and overlooked unless liver function studies are performed. Some patients with this form of vasculitis have chronic liver disease, which may progress to hepatic failure. The evaluation of a patient with polyarteritis should include a search for the hepatitis B surface antigen.

In some patients the necrotizing vasculitis appears to follow a bout of serous otitis media. The basis of this association has not been established.

TREATMENT The prognosis of periarteritis nodosa with involvement of many organ systems is grim. Hypertension and renal involvement are thought to predict rapid progression of the disease. In untreated patients one-half to two-thirds have died within a year, but these statistics are heavily biased by postmortem studies and selective inclusion of severely ill patients. Treatment with corticosteroids frequently leads to rapid symptomatic improvement (initial dose 40 to 60 mg prednisone or prednisolone per day, tapered subsequently). In one study 5-year survival in untreated patients was estimated at 13 percent. Controlled studies on the use of cytotoxic (immunosuppressive) drugs have not been recorded, but some experiences suggest that these agents may help when other drugs have failed.

ALLERGIC GRANULOMATOSIS

DEFINITION Allergic granulomatosis is separated from periarteritis nodosa because of prominent eosinophilia, the presence of perivascular granulomas, lung involvement, and the clinical association with bronchial asthma.

PATHOLOGY In allergic granulomatosis small arteries, veins, and smaller vessels are commonly involved in segmental fashion. The vascular lesion has numerous epithelioid cells, giant cells, eosinophils, and other inflammatory cells, producing a granulomatous appearance. At times extravascular granulomas are present. The organ involvement is comparable to that of periarteritis nodosa, except that pulmonary involvement is seen with granuloma formation in the vessel walls and perivascular areas.

MANIFESTATIONS Patients with allergic granulomatosis frequently give a history of an antecedent respiratory infection. Many have asthma that precedes evidence of vasculitis; fever is common. Fifty-four percent of these patients have peripheral eosinophilia, with eosinophils in excess of 1500 per cubic millimeter. The radiologic examination is not diagnostic, but parenchymal lung lesions include large nodular, interstitial, and transient patchy infiltrates. Pleural effusions are not common.

The clinical findings due to involvement of other organs is quite similar to that in periarteritis nodosa, and includes the heart, kidneys, intestine, and peripheral nerves.

TREATMENT This has not been evaluated systematically. Sporadic reports and analogy to other forms of necrotizing vasculitis indicate that corticosteroids, in the same doses used for periarteritis, are the drugs of choice. Cytotoxic (immunosuppressive) drugs might be tried in patients unresponsive to corticosteroids.

WEGENER'S GRANULOMATOSIS

See Chap. 237.

HYPERSENSITIVITY VASCULITIS (SMALL-VESSEL VASCULITIS)

DEFINITION Hypersensitivity vasculitis has been given many names because of its varied clinical picture. The role of immune mechanisms in its pathogenesis is inferred by similarity to experimental models, and in some patients with this disorder the involvement of antigen-antibody complexes is documented. Basically, the arterioles, venules, and capillaries of many organs are involved by necrotizing inflammation. All lesions tend to be of the same age. The clinical picture depends on the extent of the disease and on the primary target organ. Systemic lupus erythematosus, rheumatoid arthritis, and essential (mixed) cryoglobulinemia are excellent examples of this type of vasculitis in which immune mechanisms have been implicated in the pathogenesis of the blood vessel inflammation. Drugs and microorganisms have also been implicated as the causative agents in hypersensitivity vasculitis. An association with hepatitis B infection has been found in many patients with essential cryoglobulinemia with the identification of hepatitis B surface antigens and antibodies in the cryoprecipitates. Small-vessel vasculitis is also seen in some patients with hyperglobulinemic purpura of Waldenström. These patients have characteristic purpura of the lower extremities, marked elevation of gamma globulin on serum protein electrophoresis, and intermediate complexes on ultracentrifugation of serum.

PATHOLOGY Hypersensitivity vasculitis (small-vessel vasculitis) is the most frequently encountered form of blood vessel inflammation. The inflammation and necrosis involve arterioles and capillaries, and not medium and large arteries. In some studies the lesions have been confined to venules. As a result, the clinical symptoms do not evolve from large-vessel ischemia and infarction but result from hemorrhagic and exudative lesions and microinfarcts. Many organs may be involved, including skin, mucous membranes, brain, lungs, heart, gastrointestinal tract, kidneys, and muscle. Neutrophils accumulate in small-vessel walls and in perivascular areas. Necrosis, edema, and extravasation of blood are present. Many neutrophils are fragmented; hence some prefer to call this form of vasculitis "leukocytoclastic angiitis." Serum complement level may be low in these patients. In contrast, when the inflammatory lesions consist entirely of lymphocytes during the active phase of the disease, the serum complement levels are normal. Healing and hyalinization occur late. Focal or diffuse glomerulonephritis occurs in some patients. Characteristically all vascular lesions are in the same stage of evolution, in contrast to what occurs in periarteritis nodosa. This observation suggests episodic, rather than continuous, exposure to immune complexes, if indeed this is the mechanism of injury. Immunopathologic studies have shown deposits of immunoglobulins and complement components in vasculitic skin lesions, if examined within 24 h of their development.

CLINICAL MANIFESTATIONS The clinical manifestations and onset of hypersensitivity vasculitis are variable, and the reasons for this variability are not known. In some patients the skin manifestations are extensive; systemic manifestations and involvement of other organs predominate throughout the course of the illness in others. In some the disease follows a quick course that leads to death, but most patients survive for years and may recover without recurrences.

In youngsters and in some adults hypersensitivity vasculitis may present as the Henoch-Schönlein syndrome, with prodromal headache, anorexia, fever, abdominal pain and bleeding, arthralgias, purpuric eruptions, and evidence of renal involvement. The immune-complex deposits in blood vessels and in glomeruli of these patients contain primarily the IgA class of antibodies. In adults the criteria for the Henoch-Schönlein syndrome are not usually fulfilled.

The history of an antecedent respiratory infection may be obtained; drugs may have been ingested. (The list is long and includes penicillin, sulfonamides, other antibiotics, salicylates, phenylbutazone, phenacetin, propylthiouracil, busulfan, iodides, vaccines, and phenothiazines.) Fever is a common systemic symptom. The skin lesions include urticaria, palpable purpura, ecchymoses, papules, nodules, vesicles, and necrotic ulcerations. Lesions may occur anywhere, but they tend to have some symmetry, and the lesions predominate in lower extremities—the legs, ankles, and feet. Patients frequently complain of itching, burning, stinging, and pain in the skin lesions. They may have myalgia, arthralgia, and arthritis. The joints may be warm, red, and painful with acute effusions. However, synovitis of long duration with synovial hypertrophy is unusual, and bony erosions do not develop, unless rheumatoid arthritis is present. Pulmonary infiltrates and pleural effusions may be found on chest radiographs. Pericarditis and myocarditis may develop, accompanied by electrocardiographic abnormalities. These patients may have peripheral neuropathy and encephalopathy, manifested by confusion, delirium, and coma. Diffuse electroencephalographic abnormalities may be present. Renal involvement becomes apparent, with microscopic hematuria, proteinuria, and decreasing renal function (see Chap. 298). Abdominal pain and gastrointestinal bleeding occur.

Small-vessel vasculitis occurs with a number of recognized disease entities. In addition to small-vessel involvement, larger vessels are at times also involved, leading to clinical and histologic features similar to periarteritis nodosa, added to the underlying disorder.

Patients with *essential (mixed) cryoglobulinemia* have cutaneous vasculitis, glomerulonephritis, arthralgias, enlargement of the spleen, liver, and lymph nodes. The vasculitis may involve the peripheral and central nervous system and the gastrointestinal system. Glomerulonephritis, however, tends to be the most serious problem (see Chap. 295). The cryoglobulins in these patients consist of immune complexes containing IgM–rheumatoid factor and normal IgG, and a high proportion of the cryoglobulins also contain hepatitis B surface antigens or antibodies. Vasculitis of small blood vessels is common in patients with rheumatoid arthritis, involving the inflamed synovium. Systemic necrotizing vasculitis develops in some patients with advanced rheumatoid arthritis, involving small to medium arteries, and resulting in a clinical picture similar to periarteritis nodosa, including mononeuritis multiplex. Similarly, in patients with systemic lupus erythematosus small-vessel vasculitis with cutaneous manifestations is most common, but a few patients develop medium-size vessel inflammation. Infrequently, vasculitis develops in patients with malignancies, including chronic lymphocytic leukemia, lymphosarcoma, and Hodgkin's disease. Presumably this occurs due to the presence of circulating immune complexes. Patients with infective endocarditis may have small-vessel vasculitis, as manifested by Osler nodes, Roth spots, palpable purpura, arthralgias, and glomerulonephritis, although some of these lesions may be embolic in origin.

LABORATORY FINDINGS Elevation of the erythrocyte sedimentation rate is the most common abnormality. Mild anemia and moderate leukocytosis occur. Complement levels may be reduced, particularly when neutrophilic infiltrates predominate in the lesions. The finding of a positive test for antibodies to nuclear antigens suggests that the vasculitis is a feature of systemic lupus erythematosus. Similarly, the finding of a positive test for rheumatoid factor might indicate underlying rheumatoid arthritis, mixed cryoglobulinemia, or subacute bacterial endocarditis with vasculitis. Examination of the urinary sediment and evaluation of proteinuria and renal function are indicated for initial evaluation and follow-up of these patients. Biopsy of lesions establishes the diagnosis of vasculitis but does not distinguish among the underlying disorders.

TREATMENT The mortality figures for this disorder are variable because many series are based on autopsy findings. Spontaneous improvement occurs in some patients; in others the disease lingers. If drugs, toxins, or other environmental factors are suspected, all these exposures should be eliminated. If this disorder is immunologically mediated, then removal of the antigen would be the best treatment. Uncontrolled observations suggest that corticosteroids favorably influence the course of this disorder. The optimal dose has not been determined; 40 to 60 mg prednisone or prednisolone seems reasonable at the onset, but the dose should be reduced when symptoms, signs, and laboratory tests show improvement. The dose should be increased when flare-ups occur. By analogy to systemic lupus erythematosus and Wegener's granulomatosis, cytostatic (immunosuppressive) drugs might be used in desperate situations. However, the results of controlled clinical trials with this therapy are not yet available.

GIANT-CELL ARTERITIS AND POLYMYALGIA RHEUMATICA

DEFINITION Giant-cell arteritis (also called *temporal or cranial arteritis*) is an inflammation of arteries in elderly persons. The cause of the disorder is unknown, and the pathogenesis of arterial inflammation has not been elucidated. However, some evidence for both humoral and cellular immunity to elastic arterial tissue has been presented. Any large or medium-sized artery may be involved, including the superficial temporal artery. Giant-cell arteritis responds dramatically to treatment with corticosteroids. This entity is different from Takayasu's arteritis (see Chap. 268) since the latter occurs principally in young women and involves the aorta and its main branches. The polymyalgia rheumatica syndrome is related to giant-cell arteritis but occurs without clinical or obtainable evidence of arteritis.

PATHOLOGY The inflammatory changes of giant-cell arteritis affect the large and medium-sized arteries without involving the arterioles and capillaries. Histiocytes, epithelioid cells, multinucleated giant cells, lymphocytes, and plasma cells accumulate in the intima and media adjacent to the internal elastic lamina of medium-sized arteries. The elastic lamina is highly fragmented and absent in some areas. In large arteries and the aorta, the media tends to be prominently involved with inflammation and fragmentation of the elastic fibers. The intima is thickened more than expected from age alone. The lesions are spotty and do not involve long stretches of the arteries. Thrombosis may occur at sites of inflammation.

The segmental lesions of giant-cell arteritis may involve any arteries, including the superficial temporal artery. The aorta is frequently involved, and aneurysms and dissection have been recorded. The external and internal carotid arteries and the vertebral artery systems are involved. Inflammation and occlusion of the ophthalmic or central retinal artery lead to blindness. Involvement of iliac, femoral, mesenteric, and coronary arteries may cause ischemia and infarction in the respective sites.

CLINICAL MANIFESTATIONS Giant-cell arteritis is a disease of the elderly that affects both sexes nearly equally. This illness has rarely been diagnosed before the age of 50 or 60, and it is rare among blacks. The symptomatic involvement of arteries is frequently preceded by systemic symptoms, including fever, sweats, malaise, fatigue, anorexia, and weight loss. The fever tends to be low grade but may be striking. A fever of unknown origin in an elderly person, accompanied by a very high erythrocyte sedimentation rate, should always raise the diagnostic possibility of giant-cell arteritis.

Patients with giant-cell arteritis often have the *polymyalgia rheumatica* syndrome as described below. Headache is a frequent symptom, particularly in patients who have clinical temporal arteritis, with tender and thickened temporal arteries. The headache has no typical pattern, but marked scalp tenderness is often prominent. Furthermore, these patients may complain of intermittent claudication of the jaws and tongue upon mastication or talking.

Loss of vision is a serious complication of giant-cell arteritis. Blindness usually develops suddenly without significant warning, but mild visual disturbances may herald total visual loss. Usually for months or weeks these patients will have had other complaints suggestive of giant-cell arteritis or polymyalgia rheumatica. Aortic aneurysms, aortic dissection, mesenteric arteritis, myocardial ischemia and infarction, and claudication of the lower extremities have been attributed to giant-cell arteritis.

Polymyalgia rheumatica Polymyalgia rheumatica occurs in elderly people and has only rarely been diagnosed under the age of 50 years. Similar to giant-cell arteritis, it is a disorder with predilection for Caucasians. The characteristic complaint is an aching or pain and stiffness in the neck, upper back, shoulders, upper arms, and hip girdle areas. The onset of these complaints may be gradual or abrupt to the degree that one day the patient feels fine and next morning can hardly arise from bed. The morning stiffness can be very striking and tends to be most prominent in the shoulder and hip girdles with less stiffness in hands and feet. These patients also may have fever of varying degree; they develop anorexia and weight loss, become apathetic and depressed. In contrast to their marked complaints, these patients have relatively few physical findings. Shoulder girdle movements may be slow and difficult, but muscle weakness is not present except what is caused by the pain. Some tenderness may be present around the shoulder girdle and shoulder joint. Synovial hypertrophy is absent, but small synovial effusions may be present.

The laboratory findings of polymyalgia rheumatica and giant-cell arteritis are similar and are discussed below. A relationship exists between these disorders because some patients with giant-cell or temporal arteritis have typical symptoms of polymyalgia rheumatica and temporal artery biopsies in some patients with polymyalgia rheumatica have the typical histologic findings of giant-cell arteritis. Because of these relationships the possibility has been considered that polymyalgia rheumatica may be a precursor of or represent giant-cell arteritis without histologic proof of blood vessel involvement. This possibility is not yet fully resolved. It is clear, however, from the experience of many clinicians that most patients with polymyalgia rheumatica respond well to a low dose of corticosteroids and do not run a high risk of complications of giant-cell arteritis, such as blindness.

The differential diagnosis of polymyalgia rheumatica includes occult infections, malignancies, and other rheumatic diseases and muscle disorders since the complaints and findings are nonspecific. The aching and stiffness of viral infections (e.g., influenza) may be striking but last for days rather than weeks or months. Muscle disorders like polymyositis are distinguished by elevation of muscle enzymes or abnormal electromyogram. Patients with depression and psychogenic rheumatic complaints do not have the characteristically high erythrocyte sedimentation rate. Malignancies of the B-lymphocyte series (e.g., multiple myeloma, macroglobulinemia) can be distinguished by protein electrophoresis. Occult infections and malignancies must be sought with appropriate tests in the presence of localizing symptoms, signs, or laboratory tests. Patients with polymyalgia rheumatica who have minimal rheumatic complaints but present with fever, weight loss, or hypoproliferative anemia are a diagnostic challenge. Biopsy of a clinically uninvolved temporal artery or a therapeutic trial of low-dose steroids with dramatic and persistent response have resolved the diagnostic problem in some patients.

LABORATORY FINDINGS The significant abnormalities in laboratory tests of patients with giant-cell arteritis or patients with polymyalgia rheumatica include a very high erythrocyte sedimentation rate (ESR), mild to moderate hypoproliferative anemia, and elevation of the alpha$_2$ globulins and fibrinogen. The ESR exceeds 50 mm/h (by Westergren's method) and often reaches values above 100 mm/h. The alkaline phosphatase may be slightly elevated. Important negative findings include normal serum levels of muscle enzymes and normal electromyograms, even in the presence of severe polymyalgia. Muscle biopsies disclose no characteristic changes.

In the absence of specific diagnostic tests, the diagnosis of giant-cell arteritis or polymyalgia rheumatica has to rest on clinical findings or a positive biopsy.

TREATMENT Though patients with the polymyalgia rheumatica syndrome and giant-cell arteritis may obtain some relief from their symptoms with salicylates, indomethacin, or phenylbutazone, the basic process does not seem to improve. Patients with these disorders, however, have a remarkable response to corticosteroid treatment. The clinical symptoms abate in a few days, the ESR and the hypoproliferative anemia return toward normal within 2 weeks, and the reversal of arterial lesions has been documented by arteriography. Several dosage schedules have been recommended. For patients with proven giant-cell arteritis a daily starting dose of 60 mg prednisone is recommended. A dramatic improvement in symptoms can be expected in a few days. The dose should be reduced gradually in 3 to 4 weeks when symptoms have abated and the ESR has decreased. The maintenance dose is usually 10 mg prednisone per day or less. In patients with polymyalgia rheumatica a starting dose of prednisone from 10 to 20 mg per day can give striking relief of symptoms. Higher doses can be considered if fever, anemia, or other symptoms are debilitating to the patient. If the low dose of corticosteroids does not lead to resolution of symptoms and decrease of the ESR, a diagnosis of giant-cell arteritis should be considered and temporal artery biopsy performed. Alternate-day corticosteroids are not useful for patients with these disorders. Ultimately, corticosteroids can be discontinued in the majority of patients. The hazards of corticosteroids should be considered, and the prolonged use of high doses of corticosteroids should be discouraged.

MISCELLANEOUS VASCULITIDES

Vasculitis is present in a number of other syndromes. Mucocutaneous lymph node syndrome (Kawasaki disease) is an acute febrile illness in children but has been reported in adults (see Chap. 56). These patients have cervical lymph node enlargement, edema and erythema of the oral mucosa, conjunctivitis, erythema and desquamation of the palms and fingertips. In a few children with this disorder coronary vasculitis with arterial occlusion and myocardial infarction has been reported. Cogan's syndrome, consisting of nonsyphilitic interstitial keratitis and vestibuloauditory symptoms may be associated with systemic vasculitis. Vasculitis is also present in patients with Behçet's syndrome (see Chap. 348).

REFERENCES

CHESON BD et al: Cogan's syndrome: A systemic vasculitis. Am J Med 60:549, 1976

CHUMBLEY LC et al: Allergic granulomatosis and angiitis (Churg-Strauss syndrome): Report and analysis of 30 cases. Mayo Clin Proc 52:477, 1977

FAUCI AS et al: The spectrum of vasculitis. Clinical, pathologic, immunologic, and therapeutic considerations. Ann Intern Med 89:660, 1978

——— et al: Cyclophosphamide therapy of severe systemic necrotizing vasculitis. N Engl J Med 301:235, 1979

HAMILTON CR JR et al: Giant cell arteritis: Including temporal arteritis and polymyalgia rheumatica. Medicine 50:1, 1971

HAMRIN B: Polymyalgia arteritica. Acta Med Scand (Suppl): 533, 1973

KLEIN RG et al: Large artery involvement in giant cell (temporal) arteritis. Ann Intern Med 83:806, 1975

LEVO Y et al: Association between hepatitis B virus and essential mixed cryoglobulinemia. N Engl J Med 296:1501, 1977

MICHALAK T: Immune complexes of hepatitis B surface antigens in the pathogenesis of periarteritis nodosa. Am J Pathol 90:619, 1978

PARK JR, HAZLEMAN BL: Immunological and histological study of temporal arteries. Ann Rheum Dis 37:238, 1978

SOTER NA et al: Two distinct cellular patterns in cutaneous necrotizing angiitis. J Invest Dermatol 66:344, 1976

ZEEK PM: Periarteritis nodosa and other forms of necrotizing angiitis. N Engl J Med 148:764, 1953

70 SYSTEMIC LUPUS ERYTHEMATOSUS

MART MANNIK
BRUCE C. GILLILAND

Systemic lupus erythematosus (SLE) is a disease of unknown cause. However, abundant evidence shows that immunologic mechanisms of tissue injury are important in its pathogenesis. The clinical presentation and the course of SLE are variable. A hallmark of this disease is the presence of a number of antibodies to nuclear components, but other immunologic abnormalities exist as well. Some patients with SLE have spontaneous remissions, others respond favorably to treatment with corticosteroids, and in some patients the course is unresponsive to available medications. On the basis of detailed studies of animal models that resemble SLE, viral infections, genetic predisposition, and abnormalities of immunoregulation appear etiologically important.

PATHOGENESIS The serum of patients with SLE contains many antibodies; among them are the antibodies to double-stranded (native) or single-stranded (denatured) deoxyribonu-

cleic acid (DNA), deoxyribonucleoprotein, histones, nuclear ribonucleoprotein, the so-called Sm antigen, and other nuclear constituents. These antibodies are collectively termed antibodies to nuclear antigens (ANA). Antibodies may also be present to cytoplasmic antigens (RNA, ribosomes), to clotting factors (lupus anticoagulants), to antigens on circulating cells (red cells, neutrophils, platelets, T lymphocytes, B lymphocytes), and to cardiolipin to produce a false-positive serological test for syphilis. The enigma of this multitude of antibodies in patients with SLE was in part explained by studying the hybridoma-produced antibodies to DNA from murine lupus. The specificity of these antibodies was directed to an antigenic determinant containing diester-linked phosphate groups that are present in DNA, cardiolipin, and certain clotting factors. These findings suggest that at least some of the apparent diversity of antibodies in SLE may be explained by common chemical features among the antigens, rather than by a diversity of antibody specificities. The antibodies to nuclear antigens alone are harmless; their presence in vivo or in tissue cultures does not harm living cells, since antibodies do not penetrate the membrane of living cells. However, the ANA participate in the pathogenesis of SLE by forming antigen-antibody complexes with their specific antigens. DNA and antibodies to DNA, deoxyribonucleoprotein and antibodies to deoxyribonucleoprotein, as well as complement components, have been demonstrated in the renal glomerular basement membrane and in the vascular basement membrane of patients with SLE. Other antigen-antibody systems are most likely also involved in the disease process. During the active phase of SLE, serum complement is decreased and circulating immune complexes can be detected with sensitive techniques. For these reasons SLE has been classified as an immune-complex disease. On the other hand, neuropsychiatric manifestations of SLE may be produced by antibodies directed to neurons.

In experimental immune-complex diseases of animals and in human serum sickness, inflammation of joints, pleura, and pericardium occurs because of the presence of antigen and subsequent immune-complex formation. Similar mechanisms may well explain the multitude of clinical manifestations in patients with SLE.

ETIOLOGY The reasons for development of the antinuclear and other antibodies in SLE are not clear. Furthermore, the origin of the antigens in tissue lesions has not been elucidated—they may be autologous nuclear components, or they may originate from invading microorganisms. The hypothesis that SLE results from a viral infection in genetically predisposed persons is supported by several observations. The strongest support for this hypothesis comes from studies on the female F_1 hybrids of New Zealand black (NZB) and white (NZW) mice and other strains of mice that develop a syndrome analogous to SLE. These mice develop, among other manifestations, renal lesions, antinuclear antibodies, antibodies to DNA, and decreased serum complement. DNA and antibodies to DNA exist in the renal deposits of immune complexes. These mice also develop antibodies to the retroviral glycoprotein with molecular weight of 70,000 (termed gp 70) and form immune complexes with this antigen. In a very high percentage of patients with SLE, cytoplasmic virus-like tubuloreticular structures are found by electron microscopy in endothelial cells of glomerular and other capillaries. These structures initially were thought to represent viruses, but now are thought to represent an unidentified response to cell injury.

Similar inclusions are seen in other disorders, but with lesser frequency.

In humans and mice with SLE, abnormalities exist in the regulatory mechanisms of the immune response. A suppression of cell-mediated immunity is apparent with an enhanced activity of humoral immunity. These observations suggest a diminution of the T-cell suppressor mechanism on B-cell functions. These abnormalities may in part account for the multitude of antibodies to intracellular components as mentioned above, but the reasons for the existence of these abnormalities remain obscure.

A genetic predisposition for SLE has been suggested by the subclinical abnormalities in relatives of patients with SLE and by the high concordance of clinical SLE in monozygotic twins. On the other hand, the finding of a high prevalence of lymphocytotoxic antibodies among household contacts, including but not limited to blood relatives, raises the possibility of nongenetic transmission of SLE. The occurrence of SLE and lupus-like syndromes in patients with several inborn errors of complement (predominantly deficiencies of C1, C4, and C2) has been noted but not explained.

PATHOLOGY The pathologic changes in SLE are variable and depend on the stage of the disease. Fibrinoid deposits are commonly seen in blood vessels, among collagen fibers, and on serosal surfaces. Hematoxylin bodies are specific for SLE and are defined as hematoxylin-stained round or oblong masses in areas of inflammation. Hematoxylin bodies are thought to represent degenerated nuclei that have interacted with antibodies to nuclear antigens.

The renal lesions in patients with SLE have been classified into *mesangial, mild, or focal glomerulonephritis, diffuse glomerulonephritis,* and *membranous lupus nephritis.* In mesangial involvement the glomeruli may appear normal or show varying degrees of mesangial hypercellularity. By immunofluorescence microscopy, immunoglobulins and complement components are seen to be present in the mesangial area. By electron microscopy, deposits are seen in the mesangial matrix, and a few small deposits may be seen in the subendothelial area. In focal glomerulonephritis some glomeruli (less than 50 percent) show focal hypercellularity, accumulation of inflammatory cells, and thickening of the basement membrane. Immunofluorescence microscopy shows the presence of immunoglobulins and complement components in involved areas as well as in the mesangium of uninvolved areas. In diffuse glomerulonephritis the same changes are present in all glomeruli, but frequently in an uneven manner. The basement membrane may be considerably thickened. On immunofluorescence microscopy, extensive "lumpy-bumpy" deposits of immunoglobulins and complement components are seen along the basement membrane. On electron microscopy, the electron-dense deposits are found on the endothelial side of the basement membrane and in the mesangium. In membranous lupus nephritis, hypercellularity is not present, but the basement membrane is diffusely thickened. Immunofluorescence microscopy discloses granular deposits of immunoglobulins and complement components. By electron microscopy these deposits are localized on the epithelial side of the basement membrane and within the basement membrane. In some patients with SLE a mixed pattern of glomerular involvement is present including the deposits in mesangial, subendothelial, and subepithelial areas. The mechanisms for these differences in renal involvement have not been elucidated. The degree of thrombosis in glomerular capillary loops appeared as the best predictor of subsequent glomerular sclerosis and loss of renal function.

Over the years a number of lupus patients with normal renal function and normal urine have had renal biopsies. Histologically these specimens may be normal, show increased mesangial cellularity, or have minimal glomerulonephritis. On immunofluorescence microscopy mesangial deposits of immunoglobulins and complement components are commonly seen. By electron-microscopic examination, electron-dense deposits are in the mesangial matrix and to a small extent in the subendothelial area of the glomerular basement membrane. These observations indicate that glomerular abnormalities are ubiquitous in patients with SLE, even when renal function and urine sediment are entirely normal by the usual clinical criteria. With follow-up only some of these patients progress to overt renal involvement and renal failure.

In addition to glomerular damage, immune complexes also lead to interstitial nephritis in SLE. Over half of biopsied patients show focal or diffuse interstitial cellular infiltrates, tubular damage, or interstitial fibrosis. The finding of immunoglobulins, complement components, and electron-dense deposits along the tubular basement membrane and in the interstitium indicate that immune complexes initiate these lesions. The immune-complex interstitial nephritis is most common in patients with diffuse proliferative glomerulonephritis and less frequent in the other glomerulonephritides associated with SLE.

The pathologic findings in skin lesions vary according to the clinical stage of the lesions. The histology of the erythematous, maculopapular eruptions, as seen in the butterfly distribution on the face, are not diagnostic. Edema, extravasation of red cells, and some perivascular inflammation are early alterations. More chronic lesions show hyperkeratosis, epidermal atrophy, and small-vessel inflammation in the dermis. The lesions in discoid lupus erythematosus will show atrophy, epidermal hyperkeratosis, and keratotic plugging. The dermis is edematous and infiltrated variably with lymphocytes, plasma cells, and histiocytes. On immunofluorescent staining, the epidermal-dermal junction of patients with SLE has IgG and C3 deposits. Similar changes are frequently present in clinically uninvolved skin. The mechanism for development of these deposits has not been clarified, but antibodies to nuclear antigens, including antibodies to DNA, have been identified in these deposits.

Widespread small-vessel vasculitis may be present in many organs. Such lesions exist in the synovium and show both mononuclear and polymorphonuclear infiltration. Autopsy studies on SLE patients with central nervous system abnormalities may show necrotizing vasculitis of arterioles and capillaries in many parts of the brain. Microinfarcts of brain tissues may be apparent. In some patients abundant deposits of immunoglobulins and complement components occur at the basement membrane of vessels in the choroid plexus analogous to glomerular deposits of immune complexes. In other patients with SLE and neuropsychiatric manifestations no significant abnormalities are found histologically. The spleen shows marked intimal proliferation of penicillar and central arteries, which gives an "onion skin" appearance to these vessels. The heart valves and chordae tendineae have at times nonbacterial verrucous vegetations (Libman-Sacks endocarditis). Considerable narrowing of the coronary arteries has been found in some young women dying with SLE.

CLINICAL MANIFESTATIONS SLE is predominantly a disease of women (9 women to 1 man) in the second to fifth decades of life, but it spares neither children nor persons of advanced age. The prevalence of SLE is 2 to 3 per 100,000. Most recent estimates indicate that 77 percent of patients with SLE survive 5 years. The presence of renal disease and central nervous system involvement decrease survival. The most frequent causes of death are uremia, heart failure, hemorrhage, central nervous system disease, and intercurrent bacterial infections.

Patients with SLE may present with a variety of abnormalities, including arthritis and arthralgias, cutaneous manifestations, nephritis, fever, central nervous system manifestations, Raynaud's phenomenon, pleurisy, pericarditis, hemolytic anemia, leukopenia, or thrombocytopenia (Table 70-1).

The course of SLE is highly variable from patient to patient. The observations on outcome and prognosis are largely based on patient populations studied at medical centers and therefore would exclude patients with mild and uncomplicated disease. SLE is not always a fatal disease as was thought years ago.

Arthritis and *arthralgias* are the most frequent presenting as well as the most common complaints during the course of the illness. The arthralgias are fleeting; they involve the hands or feet and also large joints. Redness, warmth, tenderness, and synovial effusions are frequently present. However, deformities are rare, and the erosions so characteristic of rheumatoid arthritis are unusual. The synovial fluid white blood cell counts are relatively low (less than 3000 per cubic millimeter), and mononuclear cells predominate. Osteonecrosis may occur, in part because of therapy with corticosteroids. Profound muscle weakness and tenderness reflect myositis in a few patients.

Fever is frequent during the course of SLE. Fatigue, malaise, anorexia, and weight loss also occur. However, systemic complaints may be totally absent in some patients.

Cutaneous manifestations of SLE include a variety of lesions. A facial eruption, with butterfly distribution over the malar areas and bridge of the nose, consists of erythema and edema during the acute phase; atrophy and telangiectasia appear in chronic lesions. This characteristic rash occurs in about 40 percent of patients. Similar eruptions may occur in other parts of the body, particularly in the exposed areas. At times skin eruptions are precipitated or worsened by exposure to ultraviolet rays. Patchy alopecia occurs with similar frequency and may be overlooked unless sought under coiffures or wigs. Patients with SLE may have short broken hairs above the forehead, the so-called lupus hairs. Dermal vasculitis can be found in about 20 percent of patients, usually as small infarcts of the digital skin. In some patients only erythema due to excessively large or numerous capillaries around the digits and fingernails is seen. Ulcers may be encountered on nasal or oral mucous membranes. Other cutaneous manifestations include purpura, bullae, hives, and angioneurotic edema. Raynaud's phenomenon is seen in about one-fifth of patients with SLE.

Discoid lupus is a chronic skin ailment with lesions usually confined to the face, neck, arms, and scalp. Scaling is prominent, with atrophy, telangiectasia, and keratotic plugging. Deep scars remain when the lesions subside. Only a few of these patients go on to develop systemic lupus erythematosus. On the other hand, some patients with SLE also have discoid lesions.

Renal involvement is one of the most serious manifestations of SLE. Clinically detectable evidence of renal involvement is seen in about one-half of all patients with SLE. These abnormalities extend from minimal proteinuria and few red blood cell casts to massive hematuria, proteinuria, and frank nephrotic syndrome. In some patients renal involvement goes on to total renal failure; in others there is a course of exacerbations and remissions, with eventual renal failure. Some patients respond well to treatment or improve spontaneously, but minimal proteinuria and decreased creatinine clearance may persist as evidence of irreversible damage.

TABLE 70-1
Clinical manifestations during the course of systemic lupus erythematosus

Manifestation	*Cumulative percentage of patients*
Arthritis and arthralgias	92
Fever	84
Skin eruptions	72
Lymphadenopathy	59
Renal involvement	53
Anorexia, nausea, vomiting	53
Myalgia	48
Pleuritis	45
Central nervous system abnormalities	26

SOURCE: *After Dubois.*

The development of superimposed urinary tract infection should always be kept in mind, since these patients seem liable to such infections.

Cardiopulmonary abnormalities are moderately frequent in patients with SLE. Symptoms and signs of pericarditis or other cardiac abnormalities are encountered in almost 50 percent of them. Pericarditis may be the presenting complaint, with the usual physical and electrocardiographic findings. Tamponade due to SLE pericarditis is unusual. Myocarditis may occur. The nonbacterial verrucous endocarditis is rarely diagnosed clinically but should be suspected when new murmurs develop in the absence of infective endocarditis. Symptomatic or asymptomatic pleural involvement occurs in nearly half the patients. Patchy and transient parenchymal infiltrates have been noted, and occasionally severe lupus pneumonitis may occur. The cause of these abnormalities is not known, and they are difficult to distinguish from infiltrates caused by infections. Narrowing of the coronary arteries may lead to early and unsuspected death of some patients with SLE.

Neurologic manifestations represent another serious aspect of SLE. A variety of central nervous system manifestations has been noted in 20 to 50 percent of patients. Among these are convulsive disorders, followed in frequency by abnormalities in mental functions and cranial nerves and by transverse myelitis. Peripheral neuropathies are infrequent. Occasionally patients present with primarily mental dysfunction, e.g., emotional lability, psychosis, or organic brain syndrome, without other significant symptoms. Cerebrospinal fluid of patients with central nervous system involvement may show slight to moderate increase in protein concentration and mild increase in lymphocytes; usually these occur late in the disease. The electroencephalogram is abnormal, with diffuse nonspecific changes. The brain scan may show focal increased uptake of isotope during active central nervous system involvement. Computerized tomography may reveal infarcts due to cerebral vasculitis. The presence of antibodies to neuronal cells in cerebrospinal fluid has a high correlation with neuropsychiatric manifestations in SLE.

Lymph node enlargement occurs in many patients with SLE. Such abnormalities may be diffuse or local. Characteristically the nodes are not tender. Splenomegaly occurs in about 10 percent of patients. *Hepatomegaly* is found in about 25 percent of patients. Some elevation of hepatic enzymes may occur without pathologic changes in the liver. Lupoid hepatitis is a syndrome of chronic active hepatitis associated with positive tests for antibodies to nuclear antigens and extrahepatic manifestations (see Chap. 319).

LABORATORY FINDINGS A variety of abnormalities in *hematologic* and *immunologic* tests may be encountered in SLE (Table 70-2).

A mild, normochromic, normocytic *anemia* is seen frequently. Most likely this is the hypoproliferative anemia that accompanies many inflammatory processes. Less frequently patients have severe immune-hemolytic anemia that requires steroid therapy or splenectomy. *Leukopenia* is seen in over half the patients. The mechanisms for leukopenia and thrombocytopenia are not fully delineated, but intravascular immune complexes as well as antibodies directed to leukocytes and platelets may contribute to these abnormalities. A potentially serious but clinically infrequent problem is the occurrence of *clotting defects* due to antibodies to factors VII, IX, or X or to the presence of an inhibitor to prothrombin activation. Prior to a renal biopsy, the integrity of the clotting mechanism must be evaluated.

Urinalysis and renal function studies indicate that over half the patients with SLE have mild to severe damage to the kidneys. With early or focal glomerulonephritis the creatinine clearance may be normal, and only mild proteinuria and microscopic hematuria may exist. With more extensive renal involvement proteinuria may become significant (>0.5 g per day), and the urine sediment may contain abundant red and white blood cells and red blood cell casts as indicators of glomerular damage.

The serum albumin/globulin ratio becomes reversed because of an increase in immunoglobulins, particularly IgG. Serum electrophoresis reveals that the major elevation is in gamma globulin. Small amounts of cryoglobulins, reflecting the presence of immune complexes, may be present. The erythrocyte sedimentation rate (ESR) tends to be high in patients with active disease.

The most characteristic laboratory abnormalities in SLE are the autoantibodies. The presence of antibodies to nuclear antigens (ANA) in a patient with active SLE is almost a *sine qua non* for the diagnosis. The ANA are usually detected by rat or mouse liver sections (other tissues with nucleated cells may also be used); the test serum is applied to the tissue section, antibodies to nuclear antigens interact with the nuclei, other proteins are washed away, and the ANA are detected with an antiserum to human immunoglobulins (these antibodies are coupled with fluorescein isothiocyanate that permits their detection with appropriate microscopy). The ANA include antibodies to single-stranded DNA, double-stranded (native) DNA, deoxyribonucleoprotein, histones, nuclear ribonucleoprotein (abbreviated RNP), and the Sm antigen (an acidic nuclear protein). Patients with SLE also have antibodies to RNA, ribosomes, lysosomes, and other cytoplasmic constituents. Many of these antibodies persist even when the disease is quiescent, except that the titers of antibodies to native DNA tend to be higher during exacerbations of the disease. Antibodies to native DNA in high titers are most specific for SLE with a low prevalence in other disorders. Antibodies to the Sm antigen occur in about 20 percent of patients with SLE and are seldom seen in other rheumatic diseases. The lupus erythematosus cell test (LE cell test) is positive less frequently than the test for ANA because more antibodies are required for positivity. No practical reasons exist for ordering the LE cell test. The listed antibodies to nuclear antigens are not specific for SLE, but when three or more of these antibodies are present, the likelihood of SLE in a given patient is very high. In end-stage renal disease due to SLE, the tests for ANA may become negative. In normal individuals the prevalence of positive tests for ANA in relatively low titers increases with age.

During flare-ups of SLE the total serum hemolytic complement (expressed in 50 percent hemolytic units—CH_{50}) or individual components of complement are decreased owing to activation by immune complexes. Complement levels in some patients are decreased due to suppressed synthesis. The most frequently used measurements of complement components are the immunochemically determined C3 and C4 levels. These measurements are useful in following the response to therapy or for detecting exacerbations. Occasionally the complement levels remain low in spite of apparent full clinical remission; the reasons for this are not known. During clinically active disease, circulating immune complexes can be detected.

About 20 percent of patients with SLE develop positive tests for rheumatoid factors, but the titers tend to be lower than in rheumatoid arthritis. False-positive tests for syphilis are encountered, at times prior to clinical onset of SLE. Antibodies to nuclear antigens occur in many other diseases (rheumatoid arthritis, 20 percent; Sjögren's syndrome, 60 percent; scleroderma, 40 percent) and are induced by several drugs (see below).

TABLE 70-2
Laboratory abnormalities in systemic lupus erythematosus

Abnormality	*Percent of patients*
HEMATOLOGIC	
Anemia (Hb < 11 g/dl)	72
Leukopenia (WBC < 4500/mm³)	61
Thrombocytopenia (platelets < 100,000/mm³)	15
Positive direct Coombs test	14
Circulating anticoagulants	Rare
IMMUNOLOGIC	
Positive tests for ANA	99
Positive LE cell tests	60–80
Hypocomplementemia	75
Increased gamma globulin (> 1.5 g/dl)	60–77
Positive tests for rheumatoid factors	20
Biologic false-positive tests for syphilis	15

DIAGNOSIS The possibility of SLE should be considered in any young or middle-aged female in the presence of three or four of the symptoms or signs listed in Table 70-1 or in the presence of glomerulonephritis, hemolytic anemia, leukopenia, or thrombocytopenia. A positive test for ANA is essential for diagnosis. Other diseases that cause positive tests for ANA must be considered, and they must often be excluded on the basis of clinical observations alone. Major consideration must be given to rheumatoid arthritis, scleroderma, Sjögren's syndrome, and the history of ingestion of drugs that might have induced a positive test for ANA. The mixed connective tissue disease (see Chap. 362) is distinguished from SLE by sclerodermatous skin changes, active myositis, lack of significant glomerulonephritis, and cerebritis. The finding of very high titers of antibodies to nuclear ribonucleoprotein is the most helpful distinguishing characteristic. SLE is distinguished from scleroderma by the absence of the sclerodermatous skin changes and of fibrosis of internal organs, the presence of skin lesions typical of SLE, of renal disease, and of the serological findings described above. Rheumatoid arthritis is clinically characterized by persistent and often symmetrical joint involvement and absence of skin, kidney, and brain involvement. Immunologic tests can further serve to distinguish these disorders. Patients with SLE presenting principally with arthralgias and arthritis are most often not immediately diagnosed. Thrombocytopenia, hemolytic anemia, and psychosis are other presenting manifestations that may lead to erroneous diagnosis. In these groups of patients initial tests for ANA which, if positive, are followed by tests for antibodies to double-stranded DNA are useful in identifying patients with SLE along with diligent search for involvement of other organ systems characteristic of SLE. A positive test for ANA alone should never serve as the basis for the diagnosis of SLE.

Drug-induced SLE Hydralazine and procainamide induce a syndrome similar to SLE in some patients. This syndrome includes arthralgias, arthritis, myalgias, pleurisy, pericarditis, fever, skin eruptions, lymphadenopathy, and positive tests for ANA. Renal disease and central nervous system involvement are very unusual in drug-induced SLE. Prospective studies have shown that about 70 percent of patients receiving procainamide develop positive tests for ANA within weeks or months. A much smaller proportion become symptomatic. Once the drug is discontinued, the symptoms abate in a few weeks but occasionally may smolder on for months; recovery may be hastened by treatment with corticosteroids. The ANA tests revert to negative in a few months. Isoniazid alone or with *p*-aminosalicylic acid (PAS), several anticonvulsants (Dilantin, Mesantoin), phenothiazine derivatives, γ-methyldopa, and levodopa have also been associated with positive tests for ANA. In these patients the positive test for ANA is due to antibodies to histones, but similar antibodies occur also in idiopathic SLE. In some patients the administration of sulfonamides, penicillin, and oral contraceptives has been associated with exacerbations of SLE.

TREATMENT A cure for SLE is not available. However, abundant experience indicates that appropriate therapy may suppress flare-ups and prolong life. The optimal treatment programs for various manifestations of SLE have not been defined. Adequately designed studies have been difficult to perform because of the variability in the manifestations and course of the disease and the lack of adequate prognostic parameters. Corticosteroids remain the cornerstone of therapy, even though the "immunosuppressive" drugs seem to be helpful in some patients.

Arthralgias, arthritis, myalgias, and fever may respond adequately to rest and salicylates. Antimalarials have been used successfully for the same symptoms, as well as for control of skin eruptions. Chloroquine was used widely, but potential retinal toxicity has decreased its usage. Hydroxychloroquine in small dosages (200 mg per day) seems safe, but the patient should be cautioned about potential toxicity, and careful examination by an ophthalmologist should be conducted at least twice a year. Exposure to ultraviolet light should be avoided, particularly with active and recurrent skin lesions. If skin involvement becomes debilitating and does not respond to conservative therapy, corticosteroids in small to moderate doses should provide relief.

Central nervous system involvement, pericarditis, myocarditis, pleurisy, severe myositis, severe hemolytic anemia, clotting problems, significant leukopenia, and thrombocytopenia are indications for use of corticosteroids. In desperate situations, particularly in central nervous system involvement with seizures or psychosis, relatively high doses should be used (even up to 2 mg prednisone or prednisolone per kilogram of body weight). With central nervous system involvement a high (60 mg or more per day) dose of prednisone should be used up to about 2 weeks. Once improvement has occurred, the dose should be tapered and adjusted to maintain control of other symptoms. If no improvement occurs in the central nervous system manifestations, the dose should be rapidly reduced to levels that control the other manifestations of SLE. Many of the above manifestations can be controlled with 10 mg prednisone or less per day as a maintenance dose. If a flare-up occurs and is recognized by the patient and the physician, only a moderate (5 to 10 mg) increase of the prednisone dose may provide control of symptoms. Careful follow-up of patients, with judicious use of laboratory tests, is essential in treatment of the above manifestations of SLE. In the use of corticosteroids the side effects, such as increased risk of infections and osteopenia, must always be considered in relation to the anticipated benefits.

Several approaches to the treatment of SLE nephritis have been advocated, but no currently available program is useful in all patients. Renal biopsy is recommended for establishing the nature of glomerular lesions, since those with focal lupus glomerulonephritis respond to treatment well or improve spontaneously. Perhaps the most useful program is to start with 40 to 60 mg prednisone or prednisolone per day until all clinical symptoms have abated. This may take a few weeks; the urinary sediment should improve, and complement should return toward normal. Thereafter the steroid dose should be reduced gradually to the minimal dose to keep the patient free of symptoms. With severe focal involvement and with diffuse lupus glomerulonephritis or membranous glomerulonephritis, higher doses (up to 150 to 200 mg prednisone or prednisolone) have been tried and found helpful for some patients, with subsequent improvement of renal function. However, the diffuse and membranous lesions do not respond well. In some patients encouraging results have been noted with pulse therapy, using 1 g of intravenous methylprednisolone on three successive days. Other investigators have added azathioprine (1 to 2 mg per kilogram of body weight) or cyclophosphamide (100 to 150 mg per day) to prednisone. Cyclophosphamide and prednisone appear to be the most effective combination, but many serious side effects are encountered, including marrow toxicity, hemorrhagic cystitis, alopecia, and sterility; their long-term risks are not fully known. Cytotoxic drugs for treatment of SLE have not been approved by the Food and Drug Administration. The search for better combinations of drugs and new medications for treatment of severe SLE continues.

Plasmapheresis in conjunction with corticosteroids and cyclophosphamide has been beneficial in some severely ill patients with SLE who have not responded to other therapy. More information is needed to evaluate the efficacy of this expensive therapeutic intervention.

Any intercurrent infections must be recognized and treated with appropriate therapy. Patients with SLE, either because of their disease or as a consequence of treatment, are liable to bacterial infections, which are a leading cause of death among them.

Exacerbations of SLE tend to occur during the third trimester of pregnancy or in the immediate postpartum period. Nevertheless, many patients with SLE can be carried to term and successful delivery with appropriate therapy. Therefore, SLE is not an absolute indication for therapeutic abortion, but the procedure may be necessary during life-threatening active disease.

REFERENCES

Appel GB et al: Renal involvement in systemic lupus erythematosus (SLE): A study of 56 patients emphasizing histologic classification. Medicine 57:371, 1978

Bluestein HG et al: Cerebrospinal fluid antibodies to neuronal cells: Association with neuropsychiatric manifestations of systemic lupus erythematosus. Am J Med 70:240, 1981

Dubois EL (ed): *Lupus Erythematosus,* 2d ed. Los Angeles, University of Southern California Press, 1974

Jones JV et al: The role of therapeutic plasmapheresis in the rheumatic diseases. J Lab Clin Med 97:589, 1981

Kant KS et al: Glomerular thrombosis in systemic lupus erythematosus: Prevalence and significance. Medicine 60:71, 1981

Kimberly RP et al: High-dose intravenous methylprednisolone pulse therapy in systemic lupus erythematosus. Am J Med 70:817, 1981

Kunkel HG: The immunopathology of SLE. Hosp Prac 15:47, 1980

Lafer EM et al: Polyspecific monoclonal lupus autoantibodies reactive with both polynucleotides and phospholipids. J Exp Med 153:897, 1981

Lloyd W, Schur PH: Immune complexes, complement, and anti-DNA in exacerbations of systemic lupus erythematosus (SLE). Medicine 60:208, 1981

Notman DD et al: Profiles of antinuclear antibodies in systemic rheumatic diseases. Ann Intern Med 83:464, 1975

71
PRINCIPLES OF DRUG THERAPY

JOHN A. OATES
GRANT R. WILKINSON

QUANTITATIVE DETERMINANTS OF DRUG ACTION

Safe and effective therapy with drugs requires their delivery to target tissues in concentrations within the narrow range that yields efficacy without toxicity. Optimal precision in achieving concentrations of drug within this therapeutic "window" can be achieved with regimens that are based on the kinetics of the drug's availability to target sites. This chapter deals with the principles of drug elimination and distribution that form the basis for loading and maintenance regimens for the average patient and considers instances in which elimination of the drug is impaired (e.g., renal failure). The kinetic basis for optimal utilization of plasma level data is also discussed.

PLASMA LEVELS AFTER A SINGLE DOSE The levels of lidocaine in plasma following intravenous administration decline in two phases as illustrated in Fig. 71-1; such a biphasic decline is typical for many drugs. Immediately following rapid injection, essentially all of the drug is in the plasma compartment, and the high initial plasma level reflects its confinement to this small volume. Subsequently, the drug is distributed from plasma into the extravascular compartment, and the period of time during which this is occurring is referred to as the *distribution phase.* For lidocaine this distribution phase is virtually complete within 30 min; then there is a slower rate of fall, referred to as the *equilibrium phase* or the *elimination phase.* During this latter phase, the drug levels in plasma and those in the tissues of the body are in pseudoequilibrium.

Distribution phase Pharmacological events during the distribution phase depend on whether the level of drug at the receptor site closely reflects that in the plasma. If this is the case, the pharmacological effects, whether favorable or adverse, may be inordinately great during this period. For example, following a small bolus dose (50 mg) of lidocaine, antiarrhythmic effects may be evident during the early distribution phase but disappear as levels rapidly fall below those that are minimally effective and even before equilibrium between plasma and tissue is reached. Thus, larger single doses or multiple small doses must be administered in order to achieve an effect that is sustained into the equilibrium phase. The toxicity of high levels of some drugs during the distribution phase precludes administration of a single intravenous loading dose that will achieve therapeutic levels during the equilibrium phase. For example, the administration of a loading dose of the anticonvulsant, phenytoin (diphenylhydantoin), as a single intravenous bolus can cause cardiovascular collapse due to the high levels during the distribution phase. For this reason, if a loading dose of phenytoin is administered intravenously, it must be given in fractions at intervals sufficient to permit substantial distribution of the prior dose before the next is given (for example, 100 mg every 3 to 5 min). For similar reasons, the loading dose of many potent drugs that rapidly equilibrate with their receptors is divided into fractional doses for intravenous administration.

After an oral dose that delivers an equivalent amount of drug into the systemic circulation, plasma levels during the distribution phase do not rise nearly as steeply as they do after an intravenous bolus dose. Because the drug is not absorbed instantly after oral administration, it is delivered into the systemic circulation more slowly, and much of the drug is already distributed by the time absorption is complete. Thus, procainamide, which is almost totally absorbed after oral administration, can be given as a single 750-mg loading dose with little risk of hypotension; in contrast, loading of the drug by the intravenous route is more safely accomplished by giving the loading dose in fractions of about 100 mg at 5-min intervals in order to avoid the hypotension that would ensue during the distribution phase in some patients if the entire loading dose were given as a single bolus.

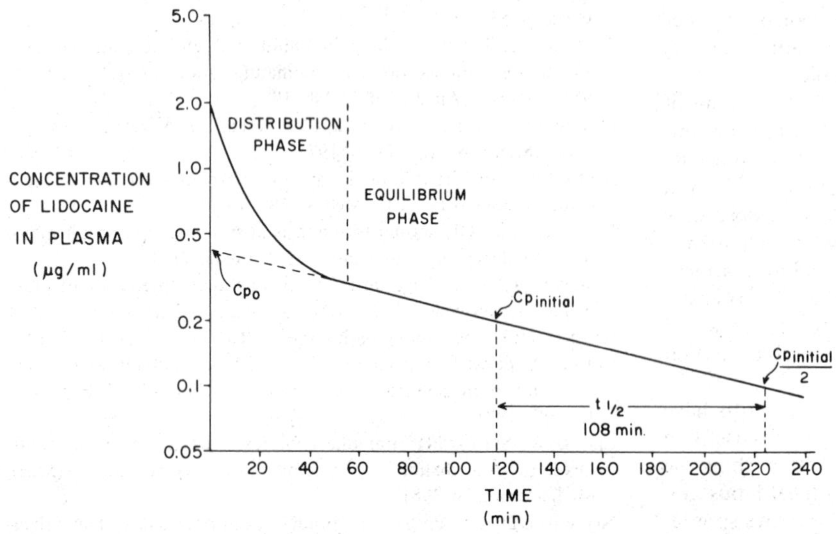

FIGURE 71-1
Concentrations of lidocaine in plasma following the administration of 50 mg intravenously. The half-life of 108 min is computed as the time required for levels to fall from any given value during the equilibrium phase ($Cp_{initial}$) to one-half that level. Cp_0 is the hypothetical concentration of lidocaine in plasma at time zero if equilibrium had been achieved instantly.

In contrast, other drugs are distributed to their sites of action only slowly during the distribution phase. For example, levels of digoxin at the receptor site (and its pharmacological effect) do not reflect plasma levels during the distribution phase. Digoxin is transported (or bound) to its cardiac receptors more slowly by a process that proceeds throughout distribution. Thus, plasma levels during a distribution phase of several hours are falling while levels at the site of action and pharmacological effect are increasing. Only at the end of the distribution phase when the drug has reached equilibrium with the receptor does the concentration of digoxin in plasma reflect pharmacological effect. For this reason, there should be a 6- to 8-h wait after the distribution phase before samples are obtained for plasma levels of digoxin that are to be used as a guide to therapy.

Equilibrium phase After distribution has proceeded to the point where the concentration of drug in plasma is in equilibrium with that in the tissues outside the vascular compartment, the levels in plasma and tissues fall in parallel as the drug is eliminated from the body. Thus, the equilibrium phase is sometimes also referred to as the *elimination phase.*

Most drugs are eliminated as a first-order process. During the equilibrium phase, a characteristic of the first-order process is that the time required for the level of drug in plasma to fall to one-half the original value (the half-life, $t_{\frac{1}{2}}$) will be the same regardless of which point on the plasma level curve is chosen as a starting point for the measurement. Another characteristic of the first-order process is that a plot of the concentrations in plasma versus time during the equilibrium phase is linear on a semilogarithmic graph. From such a plot (Fig. 71-1) it can be seen that the half-life of lidocaine is 108 min.

One can readily calculate what amount of the administered dose remains in the body at any multiple of the half-life interval following administration:

Number of half-lives	*Amount of dose remaining in the body, %*
1	50
2	25
3	12.5
4	6.25
5	3.125

In theory, the elimination process never reaches completion. From a clinical standpoint, however, elimination can be considered as being essentially complete when it has reached 90 percent. Therefore, for practical purposes, *a first-order elimination process can be said to reach completion after 3 to 4 half-lives.*

DRUG ACCUMULATION—LOADING AND MAINTENANCE DOSES With repeated administration of a drug, the amount in the body will accumulate if the elimination of the first dose is incomplete when the second dose is given, and both the amount of drug in the body and its pharmacological effect will increase with continuing administration until they reach a plateau. The accumulation of digoxin administered in repeated maintenance doses (without a loading dose) is illustrated in Fig. 71-2. As digoxin's half-life is about 1.6 days in a patient with normal renal function, 65 percent of digoxin remains in the body at the end of 1 day. Thus, the second dose will raise the amount of digoxin in the body (and average plasma level) to 165 percent of that following the first dose. Each subsequent dose will result in greater amounts in the body until a plateau is attained. At the plateau, or *steady state,* drug intake per unit of time is the same as the rate of drug elimination. For *all* drugs with first-order kinetics, the time required to accumulate to steady-state levels can be predicted from the half-life because accumulation also is a first-order process with a half-life identical to that for elimination. Hence, accumulation will reach 90 percent of steady-state levels at the end of 3 to 4 half-lives. For digoxin, with a half-life of 1.6 days (with normal renal function), accumulation thus will be practically complete in 5 days. Continuing infusion of a drug at a constant rate also will result in progressive accumulation to a steady state over a time course predictable from the elimination curve for that drug (Fig. 71-3).

When the time required to reach steady-state levels is longer than one wishes to wait, plasma levels may be achieved more rapidly by the administration of a *loading dose.* Loading entails the administration of an amount that will bring the concentration in plasma (at equilibrium) to the level present during steady state. This may be accomplished by the administration of the loading amount as a single dose, or in the case of drugs with low therapeutic indexes (the therapeutic index is the ratio of the toxic dose to the therapeutic dose) the loading amount is given in a series of fractions of the total loading amount. As the accumulation of procainamide to 90 percent of steady state by infusion would require approximately 10 h (the

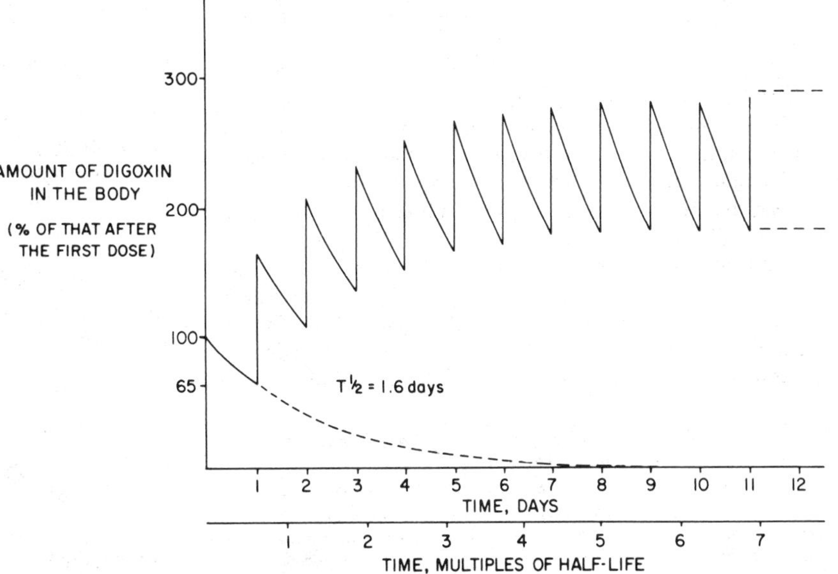

FIGURE 71-2
The time course of digoxin accumulation when a single daily maintenance dose is given without a loading dose. Note that accumulation is more than 90 percent complete by the end of 4 half-lives.

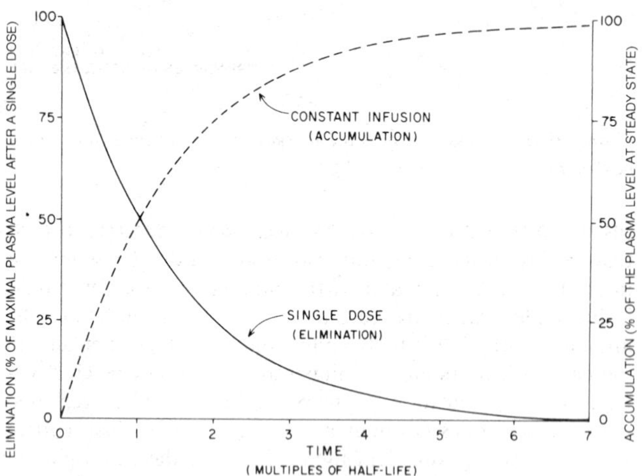

FIGURE 71-3
The time course of plasma levels of a drug following a single intravenous dose (——) compared with those during a constant intravenous infusion (----). This relationship applies to all drugs that rapidly achieve equilibrium between plasma and tissues.

$t_{\frac{1}{2}}$ is 3 h), a loading regimen is almost always desirable. The load required to suppress an arrhythmia, however, varies among individuals from 300 to 1000 mg, and rapid intravenous administration of the *average loading dose* would cause hypotension during the high plasma levels in the distribution phase in some patients. Therefore, the intravenous loading dose of procainamide is given in fractions (e.g., 100 mg every 5 min) until the arrhythmia is controlled or adverse effects such as hypotension indicate that no further drug should be given. Dividing the loading dose into fractions is appropriate for most drugs that, like procainamide, have a low therapeutic index. This permits better individualization of the loading amount and avoids needless adverse effects that might occur during the distribution phase of a single large dose.

The size of loading dose required to achieve the plasma levels present at steady state can be determined from the fraction of drug eliminated during the dosage interval and the maintenance dose (in the case of intermittent drug administration). For example, if the fraction of digoxin eliminated daily is 35 percent and the planned maintenance dose is to be 0.25 mg daily, then the loading dose to achieve steady-state levels should be 100/35 times the maintenance dose, or approximately 0.75 mg. Thus,

$$\text{Loading dose} = \frac{100}{\begin{array}{c}\text{\% of drug eliminated}\\ \text{per dosage interval}\end{array}} \times \text{maintenance dose}$$

The fraction of drug eliminated during any dosage interval can be determined from a semilogarithmic graph, in which the total amount in the body at time zero is set at 100 percent and the fraction remaining at the end of 1 half-life is 50 percent.[1] Conversely, if the loading dose is known, the maintenance dose can be similarly calculated.

Regardless of the size of the loading dose, *after maintenance therapy has been given for 3 to 4 half-lives, the amount of drug in the body is determined only by the maintenance dose.* The independence of the plasma levels at steady state from the load is illustrated in Fig. 71-3, which indicates that the elimination of any drug (elimination curve) would be practically complete after 3 to 4 half-lives.

DETERMINANTS OF PLASMA LEVELS DURING THE EQUILIBRIUM PHASE An important determinant of the level of drug in plasma during the equilibrium phase after a single dose is the extent to which the drug has distributed outside the plasma compartment. For example, if the distribution of a 3-mg dose of a large macromolecule is confined to a plasma volume of 3 liters, then the concentration in plasma will be 1 mg per liter. However, if a different drug is distributed so that 90 percent of it leaves the plasma compartment, then only 0.3 mg will remain in the 3-liter plasma volume, and the concentration in plasma will be only 0.1 mg per liter. The extent of extravascular distribution at equilibrium can be expressed by the term *apparent volume of distribution,* or V_d. More precisely, V_d expresses the constant relationship between the amount of drug in the body and the plasma concentration at equilibrium:

$$V_d = \frac{\text{amount of drug in body}}{\text{plasma concentration}}$$

The amount of drug in the body is expressed as mass (e.g., milligrams), and the plasma concentration is expressed as mass per volume (e.g., milligrams per liter). Thus V_d is a hypothetical volume into which a quantity of drug would distribute if its concentration in the entire volume were the same as that in plasma. Although it does not represent a real volume, it is an important quantity because it determines the fraction of total drug which is in the plasma and therefore the fraction available to the organs of elimination. An approximation of V_d in the equilibrium phase can be obtained by estimating the concentration of drug in plasma at time zero (Cp_0) by back-extrapolation of the equilibrium phase plot to zero time as illustrated in Fig. 71-1. Then, after intravenous administration when the amount in the body at time zero is the dose, we have

$$V_d = \frac{\text{dose}}{Cp_0}$$

For the administration of the large macromolecule mentioned above, the measured Cp_0 of 1 mg per liter after a 3-mg dose indicates a V_d that is a real volume, the plasma volume. This example is the exception, however, for the V_d of most drugs does not relate to any real volume; many drugs are so extensively taken up by cells that cellular levels greatly exceed those in plasma water. For such drugs, the hypothetical V_d will be large, even greater than the volume of body water. For example, Fig. 71-1 indicates that the Cp_0 obtained by extrapolation following 50 mg lidocaine is 0.42 mg per liter, yielding a V_d by the above equation of 119 liters.

As elimination is carried out largely by individual organs such as the kidney and liver, it is useful to consider the elimination of drugs by these organs according to the *clearance* concept. For example, in the kidney, regardless of the extent to which removal of drug is determined by filtration, secretion, or reabsorption, the net result is that drug removal results in a reduction of the concentration of drug in plasma as it passes through the organ. The extent to which the concentration is reduced is expressed as the *extraction ratio,* or *E,* which is constant as long as first-order elimination occurs.

$$E = \frac{C_a - C_v}{C_a}$$

where C_a = arterial plasma concentration
C_v = venous plasma concentration

If the extraction is complete, $E = 1$. If the total plasma flow to the kidneys is Q (ml/min), the total volume of plasma from

[1] *Alternatively, the fraction of drug lost from the body during a dosage interval can be determined nongraphically from this equation*

$$\textit{Fraction of drug lost from body} = 1 - e^{-kt}$$

Values for e^{-kt} can be obtained from a table of natural exponential functions or by a calculator, where k ($= 0.693/t_{\frac{1}{2}}$) is the fractional elimination constant (described in the next section) and t is the time interval after drug administration.

which drug is completely removed in a unit time (clearance) is determined as

$$\mathrm{Cl}_{\mathrm{renal}} = QE$$

If the renal extraction ratio of penicillin is 0.5 and renal plasma flow is 680 ml/min, then penicillin's renal clearance will be 340 ml/min. If the extraction ratio of a compound is high, as is the case for renal extraction of *p*-aminohippuric acid (PAH) or hepatic extraction of propranolol, then clearance becomes primarily a function of organ blood flow.[2]

Clearance from the total body (Cl) is the sum of clearance from all organs of elimination and is the best measure of the efficiency of the elimination processes. If a drug is removed by both renal excretion and hepatic metabolism, then

$$\mathrm{Cl} = \mathrm{Cl}_{\mathrm{renal}} + \mathrm{Cl}_{\mathrm{hepatic}}$$

Thus, if penicillin is eliminated by both renal clearance (340 ml/min) and hepatic clearance (36 ml/min) in a normal individual, total clearance will be 376 ml/min. If renal clearance is reduced to half, total clearance = 170 + 36 = 206 ml/min. In anuria, total clearance will equal hepatic clearance.

Only the drug in the vascular compartment can be cleared during each passage through an organ. To ascertain the effect of a given plasma clearance by one or more organs on the rate of removal of drug from the body, the clearance must be related to the volume of "plasma equivalents" to be cleared, that is, the volume of distribution. If the volume of distribution is 10,000 ml and clearance is 1000 ml/min, then one-tenth of the drug in the body is eliminated per minute. This fraction, Cl/V_d, is known as a *fractional elimination constant* and is designated as k:

$$k = \frac{\mathrm{Cl}}{V_d}$$

If the fraction k is multiplied by the total amount of drug in the body, the actual rate of elimination at any given time can be determined:

$$\text{Rate of elimination} = k \times \text{amount in body} = \mathrm{Cl}Cp$$

This is the general equation for all first-order processes and expresses the fact that rate is proportional to the declining quantity in a first-order process.

As half-life is a temporal expression of the exponential first-order process, half-life ($t_{\frac{1}{2}}$) can be related to k as follows:

$$t_{\frac{1}{2}} = \frac{0.693}{k}$$

$$\text{Because} \quad k = \frac{\mathrm{Cl}}{V_d}$$

$$\text{then} \quad t_{\frac{1}{2}} = \frac{0.693V_d}{\mathrm{Cl}}$$

As will be seen in the following discussion on drug dosage in renal failure, the linear relationship of k to creatinine clearance makes k a more useful parameter upon which to base calculations of the changes in drug elimination that occur with a known reduction in creatinine clearance in renal insufficiency. Half-life is not linearly related to clearance.

The important relationship

$$t_{\frac{1}{2}} = \frac{0.693V_d}{\mathrm{Cl}}$$

expresses clearly that half-life is determined by both clearance and volume of distribution. Thus, for example, half-life is shortened when phenobarbital induces the enzymes responsible for hepatic clearance of a drug, and half-life is lengthened when a drug's renal clearance is attenuated in renal failure. Also, the half-life of some drugs is shortened when their volume of distribution is reduced. If, as in the case of cardiac failure, the volume of distribution is reduced at the same time that clearance is reduced, there may be little change in drug half-life to reflect the impaired clearance, but plasma levels will be increased, as is the case with lidocaine. In treating patients after an overdose, expectations of how hemodialysis will affect the drug's elimination are dependent on its volume of distribution. When the volume of distribution is very large, as is the case with tricyclic antidepressants (V_d of desipramine equals more than 2000 liters), the removal of drug, even with a high-clearance dialyzer, will proceed slowly.

The extent to which a drug is bound to plasma protein also determines the fraction of drug extracted by the organ(s) of elimination. Altered binding will change the extraction ratio significantly, however, only when elimination is limited to the unbound (free) drug in plasma. The extent to which binding influences elimination depends on the relative affinity of the plasma binding versus the affinity of the drug for the extraction process. The high affinity of the renal tubular anion transport system for many drugs will lead to extraction of both bound and unbound drug, and the efficient process by which the liver removes propranolol will result in extraction of most of this highly bound drug from blood.

STEADY STATE With a constant infusion of drug, the infusion rate equals elimination rate at steady state. Therefore,

$$\underset{(\text{amt/unit time})}{\text{Infusion rate}} = \underset{(\text{amt/vol})}{Cp} \times \underset{(\text{vol/unit time})}{\mathrm{Cl}}$$

when the units for amount, volume, and time are consistent.

Thus, if clearance (Cl) is known, the infusion rate required to achieve a given plasma level can be calculated. An approach to estimating the clearance of a number of drugs is discussed below in the section on renal disease.

When the dose is given intermittently instead of by infusion, the above relationship between plasma concentration and the dose administered at each dosage interval can be expressed as

$$\text{Dose} = Cp_{\mathrm{av}} \times \mathrm{Cl} \times \text{dosage interval}$$

The average plasma concentration (Cp_{av}) implies that, as seen in Fig. 71-2, levels can be considerably higher and lower than the average during the dosage interval.

When a drug is given orally, only a fraction (F) of the administered dose may reach the systemic circulation. This is termed *bioavailability* and may reflect a poorly formulated dosage form that fails to disintegrate or dissolve in the gastrointestinal fluids. Regulatory standards have, however, significantly reduced the extent of this particular type of problem. Drug interactions also can impair absorption after oral dosing. Bioavailability may also be reduced due to drug metabolism in the gastrointestinal tract and/or the liver during the overall absorption process, the *first-pass effect.* This is a particular problem for drugs which are extensively extracted by these organs, and considerable interpatient variability often exists in bioavailability. Lidocaine is not administered orally for the control of arrhythmias because of the first-pass effect. It is also possible for drugs that are injected intramuscularly to have a low bioavailability, e.g., phenytoin. An unexpected drug re-

[2] *When drug is present in the formed elements of blood, then calculation of extraction and clearance from blood is more physiologically meaningful than from the plasma.*

sponse in a patient should always lead to consideration of bioavailability as a possible factor. Calculation of a dosage regimen should be corrected for bioavailability:

$$\frac{\text{Oral}}{\text{dose}} = \frac{Cp_{av} \times \text{Cl} \times \text{dosage interval}}{F}$$

DRUG ELIMINATION THAT IS NOT FIRST-ORDER The elimination of some important drugs such as phenytoin, salicylate, and theophylline does not follow first-order kinetics when amounts of drug in the body are in the therapeutic range. For these drugs, the clearance is not a constant value but changes as levels in the body fall during elimination or after changes in dose. This pattern of elimination is said to be *dose-dependent.* Accordingly, the time for the concentration to fall to one-half becomes less as plasma levels fall; this halving-time is not truly a half-life, however, because the term *half-life* applies to first-order kinetics and is a constant. The elimination of phenytoin is dose-dependent, and when very high levels are present (in the toxic range), the halving time may be longer than 72 h, whereas after the concentration in plasma has declined to lower levels, the clearance increases and the concentration in plasma will halve in 20 to 30 h. When drug is eliminated by first-order kinetics, the plasma level at steady state is directly related to the amount of the maintenance dose, and a doubling of the dose should lead to doubling of the steady-state plasma level. However, for phenytoin and other drugs with dose-dependent kinetics, increases in the dose may be accompanied by disproportionately large increases in plasma level. Thus, if the daily dose of phenytoin is increased from 300 to 400 mg, plasma levels rise by considerably more than 33 percent. Unfortunately, the extent of increase is not predictable because of the wide interpatient variability in the extent to which clearance deviates from first order. Salicylates are also eliminated by dose-dependent kinetics at high plasma levels, and in children particular caution must be taken with the administration of high doses. Ethanol metabolism also is dose-dependent, with obvious implications. The mechanisms involved in dose-dependent kinetics may include the saturation of the rate-limiting step in metabolism or a feedback inhibition of the rate-limiting enzyme by a product of the reaction.

INDIVIDUALIZATION OF DRUG THERAPY

Recognition of factors modifying drug action is essential for therapy that provides optimal benefit with minimal risk to each individual patient. Certain disease states can modify the delivery of a drug to its site of action.

ALTERATION OF DRUG DOSAGE IN RENAL DISEASE Where urinary excretion is an important route of elimination, renal failure results in decreased drug clearance and therefore slower removal of the drug from the body, so that administration according to the usual dosage regimen leads to greater accumulation and an increased likelihood of toxicity. A reasonable therapeutic goal in such cases is to modify the dosage schedule so that the average drug concentration in the plasma of the patient with renal insufficiency is the same, and steady state is reached after a similar time interval, as in the patient with normal renal function. This is particularly appropriate for drugs with long half-lives and narrow therapeutic indexes (e.g., digoxin).

One approach to dosage alteration in renal insufficiency is to calculate the *fraction of the normal dose* that is to be given at the usual dosage interval. This fraction can be determined from data on either drug clearance (Cl) or the fractional rate constant (k), based on the fact that both renal clearance and renal k are directly proportional to creatinine clearance (Cl_{cr}). Creatine clearance is best determined directly. However, serum creatinine (C_{cr}) may be used to estimate the value by the following equation which is applicable to male patients:

$$\text{Cl}_{cr} = \frac{(140 - \text{age}) \times \text{weight (kg)}}{72 \times C_{cr}\ (\text{mg/dl})}\ (\text{ml/min})$$

For females, the value should be reduced to 85 percent of that estimated by this equation. This approach to estimation of Cl_{cr} is invalid in gross renal insufficiency ($C_{cr} > 5$ mg/dl) or changing renal function.

The clearance approach Calculation of drug dosage is most accurately based on the clearance of a drug because this is a direct measure of drug removal. From data on the clearance of a drug, the dose in renal insufficiency (Dose_{ri}) may be calculated as follows:

$$\text{Dose}_{ri} = \text{Dose} \times \frac{\text{Cl}_{ri}}{\text{Cl}}$$

where ri = renal insufficiency
Cl = clearance from the whole body with normal renal function
Cl_{ri} = clearance from the whole body with renal insufficiency
Dose = maintenance dose with normal renal function ($\text{Cl}_{cr} \sim 100$ ml/min)

The normal clearance and that in renal impairment can be obtained by employing the data in Table 71-1 in the following equations:

$$\text{Cl} = \text{Cl}_{renal} + \text{Cl}_{nonrenal}$$

$$\text{Cl}_{ri} = \text{Cl}_{renal} \times \frac{\text{measured Cl}_{cr}}{100\ \text{ml/min}} + \text{Cl}_{nonrenal}$$

As the Cl_{renal} values in Table 71-1 are those found with $\text{Cl}_{cr} = 100$ ml/min, then the renal clearance of drug in renal insufficiency is obtained by multiplying Cl_{renal} by the ratio of measured Cl_{cr} (in milliliters per minute) to 100 ml/min.

For gentamicin, with a normal Cl_{renal} of 78 ml/min and $\text{Cl}_{nonrenal}$ of 3 ml/min, Cl = 81 ml/min. Therefore, with a Cl_{cr} of 12 ml/min, $\text{Cl}_{ri} = 78 \times (12/100) + 3 = 12.4$ ml/min. If the dose of gentamicin for a given infection should be 1.5 mg/kg per 8 h in the presence of normal renal function, then

$$\text{Dose}_{ri} = \frac{1.5\ \text{mg/kg}}{8\ \text{h}} \times \frac{12.4\ \text{ml/min}}{81\ \text{ml/min}} = \frac{0.23\ \text{mg/kg}}{8\ \text{h}}$$

TABLE 71-1
Clearance of drugs

Drug	*Renal clearance,* ml/min*	*Nonrenal clearance, ml/min*
Ampicillin†	340	12
Carbenicillin	68	10
Digoxin†	110	36
Gentamicin	78	3
Kanamycin	60	0
Penicillin G‡	340	36

* *The "normal" renal clearances are those associated with a clearance of creatinine of 100 ml/min.*
† *The fraction of digoxin absorbed after an oral dose (F) is approximately 0.75 and F for ampicillin is 0.5.*
‡ *One microgram of penicillin G = 1.6 units.*

In the patient with renal insufficiency, this computation will yield an average plasma level during a dosage interval that is the same as the average plasma level during the dosage interval with normal renal function; the fluctuations between peaks and troughs, however, will be less pronounced.

In some instances it may be desirable to calculate a dose that will yield a certain plasma level at steady state. This approach is most appropriate for constant intravenous infusions where 100 percent of the dose is delivered to the systemic circulation. When clearance of a drug in a patient with renal insufficiency is calculated as above, then

$$\underset{\text{(amt/unit time)}}{\text{Dose}_{ri}} = \underset{\text{(vol/unit time)}}{\text{Cl}_{ri}} \times \underset{\text{(amt/vol)}}{Cp}$$

where the time, amount, and volume terms are uniform.

If a plasma concentration of carbenicillin of 100 μg/ml is the therapeutic objective in a patient with a creatinine clearance of 25 ml/min, the infusion rate is calculated as follows. Carbenicillin clearance is

$$\text{Cl}_{ri} = 68 \times \frac{25}{100} + 10 = 27 \text{ ml/min}$$

Therefore, carbenicillin should be infused at a rate of 2700 μg/min.

Should the method of calculating dose based on the desired plasma level be applied to intermittent-dose therapy, particular attention should be given to the fact that the calculation is based on an *average* plasma level and that peak plasma levels will obviously be higher. In addition, if a drug is given orally and is not completely absorbed, the computed dose must be divided by the fraction of drug which reaches the systemic circulation following oral administration (F) (see "Steady State" above).

The fractional rate constant (k) approach For many drugs, clearance data in renal failure are not available. In these cases, the fraction of the normal dose that is required in a patient with renal failure can be approximated from the ratio of the fractional rate constant for elimination from the body in renal failure (k_{ri}) to that with normal renal function (k). This approach requires the assumption that the distribution of the drug (V_d) is not affected by renal disease. The approach is the same as that employed with clearance data:

$$\text{Dose}_{ri} = \text{Dose} \times \frac{k_{ri}}{k}$$

As the ratio k_{ri}/k is the fraction of the usual dose employed in a given degree of renal insufficiency, it is termed the *dose fraction* and may be readily estimated from the information in Table 71-2 and the nomogram (Fig. 71-4). Table 71-2 gives the fraction of the usual dose of a drug required at a creatinine clearance of zero (dose fraction$_0$). The nomogram presents the dose fraction as a linear function of creatinine clearance.

To calculate the dose fraction$_{ri}$, the dose fraction$_0$ is obtained from Table 71-2, plotted on the left ordinate of the nomogram, and connected by a straight line to the upper right-hand corner of the nomogram. This line describes the dose fraction over a range of creatinine clearances from 0 to 100 ml/min. The point of intersection between the patient's measured creatinine clearance (on the lower abscissa) with this dose fraction line is a coordinate with the dose fraction (on the left ordinate) corresponding with that particular creatinine clearance. For example, if a patient with a creatinine clearance of 20 ml/min requires penicillin G for an infection that would be treated with 10 million units daily in patients with normal renal function, then an appropriate dose would be 2.8 million units daily. This estimated dose is obtained by plotting the dose fraction$_0$ for penicillin G (0.1) on the left-hand ordinate and connecting it to the top right-hand corner of the nomogram (Fig. 71-4). On this dose fraction line for penicillin G, the coordinate for a creatinine clearance of 20 ml/min corresponds on the left ordinate with a dose fraction of 0.28. Hence, the dose is 0.28 × 10 million units daily.

The loading dose In addition to adjusting the maintenance dose in patients with renal failure, consideration must also be given to the necessity of a loading dose. Since this dose is designed to bring the plasma concentration, or more particularly the amount of drug in the body, rapidly to the level that is reached at steady state, there is no need to modify the usual loading dose, if one is normally used. For many drugs, however, their elimination is sufficiently rapid that the time required to reach steady state is not clinically significant and no loading dose is usually used. On the other hand, in renal failure

TABLE 71-2
Estimated fraction of usual dose of drug required for a patient with a creatinine clearance of zero (dose fraction$_0$) and average overall fractional elimination rate constant for a patient with normal renal function *(k)*

Drug	*Dose fraction$_0$*	*k, per hour*
ANTIBIOTICS		
Amikacin	0.01	0.4
Amoxicillin	0.15	0.7
Ampicillin	0.1	0.6
Carbenicillin	0.1	0.6
Cephalexin	0.04	0.7
Cephaloridine	0.08	0.4
Cephalothin	0.02	1.4
Cephazolin	0.06	0.35
Chloramphenicol	0.8	0.3
Clindamycin	0.8	0.2
Cloxacillin	0.25	1.2
Colistimethate	0.3	0.2
Dicloxacillin	0.5	1.2
Doxycycline	0.8	0.03
Erythromycin	0.7	0.5
Gentamicin	0.02	0.3
Isoniazid:		
Fast inactivators	0.8	0.5
Slow inactivators	0.5	0.25
Kanamycin	0.03	0.35
Lincomycin	0.4	0.15
Methicillin	0.12	1.4
Minocycline	0.9	0.06
Nafcillin	0.4	1.2
Oxacillin	0.25	1.4
Oxytetracycline	0.2	0.08
Penicillin G	0.1	1.4
Polymyxin B	0.12	0.15
Rifampin	1.0	0.25
Streptomycin	0.04	0.25
Sulfadiazine	0.45	0.7
Sulfamethoxazole	0.85	0.07
Tetracycline	0.12	0.08
Tobramycin	0.02	0.35
Tricarcillin	0.1	0.6
Trimethoprim	0.45	0.06
Vancomycin	0.03	0.12
MISCELLANEOUS DRUGS		
Chlorpropamide	0.4	0.02
Lidocaine	0.9	0.4
Sulfinpyrazone	0.55	0.3
CARDIAC GLYCOSIDES		
		k, per day
Digitoxin	0.7	0.1
Digoxin	0.3	0.45

where the half-life may be significantly prolonged, this accumulation period may become unacceptably long. In such a case, for a drug given intermittently, a loading dose may be calculated as described in "Drug Accumulation" above. For an infusion, the loading dose may be approximated (when all units are consistent)

$$\text{Loading dose}_{ri} = \frac{\text{infusion rate}_{ri}}{k_{ri}}$$

General considerations for determining dosage in renal insufficiency Because of the considerable differences in volumes of distribution and rates of metabolism, the above calculations of drug dose for patients in renal failure must be viewed as valuable approximations which prevent the use of doses that are grossly excessive or inadequate for most patients. However, *maintenance dosages are most accurate when plasma level data are employed as a feedback to enable adjustment of the dose where necessary.*

In all the above calculations, it is assumed that the nonrenal clearance and nonrenal k are constant in renal failure. In fact, when cardiac failure accompanies renal failure, metabolic clearance for many drugs is reduced. Accordingly, when a drug with a narrow therapeutic index, such as digoxin, is used in cardiac failure, an appropriate precaution would be to reduce the value for nonrenal clearance (or k) to about one-half.

Active or toxic metabolites of drugs also may accumulate in renal failure. Meperidine, for example, is cleared largely by metabolism, and its concentration in plasma is little altered by renal insufficiency. However, the plasma concentration of one of its metabolites, normeperidine, is substantially increased when its renal elimination is impaired. As normeperidine has more convulsant activity than meperidine, its accumulation in patients with renal failure probably accounts for the signs of central nervous system excitation such as irritability, twitching, and seizures that result from the administration of multiple doses of meperidine to patients in renal insufficiency.

The metabolite of procainamide, *N*-acetylprocainamide, has cardiac effects that are similar to those of the parent drug. As *N*-acetylprocainamide is eliminated almost entirely by the kidney, its concentration in plasma is increased by renal failure. Thus, the potential of procainamide to produce toxicity in patients with renal insufficiency cannot be assessed by measuring the plasma concentration of procainamide alone.

FIGURE 71-4

Nomogram for estimation of the dose fraction (k_{ri}/k) in patients with renal insufficiency. The application of the nomogram is described in the text.

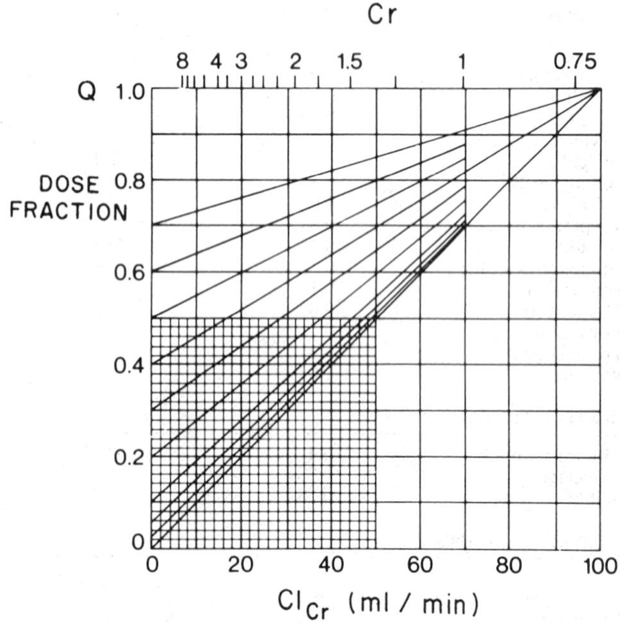

LIVER DISEASE In contrast to the predictable decline in renal clearance of drugs when glomerular filtration is reduced, it is not possible to make a general prediction of the effect of liver disease on hepatic biotransformation of drugs (Chap. 314). Rather, in hepatitis and cirrhosis there is a spectrum of changes ranging from impaired to increased drug clearance. Even when there is advanced hepatocellular disease, the magnitude of impairment in drug clearance usually is only about two- to fivefold. The extent of such changes, however, cannot be predicted by any of the commonly available tests of liver function. Consequently, even though it may be suspected that drug elimination is altered in a patient with liver disease, there is no quantitative base upon which to adjust the dosage regimen other than assessment of clinical response and concentration of drug in plasma.

Portacaval shunting creates a special situation because the effective hepatic blood flow is substantially reduced. This situation has its greatest effect on drugs that normally have a high hepatic extraction ratio so that their clearance is largely a function of blood flow; thus the clearance of such drugs (e.g., propranolol and lidocaine) will be remarkably reduced by portacaval shunting. In addition, the fraction of an administered oral dose reaching the systemic circulation will be significantly increased, because drug that is shunted around the liver during the absorption process will escape the efficient first-pass metabolism by this organ (e.g., meperidine, pentazocine).

CIRCULATORY INSUFFICIENCY—CARDIAC FAILURE AND SHOCK Under conditions leading to decreased tissue perfusion, redistribution of the cardiac output occurs to preserve blood flow to the heart and brain at the expense of other tissues (Chap. 29). As a result, the drug is distributed into a smaller volume of distribution, higher drug concentrations are present in the plasma, and the vital organs are exposed to these higher concentrations. If either the brain or heart is sensitive to the pharmacological effect of the drug, an alteration in response will occur.

Furthermore, the decreased perfusion of the kidney and liver may impair drug clearance by these organs either directly or indirectly. Thus, in severe congestive heart failure, in hemorrhagic shock, and particularly in cardiogenic shock, the response to the usual dose of the drug may be excessive, and dosage modification may be necessary. For example, the clearance of lidocaine is reduced by about 50 percent in cardiac failure, and consequently therapeutic plasma levels are achieved at infusion rates of only about half of those usually required. In cardiac failure there also is a significant reduction in lidocaine's volume of distribution which results in the requirement of a smaller loading dose. Similar situations are thought to exist for procainamide, theophylline, and possibly quinidine. Unfortunately, predictors of these types of pharmacokinetic alterations are unavailable. Therefore, loading doses should be conservative, and continued therapy should be monitored closely, following clinical indicators of toxicity and plasma levels.

DISEASE-INDUCED CHANGES IN PLASMA BINDING Many drugs circulate in the plasma partly bound to the plasma proteins and other constituents. Since only the unbound or free drug can distribute to the site of pharmacological action, the therapeutic response should be related to the free rather than the total circulating plasma drug concentration. In most cases the degree of binding is fairly constant across the therapeutic concentration range so that significant error is not caused by individualizing therapy on the basis of measuring levels of total drug in plasma. However, several clinical states such as hypoalbuminemia, liver disease, and renal disease can decrease the extent of drug binding so that at any total plasma level there is a greater concentration of free drug and a risk of increased response and toxicity. The drugs for which such changes are important are those which are normally highly bound in the plasma (> 90 percent) because a small alteration in the extent of binding produces a large relative increase in the fraction of drug in the unbound form.

The pharmacokinetic consequences of these binding changes, particularly with respect to total drug levels, depend on whether the clearance and distribution are dependent on the unbound or total drug. For many drugs, including those cited above, elimination and distribution are largely restricted to the unbound fraction, and therefore a decrease in binding leads to an increase in the clearance and distribution of the total drug. The relative magnitudes of these changes are such that the net effect is to shorten the half-life. The appropriate modification of the dosage regimen in clinical conditions with reduced drug binding is simply to administer the usual daily dose of the drug, but in divided doses at more frequent intervals. Individualization of therapy can then be based on either the clinical response or the plasma concentration of unbound drug. It is critical that the patient not be titrated into the usual therapeutic range for concentration of *total* drug in plasma since this will lead to excessive response and toxicity.

INTERACTIONS BETWEEN DRUGS

The effect of some drugs can be altered markedly by the administration of other agents. Such interactions can sabotage therapeutic intent by producing excessive drug action (with adverse effects) or decreasing the action of a drug, rendering it ineffective. Drug interactions must be considered in the differential diagnosis of unexpected responses to drugs, taking into account that ambulatory patients often come to the physician with a legacy of drugs acquired during their previous medical experiences. A meticulous drug history will minimize the unknown elements in the patient's therapeutic milieu; it should include examination of the patient's medications and calls to the pharmacist to identify prescriptions, if necessary.

There are two principal types of interactions between drugs. *Pharmacokinetic interactions* result from alteration in the delivery of drugs to their sites of action. *Pharmacodynamic interactions* are those in which the responsiveness of the target organ or system has been modified by other agents.

An index of the drug interactions discussed in this chapter is provided in Table 71-3. Included are a selected group of interactions which have verified significance in patients and a few which are of such potential danger to the patient that cognizance should be taken of experimental data or case reports suggesting their likely occurrence.

I PHARMACOKINETIC INTERACTIONS CAUSING DIMINISHED DRUG DELIVERY

***A* Impaired gastrointestinal absorption** Aluminum ions, present in antacids, form insoluble chelates with the tetracyclines, thereby preventing absorption of these drugs. Ferrous ions similarly block tetracycline absorption. Cholestyramine, an ionic exchange resin, binds thyroxine, triiodothyronine, and the cardiac glycosides with sufficiently high affinity to impair their absorption from the gastrointestinal tract. This resin probably also interferes with the absorption of other drugs, and it is safest not to give it within 2 h of their administration. Kaolin-pectin suspension binds digoxin, and when the drugs are administered together, digoxin absorption is reduced by about one-half. However, when kaolin-pectin is administered 2 h after digoxin, there is no effect on absorption of digoxin. Oral administration of *p*-aminosalicylate interferes with the absorption of rifampin by a mechanism not yet determined.

All the above instances of impaired absorption result in a reduction in the total amount of drug absorption, with reduced

TABLE 71-3
Drug interaction index

Drug	*Section of chapter describing interaction*
Acetohexamide	IIB
Allopurinol	IIA
p-Aminosalicylate	IA
Amphetamine	IC, III
Antidepressants, tricyclic (desipramine, nortriptyline, imipramine, doxepin, protriptyline, amitriptyline)	IC
Aspirin	IIB, III
Azathioprine	IIA
Barbiturates (class)	IB
Bethanidine	IC
Chloral hydrate	IIC
Chloramphenicol	IIA, III
Chlordiazepoxide	IIA
Chlorpromazine	IC
Cholestyramine	IA
Cimetidine	IIA
Clofibrate	IIA
Clonidine	IC
Cyclophosphamide	IIA
Dexamethasone	IB
Diazepam	IIA
Dicumarol	IB, IIA, IIB
Digitoxin	IA, IB, IIB
Digoxin	IA, IIB
Diphenylhydantoin (see phenytoin below)	
Disulfiram	IIA
Ephedrine	IC, III
Ethanol	IIA
Furazolidone	III
Guanethidine	IC
Indomethacin	III
Isoniazid	IIA
Kaolin-pectin	IA
Lidocaine	IIA
6-Mercaptopurine	IIA
Methotrexate	IIB
Metronidazole	IIA
Metyrapone	IB
Monoamine oxidase inhibitors	III
Pargyline	III
Phenobarbital	IB
Phenylbutazone	IIA, IIB
Phenylpropanolamine	III
Phenytoin (diphenylhydantoin)	IB, IIA
Potassium	III
Prednisone	IB
Propranolol	III
Quinidine	IB
Rifampin	IA, IB
Spironolactone	III
Tetracycline	IA, III
Thiazide diuretics	III
Tolbutamide	IIA
Triamterene	III
Warfarin	IB, IIA, IIC, III

area under the plasma level curve and reduced peak plasma levels, as well as lower steady-state concentrations of the drug involved.

B Induction of hepatic drug-metabolizing enzymes When the elimination of the drug proceeds largely via biotransformation, an increase in the rate at which it is metabolized reduces its availability to sites of action. The biotransformation of most drugs occurs largely in the liver, because of its mass, high blood flow, and concentration of enzymes that metabolize drugs. The initial step in metabolism of many drugs is executed by the mixed-function oxidase enzymes located in the hepatic endoplasmic reticulum. These enzyme systems containing cytochrome P_{450} oxidize the molecule by a variety of reactions including aromatic hydroxylations, *N*-demethylations, *O*-demethylations, and sulfoxidations. The products of these reactions are usually more polar (and more readily excreted by the kidney).

The number of mixed-function oxidase enzyme molecules in the liver can be increased by treatment with enzyme inducers, of which phenobarbital is the prototype. Almost all the barbiturates in clinical use increase the mixed-function oxidase enzymes. Induction with phenobarbital can occur with doses of as little as 60 mg daily. Mixed-function oxidases are also induced by rifampin, phenytoin, and glutethimide and by occupational exposure to chlorinated insecticides such as DDT, as well as by chronic alcohol ingestion.

The actions of a number of drugs are inhibited by treatment with inducing agents. Phenobarbital and other inducers lower plasma levels of warfarin, dicumarol, digitoxin, quinidine, dexamethasone, prednisolone (the active metabolite of prednisone), and metyrapone. These interactions all have obvious clinical significance. With the coumarin anticoagulants, the major risk occurs when an appropriate level of anticoagulation is achieved while the coumarin drug is coadministered with an inducing agent. When the inducer is discontinued, e.g., following discharge from the hospital, plasma levels of the coumarin anticoagulant will rise as the induction effect wears off, leading to excessive anticoagulation. Barbiturates have been shown to lower the plasma levels of phenytoin in some patients, but the clinical effect of reduced phenytoin levels is probably counterbalanced by the anticonvulsant effects of phenobarbital.

There is considerable variation among individuals in the extent to which drug metabolism can be induced. In some patients phenobarbital leads to marked acceleration in the rate of drug metabolism, whereas little induction is seen in others. This variability in the extent of induction of mixed-function oxidases is largely genetically determined.

In addition to inducing the mixed-function oxidase enzymes, phenobarbital has a number of other effects on hepatic function. It increases liver blood flow, bile flow, and the hepatocellular transport of organic anions. The conjugation of drugs and bilirubin is also enhanced by inducing agents.

C Inhibition of cellular uptake or binding The guanidinium antihypertensives, guanethidine and bethanidine, are transported to their site of action in adrenergic neurons by an energy-requiring membrane transport system for biogenic monoamines. Although the physiological function of the transport system is reuptake of the adrenergic neurotransmitter, it also transports a variety of ring-substituted bases, including guanethidine and bethanidine, into the adrenergic neuron against a concentration gradient. Inhibitors of norepinephrine uptake will prevent the uptake of the guanidinium antihypertensives into adrenergic neurons and will thereby block their pharmacological effects. The tricyclic antidepressants are potent inhibitors of norepinephrine uptake. Consequently, concomitant administration of clinical doses of tricyclic antidepressants including desipramine, protriptyline, nortriptyline, and amitriptyline will almost totally abolish the antihypertensive effects of guanethidine and bethanidine. Although they are less potent inhibitors of norepinephrine uptake, doxepin and chlorpromazine, when given in doses of greater than 100 mg daily, produce dose-related antagonism of the action of the guanidinium antihypertensives. In patients with severe hypertension, the loss of control of blood pressure resulting from these drug interactions can lead to serious clinical complications such as stroke and malignant hypertension.

Amphetamine also antagonizes the antihypertensive effect of guanethidine by displacing it from its site of action within the adrenergic neuron (Chap. 267). Ephedrine, a component of many drug combinations used in asthma, also antagonizes the effect of guanethidine, probably by both inhibition of uptake and displacement from the neuron.

The antihypertensive effect of clonidine in humans is partially antagonized by the tricyclic antidepressants. Clonidine lowers arterial pressure by reducing sympathetic outflow from the blood-pressure-regulating centers in the hindbrain (Chap. 267). This central hypotensive action is antagonized by the tricyclic antidepressants.

II PHARMACOKINETIC INTERACTIONS CAUSING INCREASED DRUG DELIVERY

A Inhibition of drug metabolism If the active form of a drug is cleared largely by biotransformation, inhibition of its metabolism will lead to a prolonged half-life and to accumulation of the drug during maintenance therapy. Excessive accumulation due to inhibited metabolism leads to significant adverse effects in the case of several drugs.

Cimetidine is a potent inhibitor of the oxidative metabolism of a number of drugs in humans, including warfarin, diazepam, chlordiazepoxide, theophylline, phenytoin, propranolol, and lidocaine. Excessive anticoagulation by warfarin also may result from inhibition of its metabolism by disulfiram, metronidazole, or phenylbutazone, or by concurrent and copious ingestion of ethanol.

The metabolism of phenytoin is inhibited by a number of drugs. Clofibrate, phenylbutazone, chloramphenicol, disulfiram, dicumarol, and isoniazid can raise the steady-state plasma levels of phenytoin by more than twofold. Impaired metabolism of tolbutamide with severe hypoglycemia has resulted from coadministration of clofibrate, phenylbutazone, chloramphenicol, and dicumarol. Excessive anticoagulation by warfarin may result from inhibition of its metabolism by disulfiram or phenylbutazone, or by concurrent and copious ingestion of ethanol. Warfarin is administered as a racemic mixture, and its *S*(−) isomer has five times the anticoagulant potency of the *R*(+) isomer. Phenylbutazone selectively inhibits the metabolism of the *S*(−) isomer, and only when this isomer is examined specifically can the substantial reduction in its metabolism produced by phenylbutazone be unmasked.

Azathioprine is readily converted in the body to an active metabolite, 6-mercaptopurine, which in turn is inactivated in part by xanthine oxidase which sequentially oxidizes it to 6-thiouric acid. When allopurinol, a potent inhibitor of xanthine oxidase, is administered concurrently with standard doses of azathioprine or 6-mercaptopurine, life-threatening toxicity (bone marrow suppression) can result.

B Inhibition of renal elimination A number of drugs are secreted by the renal tubular transport systems for organic ions. Inhibition of this tubular transport system can cause excessive accumulation of a drug when this is the major pathway of its elimination. Several drugs, including phenylbutazone, probenecid, salicylates, and dicumarol, will competitively inhibit this transport system. Salicylate, for example, reduces the renal clearance of methotrexate, an interaction that may lead to methotrexate toxicity. Renal tubular secretion contributes substantially to the elimination of penicillin, which can be inhibited by probenecid. The concentrations of digoxin and digitoxin in plasma are elevated substantially by quinidine, an effect that results largely from inhibition of the renal elimination of these glycosides by quinidine.

C **Inhibition of plasma protein binding** When the binding of a drug to plasma protein is reduced by another agent, more unbound drug will be made available to receptor sites for any given level of total drug. Reduction in the binding of a drug does not have significance in vivo unless the drug is very highly bound (more than 90 percent) and the volume of distribution is small. A drug may alter the binding of another by competitive displacement or by an interaction with protein (usually albumin) to decrease binding affinity.

III **PHARMACODYNAMIC AND OTHER INTERACTIONS BETWEEN DRUGS** Therapeutically useful interactions in which the combined effect of two drugs is greater than that of either drug alone are numerous. These favorable drug combinations are covered extensively in specific therapeutic sections in this text, and the following is directed toward those pharmacodynamic interactions that create unwanted effects. Two drugs may act on separate components of a common process and yield effects greater than either drug alone. For example, small doses of aspirin (less than 1 g daily) will not alter the prothrombin time appreciably in patients who are stabilized on warfarin therapy. However, the addition of aspirin to patients therapeutically anticoagulated with warfarin increases the risk of bleeding because aspirin inhibits platelet aggregation. Thus the combination of impaired functions of both the platelets and the fluid-phase clotting system increases the potential for hemorrhagic complications in patients receiving warfarin therapy.

Indomethacin and probably other nonsteroidal anti-inflammatory drugs antagonize the antihypertensive effects of both propranolol and thiazide diuretics. The administration of supplemental potassium leads to more frequent and more severe hyperkalemia when potassium elimination is reduced by concurrent treatment with spironolactone or triamterene.

VARIABLE ACTIONS OF DRUGS CAUSED BY GENETIC DIFFERENCES IN THEIR METABOLISM

ACETYLATION Isoniazid, hydralazine, procainamide, and a number of other drugs are metabolized by acetylation of a hydrazino or amino group. This reaction is catalyzed by *N*-acetyl transferase, a nonmicrosomal (soluble) enzyme in the liver that transfers an acetyl group from acetyl coenzyme A to the drug. Individuals differ markedly in the rate at which drugs are acetylated, and there is a bimodal distribution of the population into "rapid acetylators" and "slow acetylators." The rate of acetylation is under genetic control; rapid acetylation is an autosomal dominant trait.

The toxic, sometimes fatal, hepatitis that occurs in about 1 percent of patients on isoniazid occurs predominantly in rapid acetylators. The greater hepatotoxicity in rapid acetylators appears to result from the synthesis of more acetylisoniazid which is further metabolized to acetylhydrazine, a potent hepatotoxin. Acetylhydrazine exerts its toxic effect through an active metabolite that binds covalently to macromolecules in the hepatic cells that produce it. Conversely, the lupus erythematosus-like syndrome produced by hydralazine occurs only in individuals who are slow acetylators.

Because these important toxic drug effects are largely predictable from the acetylation phenotype, it may in certain instances be of value to determine the rate of acetylation in patients who are to receive isoniazid, or those who would benefit from doses of hydralazine above the 200 mg per day dose that can be safely employed in the population at large. Acetylation phenotype can be determined by measuring the ratio of acetylated to nonacetylated dapsone or sulfamethazine in plasma or urine following administration of a test dose of these acetylation substrates. The ratio of monoacetyldapsone to dapsone in plasma at 6 h after dapsone administration is less than 0.35 for slow acetylators and greater than 0.35 for rapid acetylators. At 6 h following the administration of sulfamethazine, less than 25 percent of the drug in the plasma is in the acetylated form in slow acetylators (rapid acetylators, more than 25 percent); in the urine collected in the 5- to 6-h interval after administration, less than 70 percent of the drug is in the acetylated form in slow acetylators (rapid acetylators, more than 70 percent).

METABOLISM BY MIXED-FUNCTION OXIDASES In healthy individuals taking no other medications, the major determinant of the rate of metabolism of drugs by the hepatic mixed-function oxidases is genetic. Hepatic microsomes contain a family of cytochrome P_{450} enzymes with different substrate specificities and it is likely that multiple genes control their biosynthesis. For certain drugs metabolized largely by a single oxidative reaction, there is evidence for a genetically controlled polymorphism of the oxidative enzyme. Many drugs undergo oxidative biotransformation by more than one enzyme and the steady-state concentrations of such drugs in plasma will be a function of the sum of the activities of these enzymes. When drugs are metabolized by multiple pathways, steady-state plasma concentrations tend to distribute unimodally in the population and may differ markedly (tenfold or more) between individuals, as is the case for chlorpromazine.

CONCENTRATION OF DRUGS IN PLASMA AS A GUIDE TO THERAPY

Optimal individualization of therapy is assisted by measuring the concentration of certain drugs in plasma. Genetic variation in elimination rates, interactions with other drugs, disease-induced alterations in elimination and distribution, and other factors combine to yield a wide range of plasma levels in patients given the same dose. Furthermore, the problem of noncompliance with prescribed regimens during continuing therapy is an endemic and elusive cause of therapeutic failure (see below). There are clinical indicators that assist the titration of some drugs into the desired range, and no chemical determination is a substitute for careful observations of the patient's response to treatment. However, the therapeutic and adverse effects are not precisely quantifiable for all drugs, and in complex clinical situations estimates of the action of a drug may be misleading. For example, previously existing neurological disease may obscure the neurological consequences of intoxication with phenytoin. Because clearance, half-life, accumulation, and steady-state plasma levels are difficult to predict, the measurement of plasma levels is often useful as a guide to the optimal dose. This is particularly so when there is a narrow range between the plasma levels yielding therapeutic and adverse effects.

The variability among individual responses to given plasma levels must be recognized. This is illustrated by a hypothetical population dose-response curve (Fig. 71-5) and its relationship to the therapeutic range or therapeutic "window" of desired plasma levels. The defined therapeutic window should include the levels at which the majority of patients will achieve the

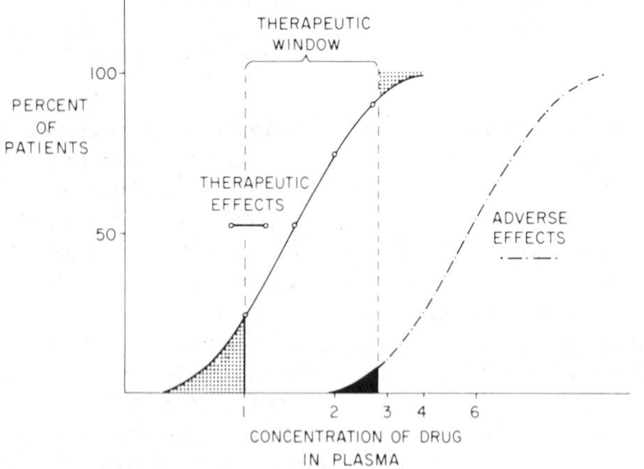

FIGURE 71-5

The cumulative percentage of patients responding to increasing levels of drug in plasma with both therapeutic and adverse effects. The therapeutic "window" defines the range of concentrations of drug that will achieve therapeutic effects in most patients with adverse effects in only a small percentage.

intended pharmacological effect. However, there are a few people who are quite sensitive to the therapeutic effects of most drugs, responding to lower levels, whereas others are sufficiently refractory as to require levels that impose an increased likelihood of adverse effects as a potential price for therapeutic benefit. For example, a few patients with strong seizure foci will require plasma levels of phenytoin exceeding 20 μg/ml in order to control their seizure disorders. Increments in dosage to achieve this effect may be appropriate.

As also illustrated in Fig. 71-5, some patients may be prone to adverse effects at levels which are well tolerated by most of the population, and therefore elevation of levels to those achieving a high probability of therapeutic effect may bring on unwanted actions in the exceptional patient. Table 71-4 presents for a number of drugs the concentrations in plasma that are associated with probable adverse and therapeutic effects in most patients. Its use within the guidelines discussed should permit more effective and safer therapy for those patients who are not "average."

TABLE 71-4

Concentrations of drugs in plasma: relation to efficacy and adverse effects

Drug	*Efficacy**	*Adverse effects†*
Amikacin	20 μg/ml	40 μg/ml
Carbenicillin	100 μg/ml‡	300 μg/ml
Carbamazepine	3 μg/ml	10 μg/ml
Digitoxin	12 ng/ml	25–30 ng/ml
Digoxin	0.8 ng/ml	2.0 ng/ml
Ethosuximide	40 μg/ml	100 μg/ml
Gentamicin	4 μg/ml§	12 μg/ml
Lidocaine	1.5 μg/ml	5 μg/ml
Lithium	0.5 meq/liter	1.3 meq/liter
Penicillin G	1–25 μg/ml¶	
Phenytoin (diphenylhydantoin)	10 μg/ml	20 μg/ml
Procainamide	4 μg/ml	8 μg/ml
Quinidine	2.5 μg/ml	6 μg/ml
Theophylline	8 μg/ml	20 μg/ml

* *The therapeutic effect is infrequent or slight at levels below these.*
† *The frequency of adverse effects increases sharply when these levels are exceeded.*
‡ *Minimal inhibitory concentration (MIC) for most strains of Pseudomonas aeruginosa. MIC for other, more sensitive, organisms is less.*
§ *Dependent on the MIC. Higher levels (up to 8 μg/ml) may be desired when host defenses are impaired.*
¶ *There is a wide range of MIC of penicillin for various organisms, and the MIC of all those for which penicillin is used is < 20. "Massive" penicillin therapy with 20 million units daily achieves levels of 20 to 25 μg/ml in patients with clearance of creatinine of 100 ml/min.*

Effective participation of the patient in therapeutic programs Measurement of the concentration of a drug in plasma is the most effective approach to determining when patients have failed to take the prescribed drug. Such "noncompliance" with recommended therapy is a frequent problem in the long-term treatment of a number of diseases such as hypertension and epilepsy, occurring in 25 percent or more of patients in therapeutic environments that lack special efforts to involve patients in the responsibility for their own health. Occasionally, noncompliance with therapeutic programs can be elicited by sympathetic, nonincriminating questioning, but more often it is diagnosed only after determining that the concentration of drug in plasma is nil or is recurrently low. Because other factors can cause plasma levels to be lower than expected, comparison with levels obtained during in-patient treatment may be required to confirm that noncompliance did, in fact, occur. Once the physician is certain of noncompliance, a nonaccusatory discussion of the problem with the patient frequently will elucidate a reason for the noncompliance and also serves as a basis for more effective participation of the patient in his or her care subsequently. Many approaches have been taken to enhance the patients' exercise of responsibility for their own treatment, most of which are based on improved communication with the patient regarding the nature of the disease and the expectations of treatment and treatment failure. This communication includes an opportunity for the patient to relate any problems associated with treatment, and it may be optimized by involving nurses and other paramedical personnel in the process. Minimizing the complexity of the regimen is helpful, both in terms of the number of drugs and the frequency of administration. Enlisting patients to take the principal role in their own health care requires a blend of the art and science of medicine.

REFERENCES

BENET LZ, SHEINER LB: Design and optimization of dosage regimens: pharmacokinetic data, in *The Pharmacological Basis of Therapeutics*, 6th ed, AG Goodman, LS Goodman, A Gilman (eds). New York, Macmillan, 1980, p 1675

CHENNAVASIN P, BRATER DC: Nomograms for drug use in renal disease. Clin Pharmacokin 6:193, 1981

DETTLI L: Elimination kinetics and dosage adjustment of drugs in patients with kidney disease. Prog Pharmacol, vol 1, no 4, 1977

SHAND DG et al: Pharmacokinetic drug interactions, in *Handbook of Experimental Pharmacology*, vol 28: *Concepts in Biochemical Pharmacology*, JR Gillette, JR Mitchell (eds). New York, Springer-Verlag, 1975, p 272

SHEINER LB, TOZER TN: Clinical pharmacokinetics: The use of plasma concentrations of drugs, in *Clinical Pharmacology: Basic Principles in Therapeutics*, 2d ed. New York, Macmillan, 1978, p 71

WILKINSON GR, SHAND DG: A physiological approach to hepatic drug clearance. Clin Pharmacol Ther 18:377, 1975

72
ADVERSE REACTIONS TO DRUGS

ALASTAIR J. J. WOOD
JOHN A. OATES

The beneficial effects of drugs are coupled with the inescapable risk that they may also cause untoward effects. The morbidity and mortality that result from these untoward effects often present diagnostic problems, for these drugs can involve every organ and system of the body.

Major advances in the investigation, development, and regulation of drugs ensure in most instances their uniformity, effectiveness, and relative safety, as well as identify their recognized hazards. However, the extremely large number and variety of drugs and drug products available over the counter (OTC) or by prescription from a physician make it impossible for patient or physician to obtain or retain the knowledge necessary to use all these drugs well. It is understandable, therefore, that many OTC drugs are used unwisely by the public and that restricted drugs may be prescribed incorrectly by physicians.

Most physicians use no more than 50 drug products in their practice, gaining familiarity with their effectiveness and safety. Most patients probably use only a limited number of OTC drugs. Nevertheless, many patients receive care and drug prescriptions from more than one physician, and surveys have shown that in any 30-day period patients may consume more than three different OTC drug products containing nine or more different chemical agents.

Twenty-five to fifty percent of patients may make errors in self-administration of prescribed medicines, and this can be responsible for adverse drug effects. Elderly patients are most likely to commit such errors. One-third or more of patients also may not take their prescribed medications. It also seems likely that many patients commit similar errors in taking OTC drugs by not reading or following the directions for use of the medicines provided on the containers. Physicians must recognize that providing directions with prescriptions does not always guarantee their patients' compliance.

Every drug can produce untoward consequences, even when used according to standard or recommended methods of administration. When used incorrectly, the drug's effectiveness may be reduced, or adverse reactions can be expected to occur more frequently. The administration of several drugs during the same period of time also may result in adverse interactions between drugs (see Chap. 71).

In the hospital all the drugs a patient is given should be under the control of a physician, and patient compliance is, in general, ensured. Errors may occur nevertheless, in that the wrong drug or dose may be given, or the drug may be given to the wrong patient, although systems improving drug distribution and administration in hospitals have reduced this problem. On the other hand, there are no means for controlling how ambulatory patients take prescription or OTC drugs.

EPIDEMIOLOGY Epidemiologic studies of adverse drug reactions have been helpful in evaluating the magnitude of the overall problem, in calculating the rate of reactions to individual drugs, and in characterizing some of the determinants of adverse drug effects.

Patients receive on the average 10 different drugs while hospitalized. The sicker the patient, the more drugs are given, and as expected, there is a corresponding increase in the likelihood of adverse drug reactions. When fewer than six different drugs are given to hospitalized patients, the probability of an adverse reaction is about 5 percent, but if more than 15 drugs are given, the probability is over 40 percent. Retrospective analysis of ambulatory patients has revealed a history of some adverse drug effects in 20 percent of them.

Thus, the magnitude of the problem posed by drug-induced disease has become exceedingly large. Two to five percent of patients are admitted to the medical and pediatric services of general hospitals because of illnesses attributed to drugs. The case/fatality ratio from drug-induced disease in hospitalized patients varies from 2 to 12 percent. A proportion of fetal or neonatal abnormalities may be due to medicines taken by the mother during pregnancy or parturition.

Women experience twice as many gastrointestinal manifestations of adverse drug effects as do men.

A small group of widely used drugs account for a disproportionate number of reactions. A number of studies have shown that aspirin, digoxin, anticoagulants, diuretics, antimicrobials, steroids, and hypoglycemic agents account for as many as 90 percent of all reactions.

ETIOLOGY Most adverse reactions to drugs may be classified into one of two groups. The most frequent are those that result from the exaggerated but predicted pharmacologic action of the drug. Other adverse reactions ensue from toxic effects on cells that result from mechanisms unrelated to the intended pharmacologic actions. These therefore are often unpredictable, are frequently severe, and result from a number of recognized as well as undiscovered mechanisms. Some of the mechanisms of extrapharmacologic toxicity include direct cytotoxicity, the initiation of abnormal immune responses, and the perturbation of metabolic processes in individuals rendered susceptible by genetic enzymatic defects.

EXAGGERATION OF THE INTENDED PHARMACOLOGIC EFFECT By prior consideration of the known factors that modify drug action, these adverse reactions often are preventable.

Abnormally high drug concentration at the receptor site (site of action) due to the pharmacokinetic variability discussed in Chap. 71 is the usual cause. For example, reduction in the volume of distribution, in the rate of metabolism, or in the rate of excretion all will result in higher than expected concentration of the drug at the receptor site with consequent increase in pharmacologic effect.

Alteration in the dose-response curve due to increased receptor sensitivity will result in an increase in drug effect at the same concentration. An example of this is seen in the excessive response to the anticoagulant warfarin at normal and lower than normal blood levels in the elderly.

The shape of the dose-response curve itself also determines the likelihood of the development of adverse drug reactions. These drugs with a steep dose-response curve are more likely to be associated with dose-related toxicity because of the small increase in dose required to produce a large change in pharmacologic effect. An increase in the dose of drugs which exhibit nonlinear kinetics, such as phenytoin (see previous chapter) may produce a proportionately greater increase in the blood level, resulting in toxicity.

Concomitant drug therapy may affect the pharmacokinetics or pharmacodynamics of other drugs. Pharmacokinetics may be affected by alterations in bioavailability, protein binding, or the rate of metabolism or excretion. Pharmacodynamics may be altered by competition for receptor sites, by prevention of the drug's reaching its site of action, or by antagonism or enhancement of the drug's pharmacologic effect. These subjects are discussed in detail in the previous chapter.

TOXICITY UNRELATED TO A DRUG'S PRIMARY PHARMACOLOGIC ACTIVITY **Cytotoxic reactions** Our understanding of these so-called idiosyncratic reactions has greatly improved recently as it has become clear that many of these reactions are due to irreversible binding of drug or metabolites to tissue macromolecules by shared electron (covalent) bonds. Some chemical carcinogens such as the alkylating agents combine directly with DNA. However, it is more commonly only after metabolic activation to chemically reactive metabolites that covalent binding occurs. This metabolic activation usually occurs in the microsomal mixed-function oxidase system, the hepatic enzyme system which is responsible for the metabolism of many drugs (Chap. 71). During the course of drug metabolism by these pathways, reactive metabolites of some drugs may be produced which covalently bind to tissue macromolecules, causing tissue damage. Because of the highly reactive nature of these metabolites covalent binding often occurs close to the site of production, such as the liver, but the mixed-function oxidase system is found in other tissues as well.

An example of this type of adverse drug reaction is the hepatotoxicity associated with isoniazid, which is metabolized principally by acetylation (Fig. 72-1) to acetylisoniazid, which is then hydrolyzed to acetylhydralazine. The further metabolism of acetylhydralazine by the mixed-function oxidase system liberates reactive metabolites which covalently bind to hepatic macromolecules, causing hepatic necrosis. The rate of acetylation shows a bimodal distribution, the population dividing into slow and fast acetylators. Fast acetylators predominate in Orientals, who have been shown to be particularly susceptible to isoniazid hepatoxicity. The administration of drugs known to increase the activity of the mixed-function oxidase system, such as phenobarbital or rifampin, together with isoniazid, is associated with the production of increased amounts of reactive metabolites, increased covalent binding, and hepatic damage.

The hepatic necrosis produced by overdosage of acetominophen is caused by the covalent binding of reactive electrophilic metabolites to hepatic macromolecules. Normally these reactive metabolites are detoxified by combining with hepatic glutathione. When glutathione becomes exhausted, the metabolites bind instead to hepatic macromolecules with resultant hepatocyte damage. The hepatic necrosis produced by the ingestion of large quantities of acetominophen can be prevented, or at least attenuated, by the administration of substances such as *N*-acetylcysteine, which reduce the binding of electrophilic metabolites to hepatic proteins with resultant hepatic necrosis. The risks of hepatic necrosis are increased in patients also receiving drugs such as phenobarbital which increase the rate of drug metabolism and rate of production of toxic metabolite(s).

It is likely, though as yet unproved, that other idiosyncratic reactions are caused by the covalent binding of reactive metabolites to tissue macromolecules, with either direct cytotoxicity or via the initiation of an immunologic response.

FIGURE 72-1
Biotransformation of isoniazid to a hepatotoxic metabolite.

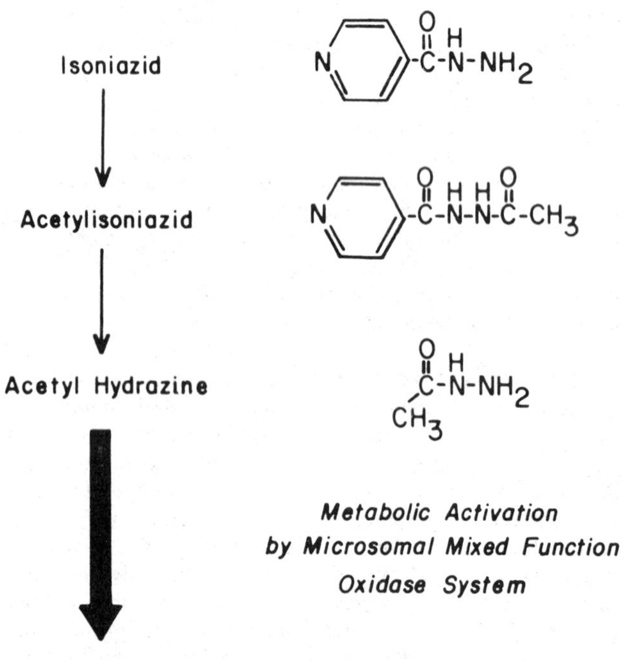

Immunologic mechanisms Most pharmacologic agents are poor immunogens since they consist of small molecules with molecular weights less than 2000. Stimulation of antibody synthesis or sensitization of lymphocytes by a drug or one of its metabolites usually requires in vivo activation and covalent linkage to protein, carbohydrate, or nucleic acid.

Drug stimulation of antibody production may mediate tissue injury by one of several mechanisms. The antibody may attack the drug affixed to a cell by covalent linkage and thereby destroy the cell, as occurs in penicillin-induced hemolytic anemia. Complexes of antibody-drug-antigen may be passively adsorbed by a bystander cell which is destroyed by activation of complement; this occurs in quinine- and quinidine-induced thrombocytopenia. Drugs or their reactive metabolites may alter host tissue, rendering it antigenic, and stimulate autoantibodies; for example, hydralazine and procainamide can chemically alter nuclear material, stimulate formation of antinuclear antibodies, and occasionally cause lupus erythematosus. Autoantibodies may be stimulated by drugs which neither interact with the host antigen nor have any chemical similarity to the host tissue; for example, alpha methyldopa frequently stimulates formation of antibodies to host erythrocytes, yet the drug does not itself attach to the erythrocyte nor share any chemical similarities with the antigenic determinants on the erythrocyte.

Serum sickness (Chap. 67) results from deposition of circulating drug-antibody complexes on endothelial surfaces. Complement activation occurs, chemotactic factors are generated locally, and an inflammatory response appears at the site of complex entrapment. Arthralgias, lymphadenopathy, glomerulonephritis, or cerebritis may result. Penicillin is the most common cause of serum sickness today. Many drugs, particularly the antimicrobial agents, induce production of IgE, which affixes to mast cell membranes. Contact with a drug antigen initiates a series of biochemical events within the mast cell and results in the release of mediators which may produce urticaria, wheezing, rhinorrhea, and occasionally hypotension characteristic of anaphylaxis.

Drugs may also excite cell-mediated immune responses. Topically administered substances may interact with sulfhydryl or amino groups in the skin and react with sensitized lymphocytes to produce the rash characteristic of contact dermatitis. Other types of rashes may also appear from the interaction of serum factors, drugs, and sensitized lymphocytes. The role of drug-activated lymphoctyes in the immune mechanisms governing destruction of visceral tissue is unknown.

Toxicity associated with genetically determined enzymatic defects In the porphyrias, drugs which increase the activity of enzymes proximal to the deficient enzyme in the biosynthetic pathway of porphyrins can increase the quantity of porphyrin precursors that accumulate proximal to the deficient enzyme (Chap. 99). These drugs are listed in Table 72-1.

Patients with a deficiency of glucose 6-phosphate dehydrogenase (G6PD) will develop hemolytic anemia on primaquine and a number of other drugs (Table 72-1) which do not cause hemolysis in patients who have adequate quantities of this enzyme (Chap. 329).

Diagnosis The manifestations of drug-induced diseases frequently resemble those associated with other diseases, and may be produced by different and dissimilar drugs. Recognition of the role of a drug or drugs responsible for illness is dependent upon appreciation of the possible implication of adverse reactions to drugs in any disease, identification of a temporal rela-

TABLE 72-1
Clinical manifestations of adverse reactions to drugs

- *I* Multisystem
  - *A* Fever
    - Penicillins
    - Novobiocin
    - *p*-Aminosalicylic acid
    - Amphotericin B
    - Antihistamines
    - Cephalosporins
    - Barbiturates
    - Phenytoin
    - Quinidine
    - Sulfonamides
    - Iodides
    - Thiouracil
    - Phenolphthalein
    - Methyldopa
    - Procainamide
  - *B* Drug-induced lupus erythematosus
    - Hydralazine
    - Procainamide
    - Isoniazid
  - *C* Serum sickness
    - Aspirin
    - Penicillins
    - Streptomycin
    - Sulfonamides
    - Propylthiouracil
  - *D* Anaphylaxis
    - Bromsulphothalein
    - Penicillins
    - Cephalosporins
    - Streptomycin
    - Dextran
    - Iron dextran
    - Procaine
    - Insulin
    - Demeclocycline
    - Iodinated drugs or contrast media
    - Lidocaine
- *II* Endocrine
  - *A* Disorders of thyroid function tests
    - Oral contraceptives
    - Bromsulphalein
    - Phenindione
    - Iodides
    - Tolbutamide
    - Chlorpropamide
    - Lithium
    - Acetazolamide
    - Gold salts
    - Dimercaprol
    - Clofibrate
    - Phenothiazines (long term)
    - Phenylbutazone
    - Sulfonamides
    - Phenytoin
  - *B* Addisonian-like syndrome
    - Busulfan
  - *C* Gynecomastia
    - Estrogens
    - Testosterone
    - Spironolactone
    - Digitalis
    - Reserpine
    - Methyldopa
    - Isoniazid
    - Ethionamide
    - Griseofulvin
  - *D* Galactorrhea (may also cause amenorrhea)
    - Methyldopa
    - Phenothiazines
    - Reserpine
    - Tricyclic antidepressants
    - Dexamphetamine
  - *E* Sexual dysfunction
    - *1* Impaired ejaculation
      - Guanethidine
      - Debrisoquin
      - Bethanidine
      - Thioridazine
    - *2* Decreased libido and impotence
      - Oral contraceptives
      - Sedatives
      - Major tranquilizers
      - Lithium
      - Methyldopa
      - Clonidine
- *III* Metabolic
  - *A* Hyponatremia
    - *1* Dilutional
      - Vincristine
      - Cyclophosphamide
      - Chlorpropamide
      - Diuretics
    - *2* Salt wasting
      - Diuretics
      - Corticosteroid (withdrawal)
      - Enemas
      - Mannitol
  - *B* Hyperkalemia
    - Spironolactone
    - Triamterene
    - Amiloride
    - Cytotoxics
    - Corticosteroid (withdrawal)
    - Succinylcholine
    - Digitalis overdose
    - Potassium salts of drugs
    - Potassium preparations including salt substitute
    - Lithium
  - *C* Hypokalemia
    - Diuretics
    - Laxative abuse
    - Corticosteroids
    - Amphotericin B
    - Alkali-induced alkalosis
    - Insulin
    - Osmotic diuretics
    - Carbenoxolone
    - Gentamicin
    - Degraded tetracycline
    - Vitamin B_{12}
  - *D* Metabolic acidosis
    - Paraldehyde (degraded)
    - Phenformin
    - Acetazolamide
    - Spironolactone
    - Salicylates
  - *E* Hypercalcemia
    - Antacids with absorbable alkali
    - Vitamin D
    - Thiazides
  - *F* Hyperuricemia
    - Thiazides
    - Chlorthalidone
    - Ethacrynic acid
    - Furosemide
    - Aspirin
    - Cytotoxics
    - Hyperalimentation
    - Fructose (IV)
  - *G* Hyperglycemia
    - Corticosteroids
    - Oral contraceptives
    - Chlorthalidone
    - Ethacrynic acid
    - Thiazides
    - Furosemide
    - Diazoxide
    - Growth hormone
  - *H* Porphyria exacerbation
    - Barbiturates
    - Chlordiazepoxide
    - Meprobamate
    - Sulfonamides
    - Estrogens
    - Oral contraceptives
    - Chlorpropamide
    - Phenytoin
    - Glutethimide
    - Griseofulvin
    - Rifampin
  - *I* Hyperbilirubinemia
    - Rifampin
    - Novobiocin
- *IV* Dermatologic
  - *A* Exfoliative dermatitis
    - Penicillins
    - Sulfonamides
    - Barbiturates
    - Phenytoin
    - Phenylbutazone
    - Gold salts
    - Quinidine
  - *B* Toxic epidermal necrolysis (bullous)
    - Barbiturates
    - Phenylbutazone
    - Phenytoin
    - Sulfonamides
    - Phenolphthalein
    - Penicillins
    - Allopurinol
    - Iodides
    - Bromides
    - Nalidixic acid
  - *C* Erythema multiforme or Steven-Johnson syndrome
    - Sulfonamides
    - Barbiturates
    - Phenylbutazone
    - Chlorpropamide
    - Thiazides
    - Sulfones
    - Phenytoin
    - Ethosuximide
    - Salicylates
    - Tetracyclines
    - Codeine
    - Penicillins
  - *D* Erythema nodosum
    - Penicillins
    - Sulfonamides
    - Oral contraceptives
  - *E* Fixed drug eruptions
    - Phenolphthalein
    - Barbiturates
    - Sulfonamides
    - Salicylates
    - Phenylbutazone
    - Quinine
    - Captopril
  - *F* Photodermatitis
    - Tetracyclines, particularly demeclocycline
    - Griseofulvin
    - Sulfonamides
    - Sulfonylureas
    - Thiazides
    - Furosemide
    - Phenothiazines
    - Nalidixic acid
    - Oral contraceptives
    - Chlordiazepoxide
  - *G* Urticaria
    - Aspirin
    - Penicillins
    - Sulfonamides
    - Barbiturates
  - *H* Nonspecific rashes
    - Ampicillin
    - Barbiturates
    - Allopurinol
    - Phenytoin
    - Methyldopa
  - *I* Pigment changes (hyperpigmentation)
    - ACTH
    - Busulfan
    - Phenothiazines
    - Hypervitaminosis A
    - Oral contraceptives
    - Gold salts
    - Chloroquine and other antimalarials
    - Cyclophosphamide
    - Bleomycin
  - *J* Alopecia
    - Cytotoxics
    - Ethionamide
    - Heparin
    - Oral contraceptives (withdrawal)
  - *K* Purpura (see also thrombocytopenia)
    - Corticosteroids
    - Aspirin
  - *L* Lichenoid eruptions
    - Chlorpropamide

TABLE 72-1 *(continued)*
Clinical manifestations of adverse reactions to drugs

Gold salts
Antimalarials
PAS
Methyldopa
Phenothiazines

M Eczema (contact dermatitis)
Topical antimicrobials
Topical local anesthetics
Topical antihistamines
Cream and lotion preservatives
Lanolin

N Acne
Anabolic and androgenic steroids
Corticosteroids
Bromides
Iodides
Oral contraceptives
Isoniazid
Troxidone

V Hematologic

A Pancytopenia (aplastic anemia)
Chloramphenicol
Phenytoin
Mephenytoin
Trimethadione
Phenylbutazone
Oxyphenbutazone
Gold salts
Mepacrine
Quinacrine
Potassium perchlorate
Cytotoxics

B Agranulocytosis (see also pancytopenia)
Chloramphenicol
Sulphonamides
Phenylbutazone
Oxyphenbutazone
Gold salts
Indomethacin
Propylthiouracil
Methimazole
Carbimazole
Phenothiazines
Cytotoxics
Tolbutamide
Cotrimoxazole
Tricyclic antidepressants
Captopril

C Thrombocytopenia platelet dysfunction (see also pancytopenia)
Quinidine
Quinine
Furosemide
Chlorthalidone
Thiazides
Gold salts
Cotrimoxazole
Aspirin
Indomethacin
Phenylbutazone
Oxyphenbutazone
Chlorpropamide
Acetazolamine
Phenytoin and other hydantoins
Methyldopa
Carbamazepine
Digitoxin
Novobiocin
Carbenacillin

D Megaloblastic anemia
Folate antagonists
Cotrimoxazole
Phenytoin
Primidone
Phenobarbital
Triamterene
Trimethoprim
Oral contraceptives

E Hemolytic anemia
Methyldopa
Levodopa
Mefenamic acid
Melphalan
Isoniazid
Rifampin
Sulfonamides
Penicillins
Cephalosporins
Insulin
Quinidine
Chlorpromazine
Phenacetin
p-Aminosalicylic acid
Dapsone

F Hemolytic anemia (in G6PD deficiency)
Antimalarials, e.g., primaquine
Chloramphenicol
Dapsone
Nalidixic acid
Nitrofurantoin
Sulfonamides
Aspirin
Phenacetin
p-Aminosalicylic acid
Quinidine
Vitamin C
Vitamin K
Cotrimoxazole
Probenecid
Procainamide

G Lymphadenopathy
Phenytoin
Primidone

H Leukocytosis
Lithium
Corticosteroids

I Eosinophilia
Erythromycin estolate
Sulfonamides
Chlorpropamide
p-Aminosalicylic acid
Imipramine
Nitrofurantoin
Procarbazine
Methotrexate

VI Cardiovascular

A Exacerbation of angina
Vasopressin
Oxytocin
Ergotamine
Methysergide
Propranolol withdrawal
Excessive thyroxin
Alpha blockers
Hydralazine

B Cardiomyopathy
Emetine
Sympathomimetics
Phenothiazines
Lithium
Sulfonamides
Daunorubicin
Adriamycin

C Pericarditis
Procainamide
Hydralazine
Methysergide
Emetine

D Fluid retention or congestive heart failure
Estrogens
Steroids
Carbenoxolone
Phenylbutazone
Indomethacin
Propranolol
Mannitol
Diazoxide
Minoxidil

E Arrhythmias
Sympathomimetics
Thyroid hormone
Digitalis
Quinidine
Procainamide
Verapamil
Atropine
Propranolol
Guanethidine
Emetine
Propellants in aerosols
Tricyclic antidepressants
Phenothiazines, particularly thioridazine
Lithium
Anticholinesterases
Papaverine
Daunomycin
Adriamycin
Lincomycin (intravenous)

F Hypotension (see also arrythmias)
Nitroglycerin
Phenothiazines
Morphine
Diuretics
Citrated blood
Levodopa

G Hypertension
Oral contraceptives
Sympathomimetics
Clonidine withdrawal
Monoamine oxidase inhibitors with sympathomimetics
Tricyclic antidepressants with sympathomimetics
Corticosteroids
ACTH
Phenylbutazone

H Thromboembolism
Oral contraceptives

VII Respiratory

A Nasal congestion
Reserpine
Guanethidine
Isoproterenol
Oral contraceptives
Decongestant abuse

B Respiratory depression
Aminoglycosides
Polymixins
Trimethaphan
Opiates
Sedatives
Hypnotics

C Airway obstruction (bronchospasm, asthma; see also anaphylaxis)
Beta blockers
Nonsteroidal anti-inflammatory drugs, e.g., aspirin, indomethacin
Cholinergic drugs
Tartrazine (drugs with yellow dye)
Penicillins
Cephalosporins
Streptomycin
Pentazocine

D Pulmonary infiltrates
Nitrofurantoin
Methysergide
Chlorambucil
Procarbazine
Busulfan
Melphalan
Cyclophosphamide
Azothioprine
Bleomycin
Methotrexate
Sulfonamides

E Pulmonary edema
Heroin
Methadone
Hydrochlorthiazide
Propoxyphene
Contrast media

VIII Gastrointestinal

A Dental discoloration
Tetracycline

B Gingival hyperplasia
Phenytoin

C Oral ulceration
Aspirin
Isoproterenol (sublingual)
Cytotoxics
Pancreatin
Gentian violet

D Taste disturbances
Penicillamine
Biguanides
Griseofulvin
Metronidazole

TABLE 72-1 *(continued)*
Clinical manifestations of adverse reactions to drugs

- Lithium
- Rifampin
- Captopril

E Dry mouth
- Anticholinergics
- Levodopa
- Tricyclic antidepressants
- Clonidine
- Methyldopa

F Swelling of salivary gland
- Phenylbutazone
- Guanethidine
- Bethanidine
- Bretylium
- Clonidine
- Iodides

G Peptic ulceration or hemorrhage
- Aspirin
- Phenylbutazone
- Indomethacin
- Ethacrynic acid
- Reserpine (large doses)

H Intestinal ulceration
- Enteric-coated potassium chloride

I Nausea or vomiting
- Digitalis
- Opiates
- Estrogens
- Levodopa
- Potassium chloride
- Ferrous sulfate
- Aminophylline
- Tetracyclines

J Diarrhea or colitis
- Lincomycin
- Clindamycin
- Broad-spectrum antibiotics
- Magnesium in antacids
- Guanethidine
- Debrisoquin
- Methyldopa
- Reserpine
- Digitalis
- Colchicine
- Purgatives
- Lactose excipients

K Constipation or ileus
- Ganglionic blockers
- Tricyclic antidepressants
- Phenothiazines
- Opiates
- Aluminum hydroxide
- Calcium carbonate
- Barium sulfate
- Ion exchange resins
- Ferrous sulfate

L Malabsorption
- Broad-spectrum antibiotics
- Neomycin
- Cholestyramine
- Colchicine
- *p*-Aminosalicylic acid
- Biguanides
- Phenytoin
- Primidone
- Phenobarbital
- Cytotoxics

M Pancreatitis
- Corticosteroids
- Thiazides
- Azathioprine
- Oral contraceptives
- Sulfonamides
- Opiates
- Furosemide
- Ethacrynic acid

N Diffuse hepatocellular damage
- Halothane
- Methoxyflurane
- Methyldopa
- Isoniazid
- Rifampin
- Aminosalicylic acid
- Ethionamide
- Phenytoin and other hydantoins
- Acetaminophen (paracetamol)
- Salicylates
- Allopurinol
- Sulfonamides
- Tetracyclines
- Erythromycin estolate
- Propylthiouracil
- Methimazole
- Oxyphenisatin
- Methotrexate
- Pyridium
- Propoxyphene
- Monoamine oxidase inhibitors
- Sodium valproate

O Cholestatic jaundice
- Phenothiazines
- Androgens
- Anabolic steroids
- Oral contraceptives
- Erythromycin estolate
- Chlorpropamide
- Gold salts
- Methimazole
- Acetohexamide

IX Renal

A Nephrotic syndrome
- Penicillamine
- Gold salts
- Phenindione
- Probenecid
- Captopril

B Tubular necrosis
- Amphotericin B
- Aminoglycosides
- Polymixins
- Cephaloridine
- Tetracyclines
- Colistin
- Sulfonamides
- Radioiodinated contrast medium
- Methoxyflurane

C Interstitial nephritis
- Penicillins, particularly methicillin
- Sulfonamides
- Phenindione
- Furosemide
- Thiazides

D Nephropathies
- Due to analgesics (e.g., phenacetin)

E Concentrating defect with polyuria (or nephrogenic diabetes insipidus)
- Vitamin D
- Lithium
- Demeclocycline
- Methoxyflurane

F Renal tubular acidosis
- Degraded tetracycline
- Amphotericin B
- Acetazolamide

G Calculi
- Acetazolamide
- Vitamin D

H Obstructive uropathy
- Intrarenal: cytotoxics
- Extrarenal: methysergide

I Hemorrhagic cystitis
- Cyclophosphamide

J Bladder dysfunction
- Anticholinergics
- Monoamine oxidase inhibitors
- Tricyclic antidepressants
- Disopyramide

X Genital (see also endocrine)

A Vaginal carcinoma
- Diethylstilbestrol (administered to mother)

B Impairment of spermatogenesis or oogenesis
- Cytotoxics

XI Neurologic

A Peripheral neuropathy
- Isoniazid
- Hydralazine
- Nitrofurantoin
- Vincristine
- Mustine
- Streptomycin
- Polymixin, colistan
- Clioquinol
- Phenelzine
- Tricyclic antidepressants
- Chloramphenicol
- Procarbazine
- Ethambutol
- Ethionamide
- Glutethimide
- Demeclocycline
- Nalidixic acid
- Tolbutamide
- Chlorpropamide
- Methysergide
- Phenytoin

B Exacerbation of myasthenia
- Aminoglycosides
- Polymixins

C Extrapyramidal effects
- Butyrophenones, e.g., haloperidol
- Phenothiazines
- Tricyclic antidepressants
- Methyldopa
- Levodopa
- Reserpine
- Metoclopramide
- Oral contraceptives

D Seizures
- Amphetamines
- Analeptics
- Phenothiazines
- Isoniazid
- Lidocaine
- Theophylline
- Penicillins
- Nalidixic acid
- Physostigmine
- Tricyclic antidepressants
- Vincristine
- Lithium

E Stroke
- Oral contraceptives

F Pseudotumor cerebri (or intracranial hypertension)
- Corticosteroids
- Oral contraceptives
- Tetracyclines
- Hypervitaminosis A

G Headache
- Hydralazine
- Bromides
- Glyceryl trinitrate
- Ergotamine (withdrawal)
- Indomethacin

XII Ocular

A Corneal opacities
- Vitamin D
- Mepacrine
- Chloroquine
- Indomethacin

B Corneal edema
- Oral contraceptives

C Cataracts
- Phenothiazines
- Corticosteroids
- Busulfan
- Chlorambucil

D Glaucoma
- Mydriatics
- Sympathomimetics

E Retinopathy
- Chloroquine
- Phenothiazines

F Optic neuritis
- Clioquinol
- Chloramphenicol
- Streptomycin
- Isoniazid
- Ethambutol
- Quinine
- Phenothiazines
- Penicillamine
- PAS
- Phenylbutazone

G Alteration in color vision
- Troxidone
- Sulfonamides
- Streptomycin

TABLE 72-1 *(continued)*
Clinical manifestations of adverse reactions to drugs

Methaqualone
Barbiturates
Digitalis
Thiazides

XIII Ear
- *A* Vestibular disorders
  - Aminoglycosides
  - Quinine
  - Mustine
- *B* Deafness
  - Aminoglycosides
  - Ethacrynic acid
  - Furosemide
  - Quinine
  - Bleomycin
  - Chloroquine
  - Mustine
  - Aspirin
  - Nortriptyline

XIV Musculoskeletal
- *A* Myopathy or myalgia
  - Corticosteroids
  - Chloroquine
  - Clofibrate
  - Oral contraceptives
  - Amphotericin B
  - Carbenoxolone
- *B* Bone disorders
  - *1* Osteoporosis
    - Corticosteroids
    - Heparin
  - *2* Osteomalacia
    - Anticonvulsants
    - Glutethemide
    - Aluminum hydroxide

XV Psychiatric disorders
- *A* Schizophrenic-like or paranoid reactions
  - Amphetamines
  - Lysergic acid
  - Levodopa
  - Tricyclic antidepressants
  - Monoamine oxidase inhibitors
  - Bromides
  - Corticosteroids
- *B* Depression
  - Centrally acting antihypertensives (reserpine, methyldopa, clonidine)
  - Propranolol
  - Corticosteroids
  - Amphetamine withdrawal
  - Levodopa
- *C* Hypomania, mania or excited reactions
  - Levodopa
  - Sympathomimetics
  - Corticosteroids
  - MAO inhibitors
  - Tricyclic antidepressants
- *D* Hallucinatory states
  - Amantadine
  - Narcotics
  - Pentazocine
  - Propranolol
  - Levodopa
  - Tricyclic antidepressants
  - Meperidine
- *E* Delirious or confusional states
  - Digitalis
  - Anticholinergics
  - Bromides
  - Sedatives and hypnotics
  - Phenothiazines
  - Antidepressants
  - Corticosteroids
  - Isoniazid
  - Levodopa
  - Amantadine
  - Penicillins
  - Aminophylline
  - Methyldopa
- *F* Sleep disturbances
  - Anorexiants
  - Levodopa
  - Monoamine oxidase inhibitors
  - Sympathomimetics
- *G* Drowsiness
  - Anxiolytic drugs
  - Major tranquilizers
  - Tricyclic antidepressants
  - Antihistamines
  - Methyldopa
  - Clonidine
  - Reserpine

tionship between drug administration and development of illness, and familiarity with the manifestations most often caused by particular drugs. Although specific reactions have been described as resulting from the use of particular drugs, there is always a "first," and any drug should be suspected of causing an adverse effect if the clinical setting is appropriate.

Illness related to a drug's pharmacologic action may be more easily recognized than illness attributable to immunologic or other mechanisms. For example, side effects such as cardiac arrhythmias in patients receiving digitalis, hypoglycemia in patients given insulin, and bleeding in patients receiving anticoagulants are more easily related to the prescribed drug than are symptoms like fever or rash, which may be caused by many drugs or by other factors.

Once an adverse reaction is suspected, discontinuance of the suspected drug followed by disappearance of the reaction is presumptive evidence of a drug-induced illness. Reappearance of the reaction upon cautious readministration of the drug may provide confirmatory evidence of the relationship if such confirmation adds useful information to the future management of the patient without entailing undue risk. With concentration-dependent adverse reactions, lowering the dosage may also be followed by disappearance of the reaction, and increasing the dose may cause it to reappear. When the reaction is thought to be allergic, however, readministration of the drug may be hazardous, since anaphylactic shock may develop. Readministration is unwise under these conditions unless alternate drugs are not available and treatment is mandatory.

If the patient is receiving many different drugs when an adverse reaction is suspected, the drugs most likely to be incriminated can usually be identified. All drugs may be discontinued at once, or if this is not practical, then drugs should be discontinued one at a time, starting with the drug under greatest suspicion, and the patient observed for signs of improvement. It must be remembered that the time taken for the disappearance of a concentration-dependent adverse effect will depend on the time taken for the concentration to fall below the range associated with the adverse effect, and this is turn will depend on the initial blood level and on the rate of elimination or metabolism of the drug. Adverse effects of drugs such as phenobarbital which have long half-lives will take a considerable time to disappear.

To assist in the identification of adverse reactions, a table of the drugs recognized as producing a number of reactions appears in this chapter (Table 72-1). This table is not intended to be exhaustive but rather includes well-documented reactions and some less well-documented reactions which are sufficiently devastating as to require their consideration. It should be used to suggest the likely causative drug, but the absence of a drug from the table should not be interpreted to mean that it is not responsible for the reaction.

Serum antibody has been demonstrated in some persons with drug allergy involving cellular blood elements, as in agranulocytosis, hemolytic anemia, and thrombocytopenia. For example, both quinine and quinidine can produce platelet agglutination in vitro in the presence of complement and the serum from a patient who has developed thrombocytopenia following this drug.

Eliciting a drug history from patients is important for diagnosis. Attention must be directed to nonprescription, or OTC, as well as to prescription drugs. Each type can be responsible for adverse drug effects, and frequently adverse interactions occur between drugs purchased by patients over the counter and those prescribed by physicians. In addition, it is common for patients to be cared for by several physicians; and duplicative, additive, counteractive, or synergistic drugs may therefore be taken if the physicians are not aware of the patients' drug histories. Every physician should determine what drugs a patient has been taking, at least during the preceding 30 days, before prescribing any medications. A history of previous adverse drug effects in patients is common. Since these patients have a predisposition to other drug-induced illnesses, familiarity with such a history should dictate added caution in prescribing drugs.

Patients with biochemical abnormalities such as erythrocyte G6PD deficiency can be identified; patients with the defect are usually blacks or of Mediterranean extraction. Drug-induced hemolytic crisis can be avoided by testing for the enzyme defect before administering these drugs. Similarly, persons with an abnormal serum pseudocholinesterase may have abnormally prolonged apnea when given succinylcholine.

General comments No drug is completely without side effects, and it is important to remember that a side effect in one patient may be the desired pharmacologic effect in another. Recent improvements in drug regulation allow physicians to prescribe drugs with considerable confidence in their purity, bioavailability, and effectiveness. However, while regulatory bodies try to ensure that drugs with serious toxic potential are not marketed, they have to constantly weigh the potential toxicity against the possible benefits. Thus toxicity which would be acceptable for an effective antineoplastic agent would not be permitted in, for example, an oral contraceptive. In addition, because of the necessarily small number of patients treated in premarketing studies, rare adverse reactions cannot be identified, so that the first responsibility for identifying and reporting these effects must rest with the practicing clinician through the use of the various national adverse reaction reporting systems, such as those operated by the Food and Drug Administration in the United States and the Committee on Safety of Medicines in Great Britain. The publication of a newly recognized adverse reaction can in a short time stimulate a very large number of similar such reports which previously had gone unrecognized.

The prevention of adverse drug reactions must first involve a high index of suspicion that the development of a new symptom or sign may be drug-related. Reduction of the dose or discontinuation of the suspected agent will usually clarify the position in concentration-dependent toxic reactions. Physicians should be familiar with the common adverse effects of the drugs they use, and if they are in doubt, should consult the literature.

REFERENCES

BÖTTINGER LE et al: Drug-induced blood dyscrasias. Acta Med Scand 205:457, 1979

———, et al: Fatal reactions to drugs. Acta Med Scand 205:451, 1979

DAVIES DM: *Textbook of Adverse Drug Reactions*, 2d ed. New York, Oxford University Press, 1981

KRAMER MS et al: An algorithm for the operational assessment of adverse drug reactions. JAMA 242(7):623, 1979

MITCHELL JR et al: Toxic drug reactions, in *Handbook of Experimental Pharmacology*, vol 28, no 3: *Concepts in Biochemical Pharmacology*, JR Gilette, JR Mitchell (eds). New York, Springer Verlag, 1975

SHAPIRO S et al: Fatal drug reactions among medical in-patients, JAMA 216:467, 1971

STEEL K et al: Iatrogenic illness on a general medical service at a university hospital, N Engl J Med 304:638, 1981

73
THE AUTONOMIC NERVOUS SYSTEM

LEWIS LANDSBERG
JAMES B. YOUNG

FUNCTIONAL ORGANIZATION OF THE AUTONOMIC NERVOUS SYSTEM

The autonomic nervous system is an efferent system that innervates vascular and visceral smooth muscle, exocrine and endocrine glands, and parenchymal cells throughout the various organ systems. Functioning below the conscious level, the autonomic nervous system responds rapidly and continuously to perturbations that threaten the constancy of the internal environment. Foremost among the many functions governed by this system are the following: the distribution of blood flow and the maintenance of tissue perfusion, the regulation of blood pressure, the regulation of the volume and composition of the extracellular fluid, the expenditure of metabolic energy and supply of substrate, and the activity of visceral smooth muscle and glands.

Autonomic responses, like those of the somatic nervous system, are induced promptly and dissipated quickly, in contrast to the slower, more prolonged effects of circulating hormones. The autonomic nervous system, like the endocrine system, regulates the rate of processes that have an intrinsic activity of their own, while the somatic nervous system initiates responses de novo. Although certain autonomic responses are highly discriminating, many are generalized and influence a variety of effectors in different organs. The interface between the autonomic nervous system and the endocrine system is exemplified by the adrenal medulla. This gland, homologous in many respects with the postganglionic sympathetic neuron, secretes a hormone (epinephrine) into the circulation to interact with adrenergic receptors throughout the body.

ANATOMIC ORGANIZATION The autonomic neurons, located in ganglia outside the central nervous system, give rise to the postganglionic autonomic nerves that innervate organs and tissues throughout the body. The activity of autonomic nerves is regulated by central neurons responsive to a diversity of afferent inputs. After central integration of afferent information autonomic outflow is adjusted to permit the smooth functioning of the major organ systems in accordance with the needs of the organism as a whole. Connections between the cerebral cortex and the autonomic centers in the brainstem coordinate autonomic outflow with higher mental functions.

The sympathetic and parasympathetic divisions The preganglionic neurons of the parasympathetic nervous system leave the central nervous system in the third, seventh, ninth, and tenth cranial nerves and in the second and third sacral nerves, while the preganglionic neurons of the sympathetic nervous system exit the spinal cord between the first thoracic and the second lumbar segments. Responses to sympathetic and parasympathetic stimulation are frequently antagonistic, as exemplified by their opposing effects on heart rate and gut motility. This antagonism reflects highly coordinated interactions within the central nervous system; the resultant changes in parasympathetic and sympathetic activity, often reciprocal, provide more precise control of autonomic responses than could be achieved by the modulation of a single system.

Neurotransmitters *Acetylcholine* (ACh) is the preganglionic neurotransmitter for both divisions of the autonomic nervous system, as well as the postganglionic neurotransmitter of the parasympathetic neurons. Those nerves which release ACh are said to be cholinergic. *Norepinephrine* (NE) is the neurotransmitter of the postganglionic sympathetic neurons; these nerves are said to be adrenergic. Within the sympathetic outflow postganglionic neurons innervating the eccrine sweat glands (and perhaps some blood vessels supplying skeletal muscle) are of the cholinergic type.

THE SYMPATHETIC NERVOUS SYSTEM AND THE ADRENAL MEDULLA

CATECHOLAMINES All three of the naturally occurring catecholamines, NE, *epinephrine* (E), and *dopamine*, function as neurotransmitters within the central nervous system. NE, the neurotransmitter of postganglionic sympathetic nerve endings, exerts its effects locally, in the immediate vicinity of its release. E, the circulating hormone of the adrenal medulla, influences processes throughout the body. Although dopamine infusion evokes responses distinct from those of E and NE, and although specific dopaminergic receptors outside the central nervous system have been described, dopamine has not been established unequivocally as a circulating hormone or neurotransmitter in the periphery.

Biosynthesis (Fig. 73-1) The biosynthesis of catecholamines proceeds from the amino acid tyrosine, which is sequentially hydroxylated to form dopa, decarboxylated to form dopamine, and hydroxylated on the beta position of the side chain to form NE. The initial step, the hydroxylation of tyrosine, is rate-limiting and is regulated so that synthesis is coupled to release. This regulation is achieved by alterations in both the activity and the amount of tyrosine hydroxylase. In the adrenal medulla, and in those central neurons utilizing E as neurotransmitter, NE is *N*-methylated to E by the enzyme phenylethanolamine-*N*-methyltransferase (PNMT). Since a major portion of the blood perfusing the adrenal medulla is enriched with corticosteroids from the adrenal cortex, and since adrenal PNMT is inducible by high concentrations of glucocorticoids, the capacity of the adrenal medulla to form E may be related to its strategic location within the adrenal cortex.

FIGURE 73-1

Catecholamine biosynthesis, release, and metabolism. Schematic representation of a peripheral sympathetic nerve ending is shown at the top; the bulbous areas on the terminal fiber represent varicosities identified by histochemical fluorescence techniques as areas of high neurotransmitter concentration. The processes of biosynthesis, release, modulation, and reuptake are shown sequentially for demonstration purposes only; in vivo they proceed concurrently. Adrenal medullary chromaffin cells are shown at the bottom of the diagram. (TH = tyrosine hydroxylase, AAD = aromatic-L-amino acid decarboxylase, DA = dopamine, DBH = dopamine-β-hydroxylase, NE = norepinephrine, PNMT = phenylethanolamine-N-methyltransferase, E = epinephrine, COMT = catechol-O-methyltransferase, NMN = normetanephrine, MAO = monoamine oxidase, DHMA = 3,4-dihydroxymandelic acid, VMA = 3-methoxy-4-hydroxymandelic acid.)

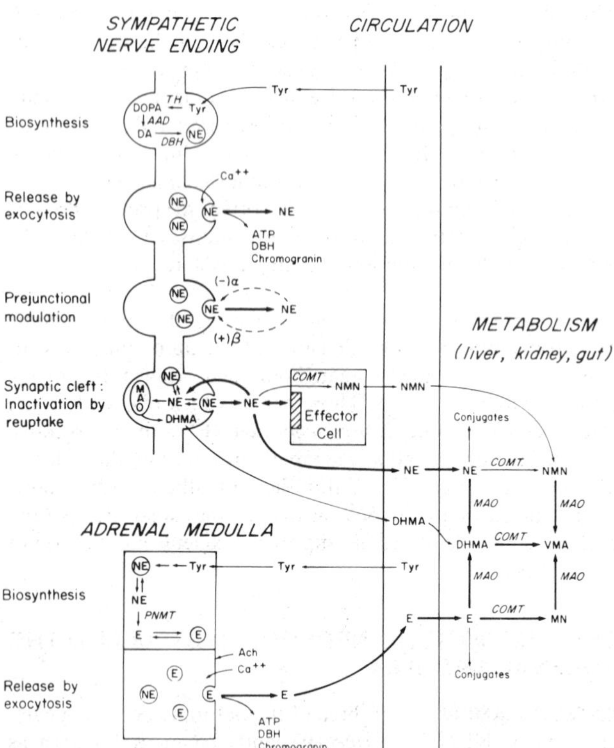

Catecholamine metabolism (Fig. 73-1) The major metabolic transformations of catecholamines involve *O*-methylation at the meta-hydroxyl group and oxidative deamination. *O*-methylation is catalyzed by the enzyme catechol-*O*-methyltransferase (COMT), and oxidative deamination is promoted by monoamine oxidase (MAO). COMT in liver and kidney is important in the metabolism of circulating catecholamines. MAO, a mitochondrial enzyme present in most tissues, including nerve endings, has a lesser role in the metabolism of circulating catecholamines but is important in regulating the catecholamine stores within the peripheral sympathetic nerve endings. The metanephrines and VMA are the major end products of catecholamine metabolism.

STORAGE AND RELEASE OF CATECHOLAMINES Catecholamines are stored in subcellular granules and released by exocytosis both in the adrenal medulla and sympathetic nerve endings. The large stores of catecholamines in these tissues provide an important physiological reserve that maintains an adequate supply of catecholamines in the face of intense stimulation.

Adrenal medulla The adrenal medullary chromaffin tissue within a pair of normal human adrenal glands weighs about 1 g and contains approximately 6 mg of catecholamines, 85 percent of which is E. Catecholamines are maintained in high concentration within the storage (chromaffin) granule by an active uptake process involving the granule membrane and by an intragranular storage complex that appears to involve ATP, calcium, and a specific granule protein (chromagranin). Catecholamine secretion, stimulated by ACh from the preganglionic sympathetic nerves, occurs after calcium influx triggers fusion of the chromaffin granule membrane and cell membrane; obliteration of the cell membrane at the point of fusion and extrusion of the entire soluble contents of the granule into the extracellular space complete the process of exocytosis (Fig. 73-1). Approximately 2 to 10 percent of the total adrenal medullary catecholamine store is turned over each day.

Peripheral sympathetic nerve endings The peripheral sympathetic nerve endings form a reticulum or ground plexus which brings the terminal fibers into close contact with effector cells. All the NE present in peripheral tissues is in the sympathetic nerve endings, and heavily innervated tissues contain as much as 1 to 2 μg/g of tissue. NE storage in the nerve endings is within discrete subcellular particles analogous to the adrenal medullary chromaffin granules. MAO within the mitochondria of the nerve endings plays an important role in regulating the local concentration of NE (Fig. 73-1). Amines within the storage vesicles are protected from oxidative deamination; amines within the cytoplasm, however, are deaminated to inactive metabolites. Release from the nerve ending occurs in response to action potentials propagated in the terminal sympathetic fibers (Fig. 73-1).

THE PERIPHERAL ADRENERGIC NEUROEFFECTOR JUNCTION Neuronal uptake The peripheral sympathetic nerve endings possess an amine transport system that actively takes up amines from the extracellular fluid. A variety of synthetic and naturally occurring amines are substrates for this process. Neuronal uptake or recapture of locally released NE terminates the action of the transmitter and contributes to the constancy of the NE stores (Fig. 73-1).

Prejunctional modulation Several mediators operating at the peripheral sympathetic nerve ending (referred to as prejunctional or presynaptic sites) appear to modify sympathetic neurotransmission by influencing the amount of NE released in response to nerve impulses. Prejunctional modulation may be either inhibitory or facilitatory. Certain modulators, such as catecholamines and ACh, may either inhibit or facilitate NE release, antagonistic effects that are mediated by different adrenergic or cholinergic receptors, respectively. Those compounds exerting an *inhibitory* effect on NE release at the prejunctional nerve ending include the following: catecholamines (alpha receptor), ACh (muscarinic receptor), dopamine, histamine (H-2 receptor), serotonin, adenosine, enkephalins, and prostaglandins. *Facilitatory* prejunctional modulators include catecholamines (beta receptor), ACh (nicotinic receptor), and angiotensin II. The overall significance of prejunctional modulation, as well as the relative importance of the various mediators, has yet to be established.

PREJUNCTIONAL ADRENERGIC RECEPTORS Catecholamines reduce NE release via prejunctional alpha receptors in a classical negative feedback system. The negative feedback system is complicated, however, by the fact that beta-receptor activation facilitates NE release. Two hypotheses have been advanced to explain how the antagonistic alpha and beta effects on NE release may be integrated in a physiologically meaningful response. One hypothesis depends upon the fact that beta-mediated effects occur at lower agonist concentrations than those mediated by the alpha receptor. During low levels of sympathetic stimulation, therefore, when NE concentrations in the synaptic cleft are low, beta-mediated positive feedback may predominate with facilitation of NE release. Conversely, at higher levels of sympathetic stimulation with increased NE concentration in the synaptic cleft, alpha-mediated negative feedback predominates and NE release is inhibited. The other hypothesis depends upon the fact that prejunctional beta receptors are more sensitive to E than NE; circulating levels of E, therefore, may stimulate the prejunctional beta receptors thereby augmenting NE release and enhancing sympathetic neurotransmission.

PREJUNCTIONAL CHOLINERGIC RECEPTORS Though both inhibitory and facilitatory effects of ACh on NE release have been described, the inhibitory effect of ACh, mediated by the muscarinic cholinergic receptor, occurs at lower ACh concentrations and is probably of greater physiological significance. This peripheral inhibitory effect of ACh on adrenergic neurotransmission may reinforce the reciprocal changes in central parasympathetic and sympathetic outflow that occur in the regulation of numerous physiological responses.

CENTRAL REGULATION OF SYMPATHOADRENAL OUTFLOW

Brainstem sympathetic centers Sympathetic outflow is initiated from groups of neurons within the reticular formation of the medulla oblongata and pons. Descending bulbospinal tracts originating in these neurons synapse in the intermediolateral cell column of the spinal cord with the preganglionic sympathetic neurons. The brainstem sympathetic centers, which have an intrinsic activity of their own, are regulated by many stimuli, including those from more rostral areas of the central nervous system (cortex, limbic lobe, hypothalamus); neural afferents which interact at the level of the brainstem centers and at the higher centers; and changes in the physical and chemical properties of the extracellular fluid, including the concentrations of hormones and substrates. The higher centers, which have connections with the brainstem, coordinate sympathetic outflow with higher mental functions, emotional reactions, and the homeostatic needs of the internal environment. Although the hallmark of intense sympathoadrenal stimulation is a global response (the fight-or-flight reaction of Cannon), sympathetic reactions are not invariably generalized; discrete changes in sympathetic outflow to different organ systems appear to be involved in the regulation of many autonomic functions.

RELATIONSHIP BETWEEN THE SYMPATHETIC NERVOUS SYSTEM AND THE ADRENAL MEDULLA The sympathetic nervous system and the adrenal medulla are often stimulated together. During periods of intense sympathetic stimulation the adrenal medulla is progressively recruited and circulating E reinforces the physiological effects of sympathetic stimulation. In other situations, however, the sympathetic nervous system and the adrenal medulla are stimulated independently. The response to upright posture, for example, involves predominantly the sympathetic nervous system while hypoglycemia stimulates only the adrenal medulla.

Sympathetic regulation of the cardiovascular system The sympathetic nervous system plays a major role in the regulation of the circulation. Stretch receptors in the systemic and pulmonary arteries and veins continuously monitor intravascular pressures; the resulting afferent impulses, after relay and integration in the brainstem, alter sympathetic activity in defense of blood pressure and blood flow to critical areas (Fig. 73-2).

ARTERIAL BARORECEPTORS An increase in blood pressure stimulates receptors in the carotid sinus and aortic arch. The ensuing afferent impulses, after relay within the nucleus of the solitary tract (NTS) in the brainstem, result in suppression of the brainstem sympathetic centers (Fig. 73-2). This baroreceptor reflex arc forms a negative feedback loop in which a rise in arterial pressure results in the inhibition of central sympathetic outflow. Interacting with the NTS is a brainstem noradrenergic pathway that participates in suppression of sympathetic outflow. This noradrenergic inhibitory pathway is stimulated by centrally acting alpha-adrenergic agonists, and may be in-

FIGURE 73-2
Sympathetic regulation of the circulation. Receptors in the venous and arterial circulations are stimulated by stretch, caused by an increase in pressure; afferent impulses from these receptors are carried to the central nervous system by the ninth and tenth cranial nerves. The net result of these afferent impulses, after relay in the brainstem, is to inhibit central sympathetic outflow. The arterial baroreceptor reflex involves a relay in the nucleus of the tractus solitarius (NTS). (+ = stimulation; − = inhibition.)

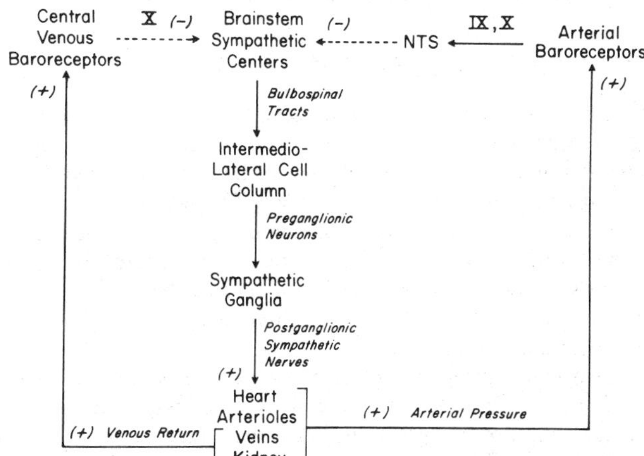

volved in the action of certain antihypertensive drugs such as clonidine, which potentiate the baroreceptor-mediated vasodepressor response (Chap. 267). In the opposite manner, when the blood pressure falls, decreased afferent impulses diminish central inhibition, resulting in an increase in sympathetic outflow and a rise in arterial pressure.

CENTRAL VENOUS PRESSURE Receptors in the low-pressure circuit in the walls of the great veins and within the atria are also involved in the regulation of sympathetic outflow. Stimulation of these receptors by high venous pressure suppresses the brainstem sympathetic centers; when central venous pressure is low, sympathetic outflow increases. The central connections are poorly understood but the afferent impulses appear to be carried in the vagus (Fig. 73-2).

ASSESSMENT OF SYMPATHOADRENAL ACTIVITY The clinical assessment of sympathoadrenal activity involves the measurement of catecholamines in plasma and of catecholamines and catecholamine metabolites in urine. Quantitation of urinary catecholamines and metabolites is useful in the diagnosis of pheochromocytoma (Chap. 113).

Plasma catecholamines The plasma NE level appears to be the best currently available index of sympathetic nervous system activity in humans. From a clinical standpoint, however, the usefulness of plasma catecholamine levels is limited to the evaluation of patients with autonomic insufficiency (Chap. 29) and, on occasion, patients with suspected pheochromocytoma (Chap. 113).

Basal plasma NE concentrations are in the range of 150 to 350 pg/ml; basal E levels are about 25 to 50 pg/ml. The half-time of disappearance of NE from the circulation is approximately 2 min. The plasma NE level is markedly affected by a variety of factors, including posture; accordingly, the conditions under which blood is obtained for assay must be carefully controlled. By convention, basal plasma NE levels are those obtained through an indwelling intravenous line after the patient has rested supine in a relaxed environment for 30 min.

PLASMA NE RESPONSE TO UPRIGHT POSTURE The predictable increase in circulating NE concentration during upright posture provides a convenient test of sympathetic nervous system function. A normal response requires an intact afferent system, appropriate central nervous system relays, and an intact peripheral sympathetic nervous system; a defect of any of these components will reduce the increment in circulating NE.

Plasma E levels have been less well studied. Change in plasma E with upright posture is usually small. Hypoglycemia and various types of mental stress, however, are associated with large increments in the plasma E level.

ADRENERGIC RECEPTORS

Catecholamines influence effector cells by interacting with specific recognition sites, or *receptors,* located on the cell surface. When stimulated by catecholamines, the adrenergic receptor initiates a series of membrane changes followed by a cascade of intracellular events that culminates in a measurable response. Compounds that elicit the response are referred to as *agonists;* those that block the interaction of the agonist with the receptor are referred to as adrenergic *receptor blocking agents* or *antagonists.*

Two major categories of response to catecholamines have long been recognized. The different types of responses reflect the activation of two populations of adrenergic receptors, designated *alpha* and *beta.* This division is clinically important because selective agonists and antagonists are available, enabling pharmacological stimulation or blockade of the physiological effects mediated by one receptor without influencing those mediated by the other. Both alpha and beta receptors may be further divided into partially distinct subtypes.

ALPHA-ADRENERGIC RECEPTORS The alpha-adrenergic receptor mediates a variety of physiological responses, including vasoconstriction, intestinal relaxation, and pupillary dilatation. E and NE are approximately equipotent as alpha-receptor agonists. Postjunctional or postsynaptic alpha-adrenergic receptors located on the effector cell (Fig. 73-1) have been designated alpha$_1$ to distinguish them from the prejunctional alpha-adrenergic receptors located on the sympathetic nerve endings; the latter receptors, designated alpha$_2$, mediate suppression of NE release from sympathetic nerve endings and inhibition of ACh release at cholinergic nerve terminals. Within the central nervous system alpha$_2$-adrenergic receptors may play a role in the action of some commonly used centrally active antihypertensive drugs. The second messenger is not known for all alpha-adrenergically mediated effects, but many responses are related to changes in intracellular calcium concentration.

BETA-ADRENERGIC RECEPTORS Physiological events associated with beta-adrenergic receptor responses include stimulation of heart rate and contractility, vasodilation, bronchodilation, and lipolysis. Beta-receptor responses have also been divided into two types. The beta$_1$ receptor responds equally to E and NE and mediates cardiac stimulation and lipolysis. The beta$_2$ receptor is much more responsive to E than to NE and induces vasodilation and bronchodilation. Isoproterenol stimulates, and propranolol blocks, both beta$_1$ and beta$_2$ receptors. Other agonists and antagonists that selectively block or stimulate the beta$_1$ or beta$_2$ receptors have been used therapeutically where the desired response involves predominantly one of the two subtypes.

The second messenger for most, if not all, beta-receptor responses is cyclic AMP (see Chap. 86). In many tissues correlations between beta-receptor occupancy and stimulation of adenylate cyclase, on the one hand, and between intracellular cyclic AMP accumulation and physiological response, on the other, have been demonstrated. While in some systems sequential enzymatic activations involving cyclic AMP–mediated protein phosphorylation or phosphomethylation are known to couple beta-receptor stimulation and physiological response, in most tissues the molecular events that mediate beta-adrenergic responses are unknown.

DOPAMINERGIC RECEPTORS Specific dopaminergic receptors, distinct from the classical alpha- and beta-adrenergic receptors, are present in the central and peripheral nervous system, and in certain nonneural peripheral tissues. Different subtypes exist; at some sites dopaminergic receptors utilize the adenylate cyclase–cyclic AMP system as a second messenger. Dopaminergic receptors stimulate renal and mesenteric vasodilation as well as relaxation of the lower esophageal sphincter. Although the physiological significance of these dopaminergic receptors is uncertain, they are of recognized pharmacological importance since dopamine is commonly employed as a pressor amine in the treatment of shock (Chap. 29) when renal and mesenteric vasodilation may be advantageous. Other dopaminergic effects of potential importance include suppression of aldosterone secretion and stimulation of renal sodium excretion.

RADIOLIGAND STUDIES OF ADRENERGIC RECEPTORS Radiolabeled adrenergic-receptor antagonists have been utilized as ligands to study the properties of adrenergic receptors. In combination with studies of peripheral tissue sensitivity these ligand studies have indicated that changes in adrenergic receptors may occur under different physiological situations. Prolonged exposure to an adrenergic agonist results in a diminished physiological response, a phenomenon known as *tachyphylaxis* or *desensitization.* Radioligand studies of adrenergic receptors indicate that this phenomenon may be attributable to a reduction in the density of adrenergic receptors on the cell surfaces. Changes in adrenergic receptors may also be involved in the altered response to catecholamines noted in many clinical situations; thyroid hormones, for example, potentiate beta-receptor-mediated responses, perhaps by increasing the density of beta-adrenergic receptors.

PHYSIOLOGY OF THE SYMPATHOADRENAL SYSTEM

Catecholamines contribute to the functional regulation of all the major organ systems. The effects induced by catecholamines take place in seconds as compared with the minutes, hours, or days that characterize the actions of the endocrine system and the other feedback loops that regulate bodily processes. The sympathoadrenal system, moreover, may respond in anticipation of a particular physiological requirement. An increase in sympathoadrenal activity prior to strenuous exercise, for example, prepares the various organ systems in advance and lessens the impact of exercise on the internal environment.

DIRECT EFFECTS OF CATECHOLAMINES Cardiovascular system Catecholamines stimulate vasoconstriction in the subcutaneous, mucosal, splanchnic, and renal vascular beds by an alpha-receptor-mediated mechanism. Since vasoconstriction in the coronary and cerebral circulations is minimal, flow to these areas is maintained. The adaptive significance of this priority given the heart and brain is clear; in both of these organs the metabolic requirements relative to blood flow are high and continuous perfusion is essential to sustain life. Skeletal muscle vasculature contains beta receptors sensitive to low circulating levels of E so that skeletal muscle blood flow is augmented during sympathoadrenal activation.

The effects of catecholamines on the heart are mediated by beta receptors and include an increase in heart rate, an enhancement of cardiac contractility, and an increase in conduction velocity. The increase in myocardial contractility is expressed physiologically by a leftward and upward shift of the ventricular function curve (Fig. 252-5) which relates cardiac work to ventricular diastolic fiber length; at any initial fiber length catecholamines increase the amount of cardiac work performed. Catecholamines also enhance cardiac output by stimulating venoconstriction, enhancing venous return, and by increasing the force of atrial contraction, thereby augmenting diastolic volume and hence fiber length. The acceleration of conduction in the junctional tissues results in a more synchronous, and hence more effective, ventricular contraction. The biological cost of cardiac stimulation is increased myocardial oxygen consumption, a factor of major importance in the pathogenesis and treatment of myocardial ischemia.

Metabolism Catecholamines increase metabolic rate. The biochemical processes involved and the sites of the increased heat production are not known with certainty, but at least in small mammals stimulation of sodium, potassium ATPase, and uncoupling of mitochondrial respiration in brown adipose tissue appear to be important.

SUBSTRATE MOBILIZATION In a variety of tissues catecholamines stimulate the breakdown of stored fuel with the production of substrate for local consumption; glycogenolysis in the

heart, for example, provides substrate for immediate metabolism by the myocardium. In addition, catecholamines accelerate fuel mobilization in liver, adipose tissue, and skeletal muscle thereby liberating substrates (glucose, free fatty acids, lactate) into the circulation for use throughout the body. Activation of enzymes involved in fuel breakdown occurs by a beta-receptor mechanism for adipose tissue lipolysis and by alpha- and beta-receptor mechanisms for hepatic glycogenolysis and gluconeogenesis. In skeletal muscle catecholamines stimulate glycogenolysis (beta receptor) with the net result of increasing lactate efflux.

Fluids and electrolytes Catecholamines contribute to the regulation of the volume and composition of extracellular fluid. By a direct action on the renal tubule, catecholamines stimulate sodium reabsorption, thereby defending extracellular fluid volume. Catecholamines also promote cellular uptake of potassium, thereby defending against the development of hyperkalemia. Regulation of calcium, magnesium, and phosphate metabolism may involve catecholamines as well.

Viscera Catecholamines affect visceral function by actions on smooth muscle and glandular epithelium. Urinary bladder and intestinal smooth muscle are relaxed while the corresponding sphincters are stimulated. Gallbladder emptying also involves sympathetic mechanisms. Catecholamine-mediated smooth-muscle contraction in the female aids ovulation and ovum transport along the fallopian tubes, and in the male provides propulsive force for the seminal fluid during ejaculation. Inhibitory alpha receptors on cholinergic neurons within the gut contribute to intestinal relaxation. Catecholamines induce bronchodilation by a beta-receptor-mediated mechanism.

INDIRECT EFFECTS OF CATECHOLAMINES The ultimate physiological response induced by catecholamines involves changes in hormone secretion and in blood flow distribution, both of which support and amplify the direct effects of catecholamines.

Endocrine system Catecholamines influence the secretion of a variety of hormones, including renin, insulin, glucagon, calcitonin, parathormone, thyroxine, gastrin, erythropoietin, progesterone, and, possibly, testosterone. Each of these hormones is governed by feedback loops that depend upon changes in the composition of the extracellular fluid or in the secretion of hypothalamic and pituitary peptides. With the exception of thyroxine and the gonadal steroids, each is a polypeptide not under the direct control of the pituitary gland. Sympathoadrenal input into the secretion of these hormones provides a mechanism for regulation by the central nervous system and ensures a rapid, coordinated hormonal response in accordance with the homeostatic needs of the organism.

RENIN The juxtaglomerular apparatus of the kidney is heavily innervated. Sympathetic stimulation increases renin release by a direct beta-receptor effect independent of vascular changes within the kidney. The renin response to volume depletion is largely sympathetically mediated and is initiated by a fall in central venous pressure. Since renin secretion activates the angiotensin-aldosterone system, angiotensin-induced vasoconstriction supports the direct effects of catecholamines on blood vessels, while aldosterone-mediated sodium reabsorption complements the direct increase in sodium reabsorption induced by sympathetic stimulation. Beta-receptor blocking agents suppress renin secretion.

INSULIN AND GLUCAGON The pancreatic islets also receive an extensive sympathetic innervation. Stimulation of pancreatic sympathetic nerves or an elevation in circulating catecholamines suppresses insulin and increases glucagon release. Inhibition of insulin secretion is mediated by the alpha receptor, while stimulation of glucagon is mediated by the beta receptor. This combination of effects on insulin and glucagon secretion supports substrate mobilization, thereby reinforcing the direct effects of catecholamines on hepatic glucose output and lipolysis. Although alpha-receptor-mediated suppression of insulin release usually appears to predominate, a potentially important beta-receptor mechanism also augments insulin secretion.

SYMPATHOADRENAL FUNCTION IN SELECTED PHYSIOLOGICAL AND PATHOPHYSIOLOGICAL STATES **Support of the circulation** The sympathetic nervous system plays a primary role in the maintenance of an adequate circulation. During upright posture and volume depletion, reduction of afferent venous and arterial baroreceptor impulse traffic diminishes an inhibitory input to the vasomotor center, thereby increasing sympathetic activity (Fig. 73-2) and reducing efferent vagal tone. As a result, heart rate is increased and cardiac output is diverted from the skin, subcutaneous tissues, mucosa, and viscera. Sympathetic stimulation of the kidney increases sodium reabsorption and sympathetically mediated venoconstriction enhances venous return. With pronounced hypotension, the adrenal medulla is recruited and E reinforces the effects of the sympathetic nervous system. A similar but less dramatic pattern of sympathetic activation occurs in the postprandial state when blood and extracellular fluid are sequestered in the splanchnic circulation and within the lumen of the gut, respectively.

CONGESTIVE HEART FAILURE The sympathetic nervous system also provides circulatory support during congestive heart failure (Chap. 253). Venoconstriction and sympathetic stimulation of the heart increase cardiac output while peripheral vasoconstriction directs blood flow to the heart and brain. The afferent signals are less clear than in simple volume depletion since the venous pressure is usually elevated. In severe heart failure depletion of cardiac NE may occur, thereby impairing the effectiveness of sympathetic circulatory support.

TRAUMA AND SHOCK In the acute phase of traumatic injury or shock, catecholamines of adrenal medullary origin are important in supporting the circulation and in mobilizing substrates. Although it is presumed that the sympathetic nervous system is activated as well, unequivocal evidence of sympathetic activation in the acute situation is lacking. In the chronic, reparative phase following injury catecholamines contribute to substrate mobilization and to the elevation in metabolic rate.

EXERCISE Sympathetic activation during muscular exertion increases cardiac output, maintains blood flow, and ensures sufficient supply of substrate to meet the increased needs of skeletal and cardiac muscle. Central neural factors, such as anticipation, and circulatory factors, such as fall in venous pressure, trigger the sympathetic response. Mild degrees of exercise stimulate the sympathetic nervous system alone; during more severe exertion the adrenal medulla is activated as well. Training or conditioning is associated with a decrease in sympathetic nervous system activity both at rest and during exercise.

Hypoglycemia Hypoglycemia elicits a marked increase in adrenal medullary epinephrine secretion. When glucose concentrations fall below overnight fasting levels, the glucose-sensitive cells within the central nervous system are stimulated and initiate a prompt increase in adrenal medullary secretion. The adrenal medullary reaction is especially intense when plasma glucose levels drop below 50 mg/dl. Under these circumstances plasma E levels increase 25 to 50 times above base line and contribute to the counterregulatory response by increasing hepatic glucose output, providing alternative substrate in the form of free fatty acids, suppressing endogenous insulin release, and inhibiting insulin-mediated glucose utilization in muscle. The clinical manifestations of hypoglycemia, such as tachycardia, palpitations, nervousness, tremor, and widened pulse pressure, are secondary to increased E secretion.

Cold exposure The sympathetic nervous system plays a critical role in the maintenance of normal body temperature during exposure to a cold environment. Receptors in the skin and central nervous system respond to a fall in temperature by activating hypothalamic and brainstem centers that increase sympathetic activity. Sympathetic stimulation leads to vasoconstriction in the superficial vascular beds, thereby diminishing heat loss. Heat production is simultaneously increased by facilitation of shivering, increased generation of metabolic heat, and enhanced substrate mobilization. Acclimatization to cold during chronic cold exposure greatly increases the capacity for metabolic heat production in response to sympathetic stimulation.

Dietary intake Although changes in sympathetic activity with changes in dietary intake have only recently been described, the evidence suggests that fasting suppresses and overfeeding stimulates the sympathetic nervous system. The reduction in sympathetic activity during fasting or starvation may contribute to the decrease in metabolic rate, bradycardia, and hypotension noted in these states. Enhanced sympathetic activity during periods of increased caloric intake may contribute to the elevation in metabolic rate associated with a chronic increase in dietary intake. The well-established associations between excessive caloric intake, hypertension, and atherosclerotic cardiovascular disease may also depend, in part, upon the relationship between dietary intake and sympathetic nervous system activity.

Hypoxia Chronic hypoxia is associated with stimulation of the sympathoadrenal system, and some of the cardiovascular changes that occur in hypoxic patients may be dependent upon catecholamines.

PARTICIPATION OF THE SYMPATHETIC NERVOUS SYSTEM IN THE PATHOGENESIS OF SELECTED DISEASE STATES

HYPERTENSION (See also Chaps. 29 and 267) As shown in Fig. 73-3, regulation of arterial pressure by the sympathetic nervous system involves blood vessels, the heart, and the kidneys. In addition to direct stimulation of the resistance vessels, the sympathetic nervous system increases peripheral resistance by activation of the renin-angiotensin system. Increased cardiac output is the result of enhanced cardiac contractility and augmented venous return, the latter a result of venoconstriction and increased renal sodium reabsorption. The effects of the sympathetic nervous system on renal sodium reabsorption are particularly important since stimulation of sodium retention diminishes the capacity of the kidney to compensate for the increase in blood pressure. Antiadrenergic agents lower blood pressure by interacting at many of the sites shown in Fig. 73-3.

The sympathetic nervous system plays at least a permissive role in the maintenance of hypertension (Chap. 29). Despite the elevated blood pressure, sympathetic nervous system activity is not suppressed in hypertensive patients and reflex control of the circulation is retained, due in part to upward resetting of the baroreceptors. In addition, peripheral sensitivity of the vasculature to NE is either normal or enhanced. The maintenance of sympathetic nervous system activity in patients with hypertension accounts for the hypotensive effects of antiadrenergic agents.

During antihypertensive treatment with vasodilators or diuretics the sympathetic nervous system may be activated in response to decreased pressure in either the venous or arterial circulation (Fig. 73-2). The heightened sympathetic activity that results, in addition to causing tachycardia, may oppose the antihypertensive therapy by activating the various effector systems shown in Fig. 73-3. Antiadrenergic agents, therefore, have a fundamental role in the therapy of most hypertensive patients.

ANGINA PECTORIS (Chap. 260) Sympathetic stimulation of the cardiovascular system increases myocardial oxygen consumption as a consequence of elevated heart rate, enhanced myocardial contractility, and increased myocardial wall tension. Clinical attacks of angina pectoris, therefore, are often precipitated by situations associated with sympathetic activation such as exercise, eating, and cold exposure. The beneficial effects of beta blockade in the treatment of angina (Chap. 29) derive from reduction in sympathetic stimulation of the heart. The possibility that alpha-adrenergically mediated coronary vasoconstriction may contribute to coronary spasm has also been raised.

HYPERTHYROIDISM (Chap. 111) Many of the peripheral manifestations of hyperthyroidism suggest a hyperadrenergic state. Beta-receptor responsiveness is enhanced in hyperthyroidism, perhaps secondary to an increase in the density of beta receptors on the cell surface. Since thyroid hormone excess does not suppress sympathetic nervous system activity (plasma NE levels are normal in thyrotoxic patients), a "normal" level of sympathetic activity may evoke an exaggerated physiological response. Many of the adrenergic manifestations of hyperthyroidism are diminished by treatment with beta-receptor blocking agents.

FIGURE 73-3
Sympathetic nervous system effects on blood pressure. Sympathetic stimulation (+) increases blood pressure by effects on the heart, the veins, the kidneys, and the arterioles. The net result of sympathetic stimulation is an increase both in cardiac output and peripheral resistance. (From JB Young, L Landsberg, in Scientific Foundations of Cardiology, P Sleight et al (eds), London, Heinemann, 1981.)

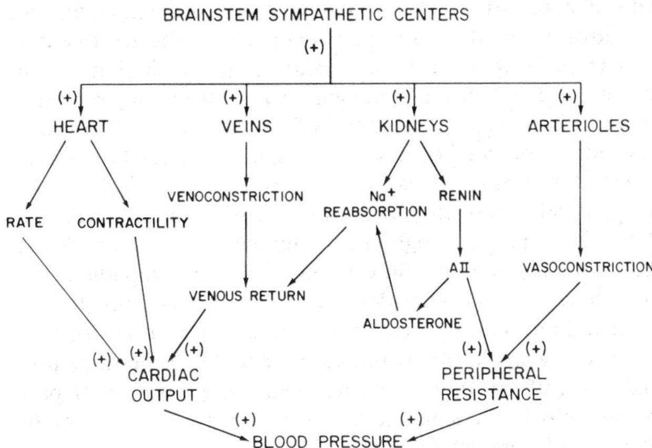

ORTHOSTATIC HYPOTENSION (Chap. 29) The maintenance of arterial pressure during upright posture depends upon an adequate blood volume, an unimpaired venous return, and an intact sympathetic nervous system. Significant postural hypotension, therefore, often reflects extracellular fluid volume depletion or dysfunction of the circulatory reflexes. Diseases of the nervous system, such as tabes dorsalis, syringomyelia, or diabetes mellitus, may disrupt these sympathetic reflexes with resultant orthostatic hypotension. Although any antiadrenergic agent may impair the postural sympathetic response, orthostatic hypotension is most prominent with drugs that block neurotransmission within the ganglia or adrenergic neurons.

The term *idiopathic orthostatic hypotension* refers to a group of degenerative diseases involving either the pre- or postganglionic sympathetic neurons. Involvement of the peripheral sympathetic nervous system is characterized by low basal NE levels, while involvement at the level of the central nervous system or preganglionic sympathetic neurons is associated with normal basal plasma NE levels. In both cases the plasma NE response to upright posture is deficient.

PHARMACOLOGY OF THE SYMPATHOADRENAL SYSTEM

A wide variety of therapeutic agents in general clinical use affect sympathetic nervous system function or interact with adrenergic receptors, making it possible to stimulate or suppress physiological effects mediated by catecholamines with some degree of specificity.

SYMPATHOMIMETIC AMINES Sympathomimetic amines may directly activate adrenergic receptors (direct acting) or release NE from the sympathetic nerve endings (indirect acting). Many of the sympathomimetic agents have both direct and indirect effects.

Epinephrine and norepinephrine The naturally occurring catecholamines are used in a number of different clinical situations; they act predominantly by the direct stimulation of adrenergic receptors. NE is employed to support the circulation and elevate the blood pressure in hypotensive or shock states (Chap. 29). Peripheral vasoconstriction is the major effect although cardiac stimulation occurs as well. E, also employed as a pressor, has special usefulness in the treatment of allergic reactions, especially those associated with anaphylaxis. The pharmacological actions of E antagonize the effects of histamine and other mediators on vascular and visceral smooth muscle. E also has an important role in the treatment of bronchospasm.

Dopamine *Dopamine* is also used widely as a pressor amine in treating of hypotension, shock (Chap. 29), and certain forms of heart failure (Chap. 253). At low infusion rates it exerts a positive inotropic effect both by a direct action on the cardiac beta$_1$ receptors and by the indirect release of NE from sympathetic nerve endings in heart. At low doses direct stimulation of dopaminergic receptors in the renal and mesenteric vasculature also results in selective regional vasodilation in the gut and kidney, and facilitates sodium excretion. At higher infusion rates interaction with alpha-adrenergic receptors results in vasoconstriction, an increase in peripheral resistance, and an elevation of blood pressure. *Dobutamine* is a congener of dopamine with relative selectivity for the beta$_1$ receptor, and with a greater effect on myocardial contractility than on heart rate; it too is used in the treatment of severe congestive heart failure, often in combination with vasodilators (Chap. 253).

Beta-receptor agonists *Isoproterenol,* a direct-acting beta-receptor agonist, stimulates the heart, decreases peripheral resistance, and relaxes bronchial smooth muscle. It raises the cardiac output and accelerates atrioventricular conduction while increasing the automaticity of ventricular pacemakers. Isoproterenol is used in the treatment of heart block and bronchoconstriction.

SELECTIVE BETA$_2$-RECEPTOR AGONISTS The cardiac stimulation caused by nonselective beta agonists, such as isoproterenol or epinephrine, is troublesome and occasionally dangerous when these agents are used in the treatment of bronchoconstriction. Selective beta$_2$ agonists (*metaproterenol, terbutaline,* and *isoetharine*) improve the therapeutic ratio by achieving bronchial dilatation with less activation of the cardiovascular system (Chaps. 273 and 279).

Alpha-adrenergic agonists *Phenylephrine* and *methoxamine* are directly acting alpha agonists that elevate blood pressure by increasing peripheral vasoconstriction. They are used primarily in the treatment of hypotension and paroxysmal supraventricular tachycardia (Chap. 255), in the latter case by increasing cardiac vagal tone through reflex baroreceptor stimulation. Phenylephrine, and a related proprietary compound, *phenylpropanolamine,* are common constituents of decongestant medications (often combined with antihistamines) for the treatment of allergic rhinitis and upper respiratory infections.

Miscellaneous sympathomimetic amines with mixed actions *Ephedrine* has both direct beta-receptor agonist properties and an indirect effect on sympathetic nerve endings, from which it releases NE, and is used primarily as a bronchodilator. *Sudephedrine,* a congener of ephedrine, is less potent at dilating bronchi and serves as a nasal decongestant. *Metaraminol* has both direct and indirect effects on sympathetic nerve endings and is employed in the treatment of hypotensive states.

ANTIADRENERGIC OR SYMPATHOLYTIC AGENTS (See also Chap. 267) **Agents inhibiting central sympathetic outflow** The antihypertensive agents *alpha methyldopa* and *clonidine* diminish central sympathetic outflow by stimulating a central alpha-adrenergic pathway (alpha$_2$ receptor) that diminishes vasomotor outflow. Central nervous system side effects such as sedation are common. When administration of clonidine is stopped abruptly, a withdrawal syndrome characterized by rebound hyperactivity of the sympathetic nervous system can produce a clinical syndrome resembling the crises of patients with pheochromocytoma. *Opiates* may also exert a central sympatholytic effect; the sympathetic excitation of morphine withdrawal responds to clonidine and vice versa. *Propranolol* and *reserpine* may exert some component of their sympatholytic effect at the level of the central nervous system.

Ganglionic blocking agents Ganglionic transmission may be antagonized by a group of drugs which block the (nicotinic) cholinergic synapse between the preganglionic and postganglionic autonomic nerves. These agents inhibit the parasympathetic as well as the sympathetic nervous system. Only *trimethaphan* is in general clinical use; its major application is in the treatment of hypertensive crises, particularly aortic dissection when controlled hypotension and decreased myocardial contractility are desirable (Chap. 268).

Agents acting at the peripheral sympathetic nerve endings Adrenergic neuron-blocking agents depress the function of the peripheral sympathetic nerves by decreasing the amount of neurotransmitter released. *Guanethidine,* the prototype of this class of drugs, is concentrated in the sympathetic nerve endings by the amine-uptake mechanism. Within the terminal it blocks the release of NE in response to nerve impulses and eventually depletes the nerve of NE by displacing it from the intraneuronal storage granules. The drug is often useful in the management of severe hypertension, although orthostatic hypotension is a common, and frequently limiting, side effect. *Bretylium,* an agent whose effects are similar to those of guanethidine, is employed in the treatment of ventricular fibrillation (Chap. 255). Both guanethidine and bretylium are antagonized by agents that affect the amine-uptake transport process including sympathomimetic amines, tricyclic antidepressants, phenoxybenzamine, and phenothiazines. The antihypertensive action of guanethidine may be rapidly reversed by these drugs.

Reserpine depletes catecholamines from the peripheral sympathetic nerve endings, the brain, and the adrenal medulla. Its antihypertensive effect in humans is usually attributed to depletion of peripheral NE stores within sympathetic nerve endings. The sedation and occasionally morbid depression attending its use result from NE depletion within the centrai nervous system.

Adrenergic-receptor blocking agents Adrenergic blocking agents antagonize the effects of catecholamines at the level of the peripheral tissue.

ALPHA-ADRENERGIC-RECEPTOR BLOCKING AGENTS *Phenoxybenzamine* and *phentolamine* are utilized principally in treating pheochromocytoma (Chap. 113). Phenoxybenzamine produces prolonged, irreversible alpha blockade while phentolamine leads to reversible, competitive blockade. Because of its rapid action and short duration, phentolamine is commonly used in the treatment of acute hypertensive paroxysms secondary to catecholamine excess, such as occur with pheochromocytoma, pressor reactions in patients receiving MAO inhibitors, and clonidine withdrawal. Both phentolamine and phenoxybenzamine antagonize alpha$_1$ and alpha$_2$ receptors although phenoxybenzamine is more potent at the alpha$_1$ receptor site. *Prazosin,* a new alpha-adrenergic blocking agent with a high degree of selectivity for the alpha$_1$ receptor, possesses pharmacological properties that resemble those of primary vasodilators and has been used increasingly in the treatment of essential hypertension. Since none of the currently used alpha-adrenergic blocking agents have much effect on the beta-adrenergic receptor, unopposed beta stimulation may result in a clinically significant tachycardia during treatment with these agents.

BETA-ADRENERGIC-RECEPTOR BLOCKING AGENTS The major clinical application of beta-blocking agents is to antagonize the cardiovascular effects of catecholamines in the treatment of angina pectoris, hypertension, and cardiac arrhythmias. The benefit of beta blockade in angina derives from the decrease in myocardial oxygen consumption following reduction in heart rate and myocardial contractility (Chap. 260). The hypotensive effect of beta blockade is well established, although not clearly understood (Chap. 267). Diminished cardiac output, decreased NE release at postganglionic sympathetic nerve endings, reduced renin secretion, and suppressed central sympathetic outflow have all been considered possible mechanisms, but the relative importance of each is uncertain. The efficacy of beta-blocking agents in the treatment of arrhythmias depends upon reduction of the rate of spontaneous depolarization of pacemaker cells in the sinus node and junctional pacemakers and slowing of conduction within the atria and atrioventricular node. Beta blockade is also effective in the management of symptomatic hyperthyroidism and the control of tachycardia and arrhythmias in patients with pheochromocytoma. The mechanism by which beta blockers reduce mortality in postmyocardial infarct patients has not been conclusively determined, but it may involve their antiarrhythmic action (Chaps. 255 and 260).

Propranolol is the prototype of the nonselective beta-adrenergic blocking agent, inducing a competitive blockade of $beta_1$ and $beta_2$ receptors. Although it also possesses significant local anesthetic properties and penetrates the central nervous system, the major effects of propranolol are generally attributed to blockade of peripheral adrenergic receptors. Other nonselective blocking agents include *nadolol* and *timolol* (approved for use in the United States), alprenolol, oxprenolol, pindolol, and sotalol (currently under investigation).

Among the adverse effects of beta-blocking agents are the precipitation of heart failure in patients in whom cardiac compensation depends upon enhanced sympathetic drive, and the aggravation of bronchospasm in asthmatic patients. These agents may also predispose to the development of hypoglycemia in insulin-requiring diabetics by blocking catecholamine-mediated counterregulation and antagonizing some of the adrenergic warning signs of impending hypoglycemia.

CARDIOSELECTIVE ($BETA_1$) ADRENERGIC-RECEPTOR BLOCKING AGENTS Cardioselective beta-adrenergic blocking drugs have the potential advantage of blocking beta-adrenergic cardiovascular effects without affecting the bronchial musculature, thereby reducing the likelihood of bronchoconstriction in individuals with reactive airways. *Metoprolol* and *atenolol* are currently available in the United States. Their major use is in the treatment of hypertension where they appear to be similar to propranolol in efficacy. The cardioselectivity of these agents is only relative, and at high doses $beta_1$-blocking agents may also precipitate bronchoconstriction in susceptible individuals.

THE PARASYMPATHETIC NERVOUS SYSTEM

ACETYLCHOLINE Acetylcholine (ACh) serves as the neurotransmitter at all autonomic ganglia, at the postganglionic parasympathetic nerve endings, and at the postganglionic sympathetic nerve endings innervating the eccrine sweat glands. The enzyme choline acetyltransferase catalyzes the synthesis of ACh from acetyl CoA, produced within the nerve ending, and from choline, actively taken up from the extracellular fluid. Within the cholinergic nerve endings ACh is stored in discrete synaptic vesicles and released in response to nerve impulses that depolarize the nerve terminals and increase calcium influx.

Cholinergic receptors Different receptors for ACh exist on the postganglionic neurons within the autonomic ganglia and at the postjunctional autonomic effector sites. Those within the autonomic ganglia and adrenal medulla are stimulated by nicotine (*nicotinic receptors*) and those on autonomic effector cells by the alkaloid muscarine (*muscarinic receptors*). Ganglionic blocking agents antagonize the nicotinic receptors while atropine blocks the muscarinic receptors.

Acetylcholinesterase Hydrolysis of ACh by the enzyme acetylcholinesterase inactivates the neurotransmitter at cholinergic synapses. This enzyme (also known as specific or true cholinesterase) is present within neurons and is distinct from butyrocholinesterase (serum cholinesterase or pseudocholinesterase). The latter enzyme is present in plasma and nonneuronal tissues and is not primarily involved in the termination of the effects of ACh at autonomic effector sites. The pharmacological effects of anticholinesterase agents are due to inhibition of neuronal (true) acetylcholinesterase.

PHYSIOLOGY OF THE PARASYMPATHETIC NERVOUS SYSTEM The parasympathetic nervous system participates in the regulation of the cardiovascular system, the gastrointestinal tract, and the genitourinary system. Tissues such as liver, kidney, pancreas, and thyroid also receive parasympathetic innervation suggesting a role for the parasympathetic nervous system in metabolic regulation as well, although cholinergic effects on metabolism are less well characterized.

Cardiovascular system Parasympathetic effects on the heart are mediated by the vagus nerve. ACh reduces the rate of spontaneous depolarization of the sinoatrial node and decreases heart rate. The heart rate achieved in different physiological states is the result of a complex and coordinated interaction between sympathetic stimulation, parasympathetic inhibition, and the intrinsic activity of the sinoatrial pacemaker. ACh also delays impulse conduction within the atrial musculature while shortening the effective refractory period, a combination of factors which may initiate or perpetuate atrial arrhythmias. At the atrioventricular node ACh reduces conduction velocity, increases the effective refractory period, and thus diminishes the ventricular response during atrial flutter or fibrillation (Chap. 255). The decrease in inotropy induced by ACh may be related to a prejunctional effect on sympathetic nerve endings as well as to a direct effect on the atrial myocardium. The ventricular myocardium is not much affected since innervation by cholinergic fibers is minimal. A direct cholinergic contribution to the regulation of peripheral resistance appears unlikely since parasympathetic innervation of the vasculature is not extensive. The parasympathetic nervous system, however, may influence peripheral resistance indirectly by inhibiting NE release from sympathetic nerves.

Gastrointestinal tract Parasympathetic innervation of the gut is via the vagus nerve and the pelvic sacral nerves. The parasympathetic nervous system increases the tone of gastrointestinal smooth muscle, enhances peristaltic activity, and relaxes the gastrointestinal sphincters. ACh stimulates exocrine secretion from the glandular epithelium as well as the secretion of a variety of gut hormones including gastrin, secretin, and insulin.

Genitourinary and respiratory systems Sacral parasympathetic nerves supply the urinary bladder and genitalia. ACh increases ureteral peristalsis, contracts the urinary detrusor muscle, and relaxes the trigone and sphincter, thereby playing a critical role in the coordination of micturition. Cholinergic stimulation is also important in producing erection of the external genitalia. The respiratory tract is innervated with parasympathetic fibers derived from the vagus nerve. ACh increases tracheobronchial secretions and stimulates bronchial constriction.

PHARMACOLOGY OF THE PARASYMPATHETIC NERVOUS SYSTEM **Cholinergic agonists** ACh itself has no therapeutic role because of its widespread effects and short duration of action. Congeners of ACh, less susceptible to hydrolysis by cholinesterase and with a narrower range of physiological effects, have been employed therapeutically. Bethanechol, the only cholinergic agonist currently in use, stimulates gastrointestinal and genitourinary smooth muscle with minimal effect on the cardiovascular system. Its major clinical application is in the treatment of urinary retention in the absence of outflow tract obstruction, and, less commonly, in gastrointestinal disorders such as postvagotomy gastric atony.

Acetylcholinesterase inhibitors Cholinesterase inhibitors enhance the effects of parasympathetic stimulation by diminishing the inactivation of ACh. The rather wide therapeutic application of these agents depends upon the role of ACh as neurotransmitter at the skeletal muscle neuroeffector junction and within the central nervous system, and includes the treatment of myasthenia gravis (Chap. 372), the termination of neuromuscular blockade following general anesthesia, and the reversal of some effects of intoxication by agents with a central anticholinergic action. With regard to the autonomic nervous system, cholinesterase inhibitors are of limited use in the treatment of intestinal and bladder smooth-muscle dysfunction such as occurs in paralytic ileus and atonic urinary bladder. Cholinesterase inhibitors induce a vagotonic response in heart and may be useful in terminating attacks of paroxysmal supraventricular tachycardia (Chap. 255).

Cholinergic-receptor blocking agents *Atropine* blocks muscarinic cholinergic receptors, with little effect on cholinergic transmission at the autonomic ganglia and the neuromuscular junctions. Many of the central nervous system actions of atropine and atropine-like drugs are attributable to blockade of central muscarinic synapses. The related alkaloid, *scopolamine,* is similar to atropine but causes drowsiness, euphoria, and amnesia, effects which make it suitable as a preanesthetic medication.

Atropine increases heart rate and enhances atrioventricular conduction, actions which may be clinically useful in combating the bradycardia or heart block associated with heightened vagal tone. In addition, atropine reverses cholinergically mediated bronchoconstriction and diminishes respiratory tract secretions. These effects on the circulation and the respiratory tract contribute to the utility of atropine as a preanesthetic medication.

Atropine also decreases gastrointestinal tract motility and secretion. Although various derivatives of atropine have been advocated in patients with peptic ulcer or with diarrheal syndromes, the chronic use of atropinics is limited by other manifestations of parasympathetic inhibition such as dry mouth and urinary retention.

REFERENCES

FRISHMAN WH: Beta-adrenoceptor antagonists: New drugs and new indications. N Engl J Med 305:500, 1981

LANDSBERG L (ed): Catecholamines, Clin Endoc Metab, vol 6, no. 3, London, Saunders, Nov 1977

LANDSBERG L, YOUNG JB: Catecholamines and the adrenal medulla, in *Metabolic Control and Disease,* 8th ed, PK Bondy, LE Rosenberg (eds). Philadelphia, Saunders, 1980

LANDSBERG L, YOUNG JB: Sympathetic nervous system and hypertension, in *Contemporary Issues in Nephrology,* B Brenner, JH Stein (eds). New York, Churchill Livingstone, 1981, vol 8

MAYER SE: Neurohumoral transmission and the autonomic nervous system, in *The Pharmacological Basis of Therapeutics,* 6th ed, AG Gilman et al (eds). New York, Macmillan, 1980

MOTULSKY JH, INSEL PA: Adrenergic receptors in many: Direct identification, physiologic regulation, and clinical alterations. N Engl J Med 307:18, 1982

section 4 | Geriatric medicine

74
THE BIOLOGY OF AGING

WILLIAM R. HAZZARD

The phenomenon of aging has always fascinated humankind, in part perhaps because until comparatively recently only a small fraction of people actually lived into old age. The concept of retirement, for example, did not really exist until the latter portion of the nineteenth century. Several forces have brought aging and its consequences into the social and scientific limelight in the last quarter of this century. Medicine has been one of the last disciplines dealing with the elderly to recognize the implications of these forces, which threaten to overwhelm health and social services unless more efficient and effective means of meeting the needs of the elderly are devised.

These forces can best be appreciated by contrasting representative longevity curves of developing and developed nations (Fig. 74-1). The former are characterized by high birth rates and high infant and childhood mortality rates; the latter are characterized by low rates in both categories. Socioeconomic development results in improved nutrition, housing, education, and personal and public hygiene, and eventually in a reduced birth rate. These trends cause increases in median age of the population and in expected longevity at birth. However, actual extension of longevity once maturity has been achieved is less pronounced, as evidenced by the similar ages at which the upper ends of the longevity curves from populations of disparate degrees of socioeconomic development intersect the abscissa, no survival beyond 115 years of age having been documented beyond question.

Hence the change in the modern era is not in the upper limit of the human life span but rather in the proportion who survive to approach that limit. Whether that limit is unchangeable is uncertain, but it should be emphasized that under optimal circumstances everyone will die, on the average, in the middle of their ninth decade. Such a demise has been called *natural death,* the inevitable result of the genetic composition of the human. When large numbers of individuals age in concert, society itself reflects the aging process. The United States is now experiencing such a redistribution of population toward an older and older median age. A steady state with equal proportions in the ages 0 to 19 and over 55, each representing about a fourth of the total, will not be reached for another half century (Fig. 75-1).

AGING AT THE CELLULAR LEVEL Clinical and epidemiological research on aging has lagged behind studies of aging at the cellular level both because of its more complicated design and also because of the difficulty in separating the effects of aging from those of the diseases that accompany aging. Hence only when reduced to its simplest unit of organization, the cell, can aging be studied independent of age-related disease. Even at this level knowledge about aging remains relatively primitive, and several theories of aging have been proposed. Research in this area was given its major impetus when human skin fibroblasts were found to have a limited potential for replication, about 50 population doublings under the most favorable conditions (the *Hayflick phenomenon*). This limit is an inherent property of the cells themselves and not of their environment and has been demonstrated repeatedly by its originator and in numerous other laboratories as well. The concept of a relatively fixed number of doublings applies to certain other cells as well, such as the arterial smooth-muscle cell. The actual number of potential doublings of a given cell in vitro is inversely related to the age of its donor. Furthermore, cells from donors with diabetes mellitus, a known concomitant of accelerated aging, and from patients with Werner's syndrome of progeria, a single gene defect that causes an even more dramatic acceleration of aging, manifest fewer doublings than do cells from age-matched controls.

As a consequence, the genetic apparatus of the cell has been examined for clues to senescence, since altered flow of information at any point in the sequence from DNA to RNA to protein synthesis and degradation could be involved. One such theory, Szilard's mutation hypothesis, holds that somatic mutations in DNA accumulate, causing chromosomal inactivation and cell death. Closely related theories suggest senescence via cumulative errors in formation of RNA or through progressive errors in translation, resulting in "error catastrophe." Such mutations have also been invoked to explain age-related increases in autoimmunity. However, the effects of mutation need not be permanent. Indeed, DNA repair capacity in fibroblasts and the amount of reserve or redundant DNA sequences have been linked with longevity of various species. Finally, the accumulation of free radicals with age has been linked to activity of superoxide dismutase and this in turn to reduced resistance to injury both intra- and extracellular.

These theories of "intrinsic" aging have been challenged not only because they are based on in vitro phenomena and hence distant from the aging whole organism but also because of differences among various cell types. For instance, while fibroblasts clearly demonstrate senescence in vitro, cells of gastrointestinal and hematopoietic origins appear capable of replication throughout the life span, and others, notably kidney and liver cells, replicate in response to nephrectomy or partial hepatectomy at all ages. Still other cells, such as those of the central nervous system and striated muscle, do not replicate in adult life. However, even cells classified as continuously mitotic do not survive indefinitely (in contrast to cancer cells). While the variation in generation time and replicative potential between cell types within a given species and within cell types between species is considerable, senescence at the cellular level appears to be a universal phenomenon of normal cells.

But do these in vitro phenomena relate to aging in vivo? Even the strongest proponents of the intrinsic school of cellular aging acknowledge that the probability that the animals age solely because one or more cell populations lose their proliferative capacity is small. Perhaps it is more likely in aging cells that decrements in functional capacities other than proliferative capacity render the organism vulnerable to death.

Alternatively, attention has been focused upon certain regulatory processes, postulating a cascade of age-related decrements that become amplified in tissues and whole organisms. Such factors have been termed *extrinsic,* since they may not be universal among all cells and tissues and can include environmental forces (or vulnerability thereto). Those systems under special scrutiny in this regard include the nervous, endocrine, and immune systems.

One school has focused upon the role of central nervous system monoamines, notably dopamine, norepinephrine, and serotonin. These neurotransmitters have come under special study in part because of known alterations in certain age-related neurological diseases. Parkinson's disease, for instance, is associated with major deficiencies of monoamines (e.g., striatal dopamine) and can be partially treated by L-dopa replacement. Furthermore, changes in catecholamine metabolism occur in the normal aging brain, and the elderly are more susceptible to development of the Parkinsonian symptoms following treatment with phenothiazines. Hence, age-related changes in dopamine uptake and catecholamine metabolism may lower the threshold for drugs that are catecholamine antagonists. Such changes could also account for the late onset of postencephalitic Parkinson's disease, in which aging unmasks an earlier viral insult. Other age-related changes attributable to alterations in central nervous system monoamines include alterations in circadian rhythms, sleep patterns, sex drive, and thermoregulation. Alternatively, changes in central nervous system cholinergic status could account for certain alterations in behavior and mental function; agents that enhance brain acetylcholine levels enjoy current vogue in the treatment of dementia.

Perhaps related to these neurotransmitter alterations are widespread changes in endocrine function with aging. For example, normal aging is accompanied by a decline in glucose tolerance, the mechanism of which has remained unresolved, and the incidence of symptomatic diabetes mellitus is increased in the aged. The higher prevalence of nonketotic hyperosmolar coma in the elderly diabetic might be due to impaired osmoregulation and thirst perception in addition to deficient insulin secretion. Clinical and subclinical thyroid deficiency are also more common, often reflecting a progressive impairment in compensation for diminished secretion of thyroid hormone. This phenomenon and perhaps the increasing incidence of diabetes may also be secondary to age-related in-

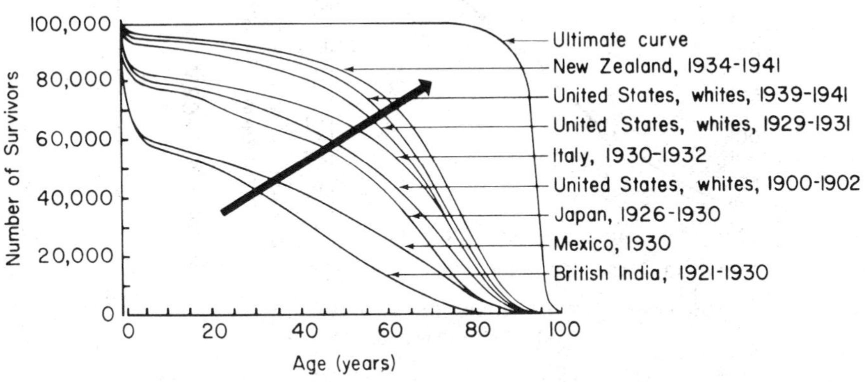

FIGURE 74-1
Survival curves in different countries varying in degree of socioeconomic development. Diagonal arrow indicates change accompanying such development. (Reprinted by permission from L Hayflick, N Engl J Med 295:1302, 1976.)

creases in autoimmune disease. Another age-related endocrine dysfunction is ovarian failure at the menopause in the female. It is not established whether the cessation of ovulation is due to some intrinsic ovarian limitation or whether changes in neuroendocrine regulation of the ovary rather than loss of oocytes per se are of primary importance in ovarian failure at the menopause. Whatever the etiology, the cascade of events including diminished estrogen secretion, diminished negative feedback control of the hypothalamus, compensating increases in FSH and LH secretion, and abnormal thermoregulation has profound secondary consequences at both psychological and physiological levels. The endocrine changes in the aging male—although less dramatic—may be of equal import and include both a decrease in mean plasma testosterone and an increase in mean plasma estrogen so that the paradox of increasing feminization in aging men parallels that of diminished estrogen production in women.

The immune system has also been suggested as an important pacemaker of the aging process. The thymus normally reaches its peak size in early childhood and begins rapid involution after puberty. Other lymphoid tissues generally reach maximum size soon after puberty and undergo gradual atrophy thereafter. This atrophy is characterized by a reduction in lymphoid cells, their replacement by connective tissue, and an even greater reduction in T-cell function than T-cell number. Other age-related changes in immune function include a decrease in the primary immune response of B cells, especially those requiring T-cell interaction. Specific functions involved include decreases in the proliferative response to mitogens such as phytohemagglutinin and concanavalin A, suppression of B lymphocytes by T cells, and cytotoxic activity of T cells. These changes may have relevance to certain diseases of the elderly. For example, the elderly have four to five times the case rate for cancer and tuberculosis and six to seven times the fatality rate from pneumonia as compared to young adults (Fig. 74-2).

The changes in neurotransmitters, endocrine function, and the immune systems with age may be interlinked. For instance, production of a thymic cell hormone may decrease with age, and this in turn may be under neuroendocrine regulation. Other endocrine changes, such as altered response to glucocorticoids or changes in glucocorticoid secretion, perhaps in turn associated with age-related stress, may directly affect the immune response.

While these regulatory systems may be of central importance in the aging of the whole organism, age-related decrements in homeostatic efficiency are measurable in nearly all physiological systems (Fig. 74-3). Such changes may produce morbid symptoms in the elderly, especially under conditions of stress and acute illness. The simultaneous deficiencies in multiple systems can explain the catastrophic cascade of complications which is often initiated by a seemingly trivial perturbation in the elderly patient and the exponential rise in death rate among the very old (e.g., above age 93) whose longevity curve suggests that death may occur almost as a random phenomenon above this age.

AGING: PHYSIOLOGICAL VS. CHRONOLOGICAL Several studies have attempted to characterize normal aging in humans through cross-sectional or longitudinal assessment of various physiological parameters in groups of healthy volunteers. One purpose of such studies has been the attempt to define physiological as opposed to chronological age (Fig. 74-3). Such studies have identified a number of parameters that correlate with chronological age (Table 74-1).

One type of study is based upon repeated measurements of anthropometric, biomedical, psychological, and psychosocial variables in the same subject over a period of many years. In these relatively healthy groups chronological age is the best predictor of change in the measured variables. These results in a healthy population, however, may not extend to all groups. For instance, similar studies of smokers and of hypertensives have suggested that functional aging is more rapid in these groups than would be predicted on the chronological age alone.

A somewhat different approach was taken in the Baltimore

FIGURE 74-2

Case rates (per 1 million) of all cancers and tuberculosis at age of diagnosis and case fatality rate (percent) at age of death from pneumonia. (From WH Adler et al.)

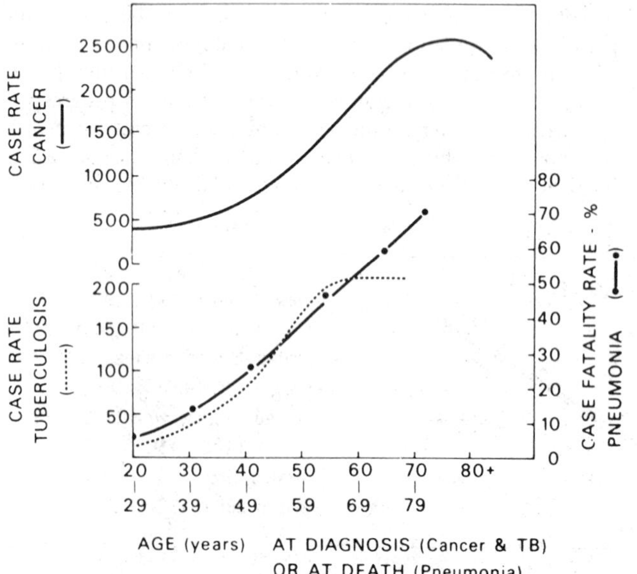

FIGURE 74-3

Decrements in physiological functions in normal men aged 30 to 80 years, expressed as percent of average values for 30-year-olds. a, fasting blood glucose; b, nerve conduction velocity, cellular enzymes; c, cardiac index (resting); d, vital capacity, renal blood flow; e, maximum breathing capacity; f, maximum work rate, maximum oxygen uptake. (From NW Shock.)

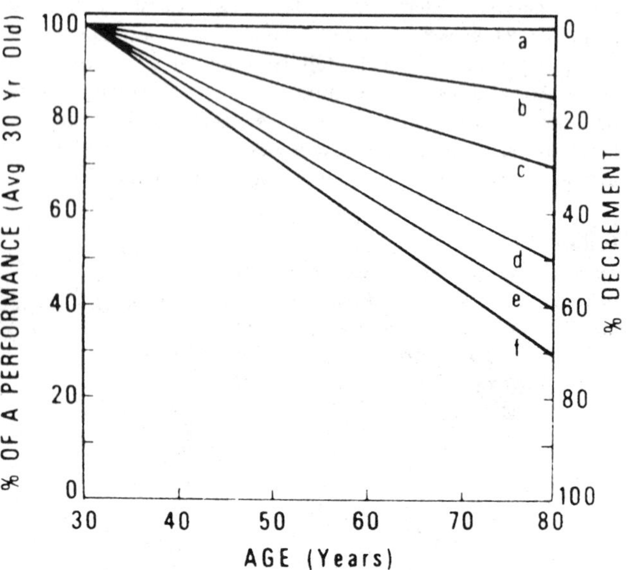

TABLE 74-1
Range of correlations with chronological age for tests used in three or more studies

	No. of studies	Correlation with chronological age	
		High	Low
Range of accommodation of the eye*	3	−0.88	−0.57
Vital capacity	8	−0.77	−0.40
Forced expiratory volume in 1.0 s	6	−0.70	−0.38
Systolic blood pressure	11	0.69	−0.16
Height	4	−0.68	−0.09
Hearing loss (4000 cps)	7	0.66	−0.42
Blood cholesterol	4	0.57	−0.23
Visual acuity	4	−0.57	−0.42
Weight	3	0.55	−0.15
Diastolic blood pressure	5	0.54	−0.10
Reaction time*	6	0.52	−0.26
Grip strength	7	−0.52	−0.21
Tapping rate	5	−0.44	−0.18

* *Regression on age is nonlinear*
SOURCE: *From Shock.*

Longitudinal Study of Aging, in which Shock examined repeatedly a self-selected, highly educated group of over 1100 apparently healthy men aged 17 to 102 years. Fifteen independent variables (from over 200 different tests and observations) correlated with chronological age. Performance profiles (Fig. 74-4) were constructed for each individual and compared with average results from participants of each age, allowing estimation as to greater or lesser "physiological age." Not surprisingly, those reporting "poorer health" appeared physiologically older than their chronological age on the basis of these profiles. Furthermore, among those who survived 5 to 10 years, the biological age at first assessment was younger on average than in those who died. While this approach seems promising for groups of aging subjects, no single test or even battery of tests can assess biological age in a given individual.

SUMMARY AND PROJECTION Aging is a universal phenomenon at the cellular level except among those cells that undergo malignant transformation. Such aging may proceed from changes in DNA, RNA, and/or protein synthesis, or from changes in intracellular metabolic regulation. While such age-related phenomena may be most readily detected in assays of cellular replication in vitro, changes affecting cell function at a more subtle level may be more relevant to aging of the whole organism. Such changes are likely to be amplified in systems that regulate metabolism and function of the whole organism, such as the neural, endocrine, and immune systems. At the level of the intact human the aging phenomenon in its entirety must be a mixture of cellular and physiological changes that are intrinsic to the species and of a series of environmental insults that interact with the intrinsic process.

Enhanced survival into old age is predominantly the result of changes in the environment that accompany socioeconomic development within societies. Such changes have resulted in increased average longevity in developed nations in the twentieth century. However, there is little evidence that the upper limit of the human life span (110 to 115 years) has been significantly altered, nor is there prospect for such a change. Hence biological aging of the human species, though poorly understood, appears relatively fixed.

Many physiological functions decline in an age-related manner after age 30, and attempts have been made to estimate physiological (as contrasted to chronological) age by application of a battery of tests to presumably healthy aging individuals. While profiles of performance on such examinations may permit a gross estimate of biological age useful in predicting outcome in groups of subjects, such batteries have no important clinical utility in dealing with individuals. Hence, while general awareness of limited reserve in many systems in elderly patients is of importance in geriatric practice, subjective estimates of physiological age are subject to wide error in the given aged patient.

REFERENCES

ADLER WH et al: Aging and immune function, in *The Biology of Aging,* JA Behnke et al (eds). New York, Plenum Press, 1978, p 221

ANDRES R: Aging and carbohydrate metabolism, in *Nutrition in Old Age, Xth Symposia of the Swedish Nutrition Foundation.* Uppsala, Sweden, Almqvist and Wiksell, 1972, p 24

BIERMAN EL: Atherosclerosis and aging. Fed Proc 37:2832, 1978

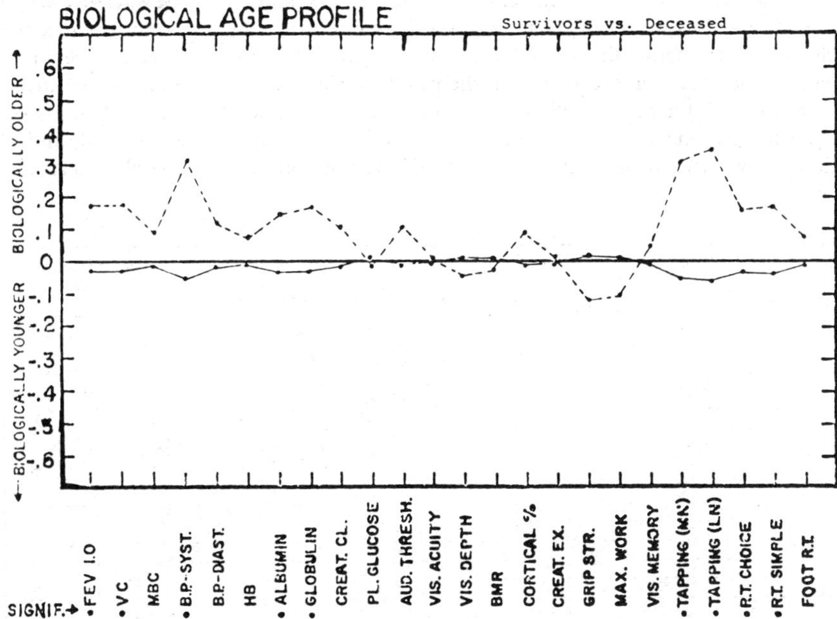

FIGURE 74-4
Average profiles of physiological function for subjects in Baltimore Longitudinal Study of Aging who died within 10 years of testing compared with profiles for survivors. Broken line = deceased; nonbroken line = survivors. (From NW Shock.)

FINCH CE: The regulation of physiological changes during mammalian aging. Quart Rev Biol 51:49, 1976

FRIES J: Aging, natural death, and the compression of morbidity. N Engl J Med 130:135, 1980

GOLDSTEIN S: The biology of aging. N Engl J Med 285:1120, 1971

HAYFLICK L: The cell biology of human aging. N Engl J Med 295:1302, 1976

MARTIN GM et al: Replicative lifespan of cultivated human cells. Effects of donor's age, tissue, and genotype. Lab Invest 23:86, 1970

SHOCK NW: Physiological and chronological age, in *Aging—Its Chemistry,* AA Dietz (ed). Washington, D.C., American Association for Clinical Chemistry, 1980, p 3

TATARYN IV et al: Luteinizing hormone, follicle-stimulating hormone, and skin temperature during the menopausal hot flash. J Clin Endocrinol Metab 49:152, 1979

75
LEADING THE HEALTH CARE TEAM FOR THE ELDERLY

WILLIAM R. HAZZARD

In the future, geriatric problems will become more and more important in the practice of general medicine because of several factors. First, continuing changes in population size and distribution by age have major demographic implications for medicine. At the beginning of this century the population of the United States was small (75 million), and life expectancy was short (47.3 years). That population was distributed by age in a triangular fashion; i.e., with the highest percentage in the very youngest age groups and an ever-decreasing proportion with increasing age, the smallest group being the very old (or "old-old," as those over 75 have come to be called). This distribution is characteristic of developing nations even today [e.g., Mexico (Fig. 75-1)].

By 1970 the population of the United States had shifted to a more rectangular distribution, approaching that of western European countries such as Sweden (Fig. 75-1). Such nations are characterized by high standards of nutrition, housing, and public health; by low infant and childhood death rates; and by a relatively low birth rate. The trend toward a lower birth rate, clearly evident before the use of birth control methods became widespread, has been accelerated in the past two decades.

Since 1970 the population of the United States has skewed toward the younger age groups, the unevenness in the distribution being attributable to the "baby boom" after World War II. However, by the year 2030 the distribution will be almost rectangular. Moreover, the difference in mortality between the sexes, especially evident in the chronic, age-related diseases (notably those proceeding from atherogenesis) will produce a progressive skewing of the elderly population toward a preponderance of women. These changes in the age distribution of the population, together with the high American birth rate until midcentury, produced a growth in the absolute number of the elderly that has exceeded their percentage growth. In 1900 4 percent of Americans (3 million in number) were 65 and over; by 1975 the percent had increased threefold (to 11 percent), and the number had increased sevenfold (to 22 million); by 2030 the percent will be 17 percent, and the number will be 46 million.

Second, the per capita utilization of health services by the elderly exceeds that of younger persons. In 1976, for instance, this figure was $1522 per elderly person, three times as high as for younger people. Moreover, a larger proportion of the total is paid from public funds (Medicare and Medicaid), and the costs of these programs have been growing faster for the elderly than for the young; hence, the greater scrutiny, criticism, and demand for cost controls and the continued reluctance to devote public funds to long-term institutional care. While institutional care is required for only 5 percent of those over 65 at any given time, nearly a quarter of the elderly require institutional care at some point in their lives, and the probability of such need increases progressively beyond the age of 75.

Third, at the same time that the practice of general internal medicine has been eroded by the growth of subspecialties, geriatric medicine has also evolved into a specialty, a pattern, for example in Great Britain, where the needs of the elderly dominate the health care system. In view of the resurgence of interest in primary health care delivery and the general nature of much of geriatric medicine, it is imperative to identify both the unique aspects of geriatric medicine and the body of knowledge, skills, and practice that it shares with general internal medicine, family medicine, and other medical specialties. On the outcome of this analysis depends the design and size of current and future training programs. If geriatric medicine is narrowly defined as a specialty, the requirement for future U.S. geriatricians has been estimated at 1500; at the other extreme, if geriatricians deliver the majority of primary care to those 75 years of age and older, as many as 8000 or more must be trained by 1990.

GERIATRIC MEDICINE: TO DEFINE OR NOT DEFINE *Geriatrics* is the discipline that relates to the care of the elderly, embracing their interrelated physical, mental, and social needs. *Geriatric medicine* is that branch of geriatrics that addresses the medical needs of the elderly. However, since the social, psychological, and physical needs of the elderly patient are intimately intertwined, the practice of geriatric medicine involves

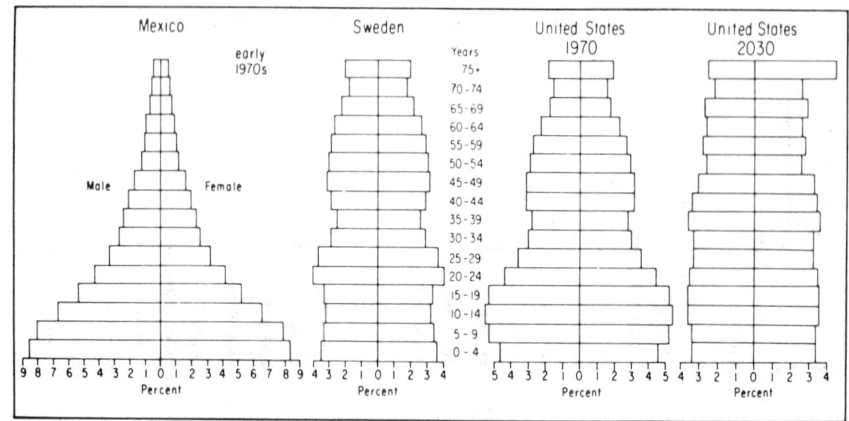

FIGURE 75-1
Comparative profiles of age and sex distribution in different populations. (From Somers.)

nonmedical as well as medical facets of life and requires mastery of a great proportion of the total body of medical knowledge. To the base of knowledge and skills (and training) in the principles and practice of medicine must be added special expertise in the management of those problems most common in the elderly, including the medical aspects of surgery and the surgical subspecialties (ophthalmology, otorhinolaryngology, urology, and orthopedics), psychiatry, physical medicine and rehabilitation, neurology, and dermatology. Finally, success in dealing with problems of the elderly requires a special interest in and understanding of chronic disease and long-term care.

An arbitrary definition of geriatric medicine strictly by age (usually at 75 years) has been defended by the special needs of those in the "old-old" category, who are especially vulnerable to social isolation and multiple disabilities. However, this definition is not really appropriate in the pluralistic medical system of the United States, which is characterized by the delivery of medical care by a single physician across a spectrum of settings.

Indeed the elderly might be better served by not attempting to define geriatric medicine. No aspect of geriatric medicine is unique. In this view, the geriatrician is one who, electively and consciously but not necessarily exclusively, cares for the elderly, notably those above 75 years of age. Such practice is delivered in the clinic, long-term care facility, home, and hospital. Hospital care comprises an important component, given the greater propensity of the elderly to develop acute illness and their generally longer period of convalescence (hospital stays for those over 75 averaging twice as long as for those under 75).

THE DIMENSIONS OF GERIATRIC MEDICINE Geriatric medicine has been defined by some as a specialty concerned with diseases that occur almost exclusively in the elderly. (Polymyalgia rheumatica is one oft-invoked example.) Other definitions concern those aspects of disease presentation or management that are different in the elderly than the young. For example, myocardial infarction may be painless, sepsis may be present without fever, and apathetic hyperthyroidism is more common. However, such contrasts are often overdrawn, since even among the very old such atypical presentations are less frequent than the more classical manifestations of these conditions.

Therefore, this discussion is focused on the assessment process and certain problem areas that are at the center of geriatric medicine: iatrogenic disorders, immobility, incontinence, (mental) incompetence, and impaired homeostasis.

Assessment of the geriatric patient Complete evaluation of the elderly patient—like that of all patients—requires systematic consideration of physical/medical, mental/psychiatric, social, financial, and functional capacities. Gathering the requisite information requires time and patience, and the staged, multivisit assessment procedure has special value in the elderly. The interview often takes longer, especially when complicated by the common barriers to effective communication (e.g., hearing loss, visual impairment, speech impediment, mental incompetence, fatigue, and general weakness). Special attention must be paid to such barriers, and attempts must be made to compensate whenever possible (hearing aids, better lighting, etc.). When necessary, information must also be gathered from family, neighbors, and prior medical records. Interviewing family and friends may also be critical to the social, functional, and financial assessment, since optimal intervention in the dependent patient may require their assistance. However, the physician must not talk with family in lieu of talking with the patient. Such would not only jeopardize the self-esteem of the patient but would also result in failure to assess mood and motivation, possible in all but the most demented. Generally, the interviews of patient and family should be held separately lest the more powerful personality, usually the caregiver from the next generation, unduly dominates the situation. This risk tends to be exaggerated in critical circumstances, such as in hospitalized patients, when it is not uncommon for the most forceful family member to exert inordinate influence in the decision-making process. Here the physician must act as a special advocate for the patient and, with other members of the care team, ensure the formulation of the most appropriate management plan possible.

Ordinarily, the physical/medical evaluation is straightforward. However, disabilities that are not discrete diseases but threaten independence may be overlooked. These include visual, auditory, and speech impairments; dental disorders; and problems with the feet.

Mental/psychiatric evaluation requires assessment of cognition, mood, and thought. The first is approached through questions to elicit date, day of the week, telephone number (or street address), age of the patient, date of birth, present and immediate past president, mother's maiden name, and subtracting 3 serially from 20. Wrong answers to three or more questions suggest significant deficit, and wrong answers to five or more indicate major cognitive impairment. Mood and ideas of reference are assessed by questions such as: Do you wake up fresh and rested most mornings? Is your daily life interesting? Have you, at times, wanted to leave home? Does it seem that no one understands you? Have you had periods of days or weeks when you couldn't get going? Is your sleep disturbed? Are you happy most of the time? Is anyone plotting against you? Do you feel useless at times? Even when you are with people, do you feel lonely much of the time? During the past few years have you been well most of the time? Do you feel weak all over much of the time? Are you troubled by headaches? Have you had difficulty in keeping your balance in walking? Are you troubled by your heart pounding or by shortness of breath?

While the answers to the questions may commonly reflect the presence of "organic" disease, it is surprising how often even the gravely disabled elderly individual without a mood disorder may perceive health as generally good. Moreover, somatic complaints frequently dominate the symptom complex in depressed older persons.

Assessment of economic and social circumstances is a necessary portion of the evaluation. The status of an individual in these spheres tends to be stable; hence repetitive assessment is usually not required. Nevertheless, a significant change in these dimensions, such as loss of a spouse, may result in changes in physical, mental, and functional status and jeopardize independence. Economic assessment requires cataloging financial resources and requirements. Social assessment focuses on living arrangements and especially the amount of personal aid and care available.

Functional assessment focuses upon the activities of daily living, such as ability to use the telephone and public or private transportation, shop, prepare meals, perform housework, take medications, handle money, eat, dress, bathe, get in and out of bed, and control urine and feces.

Having completed this assessment (with the appropriate physical and laboratory examinations and consultations), a systematic plan of management can be constructed. In such planning the input of the family and the patient are critical to assure the correctness of the process and to involve the family in a joint effort to the benefit of the patient. Whereas in acute situations an authoritarian, hierarchical role of the physician may be most efficient, in the chronic care of the elderly patient this approach may be inappropriate and ineffective. A more corporate, egalitarian approach is generally to be preferred, given that the long-term needs of the patient will be met primarily by nonphysicians. Hence, tact, diplomacy, and administrative leadership skills are requisites of optimal geriatric practice, and familiarity with and respect for the contributions of each member of the health care team is an essential part of good medical care for the elderly. Moreover, coordinating the activities of the multiple disciplines involved is a central part of geriatric practice, case conferences frequently involving nurses, social workers, nutritionists, psychologists, dentists, pharmacists, rehabilitation therapists, and other physicians.

Iatrogenic disorders The diagnostic search for the cause of any abrupt change in physical, mental, or functional status should begin with a review of the medical regimen. Given the multiple coexisting diseases and the limited physiological reserve (most apparent in circumstances of sickness or stress), it is not surprising that iatrogenic disorders are especially prevalent among the elderly, notably in the hospital environment. These disorders include problems such as falls due to lack of appropriate restraints or assistance and drug-related problems. More subtle are such phenomena as "pseudoincontinence" (when the patient cannot gain access to toilet facilities); disorientation in a foreign, threatening hospital environment; and complications from diagnostic procedures (e.g., constipation after a barium enema). Nutritional deficiency, often attributable to the underlying disease process but frequently exacerbated in the hospital environment, also represents a barrier to recovery and rehabilitation.

Drug-related disorders are of particular concern. In selection of appropriate drugs and dosages in the elderly patient special attention must be paid to drug absorption, protein binding in the plasma compartment, distribution, action at target receptors and tissues, and metabolism and excretion. Given that many aspects of drug metabolism change in the elderly due to changing body mass, body composition, and metabolic reserve, and that the therapy of many disorders involves multiple drug regimens, it is not surprising that the probability of drug reactions rises exponentially with age among the elderly. Coupled with the diminished effectiveness of many drugs in the elderly, the therapeutic index may become less than unity. Treatment of drug-related complications, withdrawal of drugs, and careful construction of alternative regimens are therefore a major part of geriatric medicine.

Immobility An axiom of geriatric medicine is that all disorders of old age are multifactorial. These include changes in the skeleton (e.g., osteoporosis, osteomalacia), supporting musculature (e.g., wasting related to nutritional deficits, disuse, abnormal innervation, or primary myopathies), joints (e.g., osteoarthritis, rheumatoid arthritis, gout), neurological regulation (e.g., peripheral neuropathy, autonomic neuropathy, amyotrophic lateral sclerosis, Parkinson's disease, stroke), and motivation (depression, Alzheimer's disease). Identifying the specific components responsible for impaired mobility in an individual patient is a challenge, because no functional decrement threatens independence more than loss of mobility, and "taking to bed" is ominous in the elderly. Conversely, identifying and correcting the reversible components of such loss represents an important and gratifying aspect of geriatric medicine. This often requires a multifaceted approach. For example, nonsteroidal anti-inflammatory drugs for the pain of osteoarthritis, withdrawal of a drug that causes postural hypotension, provision of external physical supports (cane, multipronged walking stick, etc.), retraining through physical therapy, and support and encouragement from health professionals, friends, and loved ones. Of these strategies the final one, rebuilding confidence and motivation through emotional support, is often the most crucial, and here consummate skill may be required in dealing with the patient, family, and other professionals. This process of remobilization is slow, and it is important to guard against impatience that would assign the patient to a lower level of independence than would be required after a longer period of active rehabilitation (e.g., to a nursing home, which often becomes a permanent disposition).

Mental incompetence There is no scourge more feared than loss of mental competence, and no disability of old age threatens independence more than loss of cognitive function. Rejection of the demented person by society, premature institutional incarceration, and the stereotype of the elderly as demented and dependent are common. A corollary to these attitudes is the burden placed upon the spouse or other caregiver of the demented patient.

Elderly patients present with varying degrees of what is usually a progressively disabling process. Commonly, the early symptoms of forgetfulness have been present for some time, often longer than admitted by the patient or immediate family, partly because of denial and partly because forgetfulness is often accepted as inevitable in old age (it is not). The physician should rapidly institute a workup for reversible causes of dementia (see Chap. 22). This is most likely to be rewarding in acute mental decompensation (often in the hospital setting), when treatment of (or spontaneous recovery from) other disorders may be accompanied by a dramatic return of mental competence. Differential diagnosis should focus upon delirium and depression, both of which can produce "pseudodementia." Infections, metabolic derangements, and drug toxicity are especially prone to induce acute mental derangement. Recovery from such acute insults may include improvement in mental status that is complete or, frequently, incomplete. The latter response indicates either that residual brain damage (e.g., with hypoglycemia, hypoxemia, or direct toxic insult) is present or that the acute insult unmasked marginal mental incompetence. Despite exhaustive evaluation of potentially reversible causes of dementia, the yield of such investigations (though necessary) is small, especially in the apparently stable outpatient. The value of the CT scan to assess brain size, ventricular size (of importance in the recognition of normal-pressure hydrocephalus), and other parameters (width of sulci, possible subdural hematoma, tumor, etc.) is under investigation. It is important to recognize, however, that substantial loss of brain matter can be demonstrated by CT scan in elderly persons who have perfectly normal mental status. Hence, documentation of brain atrophy is compatible with the diagnosis of irreversible dementia but is also compatible with the possibility that some reversible process is present as well.

A careful (though difficult) search for depression is also critical. This mood disorder is common in the elderly and may present as cognitive impairment (pseudodementia) or, more commonly, complicate and aggravate early dementia of the Alzheimer type. Treatment of such depression through changes in the milieu and/or antidepressants may effect remarkable improvement in patient function (a therapeutic trial of antidepressant therapy is often warranted).

Assessment of prognosis is helpful in the formulation of a management plan. The dementia proceeding from multiple small brain infarcts (as much as 15 percent of dementia in the elderly) is noted for stepwise progression. Hence, the patient may improve after such "small strokes" and suffer no further deterioration until (and if) another episode occurs.

Most commonly the fundamental process is the syndrome of primary neuronal degeneration or (senile) dementia of the Alzheimer type, a pathological diagnosis made certain only by brain biopsy or at autopsy. Even in this circumstance, prognosis is difficult to establish with accuracy, but the progression is generally inexorably downhill and is not affected by pharmacological intervention, often ending in near-complete dependency. Death, commonly within 2 years of diagnosis, is usually the result of malnutrition or intercurrent infection. The physician must support both the patient and the caregivers, serving as advocate and counselor during the course of the disease and helping with treatment of intercurrent illnesses and with the stepwise transfer of decisions and care from family to others as loved ones become unable to cope. This kind of support requires the assistance (and primary efforts) of persons other than physicians, and the effective geriatrician assures that the available resources and skills are deployed optimally for the needs of the patient and the patient's family.

Incontinence Incontinence is a special scourge of the elderly and is often the deciding determinant for institutionalization. For example, the person with Alzheimer's disease can frequently be maintained in the community until incontinence becomes an unendurable burden upon the supporters. Urinary incontinence is frequent among the elderly, especially in women, and occurs in a quarter to a third of institutionalized old people, twice the prevalence in the community. Moreover, the degree of incontinence is generally greater among the institutionalized because a substantial proportion of the problem in noninstitutionalized individuals is relatively trivial and of long standing (e.g., stress incontinence in women). Fecal incontinence, while a major problem, is uncommon without coexisting urinary incontinence and in isolation suggests a local process affecting the rectum or anus such as fecal impaction (often with paradoxical mucous diarrhea) or diarrhea of other causes.

Micturition is a complex process, resulting from the integrated actions of the bladder, its internal and external sphincters, the musculature of the pelvic floor, and neurological control over these muscles at three levels, in the bladder wall or sphincter itself, autonomic centers of the spinal cord, and the central nervous system at the level of the cerebral cortex and hypothalamus. The central influences on micturition are predominantly inhibitory, and loss of this inhibition through such diseases as stroke. Alzheimer's disease, and parkinsonism is the most frequent cause of major, permanent incontinence in the elderly. In addition, incontinence may proceed from disorders of the peripheral-autonomic nervous system (e.g., diabetes mellitus), higher centers regulating the autonomic nervous system, or the peripheral autonomic receptors (e.g., with various autonomic blocking agents).

Specific age-related changes in these structures that may contribute to incontinence in the elderly include reductions in bladder capacity, the ability to inhibit reflex bladder contractions, and urethral closing pressure, and (in men) development of prostatic hyperplasia. In each instance, the likelihood of residual urine is increased. Commonly a mixture of urological, neurological, locomotor, and psychological factors produce the incontinence, and diagnosis is addressed to sorting out the contributing factors in any given patient.

Occasionally, incontinence may be transient, as in the hospitalized patient with acute urinary tract infection in whom another acute process may have reduced mobility, caused acute confusion, or be attributable to drug-induced dysfunction. Chronic incontinence suggests dysfunction attributable to disease of the structures and functions listed above and all too often follows surgery for prostatic hyperplasia.

Evaluation includes history, physical examination, urinalysis and culture, determination of postvoiding residual urine volume, studies of urine flow (with stress voiding cystourethrogram in women), and cystoscopy. The cystometrogram is especially helpful in identifying specific points of dysfunction in the voiding process by measuring (1) residual urine, (2) bladder capacity, (3) intravesical pressure at various stages, (4) the presence of uninhibited bladder contractions, and (5) the point at which voiding desire is perceived.

Treatment is directed first at remediable causes such as prostatic hyperplasia, bladder tumor, weakness of the pelvic diaphragm, or infection. The uninhibited bladder may be approached by charting the times of incontinence and appropriate planning of timed, assisted voiding, and anticholinergic medications such as propantheline bromide (timed by reference to the incontinence chart), where contraindications such as glaucoma or cardiovascular disease do not preclude such drugs. Incontinence and retention caused by a reflex neurogenic bladder are treated with intermittent catheterization and measures such as perineal massage to trigger the sacral reflex arc. Finally, external collectors have been developed with varying degrees of sophistication (Texas catheter, sheath rubber collectors for the man, incontinence pads for the woman). Indwelling catheters represent the last resort, with their predictable complications, chiefly infection.

Impaired homeostasis As a general principle the reserve of all physiological systems is limited in the process of aging. Most apparent among the elderly are deficiencies that produce symptoms at a low threshold (e.g., of balance and cardiopulmonary function) or reflect processes that are finely regulated on a moment-to-moment basis and are frequently monitored by health practitioners with or without symptoms, e.g., blood glucose and creatinine levels. Age-related changes in these parameters reflect diminished reserve, and caution is urged in the interpretation of such values independent of age and especially in overaggressive treatment of asymptomatic, "chemical disorders."

SUMMARY AND CONCLUSIONS Geriatric medicine will become more important in the practice of internists and other general physicians as the proportion of elderly, especially the very old, increases over the next several decades. Given the complex and often subtle presentation and management of disease and dysfunction, the narrowed therapeutic index of almost any intervention, and the tendency for most disease processes to be multidimensional and chronic or progressive in the elderly, the characteristics of judgment, synthesis, patience, and compassion are necessary features of the physician who successfully cares for the elderly.

REFERENCES

Andres R: Relation of physiological changes in aging to medical change of disease in the aged. Mayo Clin Proc 42:679, 1967

Bagnall WE et al: Geriatric medicine in Hull: A comprehensive service. Br Med J 2:102, 1977

Brocklehurst JC: Great Britain, in *Geriatric Care in Advanced Societies,* JC Brocklehurst (ed). Baltimore, University Park Press, 1975, pp 5–41

Kane RL, Kane RA: Care of the aged: Old problems in need of new solutions. Science 200:913, 1978

Kane R et al: The future need for geriatric manpower in the United States. N Engl J Med 302:1327, 1980

Somers AR: Geriatric care in the United Kingdom: An American perspective. Ann Intern Med 84:466, 1976

76
NUTRITIONAL REQUIREMENTS

DANIEL RUDMAN
JULIA C. BLEIER

ESSENTIAL AND NONESSENTIAL NUTRIENTS AND THEIR THRESHOLDS (REQUIREMENTS, ALLOWANCES, AND TOLERANCES) Over the past few decades diverse factors, including increased personal income, expanded public assistance programs, and vitamin and mineral enrichment of food, have reduced the prevalence of the classic nutritional deficiency diseases in the United States. Nevertheless, malnutrition, both overt and subclinical, remains a major problem, especially among the poor, the elderly, alcoholics, the chronically ill, and hospital populations. All too often the patient's nutritional status is ignored during the initial clinical evaluation, and complete nutritional needs are not met during hospitalization. To approach nutritional care rationally, the physician must understand how disease affects nutrient thresholds, assess the preexisting nutritional status, calculate the needs for maintenance and repletion, and institute the appropriate diet therapy.

The body contains many thousands of species of organic molecules but requires for health the intake of only 23 organic compounds in addition to a source of energy and water: 9 essential amino acids, 1 fatty acid, and 13 vitamins. The vast majority of organic molecules in food, although metabolized or assimilated by the body, are "nonessential" in the sense that their deletion from the diet does not cause illness. The simplicity of the nutritional requirements of the healthy subject, compared with the complexity of his or her chemical composition, is the result of the remarkable capacity for endogenous biosynthesis.

Of the limited number of inorganic compounds in food, the majority of their constituent elements, that is 15, are believed to be nutritionally essential: calcium, phosphorus, iodine, iron, magnesium, zinc, copper, potassium, sodium, chloride, cobalt, chromium, manganese, molybdenum, and selenium.

TABLE 76-1
Recommended daily dietary allowances[a]

					Fat-soluble vitamins		
Age, years	*Weight, kg*	*Height, cm*	*Energy, kcal*	*Protein, g*	*Vitamin A RE*[b]*, μg*	*Vitamin D, μg*[c]	*Vitamin E, mg αTE*[d]
INFANTS							
0.0–05	6	60	kg × 115	kg × 2.2	420	10	3
0.5–1.0	9	71	kg × 105	kg × 2.0	400	10	4
CHILDREN							
1–3	13	90	1300	23	400	10	5
4–6	20	112	1700	30	500	10	6
7–10	28	132	2400	34	700	10	7
MALES							
11–14	45	157	2700	45	1000	10	8
15–18	66	176	2800	56	1000	10	10
19–22	70	177	2900	56	1000	7.5	10
23–50	70	178	2700	56	1000	5	10
51+	70	178	2400	56	1000	5	10
FEMALES							
11–14	46	157	2200	46	800	10	8
15–18	55	163	2100	46	800	10	8
19–22	55	163	2100	44	800	7.5	8
23–50	55	163	2000	44	800	5	8
51+	55	163	1800	44	800	5	8
PREGNANCY							
			+300	+30	+200	+5	+2
LACTATION							
			+500	+20	+400	+5	+3

[a] *The allowances are intended to provide for individual variations among most normal persons as they live in the United States under usual environmental stresses. Diets should be based on a variety of common foods in order to provide other nutrients for which human requirements have been less well defined.*
[b] *Retinol equivalents; 1 retinol equivalent = 1 μg retinol or 6 μg β-carotene.*
[c] *As cholecalciferol; 10 μg cholecalciferol = 400 IU vitamin D.*
[d] *α-Tocopherol equivalents; 1 mg d-α-tocopherol = 1 αTE.*
[e] *Niacin equivalents; 1 NE = 1 mg niacin or 60 mg dietary tryptophan.*
[f] *The folacin allowances refer to dietary sources as determined by* Lactobacillus casei *assay after treatment with enzymes ("conjugases") to make polyglutamyl forms of the vitamin available to the test organism.*

The requirement of an essential nutrient is the smallest quantity that maintains normal mass, chemical composition, morphology, and physiological functions of the body and prevents any clinical or biochemical sign of the corresponding deficiency state. In children, an additional criterion is a normal rate of growth.

Because the requirements vary among individuals due to numerous genetic and environmental circumstances, the recommended dietary allowances (RDA) provide a margin of safety sufficient to meet the needs of 90 to 95 percent of the healthy population (Tables 76-1 and 76-2). RDA is determined as follows:

1 In healthy adults the requirements of protein (or its constituent amino acids) and macrominerals (requirement greater than 100 mg) can be assessed by the elemental balance technique. Daily balance of each element equals intake minus output (urinary plus fecal). The requirement of each amino acid or macromineral is the smallest intake that maintains zero balance for nitrogen or for the mineral under study. Negative balance of any essential element, if it persists long enough, leads to illness and death.

2 In the infant or growing child the requirement of energy and essential nutrients is the smallest amount of each that maintains an optimal rate of growth while all others are fed in adequate amounts.

3 For micronutrients (requirement less than 100 mg) the requirement is the smallest daily intake that prevents eventual appearance of the nutrient-specific deficiency state.

Table 76-3 lists the amino acids required by infants and adults to illustrate the effect of age on nutrient requirements. Table 76-4 describes the main features of the illness which ensues when each essential nutrient is deficient.

Another nutritional threshold is the maximal daily tolerance of a nutrient. Just as intake of any essential nutrient below a specific level causes disease, likewise intake above a certain level for many nutrients (either essential or nonessential) disturbs body structure or function. Intakes exceeding tolerance can lead to acute reversible symptoms, acute permanent damage, or progressive systemic impairments (Table 76-5). A physiologic diet provides intakes of each nutrient between the two thresholds of minimal requirement and maximal tolerance. The recognition that tolerance for a nutrient can be exceeded is important during parenteral nutrition, when the gastrointestinal mechanisms (emesis, incomplete absorption, diarrhea) that ordinarily protect the individual at least partially from the ill effects of excessive nutrient intake are bypassed. Although allowances have been established for nutrients, the maximal tolerance for most nutrients is uncertain.

FACTORS ALTERING NUTRITIONAL THRESHOLDS Both the recommended allowances and maximal tolerance of each essential nutrient are influenced by a host of factors: rate of growth, age, exercise, pregnancy and lactation, chemical composition of the diet, diseases, drugs. In addition, the route, rate,

Water-soluble vitamins							*Minerals*					
Ascorbic Acid, mg	*Thiamin, mg*	*Riboflavin, mg*	*Niacin, mg NE*[e]	*Vitamin B_6, mg*	*Folacin, μg*[f]	*Vitamin B_{12}, μg*	*Calcium, mg*	*Phosphorus, mg*	*Magnesium, mg*	*Iron, mg*	*Zinc, mg*	*Iodine, μg*
35	0.3	0.4	6	0.3	30	0.5	360	240	50	10	3	40
35	0.5	0.6	8	0.6	45	1.5[g]	540	360	70	15	5	50
45	0.7	0.8	9	0.9	100	2.0	800	800	150	15	10	70
45	0.9	1.0	11	1.3	200	2.5	800	800	200	10	10	90
45	1.2	1.4	16	1.6	300	3.0	800	800	250	10	10	120
50	1.4	1.6	18	1.8	400	3.0	1200	1200	350	18	15	150
60	1.4	1.7	18	2.0	400	3.0	1200	1200	400	18	15	150
60	1.5	1.7	19	2.2	400	3.0	800	800	350	10	15	150
60	1.4	1.6	18	2.2	400	3.0	800	800	350	10	15	150
60	1.2	1.4	16	2.2	400	3.0	800	800	350	10	15	150
60	1.1	1.3	15	1.8	400	3.0	1200	1200	300	18	15	150
60	1.1	1.3	14	2.0	400	3.0	1200	1200	300	18	15	150
60	1.1	1.3	14	2.0	400	3.0	800	800	300	18	15	150
60	1.0	1.2	13	2.0	400	3.0	800	800	300	18	15	150
60	1.0	1.2	13	2.0	400	3.0	800	800	300	10	15	150
+20												
	+0.4	+0.3	+2	+0.6	+400	+1.0	+400	+ 400	+150	[h]	+5	125
+40	+0.5	+0.5	+5	+0.5	+100	+1.0	+400	+ 400	+150	[h]	+10	250

RDA for vitamin B_{12} in infants is based on average concentration of the vitamin in human milk. The allowances after weaning are based on energy intake (as ommended by the American Academy of Pediatrics) and consideration of other factors such as intestinal absorption.

increased requirement during pregnancy cannot be met by the iron content of habitual American diets nor by the existing iron stores of many women; therefore, the use 30 to 60 mg of supplemental iron is recommended. Iron needs during lactation are not substantially different from those of nonpregnant women, but continued plementation of the mother for 2 to 3 months after parturition is advisable in order to replenish stores depleted by pregnancy.

TABLE 76-2
Estimated safe and adequate daily dietary intakes of additional selected vitamins and minerals*,†

	Vitamins				*Trace elements*				
	Age, yr	*Vitamin K, μg*	*Biotin, μg*	*Pantothenic acid, mg*	*Copper, mg*	*Manganese, mg*	*Fluoride, mg*	*Chromium, mg*	*Selenium, mg*
Infants	0–0.5	12	35	2	0.5–0.7	0.5–0.7	0.1–0.5	0.01–0.04	0.01–0.04
	0.5–1.0	10–20	50	3	0.7–1.0	0.7–1.0	0.2–1.0	0.02–0.06	0.02–0.06
Children and adolescents	1–3	15–30	65	3	1.0–1.5	1.0–1.5	0.5–1.5	0.02–0.08	0.02–0.08
	4–6	20–40	85	3–4	1.5–2.0	1.5–2.0	1.0–2.5	0.03–0.12	0.03–0.12
	7–10	30–60	120	4–5	2.0–2.5	2.0–3.0	1.5–2.5	0.05–0.20	0.05–0.20
	11+	50–100	100–200	4–7	2.0–3.0	2.5–5.0	1.5–2.5	0.05–0.20	0.05–0.20
Adults		70–140	100–200	4–7	2.0–3.0	2.5–5.0	1.5–4.0	0.05–0.20	0.05–0.20

* *Because there is less information on which to base an allowance, these are not given in the main table of dietary allowances but are provided here in the form of ranges of recommended intakes.*
† *Because the toxic levels for many trace elements may be only several times usual intakes, the upper levels for the trace elements given in this table should not be habitually exceeded.*

and timing of alimentation influence requirements and tolerances. As the "distance" between requirement and tolerance narrows, nutritional management becomes more difficult (e.g., protein intake of a cachectic, encephalopathic, cirrhotic patient).

Physiological factors Growth, exercise, pregnancy, and lactation (Table 76-1) increase the daily requirements per unit of body weight for energy and most essential nutrients. In the aged person, energy requirements per kilogram of lean body mass are the same as those of a younger person; nevertheless, energy requirements decline with age due to the reduced lean body mass and reduced activity.

Composition of the diet Given diets with identical contents of nitrogen, digestible carbohydrates, fat, vitamins, and minerals, the metabolic availability of the nutrients may vary widely. Thus, all proteins are not equally effective in meeting the daily requirement because of differences in digestibility or in content of essential amino acids (Table 76-6). Gastrointestinal absorption of some minerals is influenced by the presence in the diet of other reactive components; the utilization of vitamins may be influenced by level of intake of organic macronutrients. Examples are given in Table 76-7.

Route, rate, and time (see Chap. 81) The allowances listed in Tables 76-1 to 76-3 apply to enteral nutrition. For some nutrients, different amounts are required for parenteral nutrition. Net gastrointestinal absorption of ingested amino acids, carbohydrates, fats, sodium, chloride, and potassium normally is greater than 90 percent (Table 76-8), and these nutrients, have the same RDAs for the intravenous as for the enteral route. For some of the remaining essential minerals, however, net absorption is only 50 percent or less (Table 76-8); consequently the intravenous requirement is only a fraction of the oral one. It is also likely that the requirements of amino acids are not identical by enteral and parenteral routes. After ingestion and absorption into the portal venous system, a portion of the absorbed amino acids is catabolized during the "first pass" through the liver, where many of the enzymes of amino acid degradation are located. Intravenously infused amino acids, in contrast, can bypass these catabolic pathways and reach sites of protein synthesis in muscle and other extrahepatic tissues.

Timing can be important. For example, some of the essential amino acids must be supplied simultaneously to support protein synthesis. If one such essential amino acid, e.g., tryptophan, is administered at a different time than the other essential and nonessential amino acids, assimilation of all into protein is curtailed. Similarly, when amino acids, glucose, lipids, and minerals are infused at separate times during the day or week, as often happens in parenteral feeding, assimilation may be impaired. Thus omission of phosphorus or potassium from central hyperalimentation solutions impairs retention of the nitrogen furnished by the same fluid. For these reasons, the requirements of several essential nutrients by the parenteral route remain uncertain.

TABLE 76-3
Recommended daily allowances of the essential amino acids per kilogram of body weight for infants, children, and adult male subjects

Amino acid	*Infants**	*Children*	*Adults*
L-Threonine	68	28	8
L-Valine	92	25	14
L-Isoleucine	83	28	12
L-Leucine	135	42	16
L-Lysine	99	44	12
L-Tryptophan	21	4	3
L-Methionine-cystine	49	22	10
L-Phenylalanine-tyrosine	141	22	16
L-Histidine	33	? †	? †

* *The preterm infant has additional requirements for arginine, tyrosine, cystine, and taurine.*
† *Essentiality has been established by long-term nitrogen balance and plasma amino acids; however, recommended levels of intake have not been established.*

Disease Nutritional requirements and tolerances may be altered by disease through at least seven mechanisms (see also Table 76-9):

1 *Increased utilization of nutrients.* Fever, infection, and trauma increase resting metabolic rate and, as a consequence, daily caloric requirement. Folate is utilized more rapidly in patients with hemolysis and increased cell turnover (hemolytic anemia, psoriasis, cancer). Many nutritional requirements are greater during repletion from cachexia than during maintenance of normal nutriture. In this respect, the repletion process in adults resembles growth in children.
2 *Malabsorption.* For each nutrient absorbed less efficiently than normal in malabsorption states, the daily requirement is increased correspondingly.
3 *Impaired ability to activate a nutrient.* The requirement for vitamin D is increased by renal disease that impairs hydroxylation of the vitamin; requirements for folate, thiamin, and pyridoxine in cirrhotics may be greater than normal because of impaired hepatic capacity to transform these vitamins into their active forms.
4 *Abnormally large losses of nutrients.* Impaired conservation of sodium, phosphorus, or amino acids because of renal disease, burns, blood loss, nasogastric suction, diarrhea, or hemodialysis leads to loss of nutrients. One criterion of normal nutriture for nitrogen and minerals in the adult is zero

	Electrolytes		
Molybdenum, mg	Sodium, mg	Potassium, mg	Chloride, mg
0.03–0.06	115–350	350–925	275–700
0.04–0.08	250–750	425–1275	400–1200
0.05–0.10	325–975	550–1650	500–1500
0.06–0.15	450–1350	775–2350	700–2100
0.10–0.30	600–1800	1000–3000	925–2775
0.15–0.50	900–2700	1525–4575	1400–4200
0.15–0.50	1100–3300	1875–5625	1700–5100

elemental balance, i.e., enteral or parenteral intake equal to urinary plus fecal output. If output of nitrogen or mineral is increased by abnormal renal or extrarenal loss, then intake must be correspondingly higher to maintain zero balance.

5 *Impaired catabolic or excretory pathways.* Metabolic defects can reduce both requirement and tolerance, because the rate of degradation or excretion of a nutrient is slowed. In children with phenylketonuria or maple syrup urine disease, the requirements for phenylalanine or branched-chain amino acids, respectively, are less than in normals. Patients with uremia have a reduced dietary requirement for nonessential amino acids.

6 *Hyperabsorption.* Increased absorption can result in a decrease in both requirement and tolerance: Examples are calcium in hyperabsorptive hypercalciuria, iron in hemochromatosis, and copper in Wilson's disease.

7 *Drugs.* Pharmacological agents can alter nutritional requirements by causing malabsorption or renal loss of a nutrient, by preventing its metabolic utilization, or by accelerating its degradation.

INDIVIDUAL ESSENTIAL NUTRIENTS **Water** A reasonable allowance is 1 ml/kcal for adults and 150 ml/kg for infants. The minimum requirement, considerably less than the customary allowance, depends on the preformed and potential solutes ingested (largely protein, sodium, chloride, and potassium), the concentrating ability of the kidney, and extrarenal losses. Normally 50 to 100 ml per day is excreted in the feces, 500 to 1000 ml is lost by exhalation and evaporation (insensible loss), and the remainder is excreted in the urine. Water intake must equal these losses to avoid under- or overhydration.

Maximal tolerance normally is more than 5 liters daily because of the kidney's large capacity for free water clearance. Water requirement and tolerance are increased by factors that cause increased losses in urine, feces, or sweat. The obligatory urinary loss is proportional to the excretion of solutes and the kidney's concentrating capacity; it is increased in proportion to intake of protein, Na^+, K^+, and Cl^-. Water requirements are increased by deficiency of antidiuretic hormone and decreased when the hormone is secreted inappropriately. Fecal loss of water may increase to over 5 liters per day in severe diarrhea. Nasogastric suction, ileostomy, gastrointestinal fistulas, and burns similarly increase daily water requirements. Water loss is excessive during fever, heavy exercise, or exposure to high environmental temperature. Each degree Celsius of fever causes an obligatory loss of about 200 ml water per day.

Energy To maintain stable weight, energy intake must equal energy output. The output can be divided in basal and activity components. Basal metabolic rate (BMR) is usually measured in the fasting, resting subject immediately after waking. Standard values are given in Table 76-10; values during sleep are about 10 percent less. After each meal, metabolic rate increases by as much as 30 percent; during each day, this "specific dynamic action" accounts for about 6 percent of the basal energy expenditure. BMR falls by 20 percent between 30 and 90 years of age; however, this decline disappears when BMR is expressed per kilogram of lean body mass.

Activity increases energy demands. Mild, moderate, or severe exercise raises energy expenditure by roughly 30, 50, or 100 (or more) percent, respectively. Energy expenditures in specific types of activity are described in Chap. 79.

The daily energy requirement equals the sum of expenditures incurred by basal metabolism, specific dynamic action, and physical activity. The requirement can be estimated by assessing basal energy expenditure per day from the subject's surface area (Table 76-10), using ideal body weight in this calculation. Subtract 10 percent from basal during the sleeping hours. Add 6 percent to the 24-h basal estimate to cover the specific dynamic action of meals. From an activity-energy chart, such as is given in Chap. 79, calculate the energy expenditure of the subject's physical activities during a typical day. The daily energy output can be estimated as the sum of basal requirements (minus correction for sleep) plus specific dynamic action plus energy requirement for physical activity. Since on average 93 percent of energy intake is utilized and 7 percent is lost in feces and urine, the estimated energy requirement for zero balance equals 107 percent of the calculated output.

In actual practice, a simpler formula can be used. The Harris-Benedict equations account for sex, weight, height, and age in estimating basal energy expenditure (Table 76-11). To this basal expenditure, 30, 50, or 100 percent is added for sedentary, moderate, or strenuous activity, respectively. Nonstressed hospitalized patients usually require 120 percent of basal energy expenditure, whereas catabolic patients usually require 150 to 200 percent of basal energy expenditure to prevent tissue breakdown or to allow anabolism. Weight is monitored weekly, and if weight increases or decreases, calories are adjusted accordingly.

Energy expenditure is increased by fever (about 13 percent over basal per degree Celsius), burns (40 to 100 percent), trauma (40 to 100 percent), and hyperthyroidism (10 to 100 percent). Hypometabolism, whether of thyroidal or other cause, lowers the energy expenditure and, therefore, the energy requirement.

Patients with severe malabsorption may absorb as little as 25 percent of their ingested calories (fat, carbohydrate, protein) compared with the normal value of over 95 percent. In these patients, the oral energy requirement is higher than normal and may prove impossible to achieve if diarrhea is aggravated by increased nutrient intake. In such patients only parenteral nutrition can prevent progressive starvation.

Protein Dietary protein provides the body a mixture of amino acids for endogenous protein synthesis and is also a metabolic fuel for energy (see Chap. 85). Healthy adults require nine essential amino acids in amounts varying from 250 to 1100 mg per day. About 7 g of nitrogen as nonessential amino acids is also required for protein synthesis. The requirement and allowance of dietary protein depend on the biologic value of the proteins ingested. Biologic value is defined as the proportion of absorbed protein retained by the body under standard test conditions. It is primarily dependent on the content of essential amino acids. Nearly optimal ratios of the 9

TABLE 76-4
Symptoms and manifestations of nutrient deficiency

Nutrient	*Disorders and symptoms of deficiency*	*Laboratory tests*
Water	Thirst, poor tissue turgor, dry mucous membranes, vascular collapse, altered mental status	Serum electrolytes ↑, serum osmolarity ↑, total body water ↓
Calories (energy)	Weakness and physical inactivity, loss of subcutaneous fat, muscle wasting, bradycardia	Weight loss, MAFA ↓, MAMA ↓, creatinine/height ↓, BMR ↓
Protein	Psychomotor change, dyspigmented, sparse, and easily plucked hair, "flaky-paint" dermatitis, edema, muscle wasting, hepatomegaly, ↓ growth	MAMA ↓, serum albumin, transferrin, retinol binding protein ↓, anemia, creatinine/height ↓, serum nonessential/essential amino acids ↑, urine urea/creatinine ↓
Linoleic acid	Xerosis, desquamation, thickening of skin	Serum ratio of triene to tetraene fatty acids ↑
Vitamin A	Xerosis of eye and skin, xerophthalmia, Bitot's spot, follicular hyperkeratosis	Plasma vitamin A ↓, dark adaptation time ↑
Vitamin D	Rickets and growth failure in children, osteomalacia in adults	Serum alkaline phosphatase concentration ↑, plasma 25-hydroxycholecalciferol ↓, serum Ca^{2+} and P ↓
Vitamin E	Anemia	Plasma α-tocopherol ↓, hemolysis of RBC in dilute H_2O_2
Vitamin K	Bleeding diathesis	Prothrombin time ↑
Vitamin C (ascorbic acid)	Scurvy, petechiae, ecchymoses, perifollicular hemorrhage, spongy and bleeding gums (if not edentulous)	Ascorbic acid concentration in plasma, platelets, whole blood, and white blood cells ↓; urinary ascorbic acid ↓
Thiamin (vitamin B_1)	Beriberi, muscle tenderness and weakness, hyporeflexia, hypesthesia, tachycardia, cardiomegaly, congestive heart failure	Erythrocyte thiamine pyrophosphate and transketolase activity ↓ and in vitro effect thereon of thiamin pyrophosphate ↑, urinary thiamin ↓, blood pyruvate and α-ketoglutarate levels ↑
Riboflavin (vitamin B_2)	Angular stomatitis (or angular scars), cheilosis, magenta tongue, atrophic lingual papillae, corneal vascularization, angular blepharitis, dyssebacia, scrotal (vulvar) dermatosis	EGR activity ↓, and in vitro effect on EGR activity of flavin adenine dinucleotide ↑, pyridoxal phosphate oxidase activity ↓ and in vitro effect thereon of riboflavin ↑, ↓ urinary riboflavin
Niacin	Pellagra, scarlet and raw tongue, atrophic lingual papillae, tongue fissuring, mental disorders, pellagrous dermatosis, diarrhea	Urinary N^1-methylnicotinamide ↓, urinary 2-pyridone/N^1-methylnicotinamide ratio ↓
Pyridoxine (vitamin B_6)	Nasolabial seborrhea, glossitis, kidney stones, peripheral neuropathy, muscular twitching, convulsions, microcytic anemia	EGOT activity ↓ and in vitro effect of pyridoxal phosphate on EGOT activity ↑, tryptophan load test ↓ (urinary excretion of xanthurenic and quinolinic acids), urinary vitamin B_6 excretion ↓
Folacin	Pallor, glossitis, stomatitis, diarrhea, anemia	Erythrocyte and serum folate concentration ↓, urine formiminoglutamic acid excretion ↑ after histidine load, macrocytic anemia, polymorphonuclear leukocytes hypersegmented, megaloblastic bone marrow
Vitamin B_{12}	Pallor, mild icterus, anorexia, diarrhea, paresthesia, ataxia, optic neuritis, mental changes	Serum vitamin B_{12} ↓, peripheral blood and bone marrow morphology
Biotin	Fatigue, depression, nausea, dermatitis, muscular pains	Urnary biotin ↓, whole blood biotin ↓
Pantothenic acid	Fatigue, sleep disturbances, impaired coordination, nausea	Urinary pantothenic acid ↓
Calcium	Stunted growth, rickets, osteomalacia, convulsions	Osteopenia by x-ray, serum Ca^{2+} ↓
Phosphorus	Weakness, osteomalacia, ↓ phagocytosis, hemolysis, ↓ cardiac function, neurological syndromes	Osteopenia by x-ray, serum P ↓
Magnesium	Growth failure, behavioral disturbances, weakness, tremor, tetany, seizures, cardiac arrhythmias	Serum, urine, and RBC Mg ↓
Iron	Pallor, weakness, reduced resistance to infection, angular stomatitis, atrophic lingual papillae, koilonychia	Plasma and marrow iron ↓, serum ferritin ↓, microcytic hypochromic anemia
Zinc	Psoriasiform rash, eczematous scaling, growth restriction, hypogonadism, delayed puberty, slow wound healing, hypogeusia, photophobia	Plasma and 24-h urine zinc ↓
Iodine	Goiter, symptoms of hypothyroidism	TSH ↑, T_4 and T_3 ↓, 24-h urine iodine ↓, RAI uptake ↑
Copper	Pallor	Neutropenia, hypochromic microcytic anemia, hypoferremia, osteopenia, plasma and urine copper ↓, ceruloplasmin ↓
Fluorine	Higher frequency of tooth decay	
Chromium	Glucose intolerance	Serum chromium ↓, urinary chromium ↓
Selenium	Cardiomyopathy, muscle pain	Plasma, RBC selenium ↓, glutathione peroxidose activity ↓
Sodium	Muscle weakness and cramps, confusion, apathy, anorexia, hypotension, oliguria	Serum Na^+ ↓, BUN/creatinine ↑
Potassium	Lassitude, polyuria, ileus, muscular weakness	Serum and urine K^+ ↓, body ^{40}K ↓, abnormal ECG
Chloride	Muscle cramps, apathy, anorexia, alkalosis	Serum Cl^- ↓

NOTES: *BMR = basal metabolism rate; BUN = blood-urea nitrogen; creatinine/height = 24-h urine creatinine/height ratio; ECG = electrocardiogram; EGOT = erythrocyte glutamic-oxaloacetic transaminase; EGR = erythrocyte glutathione reductase; MAFA = midarm fat area; MAMA = midarm muscle area; RAI = radioactive iodine; RBC = red blood cell; T_3 = triiodothyroxine; T_4 = thyroxine; TSH = thyroid-stimulating hormone.*

TABLE 76-5
Syndromes that can result from excessive intake or absorption of nutrients by oral route or from excessive infusion by parenteral route

Nutrient	*Manifestation of overnutrition*
Water	Edema, headache, nausea, hypertension
Calories	Obesity
Proteins	Exacerbation of inborn errors in amino acid catabolism or "nitrogen accumulation diseases"
Fat	In predisposed individuals, hyperlipemia
Vitamin A	Headache, vomiting, peeling of skin, anorexia, swelling of long bones, cirrhosis
Vitamin D	Hypercalcemia, nephrolithiasis, impaired renal function
Vitamin K	At high doses may cause jaundice
Ascorbic acid (vitamin C)	Hyperoxaluria
Calcium	Hypercalcemia, mental and renal dysfunction
Magnesium	Diarrhea
Iron	Siderosis, hemochromatosis
Zinc	Fever, nausea, vomiting, diarrhea
Iodine	Depression of thyroid activity, goiter, occasional hyperthyroidism
Copper	Wilson's disease, vomiting
Manganese	Generalized disease of nervous system
Fluorine	Mottling of teeth, increased bone density, neurological disturbances
Sodium chloride	Hypertension, edema, heart failure
Potassium	Muscular weakness, arrhythmia, death

TABLE 76-6
Biologic value of food proteins*

Protein source	*Biologic value*
Milk	93
Egg	93
Beef	76
Peanut meal	74
Potato	69
Oat	65
Rice	65
Corn	50
Soy flour	41
Wheat gluten	40

* *As determined from nitrogen balance studies conducted in the rat, generally at a dietary protein concentration of 5 percent. Tests in the rat at other concentrations, or in other species, give generally similar but not identical biologic values.*

TABLE 76-7
Some essential nutrients for which the daily dietary requirement is influenced by other dietary components

Nutrient	*Influence by other dietary component*
Protein	Requirement inversely related to calories when the latter are deficient
Essential amino acids	Utilization curtailed if any essential amino acid is deficient
Phenylalanine	Requirement inversely related to tyrosine intake
Methionine	Requirement inversely related to cystine intake
Valine, leucine, isoleucine	Requirement of each is increased by excess of the other branched-chain amino acid(s)
Vitamin E	Requirement proportional to intake of polyunsaturated fat
Thiamin	Requirement proportional to calories
Niacin	Requirement inversely related to tryptophan intake
Vitamin B_6	Requirement increased by protein
Folacin	Requirement increased by alcohol intake
Calcium	Urinary excretion increased by high protein intake
Calcium, magnesium, nonheme iron, zinc	Absorption decreased by phytates
Nonheme iron	Absorption improved by vitamin C or sulfur-containing amino acids
Copper	Absorption decreased by calcium, requirement increased by excess dietary zinc

TABLE 76-8
Net absorption of nutrients in normal adults on diets containing mixtures of plant and animal foods

Element	*Percent*	*Element*	*Percent*
Carbohydrate	>90	Manganese	<5
Protein	>90	Fluorine	80–90
Fat	>95	Chromium	1–3
Calcium	5–40	Selenium	>50
Phosphorus	50–60	Molybdenum	40–50
Magnesium	25–50	Cobalt	>50
Iron	5–15	Sodium	>95
Zinc	33	Potassium	80–90
Iodine	>50	Chlorine	>95
Copper	25		

TABLE 76-9
Disorders that alter nutrient requirements by the oral route

Nutrient	*Increases dietary requirement*	*Reduces dietary requirement*
Calories	Fever, hyperthyroidism, trauma, malabsorption	Coma, hypothyroidism
Protein	Fever, hyperthyroidism, trauma, azotorrhea	Nitrogen accumulation diseases, inborn errors of urea synthesis
Phenylalanine		Phenylketonuria
Branched-chain amino acids		Maple syrup urine disease
Linoleic acid and fat-soluble vitamins	Malabsorption syndromes	
Folacin	Increased cell turnover	
Calcium	Malabsorption syndromes	Hyperabsorptive hypercalciuria
Phosphorus	Malabsorption syndromes	Renal insufficiency
Magnesium	Malabsorption syndromes	
Iron	Malabsorption syndromes	Hemochromatosis
Zinc	Acrodermatitis enteropathica	
Copper	Malabsorption syndromes	Wilson's disease
Carnitine*	Advanced cirrhosis	

* *No requirement normally.*

TABLE 76-10
Basal energy requirements of normal subjects

Age, years	*Males, (cal/m²)/h*	*Females, (cal/m²)/h*
14–16	46.0	43.0
16–18	43.0	40.0
18–20	41.0	38.0
20–30	39.5	37.0
30–40	39.5	36.5
40–50	38.5	36.0
50–60	37.5	35.0
60–70	36.5	34.0
70–80	35.5	33.0

SOURCE: *EF DuBois, Basal Metabolism in Health and Disease, 3d ed. Philadelphia, Lea & Febiger, 1936, p 151*

TABLE 76-11
Calculation of basal energy expenditure (BEE) by Harris-Benedict equations

WOMEN

$$\text{BEE} = 655 + (9.6 \times W) + (1.8 \times H) - (4.7 \times A)$$

MEN

$$\text{BEE} = 66 + (13.7 \times W) + (5 \times H) - (6.8 \times A)$$

NOTE: *W = ideal body weight in kilograms, H = height in centimeters, A = age in years* essential and 11 nonessential amino acids are present in egg and milk proteins, which consequently have the highest biologic values for the diet, viz., 90 to 95 (Table 76-6). The biologic value of proteins in the world's major food products follows the general order: animal products > legumes > cereals (rice, wheat, corn) > roots. The adult RDA for protein given in Table 76-1, about 50 g per day, assumes a biologic value of about 80, a characteristic value when animal products are the major protein source. The lower the biologic value, the higher the daily protein requirement.

Plant proteins have low biologic value because one or more essential amino acids are deficient. Thus for corn (maize), lysine and tryptophan are limiting; for soy beans and grean peas, methionine; for rice, lysine and threonine; for wheat, lysine. Therefore, mixtures of two "complementary" vegetable proteins deficient in different essential amino acids have a higher biologic value than either protein separately.

While the usual reason for low biologic value of a particular protein or mixtures of proteins is the limiting content of one or more essential amino acids, a change in the proportion of amino acids or an excess of amino acids can impair the value. For example, when a mixture of amino acids lacking histidine is added to a marginally adequate protein source containing histidine, rats become anorexic and cease growing. This amino acid imbalance is corrected by adding the most limiting amino acid, histidine. An excess of certain amino acids, e.g., methionine and tyrosine, can cause toxic reactions. Requirements for other amino acids can be enhanced by an excess of a structurally similar amino acid, e.g., the branched-chain amino acids, leucine, isoleucine, and valine. These are important considerations in planning the composition of mixtures of synthetic amino acids for parenteral or enteral feeding. In addition, certain amino acids may be "spared" by chemically related amino acids. For example, cystine and tyrosine, which are synthesized from methionine and phenylalanine, respectively, exert a "sparing" effect in that 80 percent of the methionine requirement and 70 percent of the phenylalanine requirement could be met by giving cystine and tyrosine, respectively.

The daily requirement of a protein, or its constituent amino acids, is also influenced by energy intake; the values for protein allowances given in Table 76-1 assume adequate energy intake. When the energy requirement is met by nonprotein calories a substantial portion of ingested amino acids is utilized for protein synthesis. If calories are severely deficient, some amino acids are diverted from protein synthesis into pathways of oxidative metabolism and gluconeogenesis. Under these circumstances, the daily protein requirement is inversely proportional to the energy intake. Thus, energy undernutrition makes a person more vulnerable to protein starvation, an interaction which accounts for the high prevalence of the combined deficiency state protein-energy undernutrition (see Chap. 78).

The daily protein requirement per unit body weight is increased by growth, pregnancy, lactation, and repletion after cachexia, fever, infection, trauma, and malabsorption. Protein requirements may be increased in some of the elderly. Balance studies have shown that some of the aged fail to maintain nitrogen equilibrium when consuming sufficient energy to maintain body weight.

To understand how the "nitrogen accumulation diseases," hepatic and renal insufficiency, alter the requirements and tolerances of dietary protein, consider the scheme of amino acid metabolism shown in Fig. 76-1. The daily adult allowance of about 50 g protein serves to maintain reaction 2, that is, protein synthesis, at a rate equal to protein breakdown (reaction 3). Tolerance for protein is greater than 250 g per day because of the high capacity of the degradative pathway (reactions 4, 6, 7, and 9). Note that 25 to 40 percent of urea formed in the liver is hydrolyzed by microbes within the colon and recycles at least once as ammonia (reaction 8). When step 10 is blocked (uremia), the requirement for nonessential nitrogen is reduced. Urea, instead of being excreted, recycles as ammonia and remains available for synthesis of nonessential amino acids; the carbon skeletons of these acids are readily produced by the intermediary metabolism of glucose. This pathway for endogenous synthesis of nonessential amino acids is the basis for the Giovanetti diet in uremia. If the uremic patient is fed the carbon skeletons (α-keto derivatives) of the essential amino acids, the requirement of the latter nutrients (except for threonine and lysine) is also reduced because of the reversibility of transamination, i.e., reaction 5 in Fig. 76-1. Similar considerations apply in advanced cirrhosis and in hereditary disorders of urea synthesis.

Not only is the daily requirement for protein in some uremics and cirrhotics lower than normal, but the maximal tolerance is curtailed as well. As little as 20 g protein a day can precipitate or aggravate symptoms of hepatocerebral disease in the susceptible hepatic patient. Intakes of protein customary for the healthy subjects in the United States (80 to 100 g per day) can also intensify the uremic syndrome.

Fat While the average adult in the United States consumes 40 percent of calories as fat (90 g), the requirement is only 2 to 3 percent of total calories as linoleic acid for prostaglandin synthesis. The American Heart Association recommends a diet containing 35 percent fat with an increased ratio of polyunsaturated oils to saturated fats in an effort to minimize the risk of atherosclerosis.

Minerals and vitamins The daily allowances and the influence of physiological and pathological circumstances on these thresholds are listed in Tables 76-1, 76-2, 76-7, and 76-9. The deficiency syndromes corresponding to each nutrient are listed in Table 76-4, and some clinical effects of exceeding the daily tolerance are given in Table 76-5 (see also Chap. 83). It is important to realize that the mineral and vitamin requirements of the elderly have not been established and that the present recommendations are based on studies of young subjects.

Nonessential substances FIBER Dietary fiber is comprised of cellulose, hemicellulose, pectins, algae polysaccharides, and lignin and contributes 15 to 25 g to the average U.S. diet. The properties of fiber in the intestine, the hydrophilic nature, gel-forming ability, and binding capacity for ions and salts have led to many claims of the beneficial effects of fiber on diverticulosis, colonic cancer, gallstones, diabetes, and coronary artery disease. Much work is still needed in this area.

FIGURE 76-1
Overview of amino acid metabolism.

Dietary protein $\xrightarrow{1}$ blood amino acids $\underset{3}{\overset{2}{\rightleftarrows}}$ tissue protein

blood amino acids $\underset{5}{\overset{4}{\rightleftarrows}}$ α-keto acids + NH_3 + aspartic acid

NH_3 $\xrightarrow{6}$ Krebs-Henseleit cycle; aspartic acid $\xrightarrow{7}$ Krebs-Henseleit cycle

Krebs-Henseleit cycle $\xrightarrow{9}$ blood urea $\xrightarrow{10}$ urine urea

blood urea $\xrightarrow{8}$ NH_3

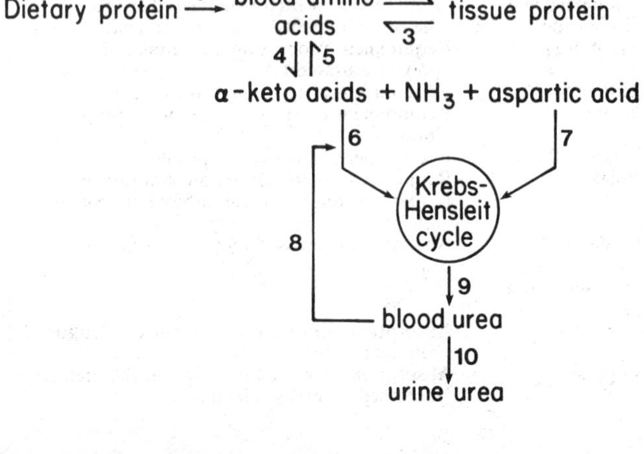

CHOLINE, CARNITINE, INOSITOL Although these organic compounds have biologic activity, they have not been considered essential vitamins because several animal species including humans have biosynthetic capabilities. However, limited biosynthesis has been documented in certain young animals and in certain genetic and acquired disorders; therefore, under these circumstances an exogenous source should be considered.

REFERENCES

FOOD AND NUTRITION BOARD: *Recommended Dietary Allowances*, Washington, D.C., National Academy of Sciences, 1979

GOODHART RS, SHILS ME (eds): *Modern Nutrition in Health and Disease*, 6th ed. Philadelphia, Lea & Febiger, 1980

HERBERT V et al: Folic acid and vitamin B_{12}, in *Modern Nutrition in Health and Disease*, 6th ed, RS Goodhart, ME Shils (eds). Philadelphia, Lea & Febiger, 1980, pp 229–259

MUNRO HN: Nutritional requirements in health. Crit Care Med 8:2, 1980

———: Nutrition and ageing. Br Med Bull 37:83, 1981

77
ASSESSMENT OF NUTRITIONAL STATUS

DANIEL RUDMAN
JULIA C. BLEIER

Undernutrition is a common contribution to morbidity and mortality rates in most hospitals. As a peculiar discrepancy, however, undernutrition rarely appears on charts in the list of diagnoses or in the progress notes. Consequently, quantitative tests of nutritional status are rare in the initial clinical workup, and the progress of the nutritional state is rarely monitored regularly during the course of illness. As a result, undernutrition tends to be recognized late, when it is severe and difficult to treat. This chapter defines feasible methods for identifying and quantifying the deficiency syndromes, for investigating their cause, and for monitoring their course.

MASS AND COMPOSITION OF THE BODY COMPARTMENTS Consideration must first be given to the normal mass and chemical composition of the major body compartments, since these compartmental properties are altered by nutritional deficiencies in characteristic ways. The body can be viewed as consisting of four compartments: extracellular fluid, protoplasm (intracellular compartment), bone, and adipose tissue. The first three make up the lean body mass.

The mass and elemental composition of the body compartments of a healthy "reference man," 70 kg in weight, 172 cm tall, 35 years old, are shown in Table 77-1. Typical masses of extracellular fluid, protoplasm, bone, and adipose tissue are 17, 35, 5, and 13 kg, respectively. Chloride is localized almost exclusively in the extracellular fluid, where its average concentration is 96 meq per liter; nitrogen and potassium are largely located in protoplasm, with normal concentrations of 27 g and 150 meq per kilogram of wet weight, respectively; calcium is found primarily in bone, where its concentration averages 260 g per kilogram of wet weight. The adipose tissue contains insignificant levels of these elements.

DIRECT AND INDIRECT METHODS FOR MEASURING MASS OF BODY COMPARTMENTS If one assumes that the concentrations of chloride, nitrogen, potassium, phosphorus, and calcium remain normal in extracellular fluid, protoplasm, and bone during a period of observation involving expansion or contraction of these compartments, and if one knows the balance (i.e., intake and output) of each element (termed Δ nitrogen, Δ phosphorus, etc.) during this period, then from the equations in Table 77-2 one can calculate the change (Δ) in the mass of each of these three compartments during the period under consideration.

The equations are based on the fact that each kilogram of extracellular fluid, protoplasm, or bone gained or lost by the body contains a characteristic amount of chloride, nitrogen, or calcium, respectively. A bedside estimate of daily nitrogen balance in grams can be made as follows:

$$\frac{\text{Daily protein intake, g}}{6.25} - (\text{24-h urine urea nitrogen, g} + 2.5\text{ g}^*)$$

Metabolic balance techniques of this type provide estimates of the change in mass of each compartment during the period of observation but provide no information about the absolute mass of the compartment at the beginning and end. Several methods capable of such absolute measurements are available: whole-body counting of potassium (total body protoplasm), measurement of total-body nitrogen by neutron activation analysis, measurement of extracellular fluid by isotope dilution, measurement of total-body water by isotope dilution, calculation of intracellular water (closely related to protoplasmic mass) as total-body water minus extracellular water, measurement of adipose mass by determining whole-body density. These various methods are largely restricted to research units. Fortunately, several indirect methods for estimating the mass of body compartments are available to the clinician:

1 In the nonedematous patient, body weight as percent of ideal is a useful indicator of adipose tissue plus lean body mass. Reduction of the body weight/ideal body weight ratio to 80 percent in nonedematous patients usually means mild protein-energy undernutrition; a reduction to 70 to 80 percent indicates moderate protein-energy undernutrition, a decline to 70 percent or less indicates severe protein-energy undernutrition.

2 Anthropometric analysis of the midarm requires only a tape measure and caliper. The principle is illustrated in Fig. 77-1;

* *Two-and-one-half grams is the approximate sum of urinary nonurea nitrogen plus fecal and integumental losses of nitrogen.*

TABLE 77-1
Approximate mass and major elemental composition of body compartments in a 70-kg healthy "reference man"

	Protoplasm	*Extracellular fluid*	*Bone*	*Adipose tissue*
Mass	35 kg	17 kg	5 kg	13 kg
Body weight	50%	24%	7%	19%
Elemental composition, kg wet wt	27 g N 97 mmol P 150 meq K	140 meq Na 96 meq Cl	260 g Ca 115 g P	

TABLE 77-2
Reifenstein equations for determining change in mass of body compartments.

ΔProtoplasm, g	= 27 × ΔN, g
ΔECF,* g	= 9.6 × ΔCl, meq
ΔBone, g	= 0.1 × ΔCa, meq
ΔAdipose tissue, g	= ΔBW, † g − [Δ protoplasm, g + ΔECF, g + Δ bone, g]

* *Extracellular fluid.*
† *Body weight.*

the arm consists of a cylinder of muscle within a sheath of adipose tissue. From the external circumference of the nondominant midarm and the width of the adipose layer (equal to one-half the triceps skin fold), midarm muscle area and midarm and fat area can be calculated. The midarm muscle and fat areas are indicators of the body's masses of skeletal muscle and adipose tissue, respectively. Normal average values for adult men and women, respectively, are midarm muscle area, 50.91 and 42.81 cm^2, and midarm fat area, 17.04 and 21.28 cm^2. By taking skin-fold measurements at the biceps, subscapular, and suprailiac sites, in addition to the triceps, one can calculate total adipose mass by the method of Durnin and Womersley. Lean body mass is derived from the difference of fat mass in kilograms and body weight.

3 Urine creatinine is related to lean body mass by the equation:

$$\text{Lean body mass, kg} = 7.138 + 0.02908 \times (\text{mg creatinine/24 h})$$

The ratio of 24-h creatinine excretion (in grams) to height (in centimeters) is considered a measure of muscle mass and can be used as an index to determine protein depletion. Three qualifying conditions should be considered: (*a*) diets containing meat influence the quantity of creatinine excreted; (*b*) impaired renal function results in falsely low creatinine excretion; and (*c*) creatinine excretion declines with age as a result of a smaller muscle mass. In normal men and women the creatinine/height ratio averages 10.5 and 5.8 mg/cm, respectively. In men, ratios in the ranges 8.4 to 9.5, 7.4 to 8.4, and less than 7.4 mg/cm signify mild, moderate, and severe degrees of protein depletion, respectively.

4 Sagittal or horizontal radiograms or CT scans of an extremity also provide quantitative information about the mass of representative skeletal muscles but are more expensive.

Skeletal muscle makes up about 30 percent of the lean body mass. This organ atrophies progressively in protein-energy starvation, the most common deficiency state in American hospitals (see Chap. 78). By monitoring the creatinine/height ratio and midarm muscle area, the clinician can identify protein-energy starvation easily and inexpensively and monitor its course.

The visceral compartment, which maintains tissue function, protein synthesis, and the immune response comprises 20 percent of the lean body mass. Under conditions of nutritional inadequacy, protein synthesis declines, metabolic pathways are altered, and the immune system becomes impaired. Certain blood proteins are sensitive indicators of these events and are used to detect malnutrition and monitor nutritional repletion. Table 77-3 lists proteins and blood concentrations that are indicative of malnutrition. Prealbumin and retinol binding protein have the shortest half-life (1 to 2 days), and thus can be used to monitor patients at high risk of developing protein-energy malnutrition and to evaluate the initial repletion. Presently, these immunoassays are expensive. Transferrin, with a half-life of 8 days, is also useful in monitoring repletion, although concurrent iron-deficiency anemia makes interpretation difficult. Albumin (half-life, 14 days) is the most useful prognostic indicator of protein-energy malnutrition. Liver disease may lower albumin synthesis; nevertheless, in undernourished cirrhotics the albumin level usually rises with nutritional repletion.

SYNDROMES OF UNDERNUTRITION When any of the 38 essential nutrient requirements (Chap. 76) are not met, undernutrition syndromes result. Undernutrition of such macronutrients as nitrogen, sodium, chloride, potassium, calcium, and phosphorus reduces the mass of one or more body compartments, often with associated abnormalities in compartmental chemistry, structure, and function. For example, deficiencies of nitrogen (protein), sodium, and calcium erode protoplasm, extracellular fluid, and bone, respectively. Undernutrition of a micronutrient tends to cause a specific morphological or functional abnormality in certain tissues without alteration in compartmental mass or elemental composition. While in theory there are 38 different types of human malnutrition, undernutrition syndromes usually occur in groups rather than in "pure" form.

Deficiency of each essential nutrient can be characterized in terms of symptoms, signs, and chemical and radiographic abnormalities, but deficiency syndromes have several principles in common:

FIGURE 77-1
Anthropometric measurement of muscle and adipose compartments of the mid-upper arm. Midarm circumference is measured with a tape measure and triceps skin fold with a caliper. (After Butterworth and Blackburn.)

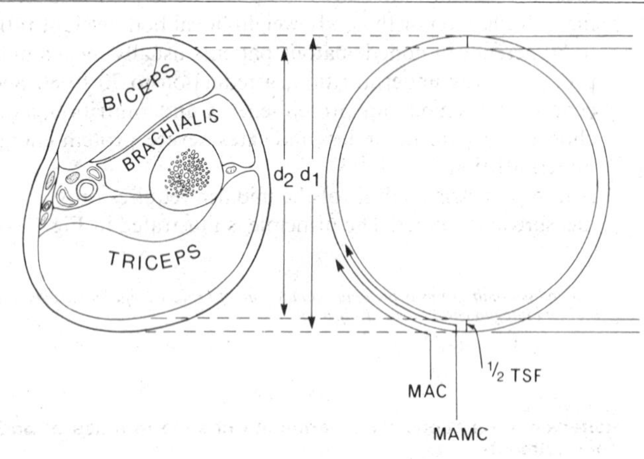

Calculation of mid upper arm muscle circumference

C_1 = mid upper arm circumference in centimeters

S = triceps skinfold in centimeters

d_1 = arm diameter

d_2 = muscle diameter

Skinfold (S) = 2 × subcutaneous fat $= d_1 - d_2$

Circumference (C_1) $= \pi d_1$

Muscle circumference $C_1 - \pi S$

$$\text{Midarm muscle area} = \frac{[C_1 - \pi S]^2}{4\pi}$$

$$\text{Midarm fat area} = \frac{(S)(C_1)}{2} - \frac{\pi(S^2)}{4}$$

Normal values (adults)	*Male*	*Female*
Triceps skinfold, mm	12.5	16.5
Midarm muscle circumference, cm	25.3	23.2
Midarm fat area, cm^2	17.0	21.3
Midarm muscle area, cm^2	50.9	42.8

1 Undernutrition can be either primary or secondary in origin. The primary form is due to inadequate supply of food containing the essential nutrients. In secondary undernutrition adequate diet is available, but because of illness or medical treatment, nutrients cannot be ingested, absorbed, or metabolized adequately, or the rate of utilization of external losses is excessive. Primary and secondary mechanisms frequently reinforce each other; for example, the hypermetabolism and anorexia of infection precipitate nutritional deficiencies more rapidly in patients who previously subsisted on marginal diets than in well-nourished individuals. To determine whether undernutrition in a particular patient is primary or secondary, the physician must obtain a dietary history, assess personal habits and living conditions, and examine the patient for organic disease.

2 Nutritional deficiency syndromes tend to evolve through three stages. Many essential nutrients are stored in the tissues of the well-nourished subject; for example, iron and vitamins B_{12}, A, and D in liver; essential fatty acids in adipose tissue; nitrogen in a labile reserve in muscle and liver. When intake falls below the daily requirement, these reserves temporarily forestall deficiency manifestations and maintain normal blood levels (stage 1). In stage 2, blood levels of the nutrient or nutrient-dependent metabolic products decline, but the patient continues to be asymptomatic. In stage 3, clinical signs and symptoms develop. Methods for assessing the nutritional status should ideally be capable of detecting all three stages of each deficiency syndrome. Available techniques, however, usually reveal only stages 2 and 3.

3 Because anorexia is a major mechanism in the current endemic of protein-energy undernutrition in hospitals in the United States, the intake of nutrients must be measured in one of three ways: by recall, by diary (outpatient), or by observation (inpatient).

4 Change in weight may be ambiguous. In the absence of edema, various proportions of weight loss are due to depletion of adipose tissue and lean body mass. In the presence of edema, body weight changes are even more difficult to interpret. Gain in weight can reflect accumulation of edema, masking erosion of protoplasm; conversely, loss of weight can reflect diuresis with simultaneous expansion of the protoplasmic compartment. An initially obese patient can lose 15 kg because of chronic wasting illness and present for the first medical examination with a normal body weight, the still substantial adipose organ masking a shrinkage in the lean body mass. In such instances, direct or indirect estimation of the size of the protoplasmic compartment is essential as described above.

5 The undernourished patient is usually deficient in several nutrients. Common patterns are deficiency of two or more water-soluble vitamins (usually including folate, vitamin C, and/or thiamine), and deficiency of both Ca^{2+} and Mg^{2+} in patients with malabsorption.

The various physical, chemical, and radiographic characteristics of each type of undernutrition are summarized in Table 76-4. The most commonly used chemical indexes of nutrient deficiency are listed in Table 77-3, which gives three average concentration ranges for each test: normal, subnormal without clinical manifestations, and subnormal with clinical signs or symptoms of deficiency. Although these tests are of value in population surveys and in following the response of patients to therapies, other influencing conditions, such as the effect of renal disease on a 24-h urinary creatinine, should be considered when these tests are used for diagnosis.

The clinician must select a reasonable number of historical, physical, and laboratory items to use as a "nutritional data base" to screen patients for undernutrition. Table 77-4 presents a selection of historical and physical items that would reveal most deficiency states in hospital patients.

TABLE 77-3
Interpretation of laboratory tests for the evaluation of nutritional status (adults)

Nutrient evaluation	*Test*	*Deficient (often with clinical manifestations)*	*Low (usually without clinical manifestations)*	*Acceptable*
Protein	Serum albumin, g/dl	<3.0	3.0–3.5	>3.5
Protein	Serum transferrin, mg/dl	<180–260		180–260
Protein	Serum prealbumin, mg/dl	<20–50		20–50
Protein	Serum retinol binding protein, μg/ml	<30–45		30–45
Protein	Creatinine/height ratio	<90% of Standard	90–95%	>95%
Protein	Nitrogen balance, g	>(−)3	(−)1–3	0–3
Protein, Fe, folacin, vitamin B_{12}	Hemoglobin, g/dl	<12	12–14	>14
Iron	Serum iron, μg/dl	<60		>60
Vitamin A	Plasma retinol, μg/dl	<10	10–20	>20
Vitamin D	Serum Ca × P product, mg/dl	<40		>40
Vitamin D	Alkaline phosphatase, King-Armstrong units/dl	>40	15–40	8–14
Vitamin C	Serum ascorbic acid, mg/dl	<0.20	0.20–0.30	>0.30
Thiamin	Erythrocyte transketolase (% thiamin disphosphate stimulation)	>20	15–20	<15
Riboflavin	Erythrocyte glutathione reductase activity coefficient	>1.40	1.20–1.40	<1.20
Niacin	*N*-Methylnicotinamide excretion, mg/g creatinine	<0.5	0.5–1.59	>1.6
Vitamin B_6	Erythrocyte aminotransferase activity coefficients:			
	EGPT	>1.25		<1.25
	EGOT	>1.5		<1.5
Vitamin B_6	Tryptophan load test (xanthurenic acid), mg/day	>50	25–50	<25
Folacin	Serum folate, ng/ml	<3	3.0–6.0	>6.0
Folacin	Erthrocyte folate, ng/ml	<140	140–160	>160
Vitamin B_{12}	Serum vitamin B_{12}, pg/ml	<150	150–200	>200
Ca	24-h urine Ca^{2+}, mg	<50	50–100	>100
P	24-h urine P, mg	<100	100–300	>300
Mg	24-h urine Mg^{2+}, meq	<4	4–8	>8
Na	24-h urine Na^{+}, meq	<20	20–40	>40
K	24-h urine K^{+}, meq	<20	20–40	>40

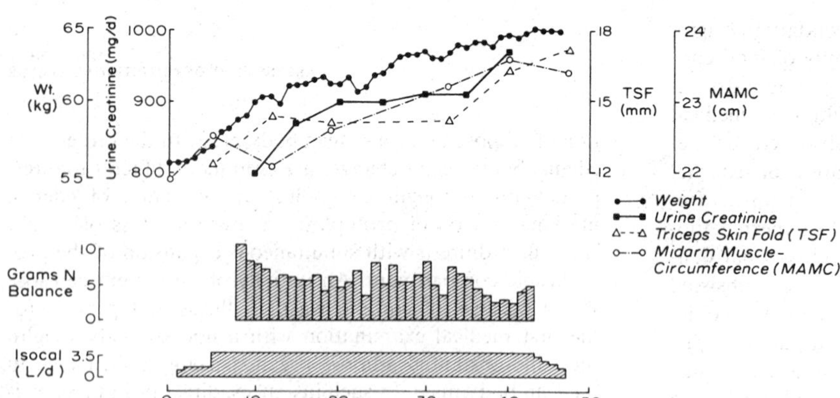

FIGURE 77-2
Monitoring the course of a patient with protein-calorie depletion during repletion by nasogastric hyperalimentation.

TABLE 77-4
Nutritional data base

HISTORY

Previous weight curve
Dietary intake by retrospective recall and prospective diary
Alcohol intake
Socioeconomic and family status, including income
Anorexia, vomiting, diarrhea
Blood loss
Pregnancy, lactation, menses
Vitamin and mineral supplements
Use of drugs that might affect nutrition

PHYSICAL EXAMINATION

General: weight as percent of ideal body weight; triceps skin fold; midarm muscle circumference
Skin: xerosis, follicular hyperkeratosis, pellagrous dermatitis, petechiae, ecchymoses, perifollicular hemorrhages, flaky paint dermatitis, pallor
Hair: dyspigmentation, easy pluckability, thinning, straightening
Head: temporal wasting, parotid enlargement
Eyes: Bitot spots, conjunctival and scleral xerosis, keratomalacia, corneal vascularization, angular palpebritis
Mouth: cheilosis, angular stomatitis, magenta tongue, atrophic lingual papillae, tongue fissuring, glossitis, spongy gums, dentition
Heart: cardiomegaly, findings of congestive heart failure
Abdomen: hepatomegaly
Extremities: edema, koilonychia
Neurological: irritability, weakness, calf tenderness, loss of deep tendon reflexes

MONITORING THE COURSE OF MALNUTRITION Besides defining the type, severity, and mechanism for the development of undernutrition, it is important to ascertain its rate of progression. This is accomplished by periodic monitoring of body weight, albumin, hematocrit, creatinine excretion, midarm muscle area, midarm fat area, and appropriate blood or urine concentrations of nutrition-dependent variables. An example of monitoring the course of progressive protein-energy malnutrition is shown in Fig. 77-2.

REFERENCES

BUTTERWORTH C, BLACKBURN G: Hospital malnutrition and how to assess the nutritional status of a patient. Nutr Today 10:8, 1974

DURNIN J, WOMERSLEY J: Body fat assessed from total body density and its estimation from skinfold thickness: Measurement on 481 men and women from 16 to 72 years. Br J Nutr 32:77, 1974

FORBES GB: Urinary creatinine excretion and lean body mass. Am J Clin Nutr 29:1361, 1976

HEYMSFIELD S: A radiographic method of quantifying protein-calorie undernutrition. Am J Clin Nutr 32:693, 1979

JELLIFFE DB: *The Assessment of the Nutritional Status of the Community.* Geneva, World Health Organization, 1966

REIFENSTEIN EC et al: The accumulation, interpretation, and presentation of data pertaining to metabolic balances, notably those of calcium, phosphorus, and nitrogen. J Clin Endocrinol Metab 5:367 1945

SAUBERLICH HE et al: *Laboratory Tests for the Assessment of Nutritional Status.* Boca Raton, Fla., CRC Press, 1979

VITERI FE, ALVARADO J: The creatinine height index: Its use in the estimation of the degree of protein depletion and repletion in protein calorie malnourished children. Pediatrics 46:696, 1970

78
PROTEIN AND ENERGY UNDERNUTRITION

DANIEL RUDMAN
JULIA C. BLEIER

RELEVANCE TO CONTEMPORARY MEDICINE Protein-energy malnutrition was described in the 1930s by physicians in developing nations. The syndrome affects structure and function of every organ in the body. The causes, manifestations, and treatment have been intensively studied in African and Asian children, in whom the prevalence of the primary form of the disorder averages 25 percent. The secondary varieties of protein-energy deficiency are common within hospital populations in developed nations. Subacutely or chronically ill patients living longer under the protection of modern therapeutics but handicapped by anorexia, hypermetabolism, or malabsorption may rapidly develop protein-energy malnutrition.

DEFINITION AND ETIOLOGY Progressive loss of both lean body mass and adipose tissue results from insufficient consumption of protein and energy, although one or the other may play the dominant role in a given individual. The inadequate intake may be primary or secondary, as discussed in Chap. 77. Synergism between the two mechanisms is common. Patients with scanty reserves of protein and energy develop clinical protein-energy starvation more rapidly than well-nourished subjects when challenged by the hypermetabolism, catabolism, and anorexia of infection or other illnesses.

On a global basis the primary mechanism predominates. Socioeconomic factors that limit the quantity and quality of the diet are paramount. Particularly important is the poor biologic value of many vegetable proteins. The problem is accentuated if energy is inadequate because a large proportion of the dietary amino acids must then be oxidized as fuel instead of used to synthesize tissue and plasma protein. In developed countries, protein-energy malnutrition is often the result of inadequate nutrient intakes due to drug or alcohol abuse, depression and isolation in the aged, or anorexia, malabsorption, or hypermetabolism in the hospitalized patient.

EPIDEMIOLOGY The prevalence of protein-energy undernutrition can be assessed by measuring percent reduction from normal in midarm fat area, midarm muscle area, 24-h urinary creatinine/height ratio, and serum albumin (see Chap. 77). Estimates of prevalence of protein-energy depletion in various population groups are given in Table 78-1. In the United States, subclinical protein deficiency is more common in the south than in the north and in blacks and Latin Americans than in whites. In contrast to developing nations, protein-energy depletion in the general population of the United States tends to be mild and subclinical. In hospitals, on the other hand, severe as well as mild deficiencies are frequent, usually associated with other types of malnutrition.

PATHOPHYSIOLOGY Energy and protein deficiencies have been studied most extensively in children of developing nations in whom inadequate or marginal diets, the augmented nutritional requirements of growth, and frequent episodes of infectious disease combine to cause florid deficiency manifestations. Two syndromes have been distinguished: (1) marasmus, manifested by stunted growth, loss of adipose tissue, and generalized wasting of lean body mass without edema; and (2) kwashiorkor, manifested by growth failure (in children), hypoalbuminemia, edema, fatty liver, and preservation of adipose tissue. Mixed forms (kwashiorkor-marasmus) are common. Similar principles apply to protein-energy malnutrition in adults.

METABOLIC AND ENDOCRINE ASPECTS **Energy deficiency** When the intake of kilocalories falls below the daily requirement, the body responds with an orderly physiologic adaptation (see Chap. 85), engineered in large part by a reduced secretion of insulin, augmented plasma levels of glucagon and cortisol, and curtailed hepatic production of triiodothyronine (T_3) from thyroxine (T_4). The fall in plasma insulin permits free fatty acids and amino acids to be mobilized from adipose tissue and muscle to provide carbon for the continuing oxidative metabolism of the body. When energy balance is negative, oxidative metabolism claims first priority in the utilization of dietary protein. During starvation, the carbon chains of amino acids also provide substrate for gluconeogenesis, since a continuing supply of glucose is required by the central nervous system. As amino acids are diverted from protein synthesis into oxidative metabolism and gluconeogenesis, protein synthesis is curtailed, particularly in muscle. The metabolic rate gradually declines, because of diminished extrathyroidal conversion of T_4 to T_3, decreased synthesis of the T_3 receptor, curtailed production and turnover of catecholamines, and loss of

TABLE 78-1
Prevalence of protein-energy malnutrition in selected groups

Group	*Criterion of deficiency*	*Prevalence of deficiency, %*
Children <5 years, 28 developing countries*	Body weight <80% (kwashiorkor) or <60% of standard (marasmus)	25
Pediatric patients, Children's Hospital Medical Center, Boston†	Weight/height <90% of standard; midarm muscle area <15th percentile	37
Cancer patients, Emory University Hospital‡	Creatinine/height <60% std., triceps skin fold <80% std.	50
General surgical patients, Boston City Hospital¶	Midarm muscle circumference, triceps skin fold, serum albumin more than two standard deviations below normal mean	48

* *J Bengou, J Trop Pediatr 13:169, 1967.*
† *R Merritt, Am J Clin Nutr 32:1320, 1979.*
‡ *D Nixon, Am J Med 68:683, 1980.*
¶ *BR Bistrian et al, JAMA 230:858, 1974.*

the specific dynamic action of the dietary components. During partial or total deprivation of calories, both lean body mass and adipose tissue contract, but the latter does so more rapidly.

During the first week of total starvation, the average patient loses 4 to 5 kg of body weight which consists of about 25 percent adipose tissue, 35 percent extracellular fluid, and 40 percent protoplasm. Losses of nitrogen, potassium, sodium, and chloride represent 3 to 8 percent of the body content of each element. Negative balances of magnesium, phosphorus, and calcium are also considerable. During ensuing weeks, as further adaptive endocrine and enzymatic adjustments occur, losses of nitrogen and other elements continue but at a slower rate. The intracellular compartment does not contract at the same rate in all tissues. The central nervous system does not lose weight. Skeletal muscle atrophies more rapidly than cardiac muscle, while gastrointestinal tract and liver lose mass more rapidly than kidneys. Mobilization of amino acids from muscle to liver permits the latter to continue to synthesize some albumin and lipoproteins; as a consequence hypoalbuminemia and fatty liver are not conspicuous.

Protein deficiency Frequently the intake of protein is more limited than that of calories. This occurs because dietary protein is more expensive than carbohydrate or fat; because protein of high biologic value (chiefly animal) is more expensive than protein of low biologic value (chiefly vegetable); because high-calorie, low-protein foods (many snack foods, ethanol, starchy root-based vegetables) are in common use in the United States and abroad; and because physicians often use glucose as the sole organic nutrient in the intravenous feeding of the patient who cannot eat. The deficiency state under these conditions is analogous to kwashiorkor in children. The reduction of insulin secretion, which is a central mechanism in the adaptation to energy starvation, is circumvented. Insulin secreted in response to the dietary or intravenous carbohydrate promotes lipogenesis and retards lipolysis; adipose tissue is well preserved, and free fatty acids are not available for oxidation in place of amino acids. The high plasma insulin also impairs mobilization and redistribution of muscle amino acids from skeletal muscle to liver. Plasma amino acids fall, and the total body rate of protein synthesis declines. Fatty infiltration of the liver is common. Two biochemical mechanisms are probably involved: (1) lack of methionine limits phospholipid synthesis, secondarily impairing lipoprotein formation; and (2) hepatic synthesis of triglycerides from glucose continues. Decreased concentrations of plasma albumin, plasma transferrin, and hemoglobin reflect severe protein starvation. Edema is characteristic of this stage.

Variable degrees of energy and protein starvation occur together.

Mineral metabolism Protein-energy undernutrition is generally associated with depletion of body minerals. In part this reflects the contraction of protoplasmic and extracellular fluid compartments with their constituent elements (nitrogen, phosphorus, potassium, and magnesium within cells; sodium and chloride in extracellular fluid) being excreted into the urine in the same proportions as in the lean body mass. However, mineral losses are often out of proportion to the contraction of lean body mass. One reason is a shift of potassium and magnesium from muscle to plasma in exchange for sodium. In addition, potassium, magnesium, phosphorus, and calcium intakes may be even less adequate than those of protein and kilocalories (e.g., during prolonged intravenous nutrition with magnesium- or phosphorus-free solutions). A reduced synthesis of transport proteins may in part account for the increased loss. Finally, renal and extrarenal losses of these elements may be significant (diuresis, diarrhea, fistulas, etc.).

STRESSED VERSUS NONSTRESSED PROTEIN-ENERGY MALNUTRITION Simple starvation in an otherwise healthy individual, as described above, involves maintenance of glucose production at the expense of muscle tissue. Unchecked protein catabolism would quickly lead to death, but a gradual metabolic adaptation mitigates the effects: (1) the need for gluconeogenesis from amino acids is reduced as the central nervous system adapts to fatty acids as a fuel source, and (2) basal energy expenditure is reduced.

Protein-energy malnutrition resulting from a metabolic stress, such as trauma, burn, or infection, presents a somewhat different series of metabolic events. The need to repair tissues and/or synthesize immune function proteins places a high demand on the body for protein synthesis. Glucose requirements are also increased by sepsis and wound healing; polymorphonuclear leukocytes and fibroblasts rely on glucose as their energy source so that basal energy expenditure may be elevated as much as 100 percent. In the face of inadequate energy or protein consumption, the body catabolizes muscle at an accelerated rate. The loss of 1.5 to 2 kg protoplasm in the first week of simple starvation should be compared to the loss of 1.0 to 2.5 kg protoplasm per day under conditions of acute metabolic stress.

CARDIOVASCULAR-RESPIRATORY AND RENAL RESPONSES The heart and kidneys lose mass progressively during the course of protein-energy starvation. These losses are generally proportional to the erosion of lean body mass, so that ratios of heart mass/lean body mass and kidney mass/lean body mass remain normal. Consequently, functional insufficiency of these two shrunken organs is not a usual feature of protein-energy depletion. Cardiac output declines in parallel with the falling metabolic rate. Blood pressure is reduced by the fall in cardiac output. The ventilatory response to hypoxia is blunted. Glomerular filtration rate and renal blood flow are lowered. The ability of the kidney to excrete an acid load or to respond to antidiuretic hormone may be impaired. Although these changes in cardiac and renal structure and function are appropriate to the reduced lean body mass and hypometabolic state, they may become important handicaps during vigorous nutritional repletion, acute infection, or other circumstances that require rapid increases in cardiac output, metabolic rate, and urinary excretion of solutes. Heart failure and death have resulted from rapid repletion of severe protein-energy malnutrition.

BLOOD Reduced blood volume, hematocrit, albumin, transferrin, and total lymphocyte count are characteristic in the wasted patient. The anemia of "pure" protein-energy depletion is normocytic and normochromic and usually results from decreased production of red blood cells, perhaps reflecting the protein requirement for globin synthesis. Frequently deficiencies of iron, folate, or pyridoxine contribute to the anemia.

STRUCTURE AND FUNCTION OF GASTROINTESTINAL TRACT AND PANCREAS The gastrointestinal tract and pancreas atrophy. In the small intestine, villous height, mitotic index, and content of disaccharidases and dipeptidases all decline. Exocrine elements of the pancreas atrophy as well, and the production of digestive enzymes is reduced. Bacterial overgrowth may occur in the small intestine. These factors combine to produce malabsorption and lactose intolerance. The structural and functional regression of the small intestine results, at least in part, from decreased oral feeding rather than systemic malnutrition, since patients fully nourished by the parenteral route exhibit the same lesion.

IMMUNE SYSTEM Lymphatic tissues atrophy. Impaired cell-mediated immunity is evident by all standard tests (blastogenic response of lymphocytes to mitogens, total lymphocyte count, and skin testing with recall antigens). Bactericidal activity of polymorphonuclear leukocytes is decreased. Plasma immunoglobin concentrations and humoral responses to antigens are preserved. Protein-energy-starved patients experience increased morbidity and mortality during common infections compared with well-nourished groups and are subject to infection by opportunistic organisms (gram-negative bacteria, *Candida,* herpes simplex). Impaired respiratory function, leading to atelectasis and pneumonia, is a common cause of death.

WOUND HEALING The fibroblastic response to surgical wounds is impaired by protein-energy depletion. Consequently incisions and enteric anastomoses heal more slowly in undernourished patients; wound dehiscence is common.

TEMPERATURE REGULATION In severe protein-energy starvation in the absence of fever, basal metabolic rate is reduced. Hypothermia is common. The underlying mechanisms are reduced heat production due to exhaustion of carbohydrate and fat reserves, low plasma T_3, possible decreased adrenergic function, and loss of thermal insulation when subcutaneous adipose tissue is gone. Hypoglycemia is occasionally seen (see Chap. 116).

REPRODUCTION Nearly every phase of the reproductive process is impaired by protein deficiency in the mother. Fertility is reduced. If implantation occurs, there is a high risk of early fetal resorption. If gestation is completed, the progeny are substandard in weight and length. Lactation is impaired so that undernutrition is common postnatally. Even if postnatal nutrition is adequate, stunted growth in the infant is in part irreversible, and life-long impairment in learning capacity may result.

CLINICAL MANIFESTATIONS **History** A primary component in the etiology can be uncovered only by reviewing the intakes of protein and kilocalories and the biologic quality of the dietary protein during the months before the clinical examination. Suggestive of a secondary etiology are the presence of a known chronic medical problem, anorexia or other gastrointestinal symptoms (including lack of teeth), or prolonged fever.

In children, failure to gain height and weight is an early sign. In adults, weight loss usually occurs. However, in the adult a body weight equal to or greater than ideal does not rule out the presence of deficiency of kilocalories, protein, or both. Thus progressive loss of protoplasm and adipose tissue may be masked by accumulating edema; or the patient may have been previously obese, and a substantial loss of lean body mass during the current illness may be masked by a residue of obesity. Listlessness, easy fatigability, sensation of coldness, swollen ankles, and dry, cracked skin are frequent symptoms in patients eating insufficient protein or kilocalories.

Physical signs The facies is drawn, temporal regions are concave and fleshless, intercostal spaces are excavated, and the skin hangs in folds on the wasted extremities. "Flaky paint" dermatitis and dyspigmentation of skin and hair are common. The patient is pale and may be edematous. Signs of deficiency of water-soluble or fat-soluble vitamins may be present. Decubiti and skin ulcers are typical in advanced stages.

Vital signs Blood pressure is decreased. Pulse is slow and extremities are cool; central temperature may be decreased.

TABLE 78-2
Undesirable practices affecting the nutritional health of hospital patients

1 Failure to record height and weight on admission
2 Lack of a weight curve in the hospital chart
3 Prolonged use of glucose and saline intravenous feedings
4 Failure to measure patient's food intake
5 Withholding meals because of diagnostic tests
6 Use of tube feedings of inadequate amount and uncertain composition
7 Ignorance of the composition of nutritional products
8 Failure to recognize increased nutritional needs due to injury or illness
9 Delay of nutrition support until the patient is in an advanced state of depletion
10 Limited availability of laboratory tests to assess nutritional status; failure to use those that are available
11 Failure to correct inadequate dentition or the edentulous state

SOURCE: *After Butterworth.*

Anthropometrics Midarm fat area and midarm muscle area are reduced in varying ratios dependent on previous nutritional state and relative severity of the energy and protein deficiencies.

Laboratory and x-ray findings The ratio of 24-h urinary creatinine/height is decreased. In the absence of renal disease, this is the most sensitive and practical clinical indicator of protein starvation and should be monitored at weekly intervals in the chronically ill hospital patient. These analyses should be done only in afebrile patients, since urinary excretion of creatinine is increased by fever. Other signs include decrease in serum albumin, serum transferrin, and hematocrit, but these changes are less specific. Nevertheless, protein depletion may be the most common cause of hypoalbuminemia in hospitalized patients, even in patients with hepatic disease. Serum essential and nonessential amino acid concentration and urine urea and creatinine levels are reduced. T-lymphocyte cell function is decreased, as revealed by cutaneous anergy and peripheral lymphopenia (absolute lymphocyte count < 1200 cells per cubic millimeter). Glucose tolerance is impaired. Plasma cortisol is often increased (in part because of retarded metabolic clearance). T_3 is decreased, reverse T_3 may be increased, and basal metabolic rate is low. Heart size is small on chest film. Echocardiography shows a small heart with decreased cardiac output. Sagittal or cross-sectional x-rays of arm show diminished muscle mass.

FIGURE 78-1
Course of a typical case of progressive protein-energy starvation.

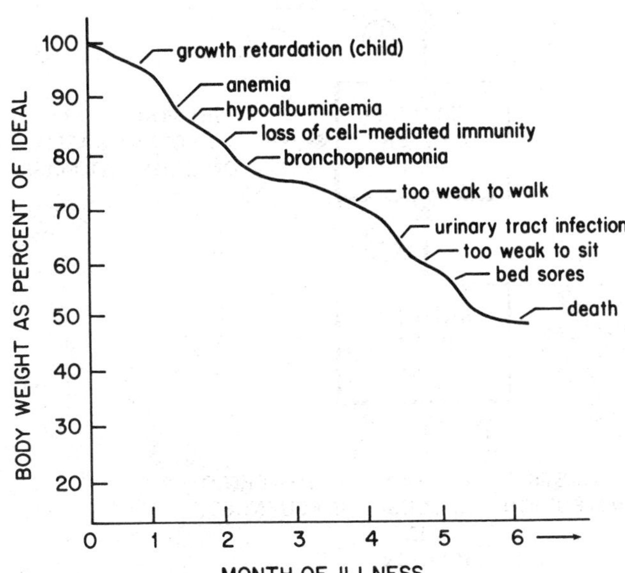

Course A typical case is illustrated in Fig. 78-1. In children, an early manifestation is slowing of growth. As the protein-energy depletion becomes more severe, pallor, fatigue, and amenorrhea appear. Loss of cell-mediated immunity predisposes to infections. The hypermetabolism and anorexia of intercurrent infection accelerate the progress of cachexia. In advanced undernutrition (midarm fat area < 2 cm^2, creatinine/height ratio < 60 percent of standard), decubiti, hypothermia, and terminal infection are the rule.

Relation to other deficiency states Usually other nutrients are also depleted. Folic acid, thiamine, riboflavin, nicotinic acid, pyridoxine, ascorbic acid, and vitamin A deficiencies are relatively common in hospital populations in the United States (see Table 78-2). Body content of most minerals is also reduced, but a distinction must be made between absolute and relative decreases. As protoplasmic protein is consumed to supply metabolic fuel and substrate for gluconeogenesis in the underfed patient, the intracellular minerals potassium, phosphorus, and magnesium and some of the microminerals are excreted in parallel with the nitrogen. Such loss is absolute but not relative, since the intracellular and extracellular concentrations of potassium, phosphorus, and magnesium usually remain normal. If the diet is specifically deficient in potassium, phosphorus, or magnesium, a further deficiency occurs with the intracellular and perhaps the extracellular and urinary concentrations becoming subnormal. Similar considerations apply to the body content of essential fatty acids. Whether the depletion of potassium, phosphorus, magnesium, or essential fatty acids is absolute or relative, repletion with a feeding solution that contains little or none of that nutrient may lead to chemical and clinical manifestations of the corresponding deficiency state within a few days. Life-threatening hypokalemia, hypophosphatemia, or hypomagnesemia can occur. By similar mechanisms, plasma levels of trace minerals regularly decline during hyperalimentation if adequate rations of these nutrients are not provided.

REFERENCES

ALLEYNE GAO et al: *Protein-Energy Malnutrition.* London, Butler & Tanner, 1977

BISTRIAN BR et al: Protein status of general surgical patients. JAMA 230:858, 1974

——— et al: Prevalence of malnutrition in general medical patients. JAMA 235:1567, 1976

BUTTERWORTH CE: The skeleton in the hospital closet. Nutr Today 9:4, 1974

———, Blackburn GL: Hospital malnutrition and how to assess the nutritional status of a patient. Nutr Today 10:8, 1975

CAHILL GF: Starvation in man. N Engl J Med 282:668, 1970

CUTHBERTSON D: Alterations in metabolism following injury: Part I. Injury 11:175, 1980

———: Alterations in metabolism following injury: Part II. Injury 11:286, 1980

LAW DK et al: Immunocompetence of patients with protein-calorie malnutrition. Ann Intern Med 79:545, 1973

LEEVY CM et al: Incidence and significance of hypovitaminemia in a randomly selected municipal hospital population. Am J Clin Nutr 17:259, 1965

STEFFEE W: Malnutrition in hospitalized patients. JAMA 244:2630, 1980

Symposium on Protein-Energy Malnutrition. Proc Nutr Soc 38:1 1979

Ten-State Nutrition Survey, 1968–1970. US Department of Health, Education and Welfare Publication (HSM) 72-8131, 1972

79 OBESITY

JERROLD M. OLEFSKY

The ability to store food energy as fat has provided significant survival value to organisms living in environments in which food supply is scarce or sporadic. Unlike glycogen or protein, triglyceride does not require water or electrolytes for storage purposes and can be retained essentially as pure fat; 1 g adipose tissue yields close to the full theoretical equivalent of 9 kcal. Because of the efficient storage of energy in adipose tissue, an individual of normal weight can survive up to 2 months of total starvation. However, western society is generally not characterized by periodic or insufficient food supply but rather by constant and abundant food. As a consequence, the ability to store fat all too frequently is of negative survival value because of overconsumption and the resulting obesity.

DEFINITION AND INCIDENCE Obesity can most easily be assessed using a subject's height and weight. One way to do this is to relate the patient's weight to an average range for his or her height and age. This measure of relative weight leads to an underestimation of the frequency of obesity, however, since in the United States the "average" individual is somewhat obese. Tables of ideal or desirable weight provide more meaningful information and are based on actuarial estimates of what is consistent with normal life expectancy. Such tables are more useful if adjusted for differences in body build. Although relative weight correlates fairly well with the degree of adiposity, excess poundage can be either lean or fat tissue. Obviously, with this measurement, heavily muscled individuals would be considered obese. More precise measurements of obesity are based on measurements of body density or isotopic dilution methods, but these are too complicated for routine clinical use. Anthropometry is a simpler method for assessing the degree of adiposity. Skin-fold thickness can be measured over various areas of the body and along with height, weight, and age can be used to assess the degree of adiposity. Triceps and subscapular skin folds are most commonly employed (see Chap. 77).

The term *obesity* implies an excess of adipose tissue, but the meaning of excess is hard to define. Aesthetic considerations aside, the clinical diagnosis of obesity can best be viewed as any degree of excess adiposity that imparts a health risk. This cutoff between normal and obese can only be approximated. The Framingham Study demonstrated that a 20 percent excess over ideal weight imparted a health risk; by use of that criterion 20 to 30 percent of men and 30 to 40 percent of women are obese.

ETIOLOGY When caloric intake exceeds expenditure the excess calories are stored in adipose tissue, and if this net positive caloric balance is prolonged, obesity results. Obviously, there are two components to weight balance, and an abnormality on either side (intake or expenditure) can lead to obesity.

The regulation of eating behavior is incompletely understood. To some extent, appetite is controlled by discrete areas in the hypothalamus: a feeding center in the ventrolateral nucleus of the hypothalamus (VLH) and a satiety center in the ventromedial hypothalamus (VMH). The cerebral cortex receives positive signals from the feeding center that stimulate eating (Fig. 79-1), and the satiety center modulates this process by sending inhibitory impulses to the feeding center. In animals destruction of the feeding center results in decreased food intake, and destruction of the satiety center leads to overeating and gross obesity. Several regulatory processes have been proposed as modulators of these hypothalamic centers. The satiety center may be activated by the surges in plasma glucose and/or insulin that follow a meal. It is of interest in this regard that the VMH contains insulin receptors and is insulin-sensitive. Meal-induced gastric distention is another possible inhibitory factor. The total adipose tissue mass may also influence the activity of the hypothalamic centers; i.e., there is a relatively fixed "set point" for the body's degree of adiposity. An elevated set point may account for the frequent recidivism in obese patients who have lost weight. How the "set point" is established and the mechanism by which the hypothalamus senses total fat stores are unknown. Glycerol release from fat cells and ascending neural impulses may be signals of adipose tissue size. Additionally, the hypothalamic centers are sensitive to catecholamines, and beta-adrenergic stimulation inhibits eating behavior. This provides at least one rationale for the anorexiant effects of amphetamines.

Ultimately, the cerebral cortex controls eating behavior, and impulses from the feeding center to the cerebral cortex are only one input. Psychological, social, and genetic factors also influence food intake. In many obese subjects these influences are overriding; indeed, obese patients usually respond to external signals such as time of day, social setting, and smell or taste of food to a greater extent than do normal persons.

Although overeating is the cause of obesity in most individuals, other factors may participate. Daily caloric needs range between 31 and 35 kcal per kilogram of body weight; this figure is somewhat higher in active and somewhat lower in sedentary individuals. Physical activity clearly modulates overall caloric balance, and obese individuals tend to be less active than normal subjects. This can be a contributory factor in the maintenance of excess weight, but decreased physical activity is unlikely to be important as a cause of major weight gain in the most obese subjects. Rather, obesity itself leads to inactivity. The modest increase in weight that often accompanies the mid-

FIGURE 79-1
The regulation of eating. The ventromedial satiety center is considered to be inhibitory, and the ventrolateral feeding center stimulatory. See text for discussion.

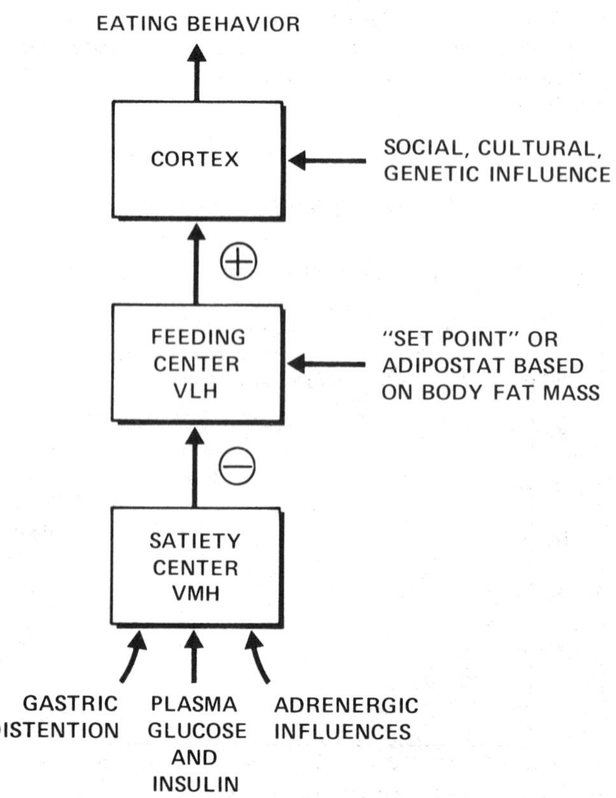

dle years may be related more directly to diminished physical activity. Injury or illness may lead to chronic restricted activity and predispose to weight gain unless caloric intake is appropriately curtailed. Perhaps the greatest factor tending to diminish the output side of the equation is simply sedentary life-style.

Decreased caloric expenditure and overefficient caloric utilization due to metabolic abnormality have also been postulated to be involved in the pathogenesis of obesity. With rare exceptions major metabolic abnormalities have not been detected in obese individuals, although more subtle defects may exist. Work performance, or calories expended per standard physical work load, can be normal or increased in obesity depending on the kind of work performed. Exercise energy expenditure is increased during weight bearing in obese compared to lean subjects due to the extra effort involved in moving or supporting an increased body mass. When this effect of increased body mass is taken into account, work performance is normal in obesity. Clearly, normal or increased caloric expenditure during physical work cannot contribute to the development of obesity.

Resting metabolic rate accounts for 60 to 75 percent of daily caloric expenditure and is measured in a thermoneutral environment while the subject is at rest following an overnight fast, several hours after any significant physical activity. Resting metabolic rate should be expressed as a function of fat-free body weight (by subtracting the subject's total adipose mass from body weight), since triglyceride mass, which is considerable in obese subjects, is metabolically inert. When expressed in this way, resting metabolic rate is normal in the usual obese subject. However, a distinction must be made between static obesity and the actual process of gaining weight. When normal subjects consume hypercaloric diets, less weight is gained than would be predicted on the basis of the excess calories ingested. This effect is most marked when carbohydrate is consumed and disappears when the excess calories consist of fat. Thus, humans can apparently partially adapt to chronic excessive carbohydrate and protein intake, and this protective effect attenuates the weight gain. Part of this adaptive response is related to an increase in thermogenesis manifested as an increase in resting metabolic rate. The mechanism of adaptive thermogenesis is unknown, but overeating of carbohydrate or mixed nutrients leads to increased plasma levels of triiodothyronine (T_3) and decreased levels of reverse T_3 (rT_3). A converse effect is seen in starvation with decreased T_3 and increased rT_3 levels. The conversion of thyroxine to T_3 occurs largely in the liver; excess food may induce adaptive thermogenesis by increasing the concentration of T_3 relative to that of T_4 and rT_3. Increased central or peripheral sympathetic outflow leading to increased catecholamine-induced caloric utilization and heat production may also play a role in the thermogenic response to overnutrition. Adaptive thermogenesis can lead to a 10 to 15 percent increase in resting metabolic rate, and this effect is seen after a 2- to 3-week period of hypercaloric intake. However, the rate of onset and the degree of adaptive thermogenesis is the same in obese and nonobese individuals when expressed on the basis of fat-free body mass. Specifically, the increase in resting metabolic rate, changes in thyroid hormone metabolism, and thermic responses to infused catecholamines are all the same in normal and obese subjects during periods of overnutrition.

Another important aspect of caloric balance is the thermic response to food. This consists of the heat, or energy, expended in the assimilation and metabolism of foodstuffs during the postprandial period. The amount of heat produced following nutrient ingestion is a form of caloric expenditure and is greater for protein and less for carbohydrate and fat. The thermic response to mixed meals can equal 10 to 15 percent of the calories ingested, and decreased thermic responses have been documented in human obesity. This difference may be due to altered flux rates through different pathways of intermediary metabolism, with more energy-efficient pathways such as those leading to caloric storage being favored in obesity. Obviously, small differences in caloric utilization maintained over years can lead to a substantial net positive caloric balance. However, although it is attractive to postulate that this decreased thermic response to food is a cause of obesity in some individuals, it should be noted that the comparisons have always been made between normal persons and subjects who are already obese. Thus, the obesity-associated changes in thermic response to food may be secondary to the obese state rather than a primary abnormality.

Still another potential regulatory process in the control of adipose tissue mass and obesity involves the enzyme lipoprotein lipase. This enzyme is present in fat, muscle, and liver, but it is the adipose tissue lipoprotein lipase (ATLPL) that is of special interest regarding obesity. This enzyme is synthesized within adipocytes and is secreted into the extracellular space where it eventually localizes on the lumenal surface of nearby endothelial cells. At this location ATLPL hydrolyzes fatty acids from the triglycerides of circulating triglyceride-rich lipoproteins. The released fatty acids are taken up locally by adipocytes where they are converted to triglycerides and stored. Thus, ATLPL provides a mechanism for the storage of excess fat calories in adipose tissue. The *lipoprotein lipase hypothesis* holds that in some obese states excessive levels of this enzyme lead to preferential deposition of fat calories into adipose tissue inducing obesity. In support of this hypothesis, ATLPL levels are increased in obese rodents and humans. Perhaps more importantly, levels of this enzyme do not return to normal following weight reduction. This latter finding is of particular interest since it represents one of the few characteristics of the obese state that is not corrected by weight reduction and may help explain the propensity obese patients have to regain their lost weight.

Certain animal models of obesity have clear-cut genetic causes, but the role of genetic influences in most instances of human obesity is difficult to evaluate because of confounding social and cultural factors.

SECONDARY OBESITY **Hypothyroidism** Obesity can result from hypothyroidism because of decreased caloric needs. However, only a minority of hypothyroid patients are truly obese, and an even smaller proportion of obese patients are hypothyroid. Indiscriminate use of thyroid hormone replacement in the treatment of obesity is to be deplored and should never be instituted without careful documentation of decreased thyroid function.

Cushing's disease Cushing's disease is a rare cause of obesity. Hyperadrenocorticism elicits a typical pattern of obesity with predominantly centripetal fat stores, characteristic rounded or moon facies, and cervical or supraclavicular fat deposits.

Insulinoma Hyperinsulinemia, secondary to an insulinoma, can occasionally cause obesity, presumably because of increased caloric intake secondary to recurrent hypoglycemia. Most patients with islet-cell tumors and hypoglycemia are not obese.

Hypothalamic disorders Froehlich's syndrome is characterized by obesity and hypogonadotrophic hypogonadism in boys with other variable features such as diabetes insipidus, visual impairment, and mental retardation. The anterior pituitary is usually normal, and the syndrome is thought to be the result of hypothalamic dysfunction. Occasionally pituitary tumors are present (as in Froehlich's original case) which may physically impair the hypothalamus. Most likely this syndrome includes a number of overlapping disorders having in common a hypothalamic lesion that leads to overeating and to hypogonadotrophism.

Other rare diseases include the Laurence-Moon-Biedl syndrome characterized by retinitis pigmentosa, mental retardation, skull deformities, polydactyly and syndactyly, and the Prader-Willi syndrome which is associated with hypotonia, mental retardation, and a predilection for diabetes mellitus. Both of these disorders also feature obesity and hypogonadism that are thought to be hypothalamic in origin.

PATHOLOGICAL SEQUELAE Increased adipose tissue stores are deposited subcutaneously, around all internal organs, throughout the omentum, and in the intramuscular spaces. Obese individuals also have an expansion of lean body mass as evidenced by increased size of the kidneys, heart, liver, and skeletal muscle mass. Fatty livers are common in extreme obesity.

Adipocyte size and number Attempts have been made to classify obese individuals on the basis of the relative degree of adipocyte hypertrophy versus hyperplasia. This classification scheme was generated as the result of experimental data indicating that in several rodent species and in humans the capacity to increase adipocyte number exists for only a limited period in early life and perhaps at the time of puberty. Thus, sometime prior to reaching adulthood, the ability to increase the number of adipocytes declines, and after this time expansion of adipose tissue mass is accompanied primarily by an increase in fat-cell size. Individuals with severe obesity have both increased adipocyte size and number, and those individuals with the greatest degree of adipocyte hyperplasia have a strong tendency toward onset of obesity early in life. Patients having mild to moderate obesity show predominantly adipocyte hypertrophy, and the onset is usually during adult life. Weight reduction leads to a decrease in adipocyte size with no change in cell number. The above observations led to the concept of the existence of a "critical period" in early life when final adipocyte number is determined and after which cell number cannot be changed. The main implication of this formulation is that alterations in adipocyte number can only be induced during this critical period. However, the concept of a strictly defined critical period for hyperplasia of the adipocytes may need to be reconsidered. When severe obesity is induced in adult rats, both adipocyte number and cell size increase. Adipocyte hypercellularity has also been documented in some patients with adult-onset obesity.

Thus, substantial overnutrition at any stage of life can probably lead to hypertrophy of individual existing adipocytes. It is also probable that there are periods during childhood and adolescence when overnutrition has an enhanced ability to induce the development of new adipocytes. Furthermore, even in adult life, if the degree of overnutrition is great enough so as to induce existing adipocytes to enlarge up to some limiting size, then the appearance of new adipocytes will occur. Whether this latter population of cells represents new cell formation or simply lipid filling of previously undetectable preadipocytes formed earlier in life cannot be determined at present. Regardless of the cause or time of development of increased adiposity (adipocyte hypertrophy with or without hyperplasia), subsequent weight reduction only leads to a decrease in the size of existing adipocytes and not a decrease in adipocyte number. Thus, once a given complement of adipocytes is attained, this number is fixed and cannot be reduced.

METABOLIC SEQUELAE Obesity has a profound impact on diabetes mellitus and various hyperlipoproteinemias primarily through its influences on insulin secretion and insulin sensitivity (see Chaps. 103 and 114).

Hyperinsulinemia: Insuiin resistance Increased insulin secretion is a well-characterized feature of obesity. It occurs in the basal state and in response to a wide variety of insulinogenic agents. A correlation exists between the degree of obesity and the magnitude of the hyperinsulinemia—particularly the basal insulin levels. Some obese patients exhibit hyperglycemia or frank diabetes in the face of hyperinsulinemia. The combination of hyper- or euglycemia and hyperinsulinemia indicates an insulin-resistant state, and decreased hypoglycemic responses to insulin are common in obese humans and animals. Insulin resistance could be due to an abnormal beta-cell product, circulating insulin antagonists, or tissue insulin insensitivity. Since abnormal islet secretory products or circulating antagonists have not been identified, it is thought that the insulin resistance of obesity is primarily due to tissue insensitivity. The initial step in the cellular action of insulin involves binding to specific cell surface receptors located in target tissues. After the formation of the plasma membrane–insulin receptor complex, insulin's biological effects are initiated. Cells from obese animals and humans contain decreased numbers of insulin receptors, and this decrease in insulin receptors doubtless plays a role in the insulin resistance of obesity. However, other factors participate. The enlarged adipocytes of obese rats have a decrease in insulin receptors but an even greater defect in the capacity to metabolize glucose, suggesting a major biochemical abnormality distal to the receptor mechanism. Since adipose tissue accounts for only a small ($<$ 5 percent) portion of total body glucose metabolism, a similar postreceptor defect presumably exists in other major insulin target tissues such as muscle and liver. In the obese human insulin resistance is due to a combination of receptor and postreceptor defects in insulin action. In those obese patients with the mildest degree of hyperinsulinemia and insulin resistance, the decrease in insulin action is predominantly due to a decreased number of insulin receptors. As the hyperinsulinemic, insulin-resistant state worsens, a postreceptor defect emerges, and in those obese patients with the most severe degree of insulin resistance, the postreceptor defect is the predominant abnormality.

Diabetes mellitus Although only a minority of obese patients are diabetic, the converse is not the case. Nonketotic, insulin-independent patients compose about 90 percent of the diabetic population in the United States, and 80 to 90 percent of nonketotic diabetics are obese. Obesity is an important contributory factor in these patients, predominantly through its influences on insulin sensitivity. Obesity exacerbates the diabetic state, and in many cases diabetes can be ameliorated by weight reduction.

Hyperlipoproteinemia (see also Chap. 103) Most plasma cholesterol circulates in the low-density lipoprotein (LDL) fraction, and, in the fasting state, very low density lipoproteins (VLDL) contain most of the circulating triglyceride. The association between obesity and elevated LDL levels is modest at best, and this is especially true when the relationship is corrected for other factors such as age. Total body cholesterol is increased in obesity, but this is mainly accounted for by adipose tissue cholesterol stores. Cholesterol turnover may be increased in obesity, leading to increased biliary excretion of cholesterol. This may contribute to the increased incidence of gallstone formation in obese individuals. Obesity has a more clear-cut and pronounced effect on VLDL metabolism. Hypertriglyceridemia is frequent, and the degree of obesity correlates with the level of hypertriglyceridemia. The increased triglyceride levels are due to increased hepatic VLDL production with no defect in the removal of VLDL from plasma. As discussed above, plasma insulin levels are greatly elevated in obesity, particularly in the portal blood. Hyperinsulinemia can promote increased hepatic VLDL synthesis and secretion. In addition, increased plasma free fatty acid (FFA) turnover exists in obesity, and FFA extracted by the liver provides an important precursor for hepatic triglyceride synthesis. Thus, the hypertriglyceridemia in obesity may be secondary to increased hepatic VLDL secretion due to hyperinsulinemia and augmented FFA availability.

MANIFESTATIONS AND COMPLICATIONS Gross obesity produces mechanical and physical stresses that aggravate or directly cause a number of disorders including osteoarthritis (especially the hips) and sciatica. Additionally, varicose veins, thromboembolism, ventral and hiatal hernias, and cholelithiasis are more common than in individuals of normal weight.

Hypertension In significantly obese persons, use of the standard size blood pressure cuff leads to readings which are erroneously high; an oversize cuff should always be used. A strong association between hypertension and obesity is observed even when accurate measurements are obtained. The mechanisms whereby obesity causes hypertension are uncertain, but peripheral vascular resistance is usually normal, while blood volume is increased. Weight loss leads to significant reductions in systemic blood pressure independent of changes in sodium balance.

Hypoventilation syndrome (Pickwickian syndrome) The obesity-hypoventilation syndrome is a heterogeneous group of disorders with differing clinical manifestations. The hypersomnolence that can occur in obesity is a manifestation of nighttime sleep apnea. In these individuals, once sleep begins, upper airway obstruction leads to hypoxemia and hypercapnia, causing arousal with return of normal respiration. Many such episodes occur each night, leading to chronic sleep deprivation and daytime somnolence. The combination of the obese habitus plus sleep-induced relaxation of the pharyngeal musculature is believed to be the cause of the intermittent upper airway obstruction. Occasionally such episodes are life-threatening (causing serious cardiac arrhythmias) and require long-term tracheostomy therapy. Chronic daytime hypoventilation is common but usually is not as severe as that occurring during sleep. Abnormalities of the respiratory control centers may also be important. Patients with hypoventilation display blunted ventilatory responses to hypercapnia and hypoxia and often develop hypercapnia and hypoxemia due to decreased basal ventilation; in addition, ventilation/perfusion mismatch due to mechanical factors may be present. In severe cases polycythemia, pulmonary hypertension, and cor pulmonale can result. Weight reduction will reverse these abnormalities if instituted before permanent cardiac damage develops. Some obese patients with sleep apnea and hypersomnolence do not have daytime hypoventilation and have normal ventilatory responses to hypoxia and hypercapnia. Progestational agents have been used therapeutically in the obesity-hypoventilation syndrome since they stimulate the ventilatory response to hypercarbia and hypoxia in normal subjects. Medroxyprogesterone increases ventilation and improves heart failure and erythrocytosis in these patients, although obstructive sleep apnea continues.

Adrenal function Although Cushing's disease can usually be distinguished from simple obesity on purely clinical grounds, laboratory testing is occasionally necessary. This can lead to confusion since 24-h urinary 17-hydroxycorticoid excretion is often elevated in obesity. Less commonly, plasma cortisol levels are also increased. Corticosteroid levels are usually suppressible with dexamethasone in obesity, but occasionally suppression is incomplete, rendering the diagnosis difficult (also see Chap. 112).

Growth hormone Secretory responses of growth hormone to a variety of stimuli such as hypoglycemia, exercise, and arginine infusion are reduced. Furthermore, the starvation-induced rise in plasma growth hormone levels is attenuated.

Atherosclerosis Obesity is a serious risk factor for the development of coronary artery disease and stroke. Most of the risk imparted by obesity is mediated through the associated hypertension, hyperlipoproteinemia, and diabetes. Nevertheless, even when these abnormalities are factored out, a residual, albeit much smaller, risk can be ascribed to obesity per se.

TREATMENT Amelioration of hyperinsulinemia, insulin resistance, diabetes, hypertension, and hyperlipidemia can occur following weight loss. These changes are significant and enduring provided the weight loss is maintained. During weight loss all adipose tissue depots diminish proportionately. Sometimes this generalized loss does not produce the attractive cosmetic effects desired. Many techniques, exercises, and other maneuvers have been proposed to effect selective adipose tissue reduction over particular regions of the body, but none is effective.

Methods of weight reduction In cases where obesity is secondary, the appropriate therapy is to treat the underlying disease. Most of the time the difficult problem of primary weight reduction must be undertaken.

Diet Caloric restriction is the cornerstone of any weight reduction program. From both the patient's and the physician's standpoint this is a frustrating and demanding undertaking. The basic principles of caloric restriction are simple. If caloric intake is less than caloric expenditure, stored calories, predominantly in the form of fat, will be consumed. In general, a deficit of 7700 kcal leads to loss of about 1 kg fat. By estimating the patient's daily caloric needs (approximately 33 kcal/kg), one can calculate the daily deficit necessary to achieve a given rate of weight loss.

Dietary restriction can range from total starvation to mild caloric deprivation, and these approaches will be discussed separately. Dietary recommendations are most effective when they are specific and geared to the patient's life-style. A dietitian or a similarly trained health professional should interview each patient and estimate his average daily caloric intake, food preferences, and eating patterns. The amount of calories the patient is to consume on the restricted diet should then be carefully explained in terms of quantities of specific foodstuffs. Frequently, the therapist must balance the degree of restriction against potential patient noncompliance. The more restrictive the diet, the more rapid the weight loss, but this often leads to a greater rate of nonadherence. It is preferable to design a diet with which the patient is happy and comfortable and that produces a modest but steady weight loss.

The process of weight reduction has become a multimillion dollar business in the United States, and there are almost as many diets as there are therapists. Each proponent claims that the presence or absence of certain foodstuffs is desirable for more effective weight loss. However, little evidence exists to support the claim that calorie for calorie one hypocaloric diet will lead to a greater weight loss than another. The relationship between the patient and the therapist, plus patient education and encouragement, are more important to success than are the specific dietary constituents. The major virtue of "fad" diets is that patients are usually motivated to try them, at least initially, and patient cooperation is often better. Provided a particular diet is not harmful, probably the best course for the therapist is to maintain flexibility in the treatment program. Nevertheless, diets markedly deficient in any major class of foodstuff are to be avoided. For example, whole-food diets that are exceedingly low in carbohydrate are by nature high in fat and, depending on the type and quantity of fat ingested, may lead to hypercholesterolemia. The major virtue of a low-carbohydrate diet is the attendant increase in ketosis. (Ketone bodies have a central anorexiant effect.) This provides part of the rationale for the widely touted liquid or powdered protein diets. These diets have been dubbed "protein-sparing modified fasts," and claims have been made that they allow drastic long-term caloric restriction without inducing negative nitrogen balance. These claims have not been substantiated, nor has it been shown that the diets lead to a greater degree of tissue weight loss than mixed hypocaloric diets of equal caloric value. Furthermore, a number of deaths have been reported in otherwise healthy individuals participating in such long-term dietary programs, even under medical supervision. Consequently, caution is required when treating obese patients with these approaches. Basically a calorie is a calorie whether it comes from protein, carbohydrate, or fat.

Prior to therapy it is wise to forewarn patients that when caloric restriction is started there is usually a marked initial weight loss, in large part due to fluid loss. The patient should be told that such rapid rates of loss will not persist. Likewise, positive shifts in fluid balance can sometimes mask real loss of adipose mass, a fact that can sometimes be demonstrated to the patient's satisfaction by keeping a record of skin-fold thickness at monthly intervals.

Total-starvation diets have been advocated for the treatment of obesity; provided underlying diseases such as gout, renal insufficiency, and ketosis-prone diabetes are not present, short-term fasts are usually well tolerated. Ketonemia and hyperuricemia regularly develop during starvation but rarely lead to acidosis or gout. Because of these potential complications, total fasting should be carried out only under medical supervision. Probably the major usefulness of total fasting is as a motivational aid at the beginning of a dietary program or when weight loss has stopped. Even though much of the weight loss during short-term fasting represents fluid, this weight loss can be encouraging to frustrated patients and motivate them to increase their compliance with the long-term weight reduction program.

The major problem in the treatment of obesity is not weight reduction but maintenance of the reduced weight. Provided the therapist works hard and long enough, most motivated patients can eventually lose weight. Unfortunately, only the rare patient maintains the weight loss permanently. Obesity is an eating disorder, and the underlying mechanisms are not reversed by limiting food intake.

Behavior modification In recognition of the problems involved, the techniques of behavior modification are being used increasingly to treat abnormal patterns of eating behavior. Many studies demonstrate that obese individuals respond less well than normal individuals to internal cues which regulate eating behavior such as gastric contractions, fear, and previous food ingestion. Conversely, obese subjects overrespond to external cues such as taste, smell, food attractiveness, abundance, and the amount of work involved in obtaining food. Given the fact that the obese individual is unusually susceptible to external stimuli, food intake may be altered by changing the pattern and nature of these external cues, and this is the major premise underlying the behavior modification approach to weight reduction.

Behavior modification begins with a detailed individual history of the patient's eating episodes with respect to time of day, length of eating period, place of ingestion (restaurant, dining table, standing in front of open refrigerator), simultaneous activities (watching television, reading, idleness), emotional state, companions (relatives, friends, or alone), and finally the kinds and quantities of foods ingested. Once this detailed record is obtained, the therapist and patient can design specific behavioral changes aimed at disrupting or aborting recurring behavior patterns which initiate or prolong abnormal eating activity. As examples: if a patient eats in response to certain emotional states, then other activities can be consciously substituted when the patient perceives such a state; if the patient snacks frequently from readily available food storage areas (refrigerators, cookie jars, etc.), then he or she is encouraged to eat only while sitting down at a table with a fixed place setting; if eating frequently occurs while watching television alone, then efforts to avoid this activity can be initiated. Obviously, many other examples of specific and general interventions could be given. Results with behavior modification techniques have been encouraging and indicate that many patients can maintain long-term weight reduction providing the new behavior patterns are truly "learned."

Exercise In any weight reduction program exercise has its place. However, the importance of exercise in terms of caloric balance must be clearly understood. Table 79-1 shows that even moderate daily exercise would not lead to a large enough increase in caloric expenditure to alter significantly the initial rate of weight reduction. This does not mean exercise is unimportant in weight reduction, since even modest increases in caloric expenditure can lead to large long-term differences in caloric balance, provided exercise is performed on a regular basis. For example, a daily increase in caloric expenditure of 300 kcal over a period of 4 months could lead to a 4.5-kg weight loss. More importantly, there is evidence that incorporation of regular exercise into the overall weight reduction program improves the chances that the patient will maintain the weight loss.

Drugs Two classes of drugs are frequently used in the treatment of obesity: anorexiants and thyroid hormone supplements. The addition of L-thyroxine or triiodothyronine to a weight reduction program is of no benefit. These drugs are ineffective in promoting adipose tissue loss and, if anything, accentuate lean tissue loss causing negative nitrogen balance. In susceptible individuals, cardiotoxicity may occur. Thus, unless clear-cut hypothyroidism is present, thyroid supplementation has no role in the treatment of obesity.

The major anorexiants are amphetamine-like agents, and these drugs presumably exert their effect at the level of the hypothalamus. It is probable that they have a modest effect in promoting short-term weight loss in certain individuals. However, they are effective for a period of only a few weeks, and problems of habituation, addiction, and generalized drug abuse limit their usefulness. Two newer anorexiants, diethylpropion and fenfluramine, may be less addictive and, therefore, somewhat more useful. However, none of these agents treats the underlying eating disorder, and they are, therefore, of little use in maintenance of weight reduction.

Injections of human chorionic gonadotropin (HCG) have been popularized as an adjunct to weight reduction, but no evidence exists to indicate a beneficial effect. The primary effectiveness of the HCG-diet program is due to the calorically restricted diet, frequent physician contact, and placebo effects.

TABLE 79-1
Energy equivalents of food calories expressed in minutes of activity

Food	Calories, kcal	Activity: Walking*	Riding bicycle†	Swimming‡	Running§	Reclining¶
Apple, large	101	19	12	9	5	78
Bacon, 2 strips	96	18	12	9	5	74
Beer, 1 glass	114	22	14	10	6	88
Bread and butter	78	15	10	7	4	60
Carbonated beverage, 1 glass	106	20	13	9	5	82
Carrot, raw	42	8	5	4	2	32
Cheese, cottage, 1 tbsp	27	5	3	2	1	21
Chicken, fried, ½ breast	232	45	28	21	12	178
Cookie, chocolate chip	51	10	6	5	3	39
Egg, fried	110	21	13	10	6	85
Ham, 2 slices	167	32	20	15	9	128
Ice cream, ⅙ qt	193	37	24	17	10	148
Mayonnaise, 1 tbsp	92	18	11	8	5	71
Milk, skim, 1 glass	81	16	10	7	4	62
Milk shake	421	81	51	38	22	324
Orange, medium	68	13	8	6	4	52
Pancake with syrup	124	24	15	11	6	95
Peas, green, ½ cup	56	11	7	5	3	43
Pizza, cheese, ⅛	180	35	22	16	9	138
Potato chips, 1 serving	108	21	13	10	6	83
Sandwiches:						
Hamburger	350	67	43	31	18	269
Tuna fish salad	278	53	34	25	14	214
Sherbet, ⅙ qt	177	34	22	16	9	136

* *Energy cost of walking for 70-kg individual = 5.2 kcal/min at 3.5 mi/h.*
† *Energy cost of riding bicycle = 8.2 kcal/min.*
‡ *Energy cost of swimming = 11.2 kcal/min.*
§ *Energy cost of running = 19.4 kcal/min.*
¶ *Energy cost of reclining = 1.3 kcal/min.*

Comparable weight loss is achieved if saline injections are substituted for HCG, suggesting a placebo or physiological effect of the act of parenteral injection.

Jejunoileal shunt Small-bowel bypass is an effective means of achieving weight reduction in morbidly obese patients. However, it is an experimental procedure and should be attempted only in institutions where a trained team is committed to regular, systematic, and long-term follow-up.

The most common operative procedures involve end-to-end or end-to-side anastomosis of about 38 cm of proximal jejunum to 10 cm of terminal ileum. Weight loss is initially rapid, reaching a plateau at 18 to 24 months. While all patients lose weight, few return to ideal weight. In several series the mean weight loss was 30 to 50 percent of initial excess weight, leaving patients still about 50 percent overweight once a steady state was reached. Although some degree of malabsorption occurs, the major portion of the weight loss is due to decreased food intake.

Most teams performing this surgery select patients who are at least 100 lb overweight and in whom adequate attempts at medical management have failed repeatedly. Because of postoperative morbidity, older patients (> 50 years) and psychologically unstable individuals are usually excluded.

Complications of jejunoileal surgery are common. The overall surgical mortality ranges from 0.5 to 7.8 percent with an average of 3.9 percent. Mortality is inversely related to the experience of the surgical team. The major postoperative morbidity is related to wound infection and thromboembolism. The common serious medical complications are cirrhosis and hepatic failure, nephrolithiasis, electrolyte imbalances, cholelithiasis, and arthritis (Table 79-2). Severe liver disease probably occurs in only 5 percent of patients, but milder degrees of hepatic dysfunction are more common. The long-range implications of mild hepatic abnormalities are unknown. Possible causes of liver damage following small-bowel bypass include (1) protein and particularly essential amino acid deficiency, (2) accumulation of hepatotoxic, secondary bile salts, and (3) release of unknown toxic substances from the excluded bowel. Hypokalemia is most likely secondary to diarrhea. Persistent calcium and magnesium deficiency can result from malabsorption and must be treated with appropriate replacement. Transient depression of plasma 25-hydroxyvitamin D levels may also contribute to abnormal mineral metabolism. Nephrolithiasis can occur in up to 30 percent of patients and is due to

TABLE 79-2
Complications of bypass surgery

Complication	*Percentage*
EARLY	
Perioperative mortality	2–6
Thromboembolic disease	1–5
Wound infection	2–5
Renal failure	3
Severe nausea, vomiting	3
Wound dehiscence	1–3
LATE	
Urinary calculi	3–10
Severe electrolyte imbalance	5–8
Acute cholecystitis	0–5
Progressive liver disease	2–4
Intestinal obstruction	2
Peptic ulcer	1–2
Osteoporosis	?
Tuberculosis	1
MINOR	
Diarrhea	100
Weakness	80
Hypokalemia	80
Hypoproteinemia	50
Vomiting	50
Thirst	50
Hypocalcemia	30
Arthralgias	15
Incisional hernias	3
Hyperuricemia	<10
Anemias (Fe, vitamin B_{12}, folate)	<10

hyperoxaluria secondary to calcium malabsorption (see Chap. 308). It can be treated by calcium supplements and a low oxalate intake. Migratory polyarthritis has been found in up to 6 percent of patients and may be due to circulating immune complexes.

This operation has been performed less frequently in recent years, in part due to the decision of many insurance companies not to render compensation for this procedure.

Gastric surgery Gastroplasty establishes a small upper gastric remnant connected to a larger lower gastric pouch by a narrow 1- to 1.5-cm channel. Gastric bypass excludes the lower 90 percent of the stomach pouch and maintains intestinal continuity of the upper 10 percent via a retrocolic gastrojejunostomy. Both of these procedures cause patients to limit food intake by delaying gastric emptying and providing a small gastric reservoir so that fullness is experienced after a small meal. Weight loss with these procedures has been comparable with that achieved with small-bowel bypass operations but without the complications related to malabsorption, diarrhea, and hepatic dysfunction. Technically this procedure is relatively easy to reverse if a decision to restore normal anatomy is made at a later time. For these reasons, gastroplasty is frequently performed for the surgical treatment of morbid obesity, especially since the number of intestinal bypass procedures is declining.

SUMMARY For most patients obesity is an eating disorder, and a major hope for effective long-term treatment of this disease lies in understanding the causes of overeating. Clearly no single etiology explains all cases, and different causes exist for different individuals. At present a variety of techniques, gimmicks, and maneuvers are available to effect initial weight loss. Unfortunately, initial weight loss is not the real therapeutic problem. Rather, the problem is that almost all obese patients eventually regain their weight. An effective means to sustain weight loss is the major challenge in the treatment of obesity today. The technique of behavioral modification, when professionally and rigorously applied, is the current best tool for this task. As information develops concerning the hypothalamic "set point," or *adipostat*, and the factors that regulate it, pharmacological and perhaps physiological methods may emerge that will effect long-term correction of abnormal eating patterns.

REFERENCES

Assimacopoulos-Jeannet F, Jeanrenaud B: The hormonal and metabolic basis of experimental obesity. Clin Endocrinol Metab 5:337, 1976

Bray GA: Current status of intestinal bypass surgery in the treatment of obesity. Diabetes 26:1072, 1977

Hashim SA, Porikos K: Food intake behavior in man: Implications for treatment of obesity. Clin Endocrinol Metab 5:503, 1976

Horton ES, Danforth E Jr: Energy metabolism and obesity, in *Diabetes Mellitus and Obesity,* SJ Bleicher, BN Brodoff (eds). Baltimore, Williams & Wilkins, 1981, p 261

Kolterman OG et al: Mechanisms of insulin resistance in human obesity. Evidence for receptor and postreceptor defects. J Clin Invest 65:1272, 1980

Mann GV: The influence of obesity on health. N Engl J Med 291:1978, 226, 1974

Olefsky JM: Insulin resistance and insulin action. An in vitro and in vivo perspective. Diabetes 30:148, 1981

Salans L: The obesities, in *Endocrinology and Metabolism,* P Felig et al (eds). New York, McGraw-Hill, 1981, p 891

80
ANOREXIA NERVOSA AND BULIMIA

DANIEL W. FOSTER

Anorexia nervosa and bulimia are eating disorders in young, previously healthy women who develop a paralyzing fear of becoming fat. The population at risk consists largely of white women from middle- and upper-class backgrounds. The disorders rarely occur in black or oriental women, are unusual in the poor, and are almost never seen in men. The driving force is the pursuit of thinness, all other aspects of life being secondary. In the anorexia nervosa syndrome this aim is achieved primarily by radical restriction of caloric intake, the end result being emaciation. In bulimia massive binge eating is followed by vomiting and excessive use of laxatives. Weight loss in bulimic subjects is not great despite the obsession with food. Some authors consider anorexia nervosa and bulimia to be distinct illnesses, while others classify bulimia as a variant of anorexia nervosa. Clearly, overlap syndromes exist since emaciated patients fulfilling the criteria of true anorexia nervosa may exhibit bulimic behavior, while subjects with bulimia often pass through a phase of anorexia. In this chapter it will be assumed that the two disorders represent different clinical expressions of a primary psychologic disturbance focused on an obsession with body weight.

PREVALENCE Estimates of prevalence for anorexia nervosa range from 0.4 to 1.5 per 100,000 population. In adolescent white girls from middle- or upper-class families rates as high as 1 per 100 have been reported. Prevalence is believed to be increasing. The incidence of bulimia is less certain; in one study of 500 patients seen in a university psychiatric clinic the diagnosis of bulimia was made 19 times.

ETIOLOGY One theory holds that an undefined disturbance in the hypothalamus is causal. Evidence for hypothalamic dysfunction includes impaired regulation of pituitary hormone secretion (especially gonadotropins), abnormal eating patterns, altered capacity to change core body temperature in response to external heat or cold, inability to concentrate urine maximally (partial diabetes insipidus), and disturbed cardiovascular function manifested by bradycardia and relative hypotension. The putative hypothalamic lesion is unlikely to be primary, however, because similar changes are seen following extreme weight loss from other causes and because the abnormalities are reversible with weight gain.

For these reasons most investigators favor a psychiatric cause for anorexia nervosa and bulimia, although there is disagreement about its nature. One view holds that the disorders begin in response to inadequate or destructive interpersonal relationships in upper middle class families that are goal-oriented and highly achieving. Despite an outward appearance of normality, interpersonal communication among family members tends to be inadequate, usually following a pattern in which the father seeks success in his work while the mother turns to her children for fulfillment and in the process becomes overdirective. Slimness and physical fitness are often emphasized as virtues even though one or both of the parents may be overweight. Much discussion centers around food. It is presumed that the fear of being fat somehow develops as a consequence of the focus on food and eating behavior. The frequent appearance of overt disease at puberty, at the time of moving away from home, or in association with death of a relative suggests that some external emotional trauma precipitates a subconscious desire within the patient to reclaim control of her body in defiance of parental dominance. The ingrained fear of fatness provides the mechanism by which this need is expressed. Despite the drive for control the sense of self is not well established, and a powerful feeling of ineffectiveness in life is characteristic.

While the preceding sequence is widely held, others believe that serious depression is the fundamental problem in anorexia-bulimia. Whatever the mechanism(s) involved, the behavioral response is obsessive and is difficult to treat.

CLINICAL PICTURE While anorexia nervosa and bulimia may exist in the same patient, the clinical pictures differ at the extremes and will be described separately.

Anorexia nervosa The anorexia nervosa syndrome usually begins before or shortly after puberty but may appear earlier or later (rarely later than the middle twenties). Many patients have been overweight in childhood. Emaciation is equivalent to that seen in the concentration camp victims of World War II. Despite profound emaciation the patients deny hunger, thinness, or fatigue. They are often physically active, and ritualized exercise programs are common. Frenzied calisthenics or running may follow food intake. There is a preoccupation with food, and elaborate meals may be prepared for others. If social circumstances require them to eat more than usual, vomiting is induced as soon as possible, often in a public restroom. Episodic binge eating may occur and is also followed by emesis. Amenorrhea is nearly always present. It usually accompanies or follows weight loss, but in a sixth of patients amenorrhea may precede anorexia. Constipation and cold intolerance are common.

In advanced cases bradycardia, hypothermia, and hypotension are present. Body fat is undetectable, and the bones visibly protrude through the skin. Interestingly, breast tissue is often preserved. The skin may be dry and scaly and may be yellow due to carotenemia, particularly visible in the palms. Body hair is often increased, usually of fine, lanugo quality, but frank hirsutism may occur. Parotid glands may be enlarged as in other forms of starvation. Edema in the absence of hypoalbuminemia is thought to be due to failure of extracellular fluid volume to diminish proportionately with body mass during weight loss. Because of edema in the legs and parotid enlargement, which gives a fullness to the face, the true state of emaciation may be masked when the patient is fully dressed. To standardize diagnosis of anorexia nervosa, sets of minimal criteria have been proposed. One such set, widely used, is shown in Table 80-1.

Laboratory abnormalities include anemia and leukopenia (with hypocellularity of the bone marrow), hypokalemia, and hypoalbuminemia. Serum β-carotene levels tend to be elevated. BUN and creatinine may be slightly increased if volume depletion is severe consequent to vomiting or laxative use. The plasma cholesterol is occasionally high. Glucose tolerance is abnormal as would be expected in any starving subject.

TABLE 80-1
Criteria for the diagnosis of anorexia nervosa

1 Onset prior to age 25
2 Anorexia with weight loss of at least 25 percent of original body weight
3 Distorted attitude toward eating, food, or weight that overrides hunger, admonitions, reassurances, and threats
4 No known medical illness that could account for the weight loss
5 No other known psychiatric disorder
6 At least two of the following manifestations:
  a Amenorrhea
  b Lanugo hair
  c Bradycardia (persistent resting pulse of 60 beats per minute or less)
  d Periods of overactivity
  e Episodes of bulimia
  f Vomiting (may be self-induced)

SOURCE: *After Feighner et al.*

A variety of endocrine abnormalities are seen. Basal luteinizing hormone (LH) and follicle-stimulating hormone (FSH) levels are low when weight loss is severe, and the LH response to luteinizing hormone–releasing hormone (LHRH) is impaired. FSH response to LHRH is quantitatively normal although time to peak increase is delayed. Studies of the 24-h circadian pattern of LH secretion show regression of the maturational stage of LH secretion to a pattern characteristic of prepubertal or early pubertal girls; i.e., episodic LH release is missing or occurs only during sleep. These findings presumably account, at least in part, for the amenorrhea. Menses return with weight gain, although the weight required for reinitiation of menstruation may be somewhat higher ($\sim$ 10 percent) than that needed for the original induction of menarche. Ovulatory menses may be induced in anorexia nervosa by prolonged treatment with LHRH, suggesting that pituitary gonadotropin release is impaired because of hypothalamic dysfunction. Prolactin levels are normal. Plasma estradiol levels are low, and plasma testosterone is in the normal range.

Growth hormone (GH) in the basal state may be normal or elevated. A rise in GH occurs after injection of thyrotropin-releasing hormone (TRH), as in other states with elevated basal levels of GH such as acromegaly, uremia, and protein-calorie malnutrition. Bioactive somatomedin concentrations are low. Plasma cortisol levels are high despite normal production rates; this is due to decreased metabolism of cortisol and prolongation of the plasma half-life. Norepinephrine concentrations in plasma are depressed.

Thyroxine (T_4) levels tend to be slightly low but free T_4 is normal. Triiodothyronine (T_3) concentrations are also reduced while reverse T_3 (rT_3) levels are increased. Thyroid-stimulating hormone (TSH) is usually normal, and TSH response to TRH is intact. The primary defect in thyroid hormone metabolism is decreased activity of the 5′-deiodinase that converts T_4 to T_3 and rT_3 to diiodothyronine in nonthyroidal tissues. These changes are characteristic of starvation and wasting diseases and are not specific for anorexia nervosa.

Bulimia Bulimia refers to the episodic ingestion of large amounts of food in uncontrollable fashion, coupled with awareness that the eating pattern is abnormal, a fear that eating cannot be stopped voluntarily, and feelings of depression at completion of the act. All bulimics have a morbid fear of becoming fat. While binge eating may occur in several types of emotional disorders, a high percentage of bulimia patients give a history of true or cryptic anorexia nervosa, suggesting that bulimia is commonly a variant of anorexia nervosa. Episodes of binge eating are followed by induced vomiting, with or without the subsequent ingestion of large quantities of laxatives. Initially vomiting is induced by placing a toothbrush or fingers in the throat, but eventually most patients learn to vomit reflexly.

Binge eating generally occurs daily in the active phase; in one series of 40 patients the mean number of episodes per week was 12, ranging from 1 to 46. The duration of the eating period averaged 1.2 h but could last as long as 8 h. The amount of food ingested can be enormous, up to 50,000 calories a day, although the mean number of calories consumed in a single episode is around 3500. High-carbohydrate foods are favored, and more than one food is usually eaten. The order of frequency in one series was: ice cream→bread→candy→donuts→soft drinks. Because of the high sugar content of the diet, dental caries are frequent.

In addition to the eating disorder, other behavioral abnormalities are common. Secrecy about the eating-vomiting sequence is characteristic; the family is often unaware. Stealing is common, being admitted by 27 of 34 subjects in one investigation. While food was the item most often stolen, clothing and jewelry were also taken. There is a high rate of alcohol and drug abuse. Depression is usual and tends to be more severe than in anorexia nervosa, making suicide a definite risk. Hysterical behavior may occur.

Despite the close relationship with true anorexia nervosa, a number of differences are noted. While most patients with bulimia are thin, weight loss to the point of emaciation is not seen; generally weight is within 15 percent of the lower limits of accepted normality as defined by life insurance tables of ideal weight. Fluctuating weight is common, with cyclical gains and losses. In contrast to anorexia nervosa, about half of the patients continue to menstruate, and a number have become pregnant during the active phase. Persistent menstruation probably reflects the absence of extreme weight loss. Sexual activity is greater in bulimic subjects than in those with anorexia.

The physical findings associated with bulimia are usually minimal, although subjects with more extensive weight loss may manifest the findings seen with anorexia nervosa.

The most common laboratory abnormality is hypokalemia with metabolic alkalosis secondary to vomiting and laxative use. Evaluation of the endocrine system has not been systematically carried out.

PROGNOSIS The course of anorexia nervosa is variable. A significant number recover and live relatively normal lives. Even so, signs of the previous illness may persist since intermittent dieting is frequent and vomiting and laxative use may periodically recur. A few become obese after recovery while some have chronic, life-long anorexia. Mortality is about 5 to 6 percent, the major causes of death being starvation and suicide. Poor prognostic signs include older age of onset, longer duration of illness, history of bulimia or vomiting, extreme weight loss, and presence of significant depression.

The prognosis in bulimia is worse than that of anorexia nervosa, probably because the accompanying psychiatric disturbances are more severe.

TREATMENT There is no specific treatment for anorexia nervosa or bulimia. Various modes of psychiatric intervention, including behavior modification and intensive psychotherapy or treatment with drugs such as Dilantin and cyproheptadine, have been tried with marginal effectiveness. The best help is probably the supportive care of an understanding physician. The patient should be seen frequently with repetitive guidance regarding diet, weight, exercise, and body image. A structured or semistructured environment, where meals are prepared by others and the patient does not eat alone, may be an important component of therapy since the drive to avoid food, gorge, or vomit is more powerful when patients are alone than when they are in a group. Hospitalization is usually recommended in bulimic subjects to interrupt the cycle of overeating, vomiting, and purging as well as to restore the potassium loss that is commonly present. When emaciation appears life-threatening, parenteral nutrition or tube feeding may be required, but it should be avoided if possible since the aim is to reestablish internal control of eating patterns.

REFERENCES

BOYAR RM et al: Anorexia nervosa: Immaturity of the 24 hour luteinizing hormone secretory pattern. N Engl J Med 291:861, 1974

DROSSMAN DA et al: Anorexia nervosa. Gastroenterology 77:1115, 1979

FEIGHNER JP et al: Diagnostic criteria for use in psychiatric research. Arch Gen Psychiatry 26:57, 1972

HALMI KA: Anorexia nervosa: Recent investigations. Annu Rev Med 29:137, 1978

MITCHELL JE et al: Frequency and duration of binge-eating episodes in patients with bulimia. Am J Psychiatry 138:835, 1981

PYLE RL et al: Bulimia: A report of 34 cases. J Clin Psychiatry 42:60, 1981

RUSSELL G: Bulimia nervosa: An ominous variant of anorexia nervosa. Psychol Med 9:429, 1979

SCHWABE AD et al: Anorexia nervosa. Ann Intern Med 94:371, 1981

VANDE WIELE RI: Anorexia nervosa and the hypothalamus. Hosp Prac 12:45, 1977

81 DIET THERAPY

JULIA C. BLEIER
DANIEL RUDMAN

Dietary modifications are indicated in many clinical situations. (1) The pathogenesis of certain chronic diseases is influenced by the long-term intake of dietary factors: sodium in hypertension, calcium in osteomalacia, and calories in obesity are examples of such situations. (2) The symptomatic stage of other disorders can be ameliorated or worsened by dietary components, for example, sodium in congestive heart failure, protein in uremia, and gluten in celiac disease. (3) Protein-energy malnutrition (PEM), the consequence of numerous subacute or chronic diseases, can often be prevented or corrected with newer techniques of nutritional support. (4) Drug therapy can modify the requirement for certain nutrients; for example, hydantoin anticonvulsants decrease serum levels of folic acid. Conversely, some foods may influence the effectiveness of drugs; for example, calcium-containing foods chelate oral tetracycline and prevent its absorption.

For these reasons, a controlled diet may be a critical aspect of a therapeutic program. The appropriate period of regulation may be temporary or permanent. In some circumstances, the physical composition and even the route of alimentation may need to be changed, with little or no alteration desired in the content of essential or nonessential nutrients. In other circumstances, a specific nutrient may need to be controlled. The physician who wishes to regulate a specific nutrient without causing deficiency or excess of other nutrients and without loss of palatability needs to understand the nutrient composition of the common foods.

This chapter aims to provide the following information:

1 The distribution of nutrients among the food groups
2 The general ways by which the diet can be modified
3 The major diet-sensitive clinical circumstances and the corresponding appropriate diet modifications
4 The principles of diet prescription

DISTRIBUTION OF NUTRIENTS AMONG FOOD GROUPS Because nutrients are not evenly distributed, a variety of foods must be eaten to achieve adequate nutrition. The average diet contains nearly 200 different food items. Isocaloric servings of meat and fruit, for example, have totally dissimilar nutrient contents.

Because of this complexity, nutritionists have arranged foods into groups of similar nutrient content. Milk-dairy products, meats-legumes, fruits-vegetables, and breads-cereals are the four food groups most commonly used (Table 81-1). The recommended number of servings from these groups meet the requirements for approximately three-fourths of the essential nutrients. Additional food selections should be made to fulfill the requirements for energy and certain vitamins and minerals.

It is often desirable to control (either increase or reduce) the intake of a specific food component or nutrient, such as sodium, potassium, lactose, or oxalate. For this purpose, lists have been compiled of foods that are the richest sources of the relevant substances (Table 81-2). In addition, for use in diabetes mellitus, an exchange food-grouping system (Table 81-3) has been adapted for the basic four food groups. This system makes it easy to exchange one food for another within a food group and allows flexibility and variety in planning a diet.

To meet therapeutic goals, food groups or specific foods can be restricted or augmented. However, such a modification may lead to deficiency or excess of other nutrients present in high concentrations in those foods that were removed from, or added to, the diet.

DIET MODIFICATION **Consistency** The consistency of the diet can be altered from solid to pureed to liquid. *Soft* denotes a general diet altered by method of food preparation to allow easier chewing. Meats, for example, can be ground. *Pureed* signifies a nutritionally adequate, general diet that has been blenderized for edentulous patients or those who have difficulty swallowing solid foods. *Full liquid* contains only liquids or foods that liquefy at room temperature. It is often used as a step in the reintroduction of foods to patients in whom oral intake has been withheld and in those recovering from oral or facial surgery. However, it is not suitable for prolonged use because it may contain large amounts of lactose and cholesterol and can be inadequate in iron, folic acid, and vitamin B_6. *Clear liquid* means liquids or frozen foods that are clear. Because there is no fiber residue, this diet is used to prepare the bowel for diagnostic workups or surgery and to serve as the initial step in progressing from nothing by mouth to solid foods. A clear liquid diet provides water, sodium, potassium, and small amounts of carbohydrate; therefore, it is usually used for short periods. When clear liquids are desired for a longer period of time, low-residue enteral feedings should be included in the diet. *Liquid formulas* are nutritionally complete (Table 81-4) and are used to provide adequate nutrition on a prolonged basis either as a supplement to solid food or as complete nutritional support via enteral tube feeding.

Residue or fiber content The residue or fiber content of a diet can be supplemented or restricted. *Dietary fiber* refers to plant material that is not digested. *Residue* signifies the fecal solids, which are made up of undigested and unabsorbed food and metabolic and bacterial products. In the normal bowel, dietary fiber is the main source of fecal residue.

Low-fiber, low-residue diet contains foods with a minimum of fiber and connective tissue. It is used to limit fecal output and prevent the formation of an obstructing bolus in patients with a narrowed intestinal lumen or with an ileostomy. Patients in an acute phase of diverticulitis, ulcerative colitis, or infectious enterocolitis may also benefit from a low-fiber diet. Low-fiber, high-residue foods (milk, prune juice) may also need to be limited.

High fiber signifies a diet with increased amounts of fiber from fruits, vegetables, and grains. It is used to (1) increase the volume of residue reaching the colon, (2) increase gastrointestinal motility, and (3) decrease intraluminal colonic pressure. Patients with chronic diverticulitis or irritable bowel syndrome may benefit from a gradual increase in dietary fiber. Increasing fiber by a mixed diet is preferred to the exclusive use of bran, which interferes with the absorption of calcium, zinc, and iron.

Omission of foods Certain foods can be omitted because they irritate the patient or interfere with certain diagnostic tests.

Bland diet previously referred to the extensive use of milk and the omission of roughage; highly seasoned foods, condiments, and spices; and caffeine. The rationale for avoiding chemical or mechanical irritation has not been supported by medical research. Therefore, the bland diet has been redefined to exclude only those items documented to cause (1) gastric irritation—red and black pepper, chili powder, caffeine, decaffeinated coffee, tea, cocoa, cola beverages, and alcohol; or (2) decreased lower esophageal sphincter (LES) pressure—tomatoes, citrus juices, chocolate, caffeine, decaffeinated coffee, peppermint, and excessively fatty foods. Individuals with gastric or duodenal ulcers or esophageal reflux may benefit from this diet and an eating pattern of frequent, small meals.

Elimination diets are useful in identifying food excitants that cause allergies. Milk, eggs, seafood, nuts, seeds, chocolate, oranges, and tomatoes, the most common excitants, are removed from the diet for a few weeks. If symptoms abate, foods are added back singly and at intervals until the offending foods are determined. Diets to control food allergies should be reviewed for nutritional adequacy.

Serotonin- and 5-hydroxyindoleacetic acid–restricted diet eliminates foods that lead to a false-positive diagnosis of malignant carcinoid tumors. Bananas, plantains, tomatoes, plums, avocados, pineapples, walnuts, and passion fruit should be omitted for 24 h prior to urine collection for such a workup.

Restriction or supplementation of foods PROTEIN MODIFICATION Protein-modified diets comprise low- and high-protein, low-ammonia, altered-amino-acid, low-purine, tyramine-free, and gluten-free diets.

Low-protein diets reduce the intake from an average of 80 to 100 g to 0 to 60 g per day by reducing high-protein items such as meat, eggs, milk, and legumes. Symptoms of nitrogen accumulation (as in hepatic encephalopathy, renal insufficiency, and genetic defects in urea synthesis) respond favorably to such restriction. Selection of proteins with high biologic value minimizes the degree of negative nitrogen balance, but prolonged use of a severely restricted diet can lead to protein malnutrition and other nutrient deficiencies.

Low-ammonia diet is used in conjunction with a low-protein diet for patients with hepatic encephalopathy or genetic disorders of urea synthesis. Gelatin, processed or cured meats, cheese, peanut butter, and brewer's yeast contain large amounts of preformed ammonia.

High-protein diets, 100 to 120 g, may be prescribed for emaciated or hypermetabolic patients. Generally, high-protein diets also have increased amounts of other nutrients and a higher energy content.

Altered-amino-acid diets are sometimes useful in the treatment of nitrogen accumulation disorders. Synthetic mixtures of amino acids reduce the accumulation of plasma amino acids and provide symptomatic treatment. However, protein adequacy must be monitored periodically. Examples of such diets include essential-amino-acid mixtures in uremia, altered ratios of branched-chain to aromatic amino acids in hepatic encephalopathy, and various altered-amino-acid mixtures in genetic errors of nitrogen metabolism.

Low-purine diets contain reduced amounts of uric acid precursors, as an adjunct in the treatment of gout and uric acid calculi. Sweetbreads, anchovies, sardines, shrimp, mackerel, liver, kidney, meat extracts, and dried legumes are excluded from the diet.

Tyramine-, dopamine-free diet eliminates foods containing tyramine or dopamine and fermented or aged foods containing bacteria capable of forming amines. Aged cheese and meats, yeast-containing products, alcoholic beverages, and bananas are omitted. This diet prevents amine-mediated hypertensive crises in patients taking monoamine oxidase inhibitors and is useful in preventing false elevations of urinary catecholamine excretion in the workup of suspected pheochromocytomas.

Gluten-free diet eliminates wheat, rye, oat, barley, and their derivatives which contain glutens. This diet provides symptomatic control of celiac disease and secondary gluten-induced enteropathy.

CARBOHYDRATE MODIFICATION Carbohydrate-modified diets restrict total carbohydrates, disaccharides, or monosaccharides.

Low total carbohydrate diets reduce carbohydrates from the customary 50 percent to 20 to 30 percent of total calories. A carbohydrate intake of less than 70 g per day is ketogenic and is helpful in certain forms of childhood epilepsy. Postgastrectomy "dumping" may also be responsive to a diet that limits the intake of osmotically active substances. Therefore, a diet containing 140 g or less of carbohydrate with restricted mono- and disaccharides and administered in small, frequent feedings is recommended.

Lactose- or sucrose-restricted diets reduce the lactose content of the diet from 25 to 30 g to 0 to 10 g per day, depending on the severity of the lactase deficiency (Table 81-2); sucrose is reduced to 5 to 15 g per day in subjects with sucrase-isomaltase deficiency. Lactose restriction requires the omission of milk and dairy products, the primary sources of calcium in the diet, and therefore calcium supplements should be given when the diet is needed on a long-term basis.

A *galactose-free diet* eliminates all sources of galactose (and thereby lactose) for the treatment of individuals with galactosemia (see Chap. 101).

The *300-g carbohydrate diet* has been advocated by some for 3 days prior to a glucose tolerance test. However, a balanced diet providing at least 150 g carbohydrate results in a valid test. Individuals on hypocaloric or low-carbohydrate diets should receive a high-carbohydrate diet for 3 days before the test.

TABLE 81-1
The nutrient content of the four food groups compared to the recommended dietary allowances (RDAs)*

Food	*Recommended servings*	*Energy, kcal*	*Protein, g*	*Fat, g*	*Carbohydrate, g*	*Vitamin A, mg RE*	*Vitamin E, mg*	*Ascorbic acid, mg*	*Thiamine, mg*	*Riboflavin, mg*	*Niacin, mg*	*Vitamin B_6, mg*	*Vitamin B_{12}, µg*	*Folacin, µg*	*Pantothenic acid, mg*
MILK GROUP															
2% low fat	2 cups	288	20	10	29	117	0.19	5	0.2	1.0	0.5	0.19	1.9	5	1.6
MEAT GROUP															
Egg	1	70	6	5	0	156	0.23	0	0.1	0.1	0.1	0.05	1.0	3	0.8
Meat, fish, poultry	4 oz.	285	31	18	0	26	0.26	0	0.3	0.2	7.3	0.59	1.6	9	0.8
VEGETABLE-FRUIT GROUP															
Leafy green and deep yellow	¼–⅓ cup	12	1	0	2	254	0.47	20	0	0.1	0.3	0.08	0	22	0.1
Other vegetables	¼–⅓ cup	19	1	0	4	35	0.16	7	0	0	0.4	0.05	0	14	0.1
Potato	1 medium	113	3	0	26	0	0.05	24	0.1	0	2.0	0.21	0	9	0.3
Citrus fruit	1 serving	44	1	0	10	12	0.04	44	0.1	0	0.3	0.03	0	3	0.2
Other fruit	1 serving	92	1	0	22	50	0.22	5	0	0	0.4	0.10	0	5	0.2
BREAD-CEREAL GROUP															
Cereal, enriched or whole grain	¾ cup	135	4	1	29	0	0.22	0	0.1	0	1.3	0.04	0	15	0.2
Bread, enriched or whole grain	3 slices	205	7	2	39	0	0.21	0	0.2	0.1	2.0	0.08	0	17	0.4
Fortified margarine	4 tsp	144	0	16	0	66	10.0	0	0	0	0	0	0	0	0
Totals		1300	75	62	161	716	12	105	1.9	1.5	14.6	1.42	4.5	102	4.7
RECOMMENDED DIETARY ALLOWANCES†															
Female (23–50 yr)		2000	44			800	12	60	1.0	1.2	13	2.0	3.0	400	4–7‡
Male (23–50 yr)		2700	56			1000	15	60	1.4	1.6	18	2.2	3.0	400	4–7‡

* *Values represent the average nutrient content of a food group.*
† *Taken from Recommended Dietary Allowances.*
‡ *Because there is less information on which to base an allowance, ranges of recommended intakes are given.*

FAT MODIFICATION Fat-modified diets may be restricted in total fat (largely triglycerides), in cholesterol, or both, and may be supplemented with medium-chain triglycerides (MCT). As shown in Table 81-6, these diets are used to treat various types of hyperlipemia (see Chap. 103) or malabsorption.

A typical *low-fat, low-cholesterol diet* for hyperlipemic states furnishes 30 to 35 percent of calories as fat, the composition of which is altered to provide more polyunsaturated and less saturated fat and less than 300 mg cholesterol per day. Some types of hyperlipemia also require restrictions of carbohydrate and calories. Increasing the polyunsaturated/saturated fatty acid ratio requires decreasing the intake of beef, pork, lamb, cheese, and egg yolks and increasing the use of chicken, turkey, veal, and fish. Skim milk is used rather than whole milk, and margarines made with polyunsaturated vegetable oils are substituted for butter. Reducing cholesterol to 300 mg per day or less involves restricting egg yolks to three per week as well as limiting fat from animal sources. Such a change in eating habits requires long-term reinforcement.

For the patient with fat malabsorption, severe chylomicronemia, or chylous ascites, long-chain triglycerides should be restricted to 20 to 50 g per day (10 percent to 25 percent of total calories). When fat intake is severely restricted, medium-chain triglycerides, which are absorbed independently of long-chain fatty acids, should be added to provide sufficient energy. To document fat malabsorption, a diet containing 100 g fat is eaten during a 3-day stool collection. Actual fat intake must be estimated to determine the extent of malabsorption.

ENERGY MODIFICATION Energy-modified diets are designed for weight reduction, weight gain, or weight maintenance. Conditions that benefit from energy-modified diets include obesity, hypertension, diabetes mellitus, arthritis, cachexia, and hypermetabolic states due to trauma, infection, and burns.

Low-kilocalorie diets usually furnish 800 to 1200 kcal for women and 1000 to 1500 kcal for men. Although a weight-reduction diet is designed to include selections from the four food groups, it may be inadequate to meet all of the recommended daily allowances if the caloric content is severely restricted; thus, vitamin and mineral supplements may be needed.

High-kilocalorie diets (2800 to 4000 kcal per day) usually are designed to provide the estimated basal energy expenditure of the individual plus an additional 100 to 200 percent for

Calcium, mg	*Phosphorus, mg*	*Magnesium, mg*	*Iron, mg*	*Zinc, mg*	*Sodium, mg*	*Potassium, mg*	*Dietary fiber, g*
698	547	62	0.5	1.9	298	854	0
24	90	6	1.1	0.5	54	57	0
14	274	33	3.1	5.4	88	430	0
34	22	13	0.6	0.3	12	127	2.0
19	22	13	0.5	0.2	30	105	1.4
11	79	14	0.8	0.3	5	614	3.5
19	17	11	0.3	0.1	1	174	0.4
10	16	13	0.6	0.2	2	176	1.5
13	75	21	1.1	0.5	303	73	3.8
68	126	38	1.9	0.8	414	143	6.4
4	12	0	0	0	200	4	0
914	1280	224	10.5	10.2	1407	2758	19
800	800	300	18	15	1100–	1875–	
800	800	350	10	15	3300‡	5625‡	

TABLE 81-2
Foods containing large amounts of certain nutrients*

SODIUM	
Salt, catsup, mustard	Cheese, buttermilk
Soy sauce, steak/barbeque sauce	Salted nuts, peanut butter
Worcestershire sauce	Self-rising flour, biscuit mixes
Bouillon cubes	Salted crackers, chips, popcorn
Commercially prepared or cured meats, fish	Pickles, olives
Canned foods (except fruit)	Commercial salad dressings
	Instant cooked cereals
POTASSIUM	
Milk	Vegetables: Artichoke, bamboo shoots, beet greens, chard, dried beans, mushrooms, potato, spinach, sweet potato, tomatoes, winter squash
Meat, fish, poultry	
Fruit: Apricots, avocado, banana, cantaloupe, dates, honeydew, orange, prunes, raisins	
OXALATE	
Spinach	Almonds, cashew nuts
Rhubarb	Chocolate, cocoa
Dandelion greens	Tea
LACTOSE	
Milk, milk products	Milk chocolate, chewing gum
Cheese	Some sugar substitutes
Commercial bread/dessert mixes	Foods with these ingredients: Milk, milk solids, dry milk, curd, whey, whey solids, demineralized whey, lactose
Commercial creamed/breaded meats	
Creamed/dehydrated soups	
Creamed, breaded, buttered vegetables	
AMMONIA	
Gelatin	Peanut butter
Processed, cured meats	Brewer's yeast
Cheese	

* *Adapted from Handbook of Clinical Dietetics and Rudman et al.*

TABLE 81-3
Diabetic exchange list

	Serving size	*Carbohydrate, g*	*Protein, g*	*Fat, g*
Milk, skim	8 oz	12	8	0
Meat	1 oz			
Lean		0	7	3
Medium fat		0	7	5
High fat		0	7	8
Bread-cereal	1 slice or $\frac{1}{2}$ cup	15	2	0
Vegetables	$\frac{1}{2}$ cup	5	2	0
Fruit	Per list	10	0	0
Fat	1 tsp	0	0	5

anabolism. If the patient is not able to consume the required caloric intake as solid food, liquid supplements can be used between meals.

Appropriate *diabetic diets* are fundamental to the treatment of diabetes mellitus with the major goals being restriction of the intake of sucrose and free glucose and achievement of ideal body weight (also see Chap. 114). Ideal body weight can be estimated from the height/weight tables of the Metropolitan Life Insurance Company or from the following simple formula: in women, 100 lb for the first 5 ft and 5 lb for every inch over 5 ft; in men, 106 lb for the first 5 ft and 6 lb for every inch over 5 ft. Energy requirements are based on the basal energy expenditure (see Chap. 73) plus an additional allowance of 25 percent, 50 percent, or 75 percent for sedentary, moderate, and strenuous activity levels, respectively. The recommended distribution of caloric intake is 50 to 60 percent from carbohydrate, 12 to 20 percent from protein, and 30 to 35 percent from fat. Three meals per day are usually planned for the obese, non-insulin-dependent diabetic. The type of insulin prescribed and the timing of insulin administration determine the meal patterns in the insulin-dependent diabetic. Usually, each of three meals and an evening snack provide three-tenths and one-tenth, respectively, of the allowed carbohydrate and caloric content. Patients receiving NPH insulin may require a midafternoon snack to avoid hypoglycemia during the peak activity of the insulin. The number of servings (exchanges) from each food group in the diabetic exchange system (Table 81-3) is comparable to the recommended intakes of the basic four food groups.

ELECTROLYTE AND MINERAL MODIFICATION Electrolyte-mineral-modified diets consist of low-sodium, low- or high-potassium, low- or high-calcium, and low-phosphorus intakes.

Low-sodium diets reduce sodium consumption from an average intake of 4 g (176 meq, 10 g NaCl) to 0.5 to 2 g (22 to 88 meq, 1.3 to 5 g NaCl). Patient compliance is poor if daily intake is restricted to less than 2 g sodium. The 2-g sodium diet eliminates the foods listed in Table 81-2 and controls the use of milk, salted breads and cereals, and salted margarines but does not require the use of salt-free milk, breads, and margarines, which are expensive and have low palatability.

Low-potassium diets reduce intake from an average of 6 g (153 meq) to 2 g (51 meq) for the patient with hyperkalemia. *High-potassium diets* provide an intake greater than 5.8 g (150 meq) and may be indicated when potassium-wasting diuretics are used (Table 81-2). *Low-calcium diets* reduce the calcium intake from an average of 800 mg to 200 to 400 mg and are used to treat hypercalcemia and some types of nephrolithiasis. The long-term consequences of a low-calcium diet on bone are unknown. *High-calcium diet* indicates a 1000-mg calcium diet which is used in the evaluation of hypercalciuria. *Low-phosphorus diet,* 700 to 800 mg per day, is used to prevent hyperphosphatemia and secondary enhancement of parathyroid hormone secretion in renal disease. *Low-oxalate diet* is designed to eliminate exogenous sources of oxalate and is useful in hyperoxaluria and in calcium oxalate nephrolithiasis.

Alteration of the feeding route The route of delivery can be changed from oral to enteral tube feeding. Technological improvements in nasoenteral tubes, formulas, and infusion pumps have improved the efficacy and safety of tube feedings. The enteral route has three advantages over intravenous feeding. (1) It maintains the integrity of the intestinal mucosa, and nutrients are handled in a more physiological manner, (2) it causes fewer metabolic and technical complications, and (3) it is less expensive than intravenous alimentation. Consequently,

TABLE 81-4
Examples of enteral formulas

Types	Example	Osmolality, mosm/kg	Kcal/ml or g	Daily volume for 100% RDA, ml	Protein		Carbohydrate	
					g/1000 kcal	Source	g/1000 kcal	Source
Elemental	Vivonex HN	810	1.00	3000	46	Amino acids	210	Glucose oligosaccharides
	Vital	460	1.00	1500	42	Peptides from whey, soy, meat, + 9 amino acids	188	Corn syrup, sucrose
	Travasorb HN	560	1.00	2000	45	Peptides from lactalbumin	175	Glucose oligosaccharides
Polymeric	Sustacal	625	1.00	1080	60	Casein, soy	138	Sucrose, corn syrup
	Ensure	450	1.06	1900	35	Casein, soy	135	Corn syrup, sucrose
	Isocal	300	1.06	1900	32	Casein, soy	125	Glucose oligosaccharides
	Portagen	354	1.00	2525	36	Casein	117	Corn syrup, sucrose
	Compleat B	300	1.07	1500	40	Beef, casein	133	Cereal, vegetable, fruit
	Ensure Plus	600	1.50	1920	37	Casein, soy	133	Corn syrup, sucrose
	Magnacal	590	2.00	1000	35	Casein	125	Maltodextrin, sucrose
Modular	Polycose	850	2.00	NA	0	NA	250	Glucose polymers
	Casec	NA	3.70	NA	230	Casein	0	NA
	MCT oil	NA	7.70	NA	0	NA	0	NA
	Product 80056	NA	4.90	NA	0	NA	146	Corn syrup, tapioca
Altered amino acids	Hepatic-Aid	1158	1.65	NA	26	Amino acids	175	Maltodextrin, sucrose
	Amin-Aid	1095	1.95	NA	10	Amino acids	187	Maltodextrin, sucrose

NOTE: *NA = not applicable.*

clinicians should consider enteral tube feeding before resorting to parenteral nutrition (see Chap. 82).

PATIENT SELECTION Oral intake can be inadequate because of anorexia or mechanical obstruction, increased nutrient losses, or hypermetabolism. Wasting disorders in which enteral feedings may be useful include cerebral vascular accidents, head and neck cancer, anorexia nervosa, trauma, and burns. Contraindications to tube feeding include intractable vomiting, upper gastrointestinal bleeding, and intestinal obstruction. Steatorrhea is a handicap but can sometimes be surmounted by the use of chemically defined "elemental" formulas or with antidiarrheal drugs.

TUBE PLACEMENT Several enteral tube placements are used: nasogastric, nasoduodenal, nasojejunal, gastrostomy, or jejunostomy. Because the latter two require surgery, the nasogastric or nasoduodenal route is most frequently chosen. Small-bore silastic or polyurethane tubing minimizes the complications of nasopharyngitis, rhinitis, otitis media, parotitis, and subsequent stricture. Insertion and maintenance of proper placement are facilitated by a removable wire stylet and a mercury-weighted tip. A properly irrigated tube may remain in place for months.

Patients who require permanent tube feedings benefit from gastrostomy for several reasons: the cosmetic problems of the nasogastric tube are avoided, and there is no need to rely on expensive formulas since the large-bore tube allows the use of blenderized foods.

Jejunal feedings may be desirable in situations in which an obstruction or fistula is proximal to the jejunum. An advantage of the jejunostomy is the reduced risk of aspiration from gastric reflux.

SELECTION OF INFUSION METHOD One of the early disadvantages of enteral tube feedings was the lack of control of the infusion rate, and as a consequence patients sensitive to large volumes or hyperosmolar solutions often developed osmotic diarrhea and cramping. Enteral infusion pumps are now available to ensure a constant drip rate. When large volumes (3000 ml) of a hyperosmolar solution (> 500 mosmol per liter) are necessary for repletion, either of two approaches can be tried. A full-strength formula can be begun at 50 ml/h for 24 h, and the rate of infusion daily can be increased as tolerated until the desired volume is achieved. Alternately, the formula can be made isotonic by dilution and infused from the start at a rate of 125 ml/h for 24 h; the concentration of the formula can then be gradually increased each day until full strength is reached. Infusion periods of less than 24 h may be preferable when aspiration is a potential problem.

FORMULA SELECTION Over 70 enteral formulas are available to meet nutritional requirements. Choosing from this array is made easier by the knowledge that the 70 products fall into 4 categories: elemental ("monomeric"), polymeric, modular, and altered amino acids (see Table 81-4).

Elemental formulas are composed of di- and tripeptides and/or crystalline amino acids, glucose oligosaccharides and vegetable oil, or medium-chain triglycerides. Residue is minimal, and little digestive action is required. An elemental formula may be of use in patients with the short-bowel syndrome, partial bowel obstruction, pancreatic insufficiency, inflammatory bowel disease, radiation enteritis, or fistulas.

Polymeric formulas are composed of complex nutrients,

Fat		*Ca, mg/1000 kcal*	*P, mg/1000 kcal*	*Na, mg/1000 kcal*	*K, mg/1000 kcal*	*Micronutrients*
g/1000 kcal	*Source*					
< 1	Safflower oil	333	333	529	1173	Yes
11	55% safflower oil 45% MCT oil	667	667	383	1167	Yes
13	MCT oil Sunflower oil	500	500	920	1170	Yes
23	Soy oil	1000	920	920	2060	Yes
35	Corn oil	511	511	708	1179	Yes
42	80% soy oil 20% MCT oil	600	500	500	1250	Yes
48	86% MCT oil 12% corn oil	936	707	468	1248	Yes
34	Beef, corn oil	625	875	625	1313	Yes
35	Corn oil	422	422	704	1267	Yes
40	Soy oil	500	500	500	625	Yes
0	NA	150	30	290	100	No
5	Milk	4312	2156	408	0	No
120	92% MCT oil	0	0	0	0	No
46	Corn oil	1102	606	147	688	Yes
22	Soy oil	0	0	0	0	No
24	Soy oil	0	0	173	0	No

e.g., protein as casein, lactalbumin, soy protein; carbohydrate as corn syrup solids or maltodextrins; and fat as vegetable oils or milk fat. There is heterogeneity with regard to lactose content, sodium content, caloric density, content of medium-chain triglycerides, and palatability. Most patients with a functional gastrointestinal tract and few specialized nutrient requirements can utilize a formula from the polymeric group.

Single nutrient modules, available for protein, carbohydrate, and fat, can be combined or added to a monomeric or polymeric formula to create a formula that meets specialized nutrient requirements. The simplest modular formula involves adding a carbohydrate source to a formula to increase caloric value. For example, a cachectic cirrhotic patient with ascites and encephalopathy may benefit from a high-caloric, low-protein, low-sodium formula.

Altered-amino-acid formulas are indicated in patients with genetic errors of nitrogen metabolism: phenylketonuria, maple syrup urine disease, homocystinuria, tyrosinemia, methylmalonic acidemia, and propionic acidemia. In the acquired disorders of nitrogen accumulation (chronic renal failure and cirrhosis) synthetic formulas are designed to limit the intake of certain amino acids and thereby provide symptomatic improvement.

TABLE 81-5
Complications of enteral hyperalimentation and their management

Type of complication	*Frequency, %*	*Management*
MECHANICAL		
Tube lumen clogged by solution	Infrequent (< 10)	Flush with water; replace tube if unsuccessful
Pulmonary aspiration of stomach contents	Rare (< 1)	Unlikely with head of bed elevated; discontinue if aspiration occurs
Esophageal erosion	Rare (< 1)	Discontinue tube
Stomal erosion	2	Discontinue tube
Wound infection	2	Treat with antibiotics
Herniation through interostomy site	Rare (< 1)	
Tube dislodgment:		
Nasoenteral	10–20	Replace tube
Gastrostomy	Rare (< 1)	Replace tube
Jejunostomy	Rare (< 1)	Use intravenous nutritional support
GASTROINTESTINAL SYMPTOMS		
Vomiting and bloating	10–15	Reduce flow rate and give 10 mg metoclopromide; add peripheral hyperalimentation if needed
Diarrhea and cramping	10–20	Reduce flow; dilute solution; consider different type solution; add antidiarrheal drug
METABOLIC, FLUID, AND ELECTROLYTE ABNORMALITIES		
Hyperglycemia and glucosuria	10–15	Reduce flow; administer insulin
Hyperosmolar coma	Rare (< 1)	Discontinue therapy
Edema	20–25	Usually none; may reduce Na content or slow hyperalimentation rate; rarely use diuretics
Volume overload in uremia	10	Dialyze more frequently
Congestive heart failure	1–5	Slow hyperalimentation; administer diuretics and digoxin
Hypernatremia, hypercalcemia	< 5	Adjust electrolyte content of hyperalimentation
Essential fatty acid deficiency	Common	Linoleic acid supplement orally or Intralipid intravenously

PATIENT MONITORING Successful enteral tube feeding requires continual, careful monitoring for possible mechanical, gastrointestinal, fluid, and electrolyte complications as detailed in Table 81-5. The guidelines given in Chap. 77 for nutritional assessment should be used to evaluate the effectiveness of the nutrition support.

INDICATIONS FOR DIET THERAPY The clinical indications for dietary modification are listed in Table 81-6. The suggested diets are those commonly used, recognizing that diet therapy must be tailored to individual needs.

DRUG REGIMENS THAT ALTER NUTRIENT REQUIREMENTS Certain foods or meal patterns can alter drug effectiveness, and certain drugs can alter nutrient requirements. Many drugs influence appetite and food intake. Hyper- and hypophagic agents are listed in Table 81-7.

Drug absorption is generally slower when taken with food, an effect that may be important when rapid onset of drug action is desired. Complete inhibition of drug absorption occurs when calcium-containing foods or iron salts chelate tetracycline, making it insoluble. Enhanced drug absorption results when lipid-soluble drugs are given with fat-containing meals or when alcohol is taken with a timed-release medicine that is alcohol soluble. Table 81-8 presents guidelines for drug administration in relation to meals.

Certain drugs adversely affect nutrient absorption by altering the intestinal lumen, chelating nutrients to form insoluble complexes or inhibiting the digestive processes. Drugs that cause malabsorption and the nutrients affected are illustrated in Table 81-9.

Drug utilization can be adversely affected by dietary components. Alcohol delays the utilization of many drugs, but the metabolism of many drugs can be accelerated in the heavy drinker due to induction of microsomal enzymes. Supplemental pyridoxine accelerates the degradation of L-dopa used in the treatment of parkinsonism. Patients receiving coumarin anticoagulants should avoid excessive consumption of foods or enteral formulas rich in vitamin K. Some of the antivitamins or antimetabolites that interfere with nutrient utilization are listed in Table 81-9.

The *urinary excretion* of drugs as weak acids or bases is influenced by urinary pH. For example, large doses of ascorbic acid can acidify the urine and decrease the half-life of weak bases. Drugs can also affect nutrient excretion by exerting a toxic effect on the renal tubules, by displacing protein-bound nutrients in the serum, or by forming a soluble drug-nutrient complex (Table 81-9).

THE PRINCIPLES OF DIET PRESCRIPTION Several considerations are involved in formulating effective diet therapy. The nature of *dietary modifications* appropriate for a given clinical situation must be delineated (change in food consistency, removal of specific foods, reduction or increase of specific nutrients, or change in route of nutrient delivery). The appropriate *degree of restriction* or supplementation should be determined, recognizing that the extreme ranges of dietary modifications may cause noncompliance. Does a cardiac patient need a 2-g or a 0.5-g sodium diet; does a dysphagic patient require a soft or pureed diet; does a patient with wasting febrile illness require a 2000- or 3000-kcal diet? When more than one dietary modification is appropriate a decision must be made as to which is the most important. Some combinations are virtually

TABLE 81-6
Some clinical disorders that benefit from appropriate diet therapy

Clinical disorder	*Recommended diet therapy*	*Comments*
GASTROINTESTINAL DISORDERS		
Dysphagia	Pureed, liquid supplements	
Reflux esophagitis	Bland, frequent small meals	
Acute gastritis	Clear liquids, bland	
Gastric ulcers	Frequent small meals	
Postgastrectomy dumping	Low-carbohydrate, frequent small meals	
Irritable bowel syndrome	High-fiber	
Crohn's disease	High-kilocalorie, high-protein	May need elemental formula
Radiation therapy to bowel	Low-fiber	
Radiation enteritis	Elemental formula	
Fat malabsorption	Low-fat—MCT supplemented	Mg and vitamin A, D, E, and K supplements
Biliary tract obstruction		
Biliary cirrhosis		In advanced cases
Enterohepatic cholestasis		
Pancreatic insufficiency		
Crohn's disease		
Jejunoileal bypass		
Short-bowel syndrome		
Bacterial overgrowth		
Postvagotomy steatorrhea		
Celiac disease	Gluten-free	
Lactose intolerance	Lactose-free	Ca supplement
Infectious enterocolitis	Low-fiber	
Acute ulcerative colitis	Low-fiber	
Acute diverticulitis	Low-fiber	
Chronic diverticulitis	High-fiber	
Chronic constipation	High-fiber, increase fluids	
HEPATIC DISORDERS		
Alcoholic liver disease:		
Alcoholic hepatitis	High-kilocalorie, high-protein	Multivitamin and folate supplements
Cirrhosis	High-kilocalorie, high-protein	Multivitamin and folate supplements
Encephalopathy	Low-protein, low-ammonia	
Ascites	Low-sodium, high-kilocalorie, high-protein	
RENAL DISORDERS		
Acute, chronic renal failure	Protein, phosphorus, sodium, potassium reduced	1,25-$(OH)_2D_3$, Ca supplements
Nephrotic syndrome	Low-sodium	
Renal osteodystrophy	Low-phosphorus	1,25-$(OH)_2D_3$, Ca supplements
Potassium wasting	High-potassium	
Hypercalciuric nephrolithiasis	Low-calcium, oxalate-free	
CARDIOVASCULAR DISORDERS		
Hyperlipemia:		
Type I	Low-fat	No alcohol
Type IIa	Low-cholesterol, low-saturated-fat, increased-polyunsaturated-fat	
Type IIb, III	Carbohydrate-controlled, low-cholesterol, low-saturated-fat	Achieve and maintain ideal body weight
Type IV	Carbohydrate-controlled, low-cholesterol, low-saturated-fat	Achieve and maintain ideal body weight
Type V	Low-fat, low-cholesterol	No alcohol, achieve and maintain ideal body weight
Hypertension	Low-sodium	Achieve and maintain ideal body weight
Congestive heart failure	Low-sodium	
Acute sickle cell crisis	Increase fluids	
Postmyocardial infarction	Low-sodium, frequent small meals	
PULMONARY DISORDERS		
Sarcoidosis	Low-calcium	If hypercalcemic
ENDOCRINE-METABOLIC DISORDERS		
Diabetes mellitus	Kilocalorie-, carbohydrate-, fat-controlled	Achieve and maintain ideal body weight
Reactive hypoglycemia	High-protein, low-carbohydrate, frequent small meals	
Obesity	Low-kilocalorie	
Osteoporosis	High-calcium	Vitamin D supplement
Gout, uric acid stones	Low-purine	
Nephrogenic diabetes insipidus	Low-sodium, protein-controlled	
Hypoparathyroidism	High-calcium	1,25-$(OH)_2D_3$ supplement
Hyperparathyroidism	Low-calcium	
Steroid therapy	Low-sodium, high-protein	
NERVOUS SYSTEM DISORDERS		
Ménière's disease	Low-sodium	
Multiple sclerosis	High-fiber	For constipation
Vascular headaches	Elimination trials	
Childhood epilepsy—Lennox-Gastaut	Low-carbohydrate, high-fat	
Acute neurological injury with dysphagia	Nasoenteral tube feeding	Progress to general diet when stable
INFECTIOUS DISEASES		
Diarrheal diseases	Fluids, glucose, electrolytes by mouth or nasoenteral tube	Progress to general diet when stable
Febrile diseases	Clear liquids, increase fluids	
PHYSICAL INJURIES		
Burns	High-kilocalorie, nasoenteral tube feeding	
GENETIC DISORDERS		
Galactosemia	Galactose-free	
Sucrose-maltose deficiency	Low-sucrose	
Cystic fibrosis	High-calorie, high-protein, low-fat—MCT supplemented	Pancreatic enzyme supplements

TABLE 81-6 *(continued)*
Some clinical disorders that benefit from appropriate diet therapy

Clinical disorder	*Recommended diet therapy*	*Comments*
GENETIC DISORDERS		
Phenylketonuria	Low-phenylalanine, tyrosine supplemented	
Maple syrup urine disease	Low-leucine, -isoleucine, -valine	Thiamine, when responsive
Homocystinuria	Low-methionine, cystine supplemented	Pyridoxine, when responsive
Adrenogenital syndrome	High-sodium	
Propionic acidemia	Low-protein	Biotin, when responsive
Methylmalonic acidemia	Low-protein	Vitamin B_{12}, when responsive
Hypophosphatemic rickets		P, 1,25-$(OH)_2D_3$ supplements
Urea cycle disorders	Low-protein, low-ammonia	
PSYCHIATRIC DISORDERS		
Anorexia nervosa	High-kilocalorie, high-protein	May need nasoenteral tube feeding
Affective disorders treated with MAO inhibitors	Tyramine- and dopamine-free	
NEOPLASTIC DISEASES		
	General	Nutritional support to prevent cancer cachexia
NUTRITIONAL DISORDERS		
Iron-deficiency anemia	Increase iron	Fe supplement
Megaloblastic anemia	Increase folate, Vitamin B_{12}	Folate supplement or vitamin B_{12} intramuscular injection depending on diagnosis
Beriberi	Increase thiamine	Multivitamin supplement
Pellagra	Increase niacin	Multivitamin supplement
Rickets, osteomalacia	Increase Ca, vitamin D	Vitamin D supplement
Scurvy	Increase ascorbic acid	Multivitamin supplement
Hypovitaminosis A	Increase vitamin A	Vitamin A supplement

incompatible, such as a low-kilocalorie, high-potassium diet; a high-calcium, lactose-free diet; or a high-protein, low-fat diet. The *duration* of the diet prescription must be estimated. Diets with severely limited nutrients should be used for as short a time as possible.

By using the type of information shown in Tables 81-1 to 81-4 and in the American Dietetic Association's *Handbook of Clinical Dietetics,* the dietitian implements the prescribed diet and reports how closely the implemented diet conforms to the desired modifications and whether undesired dietary imbalances may have been created by the prescription. Severely altered diets may be deficient or augmented in nutrients not considered in the original diet prescription; for example, a lactose-free diet is also low in calcium and riboflavin. Therefore, further manipulations may be necessary to prevent secondary deficiencies or excesses inherent in the original diet order. Three examples of prescribed diets and their implementations are given below.

TABLE 81-7
Some drugs affecting food intake

Agents that may impair appetite	*Agents that may enhance appetite*
Methyl cellulose	Antihistamines (cyproheptadine hydrochloride, buclizine, cimetidine)
Amphetamines	Tranquilizers
Biguanides	Insulin
Digitalis	Steroids
Chemotherapeutic agents	Dopamine antagonist (metoclopramide)
Narcotics	

TABLE 81-8
Optimal timing of drug administration in relation to meals

1 Drugs taken 1 h before or 2 h after a meal for more rapid absorption

Oral antibiotics
Penicillamine

2 Drugs taken ½ h before meals

Anticholinergics—to decrease gastrointestinal motility
Anorexiants—to reduce food intake
Dopamine antagonist (metoclopramide)—to prevent nausea

3 Drugs taken with meals to prevent gastric irritation or improve absorption of lipid-soluble drugs

Cimetidine	Propranolol
Corticosteroids	Hydralazine
Theophylline	Hydrochlorothiazide
Anti-inflammatory drugs	Propoxyphene
Aspirin	Griseofulvin
Oral hypoglycemic agents	Spironolactone
Potassium, iron supplements	Carbamazepine
Antituberculosis drugs	Diphenylhydantoin
Urinary antiseptics	

4 Drugs taken ½ h after meals to relieve gastric upset

Antacids

Example 1

I Diagnosis: Obesity and hypertension.
II Physician's order: 1200 kcal, 2 g Na, high potassium.
III Dietitian's response: High potassium (> 5.8 g, 150 meq) is difficult to achieve when a kilocalorie restriction is ordered. Potassium supplements may be necessary.

	*Energy, kcal**	*Na, mg**	*K, mg**
2 cups milk, skim	180	240	710
6 oz meat, lean	330	150	780
4 servings bread	280	800	180
4 servings vegetables	100	40	1440
3 servings fruit	120	0	1140
4 servings margarine, oil	180	200	40
	1190	1430 (62 meq)	4290 (110 meq)

* *Values represent the average nutrient content of a food group.*

Nutritional analysis: No deficiencies or excesses of essential nutrients.

Example 2

I Diagnosis
A Cirrhosis of the liver
1 Encephalopathy
2 Ascites

B Chronic pancreatitis
C Malnutrition

II Physician's order: 40 g protein, low ammonia, 1 g Na, low fat, increased calories.

III Dietitian's response: Increased caloric intake (> 2500 kcal) is difficult to achieve when protein and long-chain fatty acids can contribute only 610 kcal. Medium-chain triglycerides (MCT) and foods containing largely sucrose will be needed to increase kilocalories.

	*Protein, g**	*Na, mg**	*Fat, g**	*Energy, kcal**
½ cup milk, whole	4	60	4	75
3 oz meat or eggs	21	75	15	220
4 servings bread or cereal	8	800	0	280
4 servings vegetables	8	40	0	100
10 servings fruit	0	0	0	400
5 servings low-protein desserts	0	0	10	460
4 servings salt-free margarine	0	0	20	180
18 servings MCT mayonnaise	0	0	90	810
	41	975 (42 meq)	139	2525

* *Values represent the average nutrient content of a food group.*

Nutritional analysis: This diet is deficient in calcium, thiamine, riboflavin, and niacin and needs to be supplemented.

TABLE 81-9
Drugs causing nutrient malabsorption, impaired utilization, or urinary hyperexcretion

Mode of action	*Drug*	*Nutrient affected*
Malabsorption	Mineral oil	Carotene, vitamins A, D, K
	Neomycin	Fat, lactose, nitrogen, Na, K, Ca, Fe, vitamin B_{12}
	Cholestyramine, colestipol	Fat; vitamins A, D, K; folacin
	Colchicine	Fat, carotene, lactose, Na, K, vitamin B_{12}
	Phenobarbital, diphenylhydantoin	Ca
	Glucocorticoids	Ca
	Aluminum/magnesium hydroxide	P
	Tetracycline	Ca, Mg, vitamin B_{12}
	Amphoteric gels	P, Fe
	Azulfidine	Folacin
Impaired utilization	Antivitamins methotrexate, pyrimethiamine, triamterene, trimethoprim	Folacin
	Isoniazid, hydralazine, cycloserine, pyrazinamide, ethionamide, theosemicarbizones, penicillamine, L-dopa	Vitamin B_6
	Coumarin anticoagulants	Vitamin K
	Oral contraceptives	Folacin, vitamin C, riboflavin, vitamin B_6, Cu
Urinary hyperexcretion	Gentamicin	Mg, Ca, K
	Cisplatin	Mg
	Thiazides	Mg, K, Na, Zn
	Furosemide, ethacrynic acid	Mg, K, Na, Zn, Ca
	Penicillamine	Zn, Cu, vitamin B_6
	Deferoxamine mesylate	Fe
	Isoniazid, hydralazine	Vitamin B_6
	Aspirin	Vitamin C
	Digitalis, cardiac glycosides	Ca, Mg

Example 3

I Diagnosis: Same patient as in Example 2, with a fourth problem, anorexia.

II Physician's order: 40 g protein, 1 g Na, low fat, enteral tube feeding.

III Dietitian's response: Modular formula.

	Protein, g	*Na, mg*	*Fat, g*	*Energy, kcal*
750 ml Isocal	25	390	33	790
18 g Casec	15	27	0	60
360 ml Polycose	0	220	0	720
105 ml MCT oil	0	0	105	945
250 ml water				
1500 ml	40	637	138	2515

Nutritional analysis: This diet needs to be supplemented with vitamins A, D, and B_6, and folic acid, iodine, iron, and zinc.

ASSESSMENT OF DIETARY COMPLIANCE Assessment of compliance and evaluation of effectiveness are the final steps in successful diet therapy. When a "calorie count" is ordered for a hospitalized patient, the dietitian can estimate the daily intake of protein, carbohydrate, fat, and kilocalories. Some nutrients can be monitored by blood or urine analysis; for example, compliance with a low-sodium diet can be determined by urinary sodium analysis. An outpatient food intake diary is useful in assessing the home environment. Improvements in symptoms and signs of the disorder also serve as indicators of effective dietary modification.

REFERENCES

American Dietetics Association: *Handbook of Clinical Dietetics.* New Haven, Yale, 1981

Heymsfield S et al: Enteral hyperalimentation: An alternative to central venous hyperalimentation. Ann Intern Med 90:63, 1979

Recommended Dietary Allowances. National Research Council. Washington, DC, National Academy of Sciences, 1980

Nutritive Value of American Foods. Agriculture Handbook #456, Agricultural Research Service, USDA, 1975

Roe DA: *Drug-Induced Nutritional Deficiencies.* Westport, Conn., AVI, 1976

Rudman D et al: Ammonia content of food. Am J Clin Nutr 26:487, 1973

Torosian M, Rombeau J: Feeding by tube enterostomy. Surg Gynecol Obstet 150:918, 1980

Wilkerson H et al: Diagnostic evaluation of oral glucose tolerance tests in nondiabetic subjects after various levels of carbohydrate intake. N Engl J Med 262:1047, 1960

82
PARENTERAL NUTRITION

KHURSHEED N. JEEJEEBHOY
JEFFREY P. BAKER

In circumstances where, owing to disorders of the gastrointestinal tract, patients cannot eat a normal diet, do not absorb an oral diet efficiently, or deteriorate on oral feeding, partial or complete nourishment via the parenteral route is needed for varying lengths of time ranging from days to years. The particular combination of nutrients and the route of infusion vary with the needs of the patient and the duration of administration.

INDICATIONS FOR TOTAL PARENTERAL NUTRITION The indications for total parenteral nutrition (TPN) include the following situations:

1 For malnourished patients who are unable to eat or to absorb an oral diet. In such patients the diagnosis of malnutrition is based on a number of factors including previous dietary history, evidence of muscle wasting, hypoalbuminemia, edema, reduced skin fold thickness, and body weight (see Chap. 77). Weight alone is not sufficient to make the diagnosis of malnutrition because edema or previous obesity may mask the degree of nitrogen depletion actually present.

2 For bowel rest in patients with Crohn's disease, intestinal fistulas, and pancreatitis. In these patients food ingestion often results in exacerbation of symptoms with increased inflammation and high output through fistulas, preventing healing. When such patients are given nothing by mouth and receive TPN, they improve rapidly, heal fistulas without surgery, and maintain nutritional status.

3 For well-nourished patients who are unable to eat temporarily. In these cases a judgment has to be made about the probable length of time that oral diet will not be available. If the period is likely to exceed 10 to 14 days, then total parenteral nutrition should be administered to avoid undue wasting and malnutrition during starvation. This is especially important if sepsis and trauma complicate the clinical picture since both accelerate catabolism and tissue wasting.

4 For prolonged coma when tube feeding is not possible.

5 For nutritional support in patients with marked hypercatabolism, such as those with severe trauma and burns, even if some oral intake is possible.

6 For nutritional support during therapy for malignant disease. In many patients with malignancy weight loss is prominent and is accentuated by surgery, radiation, or chemotherapy. Chemotherapy is particularly prone to cause anorexia and mucosal inflammation that may limit oral intake. TPN given prior to and with chemotherapy results in an improved nutritional status in these patients.

7 For prophylactic use in malnourished patients especially those likely to undergo surgery.

NUTRIENT REQUIREMENTS DURING TPN **Energy and fluid requirements** Afebrile patients without septicemia require about 32 kcal per kilogram of ideal body weight daily for weight maintenance and 40 to 45 kcal/kg for weight gain when malnourished. The energy requirement increases to 60 kcal/kg per day with a body temperature of 40°C. While elective surgery does not increase these requirements significantly, septicemia does increase them by 50 percent; in burns exceeding 40 percent of the surface area, the requirements may increase by about 100 percent.

Basal fluid intake should be about 1 to 1.2 ml per kilocalorie infused. To this amount should be added a volume equivalent to losses from diarrhea, stomal output, nasogastric suction, and fistula drainage. In oliguric renal failure a basal intake of 750 to 1000 ml should be given plus a volume equal to that of urine and other losses. In patients with cardiac failure about 40 ml/kg can be infused provided that the sodium intake is restricted to between 20 and 50 meq per day.

Amino acid requirements The efficient functioning of the body requires maintenance of the integrity of the musculoskeletal system and viscera together with normal levels of enzymes, hormones, and plasma proteins. All are dependent on new protein synthesis to meet the demands of normal turnover, and this protein synthesis in turn requires that amino acids be available. A major objective of parenteral nutrition is to provide an adequate supply of amino acids for protein synthesis. The amount required is influenced by several factors. Severe injury, sepsis, and burns increase nitrogen losses as mentioned, making it necessary that larger amounts of amino acids be infused. The pattern of amino acids infused is important since unbalanced mixtures do not support protein synthesis. However, enrichment of amino acid mixtures with branched-chain amino acids may aid protein synthesis in septic patients. Finally, requirements are larger if amino acids are the sole energy source than if caloric demands are met by fat or carbohydrate.

In pure starvation the infusion of 100 g glucose per day reduces urinary nitrogen loss but does not produce positive nitrogen balance. Infusion of amino acids also reduces net nitrogen deficits and in large amounts (~2 g/kg per day) can induce a slight positive nitrogen balance. During starvation a fall in plasma insulin coupled with a rise in glucagon, cortisol, and catecholamines shifts body metabolism toward a fat economy by elevating plasma free fatty acid concentrations and increasing ketone body production. This elevation of plasma ketones may have a role in minimizing breakdown of muscle protein (and hence the negative nitrogen balance of prolonged starvation). Thus, it was postulated by some investigators that the infusion of glucose together with amino acids would be detrimental since a glucose-induced rise in insulin secretion would lower plasma free fatty acids and diminish plasma ketone concentrations, with the result that protein breakdown in muscle would be accelerated. While this area remains controversial, the authors believe that when amino acids are infused with glucose sufficient to meet caloric requirements, they are more efficiently used than when given alone. Significantly positive nitrogen balance is achieved in most malnourished patients (not suffering abnormal losses) by infusing only 0.5 to 1.0 g amino acids per kilogram of ideal body weight per day if nonprotein calories are optimal. Abnormal losses, such as protein-rich exudates in burns or upper gastrointestinal tract contents rich in pancreatic secretions increase requirements to between 1.5 and 2.0 g/kg per day. As the input of nonprotein energy is increased, nitrogen retention is augmented at all levels of amino acid intake until the input of nonprotein energy reaches 55 to 60 kcal per kilogram of ideal body weight. Beyond this point additional calories do not improve nitrogen retention significantly in adults.

Relation of nitrogen retention to the source of nonprotein energy Both carbohydrates and lipids can be infused with amino acids to provide sufficient nonprotein energy to meet metabolic requirements of the patient. The two types of substrate are equal in efficacy after an initial 3- to 4-day period for adaptation to the source of the energy. Hence the source of nonprotein energy chosen for use in a patient depends on factors other than its effect on nitrogen retention.

The first factor of importance is osmotic pressure. Concentrated glucose solutions are hyperosmolar and cause thrombosis when administered by peripheral vein. TPN regimens using glucose as the primary energy source thus require placement of a catheter in the superior vena cava where rapid blood flow quickly dilutes the hypertonic infusion. A second major consideration is the metabolic state of the patient. Glucose requires insulin for utilization, and hypertonic glucose solutions are probably not ideal in diabetic subjects. Conversely triglyceride emulsions might be contraindicated in hyperlipoproteinemic states. A third consideration is that infusing glucose as the sole source of calories causes increased metabolic rate and

CO_2 production. The implication is that infusing large amounts of glucose in hypermetabolic patients may accentuate ventilatory demands. In such patients giving half the nonprotein calories as fat reduces CO_2 excretion and aids protein synthesis.

Glucose infusion mixtures are simple and consist of 25 percent dextrose containing 2 percent amino acids together with necessary vitamins and minerals. Lipid emulsions are mixtures of triglyceride, phospholipid (as an emulsifying agent), and glycerol or sorbitol which is added to maintain isotonicity. Lipid can be infused with amino acid–dextrose mixtures using a Y connector to provide 50 to 80 percent of nonprotein calories. These concentrations can be given by peripheral vein without fear of thrombosis. Insulin is not required for metabolism of the fat; indeed, insulin concentrations are low, and free fatty acids and ketones are high during the administration of lipid when this is providing the major part of nonprotein calories. A valuable additional benefit is that lipid solutions can be discontinued abruptly without danger of hypoglycemia because insulin levels are not elevated. This aspect is important in critically ill patients who may require repeated and unpredictable alterations in their infusions, especially when surgery has to be carried out upon short notice. Finally, lipid infusions meet essential fatty acid requirements since linoleic acid is present in sufficient quantities if as little as 500 ml Intralipid (the commercially available triglyceride emulsion) is given daily. While essential fatty acid deficiency is rare in adults, biochemical evidence of deficiency may appear in as little as 1 week with TPN in the absence of lipid, and abnormalities of liver function and skin rash may follow.

It is also possible to carry out TPN with a 1:1 mixture of glucose and lipid calories. Substrate and hormone profiles in the blood following infusion of such a mixture are similar to those seen in the postprandial state.

Recommendations regarding source (type) of nonprotein energy In North America, in contrast to Europe and the United Kingdom, lipid-free systems were used almost exclusively in the past because triglyceride emulsions had not been approved for nonexperimental use. At the present time lipid-free systems are required only in patients with hyperchylomicronemia. The authors believe that most patients should receive lipid as a part of the regimen for total parenteral nutrition. The 80 percent lipid system can be given by peripheral vein, minimizing the threat of catheter sepsis and other catheter-related complications. The 1:1 lipid-glucose solution, given through a central venous line, simulates closely the normal diet and causes neither hyperinsulinemia nor hyperglycemia, thus almost eliminating the need for exogenous insulin.

Other requirements VITAMINS Vitamin requirements are given in Table 82-1. Amounts of vitamins sufficient to meet these needs must be added to the basic parenteral feeding solutions. It is important to avoid infusing excessive amounts of fat-soluble vitamins, in particular vitamins A and D, because of the danger of hypercalcemia and other toxic effects. A combination of 5 ml MVI with 10 ml Soluzyme plus vitamin C on alternate days will meet the requirements for vitamins A and D and will meet or exceed the need for most water-soluble vitamins. These solutions should be supplemented with vitamin K (5 mg) and vitamin B_{12} (200 μg) initially and at intervals of 3 weeks. Folate (5 mg) is given weekly. Biotin deficiency has been reported in infants on TPN, manifested by acidosis, rash, and alopecia.

ELECTROLYTES Electrolytes are an essential component of the fluids infused during total parenteral nutrition. Potassium, magnesium, and phosphorus are necessary for optimal nitrogen retention and tissue formation. In addition sodium and chloride are required to maintain osmolality and acid-base balance. Calcium is required to maintain calcium balance and prevent demineralization of bone. Recommended ranges of intake are given in Table 82-2.

TRACE ELEMENTS Trace elements, in particular zinc, copper, and chromium, are needed in courses of parenteral nutrition that exceed 1 to 2 weeks.

Zinc is essential for wound healing, for defense against infection, and for the activity of a number of enzymes. In its absence ageusia, loss of hair, night blindness, and a skin rash occur. The skin rash is often associated with superficial infec-

TABLE 82-1
Vitamin input and blood or plasma vitamin levels in six patients on long-term TPN

	Input provided by:*				*Plasma/blood vitamin level*	
Vitamin	*MVI, per 5 ml*	*Soluzyme + vitamin C, per 10 ml*	*Consequent average daily input*	*Daily (oral) recommended requirement*	*Average level observed in six patients*	*Normal range*
A	5000 IU		2500 IU	5000 IU	41.6	25–70 μg/dl
D	500 IU		250 IU	400 IU	34.4	28–42 ng/ml
E	5 mg		27.5 mg†	30 mg	0.65	0.8–1.2 ng/dl
B_1	22 mg	10 mg	16.0 mg	1.5 mg	226	10–64 ng/ml
B_2	5 mg	10 mg	7.5 mg	2.0 mg		
Niacinamide	50 mg	250 mg	150 mg	20.0 mg	16	3–6 μg/ml
Pantothenate	12 mg	45 mg	28 mg	10.0 mg	689	150–400 ng/ml
Pyridoxine	6 mg	5 mg	5.5 mg	2.5 mg	40	30–80 ng/ml
Ascorbic acid	500 mg	500 mg	500 mg	75 mg	2.0	0.4–1 mg/dl
Folic acid		5 mg	2.5 mg	0.15 mg	48	4–20 ng/dl
B_{12}		25 μg	12.5 μg	1.0 μg	872	100–900 pg/ml
Biotin				300 μg	63	200–500 pg/ml

* *Given on alternate days.*
† *Twenty-five milligrams of the average of 27.5 mg vitamin E per day is provided by infusing 500 ml Intralipid per day.*
SOURCE: *After KN Jeejeebhoy, Ann Coll Physicians Surg Can 9:287, 1976.*

tion due to staphylococci and yeast and responds only to zinc supplementation. Zinc deficiency also interferes with delayed hypersensitivity. In the absence of excessive gastrointestinal losses, 3 mg zinc per day is sufficient to meet needs. For each liter of intestinal fluids lost through fistulas, stomal output, suction, or diarrhea in patients with extensive resection of the small bowel, an additional 12 mg should be added. If the small bowel is intact, zinc losses are greater and about 17 mg zinc is required per liter of intestinal fluids lost per day.

Deficiency of *copper* causes anemia and neutropenia. The daily requirement is estimated to be between 0.3 and 0.5 mg with the larger intake to be given patients with major losses of gastrointestinal fluid. Copper should not be given to patients with obstructive jaundice.

The estimated requirement for *manganese* is about 0.8 mg per day. This element also should not be given if obstructive jaundice is present.

Deficiency of *chromium* is associated with glucose intolerance and neuropathy. The daily requirement of chromium is about 20 μg.

Deficiency of *selenium* has been associated with congestive cardiomyopathy and possibly muscle disease. Selenium requirements are probably somewhat greater than 10 μg per day.

ROUTES OF ADMINISTRATION **Central venous catheterization** This route allows infusion of fluids irrespective of osmolality and is comfortable for patients since repeated venipuncture is avoided. On the other hand, there is a risk of septicemia and thrombosis, especially if the catheter is not properly inserted and cared for during administration of the parenteral nutrition.

Basic principles of catheter insertion and care are as follows:

1 Catheters should always be placed and subsequently handled using completely aseptic technique. Face mask and sterile gloves are required.
2 The catheter should be documented radiologically to be in the superior vena cava prior to commencing TPN with hypertonic fluids. If the tip is in another central vein (e.g., the internal jugular), thrombosis may occur.
3 Catheters should always be introduced via puncture of a large central vein and not a peripheral vein.
4 The catheter used for TPN should not be used to withdraw blood or measure central venous pressure.
5 The skin puncture site should be cleansed weekly with a detergent, painted with a povidone iodine solution, and occluded with a dressing. A transparent plastic dressing is recommended since it is occlusive and easy to apply and allows for easy inspection of the insertion site for infection, drainage, bleeding, etc.
6 Barium-impregnated silicone rubber catheters (e.g., Silastic, made by Extracorporeal Medical Specialties, Inc., King of Prussia, Pennsylvania) should be used since they do not traumatize the central veins and are less likely to be surrounded with a fibrin clot.

TABLE 82-2
Recommended electrolyte intake per day, (mmol)

	Na	*K*	*Ca*	*Mg*	*P*
Basal*	100–120	80–100	10–15	10–12	12–16
Cardiac failure	20–50	80–100	10–15	10–12	12–16
Renal failure	20	†	†	†	†

* *To this basal intake, amounts of Na, K, Cl, and HCO_3 are added to meet losses from fistulas, nasogastric tube drainage, diarrhea, and stomal output.*
† *These ions are added as needed, on the basis of initial and continuing measurements of their circulating level and the clinical state of the patient.*

Peripheral venous infusion This route is safe and not as likely to be a source of sepsis or thrombotic complications. However the infused fluids must be isotonic or only mildly hypertonic. To achieve these conditions, nonprotein energy must be given mainly as lipid. A representative protocol is discussed below.

REPRESENTATIVE PROTOCOLS FOR ADMINISTRATION OF TOTAL PARENTERAL NUTRITION The three sample protocols given in Table 82-3 are designed for a 60-kg individual. They are intended to be administered throughout 24 h and provide 1 g amino acids and 40 nonprotein calories per kilogram of body weight. Proportionate modifications can be made for larger or smaller persons. Nonprotein energy is provided as (1) glucose, (2) 50 percent glucose and 50 percent lipid, or (3) 85 percent lipid and 15 percent glucose. The latter is suitable for peripheral venous administration. Preparation of the infusion materials must be carried out with great care. In most centers such preparation is done exclusively by specially trained pharmacists.

HOME PARENTERAL NUTRITION (HPN) It is now possible to administer parenteral nutrition at home in patients requiring prolonged nutritional support. A permanent silicone rubber catheter is placed in the superior vena cava via a subclavian or jugular vein and led to the outside through a subcutaneous tunnel. These catheters may be left in place for years without need for replacement. The patient receives monthly supplies of

TABLE 82-3
Representative daily protocols for total parenteral nutrition

Component solutions	*100% dextrose regimen*[a]	*50% dextrose–50% lipid regimen*[a]	*15% dextrose–85% lipid regimen*[a]
Amino acid 2.1%, dextrose 25%	3000 ml	—	—
Amino acid 4.2%, dextrose 25%	—	1500 ml	—
Amino acid 5%, dextrose 12.5%[b]	—	—	1500 ml
Lipid 10%[c,d]	—	1000 ml	1500 ml
Electrolyte mix[e]	60 ml	60 ml	60 ml
Trace element mix[f]	5 ml	5 ml	5 ml
Vitamins[g]	10 ml	10 ml	10 ml
Total volume	3075 ml	2575 ml	3075 ml
Total electrolytes:[h]			
Na^+, meq	125	125	132.5
K^+, meq	81	80	87
Ca^{2+}, meq	10	10	10
Mg^{2+}, meq	22	22	16
Cl^-, meq	193	192	148
Ac^-, meq	96	95	112.5
P, mg	582	582	693
Total protein, g	60	60	75
Total nonprotein calories, kcal	2550	2375	2286

[a] *All values represent total 24-h amount. Percentage of total calories derived from dextrose and lipid as noted.*
[b] *Obtained by mixing equal volumes of commercially available 10% amino acid and 25% dextrose.*
[c] *The triglyceride and dextrose–amino acid mixture are infused concurrently through a central venous line using a connector for continuous mixing.*
[d] *Intralipid 10% (Cutter Laboratories) or Liposyn 10% (Abbott Laboratories).*
[e] *Electrolyte mix contains 80 meq Na^+, 10 meq Ca^{2+}, 16 meq Mg^{2+}, 42 meq K^+, and 148 meq Cl^- per 60 ml.*
[f] *Trace-element mix contains 1 ml each of (1) 0.5 mg/ml elemental Cu as cupric chloride ($CuCl_2 \cdot 2H_2O$), 20 μg/ml elemental Cr as chromic nitrate [$Cr(NO_3)_3$], and 120 μg/ml of elemental Se as selenious acid (H_2SeO_3); (2) 120 μg/ml elemental I as potassium iodide (KI); (3) 3 mg/ml elemental Zn as zinc sulfate ($ZnSO_4 \cdot 7H_20$); and (4) 0.7 mg/ml elemental Mn as manganous chloride ($MnCl_3 \cdot 4H_20$).*
[g] *Vitamins include MVI injection (USV Pharmaceutical Corporation) once weekly and Soluzyme (Upjohn) six times weekly. Vitamin K is given as Synkayvite (Roche) 10 mg weekly.*
[h] *Total electrolytes are calculated on the assumption that the amino acid mixture used contains electrolytes. The total input of electrolytes in this table has been found to be capable of maintaining balance in patients without abnormal losses of gastrointestinal secretions.*

prepackaged nutrients ready for infusion. The nutrients are infused during the night while the patient is sleeping. A simple pneumatic cuff placed around the plastic bags containing the prepackaged infusion fluids is safe, inexpensive, and less cumbersome than mechanical-electrical delivery systems. The system is disconnected in the morning after a 10-h overnight infusion, and the catheter is capped and filled with a heparin solution. The patient is then free to carry out normal activities or work during the day. This method has revolutionized the life of persons who otherwise would require prolonged hospitalization for TPN.

PARTIAL PARENTERAL NUTRITION Whether amino acids should replace glucose and electrolyte solutions in the management of patients unable to eat for short periods (up to 1 week) following surgery, strokes, or other acute illnesses is debatable. In 7 days a patient has (on average) a net negative nitrogen balance of 100 to 110 g when receiving only glucose replacement. If amino acids are given at a level of 1 g/kg per day, the nitrogen loss is cut to 35 to 45 g. This difference is equal to only about 3 percent of the total nitrogen content in a 60-kg man. Since there is no evidence that such a small deficit makes any difference in clinical outcome (the nitrogen loss is quickly repleted when food intake is restored) and since amino acid solutions are expensive, amino acid infusion is not recommended for fasts of up to 1 week. Beyond 1 week, full TPN should probably be given.

In some patients oral intake is possible but the amounts ingested are inadequate for full nutrition. In such cases an estimate is made of the amount taken orally, and the deficiency is made up by parenteral means. When there is a question about how much of the ingested diet is absorbed (e.g., after bowel resection or with intestinal fistulas), the amount of nutrition given parenterally will have to be determined by trial and error, with evaluation of weight gain and other signs of clinical improvement.

REFERENCES

Anderson GH et al: Design and evaluation by nitrogen balance and blood aminograms of an amino acid mixture for total parenteral nutrition of adults with gastrointestinal disease. J Clin Invest 53:904, 1974

——— et al: Dose-response relationships between amino acid intake and blood levels in newborn infants. Am J Clin Nutr 30:1110, 1977

Batstone GF et al: Metabolic studies in subjects following thermal injury. Intermediary metabolites, hormones and tissue oxygenation. Burns 2:207, 1976

Blackburn GL et al: Protein sparing therapy during periods of starvation with sepsis or trauma. Ann Surg 177:588, 1973

Cahill GF Jr et al: Starvation in man. N Engl J Med 282:668, 1970

Craig RP et al: Intravenous glucose, amino acids and fat in the postoperative period. Lancet 2:8, 1977

Greenberg GR et al: Protein-sparing therapy in postoperative patients. Effects of added hypocaloric glucose or lipid. N Engl J Med 294:1411, 1976

Jeejeebhoy KN: Protein sparing effect of amino acids, in *Clinical Nutrition Update: Amino Acids,* HL Greene et al (eds). Chicago, American Medical Association, 1977

———: Role of measuring albumin synthesis as a way of measuring protein body repletion, ibid.

——— et al: Metabolic studies in total parenteral nutrition with lipid in man: Comparison with glucose. J Clin Invest 57:125, 1976

——— et al: Total parenteral nutrition at home: Studies in patients surviving 4 months to 5 years. Gastroenterology 71:943, 1976

Korentz RL, Meyer JH: Elemental diets—Facts and fantasies. Gastroenterology 78:393, 1980

Meng HC, Wilmore DW (eds): *Fat Emulsions in Parenteral Nutrition.* Chicago, American Medical Association, 1976

Munro HN: General aspects of the regulation of protein metabolism by diet and by hormones, in *Mammalian Protein Metabolism,* HN Munro, JB Allison (eds). New York, Academic, 1964, vol I

Rudman D et al: Elemental balances during intravenous hyperalimentation of underweight adult subjects. J Clin Invest 55:94, 1975

83
DISORDERS OF VITAMINS: DEFICIENCY, EXCESS, AND ERRORS OF METABOLISM

(For vitamin D see Chap. 340 and for the hematologic vitamins see Chap. 327)

JEAN D. WILSON

The role of specific vitamins in disease states has changed strikingly within the past few decades. Since the pathophysiology of deficiency and excess states was elucidated and nutritional education became more widespread, disorders of single vitamins are less frequent, even in developing nations. As a consequence, the disorders are now rarely endemic, and abnormalities of vitamins usually occur either as a portion of a generalized state of malnutrition, as a result of food faddism, as a complication of a more widespread disease state such as a malabsorption syndrome, as complications of complex therapy such as hemodialysis, or as the result of an inborn error of metabolism. Nevertheless, the disorders are still encountered on occasion in general hospitals, usually coexisting with other clinical problems. The biochemical means of proving a diagnosis, once suspected, are limited, and since nonspecific vitamin therapy is a constituent of standard medical supportive care, the role of vitamin deficiency in disease states is frequently not recognized. As a consequence, an understanding of the various manifestations of vitamin deficiency and a high index of suspicion in the appropriate clinical setting are essential, and in some instances demonstration of a response to replacement therapy is the most accurate way to confirm a diagnosis.

In considering the pathophysiology of vitamins several broad points are worth emphasis. One, the fact that organic compounds cannot be synthesized within the body and are required constituents of the diet of humans is the result of mutations. In some instances, such as the limited ability to synthesize thiamine, the requirement is common to many if not all animals, and the mutation must have occurred early in evolution; in others, such as the single gene defect that prevents ascorbic acid synthesis, humans share the defect only with a few other species such as the guinea pig. At any rate, the provision of vitamins in the diet is a form of therapy for an inborn error of metabolism. The feature that separates vitamins from other required organic constituents in the diet is that their requirements are small in contrast to the relatively large amounts of essential amino acids and essential fatty acids required. This is a consequence of the fact that, by and large, these organic compounds function not as major building blocks of tissue mass but rather as prosthetic groups for quantitatively minor tissue constituents or as catalytic cofactors for biological reactions; like most catalysts they are required only in relatively small amounts. Second, deficiency of some vitamins has never been clearly established in humans (e.g., pantothenic acid) implying that these vitamins are either so ubiquitous in food sources or are conserved so efficiently by the body that deficiency can become manifest, if at all, only in the context of a mixed nutritional and vitamin deficiency. Third, despite the enormous amounts of vitamins ingested in this country toxicity is common only for the fat-soluble vitamins A and D, implying either that the capacity to excrete excess water-soluble vitamins is large or that these compounds are relatively innocuous. Fourth, alcoholism is the background upon which most vitamin deficiencies develop in the United States. This is the consequence of several interlocking factors including diminished intake, impairment of absorption and storage of vitamins, and in some instances possible predisposing genetic factors. In those instances in which alcoholism is not associated with an increased frequency of disease (e.g., pellagra) the etiology of the disorder is more complicated than a simple deficiency state.

DEFICIENCY OF NIACIN (PELLAGRA)

NORMAL PHYSIOLOGY OF NIACIN Biochemistry *Niacin* is the generic term for nicotinic acid (pyridine 3-carboxylic acid) and derivatives that exhibit the nutritional activity of nicotinic acid (Fig. 83-1). In one sense niacin is not a vitamin since it can be formed from the essential amino acid tryptophan. In the human an average of about 1 mg of niacin is formed from 60 mg of dietary tryptophan. Accordingly, estimates of the adequacy of dietary intake must take into account the tryptophan content of the diet as well as the content of niacin. Many foodstuffs, especially cereals, contain bound forms of niacin from which the vitamin is not nutritionally available.

FIGURE 83-1
The structure and principle functions of some of the vitamins associated with human disorders.

VITAMIN	ACTIVE DERIVATIVE OR COFACTOR FORM	PRINCIPAL FUNCTION
Niacin 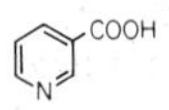 (COOH, N)	Nicotinamide Adenine Dinucleotide Phosphate (NADP) and Nicotine Adenine Dinucleotide (NAD)	Coenzymes for Oxidations and Reductions
Thiamine 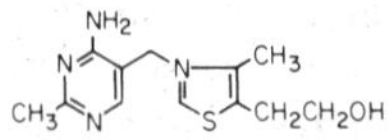 (NH_2, N, CH_3, S, CH_2CH_2OH)	Thiamine Diphosphate	Coenzyme for Cleavage of Carbon-Carbon Bands
Pyridoxine 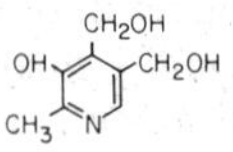 (CH_2OH, OH, CH_2OH, CH_3, N)	Pyridoxal Phosphate	Cofactor for Enzymes of Amino Acid Metabolism
Riboflavin 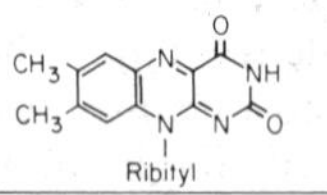 (CH_3, CH_3, N, NH, O, Ribityl)	Flavin Mononucleotide (FMN) and Flavin Adenine Dinucleotide (FAD)	Cofactor for Oxidation-Reduction Reactions and Covalently Attached Prosthetic Groups for Some Enzymes
Ascorbic Acid 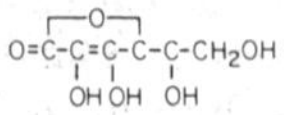 (O=C-C=C-C-C-CH2OH; OH OH OH)	Ascorbic Acid and Dehydroascorbic Acid	Participation as a Redox Ion in Many Biological Oxidation Reactions
Vitamin A 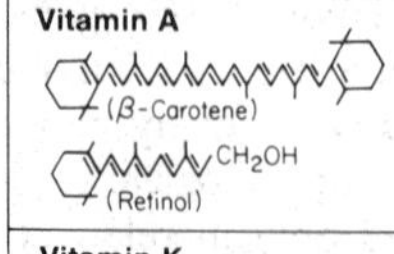 ((β-Carotene); CH_2OH (Retinol))	Retinol, Retinal, and Retinoic Acid	Formation of Carotenoid Proteins (Vision) and Glycoproteins (Epithelial Cell Function)
Vitamin K 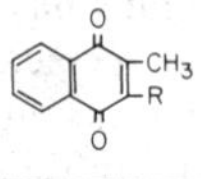 (O, CH_3, R, O)	Menaquinone	Cofactor for Post-Translational Carboxylation of Many Proteins Including Essential Clotting Factors

The absorption, tissue distribution, and metabolism of the vitamin are poorly understood. In most species approximately a fifth of the vitamin is decarboxylated, and the remainder is excreted in the urine as methylated products, largely *N*-methylnicotinamide and its derivatives.

Mechanism of action Niacin is an essential component of nicotinamide-adenine dinucleotide (NAD) and nicotinamide-adenine dinucleotide phosphate (NADP), coenzymes for many oxidation-reduction reactions. Nicotinic acid is converted to nicotinamide which subsequently reacts with phosphoribosyl pyrophosphate to form nicotinamide mononucleotide; the latter then reacts with ATP to form NAD, and the reaction with a second molecule of ATP results in the formation of NADP.

Requirements The requirements and recommended daily allowances for niacin and tryptophan are listed in Tables 76-1 and 76-2. In contrast to most vitamins there is no clear evidence that requirement for niacin is increased during pregnancy. The major factor that influences requirements may be the amino acid composition of the diet.

EXPERIMENTAL DEPLETION After the institution of a diet deficient in niacin and tryptophan, the urinary excretion of niacin metabolites decreases rapidly, reaching minimal values ($<$ 1.5 mg per day) after 1 to 2 months and remaining constant thereafter. Clinical evidence of deficiency is usually noted shortly after excretion becomes stable at a low level and consists of dermatitis, glossitis, stomatitis, diarrhea, proctitis, mental depression, heartburn, abdominal pain, vaginitis, dysphagia, and amenorrhea, findings similar to those in pellagra.

CLINICAL DEFICIENCY Frequency and clinical context Pellagra was previously an endemic disease in the American south and in many other parts of the world. Endemic pellagra is usually associated with a high intake of maize (American corn) and can be cured by the administration of niacin; nevertheless, the fact that large populations of people exist on a diet in which maize is the major source of protein but nevertheless are free of endemic pellagra implies that the relation between maize intake and the development of the disease is not straightforward. As a consequence, the concept of the pathogenesis of pellagra has evolved over the years from that of a pure vitamin deficiency or a mixed deficiency of tryptophan and available niacin in the diet to that of a more complicated disorder. Two other factors may be involved in the etiology of pellagra. First, the disorder may be due to an imbalance in dietary amino acids. This concept is based upon the fact that the niacin equivalent (available niacin and tryptophan) of maize, although low, is no lower than that of some cereals that are unassociated with endemic pellagra and that the leucine content of common varieties of maize is high. A hybrid strain of maize, opaque 2, differs from the ordinary grain in having lower leucine but similar tryptophan and niacin content. Dogs fed a diet rich in conventional maize or a diet rich in opaque 2 maize supplemented with leucine develop experimental pellagra, whereas dogs fed the opaque 2 maize alone do not. This finding presumably explains why pellagra occurs in individuals who ingest a diet rich in millet (sorghum, jowar), which has a leucine content similar to that of maize but a niacin and tryptophan content (and availability) equivalent to that of rice. Leucine is believed to inhibit the synthesis of nicotinic acid mononucleotide and consequently the synthesis of NAD and NADP. Thus, the development of symptomatic niacin "deficiency" may depend on the amino acid content of the rest of the diet as well as upon the intake of the vitamin and its precursors. The second possibility is that treatment of maize with alkali in the preparation of foods in Latin America serves both to hydrolyze bound nicotinic acid and hence enhance its bioavailability and to inactivate toxins that may accumulate in stored grain contaminated with molds. In either case the effect would be to prevent the development of pellagra.

Whatever the exact cause, endemic pellagra disappeared in the United States coincident with the improvement in nutritional education and the institution of widespread supplementation of grain cereals with niacin. However, pellagra is an occasional secondary manifestation of two disorders that profoundly affect tryptophan metabolism, the carcinoid syndrome in which up to 60 percent of tryptophan is catabolized by what is ordinarily a minor pathway of metabolism (see Chap. 131) and Hartnup disease (see Chap. 92), an autosomal recessive disorder in which several amino acids including tryptophan are absorbed poorly from the diet. In both disorders the symptoms of pellagra appear to be the consequence of diminished availability of effective niacin equivalents, and in both the symptoms and signs of pellagra can be cured by the administration of large amounts of the vitamin.

Manifestations The typical presentation of pellagra is that of a chronic wasting disease associated with dermatitis, dementia, and diarrhea. The characteristic dermatitis is bilateral, symmetrical, present in sites exposed to sunlight, and due to photosensitivity. The mental changes are less discrete; fatigue, insomnia, and apathy may precede the development of an encephalopathy characterized by confusion, disorientation, hallucination and loss of memory, and eventually, frank organic psychosis. Paresthesias and polyneuritis may be the result of coexisting deficiencies of other vitamins. The diarrhea, when it occurs, is a portion of a widespread inflammation of the mucous surfaces; other gastrointestinal manifestations include achlorhydria, glossitis, stomatitis, and vaginitis. The course is slowly progressive over a several-year period before death supervenes, usually due to secondary complications.

The exact relation between the known coenzyme functions of NAD and NADP and these various symptoms has not been defined. Levels of NAD and NADP in erythrocytes are lower in patients with pellagra than in normal individuals, but the coenzymes are essential to so many reactions in intermediary metabolism that profound deficiency of the coenzymes is incompatible with life. The mental changes in pellagra may be associated with diminished conversion of tryptophan to serotonin.

Diagnosis No biochemical test is of diagnostic value, and diagnosis must be based upon suspicion and response to replacement therapy. As would be predicted, the urinary excretion of the metabolites of nicotinic acid and tryptophan is lower than average but not lower than in patients with generalized malnutrition (Table 77-4). Plasma tryptophan and erythrocyte NAD and NADP levels may be low. Histopathology of the skin lesions is characterized by hyperkeratosis, hyperpigmentation, and desquamation.

Management The administration of small amounts of niacin (10 mg/day) in the face of limiting amounts of dietary tryptophan may be sufficient to cure endemic pellagra. Large amounts (40 to 200 mg/day) may be required in Hartnup disease and in the carcinoid syndrome.

DEFICIENCY OF THIAMINE (BERIBERI)

NORMAL PHYSIOLOGY OF THIAMINE Biochemistry Thiamine consists of a pyrimidine ring and a thiazole moiety linked by a methylene bridge (Fig. 83-1). The vitamin is synthesized by a variety of plants and microorganisms but not ordinarily by animals. However, rats and pigeons fed a thiamine-free diet

can be protected from developing symptoms of deficiency by giving large quantities of the pyrimidine and thiazole moieties, suggesting that animals have a small capacity to couple the subunits together. Limited amounts of the vitamin may also be synthesized by microorganisms in the gastrointestinal tract. Thiamine is absorbed from the diet both by an active-transport process and by passive diffusion. The capacity to absorb the vitamin in the human intestine is limited to about 5 mg/day. Approximately 25 to 30 mg is stored in the body, 80 percent as thiamine diphosphate (pyrophosphate), 10 percent as thiamine triphosphate, and the remainder as free thiamine and thiamine monophosphate. Large amounts are present in skeletal muscles (about half of body stores), heart, liver, kidneys, and brain. Three enzymes are known to participate in the formation of thiamine phosphate esters—a pyrophosphate kinase that catalyzes the formation of thiamine diphosphate from ATP and thiamine, a phosphoryl transferase that catalyzes the formation of thiamine triphosphate from ATP and the diphosphate, and a pyrophosphatase that hydrolyzes thiamine triphosphate to thiamine monophosphate. A number of thiaminase enzymes inactivate thiamine by splitting the vitamin into its two component parts. Several metabolites of thiamine are excreted in the urine, principally thiamine itself (which is secreted by the renal tubules), an acetylated metabolite, and end products of thiamine catabolism, principally derivatives of thiazole acetate and pyrimidine carboxylate.

Mechanism of action Thiamine diphosphate acts as a coenzyme for reactions that have in common the cleavage of carbon-carbon bonds—the oxidative decarboxylation of alpha keto acids (pyruvate and alpha ketoglutarate) and keto analogues of leucine, isoleucine, and valine, and the transketolase reaction in the pentose phosphate pathway. It was originally believed that the entire spectrum of changes in thiamine deficiency is the result of inhibition of these key enzymatic reactions and, in some instances, the accumulation of the proximal metabolites. However, circumstantial evidence now suggests that thiamine may have a specific role in neural conduction independent of its coenzymatic function in general metabolism. Thiamine and its esters are located in axonal membranes of nerves, and electrical stimulation of nerves results in the hydrolysis and release of both thiamine diphosphate and triphosphate.

Requirements The recommended daily allowances for thiamine are described in Tables 76-1 and 76-2. The vitamin has a widespread distribution in food and is absent only from oils, fats, cassava, and refined sugar. A large portion of the vitamin in vegetable products is in the form of thiamine itself. The outer layers of cereal grains are especially rich in the vitamin; hence, machine-milled rice is a poor source. In animal tissues thiamine is present largely in the form of phosphate esters. The esters are dephosphorylated by phosphatases in the intestine, and only the free vitamin is absorbed. A substantial loss of the vitamin takes place during cooking above 100°C.

Several factors influence the absorption and metabolism of the vitamin (and hence alter daily requirements). One is the presence of thiaminases in foods including fresh fish, clams, shrimp, mussels, and some raw animal tissues. Some microorganisms in the colon may also contain thiaminases. Thiamine requirements are also influenced by carbohydrate and caloric intake. Daily needs decrease when fat forms a large part of the diet and increase as carbohydrate intake increases. As is true for many vitamins, requirements are increased in pregnancy, during lactation, in thyrotoxicosis, and by fever. Accelerated loss of thiamine from the body may occur as the result of diuretic therapy, hemodialysis, peritoneal dialysis, and diarrhea. Defective intestinal absorption can occur in malabsorption states, alcoholism, chronic malnutrition, and in folate deficiency.

EXPERIMENTAL DEPLETION Following the institution of a thiamine-free diet in control subjects, thiamine excretion in the urine decreases to 5 percent of the control value after a week and becomes undetectable after 2 weeks. However, the excretion of the pyrimidine and thiazole catabolites of thiamine remains about 0.8 mg per day for as long as a month, indicating that the body pool is slowly utilized during a period of deficient intake.

Within a week after the institution of a deficient diet, subjects develop a resting tachycardia, followed by the onset of muscle weakness, decreased deep-tendon reflexes, and (in some) a sensory neuropathy. Subjective symptoms include generalized malaise, headache, nausea, and aching of the muscles. Development of these symptoms is paralleled by a fall in red blood cell transketolase activity. Within a week of thiamine repletion (2 mg per day) all abnormal physical findings disappear; the subjective symptoms clear after 2 weeks. (Experimental depletion in humans has never been carried to the point of development of severe cerebral or cardiovascular symptoms.)

CLINICAL DEFICIENCY **Frequency and clinical context** In most developed nations thiamine deficiency occurs in alcoholics or food faddists or in the context of special clinical situations, such as refeeding after starvation, chronic peritoneal dialysis or hemodialysis, or the administration of glucose to asymptomatic but thiamine-depleted patients. In developing countries the causes derive mainly from the consumption of milled rice and of foods containing thiaminases and (possibly) other antithiamine factors.

Factors involved in development of thiamine deficiency in chronic alcoholics include low thiamine intake, impaired thiamine absorption and storage, accelerated destruction of thiamine diphosphate, and varying degrees of energy expenditure. However, clinical manifestations of thiamine deficiency develop in only a small fraction of alcoholics and other chronically malnourished persons. Some studies suggest that genetic factors may be involved in the pathogenesis of clinical manifestations, namely in fibroblasts cultured from patients with the Wernicke-Korsakoff syndrome the thiamine-requiring transketolase binds thiamine diphosphate only a tenth as avidly as controls. This finding implies an underlying genetic abnormality that is clinically silent when the diet is adequate but becomes overt if thiamine intake is low or marginal. It is possible, therefore, that beriberi occurs against the background of an otherwise asymptomatic genetic polymorphism.

Manifestations The two major syndromes of thiamine deficiency involve the cardiovascular (wet beriberi) and nervous systems (dry beriberi and the Wernicke-Korsakoff syndrome). The typical patient has mixed symptoms involving both the cardiovascular and nervous systems, but pure cardiovascular, pure polyneuritic, and pure cerebral forms also occur. The factors that determine the relative preponderance of these manifestations are related in part to the duration and severity of the deficiency, the degree of physical exertion, and the caloric intake. Severe physical exertion, high carbohydrate intake, and a moderate degree of chronic deficiency favor wet beriberi with little or no peripheral neuritis, whereas an equal deficiency with caloric restriction and relative inactivity favors the development of dry (polyneuritic) beriberi.

Cardiovascular system Beriberi heart disease comprises three major physiologic derangements: (1) peripheral vasodilatation leading to a high-output state, (2) biventricular myocardial failure, and (3) retention of sodium and water leading to edema.

In the chronic form, the peripheral vasodilatation leads to increased arteriovenous shunting of blood, rapid circulation time, tachycardia, increased cardiac output, and a venous congestive state characterized by elevated peripheral venous pressure, elevated right ventricular end-diastolic pressure, decreased arteriovenous extraction of oxygen, sodium retention, and edema. Disordered flow of blood to the organs (decreased cerebral and renal blood flow and increased flow to muscles) is common. Cardiac output increases to such an extent that, notwithstanding the lowered peripheral vascular resistance, ventricular work, arterial blood pressure, and pulmonary wedge pressure tend to be elevated. Temporary appearance or worsening of hypertension occurs commonly during thiamine repletion, presumably due to closing of arteriovenous shunts and temporary volume overload.

In acute fulminant cardiovascular (shoshin) beriberi, the myocardial lesion appears to be the central feature in a course in which severe dyspnea, intense thirst, restlessness, and anxiety lead to acute cardiovascular collapse and death within hours to days. Physical findings include stocking-glove cyanosis, extreme tachycardia, marked cardiomegaly, hepatomegaly, arterial bruits, and neck vein distention. The venous pressure is high, and the circulation time is rapid. Because of the fulminant course edema may be minimal or absent. Administration of thiamine rapidly restores peripheral vascular resistance, but improvement in the myocardial abnormality may be delayed so that low-output failure may supervene during treatment.

Nervous system Three types of nervous system involvement occur: peripheral neuropathy, Wernicke's encephalopathy (cerebral beriberi), and the Korsakoff syndrome. The neuropathy may or may not be painful and is characterized by a symmetrical impairment of sensory, motor, and reflex function that affects the distal segments of limbs more severely than the proximal ones. The histological lesion consists of a noninflammatory degeneration of myelin sheaths. No meaningful distinction can be made between this disorder and so-called alcoholic neuropathy either on the basis of clinical or of neurologic criteria.

The symptoms of Wernicke's encephalopathy ordinarily develop in an orderly sequence and consist of vomiting, nystagmus (horizontal more commonly than vertical), palsies of the rectus muscles leading to unilateral or bilateral ophthalmoplegia (and decrease in the nystagmus), fever, ataxia, and progressive mental deterioration that eventuates in a global confusional state and may progress to coma and death. Improvement occurs after the institution of thiamine replacement, although symptoms of Korsakoff's syndrome may supervene. Thus, the eye palsies are corrected, the nystagmus improves in half, the ataxia improves or disappears in two-thirds, and the global confusion state disappears to be replaced by Korsakoff's syndrome. The latter consists of retrograde amnesia, impaired ability to learn, and (usually) confabulation. The patient is usually alert and responsive and exhibits no serious defect in behavior. Once the Korsakoff disorder supervenes, recovery (complete or partial) can be expected in only half.

In summary, the Wernicke's encephalopathy and the amnesic psychosis of the Korsakoff syndrome are not separate clinical events; instead, the changing ocular and ataxic signs, the transformation of the global confusional state into the amnesic-confabulatory syndrome, and the subsequent development of a nonconfabulatory amnesic state are successive stages in the recovery from a single disease process. The clinical spectrum, differential diagnosis, course, and pathology of cerebral beriberi are discussed in greater detail in Chap. 363.

Diagnosis Various biochemical tests based on thiamine metabolism or the biochemical functions of thiamine diphosphate have been developed to detect thiamine deficiency. These include the measurement of blood thiamine, pyruvate, α-ketoglutarate, lactate, and glyoxylate; the urinary excretion of thiamine and thiamine metabolites; a thiamine-loading test; and measurement of urinary methylglyoxal content. At present the most reliable method is the measurement of whole blood or erythrocyte transketolase activity. Any enhancement in enzymatic activity resulting from added thiamine diphosphate (TPP) is referred to as the TPP effect (expressed in percent). If the activity of the enzyme is increased more than 15 percent by the added thiamine diphosphate, then a deficiency state is probably present (Table 77-4). Due to variability in transketolase activity, measurement of isolated levels of the enzyme is not useful, but demonstration of an increase in activity after treatment coupled with a significant stimulation in vitro by added thiamine diphosphate prior to treatment suggests the presence of thiamine deficiency.

Another criterion for the diagnosis of thiamine deficiency is the assessment of clinical response to thiamine administration. Clinical improvement may be dramatic in cardiovascular beriberi, an increase in blood pressure and decrease in heart rate may be seen within 12 h after start of therapy. Diuresis and reduction in heart size may be apparent within 1 to 2 days.

Management Prompt administration of thiamine is indicated when beriberi is diagnosed or suspected. Fifty milligrams per day should be given intramuscularly for several days after which 2.5 to 5 mg per day can be administered by mouth. Larger amounts are usually not absorbed. All patients should also receive other water-soluble vitamins in therapeutic quantities.

THIAMINE-RESPONSIVE INBORN ERRORS OF METABOLISM
A number of thiamine-responsive inborn errors of metabolism have been described in which patients respond to pharmacological doses of thiamine. These include thiamine-responsive megaloblastic anemia, for which the mechanism is unknown; thiamine-responsive lactic acidosis, which is due to low activity of pyruvate carboxylase in liver; thiamine-responsive branched-chain ketoaciduria, which is due to low activity of a ketoacid dehydrogenase; and intermittent cerebellar ataxia which may result from an abnormal pyruvate dehydrogenase. In addition, it is possible that the autosomal recessive disorder known as subacute necrotizing encephalomyelopathy (Leigh's disease) may be related to a diminished amount of thiamine triphosphate in neural tissue; a factor has been isolated from urine of such patients that inhibits the enzyme that synthesizes thiamine triphosphate. The clinical response of patients with Leigh's disease to pharmacological doses of the vitamin appears to be minor, however.

PYRIDOXINE (VITAMIN B_6)

NORMAL PHYSIOLOGY OF PYRIDOXINE Biochemistry The biological activity of the vitamin B_6 group is displayed by pyridoxine, pyridoxal, and pyridoxamine and their 5-phosphate esters (Fig. 83-1). The coenzyme form is pyridoxal 5-phosphate, and the other compounds owe their enzymatic activity to conversion by tissues to pyridoxal 5-phosphate. The vitamin is widely and uniformly distributed in all foods; muscle meats, liver, vegetables, and whole-grain cereals are among the best sources.

Mechanism of action Pyridoxal phosphate acts as a cofactor for a large number of enzymes involved in amino acid metabolism, including transaminases, synthetases, and hydroxylases. In humans the vitamin is of particular importance in the metabolism of tryptophan, glycine, serine, glutamate, and the sulfur-containing amino acids. Pyridoxal phosphate is also required for the synthesis of the heme precursor δ-amino levulinic acid. A large portion of body stores of pyridoxine is in muscle phosphorylase, where it functions to stabilize the enzyme rather than catalytically. It also plays a vital (but poorly understood role) in neuronal excitability, possibly as a result of its function in transulfuration reactions or γ-amino butyric acid metabolism.

Requirements The recommended daily allowances for the vitamin are described in Tables 76-1 and 76-2. Even more than for most vitamins, the requirement is increased in pregnancy and by the ingestion of estrogens. In both conditions abnormal tryptophan metabolites are excreted in urine, and this can be prevented by supplementation with pyridoxine. Estrogens appear to inhibit selectively the role of pyridoxal phosphate in tryptophan metabolism. In addition, pyridoxine requirement may be increased by high protein intake. The ingestion of ethanol interferes with the metabolism of pyridoxal phosphate, the ethanol metabolite acetaldehyde displacing the coenzyme from proteins and thus enhancing its degradation.

EXPERIMENTAL DEPLETION The feeding of pyridoxine-deficient diets to experimental subjects leads to chemical evidence of deficiency (increased xanthurenic acid and decreased pyridoxine in urine) within a week. Electroencephalographic abnormalities appear within 3 weeks in subjects with previously normal EEGs, and some subjects subsequently have grand mal seizures. Deficiency induced with the pyridoxine antagonist desoxypyridoxine causes, in addition, seborrheic dermatitis, cheilosis, glossitis, and severe systemic symptoms such as nausea, vomiting, weakness, and dizziness.

CLINICAL DEFICIENCY Frequency and clinical context The widespread occurrence of the vitamin in food is probably the reason that a naturally occurring pure pyridoxine deficiency has never been recognized except when the pyridoxine content of food is either destroyed or converted to less available protein-bound forms during processing, as has occurred in some infant formulas. It is a paradox, therefore, that at present pyridoxine deficiency is frequent in the United States. This is because many commonly used drugs act as pyridoxine antagonists. Hydrazines such as *isoniazid* induce peripheral neuritis that can be prevented by pyridoxine supplementation; these drugs combine with pyridoxal or pyridoxal phosphate to form hydrazones. The hydrazones may act to inhibit enzymes such as pyridoxal kinase, to induce convulsions directly, and to accelerate pyridoxine loss in the urine and thus induce a vitamin deficiency. *Cycloserine* also causes an increase in the excretion of the vitamin in the urine and produces profound neurologic effects, presumably by forming a complex with pyridoxal phosphate that competes with the cofactor for apoenzymes. *Penicillamine* acts as an antagonist by forming a thiazolidine derivative with pyridoxal phosphate. In each of these instances abnormal tryptophan metabolism and convulsions can be prevented by supplementation with the vitamin.

Diagnosis Estimates of vitamin deficiency have been based upon the correction of clinical signs of deficiency following administration of the vitamin, measurement of the excretion of tryptophan metabolites after tryptophan-loading tests, measurement of various amino acid transferase activities in blood, and measurement of the excretion of pyridoxine or its metabolites or of oxalate in the urine (Table 77-4). The most commonly used index is the measurement of urinary tryptophan metabolites, particularly xanthurenic acid, following tryptophan loading. Alternatively, cystathionine can be assayed after administration of a methionine load. In vitro measurement of red blood cell glutamic pyruvic transaminase in the presence and absence of pyridoxal phosphate may be a better indicator of pyridoxine status than either loading test.

Management The appropriate management is prevention of deficiency. Supplementation of the diet with 30 mg of pyridoxine normalizes tryptophan metabolism in pregnancy, in users of contraceptives, and in patients taking isoniazid. Doses as high as 100 mg per day may be required in subjects taking penicillamine.

PYRIDOXINE-RESPONSIVE DISEASES Several genetic conditions cause abnormalities in vitamin B_6 metabolism. In one group, infants develop convulsions and brain damage and die if not provided with large daily supplements of pyridoxine; these children have an apoenzyme for glutamic acid decarboxylase that has a decreased binding affinity for pyridoxal phosphate. Consequently they do not form normal amount of γ-amino butyric acid, a physiologic inhibitor of neurologic activity in the brain. Another group of patients has pyridoxine-responsive chronic anemia; pyridoxine supplementation results in prompt hematologic improvement but does not correct the coexisting morphological abnormality in the erythrocytes.

The synthesis of cystathionine from homocystine and serine and its cleavage to cysteine and homoserine are catalyzed by two pyridoxal phosphate enzymes. The biochemical changes that occur in deficiency of these two enzymes and in xanthurenic aciduria due to kynureninase deficiency have been reviewed by Mudd. Some patients with vitamin B_6–responsive xanthurenic aciduria or cystathioninuria have a mutant apoenzyme that interacts abnormally with pyridoxal phosphate in a manner that can be largely overcome by elevated concentrations of the cofactor. In contrast, the vitamin B_6 response in patients with homocystinuria due to cystathionine synthetase deficiency is not due to restoration of the affected enzyme to normal levels but to an enhancement of the activity of the residual amount of normal enzyme present.

RIBOFLAVIN

Riboflavin in the form of the coenzymes flavin mononucleotide (FMN) and flavin adenine dinucleotide (FAD) participates in a variety of oxidation-reduction reactions (Fig. 83-1). In addition, covalently attached flavins are essential to the structure of such enzymes as succinate dehydrogenase and monoamine oxidase. The vitamin is absorbed from the gastrointestinal tract either as free riboflavin or the 5′-phosphate by a specific transport process. The requirements and recommended daily allowances are listed in Tables 76-1 and 76-2. Covalently linked vitamin accounts for less than a tenth of the tissue pool. The vitamin is excreted in urine predominantly in the free form although a small fraction of the daily turnover is the result of catabolism by microorganisms in the gastrointestinal tract.

Clinical riboflavin deficiency can be induced in human subjects by feeding a riboflavin-deficient diet and/or by the administration of riboflavin antagonists such as galactoflavin. The deficiency syndrome is characterized by sore throat, hyperemia and edema of the pharyngeal and oral mucous membranes, cheilosis, angular stomatitis, glossitis, seborrheic dermatitis, and normochromic, normocytic anemia associated with pure red cell hypoplasia of the bone marrow. These features can be rapidly and completely reversed after riboflavin administration. Thyroid hormones and adrenal steroids both act to enhance FMN and FAD synthesis whereas certain psychotropic agents (phenothiazines and tricyclic antidepressants) competitively inhibit flavin coenzyme biosynthesis, but these agents alone are not sufficient to induce a deficiency state. Indeed, riboflavin deficiency almost invariably occurs in combination with other vitamin deficiencies. Certain features of the syndrome such as glossitis and dermatitis can also result from deficiency of other vitamins as well.

DEFICIENCY OF VITAMIN C (SCURVY)

NORMAL PHYSIOLOGY OF VITAMIN C Biochemistry In most animals ascorbic acid (vitamin C) can be readily synthesized from glucose. However, humans, other primates, and the guinea pig are unable to synthesize L-ascorbic acid and require vitamin C in the diet to prevent scurvy. These species can perform the various reactions required for the biosynthesis of the vitamin from D-glucose except for one step, the conversion of L-gluconogammalactone to L-ascorbic acid. The enzyme that catalyzes this reaction (L-gluconolactone oxidase) is missing because of a mutation; thus the need for vitamin C in the diet is the result of a defect in carbohydrate metabolism.

Mechanism of action L-Ascorbic acid readily undergoes reversible oxidation and reduction as follows:

$$\text{L-Ascorbic acid} \rightleftharpoons \text{dehydro-L-ascorbic acid} + 2H^+ + 2e$$

This property of the vitamin is of paramount importance in understanding its physiologic role. Indeed, several systems have been characterized in animal tissues in which L-ascorbic acid is coupled with other redox agents. However, the vitamin does not act as a conventional cofactor since its requirement can usually be replaced by other compounds with similar redox properties. The most clearly established functional role of the vitamin is in the synthesis of collagen; absence of the vitamin in vitro leads to impairment of peptidyl hydroxylation of procollagen and a reduction in collagen formation and excretion by the connective tissue cell. Nonhydroxylated collagen is unstable and cannot form the triple helix required for participation in normal tissue structure. Many of the clinical findings in scurvy result from this defect in collagen synthesis, including the capillary fragility that underlies the hemorrhagic features, the poor healing of wounds, and (in part) the bony abnormalities of children. Collagens that normally have the highest content of hydroxyproline are most affected, accounting for the characteristic early disruption of blood vessel adventitia, media, and basal laminae. Ascorbic acid also functions to prevent oxidation of tetrahydrofolate and thus protect the active folic acid pool and to regulate iron distribution and storage, probably by influencing the valence of stored iron and maintaining a normal ratio of ferritin to hemosiderin. Scorbutic patients excrete incompletely oxidized products of tyrosine metabolism, but the clinical significance of these metabolites is not clear.

Requirements The recommended daily allowances for vitamin C are described in Tables 76-1 and 76-2. The vitamin is present in milk and some meats (kidney, liver, fish) and is widely distributed in a variety of fruits and vegetables. A portion of the vitamin is lost after prolonged storage of unprocessed fruits and vegetables (for example, potatoes), but it is partially preserved (half or greater) by most means of food processing (boiling, steaming, pressure cooking, preserving jams and jellies, freezing, dehydration, and canning). As a consequence, it is easy to fulfill the recommended daily allowances with even a modest intake of fruits or vegetables. The utilization of the vitamin is increased during pregnancy and lactation and in thyrotoxicosis, and absorption is decreased in diarrheal states and in achlorhydria.

EXPERIMENTAL DEPLETION The total-body pool of vitamin C varies from 1.5 to 3 g, and when a deficient diet is instituted the pool is depleted at a constant rate, which varies among individuals but may be as high as 4 percent per day. In monkeys the major catabolic pathway involves oxidation of the alcohol at carbon 6 to an aldehyde and then to an acid. Because of differences in initial pool size and rates of turnover, variability in the completeness of deficiency in different experimental diets, and variation among normal subjects at the cellular or enzymatic level as well, the time required for the appearance of symptoms ranges from 1 to 3 months in different studies. Symptoms of deficiency correlate better with the total pool size than with plasma or blood levels. The first symptoms (petechial hemorrhages and ecchymoses) develop when the pool size is less than 0.5 g; with further depletion (pool size 0.1 to 0.5 g) additional abnormalities including gum involvement, hyperkeratosis, congested hair follicles, arthralgias, the sicca syndrome, coiled hairs, and joint effusions develop. When depletion is extreme (pool size < 0.1 g), dyspnea, edema, oliguria, and neuropathy supervene. Clinical progress of the disease may then be rapid.

Symptoms do not improve until the normal pool is repleted, and the larger the therapeutic dose the more rapid the repletion. However, with doses as small as 6.5 mg per day the body pool eventually returns to normal, and amelioration of symptoms follows.

CLINICAL DEFICIENCY Frequency and clinical context Clinical scurvy is now unusual. It occurs for the most part in areas of urban poverty, and patients are admitted from time to time to municipal hospitals. An increased incidence occurs at 6 to 12 months of age in infants whose processed milk formulas are unsupplemented with citrus fruit or vegetables as the result of maternal error or neglect. Another peak occurs in middle and old age; edentulous *men* who live alone and cook for themselves are particularly prone to develop scurvy. Clinical scurvy is more severe than the experimental disease, doubtlessly because affected individuals usually have deficiencies of other dietary constituents as well and because the groups at risk (infants and the elderly) are especially vulnerable. The disorder has different clinical features in adults and children.

Manifestations In adults the characteristic features include perifollicular hyperkeratotic papules in which hairs become fragmented and buried; perifollicular hemorrhages; purpura beginning on the backs of the lower extremities coalescing to become ecchymoses (Fig. 83-2); hemorrhage into the muscles of the arms and legs with secondary phlebothromboses; hemorrhages into joints; splinter hemorrhages in the nail beds; gum involvement (only in people with teeth) that includes swelling, friability, bleeding, secondary infection, and loosening of the teeth; poor healing of wounds and breakdown of recently healed wounds; petechial hemorrhages in the viscera and emotional changes. Symptoms resembling those of the sicca syndrome may occur. Terminally, icterus, edema, and fever are common, and convulsions, shock, and death may occur abruptly.

In infancy and childhood, hemorrhage into the periosteum of long bones causes painful swellings and may result in epiphyseal separation. The sternum may sink inwardly, leaving a sharp elevation at the rib margins (scorbutic rosary). Purpura and ecchymoses may develop in the skin, and gum lesions occur if the teeth have erupted. Retrobulbar, subarachnoid, and intracerebral hemorrhages eventuate in a rapidly progressive illness culminating in death if treatment is delayed.

Severe to moderate anemia is common both in children and in adults, is characteristically normochromic and normocytic, and is due to bleeding into tissues. The anemia may be macrocytic and/or megaloblastic (a fifth of patients in one series). Many foods that contain vitamin C also contain folate, and diets that cause scurvy may also cause folate deficiency. However, folate metabolism is also altered in scurvy; ascorbic acid deficiency results in an increased oxidation of formyl tetrahydrofolic acid to inactive folate metabolites and may cause a decrease in the active folate pool. Whether changes in iron distribution and storage are involved in the pathogenesis of the anemia is unclear. Whatever the mechanism, the anemia is cor-

FIGURE 83-2
Hemorrhages and ecchymoses in a patient with scurvy. (Photograph courtesy of Dr. Leonard L. Madison.)

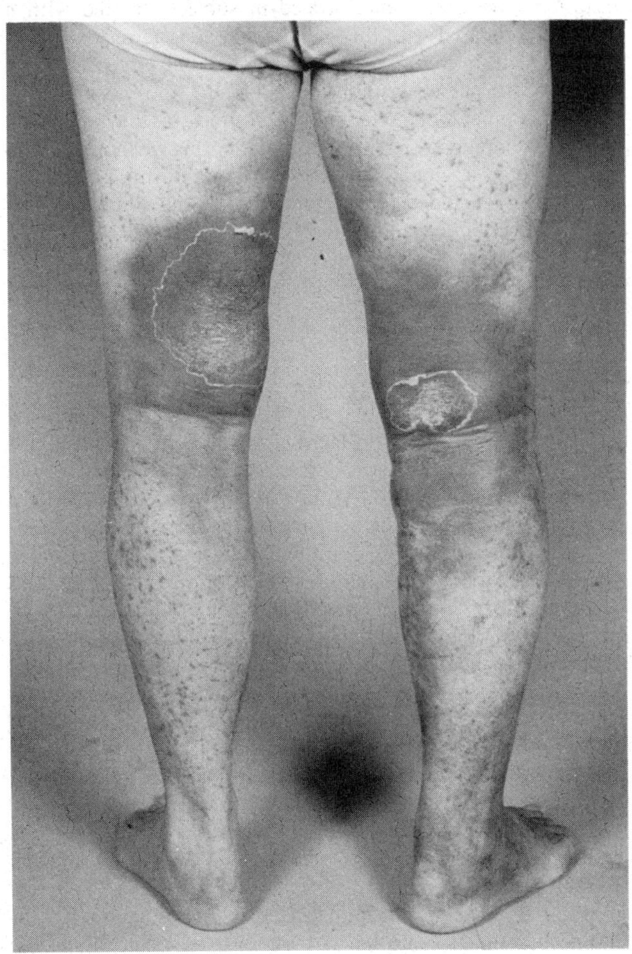

rected with refeeding and replenishment of vitamin C and the institution of a balanced diet.

Diagnosis In some hospitals platelet ascorbic acid levels are useful in diagnosing scurvy and are usually less than a fourth of the normal value (52 ± 22 μg per 10^{10} platelets). Plasma levels of the vitamin correlates less well with the clinical state (Table 77-4). In infants x-ray changes of the bones may be diagnostic. Indirect bilirubin is frequently elevated. Capillary fragility is abnormal. The remainder of the laboratory tests are nondiagnostic.

Management Scurvy is potentially fatal; if the diagnosis is suspected blood should be obtained and ascorbic acid therapy should be initiated promptly. The usual dose in adults is 100 mg 3 to 5 times a day by mouth until 4 g has been administered, then 100 mg per day. In infants and children 10 to 25 mg 3 times a day is adequate. A diet rich in vitamin C should be initiated simultaneously. Spontaneous bleeding usually ceases within 24 h, muscle and bone pains subside quickly, and the gums begin to heal within 2 to 3 days. Even large ecchymoses and hematomas resolve in 10 to 12 days, although pigmentary changes in areas of extensive hemorrhage may persist for months. Serum bilirubin becomes normal within 3 to 5 days, and the anemia is ordinarily corrected within 2 to 4 weeks.

THE MEGAVITAMIN QUESTION Considerable controversy has risen over the claim that large doses of vitamin C (a gram or greater per day) are effective in preventing or minimizing the symptoms of the common cold. However, in controlled studies, no significant differences in occurrence, severity, or duration have been demonstrated in subjects treated with a placebo compared with the vitamin. The long-term toxicity of ascorbic acid in these doses is not known, but large doses can interfere with the absorption of vitamin B_{12}, and by enhancing the development of metabolizing enzymes in the fetus may cause development of scurvy in the offspring of mothers who have ingested large amounts of the vitamin during pregnancy. It must be concluded that common use of the vitamin in this way is unwarranted and probably unwise. However, pharmacological doses (200 mg daily) may correct leukocyte abnormalities in patients with the Chédiak-Higashi syndrome (see Chap. 57).

DEFICIENCY AND EXCESS OF VITAMIN A

NORMAL PHYSIOLOGY Biochemistry Vitamin A (retinol) can either be ingested or synthesized within the body from plant carotenoids (Fig. 83-1). Preformed vitamin A is present in animal tissues, and the best sources are liver, milk, and kidney, where it occurs largely in the form of fatty acid esters. The esters are hydrolyzed during the process of digestion, absorbed in the free form, reesterified with fatty acids within the intestinal mucosa, and enter the circulation in association with lymph chylomicrons. The carotenoid substrates for synthesis of vitamin A, mainly β-carotenes, are widely distributed in plants. β-Carotene can either be absorbed intact or cleaved at the central double bond by a dioxygenase enzyme in the intestinal mucosa (or lumen) to form two molecules of retinaldehyde. Retinaldehyde is subsequently reduced by an aldehyde reductase to retinol. Retinol from whatever source is stored as retinyl esters in the parenchymal cells of the liver. The body retinol pool in normal subjects varies from 300 to 900 mg.

Prior to release from the liver the retinyl esters are hydrolyzed, and the free alcohol is mobilized bound to a specific transport protein, retinol-binding protein (RBP), for transport to peripheral tissues. In vitamin A deficiency the release of RBP from the liver is inhibited, and the protein accumulates in liver; with repletion rapid release of the protein from preformed stores occurs. The pathway by which retinol is catabolized and excreted has not been defined; approximately equal amounts are excreted in the bile and urine.

Mechanism of action The best-defined function of vitamin A is its role in vision; in the retina vitamin A constitutes the prosthetic group of a series of carotenoid proteins that provide the molecular basis for visual excitation. In addition to its role in the visual cycle, vitamin A is known to be required for growth, reproduction, and the maintenance of life. Retinol-phosphate-mannose glycolipid is present in a variety of cell membranes, and the vitamin plays a primary role in sugar transfer reactions involved in the synthesis of glycoproteins. The importance of glycoprotein to every cell implies that this may be a second major function of the vitamin.

Requirements The recommended daily allowances for vitamin A are listed in Tables 76-1 and 76-2. The assumed utilization efficiency for the conversion of β-carotene to vitamin A in the human is one-sixth (0.167). Other carotenoids with provitamin A activity have, on the average, half the activity of β-carotene. Pregnancy and disease states in which there is impaired absorption or storage, excessive utilization, or increased excretion of vitamin A may lead to increased requirements.

EXPERIMENTAL DEPLETION When experimental subjects are fed a diet deficient in both retinol and carotene, plasma levels fall progressively to less than 10 μg/dl, and the body pool shrinks to less than half the control value. An overt deficiency supervenes, manifested by follicular hyperkeratosis, impaired dark adaptation, and abnormalities of the electroretinogram. These changes are corrected after supplementation with 150 μg of retinol or 300 μg of β-carotene per day.

CLINICAL DEFICIENCY Frequency and clinical context Endemic deficiency results from inadequate amounts of the vitamin and the carotene provitamins in the diet and probably never occurs except in conjunction with deficiency of other nutrients or complicating diseases. In some developing countries vitamin A deficiency is a major cause of blindness in the young as a consequence of failure to incorporate green leafy vegetables or other sources of the provitamin or vitamin into the diet. Vitamin A deficiency may also accompany protein-calorie mulnutrition, and here the deficiency is due to a defective release mechanism from the liver secondary to inadequate retinol-binding protein. In most developed nations, including the United States, vitamin A deficiency is almost always due either to intestinal malabsorption (in sprue or following intestinal bypass surgery), abnormal storage (liver disease), or enhanced destruction or excretion of the vitamin (proteinuria). Vitamin A deficiency has also been described in patients receiving total parenteral nutrition because of loss of vitamin A after prolonged storage of intravenous fluids.

Manifestations Night blindness is the earliest symptom of deficiency, followed by degenerative changes in the retina. The bulbar conjunctiva becomes dry (xerosis), and small gray plaques with foamy surfaces develop (Bitot's spots). These lesions are reversible with vitamin A. The more serious effects of vitamin A deficiency are ulceration and necrosis of the cornea (keratomalacia), leading to perforation, endophthalmitis, and blindness. Patients may also have dryness and hyperkeratosis of the skin.

Diagnosis Vitamin A levels in plasma are not reliable for the assessment of stores in individual cases. Measurements of dark adaptation, rod scotometry, and electroretinography are reliable indicators of vitamin A stores but require trained personnel and expensive equipment; consequently, the diagnosis is usually based upon a high index of suspicion in malnourished children or in patients with known predisposing factors for its development.

Management Night blindness and the milder conjunctional changes respond well to 30,000 IU of vitamin A daily for a week. Corneal damage constitutes a therapeutic emergency, and the usual treatment is 20,000 IU per kilogram of body weight per day for 5 days.

OVERDOSAGE Carotenemia Carotenemia results from excessive intake of carotene-containing foods, principally carrots. Excess carotene is not injurious apart from the cosmetic effect; the fact that carotenemia does not cause hypervitaminosis A indicates that the conversion of carotene to vitamin A must be regulated. Carotenemia is manifested by yellowing of the skin with greatest intensity on the palms and soles and by a corresponding yellowness of serum. The yellowing of the skin can be distinguished from jaundice in that the scleras remain white. Hypothyroid patients are particularly susceptible. The omission of carrots from the diet leads to the rapid disappearance of the pigmentation. Yellowness of the skin can also result on occasion from the consumption of excessive amounts of other colored fruits and vegetables.

Vitamin A toxicity Hypervitaminosis A can result from accidental overingestion by hunters or explorers (polar bear liver), as the result of food faddism (usually caused by overly solicitous parents), or as a side effect of inappropriate therapy. Acute toxicity from a single massive dose consists of abdominal pain, nausea, vomiting, severe headaches, dizziness, sluggishness, and irritability followed within a few days by generalized desquamation of the skin and recovery. Chronic toxicity occurs following ingestion of 40,000 units or more daily for protracted periods and is characterized by bone and joint pain, hair loss, dryness and fissures of the lips, anorexia, benign intracranial hypertension, weight loss, and hepatomegaly. The only diagnostic laboratory finding is elevation of the vitamin in serum, chiefly in the form of retinyl esters. The concentration of retinol-binding protein is normal, and the excess vitamin A circulates in association with lipoprotein. Relief is prompt on withdrawal of the vitamin from the diet.

VITAMIN K

Vitamin K consists of a quinone ring attached to a side chain (labeled R in Fig. 83-1) that varies depending on the source of the vitamin. Vitamin K_1 (phylloquinone) is present in most edible vegetables, particularly in green leaves, and vitamin K_2 is produced by intestinal bacteria. The many compounds with vitamin K activity are structurally related to the simpler compound, 2-methyl-1,4-naphthoquinone (menadione). Menadione is formed in the gut by the removal of the side chain from the vitamin by intestinal bacteria. After absorption, menadione is converted in the body to the active menaquinone. The vitamin is a component of a specialized microsomal electron-transport system coupled to a carbon dioxide fixation that effects the posttranslation γ-carboxylation of glutamic acid in several proteins of the plasma, bone, kidney, and urine, including the precursor proteins for the clotting factors VII, IX, X, and possibly V. It is presumed that in deficiency states death from hemorrhage ensues before deficiency of the other carboxylated proteins becomes manifest.

Under ordinary circumstances about 80 percent of vitamin K is absorbed from the small bowel into the intestinal lymph. Because the naturally occurring forms of vitamin K are fat-soluble and are poorly stored in the body, a conditioned deficiency can occur in association with diseases that interfere with fat absorption. In addition, long-term treatment with certain antimicrobial drugs may temporarily eliminate intestinal bacteria as a source for vitamin K. The warfarin anticoagulant drugs induce hypoprothrombinemia by inhibiting the γ-carboxylation of the precursor protein.

Newborn infants tend to be deficient in vitamin K and have low plasma levels of several coagulation factors in the prothrombin complex. Such deficiencies result from minimal stores of vitamin K at birth, lack of an established intestinal flora, and a limited dietary intake of the vitamin.

Routine determination of prothrombin should be performed before all surgical procedures and deliveries. Subjects with levels below 70 percent of normal should receive therapy with vitamin K. Vitamin K deficiency can be separated from hypoprothrombinemia of liver disease by measurement of the noncarboxylated prothrombin precursor that accumulates in plasma in the vitamin deficiency.

REFERENCES

Niacin

CASTIELLO RJ, LYNCH PJ: Pellagra and the carcinoid syndrome. Arch Derm 105:574, 1972

DARBY WJ et al: Niacin. Nutr Rev 33:289, 1977

DE LANGE DJ, JOUBERT CP: Assessment of nicotinic acid status of population groups. Am J Clin Nutr 15:169, 1964

GOLDSMITH GA: Experimental niacin deficiency. J Am Dietetic Assoc 32:312, 1956

GOPALAN C, RAO KSJ: Pellagra and amino acid imbalance, in *Vitamins and Hormones,* PL Munson et al (eds). New York, Academic, 1975, vol 33, p 505

JEPSON JB: Hartnup disease, in *The Metabolic Basis of Inherited Disease,* 4th ed, JB Stanbury et al (eds). New York, McGraw-Hill, 1978, p 1563

SCHOENTAL R: Moundy grain and the aetiology of pellagra: The role of toxic metabolites of *Fusarium.* Biochem Soc Trans 8:147, 1980

Thiamine

BLASS JP, GIBSON GE: Abnormality of a thiamine-requiring enzyme in patients with Wernicke-Korsakoff syndrome. N Engl J Med 297:1367, 1977

BROWN GM: Biogenesis and metabolism of thiamine, in *Metabolic Pathways,* 3d ed, DM Greenberg (ed). Academic, New York, 1970, p 369

HOYUMPA AM: Mechanisms of thiamin deficiency in chronic alcoholism. Am J Clin Nutr 33:2750, 1980

KAWAI C et al: Reappearance of beriberi heart disease in Japan. Am J Med 69:383, 1980

KOZAM RL et al: Cardiovascular beriberi. Am J Cardiology 30:418, 1972

KURIYAMA M et al: Blood vitamin B_1, transketolase, and thiamine pyrophosphate (TPP) effect in beriberi patients. Clin Chim Acta 108:159, 1980

PINCUS JH et al: Thiamine derivatives in subacute necrotizing encephalomyelopathy. Pediatrics 51:716, 1973

SCRIVER CR: Vitamin-responsive inborn errors of metabolism. Metabolism 22:1319, 1973

VICTOR M et al: *The Wernicke-Korsakoff Syndrome.* Philadelphia, Davis, 1971

ZIPORIN ZZ et al: Excretion of thiamine and its metabolites in the urine of young adult males receiving restricted intakes of the vitamin. J Nutr 85:287, 1965

Pyridoxine

FRIMPTER GW et al: Vitamin B_6-dependency syndromes: New horizons in nutrition. Am J Clin Nutr 22:794, 1969

GERSHOFF SN: Vitamin B_6, in *Nutrition Reviews' Present Knowledge in Nutrition,* 4th ed, DM Hegsted et al (eds). Washington, DC, The Nutrition Foundation, 1976, p 149

HARRIS JW, HORRIGAN DL: Pyridoxine-responsive anemia-prototype and variations on the theme, in *Vitamins and Hormones,* RS Harris et al (eds). New York, Academic, 1964, vol 22, p 721

JAFFE IA: The antivitamin B_6 effect of penicillamine: Clinical and immunological implications, in *Advances in Biochemical Psychopharmacology,* MS Ebodi et al (eds). New York, Raven, 1972, vol 4

LUHBY AL et al: Vitamin B_6 metabolism in users of oral contraceptive agents: I. Abnormal urinary xanthurenic acid excretion and its correction by pyridoxine. Am J Clin Nutr 24:684, 1971

MUDD SH: Pyridoxine-responsive genetic disease. Fed Proc 30:970, 1971

SAUBERLICH HE et al: Biochemical assessment of the nutritional status of vitamin B_6 in the human. Am J Clin Nutr 25:629, 1972

Riboflavin

MERRILL AH JR et al: Formation and mode of action of flavoproteins. Ann Rev Nutr 1:281, 1981

PINTO J et al: Inhibition of riboflavin metabolism in rat tissue by chlorpromazine, imipramine, and amitriptyline. J Clin Invest 67:1500, 1981

RIVLIN RS: Hormones, drugs, and riboflavin. Nutr 37:241, 1979

Ascorbic acid

BAKER EM et al: Ascorbic acid metabolism in man. Am J Clin Nutr 19:371, 1966

BARNES MJ, KODICEK E: Biological hydroxylations and ascorbic acid with special regard to collagen metabolism, in *Vitamins and Hormones,* P Munson et al (eds). New York, Academic, 1972, vol 30, p 1

BARNESS LA: Nutritional aspects of vegetarianism, health foods and fad diets. Nutr Rev 59:153, 1977

BOXEN LA et al: Correction of leucocyte function in Chédiak-Higashi syndrome by ascorbate. N Engl J Med 295:1041, 1976

CHALMERS TC: Effects of ascorbic acid on the common cold. Am J Med 58:532, 1975

HODGES RE et al: Clinical manifestations of ascorbic acid deficiency in man. Am J Clin Nutr 24:432, 1971

SATO P, UDENFRIEND S: Studies on ascorbic acid related to the genetic basis of scurvy, in *Vitamins and Hormones,* P Munson et al (eds). New York, Academic, 1978, vol 36, p 33

TOLBERT BM et al: New information on synthesis and metabolism of ascorbic acid. Nutr Rev 35:22, 1977

VILTER RW: Effects of ascorbic acid deficiency in man, in *The Vitamins,* WH Sebrell Jr et al (eds). New York, Academic, 1967, vol 1, p 457

WALLERSTEIN RO, WALLERSTEIN RO JR: Scurvy. Sem Hematol 13:211, 1976

Vitamin A

DELUCA LM: The direct involvement of vitamin A in glycosyl transfer reactions of mammalian membranes, in *Vitamins and Hormones,* PL Munson et al (eds). New York, Academic, 1977, vol 35, p 1

Howard L et al: Vitamin A deficiency from long term parenteral nutrition. Ann Intern Med 93:576, 1980

LOMBAERT A, CARTON H: Benign intracranial hypertension due to A-hypervitaminosis in adults and adolescents. Eur Neurol 14:340, 1976

SAUBERLICH HE et al: Vitamin A metabolism and requirements in the human studied with the use of labeled retinol, in *Vitamins and Hormones,* RS Harris et al (eds). New York, Academic, 1974, vol 32

SMITH FR, GOODMAN DS: Vitamin A transport in human vitamin A toxicity. N Engl J Med 294:805, 1976

———, ———: Vitamin A metabolism and transport, in *Present Knowledge in Nutrition,* 4th ed, DM Hegsted et al (eds). Washington, DC, The Nutrition Foundation, 1976

SOMER A et al: Clinical characteristics of vitamin A responsive and nonresponsive Bitot's spots. Am J Ophthalmol 90:160, 1980

SRIKANTIA SG: Human vitamin A deficiency, in *World Review of Nutrition and Dietetics,* GH Bourne (ed). Basel, S Karger, 1975, vol 20, p 185

WALD G: Molecular basis of visual excitation. Science 162:230, 1968

Vitamin K

BERTINA RM et al: New method for the rapid detection of vitamin K deficiency. Clin Chim Acta 105:93, 1980

DOISY EA JR, MATSCHINER JT. Biochemistry of vitamin K, in *Fat-Soluble Vitamins,* RA Morton (ed). Pergamon, 1970, vol 9, p 293

OLSON RE, SUTTIE JW: Vitamin K and α-carboxyglutamate biosynthesis, in *Vitamins and Hormones,* PL Munson et al (eds). New York, Academic, 1977, vol 35, p 59

SHEARER MJ et al: Studies on the absorption and metabolism of phylloquinone (vitamin K) in man, in *Vitamins and Hormones,* RS Harris et al (eds). New York, Academic, 1974, vol 32, p 513

SUTTIE JW: *Vitamin K Metabolism and Vitamin K-Dependent Proteins.* Baltimore, University Park Press, 1980

84 DISTURBANCES IN TRACE ELEMENT METABOLISM

DAVID D. ULMER

Inorganic ions are crucial to virtually all biochemical and physiologic processes. Some, present in tissues only in minute quantity, micrograms to picograms per gram of wet organ, are arbitrarily designated *trace elements.* Of these, iron, iodine, cobalt, copper, manganese, molybdenum, selenium, chromium, fluorine, silicon, nickel, zinc, tin, and vanadium are now thought to be essential for animal life.

The functions of trace elements have been defined at levels of biologic complexity ranging from isolated enzymes to intact animals. Thus, many metals participate in enzymic catalysis through substrate binding, activation of the enzyme-substrate complex, or by formation of a tight coordination complex with the enzyme such that the two are isolated together as a unit, i.e., *metalloenzyme.* Metals appear to play a role in the synthesis of both proteins and nucleic acids. Trace elements are also involved in the function of organized subcellular systems, such as mitochondria, in regulation of intracellular heme concentrations, in both cellular and humoral immunity, and in membrane transport, nerve conduction, and muscle contraction. Critical biologic functions in animals are disrupted by deprivation of essential metals resulting in discrete deficiency states. Toxic manifestations owing to grossly excessive exposure to metals are also recognized. The biologic effects of metals, both essential and toxic, are often conditioned by *metal-ion antagonism;* i.e., one metal induces a biologic effect by altering the requirement for another, usually through competition for the same biochemical sites. As a consequence, such metal-ion *imbalances* are likely among the most common and certainly the most elusive sources of either metal-deficiency or intoxication states. This phenomenon complicates investigative efforts and helps to account for the fact that proven manifestations of trace-element deficiency in human beings, except for those due to iron and iodine, are rare despite extensive documentation of deficiency syndromes in animal species. However, during the past decade, trace-metal deficiencies have been more frequently recognized and better delineated owing to extensive use of total parenteral nutrition.

ZINC The average adult human body contains 1.4 to 2.3 g zinc; highest concentrations are in liver, voluntary muscle, bone, prostate, and eye. The minimum daily requirement (about 15 mg) is easily attained in most diets since the element is widely distributed in food, particularly meat, shellfish, liver, gelatin, bread, cereals, lentils, peas, beans, and rice. However, *phytic acid* in the diet binds zinc tightly, limits its absorption, and operates as a conditioning factor to induce zinc deficiency. Zinc is crucial to growth, development, and normal function of all living forms. It is an essential component of many enzymes in the liver, pancreas, and other organs, and its importance may be surmised from the fact that both DNA and RNA polymerases are zinc metalloenzymes. While marked changes in the zinc content of tissues, blood, and urine accompany many different diseases, the relationship of such alterations to the underlying conditions are, for the most part, poorly understood.

Spontaneous or experimental zinc deficiency in animals results in anorexia, retarded growth, gonadal atrophy, hyperkeratotic dermatitis, loss of hair, parakeratosis of tongue and esophagus, diarrhea, thymic hypoplasia, and impaired immunity. Two human syndromes exhibit features observed in zinc-deficient animals. Hypogonadal dwarfism, sometimes accompanied by hepatosplenomegaly, anemia, and geophagia, has been described in rural Iranian and Egyptian boys subsisting on diets consisting largely of bread and beans and nearly devoid of animal protein. The youths have decreased zinc concentrations in plasma, red cells, and hair and decreased activity of serum alkaline phosphatase, a zinc-dependent enzyme. Oral zinc supplements enhance growth and sexual maturation beyond that observed with administration of an adequate diet alone. However, the anemia is improved only by correction of concomitant iron deficiency. Delayed growth and sexual maturation accompanied by moderate decreases in serum zinc concentration have also been observed in this country in youths afflicted with chronic illnesses such as intestinal malabsorption and sickle cell anemia. It is postulated that such patients may have an incomplete form of the hypogonadal dwarf syndrome.

In recent years, *acrodermatitis enteropathica* has been characterized as the first inherited human zinc-deficiency disease. This autosomal recessive disorder is manifested by severe chronic diarrhea, wasting, alopecia, and roughened, thickened, and ulcerated skin about body orifices and on the extremities. Patients exhibit a profound decrease in zinc concentrations in serum and hair and defective leukocyte chemotaxis. They improve quickly upon administration of zinc. Whether the zinc deficiency results from an intestinal absorptive defect, excessive losses, or other factors is not yet clear. Acrodermatitis enteropathica owing to acquired zinc deficiency has also been observed in adults maintained on long-term parenteral nutrition or after intestinal bypass operations. Such patients may manifest T-lymphocyte dysfunction and anergy. Both acrodermatitis and the altered cellular immunity respond dramatically to administration of zinc.

Demonstration of the value of zinc replacement in patients with acrodermatitis enteropathica has prompted renewed interest in the role of this element in promoting healing of surgical wounds and chronic skin ulcers. Several investigations suggest that wound healing is delayed in patients with zinc

deficiency and is restored to normal by oral administration of zinc. However, controlled studies indicate that zinc has no effect in wound-healing in normal persons.

Zinc has been postulated to play a role in the maintenance of normal taste, and patients with decreased taste acuity (hypogeusia) may improve with oral administration of zinc sulfate.

Zinc toxicity may result from excessive ingestion of the element in food or drink, although the margin of safety is large. Nausea, vomiting, colic, and diarrhea are predominant manifestations. Toxicity also results from inhalation of high concentrations of zinc oxide fumes, leading to *metal-fume fever* or *brass chills.* Once a fairly common industrial hazard, this self-limited, acute illness is accompanied by fever, shaking chills, excessive salivation, headache, cough, malaise, and pronounced leukocytosis.

COPPER Copper is an essential nutrient for animals and is critical to such diverse activities as heme synthesis, connective tissue metabolism, bone development, and nerve function. Experimental copper deficiency is manifested by severe anemia; abnormalities of hair and skin pigmentation; defective elastic tissue in great vessels resulting in arterial rupture; faulty development of bone and nervous tissue; an impaired, humoral-mediated, immune response; and decreased concentrations of plasma copper and the serum copper protein, *ceruloplasmin (ferroxidase).* Ceruloplasmin catalyzes oxidation of ferrous to ferric ions and is postulated to control the rate of iron uptake by transferrin—hence, availability to reticulocytes of iron for heme synthesis. Copper is also a component of a number of other critical metalloenzymes, e.g., cytochrome oxidase, lysine oxidase, polyphenol oxidases, amine oxidases, and the cupreins—cuprozinc proteins in liver, red cells, and brain which appear to function as superoxide dismutases and may also serve in quenching highly reactive singlet oxygen in cells. Copper is important to mitochondrial function and is found frequently as a component of ribonucleic acid.

The copper concentration in adult human beings averages 1.5 to 2.4 μg per gram of fat-free tissue; the metal concentrates in liver, heart, brain, kidneys, and hair; for example, to 18 to 45 μg per gram of dry weight in liver. Balance is maintained on an average intake of 2 to 5 mg copper daily, obtained readily from meats, particularly liver and kidney, shellfish, raisins, whole-grain cereals, dried legumes, and nuts. Bile constitutes a major route of excretion.

Elevated concentrations of copper in serum are observed in a large number of acute and chronic diseases and appear to be a manifestation of response to stress. Hypocupremia is a more specific finding and is associated primarily with hepatolenticular degeneration (Wilson's disease), certain dysproteinemias of infancy, the nephrotic syndrome (secondary to renal loss of copper proteins), intestinal malabsorption, and kwashiorkor. Acute poisoning owing to ingestion of metallic copper manifests as nausea, vomiting, hematemesis, and melena, and may be accompanied by centrilobular liver necrosis. Rapid absorption of copper sulfate through the skin, as employed for therapy of burns, or through use of copper-containing dialysis equipment, has resulted in acute hemolytic anemia. Increased copper accumulation is observed in Wilson's disease (see Chap. 98), primary biliary cirrhosis (Chap. 320), and prolonged extrahepatic biliary tract obstruction (Chap. 323).

Frank copper deficiency is rare in human beings, but has been reported in severely malnourished infants, premature infants, and in children and adults receiving prolonged intravenous hyperalimentation (see Chap. 82). Anemia, leukopenia, and neutropenia are observed, and the bone marrow is megaloblastoid, contains increased sideroblasts, and shows a predominance of early granulocytes and cytoplasmic vacuolization of erythroid and myeloid elements (maturation arrest). The hematologic abnormalities are reversed by oral copper therapy.

An abnormality in copper transport by intestinal cells has been described in *Menkes kinky hair disease,* a rare X-linked syndrome manifested by rapid central nervous system and arterial degeneration, bony abnormalities, and hypothermia in male infants. As is also observed in copper-deficient animals, the hair of affected patients has less crimp and has a steely texture (pili torti), presumably owing to impaired disulfide bond formation. Concentrations of serum copper and ceruloplasmin are markedly decreased and can be restored to normal by intravenous but not oral administration of copper. Thus far, however, therapeutic efforts to replace copper and prevent early death have failed.

COBALT Although cobalt deficiency occurs in ruminants, the physiologic significance of cobalt to most other animals and humans is limited to its participation in reactions of vitamin B_{12}, of which it is a component (see Chap. 327). Acute cobalt poisoning in humans is manifested by nausea, vomiting, diarrhea, tinnitus, and loss of hearing, while chronic administration of cobalt induces polycythemia and, by blocking iodine uptake, may produce goiter, especially in children. At one time, cobalt added to beer as an antifoaming agent produced several localized epidemics of an extraordinary cardiomyopathy, often accompanied by pericardial effusion, frequently with fatal outcome.

SELENIUM Selenium deficiency in animals results in liver necrosis, striking pallor, and degeneration of skeletal muscle, *white-muscle disease,* occasionally involving the heart. These alterations resemble certain of the manifestations of vitamin E deficiency in animals and can be ameliorated by dietary supplementation with sulfur-containing amino acids. The nature of these interrelationships has been partially clarified recently by findings that selenium is a component of glutathione peroxidase in red blood cells and likely other tissues. Hence, selenium, like vitamin E, appears to help protect against damage from complex intracellular peroxides.

Selenium deficiency in humans may cause features similar to those in animals. Dietary selenium supplementation reduces the incidence of Keshan disease, a fatal, congestive cardiomyopathy affecting mainly children and young women in rural areas of China where the soil has a low selenium content. Moreover, cardiomyopathy and skeletal muscle dysfunction have been described in patients maintained on long-term parenteral nutrition who develop low red cell selenium concentrations and reduced glutathione peroxidase activity. Precise delineation of the selenium-deficient state in humans awaits further studies.

MANGANESE Manganese activates a host of critical intracellular enzymes; among these, mitochondrial pyruvate carboxylase and superoxide dismutase from chicken liver have recently been identified as manganese metalloenzymes. The metal appears to play a role in oxidative phosphorylation, fatty acid metabolism, and the synthesis of proteins, mucopolysaccharides, and cholesterol. Experimental manganese deficiency has not been described in humans. Manganese intoxication, an occupational hazard in mines and mills, induces extrapyramidal signs similar to those observed in Parkinson's disease, and patients improve upon treatment with L-dopa.

NICKEL Nickel is firmly bound to RNA from several tissues and may act to stabilize nucleic acid structure. The metal is also postulated to play a role in the maintenance of membrane structure and function. A nickel-containing $alpha_2$ macroglobulin, nickeloplasmin, has been isolated from both human and rabbit serum, but its significance is uncertain. Nickel carbonyl, formed from nickel and carbon monoxide, produces severe lung inflammation and liver necrosis. Chronic excess industrial exposure to nickel is associated with an increased incidence of lung and nasal carcinomas.

SILICON (AND SILICA) Silicon is a component of many mucopolysaccharides and may contribute to connective tissue structure by bridging polysaccharide chains or linking polysaccharides to proteins. Inhalation of fine particles of free crystalline silica (SiO_2) produces a pulmonary inflammatory response, granuloma formation, and chronic fibrosis (silicosis) (see Chap. 275).

FLUORINE In pharmacologic doses, fluorine exerts anticariogenic effects, promotes stabilization of newly synthesized bone matrix, and inhibits bone resorption, providing a rationale for its use in treatment of osteoporosis (see Chap. 341). Chronic ingestion of fluorides in moderate amounts produces mottling of dental enamel (fluorosis); in larger amounts, e.g., from ingestion of insect poisons, fluorides cause nausea, vomiting, abdominal pain, diarrhea, and tetany often resulting in death from cardiovascular collapse (see Chap. 238).

CHROMIUM Chromium, in the form of a low-molecular-weight organic complex, *glucose tolerance factor,* present in brewer's yeast, animal meats, and grains, is required for normal glucose metabolism in several animal species. The ability of mammals to synthesize glucose tolerance factor appears to be limited, and, in humans, marginal chromium deficiency may possibly accompany protein-caloric malnutrition, pregnancy, and old age. Glucose intolerance, reversed by chromium supplementation, has been reported in patients receiving long-term total parenteral nutrition. The precise relation of this metal to diabetes remains uncertain.

REFERENCES

ALLEN JI et al: Severe zinc deficiency in humans: Association with a reversible T-lymphocyte dysfunction. Ann Intern Med 95:154, 1981

AMERICAN MEDICAL ASSOCIATION, DEPARTMENT OF FOODS AND NUTRITION: Guidelines for essential trace element preparations for parenteral use. JAMA 241:2051, 1979

BURCH RE, SULLIVAN JF (eds): Symposium on trace elements. Med Clin Am 60:653, 1976

EVANS GW: Normal and abnormal zinc metabolism in man and animals: The tryptophan connection. Nutr Rev 38:137, 1980

MILLS CF (ed): *Biological Roles of Copper.* Ciba Foundation symposium 79, Amsterdam, Excerpta Medica, 1980

SOLOMONS NW: On the assessment of zinc and copper nutriture in man. Am J Clin Nutr 32:856, 1979

ULMER DD: Trace elements. N Engl J Med 297:318, 1977

WALDRON HA (ed): *Metals in the Environment.* London, Academic Press, 1980

WEISMANN K et al: Acquired zinc deficiency dermatosis in man. Arch Dermatol 114:1509, 1978

YOUNG VR: Selenium: A case for its essentiality in man. N Engl J Med 304:1228, 1981

section 6 | Metabolic pathways

The interface between basic science and clinical medicine shifts constantly, and the delineation of those aspects of basic science that have immediate import for understanding the disease process constitutes a special challenge. Recent developments in several arenas of molecular biology and biochemistry receive special attention in this section—the adenylate cyclase system, receptor-mediated endocytosis, the arachidonic acid metabolites, and the endogenous opioid peptides. Advances in each field have provided insight into the pathogenesis of diseases that span the spectrum from infectious processes to clinical pharmacology to rare inborn errors of metabolism. As before, the chapters in this section are referred to frequently throughout the book.

85 RECEPTOR-MEDIATED ENDOCYTOSIS AND THE CELLULAR UPTAKE OF TRANSPORT PROTEINS, HORMONES, ENZYMES, VIRUSES, AND TOXINS

JOSEPH L. GOLDSTEIN
RICHARD G. W. ANDERSON
MICHAEL S. BROWN

All nucleated human and animal cells have the capacity to ingest certain proteins from the extracellular fluid by a process called *receptor-mediated endocytosis.* The first step is the binding of the protein to its receptor on the surface of the plasma membrane. The protein enters cells when the membrane to which it is bound folds inward and pinches off to form an endocytic vesicle. Receptor-mediated endocytosis is the mechanism by which protein-bound nutrients [such as cholesterol (Chap. 103), iron (Chap. 326), and vitamin B_{12} (Chap. 327)] are delivered to cells. In addition, this mechanism accounts for the cellular uptake and degradation of certain plasma proteins (such as glycoproteins and alpha$_2$ macroglobulin). Receptor-mediated endocytosis also operates on protein hormones (such as insulin, chorionic gonadotropin, and epidermal growth factor) that bind to receptors on cell surfaces (see Chap. 108). Finally, receptor-mediated endocytosis is a route by which protein toxins [such as pseudomonas toxin and diphtheria toxin (Chap. 165)] and viruses [such as Semliki Forest virus and certain strains of influenza virus (Chap. 196)] gain entry to animal cells. The relevance of receptor-mediated endocytosis to human disease is further underscored by the observation that a genetic defect in one of the receptors leads to a failure of cells to take up cholesterol-carrying plasma lipoproteins, producing a common disease, familial hypercholesterolemia (Chap. 103).

GENERAL CHARACTERISTICS OF RECEPTOR-MEDIATED ENDOCYTOSIS Receptor-mediated endocytosis has four characteristics that distinguish it from other cellular uptake mechanisms. First, the receptors are proteins embedded in the bilayer of the plasma membrane; they bind extracellular proteins with high affinity and specificity. Extracellular proteins that do not bind to receptors are not taken up with high efficiency. Second, internalization of the ligand is efficiently coupled to binding. The half-time for internalization of receptor-bound ligands is less than 10 min. Third, in all cases for which ultrastructural data are available, the receptor-bound proteins enter cells through *coated pits,* which are specialized regions of the surface membrane that invaginate rapidly into the cell during endocytosis to form coated endocytic vesicles (see below). Fourth, the internalized proteins are usually delivered to lysosomes where they are degraded completely to amino acids; occasionally, the proteins are delivered to cellular compartments other than lysosomes.

To date, at least 22 proteins and macromolecular complexes are known to be taken up by cells via receptor-mediated endocytosis. These ligands are listed in Table 85-1.

THE COATED PIT AS A MECHANISM FOR RECEPTOR-MEDIATED ENDOCYTOSIS Receptor-mediated endocytosis takes place in discrete regions of the plasma membrane called *coated pits,* which occupy about 2 percent of the surface of most cells. The pits are regions in which the plasma membrane is indented and coated on its cytoplasmic surface by a lattice-like structure composed of a protein called *clathrin* (Fig. 85-1*A* and *B*). The coated pits continually fold inward and pinch off to form coated vesicles, which are membrane-bound sacs surrounded by clathrin (Fig. 85-1*C* and *D*, and Fig. 85-2). Ligands are internalized when their receptors migrate laterally in the plane of the membrane and become trapped in the membrane of a coated pit. Certain receptors move to coated pits spontaneously, even when the ligand is not bound. This is particularly true of the receptors for plasma low-density lipoprotein (LDL) and plasma asialoglycoproteins. Other receptors seem to occupy random locations on the plasma membrane, and the receptor-ligand complexes move laterally to coated pits only after the ligand attaches to these receptors. Such ligand-induced movement occurs in the case of receptors for epidermal growth factor, insulin, and certain viruses.

After the coated pit pinches off from the plasma membrane, the clathrin coat is detached from the vesicle and the uncoated endocytic vesicle migrates through the cytoplasm (Fig. 85-1*E* and *F*). Each vesicle appears to contain sufficient information to direct it to a specific cellular site. Most endocytic vesicles are directed toward lysosomes. The membranes of the endocytic vesicle and the lysosome fuse, creating a common vesicular compartment that exposes the ligands to an acid pH and to

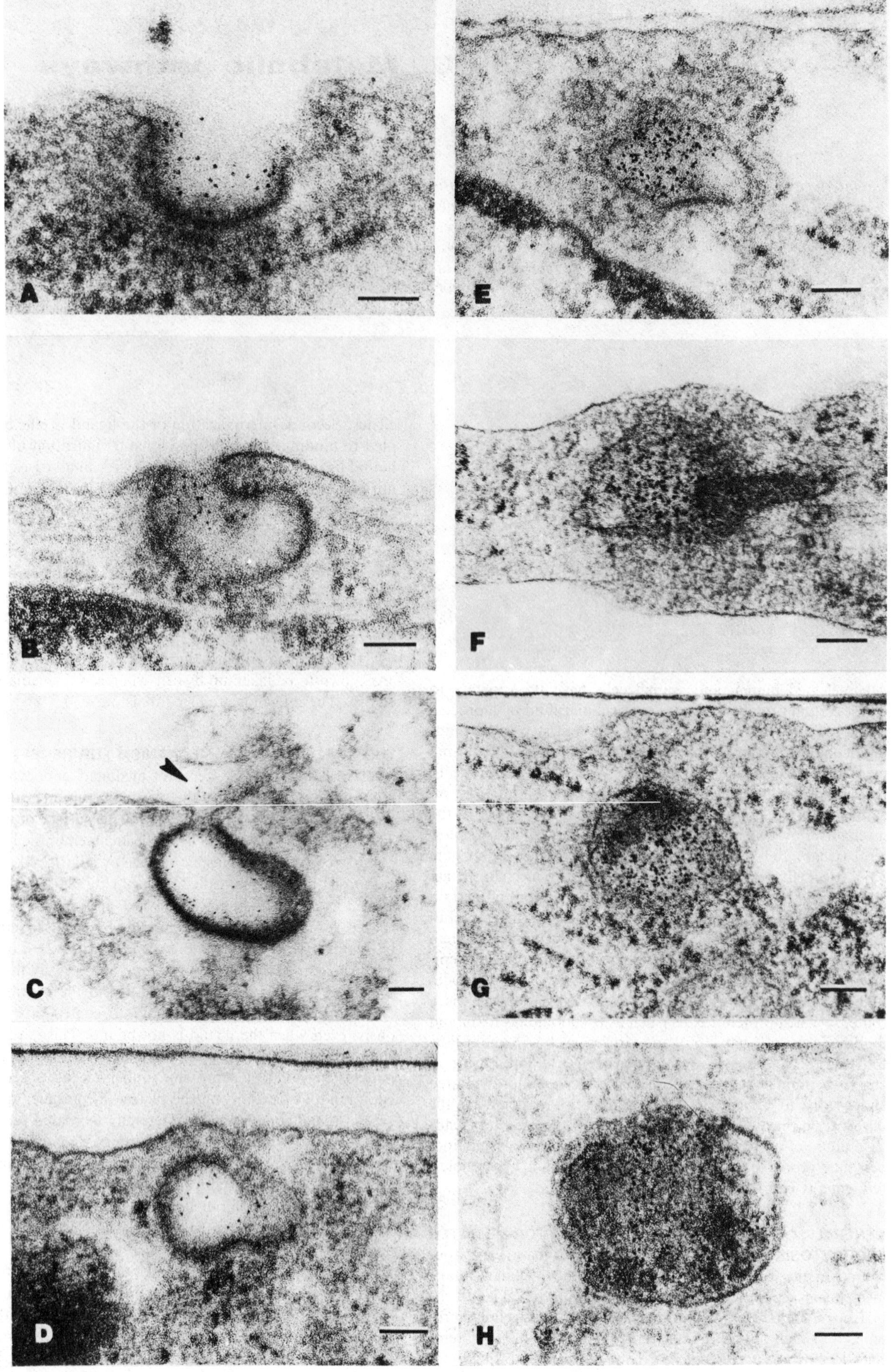
A
E
B
F
C
G
D
H

the hydrolytic action of multiple lysosomal hydrolase enzymes (Fig. 85-1*G* and *H*).

Figure 85-2 shows a stereoscopic view of the proposed structure of the protein network that forms the coat of a coated vesicle. In this vesicle, the protein coat is organized in a network of 12 pentagons and 8 hexagons. Each vertex of a hexagon or pentagon is formed by the union of three clathrin molecules, making a total of 108 molecules of clathrin. Coated vesicles having other sizes and shapes are believed to be constructed similarly with each vesicle containing 12 pentagons plus a variable number of hexagons. The structural properties of each clathrin molecule (180,000 mol wt) are ideally suited to its function. For example, under specified in vitro conditions, molecules of clathrin spontaneously aggregate to form trimeric structures (called *triskelions*) that represent the vertices. The triskelions spontaneously form a basket-like network of hexagons and pentagons similar to those that surround coated pits and vesicles in vivo.

In some cases endocytic vesicles are directed to subcellular structures other than lysosomes. For example, endocytic vesicles containing nerve growth factor are transported retrograde in axons to the nucleus of the nerve cell. Plasma lipoproteins that are taken up by this mechanism in chicken oocytes are delivered to the yolk granules where the lipids are liberated from the proteins for storage. Maternal immunoglobulins are transported in endocytic vesicles that traverse the trophoblasts of the placenta and also the epithelial cells of the neonatal gut, being discharged intact on the opposite side. In each case the uptake mechanism appears to be via receptor-mediated endocytosis, but the vesicles are targeted to sites other than lysosomes.

In many of the systems listed in Table 85-1, the receptors are not destroyed in lysosomes, but rather they, together with clathrin, are returned to the plasma membrane where they again bind another molecule of ligand. In the case of the LDL receptor (see below), each receptor molecule is believed to cycle through the cell membrane at least 100 times during its lifetime. This process is termed *receptor recycling.*

Figure 85-3 shows a schematic diagram illustrating the sequential steps in receptor-mediated endocytosis.

FIGURE 85-1

Electron micrographs showing representative stages in the receptor-mediated endocytosis of LDL and its subsequent delivery to lysosomes. Panel A shows a coated pit in the plasma membrane of a human fibroblast in tissue culture. The outer surface of the pit is lined with receptors for many plasma proteins and hormones, including the cholesterol transport protein LDL. The black dots above the surface of the coated pit are particles of LDL that have been coupled to the electron-dense protein ferritin, so that the LDL can be seen in the micrographs. In this series of micrographs, human fibroblasts were incubated with LDL-ferritin at 4°C, a temperature at which binding occurs but internalization does not. The cells were washed extensively, and then warmed to 37°C for various times. A. A typical coated pit (time at 37°C, 1 min). B. A coated pit undergoing transformation into an endocytic vesicle with LDL-ferritin included (time at 37°, 1 min). C. Formation of a coated vesicle. As the plasma membrane begins to fuse to form the vesicle, some of the LDL-ferritin is excluded from the interior and is left on the surface of the cell (arrow) (time at 37°C, 1 min). D. A fully formed coated vesicle that appears to be losing its cytoplasmic coat on the right side (time at 37°C, 2 min). E. An endocytic vesicle that has completely lost its cytoplasmic coat. Note the irregular shape of this vesicle (time at 37°C, 2 min). F. An irregularly shaped endocytic vesicle that contains abundant LDL-ferritin (time at 37°C, 6 min). G. An endocytic vesicle similar to F with more electron-dense material in the lumen (time at 37°C, 6 min). H. A lysosome that contains LDL-ferritin (time at 37°C, 8 min). Magnifications, × 38,000 to 53,000. (From RGW Anderson et al, Cell 10:351, 1977.)

EXAMPLES OF RECEPTOR-MEDIATED ENDOCYTOSIS **Low-density lipoprotein (LDL)** LDL is the major cholesterol transport protein in human plasma. The bulk of cholesterol in LDL is contained in a central core in which each cholesterol molecule is esterified with a long-chain fatty acid. The LDL particle, containing a core of approximately 1500 molecules of cholesteryl ester, is internalized by cells after binding to the LDL receptor. Within lysosomes the protein component of LDL is degraded completely to amino acids. The cholesteryl esters of LDL are also hydrolyzed by a lysosomal acid lipase enzyme. The liberated cholesterol crosses the lysosomal membrane and enters the cytosol where it is used for several metabolic purposes, e.g., the synthesis of plasma membranes in most tissues and the synthesis of steroid hormones in the adrenal gland. Fig. 85-1 shows a series of electron micrographs illustrating the receptor-mediated endocytosis of LDL.

The importance of the LDL receptor system to medicine lies in the fact that genetic defects affecting the structure of the receptor are responsible for a common autosomal dominant disease, familial hypercholesterolemia (see Chap. 103). Heterozygotes for this condition express about half the normal number of LDL receptors. Homozygotes express no LDL receptors or only a very small number. Since LDL cannot be taken up and degraded normally by cells with decreased receptors, the lipoprotein accumulates in the plasma of these patients and produces hypercholesterolemia. Eventually, the elevated plasma LDL deposits in the arterial wall, and atherosclerosis occurs.

Transferrin The plasma transport protein transferrin delivers iron to erythroblasts and reticulocytes, which require large amounts of iron for hemoglobin synthesis (see Chap. 326). Transferrin also delivers smaller amounts of iron to cells that require iron for the synthesis of certain enzymes and cytochromes. In the delivery process, transferrin binds to receptors and is internalized by receptor-mediated endocytosis. The acid pH of the lysosome causes the iron to dissociate from the transferrin. Unlike the protein component of LDL, the transferrin protein is not destroyed within the lysosome. Rather, it reenters the plasma where it can bind another molecule of iron and again deliver it to cells.

Transcobalamin II Vitamin B_{12} is transported in plasma bound to a transport protein called *transcobalamin II* (see Chap. 327). This protein binds to receptors on cell surfaces, is internalized by receptor-mediated endocytosis, and is degraded in lysosomes where the vitamin B_{12} is liberated for use by the cell. Once inside the cell, the vitamin B_{12} (cyanocobalamin) is activated to either adenosylcobalamin (an essential cofactor in the conversion of methylmalonyl enzyme A to succinyl coenzyme A) or methylcobalamin (an essential cofactor in the conversion of homocysteine to methionine).

Protein hormones Among the protein hormones, the best-documented example of receptor-mediated endocytosis occurs in the case of epidermal growth factor. This polypeptide hormone (6000 mol wt) appears structurally identical to human urogastrone. Epidermal growth factor stimulates the growth and differentiation of epidermal tissues during embryogenesis. After binding to its receptor on target cells, epidermal growth factor stimulates the phosphorylation of a plasma membrane protein and ultimately enhances cell growth. In a parallel reaction the receptor-bound epidermal growth factor is taken into the cell by receptor-mediated endocytosis, and both the receptor and the hormone are degraded in lysosomes. The lysosomal degradation of the receptor limits the response to epidermal growth factor so that each receptor molecule can only function once.

Insulin is a polypeptide hormone (6000 mol wt) that has multiple actions: it stimulates glucose and amino acid uptake by cells, it regulates key enzymes of carbohydrate, lipid, and amino acid metabolism, and like epidermal growth factor it stimulates growth of certain cells (see Chap. 114). Insulin is internalized by cells in a manner similar to that of epidermal growth factor. In the case of insulin, the internalized receptor is not immediately degraded. Rather, the receptor appears to recycle and be reutilized after the insulin is degraded. The role of the internalization and degradation reactions in the action of insulin and epidermal growth factor are not known. These processes may merely function to dispose of the hormone after

TABLE 85-1
Proteins that undergo receptor-mediated endocytosis

Protein	*Major target cell*	*Internalization via coated pits and coated vesicles*	*Fate of internalized protein*	
			Degraded in lysosomes	*Other*
TRANSPORT PROTEINS				
LDL	Fibroblasts, hepatocytes, adrenocortical cells, lymphocytes, other nonmacrophage cells	Yes	Yes; cholesterol retained by cells	
Chylomicron remnants	Hepatocytes	Data not available	Yes; cholesterol retained by cells	
Yolk proteins (lipovitellin)	Oocytes (chicken, mosquito)	Yes	No	Delivered to yolk granules
Transcobalamin II	Kidney cells, hepatocytes, fibroblasts	Yes	Yes; vitamin B_{12} retained by cells	
Transferrin	Erythroblasts, reticulocytes, fibroblasts	Yes	Iron dissociates from transferrin in lysosomes; apotransferrin is discharged intact from cells, while iron is retained	
PROTEIN HORMONES				
Epidermal growth factor	Fibroblasts, hepatocytes	Yes	Yes	
Nerve growth factor	Sympathetic ganglion cells	Data not available	Data not available	Carried in vesicles retrograde up the axon
Insulin	Hepatocytes, lymphocytes, adipocytes, fibroblasts	Yes (for some cell types)	Yes	Also may be delivered to Golgi region
Chorionic gonadotropin	Leydig cells, ovarian luteal cells	Data not available	Yes	
β-Melanotropin	Melanoma cells	Data not available	Data not available	Delivered to Golgi region and melanosomes
Prolactin	Breast cells, hepatocytes	Data not available	Yes	Also may be delivered to Golgi region
GLYCOPROTEINS				
Asialoglycoproteins (galactose)*	Hepatocytes	Yes	Yes	
Lysosomal enzymes (mannose 6-phosphate)*	Fibroblasts	Yes	No	Delivered to lysosomes and Golgi region, enzymes remain active for many days
Glycoproteins (mannose or glucose)*	Macrophages	Data not available	Yes	
OTHER PLASMA PROTEINS				
Alpha$_2$-macroglobulin	Macrophages, fibroblasts	Yes	Yes	
Maternal immunoglobulins (IgG)	Placenta, fetal yolk sac, neonatal intestinal epithelial cells	Yes	No	Transferred intact in coated vesicles to basal surface of cells where IgG is discharged into fetal or neonatal circulation
Immune complexes (Fc domain)†	Macrophages	Yes	Yes	
Chemotactic peptide	Neutrophils, macrophages	Data not available	Yes	
VIRUSES AND TOXINS				
Semliki Forest virus	Fibroblasts	Yes	Acidic pH of lysosome allows fusion between viral membrane and lysosomal membrane, releasing viral nucleocapsid into cytosol	
Diphtheria toxin	Fibroblasts, kidney cells	Data not available	Yes	Some of the A chains escape lysosomal degradation and inhibit protein synthesis in cytosol
Pseudomonas toxin	Fibroblasts	Yes	Yes	
Ricin toxin	Fibroblasts	Data not available	Yes	

* *Carbohydrate moiety that is recognized by cell surface receptor.*
† *Portion of antibody component of immune complex that is recognized by cell surface receptor.*

it has acted; they may also play a role in regulating the number of receptors on the cell surface.

Chorionic gonadotropin is a glycoprotein hormone that acts by binding to a cell surface receptor and thereby stimulates the activity of adenylate cyclase in the plasma membrane (see Chaps. 86 and 108). After it achieves this effect, the chorionic gonadotropin does not dissociate from its receptor. Rather, the receptor-bound hormone is taken into the cell and degraded. Again, the function of this degradation may play a role in regulating plasma levels of the hormone and the number of receptors on the cell surface.

Lysosomal enzymes Many lysosomal enzymes contain covalently bound chains of carbohydrate that include residues of mannose 6-phosphate. During normal endocytosis some of these lysosomal enzymes leak out of cells into the extracellular space. Rather than being lost, these enzymes are reclaimed by cells because they bind to plasma membrane receptors that recognize the mannose 6-phosphate residues. The receptors allow the cells to take up the lysosomal enzymes by receptor-mediated endocytosis and return them to lysosomes where they remain catalytically active. The same receptor is also believed to function within the cell where it directs newly synthesized lysosomal enzymes from their sites of synthesis in the endoplasmic reticulum to their residence in the lysosome. In one human disease, *I-cell disease,* an enzyme required for the formation of mannose 6-phosphate on the carbohydrate chain of the lysosomal enzymes is genetically deficient. As a result, lysosomal enzymes of patients with I-cell disease lack this recognition marker. The enzymes cannot be incorporated properly into lysosomes; consequently, they leak out into the plasma and are excreted in the urine. Affected individuals suffer from a deficiency of a number of lysosomal hydrolases and develop a devastating generalized lysosomal storage disease (see Chap. 104).

Asialoglycoproteins Most of the proteins that circulate in plasma are glycoproteins that contain covalently bound chains of sugar residues. The terminal sugar in many of the chains is sialic acid (*N*-acetylneuraminic acid). When the sialic acid is removed from these proteins, an underlying galactose residue is exposed. Liver cells contain a receptor that recognizes this galactose but only when it is exposed. In their native form, plasma glycoproteins (such as alpha$_1$ antitrypsin and ceruloplasmin) do not bind to this receptor and circulate for long periods in plasma. However, once the terminal sialic acid is removed and the galactose is exposed, the proteins bind to the liver receptor. Within minutes they are removed from the circulation and degraded in lysosomes. This receptor system is believed to play a role in the removal of circulating glycoproteins from plasma.

Viruses Certain viruses that are surrounded by a lipid envelope bind to the plasma membrane of target cells by attaching to specific proteins on the cell surface. These viruses are then internalized by receptor-mediated endocytosis and delivered to lysosomes. At acid pH the membrane surrounding the virus fuses with the membrane of the lysosome, allowing the nucleic acid of the virus to cross the lysosomal membrane and enter the cytoplasm where the virus replicates. Infection of tissue culture cells by these viruses (such as Semliki Forest virus, vesicular stomatitis virus, and certain strains of influenza virus) can be prevented by chloroquine, an agent that blocks the function of lysosomes. Chloroquine is a weak base that diffuses into lysosomes and becomes protonated, raising the pH and the ionic strength of the lysosome. When the pH rises, the lysosomal enzymes fail to function. Viruses that require acid pH to fuse with cell membranes can no longer do so in the presence of chloroquine, and the cells are protected from infection. Amantidine, which is used clinically in the prevention and symptomatic treatment of infections caused by influenza A virus, prevents viral infection in vitro by a mechanism simi-

FIGURE 85-2
Schematic depiction of the cagelike network of proteins that forms the coat of a coated vesicle. This drawing was made on the basis of stereoscopic views of isolated coated vesicles studied by electron microscopy after negative staining. In this particular coated vesicle, the protein coat is composed of 108 clathrin molecules organized in a network of 12 pentagons and 8 hexagons. The membrane vesicle is enclosed within this cage. (Redrawn from BF Pearse, Proc Nat Acad Sci USA 73:1255, 1976.)

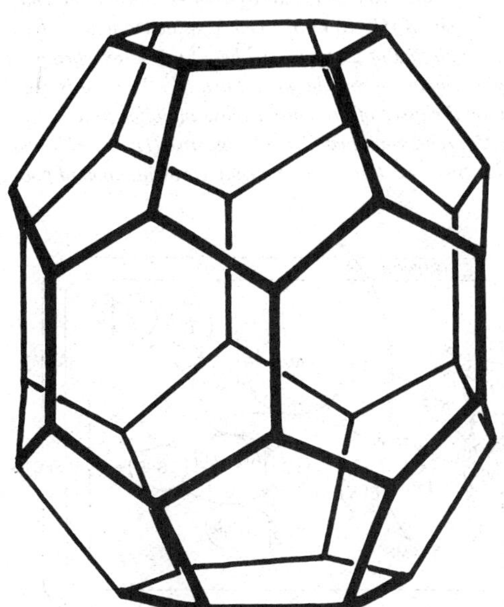

FIGURE 85-3
Schematic illustration of the proposed pathway by which certain cell surface receptors (such as LDL receptors) become localized to clathrin-containing coated pits on the plasma membrane of cells. The sequential steps are as follows: (1) synthesis of receptors on polyribosomes; (2) insertion of receptors as integral membrane proteins at random sites along noncoated segments of plasma membrane; (3) clustering together of receptors in coated pits; (4) internalization of receptors and their bound ligands when coated pits invaginate to form coated endocytic vesicles, followed by delivery of the ligands to lysosomes; and (5) recycling of internalized receptors and clathrin back to the plasma membrane. (Redrawn from MS Brown et al, Cold Spring Harbor Symp Quant Biol 46:713, 1982.)

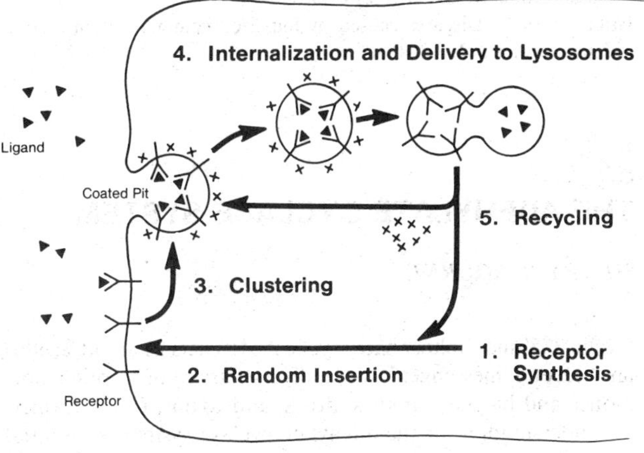

lar to that described for chloroquine. Certain other lipid-envelope viruses can enter cells by penetrating through the plasma membrane without a requirement for endocytosis (see Chap. 196).

Toxins Bacteria and plants produce and secrete a large number of proteins (exotoxins) that are toxic to animal cells. One class of toxins consists of protein molecules that have two subunits. One subunit, the B chain, binds to a cell surface receptor, and the other subunit, the A chain, enters the cell, where it inhibits protein synthesis. In several instances the penetration of the active subunit into the cytoplasm occurs only after receptor-mediated endocytosis. For example, the proteins responsible for the toxicity of diphtheria, pseudomonas, and ricin bind to a receptor on the cell surface and are taken into a vesicle by receptor-mediated endocytosis before the active subunit can cross the cell membrane (see Chap. 165). Other toxins, such as cholera toxin, penetrate the plasma membrane directly without a requirement for endocytosis and act by stimulation of adenylate cyclase (see Chap. 86).

RECEPTOR-MEDIATED ENDOCYTOSIS IN MACROPHAGES In addition to the capacity to ingest particulate matter (such as opsonized bacteria) by phagocytosis, macrophages can also take up soluble macromolecules by receptor-mediated endocytosis. Indeed, the macrophage surface contains a variety of receptors that perform this function. These include (1) receptors for the Fc portion of immunoglobulins that are responsible for the uptake of soluble immune complexes, (2) receptors for mannose- or glucose-terminal residues of glycoproteins, (3) receptors for the plasma protein alpha$_2$ macroglobulin that mediate the uptake of this protein when it is complexed with proteases, and (4) receptors for chemically altered proteins, such as acetylated low-density lipoprotein. Collectively, these receptors allow macrophages to scavenge and destroy partially degraded, complexed, or chemically altered proteins so as to prevent their accumulation in extracellular fluids. A decrease in one of these receptors, namely the Fc receptor, is believed to be responsible in part for the low rate of clearance of circulating immune complexes in patients with systemic lupus erythematosus, with consequent deposition of immune complexes in various tissues. Macrophage receptors for chemically modified lipoproteins have been postulated to play a role in the accumulation of cholesterol within macrophages of the artery wall during the formation of atherosclerotic plaques.

REFERENCES

GOLDSTEIN JL et al: Coated pits, coated vesicles, and receptor-mediated endocytosis. Nature 279:679, 1979

KAPLAN J: Polypeptide-binding membrane receptors: Analysis and classification. Science 212:214, 1981

RUBENSTEIN E: Diseases caused by impaired communication among cells. Sci Am 242:102, 1980

86
THE ADENYLATE CYCLASE SYSTEM

HENRY R. BOURNE

Cyclic 3′,5′-monophosphate (cyclic AMP) acts as an intracellular "second messenger" for a diverse array of peptide hormones and biogenic amines, drugs, and toxins. Consequently, an understanding of the adenylate cyclase system is essential for understanding the pathophysiology and management of many diseases. For example, investigation of the second messenger role of cyclic AMP has advanced our understanding of endocrine, neural, and cardiovascular regulation. Conversely, research aimed at unravelling the biochemical basis of certain diseases has contributed to understanding the molecular mechanisms by which the synthesis of cyclic AMP is regulated. This chapter will review the biochemistry and biological role of cyclic AMP, with particular emphasis on normal and pathologic functioning of the pivotal regulatory enzyme, hormone-sensitive adenylate cyclase.

BIOCHEMISTRY The enzymatic steps involved in the actions of hormones (first messengers) that work via cyclic AMP are depicted in Fig. 86-1, and the hormones that work via this mechanism are listed in Table 86-1. These hormones initiate their actions by binding to specific receptors on the external surface of the plasma membrane. The hormone-receptor complex activates the membrane-bound enzyme, adenylate cyclase,

FIGURE 86-1
Cyclic AMP as an intracellular second messenger for hormones. The diagram depicts an idealized cell containing the protein molecules (enzymes) involved in mediating the actions of hormones that work via cyclic AMP. The first three classes of these proteins are embedded in the plasma membrane: Hormone receptors (Rec), oriented toward the membrane's outer face, bind specific hormonal agonists. The diagram shows two receptors, Rec 1 and Rec 2, capable of binding two different hormones, H_1 and H_2, to emphasize the fact that a cell may respond to more than one kind of extracellular hormonal signal through a common adenylate cyclase system. The guanine nucleotide-binding regulatory protein (N protein), oriented toward the cytoplasm, interacts with receptors to mediate hormonal stimulation of cyclic AMP synthesis. Catalytic adenylate cyclase (AC), also exposed to the cytoplasm, is activated by the N protein, and converts ATP to cyclic AMP and pyrophosphate (PP_i). The intracellular concentration of cyclic AMP is dependent upon a balance between its rate of synthesis and two processes that remove it from the cell: degradation by cyclic nucleotide phosphodiesterases (PDE), which convert cyclic AMP to 5′-AMP, and extrusion from the cell by an energy-dependent transport system. The intracellular actions of cyclic AMP are mediated or regulated by at least five additional classes of proteins. The first of these, the cyclic AMP–dependent protein kinases (RC), are composed of regulatory (R) and catalytic (C) subunits. In the RC holoenzyme the C subunit is catalytically inactive (inhibited by R). Cyclic AMP acts by binding to the R subunits, freeing C from the cyclic AMP-R complex. Free catalytic subunits (C) catalyze transfer of the terminal phosphate of ATP to specific protein substrates (S), e.g., phosphorylase kinase. In the phosphorylated state (S∼P) these substrate proteins (usually enzymes) initiate the characteristic actions of cyclic AMP within the cell (e.g., activation of glycogen phosphorylase, inhibition of glycogen synthetase). The proportion of the kinase substrate proteins in the phosphorylated (S∼P) state is regulated by two additional classes of proteins: Kinase inhibitor protein (IP) binds reversibly to C*, rendering it catalytically inactive (IP-C). Phosphatases (P'ase) recycle S∼P back to S by removing covalently bound phosphate.*

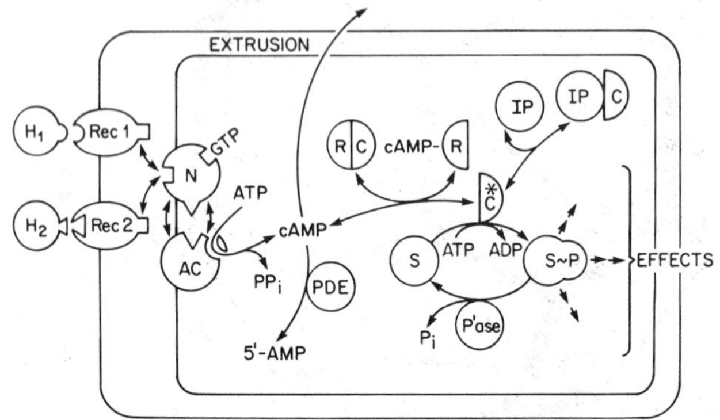

which synthesizes cyclic AMP from intracellular ATP. Within the cell cyclic AMP relays the hormonal message by combining with its own receptor, cyclic AMP–dependent protein kinase. Activated by cyclic AMP, the protein kinase transfers the terminal phosphate of ATP to specific protein substrates (usually enzymes). Phosphorylation of these enzymes enhances (or in some cases, inhibits) their catalytic activities. Altered activities of these enzymes produce the characteristic effects of the hormone on its target cell.

Additional biochemical mechanisms decrease or turn off the synthesis, intracellular accumulation, or actions of the second messenger. Most of these inhibitory mechanisms are themselves subject to regulation by hormones. Such regulation allows fine tuning the hormonal responsiveness of cells by additional neural and endocrine pathways. Other mechanisms that limit the actions of cyclic AMP (see Fig. 86-1) include degradation of cyclic AMP to 5′-AMP by cyclic nucleotide phosphodiesterases, extrusion of cyclic AMP through the plasma membrane into the extracellular fluid, inhibition of cyclic AMP–dependent protein kinase by specific proteins that bind to the catalytic subunit of the enzyme, and specific phosphatases that remove the phosphate from substrate proteins phosphorylated by cyclic AMP–dependent protein kinases and in this way reverse changes in enzymatic activity caused by phosphorylation.

Biological role of cyclic AMP Each of the protein molecules involved in the intricate push-pull mechanisms of Fig. 86-1 represents a potential site for regulation of hormonal responsiveness, for therapeutic and toxic actions of drugs, and for pathologic alterations in disease. Specific instances of such interactions are discussed in later sections of this chapter. To set these in context, the general biological functions of cyclic AMP as a second messenger should be considered. These functions are conveniently illustrated by reference to the regulation of the release of glucose from hepatic glycogen stores (the biochemical system in which cyclic AMP was discovered) by glucagon and other hormones.

TABLE 86-1
Hormones that utilize cyclic AMP as a second messenger

Hormone	*Target organ/tissue*	*Characteristic effect*
Adrenocorticotropic hormone	Adrenal cortex	Cortisol production
Calcitonin	Bone	↓Serum calcium
Catecholamines (beta-adrenergic)	Heart	↑Rate, contractility
Chorionic gonadotropin	Ovary, testis	↑Production of sex steroids
Follicle-stimulating hormone	Ovary, testis	↑Gametogenesis
Glucagon	Liver	Glycogenolysis, release of glucose
Luteinizing hormone	Ovary, testis	↑Production of sex steroids
Luteinizing hormone-releasing hormone	Pituitary	↑Release of luteinizing hormone
Melanocyte-stimulating hormone	Skin (melanocytes)	↑Pigmentation
Parathyroid hormone	Bone, kidney	↑Serum calcium, ↓serum phosphate
Prostacyclin, prostaglandin E_1	Platelets	↓Platelet aggregation
Thyrotropin	Thyroid	↑Production and release of T_3, T_4
Thyrotropin-releasing hormone	Pituitary	↑Release of thyrotropin
Vasopressin	Kidney	↑Concentration of urine

NOTE: *Only the best-documented cyclic AMP–mediated effects are listed here, although many of these hormones produce multiple effects in several target organs.*

TRANSDUCTION OF HORMONAL SIGNALS ACROSS THE PLASMA MEMBRANE The biological stability and structural complexity of peptide hormones like glucagon make them useful carriers of diverse hormonal messages between cells but impair their ability to penetrate cell membranes. Hormone-sensitive adenylate cyclase allows the information content of the hormonal signal to cross the membrane, although the hormone itself may not.

AMPLIFICATION By binding to a few specific receptors (probably less than 1000 per cell), glucagon stimulates synthesis of a much larger number of cyclic AMP molecules. These cyclic AMP molecules stimulate cyclic AMP–dependent protein kinase, which causes activation of thousands of molecules of hepatic phosphorylase (the enzyme that limits glycogen breakdown) and subsequent release of millions of glucose molecules from a single cell.

METABOLIC COORDINATION AT THE LEVEL OF A SINGLE CELL In addition to stimulating phosphorylase and causing degradation of glycogen to glucose, cyclic AMP–dependent protein phosphorylation simultaneously deactivates the enzyme that synthesizes glycogen (glycogen synthase) and stimulates enzymes responsible for hepatic gluconeogenesis. Thus, a single chemical signal, glucagon, mobilizes energy reserves via more than one metabolic pathway.

TRANSDUCTION OF DIVERSE MESSAGES INTO A SINGLE METABOLIC PROGRAM Because hepatic adenylate cyclase can be stimulated by epinephrine (acting through beta-adrenergic receptors) as well as glucagon, cyclic AMP allows regulation of hepatic carbohydrate metabolism by two chemically distinct hormones. If the second messenger did not exist, each of the regulatory enzymes involved in hepatic mobilization of carbohydrates would have to be able to recognize both glucagon and epinephrine.

COORDINATED REGULATION OF DIFFERENT CELLS AND TISSUES BY A FIRST MESSENGER In the classic "fight-or-flight" response to stress, catecholamines bind to beta-adrenergic receptors in heart, adipose tissue, blood vessels, and many other tissues besides the liver. If cyclic AMP were not available to mediate most of the responses to beta-adrenergic catecholamines (e.g., increased heart rate and contractility, dilatation of vessels supplying skeletal muscle, mobilization of energy from carbohydrate and lipid stores), a huge panoply of distinct enzymes in these tissues would have to possess specific binding sites for regulation by catecholamines.

Similar examples of the biological functions of cyclic AMP could be adduced from the other first messengers listed in Table 86-1. Cyclic AMP acts as an intracellular symbol for each of these hormones, signifying their presence on the cell surface. Like all good symbols, cyclic AMP provides a simple, economical, and highly specific way of communicating diverse and complex messages.

HORMONE-SENSITIVE ADENYLATE CYCLASE The pivotal enzyme that mediates this system is hormone-sensitive adenylate cyclase. This enzyme is composed of at least three separable protein components, each embedded in the lipid bilayer of the plasma membrane (Fig. 86-2).

Hormone receptors (Rec), exposed on the outer surface of the cell membrane, contain binding sites that specifically recognize individual hormones which stimulate cyclic AMP synthesis.

The catalytic unit of adenylate cyclase (AC), exposed on the cytoplasmic face of the plasma membrane, converts intracellular ATP to cyclic AMP and pyrophosphate. The guanine nucleotide-binding regulatory component (N protein), also exposed to the cytoplasm, functionally couples Rec and AC and is essential for hormonal stimulation of cyclic AMP synthesis.

The coupling function of the N protein depends upon its capacity to bind guanosine triphosphate (GTP) (Fig. 86-2). When GTP is bound to it, the N protein can bind to AC and activate cyclic AMP synthesis. Binding and activation of AC are not permanent; instead, the terminal phosphate of GTP in the N-GTP-AC complex is eventually hydrolyzed, and N-GDP dissociates from AC. Because N-GDP is a poor activator of AC, sustained elevation of adenylate cyclase activity requires continued recycling of N-GDP to N-GTP. Hormone-receptor (HRec) complexes function to accelerate the exchange of GDP for GTP. In the presence of hormone (outside the cell) and GTP (supplied by intracellular metabolism), N shuttles back and forth between HRec and AC. In effect, N-GTP acts as a second messenger for HRec, mediating hormonal activation of AC. This mechanism temporally and spatially separates the binding of hormone to Rec from the activation of cyclic AMP synthesis and uses the energy stored in the terminal phosphate bond of GTP to amplify the stimulatory effect of HRec.

FIGURE 86-2

Molecular mechanism of activation of adenylate cyclase by hormones. In the basal, unstimulated state (upper left in the figure) the three protein components are separate. Receptors (Rec) are exposed on the extracellular face of the membrane, while the nucleotide-binding protein (N), bound to GDP, and the inactive adenylate cyclase unit (AC) are oriented toward the cytoplasm. Binding of hormonal agonist (H) to Rec (upper right) induces a conformational change in the receptor, which in turn binds to the N protein and causes release of bound GDP. Then (lower portion of diagram) hormone and receptor dissociate from N and the nucleotide binding site is filled by GTP (which is more abundant than GDP in cells); the activated N-GTP complex now binds to and activates AC, resulting in synthesis of cyclic AMP from intracellular ATP. The N-GTP-AC complex possesses intrinsic GTPase activity, which eventually hydrolyzes the terminal phosphate of the bound GTP; then N-GDP and (inactive) AC dissociate to return to the basal state (upper left). Note that the role of hormone-receptor complex (HRec) is catalytic—i.e., HRec causes activation of N by promoting replacement of GDP by GTP at the nucleotide binding site, with resulting activation of cyclic AMP synthesis. Thus the role of hormone is to activate adenylate cyclase and to reactivate it after the GTPase reaction, but hormone need not be bound to Rec while AC is making cyclic AMP. The activating effect of cholera toxin is quite different from that of hormones. ADP-ribosylation of N by cholera toxin inhibits the GTPase activity of the N-GTP-AC complex, stabilizing this complex in the active (cyclic AMP–synthesizing) form.

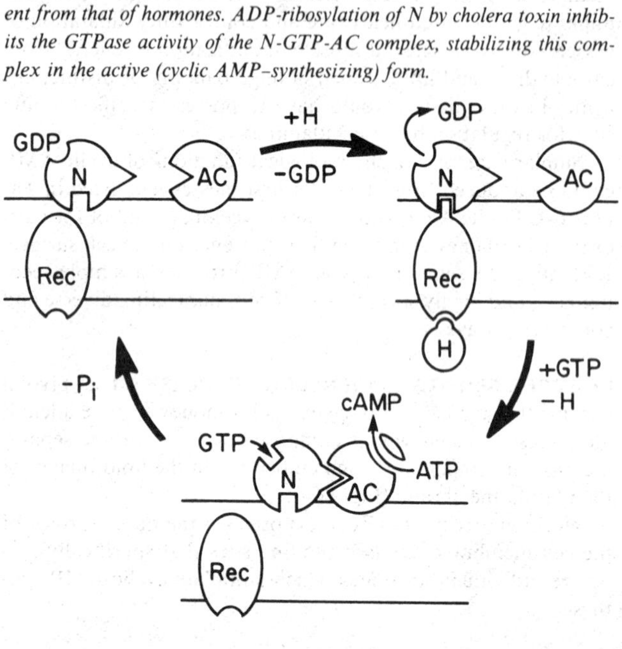

This scheme explains how several different hormones can stimulate cyclic AMP synthesis within a single cell. Because receptors are physically distinct from adenylate cyclase, the array of receptors expressed on a cell surface determines the cell's specific pattern of responsiveness to external chemical signals. An individual cell may express one or as many as six or seven different surface receptors, all capable of stimulating adenylate cyclase. In contrast, all cells appear to contain similar (perhaps identical) N and AC components.

The molecular components of hormone-sensitive adenylate cyclase provide control points for changing the sensitivity of a given tissue to hormonal stimulation. Both R and N are critical in physiological regulation of hormonal sensitivity, and alterations of the N protein are implicated as the primary lesion of certain clinical disorders discussed below.

Regulation of sensitivity to hormones (also see Chap. 73) Repeated administration of a hormone or drug often causes gradually increasing resistance to its effects. This phenomenon is variously termed desensitization, refractoriness, tachyphylaxis, or tolerance. Investigation of endocrine and neural responses mediated by cyclic AMP has uncovered the molecular mechanisms that underlie changes in sensitivity to hormones and helps to explain certain manifestations of disease and consequences of drug therapy.

Hormones or neurotransmitters may induce desensitization that is receptor-specific or "homologous." For example, administration of beta-adrenergic catecholamines induces specific refractoriness of heart muscle to readministration of the same amines but not to drugs that do not act via beta-adrenergic receptors. Receptor-specific desensitization involves at least two separate mechanisms. The first, which develops rapidly (within minutes) and is rapidly reversed upon removal of the hormone, functionally "uncouples" receptors from the N protein and therefore reduces their ability to stimulate adenylate cyclase. The second process involves actual reduction in the number of receptors on the cell membrane, a process termed *receptor down-regulation.* The down-regulation process requires interaction of receptors with the N protein. It may require hours to occur and is not readily reversible.

These desensitization processes are part of normal regulation. Removal of normal physiological stimuli may result in increased sensitivity of a target tissue to pharmacologic stimulation, as in denervation supersensitivity. A potentially important clinical correlate of this increase in receptor number may occur in patients in whom therapy with propranolol, a beta-adrenergic blocking agent, is abruptly withdrawn. Such patients often have transient signs of elevated sympathetic tone (tachycardia, elevation of blood pressure, headaches, tremor, etc.) and may develop symptoms of coronary insufficiency. Peripheral blood leukocytes of subjects receiving propranolol exhibit elevated numbers of beta-adrenergic receptors, and receptor number returns slowly to normal when propranolol is withdrawn. Although the increased number of receptors in leukocytes certainly does not mediate the cardiovascular symptoms and signs of propranolol withdrawal, it is possible that receptors in myocardium and other tissues undergo similar changes.

Sensitivity of cells and tissues to hormones may also be regulated in a "heterologous" fashion—i.e., the sensitivity to one hormone is regulated by a second hormone, acting through a different set of receptors. Regulation of cardiovascular sensitivity to beta-adrenergic amines by thyroid hormones is the most prominent clinical example of heterologous regulation. Thyroid hormones cause an accumulation of an increased number of beta-adrenergic receptors in heart muscle. This increase in receptors partially accounts for the increased cardiac sensitivity of thyrotoxic patients to catecholamines. However, the fact that in experimental animals the increase in number of beta-adrenergic receptors produced by administration of thyroid hormones is not sufficient to account for the increased cardiac sensitivity to catecholamines suggests that thyroid hormones also affect components of the hormone response distal to receptors, possibly including, but not limited to, the N protein. Other examples of heterologous regulation include regulation by estrogen and progesterone of uterine sensitivity to relaxation by beta-adrenergic agonists and the increased responsiveness of many tissues to epinephrine that is produced by glucocorticoids.

A second type of heterologous regulation involves inhibition of hormonal stimulation of adenylate cyclase by agents that act directly on membranes. Three classes of inhibitory agents—acetylcholine, opiates, and alpha-adrenergic catecholamines—act through distinct receptors (muscarinic, opioid, and alpha-adrenergic) to decrease the sensitivity of adenylate cyclase in some tissues to stimulation by other hormones. These inhibitory effects involve GTP and may be mediated either directly through the N protein or through a second kind of guanine nucleotide regulatory protein. The clinical importance of this type of heterologous regulation is not established, but inhibition of cyclic AMP synthesis by morphine and other opiates could account for some aspects of tolerance to opiates. Similarly, relief of such inhibition may be involved in producing the syndrome that follows withdrawal of opiates.

Cholera (also see Chap. 166) Elevated cyclic AMP in intestinal mucosal cells causes the massive secretion of water and electrolytes that results in the diarrhea of cholera. Pathogenic *Vibrio cholerae* produce a protein exotoxin that can stimulate cyclic AMP synthesis in virtually all animal cells. Intestinal mucosa are the only tissues affected in the clinical disease because the toxin is not absorbed from the gastrointestinal tract. As a consequence, other tissues are not accessible to the toxin produced by bacteria growing in the intestinal lumen.

Unlike stimulation of adenylate cyclase by hormones, the effect of cholera toxin is slow in onset and does not disappear immediately when the toxin is removed. The reason for this difference is that cholera toxin does not act by reversible binding to a stimulatory receptor but instead acts as an enzyme, producing a stable covalent modification of the N protein component of adenylate cyclase. Following binding of the toxin to cells, one of its peptide subunits penetrates the cell membrane, where it catalyzes ADP-ribosylation of the N protein, using intracellular nicotinamide adenine dinucleotide (NAD^+) as a substrate:

$$N + NAD^+ \xrightarrow{\text{toxin}} \text{N-ADP-ribose} + \text{nicotinamide} + H^+$$

ADP-ribosylation of the N protein increases cyclic AMP synthesis, apparently by decreasing the rate of hydrolysis of GTP in the N-GTP-C complex that synthesizes cyclic AMP (Fig. 86-2)

This biochemical mechanism may explain why the diarrhea of cholera can be produced by a relatively small number of pathogenic organisms and why the diarrhea persists for some time after the organisms have been eradicated. The first phenomenon stems from the fact that the toxin is an enzyme, so that small numbers of toxin molecules suffice to ADP-ribosylate a substantial fraction of the N molecules in a cell. Persistently elevated cyclic AMP synthesis after removal of the toxin, at least in experimental studies, correlates with stability of N-ADP-ribose. Most cells apparently lack enzymes capable of removing ADP-ribose from N, so that the effect of the toxin disappears only when the N-ADP-ribose molecules are replaced by newly synthesized N molecules. Recovery from the clinical disease may even require replacement of the mucosal cells themselves. Elucidation of the molecular basis for the action of cholera toxin served as a valuable tool in the discovery and characterization of the N protein and advanced our understanding of the biochemical basis of hormone action.

Pseudohypoparathyroidism (also see Chap. 339) A genetic defect involving the N component of adenylate cyclase is the molecular basis of pseudohypoparathyroidism, type I (PHP-I). This rare inherited disease is characterized by hypocalcemia and hyperphosphatemia, elevated serum parathyroid hormone (PTH), and resistance to the metabolic effects of exogenously administered PTH.

PTH regulates calcium homeostasis at least in part by stimulating adenylate cyclase in kidney and bone. Administration of PTH to normal subjects (and to patients with idiopathic or surgical hypoparathyroidism) causes greatly increased excretion of cyclic AMP in urine. In contrast, PTH causes little or no increase in the urinary cyclic AMP of PHP-I patients. This finding initially raised the possibility that PHP-I is caused by a defect in the PTH receptor, rendering it less capable of stimulating cyclic AMP synthesis.

A defect confined to the PTH receptor, however, could not account for recent observations that many PHP-I patients are also partially resistant to effects of other hormones, including thyrotropin (TSH), antidiuretic hormone, glucagon, and gonadotropins. Many PHP-I patients require replacement therapy for symptomatic hypothyroidism, because of thyroid resistance to TSH. Resistance to the action of the other hormones is for the most part clinically silent and can be detected only with specialized tests.

The fact that these hormones utilize cyclic AMP as a second messenger suggests that PHP-I is caused by a defect distal to hormone receptors, affecting some component common to all cyclic AMP–mediated responses. For many PHP-I patients that component is the N protein. Activity of the N protein is reduced by about 50 percent in erythrocytes, platelets, and skin fibroblasts of most PHP-I patients. Its activity is therefore probably reduced in their endocrine target cells as well, including kidney, bone, thyroid, liver, etc.

If N deficiency is generalized in PHP-I, why are most of its important clinical consequences related to resistance to a single hormone, PTH? While this question cannot be answered with certainty, it appears that most hormone responses mediated by cyclic AMP are maintained—in spite of partial N deficiency—by a variety of compensatory mechanisms, including elevation of circulating concentrations of the stimulating hormone. Elevated circulating PTH does not suffice to maintain normal calcium homeostasis in PHP-I, however, presumably because the actions of PTH are more critically dependent upon normal activity of the N protein. Fortunately, the defect in PTH responsiveness can be bypassed by treatment with vitamin D, which restores serum calcium and phosphate to normal.

CYCLIC AMP IN CLINICAL MEDICINE A large number of hormones and neurotransmitters act by stimulating adenylate cyclase, and several pharmacologic antagonists act by blocking their binding to specific receptors—e.g., propranolol at beta-adrenergic receptors and cimetidine at H_2-histamine receptors. The therapeutic actions of these agents depend upon elevations or decreases in cyclic AMP content of target cells and tissues in patients. In addition, the methylxanthines (caffeine and theophylline) block cyclic nucleotide phosphodiesterases and may produce some of their therapeutic effects (e.g., bronchodilatation) by elevating cellular cyclic AMP.

In clinical practice, measurements of cyclic AMP in the urine are useful in diagnosing disorders that involve PTH and calcium homeostasis. This is because a substantial fraction of urinary cyclic AMP is made in the kidney itself, in proximal tubular cells responding to circulating PTH. Thus, urinary cyclic AMP provides a convenient "window" for assessing effects of PTH on the kidney and can reflect elevated PTH (in hyperparathyroidism), decreased PTH (in hypoparathyroidism), or end-organ resistance to PTH (in pseudohypoparathyroidism, type I) (see Chap. 339).

At present, however, the real importance of cyclic AMP for medicine is as a tool in understanding normal and pathologic regulation and in developing new drugs. Adenylate cyclase assays are now routinely used to screen new compounds for their ability to stimulate or block adrenergic, histaminergic, and many peptide receptors. Hormone receptors are not the only critical and specific control points in regulation mediated by cyclic AMP; it seems likely that the other proteins depicted in Fig. 86-1 will serve as targets of useful therapeutic agents in the future.

OTHER SECOND MESSENGERS Although cyclic AMP is the most thoroughly studied hormonal second messenger, some hormones act by increasing intracellular concentrations of other chemical signals, including calcium ion and cyclic guanosine 3',5'-monophosphate (cyclic GMP). Certain effects of alpha-adrenergic and cholinergic (muscarinic) agents, for example, appear to be mediated by elevated cytoplasmic concentrations of calcium. Many cell types contain guanylate cyclase, cyclic GMP phosphodiesterases, and protein kinases that are specifically stimulated by cyclic GMP. Nonetheless, the role of this second cyclic nucleotide in normal and pathologic regulation is not well defined.

REFERENCES

FARFEL Z et al: Defect of receptor-cyclase coupling protein in pseudohypoparathyroidism. N Engl J Med 303:237, 1980

HAMET P, SANDS H (eds): *Pathophysiological Aspects of Cyclic Nucleotides,* vol 12: *Advances in Cyclic Nucleotide Research,* P Greengard, GA Robison (eds), New York, Raven, 1980

87

PROSTANOIDS AND EICOSANOIDS: ARACHIDONIC ACID METABOLITES RELEVANT TO MEDICINE

R. PAUL ROBERTSON

This chapter focuses on the formation and mechanism of action of the physiologically active metabolites of arachidonic acid and on the biological phenomena in which these compounds may be involved.

FORMATION OF THE PROSTANOIDS AND EICOSANOIDS Prostaglandins, the first arachidonic acid metabolites to be recognized, were so named because they were originally identified in seminal fluid and thought to be secreted by the prostate. Other active metabolites were characterized subsequently, and it was established that they are formed by one of two synthetic pathways—the cyclooxygenase or the lipoxygenase system. These synthetic pathways are summarized schematically in Fig. 87-1, and structures of representative metabolites are shown in Fig. 87-2. The products of the cyclooxygenase pathway—the prostaglandins and the thromboxanes—are collectively termed *prostanoids,* and the products of the lipoxygenase pathway are called *eicosanoids.*

The initial synthetic step for both pathways involves the cleavage of arachidonic acid from phospholipid in the plasma membrane of cells. Free arachidonic acid can then be metabolized by the cyclooxygenase or lipoxygenase pathway. The first product of the cyclooxygenase pathway is the cyclic endoperoxide PGG_2, which is then converted to PGH_2. PGG_2 and PGH_2 are the key intermediates in the formation of the classical prostaglandins (PGA_2, PGD_2, PGE_2, and $PGF_{2\alpha}$), prostacyclin (PGI_2), and thromboxane A_2 (TXA_2). The first product of the lipoxygenase pathway is hydroperoxyeicosatetraenoic acid (HPETE) which is an intermediate in the formation of 5-hydroxyeicosatetraenoic acid (HETE) and the leukotrienes (LTA, LTB, LTC, and LTD). Two fatty acids other than arachidonic acid [3,11,14-eicosatrienoic acid (dihomo-γ-linolenic acid) and 5,8,11,14,17-eicosapentaenoic acid] can be converted to metabolites closely related to the prostanoids and eicosanoids. Products of the former substrate carry the subscript 1, whereas those of the latter have the subscript 3. Arachidonic acid forms products with the subscript 2. (The subscripts designate the number of double bonds between carbon atoms in the side chains.)

All cells have the necessary substrates and enzymes to form some of the metabolites of arachidonic acid, but tissues differ widely in the amounts of the various enzymes and consequently in the amounts of the various products formed. The prostanoids and eicosanoids are synthesized according to immediate need and are not stored in significant amounts for later release.

The classical prostaglandins Prostaglandins A_2, D_2, E_2, and $F_{2\alpha}$ are formed from the cyclic endoperoxides PGG_2 and PGH_2. Of these, PGE_2 and $PGF_{2\alpha}$ appear to be physiologically important. Although PGA_2, a degradation product of PGE_2, has strong vasodepressor actions, its physiologic relevance is uncertain. Similarly, a role for PGD_2 in platelet aggregation has been postulated but not documented.

Prostacyclin (PGI_2) Formation of PGI_2 from PGH_2 is the dominant pathway of arachidonic acid metabolism in the endothelial cells of vessel walls. Nonvascular tissues also synthesize PGI_2. Prostacyclin is a vasodilator as well as an inhibitor of platelet aggregation.

Thromboxanes Thromboxane synthetase catalyzes the incorporation of an oxygen atom into the ring of the endoperoxide PGH_2 to form the thromboxanes. TXA_2 is synthesized by platelets and acts to enhance platelet aggregation.

Eicosanoids The eicosanoids (HETE and the leukotrienes) are the end products of the lipoxygenase pathway of endoperoxide metabolism. The leukotrienes have histamine-like actions, including induction of increased vascular permeability and of bronchospasm. In addition, LTC and LTD have been identified as slow-reacting substances of anaphylaxis (SRS-A). (The pathophysiology of the leukotrienes is discussed in detail in Chap. 273.)

EFFECTS OF DRUGS ON THE SYNTHESIS OF PROSTANOIDS AND EICOSANOIDS Many drugs block the synthesis of prostanoids and eicosanoids by inhibiting one or more enzymes in the biosynthetic pathway. Glucocorticoids and several antima-

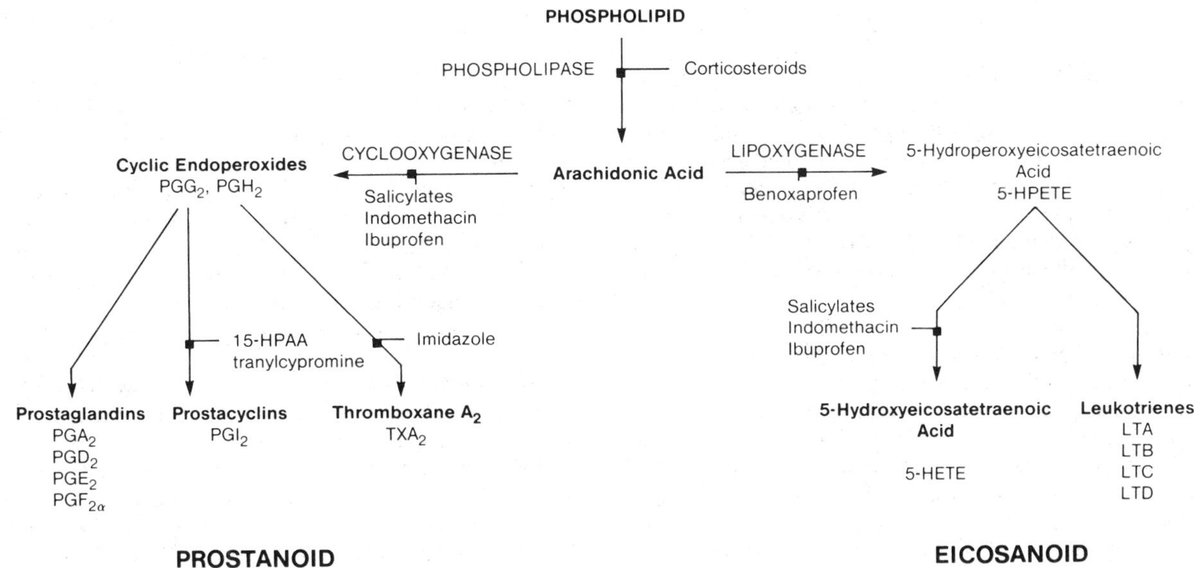

FIGURE 87-1

Scheme of arachidonic acid metabolism. The various drugs act at the enzymatic steps as indicated to inhibit formation of the metabolites. Five major groups of metabolites are formed: the prostanoids (prostaglandins, prostacyclins, and thromboxanes) via the cyclooxygenase pathway and the eicosanoids (5-HETE and the leukotrienes) via the lipoxygenase pathway.

larial drugs interfere with the cleavage of arachidonic acid from phospholipids (Fig. 87-1). Cyclooxygenase, the initial enzyme in the pathway, is directly inhibited by nonsteroidal anti-inflammatory drugs including the salicylates, indomethacin, and ibuprofen. These same three drugs also inhibit the peroxidase-mediated step that converts HPETE to HETE. Benoxaprofen, another nonsteroidal anti-inflammatory drug, inhibits the lipoxygenase-mediated conversion of arachidonic acid to HPETE. 15-Hydroperoxyarachidonic acid (15-HPAA), an arachidonic acid analogue, and tranylcypromine, an antidepressant drug, inhibit the conversion of cyclic endoperoxides to PGI_2, and imidazole inhibits thromboxane synthesis.

Most of these drugs inhibit early reactions in the synthetic pathways and therefore block the formation of more than one product. Imidazole and 15-HPAA are exceptions to this rule but are not available for clinical use. No specific inhibitors of the conversion of HPETE to the leukotrienes or of the specific actions of individual arachidonic acid metabolites have been identified. The lack of such antagonists is a barrier to elucidating the role of these metabolites in physiologic and pathophysiologic processes.

The fact that a drug inhibits the synthesis of a certain compound does not mean that a given drug effect is the direct result of a deficiency of that compound. For example, indomethacin not only inhibits formation of cyclic endoperoxides by cyclooxygenase but also disrupts calcium flux across membranes, inhibits cyclic AMP–dependent protein kinase and phosphodiesterase, and inhibits one of the enzymes responsible for degradation of PGE_2.

FIGURE 87-2

Structures of representative biologically active metabolites of arachidonic acid.

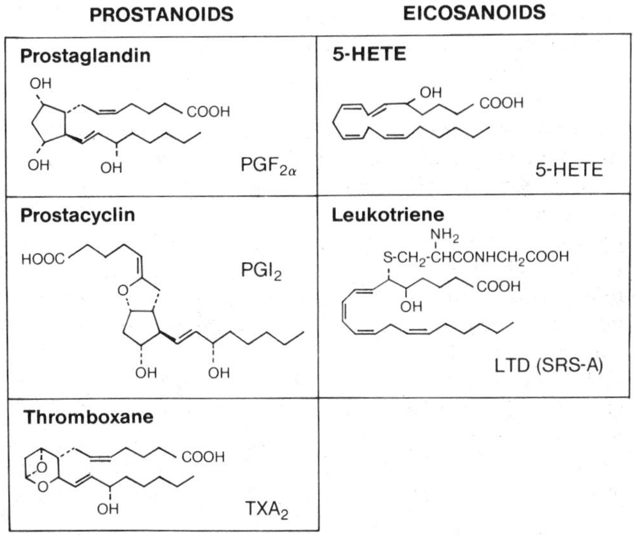

PROSTANOIDS	EICOSANOIDS
Prostaglandin OH, COOH, OH, OH — $PGF_{2\alpha}$	**5-HETE** OH, COOH — 5-HETE
Prostacyclin HOOC, O, OH, OH — PGI_2	**Leukotriene** NH_2, S-CH_2-CHCONHCH_2COOH, COOH, OH — LTD (SRS-A)
Thromboxane O, O, COOH, OH — TXA_2	

METABOLISM AND ASSAY OF PROSTANOIDS AND EICOSANOIDS Arachidonic acid metabolites are catabolized rapidly in vivo. Prostaglandins of the E and F series, although chemically stable, are almost completely degraded during a single passage through the liver and the lung. As a consequence, nearly all nonmetabolized PGE measurable in urine is derived from renal and seminal vesicle secretion, whereas PGE metabolites in urine represent PGE synthesis by other organs. PGI_2 and TXA_2 are chemically unstable and also are rapidly catabolized. PGI_2 is converted to 6-keto-$PGF_{1\alpha}$, and TXA_2 is converted to TXB_2. Because both PGI_2 and TXA_2 are short-lived in vivo, measurement of their inactive metabolites is commonly used as an index of the rates of their formation. The degradative pathways of HETE and the leukotrienes have not been characterized in humans.

Five methods are currently used to measure arachidonic acid metabolites in physiologic fluids: bioassay, radioimmunoassay, chromatography, receptor assay, and mass spectrometry. With each method certain precautions must be taken in handling samples during and after collection because prostaglandin synthesis in biological samples may be enhanced during the collection procedure. For example, if blood is allowed to clot or if platelets are not carefully separated from plasma, large amounts of PGE and thromboxanes may be generated during processing and lead to erroneous results. Use of an inhibitor of prostaglandin synthesis in the collection tube may minimize this problem.

Prostaglandins have specific receptor sites on the plasma membranes of cells such as liver, corpus luteum, adrenal gland, adipocytes, thymocytes, uterus, pancreatic islets, and platelets.

Most of the binding sites have specificity for prostaglandins of a given type. For example, one liver plasma membrane receptor binds PGE_1 and PGE_2 with high affinity but not prostaglandins of the A, F, and I configurations. Platelets contain one receptor that recognizes PGI_2 and PGE_2 and a separate binding site for PGD_2 that does not readily recognize either PGE_2 or PGI_2. The mechanisms by which the binding of the prostaglandins influences cell function have not been identified.

PHYSIOLOGY No convincing evidence has been obtained that the normal physiologic actions of prostanoids and eicosanoids are mediated by changes in plasma levels of the metabolites. Consequently, it is believed that both prostanoids and eicosanoids act as local, intracellular modulators of biochemical activity in the tissues in which they are formed (e.g., a paracrine function). Most are short-lived in the circulation because of chemical instability and/or rapid degradation.

Lipolysis PGE_2 is synthesized by adipocytes and is a potent endogenous inhibitor of lipolysis. Since the formation of cyclic adenosine monophosphate (cAMP) is necessary in the action of hormones that stimulate lipolysis, the interactions between PGE and adenylate cyclase have been examined in considerable detail. PGE inhibits lipolysis by decreasing the formation of cAMP in response to epinephrine, adrenocorticotropic hormone (ACTH), glucagon, and thyroid-stimulating hormone (TSH). Consequently, PGE may act as an endogenous antilipolytic substance by interfering with the stimulation of cAMP formation by hormones.

Insulin and PGE may act independently during their antilipolytic actions on the adipocyte. For example, insulin but not PGE inhibits the stimulation of lipolysis by exogenous cAMP in isolated adipocytes, but both agents inhibit hormone-stimulated generation of cAMP. This suggests a site of action of insulin distal to the stimulation of adenylate cyclase. In some adipocytes PGE inhibits glucagon-induced lipolysis whereas insulin does not.

Sodium and water balance The renin-angiotensin-aldosterone system is a major regulator of sodium homeostasis, and vasopressin exerts the principal control over water balance. Arachidonic acid metabolites influence both systems. PGE_2 and PGI_2 stimulate renin secretion, and inhibitors of prostaglandin synthesis have the opposite effect. PGI_2 decreases renal vein resistance and increases blood flow; this results in redistribution of blood flow from the outer renal cortex to the juxtamedullary region of the kidney. Conversely, two inhibitors of prostaglandin synthesis, indomethacin and meclofenamate, decrease total renal blood flow and shunt the remaining flow to the outer cortex.

In dogs, indomethacin also increases sensitivity to exogenous vasopressin. Conversely, PGE_2 decreases vasopressin-stimulated water transport. Since this effect of PGE_2 is circumvented by the administration of dibutyryl-cAMP, PGE_2 most likely interferes with the stimulation of adenylate cyclase by vasopressin. Sulfonylurea drugs such as chlorpropamide used to treat partial diabetes insipidus may act by decreasing PGE_2 synthesis, thereby augmenting vasopressin-induced water transport.

Platelet aggregation Platelets synthesize PGE_2, PGD_2, and TXA_2. Although a physiologic role has not been established for PGE_2 and PGD_2 in platelet function, TXA_2 is a potent stimulator of platelet aggregation; in contrast PGI_2, formed by the endothelial cells of blood vessel walls, is a potent antagonist of platelet aggregation. Since decreases in cAMP are associated with platelet aggregation, TXA_2 and PGI_2 may exert their opposing effects by influencing platelet generation of cAMP.

Inhibitors of endogenous prostaglandin synthesis interfere with platelet aggregation. For example, a single dose of aspirin can suppress normal platelet aggregation for 48 h. This effect is presumed to be the result of suppression of cyclooxygenase-mediated TXA_2 synthesis. Cyclooxygenase inhibition by a single dose of aspirin or indomethacin is of longer duration in platelets than in other tissues, probably because the platelet, in contrast to nucleated cells that can synthesize new proteins, does not have the necessary machinery to form new enzymes. Consequently, the effect of the prostaglandin synthesis inhibitors persists until newly formed platelets have been released. Endothelial cells on the other hand rapidly recover cyclooxygenase activity following discontinuation of treatment with inhibitors of prostaglandin synthesis, and PGI_2 production is restored; this is one reason that patients taking these drugs are not predisposed to excessive formation of platelet thrombi. Another possible explanation is that the platelet is more sensitive than the endothelial cell to drugs that inhibit cyclooxygenase.

Endothelial damage may lead to platelet aggregation along the blood vessel wall by causing a local decrease in PGI_2 synthesis, thereby allowing unbridled platelet aggregation at the site of vessel wall damage.

Vascular effects The vasoactive properties of arachidonic acid metabolites are among their most physiologically important actions. Prostaglandins of the E and A series and PGI_2 are vasodilators where $PGF_{2\alpha}$ and TXA_2 are vasoconstrictors. These effects appear to be the result of direct action on the smooth muscle of the vessel wall. Provided that systemic blood pressure is maintained, the vasodilatory arachidonic acid metabolites act to increase blood flow. If blood pressure falls, however, blood flow decreases even though the arterial bed is dilated since with systemic hypotension catecholamine-induced vasoconstriction offsets the vasodilatory effect of the prostaglandins. For these reasons, significant alterations in systemic blood pressure must be excluded when evaluating the effects of arachidonic acid metabolites on organ blood flow.

Gastrointestinal effects Prostaglandins of the E series influence gastrointestinal function. Infusion of either PGI_2 or PGE_2 into the gastric artery of dogs causes increases in blood flow and inhibition of acid output, and several PGE analogues inhibit gastric acid output when taken orally. Oral PGE also protects the gastrointestinal mucosa from several forms of injury, possibly due to direct effects rather than to inhibition of gastric acid secretion. In in vitro experiments prostaglandins stimulate gastrointestinal smooth muscle and thereby increase motility, but it is not clear whether these actions are physiologically important.

Neurotransmission PGE inhibits egress of norepinephrine from sympathetic nerve terminals. The PGE effect on norepinephrine secretion appears to be prejunctional, i.e., at a site on the nerve terminal proximal to the synaptic cleft, and can be reversed by increases in calcium concentration in the perfusing medium. Therefore, PGE_2 may inhibit norepinephrine release by blocking calcium influx. Inhibitors of PGE_2 synthesis augment norepinephrine release in response to stimulation of adrenergic nerves.

In contrast, catecholamines can release PGE_2 from a variety of tissues, probably by an alpha-adrenergic-mediated mechanism. For example, in innervated tissues such as the spleen, nerve stimulation or injection of norepinephrine causes release of PGE_2. This release is blocked after denervation or administration of alpha-adrenergic blockers. A stimulus that activates the nerve causes release of norepinephrine, which in turn stimulates synthesis and release of PGE_2; PGE_2 then feeds back at the prejunctional level of the nerve terminal to decrease the amount of norepinephrine released.

Pancreatic endocrine function PGE has both stimulatory and inhibitory effects on insulin secretion by the pancreatic beta cell in vitro. However, insulin secretion, specifically the acute insulin response to intravenous glucose, is inhibited by PGE when infused into animals and humans. This inhibitory effect appears to be specific for glucose because the responses of plasma insulin to several other secretagogues are not influenced by PGE. PGI_2 and TXA_2 do not appear to affect insulin secretion. In vivo studies with inhibitors of prostaglandin synthesis support the concept that endogenous prostaglandins inhibit insulin secretion. In general these drugs augment insulin secretion and improve carbohydrate tolerance. An exception is indomethacin, which inhibits glucose-induced insulin secretion and can cause hyperglycemia. The discordant results with indomethacin are likely due to some effect other than inhibition of cyclooxygenase.

Luteolysis In sheep hysterectomy during the luteal phase results in maintenance of the corpus luteum, suggesting that the uterus normally produces a luteolytic substance. A candidate for this substance is $PGF_{2\alpha}$ since it can cause luteal regression.

PATHOPHYSIOLOGY Most postulated roles for arachidonic acid metabolites in disease involve excessive production, but a few disorders may be the result of decreased production. The latter could result from dietary deficiency of arachidonic acid (an essential fatty acid), damage to a tissue required for prostaglandin synthesis, or from therapy with drugs that inhibit enzymes in the synthetic pathway.

Bone resorption: Hypercalcemia of malignancy (see also Chap. 339) Hypercalcemia occurs in association with nonparathyroid malignancies of many different types. Parathyroid hormone excess, as the result either of autonomous production by parathyroid tissue or ectopic formation by the tumor itself, causes a portion of these cases. However, most patients with hypercalcemia of malignancy do not have elevated plasma levels of parathyroid hormone, and the etiology of the hypercalcemia has been the subject of considerable interest.

Prostaglandin E_2 is a potent inducer of bone resorption and of calcium release from bone, and PGE_2 production is elevated in certain hypercalcemic animals with transplantable tumors. Treatment of these animals with inhibitors of PGE synthesis causes reduction of PGE levels and a concomitant decrease in hypercalcemia. Likewise, some patients with hypercalcemia and malignancy have excessive amounts of PGE in plasma and of PGE metabolites in urine, whereas elevated levels have not been observed in normocalcemic patients with otherwise similar malignancies. Drugs that inhibit prostaglandin synthesis decrease circulating calcium levels in some patients with hypercalcemia of malignancy. Patients whose plasma calcium decreases in response to these drugs have elevated PGE production, whereas those with normal PGE production do not respond. Thus, a subset of approximately 10 percent of patients with hypercalcemia and malignancy have elevated PGE production and can be treated with drugs that inhibit prostaglandin synthesis.

The source of the excess PGE in these patients has not been identified. Increased liver and lung degradation of PGE would be expected if large amounts of PGE were present in the circulation. It is possible, of course, that such large amounts of PGE are released by a tumor into the circulation that liver and lung

degradation cannot handle the load. Alternatively, if lung metastases are present, the venous drainage from the tumors could arrive at bone directly. A third possible mechanism involves metastatic seeding of bone. Tumor cells synthesize PGE in culture, and metastatic tumor cells in bone could synthesize PGE that acts locally to cause bone resorption. Hypercalcemia of malignancy can occur in the absence of demonstrable bone metastases, but the clinical tools for excluding such metastases, such as radioisotope scans, may not be sensitive enough to detect many small lesions.

Bone resorption: Rheumatoid arthritis and dental cysts (see Chap. 346) Overproduction of PGE_2 has been postulated as a cause of the juxtaarticular osteoporosis and bony erosions seen in some patients with rheumatoid arthritis. Rheumatoid synovia synthesize PGE_2 in tissue culture, and media from these cultures promote bone resorption; moreover, the inclusion of indomethacin in the culture medium blocks this bone-resorptive capacity. Since indomethacin does not prevent bone resorption due to preformed PGE_2, the PGE_2 produced by the synovia may be responsible for the resorptive activity.

Cells from benign dental cysts also cause bone resorption and synthesize PGE_2 in tissue culture. Again, bone resorption caused by the culture medium from such cells is decreased if indomethacin is added prior to the incubation. A related problem is that of alveolar bone resorption in patients with periodontal disease. PGE_2 levels in inflamed gingiva are greater than in healthy gingival tissue, and alveolar resorption may be due, in part at least, to local overproduction of these metabolites.

Bartter's syndrome (see Chap. 299) Bartter's syndrome is characterized by elevated levels of plasma renin, aldosterone, and bradykinin; resistance to the pressor effect of angiotensin infusion; hypokalemic alkalosis; and renal potassium wasting in the presence of normal blood pressure. The basis for the postulated role of prostaglandins in Bartter's syndrome is that PGE_2 and PGI_2 stimulate the release of renin and that the pressor response to infused angiotensin is blunted by the vasodilator effects of the prostaglandin. The increase in renin release leads to increased aldosterone secretion, which in turn can increase urinary kallikrein activity.

In keeping with this postulate, elevated levels of PGE_2 and 6-keto-$PGF_{1\alpha}$ have been documented in urine from patients with the syndrome. Hyperplasia of renal medullary interstitial cells (which synthesize PGE in culture) has also been demonstrated. These findings led to therapeutic trials of inhibitors of prostaglandin synthesis in the disorder. Indomethacin (and other inhibitors) reversed virtually all the abnormalities except for hypokalemia, suggesting that a prostaglandin, probably PGE_2 or PGI_2, is responsible for mediating many but not all of the manifestations of Bartter's syndrome.

Diabetes mellitus (see Chap. 114) Glucose administration to a normal individual causes an acute or first-phase increase in secretion of insulin into plasma. If a large amount of glucose is given, the first-phase increase is followed by a slower, more prolonged response termed second-phase insulin secretion. Patients with non-insulin-dependent (adult-onset) diabetes mellitus have subnormal first-phase insulin release in response to glucose administration and a variable decrease in the second phase of insulin secretion; insulin response to other secretagogues, such as arginine, isoproterenol, glucagon, and secretin, is preserved. Diabetics appear to have a specific defect that interferes with normal perception of glucose signals (the glucoreceptor hypothesis). Since PGE inhibits glucose-induced insulin secretion in normal individuals, inhibitors of endogenous prostaglandin synthesis have been given to patients with non-insulin-dependent diabetes mellitus to ascertain whether insulin secretion can be improved. Both sodium salicylate and aspirin partially restore the acute insulin response and improve glucose disposal.

Essential hypertension After the vasodilator roles of PGA and PGE were characterized, it was suggested that a deficiency of either might be involved in the pathogenesis of essential hypertension. In keeping with this possibility, patients with essential hypertension excrete smaller amounts of PGE in urine (derived from renal production of PGE) than do subjects with renovascular hypertension or primary aldosteronism.

Patent ductus arteriosus (see Chap. 256) The ductus arteriosus in sheep is sensitive to the vasodilatory properties of PGE, and PGE-like material is present in the ductal wall. It is believed, therefore, that enhanced endogenous PGE might maintain prenatal patency of the ductus. Since inhibitors of prostaglandin synthesis cause constriction of the ductus of fetal lambs, trials with indomethacin were undertaken in premature human infants with patent ductus arteriosus. Such treatment for several days is followed by closure of the vessel in the majority of patients, although some require a second course of therapy and a minority eventually require surgical ligation. Infants under 35 weeks of age are most likely to respond.

Patients with certain types of congenital heart disease require a patent ductus arteriosus to survive. *Ductus-dependent pulmonary blood flow* is essential under circumstances in which the ductus is the major channel by which nonoxygenated blood reaches the lungs from the aortic arch, for example, in pulmonary atresia and tricuspid atresia. Since PGE relaxes the smooth muscle in the lamb ductus arteriosus, clinical trials of intravenous infusion of PGE were undertaken to attempt to maintain patency of the ductus in such patients as an alternative to emergency surgery. Such PGE infusions for a short time cause a temporary increase in blood flow to the lungs and improve arterial oxygen saturation until the necessary corrective heart surgery can be performed. The large right-to-left shunt in these cardiac malformations allows the intravenously infused PGE_2 to escape pulmonary degradation before arriving at the ductus. In this instance, the disease process itself facilitates delivery of the therapeutic agent.

Peptic ulcer disease (see Chap. 306) Gastric acid secretion is excessive in patients with peptic ulcer disease and may be involved in damaging the intestinal mucosa. Various analogues of PGE_2 that inhibit gastric acid secretion appear to be cytoprotective. In several studies these agents were more effective than placebos in relieving pain and decreasing gastric acid secretion in patients with peptic ulcer disease. Moreover, acceleration of the healing of ulcer craters as assessed by endoscopic criteria has been reported in patients receiving PGE analogues as compared with placebo-treated groups.

Dysmenorrhea (see Chap. 118) Dysmenorrhea is usually associated with increased uterine contractions. The fact that some analgesics used in the disorder also inhibit prostaglandin synthesis led to the suggestion that arachidonic acid metabolites may play a role in the pathogenesis of dysmenorrhea. Prostaglandins of the E and F series are present in human endometrium. Intravenous infusion of either produces uterine contractions and can potentially alter blood flow to the uterus. Also, PGF and PGE levels in menstrual blood are decreased by administration of prostaglandin synthesis inhibitors. Controlled trials comparing inhibitors of prostaglandin synthesis with placebo in women with dysmenorrhea suggest that symptomatic improvement is greater following drug therapy. However, a cause-and-effect relationship has not been established between uterine production of prostaglandins and dysmenorrhea.

Asthma See Chap. 273.

Inflammatory response and immune response Drugs such as aspirin have long been used as antipyretics and anti-inflammatory agents as well as analgesics. Several arguments have been marshaled to support a relation between inflammation and the arachidonic acid metabolites: (1) Inflammatory stimuli such as histamine and bradykinin release endogenous prostaglandins in parallel. (2) Several arachidonic acid metabolites cause vasodilatation and hyperalgesia. (3) Prostaglandins are present in areas of inflammation, polymorphonuclear cells release PGE during phagocytosis, and PGE is chemotactic for leukocytes. (4) Some arachidonic acid metabolites cause increased vascular permeability, a feature of the inflammatory response that gives rise to local edema. (5) Vasodilatation induced by PGE is not abolished by atropine, propranolol, methysergide, or antihistamines, known antagonists of other possible mediators of the inflammatory response. These findings suggest that PGE may have a direct inflammatory effect, and some potential mediators of inflammation may act by influencing PGE release. (6) Various arachidonic acid metabolites can cause pain in appropriate animal models and hyperalgesia or an increased sensitivity to pain in humans. (7) PGE can cause fever, usually after injection into the cerebral ventricles or into the hypothalamus of experimental animals. (8) Pyrogens cause increased concentrations of prostaglandins in cerebrospinal fluid, whereas prostaglandin synthesis inhibitors decrease fever and decrease release of prostaglandins into cerebrospinal fluid.

Arachidonic acid metabolites have also been postulated to play a role in the immune response. Small amounts of PGE can suppress stimulation of human lymphocytes by mitogens such as phytohemagglutinin. This observation and the fact that the inflammatory response is associated with the local release of arachidonic acid metabolites have led to the hypothesis that these substances act as negative modulators of lymphocyte function. The release of PGE by mitogen-stimulated lymphocytes may constitute a portion of a negative feedback control mechanism by which lymphocyte activity is regulated. Sensitivity of lymphocytes to the inhibiting effects of PGE_2 increases with age, and indomethacin augments lymphocyte responsiveness to mitogens to a greater degree in the elderly. Lymphocytes cultured from patients with Hodgkin's disease release more PGE_2 after the addition of phytohemagglutinin, and lymphocyte responsiveness is enhanced by indomethacin. When suppressor T cells are removed from the cultures, the amount of PGE_2 synthesized is diminished, and the responsiveness of the lymphocytes from the Hodgkin's patients and controls is no longer different. Depressed cellular immunity in patients with Hodgkin's disease may be the result of PGE inhibition of lymphocyte function.

REFERENCES

FICHMAN MP et al: Role of prostaglandins in the pathogenesis of Bartter's syndrome. Am J Med 60:785, 1976

FLOWER RJ: Drugs that inhibit prostaglandin biosynthesis. Pharmacol Rev 26:33, 1974

GOODWIN JS et al: Prostaglandin-producing suppressor cells in Hodgkin's disease. N Engl J Med 297:963, 1977

METZ SA et al: Prostaglandins as mediators of paraneoplastic syndromes: Review and update. Metabolism 30:299, 1981

PELUS LM, STRAUSSER HR: Prostaglandins and the immune response. Life Sci 20:903, 1977

PULKKINEN MO, CSAPO AI: Effect of ibuprofen on menstrual blood prostaglandin levels in dysmenorrheic women. Prostaglandins 18:137, 1979

ROBERTSON RP: Review: Prostaglandins as modulators of pancreatic islet function. Diabetes 28:943, 1979

——— : Prostaglandins, thromboxanes, and eicosanoids: Arachidonic acid metabolites relevant to medicine, in *Update I: Harrison's Principles of Internal Medicine,* KJ Isselbacher et al (eds). New York, McGraw-Hill, 1981, p 191

ROBINSON DR et al: Prostaglandin-stimulated bone resorption by rheumatoid synovia. J Clin Invest 56:1181, 1975

SAMUELSSON B et al: Prostaglandins. Annu Rev Biochem 44:669, 1975

SEYBERTH HW et al: Prostaglandins as mediators of hypercalcemia associated with certain types of cancer. N Engl J Med 293:1278, 1975

WILSON DE et al: Inhibition of stimulated gastric secretion by an orally administered prostaglandin capsule. Ann Intern Med 84:688, 1971

ZUSMAN RM et al: Inhibition of vasopressin-stimulated prostaglandin E biosynthesis by chlorpropamide in the toad urinary bladder. J Clin Invest 60:1348, 1977

88
ENDOGENOUS OPIOID PEPTIDES

ELI IPP
ROGER H. UNGER

The discovery of the physiological opioid peptides initiated a period of far-reaching research with major implications for physiology, medicine, and psychiatry. This chapter is designed to provide a general background in this rapidly evolving area of investigation.

BACKGROUND Morphine has been in clinical use for almost 200 years, but the mechanism of its action has only recently been clarified. In 1973, several groups established that these alkaloids exert their effects within the central nervous system by binding to specific receptors. Such receptors are present in high concentrations in those regions of the brain where opiates are known to have biological effects, including the regions of pain perception. This discovery suggested that the receptor system probably functions under physiological conditions to mediate the action of an endogenous substance (or substances) resembling opiate drugs.

Endogenous opioid activity in brain and pituitary extracts was described soon after the discovery of the opiate receptors. Two pentapeptides with opioid activity were extracted from the brain, isolated, and characterized. These peptides were termed *enkephalins.* The amino acid sequence of one (Met-enkephalin) was identical to amino acid residues 61 to 65 of the β-lipotropin molecule, a 91-amino acid pituitary polypeptide which had been characterized some 10 years earlier and which is devoid of opioid activity. This observation stimulated interest in other fragments of β-lipotropin in the hope that additional peptides with opioid activity would be found. Subsequently, several *C*-terminal portions of the β-lipotropin molecule were shown to have such activity. These polypeptides were collectively termed *endorphins,* an abbreviation for *endogenous morphine.* Common to all of them was the Met-enkephalin sequence, namely, residues 61 to 65 of β-lipotropin.

NOMENCLATURE *Endorphin* was originally used synonymously with the term *opioid peptides* to designate any polypeptide with biological activities similar to those of the opiate

drugs; increasingly, however, the term *endorphin* is being limited to the opioid peptides larger in molecular size than the enkephalins. The term *enkephalin* is applied to the two pentapeptides, Met-enkephalin and Leu-enkephalin.

STRUCTURE AND BIOSYNTHESIS The amino acid sequence of the β-lipotropin molecule is shown in Fig. 88-1. The amino acid sequence of all peptides with biological opioid activity is identical to one or more sections of the *C*-terminal region of β-lipotropin (also see Chap. 109).

The biologically active peptides thus far identified include β-endorphin, which is the most abundant and which comprises the amino acid residues 61 to 91 of the β-lipotropin molecule, α-endorphin, consisting of residues 61 to 76 of β-lipotropin, γ-endorphin, made up of β-lipotropin residues 61 to 77, and δ-endorphin, which includes residues 61 to 87 of β-lipotropin. Enkephalins are the smallest molecules with opioid bioactivity. Leu-enkephalin has a leucine residue in place of the methionine residue of Met-enkephalin but is otherwise identical. The pentapeptide appears to be the minimum sequence necessary for opioid activity, and lengthening the chain both alters potency and influences biological effects. The Met- or Leu-enkephalin pentapeptide sequence, common to all the opioid peptides, has conformational similarities to the opiate alkaloids, which probably explains the fact that two such different substances can bind to the same receptors.

Since the opioid peptides share a common sequence with β-lipotropin, it is logical to consider the larger molecule as their possible precursor. Brain tissue can generate opioid activity from β-lipotropin in vitro, and pulse-chase studies indicate that β-lipotropin is an obligatory precursor of β-endorphin but not the enkephalins. Although the Met-enkephalin sequence could theoretically be derived from β-lipotropin, Leu-enkephalin could not be, since no β-lipotropin with a leucine in position 65 has been isolated. Furthermore, enkephalin and β-endorphin are present in different neurons in the brain. β-lipotropin tends to be found in the same sites in brain as β-endorphin but not in the same sites as the enkephalins. These findings suggest that Met- and Leu-enkephalin are synthesized by some other mechanism, possibly involving other precursor proteins. Other bioactive Met- or Leu-enkephalin-related peptides with a *C*-terminal extension of one, two, or eight amino acid residues have also been described (Fig. 89-1). These peptides appear to comprise another distinct family of enkephalin-related opioid peptides, whose synthetic pathway has also not been identified.

The biosynthesis of certain other peptide hormones is linked to the formation of the opioid peptides. The β-lipotro-

FIGURE 88-1
The relationship of the 91-amino acid β-lipotropin molecule to the known opioid peptides with amino acid sequences identical to segments of β-lipotropin.

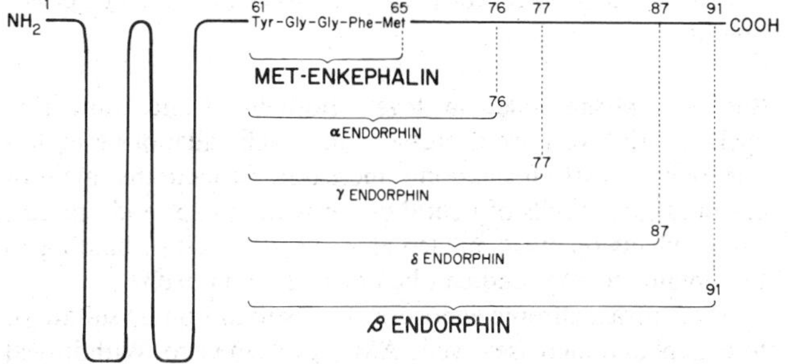

pin molecule isolated from normal pituitary or pituitary tumors is a part of a larger molecule of about 31,000 mol wt termed *pro-opiocortin* since it also contains the full sequence of adrenocorticotropic hormone (ACTH) (see Chap. 109). (Messenger RNA that codes for pro-opiocortin has also been isolated.) The finding of a common biosynthetic precursor for ACTH and β-lipotropin explains why these two polypeptides are present in the same secretory granules of the same cells of the pituitary and why β-endorphin and ACTH are simultaneously released in equimolar amounts from the pituitary gland under various conditions.

DISTRIBUTION OF THE ENDOGENOUS PEPTIDES β-Endorphin is present in the porcine hypothalamus and pituitary gland and in the brain is localized in discrete nerve fibers, consisting of single hypothalamic cells with long ascending and descending processes. The concentration in brain is lower than in the pituitary. Since β-endorphin persists in the brain after hypophysectomy, it is likely synthesized in the brain as well as in the pituitary. β-endorphin is also present in the human placenta.

The enkephalins are distributed more widely in nervous tissue. High concentrations are present in the dorsal columns of the spinal cord, the amygdala, and the medial hypothalamus. The ratio of Met- to Leu-enkephalin in the brain varies in different species. Immunohistologic studies reveal systems of enkephalin-containing nerve terminals, a finding suggesting a possible neurotransmitter role for the peptides. Enkephalins are also present in the gastrointestinal tract; indeed, the content of enkephalin in the myenteric plexus of the longitudinal muscles of the gut is higher than in the brain. Enkephalin-containing cells and nerve fibers have also been identified in the adrenal medulla.

MECHANISM OF ACTION **The opiate receptors** As is true for many hormones, the first step in the biological action of opioid hormones is binding to a specific receptor on target cells. Cell surface receptors for peptide hormones permit recognition of the particular peptide and result in the formation of a hormone-receptor complex capable of initiating a biological response (see Chap. 87). The finding that opioid receptors are heterogeneous may explain the different effects of various peptides in different tissues.

Naloxone The morphine antagonist naloxone is a congener of the opiate family that has no known opiate-like actions of its own. The fact that the drug binds to the opiate receptor, competing with and displacing morphine and other opiates, has been used to establish the specificity of binding by the opiates and opioid peptides. By using this drug to inhibit opiate actions, one can determine whether a particular biological phenomenon is mediated by an endogenous opioid peptide. For example, the fact that naloxone blocks the analgesic effects of electrical stimulation of the periaqueductal gray area provides strong evidence that endogenous opioid peptides mediate analgesia in this area of the brain. Thus, naloxone is a powerful tool in delineating the physiological roles of the endogenous opioids.

Response at the molecular level Both basal and stimulated cyclic AMP levels are decreased, and cyclic guanosine monophosphate (GMP) formation is increased by acute treatment of cultured tumor cells of neural origin with opiates and opioids. These effects on cyclic nucleotides are the result of binding to the opiate receptor and can be blocked by naloxone.

By contrast chronic exposure of cells to morphine sulfate or to enkephalin increases cyclic AMP levels in vitro. Withdrawal of the opioid or opiate results in a further increase in cyclic AMP in these cells. These changes may be implicated in certain aspects of drug abuse, such as addiction, tolerance, and the withdrawal syndrome.

Anatomic location of opioid receptors Opioid receptors are most abundant in those areas of the central nervous system in which opiates exert a biological effect and generally correspond with regions in which the enkephalins are present in high concentrations. In addition to the periaqueductal gray area high concentrations of receptors have been found in the following locations:

1 The *medial hypothalamus,* which mediates emotionally influenced deep pain, the pain most responsive to opiates. (The lateral hypothalamus mediates somatotrophic pain, is minimally affected by morphine, and has few opiate receptors.)
2 The *substantia gelatinosa* in the spinal cord, which integrates sensory information.
3 The *solitary nuclei receiving visceral sensory fibers from the vagus and glossopharyngeal nerve;* these are involved in cough reflexes, postural changes in blood pressure, and gastric secretion, all functions that are influenced by opiates.
4 The *amygdala,* the area with the highest density of opiate receptors; this region is thought to be involved in various forms of emotional behavior.
5 The *area postrema,* in which opioids produce nausea and vomiting.
6 The *gastrointestinal tract,* an organ well known to respond to opiate alkaloids.

POSSIBLE PHYSIOLOGICAL AND PATHOPHYSIOLOGICAL ROLES Most work on opioid peptides has been performed in experimental animals, and extrapolation of the results to humans may be invalid. Nevertheless, as indicated above, the enkephalins are present in high concentrations in those regions of the central nervous system concerned with deep pain, emotional behavior, nausea and vomiting, cough reflexes, respiration, blood pressure, thermoregulation, and gastrointestinal function. It is reasonable to postulate that the endogenous opioids in some of or all these areas function as neurotransmitters or neuromodulators and subserve physiological roles.

Actions on the brain: Role in nonpharmacological analgesia (acupuncture, hypnosis, electric shock) The biological actions of the various endorphins vary somewhat when injected into the brain of rats. The observed effects include analgesia, hypothermia, hyperthermia, tranquilization, irritability, agitation, and, in high doses, violent behavior, catalepsy, narcolepsy, and catatonia. These effects disappear without sequelae and can be reversed or prevented by naloxone. The role of the endogenous opioids in influencing pain is uncertain because of conflicting results in tests of the influence of naloxone on various forms of pain. Naloxone appears to intensify certain forms of pain in humans, for example, that produced by dental extraction. Some workers have failed to observe an antagonistic effect upon analgesia produced by electric shock and hypnosis. However, studies in patients with persistent pain reveal that analgesia produced by electrical stimulation of periventricular brain sites is accompanied by a rise in ventricular enkephalin-like and β-endorphin-like activity and that this analgesia is blocked by naloxone, suggesting that the analgesia is mediated by endogenous opioid peptides. The opioid peptides may also be involved in the analgesic effects of acupuncture; acupuncture analgesia in mice is blocked by naloxone and abolished by hypophysectomy. The opioid peptides may also mediate placebo-induced analgesia. In those subjects who benefit from placebos tolerance and dependence on the placebos may develop, and the analgesic effects have been blocked by naloxone.

Role in thermogenesis The opioid peptides are believed to be physiological determinants of the adaptive responses to heat. For example, after acute and chronic exposure of rats to high temperatures, the administration of naloxone causes a rapid increase in temperature.

Effects on the endocrine system Morphine and the opioid peptides have similar actions, namely stimulating the secretion of growth hormone, prolactin, and antidiuretic hormone and inhibiting ovulation and the secretion of luteinizing hormone (LH). These effects are not mediated by direct action on the pituitary gland but involve a centrally mediated mechanism, possibly an effect on the formation or action of the releasing factors for pituitary hormones. (Enkephalins are capable of inhibiting dopamine-induced LHRH release from the hypothalamus.)

Although β-lipotropin has no opioid activity in vitro, aldosterone-stimulating activity has now been described.

Role in stress Hypothalamic opioid peptides appear to be implicated in certain stress-mediated phenomena. In experimental animals naloxone prevents the stress-induced increase in serum prolactin as well as stress-induced eating. Opioid peptides of the anterior pituitary may also have a role in stress. β-Endorphin is secreted concomitantly with ACTH during acute stress and after adrenalectomy, and, like ACTH, β-endorphin release is stimulated by corticotropin-releasing factor and inhibited by glucocorticoids. However, the target organs of circulating β-endorphin remain to be identified.

Role in feeding β-Endorphin in rats increases eating. The pituitaries of congenitally obese mice also contain higher concentrations of β-endorphin than do those of lean littermates; the finding that naloxone abolishes overeating in these mice raises the possibility that this opioid peptide may play a role in the physiological control of appetite and possibly in overeating and obesity.

Actions in digestive organs The presence of enkephalins in endocrine cells as well as nerve fibers of the myenteric plexus of the gastrointestinal tract implies a role of gastrointestinal function. It seems likely that the enkephalins serve an opioid function (an endogenous paregoric-like role) since they diminish gastrointestinal propulsion, perhaps by inhibiting the firing of neurons in the myenteric plexus. Enkephalin analogues also stimulate gastric acid secretion and mucosal blood flow.

Enkephalins appear to have a role in the function of the endocrine and exocrine pancreas. Insulin and glucagon secretion are stimulated, and somatostatin secretion is inhibited by opiates and opioid peptides. These effects are blocked by naloxone. Morphine and enkephalin also inhibit the secretion of bicarbonate and enzymes by the exocrine pancreas.

POTENTIAL CLINICAL IMPLICATIONS The endogenous opioid peptides may play a role in the pathophysiology of several disease processes.

Psychiatric diseases The possibility that abnormalities in endogenous opioids may be present in psychiatric disorders is suggested by the finding that β-endorphin levels are elevated in the cerebrospinal fluid of schizophrenics. Naloxone does not appear to alter experimental pain or mood in humans, and beneficial effects of β-endorphin or naloxone in schizophrenic or depressive states have not been observed consistently. Chronic treatment of rats with lithium, an agent used in the treatment of mania and depression, increases Met-enkephalin levels in the striatum in proportion to the serum lithium levels. This increase has been attributed to a reduced rate of release of Met-enkephalin from the striatum.

Drug addiction and analgesia The proposal has been made that the chronic abuse of narcotics either suppresses the biosynthesis or accelerates the degradation of endogenous opioids and that the manifestations of narcotic withdrawal are due to the uncovering of a secondary endogenous opioid deficiency throughout the body. Alternatively, a genetically predetermined opioid deficiency may predispose certain people to narcotic addition. Although it was originally hoped that endogenous opioids might be free of addictive properties, a similar tolerance and dependence is produced by chronic injections of β-endorphin or chronic infusion of enkephalins into the brain as is seen with morphine-like drugs. Thus, it seems unlikely that the development of analogues of the opioid peptides will lead to the production of analgesics with nonaddicitve properties. However, drugs may be developed with a different spectrum of activity compared with the presently known analgesic narcotics.

Clinical endocrinology The effects of opioids on hormone secretion in the human are not identical to those in experimental animals. Thus, endorphin does not stimulate the release of growth hormone or ACTH. On the basis of studies with naloxone, however, opioids appear to play a role in the modulation of gonadotropin, vasopressin, and possibly ACTH secretion and, to a lesser extent, in the release of prolactin, growth hormone, and thyrotropin as well. For example, naloxone increases LH secretion in the luteal phase of the menstrual cycle and inhibits the rise in vasopressin induced by an orthostatic stimulus.

The release of β-endorphin from the anterior pituitary and the control of its secretion appear to be similar to that of ACTH in humans. Elevated levels are found in patients with Cushing disease, Nelson syndrome and adrenal insufficiency. In Cushing disease the ratio of plasma endorphin to β-lipotropin is increased, suggesting altered processing of pro-opiocortin. Whether this relative increase in endorphin concentrations has diagnostic value is not yet clear. Enkephalin immunoreactivity is present in human plasma, but the sources, control, and biological role of plasma enkephalins have not been defined.

Other diseases A number of disease states in which opioid peptides potentially play a pathogenetic role have been tested with naloxone in an attempt to reverse some of the manifestations of the disease. Naloxone had a beneficial effect upon blood pressure in experimental endotoxic, hypovolemic, and spinal shock and in septic shock in humans. These studies suggest that endogenous opioid peptides may be involved in the control of blood pressure. A previously undescribed hypothalamic syndrome has been reported in which transient reversal of analgesia, restoration of hormonal responses, and correction of neurological features occurred following administration of naloxone. Long-acting opiate antagonists may play a therapeutic role in such situations.

BIOLOGICAL IMPLICATIONS Physiology Many so-called drug receptors may represent binding sites for endogenous factors that, through a coincidence of chemistry, cross react with a foreign substance. Indeed, it seems unlikely that nature would have endowed animals and humans with receptors to opium, a substance found in poppies. It is predictable that certain other pharmacologically active drugs are, like morphine, coincidental ligands to receptors intended to receive other, still undiscovered, endogenous substances.

Hormone biosynthesis The idea that opioid peptides may be derived from a precursor that contains the full sequence of other peptide hormones altered our concepts of peptide hormone biosynthesis. At least some of the opioid peptides are derived from a single 31,000 mol wt precursor of β-lipotropin, and ACTH (and perhaps other hormones) is also derived from this preprohormone. This finding raises the possibility that other peptide hormones may be derived from a small number of primary gene products containing the sequence of such hormones and serving as an uncommitted precursor. According to this concept, the final secretory product or products of a particular cell type is determined in part by the way such large polypeptides are cleaved by the cell as well as through synthesis of distinct amino acid sequences by different cells. For example, functionally distinct cells producing such peptides as MSH, ACTH, opioid peptides, and perhaps other hormones might all synthesize the same primary gene product, but the final hormone released by each cell type is determined by enzymatic machinery that excises a particular amino acid sequence from the common precursor protein. Perhaps this might explain why certain endocrine and nonendocrine neoplasms appear to produce seemingly inappropriate hormones and hormone precursors. Support for this contention is found in the observed differences in the processing of pro-opiocortin in different tissues. While β-lipotropin and ACTH are major end products in the anterior pituitary, in the hypothalamus and intermediate lobe of the pituitary (of animals) the precursor is processed further, and α-MSH and β-endorphin are present in higher concentrations.

Relationships among brain, gut, and pancreas The discovery of the opioid peptides has extended our concepts of relationships among the cells of the brain, an organ whose principal function is to transmit signals from one cell to another, and endocrine cells, located outside the central nervous system but serving the same purpose. Certain of the peptide-secreting endocrine cells, particularly those in the endocrine pancreas and the gastrointestinal tract, have an ontological origin in common with the central nervous system. The fact that opioid peptides are present in the central nervous system, pituitary glands, gastrointestinal tract, and pancreas adds another polypeptide family to the growing group of substances, including somatostatin, ACTH, growth hormone, thyrotropin-releasing factor, cholecystokinin, substance P, neurotensin, vasoactive intestinal polypeptide (VIP), and many others, that have been identified by immunologic techniques both in and outside the central nervous system. It is difficult to understand why thyrotropin-releasing hormone, for example, should be present in the islets of Langerhans or why cholecystokinin is the most abundant polypeptide hormone in the brain. Perhaps in the course of evolution the brain, the primary organ for generation of signals to coordinate cellular activities of the entire organism, was compelled by the sheer increase in complexity of evolving organisms to develop alternative pathways of signal transmission by using avenues other than axonal neurotransmission. Nonaxonal, nonsynaptic routes for transmission of signals may, therefore, have evolved, exploiting pathways not specifically designed for this purpose, i.e., the vascular and interstitial spaces, through which the number of signals that could be relayed would theoretically be unlimited. Extraneural sites of signal biosynthesis, the endocrine cells (believed to be of neuroectodermal origin), evolved in anatomically propitious regions of the body such as the pancreas and the gastrointestinal tract to serve such a function. Polypeptide signals released from these cells would still be under the influence of the central nervous system and thus would amplify its control function by nonneuronal means.

REFERENCES

Beaumont A, Hughes J: Biology of opioid peptides. Ann Rev Pharmac Toxicol 19:245, 1979

Bunney WE Jr et al: Basic and clinical studies of endorphins. Ann Intern Med 91:239, 1979

Krieger DT, Martin JB: Brain peptides. N Engl J Med 304:876, 944, 1981

Morley JE: The endocrinology of the opiates and opioid peptides. Metabolism 30:195, 1981

Snyder SH: Opiate receptors in the brain. N Engl J Med 296:266, 1977

89 INTERMEDIARY METABOLISM OF CARBOHYDRATES, LIPIDS, AND PROTEINS

DANIEL W. FOSTER
J. DENIS McGARRY

Fuel metabolism is a complicated and finely regulated process. In this chapter the general principles of the intermediary metabolism of carbohydrates, lipids, and proteins will be briefly reviewed. Emphasis is placed on the physiology of substrate flow under the influence of the endocrine system rather than on the molecular biochemistry of the various pathways.

It is helpful to consider intermediary metabolism in two phases—*anabolic* and *catabolic*. Under ordinary circumstances energy needs of the body are met by exogenous substrate derived from food. In simple terms, oxidation of the constituent molecules of absorbed foodstuffs to carbon dioxide and water is accompanied by the generation of adenosine triphosphate (ATP), the principal high-energy compound of the body (Fig. 89-1). In one sense life can be defined as the continued ability to generate ATP (and related high-energy nucleotides) for the preservation of cellular integrity in all its manifestations.

When caloric intake is greater than immediate oxidative needs, as after the usual meal, excess substrate is stored as fat, structural protein, and glycogen. This stored substrate is readily mobilized for use by the various tissues of the body during fasting or caloric restriction (Fig. 89-2). From conception to adult life net substrate flux is in the anabolic direction (caloric balance is positive) to allow body growth. At maturity anabolic and catabolic cycles ideally balance such that weight is maintained constant. Deviation in a positive direction results in obesity, while prolonged fasting or semistarvation leads to flow over the catabolic pathway and weight loss.

Anabolic and catabolic phases of metabolism are hormonally determined, and transition from one to the other is smoothly integrated. Insulin is the primary hormone mediating the anabolic phase, while a rise in plasma glucagon, coupled with a fall in insulin, initiates catabolism. Epinephrine, cortisol, and growth hormone likewise increase during the catabolic phase and doubtless contribute to the metabolic pattern. A summary of the feeding-fasting cycle is given in Table 89-1.

ANABOLIC PHASE

When food is ingested the absorptive process begins through the action of intraluminal and brush border enzymes in the intestine which break down complex carbohydrates, lipids, and proteins to constituent sugars, fatty acids, and amino acids. The normal diet is a mixture of all three components, and absorption and metabolism of carbohydrate, fat, and protein occur simultaneously. For descriptive purposes, however, each will be discussed separately.

CARBOHYDRATE Following a carbohydrate meal, absorbed sugars pass into the portal vein for transport to the liver and peripheral tissues. As plasma glucose concentrations rise, insulin release from the pancreas is stimulated and glucagon levels fall. The magnitude of the insulin response to glucose is increased through the action of other gastrointestinal hormones secreted following food intake. The latter account for the fact that glucose taken by mouth results in greater insulin release than equivalent amounts given intravenously. The major gastrointestinal hormone appears to be gastric inhibitory polypeptide (GIP), a hormone released into plasma during food absorption. The newly released insulin accelerates the disposal of glucose in muscle and adipose tissue. In muscle a portion of the glucose taken up is oxidized, and the remainder is stored as glycogen. In adipose tissue glucose is utilized for de novo synthesis of long-chain fatty acids, which, in turn, are esterified with glucose-derived glycerol to form triglycerides. Although glucose is metabolized in peripheral tissues, most of the ingested load (> 60 percent) is directly or indirectly taken up by the splanchnic bed (primarily liver) where it is utilized for the formation of glycogen and triglycerides. The former is stored

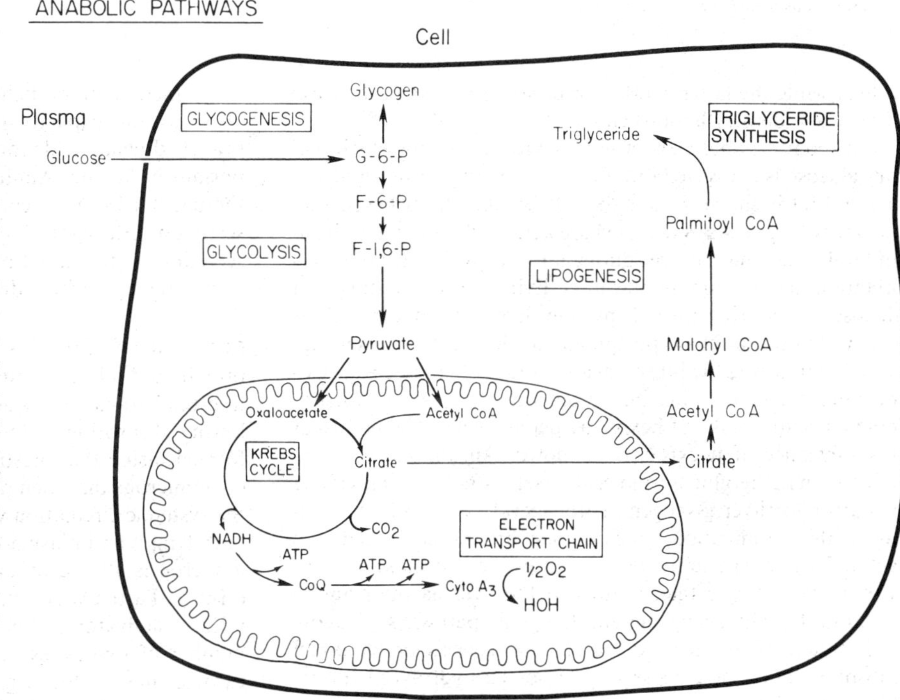

FIGURE 89-1
Anabolic pathways. Simplified scheme showing a hepatic cell with a mitochondrion. Transport systems and enzymatic details are omitted. Following a meal, a portion of ingested food is used directly to generate energy in the form of ATP while the remainder is available for storage. In the example shown glucose is oxidized via the glycolytic pathway and Krebs cycle, serves as substrate for glycogen synthesis, and is transformed to fat following conversion to citrate in the mitochondrion. Citrate is transported to the cytosol and hydrolyzed to acetyl CoA, the substrate from which malonyl CoA is formed, and oxaloacetate, which then is transported back into the mitochondrion (not shown). Exogenous amino acids and fatty acids are stored as protein and triglyceride in muscle cells and adipocytes, respectively. G-6-P, glucose 6-phosphate, F-6-P, fructose 6-phosphate, F-1,6-P, fructose 1,6-diphosphate; NADH, nicotinamide adenine dinucleotide; ATP, adenosine triphosphate; CoQ, coenzyme Q; Cyto A_3, cytochrome A_3; CoA, coenzyme A.

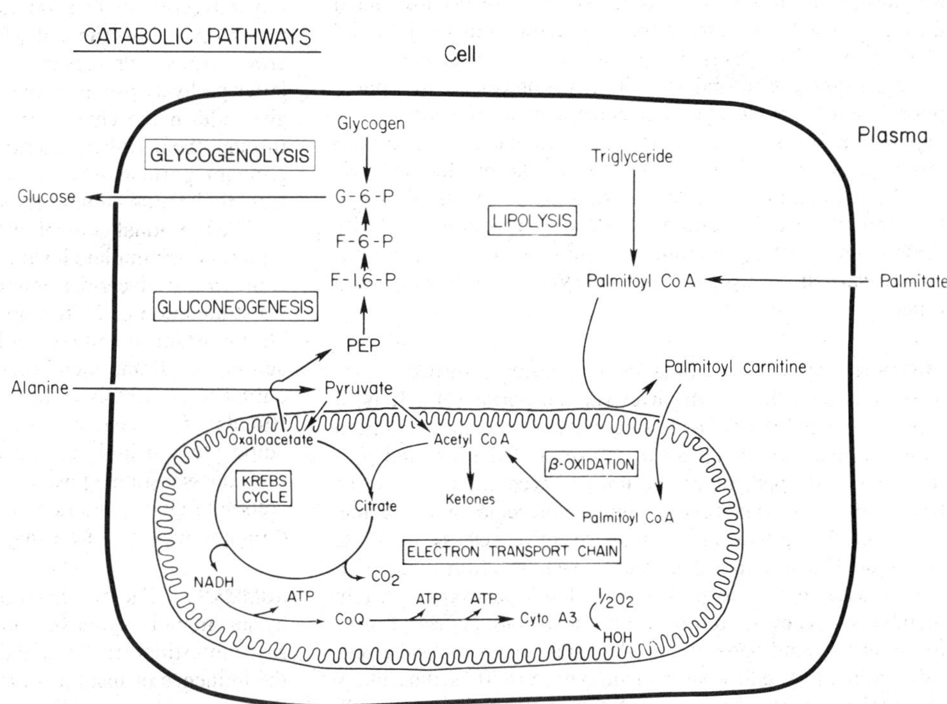

FIGURE 89-2
Catabolic pathways. Simplified scheme showing a hepatic cell with a mitochondrion. Transport systems and enzymatic details are omitted. In the postabsorptive state hepatic glucose production is derived from glycogen breakdown and gluconeogenesis. The latter is largely dependent on amino acids and lactate moving to the liver from the periphery. The energy for gluconeogenesis (ATP) comes primarily from oxidation of long-chain fatty acids released from adipose tissue and from hepatic triglycerides. Fatty acids are also the substrate for ketone body synthesis (see text). PEP, phosphoenolpyruvate; other abbreviations as defined for Fig. 89-1.

TABLE 89-1
The feeding-fasting cycle

Phase	*Primary hormone*	*Plasma substrates*	*Substrate flux*	*Active process*
Anabolic*	Insulin	↑ Glucose ↑ Triglycerides ↑ Branched-chain amino acids ↓ Free fatty acids ↓ Ketones	Splanchnic bed → storage and utilization sites	Glycogen storage Protein synthesis Triglyceride formation
Catabolic†	Glucagon	↓ Glucose ↓ Triglycerides ↑ Alanine and glutamine‡ ↑ Free fatty acids ↑ Ketones	Storage sites → liver and utilization sites	Glycogenolysis Gluconeogenesis Proteolysis Lipolysis Ketogenesis

* *Expected findings during the first several hours after ingestion of a mixed meal of fat, carbohydrate, and protein.*
† *The major catabolic phase occurs during the overnight fast, although partial catabolic cycles occur between meals.*
‡ *Arrows indicate plasma concentrations except for alanine and glutamine. While arterial concentrations of these amino acids are relatively constant, uptake by the liver and intestine is increased in the catabolic phase.*

in liver while the latter is transported to fat depots in the form of very low density lipoproteins.

The conventional view of intrahepatic events by which dietary glucose is converted into the stored energy forms of glycogen and fat is shown in Fig. 89-1. It is generally believed that the anabolic pathways depicted are activated by the high insulin levels reaching the liver during a meal. However, this interpretation may require modification. Evidence is mounting that glucose is poorly utilized by the liver at concentrations achieved in portal blood postprandially. Thus, it has been suggested that during the intestinal absorption of glucose a gastrointestinal factor (not insulin) is generated that serves to promote efficient uptake of hexose by hepatic cells. The nature of this substance, if it exists, is unknown. An alternative viewpoint is that the glucose molecule itself is not the immediate precursor for liver glycogen or triglyceride synthesis. According to this formulation, glucose must first be converted into lactate by nonhepatic tissues (e.g., intestine and muscle). Glucose-derived lactate then returns to the liver as the primary substrate for gluconeogenic and lipogenic pathways. Glucose 6-phosphate (G6P) formed via gluconeogenesis or by direct phosphorylation of glucose may either be hydrolyzed for release into plasma as free glucose or converted to glycogen. Since plasma glucose levels rise following a meal (i.e., there is no glucose "need") while glycogen stores have been depleted during the preceding fast, glycogen synthesis is favored. "Pull" of G6P into glycogen is thought to result from activation of glycogen synthase secondary to inactivation of glycogen phosphorylase by an elevated free-glucose concentration in the hepatocyte. It is attractive to speculate that glucose 6-phosphatase activity might likewise be blunted as plasma glucose levels rise following a meal, further contributing to enhanced flux of G6P into glycogen. Additional work will be required to clarify these issues. Dietary fructose and amino acids may also contribute carbon to glycogen and fat synthesis following food intake.

PROTEIN After a protein-containing meal, absorbed amino acids also pass first to the liver via the portal vein. It is of interest that the amino acids entering the systemic circulation from the liver do not reflect the makeup of the ingested protein; about 60 percent of the total is accounted for by the branched-chain components valine, isoleucine, and leucine. The precise mechanism whereby selective release of these amino acids is accomplished is unknown. The branched-chain amino acids appear to play a pivotal role in overall protein metabolism. They are responsive to the anabolic effect of insulin in muscle, and one of them—leucine—seems to have a specific stimulatory effect on protein synthesis. It is thus likely that replenishment of protein stores in muscle following a meal is a function of branched-chain amino acid uptake. Muscle also has the capacity (not shared by liver) to oxidize the branched-chain acids for energy purposes. This capacity is important in fasting. Amino acids stimulate insulin release from the pancreas but, in contrast to glucose, also cause glucagon secretion. Glucagon may prevent hypoglycemia when insulin secretion is stimulated by a protein meal under circumstances where dietary carbohydrate is absent or limited.

FAT Fat absorption is slower than that of carbohydrate or protein and follows a different course. The rate-limiting step is intestinal transport, which may take hours to complete. Following absorption of long-chain fatty acids, triglyceride is reformed inside the intestinal cell and packaged in the form of chylomicrons that then pass into the lymph channels and reach the systemic circulation via the thoracic duct. During transit in both lymph and plasma the apolipoprotein content of the chylomicron is altered by exchange with high-density lipoprotein (HDL). Particularly important is an increase in apoprotein CII, an activator of lipoprotein lipase. In the capillaries of a number of tissues, especially adipose tissue and skeletal and cardiac muscle, the triglycerides of chylomicrons are broken down to free fatty acids and 2-monoglycerides by lipoprotein lipase. Subsequently, the monoglyceride is hydrolyzed by a monoglyceridase. The free fatty acids liberated by the two reactions pass into the cell where they may be oxidized for energy purposes or reesterified for storage as triglyceride. The latter pathway predominates in the adipocyte. Most of the triglyceride in the chylomicron is removed in a single passage through the peripheral capillary bed. The cholesterol ester–rich remnant particle then passes to the liver where it serves to regulate hepatic cholesterol synthesis.

The hormonal control of lipid metabolism is complex. Pure fat does not stimulate insulin release. However, if carbohydrate is present, triglycerides enhance the insulin response, probably via stimulation of gastric inhibitory polypeptide. Insulin plays an important, if indirect, role in the transport of triglyceride across the plasma membrane of peripheral cells since it is required for synthesis of lipoprotein lipase. Insulin also acts to stimulate fatty acid synthesis and triglyceride formation in the adipocyte and inhibits lipolysis catalyzed by the intracellular hormone-sensitive lipase. In animals triglyceride stimulates secretion of glucagon and enteric glucagon-like material, but this does not appear to be a major response in humans.

SUMMARY The first few hours after a meal are characterized by an anabolic state in which ingested foods pass from the gastrointestinal tract to the liver and peripheral tissues. Under the influence of insulin some substrate is utilized immediately for energy purposes, but significant quantities are stored as glycogen, structural protein, and fat to be used as needed in the postabsorptive state or during more prolonged fasting.

CATABOLIC PHASE

Postabsorptively[1] a series of metabolic adaptations ensure adequate fuels for body tissues in the absence of exogenous substrate. Since the brain and other parts of the central nervous system can utilize only glucose or ketone bodies for energy purposes, it is obvious that during a fast plasma glucose concentrations must be sustained in a safe range until acetoacetate and β-hydroxybutyrate concentrations rise to protective levels. Three major processes are involved: (1) The liver is transformed from an organ of glucose storage to one of net glucose production. Initially the bulk of glucose released comes from glycogen breakdown, while in later stages new glucose production is derived from peripheral precursors via gluconeogenesis. (2) Free fatty acids are mobilized from adipose tissue to be utilized directly for oxidative purposes in many tissues and to serve as substrate for ketone body synthesis in the liver. Importantly, free fatty acids also provide the energy required for gluconeogenesis in the liver although they are not themselves substrates for glucose formation. (3) Hepatic ketogenic machinery is activated. As a result of the latter two processes, after only a few days of fasting most tissues of the body utilize free fatty acids and ketones for energy, sparing glucose for the central nervous system. Under these circumstances the enhanced endogenous production of glucose by the liver is adequate to avoid hypoglycemia. In addition the ketone bodies themselves become a major substrate for the brain, sufficient to maintain central nervous system function if for any reason glucose production is impaired. An outline of glucose homeostasis during fasting is given in Table 89-2.

All three of the adaptive processes described above are hormonally induced. In the postabsorptive state there is a fall in insulin release, probably primarily as the consequence of a decline in plasma glucose concentration. Concomitantly there is a rise in four key counterregulatory hormones: epinephrine, glucagon, cortisol, and growth hormone. From studies of experimental hypoglycemia, glucagon appears to be responsible for maintenance of the plasma glucose in the early stages of a fast. Blockade of glucagon release by somatostatin impairs recovery from insulin-induced hypoglycemia even though catecholamine levels increase normally. Epinephrine contributes to counterregulation, however, as evidenced by a further delay in recovery from hypoglycemia when adrenergic blockade is superimposed on the somatostatin infusion. Growth hormone and cortisol concentrations increase late following hypoglycemia, but immediate effects on plasma glucose are minimal. Doubtless their major role is to enhance gluconeogenesis; i.e., they exert counterregulatory effects primarily during prolonged fasting. Lipolysis is the consequence of insulin deficiency but is also stimulated by catecholamines. The ketogenic capacity of liver is induced by the rise in plasma glucagon concentration relative to that of insulin.

[1] *The term* postabsorptive *is used in the literature to indicate an overnight (10- to 12-h) fast. In this discussion it is used to indicate the end of the anabolic phase, which may occur earlier.*

TABLE 89-2
Maintenance of plasma glucose during fasting

Length of fast	*Source of plasma glucose*	*Mechanism*	*Tissues using glucose*	*Primary fuel of brain*
3–4 h	Diet	Intestinal absorption	All	Glucose
4–16 h	Liver	Glycogenolysis	All except liver (↓ rates in muscle and adipose tissue)	Glucose
16–48 h	Liver	Gluconeogenesis (± glycogen-olysis)	All except liver (further ↓ rates in muscle and adipose tissue)	Glucose
2–24 days	Liver, kidney	Gluconeogenesis	Brain, RBC, renal medulla	Glucose Ketones
>4 weeks	Liver, kidney	Gluconeogenesis	Brain, RBC, renal medulla (↓ rates)	Ketones Glucose

SOURCE: *After Ruderman et al.*

GLYCOGENOLYSIS AND GLUCONEOGENESIS At the level of the liver the starvation-induced reversal in the direction of glucose metabolism (compare Figs. 89-1 and 89-2) appears to be triggered by a fall in the circulating insulin that allows glucagon to act in unrestrained fashion. The result is a rise in hepatic cyclic adenosine monophosphate (cyclic AMP) concentration that has far-reaching effects. Breakdown of glycogen into glucose begins immediately. This is accompanied by suppression of glycolysis (the oxidation of G6P to pyruvate) and stimulation of the gluconeogenic pathway. The biochemical events underlying the cyclic AMP–mediated acceleration of glycogenolysis (activation of glycogen phosphorylase with concomitant inactivation of glycogen synthase) are well established. The mechanisms by which carbon flow between G6P and pyruvate is blocked have only recently come to light. The key regulatory enzyme in glycolysis, phosphofructokinase (PFK), which catalyzes the conversion of fructose 6-phosphate into fructose 1,6-diphosphate, exists in both nonphosphorylated and phosphorylated forms. The former, but not the latter, is able to bind an "activation factor," fructose 2,6-diphosphate (F2,6P), with a manyfold increase in catalytic capacity. F2,6P also inhibits fructose diphosphatase (FDPase), a key enzyme in the reverse pathway of gluconeogenesis. The effect of cyclic AMP on this system is twofold: first, it promotes the phosphorylation of phosphofructokinase, thus reducing its affinity for F2,6P; second, it inhibits the kinase responsible for the production of F2,6P from F6P. The net result is a profound fall in the level of PFK activity and stimulation of FDPase such that glycolysis is inhibited and gluconeogenesis is activated. A second regulatory site in the glycolytic pathway is the pyruvate kinase reaction, which effects the conversion of phosphoenolpyruvate into pyruvate. This enzyme is also subject to cyclic AMP–mediated phosphorylation and inactivation, contributing to the block in glycolysis that occurs in the catabolic phase.

In quantitative terms hepatic glucose production in the immediate postabsorptive state is due almost exclusively to breakdown of preformed glycogen. Ordinarily the liver contains sufficient glycogen to maintain the plasma glucose for only 12 to 24 h (depending on activity and caloric demands). Beyond this period gluconeogenesis is required if hypoglycemia is to be avoided. The gluconeogenic substrates are lactate, glycerol, and amino acids. Lactate derived from glucose not completely oxidized in peripheral tissues normally returns to the liver and after an overnight fast accounts for up to 20 percent of hepatic glucose production (Cori cycle). This does not result in net glucose synthesis, however, since the lactate was originally derived from glucose passing to muscle and other tissues. Net glucose synthesis from lactate (as opposed to the recycling sequence) requires the latter's production from stored muscle glycogen. Glycerol utilized for gluconeogenesis comes from triglycerides hydrolyzed in adipose tissue. Its contribution to overall glucose production is relatively minor. Amino acids represent the major substrate for gluconeogenesis, but amino acid metabolism during fasting is complicated. While there is net release of all amino acids, the output of alanine and glutamine is out of proportion to their relative concentrations in muscle protein. Glutamine is preferentially utilized by extrahepatic splanchnic tissues, while alanine uptake by the liver is greater than that of any other amino acid, suggesting that it plays a prime role in the gluconeogenic process. Moreover, alanine extraction by the liver increases during fasting. Glutamine is also taken up by the kidney, serving as substrate for NH_3 generation and renal gluconeogenesis. While liver is the primary gluconeogenic organ, measurable glucose production occurs in the kidney during prolonged fasting.

It is now thought that the bulk of the alanine released from muscle is derived from transamination of pyruvate which, in turn, is produced from muscle glycogen, glucose from plasma, and possibly directly from amino acids themselves. The source of nitrogen for the transamination of pyruvate is likely the branched-chain amino acids that are released from the breakdown of muscle protein. Following transamination, the α-keto analogues of these acids are oxidized to provide energy for the muscle. The end result is that muscle protein becomes the major source of new glucose formation by the liver, transported to that organ in the form of alanine. Presumably the advantage of alanine resides in its ready ability to enter the hepatocyte and the gluconeogenic pathways.

The amino acids utilized in gluconeogenesis come from structural protein of muscle rather than from nonfunctional storage pools. As a consequence they represent enzymes, transport molecules, and membrane proteins, all of which are vital to cellular integrity (in contrast to loss of glycogen and triglyceride which are not essential to the cell). For this reason when starvation is extended beyond a few days, limitation of protein loss becomes critical. After several weeks of total starvation (in obese subjects) nitrogen excretion in the urine decreases. At this stage essentially all tissues of the body are sustained by the oxidation of fat—either as free fatty acids or ketone bodies. As a result the demand for glucose (and thus the demand for protein as gluconeogenic substrate) diminishes, and the negative nitrogen balance of starvation is blunted. It was suggested that the ketone bodies somehow signaled the muscle to damp amino acid release, based on the observation that infusion of sodium β-hydroxybutyrate into fasted subjects lowered plasma alanine concentration and diminished urinary nitrogen content. However, subsequent studies have cast considerable doubt on this formulation. On clinical grounds the hypothesis was also suspect since massive negative nitrogen balance occurs in diabetic ketoacidosis in the face of plasma concentrations of ketones far higher than maximal levels attained in prolonged starvation. Thus, the cause of the secondary decline in nitrogen loss remains unknown. Changes in availability of other substrates (e.g., pyruvate, which might limit alanine transport from muscle to liver) with or without small secondary changes in the ratio of anabolic/catabolic hormones conceivably could constitute the damping signal(s).

LIPOLYSIS The hydrolysis of adipose tissue triglycerides to free fatty acids and glycerol is mediated by an intracellular, hormone-sensitive lipase which is distinct from the extracellular lipoprotein lipase previously mentioned. This lipase is susceptible to both positive and negative regulation. Insulin in low concentrations can effectively block lipolysis, while catecholamines activate the process. A number of hormones that increase triglyceride breakdown in rat adipose tissue (e.g., glucagon, growth hormone, adrenocorticotropin) appear to be less effective in human adipocytes. Activation is thought to involve cyclic adenosine monophosphate acting via a protein kinase that phosphorylates the hormone-sensitive lipase. On the negative side both the ketone bodies and adenosine, in addition to insulin, have been suggested to deactivate lipolysis. Free fatty acids rise early in the postabsorptive state and usually reach a maximum of about 1 m*M* in prolonged fasting.

The importance of lipolysis resides in the fact that body fat represents the organism's primary defense against starvation. This is true because its energy value per gram (about 9 cal) is twice that of protein and carbohydrate (about 4 cal/g) and because its mass is large. The average-size person has approximately 140,000 cal stored as fat compared with 24,000 cal as protein and 300 cal as glycogen. If adipose tissue is depleted (because of disease or famine) or if fatty acids cannot be normally oxidized (see Chap. 116), fatal hypoglycemia or death from protein deficiency may occur.

KETOGENESIS As noted, the ketone bodies play a critical role in the catabolic response to food deprivation. They represent an energy source that can be used by almost every tissue in the body, and they are the only effective alternative substrate for brain metabolism. Interestingly, when total ketones reach concentrations of 4 to 6 m*M*, hypoglycemia sufficient to cause adrenergic response and mental confusion in a nonketotic individual produces no symptoms. Under these circumstances acetoacetate and β-hydroxybutyrate can meet the metabolic demands of the central nervous system despite inadequate glucose.

Significant ketosis requires changes in both liver and adipose tissue. In the fed state the capacity for fatty acid oxidation in the liver is low. Most of the fatty acid taken up by the hepatocyte is reesterified to triglyceride and either stored or released as a very low density lipoprotein particle. The rate of hepatic fatty acid oxidation is governed by the activity of the carnitine acyltransferase system of enzymes that transports fatty acids into the mitochondria. In the fed state malonyl CoA, a potent inhibitor of carnitine acyltransferase I, keeps the system inactive. This inhibition is removed during fasting through the action of glucagon which lowers the malonyl CoA concentration and simultaneously increases the carnitine content of liver. With these changes the capacity for fatty acid oxidation and ketogenesis is maximally activated in the hepatocyte. (For a more detailed explanation, see Chap. 114.) Once the liver is activated, the rate of ketone body production is determined solely by the rate of delivery of free fatty acids from the periphery; i.e., the higher the free fatty acid concentration in plasma, the greater the hepatic production of acetoacetate and β-hydroxybutyrate until maximal rates are obtained.

Quantitative estimates of substrate flux after a 24-h fast are shown in Table 89-3.

SUMMARY The catabolic changes that occur in the absence of food vary with the duration of the fast. In the first few hours glycogenolysis predominates, while the adaptive response after the first day involves gluconeogenesis and protein breakdown together with acceleration of fat catabolism. If the fast is prolonged, a fat economy is established with diminution of gluco-

TABLE 89-3
Substrate flux during fasting (per 24 h)*

Amino acids released	75 g
Free fatty acids released	160 g
Used directly	120 g
Converted to ketones	40 g
Glucose produced	180 g
Ketones produced	60 g

* *Fluxes calculated after 24 h of fasting in a subject with basal energy requirements of 1800 cal.*
SOURCE: *After Cahill.*

neogenesis and nitrogen wastage. If adipose tissue stores are adequate, prolonged survival can occur in the absence of food.

STARVATION AND DIABETIC KETOACIDOSIS

Diabetic ketoacidosis is a catabolic illness that resembles an accelerated state of starvation. In this situation hepatic gluconeogenesis is markedly increased, plasma free fatty acids are high (2 to 4 m*M*), acetoacetate and β-hydroxybutyrate concentrations are sufficient (18 to 20 m*M*) to cause acidosis, and protein wastage is massive. The quantitative differences between starvation and diabetic ketoacidosis can be accounted for primarily by the almost complete absence of insulin in ketoacidosis-prone diabetes. As outlined above, normal persons subjected to fasting show a modest fall in plasma glucose which results in diminished insulin release from the pancreatic islets. The fall in insulin concentration, coupled with release of glucagon and other counterregulatory hormones, activates glycogen breakdown, gluconeogenesis, lipolysis, and ketogenesis. Since both ketone bodies and free fatty acids can stimulate insulin release from the beta cell, a protective feedback loop is available during fasting in the normal subject that prevents the occurrence of ketoacidosis; i.e., when total ketones and free fatty acids approach levels sufficient to produce a significant acidosis, insulin release is stimulated (or further fall in insulin is prevented), resulting in modulation of adipose tissue lipolysis and limitation of ketone formation by restriction of fatty acid flow to the liver. In the absence of an adequate insulin feedback loop, as in the juvenile diabetic, lipolysis is unrestrained and ketogenesis becomes maximal, resulting in life-threatening ketoacidosis. Ketoacidosis and the major catabolic responses so characteristic of the uncontrolled insulin-dependent patient do not occur in maturity-onset diabetes. The difference resides in the fact that insulin deficiency is not as complete in the latter state. A comparison of laboratory values in fasting and diabetic ketoacidosis is shown in Table 89-4.

TABLE 89-4
Typical laboratory values in fasting and diabetic ketoacidosis

	48-h fast	*Ketoacidosis*
Glucose, mg/dl	65	475
Free fatty acids, m*M*	0.9	2.1
Acetoacetate, m*M*	0.8	4.8
β-Hydroxybutyrate, m*M*	2.2	13.7
Lactate, m*M*	0.7	4.6
Blood urea nitrogen, mg/dl	16	25
Urinary nitrogen, g per 24 h	12	20
HCO_3^-, m*M*	22	5
pH	7.35	7.05
Insulin, μU/ml	10	<5
Glucagon, pg/ml	200	400

REFERENCES

BROWN MS et al: Regulation of plasma cholesterol by lipoprotein receptors. Science 212:628, 1981

BOYD ME et al: In vitro reversal of the fasting state of liver metabolism in the rat. Reevaluation of the roles of insulin and glucose. J Clin Invest 68:142, 1981

BUSE MG, REID SS: Leucine. A possible regulator of protein turnover in muscle. J Clin Invest 56:1250, 1975

CAHILL GF JR: Starvation in man. N Engl J Med 282:668, 1970

FELIG P: Amino acid and protein metabolism in diabetes mellitus. Arch Intern Med 137:507, 1977

HAYMOND MW, MILES JM: Branched chain amino acids as a major source of alanine nitrogen in man. Diabetes 31:86, 1982

KHOO JC et al: The mechanism of activation of hormone-sensitive lipase in human adipose tissue. J Clin Invest 53:1124, 1974

MCGARRY JD, FOSTER DW: Regulation of hepatic fatty acid oxidation and ketone body production. Ann Rev Biochem 49:395, 1980

RIZZA RA et al: Role of glucagon, catecholamines, and growth hormone in human glucose counterregulation. Effects of somatostatin and combined α- and β-adrenergic blockade on plasma glucose recovery and glucose flux rates after insulin-induced hypoglycemia. J Clin Invest 64:62, 1979

RUDERMAN NB et al: Gluconeogenesis and its disorders in man, in *Gluconeogenesis: Its Regulation in Mammalian Species,* RW Hanson, MA Mehlman (eds). New York, Wiley, 1976, pp 512–532

UNGER RH, ORCI L: Glucagon and the A cell. Physiology and pathophysiology. N Engl J Med 304:1518, 1575, 1981

UYEDA K et al: The effect of natural and synthetic D-fructose 2,6-bisphosphate on the regulatory kinetic properties of liver and muscle phosphofructokinases. J Biol Chem 256:8394, 1981

WALSER M, WILLIAMSON JR (eds): *Metabolism and Clinical Implications of Branched Chain Amino and Ketoacids.* New York, Elsevier/North-Holland, 1981

section 7 | Metabolic disorders

Disorders of amino acid metabolism

90
OVERVIEW OF INHERITED METABOLIC DISEASES

LEON E. ROSENBERG

GENE-ENVIRONMENT INTERACTION Metabolism, by definition, comprises all the processes by which living matter is built up (anabolism) or broken down (catabolism). These processes begin with the earliest chemical reactions leading to the formation of the sperm and egg; continue throughout growth, maturation, and senescence; and end inexorably with the death of cell, tissue, organ, and finally the individual. Metabolic processes are controlled by two integrated inputs: the *genes,* which delimit the capacity of any given cell (and pari passu of any organism), and the *environment,* which determines how those genes will be expressed. It follows that all metabolic disorders result from some disturbance in the interaction between genetic and environmental factors, and, in the strictest sense, that no metabolic disorder can be classified as either purely *inherited* or *acquired.* When we have little or no information about the genetic determinants of a disease, as in susceptibility to tuberculosis or to traumatic fractures of bones, we think of the condition as acquired. Conversely, when a metabolic disorder is due to a primary abnormality of a specific protein (and hence to a mutation of a specific gene) and when this abnormality is inherited as a simple mendelian dominant or recessive trait (as in acute intermittent porphyria or phenylketonuria), we consider the metabolic derangement inherited. In fact neither acute intermittent porphyria nor phenylketonuria would be significant clinically were it not for precipitating and modifying factors in the environment (drugs and hormones in porphyria; dietary phenylalanine in phenylketonuria). Appreciation of this gene-environment continuum is of more than nosologic interest. Thus, identification of genes controlling susceptibility to tuberculosis will, one day, enable us to identify individuals and groups at risk; and additional information about age-related dietary phenylalanine requirements will permit more effective nutritional treatment of phenylketonuria.

CHARACTER OF INBORN ERRORS In the chapters of the section to follow, those metabolic disorders with an "inherited" etiology are emphasized. Literally hundreds of such inherited metabolic diseases or, as they were originally designated by Garrod, "inborn errors of metabolism," are now recognized, and new ones continue to be described at a rapid rate. As a group, these conditions affect all phases of metabolism and have contributed enormously to the understanding of normal metabolic pathways (confirming the wisdom of the dictum "treasure your exceptions"). They share only the two common features mentioned earlier: each is inherited as a simple mendelian trait and each has been traced (or is attributed) to a functional abnormality of a specific protein. In other ways the features are diverse. Most are inherited as autosomal recessive traits, implying that a double dose of the mutant gene is required for the disorder to be phenotypically manifest (see Chap. 58); others are inherited as X-linked or autosomal dominant traits. Some have an incidence as high as 1:500 (familial hypercholesterolemia); others have an incidence as low as 1:1,000,000 (alcaptonuria). Some demonstrate prominent racial or ethnic clustering, and others appear to be uniformly distributed in races and groups. Some produce clinical manifestations at birth (or even before), others only in adult life (or not at all). Some are uniformly lethal regardless of treatment; others are compatible with a normal life span and health.

LEVELS OF UNDERSTANDING Since it is generally assumed that the clinical and chemical abnormalities observed in patients with a given inherited metabolic disease reflect the mutational disturbance of a specific gene, it is theoretically possible to understand each inborn error at four levels: the gene, the protein coded for by the gene, the metabolic step at which the protein works, and the clinical or chemical phenotype produced by abnormalities at that step. A number of defects in globin-chain synthesis (the thalassemias and hemoglobinopathies) have now been explored at each of these levels (see Chap. 330). In hemoglobin S disease (sickle cell anemia), for example, the specific nucleotide base change in the structural gene for β globin and the precise amino acid substitution in the β-globin polypeptide have been identified. Furthermore, physicochemical studies with hemoglobin S have shown why this mutant protein has a tendency to gel in the deoxygenated state and form the tactoids that distort the erythrocyte and lead to the hyperviscosity, sludging, tissue infarction, and hemolysis characteristic of this disorder. Until recently, information at the level of the gene was available only for disorders of globin-chain synthesis. The development of recombinant DNA technology has led to an explosive increase in the number of human genes which have been probed or isolated (see Chap. 59). This list, which now includes loci coding for such proteins as collagen, growth hormone, HLA antigens, insulin, interferon, prolactin, and placental lactogen, will undoubtedly increase rapidly. For most loci, however, understanding stops at the level of the gene product and, even there, in an incomplete way. For example, in one form of galactosemia the activity of galactose 1-phosphate uridyltransferase is deficient; this deficiency leads to accumulation of galactose and galactose 1-phosphate, which results in serious hepatic and central nervous system dysfunction. However, we know little about either the molecular nature of the transferase deficiency or the means by which metabolite accumulation leads to cirrhosis and mental retardation. In other instances, such as Wilson's disease or cystinosis, the particular protein whose function is deranged is unknown, although it is recognized that copper and cystine, respectively, accumulate in tissues of affected patients. Even more primitive is our understanding of Huntington's disease, which can only be described clinically as an autosomal dominant disease without a known biochemical "handle" with which to grapple with the diagnostic and prognostic dilemmas. Much has been learned about inherited metabolic disorders in the past 25 years. A quantum jump in our knowledge can be anticipated in the coming decade.

PROTEINS AS GENE PRODUCTS

SPECTRUM OF MUTANT PROTEINS Genes and messenger RNAs are polymers of nucleic acids often referred to as "informational macromolecules." Along similar lines proteins and polypeptides can be called "functional macromolecules." These linear polymers of amino acids convert the informational potential of genes and messengers into chemical and physiologic work. Proteins are ubiquitous. They are a vital constituent of the membranes that separate tissues, cells, and organelles from one another. In the blood, lymph, and cerebrospinal fluid they maintain osmotic pressure and selectively bind and transport a large number of small molecules. As enzymes and hormones, whether extracellular or intracellular, they catalyze or regulate reactions that allow anabolic and catabolic pathways to proceed. Proteins display almost limitless variation in size, shape, and function. Molecular weights vary from a few hundred for the pituitary hormone releasing factors to more than a million for gamma macroglobulin. Some are monomeric; others are oligomers of two, three, four, or more like or unlike polypeptide chains. Some are globular while others are helical; still others have both globular and helical regions. Some have metal ions as prosthetic groups or cofactors, while others require organic constituents for activity. Each, however, owes its unique structural features and functional specificity to a single feature—the primary amino acid sequence. Since this primary sequence is dependent on the nucleotide sequence of the gene and messenger RNA that codes for the polypeptide, inherited variations in protein structure or function are the visible expression of gene mutation. Mutations occur in all genes, and hence variation must occur in all proteins. Some variants are detected easily because they lead to obvious chemical or clinical disturbance. Others are detected with great difficulty, either because they produce early lethality or because they are clinically or chemically silent.

In general, mutations responsible for inherited metabolic disorders affect the structural genes that code for the *primary structure* of the protein (see Chap. 58). Single codon changes usually lead to single amino acid substitutions and are referred to as *missense* mutations. Other point mutations (those leading to inappropriately placed terminator codons) as well as deletions and insertions (of codons, segments, or entire genes) produce *nonsense* mutations that result in complete absence of the gene product or one so incomplete or distorted as to be essentially functionless. Alternatively, mutations can modify the *rate* at which a protein is made. Such rate control may be exerted either by modifying control genes or by changing codons in structural genes in a way that leads to accelerated or retarded transcription or translation. Finally, mutations can influence the posttranslational modification of proteins. Since most proteins destined for secretion, for membrane insertion, or for transport to such organelles as lysosomes or mitochondria are synthesized as precursors which must be processed, trimmed, or glycosylated as part of their delivery system, we can expect to find mutations that alter such "traffic." In fact, hyperproinsulinemia and I-cell disease are known examples of human phenotypes resulting from defective processing of secretory and lysosomal proteins, respectively.

Inborn errors have been described for all types of proteins. In their seminal contributions, Garrod, Beadle, Tatum, and associates stressed enzymatic defects that produce a block in an anabolic or catabolic pathway. More than 100 examples of this type of defect are known (see subsequent chapters), and new enzymatic deficiencies are currently being described at a rate of about 10 per year. Although dysfunction of these intracellular catalysts provides the largest body of data concerning the impact of inherited variation on homeostasis, they do not reflect the full scope of functional changes produced by genetic alterations. For example, numerous inherited disorders of cell membrane function have been described. Inborn errors of transport affecting gut and kidney may selectively impair transmembrane movement of sugars, amino acids, phosphate, vitamins, or water (see Chap. 93). Disorders like cystinuria or glycosuria are thought to reflect deficiency of specific membrane carrier proteins required for transepithelial movement of dibasic amino acids or glucose, respectively. Other transport defects lead to abnormal binding of hormones to membrane receptors as in vasopressin-resistant diabetes insipidus or of protein-ligand complexes as in the cell surface receptor defect for low-density lipoprotein in familial hypercholesterolemia (see Chap. 103). Still other mutations alter circulating proteins rather than membrane constituents or intracellular enzymes. Analbuminemia, transcobalamin II deficiency, and abetalipoproteinemia are examples of such deficiencies.

FUNCTIONAL DERANGEMENTS **Increased activity** Simply put, metabolic disorders can be thought of as resulting from too much or too little of a specific protein (or of that protein's activity). Variant forms of G6PD, pseudocholinesterase, and phosphoribosylpyrophosphate synthetase have been described in which enzyme activity is *increased.* In these instances, mutations result in an increase in intracellular enzyme content either because the mutant protein is synthesized more rapidly than normal or is degraded more slowly. In acute intermittent porphyria and familial hypercholesterolemia, rate-controlling enzymes are increased as well (see Chaps. 99 and 103). In the latter disorders, however, enzyme overactivity is a secondary event, reflecting impaired feedback regulation produced by other primary genetic disturbances.

Decreased activity All other inborn errors that have been analyzed in detail are associated with decreased activity (or content) of a protein. The deficiency may be *virtually complete* (as in the classical forms of phenylketonuria and galactosemia) or *partial* (as in the benign variants of those disorders). It should be emphasized that complete loss of enzyme activity cannot be equated with complete absence of a protein. For example, in classic galactosemia, no galactose 1-phosphate uridyltransferase activity can be detected in tissues of affected patients, but immunochemical analyses have shown that such tissues contain a protein that cross-reacts with antibody to the native transferase molecule. Numerous examples of cross-reacting material positive (CRM^+) abnormalities are now recognized. They indicate that the mutation has resulted in the synthesis of a protein that has lost catalytic activity but retains antigenic specificity. Other metabolic disorders characterized by complete enzyme deficiency such as muscle phosphorylase deficiency or von Willebrand disease are CRM^-, implying either that no protein is made or that the gene product is so altered that both catalytic and antigenic functions have been lost.

As increasingly sensitive methods of enzyme assay have been developed, it has become apparent that most inborn errors are characterized by partial, rather than complete, loss of activity. Such partial deficiency may result from several different mechanisms. First, it may reflect reduced rate of synthesis of normal or abnormal enzyme molecules. Second, it may result from accelerated destruction of a structurally altered enzyme. Third, reduced activity may reflect reduced affinity of the active enzyme for substrate or cofactor. Fourth, for oligomeric enzymes, reduced activity could result from impaired interaction of identical or nonidentical subunits. Fifth, for those enzymes in which more than a single isoenzyme exists in a tissue, reduced activity could reflect isolated loss of one form of the enzyme. Examples of each of these mechanisms exist among inherited metabolic disorders in humans. Moreover, the same phenotypic manifestations can result from different mechanisms. For example, some G6PD variants exhibit increased lability, others abnormal affinity for substrate, and still others impaired oligomer formation. All these abnormalities result from different structural alterations in a single polypeptide chain.

CONSEQUENCES OF TRANSPORT OR ENZYMATIC DEFECTS

The effect of any given genetic alteration on cellular metabolism and clinical status depends on the role that the mutant protein plays and the severity of the defect. As mentioned earlier, most inborn errors are the result of intracellular enzymatic defects or of membrane transport abnormalities. Since these kinds of mutations are discussed repeatedly in the following chapters, it is appropriate to summarize the possible consequences of inherited transport or enzyme defects. The model reaction sequence shown in Fig. 90-1 is used for illustrative purposes. A, B, C, D, F, and G are substrates or products of a series of enzymatic reactions; T_A, E_{AB}, E_{BC}, and E_{CD} refer to specific transport systems or enzymes catalyzing specific reactions in this sequence. The major pathway involves the conversion of A to D via intermediates B and C. F and G are products of an alternate metabolic pathway. The arrow from D to E_{AB} represents negative feedback control of the first enzyme in the pathway by the final product of the sequence. Wherever possible, examples of specific inborn errors that illustrate specific consequences of transport or enzyme defects will be cited.

PRECURSOR DEFICIENCY If T_A, the receptor or carrier system that transports A into the cell, is defective, the intracellular concentration of A may be so low that E_{AB} will not be saturated with its substrate. This could slow the entire reaction sequence and result in inadequate formation of B, C, and D. In Hartnup disease (see Chap. 93), intestinal transport of tryptophan is defective. This transport defect has important chemical and clinical consequences, since tryptophan is converted to nicotinamide intracellularly. Patients with this disorder may exhibit cerebellar ataxia and temporary or permanent dementia due to nicotinamide deficiency if they do not receive supplements of niacin in the diet. Similarly, patients with inherited defects in intestinal absorption of vitamin B_{12} develop megaloblastic anemia unless the vitamin is supplied parenterally. Precursor or substrate deficiency may also occur if the defect involves a circulating protein that transports substance A in the blood and carries it to the cell surface.

PRECURSOR ACCUMULATION Let us next consider the effect of reduced activity of one of the intracellular enzymes (E_{AB}, E_{BC}, or E_{CD}). Such a defect might lead to intracellular and extracellular accumulation of the immediate or remote precursors of the reaction. If E_{AB} is defective, only A will accumulate. Such a result is illustrated by the marked increase in lysosomal glucocerebroside content in Gaucher's disease (see Chap. 104) and of blood galactose concentration in galactokinase deficiency (see Chap. 101). Defects of E_{BC} may result in accumulation of A as well as B, and a defect of E_{CD} could lead to the pileup of A, B, and C. In homocystinuria due to cystathionine synthase deficiency, methionine, a remote precursor, accumulates, as does homocystine, the immediate precursor of the blocked reaction (see Chap. 91).

ALTERNATE PATHWAY UTILIZATION If the conversion of A to B is impaired by deficiency of E_{AB}, not only will A accumulate, but the usually minor, alternate pathway to F and G may become prominent. Phenylketonuria represents an excellent example of this phenomenon. The absence of phenylalanine hydroxylase activity leads to gross overproduction and excretion of phenylpyruvic, phenylacetic, and phenyllactic acids, compounds not usually detectable in blood or urine (see Chap. 91). Such alternate pathway augmentation may have important physiologic significance if the products of the alternate pathway interfere with cell processes when present in more than minute concentrations.

PRODUCT DEFICIT If D is the physiologically active product of the hypothetical reaction sequence, a block at any of the steps from A to D results in inadequate synthesis of D. The formation of thyroxine in the thyroid gland proceeds through just such a series of reactions, involving first the transport of iodide into the gland and then its subsequent oxidation and organification. Several enzymatic defects lead to goitrous cretinism due to impaired synthesis of thyroxine. Similarly, in some patients with congenital adrenal hyperplasia due to a defect in hydroxylation on carbon 21 of the steroid nucleus, aldosterone production is impaired, leading to renal salt wasting and hyponatremic crises. Deficient synthesis of product may cause overproduction of precursors, as in acute intermittent porphyria, because of loss of feedback control (D → E_{AB}).

FIGURE 90-1
Schematic representation of metabolic pathway including transport system, enzymes, alternate route, and feedback regulation. (From Rosenberg.)

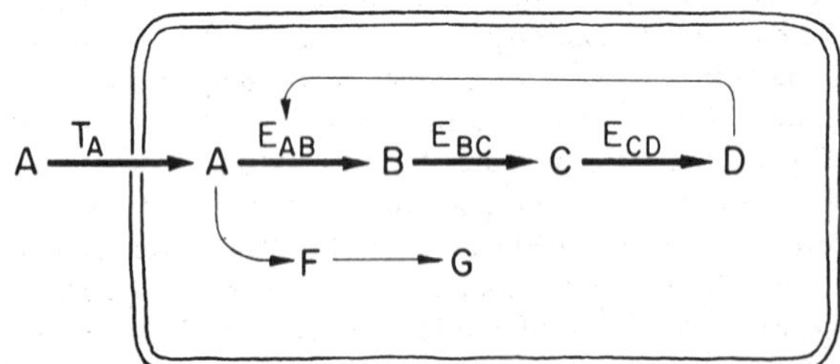

A, B, C, D - Substrate and Products of Major Pathway
F, G - Products of Minor Pathway
T_A - Transport System for A
E_{AB}, E_{BC}, E_{CD} - Enzymes Catalyzing Conversion of A to B, B to C, and C to D
‖ - Cell Membrane

PRODUCT EXCESS As shown in Fig. 90-1, the end product of the reaction sequence D is presumed to regulate the activity of E_{AB}, the first enzyme in this biosynthetic pathway. The phenomenon of end-product inhibition (commonly called feedback inhibition) was first described in microbial systems but is now known to exist for pathways in mammalian cells as well. Several inborn errors demonstrate abnormalities in feedback regulation, but the biochemical events involved are not well understood. In some patients with primary gout, urate is overproduced, presumably because the first enzyme in the purine pathway is defective and does not respond to its normal feedback inhibitors, hypoxanthine and adenine. Abnormal feedback control occurs in the congenital adrenal hyperplasias and congenital goitrous cretinism as well, presumably by different chemical mechanisms. In these disorders the formation or release of ACTH and TSH, respectively, is not impeded by their usual "servo" regulators, cortisol and thyroxine, resulting in hyperplasia and functional disturbances in the two target glands.

Faulty feedback control is not the only mechanism capable of producing product excess. In those disorders characterized by enzyme excess, such as hyperuricemia resulting from increased PRPP synthetase activity (see Chap. 94), product excess can be explained simply by accelerated conversion of precursor to product.

GENETIC HETEROGENEITY

It is well recognized that a given abnormal phenotype may be produced by more than one genotype. This situation, referred to as genetic heterogeneity, is ubiquitous and important. Clinically, an appreciation of genetic heterogeneity has important diagnostic implications, and since diagnosis defines our approach to treatment and counseling, it is important in these matters as well. Scientifically, elucidation of the mechanisms of heterogeneity is imperative for understanding the ways in which the human genome can be modified and how such genetic manifestations can be expressed phenotypically. As noted in Table 90-1, heterogeneity has been discerned using three general methodologic approaches: clinical, biochemical, and genetic.

TABLE 90-1
Methods of demonstrating genetic heterogeneity

1 Clinical analysis
- *a* Age of onset
- *b* Severity
- *c* Specific features

2 Biochemical analysis
- *a* Constituents of blood, urine, and cerebrospinal fluid
- *b* Enzymatic activity
- *c* Protein characterization
- *d* DNA-RNA or DNA-DNA hybridization

3 Genetic analysis
- *a* Chance matings
- *b* Mode of inheritance
- *c* Manifestations in heterozygotes
- *d* Linkage relationships
- *e* Complementation in mixed cells or heterokaryons

CLINICAL EVIDENCE In the absence of independent biochemical or genetic information, it is often impossible to determine whether subtle variations in clinical expression of a given metabolic disorder in any two affected individuals reflect the presence of different mutations or result from modification of an identical mutation by other genetic and environmental influences. However, on the basis of information gleaned from biochemical techniques, such clinical evidence suggesting heterogeneity becomes interpretable. For example, it is likely that patients with juvenile Gaucher's disease have an earlier age of onset and a more rapidly progressive downhill course than do those with adult Gaucher's disease because the mutant glucocerebrosidase in cells from the former group is distinct from and retains less catalytic activity than that in cells from the latter (see Chap. 104). It follows that tissue glucocerebroside content will increase more rapidly if glucocerebrosidase activity is 3 percent of normal than if it is 15 percent of normal. Similarly, the reason that patients with Hunter's disease do not have corneal clouding, whereas patients with the phenotypically similar Hurler's disease do, almost certainly depends on the different enzymatic dysfunctions in the two disorders: iduronate sulfatase deficiency in Hunter's, α-L-iduronidase deficiency in Hurler's.

BIOCHEMICAL TECHNIQUES More often, heterogeneity is first defined through chemical or biochemical assays. Such assays vary greatly in design and complexity—from identification of compounds in blood, urine, or CSF to molecular hybridization analyses. Illustrative examples of disorders shown to be heterogeneous by each of the four kinds of biochemical assays noted in Table 90-1 are as follows. First, the "ketotic hyperglycinemia" syndrome, characterized by episodic ketoacidosis, protein intolerance, and hyperglycinemia, was shown by chemical analyses of blood and urine to be a feature of several different disturbances of organic acid metabolism — α-methylacetoacetic acidemia, propionic acidemia, and methylmalonic acidemia. Second, patients from different families with an entity originally called "congenital, nonspherocytic hemolytic anemia" were found to have different deficiencies in glycolytic enzymes when assays were carried out with erythrocyte hemolysates. Third, the nature of the heterogeneity in patients with G_{M2} gangliosidosis did not become apparent until the lysosomal hexoseaminidases were subdivided into A and B isoenzymes whose activities could be measured individually in patients with Tay-Sachs or Sandhoff's disease. The fourth approach is directed at the gene rather than the gene product. Molecular hybridization experiments employing DNA and RNA provided the evidence for two general categories of β thalassemia: β^0, characterized by the apparent absence of β-globin mRNA, and β^+, characterized by reduced but clearly detectable amounts of β-globin message. Such hybridization studies were also useful in defining heterogeneity in α thalassemia and in those conditions characterized by hereditary persistence of fetal hemoglobin.

GENETIC METHODS Genetic methods have also been important in demonstrating heterogeneity (Table 90-1). One of the earliest and most convincing evidences of such heterogeneity came from the chance mating of two individuals each affected with autosomal recessively inherited nerve deafness. None of their progeny was deaf, demonstrating conclusively that the mutations that produced deafness in the parents were different and likely nonallelic. In several instances heterogeneity was suggested by different modes of inheritance of phenotypically similar (or identical) disorders. For example, Hunter's and Hurler's diseases were differentiated early because the former is inherited as an X-linked trait, the latter as an autosomal recessive. Similarly, at least three forms of spastic diplegia are now recognized: one inherited as an autosomal dominant, a second as an autosomal recessive, and a third as an X-linked trait. In a few instances heterogeneity was first appreciated by studying obligate heterozygotes for a recessive phenotype. Thus, cystinuria was shown to be heterogeneous by the observation that all obligate heterozygotes in some families excreted increased amounts of cystine and lysine, whereas in other pedigrees urinary findings in obligate heterozygotes could not be distinguished from controls. A fourth genetic tool that has revealed heterogeneity is classical linkage analysis. Through this type of investigation hereditary elliptocytosis was divided into two forms — one closely linked to the Rh blood group locus, the other not. Finally, heterogeneity has been demonstrated in a number of instances by application of complementation analyses as first worked out in bacteria and neurospora. The general strategy of such studies is simple. Cultured fibroblasts from two affected individuals are cocultivated in the same dish or are fused into heterokaryons with Sendai virus or polyethylene glycol. If the abnormal phenotype expressed in both parental strains remains in the mixed culture, the defect in the two patients is assumed to be identical; if correction occurs in the mixed culture, the defects in the original strains must be different. This approach has been used to define heterogeneity in a wide variety of disorders, including the mucopolysaccharidoses, the G_{M2} gangliosidoses, the methylmalonic acidemias, the propionic acidemias, xeroderma pigmentosum, and branched-chain ketoaciduria. Theoretically, positive complementation tests could reflect either of two general mechanisms: intergenic complementation, in which two different loci are involved, or interallelic complementation, in which two different mutations at the same locus are mutally corrective. It seems likely that the vast majority of positive complementation tests reflect the intergenic mechanism.

COMPOUND HETEROZYGOTES One of the important conclusions drawn from these biochemical and genetic demonstrations of heterogeneity is that in some instances individuals with a given metabolic disorder are "compound heterozygotes" rather than true homozygotes. Compound heterozygotes are individuals who have received a different mutant allele at a given locus from each parent rather than identical mutant alleles. Patients with hemoglobin SC disease were the first compounds identified, having inherited the gene for hemoglobin S from one parent and that for hemoglobin C from the other. These individuals have a double dose of a mutation for β-globin-chain synthesis and thus make no normal β chains. They are clinically and chemically distinct from true SS or CC homozygotes. More recently, compound heterozygotes have been identified in patients with cystinuria, iminoglycinuria, galactose 1-phosphate uridyltransferase deficiency, and L-iduronidase deficiency. Some, but not all, compounds are as severely affected as true homozygotes, depending on the nature of the mutant alleles inherited.

DIAGNOSTIC TECHNIQUES AND TARGETS

PHYSIOLOGIC FLUIDS Most of the early information concerning the mechanisms of the inborn errors and their mode of detection came from chemical studies of blood or urine. Such chemical determinations did more than point out specific biochemical abnormalities; they provided the clues in many instances for the more elegant enzymatic studies that clarified the specific defect involved. They also allowed large populations to be screened for specific disorders, thereby facilitating the detection of affected subjects prior to the onset of overt clinical problems. The use of screening tests in blood and urine has allowed the detection of heterozygous carriers for many conditions. They are also often useful in monitoring the effects of specific dietary, drug, or replacement therapy.

TISSUE ANALYSES Enzymatic assays and biochemical studies using human tissue obtained by biopsy made a great impact on the definition and detection of the inborn errors. Analyses of liver, muscle, brain, gut mucosa, kidney, erythrocytes, leukocytes, stratum corneum, and spleen have revealed specific enzymatic defects in more than a hundred metabolic diseases. Membrane transport defects have also been demonstrated in vitro in such disorders as hereditary spherocytosis, cystinuria, and the glucose-galactose malabsorption syndrome by the use of erythrocytes, kidney cortex, and gut mucosa, respectively. These assays have often identified the biochemical and genetic heterogeneity characteristic of the inborn errors, in addition to documenting specific gene product abnormalities. Tissue studies do not lend themselves to population surveys and have the greatest impact when combined with investigations of detectable abnormalities in blood and urine.

CELL CULTURE Human fibroblasts grown in tissue culture have also yielded important insights into the biochemistry and genetics of numerous inborn metabolic disorders. In some instances (acatalasia, galactosemia, glucose 6-phosphate dehydrogenase deficiency, glycogen storage disease type II, branched-chain ketoaciduria, and orotic aciduria) enzymatic defects initially described in other tissues were confirmed in cultured fibroblasts. In citrullinemia and Refsum's disease, specific enzymatic defects were first demonstrated in fibroblasts, while in the Lesch-Nyhan syndrome defective hypoxanthine-guanine phosphoribosyl transferase activity was demonstrated coincidently in erythrocytes, leukocytes, and cultured fibroblasts. Cultured cells are not only of value in defining biochemical abnormalities in affected patients; abnormalities found in cells from heterozygous carriers have also been of significance. For example, the study in obligate heterozygotes of several X-linked traits provided evidence confirming the validity of the Lyon hypothesis.

HETEROZYGOTE DETECTION The detection of heterozygous carriers contributes to the study of inborn errors in two important ways. First, such detection provides the most convincing evidence for a recessive mode of inheritance of a disorder, whether the mutation is autosomal or X-linked. Second, the identification of heterozygous carriers in a single pedigree provides valuable information for counseling family members. Counseling relates to such problems as family planning or the choice of a marriage partner. In those diseases in which clinical manifestations may be observed in the carriers (i.e., in dominantly inherited conditions such as acute intermittent porphyria or familial hypercholesterolemia) heterozygote detection has direct clinical relevance.

Identification of heterozygotes requires many of the same methods employed for the recognition of chemical or enzymatic defects in affected subjects. In a few instances, simple blood or urine screening techniques may be sufficient to detect carriers. Enzymatic assays using blood cells or serum have been helpful in several other conditions. In some disorders blood or urine analyses fail to discriminate between normal subjects and heterozygous carriers, but carriers can be detected after administration of oral or parenteral loads of the metabolic precursor involved in the chemical defect. Thus, heterozygotes for galactosemia and phenylketonuria respond to oral loads of galactose and phenylalanine, respectively, with higher plasma concentrations of these substances than observed in normal subjects.

Finally, carriers for an increasing number of diseases have been detected only by enzymatic assays or phenotypic appearance of cells in biopsy material. These techniques for carrier detection have usually been worked out and utilized in one laboratory or, in some instances, a few centers. Because of their complexity, they have not been employed for carrier detection in large populations.

PRENATAL DETECTION There is now considerable interest in the detection of genetic diseases in utero (see Chap. 58). More than 30 inherited metabolic disorders have been identified by chemical examination of amniotic fluid or enzymatic assays on amniotic fluid cells. The largest group of disorders so detected are those mucopolysaccharide or lipid storage diseases due to deficiency of particular lysosomal hydrolases, but a growing list of disorders of amino acid, organic acid, carbohydrate, and purine metabolism have been identified as well. A few inborn errors have been diagnosed by examination of fetal blood obtained by placental puncture or under fetoscopic control. Sickle cell anemia, β thalassemia, and hemophilia have been detected in this way. Whereas the above techniques examine gene products or metabolites, diagnosis of certain hemoglobinopathies and thalassemia syndromes has been accomplished using nucleic acid probes that hybridize directly with nucleotide sequences of specific genes. This technique holds great promise because it can be used on such easily available but poorly differentiated cells such as cultured amniotic fluid cells which contain, but do not express, the genes for many highly differentiated functions including globin and polypeptide hormone synthesis.

GENETIC SCREENING

Genetic screening is the search in a population for persons possessing certain genotypes that are known to be associated with or to predispose to disease in the individuals or their descendants. As a research tool, screening can define the incidence of a particular genotype in the population and can be used to search for polymorphism. In the context of this discussion of inherited metabolic diseases, however, screening has two important applications: early identification of at-risk patients with treatable disease prior to onset of clinical symptoms and identification of at-risk couples who may benefit from appropriate genetic counseling. The prototypic example of the former application is neonatal screening for phenylketonuria. The features of this screening application include a relatively common disease (about 1:10,000 in Caucasians) with serious clinical consequences (severe mental retardation); clear evidence that institution of dietary phenylalanine restriction by age 30 days can return blood phenylalanine concentrations to values commensurate with normal or near normal development; and a simple, sensitive, and specific assay that can be performed in the neonatal period. More than 90 percent of neonates in North America and western Europe are currently being screened for phenylketonuria using the bacterial inhibition assay. The human and monetary savings of this screening program have been enormous and have prompted extension to neonatal detection of other treatable diseases such as galactosemia, hypothyroidism, and homocystinuria. Such "secondary" prevention emphasizes the interaction between environment and heredity and raises no serious ethical problems.

That statement, however, cannot be made with regard to the other screening application—identification of couples at risk for having offspring with untreatable (or nearly untreatable) disorders. The prototype is Tay-Sachs disease in Ashkenazi Jews. When two Ashkenazim marry, there is a 1:900 chance that both individuals are carriers for the Tay-Sachs gene. Theoretically, if all Ashkenazim were screened before marriage, if all pregnancies in at-risk couples were monitored by prenatal diagnosis and if all affected fetuses were aborted, the incidence of Tay-Sachs disease could be decreased to zero. However, mandatory screening is not a possibility, and compliance for voluntary testing is poor. Education, motivation, and effective follow-up are crucial to the success of such a venture. Similar programs have been mounted in the black community, where 1:100 couples are at risk for having children with sickle cell anemia. Early results were not only ineffective but indeed counterproductive, owing to inadequate pretesting educational programs, misunderstanding about the difference between sickle trait and sickle cell disease, and penalties for diagnosis levied by employers and insurance companies. This debacle points out the importance of ethical and social issues in such screening programs.

TREATMENT

A pessimistic approach to the treatment of inherited metabolic disorders is no longer warranted. Effective therapy is available for many of these disorders, particularly those in which the biochemical abnormalities have been defined. As more is learned about the mutational events responsible for specific disorders and about the chemical consequences of the mutations, other inborn errors will surely be controlled or modified by specific therapeutic programs. Two potential levels of treatment exist: the first is directed to means by which the basic genotype of the affected subject can be altered; the second aims to manipulate the environment so as to lessen or eradicate the harmful effect of the mutant phenotype. Successful therapy of the inborn errors has, thus far, been achieved only at the latter level. Although there is great interest in the possibility of genotypic alteration in humans, clinical application remains only a distant hope.

Several prerequisites are necessary for successful therapy. The correct diagnosis must be established. Some inborn errors such as phenylketonuria have harmless phenocopies that produce transient but similar biochemical abnormalities in the newborn. Whereas a low-phenylalanine diet mitigates the central nervous system complications of true phenylketonuria, such a diet may have catastrophic effects on the growth and development of a newborn with transient hyperphenylalaninemia due to delayed maturation of phenylalanine hydroxylase. Next, the physician must be convinced that the disorder is harmful and requires therapy. As stated earlier, some well-defined inborn errors such as pentosuria or iminoglycinuria do not appear to cause any significant clinical pathology and require no treatment. Finally, any therapeutic program must be continually scrutinized for evidence of harmful effects as well as for documentation of beneficial effects of therapy. These may be difficult parameters to dissociate. Penicillamine is an effective drug in Wilson's disease because of its ability to chelate copper; it is also efficacious in solubilizing and preventing the formation of cystine stones in cystinuria. Unfortunately, penicillamine also causes several untoward effects that limit its usefulness and demand careful medical follow-up.

MODALITIES EMPLOYED Phenotypic modification has been approached in many ways, depending on the nature of the defect and the timing of its deleterious effects. Both medical and surgical modalities have been employed, the range and experience with the former far exceeding the latter. Five medical modalities have been used and will be described briefly.

Avoidance For several disorders, clinical consequences can be mitigated or forestalled entirely by avoiding exposure to particular environmental influences. For example, the hemolytic episodes in patients with G6PD deficiency can be modified significantly by avoiding exposure to such drugs as primaquine or sulfa and to such foods as fava beans. Similarly, the prolonged apnea that occurs after succinylcholine administration in individuals deficient in pseudocholinesterase activity will not occur if this anesthetic is not used. Avoiding barbiturates and many other drugs in acute intermittent porphyria and cigarettes and other noxious fumes in alpha$_1$-antitrypsin deficiency is another example of this approach.

Restriction There are numerous disorders in which the phenotypic abnormalities result from the accumulation of a specific substrate or its metabolic by-products. Such disorders may respond to restriction of intake of the injurious substrate or its precursors, providing that the substrate is essential in the dietary sense and thus cannot be manufactured by the organism. Phenylketonuria, branched-chain ketoaciduria, homocystinuria, galactosemia, essential fructosuria, and Refsum's disease are examples of inborn errors that have been effectively treated in this way. Similarly, patients with the glucose-galactose malabsorption syndrome who develop profound diarrhea when fed lactose-containing foods do well if their source of dietary carbohydrate is changed. In contrast, dietary restriction is of no value in hyperprolinemia, hydroxyprolinemia, or citrullinemia, because these amino acids are synthesized extensively de novo. Even in those conditions in which dietary restriction is of value, doubt exists about the needed duration of such restriction. The injurious effects of excess phenylalanine, galactose, or branched-chain amino acids or keto acids may be limited to the early years of life when brain development and organization are proceeding at a maximal rate. If this is so, it should be possible to modify or even discontinue dietary restrictions after a given age. There is still considerable uncertainty regarding this matter, however, and more experience is needed before meaningful recommendations can be made.

Replacement Many disorders caused by the failure to make a specific protein or small-molecular-weight product have responded dramatically to replacement therapy. Hemophilia and agammaglobulinemia are examples of inborn errors that respond to parenteral protein replacement. These disorders are amenable to such replacement because the proteins involved normally circulate in abundance. In most instances, however, the missing protein or enzyme is confined to some intracellular organelle and is present in very small amounts. Replacement therapy in these instances may be difficult or impossible for three reasons: first, because large amounts of the protein are difficult to purify or synthesize; second, because parenteral administration of the protein will not increase its entry into the cell where it is required; and third, because the protein may initiate unfavorable immunologic reactions. Despite these drawbacks, attempts along these lines are being made. Pure human glucocerebrosidase has been administered intravenously to a few patients with Gaucher's disease. Tissue glucocerebroside content fell modestly in these patients, suggesting that some enzyme was being taken up by cells and was active intracellularly. More striking success has been reported in combined immunodeficiency due to adenosine deaminase deficiency. Administration of frozen, irradiated, normal erythrocytes led to prolonged and dramatic improvement in immune status.

The clinical stigmata of a disorder may be related not to the protein whose synthesis is defective but rather to the product of the blocked pathway. Cortisol synthesis is blocked in several variants of congenital adrenal hyperplasia, and replacement therapy with this steroid produces dramatic improvement. Similarly, administration of thyroid hormone and uridine reverses the serious clinical disturbances in familial goitrous cretinism and orotic aciduria, respectively.

Supplementation A growing list of metabolic disorders respond clinically and/or chemically to supplementary amounts of specific vitamins. Infants with seizures controlled only by supraphysiologic amounts of pyridoxine provided the first evidence for this phenomenon. Now more than 20 different disorders are known to respond to supplements of a single vitamin. Most of these disorders are caused by primary enzymatic disturbances that result in impaired affinity for cofactor. A growing list, however, are caused by primary abnormalities in the pathway of coenzyme or metabolite synthesis from vitamin precursors. Several disorders responsive to cobalamin (vitamin B_{12}), folate, or vitamin D can now be included in this category. Long-term experience with such vitamin supplements is limited but promising.

Drug administration Clinical disturbances in several inherited metabolic disorders result from deposition of a specific substance in one or more tissues. Successful treatment of these conditions may be achieved by enhancing the excretion of the stored chemical or by preventing its formation. Copper deposition in Wilson's disease can be controlled by drugs such as D-penicillamine, which chelates copper and markedly enhances its urinary excretion. The excretion of iron in hemochromatosis is augmented by phlebotomy and by the administration of desferrioxamine B. D-Penicillamine is also effective in solubilizing cystine calculi in cystinuria by reacting with cystine to form the more soluble cysteine-penicillamine disulfide. In this instance, the amount of cystine excreted is not changed, but its chemical form is altered in a therapeutically advantageous fashion. Uric acid deposition in gout responds both to drugs that enhance its excretion, such as sulfinpyrazone and probenecid, and to metabolic inhibitors like allopurinol that inhibit uric acid biosynthesis.

Surgical intervention At present, surgery is of limited value in the treatment of the inborn errors. Its use is restricted to a few conditions, such as gout, cystinuria, and oxalosis, in which nephrolithotomy or ureterolithotomy may provide important symptomatic relief while other programs of therapy are initiated. Several reports indicate that tissue transplants may be beneficial in some diseases. Thus, kidney transplants have been undertaken in cystinosis, hyperoxaluria, and Fabry's disease. Here the aim is restoration of renal function in conditions which produce progressive, and ultimately lethal, renal injury. Results have been variable. In hyperoxaluria, the transplanted kidney has been destroyed by oxalate deposition. In cystinosis, this has not occurred. A second, and quite different, goal of transplantation involves restitution of normal function. Thus, in combined immune deficiency, administration of fetal liver cells has produced clinical improvement. Similar beneficial results of bone marrow transplantation have been reported in other immune deficiency diseases. In the future, spleen transplantation may provide lasting benefit to patients with hemophilia or agammaglobulinemia by providing a constant source of antihemophilic globulin or gamma globulin, respectively. It is likewise possible that hepatic homografts may supply specific enzymes in phenylketonuria, branched-chain ketoaciduria, or the glycogen storage diseases and thus prevent the accumulation of toxic substances that lead to clinical abnormalities.

REFERENCES

HARRIS H: *The Principles of Human Biochemical Genetics,* 3d ed. Amsterdam, North-Holland, 1980

ROSENBERG LE: Inborn errors of metabolism, in *Metabolic Control and Disease,* 8th ed, PK Bondy, LE Rosenberg (eds). Philadelphia, Saunders, 1980

STANBURY JB et al: Inherited variation and metabolic abnormality, in *The Metabolic Basis of Inherited Disease,* 5th ed, JB Stanbury et al (eds). New York, McGraw-Hill, 1983, p 3

91
INHERITED DISORDERS OF AMINO ACID METABOLISM

LEON E. ROSENBERG

All polypeptides and proteins are polymers of 20 different amino acids. Eight of these, referred to as *essential,* cannot be synthesized by humans and must be obtained from dietary sources. The others are formed endogenously by a variety of chemical rearrangements. Although the vast bulk of the body's amino acids are "tied up" in proteins, small but critical pools of *free* amino acids are found intracellularly, and these pools are in equilibrium with extracellular reservoirs in plasma, cerebrospinal fluid, and the lumina of the gut and kidney. Physiologically, amino acids are more than mere "building blocks." Some (glycine, γ-aminobutyric acid) are neurotransmitters. Others (phenylalanine, tyrosine, tryptophan, glycine) are precursors of hormones, coenzymes, pigments, purines, or pyrimidines. Each has a unique and complicated degradative pathway by which its nitrogen and carbon components are used for the synthesis of other amino acids, carbohydrates, and lipids.

Current concepts of inherited metabolic diseases depend to a considerable degree on investigations of amino acid disorders. Three of the conditions analyzed by Garrod in his seminal descriptions of "inborn errors of metabolism" in the first decade of this century involved amino acids (alkaptonuria, albinism, and cystinuria). Although not appreciated at the time, these three conditions contain examples of the two general classes of "aminoacidopathies" now recognized: enzymatic defects in amino acid catabolism and disorders of transmembrane transport. More than 70 inherited aminoacidopathies are now known, the catabolic defects (approximately 60) discussed in this and the following chapter far outnumbering the transport abnormalities (approximately 10) considered in Chap. 93. Each of these disorders is rare—their incidences range from 1 in 10,000 for phenylketonuria to 1 in 200,000 for alkaptonuria. Collectively, however, they occur in perhaps 1 in 500 to 1 in 1000 live births.

The salient features of inherited disorders of amino acid catabolism, arranged according to structural classes of the respective amino acids, are presented in Table 91-1. In general, these disorders are named for the compound which accumulates to highest concentration in blood (*-emias*) or urine (*-urias*). For many conditions the parent amino acid is found in excess; for others, products in the catabolic pathway accumulate. Which process takes place depends, of course, on the site of the enzymatic block, the reversibility of the reactions proximal to the lesion, and the existence of alternate pathways of metabolic "run-off." For some amino acids, such as the sulfur-containing or branched-chain molecules, defects at nearly each step in the catabolic pathway have been described. For others numerous gaps in our knowledge remain but are being filled rapidly as biochemical screening programs expand and interest in the field grows. Biochemical and genetic heterogeneity abounds among the aminoacidopathies. At least four distinct forms of hyperphenylalaninemia, three variants of homocystinuria, and five types of methylmalonic acidemia are recognized—variants of both chemical and clinical interest.

The manifestations of these conditions differ widely as noted in Table 91-1. Some, such as sarcosinemia or hyperprolinemia, appear to produce no clinical consequences. At the other extreme, uniform neonatal lethality occurs in the untreated patient with complete deficiency of ornithine transcarbamylase or of branched-chain keto acid dehydrogenase. Central nervous system dysfunction, in the form of developmental retardation, seizures, alterations in sensorium, or behavioral disturbances, occurs in more than half of the disorders. Protein-induced vomiting, neurological dysfunction, and hyperammonemia occur in many disorders of urea cycle intermediates. Metabolic ketoacidosis often accompanied by hyperammonemia is a frequent presenting finding in the disorders of branched-chain amino acid metabolism. Occasional disorders produce focal tissue or organ involvement such as liver disease, renal failure, cutaneous abnormalities, or ocular lesions.

The clinical manifestations in many of these conditions can be prevented or mitigated significantly if diagnosis is achieved early and appropriate treatment (i.e., dietary protein or amino acid restriction or vitamin supplementation) is instituted promptly. For this reason, aminoacidopathies are screened for in mass newborn surveys which analyze blood or urine with an array of chemical and microbiological techniques. Once a presumptive diagnosis is made, confirmation can be provided by direct enzyme assay on extracts of leukocytes, erythrocytes, cultured fibroblasts, or liver. Several (cystinosis, branched-chain ketoaciduria, propionic acidemia, and methylmalonic acidemia) have been diagnosed in utero by chemical analysis on cultured amniotic fluid cells. The remainder of this and the subsequent chapter are focused on selected disorders that illustrate the problems posed by aminoacidopathies.

THE HYPERPHENYLALANINEMIAS

DEFINITION The hyperphenylalaninemias are a group of disorders (Table 91-1), each resulting from impaired conversion of phenylalanine to tyrosine. The most important is phenylketonuria, which in the untreated state is characterized by an increased concentration of phenylalanine in blood, increased concentrations of phenylalanine and its by-products (notably phenylpyruvate, phenylacetate, phenyllactate, and phenylacetylglutamine) in urine, and severe mental retardation.

ETIOLOGY AND PATHOGENESIS Each of the hyperphenylalaninemias results from reduced activity of the enzyme complex called *phenylalanine hydroxylase.* This system is found in appreciable amounts only in liver and kidney. Phenylalanine and molecular oxygen are substrates for the apoenzyme which requires a reduced pteridine, tetrahydrobiopterin, as a cofactor. Tyrosine and dihydrobiopterin are the products of this catalytic system, the latter being reconverted to tetrahydrobiopterin by a second enzyme, dihydropteridine reductase. In classic phenylketonuria activity of the hydroxylase apoenzyme is almost totally deficient. Benign hyperphenylalaninemia results from a less complete deficiency, whereas transient hyperphenylalaninemia (sometimes called transient phenylketonuria) is caused by a delayed maturation of the hydroxylase apoenzyme. In two variant forms of phenylketonuria, however, persistently impaired hydroxylating activity results not from abnormality in the apohydroxylase but from a lack of tetrahydrobiopterin. The tetrahydrobiopterin deficiency has two distinct metabolic bases: a block in the pathway by which biopterin is synthesized from its precursors, or deficiency of dihydropteridine reductase, the enzyme that regenerates tetrahydrobiopterin from dihydrobiopterin.

As a group the hyperphenylalaninemias occur in about 1 in 10,000 births. Classic phenylketonuria, which accounts for nearly half of these, is inherited as an autosomal recessive trait

and is widely distributed among Caucasian ethnic groups and Orientals. It is rare in blacks. Phenylalanine hydroxylase activity in obligate heterozygotes is distinctly less than normal but higher than in homozygotes. Heterozygous carriers are clinically well but usually have slightly increased phenylalanine concentrations in postprandial blood plasma. Each of the other hyperphenylalaninemias also appears to be inherited as an autosomal recessive.

Phenylalanine accumulation in blood and urine and reduced tyrosine formation are direct consequences of the impaired hydroxylation. In untreated phenylketonuria and in its tetrahydrobiopterin-deficient variants, plasma concentrations of phenylalanine become sufficiently high (greater than 20 mg/dl) to activate alternate pathways of metabolism and lead to formation of phenylpyruvate, phenylacetate, phenyllactate, and other derivatives that are rapidly cleared by the kidney and excreted in urine. Plasma concentrations of several other amino acids are moderately reduced, probably secondary to inhibition of gastrointestinal absorption or impairment of renal tubular reabsorption by the excess phenylalanine in body fluids. The severe brain damage observed in untreated phenylketonuria appears to be related to several consequences of phenylalanine accumulation: deprivation of other amino acids required for protein synthesis, impaired polyribosome formation or stabilization, reduced myelin synthesis, and inadequate formation of norepinephrine and serotonin. Phenylalanine is a competitive inhibitor of tyrosinase, a key enzyme in the pathway of melanin synthesis. This block plus reduced availability of the melanin precursor, tyrosine, accounts for the hypopigmentation of hair and skin.

CLINICAL MANIFESTATIONS No abnormalities are apparent at birth. Untreated children with classic phenylketonuria fail to attain early developmental milestones and demonstrate progressive impairment of cerebral function with IQ scores usually less than 50. Most require chronic institutionalization within a few years of birth because of the hyperactivity and seizures that accompany the severe mental retardation. Electroencephalogram abnormalities, "mousy" odor of skin, hair, and urine (due to phenylacetate accumulation), and a tendency to hypopigmentation and eczema complete the devastating clinical picture. In contrast, children who are detected at birth and treated promptly show none of these abnormalities. Children with transient hyperphenylalaninemia or with the benign variant are not at risk for any of the clinical consequences seen in untreated classic phenylketonuria. Those children with tetrahydrobiopterin deficiency, however, are the most unfortunate. Seizures appear early, followed by progressive cerebral and basal ganglia dysfunction (rigidity, chorea, spasms, hypotonia). Each has succumbed to secondary infection within a few years despite early diagnosis and standard treatment.

Occasionally, women with untreated classic phenylketonuria have reached adulthood and had children. More than 90 percent of the offspring are markedly retarded, and many have exhibited other congenital anomalies such as microcephaly, growth retardation, and congenital heart defects. Since these children are heterozygous, not homozygous for the phenylketonuria mutation, their clinical manifestations must be attributed to intrauterine damage produced by the elevated maternal concentrations of phenylalanine to which they have been exposed.

DIAGNOSIS Plasma phenylalanine concentrations may be normal at birth in all the hyperphenylalaninemias but rise rapidly after institution of protein feedings and are usually markedly abnormal by day 4. Since diagnosis and initiation of die-

TABLE 91-1
Inherited disorders of amino acid catabolism

Amino acid(s) affected	*Disorder or condition*	*Enzyme defect*	*Clinical manifestations** *Mental retardation*	*Neuropsychiatric dysfunction*	*Protein intolerance*	*Metabolic ketoacidosis*
AROMATIC—HETEROCYCLIC						
Phenylalanine	Classic phenylketonuria	Phenylalanine hydroxylase	+	+	−	−
	Benign hyperphenylalaninemia	Phenylalanine hydroxylase	−	−	−	−
	Transient hyperphenylalaninemia	Phenylalanine hydroxylase	−	−	−	−
	Variant phenylketonuria	Dihydropteridine reductase	+	+	−	−
	Variant phenylketonuria	Dihydrobiopterin synthetase (?)	+	+	−	−
Tyrosine	Hypertyrosinemia	Tyrosine aminotransferase (cytosol)	+	−	−	−
	Tyrosinosis	Tyrosine aminotransferase (?)	−	−	−	−
	Hereditary tyrosinemia	Unknown	−	−	−	−
	Alkaptonuria	Homogentisic acid oxidase	−	−	−	−
	Albinism (oculocutaneous)	Tyrosinase	−	−	−	−
	Albinism (ocular)	Unknown	−	−	−	−
Tryptophan	Tryptophanuria	Tryptophan pyrrolase	+	+	−	−
	Xanthurenic aciduria	Kynureninase	?	−	−	−
Histidine	Histidinemia	Histidine-ammonia lyase	±	±	−	−
	Urocanic aciduria	Urocanase	+	+	−	−
	Formiminoglutamic aciduria	Formiminotransferase	?	+	−	−
GLYCINE-IMINO ACIDS						
Glycine	Hyperglycinemia	Glycine cleavage	+	+	−	−
	Sarcosinemia	Sarcosine dehydrogenase	−	−	−	−
	Hyperoxaluria (type I)	α-Ketoglutarate: glyoxylate carboligase	−	−	−	−
	Hyperoxaluria (type II)	D-Glyceric acid dehydrogenase	−	−	−	−
Imino acids	Hyperprolinemia (type I)	Proline oxidase	−	−	−	−
	Hyperprolinemia (type II)	Δ'-Pyrroline dehydrogenase	−	−	−	−
	Hyperhydroxyprolinemia	Hydroxyproline reductase	−	−	−	−
	Iminopeptiduria	Prolidase	+	−	−	−
SULFUR-CONTAINING						
Methionine	Hypermethioninemia	Methionine adenosyltransferase	−	−	−	−
Homocystine	Homocystinuria	Cystathionine β-synthase	±	±	−	−
	Homocystinuria	5,10-Methylenetetrahydrofolate reductase	±	±	−	−
	Homocystinuria and methylmalonic acidemia (cbl C, D)‡	Cobalamin (vitamin B_{12}) reductase (cytosol) (?)	±	±	−	−
Cystathionine	Cystathioninuria	Cystathionase	±	−	−	−
Cystine	Cystinosis	Unknown	−	−	−	−
S-Sulfo-L-cysteine	S-Sulfo-L-cysteine, sulfite, and thiosulfaturia	Sulfite oxidase	+	+	−	−
CATIONIC						
Lysine	Hyperlysinemia (type I)	Lysine dehydrogenase	−	+	+	−
	Hyperlysinemia (type II)	Lysine: α-ketoglutarate reductase	±	±	−	−
	Saccharopinuria	Saccharopine dehydrogenase	−	−	−	−
	Hydroxylysinemia	Unknown	+	−	−	−
	Pipecolic acidemia	Unknown	+	+	−	−
	α-Ketoadipic aciduria	α-Ketoadipic acid decarboxylase	±	±	−	−
	Glutaric aciduria (type I)	Glutaryl CoA dehydrogenase	−	+	−	−
	Glutaric aciduria (type II)	Medium-chain acyl CoA dehydrogenase (?)	−	+	−	−

* *+, regularly present; ±, sometimes present; −, absent; ?, uncertain; all designations refer to manifestations in untreated disorder.*
† *AR, autosomal recessive; XL, X-linked; (AR), probably autosomal recessive.*
‡ *Designations in parentheses refer to complementation groups assigned by genetic analysis with cultured cells.*

Ammonia intoxication	*Other*	*Inheritance pattern*†
–	Hypopigmented skin and hair, eczema	AR
–		AR
–		(AR)
–		(AR)
–		(AR)
–	Palmar keratosis, corneal dystrophy	(AR)
–	Myasthenia gravis	?
–	Cirrhosis, hepatic failure, renal tubular dysfunction	AR
–	Ochronosis, arthritis	AR
–	Hypopigmentation of hair, skin, and optic fundus	AR
–	Hypopigmentation of optic fundus	XL
–	Photosensitive skin rash	AR
–		?
–	Hearing and speech deficit	AR
–		?
–		(AR)
–		AR
–		AR
–	Renal failure	AR
–	Calcium oxalate nephrolithiasis, renal failure	AR
–		AR
–		AR
–		AR
–	Crusting, erythematous, ecchymotic dermatitis	AR
–		?
–	Dislocated lenses, osteoporosis, thrombotic vascular disease	AR
–		(AR)
–	Megaloblastic anemia	(AR)
–		AR
–	Fanconi syndrome, renal failure, photophobia	AR
–	Dislocated lenses	AR
+		?
–		AR
–		?
–		(AR)
–	Hepatomegaly, dysplastic optic disks	?
–		?
–		AR
–	Hypoglycemia	?

(Table continues next page)

tary treatment of classic phenylketonuria must be completed before 30 days of age if developmental retardation is to be prevented, most newborns in North America and Europe are screened by determinations of blood phenylalanine concentration using the Guthrie bacterial inhibition assay. Infants with abnormal values are followed up with more quantitative fluorometric or chromatographic assays. In classic phenylketonuria and in tetrahydrobiopterin deficiency, values greater than 20 mg/dl are regularly observed. In transient or benign hyperphenylalaninemia concentrations are usually lower but still above control values of less than 1 mg/dl. Distinction of classic phenylketonuria from its benign variants depends on following serial plasma phenylalanine concentrations as a function of age and dietary restriction. In transient hyperphenylalaninemia plasma values return to normal within 3 to 4 months. In benign hyperphenylalaninemia dietary restriction produces a more profound fall in plasma phenylalanine than that observed in classic phenylketonuria. Deficiency of tetrahydrobiopterin must be considered in any child with hyperphenylalaninemia who develops progressive neurological impairment despite prompt diagnosis and dietary treatment. Diagnostic confirmation of these variants, which may account for 1 to 5 percent of phenylketonuric children, can be achieved by enzyme assay on extracts of cultured fibroblasts. Of potentially greater therapeutic value, however, is the observation that administration of oral tetrahydrobiopterin loads can distinguish children with classic phenylketonuria (who show no chemical response) from those with tetrahydrobiopterin deficiency (who exhibit a sharp fall in plasma phenylalanine).

TREATMENT Classic phenylketonuria was the first inherited metabolic disease in which it was demonstrated that mitigating the accumulation of the offending metabolite prevented the clinical abnormalities. This is accomplished by a special diet in which the bulk of protein is replaced by an artificial amino acid mixture low in phenylalanine. By supplementing this formula with a small amount of natural foods, an amount of dietary phenylalanine is provided that is sufficient for normal growth but is insufficient to produce markedly increased quantities of phenylalanine in blood. Ordinarily, plasma phenylalanine concentrations are maintained between 3 and 12 mg/dl.

Until it is determined whether dietary treatment can be terminated safely after 6 to 8 years, dietary restriction in classic phenylketonuria should be continued indefinitely. The transient and benign forms of hyperphenylalaninemia do not require long-term dietary restriction. As mentioned earlier, children with tetrahydrobiopterin deficiency deteriorate despite dietary phenylalanine restriction; efficacy of pteridine cofactor replacement is under study.

THE HOMOCYSTINURIAS

The homocystinurias are three biochemically and clinically distinct disorders (Table 91-1), each characterized by increased concentration of the sulfur-containing amino acid, homocystine, in blood and urine. The most common form results from markedly reduced activity of cystathionine β-synthase, an enzyme catalyzing a key step in the transsulfuration pathway by which methionine is converted to cysteine. The two other forms are the result of impaired conversion of homocysteine to methionine, a reaction catalyzed by homocysteine: methyltetrahydrofolate methyltransferase and two essential cofactors methyltetrahydrofolate and methylcobalamin (methyl-vitamin B_{12}). Depending on the underlying disorder, some patients with each of the homocystinurias show chemical and, in some

TABLE 91-1 *(continued)*
Inherited disorders of amino acid catabolism

			*Clinical manifestations**			
Amino acid(s) affected	*Disorder or condition*	*Enzyme defect*	*Mental retardation*	*Neuropsychiatric dysfunction*	*Protein intolerance*	*Metabolic ketoacidosis*
CATIONIC *(continued)*						
Ornithine	Hyperornithinemia (type I)	Ornithine decarboxylase	+	+	+	−
	Hyperornithinemia (type II)	Ornithine aminotransferase	−	−	−	−
UREA CYCLE						
Carbamylphosphate	Hyperammonemia (type I)	Carbamylphosphate synthetase I	+	+	+	−
Ornithine	Hyperammonemia (type II)	Ornithine transcarbamylase	±	+	+	−
Citrulline	Citrullinemia	Argininosuccinate synthetase	+	+	+	−
Argininosuccinic acid	Argininosuccinic aciduria	Argininosuccinase	+	+	+	−
Arginine	Argininemia	Arginase	+	+	+	−
BRANCHED-CHAIN						
Valine	Hypervalinemia	Valine aminotransferase	+	+	+	−
Leucine, isoleucine	Hyperleucine-isoleucinemia	Leucine-isoleucine aminotransferase	+	+	+	−
Valine, leucine, isoleucine	Classic branched-chain ketoaciduria	Branched-chain ketoacid dehydrogenase	+	+	+	+
	Intermittent branched-chain ketoaciduria	Branched-chain ketoacid dehydrogenase	±	−	+	+
Leucine	Isovaleric acidemia	Isovaleryl CoA dehydrogenase	±	±	+	+
	β-Methylcrotonyl glycinuria	β-Methylcrotonyl CoA carboxylase	+	+	−	+
	β-Hydroxy-β-methylglutaric aciduria	β-Hydroxy-β-methylglutaryl CoA lyase	−	+	+	+
Isoleucine, valine	α-Methylacetoacetic aciduria	β-Ketothiolase	±	±	+	+
	Propionic acidemia (pcc A, B, C)‡	Propionyl CoA carboxylase	±	±	+	+
	Propionic acidemia (bio)‡	Holocarboxylase synthetase (?)	+	±	+	+
	Methylmalonic acidemia (mut)‡	Methylmalonyl CoA mutase	±	±	+	+
	Methylmalonic acidemia (cbl A)‡	Cobalamin (vitamin B_{12}) reductase (mitochondrial) (?)	±	±	+	+
	Methylmalonic acidemia (cbl B)‡	Cobalamin (vitamin B_{12}): ATP adenosyltransferase	±	±	+	+
DICARBOXYLIC						
Glutamic acid	Glutathionemia	γ-Glutamyltranspeptidase	+	−	−	−
	5-Oxoprolinuria	Glutathione synthetase	±	±	±	+

* *+, regularly present; ±, sometimes present; −, absent; ?, uncertain; all designations refer to manifestations in untreated disorder.*
† *AR, autosomal recessive; XL, X-linked; (AR), probably autosomal recessive.*
‡ *Designations in parentheses refer to complementation groups assigned by genetic analysis with cultured cells.*

instances, clinical improvement following administration of specific vitamin supplements (pyridoxine, folate, or cobalamin).

CYSTATHIONINE β-SYNTHASE DEFICIENCY **Definition** Deficiency of this enzyme leads to increased concentrations of methionine and homocystine in body fluids and to decreased concentrations of cysteine and cystine. The clinical hallmark is dislocated optic lenses. Mental retardation, osteoporosis, and thrombotic vascular disease are frequent.

Etiology and pathogenesis The sulfur atom of the essential amino acid methionine is transferred ultimately to cysteine by a series of reactions designated as the transsulfuration pathway. In one of these steps, homocysteine condenses with serine to form cystathionine. This reaction is catalyzed by the pyridoxal phosphate–dependent enzyme, cystathionine β-synthase. Since 1964 more than 200 patients have been described with deficiency of this enzyme. The condition is common in Ireland (1 in 40,000 births) but rare elsewhere (less than 1 in 200,000 births).

Homocysteine and methionine accumulate in cells and body fluids; cysteine synthesis is impaired, resulting in reduced concentrations of this amino acid and its disulfide form, cystine. In approximately half of patients synthase activity in liver, brain, leukocytes, and cultured fibroblasts is absent. In

Ammonia intoxication	*Other*	*Inheritance pattern*[†]
+		(AR)
−	Gyrate atrophy of choroid and retina	AR
+		AR
+		XL
+		AR
+		AR
+		AR
−		?
−		?
−	"Maple syrup" odor	AR
−		AR
±	"Sweaty feet" odor	AR
−	"Cat's urine" odor	AR
−		?
+		AR
+		AR
−		?
+		AR
+		AR
+		AR
−		(?)
−		AR

the remaining patients, tissues retain 1 to 5 percent of normal activity. Heterozygous carriers of this autosomal recessive trait show no chemical abnormalities in body fluids but have reduced tissue synthase activity.

Homocysteine interferes with the normal cross-linking of collagen, an effect that likely plays an important role in the ocular, skeletal, and vascular complications.

Altered collagen in the suspensory ligament of the optic lens and in bone matrix may account for the dislocated lenses and osteoporosis. Similarly, interference with normal ground substance metabolism in vascular walls may predispose to the arterial and venous thrombotic diathesis. Recurrent cerebrovascular accidents secondary to thrombotic disease may account for the mental retardation, but direct chemical effects on cerebral cell metabolism have not been excluded.

Clinical manifestations More than 95 percent of patients have dislocated optic lenses. This abnormality usually appears by 3 to 4 years of age and often results in acute glaucoma as well as impaired visual acuity. Mental retardation occurs in less than 50 percent, often accompanied by ill-defined behavioral disturbances. Osteoporosis is a common radiological finding but rarely causes clinical disease. Life-threatening vascular complications, probably initiated by damage to vascular endothelium, are the major cause of morbidity and mortality. Occlusion of coronary, renal, and cerebral arteries with attendant tissue infarction can occur during the first decade of life. Many patients die of vascular disease before age 30. These vascular complications seem to be exacerbated by angiographic procedures.

Diagnosis The cyanide-nitroprusside test is a simple way of demonstrating increased excretion of sulfhydryl-containing compounds in urine. Since cystine and *S*-sulfocysteine also give a positive test, other disorders of sulfur metabolism must be excluded, but this is usually simple on clinical grounds. Distinction of cystathionine β-synthase deficiency from other causes of homocystinuria can usually be accomplished by measurements of plasma methionine, which tend to be markedly increased in synthase-deficient patients and normal or low in those with impaired methionine formation (see below). Diagnostic confirmation depends on measurements of synthase activity in tissue extracts.

Treatment As with classic phenylketonuria, effective treatment depends on early diagnosis. A few infants diagnosed in the newborn period have been treated successfully with methionine-restricted, cystine-supplemented diets. Their clinical course has, thus far, been benign compared with that of untreated affected siblings. In approximately half of patients, oral supplements of pyridoxine (25 to 500 mg per day) produce a marked fall in plasma and urinary methionine and homocystine and an increase in cystine concentration in body fluids. This effect probably reflects a modest increase in synthase activity in cells of patients in whom the enzymatic defect is characterized by either reduced affinity for cofactor or accelerated degradation of mutant enzyme. Since such vitamin supplementation is simple and apparently harmless, it should be tried in all patients. There are no reports of the effect of pyridoxine supplementation therapy that has been initiated soon after birth.

5,10-METHYLENETETRAHYDROFOLATE REDUCTASE DEFICIENCY Definition In this form of homocystinuria, methionine concentrations in body fluids are normal or decreased because deficiency of 5,10-methylenetetrahydrofolate reductase leads to impaired synthesis of 5-methyltetrahydrofolate, a cofactor in the enzymatic formation of methionine from homocysteine. Central nervous system dysfunction occurs in most patients.

Etiology and pathogenesis 5-Methyltetrahydrofolate:homocysteine methyltransferase catalyzes the conversion of homocysteine to methionine. The methyl group transferred in this reaction comes from 5-methyltetrahydrofolate, which is converted to tetrahydrofolate in the process. 5-Methyltetrahydrofolate, in turn, is synthesized enzymatically from 5,10-methylenetetrahydrofolate by another folate cycle enzyme, 5,10-methylenetetrahydrofolate reductase. Thus, reductase activity controls both methionine synthesis and tetrahydrofolate generation. This series of reactions is critical to normal DNA and RNA synthesis. A primary defect in the reductase activity results, secondarily, in deficient methyltransferase activity and impaired conversion of homocysteine to methionine. Although the mechanism of the central nervous system dysfunction is unknown, methionine deficiency and impaired nucleic acid synthesis are likely explanations. The disorder appears to be inherited as an autosomal recessive trait.

Clinical manifestations Fewer than 10 children with homocystinuria due to reductase deficiency have been reported. The most severely affected have presented with profound developmental retardation and cerebral atrophy early in life. Others manifested prominent behavioral disturbances (catatonia) during the second decade. In the remainder, mild retardation has been observed. Presumably the severity of the clinical manifestations reflects the severity of the reductase deficiency.

Diagnosis and treatment The combination of increased concentrations of homocystine in body fluids with normal or decreased concentrations of methionine should suggest this entity. Serum folate concentrations are low in some patients. Confirmation requires direct reductase assays in tissue extracts (brain, liver, cultured fibroblasts). Although therapeutic experience is limited, one teenage girl with a catatonic psychosis responded dramatically, both chemically and clinically, to folate supplements (5 to 10 mg per day). When the folate was withdrawn, behavior worsened. This observation suggests that early diagnosis followed by folate supplementation may forestall neurological or psychiatric disturbances.

DEFICIENCY OF COBALAMIN (VITAMIN B_{12}) COENZYME SYNTHESIS **Definition** This form of homocystinuria also reflects impaired conversion of homocysteine to methionine. The primary defect is in the synthesis of methylcobalamin, a cobalamin (vitamin B_{12}) coenzyme required by methyltetrahydrofolate:homocysteine methyltransferase. Methylmalonic acid accumulates in body fluids as well because synthesis of a second coenzyme, adenosylcobalamin, required for isomerization of methylmalonyl coenzyme A (CoA) to succinyl CoA is also impaired.

Etiology and pathogenesis As with 5,10-methylenetetrahydrofolate reductase deficiency, this disorder involves remethylation of homocysteine. The primary defect concerns deficient synthesis of cobalamin coenzymes from precursor vitamin. Since methylcobalamin is required for methyl-group transfer from methyltetrahydrofolate to homocysteine, impaired cobalamin metabolism leads to deficient methyltransferase activity. The precise defect responsible for impaired synthesis of methylcobalamin is unknown but involves some early step in lysosomal or cytosolic activation of the vitamin precursor. Somatic cell genetic studies indicate that two distinct lesions underlie deficient coenzyme formation, each of which appears to be inherited as an autosomal recessive trait.

Clinical manifestations The first reported patient died of infection at age 6 weeks following severely arrested development. Clinical manifestations in the other affected children vary: two had megaloblastic anemia and pancytopenia; three had significant spinocerebellar neurological impairment; one exhibited little clinical abnormality.

Diagnosis and treatment Homocystinuria, hypomethioninemia, and methylmalonic aciduria are the chemical hallmarks. These findings may also be present in juvenile or adult onset pernicious anemia in which intestinal cobalamin absorption is impaired. Measurement of serum cobalamin concentrations, low in pernicious anemia and normal in patients with defective conversion of cobalamin vitamin to coenzymes, helps in the differential diagnosis. Definitive diagnosis depends on demonstrating impaired coenzyme synthesis in cultured cells. Treatment of affected children with cobalamin supplements (1 to 2 mg per day) shows promise: homocystine and methylmalonate excretion fall to near normal values; the hematologic and neurological deficits have also lessened to a more variable degree.

REFERENCES

LENKE RR, LEVY HL: Maternal phenylketonuria and hyperphenylalaninemia. N Engl J Med 303:1202, 1980

MCKUSICK VA: Homocystinuria, in *Heritable Disorders of Connective Tissue,* 4th ed. St. Louis, Mosby, 1972, pp 224–281

MUDD SH, LEVY HL: Disorders of transsulfuration, in *The Metabolic Basis of Inherited Disease,* 5th ed, JB Stanbury et al (eds). New York, McGraw-Hill, 1983, chap 25

NYHAN WL (ed): *Heritable Disorders of Amino Acid Metabolism.* New York, Wiley, 1974

ROSENBERG LE, SCRIVER CR: Disorders of amino acid metabolism, in *Metabolic Control and Disease,* 8th ed, PK Bondy, LE Rosenberg (eds). Philadelphia, Saunders 1980, pp 583–776

———, TANAKA K: Disorders of amino acid and organic acid metabolism, in *The Year in Metabolism 1977,* N Freinkel (ed). New York, Plenum, 1978, pp 219–246

SCRIVER CR, CLOW CL: Phenylketonuria: Epitome of human biochemical genetics. N Engl J Med 303:1336, 1394, 1980

92
STORAGE DISEASES OF AMINO ACID METABOLISM

LEON E. ROSENBERG

A number of inherited metabolic disorders are characterized by deposition or storage of particular metabolites in tissues. In most, storage reflects impaired degradation of the substance in question; in others, the mechanism is unknown. Many storage diseases involve large molecules such as glycogen, sphingolipids, mucolipids, cholesterol esters, and mucopolysaccharides (see Chaps. 100, 103, and 104); in others, metals such as iron and copper are deposited (see Chaps. 97 and 98). Finally, there is a group of storage diseases in which relatively small organic molecules are deposited. These include gout (see Chap. 94) and a group of disorders of amino acid metabolism.

ALKAPTONURIA

DEFINITION Alkaptonuria is a rare disorder of tyrosine catabolism. Deficiency of the enzyme homogentisic acid oxidase leads to excretion of large amounts of homogentisic acid in urine and to accumulation of oxidized homogentisic acid pigment in connective tissues (ochronosis). After many years ochronosis produces a distinctive form of degenerative arthritis.

ETIOLOGY AND PATHOGENESIS Homogentisic acid is a normal intermediate formed during the catabolism of tyrosine to fumarate and acetoacetate. Activity of homogentisic acid oxidase, the enzyme that catalyzes the opening of the phenolic ring yielding maleylacetoacetic acid, is virtually absent in liver and kidney of patients with alkaptonuria, and homogentisic acid accumulates in cells and body fluids. Patients have minimally increased concentrations of homogentisic acid in blood because it is rapidly cleared by the kidney. As much as 3 to 7 g homogentisic acid may be excreted in the urine per day, but this is of little pathophysiologic significance. However, homogentisic acid and its oxidized polymers bind to collagen, leading to the progressive deposition of a gray to bluish-black pigment. The mechanism(s) by which degenerative changes develop in cartilage, intervertebral disk, and other connective tissues is unknown but may involve direct chemical irritation or inhibition of one or more enzyme systems involved in normal connective tissue metabolism.

Alkaptonuria was the first human disease shown to be inherited as an autosomal recessive trait. Affected homozygotes occur with a frequency no greater than 1 in 200,000. Heterozygous carriers are clinically well and excrete no homogentisic acid in urine, even after loading doses of tyrosine.

CLINICAL MANIFESTATIONS Alkaptonuria often goes unrecognized until middle life when degenerative joint disease appears in the majority. Prior to this time the tendency of the patient's urine to darken on standing may go unnoticed, as may slight discoloration of the sclerae and external ears. The latter manifestations of homogentisic acid deposition in tissue are generally the earliest external evidence of the disorder with appearance after age 20 to 30. Foci of gray-brown scleral pigment and generalized darkening of the concha, antihelix, and, finally, helix of the ear are typical. Ear cartilages may feel irregular and thickened. *Ochronotic arthritis* is heralded by pain, stiffness, and some limitation of motion of the hips, knees, and shoulders. Intermittent periods of acute arthritis, which may resemble rheumatoid arthritis, occur, but small joints are usually spared. Limitation of motion and ankylosis of the lumbosacral spine are common late manifestations. Pigmentation of heart valves, larynx, tympanic membranes, and skin occurs, and occasional patients develop pigmented renal or prostatic calculi. An increased incidence of degenerative cardiovascular disease has been reported in older patients, but a clear relationship between these findings and ochronosis has not been established.

DIAGNOSIS A patient whose urine darkens to blackness on standing must be suspected of having alkaptonuria, but because of modern plumbing conditions this finding is not often observed. The diagnosis is usually made from the triad of degenerative arthritis, ochronotic pigmentation, and urine which turns black upon alkalinization. Homogentisic acid in urine may be identified presumptively by other tests: upon addition of ferric chloride, a purple-black color is observed; treatment with Benedict's reagent yields a brown color; and addition of a saturated silver nitrate solution produces an immediate black color. These screening tests can be confirmed by chromatographic, enzymatic, or spectrophotometric determinations of homogentisic acid. X-rays of the lumbar spine are virtually pathognomonic. They show degeneration and dense calcification of the intervertebral disks and narrowing of the intervertebral spaces.

TREATMENT There is no specific treatment for ochronotic arthritis. It is conceivable that joint manifestations could be mitigated if homogentisic acid accumulation and deposition could be curbed by dietary restriction of phenylalanine and tyrosine, but the long course of the disease has discouraged such therapeutic attempts. Since ascorbic acid impedes oxidation and polymerization of homogentisic acid in vitro, its use has been suggested as a possible means of decreasing pigment formation and deposition. The efficacy of this form of treatment has not been established. Symptomatic treatment is similar to that for osteoarthritis (Chap. 351).

CYSTINOSIS

DEFINITION Cystinosis is a rare disorder characterized by the intralysosomal accumulation of free cystine in body tissues. This results in the appearance of cystine crystals in the cornea, conjunctiva, bone marrow, lymph nodes, leukocytes, and internal organs. Three clinical forms have been identified: an infantile (nephropathic) form leading to the Fanconi syndrome and renal insufficiency in the first decade; a juvenile (intermediate) form in which renal disease becomes manifest during the second decade; and an adult (benign) form characterized by deposition of cystine in the cornea but not in the kidney.

ETIOLOGY AND PATHOGENESIS The basic defect has not been identified. Numerous studies of enzymes concerned with cystine metabolism have not yielded any consistent abnormality, nor have investigations of cystine or cysteine transport. The cystine content of tissues in the infantile form may be more than 100 times normal, that in the adult form more than 30 times normal. Intracellular cystine appears to be located only in lysosomes and does not exchange with other intracellular or extracellular pools of this amino acid. Neither plasma nor urinary concentrations of cystine are particularly elevated.

The extent of cystine crystal deposition varies considerably from patient to patient, depending on both the form of the disease and the methods used to prepare pathological specimens. In the kidney cystine accumulation causes renal insufficiency in the infantile and juvenile forms. The kidneys are pale and shrunken, the capsule is adherent, and the corticomedullary junction is obscured. Microscopically, nephron organization is interrupted, glomeruli are hyalinized, connective tissue is increased, and the normal epithelium of the tubules is replaced by cuboidal cells. Narrowing and shortening of the proximal tubule produces the so-called swan neck deformity now known not to be specific for cystinosis. Patchy depigmentation of the peripheral retina occurs in the infantile and juvenile forms. This retinal degeneration is to be distinguished from the deposition of cystine crystals in the ocular conjunctiva or uvea.

Each form of cystinosis appears to be inherited as an autosomal recessive trait. Obligate heterozygotes have intracellular cystine contents intermediate between those of normal persons and affected patients but are free of clinical abnormalities.

CLINICAL MANIFESTATIONS In the infantile form abnormalities are usually apparent by 4 to 6 months of age. Growth retardation, vomiting, fever, vitamin D–resistant rickets, polyuria, dehydration, and metabolic acidosis are prominent. Generalized proximal tubular dysfunction (the Fanconi syndrome) leads to hyperphosphaturia and hypophosphatemia, renal glycosuria, generalized aminoaciduria, hypouricemia, and often hypokalemia. Pyelonephritis is common and may contribute, along with interstitial fibrosis, to progressive glomerular insufficiency. Death due to uremia or intercurrent infection usually occurs before age 10. Ocular manifestations are also prominent. Photophobia is usually demonstrable within the first few years of life due to cystine deposits in the cornea, and retinal degeneration may appear even earlier.

In contrast, patients with the adult form manifest only ocular abnormalities. Photophobia, headache, and burning or itching of the eyes are major complaints. Glomerular and tubular function and the integrity of the retina are preserved. The findings in the juvenile variant fall between these extremes. These patients have both ocular and renal manifestations, but the latter do not become significant until the second decade. The renal lesion, albeit milder than that seen in the infantile form, eventually leads to renal insufficiency.

DIAGNOSIS Cystinosis must be considered in any child with vitamin D–resistant rickets, the Fanconi syndrome, or glomerular insufficiency. Hexagonal or rectangular cystine crystals are most easily detected in the cornea (by slit-lamp examination), in unstained preparations of leukocytes from peripheral blood or bone marrow, or in biopsies of rectal mucosa. Diagnosis can be confirmed by quantitative determination of cystine in extracts of peripheral blood leukocytes or cultured fibroblasts. The infantile form of cystinosis has been diagnosed prenatally by the demonstration of vastly increased cystine content in cultured amniotic fluid cells.

TREATMENT The adult form of cystinosis is benign and requires no treatment. Symptomatic treatment of renal disease in patients with the infantile or juvenile form of cystinosis does not differ from that of other forms of chronic renal insufficiency: maintenance of adequate fluid intake to prevent dehydration; administration of sodium citrate or sodium bicarbonate to correct the metabolic acidosis; and ingestion of supplementary calcium, phosphate, and vitamin D to heal the rickets. Such measures are critical in maintaining growth, development, and well-being in affected children for a time. Two types of more specific therapy have been attempted without much success. Cystine-restricted diets are difficult to prepare and have not prevented progression of renal disease. Likewise, the use of sulfhydryl reagents (D-penicillamine, dimercaprol) and reducing agents (vitamin C) have yielded no long-term benefit.

The most promising form of therapy for nephropathic cystinosis is renal transplantation. More than 20 affected children with end-stage renal disease have been so treated. Those patients who tolerated the procedure and did not develop immunologic problems have shown return of kidney function toward normal. Several patients have been followed for 3 or more years after transplantation. The transplanted kidneys have not developed the functional abnormalities typical of cystinosis (i.e., the Fanconi syndrome or glomerular insufficiency). They may, however, reaccumulate some cystine, apparently owing to migration of interstitial or mesangial cells from the host. This experience justifies offering renal transplantation to patients with terminal renal failure.

PRIMARY HYPEROXALURIA

DEFINITION Primary hyperoxaluria is the designation for two rare disorders characterized by chronic excessive urinary excretion of oxalic acid and by calcium oxalate nephrolithiasis and nephrocalcinosis. Typically, patients with either form develop renal insufficiency early in life and die of uremia. At postmortem examination, calcium oxalate deposits are generally widespread in renal and extrarenal tissues, a condition referred to as *oxalosis.*

ETIOLOGY AND PATHOGENESIS Since both types of primary hyperoxaluria result from increased oxalate synthesis and since glyoxylate is the only significant precursor of oxalate in humans, the metabolic basis for the primary hyperoxalurias logically involves pathways of glyoxylate metabolism. In type I hyperoxaluria, urinary excretion of oxalate, the oxidized form of glyoxylate, and glycolic acid, the reduced form, is increased. The excessive synthesis of these substances in this condition results from a block in one of the routes of metabolism of glyoxylate. Activity of the cytosolic enzyme α-ketoglutarate:glyoxylate carboligase, which catalyzes the formation of α-hydroxy-β-ketoadipic acid, is markedly reduced in extracts of liver, kidney, and spleen. The resulting expansion of the glyoxylate pool behind this metabolic block leads to oxidation of glyoxylate to oxalate and to reduction of glyoxylate to glycolate. Each of these 2-carbon acids is then excreted in excess in the urine. In type II hyperoxaluria, L-glyceric acid is excreted in excess along with oxalate. In this condition, activity of D-glyceric acid dehydrogenase, an enzyme that catalyzes the reduction of hydroxypyruvate to D-glyceric acid in the catabolic pathway of serine metabolism, is absent in leukocytes (and presumably other tissues). The accumulated hydroxypyruvate is instead reduced by lactic dehydrogenase to the L-isomer of glycerate, which is excreted in the urine. Apparently the reduction of hydroxypyruvate is coupled in some way to the oxidation of glyoxylate to oxalate, thus causing the formation of increased oxalate.

Both disorders appear to be inherited as autosomal recessive traits. Heterozygotes are asymptomatic. Partial enzyme deficiency has been observed in heterozygotes for type II hyperoxaluria, but no studies with type I heterozygotes have been reported.

The pathogenesis of stone formation, nephrocalcinosis, and oxalosis relates directly to the insolubility of calcium oxalate. Extrarenal deposits of oxalate have been most widely reported in the heart, walls of arteries and veins, male urogenital tract, and bone.

CLINICAL MANIFESTATIONS Nephrolithiasis and oxalosis may become manifest during the first year of life. Most patients experience initial symptoms of renal colic or hematuria between ages 2 and 10 and succumb to uremia before age 20. With the onset of uremia, patients may develop severe peripheral arterial spasm and necrosis with resulting vascular insufficiency. In patients with delayed onset of symptoms, survival to age 50 or 60 has been reported, despite recurrent attacks of nephrolithiasis.

DIAGNOSIS Oxalate excretion in normal children or adults is less than 60 mg per 1.73 m^2 per day. Patients with type I or type II hyperoxaluria generally excrete two to four times this amount. Distinction between the two types of primary hyperoxaluria depends on measurements of the other organic acids that identify them: glycolic acid in type I and L-glyceric acid in type II. Since patients with pyridoxine deficiency or chronic ileal disease may excrete excessive amounts of oxalate, these conditions must be excluded.

TREATMENT There is no satisfactory treatment for primary hyperoxaluria. Urinary oxalate concentration can be reduced by increasing the urinary flow rate, but success is transient. Large doses of pyridoxine (100 mg per day) may reduce urinary oxalate in some patients, but long-term effects are not dramatic. A diet high in phosphate content seems to reduce the frequency of attacks of renal colic, but oxalate excretion is unaffected. Finally, renal transplantation has been attempted several times, but in each instance renal function was lost because of calcium oxalate deposition in the transplanted kidney.

REFERENCES

BOQUIST L et al: Primary oxalosis. Am J Med 54:673, 1973

LADU NB: Alcaptonuria, in *The Metabolic Basis of Inherited Disease,* 4th ed, JB Stanbury et al (eds). New York, McGraw-Hill, 1978, pp 268–282

O'BRIEN W et al: Biochemical, pathologic and clinical aspects of alcaptonuria, ochronosis and ochronotic arthropathy. Am J Med 34:813, 1963

SCHNEIDER JA, SCHULMAN, JD: Cystinosis, in *The Metabolic Basis of Inherited Disease,* 5th ed, JB Stanbury et al (eds). New York, McGraw-Hill, 1983, chap 85

SCHULMAN JD (ed): *Cystinosis,* US Department of Health, Education, and Welfare Publication (NIH) 72–249, 1972

WILLIAMS HE, SMITH LH JR: Primary hyperoxaluria, in *The Metabolic Basis of Inherited Disease,* 5th ed, JB Stanbury et al (eds). New York, McGraw-Hill, 1983, chap. 10

93 INHERITED DEFECTS OF MEMBRANE TRANSPORT

LEON E. ROSENBERG
ELIZABETH M. SHORT

The passage of certain large and small molecules across mammalian plasma cell membranes depends on the existence of specific transport systems that owe their specificity to a variety of membrane receptor and "carrier" proteins. These specific membrane constituents recognize individual substrates or a group of structurally related ones and catalyze their transmembrane movement by mechanisms poorly understood. The disorders considered in this chapter have three features in common: each is characterized by a specific defect in the transport of one or more compounds; each is inherited as a dominant or recessive, implying that a single genetic locus is involved; and each is presumed to reflect a primary alteration in a specific membrane protein. Many of these defects have been well characterized physiologically, but in none has the putative mutant transport protein been isolated.

More than 20 inherited disorders of membrane transport have been described in humans (Table 93-1). Most affect the gut and/or kidney only. Numerous classes of substrates are represented, including amino acids, hexoses, cations, anions, vitamins, and water. Some are discussed elsewhere in this text. Those impairing the transport of amino acids, hexoses, urate, and chloride are discussed here as examples of the range and significance of the abnormalities encountered.

DISORDERS OF AMINO ACID TRANSPORT

As noted in Table 93-1, 10 distinct disorders of amino acid transport have been described. Five of these (cystinuria, dibasicaminoaciduria, Hartnup disease, iminoglycinuria, and dicarboxylicaminoaciduria) show transport abnormalities for groups of structurally related amino acids, thereby implying the existence of group-specific membrane receptors or carriers. With the exception of iminoglycinuria and dicarboxylicaminoaciduria, these defects have important clinical consequences. The remaining five disorders affect the transport of only one amino acid, implying the existence of substrate-specific as well as group-specific transport systems. Each of these conditions affects transport in the kidney, gut, or both; none has been shown to alter transport in other tissues.

CYSTINURIA **Definition** Cystinuria is the most common inborn error of amino acid transport. It is characterized by excessive urinary excretion of the dibasic amino acids: lysine, arginine, ornithine, and cystine. This aminoaciduria results from impaired tubular reabsorption of these amino acids. A similar transport defect exists in the intestinal mucosa. Because cystine is the least soluble of the naturally occurring amino acids, its overexcretion predisposes to the formation of renal, ureteral, and bladder calculi. Such calculi are responsible for the signs and symptoms in affected patients.

Etiology and pathogenesis Massive excretion of cystine and the other dibasic amino acids occurs only in classic cystinuria. The disorder, inherited as an autosomal recessive trait, is believed to result from alterations in a membrane carrier protein essential for transport of this group of amino acids in the apical brush border of proximal renal tubule and small intestinal cells. Renal clearance studies indicate that the putative protein has a greater affinity for ornithine and arginine than for lysine and cystine. Although the endogenous renal clearance of all four amino acids is increased in homozygotes, the presence of some residual transport capacity for these compounds plus the existence of three other disorders marked by selective excretion of members of this group (dibasicaminoaciduria, hypercystinuria, lysinuria) argues for the existence of at least three discrete renal transport systems for these amino acids: one for each amino acid alone; one shared by lysine, arginine, and ornithine; and one for all four amino acids.

Whereas urinary excretion patterns and renal clearance abnormalities in all homozygotes are similar, evidence for three allelic variants has come from studies of intestinal transport in homozygotes and of urinary excretion in obligate heterozygotes. These variants have been designated types I, II, and III. Type I homozygotes lack mediated intestinal transport of cystine, lysine, arginine, and ornithine; their heterozygous relatives have normal urinary amino acid excretion patterns. Type II homozygotes lack mediated lysine transport in the gut but retain some capacity for cystine transport; heterozygotes have moderately increased urinary excretion of each of the four amino acids. Type III homozygotes retain some capacity for mediated intestinal transport of the four involved substrates; heterozygotes have modestly increased urinary lysine and cystine.

Clinical manifestations Cystinuria is among the most common inborn errors, homozygotes occurring with a frequency of 1 in 10,000 to 1 in 15,000 in many ethnic groups. Cystine stones account for 1 to 2 percent of all urinary tract calculi. The maximum solubility of cystine in the physiological urinary pH range of 4.5 to 7.0 is about 300 mg per liter. Since affected homozygotes regularly excrete 600 to 1800 mg per day, crystalluria and calculus formation are a constant threat. Cystine stone formation usually becomes manifest in the second or third decade but has been reported as early as the first year of life. Symptoms and signs are those typical of urolithiasis regardless of etiology: hematuria, flank pain, renal colic, obstructive uropathy, and infection. Recurrent episodes of urolithiasis may lead to progressive renal insufficiency.

Diagnosis The presence of cystine in a urinary tract stone is pathognomonic of cystinuria. However, since 50 percent of the stones excreted by cystinuric subjects are of mixed composition and since as many as 10 percent may contain *no* detectable cystine, a urinary nitroprusside test should be done on all patients with urolithiasis to exclude this diagnosis. The nitroprusside test is also positive (appearance of a cherry red color) in some heterozygotes for cystinuria, in patients with hypercystinuria, homocystinuria, and cysteine β-mercaptolactate disulfiduria, and in the presence of acetone in the urine. When cystine content exceeds 250 mg per liter, cystine crystals may be seen in the sediment of acidified, concentrated, chilled urine. These crystals, in the form of hexagonal plates, are pathogno-

TABLE 93-1
Genetic disorders of membrane transport

Class of substance and disorder	*Individual substrates*	*Tissues manifesting transport defect*	*Proposed molecular basis of defect*	*Major clinical manifestations*	*Mode of inheritance*	*Location of discussion*
AMINO ACIDS						
Classic cystinuria	Cystine, lysine, arginine, ornithine	Proximal renal tubule, jejunal mucosa	Mutation of shared dibasic-cystine transport protein	Cystine nephrolithiasis	Autosomal recessive	Chap. 93
Dibasicaminoaciduria	Lysine, arginine, ornithine	Proximal renal tubule, jejunal mucosa	Mutation of dibasic transport protein	Type I: Moderate retardation Type II: Protein intolerance, hyperammonemia, retardation	Autosomal recessive	Chap. 93
Hypercystinuria	Cystine	Proximal renal tubule	Mutation of cystine transport protein	Some risk of cystine nephrolithiasis	Autosomal recessive	Chap. 93
Lysinuria	Lysine	Proximal renal tubule, jejunal mucosa	Mutation of lysine transport protein	Seizures, physical and mental retardation	Possible autosomal recessive	Chap. 93
Hartnup disease	Neutral amino acids	Proximal renal tubule, jejunal mucosa	Mutation of neutral amino acid–shared transport protein	Constant neutral aminoaciduria, intermittent symptoms of pellagra	Autosomal recessive	Chap. 93
Tryptophan malabsorption	Tryptophan	Jejunal mucosa	Mutation of tryptophan transport protein	Indoluria, ?hypercalcemia, ?nephrocalcinosis	Probable autosomal recessive	Chap. 93
Methionine malabsorption	Methionine	Jejunal mucosa	Mutation of methionine transport protein	α-Hydroxybutyricaciduria, white hair, mental retardation, convulsions, hyperpneic attacks, edema	Probable autosomal recessive	Chap. 93
Histidinuria	Histidine	Proximal renal tubule, jejunal mucosa	Mutation of histidine transport protein	Mental retardation	Autosomal recessive	Chap. 93
Iminoglycinuria	Glycine, proline, hydroxyproline	Proximal renal tubule, jejunal mucosa	Mutation of shared glycine–imino acid transport protein	None	Autosomal recessive	Chap. 93
Dicarboxylicaminoaciduria	Glutamic acid, aspartic acid	Proximal renal tubule, jejunal mucosa	Mutation of shared dicarboxylic amino acid transport protein	None	Probable autosomal recessive	Chap. 93
HEXOSES						
Renal glycosuria	D-Glucose	Proximal renal tubule	Mutation of D-glucose transport protein	Glycosuria with normal blood glucose	Autosomal recessive	Chap. 93
Glucose-galactose malabsorption	D-Glucose D-Galactose	Jejunal mucosa, proximal renal tubule	Mutation of shared glucose-galactose transport protein	Watery diarrhea on feeding glucose, lactose, sucrose, or galactose	Autosomal recessive	Chaps. 93, 308
LIPIDS						
Familial hypercholesterolemia	Cholesterol	Fibroblasts, lymphoid lines, leukocytes	Mutation of membrane LDL-cholesterol receptor protein	Hypercholesterolemia, tendon xanthomas, arcus corneae, coronary artery atherosclerosis	Autosomal dominant	Chap. 103
URATE						
Hypouricemia	Uric acid	Proximal renal tubule	Mutation of urate transport protein	Hypouricemia, hyperuricosuria, ?hypercalcinuria	Autosomal recessive	Chap. 93
ANIONS						
Familial hypophosphatemic rickets	Inorganic phosphate	Proximal renal tubule, jejunal mucosa	Mutation of inorganic phosphate transport protein	Hypophosphatemia, phosphaturia, phosphatopenic rickets/osteomalacia	X-linked dominant	Chap. 341

TABLE 93-1 *(continued)*
Genetic disorders of membrane transport

Class of substance and disorder	*Individual substrates*	*Tissues manifesting transport defect*	*Proposed molecular basis of defect*	*Major clinical manifestations*	*Mode of inheritance*	*Location of discussion*
ANIONS *(continued)*						
Congenital chloridorrhea	Chloride	Ileal and colonic mucosa	Mutation of Cl^-/HCO_3^- exchange pump carrier protein	Hydramnios, watery diarrhea, elevated fecal chloride, achloriduria, metabolic alkalosis with volume depletion, hyperaldosteronism	Autosomal recessive	Chaps. 93, 308
Familial goiter	Inorganic iodide	Thyroid gland, salivary gland, gastric mucosa	Mutation of iodide transport protein	Congenital hypothyroidism (cretinism), goiter	Probable autosomal recessive	Chap. 111
CATIONS						
Distal renal tubular acidosis (type I—gradient)	Hydrogen ion	Distal renal tubule	Mutation of distal tubule H^+ pump carrier protein	Hyperchloremic acidosis, hypokalemia, acquired nephrocalcinosis, and hypercalcinuria	Autosomal dominant	Chap. 299
Proximal renal tubular acidosis (type II—HCO_3 wasting)	Hydrogen ion	Proximal renal tubule	Mutation of proximal tubule H^+ pump carrier protein	Hyperchloremic acidosis, bicarbonate wasting	Probable autosomal recessive	Chap. 299
Menkes' disease	Copper	Duodenal and jejunal intestinal cells	Possible serosal transport protein or intracellular transport defect	Severe mental retardation, pili torti (kinky hair), typical facies, arterial tortuosity, excess Wormian bones, thermal instability	X-linked recessive	Chap. 84
Hereditary Spherocytosis Elliptocytosis Ovalocytosis Stomatocytosis	Sodium	Red blood cell (RBC) membranes	Mutation of membrane structure (? lipid or protein) resulting in increased sodium permeability	Increased RBC fragility resulting in variable degrees of hemolytic anemia, splenomegaly, and jaundice; RBC shape respectively spherocytic, elliptocytic, ovalocytic, or stomatocytic (target-shaped)	Each of these diseases of RBC morphology is a separately inherited autosomal dominant	Chap. 329
WATER						
Nephrogenic diabetes insipidus (ADH-resistant)	Water	Distal renal tubule	Lack of activation of ADH-responsive luminal membrane adenylate cyclase, possible defect in receptor or enzyme protein	Polyuria, polydipsia, hyposthenuria	X-linked recessive	Chap. 299
VITAMINS						
Juvenile pernicious anemia	Cobalamin (vitamin B_{12})	Ileal mucosa	Mutation of receptor for intrinsic factor–cobalamin complex	Megaloblastic anemia	Autosomal recessive	Chap. 327
Folate malabsorption	Folic acid	Small bowel	Mutation of folate transport protein	Megaloblastic anemia	Autosomal recessive	Chap. 327
Multiple carboxylase deficiency (type II)	Biotin	Small bowel	Mutation of biotin transport protein	Ketoacidosis, alopecia, eczematoid eruption	Undefined	

monic of cystine overexcretion in patients not taking sulfonamides.

Diagnostic confirmation of cystinuria depends upon the demonstration of the characteristic amino acid excretion pattern in the urine. Selective excretion of cystine, lysine, arginine, and ornithine can be demonstrated by paper chromatography or electrophoresis, and quantitative determinations can be made by column chromatography. Quantitation becomes important in differentiating some heterozygotes from homozygotes and in documenting the reduction of free cystine excretion during therapy.

Treatment Medical management of cystinuria is aimed at reducing the concentration of cystine in urine. The single most important aspect of this treatment is maintenance of a large urine volume. Fluid ingestion in excess of 4 liters per day is essential, and 5 to 7 liters per day is optimal. Stones can be prevented and even dissolved by such vigorous hydration. It must be made clear to the cystinuric subject that water is a drug. Solubility of cystine rises sharply in urine above pH 7.5, and various regimens of urinary alkalinization have been used therapeutically. Vigorous administration of sodium bicarbonate, Diamox, and polycitrates is required to maintain a persistently alkaline pH, but this measure introduces the danger of inducing formation of other "alkaline" stones (calcium oxalate, calcium phosphate, magnesium ammonium phosphate) and even of producing nephrocalcinosis.

Another medical approach to treatment involves administration of D-penicillamine (β,β-dimethylcysteine) which undergoes sulfhydryl-disulfide exchange with cystine to form the mixed disulfide of penicillamine and cysteine. Since this disulfide is more than 50 times as soluble as cystine, D-penicillamine (in doses of 1 to 3 g per day) has the capacity to reduce free cystine excretion markedly, thereby preventing new stone formation and promoting dissolution of existing calculi. Unfortunately D-penicillamine is immunogenic, and allergic manifestations include acute serum sickness, agranulocytosis, pancytopenia, immune glomerulitis, and the Goodpasture syndrome. Thus, its use should be reserved for patients who fail to respond to hydration alone or who are in a particularly high-risk category (one remaining kidney, renal insufficiency). When medical management fails, urologic surgery is required. An occasional patient may require renal transplantation because of renal failure.

DIBASICAMINOACIDURIA A number of families have been described in which affected members have a defect in renal tubular reabsorption of lysine, arginine, and ornithine but *not* of cystine. The disorder almost surely reflects mutations in the genes coding for a renal transport protein used by the three dibasic amino acids only. Two clinically distinct variants have been observed, each apparently inherited as an autosomal recessive trait. Clinical manifestations appear to be related to the significant losses of ornithine, arginine, and perhaps lysine.

In the common form of dibasicaminoaciduria (type II), homozygotes show defective intestinal transport of dibasic amino acids as well as exaggerated renal losses. A defect in hepatic cell uptake of these substances has also been proposed. Affected patients present in childhood with hepatosplenomegaly, protein intolerance, and episodic ammonia intoxication. Plasma concentrations of lysine, arginine, and ornithine are reduced. The clinical findings have been attributed to hyperammonemia resulting from insufficient amounts of arginine and ornithine to maintain proper function of the Krebs-Henseleit urea cycle. Treatment includes dietary protein restriction and supplementation with arginine and ornithine. Obligate heterozygotes are clinically well and show no excess urinary loss of dibasic amino acids.

Type I dibasicaminoaciduria has been described in only one homozygote. She was moderately mentally retarded but had no clear history of protein intolerance or hyperammonemia. Her urinary losses of dibasic amino acids were not as great as those seen in type II homozygotes. The condition was distinguished from type I by the presence of modest excesses of dibasic amino acids in urine of both asymptomatic parents. Other pedigrees containing asymptomatic heterozygotes have been identified by urinary screening programs.

HARTNUP DISEASE Pellagra-like skin lesions, variable neurological manifestations, and a constant renal aminoaciduria for the monoaminomonocarboxylic amino acids with neutral or aromatic side chains characterize Hartnup disease. Alanine, serine, threonine, valine, leucine, isoleucine, phenylalanine, tyrosine, tryptophan, glutamine, asparagine, and histidine are excreted in urine in quantities from 5 to 10 times normal, and an intestinal transport defect for these same amino acids has been demonstrated. The clinical spectrum appears to relate solely to nutritional deficiency of the essential amino acid tryptophan, caused by the combination of intestinal malabsorption and renal loss. Disease manifestations are episodic, related, at least in part, to metabolic demands for tryptophan.

The major catabolic pathway of tryptophan metabolism leads to the synthesis of niacin and nicotinamide-adenine dinucleotide (NAD). This pathway supplies about 50 percent of daily niacin needs. In patients with Hartnup disease, the renal and intestinal transport defect for neutral and aromatic amino acids, including tryptophan, leads to niacin deficiency. The transport defect likely reflects abnormalities of a group-specific system for neutral amino acids. Renal clearance studies show some residual reabsorptive capacity for each involved amino acid. This suggests that they are transported by other carrier systems as well, a conclusion supported by the subsequent description of patients with substrate-specific transport errors for tryptophan, methionine, and histidine.

Hartnup disease is inherited as an autosomal recessive trait. Homozygotes occur with a frequency of about 1 in 16,000 births. Heterozygotes exhibit no clinical or chemical abnormalities.

Pellagra is the clinical syndrome produced by dietary niacin deficiency, and its clinical features of diarrhea, dementia, and dermatitis are those which characterize Hartnup disease (see Chap. 83). The diagnosis should be suspected in any patient with pellagra without a history of severe dietary niacin deficiency. The neurological and psychiatric manifestations range from attacks of cerebellar ataxia to mild emotional lability to frank delirium and usually accompany exacerbations of the erythematous, eczematoid skin rash. Fever, sunlight, stress, and sulfonamide therapy provoke clinical relapses. Diagnosis is made by detection of the pathological neutral aminoaciduria which does not occur in dietary niacin deficiency. Treatment is directed at niacin repletion and includes a high-protein diet and daily nicotinamide supplementation (50 to 250 mg).

IMINOGLYCINURIA This trait is characterized by excessive urinary excretion of glycine and the imino acids proline and hydroxyproline. Homozygotes for this autosomal recessive disorder occur with a frequency of about 1 in 16,000. The exaggerated renal clearance of glycine, proline, and hydroxyproline reflects a defect in the tubular transport system shared by these three compounds. An intestinal transport defect has been demonstrated in some. This suggests that more than one mutation may lead to persistent iminoglycinuria, a thesis corroborated by studies of urinary amino acid excretion in obligate heterozygotes from different families. No consistent clinical abnormalities have been reported in homozygotes, who are usually detected by urinary amino acid screening programs. Individuals with iminoglycinuria should be reassured as to the benign nature of the disturbance.

DICARBOXYLICAMINOACIDURIA Selective urinary loss and exaggerated endogenous renal clearance of glutamic and aspartic acids have been described in two unrelated children. Intestinal absorption of these dicarboxylic amino acids was impaired in one but not in the other. The former suffered from recurrent hypoglycemia; the latter was asymptomatic. It remains to be determined whether this defect is of clinical significance.

SUBSTRATE-SPECIFIC DEFECTS IN AMINO ACID TRANSPORT Rare pedigrees exist in which individuals have defective renal tubular reabsorption and/or impaired intestinal absorption of a single free amino acid. These disorders, each apparently inherited as an autosomal recessive trait, provide the strongest evidence that transmembrane transport of amino acids is catalyzed by substrate-specific as well as group-specific transport mechanisms.

Hypercystinuria Two siblings exhibited modest cystinuria without excessive urinary excretion of lysine, arginine, or ornithine. Fractional tubular reabsorption of cystine was reduced to about 80 percent of the filtered load, and up to 250 mg per day was excreted in the urine. Neither showed any abnormality in intestinal absorption of cystine. Both were clinically well, although their cystine excretion would appear to place them at some risk for cystine urolithiasis. Urinary cystine excretion by both parents was unremarkable.

Lysinuria Only a single child with selective impairment of renal tubular reabsorption of lysine has been described. Endogenous lysine clearance was increased; intestinal transport was impaired; plasma lysine was reduced. Severe mental and growth retardation and seizures were present. A lysine-supplemented diet appeared to stimulate growth. Urinary excretion of lysine was normal in the parents.

Histidinuria Two siblings, each with moderate mental retardation, exhibited a renal transport defect for histidine only. Urinary loss of histidine approached 40 to 50 percent of the filtered load, and an intestinal transport defect for histidine was also present. The clinically normal parents had normal urinary excretion but a modest defect in intestinal absorption of histidine.

Methionine malabsorption Single children from two pedigrees have shown an intestinal transport defect for methionine. One may have had a renal transport defect as well. This disorder was detected because of urinary excretion of α-hydroxybutyric acid, a distinctive by-product of the intestinal bacterial breakdown of the unabsorbed methionine. This compound, which gives an unusual odor resembling malt or dried celery to the urine, appears to be responsible for the white hair, attacks of hyperpnea, convulsions, edema, and mental retardation. Treatment of one of these children with a methionine-restricted diet was followed by improvement in all clinical manifestations.

Tryptophan malabsorption An isolated defect in intestinal absorption of tryptophan has been described in two siblings. The renal tubular reabsorption of tryptophan was normal. A variety of indoles were excreted in stool and urine. These compounds result from chemical degradation of unabsorbed tryptophan by intestinal bacteria and have been described in patients with Hartnup disease as well. Because of concomitant

renal parenchymal disease, hydrolytic enzymes were released into the urine, acted upon the indoles found there, and led to the formation of a blue pigment, indigotin. This sequence of events earned this condition the sobriquet "blue-diaper syndrome." No pellagra-like symptoms were described. The patients' mother also excreted modest excesses of indole compounds, suggesting that she is a carrier of this trait.

DISORDERS OF HEXOSE TRANSPORT

Nondiabetic melituria occurs in a number of conditions. Pentoses, hexoses, heptoses, and disaccharides have been identified in the urine; all except sucrose yield a positive test for reducing substances. Some meliturias result from diffuse renal injury, others from ingestion of nonmetabolizable sugars. In still others the sugars accumulate in blood due to deficient activity of catabolizing enzyme systems and "spill" into the urine. Only among the hexoses have specific inherited disorders of sugar transport been identified. The existence of renal glycosuria and intestinal glucose-galactose malabsorption as heritable, autosomal recessive disorders points to the existence of at least two specific carrier proteins for hexoses in human jejunal and renal brush border membranes: one for glucose and one shared by glucose and galactose.

RENAL GLYCOSURIA To avoid confusion with diabetes mellitus, Marble's criteria for the diagnosis of renal glycosuria should be followed: (1) glycosuria in the absence of hyperglycemia, (2) constant glycosuria with little fluctuation related to diet, (3) normal (or slightly flat) oral glucose tolerance test, (4) identification of urinary reducing substance as glucose, and (5) normal storage and utilization of carbohydrates. The Fanconi syndrome, in which renal glycosuria occurs as part of generalized proximal tubular dysfunction, should also be excluded. The incidence is less than 1 in 500. The condition is benign, but occasionally glycosuria may be great enough to cause polyuria and polydipsia. Even more rarely, dehydration or ketosis may develop under conditions of stress such as pregnancy or starvation.

In normal persons glucose is present in the glomerular filtrate at a concentration equal to that in plasma water and is actively reabsorbed throughout the proximal renal tubule by a sodium-dependent, phlorizin-inhibitable transport process. Reabsorptive capacity exceeds normal plasma glucose concentration. Thus, glucose does not appear in the urine until the threshold for reabsorption is reached. Titration studies suggest that the plasma concentration at which some filtered glucose begins to escape proximal tubular reabsorption is 200 to 240 mg/dl. Maximal renal reabsorptive capacity is exceeded at a filtered load of 325 ± 36 mg/min per 1.73 m^2, and this value is defined as the tubular maximum for glucose (TmG).

Titration studies in subjects with renal glycosuria have shown two patterns of glycosuria: type A characterized by a reduced tubular maximum reabsorptive capacity and type B showing a reduced threshold for glycosuria, an increased "splay" in the titration curve, and a normal TmG. Marked renal glycosuria occurs in individuals homozygous for either of these recessively inherited mutations of the specific membrane transport process for glucose and in genetic compounds for these presumably allelic mutations. Modest reduction in renal threshold or TmG has been demonstrated in obligate heterozygotes in some pedigrees; modest glycosuria can be expected in such family members when plasma glucose is elevated.

GLUCOSE-GALACTOSE MALABSORPTION In this condition, infants develop a profuse, watery diarrhea when fed milk or foods containing lactose, sucrose, glucose, or galactose. Fructose or carbohydrate-free formulas are well tolerated. A specific defect in intestinal absorption of glucose and galactose can be demonstrated by oral tolerance tests that produce little or no increase in plasma glucose or galactose. Treatment with a glucose- and galactose-free diet leads to resolution of symptoms in childhood. Although the basic transport defect can be demonstrated throughout life, most patients show an improved tolerance for glucose and galactose as they get older.

Intestinal transport studies performed in vitro on small biopsy specimens of jejunal mucosa have shown a complete absence of active D-glucose and D-galactose transport in affected children and intermediate transport capacity in their parents. These findings confirm the specificity of the mutation for these two sugars and the autosomal recessive inheritance of this transport disorder.

A number of these patients have renal glycosuria at normal plasma glucose concentrations. Renal titration studies generally demonstrate a reduced threshold for glucose reabsorption (type B renal glycosuria) with a normal TmG. Urinary glucose loss is not as severe as in isolated renal glycosuria. This finding suggests the presence of multiple glucose transport proteins in the kidney. One, responsible for the bulk of glucose reabsorption and specific for glucose only, is affected in renal glycosuria; another, shared by glucose and galactose and responsible for transporting less of the filtered load of glucose, is affected in glucose-galactose malabsorption. Either the former is not present in intestinal mucosa or the shared system is more important in that tissue. In both disorders transport of sugars in all other tested tissues is normal, reflecting the multiplicity and tissue specificity of membrane transport proteins.

DEFECTIVE URATE TRANSPORT: HYPOURICEMIA

A small number of pedigrees have been described containing individuals with a selective defect in renal tubular reabsorption of sodium urate. These subjects are identified by the presence of marked hypouricemia. Since little serum urate is bound to plasma proteins, failure to reabsorb filtered urate results in a serum urate ranging from 0.2 to 1.8 mg/dl. No disease is associated with this isolated defect, although the risk of uric acid nephrolithiasis is theoretically present.

Renal urate clearance normally averages 15 percent of glomerular filtration rate, and the excreted urate is composed both of filtered urate that has escaped reabsorption and secreted urate. Subjects with isolated hypouricemia have urate clearances averaging from 33 to 85 percent of the filtration rate; in some, urate clearance exceeds the glomerular filtration rate. Studies with probenecid, which blocks tubular reabsorption of urate, and pyrazinamide, which blocks tubular secretion, suggest that the disorder is due to a partial defect in proximal tubular reabsorption. In two families hypercalcinuria due to enhanced intestinal calcium absorption was also present, but in all others only uricosuria has been demonstrated. The defect is inherited as an autosomal recessive. Urate transport has not been studied in nonrenal tissue or in obligate heterozygotes. The defect is presumed to reflect mutation of a proximal renal tubular membrane protein that selectively transports sodium urate.

DEFECTIVE ANION TRANSPORT: CHLORIDORRHEA

This rare, autosomal recessive disease results from impairment of active transport of chloride in the ileum and colon. Absence of the chloride-bicarbonate ion exchange "pump" causes profound symptoms even before birth (polyhydramnios and absence of meconium). Massive watery diarrhea is apparent from the first days of life. This fluid loss, with its attendant impairment of electrolyte homeostasis, is life-threatening. A hypokalemic, hypochloremic, hyponatremic metabolic alkalosis develops with dehydration and secondary hyperaldosteronism. Fecal fluid contains an excess of chloride ion over the sum of the accompanying cations, sodium and potassium. Fecal chloride concentration always exceeds 90 mmol per liter when volume and serum electrolyte disturbances are corrected, and this chloridorrhea is diagnostic. Renal chloride transport is normal. Decreased urine chloride results from the kidney's attempts to conserve salt and water.

Treatment necessitates adequate, life-long repletion of electrolyte and fluid losses, since no way has yet been found to mitigate the transport disorder. Exact replacement of water, sodium chloride, and potassium chloride can prevent the growth and psychomotor retardation and the development of progressive renal damage. The renal lesion, with hyalinized glomeruli, juxtaglomerular hyperplasia, calcifications, and arteriolar changes, is probably a result of chronic volume depletion.

REFERENCES

Elsas LJ, Rosenberg LE: Renal glycosuria, in *Strauss and Welt's Diseases of the Kidney,* 3d ed, LE Earley, CW Gottschalk (eds). Boston, Little, Brown, 1979, pp 1021–1028

Gorden P, Levitin H: Congenital alkalosis with diarrhea; a sequel to Darrow's original description. Ann Intern Med 87:876, 1973

Holmberg C et al: Congenital chloride diarrhoea. Arch Dis Child 52:255, 1977

Krane SM: Renal glycosuria, in *The Metabolic Basis of Inherited Disease,* 4th ed, JB Stanbury et al (eds). New York, McGraw-Hill, 1978, pp 1607–1617

Rosenberg LE: Intestinal hexose transport in familial glucose-galactose malabsorption, in *Membranes and Disease,* L Bolis et al (eds). New York, Raven Press, 1976, pp 253–262

———, Scriver CR: Disorders of amino acid metabolism, in *Metabolic Control and Disease,* 8th ed, PK Bondy, LE Rosenberg (eds). Philadelphia, Saunders, 1980, pp 616–645

Short EM, Rosenberg LE: Renal aminoaciduria, in *Strauss and Welt's Diseases of the Kidney,* 3d ed, LE Earley, CW Gottschalk (eds). Boston, Little, Brown, 1979, pp 975–1020

Thier SO, Segal S: Cystinuria, in *The Metabolic Basis of Inherited Disease,* 5th ed, JB Stanbury et al (eds). New York, McGraw-Hill, 1983, chap 80

Wyngaarden JB, Kelley WN: *Gout and Hyperuricemia.* New York, Grune & Stratton, 1976, pp 411–420

Disorders of nucleic acid metabolism

94
GOUT AND OTHER DISORDERS OF PURINE METABOLISM

WILLIAM N. KELLEY

Gout is a term representing a heterogeneous group of diseases found exclusively in humans, which in their full development are manifested by (1) an increase in the serum urate concentration; (2) recurrent attacks of a characteristic type of acute arthritis, in which crystals of monosodium urate monohydrate are demonstrable in leukocytes of synovial fluid; (3) aggregated deposits of monosodium urate monohydrate (tophi) chiefly in and around the joints of the extremities and sometimes leading to severe crippling and deformity; (4) renal disease involving interstitial tissues and blood vessels; and (5) uric acid nephrolithiasis. These may occur singly or in combination.

PREVALENCE AND EPIDEMIOLOGY The serum urate value is elevated in an absolute sense when it exceeds the limit of solubility of monosodium urate in serum. At 37°C the saturation value of urate in plasma is about 7.0 mg/dl; a value above this represents supersaturation in a physicochemical sense. The serum urate concentration is relatively elevated when it exceeds the upper limit of an arbitrary normal range, usually defined as the mean serum urate value plus 2 standard deviations in a healthy population matched for age and sex. In most epidemiological studies the upper limit is about 7.0 mg/dl in men and 6.0 mg/dl in women. In epidemiological terms a serum urate value in excess of 7.0 mg/dl carries an increased risk of gouty arthritis or renal stones.

Sex and age influence urate levels. The serum urate concentration before puberty in both boys and girls averages approximately 3.6 mg/dl. After puberty, levels increase in boys more than in girls. Values in men reach a plateau in the early twenties and are essentially stable thereafter. Values in women are constant from age 20 through 40, but with menopause the values rise and approach or equal those in men. These age and sex differences are thought to be related to differences in the renal clearance of urate, perhaps determined by the levels of estrogens and androgens. Other factors, including warm ambient temperature, obesity, high social status, and achievement or intelligence also appear to correlate with a higher serum urate concentration.

Hyperuricemia by one or more of the above definitions is present in 2 to 18 percent of the population. In one hospitalized group, 13 percent of adult men exhibited a serum urate concentration in excess of 7.0 mg/dl.

The prevalence of gout is less than that of hyperuricemia and is different around the world. In most of the western world it ranges from 0.13 to 0.37 percent of the population. Gout is primarily a disease of adult men, and only about 5 percent of cases occur in women; it occurs rarely in the prepubertal child of either sex. The usual form of gout is uncommon before the third decade, and the peak incidence is in the fifth decade.

INHERITANCE In the United States a family history of gout is obtained in 6 to 18 percent of gouty subjects, and figures as high as 75 percent are noted after persistent questioning. A precise definition of the inheritance of gout is complicated by the numerous environmental factors that alter the serum urate concentration. In addition, the identification of several specific genetic causes of gout has established that gout is the common clinical manifestation of a heterogeneous group of diseases. Accordingly, study of the inheritance of hyperuricemia and gout in the population or even within families is difficult. Two specific enzymatic causes of gout, hypoxanthine-guanine phosphoribosyltransferase deficiency and 5-phosphoribosyl-1-pyrophosphate (PRPP) synthetase overactivity, are X-linked. Other pedigrees have been reported in which the inheritance is consistent with an autosomal dominant mode. More commonly, genetic studies suggest multifactorial inheritance.

CLINICAL FEATURES The full natural history of gout comprises four stages: asymptomatic hyperuricemia, acute gouty arthritis, intercritical gout, and chronic tophaceous gout. Nephrolithiasis may occur in any stage but the first.

Asymptomatic hyperuricemia Asymptomatic hyperuricemia is that stage in which the serum urate level is raised but arthritic symptoms, tophi, or uric acid stones have not yet appeared. In men vulnerable to classic gout hyperuricemia begins at puberty, whereas in women at risk hyperuricemia is usually delayed until menopause. In contrast, patients with certain of the enzyme defects to be described later may be hyperuricemic from birth. While asymptomatic hyperuricemia may last throughout the lifetime with no recognizable consequences, the tendency toward acute gouty arthritis increases as a function of serum urate concentration and the duration of hyperuricemia. The risk of nephrolithiasis also increases as serum urate values increase and correlates with the magnitude of uric acid excretion. While virtually all gouty subjects are hyperuricemic, perhaps no more than 5 percent of hyperuricemics ever develop gout.

The phase of asymptomatic hyperuricemia ends with the first attack of gouty arthritis or nephrolithiasis. In most, gout comes before stone, usually after at least 20 to 30 years of sustained hyperuricemia. However, between 10 and 40 percent of gouty subjects have renal colic prior to the first episode of arthritis.

Acute gouty arthritis The primary manifestation of acute gout is exquisitely painful arthritis, at first usually monoarticular and associated with few constitutional symptoms but later often polyarticular and accompanied by fever. Attacks last a variable but limited period of time and are separated by intervals of freedom from all symptoms. About 90 percent of first attacks occur in a single joint, and in at least half the initial attack occurs in the first metatarsal phalangeal joint. Ultimately, 90 percent of patients experience an acute attack in the great toe (podagra).

Acute gouty arthritis is predominantly a disease of the lower extremities. The more distal the site of involvement the more typical are the attacks. Following the toe in order of frequency as sites of initial involvement are the insteps, ankles, heels, knees, wrists, fingers, and elbows. While acute attacks may occur in other joints, such as shoulder, hips, spine, sacroiliac, sternoclavicular, and mandibular joints, these sites are rare except in patients with established, severe disease. The patient may report trivial episodes of pain preceding the first dramatic gouty attack. Commonly, the major attack begins at night, is exquisitely painful with inflamed joints, and may be triggered by a specific event such as trauma, alcohol ingestion, certain drugs, dietary excess, or surgery. It is difficult to improve upon Syndenham's classical description:

The victim goes to bed and sleeps in good health. About two o'clock in the morning he is awakened by a severe pain in the great toe; more rarely in the heel, ankle or instep. This pain is like that of a dislocation, and yet the parts feel as if cold water were poured over them. Then follow chills and shivers, and a little fever. The pain, which was at first moderate, becomes more intense. With its intensity the chills and shivers increase. After a time this comes to its height, accommodating itself to the bones and ligaments of the tarsus and metatarsus. Now it is a violent stretching and tearing of the ligaments—now it is a gnawing pain and now a pressure and tightening. So exquisite and lively meanwhile is the feeling of the part affected, that it cannot bear the weight of bedclothes nor the jar of a person walking in the room. The night is passed in torture, sleeplessness, turning of the part affected, and perpetual change of posture; the tossing about of the body being as incessant as the pain of the tortured joint, and being worse as the fit comes on. Hence the vain effort by change of posture, both in the body and the limb affected, to obtain an abatement of the pain.

Intercritical period The attack of gout may last only a day or two or up to several weeks but characteristically subsides spontaneously. An asymptomatic phase termed the *intercritical period* then commences. The patient is totally free of symptoms during this stage, a feature that is diagnostically important. While approximately 7 percent never have a second attack, most experience a recurrence within 1 year. However, the intercritical period may last up to 10 years. Later attacks tend to be polyarticular, more severe, more prolonged, and associated with fever. In this stage gout may be difficult to differentiate from other types of polyarticular arthritis such as rheumatoid arthritis. Rare patients progress directly from the initial acute attack to chronic polyarticular disease with no remissions.

Tophi and chronic gouty arthritis In the untreated patient the urate pool expands, and crystal deposits of monosodium urate eventually appear in cartilage, synovial membranes, tendons, and soft tissues. The rate of formation of these tophaceous deposits is a function of the degree and duration of hyperuricemia and of the severity of renal disease. The classic location of a tophus is the helix or antihelix of the ear (Fig. 94-1). Tophi also commonly occur along the ulnar surface of the forearm, as saccular distensions of the olecranon bursae (Fig. 94-2), as enlargements of the Achilles tendon, or at other pressure points. Patients with the most severe tophi, interestingly, often have sparing of the helix and antihelix of the ear.

Tophi are difficult to differentiate from rheumatoid nodules and other types of subcutaneous nodules. They may ulcerate and exude chalky or pasty material rich in monosodium urate crystals. In contrast to other subcutaneous nodules, tophi are rarely transient although they may resolve slowly in response to treatment of hyperuricemia. For reasons that are unclear, it is rare for a tophus to become infected. Patients with severe tophaceous disease appear to have milder and less frequent attacks of acute gouty arthritis than do nontophaceous subjects. Chronic tophaceous gout rarely occurs prior to the onset of gouty arthritis.

Since the advent of effective antihyperuricemic therapy, only a minority of patients develop visible tophi, permanent joint changes, or chronic symptoms. Thus, effective therapy alters the natural history of the disease.

Nephropathy Some renal dysfunction occurs in up to 90 percent of subjects with gouty arthritis. Prior to the advent of chronic hemodialysis, renal failure accounted for 17 to 25 percent of deaths in the gouty population. The initial manifestation of renal involvement may be albuminuria or isosthenuria. If the patient presents in an advanced stage of renal failure it may be difficult to determine whether renal failure is a consequence of hyperuricemia or hyperuricemia is the result of renal disease.

Several types of parenchymal renal damage have been described. The first, urate nephropathy, has been attributed to the deposition of monosodium urate crystals in the renal interstitial tissue. The second, obstructive uropathy, is due to the

FIGURE 94-1
Tophus of the helix of the ear adjacent to the auricular tubercle.

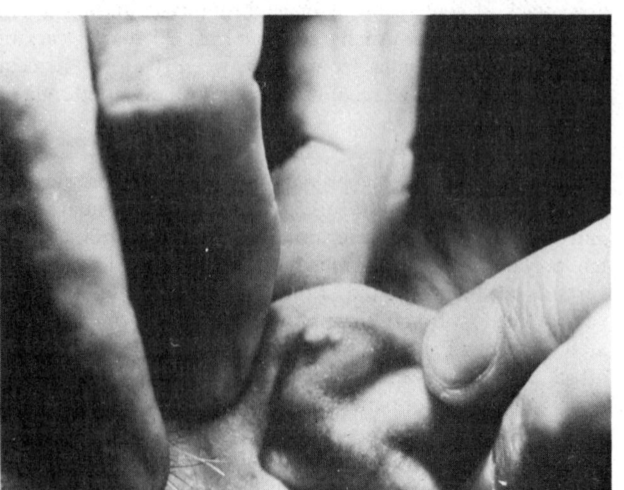

FIGURE 94-2
Effusions of olecranon bursae of patient with gout. Note also the cutaneous deposits of urate and the minimal inflammatory response.

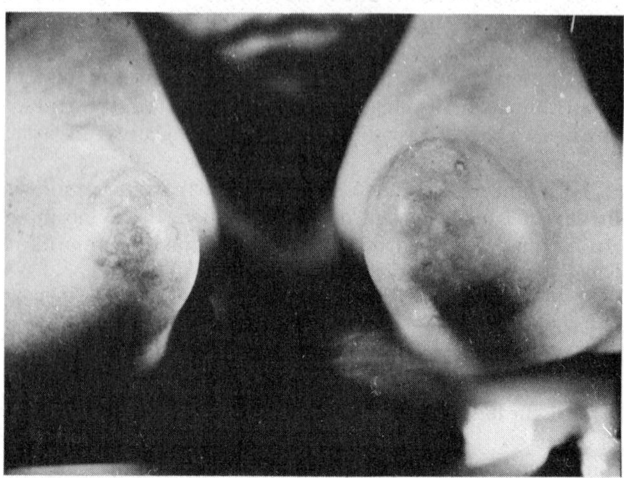

formation of uric acid crystals in the collecting tubules, renal pelvis, or ureter, with resulting blockage of urine flow.

There is considerable controversy over the pathogenesis of urate nephropathy. While crystals of monosodium urate have been demonstrated in the interstitium of kidneys from gouty subjects, such crystals are not demonstrable in the kidneys of most people with gout. Further, there is a close correlation between the development of renal disease and the presence of hypertension in patients with gout. It is not clear, therefore, whether the hypertension causes the renal disease or the gouty renal disease is the cause of the hypertension.

Acute obstructive uropathy is a severe form of acute renal failure due to the precipitation of uric acid crystals in collecting ducts and ureters. This condition occurs most commonly in (1) patients with profound overproduction of uric acid, particularly subjects with leukemia or lymphoma who are subjected to aggressive chemotherapy, (2) patients with gout and marked hyperuricaciduria, and (3) (possibly) patients following severe exercise or convulsions. Postmortem studies reveal intraluminal precipitates of uric acid with dilatation of proximal tubules. Therapy designed to decrease the formation of uric acid, accelerate urine flow, and increase the fraction of uric acid present as the more soluble ionized form, monosodium urate, is effective in the reversal of this process.

Nephrolithiasis While the prevalence of uric acid stones in the United States is about 0.01 percent, the prevalence in gouty subjects ranges from 10 to 25 percent. The major factor favoring formation of uric acid stones is the increased urinary excretion of uric acid. When the urinary uric acid exceeds 1100 mg per day the incidence reaches 50 percent. There is also correlation with increasing serum urate concentrations, the prevalence reaching approximately 50 percent at a serum urate value of 13 mg/dl or above. Other factors contributing to the formation of uric acid stones include (1) undue acidity of the urine, (2) increased urine concentration, and (3) (perhaps) abnormalities of urinary constituents that affect the solubility of uric acid itself.

Gouty subjects also have an increased frequency of calcium-containing stones; the occurrence in gout is 1 to 3 percent, while that in the general population is about 0.1 percent. While the mechanisms for this association are unclear, there is a high frequency of hyperuricemia and hyperuricaciduria in patients seen because of calcium stones. It is possible that uric acid crystals serve as a nidus for calcium stone formation.

Associated conditions Obesity, hypertriglyceridemia, and hypertension are common. The hypertriglyceridemia of primary gout is strongly associated with obesity or alcohol ingestion and not with hyperuricemia itself. The incidence of hypertension in the nongouty population is correlated with age, sex, and obesity; when these factors are appropriately scored there appears to be little or no direct relationship between hyperuricemia and hypertension. The increased frequency of diabetes is also probably related to factors such as age and obesity and not to hyperuricemia itself. Finally, the increased incidence of atherosclerosis has been attributed to the concomitant obesity, hypertension, diabetes, and hypertriglyceridemia.

Independent analysis of these variables suggests that obesity is most important. Hyperuricemia in the obese subject appears to be related to both increased production and reduced excretion of uric acid.

DIAGNOSIS AND DIFFERENTIAL DIAGNOSIS The diagnosis of acute gouty arthritis can be established by demonstration of monosodium urate crystals in white cells of synovial fluid obtained from the inflamed joint by compensated polarized light microscopy (Fig. 94-3). Such crystals can be identified in synovial fluid from virtually every patient with acute gouty arthritis. Failure to demonstrate urate crystals in synovial fluid after careful search under appropriate conditions makes the diagnosis unlikely. Demonstration of intracellular urate crystals establishes the diagnosis but does not exclude the possibility that another type of arthropathy is present concurrently.

Synovial fluid analysis may also be helpful in other ways. The total leukocyte count may range from 1000 to more than 70,000 per milliliter. The predominant cell type is the polymorphonuclear leukocyte. As with other inflammatory fluids, the mucin clot is fair to poor. The concentrations of glucose and uric acid are the same as in serum.

In the patient in whom synovial fluid cannot be obtained or in whom intracellular crystals cannot be demonstrated, a presumptive diagnosis of gout can be seriously entertained if the patient has (1) hyperuricemia, (2) the classical clinical features described above, and (3) a dramatic response to colchicine. In the absence of crystals or this highly suggestive triad, the diagnosis of gout should be considered tentative. While a dramatic therapeutic response to colchicine is strongly suggestive of the diagnosis of gouty arthritis, it is not pathognomonic by itself.

Acute gouty arthritis must be differentiated from other conditions in which monoarticular or polyarticular arthritis occurs. The most common initial presentation in the gouty patient is podagra, but many conditions mimic the painful, swollen big toe characteristic of the disease. These include soft tissue infection, inflamed bunions, local trauma, rheumatoid arthritis, degenerative arthritis with acute inflammation, acute sarcoidosis, psoriatic arthritis, pseudogout, acute calcific tendonitis, palindromic rheumatism, Reiter's disease, and sporotrichosis. Rarely, confusion may be caused by cellulitis, gonorrhea, fibrosis of the sole and heel, hematoma, and subacute

FIGURE 94-3
Crystals of monosodium urate monohydrate in joint aspirate.

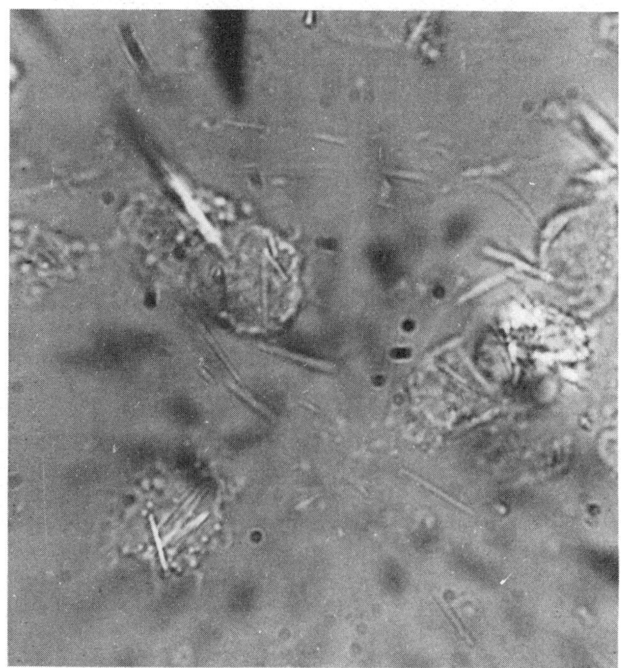

bacterial endocarditis with embolization or suppurative arthritis. Gouty involvement of other joints such as the knee must also be differentiated from acute rheumatic fever, serum sickness, hemarthrosis, and the peripheral joint involvement of ankylosing spondylitis or inflammatory bowel disease.

PATHOPHYSIOLOGY OF HYPERURICEMIA Classification The biochemical hallmark and prerequisite of gout is hyperuricemia. The concentration of uric acid in body fluids is determined by the balance between rates of production and elimination. Uric acid is formed by oxidation of purine bases, which may be exogenous or endogenous in origin. About two-thirds of uric acid is excreted into the urine (300 to 600 mg per day), and approximately one-third is excreted into the gastrointestinal tract, where it is ultimately destroyed by bacteria. Hyperuricemia may be due to an excessive rate of uric acid production, a decrease in the renal excretion of uric acid, or a combination of both events.

Hyperuricemia and gout may be classified as metabolic or renal (Table 94-1). In those patients with hyperuricemia of metabolic origin, there is an increased production of uric acid, whereas in those with hyperuricemia of renal origin, decreased renal excretion of uric acid causes the hyperuricemia. In the classification used here *primary* refers to those cases in which gout or hyperuricemia is the central manifestation of the disease, namely, gout that is neither secondary to another acquired disorder nor a subordinate manifestation of an inborn error that leads initially to a major disease unlike gout. While some cases of primary gout have a defined genetic basis, others do not. *Secondary* hyperuricemia or gout refers to those cases which develop in the course of another disease or as a consequence of drugs.

Overproduction of uric acid Overproducers of uric acid by definition excrete in excess of 600 mg per day after a 5-day period of dietary purine restriction; such patients probably represent less than 10 percent of the gouty population. In these patients there is an acceleration in the rate of purine biosynthesis de novo or an increased turnover of purines. Understanding the basic mechanisms responsible for these abnormalities requires an understanding of purine metabolism (Fig. 94-4).

The purine nucleotides, adenylic acid (AMP), inosinic acid (IMP), and guanylic acid (GMP), are the end products of purine biosynthesis. They can be synthesized in one of two ways: either directly from the purine bases, e.g., guanine to GMP, hypoxanthine to IMP, and adenine to AMP; or they may be synthesized de novo, beginning with nonpurine precursors and progressing through a series of steps to the formation of IMP, which is the common intermediate purine nucleotide. IMP can be converted either to AMP or to GMP. Once the purine nucleotides are formed, they are utilized for the synthesis of nucleic acids, cyclic AMP, cyclic GMP, ATP, and certain cofactors.

The various purine components are degraded to the purine nucleotide monophosphates. GMP is degraded via guanosine, guanine, and xanthine to uric acid. IMP is degraded through inosine, hypoxanthine, and xanthine to uric acid. AMP can be deaminated to IMP and further catabolized through inosine to uric acid, or it may be degraded to inosine by an alternate pathway with the intermediate formation of adenosine.

While the purine pathway is regulated in a complex manner, the intracellular concentration of 5-phosphoribosyl-1-pyrophosphate (PRPP) appears to be a major determinant of the rate of synthesis of uric acid in humans. Generally, when the concentration of PRPP in the cell is elevated, uric acid synthe-

FIGURE 94-4
Outline of purine metabolism: (1) amidophosphoribosyltransferase; (2) hypoxanthine-guanine phosphoribosyltransferase; (3) PRPP synthetase; (4) adenine phosphoribosyltransferase; (5) adenosine deaminase; (6) purine nucleoside phosphorylase; (7) 5′-nucleotidase; (8) xanthine oxidase.

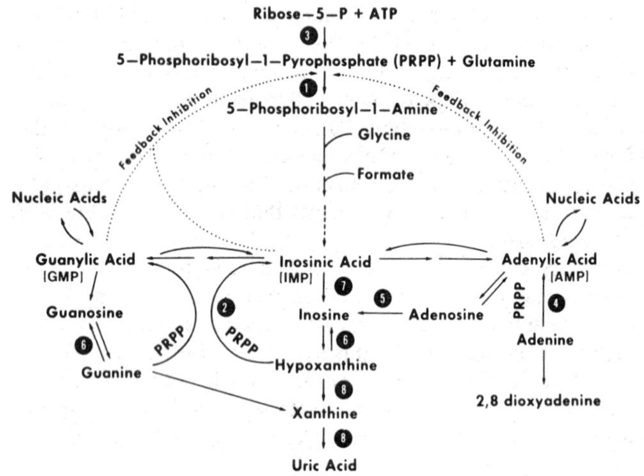

TABLE 94-1
Classification of hyperuricemia and gout

Type	*Metabolic disturbance*	*Inheritance*
Metabolic (10%):		
Primary		
Molecular defects undefined	Not established	Polygenic
Associated with specific enzyme defects		
P-ribose-PP synthetase variants, increased activity	Overproduction of P-ribose-PP and of uric acid	X-linked
Hypoxanthine-guanine phosphoribosyltransferase deficiency, partial	Overproduction of uric acid, increased purine biosynthesis de novo driven by surplus P-ribose-PP	X-linked
Secondary		
Associated with increased purine biosynthesis de novo		
Glucose 6-phosphatase deficiency or absence	Overproduction plus underexcretion of uric acid; glycogen storage disease, type I (von Gierke)	Autosomal recessive
Hypoxanthine-guanine phosphoribosyltransferase deficiency, "virtually complete"	Overproduction of uric acid; Lesch-Nyhan syndrome	X-linked
Associated with increased nucleic acid turnover	Overproduction of uric acid	
Renal (90%):		
Primary		
Secondary		

sis is elevated; when the concentration of PRPP is reduced, the synthesis of uric acid is also reduced. Although exceptions are recognized, this concept is applicable to most situations.

From 5 to 10 percent of adult gouty subjects with overproduction of uric acid have a partial deficiency of hypoxanthine-guanine phosphoribosyltransferase, the enzyme that catalyzes the conversion of hypoxanthine to inosinic acid and guanine to guanylic acid (reaction 2, Fig. 94-4). The deficiency of hypoxanthine-guanine phosphoribosyltransferase leads to a decreased consumption and increased accumulation of PRPP, thus accelerating purine biosynthesis and the production of uric acid. These patients typically have the onset of gouty arthritis at a young age (15 to 30 years), a high incidence of uric acid stones (75 percent), and the occasional occurrence of mild neurologic dysfunction characterized by dysarthria, hyperreflexia, incoordination, and/or mental retardation. This disease is inherited in an X-linked manner so that males are affected through carrier females. A more severe deficiency of the same enzyme leads to the development of the Lesch-Nyhan syndrome.

Several families are described in which there is increased activity of the enzyme PRPP synthetase (reaction 3, Fig. 94-4). The mutant enzymes, of which three different types are recognized, all exhibit increased activity, resulting in increased intracellular concentrations of PRPP, accelerated purine biosynthesis, and elevated excretion of uric acid. The inheritance pattern in this disease is also X-linked. These patients, like those with partial hypoxanthine-guanine phosphoribosyltransferase deficiency, generally develop gout in the second or third decade and have a high incidence of uric acid stones.

These two inborn errors of purine metabolism, hypoxanthine-guanine phosphoribosyltransferase deficiency and PRPP synthetase overactivity, account for less than 15 percent of all patients with what is now considered to be primary hyperuricemia associated with an overproduction of uric acid. The cause of the overproduction in the majority of patients has not been defined.

There are numerous causes of secondary hyperuricemia associated with an increased production of uric acid. In some, the increased excretion of uric acid is related, as it is in primary gout, to an accelerated rate of purine biosynthesis de novo. Patients with glucose 6-phosphatase deficiency (type I glycogen storage disease) uniformly exhibit an increased production of uric acid as well as an accelerated rate of purine biosynthesis de novo (see Chap. 100). It is postulated that patients with this enzyme defect also have an increased concentration of PRPP, which in turn is responsible for the accelerated rate of purine biosynthesis and uric acid overproduction. Patients with the Lesch-Nyhan syndrome, which is due to a virtually complete deficiency of hypoxanthine-guanine phosphoribosyltransferase, also uniformly exhibit a profound overproduction of uric acid and an accelerated rate of purine biosynthesis de novo. In these patients, as in those with gout due to a partial deficiency of hypoxanthine-guanine phosphoribosyltransferase, the basic mechanism is thought to be related to a decreased consumption of PRPP.

In the majority of patients with secondary hyperuricemia due to an overproduction of uric acid, the predominant abnormality appears to be an increased turnover of nucleic acids. A number of diseases, including the myeloproliferative and lymphoproliferative disorders, multiple myeloma, secondary polycythemia, pernicious anemia, certain hemoglobinopathies, thalassemia, other hemolytic anemias, infectious mononucleosis, and some carcinomas may be associated with increased marrow activity or increased cell turnover at other sites and an associated increased turnover of nucleic acids. The increased

turnover in nucleic acids leads in turn to hyperuricemia, hyperuricaciduria, and a compensatory increase in the rate of purine biosynthesis de novo.

Reduced excretion A large proportion of gouty subjects require a plasma urate value of 1 to 2 mg/dl higher than normal subjects to achieve a given rate of uric acid excretion (Fig. 94-5). This abnormality is most prominent in the gouty subject with a normal production of uric acid and is not present in most subjects with overproduction of uric acid.

The excretion of urate is dependent on glomerular filtration, tubular reabsorption, and tubular secretion. Uric acid appears to be completely filtered at the glomerulus and reabsorbed in the proximal tubule (i.e., presecretory reabsorption). Uric acid secretion then occurs in a subsequent segment of the proximal tubule, and partial reabsorption takes place at a second reabsorptive site in the distal portion of the proximal tubule (i.e., postsecretory reabsorption). While some uric acid reabsorption may also occur in the ascending limb of the loop of Henle and in the collecting duct, these latter two sites are thought to be quantitatively less important. Attempts to define further the location and nature of these latter sites and to quantify their contribution to uric acid transport in normal humans or in various disease states have been largely unrewarding.

Theoretically, the altered renal excretion of uric acid exhib-

FIGURE 94-5

Rate of uric acid excretion at various plasma urate levels in nongouty (solid symbols) and gouty (open symbols) subjects. Large symbols represent mean values; small symbols represent individual data of a few mean values selected to illustrate the degree of scatter within groups. Studies were conducted under basal conditions, after RNA feeding, and after infusions of lithium urate. (From Wyngaarden. Reproduced by permission of Academic Press.)

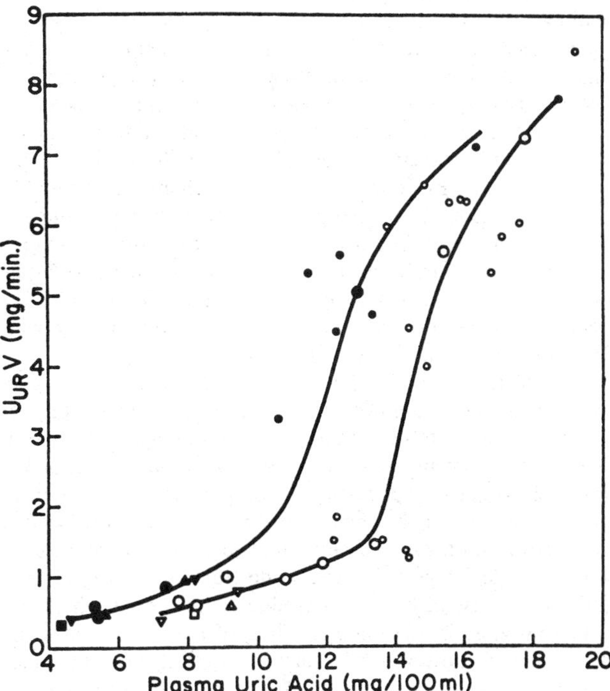

ited by most patients with gout could be due to (1) reduced filtration of uric acid, (2) enhanced reabsorption, or (3) decreased secretion. While there are no unequivocal data to establish any one of these mechanisms as the basic defect, it is likely that all three are operative within the gouty population.

Numerous secondary causes of hyperuricemia and gout can also be attributed to a decrease in the renal excretion of uric acid. A reduction in the glomerular filtration rate leads to a decrease in the filtered load of uric acid and thus to hyperuricemia; patients with renal disease are hyperuricemic on this basis. Other factors, such as decreased secretion of uric acid, have been postulated in patients with some types of renal disease (e.g., polycystic kidney disease and lead nephropathy). Gout is a rare complication of the secondary hyperuricemia due to renal disease.

Diuretic therapy is one of the most important causes of secondary hyperuricemia. Diuretic-induced volume depletion leads to enhanced tubular reabsorption of uric acid as well as decreased uric acid filtration. Decreased secretion of uric acid has also been postulated as a possible mechanism in diuretic-induced hyperuricemia. A number of other drugs lead to hyperuricemia by undefined renal mechanisms; these agents include low-dose aspirin, pyrazinamide, nicotinic acid, ethambutol, and ethanol.

Impaired renal excretion of uric acid is thought to be an important mechanism for the hyperuricemia associated with several disease states. Volume depletion may be important in patients with hyperuricemia associated with adrenal insufficiency and nephrogenic diabetes insipidus. In some situations hyperuricemia has been attributed to competitive inhibition of uric acid secretion by excess organic acids thought to be secreted by the same renal tubular mechanism responsible for uric acid secretion. Examples include starvation (ketosis and free fatty acids), alcoholic ketosis, diabetic ketoacidosis, maple syrup urine disease, and lactic acidosis of any cause. Hyperuricemia in conditions such as hyperparathyroidism, hypoparathyroidism, pseudohypoparathyroidism, and hypothyroidism may also have a renal basis, but the mechanism is unclear.

PATHOGENESIS OF ACUTE GOUTY ARTHRITIS The events leading to the initial crystallization of monosodium urate in a joint after an average of 30 years of asymptomatic hyperuricemia are not completely understood. Sustained hyperuricemia leads eventually to the development of microtophi in the synovial lining cells and perhaps to an accumulation of monosodium urate in cartilage on proteoglycans that have a high affinity for urate. By one of several mechanisms, probably including trauma with disruption of the microtophi and increased turnover of the cartilage proteoglycans, there is an episodic release of urate crystals into the synovial fluid. Other factors, such as a lower temperature in the joint space or an unequal reabsorption of water and urate from the synovial fluid, may accelerate urate precipitation.

A sufficient number of crystals in the joint space triggers the acute attack by a process that appears to include (1) phagocytosis of the crystals by leukocytes with the rapid release of a chemotactic protein from the leukocytes, (2) activation of the kallikrein system, (3) activation of complement with the consequent formation of the chemotactic complement components, and (4) the ultimate urate-mediated disruption of lysosomes within the leukocytes, leading to destruction of white blood cells and release of lysosomal products into the synovial fluid. While progress in the understanding of acute gouty arthritis has occurred, questions about factors responsible for spontaneous resolution of the acute attack and the effect of colchicine remain to be completely answered.

TREATMENT The therapeutic aims in gout are (1) to terminate the acute attack as promptly and gently as possible; (2) to prevent recurrences of acute gouty arthritis; (3) to prevent or reverse complications of the disease resulting from deposition of monosodium urate crystals in joints, kidneys, and other sites; (4) to prevent or reverse associated features such as obesity, hypertriglyceridemia, or hypertension; and (5) to prevent formation of uric acid kidney stones.

Treatment of the acute gouty attack Acute gouty arthritis is treated with an anti-inflammatory agent. Colchicine is the drug most frequently employed. Standard therapy involves administration of 0.5 mg each hour or 1.0 mg every 2 hours by mouth until one of three things occurs: (1) the patient improves, (2) gastrointestinal side effects develop, or (3) a maximum of 6 mg is taken without relief. Colchicine is most effective if therapy is begun shortly after the onset of symptoms. Over 75 percent of patients with gout show major improvement in symptoms within the first 12 h of treatment. However, as many as 80 percent of patients are unable to tolerate an optimal dose because of gastrointestinal side effects, which may precede or coincide with clinical improvement. Intravenous administration of colchicine eliminates the gastrointestinal side effects for the majority and also provides a more rapid response.

Colchicine levels become high in leukocytes, remain constant for 24 h, and are detectable for over 10 days after a single intravenous infusion. As an initial dose 2 mg should be given intravenously, followed by two additional doses of 1 mg at 6-h intervals if needed. Special care must be taken in the intravenous administration of colchicine. The drug is irritative and can lead to severe pain and necrosis if allowed to extravasate to surrounding tissues. It is important to make certain that the intravenous route is secure and that the drug is diluted with 5 to 10 volumes of normal saline and infused over a period of no less than 5 min. Colchicine by either oral or parenteral route may cause bone marrow depression, alopecia, hepatocellular failure, mental depression, seizures, ascending paralysis, respiratory depression, and death. Toxic effects are more likely in patients with significant hepatic, bone marrow, or renal disease and in those subjects on prophylactic maintenance colchicine. The dosage should be reduced for these individuals, and the drug should not be used in neutropenic patients.

Other anti-inflammatory agents, including indomethacin, phenylbutazone, naproxen, and fenoprofen, are also effective in the treatment of acute gouty arthritis. Indomethacin may be given at a dose of 75 mg orally, followed by 50 mg every 6 h and continued at that dose for 24 h after relief is obtained. The drug is then tapered to 50 mg every 8 h for three doses, and then to 25 mg every 8 h for three doses. Side effects of indomethacin include gastrointestinal toxicity, sodium retention, and complaints referable to the central nervous system. While the incidence of side effects may be as high as 60 percent in patients taking the doses described above, the drug is generally better tolerated than colchicine and probably is the treatment of choice in the patient with a well-established diagnosis of acute gouty arthritis. To improve the therapeutic response and thus diminish morbidity of the disease, the patient may be instructed to begin therapy with an anti-inflammatory agent at the first twinge of an acute attack.

Prophylaxis Once the acute episode has resolved, a number of measures can reduce the likelihood of recurrence: (1) the institution of prophylactic daily colchicine or indomethacin, (2) controlled weight reduction for the obese patient, (3) avoidance of known precipitating factors such as heavy alcohol consumption or a diet rich in purines, and (4) the institution of antihyperuricemic therapy.

The administration of small daily doses of colchicine is effective prophylaxis against further acute attacks. A program of 1 to 2 mg colchicine a day is completely successful in about three-fourths of patients with gout and fails completely in only about 5 percent. In addition, this program is safe and essentially free of side effects. However, unless serum urate is maintained at normal levels, the patient is spared only acute arthritis and may well proceed to develop other manifestations of gout. Maintenance colchicine therapy is particularly helpful during the first year or two after institution of antihyperuricemic drugs.

Prevention or reversal of the deposition of monosodium urate in tissues Antihyperuricemic agents are effective in reducing serum urate concentration and should be used in patients with (1) one or more attacks of acute gouty arthritis, (2) one or more tophi, and (3) uric acid nephrolithiasis. The aim of antihyperuricemic therapy is to maintain the serum urate below 7.0 mg/dl, the minimal concentration at which urate saturates the extracellular fluid. Reduction to these levels may be achieved by use of drugs that increase the renal excretion of uric acid or decrease uric acid production. Antihyperuricemic drugs generally do not have anti-inflammatory properties. Uricosuric agents reduce serum urate by enhancing the renal excretion. While a large number of drugs exhibit this property, the most effective agents available in the United States are probenecid and sulfinpyrazone. Probenecid is usually started in doses of 250 mg twice a day; it is increased over a period of several weeks to the dose necessary to achieve effective reversal of the hyperuricemia. A total dose of 1 g per day is appropriate for half of patients; the maximum dose should not exceed 3.0 g per day. Because the half-life is 6 to 12 h, it should be given in two to four evenly spaced doses per day. Hypersensitivity, skin rash, and gastrointestinal complaints are the major side effects. Although serious toxicity is rare, side effects may cause up to a third of the patients to discontinue probenecid.

Sulfinpyrazone is a metabolite of phenylbutazone with no anti-inflammatory activity. The drug is usually started at a dose of 50 mg twice a day and gradually increased to a maintenance level of 300 to 400 mg per day given in three or four divided doses. The maximum effective daily dose is 800 mg. Side effects are similar to those with probenecid, although the incidence of bone marrow toxicity may be higher. Approximately a fourth of patients stop the drug for one reason or another.

Probenecid and sulfinpyrazone are effective in most patients with hyperuricemia and gout. In addition to intolerance, failures can result from poor patient compliance, concomitant salicylate ingestion, or impaired renal function. Aspirin at any dose blocks the uricosuric effect of probenecid and sulfinpyrazone. These agents begin to lose effectiveness as the creatinine clearance falls below 80 ml/min and are completely ineffective when clearance reaches 30 ml/min.

During the negative urate balance induced by uricosuric therapy, the serum urate value drops, and urinary uric acid excretion is elevated above pretreatment levels. With continuation of therapy excess urate is mobilized and eliminated, the serum urate falls, and uric acid excretion returns essentially to pretreatment levels. The transient increase in uric acid excretion, which usually lasts for only a few days, may lead to the development of renal calculi in a tenth of patients so treated. To avoid this complication uricosuric agents should be started at low doses and gradually increased as described. Maintaining an ample urine flow with adequate hydration and alkalinizing the urine with oral sodium bicarbonate alone or in combination with acetazolamide reduce the likelihood of stone formation. The ideal candidate for uricosuric agents is under 60 and has normal renal function, uric acid excretion of less than 700 mg per day on a general diet, and no history of renal stones.

Hyperuricemia may also be controlled by allopurinol, a drug that decreases uric acid synthesis. Allopurinol inhibits xanthine oxidase (reaction 8, Fig. 94-4), the enzyme that catalyzes the oxidation of hypoxanthine to xanthine and xanthine to uric acid. While allopurinol has a half-life in vivo of only 2 to 3 h, it is metabolized largely to oxipurinol, which also is an effective inhibitor of xanthine oxidase and has a half-life ranging from 18 to 30 h. In most patients 300 mg per day is an effective antihyperuricemic dose. Because of the long half-life of the major metabolite the drug may be administered once a day. Since oxipurinol is largely excreted in the urine, its half-life is prolonged in patients with renal insufficiency. The dose of allopurinol should, therefore, be reduced by half in patients with significant renal dysfunction.

Significant side effects of allopurinol include gastrointestinal distress, skin rashes, fever, toxic epidermal necrolysis, alopecia, bone marrow suppression, hepatitis, jaundice, and vasculitis. The overall incidence of side effects is about 20 percent and more common in the presence of renal insufficiency. In only 5 percent of patients are the side effects sufficient to force discontinuation of the drug. Important drug-drug interactions involving allopurinol include prolongation of the half-lives of mercaptopurine and azathioprine and enhancement of the toxicity of cyclophosphamide.

Specific indications for choosing allopurinol over a uricosuric drug include (1) an increased urinary uric acid excretion (greater than 700 mg per day on a general diet), (2) impairment of renal function with a creatinine clearance less than 80 ml/min, (3) tophaceous gout regardless of renal function, (4) uric acid nephrolithiasis, and (5) gout not controlled by uricosuric agents because of ineffectiveness or intolerance. Allopurinol and a uricosuric drug may be used simultaneously in the rare patient who cannot be controlled by a single medication. Such combination therapy requires no modification in the dosage of either agent and usually results in further lowering of the serum urate concentration.

Acute gouty arthritis may occur whenever there is a rapid and substantial change in the serum urate concentration. Thus, the initiation of antihyperuricemic therapy with any agent may precipitate acute gouty arthritis. In addition, recurrent attacks may occur for a year or longer when large tophaceous deposits are present, even if hyperuricemia is controlled. For these reasons, it is prudent to begin prophylactic therapy with colchicine prior to initiation of antihyperuricemic drugs and to continue it until the serum urate is controlled for at least a year or until all tophi have resolved. Patients should be warned of the possibility of flare-up during the early phase of therapy. While it is not necessary in most gouty patients, strict dietary purine restriction should be instituted in patients with severe tophaceous gout and/or renal failure.

Prevention and treatment of acute uric acid nephropathy Immediate and vigorous therapy is essential for acute uric acid nephropathy. The first step is to increase urine flow by vigorous hydration coupled with administration of a potent diuretic such as furosemide. The urine should be alkalinized to achieve conversion of uric acid to the more soluble monosodium urate. Alkalinization can be accomplished by the administration of sodium bicarbonate alone or in combination with acetazolamide. Allopurinol should also be administered to reduce uric acid formation. The initial dose in this setting should be 8 mg/kg per day given as a single daily dose. The dose should be decreased after 3 or 4 days to 100 to 200 mg per day if renal insufficiency persists. Treatment for uric acid kidney stones is similar to that for acute uric acid nephropathy. In most cases allopurinol combined only with high fluid intake is effective.

WORKUP OF THE HYPERURICEMIC PATIENT Evaluation of the patient with hyperuricemia is directed toward (1) defining the cause of the hyperuricemia (which may disclose an important disease other than gout), (2) assessing the presence and extent of damage to tissues and organs, and (3) identifying associated abnormalities. From a practical standpoint these inquiries are pursued simultaneously, since decisions about the significance of hyperuricemia and about therapy depend on the answers to all of these.

The most important single test in the hyperuricemic patient is analysis of the urine for uric acid. If a history of stone disease is present, a flat plate of the abdomen and intravenous pyelogram may be indicated. If a renal stone is recovered, analysis for uric acid and other constituents is useful. If joint disease is present, synovial fluid analysis and x-rays of the involved joints are helpful. If there is a history of exposure to lead, measurement of urinary lead excretion after an infusion of calcium EDTA may be useful in documenting the presence of gout due to lead exposure. In cases where the patient appears to be an overproducer, measurement of erythrocyte hypoxanthine-guanine phosphoribosyltransferase and PRPP synthetase levels may be indicated.

Management of asymptomatic hyperuricemia There is considerable controversy about the indications for therapy of the patient with asymptomatic hyperuricemia. Generally, treatment should be withheld unless the patient (1) becomes symptomatic; (2) has a strong family history for gout, nephrolithiasis, or renal failure; or (3) is excreting large quantities of uric acid (greater than 1100 mg per day).

OTHER DISORDERS OF PURINE METABOLISM Lesch-Nyhan syndrome The Lesch-Nyhan syndrome is an X-linked disorder which was described in 1964. Affected patients have hyperuricemia and a profound overproduction of uric acid. In addition, they have a bizarre neurologic disorder characterized by self-mutilation, choreoathetosis, spasticity, and retardation of growth and mental function. The incidence is estimated at 1:100,000 births. The characteristic biochemical abnormality is a profound deficiency of the enzyme hypoxanthine-guanine phosphoribosyltransferase (reaction 2, Fig. 94-4).

Adenine phosphoribosyltransferase deficiency Adenine phosphoribosyltransferase catalyzes the conversion of adenine to AMP (reaction 4, Fig. 94-4). The first subjects described with a deficiency of this enzyme were heterozygous for deficiency of the enzyme and had no associated disease. It subsequently became apparent that heterozygosity for this deficiency is common, perhaps as frequent as 1:100. A homozygous deficiency of this enzyme has now been described in 11 patients with a history of renal stones composed of 2,8-dioxyadenine. Because of chemical similarity, 2,8-dioxyadenine may be confused with uric acid, and in each of these patients an incorrect diagnosis of uric acid nephrolithiasis was made initially.

Adenosine deaminase deficiency and purine nucleoside phosphorylase deficiency See Chap. 95.

Xanthine oxidase deficiency Xanthine oxidase catalyzes the oxidation of hypoxanthine to xanthine, xanthine to uric acid, and adenine to 2,8-dioxyadenine (reaction 8, Fig. 94-4). Xanthinuria, the first inborn error of purine metabolism to be defined at the enzyme level, is due to a deficiency of xanthine oxidase. As a result, affected patients with xanthinuria have hypouricemia and hypouricaciduria as well as an increased urinary excretion of the oxypurines, hypoxanthine, and xanthine. Half are asymptomatic and a third have urinary xanthine stones. Several patients have been noted to have a myopathy and one patient with polyarthritis has been reported. Precipitation of xanthine is thought to be the important factor in the development of each of these clinical manifestations.

REFERENCES

KELLEY WN: Crystal-induced arthropathies, in *The Clinics in Rheumatic Diseases.* Philadelphia, Saunders, 1977, vol 3, pp 1–171

——— et al: Hypoxanthine-guanine phosphoribosyltransferase deficiency in gout. Ann Intern Med, 70:155, 1969

SEEGMILLER JE: Diseases of purine and pyrimidine metabolism, in *Duncan's Diseases of Metabolism,* 8th ed, PK Bondy, LE Rosenberg (eds). Philadelphia, Saunders, 1980, p 777

TALBOTT JH, YU TF: *Gout and Uric Acid Metabolism.* New York, Stratton, 1976

WYNGAARDEN JB: Gout, in *Advances in Metabolic Disorders,* R Levine, and R Luft (eds). New York, Academic, 1965, vol 2, pp 2–78

———, KELLEY WN: *Gout and Hyperuricemia.* New York, Grune & Stratton, 1976

———, ———: Gout, in *The Metabolic Basis of Inherited Diseases,* 5th ed, JB Stanbury et al (eds). New York, McGraw-Hill, 1983

95
DISORDERS OF PURINE METABOLISM THAT LEAD TO IMMUNODEFICIENCY

BEVERLY S. MITCHELL
WILLIAM N. KELLEY

Deficiencies of either of two enzymes in the purine metabolic pathway cause disorders of the immune system. Adenosine deaminase deficiency is associated with loss of both T and B lymphocytes, while purine nucleoside phosphorylase deficiency causes a relatively pure T-cell deficit. These two conditions represent the first enzyme defects identified in the immunodeficiency diseases. As such they have provided important clues to understanding the metabolic basis of lymphocyte dysfunction (also see Chap. 64).

ADENOSINE DEAMINASE DEFICIENCY Clinical features Within the first 6 months of life children with adenosine deaminase deficiency develop severe, recurrent infections involving the respiratory tract, skin, and gastrointestinal tract. Pathogenic agents include fungi, protozoa, viruses, and bacteria. Vomiting, diarrhea, and failure to thrive are also common. Lymphopenia with marked depletion of T lymphocytes and absence of appropriate delayed hypersensitivity reactions are usual, and B lymphocytes and immunoglobulin levels are frequently depressed as well. The thymic shadow is either absent on chest x-ray or gradually diminishes in size. Several associated bony abnormalities suggest, but are not pathognomonic of, the disease. These include cupping of the ribs at the costochondral junctions, abnormal metaphyses, and short extremities. The disease has an incidence of less than 1 in 100,000 live births but accounts for a third or more of cases of autosomal recessive severe combined immunodeficiency disease. Death from infection usually occurs within the first several years of life.

Diagnosis Since the clinical features overlap with those in other immunodeficiency states, the diagnosis is established by demonstrating deficiency of the enzyme in red blood cells and/

or fibroblasts cultured from children with defective cellular and humoral immunity. The enzyme defect is inherited as an autosomal recessive trait, and erythrocytes from most obligate heterozygotes have intermediate levels of the enzyme. Prenatal diagnosis has been made in cultured amniotic fluid cells.

The enzyme defect is usually demonstrable in all tissues. However, four individuals with markedly decreased erythrocyte adenosine deaminase had measurable enzyme in lymphocytes and normal immune function. These cases appear to represent a different mutation than is present in the usual patient.

Pathogenesis Adenosine deaminase catalyzes the irreversible deamination of adenosine and 2′-deoxyadenosine to inosine and 2′-deoxyinosine, respectively (Fig. 95-1). Affected children excrete increased amounts of 2′-deoxyadenosine in urine and have elevated levels of the 2′-deoxyadenosine metabolite dATP in erythrocytes. These findings have led to the hypothesis that accumulation of the substrate 2′-deoxyadenosine may mediate the lymphocyte toxicity as a consequence of its conversion in cells to dATP, a known inhibitor of DNA synthesis. Two observations support this view. First, the kinase activity responsible for phosphorylating deoxyadenosine is located predominantly in lymphoid cells. Secondly, 2′-deoxyadenosine itself is toxic to cultured T lymphoblasts but not to B lymphoblasts, and the toxicity correlates with the accumulation of dATP. This hypothesis thus accounts for the selective involvement of the immune system in general and of T cells in particular. Increased levels of adenosine or 2′-deoxyadenosine may also inhibit essential methylation reactions in lymphocytes by causing an accumulation of *S*-adenosylhomocysteine, a known inhibitor of *S*-adenosylmethionine-mediated methylation.

Treatment The optimal treatment of adenosine deaminase deficiency is bone marrow transplantation with engraftment of donor lymphocyte precursors. In the absence of an appropriate donor for this procedure, enzyme replacement therapy consisting of repeated transfusions of red blood cells containing normal adenosine deaminase activity has resulted in improvement in lymphocyte number and function in approximately half of patients. Both adenosine and 2′-deoxyadenosine readily diffuse through the red cell membrane and may be deaminated by the transfused cells. A good response to the transfusion regimen appears to depend on the continued presence of viable lymphocyte precursors that can be rescued by accelerating removal of the toxic metabolites. Fetal liver and thymic transplants have been performed on an experimental basis.

PURINE NUCLEOSIDE PHOSPHORYLASE DEFICIENCY Individuals with purine nucleoside phosphorylase deficiency appear normal at birth but experience a progressive depletion of T lymphocytes, leading to recurrent infections beginning between the first and second year of life. The numbers of B cells and the levels of plasma immunoglobulins are generally normal. Some also have an autoimmune hemolytic anemia, and some have multiple abnormal laboratory tests suggestive of a connective tissue disease. Partial deficiency of the enzyme may result in a milder clinical syndrome.

Purine nucleoside phosphorylase deficiency is a rare autosomal recessive disorder (only six families having been described) and is diagnosed by demonstrating a deficiency of the enzyme in red blood cells. Affected homozygotes also have reduced levels of uric acid in the serum and urine and increased excretion of purines in urine.

Purine nucleoside phosphorylase catalyzes the conversion of inosine and 2′-deoxyinosine to hypoxanthine and of guanosine and 2′-deoxyguanosine to guanine (Fig. 95-1); deficiency of this enzyme leads to increased circulating levels and urinary excretion of these substrates and to an increased level of dGTP in the red cells. The increase in dGTP is analogous to the accumulation of dATP in adenosine deaminase deficiency and may similarly impair DNA synthesis in these cells.

Red cell transfusions have resulted in transient improvements in T-cell function, in conjunction with diminished excretion of the purine substrates and increased serum uric acid levels.

FIGURE 95-1

Inborn errors of purine metabolism associated with immunodeficiency diseases: (1) adenosine deaminase, (2) purine nucleoside phosphorylase; (d) indicates the 2′-deoxy compounds.

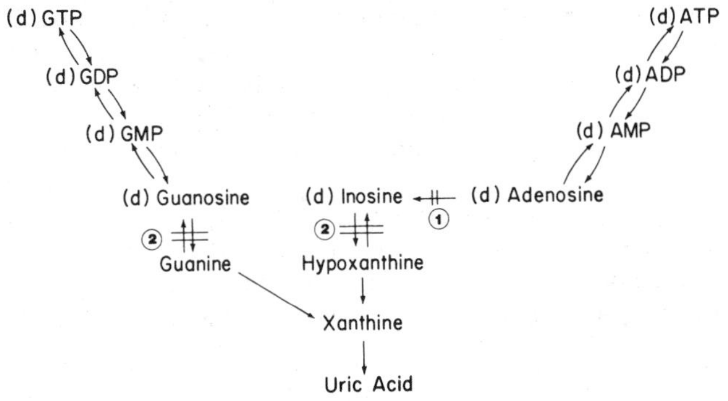

IMPLICATIONS The causal relationship between these two inborn errors of purine metabolism and the selective depletion of lymphocytes has suggested that inhibitors of adenosine deaminase or purine nucleoside phosphorylase may be effective immunosuppressive and chemotherapeutic agents. Pharmacologic inhibition of adenosine deaminase in the human does result in toxicity to both normal and neoplastic lymphocytes but also causes undesirable side effects. An inhibitor of purine nucleoside phosphorylase, 8-aminoguanosine, potentiates 2′-deoxyguanosine toxicity for cultured T cells and may be more selectively lymphocytotoxic in vivo. An alternative approach is the development of analogues of 2′-deoxyadenosine or 2′-deoxyguanosine that could be phosphorylated to toxic metabolites exclusively in lymphoid cells.

REFERENCES

ELLIOTT K, WHELAN J (eds): *Enzyme Defects and Immune Dysfunction, Ciba Foundation Symposium.* Amsterdam, Excerpta Medica, 1979

GIBLETT ER et al: Adenosine deaminase deficiency in two patients with severely impaired cellular immunity. Lancet 2:1067, 1972

——— et al: Nucleoside phosphorylase deficiency in a child with defective T-cell immunity and normal B-cell immunity. Lancet 1:1010, 1975

KAZMERS IS et al: Inhibition of purine nucleoside phosphorylase by 8-aminoguanosine: Selective toxicity for T lymphoblasts. Science (in press)

MARTIN DW, GELFAND EW: Biochemistry of diseases of immunodevelopment. Ann Rev Biochem 50:845, 1981

MITCHELL BS, KELLEY WN: Purinogenic immunodeficiency diseases: Clinical features and molecular mechanisms. Ann Intern Med 92:826, 1980

96
HEREDITARY OROTIC ACIDURIA

WILLIAM N. KELLEY

Hereditary orotic aciduria is a rare disorder of pyrimidine metabolism characterized by retarded growth and development, hypochromic anemia associated with a megaloblastic marrow unresponsive to usual therapy, and excessive urinary excretion of orotic acid. The first patient was reported by Huguley and coworkers in 1959. Eight additional cases have been described.

PATHOGENESIS The synthesis of pyrimidine nucleotides de novo is outlined in Fig. 96-1. Orotic aciduria occurs when the rate of synthesis of orotic acid exceeds the rate at which it is converted to orotidine 5′-monophosphate in the reaction catalyzed by orotate phosphoribosyltransferase. Patients with hereditary orotic aciduria have a genetically determined deficiency of orotate phosphoribosyltransferase and orotidine 5′-phosphate decarboxylase (type 1) or of orotidine 5′-phosphate decarboxylase alone (type 2). In the former the capacity of the cell to convert orotic acid to orotidine 5′-monophosphate is reduced. In the latter it is assumed that orotidine 5′-phosphate accumulates and thus inhibits orotate phosphoribosyltransferase activity. The two enzymes, orotate phosphoribosyltransferase and orotidine 5′-phosphate decarboxylase, are intimately associated in a complex. In patients with the double enzyme defect, it has been proposed that a mutation affecting the structure of orotate phosphoribosyltransferase destabilizes the complex, leading to the concomitant loss of orotidine 5′-phosphate decarboxylase activity.

Patients with both types of hereditary orotic aciduria excrete 600 to 1500 mg orotic acid in the urine per day, 3000 to 5000 times normal. In addition, patients excrete 15 to 30 mg orotidine per day, 20 to 40 times normal.

The clinical manifestations of hereditary orotic aciduria are due to (1) increased excretion of orotic acid and (2) pyrimidine nucleotide deficiency. Accumulation of orotic acid per se is harmful in that it may crystallize in the urine and obstruct urine flow. Orotidine is more soluble than orotic acid and does not form stones. The remaining clinical features of hereditary orotic aciduria are due to deficiency of nucleic acid precursors.

FIGURE 96-1

Pyrimidine biosynthesis de novo. (1) Carbamyl phosphate synthetase, (2) aspartate transcarbamylase, (3) dihydroorotase, (4) dihydroorotic acid dehydrogenase, (5) orotate phosphoribosyltransferase, and (6) orotidine 5′-monophosphate decarboxylase.

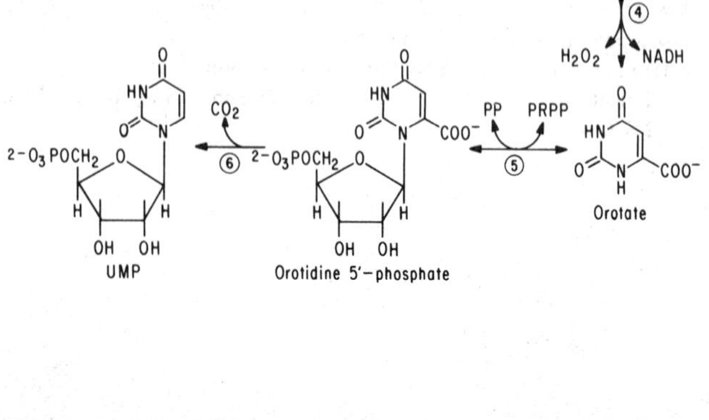

CLINICAL FEATURES The most specific early finding is severe hypochromic anemia with marked anisocytosis and poikilocytosis, associated with erythroid hyperplasia and atypical megaloblastic changes in the bone marrow. Leukopenia but not thrombocytopenia is also a consistent finding. The megaloblastosis probably results from a selective defect of DNA synthesis which interferes with mitosis. The megaloblasts in hereditary orotic aciduria are not as large as in pernicious anemia or folic acid deficiency, and the cellular abnormalities in orotic aciduria are more pronounced in the more mature red blood cell precursors. The degree of microcytosis and hypochromia in circulating erythrocytes also differentiates this from other megaloblastic anemias. Typically, poor growth and development are evident during the first few months of life with lassitude, pallor, and nonspecific failure to thrive. While no characteristic neurological picture exists, most patients appear to have some mental retardation. Orotic acid crystalluria is uniformly present, and urinary tract obstruction occurs in about half.

GENETICS Orotic aciduria is transmitted as an autosomal recessive disease. Heterozygotes are asymptomatic and excrete only slightly increased amounts of orotic acid in the urine.

TREATMENT The hematologic abnormalities and the retardation of growth and development respond promptly and completely to doses of uridine in the range of 100 to 150 mg/kg per day. Uridine is converted directly to uridine 5′-phosphate in the reaction catalyzed by the enzyme uridine kinase, thus bypassing the enzymatic defect and correcting the pyrimidine nucleotide deficiency and the deficiency in nucleic acid synthesis. Uridine therapy also produces a substantial decrease in the urinary excretion of orotic acid, probably by virtue of the increased levels of pyrimidine nucleotides and the consequent inhibition of pyrimidine biosynthesis de novo. The fatal outcome of untreated hereditary orotic aciduria and the residual impairment of mental function that may occur serve to emphasize the importance of early diagnosis and treatment.

Glucocorticoid therapy causes partial hematologic remission without reversal of the megaloblastic changes in the bone marrow. Oral administration of a mixture of yeast nucleotides has also been associated with rapid improvement in the general clinical state with hematologic remission and a decrease in urinary orotic acid. This preparation, however, is not well tolerated because of gastrointestinal side effects.

OTHER CAUSES OF OROTIC ACIDURIA Drugs such as allopurinol, oxipurinol, and azauridine produce modest orotic aciduria and orotidinuria. In each case one or more nucleotide derivatives of the drug are potent inhibitors of orotidine 5′-phosphate decarboxylase. There is no evidence that patients so treated develop a significant deficiency of pyrimidine nucleotides.

5-Phosphoribosyl-1-pyrophosphate (PRPP) is an essential and rate-limiting substrate for the orotate phosphoribosyltransferase reaction. A low intracellular level of PRPP as, for example, in a patient unable to synthesize PRPP due to PRPP synthetase deficiency is also associated with orotic aciduria, megaloblastic anemia, and mental retardation.

Several disorders of the urea cycle, including ornithine transcarbamylase deficiency, argininosuccinic aciduria, and citrullinemia, lead to orotic aciduria (see Chap. 91). In each of these diseases, carbamyl phosphate utilization in the urea cycle is reduced, and its availability for pyrimidine biosynthesis is enhanced. This shift in carbamyl phosphate utilization to the pyrimidine pathway appears to enhance the rate of pyrimidine biosynthesis de novo up to at least the step of orotic acid formation.

REFERENCES

HUGULEY CM et al: Refractory megaloblastic anemia associated with excretion of orotic acid. Blood 14:615, 1959

KELLEY WN, SMITH LH: Hereditary orotic aciduria, in *The Metabolic Basis of Inherited Diseases*, 5th ed, JB Stanbury et al (eds). New York, McGraw-Hill, 1983

Disorders of metals and metalloproteins

97 HEMOCHROMATOSIS

LAWRIE W. POWELL
KURT J. ISSELBACHER

DEFINITION Hemochromatosis is an iron-storage disorder in which an inappropriate increase in intestinal iron absorption results in deposition of iron in parenchymal cells with eventual tissue damage and functional insufficiency of the organs involved, especially the liver, pancreas, heart, and pituitary. In 1889, von Recklinghausen named the disease *hemochromatosis* and the iron-storage pigment *hemosiderin* because he believed that the pigment was derived from the blood. Although there is still debate about the most appropriate definitions, in view of the recent confirmation of a genetic basis for "idiopathic hemochromatosis" it seems logical to use the following terminology: (1) *genetic hemochromatosis*—the inherited disease now known to be associated with an abnormal iron-loading gene tightly linked to the A locus of the HLA complex on chromosome 6, (2) *acquired hemochromatosis*—gross iron overload with tissue injury arising secondarily to other disease, usually thalassemia or sideroblastic anemia. It should be emphasized, however, that in these acquired iron-loading disorders massive iron deposits in parenchymal tissues can lead to the same clinical and pathological features that are seen in genetic hemochromatosis.

The metabolic defect leading to increased iron absorption in hemochromatosis is unknown. The genetic disease is now increasingly recognized during its early stages when the iron overload is of lesser degree and organ damage minimal. At this stage the disease is best referred to as *latent* or *precirrhotic hemochromatosis* (see Fig. 97-1).

PREVALENCE Fully developed, genetic hemochromatosis is an uncommon disease. Estimates of its prevalence have ranged from 2.5 per 10,000 autopsies to 1 in 10,000 of the white Anglo-Saxon population. It is observed 5 to 10 times more frequently in males than in females. Nearly 70 percent of all patients develop their first symptoms between ages 40 and 60. The disease is rarely clinically evident below age 20, although with family screening (see below) asymptomatic subjects with iron overload are being increasingly recognized, including young menstruating women. Thus, the actual prevalence of the disease is probably much greater.

PATHOGENESIS Normally the body iron content of 3 to 4 g is maintained such that intestinal mucosal absorption of iron is equal to loss. This amount is approximately 1 mg per day in men and 1.5 mg per day in menstruating women. In hemochro-

FIGURE 97-1
Sequence of events in genetic hemochromatosis and their correlation with the serum ferritin concentration. Increased iron absorption is present throughout life. Overt, symptomatic disease usually develops between ages 40 and 60, but latent precirrhotic disease can be detected long before this.

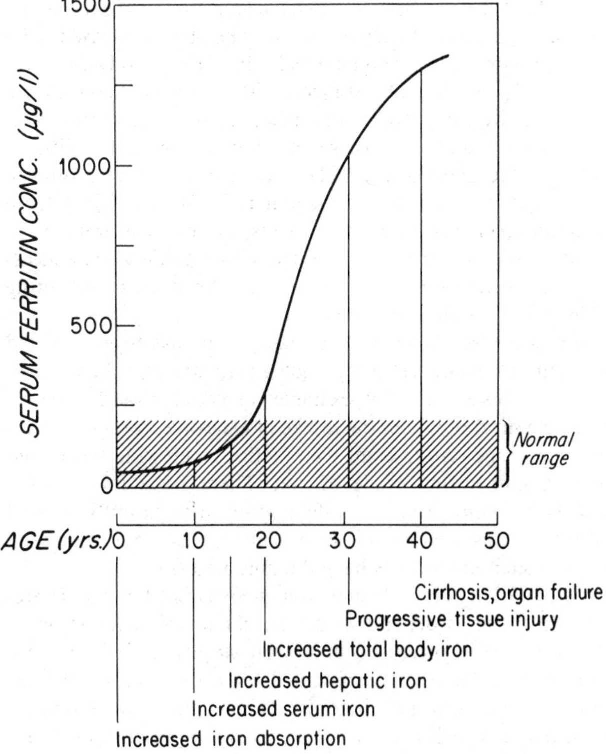

matosis mucosal absorption is inappropriate to body needs, amounting to 4 mg per day or more. The resulting progressive accumulation of iron is reflected in an early elevation in the plasma iron and an increased percentage saturation of transferrin. In advanced disease, the tissues may contain over 20 g iron. This excess iron is deposited mainly in parenchymal cells of the liver, pancreas, and heart. Iron in the liver and pancreas increases 50 to 100 times; in the heart, 5 to 25 times; in the spleen, kidney, and skin, about 5 times. Tissue injury may result from disruption of iron-laden lysosomes and lipid peroxidation of subcellular organelles by excess iron. The recent demonstration of an association between hemochromatosis and the histocompatibility antigens HLA-A3, HLA-B14, and HLA-B7 has confirmed the genetic basis for the disease. The mode of inheritance is either autosomal recessive or intermediate, with homozygotes usually developing severe iron overload and symptomatic disease and heterozygotes developing only minor derangements in iron metabolism without progressive iron overload or clinical evidence of the disease.

Gross parenchymal iron overload leading to acquired hemochromatosis is observed in association with chronic disorders of erythropoiesis, particularly in those with a defect in hemoglobin synthesis and ineffective erythropoiesis. In this group of disorders the absorption of iron is increased, and in addition these patients are also frequently treated with iron and blood transfusions. Such iron loading is observed primarily in patients with sideroblastic anemia and thalassemia. Porphyria cutanea tarda, a disorder characterized by a defect in porphyrin biosynthesis (Chap. 99), is also sometimes associated with excessive parenchymal iron deposits; however, the magnitude of the iron load is usually insufficient to produce tissue damage.

Alcoholic subjects with chronic liver disease may show evidence of increased tissue iron stores. They can be divided into two groups. The first group comprises patients who have a mild to moderate increase in stainable hepatic iron but relatively normal body iron stores. These patients have alcoholic liver disease (usually cirrhosis) but not hemochromatosis. The reason for their increased stainable iron is unknown. It may be related in part to cell necrosis and uptake of iron released from adjacent Kupffer and parenchymal cells. The second (less common) group of alcoholic subjects with increased hepatic iron have gross iron deposition and increased body iron stores and are usually found to have genetic hemochromatosis with or without superimposed alcoholic liver disease. Hemochromatosis occurring in a heavy drinker may be distinguished from alcoholic liver disease by two means: (1) by measurement of hepatic iron concentration (see below and Table 97-1) and (2) by studying relatives for evidence of the disease, including HLA typing of all family members.

Excessive iron ingestion over many years has been reported to result in the clinical and pathological features of hemochromatosis. This occurs, for example, in certain South African blacks (Bantu) in whom the intake of excessive iron in an alcoholic beverage results from the practice of brewing fermented beverages in vessels made of iron. There are a few isolated reports of hemochromatosis developing in apparently normal subjects taking medicinal iron over many years, but it is possible that such individuals have the inherited trait.

The basic defect in hemochromatosis is not known. Therefore, diagnosis is dependent on the phenotypic expression of the disease (i.e., increased body iron stores), and the phenotypic expression may be modified by other factors such as blood loss and oral iron ingestion. The common denominator in all patients with hemochromatosis is the presence of *excessive amounts of iron in parenchymal tissues*. Parenteral administration of iron in the form of transfusions or iron preparations results in predominantly *reticuloendothelial cell* iron overload. This appears to lead to less tissue damage than iron loading of parenchymal cells.

PATHOLOGY At autopsy the enlarged, nodular liver and pancreas present a striking ochre color. Histologically iron is found in increased amounts in many organs, particularly in the liver and pancreas and to a lesser extent in the endocrine glands and the heart. A notable exception is the testis, the iron content of which is relatively low despite the fact that gonadal failure is a characteristic and early feature of the disease. In contrast, the pituitary gland is almost always involved. The epidermis of the skin is thin, and increased *melanin* is found in the cells of the basal layer. Deposits of iron are observed around the synovial lining cells of the joints, and calcium pyrophosphate crystals may be seen to lie within deposits of calcium embedded in the synovial tissue.

The parenchymal deposits of iron in the liver of patients with genetic hemochromatosis are in the form of ferritin and hemosiderin. In the early stages, these deposits are found in the periportal parenchymal cells, especially within lysosomes in the pericanalicular cytoplasm of the hepatocytes. This stage progresses to perilobular fibrosis and deposition of iron in bile duct epithelium, Kupffer cells, and fibrous septa. Inflammatory cells are few in contrast to prominent proliferation of bile ductules. Wedge biopsy specimens show a characteristic pattern of fibrosis with dense fibrous septa surrounding groups of lobules somewhat analogous to the pattern seen in chronic biliary disease. In the advanced stage, a macronodular or mixed macro- and micronodular cirrhosis develops.

CLINICAL MANIFESTATIONS The symptoms and signs of hemochromatosis include skin pigmentation, diabetes, liver and cardiac impairment, arthropathy, and hypogonadism. The initial symptoms most frequently encountered are weakness, lassitude, weight loss, change in skin color, abdominal pain, loss of libido, and symptoms related to the onset of diabetes. Hepatomegaly, pigmentation, spider angiomas, splenomegaly, arthropathy, ascites, cardiac arrhythmias, congestive heart failure, loss of body hair, testicular atrophy, and jaundice are the most prominent physical signs in the fully established disease.

The *liver* is usually the first organ to be affected, and hepatomegaly is present in more than 95 percent of symptomatic cases. Hepatic enlargement may exist in the absence of symptoms or in the presence of normal liver function tests. Indeed, over half the patients with symptomatic hemochromatosis have little or no laboratory evidence of functional impairment of the liver, in spite of hepatomegaly and fibrosis. Loss of body hair, palmar erythema, testicular atrophy, and gynecomastia are often seen. Manifestations of portal hypertension and esophageal varices may occur but are less commonly observed than in Laennec's cirrhosis. Splenomegaly is present in approximately half the cases. Hepatocellular carcinoma develops in about 30 percent. The incidence of this last complication increases with age and is now the most common cause of death in treated patients. However, it appears to occur only in cirrhotic patients; hence the importance of early diagnosis and therapy.

Excessive *skin pigmentation* is present in about 90 percent of symptomatic patients at the time the diagnosis is established. The melanin deposition in the skin usually gives rise to bronzing. The characteristic metallic gray hue is believed to result from the presence of increased melanin or both melanin and iron in the dermis. Pigmentation usually is diffuse and generalized, but frequently it is deeper on the face, neck, extensor aspects of the lower forearms, dorsa of the hands, lower legs, genital regions, and in scars. In only 10 to 15 percent of cases is there demonstrable pigmentation of the oral mucosa. Pigmentation of the hard palate and retina has been described.

Diabetes mellitus and symptoms therefrom develop in about 65 percent of patients. Diabetes is more likely to develop in patients with a family history of diabetes. The presence of a family history of diabetes, the existence of liver disease, and direct damage to the pancreas by iron deposition may all contribute to the development of diabetes in hemochromatosis. The management of the diabetes is similar to that of other types of idiopathic diabetes mellitus except for a higher incidence of insulin resistance and of insulin fat atrophy. Late degenerative sequelae are the same as in diabetes mellitus.

Arthropathy, which differs from osteoarthritis and rheumatoid arthritis, develops in 25 to 50 percent of patients. It most commonly occurs after the age of 50 but may occur at any time in the course of the disease, even as a first manifestation or long after therapy. The small joints of the hands, especially the second and third metacarpophalangeal joints, are usually the first joints to be involved. A progressive polyarthritis involving wrists, hips, and knees may ensue. Acute brief attacks of synovitis may occur, associated with deposition of calcium pyrophosphate (chondrocalcinosis or pseudogout), chiefly in the knees. Roentgenologic manifestations consist of cystic changes of sclerosis of the subchondral bones, loss of articular cartilage with narrowing of the joint space, diffuse demineralization, hypertrophic bone proliferation, and calcification of the synovium. The mechanism of these abnormalities and their relationship to iron metabolism is not known.

Cardiac involvement is the presenting manifestation in about 15 percent of patients. The most common cardiac manifestation is congestive heart failure. It is observed in about 10 percent of young adults with the disease. Symptoms of congestive failure may develop suddenly, with rapid progression to death if untreated. The heart is diffusely enlarged, and such cases may be misdiagnosed as idiopathic cardiomyopathy if other overt manifestations are absent. A variety of cardiac arrhythmias may be present, particularly supraventricular beats and paroxysmal tachyarrhythmias. Atrial flutter, atrial fibrillation, and varying degrees of atrioventricular block have also been described.

Loss of libido and *testicular atrophy* are common in hemochromatosis. The former may antedate the other clinical manifestations of the disease. Testicular atrophy is probably due to the decreased production of gonadotropins associated with impaired hypothalamic-pituitary-gonadal function due to iron deposition. Addison's disease, hypothyroidism, and hypoparathyroidism have been described but are rare.

DIAGNOSIS The association of (1) hepatomegaly, (2) skin pigmentation, (3) diabetes mellitus, (4) heart disease, (5) arthritis, and (6) evidence of hypogonadism should suggest the diagnosis of hemochromatosis. However, a parenchymal iron overload of comparatively short duration or modest degree may exist without any of these clinical manifestations, or with only some of them [e.g., in young subjects (see Fig. 97-1)]. Therefore, the diagnosis should be considered in any patient with unexplained hepatomegaly, idiopathic cardiomyopathy, abnormal skin pigmentation, loss of libido, diabetes, or arthritis.

The history should be particularly detailed in regard to disease in other members of the family, alcohol ingestion, and iron intake and the ingestion of large doses of ascorbic acid which promotes iron absorption. The blood should be examined for evidence of anemia and abnormal erythropoiesis to rule out iron loading secondary to a hematologic disorder. Confirmation of the presence of liver, pancreatic, cardiac, and joint disease should be obtained by physical examination, roentgenologic examination, and routine function tests of these organs. It then remains to be demonstrated that there is an increase in total body iron stores and, in particular, an increased parenchymal iron concentration associated with tissue damage.

The methods available for the demonstration of excessive parenchymal iron stores include (1) measurement of serum iron, (2) determination of percent saturation of transferrin, (3) estimation of chelatable iron stores using the agent desferrioxamine, (4) measurement of serum ferritin concentration, and (5) liver biopsy (Table 97-1). Each has its inherent advantages and limitations. The serum iron level and percent saturation of transferrin are elevated early in the course of the disease, but their specificity is reduced by relatively high false-positive and false-negative rates. In particular, an increased serum iron concentration may be present in patients with alcoholic liver disease without iron overload; in this situation, however, the iron-binding capacity is usually not decreased as in hemochromatosis.

The serum ferritin concentration is usually a good index of body iron stores, whether they are decreased or increased. In untreated patients with hemochromatosis, the serum ferritin level is greatly increased (Table 97-1). This test is also useful as a noninvasive screening test for the diagnosis of early disease, since it is usually abnormal before there is any morphological evidence of liver damage and the ferritin concentration correlates with the magnitude of body iron stores. It has, therefore, replaced the more cumbersome screening tests involving urinary iron excretion. However, it should be noted that in patients with infection and hepatocellular necrosis serum ferritin levels may be elevated out of proportion to body iron stores. Also, some families have been reported in whom serum ferritin levels in symptomatic relatives have been normal despite increased iron stores; the reason for this finding is unclear but would appear to be unusual. In clinical practice, the *combined measurements* of the (1) serum iron concentration, (2) percent transferrin saturation, and (3) serum ferritin level provide the simplest and most reliable screening test for hemochromatosis, including the precirrhotic phase of the disease. If any of these tests are abnormal, liver biopsy should be performed since it is the *definitive* test for the diagnosis of hemochromatosis. It permits histochemical estimation of tissue iron, measurement of hepatic iron concentration, and assessment of the extent of tissue damage.

It is of particular importance to examine family members when the diagnosis of hemochromatosis is established. Asymp-

TABLE 97-1
Representative iron values in normal subjects and in patients with hemochromatosis

Determination	*Normal subjects*	*Patients with symptomatic hemochromatosis*	*Homozygous subjects with early, asymptomatic hemochromatosis*
Plasma iron, μg/dl	50–150	180–300	Usually elevated
Total iron-binding capacity, μg/dl	250–370	200–300	200–300
Percent transferrin saturation, μg/dl	22–46	50–100	50–100
Serum ferritin, ng/ml	10–200	900–6000	200–500
Urinary iron,* mg/24 h	0–2	9–23	2–5
Liver iron, μg/100 mg dry wt	30–140	600–1800	200–400

* *After intramuscular administration of 0.5 g desferrioxamine.*

tomatic as well as symptomatic family members with the disease will usually have an increase in plasma iron, a decrease in total iron-binding capacity, an increased saturation of transferrin, and an increased or increasing serum ferritin concentration. These changes occur even before the iron stores are greatly increased. A liver biopsy should then be performed, since it is imperative to establish the diagnosis and begin therapy before tissue damage occurs. HLA typing may be helpful in diagnosis of families with the disease. Affected siblings usually have both HLA haplotypes identical with those of the proband, and where children are affected a homozygous-heterozygous mating probably occurred.

The distinction between hemochromatosis and alcoholic cirrhosis associated with increased tissue iron is discussed above.

TREATMENT The therapy of genetic hemochromatosis involves the removal of the excess body iron and supportive treatment of damaged organs.

Iron is best removed from the body by weekly or twice weekly phlebotomy of 500 ml. Although there is an initial modest decline in the volume of packed red blood cells to about 35 ml/dl, the anemia stabilizes after several weeks. The plasma iron concentration remains increased until the available iron stores are depleted. Since one 500-ml unit of blood contains from 200 to 250 mg iron and about 25 g iron must be removed, 2 or 3 years of weekly phlebotomy are usually required. When the plasma iron level becomes normal, phlebotomies are performed at such time intervals as are required to maintain a plasma iron concentration of less than 150 μg/dl. Usually one phlebotomy every 3 months will suffice. The adequacy of the therapy may be evaluated at any time by measuring the plasma iron, the percentage of saturation of transferrin with iron, or the serum ferritin concentration. These measurements become abnormal promptly with iron reaccumulation.

Chelating agents such as desferrioxamine, when given parenterally, remove 10 to 20 mg iron per day, less than half that mobilized by one weekly phlebotomy. Phlebotomy is not only a more effective but also a less expensive, more convenient, and safer treatment for patients with genetic hemochromatosis. Chelating agents may be used as a substitute method for iron removal when anemia or hypoproteinemia is severe enough to preclude phlebotomy. Subcutaneous infusions of desferrioxamine using a portable slow pump are most effective.

The management of the hepatic failure, cardiac failure, and diabetes differs little from conventional management of these conditions. Loss of libido and change in secondary sex characteristics are partially relieved by testosterone therapy or gonadotropin therapy.

PROGNOSIS The principal causes of death in *untreated* patients are cardiac failure (30 percent), hepatocellular failure or portal hypertension (25 percent), and hepatocellular carcinoma (30 percent).

Life expectancy of symptomatic patients is extended to an average of more than 8 years by removal of the excessive stores of iron and maintenance of these stores at near-normal levels. The 5-year survival rate with therapy is increased from 33 to 89 percent. With removal of iron by repeated phlebotomy, the liver and spleen decrease in size, liver function studies return to normal, pigmentation of skin decreases, and cardiac failure is reversed. Carbohydrate tolerance improves in about 40 percent of cases. The fibrosis in the liver may decrease, but cirrhosis is irreversible. Removal of excess iron has little or no effect on hypogonadism or arthropathy. Hepatocellular carcinoma occurs as a late sequela in about one-third of the patients despite adequate iron removal. The apparent increase in its incidence in treated patients is probably related to their increased life span. This complication does not appear to develop if the disease is treated in the precirrhotic stage. Hence, the importance of family screening and early therapy cannot be emphasized too strongly. Asymptomatic subjects who are detected by family studies should have phlebotomy therapy if iron stores are moderately to severely increased. Screening for increasing iron stores at appropriate intervals is also important. With this approach most manifestations of the disease can be prevented.

REFERENCES

BASSETT ML et al: HLA typing in idiopathic hemochromatosis: Distinction between homozygotes and heterozygotes with biochemical expression. Hepatology 1:120, 1981

EDWARDS CQ et al: Hereditary hemochromatosis. N Engl J Med 297:7, 1977

FINCH CA, HUEBERS H: Perspectives in iron metabolism. N Engl J Med 306:1520, 1982

GRACE ND, POWELL LW: Iron storage disorders of the liver. Gastroenterology 64:1257, 1974

HALLIDAY JW et al: Serum ferritin in the diagnosis of early haemochromatosis: A study of 43 families. Lancet 2:621, 1977

LESAGE GD et al: Hemochromatosis: Genetic or alcohol induced? Hepatology (in press)

POWELL LW, KERR JFR: The pathology of liver in hemochromatosis, in *Pathobiology Annual*, H Joacim (ed). New York, Appleton-Century-Crofts, 1975

SIMON M et al: Idiopathic hemochromatosis and iron overload in alcoholic liver disease: Differentiation by HLA phenotype. Gastroenterology 73:655, 1977

——— et al: Idiopathic hemochromatosis. Demonstration of recessive transmission and early detection by family HLA typing. N Engl J Med 297:1017, 1977

98
WILSON'S DISEASE

I. HERBERT SCHEINBERG

Wilson's disease is an inherited autosomal recessive abnormality in the hepatic excretion of copper that results in toxic accumulations of the metal in liver, brain, and other organs. Deficiency of the plasma copper-protein ceruloplasmin is a characteristic feature.

NATURAL HISTORY Normal babies have low levels of plasma ceruloplasmin and high concentrations of hepatic copper. During the first year of life ceruloplasmin values rise, and hepatic copper concentrations fall to normal adult levels. In contrast, serum ceruloplasmin changes very little in Wilson homozygotes, and the concentration of hepatic copper increases steadily with age. However, clinical manifestations of copper excess are rare before age 6, and half of untreated patients remain asymptomatic to age 16.

Wilson's disease presents with hepatic involvement in somewhat less than half of patients. The toxic effects of copper in the liver may be manifest as acute hepatitis, cirrhosis of the liver, or asymptomatic hepatosplenomegaly. The acute hepatitis is similar to viral hepatitis, can be mistaken for infectious mononucleosis, and may evolve in three different ways. The first is a fulminant, sometimes lethal disease characterized by jaundice, malaise, and at times ascites, hypoalbuminemia, and elevated levels of liver enzymes in plasma. In the acute phase sufficient copper may be released into plasma to cause a hemolytic anemia. The disease may not be diagnosed until autopsy or until the diagnosis in a younger sibling leads to retrospective analysis of preserved tissues. Second, there may be insidious development of parenchymal liver disease resulting in a clinical and histological picture indistinguishable from chronic active hepatitis. Third, patients may apparently recover from the hepatitis. Years or decades may elapse with no sign or symptom of disease. In these patients the past history of an episode of hepatitis can be overlooked unless they are questioned carefully.

More frequently, the copper-induced hepatic disease evolves to cirrhosis without any recognized overt indication of hepatitis. In these patients the initial manifestations are extrahepatic. Neurological or psychiatric disturbances are the first clinical signs in most of this group and are always accompanied by Kayser-Fleischer rings (Plate 8-8). These green or golden deposits of copper in Descemet's membrane of the cornea never interfere with vision but indicate that hepatic copper has been released and caused the brain damage. Rarely Kayser-Fleischer rings may be accompanied by sunflower cataracts. If a patient with frank neurological or psychiatric disease does not have Kayser-Fleischer rings when examined by a trained observer using a slit-lamp, the diagnosis of Wilson's disease can be excluded.

The primary neurological manifestation is that of a movement disorder, particularly resting and intention tremors. Spasticity, rigidity, chorea, drooling, dysphagia, and dysarthria are common. Babinski responses and absent abdominal reflexes are occasionally noted; sensory changes are extremely rare. Psychiatric disturbances, in part due to the toxic effects of copper on the brain and in part to the reactions to a life-threatening disease, are evident in most patients with symptomatic disease. Syndromes indistinguishable from schizophrenia, manic-depressive psychoses, and classic neuroses may occur, and some bizarre behavioral disturbances defy classification. Improvement in the psychiatric state can occur with pharmacological reduction of the copper excess, but psychotherapy is often also required.

In occasional patients the clinical onset reflects neither a hepatic nor a central nervous system disturbance. For example, primary or secondary amenorrhea may be the first evidence of disease in some young women; in others, repeated spontaneous abortions may result from excess free copper in intrauterine secretions. Routine ophthalmologic examination in patients without symptomatic liver or neurological disease occasionally reveals Kayser-Fleischer rings, leading to the diagnosis. Cirrhosis may be observed incidentally at surgery.

PATHOGENESIS The metabolic defect in Wilson's disease is an inability to maintain a near-zero balance of copper. Excess copper accumulates possibly because hepatic lysosomes lack the normal mechanism to excrete into bile the copper that has been catabolically cleaved from ceruloplasmin. This may cause deficiency of ceruloplasmin since a stoichiometric excess of copper inhibits the formation of ceruloplasmin from apoceruloplasmin and copper. The capacity of hepatocytes to store copper is eventually exceeded, and release into blood and uptake in extrahepatic sites occurs (Table 98-1).

Under normal circumstances essentially all tissue copper is present as the prosthetic element of copper proteins such as cytochrome oxidase, tyrosinase, superoxide dismutase, and ceruloplasmin. There is normally little or no free (non-protein-bound) copper. In Wilson's disease more copper is present than can be bound by specific copper proteins; such copper is as toxic as excess iron, zinc, mercury, or lead. Toxicity of these cations is probably effected in large degree by pathological combinations with proteins that ordinarily do not contain metal.

The pathological consequences of the accumulated copper occur first in the liver. Abnormal fat and glycogen deposits are the earliest findings by light microscopy (Fig. 98-1). With electron microscopy mitochondrial abnormalities are observed early and appear to be specific for Wilson's disease (Fig. 98-2).

FIGURE 98-1
Fatty changes, glycogen deposits, and cellular infiltrates in a hematoxylin and eosin–stained section of liver from an asymptomatic boy with Wilson's disease.

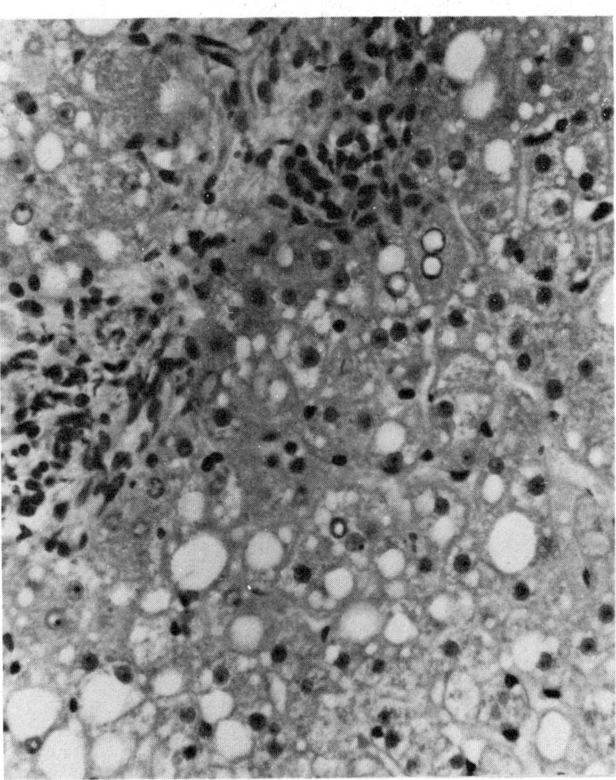

TABLE 98-1
Summary of analytical data in patients with Wilson's disease, heterozygous carriers, and control subjects

	Serum ceruloplasmin			*Hepatic copper concentration*		
Group	*No. of patients*	*Range, mg/dl*	*Mean ± SD, mg/dl*	*No. of patients*	*Range, μg/g dry weight*	*Mean ± SD, μg/g dry weight*
Wilson's disease:						
Asymptomatic	31	0–19.5	3.6±5.3	36	152–1828	983.5±368
Symptomatic	84	0–43.0	5.9±7.1	33	94–1360	588.3±304
Heterozygous carriers	95*	1–50.1	28.4±8.5	14	39–213	117.0±51
Normal subjects	180	18.5–65.9	30.7±3.5	16	20–45	31.5±6.8

* *71 parents of patients with Wilson's disease and 24 children, each of whom had one parent with Wilson's disease.*
SOURCE: *Sternlieb and Scheinberg, 1968.*

Later, necrosis, inflammation, fibrosis, bile duct proliferation, and cirrhosis occur. Abnormalities in liver function tests develop later than the histological changes.

Death can occur from the effects of copper toxicosis in the central nervous system with little or no evidence of liver dysfunction, but in most subjects significant liver disease becomes apparent sometime during the course. Patients with prolonged survival always show hepatic cirrhosis.

In the brain the excess copper is distributed ubiquitously. Necrosis of neurons with cavitation may be preceded by the appearance of Opalski and Alzheimer type II cells; however, neither is specific for Wilson's disease.

Increased copper in the kidney produces little if any structural change and commonly does not alter renal function. Hematuria, proteinuria, the Fanconi syndrome, and renal tubular acidosis occur rarely. Pathological effects in other organs and tissues are minor.

DIAGNOSIS The diagnosis is easy *provided it is suspected.* Wilson's disease should be considered in any patient under the age of 40 with an unexplained disorder of the central nervous system, signs or symptoms of chronic active hepatitis, unexplained persistent elevations of serum transaminase, acquired hemolytic anemia (particularly in the presence of hepatitis), or unexplained cirrhosis, or in any patient who has a relative with Wilson's disease.

FIGURE 98-2
Electron micrograph showing portions of two hepatocytes from the liver biopsy of a young asymptomatic woman with Wilson's disease. There are lipid droplets (L) and grossly abnormal mitochondria (M) in the cytoplasm. N, nucleus; P, peroxisome. (Courtesy of Dr I Sternlieb.)

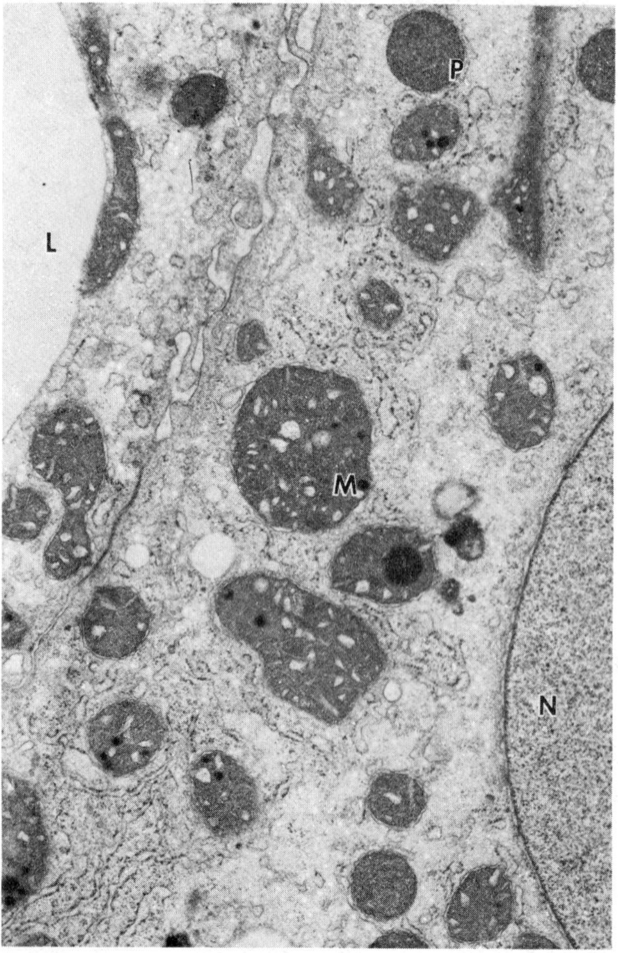

The diagnosis is confirmed in suspected cases by the demonstration either of (1) a serum concentration of ceruloplasmin less than 20 mg/dl and Kayser-Fleischer rings, or (2) a serum ceruloplasmin less than 20 mg/dl and a concentration of copper in a liver biopsy sample greater than 250 μg per gram of dry weight. Most patients also excrete more than 100 μg copper per day in urine and exhibit histological abnormalities on liver biopsy.

About 5 percent of patients have a serum concentration of ceruloplasmin greater than 20 mg/dl, and some patients with other hepatic disorders have elevated hepatic copper and Kayser-Fleischer rings. In either circumstance measurement of the ability to incorporate radioactive copper into ceruloplasmin is useful as a discriminating test. Even in the presence of a normal concentration of ceruloplasmin, patients with Wilson's disease incorporate little or no isotope into the protein, while patients with other liver disorders and elevated hepatic copper incorporate the isotope normally.

TREATMENT Treatment consists of removing the deposits of copper as rapidly as possible and should be instituted once the diagnosis is secure whether the patient is ill or asymptomatic. The drug of choice is D-penicillamine. It is administered orally in an initial dose of 1 g daily, usually in divided doses before meals and at bedtime. Since penicillamine has an antipyridoxine effect in animals, 25 mg per day of vitamin B_6 is also given. Effectiveness of therapy should be assayed chemically and clinically. Initially, the patient's 24-h urinary excretion of copper should increase fivefold or more over the pretreatment level, and 1 to 3 mg copper per day may be excreted during the first months of therapy.

White blood cell and platelet counts, urinalysis, and body temperature should be monitored several times weekly for the first month of therapy and at intervals thereafter. Sensitivity to penicillamine usually appears within the first 14 days of treatment and may cause rash, fever, leukopenia, thrombocytopenia, lymphadenopathy, or proteinuria. Discontinuation of treatment is required if sensitivity develops. Therapy can often be resumed if the drug is reinstituted in small and gradually increasing dosage; alternatively, 20 mg prednisone can be given daily for the first 2 weeks of penicillamine treatment and subsequently gradually discontinued. Reactions requiring a desensitizing regimen may recur several times before penicillamine can be administered without a steroid.

Lifelong treatment is required. Inadequate treatment or interruption of therapy causes relapse that may be irreversible. Reinstitution of penicillamine after temporary interruption of therapy may be accompanied by the appearance or reappearance of sensitivity reactions. At any time—even after years of uneventful administration—granulocytopenia (or agranulocytosis), thrombocytopenia, the nephrotic syndrome, the Goodpasture syndrome, systemic lupus erythematosus, severe arthralgias, or myasthenia gravis may supervene. Toxicity is sometimes dose-related, and reduction of the dose to a level that is therapeutically effective but nontoxic may be possible. Continued low dosage of steroids may control penicillamine-associated lupus or arthralgias. After temporary interruption of the drug in patients with the nephrotic syndrome, it is sometimes possible to reinstitute therapy without recurrence of proteinuria. However, although irreversible intolerance to D-penicillamine is rare, the toxicity may be such that the drug must be withdrawn permanently. The lifelong administration of dimercaprol by injection is impractical, and the only other alternative mode of therapy is an investigational drug, triethylene tetramine.

After therapy with penicillamine has been successfully instituted, the patient should be seen indefinitely at 1- to 3-month intervals to detect drug toxicity and manage the disease. Physical examination, including relevant neurological assessment and inspection of the corneas with a slit-lamp, together with the patient's own evaluation, provides the best indicator of the efficacy of treatment. Serial determinations of serum transaminase levels, albumin, and bilirubin are useful in following the course of liver function. Lack of clinical improvement or worsening of the disease may be due to irreversible damage present before therapy was begun, to poor patient compliance, or to inadequate dosage of penicillamine. Quantitative determinations of urinary copper excretion and of free copper in serum (total serum copper minus ceruloplasmin-bound copper) can help determine which is the case. After treatment for long periods, urinary copper should be lower than at the onset of therapy and rarely exceeds 1.5 mg per day. Even more helpful, an adequately treated patient generally has a concentration of free serum copper less than 10 μg/dl. After a patient has remained asymptomatic with no laboratory evidence of liver dysfunction for a year and in patients with minimal residual disease that has not changed, the dose of penicillamine may be reduced to 0.75 g per day.

Treatment of more than 100 asymptomatic patients with a confirmed diagnosis has established that continued administration of D-penicillamine can prevent virtually every manifestation of this disease.

REFERENCES

CARTWRIGHT GE: The diagnosis of treatable Wilson's disease. N Engl J Med 298:1347, 1978

Copper: Report of the Committee on Medical and Biologic Effects of Environmental Pollutants. Washington, DC, National Academy of Sciences, 1977

STERNLIEB I: Evolution of the hepatic lesion in Wilson's disease (hepatolenticular degeneration), in *Progress in Liver Diseases,* vol IV, H Popper et al (eds). New York, Grune & Stratton, 1972

———, SCHEINBERG IH: Prevention of Wilson's disease in asymptomatic patients. N Engl J Med 278:352, 1968

———, ———: Chronic hepatitis as a first manifestation of Wilson's disease. Ann Intern Med 76:59, 1972

WALSHE JM: Wilson's disease (hepatolenticular degeneration), in *Handbook of Clinical Neurology,* vol 27, PJ Vinken et al (eds). New York, American Elsevier, 1976

99 PORPHYRIAS

URS A. MEYER

The porphyrias are a group of diseases associated with inherited or acquired disturbances in heme biosynthesis. Porphyrins are tetrapyrrole pigments that serve as intermediates in this pathway. They are formed from the precursors δ-aminolevulinic acid (ALA) and porphobilinogen. Heme, the ferrous iron complex of protoporphyrin IX, functions as a prosthetic group for hemoproteins such as hemoglobin, microsomal and mitochondrial cytochromes, catalase, tryptophan oxygenase, and others. Heme biosynthesis involves a pathway essential to life and is operative in all aerobic cells.

Each of the porphyrias is characterized by a unique pattern of overproduction, accumulation, and excretion of intermediates of heme biosynthesis. These patterns are the metabolic expression of deficiencies of specific enzymes of the heme biosynthetic pathway (Table 99-1).

The main clinical manifestations are intermittent attacks of nervous system dysfunction and sensitivity of the skin to sunlight. The *neurological syndrome* is characteristically precipitated by drugs such as barbiturates and results in abdominal pain, peripheral neuropathy, and mental disturbance. These neuropsychiatric symptoms occur only in those porphyrias in which there is great overproduction of the porphyrin precursors ALA and porphobilinogen. The pathogenesis of the neurological lesion is unclear. The *skin photosensitivity* is related directly to increased porphyrin accumulation, although the lesions differ among diseases. The photosensitivity is due to the photodynamic action of porphyrins and is probably mediated through the formation of singlet-oxygen with consequent destructive processes such as the peroxidation of lipids in the membranes of lysosomes. The dominantly inherited human porphyrias exhibit variable expressivity. In many patients only the biochemical or enzymatic abnormalities are apparent. Exacerbations in ordinarily asymptomatic patients can be precipitated by factors such as drugs, hormones, or liver disease. Clinically or chemically latent disease may occur as a phase or persist throughout life.

CLASSIFICATION The porphyrias are usually divided into two main groups, erythropoietic and hepatic, according to the two major sites of heme synthesis where the error of metabolism is expressed (Table 99-1). The only pure erythropoietic form of porphyria is the rare *congenital erythropoietic porphyria* (CEP). In *protoporphyria* (PP) porphyrins accumulate in both erythropoietic and hepatic tissue. In *intermittent acute porphyria* (IAP), *hereditary coproporphyria* (HCP), and *variegate porphyria* (VP), dominantly inherited enzyme deficiencies impair heme biosynthesis predominantly in the liver, apparently without affecting hemoglobin formation. *Porphyria cutanea tarda* (PCT) was previously considered to be an acquired hepatic porphyria. However most if not all patients with this disease have been found to have hereditary deficiency of uroporphyrinogen decarboxylase. Toxic acquired porphyria resembling PCT occurs in individuals accidentally exposed to polychlorinated hydrocarbons and in association with hepatic tumors. Poisoning with lead produces well-recognized abnormalities in porphyrin and heme synthesis (see Chap. 239). Increased urinary excretion of porphyrins or precursors and accumulation of porphyrins in erythrocytes may also occur in numerous clinical conditions; these are secondary phenomena which do not produce symptoms or signs of porphyria.

BIOCHEMICAL CONSIDERATIONS A schematic outline of heme biosynthesis is presented in Fig. 99-1. The sequence of reactions that leads from the simple substrates glycine and succinyl coenzyme A to ALA, porphobilinogen (PBG), and finally heme is composed of four mitochondrial and four cytosolic enzymes. Differences exist in the regulation of heme biosynthesis among tissues.

In the liver ALA synthase catalyzes the rate-limiting reaction for heme formation under physiological conditions. The enzymes subsequent to ALA synthase are present in excess. The principal regulation of ALA synthase is feedback repression by heme, the end product of the pathway. Increased demands for heme are met by the synthesis of ALA synthase. Hepatic ALA synthase can be induced by a large number of lipid-soluble drugs, steroids, and chemicals that are substrates and inducers of cytochrome P_{450} hemoproteins, the terminal oxidases in microsomal drug metabolism. This induction is

TABLE 99-1
Characteristics of the porphyrias

	Erythropoietic porphyria	*Hepatic porphyrias*				*Erythrohepatic porphyria*
	Congenital erythropoietic porphyria (CEP)	*Intermittent acute porphyria (IAP)*	*Hereditary coproporphyria (HCP)*	*Variegate porphyria (VP)*	*Porphyria cutanea tarda (PCT)*	*Protoporphyria (PP)*
Enzyme deficiency	Uroporphyrinogen I synthase and/or uroporphyrinogen III cosynthase (?)	Uroporphyrinogen I synthase	Coproporphyrinogen oxidase	Protoporphyrinogen oxidase or ferrochelatase (?)	Uroporphyrinogen decarboxylase	Ferrochelatase
Inheritance	Autosomal recessive	Autosomal dominant	Autosomal dominant	Autosomal dominant	Autosomal dominant	Autosomal dominant
Metabolic expression	Erythroid cells	Liver	Liver	Liver	Liver	Erythroid cells and liver
Signs and symptoms:						
Photosensitive cutaneous lesions	Yes	No	Infrequent	Yes	Yes	Yes
Attacks of abdominal pain, neuropsychiatric syndrome	No	Yes	Yes	Yes	No	No
Laboratory abnormalities:						
Red blood cells:						
Uroporphyrin	+++	N	N	N	N	N
Coproporphyrin	++	N	N	N	N	+
Protoporphyrin	(+)	N	N	N	N	+++
Urine:						
δ-Aminolevulinic acid	N	(+++)	(+++)	(+++)	N	N
Porphobilinogen	N	(+++)	(+++)	(+++)	N	N
Uroporphyrin	+++	++	+	+	+++	N
Coproporphyrin	++	N	++	++	+	(+)
Feces:						
Coproporphyrin	+	N	+++	+	(+)	(+)
Protoporphyrin	+	N	+	+++	N	++

NOTE: *N, normal;* +, *increased levels or excretion;* ++, *moderately increased;* +++, *markedly increased;* (+), *increased in some patients only;* (+++), *frequently increased only during acute attacks.*

modulated by multiple genetic, metabolic, and environmental factors. The interdependence of heme synthesis and microsomal drug oxidation is important in some hepatic porphyrias where clinical symptoms are precipitated by these inducing drugs.

In the bone marrow ALA synthase is also rate-limiting in cells with fully expressed heme synthesis, but little is known of the role of the enzyme in overall heme synthesis during division, differentiation, and maturation of erythroid cells. With maturation of erythroid cells the nuclei and mitochondria are extruded, and the mitochondrial enzymes of heme synthesis disappear, while the cytosolic enzymes catalyzing the reactions between ALA and coproporphyrinogen persist. Therefore, erythrocytes can be used for the diagnosis and study of porphyrias provided the deficiency is in a cytosolic enzyme.

Control of heme synthesis differs in bone marrow and liver. The level of ALA synthase is the major determinant of heme formation in the liver, while heme synthesis in the bone marrow is triggered by the complex process of erythroid differentiation. These considerations probably explain the different phenotypic expression of specific enzyme defects of heme synthesis in erythroid cells and liver.

The porphyrinogens, reduced forms of porphyrins, serve as intermediates between porphobilinogen and protoporphyrin. Porphyrinogens are colorless and nonfluorescent. Porphyrins are by-products that have escaped from the biosynthetic path by irreversible oxidation of the corresponding porphyrinogen. Porphyrins do not possess physiological function but are responsible, through their pigment and fluorescent properties, for the spectacular appearance of urine and erythrocytes in some patients.

The arrangement of two substituent side chains on the pyrrole ring of porphyrins determines the structural isomer types, numbered I to IV. In nature only types I and III have been identified, and only type III serves as substrate for the terminal steps of the pathway leading to protoporphyrin IX and heme. The catabolism of heme does not lead to porphyrins but to noncyclic tetrapyrroles referred to as *bile pigments.*

CONGENITAL ERYTHROPOIETIC PORPHYRIA

DEFINITION Congenital erythropoietic porphyria (CEP; Günther's disease, congenital photosensitive porphyria, erythropoietic uroporphyria) is a rare, recessively inherited defect that causes chronic photosensitivity with severe, mutilating skin lesions and hemolytic anemia.

GENETICS, INCIDENCE, AND PATHOGENESIS About 80 cases have been reported. Affected individuals are homozygous for an autosomal recessive gene; heterozygotes rarely have demonstrable abnormalities in porphyrin metabolism and appear normal. The underlying enzyme abnormality has not been entirely elucidated, but there appears to be a functional imbalance between the activities of uroporphyrinogen I synthase and uroporphyrinogen III cosynthase. The defect is expressed solely in maturing erythroid cells and results in massive overproduction of uroporphyrinogen I while the overall production of uroporphyrinogen III is normal or slightly increased. Uroporphyrinogen I cannot be used for heme synthesis but is converted to coproporphyrinogen I which cannot be metabolized further. Uroporphyrin I, coproporphyrinogen I, and coproporphyrin I accumulate in tissues and are excreted in excess amounts in urine and feces.

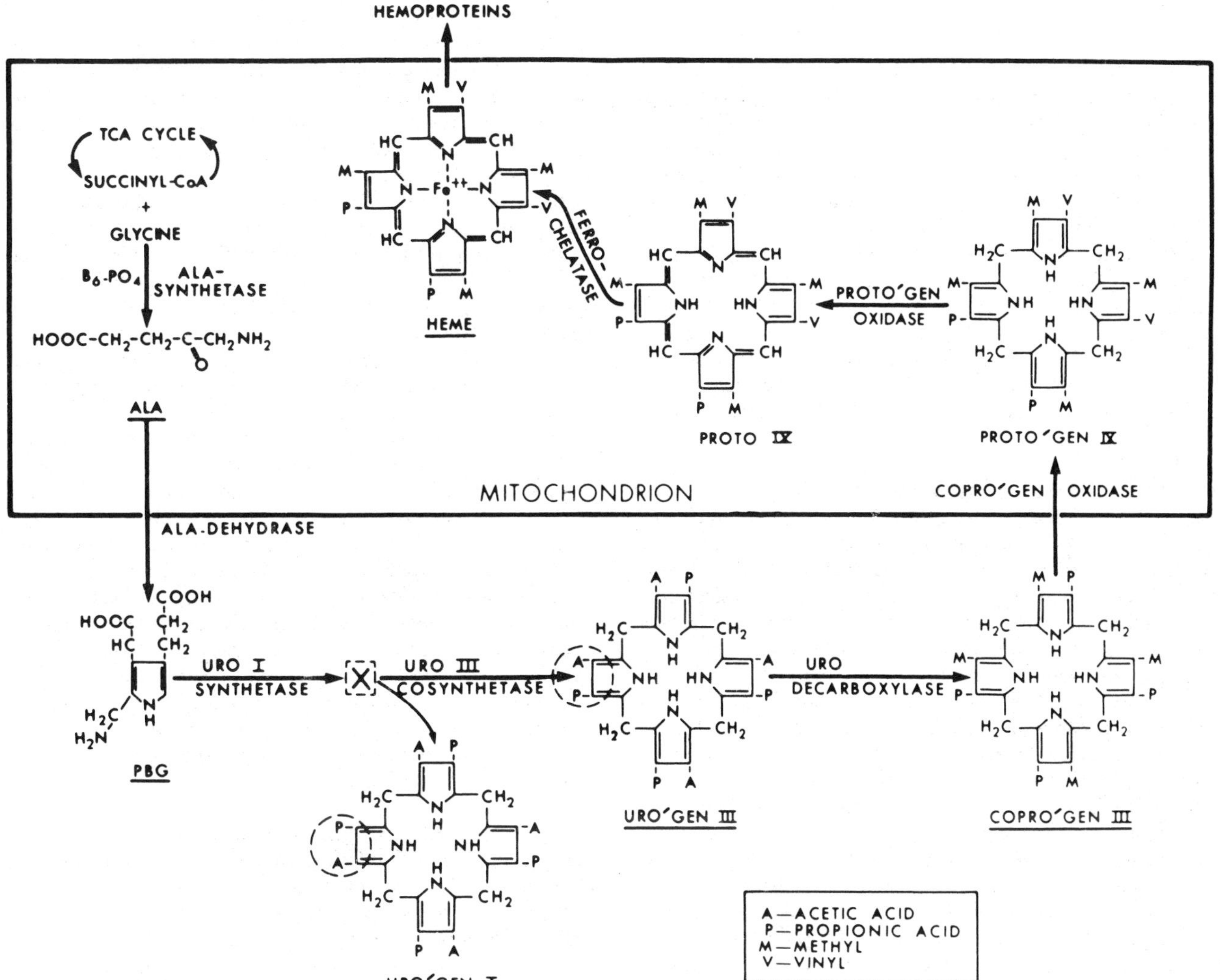

FIGURE 99-1

Outline of heme biosynthesis. (ALA, δ-aminolevulinic acid; PBG, porphobilinogen; URO, uroporphyrin; UROgen, uroporphyrinogen; COPROgen, coproporphyrinogen; PROTOgen, protoporphyrinogen; PROTO, protoporphyrin; X, postulated intermediate.)

CLINICAL PRESENTATION AND DIAGNOSIS Porphyrins accumulate in affected individuals during fetal development. Excretion of pink or red urine usually begins at or shortly after birth, whereas cutaneous photosensitivity, intermittent hemolysis, and splenomegaly may not be detected until later. Hypertrichosis and red discoloration of the teeth and bones are common. Death may occur in childhood. With longer survival, severe scarring and mutilation occur, mostly affecting fingers, nose, and ears. The urine contains high concentrations of uroporphyrin I and increased amounts of coproporphyrin as well as porphyrins with seven, six, five, and three carboxyl groups, whereas the excretion of ALA and PBG is normal. Large amounts of coproporphyrin I are found in the feces. Normoblasts, reticulocytes, and erythrocytes contain large quantities of uroporphyrin I and lower concentrations of coproporphyrinogen I. Normoblasts and reticulocytes exhibit intense red fluorescence. In accordance with the normal excretion of ALA and PBG, neurological disturbance does not occur in CEP.

TREATMENT Exposure to sunlight should be avoided. In some cases, splenectomy has ameliorated hemolytic anemia, porphyrin excretion, and photosensitivity. The use of hematin infusions and oral β-carotene remains experimental.

HEPATIC PORPHYRIAS

Three hepatic porphyrias, intermittent acute porphyria (IAP), hereditary coproporphyria (HCP), and variegate porphyria (VP), have many features in common. All are transmitted as autosomal dominants. Acute attacks of a life-threatening neurological syndrome are precipitated by a variety of drugs, hormones, and other agents. During acute attacks excessive urinary excretion of the porphyrin precursors ALA and PBG occurs in all, but the patterns of porphyrins excreted in urine and feces differ (Fig. 99-2).

INTERMITTENT ACUTE PORPHYRIA Definition Intermittent acute porphyria [IAP, acute intermittent porphyria (AIP), pyrroloporphyria] is characterized by recurrent attacks of neurological and psychiatric dysfunction. Photosensitivity does not occur. The primary defect is in uroporphyrinogen I synthase.

Genetics, incidence, and pathogenesis IAP is an autosomal dominant trait with variable expressivity. The frequency of the abnormal gene is estimated to be between 1 in 10,000 and 1 in 50,000, but in certain regions the incidence may be higher. Homozygous cases of IAP have not been observed. The defect consists of a partial (50 percent) deficiency of uroporphyrinogen I synthase, the enzyme that converts PBG to uroporphyrinogen I. In the liver this leads to increased activity and/or inducibility of ALA synthase by drugs and other factors and, consequently, to increased formation and urinary excretion of ALA and PBG. Preformed porphyrins do not accumulate, and, therefore, cutaneous photosensitivity does not occur. Decreased uroporphyrinogen I synthase activity has been demonstrated in liver, erythrocytes, cultured skin fibroblasts, lymphocytes, and amniotic cells of patients with IAP. Thus, the enzymatic defect of IAP is present, albeit metabolically unexpressed, in tissues other than liver. Deficiency of uroporphyrinogen I synthase does not necessarily result in clinical manifestations of acute porphyria without additional acquired factors, and families with many phenotypically normal carriers of the genetic defect have been found (latent porphyria). The relation between the genetic defect and the neurological lesions is unknown.

Clinical presentation and diagnosis Symptoms rarely occur before puberty. Abdominal pain is frequently the initial and most prominent symptom of the porphyric attack. It may be moderate or severe, colicky, localized or generalized; radiation to the back or loins may occur. The pain probably results from autonomic neuropathy causing disturbed gastrointestinal motility with alternate areas of spasm and dilatation. The abdomen is usually soft, and tenderness is not marked. Because it is often accompanied by fever and leukocytosis, the acute porphyric attack can mimic any inflammatory abdominal disease. Severe vomiting and persistent constipation are common. Neurological manifestations and mental disturbance are variable. Peripheral nerves, the autonomic nervous system, brainstem, cranial nerves, or cerebral function may be involved. Sinus tachycardia and labile hypertension with postural hypotension, urinary retention, and excessive sweating are frequent during the acute attack. Hypertension and tachycardia correlate with increased excretion of catecholamines. Peripheral neuropathy is usually predominantly motor, but sensory components may be present. Deep tendon reflexes are diminished or absent. Neuritic pain in the extremities, areas of hypesthesia and paresthesia, and foot and wrist drop are typical. Paraplegia or complete flaccid quadriplegia may ensue. In the past, complications due to respiratory paralysis were a leading cause of death. Cranial nerve involvement may lead to optic nerve atrophy, ophthalmoplegia, and dysphagia. With more severe CNS involvement, delirium, coma, and seizures occur. Although the neuropathy is reversible to a surprising degree, residual paresis may last for several years following an acute attack. Many patients have a long history of vague nervousness, emotional instability, and functional disturbances. Significant signs of mental disturbance occur in one-third, and an organic brain syndrome with restlessness, disorientation, and visual hallucinations may supervene. During attacks hyponatremia can be severe. Multiple mechanisms (including gastrointestinal loss of sodium, imprudent fluid therapy, and a sodium-losing nephropathy related to a toxic effect of ALA) have been implicated, but the major mechanism appears to be inappropriate release of antidiuretic hormone.

Acute attacks may last from several days to several months and vary in frequency and severity. In periods of remission symptoms may be slight or completely absent. Clinical (and biochemical) manifestations may be precipitated by usual therapeutic doses of several drugs including barbiturates, anticonvulsants, estrogens, contraceptives, and alcohol. All these drugs are oxidized by hemoproteins of the cytochrome P_{450} system. Impaired hepatic metabolism of some of these drugs has been demonstrated during acute attacks of IAP. In some women, exacerbations are correlated with the menstrual cycle, and latent porphyria may become clinically manifest late in pregnancy or shortly after delivery. Prolonged periods of decreased caloric intake (deliberate fasting) and infections may also provoke attacks.

LABORATORY FINDINGS Excessive excretion of ALA and PBG in the urine is characteristic during acute attacks. It does not differentiate IAP from HCP and VP, and the levels do not correlate with the severity of the symptoms. The qualitative determination of porphobilinogen in the urine by the Watson-Schwartz or the Hoesch test is a simple and valuable screening aid for the diagnosis of an acute attack in IAP, HCP, and VP. These tests are almost always positive during episodes of neuropsychiatric dysfunction. However, both screening tests become positive only when the concentration of PBG in the urine

FIGURE 99-2
Patterns of urinary porphyrin and porphyrin precursor excretion in the hepatic porphyrias in relation to the pathway of heme biosynthesis. Intermediates of the pathway excreted excessively during the acute phase of each of the hepatic porphyrias are within the respective brackets. (ALA, δ-aminolevulinic acid; PBG, porphobilinogen; UROgen, uroporphyrinogen; COPROgen, coproporphyrinogen; PROTOgen, protoporphyrinogen.)

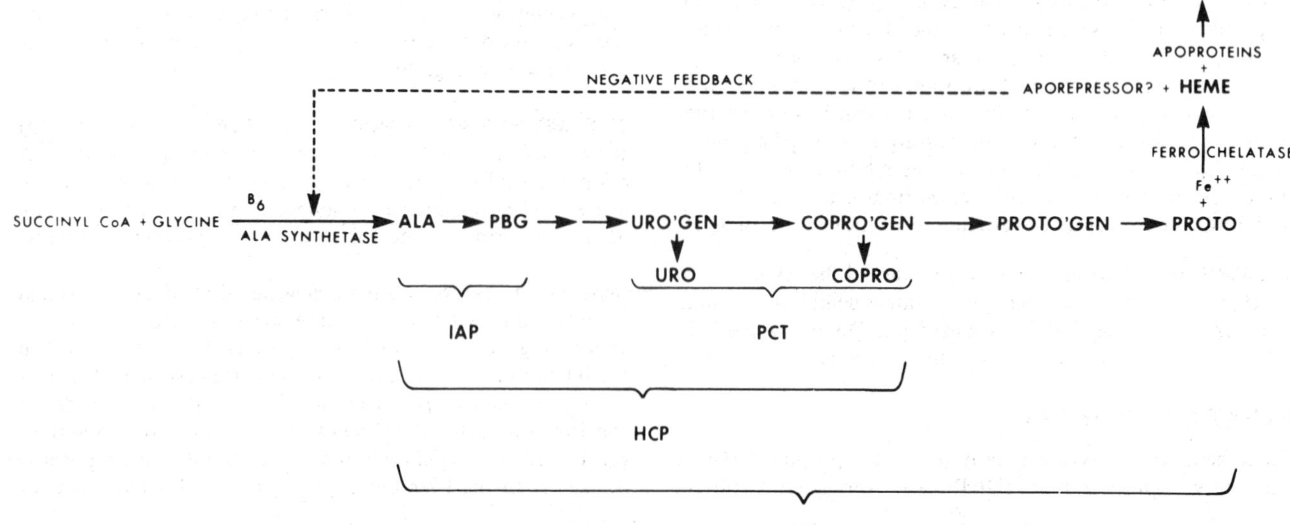

is three to five times the upper limit of normal; as a consequence, they may be negative in latent cases and in patients in whom urinary excretion of PBG becomes normal following recovery from an acute attack. In these instances urinary ALA and PBG excretion should be measured quantitatively by chromatographic methods. In latent IAP with normal excretion of ALA and PBG, diagnosis is possible only by measuring the activity of uroporphyrinogen I synthase in erythrocytes, lymphocytes, or cultured skin fibroblasts.

In IAP the porphyrin precursors ALA and PBG are excreted in increased amounts, consistent with the enzymatic defect. Freshly passed urine is, therefore, usually colorless and contains little preformed uro- or coproporphyrin. The urine may darken on standing because PBG polymerizes spontaneously to uroporphyrin and porphobilin, a dark brown pigment of unknown structure. However, some patients have enough nonenzymatically formed pigments to impart a dark-red appearance to freshly voided urine. The fecal porphyrin concentration is usually normal. In the other two hepatic porphyrias associated with acute neuropsychiatric attacks, increased amounts of preformed porphyrins are excreted in urine and feces.

Conventional liver function tests are normal except for increased Bromsulphalein (BSP) retention. A moderate reduction in red blood cell mass and blood volume or a transient normochromic, normocytic anemia are the only hematologic disturbances. Numerous metabolic abnormalities may be associated with acute attacks including hypercholesterolemia with increased low-density lipoprotein levels, increased serum thyroxine (without hyperthyroidism), abnormal glucose tolerance, and defective 5α reduction of testosterone in liver. The relationship of these abnormalities to the genetic defect is unknown.

Treatment The treatment of the acute attack is identical in IAP, HCP, and VP. Some acute attacks seemingly can be aborted by administration of large quantities (500 g per day) of carbohydrates (glucose effect), although no objective study of the efficacy of this therapy has been performed. Intravenous administration of glucose at a rate of 20 g/h is recommended. If the patient does not improve within 48 h of continued glucose infusion or if neuropsychiatric symptoms progress, intravenous infusion of hematin (4 mg per kilogram of body weight infused over 10 to 15 min every 12 h) should be tried. Both hematin and glucose effectively prevent the induction of hepatic ALA-synthase in experimental animals, and both appear to reverse the biochemical abnormalities and cause clinical improvement within 48 h in many patients. Supportive treatment with careful monitoring of fluid and electrolytes is important because hyponatremia, hypomagnesemia, and azotemia commonly occur. Tachycardia and hypertension should be treated with beta-adrenergic blocking drugs. A list of agents considered to be "safe" or "probably safe" in patients with latent and acute IAP, HCP, and VP is given in Table 99-2. The most important measure in the management is prevention of acute attacks by instructing the patient about the avoidance of provocative factors, namely drugs, steroids, alcohol excess, and deliberate fasting. With early recognition of the condition, immediate withdrawal of provocative agents, careful fluid and electrolyte therapy, and the use of glucose and/or hematin infusions most attacks are reversible, and fatalities are rare.

HEREDITARY COPROPORPHYRIA Definition and genetics Hereditary coproporphyria (HCP) is a hepatic porphyria characterized by acute attacks of neuropsychiatric dysfunction identical to those of IAP and VP. In addition, photosensitivity occurs in some. The primary genetic defect is a deficiency of coproporphyrinogen oxidase. The disease is inherited as an autosomal dominant trait. Accurate assessment of the incidence of HCP is difficult since over half of affected individuals remain asymptomatic.

Pathogenesis and clinical picture Biochemically, HCP is characterized by the excretion of large amounts of coproporphyrin III, mainly in feces but also in urine. Excretion of ALA and PBG is increased during acute attacks (positive Watson-Schwartz or Hoesch test) but usually returns to normal during remission. Acute attacks are indistinguishable from those of IAP and VP and are precipitated by the same factors. Skin photosensitivity occurs in approximately one-third of patients with overt HCP. Its onset is frequently associated with intercurrent hepatic disease. A partial deficiency of coproporphyrinogen oxidase can be demonstrated in leukocytes and cultured skin fibroblasts.

Treatment Treatment is identical to that described for IAP.

VARIEGATE PORPHYRIA Definition Variegate porphyria (VP; South African genetic porphyria) is characterized by both acute attacks of neuropsychiatric dysfunction and chronic skin sensitivity to sunlight and to mechanical trauma. The primary enzymatic lesion in heme biosynthesis has not been unequivocally identified.

Genetics, incidence, and pathogenesis VP is inherited as an autosomal dominant trait. The disease is particularly common among the white population of South Africa, where its incidence is estimated at 1 in 400, and many cases can be identified as descendants of a woman who emigrated to Cape Town from the Netherlands in 1688. Elsewhere the disease is less frequent, but VP has been recognized in many countries. The defect leads to the excretion of large amounts of protoporphyrin in bile and feces (with lesser increases in the fecal excretion of coproporphyrin) and to markedly increased urinary excretion of ALA, PBG, and coproporphyrin during acute attacks.

TABLE 99-2

Drugs considered to be safe (or probably safe) in patients with intermittent acute porphyria, hereditary coproporphyria, and variegate porphyria

Analgesics:
- Salicylates
- Morphine and related opiates (pethidine)

Antibiotics:
- Penicillins
- Furadantin
- Mandelamine

Psychoactive drugs:
- Phenothiazines (chlorpromazine)

Antihistamines:
- Diphenhydramine

Antihypertensives:
- Guanethidine
- Propranolol
- Reserpine

Miscellaneous:
- Atropine
- Neostigmine
- Propanidid
- Procaine
- Succinylcholine
- Ether
- Nitrous oxide
- Corticosteroids
- Oxazepam
- Chlordiazepoxide

The excretion pattern suggests a deficiency either of protoporphyrinogen oxidase or ferrochelatase, but study of these enzymes in VP patients so far has given conflicting results.

Clinical presentation and diagnosis Overt cases with VP usually present in the second or third decade. The clinical picture includes acute attacks of abdominal pain and neuropsychiatric symptoms, coupled with photocutaneous lesions. Neurological and cutaneous manifestations may occur simultaneously or at different times. More than 80 percent of the South African patients have signs of cutaneous involvement, consisting of dermal abrasions, superficial erosions, and blister formation after trivial mechanical trauma. The mechanical fragility usually is limited to light-exposed parts of the skin. The lesions often leave depigmented or pigmented scars. Secondary infection frequently delays healing. Hyperpigmentation of the face and hands is common, and women often have hirsutism. The skin lesions are indistinguishable from those of porphyria cutanea tarda (PCT). Severe exacerbations of the cutaneous lesions sometimes are associated with intercurrent hepatic disease, presumably related to decreased fecal excretion and a concomitant increase in the urinary excretion of porphyrins. Acute attacks of neuropsychiatric dysfunction are indistinguishable from those of IAP and HCP and are precipitated by the same factors. The characteristic chemical finding in VP is the continuous excretion of large amounts of proto- and coproporphyrin, even when clinical manifestations are minimal or absent. The levels of protoporphyrin exceed those of coproporphyrin, the reverse of the situation in HCP. Urinary excretion of ALA, PBG, and porphyrins is either normal or moderately increased in asymptomatic patients or those who have only skin symptoms. During acute attacks the urinary excretion of ALA and PBG is increased (positive Watson-Schwartz or Hoesch test), and there also is increased urinary excretion of coproporphyrin and uroporphyrin. Erythrocyte porphyrins are normal, allowing distinction from protoporphyria.

Treatment Prophylactic measures and treatment of the acute attack with glucose and possibly hematin infusions are the same as for IAP and HCP, although the experience with hematin in VP is limited. Avoidance of exposure to direct sunlight and use of protective clothing (gloves, hats) are advocated.

PORPHYRIA CUTANEA TARDA **Definition** Porphyria cutanea tarda (PCT; symptomatic cutaneous hepatic porphyria, symptomatic porphyria) is the most common form of porphyria. The disease is characterized by chronic skin lesions, the frequent presence of hepatic disease (and hepatic siderosis), and a distinct pattern of urinary excretion of porphyrins. The disorder is probably caused by an inherited or acquired deficiency of hepatic uroporphyrinogen decarboxylase. Neurological manifestations are absent.

Genetics, incidence, and pathogenesis PCT was considered to be an acquired disorder because of its sporadic (and usually nonfamilial) occurrence late in life and its common association (in most series more than 70 percent of patients) with alcoholic liver disease and hepatic siderosis.

The true incidence of the disease has not been evaluated, but PCT is frequent where both alcoholism and iron overload are common, as among the Bantus in South Africa. Recent studies suggest that PCT can be a familial disease, inherited in an autosomal dominant fashion with variable expressivity. The inherited defect consists of a decrease in hepatic and erythrocyte uroporphyrinogen decarboxylase activity; clinically and chemically latent carriers of the defect have been identified. It is not clear whether in some patients PCT also may occur as a consequence of an acquired (or toxic) decrease in hepatic uroporphyrinogen decarboxylase activity. Deficiency (of whatever etiology) in uroporphyrinogen decarboxylase, which catalyzes the conversion of uroporphyrinogen to coproporphyrinogen, leads to a disturbance of hepatic heme synthesis and consequent skin photosensitivity only in the presence of additional factors such as iron overload, usually in association with liver disease and the prolonged administration of estrogens. The mechanism by which iron overload and hormones cause clinical expression of latent PCT is unknown. In contrast to IAP, HCP, and VP, the enzymatic defect in PCT does not result in altered regulation of the hepatic heme synthetic pathway, and ALA synthase activity remains normal or only minimally increased even in overt cases. This probably accounts for the absence of acute neuropsychiatric attacks, the usually normal urinary ALA and PBG, and the lack of sensitivity to drugs such as barbiturates.

Clinical presentation and diagnosis Photosensitivity is the only major manifestation of PCT. The skin lesions are indistinguishable from those in VP. Skin symptoms usually begin insidiously, most often in men age 40 to 60, and consist of enhanced facial pigmentation, increased fragility to trauma, erythema, and vesicular and ulcerative lesions. Sclerodermatous changes and increased hair on the forehead, malar region, or forearms are common.

Liver disease, frequently related to alcohol, is common, and hepatic siderosis is an almost constant finding, although the degree of iron deposition is variable and rarely severe. Spontaneous remission may occur. Occasionally, estrogens (including contraceptive pills) or known hepatotoxic drugs precipitate the clinical disease. The incidence of diabetes mellitus is increased in PCT, and association with systemic lupus erythematosus and other autoimmune syndromes has been noted.

The excretion of uroporphyrin and, to a lesser extent, coproporphyrin in the urine is increased. The urine may be pink or brown. The excretion of ALA and PBG in the urine is usually normal (negative Watson-Schwartz or Hoesch test). Although uroporphyrin is the major porphyrin in the urine, intermediary porphyrins (particularly heptacarboxylic porphyrin) are also found. Increases in fecal porphyrins are less striking and usually restricted to the coproporphyrin fraction. The diagnosis of PCT is established by the combined presence of skin photosensitivity, liver disease, increased urinary uroporphyrin excretion, the lack of an increase in porphyrin precursors (ALA, PBG), and absence of a history of neuropsychiatric attacks.

Toxic acquired porphyria resembling PCT has occurred in individuals accidentally exposed to hexachlorobenzene, polychlorinated biphenyls, tetrachlorodibenzo-*p*-dioxin (TCDD), and other polychlorinated hydrocarbons. Moreover, several instances of benign or malignant primary tumors of the liver have been observed in association with PCT.

Treatment Abstinence in alcoholic patients usually leads to improvement of PCT. Removal of hepatic iron by repeated phlebotomy is effective and may lead to long-lasting remissions. Alternatively, chelation therapy with desferoxamine may be tried. The administration of small doses of chloroquine apparently removes uroporphyrins from the liver and has been successful in some patients. However, its use is inadvisable because of the risk of hepatic necrosis.

PROTOPORPHYRIA

DEFINITION Protoporphyria (PP; erythropoietic protoporphyria, erythrohepatic protoporphyria), a disorder in which mild skin photosensitivity is associated with high concentrations of protoporphyrin in erythrocytes, is due to a deficiency of ferrochelatase. Protoporphyrin also accumulates in the liver in some patients.

GENETICS, INCIDENCE, AND PATHOGENESIS PP is inherited as an autosomal dominant trait with variable expressivity. Several hundred cases have been reported. Deficient activity of ferrochelatase, the mitochondrial enzyme that catalyzes the incorporation of ferrous iron into protoporphyrin, can be demonstrated in bone marrow, peripheral blood, liver, and cultured skin fibroblasts of patients with PP. This generalized enzyme deficiency results in the excessive accumulation of protoporphyrin in late normoblasts, reticulocytes, and young erythrocytes; protoporphyrin leaks into the plasma from erythrocytes as they age. Photosensitivity is mediated by protoporphyrin in plasma and skin and is evoked by visible light (380 to 560 nm). The liver participates in excess porphyrin production in some patients or, alternatively, may take up protoporphyrin from plasma. Many carriers of the defect remain clinically (and chemically) asymptomatic, and detection may be possible only through enzymatic studies. Skin photosensitivity in symptomatic patients shows seasonal variability.

CLINICAL PRESENTATION AND DIAGNOSIS Mild photosensitivity usually begins in childhood. Exposure to sunlight is rapidly followed by pruritus, erythema, and occasional edema (solar urticaria). The lesions subside over hours or days without scarring. In some patients, cutaneous manifestations occur only after prolonged exposure to sunlight; in others the initial skin lesions progress to a chronic eczematous phase (solar eczema). There is no abnormal mechanical fragility or blister formation in skin as is characteristic for VP and PCT. Erythrodontia, hypertrichosis, and hyperpigmentation are absent. Attacks of neuropsychiatric dysfunction do not occur.

PP is generally benign, but patients have been reported who have associated abnormalities of liver, biliary tract, or blood. The incidence of cholelithiasis is increased, and the gallstones contain protoporphyrin. In rare cases, liver disease due to massive deposition of protoporphyrin may progress to fatal cirrhosis. Many patients have mild anemia.

PP is diagnosed by the detection of high concentrations of protoporphyrin in erythrocytes. When a smear of blood from a patient is examined under the fluorescent microscope, large numbers of red-fluorescing erythrocytes are seen. Protoporphyrin may also be elevated in plasma and feces, while urinary porphyrins, ALA, and PBG are usually normal.

TREATMENT Topical sunscreens are ineffective. Orally administered β-carotene (usually as a mixture of β-carotene and canthaxanthine) substantially improves the tolerance to sunlight.

REFERENCES

Dean G: *The Porphyrias,* 2d ed. London, Pitman Medical Publishing Company, 1972

Elder GH: The porphyrias: Clinical chemistry, diagnosis and methodology. *Clinics in Hematology,* vol 9, no 2, p 371, June 1980

Meyer UA, Schmid R: The porphyrias, in *The Metabolic Basis of Inherited Disease,* 4th ed, JB Stanbury et al (eds). New York, McGraw-Hill, 1978, p 1166

Pierach CA et al: Hematin therapy in porphyric attacks. Klin Wochenschr 58:829, 1980

Tschudy DP, Lamon JM: Porphyrin metabolism and the porphyrias, in *Duncan's Diseases of Metabolism,* 8th ed, PK Bondy, LE Rosenberg (eds). Philadelphia, Saunders, 1980, p 939

Disorders of carbohydrate metabolism

100
THE GLYCOGEN STORAGE DISEASES

ARTHUR L. BEAUDET

The glycogen storage diseases are a group of genetic disorders involving the pathways for storage of carbohydrate as glycogen and for its utilization to maintain blood sugar and to provide energy. Some are not associated with actual increases in glycogen content in tissues.

Glycogen is a highly branched polymer of glucose with the majority of residues in 1,4 linkage and with 7 to 10 percent of residues in 1,6 linkage. The treelike structure undergoes addition and removal of residues at its periphera. Glycogen molecules have molecular weights of many millions, and molecules may aggregate to form structures recognizable by electron microscopy. Liver tissue generally contains less than 70 mg glycogen per gram of tissue, and muscle usually contains less than 15 mg/g, but these levels fluctuate as a consequence of feeding and hormonal stimuli. Abnormalities of glycogen structure can result either from decreased or increased branching.

The metabolic pathways involved in glycogen synthesis and breakdown are outlined in Fig. 100-1. These pathways differ among tissues; for example, certain reactions are active in liver but trivial or absent in muscle, and some enzyme functions are encoded by different genes in muscle and liver. Plasma glucose enters the cell and is phosphorylated by glucokinase or hexokinase. The former enzyme is found in liver where it accomplishes the majority of phosphorylation of glucose, while multiple hexokinases are distributed more widely in tissues. Glucose 6-phosphate (G6P) is converted to glucose 1-phosphate (G1P) in a reversible reaction catalyzed by phosphoglucomutase. Uridine diphosphate glucose (UDPG) is synthesized from G1P and UTP by UDPG pyrophosphorylase. Genetic deficiency has not been documented for any of the hepatic enzymes up to this point. Glycogen is then elongated by the addition from UDPG of individual glucose residues to an existing polymer. This reaction is catalyzed by glycogen synthase, which exists in an active dephosphorylated form and in an inactive phosphorylated form. Synthesis of a normally branched glycogen structure also requires the action of a branching enzyme (1,4-α-glucan:1,4-α-glucan 6-glucosyltransferase) which transfers a 1,4-linked oligosaccharide to a 1,6-linkage position.

Glucose is mobilized from glycogen by a complex group of enzyme reactions. Glycogen is acted upon directly by the active form of phosphorylase, phosphorylase *a*, to remove individual glucose units and yield G1P. Phosphorylase is encoded by different gene products in muscle and in liver. In both tissues, the enzyme can exist in an active phosphorylated form and in an inactive dephosphorylated form. The inactive phosphorylase *b* is converted to the active form by phosphorylase *b* kinase. Phosphorylase *b* kinase also exists in an active phosphorylated form and in an inactive dephosphorylated form. The rate of glucose mobilization by this system is regulated by a cascade of kinase reactions, ultimately under the control of cAMP. Epinephrine and glucagon act to increase blood sugar via this cascade system by activation of phosphorylase and simultaneous inactivation of glycogen synthase. Glycogen also is acted upon directly by a debranching enzyme which carries out the debranching process by first transferring an oligosaccharide from a branch point to leave a single 1,6-linked glucose residue and then hydrolyzing the 1,6 linkage. Thus, the debrancher enzyme has both glucan transferase activity (oligo-1,4 → 1,4-transferase) and a glucosidase (amylo-1,6-glucosidase) activity and yields a single residue of glucose for each branch point removed. The G1P generated by phosphorylase, as mentioned above, must be further metabolized to G6P by phosphoglucomutase. In the liver, G6P is thought to be transported by a specific translocase to the inner surface of the endoplasmic reticulum for hydrolysis by glucose 6-phosphatase. Glucose is then free to exit the hepatic cell to maintain blood levels. Many genetic deficiencies occur in the enzymes required for the conversion of glycogen to free glucose in the liver, and these cause the hepatic-hypoglycemic forms of glycogen storage disease.

If glycogen is used as a direct energy source, as in muscle, G6P and G1P must enter the pathways for glycolysis. Again, numerous enzymes are required in muscle for proper break-

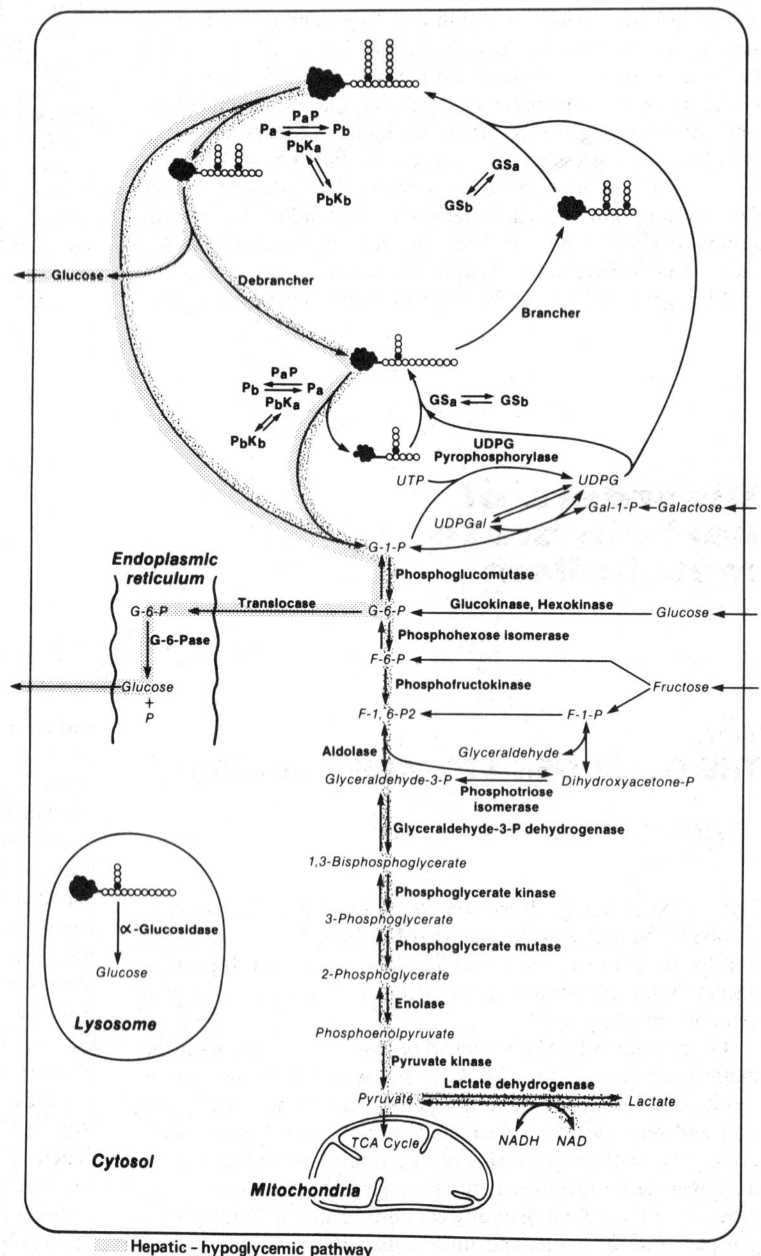

FIGURE 100-1
Metabolic pathways related to glycogen storage disease. A hypothetical composite cell is shown depicting both hepatic and muscle pathways. The shaded areas depict pathways that are blocked in the hepatic-hypoglycemic diseases or in the muscle-energy diseases. Nonstandard abbreviations are as follows: GS_a*, active glycogen synthase;* GS_b*, inactive glycogen synthase;* P_a*, active phosphorylase;* P_b*, inactive phosphorylase;* P_aP*, phosphorylase a phosphatase;* P_bK_a*, active phosphorylase b kinase;* P_bK_b*, inactive phosphorylase b kinase.*

down of glycogen and entry into the glycolytic pathway and TCA cycle. The enzymatic steps known to be associated with genetic deficiency states in muscle include muscle phosphorylase, debranching enzyme, muscle phosphofructokinase (PFK), and probably muscle phosphoglycerate mutase (PGAM) and lactate dehydrogenase (LDH) M subunit.

The lysomal enzyme, α-glucosidase, which is structurally and metabolically separate from the above-described pathways, is capable of degrading both 1,4 and 1,6 linkages in glycogen to give free glucose. This enzyme has widespread distribution in tissues, but its deficiency affects primarily skeletal and cardiac muscle.

CLASSIFICATION The clinical manifestations, diagnostic criteria, and therapy for glycogen storage diseases can be formulated in terms of the metabolic pathway outlined above (Table 100-1). According to this schema, two broad categories of disease can be delineated—the hepatic-hypoglycemic disorders and the muscle-energy diseases.

The hepatic-hypoglycemic disorders include type Ia (glucose 6-phosphatase deficiency), type Ib (possibly due to a defect in microsomal G6P transport), type III (debranching enzyme deficiency), type VI (hepatic phosphorylase deficiency), and phosphorylase *b* kinase deficiency. Within this group, a distinction can be made between those disorders in which G6P and its metabolites are likely to be elevated (types Ia and Ib) and those disorders where G6P and related metabolites are likely to be decreased. This explains why increased glycolysis and lactic acidosis occur in types Ia and Ib disease but not in other forms of hepatic-hypoglycemic disease. Likewise, types Ia and Ib disease are distinct because gluconeogenesis, galactose, and fructose cannot contribute effectively to maintenance of blood sugar, in contrast to the other forms of hepatic-hypoglycemic disease. The glycemic response to epinephrine or glucagon tends to be blunted in the hepatic-hypoglycemic disorders. Dietary therapy with frequent feeding is a rational approach to the hepatic-hypoglycemic disorders and is tailored to reduce protein and to eliminate sources of galactose and fructose in types Ia and Ib disease.

The muscle-energy disorders include type V (muscle phosphorylase deficiency), type VII (phosphofructokinase deficiency), phosphoglycerate mutase deficiency and LDH M-subunit deficiency. The clinical picture is one of muscle pain, myoglobinuria, and elevation of muscle enzymes in serum following vigorous exercise. The interruption of the pathway from glycogen to lactate with the accompanying failure to oxidize NADH is the unifying theme in these disorders. The failure of blood lactate to increase in response to exercise is a useful diagnostic test for the muscle-energy deficiency disorders. Debrancher enzyme deficiency constitutes an overlap syndrome; it presents primarily as a hepatic-hypoglycemic disorder, and the glucose released by phosphorylase appears to be sufficient to prevent myoglobinuria but not to prevent skeletal myopathy and weakness.

Two other disorders are best considered individually. Deficiency of lysosomal α-glucosidase is a lysosomal storage disease without major impact on either carbohydrate metabolism or maintenance of blood sugar (see Chap. 104). The major pathologic process in branching enzyme deficiency is a severe hepatic cirrhosis, possibly due to the harmful effects of the abnormal glycogen that accumulates. Glycogen content is generally normal, and the ability to maintain a normal blood sugar is not impaired. Other less well characterized disorders will be discussed briefly.

HEPATIC-HYPOGLYCEMIC DISEASES Type Ia, glucose 6-phosphatase deficiency CLINICAL FEATURES Type Ia, or von Gierke disease, is an autosomal recessive genetic disorder with an incidence of 1 in 100,000 to 400,000. The disorder is usually

manifested during the first 12 months of life by symptomatic hypoglycemia or by the recognition of hepatomegaly. Occasional patients experience hypoglycemia in the immediate neonatal period, and rare patients never have hypoglycemia. Characteristic physical findings include a full-cheeked, rounded facial appearance; a protuberant abdomen due to marked hepatomegaly; and thin extremities. Hyperlipidemia with eruptive xanthomas and lipemia retinalis may occur. Splenomegaly is usually mild or absent, although massive enlargement of the left lobe of the liver may be mistaken for enlargement of the spleen. Growth is usually normal for the first few months of life; growth retardation then supervenes and adolescence is delayed. Mental development is usually normal.

The characteristic profound symptomatic hypoglycemia may be associated with blood glucose levels below 15 mg/dl. Liver enzymes are mildly elevated if at all. The presence of lactic acidosis is helpful in diagnosing this disorder, although blood lactate may be normal in the fed state in young infants. However, these patients are relatively resistant to development of ketosis. Hyperlipidemia is frequent and involves elevation of both cholesterol and triglycerides. Hypertriglyceridemia can be extreme with levels as high as 5000 to 6000 mg/dl. Hyperuricemia due both to decreased renal excretion and increased production is frequent and often becomes more severe after adolescence. The rise in plasma glucose following administration of epinephrine or glucagon is impaired, as is the rise in blood glucose following administration of galactose by mouth. Renal enlargement can be demonstrated by radiologic or sonographic techniques. Mild renal tubular dysfunction or the Fanconi syndrome may occur. Moderate anemia is usually due to recurrent nose bleeds and chronic acidosis, but may become severe after prolonged acidosis. A bleeding diathesis is due to a platelet dysfunction.

Once type Ia disease is suspected clinically, the diagnosis is established by liver biopsy. The diagnosis is suggested by lactic acidosis, an abnormal galactose tolerance test, or renal enlargement. Immediate processing of fresh tissue is desirable to distinguish types Ia and Ib, and sufficient material for enzyme assay may be obtained by needle biopsy provided the bleeding time is normal. Alternatively, open liver biopsy provides more abundant tissue for analysis. Microscopic examination of liver reveals increased glycogen in cytoplasm and nuclei; lipid vacuoles in hepatocytes are prominent, and fibrosis is usually absent. Specific glucose 6-phosphatase deficiency can be demonstrated in fresh or frozen biopsy material from liver or the mucosa of the small intestine.

The hypoglycemia and lactic acid acidosis may be life-threatening. Other troublesome features include short stature, delayed adolescence, and hyperuricemia. During adult years uric acid nephropathy and hepatic adenomata may develop. The latter lesions are often large and either palpable or demonstrable by radioisotopic scan. There is a significant risk of malignant degeneration, often during the third decade, and subjects who live long enough are probably at increased risk for development of atherosclerosis.

TREATMENT The mainstay of management is frequent feeding. The most widely used approach in children is the combination of frequent daytime feeding by mouth and continuous nighttime feeding by nasogastric tube (see Chap. 81). The regimen should include approximately 60 percent carbohydrate, and no significant portion of carbohydrate should come from sources containing galactose or fructose, which cannot be utilized effectively to maintain blood sugar. The ability of a family to carry out such a program is a significant variable, but in

TABLE 100-1
Glycogen storage diseases

Type	*Basic defect*	*Clinical findings*	*Laboratory*	*Diagnosis*	*Treatment*	*Comments*
HEPATIC-HYPOGLYCEMIC DISEASES						
Ia	Glucose 6-phosphatase	Hypoglycemia, hepatomegaly, bleeding diathesis, short stature, delayed adolescence, hepatic adenomas, enlarged kidneys.	Increased lactate, cholesterol, triglyceride, and uric acid	Enzyme assay on liver or intestine, increased glycogen with normal structure in liver	Frequent feeding, nighttime tube feeding, 60–70% carbohydrate, restrict sucrose and lactose, bicarbonate and allopurinol as needed	Common, severe, autosomal recessive
Ib	?G6P microsomal translocase	As for Ia with addition of neutropenia and recurrent infection.	As for Ia	Enzyme assay on liver with and without detergent	As for Ia	Rare, severe, autosomal recessive
III	Debrancher	Hypoglycemia, hepatomegaly, some short stature and delayed adolescence, mild myopathy worsening in some adults.	Normal lactate and uric acid; increased cholesterol, triglyceride, and SGOT	Enzyme assay on liver, muscle, or fibroblasts; leukocytes variable; increased glycogen with abnormal structure in liver and muscle	Frequent feeding, nighttime tube feeding, 50% carbohydrate and 15–20% protein	Common, intermediate severity, some hepatic fibrosis
VI	Hepatic phosphorylase	Hepatomegaly, variable hypoglycemia.	Minimal changes, ? hyperlipidemia	Enzyme assay on liver, increased hepatic glycogen with normal structure	Dietary therapy as for type III, often little treatment required	Rare and poorly characterized; ? autosomal recessive
Formerly VIb, VIII, or IX	Hepatic phosphorylase *b* kinase	Hepatomegaly, variable hypoglycemia, occasional findings in heterozygous females.	Minimal changes	Enzyme assay on leukocytes, fibroblasts, or liver; increased hepatic glycogen with normal structure	Dietary therapy as for type III, often little treatment required	Very mild but may be fairly common, X-linked
MUSCLE-ENERGY DISEASES						
V	Muscle phosphorylase	Pain, cramps, and myoglobinuria on strenuous exercise.	Increased CPK with episodes, deficient lactate production with ischemic exercise test	Muscle enzyme assay, increased muscle glycogen with normal structure	Avoid exercise, glucose or fructose before exercise	Some clearly autosomal recessive, male preponderance

some instances the metabolic abnormalities and the rate of growth have improved substantially. Optimal management requires a team attentive to the dietary and psychosocial needs of patient and family. If metabolic acidosis is not corrected by dietary therapy, bicarbonate supplementation may be added. Control of elevated plasma urate may require the addition of allopurinol. This regimen provides a reasonably optimistic short-term prognosis, but it is not known whether the long-term risks of hepatic malignancy and atherosclerosis are ameliorated. Portocaval anastomosis was previously used in the management of some forms of glycogen storage disease, but the enthusiasm for the procedure has declined. Prenatal diagnosis is not possible at present.

Type Ib glycogen storage disease Type Ib glycogen storage disease, sometimes referred to as *pseudo type I,* has an incidence of perhaps one-tenth or less that of type Ia. The clinical features are similar to those in type Ia, but unique features include neutropenia, impaired neutrophil migration, and recurrent pyogenic infections; in general, type Ib is more severe than Ia. Laboratory findings, responses to tolerance tests, and management are similar in the two disorders.

Type Ib disease was initially distinguished from type Ia by the presence of normal glucose 6-phosphatase activity on assay of biopsy tissue in the presence of detergent. However, glucose 6-phosphatase activity is low in type Ib disease when fresh tissue is homogenized and assayed in the absence of detergent. These results have been interpreted to imply a genetic deficiency of a microsomal glucose 6-phosphate transport system as a primary defect in type Ib glycogen storage disease. The cause for the neutropenia and abnormal neutrophil migration is unknown.

Type III, debrancher deficiency CLINICAL FEATURES Type III glycogen storage disease, also known as *Cori* or *Forbes disease,* is an autosomal recessive disorder and is one of the more frequent forms of glycogen storage diseases, occurring with a particularly high frequency in North African Jews. Symptomatic disease in the newborn period is unusual, and patients usually present with hypoglycemia or hepatomegaly during the first year of life. The physical findings are similar to those in type Ia, except that splenomegaly is more prominent, but the clinical course tends to be less severe. The skeletal myopathy is usually mild or insignificant in childhood but may be disabling and progressive in adults. Some patients with myopathy are first diagnosed as adults because the features in childhood were mild and overlooked.

Fasting hypoglycemia occurs in about 80 percent of patients. The glucose response after glucagon or epinephrine is abnormal in the fasting state but may be normal shortly after eating since the terminal glucose residues in glycogen can be mobilized. The galactose tolerance test is usually normal. Ketosis is prominent, and blood lactate is normal. Serum transaminase is elevated, and further increases may occur with mi-

TABLE 100-1 *(continued)*
Glycogen storage diseases

Type	*Basic defect*	*Clinical findings*	*Laboratory*	*Diagnosis*	*Treatment*	*Comments*
MUSCLE-ENERGY DISEASES *(continued)*						
VII	Muscle phosphofructo-kinase	As for type V, mild hemolytic anemia.	As for type V	Muscle enzyme assay, increased muscle glycogen with normal structure	As for type V	Rare, autosomal recessive
	Muscle phosphoglyc-erate mutase	As for type V.	As for Type V	Muscle enzyme assay, normal glycogen content	? As for type V	Based on one affected male
	LDH-M subunit	As for type V.	Increased CPK with episodes; pyruvate but not lactate rises with ischemic exercise test	LDH isozymes on serum, erythrocytes or leukocytes; enzyme assay on muscle; ? glycogen content normal	? As for type V	Based on sibship of 3 males and 1 female affected
UNCLASSIFIED						
II	Lysosomal α-glucosidase	*Infantile:* hypotonia, muscle weakness, cardiac enlargement and failure, enlarged tongue, fatal early. *Juvenile:* progressive skeletal muscle weakness. *Adult:* progressive skeletal msucle weakness, pulmonary insufficiency presentation.	Increased CPK, no hypoglycemia	Enzymes assay on muscle or fibroblasts, enzyme assay on leukocytes possible but pitfalls are serious	No effective treatment	Common, autosomal recessive, prenatal diagnosis available and widely utilized in infantile
IV	Brancher enzyme	Infantile failure to thrive, cirrhosis and liver failure, extreme hypotonia and weakness in some, fatal early.	No hypoglycemia, changes of liver disease	Enzyme assay on liver, muscle, leukocytes or fibroblasts; glycogen content not remarkable but structure abnormal	No effective treatment	Very rare, autosomal recessive

nor illnesses. Blood cholesterol and triglyceride are elevated in about two-thirds. Hyperuricemia is rare.

Two diagnostic modalities are used to establish the diagnosis—analysis of glycogen and measurement of debranching enzyme in tissue samples. The glycogen content of red blood cells and liver is increased in almost all, whereas glycogen content of muscle is increased only in some. Documentation of abnormal structure of glycogen with the use of spectrophotometric techniques is a more consistent finding than the increase in glycogen content. The establishment of the diagnosis by enzymatic assay is complicated both by methodological problems and what is believed to be genetic heterogeneity. Both debrancher functions—the glucan transferase activity and glucosidase activity—are believed to reside in a single polypeptide, but as many as six subtypes of the disease may occur. While the diagnosis can be made in some patients using red cells, leukocytes, or fibroblasts, it is generally preferable to document the abnormal glycogen structure and the enzyme deficiency directly in biopsy material from liver or muscle. The pathologic findings in liver are similar to those in type Ia except for less lipid deposition and more prominent fibrous septae.

The course is one of progressive improvement following adolescence, in regard to growth retardation and abdominal protuberance, so that the adult appearance may be normal and hypoglycemia is less frequent. Liver tumors do not occur, and there is no information regarding the long-term risks of hyperlipidemia. The percent of adult patients who develop a debilitating myopathy is probably low. Affected patients have had children.

TREATMENT Frequent feeding is also the mainstay of therapy for type III in childhood. Gluconeogenesis is normal, and as described above patients can ingest galactose, fructose, or protein to help maintain blood glucose. Thus, dietary therapy can include a larger percentage of calories as protein, but carbohydrate intake should be 40 to 50 percent of the total. An evening feeding is often sufficient to avoid hypoglycemia, but nighttime nasogastric tube feeding may be required in severely affected children. Attempts to lower blood lipids using dietary means are desirable.

Type VI, hepatic phosphorylase deficiency The diagnosis of type VI, or Hers disease, was previously applied to a diverse group of patients with reduced hepatic phosphorylase levels due to a variety of causes but is now limited to patients in whom deficiency of hepatic phosphorylase is the primary defect. This nosologic difficulty is a consequence of the fact that phosphorylase exists in both active and inactive forms, and many factors may inhibit the activation of the enzyme secondarily. Consequently, diagnosis requires documentation that phosphorylase is in fact absent and that the phosphorylase *b* kinase responsible for its activation is normal. The disorder is probably due to an autosomal recessive mutation.

Most patients have features similar to those in type III but in a milder form. The diagnosis is suspected because of hepatomegaly or hypoglycemia, and patients generally respond to dietary management similar to that employed in type III disease.

Phosphorylase *b* kinase deficiency Phosphorylase *b* kinase deficiency, now known to be a separate entity, was previously included in the type VI category. Various authors have designated this disorder as type VIa, type VIII, or type IX, but it is most commonly termed *phosphorylase b kinase deficiency.* This relatively benign disorder is inherited as an X-linked trait, manifested in affected males by hepatomegaly, occasional fasting hypoglycemia, and some growth retardation, all of which tend to resolve spontaneously at the time of adolescence. Mild hepatomegaly may occur in female carriers of the trait. The diagnosis can be established by specific enzyme assay of leukocytes, cultured skin fibroblasts, or liver. Muscle phosphorylase *b* kinase is believed to be normal in this condition. Dietary management similar to that employed in type III can be employed for hypoglycemia or growth retardation. It is possible that this condition is relatively common and is undiagnosed. Healthy adults with a history of abdominal protuberance in childhood are often identified during family studies of patients with this condition.

MUSCLE-ENERGY DISEASES (See also Chap. 374) In recognizing the various glycogen storage diseases that affect muscle, the *ischemic exercise test* is of particular use in the initial evaluation. A blood pressure cuff is inflated above arterial pressure, and the ischemic hand is exercised to maximum effort. The pressure cuff is released, and blood is drawn from the other arm at 2, 5, 10, 20, and 30 min for assay of lactate and pyruvate, muscle enzymes, and myoglobin.

Type V, myophosphorylase deficiency Myophosphorylase deficiency or McArdle disease is uncommon, less than 50 cases having been reported. Symptoms of pain and cramps after exercise are usually detected during the second or third decade. A history of myoglobinuria is present in most, and on occasion myoglobinuria can cause renal failure. Affected individuals are otherwise healthy, without evidence of hepatic, cardiac, or metabolic disturbance. Performance of an ischemic exercise test usually causes painful cramping, which is helpful diagnostically. In addition, blood lactate does not rise whereas serum creatine phosphokinase is markedly elevated after strenuous exercise.

The diagnosis is established by documentation of elevated glycogen content and reduced phosphorylase activity in biopsied muscle tissue. The increased glycogen deposition is usually demonstrable histologically in subsarcolemmal regions of the muscle. Myophosphorylase deficiency is thought to be an autosomal recessive disorder; however, the fact that there is an excess of male patients and the fact that muscle phosphorylase *b* kinase in the mouse is X-linked raise the possibility that the disorder, like hepatic phosphorylase deficiency, may be genetically heterogeneous. A fatal infantile form of hypotonia in association with myophosphorylase deficiency also has been described.

Management of myophosphorylase deficiency requires the avoidance of strenuous exercise. Glucose or fructose ingestion prior to exercise can reduce symptoms.

Type VII, muscle phosphofructokinase deficiency There are two genetically distinct forms of phosphofructokinase. All activity in muscle is due to a distinct muscle isoenzyme, whereas activity in red cells is due both to a red cell isoenzyme and to the muscle form of the enzyme. A small number of families have been identified with deficiency of the muscle isoenzyme. Symptoms similar to those in myophosphorylase deficiency were present with pain and cramps, myoglobinuria, and elevated muscle enzymes in serum after strenuous exercise. Lactate production was impaired. In addition, such patients have a mild nonspherocytic hemolytic anemia. Other patients have the anemia but no muscle symptoms; the latter phenomenon might be due to a qualitatively abnormal, unstable enzyme that rapidly disappears from the anucleate red cell but is replaced effectively in muscle cells and consequently prevents muscle symptoms.

Other muscle-energy diseases A group of even rarer familial metabolic disorders must be considered in the differential diagnosis of patients with myoglobinuria and elevated muscle enzymes in serum after exercise. These include phosphoglycerate mutase deficiency, LDH M-subunit deficiency, and carnitine palmityl transferase deficiency. (Older reports of phosphoglucomutase deficiency and phosphohexoseisomerase deficiency seem inconclusive by current standards.) When myophosphorylase, phosphofructokinase, or phosphoglycerate mutase are deficient, neither lactate nor pyruvate rises following exercise, whereas in deficiency of LDH M subunit there is a rise in pyruvate in the face of a failure of lactate production. Carnitine palmityl transferase deficiency is a disorder of lipid metabolism and is discussed in Chap. 116. Definitive diagnosis of these disorders must be established by enzyme assay of muscle tissue. Some patients with this clinical presentation have none of the above-mentioned enzyme deficiencies, and identification of other defects in muscle metabolism is likely in the future.

UNCLASSIFIED DISORDERS Type II, α-glucosidase deficiency Type II, or Pompe disease, is a lysosomal storage disease, and the pathophysiology is discussed in Chap. 104. The incidence is not known but may exceed 1 in 100,000. The disorder is not associated with hypoglycemia, ketosis, or other abnormalities of intermediary metabolism.

The infantile form presents within the first 6 months of life and may be recognized at birth. Clinical features include skeletal muscle hypotonia and weakness, massive cardiac enlargement, enlargement of the tongue, and varying degrees of hepatomegaly. Muscle enzymes such as creatine phosphokinase and aldolase are usually elevated, and the ECG may show large QRS complexes and a shortened PR interval. Motor weakness and developmental delay may be present. Death occurs in the first 2 to 3 years in most cases due to the cardiac involvement.

The juvenile form has features suggestive of a progressive form of muscular dystrophy. These patients have gait abnormalities but no cardiac symptoms. Plasma creatine phosphokinase and aldolase are elevated, and the length of survival is variable. An even milder adult form presents as skeletal muscle weakness in the third to the fifth decade. Again, cardiac symptoms are absent, and serum muscle enzymes are elevated. Some patients have respiratory failure due to involvement of the muscles of respiration and are often misdiagnosed as having some form of muscular dystrophy.

Vacuolization of muscle and increased glycogen content are demonstrable on muscle biopsy. Electron-microscopic studies demonstrate membrane-bound vacuoles containing glycogen, a finding strongly suggestive of the disorder. Excessive glycogen is also found in other tissues including liver and central nervous system, particularly in the anterior horn cells of the spinal cord. Specific diagnosis is made by enzyme assay in biopsy material from muscle or liver or in cultured skin fibroblasts. In general, some residual enzyme activity can be demonstrated in patients with the adult form of disease, but the exact level is not of prognostic significance. Prenatal diagnosis is reliable, particularly for the infantile form. Various forms of enzyme infusion therapy have been tried but are ineffective.

Type IV, brancher deficiency Type IV, or Andersen disease, is a rare, autosomal recessive disorder, less than 20 patients having been reported. Features in infants include hepatomegaly, failure to thrive, and hypotonia in the first few months of life with subsequent development of progressive cirrhosis. In other patients the predominant feature is cardiac involvement and/or extreme hypotonia similar to that observed in spinal muscular atrophy and anterior horn-cell degeneration. Death occurs within the first 2 or 3 years.

The symptoms are thought to be related primarily to the abnormal glycogen structure that results from a generalized deficiency of brancher enzyme. The presence of long outer chains on the glycogen molecules has led to the designation of the disease as amylopectinosis. The laboratory findngs are generally those associated with severe liver disease except that hypoglycemia usually does not occur. The absence of hypoglycemia and the presence of normal glycogen content in the liver make the diagnosis difficult to establish. The diagnosis is suggested by finding abnormally structured glycogen in biopsy material and is established by direct assay of the enzyme in liver, leukocytes, or cultured skin fibroblasts. No effective treatment is known, but prenatal diagnosis may be possible in cultured amniotic cells.

Other possible disorders of glycogen metabolism Deficiency of glycogen synthase has been reported in a small number of families. Affected patients usually have fasting hypoglycemia, seizures, and some degree of mental impairment. The presence of some hepatic glycogen, the increase in plasma glucose in response to glucagon or galactose, and the known lability of the activation system for glycogen synthase have all led to skepticism as to whether such a disorder actually exists. This syndrome may be confused with ketotic hypoglycemia of childhood (see Chap. 116).

There are also reports of more than one enzyme defect in the same patient and of different enzyme defects among siblings. Many of these reports may be related to difficulties inherent in measuring enzymes of glycogen metabolism in human pathologic tissue. At present no specific syndrome of multiple primary enzyme deficiency is documented.

REFERENCES

Fernandes J: Hepatic glycogen storage diseases, in *The Treatment of Inherited Metabolic Disease,* DN Raine (ed). New York, American Elsevier, 1974

Greene HL et al: Type I glycogen storage disease: A metabolic basis for advances in treatment. Adv Pediatr 26:63, 1979

Howell RR, Williams J: The glycogen storage diseases, in *The Metabolic Basis of Inherited Disease,* 5th ed, JB Stanbury et al (eds). New York, McGraw-Hill, 1982

Moses SW, Gutman A: Inborn errors of glycogen metabolism. Adv Pediatr 19:95, 1972

101 GALACTOSEMIA

KURT J. ISSELBACHER

DEFINITION Galactosemia refers to an inborn error of metabolism associated with an impairment in the metabolism of galactose. Two disorders are currently recognized. "Classic" galactosemia is due to the deficiency of the enzyme galactose 1-phosphate uridyl transferase; it is typically associated with cataract formation, mental retardation, and cirrhosis. The second disorder, first described in 1965, is due to galactokinase deficiency and leads primarily to cataract formation.

PATHOGENESIS Lactose, the main carbohydrate in milk, is a disaccharide containing galactose and glucose; when ingested it is hydrolyzed by intestinal lactase. Normally the absorbed galactose is converted in the liver to glucose. The first reaction in this pathway involves the phosphorylation of galactose to galactose 1-phosphate by galactokinase:

$$\text{Galactose} + \text{ATP} \xrightarrow{\text{galactokinase}} \text{galactose 1-phosphate}$$

The gene for galactokinase has been assigned to chromosome 17. The next step involves the conversion of galactose 1-phosphate to glucose 1-phosphate. The enzyme involved is galactose 1-phosphate uridyl transferase (GALT), the gene for which is located on chromosome 9. GALT catalyzes a reaction involving the participation of uridine diphosphate (UDP) sugars as follows:

$$\text{Galactose 1-phosphate} + \text{UDP-glucose} \xrightarrow{\text{GALT}} \text{UDP-galactose} + \text{glucose 1-phosphate}$$

The UDP sugars can be reversibly interconverted by an epimerase reaction:

$$\text{UDP-galactose} \xrightleftharpoons{\text{epimerase}} \text{UDP-glucose}$$

Several alternate pathways of galactose metabolism appear to exist. Galactose can be converted (reduced) in the presence of NADPH (or NADH) to galactitol (dulcitol) by aldose reductase, an enzyme which occurs especially in the lens. Galactose can be oxidized to a limited extent by galactose dehydrogenase leading eventually to the formation of galactonic acid, xylulose, and CO_2. There is also a pyrophosphorylase reaction involving the interaction of galactose 1-phosphate with uridine triphosphate to form UDP-galactose. One or more of these pathways may account for a limited galactose metabolism in some patients with galactosemia.

In galactokinase deficiency, galactose accumulates in the blood and tissues. In the lens galactose is converted by aldose reductase to galactitol, a sugar to which the lens is impermeable. As a consequence, excessive hydration occurs which, together with a decrease in lenticular glutathione, leads to cataract formation.

In classic galactosemia, GALT deficiency leads to tissue accumulation of galactose 1-phosphate and galactose. As in galactokinase deficiency, cataracts develop secondary to galactitol accumulation in the lens. It is assumed but not proved that the cirrhosis and mental retardation of classic galactosemia are in some manner related to increased amounts of galactose 1-phosphate in these tissues. Elevated blood galactose levels may lead to a decreased hepatic output of glucose and hypoglycemia. In the kidney and intestine, accumulation of galactose and galactose 1-phosphate appears to lead to an inhibition of amino acid transport. In some women ovarian malfunction develops in association with hypergonadotrophic hypogonadism; the pathogenesis of this is unclear.

Both galactokinase- and GALT-deficiency galactosemia are transmitted as autosomal recessive traits. Heterozygotes for these disorders have half-normal enzyme levels but are asymptomatic. Maternal deficiency of galactokinase, together with a significant lactose intake during pregnancy, may contribute to cataract formation during fetal development. However, not all persons with half-normal GALT enzymes in their cells are carriers of galactosemia. Some individuals homozygous for another gene, called the Duarte variant, normally have only half-normal GALT levels. This group can be differentiated from galactosemia heterozygotes on the basis of the electrophoretic properties of the mutant enzyme. In both types of galactosemia, the disorder is due either to the functional deficiency or absence of the involved enzyme. In the classic type of galactosemia there is evidence that the disorder is due to a structural gene mutation and that the enzyme (GALT) protein is present but structurally altered and not functioning normally. Several other clinical variants with altered enzyme electrophoretic mobility have been described.

The exact incidence of classic galactosemia is still unclear. Estimates range from 1 in 18,000 to 1 in 100,000 births. Population studies indicate that 0.8 to 1.3 percent of the population are heterozygous for the galactosemia gene and about 10 percent carry the Duarte variant.

CLINICAL FEATURES Symptoms of classic galactosemia usually begin within days to several weeks after birth. The infant usually is reluctant to ingest breast milk or milk formulas, develops vomiting, shows poor nutrition, and fails to thrive. Jaundice, hepatomegaly, and evidence of liver disease may then develop. Cataracts are usually not present at birth but occur gradually over a period of weeks to months. Mental retardation may be difficult to detect but becomes evident after 6 or 12 months. Infants with classical galactosemia are subject to bacterial sepsis (especially with *Escherichia coli*), and this may be the primary cause of death in the neonatal period. The only consistent complication of galactokinase deficiency is cataract formation, but several cases of mental retardation have been reported.

DIAGNOSIS Galactokinase deficiency should be suspected in infants or children with cataract formation who have non-glucose-reducing substances in their urine. The diagnosis is made by demonstrating the deficiency of galactokinase in red blood cells.

Classic galactosemia must be considered when one or more of the clinical features described above are found. If the patient is ingesting milk, reducing sugar may be found in the urine, which gives a negative glucose oxidase reaction (i.e., is not glucose) and is identified as galactose by other techniques, such as chromatography. If the child is vomiting, has a poor food intake, or is on intravenous glucose feedings, galactose may not be present in the urine. The definitive diagnosis consists of demonstrating a lack or deficiency of red cell GALT. A variety of assay techniques have been described. The disease can also be diagnosed prenatally either by enzyme studies on cultured cells obtained by amniocentesis or by demonstrating increased galactitol in amniotic fluid.

In the neonatal period galactosemia needs to be differentiated from primary liver disease. With liver damage, galactose removal from the blood is impaired, and elevated blood galactose levels as well as galactosuria may occur. However, in hepatitis or cirrhosis the GALT levels will be normal.

TREATMENT The treatment of galactosemia consists of the removal of galactose-containing foods from the diet, especially milk. In infants, milk substitutes such as DextriMaltose and Nutramigen are often used. Soybean preparations have also been used in the past, but their polysaccharides contain some galactose and they should be avoided.

The institution of a galactose-free diet usually leads to a dramatic improvement in the patient; in fact, all clinical features except for mental retardation may improve or disappear. In general, patients are kept on galactose-free diets indefinitely or at least until they have reached adequate physical and neurologic development.

REFERENCES

ALLEN JT et al: Evidence of galactosemia in utero. Lancet 1:603, 1980

BURMAN D et al (eds.): *Inborn Errors of Carbohydrate Metabolism.* Lancaster, MTP Press, 1979

KAUFMAN F et al: Ovarian failure in galactosemia. Lancet 2:737, 1979

GITZELMANN R et al: Galactose metabolism in a patient with hereditary galactokinase deficiency. Eur J Clin Invest 4:79, 1974

SEGAL S: Disorders of galactose metabolism, in *The Metabolic Basis of Inherited Disease,* 5th ed, JB Stanbury et al (eds). New York, McGraw-Hill, 1983

102 HEREDITARY FRUCTOSE INTOLERANCE

DANIEL W. FOSTER

Hereditary fructose intolerance is an autosomal recessive disorder characterized by vomiting and hypoglycemia following the ingestion of fructose-containing foods. The underlying molecular defect is a deficiency of the enzyme fructose 1-phosphate aldolase.

CLINICAL PICTURE Clinical manifestations of fructose intolerance vary with age, the most severe form occurring in infants. Characteristically the baby is normal when breast fed but develops symptoms once fructose-containing formulas or foods are ingested. The primary response to fructose is severe vomiting and diarrhea with consequent failure to thrive. Hepatic disease is invariable; hepatomegaly is accompanied by hyperbilirubinemia, elevated levels of hepatic enzymes in plasma, hypoalbuminemia, and even ascites. Hemorrhage may be a major problem due to deficiencies of prothrombin, fibrinogen, and other clotting factors. Postprandial hypoglycemia may lead to loss of consciousness or convulsions. Albuminuria and renal tubular acidosis of the proximal type with aminoaciduria and bicarbonate wastage are common. The children are vulnerable to lactic acidosis.

Older children and adults have a less severe syndrome, often because they learn spontaneously to avoid sweets. The usual picture is that of abdominal pain, nausea, bloating, and diarrhea with or without signs of hypoglycemia following the ingestion of foods containing fructose, sucrose, or sorbitol (which is converted to fructose in the body). Hyperuricemia and uricosuria are common, and kidney stones may be present. Dental caries are unusual because of diminished sugar intake. Hepatic disease is less severe in the adult.

If the diagnosis is made early and effective treatment is initiated, all manifestations of the disease disappear; i.e., the renal and hepatic lesions are reversible. Prolonged exposure to fructose in infants may result in permanent liver damage with changes of portal or biliary cirrhosis evident on pathological examination.

PATHOPHYSIOLOGY The disorder is due to deficiency of fructose 1-phosphate aldolase. When fructose is ingested, the first step in its metabolism is the formation of fructose 1-phosphate, a reaction catalyzed by the enzyme fructokinase. Fructose 1-phosphate is then split to form the trioses glyceraldehyde and dihydroxyacetone phosphate by fructose 1-phosphate aldolase. A deficiency of the enzyme results in the accumulation of fructose 1-phosphate in the tissues following ingestion of fructose and sorbitol. This intermediate is presumably directly responsible for hepatic and renal tubular damage. Fructose 1-phosphate also secondarily inhibits other enzymes. Inhibition of fructokinase accounts for fructosemia and fructosuria, while postprandial hypoglycemia is presumably due to inhibition of hepatic glycogen phosphorylase activity, an impairment that accounts for glucagon unresponsiveness in the syndrome. Fructose 1-phosphate also inhibits fructose 1,6-diphosphate aldolase, thereby blocking gluconeogenesis. While the block in glycogen breakdown is the primary reason for postprandial hypoglycemia, impairment of gluconeogenesis plays a contributing role. Sharp falls in tissue and plasma inorganic phosphate concentrations occur with fructose ingestion and presumably account for the depletion of tissue adenosine triphosphate that characteristically follows. Hyperuricemia is due to increased turnover of purine nucleotides. The mechanism is thought to be an activation of adenosine deaminase, the limiting enzyme in hepatic adenine nucleotide breakdown, by a fructose-induced decrease in inorganic phosphorus and GTP.

DIAGNOSIS The diagnosis is usually suggested by history. In infants the differential lies between hereditary fructose intolerance, galactosemia, and tyrosinosis. The latter two syndromes are also associated with postprandial vomiting and failure to thrive and are due to the ingestion of galactose and tyrosine, respectively. If symptoms are immediately relieved by the intravenous infusion of glucose and do not return when a sucrose- and fructose-free diet is consumed, the diagnosis is clear. Confirmation requires testing with fructose. While normal persons develop hypoglycemia with large fructose loads, the administration of small doses of the hexose (0.25 g/kg in adults, 3 g per square meter of body surface area in children) produces symptoms and a fall in plasma glucose and phosphorus concentrations only in subjects with the disease.

TREATMENT Treatment consists of eliminating sucrose, fructose, and sorbitol from the diet.

REFERENCES

Gitzelmann R et al: Essential fructosuria, hereditary fructose intolerance, and fructose-1,6-diphosphatase deficiency, in *The Metabolic Basis of Inherited Disease,* 5th ed, JB Stanbury et al (eds). New York, McGraw-Hill, 1982

Odièvre M et al: Hereditary fructose intolerance in childhood. Am J Dis Child 132:605, 1978

Richardson RMA et al: Pathogenesis of acidosis in hereditary fructose intolerance. Metabolism 28:1133, 1979

Steiner G et al: Studies of glucose turnover and renal function in an unusual case of hereditary fructose intolerance. Am J Med 62:150, 1977

Disorders of lipid metabolism

103

THE HYPERLIPOPROTEINEMIAS AND OTHER DISORDERS OF LIPID METABOLISM

MICHAEL S. BROWN
JOSEPH L. GOLDSTEIN

The *hyperlipoproteinemias* are disturbances of lipid transport that result from abnormalities in the synthesis or degradation of plasma lipoproteins. The clinical importance of the elevated plasma lipoprotein level derives from the ability of plasma lipoproteins to cause two life-threatening diseases: atherosclerosis and pancreatitis. Some hyperlipoproteinemias are the direct result of *primary* defects in the metabolism of lipoprotein particles. Other hyperlipoproteinemias are *secondary,* that is, the elevated plasma lipoprotein level occurs as part of a constellation of abnormalities caused by an underlying disorder in a related metabolic system, such as thyroid hormone deficiency or insulin deficiency. The primary hyperlipoproteinemias can be divided into two broad categories: (1) *single-gene disorders* that are transmitted by simple dominant or recessive mechanisms and (2) *multifactorial disorders* with complex inheritance patterns in which multiple variant genes interact with environmental factors to produce varying degrees of hyperlipoproteinemia in members of a family.

PHYSIOLOGIC ROLE OF LIPOPROTEINS IN LIPID TRANSPORT

The lipoproteins are globular particles of high molecular weight that transport nonpolar lipids (primarily *triglycerides* and *cholesteryl esters*) through the plasma. A general model for the structure of a lipoprotein particle is shown in Fig. 103-1. Each lipoprotein particle contains a nonpolar *core,* in which many molecules of hydrophobic lipid are packed to form an oil droplet. This hydrophobic core, which accounts for most of the mass of the particle, consists of triglycerides and cholesteryl esters in varying proportions. Surrounding the core is a polar *surface coat* of phospholipids that stabilize the lipoprotein particle so that it can remain in solution in the plasma. In addition to phospholipids, the polar coat contains small amounts of unesterified cholesterol. Each lipoprotein particle also contains specific proteins (termed *apoproteins*) that are partly exposed at the surface. The apoprotein binds to specific enzymes or transport proteins on cell membranes, thus directing the lipoprotein to its sites of metabolism.

Table 103-1 describes the characteristics of the five major classes of lipoproteins that normally circulate in human plasma. These lipoprotein classes differ in the composition of the nonpolar lipids in the core; in the composition of the apoproteins; and in density, size, and electrophoretic mobility.

Lipid transport: The exogenous pathway Figure 103-2 shows the pathways by which lipoproteins transport lipids in plasma. The largest amounts of lipoproteins are involved in the transport of dietary fat, which amounts to more than 100 g triglyceride and about 1 g cholesterol per day. Within intestinal epithelial cells, dietary triglycerides and cholesterol are incorporated into large lipoprotein particles called *chylomicrons.* The chylomicrons are secreted into the intestinal lymph and pass into the general circulation for transport to the capillaries of adipose tissue and skeletal muscle, where they adhere to binding sites on the capillary walls. While bound to these endothelial surfaces, the chylomicrons are exposed to the enzyme *lipoprotein lipase.* The chylomicrons contain an apoprotein, apoprotein CII, that activates the lipase, liberating free fatty acids and monoglycerides (Fig. 103-3). The fatty acids pass through the endothelial cells and enter the underlying

A. TYPICAL LIPOPROTEIN PARTICLE

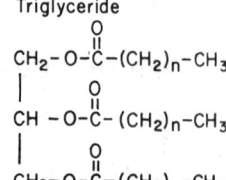

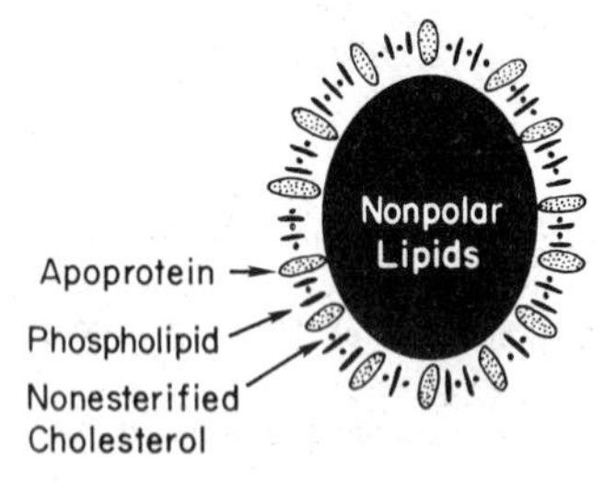

B. NONPOLAR LIPIDS

Triglyceride

$CH_2-O-\overset{O}{\overset{\|}{C}}-(CH_2)_n-CH_3$

$CH-O-\overset{O}{\overset{\|}{C}}-(CH_2)_n-CH_3$

$CH_2-O-\overset{O}{\overset{\|}{C}}-(CH_2)_n-CH_3$

Cholesteryl Ester

$CH_3-(CH_2)_n-\overset{O}{\overset{\|}{C}}-O-$

FIGURE 103-1

A. Diagrammatic representation of the structure of a typical plasma lipoprotein particle. The core *of the spherical lipoprotein particle is composed of two nonpolar lipids, triglyceride and cholesteryl ester, which are present in different lipoproteins in varying amounts. The nonpolar core is surrounded by a* surface coat *composed primarily of phospholipids. Apoproteins are exposed at the surface and extend into the core. Variable amounts of unesterified cholesterol are interdigitated with the phospholipids of the surface coat. The qualitative composition of each of the five major classes of lipoprotein particles in human plasma is summarized in Table 103-1. B. Structures of the two nonpolar lipids, triglyceride and cholesteryl ester. In order for these nonpolar lipids to be assimilated into tissues, the ester bonds between the fatty acids and either glycerol (triglycerides) or cholesterol (cholesteryl esters) must be broken by lipoprotein lipase and the lysosomal cholesterol esterase, respectively.*

adipocytes or muscle cells, where they are either reesterified to triglycerides or oxidized.

After the core triglycerides have been removed, the remainder of the chylomicron dissociates from the capillary endothelium and reenters the circulation. It has now been transformed into a particle that is relatively poor in triglyceride and enriched in cholesteryl esters. It has also undergone an exchange of apoproteins with other plasma lipoproteins. The net result is the conversion of the chylomicron to a *remnant particle,* enriched in cholesteryl esters and apoproteins B, CIII, and E. This remnant travels to the liver, where it is taken up with great efficiency. This uptake is mediated by the binding of apoprotein E to specific receptors on the surface of the hepatocytes. The surface-bound remnants are taken into the cell and degraded within lysosomes by a process called receptor-mediated endocytosis (Fig. 103-3 and Chap. 85). The overall result of the chylomicron transport process is to deliver dietary triglyceride to adipose tissue and cholesterol to the liver.

Some of the cholesterol that reaches the liver is converted to bile acids, which are excreted into the intestine to act as detergents and facilitate the absorption of dietary fat. In addition, some cholesterol is excreted into the bile without metabolism to bile acids. The liver also distributes cholesterol to other tissues (discussed below).

FIGURE 103-2

Model for plasma triglyceride and cholesterol transport in humans. The details of this model are discussed in the text. VLDL, very low density lipoprotein; LDL, low-density lipoprotein; HDL, high-density lipoprotein; LCAT, lecithin:cholesterol acyltransferase.

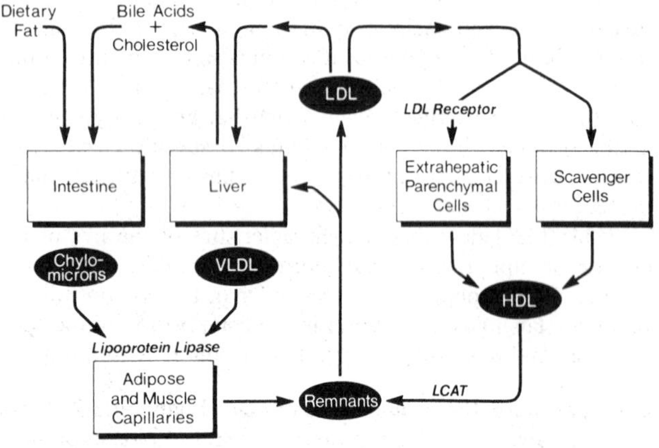

Lipid Transport: The endogenous pathway Triglyceride synthesis in the liver is enhanced when the diet contains excess carbohydrates. The liver converts the carbohydrate to fatty acids, esterifies the fatty acids with glycerol to form triglycerides, and secretes the triglyceride into the bloodstream in the core of *very low density lipoproteins* (*VLDL*). The VLDL particles are relatively large, carry 5 to 10 times more triglycerides than cholesteryl esters, and contain apoproteins that are similar to those of chylomicrons (Table 103-1).

The VLDL particles are transported to tissue capillaries, where they interact with the same lipoprotein lipase enzyme that catabolizes chylomicrons. The core triglycerides of the VLDL are hydrolyzed, and the fatty acids are used for triglyceride synthesis within adipose tissue. The remnants generated from the action of lipoprotein lipase on VLDL are similar to those formed from chylomicrons. However, in contrast to chy-

TABLE 103-1

Characteristics of the major classes of lipoproteins in human plasma

Lipoprotein class	*Major core lipids*	*Major apoproteins*	*Density, g/ml*	*Diameter, Å*	*Electrophoretic mobility*
Chylomicrons	Dietary triglycerides	AI, AII, B, CI, CII, CIII	<1.006	800–5000	Remains at origin
VLDL	Endogenous triglycerides	B, CI, CII, CIII, E	<1.006	300–800	Pre-β
Remnants	Cholesteryl esters, triglycerides	B, CIII, E	<1.019	250–350	Slow pre-β
LDL	Cholesteryl esters	B	1.019–1.063	180–280	β
HDL	Cholesteryl esters	AI, AII	1.063–1.210	50–120	α

FIGURE 103-3

Comparison of the mechanisms by which triglyceride-rich lipoproteins and cholesterol-rich lipoproteins deliver their core lipids to target tissues. Triglycerides are hydrolyzed by an extracellular enzyme (LPL) that is attached to endothelial cells and operates at the endothelial surface. Cholesteryl esters are hydrolyzed by an intracellular enzyme, acid lipase, that is located in lysosomes and cleaves the esters that enter cells via receptor-mediated endocytosis. TG, triglycerides; FFA, free fatty acids; LPL, lipoprotein lipase; VLDL, very low density lipoproteins; CE, cholesteryl esters; LDL, low-density lipoproteins. The apoproteins responsible for the interactions (CII, B, and E) are indicated.

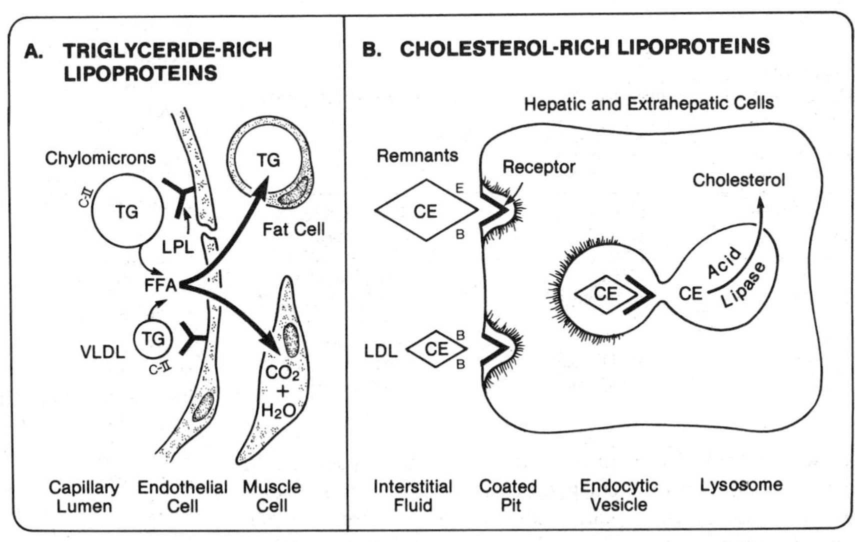

lomicron remnants, a portion of the VLDL remnants are catabolized by the liver and the remaining VLDL remnants undergo a further transformation in which nearly all the residual triglycerides are removed and replaced with cholesteryl esters. During this conversion, all the apoproteins are removed from the particle with the exception of apoprotein B. The result is the transformation of the VLDL remnant particle into the cholesterol-rich *low-density lipoprotein* (*LDL*). The core of LDL is composed almost entirely of cholesteryl esters, and the surface coat contains only one apoprotein, apoprotein B. About three-fourths of the total cholesterol in normal human plasma is contained within LDL particles.

The function of LDL is to supply cholesterol to a variety of extrahepatic parenchymal cells, such as adrenal cortical cells, lymphocytes, muscle cells, and renal cells.

These cells have *LDL receptors* localized on the cell surface. LDL that binds to this receptor is taken up by receptor-mediated endocytosis and digested by lysosomes within the cells (Fig. 103-3). The cholesteryl esters of LDL are hydrolyzed by a lysosomal cholesteryl esterase (acid lipase), and the liberated cholesterol is used both for membrane synthesis and as a precursor for steroid hormone synthesis. This LDL receptor pathway serves as the major route for the degradation of LDL.

In addition to its degradation by the LDL pathway in extrahepatic parenchymal cells, some of the LDL is degraded by a scavenger cell system that consists of phagocytic cells in the reticuloendothelial system. In contrast to the receptor-mediated pathway for LDL degradation, the scavenger cell pathway is thought to function solely to degrade LDL when the lipoprotein reaches high concentrations in plasma rather than to supply cholesterol to cells.

As the membranes of parenchymal and scavenger cells undergo turnover and as cells die and are renewed, unesterified cholesterol is released into plasma, where it binds initially to *high-density lipoprotein* (*HDL*). This unesterified cholesterol is then coupled to a fatty acid in an esterification reaction catalyzed by the plasma enzyme *lecithin:cholesterol acyltransferase* (*LCAT*). The cholesteryl esters that are formed on the surface of HDL are transferred to VLDL and eventually appear in LDL. This establishes a cycle by which LDL delivers cholesterol to extrahepatic cells and by which cholesterol is returned to LDL from extrahepatic cells via HDL. Some of the cholesterol released from extrahepatic tissues is transported to the liver for excretion in the bile. The mechanism by which the liver takes up this cholesterol is unknown, but it is possible that hepatic LDL receptors are involved.

DIAGNOSIS OF HYPERLIPOPROTEINEMIA A variety of diseases cause elevations in the concentrations of one or more lipoprotein classes in plasma. In general, these abnormalities are detected by the finding of an elevated concentration of triglycerides or cholesterol in fasting plasma, a condition called *hyperlipidemia.* The value for plasma cholesterol represents the total cholesterol, which includes both cholesteryl esters and unesterified cholesterol. The absolute and relative values for the plasma cholesterol and triglyceride levels provide information regarding the nature of the lipoprotein particle that is increased. An isolated elevation in plasma triglycerides indicates that the concentrations of chylomicrons, VLDL, and/or remnants are increased. On the other hand, an isolated elevation of plasma cholesterol nearly always indicates that the concentration of LDL is increased. Frequently, both triglycerides and cholesterol are elevated. Such a combined abnormality may be produced by a marked elevation in chylomicrons or VLDL, in which case the ratio of triglyceride to cholesterol in plasma will be greater than 5:1. Alternatively, there may be an elevation of both VLDL and LDL, in which case the triglyceride/cholesterol ratio in plasma is less than 5:1.

The definition of hyperlipoproteinemia is arbitrary because plasma lipid and lipoprotein levels exhibit a bell-shaped distribution in the population, without clear separation between normal and abnormal values. Since lipoprotein concentrations are influenced by diet and other environmental factors, standards must be established for the population under consideration. What is usually done is to set arbitrary statistical limits of normal concentrations based on the examination of a large number of healthy-appearing subjects of different ages. The cut-off limit that is usually used is the upper 5 to 10 percent of values found in apparently healthy individuals (i.e., the 90th to 95th percentile values). However, a vast amount of epidemiologic data from both industrialized and more agrarian cultures indicate that lipid and lipoprotein concentrations that are "normal" in a statistical sense are not necessarily healthy. As a working rule, clinically significant hyperlipoproteinemia is considered to be present in any individual below the age of 20 whose total plasma cholesterol level exceeds 200 mg/dl or whose triglyceride level exceeds 140 mg/dl. In individuals above the age of 20, significant hyperlipoproteinemia exists whenever the plasma cholesterol level exceeds 240 mg/dl or the triglyceride level exceeds 200 mg/dl.

The various combinations of elevated lipoproteins that occur in disease states have been divided into six lipoprotein types or patterns. These are summarized in Table 103-2. As

TABLE 103-2
Patterns of lipoprotein elevation in plasma (lipoprotein types)

Lipoprotein pattern	*Major elevation in plasma*	
	Lipoprotein	*Lipid*
Type 1	Chylomicrons	Triglycerides
Type 2a	LDL	Cholesterol
Type 2b	LDL and VLDL	Cholesterol and triglycerides
Type 3	Remnants	Triglycerides and cholesterol
Type 4	VLDL	Triglycerides
Type 5	VLDL and chylomicrons	Triglycerides and cholesterol

shown in Table 103-3, most of the lipoprotein types can be caused by several different genetic diseases; conversely, some genetic diseases can produce more than one lipoprotein pattern. In addition, each of the abnormal lipoprotein types can occur as a secondary consequence of another metabolic disease (Table 103-4). Hence, the lipoprotein type is a shorthand notation to describe an abnormal lipoprotein pattern in plasma and not a designation of a specific disease state.

Ordinarily, the simple measurement of plasma lipid levels, coupled with a clinical assessment, is sufficient to classify the type of lipoprotein abnormality present (Table 103-2). Occasionally, paper electrophoresis of the plasma is useful either when an elevation in remnant particles is suspected (type 3 lipoprotein pattern giving a "broad beta" band on electrophoresis) or when chylomicronemia is a possibility (type 1 pattern). Recently, there has been interest in the measurement of HDL levels, since high levels of this lipoprotein class are statistically associated with a decreased risk of myocardial infarction (see Chap. 266). The level of HDL can be estimated in clinical laboratories using standardized lipoprotein separation techniques, but the value of such measurement for predicting the occurrence of myocardial infarction in the individual patient has not been established.

PRIMARY HYPERLIPOPROTEINEMIAS RESULTING FROM SINGLE-GENE MUTATIONS

FAMILIAL LIPOPROTEIN LIPASE DEFICIENCY This is a rare autosomal recessive disorder due to the absence or marked reduction in the activity of the enzyme lipoprotein lipase. This deficiency leads to a metabolic block in the metabolism of chylomicrons, causing these lipoproteins to accumulate to massive levels in plasma.

Clinical features The disease usually presents in infancy or childhood with recurrent attacks of abdominal pain. The pain is due to pancreatitis occurring as a consequence of the massive elevation of chylomicrons in plasma. Affected individuals intermittently develop eruptive xanthomas, small yellowish papules, frequently surrounded by an erythematous base, that appear predominantly on the buttocks and other pressure-sensitive surfaces. The xanthomas are caused by the deposition of large amounts of chylomicron triglycerides in cutaneous histiocytes. Triglycerides are also deposited at widespread sites in phagocytes of the reticuloendothelial system, producing hepatomegaly, splenomegaly, and foam-cell infiltration of the bone marrow. When the level of chylomicrons in the blood is massively elevated (i.e., plasma triglyceride level greater than 2000 mg/dl), the blood appears pale and creamy and is said to be *lipemic*. When viewed with the ophthalmoscope, the retina appears pale, and the retinal vessels are white, producing the classic appearance of lipemia retinalis. Despite the massive elevation of triglycerides in the bloodstream, accelerated atherosclerosis does not occur in this disorder.

Pathogenesis Affected individuals are homozygous for a mutation that prevents normal expression of lipoprotein lipase activity. The primary genetic defect appears to involve the structure of the enzyme itself; the activator of lipoprotein lipase, apoprotein CII, is present in normal amounts. The parents are obligate heterozygotes for this defect, but they are clinically normal. As a result of the deficiency of lipoprotein lipase, chylomicrons cannot be metabolized normally and the level of chylomicrons in the blood rises to high levels after a fat meal. In normal individuals chylomicrons disappear from the blood after a 12-h fast. However, in affected patients high levels of chylomicrons are found in the plasma even after several days of fasting or ingestion of a fat-free diet.

The circulating chylomicrons inflame the pancreas when they pass through its capillaries. Within the capillary lumen in the pancreas, chylomicrons are exposed to small amounts of pancreatic lipase that leaks from the tissue. Partial hydrolysis of the triglycerides and phospholipids of the chylomicron pro-

TABLE 103-3
Characteristics of the primary hyperlipoproteinemias resulting from single-gene mutations

Genetic disorder	Primary biochemical defect	Plasma lipoprotein elevation	Lipoprotein pattern	*Typical clinical findings*			Lipoprotein pattern in affected relatives
				Xanthomas	*Pancreatitis*	*Premature atherosclerosis*	
Familial lipoprotein lipase deficiency	Deficiency of lipoprotein lipase	Chylomicrons	1	Eruptive	+		1
Familial apoprotein CII deficiency	Deficiency of apoprotein CII	Chylomicrons and VLDL	1 or 5		+		1 or 5
Familial dysbetalipoproteinemia	Abnormal apoprotein E of VLDL	Remnants	3	Xanthelasma; tuberous; palmar creases		+	3, 2a, 2b, or 4
Familial hypercholesterolemia	Deficiency of LDL receptor	LDL	2a (rarely 2b)	Xanthelasma; tendon		+	2a (rarely 2b)
Familial hypertriglyceridemia	Unknown	VLDL (rarely chylomicrons)	4 (rarely 5)	(Eruptive)	(+)	+	4 (rarely 5)
Multiple lipoprotein-type hyperlipidemia (familial combined hyperlipidemia)	Unknown	LDL and VLDL	2a, 2b, or 4 (rarely 5)			+	2a, 2b, or 4 (rarely 5)

duces toxic products, including fatty acids and lysolecithin, that break down tissue membranes and cause further leakage of lipase from the pancreatic acinar cells. This produces a vicious cycle that eventually causes fulminant pancreatitis.

Diagnosis The diagnosis of familial lipoprotein lipase deficiency is suggested by the finding of lipemic plasma in a young individual who has been fasting for at least 12 h. This lipemic plasma, when collected in the presence of EDTA, has a characteristic appearance after it has incubated overnight in a refrigerator at 4°C. A white layer of cream (which consists of chylomicrons) appears at the top of the tube. The layer beneath the cream is clear. The diagnosis of familial lipoprotein lipase deficiency is supported by the finding of a type 1 pattern on lipoprotein electrophoresis. It is confirmed by the demonstration that lipoprotein lipase levels in plasma fail to increase following the infusion of heparin. Gel electrophoresis of VLDL apoproteins shows a normal amount of activator apoprotein CII. In normal individuals, intravenous heparin releases lipoprotein lipase from its binding sites within the capillary endothelium, and increased amounts of enzyme can then be assayed in the plasma. Patients with familial lipoprotein lipase deficiency need to be distinguished from those with the related disorder, familial apoprotein CII deficiency (see below).

Treatment All the symptoms and signs of the disease recede when the patient is placed on a fat-free diet. Every attempt should be made to maintain the fasting plasma triglyceride level below 1000 mg/dl to prevent pancreatitis. It has been found empirically that the chronic fat intake in affected adults must be less than 20 g per day to prevent symptomatic hyperlipemia. Since medium-chain triglycerides are not normally incorporated into chylomicrons, they have been employed to help achieve normal caloric intake. The diet should be supplemented with fat-soluble vitamins.

FAMILIAL APOPROTEIN CII DEFICIENCY This rare autosomal recessive disorder is due to the absence of apoprotein CII, an essential cofactor for lipoprotein lipase. Deficiency of this peptide creates a functional lipoprotein lipase deficiency, thus producing a clinical syndrome that is similar but not identical to familial lipoprotein lipase deficiency (see above). Because of the apoprotein CII deficiency, lipoprotein lipase is not activated, and its two substrate lipoproteins, chylomicrons and VLDL, accumulate in the blood, thus causing hypertriglyceridemia (type 1 or type 5 lipoprotein pattern). The disorder is diagnosed in children or adults on the basis of recurrent attacks of pancreatitis or by milky plasma detected by chance. The diagnosis is made by showing an absence of apoprotein CII on gel electrophoresis of VLDL apoproteins. Transfusion of normal plasma (which contains abundant apoprotein CII) into the patient is followed by a dramatic fall in plasma triglyceride levels. Heterozygotes, who have 50 percent reduction in apoprotein CII levels, may exhibit slightly elevated triglyceride concentrations, but they do not have pancreatitis. Treatment involves use of a fat-restricted diet throughout life. In case of severe pancreatitis, transfusion of one or two units of normal plasma is helpful. As compared with patients with familial lipoprotein lipase deficiency, the homozygous apoprotein CII–deficient subjects are generally detected at a later age, accumulate significantly more VLDL in their plasma, and rarely show cutaneous eruptive xanthomas. The reason for these clinical differences in the two syndromes is not known.

FAMILIAL DYSBETALIPOPROTEINEMIA This is an inherited disorder in which the plasma concentrations of cholesterol and triglycerides are both elevated owing to the accumulation in plasma of remnant-like particles derived from the partial catabolism of VLDL. Also called familial type 3 hyperlipidemia,

the disorder is transmitted by a single-gene mechanism, but its expression appears to require the presence of contributory environmental and/or genetic factors (discussed below).

Clinical features Affected individuals characteristically do not manifest hyperlipidemia or any of the other clinical features of the disease until after age 20. A unique clinical feature of the disorder is the occurrence of two types of cutaneous xanthomas. These are xanthoma striata palmaris, which appear as orange or yellow discolorations of the palmar and digital creases, and tuberous or tuberoeruptive xanthomas, which are bulbous cutaneous xanthomas that may vary from pea to lemon size. These tuberous xanthomas are characteristically located over the elbows and knees. Xanthelasmas of the eyelids also occur, but these are not unique to this disorder (see "Familial Hypercholesterolemia" below).

Severe and fulminant atherosclerosis involving the coronary arteries, the internal carotids, and the abdominal aorta and its branches is also a prominent feature. The clinical sequelae include the occurrence of premature myocardial infarctions, strokes, intermittent claudication, and gangrene of the lower extremities. Patients who develop clinical manifestations of dysbetalipoproteinemia often have hypothyroidism, obesity, or diabetes mellitus.

Pathogenesis The hyperlipidemia is caused by the accumulation of large lipoprotein particles that contain both triglycerides and cholesteryl esters. These particles are remnants that are normally produced from the catabolism of VLDL and chylomicrons through the action of lipoprotein lipase. In normal subjects, chylomicron remnant particles are rapidly taken up by the liver, and hence they are barely detectable in plasma. A portion of the VLDL remnants is also taken up by the liver while the rest is converted to LDL. In patients with familial dysbetalipoproteinemia the uptake of VLDL and chylomicron remnants by the liver is blocked, and these lipoproteins accumulate to high levels in plasma and tissues, producing xanthomas and atherosclerosis.

The mutation responsible for this disease involves the gene that encodes the structure of apoprotein E, a protein normally found in VLDL and chylomicron remnants. This protein binds to liver receptors and thus mediates the uptake of remnants by the liver. The gene for apoprotein E is polymorphic in the population. There are three common alleles, designated E^2, E^3, and E^4, with approximate frequencies of 0.12, 0.75, and 0.13 in the population. Each allele specifies a distinctive form of apoprotein E that can be detected by isoelectric focusing. The three alleles create six genotypes: E^2/E^2, E^3/E^3, E^4/E^4, E^2/E^3, E^2/E^4, and E^3/E^4. Familial dysbetalipoproteinemia occurs only in individuals who are homozygous for the E^2 allele (genotype, E^2/E^2). The protein produced by the E^2 allele is defective in its ability to bind to the liver receptor that mediates uptake of remnant lipoproteins, and this causes the remnants to accumulate in plasma.

The frequency of the E^2/E^2 genotype in the population is about 1 in 100. Yet the frequency of familial dysbetalipoproteinemia is only about 1 in 10,000. Thus, only 1 percent of the individuals having genotype E^2/E^2 have symptomatic familial dysbetalipoproteinemia. It seems that most homozygotes for the E^2 allele are able to compensate for the abnormal apoprotein E, perhaps by using an alternate receptor system to deliver remnant lipoproteins to the liver. Familial dysbetalipoproteinemia occurs only in those individuals who are homozygous for the E^2 allele and who are also unable to compensate for the abnormal function of the E protein. The inability to compen-

TABLE 103-4
Clinical disorders associated with secondary hyperlipoproteinemia

Underlying disorder	*Plasma lipoprotein elevation*				*Lipoprotein type*	*Proposed mechanism for hyperlipoproteinemia*	*Associated abnormality of carbohydrate metabolism*
	Chylomicrons	*Remnants*	*VLDL*	*LDL*			
ENDOCRINE AND METABOLIC							
Diabetes mellitus	+		+++		4 (rarely 5)	Increased secretion of VLDL Decreased catabolism of VLDL and chylomicrons due to reduced lipoprotein lipase activity	Insulin deficiency or resistance
von Gierke's disease (glycogenosis, type I)	+		+++		4 (rarely 5)	Increased secretion of VLDL Decreased catabolism of VLDL and chylomicrons due to reduced lipoprotein lipase activity	Hypoglycemia with decreased insulin secretion
Lipodystrophies (congenital and acquired forms)			++		4	Increased secretion of VLDL	Insulin resistance
Cushing's syndrome			+	++	2a or 2b	Increased secretion of VLDL with conversion to LDL	Insulin resistance
Sexual ateliotic dwarfism (isolated growth hormone deficiency)			++	++	2b	Increased secretion of VLDL with conversion to LDL	Insulin deficiency or resistance
Acromegaly			+		4	Increased secretion of VLDL	Insulin resistance
Hypothyroidism		+		+++	2a (rarely 3)	Decreased catabolism of LDL and remnants	
Anorexia nervosa				++	2a	Reduced biliary excretion of cholesterol and bile acids	
Werner's syndrome				++	2a	Unknown	Insulin resistance
Acute intermittent porphyria				++	2a	Unknown	
DRUG-INDUCED							
Alcohol	+		+++		4 (rarely 5)	Increased secretion of VLDL in individuals genetically predisposed to hypertriglyceridemia	
Oral contraceptives	+		+++		4 (rarely 5)	Increased secretion of VLDL in individuals genetically predisposed to hypertriglyceridemia	Insulin resistance
Glucogenic corticosteroids			+	++	2a or 2b	Increased secretion of VLDL with conversion to LDL	Insulin resistance

sate may be caused by the independent inheritance of another defect in lipoprotein metabolism, such as familial hypercholesterolemia or multiple lipoprotein-type hyperlipoproteinemia (see below). When an individual is a heterozygote for one of these dominant diseases and is also homozygous for the E^2 allele, he or she expresses the syndrome of familial dysbetalipoproteinemia. The expression of dysbetalipoproteinemia is also brought out when an individual of genotype E^2/E^2 develops hypothyroidism, diabetes mellitus, or obesity. It should be emphasized that heterozygotes for the E^2 allele do not show the clinical syndrome of familial dysbetalipoproteinemia.

The high frequency of the E^2 allele in the population gives rise to pedigrees in which symptomatic familial dysbetalipoproteinemia occurs in several generations of the same family. Such a pseudodominant inheritance pattern arises because an individual homozygous for the E^2 allele has a 12 percent chance of marrying a heterozygote for the E^2 allele. In such a mating half the children are homozygous for the E^2 allele, and thus a recessive trait occurs in a parent and a child, simulating autosomal dominant inheritance.

Diagnosis The diagnosis is suggested by the finding of palmar or tuberous xanthomas in a patient with elevated plasma levels of both cholesterol and triglyceride. Approximately 80 percent of symptomatic patients exhibit these xanthomas. The diagnosis is also suggested when a moderate elevation in the plasma concentration of both cholesterol and triglyceride occurs in such a way that the absolute concentrations of cholesterol and triglyceride are nearly equal (e.g., the plasma cholesterol and triglyceride level are both about 300 mg/dl). However, this finding does not always hold true and becomes especially unreliable when the disease is in severe exacerbation, in which case the plasma triglyceride tends to rise higher than cholesterol.

The diagnosis is supported by the finding of a so-called broad beta band on lipoprotein electrophoresis (type 3 pat-

TABLE 103-4 *(continued)*
Clinical disorders associated with secondary hyperlipoproteinemia

Underlying disorder	Plasma lipoprotein elevation: Chylo-microns	Remnants	VLDL	LDL	Lipoprotein type	Proposed mechanism for hyperlipoproteinemia	Associated abnormality of carbohydrate metabolism
RENAL							
Uremia			+++		4	Decreased catabolism of VLDL due to reduced lipoprotein lipase activity	Insulin resistance
Nephrotic syndrome			++	+++	2a or 2b	Increased secretion of VLDL Direct secretion of LDL from liver Decreased catabolism of VLDL and LDL	
HEPATIC							
Primary biliary cirrhosis and extrahepatic biliary obstruction					↑ Cholesterol ↑ Phospholipids ↑ Lipoprotein X	Diversion of biliary cholesterol and phospholipids into bloodstream	
Acute hepatitis (nonfulminant)			+++		4	Decreased hepatic secretion of lecithin: cholesterol acyltransferase (LCAT)	
Hepatoma				++	2a	Lack of feedback inhibition of hepatic cholesterol synthesis by dietary cholesterol	
IMMUNOLOGIC							
Systemic lupus erythematosis	++				1	Presence of IgG or IgM that binds heparin, thereby decreasing activity of lipoprotein lipase	
Monoclonal gammopathies (myeloma, macroglobulinemia, lymphoma)		++	++		3 or 4	Presence of IgG or IgM that forms immune complex with remnants and/or VLDL, thereby decreasing their catabolism	
STRESS-INDUCED							
Emotional stress, acute myocardial infarction, extensive burns, acute gram-negative sepsis			++		4	Increased secretion and decreased catabolism of VLDL	

tern). This appearance results from the presence of the remnant particles that migrate between β and pre-β lipoproteins and cause a distinctive smear of this region of the electrophoretogram. The diagnosis can be established in specialized laboratories by two procedures. First, the plasma can be subjected to ultracentrifugation, and the chemical composition of the VLDL fraction can be measured. In affected patients, the VLDL fraction contains the abnormal remnant particles and has a relatively high ratio of cholesterol to triglyceride. Second, the diagnosis can be confirmed by the finding of homozygosity for the E^2 allele on isoelectric focusing of the proteins extracted from the remnant particles.

Treatment A vigorous search for occult hypothyroidism should be made, including measurement of plasma thyroid stimulating hormone levels. If hypothyroidism exists, L-thyroxine should be instituted. Patients who have hypothyroidism show a dramatic lowering of lipid levels with treatment. In addition, attempts should be made to control obesity and diabetes mellitus through diet and insulin treatment. If these measures are not successful, patients with familial dysbetalipoproteinemia should be treated with clofibrate. Affected patients usually show a dramatic and sustained reduction in plasma lipid levels when treated with this drug.

FAMILIAL HYPERCHOLESTEROLEMIA This common autosomal dominant disorder affects approximately 1 in 500 persons in the general population. Heterozygotes manifest a two- to threefold elevation in the concentration of total plasma cholesterol which is attributable to an elevation in the level of LDL. Patients with the homozygous form have six- to eight-fold elevations in plasma LDL-cholesterol levels.

Clinical features Heterozygotes with familial hypercholesterolemia can often be diagnosed at birth because their umbilical cord blood contains a two- to threefold increase in the concentration of LDL cholesterol. The elevated levels of plasma LDL persist throughout life, but symptoms typically do not develop until the third or fourth decade. The most important clinical feature is the occurrence of premature and accelerated coronary atherosclerosis. Myocardial infarctions begin to occur in affected men in the third decade and show a peak incidence in the fourth and fifth decades. By age 60, approximately 85 percent have experienced a myocardial infarction. In women the incidence of myocardial infarction is also elevated, but the mean age of onset is delayed 10 years as compared with males. Heterozygotes for this disorder constitute about 5 percent of all patients who have a myocardial infarction.

Xanthomas of the tendons constitute the second major clinical manifestation of the heterozygous state. These xanthomas are nodular swellings that typically involve the Achilles and other tendons about the knee, elbow, and dorsum of the hand. They are formed by the deposition of LDL-derived cholesteryl esters in tissue macrophages located in interstitial spaces. The macrophages are swollen with lipid droplets and form foam cells. Cholesterol is also deposited in the soft tissue of the eyelid, producing xanthelasma, and within the cornea, producing arcus corneae. Whereas tendon xanthomas are essentially diagnostic of familial hypercholesterolemia, xanthelasma and arcus corneae are not specific. The latter abnormalities also occur in many adults with normal plasma lipid levels. The incidence of tendon xanthomas in familial hypercholesterolemia increases with age, and up to 75 percent of affected heterozygotes display this sign. The absence of tendon xanthomas does not rule out familial hypercholesterolemia.

Approximately 1 in 1 million persons in the general population inherits two copies of the familial hypercholesterolemia gene and is a homozygote for the disorder. These individuals have marked elevations in the plasma level of LDL from birth. A unique type of planar cutaneous xanthoma is often present at birth and always develops within the first 6 years of life. These characteristic xanthomas are raised, yellow, plaque-like lesions that occur at points of cutaneous trauma, such as over the knees, elbows, and buttocks. Xanthomas are almost always present in the interdigital webs of the hands, particularly between the thumb and index finger. Tendon xanthomas, arcus corneae, and xanthelasma are also characteristic. Coronary artery atherosclerosis frequently has its clinical onset in homozygotes before age 10, and myocardial infarction has been reported as early as 18 months of age. In addition to coronary atherosclerosis homozygotes frequently develop cholesterol deposition in the aortic valve, producing symptomatic aortic stenosis. Homozygotes usually succumb to the complications of myocardial infarction before age 20.

Obesity and diabetes mellitus do not occur with increased frequency in familial hypercholesterolemia. A slender body habitus is the rule.

Pathogenesis The primary defect resides in the gene for the LDL receptor. Studies of cultured cells suggest that three classes of mutant alleles occur at this locus. The most common, designated receptor-negative or R^{b0}, specifies a gene product that is nonfunctional. The second most frequent mutant, designated receptor-defective or R^{b-}, produces a receptor that has 1 to 10 percent of normal LDL binding activity. The third type, designated $R^{b+,i0}$, produces a receptor that binds LDL normally but is unable to transport the receptor-bound lipoprotein into the cell. This very rare allele produces the so-called internalization defect.

Phenotypic homozygotes possess two mutant alleles at the LDL receptor locus, and hence their cells show a total or near-total inability to bind or take up LDL. Heterozygotes have one normal allele and one of the three mutant alleles at the LDL receptor locus, and hence their cells are able to bind and take up LDL at approximately half the normal rate.

Because of the reduction in LDL receptor activity, LDL catabolism is blocked and the level of LDL in plasma rises in a manner that is inversely proportional to the reduction in LDL receptors. In addition to the impaired catabolism of LDL, an increased production of LDL has also been noted in homozygotes. Enhanced production of LDL has been attributed to the lack of an LDL receptor on liver cells such that the liver fails to sense the adequacy of the plasma LDL level. In contrast to normal individuals in whom all plasma LDL appears to be derived from VLDL, in FH homozygotes a large fraction of circulating LDL is secreted directly from the liver into the plasma. This overproduction of LDL, together with its inefficient catabolism, accounts for the high concentrations seen in affected patients. The elevated LDL levels cause an increase in the uptake of LDL by scavenger cells, which accumulate at various sites in the body, producing xanthomas.

The accelerated coronary atherosclerosis in familial hypercholesterolemia also results from the high LDL levels, which lead to an enhanced infiltration of LDL into the artery wall following episodes of endothelial damage. The large amounts of LDL that penetrate the artery wall are greater than can be cleared from the interstitial space by the scavenger cells, and atherosclerosis ultimately results. Evidence also indicates that the high LDL levels may act to accelerate platelet aggregation at sites of endothelial injury, thereby enhancing the growth of the atherosclerotic plaque (see Chap. 266).

Diagnosis The diagnosis of heterozygous familial hypercholesterolemia is suggested by the finding of an isolated elevation of plasma cholesterol, with a normal concentration of plasma triglycerides. In nearly all cases, such an isolated elevation in plasma cholesterol is due to an elevation in the plasma concentration of LDL alone (type 2a pattern). However, most individuals in the general population with type 2a hyperlipoproteinemia do not have familial hypercholesterolemia. Rather, they have a form of polygenic hypercholesterolemia that puts them on the upper end of the bell-shaped curve for the general population (see "Polygenic Hypercholesterolemia" below). Type 2a hyperlipoproteinemia is also caused by multiple lipoprotein-type hyperlipidemia (discussed below). In addition, a variety of metabolic disorders, including hypothyroidism and nephrotic syndrome, can cause type 2a hyperlipoproteinemia (Table 103-4).

Among individuals who have a type 2a lipoprotein pattern, those with heterozygous familial hypercholesterolemia can be distinguished from those with polygenic hypercholesterolemia and multiple lipoprotein-type hyperlipidemia on several grounds. (1) In familial hypercholesterolemia the plasma cholesterol level tends to be higher. A plasma cholesterol level in the range of 350 to 400 mg/dl is more suggestive of heterozygous familial hypercholesterolemia than of the other disorders. However, many patients with heterozygous familial hypercholesterolemia have cholesterol levels of 285 to 350 mg/dl, a range in which the other disorders cannot be excluded. (2) The occurrence of tendon xanthomas virtually establishes the diagnosis of familial hypercholesterolemia, since such xanthomas usually do not occur in patients with other forms of hyperlipidemia. (3) In cases in which the diagnosis is in doubt, other family members should be surveyed. In familial hypercholesterolemia half of first-degree relatives show an elevated plasma cholesterol level. Hypercholesterolemia is particularly informative when it occurs in relatives who are children, since elevated levels of cholesterol in childhood are characteristic of familial hypercholesterolemia but not of any of the other aforementioned disorders.

Approximately 10 percent of heterozygotes with familial hypercholesterolemia have a concomitant elevation in plasma triglyceride levels (type 2b pattern). In these cases, the disease is difficult to differentiate from multiple lipoprotein-type hyperlipidemia. The finding of a tendon xanthoma or a hypercholesterolemic child in the family favors the diagnosis of familial hypercholesterolemia.

The diagnosis of homozygous familial hypercholesterolemia ordinarily affords no problem, providing the physician is familiar with the clinical picture. Most patients are first seen by dermatologists in childhood because of the cutaneous xanthomas. Occasionally, the presentation is delayed until the onset of angina pectoris or until the child suffers a syncopal episode owing to the xanthomatous aortic stenosis. The finding of a cholesterol level greater than 600 mg/dl with normal triglyceride values in a nonjaundiced child is highly suggestive of the diagnosis. Both parents should have moderately elevated cholesterol levels and other features of heterozygous familial hypercholesterolemia.

In specialized laboratories the diagnosis of both heterozygous and homozygous familial hypercholesterolemia can be made by direct measurement of the number of LDL receptors on cultured skin fibroblasts or freshly isolated blood lymphocytes. Homozygous familial hypercholesterolemia has been diagnosed in utero by the absence of LDL receptors on cultured amniotic fluid cells.

Treatment Inasmuch as the atherosclerosis in this disorder is a consequence of the long-standing elevation in plasma LDL levels, every effort should be made to lower the plasma LDL level into the normal range. Patients should be placed on a diet that is low in cholesterol, low in saturated fats, and high in polyunsaturated fats. This generally means the avoidance of milk, butter, cheese, chocolate, shellfish, and fatty meats and the addition of polyunsaturated cooking oils such as corn oil and safflower oil. With such a diet heterozygotes usually show a 10 to 15 percent drop in plasma cholesterol level.

Bile acid–binding resins, such as cholestyramine, should be added to the regimen when dietary therapy fails to lower the cholesterol levels to the normal range. These resins trap the bile acids excreted by the liver into the intestine and carry them into the feces. The liver responds to bile acid depletion by converting additional cholesterol into bile acids. This leads to an enhanced production of LDL receptors by the liver, which in turn lowers the plasma level of LDL. However, affected subjects respond to bile acid depletion by enhancing cholesterol synthesis in the liver, and this compensatory response ultimately limits the long-term success of therapy. With the combination of diet and bile acid–binding resins, the extent of reduction in plasma cholesterol level usually is in the range of 25 percent in heterozygotes. The addition of nicotinic acid may help to block the compensatory increase in hepatic cholesterol synthesis, thus allowing a further lowering of the cholesterol. Major side effects of bile acid–binding resins include gastrointestinal bloating, cramps, and constipation. The major side effect of nicotinic acid is hepatotoxicity; it also produces flushing and headaches in most patients. Probucol has also been used for the treatment of familial hypercholesterolemia, but its efficacy has not been established.

Heterozygotes often show a moderate to marked lowering of plasma cholesterol level in response to the creation of an intestinal anastomosis that bypasses the ileum. This operation has the same functional effect as bile acid–binding resins, i.e., it accelerates the loss of bile acids in the stool. In certain patients in whom drug therapy is not tolerated, the creation of an ileal bypass may be indicated.

Homozygotes tend to be more resistant to treatment, probably because they are unable to increase production of LDL receptors. In general, combination therapy consisting of diet, a bile acid–binding resin, and nicotinic acid has little effect. Ileal bypass is uniformly ineffective. Several children have responded to surgical creation of a portacaval anastomosis. However, this procedure is still experimental. The use of a continuous-flow blood cell centrifuge to perform plasma exchanges at monthly intervals is one treatment that will lower the cholesterol in all homozygotes. After each plasma exchange, the plasma cholesterol level drops to about 300 mg/dl and then gradually rises over the ensuing 4 weeks to the pretreatment level. If facilities are available, plasma exchange is the treatment of choice for homozygotes.

FAMILIAL HYPERTRIGLYCERIDEMIA This is a common autosomal dominant disorder in which the concentration of VLDL is elevated in the plasma, causing hypertriglyceridemia.

Clinical features Affected individuals do not usually express hypertriglyceridemia until puberty or early adulthood. Thereafter, the fasting plasma triglyceride level tends to be moderately elevated in the range of 200 to 500 mg/dl (type 4 lipoprotein pattern). The typical affected patient exhibits a clinical triad consisting of obesity, hyperglycemia, and hyperinsulinemia. In addition, hypertension and hyperuricemia are frequent.

The incidence of atherosclerosis is increased. In one study affected patients constituted 6 percent of all individuals with myocardial infarction. However, it has not been established that the hypertriglyceridemia per se causes the increased atherosclerosis. As discussed above, many patients with this disease have diabetes, obesity, and hypertension. Each of these disorders by itself may predispose to atherosclerosis. Xanthomas are not a characteristic feature of familial hypertriglyceridemia.

Affected patients ordinarily have mild to moderate hypertriglyceridemia but can develop a severe exacerbation when exposed to a variety of precipitating factors. These include poorly controlled diabetes mellitus, excessive consumption of alcohol, ingestion of birth control pills containing estrogen, and the development of hypothyroidism. In response to any of these stimuli, the plasma triglyceride level can rise to more than 1000 mg/dl. Under these conditions, large triglyceride-laden particles with the characteristics of chylomicrons appear in plasma. During exacerbations such patients develop *mixed hyperlipidemia;* that is, they show an elevation in the concentration of both VLDL and chylomicrons (type 5 lipoprotein pattern). Whenever the concentration of chylomicrons rises to high levels, patients are predisposed to the formation of eruptive xanthomas and the development of pancreatitis. With treatment of the exacerbating condition, the chylomicron-like particles disappear from plasma, and the concentration of triglycerides returns to the moderately elevated basal condition.

In certain families some patients exhibit a severe mixed hyperlipidemia, even in the absence of known exacerbating factors. This is the so-called familial type 5 hyperlipidemia. Other individuals in the same family may have only the mild form of the disease with moderate hypertriglyceridemia and no hyperchylomicronemia (type 4 pattern).

Pathogenesis Familial hypertriglyceridemia is transmitted as an autosomal dominant trait, implying a mutation in a single gene. However, the nature of the mutant gene and the mechanism by which it produces hypertriglyceridemia have not been identified. It is likely that the disorder is genetically heterogeneous; that is, the hypertriglyceridemia phenotype in different families may result from different mutations.

Some affected patients have an elevated production rate of VLDL, especially when they ingest diets high in carbohydrate.

However, many of these patients have obesity and diabetes mellitus. Other individuals with obesity and diabetes mellitus, who have normal plasma VLDL levels, also overproduce VLDL. Thus, patients with familial hypertriglyceridemia may have an underlying defect in the ability to catabolize the triglycerides of VLDL. When VLDL production rates become elevated due to obesity or diabetes, they are unable to increase the catabolism of VLDL proportionately and hypertriglyceridemia results. However, lipoprotein lipase activity increases normally in plasma after the administration of heparin, and no abnormalities of lipoprotein structure have been identified.

The increased prevalence of diabetes and obesity in this syndrome is believed to be fortuitous, owing to the fact that both conditions tend to increase VLDL production and hence to exacerbate hypertriglyceridemia. Thus, in family studies, one can find relatives who have diabetes without hypertriglyceridemia and relatives who have hypertriglyceridemia without diabetes, indicating that the two are inherited by independent mechanisms. When an individual inherits both the gene(s) for diabetes and the gene for hypertriglyceridemia, the hypertriglyceridemia is more severe, and such a person is more apt to come to medical attention. Similarly, an individual with familial hypertriglyceridemia who has a normal weight usually has mild hypertriglyceridemia and is less likely to come to medical attention. However, if obesity develops, the hypertriglyceridemia worsens, and a diagnosis is more likely to be made.

Diagnosis The finding of a moderate elevation in plasma triglyceride level, together with a normal cholesterol level, raises the possibility of familial hypertriglyceridemia. In most patients, the plasma is clear to somewhat cloudy on inspection. Chylomicrons typically are not found at the top of the plasma after overnight refrigeration. Electrophoresis of the plasma reveals an increase in the pre-β fraction (type 4 lipoprotein pattern). As mentioned above, an occasional patient exhibits severe hypertriglyceridemia with an elevation in both chylomicrons and VLDL. In this case, a cream layer develops on top (chylomicrons) and a cloudy infranatant (VLDL) is present after overnight storage of plasma in the refrigerator (type 5 lipoprotein pattern).

Given an individual who has an elevation in VLDL levels with or without an elevation in chylomicrons, no simple test exists to determine whether this subject has familial hypertriglyceridemia or hypertriglyceridemia due to some other genetic or acquired cause, such as multiple lipoprotein-type hyperlipidemia or sporadic hypertriglyceridemia. In a typical case of familial hypertriglyceridemia, half of the first-degree relatives have hypertriglyceridemia and no relatives with isolated hypercholesterolemia should be found. Measurement of plasma lipid levels in children is not helpful inasmuch as the disease is typically not manifest until the time of puberty.

Treatment Attempts should be made to control all the exacerbating conditions. Caloric restriction is required in the obese subject. The dietary content of saturated fat should also be limited. Alcohol and oral contraceptives should be avoided. Diabetes mellitus, if present, should be treated vigorously. Thyroid function should be checked, and hypothyroidism treated if found. If the above measures fail, patients respond to the administration of clofibrate, a drug whose mechanism of action is unknown.

MULTIPLE LIPOPROTEIN-TYPE HYPERLIPIDEMIA This common disorder, which is also called familial combined hyperlipidemia, is inherited as an autosomal dominant trait. Affected individuals in a single family characteristically show one of three different lipoprotein patterns: hypercholesterolemia (type 2a), hypertriglyceridemia (type 4), or both hypercholesterolemia and hypertriglyceridemia (type 2b).

Clinical features Hyperlipidemia is not ordinarily present in childhood. Elevations in the plasma cholesterol and/or triglyceride level begin to appear at puberty and continue throughout life. The lipid elevations tend to be mild and vary from time to time so that affected individuals may have a mildly elevated cholesterol level at one examination and/or a mildly elevated triglyceride level at another time. Xanthomas are not a feature. However, premature atherosclerosis occurs, and the incidence of myocardial infarction in middle age is elevated in affected women as well as men.

Patients usually have a strong family history of premature coronary artery disease. This disorder is found in about 10 percent of all patients who have a myocardial infarction. The frequency of obesity, hyperuricemia, and glucose intolerance is increased in affected individuals, especially those with hypertriglyceridemia. However, this association is not as striking as in familial hypertriglyceridemia.

Pathogenesis The disease is transmitted within families as an autosomal dominant trait, implying a mutation in a single gene. Family studies show that about half of the first-degree relatives of an affected individual have hyperlipidemia. However, blood lipid levels are variable among affected individuals in the same family as well as in the same individual at different times. About one-third of hyperlipidemic relatives have hypercholesterolemia (type 2a lipoprotein pattern), one-third hypertriglyceridemia (type 4), and one-third both hypercholesterolemia and hypertriglyceridemia (type 2b). In most affected relatives the plasma lipid levels tend to be just above the 95th percentile for the population and to dip into the normal range intermittently.

While the extent (if any) of the genetic heterogeneity and the nature of the underlying biochemical mechanisms are not known, it has been postulated that affected individuals have an elevated secretion rate of VLDL by the liver. Depending on the interplay of factors governing the efficiency of conversion of VLDL to LDL and the efficiency of catabolism of LDL, this overproduction of VLDL may manifest itself alternatively as an elevation in plasma VLDL levels (hypertriglyceridemia), an elevation in LDL levels (hypercholesterolemia), or both. The hyperlipidemia is worsened by diabetes, alcoholism, and hypothyroidism.

Diagnosis No clinical or laboratory methods exist by which to determine whether an individual with hyperlipidemia has the multiple lipoprotein-type disorder. The 2a, 2b, and 4 lipoprotein patterns can each occur in patients with several other diseases (see Tables 103-3 and 103-4). However, this disorder should be suspected in any individual whose hyperlipoproteinemia is mild and whose lipoprotein type changes with time. The diagnosis is supported by the finding of multiple abnormal lipoprotein types in relatives. The diagnosis can be ruled out by the finding of tendon xanthomas in the patient or his relatives or by the finding of hypercholesterolemia in a relative under the age of 10 years.

Treatment Therapy should be directed at the predominant lipid elevated at the time of examination. General measures such as weight reduction, restriction of dietary saturated fat and cholesterol, and avoidance of alcohol and oral contraceptives are useful. Triglyceride elevations may respond to clofibrate. When only the cholesterol level is elevated, a bile acid–binding resin should be given. However, in some individuals the lowering of cholesterol levels with such a drug is accompanied by an increase in triglyceride levels.

PRIMARY HYPERLIPOPROTEINEMIAS OF UNKNOWN ETIOLOGY

POLYGENIC HYPERCHOLESTEROLEMIA By definition, 5 percent of individuals in the general population have LDL-cholesterol levels that exceed the 95th percentile and therefore have hypercholesterolemia (type 2a or type 2b lipoprotein patterns). On the average, among every 20 such hypercholesterolemic persons, 1 person has the heterozygous form of familial hypercholesterolemia, and 2 have multiple lipoprotein-type hyperlipidemia. The remaining 17 have a form of hypercholesterolemia, designated polygenic hypercholesterolemia, that owes its origin not to a single mutant gene but rather to a complex interaction of multiple genetic and environmental factors.

Most of the factors that place an individual in the upper part of the bell-shaped curve for cholesterol levels are not known. It is likely that subtle genetic differences exist among people with regard to many processes governing cholesterol metabolism. For example, among normal people there may be genetic polymorphisms in the proteins that govern the rates of intestinal cholesterol absorption, bile acid synthesis, cholesterol synthesis, and LDL synthesis or catabolism. Certain unfavorable combinations of these mildly altered proteins, coupled with an environmental challenge, such as a diet high in cholesterol or saturated fat, may raise the plasma cholesterol level.

Clinically, polygenic hypercholesterolemia can be distinguished from familial hypercholesterolemia and multiple lipoprotein-type hyperlipidemia in two ways: (1) family studies (hyperlipidemia is present in no more than 10 percent of first-degree relatives in polygenic hypercholesterolemia in contrast to 50 percent in the other two disorders) and (2) examination for tendon xanthomas (absent in both polygenic hypercholesterolemia and multiple lipoprotein-type hyperlipidemia but present in about 75 percent of adult heterozygotes with familial hypercholesterolemia).

Certain patients with polygenic hypercholesterolemia respond well to dietary restriction of saturated fat and cholesterol. Other patients require drug therapy to achieve a significant lowering of plasma cholesterol levels. Clofibrate is sometimes effective in this latter group. Cholestyramine may also be used.

SPORADIC HYPERTRIGLYCERIDEMIA In addition to the forms of primary hypertriglyceridemia that show familial aggregation, endogenous hypertriglyceridemia with or without hyperchylomicronemia is sometimes seen in individuals whose relatives do not manifest hyperlipidemia. For purposes of classification, this disorder is called sporadic hypertriglyceridemia. Affected patients comprise a heterogeneous group. Some would undoubtedly be classified under one of the genetic disorders described above if a larger number of relatives were available for lipid measurements. Other than an absence of hyperlipidemic relatives, patients with sporadic hypertriglyceridemia cannot be distinguished clinically from patients with the single-gene forms of primary hypertriglyceridemia. Inasmuch as patients with sporadic hypertriglyceridemia may develop hyperchylomicronemia and pancreatitis, they should be treated with diet and drugs as in the familial disease.

FAMILIAL HYPERALPHALIPOPROTEINEMIA This entity is characterized by elevated plasma levels of HDL, also called alpha lipoprotein. The plasma levels of LDL, VLDL, and triglycerides are normal. The elevated HDL causes a slight elevation in the total plasma cholesterol level. Although a selective elevation in plasma HDL cholesterol can be observed in individuals after exposure to chlorinated hydrocarbon pesticides, in alcoholism and after administration of exogenous estrogen, most cases of hyperalphalipoproteinemia have a genetic basis. In some hyperalphalipoproteinemia is inherited as an autosomal dominant trait, while in others a multifactorial or polygenic basis is suspected.

Individual subjects with familial hyperalphalipoproteinemia show no distinctive clinical features.

Statistical studies suggest that the hyperalphalipoproteinemia is associated with a slightly increased longevity and an apparent protection against myocardial infarction. The mechanism for the increase in plasma HDL levels in this disorder has not been determined.

SECONDARY HYPERLIPOPROTEINEMIAS

A variety of clinical disorders produce secondary hyperlipoproteinemias. These are summarized in Table 103-4 (see references). The most frequently encountered forms of secondary hyperlipoproteinemia occur in association with diabetes mellitus, consumption of alcohol, and ingestion of oral contraceptives.

DIABETES MELLITUS Three distinct patterns of hypertriglyceridemia occur in patients with diabetes mellitus. Classical "diabetic hyperlipemia" consists of a massive elevation in the plasma triglyceride level that occurs in patients who have suffered from insulin deficiency or insulin resistance for many weeks or months. Such insulin-deprived patients develop a progressive increase in concentration of plasma VLDL and eventually of chylomicrons as well. Triglyceride levels as high as 25,000 mg/dl are seen. Eruptive xanthomas, lipemia retinalis, and hepatomegaly can occur. Ketosis is frequently present, but severe acidosis is not characteristic. This form of massive hyperlipemia is only seen in partial insulin deficiency. Patients with this form of diabetic hyperlipidemia usually respond to a fat-free diet and to the administration of insulin, although triglyceride levels may not return entirely to normal.

The second type of hypertriglyceridemia in diabetics is associated with acute ketoacidosis. Such patients usually exhibit a mild hyperlipidemia with elevations of VLDL but not chylomicrons. On occasion, however, marked elevations of triglyceride are seen with lipemia retinalis. In this case both VLDL and chylomicrons are present.

The third type of hypertriglyceridemia is a mild to moderate elevation in plasma VLDL that persists even when patients appear to be adequately treated for their diabetes. This chronic triglyceride elevation generally occurs in patients who are obese. Inasmuch as most patients with well-controlled diabetes have normal plasma triglyceride levels, the occasional patient with persistent hypertriglyceridemia is likely to have an underlying familial hyperlipoproteinemic disorder. Indeed, family studies indicate that many of these patients have inherited the trait for familial hypertriglyceridemia in a pattern independent of the inheritance of diabetes mellitus.

The insulin deficiency or insulin resistance of diabetes produces a high VLDL level by two mechanisms. With acute insulin deprivation there is an increase in VLDL secretion from the liver as a secondary response to the increased mobilization of free fatty acids from adipose tissue. As the state of insulin deprivation becomes prolonged, the rate of removal of VLDL and chylomicrons from the circulation declines because lipoprotein lipase activity becomes diminished.

ALCOHOL CONSUMPTION In any individual the daily consumption of large amounts of ethanol can produce a mild, asymptomatic elevation in the plasma triglyceride level due to an elevation of VLDL. However, in a subgroup ethanol ingestion regularly produces massive and clinically significant hyperlipidemia with elevations in both VLDL and chylomicrons (type 5 lipoprotein pattern). In most of this group, the VLDL level remains mildly elevated (type 4 lipoprotein pattern), even in the basal state after recovery from the severe alcoholic hyperlipidemia. This suggests that these individuals have a form of familial hypertriglyceridemia or multiple lipoprotein-type hyperlipidemia that is exacerbated and converted to a type 5 pattern by the ethanol ingestion.

Ethanol elevates the plasma triglyceride level primarily because it inhibits fatty acid oxidation and enhances fatty acid synthesis in the liver. The excess fatty acids are esterified to triglyceride. Some of this excess triglyceride accumulates in the liver, producing the characteristic enlarged fatty liver of alcoholics. The remainder of the newly formed triglyceride is secreted into plasma, resulting in an increased secretion of VLDL. In those who develop massive alcoholic hyperlipidemia, there appears to be a partial defect in the catabolism of these VLDL particles. As the concentration of VLDL increases, the lipoprotein begins to compete with chylomicrons for hydrolysis by lipoprotein lipase, and the plasma concentration of chylomicrons also rises.

In severe alcoholic hyperlipidemia, eruptive xanthomas and lipemia retinalis are frequently present. The most serious complication is pancreatitis. Pancreatitis may be difficult to diagnose, since elevated triglyceride levels can interfere with the estimation of serum amylase. There is no solid evidence to indicate that pancreatitis itself can cause hyperlipidemia; rather the hyperlipidemia is the cause of the pancreatitis.

Plasma from patients with alcoholic hyperlipidemia is creamy in appearance. If a blood sample is drawn in EDTA and the plasma placed in the refrigerator at 4°C overnight, the chylomicrons float to the top, and the infranatant layer is turbid, owing to the combined elevation of VLDL and chylomicrons (type 5 pattern).

ORAL CONTRACEPTIVES The ingestion of estrogen-containing birth control pills is regularly associated with an increase in the VLDL secretion rate from the liver. In most women the catabolism of VLDL also increases, so that the overall increase in plasma triglyceride level is only modest. However, in women who have an underlying genetic disorder (such as familial hypertriglyceridemia or multiple lipoprotein-type hyperlipidemia) the plasma VLDL-triglyceride level can increase markedly, and hyperchylomicronemia can develop when estrogen-containing medications are taken. These women generally have mild to moderate hypertriglyceridemia prior to the institution of oral contraceptive therapy, and they presumably are unable to increase VLDL catabolism in response to the stimulation of VLDL production. As the plasma VLDL concentration rises, the elevated VLDL prevents the normal catabolism of chylomicrons by lipoprotein lipase, and secondary hyperchylomicronemia ensues. When the latter develops, severe pancreatitis can occur.

Ingestion of oral contraceptives has also been implicated as a risk factor in promoting thromboembolic disease in young women, especially those with preexisting hypercholesterolemia.

TABLE 103-5
Rare autosomal recessive disorders of lipid metabolism

Disorder	*Typical age of onset*	*Plasma lipid abnormality*	*Major clinical manifestations*	*Pathogenesis*	*Treatment*
Abetalipoproteinemia	Early childhood	Cholesterol, ~ 50 mg/dl; triglycerides, < 10 mg/dl	Malabsorption of fat, ataxia, neuropathy, retinitis pigmentosa, acanthocytosis	Defective synthesis of apoprotein B leads to absence of chylomicrons, VLDL, and LDL in plasma	Vitamin E
Tangier disease	Childhood	Cholesterol, 40 to 125 mg/dl; triglycerides, normal to slightly elevated	Large orange tonsils, corneal opacities, relapsing polyneuropathy No premature atherosclerosis	Absence of HDL from plasma leads to generation of abnormal chylomicron remnants, which are taken up and stored as cholesteryl esters in phagocytic cells	None
Lecithin:cholesterol acyltransferase (LCAT) deficiency	Young adult	Total plasma cholesterol level variable with marked decrease in esterified cholesterol and increase in unesterified cholesterol; elevated VLDL level Structure of all lipoproteins is abnormal	Corneal opacities, hemolytic anemia, renal insufficiency, premature atherosclerosis	Decreased LCAT activity in plasma leads to accumulation of excess unesterified cholesterol in plasma and body tissues	Fat-restricted diet, kidney transplantation
Cerebrotendinous xanthomatosis	Young adult	None	Progressive cerebellar ataxia, dementia and spinal cord paresis, subnormal intelligence, tendon xanthomas, cataracts	Defective synthesis of primary bile acids in liver leads to increased hepatic synthesis of cholesterol and cholestanol, which accumulate in brain, tendons, and other tissues	None
Sitosterolemia	Childhood	Elevated levels of plant sterols in plasma, elevated or normal levels of cholesterol, normal triglyceride levels	Tendon xanthomas	Increased intestinal absorption of dietary sitosterol and other plant sterols with accumulation in plasma and tendons	Diet low in plant sterols

Thus, it is important to measure the plasma cholesterol and triglyceride levels prior to the institution of birth control therapy. The finding of hyperlipidemia is a contraindication to the use of these drugs.

RARE DISORDERS OF LIPID METABOLISM

Table 103-5 summarizes the clinical and pathophysiological features of five rare disorders of lipid metabolism, each of which is inherited as an autosomal recessive trait. In two—abetalipoproteinemia and Tangier disease—the major effect of the abnormality is to cause a decrease in lipid levels in plasma. In two—cerebrotendinous xanthomatosis and sitosterolemia—the major effect of the inborn error is to cause an accumulation of unusual sterols in tissues. In LCAT deficiency, the underlying mutation produces both an abnormal pattern of lipoproteins in plasma and an accumulation of unesterified cholesterol in tissues.

REFERENCES

Brown MS et al: Familial type 3 hyperlipoproteinemia, in *The Metabolic Basis of Inherited Disease,* 5th ed, JB Stanbury et al (eds). New York, McGraw-Hill, 1983, chap 32

——— et al: Regulation of plasma cholesterol by lipoprotein receptors. Science 212:728, 1981

Goldstein JL, Brown MS: Familial hypercholesterolemia, in *The Metabolic Basis of Inherited Disease,* 5th ed, JB Stanbury et al (eds). New York, McGraw-Hill, 1983, chap 33

Havel RJ et al: Lipoprotein and lipid transport, in *Metabolic Control and Disease,* 8th ed, PK Bondy, LE Rosenberg (eds). Philadelphia, Saunders, 1980, chap 7

Levy RI: Drugs used in the treatment of hyperlipoproteinemias, in *The Pharmacological Basis of Therapeutics,* 6th ed, AG Gilman et al (eds). New York, Macmillan, 1980, chap 34

Nikkila E: Familial lipoprotein lipase deficiency and related disorders of chylomicron metabolism, in *The Metabolic Basis of Inherited Disease,* 5th ed, JB Stanbury et al (eds). New York, McGraw-Hill, 1983, chap 30

Stanbury JB et al (eds): *The Metabolic Basis of Inherited Disease,* 5th ed. New York, McGraw-Hill, 1983, chaps 29, 31, 34

104 LYSOSOMAL STORAGE DISEASES

ARTHUR L. BEAUDET

GENERAL FEATURES

DEFINITION Lysosomes are cytoplasmic organelles which enclose an acidic environment containing numerous enzymes capable of hydrolyzing most biological macromolecules (Fig. 104-1). Primary lysosomes, the original bodies derived from the Golgi apparatus, may fuse with other membrane-bound vesicles to form secondary lysosomes. Secondary lysosomes contain material derived from outside the cell through endocytosis or material from within the cell through autophagy. A major function of the lysosome is degradation of used macromolecules related to normal turnover and tissue remodeling. The lysosomal storage diseases emphasize the physiological significance of this disposal role. Recent studies of lipoprotein and vitamin B_{12} metabolism suggest that the lysosome is important not only in the processing of used macromolecules but also in the acquisition of essential compounds from the exterior of the cell through the process of endocytosis and degradation of carrier proteins. The lysosomal enzymes are glycoproteins which are synthesized within the endoplasmic reticulum. The initial products of translation undergo extensive modification including proteolytic cleavage, addition of complex oligosaccharides, synthesis of recognition markers (mannose 6-phosphate in some instances), and compartmentalization into primary lysosomes. These processes occur in the endoplasmic reticulum, in the Golgi apparatus, and probably in the primary, if not secondary, lysosomes as well.

The concept of lysosomal storage diseases arose from the studies of type II (Pompe) glycogen storage disease. The demonstration of lysosomal accumulation of glycogen as the result of α-glucosidase deficiency and data from other disorders led Hers to define an inborn lysosomal disease as one in which (1) a single lysosomal enzyme is deficient and (2) abnormal deposits (of substrate) lie within vacuoles related to lysosomes. This definition can be modified to include single gene defects affecting one or more lysosomal enzymes and thus encompass disorders such as the mucolipidoses and multiple sulfatase deficiency.

The lysosomal storage diseases include most of the lipid storage disorders, the mucopolysaccharidoses, the mucolipidoses, glycoprotein storage diseases, and others, as indicated in Table 104-1. The enzyme deficiencies have an autosomal recessive basis with the exception of Hunter mucopolysaccharidosis II (MPS II), which is X-linked recessive, and Fabry disease, which is X-linked with frequent manifestations in females. The target organs are determined by the usual sites of degradation

FIGURE 104-1

Biology of lysosomes. E represents lysosomal enzymes, including precursor forms. Lysosomal enzymes are synthesized in the endoplasmic reticulum and then undergo posttranslational processing that allows packaging into the primary lysosomes. The primary lysosomes can then undergo any of the several fates outlined.

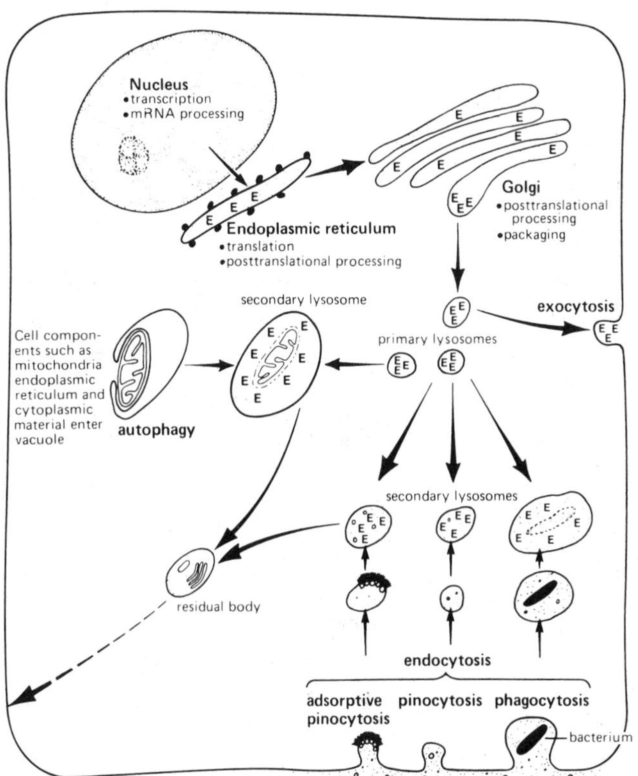

TABLE 104-1
Summary of lysosomal storage diseases

Disorder	*Heterogeneity (onset)*	*Enzyme deficiency*	*Stored material*	*Neurological*
G_{M1} gangliosidosis	Infantile (birth) Juvenile (6–20 mo) Adult	β-Galactosidase	G_{M1} ganglioside Glycoproteins Keratan sulfate	Mental retardation, seizures, blindness; later in juvenile form, variable in adults
Tay-Sachs and variants, G_{M2} gangliosidosis	Infantile (3–6 mo) Juvenile Adult forms	Hexosaminidase A	G_{M2} ganglioside	Mental retardation, seizures, blindness; later in juvenile form
Sandhoff, G_{M2} gangliosidosis	Infantile (3–6 mo)	Hexosaminidase A and B	G_{M2} ganglioside Globoside	Mental retardation, seizures, blindness
G_{M2} gangliosidosis, AB variant	Findings similar to Tay-Sachs except primary defect thought to be activator protein			
Krabbe, galactosylceramide lipidosis	Infantile (2–6 mo) Late onset	Galactosylceramide β-Galactosidase	↑ Galactoscerebroside/sulfatide ratio	Mental retardation, leukodystrophy; variable in late onset
Metachromatic leukodystrophy, sulfatide lipidosis	Late infantile (1–4 yr) Juvenile (4–20 yr) Adult	Arylsulfatase A (cerebroside sulfatase)	Galactosyl sulfatides	Mental retardation, leukodystrophy, psychosis and dementia in adults
Niemann-Pick, sphingomyelin lipidosis	Infantile neuropathic (1–4 mo) Late onset neuropathic Visceral	Sphingomyelinase ? Specific isozymes in some	Sphingomyelin	Mental retardation, 2594ia, and seizures in neuropathic forms
Gaucher, glucosylceramide lipidosis	Infantile (1–12 mo) Juvenile (2–6 yr) Adult	β-Glucocerebrosidase	Glucosylceramide	Mental retardation; spastic, later flaccid, ataxia in juvenile; no neurological symptoms in adult form
Fabry, trihexosyl ceramidosis	Hemizygous males Heterozygous females	α-Galactosidase A	Trihexosylceramide	Painful neuropathy
Acid lipase deficiency	Infantile Wolman disease (0–3 mo) Late onset cholesteryl ester storage disease	Acid lipase	Cholesteryl ester Triglyceride	Mental retardation but mild related to growth failure in Wolman; none in CESD
Farber, ceramide deficiency	Infantile (0–4 mo) Rare juvenile	Ceramidase	Ceramide	Occasional mental retardation, but may be secondary to somatic features
Pompe, glycogen storage type II	Infantile (0–6 mo) Juvenile Adult	Acid maltase (α-1,4- and 1,6-glucosidase)	Glycogen	Probably normal mentally
Acid phosphatase deficiency	Infantile (0–3 mo)	Acid phosphatase	Not characterized	Mental retardation

* *AR = autosomal recessive.*

Liver and/or spleen enlargement	*Skeletal dysplasia*	*Ophthalmic*	*Hematologic*	*Genetics*	*Unique manifestations*	*References*
++++ Less in juvenile, variable in adult	++++ Variable in juvenile and adult forms	Cherry red spot in 50% of infantile; corneal clouding variable but more in adults	Foam cells Vacuolated lymphocytes	AR*	Coarse facies, edema, macroglossia, mucopolysacchariduria; early blindness in infantile, milder in juvenile; in adults often spondyloepiphyseal dysplasia +/− mucopolysacchariduria	Hers and Van Hoof, chap 12 Stanbury et al, chap 46 Ho et al
0	0	Cherry red spot in infantile form, rare in juvenile	0	AR	Macrocephaly, hyperaucusis in infantile; increased in Ashkenazi Jews	Hers and Van Hoof, chap 13 Stanbury et al, chap 46 Ho et al
0	0	Cherry red spot	0	AR	Macrocephaly, hyperaucusis, visceral histiocytosis	Hers and Van Hoof, chap 14 Stanbury et al, chap 46 Ho et al
0	0	Optic atrophy	0	AR	Extreme irritability, ↑ CSF protein, fever, globoid cell neuropathology	Hers and Van Hoof, chap 17 Stanbury et al, chap 43 Ho et al
0	0	Optic atrophy, less in juvenile and adult forms	0	AR	↑ CSF protein and early gait abnormalities in late infantile; peripheral neuropathy	Hers and Van Hoof, chap 18 Stanbury et al, chap 44
++++ Less prominent in late onset forms	0	Macular degeneration and cherry red spot in neuropathic forms	Distinctive foam cell Vacuolated lymphocytes	AR	Pulmonary infiltrates, brownish skin, infantile neuronopathic form increased in Ashkenazi Jews, sea blue histiocytes	Hers and Van Hoof, chap 19 Stanbury et al, chap 41
++++ Hypersplenism common	++	Usually normal	Distinctive foam cell	AR	Adult form includes ↑ acid phosphatase, pathologic fractures; Ashkenazi Jewish predilection	Hers and Van Hoof, chap 16 Stanbury et al, chap 42 Ho et al
0	0	Corneal dystrophy, vascular lesions, cataracts	0	X-linked dominant	Cutaneous angiokeratoma, vascular thromboses, hypohidrosis	Hers and Van Hoof, chap 15 Stanbury et al, chap 45 Ho et al
+++	0	0	Foam cells Vacuolated lymphocytes	AR	Adrenal calcification, anemia, vomiting and poor growth in Wolman; hepatic fibrosis and ↑ blood cholesterol in CESD	Hers and Van Hoof, chap 20 Stanbury et al, chap 39
+/−	?	Mild macular degeneration	0	AR	Arthropathy—subcutaneous, periarticular and visceral nodules (lipogranulomatosis); ↑ CSF protein	Hers and Van Hoof, chap 24 Stanbury et al, chap 40 Ho et al
Mild hepatomegaly	0	0	0	AR	Lethal skeletal and cardiac myopathy in infantile; primarily skeletal myopathy in adults	See chap 97 Hers and Van Hoof, chap 7 Stanbury et al, chap 6
++	0	0	0	AR?	Lethal disorders described in two families	Hers and Van Hoof, chap 21 Hirschhorn and Weissmann

TABLE 104-1 *(continued)*
Summary of lysosomal storage diseases

Disorder	*Heterogeneity (onset)*	*Enzyme deficiency*	*Stored material*	*Neurological*
Fucosidosis	Infantile (3–12 mo) Juvenile	α-Fucosidase	Glycopeptides Glycolipids Oligosaccharides	Mental retardation
Mannosidosis	Infantile (6–18 mo) Milder form	α-Mannosidase	Oligosaccharides	Mental retardation
Aspartylglucosaminuria	Young adult onset	Aspartylglucosamine amidase	Aspartylglucosamine Glycopeptides	Mental retardation
Mucopolysaccharidosis 1H and 1S	Infantile Hurler (6–12 mo) Intermediate Adult Scheie	α-Iduronidase	Dermatan sulfate Heparan sulfate	Mental retardation, absent in Scheie
Hunter, mucopolysaccharidosis II	Severe infantile (6–12 mo) Mild juvenile	Iduronosulfate sulfatase	Dermatan sulfate Heparan sulfate	Mental retardation, less in mild form
Sanfilippo A, mucopolysaccharidosis III A	Late infantile (1–4 yr)	Heparan *N*-sulfatase (sulfamidase)	Heparan sulfate	Severe mental retardation
Sanfilippo B, mucopolysaccharidosis III B		*N*-Acetyl-α-glucosaminidase		
Sanfilippo C, mucopolysaccharidosis III C		Acetyl-CoA:α-glucosaminide *N*-acetyltransferase		
Sanfilippo D, mucopolysaccharidosis III D		*N*-Acetylglucosamine 6-sulfate sulfatase		
Morquio, mucopolysaccharidosis IV	Some variation	*N*-Acetylgalactosamine 6-sulfate sulfatase	Keratan sulfate	0
Maroteaux-Lamy, mucopolysaccharidosis VI	Variation in severity and cardiovascular involvement	*N*-Acetylhexosamine 4-sulfate sulfatase (arylsulfatase B)	Dermatan sulfate	0
β-Glucuronidase deficiency, mucopolysaccharidosis VII	Few patients; infantile to adult forms	β-Glucuronidase	Dermatan sulfate ? Heparan sulfate	Mental retardation ? absent in some adults
Multiple sulfatase deficiency	Late infantile (1–4 yr)	Arylsulfatases A, B, and C Other sulfatases	Sulfatides Mucopolysaccharides	Mental retardation
Sialidosis	Congenital, infantile, juvenile, cherry red spot myoclonus	Glycoprotein neuraminidase (sialidase)	Sialyloligosaccharides	Mental retardation, myoclonus
Mucolipidosis II, I cell disease	Infantile (0–3 mo)	UDP-*N*-acetylglucosamine (GlcNAc):glycoprotein GlcNAc1-phosphotransferase	Glycoproteins Glycolipids	Mental retardation
Mucolipidosis III, pseudo-Hurler polydystrophy	Late infantile (>2 yr)		Glycoproteins Glycolipids	Mild mental retardation
Mucolipidosis VI	Infantile	? Ganglioside neuraminidase	? Multiple	Mental retardation
Neuronal ceroid lipofuscinoses	Late infantile Juvenile Adult	Unknown	"Ceroid" "Lipofuscin"	Mental retardation, dementia variable in adults, seizures

Liver and/or spleen enlargement	*Skeletal dysplasia*	*Ophthalmic*	*Hematologic*	*Genetics*	*Unique manifestations*	*References*
++	++	0	Vacuolated lymphocytes Foam cells	AR	Coarse facies, increased sweat electrolytes, angiokeratoma in juvenile	Hers and Van Hoof, chap 11 Ho et al Stanbury et al, chap 38
+++	++	Cataracts, corneal clouding	Vacuolated lymphocytes Granulated neutrophils	AR	Coarse facies, enlarged tongue	Hers and Van Hoof, chap 11 Stanbury et al, chap 38
0	++	Lens opacities	Vacuolated lymphocytes	AR	Coarse facies, detectable by urine amino acid analysis	Hers and Van Hoof, chap 24 Stanbury et al, chap 38
+++	++++	Corneal clouding	Granulated lymphocytes	AR	Coarse facies, cardiovascular involvement, joint stiffness	Hers and Van Hoof, chaps 8 and 9 Stanbury et al, chap 36 McKusick
+++	++++	Retinal degeneration, no significant corneal clouding	Granulated lymphocytes	X-linked	Coarse facies, cardiovascular involvement, joint stiffness	
+	+	0	Granulated lymphocytes	AR	Mild coarsening of facies	
+	Severe, distinctive	Corneal clouding	Granulated neutrophils	AR	Severe deformity, odontoid hypoplasia, aortic regurgitation	
++	++++	Corneal clouding	Granulated neutrophils and lymphocytes	AR	Mild coarsening of facies, joint stiffness, valvular heart disease	
+++	+++	Corneal clouding	Granulated neutrophils	AR	Coarse facies, ↑ vascular involvement	
+	MPS features	Retinal degeneration	Vacuolated and granulated cells	AR	Icthyosis, combined MPS and metachromatic leukodystrophy phenotype	Hers and Van Hoof, chaps 8 and 18 Stanbury et al, chap 44
++ Less in late form	++ Less or absent in late form	Cherry red spot	Vacuolated lymphocytes	AR	MPS phenotype in all but cherry red spot myoclonus	Hers and Van Hoof, chap 8 Stanbury et al, chap 38
0/+	++++	Corneal clouding	Vacuolated and granulated neutrophils	AR	Coarse facies, inclusions in cultured fibroblasts, normal mucopolysacchariduria	Hers and Van Hoof, chap 8 Stanbury et al, chap 37
0	+++	Corneal clouding	Vacuolated plasma cells	AR	Coarse facies, inclusions in cultured fibroblasts, joint contractures, valvular heart disease, normal mucopolysacchariduria	
0	0	Corneal clouding, retinal degeneration	0	AR	Diagnosis based on electron microscopy; ? Ashkenazi Jewish predilection	Stanbury et al, chap 37
0	0	Optic atrophy, macular degeneration, retinitis pigmentosa	Vacuolated lymphocytes Granulated neutrophils	AR AR	Electron microscopy helpful, degree of genetic heterogeneity unknown	Hers and Van Hoof, chap 23

for a macromolecule. For example, cerebral white matter is affected in patients with defects in degradation of myelin, hepatosplenomegaly develops in those with defects in degradation of glycolipids from red cell stroma, and generalized tissue involvement may occur in patients with defects in the degradation of ubiquitous mucopolysaccharides. The accumulated material often causes visceromegaly or macrocephaly, but secondary atrophy also can occur, particularly in brain or muscle. In simple terms, the symptoms appear to be due to damage from stored material, but exactly how this causes cell death or dysfunction often is unclear. All the disorders are progressive, and many are fatal in childhood or adolescence. Definitive diagnosis is accomplished best by specific enzyme assays on serum, leukocytes, or cultured skin fibroblasts, selecting the appropriate tests on clinical grounds. There is extensive phenotypic variation within disorders with infantile, juvenile, and adult forms of many entities. In addition, varying combinations of visceral, skeletal, and neurological involvement can occur within a single enzyme disorder.

DIAGNOSIS A lysosomal storage disease is usually suspected on the basis of progressive neurological dysfunction, visceromegaly, skeletal dysostosis, or some more specific finding, as outlined in Table 104-1. Progressive or degenerative disease is the hallmark of these disorders. The superimposition of degeneration upon normal childhood development results in a slowing of progress prior to loss of previously acquired abilities. The history should focus on the course of childhood development, neurological symptoms, including seizures and visual or auditory impairment, the course of physical growth, and more specific findings such as coarsening facies, corneal clouding, exaggerated startle response, abdominal distention, joint pain, joint stiffness, hernias, and recurrent infection. The family history may reveal similarly affected siblings or consanguinity in autosomal recessive disease or other affected male family members in X-linked disorders. Ethnic background may be helpful since several lipid storage diseases are more frequent in Ashkenazi Jews and since disorders such as mannosidosis and aspartylglucosaminuria may occur with increased frequency in Scandinavian populations. The juvenile form of sialidosis is frequent in the Japanese.

On physical examination the head circumference may be enlarged. Gigantism occurs early in the course of some MPS disorders and glycoprotein storage diseases, while short stature is a later finding in many disorders. Ophthalmologic examination should include slit-lamp and careful funduscopic examination. Enlargement of the tongue, coarsening of the facies, and hepatosplenomegaly may occur. Skeletal findings may include gibbus deformity, broadening of the long bones, and joint stiffness. Cutaneous findings are rare except in fucosidosis, sialidosis, Fabry disease, and Hunter disease. Careful neurological examination should attempt to distinguish the extent of involvement of gray matter, white matter, and peripheral nerves. Preliminary diagnostic studies should include examination of the peripheral blood smear for vacuolated or granulated leukocytes, urinary spot test for mucopolysaccharide, and radiological bone survey. The preferred method of diagnosis is to use the above information to select specific enzyme assays in serum, leukocytes, or cultured skin fibroblasts. If a mucopolysaccharide screening test is positive or if clinical findings are suggestive, quantitative mucopolysaccharide analysis can be carried out. If a specific diagnosis is not readily established, biopsy of skin, bone marrow, rectal mucosa, liver, peripheral nerve, conjunctiva, or other tissue for light and electron microscopy can be helpful. Electron-microscopic findings can direct one toward or away from the general category of lysosomal storage diseases based on the presence or absence of engorged lysosomes. When significant evidence favors a lysosomal storage disease but no enzyme deficiency is demonstrable, chemical analysis of biopsy tissue from liver or brain is an appropriate investigative starting point.

HETEROGENEITY There is extensive clinical and biochemical heterogeneity within the lysosomal storage diseases. The biochemical genetic principles underlying this heterogeneity are reviewed in Chaps. 58 and 90. In general, a structural gene for lysosomal enzyme produces a product which acts to degrade one or more macromolecules. Most or all of the lysosomal enzymes undergo posttranslational modification to become glycoproteins, often resulting in a series of electrophoretic variants or isozymes. These isozymes may hydrolyze one or a variety of substrates, and the substrate specificity of particular isozymes may vary. Differences in substrate specificity also arise from the occurrence of similar but genetically distinct enzymes, for example, the β-galactosidases. Mutations within a gene may totally eliminate or reduce enzyme activity, alter the ability of the enzyme to undergo posttranslational modification, or alter the activity of the enzyme for specific substrates.

In most instances different mutations within the structural genes for lysosomal enzymes probably account for varying degrees of severity from individual to individual as well as for the diverse combinations of visceral, skeletal, neurological, ocular, and other manifestations. The heterogeneity is increased further by the recessive nature of most of the conditions in that each affected individual must have two mutant genes at the same locus. The exact mutation may vary in the two copies of the gene, making the patient a genetic compound heterozygote. In this instance either one or both genes may encode some form of residual enzyme activity for one or more substrates. An excellent example of a genetic compound is MPS I, to be discussed below. Although it is useful to characterize clinical phenotypes as infantile, juvenile, adult, neuropathic, or nonneuropathic, the existence of different mutant alleles and of genetic compounds provides an explanation for those occasional patients who appear aberrant or intermediate as compared with the usual phenotype. Another type of heterogeneity is illustrated by MPS III A, B, C, and D, which are relatively indistinguishable clinical disorders caused by different gene defects. Thus these genocopies demonstrate that biochemical heterogeneity can underlie apparent clinical homogeneity.

Further complexity results from the fact that certain enzyme activities are derived from complexes of nonidentical subunits. As a consequence, different mutations can cause deficiency of the same enzyme, as for example, hexosaminidase A deficiency in Tay-Sachs and Sandhoff diseases, and can explain multiple enzyme deficiencies due to a single gene defect as in Sandhoff disease. Genetic disorders involving the posttranslational modification of lysosomal enzymes and general defects in the integrity and function of the lysosome may also cause lysosomal storage diseases. The mucolipidoses II and III appear to represent situations in which a single gene defect alters the ability of a number of lysosomal enzymes to enter the lysosome. Thus, mutations outside the structural genes for the enzymes themselves can account for further heterogeneity. Better biochemical understanding of the identity, subunit structure, posttranslational processing, and substrate specificities of lysosomal enzymes should provide further insight into phenotypic and genotypic heterogeneity.

Clinical diagnosis is facilitated but also somewhat complicated by the widespread use of synthetic substrates for measuring lysosomal enzyme activities. These substrates often measure a group of related activities attributable to different enzymes. Thus, the activity of β-galactosidase using an artificial substrate may represent the sum of various β-galactosidases encoded by different structural genes and having different substrate specificities. Clinical reliability generally is achieved by manipulating in vitro conditions to reflect that enzyme activity whose deficiency is characteristic of a clinical disorder. Genetic heterogeneity has, however, resulted in individuals with mutant enzyme that either hydrolyzes the natural substrate and not the artificial substrate, or vice versa. This is exemplified by the normal individuals who have hexosaminidase A deficiency using artificial substrate and by patients with Tay-Sachs disease who have substantial levels of hexosaminidase A activity with artificial substrates. The presence or absence of disease correlates with ability to hydrolyze the natural G_{M2} ganglioside substrate. These phenomena have considerable significance for identification of affected patients, for heterozygote screening, and for prenatal diagnosis. They indicate the need to go beyond artificial substrate enzyme assays if normal results occur in the face of overwhelming clinical, electron-microscopic, or chemical evidence of a storage disease.

MANAGEMENT AND PREVENTION Specific therapy is not effective in lysosomal storage diseases at present, and care is largely symptomatic. The relentless, progressive course in many instances represents a tragic burden. Transplantation is effective in reversing the renal failure that commonly occurs in Fabry disease, and splenectomy frequently is helpful in adult Gaucher disease. Considerable attention has been focused on enzyme replacement for lysosomal storage diseases using organ or fibroblast transplantation or the infusion of either plasma, leukocytes, purified enzyme itself, or enzyme trapped in erythrocytes or liposomes. Although these approaches offer promise for treatment of manifestations outside the central nervous system, they are not of proved efficacy. The most distressing aspects of lysosomal storage diseases involve the central nervous system, where the blood-brain barrier presents an additional obstacle to the development of effective enzyme replacement therapy.

Genetic counseling is important in the management of these disorders. All the lysosomal storage diseases in which the specific enzyme deficiency is known either have been or presumably could be diagnosed in utero, since lysosomal enzyme activities appear to be expressed in cultured amniotic fluid cells as well as in cultured skin fibroblasts. Artificial insemination is an alternative for couples who have children affected with an autosomal recessive disease. Heterozygote detection in close relatives is frequently possible, although feasibility varies for the disease, and it can be difficult to achieve the statistical confidence desired for such determinations. Heterozygote detection is further complicated by lyonization for X-linked diseases, but counseling of females at risk in such families should be pursued vigorously. More effective approaches to prevention require identification of heterozygous couples prior to the birth of an affected offspring. The feasibility of this approach has been demonstrated by heterozygote testing programs for Tay-Sachs disease. Such programs could result in a decreased frequency of these disorders through extensive testing and appropriate reproductive decisions on the part of the rare couples identified as being at risk for having affected offspring; the high frequency of the heterozygous state in Ashkenazi Jews and favorable biochemical aspects of carrier detection for Tay-Sachs disease have facilitated this program. Efficient, accurate heterozygote detection methods would be needed to apply this approach to other diseases and to populations with lower heterozygote frequencies. Even under optimal conditions genetic variants might cause false-positive or false-negative results in any screening process.

SPECIFIC DISORDERS

SPHINGOLIPIDOSES **G_{M1} gangliosidosis** G_{M1} gangliosidosis was recognized in 1965 in infants with features of Tay-Sachs disease and mucopolysaccharidosis and is due to deficiency of β-galactosidase. Prominent features of the infantile form are the presence of abnormalities at or near birth, developmental delay, seizures, coarse facies, edema, hepatosplenomegaly, macroglossia, ocular cherry red spot, and a distinctive mucopolysaccharidosis-like dysostosis multiplex. Death usually occurs in the first or second year of life. The juvenile form is characterized by a later onset, survival to the latter half of the first decade, neurological impairment and seizures, and milder skeletal and ocular findings. In the adult form of spondyloepiphyseal dysplasia similar to MPS IV, corneal clouding and normal intelligence are common. Joint pain and limitation of motion, particularly at the hips, can be disabling in these patients. Prominent spasticity and ataxia with mild bony abnormalities have occurred in other adult patients. A high index of suspicion is necessary to recognize the diverse phenotypes caused by β-galactosidase deficiency in juvenile and adult patients, since almost any combination of skeletal, ocular, neurological, and visceral findings can occur. Isozymes of β-galactosidase occur, but evidence suggests that these derive from a single gene on chromosome 22. Thus, the diversity of phenotypes is due to different mutations in the structural gene. All forms of G_{M1} gangliosidosis have an autosomal recessive inheritance. There is no ethnic predilection. The frequency of the disease is low, with less than 50 patients reported for any given phenotype. Some patients originally reported to have β-galactosidase deficiency were subsequently shown to have sialidosis, and the β-galactosidase deficiency is now interpreted to be a secondary effect.

G_{M2} gangliosidosis Tay-Sachs disease, first recognized in 1881, is a relatively common inborn error of metabolism with thousands of documented cases. Although it is clinically very similar to Sandhoff disease, the two are genetically distinct with deficiency of hexosaminidase A in the former and hexosaminidase A and B in the latter. An additional disorder, called the AB variant of G_{M2} gangliosidosis, occurs with normal hexosaminidase A and B activity. This variant may be due to a deficiency of a protein factor (activator) necessary for activity of the enzyme against natural substrate. The presenting features are similar in all of the infantile disorders and include a developmental delay beginning in the third to sixth month with subsequent, rapidly progressive neurological deterioration. Macrocephaly, seizures, retinal cherry red spot, and an augmented startle response to sound suggest the diagnosis. The diagnosis is confirmed by enzyme assay. Most juvenile-onset patients with hexosaminidase deficiency present with dementia, seizures, and ocular findings, and some have an atypical spinocerebellar degeneration.

Sandhoff disease is nonallelic with Tay-Sachs disease, but the juvenile forms of hexosaminidase deficiency likely are allelic with Tay-Sachs disease. Tay-Sachs disease is the most frequent form of hexosaminidase deficiency, the risk being about 100 times higher in Ashkenazi Jews compared with other ethnic groups. All forms of G_{M2} gangliosidosis are autosomal recessive. There is evidence that hexosaminidase B is composed of β subunits whose structural locus is on chromosome 5, while hexosaminidase A is composed of α and β subunits with the structural locus for the α subunit on chromosome 15. Thus there is a defect in the α subunit in Tay-Sachs disease and in the β subunit in Sandhoff disease.

Although no specific therapy is available, extensive programs for heterozygote detection to prevent Tay-Sachs disease have been carried out throughout the world. As of 1979, more than 250,000 people had been tested, and more than 10,000 heterozygotes and 210 couples at risk for Tay-Sachs in their offspring had been identified. Four hundred forty-one pregnancies had been monitored by prenatal diagnosis because of a previous affected child, and 182 pregnancies had been monitored based on results of carrier screening by 1979.

LEUKODYSTROPHIES Krabbe galactosylceramide lipidosis or globoid cell leukodystrophy is an infantile disease due to deficiency of galactosylceramide β-galactosidase. The disorder is characterized by onset at 2 to 6 months of age, with irritability, hyperesthesia, hypersensitivity to external stimuli, unexplained fever, optic atrophy, and sometimes seizures. Spinal fluid protein is usually increased. Initially there is hypertonicity and increased deep tendon reflexes with progression to a hypotonic state. Rapid neurological deterioration and death occur within 1 to 2 years of onset. Premortem diagnosis is accomplished by enzyme assay. The presence of globoid cells on neuropathologic examination is characteristic and possibly specific for this enzyme deficiency. Galactosylceramide β-galactosidase functions in the degradation of sulfatides derived from myelin. Myelin synthesis is so impaired by tissue damage that the absolute amount of the galactocerebroside substrate is usually not increased in postmortem tissue. Galactosylceramide β-galactosidase is genetically distinct from the β-galactosidase that is deficient in G_{M1} gangliosidosis.

Krabbe disease is relatively rare, with about 150 reported cases and numerous unreported cases. It has an autosomal recessive genetic basis and is present in all ethnic groups with a possible increased frequency in the Scandinavian countries. Although no specific therapy is available, prenatal diagnosis has been accomplished.

Deficiency of arylsulfatase A (cerebroside sulfatase) is the basis of metachromatic leukodystrophy, a lipid storage disease with a frequency of 1 in 40,000. The age of onset is later than that in Tay-Sachs disease or Krabbe disease. Patients develop the ability to walk and frequently present with gait abnormalities in the second to fourth year of life. Initially the patients may be hypotonic with decreased deep tendon reflexes, the latter reflecting peripheral nerve involvement. The disease progresses over the first decade to include ataxia, increased muscle tone, decorticate or decerebrate posturing, and eventual loss of all contact with surroundings. Duration of survival depends on nursing care and support such as nasogastric or gastrostomy feeding.

Although some diagnostic studies have been performed on urine, leukocytes or fibroblasts are preferable for diagnostic enzyme assay. Changes demonstrable on metachromatic staining of nerve tissue are nonspecific and not an adequate substitute for enzyme assay. Rare patients with a juvenile form of metachromatic leukodystrophy are described with an onset between 4 and 20 years of age and a slower progression. The adult form of this disease deserves special mention as an example of the difficulties presented by subtle, slowly progressive forms of lysosomal storage diseases. The onset is in the second to fifth decade with a slowly progressive dementia. Emotional difficulties, motor dysfunction, and indistinct speech are often present. Even though conduction velocity in peripheral nerves is usually diminished, the deep tendon reflexes are often increased. Typical premortem diagnoses include organic dementia, schizophrenia, and multiple sclerosis; a correct premortem diagnosis has been made in only a minority.

Arylsulfatase A is routinely measured using artificial substrate, and complexities involving low levels of activity in normal individuals and moderate levels of residual activity in symptomatic patients have been described. Heterogeneity involving mutations in multiple components of the cerebroside sulfatase activity may exist, but the majority of patients probably have simple allelic disorders on an autosomal recessive basis. A few cases of sulfatide lipidosis with normal arylsulfatase A activity may represent deficiency of some other required factor. Arylsulfatase A deficiency also occurs in multiple sulfatase deficiency discussed below.

NIEMANN-PICK DISEASE Niemann-Pick disease is a sphingomyelin lipidosis. In type A and B disease, there is a clear deficiency of sphingomyelinase, an enzyme that hydrolyzes sphingomyelin to yield ceramide and phosphorylcholine. The most common disorder, Niemann-Pick A, is an infantile neuropathic disorder which begins shortly after birth with hepatosplenomegaly, failure to thrive, and neurological impairment. Retinal cherry red spots occur, but seizures and hypersplenism are rare. The diagnosis can be made with considerable confidence by recognition of the distinctive Niemann-Pick cell in the bone marrow but should be confirmed by enzyme assay. Niemann-Pick B disease is a relatively benign disorder with hepatosplenomegaly, sphingomyelinase deficiency, and sometimes pulmonary infiltrates; but there is no neurological involvement. Niemann-Pick C disease is characterized by sphingomyelin lipidosis, progressive neurological deterioration in childhood, and substantial or normal sphingomyelinase activity. Niemann-Pick D disease resembles type C but is separated primarily on the basis of occurrence in a Nova Scotian population. Niemann-Pick E disease describes a group of patients with visceral sphingomyelin lipidosis without neurological involvement and without sphingomyelinase deficiency. The biochemical basis for Niemann-Pick types C, D, and E is not understood. Many patients described with the sea blue histiocyte syndrome may have had sphingomyelinase deficiency; other patients with the sea blue histiocyte syndrome may represent unique disorders not yet biochemically characterized.

GAUCHER DISEASE Gaucher disease is a glucosylceramide lipidosis caused by deficiency of glucosylceramidase. An infantile form is characterized by early onset, marked hepatosplenomegaly, and severe neurological progression to early death. A juvenile form with milder neurological involvement exists. The adult form of the disease may be the most commonly encountered lysosomal storage disease. Patients with juvenile and adult Gaucher disease have been observed within the same family but not within the same sibships, suggesting that these are allelic disorders.

All forms of Gaucher disease have an autosomal recessive genetic basis. The disorder is about 30 times more frequent in Ashkenazi Jews, with an incidence in this ethnic group of about 1 in 2500 births. Although commonly termed "adult Gaucher disease," this variant frequently has its onset in childhood. Absence of neurological involvement is the criterion for inclusion in this category. Manifestations include hepatosplenomegaly, hypersplenism, bleeding diathesis, bone pain, pathological fractures, and pulmonary involvement with associated pneumonia. Serum acid phosphatase is characteristically elevated. A distinctive storage cell occurs in the bone marrow in all forms of Gaucher disease, but enzyme assay should be performed because the Gaucher cell may also be found in patients with granulocytic leukemia and myeloma.

The clinical course is variable; pulmonary involvement may lead to early death, but in many patients life span is not shortened by the disease. Bleeding secondary to thrombocytopenia frequently responds to splenectomy with considerable benefit. Because of the frequency of the disease and the lack of neurological involvement, the adult form of Gaucher disease is particularly worthy of research efforts to develop enzyme replacement therapy.

FABRY DISEASE Fabry disease involves the accumulation of a trihexoside, galactosylgalactosylglucosylceramide due to deficiency of α-galactosidase A. The disorder is X-linked, and the most severe symptoms are in affected males. Onset is in childhood with periodic crises of severe pain in the extremities, cutaneous angiokeratomas, a characteristic corneal dystrophy, hypohidrosis, vascular thromboses, and progressive renal impairment. Death most often results from renal failure, typically in the third to fifth decade. Heterozygous females are affected more mildly. Corneal dystrophy is the most frequent finding, but all other manifestations may be seen also. Life expectancy is greater in women, although fatal complications can occur rarely. Renal failure can be treated by chronic dialysis or transplantation. Enzyme replacement therapy has been attempted in this disease. In addition, patients undergoing transplantation presumably derive normal enzyme from the transplanted kidney. Administration of phenytoin sodium (Dilantin) has been used in treatment of the painful neuropathy.

The α-galactosidase A structural gene may reside on the X chromosome, although alternative explanations involving regulatory components have been suggested. Clinically the disorder should be considered as an X-linked dominant, since heterozygous females usually manifest the condition.

ACID LIPASE DEFICIENCY Acid lipase deficiency is the basis for two disorders with different phenotypic features. Wolman disease is a severe disorder of early onset, with prominent hepatosplenomegaly, anemia, vomiting, failure to thrive, and characteristic adrenal calcification. Neurological involvement is minimal compared with the severe somatic handicap. Cholesteryl ester storage disease is a rare disorder with mild phenotypic features by comparison. The most constant features are hepatosplenomegaly and increased plasma cholesterol. Hepatic fibrosis, esophageal varices, and poor growth have occurred. One reported sibship may represent an intermediate phenotype, since two females died at 7 and 9 years of age with unexplained acute hepatic failure, and a third sibling developed adrenal calcification and pulmonary hypertension early in life. Tissues from patients with acid lipase deficiency demonstrate inability to hydrolyze triglycerides as well as cholesteryl esters. Possibly a single enzyme hydrolyzes multiple substrates, but the subunit structure and hydrolytic capacities of various lysosomal lipases are not well studied. Deficiency of acid lipase results in impairment of the LDL pathway as described in Chap. 103 and may be associated with premature atherosclerosis. Both Wolman and cholesteryl ester storage diseases have an autosomal recessive basis.

GLYCOPROTEIN STORAGE DISORDERS Fucosidosis, mannosidosis, and aspartylglucosaminuria are rare, autosomal recessive disorders involving hydrolases that degrade polysaccharide linkages. Glycolipids as well as glycoproteins are accumulated in fucosidosis. All are characterized by neurological impairment and varying somatic involvements, as outlined in Table 104-1. Fucosidosis and mannosidosis are most often lethal disorders in childhood, while aspartylglucosaminuria presents as a late-onset lysosomal storage disease with prominent mental retardation and a prolonged course. Abnormal sweat electrolytes and cutaneous angiokeratomas are distinctive in fucosidosis, and an unusual cartwheel-type cataract occurs in mannosidosis. Aspartylglucosaminuria is remarkable in that urinary amino acid analysis is diagnostic with an increase of aspartylglucosamine; it is more frequent in the Finnish population. Sialidosis encompasses a group of phenotypes associated with glycoprotein neuraminidase (sialidase) deficiency. The phenotypes include an adult cherry red spot myoclonus syndrome, infantile and juvenile presentations with mucopolysaccharidosis-like phenotypes, and a congenital presentation with hydrops fetalis. Many patients previously classified as mucolipidosis I have been proved to have mannosidosis or sialidosis. Some patients with sialidosis have β-galactosidase deficiency as well as neuraminidase deficiency. The former defect is thought to be secondary but led to some sialidosis patients being reported initially as having G_{M1} gangliosidosis. Each of the glycoprotein storage diseases can be diagnosed by appropriate enzyme assay.

MUCOPOLYSACCHARIDOSIS (MPS) The mucopolysaccharidoses represent a broad spectrum of disorders due to deficiencies of one of a group of enzymes which degrade three classes of mucopolysaccharides: heparan sulfate, dermatan sulfate, and keratan sulfate. The general MPS phenotype includes coarse facies, corneal clouding, hepatosplenomegaly, joint stiffness, hernias, dysostosis multiplex, mucopolysaccharide excretion in the urine, and metachromatic staining in peripheral leukocytes and bone marrow. Various components of the MPS phenotype are also found in the mucolipidoses, glycoprotein storage disorders, and other lysosomal storage diseases. Detailed clinical and radiologic evaluation and identification of the type of MPS excreted in the urine help to narrow the diagnostic possibilities. Definitive diagnosis requires assay of specific enzymes in various tissues such as cultured skin fibroblasts.

The Hurler or MPS IH disorder is the prototype MPS. Virtually all the components of the phenotype mentioned above are present and expressed in a severe degree. Nasal congestion and grossly visible corneal clouding are early features. Excessive growth during the first year of life is followed by poor growth late in the course. Radiologic features include enlargement of the sella turcica with a distinctive "shoe-shaped" fossa, broadening and shortening of the long bones, and hypoplasia and beaking of the vertebrae in the lumbar area. The vertebral beaking gives rise to an accentuated kyphosis or gibbus deformity. Death occurs within the first decade; postmortem findings include hydrocephalus and cardiovascular disease due to occlusion of the coronary arteries. The biochemical defect is α-iduronidase deficiency with accumulation of heparan sulfate and dermatan sulfate.

MPS IS, or Scheie syndrome, a clinically distinct disorder with childhood onset but adult survival, is characterized by joint stiffness, corneal clouding, aortic regurgitation, and usually normal intelligence. Surprisingly, this much milder disorder is also the result of α-iduronidase deficiency; it is allelic with the Hurler syndrome, as shown by lack of cross-correction of enzyme activity in cocultures of skin fibroblasts. Phenotypes occur that are clearly intermediate between Hurler and Scheie syndromes. It is believed that patients with an intermediate phenotype represent genetic compounds with one Hurler allele and one Scheie allele. Although genetic compounds must occur, in any one case their existence is difficult to distinguish from still other mutations of intermediate severity.

The Hunter or MPS II syndrome is distinguishable from the Hurler phenotype by the absence of gross corneal clouding and the X-linked recessive inheritance. The infantile form resembles the Hurler phenotype, and a milder form allows survival into adulthood. The severe and mild forms may be allelic, since both are sex-linked and share the same enzyme deficiency (iduronosulfate sulfatase).

The Sanfilippo mucopolysaccharidoses (MPS IIIA, IIIB, IIIC, and IIID) are distinguished by the accumulation of heparan sulfate without dermatan or keratan sulfate and by the marked central nervous system involvement with milder somatic involvement. Because the somatic features of this MPS are mild, the condition can be overlooked in the evaluation of an apparently isolated central nervous system problem. Death usually occurs during the second or third decade. The MPS III disorders are approximate genocopies. That is, four different enzyme deficiencies give rise to relatively indistinguishable clinical phenotypes with the same storage product. The four MPS III disorders can be diagnosed and distinguished by enzyme assay (Table 104-1).

The Morquio or MPS IV syndrome is distinguished by the absence of mental retardation and the presence of a distinctive bony dystrophy which can be classified as a spondyloepiphyseal dysplasia. Marked hypoplasia of the odontoid process can cause cervical dislocation and usually leads to some degree of spinal cord compression. Aortic regurgitation is frequent. The deficiency of *N*-acetylgalactosamine 6-sulfate sulfatase is the basis for this condition. Bone changes somewhat suggestive of the Morquio syndrome may also occur in β-galactosidase deficiency and in other forms of spondyloepiphyseal dysplasia. The Maroteaux-Lamy or MPS VI disorder is characterized by prominent osseous involvement, corneal clouding, and normal intellect. Allelic forms with variable severity but the same deficiency of arylsulfatase B (*N*-acetylhexosamine 4-sulfate sulfatase) have been described. MPS VII, or β-glucuronidase deficiency has been described in only a few patients with a rather complete MPS phenotype. Extreme variability from a lethal infantile form to a mild adult disease occurs.

MULTIPLE SULFATASE DEFICIENCY Multiple sulfatase deficiency is a unique disorder, which, although autosomal recessive, is characterized by deficiency of five or more cellular sulfatases. Arylsulfatase A, arylsulfatase B, other mucopolysaccharide sulfatases, and a nonlysosomal placental sulfatase are deficient in this condition. The clinical picture combines features of metachromatic leukodystrophy, an MPS phenotype, and ichthyosis. The last feature presumably relates to the placental sulfatase deficiency which also occurs as an isolated X-linked enzyme deficiency characterized by abnormal parturition and ichthyosis. Biochemical studies of this condition should provide further insight into biochemical and clinical genetic heterogeneity.

MUCOLIPIDOSES Mucolipidosis is a general term for lysosomal storage diseases involving some combination of MPS, glycoprotein, oligosaccharide, and glycolipids. The category of mucolipidosis I probably can be abandoned since most or all of these patients actually have a specific glycoprotein storage disease.

Mucolipidosis II, or I-cell disease, is an early-onset disorder with mental retardation and an MPS phenotype. The distinctive features are striking inclusions in cultured skin fibroblasts and markedly elevated serum levels of lysosomal enzymes. The disorder has an autosomal recessive basis and is thought to involve a defect in the processes for entry into, or maintenance of, lysosomal enzymes within that organelle. Mucolipidosis III or pseudo-Hurler polydystrophy is a milder disorder with many aspects of the MPS phenotype, particularly dysostosis multiplex. The disorder presents in the first decade with joint stiffness, the diagnosis of rheumatoid arthritis often being considered. The major handicaps are progressive physical disabilities, particularly claw hand deformity and hip dysplasia. Mild mental retardation is common. Aortic and/or mitral valvular disease is routinely present, although often not functionally significant. Survival into adult life with possible stabilization of the condition is characteristic, with greater disability in males than in females. Inclusions in cultured skin fibroblasts and elevation of serum lysosomal enzymes are essentially identical with the findings in mucolipidosis II, suggesting that these may be allelic disorders. The primary defect in mucolipidosis II and III appears to be deficiency of UDP-*N*-acetylglucosamine (GLcNAc):glycoprotein GLcNAc 1-phosphotransferase, an enzyme involved in posttranslational synthesis of the oligosaccharide portion of the lysosomal enzymes.

Mucolipidosis IV is a disorder with mental retardation, corneal clouding, and retinal degeneration without other somatic features. Diagnosis has been made primarily on electron-microscopic findings. A small number of patients, all of Ashkenazi Jewish origin, have been described. The disorder may be due to deficiency of a neuraminidase which is active against ganglioside substrates.

NEURONAL CEROID LIPOFUSCINOSES The neuronal ceroid lipofuscinosis group of disorders includes a wide clinical spectrum with onset in childhood, juvenile, or adult periods. It is uncertain if these disorders are true lysosomal storage diseases, indeed whether single or multiple biochemical genetic disorders are present in the patients reported. The clinical features include central nervous system deterioration with cerebral atrophy, usually commensurate with degree of impairment. Seizures, particularly myoclonic jerks, are a prominent feature. Ocular involvement with optic atrophy, retinitis pigmentosa, and macular degeneration is present in the infantile and juvenile disorders but often absent in adult forms. Autosomal recessive inheritance is likely in most instances. The neuropathologic findings form the basis of the descriptive term for the disease. Electron microscopy demonstrates abnormal inclusions within lysosomes throughout a wide variety of tissues, despite the rather isolated neurological clinical involvement. The presence of curvilinear bodies, electron-dense material, and fingerprint profiles on electron microscopy of white blood cells, liver biopsy, or muscle biopsy can be helpful diagnostically.

OTHER LYSOSOMAL STORAGE DISEASES Glycogen storage disease type II (Pompe disease) is the prototype lysosomal storage disease. The predominant clinical features of skeletal and cardiac myopathy are described in Chap. 100. Acid phosphatase deficiency and Farber lipogranulomatosis are included in Table 104-1. Lactosyl ceramidosis appears to represent a variant of Niemann-Pick disease; in vitro hydrolysis of lactosyl ceramide is accomplished by those enzymes that are deficient in G_{M1} gangliosidosis or in Krabbe disease, depending upon the in vitro conditions used. Reports of *N*-acetylglucosamine 6-sulfate sulfatase deficiency causing a type VIII mucopolysaccharidosis may be incorrect. Adrenoleukodystrophy is identifiable as a distinct X-linked disorder with accumulation of long-chain fatty acid cholesteryl esters in tissues, but it may not represent a lysosomal storage disease. The recognition of females with the Hunter MPS II phenotype and identical enzyme deficiency has raised the possibility of an autosomal recessive form of the Hunter syndrome. Such could occur if the enzyme in question had nonidentical subunits coded for by one autosomal and one X-linked gene, or if regulatory genetic elements were invoked. On the other hand females with phenotypic manifestations could occur, owing to X-chromosome inactivation. One family has been described with G_{M3} gangliosidosis. This is not a lysosomal storage disease but does possibly represent a defect in ganglioside synthesis. The clinical features are similar to those seen in lysosomal storage diseases, but inconsistencies between siblings leave question of whether this is a unique genetic disorder. Other neurodegenerative diseases may eventually become classifiable as lysosomal storage diseases. Disorders such as juvenile dystonic lipidosis, neuroaxonal dystrophy, Hallervorden-Spatz disease, Pelizaeus-Merzbacher disease, and other candidates exist. In addition, it is not unusual to identify patients with distinctive clinical features suggestive of lipidosis, mucolipidosis, or mucopolysaccharidosis, in which none of the present biochemically identifiable disorders can be identified. For these reasons, the number of distinct lysosomal storage diseases is likely to continue to increase.

REFERENCES

HERS HG, VAN HOOF F (eds): *Lysosomes and Storage Diseases.* New York, Academic, 1973

HIRSCHHORN R, WEISSMANN G: Genetic disorders of lysosomes, in *Progress in Medical Genetics,* AG Steinberg et al, (eds). Philadelphia, Saunders, 1976, vol 1

HO MW et al: Glycosphingolipid hydrolases: Properties and molecular genetics. Mol Cell Biochem 17:125, 1977

MCKUSICK VA: *Heritable Disorders of Connective Tissue,* 4th ed. St Louis, Mosby, 1972

O'BRIEN JS: Neuraminidase deficiency in the cherry red spot–myoclonus syndrome. Biochem Biophys Res Comm 79:1136, 1977

STANBURY JB et al (eds): *The Metabolic Basis of Inherited Disease,* 5th ed. New York, McGraw-Hill, 1983

105
THE LIPODYSTROPHIES AND OTHER RARE DISORDERS OF ADIPOSE TISSUE

DANIEL W. FOSTER

This chapter is concerned with syndromes characterized by abnormalities in adipose tissue. The disorders are rare, the pathophysiology is frequently not clear, and only clinical descriptions can be given.

THE LIPODYSTROPHIES

The lipodystrophies are characterized by generalized or partial loss of body fat and a series of metabolic abnormalities, including insulin resistance, hyperglycemia, and hypertriglyceridemia.

GENERALIZED LIPODYSTROPHY Generalized lipodystrophy (also called lipoatrophic diabetes) may be either congenital or acquired. The congenital form is transmitted as an autosomal recessive trait. Rates of parental consanguinity are high. Loss of fat is obvious at birth, but the rest of the clinical picture may not develop until later. The acquired disease often develops after some other illness. Infections such as measles, chicken pox, whooping cough, or infectious mononucleosis are common precipitating events, but hypothyroidism, hyperthyroidism, and pregnancy have also been implicated. Some cases begin with the appearance of painful nodular swellings of adipose tissue resembling acute panniculitis (see below). While certain differences exist, the congenital and acquired forms are similar in clinical manifestations (Table 105-1).

Fat atrophy Loss of body fat is the characteristic finding. In congenital cases the skin of the face is tightly drawn over the bony structures, and the entire body is devoid of adipose tissue. Rarely, a small amount of breast fat remains. In the acquired form the face may be spared, but all other fat disappears. Adipose tissue cells can be identified microscopically, but they contain no triglyceride stores. Paradoxically the liver is stuffed with fat, and the reticuloendothelial system contains lipid-laden macrophages (foam cells). The cause of the fat atrophy is not known. No uniform abnormality in triglyceride transport, triglyceride synthesis, or lipolysis has been found. Fat-mobilizing polypeptides have been reported in the urine of patients with generalized lipodystrophy, but their role in the disease is uncertain. Release of free fatty acids into plasma following norepinephrine infusion is impaired, but this may simply reflect the depleted triglyceride stores. Adipose tissue from a dystrophic site in a patient with partial lipodystrophy accumulates fat when transplanted into a normal region of the body, while fat from an uninvolved region loses its triglyceride on transplantation to a dystrophic area, suggesting a localized (neuropathic?) cause for fat atrophy.

Growth and maturation Linear growth is accelerated in the first few years of life in the congenital disorder and in acquired disease that begins early in childhood. Epiphyses close early, however, so that the final height in most patients is normal. True muscular hypertrophy is present, and patients may have an acromegalic appearance with coarse facial features and large hands and feet. The ears tend to be prominent in the congenital form. Many viscera are enlarged, and generalized lymphadenopathy may be present.

Liver The liver is uniformly enlarged, and as a consequence the abdomen is protuberant. Fatty liver may progress to cirrhosis, especially in the acquired form. Several patients have died from bleeding esophageal varices. Splenomegaly probably does not occur in the absence of portal hypertension.

Kidneys The kidneys are usually enlarged. Subjects with the acquired disorder may have proteinuria and the nephrotic syndrome, although not as frequently as in partial lipodystrophy. Moderate hypertension is common.

Genitalia The external genitalia (penis and testes in males, clitoris in females) are usually hypertrophied in congenital disease. In women polycystic ovaries are common, resulting in the clinical picture of Stein-Leventhal syndrome.

TABLE 105-1
Characteristics of the lipodystrophies

Finding	*Congenital general*	*Acquired general*	*Acquired partial*	*Dominant partial*
Inheritance	Autosomal recessive	Sporadic	Usually sporadic	Autosomal dominant
Age of onset	Infancy	Childhood to adult	Childhood to adult	Puberty
Sex incidence	Males and females equal	Female preponderance	Female preponderance	Female preponderance
Lipoatrophy	Face, trunk, limbs	Face, trunk, limbs	Face, upper trunk, upper limbs	Trunk and limbs
Liver involvement	+	++	Rare	0
Renal disease	+	+	++	0
Insulin resistance	+	+	+	+
Hyperglycemia	+	+	+	+
Hypertriglyceridemia	+	+	+	+
Acanthosis nigricans	+	+	Rare	+
Genital hypertrophy	+	+	Rare	+
Bone age	Accelerated	Normal to accelerated	Normal	Normal

Skin Acanthosis nigricans is present in most. Hypertrichosis of face, neck, trunk, and limbs is frequent. Scalp hair is usually thick and curly, particularly early in life.

Central nervous system Mental retardation is present in about half the congenital cases. Dilatation of the third ventricle and basal cisterns has been demonstrated by pneumoencephalography. Central nervous system involvement is less marked in the acquired disease, although two patients had astrocytomas arising in the floor of the third ventricle.

Metabolic and endocrine abnormalities Three major metabolic disturbances are characteristic.

1 *Severe insulin resistance with hyperglycemia.* The nature of the insulin resistance is not known. Diminished binding of insulin to its receptor has been reported in monocytes from affected individuals, but in cultured fibroblasts the issue is less clear, at least two studies reporting normal binding characteristics. In one report impaired insulin action on intracellular chemical sequences was found despite apparently normal receptor function, suggesting that the insulin resistance was postreceptor in type. Despite profound insulin resistance, ketoacidosis does not occur, even in the face of severe hyperglycemia. The capillary basement membranes in skeletal muscle are not thickened, differentiating this condition from the common forms of diabetes mellitus.
2 *Hypertriglyceridemia with accumulation of both chylomicrons and very low density lipoproteins in the blood.* Eruptive xanthoma and recurrent pancreatitis may be seen, presumably precipitated by hypertriglyceridemia. Cause of the hyperlipemia is not known, although it has been speculated that insulin resistance leads to a defect in clearance of lipoproteins from plasma.
3 *A hypermetabolic state with normal thyroid function.* Basal metabolic rates are usually markedly elevated although thyroid hormone values (T_4, T_3, rT_3) are normal. Patients do not gain weight with excessive caloric intake, indicating a facile capacity to waste calories as heat. Thyroidectomy in one patient decreased but did not normalize the basal metabolic rate; symptoms and signs of hypothyroidism supervened in this patient, requiring treatment with thyroid hormone despite continued high metabolic rates. It thus seems clear that hypermetabolism is not due to hyperthyroidism.

Endocrine status has not been systematically evaluated. In one patient basal concentrations of LH, FSH, TSH and growth hormone were normal while prolactin and ACTH levels were high. Response of TSH to stimulation by thyrotropin-releasing hormone (TRH) was increased while suppression of ACTH by dexamethasone was impaired. Galactorrhea and amenorrhea developed following plasmapheresis for treatment of hypertriglyceridemia. The extent to which these findings apply to other cases is not known.

ACQUIRED PARTIAL LIPODYSTROPHY This is the most common of the lipodystrophies and usually affects women. Fat atrophy occurs in the upper half of the body, including the face, but spares the lower extremities. Rarely the lower half of the body is affected, leaving the upper torso intact. Occasionally the lesion affects only one side. The other anatomic features of generalized lipodystrophy are usually absent, and liver disease appears to be rare. Proteinuria, with or without the nephrotic syndrome, occurs much more frequently than in other forms. The complement system is abnormal, and C_3 levels tend to be low. C_3 nephritic factor, a polyclonal IgG immunoglobulin which interacts with alternative pathway convertase to augment C_3 activation, is found in the serum of affected subjects. C_3 levels may be low in unaffected first-degree relatives, but C_3 nephritic factor is absent. Dermatomyositis and Sjögren's syndrome occur in some patients. Rarely partial lipodystrophy converts or progresses to the generalized form of the disease.

LIPODYSTROPHY WITH DOMINANT TRANSMISSION This variant is characterized by fat atrophy of the limbs and trunk with sparing of the face, which may actually be rounded. The neck may also be exempt. The disease usually begins at puberty but may not appear until middle age. Males are rarely affected. Insulin resistance and hyperglycemia are usual, and severe hypertriglyceridemia with eruptive xanthoma may occur. The labia majora are hypertrophied, and polycystic ovaries may be seen. Acanthosis nigricans is usually present. Liver and renal disease do not occur.

MULTIPLE SYMMETRIC LIPOMATOSIS

This disease is characterized by the formation of multiple, nonencapsulated lipomas in the nape of the neck, supraclavicular, and deltoid regions to produce an extraordinary bull-necked appearance (sometimes called *Madelung collar*). Lipomas can also appear elsewhere in the body. Expansion of the lipomas with infiltration between fascial planes can cause tracheal, laryngeal, and mediastinal compression. Most cases occur in alcoholics for reasons that are not clear. Hypertriglyceridemia, hyperuricemia, hyperinsulinemia, and renal tubular acidosis have been reported in some subjects.

The etiology is not known. Fat cells in the tumors are small, suggesting new formation of adipocytes rather than a defect in triglyceride storage. Catecholamine-induced lipolysis is impaired in tumor tissue, but this may be a result rather than the cause of the lesion. A significant amount of the adipose tissue in the lipomas has the characteristics of brown rather than white fat, but the meaning of this finding is unclear.

In the familial form of multiple lipomatosis the distribution of lipomas is much more general; i.e., lesions are not limited to the neck region. Inheritance appears to be autosomal dominant in nature. It is not known whether this condition is a variant of multiple symmetric lipomatosis or a different disease.

ADIPOSIS DOLOROSA

Adiposis dolorosa is characterized by the presence of painful, circumscribed fatty deposits in the subcutaneous tissue of the extremities and occasionally elsewhere in the body. The face is not involved. Pain may occur spontaneously or upon pressure. Involved areas vary in size from 0.5 to 5.0 cm. Affected subjects are usually obese, postmenopausal women who have weakness and asthenia. Epilepsy has been noted in a number of cases, and emotional instability or frank dementia may be present. Most cases probably are sporadic, but familial inheritance in a dominant pattern has been noted. Microscopic examination of involved adipose tissue shows granulomas with giant-cell formation. Fat necrosis is unusual, thus separating the condition from acute panniculitis.

Treatment is unsatisfactory, possibly because many of the complaints are functional. Oral analgesics and injection with local anesthetics have been tried. The intravenous infusion of lidocaine has been reported to provide symptomatic relief.

ACUTE PANNICULITIS (NODULAR FAT NECROSIS)

The appearance of single or multiple crops of tender nodules in subcutaneous fat with a histologic picture of fat-cell necrosis, infiltration of inflammatory cells, and development of fat-filled macrophages (foam cells) is the hallmark of acute panniculitis. The nodules range in size from 0.5 to 10 cm and may be firm or fluctuant. On occasion they drain an oily solution, and suppuration may occur. Individual lesions last from 1 to 8 weeks before disappearing, and a pigmented depressed area may be left at the involved site. While some patients have only nodular panniculitis, which may or may not be relapsing, others develop a systemic syndrome that includes fever, abnormal liver function, involvement of the bone marrow with leukemoid response or bleeding tendencies, nodular pulmonary lesions, and evidence of pancreatic disease with elevated plasma amylase and lipase levels. In the past this constellation of findings was called *Weber-Christian disease.* However, since painful or nonpainful panniculitis may result from a variety of conditions, Weber-Christian disease is not a specific entity, and the term should probably be abandoned.

While the pathophysiology of acute panniculitis has not been well worked out, some general associations can be identified. Physical causes include direct trauma to subcutaneous fat and cold exposure. The former includes factitious panniculitis wherein patients traumatize themselves. Cold exposure may produce generalized or local lesions. One variant, equestrian cold panniculitis, occurs in the outer thighs of subjects who ride horseback for several hours in icy weather. Subcutaneous fat necrosis of the newborn has been attributed to a combination of hypothermia and obstetrical trauma, but the etiology is actually unknown. The condition resolves spontaneously. Cold agglutinins or cryoglobulins have not been demonstrated in cold-induced fat necrosis. Systemic signs are usually absent with these forms of panniculitis.

The histologic picture of acute panniculitis may also be seen with erythema nodosum (of a variety of causes), erythema induratum (probably a localized hypersensitivity vasculitis, although it may have a granulomatous component), or collagen-vascular diseases (lupus, polyarteritis, subcutaneous morphea, or rheumatoid arthritis).

Acute panniculitis is also associated with lymphoproliferative diseases such as lymphomas and histiocytosis. One variant, histiocytic, cytophagic panniculitis, is characterized by a severe hemorrhagic diathesis and a high mortality rate.

Finally, acute panniculitis can be caused by enzymatic disorders such as alpha$_1$-antitrypsin deficiency and by severe pancreatic disease leading to release of digestive enzymes into plasma. The latter condition, usually designated metastatic fat necrosis, is discussed below.

In summary, acute panniculitis can only be diagnosed histologically. Once the lesion is identified, a search must be made for the underlying cause. If a rapid downhill course with systemic symptoms accompanies the panniculitis, the diagnosis is likely collagen-vascular disease, pancreatic disease, or a lymphoproliferative disorder. Treatment depends on the diagnosis. Steroids are frequently tried but usually are unsatisfactory.

METASTATIC FAT NECROSIS

Metastatic fat necrosis is a syndrome of extensive adipose tissue inflammation and cell death resembling or identical with acute nodular panniculitis. It is accompanied by fever, destructive polyarthritis (which may cause flail joints), lytic bone lesions, pleural and pericardial effusions, ascites, and elevation of lipase and amylase levels in the plasma. Eosinophilia occurs in some patients. Pancreatic disease is invariably present. About two-thirds of patients have pancreatitis, while the remainder have a carcinoma of the pancreas, usually acinar. The cause of the syndrome is unknown. Fat necrosis has been speculated to be due to pancreatic lipase acting at multiple sites in the body, but the picture may result from an autoimmune phenomenon. Complement levels are low, and involved tissues show immunofluorescent staining for IgG and the third component of complement. Prognosis is poor, and death often occurs within a few months whether or not the underlying cause is cancer.

REFERENCES

Lipodystrophy

DUNNIGAN MG et al: Familial lipoatrophic diabetes with dominant transmission. Q J Med 169:33, 1974

HOWARD BV et al: Cell culture studies of a patient with congenital lipoatrophic diabetes—Normal insulin binding with alterations in intracellular glucose metabolism and insulin action. Metabolism 30:845, 1981

SEIP M: Generalized lipodystrophy. Ergeb Inn Med Kinderheilkd 31:59, 1971

SOLER NG et al: Lipoatrophic diabetes: Endocrine dysfunction and the response to control of hypertriglyceridemia. Metabolism 31:19, 1982

Multiple symmetric lipomatosis

ENZI G et al: Multiple symmetric lipomatosis. A defect in adrenergic-stimulated lipolysis. J Clin Invest 60:1221, 1977

SULLY L, MCGROUTHER DA: Brown fat in benign symmetrical lipomatosis. Br J Plast Surg 32:331, 1979

Adiposis dolorosa

BLOMSTRAND R et al: Adipose dolorosa associated with defects of lipid metabolism. Acta Derm Venereol 51:243, 1971

CANTU JM et al: Autosomal dominant inheritance in adiposis dolorosa (Dercum's disease). Humangenetik 18:89, 1973

Acute panniculitis

FÖRSTRÖM L, WINKELMANN RK: Acute panniculitis. A clinical and histopathologic study of 34 cases. Arch Dermatol 113:909, 1977

WINKELMANN RK, BOWIE EJW: Hemorrhagic diathesis associated with benign histiocytic, cytophagic panniculitis and systemic histiocytosis. Arch Intern Med 140:1460, 1980

Metastatic fat necrosis

PHILLIPS RM JR et al: Inflammatory arthritis and subcutaneous fat necrosis associated with acute and chronic pancreatitis. Arth Rheum 23:355, 1980

POTTS DE et al: Syndrome of pancreatic disease, subcutaneous fat necrosis and polyserositis. Case report and review of literature. Am J Med 58:417, 1975

Genetic disorders affecting multiple organ systems

106
DISORDERS OF CONNECTIVE TISSUE

PHILIP J. FIALKOW

Elastin, collagen, glycoproteins, and proteinpolysaccharides are the major extracellular macromolecules of connective tissue. An inherited abnormality in connective tissue may affect any one of the numerous steps in the biosynthesis and the metabolism of these substances or the processes by which the macromolecules are physically organized and oriented to one another.

Heritable, generalized disorders of connective tissue may be classified as primary or secondary. The former group includes those diseases caused by mutations in genes that directly involve the synthesis or metabolism of elements such as collagen or elastin. In secondary disorders, mutant genes affect metabolism exogenous to connective tissue pathways, resulting in the accumulation of a product that damages connective tissue (e.g., homocystinuria, Chap. 91).

The heritable disorders discussed in this chapter are thought to involve collagen or elastic fibers. With some exceptions the basic defects are undefined, and it is not known whether the mutations affect connective tissue primarily or secondarily. In some cases it is not certain whether the abnormalities involve collagen, elastin, or other connective tissue components. All the disorders are genetically heterogeneous, i.e., two or more different mutations produce clinically similar diseases. Diseases primarily affecting mucopolysaccharides are described in Chap. 104.

THE EHLERS-DANLOS SYNDROME

The Ehlers-Danlos syndrome (EDS) constitutes a group of heritable, generalized disorders of connective tissue whose major features include fragile and hyperextensible skin (Fig. 106-1), easy bruising, and loose-jointedness. There are at least eight distinct types that vary in clinical manifestations and in severity. The patterns of inheritance include autosomal dominant and recessive and X-linked recessive. The prevalence is uncertain.

The biochemical abnormalities are known in several types of the EDS, and in each of these collagen is affected. The basic building block of the collagen fiber, the collagen monomer, is a triple helix of three α chains. The extracellular collagen molecules aggregate into fibrils which in turn form the fibers that are visible with the light microscope. At least five types of collagen, each of which contains a genetically distinct type of α chain, have been identified. The ubiquitous molecule (type I) is a triple helix containing two different α chains and is found in skin, tendon, ligament, bone, blood vessels, dentin, and other organs. Abnormalities in type I collagen are found in EDS VI and EDS VII. Type II collagen is found primarily in cartilage and consists of three α chains similar to, but not identical with, those found in type I. Type III collagen, the molecule thought to be involved in EDS IV, has three identical α chains which differ from those found in types I and II. It has a similar tissue distribution to type I but is not found in bone or dentin.

EDS I, GRAVIS TYPE This is the classical EDS, which, because of its severe clinical manifestations, is termed *gravis.*

Clinical manifestations SKIN The skin is soft, velvety, and hyperextensible. It can be pulled far away from the underlying structures, but upon release it promptly returns to its original position (Fig. 106-1). With advancing age focal losses of elasticity may cause the skin over some areas such as the palms to become lax. The skin is fragile and easily bruised. Minor trauma often produces a gaping, fish-mouth wound that is hard to suture but does not bleed extensively. Paper-thin scars develop with healing. Minor injury often results in purpura or hematomas which may organize, calcify, and resemble a neoplasm. Another type of pseudotumor develops over pressure points such as the knees and elbows. These smaller, subcutaneous pea-sized "spherules" calcify and are visible on roentgenograms.

MUSCULOSKELETAL SYSTEM Hyperextensible joints may allow patients to perform unusual contortions (e.g., "India rubber man," "human pretzel"). Because of joint instability, these patients are prone to develop effusions or recurrent dislocations of the hip, patella, shoulder, and other joints. Hemarthroses sometimes occur. Backward curvature of the knees (genu recurvatum), flatfeet, kyphoscoliosis, and looseness of the clavicles at their sternal ends are common. Joint hyperextensibility

FIGURE 106-1
Hyperextensible skin in a patient with an unclassified form of Ehlers-Danlos syndrome.

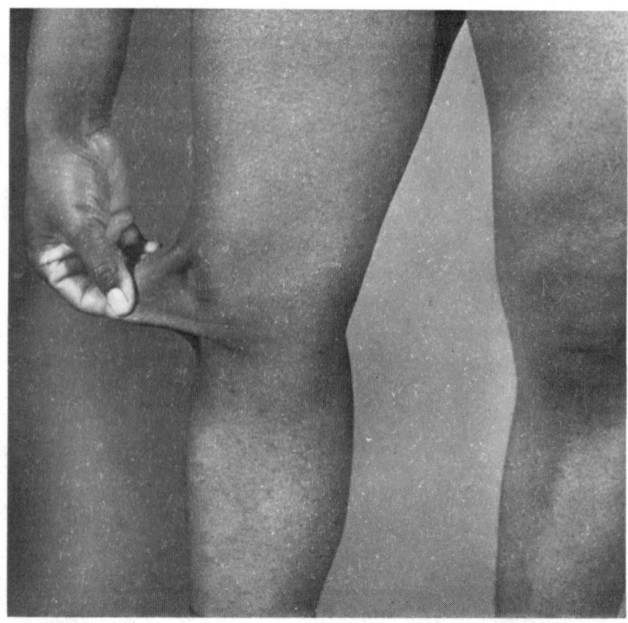

may decrease somewhat with advancing age. Spondylolisthesis may be seen, and high-arched palate and "pigeon breast" are occasionally found. Muscle hypotonia, dental abnormalities, and nocturnal leg cramps are frequent.

BLEEDING This may occur into the skin and joints as described above. Severe gastrointestinal or respiratory tract bleeding occasionally occurs. The gums may bleed with minor trauma (e.g., brushing of the teeth), and bleeding may complicate tooth extraction or tonsillectomy. Weakness of vessel walls or abnormal interactions of platelets with collagen apparently underlies the hemorrhagic diathesis; consistent abnormalities in clotting factors have not been described.

EYES Blue sclerae are occasionally seen. Epicanthal folds are frequent in younger patients. In older patients the eyes may appear widely spaced.

CARDIOVASCULAR SYSTEM Mitral valve prolapse occurs in this and other forms of EDS, especially types II and III. Right bundle branch block or other conduction abnormalities are found in some patients with EDS. Aortic valve regurgitation and dissecting aneurysm of the aorta are rare complications.

Congenital cardiac anomalies have also been reported, but their prevalence may not be higher in EDS than in the general population. Vascular complications such as spontaneous rupture of the large arteries and rupture of intracranial aneurysms leading to cerebral vascular accidents are rare and are more likely to be seen in EDS IV. Because the arteries may be friable, cerebral angiography and other diagnostic arterial invasions should be performed cautiously.

OTHER MANIFESTATIONS Generalized tissue fragility makes surgery and subsequent wound healing difficult and may lead to pneumothorax. Spontaneous rupture of the bowel is rare and more likely to be seen in EDS IV. Premature birth due to early rupture of the fetal membranes is common. Diaphragmatic and other hernias and gastrointestinal tract diverticula occur with increased frequency.

Inheritance EDS I is inherited as an autosomal dominant and may itself be genetically heterogeneous.

Pathogenesis The basic defect in EDS I is unknown. Dermal collagen bundles often appear fragmented, and collagen fibrils are abnormal on electron microscopy.

EDS II, MITIS TYPE Clinical manifestations are similar to those of EDS I but are less severe. Hence EDS II is termed *mitis* type. Skin and joint changes are mild, and hyperextensibility may be limited to joints of the hands and feet. Tissue friability is not a problem, and internal manifestations are uncommon with the exception of mitral valve prolapse. As in EDS I, this form of EDS is inherited as an autosomal dominant and may be genetically heterogeneous. Ultrastructural findings are similar to those in EDS I. The biochemical defect is unknown.

EDS III, BENIGN HYPERMOBILE TYPE This may be the most common type of EDS. Patients have generalized small and large joint hypermobility with an increased risk for joint dislocations and effusions and eventual degenerative arthritis. Cutaneous manifestations are minimal. Mitral valve prolapse may occur. EDS III is transmitted as an autosomal dominant, is probably genetically heterogeneous, and may show variable clinical manifestations even in affected relatives.

EDS IV, ECCHYMOTIC OR ARTERIAL TYPE In this rare form of EDS, the skin is fragile, thin, and translucent, allowing easy visualization of subcutaneous veins. In contrast to other types of the EDS, the skin is not hyperextensible and may even be tight. Severe bruising occurs easily. Joint hypermobility is usually found only in the digits. Severe complications which may lead to premature death are rupture of hollow viscera (usually the colon), large arteries, or the gravid uterus near term. This form of EDS is genetically heterogeneous, and families with autosomal dominant or recessive inheritance have been described. The recessive varieties are more severe and are associated with a decrease in life expectancy. The life expectancy in the dominant variety is not always reduced. Normal blood vessels are especially rich in type III collagen, and the tissue content of this type of collagen is decreased in EDS IV. The precise biochemical defects are unknown, but it is likely that several different abnormalities in the structure or processing of type III collagen are associated with EDS IV.

EDS V, X-LINKED TYPE The most striking feature is hyperextensible skin with moderate fragility, thin scars, and bruising. Joint hypermobility is mild. These features are similar to those of EDS II, and EDS V is distinguished more by its pattern of inheritance (X-linked recessive) than by its clinical manifestations. In some patients with apparently X-linked recessive EDS, short stature and severe joint hypermobility occur. The biochemical defect is unknown.

EDS VI, OCULAR TYPE Hyperextensible skin and joints with the ensuing complications are present, but the distinctive features of this type of EDS are the ocular manifestations, severe scoliosis, and mild to moderate arachnodactyly. The cornea may be abnormal in size or shape and, like the sclera, is fragile and prone to rupture from even mild trauma. Glaucoma and retinal detachment also occur.

The primary abnormality in this autosomal recessive disorder is deficient activity of lysyl hydroxylase. The tensile strength of collagen fibrils in tissues depends upon the formation of interchain cross-links, which in large part result from interactions involving lysyl- or hydroxylysyl-derived aldehydes. With deficient lysyl hydroxylase activity, the hydroxylysine residue content of collagen is markedly decreased, hydroxylysine interchain cross-links are diminished, tensile strength is decreased, and the clinical manifestations ensue.

EDS VII, ARTHROCHALASIS MULTIPLEX CONGENITA This rare form of EDS is characterized by marked joint hypermobility with only mild skin hyperextensibility and minimal bruising. Congenital bilateral hip dislocation and postnatal dislocations of other joints are found. EDS VII may be genetically heterogeneous: both autosomal recessive and autosomal dominant varieties have been postulated. The primary defect in the autosomal recessive EDS VII is deficient activity of a protease involved in the formation of collagen from its precursor, procollagen. Other patients, presumably with autosomal dominant inheritance, may have structural abnormalities in procollagen.

EDS VIII, PERIODONTAL TYPE Hyperextensible joints and hyperextensible and fragile skin with the ensuing complications are present, but the distinctive feature of this type of EDS is progressive periodontal disease resulting in gum and alveolar process resorption with loss of teeth in the second or third decade. EDS VIII is inherited as an autosomal dominant; the primary defect is unknown.

DIFFERENTIAL DIAGNOSIS Congenital joint hypermobility occurs as an isolated finding, sometimes in more than one relative, and is probably a distinct entity from the EDS. Loose-jointedness also occurs in the Marfan and Noonan syndromes, many of the chondrodystrophies, some of the mucopolysaccharidoses, and in osteogenesis imperfecta. In cutis laxa the skin is not only hyperextensible, but it is also lax, i.e., it has decreased elasticity and may hang in loose folds. Late in the course of EDS the skin in localized areas may resemble that seen in cutis laxa.

TREATMENT AND PROGNOSIS No specific therapy is known. Trauma to skin and joints should be avoided. In moderate and severe forms of the EDS, surgery should be undertaken with caution because of the fragility of skin, arteries, and internal organs. Wound dehiscence is frequent, and sutures should be left in place longer than usual.

Pregnancy may be accompanied by increased bruisability and exacerbation of joint manifestations and carries increased risk for development of abdominal herniae; leg and vulva varicosities; complications of episiotomy and cesarean section; and premature delivery in type I EDS and uterine rupture in type IV EDS.

Death from arterial rupture is relatively frequent in patients with the severe variety of EDS IV. In other types of EDS death may occasionally occur from internal complications, but the prognosis for normal life expectancy is good. Some patients experience considerable morbidity from cutaneous and joint abnormalities.

MARFAN SYNDROME

The Marfan syndrome is an inherited, generalized disorder of connective tissue with ocular, skeletal, and cardiovascular manifestations. There is wide variability in clinical expression, and some patients have findings in only one or two systems. The prevalence of the disorder has been estimated to be more than 1 in 50,000, perhaps 1 in 10,000 persons.

Clinical manifestations These result from abnormalities in the supporting tissues of the ocular, cardiovascular, and skeletal systems. Although the diagnosis may be apparent during infancy, ordinarily it is not made until the second decade or later.

EYES Weakness and redundancy of the supporting tissues of the lens is the cause of the most characteristic finding in the Marfan syndrome, bilateral subluxation or dislocation of the lens (ectopia lentis). This occurs in over 60 percent of patients, and its presence may be signaled by tremulousness of the iris (iridodenesis). The lens dislocation is most frequently in an upward and outward direction, but this is not a pathognomic feature. Complications of lens subluxation include reduced visual acuity, retinal detachment, uveitis, glaucoma, and cataracts. Subtle dislocation is frequent and can be detected only by careful slit-lamp examination through a dilated pupil. High-grade myopia and relatively flat corneas are also common; some patients have blue sclerae.

CARDIOVASCULAR SYSTEM About 90 percent of patients have cardiovascular abnormalities, some of which may be evident only with sensitive diagnostic modalities such as echocardiography. Weakness in the media of the aorta causes the most life-threatening abnormality in the Marfan syndrome, progressive dilatation, and dissecting aneurysm of the proximal portion of the ascending aorta. Clinical manifestations such as diastolic murmur or roentgenographic evidence of aortic dilatation may be detected in infancy or as late as in the fifth or sixth decades. The predilection for involvement of the ascending aorta is not surprising in view of the hemodynamic stresses that occur there.

Although *severe* mitral valve regurgitation is less common than *severe* aortic valve disease, echocardiographic studies reveal some abnormality of the mitral valve, including mitral valve prolapse, in most patients (the "click murmur" syndrome, Chap. 258). Echocardiography is also useful in detecting and following patients with aortic root and valve abnormalities. Bacterial endocarditis may involve heart valves with only minor antecedent alterations. Coarctation of the aorta and abnormalities in the conduction system have also been reported.

SKELETAL SYSTEM Increased length of the tubular bones is the most conspicuous external feature of the disease (Fig. 106-2). The extremities are long and thin (dolichostenomelia); almost all patients are tall, either absolutely or relatively when their heights are assessed against the background of their families.

Abnormal body proportions are even more specific. The distance from the top of the pubic symphysis to the sole of the foot ("lower segment") is increased in patients with the Marfan syndrome, causing a low ratio of the upper segment (pubic symphysis to crown) to the lower segment of the body. In normal postpubertal whites this ratio is 0.92 ± 0.04, and in normal blacks it is 0.85 ± 0.03. A significant decrease in these

FIGURE 106-2

A 16-year-old boy with the Marfan syndrome. Manifestations include dislocated lens, long, thin face, long fingers (arachnodactyly) and extremities (dolichostenomelia), and inward displacement of the sternum (pectus excavatum). (Courtesy of JG Hall.)

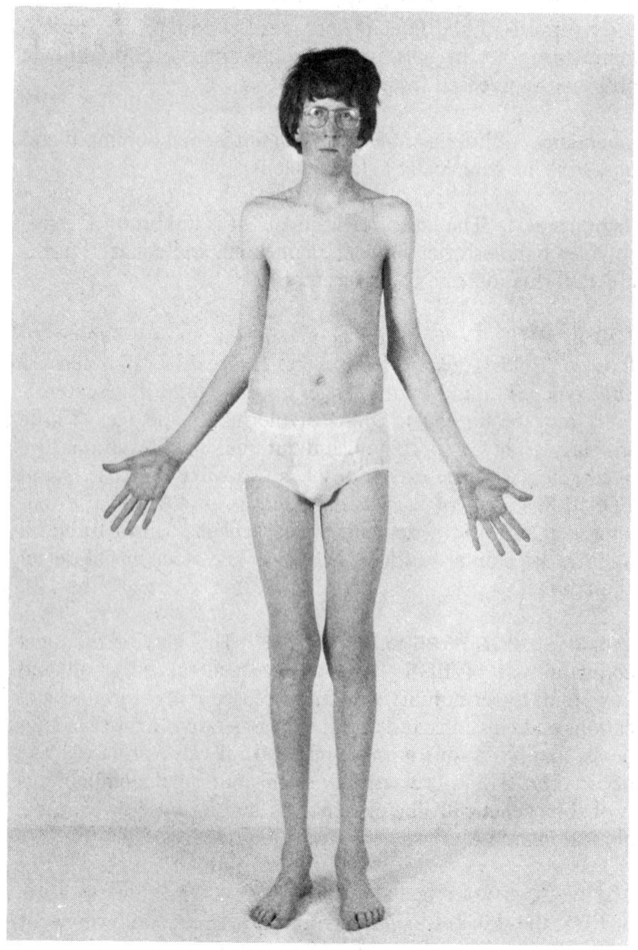

values is helpful in establishing the diagnosis. The arm span may be greater than the height.

Excessively long finger bones (arachnodactyly, "spider fingers") are found in most patients. When this is subtle, roentgenograms of the hands with calculation of the "metacarpal index" may be helpful. The length of each of the last four metacarpal bones is divided by the width at its midpoint, and the values are averaged. In patients with the Marfan syndrome the index is often greater than 8.4; in normal individuals it is usually less than 8. Sternal displacement upward causes "pigeon breast" (pectus carinatum), and sternal displacement inward causes pectus excavatum. The palate is often high and arched, and the facies long and narrow.

Weakness and redundancy of the ligaments and other supporting tissues of the joints lead to loose- or "double-jointedness," flatfeet, backward curvature of the knees (genu recurvatum), kyphoscoliosis, and recurrent dislocations, especially of the hip and patella. Inguinal or femoral hernias are frequent.

OTHER MANIFESTATIONS Many patients have sparse subcutaneous fat and muscle hypotonia. Striae may be present, especially in the skin of the pectoral, deltoid, and thigh areas. Lung cysts with spontaneous pneumothorax occasionally occur.

Inheritance The Marfan syndrome is inherited as an autosomal dominant. There is wide variability in clinical expression ("variable expressivity"), and an affected relative may have only mild manifestations confined to one system (e.g., dislocated lenses detected only by slit-lamp examination). Rarely, an individual genetically proved to possess the Marfan gene (e.g., a person with an affected parent and offspring) does not have any detectable expression. Perhaps 15 percent of cases are sporadic and presumably the result of a fresh mutation in a parental germ cell. Elevated paternal age is considered a factor in the occurrence of fresh mutations.

Pathology and pathogenesis The basic biochemical abnormality is unknown. Defective collagen cross-linking is possible, but unproven. The early aortic changes are those of cystic medial necrosis (Chap. 268). Later findings are loss of elastic fibers and scarring with irregular whorls of smooth muscle. No histological changes or electron microscopic abnormalities in collagen have been reported in ligaments or tendons.

Differential diagnosis Because the disorder displays wide variability in clinical expression and because there is no specific test, the diagnosis may be difficult to establish in patients without the classical tetrad of dislocated lens, aortic dilatation or aneurysm, excessive length of tubular bones, and family history consistent with autosomal dominant inheritance. In such cases careful examination of close relatives and exclusion of disorders resembling the Marfan syndrome can be helpful. It may be impossible to establish the diagnosis definitively in a patient with skeletal or cardiac abnormalities who does not have a dislocated lens or a clearly affected relative.

The homocystinurias, inborn errors of methionine metabolism with secondary effects on connective tissue (Chap. 91), are the principal diseases to be distinguished from the Marfan syndrome. The disorders have dislocated lens and skeletal deformities in common but differ in other clinical manifestations and in their pattern of inheritance (Table 106-1). As its name implies, there is a specific laboratory test for homocystinuria.

A "marfanoid hypermobility" syndrome is characterized by hyperextensible joints and skin changes similar to those seen in Ehlers-Danlos syndrome as well as by arachnodactyly, pectus deformity, and regurgitation of the aortic and mitral valves.

Congenital contractural arachnodactyly, an autosomal dominant disorder associated with severe kyphoscoliosis, generalized osteopenia, and arachnodactyly, is distinguished from the Marfan syndrome by the presence of congenital contractures of the fingers and abnormally shaped ears. It has been suggested that congenital contractural arachnodactyly and the marfanoid hypermobility disorder are forms of, and reflect genetic heterogeneity of, the Marfan syndrome. It has also been postulated that the more typical cases of the Marfan syndrome can be subdivided into at least two types: asthenic, mainly in children, and nonasthenic.

Dislocation of the lens is a feature of another genetic disorder of connective tissue, the Weill-Marchesani syndrome, but the skeletal abnormalities in this autosomal recessive disorder are short stature and stiffness of joints. Ectopia lentis can also occur without skeletal or cardiac involvement as an autosomal dominant disorder.

Treatment and prognosis Estrogen therapy in girls and androgen treatment in boys may reduce adult height in children who are already tall in the prepubertal period and may also prevent severe kyphoscoliosis. The potential benefits of the sex steroids must be weighed against their possible complications, including the psychological and physical effects of inducing precocious pubertal development. Prophylactic administration of drugs like propranolol which decrease myocardial contractility and diminish the stress on the aorta has been suggested, but thus far it has not been documented to be beneficial in patients with early aortic changes. The risks of surgery for aortic or valvular disease are high, primarily because the abnormal

TABLE 106-1
Comparison of the Marfan syndrome with homocystinuria

			Clinical manifestations					
				Skeletal				
Disorder	*Mode of inheritance*	*Basic biochemical defect*	*Ectopia lentis*	*Arachnodactyly*	*Pectus deformities*	*Cutaneous and subcutaneous*	*Cardiovascular*	*Mental retardation*
Marfan syndrome	Autosomal dominant	Unknown	+++ (usually upward)	++++	+++	Striae; sparse subcutaneous fat	Mitral valve prolapse Aorta: regurgitation/dissecting aneurysm	−−
Homocystinuria	Autosomal recessive	Usually decreased cystathionine synthase activity	++++ (usually downward)	++	++	Malar flush	Vascular thrombosis	++

connective tissue may not hold sutures well. However, therapy is often successful. All patients with Marfan syndrome are at risk for endocarditis; therefore, antibiotic prophylaxis with dental procedures and genitourinary instrumentation has been recommended.

The major threats to life, severe cardiovascular complications, may occur anytime from infancy to the seventh decade. These complications include dilatation, dissection, or rupture of the aorta and severe regurgitation of the aortic or mitral valve. In one series, the mean age at death was 43 for men and 46 for women. Pregnancy may be particularly hazardous for women with aortic disease, but is usually uneventful for women with normal aortas. Echocardiography is useful for detecting preclinical aortic root disease early in pregnancy.

Patients with the Marfan syndrome may be disabled by profound kyphoscoliosis; recurrent joint dislocations; recurrent pneumothorax; or serious visual impairment from myopia, retinal detachment, or the uveitis and glaucoma that result from subluxation of the lens.

OSTEOGENESIS IMPERFECTA

Osteogenesis imperfecta (OI; fragilitas ossium, maladie de Lobstein) comprises a group of heritable, generalized disorders of connective tissue with clinical manifestations in the skeleton, ear, joints and ligaments, teeth, sclera, and skin. Biochemical studies suggest that the defects in OI involve collagen, but the basic defects are unknown. The frequency of OI has been estimated at more than 1 in every 20,000 births.

It has been proposed that there are at least four distinct types of OI that each have specific clinical features and natural histories and different modes of inheritance. Although the delineation of precise biochemical abnormalities necessary to confirm this subdivision of OI has not been described, the concept is valuable to the clinician who is evaluating and counseling patients with OI; therefore the proposed classification is given here.

OI TYPE I, DOMINANT WITH BLUE SCLERAE This is the most prevalent type of OI.

Clinical manifestations The cardinal features are blue sclerae, hearing impairment, and multiple fractures after birth. Abnormalities of the teeth (dentinogenesis imperfecta) occur in some families.

SKELETON Bone fragility may be present at birth, but fractures do not usually occur until the child begins to stand or walk. The fractures may occur with minor trauma and frequently involve the long bones of the legs. Most often susceptibility to fractures decreases after puberty, but it may return later, especially with inactivity, pregnancy, or menopause. Roentgenograms may show wormian bones in the skull, a finding that may help establish the diagnosis. Osteoporosis is usually present, even in infancy. Skeletal deformity is unusual and stature is generally near normal.

EYES The sclerae appear translucent, thin, and blue, owing to partial visualization of the underlying choroid. This is probably the most frequent manifestation of OI type I.

EARS Progressive hearing impairment from otosclerosis may begin in childhood, but deafness usually does not develop until adulthood.

JOINTS Abnormalities in the ligaments and tendons lead to loose-jointedness, which causes in turn the increased frequency of kyphoscoliosis, flatfeet, and recurrent joint dislocations. Joint laxity usually decreases after puberty.

TEETH Hypoplasia of dentine and pulp causes the characteristically small, misshapen, blue-yellow teeth (dentinogenesis imperfecta). These dental abnormalities are probably present only in patients with a subtype of OI I.

Inheritance OI type I is inherited as an autosomal dominant and is almost certainly heterogeneous. There may be two distinct subtypes, one with and the other without dental abnormalities. The latter may itself exist in two genetically distinct forms, one more severe and associated with mild short stature and occasional skeletal deformity. It has been suggested that fetal roentgenograms should be made near term in pregnancies at risk for the birth of a child with OI type I so that delivery by cesarean section can be considered if the fetus is found to have the disease.

OI TYPE II, LETHAL PERINATAL This is the most common type of OI and is uniformly lethal.

Clinical manifestations Infants with OI type II are either stillborn or die within days to weeks after birth. Short stature, marked deformity of limbs, and virtual absence of calvarium ossification are present. Almost all bones break in utero. Characteristically the ribs are "beaded" due to recurrent fracturing and healing. Connective tissue abnormalities may be so severe that limbs become detached during birth. Sclerae are dark blue.

Inheritance OI type II is probably heterogeneous. In some families, it is apparently inherited as an autosomal recessive, but in many of the sporadically occurring cases the disease may be dominant and result from a fresh mutation in a parental germ cell or have another cause.

Prenatal diagnosis can be made in OI type II. One suggested regimen is to do ultrasonography at 16, 20, and 23 weeks of gestation to detect skeletal abnormalities. However, before termination of the pregnancy the diagnosis should be confirmed with roentgenograms.

OI TYPE III, PROGRESSIVE DEFORMING This type of OI is characterized by multiple bone fractures, growth retardation, and progressive skeletal deformity. Numerous fractures are often present at birth, but the bones are better developed than in OI type II. Birth weight and length are usually normal, but almost all children who survive infancy have very short stature. Bone deformity is progressive and may occur without fractures. Severe kyphoscoliosis is often present by the time of puberty. Sclerae may be pale blue in infancy but thereafter are white. Hearing loss is rare; dentinogenesis imperfecta is common. Inheritance in some patients appears to be autosomal recessive but is undoubtedly genetically heterogeneous.

OI TYPE IV, DOMINANT WITH NORMAL SCLERAE This type of OI is distinguished from OI type I by the presence of normal sclerae. It is probably heterogeneous. In some families the disorder seems to be mild and similar to OI type I, but in others it resembles OI type III and is distinguished from it by the pattern of inheritance. The presence or absence of dentinogenesis imperfecta also may define subtypes.

Differential diagnosis Without a clear family history, it may be difficult to distinguish OI early in its course from "idiopathic" osteoporosis. The same is true after the menopause in women with OI type I who have experienced few fractures earlier in life. When the legs are short and the head appears large,

OI may resemble achondroplasia. OI manifest in infancy must also be distinguished from hypophosphatasia.

Treatment and prognosis No specific therapy is known. Careful orthopedic management is necessary, and immobilization should be avoided. Infants with OI type II are born dead or die in infancy. OI types I and IV are more benign disorders, but disability may occur from multiple fractures, skeletal deformities, or deafness. Nonetheless, many patients adjust to their disease and lead normal lives. The frequency of fractures generally decreases after puberty but may again increase later in life. Deafness is present in about 35 percent of patients with OI type I in the fourth decade and in about 50 percent in the sixth decade.

PSEUDOXANTHOMA ELASTICUM

Pseudoxanthoma elasticum (PXE; Groenblad-Strandberg syndrome) constitutes a group of genetically heterogeneous disorders with protean clinical manifestations most frequently involving the skin, eyes, and arteries. The basic pathogenetic abnormality is unknown but probably involves elastic fibers. Clinical changes usually first appear in the second or third decade and thereafter are progressive. The prevalence of PXE has been estimated at between 1 in 200,000 and 1 in 50,000 adults.

Clinical manifestations SKIN PXE derives its name from the characteristic yellow xanthoma-like papular and reticulated skin lesions. Skin changes are usually evident in the second or third decade and in later life are found in virtually all patients.

The changes are most notable in the neck and axillae, and the antecubital fossae, periumbilical area, groin, and penis may also be involved. The abnormalities range from a few yellow papules confined to one or two areas (usually the neck, axilla, or both) to confluent yellow papules and plaques that cause redundant folds of lax skin over flexural surfaces. The skin around the mouth, chin, and nasolabial folds may be thickened as well as lax.

The extent of changes detected histologically correlates with the severity of clinical cutaneous lesions, but occasionally changes of PXE may be seen in a biopsy from a patient without obvious clinical alterations.

EYES Angioid streaks are breaks in Bruch's membrane and are usually first noted during the second or third decade and found thereafter in all but a very few patients. The streaks are bilateral. They are flat, lie beneath the retinal vessels, and are usually three to five times the diameter of retinal veins, red-brown, and most numerous around the optic discs from which they appear to emanate. Subretinal neovascularization can cause hemorrhage and chorioretinal scarring which may obscure the angioid streaks and also may result in significant visual loss in one or both eyes.

VASCULAR SYSTEM Most patients with PXE have some combination of peripheral, cardiac, or cerebrovascular abnormalities. Involvement of peripheral arteries results in weak or absent pulses and often in calcification. Easy fatigability of the limbs and intermittent claudication are common. Some patients develop early-onset hypertension or coronary artery disease that usually presents as angina or an altered ECG. Cerebrovascular symptoms are less frequent and may be rare in the absence of hypertension. Hypothyroidism, perhaps from altered thyroid vasculature, may occur.

Upper gastrointestinal tract bleeding is frequent, often severe, and occasionally the presenting manifestation. The hemorrhage is probably from arterial disease in the gastrointestinal tract. Sometimes peptic ulcer or hiatus hernia is present, but in many patients the source of the bleeding is not detected. Uterine bleeding may be severe. Hemorrhage may also occur in the urinary and upper respiratory tracts.

Inheritance PXE is a genetically heterogeneous disorder. In most families it is autosomal recessive, but autosomal dominant inheritance also occurs. There may be at least two varieties of autosomal dominant PXE. Type I is characterized by classic orange-peel-like skin changes, severe vascular manifestations, and ocular manifestations. Patients with the more frequent type II have a much milder disease. The skin is hyperextensible, and the rash is macular or focal. Other manifestations such as high-arched palate, blue sclerae, and loose-jointedness may also occur in patients with type II.

Pathology and pathogenesis The basic defect in PXE is unknown, but probably involves, either primarily or secondarily, elastic fibers in the dermis, media of arteries, and Bruch's membrane which lies between the retina and choriocapillaries. Early skin changes are small patchy areas of swollen, fragmented, and irregularly clumped basophilic elastic fibers in the middermis.

These altered areas have affinity for calcium, and von Kossa staining (for calcium) may be valuable in confirming subtle lesions. Later in the disease all the elastic fibers of the mid and lower dermis are affected. Studies with the electron microscope indicate that the principal alterations are in the elastin moiety of the elastic fibers.

Differential diagnosis Virtually all patients with PXE have characteristic cutaneous changes, and the diagnosis can be confirmed with a skin biopsy. Actinic (or "senile") elastosis may cause confusion in some patients; however, the changes are limited to exposed sites, and the disorder is histologically distinguishable from PXE. Angioid streaks are present in the great majority of patients with PXE, and while it is estimated that about two-thirds of people with them have PXE, they are also found in other disorders such as sickle cell anemia and Paget's disease.

Treatment and prognosis No specific treatment for PXE is known. Skin changes may be a cosmetic problem. Subretinal neovascularization may be treatable in some patients before significant visual loss occurs. Early death may occur from hemorrhage, cardiac disease, or cerebrovascular accidents, but some patients have a normal life span.

REFERENCES

HOLLISTER DW et al: Genetic disorders of collagen metabolism, in *Advances in Human Genetics*, H Harris, K Hirschhorn (eds). New York, Plenum Press (in press)

MCKUSICK VA: *Heritable Disorders of Connective Tissue*, 4th ed. St Louis, Mosby, 1972

PYERITZ RE, MCKUSICK VA: The Marfan syndrome: Diagnosis and management. N Engl J Med 300:772, 1979

SILLENCE DO et al: Genetic heterogeneity in osteogenesis imperfecta. J Med Gen 16:101, 1979

107
NOONAN SYNDROME AND OTHER DISORDERS INVOLVING MULTIPLE ORGAN SYSTEMS

PHILIP J. FIALKOW

The pathophysiology of many clinically important genetic diseases is unknown. Most of these disorders are described under the principal organ systems affected. Some others involving multiple organ systems are discussed here.

NOONAN SYNDROME

The Noonan syndrome probably comprises several distinct but as yet undefined disorders. It shows wide phenotypic variability. Many patients have characteristic facies with ptosis, webbing of the neck, congenital heart disease with predominantly right-sided lesions, short stature, and intellectual impairment. The prevalence, clinical spectrum, natural history, pathogenesis, and mode of inheritance are poorly delineated. Furthermore, only within the last 10 to 15 years has it been appreciated that the Noonan syndrome is distinct from the Turner syndrome (gonadal dysgenesis), which is due to a partial or complete absence of one X chromosome. It is likely that most patients previously described as Ullrich, male Turner, or female pseudo-Turner syndromes and as Turner, Ullrich, or Bonnevie-Ullrich phenotype with normal chromosomes fall within the spectrum of the Noonan syndrome.

CLINICAL MANIFESTATIONS Definition of the Noonan syndrome phenotype has been hampered by "lumping" together what are certainly several distinct disorders. Furthermore, since few family studies have been performed, the spectrum and prevalence of individual abnormalities given here cannot be regarded as definitive.

Facies Patients with the Noonan syndrome have a characteristic appearance, including a flattened midface and small mandible with triangular-shaped mouth, epicanthic eye folds, hypertelorism, ptosis, downward ("antimongoloid") slant of the eyes, and ears that are prominent, fleshy, low-set and posteriorly rotated (Fig. 107-1). Webbing of the neck and a low posterior hairline are found in about half of patients.

Skin Multiple pigmented nevi and dystrophic nails are frequent. Patients may have congenital lymphangiectatic edema of the hands and feet which sometimes persists into adulthood. Keloid formation is frequent. The skin may be hyperelastic. Dermatoglyphic patterns may be abnormal but are nonspecific.

Skeletal system Most patients are short. Others have normal stature but are not as tall as would be expected for their genetic background. Mild skeletal abnormalities are common and include high-arched palate, dental malocclusion, increased carrying angle of the elbow (cubitus valgus), shield-shaped chest with wide-spaced nipples, pectus deformities, and kyphoscoliosis. Anomalies of the sternum, vertebrae, limbs, or skull may be seen radiographically. Often the pectus deformity is distinctive in that the upper portion of the sternum is displaced outward and the lower portion is displaced inward; that is, pectus carinatum and excavatum are both present in the same patient. The joints may be hyperextensible.

Intellectual development Intelligence ranges from superior to profoundly retarded, but most have mild or borderline mental retardation, as compared with nonaffected family members. From 25 to 50 percent of patients have normal intelligence.

Heart The true prevalence of congenital heart disease is unknown but may be between 30 and 50 percent. The most frequent finding is valvular pulmonic stenosis, alone or in combination with septal defects (especially atrial), asymmetric septal hypertrophy, or pulmonary artery branch stenosis. The last three abnormalities are less frequent in the absence of valvular pulmonic stenosis. In contrast to the Turner syndrome coarctation of the aorta is rare.

Sexual development Penile size may be normal or decreased; more than half of the males have cryptorchidism. Fertility is rare in men with the Noonan syndrome. In contrast, most affected females apparently are fertile.

Other manifestations Hydronephrosis with pyeloureteral obstruction and other renal anomalies occur, but the prevalence is unknown. Other abnormalities include thyroiditis, hypothyroidism, and hepatosplenomegaly in the absence of cardiac failure.

INHERITANCE Clinical and genetic heterogeneity clearly occurs. There are likely to be several "cardiofacial" syndromes which have in common unusual facies and congenital cardiac abnormalities. Among these is the typical Noonan syndrome.

No chromosomal abnormality has been found in patients with the Noonan syndrome. Autosomal dominant inheritance, described in some families, may be the mode of transmission for many patients. The relatively high proportion of sporadic cases (theoretically representing new mutations) would not be unusual for an autosomal dominant disorder often accompa-

FIGURE 107-1
A 14-year-old boy with the Noonan syndrome. Manifestations include downward ("antimongoloid") slant of the eyes, epicanthic eye folds, midface hypoplasia, prominent ears, broad neck, and upturned nose. (Courtesy of JG Hall.)

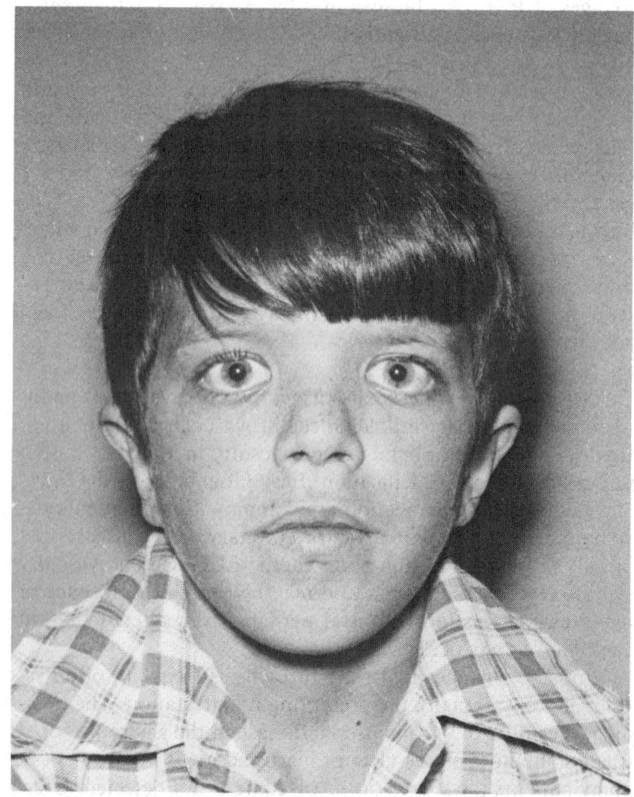

nied by infertility. In some families "unaffected" relatives have mild signs of the disorder.

Genetic counseling should include a discussion not only of disease recurrence risks but also of the wide range of clinical expression, especially as it pertains to cardiac anomalies, intelligence, stature, and fertility. Until the presumed heterogeneity is better defined, prognosis and recurrence risks are difficult to estimate and should be based largely on individual findings in the patient and family. The risk of severe disease in a patient's sibling or child is higher if the patient is severely affected. If the parents are unaffected, the recurrence risk is very low.

DIFFERENTIAL DIAGNOSIS Noonan syndrome must be distinguished from the Turner syndrome (gonadal dysgenesis) (Chap. 120). Shortness of stature and anomalies of the skeleton, skin, and integument are common in both disorders. Although the characteristic facies is seen to some extent in every Noonan patient, it alone is not distinctive enough to exclude the Turner syndrome. Clinical features that help identify the Turner syndrome include normal intelligence, infertility, and negative family history for other affected individuals. Pulmonic stenosis is common in the Noonan but infrequent in the Turner syndrome, whereas the reverse is true for coarctation of the aorta. Finally, chromosome studies with banding techniques must be done in patients of either sex and will usually allow the definitive diagnosis of the Turner syndrome.

The Aarskog syndrome (faciogenital dysplasia) is also associated with shortness of stature and facial anomalies but is further characterized by its X-linked recessive pattern of inheritance and by the fact that the scrotum often overhangs the penis ("shawl/saddlebag scrotum"). The fetal alcohol, fetal hydantoin, and Williams syndromes, all characterized by growth retardation, mild to moderate mental retardation and craniofacial abnormalities, must also be distinguished from the Noonan syndrome. In Noonan patients with hyperelastic skin and loose-jointedness, an erroneous diagnosis of Ehlers-Danlos syndrome may be made.

TREATMENT AND PROGNOSIS Therapy is directed toward correcting debilitating and life-threatening anomalies. Decisions to operate on patients for ptosis and webbing of the neck must be tempered by the reports of increased predilection to keloid formation. Surgical correction of valvular pulmonic stenosis should be performed when indicated, but results may be unsatisfactory because both the valve and contiguous tissue may be dysplastic. Orchiopexy for undescended testes should be attempted but is frequently unsuccessful. Although poorly defined, the life span in the Noonan syndrome, excluding cardiovascular problems and a possible increased frequency of neoplasia, is probably normal.

LAURENCE-MOON-BIEDL SYNDROME

The Laurence-Moon-Biedl (LMB) syndrome (Laurence-Moon-Biedl-Bardet syndrome, Bardet-Biedl syndrome, Biedl-Bardet syndrome) is an autosomal recessive disorder characterized by obesity, mental retardation, digital anomalies, hypogonadism, retinal dystrophy, and nephropathy. The basic defect and the prevalence of the LMB syndrome are unknown. Over 400 cases have been recorded.

CLINICAL MANIFESTATIONS **Obesity** Usually truncal in location, obesity is present in at least 80 percent of patients with the LMB syndrome. It begins in childhood and increases in severity with advancing age.

Eyes Retinal dystrophy occurs in over 90 percent of patients and differs from "typical" retinitis pigmentosa. The earliest symptom may be deficient dark adaptation ("night blindness"), but many patients have reduced acuity in childhood. Pigmentary disturbance of the retina may be minimal. Therefore, the electroretinogram, which is a sensitive test of retinal function, is helpful in establishing the diagnosis in questionable cases. The retinal degeneration is progressive and usually results in total blindness by the third or fourth decade. As in all retinal dystrophies, posterior subcapsular cataracts are common.

Gonads Hypogonadism is present in at least 75 percent of males but is rare in females. In many instances gonadotropin levels are low, but primary gonadal failure also occurs.

Digits Anomalies are noted in about 80 percent. The most frequent finding is postaxial polydactyly of one or more extremities. Some patients have only syndactyly of toes two and three or generalized shortening of the digits (brachydactyly).

Mental retardation Mild to moderate intellectual impairment is the usual finding. About a fifth of patients have severe retardation, and another tenth have normal intelligence.

Kidney Nephropathy is a significant feature. The renal lesion varies from mesangial proliferative glomerulopathy to medullary cystic disease (nephronophthisis) to focal areas of dysplasia. Patients often present with hypochromic microcytic anemia associated with polyuria and polydypsia. The nephropathy then progresses to renal failure despite normal urinary sediment. Blood pressure often remains normal.

Other manifestations Hip dysplasia may occur. In contrast to the Alstrom syndrome, diabetes mellitus and nerve deafness are not features of the LMB syndrome.

INHERITANCE The LMB syndrome is transmitted as an autosomal recessive disorder. There may be genetic heterogeneity.

DIFFERENTIAL DIAGNOSIS Since there is no specific test, the diagnosis must be established clinically. This can be done with little difficulty in the presence of the five cardinal manifestations (obesity, mental retardation, polydactyly, retinal dystrophy, and hypogonadism). However, the limits of the syndrome are poorly defined, and the diagnosis is often extended to patients with only some of these components. Variability in clinical expression occurs even among patients within the same family.

The LMB syndrome must be distinguished from syndromes bearing the eponyms Senior (retinal-renal dysplasia), Jeune (asphyxiating thoracic dystrophy), and Alstrom (described in the following section) in which eye and renal lesions similar to those of the LMB syndrome occur.

ALSTROM SYNDROME

The Alstrom syndrome is a rare inherited disease with major involvement of the retina, ear, kidney, and endocrine glands. In childhood, the typical patient has obesity, moderately severe nerve deafness, and retinal degeneration with later pigmentary changes ("atypical retinitis pigmentosa") and blindness. In adulthood, carbohydrate intolerance and slowly progressive renal disease develop; obesity may disappear. Males often have an unusual form of primary hypogonadism in which normal secondary sex characteristics occur, despite small testes, low plasma testosterone, and elevated gonadotropin levels. Females lack evidence of hypogonadism, but menses are irregular. Other clinical manifestations include hyperuricemia, hypertriglyceridemia, acanthosis nigricans, baldness, scoliosis, and hyperostosis frontalis. Although signs and symptoms appear early in life, the correct diagnosis is usually not made until the third decade. Before that time cases may be classified as congenital blindness or deafness or the Laurence-Moon-Biedl syndrome.

Although the Alstrom and the Laurence-Moon-Biedl syndromes both have retinal degeneration, childhood obesity, and nephropathy, they can be distinguished clinically. Most noteworthy are the rarity of mental retardation and digital anomalies in the Alstrom syndrome and the rarity of nerve deafness and diabetes mellitus in the Laurence-Moon-Biedl syndrome. Furthermore, total blindness occurs in the Alstrom syndrome at about 7 years and in the Laurence-Moon-Biedl syndrome at about 30 years.

Although the Alstrom syndrome is inherited as an autosomal recessive, suggesting an abnormality in a single enzyme, the primary biochemical defect is unknown. Membrane thickening and hyalinization in the kidney, testes, and skin suggest that the basic abnormality involves an element in membranes common to these organs, the retina, neural apparatus of the ear, and perhaps, adipose tissue. Patients with the Alstrom syndrome are resistant to the action of at least three polypeptide hormones: insulin, vasopressin, and gonadotropins. This resistance may reflect membrane changes or degeneration of cells in the target organs (see Chap. 123).

REFERENCES

COLLINS E, TURNER G: The Noonan syndrome. J Pediatr 83:941, 1973

GOLDSTEIN J, FIALKOW PJ: The Alstrom syndrome. Medicine 52:53, 1973

KLEIN D, AMMANN F: The syndrome of Laurence-Moon-Bardet-Biedl and allied diseases in Switzerland. Clinical, genetic and epidemiological studies. J Neurol Sci 9:479, 1969

HURLEY R et al: The renal lesion of the Laurence-Moon-Biedl syndrome. J Pediatr 87:206, 1975

section 8 | Endocrine diseases

108 PRINCIPLES OF ENDOCRINOLOGY

JEAN D. WILSON

The functional capacities of cells are determined ultimately by genetic factors, but the rates of the metabolic pathways in cells are regulated in large part by two interlocking and coordinated systems, the endocrine system and the nervous system. As originally formulated, these two regulatory systems were considered distinct, information being carried by neural impulses for the nervous system and by chemical mediators in the blood for the endocrine system. It is now clear that this conception is incomplete. Not only may neurotransmitters such as norepinephrine circulate in blood as hormones, but neural impulses have major effects on the release of chemical mediators such as testosterone and insulin. This interlocking relationship is most apparent in the hypothalamus, which serves as the highest integrative center for the two systems. Hence, one neuroendocrine system has evolved to integrate and coordinate the metabolic activities of the organism. Endocrinology deals largely with the chemical mediators in this system, but proper understanding of the role of hormones requires knowledge of both the autonomic nervous system (Chap. 73) and the metabolic capacities of cells (Chaps. 85–89).

The original formulation of endocrinology has been blurred in additional ways. The term *hormone* was originally applied to substances that are secreted into the circulation and act as chemical effectors in other tissues. However, the capacity to form such chemical mediators is not limited to so-called endocrine organs. Some hormones such as angiotensins II and III are formed from precursors in the circulation itself. Others such as testosterone in the female and dihydrotestosterone and estradiol in the male are formed largely in peripheral tissues from circulating precursors, so-called prohormones. Still other chemical mediators circulate only in restricted compartments such as the hypothalamic-pituitary portal system and do not reach the systemic circulation in appreciable quantities. Finally, certain hormones such as insulin and dihydrotestosterone have actions in the same tissues in which they are formed, so-called paracrine functions. Therefore, the action as well as the origins should be considered when deciding whether or not a given effector should be classified as a hormone.

BIOCHEMISTRY Synthesis The mammalian hormones, now recognized to be greater than 50 in number, fall into three general categories—peptides or peptide derivatives, steroids, and amines. These hormones are formed by two types of synthetic processes. In the case of peptide hormones, genes code for messenger RNA which is then translated into protein precursors. These proteins undergo posttranslational cleavage (preproparathyroid hormone → proparathyroid hormone → parathyroid hormone and proinsulin → insulin) and/or processing (thyroglobulin → thyroxine → triiodothyronine) to form the active hormone recognized by the target tissue. The distinct feature of peptide hormones is that one (or a few) genes code for the amino acid sequence of the peptide while other genes are responsible for the alteration of the peptide to its final form. In the case of hormones with subunits, the subunits may either be derived from a single precursor (insulin) or from separate precursors [luteinizing hormone (LH)]. Furthermore, the same peptide hormone (somatostatin) can be formed from different prohormones encoded by distinct genes and that individual prohormones such as pro-opiocortin can be metabolized to different hormone products in different cells, depending on the processing enzyme complement of the cell in question (see Chap. 88). Whether the various small peptide-releasing factors of the hypothalamus such as thyrotropin-releasing hormone (TRH) and gonadotropin-releasing hormone (LHRH) are cleaved from prohormones or synthesized de novo is unknown. Peptide hormones can also be formed ectopically in dedifferentiated tissues of nonendocrine origin such as carcinoma of the lung (see Chap. 122). The smaller the number of genes involved in controlling synthesis of a hormone, the more likely is such ectopic production to occur in malignant tissues.

In the case of steroid hormones the fundamental precursor—cholesterol (for most steroid hormones) or 7-dehydrocholesterol (for vitamin D metabolites)—undergoes a series of enzymatic transformations to form the final products. A minimum of six enzymes (or enzyme complexes) and consequently six or more genes is required to transform cholesterol to estradiol. Because of the large number of enzymes required for the formation of steroid hormones the synthesis of steroids from cholesterol in malignancies of nonendocrine tissues is unusual, even rare. However, many tissues that lack the capacity to form steroid hormones de novo from cholesterol do contain enzymes that convert circulating steroids to other hormones, for example, the conversions of androgens to estrogens by trophoblastic tumors and the conversion of progesterone to deoxycorticosterone by the kidney.

The amine hormones are synthesized by a similar but simpler series of reactions to those involved in steroid hormone synthesis except that the precursors are amino acids. For example, tyrosine is the precursor for epinephrine and norepinephrine (see Chap. 73).

Storage Most tissues that synthesize hormones have a limited capacity to store the completed product. For example, the normal adult testes contain only about a sixth of the quantity of testosterone needed for daily turnover, and consequently the testicular pool turns over several times to provide the normal daily output of hormone. Even when tissues have special storage organelles for hormone the amount of hormone stored is usually limited. For example, the insulin granules in the pancreatic beta cell ordinarily contain amounts of insulin sufficient only for short-term, reserve needs, whereas nerve endings may contain a several-day supply of norepinephrine. The limited capacity to store hormones is a chemical consequence of their unsuitability for incorporation into any of the three main storage compartments of the body (lipids, glycogen, or protein). For example, most steroid hormones are too polar to be stored in large quantities in lipid compartments, and peptide and amine hormones are unsuitable for incorporation into proteins. As a consequence of these factors the body pools of most hormones tend to be small. The major exceptions to this rule are those instances in which the precursor forms of hormone can be stored either as protein or in neutral lipid compartments; the normal thyroid gland contains the equivalent of a 2-week supply of thyroid hormones in the form of the protein thyroglobulin, and the precursor and intermediate forms of vitamin D can be stored in considerable quantity in hepatic lipid.

Release The biochemical mechanisms involved in the release process are poorly understood. In some instances they are thought to involve conversion of insoluble to soluble derivatives (proteolysis of thyroglobulin to thyroid hormones). In others, release is due to exocytosis of storage granules (insulin, glucagon, prolactin, growth hormone). Finally, release may involve passive diffusion of newly synthesized molecules down activity gradients into plasma (steroid hormones).

Because of the limited capacity for storage, most hormones are released into plasma as a reflection of the rates of formation. For example, the pituitary trophic hormones (ACTH, LH, FSH, TSH) act in their target tissues to influence rates of both hormone synthesis and release. Even in the case of peptide hormones stored in granules, initial release of the stored material is followed by an enhanced rate of synthesis (as for example the two-phase release of insulin induced by glucose infusion). For some hormones, there are in addition major diurnal, sleep-related, developmental, and neural influences on hormone release; again it is assumed that in most of these instances synthesis and release are tightly linked.

In many instances, the regulation of hormone release on a short-term basis is poorly understood. The release of some hormones is pulsatile with bursts of output occurring in a repetitive pattern; whether this intermittent release is accomplished by alterations in synthetic rates, alterations in blood flow, or by other mechanisms is uncertain. Although the physiological significance of pulsatile release is not established, changes either in frequency or in amplitude of the release pattern may characterize specific disease states.

Transport Hormones are transported from sites of synthesis to sites of cellular action and ultimately of metabolic inactivation and degradation via lymph, blood, and extracellular fluids. The plasma is probably a passive diluent for most peptide and amine hormones but provides specific proteins for binding and transport of certain steroid and thyroid hormones. The generalization can be made that the more insoluble a hormone in water, the more important the role of transport proteins. No transport protein yet characterized is exclusive; for example, testosterone can be transported both by a specific binding protein and by albumin; thyroxine can be transported both by prealbumin and by thyroxine-binding globulin (TBG). Protein-bound hormone (HP) cannot enter most cellular compartments and serves as a reservoir from which free hormone (H) is liberated in sufficient quantities for diffusion into intracellular compartments:

$$H + P \rightleftharpoons HP$$

Distribution of bound and free hormone in plasma is determined by the amount of hormone, the amount of binding protein, and the binding affinity of hormone for the protein. However, in the intact organism the effective level of free hormone is influenced by additional factors. When the rate of dissociation of a hormone from a binding protein is rapid (less than the capillary transit time for a specific organ), then the apparent free fraction in vivo is also a function of capillary transit time and membrane permeability.

Understanding the relation between free and bound hormone is essential for assessment of endocrine function. First, the free (dialyzable) fraction in vitro is generally less than the potential or apparent free fraction that is available for transport in vivo; this is because the portion of hormone bound to weak binding proteins such as albumin (in contrast to that portion bound to specific, high-affinity binding proteins) rapidly dissociates from the albumin as the free fraction diffuses from the capillary; consequently the albumin-bound hormone usually acts in vivo as a free fraction. Under most conditions, measurement of the dialyzable fraction does provide a useful index of the in vivo apparent free fraction. However, in hypoalbuminemic states, the free (dialyzable) fraction may increase under circumstances in which the in vivo free hormone level is diminished. In addition, in those tissue compartments such as liver in which protein-bound hormone is cleared (in contrast to the situation in peripheral tissues in which only the free hormone enters the cell) free hormone levels have minimal effects on hormone uptake by the tissue.

Second, the net distribution of hormones between plasma and tissue is a function of the balance between tissue binding proteins and plasma binding proteins. Therefore, measurement of true or apparent free hormone cannot necessarily be expected to predict the hormone within cells.

Third, only the plasma free hormone interacts with peripheral cells and participates in the regulatory feedback mechanisms that control the rates of hormone synthesis. As a consequence, changes in the amount of transport protein alone (e.g., changes in the free hormone level) cannot cause endocrine pathology in the steady state, provided the remainder of the endocrine feedback loop is intact. For example, profound elevations or decreases in thyroid binding globulin (either because of genetic or other factors) are both compatible with a euthyroid state. To illustrate, a sudden increase in TBG lowers the level of free (dialyzable) hormone and of the amount bound to albumin; as a consequence TSH secretion increases, and the output of thyroxine by the thyroid is increased *until* TBG is again saturated so that the level of free hormone returns to the normal range, at which time TSH levels and thyroid hormone secretion also return to normal. Likewise, a decrease in TBG temporarily increases the level of free hormone, and TSH secretion and thyroxine output fall until the free level returns to normal. To summarize, a change in a specific, high-affinity binding protein can cause profound alterations in hormone levels but by itself cannot cause either a steady-state hormone excess or deficiency, provided the regulatory feedback control mechanisms are intact. However, alteration of the amount of a binding protein may cause endocrine pathology in those instances in which hormone formation is not regulated by ordinary feedback control mechanisms. For example, testosterone production in women is not regulated directly by testosterone levels, and alterations in testosterone-binding globulin (TeBG) levels in women may alter the levels of free testosterone indefinitely.

Degradation and turnover The plasma level (PL) of any hormone is dependent on two factors—the secretion rate (SR) of the hormone and the overall rates by which it is metabolized and excreted, the so-called metabolic clearance rate (MCR):

$$PL = \frac{SR}{MCR} \quad \text{or} \quad SR = MCR \times PL$$

There is considerable variation in the mechanisms by which the metabolic clearance of hormones is accomplished. Only small fractions of hormones are excreted intact in urine or bile. Degradation and inactivation of the hormone can take place in target tissues, in other organs such as liver and kidneys, or in both target and nontarget tissues. In many instances hormone metabolism facilitates excretion by rendering the hormone soluble in urine or bile. Peptide hormones are in general inactivated by proteases, largely in target tissues. Thyroid hormones are deiodinated, deaminated, and deconjugated primarily by the liver. Steroid hormones are reduced, hydroxylated, and converted into glucuronide and sulfate conjugates. On occasion biliary conjugates may be hydrolyzed in the gastrointestinal tract and reabsorbed into the circulation. The degradative mechanisms for different hormones have one common feature, namely, that alternative pathways exist for the catabolism of all hormones described to date.

Because of the nature of the feedback mechanisms involved in the regulation of hormone secretion, changes in rates of hormone degradation alone do not cause endocrine pathology, provided the feedback loops that regulate synthesis are intact. For example, in severe liver disease and in myxedema, the degradation of glucocorticoids by the liver is impaired; as a consequence the turnover of the hormone slows, but the plasma level does not rise because secretion of ACTH is inhibited. Thus, a normal level of free hormone is maintained by decreasing the rate of secretion of glucocorticoid. The opposite is the case when glucocorticoid degradation is enhanced (as in thyrotoxicosis); here glucocorticoid secretion rises to keep the level of the hormone normal.

Although changes in rates of hormone degradation alone do not result in hormone deficit or excess, such changes may cause profound alterations in endocrine pharmacology. Thus, it is necessary to recognize that ordinary doses of glucocorticoids may cause the Cushing syndrome in patients with myxedema or liver disease, and consequently glucocorticoid dosage must be reduced in both conditions. Likewise, doses of glucocorticoids may have to be increased in the presence of hyperthyroidism. In addition, the development of hyperthyroidism in a patient with inadequate adrenal reserve might precipitate an adrenal crisis by accelerating the rate of glucocorticoid catabolism. Thus, in circumstances in which the normal servomechanisms that regulate hormone synthesis are either circumvented or inoperative, changes in rates of hormone degradation may aggravate or cause pathology.

REGULATION OF HORMONE PRODUCTION As stated above, fluctuations of hormone levels in the normal person are determined primarily by changes in production. A unifying feature of all endocrine systems is the fact that the production of each hormone is regulated directly or indirectly by the metabolic activity of the hormone itself. This regulation is accomplished through a series of negative feedback loops (Fig. 108-1). In many cases a fairly constant blood level of hormone is required, and some sensing device must exist to monitor either the hormone level itself or some related function such as plasma osmolality, blood glucose, plasma calcium, or body sodium content. For example, hormones produced in response to pituitary trophic hormones (cortisol, thyroxine, gonadal steroids) feed back into the hypothalamic-pituitary system to regulate the secretion of additional hormone. Similarly, parathyroid hormone and insulin are secreted in response to feedback signals from serum calcium and glucose levels, respectively. Feedback systems are generally more complex than this description indicates, sometimes operating indirectly by several steps; in those instances in which the hormone itself acts as the direct regulator of feedback (testosterone on the pituitary), the effect is mediated by the same cellular machinery by which the action of the hormone is accomplished in other target tissues.

Both negative and positive feedback can occur; an example of positive feedback is the stimulation of LH release by estradiol prior to ovulation. Nonhormonal and environmental factors may alter either positive or negative feedback control mechanisms or the response to such control.

A common feature of the feedback systems is rapidity of action; indeed, most respond within minutes or hours to vary-

FIGURE 108-1
Feedback control of an endocrine organ such as the adrenal, thyroid, or gonads by the pituitary.

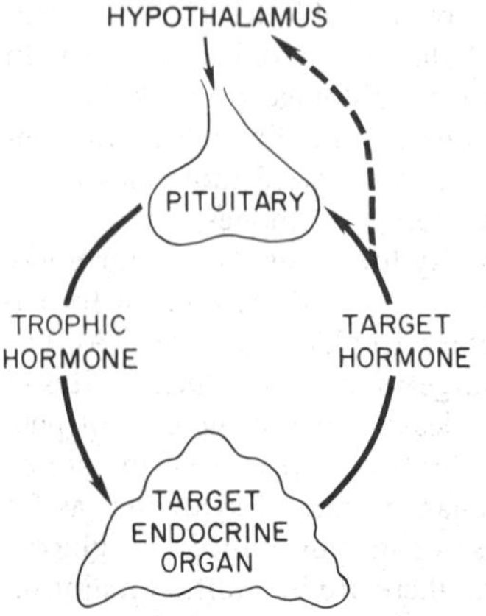

ing metabolic demands to maintain homeostatic control within a narrow range. The main exceptions relate to gametogenesis in the ovary and testis (see Chaps. 117 and 118). In both instances, a complex differentiative process is involved. The steady-state operation of these systems is such that sperm production tends to be relatively constant from day to day whereas ovulation is cyclic. However, spermatogenesis requires approximately a month to complete so that changes in FSH levels may not be manifested by altered rates of sperm production for long periods.

The fact that the secretion of all hormones is under regulatory control has several important clinical implications. First, the clinical significance of plasma levels of hormones may be interpretable only if the appropriate regulatory factors are taken into account (Fig. 108-2). The meaning of a borderline low testosterone value may only become clear when LH is measured simultaneously; likewise, plasma insulin and parathyroid hormone levels may be interpretable only in conjunction with simultaneous measurements of plasma glucose and calcium, respectively. Second, the finding of simultaneous elevations of hormone pairs (or hormone-regulatory factor pairs) in the absence of signs of hormone excess suggests the presence of a hormone-resistance state. For example, simultaneous elevation of plasma glucose and insulin is indicative of insulin resistance; simultaneous elevation of LH and testosterone suggests androgen resistance, etc. Third, insight into the regulatory control of hormone secretion is the basis for the various dynamic tests of hormone reserve and hormone secretion.

MECHANISMS OF HORMONE ACTION The first step in hormone action is thought to involve the interaction of the hormone with specific macromolecules in the cell, so-called hormone receptors. Two general classes of hormone receptors are now recognized, those on the plasma membrane of the cell surface and those that are intracellular.

Hormones with cell surface receptors The hormones of the first type bind to surface receptors localized on the plasma membrane (Fig. 108-3). At least three categories of plasma membrane–hormone interaction can be distinguished. In the first category (H_1 in Fig. 108-3) the hormone-receptor complex on the cell surfaces causes the production of a so-called second messenger, cyclic adenosine 3′,5′-monophosphate (cAMP), and the subsequent actions of the hormone are mediated by cAMP (see Chap. 86). This mechanism applies to several protein hormones and to the biogenic amines. In the second category (H_2 in Fig. 108-3) the cell surface receptor causes the production or release of other second messengers, for example, calcium. This mechanism applies to certain neurotransmitters and TRH. The precise mechanism of calcium release and action in such systems is not known; the latter may involve binding of calcium to the enzyme-regulating protein calmodulin. In the third category (H_3 in Fig. 108-3) the cell surface receptor–hormone complex is internalized within the cell, but the subsequent events have not been defined clearly. A hormone of the latter category is insulin (see Chap. 85).

The best understood of these systems is that in which cAMP serves as the second messenger (Fig. 108-3). Cellular concentration of cAMP is controlled by two enzymes with opposite activities. Adenylate cyclase (AC), localized in the plasma membrane, converts adenosine triphosphate (ATP) into cAMP. Phosphodiesterase (PDE) found largely in the cell cytosol, inactivates cAMP by converting it to 5′-adenosine monophosphate (5′-AMP). Hormones (H_1) that act at the cell surface form a reversible complex with specialized membrane protein receptors (R_1). These proteins bind the hormone with high affinity but limited capacity. The formation of the hormone-receptor complex is coupled to a stimulation of the adenylate cyclase. The H_1R_1 complex binds the N subunit of the adenylate cyclase (a protein that also binds GTP) and activates the catalytic subunit of the enzyme (AC), thus stimulating cAMP synthesis. Phosphorylating enzymes—known as protein kinases—appear to play an important role in the overall process; these kinases are composed of catalytic (C) and regulatory (R) subunits. Binding of cAMP to the regulatory subunit frees the catalytic subunit and allows phosphorylation of various proteins (S) with consequent activation or inactivation.

Hormones with intracellular receptors Steroid and thyroid hormones are transported in plasma bound to carrier proteins (Fig. 108-4). The protein-bound hormones (HP) are in dynamic equilibrium with small amounts of free hormones (H)

FIGURE 108-2
Relation between target hormone level and trophic hormone level in normal and disease states (e.g., TSH and thyroid hormones, ACTH and cortisol, LH and testosterone).

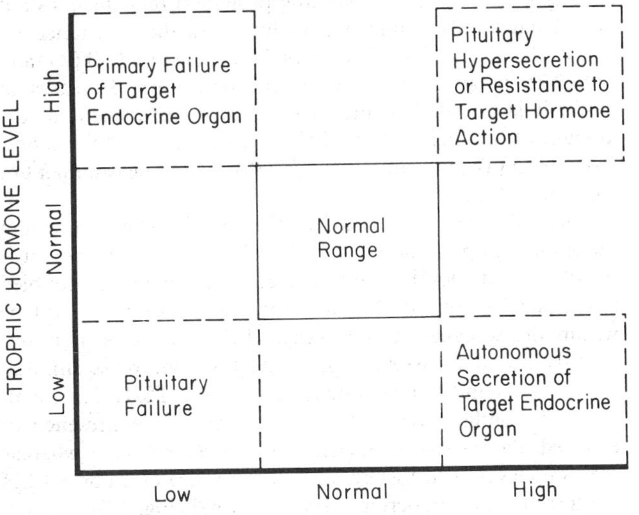

FIGURE 108-3
Schema of action of hormones with cell surface receptors. H = hormone; R = receptor; C = catalytic subunit; R = cAMP-binding subunit of protein kinase; cAMP = cyclic AMP; AC = adenylate cyclase.*

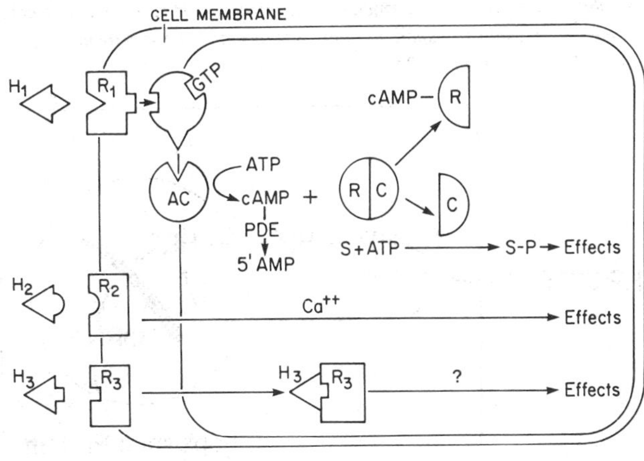

that diffuse by a passive mechanism into cells where they act by fundamentally different mechanisms than do the peptide hormones. Inside the cells some of these hormones (thyroxine, testosterone) undergo chemical conversion to more active forms such as triiodothyronine and dihydrotestosterone. In other instances the principal form of the hormone secreted into plasma (cortisol, progesterone, aldosterone, estradiol) undergoes no further metabolism within the cell, and the molecular species that circulates in plasma is the molecule that is ultimately responsible for hormone action within the target cell.

H then binds to specific receptor proteins (R) in the cytoplasm of the cell to form a hormone-receptor complex (HR). The hormone-receptor complex undergoes transformation by a poorly understood, temperature-dependent process to form an activated complex (HR*). The activated hormone-receptor complex has the capacity to bind chromatin. As the result of this binding a series of new messenger RNAs (mRNAs) is formed, and the subsequent synthesis of cytoplasmic proteins is enhanced. These proteins in turn mediate the effects of the hormone. In some instances (triiodothyronine and possibly certain steroids) the unoccupied receptor proteins appear to be located predominately in nuclei; in such cases the unbound hormone enters the nucleus where the active hormone–receptor complex is formed and attaches to the chromatin in a similar fashion.

ASSESSMENT OF HORMONE FUNCTION In routine practice endocrine status is assessed either by measuring plasma levels of a hormone, the urinary excretion of a hormone or of some metabolite, the rates of secretion of hormones into the circulation, dynamic tests of hormone reserve and regulation, hormone receptors, selected effects of hormone action in target tissues, or appropriate combinations of these tests. Each of these techniques is useful in certain clinical situations.

Plasma levels The plasma levels of steroid and thyroid hormones range between 1 n*M* and 1 μ*M*, while those of peptide hormones are generally in the range of 1p*M* to 0.1 n*M*. The application of modern chemical, chromatographic, radioreceptor, and radioimmunoassay techniques for the assessment of plasma constituents in low concentrations constitutes one of the significant advances of modern medicine and has transformed endocrinology from a largely descriptive discipline to a more quantitative one. In the case of hormones whose plasma levels are relatively constant from moment to moment and day to day (thyroxine and triiodothyronine), the measurement of

FIGURE 108-4

Mechanism of action of hormones with intracellular receptors. H=hormone; P=plasma transport protein; R=receptor; R=activated receptor; mRNA=messenger RNA.*

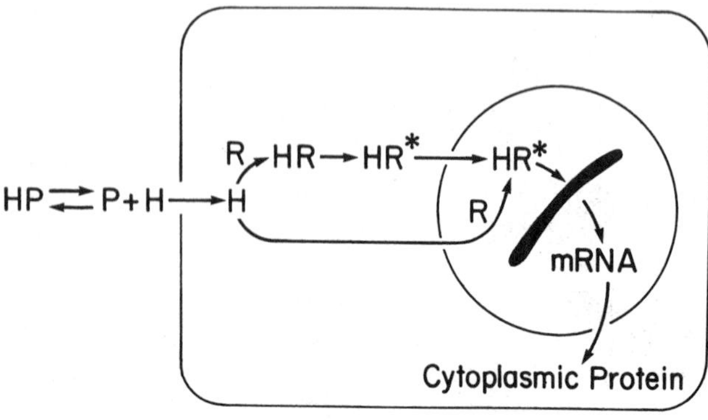

isolated plasma levels alone provides a reliable assessment of the hormone status in the vast majority of clinical situations.

For several reasons, however, care must be exercised in assessing isolated plasma levels. First, for hormones with relatively simple structures (steroid and thyroid hormones) chemical and radioimmunoassay techniques are reliable so that measured values usually reflect the plasma levels as of a given moment. In the case of the more complex peptide hormones, however, considerable variability may exist in the structure of physiologically active hormone molecules in the circulation, some of which may be measured poorly in specific radioimmunoassay procedures; for example, standard radioimmunoassays for LH and for parathyroid hormone may on occasion either underestimate or overestimate the amount of biologically active hormone in plasma.

Second, in the case of hormones that undergo pulsatile secretion (LH, testosterone) a single value may or may not be representative of mean plasma levels. In these instances it is necessary either to measure levels in several samples drawn at random or to pool aliquots of three or more samples of plasma drawn at 20-to 30-min intervals for a single determination.

Third, when plasma levels exhibit a characteristic, predictable fluctuation such as the diurnal variation of plasma cortisol, the timing of plasma sampling can be designed to provide a useful index of the hormone status. Even here, however, it is important to recognize that plasma levels may exhibit diurnal variation only during certain phases of life (plasma LH levels in early puberty). In women during the reproductive years appropriate interpretation of plasma gonadotropins, progesterone, and estradiol requires reference to the corresponding phase of the ovulatory and menstrual cycles, and in most instances it is necessary to obtain sequential studies over several days to provide interpretable data. Although seasonal variations occur in the levels of certain hormones (such as thyroxine and testosterone), these changes are generally of such a small magnitude as to have no significance in the interpretation of individual values.

Fourth, in the case of the steroid and thyroid hormones, which are transported in plasma largely bound to proteins, it is essential to remember that measurement of total hormone concentration provides an index of endocrine status *only* to the extent that it allows a deduction of the level of the free or unbound hormone. Indeed, direct measurements of the free (dialyzable) levels of these hormones (usually 1 percent or less of the total) can be done only in a few labs. Since the amount of free hormone is a function of the amount and the affinity of binding of transport proteins and the amount of hormone, the total hormone level reflects the amount of free hormone only as long as the amount of binding protein(s) remains constant or fluctuates only within narrow limits. In those instances in which the level of binding protein is increased (TBG and TeBG in pregnancy) or decreased (hereditary decreases in TBG) it is essential to utilize some other assessment of the amount of binding protein to allow deduction of the free hormone level (T_3 resin uptake for TBG or direct measurement of TBG or TeBG).

Fifth, the range of plasma levels of most hormones within the normal population is fairly broad. As a consequence, it is possible for the level in an individual to be halved or doubled (and thus be grossly abnormal for that person) but still be within the so-called normal range. For this reason it is frequently useful to assess appropriate hormone pairs simultaneously (LH and testosterone, thyroxine and TSH). For example, a borderline low testosterone level in the presence of elevated plasma LH is indicative of testicular failure, whereas the same level of testosterone in the presence of a normal LH implies that the endocrine status is normal (Fig. 108-2). Likewise, in women with increased testosterone production and secondary decrease in TeBG, a normal plasma testosterone concentration may be found despite the increased production of the hormone.

Urinary excretion The measurement of urinary excretion of a hormone or some hormone metabolite that reflects either plasma levels or secretory rates offers certain advantages over the measurement of isolated plasma levels, e.g., the urinary excretion reflects average plasma levels and hence average production rates over the time of collection. Thus, a 24-h urine 17-hydroxycorticoid value may provide a better estimate of the function of the adrenal cortex than isolated measurements of plasma cortisol. Again, however, certain limitations of the use of urinary measurements must be kept in mind. (1) Creatinine determinations should be done routinely to document the adequacy of the urine collection. Women excrete on average about 1 g, while men excrete about 1.8 g per day. Day-to-day variation should not exceed 20 percent. (2) The excretion of individual metabolites may not reflect changes in hormone secretion under all conditions. For example, the formation of the 18-oxo derivative of aldosterone may be influenced by drugs that do not influence secretion or plasma levels of the hormone. (3) Urine values are obviously meaningless for those hormones (thyroxine, triiodothyronine) excreted into bile. Of more importance is the fact that peptide hormones such as gonadotropins can be metabolized differently in different individuals prior to excretion into the urine so that establishment of the range of normal is difficult. (4) Hormones from more than one source may be excreted as common metabolites; urinary 17-ketosteroids are derived from both adrenal and gonadal androgens, and consequently their measurement is of little value in assessing testicular androgen production in men. (5) Changes in renal function may influence rates of hormone excretion into urine. Such changes can be in part corrected by measurement of urine creatinine, but in the case of metabolites or conjugates formed in the kidney itself excretion patterns may be distorted out of proportion to the decrease in creatinine clearance.

Secretion and production rates The measurement of the actual secretion rate of a hormone circumvents virtually all the problems inherent in measurement of plasma levels and urinary excretion. Such measurements involve the administration of radioactive hormone and measuring the dilution that such a hormone undergoes as a consequence of mixture with endogenously secreted, nonradioactive hormones over a fixed period of time. In practice a unique metabolite of the hormone from urine or the plasma hormone itself is isolated, purified to radiochemical homogeneity, and used to calculate the amount of the hormone secreted during the time of study. In the case of hormones formed principally in peripheral tissues (estradiol and dihydrotestosterone in men, triiodothyronine in both sexes) radioactive precursors can be administered, and the rates of conversion to the metabolites in question can be measured for assessment of overall production rates. Alternatively, as described above, clearance rates of hormones can be measured and, together with mean plasma levels, used to estimate secretion rates. Unfortunately, these various techniques are technically difficult, are expensive to perform, require administration of radioactive isotopes, and can be done in only a few centers.

Dynamic tests of hormone reserve and regulation When hypo- or hyperfunction is severe, measurement of the level of hormone in blood or urine may be satisfactory for making a diagnosis, particularly when the tests demonstrate normal feedback relationships. e.g., low plasma testosterone coupled with high plasma LH indicates primary testicular failure. In less clear-cut instances, however, stimulation tests are useful in establishing the significance of borderline low values. Likewise, suppression tests are used to document the presence of hyperfunction of endocrine systems. All such dynamic tests are designed to take advantage of the known feedback control mechanisms for various hormones (Fig. 108-1).

Two types of stimulation tests are in common usage. In one, endogenous hormone production or action is blocked (cortisol production by metyrapone, estradiol action by clomiphene), and the capacity of the pituitary to respond by increasing endogenous production of the trophic hormone and/or the capacity of the target tissue to respond are then assessed; ideally such tests measure the integrity of an entire hypothalamic–pituitary–target tissue system. In the other type of stimulation test, the trophic hormone itself is administered under some standardized regimen, and the capacity of the target tissue to respond is determined (cortisol levels before and after ACTH administration). Stimulation tests are particularly useful in four situations: (1) assessment of hormone status when precise quantification of plasma levels is difficult or imperfect (ACTH), (2) assessment of endocrine status when static tests are borderline low, (3) distinguishing primary from secondary (pituitary) causes of endocrine failure, and (4) assessing gonadal reserve in prepubertal patients in whom plasma gonadotropins and gonadal steroids are difficult to interpret.

Suppression tests are useful for the diagnosis of hyperfunction because the hyperfunctioning gland by definition does not operate under normal control mechanisms. Suppression can either be quantitatively or qualitatively abnormal. For example, the feedback control of the pituitary may be reset to respond to high levels of the suppressing hormone (pituitary ACTH secretion in Cushing's disease), or secretion can be autonomous and without any control (ACTH secretion by an oatcell carcinoma of the lung). In principle, the feedback regulator is administered, and the capacity of the hormone to be inhibited is assessed for the endocrine system in question (change in ^{131}I uptake after administration of thyroid hormones, change in cortisol secretion after the administration of potent exogenous glucocorticoids, suppressibility of plasma growth hormone by glucose).

These dynamic tests continue to be of critical importance in certain clinical states; however, in circumstances in which hormone pairs can be measured accurately (TSH and thyroxine in evaluating hypothyroidism, testosterone and LH in hypogonadal states) such tests are required only occasionally.

Hormone receptors and antibodies The measurement of hormone receptors in biopsy material from target tissues or in fibroblasts propagated from biopsy material is useful—particularly in the diagnosis of partial hormone-resistance states such as rickets due to vitamin D resistance, hyperglycemia and hyperinsulinemia associated with insulin resistance, and male pseudohermaphroditism due to androgen resistance. Likewise, under selected conditions measurement of antibodies to hormones (such as antibodies to thyroid hormones that can cause hypothyroidism) or antibodies to target tissues (adrenal gland, gonads, thyroid) may be essential for the assessment of endocrine status. With certain exceptions (antibodies to thyroid tissue) these tests are not widely available.

Tissue effects The ideal hormone test perhaps is the measurement of the peripheral end result of hormone action in the target tissues for the hormone. For example, demonstration of the capacity to concentrate urine maximally following water restriction indicates that the hypothalamic control mechanisms are intact, that the posterior pituitary has a normal capacity to secrete vasopressin, that the vasopressin receptor is intact, and the postreceptor effector mechanisms for the hormone are operative. Optimally such a test assesses the function of the entire pathway of hormone secretion and action. In practice, many such tests are imperfect. For example, even though vasopressin secretion is normal, intrinsic renal disease can result in a fixed low urine osmolality and thus distort the interpretation of the functional test of vasopressin action. In other instances the tests are difficult to perform and subject both to artifact and to influences from diverse parameters (for example, the metabolic rate is increased by fever even when thyroid function is normal). For these reasons, the identification of additional specific tissue markers for hormone action would be very useful.

CLINICAL SYNDROMES At the clinical level, endocrinopathy can result from hormone deficiency, hormone excess, or resistance to hormone action. It is increasingly clear that abnormalities in more than one endocrine system commonly coexist in the same individual.

Deficiency states With few exceptions (calcitonin, melatonin) hormone deficiency results in pathological manifestations. The elucidation of clinical disorders that results from hormone deficiency or absence played an important role in the evolution of endocrinology as a discipline. Such studies were followed by attempts to extract the responsible hormone from normal endocrine tissues, characterize its chemical nature (and ultimately synthesize it), and administer the hormone to replace the deficit. Thus, the routine treatment of hypothyroidism by the administration of thyroid hormone is probably as successful as any therapeutic measure in medicine. Because clinical deficiency states can be induced in experimental animals by appropriate destruction or removal of the endocrine organ, an enormous amount is known about the pathophysiology of the deficiency states (diabetes mellitus, pituitary and adrenal insufficiency, hypothyroidism, and hypogonadism).

The pathogenesis of the destructive processes involved in the failure of the endocrine organs is also understood in many instances; these include infections (adrenal insufficiency due to tuberculosis), infarction (postpartum pituitary failure) and tissue death of other causes (diabetes secondary to pancreatitis), tumors (chromophobe adenomas of the pituitary), autoimmune processes (Hashimoto's thyroiditis), dietary inadequacy (hypothyroidism due to iodine deficiency), and hereditary defects (pituitary dwarfism). In certain forms of diabetes mellitus, the cause may be a hereditary predisposition that renders the pancreas subject to destruction by several mechanisms (see Chap. 114). In other endocrine-deficiency diseases the etiology of the underlying defect is unidentified (ordinary myxedema and congenital anorchia).

Hormone excess With few exceptions (testosterone in men, progesterone in men and women) hormone excess causes pathological effects. Four general types of hormone excess are recognized. In one, the hormone is overproduced by the gland that is the usual site of its production (hyperthyroidism, acromegaly, Cushing's disease); in every instance such excess production results from failure or circumvention of the feedback control mechanisms that regulate production of the hormone in the normal state, but the underlying mechanism is often obscure because animal models for the diseases are rare. The second type of hormone excess results when a hormone is produced by a tissue (usually malignant) that ordinarily is not an endocrine organ (for example, ACTH production in oat-cell carcinoma of the lung, thyroid hormone secretion in struma ovarii). Such hormone-excess states have been described for many hormones. A third type of hormone-excess state involves the overproduction of hormones in peripheral tissues from circulating prohormones; for example, overproduction of estrogen in liver disease can result from diversion of the precursor androstenedione from its usual sites of catabolism in the liver to sites of peripheral metabolism. Finally, hormone excess all too commonly results from iatrogenic causes; for example, the complications resulting from the administration of glucocorticoids constitute a major clinical problem (see Chap. 112).

Excess of a given hormone may result from more than one cause. For example, thyrotoxicosis can result from overproduction of hormone by the thyroid as a result of overproduction of TSH (rare), from stimulation by extrapituitary thyroid-stimulating factors, from autonomous thyroid hyperfunction; from leakage of preformed hormone from the thyroid due to an inflammatory injury; or from excess hormone from sources other than the thyroid itself, as in thyroid hormone overdosage or struma ovarii (see Chap. 111). The unraveling of the cause of specific hormone-excess states can be one of the most challenging problems of clinical endocrinology.

Hormone resistance The concept that an endocrinopathy could result because the tissues cannot respond to normal (or increased) levels of a hormone evolved from the deduction by Fuller Albright and his colleagues that pseudohypoparathyroidism is due to peripheral resistance to the action of parathyroid hormone (see Chaps. 86 and 339). This concept has had far-reaching implications for endocrinology. First, the concept of hormone resistance has served as a major stimulus for the study of how hormones act within cells. Second, more and more forms of hormone resistance have been identified so that diseases are now recognized to result from resistance to many hormones. Such hormone resistance is frequently due to hereditary causes. Third, hormone resistance is now known to result from a variety of mechanisms, including defects in receptors and in postreceptor effector mechanisms for hormones, the formation of incomplete or abnormal forms of hormones, development of antibodies to hormones or hormone receptors, and the absence of target cells. Fourth, abnormalities of receptors are now implicated in the pathogenesis of diseases outside the endocrine domain, such as myasthenia gravis and familial hypercholesterolemia.

A common feature of hormone-resistance states is the presence of a normal or *elevated* level of the hormone in the circulation of a patient with evidence of deficient hormone action. This feature is a consequence of the fact that every hormone is under regulatory feedback control, and failure of hormone action usually leads to increased hormone production.

However, hormone resistance does not necessarily involve equally all target tissues for the hormone. For example, selective resistance to thyroid hormone has been described in which the defect in hormone action appears to be restricted to the pituitary itself, and a form of androgen resistance has been characterized in which androgen action is impaired more completely in the testis than in other target tissues. Elucidation of the pathogenesis of these selective defects will doubtlessly provide valuable insight into the factors that determine the nature of "target tissues" for hormones in the normal state.

Diseases affecting multiple endocrine systems The fact that disorders can affect more than one endocrine system has been known since the description of panhypopituitarism in the nineteenth century. However, the disorders affecting more than one endocrine system are more common than previously thought and encompass diverse etiologies including autoimmunity (Schmidt syndrome), receptor abnormalities (gonadotropin and thyrotropin resistance in pseudohypoparathyroidism), tumors (multiple endocrine neoplasia or MEN), and hereditary disorders of unknown etiology (lipodystrophies). They may include both hypo- and hyperfunctioning states, and some clinical syndromes may occur in the context of more than one polyendocrine state (pheochromocytoma in MEN II and MEN III, diabetes in Schmidt syndrome and in lipodystrophy).

Because each endocrinopathy that occurs as the part of such a constellation can also occur alone it is essential that all endocrine patients be approached with a high index of suspicion for abnormalities of multiple systems. This is of particular importance because treatment of one condition may cause worsening of another (surgical procedures in patients with unrecognized pheochromocytoma) and because in certain of the familial syndromes it is mandatory to make systematic searches for the disease in potentially affected family members.

REFERENCES

BAXTER JD, MACLEOD KM: Molecular basis for hormone action, in *Metabolic Control and Disease,* 8th ed, PK Bondy, LE Rosenberg (eds). Philadelphia, Saunders, 1979

FEDERMAN DD: General principles of endocrinology, in *Textbook of Endocrinology,* RH Williams (ed). Philadelphia, Saunders, 1982, pp 1–14

GRODY WW et al: Activation, transformation, and subunit structure of steroid hormone receptors. Endocr Rev 3:141, 1982

HAEBENER JF: Hormone biosynthesis and secretion, in *Endocrinology and Metabolism,* P Felig et al (eds). New York, McGraw-Hill, 1982, p 29

PARTRIDGE WM: Transport of protein-bound hormones into tissues *in vivo.* Endocr Rev 2:103, 1981

VERHOEVEN GFM, WILSON JD: The syndromes of primary hormone resistance. Metabolism 28:253, 1979

109 DISEASES OF THE HYPOTHALAMUS AND ANTERIOR PITUITARY

PETER O. KOHLER

ANATOMY AND PHYSIOLOGY

The hypothalamus and pituitary form a control unit that regulates growth, lactation, the function of the thyroid, adrenals, and gonads, and the state of hydration. Disorders of the hypothalamus are frequently expressed as abnormalities of pituitary hormone secretion. Understanding the functional relationship of the hypothalamus to the pituitary requires an appreciation of the anatomic relationships. The hypothalamus is a small, specialized area at the base of the brain lying superior and posterior to the optic chiasm and superior to the pituitary gland. The inferior portion of the hypothalamus, or tuber cinereum, has a central projection called the *median eminence* which forms the base of the third ventricle of the brain.

The pituitary is located below the base of the brain and is connected to the median eminence of the hypothalamus by the pituitary stalk. The pituitary is located within a bony structure which resembles a Turkish saddle, hence the name *sella turcica.* The stalk passes through the center of a thick reflection of dura called the *diaphragma sellae,* which separates the pituitary from the brain. Embryologically, the posterior lobe of the pituitary (neurohypophysis) develops as a downward projection of neuroectoderm from the base of the brain. The larger anterior lobe (adenohypophysis) develops separately as an upwardly displaced group of cells from the primitive buccal endothelium. A third section of the pituitary, the intermediate lobe, is present in many animals but is poorly developed in humans. The normal pituitary weighs 0.5 to 1.0 g and measures approximately 6 to 13 mm in each dimension.

Functions of the anterior and posterior pituitary are regulated by the hypothalamus but by different mechanisms (Fig. 109-1). The neurohypophysis is an extension of large neurons originating in the supraoptic and paraventricular nuclei of the hypothalamus. The neurohypophyseal hormones, vasopressin [antidiuretic hormone (ADH)] and oxytocin, are produced by neurons in the supraoptic and paraventricular neurosecretory cells of the hypothalamus. These hormones are transported in vesicles into the posterior lobe of the pituitary in association with specific carrier (and possibly precursor) proteins called *neurophysins.* In response to appropriate stimuli depolarization of these large neurons occurs, and vasopressin or oxytocin is released by the neurohypophysis into systemic circulation.

In contrast to this direct form of control, the anterior pituitary hormones are synthesized within the adenohypophysis, and secretion is regulated by hypothalamic peptides and possibly other factors formed in the hypothalamus. The regulatory

FIGURE 109-1
Schematic representation of the relationship between the hypothalamus and pituitary. The neurohypophysis or posterior lobe of the pituitary is a downward projection of the hypothalamus. The posterior pituitary hormones, antidiuretic hormone (ADH, vasopressin) and oxytocin, are synthesized in neurons in the hypothalamus and are transported down the axons from these neurons into the posterior lobe. In contrast, the anterior pituitary develops embryologically from different tissue and has no direct neural connection with the hypothalamus. The control of the anterior pituitary hormones is through a combination of factors including feedback inhibition by target organ hormones such as the thyroid, adrenal, and gonadal hormones. The hypothalamus exerts control over the anterior lobe by hypothalamic factors such as thyrotropin-releasing hormone (TRH), luteinizing hormone–releasing hormone (LHRH), and prolactin-inhibiting factor (PIF). These factors are released into capillaries of the pituitary portal system, reach the anterior pituitary cells via portal blood, and regulate the secretion of the anterior pituitary hormones. The intermediate lobe of the pituitary is essentially vestigial in humans.

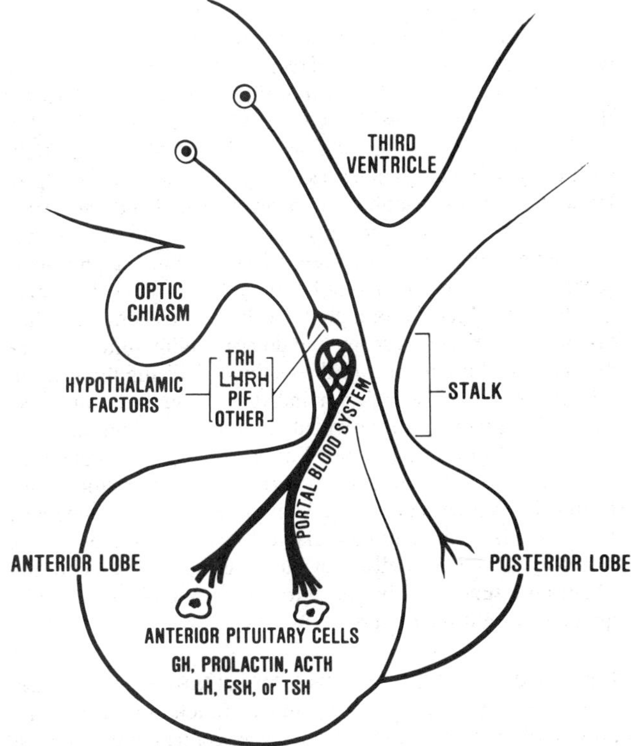

factors are released into the capillaries of a portal venous system that connects the hypothalamus and anterior lobe of the pituitary. The blood supply to the median eminence comes from the superior hypophyseal arteries which arise from the internal carotid arteries. The capillary system from the hypothalamus drains into the long portal veins that traverse the pituitary stalk to supply the anterior lobe with portal venous blood. A small amount of blood may reach the anterior pituitary through the small arteries contained in a band of connective tissue on the superior portion of the anterior lobe (the trabecula) or from branches of the inferior capsular or inferior hypophyseal arteries. However, the major supply to the adenohypophysis is through the portal venous system. Blood may also travel in a retrograde fashion from the pituitary to the hypothalamus. The fact that the perfusion pressure of the anterior pituitary is that of the venous system may be one reason that the enlarged pituitary of pregnancy is susceptible to infarction during hypovolemic shock (see Sheehan's syndrome under "Infarction and Vascular Disorders" below). In contrast to the anterior lobe, the neurohypophysis has a direct arterial supply from the inferior hypophyseal branches of the internal carotid arteries.

Another unusual feature of the blood supply to the hypothalamus is important with regard to function. The blood-brain barrier is incomplete in the median eminence where the major plexus of the portal system originates, and the capillary loops of the plexus in this area exhibit endothelial fenestration. As a consequence large molecules such as hormones may cross the blood-brain barrier, gain access to the hypothalamus and pituitary, and provide feedback regulation of pituitary function.

The hypothalamus has multiple connections with other areas of the brain providing control from higher centers. In addition to the regulation of pituitary function, the hypothalamus has an important role in several nonendocrine homeostatic and physiological functions. These include (1) thirst, which is regulated by osmoreceptors different from those involved with vasopressin release, (2) appetite and caloric intake, (3) sleep-wake behavior, (4) emotions such as rage and apathy, (5) autonomic balance, and (6) cognition.

Histologically, the anterior pituitary cells are arranged in cords or acinar-like structures surrounded by an extensive network of capillary sinusoids. Traditionally, the anterior pituitary cells have been divided into three types on the basis of their staining characteristics with hematoxylin and eosin, Mallory's trichrome, and periodic acid Schiff (PAS) stains. Cells with eosin-staining granules secrete growth hormone and prolactin. Cells with basophilic granules, which also demonstrate positive PAS staining for glycoprotein, secrete thyrotropin (thyroid-stimulating hormone, TSH), luteinizing hormone (LH), and follicle-stimulating hormone (FSH) as well as corticotropin (ACTH). Chromophobic cells do not contain visible granules by light microscopy and do not exhibit affinity for the usual stains. Immunochemical techniques utilizing fluorescent-labeled antibodies specific for individual hormones and electron microscopy have provided additional insight into the function of specific cell types. For example, eosinophilic cells containing growth hormone granules can now be distinguished from cells that contain prolactin granules, and it is now clear that essentially all the glandular cells contain some type of secretory granules. Cells previously designated as chromophobes are functional but have too few granules to stain adequately by light microscopy.

PHYSIOLOGICAL REGULATION OF PITUITARY HORMONE SECRETION The regulation of pituitary function requires integration of numerous stimuli from higher centers in the brain as well as those acting directly on the hypothalamus and pituitary. One important mechanism in this regulation is feedback control. Anterior pituitary hormone secretion is suppressed by the products of target endocrine glands such as thyroid, adrenal, and gonads. This feedback control is powerful; for example, even a slight excess of thyroid hormone blocks the release of thyrotropin by the pituitary in response to the specific releasing hormone. Some hormones such as prolactin and growth hormone may regulate their own secretion directly by acting on the hypothalamus (short-loop feedback). Essentially all anterior pituitary hormones are preferentially discharged during sleep, but the reasons for these nocturnal surges have not been elucidated.

Neurohypophysis Oxytocin and vasopressin are stored in the posterior lobe in granules in association with hormone-specific carrier proteins, the neurophysins. After appropriate stimuli, vasopressin, oxytocin, and the specific neurophysin are released into systemic circulation via the capillaries of the neurohypophysis.

VASOPRESSIN (ANTIDIURETIC HORMONE, ADH) (see also Chap. 110) The major action of ADH is to cause concentration of the urine by permitting free water reabsorption from the hypotonic tubular fluid in the distal nephron. Without ADH the distal convoluted tubule is essentially impermeable to water, although solutes are actively reabsorbed. In the presence of ADH, the tubule and collecting duct are permeable to water, which diffuses from the hypotonic tubular fluid to the hypertonic interstitium. This allows concentration of the tubular fluid and, therefore, of the urine. ADH interacts with specific membrane receptors in the renal tubule and acts through a mechanism involving induction of adenylate cyclase and generation of cyclic adenosine monophosphate (AMP).

The primary control for release of the hormone is the osmolality of blood reaching the hypothalamus. Supraoptic neurons appear to act as osmoreceptors, and their rates of discharge are increased when the osmolality of the perfusing blood is increased. This same mechanism prevails normally during dehydration, resulting in release of ADH and maximal concentration of the urine. Although blood osmolality is the major regulator of ADH release, a fall in blood pressure, as produced by hemorrhage, also causes ADH secretion, even when blood osmolality is normal or low. This pressor control mechanism is mediated by volume receptors in the carotid sinus, left atrium, and aortic arch. In addition, nicotine, various forms of stress, head trauma, and certain types of anesthesia and drugs may stimulate ADH release.

OXYTOCIN Oxytocin has a role in the induction of labor, although delivery can occur in patients with posterior pituitary deficiency. The sensitized uterus of the pregnant woman at term is stimulated to contract by oxytocin. The other major function of oxytocin is the stimulation of the myoepithelial cells of the acini of the lactating breast. Myoepithelial cell contraction forces the acinar content into the duct system so that milk accumulates in the nipples. Oxytocin release occurs after nipple stimulation. Spinal cord or brainstem lesions can abolish this neural reflex arc, and ethanol or emotional stress can inhibit the oxytocin response. Control of oxytocin secretion is separate from that of ADH. For example, release of the oxytocin-specific neurophysin is stimulated by estrogens, while ADH-specific neurophysin is released after nicotine. Also, water loading inhibits the release of ADH without affecting oxytocin-induced milk ejection.

Anterior pituitary HYPOTHALAMIC REGULATORY HORMONES When the pituitary stalk is severed, secretion of most pituitary hormones decreases substantially. An exception is prolactin secretion, which increases greatly when the hypothalamus is destroyed or the portal system is interrupted. Thus, the hypothalamus provides a net stimulatory influence on the secretion of all major anterior pituitary hormones except prolactin, which is primarily under inhibitory control by the hypothalamus. In addition, crude hypothalamic extracts of the median eminence release anterior pituitary hormones when injected into laboratory animals or added to isolated pituitary tissue in vitro. To date, three hypothalamic regulatory factors have been isolated, chemically characterized, synthesized, and tested in man. These are thyrotropin-releasing hormone (TRH), luteinizing hormone–releasing hormone (LHRH), and somatostatin. Presumptive evidence exists for several other hypothalamic hormones, including a growth hormone–releasing hormone and a prolactin-releasing hormone. Vasopressin has the capacity to release ACTH but is not believed to be a major corticotropin-releasing hormone. An ovine peptide that stimulates secretion of ACTH and beta endorphin has been characterized recently and may be available for human use in the future. Dopamine inhibits prolactin release in vitro and in vivo and may either be the prolactin inhibitory factor (PIF) or cause PIF release by the hypothalamus.

THYROTROPIN-RELEASING HORMONE (TRH) When given intravenously to humans, a small quantity of TRH (pyroglutamylhistidylprolinamide) releases TSH from the pituitary with a peak seen at about 20 min. The thyrotropin response is blocked by excess circulating triiodothyronine or thyroxine as in hyperthyroidism.

TRH also stimulates prolactin release by a direct effect on the lactotrophs. Although TRH appears to be a physiological prolactin-releasing factor, another release mechanism separate from TRH must exist since several physiological stimuli for prolactin secretion do not cause a rise in TSH. These include breast feeding, stress, and the nocturnal rise in prolactin. Alternatively, prolactin release could occur as a result of a decrease in the hypothalamic PIF. Both the prolactin and TSH responses to TRH are modulated by negative feedback of thyroid hormone on the pituitary, but prolactin release is less sensitive than that of thyrotropin. Hypothyroid patients have high basal prolactin levels and an exaggerated prolactin response to TRH.

Other hormones also modulate the TRH effect. Somatostatin and high doses of glucocorticoids reduce the thyrotropin response to TRH. Estrogens increase thyrotropin and prolactin release in response to TRH through unknown mechanisms. TRH does not normally cause the release of growth hormone (GH), ACTH, LH, or FSH. However, in patients with acromegaly, depression, anorexia nervosa, hypothyroidism, or uremia, TRH may stimulate GH secretion. TRH is present in many areas of the brain outside the hypothalamic-pituitary axis; its function in these areas is unknown.

LUTEINIZING HORMONE–RELEASING HORMONE (LHRH) Since the secretion rates of gonadotropins vary independently, it was expected that separate releasing factors might be found for LH and FSH. However, in 1971, a linear peptide containing 10 amino acids was isolated and shown to cause release of both LH and FSH in rats. Its composition is identical in sheep and pigs and on the basis of immunologic evidence appears to be the same in humans. Since the effect on LH release is more dramatic than its effect on FSH, this decapeptide is often referred to as luteinizing hormone–releasing hormone (LHRH) or gonadotropin–releasing hormone (GnRH). The differences in the secretion of LH and FSH following intravenous administration of LHRH are believed to result from differential negative and positive feedback of gonadal hormones on the hypothalamic-pituitary system that alter the response of the gonadotroph cells to the single releasing hormone.

Catecholamines serve as mediators of the signals from higher centers in the brain to the hypothalamus in regulating LHRH release. Both norepinephrine and dopamine may be involved in LHRH regulation. Although LHRH appears to be located primarily in the hypothalamus, immunoreactive LHRH is also present in other areas of the brain and even in the peripheral circulation.

Intravenous administration of LHRH at doses of 100 to 150 μg to men or women causes a rapid release of LH and FSH with peak levels of LH at 15 to 30 min and a maximal response of FSH at about 120 min. Gonadal steroids exert both a positive and negative feedback on the pituitary response to LHRH depending on the levels of the steroid hormone in the blood. Prolonged treatment of hypogonadal, castrate, or postmenopausal women with estrogen reduces both the elevated basal levels of LH and FSH and the acute response of the gonadotropins to LHRH through a negative feedback mechanism. However, in normal women the LH and FSH responses to LHRH are increased by higher estrogen concentrations. The integrated or total LH response to LHRH is greater in the late follicular (high estrogen) phase of the menstrual cycle than in the early (low estrogen) follicular phase. This variable response may explain some of the seemingly paradoxical events of the normal menstrual cycle such as the increased plasma LH following the ovarian estrogen surge. In castrate or hypogonadal men, testosterone suppresses the LH response to LHRH apparently through a direct effect at the hypothalamic-pituitary axis. LHRH does not release GH, prolactin, TSH, or ACTH in normal people, but acromegalic patients may have an abnormal GH release to LHRH as well as to TRH.

SOMATOSTATIN (SOMATOTROPIN-RELEASE-INHIBITING FACTOR, SRIF) The dominant hypothalamic control over GH production is positive since hypothalamic lesions, stalk section, or pituitary transplantation all result in decreased GH secretion. However, an inhibitory peptide for growth hormone release has been isolated from the hypothalamus and named *somatostatin*. This 14-amino acid peptide blocks GH release to all stimuli in normal humans and lowers the increased GH secretion in acromegalic patients. Unfortunately, somatostatin is degraded rapidly in vivo so that a constant intravenous infusion is necessary for sustained inhibition of GH secretion.

Although somatostatin decreases the TSH response to TRH, it does not alter the secretion of ACTH, LH, or FSH. Secretion of insulin and glucagon is inhibited by somatostatin (see Chap. 114), as is the secretion of gastrin and vasoactive intestinal peptide (VIP). Somatostatin is present in the D cells of the pancreatic islets, in the duodenum and antrum of the stomach, and in areas of the brain other than the hypothalamus.

Anterior pituitary hormones The regulation and physiological effects of the various anterior pituitary hormones are so different that each must be considered separately.

PROLACTIN Prolactin is secreted by the lactotrophs. Both the number and size of lactotrophs and the pituitary content of prolactin increase during pregnancy. Human prolactin has a molecular weight of approximately 22,500. Similarities and homologies exist among human prolactin, growth hormone, and placental lactogen, but sensitive and specific radioimmunoassays for prolactin are now available.

The only clearly established physiological function of prolactin in humans relates to lactation, although receptors for prolactin are present in the kidney, liver, adrenal, heart, and gonads. The exact mechanism of prolactin action on the breast is not known. Whether the hormone has any physiological function in males is also unknown. Over 85 actions of prolactin have been described in other animals, many of which relate to actions on the gonad or to synergism with steroid hormones from the gonads or adrenal glands. However, prolactin also has a clear osmoregulatory function in some fish and appears to affect organ growth in some animals.

The normal range for plasma prolactin is 1 to 25 ng/ml for women and 1 to 20 ng/ml for men. The higher mean levels in women are probably the result of the stimulatory effect of estrogens on prolactin secretion. Prolactin concentration in plasma gradually increases during pregnancy. Secretion of prolactin is episodic, and the half-time in the blood is approximately 20 min, resulting in oscillations of blood levels during the day. The nocturnal peak of prolactin secretion is not synchronous with nocturnal growth hormone release. Prolactin elevations appear to be related to sleep itself rather than to an intrinsic circadian rhythm. Nipple or breast stimulation, particularly during nursing, causes a rapid rise in serum prolactin levels. This response requires the presence of afferent neural pathways from the breast to the brain. Other factors that cause prolactin release are stress (including hypoglycemia), strenuous exercise, surgery, and sexual intercourse (in women). Prolactin levels may be increased in hypothyroidism and renal failure.

The importance of the dopaminergic control of prolactin secretion is demonstrated by the striking effects of several drugs. L-Dopa which is converted to dopamine lowers prolactin levels in both normal and abnormal conditions. The dopamine agonists apomorphine and bromocriptine also reduce prolactin secretion. Conversely, drugs such as phenothiazines and butyrophenones, which inhibit dopaminergic transmission by blocking dopamine receptors, produce elevation of serum prolactin. Morphine, β-endorphin, and the enkephalins also increase prolactin levels.

GROWTH HORMONE (GH, SOMATOTROPIN) Human GH is a linear polypeptide with 191 amino acids and contains two intrachain disulfide bridges. Growth hormone has many amino acid sequences in common with prolactin and placental lactogen, suggesting evolution from a similar structural gene. Although there are similarities and homologous amino acid sequences in the growth hormones from different species, there is considerable interspecies variability in immunologic and biological activity. Only primate growth hormone has appreciable biological activity in humans.

The major biological effect of somatotropin is to promote growth. The organ systems affected include the skeleton, connective tissue, muscles, and viscera such as liver, intestine, and kidneys. Many effects of GH are exerted through induction of somatomedins produced in the liver. The somatomedins (initially called *sulfation factor*) are small peptides which are transported in the blood by carrier proteins. Somatomedins may be responsible for some of the insulin-like activity of serum that cannot be neutralized by antibodies to insulin (nonsuppressible insulin-like activity, NSILA). Plasma somatomedin activity falls after hypophysectomy and is restored by growth hormone injection.

Growth hormone exerts its action through interaction with specific receptors on cell membranes. One variety of dwarfism (Laron dwarfism) occurs in patients in whom growth hormone is present but in whom receptors appear to be defective or absent so that somatomedin generation does not occur. The net metabolic effects of growth hormone (and somatomedins) include stimulation of nucleic acid and protein synthesis, induction of positive nitrogen balance, stimulation of lipolysis, and a decrease in urea excretion. Chronic growth hormone stimulation results in insulin resistance and a tendency to elevated blood glucose. The stimulation of connective tissue produces increased collagen synthesis and increased hydroxyproline excretion. Calcium and phosphorus metabolism are altered with increased calcium absorption, a tendency to hypercalciuria, increased serum inorganic phosphate, and increased renal tubular reabsorption of phosphate. Alkaline phosphatase may also be elevated.

A specific growth hormone–releasing factor has not been isolated. Somatostatin can suppress growth hormone levels, but its role in the physiological control of growth hormone is not known. A "short-loop feedback" whereby growth hormone itself feeds back on the hypothalamus has been suggested as one potential control mechanism.

A number of drugs that alter monamine turnover or receptors in the hypothalamus also affect growth hormone release. Neuropharmacological studies indicate that the neurotransmitters dopamine, norepinephrine, and serotonin each control certain aspects of GH secretion. L-Dopa releases growth hormone, apparently after conversion to dopamine. The GH rise which occurs with many stimuli is enhanced by beta blockers and is blunted by blockade of alpha receptors, suggesting that alpha-adrenergic mechanisms may play a role. Serotonin precursors also increase growth hormone secretion, but the significance of this action is not known.

During the normal rapid growth phase of childhood and adolescence, total growth hormone secretion is increased primarily because of increased nocturnal secretion of the hormone. Sleep results in growth hormone release after about 90 min, earlier than the sleep-related prolactin release. Either physical or emotional stress, if severe enough, may cause growth hormone release in the lean patient. Obesity blunts or prevents growth hormone response to most stimuli.

Various alterations in metabolic fuels also affect growth hormone levels. Hypoglycemia may increase growth hormone release, and hyperglycemia suppresses growth hormone secretion in normal subjects. Amino acids such as arginine infused intravenously release growth hormone. The stimulation of growth hormone release after exercise and the increased levels seen in patients with cirrhosis, renal failure, and some diabetics may also be the consequence of alterations in metabolic fuels.

Other hormones also influence growth hormone levels. Estrogens increase growth hormone responses to provocative tests and upright posture. Part of this effect may relate to inhibition of somatomedin generation by the liver or result from peripheral resistance to growth hormone. Pretreatment of men and prepubertal children with estrogen enhances the growth hormone responses to stimulation tests. Glucocorticoids in high doses tend to suppress growth hormone release, although the major growth-retarding effect of glucocorticoids involves somatomedin production and a peripheral tissue effect rather than direct inhibition of growth hormone release. Vasopressin in pharmacological doses and glucagon also cause growth hormone secretion.

PITUITARY GONADOTROPINS Both LH and FSH are glycoproteins. These gonadotropins have similarities with TSH as well as the placental hormone human chorionic gonadotropin (HCG). In fact, all four have a molecular weight of approximately 30,000 and are composed of an alpha and a beta subunit. The alpha subunits of these four hormones are nearly identical, and the specificity of each hormone is conferred by the beta subunit. Both LH and FSH can be measured easily in blood by radioimmunoassays. Urine can also be extracted and used for a variety of assays of biological activity.

In contrast to the apparent specificity of cell type for most pituitary hormones, some pituitary cells appear to synthesize both LH and FSH, although cells containing only LH or FSH are also present. There is, however, apparent specificity of action of LH and FSH. LH in men appears to act on the Leydig or interstitial cells to cause the increased synthesis of testosterone. LH in women also acts on the interstitial cells resulting in synthesis of androgens, estrogens, and progestins depending on other local factors. LH binds to specific hormone receptors on the cell membrane and acts through a mechanism involving activation of adenylate cyclase and induction of cyclic adenosine monophosphate (AMP) levels. The subsequent steps appear to involve cyclic AMP–dependent protein kinases, but the specific substrates have not yet been identified.

FSH appears to control gametogenesis in both men and women. The specific target cell for FSH in the male appears to be the Sertoli cell which has a supportive function for the developing spermatozoa. The target cell in the ovary is the granulosa cell of the ovarian follicle. FSH is also believed to act synergistically with estrogen and LH to cause follicle growth and maturation. FSH appears to increase LH receptors in the interstitial cells and to stimulate the aromatization of androgen to estradiol in the granulosa and Sertoli cells.

The regulation of gonadotropin secretion is still not fully understood. LHRH stimulates LH and FSH synthesis and release. The gonadal hormones, stimulated by LH and FSH, in turn feed back on the pituitary and hypothalamus. Puberty appears to occur as a result of a decreased sensitivity of the hypothalamus and pituitary to feedback inhibition by low levels of gonadal steroids, resulting in increased pulsatile secretion of LH during sleep. In both men and women primary hypogonadism results in an elevation of basal LH and FSH levels in the blood to approximately twice the normal concentrations.

Testosterone appears to suppress LH synthesis, while testosterone and inhibin, a peptide which is derived from the testis, are thought to suppress FSH (see Chap. 117). Inhibin has not been well characterized, but it is presumably produced by the Sertoli cells. Its release appears to be impaired when spermatogenesis is decreased. This separate feedback by inhibin probably explains the isolated elevation of FSH seen in patients who have decreased spermatozoa but normal LH and testosterone levels. Pharmacological doses of testosterone or of estrogen plus progesterone suppress both gonadotropins and spermatogenesis in the male.

In women, the regulation of the menstrual cycle is more complex (see Chap. 118). However, the differential inhibitory and stimulatory effects of ovarian steroids on the hypothalamus and pituitary appear to be critical. Inhibin may be important in women as well as men. A surge of ovarian estrogen at the end of the follicular phase of the cycle ultimately causes the release of LH and FSH, presumably through LHRH release from the hypothalamus. The normal cyclic release of gonadotropin is eliminated by estrogen-progestin combinations used in oral contraceptives. Normal menses usually resume within a few months after these medications are discontinued.

THYROTROPIN (THYROID-STIMULATING HORMONE, TSH) TSH is a glycoprotein hormone with a molecular weight of approximately 30,000. The major function of TSH is the stimulation of thyroid hormone synthesis by the thyroid. This stimulation is accompanied by increases in the rate of synthesis of protein and RNA, phospholipid production, iodine uptake, and colloid droplet formation by the thyroid.

The action of TSH involves interaction with specific TSH receptors on the cell membrane of the thyroid, activation of adenylate cyclase, and increased cyclic AMP formation. TSH has a half-life in blood of about 50 min. The pituitary apparently secretes an amount of TSH equivalent to its total content daily. TSH is easily measured in plasma or serum by radioimmunoassays, although most assays are unable to distinguish normal from low levels of the hormone.

The regulation of TSH secretion involves stimulation of TSH release by TRH and feedback inhibition of TSH secretion by triiodothyronine (T_3) and thyroxine at the level of the pituitary. This feedback regulation is so finely adjusted that a minimal thyroid deficiency results in elevated TSH levels. Therefore, assessment of serum TSH is useful in testing for mild primary hypothyroidism and in differentiating primary from hypothalamic-pituitary hypothyroidism (Fig. 109-2). Minimal elevations of thyroid hormones in the blood prevent the TSH release following administration of TRH (see Chap. 111). Chronic administration of excess thyroid hormone causes prolonged suppression of TSH secretion. In normal subjects this suppression is reversible, and normal TSH secretion occurs within 3 to 4 weeks after thyroid hormone treatment is stopped.

CORTICOTROPIN (ACTH) Human ACTH is a single polypeptide composed of 39 amino acids and has a molecular weight of approximately 4500. ACTH is derived from a large glycoprotein prohormone which is cleaved to give rise to ACTH and also to β-lipotropin (see Chap. 88). The latter contains the sequences of β-melanocyte-stimulating hormone (β-MSH) and the opioid peptides β-endorphin and enkephalin. β-Endorphin appears to be cosecreted with ACTH. β-Lipotropin is secreted by some pituitary tumors and at times in normal individuals during stress. β-MSH was previously thought to play a role in human skin pigmentation, but the belief now is that the hormone is an artifact of β-lipotropin degradation during extraction and that it does not normally circulate in humans.

FIGURE 109-2
Serum thyrotropin (TSH) levels in normal subjects, primary myxedema, hyperthyroidism, and hypopituitarism. The high levels of TSH in primary myxedema indicate the usefulness of this test in diagnosing primary disease of the thyroid. (After JM Hershman, JA Pittman, Ann Intern Med 74:481, 1971.)

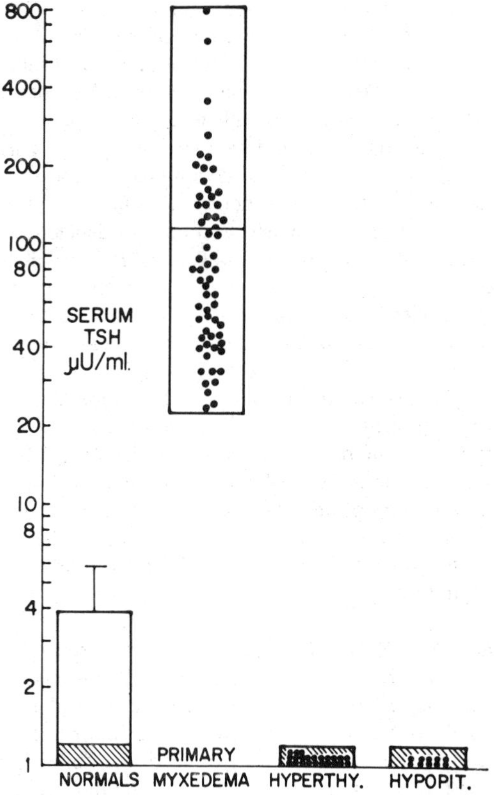

The major biological function of ACTH is maintenance of adrenal function. Although ACTH stimulates production of all three major types of adrenal steroids, i.e., glucocorticoids, androgens, and mineralocorticoids, the predominant control of aldosterone is mediated by the renin-angiotensin system. The major physiological role of ACTH is the control of cortisol secretion. Both ACTH and β-lipotropin play a role in alteration of skin pigmentation that occurs in primary adrenal insufficiency. Like TSH and the gonadotropins, ACTH appears to act through specific cell membrane receptors to induce adenylate cyclase activity and cyclic AMP synthesis.

ACTH secretion is controlled at several levels. These include a basal diurnal variation, feedback inhibition by adrenal steroids, and a rapid release in response to stress. The physiological secretion of ACTH follows a diurnal rhythm; levels peak in the early morning and gradually decrease during the day. Like other anterior pituitary hormones, ACTH is secreted episodically. Cortisol is the major glucocorticoid that provides a negative feedback control on the hypothalamic-pituitary unit. Reduction of steroid synthesis and secretion by drugs or by removing adrenal tissue increases ACTH levels. Exogenous steroid administration prevents the normal morning ACTH release. After chronic excess exogenous steroid administration the hypothalamic-pituitary axis is suppressed, and recovery of normal ACTH secretion may not occur for up to 6 months after initial attempts to withdraw the steroids. Stressful stimuli that cause ACTH release such as insulin-induced hypoglycemia, pyrogen, or surgery provide additional control mechanisms. The ACTH response to stress is critical in conditions such as anesthesia and surgery (see Chap. 112).

DISEASES OF THE HYPOTHALAMUS AND ANTERIOR PITUITARY GLAND

Anterior pituitary disorders usually present to the clinician with one or more of four types of problems: (1) enlargement of the sella turcica with or without other evidence of a space-occupying lesion, (2) visual disorders, (3) symptoms and signs of hypopituitarism, and (4) evidence of pituitary hormone hypersecretion. At times all four presentations may be found together, as in a patient with acromegaly in whom a growth hormone–producing pituitary tumor has compromised other normal anterior pituitary functions sufficient to cause hypopituitarism, to enlarge the sella, and to impinge on the optic chiasm and cause visual field defects. Hypothalamic disorders may also present as pituitary hypofunction. This has given rise to the concept of primary, secondary, and tertiary deficiencies for target glands such as the thyroid and gonads. Primary deficiencies occur as a result of disease of the target gland itself, secondary deficiencies result from pituitary lesions, and tertiary deficiencies occur as a consequence of hypothalamic disorders.

Theoretically, a decreased sensitivity of the hypothalamus to feedback inhibition by circulating hormones could also result in pituitary hormone overproduction. For example, it has been proposed that the ACTH excess in pituitary Cushing's disease is due to inappropriately high setting for the feedback regulatory system. Adenomas of the pituitary corticotrophs are often found in this disorder, and evidence for a hypothalamic etiology is still indirect.

ENLARGEMENT OF THE SELLA TURCICA An increase in size or apparent erosion of the sella turcica is often the presenting problem in patients referred for pituitary evaluation. Enlargement of the sella is frequently encountered in routine skull series obtained in patients complaining of headache, following an accident, or for various other indications. The differential diagnosis of the enlarged sella includes pituitary adenomas (which constitute approximately 10 percent of all intracranial neoplasms), craniopharyngiomas, meningiomas, epithelial and other cysts occurring in the area of the sella, metastatic tumor as from breast carcinoma, and granulomas. Perhaps more common than any of these neoplasms is the nontumorous enlargement of the sella turcica or "empty sella syndrome." Sella enlargement occurs occasionally in children and rarely in adults with primary hypothyroidism. This enlargement is presumably the result of hyperplasia of the thyrotrophs and is accompanied by elevated thyrotropin levels. Sella enlargement as an apparent consequence of similar hyperplasia of gonadotrophs has been reported in a few adults with hypogonadism and high gonadotropin levels. It should also be remembered that the sella turcica represents a weak area in the bony structure of the skull and that rarely the sella may acutely increase in size secondary to rapid increases of intracranial pressure, as with a brain tumor such as glioblastoma multiforme.

Diagnostic studies useful in patients with suspected pituitary disease fall into three types: radiological, neuroophthalmologic, and endocrine. The extent to which each type of testing is used depends on the presenting manifestations. In general, radiological evaluation is most important in any patient with an enlarged sella and is critical to any therapeutic decision. The visual-field examination provides important evidence of suprasellar disease, while endocrine evaluation is necessary for the assessment of the type and severity of the hypothalamic or pituitary lesion.

Radiological studies The development of computerized tomography (CT) scanning has improved the diagnostic accuracy of noninvasive techniques, and has essentially replaced pneumoencephalography. The addition of contrast material such as intrathecal metrizamide to the CT scan may be useful in identifying many marginal lesions and in situations in which an intermediate-size intrasellar tumor with possible minimal extension above the sella must be differentiated from the empty sella syndrome (see below).

Initial radiographic studies should include high-quality plain skull films, preferably with a coned-down lateral and frontal view of the sella turcica. Enlargement of the sella is indicative of a disease process such as tumor or empty sella. On a correctly performed lateral skull x-ray the anterior clinoid processes are superimposed. Modified anteroposterior films to show the sellar floor are also useful, but considerable experience is needed for accurate assessment. A particularly useful finding in the patient with a suspected microadenoma on lateral skull films is a double density of the floor of the sella. This may be a normal variant in up to 30 percent of the population due to sloping of the sella floor or improper positioning during x-ray. However, the appearance of a double contour or erosion of the floor is an indication to proceed to tomography or CT scanning. Tomography has been particularly useful in differentiating microadenomas from normal variants and in detecting small areas of erosion by a tumor. Lateral tomography alone is frequently adequate, but anteroposterior tomography may be helpful if definite findings are not apparent on the lateral projections. However, improved CT scanning techniques are replacing the need for tomography.

Delineation of the extent of a pituitary lesion can be determined by CT scanning, usually combined with intravenous injection of contrast material. The CT scan can show lesions at or above the diaphragma sellae, but intrasellar lesions are less well defined. Metrizamide CT cisternography or pneumoencephalography with tomography can define lesions in the area of the diaphragma sellae. With adequate positioning, these studies identify the empty sella (see below). Pneumoencephalography usually results in a stress type of ACTH release and subsequent cortisol elevation in normal patients. This study is relatively uncomfortable and tolerated poorly by patients with ACTH and TSH deficiencies. Cortisol (100 mg parenterally several hours prior to the study) should be given prophylactically if there is any suspicion of ACTH deficiency. Arteriography is sometimes indicated prior to surgery to exclude the possibility of an aneurysm in the pituitary fossa or adjacent area.

Empty sella syndrome This term describes a nontumorous enlargement of the sella turcica that may be misdiagnosed as a pituitary neoplasm. The enlarged sella contains cerebrospinal fluid rather than a tumor (Fig. 109-3). Up to 30 percent of normal persons have some cerebrospinal fluid below the diaphragma sellae in a small arachnoid diverticulum extending through the foramen where the stalk passes through the diaphragm. The primary empty sella syndrome occurs when the arachnoid diverticulum enlarges to such a degree that the sella becomes enlarged and the pituitary is compressed against the floor of the sella. Some empty sellas develop as a secondary process after spontaneous infarction or regression of a tumor which previously enlarged the sella. However, the majority of patients with the empty sella syndrome appear never to have had a tumor and have no abnormalities of pituitary function. The enlarged sella, therefore, causes difficulty primarily because it may be misinterpreted as a pituitary tumor.

Approximately 90 percent of patients with the empty sella syndrome are women. The enlargement of the pituitary during pregnancy with subsequent regression in size may play some role in the pathogenesis. Headache is a common complaint. Obesity is present in about 80 percent and hypertension in 30 percent of these patients. On x-ray the sella often appears ballooned. There is usually no evidence of erosion as in tumorous enlargement, although cerebrospinal fluid rhinorrhea occurs in up to 10 percent in some series. Clinical endocrine deficiencies are rare, and laboratory studies are usually normal. Visual field defects are also rare, although on occasion the optic chiasm may prolapse into the sella and cause field deficits. In patients who have had infarction of a pituitary tumor with subsequent development of the empty sella syndrome, visual field and endocrine abnormalities are more common. Diagnosis can often be made at tomography which shows the characteristic ballooned appearance without erosive changes in the floor. The diagnosis can be confirmed by CT scanning with or without metrizamide. Occasionally pneumoencephalography with appropriate rotation of the patient so that air fills the arachnoid cavity below the diaphragm may be necessary. The major clinical significance of the empty sella syndrome is to avoid the mistake of diagnosing pituitary tumor. No treatment other than weight loss or control of hypertension is required unless cerebrospinal fluid rhinorrhea is present.

Endocrine evaluation in patients with enlargement of the sella turcica The extent of the endocrine evaluation depends largely on the management plan. Base-line studies should include assessment of peripheral thyroid and adrenal hormone levels and a screen for diabetes insipidus such as the ability to concentrate on overnight urine. Measurement of basal prolactin values is helpful since approximately half of pituitary tumors appear to secrete prolactin. Basal gonadotropin levels and basal testosterone values in men are useful. Patients with evidence of hypopituitarism should have a more extensive evaluation (see below).

In many centers more extensive endocrine studies are omitted prior to surgical treatment of large pituitary tumors or vascular lesions. These patients are treated with thyroid replacement if needed and with parenteral glucocorticoids equivalent to 300 mg cortisol on the day of surgery with gradual tapering of the steroid replacement over several days following the procedure. Endocrine evaluation may then be performed to determine the extent of endocrine deficiencies. However, if the patient is to be followed without treatment or treated with radiation or selective transsphenoidal microsurgery, more extensive endocrine evaluation is indicated.

VISUAL DISORDERS AND OPHTHALMOLOGIC EVALUATION
Patients with radiographic abnormalities of the sella deserve a careful ophthalmologic examination. Visual disorders were previously the most frequent presenting complaint in patients with large pituitary tumors (Table 109-1), but because of the capacity to diagnose smaller pituitary adenomas, the frequency of visual disorders as a presenting complaint has decreased substantially. Large visual field defects can be identified at the bedside, but formal visual field examination by tangent screen or Goldman perimetry is advised.

The classic bilateral homonymous hemianopsia or superior quadrantic defects are expected when a pituitary tumor extends upward from the diaphragma sellae and compresses the optic chiasm lying above the sella turcica. In actual practice

TABLE 109-1
Initial complaints in 1000 patients with large pituitary tumors

Visual	421	Cushing's disease	29
Headache	137	Incidental finding	15
Acromegaly	136	Diabetes insipidus	10
Hypopituitarism	95	ENT complaints	6
Amenorrhea	48	CSF rhinorrhea	5
Diplopia	7	Multiple endocrine adenomas	4
CNS*	24	Undetermined	19
Pain (not headache)	44		

* *Syncope, 5; seizures, 5; dizziness, 9; confusion, 4; inappropriate ADH syndrome, 1.*
SOURCE: *After RW Hollenhorst, in Diagnosis and Treatment of Pituitary Tumors, PO Kohler, GT Ross (eds). New York, American Elsevier, 1973.*

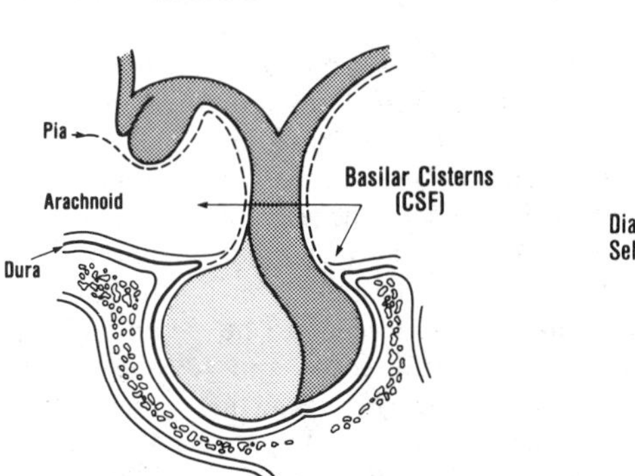

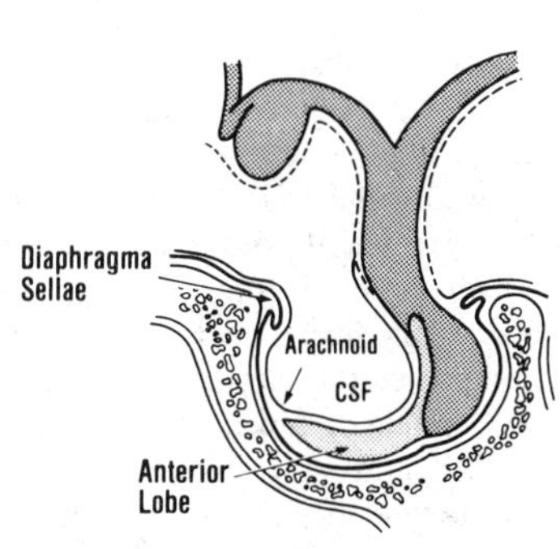

FIGURE 109-3
Diagram indicating the findings in patients with the nontumorous enlargement of the sella turcica or the primary empty sella syndrome. The left panel shows the normal anatomic relationships. In patients with the empty sella syndrome an arachnoid diverticulum herniates through an incompetent diaphragm into the sella. Ballooning of the sella may occur causing enlargement suggesting a pituitary tumor. The pneumoencephalogram will show excessive air entering the sella. (After RM Jordan et al, Am J Med 62:569, 1977.)

the defects produced by large tumors vary from no defects to combinations of unilateral or bilateral field defects in all quadrants. Reasons for the irregular patterns include variations in the position of the chiasm above the sella and variable compromise of blood vessels supplying the optic chiasm. Other tumors such as craniopharyngiomas may also cause visual field loss advancing to optic atrophy and total blindness. Careful visual field and visual acuity examinations should be obtained before and after surgery in order to document any subsequent change in vision. Patients with defects should have visual field examinations at least annually.

HYPOPITUITARISM Deficiencies of anterior pituitary hormones may occur as isolated or combined deficits. The presentation of the patient depends on the number and extent of hormone deficiencies. Patients may complain of weakness, fatigue, headaches, loss of sexual function, and cold intolerance. Hypogonadotropism is the most common symptomatic endocrine deficiency encountered in adults with either pituitary tumors or craniopharyngiomas. Children present more commonly with growth retardation secondary to inadequate growth hormone. Provocative tests indicate that growth hormone is usually deficient in adults, but this deficiency does not cause symptoms in a patient who has experienced the normal pubertal growth period.

The adult with panhypopituitarism may have a striking appearance: absence of axillary and pubic hair, genital and breast atrophy, pallor of the skin and nipples, fine wrinkling (particularly on the face), and poor muscle development. Short stature may be present if the pituitary disease occurred before puberty, and there is often the appearance of premature aging. Men with hypopituitarism and hypogonadism have a juvenile pattern of scalp hair without temporal recession or baldness. In contrast to the original description of cachexia in hypopituitarism by Simmonds, patients with advanced disease may be somewhat puffy and slightly overweight as if hypothyroidism were the prevalent feature. The presence of diabetes insipidus (see Chap. 110) suggests hypothalamic involvement since only massively enlarged anterior pituitary lesions cause disruption of ADH release by the neurohypophysis. The clinical presentation of the patient with hypopituitarism is often a composite of several hormone deficiencies. Manifestations of each individual hormone deficiency will be considered separately.

PROLACTIN DEFICIENCY Failure to lactate after parturition is the only clinical consequence of prolactin deficiency. This has classically been associated with hemorrhage and shock in women with postpartum pituitary necrosis (Sheehan's syndrome). The incidence of prolactin deficiency in other pituitary diseases is not known. Failure to respond to prolactin provocative tests has been noted in some patients with advanced pituitary disease, but some normal individuals also have blunted responses to stimulation tests.

GROWTH HORMONE DEFICIENCY Inadequate growth hormone in the child causes retardation of growth, epiphyseal development, and bone age. Hypopituitary dwarfs tend to have increased truncal fat and a puffy appearance to the skin even in the presence of normal levels of thyroid hormone. The legs are longer in relation to the trunk than those of a normal child. Secondary sexual characteristics are retarded or absent. Development of the larynx is impaired, and the voice tends to be high pitched. Since growth does not ordinarily cease completely and since gonadal maturation is delayed, growth hormone-deficient patients may continue to grow slowly past the usual age of puberty. Hypoglycemia may occur in very young children or infants with growth hormone deficiency. All these changes can be reversed with growth hormone treatment.

In the adult the onset of growth hormone deficiency appears to be a "silent" lesion without hypoglycemia or other clinical manifestations. However, a failure to evoke a growth hormone response to provocative tests is still the most common hormone deficiency in hypothalamic-pituitary lesions. Therefore, growth hormone evaluation is useful in the patient with suspected pituitary disease.

GONADOTROPIN DEFICIENCY Hypogonadism is the most common clinical endocrine manifestation of hypothalamic-pituitary deficiency in the adult. Gonadotropin deficiency prior to puberty results in a eunuchoid appearance with lack of development of secondary sexual characteristics and infertility. Boys with hypogonadism fail to develop a beard, an adult male scalp hair pattern, a normal adult voice, or normal enlargement of the genitalia. Girls with prepubertal hypogonadism lack normal breast development and menstruation. Both sexes may have decreased or absent pubic and axillary hair, although growth of sexual hair is also dependent on adrenal function. If growth hormone secretion is adequate, prepubertal hypogonadal patients may have a tall stature because continued growth of the long bones occurs in the absence of sufficient gonadal steroids to cause epiphyseal fusion. Gonadotropin insufficiency in the premenopausal woman is manifested by secondary amenorrhea. In advanced deficiency the breasts and uterus atrophy, and vaginal cornification is diminished because of diminished ovarian estrogen production. In the adult man, secondary testicular atrophy is accompanied by decrease in libido, potency, muscle tone, and beard growth. In some patients with hyperprolactinemia and hypogonadotropinism prolactin may have an antigonadal effect, but the relationship is inconstant.

THYROTROPIN DEFICIENCY Hypothalamic or pituitary hypothyroidism is similar to primary hypothyroidism but frequently is less severe. Lethargy, fatigue, and pallor of the skin are common. Isolated TSH deficiency is rare, and growth hormone and gonadotropin deficiency are usually present when thyrotropin deficiency is expressed, thus facilitating the separation of hypothalamic-pituitary disease (tertiary or secondary) from primary hypothyroidism. The skin in pituitary hypothyroidism often shows a fine wrinkling, particularly on the face, which may be related in part to an associated gonadal deficiency. Associated findings such as visual field defects or loss of secondary sexual characteristics are helpful in identification of pituitary hypothyroidism. The hair is dry but less coarse in the pituitary form of hypothyroidism than in primary disease. Tongue enlargement may occur in severe primary hypothyroidism but is usually not present in pituitary hypothyroidism. The menstrual history is useful in premenopausal women in that menorrhagia may occur with primary hypothyroidism, whereas amenorrhea is expected in pituitary disease. Laboratory evaluation makes it possible to separate primary from secondary hypothyroidism.

ACTH DEFICIENCY This is the most serious endocrine deficiency in patients with pituitary disease. While ACTH deficiency usually occurs only in massive pituitary lesions, it must be looked for in all patients with evidence of pituitary disease. Most patients with ACTH deficiency have evidence of other hormone loss. There may be a history of inadequate response to stress with nausea, vomiting, and collapse. Hypovolemia and hyperkalemia are unusual in the absence of vomiting, diarrhea, or diabetes insipidus because aldosterone secretion is maintained to a large degree by the renin-angiotensin system. Patients with ACTH deficiency may have hyponatremia from an inappropriate ADH-type syndrome with volume expansion.

Decreased skin and nipple pigmentation may be useful in differentiating the pituitary hypoadrenal patient from the more darkly pigmented patient with primary adrenal disease. Patients with any form of adrenal insufficiency tolerate stress poorly and should be treated with additional corticosteroids during surgery or intercurrent illness.

Disorders producing hypopituitarism Lesions in either the hypothalamus or pituitary may produce hypopituitarism (Table 109-2).

NEOPLASMS Although a variety of primary and metastatic tumors may rarely occur in the hypothalamic-pituitary area, the most common neoplasms are craniopharyngiomas in children and primary pituitary tumors in adults.

CRANIOPHARYNGIOMAS These squamous cell tumors develop from remnants of Rathke's pouch. They usually occur in a suprasellar location but may arise in or extend into the sella turcica. Most are cystic to some degree, and about half are multicystic. The cysts are filled with a yellow to brown fluid that resembles motor oil. The peak incidence is in the second decade of life. Although children often present with evidence of increased intracranial pressure, the most common problems in adults are visual disorders such as optic atrophy, visual field defects, or papilledema. Over half of adults have endocrine deficits, the most common endocrinopathy being hypogonadism secondary to LH and FSH deficiencies. Diabetes insipidus and short stature with delayed bone maturation (due to growth hormone deficiency and hypogonadism) are also common. Complete hypopituitarism occurs in 5 to 10 percent of patients. Occasionally, hypothalamic syndromes such as obesity, anorexia, somnolence, or hyperkinetic behavior may be present. The tumor is calcified and thus visible on skull films in about 75 percent of children and 35 percent of adults. Although other tumors such as meningiomas and granulomas may also calcify, craniopharyngiomas are the most common cause of suprasellar or intrasellar calcification.

TABLE 109-2
Etiologies of pituitary disease

I Neoplasms
- *A* Hypothalamic disorders
  - *1* Craniopharyngioma
  - *2* Metastatic neoplasms
  - *3* Other (meningioma, hamartoma, teratoma, ectopic pinealoma, leukemia, lymphoma)
- *B* Pituitary tumors
  - *1* Pituitary adenomas
  - *2* Meningioma
  - *3* Other (metastatic, glioma, chordoma, primary malignant, cysts)

II Congenital or hereditary conditions
- *A* Idiopathic growth hormone deficiency
- *B* Idiopathic corticotropin deficiency
- *C* Idiopathic gonadotropin deficiency
- *D* Idiopathic thyrotropin deficiency (hypothalamic)
- *E* Multiple hormone deficiencies (idiopathic)
- *F* Hypothalamic hypogonadism (Kallmann's syndrome)

III Vascular disorders
- *A* Pituitary infarction
- *B* Postpartum necrosis (Sheehan's syndrome)
- *C* Aneurysm
- *D* Vasculitis

IV Infections or granulomas
- *A* Sarcoidosis
- *B* Tuberculosis
- *C* Other (meningitis, luetic, mycotic, pyogenic, Wegener's granulomatosis)

V Physical agents
- *A* Radiation
- *B* Surgery
- *C* Head trauma

VI Miscellaneous
- *A* Histiocytosis X
- *B* Hemochromatosis
- *C* Emotional deprivation (children)
- *D* Tay-Sachs disease
- *E* Drugs

CT scan is a valuable diagnostic technique in identifying these cystic tumors. Treatment consists of surgical extirpation. Unfortunately, complete removal is frequently difficult. Although craniopharyngiomas are relatively resistant to irradiation, radiotherapy may be useful in patients who cannot be cured by surgery. Replacement of hormone deficiencies may also be necessary.

PITUITARY ADENOMAS Over 10 percent of all intracranial tumors are pituitary adenomas. Essentially all primary pituitary tumors arise in the anterior lobe, tumors of the posterior lobe being extremely rare. In the past, most pituitary tumors were assumed to be nonfunctional chromophobe adenomas. However, widespread use of the prolactin radioimmunoassay has shown that plasma prolactin levels are elevated in 50 percent of cases. This is usually the result of prolactin secretion by the tumor but may also be the consequence of interference by the tumor mass with the normal inhibitory influence of the hypothalamus on prolactin secretion. Prolactin secretion in such cases may be clinically inapparent, and these tumors therefore present in a manner identical to nonfunctioning tumors. Many pituitary tumors exhibit no detectable hormone secretion.

Patients with pituitary tumors may rarely have Wermer's syndrome, or multiple endocrine neoplasia, type I (see Chap. 123). In this condition, which is inherited as an autosomal dominant trait, patients have a predisposition to develop tumors of the pituitary, parathyroid glands, and pancreas. For this reason, all patients with pituitary adenomas should be questioned carefully with regard to the family history and should be considered for the possibility of hyperparathyroidism, gastrinoma, or other functional pancreatic neoplasm.

NONFUNCTIONING PITUITARY TUMORS Patients with nonfunctioning tumors present with signs and symptoms of a space-occupying lesion or evidence of hypopituitarism (Table 109-1). The loss of vision was the most common complaint in the past. Bitemporal hemianopsia is the classic manifestation of a large pituitary tumor compressing the optic chiasm, although any type of visual defect may occur. Patients with tumors large enough to cause visual disorders usually have associated trophic hormone deficiencies. The most common of these is an inadequate growth hormone response to provocative tests. The next most common hormone deficiency is hypogonadotropinism which occurs in about 75 percent of patients with large tumors. ACTH and TSH deficiencies are less common, each occurring in 40 to 50 percent of patients with extensive tumors. Patients with small pituitary tumors may have no evidence of hypopituitarism. The natural history of nonfunctioning tumors is not entirely clear. The fact that up to 25 percent of people without known pituitary disease have small pituitary adenomas at autopsy suggests that small tumors often cause no clinical disease. Once patients develop visual or endocrine disorders, however, treatment is indicated.

ISOLATED HORMONE DEFICIENCIES Isolated deficiencies of any of the pituitary hormones may occur. The mechanisms by which these isolated deficiencies occur are not known. Isolated growth hormone deficiency is one of the most common causes of growth retardation in children. Growth hormone failure in children may also be associated with other anterior pituitary hormone deficiencies of unknown etiology.

The most common form of isolated hypogonadotropic hypogonadism in both men and women is the *Kallmann syndrome* (see also Chap. 117). This is a familial condition in which gonadotropin deficiency secondary to inadequate LHRH secretion is frequently associated with anosmia or hyposmia due to hypoplasia of the olfactory lobes. Other midline developmental defects such as harelip, cleft palate, and facial fusion abnormalities may be present, and unilateral renal agenesis is occasionally seen. A history of undescended testes is obtained in about a third of affected males. These patients are often identified at the time of expected puberty when secondary sexual characteristics fail to develop. Careful testing of the sense of smell is indicated because affected individuals may be unaware of hyposmia. The mode of inheritance appears to vary, but in some families it appears to be an autosomal dominant trait with variable phenotypic expression. Fertility can be accomplished by treatment with human gonadotropins.

Deficiencies of LH and FSH may occur in men who present with evidence of hypoandrogenization such as a eunuchoid appearance and scanty beard growth, but who have some degree of spermatogenesis. This has been called the "fertile eunuch syndrome" but probably is just a partial form of LHRH deficiency (i.e., an incomplete variant of Kallmann's syndrome). Patients with apparent unrelated isolated deficiency of FSH have also been described.

INFECTIOUS AND GRANULOMATOUS LESIONS In the past, tuberculous meningitis, granulomas, and syphilis occasionally caused hypopituitarism. Sarcoidosis may involve the hypothalamus or pituitary and cause diabetes insipidus or anterior pituitary hormone deficiency.

PHYSICAL AGENTS Hypopituitarism may result from head trauma, and any surgery in the infratentorial region of the brain may produce variable degrees of hypopituitarism depending on the extent of procedures. Another cause of hypopituitarism is external radiation in the hypothalamic-pituitary area for malignancies of the nasopharynx. These patients usually have subclinical deficiencies of growth hormone, ACTH, and TSH, but overt disease may develop rarely. Basal prolactin levels may be elevated. Thus, patients who have received radiation for head or neck tumors may require evaluation for hypothalamic-pituitary insufficiency.

INFARCTION AND VASCULAR DISORDERS The most common clinically significant cause of infarction of the normal pituitary has been postpartum pituitary necrosis (Sheehan syndrome) secondary to hemorrhagic shock. The anterior pituitary gland is enlarged during pregnancy and, lacking a direct arterial blood supply, is vulnerable to infarction during shock from excessive uterine bleeding at parturition. The severity of the syndrome varies from an unrecognized contributory cause of morbidity at the time of the initial insult to failure to lactate after delivery or failure to resume menses. Some patients develop evidence of other anterior pituitary hormone loss years after the insult. The incidence of Sheehan's syndrome appears to be decreasing with improved obstetric techniques.

Although small areas of intrapituitary hemorrhage are commonly found postmortem, major infarctions are unusual. *Pituitary apoplexy* may occur in pituitary tumors that infarct, in diabetics with cerebrovascular disease, and rarely in patients with sickle cell disease. Such patients present with excruciating headaches, often bitemporal in location, fever, visual field deficits, and oculomotor palsies. They may have photophobia, stiff neck, altered consciousness, convulsions, and localizing neurological signs. Papilledema may develop, and the cerebrospinal fluid may be bloody.

The CT scan is a valuable, rapid, noninvasive technique for evaluating the possibility of hemorrhage or enlargement of an infarcted tumor mass above the diaphragma sellae. Pituitary apoplexy is a medical emergency requiring administration of glucocorticoids and radiological evaluation for possible compression of structures in the area of the pituitary. Surgical decompression may be required, although this is not always necessary. At times patients with prolactin- or growth hormone–secreting tumors improve after infarction of the tumor mass. Rarely, hypopituitarism is produced by aneurysm of the internal carotid artery in the absence of hemorrhage, by systemic lupus erythematosus, or by other forms of vasculitis.

MISCELLANEOUS CAUSES OF HYPOPITUITARISM Histiocytosis X or the multifocal type eosinophilic granuloma, also called Hand-Schüller-Christian disease, is a nonneoplastic histiocytic reaction to unknown stimuli. Approximately half of these patients have diabetes insipidus, and a fourth have growth hormone deficiency from hypothalamic involvement. The anterior pituitary is usually free of histiocytes, and other anterior pituitary hormone deficiencies are rare. The classic triad in this disease includes punched-out skull lesions, exophthalmos (from histiocytic invasion of the retroorbital space), and diabetes insipidus. The disease is usually responsive to radiation and treatment with prednisone or vinblastine, although reversal of the ADH and growth hormone deficiencies does not occur. Other rare causes of pituitary deficiency include hemochromatosis, Tay-Sachs disease, and Wegener's granulomatosis. Patients with acute intermittent porphyria may have evidence of abnormal hypothalamic-pituitary function such as inappropriate ADH secretion or inappropriate release of growth hormone after glucose ingestion.

Evaluation In the evaluation of patients with suspected hypopituitarism, the history and physical examination may be helpful with regard to etiology. A recent or remote history of postpartum hemorrhage with shock, particularly if combined with failure to lactate, suggests the Sheehan syndrome. Visual field defects usually indicate a tumor large enough to impinge on the optic chiasm. Anosmia or developmental defects such as harelip or cleft palate in a man or woman with hypogonadism suggests the hypothalamic lesion of the Kallmann syndrome. Evidence of lactation or of acral growth suggests a pituitary tumor producing prolactin or growth hormone. As discussed below, hypothalamic or stalk lesions may also cause hyperprolactinemia.

In the differential diagnosis of hypopituitarism, anorexia nervosa (see Chap. 80) and severe malnutrition should be considered since amenorrhea is a common feature. Blood glucose, serum thyroxine, and urinary steroid excretion may be low in anorexia nervosa. However, serum cortisol levels are usually normal, and growth hormone reponses to stimuli may be supranormal. There is evidence for a functional disorder of the hypothalamus in this disorder.

DIAGNOSTIC STUDIES Laboratory evaluation will differentiate between target organ failure and disease of the hypothalamic-pituitary system.

Unfortunately, the separation of hypothalamic from pituitary lesions by endocrine testing is more difficult unless the lesion can be located by radiographic studies.

ENDOCRINE EVALUATION Endocrine evaluation in patients with suspected hypothalamic-pituitary lesions is important for two reasons: (1) documentation of specific endocrine deficits, including those potentially life-threatening deficiencies such as ACTH and TSH, and (2) evaluation of progression of a known lesion or the response to therapy. The initial endocrine evaluation usually should include tests for hyposecretion of each of the anterior pituitary hormones as well as determination of adequate ADH secretion. Evaluation of hypersecreting pituitary adenomas will be discussed later under specific hypersecretory syndromes.

Although base-line hormone levels can provide much information, the pulsatile nature of anterior hormone secretion often makes interpretation of basal hormone levels difficult to evaluate. It is particularly difficult to distinguish between normal and low blood levels of these hormones. For this reason, various provocative tests are used to examine the adequacy of hypothalamic-pituitary response to various challenges such as stress, administration of releasing factors, and blockade of feedback inhibition. Twenty-four hour urine collections for measurement of gonadotropins or steroid secretion are valuable in that they represent an integration of hormone secretion over a relatively long period of time.

TESTS FOR PROLACTIN DEFICIENCY Although prolactin levels in the blood vary in response to physiological stimuli, the basal morning levels are relatively well standardized with a normal range of 1 to 20 ng/ml in men and 1 to 25 ng/ml in women. Measurements of basal prolactin levels are useful in suspected hypothalamic or pituitary disease because elevated prolactin may occur in patients with hypothalamic or stalk lesions or prolactin-producing tumors. Patients with large pituitary lesions may have low prolactin values and show a deficient response to provocative tests such as TRH, chlorpromazine, or metoclopramide. However, testing for prolactin deficiency is rarely necessary.

TESTS FOR GROWTH HORMONE RESERVE Growth hormone (GH) values vary during the day in response to fluctuations in metabolic fuels, stress, and other stimuli. A glucose load (as occurs after eating a normal meal) will suppress GH levels. As the blood sugar falls several hours after a meal, GH will rise. Basal morning growth hormone values tend to be low, making it difficult to distinguish between normal and pathologically low values. As a consequence, provocative tests are required to demonstrate adequate GH response. Once GH deficiency has developed, it is rarely reversed by therapy, and therefore continued testing is unnecessary.

Multiple provocative tests have been developed to test GH release. These include measurement of the normal growth hormone release during sleep or in response to exercise. A normal GH reserve may often be documented in the office or clinic by asking a patient to arrive fasting and then to exercise by climbing several flights of stairs. If the GH level in blood drawn after the exercise is greater than 6 ng/ml, the GH reserve can be assumed to be normal. When this is not an adequate challenge, specific provocative GH testing must be performed. The two most frequently used tests are insulin-induced hypoglycemia and L-dopa administration. The insulin test is performed by giving 0.1 unit of regular insulin per kilogram of body weight as a bolus to a fasting patient via an intravenous saline drip. Blood is drawn prior to injection and at 30-min intervals for 2 h for measurement of glucose and GH. A fall in plasma glucose to half the normal fasting level or to below 45 mg/dl should provide an adequate stimulus for GH release. If hypoglycemia is inadequate, 0.15 to 0.2 unit of regular insulin per kilogram may be used. ACTH, cortisol, glucagon, and epinephrine are also released in response to this challenge. If hypoglycemic symptoms occur, they can be rapidly reversed by intravenous glucose. A normal GH response is an elevation to greater than 6 to 8 ng/ml during the test. The peak GH values usually occur at 30 to 60 min (Fig. 109-4). This test should not be performed in the elderly or in patients with cerebrovascular or cardiovascular disease. The ACTH response to stress can be measured at the same time, but in view of the expense involved in measuring ACTH, serum cortisol is often measured and used as evidence of ACTH release. A typical normal response to hypoglycemia is shown in Fig. 109-4.

In the patient who is not a candidate for insulin-induced hypoglycemia, the L-dopa test is an effective alternative. The ingestion of L-dopa (500 mg per 70 kg) provokes a GH release in about 30 to 60 min in 90 to 95 percent of normal lean adults. A normal response is a GH level of above 6 to 8 ng/ml at some point during the test. L-Dopa causes side effects such as nausea and occasional vomiting in some patients; it does not release ACTH or other anterior pituitary hormones but does lower prolactin levels.

Other stimuli used to test GH reserve include sleep, arginine infusion, vasopressin, glucagon, pyrogen, and nicotinic acid. Pyrogen provokes both GH and ACTH release but is rarely used because of side effects. Arginine, which has almost

FIGURE 109-4
Effect of intravenous insulin, 0.1 unit per kilogram of body weight, on blood sugar, plasma growth hormone (HGH), and plasma cortisol. This insulin tolerance test permits evaluation of both growth hormone and ACTH in patients with pituitary disease. (After KJ Catt, Lancet 1:933, 1970.)

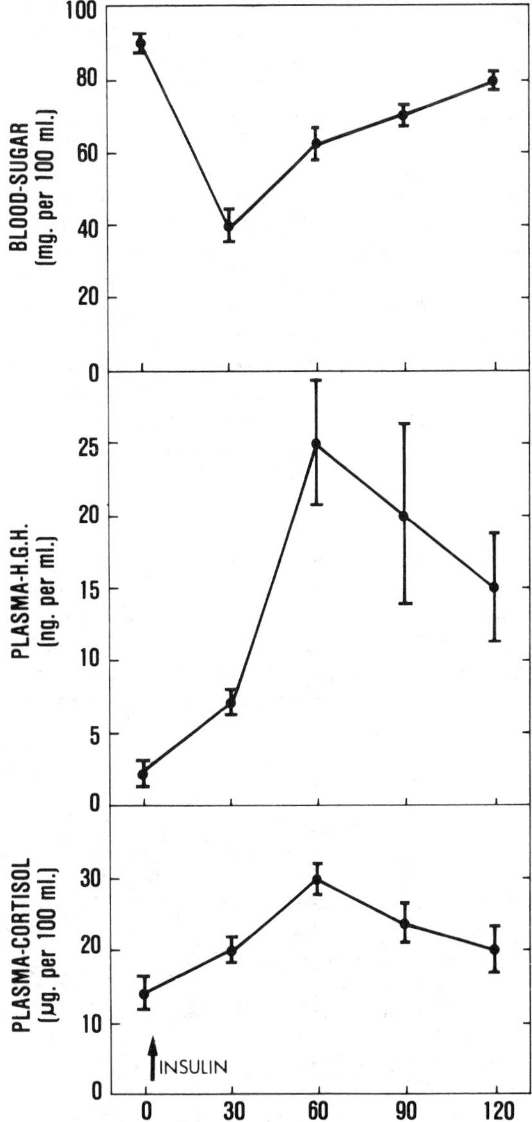

no side effects, or vasopressin may be useful in some circumstances. All stressful GH-provocative tests should be performed only after demonstrating that there is no severe deficiency of ACTH or TSH. If ACTH or TSH is deficient, GH will also usually be deficient. In these instances the patient should be on adrenal and/or thyroid replacement therapy before provocative tests are administered.

There are other important considerations in interpreting the response to provocative tests. The GH responses to all stimuli are blunted or abolished and should be interpreted with caution in the obese patient. In addition, since glucose normally suppresses GH, all tests should be performed fasting, although the response to certain types of stress such as pyrogen may occur despite hyperglycemia. Glucocorticoids in high doses may also blunt the GH response. Finally, estrogens appear to increase the GH response to various stimuli, particularly exercise. For this reason, estrogen pretreatment has occasionally been used prior to testing, particularly in pediatric patients who are candidates for GH replacement therapy.

TESTS OF LH AND FSH RESERVE It is important to emphasize that evidence of normal gonadal function in the absence of hormonal treatment indicates normal hypothalamic-pituitary-gonadal function. Thus, normal cyclic menses in women and normal sperm counts in men essentially exclude hypogonadotropism. The serum testosterone in men provides a useful index of Leydig cell function. Serum estradiol fluctuates considerably during the normal menstrual cycle and has limited usefulness as an index of ovarian function (see Chap. 118).

Measurement of basal LH and FSH levels provides valuable information as to whether gonadal insufficiency is primary or secondary-tertiary. Patients with primary gonadal problems have elevated gonadotropin levels from lack of feedback inhibition. LH elevation appears to occur as a result of testosterone or estrogen deficiency and FSH elevation as a result of decreased gametogenesis. The degree of LH or FSH elevation depends on the degree of gonadal failure. Hypogonadal patients with hypothalamic or pituitary lesions have low or low normal basal gonadotropin levels. Because gonadotropin secretion is pulsatile, three basal blood samples should be drawn 30 min apart and pooled, or the average taken of the separate LH and FSH determinations for an accurate evaluation.

FIGURE 109-5

The effect of 150 μg LHRH intravenously on plasma luteinizing hormone (LH) in patients with pituitary tumors and hypogonadotropic hypogonadism. The shaded area represents the range of responses in normal subjects. Open circles indicate values in postmenopausal women, and the closed circles represent younger women and men. A few patients exhibit a normal response in spite of clinical hypogonadotropinism. (After AM Coscia et al, J Clin Endocrinol Metab 38:83, 1974.)

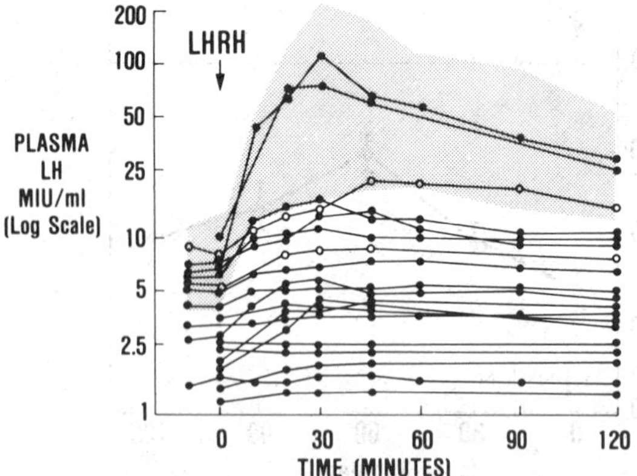

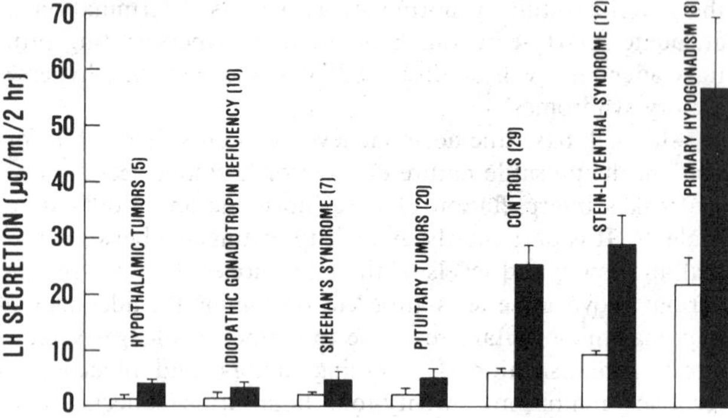

FIGURE 109-6

The effect of 100 μg LHRH intravenously on luteinizing hormone (LH) secretion in various clinical conditions. The clear bars show mean integrated levels of basal LH, and the solid bars show mean integrated levels for 2 h after administration of LHRH. The indices of basal and response LH were derived by computing areas under the curves formed by basal and response LH. The brackets indicate the standard error of the mean. The magnitude of the LH response in the various conditions appears to be related to basal LH levels. (After RH Mortimer et al, J Clin Endocrinol Metab 43:1240, 1978.)

The luteinizing hormone–releasing hormone (LHRH) test may also be used to assess pituitary gonadotropin reserve. LHRH (usually 100 or 150 μg) is injected intravenously, and blood LH (FSH optional) values are determined at base line and 20- to 30-min intervals. In normal patients the peak LH response occurs at 20 to 30 min (Fig. 109-5). Although the LHRH test may be useful in following a given patient, the magnitude of the LHRH integrated response can usually be predicted from the basal gonadotropin levels (Fig. 109-6). Therefore, the LHRH test is usually not necessary in the evaluation of patients with pituitary disease unless the patient is undergoing special studies. Another potential use for the LHRH test, i.e., differentiation between hypothalamic and pituitary disease, has also failed to be as useful as anticipated. Theoretically, patients with hypothalamic lesions lacking LHRH might have a normal LH and FSH release from the pituitary, while patients with pituitary lesions (secondary deficiencies) would fail to respond. However, the pituitary response is variable in both conditions, and LHRH appears to have a trophic effect on gonadotropin synthesis. Patients with definite hypothalamic lesions may initially have a poor response to LHRH, but after repeated stimulation gonadotropin response improves dramatically.

The integrity of the hypothalamus and pituitary together may be tested with clomiphene citrate, an estrogen antagonist which blocks the feedback of gonadal steroids on the hypothalamus in both men and women and which is also used for induction of ovulation in women. In men, the administration of clomiphene citrate 50 mg bid for 7 to 10 days usually produces a doubling of the LH and testosterone levels and a smaller increase in FSH values. For a normal response, both the hypothalamus and pituitary must function normally.

The measurement of urinary gonadotropins by bioassay or radioimmunoassay may be useful in selected patients. However, at times normal persons have no measurable gonadotropin excretion by bioassay, and the blood tests are more reliable.

TESTS OF THYROTROPIN (TSH) RESERVE Measurement of peripheral thyroid hormone levels is useful in identifying hypothalamic or pituitary hypothyroidism as well as primary thyroid deficiency. Chronic illness may be associated with low triiodothyronine and occasionally low thyroxine values in the absence of true hypothyroidism (see Chap. 111). Basal levels of

TSH are useful in differentiating primary thyroid gland deficiency from pituitary insufficiency. In primary hypothyroidism, serum TSH is elevated from lack of feedback inhibition by thyroid hormone. Patients with hypothalamic or pituitary disease have TSH values in the low or normal range. Unfortunately, most clinically available radioimmunoassays for TSH cannot distinguish between low and normal levels.

It is sometimes useful to measure the TSH response to thyrotropin-releasing hormone (TRH), particularly when evaluation of prolactin values is also desired. After the intravenous injection of 400 to 500 μg TRH, the normal peak TSH response occurs at 20 to 30 min and is approximately a doubling of base-line values (Fig. 109-7). Normally, prolactin values increase two- to eightfold. Unfortunately, the TRH test is similar to the LHRH test in that it does not always clearly differentiate between hypothalamic and pituitary disease. In addition, a few patients with large pituitary tumors have a normal TSH response to TRH even when they appear mildly hypothyroid. Other patients who are euthyroid and all patients who are hyperthyroid (Chap. 111) fail to respond to TRH. These occasional inconsistent responses limit the value of the test in differentiating hypothalamic and pituitary disease. No clinically useful feedback inhibition test for TSH is available at the present time.

TESTS FOR ACTH DEFICIENCY In patients suspected of having severe pituitary-adrenal insufficiency, basal morning plasma cortisol or 24-h urine 17-hydroxysteroid excretion should be measured prior to strenuous provocative tests such as the insulin tolerance test. Patients with adrenal insufficiency are very sensitive to insulin. These patients may be treated with replacement doses of a synthetic glucocorticoid such as 0.5 mg dexamethasone daily, which allows the patient to tolerate stress without ablating the ACTH response. Hypoglycemia during the insulin tolerance test normally provokes ACTH release and subsequent rise in plasma ACTH and cortisol levels. A cortisol rise of 5 to 7 μg/dl above base line or an absolute value above 15 μg/dl during the insulin tolerance test in a patient with normal corticotropin-binding globulin indicates a normal ACTH response.

FIGURE 109-7
Effect of 500 μg TRH on plasma thyrotropin (TSH) values in patients with pituitary tumors who are clinically euthyroid. The shaded area represents the range of responses in normal subjects. The TSH response in these patients varies from normal to none. Patients with large pituitary lesions producing TSH deficiency tend to have an absent TSH response although the TSH response occasionally may be normal. Patients with hypothalamic lesions and a normal pituitary (tertiary or hypothalamic hypothyroidism) may have a late sustained TSH response to exogenous TRH. Excess thyroid hormones will ablate the TSH response to TRH. (After N Fleischer et al, J Clin Endocrinol Metab 34:617, 1972.)

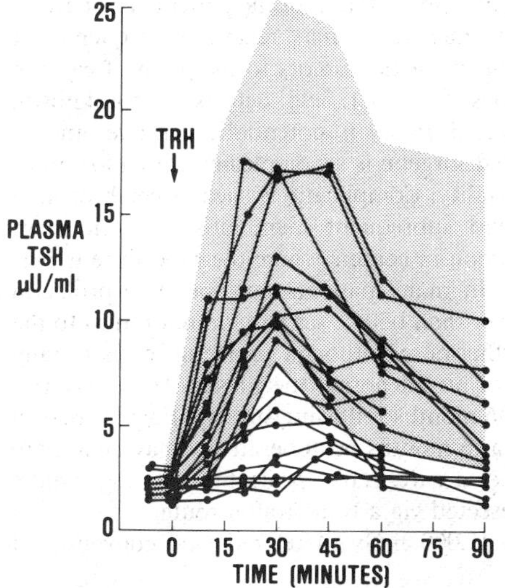

Patients who are not candidates for the insulin tolerance test (see above) may be tested with metyrapone, a blocker of the 11β-hydroxylation step of cortisol synthesis. This block induces ACTH elevations by preventing the normal cortisol feedback inhibition on the hypothalamic-pituitary unit. Exogenous steroid treatment precludes the use of this test. A normal response to oral or intravenous metyrapone may be determined from a rise of 11β-deoxycortisol (compound S) in the blood or by a rise in urinary 17-hydroxycorticosteroids, reflecting increased excretion of metabolites of 11-deoxycortisol. A patient who fails to respond to metyrapone should have documentation that the adrenals respond to exogenous ACTH. Some patients have normal ACTH and cortisol response to hypoglycemia but not to metyrapone. These patients usually do not need steroid replacement but should be carefully followed for the development of severe ACTH deficiency.

TESTS FOR ADH DEFICIENCY Evaluation of the patient with suspected diabetes insipidus is described in Chap. 110. The presence of diabetes insipidus usually indicates either vasopressin resistance or a hypothalamic lesion such as craniopharyngioma since ADH is synthesized in the hypothalamus. Lesions restricted to the pituitary usually do not cause diabetes insipidus until stalk or hypothalamic damage occurs. A simple screening test for diabetes insipidus is the determination of the urine osmolality after overnight water deprivation. If the osmolality is below 350 mosmol/kg, a full-scale dehydration test may be indicated.

Treatment Patients with space-occupying lesions such as craniopharyngioma or pituitary tumors are candidates for surgery and/or irradiation, particularly if there are visual field deficits. Craniopharyngiomas are usually approached by the transfrontal route, as are very large pituitary tumors that extend any distance above the optic chiasm. Transsphenoidal microsurgery is the usual choice in tumors confined to the sella. If tumor removal is incomplete or if the patient is not a candidate for surgery, irradiation with 4500 rads is usually indicated. The use of postoperative irradiation in patients in whom complete removal of a pituitary tumor is not possible may delay or prevent continued growth of the tumor. Patients should have an endocrine evaluation following treatment to determine the need for replacement therapy.

Patients with tumors who have received surgical or radiation treatment should be reevaluated at least annually for progression of their disease. Radiographic evaluation should minimally consist of coned-down views of the sella turcica. Visual fields should be determined, and an endocrine evaluation should include as a minimum measurement of thyroid and adrenal hormone levels in the blood or urine. More extensive tests including provocative tests such as the insulin tolerance or metyrapone tests and evaluation of gonadal function are frequently desirable. Patients with low thyroid or adrenal hormone values or patients who fail to respond to provocative tests should be started on hormone replacement. Once an endocrine deficiency such as TSH or ACTH is documented, return of function is unlikely, and continued testing for that hormone is unnecessary.

Hormone replacement in hypopituitary patients depends on the type and extent of the lesion and the degree of hormone deficit. Human growth hormone is usually given in three intramuscular injections per week to GH-deficient prepubertal children. TSH deficiency is corrected by treatment with oral L-thyroxine 100 to 200 μg daily. Pituitary-adrenal insufficiency can be treated with oral prednisone 5 to 7.5 mg daily in a single dose or hydrocortisone 20 to 30 mg daily in divided doses. Mineralocorticoid replacement is not necessary in hypopituitary patients with normal adrenal glands because aldosterone secretion is maintained in a functionally adequate range. Patients with diabetes insipidus can be controlled with the synthetic vasopressin analogue, 1-desamino-8-D-arginine vasopressin (DDAVP) intranasally or with intramuscular pitressin tannate in oil (see Chap. 110). Partial diabetes insipidus can be treated with chlorpropamide, clofibrate, or thiazide diuretics.

The most difficult form of replacement is that of gonadotropin in infertile patients desiring children. If fertility is not an objective, men may be treated with a long-acting parenteral testosterone preparation such as testosterone enanthate 200 mg every 2 weeks. This will preserve libido, potency, and secondary sexual characteristics such as beard growth. Women may be treated with cyclic estrogen and progesterone. Men or women who desire children must be treated with human gonadotropin preparations including extracts from human urine (containing both FSH and LH activity) and chorionic gonadotropin, which has primarily LH-like activity (see Chaps. 117 and 118). LHRH over long periods has also been used successfully in some patients.

DISEASES OF ANTERIOR PITUITARY HORMONE HYPERSECRETION Disorders of pituitary hormone hypersecretion occur in patients with functioning adenomas producing either prolactin (galactorrhea-amenorrhea syndrome), growth hormone (acromegaly), or ACTH (Cushing's disease). For unknown reasons, functional adenomas of cells synthesizing the glycoprotein pituitary hormones TSH, LH, and FSH rarely develop. The adenomas responsible for excess prolactin secretion in women are often small and are classified as microadenomas, being less than 10 mm in diameter. ACTH-producing adenomas are also often quite small, while growth hormone–producing tumors and prolactin-producing tumors in men are often large enough to enlarge the sella turcica.

Hyperprolactinemia Recognition and treatment of prolactin-secreting pituitary microadenomas have resulted in major diagnostic and therapeutic advances in the area of pituitary disease. Traditionally, prolactinomas have been associated with the amenorrhea-galactorrhea syndrome in women. However, these hypersecretory adenomas do not always cause either amenorrhea or galactorrhea. Men with prolactin-secreting tumors may but usually do not have galactorrhea because the male breast lacks adequate development of acini. (For discussion of the differential diagnosis of galactorrhea see Chap. 119.) Prolactin-producing tumors in men usually present as space-occupying lesions, often with hypogonadism. A basal serum prolactin determination in patients with suspected hypothalamic or pituitary disease is useful because (1) prolactin-secreting adenomas are the most common form of pituitary tumor and (2) hypothalamic lesions may cause hyperprolactinemia.

Women with prolactin-producing microadenomas frequently present during the reproductive years. These patients may have galactorrhea, amenorrhea, or both. Prolactinomas have been reported to be the etiology of 20 to 25 percent of cases of secondary amenorrhea in some series. Libido may be depressed, and some have evidence of decreased estrogens and hirsutism. This has been thought to represent either a depression of ovarian function or stimulation of adrenal androgen secretion. Other clinical manifestations depend on the extent of other anterior pituitary hormone deficiencies. Prolactinomas are frequently detected in women before other hormone deficiencies develop.

In men, recognition of prolactin-secreting tumors usually occurs only after the tumor has reached a large size and produced the same signs and symptoms as a nonfunctioning tumor (see above). However, small adenomas have been reported in men who present with decreased libido and/or infertility. In some, these symptoms have improved after removal of the adenoma.

DIAGNOSTIC TESTS The diagnostic evaluation of patients with galactorrhea is performed with the goal of detecting patients with pituitary adenoma or other space-occupying lesions. Basal prolactin levels are a critical part of the evaluation. In general, the higher the basal prolactin level, the more likely the patient has a pituitary tumor. Values above 100 to 150 ng/ml usually indicate tumor. Dynamic tests have been used in an effort to distinguish pituitary adenomas from other types of hyperprolactinemia. TRH, which stimulates the lactotrophs, and chlorpromazine, which interferes with PIF activity, have been used to stimulate prolactin release. Both TRH (400 μg intravenously) and chlorpromazine (CPZ) (25 to 50 mg intramuscularly) cause an increase of prolactin levels to more than double basal values in normal adults. Metoclopramide, a dopaminergic antagonist that is a potent stimulus for prolactin release in normal subjects, has also been used (10 mg intravenously) as a testing agent. Responses to all three agents are blunted in patients with high basal levels owing to pituitary adenomas. Many patients with idiopathic galactorrhea give a similar response. An occasional patient with a pituitary tumor and high basal prolactin values is stimulated by TRH, indicating apparent storage of prolactin in the tumor. Patients with other causes of galactorrhea tend to show variable stimulation after either test. L-Dopa suppresses prolactin secretion regardless of etiology and therefore is not useful in determining which patients have adenomas. High basal levels should arouse the suspicion of a pituitary tumor. The metoclopramide and TRH tests may be useful in confirming this impression. However, after demonstration of an elevated prolactin, the most useful diagnostic studies are radiological. Coned-down views of the sella, CT scanning, or polytomography should be performed. These usually distinguish between normal irregularities of the sella floor contour, such as the carotid groove, and a defect produced by a microadenoma. Visual field examinations should also be obtained. However, since prolactin-secreting microadenomas in young women are ordinarily detected while still small, the visual fields are usually normal.

TREATMENT The type of treatment depends on the lesion involved and the original presentation of the patient. The natural history of pituitary microadenomas regarding frequency of subsequent enlargement of the tumors to the point of causing hormone deficiencies or visual field defects is not known. Transsphenoidal microsurgery is potentially curative, and in the hands of a skilled surgeon is accomplished with a low morbidity and low mortality. Complications such as cerebrospinal fluid rhinorrhea and subsequent meningitis or optic-nerve damage are uncommon in centers where the procedure is performed frequently. In many patients postoperative prolactin levels, although lower than before surgery, do not return to the normal range. Furthermore, although prolactin levels usually fall after removal of an adenoma, the plasma level may rise gradually for up to 6 months following surgery. For this reason the prolactin level at 6 months postoperatively may be a more reliable indication of a cure. Large prolactin-secreting tumors often have to be resected via a transfrontal route.

Radiation with 45,000 mGy (4500 rads) by conventional

supravoltage technique has also been successful in lowering prolactin levels. This treatment requires more time for the beneficial effect to occur and is therefore less commonly used.

Medical treatment of hyperprolactinemia and galactorrhea is promising. After L-dopa was shown to reduce prolactin levels, the drug was tried in the treatment of patients with galactorrhea and amenorrhea. Unfortunately, L-dopa, to be effective, had to be given frequently and in large doses resulting in nausea and other unpleasant side effects. However, other dopamine agonists such as bromocriptine, an ergot derivative, are now available and reduce hyperprolactinemia of all etiologies. Women with galactorrhea-amenorrhea frequently have a cessation of galactorrhea, resumption of menses, and restoration of fertility after oral bromocriptine 2.5 mg bid or tid. This drug also has an antitumor effect with shrinkage of the prolactinoma. However, hyperprolactinemia usually recurs when therapy is stopped, and rapid expansion of the adenoma may ensue. Patients with pituitary tumors who become pregnant after bromocriptine treatment may have enlargement of the pituitary to the point of compression of the optic chiasm. However, some patients have been followed through pregnancy without permanent visual loss. The U.S. Food and Drug Administration has not yet approved bromocriptine for use in patients with documented pituitary tumors, although the drug is widely used for this purpose outside the United States.

Disorders of growth hormone excess Both gigantism and acromegaly are the consequence of excess growth hormone secretion by pituitary adenomas. There is also evidence of disordered hypothalamic control or pituitary responsiveness in these patients (e.g., abnormal GH release after TRH or LHRH and the occasional paradoxical increase of GH after glucose). These abnormalities in GH control plus the fact that acromegaly may appear before a pituitary adenoma is demonstrable have suggested that GH-secreting tumors may be the result of hypothalamic stimulation. However, microadenoma without sellar enlargement may also cause acromegaly. The tumors are usually eosinophilic on light microscopy and can be demonstrated to contain growth hormone granules on electron microscopy.

GIGANTISM When growth hormone hypersecretion occurs prior to puberty and fusion of the epiphyses, gigantism develops. These patients may reach enormous proportions because of massive growth of the skeleton. One was 8 ft 11 in tall and weighed 475 lb prior to his death at age 22. The soft tissues, including the peripheral nerves, are enlarged. Early in the course of the disease, patients may be unusually strong. However, they later may develop pituitary insufficiency with weakness and hypogonadism. Myopathy and severe peripheral sensory and motor neuropathy with findings such as weakness, foot drop, and Charcot-type arthropathy may be prominent in extreme gigantism.

ACROMEGALY When growth hormone–secreting tumors develop after puberty, acromegaly results. The disorder occurs equally in men and women. Approximately 10 to 15 percent of all large pituitary tumors secrete growth hormone and cause acromegaly. Because of the slow progression of the disease, the changes in physical features, which often begin between the second and fourth decades, are frequently not recognized for 10 to 20 years. Since linear growth of the long bones is not possible after epiphyseal fusion, enlargement is most apparent in the acral parts including the hands, feet, nose, and mandible; hence the name *acromegaly*. The extent and course of the clinical disease does not always correlate precisely with GH or somatomedin C levels. The clinical manifestations of acromegaly are protean and are the result of the excessive secretion of

growth hormone combined with the mass effect of the pituitary tumor (Table 109-3).

The patient with acromegaly may note progressive increase in ring, shoe, glove, and hat size after puberty. Increased soft-tissue growth is almost invariably present but may go unnoticed by the patient or family for long periods of time. The increased size of the nose, lips, and soft tissue of the face results in a characteristic coarsening of the facial features (Fig. 109-8). Enlargement of the mandible may be manifested as prognathism with underbite and increased spacing of the lower teeth. The large nose, thick lips, accentuated nasolabial folds, and coarse features cause a characteristic facial appearance in acromegalic patients. The forehead and orbital ridges are prominent in part because of a characteristic enlargement of the frontal sinuses. The tongue enlarges and may show indentations from the teeth. The voice often develops a characteristic deep, cavernous, and husky quality. The feet and hands are fleshy and often grossly enlarged. The broad hands with thick, large fingers have been described as spade-like in appearance. The feet are also characteristically broad, causing a need for extra-wide shoes.

Patients with acromegaly have an increased metabolic rate and usually note increased sweating and sebaceous activity. The skin is warm, moist, and thickened. Other cutaneous changes include small papillomatous lesions over the trunk called *fibromata mollusca,* increased skin pigmentation, and oc-

TABLE 109-3
Manifestations of acromegaly

	*Series 1,** %	*Series 2,†* %
PRIMARILY FROM GROWTH HORMONE HYPERSECRETION		
Acral enlargement (hands, feet, nose, jaw)	100	96
Soft-tissue overgrowth (heel pad > 22 mm on x-ray)		98
Excessive perspiration	60	88
Joint pain		76
Weight gain	39	76
Hypertrichosis	53	
Voice change		50
Paresthesias	30	62
Cutaneous pigmentation	46	
Acanthosis nigricans		26
Fibromata mollusca	27	38
Enlarged thyroid	25	18
Glucose intolerance		56
Glycosuria	25	
Clinical diabetes mellitus	12	8
Hypertension		23
Cardiac symptoms		12
Lactation	4	8
PRIMARILY FROM PITUITARY TUMOR ENLARGEMENT		
Enlargement of sella on x-ray	93	90
Headache	87	64
Visual disturbances	62	
Photophobia	12	46
COMBINED EFFECTS INCLUDING HYPOPITUITARISM		
Drowsiness, fatigue, and lethargy	42	82
Amenorrhea‡	73	32
Decreased libido	38	27
Asthenia	33	

* *From a series of 100 patients reported by L Davidoff, Endocrinology 10:461, 1926.*

† *From a series of 50 patients reported by S Levin, Calif Med 116:57, 1972, and Am J Med 57:526, 1974.*

‡ *Percent of women.*

casionally acanthosis nigricans. Frequently, acromegalic patients have an increased growth of coarse body hair.

Joint complaints are relatively common. Early in the course of the disease there is widening of the joint spaces as a consequence of growth of the cartilage and soft tissues. Later, osteoarthritis with pain and limitation of joint motion may occur in several joints including the temporomandibular joint. Degenerative changes in the spine may cause nerve root or cord compression. Prominent muscular development usually occurs as part of the soft-tissue growth. Myopathy and peripheral neuropathy with weakness may occur later in the disease. Paresthesias are a frequent complaint. A carpal tunnel syndrome may be present in about a third of patients because of pressure on the median nerve from tissue enlargement, but not all paresthesias can be explained by this mechanism.

Hypertension is present in about 25 percent, and patients may have cardiac enlargement as a result of the GH excess as well as hypertension. Congestive heart failure may occur. Visceral enlargement also involves the liver, spleen, kidneys, and occasionally the thyroid and adrenals. Glomerular filtration rate in the enlarged kidneys is increased. Thyroid and adrenal function are usually in the normal range.

Glucose intolerance is present in approximately half of acromegalics because hypersecretion of GH causes an insulin-resistant state. Insulin levels are commonly elevated and return to normal after successful treatment and reduction of GH levels. The hyperglycemia of acromegaly is usually well tolerated, although clinical diabetes may occur in patients with a genetic predisposition to the disease. Glycosuria, polydipsia, and polyphagia are found in about 25 percent of patients with advanced illness. The polydipsia is probably best correlated with glycosuria, although diabetes insipidus may rarely be present. Hypermetabolism and hyperhidrosis contribute to both the polydipsia and polyphagia.

The pituitary enlargement produces symptoms and signs similar to other space-occupying lesions of the sella. Headaches are extremely common and may be bitemporal or variable in location. Visual complaints are frequent and include decreased vision and photophobia. As the GH-secreting tumor enlarges, normal pituitary function is often compromised. Asthenia, fatigue, lethargy, amenorrhea, and decreased libido probably are the consequence of several factors including the metabolic effects of GH, myopathy, neuropathy, and variable degrees of hypopituitarism.

Other endocrine diseases may be associated with acromegaly. The autosomal dominant syndrome of multiple endocrine neoplasia, type I (Wermer syndrome), consisting of adenomas of the pituitary, pancreas, and parathyroids may be manifest as acromegaly (see Chap. 123). Galactorrhea may be present in women with tumors that secrete both GH and prolactin. The hypermetabolism and thyroid enlargement of acromegaly are usually the result of GH excess alone. However, true thyrotoxicosis occasionally occurs.

The x-ray changes are often striking. In the past, approximately 90 percent of patients with acromegaly had an enlarged sella turcica at the time of diagnosis. The combination of frontal sinus enlargement with an increased sella size is suggestive of the diagnosis. Radiological evaluation should therefore include careful studies of the sella including tomograms, CT scan, or pneumoencephalogram to evaluate the possibility and extent of suprasellar extension and extension into the sphenoid sinuses. Another useful radiographic finding is thickening of the soft tissue of the heel pad which usually exceeds 22 mm in acromegalic patients. Late in the disease the ends of the distal phalanges of the hands may develop a tufted appearance on x-ray which resembles an arrowhead. The bony enlargement of the hands and feet may be combined with decreased bone density that is particularly apparent in the metatarsals. Osteophyte formation and osteoarthritis are prominent changes which increase with age.

Careful visual fields and full ophthalmologic examination should be performed because of the relatively high frequency of visual field abnormalities. The classic bitemporal hemianopsia from compression of the optic chiasm by the tumor mass may be present. However, as is true for all pituitary tumors, visual field defects may vary from a unilateral small quadrantic defect to extensive bilateral defects. Occasionally papilledema or optic atrophy may be present in patients with extensive tumors.

The diagnosis of acromegaly is made on the basis of the characteristic clinical and radiographic features combined with inappropriately elevated growth hormone levels. A useful laboratory test is the measurement of growth hormone during the glucose tolerance test. In normal persons growth hormone values at 30 to 90 min after the ingestion of 100 g glucose are suppressed to less than 5 ng/ml. Acromegalic patients do not suppress and occasionally show a paradoxical increase in growth hormone after glucose. Patients with diabetes, uremia, chronic starvation, or acute intermittent porphyria also may show a poor GH suppression after glucose. Another diagnostic test is the growth hormone response to TRH. Normal patients have no GH response to TRH, whereas acromegalic patients have an abnormal release. Patients with anorexia nervosa, depression, uremia, hypothyroidism, and protein-calorie deprivation may also have an abnormal GH response to TRH, but the diagnosis is usually obvious. Plasma somatomedin C level as measured by radioimmunoassay is usually elevated in active acromegaly and may be useful to confirm the diagnosis. Evaluation of other anterior pituitary hormones including the gonadotropins, TSH, and ACTH should be performed as described previously.

The routine laboratory evaluation of the patient with acro-

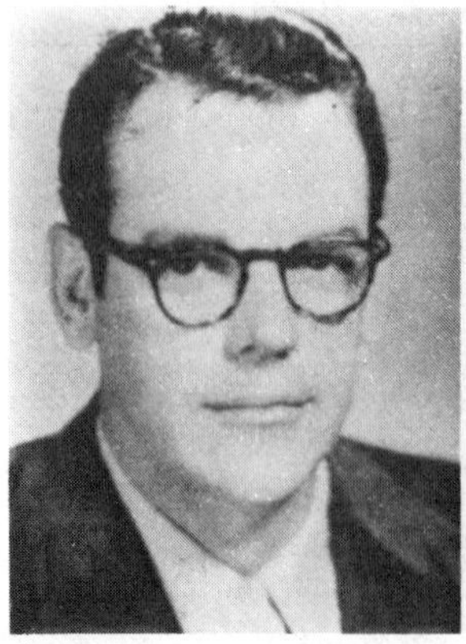
A

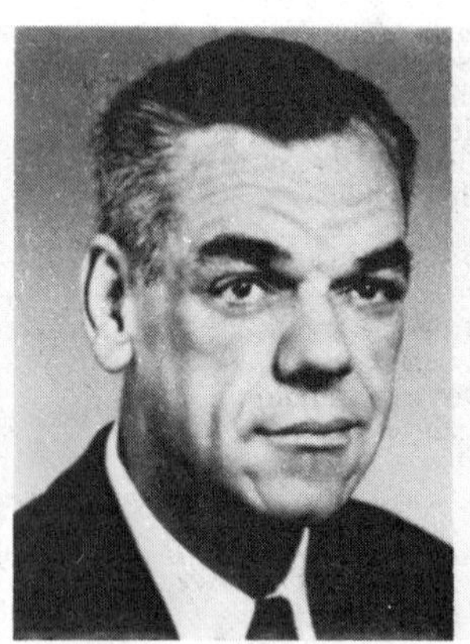
B

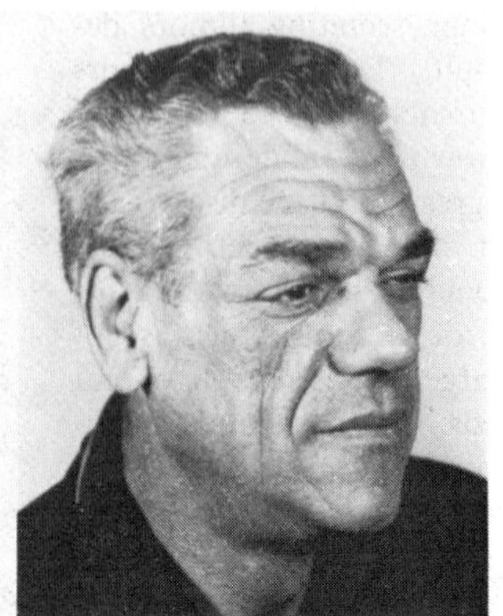
C

FIGURE 109-8
Progressive development of acromegalic features. A. Age 30. B. Age 37. C. Age 40. (Courtesy of N Kaplan.)

megaly may disclose hyperglycemia and glycosuria. Overt diabetes mellitus is present in only about 10 percent of patients and usually is limited to those with a positive family history for diabetes. The serum phosphate may be elevated from the excess growth hormone.

TREATMENT Although acromegaly is a slowly progressive disorder, there is an increased incidence of cardiovascular complications, and treatment is indicated. There are several methods for treating the pituitary tumor. Transfrontal surgery may be required for large tumors, while transsphenoidal microsurgery is successful in removing small adenomas. Growth hormone levels fall rapidly to normal after successful surgery. The other major type of treatment is radiation. Both proton beam or heavy-particle treatment and conventional supravoltage radiation can reduce growth hormone values in 90 percent of patients, although the latter method may require several years for a full therapeutic effect. Both surgery and radiation may be necessary to control tumor growth. Patients should be monitored at 6- to 12-month intervals for the possible development of other anterior pituitary hormone deficiencies.

Several medical treatments for acromegaly such as estrogen, medroxyprogesterone, and chlorpromazine have been attempted in the past with limited success. Somatostatin lowers growth hormone levels, but, since it must be infused to sustain this effect, it is not useful in treatment. However, dopamine agonists such as bromocriptine lower growth hormone levels in many patients. This does not represent definitive therapy but may be useful as adjunctive treatment in patients with galactorrhea, diabetes mellitus, or cardiovascular complications who are not candidates for surgery and whose growth hormone levels do not fall promptly after radiation.

ACTH hypersecretion (see also Chap. 112) Cushing's disease is the consequence of oversecretion of ACTH by the pituitary. This should not be confused with Cushing's *syndrome,* which is a nonspecific term indicating increased glucocorticoid levels from any source, including iatrogenic steroid administration. ACTH secretion tends to be sustained throughout the day in patients with Cushing's disease with loss of the usual diurnal variation of plasma ACTH and cortisol levels. ACTH release is impaired after stress such as insulin-induced hypoglycemia, and there is a decreased sensitivity of ACTH secretion to steroid feedback inhibition; i.e., glucocorticoids in physiological amounts do not suppress ACTH secretion, although supraphysiological steroid levels are effective. The dexamethasone-suppresion test is designed to test for this abnormal feedback sensitivity. Most patients with Cushing's disease do not show suppression of glucocorticoids in plasma or urine after dexamethasone (2 mg per day given as 0.5 mg every 6 h) equivalent to more than twice the normal glucocorticoid requirement. However, suppression of plasma cortisol to < 5 μg/dl or urinary 17-hydroxysteroids to < 3 mg per gram of creatinine may occur with amounts of dexamethasone (8 mg per day given as 2 mg every 6 h) approximately 10 times the normal replacement equivalent of cortisol. While the hypothalamic-pituitary axis remains partially responsive to feedback control (albeit at an abnormal level), most patients with Cushing's disease have identifiable pituitary adenomas. This raises the possibility that the adenomas develop as a result of abnormal hypothalamic stimulation. If large pituitary adenomas are present, suppression of ACTH secretion can be demonstrated only after much larger doses of dexamethasone, if at all. Some patients with a primary psychiatric depression have elevated serum and urinary cortisol levels with a loss of normal diurnal variation and may have abnormal response to dexamethasone suppression as well. Since patients with Cushing's disease often have depression, this may cause confusion. However, patients with depression tend to have a normal ACTH release to stress, while patients with Cushing's disease do not.

The pituitary adenomas in Cushing's disease are usually small, and less than 10 percent of patients have an enlarged sella turcica. The approach to diagnosis of Cushing's disease is discussed in Chap. 112. Cushing initially treated patients by hypophysectomy, but subsequently this procedure was replaced by bilateral adrenalectomy. However, although adrenalectomy is appropriate in some patients with severe disease, the primary problem is not in the adrenals but in the hypothalamus or pituitary. A few patients who have had adrenalectomy without pituitary treatment develop *Nelson's syndrome.* This is a more aggressive ACTH-secreting tumor that may be locally invasive and difficult to manage. Patients with Nelson's syndrome frequently develop severe visual field defects from the enlarging tumor and usually have hyperpigmentation from ACTH or β-lipotropin hypersecretion.

The recent advances in transsphenoidal microsurgery have reestablished pituitary surgery in the treatment of Cushing's disease. Selective removal of the adenoma can be accomplished in many instances with good clinical results. Proton beam or conventional supravoltage radiation has also been used successfully in many patients. Adrenalectomy is still required in patients with severe disease and in patients who do not respond to other measures. In patients undergoing adrenalectomy, prophylactic pituitary radiation has been advocated to prevent the development of Nelson's syndrome, but the latter has occurred in some patients despite radiation. Medical treatment of the glucocorticoid hypersecretion may be attempted with metyrapone, which blocks 11β-hydroxylation, with *o,p'*-DDD (mitotane), which has a direct toxic effect on the adrenal, or with cyproheptadine, which acts through a central mechanism to decrease ACTH secretion. Although medical treatment may be useful in the patient who is a poor candidate for surgery or radiation, definitive therapy is ultimately required. The choice depends to some degree on the surgical expertise and equipment available. Although proton beam radiation is frequently successful and conventional radiation reduces ACTH to normal levels in about 25 percent of patients, transsphenoidal selective microsurgery is the treatment of choice in most medical centers.

MISCELLANEOUS HYPERSECRETORY SYNDROMES In contrast to prolactin, growth hormone, and ACTH, hypersecretion of the glycoprotein hormones TSH, LH, and FSH by pituitary tumors rarely occurs. The few reported LH- and FSH-secreting pituitary tumors developed in patients with gonadal insufficiency who may have had a stimulus to increased gonadotropin secretion from lack of feedback inhibition. Autonomous production apparently occurred subsequent to compensatory hypersecretion. TSH-producing pituitary tumors causing hyperthyroidism have been documented in only a few patients.

Ectopic secretion of essentially all pituitary hormones by carcinomas of nonendocrine tissues has been reported (see Chap. 122). Ectopic ACTH production is not uncommon, particularly by carcinomas of the lung. This must be considered in the differential diagnosis of hypersecretion of adrenal steroids. Because of the rapid progression and short duration of the illness, such patients usually present with wasting and with metabolic effects such as hypokalemia rather than the typical cushingoid appearance. Ectopic gonadotropin secretion is also common in malignancies of the lung, gastrointestinal tract, and testis. Male patients may present with gynecomastia. However, the gonadotropin usually has the characteristics of HCG rather than pituitary LH or FSH. Ectopic secretion of alpha subunit that is common for LH and HCG also occurs without causing clinical manifestations and may be used as a tumor marker. Ectopic secretion of growth hormone, LH, FSH, or prolactin may be difficult to detect because of the continuous pituitary secretion of these hormones.

REFERENCES

Banna M: Craniopharyngioma: Based on 160 cases. Br J Radiol 49:206, 1976

Boyd AE III et al: Galactorrhea-amenorrhea syndrome: Diagnosis and therapy. Ann Intern Med 87:165, 1977

Burger HG, Patel YC: Thyrotropin releasing hormone—TRH. Clin Endocrinol Metab 6:83, 1977

Child DF et al: Prolactin studies in "functionless" pituitary tumors. Br Med J 1:604, 1975

Cowden EA et al: Tests of prolactin secretion in diagnosis of prolactinomas. Lancet 1:1155, 1979

del Pozo E, Lancranjan I: Clinical use of drugs modifying the release of anterior pituitary hormone, in *Frontiers in Neuroendocrinology*, vol 5, WF Ganong, L Martini (eds). New York, Raven Press, 1978

Frantz A: Prolactin. N Engl J Med 298:201, 1978

Hardy J: Transsphenoidal surgery of hypersecreting pituitary tumors, in *Diagnosis and Treatment of Pituitary Tumors*, PO Kohler, GT Ross (eds). New York, American Elsevier, 1973, p 179

Jordan RM et al: The primary empty sella syndrome. Am J Med 62:569, 1977

Kleinberg DL et al: Galactorrhea: A study of 235 cases, including 48 with pituitary tumors. N Engl J Med 296:589, 1977

Kohler PO, Ross GT (eds): *Diagnosis and Treatment of Pituitary Tumors*. New York, American Elsevier, 1973

Kreiger DT, Glick SM: Growth hormone and cortisol responsiveness in Cushing's syndrome. Am J Med 52:25, 1972

Lin T, Tucci JR: Provocative tests of growth hormone release. Ann Intern Med 80:464, 1974

Martin JB et al (eds): *Clinical Neuroendocrinology*. Philadelphia, Davis, 1977

Mortimer RH et al: Correlation between integrated LH and FSH levels and the response to luteinizing hormone releasing factor (LRF). J Clin Endocrinol Metab 43:1240, 1976

Neelon FA et al: The primary empty sella: Clinical and radiographic characteristics and endocrine function. Medicine 52:73, 1973

Nelson DH et al: ACTH-producing pituitary tumors following adrenalectomy for Cushing's syndrome. Ann Intern Med 52:560, 1960

Reichlin S: Regulation of the hypophysiotropic secretions of the brain. Arch Intern Med 135:1350, 1975

Reichlin S et al (eds): *The Hypothalamus*. New York, Raven Press, 1978

Smith LH, Levin SR: Manifestations and treatment of acromegaly. Calif Med 116:57, 1972

Spark RF, Dickstein G: Bromocriptine and endocrine disorders. Ann Int Med 90:949, 1979

Tucker H St G et al: Galactorrhea-amenorrhea syndrome: Follow-up of forty-five patients after pituitary tumor removal. Ann Int Med 94:302, 1981

Tyrell JB et al: Cushing's disease: Selective trans-sphenoidal resection of pituitary microadenomas. N Engl J Med 298:753, 1978

Vale W et al: Characterization of a 41-residue ovine hypothalamic peptide that stimulates secretion of corticotropin and beta endorphin. Science 213:1394, 1981

Yen SSC, Jaffee RB (eds): *Reproductive Endocrinology*. Philadelphia, Saunders, 1978

110 DISORDERS OF THE NEUROHYPOPHYSIS

DAVID H. P. STREETEN
ARNOLD M. MOSES
MYRON MILLER

There are two largely independent hypothalamic-neurohypophyseal systems composed of neurons in the supraoptic and paraventricular nuclei, from which axons extend through the pituitary stalk to the posterior pituitary. Hormones (vasopressin and oxytocin) formed within separate ganglion cells, migrate in association with carrier proteins, neurophysins, down the axons and are stored in secretory granules within the nerve terminals located in the neurohypophysis. By the process of exocytosis, the hormones are released with their neurophysins from the granules into the bloodstream. Vasopressin or antidiuretic hormone (AVP or ADH) is predominantly concerned with the control of water conservation. Release of vasopressin is closely coordinated with the activity of the thirst center which regulates fluid intake. Oxytocin stimulates uterine contractions and milk ejection.

VASOPRESSIN RELEASE AND ACTION

CHEMISTRY Arginine vasopressin (AVP) is a nonapeptide which comprises six amino acids in a ring attached to a side chain of three amino acids, including arginine in humans.

ACTIONS ADH acts to conserve water and concentrate urine by enhancing the hydroosmotic flow of water from the luminal fluid through the cells of the collecting tubule of the kidney to the medullary interstitium. This action of ADH assists in maintaining constancy of the osmolality and volume of body fluids. High concentrations of ADH can cause vasoconstriction, as may occur in response to severe hypotension or to infusion of vasopressin for treatment of bleeding esophageal varices.

There is evidence that ADH, perhaps released from axons which terminate in the cerebrum, may play a role in learning and memory. ADH released from fibers terminating in the median eminence may influence corticotropin secretion.

ASSAY ADH is assayed biologically by measuring its antidiuretic or pressor action in experimental animals. More recently ADH has been quantitated in blood and urine by radioimmunoassay. The results may be expressed as units or fractions of units based on pressor activity in the rat, or in terms of weight of purified vasopressin. Arginine vasopressin has a biological activity of approximately 400 units per milligram (1 μU = 2.5 pg). The human neurohypophysis under conditions of random fluid intake contains approximately 8 units of ADH. Under the same conditions peripheral plasma ADH concentration in humans ranges from 1 to 3 μU/ml. The ADH concentration of blood fluctuates, with a maximum late at night and in the early morning and a minimum in the early afternoon. Under conditions of normal hydration, healthy subjects excrete approximately 10 to 35 mU ADH in 24 h, while releasing 400 to 550 mU from the pituitary. During 24 to 28 h of dehydration the amount released increases three to five times with corresponding increases in plasma and urinary ADH levels.

METABOLISM Inactivation of ADH occurs largely in liver and kidneys, a major mechanism being the cleavage of the terminal glycinamide to produce a biologically inactive substance. Approximately 10 percent of secreted ADH is excreted in the urine as active hormone.

CONTROL OF ADH RELEASE The release of ADH into the circulation is influenced by a number of stimuli (Fig. 110-1).

Osmoregulation Under normal conditions ADH release is primarily regulated by osmoreceptors in the hypothalamus. Changes in the concentrations of plasma solutes to which the cellular membrane is impermeable cause alterations in the volume of the osmoreceptor cells. These cellular volume changes alter the electrical activity of the neurons and in this way control ADH release. There is evidence from animal studies that osmotic changes which stimulate release also enhance production of ADH. The servomechanism between effective plasma osmolality and vasopressin release normally maintains plasma osmolality within a very narrow range. The mean plasma osmolality of normal subjects following a water load of 20 ml per kilogram of body weight is 281.7 mosmol/kg, while that which initiates ADH release following infusion of hypertonic saline into water-loaded subjects is 287.3 mosmol/kg. Thus the increase in plasma osmolality from full diuresis to the initiation of antidiuresis by hypertonic saline is only 5.6 mosmol/kg, or 2 percent.

The infusion of hypertonic saline at a constant rate into water-loaded human subjects causes a linear rise in plasma osmolality with time. After an interval which depends on the infusion rate and the concentration of the saline, there is an abrupt, progressive fall in free water clearance without a significant change in solute or creatinine excretion. We have defined the osmotic threshold for ADH release as the plasma osmolality at the onset of antidiuresis under these conditions. In 73 normal subjects, this occurred at a mean plasma osmolality of 287 mosmol/kg. The plasma osmolality at which ADH release is initiated was determined by Robertson from measurements of the rising plasma ADH level in response to increasing plasma osmolality during hypertonic saline infusions and was found to range from 280 to 291 mosmol/kg, similar to the above value.

FIGURE 110-1
Schematic representation of control of ADH release and cellular action of ADH.

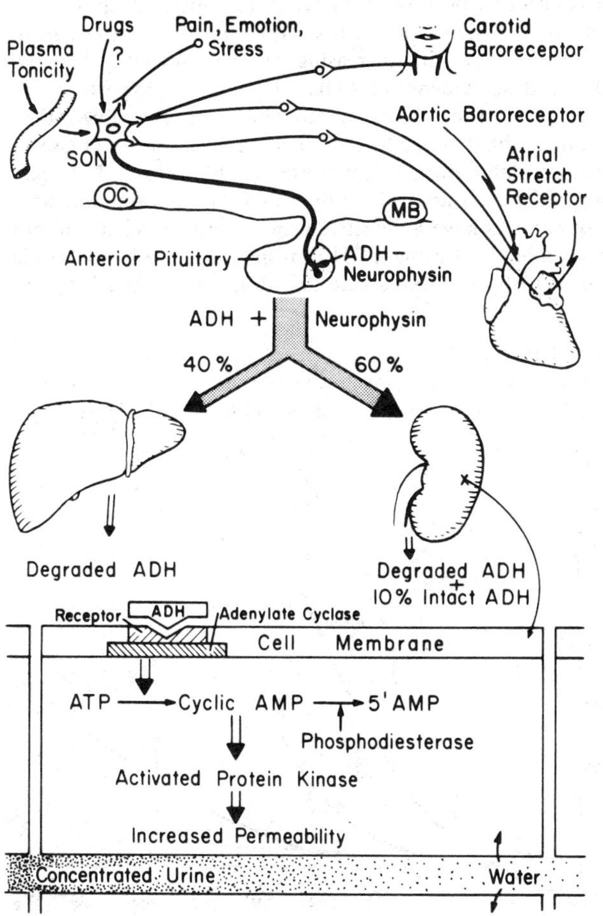

Volume regulation Decreases in plasma volume, through effects on stretch receptors in the left atrium and perhaps the pulmonary veins, stimulate the release of ADH by reducing the tonic inhibitory impulses from the left atrium to the hypothalamus. The neural impulses travel via the vagi to the reticular formation of the midbrain and diencephalon and thence to the supraoptic and paraventricular nuclei, where they are integrated with the other stimuli which affect ADH release. Positive pressure breathing, quiet standing, and vasodilatation due to heat may activate this mechanism, which serves to restore plasma volume, even at times overriding osmotic inhibition of ADH release. Following volume stimulation circulating ADH concentrations may reach 10 times the levels induced by hypertonicity. Increased plasma volume inhibits ADH release by the reverse mechanisms leading to a diuresis and the correction of the hypervolemia. Negative pressure breathing, recumbency, lack of gravitational force as occurs in space travel, submersion in water, and exposure to cold may activate this mechanism.

Baroreceptor regulation Activation of carotid and aortic baroreceptors in response to hypotension causes the release of ADH. Hypotension due to blood loss is the most potent stimulus to ADH release and may raise plasma levels of ADH to approach 1000 μU/ml at times. These very high concentrations of ADH may cause marked vasoconstriction, which probably plays a role in the restoration of blood pressure.

Neural regulation Recent evidence indicates that peptide neurotransmitters and neuromodulators such as angiotensin II and beta endorphin may mediate stimulatory and inhibitory input into the hypothalamus. Acetylcholine appears to be the final link connecting neural pathways to the supraoptic neurons involved in ADH release. Both cholinergic and beta-adrenergic stimuli release ADH, while atropine and alpha-adrenergic stimulation inhibit ADH release, apparently by actions on the hypothalamus. Emotional stress, emesis, and pain may overcome a diuresis. A diuresis may follow hypnotic suggestion, psychologic conditioning, and inhalation of carbon dioxide. The above observations indicate that higher neural centers may alter ADH release.

Pharmacologic influences Pharmacologic agents which may stimulate ADH release include nicotine, morphine, barbiturates, vincristine, vinblastine, cyclophosphamide, clofibrate, chlorpropamide, and some of the tricyclic anticonvulsants and antidepressants. Ethanol has long been recognized to have diuretic properties and to inhibit neurohypophyseal function under a variety of conditions. Some narcotic antagonists have also been found to inhibit ADH release. Experimentally chlorpromazine, reserpine, and diphenylhydantoin all diminish the depletion of pituitary vasopressin and the rise in urinary excretion of ADH, resulting from water deprivation. In humans, diphenylhydantoin and chlorpromazine may inhibit ADH release and produce diuresis.

ADH RESPONSE TO WATER DEPRIVATION AND TO WATER LOAD Water deprivation provides both an osmotic and a volume stimulus to vasopressin release by increasing plasma osmolality and decreasing plasma volume. The maximum urinary osmolality reached after water deprivation varies considerably, depending on renal medullary osmolality and other intrarenal factors. In response to fluid deprivation for 18 to 24 h in normal individuals, plasma osmolality rarely rises above 292 mosmol/kg. The resultant stimulation of ADH release increases plasma ADH concentration to 6 to 10 μU/ml.

The administration of water lowers plasma osmolality and expands blood volume, inhibiting the release of ADH via both the osmoreceptor and the atrial volume receptor mechanisms. An oral water load of 20 ml/kg in normal adults, which results in a fall in plasma osmolality to a mean of 281.7 mosmol/kg, causes a maximum diuresis in approximately 1 to $1\frac{1}{2}$ h with the free water clearance rising to approximately 12 ml/min and the urine osmolality falling to 40 to 60 mosmol/kg. The delay in reaching maximal diuresis is accounted for by the time involved in absorption of water from the gut, in metabolizing previously secreted vasopressin, and in renal recovery from the action of vasopressin.

INTERACTION OF OSMOTIC AND VOLUME INFLUENCES ON ADH RELEASE Under conditions of water deprivation and of water loading, volume and osmotic influences on ADH release act in parallel. In other circumstances, when volume and osmotic influences on ADH release may be competitive, minor changes in plasma volume can significantly modify hypertonic stimuli to ADH release. Under the relatively nonstressful conditions of daily life, osmotic factors probably predominate to maintain plasma osmolality within a very narrow range. Larger changes in blood volume, such as those induced by hemorrhage, may blunt and eventually overcome the osmotic influences. Hypotension leading to the activation of arterial baroreceptors exerts a powerful stimulus to the elaboration of ADH which may override simultaneous inhibiting influences.

EFFECTS OF GLUCOCORTICOIDS The antagonism between the hormones of the adrenal cortex and the posterior pituitary on water excretion has been recognized for years. Glucocorticoids protect against water intoxication and overcome the impaired response to water loading in adrenal insufficiency. Cortisol elevates the osmotic threshold for ADH release elicited by hypertonic saline infusion in water-loaded normal subjects.

The subnormal ability to dilute the urine manifested by patients with adrenal insufficiency may in part be due to excessive circulating ADH. However, there is also evidence that glucocorticoids can act directly on the renal tubules to decrease water permeability and to increase solute-free water in the absence of ADH.

CELLULAR MECHANISM OF ADH ACTIVITY Our present understanding of the biochemical basis for the action of ADH on the renal tubule (Fig. 110-1) is that (1) ADH binds to specific contraluminal receptor sites; (2) the receptor-hormone complex is coupled to and activates the adenylate cyclase in the same contraluminal membrane via a guanine nucleotide regulatory protein (see Chap. 86); (3) the production of cyclic AMP from ATP is increased; (4) the cyclic AMP is translocated to the luminal cell membrane where it causes the activation of membrane-bound protein kinase; (5) the activated protein kinase causes the phosphorylation of membrane proteins; and (6) permeability of the luminal membrane to water is increased. The ADH-generated cyclic AMP may be inactivated by cytosolic cyclic AMP phosphodiesterase which converts cyclic AMP to 5′-AMP. ADH stimulates prostaglandin E_2 production which, in turn, acts as a feedback inhibitor of adenylate cyclase activation.

The entire sequence of events leading to the transtubular movement of water depends on the integrity of the microtubular system of the epithelial cells. The above biochemical events lead to the passive flow of water along an osmotic gradient across the collecting tubule. The physiologic effect of vasopressin is accompanied by anatomic changes, including cell swelling, vacuolization, expansion of the medullary interstitium, and widening of the lateral intercellular spaces of the collecting ducts. The latter changes indicate that fluid resorption during ADH-induced antidiuresis occurs in part by way of lateral intercellular channels.

Various cations and drugs can influence the action of ADH. Calcium and lithium inhibit the adenylate cyclase response to vasopressin. Lithium also interferes with a subsequent biochemical action, as does potassium deficiency. Demethylchlortetracycline inhibits adenylate cyclase stimulation by ADH and also inhibits the cyclic AMP–dependent protein kinase. In contrast, chlorpropamide increases the ADH-induced activation of adenylate cyclase.

DEFICIENCY OF VASOPRESSIN: DIABETES INSIPIDUS

Diabetes insipidus is a disorder due to impaired renal conservation of water which results from low blood levels of ADH, reflecting deficient vasopressin release in response to normal physiologic stimuli.

PATHOPHYSIOLOGY Deficiency of vasopressin release in response to the appropriate stimuli may result from lesions at several functional sites in the physiologic chain of events which culminates in discharge of the hormone into the bloodstream. For conceptual purposes four types of diabetes insipidus can be defined. Patients of the first type show very little rise in urine osmolality with increasing plasma osmolality (1, Fig. 110-2) and no evidence of ADH release during hypertonic saline infusion. They are essentially devoid of releasable ADH. In patients of the second type there is an abrupt increase in urine osmolality during dehydration (2, Fig. 110-2), but there is no evidence of an osmotic threshold during saline infusion. These patients have a defective osmoreceptor mechanism, but are capable of releasing ADH in response to the hypovolemic stimulus resulting from severe dehydration. The third type of

FIGURE 110-2
Relation of plasma and urinary osmolality in normal adult subjects (shaded area) and in four types of patients with diabetes insipidus.

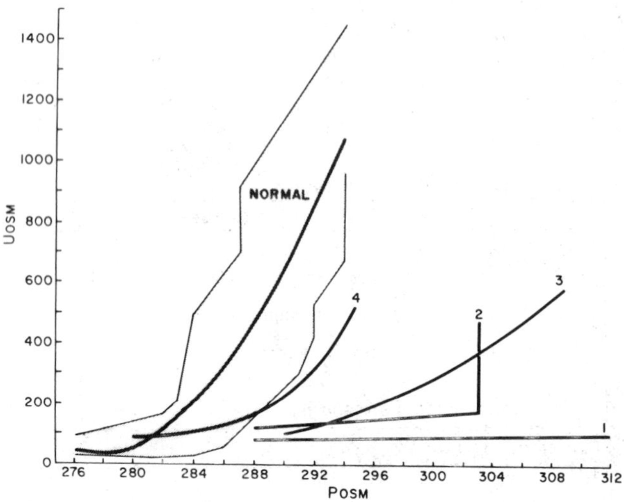

patient has some rise in urine osmolality with increasing plasma osmolality (3, Fig. 110-2) and has an elevated osmotic threshold for ADH release. These patients have a sluggish ADH release mechanism and may be said to have a high-set osmoreceptor. The fourth type of patient has urine and plasma osmolality coordinates just to the right of normal (4, Fig. 110-2) and a normal osmotic threshold. ADH release in these patients is initiated at a normal plasma osmolality but is subnormal in amount.

The second to fourth types of patients may develop a good antidiuresis in response to nausea, nicotine, acetyl-β-methylcholine (Mecholyl), chlorpropamide, or clofibrate, indicating that there is sufficient synthesis and storage of ADH to allow for adequate urinary concentrating ability in the presence of an appropriate stimulus to ADH release. In rare instances patients of the second to fourth types may have largely asymptomatic hypernatremia associated with loss of thirst and mild or absent evidence of diabetes insipidus.

ETIOLOGY The causes of diabetes insipidus in 100 consecutive patients who satisfied the criteria described under "Diagnostic Tests" (below) and who had had diabetes insipidus for at least 6 months, are shown in Table 110-1. It is evident that diabetes insipidus frequently starts in childhood or early adult life (median age of onset 21 years) and is slightly more common in males than females. The major causes are as follows: (1) *neoplastic or infiltrative lesions* of the hypothalamus or pituitary, including chromophobe adenomas, craniopharyngiomas, pinealomas, metastatic tumors, leukemia, histiocytosis X, and sarcoidosis (32 patients in groups 1, 3, 7, and 9 in Table 110-1). In approximately 60 percent of these patients evidence of partial or complete loss of adenohypophyseal function was present. (2) *Pituitary or hypothalamic surgery or isotopic ablative therapy* caused diabetes insipidus in 20 patients and this was associated with anterior hypopituitarism in almost 90 percent of the patients. Surgically induced diabetes insipidus usually appears between 1 and 6 days after the operation and often disappears after a few days and may remain absent or may recur and become chronic after an "interphase" of 1 to 5 days. Removal of the posterior lobe of the pituitary induces permanent diabetes insipidus only when the pituitary stalk is sectioned high enough to induce retrograde degeneration of most of the neurons of the supraoptic nucleus. (3) *Severe head injuries* usually associated with fractures of the skull caused diabetes insipidus in 17 patients and were associated with anterior hypopituitarism in only about 15 percent of these patients. Spontaneous remissions of traumatic diabetes insipidus occurred in a fourth, presumably because of regeneration of disrupted axons within the pituitary stalk. (4) *Vascular lesions* causing cerebral ischemia were a rare cause of diabetes insipidus (4 patients). Three of these patients were found to have diabetes insipidus associated with cerebral malacia resulting from cardiac asystole followed by resuscitation. (5) *Idiopathic diabetes insipidus* in 27 patients usually started in childhood and was seldom (<20 percent) associated with adenohypophyseal deficiencies. This diagnosis can be made only after a careful search has failed to reveal evidence of a tumor, infiltrative lesion, vascular, or other presumptive cause of the vasopressin deficiency. The presence of anterior hypopituitarism or hyperprolactinemia or radiological suspicions of lesions within or above the sella should stimulate a continuing search for a causative lesion at 3- to 12-month intervals. The diagnosis of idiopathic diabetes insipidus is made with increasing confidence as the duration of negative findings on follow-up increases. A striking decrease in the number of neurons in the supraoptic and paraventricular nuclei has been reported occasionally in idiopathic diabetes insipidus. Dominant inheritance of idiopathic diabetes insipidus has been documented.

TABLE 110-1
Characteristics of 100 consecutive patients with permanent diabetes insipidus

	Age of onset, years				
	*Median**	*Range*	*Total number*	*Males*	*Females*
1. Histiocytosis X	1.5	1–20	4	2	2
2. Idiopathic	12	Infancy–66	27	16	11
3. Primary tumor of brain or pituitary	17.5	3–58	18	15	3
4. Trauma	22	5–48	17	11	6
5. Following pituitary surgery	24	6–68	20	7	13
6. Ruptured intracranial aneurysm	39		1	1	
7. Sarcoidosis	42		1		1
8. Cerebral hypoperfusion	49	37–73	3	1	2
9. Metastatic tumors including leukemia	57	44–71	9	5	3
Totals			100	59	41

* *Median age of onset for all 100 patients = 21.*
NOTE: *Evaluated by authors at SUNY, Upstate Medical Center, Syracuse, New York (arranged in order of increasing median age of onset).*

CLINICAL MANIFESTATIONS *Polyuria, excessive thirst,* and *polydipsia* are the only clinical features that are almost invariably present in diabetes insipidus. Characteristically these symptoms are sudden in onset, both when the disorder first presents itself and whenever the effects of administered vasopressin disappear during the long-term therapy of patients with the disorder. In severe cases, the urine is pale in color, and its volume may be immense (up to 16 to 24 liters per day), requiring micturition at intervals of 30 to 60 min throughout the day and night. More frequently, however, the urine volume is only mildly to moderately excessive (2.5 to 6 liters per day), and very occasionally it may be less than 2 liters per day, causing no complaints on the part of the patient. Urinary concentration (less than 290 mosmol/kg, specific gravity less than 1.010) is well below that of the serum in severe cases but may be higher (290 to 600 mosmol/kg) in patients with mild diabetes insipidus.

The slight rise in serum osmolality resulting from hypotonic polyuria stimulates thirst. Large volumes of fluid are imbibed, and cold drinks are preferred, the patients often going to great trouble to secure refrigerated fluids. Although thirst is probably secondary to loss of water in this disorder, the administration of vasopressin often relieves or reduces thirst, even in the absence of fluid intake by the patient.

Normal function of the thirst center ensures that polydipsia closely matches polyuria, so that dehydration is seldom detectable except by the frequently observed mild elevation of serum sodium concentration. However, when adequate replenishment of water lost by excretion is interfered with, dehydration may become severe, causing weakness, fever, psychic disturbances, prostration, and even death. These clinical features are associated with a rising serum osmolality and serum sodium concentration, the latter sometimes exceeding 175 meq per liter. Adipsia is not found in idiopathic diabetes insipidus but it may result from impaired function of the hypothalamic thirst center because of extension of the same abnormality that caused the diabetes insipidus. More frequently, dehydration occurs during unconsciousness produced by surgical anesthesia, head trauma, or other causes. It is particularly hazardous to administer large volumes of isotonic saline intravenously or of hyperosmolar protein preparations by nasogastric tube unless adequate amounts of water or hypotonic fluids are administered simultaneously during unconsciousness in patients with untreated diabetes insipidus.

Hydronephrosis is a rare complication of the polyuria, especially in patients who fail to empty their bladders adequately because of uretheral strictures or for other reasons.

DIAGNOSTIC TESTS The principle that underlies diagnostic tests for diabetes insipidus is that elevation of the plasma osmolality by fluid deprivation or hypertonic saline infusion elicits subnormal ADH release. This may be documented by plasma or urinary ADH measurements or by demonstrating that urinary osmolality fails to rise to the extent which occurs when exogenous vasopressin is administered in supramaximal amounts. Measurements of plasma and urinary osmolalities are so simple and reliable that ADH measurements are seldom needed in clinical practice.

Assessment of the relation of plasma to urine osmolality The normal relationship between plasma osmolality (assuming no increase in blood urea or glucose) and urine osmolality is indicated in Fig. 110-2. If several simultaneously determined plasma and urine osmolalities in a patient with polyuria fall substantially to the right of the shaded area, the patient has diabetes insipidus or nephrogenic diabetes insipidus. The latter diagnosis can be made if plasma ADH concentration is increased or if the response to injected vasopressin is subnormal (see "Dehydration Test" below). The practice of relating plasma to urine osmolality is useful, particularly in postoperative neurosurgical cases or after head trauma, where its use can lead quickly to the differentiation of diabetes insipidus from parenteral fluid excess. In such patients, intravenous hydration can be slowed temporarily, and repeated plasma and urine osmolalities can be obtained and plotted as in Fig. 110-2, to determine whether their relationship is normal.

Dehydration test Comparison of the urinary osmolality reached after dehydration with that attained after vasopressin administration is a simple and reliable way of diagnosing diabetes insipidus and of differentiating vasopressin deficiency from other causes of polyuria.

The maximal urinary concentrating capacity varies widely between individuals (see Fig. 110-3), and no absolute lower limits of "normal" can be defined in patients with nonspecific illnesses in whom vasopressin is produced in adequate amounts. It is impossible to distinguish between deficiency and sufficiency of vasopressin release solely by the absolute level of the urinary osmolality attained after specified periods of water deprivation. On the other hand, if after prolonged dehydration vasopressin administration induces a further rise in urinary osmolality, there is a strong implication that vasopressin deficiency exists.

PROCEDURE

1 Fluids are withheld long enough to result in stable hourly urinary osmolalities (an hourly increase of <30 mosmol/kg for at least three successive hours). This is usually associated with a loss in body weight of at least 1 kg. In patients whose daily urinary volumes exceed 10 liters, the fluid deprivation should begin between 4 A.M. and 6 A.M. so that the patient can be carefully watched and the test terminated if weight loss exceeds 2 kg or the clinical condition deteriorates. In most other polyuric patients whose urinary volumes are less than 10 liters per day, it is preferable to start fluid deprivation between 6 P.M. and midnight and to continue to withhold fluids until noon the following day.

2 Urine specimens are collected hourly for osmolality measurements from 6 A.M. at least until noon and preferably until the osmolality has been stable for three consecutive hours.

3 At 11 A.M. (if dehydration started at 6 P.M.) or after the third hour of stable urinary osmolalities, the patient is given vasopressin as 5 units aqueous Pitressin by subcutaneous injection.

4 Plasma osmolality is determined immediately before the injection of vasopressin, and urinary osmolality is measured on the specimen collected during the hour after the injection.

Vital signs should be monitored during the dehydration procedure, but when the test has been performed as described, adverse effects are rare.

INTERPRETATION In subjects with normal neurohypophyseal function, urinary osmolality does not rise by more than 9 percent after the injection of Pitressin, whatever the maximal urinary osmolality might be after dehydration alone (Fig. 110-3). In diabetes insipidus of central origin, the rise in urinary osmolality after Pitressin exceeds 9 percent. To ensure adequacy of dehydration, plasma osmolality before the vasopressin injection should be above 288 mosmol/kg. Patients who have polyuria resulting from renal diseases, potassium depletion, or nephrogenic diabetes insipidus (see below) usually show little rise in urinary osmolality with dehydration and no further rise after Pitressin injection. Patients with compulsive water drinking (primary polydipsia) often require prolonged water deprivation before plasma osmolality reaches 288 mosmol/kg and before a plateau in urinary osmolality has been reached. Their urinary osmolality fails to rise by >9 percent after the administration of exogenous vasopressin.

Hypertonic saline infusions Assessment of the renal response to hypertonic saline infusion is required to determine whether ADH deficiency is or is not due entirely to a defect in osmoreceptor function. It is important to measure urinary and plasma

FIGURE 110-3

Dehydration studies in four subjects with normal ADH production, demonstrating that the maximum urinary osmolality varies from approximately 500 to 1400 mosmol/kg, and that the injection of ADH causes no further increase. [From AM Moses, M Miller, in Current Therapy 3, H Conn, R Conn (eds), Philadelphia, Saunders, 1971.]

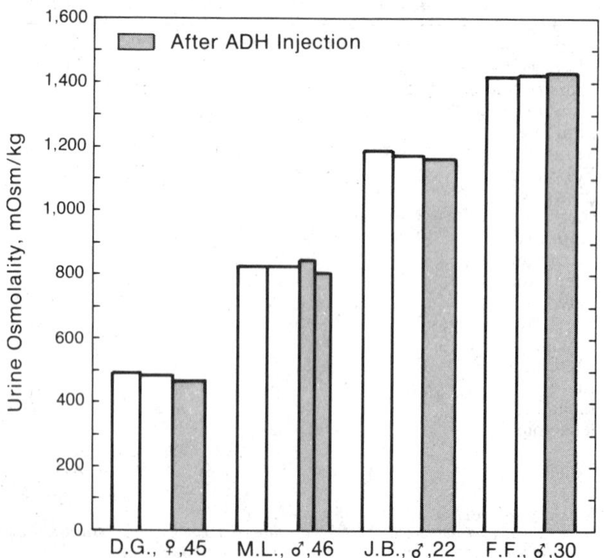

osmolality in at least one urine specimen before and immediately after the 5% saline infusion, in order to calculate changes in free water clearance so as to obtain conclusive results from this procedure (Fig. 110-4). The test is dangerous in patients who are unable to tolerate a saline load.

PROCEDURE

1 Administer a water load (20 ml/kg by mouth), and subsequently replace the urine voided every 15 min by an equal volume of water by mouth.
2 Infuse 5% sodium chloride solution intravenously into one arm, preferably by infusion pump, at approximately 0.5 ml/min—to replace solute lost in the urine—until urine flow rate has stabilized, usually at 8 to 20 ml/min, for at least four 15-min periods.
3 Increase the rate of 5% saline infusion to 0.05 (ml/kg)/min and continue the infusion until urine flow rate has shown an abrupt, sustained fall lasting for at least two 15-min periods, or until ten 15-min periods of the more rapid infusion have elapsed, or until headache, nausea, or other unpleasant symptoms have supervened, whichever comes first.
4 Draw blood through an indwelling cannula or needle in a vein in the other arm every 15 min, starting at least 15 min before the onset of the more rapid rate of infusion.
5 Measure urinary and plasma (or serum) osmolality in all specimens. Calculate free water clearances and plot the data.

INTERPRETATION Inspection of the data will show whether a sudden, clear-cut onset of a progressive fall in free water clearance can be identified. The osmotic threshold for ADH release is the plasma osmolality deduced by interpolation on the best straight line representing plasma osmolality measurements, at the onset of the fall in free water clearance (Fig. 110-4). When defined in this way in water-loaded subjects, the osmotic threshold is normally 287.3 ± 3.3 mosmol/kg (mean ± standard deviation). In most patients with diabetes insipidus there

is no detectable osmotic threshold, i.e., no fall in free water clearance even after elevating plasma osmolality well above 300 mosmol/kg (Fig. 110-4). However, some patients may have a high or normal osmotic threshold and yet have diabetes insipidus (3 and 4, Fig. 110-2).

DIFFERENTIAL DIAGNOSIS Diabetes insipidus has to be distinguished from several other types of polyuria (Table 110-2), in all of which there is loss of the renal tubular response to endogenous vasopressin. These other types of polyuria can, therefore, be recognized by failure of response to administered ADH. Among the types of polyuria listed in the table, several are easily distinguishable from spontaneous diabetes insipidus by the history [e.g., recent lithium or mannitol administration, recent surgery under methoxyflurane (Penthrane) anesthesia, or recent renal transplantation]. In others the physical examination or simple laboratory procedures will indicate the diagnosis (evidence of glycosuria, renal disease, sickle cell anemia, hypercalcemia, or potassium depletion, including such causes as primary aldosteronism).

Nephrogenic diabetes insipidus is a rare, usually inherited, form of polyuria resulting from unresponsiveness to ADH. It is usually evident from the lack of a reduction in polyuria or rise in urinary osmolality after an injection of vasopressin, as described in the "Dehydration Test" above. These patients can be distinguished from patients with vasopressin-deficient diabetes insipidus by the usual evidence of inheritance of the renal disorder (rare in diabetes insipidus) and by lack of the dramatic reduction in daily urine volume which is invariably seen when vasopressin or DDAVP is administered to patients with vasopressin-deficient diabetes insipidus. Occasionally patients with nephrogenic diabetes insipidus respond to vasopressin with a 40 to 50 percent increase in urinary osmolality, which is

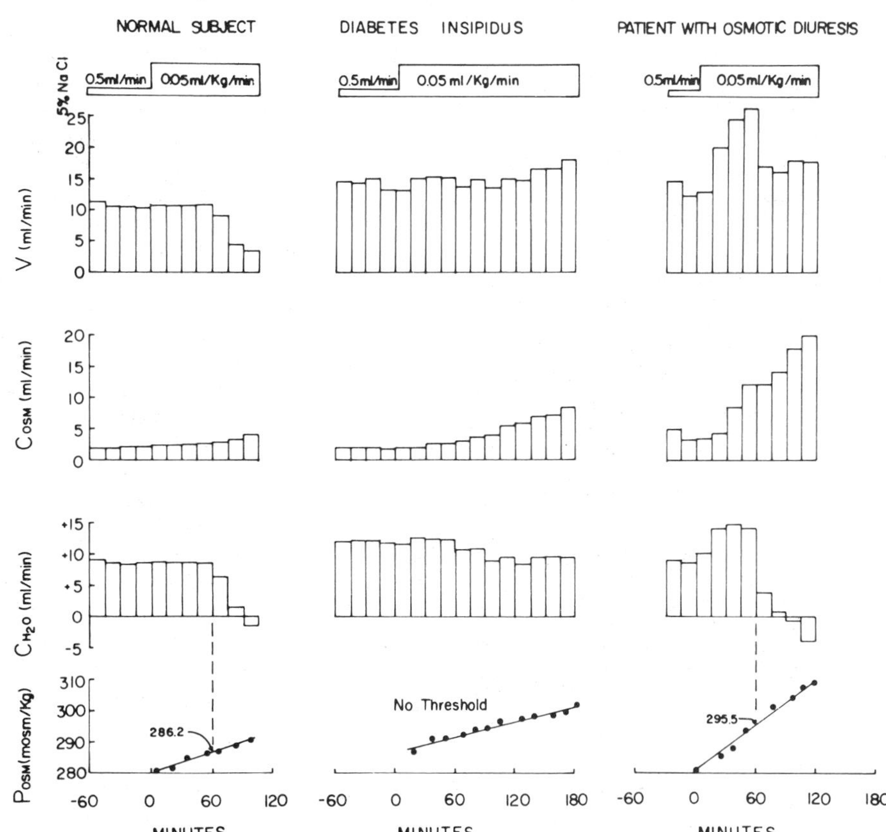

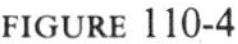
FIGURE 110-4
Diagnostic use of responses to 5% saline infusion *in subjects preloaded with water (20 ml/kg). In the* normal subject *(left) 5% NaCl, infused at 0.05 (ml/kg)/min, caused a gradual rise in osmolal clearance (Cosm) and an abrupt fall in urine flow rate (V) and free water clearance (C_{H_2O}) when the plasma osmolality (Posm) had been raised to the osmotic threshold for ADH release (286.2 mosm/kg). In the* patient with diabetes insipidus *(middle), 5% NaCl infusion failed to cause a fall in V or C_{H_2O} despite elevation of Posm above 300 mosm/kg. In the third subject (right) 5% NaCl infusion induced a rapid rise in Cosm resulting from* osmotic diuresis *which prevented a fall in V. This finding might have suggested diabetes insipidus but the fall in C_{H_2O} indicated ADH release at an osmotic threshold (295.5 mosm/kg) which was elevated because of steroid therapy. (From AM Moses, DHPS Streeten, Am J Med 42:368, 1967.)

intermediate between the responses of patients with mild and severe diabetes insipidus. In those rare instances in which nephrogenic and central diabetes insipidus cannot be differentiated with certainty by these procedures, measurement of an elevated plasma or urinary ADH concentration after water deprivation for 6 to 12 h will establish the diagnosis of nephrogenic diabetes insipidus.

Primary polydipsia One condition that is occasionally difficult to differentiate from diabetes insipidus is primary or psychogenic polydipsia. This may occur in two forms. First and more common is chronic overingestion of water resulting in hypotonic polyuria and often confused with diabetes insipidus. The second variant is intermittent ingestion of very large volumes of water, which may lead to water intoxication even though a very dilute urine is excreted.

Polydipsia and polyuria in this disorder are usually somewhat erratic in contrast to the sustained polydipsia and polyuria of diabetes insipidus. These patients usually have no nocturnal polyuria. Polyuria of long duration may result in the development of large bladder capacities and consequently infrequent urination. The patients are often emotionally disturbed. The syndrome may be seen in occasional patients with anorexia nervosa, who may drink huge quantities of water while eating very little. Fluid intake may decrease markedly when food intake increases. Rarely, a patient with chronic fluid overingestion may have a central nervous system lesion, although adipsia or hypodipsia from central nervous system lesions is more common.

The intermittent ingestion of large quantities of fluid may lead to water intoxication and dilutional hyponatremia even though there is normal urinary diluting capacity. This phenomenon is rare because normal adults can excrete between 10 and 14 ml/min of solute-free water, and it is an unusual circumstance which results in the ingestion of sufficiently more water than this to cause dilutional hyponatremia. The syndrome of water intoxication with normal diluting capacity has been reported in persons who take large enemas, drink excessive amounts of beer, or are given thioridazine (Mellaril). The phenothiazine drugs have parasympathetic effects and may cause dryness of the mouth, which aggravates tendencies toward compulsive water drinking. It is also possible that thioridazine may directly stimulate the thirst center.

The diagnosis is usually evident from the combination of low plasma and urinary osmolalities. When plasma osmolality is normal, the diagnosis can be made by a normal response to the dehydration test, or by determining plasma and urinary osmolality coordinates (see Fig. 110-2). However, the patients may be so overhydrated that it may require at least 18 h of dehydration before hourly urinary osmolalities become constant.

TABLE 110-2
Major polyuric syndromes

I Primary disorders of water intake or output
- *A* Excessive water intake
  - *1* Psychogenic polydipsia
  - *2* Hypothalamic disease: histiocytosis X, sarcoidosis
  - *3* Drug-induced polydipsia
    - *a* Thioridazine
    - *b* Chlorpromazine
    - *c* Anticholinergic drugs (dry mouth)
- *B* Inadequate tubular reabsorption of filtered water
  - *1* Vasopressin deficiency
    - *a* Central diabetes insipidus
    - *b* Drug-induced inhibition of ADH release
      - *(1)* Narcotic antagonists
  - *2* Renal tubular unresponsiveness to ADH
    - *a* Nephrogenic diabetes insipidus (congenital and familial)
    - *b* Nephrogenic diabetes insipidus (acquired)
      - *(1)* Several chronic renal diseases, after obstructive uropathy, unilateral renal arterial stenosis, after renal transplantation, after acute tubular necrosis
      - *(2)* Potassium deficiencies, including primary aldosteronism
      - *(3)* Chronic hypercalcemias, including hyperparathyroidism
      - *(4)* Drug-induced: lithium, methoxyflurane anesthesia, demethylchlortetracycline
      - *(5)* Various systemic disorders: multiple myeloma, amyloidosis, sickle cell anemia, Sjögren's syndrome

II Primary disorders of renal absorption of solutes (osmotic diuresis)
- *A* Glucose: diabetes mellitus
- *B* Salts, especially sodium chloride
  - *1* Various chronic renal diseases, especially chronic pyelonephritis
  - *2* After various diuretics, including mannitol

TREATMENT (See Table 110-3) Diabetes insipidus can be treated by hormone replacement. As is true of most peptides, oral administration of vasopressin is ineffective. Aqueous vasopressin (Pitressin) may be administered subcutaneously in doses of 5 to 10 units and usually has a duration of action of 3 to 6 h. The main use of this preparation is in initial management of unconscious patients with acute onset of diabetes insipidus following head trauma or a neurosurgical procedure. The short duration of its action allows recognition of the return of neurohypophyseal function and prevents the development of water intoxication in patients who may be receiving intravenous fluids.

Desmopressin (1-deamino-8-arginine vasopressin; DDAVP) has prolonged antidiuretic activity and is almost completely devoid of pressor effects. When used intranasally in amounts between 10 and 20 μg (0.1 to 0.2 ml), it has an antidiuretic action for 12 to 24 h in most patients. At present this analogue is the drug of choice in the treatment of most patients with diabetes insipidus. Lypressin (Diapid) is a solution of synthetic 8-lysine vasopressin used as a nasal spray. A single application may result in an antidiuresis lasting approximately 4 to 6 h. Nasal absorption of both analogues of vasopressin may be markedly decreased in the presence of an upper respiratory infection or allergic rhinitis with edema of the nasal mucosa. The use of these nasal sprays in the unconscious patient with diabetes insipidus is difficult.

In the past, patients with an established diagnosis of diabetes insipidus have usually been treated with intramuscular injections of vasopressin (Pitressin) tannate in oil (5 units per milliliter). A single injection of 2.5 or 5 units has an antidiuretic effect for 24 to 72 h. Since this material is a suspension of vasopressin tannate in peanut oil, it is essential that the ampul be warmed and then thoroughly shaken or inverted repeatedly until the brownish deposit of pituitary powder in the ampul is evenly distributed as a slightly cloudy suspension in the oil. A perfectly dry syringe should always be used. Erratic or poor response to treatment with this agent is usually due to failure to shake the ampul properly.

Patients with diabetes insipidus who have some residual releasable ADH (types 2 to 4) may respond to oral treatment with several nonhormonal agents. The sulfonylurea, chlorpropamide, has been shown both to stimulate ADH release from the neurohypophysis and to potentiate the action of submaximal amounts of ADH on the renal tubule. These properties of the drug have allowed it to be used successfully in many patients with diabetes insipidus. Doses of 200 to 500 mg, usually taken once daily, are sufficient for an antidiuretic response. Its action starts within several hours of administration and usually lasts for 24 h. Chlorpropamide may restore thirst perception and thus be useful in patients with thirst center defects. Hypoglycemia may occur but can often be avoided by adherence to a regular schedule of meals. The hypolipidemic agent, clofibrate, is capable of stimulating ADH release from the neurohypophysis and has been used in the treatment of diabetes

TABLE 110-3
Agents used in treatment of diabetes insipidus

	Dose form	Usual dose	Duration of action, h
CENTRAL DIABETES INSIPIDUS			
Hormone replacement:			
Aqueous vasopressin (Pitressin)	10 or 20 units/ampul	5–10 units subcutaneously	3–6
Desmopressin (DDAVP)	2.5-ml bottle, 0.1 mg/ml	10–20 μg intranasally	12–24
Lypressin (Diapid)	5-ml bottle, 50 units/ml	2–4 units intranasally	4–6
Vasopressin tannate in oil (Pitressin)	5 units/ampul	5 units intramuscularly	24–72
Nonhormonal agents:			
Chlorpropamide	100- and 250-mg tablets	200–500 mg daily	
Clofibrate	500-mg capsules	500 mg four times daily	
Carbamazepine	200-mg tablets	400–600 mg daily	
NEPHROGENIC DIABETES INSIPIDUS			
Hydrochlorothiazide	50-mg tablets	50–100 mg daily	
Chlorthalidone	50-mg tablets	50 mg daily	

insipidus. Doses of 500 mg four times a day often result in a prompt and sustained antidiuresis. In some patients, combined treatment with chlorpropamide and clofibrate results in complete restoration of water regulation to normal. Carbamazepine, used in the treatment of tic douloureux and diabetic neuropathy, has also been observed to produce an antidiuresis in patients with diabetes insipidus. This effect is mediated by stimulation of ADH release. Doses of 400 to 600 mg daily are effective, but the drug has not been widely used owing to toxicity involving the central nervous system, bone marrow, and liver.

All the therapeutic agents discussed thus far are effective only in central diabetes insipidus. In nephrogenic diabetes insipidus the only agents of clinical value are thiazides and other diuretics. By producing sodium depletion, the diuretics cause a fall in glomerular filtration rate with enhanced reabsorption of fluid in the proximal portion of the nephron. This results in decreased delivery of sodium to the ascending limb of the loop of Henle and consequently reduces capacity to dilute the urine. The therapeutic effect of diuretics in patients with nephrogenic diabetes insipidus is lost unless sodium intake is restricted.

PROGNOSIS The long-term prospects of a patient with diabetes insipidus are dependent primarily upon the underlying cause. In the absence of brain tumor or systemic disease, ready access to water and proper treatment of the polyuria usually lead to a normal life with a virtually normal life expectancy. Early recognition and treatment are important to prevent bladder distention, hydroureter, and hydronephrosis which may develop in patients with long-standing polyuria, particularly in patients with nephrogenic diabetes insipidus. The rare patient with adipsia or hypodipsia in association with diabetes insipidus is in danger of developing severe dehydration, which may lead to vascular collapse or central nervous system damage. Similarly severe complications may occur in patients with diabetes insipidus who develop impairment of consciousness. For this reason, all patients with diabetes insipidus should carry identification indicating the presence of the disorder and the necessity for treatment and fluid administration.

SYNDROME OF INAPPROPRIATE ADH SECRETION

The syndrome of inappropriate ADH secretion (SIADH) is a disorder characterized by hyponatremia which results from water retention attributable to ADH release. In SIADH the vasopressin is released either autonomously or in response to potent stimuli which override the inhibitory influence of hypo-osmolality. Since patients with the syndrome are unable to excrete a dilute urine, ingested fluids are retained, with consequent expansion of the extracellular fluid volume without edema. The amount of ADH released and the elevation of urinary osmolality which it produces are considered to be inappropriate only in relationship to the level of plasma osmolality or serum sodium concentration. The hallmark of SIADH is, thus, hyponatremia due to water retention, in the presence of urinary osmolality above plasma osmolality. Rarely, when solute intake is markedly restricted, urinary osmolality may be somewhat less than plasma osmolality.

Water retention can be mediated by ADH as a result of excessive ADH secretion or as a consequence of enhanced renal action of ADH. It can also result from mechanisms unrelated to ADH. A fall in renal blood flow or glomerular filtration rate can increase the percentage reabsorption of sodium and water in the proximal portion of the nephron, with consequent decrease in delivery of sodium and water to the diluting segment. This leads to impaired ability to dilute the urine and water retention.

ETIOLOGY AND PATHOPHYSIOLOGY The various causes of SIADH operate through three pathophysiological mechanisms (Table 110-4).

In the first of these, ADH is synthesized, stored, and autonomously released from tumor tissue, in amounts which are apparently determined largely by the tumor mass and not by osmolal, volume, pressure, or known chemical stimuli. Small-cell or oat-cell carcinoma of the lung accounts for 80 percent of the patients of this type. In prospective studies of patients with oat-cell carcinoma, more than 50 percent have impaired water excretion and elevated plasma ADH levels, even though many do not have evident hyponatremia. Chemical and biological analyses have shown that the ADH produced by the neoplasms is identical with arginine vasopressin produced by the normal neurohypophyseal system and may be associated with a carrier protein or neurophysin. Other malignancies which have been associated with SIADH include pancreatic and duodenal carcinomas, lymphosarcoma, reticulum cell sarcoma, Hodgkin's disease, and thymoma.

In the second pathophysiological type of SIADH, nontumorous lung tissue acquires the capacity to synthesize and release ADH autonomously during inflammatory diseases, especially resulting from tuberculous or staphylococcal infections. This process probably accounts for the hyponatremia which has long been known to be a common feature of pulmonary tuberculosis. ADH has been demonstrated in tuberculous lung tissue but not in uninvolved lung or in suspensions of tubercle bacilli.

The third type of SIADH involves release of ADH from the patient's neurohypophysis in consequence of neighboring infectious, inflammatory, neoplastic, or vascular lesions (group III, Table 110-4) or of drugs (group IV, Table 110-4), and independently of the normal stimuli.

Chlorpropamide (Diabinese) stimulates ADH release and enhances the antidiuretic action of submaximal concentrations of ADH. Many cases of chlorpropamide-induced water intoxication have been reported in patients with diabetes mellitus. The antineoplastic drugs, vincristine, vinblastine, and cyclophosphamide, produce the clinical picture of SIADH by causing release of ADH from the neurohypophysis. The tendency to water retention in these patients is aggravated by the common practice of recommending large fluid intake to prevent formation of uric acid calculi and the occurrence of chemical cystitis. Carbamazepine, used in treatment of tic douloureux, has caused water intoxication by stimulating ADH release. There are isolated instances of other drugs, particularly tricyclic compounds, producing SIADH. Clofibrate is capable of stimulating ADH release, but only rarely causes SIADH. Oxytocin possesses inherent antidiuretic activity and, when administered in large amounts to obstetrical patients, may cause water intoxication. Patients who have been exposed to general anesthetics or narcotics in association with surgical procedures may release excessive amounts of ADH. Elevated plasma ADH concentrations may be found in some conditions in which ADH release is probably an appropriate response to hypovolemia: sodium depletion (such as after diuretic therapy), adrenal insufficiency, and perhaps congestive heart failure. To consider these conditions as types of SIADH might be technically correct but is disadvantageous since it may lead to the misguided use of fluid restriction.

The excessive ADH released in this syndrome, in combination with water intake in amounts greater than can be excreted at the existing level of urinary osmolality, results in water retention and extra- and intracellular hypotonicity. Sodium excretion is enhanced because of increased glomerular filtration rate and, probably, suppression of aldosterone secretion. Excessive sodium losses aggravate the hypotonicity of body fluids.

TABLE 110-4
Causes of SIADH

I Malignancy
- *A* Oat-cell carcinoma of lung
- *B* Carcinoma of pancreas
- *C* Lymphosarcoma, reticulum cell sarcoma, Hodgkin's disease
- *D* Carcinoma of duodenum
- *E* Thymoma

II Nonmalignant pulmonary disease
- *A* Tuberculosis
- *B* Lung abscess
- *C* Pneumonia
- *D* Viral pneumonitis
- *E* Empyema
- *F* Chronic obstructive airways disease

III Central nervous system disorders
- *A* Skull fracture
- *B* Subdural hematoma
- *C* Subarachnoid hemorrhage
- *D* Cerebral vascular thrombosis
- *E* Cerebral atrophy
- *F* Acute encephalitis
- *G* Tuberculous meningitis
- *H* Purulent meningitis
- *I* Guillain-Barré syndrome
- *J* Lupus erythematosus
- *K* Acute intermittent porphyria

IV Drugs
- *A* Chlorpropamide
- *B* Vincristine
- *C* Vinblastine
- *D* Cyclophosphamide
- *E* Carbamazepine
- *F* Oxytocin
- *G* General anesthesia
- *H* Narcotics
- *I* Tricyclic antidepressants

V Miscellaneous
- *A* Hypothyroidism
- *B* Positive pressure respiration

CLINICAL AND LABORATORY FEATURES Patients with SIADH may present with weight gain, weakness, lethargy, and mental confusion, ultimately progressing to convulsions and coma. Rarely do they have evident edema or hypertension. Laboratory features include low levels of BUN and serum creatinine, uric acid, and albumin concentrations. The serum sodium concentration is generally less than 130 meq per liter, and the plasma osmolality is below 270 mosmol/kg. The urine is almost always hypertonic to plasma. Urinary sodium concentration is usually more than 20 meq per liter but may initially be less in patients who have been chronically sodium depleted due to poor intake or excessive losses.

DIAGNOSIS SIADH should be suspected in any patient with hyponatremia who excretes urine which is hypertonic relative to plasma. The finding that urinary sodium concentration is greater than 20 meq per liter provides further support for the diagnosis. To make the diagnosis of SIADH it is essential to exclude (1) depletional hyponatremias, especially due to adrenal insufficiency, salt-losing nephritis, diarrhea, and previous diuretic therapy; (2) hyponatremic edema states (congestive heart failure, cirrhosis, nephrosis); (3) pseudohyponatremia (associated with hyperlipemia); (4) severe hyperglycemia; and (5) primary polydipsia, in which the urine is invariably dilute. In contrast with patients who have SIADH, patients with depletional hyponatremia are often clearly dehydrated and usually have elevated BUN levels, hemoconcentration, and urinary sodium concentrations below 20 meq per liter (see Chap. 43). Since SIADH is associated with hypervolemia, while primary sodium depletion usually lowers plasma volume, orthostatic hypotension is not a feature of SIADH and is commonly seen in depletional hyponatremia. For the same reason, plasma renin activity and plasma aldosterone concentrations are low in SIADH and usually elevated in states of sodium depletion except in adrenal insufficiency where PRA may be high but plasma aldosterone level is usually low. When severe hypertension accompanies hyponatremia, this may be due to high plasma angiotensin II levels resulting from renovascular stenosis or other forms of angiotensinogenic hypertension, which may increase ADH release. Hypokalemia may occur but is uncommon in SIADH.

In patients with the features of SIADH in whom central nervous system disease and the use of drugs capable of causing water retention can be excluded, the possibility of malignancy must be seriously considered, especially oat-cell carcinoma of the lung. Water retention and hyponatremia may occur before evidence of malignancy can be detected on chest x-ray.

The response to water loading is a useful means of establishing the diagnosis of SIADH. Before water loading is carried out, the serum sodium must be brought to a safe level, generally above 125 meq per liter, by appropriate fluid restriction and sodium administration (if necessary), and the patient must be free of symptoms of hyponatremia. An oral water load of 20 ml per kilogram of body weight is given over a period of 15 to 20 min, and urine is collected hourly for the next 5 h while the patient is recumbent. In normal individuals given such a water load, more than 80 percent of the water is excreted by the fifth hour and the urinary osmolality falls to less than 100 mosmol/kg (specific gravity 1.005). Patients with hyponatremia who excrete the water load normally may be considered to have a low-set osmoreceptor, such as occurs in chronic ill health. In contrast, patients with SIADH have impaired excretion of the water load (often excreting less than 40 percent in 5 h) and fail to dilute the urine to hypotonic levels. When a water load has been given to a patient with SIADH, no further water intake should be permitted over the next 24 h or until the serum sodium concentration has returned to the pretest value. In this way, production of symptomatic water intoxication can be prevented. Adrenal insufficiency cannot be distinguished from SIADH by the water load test.

Measurements of ADH in patients with SIADH have revealed persistence of inappropriately elevated levels of ADH in plasma and urine when hypoosmolality should normally have inhibited ADH release. In response to further reduction of plasma osmolality after a water load, ADH has remained detectable in plasma and urine, confirming that indeed the ADH secretion is inappropriate relative to plasma osmolality.

It should be emphasized that SIADH cannot be diagnosed with confidence in the presence of severe "stress," pain, hypovolemia, hypotension, and other stimuli which may evoke physiologic release of ADH, even in the presence of hypotonicity.

TREATMENT Patients with mild or moderate symptoms of water intoxication should be treated by restricting fluid intake to about 800 to 1000 ml daily. If water restriction is adequate, a steady increase in serum sodium concentration or osmolality occurs as body weight decreases. Occasional patients with severe water intoxication associated with mental confusion, convulsions, or coma must be treated more vigorously. Intravenous administration of 200 to 300 ml of 5% saline solution over several hours is usually sufficient to raise the serum sodium to a level at which the symptoms will improve. When there is the possibility of congestive heart failure due to the fluid overload, the simultaneous administration of large doses of furosemide usually causes a diuresis sufficient to reduce cardiac overload. When furosemide is given, careful attention must be paid to correction of potassium and other electrolyte losses induced by the drug. If, for any reason, intravenous fluid administration is considered necessary when the serum sodium has been raised to an appropriate level, isotonic saline and not 5% dextrose solution should be infused slowly to maintain normality of the serum sodium concentration.

Once the initial hyponatremia is improved, careful adherence to a regimen of fluid restriction is necessary to prevent recurrence of water intoxication. Treatment should be directed at the underlying problem. The withdrawal of drugs which might have been causing water retention usually results in prompt clearing of SIADH. The SIADH occurring with central nervous system disorders is usually transient and clears with improvement of the underlying disease. Treatment of pulmonary tuberculosis with appropriate antituberculous therapy results in gradual disappearance of SIADH. Similarly, antibiotic treatment of lung abscess or pneumonia results in resolution of SIADH.

In patients with SIADH due to malignancy, surgical resection, irradiation, or chemotherapy may be successful in alleviating water retention. Sometimes, these measures should be carried out even when there is little likelihood of curing the malignancy, since such treatment may correct life-threatening water intoxication and prevent the necessity for rigid fluid restriction. In patients in whom treatment is judged to have been curative, the disappearance of SIADH may confirm the success of treatment. Periodic water load tests may be valuable in following such patients for evidence of recurrence of malignancy.

At present, no drugs are available which are clinically useful in suppressing ADH release from the neurohypophyseal system or from a tumor. Diphenylhydantoin inhibits ADH release but is clinically ineffective. Several narcotic antagonists, such as naloxone and butorphanol, are capable of inhibiting ADH release from the neurohypophysis. Their role in the treatment of SIADH remains to be determined. Drugs capable of blocking ADH effect on the renal tubule may be of value in the chronic management of patients with hyponatremia. Lithium salts can interfere with the antidiuretic action of ADH on the kidney but are too toxic for use in SIADH. Demethylchlortetracycline is effective in interfering with the renal action of ADH. Administration of the drug in doses of 900 to 1200 mg per day to patients with SIADH due to lung malignancy has resulted in diuresis with excretion of an isotonic or hypotonic urine and improvement in hyponatremia. The only untoward effect has been azotemia without other evidence of renal toxicity, which has disappeared promptly on discontinuation of the drug. Thus, demethylchlortetracycline may be a useful agent in the management of SIADH in the ambulatory patient in whom fluid restriction is difficult to accomplish.

PROGNOSIS The prognosis of a patient with SIADH depends on the underlying cause of the syndrome. Transient or reversible SIADH as in central nervous system disorders or following use of water-retaining drugs is usually benign as long as proper treatment of acute water intoxication is effectively carried out. SIADH in association with malignancy has ominous implications, since the malignancies most commonly associated are oat-cell carcinoma of the lung and adenocarcinoma of the pancreas, both usually associated with rapid spread and early death. In patients in whom SIADH is not correctable by surgery, irradiation, or chemotherapy, long-term fluid restriction is necessary to prevent symptomatic water intoxication.

PARAVENTRICULAR-NEUROHYPOPHYSEAL SYSTEM AND OXYTOCIN

CHEMISTRY AND PHYSIOLOGY Oxytocin is a nonapeptide which differs by two amino acids from vasopressin. Oxytocin is produced predominantly in the cell bodies of the paraventricular nuclei, and to a lesser extent in those of the supraoptic nuclei. It is synthesized and transported in neurosecretory granules by way of nerve tracts to the neurohypophysis, where it is stored or released, in conjunction with an oxytocin-specific neurophysin. Oxytocin release results from nerve impulses originating in the hypothalamus, which cause depolarization of the neurosecretory terminals of the posterior pituitary, and subsequent release of oxytocin through a calcium-dependent process, similar to the mechanism for vasopressin. The secretion of oxytocin, as well as of vasopressin, is inhibited by ethanol. Some stimuli such as pain apparently release oxytocin and vasopressin simultaneously, but most stimuli release the two hormones independently. Oxytocin is primarily liberated during suckling, whereas after an osmotic stimulus or hemorrhage, vasopressin is released in much greater quantities than is oxytocin. Manipulation or distention of the female genital tract, artificially or during parturition, appears to be a more effective stimulus to oxytocin release than is suckling.

Oxytocin acts on the excitable membranes surrounding the myometrial and myoepithelial cells and results in an increased force of contraction. Sensitivity of the myometrium to oxytocin increases with the duration of pregnancy, but it is not known if oxytocin per se is responsible for the initiation and maintenance of labor. Oxytocin may have survival value to the offspring since it may hasten the final stages of birth and lessen the chances of anoxia. Oxytocin continues to exert a contractile action on the myometrium post partum. Circulating oxytocin contracts the myoepithelial cells of the mammary alveoli, causing them to expel milk from the secretory tissue to the nipple. Oxytocin is 100 times more potent than vasopressin in its milk-ejecting activity in the human. In contrast, the antidiuretic potency of oxytocin relative to vasopressin is about 1:200.

It is unlikely that oxytocin exerts any significant physiologic effect other than on the uterus and breast.

One milligram of purified preparation of oxytocin contains 450 IU of hormone, and the amount of oxytocin in the posterior pituitary ranges from 10 to 15 units per lobe. In spite of the fact that there is no known role of oxytocin in the male, the male neural lobe stores oxytocin in amounts similar to those in the female. Plasma oxytocin concentration in both men and women exhibits episodic increases, with values ranging from a low of approximately 0.5 to a high of 2.0 μU/ml. There is no evidence of a diurnal secretion pattern. In normal women there is a midcycle increase in plasma oxytocin concentration from a preovulatory value of approximately 1.0 μU/ml to a peak value of 2 to 4 μU/ml at the time of ovulation. During labor, plasma oxytocin concentrations may reach several hundred microunits per milliliter, with a rapid fall to prepartum levels after delivery. During suckling, plasma oxytocin levels of the mother vary widely but are usually about 5 to 10 μU/ml. The half-life of oxytocin in plasma is about 3 to 5 min. Removal of oxytocin from the circulation is mainly by the kidneys and liver, although the uterus and mammary gland may remove some.

CLINICAL USE OF OXYTOCIN The clinical use of oxytocin is limited to the induction of labor, control of hemorrhage following incomplete abortion and curettage, and treatment of impaired milk ejection. For a detailed discussion of the obstetrical uses of oxytocin, the reader is referred to textbooks on obstetrics. Care must be taken in the use of oxytocin because it may cause uterine rupture and fetal death. The antidiuretic action of oxytocin can be elicited with single intravenous doses of as little as 100 mU. Maximal antidiuresis is reached with 40 to 50 mU/min. Since 10 to 40 units of oxytocin per liter of dextrose is often used in obstetrical practice, it is apparent that water intoxication may result. The vasodilatory action of oxytocin may cause sudden death of obstetrical patients with heart disease because of hypotension, tachycardia, and arrhythmias. Anesthetics may modify the cardiovascular responses to oxytocin. For instance, in patients under cyclopropane anesthesia, oxytocin produces more hypotension but less tachycardia than in unanesthetized subjects. The vasodilatory effect of oxytocin can be blocked by vasopressin.

REFERENCES

BARTTER FC, SCHWARTZ WB: The syndrome of inappropriate secretion of antidiuretic hormone. Am J Med 42:790, 1967

KNOBIL E, SAWYER WH (eds): The pituitary gland—its neuroendocrine control, part I, in *Handbook of Physiology*, sec 7: *Endocrinology*, vol IV. Washington, American Physiological Society, 1974

MILLER M et al: Recognition of partial defects in antidiuretic hormone secretion. Ann Intern Med 73:721, 1970

MOSES AM et al: Pathophysiologic and pharmacologic alterations in the release and action of ADH. Metabolism 25:697, 1976

ROBERTSON GL: The regulation of vasopressin function in health and disease. Rec Progr Hormone Res 33:333, 1977

111 DISEASES OF THE THYROID

SIDNEY H. INGBAR
KENNETH A. WOEBER

The normal function of the thyroid gland is to secrete L-thyroxine (T_4) and 3,5,3′-triiodo-L-thyronine (T_3), iodinated amino acids that are the active thyroid hormones and that influence a diversity of metabolic processes (Fig. 111-1). Diseases of the thyroid gland are manifested by qualitative or quantitative alterations in hormone secretion, enlargement of the thyroid (goiter), or both. Insufficient hormone secretion results in the syndrome of *hypothyroidism* or *myxedema*, in which decreased oxygen consumption (hypometabolism) is a classic manifestation. Conversely, excessive secretion of active hormone results in hypermetabolism and other features of a syndrome termed *hyperthyroidism* or *thyrotoxicosis*. Enlargement of the thyroid gland (normally 15 to 25 g in adults) may be generalized or focal. Generalized enlargements may not be absolutely symmetric, however, the right lobe tending to enlarge more than the left. They are associated with increased, normal, or decreased hormone secretion, depending upon the underlying disturbance. Truly focal enlargement usually reflects neoplastic transformation, either benign or malignant, the former sometimes being responsible for hypersecretion of hormone and hyperthyroidism, the latter very rarely so. Either type of goiter may result in compression of adjacent structures in the neck or mediastinum.

EMBRYOLOGY, ANATOMY, AND HISTOLOGY

The human thyroid originates embryologically from an evagination of the pharyngeal epithelium with some cellular contributions from the lateral pharyngeal pouches. Progressive descent of the midline thyroid anlage gives rise to the thyroglossal duct, which extends from the foramen cecum near the base of the tongue to the isthmus of the thyroid. Remnants of tissue may persist along the course of this tract as "lingual thyroid," as thyroglossal cysts or nodules, or as a structure

FIGURE 111-1
Structural formulas of thyroxine, its precursors, and certain of its metabolites.

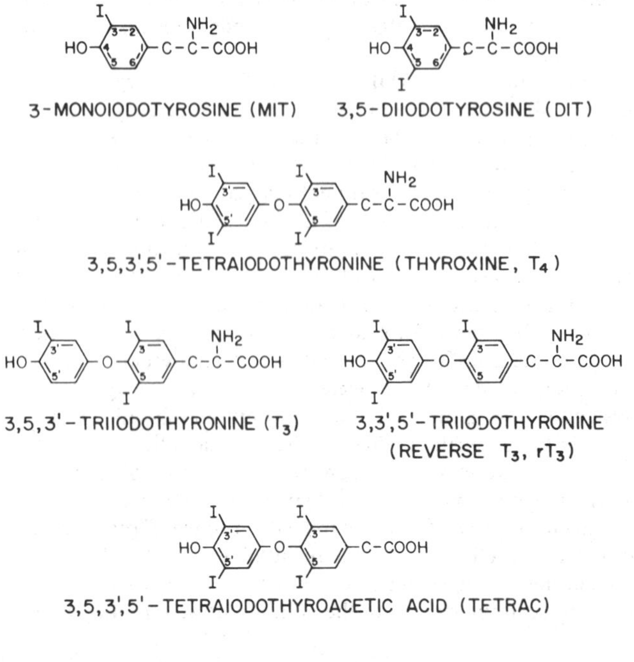

3-MONOIODOTYROSINE (MIT)

3,5-DIIODOTYROSINE (DIT)

3,5,3′,5′-TETRAIODOTHYRONINE (THYROXINE, T_4)

3,5,3′-TRIIODOTHYRONINE (T_3)

3,3′,5′-TRIIODOTHYRONINE (REVERSE T_3, rT_3)

3,5,3′,5′-TETRAIODOTHYROACETIC ACID (TETRAC)

contiguous with the thyroid isthmus called the *pyramidal lobe.* The latter is usually not discernible, except when the remainder of the gland is goitrous. In some individuals, lingual thyroid may be the sole functioning thyroid tissue. In such cases, its secretion may or may not be sufficient to maintain a normal metabolic (euthyroid) state. Thyroid aplasia and functional failure of ectopic thyroid tissue are causes of sporadic neonatal hypothyroidism, an important disorder because of its frequency (1 in every 4000 or 5000 newborns) and response to early treatment.

Knowledge of the ontogenetic sequence in human thyroid development is limited by the availability of specimens for analysis. It is clear, however, that the fetal thyroid acquires the capacity to collect and organify iodine at about 10 weeks gestation. Both T_4 and thyroid-stimulating hormone (thyrotropin, TSH) are detectable in the blood soon thereafter and increase progressively in concentration during the second trimester. The increase in serum T_4 is due both to increasing thyroid secretion and to the appearance in plasma of thyroxine-binding globulin (TBG), whereas the increase in TSH is a reflection of the maturation of the fetal hypothalamus with resulting secretion of thyrotropin-releasing hormone (TRH). Maternal TRH readily crosses the placenta and therefore could play a role in the development of the fetal pituitary-thyroid axis. Maternal TSH, by contrast, does not cross the placenta. T_3 becomes detectable in the blood later during the second trimester, but its concentration in blood and amniotic fluid remains very low until shortly after parturition. By contrast, the concentration of its isomer, 3,3′,5′-triiodo-L-thyronine (reverse T_3, rT_3), in fetal blood and amniotic fluid is increased relative to that in maternal blood (Fig. 111-1). These differences are due to qualitative alterations in T_4 metabolism in the fetus that are discussed more fully later. In any event, the very low T_3 concentration in fetal blood and amniotic fluid in the face of a high maternal concentration indicates that maternal-fetal transfer of T_3 is minimal and that the maintenance of a eumetabolic state in the fetus is accomplished through secretion of T_4 by the fetal thyroid. Except for the possible effect of maternal TRH, therefore, the fetal pituitary-thyroid axis is a functional unit distinct from that of the mother.

The normal adult thyroid is a vascular organ, comprising two lobes joined by an isthmus and lying just anterior and slightly caudad to the cartilages of the larynx. Fibrous septa divide the gland into pseudolobules which, in turn, are comprised of vesicles, called *follicles* or *acini,* surrounded by a capillary network. Normally, the follicle walls are composed of cuboidal epithelium. Their lumen is filled with a proteinaceous material termed *colloid,* which contains a protein peculiar to the thyroid, *thyroglobulin,* within the peptide sequence of which T_4 and T_3 are synthesized and stored. In addition to follicular cells, the thyroid contains another population of cells, the C cells. They are the source of calcitonin and give rise to medullary thyroid carcinoma when they undergo malignant transformation.

HORMONE SYNTHESIS, SECRETION, AND METABOLISM

SYNTHESIS AND SECRETION Thyroid hormone synthesis that is both qualitatively and quantitatively normal depends on entry into the thyroid of adequate quantities of iodine, a constituent of the active hormones, T_4 and T_3; normality of pathways for iodine metabolism within the gland; and concurrent synthesis of a normal receptor protein for iodine, thyroglobulin. Secretion of normal quantities of hormone, in turn, requires both a normal rate of hormone synthesis and the integrity of processes within the gland by which thyroglobulin is hydrolyzed and the hormonally active iodoaminoacids thereby liberated. Iodine enters the thyroid from the bloodstream in the form of inorganic or ionic iodide whose source is twofold: iodide derived either from the deiodination of thyroid hormones or from iodinated agents that the patient may have been given and iodide ingested in food, water, or medication. Formerly, a dietary iodine intake of approximately 200 μg was considered normal within the continental United States, and this was sufficient to sustain a plasma iodide concentration of approximately 0.5 μg/dl. However, owing largely to enrichment of bread with iodine, and to the widespread use of iodine in drugs, vitamin preparations, and antiseptic agents, the average iodine intake has increased substantially, to values as high as 1000 μg daily, with corresponding increases in plasma iodide concentration. Iodide is removed from the plasma by the thyroid, kidneys, and salivary and gastrointestinal glands, but since iodide that enters gastrointestinal secretions is reabsorbed, net clearance is effected only by the thyroid and kidneys. In effect, the thyroid and kidneys compete for plasma iodide. However, since renal clearance is largely a function of glomerular filtration rate and is not influenced by humoral factors or plasma iodide concentration, the kidney is normally a passive participant in this competition. Hence, adjustments in the rate of entry of iodide into the thyroid relative to the rate of urinary excretion are mediated by changes in thyroid, rather than renal, avidity.

The reactions involved in the synthesis and secretion of the active thyroid hormones can be divided into four sequential steps (Fig. 111-2). The first involves active inward transport of iodide from the plasma into the thyroid cell and follicular lumen. This occurs at a rate that exceeds passive diffusion of iodide from the gland, with the result that the thyroid is capable of maintaining concentration gradients for iodide (thyroid/plasma concentration ratios) of substantial magnitude (up to 500, or more, under certain physiologic or pathologic conditions). Energy for iodide transport is phosphate bond–derived and therefore depends upon oxidative metabolism within the gland. The second step in hormone biosynthesis involves oxidation of iodide to a higher valence form, as yet undetermined, that is capable of iodinating tyrosyl residues in thyroglobulin, a glycoprotein of approximately 650,000 mol wt that is synthesized within the follicular cell. Oxidation of iodide is effected by an iodide peroxidase, which utilizes hydrogen peroxide generated during the course of oxidative metabolism within the gland. Organic iodinations, which occur at the cell-colloid interface, result in the formation of the peptide-bound, hormonally inactive precursors, monoiodotyrosine (MIT), and diiodotyrosine (DIT). Subsequently, these iodotyrosines undergo oxidative condensation, again through the mediation of peroxidase. This so-called coupling reaction occurs within the thyroglobulin molecule and yields a variety of iodothyronines, including T_4 and T_3. Although minute quantities of thyroglobulin are detectable in the blood of normal patients and those with thyroid disease, the vast bulk of thyroglobulin is retained for a time within the gland, serving as a storage form of thyroid hormone, or "prohormone." Liberation of the active hormones into the blood, the third step in hormone synthesis and release, involves pinocytosis of follicular colloid at the apical margin of the cells to form colloid droplets. Functioning microtubules are necessary for this process. The colloid droplets fuse with thyroid lysosomes to form "phagolysosomes," in which thyroglobulin is hydrolyzed by proteases and peptidases. The final step is release of the free iodothyronines, T_4 and T_3, into the blood. The thyroid gland is the only source of endogenous T_4; in contrast, in the normal individual, thyroid secretion accounts for only about 20 percent of the T_3 produced, the remaining 80 percent being generated in peripheral tissues by the enzymatic removal of the 5′-iodine from the outer ring of T_4. Inactive iodotyrosines liberated by the hydrolysis of thyroglobulin are stripped of their iodine by an intrathyroidal enzyme, iodotyrosine dehalogenase. Normally, iodide liberated thereby is largely reutilized in the synthesis of hormone, but a small proportion is lost into the blood (iodide leak); this proportion may become large in abnormal circumstances.

As with iodide, the thyroid is capable of concentrating other monovalent anions. Notable among these is the pertechnetate ion, which is available as the radioactive isotope, sodium [^{99m}Tc]pertechnetate. Unlike iodide, little pertechnetate is organically bound; hence, its duration of stay within the thyroid is short. This property, together with its short physical half-life, makes pertechnetate a valuable radionuclide for imaging the thyroid with scintillation scanning techniques.

The foregoing reactions are subject to inhibition by a variety of chemical compounds. Such agents are generally termed *goitrogens,* since, by virtue of their ability to inhibit hormone synthesis and indirectly stimulate TSH secretion, they induce goiter formation. Certain inorganic anions, notably perchlorate and thiocyanate, inhibit the iodide transport mechanism and thereby reduce available substrate for hormone formation. The goiter and hypothyroidism that follow, however, can be prevented or relieved, by doses of iodide sufficiently large to enable adequate quantities to enter the gland by simple diffusion. The commonly employed antithyroid agents, such as the derivatives of thiourea and mercaptoimidazole, exert more complex actions upon pathways of hormone biosynthesis. These agents, as well as certain aniline derivatives, inhibit the initial oxidation (organic binding) of iodide, decrease the proportion of DIT relative to MIT, and block coupling of iodotyrosines to form the hormonally active iodothyronines. The latter reaction is the most sensitive. Thus, it is possible for the synthesis of hormonally active iodothyronines to be decreased greatly, although the total incorporation of iodine by the thyroid is inhibited but little. In contradistinction to the effect of the monovalent anions, the goitrogenic action of inhibitors of organic binding is not overcome by large quantities of iodine. Indeed, certain weak goitrogens, such as sulfonamides and antipyrine, are rendered more potent when given with iodide, an effect not clearly understood. Iodine itself, when given acutely in large doses, is capable of blocking the organic-binding and coupling reactions. This action (Wolff-Chaikoff effect) is normally transient. In a small proportion of seemingly normal individuals, however, prolonged administration of iodide is associated with continued inhibition of hormone synthesis and development of goiter, with (iodide myxedema) or without hypothyroidism. A large proportion of patients with Graves' disease, especially after treatment with radioiodine or surgery, and also patients with Hashimoto's disease are inordinately sensitive to the blocking effect of iodide and, when given iodides chronically, develop hypothyroidism. The fetal thyroid is similarly sensitive, and consequently pregnant women should not be given iodide in large doses because of the danger of inducing goitrous hypothyroidism in the fetus. Iodide in large doses is capable of inhibiting proteolysis of thyroglobulin and hormone release, an effect which is most readily demonstrable in hyperfunctioning thyroids and which is responsible for the rapid ameliorative action of iodides in most patients with hyperthyroidism. Lithium, which is administered as the carbonate salt in some patients with depressive states, has a variety of effects on intrathyroidal iodine metabolism. Among these is an action to inhibit hormone release. Finally, dexamethasone in large doses is also capable of inhibiting hormone release and thus, in conjunction with iodide, can be employed to effect a rapid reduction in the degree of thyrotoxicosis in patients with this syndrome.

FIGURE 111-2
Schema depicting pathways in the synthesis and secretion of thyroid hormones and mechanisms for the suprathyroidal and intrathyroidal regulation of thyroid function. Small, solid arrows indicate pathways of iodine metabolism; open arrows indicate stimulation; crosshatched arrows indicate inhibitory influences. TRH, thyrotropin-releasing hormone; TSH, thyroid-stimulating hormone; IPO, iodide peroxidase; prot., thyroid protease; peptid., thyroid peptidase; MIT, monoiodotyrosine; DIT, diiodotyrosine; T_4, thyroxine; T_3, 3,5,3′-triiodothyronine.

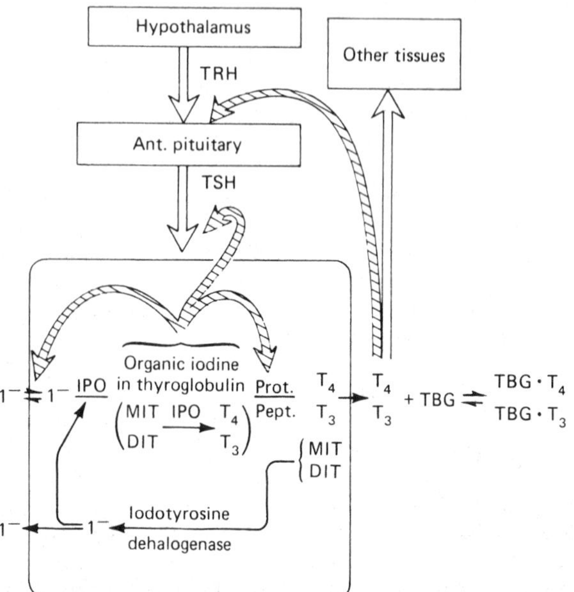

TRANSPORT AND METABOLISM In the blood, T_4 and T_3 are almost entirely bound to plasma proteins. Electrophoretic analyses indicate that T_4 is bound, in decreasing order of intensity, to an inter-alpha globulin, termed thyroxine- or thyronine-binding globulin (TBG), to a T_4-binding prealbumin (TBPA), and to albumin. By virtue of its intense affinity for T_4, TBG is the major determinant of overall binding intensity. The interaction between T_4 and its binding proteins conforms to a reversible binding equilibrium in which the majority of the hormone is bound and a small proportion (normally about 0.03 percent) is free. T_3 is not significantly bound by TBPA and is bound less firmly than T_4 by TBG. As a consequence, the normal proportion of free T_3 (approximately 0.3 percent) is 8 to 10 times greater than that of T_4. It appears likely that only the free or unbound hormone is available to tissues; therefore, the metabolic state of the patient correlates more closely with the concentration of free than with the total concentration of hormone in plasma, and homeostatic regulation of thyroid function is directed toward maintenance of a normal concentration of free rather than total hormone. Moreover, the relatively weak binding of T_3 accounts for its failure to contribute materially to the total hormonal iodine concentration in the blood and possibly for its more rapid onset and offset of action. Disturbances of the thyroid hormone–plasma protein interaction are of two general types (see Table 111-1). In the first, the thyroid-pituitary axis is intrinsically normal, and the homeostatic control of thyroid hormone secretion is intact. Under these circumstances, disordered binding interactions result from primary alterations in the concentration of TBG. For example, an increase in TBG initially lowers the concentration of free hormone and thus diminishes the quantity of hormone available to tissues. Total hormone concentration in serum then increases until the concentration of free hormone is restored to normal. At this time, the proportions of T_4 and T_3

TABLE 111-1
Classification of the varieties of disordered thyroid hormone–plasma protein interactions

Type of abnormality	*Serum T_4 and T_3*	*Percent FT_4 and FT_3 or RT_3U*	*FT_4 and FT_3 or FT_4I and FT_3I*
I Primary abnormality in thyroxine-binding proteins			
A Increased concentration	↑	↓	N
B Decreased concentration	↓	↑	N
II Primary disorder of thyroid function			
A Hypothyroidism	↓	↓	↓
B Hyperthyroidism	↑	↑	↑

NOTE: FT_4 = free T_4; FT_3 = free T_3; FT_4I = free T_4 index; FT_3I = free T_3 index; RT_3U = resin-T_3 uptake.

that are free will be decreased. The increase in total hormone concentration counterbalances the decrease in the free proportion; as a result, the absolute concentration of free hormone is normal, and the metabolic state of the patient is unchanged. Converse changes occur when the concentration of TBG declines. Table 111-2 summarizes those states associated with primary alterations in the concentration of TBG.

The second type of disturbance of thyroid hormone–binding interactions results from a primary alteration in the concentration of thyroid hormones in the blood, such as occurs in hypothyroidism or thyrotoxicosis. Here, normal homeostatic control of thyroid hormone secretion is lost, either because of disease within the control mechanism itself or because the appropriate response of a normal control mechanism is incapable of overcoming the effects of disease elsewhere. Under these circumstances, the concentration of TBG is changed little, if at all, and the concentration of free hormone varies directly with the total concentration of hormone. Since homeostatic mechanisms cannot restore the concentration of free hormone to normal, primary changes in thyroid function are associated with persistent changes in the concentration of both total and free hormone, and, consequently, with alterations in the metabolic state of the patient. In these disorders, the relative change in the concentration of free hormone is greater than the change in total hormone concentration so that the proportion of free hormone changes in a direction similar to that of the change in hormone supply.

Following their penetration into the cell, T_4 and T_3 undergo a variety of reactions which lead ultimately to their excretion or inactivation. As judged from experiments with isotopically labeled hormones, thyroid hormones undergo metabolism mainly through the sequential removal of single iodine atoms (monodeiodinations) that ultimately yields the thyronine nucleus stripped of its iodine content. Deiodinative pathways are present in all tissues tested and account for approximately 70 percent of labeled T_4 and T_3 disposal. Substantial quantities of T_4, T_3, and their metabolites are excreted in the bile, principally as conjugates with glucuronate and sulfate, and are presumably available for reabsorption, probably after hydrolysis of the conjugates. However, the magnitude of the enterohepatic circulation of T_4 and T_3 in humans is unknown. Reabsorption is incomplete at best, since fecal excretion of T_4, T_3, and their iodine-containing metabolites accounts for approximately 20 percent of hormone disposal. A small proportion of the hormones (approximately 10 percent) undergoes oxidative deamination and decarboxylation of the alanine side chain to yield the acetic acid analogues of T_4 and T_3, tetra- and triiodothyroacetic acids. The most important initial product of T_4 metabolism is T_3 itself. Since T_3 appears to be approximately three times more potent than T_4 in most respects, this process yields a product of enhanced potency. Approximately 30 percent of T_4 is initially monodeiodinated in the 5′ position of its outer ring to yield T_3. This source normally accounts for about 80 percent of the T_3 produced, the remainder being derived through direct thyroid secretion. A major clinical implication is that athyreotic or hypothyroid patients maintained with synthetic levothyroxine so that serum T_4 concentration is normal have, in addition, nearly normal concentrations of T_3 in their blood. However, direct thyroid secretion accounts for a greater proportion of overall T_3 production in hyperthyroidism; in early thyroid failure, in which the gland is under intense stimulation by TSH; and in iodine deficiency. The remaining approximately 40 percent of T_4 disposal is accounted for by monodeiodination of T_4 at the 5 position of its inner ring to yield 3,3′,5′-triiodo-L-thyronine (reverse T_3, rT_3); this process accounts for almost all of the rT_3 produced. Unlike T_3, rT_3 has little if any metabolic potency; therefore, the relative poise between outer- and inner-ring monodeiodination of T_4 could represent a regulatory mechanism for modulating the quantity of metabolically active hormone at the tissue level. Impairment of the peripheral conversion of T_4 to T_3 is responsible for the decreased serum total and free T_3 concentrations that occur in various physiologic and pathologic states (Table 111-3). In these states of low serum T_3 concentration ("low T_3 syndrome") serum total and free T_4 concentrations are usually normal or marginally increased, but in the most severely ill patients serum total T_4 concentrations may be well below normal in the absence of intrinsic thyroid disease. In almost all patients with the low T_3 syndrome, serum rT_3 concentration is distinctly increased. This increase cannot be accounted for by an increase in the production of rT_3 from T_4. Rather, it appears to be due, at least largely, to a decrease in the 5′-deiodination of rT_3 to yield 3,3′-diiodothyronine (3,3′-T_2). In these states, therefore, both the decreased conversion of T_4 to T_3 and the decreased degradation of rT_3 can be ascribed to a selective impairment of 5′-monodeiodinations. This impairment has been variously attributed to enzyme inhibition, cofactor deficiency, or decreased enzyme concentration. It is not known whether the tissues of patients with the low T_3 syndrome are subject to a decreased supply of active thyroid hormone. Since

TABLE 111-2
Circumstances associated with altered concentration of TBG

Increased TBG	*Decreased TBG*
Pregnancy	Androgenic and anabolic steroids
Newborn state	Large doses of glucocorticoid
Oral contraceptives and other sources of estrogen	Chronic liver disease
Acute intermittent porphyria	Severe systemic illness
Chronic liver disease	Active acromegaly
Acute hepatitis	Nephrosis
Genetically determined	Genetically determined

TABLE 111-3
States associated with decreased peripheral conversion of T_4 to T_3

I Physiologic
- *A* Fetal and early neonatal life
- *B* ? Old age

II Pathologic
- *A* Fasting
- *B* Malnutrition
- *C* Systemic illness
- *D* Physical trauma
- *E* Postoperative state
- *F* Drugs (propylthiouracil, dexamethasone, propranolol, Amiodarone)
- *G* Radiographic contrast agents (Oragrafin, Telepaque)

neither basal values for serum TSH nor the responsiveness of TSH to TRH are increased, it must be that there is a downward resetting of the threshold for feedback inhibition of TSH secretion or that conversion of T_4 to T_3 within the pituitary continues at a normal rate despite the impaired conversion in the peripheral tissues. Thus, the absence of increased TSH secretion need not necessarily exclude an insufficiency of thyroid hormone in the other peripheral tissues. Such a peripheral hypothyroid state could provide a means for conserving critical energy resources as an adaptation to severe illness.

Under certain circumstances, changes in the activity of cellular processes involved in hormone accumulation and metabolism may be the major determinant of changes in the rates of metabolic clearance of T_4 and T_3. Both phenobarbital and diphenylhydantoin increase the metabolic clearance of thyroid hormones without increasing the proportion of free hormone in the blood. Indeed, in the case of diphenylhydantoin, both total and free T_4 concentrations are diminished. Nevertheless, a normal metabolic state is maintained. The effects of these agents are doubtless related to the hypertrophy of smooth endoplasmic reticulum and increased activity of various microsomal enzymes that they induce.

REGULATION OF THYROID FUNCTION Regulation of thyroid function is effected by two general mechanisms, one suprathyroid and one intrathyroid in locus (Fig. 111-2). The proximate mediator of suprathyroid regulation is thyrotropin or thyroid-stimulating hormone (TSH), a glycoprotein secreted by basophilic cells in the anterior pituitary. TSH stimulates thyroid hypertrophy and hyperplasia; accelerates most aspects of glandular intermediary metabolism; enhances synthesis of nucleic acid and protein, including thyroglobulin; and stimulates all steps in thyroid iodine metabolism leading to the synthesis and secretion of thyroid hormones. These actions of TSH result from binding of the hormone to specific receptors in the surface of the follicular cell and subsequent activation of the plasma membrane enzyme adenylate cyclase. The resulting increase in the cellular cyclic 3′,5′-adenosine monophosphate (cyclic AMP) concentration initiates the responses that characterize the action of TSH.

Regulation of TSH secretion, in turn, is effected by two opposing influences interacting at the level of the pituitary thyrotroph. Thyrotropin-releasing hormone (TRH), a tripeptide of hypothalamic origin, stimulates the secretion and synthesis of TSH, while thyroid hormones both inhibit the TSH secretory mechanism directly and antagonize the action of TRH. Thus, homeostatic control of TSH secretion is exerted in a negative-feedback manner by thyroid hormones, and the threshold for feedback inhibition is apparently set by TRH. TRH is synthesized by neurons in the ventromedial hypothalamus, reaches the pituitary via the hypophyseal portal blood system, and binds to specific receptors on the plasma membrane of the thyrotroph cell. The ensuing activation of the adenylate cyclase–cyclic AMP system then initiates TRH action. To what extent, if any, suprahypothalamic centers affect the secretion of TRH is uncertain. The negative-feedback effect of the thyroid hormones appears to take place entirely at the level of the thyrotroph. Thyroid hormones do not directly affect the hypothalamic secretion of TRH but reduce the number of TRH receptors on the thyrotrophic cell, thus impairing its responsiveness to TRH. The negative-feedback action of the thyroid hormones is apparently mediated by an inhibitory protein whose synthesis is induced by binding of the hormones to specific receptors in the nucleus of the thyrotrophic cell. The principal arbiter of thyroid hormone action within the pituitary is T_3 that is both generated locally from the free T_4 that has entered from the plasma and derived from the pool of free T_3 in the plasma. To what extent T_4 itself is effective within the pituitary is uncertain, but several other factors modify the secretion of TSH and its response to TRH. Both somatostatin and dopamine appear to be physiologic inhibitors of TRH secretion. Estrogens enhance responsiveness to TRH, whereas glucocorticoids have a damping effect on this function.

Intrathyroid regulation of thyroid function is less well understood but is nevertheless important. In some manner, changes in glandular organic iodine content are associated with reciprocal changes in thyroid iodide transport activity, as well as in growth, glucose metabolism, and nucleic acid synthesis. Although these influences are evident in the absence of TSH stimulation, and hence may be termed *autoregulatory,* their most important role is to modify (iodine-enrichment inhibiting, and iodine-depletion enhancing) the response of these functions to TSH, probably by modifying the generation of cyclic AMP consequent to TSH stimulation.

LABORATORY TESTS Laboratory tests of thyroid hormone economy can be divided into five major categories: direct tests of thyroid function, tests related to the concentration and binding of thyroid hormones in blood, metabolic indexes, tests of the homeostatic control of thyroid function, and tests that do not fit into other categories.

Direct tests of thyroid function Among all tests designed to assess thyroid status, only those that involve in vivo administration of radioactive iodine test glandular function per se, and measurement of the *thyroid radioactive iodine uptake* (RAIU) is the most commonly used among them. Although ^{131}I has been used for this purpose for decades, ^{123}I is preferable because of the lower radiation dose that it delivers. The administered radioiodine mixes uniformly with the endogenous iodide in the extracellular fluid and, in the steady state, can be used to assess what percentage of the iodide entering and leaving the extracellular space per unit time is accumulated by the thyroid. The RAIU is usually measured 24 h after administration of the isotope since it has usually reached a plateau value at this time. The RAIU varies inversely with the plasma iodide concentration and directly with the functional state of the thyroid. At usual levels of iodine intake in the United States (up to 1000 μg per day), the normal range for the 24-h RAIU is approximately 5 to 30 percent of the administered dose. Consequently, this test discriminates poorly between normal and hypothyroid states. Values above the normal range, however, indicate thyroid hyperfunction, and remain useful, therefore, in the diagnosis of hyperthyroidism. The RAIU is also used as part of the thyroid suppression test.

Certain causes of thyrotoxicosis can be diagnosed by the demonstration of a low value of the RAIU. These include not only iodine-induced hyperthyroidism and thyrotoxicosis factitia but also the spontaneously resolving thyrotoxicosis that is associated with either a painless chronic thyroiditis or the classic painful, subacute thyroiditis.

Tests related to hormone concentration and binding in blood Measurement of the concentration of one or both thyroid hormones in serum, T_4 and T_3, in conjunction with some assessment of hormone binding, is generally the most reliable means of confirming a diagnosis of hyperthyroidism or hypothyroidism. Highly specific and sensitive radioimmunoassays are used to measure *serum T_4* and *T_3* concentrations, and a specific radioimmunoassay is available for measuring *serum rT_3* concentration as well. The approximate normal ranges are 4 to 12 $\mu g/dl$ for T_4, 80 to 100 ng/dl for T_3, and 10 to 40 ng/dl for rT_3.

Measurements of serum *protein-bound iodine* (PBI) were once used as an indirect means of assessing serum T_4 concentration. At present, the serum PBI is occasionally measured as a means of detecting release from the thyroid of abnormal iodoproteins, such as occurs in various forms of thyroiditis or as the result of an intrathyroid biosynthetic defect.

As mentioned in a previous section, alterations in the concentration of TBG, as well as alterations in hormone secretion, influence the total concentration of hormone in the blood. However, only alterations in hormone secretion will lead to steady-state alterations in the concentration of free hormone. The *percent of free hormone* (*percent FT_4* or *percent FT_3*) can be measured by equilibrium dialysis of serum enriched with a tracer quantity of the labeled hormone, and the product of this value and the serum T_4 or serum T_3 yields the *concentration of free hormone* (*FT_4* or *FT_3*). Measurement of percent FT_4 or percent FT_3 is cumbersome. Hence, for clinical purposes, the *in vitro uptake test* is employed, as it is simple to perform and yields qualitatively the same information. Here, the serum is enriched with labeled hormone and then incubated with an insoluble, particulate material, such as resin or charcoal, that binds hormone. The percent of labeled hormone taken up by the particulate material varies inversely with the concentration of unoccupied binding sites on TBG. Labeled T_3 is employed in preference to labeled T_4 since it is less strongly bound by the serum and hence yields higher and therefore more accurate uptake values. Normal values for the *resin-T_3 uptake* (*RT_3U*) range from 25 to 35 percent. Results may also be expressed as the quotient of the RT_3U value in the patient's serum and that obtained in a normal control specimen (*RT_3U ratio*). The product of the serum T_4 or serum T_3 concentration and the RT_3U is the so-called *free T_4 index (FT_4I)* or *free T_3 index (FT_3I)*. Analogous calculations in which the RT_3U ratio, rather than the RT_3U, is used yield values for the *normalized FT_4I* or *normalized FT_3I*. Primary alterations in hormone binding (Table 111-2) produce *reciprocal* alterations in RT_3U and serum T_4 and T_3; as a result the FT_4I and FT_3I remain normal. By contrast primary alterations in T_4 secretion produce changes in RT_3U that are in the same direction as those in serum T_4. Hence, the FT_4I affords a better discrimination from normal values than either of its components alone. Recently introduced radioimmunoassay methods for the *direct measurement of the FT_4 concentration* appear promising and may supplant measurements of the FT_4I.

Some states are associated with an increased thyroid secretion of T_3, at least relative to the secretion of T_4. As a result, the serum T_3 concentration is disproportionately high relative to the prevailing serum T_4 concentration. This is apparently a consequence of hyperfunction of the follicular cell, since it is seen in all varieties of hyperthyroidism, as well as in early thyroid failure, in which the gland is exposed to enhanced stimulation by TSH. Accordingly, the serum T_3 concentration and the derived FT_3I are generally superior to the corresponding values for T_4 in the diagnosis of hyperthyroidism. In *early* hypothyroidism, by contrast, the serum T_3 concentration and FT_3I may be normal despite subnormal values for the serum T_4 concentration and FT_4I. Measurement of the serum rT_3 concentration is especially valuable in differentiating the low T_3 syndrome from intrinsic hypothyroidism; in the former state, the serum rT_3 concentration is increased, whereas in the latter it is usually subnormal.

Metabolic indexes These tests measure the metabolic impact of thyroid hormone in the peripheral tissues. The *basal metabolic rate* (*BMR*) measures energy expenditure in terms of the amount of O_2 consumed in the basal state. Values are expressed as a percentage difference from the mean value of normal individuals of the same age, sex, and body surface area. The normal range is approximately -15 to $+5$ percent. Owing to the variety of nonthyroidal factors that affect the BMR, however, this test is of limited diagnostic value. Increases in the *serum cholesterol concentration* are suggestive of hypothyroidism of thyroid origin; however, decreases in serum cholesterol are of little value in the diagnosis of thyrotoxicosis. *Systolic time indexes,* such as the preejection period and pulse-wave arrival time, are prolonged in hypothyroidism and shortened in hyperthyroidism. They are of value in monitoring thyroid replacement therapy in elderly patients or in patients with coexisting heart disease.

Tests of homeostatic control Measurement of the basal *serum TSH concentration* has become an important tool in the diagnosis of both frank and subclinical hypothyroidism. The latter state represents a stage in the evolution of hypothyroidism, in which a structural or functional abnormality that impairs hormone synthesis is compensated for by hypersecretion of TSH and activation of the thyroid. Serum TSH concentration is measured by radioimmunoassay. The normal range is less than 5 μU/ml; current sensitivity does not generally permit distinction between normal and low values. Measurement of serum TSH affords the best means of distinguishing between untreated hypothyroidism of thyroid origin, in which the values are invariably increased, and pituitary or hypothalamic hypothyroidism, in which the values are usually undetectable or within the normal range. In thyrotoxicosis, serum TSH is undetectable, except in rare cases of TSH-induced hyperthyroidism, usually the result of a pituitary tumor. Occasional patients with hypothyroidism of hypothalamic or pituitary origin secrete a form of TSH that is immunoactive but not bioactive. Here, serum TSH concentrations may be slightly elevated, rather than depressed.

The *thyrotropin-releasing hormone* (*TRH*) *stimulation test* assesses the functional state of the TSH-secretory mechanism, and has, as a consequence, value for diverse diagnostic purposes. Following the intravenous injection of TRH in normal subjects, the serum TSH begins to increase at 10 min, reaches a maximum between 20 and 45 min, and then rapidly declines. When the TSH-secretory mechanism is impaired by intrinsic pituitary disease, a subnormal response to TRH may be expected. Further, the response of the thyrotroph to TRH is finely attuned to slight deficiency or excess of thyroid hormone. As a result, a supranormal response occurs in patients with hypothyroidism of thyroid origin, whereas little or no response occurs in patients with thyrotoxicosis. The sensitivity of TRH responsiveness to feedback inhibition apparently accounts for the subnormal responses to TRH that commonly occur in clinically euthyroid patients with autonomously functioning adenomas and possibly in some with apparently euthyroid Graves' disease. Responses to TRH are often decreased in elderly individuals, especially men. Despite these exceptions, a subnormal or absent response to TRH serves as an excellent confirmatory test for thyrotoxicosis. This test is also of value in the recognition and differential diagnosis of pituitary and hypothalamic hypothyroidism. In the former, but not the latter, no response to TRH would be expected, though those patients in the former group whose pituitaries secrete a biologically inactive TSH may show some response (see also Chap. 109).

The *thyroid suppression test* is used to assess whether thyroid function is controlled by normal homeostatic mechanisms. Normally, exogenous thyroid hormone suppresses pituitary TSH secretion, resulting in a decrease in the RAIU. Since liothyronine is usually employed (100 μg daily for 10 days), the resulting decline in serum T_4, as well as in the RAIU, can serve as an index of suppression. A normal suppressive response is a decrease of the RAIU to less than half of the control value and a decline of the serum T_4 to low normal or subnormal values. An abnormal suppression test is always present in hyperthyroidism, irrespective of the underlying cause; this indicates either autonomy of thyroid function, the presence of an abnormal stimulator, or unremitting hypersecretion of TSH. A normal suppression test, on the other hand, is incompatible with, and excludes the presence of, hyperthyroidism. An abnormal suppression test is not pathognomonic of hyperthyroidism, however, since it is seen after treatment of hyperthyroidism in Graves' disease, in about half of the euthyroid patients with the ophthalmopathy of Graves' disease, and in seemingly euthyroid patients in whom autonomous hyperfunctioning adenomas suppress the remainder of the gland.

Because of the risk of adverse effects of exogenous thyroid hormone in elderly patients and in those with cardiovascular disease, and since the TRH test is almost entirely devoid of undesirable side effects, the latter test has almost entirely supplanted the thyroid suppression test as an aid in the diagnosis of hyperthyroidism.

Miscellaneous tests A variety of tests that do not assess thyroid function are of value in defining the nature of the thyroid disorder or in planning therapy. For example, high titers of *antimicrosomal antibodies* or *antithyroglobulin antibodies* are found in the serum of most adult patients with Hashimoto's disease and in many patients with primary thyroprivic hypothyroidism or Graves' disease. In the latter, the serum also contains immunoglobulins that are capable of inhibiting the binding of TSH to its receptors in human thyroid plasma membranes (TSH-binding inhibitory immunoglobulins, TBII) and of stimulating the production of cyclic AMP therein (thyroid-stimulating immunoglobulins, TSI). In a clinical setting, the principal utility of tests for TSI and TBII stems from the fact that the disappearance of these factors from the serum during treatment with antithyroid agents implies the likelihood of a long-term remission when therapy is withdrawn.

Imaging by *scintiscanning* permits localization of sites of radioiodine or sodium [^{99m}Tc]pertechnetate accumulation. This technique is useful for defining areas of increased or decreased function within the thyroid and for detecting retrosternal goiter, ectopic thyroid tissue, hemiagenesis of the thyroid, and functioning metastases of thyroid carcinoma. Ultrasonic examination of the thyroid is also a valuable technique for differentiating cystic nodules from those that are solid. Since ultrasonic scans provide an accurate indication of size, are noninvasive, and apparently have no injurious effects, sequential scans can be employed to assess changes in the size of the thyroid as a whole or of discrete nodules over time or in response to treatment.

Along with several other thyroid disorders, differentiated carcinomas of the thyroid release thyroglobulin into the bloodstream. As a consequence, measurements of the *serum thyroglobulin concentration* by radioimmunoassay have value, not in the initial diagnosis of thyroid carcinoma, but in assessing the adequacy of initial therapy and in monitoring for recurrence or dissemination of the disease.

SIMPLE (NONTOXIC) GOITER

There is considerable confusion about the descriptive terms *endemic* and *sporadic* goiter. *Endemic* implies an etiologic factor or factors common to a particular geographic region. The term has been defined as indicating the presence of generalized or localized thyroid enlargement in over 10 percent of the population. The connotation of *sporadic* is that goiter arises in nonendemic areas as a result of a stimulus that does not affect the population generally. Since these terms fail to define or distinguish the causes of such goiters and since thyroid enlargement of diverse etiology may exist in both endemic and nonendemic regions, it seems prudent to employ a general term such as simple or nontoxic goiter. This all-inclusive category can be further subdivided into specific etiologic groups as defined by objective procedures. Simple or nontoxic goiter may be defined as any enlargement of the thyroid gland that does not result from an inflammatory or neoplastic process and is not initially associated with thyrotoxicosis or myxedema.

ETIOLOGY AND PATHOGENESIS Although the causes of simple goiter are manifold, their clinical manifestations are thought to reflect the operation of a common pathophysiologic mechanism. Simple goiter results when one or more factors impair the capacity of the thyroid gland in the basal state to secrete quantities of active hormones necessary to meet the needs of the peripheral tissues. Although this has been presumed to lead to increased secretion of TSH, concentrations of TSH in the serum of patients with established simple goiter are usually normal. Hence, some other mechanism of goitrogenesis may be operative. A likely possibility is that depletion of glandular organic iodine accompanying impaired hormone synthesis increases the responsiveness of thyroid structure and function to basal levels of TSH. The resulting increases in both functioning thyroid mass and cellular activity are sufficient to overcome mild or moderate impairment of hormone synthesis; thus, the patient remains metabolically normal, though goitrous. When, however, the underlying disorder is severe, compensatory responses, now including hypersecretion of TSH, are inadequate to overcome the impairment, and the patient is both goitrous and more or less severely hypothyroid. Thus, the entity simple goiter cannot be separated clearly, in the pathogenetic sense, from goitrous hypothyroidism. Specific causes of simple goiter are included in Table 111-4 and may exist with or without hypothyroidism. Defective iodination of thyroglobulin may be an important pathogenetic factor in many patients with the sporadic variety of simple goiter.

PATHOLOGY The histopathology of the thyroid in simple goiter varies with the severity of the etiologic factor and the stage at which the examination is made. In its initial stages, the gland reveals a uniform hypertrophy, hyperplasia, and hypervascularity. As the disorder persists or undergoes repeated exacerbations and remissions, uniformity of thyroidal architecture is usually lost. Occasionally, the greater part of the gland may display a reasonably uniform degree of involution or hyperinvolution with colloid accumulation. More often such areas are interspersed with patchy areas of focal hyperplasia. Fibrosis may demarcate a variable number of nodules, which may be hyperplastic or involuted. These may resemble, but do not really represent, true neoplasms (adenomas). Areas of hemorrhage and irregular calcification may be present. The evolution of the multinodular stage is often accompanied by the development of functional autonomy. As a result, hyper-

TABLE 111-4
Classification of the causes of hypothyroidism

I Thyroid
- *A* Thyroprivic
  - *1* Congenital development defect
  - *2* Primary idiopathic
  - *3* Postablative (radioiodine, surgery)
  - *4* Postradiation (lymphoma)
- *B* Goitrous
  - *1* Heritable biosynthetic defects
  - *2* Maternally transmitted (iodides, antithyroid agents)
  - *3* Iodine deficiency
  - *4* Drug-elicited (*p*-aminosalicylic acid, iodides, phenylbutazone, iodoantipyrine, lithium)
  - *5* Chronic thyroiditis (Hashimoto's disease)

II Suprathyroid (trophoprivic)
- *A* Pituitary
- *B* Hypothalamic

thyroidism may ensue spontaneously (toxic multinodular goiter) or be induced by large quantities of iodide (jodbasedow phenomenon).

CLINICAL MANIFESTATIONS In simple goiter the clinical manifestations arise solely from enlargement of the thyroid since the metabolic state of the patient is normal. In goitrous hypothyroidism, symptoms caused by thyromegaly are similarly present but are accompanied by signs and symptoms of hormonal insufficiency. Mechanical sequelae include compression and displacement of the trachea or esophagus, occasionally with obstructive symptoms if the goiter becomes sufficiently large. Superior mediastinal obstruction may occur with large retrosternal goiters. Signs of compression can be induced in the case of large retrosternal goiters when the patient's arms are raised above the head (Pemberton's sign); suffusion of the face, giddiness, or syncope may result from this maneuver. Compression of the recurrent laryngeal nerve leading to hoarseness is rare in simple goiter and suggests neoplasm. Sudden hemorrhage into a nodule may lead to an acute, painful swelling in the neck and may produce or enhance compressive symptoms. Hyperthyroidism not uncommonly supervenes in long-standing multinodular goiter (toxic multinodular goiter). In both endemic and sporadic multinodular goiter, the ingestion of excess iodide may result in the development of thyrotoxicosis (jodbasedow phenomenon).

In geographic regions where iodine deficiency is severe, acquired goitrous enlargement may also be associated with varying degrees of hypothyroidism. Cretinism, both goitrous and nongoitrous, occurs with increased frequency in the children of goitrous parents and contributes a significant sector of the socially dependent population in many countries where goiter is common. Although iodine deficiency is doubtless a necessary factor in the etiology of endemic goiter, the frequency of goiter may differ greatly among areas of equally severe iodine deficiency. In such instances, dietary or water-borne goitrogens appear to be important conditioning factors.

DIAGNOSIS The diagnosis of simple goiter requires, first, demonstration of a normal metabolic state and, second, differentiation of the goitrous condition from Hashimoto's disease or thyroid neoplasia. Physical examination alone cannot serve to make the diagnosis. A careful history is important, particularly with respect to the occurrence of thyroid pain or tenderness, rapid change in size, hoarseness, or previous drug ingestion. High titers of circulating antimicrosomal or antithyroglobulin antibodies indicate Hashimoto's disease. In patients with simple goiter, the serum T_4 and T_3 concentrations are generally within the normal range, but the ratio of T_3 to T_4 is often increased, reflecting defective iodination of thyroglobulin. In many patients, the serum thyroglobulin concentration is increased. The RAIU is usually normal but may be increased in the presence of iodine deficiency or a biosynthetic defect. The functional autonomy that may accompany long-standing multinodular goiter often results in diminished or absent responsiveness of serum TSH to the administration of TRH.

TREATMENT The object of treatment is to reverse the thyroid hyperplasia, either by relieving external encumbrances to hormone formation or by providing sufficient quantities of exogenous hormone to inhibit TSH secretion and thereby put the thyroid gland almost completely at rest. In disorders characterized by decreased thyroid iodide stores, such as iodine deficiency or impairment of the thyroid iodide-concentrating mechanism, small doses of iodide may prove effective. Occasionally, a known extrinsic goitrogen can be withdrawn. Most commonly, however, no specific etiologic factor can be detected, and suppressive thyroid therapy is required. For this purpose, sodium L-thyroxine (levothyroxine) is the agent of choice. In the younger patient with the early diffuse stage of simple goiter, treatment can be instituted with 100 μg of levothyroxine daily, and the dose is increased over the next month or so to a maximum of 150 or 200 μg daily. Adequacy of suppression can be assessed by measuring the RAIU, which should have decreased to less than 5 percent of the administered dose at 24 h. Lesser decreases indicate only partial suppression, reflecting the presence of autonomous foci demonstrable by scanning techniques. In the elderly patient or the patient with long-standing multinodular goiter, a TRH stimulation test should be undertaken before initiating treatment with levothyroxine to determine whether or not functional autonomy has supervened. If such is indicated by diminished or absent TSH responsiveness to TRH, suppressive therapy with levothyroxine is contraindicated since such patients are or will eventually become thyrotoxic. Rather, consideration should be given to radioiodine ablation of the autonomous foci (see later section on "Toxic Multinodular Goiter"). On the other hand, if the TSH response to TRH is normal, excluding significant functional autonomy, treatment with levothyroxine can be initiated. In the elderly patient, the initial dose should not exceed 50 μg daily, and the dosage should be gradually increased, partial rather than complete suppression of the value for the RAIU being the end point.

Reported results of therapy vary widely. There is general agreement that the early diffuse, hyperplastic goiter responds well, with regression or disappearance in 3 to 6 months. In the authors' experience, the later, nodular stage responds less favorably, and significant reduction in gland size is achieved only in about one-third of the cases; however, in the remainder, suppressive treatment probably forestalls further glandular growth. Internodular tissue regresses more often than do nodules themselves. The latter may therefore become more prominent during treatment. After maximum regression of the goiter, suppressive medication may be maintained for prolonged periods, reduced to minimal levels, or at times withdrawn. In an unpredictable manner, goiter will in some cases remain relieved while in others it will recur. In the latter instances, suppressive therapy should be reinstituted and should be continued indefinitely.

In areas of endemic iodine deficiency, the size and prevalence of goiter, and probably the frequency of cretinism, can be reduced by the provision of iodized salt or water or the infrequent injection of iodized oil.

Surgical therapy of simple goiter is physiologically unsound, but it may occasionally be necessary to relieve obstructive symptoms, especially those which persist after a conscientious trial of medical therapy. Surgical exploration of nodular goiter may be indicated in some individuals when evidence suggests carcinoma. However, the suggestion that subtotal resection of multinodular nontoxic goiter affords effective prophylaxis against the development of thyroid carcinoma is unsound. If for some reason subtotal thyroidectomy has been performed, levothyroxine in a usual dose of about 150 μg daily is recommended to inhibit regenerative hyperplasia and further goitrogenesis.

HYPOTHYROIDISM

Hypothyroidism may result from any of a variety of structural or functional abnormalities that lead to insufficient synthesis of thyroid hormone. Hypothyroidism dating from birth and resulting in developmental abnormalities is termed *cretinism.* The term *myxedema* connotes severe hypothyroidism in which there is accumulation of hydrophilic mucopolysaccharides in the ground substance of the dermis and other tissues, leading to thickening of the facial features and doughy induration of the skin.

ETIOLOGY AND PATHOGENESIS A classification of the causes of hypothyroidism is presented in Table 111-4. Overall, the thyroid varieties account for approximately 95 percent of cases, only 5 percent or less being suprathyroid in origin. In thyroprivic hypothyroidism, loss of thyroid tissue leads to inadequate synthesis of thyroid hormone, despite maximum stimulation of any thyroid remnant by TSH. The most common cause of thyroprivic hypothyroidism is surgical or radioiodine ablation of the thyroid gland in the treatment of Graves' disease. Thyroprivic hypothyroidism may also occur as a primary idiopathic phenomenon. Primary hypothyroidism is frequently associated with circulating antithyroid antibodies and may coexist with a wide variety of other diseases in which circulating autoantibodies are found. These diseases include pernicious anemia, systemic lupus erythematosus, rheumatoid arthritis, Sjögren's syndrome, and chronic hepatitis. In addition, hypothyroidism can be one manifestation of a polyglandular endocrine deficiency state in which autoantibodies cause variable insufficiency of thyroid, adrenal, parathyroid, and gonadal function (see Chap. 123). All these diseases, including isolated primary hypothyroidism, are associated with an increased frequency of specific HLA haplotypes and may be diverse reflections of disordered immune regulation. Finally, a developmental defect may result in failure of the gland to function adequately, leading to sporadic nongoitrous cretinism or juvenile hypothyroidism.

A purely functional impairment in the ability to synthesize adequate quantities of thyroid hormone leads to hypersecretion of TSH and hence goiter. If this compensatory response is inadequate, goitrous hypothyroidism ensues. The commonest cause in North America is Hashimoto's disease, in which defective organic binding of iodide and abnormal secretion of iodoproteins are frequent biosynthetic abnormalities. Iodide-induced goiter with or without hypothyroidism appears often to arise from an intrinsic defect in the organic binding mechanism, which permits a persistent Wolff-Chaikoff effect. Patients with Graves' disease, especially after radioiodine treatment, those with Hashimoto's disease, and the normal fetus are particularly susceptible to iodide-induced goiter. In view of the susceptibility of the fetal thyroid to iodide, with resulting goiter and hypothyroidism, women should not be given iodine in large doses during pregnancy. Less common causes of goitrous hypothyroidism are heritable defects in pathways of hormone biosynthesis and ingestion of drugs which induce defects in hormone biosynthesis, such as *p*-aminosalicylic acid and lithium carbonate. Finally, in many areas of the world where there is environmental iodine deficiency, goitrous cretinism and hypothyroidism occur on an endemic basis. Diminished thyroid reserve occurs as a stage in the evolution of both thyroprivic and goitrous hypothyroidism.

In hypothyroidism of suprathyroid origin, the thyroid is intrinsically normal but is deprived of stimulation by TSH. Deprivation of TSH, most commonly the result of postpartum pituitary necrosis or a tumor of the pituitary or adjacent regions, results in pituitary hypothyroidism. Hypothalamic hypothyroidism appears to be less common and results from inadequate secretion of TRH.

CLINICAL PICTURE The general appearance of children with hypothyroidism varies, depending on the age at which the deficiency began and the promptness with which replacement therapy was instituted. Manifestations of cretinism may be present at birth but are more commonly evident within the first several months, depending upon the extent of thyroid failure. During the neonatal period, the abnormally long persistence of physiologic jaundice, hoarse cry, constipation, somnolence, and feeding problems should call attention to the diagnosis. In later months, delay in reaching the normal milestones of development becomes evident, and the physical characteristics of the cretin appear. These include short stature, coarse features with protruding tongue, broad flat nose, widely set eyes, sparse hair, dry skin, and protuberant abdomen with an umbilical hernia. X-ray examination reveals retarded bone age, epiphyseal dysgenesis, and delayed dental development. Mental development is retarded; eventual intellectual attainment depends upon how soon full replacement therapy is instituted. Consequently, it is fortunate that neonatal hypothyroidism can readily be diagnosed from measurements of the serum T_4 or serum TSH in either cord blood or infant's blood. Extensive surveys using these techniques have revealed an approximate frequency of this disorder of 1 in every 5000 births. Hence, every newborn should undergo screening for hypothyroidism so that treatment of those who are hypothyroid can be begun as soon as possible.

In the older child with hypothyroidism, the clinical manifestations are intermediate between those of infantile and adult hypothyroidism. Retardation of linear growth results in shortness of stature, and retardation of sexual maturation results in delay in the onset of puberty. Poor performance at school may call attention to the diagnosis. The manifestations of adult hypothyroidism are present to a variable degree. X-ray examination reveals delayed union of the epiphyses.

In the adult, early symptoms of hypothyroidism are nonspecific and of insidious onset. They may include lethargy, constipation, cold intolerance, and menorrhagia. Over the succeeding months, slowing of intellectual and motor activity appears, appetite declines, and modest weight gain occurs. The hair becomes dry and tends to fall out. The patient may complain of dry skin and of stiff aching muscles. The voice becomes deeper and hoarse and auditory acuity may deteriorate. Ultimately, the clinical picture of florid myxedema appears, with dull expressionless face, sparse hair, periorbital puffiness, large tongue, and pale, cool skin which feels rough and doughy. Thyroid tissue is not readily palpable, except in the goitrous variety of hypothyroidism. The heart is enlarged owing to both dilation and pericardial effusion; if the heart is small, pituitary hypothyroidism should be considered. Adynamic ileus may occur, producing the clinical picture of megacolon. Rarely, psychiatric reactions or cerebellar ataxia may dominate the clinical picture. The relaxation phase of the deep tendon reflexes is characteristically prolonged, the so-called hung-up reflex. If left untreated, the patient with severe longstanding hypothyroidism may pass into a hypothermic, stuporous state (*myxedema coma*), which is frequently fatal. Respiratory depression is an important component of this state, and hence an increased arterial P_{CO_2} is of premonitory value. Factors that predispose to myxedema coma include cold exposure, trauma, infection, and administration of central nervous system depressants. Dilutional hyponatremia is common in severe hypothyroidism and results from diminished renal perfusion leading to impaired water excretion, as well as from disordered regulation of vasopressin secretion.

LABORATORY TESTS A decrease in serum T_4 and in the FT_4I is common to all varieties of hypothyroidism, as is a decrease in BMR. In the thyroidal varieties, the serum T_3 may be decreased to a lesser extent than is the serum T_4, the presumption being that the compensatory hypersecretion of TSH leads to a relative preponderance of T_3 secretion. In thyroprivic hypothyroidism the RAIU is decreased, but this is of limited diagnostic utility because of the low value for the lower limit of the normal range. In goitrous hypothyroidism, the RAIU may be increased or may display an abnormal pattern of accumulation or retention. The serum TSH is invariably increased in the thyroprivic and goitrous varieties and is usually normal or undetectable in pituitary or hypothalamic hypothyroidism. In the latter instances, in addition to possible evidence of intracranial disease, hyposecretion of TSH is accompanied by hyposecretion of other pituitary hormones; this is amenable to laboratory testing (see Chap. 109). A subnormal response of the serum TSH to the administration of TRH confirms the presence of pituitary hypothyroidism.

Other frequent, but not invariable, manifestations of the hypothyroid state include an increased serum cholesterol in hypothyroidism of thyroid (but not pituitary) origin and increased concentrations in serum of creatine phosphokinase, glutamic oxaloacetic transaminase, and lactic dehydrogenase. Systolic time intervals are altered in that the preejection period is distinctly prolonged and the ratio of the preejection period to left ventricular ejection time is increased. Electrocardiographic changes are common and include bradycardia, low amplitude QRS complexes, and flattened or inverted T waves. In primary thyroprivic hypothyroidism, overt pernicious anemia reportedly occurs in about 12 percent of patients; histamine-fast achlorhydria and the presence of circulating antigastric parietal cell antibodies are even more common.

In addition to patients who are clinically hypothyroid, some patients who appear clinically euthyroid display laboratory evidence of early thyroid failure (subclinical hypothyroidism). In mild cases serum TSH and its response to TRH administration are increased while serum T_4 and T_3 concentrations are normal. When there is a greater degree of thyroid failure, serum T_4 concentration is decreased, but the serum T_3 concentration is normal or nearly so owing to TSH-induced hypersecretion of T_3 relative to T_4. These varieties of subclinical hypothyroidism are most often seen in patients with Hashimoto's disease or those with Graves' disease who have been treated with ^{131}I or surgery and, at least in some, are stages in the evolution of frank hypothyroidism.

DIFFERENTIAL DIAGNOSIS Little difficulty will be experienced in diagnosing the classic picture of cretinism or juvenile and adult hypothyroidism. Occasionally, an infant with Down syndrome may be confused with a cretin. However, the characteristic mongoloid eyes, Brushfield's spots in the iris, hyperextensibility of the joints, and normal skin and hair texture distinguish Down syndrome from hypothyroid cretinism. Chronic nephritis and especially the nephrotic syndrome may simulate myxedema, particularly because of the facial puffiness and pallor. The nephrotic patient may also display anemia, hypercholesterolemia, and anasarca. In addition, the serum T_4 concentration may be decreased if there is significant loss of TBG into the urine, but the FT_4I is normal or increased. The serum T_3 concentration is often subnormal as it might be in any severe systemic illness owing to impaired peripheral generation from T_4, but the serum TSH concentration is not increased.

TREATMENT Two general types of preparation are available for the treatment of hypothyroidism, synthetic hormone and thyroprotein derived from animal thyroids. Synthetic hormones include L-thyroxine sodium (levothyroxine), L-triiodothyronine sodium (liothyronine), and a combination of the two (liotrix). The preparation of natural origin most commonly used is thyroid extract, USP. The approximate therapeutic equivalence of these drugs is presented in Table 111-5. Because of their uniform potency, the authors prefer the synthetic preparations, and of these the authors prefer levothyroxine. Unlike liothyronine, liotrix, and even thyroid extract, ingestion of levothyroxine does not lead to abrupt increases in serum T_3 concentration, which could be dangerous in the older patient or in the patient with coexisting heart disease. Rather, a stable T_3 concentration is attained through continuous generation from administered T_4.

In most instances, restoration of a normal metabolic state should be undertaken gradually, especially in the elderly or the patient with heart disease, since sudden increases in metabolic rate may tax cardiac reserve. In adults, an initial daily dose of 25 μg levothyroxine is recommended, and this can be increased by 25- to 50-μg increments at 2- to 3-week intervals, until a normal metabolic state is attained. The daily dose usually necessary to sustain a normal metabolic state is about 150 μg, and this is usually accompanied by a serum T_4 at or somewhat above the upper limit of the normal range. Because of its long half-life, levothyroxine is generally administered as a single daily dose. The optimum dose for the individual patient should be based on clinical criteria, the serum TSH or T_3 concentration being employed only as a confirmatory test.

In cretinism and juvenile hypothyroidism it is essential that full replacement therapy be begun as soon as possible; otherwise the chances of normal intellectual development and growth are poor. Infants and children require doses of levothyroxine that are disproportionately large in relation to body size. *In known or strongly suspected pituitary and hypothalamic hypothyroidism, thyroid replacement should not be instituted until treatment with hydrocortisone has been initiated,* since acute adrenocortical insufficiency may be precipitated by an increase in metabolic rate.

In some patients, it is important that hypothyroidism be treated rapidly. This includes patients with myxedema coma and, because of the extreme sensitivity to central nervous system depressants, hypothyroid patients being prepared for emergency surgery. Here, intravenous administration of levothyroxine, in conjunction with the use of hydrocortisone, is indicated.

THYROTOXICOSIS

The term *thyrotoxicosis* denotes the complex of clinical, physiologic, and biochemical findings that results when the tissues are exposed to, and respond to, an excess supply of active thyroid hormone. Rather than a specific disease, thyrotoxicosis is a clinical syndrome that can originate in a variety of ways. In general, three main categories of disorder can produce the thyrotoxic state (Table 111-6). The first, and most important, encompasses those diseases that lead to sustained overproduction of hormone by the thyroid gland itself. Here, hyperfunction of the gland variously results from excessive secretion of TSH, a rare cause usually associated with pituitary tumor; the action of an abnormal, homeostatically unregulated thyroid stimulator of extrapituitary origin, as in patients with Graves' disease or trophoblastic tumors; or the development of one or more areas of autonomous hyperfunction within the gland itself. The second category encompasses the thyrotoxic states associated with subacute thyroiditis and the syndrome termed *chronic thy-*

TABLE 111-5
Approximate therapeutic equivalence of various thyroid hormone preparations

Preparation	*Average daily oral maintenance dose*	*Serum T_4*
Thyroid extract, USP	120–180 mg	Normal
Levothyroxine	150 μg	Normal or slightly increased
Liothyronine	50 μg	Decreased
Liotrix (T_4/T_3 = 4:1)	2 units	Normal

roiditis with spontaneously resolving thyrotoxicosis; an excess of preformed hormone leaks from the gland owing to the presence of inflammatory disease. New hormone formation is decreased, however, owing to the suppression of TSH secretion by the hormone excess, and in some cases to the inflammatory injury itself. Since the inflammatory disorders are transitory and since stores of preformed hormone are ultimately depleted, the thyrotoxicosis in these disorders is self-limited and is often followed by a transient period of thyroid hormone insufficiency. The third category of thyrotoxic state is one in which the source of excess hormone is outside of the thyroid gland itself, as in thyrotoxicosis factitia, the rare functioning metastatic thyroid carcinoma, or struma ovarii.

Although all of the foregoing disorders are associated with thyrotoxicosis, not all are associated with hyperthyroidism, a term which should be used to denote only those conditions in the first category described above, i.e., those in which sustained hyperfunction of the thyroid leads to thyrotoxicosis. Thus, thyrotoxic states can be classified according to whether or not they are associated with hyperthyroidism. This distinction has practical implications from both the diagnostic and therapeutic standpoints. In hyperthyroidism, hyperfunction of the thyroid is reflected in an increased RAIU, whereas in the nonhyperthyroid thyrotoxic states, thyroid function including the RAIU is subnormal. Further, treatment of thyrotoxicosis by means intended to decrease hormone synthesis (antithyroid agents, surgery, or radioiodine) is appropriate in hyperthyroidism but is inappropriate and ineffective in other forms of thyrotoxicosis.

Though the specific diseases that cause thyrotoxicosis each make their own imprint on the clinical picture, the manifestations of the thyrotoxic state are largely the same. In the discussion that ensues, the major diseases that lead to a thyrotoxic state are individually described. Since the first considered and most important is Graves' disease, the common manifestations of thyrotoxicosis are described in relation to Graves' disease.

GRAVES' DISEASE Graves' disease, also known as Parry's or Basedow's disease, is a disorder of unknown etiology with a characteristic triad of major manifestations: hyperthyroidism with diffuse goiter, ophthalmopathy, and dermopathy. Although considered part of the same disease complex, the three major manifestations need not appear together. Indeed, one or two need never appear, and moreover, the three tend to run courses that are largely independent of one another.

Prevalence Graves' disease is a relatively common disorder which may occur at any age but especially in the third and fourth decades. The disease is more frequent in women than in men. In nongoitrous areas the ratio of predominance in women may be as high as 7:1. In endemic goitrous areas the ratio is lower. Genetic factors play an important role; among patients with this disease, studies have revealed an inordinate frequency of haplotypes HLA-B8 and DRw3 in Caucasians, HLA-Bw36 in Japanese, and HLA-Bw46 in Chinese. Not surprisingly, there is a distinct familial predisposition to Graves' disease; in addition, among family members of patients with Graves' disease, a clinical and immunological overlap exists with respect to Hashimoto's disease, primary thyroprivic hypothyroidism, and pernicious anemia, and probably with respect to other diseases in which autoimmune features are prominent. In occasional patients, the disease picture may change from one of Graves' disease to one of Hashimoto's disease, or vice versa, and rarely patients with proven primary myxedema have later become hyperthyroid. Thus, it is proper to include Graves' disease, Hashimoto's disease, and primary myxedema in a broad category of closely related autoimmune thyroid diseases.

Etiology and pathogenesis The cause of Graves' disease is unknown. In view of the varied manifestations of Graves' disease and their differing courses, it is possible, and indeed likely, that no single factor is responsible for the entire syndrome. With respect to hyperthyroidism, it is apparent that central to this disorder is a disruption of homeostatic mechanisms that normally adjust hormone secretion to meet the needs of peripheral tissues; if such were able to operate, hyperthyroidism could not be sustained. There is now compelling evidence to suggest that this homeostatic disruption results from the presence in plasma of an abnormal thyroid stimulator. The existence of such was recognized more than 20 years ago when it was shown that the sera of patients with Graves' disease released radioiodine from the prelabeled guinea pig or mouse thyroid. In view of its prolonged duration of action relative to TSH in this bioassay system, this material was designated the long-acting thyroid stimulator (LATS). LATS was demonstrated to reside in one or more immunoglobulins of the class IgG that are elaborated by lymphocytes of patients with Graves' disease. It soon became apparent, however, that LATS could be detected only in about half of patients with this disorder, and consequently its pathogenetic role was seriously questioned. More recently, it has been demonstrated that this failure to detect LATS in many patients with Graves' disease is due to the fact that the stimulator in human serum has variable cross-reactivity in other species and may not be detectable, therefore, in the conventional LATS assay. When human thyroid tissue is used as the assay system, however, one or more of a variety of in vitro responses can be demonstrated to immunoglobulin G derived from the plasma of most patients. These responses and the corresponding names given to the responsible factors are as follows: prevention of the adsorption of LATS activity by human thyroid particulate fractions (LATS-protector, LATS-p), stimulation of colloid droplet or cyclic AMP generation in human thyroid slices or membranes (thyroid-stimulating immunoglobulins, TSI), and inhibition of the binding of TSH to its receptors in human thyroid tissue (TSH-binding inhibitory immunoglobulins, TBII). The underlying nature of these factors, their number, and their relationship to one another are uncertain, but they are thought by some to be one or more antibodies directed against some component of the thyroid plasma membrane, perhaps the TSH receptor itself. Activities of this type are also found in sera of some patients with euthyroid ophthalmic Graves' disease, an occasional patient with Hashimoto's disease, and some euthyroid relatives of patients with Graves' disease, though the reason for the absence of thyrotoxicosis in such instances is uncertain. It appears that disappearance of these stimulatory factors from the serum during antithyroid treatment augurs well for long-term remission after

TABLE 111-6
Varieties of thyrotoxic states

I Disorders associated with thyroid hyperfunction*
- *A* Excess production of TSH (rare)
- *B* Abnormal thyroid stimulator
  - *1* Graves' disease
  - *2* Trophoblastic tumor
- *C* Intrinsic thyroid autonomy
  - *1* Hyperfunctioning adenoma
  - *2* Toxic multinodular goiter

II Disorders not associated with thyroid hyperfunction†
- *A* Disorders of hormone storage
  - *1* Subacute thyroiditis
  - *2* Chronic thyroiditis with transient thyrotoxicosis
- *B* Extrathyroid source of hormone
  - *1* Thyrotoxicosis factitia
  - *2* Ectopic thyroid tissue
    - *a* Struma ovarii
    - *b* Functioning follicular cacinoma

* *Associated with increased RAIU unless body iodine burden is excessive.*
† *Associated with decreased RAIU.*

treatment is withdrawn. Thus, while the basic cause of Graves' disease is not understood, there is good evidence that an immunoglobulin G or family of immunoglobulins directed against some component of the thyroid is pathogenetically involved in mediating the thyroid stimulation of Graves' disease. It has been proposed that a heritable abnormality in immune surveillance may permit a particular clone of lymphocytes to survive, proliferate, and secrete the stimulatory immunoglobulins in response to some precipitating factors.

The pathogenesis of the ophthalmic component of Graves' disease is even more enigmatic. One proposed mechanism invokes the activity of a fragment of the TSH molecule, which, in conjunction with an immunoglobulin, binds to and produces edema of retroorbital tissue. A second postulate invokes cephalad lymphatic transport of thyroglobulin from the thyroid to retroorbital tissues, at which site an immune response is evoked. Nothing is known of the pathogenesis of the dermopathy of Graves' disease.

Pathology In Grave's disease, the *thyroid gland* is diffusely enlarged, soft, and vascular. The essential pathology is that of parenchymatous hypertrophy and hyperplasia, characterized by increased height of the epithelium and redundancy of the follicular wall, giving the picture of papillary infoldings and cytologic evidence of increased activity. Such hyperplasia is usually accompanied by lymphocytic infiltration that reflects the immune aspect of the disease and its attendant chronic thyroiditis and that correlates in severity with titers of antithyroid antibodies in the blood. Following iodine medication, there is colloid storage, which sometimes causes enlargement and increased firmness of the gland. Grave's disease is associated with generalized lymphoid hyperplasia and infiltration, and occasionally with enlargement of the spleen or thymus. Thyrotoxicosis may lead to degeneration of skeletal muscle fibers, enlargement of the heart, fatty infiltration or diffuse fibrosis of the liver, decalcification of the skeleton, and loss of body tissue (including fat deposits, osteoid, and muscle).

The *ophthalmopathy* of Graves' disease is characterized by an inflammatory infiltrate of the orbital contents, exclusive of the globe, with lymphocytes, mast cells, and plasma cells being the predominant cellular components. The orbital musculature is mainly involved and often is greatly enlarged, largely accounting for the increased volume of the orbital contents that causes the globe to protrude. Muscle fibers show degeneration and loss of striations, with ultimate fibrosis.

The *dermopathy* of Graves' disease is characterized by thickening of the dermis, which is infiltrated with lymphocytes and with hydrophilic, metachromatically staining mucopolysaccharides.

Clinical manifestations The clinical manifestations comprise those that reflect the associated thyrotoxicosis and those specifically related to Graves' disease. The former vary in intensity with the severity of the thyrotoxicosis but are also modified by the age of the patient and the presence of disease in other organs, such as the heart.

MANIFESTATIONS OF THYROTOXICOSIS Common symptomatic manifestations of thyrotoxicosis include nervousness, emotional lability, inability to sleep, tremors, excessive sweating, and heat intolerance. Weight loss is frequent, usually despite a well-maintained or increased appetite. Loss of strength is often manifested by difficulty in climbing stairs. In premenopausal women, oligomenorrhea and amenorrhea tend to occur. Dyspnea, palpitations, and, in patients over the age of 40, enhancement of angina pectoris or cardiac failure may occur. In general, nervous symptoms dominate the clinical picture in younger individuals, whereas cardiovascular and myopathic symptoms predominate in older subjects.

Usually, the patient appears anxious and restless or fidgety. The skin is warm and moist with a velvety texture, and palmar erythema is often found. Separation of the fingernail from the nailbed (Plummer's nail) is often seen, especially on the ring finger. The hair is fine and silky. A fine tremor of the fingers and tongue, together with hyperreflexia, is characteristic. *Ocular signs* include a characteristic stare with widened palpebral fissures, infrequent blinking, lid lag, and failure to wrinkle the brow on upward gaze. These signs are thought to result from sympathetic overstimulation and usually subside when the thyrotoxicosis is corrected. They are to be distinguished from the *infiltrative ophthalmopathy* characteristic of Graves' disease, discussed below.

Cardiovascular findings include a wide pulse pressure, sinus tachycardia, atrial arrhythmias (especially atrial fibrillation), systolic murmurs, increased intensity of the apical first sound, cardiac enlargement, and, at times, overt heart failure. A to-and-fro, high-pitched sound may be audible in the pulmonic area and may simulate a pericardial friction rub (Means-Lerman scratch).

MANIFESTATIONS OF GRAVES' DISEASE The three major manifestations of Graves' disease, diffuse hyperfunctioning goiter, ophthalmopathy, and dermopathy, appear in varying combinations and with varying frequency, goiter being the most common. Premature graying of the hair and patchy vitiligo are often seen but are not specific to Graves' disease per se since they are also common in other autoimmune disorders, whether of the thyroid or other organ systems.

The *diffuse toxic goiter* may be asymmetric and lobular. Often a bruit is heard directly over the gland. When heard, it usually signifies that the patient is thyrotoxic, but it may also rarely be present in association with other disorders in which the thyroid is markedly hyperplastic. Venous hums and carotid souffles should be distinguished from true thyroid bruits. A hyperplastic pyramidal lobe of the thyroid may often be palpable.

The clinical signs associated with the *ophthalmopathy* of Graves' disease may be divided into two components: the spastic and the mechanical. The former includes the stare, lid lag, and lid retraction that accompany thyrotoxicosis and account for the "frightened" facies and classic eye signs previously described. These findings need not be associated with actual proptosis and usually return to normal after appropriate correction of thyrotoxicosis. The mechanical component includes proptosis of varying degrees with ophthalmoplegia and congestive oculopathy characterized by chemosis, conjunctivitis, periorbital swelling, and the resultant complications of corneal ulceration, optic neuritis, and optic atrophy. When exophthalmos progresses rapidly and becomes the major concern in Graves' disease, it is usually referred to as *progressive,* and if severe, *malignant exophthalmos.* The term *exophthalmic ophthalmoplegia* refers to the ocular muscle weakness that so commonly accompanies this disorder and results in strabismus with varying degrees of diplopia. Exophthalmos may be unilateral early in the course of the disorder but usually progresses to bilateral involvement.

The *dermopathy* of Graves' disease usually occurs over the dorsum of the legs or feet and is termed *localized* or *pretibial myxedema.* It occurs in patients with past or present Graves' disease and is not a manifestation of hypothyroidism. About half of cases occur during the active stage of thyrotoxicosis; in the remainder the lesions develop after treatment. The affected area is usually well demarcated from normal skin by the fact that it is raised, thickened, has a *peau d'orange* appearance, and may be pruritic and hyperpigmented. The lesions are usually discrete, assuming a plaque-like or nodular configuration, but in some instances the lesions become widely confluent. Clubbing of the fingers and toes with characteristic bony changes differentiable from those of hypertrophic pulmonary osteoarthropathy may accompany the dermal changes (*thyroid acropachy*). This disorder is usually self-limited.

Diagnosis When severe, Graves' disease presents little difficulty in diagnosis. Florid thyrotoxicosis is manifested by weakness, weight loss despite good appetite, nervous instability, tremor, intolerance to heat, hyperhydrosis, palpitations, and hyperdefecation. When associated with diffuse thyroid enlargement, often accompanied by a bruit, and particularly when associated with ophthalmopathy, Graves' disease presents a clinical picture that is virtually unique. In such instances, laboratory tests, which reveal increased RAIU, serum T_4 and T_3, RT_3U, and FT_4I serve mainly as base lines for evaluation of therapy, rather than necessary diagnostic aids. Occasionally, laboratory tests reveal a normal RAIU, serum T_4, and RT_3U, the serum T_3 and FT_3I alone being increased (T_3 toxicosis).

In less severe cases, particularly when ophthalmopathy is lacking, the diagnosis may be more difficult, since the symptoms of mild thyrotoxicosis are similar to those of other disorders (see "Differential Diagnosis" below). Presence of a goiter makes the diagnosis of hyperthyroidism likely, but careful palpation is necessary to determine whether toxic multinodular goiter, toxic adenoma, or subacute thyroiditis is present, since treatment of these disorders may differ from that of diffuse toxic goiter. Absence of thyroid enlargement makes the diagnosis of Graves' disease unlikely but does not exclude it. In mild cases, confirmatory laboratory tests assume great importance. Unfortunately, mild thyrotoxicosis is often associated with marginal abnormalities in laboratory tests, and values may in fact lie within the upper limit of the normal range. In such instances the thyroid suppression test or the TRH stimulation test assumes crucial importance.

In a few patients, the clinical picture may be one of apathy rather than hyperactivity, and evidence of hypermetabolism may be slight. In such patients, myopathic features may be pronounced. More often, cardiovascular manifestations predominate since, in patients with underlying heart disease, even mild hyperthyroidism may produce severe disability. Hence, *all patients with unexplained cardiac failure or irregularities in rhythm, especially if atrial in origin, should be examined for thyrotoxicosis.* Clues to the diagnosis include a relatively rapid circulation time and resistance to the usual doses of digitalis, but laboratory confirmation is required.

Differential diagnosis Signs and symptoms in a number of nonthyroid disorders may simulate certain aspects of the thyrotoxic syndrome. Anxiety is a prominent feature of thyrotoxicosis, and there is thus some overlap in the symptomatology of this disorder with that of anxiety states of emotional origin. Such symptoms as tachycardia, tremulousness, irritability, weakness, and fatigue are common to the anxiety of both disorders. In anxiety of emotional origin, however, the peripheral manifestations of excessive thyroid hormones are absent; the skin of the extremities is usually cold and clammy rather than warm and moist. Weight loss, when present in emotional anxiety, is characteristically accompanied by anorexia, whereas in thyrotoxicosis it is generally, but not invariably, accompanied by excessive appetite. Thyrotoxicosis can occasionally be confused with such disorders as metastatic carcinoma, cirrhosis of the liver, hyperparathyroidism, sprue, and neuromyopathies such as myasthenia gravis and muscular dystrophy. Hypokalemic periodic paralysis is more common in thyrotoxic patients, especially in the case of Oriental males. Signs and symptoms of thyrotoxicosis may overlap with those of pheochromocytoma, which may present with heat intolerance, excessive perspiration, tachycardia with palpitations, and a hypermetabolic state that may be severe. In all the above disorders, as well as other conditions considered in the differential diagnosis, judiciously applied laboratory tests usually suffice to differentiate them from thyrotoxicosis.

When bilateral ophthalmopathy is accompanied by goiter and thyrotoxicosis, the origin of the ophthalmopathy in the process is virtually certain. The presence of unilateral ophthalmopathy, even when associated with thyrotoxicosis, should alert the physician to the possibility of some other intraorbital or intracranial disease. In the patient who is not thyrotoxic, it is more difficult to ascribe ophthalmopathy to Graves' disease, and other causes must be excluded. Among the local causes of unilateral or bilateral exophthalmos are cavernous sinus thrombosis, sphenoidal ridge meningioma, and retrobulbar tumors, including leukemic deposits, as well as the rare granulomatous disorder, pseudotumor oculi. Exophthalmos may also be seen in some patients with certain systemic disorders, such as uremia, accelerated hypertension, chronic alcoholism, chronic obstructive pulmonary disease, superior mediastinal obstruction, and Cushing's syndrome. Ophthalmoplegia in the absence of overt infiltrative manifestations can be confused with that which occurs in diabetes mellitus, myasthenia gravis, and myopathies. When doubt exists about the cause of ophthalmopathy, the demonstration of an abnormal thyroid suppression test or TRH stimulation test suggests that the cause is Graves' disease, though not all patients with "euthyroid Graves' disease" will demonstrate abnormal responses. In such cases, ultrasonography or computerized axial tomography of the orbits is valuable in demonstrating characteristic thickening of the extraocular muscles.

When a thyrotoxic state occurs in a patient lacking the characteristic ophthalmopathy of Graves' disease, other causes of thyrotoxicosis must be considered. Careful palpation of the thyroid and studies with radioactive iodine are important in this regard. A symmetric, diffuse goiter of moderate or large size almost surely establishes a diagnosis of Graves' disease, especially if a bruit is present. However, the uncommon patient whose hyperthyroidism is secondary to an excess of TSH (usually associated with a *pituitary tumor*) or an abnormal stimulator of trophoblastic origin (*hydatidiform mole* or *choriocarcinoma of uterus or testis;* see Chap. 122) may present in this way. A single, prominent thyroid nodule or multiple nodules suggest *toxic adenoma* or *toxic multinodular goiter,* respectively. Tenderness of the thyroid associated with firm nodularity strongly suggests *subacute thyroiditis,* while a small, firm, nontender goiter is consistent with the syndrome of chronic thyroiditis with spontaneously resolving thyrotoxicosis. The foregoing disorders are discussed more fully in later sections. Absence of a palpable thyroid gland suggests an extrathyroid source of hormone, such as ectopic thyroid tissue *(struma ovarii)* or, more commonly, self-administration of hormone *(thyrotoxicosis factitia).* Studies with radioactive iodine are also helpful. Except when hormone overproduction is secondary to increased iodine intake, values of the RAIU are increased in all disorders producing hyperthyroidism, and scintillation scanning may aid in differentiating among them. Conversely, those forms of thyrotoxicosis that are not the result of hyperthyroidism are characterized by subnormal values of the RAIU. Among them, subacute thyroiditis and chronic thyroiditis with spontaneously resolving thyrotoxicosis are the more common. Ectopic thyroid tissue producing thyrotoxicosis is rare. Here, the RAIU, as measured over the thyroid, is low since TSH secretion is suppressed, but despite this, urinary excretion of the dose of ^{131}I is also low, owing to accumulation of ^{131}I by the ectopic tissue. Functioning ectopic tissue can be located by direct counting or scintillation scanning. Thyrotoxicosis factitia most frequently occurs in medical or paramedical personnel or in those who have easy access to thyroid hormone preparations. Physiologically, it resembles thyrotoxicosis caused by ectopic thyroid tissue in that the patient's thyroid gland is suppressed. By contrast, however, most of an administered dose of ^{131}I is excreted in the urine. When the disorder is caused by ingestion of preparations containing T_4, such as levothyroxine or thyroid extract, the serum T_4 is increased. On the other hand, when caused by liothyronine, the serum T_4 is subnormal. Irrespective of the preparation, the serum T_3 is increased but more so when liothyronine is the offending agent.

The demonstration of elevated titers of antithyroid antibodies or of TSI or TBII activity in the blood also provides strong evidence that Graves' disease is the cause of thyrotoxicosis.

Treatment HYPERTHYROIDISM The hyperthyroidism in Graves' disease is often characterized by cyclic phases of exacerbation and remission, each of unpredictable onset and duration. Moreover, in many patients, long-standing disease is associated with progressive thyroid failure, probably consequent to chronic thyroiditis, with the result that hypothyroidism or decreased thyroid reserve supervenes. These characteristics of Graves' disease have important implications in the choice of and response to therapy.

There are two major approaches to the treatment; both are directed to limiting the quantity of thyroid hormones the gland can produce. The first major therapeutic modality, the use of antithyroid agents, interposes a chemical blockade to hormone synthesis, the effect of which is operative only as long as the drug is administered or until a spontaneous remission occurs. Thus, the agents can control a given phase of active thyrotoxicity but probably do not prevent exacerbation at some subsequent period. The second major approach is ablation of thyroid tissue, thereby limiting hormone production. This may be achieved either surgically or by means of radioactive iodine. Since these procedures induce permanent anatomic alterations of the thyroid, they can control the individual active phase and are more likely to prevent recurrence of thyrotoxicity during a later exacerbation. On the other hand, the permanency of the effects of surgery or radiation makes these modes of therapy capable of leading to hypothyroidism, either shortly after treatment or with the passage of years.

Each therapy has advantages and disadvantages, indications and contraindications. The latter are more often relative than absolute. In general, a trial of long-term antithyroid therapy is desirable in children, adolescents, young adults, and pregnant women but may also be employed in older patients. Indications for ablative procedures include relapse or recurrence following drug therapy, a large goiter, drug toxicity, and failure of the patient to follow a medical regimen or to return for periodic examinations. Subtotal thyroidectomy is usually elected for patients under the age of 40 in whom ablative therapy is required; however, opinions differ, and some authorities employ radioactive iodine in the treatment of patients in the second or third decades. With older patients, radioactive iodine is clearly the ablative procedure of choice, as it is for patients who have had previous thyroid surgery or those in whom serious systemic disease contraindicates elective surgery.

In those patients selected for *long-term antithyroid therapy,* satisfactory control can almost always be achieved if a sufficient dosage of the drug is administered. Most patients can be managed successfully with propylthiouracil, 100 to 150 mg every 6 or 8 h. In occasional patients whose disease is severe, larger doses are required for initial control. Methimazole is at least as effective as propylthiouracil when administered in one-tenth the dosage. Once euthyroidism is achieved, the daily dosage may be reduced to the smallest doses that control the thyrotoxicosis fully. In some clinics, however, the initial dose is continued and is supplemented with levothyroxine. By this latter regimen, hypothyroidism resulting from overdosage of antithyroid drugs can be prevented. The undesirable consequences of hypothyroidism, such as enhancement of ophthalmopathy and enlargement of the goiter, may thereby be forestalled. The precise duration of therapy is difficult to predict in the individual patient and may be a function of the spontaneous course of the disease itself. If this is the case, the longer the course of therapy, the more likely it is that the patient will remain well when the drug is discontinued, and recent studies have shown this to be the case. In general, however, a 12- to 24-month course is employed, following which about one-third or one-half of the patients remain well for a prolonged period or indefinitely. The likelihood of a prolonged remission is increased by a lessening of goiter size, reversion of the thyroid suppression test to normal, or disappearance of Graves' disease–related immunoglobulins (TSI and TBII) from the serum during treatment.

Leukopenia is the principal undesirable side effect of antithyroid drugs. Mild transient leukopenia may occur in approximately 10 percent of patients treated and is not necessarily an indication for discontinuing therapy. When the absolute number of polymorphonuclear leukocytes reaches 1500 or less, antithyroid medication should be discontinued. Allergic rashes and drug sensitivity develop in a small percentage of patients. These may disappear with antihistamine therapy at the same or reduced dosage of antithyroid agent, but it is probably preferable when sensitivity reactions occur to change to another drug. On rare occasions (in less than 0.2 percent), agranulocytosis may occur. This may be sudden in onset. Hepatitis, drug fever, and arthralgias are occasional adverse reactions to antithyroid agents. In the authors' view, such severe sensitivity reactions, including, of course, agranulocytosis, dictate the abandonment of antithyroid therapy, rather than recourse to an alternate drug.

Iodide inhibits the release of hormones from the hyperfunctioning thyroid gland, and its ameliorative effects occur more rapidly than those of agents that merely inhibit hormone synthesis. Hence, its main use is in patients with actual or impending thyrotoxic crisis or in patients with severe thyrocardiac disease. However, the response to iodide is often incomplete and transient. Furthermore, by expanding the thyroid store of hormone, iodide may prolong greatly the latency of response to subsequently instituted antithyroid therapy. Therefore, iodide should be used in conjunction with the antithyroid agents. If the clinical course of the patient is sufficiently severe to require iodide administration, antithyroid drugs will usually be the primary therapeutic agents and should be given in large doses prior to iodide. Since iodide appears to synergize with radiation in the thyroid, it is also useful in controlling thyrotoxicosis following ^{131}I administration, during the period in which the therapeutic effect of radioiodine has not yet taken place. By a poorly understood mechanism, large doses of *glucocorticoids* (2 mg of dexamethasone every 6 h) sharply reduce the serum T_4 concentration, and should be added to the regimen when relief of thyrotoxicosis is urgent.

Owing to the pronounced adrenergic component in thyrotoxicosis, various *adrenergic antagonists* have been employed in the management of this disorder. Of these, propranolol appears to be the agent of choice because of its relative freedom from side effects. In doses of 40 to 120 mg daily, propranolol alleviates such adrenergic manifestations as sweating, tremor, and tachycardia and may reduce to some extent the conversion of T_4 to T_3. However, propranolol should be used only as adjunctive therapy rather than sole therapy, as some have suggested, since the underlying metabolic abnormalities are not significantly affected. Moreover, although the diminution in heart rate and cardiac work that propranolol induces may be beneficial, the withdrawal of adrenergic support of myocardial contractility contraindicates its use in the patient with coexisting heart failure, unless rate- or rhythm-related. As adjunctive therapy, propranolol has its major usefulness in the period during which the response to conventional antithyroid agents or to radioiodine therapy is being awaited and in the management of thyrotoxic crisis. It has also been employed as the sole agent in preparation for thyroidectomy. However, since it does not render the patient euthyroid, with a likely greater risk of surgically induced crisis, its use in this setting is not recommended.

Radioactive iodine (*^{131}I*) affords a relatively simple, effective, and economical means of treating thyrotoxicosis. Its major advantage is that it can produce the ablative effects of surgery without the immediate operative and postoperative complications. The principal disadvantage of ^{131}I therapy, in the dosage which has usually been employed, is its tendency to produce hypothyroidism with a frequency that increases progressively with time. As many as 40 to 70 percent of patients may develop this complication by 10 years after treatment. Although hypothyroidism is readily treated, once diagnosed, the insidious onset of the disorder may obscure the diagnosis until serious complications have developed. Hence, some recommend that all patients be treated with large doses of ^{131}I to ensure relief of thyrotoxicosis and then be placed on permanent physiologic replacement doses of thyroid hormone.

Studies to the point have provided no evidence of carcinogenic or leukemogenic effects of radioiodine when it is given to adults in the doses commonly used in treating hyperthyroidism. There is, however, some question of whether the susceptibility to carcinogenesis is increased in the thyroids of children. Mutagenic effects have not been reported but are difficult to evaluate. For these reasons, many physicians prefer to reserve radioiodine therapy for patients over 30 years of age or those unlikely to have children subsequently. Moreover, the longer the patient's life expectancy after ^{131}I therapy, the greater the likelihood that hypothyroidism will develop. Among younger patients, therefore, those with recurrent thyrotoxicosis following surgery, those who refuse surgery, and those with complicating illness that contraindicates surgery are candidates for radioiodine therapy. In elderly patients, treatment with large doses of radioiodine is the general method of choice, so that the undesirable effects of incomplete treatment or recurrence can be avoided.

The usual therapeutic dose of ^{131}I [approximately 5.92 MBq (160 μCi) per gram of estimated gland weight] is the dose that has led to the disturbingly high frequency of hypothyroidism. As a result, though continuing to use this dose, some authorities regularly administer prophylactic replacement doses of thyroid hormone. On the other hand, others have been led to administer smaller doses [approximately 2.96 MBq/g (80 μCi/g)]. However, this does not diminish the frequency of late hypothyroidism but merely delays its onset. Moreover, the smaller dose is less likely to relieve thyrotoxicosis within a relatively short period. Antithyroid agents can be employed, however, to speed the attainment of a eumetabolic state, and propranolol can be given to relieve symptoms, while the effect of the ^{131}I is taking hold. There is general agreement that patients with thyrocardiac disease should receive ^{131}I in large doses in view of the hazard of recurrent thyrotoxicosis.

Radiation thyroiditis is an occasional immediate complication of ^{131}I therapy. When present, it commonly appears within 7 to 10 days and is associated with excessive release of hormone into the blood. For this reason, patients with severe hyperthyroidism or underlying heart disease should be rendered eumetabolic with antithyroid agents before ^{131}I is administered. Interruption of antithyroid therapy for several days before and after ^{131}I treatment suffices to permit adequate accumulation and retention of administered ^{131}I. Propranolol may be used as an adjunct both before and after ^{131}I administration but should not be relied upon to provide adequate prophylaxis if given alone. The swelling that accompanies radiation thyroiditis may contraindicate the use of large doses of ^{131}I in patients with large retrosternal goiters.

Before radioactive iodine was introduced, *subtotal thyroidectomy* was the standard form of ablative therapy, and it is still widely employed in younger patients in whom antithyroid therapy is unsuccessful. Although precise preoperative programs differ, several general principles should be emphasized. Patients should first be rendered fully euthyroid by means of antithyroid agents. Only then should iodide (five drops of Lugol's solution a day for approximately 10 days) be administered concomitantly to effect an involutional response in the gland. Antithyroid drugs should not be discontinued merely because treatment with iodide is instituted. The response of the patient, and not the calendar, should dictate when surgery is performed.

Hazards of subtotal thyroidectomy include immediate complications, such as anesthetic accidents, hemorrhage sometimes leading to respiratory obstruction, and damage to the recurrent laryngeal nerve leading to vocal cord paralysis. Later complications include wound infection, hemorrhage, hypoparathyroidism, or hypothyroidism. In experienced hands, surgery is an effective and relatively safe mode of therapy. Postoperative recurrences are quite uncommon. However, carefully conducted follow-up studies reveal that hypothyroidism follows surgery more frequently than previously suspected, although not as commonly as following treatment with ^{131}I.

The *treatment of hyperthyroidism during pregnancy* is a subject of some disagreement. Most physicians believe that antithyroid therapy is preferable to surgery, which should not be performed in any event during the first and third trimesters. The major disadvantage of antithyroid therapy is the possibility of inducing hypothyroidism in the fetus, since antithyroid agents readily traverse the placenta. T_4 and T_3 traverse the human placenta from mother to fetus only slowly, if at all, and simultaneous administration of thyroid hormone and antithyroid drugs to the mother will not protect the fetus from developing hypothyroidism. Hence, the cardinal rule in using the antithyroid agents in pregnancy is that the dosage should be the smallest necessary to control hyperthyroidism in the mother. From the laboratory standpoint, the physician should aim to keep the serum FT_4 concentration or the FT_4I well within the normal limits, remembering that pregnancy is normally associated with some elevation of the serum total T_4, owing to an increase in serum TBG concentration. Since pregnancy appears to attenuate the severity of hyperthyroidism, this can often be achieved with maintenance doses of 200 mg of propylthiouracil daily or less. At this dose level, fetal goiter or hypothyroidism has not been a problem. Patients who require doses of 300 mg daily or more during the first trimester should probably be treated by subtotal thyroidectomy during the middle trimester. Although some would disagree, the authors believe that patients carried through pregnancy on antithyroid agents should not be given propranolol as adjunctive treatment, in view of reports of fetal growth retardation and neonatal depression. Radioiodine should never be administered to a pregnant woman, and the authors believe that all women of childbearing age who are about to receive a therapeutic dose of ^{131}I should have a pregnancy test performed first.

OPHTHALMOPATHY, DERMOPATHY When severe and progressive, ophthalmopathy is the most difficult component of Graves' disease to treat satisfactorily. Fortunately, however, in most patients the disorder runs a benign course that is largely independent of the course of the hyperthyroid component. In most instances, the activity of even moderately severe disease declines and disappears with time, although some exophthalmos and ophthalmoplegia may persist. In mild disease, considerable benefit may be obtained from simple measures, such as elevating the head at night, administering diuretics to reduce edema, and providing tinted glasses for protection from sun, wind, and foreign bodies. A 1% solution of methylcellulose or plastic shields may help to prevent corneal drying in patients unable to oppose the lids during sleep. In more severe cases, as evidenced by progressive exophthalmos, chemosis, ophthalmoplegia, or loss of vision, large doses of prednisone (120 to 140 mg daily) should be administered, since this is usually effective in reducing the edematous and infiltrative components. With improvement, the dosage is reduced to the lowest effective level, since prolonged administration of large doses leads to adverse accompaniments of glucocorticoid excess. Orbital radiation may be helpful in some patients with acute, severe infiltrative manifestations. In cases that progress despite these measures, orbital decompression, i.e., removal of part of the bony orbit to relieve intraorbital pressure, usually halts progression of the disease. The management must always be conducted in concert with an ophthalmologist.

In general, treatment of associated hyperthyroidism should be carried out much as would be the case were ophthalmopathy not present, since there is no convincing evidence that the mode of treatment of the hyperthyroidism influences the course of the ocular disease. The suggestion that total thyroid ablation by surgery and large doses of ^{131}I is beneficial to the ophthalmic disease has not been borne out. It is agreed, however, that hyperthyroidism should be treated and that hypothyroidism be avoided.

Severe dermopathy can be alleviated by the topical application of glucocorticoids.

TOXIC MULTINODULAR GOITER

Toxic multinodular goiter is a not infrequent consequence of long-standing simple goiter, although the exact proportion of cases in which this complication arises is uncertain. In areas of nonendemicity, the specific etiology of nontoxic multinodular goiter is usually indeterminate. Hence, it is unclear whether a specific etiologic factor underlies those cases of nontoxic multinodular goiter that progress to thyrotoxic phase. Common to many nontoxic multinodular goiters, even in areas of iodine sufficiency, is a decrease in the iodine content of thyroglobulin, suggesting either a conditioned deficiency of iodine or an impairment of pathways for its normal incorporation into iodinated amino acids. Pathologically, there is nothing to distinguish the nontoxic from the toxic multinodular goiter. Functionally, however, the transition from nontoxic to toxic nodular goiter involves the development of autonomy, i.e., independence from TSH stimulation in one or more areas of the gland. Even among seemingly euthyroid patients with nontoxic nodular goiter, approximately a fourth display, as evidence of functional autonomy, subnormal or absent responses to TRH administration. As judged from radioautographic and scintillation scanning studies, functional patterns may be of two types. In the first and more common, iodine accumulation occurs diffusely but in patchy foci throughout the gland. Histologically, associated areas reveal cellular hyperplasia. The second, less common, pattern is that of iodine accumulation in one or more discrete nodules within the gland, the remainder being essentially nonfunctional. Whether the former represent true adenomas or are merely colloid nodules that have developed functional autonomy is also uncertain. In both endemic and sporadic nontoxic multinodular goiter, administration of iodides may lead to the development of thyrotoxicosis, implying that areas of potentially autonomous function had been present.

Because it arises in long-standing simple goiter, toxic multinodular goiter is a disease of the aging or elderly. For this reason and because of the nature of the underlying disease, the clinical presentation differs from that in Graves' disease. Ophthalmopathy is rare and would signal the emergence of Graves' disease superimposed on simple goiter. Some patients may present with quite typical thyrotoxicosis. Often, however, the degree of thyrotoxicosis is less severe than that seen in Graves' disease, although its physiologic impact upon specific organ systems may be great. Notable among these is the cardiovascular system, in which arrhythmias or congestive failure may be precipitated or accentuated by thyrotoxicosis that not infrequently is manifested only by subtle findings in other areas (apathetic hyperthyroidism). Weakness and wasting may predominate, frequently with loss of appetite rather than hyperphagia, suggesting the presence of a carcinoma.

A nodular goiter that is readily visible or palpable will establish the diagnosis. In some instances, however, the thyroid gland is not detectably enlarged. Nevertheless, if suggestive clinical findings are present, the physician is obligated to establish or to exclude the presence of thyrotoxicosis. This is often difficult, since results of conventional laboratory tests are frequently in the borderline range, consistent with the mild degree of thyrotoxicity. However, a value for the serum T_3 that would be considered normal for a young adult may represent an increase in the elderly patient, since values for serum T_3 usually decline with age. Despite their great value in situations such as this, thyroid suppression tests should not be undertaken in the elderly patient because of the hazard of adverse cardiovascular responses. Unfortunately, although a normal response to TRH would exclude a diagnosis of thyrotoxicosis in a patient with a nodular goiter, subnormal responses do not establish the diagnosis. Not only do responses to TRH decline in the elderly, especially in men, but a high proportion of patients with nodular goiter who otherwise seem quite euthyroid also respond subnormally to TRH as a reflection of at least partial functional autonomy of the thyroid gland. When laboratory findings do not permit a clear diagnosis of thyrotoxicosis but suggestive clinical findings are present, a therapeutic trial of antithyroid drugs is indicated.

Radioactive iodine is the treatment of choice for toxic multinodular goiter, once the diagnosis has been established. Large doses [740 to 1110 MBq (20 to 30 mCi)] are usually required, owing to the generally lower RAIU and to the variable degree of function throughout the gland. Moreover, the physiologic instability of the elderly patient makes definitive treatment desirable. For the same reason, it is usually wise to initiate therapy with antithyroid agents, withholding radioiodine until a euthyroid state has been achieved and thereby forestalling an exacerbation of thyrotoxicosis, should radiation thyroiditis occur. Unless contraindicated, propranolol is often useful in controlling manifestations of thyrotoxicosis both before and after radioiodine therapy, while its therapeutic effect is awaited. Hypothyroidism is an uncommon consequence of radioiodine treatment of toxic multinodular goiter, owing to the variable activity of differing portions of the gland, which permits previously quiescent areas to replace functionally those that have been destroyed by ^{131}I.

T_3 TOXICOSIS T_3 toxicosis is thyrotoxicosis in which serum T_4 is normal or low in the absence of a deficiency of TBG, while the serum T_3 is increased. Although the production rate of T_3 is disproportionately increased relative to that of T_4 in all patients with hyperthyroidism, in some this discrepancy is greatly exaggerated. This may occur in association with Graves' disease, multinodular goiter, or hyperfunctioning adenoma. The diagnosis should be suspected in a patient with clinical manifestations of thyrotoxicosis in whom the serum T_4 and FT_4 are normal or low and the RAIU is normal or increased. This, together with the frequently palpable goiter, serves to differentiate this disorder from liothyronine-induced thyrotoxicosis factitia. In contradistinction from patients with nonthyroidal disorders mimicking thyrotoxicosis, patients with this disorder, as would be expected, demonstrate nonsuppressibility of thyroid function in response to exogenous T_3 and blunted or absent responses to TRH. In some patients, thyrotoxicosis with increased serum T_3 and normal serum T_4 antecedes emergence of typical increases in both, either during an initial episode of hyperthyroidism or more commonly during recurrence after previous treatment. In some patients in whom symptoms of thyrotoxicosis fail to regress completely during antithyroid therapy despite normalization of the serum T_4 concentration, the serum T_3 concentration is persistently elevated.

T_4 TOXICOSIS In most patients with hyperthyroidism, the serum T_3 is increased to a relatively greater extent than is the serum T_4. This reflects the fact that in hyperthyroidism T_3 generated from T_4 peripherally is supplemented by release of substantial quantities of T_3 from the thyroid. However, patients are sometimes seen in whom thyrotoxicosis is associated with a clear elevation of serum T_4 and a seemingly normal serum T_3 concentration. This syndrome of *T_4 toxicosis* has been reported most commonly in patients who are elderly, ill, or both, and who are, therefore, commonly seen in a hospital setting. Presumably, the combination of high serum T_4 and normal serum T_3 concentration reflects inhibition of peripheral T_3 generation from T_4, with persistence of T_3 secretion along with T_4 from the thyroid.

JODBASEDOW PHENOMENON This term refers to the induction of thyrotoxicosis in a previously euthyroid patient as a result of exposure to increased quantities of iodine. Classically, it occurs in areas of endemic iodine deficiency when measures to increase iodine intake or body iodine stores are implemented. The presumption is that the supplemental iodine permits functionally autonomous thyroid tissue to produce and secrete excessive hormone. A similar phenomenon can occur in areas of environmental iodine sufficiency in patients with nontoxic multinodular goiter who have received large doses of iodide. Since such patients tend to be elderly with the danger of serious cardiovascular manifestations should thyrotoxicosis ensue, large doses of iodine should not be given to those with multinodular goiter. Similarly, in such patients, pharmaceuticals containing iodine, such as x-ray contrast media, should be used only when indicated and with consideration of the possible hazard of inducing the jodbasedow phenomenon. Some patients may develop hypothyroidism following exposure to large quantities of iodine despite the fact that after iodine is withdrawn and they have recovered, their thyroid function appears to be entirely normal and evidence of functional autonomy is lacking.

MAJOR COMPLICATIONS OF THYROTOXICOSIS

THYROCARDIAC DISEASE Thyrotoxicosis imposes a variety of burdens upon the heart. Hypermetabolism of the peripheral tissues increases both the metabolic and nonmetabolic (heat-loss) circulatory load, while direct effects of thyroid hormone on the myocardium increase the force, velocity, and rate of ventricular contraction. As a result, cardiac work and cardiac output are increased. Moreover, atrial irritability is enhanced, leading to tachydysrhythmias, most importantly atrial fibrillation. In the patient with a normal heart, these burdens are usually, but not invariably, tolerated. In the patient with underlying heart disease, however, cardiac insufficiency may be precipitated or aggravated. As would be expected, this complication is more common in the elderly patient and is usually seen, therefore, in the patient with toxic multinodular goiter, not infrequently as the most prominent manifestation of the thyrotoxic state.

In patients with cardiac insufficiency, clues to the presence of thyrotoxicosis include atrial fibrillation, relatively rapid circulation time, increased cardiac output (high-output failure), and resistance to the usual therapeutic doses of digitalis.

Treatment is directed at both rapid alleviation of thyrotoxicosis and restoration of cardiac compensation. The former objective is best met by initiation of treatment with large doses of an antithyroid agent, followed by iodine if the clinical situation is urgent. In less severe cases, radioiodine treatment is anteceded by antithyroid drug treatment alone. Management of the cardiac decompensation is carried out in the usual manner, employing larger than usual doses of digitalis but with care to avoid digitalis intoxication as the thyrotoxicosis is alleviated. Adrenergic antagonists should not be employed in the presence of cardiac failure, unless it is felt that failure is the consequence primarily of disturbance of cardiac rate or rhythm.

THYROTOXIC CRISIS The clinical picture of thyrotoxic crisis or storm is that of a fulminating increase in all the signs and symptoms of thyrotoxicosis. In the past, this disturbance was most often observed postoperatively in patients poorly prepared for surgery. However, with the preoperative use of antithyroid drugs and iodide and with appropriate measures directed to control of metabolic factors, weight, and nutritional status, postoperative thyrotoxic crisis should not occur. At present, so-called medical storm is more common and occurs in untreated or inadequately treated patients. It is precipitated by surgical emergency or complicating medical illness, usually sepsis. The syndrome is characterized by extreme irritability, delirium or coma, fever to 41.1°C (106°F) or more, tachycardia, restlessness, hypotension, vomiting, and diarrhea. Rarely, the clinical picture may be more subtle, with apathy, severe prostration, and coma, but with only slight elevation of temperature. Such postoperative complications as sepsis, septicemia, hemorrhage, and transfusion or drug reactions may mimic thyrotoxic crisis. It is thought that in some patients thyrotoxic crisis is associated with or precipitated by adrenocortical insufficiency. The possibility of this complication gains support from evidence indicating increased adrenocortical hormone requirements in thyrotoxicosis and from evidence of reduced adrenocortical reserve in this disorder.

Treatment of this most serious disorder consists in providing general supportive therapy while undertaking measures for alleviating thyrotoxicosis as rapidly as possible. Supportive therapy includes treatment of dehydration and the intravenous administration of glucose and saline, vitamin B complex, and glucocorticoids. Patients should be placed in a cooled, humidified oxygen tent, and, if hyperpyrexia is present, a cooling blanket should be used. Digitalization is required in the presence of cardiac failure. If shock exists, intravenous pressor agents should be employed. Therapy of the hyperthyroidism consists of induction of blockade of hormone synthesis by the immediate and continued administration of large doses of an antithyroid agent (e.g., 100 mg propylthiouracil every 2 h). If the patient is unable to swallow the medication, the tablets should be triturated and given by nasogastric tube, as parenteral preparations are unavailable. Following initiation of antithyroid therapy, inhibition of hormone release is sought through the administration of large doses of iodine intravenously or by mouth. Adrenergic antagonists are an important, and perhaps critical, part of the therapeutic regimen, in the absence of cardiac failure. The beta-adrenergic blocking agent propranolol can be administered in doses of 40 to 80 mg every 6 h. If medications cannot be taken orally, 2 mg of propranolol may be given intravenously, with careful electrocardiographic monitoring. Large doses of dexamethasone (e.g., 2 mg every 6 h) should also be administered, since they have been shown both to inhibit hormone release and to impair the peripheral generation of T_3 from T_4, in addition to providing adrenal support. Indeed, the combined use of propylthiouracil, iodine, and dexamethasone will generally normalize the serum T_3 concentration within 24 to 48 h. Antithyroid therapy, iodine, and dexamethasone must be continued until a normal metabolic state is approached, at which time iodine is progressively withdrawn and plans for a definitive regimen of treatment made.

NEOPLASMS

THYROID ADENOMAS True adenomas, as contrasted with localized adenomatous areas, are encapsulated and usually compress contiguous tissue. Adenomas vary greatly in size and histologic characteristics and are often classified into three major types: papillary, follicular, and Hürthle cell. The follicular adenomas can be subdivided according to the size of the follicles into colloid or macrofollicular, fetal or microfollicular, and embryonal varieties. There is considerable variation in physiologic differentiation, as judged by their ability to concentrate radioiodine. The more highly differentiated adenomas (follicular) are the most common and are the most likely to mimic the function of normal thyroid tissue. Though their function may be responsive to TSH stimulation, it differs from that of normal thyroid tissue in being autonomous, i.e., the basal activity is independent of TSH stimulation. Adenomas of this type are usually unifocal, presenting as a single nodule. Often the patient reports that the nodule has been growing slowly over many years. Initially, its function is insufficient to disturb hormonal equilibrium though its capacity to accumulate radioiodine is evident in scintiscans as an area of increased density within the still-functioning extranodular tissue (*"warm" nodule*). At this stage, demonstration of the inherent autonomy of the nodule's function requires scintiscanning while the patient is receiving suppressive doses of exogenous thyroid hormone (suppression scan). With time the nodule grows larger, its function increasing until it is sufficient to suppress TSH secretion. Consequently, the remainder of the gland undergoes atrophy and loss of function, and the scintiscan then reveals radioiodine accumulation only in the region of the nodule (*"hot" nodule*). At this time, the patient may or may not appear overtly thyrotoxic, but frank thyrotoxicosis usually supervenes eventually (*toxic adenoma*). Relative to its overall rate of occurrence, hyperfunctioning adenoma is a frequent cause of T_3 toxicosis. Hyperfunctioning adenomas are readily amenable to ablation by surgery or ^{131}I. Large doses of the latter are usually required to bring about prompt cure. Before such treatment it is desirable to administer TSH and demonstrate by scintiscan the latent functional capacity of the extranodular tissue. Although it has been thought that radiation damage would be confined solely to the hyperfunctioning nodule being treated with ^{131}I, the remaining tissue being spared, this may not always be the case, since some patients with hyperfunctioning adenoma become euthyroid after treatment with ^{131}I only to become hypothyroid years later.

Hyperfunctioning nodules are only rarely the seat of carcinoma. However, hyperfunctioning adenomas not infrequently undergo hemorrhagic necrosis; this results in loss of function and the appearance of a *"cold" nodule* on scintiscanning, since the remainder of the thyroid will have resumed function. When this happens, the nodule is likely to be mistaken for a carcinoma. Indeed, hypofunctioning, hemorrhagic adenomas account for the majority of cold nodules initially suspected of being carcinomas.

THYROID CARCINOMAS Thyroid carcinoma may be classified into two varieties, depending upon whether the lesion arises in thyroid follicular epithelium or whether it arises from the parafollicular or C cells. Since the latter disorder, medullary thyroid carcinoma, has distinctive physiologic and clinical characteristics, it is discussed separately (see Chap. 123). The thyroid may also be the site of one or another of the lymphoproliferative diseases or of carcinoma metastatic from a diagnosed or undiagnosed primary tumor elsewhere.

Carcinomas of follicular epithelium These are of three general histologic types which differ in their clinical course. The least common is *anaplastic carcinoma,* which is histologically undifferentiated, usually afflicts the elderly, and is highly malignant. Usually the lesion is rapidly fatal, owing to extensive local invasion which is refractory to radiation. The second type of tumor, *follicular carcinoma,* is also uncommon and histologically closely mimics normal thyroid tissue. This lesion usually undergoes early hematogenous spread, and hence the patient may present with a distant metastasis, usually in lung or bone. Follicular carcinoma or follicular elements in papillary carcinoma are responsible for those instances in which thyroid carcinoma, in situ or in metastases, accumulates significant quantities of ^{131}I. The third and most common type of tumor, *papillary carcinoma,* has a bimodal frequency, peaks occurring in the second or third decades and again in later life. This lesion is usually slowly growing and typically spreads to the regional lymph nodes, where it may remain indolent for many years. Although more common in the older patient, acceleration of the disease may take place at any time. Follicular elements are usually present in both the primary lesion and its metastases.

DIAGNOSIS AND MANAGEMENT The diagnosis and management of thyroid carcinoma are closely interwoven with the management of the nodular goiter. In the past, this subject has been one that evoked a wide disparity of views among authorities, stemming largely from seemingly contradictory data. On the one hand, surgically excised specimens of thyroid nodules, particularly solitary nodules, revealed a high frequency of carcinoma (as much as 20 percent in some series). On the other hand, despite the frequency of nodular goiter in the general population (approximately 4 percent), the frequency of thyroid carcinoma, either newly diagnosed or as a cause of death, is very low. These respective data led to either vigorous or conservative approaches to the management of nodular goiter. It now appears that this discordance can be explained, by the ability of the physician, even then, to select for surgery those patients who were at high risk of harboring thyroid carcinoma, with consequent weighting of statistics derived from surgical series. This capability has increased still further, the as yet unrealized aim being to operate on only those patients whose thyroids harbor carcinoma and to avoid surgery in patients whose thyroids do not.

The clinical features that suggest the presence of thyroid carcinoma are rather well defined. Recent growth of a thyroid nodule or mass, especially if rapid and unaccompanied by tenderness and hoarseness, are sources of suspicion. Of particular importance is a history of x-ray to the head or neck or upper mediastinum in infancy or childhood, since this is associated with a high incidence of thyroid disease, including carcinoma, later in life. Nodular disease is particularly common in individuals so exposed, being found in approximately 20 percent of patients at risk, and may not be apparent until 30 years or more after the radiation exposure. Among patients in this group who have palpable nodules, approximately a third have thyroid carcinoma at surgery, often multicentric and sometimes metastatic.

Skillful palpation of the thyroid provides crucially important information. A nodule in an otherwise normal gland (solitary nodule) creates far more suspicion of thyroid tumor than does one nodule among many, since the latter is more likely to be part of a diffuse process, such as simple goiter. In addition, carcinomas are usually very firm or hard in consistency and nontender. Fixation to surrounding structures and lymphadenopathy are late features. Since purely cystic lesions, especially those that are less than a few centimeters in diameter, are less likely to reflect malignancy than solid lesions, transillumination is sometimes helpful, but ultrasonograms (see below) are particularly so. Age and sex of the patient also influence the clinical decision. Benign nodular lesions are more common in women than in men, malignant nodular lesions less so. Hence, nodular lesions in men create more suspicion of carcinoma than in women. Further, multinodular goiter is a disease of older age and predominantly of women. Thus, a solitary nodule is particularly suspect, especially if it occurs in a young woman or in a man of any age, except the most elderly.

Laboratory tests are of little assistance in differentiating between malignant and nonmalignant thyroid nodules. Overall thyroid function is usually normal. Except in patients with medullary thyroid carcinoma, in whom serum calcitonin concentrations may be elevated, tumor markers are of little value. Elevations of serum thyroglobulin are present in many patients with differentiated thyroid carcinoma but are not useful in the initial diagnosis, since they are often elevated in patients with benign adenoma, simple goiter, or Graves' disease. Soft-tissue x-rays of the neck may be of assistance, since finely stippled calcification within the thyroid suggests the presence of psammoma bodies within a papillary carcinoma.

Scintillation scanning is a keystone in the approach to the management of the patient with nodular goiter. Although only approximately 20 percent of nonfunctioning thyroid nodules prove to be malignant, demonstration that a nodule is cold adds substantial weight to the other factors suggesting carcinoma. On the other hand, nodules that are hyperfunctioning are rarely malignant. Ultrasonograms of the thyroid have value in demonstrating whether nodules are cystic, solid, or a mixture of the two. Cystic nodules can be aspirated, a procedure that is often curative, but their contents should be subjected to cytopathologic examination. Solid or mixed lesions are consistent with tumor but may be either benign or malignant.

At this point in the evaluation, the physician must decide whether to continue to observe the patient; whether to administer suppressive doses of thyroid hormone in the hope that the suspect nodule will shrink or disappear, a hope that in the authors' experience is usually unrealized; whether to obtain a closed biopsy; or whether to proceed to excisional biopsy and thyroidectomy. There are some patients in whom the authors choose the latter course. In general, these include patients with a history of radiation to the thyroid and one or more clearly palpable nodules, as well as young men and women with solitary cold nodules, particularly if hard, nontender, and changing rapidly in size. In the remainder, the authors recommend either aspiration or cutting-needle biopsy. The former is simpler to learn, free of complications, and applicable to smaller nodules. Optimum application of that technique rests upon the availability of experienced histopathologic interpretation of the specimen obtained. When such is available, aspiration biopsy provides a reliable means of differentiating between benign and malignant nodules in all except highly cellular lesions or follicular lesions, where evidence of vascular invasion may be required to differentiate benign from malignant forms. Despite the occasional occurrence of false-positives and -negatives, the procedure can reduce the number of operations performed for nodules that prove to be benign. Further, a diagnosis of carcinoma permits planning of the surgery to be undertaken preoperatively and is often useful in providing an impetus to surgery when the patient or physician is uncertain if surgery should be performed.

Surgery for thyroid carcinoma should be performed by a surgeon experienced in the field. Several weeks of suppressive therapy with levothyroxine is sometimes recommended preoperatively to facilitate the operative procedure and possibly to reduce the likelihood of tumor dissemination. In patients in whom a definitive preoperative diagnosis, as by biopsy, has not been made, the suspected lesion is removed en bloc with a wide margin of surrounding tissue and is examined by frozen section. A diagnosis of carcinoma is an indication for a near-total thyroidectomy in view of the evidence both of frequent seeding of carcinoma through the gland by transglandular lymphatic spread and of a lower recurrence rate after this procedure than after simple lobectomy. Regional lymph nodes should be explored and removed if there is evidence of involvement, but radical neck dissection is not justified. If permanent sections reveal carcinoma when frozen section had failed to do so, secondary surgery should be undertaken to remove residual thyroid tissue. Shortly after surgery, liothyronine (75 to 100 μg daily) is substituted for levothyroxine, since it permits a more rapid return of TSH secretion. Two or three weeks later, a large scanning dose of ^{131}I [37–74 MBq (1 to 2 mCi)] is administered. If residual thyroid tissue is found, as is usually the case, a thyroid ablating dose of 1850 MBq (50 mCi) of ^{131}I is administered, but if functioning metastases are present, the dose is increased to 3700 MBq (100 mCi) of ^{131}I. Suppressive therapy with levothyroxine is reinstituted 24 to 48 h later. At yearly intervals, suppressive therapy is withdrawn according to the regimen described above and the scanning procedure is repeated. If functioning metastases are found, a further therapeutic dose of ^{131}I is administered. In the patient with known differentiated thyroid carcinoma, in whom the lesion and the thyroid have been excised, serum thyroglobulin measurements should be made at the time of each follow-up examination, as they may signal recurrence even if no functioning metastases are found. Discrete palpable lymph nodes that emerge during suppressive therapy are often best treated by surgical excision, regardless of whether or not they accumulate radioiodine. The foregoing procedures are repeated during ensuing years until the disease appears to have been eradicated. There is now clear evidence that a program of this nature, involving near-total thyroidectomy, long-term suppressive therapy, and treatment of functioning metastases with radioiodine reduces the recurrence rate and prolongs survival in patients with papillary carcinoma of the thyroid. Follicular carcinoma should be treated with at least equal vigor, though the results are generally less favorable. Treatment of anaplastic carcinoma is largely palliative; most patients with this disease die within 6 months from the time of diagnosis.

THYROIDITIS

Thyroiditis embraces several disorders of differing etiology. Two are exceedingly uncommon, *pyogenic thyroiditis* and *chronic fibrosing* (*Riedel's*) *thyroiditis.* Pyogenic thyroiditis is usually anteceded by a pyogenic infection elsewhere and is characterized by tenderness and swelling of the thyroid, redness and warmth of the overlying skin, and constitutional signs of infection. Treatment consists of antibiotic therapy, along with incisional drainage if a fluctuant area within the thyroid should occur. Riedel's thyroiditis is a rare disorder in which intense fibrosis of the thyroid and surrounding structures, leading to induration of the tissues of the neck, may be associated with mediastinal and retroperitoneal fibrosis. The principal importance of this disorder is that it requires differentiation from thyroid neoplasia.

SUBACUTE THYROIDITIS This disorder, which is also termed *granulomatous, giant-cell,* or *de Quervain's thyroiditis,* is a distinct disease that appears to be viral in origin.

Symptoms of thyroiditis usually follow those of an upper respiratory infection and most commonly comprise pronounced asthenia, malaise, and symptoms referable to stretching of the thyroid capsule, principally pain over the thyroid or pain referred to the lower jaw, ear, or occiput. Referred, rather than local, pain may predominate. These symptoms may smolder for many weeks before the correct diagnosis is suspected. Less commonly, the onset is acute, with severe pain over the thyroid, accompanied by fever and occasionally symptoms of thyrotoxicosis. Cardinal physical findings include exquisite tenderness and nodularity over the thyroid, which may be predominantly unilateral but which usually involves other areas of the gland. Although local or referred pain is the commonest symptom of subacute thyroiditis, occasional patients manifest other typical features of the disease but have no pain.

Two tests provide the hallmark of the disease from the laboratory standpoint: an inordinately increased erythrocyte sedimentation rate (ESR) and a markedly depressed RAIU. Values for the remaining tests depend upon the stage of the disease in which they are obtained. Early, many patients are at least mildly thyrotoxic owing to leakage of hormone from the gland. The serum T_4 and T_3 are high. Later in the disease, as glandular hormone is depleted, the patient may pass through a hypothyroid phase, in which serum T_4 and T_3 are low and TSH increased. Diagnosis of the thyrotoxic phase is especially troublesome in patients with the painless variant of the disorder, since the patient may be thought to have Graves' disease or toxic nodular goiter and therapy inappropriate for subacute thyroiditis may be instituted. Demonstration of a low RAIU serves to differentiate subacute thyroiditis from these other causes of hyperthyroidism in most instances. Differentiation of painless subacute thyroiditis from the syndrome of chronic thyroiditis with transient thyrotoxicosis is discussed in the section that follows.

If left untreated, the disorder may smolder for months, but eventually subsides with a return of normal thyroid function. In mild cases, aspirin suffices to control the symptoms. In more severe cases, glucocorticoid (prednisone, 20 to 40 mg daily) is generally effective. Propranolol can be used to control hyperthyroidism. Return of the RAIU to normal indicates the time at which therapy can be withdrawn without recurrence of symptoms.

CHRONIC THYROIDITIS WITH TRANSIENT THYROTOXICOSIS This term denotes a disorder in which a self-limited bout of thyrotoxicosis is associated with a histologic picture of chronic lymphocytic thyroiditis that differs from that of Hashimoto's disease. This syndrome has been variously designated as painless thyroiditis, silent thyroiditis, hyperthyroiditis, chronic thyroiditis with spontaneously resolving hyperthyroidism, or, as the authors prefer, chronic thyroiditis with transient thyrotoxicosis (CT/TT). Designations that imply the existence of hyperthyroidism are inappropriate, since ongoing production of thyroid hormone is negligible and the RAIU is greatly decreased.

The syndrome occurs in patients of any age, and although it occurs mainly in women, the female/male ratio is not as high as in Graves' disease. The disorder is characterized by manifestations of thyrotoxicosis that are usually mild but may be severe. The thyroid is nontender, firm, symmetrical, and enlarged only slightly or moderately, if at all. Laboratory features include elevations of the serum T_4 and T_3 concentrations consonant with the thyrotoxicosis but associated with a markedly depressed RAIU. The ESR is normal or only slightly elevated, rarely exceeding 50 mm/h, and antithyroid antibodies, when present, are present in low titer.

The etiology, pathogenesis, and pathophysiology of this disorder are unclear. Viral antibody titers show no characteristic patterns. It is presumed that thyrotoxicosis results from leakage of hormone from the gland, as in subacute thyroiditis. Low values for the RAIU are, in turn, thought to reflect mainly a resulting suppression of TSH secretion, since urinary iodine excretion is not elevated. Some degree of intrinsic malfunction is indicated, however, by failure of the RAIU to respond briskly to exogenous TSH stimulation.

Thyrotoxicosis in CT/TT is self-limited, usually abating within 2 to 5 months. Many patients have recurrent episodes of thyrotoxicosis of similar nature, sometimes following pregnancy. The thyrotoxic phase may be followed in several months by a phase of self-limited hypothyroidism. The latter, which has been noted particularly in the postpartum period, may be the only component of the disease that is diagnosed.

This disorder, in the thyrotoxic phase, needs differentiation, first from Graves' disease; this can be accomplished by demonstration of a depressed RAIU and absence of increased urinary iodine excretion. The latter serves also to exclude the jodbasedow syndrome. When these data are available, the disorder must be differentiated from other causes of thyrotoxicosis with a low RAIU, principally subacute thyroiditis. Lack of tenderness or nodularity of the thyroid and absence of marked elevation of the ESR tend to exclude the latter diagnosis. Patients with functioning ectopic thyroid tissue and thyrotoxicosis factitia characteristically respond to exogenous TSH stimulation with a brisk increase in RAIU. Definitive diagnosis of CT/TT can be made by thyroid biopsy.

Since the thyroid is not hyperfunctioning in this disorder, measures used in the treatment of hyperthyroidism are useless. Symptomatic treatment with propranolol or mild sedatives is administered until the thyrotoxicosis abates. In patients with frequently recurrent disease, thyroid ablation with ^{131}I during a period of remission followed by long-term replacement therapy has been advocated by some.

HASHIMOTO'S DISEASE This disorder, also termed *lymphadenoid goiter,* is a common chronic inflammatory disease of the thyroid in which autoimmune factors play a prominent role, occurring most frequently in women of middle age. It is, in addition, the most common cause of sporadic goiter in children. Evidence of the participation of autoimmune factors includes the lymphocytic infiltration of the gland, as well as the presence in the serum of increased concentrations of immunoglobulins and of antibodies directed against several components of thyroid tissue. Of these, the most important from the clinical standpoint are the antithyroglobulin antibody detected by the tanned red cell agglutination technique and the antimicrosomal antibody detected by immunofluorescence or complement fixation techniques. This disorder also coexists with inordinate frequency with other diseases of a presumed autoimmune nature, including pernicious anemia, Sjögren's syndrome, chronic active hepatitis, systemic lupus erythematosus, rheumatoid arthritis, nontuberculous Addison's disease, diabetes, and Graves' disease itself (see Chap. 123). These disorders, as well as Hashimoto's disease itself, also appear with unusual frequency in family members of patients with Hashimoto's disease.

Goiter is the outstanding feature. The enlargement involves the entire gland but not necessarily symmetrically. Typically, the consistency is rubbery, the margins are scalloped, and the general outline of the gland is preserved. The pyramidal lobe may be prominent. Early in the disease the patient is metabolically normal; however, even then decreased thyroid reserve is often manifest in an increase in serum TSH. The RAIU may be elevated early in the disease, reflecting the secretion of calorigenically inactive iodoproteins, but the serum T_4 and T_3 are normal and the patient is euthyroid. As the disease progresses, thyroid failure, at first subclinical, gradually supervenes owing to progressive replacement of thyroid parenchyma by lymphocytes or fibrous tissue. The thyroid failure is evident first in a rise in serum TSH concentration. With time, the serum T_4 concentration declines though the serum T_3 remains normal. Eventually, the serum T_3 concentration falls below normal, and the patient is frankly hypothyroid. High titers of antimicrosomal antibody are almost always present. High titers may also occur in other thyroid disorders, particularly primary thyroprivic hypothyroidism and Graves' disease but with lesser frequency. Although the foregoing findings usually suffice to permit a diagnosis, histologic confirmation by needle biopsy is occasionally required. In view of the frequency with which hypothyroidism is either present or eventually develops, treatment with replacement doses of levothyroxine is indicated. In some patients, such therapy is associated with regression of goiter.

REFERENCES

INGBAR SH, BORGES M: Peripheral metabolism of the thyroid hormones, in *Free Thyroid Hormones,* R Ekins et al (eds). Amsterdam, Excerpta Medica, 1979, p 17

KIDD A et al: Immunologic aspects of Graves' and Hashimoto's diseases. Metabolism 29:80, 1980

MAZZAFERRI EL et al: Papillary thyroid carcinoma: The impact of therapy in 576 patients. Medicine 56:171, 1977

MILLER JM et al: Diagnosis of thyroid nodules. Use of fine-needle aspiration and needle biopsy. JAMA 241:481, 1979

STERLING K: Thyroid hormone action at the cell level. N Engl J Med 300:117, 173, 1979

WITT JR et al: The approach to the irradiated thyroid. Surg Clin N Amer 59:45, 1979

112 DISEASES OF THE ADRENAL CORTEX

GORDON H. WILLIAMS
ROBERT G. DLUHY

BIOCHEMISTRY AND PHYSIOLOGY

STEROID NOMENCLATURE Steroids contain as their basic structure a cyclopentenoperhydrophenanthrane nucleus consisting of three 6-carbon hexane rings and a single 5-carbon pentane ring (D). The carbon atoms are numbered in a predetermined sequence beginning with ring A (Fig. 112-1). Adrenal steroids contain either 19 or 21 carbons. The C_{19} steroids have methyl groups at positions C-18 and C-19. C_{19} steroids that also have a ketone group at C-17 are termed *17-ketosteroids.* The C_{19} steroids have predominant androgenic activity. The C_{21} steroids are those which have a 2-carbon side chain (C-20 and C-21) attached at position 17 of the D ring and, in addition, have substituent methyl groups at C-18 and C-19. C_{21} steroids that also possess a hydroxyl group at position 17 are termed *17-hydroxycorticosteroids* or *17-hydroxycorticoids.* The C_{21} steroids may have either predominant glucocorticoid or mineralocorticoid properties. *Glucocorticoid* signifies a C_{21} steroid with predominant action on intermediary metabolism, and *mineralocorticoid* indicates a C_{21} steroid with predominant action on the metabolism of sodium and potassium.

BIOSYNTHESIS OF ADRENAL STEROIDS Cholesterol, derived from the diet and from endogenous synthesis via acetate, is the principal starting compound in steroidogenesis. The three major adrenal biosynthetic pathways lead to the production of glucocorticoids (cortisol), mineralocorticoids (aldosterone), and adrenal androgens (dehydroepiandrosterone). Separate zones of the adrenal cortex synthesize specific hormones, reflecting the capacity of each zone to carry out certain transformations and hydroxylations mediated by specific enzymes (Fig. 112-2). The outer (glomerulosa) zone is mainly involved in aldosterone biosynthesis, and the inner (fasciculata-reticularis) zone is mainly involved in cortisol and androgen biosynthesis.

STEROID TRANSPORT Some of the steroid hormones, e.g., testosterone and cortisol, appear to circulate to a considerable extent bound to plasma proteins. Cortisol occurs in the plasma in three forms: free cortisol, protein-bound cortisol, and cortisol metabolites. *Free cortisol* refers to that quantity which is physiologically active but not protein-bound and, therefore, represents a form of cortisol acting directly on tissue sites. Normally, less than 5 percent of circulating cortisol is free. The diffusible fraction is estimated to range between 0.7 and 1.0 μg/dl. Only the unbound cortisol and its metabolites are filtrable at the glomerulus. Greater than normal quantities of free steroid are excreted in the urine in states characterized by hy-

FIGURE 112-1
Basic steroid structure and nomenclature.

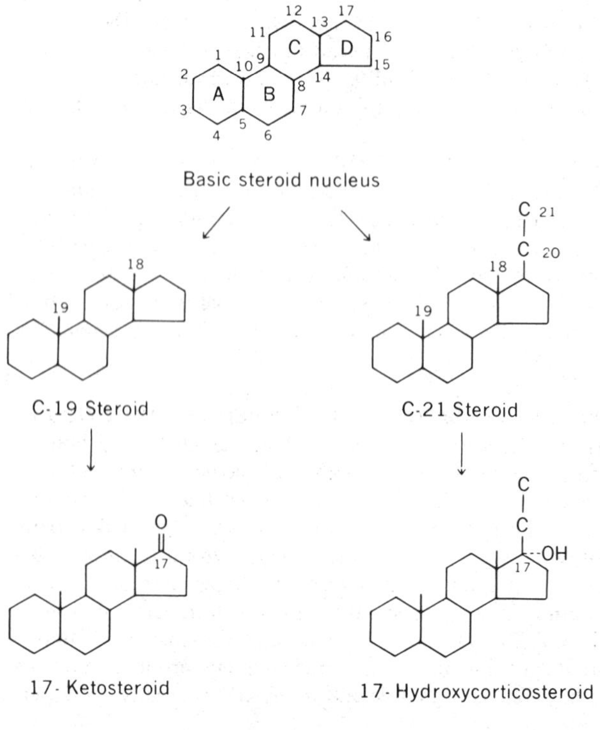

Basic steroid nucleus

C-19 Steroid

C-21 Steroid

17- Ketosteroid

17- Hydroxycorticosteroid

persecretion of cortisol, as the unbound fraction of plasma cortisol rises. *Protein-bound cortisol* is that portion of cortisol which is reversibly bound to circulating plasma proteins. There are two distinct cortisol-binding systems of plasma. One is a high-affinity, low-capacity alpha$_2$ globulin termed *transcortin* or *cortisol-binding globulin* (CBG), and the other is a low-affinity, high-capacity protein, albumin. Cortisol-binding globulin in normal humans can bind approximately 20 to 25 μg cortisol per deciliter of plasma. As the amounts of cortisol released by the adrenal gland exceed this level, the excess becomes bound in part to albumin and a greater proportion circulates unbound. The CBG level is increased in high-estrogen states (e.g., pregnancy, oral contraceptive administration). The endogenous rise in CBG is accompanied by a parallel rise in protein-bound cortisol, with the result that the plasma cortisol concentration is elevated. However, the free-cortisol levels probably remain normal, and signs and symptoms of glucocorticoid excess are absent. Most synthetic glucocorticoid analogues bind less efficiently to CBG (approximately 70 percent binding). This may explain the propensity of some synthetic analogues to produce cushingoid side effects at low dosage. *Cortisol metabolites* are biologically inactive and bind only weakly to circulating plasma proteins.

Aldosterone is bound to proteins to a smaller extent than either testosterone or cortisol with an ultrafiltrate of plasma containing as much as 50 percent of the circulating aldosterone. The limited binding of aldosterone by plasma protein is significant in the metabolism of this hormone.

STEROID METABOLISM AND EXCRETION **Glucocorticoids** The daily secretion of cortisol ranges between 15 and 30 mg, with a pronounced diurnal cycle. Cortisol is distributed in a volume of body fluids approximating the total extracellular fluid space. The total plasma concentration of cortisol in the morning hours is approximately 15 μg/dl, with more than 90 percent in the protein-bound fraction. The plasma concentration of cortisol is determined by the rate of secretion, the rate of inactivation, and the rate of excretion of free cortisol. The

FIGURE 112-2
Biosynthetic pathways for adrenal steroid production. Major pathways to mineralocorticoids, glucocorticoids, and androgens. Circled letters and numbers denote specific enzymes: DE = debranching enzyme; 3β = 3β-ol-dehydrogenase with $\Delta^{4,5}$-isomerase; 11 = C-11 hydroxylase; 17 = C-17 hydroxylase; 21 = C-21 hydroxylase.

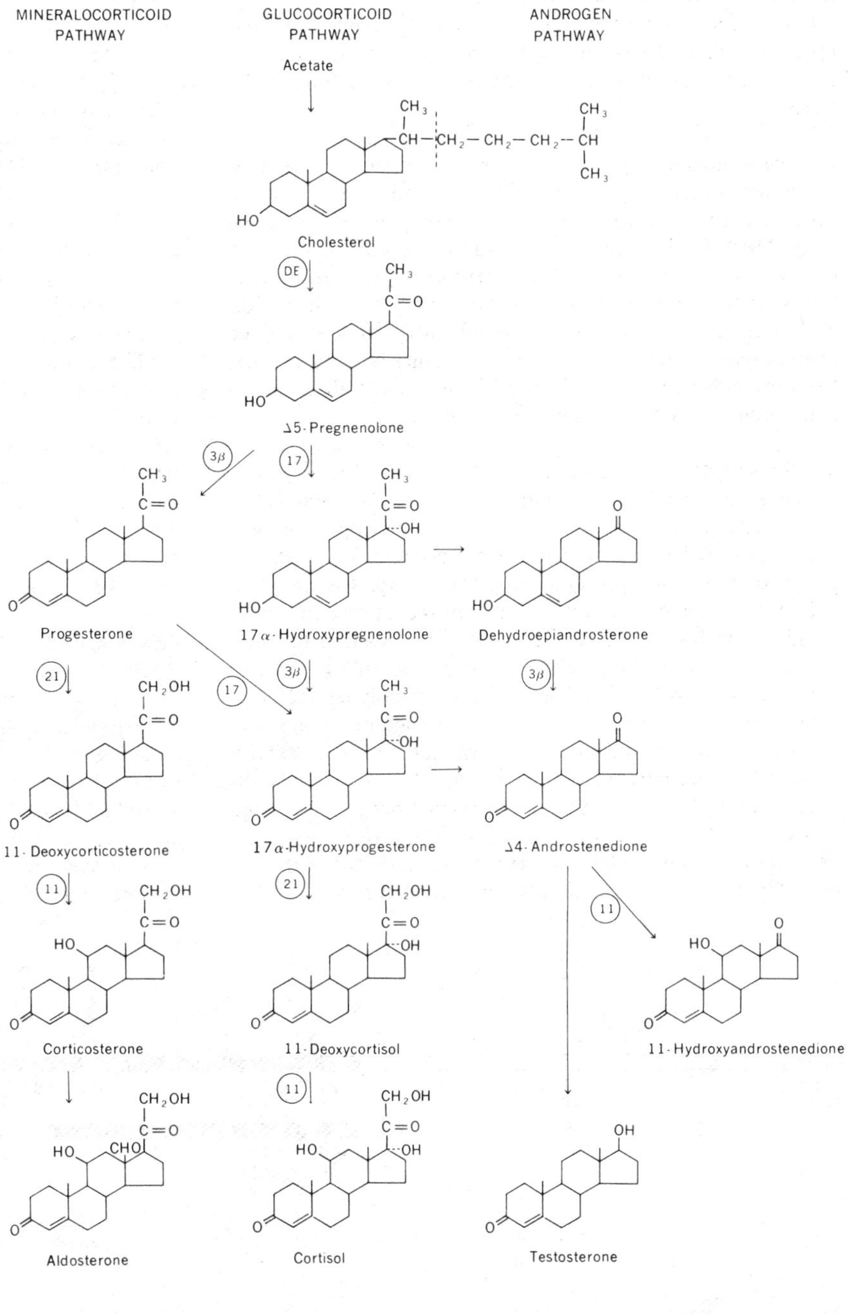

liver is the major organ responsible for steroid inactivation by reduction of ring A and conjugation of the reduced products with glucuronic acid at position C-3 to form water-soluble compounds. The 11-dehydrogenase system converting cortisol to the inactive cortisone is influenced by the level of circulating thyroid hormone, the oxidative reaction being increased in hyperthyroidism.

Mineralocorticoids In normal subjects on a normal salt intake, the average daily secretion of aldosterone ranges between 50 and 250 μg, and the plasma concentration ranges between 5 and 15 ng/dl. Since aldosterone is only weakly bound to proteins, its volume of distribution is larger than that of cortisol and approximates 35 liters. More than 75 percent of circulating aldosterone is normally inactivated during a single passage through the liver by ring A reduction and conjugation with glucuronic acid. However, under certain conditions, such as congestive failure, this percentage is markedly reduced.

From 7 to 15 percent of aldosterone appears in the urine as a glucuronide conjugate, from which free aldosterone is released on standing at pH 1. This *acid-labile conjugate* appears to be formed both in the liver and in the kidney. For average salt intake, the 24-h urine excretion of the acid-labile conjugate ranges from 2 to 20 μg, that of the reduced derivative from 25 to 35 μg, and that of the nonconjugated, nonreduced free aldosterone from 0.2 to 0.6 μg.

Adrenal androgens The major androgen secreted by the adrenal is dehydroepiandrosterone (DHEA) and its C-3 sulfuric acid ester. From 15 to 30 mg of these compounds is secreted daily. Much smaller amounts of Δ^4-androstenedione and 11β-hydroxyandrostenedione and testosterone are secreted. DHEA serves as the major precursor of the urinary 17-ketosteroids. Two-thirds of the urine 17-ketosteroids in the male is derived from adrenal metabolites, and the remaining one-third comes from testicular androgens. In the female, almost all urine 17-ketosteroids are derived from the adrenal.

ACTH PHYSIOLOGY Adrenocorticotropin (ACTH; see Chap. 109) is an unbranched polypeptide containing 39 amino acids. ACTH and a number of other peptides (lipotropins, endorphins, and MSHs) are processed from a larger 31,000-dalton precursor molecule—pro-opiocortin (see Chap. 109 and Fig. 112-3). It is stored in and released from the anterior pituitary gland, where histologically it appears to be localized to basophil cells. Much of the potential for producing the corticotropic actions of ACTH is present in smaller polypeptide fragments; the *N*-terminal 18-amino-acid structure retains full biologic potency, while shorter *N*-terminal fragments exhibit reduced biologic activity. The biologic half-life of ACTH is less than 10 min. Release of ACTH and related peptides as noted above from the anterior pituitary gland is governed by a "corticotropin-releasing center" in the median eminence of the hypothalamus, which upon stimulation releases a peptide with a chain of 41 amino acids (corticotropin-releasing factor, CRF) that travels via the pituitary-stalk portal bloodstream to the anterior pituitary gland, where it effects the release of stored ACTH (Fig. 112-3). It appears that the related lipotropin peptides are released in equimolar concentrations with ACTH suggesting enzymatic cleavage prior to or concomitant with the secretory process from the parent molecule.

Three major factors control CRF and ACTH release: plasma free-cortisol concentration, stress, and the sleep-wake cycle (Fig. 112-4). The plasma level of ACTH varies sporadically during the day but roughly follows a diurnal pattern, with a peak occurring just prior to awaking and a nadir shortly before retiring. After several days on a new sleep-wake cycle, the pattern is altered to conform to the new cycle. Stress (e.g., pyrogens, surgery, hypoglycemia, exercise, severe emotional trauma) can also affect ACTH release. The secretion of ACTH following stress and the diurnal ACTH release are under neural regulation by CRF, the so-called open feedback loop. CRF is probably also influenced by the hypothalamic monoaminergic neurotransmitters with the serotoninergic and cholinergic systems known to stimulate the secretion of CRF and ACTH. Finally, ACTH release is regulated by the plasma free-cortisol level. Cortisol decreases the responsiveness of the anterior pituitary adrenocorticotropic cells to CRF; i.e., in the presence of cortisol, more CRF is required to produce a given increment of ACTH than in its absence. Thus, in the presence of a constant CRF level, this *negative feedback* relationship causes decreased ACTH release when cortisol levels are high. This servomechanism establishes the primacy of blood cortisol concentration. The inhibition of ACTH secretion occurs in two phases: (1) an early fast feedback, a possible membrane effect, and (2) a delayed-feedback response, probably due to inhibition of synthesis of the precursor protein. It also appears that cortisol feeds back on the hypothalamus (CRF), higher brain centers (hippocampus, reticular system, septum), and perhaps on the adrenal cortex as well (Fig. 112-4).

The action of ACTH on the adrenal is rapid; within minutes of its release, there is an increased concentration of steroids in the adrenal venous blood. The mechanism by which ACTH stimulates steroidogenesis is via activation of the membrane-bound adenyl cyclase. This increases the level of cyclic adenosine 3′,5′-monophosphate (cAMP), which then activates adrenocortical protein kinase enzymes. This results in the phosphorylation of proteins which in some way activate steroid biosynthesis.

RENIN-ANGIOTENSIN PHYSIOLOGY (See also Chap. 267.) Renin is a proteolytic enzyme which is produced and stored in the granules of the juxtaglomerular cells surrounding the afferent arterioles of the cortical glomeruli. Renin exists not only as an active enzyme but also as a large-molecular-weight inactive form. Whether this larger form is a precursor ("prorenin") or is a product formed after release is uncertain. The juxtaglomerular apparatus consists of both the juxtaglomerular cells and the cells of the macula densa. Renin acts on the basic substrate angiotensinogen (a circulating alpha$_2$ globulin), made in the

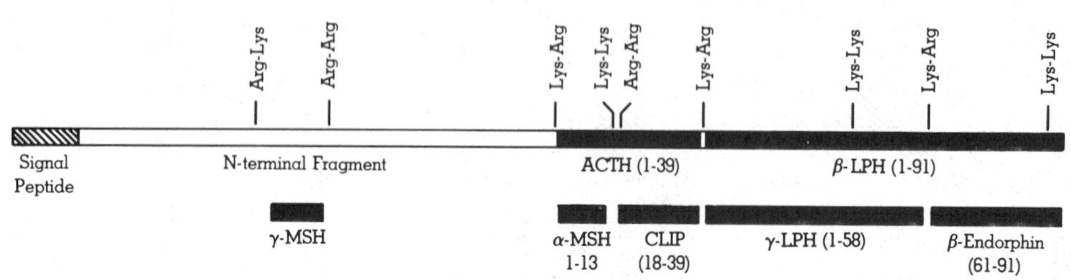

FIGURE 112-3 *Schematic representation of the probable structure of the 31,000-dalton ACTH precursor molecule—pro-opiocortin. (From DT Krieger, JB Martin, N Engl J Med 304:880, 1981. By permission of the New England Journal of Medicine.)*

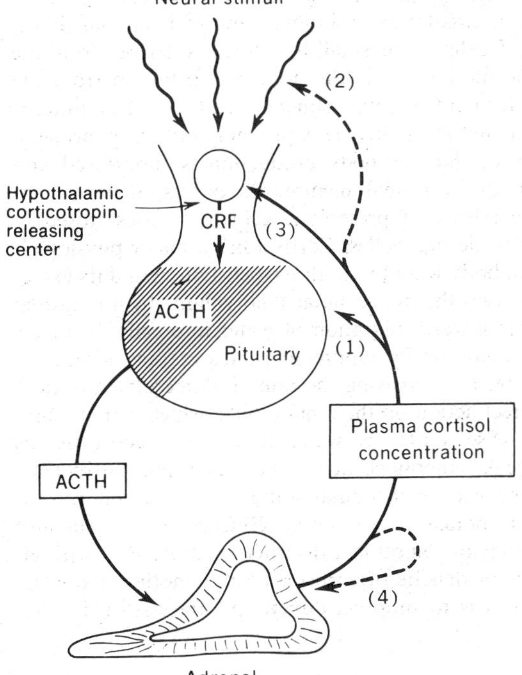

FIGURE 112-4
Hypothalamic-pituitary-adrenal axis. (1) Dominant feedback control on the pituitary gland; (2) possible feedback of plasma cortisol on higher nerve centers, (3) on the hypothalamus, and/or (4) the adrenal gland itself. CRF = corticotropin-releasing factor.

liver, to form the decapeptide angiotensin I (Fig. 112-5). Angiotensin I is then enzymatically converted by converting enzyme to the octapeptide angiotensin II by splitting off the two *C*-terminal amino acids. Angiotensin II is the most potent pressor compound (on a mole-for-mole basis) made in the body, and it exerts this pressor action by a direct effect on arteriolar smooth muscle. In addition, angiotensin II is a potent direct stimulus to the production of aldosterone by the zona glomerulosa of the adrenal cortex. Recent studies suggest that the nonapeptide, angiotensin III, can also stimulate aldosterone production. However, this hypothesis is still controversial. Angiotensinases rapidly destroy angiotensin II (half-life approximately 1 min), while the half-life of renin is more prolonged (10 to 20 min). Finally, other tissues, such as uterus, vascular tissue, brain, and salivary glands, also produce renin-like substances. The significance of these so-called isorenins is not understood.

Renin release is controlled by four major factors. For the most part, these are interdependent, and the amount of renin released is a composite of the input of all four. The *juxtaglomerular cells,* which are specialized myoepithelial cells cuffing the afferent arterioles, act as miniature pressure transducers, sensing renal perfusion pressure and corresponding changes in afferent arteriolar perfusion pressures. The changes in pressure are perceived as distortions in the existing stretch on the arteriolar walls. For example, under conditions of a reduction in circulating blood volume, there is a corresponding reduction in renal perfusion pressure and, therefore, in afferent arteriolar pressure (Fig. 112-5). This is perceived by the juxtaglomerular cells as a decreased stretch exerted on the afferent arteriolar walls. The juxtaglomerular cells then release increasing quantities of renin within the kidney circulation. This results in the formation of angiotensin I, which is converted in the kidney and peripherally to angiotensin II by a peptidyldipeptide hydrolase (so-called converting enzyme). Angiotensin II stimulates the adrenal cortex to release increasing quantities of aldosterone. Increasing plasma levels of aldosterone lead to increasing renal sodium retention and thus result in expansion of extracellular fluid volume, which, as it is completed, dampens the initiating signal for renin release. Within this context, the renin-angiotensin-aldosterone system subserves volume control by appropriate modifications of renal tubular sodium transport.

A second control mechanism for renin release centers in the *macula densa* cells, a group of distal convoluted tubular epithelial cells found in direct apposition to the juxtaglomerular cells. They may function as chemoreceptors, monitoring the sodium (or chloride) load presented to the distal tubule, and such information, while it is being monitored, may be directly fed back to the juxtaglomerular cells, where appropriate modifications in renin release take place. Under conditions of increased delivery of filtered sodium to the macula densa, feedback occurs to the juxtaglomerular apparatus, resulting in a release of increasing quantities of renin, which are capable of decreasing glomerular filtration rate, thereby reducing the filtered load of sodium. The evidence for this hypothesis is conflicting.

The *sympathetic nervous system* is the predominant factor regulating the release of renin in response to assuming the upright posture. The mechanism is either a direct effect on the juxtaglomerular cell to increase adenyl cyclase activity or an indirect effect on either the juxtaglomerular or the macula densa cells by way of a vasoconstrictive action on the afferent arteriole.

Finally, a number of circulating factors may alter renin release. Increasing dietary *potassium* directly decreases renin release; decreasing potassium intake increases renin release. The

FIGURE 112-5
The interrelationship of the volume and potassium feedback loops on aldosterone secretion. Integration of signals from each loop determines the level of aldosterone secretion.

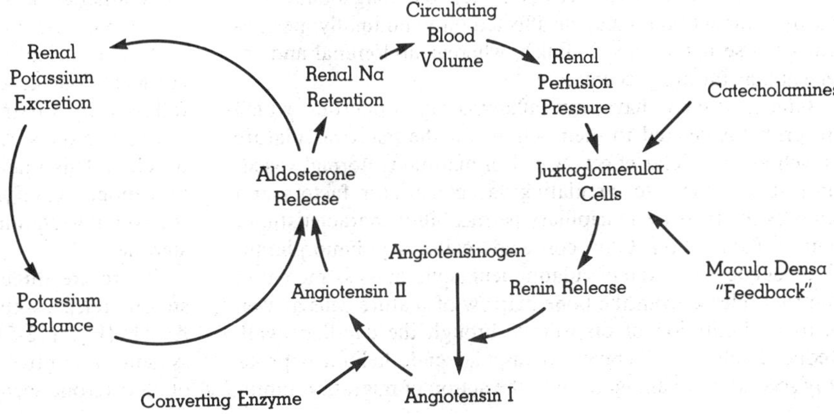

significance of this potassium effect is unclear. *Angiotensin II* itself can exert a negative feedback control on renin release independent of alterations in renal blood flow, pressure, or aldosterone secretion. Thus, the control of renin release is complex, consisting of both *intrarenal* (pressor receptor and macula densa) and *extrarenal* (sympathetic nervous system, potassium, angiotensin, etc.) mechanisms. A given level of renin secretion probably reflects all these factors, with the intrarenal mechanism predominating.

GLUCOCORTICOID PHYSIOLOGY The division of adrenal steroids into glucocorticoids and mineralocorticoids is somewhat arbitrary in that most glucocorticoids have some mineralocorticoid-like properties, and vice versa. The descriptive term *glucocorticoid* is applied to those adrenal steroids having a predominant action on intermediary metabolism. The principal glucocorticoid is cortisol (hydrocortisone). Cortisol enters the target cell by diffusion, combines with a specific high-affinity cytoplasmic receptor protein, and is transferred to a specific acceptor site on the chromatin tissue of the nucleus, which then produces an increase in RNA synthesis and later in protein synthesis. Thus, an alternative way of defining a glucocorticoid effect is one mediated by a class of high-affinity cytoplasmic receptors (glucorticoid receptors) (see Chap. 108). The physiological actions of the glucocorticoids on intermediary metabolism are predominantly anti-insulin and include the regulation of protein, carbohydrate, lipid, and nucleic acid metabolism. Their actions appear mainly to be catabolic in effect, with an increased protein breakdown and nitrogen excretion. Glucocorticoids increase hepatic glycogen content and promote the hepatic synthesis of glucose (gluconeogenesis). These actions are in large part explained by the mobilization of glycogenic amino acid precursors from peripheral supporting structures, such as bone, skin, muscle, and connective tissue due to protein breakdown as well as to the inhibition of protein synthesis and amino acid uptake. Glucocorticoid-induced hyperaminoacidemia also indirectly facilitates gluconeogenesis by stimulating glucagon secretion. In addition, glucocorticoids have a direct action on the liver to stimulate the synthesis of hepatic enzymes, such as tyrosine amino transferase and tryptophan pyrrolase. Inhibition of extrahepatic protein synthesis and stimulation of hepatic enzyme synthesis are reflected in the actions of glucocorticoids on nucleic acid metabolism. Corticoids inhibit the synthesis of nucleic acids in most body tissues, but in the liver ribonucleic acid (RNA) synthesis is stimulated. Glucocorticoids are necessary for fatty acid mobilization by permitting and enhancing activation of cellular lipase by lipid-mobilizing hormones (e.g., catecholamines and pituitary peptides).

The actions of cortisol on structural protein and adipose tissue vary in different parts of the body. For example, pharmacological doses of cortisol may deplete the protein matrix of the vertebral column (trabecular bone), but long bones (primarily compact bone) may be affected only minimally; peripheral adipose tissue may diminish, whereas abdominal and interscapular fat may accumulate.

Glucocorticoids have anti-inflammatory properties, which are probably related to their actions on the microvasculature as well as to cellular effects. Cortisol maintains normal vascular responsiveness to circulating vasoconstrictor factors and opposes the increase in capillary permeability characteristic of acute inflammation. Glucocorticoids cause a polymorphonuclear leukocytosis; the circulating leukocyte mass is increased due to a release from the bone marrow of mature cells as well as to an inhibition of diapedesis through the capillary wall. Reduced cellular adherence to vascular endothelium is probably secondary to antagonism to the action of migration-inhibiting factor (MIF) by glucocorticoids. Glucocorticoids produce a depletion of circulating eosinophils and of lymphoid tissue, specifically, T cells or the small lymphocytes derived from the thymus. The mechanism is due to a redistribution from the circulation into other compartments. Thus, cortisol impairs cellular-mediated immunity. It is probably only at pharmacological dosages that antibody production is suppressed and stabilization of lysosomal membranes occurs, thereby suppressing the release of proteolytic acid hydrolases stored in these cytoplasmic organelles. Cortisol has a major physiological action on body water, in both its distribution and its excretion. It subserves the extracellular fluid volume by a retarding action on the inward migration of water into cells. It affects renal water excretion by suppressing the secretion of antidiuretic hormone, by increasing the rate of glomerular filtration, and by a direct action on the renal tubule, which actions summate to increase solute-free water clearance. Glucocorticoids also have weak mineralocorticoid-like properties, but increasing doses produce renal tubular sodium reabsorption and increased urine potassium excretion. Glucocorticoids can also influence behavior; emotional disorders may be seen with either excesses or deficits of cortisol. Lastly, another major action of cortisol is to suppress directly pituitary ACTH secretion.

MINERALOCORTICOID PHYSIOLOGY The major mineralocorticoid produced by the human adrenal is aldosterone. Aldosterone has two important activities: (1) it is a major regulator of extracellular fluid volume, and (2) it is a major determinant of potassium metabolism. These mineralocorticoid effects are mediated by binding of aldosterone to specific, high-affinity mineralocorticoid receptor proteins in target tissues. It regulates volume through a direct effect on the renal tubular transport of sodium. Aldosterone acts predominantly at the site of the distal convoluted tubule, where it causes a decrease in the excretion of sodium with an increase in excretion of potassium. The reabsorption of positively charged sodium ions causes a fall in the transmembrane potential, thus producing an environment favorable for the flow of positive ions out of the cell into the lumen. The major singly charged positive ion present intracellularly is potassium. Since its concentration in the cell is forty- to eightyfold greater than in the lumen, it passively follows this relative electrical gradient to restore the normal positive charge to the lumen. The reabsorbed sodium ions are then transported out of the tubular epithelial cells into the interstitial fluid of the kidney and from there into the renal capillary circulation. Water passively follows the aldosterone-mediated transported sodium.

Hydrogen ion is also abundant in the tubular epithelial cell. Since its concentration in the lumen is greater than in the cell, it is actively secreted, but the reduced intraluminal positivity allows more hydrogen to be secreted with the same amount of energy. Aldosterone and other mineralocorticoids also act on the epithelium of the salivary ducts and sweat glands and on the epithelial cells of the gastrointestinal tract to cause reabsorption of sodium in "exchange" for potassium ions.

When normal individuals are given aldosterone (or deoxycorticosterone acetate), an initial period of sodium retention is followed by a natriuresis, and sodium balance is reestablished after 3 to 5 days. As a result, clinical edema formation does not develop. This phenomenon is referred to as the "escape phenomenon," signifying an "escape" by the renal tubules from the sodium-retaining action of chronically administered aldosterone.

There are three well-defined *control* mechanisms for aldosterone release—the renin-angiotensin system, potassium, and ACTH (Fig. 112-5). The renin-angiotensin system is the major system for control of extracellular fluid volume, via regulation of aldosterone secretion. In effect, the renin-angiotensin system attempts to maintain the circulating blood volume constant by causing aldosterone-induced sodium retention during periods registered as volume deficiencies, and by decreasing aldosterone-dependent sodium retention under conditions in which volume is registered as being ample.

Potassium ions directly regulate aldosterone secretion independently of the renin-angiotensin system. In normal humans, oral potassium loading increases aldosterone excretion, secretion, and plasma levels. In addition, systemic infusion of potassium ions under certain circumstances increases plasma aldosterone levels with as small as a 0.1 meq per liter increase in serum potassium. Potassium may alter aldosterone secretion owing to changes in serum potassium levels, to changes in intracellular potassium concentration, or to change in the flux of potassium across the adrenal cortical cell membrane.

Physiological amounts of ACTH acutely stimulate aldosterone secretion, but this action is not sustained if ACTH is continuously infused for periods greater than 10 to 12 h. However, other studies seem to relegate ACTH to a minor role in the control of aldosterone in normal humans. For example, subjects on high-dose steroid therapy for several years and with presumably complete suppression of ACTH have normal aldosterone-secretory responses to sodium restriction. Therefore, chronic ACTH deficiency per se does not alter glomerulosa cell responsiveness.

The prior dietary intake of both potassium and sodium can alter the magnitude of the aldosterone response to acute stimulation. Increasing potassium intake or decreasing sodium intake sensitizes the response of the glomerulosa cells to acute stimulation by ACTH, angiotensin II, and/or potassium.

Neurotransmitters (dopamine and serotonin) and unidentified peptides may also participate in the regulation of aldosterone secretion.

ANDROGEN PHYSIOLOGY Androgens are substances that stimulate male secondary sexual characteristics. They produce these actions also by binding to high-affinity cytoplasmic receptors. The secondary sexual characteristics are affected through inhibition of the female characteristics (defeminization) and accentuation of the male characteristics (masculinization). These are seen clinically as hirsutism and virilization in the female with amenorrhea, atrophy of the breasts and uterus, enlargement of the clitoris, deepening of the voice, acne, increased muscle mass, increased sexual drive, and receding hairline (Chap. 48).

Steroids with predominant androgenic activity have 19 carbon atoms (Fig. 112-1). The principal adrenal androgens are dehydroepiandrosterone (DHEA), androstenedione, and 11-hydroxyandrostenedione. DHEA and its sulfate are *quantitatively* the major androgens secreted by the adrenal. DHEA, androstenedione, and 11-hydroxyandrostenedione are weak androgens, but all are peripherally interconvertible with the potent androgen, testosterone.

The release of adrenal androgens is stimulated by ACTH, not by gonadotropins. With ACTH stimulation, 17-ketosteroids increase but to a lesser extent than do urine 17-hydroxycorticosteroids. It follows that adrenal androgens are suppressed by exogenous glucocorticoid administration.

LABORATORY EVALUATION OF ADRENOCORTICAL FUNCTION

The basic assumption in the measurement of plasma levels or the urinary excretion of steroid metabolites is that they accurately reflect adrenal *secretory* rates of that steroid. A disadvantage of urine *excretion* values is that they may not truly reflect the secretion rate because of improper collection or altered metabolism. Measurement of the actual adrenal secretory rate of a given steroid would be preferable but is more difficult, involving isotope dilution techniques following administration of a radioactive steroid. Plasma levels reflect the level of secretion only at the time of measurement. The plasma level (PL) is dependent on two factors: the secretion rate (SR) of the hormone and the rate at which it is metabolized, i.e., its metabolic clearance rate (MCR). These three factors can be related mathematically as follows:

$$\text{PL} = \frac{\text{SR}}{\text{MCR}} \quad \text{or} \quad \text{SR} = \text{MCR} \times \text{PL}$$

BLOOD LEVELS See Table 112-1.

Peptides ACTH and angiotensin II can be measured by radioimmunoassay. ACTH is secreted episodically during the day, with a trend for plasma levels to vary diurnally, with lower levels in the early evening than in the morning. Angiotensin II levels also vary diurnally but are influenced in addition by dietary sodium intake and posture. Both upright posture and sodium restriction elevate angiotensin II levels.

The majority of clinical determinations of the renin-angiotensin system, however, involve measurements of peripheral "plasma renin activity" (PRA) in which the renin activity is gauged by the generation of angiotensin I during a standardized incubation period. This method depends on the presence of sufficient angiotensinogen in the patient's plasma as substrate. The generated angiotensin I is then measured by radioimmunoassay. Plasma renin activity depends on dietary sodium intake and whether the patient is ambulatory. In normal recumbent or upright humans, a diurnal rhythm for plasma renin activity is characterized by peak values in the morning with decreases in activity in the afternoon.

Steroids Cortisol and aldosterone are both secreted episodically, but levels generally decline during the day, with peak

TABLE 112-1
Range of normal values for tests of adrenal function

Test	*Normal value, range*
Plasma cortisol, μg/dl:	
8 A.M.	9–24
4 P.M.	3–12
Cortisol secretory rate, mg/24 h	5–25
Urine free cortisol, μg/24 h	20–100
17-Hydroxycorticoids, mg/24 h	2–10
Plasma testosterone, μg/dl:	
Males	0.3–1.0
Females	0.01–0.1
17-Ketosteroids, mg/24 h:	
Males	7–25
Females	4–15
Plasma dehydroepiandrosterone (DHEA) μg/dl	0.2–0.9
Plasma DHEA sulfate, μg/dl	50–250
Plasma 11-deoxycortisol (S), μg/dl	<1.0
Plasma 17αOH progesterone, ng/dl:	
Female	
Follicular phase	6–110
Luteal phase	50–350
Male	6–300
Plasma aldosterone, ng/dl (100 meq Na, 60–100 meq K, supine, 8 A.M.)	1–5
Aldosterone secretion, μg/24 h (100 meq Na, 600–100 meq K)	50–250
Aldosterone excretion, μg/24 h (100 meq Na, 60–100 meq K)	2–10
Plasma renin activity, (ng/ml)/h (100 meq Na, 60–100 meq K, supine, 8 A.M.)	1–2.5
Plasma angiotensin II, pg/ml (100 meq Na, 60–100 meq K, supine, 8 A.M.)	10–30
Plasma ACTH, pg/ml (8 A.M.)	<80

values in the morning and low levels in the evening. In addition, the plasma level of aldosterone, but not of cortisol, is increased by dietary potassium loading, sodium restriction, or assuming the upright posture. Measurement of the sulfate conjugate of DHEA is a useful index of adrenal androgen secretion since little is secreted by the gonads and the half-life is prolonged (7 to 9 h).

URINE LEVELS The urine *17-hydroxycorticoids* are determined as Porter-Silber chromogens; this reaction is specific for steroids with a "dihydroxyacetone" C-17 side chain, i.e., with hydroxyl groups on C-17 and C-21 and a ketone group on C-20. Therefore, this determination includes cortisol, cortisone, tetrahydrocortisol, tetrahydrocortisone, and 11-deoxycortisol (Fig. 112-2). Normally, daytime (7 A.M. to 7 P.M.) excretion exceeds night values (7 P.M. to 7 A.M.).

The urine *17-ketosteroids* are those containing a ketone group at C-17 (Fig. 112-1). They originate either in the adrenal gland or the gonad. In normal women, 90 percent or more of total urinary 17-ketosteroids is derived from the adrenal gland, while in men, only 60 to 70 percent is of adrenal origin. Urine 17-ketosteroid values are highest in young adults and decline with age.

The determination of urine free cortisol is useful since elevated excretion values correlate well with states of hypercortisolism, reflecting changes in the unbound, physiologically active, circulating levels of cortisol.

A carefully timed urine collection is a prerequisite for all excretory determinations. Simultaneous creatinine determinations are of importance to demonstrate the accuracy and adequacy of the collection procedure. Adjustments for body size can be made; e.g., normal subjects excrete 3 to 7 mg 17-hydroxycorticosteroids per gram of creatinine.

STIMULATION TESTS Stimulation tests are useful in documenting the existence of a hormonal deficiency state. A standardized and specific stimulus for the production and release of a given hormone is applied, and the quantity of the released hormone can then be measured.

Tests of glucocorticoid reserve Within minutes after initiation of an infusion of ACTH, increased cortisol levels are noted in adrenal venous blood. This responsiveness of the adrenal gland to ACTH is utilized as an index of the "functional reserve" of the gland to produce cortisol. Under maximal ACTH stimulation the cortisol secretion increases tenfold to 300 mg per day. Such maximal stimulation can be obtained only with prolonged ACTH infusions. For clinical purposes, the functional adrenal reserve for cortisol production is standardized with a 24-h ACTH infusion. Synthetic α^{1-24}-ACTH (cosyntropin) is usually used because of its greater purity and given in 500 to 1000 ml normal saline at a rate of 2 units per hour for 24 h. Normal subjects increase 17-hydroxysteroid excretion rates to at least 25 mg per 24 h, and plasma cortisol levels exceed 40 μg/dl. In patients with secondary adrenal insufficiency, the maximal 17-hydroxysteroid excretion rate is 3 to 20 mg per 24 h, and the plasma cortisol value at 24 h ranges between 10 and 40 μg/dl. Patients with primary adrenal insufficiency have smaller responses.

A rapid screening test is to administer 25 units (0.25 mg) cosyntropin intravenously or intramuscularly and measure plasma cortisol levels before and 30 and 60 min later. An increment of at least 7 μg/dl above base line is observed in normal subjects.

Tests of mineralocorticoid reserve and stimulation of the renin-angiotensin system Stimulation tests have been devised utilizing a protocol of programmed volume depletion, such as sodium restriction, diuretic administration, or upright posture. A simple potent stimulation test consists of severe sodium restriction and upright posture. After 3 to 5 days of a 10-meq sodium intake, aldosterone secretion or excretion rates should exhibit a two- to threefold increase over control. Supine morning plasma aldosterone levels usually increase three- to sixfold. In addition, plasma levels increase two- to fourfold in response to 2 to 3 h of upright posture.

Stimulation tests on normal dietary sodium intake may also be carried out by the administration of a potent diuretic, such as 40 to 80 mg furosemide, followed by 2 to 3 h of upright posture. The normal response is a two- to fourfold rise in plasma aldosterone levels.

SUPPRESSION TESTS Suppression tests are used to document hypersecretion of adrenocortical hormones and are based on the demonstration of a decrease in the target hormone following standardized suppression of its tropic hormone. Thus, suppression testing for cortisol hypersecretion involves suppression of ACTH release, with documentation of an appropriately normal decrease in cortisol production, while suppression testing of aldosterone involves demonstration of a decrease in aldosterone secondary to suppression of the renin-angiotensin system.

Tests of pituitary-adrenal suppressibility The hypothalamo-pituitary ACTH release mechanism is sensitive to the circulating blood level of glucocorticoids. When such blood levels are increased in the normal individual, less ACTH is released from the anterior pituitary, and secondarily, less steroid is produced by the adrenal gland. The integrity of this feedback mechanism can be tested clinically by giving a potent glucocorticoid and judging suppression of ACTH secretion by analysis of urine steroid excretory values and/or plasma cortisol and ACTH levels. A potent glucocorticoid such as dexamethasone is utilized in order that the administered compound may be given in such small amounts as not to contribute significantly to the steroids to be analyzed.

The best *screening* procedure is the overnight dexamethasone suppression test. This involves the measurement of plasma cortisol levels at 8 A.M. following the oral administration of 1 mg dexamethasone the previous midnight. The 8 A.M. value for plasma cortisol in normal subjects should be less than 5 μg/dl.

The definitive test of adrenal suppressibility is to administer 0.5 mg dexamethasone every 6 h for two successive days while collecting urine over a 24-h period for determination of creatinine, 17-hydroxysteroids and/or free cortisol and/or measuring plasma cortisol levels. In patients with a normal hypothalamic pituitary ACTH release mechanism, a fall in the urine 17-hydroxycorticoids to less than 3 mg a day on the second day of dexamethasone administration, free cortisol to less than 30 μg per day, or a plasma cortisol to less than 5 μg/dl is seen.

Normal responses to either of the suppression tests implies that the ACTH control of the adrenal glands is physiologically normal. However, an isolated abnormal result, particularly when the overnight suppression test is being used, does not in itself imply pituitary and/or adrenal disease.

Tests of mineralocorticoid suppressibility Mineralocorticoid suppression testing procedures have been devised using saline infusions, oral salt loading, or deoxycorticosterone acetate (DOCA) administration as the means for expansion of the extracellular fluid volume. With expansion of extracellular fluid volume, there is a decrease in renal renin release, a decrease in circulating plasma renin activity, and a decrease in aldosterone secretion and/or excretion. Various tests differ in the rate at which extracellular fluid volume is expanded. One convenient suppression test is the intravenous infusion of 500 ml normal saline per hour for 4 h which normally suppresses plasma aldosterone levels to < 8 ng/dl on a sodium-restricted diet or to < 5 ng/dl on a normal sodium intake. This test should not be performed in potassium-depleted subjects.

TESTS OF PITUITARY-ADRENAL RESPONSIVENESS A number of stimuli, such as insulin hypoglycemia, arginine vasopressin, and pyrogen, cause release of ACTH from the pituitary by an action on higher nerve centers, the hypothalamus, or the pituitary itself. By measuring plasma ACTH or blood glucocorticoids the status of pituitary ACTH can be evaluated. Insulin-induced hypoglycemia is particularly useful since the release of growth hormone as well as ACTH is stimulated. In this test 0.05 to 0.1 unit of crystalline insulin per kilogram of body weight is administered intravenously as a bolus to reduce fasting glucose levels at least 50 percent below basal. The normal cortisol response is a doubling above control levels within 30 to 60 min.

Metyrapone is a drug that inhibits 11β-hydroxylase in the adrenal gland. As a result, the conversion of 11-deoxycortisol (compound S) to cortisol is interfered with, and increased amounts of 11-deoxycortisol accumulate while blood levels of cortisol decrease (Fig. 112-2). The anterior pituitary responds to the declining cortisol blood levels by releasing larger quantities of ACTH in an attempt to stimulate the adrenal gland to release additional cortisol, which attempt, however, is thwarted by the metyrapone-induced enzymatic blockade. The metabolites of 11-deoxycortisol are excreted in increasing amounts in the urine, where they are measured as 17-hydroxycorticoids. Alternatively, changes in plasma 11-deoxycortisol levels can be measured. *Note that the adrenal glands must be capable of being stimulated by ACTH, since assessment of the response depends on adrenal steroid production.*

The metyrapone test involves administering orally 750 mg of the drug every 4 h over a 24-h period and comparing the control and the post-metyrapone 17-hydroxysteroid excretion rates and/or plasma 11-deoxycortisol levels. Normal individuals respond with at least a doubling of their basal 17-hydroxysteroid excretion; 11-deoxycortisol levels in the blood should exceed 10 μg/dl following metyrapone administration. The metyrapone test does not accurately reflect ACTH reserve if subjects are ingesting exogenous glucocorticoids or drugs that accelerate the metabolism of metyrapone (e.g., phenytoin).

A test that distinguishes between primary and secondary adrenal insufficiency takes advantage of the preservation of relatively normal aldosterone secretion in secondary adrenal insufficiency. Thus, when ACTH is administered, neither group has a normal rise in cortisol levels (distinguishing them from normal subjects), but patients with primary adrenal insufficiency also fail to have a normal aldosterone response. Twenty-five units synthetic α^{1-24}-ACTH (cosyntropin) is given intravenously or intramuscularly, and plasma cortisol and aldosterone levels are obtained before and 30 and 60 min later. Neither group shows the normal cortisol increment of greater than 7 μg/dl, but only patients with primary insufficiency fail to increase aldosterone levels above control by at least 5 ng/dl.

HYPERFUNCTION OF THE ADRENAL CORTEX

Distinct clinical syndromes are produced when excess amounts of the principal adrenocortical hormones are secreted. Thus, excess production of cortisol is associated with Cushing's syndrome; excess production of aldosterone with clinical and chemical signs of aldosteronism; excess production of adrenal androgens with adrenal virilism. As would be expected, these syndromes do not always occur in the "pure" form but may have overlapping features.

CUSHING'S SYNDROME **Etiology** Harvey Cushing, in 1932, described a syndrome characterized by truncal obesity, hypertension, fatigability and weakness, amenorrhea, hirsutism, purplish abdominal striae, edema, glucosuria, and osteoporosis. As awareness of this syndrome increased and as clinical tests of adrenocortical function became standardized and readily available, the diagnosis of Cushing's syndrome has been broadened into the classification shown in Table 112-2. It is apparent that, regardless of etiology, all cases of Cushing's syndrome are due to increased production of cortisol by the adrenal gland. The majority of cases are due to *bilateral adrenal hyperplasia,* secondary to adrenocortical stimulation by hypersecretion of pituitary ACTH or the production of ACTH by nonendocrine tumors. It was originally hypothesized that the elaboration of increased amounts of ACTH in the presence of a radiographically normal sella turcica was a result of pituitary-hypothalamic dysfunction, whereby ACTH secretion is reset to respond to a higher level of circulating cortisol. However, many patients with bilateral hyperplasia have ACTH-producing microadenomas which are sometimes detected only by careful radiographic evaluation of the sella turcica. Thus, the frequency of pituitary adenomas as the cause of Cushing's syndrome is still uncertain. The incidence of pituitary ACTH-dependent adrenal hyperplasia in women is three times that in men, with the most frequent age of onset being the third or fourth decade.

Nonendocrine tumors that secrete polypeptides biologically, chemically, and immunologically indistinguishable from ACTH are also responsible for Cushing's syndrome secondary to bilateral adrenal hyperplasia (see also Chap. 122). Hypokalemic alkalosis is often prominent in such cases, whereas many of the distinctive physical findings usually associated with Cushing's syndrome may be absent.

Approximately 20 to 25 percent of patients with Cushing's syndrome have *primary* overproduction of cortisol and other adrenal steroids due to an adrenal neoplasm. These tumors are almost invariably unilateral, and about half are malignant.

Clinical signs and symptoms The frequency of clinical findings is listed in Table 112-3. Many of the signs and symptoms logically follow from the known action of glucocorticoids. As a result of mobilization of peripheral supportive tissue, there are muscle weakness and fatigability, osteoporosis, and cutaneous striae. The latter involve a weakening and rupture of collagenous fibers in the dermis, so that the heavily vascularized subcutaneous tissues are exposed. Likewise, because of the loss of perivascular supporting tissue, there is easy bruisability, and ecchymoses often appear at sites of mild trauma. The osteoporosis may be so severe that collapse of vertebral bodies and pathological fractures of other bones are frequently encoun-

TABLE 112-2
Causes of Cushing's syndrome

I Adrenal hyperplasia
- *A* Secondary to pituitary ACTH overproduction
  - *1* Pituitary-hypothalamic dysfunction
  - *2* Pituitary ACTH-producing micro- or macroadenomas
- *B* Secondary to ACTH-producing nonendocrine tumors (bronchogenic carcinoma, thymoma, pancreatic carcinoma, bronchial adenoma)

II Adrenal nodular hyperplasia

III Adrenal neoplasia
- *A* Adenoma
- *B* Carcinoma

IV Exogenous, iatrogenic
- *A* Prolonged use of glucocorticoids
- *B* Prolonged use of ACTH

tered. As a result of increased hepatic gluconeogenesis and insulin resistance, impaired glucose tolerance is common. Frank diabetes occurs in less than 20 percent of patients, probably in individuals with a familial predisposition to this disorder. Hypercortisolism promotes the deposition of adipose tissue in characteristic sites. This is observed most notably in the upper part of the face, the classic "moon" facies; in the interscapular area, the "buffalo" hump; and in the mesenteric bed, where it produces the classic "truncal" obesity (Fig. 112-6). Rarely, there may be episternal fatty tumors and mediastinal widening secondary to fat accumulation. The reason for this peculiar distribution of lipid is not known. The face also appears plethoric, even in the absence of any increase in red blood cell concentration. Hypertension is commonly present, and frequently there are profound emotional changes, ranging from irritability or emotional lability to severe depression, confusion, or even frank psychosis. If adrenal androgen secretion is increased, acne and hirsutism are frequent in women. Likewise, oligomenorrhea or amenorrhea is frequent.

Laboratory findings Plasma and urine cortisol and urinary 17-hydroxycorticoid levels are variably elevated. Patients characteristically show a mild neutrophilic leukocytosis and occasionally erythremia with higher hematocrits. Serum sodium concentration is usually normal; however, with marked excess secretion of cortisol, there may be hypokalemia, hypochloremia, and metabolic alkalosis. X-ray studies may reveal generalized osteoporosis, usually most marked in the spine and pelvis but also in the skull.

The preferred radiographic study to visualize the adrenals is computerized tomography (CT scan) of the abdomen (Fig. 112-7). This procedure has largely replaced previous invasive procedures (such as selective adrenal arteriography and venography) and 19-[^{131}I]iodocholesterol scanning and is of value in localizing adrenal tumors and differentiating them from bilateral hyperplasia.

Diagnosis The diagnosis of Cushing's syndrome depends on the demonstration of increased cortisol production, the ab-

FIGURE 112-6
A 20-year-old female with Cushing's syndrome due to a right adrenal cortical adenoma. A. Two years prior to surgery, age 18. B. One month prior to surgery, age 20. C. One year after surgery, age 21.

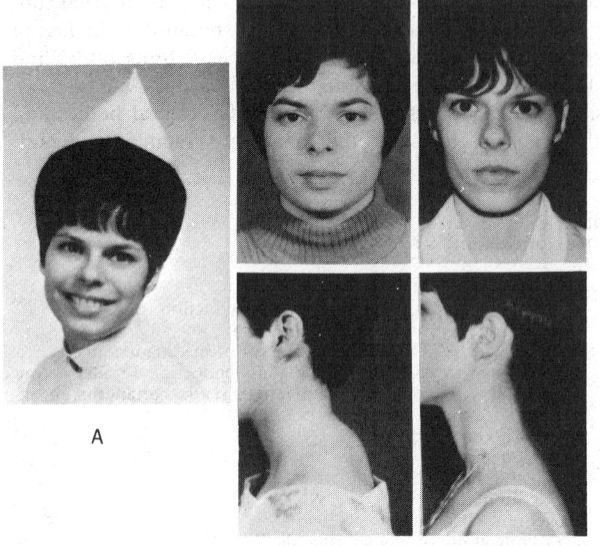

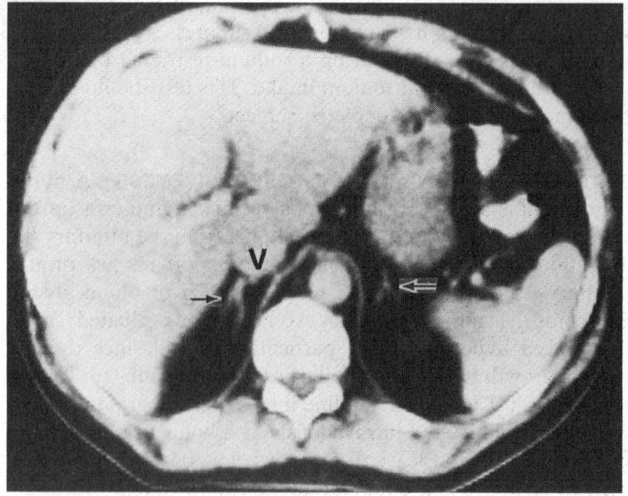

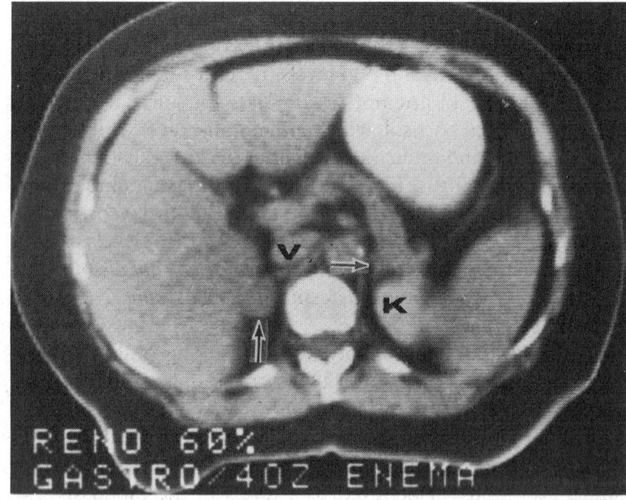

FIGURE 112-7
Computerized tomography is an excellent method for visualizing the adrenal glands. The adrenal glands are indicated by arrows. A. Note the position of the normal right adrenal gland adjacent to the inferior vena cava (V) as it emerges from the liver. Approximately 90 percent of right adrenal glands appear as linear structures extending posteriorly from the inferior vena cava into the space between the right lobe of the liver and the crus of the diaphragm. The normal left adrenal gland is seen lateral to the left crus of the diaphragm and below the stomach. The majority of left adrenal glands are shaped like an inverted V or Y. B. The normal left adrenal gland is seen in its more characteristic position, posterior to the tail of the pancreas and on the anterior surface of the superior pole of the left kidney (K). An adrenal mass replacing the right gland is seen in the usual location of the adrenal posterior to the inferior vena cava (V).

TABLE 112-3
Incidence of signs and symptoms in Cushing's syndrome, percent

Typical habitus	97	Amenorrhea	77
Increased body weight	94	Cutaneous striae	67
Fatigability and weakness	87	Personality changes	66
		Ecchymoses	65
Hypertension (> 150/90)	82	Edema	62
		Polyuria, polydipsia	23
Hirsutism	80	Hypertrophy of clitoris	19

sence of normal diurnal rhythmicity of hormonal secretion, and, most importantly, the failure to suppress endogenous cortisol secretion normally when the glucocorticoid dexamethasone is administered exogenously. Once the diagnosis is established, further testing is designed to determine the etiology of the hypercortisolism (see Fig. 112-8).

For initial screening, the overnight dexamethasone suppression test is recommended (see above). An additional measurement that may be useful in difficult cases (e.g., obesity) is finding a urine free-cortisol excretion rate greater than 100 μg per day. The definitive diagnosis is then established by failure to suppress 17-hydroxysteroid excretion to less than 3 mg per 24 h, urinary free cortisol to less than 30 μg per day, or plasma cortisol to less than 5 μg/dl after a standard low-dose (0.5 mg every 6 h for 48 h) dexamethasone suppression test.

Owing to diurnal variability, plasma cortisol determinations are not meaningful when performed in isolated fashion, but demonstration that the expected normal fall in the bedtime blood levels does not occur may be useful.

Specific diagnosis of the type of Cushing's syndrome can be aided by high-dose dexamethasone suppression testing. When patients with "inappropriate" pituitary ACTH secretion are given high doses of dexamethasone (2 mg every 6 h), suppression of urine 17-hydroxysteroid or free-cortisol levels to less than half the base-line levels can frequently be demonstrated. This is consistent with the view that a pituitary microadenoma is present or that the hypothalamic pituitary axis is reset upward and is responsive only to higher blood levels of glucocorticoids, at which point an appropriate decline in ACTH release occurs. In patients with adrenal hyperplasia secondary to an ACTH-producing tumor, such as an oat-cell bronchogenic carcinoma, or in patients with adrenal neoplasms, usually no suppression occurs after low or high dexamethasone administration. In some instances, ACTH release by nonendocrine tumors can be suppressed by glucocorticoid administration.

The diagnosis of cortisol-producing *adrenal adenoma* is suggested by disproportionate elevations in base-line urine 17-hydroxycorticoid or free-cortisol levels with only modest rises or suppression of urinary 17-ketosteroids or plasma DHEA sulfate. Adrenal androgen secretion is usually reduced in these patients owing to the cortisol-induced suppression of ACTH and subsequent involution of the androgen-producing zona reticularis. Another entity in the differential diagnosis is multinodular ("adenomatous") adrenal hyperplasia, which is an uncommon condition characteristically having features of both hyperplasia and adenomas. Response to ACTH stimulation is variable, but patients with multinodular adrenal hyperplasia most often do not show suppression with the standard doses of dexamethasone. However, with large doses, such as 4 to 8 mg every 6 h, suppression often occurs.

Metyrapone testing is useful in differentiating adrenal tumors (adenoma or carcinoma) from adrenal hyperplasia, since the autonomous adrenal tumors suppress the ACTH-releasing capacity of the pituitary, with the result that on metyrapone challenge testing the pituitary fails to release ACTH in an appropriate manner. This finding of impaired response to metyrapone challenge separates adrenal tumors from adrenal hyperplasia secondary to pituitary ACTH secretion, in which normal or hyperactive responses occur.

The diagnosis of *adrenal carcinoma* as a cause of Cushing's syndrome is suggested by a palpable abdominal mass and by *markedly* elevated base-line values of *both* urine 17-hydroxycorticoids and 17-ketosteroids and plasma DHEA sulfate. Plasma and urine cortisol levels are variably elevated. Adrenal carcinoma is usually resistant to both ACTH stimulation and dexamethasone suppression because of the autonomy of the tumor tissue itself and because of atrophy of the normal remaining adrenal tissue. Markedly elevated adrenal androgen secretion often leads to virilization in the female. Feminizing estrogen-producing adrenocortical carcinoma in the male usually presents with gynecomastia. These adrenal tumors secrete increased amounts of androstenedione which is peripherally converted to the estrogens, estrone and estradiol (see Chap. 119). Functioning adrenal carcinomas that produce Cushing's syndrome are most often associated with elevated values for the intermediates of steroid biosynthesis (especially 11-deoxycortisol), suggesting inefficient conversion of the intermediates to the final product. This is in contrast to Cushing's syndrome associated with adrenocortical hyperplasia, in which the elevation of urine steroids is largely accounted for by cortisol metabolites. It is also important to recognize that 20 percent of adrenal carcinomas are not associated with endocrine syndromes and are presumed to be nonfunctioning or associated with the production of biologically inactive steroid precursors. Finally, the excessive production of sex steroids is not detect-

FIGURE 112-8
Diagnostic flowchart for evaluating patients suspected of having Cushing's syndrome.

**The 17-hydroxycorticosteroid response to metyrapone (750 mg given orally every 4 h for six doses) may be used as an alternative test to the high-dose dexamethasone test (2 mg given orally every 6 h). Increased urinary 17-hydroxycorticosteroid excretion following metyrapone occurs in the majority of patients with adrenal hyperplasia secondary to pituitary ACTH secretion; no response suggests an adrenal neoplasm or adrenal hyperplasia secondary to a nonendocrine ACTH-producing tumor.*

***This group of patients probably contains subjects with both pituitary-hypothalamic dysfunction and pituitary microadenomas. In some instances, a pituitary microadenoma may be visualized by radiographic study, such as CT scanning of the sella turcica.*

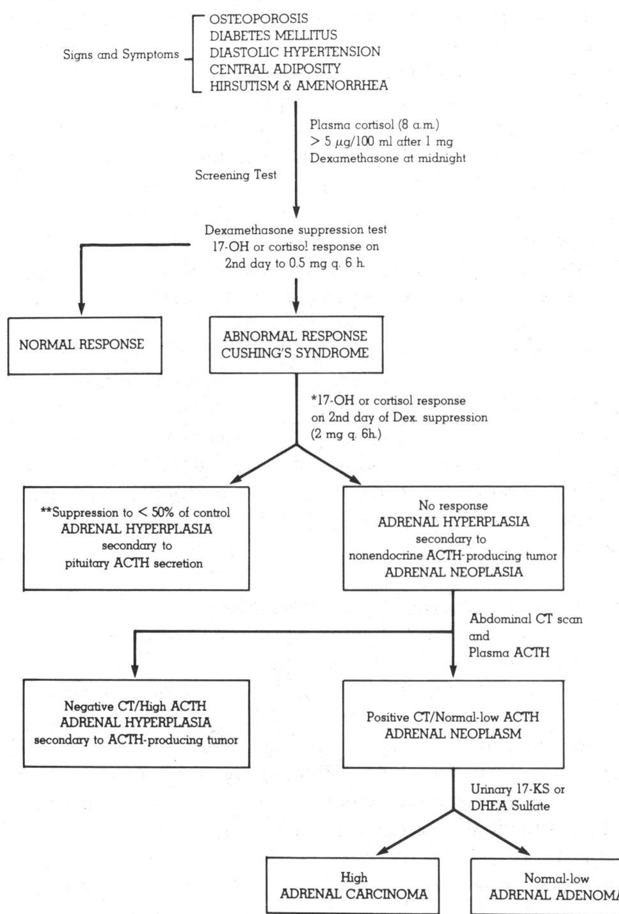

able in certain situations (e.g., androgens in adult male patients), leading to differing rates of occurrence of clinical syndromes in male and female subjects (Table 112-4).

Cushing's syndrome also results from the autonomous production of ACTH by *nonendocrine tumors,* with the resultant development of adrenal hyperplasia. The majority of these cases have been associated with the primitive small-cell type of bronchogenic carcinoma, and the remainder have been reported chiefly with tumors of the thymus, pancreas, or ovary, medullary carcinoma of the thyroid, or bronchial adenomas. The onset of Cushing's syndrome is distinctively sudden in these patients, and this partly accounts for their failure to exhibit all the classic physical findings of the syndrome. (See also Chap. 122.) The secretion of ACTH by nonendocrine tumors is also accompanied by the accumulation of circulating ACTH fragments as well as elevated levels of the larger-molecular-weight species (e.g., β-lipotropin). Since such tumors may produce large amounts of ACTH, base-line urine steroid values are usually markedly elevated, and increased skin pigmentation is usually present. Production of CRF-like material by such tumors has also been reported to cause hypercortisolism. Hypokalemic alkalosis, edema, and hypertension are more common in these patients than in Cushing's syndrome from other causes and are attributed to extremely high levels of cortisol secretion. *Failure to suppress with dexamethasone* and no increment in urine 17-hydroxycorticoid excretion after metyrapone administration are the rule but exceptions have been noted (e.g., bronchial carcinoids). Plasma ACTH levels are often *markedly* elevated in these patients, a helpful diagnostic finding, since plasma ACTH levels in other categories of Cushing's syndrome are at most modestly elevated.

Hyperpigmentation in patients with Cushing's syndrome always points to an extraadrenal tumor, either in an extracranial location, as discussed in the previous paragraph, or within the cranium. Ten to twenty percent of patients undergoing bilateral adrenalectomy for Cushing's syndrome over subsequent months or years develop chromophobe adenomas with progressive cutaneous hyperpigmentation and erosion of the sella turcica (Nelson's syndrome) (see Chap. 109). ACTH and related peptide levels in these patients are extremely high. These tumors may be locally invasive and may impinge on the optic chiasm or extend into the cavernous or sphenoid sinuses. Since intrasellar microadenomas may be present prior to operation in many patients *without* sellar enlargement, a decisive opinion as to their role in the genesis of Cushing's syndrome or in the sequelae of Nelson's syndrome must be withheld. Clinically, all patients documented to have Cushing's syndrome must be carefully examined for pituitary tumor by sella tomography and computerized tomography of the skull. Following bilateral adrenalectomy, patients should be followed for evidence of progressive hyperpigmentation. Periodic but indefinite radiographic evaluation of the sella turcica and serial ACTH levels are important parameters to follow. A diagnostic flowchart for evaluation of patients suspected of having Cushing's syndrome is presented in Fig. 112-8.

TABLE 112-4
Clinical features of adrenal carcinoma in adults

	Male	*Female*
Cushing's syndrome	++	++
Cushing's syndrome plus virilization	0	++++
Virilization	0	+++
Feminization	+	0
Primary aldosteronism	±	±
No endocrine syndrome	+++	++

NOTE: *0, not detectable; +, least common; ++++, most common.*

Differential diagnosis PSEUDOCUSHING'S SYNDROME Three patient groups may present problems in diagnosis: obesity, chronic alcoholism, and depression. Extreme *obesity* is uncommon in Cushing's syndrome; furthermore, with exogenous obesity, the adiposity is generalized, not truncal. On adrenocortical testing, abnormalities in patients with exogenous obesity are usually only modest. Basal urine steroid excretion levels in obese patients are either normal or slightly elevated, a finding similar to their cortisol secretory values. Some patients demonstrate elevated conversion of secreted cortisol into excreted metabolites. *Urinary free* and *blood cortisol* levels are normal, and a normal diurnal pattern in blood and urine levels is seen. It appears that exogenous obesity may *cause* alterations in the secretion and metabolism of steroids, pointing up the secondary nature of altered steroid testing patterns sometimes encountered. Patients with *chronic alcoholism* and *depression* share similar abnormalities in steroid output: elevated urinary 17-hydroxycorticoids, absent diurnal variation, and resistance to suppression with dexamethasone (overnight and low dose). In contrast to alcoholic subjects, depressed patients do not have clinical signs and symptoms of Cushing's syndrome. Following discontinuation of alcohol and/or improvement of the emotional status, steroid testing often returns to normal. A normal cortisol response to insulin hypoglycemia may distinguish these patients from subjects with Cushing's syndrome.

Iatrogenic Cushing's syndrome, induced by the administration of either glucocorticoids or ACTH, is indistinguishable by physical findings from the endogenous forms of adrenocortical hyperfunction. On occasion one may wish to rule out an underlying endogenous form of Cushing's syndrome that may be clinically magnified by exogenous therapy. This is accomplished by changing the therapy to 1 mg dexamethasone daily while collecting urine for corticosteroid analysis. Patients with a pure exogenous form of Cushing's syndrome due to prolonged suppression of the hypothalamic-pituitary axis by administered steroid demonstrate low base-line steroid excretion, a finding in distinct contrast to that in patients with endogenous Cushing's syndrome. Patients receiving long-term ACTH therapy, in addition to the features of glucocorticoid excess, may also have skin pigmentation and hirsutism. The production of iatrogenic Cushing's syndrome is related both to the total steroid dose and to the duration of therapy. Also, patients on afternoon and evening doses of steroid develop Cushing's syndrome more readily on smaller daily steroid doses than do patients on a steroid program limited to morning doses only. In addition, there appears to be a marked difference among patients in the enzymatic disposition and binding (e.g., low albumin) of administered steroid. Several cases have been reported in which a spontaneous remission of Cushing's syndrome occurred; some have been characterized by intermittent abnormalities in adrenal function tests. It is difficult to know whether such abnormalities are functional in nature or true pathophysiological processes.

Evaluation of asymptomatic adrenal masses With the introduction of abdominal CT scanning, many patients with adrenal masses are being discovered. This is not surprising since 10 to 20 percent of subjects at autopsy have adrenal cortical adenomas. The differential diagnosis of this radiographic finding includes Cushing's syndrome (see Figs. 112-7 and 112-8), primary aldosteronism (Fig. 110-9), pheochromocytoma (see Chap. 113), metastatic carcinoma, adrenal cyst, myelolipoma, and nonfunctioning adrenal adenoma, or carcinoma. Further diagnostic or therapeutic intervention is not required in patients with known metastatic disease, or upon demonstration that the lesion is an adrenal cyst or a myelolipoma by CT scanning. The remaining patients should be evaluated for functioning adrenal tumors by appropriate screening procedures; functional tumors should be surgically removed after appropriate presurgical preparation (e.g., see Chap. 113). Nonfunctioning tumors raise difficult therapeutic options. Since 20 percent of adrenal carcinomas are nonfunctioning one could argue that all such lesions should be removed. However, since the frequency of adrenal carcinoma is low compared to the frequency of benign cortical adenoma (less than 1 percent), it is unclear whether surgery is indicated in most cases. If surgery is not performed, a repeat CT scan in 3 to 6 months is required.

Therapy ADRENAL NEOPLASMS When an adenoma or carcinoma is radiographically confirmed, adrenal exploration is performed with excision of the tumor. Because of the possible atrophy of the contralateral adrenal, the patient is treated pre- and postoperatively for total adrenalectomy even when a unilateral lesion is suspected, the routine being similar to that for an Addisonian patient undergoing elective surgery (Table 112-10).

Despite operative intervention, most patients with adrenal carcinoma die within 3 years of diagnosis. Metastases occur most often to liver and lung. The principal antitumor drug used to treat metastatic adrenocortical carcinoma is *o,p′*-DDD [2,2-bis(2-chlorophenyl-4-chlorophenyl)-1,1-dichloroethane], an isomer of the insecticide DDT. This drug suppresses cortisol production and decreases plasma and urine steroid levels. Although its cytotoxic action is relatively selective for the glucocorticoid-secreting zone of the adrenal cortex, the zona glomerulosa (site of aldosterone biosynthesis) may also be inhibited. *o,p′*-DDD also alters the extraadrenal metabolism of cortisol, resulting in a smaller percent excreted in the urine as 17-OHCS. Therefore, *plasma or urinary free-cortisol* levels must be followed to determine the effect of *o,p′*-DDD on the hypercortisolism. *o,p′*-DDD is given in divided doses three to four times daily. The dose is gradually increased to 8 to 10 g daily or the highest dose tolerated by the patient. Almost all patients experience gastrointestinal (anorexia, diarrhea, or vomiting) or neuromuscular (lethargy, somnolence, dizziness) side effects. All patients should be placed on long-term maintenance glucocorticoid; in some instances mineralocorticoid replacement therapy should also be instituted. In approximately one-third of patients regressions of both tumor and metastases occur, but long-term survival is limited. The mean duration of life from onset of treatment is approximately 8 months. In many patients, *o,p′*-DDD only inhibits steroidogenesis and does not produce regression of tumor metastases. Osseous metastases are usually refractory to *o,p′*-DDD; radiation should be used to treat these lesions.

BILATERAL HYPERPLASIA All patients with hyperplasia have a relative or absolute increase in ACTH levels. Primary therapy would logically be directed at correcting this abnormality. Thus, ideally, treatment of nonendocrine, ACTH-producing tumors is surgical removal of the neoplasm. Often this is not possible because the neoplastic disease is far advanced. In this situation "medical" or surgical adrenalectomy may be indicated to correct the hypercortisolism.

Three therapeutic modalities have been employed to reduce pituitary ACTH hypersecretion (Table 112-5). Initial efforts should be directed at radiographically assessing whether a pituitary tumor is present (sella tomography and CT of the sella turcica). If an abnormality is found, transsphenoidal microdissection is the treatment of choice in most centers. Rarely a craniotomy may be necessary if the tumor is large with significant suprasellar and/or lateral extension. If radiographic studies are normal, a microadenoma may still be present. Thus, controversy exists as to whether these patients should be surgically "explored." Complications of surgical therapy included cerebrospinal fluid rhinorrhea, optic nerve injury, diabetes insipidus, and panhypopituitarism. In addition, it is not certain whether these neoplasms will recur over time if the fundamental abnormality is hypothalamic dysfunction.

In some centers, pituitary radiation is the primary treatment. There are two major methods of directing radiotherapy at the pituitary gland. (1) The classic approach is the use of conventional external radiation at a dose of 50,000 mGy (5000 rads) delivered over 3 weeks. Total dosage is limited by possible damage to surrounding neural structures and by the loss of additional pituitary tropic function. Treatment has been successful in fewer than one-third of patients with Cushing's syndrome treated solely by this method. (2) The alpha particle or proton beam has also been used as a source of external radiation. By this method as much as 120,000 mGy (12,000 rads) can be directed at the pituitary gland without evident damage to surrounding structures, because the beam can be focused more sharply than the more commonly used technique and because multiple portals of entry can be used. However, with proton-beam therapy, there may be an increased incidence of ocular motor palsies and hypopituitarism. The long lag time between treatment and remission and the fact that the remission rate is less than 50 percent contraindicate the use of external pituitary irradiation in the presence of rapidly progressing or severe Cushing's disease.

Successful reduction in steroid output in bilateral hyperplasia has also been reported with the chronic administration of the serotonin antagonist, cyproheptadine. Cyproheptadine may block the stimulating effect of hypothalamic serotonin on the release of CRF, thereby reducing pituitary ACTH secretion.

If ACTH levels cannot be successfully lowered by either of these treatment modalities, then medical or surgical adrenalectomy may be indicated (Table 112-5). Chemical adrenalectomy may be accomplished by administration of *o,p′*-DDD (2 to 3 g per day) and/or aminoglutethimide (1 g per day) and metyrapone (2 to 3 g per day).

In patients with *severe* Cushing's syndrome due to adrenal hyperplasia, with features of hypertension, overt diabetes, psychosis, and osteoporosis with pathological fractures and with normal radiographic evaluation of the sella turcica, a complete total bilateral adrenalectomy may be required. Since at least a tenth of these patients develop pituitary tumors after surgery, pituitary irradiation and/or transsphenoidal surgery may also be indicated in any patient who develops increased pigmentation, rising ACTH levels, or in whom the size of the sella turcica increases postoperatively. If Cushing's syndrome redevelops after bilateral adrenalectomy, excessive stimulation of a remnant of adrenocortical tissue may be occurring. In rare in-

TABLE 112-5
Treatment modalities for patients with adrenal hyperplasia secondary to pituitary ACTH hypersecretion

I Reduce pituitary ACTH production
- *A* Transphenoidal resection of microadenoma
- *B* Radiation
- *C* Treatment with hypothalamic serotonin antagonist (cyproheptadine)*

II Reduce or eliminate adrenocortical cortisol secretion
- *A* Bilateral adrenalectomy
- *B* Medical adrenalectomy (metyrapone, *o,p′*-DDD, aminoglutethimide)*

* *Not curative but effective as long as chronically administered in selected patients.*

stances an embryologic extraadrenal remnant may be stimulated to produce excess cortisol. Surgical exploration is difficult because adrenocortical remnants are small. Measurement of cortisol levels from various points along the inferior vena cava may locate the remnant tissue. The use of 19-[^{131}I]iodocholesterol scintillation scanning offers interesting possibilities.

ALDOSTERONISM Aldosteronism is a syndrome associated with hypersecretion of the major adrenal mineralocorticoid aldosterone. *Primary* aldosteronism signifies that the stimulus for the excessive aldosterone production resides within the adrenal gland; in *secondary* aldosteronism the stimulus is of extraadrenal origin.

Primary aldosteronism The constellation of signs and symptoms of excessive inappropriate aldosterone production was first summarized by Conn in 1956. In the original case and in a number of subsequent cases, the disease was the result of an *aldosterone-producing adrenal adenoma* (Conn's syndrome). The majority of cases involved a unilateral adenoma, usually small and occurring with equal frequency on either side. Rarely primary aldosteronism has been reported in association with adrenal carcinoma. It is twice as common in women as in men, presenting between the ages of 30 and 50 and occurring in approximately 1 percent of unselected hypertensive patients. Many cases have been reported with clinical and biochemical characteristics previously considered diagnostic of primary aldosteronism, but a solitary adenoma was not found at surgery. Instead, these patients have *bilateral cortical nodular hyperplasia.* The cause of this hyperplasia is unknown. In the literature this disease has been alternatively termed "pseudo" primary aldosteronism, idiopathic hyperaldosteronism, or nodular hyperplasia.

SIGNS AND SYMPTOMS The continual hypersecretion of aldosterone increases the renal distal tubular exchange of intratubular sodium for secreted potassium and hydrogen ions, with progressive depletion of body potassium and development of hypokalemia. Almost all patients have diastolic hypertension, usually not of marked severity, and complain of headaches. The hypertension is probably due to the increased sodium reabsorption and extracellular volume expansion. *Potassium depletion* is responsible for the muscle weakness and fatigue and is related to the effect of intra- and extracellular potassium ion depletion on muscle membrane. The polyuria results from impairment of concentrating ability and is often associated with polydipsia. These patients may have electrocardiographic and roentgenographic signs of left ventricular enlargement which is secondary to their hypertension. Electrocardiographic signs of potassium depletion such as prominent U waves, cardiac arrhythmias, and premature contractions are not uncommon. In the absence of associated congestive heart failure, renal disease, or preexisting abnormalities (such as thrombophlebitis), edema is characteristically absent in these patients.

In cases of long duration, nephropathy with azotemia may occur, and in some instances it is associated with congestive heart failure and edema.

LABORATORY FINDINGS Laboratory findings are dependent on both the duration and the severity of the potassium depletion. An overnight concentration test often reveals impaired ability to concentrate the urine. Urine pH is neutral to alkaline, because of excessive secretion of ammonium and bicarbonate ions to compensate for a metabolic alkalosis. Tests of glucocorticoid and androgen secretion are always within the normal range in patients with aldosteronomas.

Hypokalemia may be severe (less than 3 meq potassium per liter) and reflects significant body potassium depletion, usually in excess of 300 meq. *Hypernatremia* is due to both sodium retention and a concomitant water loss from polyuria. Metabolic alkalosis and elevation of serum bicarbonate are a result of hydrogen ion loss into the urine and migration into potassium-depleted cells. The alkalosis is perpetuated with potassium deficiency, since such deficiency increases the capacity of the proximal convoluted tubule to reabsorb filtered bicarbonate. If hypokalemia is severe, serum magnesium levels are also reduced. In the absence of azotemia, serum uric acid concentration is normal.

Total body sodium content and total exchangeable sodium are increased while total exchangeable body potassium is usually reduced. The expanded extracellular fluid volume is thought to be responsible for the reversed diurnal excretory pattern for salt and water that many of these patients exhibit, with predominant salt and water excretion occurring during the night.

DIAGNOSIS The diagnosis is suggested by the presence of persistent hypokalemia in a nonedematous patient on a normal sodium intake who is not receiving potassium-wasting (furosemide, ethacrynic acid, thiazides) or potassium-sparing (triamterene, spironolactone) diuretics. If hypokalemia is discovered in a hypertensive patient on a potassium-wasting diuretic, the diuretic should be discontinued, and the patient should be given potassium supplements. After 1 to 2 weeks the potassium level should be remeasured, and if hypokalemia persists, the patient should be evaluated for a mineralocorticoid excess syndrome (Fig. 112-9).

The criteria that subsequently permit the clinician to derive a diagnosis of primary aldosteronism are (1) diastolic hypertension without edema, (2) hyposecretion of renin (as judged by low plasma renin activity levels) which fails to increase appropriately during volume depletion (upright posture, sodium depletion), and (3) hypersecretion of aldosterone which fails to be suppressed appropriately during volume expansion (salt loading).

Patients with primary aldosteronism characteristically *do not have edema,* since they are exhibiting a perpetuated "escape" phenomenon from the sodium-retaining aspects of mineralocorticoids. Rarely in patients with associated nephropathy and azotemia, pretibial edema may be present.

The estimation of plasma renin activity has been of limited value in separating patients with primary aldosteronism from those with other causes of hypertension. While the failure of plasma renin activity to rise normally during volume-depletion maneuvers is a diagnostic criterion for primary aldosteronism, suppressed renin activity also occurs in about 25 percent of patients with essential hypertension.

Since the determination of plasma renin responsiveness is not sufficient, the demonstration of lack of suppression of aldosterone secretion is necessary to diagnose primary aldosteronism (Fig. 112-9). The autonomy exhibited by aldosterone tumors in these patients refers only to their resistance to suppression of secretion during volume expansion; such tumors can and do respond either in normal or supernormal fashion to the stimuli of potassium loading or ACTH infusion.

Once hyposecretion of renin and failure to suppress aldosterone secretion are demonstrated, then localization of aldosterone-producing adenomas should be determined preoperatively by abdominal CT scan or the technique of percutaneous transfemoral bilateral adrenal vein catheterization with simultaneous adrenal venography. The latter technique permits radiological localization, and, in addition, the adrenal vein sampling may demonstrate a two- to threefold increase in plasma aldosterone concentration on the involved side compared with the uninvolved side. In cases of hyperaldosteronism secondary to cortical nodular hyperplasia, no localization is found. It is important for samples to be obtained simultaneously if possible and for cortisol levels to be measured to ensure that false localization does not reflect an ACTH- or stress-induced rise in aldosterone levels.

DIFFERENTIAL DIAGNOSIS Patients with hypertension and hypokalemia may have primary or secondary hyperaldosteronism (see Fig. 112-10). A useful maneuver to distinguish between them is the measurement of plasma renin activity. In patients with accelerated hypertension and secondary aldosteronism, the aldosteronism is secondary to elevated plasma renin levels; in contrast, patients with primary aldosteronism have suppressed plasma renin levels.

Primary aldosteronism must also be distinguished from other *hypermineralocorticoid states.* The most common problem is to distinguish between hyperaldosteronism due to an adenoma and that due to idiopathic bilateral nodular hyperplasia. This is of considerable importance, since the hypertension associated with idiopathic hyperplasia is usually not benefited by bilateral adrenalectomy. In contrast, the hypertension associated with aldosterone-producing tumors is usually improved or cured following removal of the adenoma. Although patients with idiopathic bilateral nodular hyperplasia tend to have less severe hypokalemia, lower aldosterone secretion, and higher plasma renin activity than patients with primary aldosteronism, differentiation is impossible solely on clinical and/or biochemical grounds. An anomalous postural decrease in plasma aldosterone has also been reported in the majority of patients with a unilateral lesion, but this test is of limited diagnostic value in the individual patient. A definitive diagnosis is best made by radiographic studies as noted above.

FIGURE 112-9
Diagnostic flowchart for evaluating patients with suspected primary aldosteronism.

**Serum K^+ may be normal in some patients with hyperaldosteronism who are taking potassium-sparing diuretics (spironolactone, triamterene) or ingesting low sodium–high potassium intakes.*

†This step should not be taken if hypertension is severe (diastolic > 115 mmHg) or if cardiac failure is present. Also, serum potassium levels should be corrected before the infusion of saline. Alternative methods producing comparable suppression of aldosterone secretion include oral sodium loading (200 meq per day for 3 days) or 10 mg deoxycorticosterone acetate (DOCA) intramuscularly every 12 h for 3 days.

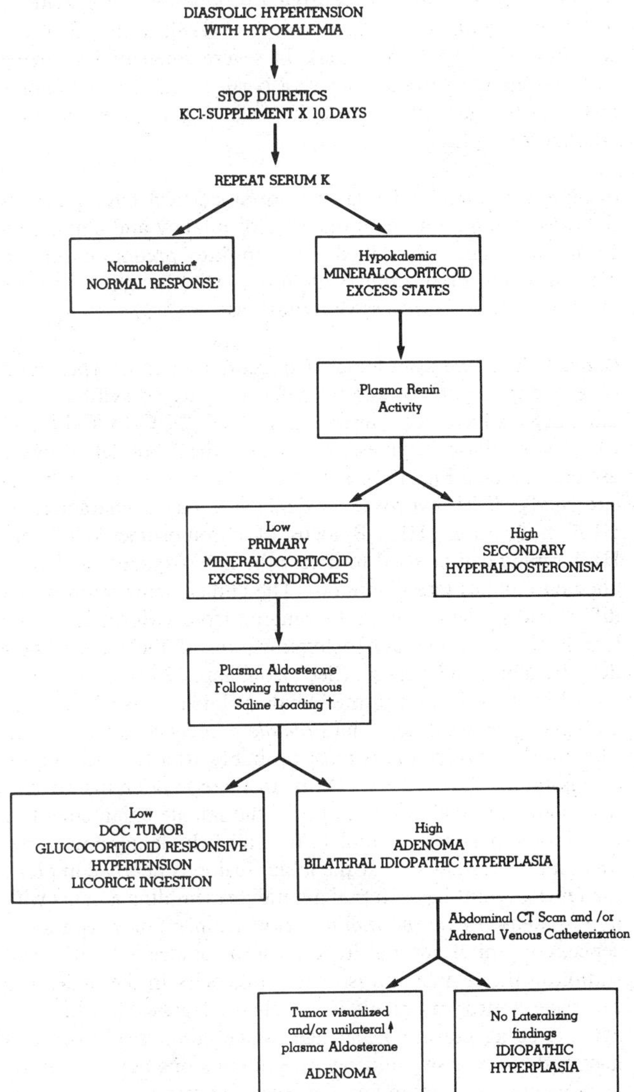

In a few instances, hypertensive patients with hypokalemic alkalosis have been found to have deoxycorticosterone (DOC)-secreting adenomas. Such patients have reduced plasma renin activity levels, but aldosterone measurements are either normal or reduced, suggesting the diagnosis of mineralocorticoid excess due to a hormone other than aldosterone. Rare cases of hypermineralocorticoidism due to a defect in cortisol biosynthesis, specifically 11- or 17-hydroxylation, have also been reported. ACTH levels are increased, with a resultant increase in the production of the mineralocorticoid 11-deoxycorticosterone. *Hypertension and hypokalemia can be corrected by glucocorticoid administration.* The definitive diagnosis is made by demonstrating an elevation of precursors of cortisol biosynthesis in the blood or urine. Occasionally, glucocorticoid administration produces normotension and normokalemia although a hydroxylase deficiency cannot be identified (Fig. 112-9).

The ingestion of candies or chewing tobacco containing certain forms of licorice produces a syndrome mimicking primary aldosteronism. The sodium-retaining principle in such agents is glycyrrhizinic acid, which, in addition to sodium retention, causes expansion of the extracellular fluid volume, hypertension, depressed plasma renin levels, and suppressed aldosterone levels. The diagnosis is established or excluded by a careful history.

TREATMENT Primary aldosteronism due to an adenoma is usually treated by surgical excision. However, dietary sodium restriction and the administration of the aldosterone antagonist, spironolactone, are also effective in many cases. Hypertension and hypokalemia are usually controlled by doses of 25 to 100 mg spironolactone every 8 h. Some patients have been successfully managed medically for years, but chronic therapy in men is usually limited by the common occurrence of gynecomastia, decreased libido, and impotence.

When bilateral hyperplasia is suspected, surgery is indicated only when significant, symptomatic hypokalemia cannot be controlled with medical therapy, e.g., spironolactone, triamterene, or amiloride. Hypertension associated with idiopathic hyperplasia is usually not benefited by bilateral adrenalectomy.

Secondary aldosteronism Secondary aldosteronism refers to an appropriately increased production of aldosterone by the adrenal gland in response to activation of the renin-angiotensin system (Fig. 112-10). The adrenal production rates of aldosterone are often higher in patients with secondary aldosteronism than in those with primary aldosteronism. Most patients with secondary aldosteronism exhibit this syndrome either as an associated feature of the accelerated phase of hypertension (regardless of the primary disease) or on the basis of an underlying edema disorder. On the other hand, secondary aldosteronism in pregnancy is a normal physiological response to estrogen-induced increases in circulating levels of renin substrate and plasma renin activity, as well as the antialdosterone actions of the progestins.

Secondary aldosteronism in hypertensive states either is secondary to a primary overproduction of renin (primary reninism) or is caused by an overproduction of renin which is secondary to a decrease in renal blood flow and/or perfusion pressure (Fig. 112-5). Secondary hypersecretion of renin could be due to a narrowing of one or both of the major renal arteries either by an atherosclerotic plaque or by fibromuscular hyperplasia. Overproduction of renin from both kidneys also occurs in association with severe arteriolar nephrosclerosis (malignant hypertension) or secondary to profound renal vasoconstriction (accelerated phase of hypertensive disease). These patients exhibit a secondary aldosteronism characterized by hypokalemic alkalosis, moderate to severe increases in plasma renin activity, and moderate to marked increases in aldosterone levels (see Chap. 267).

Secondary aldosteronism with hypertension is also associated with the rare renin-producing tumor, so-called primary reninism. These patients have all the biochemical characteristics of renal vascular hypertension; however, the primary defect is not a decrease in renal blood flow and/or perfusion pressure but renin secretion by a juxtaglomerular-cell tumor. The diagnosis can be made by the absence of changes in renal vasculature and/or demonstration of a space-occupying lesion by radiographic techniques and unilateral increases in renal vein renin activity.

Secondary aldosteronism is present in many *edema* disorders. Increased aldosterone secretion rates have been documented in patients with edema as a result of either cirrhosis or the nephrotic syndrome. In congestive heart failure, however, elevated aldosterone secretion is a variable finding dependent on the severity of cardiac decompensation. The stimulus for aldosterone release in these clinical conditions appears to be *arterial hypovolemia* and/or hypotension. Diuretic therapy often exaggerates the features of secondary aldosteronism via the mechanism of acute volume depletion; when this happens hypokalemia and on occasion alkalosis become prominent features.

Secondary hyperaldosteronism may rarely occur without edema or hypertension (Bartter's syndrome). This syndrome is characterized by the signs of severe hyperaldosteronism (hypokalemic alkalosis) with moderate to marked increases in renin activity but normal blood pressure and absence of edema. Renal biopsy shows juxtaglomerular hyperplasia. The pathogenesis of this syndrome may be a defect in the renal conservation of sodium or chloride. The renal loss of sodium is thought to stimulate renin secretion and subsequently aldosterone production. Hyperaldosteronism produces potassium depletion, with the hypokalemia further elevating plasma renin activity. In some cases, the hypokalemia may be potentiated by a defect in renal conservation of potassium. One associated abnormality is an increased production of prostaglandins.

FIGURE 112-10
Responses of the renin-aldosterone volume control loop in primary versus secondary aldosteronism.

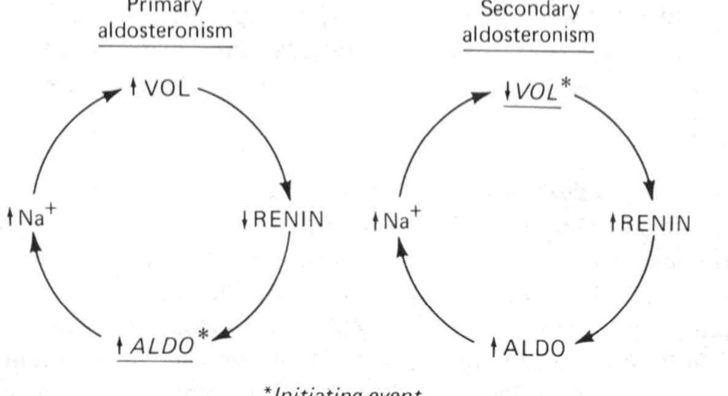

ADRENAL VIRILISM AND CONGENITAL ADRENAL HYPERPLASIA The adrenal virilizing syndromes result from excessive production of adrenal androgens, such as dehydroepiandrosterone and androstenedione, which are converted to testosterone; the elevated testosterone levels account for most of the virilization. As in other states of adrenocortical hyperfunction, the syndrome may result from hyperplasia, adenoma, or carcinoma. Adrenal virilization may arise in a congenital form, termed *congenital adrenal hyperplasia,* due to enzymatic deficits. The adrenal virilizing syndromes may be associated with secretions of greater or smaller amounts of other adrenal hormones and may, therefore, present as "pure" syndromes of virilization or as "mixed" syndromes associated with excessive production of glucocorticoid and some of the characteristics of Cushing's syndrome. In *congenital* adrenal hyperplasia the virilizing syndromes are associated with increased adrenal androgen production and either excessive or decreased secretion of mineralocorticoid or decreased production of glucocorticoid.

Since in humans cortisol is the principal adrenal steroid regulating ACTH elaboration and since ACTH stimulates both cortisol and adrenal androgen production, an enzymatic interference with cortisol synthesis may result in the enhanced secretion of adrenal androgens. In severe congenital virilizing hyperplasia, the adrenal output of cortisol may be so compromised as to cause glucocorticoid deficiency despite anatomic adrenal hyperplasia.

Incidence Congenital bilateral adrenocortical hyperplasia is the most common adrenal disorder of infancy and childhood. It has also been described later in life, predominantly in women. Congenital adrenal hyperplasia is thought to be the result of autosomal recessive mutations.

Clinical signs and symptoms Congenital adrenal hyperplasia is secondary to one of several defects in steroid synthesis. To date, defects have been described in the C-21, C-18, C-17, and C-11 hydroxylase enzymes, as well as in the 3β-ol-dehydrogenase enzyme (see Fig. 112-2). These enzyme deficits usually occur singly. C-21 hydroxylase deficiency has a characteristic HLA association (HLA-B locus of chromosome 6) so that HLA typing can be used to detect the heterozygous carriers in affected families (see Chap. 60). The clinical expression in the different disorders is variable, ranging from virilization of the female (C-21 deficiency) to feminization of the male (3β-ol-dehydrogenase deficiency). (See also Chap. 120.)

Adrenal virilization in the female at birth is associated with ambiguous external genitalia (*female pseudohermaphroditism*). The onset of virilization is most probably after the fifth month of embryonic development. At birth there may be macrogenitosomia in the male infant, and in the female enlargement of the clitoris, partial or complete fusion of the labia, and sometimes a urogenital sinus. If the labial fusion is nearly complete, the female infant has external genitalia resembling a penis with hypospadias. In the *postnatal* period from infancy to adolescence, congenital adrenal hyperplasia is associated with virilization in the female and isosexual precocity in the male. The excessive androgens result in accelerated growth, with bone age exceeding chronological age. Since epiphyseal closure is hastened by excessive androgens, growth stops but truncal development continues, giving the characteristic appearance of a child of short stature with well-developed trunk. Incomplete variants of congenital adrenal hyperplasia sometimes become manifest only in adult life with virilization or hirsutism in the female.

In the adult woman, regardless of the cause of the condition, the clinical signs and symptoms are those anticipated from excessive androgen production. These include hirsutism, acne, increased sebum production, temporal baldness, deepening of voice, increased muscle mass and strength, decreased breast size, amenorrhea, enlargement of the clitoris, increased sexual drive, and development of a male habitus. The clinical distinction between excessive hair growth (hirsutism) and virilization is useful. Virilization signifies that multiple signs of androgen excess are present in addition to hirsutism; one of the more easily recognized of these signs is hypertrophy of the clitoris.

The most common form of congenital adrenal hyperplasia (95 percent of cases) is a result of impairment of *C-21 hydroxylation.* In addition to cortisol deficiency, in approximately one-third of the patients, there is an associated reduction in aldosterone secretion. Thus, with congenital adrenal hyperplasia secondary to C-21 hydroxylase deficiency, adrenal virilization is present with or without an associated salt-losing tendency due to aldosterone deficiency (see Fig. 112-2).

With *C-11 hydroxylase* deficiency a "hypertensive" variant of congenital adrenal hyperplasia develops. Hypertension and hypokalemia occur because of the impaired conversion of 11-deoxycorticosterone to corticosterone, resulting in the accumulation of 11-deoxycorticosterone, a potent mineralocorticoid. Increased shunting again occurs into the androgen pathway.

The *C-17 hydroxylase* deficiency is characterized by hypogonadism, hypokalemia, and hypertension. In patients with this rare deficiency there is decreased production of cortisol and shunting of precursors into the mineralocorticoid pathway with hypokalemic alkalosis, hypertension, and suppressed plasma renin activity. In most patients, 11-deoxycorticosterone production is elevated. Because C-17 hydroxylation is required for biosynthesis of adrenal androgens as well as for biosynthesis of gonadal testosterone and estrogen, this defect is associated with sexual immaturity, high urinary gonadotropin levels, and low urinary 17-ketosteroid excretion. Female patients have primary amenorrhea and lack of development of secondary sexual characteristics. Because of deficient androgen production, male patients either have ambiguous external genitalia or a female phenotype (male pseudohermaphroditism). Exogenous glucocorticoids can correct the hypertensive syndrome, but treatment with appropriate gonadal steroids is necessary to produce sexual maturation.

With 3β-ol-dehydrogenase deficiency, there is impaired conversion of pregnenolone to progesterone, with the result that pathways to both cortisol and aldosterone are "blocked," with shunting then occurring into the adrenal androgen pathway via 17α-hydroxypregnenolone to dehydroepiandrosterone. Since dehydroepiandrosterone is a weak androgen and because this enzyme deficiency is also present in the gonad, the genitalia of the male fetus may be incompletely virilized or feminized. Conversely, in the female, overproduction of dehydroepiandrosterone may produce partial virilization.

Diagnosis The diagnosis of *congenital adrenal hyperplasia* should be considered in all infants exhibiting "failure to thrive," particularly those having episodes of acute adrenal insufficiency or salt-wasting, or showing sustained hypertension. The diagnosis is further suggested by the finding of hypertrophy of the clitoris, fused labia, or urogenital sinus in the female and isosexual precocity in the male. In infants and children with a *C-21 hydroxylation block,* increased urine 17-ketosteroid excretion and plasma DHEA sulfate are typically associated with an increase in the blood levels of 17α-hydroxyprogesterone and the urinary excretion of the metabolite of this steroid, pregnanetriol.

The diagnosis of a *salt-losing form of congenital* adrenal hyperplasia due to defects in C-21 hydroxylase enzyme is suggested by episodes of acute adrenal insufficiency with hyponatremia, hyperkalemia, dehydration, and vomiting. These infants and children often "crave" salt and exhibit laboratory signs of concomitant deficits in both cortisol and aldosterone secretion.

With the *hypertensive form* of congenital adrenal hyperplasia due to impaired C-11 hydroxylation, 11-deoxycorticosterone (a potent mineralocorticoid) and 11-deoxycortisol accumulate. Both urine 17-ketosteroid and 17-hydroxycorticoid excretion may be elevated since 11-deoxycortisol is included in the analysis of Porter-Silber chromogens. The diagnosis is secured by demonstrating increased levels of 11-deoxycortisol in the blood or increased amounts of tetrahydro-11-deoxycortisol in the urine.

The finding of very high levels of urine dehydroepiandrosterone with low levels of pregnanetriol and of cortisol metabolites is characteristic of patients with congenital adrenal hyperplasia due to 3β-ol-dehydrogenase deficiency. These patients also exhibit marked salt wasting.

The *C-17 hydroxylase* deficiency results in the accumulation of progesterone and its metabolite, pregnanediol. The excretion of deoxycorticosterone and of corticosterone is increased, while aldosterone production is usually subnormal.

The adrenal virilizing syndrome in adults is most often due to acquired causes—namely, tumor or adrenal hyperplasia. *Adrenal adenomas* and *carcinomas* may cause a pure or mixed virilizing syndrome (Table 112-4). Since adrenal androgens are weak compared with gonadal androgens, adrenal virilization is characterized by *large increments in urine 17-ketosteroid excretion.* Virilizing adrenocortical adenomas are rare. *Virilizing adrenal carcinomas* are the most common adrenal tumor causing virilization. They are associated with high plasma DHEA sulfate levels and high urinary 17-ketosteroid excretion rates; cortisol levels and 17-hydroxycorticosteroid excretion are normal or moderately elevated. Clinical differentiation between virilizing adrenal adenoma and carcinoma cannot be made with certainty preoperatively.

Some patients with hirsutism may have a mild form of congenital adrenal hyperplasia. Mild hirsutism usually appears after puberty and is characterized by normal or moderately elevated urinary 17-ketosteroids and plasma DHEA sulfate. With ACTH stimulation, there may be a brisk rise in the urinary 17-ketosteroids, DHEA sulfate, and one or more precursors of cortisol biosynthesis (e.g., 11-deoxycortisol, 17α-hydroxyprogesterone). Baseline 17-ketosteroids are easily suppressed by daily administration of 2 mg dexamethasone.

Differential diagnosis In the female, the differential diagnosis of hirsutism and virilization is between adrenal and ovarian etiologies (Table 112-6). *Sudden onset of progressive hirsutism and virilization* suggests an adrenal or ovarian neoplasm. Since adrenal tumors secrete weak androgens (such as DHEA), virilizing adrenal neoplasms are characterized by high urine 17-ketosteroid excretion, usually in excess of 30 to 40 mg per 24 h, and high plasma DHEA sulfate levels. Failure to reduce 17-ketosteroid levels and plasma DHEA sulfate levels to normal following dexamethasone suppression (0.5 mg given orally every 6 h for 7 days) supports a diagnosis of virilizing adrenal tumor and excludes congenital adrenal hyperplasia. The most common *ovarian tumor* causing virilization is the arrhenoblastoma, but other ovarian tumors, such as adrenal rest tumor,

TABLE 112-6
Causes of hirsutism in women

I Familial
II Idiopathic
III Ovarian
  A Polycystic ovaries; hilus-cell hyperplasia
  B Tumor; arrhenoblastoma, hilus cell, adrenal rest
IV Adrenal
  A Congenital adrenal hyperplasia
  B Noncongenital adrenal hyperplasia (Cushing's)
  C Tumor: virilizing carcinoma or adenoma

granulosa-cell tumor, hilar-cell tumors, and Brenner tumors have been associated with virilization. Virilization due to ovarian tumors is usually characterized by normal levels of urinary 17-ketosteroids and DHEA sulfate, since the neoplasm usually secretes the potent androgen testosterone. Occasionally increases in 17-ketosteroid excretion occur in some patients with ovarian neoplasms, but base-line 17-ketosteroid excretion in excess of 30 mg per day is rare with the exception of adrenal rest tumors. Like adrenal neoplasms, ovarian tumors fail to be suppressed by dexamethasone. With the exception of adrenal rest tumors, they are largely independent of ACTH stimulation. Elevations of plasma testosterone or urinary testosterone excretion do not localize the neoplasm to the ovary, since testosterone can be elevated subsequent to peripheral conversion of adrenal precursors, such as DHEA (see Chap. 118).

Hirsutism without virilization beginning after puberty and associated with normal ovarian and adrenal function is diagnostic of idiopathic or familial hirsutism. In another group of patients, hirsutism is seen in association with sclerocystic or polycystic ovaries. Oligomenorrhea, anovulatory bleeding, and/or amenorrhea commonly occur in these patients. The ovaries may be palpably enlarged bilaterally; unilateral enlargement suggests an ovarian neoplasm. The presence of polycystic ovaries at laparoscopy does not establish an ovarian causation since polycystic ovaries have been described in association with adrenal virilization. 17-Ketosteroid excretion values and DHEA levels in hirsute females with polycystic ovary disease are usually normal or slightly elevated. *Plasma testosterone* levels tend to be higher in females with polycystic ovary disease than in normal females, and in 20 percent of cases testosterone levels are greater than the upper limit of normal. In some instances where the testosterone levels are normal, the free or unbound fraction has been found to be elevated. Luteinizing hormone (LH) levels are tonically elevated in some patients with polycystic ovary disease. The laboratory findings in patients with hirsutism-virilizing syndromes are summarized in Table 112-7.

Treatment Treatment of adrenal virilism is dictated by the type of lesion suspected. Patients with *congenital adrenal hyperplasia* have a fundamental defect of cortisol deficiency with resultant excessive ACTH stimulation, producing hyperplasia of the adrenal glands and causing additional "shunting" into the adrenal androgen pathway. Therapy in these patients consists of daily administration of glucocorticoids to suppress pituitary ACTH secretion. Because of its cost and intermediate half-life, prednisone is the drug of choice except in infants, when hydrocortisone is usually used. The amount of steroid required to manage patients with congenital adrenal hyperplasia is equivalent to approximately 1 to 1.5 times the normal cortisol production rate of 12 to 13 mg cortisol per square meter of body surface area per day and is given in divided doses two or three times a day. In some patients, a single bedtime dose of a long-acting glucocorticoid may suffice. As the patient grows, the maintenance dose obviously should be increased. The dosage schedule is governed by repetitive analysis of the urinary 17-ketosteroids, plasma DHEA sulfate, and/or precursors of cortisol biosynthesis. Skeletal growth and maturation must also be closely monitored since overtreatment with glucocorticoid replacement therapy retards linear growth. In children, glucocorticoids not only suppress urinary ketosteroid excretion but also end virilization and the associated problems of hyperandrogenicity. Some infants and children with the associated defect of salt wasting require vigorous correction of salt deficits in conjunction with small doses of a potent mineralocorticoid such as 9α-fluorohydrocortisone. Children with abnormalities of external genitalia may require surgical correction of labial fusion, urogenital sinus, etc. Diagnosis of the adrenogenital syndrome in the newborn with ambiguous external genitalia is crucial to avoid errors in the assignment of sex (see Chap. 120). Response of these children to steroid therapy is gratifying in that normal growth and development occur and the menarche and onset of spermatogenesis occur at the appropriate age. Many females with this disorder have married and have borne children. Steroid therapy is indicated throughout life, and dosages should be periodically adjusted for major stress as in the Addisonian patient.

HYPOFUNCTION OF ADRENAL CORTEX

Adrenocortical hypofunction includes all conditions in which the secretion of adrenal steroid hormones falls below the requirements of the body. Adrenal insufficiency may be divided into two general categories: (1) those associated with primary inability of the adrenal to elaborate sufficient quantities of hormone and (2) those associated with a secondary failure due to a primary failure in the elaboration of ACTH (Table 112-8).

PRIMARY ADRENOCORTICAL DEFICIENCY (ADDISON'S DISEASE) Addison's description in 1855, namely, "general languor and debility, remarkable feebleness of the heart's action, irritability of the stomach, and a peculiar change of the color of the skin," summarizes the dominant clinical features of the

TABLE 112-7
Laboratory evaluation of hirsutism-virilizing syndromes

	Ovarian		*Adrenal*			
	PCO	*Ovarian tumor*	*CAH*	*Adrenal neoplasm*	*Cushing's syndrome*	*Idiopathic*
Urinary 17-ketosteroids, plasma DHEA sulfate	N↑	N	N↑	↑↑↑	N↑	N
Plasma testosterone	N↑	↑↑	N↑	N↑	N↑	N
Serial LH levels	N↑	N	N	N	N	N
Precursors of cortisol biosynthesis:						
Basal	N	N	N↑	N↑	N	N
Following ACTH infusion	N	N	↑↑	N↑	N	N
Cortisol following overnight dexamethasone suppression test	N	N	N	↑	↑	N

NOTE: *N, normal; CAH, congenital adrenal hyperplasia; PCO, polycystic ovary syndrome; LH, luteinizing hormone.*

TABLE 112-8
Classification of adrenal insufficiency

I Primary adrenal insufficiency
  A Anatomic destruction of gland (chronic and acute)
    1 "Idiopathic" atrophy (autoimmune)
    2 Surgical removal (metastatic breast cancer)
    3 Infection (tuberculous, fungous)
    4 Hemorrhage
    5 Invasion: metastatic
  B Metabolic failure in hormone production
    1 Congenital adrenal hyperplasia
    2 Enzyme inhibitors (metyrapone)
    3 Cytotoxic agents (*o,p*′-DDD)
II Secondary adrenal insufficiency
  A Hypopituitarism due to pituitary disease
  B Suppression of hypothalamic-pituitary axis
    1 Exogenous steroid
    2 Endogenous steroid from tumor

disease. Advanced cases are usually easy to diagnose, but recognition of the disease in its earlier phases may present a real challenge. Early diagnosis is important, since present-day therapy completely corrects the metabolic derangement.

Incidence Primary adrenocortical insufficiency is relatively rare. It may occur at any age and affects both sexes with equal frequency. Because of increasing therapeutic use of exogenous steroids, secondary adrenal insufficiency is seen with increasing frequency.

Etiology and pathogenesis Addison's disease results from progressive adrenocortical destruction, which must involve more than 90 percent of the glands before clinical signs of adrenal insufficiency appear. The adrenal is a frequent site for chronic infectious diseases of the granulomatous variety, predominantly tuberculosis but also including fungal infections, such as histoplasmosis, coccidioidomycosis, and cryptococcosis. In previous years, tuberculosis was found at postmortem examination in 70 to 90 percent of cases; however, the most frequent finding at present is *idiopathic* atrophy, and an autoimmune mechanism is probably responsible. Rarely, other lesions are encountered, such as bilateral tumor metastases, amyloidosis, or sarcoidosis.

The possibility that some patients may have primary adrenal insufficiency on an *autoimmune basis* is strengthened by the finding that half of patients with Addison's disease have circulating adrenal antibodies. Certain of these patients also have additional circulating antibodies to thyroid, parathyroid, and/or gonadal tissue (see also Chap. 123). There is also an increased incidence of chronic lymphocytic thyroiditis (Hashimoto's disease) in patients with nontuberculous, idiopathic adrenal insufficiency (Schmidt's syndrome). Idiopathic hypoparathyroidism is also seen with increased frequency in patients with Addison's disease (Chap. 123). Concomitant parathyroid and adrenal insufficiency and mucocutaneous moniliasis constitutes a distinct familial, autosomal recessive syndrome. Diabetes mellitus, ovarian failure, and pernicious anemia are also seen in association with idiopathic Addison's disease and chronic thyroiditis. The mechanisms by which genetic predisposition and/or autoimmunity interact in the pathogenesis of these diseases is unknown. Recent reports also indicate a greater incidence of these endocrine deficiency states in patients with specific human leukocyte antigens (B8 and Dw3).

Clinical signs and symptoms Adrenocortical insufficiency is characterized by an insidious onset of slowly progressive fatigability, weakness, anorexia, nausea and vomiting, weight loss, cutaneous and mucosal pigmentation, hypotension, and occasionally hypoglycemia (Table 112-9). However, the spectrum may vary, depending on the duration and degree of adrenal hypofunction, from a complaint of mild chronic fatigue to the fulminating shock associated with acute massive destruction of the glands in the type of syndrome described by Waterhouse and Friderichsen.

Asthenia is the cardinal symptom of Addison's disease. Early it may be sporadic, usually most evident at times of stress; as adrenal function becomes more impaired, the weakness progresses until the patient is continuously fatigued, necessitating bed rest.

Hyperpigmentation may be a striking sign of the disease, but its absence does not exclude this diagnosis. It commonly appears as a diffuse brown, tan, or bronze darkening of both exposed and unexposed parts such as elbows or creases of the hand and in areas normally pigmented such as the areolas about the nipples. In many patients, bluish-black patches appear on the mucous membranes. Some patients develop dark freckles, and occasionally irregular areas of vitiligo may appear paradoxically. As an early sign, patients may notice an unusually persistent tanning following exposure to the sun.

Arterial hypotension is frequent, and in severe cases blood pressures may be in the range of 80/50 or less. Postural accentuation is common.

Abnormalities of gastrointestinal function often are the presenting complaint. Symptoms may vary from mild anorexia with weight loss to fulminating nausea, vomiting, diarrhea, and ill-defined abdominal pain, which at times may be so severe as to be confused with an acute abdomen. In addition, patients with adrenal insufficiency frequently have marked personality changes, usually in the form of excessive irritability and restlessness. Enhancement of the sensory modalities of taste, olfaction, and hearing is often present and is reversible with therapy. A decrease in axillary and pubic hair is common in female patients due to loss of adrenal androgen production.

Laboratory findings In the milder forms, there may be no demonstrable abnormalities in any of the parameters measured in the routine laboratory, and even plasma and urinary steroid determinations may indicate values relatively low yet within normal range. However, studies of adrenal stimulation with ACTH show abnormalities even in this stage of the disease. In the more advanced stages, levels of serum sodium, chloride, and bicarbonate are reduced while serum potassium is elevated. The hyponatremia is due to extravascular loss of sodium both into the urine (due to aldosterone deficiency) and into the intracellular compartment. This extravascular sodium loss depletes extracellular fluid volume and accentuates hypotension. Elevated plasma vasopressin and angiotensin II levels may be contributing factors to hyponatremia through impairment of free-water clearance. The hyperkalemia is due to a combination of factors, including aldosterone deficiency, impaired glomerular filtration, and acidosis. Mild to moderate hypercalcemia is seen in 10 to 20 percent of patients; the reason for this is not understood. The electrocardiogram may show nonspe-

TABLE 112-9
Incidence of symptoms and signs in Addison's disease, percent

Symptom/sign	%	Symptom/sign	%
Weakness	99	Hypotension (<110/70)	87
Pigmentation of skin	98	Abdominal pain	34
Pigmentation of mucous membranes	82	Salt craving	22
Weight loss	97	Diarrhea	20
Anorexia, nausea, and vomiting	90	Constipation	19
		Syncope	16
		Vitiligo	9

cific changes, and the electroencephalogram exhibits a generalized reduction and slowing. There may be a normocytic anemia, a relative lymphocytosis, and usually a moderate eosinophilia.

Diagnosis The diagnosis of adrenal insufficiency should be made only with ACTH stimulation testing to assay the adrenal reserve capacity for steroid production (see above for ACTH test protocols).

In cases of severe *adrenal insufficiency* the cortisol secretory rate is markedly decreased, and this may be ascertained indirectly by the finding of low to absent 24-h urine cortisol, 17-hydroxycorticoids, and 17-ketosteroids. With mild or moderate adrenal insufficiency, urine steroid excretion values overlap into the normal range; because of this, a diagnosis of adrenal insufficiency should never be excluded solely on the basis of normal basal urine steroid determinations. Plasma cortisol values vary from zero to the lower range of normal. Aldosterone secretion is usually low, resulting in salt wasting and secondary rises in plasma renin levels. In patients with primary adrenal insufficiency, plasma ACTH and associated peptides are elevated because of loss of the usual cortisol-hypothalamic-pituitary feedback relationship, whereas in secondary adrenal insufficiency, plasma ACTH values are low, or "inappropriately" normal (Fig. 112-11).

Differential diagnosis Since weakness and fatigue are common complaints, clinical diagnosis of early adrenocortical insufficiency is frequently difficult. However, mild gastrointestinal distress with weight loss, anorexia, and a suggestion of increased pigmentation make mandatory ACTH stimulation testing to rule out adrenal insufficiency, particularly before steroid treatment is begun. Weight loss is useful in evaluating the significance of weakness and malaise. Weight gain associated with lassitude is more characteristic of depressive syndromes. Racial pigmentation in many individuals may be a problem, but a *recent* and progressive *increase* is usually reported by the Addisonian patient. Hyperpigmentation in other diseases may also present a problem, but the appearance and distribution of pigment in Addison's disease are usually characteristic. When doubt exists, measurement of ACTH levels and testing of adrenal reserve with the infusion of ACTH provide clear-cut differentiation.

Treatment All patients with Addison's disease should receive specific hormone replacement. Like diabetics, these patients require careful and persistent education in regard to their disease. Since the adrenal gland elaborates three general classes of hormone, of which two, glucocorticoids and mineralocorticoids, are of primary clinical importance, replacement therapy should correct both deficiencies. Cortisone (or cortisol) is the mainstay of treatment; however, its mineralocorticoid effect, when it is given in sufficient dosage to replace the endogenous cortisol deficiency, is inadequate for complete electrolyte balance; therefore, the patient usually requires other supplementary therapy. Cortisone dosage varies from 12.5 to 50 mg daily, with the majority of patients taking 25 to 37.5 mg in divided doses. Cortisol (30 mg daily) or prednisone (7.5 mg daily) in divided doses may also be given for substitution therapy. Because of its direct local effect on gastric mucosa, patients are advised to take their cortisone with meals or, if this is impractical, with milk or an antacid preparation. In addition, the larger proportion of the dose (25 mg) is taken in the morning and the remainder (12.5 mg) in the late afternoon, to simulate the normal diurnal adrenal rhythm. Some patients may exhibit insomnia, irritability, and mental excitement after initiation of therapy; in these, the dosage should be reduced. Other indications for maintaining the patient on smaller amounts of glucocorticoids are hypertension, diabetes, or active tuberculosis.

Since this amount of cortisone or cortisol fails to replace the mineralocorticoid component of the adrenal gland, supplementary hormone is usually needed. This is accomplished by the daily oral administration of 0.05 to 0.1 mg 9α-fluorohydrocortisone. If parenteral administration is indicated, a dosage of 2 to 5 mg deoxycorticosterone acetate in oil may be given every day intramuscularly.

Complications of glucocorticoid therapy, with the exception of gastritis, are *rare* in the dosage used in the treatment of Addison's disease. Complications of mineralocorticoid therapy occur more frequently and include hypokalemia, edema, hypertension, cardiac enlargement, or even congestive failure due to sodium retention. In the management of patients with Addison's disease, periodic measurements of body weight, serum potassium, and blood pressure are useful.

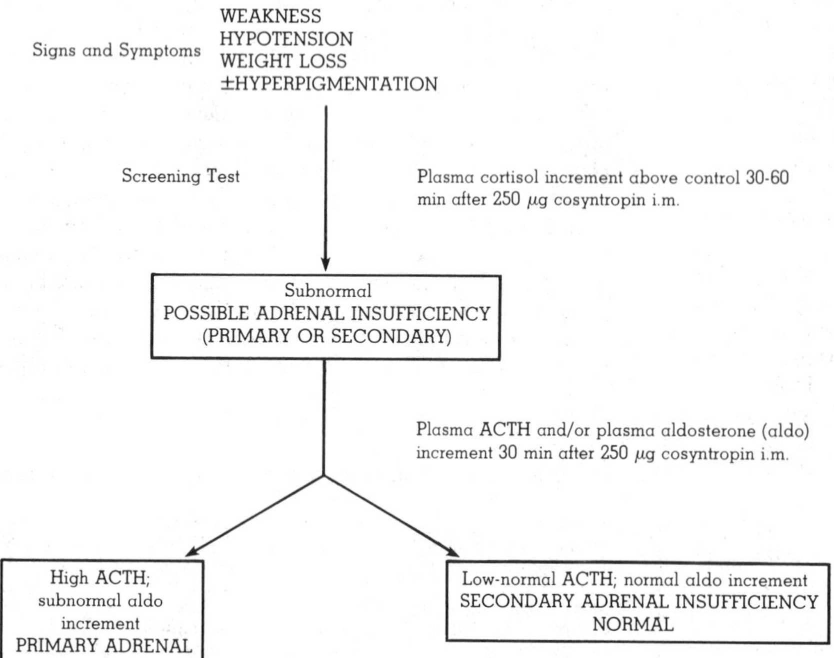

FIGURE 112-11
Diagnostic flowchart for evaluating patients with suspected adrenal insufficiency. Plasma ACTH levels are low in secondary adrenal insufficiency. In adrenal insufficiency secondary to pituitary tumors or idiopathic panhypopituitarism, other pituitary hormone deficiencies are present. On the other hand, ACTH deficiency may be isolated, as seen following prolonged use of exogenous glucocorticoids.

Since the isolated blood levels obtained in these screening tests may not be definitive in certain patients, the diagnosis should always be confirmed by a continuous 24-h ACTH infusion. Normal subjects and patients with secondary adrenal insufficiency may be distinguished by insulin tolerance or metyrapone testing.

Some female patients with Addison's disease experience a persistent decline in libido even after optimal treatment with glucocorticoids and mineralocorticoids, possibly related to subnormal adrenal androgen production. Small doses of intramuscular depo-testosterone (e.g., 25 mg every 4 to 6 weeks) may be used to advantage, but overtreatment leading to masculinizing side effects must be avoided.

All patients with adrenal insufficiency, including bilaterally adrenalectomized patients, should carry medical identification, should be instructed in the parenteral self-administration of steroids, and should be registered with a national medical alerting system.

Special therapeutic problems During periods of intercurrent illness, the dose of cortisone or cortisol should be increased to levels of 75 to 150 mg per day. When oral administration is not possible, parenteral routes should be employed. Likewise, before surgery or dental extractions, supplemental glucocorticoids should be administered. For a representative program of steroid therapy for an Addisonian patient or an adrenalectomized patient undergoing a major operation, see Table 112-10. This schedule is designed to mimic the maximal output of cortisol in normal individuals undergoing prolonged major stress with presumed continuous ACTH stimulation (10 mg/h, 250 to 300 mg per 24 h). Patients should also be advised to increase the dose of 9α-fluorohydrocortisone and add excess salt to their otherwise normal diet during periods of excessive exercise with sweating, during extremely hot weather, or during periods of gastrointestinal upsets.

SECONDARY ADRENOCORTICAL INSUFFICIENCY Pituitary ACTH deficiency causes *secondary* adrenocortical insufficiency. ACTH deficiency may be selective, as is seen following prolonged administration of excess glucocorticoids, or may occur in association with multiple pituitary tropic hormone deficiencies (panhypopituitarism) (see Chap. 109). Patients with secondary adrenocortical hypofunction may have many symptoms and signs in common with Addisonian patients but are *characteristically not hyperpigmented* since ACTH and related peptide levels are low. In fact, plasma ACTH levels distinguish between primary and secondary adrenal insufficiency, since they are elevated in the former and decreased to absent in the latter. Patients with total pituitary insufficiency also have signs and symptoms suggestive of multiple hormone deficiencies. An additional feature distinguishing primary from secondary adrenocortical insufficiency is the *near-normal level of aldosterone secretion* seen in the presence of pituitary and/or isolated ACTH deficiencies (Fig. 112-11). Patients with pituitary insufficiency may present with hyponatremia, which may be dilutional or secondary to subnormal increments in aldosterone secretion in response to severe sodium restriction. However, the findings of severe dehydration, *hyponatremia,* and *hyperkalemia* are characteristic of severe mineralocorticoid insufficiency and favor a diagnosis of primary adrenocortical insufficiency.

Patients receiving long-term steroid therapy, despite physical findings of Cushing's syndrome, develop adrenal insufficiency both because of prolonged pituitary-hypothalamic suppression and because of adrenal atrophy secondary to the loss of endogenous ACTH. Thus, these patients acquire two deficits, a loss of adrenal responsiveness to ACTH and a failure of pituitary ACTH release. These patients are characterized by low blood cortisol and ACTH levels, low base-line steroid excretion, and abnormal ACTH and metyrapone test results. Most patients with steroid-induced adrenal insufficiency eventually recover normal hypothalamic-pituitary-adrenal responsiveness, but individual response time is variable, ranging from days to months. The rapid ACTH test can be used as a convenient and valuable assessment of recovery of hypothalamic-pituitary-adrenal function. Since the plasma cortisol concentrations after injection of cosyntropin and during insulin-induced hypoglycemia correlate closely, the rapid ACTH test assesses the integrated hypothalamic-pituitary-adrenal function. Additional testing to assess endogenous pituitary ACTH reserve includes the standard metyrapone and the insulin tolerance tests.

Substitution glucocorticoid therapy in patients with secondary adrenocortical insufficiency does not differ from that outlined for Addisonian patients. Mineralocorticoid replacement therapy is usually not necessary, since aldosterone secretion is preserved. Otherwise, the basic principles outlined for replacement should be applied to patients with secondary adrenocortical insufficiency.

ACUTE ADRENOCORTICAL INSUFFICIENCY Acute adrenocortical insufficiency may result from several processes. One of these, termed *adrenal crisis,* is a rapid and overwhelming intensification of chronic adrenal insufficiency, usually precipitated by sepsis or surgical stress. Another involves an acute hemorrhagic destruction of both adrenal glands, usually associated with an overwhelming septicemia. Adrenal hemorrhage associated with anticoagulant therapy in stressed patients with increased adrenocortical activity has also been reported. A third, and probably the most frequent, cause of acute insufficiency results from the rapid withdrawal of steroids from patients with adrenal atrophy secondary to chronic steroid administra-

TABLE 112-10
Steroid therapy schedule for Addisonian patient undergoing a major operation*

	Cortisone acetate (intramuscularly)		*Cortisol infusion, **continuous**, mg/h*	*Cortisone acetate (orally)*		*Fluorohydrocortisone (orally),*
	7 A.M.	*7 P.M.*		*8 A.M.*	*4 P.M.*	*8 A.M.*
Routine daily medication				25	12.5	0.1
Day before operation		50		25	12.5	0.1
Day of operation	50	50	10			
Postoperative:						
Day 1	50	50	5–7.5			
Day 2	50	50	2.5–5			
Day 3	50	50				
Day 4	50				25	0.1
Day 5				37.5	25	0.1
Day 6				25	25	0.1
Day 7				25	12.5	0.1

* *All steroid doses are given in milligrams.*

tion. In the presence of severe stress, acute adrenocortical insufficiency may also occur in patients with congenital adrenal hyperplasia and those receiving pharmacological agents which are capable of inhibiting steroid synthesis by the gland (such as *o,p′*-DDD).

Adrenal crisis The long-term survival of patients with Addison's disease largely depends upon prevention and treatment of adrenal crisis. Consequently, the occurrence of infection, trauma (including surgery), gastrointestinal upsets, or other forms of stress requires an immediate increase in hormone. In previously untreated patients, preexisting symptoms are intensified. Nausea, vomiting, and abdominal pain may become intractable. Fever is frequently severe but may be absent. Lethargy deepens into somnolence, and the blood pressure and pulse fail as hypovolemic vascular shock ensues. In contrast, patients previously maintained on chronic glucocorticoid therapy may not exhibit severe dehydration or hypotension until preterminally, since mineralocorticoid secretion is usually preserved.

In all patients in crisis, a precipitating cause should be sought. Intercurrent infection associated with omission or failure to increase maintenance therapy is a common setting.

Treatment is primarily directed toward the rapid elevation of circulating glucocorticoid and the immediate replacement of the sodium and water deficits. Hence, an intravenous infusion of 5% glucose in normal saline solution should be immediately started with a bolus intravenous infusion of 100 mg cortisol followed by a continuous infusion of cortisol at a rate of 10 mg/h. It is also advisable to administer 50 mg cortisone acetate intramuscularly in case the infusion becomes infiltrated or inadvertently stopped. Effective treatment of hypotension consists primarily of aggressive repletion of sodium and water deficits. If the crisis was preceded by prolonged nausea, vomiting, and dehydration, several liters of saline may be required within the first few hours. Vasoconstrictive agents (such as dopamine) may be indicated in extreme conditions as adjuncts to volume replacement. With large doses of steroid, as, for example, 100 to 200 mg cortisol, the patient receives a maximal mineralocorticoid effect, and supplementary mineralocorticoid is superfluous. Following improvement, the patient can be offered oral fluids and the steroid dosage is tapered over the next few days to maintenance levels, with reinstitution of supplementary mineralocorticoid if needed (Table 112-10).

Adrenal hemorrhage Adrenal hemorrhage (adrenal apoplexy) is usually associated with overwhelming septicemia (Waterhouse-Friderichsen syndrome); however, it may also occur in the absence of sepsis. Occasionally, massive bilateral adrenal hemorrhage results from birth trauma. The infant may be stillborn or die after birth of shock and hyperpyrexia. Adrenal hemorrhage also occurs during pregnancy, following idiopathic adrenal vein thrombosis, during convulsions in epilepsy or electroconvulsive therapy, with excessive anticoagulant therapy, after trauma or surgery, and as a complication of adrenal venography (e.g., infarction of an adenoma). Pain in the flank and epigastrium is frequent, and if the hemorrhagic process ruptures into the abdomen, signs of peritoneal inflammation are present. Acute adrenal insufficiency should also be considered in the differential diagnosis of hypotension in patients maintained on anticoagulant therapy in the period immediately following a myocardial infarction.

The adrenal hemorrhage associated with septicemia is most frequent with meningococcemia but is also seen with overwhelming infections due to pneumococcus, staphylococcus, or *Hemophilus influenzae*. The onset is often explosive, with a shaking chill, violent headache, vertigo, vomiting, and prostration. A petechial rash appears on the skin and mucous membranes and progresses rapidly to a confluent, extensive purpura. Large areas of skin may become grossly hemorrhagic. Body temperature may be subnormal but is usually markedly elevated. Circulatory collapse rapidly ensues, and death may occur within 6 to 48 h. Specific diagnosis requires immediate identification of the organism. Frequently, the septicemia is so massive that organisms may be seen in peripheral blood smears or petechial scrapings. Since shock may also be associated with massive septicemia without adrenal hemorrhage, one is never completely certain whether adrenal insufficiency is contributing to the patient's decompensation. Sufficient time is not available for assessment of adrenal function; however, a plasma sample for later determination of cortisol level may be of interest.

Treatment must be immediate and intensive. Control of the infection by vigorous administration of intravenous antibiotics is indicated. Intravenous dopamine may also be required to maintain vascular tone. Steroid treatment should also be administered at the earliest possible point in all patients in whom fulminating septicemia is associated with shock. The dose range administered in such patients is usually massive (e.g., 1 to 2 g cortisol daily). However, available data are inconclusive that such doses of steroid improve mortality in septic shock.

HYPOALDOSTERONISM

Isolated aldosterone deficiency accompanied by normal cortisol production has been reported in association with hyporeninism; as a congenital biosynthetic defect; postoperatively, following removal of aldosterone-secreting adenomas; during protracted heparin or heparinoid administration; in pretectal disease of the nervous system; and in severe postural hypotension.

The feature common to all patients with hypoaldosteronism is the inability to increase aldosterone secretion appropriately during salt restriction. Most cases present as unexplained hyperkalemia often exacerbated by restriction of dietary sodium intake. In severe cases urine sodium wastage occurs on a normal salt intake, whereas in milder forms excessive losses of urine sodium occur only during salt restriction.

Most cases of isolated hypoaldosteronism occur in patients with a deficiency in renin production (so-called hyporeninemic hypoaldosteronism). This syndrome is most commonly seen in adult subjects with mild renal failure and diabetes mellitus in association with hyperkalemia and metabolic acidosis disproportionately severe to the state of renal impairment. Plasma renin levels fail to rise normally following sodium restriction and postural changes. The pathogenesis of the hyporeninism is uncertain. Possibilities include renal disease (most likely), autonomic nephropathy, extracellular fluid volume expansion, and a defect in conversion of so-called renin precursors into active renin. Aldosterone levels also fail to rise normally following salt restriction and volume contraction, probably related to the hyporeninism since biosynthetic defects in aldosterone secretion cannot usually be demonstrated. In these patients, aldosterone secretion increases promptly following ACTH stimulation, but it is uncertain as to whether the magnitude of the response is normal. On the other hand, the level of aldosterone appears to be subnormal in relationship to the hyperkalemic status of these subjects.

Hypoaldosteronism can also be associated with high renin levels. In many of these subjects, a biosynthetic defect has been noted where there is an inability to transform the angular C-18 methyl group of corticosterone to the C-18 aldehyde grouping of aldosterone due to a deficiency of the enzyme 18-hydroxysteroid dehydrogenase. These patients not only manifest low to absent aldosterone secretion and elevated plasma renin levels but also elevated values for the intermediates of aldosterone biosynthesis (corticosterone and 18-hydroxycorticosterone).

Before considering the diagnosis of isolated hypoaldosteronism in a patient with hyperkalemia, "pseudohyperkalemia" (e.g., hemolysis, thrombocytosis) should be excluded by measuring a plasma potassium level. The next step is to demonstrate a normal cortisol response to ACTH stimulation. Then stimulated (upright posture, sodium restriction) renin and aldosterone levels are obtained. Low renin–low aldosterone levels establish a diagnosis of hyporeninemic hypoaldosteronism. High renin–low aldosterone levels are consistent with an aldosterone biosynthetic defect or a selective unresponsiveness of the glomerulosa to angiotensin II. Finally, elevated renin and aldosterone levels suggest primary renal unresponsiveness to aldosterone, so-called pseudohypoaldosteronism.

Treatment of patients with isolated hypoaldosteronism would logically be to replace the mineralocorticoid deficiency. For practical purposes, the oral administration of 9α-fluorohydrocortisone in a dose of 0.1 to 0.2 mg daily should restore electrolyte balance. However, patients with hyporeninemic hypoaldosteronism, usually require greater doses of mineralocorticoid to normalize the hyperkalemia. This poses a risk in these patients who usually have hypertension and mild renal insufficiency. Therefore, an alternative approach is to administer furosemide which can ameliorate the acidosis and the hyperkalemia. Occasionally a combination of these two approaches may be efficacious.

NONSPECIFIC USE OF ADRENAL STEROIDS AND ACTH IN CLINICAL PRACTICE

The widespread utilization of glucocorticoids and ACTH in clinical practice emphasizes the need for a thorough understanding of the metabolic effects of these agents when used nonspecifically, if optimum effectiveness is to be obtained and if undesirable side reactions are to be minimized. Before instituting adrenal hormone therapy, a physician should weigh carefully the gains that can reasonably be expected versus the potentially undesirable metabolic actions of pharmacological doses of hormone.

HOW SERIOUS IS THE DISORDER? In a patient whose life is threatened by unexplained shock, or in whom other measures have failed, the physician need not hesitate to employ large-dosage steroid therapy. On the other hand, one should exercise restraint in administering steroids to a patient with early rheumatoid arthritis who as yet has not been exposed to the possible benefits of physiotherapy, analgesics, and a well-organized program of general medical care.

HOW LONG WILL GLUCOCORTICOID THERAPY BE REQUIRED? The use of intravenously administered steroids for a period of 24 to 48 h in the treatment of such life-threatening situations as status asthmaticus or pseudotumor cerebri has little or no contraindication, in contrast to the initiation of a program of chronic steroid therapy for asthma, arthritis, or psoriasis. In the latter instances, the almost certain complication of a Cushing's syndrome of some degree must be weighed against the potential benefit to the patient. The need for minimizing these side effects by a careful choice of steroid preparations, alternate-day or interrupted therapy programs, and the judicious use of supplementary adjuvants is evident.

WHICH ADRENAL PREPARATION IS PREFERABLE? At least five considerations need to be taken into account in deciding which steroid preparation to use:

1 The biological half-life of the particular compound. The rationale behind every-other-day therapy is to decrease the metabolic effects of the steroids for a significant amount of time over the 2-day period, yet at the same time to produce pharmacological suppression of sufficient duration to maintain the disease in remission. Too long a half-life would defeat the first purpose, and too short a half-life would defeat the second. In general, the more potent the steroid, the longer its biologic half-life tends to be.

2 The importance of the mineralocorticoid effects of the steroid. Synthetic steroids have less mineralocorticoid effect relative to their glucocorticoid effect than cortisol or cortisone (Table 112-11). This may be an important consideration in certain disease states.

3 Cortisone and prednisone, in contrast to the other glucocorticoids, have to be converted to their biologically active equivalents before any anti-inflammatory effects can occur. Because of this, in a clinical condition in which steroids are known to be effective and in which an adequate dose has been given without any response, one should consider substituting cortisol or prednisolone for cortisone or prednisone.

4 The cost of the medication. This is a serious consideration if chronic administration is to be undertaken. Prednisone is the least expensive of available steroid preparations.

5 The appreciable variation in the manner in which commercial preparations of glucosteroids are formulated. This factor may significantly modify absorption. Thus it is advisable for a patient whose steroid dosage has been standardized to continue to utilize the same pharmaceutical preparation to avoid relapse or overdosage.

ACTH VERSUS STEROIDS In general, adrenal steroid therapy is effective by mouth and can be regulated more accurately than ACTH therapy. The latter fluctuates considerably in the amount of steroid produced from day to day, depending on the rate and extent of absorption of ACTH and on the state

TABLE 112-11
Glucocorticoid preparations

	Estimated potency†	
*Commonly used name**	*Glucocorticoid*	*Mineralocorticoid*
SHORT-ACTING		
Cortisol	1	1
Cortisone	0.8	0.8
INTERMEDIATE-ACTING		
Prednisone	4	0.25
Prednisolone	4	0.25
Methylprednisolone	5	±
Triamcinolone	5	±
LONG-ACTING		
Paramethasone	10	±
Betamethasone	25	±
Dexamethasone	30–40	±

* *The steroids are divided into three groups according to the duration of biologic activity. Short-acting preparations have a biologic half-life of less than 12 h; long-acting, greater than 48 h; and intermediate, between 12 and 36 h. Triamcinolone has the longest half-life of the intermediate-acting preparations.*

† *Relative milligram comparisons with cortisol, setting the glucocorticoid and mineralocorticoid properties of cortisol as 1. Sodium retention is insignificant in usual doses employed of methylprednisolone, triamcinolone, paramethasone, betamethasone, and dexamethasone.*

of the adrenal cortex. ACTH therapy stimulates the secretion of adrenal androgens as well as hydroxysteroids. Sodium retention with ACTH is often more marked than with cortisone or, particularly, with prednisone therapy.

While some studies imply that ACTH may be superior to oral steroid therapy in the treatment of certain disorders such as dermatomyositis and multiple sclerosis, it is now generally believed that the two agents are equally effective (or ineffective). Both ACTH and steroid therapy induce hypothalamo-pituitary suppression; however, in ACTH therapy adrenal gland size and activity are maintained, in contrast to the adrenal atrophy usually associated with steroid therapy.

EVALUATION OF PATIENT PRIOR TO INITIATING STEROID THERAPY See Table 112-12.

Chronic infection Three problems demand attention. (1) Any active infection, particularly tuberculosis, should be identified. If tuberculosis is present, steroid therapy can be employed, if indicated, in conjunction with antituberculous chemotherapy. (2) The chest film and tuberculin test provide base-line information for future comparison. Since high-dosage steroids minimize the tuberculin reaction, serial chest roentgenograms may be indicated. (3) Infection due to "opportunistic" low-virulence pathogens should be constantly considered in patients on high steroid dosage, especially when steroid therapy is combined with other immunosuppressive agents.

Diabetes mellitus Prolonged glucocorticoid therapy may unmask latent diabetes mellitus or aggravate preexisting disease. For this reason a careful history is important to exclude familial incidence of diabetes. Obviously the presence of frank diabetes mellitus or the demonstration of impaired glucose tolerance affects the physician's decision to institute adrenal hormone therapy.

Osteoporosis All patients receiving long-continued steroid therapy are likely to develop some degree of osteoporosis. For patients at high risk (postmenopausal females, elderly individuals, and patients whose basic disease process results in restricted physical activity) initial films of the thoracolumbar segment of the spine are mandatory because osteoporosis, with vertebral fractures or compression, is one of the most serious potential hazards of long-term steroid therapy. Adjunctive therapies with vitamin D and calcium may be effective in steroid osteoporosis, although alternate-day or interrupted steroid therapy minimizes this important complication (Table 112-13).

Peptic ulcer, gastric hypersecretion, or esophagitis In conventional therapeutic doses (equivalent to 25 mg prednisone per day or less) glucocorticoids probably do not cause peptic ulceration; whether higher doses are associated with increased incidence of peptic ulcer disease is not established and probably depends on duration of treatment (as well as dose) and the

TABLE 112-12
A "checklist" for use prior to the administration of glucocorticoids in pharmacological dosages

1 Presence of tuberculosis or other chronic infection (chest x-ray, tuberculin test)
2 History of diabetes mellitus in family
3 Evidence of preexisting osteoporosis (spine x-ray in post-menopausal patients)
4 History of peptic ulcer, gastritis, or esophagitis (stool guaiac test)
5 Evidence of hypertension or cardiovascular disease
6 History of psychological disorders

TABLE 112-13
Supplementary measures designed to minimize undesirable metabolic effects of glucocorticoids

1 Monitor caloric intake to prevent weight gain.
2 Restrict sodium intake to prevent edema and minimize hypertension and potassium loss.
3 Potassium supplementation if necessary.
4 Antacid therapy.
5 Alternate-day steroid schedule if possible. Patients on steroid therapy over a prolonged period should be protected by an appropriate increase in hormone level during periods of acute stress. A rule of thumb is to *double* the maintenance dose.
6 To minimize osteopenia (not proved effective):
  a Estrogen therapy for postmenopausal women; 0.625–1.25 mg conjugated estrogens, equine may be given "cyclically." Regular Papanicolaou smear and breast examination mandatory (see Chap. 118).
  b Consider supplementary vitamin D and calcium.

presence of predisposing factors such as hypoalbuminemia or cirrhosis. However, even in conventional doses patients with a history of ulcer may experience aggravation of symptoms while receiving glucocorticoids. Consequently, all individuals with a positive history or with known risk factors should be given a vigorous "ulcer combating" program (antacids, cimetidine) along with glucocorticoids. *The development of anemia in a patient receiving glucocorticoids should suggest gastrointestinal bleeding as a cause, and patients should be cautioned to note black stools.*

Hypertension or cardiovascular disease In general, the sodium-retaining propensity of many adrenal steroid preparations requires that caution be used when they are given to patients with preexisting hypertension or cardiovascular or renal disease. Use of preparations in which sodium-retaining activity is minimal, restriction of dietary sodium intake, and the use of diuretic agents and supplementary potassium salts will minimize the mineralocorticoid actions of steroid therapy. However, hypertension may still be exacerbated by steroid-induced increases in renin substrate and consequently angiotensin II levels.

Psychological difficulties Steroid therapy may be complicated by severe psychological disturbances; less severe abnormalities are relatively frequent. In general, serious psychological disturbances are more closely related to the patient's personality structure than to the actual dose of hormone, although, as might be anticipated, larger doses of hormone are associated with more frequent serious reactions. At present there is no reliable method of determining beforehand a patient's psychological reaction to steroid therapy; moreover, previous tolerance of steroids does not necessarily ensure immunity to subsequent courses of therapy. Untoward psychological reactions on one occasion do not invariably mean that the patient will respond unfavorably to a second course of treatment; however, prophylactic treatment with lithium may be indicated.

Sleeplessness is a well-known complication of glucocorticoid therapy. This can be minimized by using the shorter-acting steroids and by prescribing the total dose as a single early-morning medication.

ALTERNATE-DAY STEROID THERAPY The single most effective measure in minimizing the cushingoid effects of glucocorticoid therapy is to administer the total 48-h dose as a *single* dose, of *intermediate-acting steroid* in the morning, *every other day.* If symptoms of the underlying disorder can be controlled by this technique, the physician can be assured that the therapeutic program is offering a distinct advantage to the patient. Three special considerations deserve mention. (1) The alternate-day schedule may be approached through a series of transition dose schedules which permit the patient an opportunity to adjust successfully to the ultimate program. (2) The physician should provide the patient with supplementary nonsteroid medications, if required, on the "off day" to minimize symptoms of the underlying disorder. (3) The physician and the patient should recognize that many symptoms noted during the off day (e.g., fatigue, joint pain, muscle stiffness or tenderness, and fever) are those of relative adrenal insufficiency, rather than an exacerbation of the underlying disease. Knowing this is of vital importance, since the physician can reassure the patient and avoid giving up the program on the basis of a misconception.

The alternate-day concept capitalizes on the fact that cortisol secretion and plasma levels normally are highest in the early morning and lowest in the evening. The normal pattern is mimicked by administering an intermediate-acting steroid in the morning (7 to 8 A.M.) (Table 112-11).

Initially the steroid program usually requires daily or more frequent doses of steroid to accomplish the desired anti-inflammatory or immunity-suppressing action. *Only after this desired effect has been achieved is an attempt made to switch over to an alternate-day program.* A number of programs may be employed for transferring a patient from a daily to an alternate-day program. The key points to be considered are flexibility in arranging a program and the use of supportive measures on the off day. One may attempt a transition by a series of gradations rather than by an abrupt complete changeover. One approach is to keep the steroid dose constant on one day and gradually reduce the level on the alternate day. Alternatively, the steroid dose can be increased on one day while being reduced on the alternate day. In any case it is important to anticipate that the patient will experience some increase in pain or discomfort between the 36 to 48 h following the last dose of steroid.

The general principles advocated in the long-term use of steroids and in implementing an alternate-day schedule are as follows:

1 Utilize intermediate-acting steroids such as prednisone or prednisolone.
2 Give the total daily steroid as a single morning dose.
3 Begin a transition program as soon as the manifestations of the diseases are under reasonable control.
4 If possible, eliminate steroid medication on the alternate day.

WITHDRAWAL OF CORTICOSTEROIDS FOLLOWING THEIR LONG-TERM USE AS PHARMACOLOGICAL AGENTS Complete withdrawal of steroids should be initiated by implementing an alternate-day schedule. Patients on an alternate-day program for a month or more experience less difficulty as far as pituitary-adrenal function is concerned. The dosage is gradually reduced and finally discontinued after a normal replacement dosage has been reached (e.g., 5 to 7.5 mg prednisone). Complications rarely ensue unless undue stress is experienced, and patients should understand that for 1 year or longer after the complete withdrawal from long-term high-dosage steroid therapy, they should receive supplementary hormone in the presence of serious infection, operation, or injury.

In patients on high-dose daily steroid therapy, it is frequently advised to reduce total steroid dosage to approximately 20 mg prednisone daily before beginning the transition to every-other-day therapy. If a patient cannot tolerate an alternate-day program, it is debatable as to whether complete discontinuance should be considered. Under these circumstances a daily dose of steroid could be continued, and at some future date another trial of gradual transition to the alternate-day schedule should be attempted. In patients with life-threatening disorders, it may be desirable to consider life-long daily maintenance therapy at an Addisonian replacement dosage. These patients will not require mineralocorticoid therapy, as aldosterone secretion is usually adequate.

REFERENCES

Bloom E et al: Nuclear binding of glucocorticoid receptors: Relations between cytosol binding, activation in the biologic response. J Steroid Biochem 12:175, 1980

Edelman IS, Marver D: Mediating events in the action of aldosterone. J Steroid Biochem 12:219, 1980

Eisenbarth GS et al: The polyglandular failure syndrome: Disease inheritance, HLA-type and immune function. Ann Intern Med 91:528, 1979

Finkelstein M, Shaefer JM: Inborn errors of steroid biosynthesis. Physiol Rev 59:353, 1979

Gwinup B et al: Clinical testing of the hypothalamic-pituitary-adrenal cortical system in states of hypo- and hypercortisolism. Metabolism 24:777, 1975

Knox FG et al: Escape from the sodium retaining effects of mineralocorticoids. Kidney Int 17:263, 1980

Korobkin M et al: Computed tomography in the diagnosis of adrenal disease. Am J Roentgenol 132:231, 1979

Kramer RE et al: Action of angiotensin II on aldosterone biosynthesis in the rat adrenal cortex. J Biol Chem 255:3442, 1980

Lamberts SWJ: Hormone secretion in alcohol induced pseudoCushing's syndrome: Differential diagnosis with Cushing's disease. JAMA 242:1640, 1979

Lindholm J et al: Reliability of the 30 minute ACTH test in assessing hypothalamic-pituitary-adrenal function. J Clin Endocrinol Metab 47:272, 1978

Luton JP et al: Treatment of Cushing's disease by *o,p'*-DDD: Survey of 62 cases. N Engl J Med 300:459, 1979

Moore TJ et al: Nelson's syndrome: Frequency, prognosis, and effect of prior pituitary radiation. Ann Intern Med 85:731, 1976

Parrillo JE, Fauci AS: Mechanisms of glucocorticoid action on immune processes. Ann Rev Pharmacol Toxicol 19:179, 1979

Pedersen RC et al: Pro-adrenocorticotropin/endorphin-derived peptides: Coordinated action on adrenal steroidogenesis. Science 208:1044, 1980

Pollack MS et al: Prenatal diagnosis of congenital adrenal hyperplasia (21-hydroxylase deficiency) by HLA typing. Lancet 1:1107, 1979

Rosenfield RL: Plasma free androgen patterns in hirsute women and their diagnostic implications. Am J Med 66:417, 1979

Schambelan M et al: Prevalence, pathogenesis and functional significance of aldosterone deficiency in hyperkalemic patients with chronic renal insufficiency. Kidney Int 17:89, 1980

Tyrrel JB et al: Cushing's disease: Selective transsphenoidal resection of pituitary adenomas. N Engl J Med 298:753, 1978

Vale W et al: Characterization of a 41-residue ovine hypothalamic peptide that stimulates secretion of corticotropin and β-endorphin. Science 213:1394, 1981

Williams GH, Braley LM: Effective dietary sodium intake and potassium intake in acute stimulation of aldosterone output by isolated human cells. J Clin Endocrinol Metab 45:55, 1977

113 PHEOCHROMOCYTOMA

LEWIS LANDSBERG
JAMES B. YOUNG

Pheochromocytomas are tumors that produce, store, and secrete catecholamines. Also known as chromaffin tumors, pheochromocytomas are derived most often from the adrenal medulla. Tumors developing outside the adrenal arise from chromaffin cells in or about sympathetic ganglia and are known as extraadrenal pheochromocytomas or paragangliomas.

The clinical features and morbidity are due predominantly to the release of catecholamines. Hypertension is the most common clinical manifestation. Paroxysms or crises, often spectacular and alarming, occur in over half the cases. Related tumors that may secrete catecholamines and produce similar clinical syndromes include chemodectomas derived from the carotid body and ganglioneuromas derived from the postganglionic sympathetic neurons.

Pheochromocytoma is a rare tumor occurring in approximately 0.1 percent of the hypertensive population. It is, however, an important correctable cause of high blood pressure. Properly diagnosed and treated, pheochromocytoma is usually curable; undiagnosed or mistreated it is commonly fatal. Postmortem series indicate that over one-third of pheochromocytomas are unsuspected clinically and that in most of these cases the tumor is related to the fatal outcome.

PATHOLOGY **Location and morphology** Approximately 80 percent occur as a solitary lesion in or about a single adrenal, 10 percent are bilateral, and approximately 10 percent are extraadrenal. In children a fourth of tumors are bilateral, and an additional fourth are extraadrenal. Solitary lesions inexplicably favor the right side. Although pheochromocytomas may grow to large size (over 3 kg) most weigh less than 100 g and are less than 10 cm in diameter. These tumors are highly vascularized with an arterial supply derived from any of the three arteries that normally supply the adrenal.

Microscopically the tumor is comprised of large, polyhedral, pleomorphic chromaffin cells. Less than 10 percent are malignant. As with other endocrine tumors malignancy cannot be determined by the histologic appearance; local invasion of surrounding tissues or distant metastases indicate malignancy.

FAMILIAL PHEOCHROMOCYTOMA In approximately 5 percent of cases pheochromocytoma is inherited as an autosomal dominant trait either alone or in combination with other abnormalities. The familial occurrence is associated with multiple endocrine neoplasia (MEN) type II (Sipple's syndrome) or type III (mucosal neuroma syndrome) (see Chap. 123), von Recklinghausen's neurofibromatosis, and von Hippel–Lindau's retinal cerebellar hemangioblastomatosis. Bilateral adrenal pheochromocytomas are more common in the familial syndromes and may be present in over half of MEN.

EXTRAADRENAL PHEOCHROMOCYTOMAS Extraadrenal pheochromocytomas have an average weight of 20 to 40 g and are usually less than 5 cm in diameter. Most are located within the abdomen in association with the celiac, superior mesenteric, and inferior mesenteric ganglia. Approximately 1 percent are located within the thorax in relation to the paravertebral sympathetic ganglia, 1 percent are located within the urinary bladder, and less than 1 percent are within the neck, usually in association with the sympathetic ganglia or the extracranial branches of the ninth or tenth cranial nerves.

Catecholamine synthesis, storage, and release Pheochromocytomas synthesize and store catecholamines by processes resembling those of the normal adrenal medulla (Chap. 73). Little is known about the mechanisms of catecholamine release from pheochromocytomas, but changes in blood flow and necrosis within the tumor may be the cause in some instances. These tumors are not innervated, and catecholamine release does not result from neural stimulation.

EPINEPHRINE, NOREPINEPHRINE, AND DOPAMINE Most pheochromocytomas contain and secrete both norepinephrine and epinephrine, and the percentage of norepinephrine is usually greater than in the normal adrenal. Most extraadrenal pheochromocytomas contain and secrete norepinephrine exclusively. Rarely, pheochromocytomas produce epinephrine alone, particularly in association with MEN. Although epinephrine-producing tumors are occasionally associated with a preponderance of metabolic and beta-receptor effects, in general the predominant catecholamine cannot be predicted from the clinical presentation. Increased production of dopamine and homovanillic acid (HVA) is uncommon; although an increase in the excretion of these precursors has been noted in some patients with malignant pheochromocytoma, measurement of dopamine and HVA are not useful in excluding or predicting malignancy.

CLINICAL FEATURES Pheochromocytoma occurs in all age groups but is most common in young to midadult life. Some series show a slight female preponderance. Although the presentation is characteristically unpredictable, the majority of patients come to medical attention as a result of hypertensive crisis, paroxysmal symptoms suggestive of seizure disorder or anxiety attacks, or hypertension that responds poorly to conventional treatment. Less commonly, unexplained hypotension or shock in association with surgery or trauma will suggest the diagnosis.

Hypertension Hypertension is the most common clinical manifestation of pheochromocytoma. In approximately 60 percent of cases the hypertension is sustained, although significant blood pressure lability is usually present and half of patients with sustained hypertension have distinct crises or paroxysms. The other 40 percent have blood pressure elevations only during an attack. The hypertension is often severe, occasionally malignant, and usually resistant to treatment with drugs that are effective in essential hypertension.

Paroxysms or crises The paroxysm or crisis is the classic manifestation of pheochromocytoma, occurring in over half of patients. In an individual patient the symptoms are often similar with each attack. In most patients the paroxysms are frequent, but in some the attacks are sporadic and recur at intervals as long as weeks or months. Over the course of time the paroxysms commonly increase in frequency, duration, and severity.

The attack usually has a sudden onset. It may last from a few minutes to several hours and on occasion even longer. Headache is a prominent feature. Profuse sweating, palpitations, and apprehension, often with a sense of impending doom, are common. Pain in the chest or abdomen may occur and occasionally is associated with nausea and vomiting. Either pallor or flushing may be noted during the attack. The blood pressure is elevated, often to alarming levels, and is usually accompanied by tachycardia.

The paroxysm may be precipitated by any activity that displaces the abdominal contents. In some cases a particular stimulus may reproduce an attack in a characteristic fashion, but in many patients no clearly defined precipitating event can be found. Although anxiety may accompany the attacks, mental stress or psychological tension does not usually provoke a crisis.

Other distinctive clinical features Symptoms and signs of an increased metabolic rate, such as profuse sweating, and mild to moderate weight loss are common. Orthostatic hypotension, probably a consequence of diminished plasma volume and blunted sympathetic reflexes, is frequent. Both of these factors may predispose the patient with unsuspected pheochromocytoma to severe hypotension or shock during surgery or major trauma.

CARDIAC MANIFESTATIONS Sinus tachycardia, sinus bradycardia, supraventricular arrhythmias, and ventricular premature contractions have all been noted. Angina and acute myocardial infarction may occur even in the absence of coronary artery disease. Catecholamine-induced increase in myocardial oxygen consumption and, perhaps, coronary spasm may be involved in the pathogenesis of these ischemic events. Electrocardiographic changes, including nonspecific ST-T wave changes, left ventricular strain, and right and left bundle branch block do not necessarily imply ischemia or infarction. Cardiomyopathy, either congestive with myocarditis and myocardial fibrosis or hypertrophic with concentric or asymmetric hypertrophy, may be associated with heart failure and cardiac arrhythmias.

CARBOHYDRATE INTOLERANCE Over half of patients have impaired carbohydrate tolerance, an apparent consequence of suppression of insulin and stimulation of hepatic glucose output. The impaired glucose tolerance almost never requires specific treatment and disappears after removal of the tumor.

HEMATOCRIT Patients with pheochromocytoma may have an elevated hematocrit secondary to diminished plasma volume. Rarely erythropoietin production by the pheochromocytoma may cause a true erythrocytosis.

PHEOCHROMOCYTOMA OF THE URINARY BLADDER When pheochromocytoma arises within the wall of the urinary bladder paroxysms typically occur in relation to micturition. The unique location of these tumors within the bladder wall is responsible for the production of symptoms while the tumors are quite small, and consequently, urinary catecholamine excretion may be normal or only minimally elevated. Hematuria is present in over half, and the tumor can often be visualized at cystoscopy.

Adverse drug interactions Severe and occasionally fatal paroxysms have been induced by opiates, histamine, ACTH, saralasin, and glucagon. These agents appear to release catecholamines directly from the tumor. Indirect-acting sympathomimetic amines, including methyldopa (when administered intravenously) may cause an unpredictable increase in blood pressure by releasing catecholamines from the augmented stores within nerve endings. Drugs that block neuronal uptake of catecholamines, such as tricyclic antidepressants or guanethidine, may enhance the physiological effects of circulating catecholamines. These drugs should be avoided in patients with known or suspected pheochromocytoma; indeed all medications should be carefully considered and cautiously administered in such patients.

Associated diseases Pheochromocytoma is associated with medullary carcinoma of the thyroid in the familial MEN syndromes types II and III and with hyperparathyroidism in MEN II (see Chap. 123). Hypercalcemia, resolving after tumor resection, has also been described in patients with pheochromocytoma in the absence of parathyroid disease. Every member of a MEN kindred should be screened periodically for pheochromocytoma by assay of a 24-h urine sample for catecholamines, including specific measurement of epinephrine. Pheochromocytoma should be excluded or removed before thyroid or parathyroid surgery.

The association of pheochromocytoma and neurofibromatosis is established but uncommon. Since incomplete forms of von Recklinghausen's disease may be associated with pheochromocytoma, minor manifestations such as five to six café au lait spots, vertebral abnormalities, or kyphoscoliosis should increase the suspicion of pheochromocytoma in a patient with hypertension. The incidence of pheochromocytoma in some kindreds with von Hippel–Lindau disease may be as high as 10 to 25 percent. Many of these are unsuspected clinically and diagnosed postmortem.

The incidence of cholelithiasis is about 15 to 20 percent in patients with pheochromocytoma. Cushing's syndrome is rarely associated with pheochromocytoma, usually a consequence of ectopic secretion of ACTH either by the pheochromocytoma or, less commonly, by a coexistent medullary carcinoma of the thyroid.

DIAGNOSIS The diagnosis of pheochromocytoma is established by the demonstration of increased amounts of catecholamines or catecholamine metabolites in a 24-h urine collection. In the majority the diagnosis can be confirmed by the analysis of a single 24-h urine sample, provided the patient is hypertensive or symptomatic at the time the collection is obtained.

Biochemical tests The determinations employed in the diagnosis of pheochromocytoma include vanillylmandelic acid (VMA), the metanephrines, and unconjugated or "free" catecholamines (Chap. 73). Although much has been written about the relative specificity and sensitivity of the different measurements, they are probably equivalent provided the assays are properly performed. Accuracy of diagnosis is improved when two of the three determinations are employed, although this is not essential as a screening procedure in every case. The following general considerations apply to all the urinary tests. (1) Despite claims for the adequacy of determinations made on random urine samples and expressed per milligram of creatinine, analysis of a full 24-h urine sample is preferable. Creatinine should be determined as well to assess the adequacy of collection. (2) Where possible the collection should be obtained when the patient is at rest, on no medication, and without recent exposure to radiographic contrast media. Where it is not practical to discontinue all medications, those drugs known specifically to interfere in the assays should be avoided. Thiazide diuretics, propranolol, and hydralazine usually cause no interference. (3) The urine collection should be properly acidified and kept cold during and after collection. (4) With specific high-quality assays dietary restrictions are minimal; the physician should follow the recommendations of the laboratory performing the analyses. (5) Although the majority of patients with pheochromocytoma excrete increased quantities of catecholamines and catecholamine metabolites each day, in patients with paroxysmal hypertension the yield is increased if a 24-h urine collection is initiated when the patient experiences a crisis.

FREE CATECHOLAMINES The upper limit of normal for total catecholamines is between 100 and 150 μg per 24 h. In most patients with pheochromocytoma values in excess of 250 μg per day are obtained. Specific measurement of epinephrine is often of value since increased epinephrine excretion (over 50 μg per 24 h) is usually associated with an adrenal lesion and may be the only abnormality in MEN cases. False-positive increases in catecholamine excretion result from exogenous catecholamines such as methyldopa, L-dopa, and sympathomimetic amines, which may elevate catecholamine excretion for up to 2 weeks. Endogenous catecholamines from excessive stimulation of the sympathoadrenal system may also increase urinary catecholamine excretion and result in a false-positive test. The relevant clinical situations include hypoglycemia, strenuous exertion, central nervous system disease with increased intracranial pressure, and clonidine withdrawal.

METANEPHRINES AND VMA In most laboratories the upper limit of normal is 1.3 mg of total metanephrine excretion and 7.0 mg VMA per 24 h. In most patients with pheochromocytoma the increase in excretion of these catecholamine metabolites is considerable, often in excess of three times the normal range. Metanephrine excretion is increased by exogenous and endogenous catecholamines and by treatment with monoamine oxidase inhibitors. VMA is less affected by endogenous and exogenous catecholamines but is increased in a nonspecific fashion by a variety of drugs. VMA excretion is decreased by MAO inhibitors.

PLASMA CATECHOLAMINES Measurement of plasma catecholamines has a limited application in the diagnosis of pheochromocytoma. The care required in obtaining basal catecholamine levels (Chap. 73); the lack of readily available, reliable plasma catecholamine assays; and the satisfactory results obtained with urinary determinations make measurement of plasma catecholamines unnecessary in most cases. In occasional problem patients, in whom the clinical features strongly suggest pheochromocytoma and in whom the urinary assays are borderline, measurement of plasma catecholamines may be worthwhile. Basal levels of total catecholamines over 2000 pg/ml support the diagnosis.

Pharmacological tests Reliable methods for the demonstration of catecholamines and catecholamine metabolites in urine have rendered obsolete both the provocative and adrenolytic tests which are nonspecific and entail considerable risk. A modified version of the adrenolytic test may be of some use, however, when employed as a therapeutic trial in a patient presenting in hypertensive crisis with clinical features suggestive of pheochromocytoma. A positive response to phentolamine (5 mg bolus after a 0.5-mg test dose) is a reduction in blood pressure of at least 35/25 mmHg that becomes maximal after 2 min and persists for 10 to 15 min. The response to a pharmacological agent is never diagnostic, and biochemical confirmation must always be obtained. Provocative tests in normotensive patients are potentially dangerous and almost never indicated.

Differential diagnosis Since the manifestations of pheochromocytoma may be protean the diagnosis must be considered and excluded in many patients with suggestive clinical features. In patients with essential hypertension and "hyperadrenergic" features such as tachycardia, sweating, and increased cardiac output, and in patients with anxiety attacks associated with blood pressure elevations, analysis of a 24-h urine collection is usually decisive in excluding the diagnosis. Repeated determinations on urine collected during attacks may be necessary, however, before the diagnosis can be excluded with certainty. Pressor crises associated with clonidine withdrawal or the use of MAO inhibitors (Chap. 73) may closely resemble the paroxysms of pheochromocytoma. Factitious crises may be produced by self-administration of sympathomimetic amines in psychiatrically disturbed patients, particularly among those employed in the health-care professions.

Intracranial lesions, particularly posterior fossa tumors or subarachnoid hemorrhage, may be associated with hypertension and increased excretion of catecholamines or catecholamine metabolites. While this is most common in patients who have suffered an obvious neurological catastrophe, the possibility of subarachnoid or intracranial hemorrhage secondary to pheochromocytoma should be considered. Diencephalic or autonomic epilepsy may be associated with paroxysmal spells, hypertension, and increased plasma catecholamine levels. This rare entity may be difficult to distinguish from pheochromocytoma, but an aura, an abnormal EEG, and a beneficial response to anticonvulsant medications will often suggest the proper diagnosis.

MANAGEMENT **Preoperative management** The induction of stable alpha-adrenergic blockade is the basis of preoperative management and provides the foundation for successful surgical treatment. Once the diagnosis of pheochromocytoma is established the patient should be placed on phenoxybenzamine to induce a long-lived, noncompetitive alpha-receptor blockade. The usual initial dose is 10 mg every 12 h with increments of 10 to 20 mg added every few days until the blood pressure is controlled and the paroxysms disappear. Because of the long duration of action the therapeutic effects are cumulative and the optimal dose must be achieved gradually with careful monitoring of supine and upright blood pressure. Most patients require between 40 and 80 mg of phenoxybenzamine per day although in some cases 200 mg or more may be necessary. Phenoxybenzamine should be administered for at least 10 to 14 days prior to surgery. Over this time the combination of alpha-receptor blockade and a liberal salt intake will restore the contracted plasma volume to normal. Before adequate alpha-adrenergic blockade with phenoxybenzamine is achieved, paroxysms may be treated with intravenous phentolamine. Nitroprusside is the only other antihypertensive agent that reliably reduces blood pressure in patients with pheochromocytoma and may be useful on occasion.

Beta-adrenergic receptor blocking agents should be given only after alpha blockade has been established, since prior administration may cause a paradoxical increase in blood pressure by antagonizing beta-mediated vasodilatation in skeletal muscle. Beta blockade is usually initiated when tachycardia develops during the induction of alpha-adrenergic blockade. Low doses often suffice and a reasonable starting dose is 10 mg propranolol 3 to 4 times per day, increased as needed to control the pulse rate. Beta blockade is effective treatment for catecholamine-induced arrhythmias, particularly those potentiated by anesthetic agents.

Preoperative localization of the tumor Surgical removal of pheochromocytoma is facilitated if the location of the tumor, or tumors, can be established preoperatively. Adrenal lesions are well demonstrated by CT scan. Angiographic studies may still be required to demonstrate extraadrenal pheochromocytomas within the abdomen. Tumors within the thorax can often be demonstrated by conventional chest roentgenography with oblique views of the chest and tomographic cuts as needed. Venous catheterization with analysis of plasma catecholamines from different regions may be helpful in localizing extraadrenal pheochromocytomas but is of limited usefulness in the localization of intraadrenal tumors. Invasive angiographic procedures should never be performed in patients with known or suspected pheochromocytoma until alpha-adrenergic blockade has been achieved.

Surgery Surgery is best performed in centers with experience in the preoperative, anesthetic, and intraoperative management of pheochromocytoma patients. In experienced hands surgical mortality is below 2 or 3 percent.

Adequate monitoring during the surgical procedure is critical and should include continuous recording of arterial pressure, central venous pressure, and electrocardiogram; if congestive failure develops, pulmonary capillary wedge pressure should be monitored as well. Adequate fluid replacement is crucial. Intraoperative hypotension responds better to volume replacement than to the administration of vasoconstrictors.

Hypertension and cardiac arrhythmias are most likely to occur during induction of anesthesia, intubation, and manipulation of the tumor. Intravenous phentolamine is usually sufficient to control the blood pressure, but nitroprusside may be required on occasion. Propranolol may be given in the treatment of tachycardia or ventricular ectopy.

PHEOCHROMOCYTOMA IN PREGNANCY Spontaneous labor and vaginal delivery in unprepared patients are usually disastrous for mother and fetus. In early pregnancy it seems reasonable to prepare the patient with phenoxybenzamine and remove the tumor as soon as the diagnosis is confirmed. The pregnancy need not be terminated but the operative procedure itself may result in spontaneous abortion. In the third trimester, treatment with adrenergic blocking agents should be undertaken; when the fetus is of sufficient size cesarean section followed by extirpation of the tumor may be successfully performed. Although the safety of adrenergic blocking drugs in pregnancy has not been established, these agents have been administered in several cases without obvious adverse effect.

UNRESECTABLE TUMOR In cases of metastatic or locally invasive tumor or in patients with intercurrent illness that contraindicates surgery, long-term medical management is required. When the manifestations of pheochromocytoma cannot be adequately controlled by the chronic administration of adrenergic blocking agents, the concomitant administration of alpha methyltyrosine may be required. This agent, which inhibits tyrosine hydroxylase, diminishes catecholamine production by the tumor and often simplifies chronic management. At present there are no practical ways of destroying the tumor by radiotherapy or chemotherapy.

PROGNOSIS In the usual case of benign pheochromocytoma the 5-year survival after surgery is over 95 percent, and the recurrence rate is less than 10 percent. After successful surgery catecholamine excretion returns to normal in about 1 week and should be measured to ensure complete tumor removal. In malignant pheochromocytoma the 5-year survival is less than 50 percent.

Complete removal of the pheochromocytoma cures the hypertension in approximately three-fourths. In the remainder hypertension recurs but is usually well controlled by standard antihypertensive agents. In this group either underlying essential hypertension or irreversible vascular damage induced by catecholamines may cause the persistence of the hypertension.

REFERENCES

BROWN MJ et al: Increased sensitivity and accuracy of phaeochromocytoma diagnosis achieved by use of plasma-adrenaline estimations and a pentolinium-suppression test. Lancet i:174, 1981

ENGELMAN K: Phaeochromocytoma. Clin Endocrinol Metab 6:769, 1977

FUDGE TL et al: Current surgical management of pheochromocytoma during pregnancy. Arch Surg 115:1224, 1980

GLUSHIEN AS et al: Pheochromocytoma: Its relationship to the neurocutaneous syndromes. Am J Med 14:318, 1953

HAMILTON BP et al: Measurement of urinary epinephrine in screening for pheochromocytoma in multiple endocrine neoplasia type II. Am J Med 65:1027, 1978

HORTON WA et al: Von Hippel-Lindau disese: Clinical and pathological manifestations in nine families with 50 affected members. Arch Intern Med 136:769, 1976

JONES DH et al: The biochemical diagnosis, localization and followup of phaeochromocytoma: The role of plasma and urinary catecholamine measurements. Q J Med 49:431, 1980

KHAIRI MRA et al: Mucosal neuroma, pheochromocytoma and medullary thyroid carcinoma: Multiple endocrine neoplasia type 3. Medicine 54:89, 1975

LAURSEN K, DAMGAARD-PEDERSON K: CT for pheochromocytoma diagnosis. AJR 134:277, 1980

MANGER WM, GIFFORD RW JR: *Pheochromocytoma.* New York, Springer-Verlag, 1977

ROSS EJ et al: Preoperative and operative management of patients with pheochromocytoma. Br Med J 1:191, 1971

STEINER AL et al: Study of a kindred with pheochromocytoma, medullary thyroid carcinoma, hyperparathyroidism and Cushing's disease: Multiple endocrine neoplasia, type 2. Medicine 47:371, 1968

114 DIABETES MELLITUS

DANIEL W. FOSTER

Diabetes mellitus is the most common of the serious metabolic diseases of humans. The true frequency in the general population is difficult to ascertain because of differing standards of diagnosis but probably is somewhere around 1 percent. The disease is characterized by a series of hormone-induced metabolic abnormalities; by long-term complications involving the eyes, kidneys, nerves, and blood vessels; and by a lesion of the basement membranes demonstrable by electron microscopy. In recent years it has become clear that a variety of syndromes are subsumed under the general term *diabetes* and that they differ both in clinical manifestations and in patterns of inheritance. In this chapter primary hyperglycemic states exhibiting the triad of findings listed above will be considered under the umbrella term *diabetes mellitus.* It should be stated at the outset that many controversies exist in this field. In the discussion that follows, an attempt has been made to identify the major questions at issue and to give the author's interpretation of the available data.

DIAGNOSIS AND CLASSIFICATION The diagnosis of symptomatic diabetes is not difficult. When a patient presents with signs and symptoms attributable to an osmotic diuresis and is found to have hyperglycemia, essentially all physicians agree that diabetes is present. There likewise would be little disagreement about an asymptomatic patient with persistently elevated fasting plasma glucose concentrations. The problem arises with the asymptomatic patient who for one reason or another is considered to be a potential diabetic but has a normal fasting glucose concentration in plasma. Such patients are often given an oral glucose tolerance test, and, if abnormal values are found, diagnosed as having "chemical" diabetes. There seems to be little question that normal glucose tolerance is strong evidence against the presence of diabetes. Less certain is the predictive value of a positive test. Much evidence suggests that the standard oral glucose tolerance test overdiagnoses diabetes to a remarkable degree, probably because stress of a variety of kinds can produce an abnormal response. The operative mechanism is thought to be epinephrine discharge. Epinephrine is known to block insulin secretion, stimulate glucagon release, activate glycogen breakdown, and impair insulin action in target tissues such that hepatic glucose production is increased and the capacity to dispose of an exogenous glucose load is impaired. Even anxiety over the necessary venipunctures may generate sufficient epinephrine to produce an abnormal test. Concomitant illness, inadequate diet, and lack of physical exercise also contribute to the high incidence of false-positive examinations.

In an attempt to deal with these problems, the National Diabetes Data Group of the National Institutes of Health has recommended new criteria for the diagnosis of diabetes following a challenge with oral glucose. These criteria, which are similar to those of the World Health Organization, are as follows:

1 *Fasting (overnight)*: Venous plasma glucose concentration $\geq$ 140 mg/dl on at least two separate occasions.
2 *Following ingestion of 75 g of glucose:* Venous plasma glucose concentration $\geq$ 200 mg/dl at 2 h and at least one other occasion during the 2-h test (i.e., *two* values $\geq$ 200 mg/dl must be obtained for diagnosis).

If the 2-h value is between 140 and 200 mg/dl and one other value during the 2-h test period is equal to or greater than 200 mg/dl, a diagnosis of "impaired glucose tolerance" is suggested. The interpretation would be that persons in this category are at increased risk for the development of fasting hyperglycemia or symptomatic diabetes relative to persons with normal glucose tolerance but that such progression is not predictable in an individual patient. Several large studies suggest that most patients (~75 percent) with impaired glucose tolerance never develop diabetes. Even subjects diagnosed as having diabetes by the second criterion may never manifest fasting hyperglycemia or symptomatic deterioration. For these reasons the author believes the glucose tolerance test to be unhelpful in clinical practice although it may still have a place in research studies. (*Note:* In evaluating older studies by the criteria of the National Diabetes Data Group, plasma glucose concentrations measured in whole blood must be increased 15 percent to be equivalent to plasma concentrations. A similar correction is recommended for capillary blood in the fasting state but not after glucose ingestion.)

Classification of diabetes is given in Table 114-1. The basic categories are those recommended by the National Diabetes Data Group except for division into primary and secondary types. The former indicates that no associated disease is present while in the latter some other identifiable condition presumably causes or allows a diabetic syndrome to develop. Insulin dependence in this classification is not equivalent to insulin therapy. Rather, the term means that the patient is at risk for ketoacidosis in the absence of insulin. Many patients classified as non-insulin-dependent require insulin for control of hyperglycemia although they do not become ketoacidotic if insulin is withdrawn or intercurrent disease induces severe stress. The terms *type 1 diabetes* or *IDDM* are often used for the insulin-dependent state, while the equivalent synonyms for non-insulin-dependent diabetes are *type 2 diabetes* and *NIDDM.* Non-insulin-dependent subjects are subclassified as obese and nonobese. Insulin resistance plays a major role in subjects within this category of the disease, especially in the obese, but this does not imply that insulin synthesis and secretory patterns are intact (see below).

TABLE 114-1
Classification of diabetes

A *Primary*
- *1* Insulin-dependent diabetes mellitus (IDDM, type 1)
- *2* Non-insulin-dependent diabetes mellitus (NIDDM, type 2)
  - *a* Nonobese NIDDM
  - *b* Obese NIDDM
  - *c* Maturity-onset diabetes of the young (MODY)

B Secondary
- *1* Pancreatic disease
- *2* Hormonal abnormalities
- *3* Drug or chemical induced
- *4* Insulin receptor abnormalities
- *5* Genetic syndromes
- *6* Other

Secondary forms of diabetes encompass a host of conditions. *Pancreatic disease,* particularly chronic pancreatitis in alcoholics, is a common cause. Destruction of the beta-cell mass is the etiologic mechanism. *Hormonal abnormalities* include diseases such as pheochromocytoma, acromegaly, and the Cushing syndrome or arise consequent to therapeutic administration of steroid hormones. "Stress hyperglycemia," associated with severe burns, acute myocardial infarctions, and other life-threatening illnesses, is due to endogenous release of glucagon and catecholamines. Mechanisms of hormonal hyperglycemia include both impairment of insulin release and induction of insulin resistance in varying combinations. A large number of *drugs* can lead to hyperglycemia, but most simply produce impaired glucose tolerance. Hyperglycemia and even ketoacidosis may occur as a result of abnormalities at the level of the *insulin receptor.* The dysfunction may be due to quantitative or qualitative defects in the receptor itself or to antibodies directed against it. The mechanism is essentially pure insulin resistance. A number of *genetic syndromes* are associated with impaired glucose tolerance or hyperglycemia. The three most common are the lipodystrophies, myotonic dystrophy, and ataxia-telangiectasia. The final category, *other,* is poorly defined and is meant to include any condition which does not fit elsewhere in the etiologic scheme. The appearance of abnormal carbohydrate metabolism in association with any of the above secondary causes does not necessarily indicate the presence of underlying diabetes although in some cases a mild, asymptomatic primary diabetes may be made overt by the secondary illness.

PREVALENCE Prevalence of diabetes is difficult to determine because numerous standards, many now no longer acceptable, have been used in diagnosis. As noted above the overall prevalence in western societies is thought to be about 1 percent. Estimates for insulin-dependent diabetes are more reliable than for the non-insulin-dependent form since most young patients are diagnosed after the abrupt appearance of symptoms. In England prevalence of the type 1 illness has been estimated to be 0.22 percent by age 16, and in the United States a study in Allegheny County, Pennsylvania, suggested a prevalence of 0.26 percent by age 20. If the prevalence of diabetes is actually 1 percent, it follows that about one-fourth of cases have insulin-dependent disease while three-fourths are non-insulin-dependent. Obviously ratios of type 1 to type 2 disease vary with age, being higher if a young population is studied and lower in the older age range.

GENETICS It has long been known that diabetes aggregates in families. The genetics of the disease has undergone intense scrutiny, but major disagreement exists regarding interpretation of the data. It is probable that diabetes is genetically heterogeneous and that similar diabetic phenotypes may result from differing genotypes. It is also possible that a single genetic defect may produce differing clinical syndromes. Unfortunately no specific genetic marker for the presence of the disease is available. It was hoped that thickening of the capillary basement membrane in muscle might be such a marker, but this now seems unlikely. The fact that some authors have equated abnormal glucose tolerance with diabetes while others have studied only overtly hyperglycemic subjects adds to the difficulty of deciphering genetic studies. Despite these problems, certain conclusions appear firm:

1 Genetic factors play a role in all primary forms of diabetes mellitus, but their importance varies. In insulin-dependent disease the genetic factor(s) may be largely permissive while in non-insulin-dependent diabetes they may be more nearly causal. This conclusion is based on extensive studies in monozygotic twins. When twins below the age of 40 were studied (most presumably having type 1 disease) the presence of diabetes in one twin was unaccompanied by diabetes in the other more than 50 percent of the time in contrast to the expected concordance of 100 percent for a purely genetic disorder. This finding suggests the necessity of some extragenetic (environmental) agent for induction of diabetes in most subjects with insulin-dependent disease but does not exclude the possibility that some patients may develop the illness in the absence of an environmental insult. In twins over 40 (mostly type 2 disease) concordance rates approach 100 percent suggesting that the genetic factor dominates in causing the illness.

2 The predisposing gene(s) in IDDM likely resides on the sixth chromosome in view of strong associations between diabetes and certain human leukocyte antigens (HLA) coded by the major histocompatibility region on this chromosome. Four loci designated by the letters A, B, C, and D are recognized with alleles at each site identified by numbers. Major alleles conferring enhanced risk for IDDM are HLA-DR3, HLA-Dw3, HLA-DR4, HLA-Dw4, HLA-B8 and HLA-B15. (DR refers to a serologic test for D-locus antigens while Dw alleles are determined by mixed lymphocyte cultures. A small w means that the antigen has been provisionally accepted by the International Histocompatibility Workshop. The w is removed once identification is considered definite.) The D locus is considered of primary importance with the B and A loci being involved through nonrandom associations with D (*linkage disequilibrium*). When compared with the general population the risk for IDDM imposed by the presence of DR3 or DR4 is 4 to 10 times. If the comparison is made not against a control population but against a subset of persons not bearing the predisposing antigen, relative risks as high as thirtyfold are obtained. Antigens B7 and DR2 (Dw2) have been called "protective" since they are found with much less frequency in diabetics than in the general population. It is likely, however, that they are acutally "low-risk" alleles (rather than protective) because they are present in inverse relationship with DR3/DR4; i.e., if DR2, Dw2 is present, high-risk alleles will be absent. The HLA genes themselves are not thought to confer susceptibility to diabetes but to be located near the putative diabetic gene(s). This accounts for the fact that IDDM may develop in the absence of any high-risk HLA alleles and that HLA associations vary from population to population. No HLA relationships are known for non-insulin-dependent diabetes except in the Xhosa tribe of South Africa.

3 The location of the predisposing gene(s) for NIDDM is not known, but speculation has focused on the eleventh chromosome which bears, on its short arm, the structural gene for insulin. This follows from the observation that a number of persons have an insertion of extra DNA located some 500 base pairs to the left (on the 5′ flank) of the insulin structural gene. This insertion, about 1.5 to 3.4 kilobases in length, has been reported to be more frequent in NIDDM than in normal controls or in patients with IDDM, although not all laboratories have been able to confirm the finding. Should the insert (or some specific variant of the insert) prove to be a reliable marker of type 2 disease, it should be possible to dissect inheritance patterns since identification of the inserts is possible utilizing leukocyte DNA from only 10 to 25 ml of whole blood. Homozygous and heterozygous states for the insert can be distinguished by current techniques.

4 The pattern of inheritance is known for only one type of primary diabetes, *maturity-onset diabetes of the young* (MODY). This disease is manifested by mild hyperglycemia in young persons who are resistant to ketosis. Four lines of evidence suggest that it is transmitted as an autosomal dominant trait. First, three-generation direct transmission has been demonstrated in over 20 families. Second, a 1:1 ratio of diabetic to nondiabetic children is found when one parent has the disease. Third, about 90 percent of obligate carriers have diabetes. Fourth, direct male-to-male transmission has been observed, ruling out X-linked inheritance.

While all types of inheritance have been postulated for IDDM, the chances that it is an autosomal dominant disorder appear vanishingly small. The strongest argument for autosomal recessive inheritance comes from studies of HLA associations in families having more than one sibling with diabetes. A high frequency of HLA identity (two shared haplotypes) exists in concordant siblings with type 1 disease as would be predicted by the recessive hypothesis. On the other hand only about half of siblings haploidentical for the D locus are concordant. This variable expressivity might reflect the fact that in IDDM both a genetic predisposition and an environmental insult are required for full clinical expression of diabetes, a conculsion compatible with cited studies in identical twins. A confounding observation is that homozygosity for a high-risk allele (e.g., Dw3/Dw3) does not incur increased risk for diabetes while the simultaneous presence of two positively associated alleles (e.g., Dw3/Dw4) more than additively increases susceptibility to disease. This has led to development of an intermediate model of inheritance (neither dominant nor recessive) in which at least two different genes confer susceptibility to diabetes. The putative genes could either be alleles at the same site or nonallelic. The intermediate model is most widely held at the time of this writing but cannot be considered proven.

Only two patterns of inheritance have been seriously considered for NIDDM: autosomal recessive and multifactorial. An autosomal recessive single-gene mutation would require the appearance of diabetes in all offspring when both parents have type 2 disease. However, study of a large number of such matings indicates that diabetes in the offspring is rare, suggesting either that inheritance is polyfactorial or that expressivity is variable.

5 Despite the cited evidence for a major genetic component in both forms of primary diabetes, analysis of pedigrees shows a surprisingly low prevalence of direct vertical transmission of the disease. In one series of 35 families in which there was a child with classic insulin-dependent diabetes only 4 of the index cases had a parent with diabetes while 2 had a diabetic grandparent. Of the 99 siblings of these diabetic children only 6 had overt disease. The figures for NIDDM, while somewhat higher, are still remarkably low given the major genetic component postulated from studies in identical twins. Approximately a third of the offspring of a type 2 diabetic parent develop the disorder while 26 percent of siblings of index cases reportedly acquire diabetes. When both parents have type 2 diabetes the trait has been reported to occur in 3 to 30 percent of offspring. These percentages should be treated with caution because diagnosis of diabetes in families with NIDDM was often based on glucose tolerance testing rather than the appearance of overt fasting hyperglycemia as is usually the case in IDDM. For this reason actual incidence may be considerably lower than the figures given. Low rates of transmission make it difficult to discern mechanisms of inheritance through study of families but is reassuring to diabetic parents who may wish to have children.

EPIDEMIOLOGY As noted above, studies in identical twins suggest the necessity for an interaction between genetic and environmental factors for development of insulin-dependent diabetes. It is now widely believed that the environmental factor in most cases is a virus capable of infecting the beta cell. A viral etiology was originally suggested by seasonal variations in the onset of the disease and what appeared to be more than a chance relationship between appearance of diabetes and preceding episodes of mumps, hepatitis, infectious mononucleosis, congenital rubella, and Coxsackie virus infections. The viral hypothesis gained support from studies showing that certain strains of encephalomyocarditis virus cause diabetes in susceptible strains of mice. The isolation of a coxsackievirus B4 from the pancreas of a previously healthy boy who died following an episode of ketoacidosis and the induction of diabetes in experimental animals inoculated with the isolated virus strongly suggest that viruses can cause diabetes in humans. A second clue to pathogenesis came from the observation that most patients with type 1 diabetes have circulating antibodies directed against the beta cell if studied soon after onset of symptoms. One type of antibody binds to cytoplasmic components while the other is directed against the plasma membrane of beta cells (*islet-cell surface antibodies*). The latter are cytotoxic in the presence of complement. Islet-cell antibodies have also been noted in rats given subdiabetogenic doses of streptozotocin and in humans who develop diabetes following ingestion of the rat poison Vacor for suicidal purposes. They likewise are found in the BB rat, an animal that spontaneously develops diabetes resembling IDDM. In humans, titers of these antibodies fall with time in most patients but persist in a small subset of patients, many of whom demonstrate the HLA-DR3, Dw3, B8 haplotype. This is of particular interest because these alleles are known to be associated with the immune endocrinopathy syndrome and because there is an established relationship between diabetes and immunologically induced endocrine disease (e.g., Schmidt's syndrome) (see Chap. 123). Taken together, these observations have led to the following formulation for the epidemiology of IDDM. In most (but not all) cases a predisposition to diabetes is inherited that permits beta-cell injury, usually by a virus but conceivably also by chemical agents in the environment. Subsequent to the beta-cell insult antigens are released into the blood with induction of autoantibodies. These autoantibodies then attack the beta cell in destructive fashion to complete the sequence. A shorthand construction would be genetic predispostion → viral injury to the islets → immune response → completed destruction of beta cells. In some cases the disease might be truly autoimmune with cytotoxic antibodies arising spontaneously rather than in response to antigen leakage from beta-cell injury. In this form of the disease, antibodies to other endocrine tissues would be expected to be common. The genetic factor could operate at several levels singly or in combination: e.g., by determining susceptibility to viral infection, by specifying the extent of the inflammatory reaction to injury in the beta cell (insulitis), or by regulating the immune-response system.

The chain of events leading to symptomatic hyperglycemia in NIDDM is not completely understood. Insulin resistance plays a major role as evidenced by the fact that hyperglycemia can be reversed by diet or weight loss sufficient to restore sensitivity to the beta-cell hormone. However, a defect in insulin synthesis or release is also required since many massively obese people with severe insulin resistance do not have hyperglycemia or diabetes. This indicates that a normal pancreas has sufficient reserve to compensate for insulin resistance imposed by obesity or other factors while the pancreas in type 2 diabetic subjects does not. In this sense the primary defect can be considered to be a dysfunctional beta cell although the abnormality would not be recognized in most patients without the addition of an insulin-resistant state. Presumably those patients with overt NIDDM who are not obese have a more severe defect in insulin synthesis or release. An interesting case has been reported of non-insulin-dependent diabetes due to production of an abnormal insulin that does not bind well to insulin receptors, but diabetes due to abnormal insulins must be very rare.

CLINICAL PICTURE While there are several dozen diseases and syndromes associated with hyperglycemia, it has been traditional to classify all forms of diabetes as either insulin-dependent or non-insulin-dependent on functional grounds. Such a classification is probably acceptable as a clinical shorthand although overlap syndromes occur. In all cases the metabolic abnormalities appear to be caused by relative or absolute insulin deficiency coupled with relative or absolute glucagon excess. Insulin resistance probably also plays a role in most patients. While obesity-associated resistance has received most emphasis, prolonged insulin deficiency per se can induce an insulin-resistant state accounting for the fact that there is impedance to hormone action in patients with type 1 disease who are not fat. Insulin-deficient insulin resistance disappears with aggressive insulin therapy. Interestingly, up to a third of patients with NIDDM appear to have insulinopenic insulin resistance which is reversible with improved control of diabetes in the absence of weight loss. Data in experimental animals suggest that insulin resistance due to insulin deficiency is associated with depletion of intracellular, microsome-bound glucose transport units that normally are recruited into the plasma membrane in response to insulin.

Insulin-dependent diabetes Insulin-dependent diabetes usually begins before the age of 40, often in childhood or adolescence. Onset of symptoms may be abrupt, with thirst, excessive urination, increased appetite, and weight loss developing over a several-day period. In some cases the disease is heralded by the appearance of ketoacidosis during an intercurrent illness or following surgery. As outlined in Table 114-2, type 1 patients are not obese (and may be wasted), depending on the length of time between onset of symptoms and start of treatment. Characteristically the plasma insulin is low or immeasurable. Glucagon levels are elevated but suppressible with insulin. Once symptoms have developed, insulin therapy is required. Occasionally an initial episode of ketoacidosis is followed by a symptom-free interval (the "honeymoon" period) during which no treatment is required. The likely explanation for this phenomenon is shown in Fig. 114-1.

Non-insulin-dependent diabetes This form of the disease usually begins in middle life or beyond. The typical patient is overweight. Symptoms begin more gradually than in IDDM, and the diagnosis is frequently made when an asymptomatic person is found to have an elevated plasma glucose on routine laboratory examination. In contrast to type 1 disease, plasma insulin levels are normal to high in absolute terms, although they are lower than predicted for the level of the plasma glucose; i.e., relative insulin deficiency is present. In other words,

TABLE 114-2
General characteristics of IDDM and NIDDM diabetes

	IDDM	*NIDDM*
Genetic locus	Chromosome 6	Chromosome 11 (?)
Age of onset	< 40	> 40
Body habitus	Normal to wasted	Obese
Plasma insulin	Low to absent	Normal to high
Plasma glucagon	High, suppressible	High, resistant
Acute complication	Ketoacidosis	Hyperosmolar coma
Insulin therapy	Responsive	Responsive to resistant
Sulfonylurea therapy	Unresponsive	Responsive

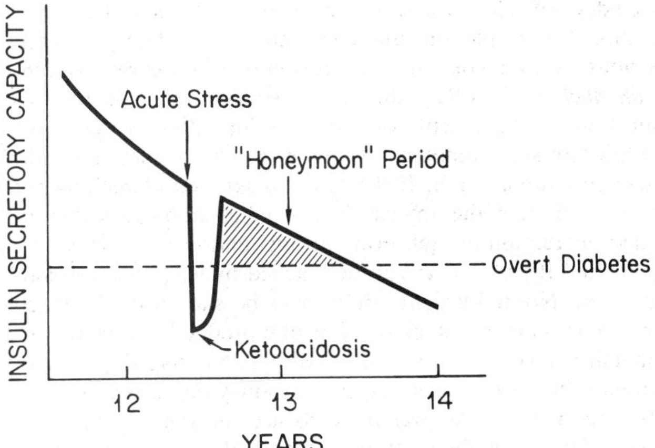

FIGURE 114-1
Schematic representation of the "honeymoon" period. In this graph insulin secretory capacity is shown gradually decreasing in a patient destined to develop diabetes. At approximately 13½ years insulin would become insufficient to maintain plasma glucose in the normal range. An initial episode of ketoacidosis, for example, in association with acute appendicitis, is shown occurring in the twelfth year. Presumably stress-induced epinephrine release blocks insulin secretion and causes the syndrome. In normal subjects insulin reserve is such that hormone release is adequate, even in the face of stress. Following recovery from the stressful episode insulin secretory capacity returns to the previous level and remains sufficient for an additional year as indicated by the shaded area—the "honeymoon" period.

if plasma glucose were raised to equivalent levels in a nondiabetic subject, the increase in plasma insulin would be higher than in the maturity-onset diabetic. Obesity is assumed to be the major cause of the higher insulin concentrations seen before and after the development of hyperglycemia. Support for this belief comes from the observation that weight reduction in the obesity-hyperglycemia syndrome may cause disappearance of hyperglycemia and return of insulin responsiveness. Insulin resistance in obesity involves both a decreased number of insulin receptors in target tissues and a postreceptor defect that has not been precisely identified. Primary insulin resistance not due to obesity may play a role as noted above. Glucagon metabolism in maturity-onset patients is complex. While the elevated fasting plasma concentrations can be lowered by large amounts of insulin, the exaggerated glucagon response to ingested nutrients cannot be suppressed; i.e., alpha-cell function remains abnormal. For unknown reasons maturity-onset diabetics do not develop ketoacidosis. In the decompensated state they are susceptible to the syndrome of hyperosmolar, nonketotic coma. If weight loss can be induced, patients may be managed by diet alone. The majority of patients failing dietary therapy respond to sulfonylureas, but improvement of hyperglycemia in many is not sufficient to meet current standards for control of diabetes. For this reason a high percentage of patients with NIDDM are now treated with insulin.

TREATMENT Diet (See also Chap. 81) Modification of the diet is the first line of therapy in diabetes. An appropriate diet stabilizes body weight at near-ideal levels, minimizes hyperglycemia, and protects against hypoglycemia in patients requiring insulin. Saturated fat intake has been lowered in diabetic diets with concomitant increase in polyunsaturated fatty acid content in an attempt to delay the appearance of atherosclerosis. Increased amounts of dietary fiber may also improve diabetic control. Detailed dietary planning is beyond the scope of this chapter and ideally should utilize the talents of a professional dietitian. Few measures are more important. If no dietitian is available in the community, referral to a medical center dietitian for initial instruction is recommended since most physicians do not have the time necessary for adequate dietary counseling.

The first step in formulating a dietary prescription is to determine optimal caloric content. Since the activity component of daily caloric needs can only be roughly estimated, an element of trial and error is involved. Basal metabolic requirements can be met by giving approximately 22 kcal per kilogram of body weight per day. Rough estimates of the additional caloric demands for activity are 30, 50, and 100 percent of the basal requirements in sedentary, moderately active, and briskly exercising individuals. Upward or downward adjustments are necessary if the goal is weight gain or weight loss. The latter is more commonly required (and much more difficult). Since the basal metabolic rate is about 1500 kcal per day in a normal adult, caloric restriction to less than this amount should cause weight loss, even in a sedentary individual. In practice, most obese patients do not adhere to reducing diets even under the threat of diabetes.

The minimal protein requirement for good nutrition is about 0.9 g per kilogram of body weight per day. The recommended carbohydrate content of the diabetic diet is 40 to 50 percent of the total calories, with fat making up the remainder. Carbohydrate intakes of up to 85 percent of total calories have been given, however, and under experimental conditions may actually improve diabetic control. This fact is mentioned to indicate that carbohydrate need not be rigidly limited to the lower figure of 40 percent. Sucrose and sucrose-containing foods are ordinarily not allowed because of rapid digestion and absorption.

The desirable degree of dietary restriction varies from patient to patient. Some overweight patients with asymptomatic hyperglycemia require only simple caloric limitation to control their disease. Most symptomatic diabetics, on the other hand, must learn to estimate food values using the exchange list technique.[1] A brief summary of the typical exchanges is shown in Table 114-3. Basically one decides how many calories are needed and the desired distribution between fat, carbohydrate, and protein. The necessary exchanges are then outlined. For example, a 2200-cal diet with 50 percent of the calories as carbohydrate and 1 to 1.5 g protein per kilogram of body weight can be met by providing 2 milk exchanges, 7 fruit exchanges, 12 bread exchanges, 8 meat exchanges, 4 fat exchanges, and unlimited type A vegetables (Table 114-4). In practice, precal-

[1] *Copies of* Exchange Lists for Meal Planning *may be ordered from the American Diabetes Association, 2 Park Avenue, New York, NY 10016, or from any local affiliate of the association.*

TABLE 114-3
Composition of food exchanges*

Exchange	*Calories*	*Carbohydrate, g*	*Fat, g*	*Protein, g*
Milk	170	12	10	8
Vegetable†	35	7	—	2
Fruit	40	10	—	—
Bread	70‡	15	—	2
Meat	75‡	—	5	7
Fat	45	—	5	—

* *Composition listed for one exchange.*
† *Type A vegetables contain little carbohydrate, fat, or protein and can be eaten in any amount. Exchange values are for type B vegetables.*
‡ *Calculated value for bread exchange is 68 cal and for meat exchange is 73 cal using 4 kcal/g for carbohydrate and protein and 9 kcal/g for fat. The values 70 and 75 cal were adapted to facilitate computations.*

culated diets of given caloric content prepared by the American Diabetes Association are usually used. Alterations in distribution of protein, fat, and carbohydrate can be easily accomplished by minor shifts of exchanges. Care must be taken to emphasize foods the patient likes and can obtain. Initially it is helpful to weigh and measure foods until visual estimates can be made accurately. As in any dietary regimen it is important to emphasize that it is the long-term, overall dietary pattern which counts. Deviation for one meal or two meals does not matter much. Thus a teenage diabetic on a date may be allowed to eat a dessert, ordinarily forbidden, as a special treat with the understanding that resumption of the diet will be necessary the next day. Even in adults the "treat" technique often ensures better dietary cooperation than more rigid demands.

In insulin-requiring diabetics the distribution of calories is also important if hypoglycemia is to be avoided. A typical pattern might include 20 percent of the total calories for breakfast, 35 percent for lunch, 30 percent for dinner, and 15 percent as a late-evening feeding. Occasionally a midafternoon snack is necessary. Different distributions may be required for different life-styles; i.e., a person employed on a late-evening or night shift would not eat the major meal at noon.

Insulin Insulin is required for treatment of all type 1 patients and many patients with non-insulin-dependent disease. If the physician does not use oral drugs (see below), all diet-unresponsive NIDDM subjects must be given the hormone. It is fairly easy to control the symptoms of diabetes with insulin, but it is difficult—probably impossible—to normalize the blood sugar throughout 24 h utilizing traditional insulin therapy given as 1 or 2 injections a day. Nondiabetic subjects maintain the plasma glucose concentration within a narrow range at all times despite episodic food intake. When a meal is eaten, a prompt rise in insulin release occurs such that absorbed carbohydrate is rapidly transported into the liver and other tissues (see Chap. 89). Even after meals, therefore, the plasma glucose does not rise into the hyperglycemic or glycosuric range. As the plasma glucose falls under the influence of insulin, release of the hormone is damped and simultaneously counterregulatory hormones enter the circulation to prevent hypoglycemia, ensuring smooth control of plasma glucose throughout the absorptive process. The diabetic treated with insulin by injection cannot reproduce these physiologic responses. If enough insulin is given to keep the postprandial glucose within the range of normal, inevitably too much insulin will be present during the postabsorptive phase and hypoglycemia will result.

Because of accumulating evidence that some of the complications of diabetes may be prevented or partially reversed by normalization or near normalization of plasma glucose concentrations throughout the day, alternative forms of therapy have been devised. Three treatment regimens will be described: conventional, multiple subcutaneous injections (MSI), and continuous subcutaneous insulin infusion (CSII). *Conventional insulin therapy* involves the administration of one or two injections a day of lente or NPH insulin with or without the addition of small amounts of regular insulin to the intermediate-acting preparation. If the newly diagnosed diabetic is not in acute distress, therapy can be started as an outpatient, provided instruction in diet, urine testing, and insulin use is adequate and the physician can be reached by telephone for consultation. Normal-weight adults may be started on 15 to 20 units a day (the estimated daily insulin production rate in nondiabetic subjects of normal size is about 25 units a day). Obese patients, because of insulin resistance, may be started on 25 to 30 units a day. It is preferable to use the same quantity of insulin for several days before changing, the one exception being the hypoglycemic patient, for whom the dose should be immediately decreased unless a clearly evident nonrecurrent cause of hypoglycemia (such as excessive exercise) is present. Generally changes should be no more than 5 or 10 units per step. Poorly controlled patients should be tried on split therapy with about two-thirds of the total insulin given before breakfast and the remainder before supper. Two injections are almost always used when the total dose reaches 50 or 60 units a day but may actually be helpful at smaller doses as well since the peak action of intermediate insulins appears to be dose-related, i.e., a low dose may exhibit maximal activity earlier and disappear sooner than a large dose. It also is frequently helpful in difficult cases to add small amounts of regular insulin to the intermediate preparation. For example, if the urine glucose pattern shows glycosuria before lunch and in the early afternoon but no glycosuria at night, 5 to 10 units of regular insulin in the morning may solve the problem. All patients should be taught to reduce the insulin dose by 5 to 10 units when extra activity is anticipated. Similarly a small amount of extra regular insulin can be taken before a meal that contains extra calories or food ordinarily not allowed (e.g., when the diabetic must eat out at a banquet or the teenager goes out on a date). Patients with complicated control problems may require hospitalization, whereby frequent plasma and urine glucose determinations can guide therapy.

During surgical procedures or delivery of the pregnant diabetic it is desirable to omit depot insulin and administer regular insulin. A reasonable approach is to give 10 units of insulin prior to induction of anesthesia and to infuse 10% dextrose in water during the procedure. Plasma glucose and urine ketones should be monitored frequently, and additional insulin or glucose should be given as needed. Maintenance of mild hyperglycemia via the glucose infusion prevents hypoglycemia in the unconscious patient.

To follow the effectiveness of conventional therapy urine glucose and ketone concentrations are checked semiquantitatively before breakfast, lunch, supper, and retirement. A double-voiding technique in which the bladder is emptied and 30 min later a urine specimen is obtained for testing is mandatory for the early-morning sample and helpful at other times to minimize lag between plasma glucose and urine values. In addition, an estimate of urine volume should be obtained. A 4+ urine glucose means little if the patient has infrequent urination during the day and no nocturia, while the same chemical reading in a patient urinating large volumes five times a night indicates massive glucose wastage. It should be noted that some diabetics drink large volumes of water by habit, even after hyperglycemia has been brought under control. If the patient complains of continued nocturia when plasma glucose concentrations are in the acceptable range, a late-night specimen should be checked for glucose. A negative test suggests a water-drinking habit. Once the patient is stabilized, urine testing can be limited to once or twice daily. With the advent of

TABLE 114-4
A 2200-cal diabetic diet (50 percent carbohydrate)

Exchange	*No.*	*Calories*	*Carbohydrate, g*	*Fat, g*	*Protein, g*
Milk	2	340	24	20	16
Vegetable*		Unlimited amounts of type A vegetables			
Fruit	7	280	70	—	—
Bread	12	840	180	—	24
Meat	8	600	—	40	56
Fat	4	180	—	20	—
Total		2240	274 (50%)	80 (33%)	96 (17%)

* *Type B vegetables include beets, carrots, onions, green peas, pumpkin, rutabagas, winter squash, and turnips. If these are desired, ½ to 1 cup can be substituted for one fruit exchange. All other common vegetables can be eaten as desired.*

home glucose monitoring and measurement of glycosylated hemoglobin (see below) it is now recognized that urine testing gives only a crude estimate of control.

The *multiple subcutaneous insulin injection technique* most commonly involves administration of intermediate insulin in the evening as a single dose together with regular insulin prior to each meal. Home glucose monitoring by the patient is necessary if near normalization of the plasma glucose is the goal, although some patients under less stringent control have been treated without home monitoring. One approach to initiation of therapy involves administration of 25 percent of the previous daily insulin dose in the patient's conventional regimen at bedtime as intermediate insulin (NPH or lente) with the other 75 percent given as regular insulin divided such that 40, 30, and 30 percent are given 30 min before breakfast, lunch, and supper, respectively. Adjustments of dosage depend on response of the plasma glucose. A number of different protocols have been utilized, all of which represent sliding scales of insulin based on the plasma glucose. [For specific details see one of the published papers using the technique (e.g., Schiffrin and Belmonte).] MSI can be very effective in controlling the plasma glucose, and in some studies it appears as effective as CSII. For patients who dislike the multiple injections it is possible to insert a subcutaneous butterfly catheter into the anterior abdominal wall through which insulin can be injected. To ensure full delivery of insulin the tubing must be flushed with physiologic saline following each injection of the hormone. The catheters can be used for 3 to 5 days before being changed.

Continuous subcutaneous insulin infusion involves use of a small battery-driven pump that delivers insulin subcutaneously into the abdominal wall, usually through a 27-gauge butterfly needle. With CSII insulin is delivered at a basal rate continuously throughout the day with increased rates programmed prior to meals. Adjustments in dosage are made in response to measured capillary glucose values in a fashion similar to that used in MSI. Ordinarily about 40 percent of the total daily dose is given at the basal rate, the remainder being administered as preprandial bursts. There is little question that CSII can improve diabetic control relative to conventional therapy. Most patients report positive feelings of well-being as control improves. Nevertheless, although insulin infusion pumps have caught the attention of the public and many physicians, they should not be used indiscriminately. Mechanical failure resulting in administration of too much or too little insulin is not uncommon, and adequate warning mechanisms for dysfunction are not yet available even in second-generation pumps. The danger of hypoglycemia is real, especially during the night in patients who maintain the plasma glucose consistently below 100 mg/dl. A fall in plasma glucose of 50 mg/dl may not be important if the starting value is 150 mg/dl but may be fatal if it occurs against a steady-state level of 60 mg/dl. Several deaths from hypoglycemia have occurred in pump users. In the author's opinion pumps should be prescribed only in highly disciplined and motivated patients who are followed by physicians with extensive experience in their use. Apart from problems of hypoglycemia, local insulin reactions and abscess formation cause difficulty in a significant fraction of patients.

In one or two centers catheters for the insulin infusion pumps have been placed intravenously rather than subcutaneously. While few difficulties have been reported, this procedure appears unwise for routine use. Implantable insulin pumps with reservoirs refillable from outside the body have now been used in a few patients but must be considered strictly experimental; at present no advantage is apparent except that a pump does not have to be worn externally.

Types of insulin A variety of insulins are available for use in the treatment of diabetes. Rapidly acting preparations are always indicated in diabetic emergencies and in CSII and MSI

programs. Intermediate preparations are used in conventional and MSI regimens, and long-acting formulations are used rarely. It is not possible to delineate precisely the biologic responses to the various preparations because peak effects and duration vary from patient to patient and depend not only on route of administration but on dose. Further, hypoglycemic effects in insulin-treated diabetics appear to be delayed relative to normal subjects, probably because of the presence of anti-insulin antibodies in plasma. In one study in diabetics, regular insulin given subcutaneously had its onset of action at about 1 h, reached a peak at 6 h, and had measurable effects on average for 16 h, whereas in normal persons onset is within minutes, maximal action is around 2 h, and duration is only 6 to 8 h. With NPH insulin, diabetics exhibited an onset of action at 2.5 h, a peak at 11 h, and a total period of action of 25 h, more closely approximating values in normal subjects.

Commercial insulins are prepared in concentrations of 100 units per milliliter (U100) although higher concentrations can be obtained (e.g., U500). In terms of contamination by proinsulin, USP (generic) insulin normally has a purity of $<10{,}000$ parts per million (ppm) (proinsulin/insulin), although it can be higher. "Improved single-peak" insulin contains <50 ppm, while "purified" insulin has a contamination of <10 ppm, with some preparations containing as little as 1 ppm. Purified pork, beef, and beef-pork mixtures are now marketed. The various insulins are available as rapid (regular, semilente), intermediate (NPH, lente, globin), and long-acting (PZI, ultralente) preparations, although not all manufacturers offer all varieties. Lente and NPH insulin are used in most conventional therapy and are roughly equivalent in biologic effects, although lente appears to be slightly more immunogenic and to mix less well with regular insulin than does NPH. Insulin with structural identity to the human molecule has been prepared in bacteria utilizing recombinant DNA technology but is still undergoing clinical trials at the time of this writing.

Should the purified insulins be routinely prescribed in diabetic patients? The answer to this question is not clear. It is reported that purified pork insulin (which is structurally almost identical with human insulin, differing only in the terminal amino acid of the beta chain) results in less anti-insulin antibody formation; it also appears to have a lesser incidence of local insulin allergy, fat atrophy, and fat hypertrophy. However, since purified preparations are more expensive than other insulins they probably do not need to be used in patients with uncomplicated diabetes. As the price differential narrows, most patients will probably be switched to the purer hormone. Care must be taken to avoid hypoglycemia when changing to purified insulin since daily requirements may fall 10 to 20 percent relative to less pure forms, especially if pure pork insulin is chosen.

Hypoglycemia and the Somogyi effect (See also Chap. 116) The problem of hypoglycemia is common in insulin-dependent diabetics, particularly when aggressive efforts are made to normalize not only the fasting plasma glucose but also postprandial hyperglycemia. Hypoglycemia may be caused by missing a meal or doing unexpected exercise but can occur in the absence of known precipitating events. Daytime episodes of hypoglycemia are usually recognized by adrenergic symptoms, such as sweating, nervousness, tremor, and hunger. Hypoglycemia occurring during sleep may produce no symptoms or cause night sweats, unpleasant dreams, or early-morning headache. In one study of insulin-dependent diabetic children monitored throughout 24 h, 18 percent had asymptomatic noctural hypoglycemia. If hypoglycemia is not aborted by ingestion of carbohydrate, central nervous system symptoms ensue: confusion, abnormal behavior, loss of consciousness, or convulsions. As diabetes progresses, particularly with the development of neuropathy, epinephrine-induced symptoms become blunted and may lose their effectiveness as warning signals, with the consequence that central nervous system signs predominate.

Hypoglycemia is potentially harmful in several ways. It may produce permanent neurologic damage or lead to injury via accident. Moreover, hypoglycemia results in worsening of diabetic control, since release of counterregulatory hormones results in rebound hyperglycemia, occasionally with mild ketosis. This phenomenon, called the *Somogyi effect,* should be suspected whenever wide swings in the plasma glucose or urine sugars are seen over short time intervals even if symptoms are not reported. Thus, a plasma glucose of 70 mg/dl before breakfast and 400 mg/dl before lunch suggests early-morning hypoglycemia with postbreakfast hyperglycemia due to counterregulatory hormone activity. Such rapid changes contrast with the alterations seen following insulin withdrawal in previously well-controlled diabetic patients in whom hyperglycemia and ketosis develop gradually and smoothly over a 12- to 24-h period. Excessive hunger and weight gain occurring in the context of worsening hyperglycemia are clues that the insulin dosage may be too high, since poor control due to underinsulinization usually results in weight loss (because of osmotic diuresis and glucose wastage). If the Somogyi phenomenon is suspected, the insulin dose should be decreased as a trial, even when specific symptoms of overinsulinization are absent. The Somogyi phenomenon probably occurs less frequently in patients utilizing insulin infusion pumps than in those treated by conventional or multiple injections of insulin as a bolus. As noted earlier, however, hypoglycemia is not uncommon with CSII, particularly if mean plasma glucose levels are kept below 100 mg/dl. *Despite assumptions to the contrary, hypoglycemic attacks are dangerous, and if frequent portend a serious and occasionally fatal outcome.*

It is not unusual for a previously stable, well-controlled diabetic to develop insulin sensitivity and hypoglycemia in the absence of change in weight, diet, or exercise. The most common cause is the appearance of diabetic renal disease. Occasionally the hypoglycemia may be due to the development of autoimmune adrenal insufficiency as part of the Schmidt syndrome (see Chap. 124), which is more frequent in diabetics than in the population as a whole. Some patients develop hypoglycemia in association with high levels of circulating insulin antibodies. The exact mechanism has not been established. Occasionally an insulinoma may develop in a diabetic patient. Very rarely, permanent remission of apparently typical diabetes occurs. The reason is not known.

Oral agents Non-insulin-dependent diabetes that cannot be controlled by careful dietary management often responds to sulfonylureas. The drugs are easy to use and appear to be safe. Fear that sulfonylureas might increase deaths from heart attacks, prompted by reports of the University Group Diabetes Program (UGDP), have largely dissipated because of questions about the design of that study. On the other hand use of the oral drugs has decreased concomitant with the emphasis on better control as a possible means of slowing the development of late complications. While some patients with relatively mild disease have near normalization of plasma glucose on oral drugs, those with significant hyperglycemia tend to improve but do not approach normality. Thus a high percentage of non-insulin-dependent diabetics are now treated with insulin.

Sulfonylureas act primarily by stimulating release of insulin from the beta cell. They also have the capacity to increase the number of insulin receptors in target tissues and enhance insulin-mediated glucose disposal. Since mean levels of plasma insulin do not increase following treatment with sulfonylureas despite significantly improved mean plasma glucose concentrations, extrapancreatic effects of the drugs have received increasing attention. However, the paradox of improved glucose metabolism in the absence of higher steady-state levels of insulin has been resolved by studies which show that elevation of plasma glucose to pretreatment values results in a rise of plasma insulin to levels higher than those seen pretreatment. Thus, the initial action of the drugs is to increase insulin release with lowering of the plasma glucose. As glucose concentrations fall insulin levels also decrease since plasma glucose is the major stimulus to insulin release, thereby masking the initial stimulatory effect. The insulinogenic effect can then be unmasked by raising the plasma glucose to the previous elevated levels. The fact that sulfonylureas are ineffective in IDDM, where beta-cell mass is markedly diminished, strongly supports the pancreatic effect as primary, although extrapancreatic mechanisms doubtless play a role.

Four major forms of sulfonylureas are available. Tolbutamide and tolazamide have relatively short half-lives and must be given in divided doses. They are inactivated by the liver. Acetohexamide undergoes hepatic metabolism, but the major hepatic metabolite retains hypoglycemic activity. Renal excretion is, therefore, the primary disposal route for acetohexamide, as well as for chlorpropamide which is only minimally metabolized in the body. Patients with renal disease are vulnerable to hypoglycemia with the latter two drugs. Chlorpropamide has a long half-life and can be given as a single dose but may cause water retention in some patients through its capacity to sensitize the renal tubule to antidiurectic hormone. Second-generation sulfonylureas (e.g., glipizide) are widely used in Europe but are not yet licensed for use in the United States. The dosage range of the sulfonylureas in grams per day is as follows:

Acetohexamide	0.25–1.5 g
Chlorpropamide	0.1–0.5 g
Tolazamide	0.1–1 g
Tolbutamide	0.5–3 g

Hypoglycemia is less common with oral agents than with insulin, but when it occurs it tends to be severe and prolonged. Some patients have required massive glucose infusions for days following the last dose of sulfonylurea. For this reason hospitalization is mandatory in patients with sulfonylurea-induced hypoglycemia.

The only other oral agents effective in the treatment of maturity-onset diabetes are the biguanides. They presumably lower plasma glucose by inhibiting gluconeogenesis in the liver although it has also been reported that phenformin increases the number of insulin receptors in some tissues. The drugs are ordinarily used only in combination with sulfonylureas under circumstances in which control is inadequate with sulfonylurea alone. Because of many reports linking phenformin to the appearance of lactic acidosis, the Food and Drug Administration removed the agent from clinical use in the United States except for certain special patients who continue to take it as an investigational drug. Metformin and buformin were never approved in the United States. Phenformin and other biguanides are still widely used elsewhere in the world. If prescribed, the maximum dose of phenformin should be 100 mg a day. Biguanides should not be given to patients with renal disease and should be immediately stopped should nausea, vomiting, diarrhea, or any intercurrent illness appear.

Potential treatments Efforts continue to develop an effective antiglucagon agent for use in the treatment of diabetes. Such an agent could be directed at lowering glucagon secretion by the alpha cell or antagonizing its action in target tissue. A somatostatin analogue that could be taken orally, that had an extended biologic half-life, and that inhibited growth hormone secretion only minimally would be an ideal candidate. Another goal is development of methods to allow oral absorption of insulin. In rats administration of insulin with 5-methoxysalicylate has been reported to allow rapid absorption of 15 percent of hormone placed in the intestine, but no studies have been carried out in humans.

Transplantation of insulin-producing islet tissue continues to be of interest. Use of the vascularized distal half of whole pancreas is technically feasible and can normalize metabolic abnormalities, but perioperative mortality is significant and complications from the required immunosuppression are frequent. For this reason the transplantation of isolated islets of Langerhans has been tried. Experimentally, islets can be transplanted across genetic barriers provided they are cultured in vitro prior to injection. The presumption is that the period of culture removes "passenger" leukocytes (T cells and macrophages) that induce rejection. Beta cells themselves apparently do not trigger rejection. While these results are encouraging, much work remains to be done before the technique can be used in humans. Apart from rejection, the problem of obtaining sufficient human islets is enormous. This difficulty would be resolved if animal islets could be rendered nonimmunogenic in humans.

Monitoring diabetic control Measurement of urine glucose is not sufficient to assess diabetic control when attempts are being made to bring mean plasma glucose values into the near-normal range since the urine will be free of glucose when the plasma concentration is less than 180 mg/dl. For this reason "home glucose monitoring" is used in those patients treated by CSII or MSI techniques. Such monitoring requires capillary blood, which can be obtained almost painlessly by a small spring-triggered device (Autolet, Ulster Scientific Inc.) equipped with disposable lancets. Glucose is analyzed utilizing chemically impregnated strips that are then read in a commercially available reflectance meter. When care is taken in calibration of the instrument, the technique gives values approximating those obtained in samples simultaneously assayed in a glucose analyzer. One reagent strip, Chemstrip bG (Bio-Dynamics), gives satisfactory values by visual inspection (utilizing a dual-color scale), eliminating the need to purchase a reflectance meter. Frequent measurement of the plasma glucose (a fairly standard program utilizes seven or eight assays over 24 h) allows a reasonable assessment of mean plasma glucose levels during the day and guides adjustment of insulin dosage.

Longer-term, objective assessment of the degree of diabetic control utilizes periodic measurement of hemoglobin A_{1c}, a fast-moving minor hemoglobin component, which is present in normal persons but increases severalfold in the presence of hyperglycemia. The change in mobility is due to nonenzymatic glycosylation of the amino acids valine and lysine. The reaction is as follows:

$$\beta\text{-NH}_2 + \begin{array}{c} \text{HC=O} \\ | \\ \text{HCOH} \\ | \\ \text{HOCH} \\ | \\ \text{HCOH} \\ | \\ \text{HCOH} \\ | \\ \text{CH}_2\text{OH} \\ \text{Glucose} \end{array} \rightleftharpoons \begin{array}{c} \text{HC=N}-\beta\text{A} \\ | \\ \text{HCOH} \\ | \\ \text{HOCH} \\ | \\ \text{HCOH} \\ | \\ \text{HCOH} \\ | \\ \text{CH}_2\text{OH} \\ \text{Aldimine} \\ \text{(Schiff base)} \end{array} \longrightarrow \begin{array}{c} \text{CH}_2-\text{N}^+\text{H}_2-\beta\text{A} \\ | \\ \text{C=O} \\ | \\ \text{HOCH} \\ | \\ \text{HCOH} \\ | \\ \text{HCOH} \\ | \\ \text{CH}_2\text{OH} \\ \text{Ketoamine} \end{array}$$

$$\text{Hb A} \underset{}{\overset{\textit{Rapid}}{\rightleftharpoons}} \text{pre A}_{1c} \overset{\textit{Slow}}{\longrightarrow} \text{Hb A}_{1c}$$

In this scheme β-NH_2 stands for the terminal valine of the β chain of hemoglobin. Aldimine formation is reversible so that pre-A_{1c} is labile while ketoamine formation is irreversible and thus stable. Pre-A_{1c} levels depend on the ambient glucose concentrations and do not reflect long-term control although they are measured in chromatographic methods for determining hemoglobin A_{1c}. Pre-A_{1c} must thus be removed to assess true Hb A_{1c} values accurately; this can be done by incubating red blood cells in saline, dialyzing hemolysates, or treating chemically with semicarbazide and aniline. A colorimetric method, utilizing thiobarbituric acid, can be done simply and inexpensively and has the advantage that it does not measure the labile pre-A_{1c} fraction. When properly assayed, the percent of glycosylated hemoglobin gives an estimate of diabetic control for the preceding 6 to 10 weeks. Normal values must be obtained for each lab; on average nondiabetic subjects have Hb A_{1c} values of around 6 percent, while levels in poorly controlled diabetics may reach 10 to 12 percent.

Glucose-lysine adducts also occur in other proteins in the body such as plasma albumin, low-density lipoprotein, erythrocytic membranes, lens protein, and basic myelin protein. Measurement of glycosylated albumin, because of its short half-life, can be used to monitor diabetic control over a 1- to 2-week period.

ACUTE METABOLIC COMPLICATIONS In addition to hypoglycemia, diabetics are susceptible to two major acute metabolic complications: diabetic ketoacidosis and hyperosmolar, nonketotic coma. The former is a complication of insulin-dependent diabetes, while the latter usually occurs in the setting of non-insulin-dependent disease. Ketoacidosis rarely, if ever, develops in type 2 diabetes.

Diabetic ketoacidosis The pathophysiology of diabetic ketoacidosis is now reasonably clear. Initiation appears to require insulin deficiency coupled with a relative or absolute increase in glucagon concentration. It is often caused by cessation of insulin intake but may result from physical (e.g., infection, surgery) or emotional stress despite continued insulin therapy. In the former case the concentration of glucagon rises secondary to insulin withdrawal, while in stress the operative stimulus is probably epinephrine release. In addition to stimulating glucagon secretion epinephrine presumably blocks release of the small amount of residual insulin found in some subjects with IDDM and inhibits insulin-induced glucose transport in peripheral tissues. These hormonal changes have multiple effects, but two are critical: (1) They induce maximal gluconeogenesis and impair peripheral utilization of glucose, causing severe hyperglycemia. It is thought that glucagon facilitates gluconeogenesis by inducing a fall in fructose 2,6-diphosphate (fructose 2,6-bisphosphate), an important intermediate which serves to stimulate glycolysis through activation of phosphofructokinase and to block gluconeogenesis by inhibiting fructose diphosphatase (see Chap. 89). The resultant osmotic diuresis leads to the volume depletion and dehydration that characterize the ketoacidotic state. (2) They activate the ketogenic process and thus initiate development of metabolic acidosis. For ketosis to occur, changes must be produced in both adipose tissue and the liver. Free fatty acids from adipose stores represent the primary substrate for ketone body formation, and plasma levels of free fatty acids must rise if high rates of ketogenesis are to develop. However, fatty acids delivered to the liver are simply reesterified and stored as hepatic triglyceride or converted into very low density lipoproteins and transported back into

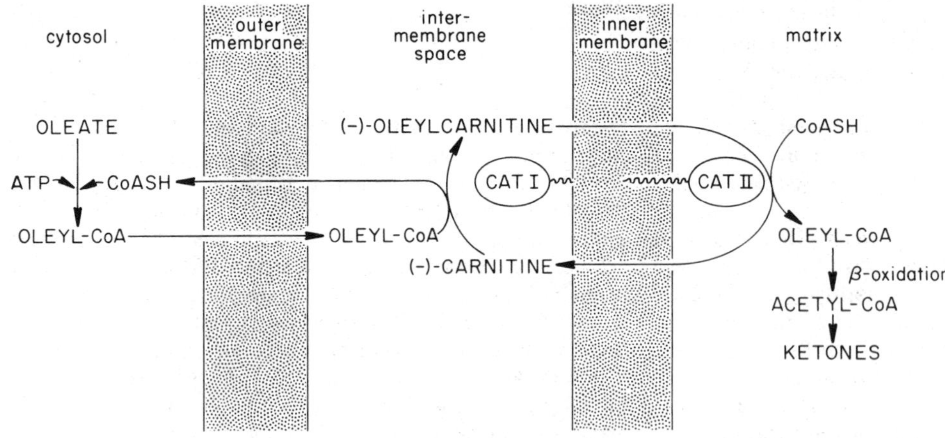

FIGURE 114-2
The carnitine acyltransferase system for the transfer of long-chain fatty acids into the mitochondria. CAT I = carnitine acyltransferase I; CAT II = carnitine acyltransferase II. (From JD McGarry et al, J Clin Invest 55:1202, 1975. Used by permission.)

the circulation unless the hepatic oxidative machinery for fatty acids is activated.

While free fatty acid release is enhanced directly by insulin deficiency, accelerated fatty acid oxidation in the liver is primarily induced by glucagon, via action on the carnitine acyltransferase system of enzymes responsible for the transport of fatty acids into the mitochondria following their esterification to coenzyme A. As shown in Fig. 114-2 carnitine acyltransferase I transesterifies fatty acyl CoA to fatty acylcarnitine, which then freely traverses the inner mitochondrial membrane. Reversal of the reaction occurs internally under the influence of carnitine acyltransferase II. In the fed state carnitine acyltransferase I is inactive, and, as a consequence, long-chain fatty acids cannot reach the β-oxidative enzymes for ketone body production. During starvation or uncontrolled diabetes the system is activated; under these circumstances the rate of ketogenesis is a first-order function of the concentration of fatty acids reaching transferase I.

The mechanism by which glucagon (or a change in the glucagon/insulin ratio) activates the transport system is twofold. First, glucagon causes a rapid fall in hepatic malonyl CoA content. Malonyl CoA, the first committed intermediate in the synthesis of fatty acids from glucose, is a powerful competitive inhibitor of carnitine acyltransferase I, and the fall in its concentration is critical to the ketogenic process. Second, glucagon causes a rise in hepatic carnitine concentration, which then drives the reaction toward fatty acylcarnitine formation by mass action. These events are summarized schematically in Fig. 114-3. At high plasma fatty acid concentrations hepatic uptake is sufficient to saturate both oxidative and esterifying pathways, resulting in fatty liver and hypertriglyceridemia as well as ketoacidosis. Overproduction of ketones by the liver is the primary event in ketotic states, but limitation of peripheral utilization also plays a role at high concentrations of acetoacetate and β-hydroxybutyrate.

Clinically ketoacidosis begins with anorexia, nausea, and vomiting, coupled with increased urine formation. Abdominal pain may be present. If untreated, altered consciousness or frank coma may occur. Initial examination usually shows Kussmaul respiration, together with signs of volume depletion. Rarely the latter is sufficient to cause vascular collapse and renal shutdown. Body temperature is normal or slightly below normal in uncomplicated ketoacidosis, and fever suggests the presence of infection. Leukocytosis, frequently very marked, is a feature of diabetic acidosis per se and may not indicate infection.

The characteristic metabolic abnormalities of diabetic coma are shown in Table 114-5. Several features deserve comment. The metabolic acidosis and anion gap are almost totally accounted for by the elevated plasma levels of acetoacetate and β-hydroxybutyrate, although other acids (e.g., lactate, free fatty acids, phosphates) contribute modestly. Despite initial potassium concentrations that are normal to high, there is a total body potassium deficit of several hundred millimoles. Similarly, initial serum phosphorus may be high despite depletion of body stores. Magnesium deficiency may also be present.

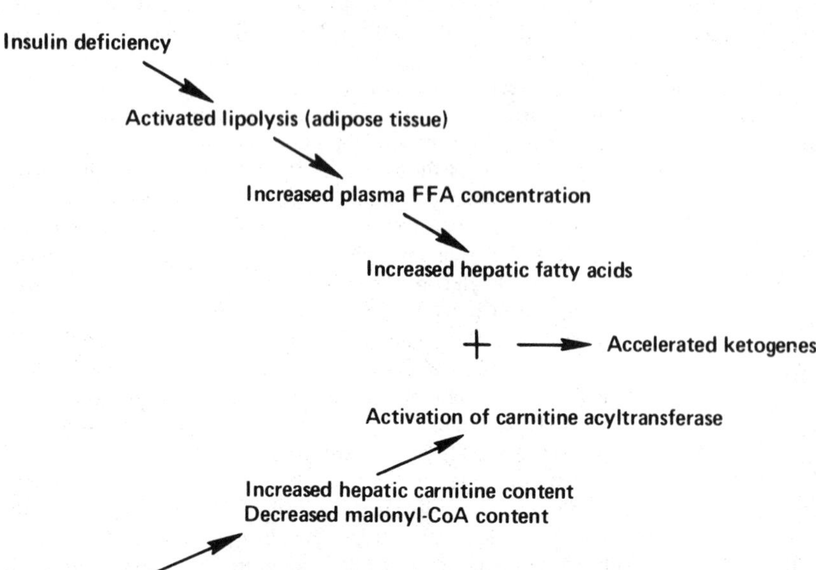

FIGURE 114-3
The regulation of ketogenesis. Significant production of acetoacetate and β-hydroxybutyrate by the liver requires provision of adequate free fatty acid substrate and activation of fatty acid oxidation. Lipolysis is primarily increased by insulin deficiency while the fatty acid oxidative sequence is activated primarily by glucagon. The immediate signal for oxidation is a fall in malonyl CoA content. (After JD McGarry, DW Foster, Am J Med 61:9, 1976.)

The serum sodium concentration tends to be low in the face of modest osmolar concentration because of the hyperglycemia which draws intracellular water into the plasma space. A very low serum sodium (e.g., 110 meq per liter) suggests an artifact due to severe hypertriglyceridemia. The latter is common in ketoacidosis and is likely the consequence of both impaired activity of lipoprotein lipase (a disposal defect) and the hepatic overproduction of very low density lipoproteins. If a fat meal has been ingested prior to the onset of ketoacidosis, chylomicrons may make up a major portion of the circulating fat. Lipemia is usually visible if triglyceride concentration is above 400 mg/dl. True hyponatremia may also occur if the patient has vomited repeatedly and continued to drink water. Prerenal azotemia, reflecting volume depletion, is common but usually is modest in degree and completely reversible with treatment. The serum amylase may be elevated and frank pancreatitis can occur.

The diagnosis of ketoacidosis in a known diabetic is not difficult. Its appearance in a patient not previously known to have diabetes requires differentiation from the other common causes of metabolic acidosis with an anion gap: lactic acidosis, uremia, alcoholic ketoacidosis, and certain poisonings. The first step is to test the urine for glucose and ketones. If urine ketones are negative, another cause for the acidosis is likely. If positive, plasma examination is required to be certain that something more than starvation ketosis is present. Since quantitative determinations of acetoacetate and β-hydroxybutyrate are not routinely available, semiquantitative tests must be done using ketone reagent strips (Ketostix) or tablets (Acetest). If the latter are used, the tablet should be crushed and results read at 2 min. Serial dilutions of plasma can be made and tested. A strong test may occur in undiluted plasma owing to starvation alone; a strong reaction beyond 1:1 dilution is presumptive evidence for ketoacidosis. Apart from diabetes the only other common ketoacidotic state is alcoholic ketoacidosis. This syndrome, which by definition occurs in chronic alcoholics, usually follows a debauch, but the patient may not have had alcohol for 24 h or longer. It never occurs in the absence of starvation and frequently is associated with severe vomiting and abdominal pain. Pancreatitis is present in up to 75 percent of patients. A plasma glucose of less than 150 mg/dl was found in three-fourths of reported cases and in 16 percent was less than 50 mg/dl on arrival at the hospital. Hyperglycemia may occur but is usually mild and rarely, if ever, above 300 mg/dl. Plasma free fatty acid concentrations are much higher (mean 2.9 m*M*) than in normal starvation (range 0.7 to 1.0 m*M*), reaching levels seen in diabetic ketoacidosis. Presumably the liver is activated for ketogenesis by starvation in these patients and driven to maximal rates of ketone formation by the high fatty acid levels. Why some alcoholics mobilize fatty acids excessively is not known. In contrast to diabetic acidosis, the syndrome is rapidly reversible by the intravenous administration of glucose. As in all alcoholics given glucose, thiamine should be supplied to avoid precipitation of acute beriberi. (Other water-soluble vitamins, though not as critical, should also be infused.) Insulin is required only if hyperglycemia persists during therapy.

TABLE 114-5
Initial laboratory findings in diabetic ketoacidosis

Series	*Dallas**	*Los Angeles†*	*Washington‡*
Age	38	36	43
Glucose, mg/dl	475	675	733
Sodium, m*M*	132	131	132
Potassium, m*M*	4.8	5.3	6.0
Bicarbonate, m*M*	<10	6	10
BUN, mg/dl	25	32	42
Acetoacetate, m*M*	4.8	—	—
β-Hydroxybutyrate, m*M*	13.7	—	—
Free fatty acids, m*M*	2.1	—	2.3
Lactate, m*M*	4.6	—	—
Osmolarity, mosmol/liter	310	323	331

* *Eighty-eight consecutive episodes of ketoacidosis at Parkland Memorial Hospital (DW Foster, unpublished observations).*
† *Mean data from 308 episodes of nonfatal ketoacidosis (PM Beigelman, Diabetes 20:490, 1971).*
‡ *Mean data from 10 episodes of ketoacidosis (JE Gerich et al, Diabetes 20:228, 1971).*

The treatment of diabetic ketoacidosis is controversial. All agree that insulin should be given, but the amount to be administered is at issue. "Low-dose insulin" schedules have become popular in recent years. It is claimed that they produce less hypoglycemia and hypokalemia during treatment than standard forms of therapy. By "low-dose insulin" most authors mean 6 to 8 units per hour given intravenously as opposed to the 50 to 100 units per hour recommended previously. Most diabetic acidosis can be reversed adequately with low-dose treatment. A small fraction of patients, however, are insulin-resistant. This resistance is probably primarily due to insulin antibodies, although it can also be seen in patients who have never received insulin. The problem is that resistant subjects cannot be identified prospectively. For this reason it is probably preferable to treat ketoacidosis with 25 to 50 units of regular insulin intravenously hourly until the acidosis is reversed. There are no known toxic effects of larger insulin doses, since maximal physiologic response is obtained once insulin receptors are saturated regardless of how much insulin is given. The advantage of the higher dosage schedule is that it assures saturation of the receptors in the face of competing antibodies or other resistance factors. If physicians choose to use the low-dose insulin schedule, they should be alert to the possibility of resistance. Should acidosis persist unabated after several hours of treatment, larger amounts of insulin are clearly indicated. Ketoacidosis can also be adequately treated with intramuscular (but not subcutaneous) insulin.

Therapy of ketoacidosis requires intravenous fluids. The usual fluid deficit is 3 to 5 liters, and both salt solutions and free water are needed. One to two liters of isotonic saline or Ringer's lactate should be given rapidly intravenously on arrival, with additional amounts determined by urine output and clinical assessment of the fluid state. Five percent glucose solutions should be given when the plasma glucose falls to about 300 mg/dl, both as a source of free water and as a prophylactic measure to prevent the late cerebral edema syndrome. The latter is a rare complication of ketoacidosis occurring most often in children. It is suspected when the patient remains comatose or lapses into coma following reversal of acidosis. The syndrome is probably related to osmotic disequilibrium between brain and plasma produced when plasma glucose concentrations are rapidly lowered. Once developed, treatment requires large doses of dexamethasone and hypertonic mannitol infusions.

Potassium replacement is always necessary, but the time of administration will vary. The initial potassium is often high despite a total body deficit because of the severe acidosis. In this case the cation will ordinarily not be needed until 3 to 4 h after initiation of therapy, when reversal of acidosis and the action of insulin cause a shift of K^+ into intracellular water. On the other hand if the admission value is normal or low, potassium should be given early, since plasma concentrations fall rapidly during therapy, predisposing the patient to cardiac arrhythmias. In view of the phosphate depletion of ketoacidosis, potassium should be administered initially as the phosphate salt rather than as potassium chloride.

Bicarbonate therapy is indicated in severely acidotic patients (pH 7.0 or below) but is not used routinely in less acutely ill subjects since rapid alkalinization may have detrimental effects on oxygen delivery to tissues. The hemoglobin-oxygen dissociation curve is normal in diabetic ketoacidosis because of the opposing effects of acidosis and deficiency of red blood cell 2,3-diphosphoglycerate (2,3-DPG). If the acidosis is rapidly reversed, the deficiency of 2,3-DPG becomes manifest, increasing the avidity with which hemoglobin binds oxygen and impairing the release of oxygen in peripheral tissues. In a volume-depleted patient with poor tissue perfusion such a change theoretically could predispose to the development of lactic acidosis. If bicarbonate is given, the infusion should be stopped when the pH reaches 7.2 to minimize effects on oxygen binding by hemoglobin and to prevent metabolic alkalosis as circulating ketones are metabolized to bicarbonate with reversal of ketoacidosis.

In following the response to treatment, two points should be emphasized. (1) Plasma glucose invariably falls more rapidly than plasma ketones. Insulin should not be stopped because glucose concentrations approach normal; rather, as mentioned, glucose should be infused and insulin continued until the ketosis has cleared. (2) Plasma ketone values as determined by nitroprusside reagent cannot be used to evaluate response to therapy. The testing materials measure acetoacetate and acetone but not β-hydroxybutyrate. Since β-hydroxybutyrate must be oxidized to acetoacetate prior to utilization, it is characteristic for the plasma ketones measured by nitroprusside to remain stable or even rise early in therapy at a time when total ketone concentration (acetoacetate plus β-hydroxybutyrate) is steadily falling. For this reason bicarbonate content and pH have to be assessed to evaluate reversal of the acidosis. Because β-hydroxybutyrate and acetoacetate represent a redox couple in equilibrium with mitochondrial NADH/NAD concentrations, vascular collapse or severe hypoxia may mask the presence of ketoacidosis as acetoacetate is reduced to β-hydroxybutyrate. Under these circumstances the β-hydroxybutyrate/acetoacetate ratio, normally about 3:1, may reach 7:1 or 8:1. Paradoxically, in such a situation, ketosis measured by Acetest tablet or Ketostix may seem to worsen as the patient gets better because of conversion of β-hydroxybutyrate to acetoacetate when the circulation is reestablished and tissue oxygenation is restored. A flow sheet outlining insulin given, fluid therapy, urine volume, and blood and urine chemistries should be maintained throughout the treatment. Without such a record therapy tends to become chaotic.

Most patients with diabetic ketoacidosis recover when properly treated. While mortality in large series is reported to be around 10 percent, the majority of deaths result from late complications rather than from ketoacidosis itself. The major causes are myocardial infarction and infection, particularly pneumonia. Poor prognostic signs on admission include hypotension, azotemia, deep coma, and associated illness.

Hyperosmolar coma Hyperosmolar nonketotic diabetic coma is usually a complication of non-insulin-dependent diabetes. It is a syndrome of profound dehydration resulting from a sustained hyperglycemic diuresis under circumstances in which the patient is unable to drink sufficient water to keep up with urinary fluid losses. Commonly an elderly diabetic—often living alone or in a nursing home—develops a stroke or infection, which worsens hyperglycemia and prevents adequate water intake. The full-blown syndrome probably does not occur until volume depletion has become severe enough to diminish urine output. Hyperosmolar coma has also been precipitated by therapeutic procedures such as peritoneal dialysis or hemodialysis, tube feeding of high-protein formulas, high-carbohydrate infusion loads, and the use of osmotic agents such as mannitol and urea. Phenytoin sodium, steroids, immunosuppressive agents, and diuretics have also been reported to initiate the disorder.

The absence of ketoacidosis is important in the pathophysiology. When ketoacidosis occurs in an insulin-dependent diabetic, nausea, vomiting, and air hunger bring the patient to the physician before extreme dehydration can occur. Such a protective mechanism is not operative in the ketoacidosis-resistant, maturity-onset diabetic. Interestingly, hyperosmolar coma can occur in insulin-dependent diabetic patients given sufficient insulin to prevent ketosis but insufficient to control hyperglycemia. While rare, there are reports of the same patient presenting on one occasion with ketoacidosis and the next with hyperosmolar coma.

The reason for the absence of ketoacidosis in maturity-onset diabetics is not known. The hepatic ketogenic machinery is not impaired since the patients frequently have ketone concentrations in the starvation range (4 to 6 m*M*). Free fatty acid levels are lower in hyperosmolar coma than in ketoacidosis, and it has been suggested that substrate deficiency limits ketone formation. That this is the sole mechanism seems unlikely since some patients with hyperosmolar coma have been found to have extremely high levels of free fatty acids in their plasma. A more likely explanation is that insulin concentrations in the portal vein of type 2 diabetics are higher than those of insulin-dependent subjects and prevent full activation of the hepatic carnitine acyltransferase system.

Clinically patients present with extreme hyperglycemia, hyperosmolality, and volume depletion, coupled with central nervous system signs ranging from clouded sensorium to coma. Seizure activity—sometimes Jacksonian in type—is not unusual, and transient hemiplegia may also be seen. Infections, particularly pneumonia and gram-negative sepsis, are common and indicate a grave prognosis. Pneumonia is often due to gram-negative organisms. A high index of suspicion for infection should be maintained, and routine culture of the blood and spinal fluid is indicated. Because of the extreme dehydration plasma viscosity is high, and widespread in situ thrombosis has been found at post mortem. Bleeding, probably the consequence of disseminated intravascular coagulation, has also been reported. Acute pancreatitis may accompany the illness.

The laboratory findings in two large series are shown in Table 114-6. Plasma glucose is generally around 1000 mg/dl, about twice the value seen in ketoacidosis. The serum osmolality is extremely high, but because of the hyperglycemia the absolute serum sodium concentration is often not elevated.[2] Prerenal azotemia with marked elevation of BUN and creatinine is characteristic. A mild metabolic acidosis is present, plasma bicarbonate on the average being about 20 meq per liter. The acidosis is due to a combination of starvation ketosis, retention of inorganic acids secondary to the azotemia, and modest elevation of plasma lactate, the latter the consequence of volume depletion. If the bicarbonate is less than 10 meq per liter and plasma ketones are not elevated, it can be assumed that lactic acidosis is present.

The mortality rate in hyperosmolar coma is very high ($>$ 50 percent). As a consequence immediate treatment is urgent. The most important measure is rapid administration of large amounts of intravenous fluids to reestablish the circulation and

[2] *Serum osmolality can be accurately estimated from the formula*

Serum osmolality (mosmol/liter)

$$= 2([Na^+] + [K^+]) + \frac{\text{glucose (mg/dl)}}{18} + \frac{\text{BUN (mg/dl)}}{2.8}$$

In practice the contribution of the BUN is often ignored since it contributes to total osmolality but does not reflect the free water deficit. There are situations in clinical medicine in which an increased osmolality is not equivalent to dehydration. Severe alcohol intoxication is the classic example, the ethanol itself providing the measured milliosmoles.

TABLE 114-6
Initial laboratory findings in hyperosmolar coma

Series	*Brooklyn**	*Washington*†
Age	60	57
Glucose, mg/dl	1166	976
Sodium, m*M*	144	142
Potassium, m*M*	5	5
Chloride, m*M*	99	98
Bicarbonate, m*M*	17	22
BUN, mg/dl	87	65
Creatinine, mg/dl	5.5	—
Free fatty acids, m*M*	0.73	0.96
Osmolarity, mosmol/liter	384	374

* *Mean data from 33 episodes of hyperosmolar coma (AA Arieff, HJ Carroll, Medicine 51:73, 1972).*
† *Mean data from 20 episodes of hyperosmolar coma (JE Gerich et al, Diabetes 20:228, 1971).*

urine flow. The average fluid deficit is 10 liters. While free water will ultimately be needed, initial therapy should be with isotonic salt solutions, and 2 to 3 liters should be given over the first 1 to 2 h. Subsequently half-strength saline can be used. As the plasma glucose approaches normal levels, 5% dextrose can be given as a vehicle for free water. While hyperosmolar coma may be reversed by fluids alone, insulin should be given to control the hyperglycemia more rapidly. Many authors recommend small doses of insulin, but larger amounts may be necessary, particularly in the obese patient. It should be noted that potassium salts are usually required earlier in the treatment of hyperosmolar coma than in ketoacidosis because the intracellular shift of plasma K^+ during therapy is accelerated in the absence of acidosis. If lactic acidosis is present, sodium bicarbonate should be given until tissue perfusion can be reestablished (see Chap. 115). Antibiotics are required if infection complicates the picture.

LATE COMPLICATIONS OF DIABETES The diabetic patient is, unfortunately, susceptible to a series of complications that cause morbidity and premature mortality. While some patients may never develop these problems and others note their onset early, on the average symptoms develop 15 to 20 years following the appearance of overt hyperglycemia. A given patient may experience several complications simultaneously, or a single problem may dominate the picture.

Circulatory abnormalities Arteriosclerosis of the type seen in nondiabetics is a common problem in diabetes and occurs more extensively and earlier than in the general population. The cause for this accelerated atherosclerosis is not known, although it has been suggested that alterations in the ratio of high-density to low-density lipoproteins in plasma may play a role. Unproven etiologic factors for which there is some evidence include abnormally functioning low-density lipoprotein (glycosylated) and diminished prostacyclin formation. Atherosclerotic lesions produce symptoms in a variety of sites. Peripheral deposits may cause intermittent claudication, gangrene, and, in men, organic impotence on a vascular basis. Surgical repair of large vessel lesions may be unsuccessful because of the simultaneous presence of widespread disease of the small vessels. Coronary artery disease and stroke are common. Silent myocardial infarction is known to occur in diabetics and should be suspected whenever symptoms of left ventricular failure appear suddenly. Diabetes may also be associated with the clinical picture of cardiomyopathy, in which heart failure occurs in the face of angiographically normal coronary arteries and the absence of other identifiable causes of heart disease. As in nondiabetics, smoking is a major risk factor for both coronary and peripheral vascular disease and should be avoided.

Retinopathy Diabetic retinopathy is a leading cause of blindness in the United States. On the other hand, most diabetics never become blind. Retinopathic lesions are divided into two large categories, *simple* (background) and *proliferative* (Table 114-7). The earliest sign of retinal change is an increased capillary permeability that is evidenced by leakage of dye into the vitreous humor after fluorescein injection. Occlusion of retinal capillaries follows, with subsequent formation of saccular and fusiform aneurysms. Arteriovenous shunts also occur. The vascular lesions are accompanied by proliferation of lining endothelial cells and a loss of the pericytes that surround and support the vessels. Hemorrhages into the inner retinal areas appear dot-shaped, while bleeding into the more superficial nerve fiber layer causes flame-shaped, blot, or linear lesions. Preretinal hemorrhages characteristically have a boat-shaped appearance. Exudates are of two types. Cotton-wool spots can be shown by angiography to be microinfarcts—nonperfused areas surrounded by a ring of dilated capillaries. A sudden increase in the number of cotton-wool spots represents an ominous prognostic sign and may herald the appearance of rapidly advancing retinopathy. Hard exudates are more common than cotton-wool spots and probably represent leakage of protein and lipids from damaged capillaries.

The fundamental characteristics of proliferative retinopathy are new vessel formation and scarring. The stimulus for neovascularization is unknown, although it is believed that hypoxia secondary to capillary or arteriolar occlusion may be the primary cause. Two serious complications of proliferative retinopathy are vitreal hemorrhage and retinal detachment. A sudden loss of vision in one eye is almost always due to one or the other of these two lesions.

The frequency of diabetic retinopathy appears to vary with the age of onset as well as the duration of the disease. Approximately 85 percent of patients eventually develop retinopathy, but some never develop ophthalmoscopically visible lesions even after 30 years of disease. Retinopathy appears to develop earlier in older patients, but proliferative retinopathy is less common. It has been estimated that 10 to 18 percent of patients with simple retinopathy progress to proliferative disease in a 10-year period. Visual prognosis in patients with and without retinopathy in one large series is shown in Table 114-8.

The treatment of choice for diabetic retinopathy is photocoagulation. Three types of light source are used. The xenon arc produces white light that is absorbed largely by the pigment epithelium and can destroy both intraretinal and surface new vessels. Its disadvantage is that without special equipment it cannot produce lesions smaller than 500 μm. The ruby laser gives monochromatic red light and can make smaller lesions.

TABLE 114-7
Lesions of diabetic retinopathy

BACKGROUND
Increased capillary permeability
Capillary closure and dilatation
Microaneurysms
Arteriovenous shunts
Dilated veins
Hemorrhages (dot and blot)
Cotton-wool spots
Hard exudates
PROLIFERATIVE
New vessels
Scar (retinitis proliferans)
Vitreal hemorrhage
Retinal detachment

The argon laser produces blue-green light that can coagulate a moving column of blood, makes small lesions (< 50 μm), and can be used to obliterate vessels extending into the retrovitreal space. The cooperative trial of the Diabetic Retinopathy Study Research Group, with an enrollment of 1700 patients, established that photocoagulation with either xenon arc or argon laser improved visual prognosis in diabetic retinopathy. All patients with neovascularization and hemorrhage should, therefore, be followed by an ophthalmologist trained in these techniques. Indications for treatment by photocoagulation include:

1 Moderate or severe new vessels on or within one disk diameter of the optic disk.
2 Mild new vessels on or within one disk diameter of the optic disk if fresh hemorrhage is present.
3 Moderate or severe new vessels elsewhere if fresh hemorrhage is present.

Whether milder forms of retinopathy should be treated with focal or panretinal photocoagulation is not yet clear. Complications of photocoagulation include vitreal hemorrhage, vitreal contraction with retinal detachment, macular edema, and visual field loss. Occasionally iritis and keratitis develop.

The role of pars plana vitrectomy in diabetic retinopathy is uncertain because of the high incidence of postoperative complications (25%) and the difficulty of assessing residual retinal function prior to surgery. It has a definite role in treatment of traction detachment of the retina and nonresolving vitreal hemorrhage.

Hypophysectomy, once widely used, is no longer recommended because photocoagulation is safer and equally or more effective. A rare exception might be the so-called florid diabetic retinopathy ("rapid, bleeding, blinding") in which widespread new vessel formation has occurred but no scar is present.

Diabetic nephropathy Renal disease is a common complication and a leading cause of death in diabetes. The pathology is complicated, with four types of lesions generally described: (1) glomerulosclerosis, (2) arteriolosclerosis of efferent and afferent arterioles, (3) arteriosclerosis of the renal artery and its intrarenal branches, and (4) peritubular deposits of glycogen, fat, and mucopolysaccharides. The glomerular lesions have received the most emphasis, probably because of their early description. Nodular glomerulosclerosis, the classical Kimmelstiel-Wilson lesion, consists of a periodic acid Schiff (PAS)–positive, rounded hyaline mass appearing near the periphery of the glomerulus. Nuclei may be embedded in the mass, and often a nonoccluded capillary runs over the surface. Diffuse glomerulosclerosis may also be present and represents thickening of the basement membrane of the capillaries. Subsequently the intercapillary or mesangial region also becomes thickened. Finally, an exudative lesion, acidophilic in staining characteristics, may develop. If located over a glomerular loop or attached to the inside of Bowman's capsule, it is called a "fibrin cap." All these changes are visible by light microscopy. Utilizing the electron microscope, thickening of capillary basement membranes in the glomerulus may be discernible before the other changes are seen. It has also been shown that glomerular and tubular basement membranes are lined with IgG and albumin in diabetic nephropathy. Whether these changes are primary or secondary has not yet been established. The pathophysiology underlying the histologic abnormalities remains unknown, but some workers feel that it may be related to the increased glomerular filtration rate and renal hypertrophy that characterize the early stages of both human and experimental diabetes.

There is no close correlation between histologic lesions and clinical renal disease: i.e., on biopsy the changes of diabetes may be seen in patients with apparently normal renal function. On the other hand if clinical renal disease is present, it can be assumed that the histologic architecture will be abnormal. Originally the term "Kimmelstiel-Wilson syndrome" referred to the presence of edema, hypertension, proteinuria, and renal failure in a diabetic patient. Many physicians now use the notation *Kimmelstiel-Wilson disease* loosely to refer to any manifestation of diabetic nephropathy, although this is both pathologically and clinically inexact. Diabetic renal disease is protean in its manifestations and may vary from a change in the renal threshold for glucose (such that glucosuria does not appear until plasma glucose is elevated considerably above the normal threshold value of 180 to 200 mg/dl) to the insidious onset of hypertension or uremia. Proteinuria may or may not be present, but the full-blown nephrotic syndrome is relatively rare. Early studies of diabetic nephropathy indicated that death followed the appearance of proteinuria after only 1 to 2 years. It is now known that heavy and persistent proteinuria (> 3 g per 24 h) is prognostically ominous but that patients with lesser degrees of protein loss may live for much longer periods—occasionally more than 10 years. A very high percentage of patients with nephropathy have simultaneous retinopathy, but many patients with retinopathy have no overt signs of renal disease.

The appearance of increasing insulin sensitivity may occasionally herald the presence of diabetic nephropathy. While insulin half-life is prolonged in renal failure, the precise mechanism for the increased sensitivity is not known. It appears to be more than a simple diminution of glycosuria secondary to the aforementioned change in renal threshold, since hyperglycemia also diminishes. Uremia affects the metabolism of glucagon and other hormones as well as altering hormone receptor function. It is probable, therefore, that increased insulin sensitivity is multifactorial in origin. Whatever the mechanism, it is frequently necessary to decrease insulin dosage in patients with nephropathy.

In the past, treatment of renal failure in the diabetic was limited to protein restriction, maintenance of fluid balance, and alkalinization to control the uremic acidosis. Renal transplantation and chronic dialysis are now commonly carried out. Originally it was thought that chronic dialysis in the diabetic was an ineffective long-term measure; however, this viewpoint is changing, and in a number of centers there is no hesitancy about entering a diabetic into a dialysis program. While it has been suggested that transplantation in the diabetic be undertaken at creatinine levels of around 6 mg/dl in an attempt to preserve eyesight, the question of whether and when to do a transplant in the individual patient remains a difficult question. Careful consultation between the physician, nephrologist, and transplant surgeon is required.

Diabetic neuropathy Diabetic neuropathy may affect every part of the nervous system with the possible exception of the brain. While it is rarely a direct cause of death, it is a major

TABLE 114-8
Prognosis for vision in diabetes*

Group†	*Good to impaired*	*Good to blind*	*Impaired to blind*
Control	2.4	0.31	1.3
Retinopathy	7.5	3.0	13.1

* *Numbers indicate the percentage of patients progressing to a worse level of vision per year.*
† *Control patients had no retinopathy when first examined. Control patients with impaired vision at entry had other eye problems. Good vision was defined as a visual acuity of 6/18 or better; impaired vision, acuities of 6/24 to 6/60; and blind, a visual acuity of less than 6/60. It should be noted that factors other than retinopathy contributed to visual loss in some patients (e.g., glaucoma).*
SOURCE: *Data adopted from FI Caird, CJ Garrett, Diabetes 12:389, 1963.*

cause of morbidity. Distinct syndromes can be recognized, and often several different types of neuropathy are present in the same patient. The most common picture is that of *peripheral polyneuropathy*. Usually bilateral, the symptoms include numbness, paresthesias, severe hyperesthesias, and pain. The pain, which may be deep-seated and severe, is often worse at night. It is occasionally lancinating or lightning in type, resembling tabes dorsalis (pseudotabes). Fortunately extreme pain syndromes are usually self-limited, lasting from a few months to a few years. Involvement of proprioceptive fibers leads to abnormalities of gait and development of typical Charcot joints, particularly in the feet. Loss of arch with multiple fractures of tarsal bones is a common finding by x-ray. On physical examination absent stretch reflexes and loss of vibratory sense are frequent early signs. Diabetic neuropathy may also cause delay in return of the ankle reflex identical with the lesion seen in hypothyroidism. *Mononeuropathy*, though less common than polyneuropathy, may also occur. Characteristically there is a sudden wrist drop, foot drop, or paralysis of the third, fourth, or sixth cranial nerves. Other single nerves, including the recurrent laryngeal, have been reported to be involved. Mononeuropathy is characterized by a high degree of spontaneous reversibility, usually over a several-week period. *Radiculopathy* is a sensory syndrome in which pain occurs over the distribution of one or more spinal nerves, usually in the chest wall or abdomen. The severe pain may mimic herpes zoster or an acute surgical abdomen. Like mononeuropathy, the lesion is usually self-limited. *Autonomic neuropathy* may present in a variety of ways. The gastrointestinal tract is a prime target, and there may be esophageal dysfunction with difficulty in swallowing, delayed gastric emptying, or diarrhea. The latter is often nocturnal. Patients may suffer from orthostatic hypotension and frank syncope. Cardiorespiratory arrest and sudden death, thought to be due solely to autonomic neuropathy, have also been reported. Bladder dysfunction or paralysis is particularly distressing and often leads to the necessity of chronic catheter drainage. Impotence and retrograde ejaculation are additional manifestations in the male. Diabetic *amyotrophy* is likely a form of neuropathy, although atrophy and weakness of the large muscles in the upper leg and pelvic girdle resemble primary muscle disease.

The cause of diabetic neuropathy is unknown. Biochemical changes have been demonstrated in the nerves of animals with experimental diabetes, but their relation to human neuropathy is uncertain. Considerable interest has focused on the fact that a neuropathy can be induced in rats made diabetic with streptozotocin which exhibits prolonged conduction times similar to those seen in human diabetes. The involved nerves were found to have a marked decrease in myoinositol content that could be reversed either by insulin treatment or by feeding myoinositol. Whether a similar defect exists in the neuropathy of humans remains to be seen.

Treatment of diabetic neuropathy is unsatisfactory in most respects. When pain is severe, it is easy for the patient to become habituated or addicted to narcotics or nonnarcotic analgesics. If the pain requires something more powerful than aspirin or acetaminophen, codeine is the drug of choice. Phenytoin sodium is believed to be useful by some physicians, but others have not found it very helpful. Carbamazepine, another anticonvulsant, may benefit some patients. The usual dose is 200 mg three times daily. Combination therapy with amitriptyline and fluphenazine hydrochloride has been reported to cause dramatic relief of pain over a several-day period. The recommended dosage is 75 mg amitriptyline at bedtime and 1 mg fluphenazine three times a day. The long-term effectiveness of this treatment is not yet known. Mononeuropathies and radiculopathies usually require no specific therapy since they are self-limited. Diabetic diarrhea often responds to treatment with diphenoxylate and atropine or loperamide. Orthostatic hypotension is best treated by having the patient sleep with the head of the bed elevated, avoidance of sudden assumption of the upright position, and the use of full-length elastic stockings. Occasionally volume expansion with fludrocortisone acetate is required as in other forms of orthostatic hypotension.

Reports have appeared indicating subjective improvement in symptoms of neuropathy utilizing oral myoinositol or treatment with an inhibitor of aldose reductase, the enzyme responsible for formation of sorbitol in tissues. (Sorbitol is thought by some to be a cytotoxic metabolite in diabetes.) These approaches remain experimental.

Diabetic foot ulcers A special problem in the diabetic is the development of ulcers of the feet and lower extremities. The ulcers appear to be primarily due to abnormal pressure distribution secondary to diabetic neuropathy. The problem is accentuated when there is bony distortion in the feet. Callus formation is usually the initial abnormality. Alternatively the ulcer may be initiated by ill-fitting shoes which cause blister formation in patients whose sensory deficits preclude recognition of pain. Cuts and punctures from foreign bodies such as needles, tacks, and glass are common, and frequently a foreign body of which the patient is completely unaware will be found in the soft tissue. For this reason all patients with ulcers should have x-rays made of the feet. Vascular disease with diminished blood supply contributes to development of the lesion, and infection is common, often with multiple organisms. While no specific therapy is available for diabetic ulcers, aggressive supportive treatment can often lead to salvation of the leg without amputation. One approach is to simply put the patient to bed using frequent foot soaks and debridement to remove nonviable tissue. Others recommend casting the leg with plaster to remove weight bearing and protect the lesion.

All diabetics should be instructed about proper foot care in an attempt to prevent ulcers. Feet should be kept clean and dry at all times. Patients with neuropathy should not be allowed to walk barefoot, even in the home. Properly fitted shoes are essential. This is a particular problem with women, since an adequate shoe for the diabetic is not often stylish. The feet should be carefully inspected daily for callus, infection, abrasions, or blisters and the physician consulted for any potentially troublesome lesion.

THE QUESTION OF CONTROL AND THE DEVELOPMENT OF COMPLICATIONS The critical question in diabetic therapy is whether hyperglycemia or some associated metabolic disorder causes or accelerates the development of the long-term complications just discussed. The alternative possibility is that complications are primarily determined by genetic factors independent of hyperglycemia. The fact that many proteins can be glycosylated nonenzymatically and that the degree of glycosylation is directly correlated with the mean level of the plasma glucose has provided an attractive hypothesis as to mechanism. It is presumed that the glycosylated peptides might cause abnormal structure and function of vascular and other tissues. For example, glycosylated low-density lipoprotein (LDL) molecules circulate in excess quantity in diabetic patients, and these altered molecules do not bind to LDL receptors or shut off intracellular cholesterol synthesis in normal fashion. Perhaps the strongest evidence that the metabolic environment per se causes complications comes from the observation that kidneys from donors who have neither diabetes nor a family history of diabetes develop characteristic lesions of diabetic nephropathy within 3 to 5 years after transplantation into a diabetic recipient. While this suggests that some factor in the metabolic environment of the diabetic subjects causes the appearance of renal disease, there is no proof that hyperglycemia is the inciting agent. Attempts to relate appearance of complications to degree of diabetic control have been inconclusive because reliable objective methods of assessing control have only recently become available. It has been possible to show partial reversal of some abnormalities accompanying diabetes by aggressive insulin therapy. These include capillary leakage of fluorescein in the retina, delayed motor nerve conduction velocity, hyperlipoproteinemia, and microalbuminuria (albumin in the urine below the limits demonstrable by routine chemical assay but detectable by radioimmunoassay). Perinatal morbidity and mortality in offspring of diabetic mothers can be minimized by aggressive treatment of diabetes, although congenital abnormalities are not prevented. In experimental animals even birth defects can be prevented provided near normoglycemia is maintained throughout pregnancy. The same might prove true in humans if hyperglycemia could be abolished in the very earliest stages of pregnancy. The problem is that pregnancy is often not recognized until a month or longer after conception, while it is in the early weeks of gestation that risk for malformation occurs.

While the above evidence suggests a possible relationship between control and complications, there is also evidence against. For example, there are a number of reports in the literature of patients who already have diabetic complications at the time of diagnosis; e.g., a young person previously well presents with ketoacidosis and is found to have retinopathy. Conversely, a significant number of patients never develop complications despite the absence of meticulous diabetic control. Thickening of the capillary basement membrane in muscle is a characteristic finding in adult diabetics with either insulin-dependent or non-insulin-dependent disease. While a subject of controversy, the lesion may represent a fundamental component of diabetic microangiopathy. It has been reported to be present in a significant number of normoglycemic children of two parents with overt diabetes. Moreover, basement membrane thickening has been found in asymptomatic parents of children with type 1 diabetes where it appears to be related to the presence of HLA-DR4. If these findings are confirmed and if basement membrane thickening is in fact a marker of diabetes-related complications, then it would seem unlikely that complications occur exclusively as a consequence of poor diabetic control.

On balance it must be concluded that a causal relationship between hyperglycemia and development of complications can at present neither be proved nor disproved. Until the issue is clarified it would appear prudent to maintain the plasma glucose as near normal as possible in all diabetic patients. About this there appears to be no disagreement. The only question is whether aggressive insulin therapy should be pushed routinely to the point of overt hypoglycemia. A mild insulin reaction consisting of nervousness, tremor, hunger, and sweating that is rapidly interrupted by carbohydrate intake is probably not harmful except for the possibility of worsening diabetic control via the Somogyi reaction. Unfortunately, as stated, many diabetics, particularly those with long-standing disease and autonomic neuropathy, do not have or do not recognize the usual warning signals and progress to altered central nervous system function with abnormal behavior, loss of consciousness, or even convulsions. The latter reactions are dangerous for both patient and society. Every effort should be made to control hyperglycemia, but the limit of therapy should be the appearance of hypoglycemic reactions. It does not seem wise to induce a condition that can cause immediate and irreversible damage to a patient in the unproved hope that late complications might be prevented.

INSULIN RESISTANCE Insulin resistance in the diabetic is arbitrarily said to exist when more than 200 units per day are required to control hyperglycemia and prevent ketosis. Relative insulin resistance is present with much lower insulin requirements, but therapy for the resistant state is usually not considered necessary below the 200-unit level. Insulin antibodies of IgG type are present in essentially all diabetics within 60 days of the initiation of insulin therapy. The titer of these antibodies fluctuates for reasons that are not clear. Although the correlation between antibody titer and functional resistance is not close, it is presumed that insulin binding by high levels of antibody is the primary mechanism in most cases. Probably less than 0.1 percent of insulin-treated diabetics ever have functionally significant resistance. The problem may appear within a few weeks of the start of therapy or many years later. The onset may be abrupt, resulting in ketoacidosis, but usually is gradual, with uncontrollable hyperglycemia being the major problem. About 20 to 30 percent of patients have concomitant insulin allergy. Therapy of the syndrome requires prednisone in large amounts—80 to 100 mg per day initially. Response often occurs in 48 to 72 h, but may take longer. If no improvement has resulted after 3 to 4 weeks it can be assumed that steroids will not be effective. Once insulin requirements begin to fall, prednisone dosage can be rapidly decreased by 10 to 20 mg every 3 to 7 days until a maintenance level of 5 to 10 mg per day is reached. These levels may be required for many months. Whether remission has occurred, allowing cessation of therapy, can only be determined by trial. On rare occasions insulin resistance in diabetics appears to be due to enhanced destruction of the hormone at the subcutaneous injection site. Such patients tend to respond normally to insulin given intravenously.

Insulin resistance may be seen in diseases other than diabetes. The physiologic consequences can be minor or severe. A variety of insulin-resistant syndromes are associated with *acanthosis nigricans,* a brown to black, velvety hyperpigmentation of the skin in the axilla, groin, neck, umbilicus, and other areas. Although acanthosis nigricans may be a sign of occult malignancy, it is not associated with neoplasia in the insulin-resistant states. A classification of insulin resistance based on the absence or presence of acanthosis nigricans is given in Table 114-9. *Obesity* and *antibodies* to insulin are by far the most common causes of insulin resistance, and neither is accompanied by acanthosis. Obesity is associated with diminished insulin receptor number and affinity but also has postreceptor hormone resistance. *Werner's syndrome* is an autosomal recessive illness with a high incidence of hyperglycemia despite elevated concentrations of plasma insulin. There is little response to exogenous hormone. Other features include growth retardation, alopecia or premature graying of the hair, cataracts, hypogonadism, leg ulcers, atrophy of muscle, fat, and bone, soft-tissue calcification, and a high frequency of sarcomas and meningiomas.

TABLE 114-9
Insulin-resistant states

I Insulin resistance without acanthosis nigricans
- *A* Obesity
- *B* Diabetes mellitus with insulin antibodies
- *C* Werner's syndrome

II Insulin resistance with acanthosis nigricans
- *A* Insulin resistance with receptor abnormality
  - *1* Receptor deficiency (type A abnormality)
  - *2* Antibody to insulin receptor (type B abnormality)
- *B* Lipodystrophic states
  - *1* Generalized lipodystrophy (congenital or acquired)
  - *2* Partial lipodystrophy (congenital or acquired)
- *C* Syndrome of familial insulin resistance, somatic abnormalities, and pineal hyperplasia
- *D* The Alström syndrome
- *E* Ataxia telangiectasia

Of the rare conditions associated with acanthosis nigricans, women with *insulin receptor abnormalities* have attracted the greatest interest. Type A patients are tall young females with a tendency to hirsutism and abnormalities of the reproductive tract who most probably have polycystic ovaries. The absolute number of insulin receptors is markedly diminished. Type B subjects are older women with evidence of immunologic disease. The clinical picture includes arthralgias, alopecia, enlarged salivary glands, proteinuria, leukopenia, and antinuclear and anti-DNA antibodies. Insulin resistance in these patients is due to blocking antibodies to the insulin receptor (not to insulin itself). Both A and B patients have high plasma insulin concentrations.

Generalized and *partial lipodystrophies* are fat depletion syndromes differing primarily in the extent of fat atrophy. In the generalized form essentially all body fat is missing, while the more common partial type exhibits atrophy of fat in the face and trunk with normal or increased adiposity in the lower half of the body. The disease can be either congenital or acquired. Typically the patients develop hyperglycemia at puberty, but ketoacidosis never occurs. Marked hypertriglyceridemia with eruptive xanthoma is a frequent feature. Characteristically present are hepatomegaly, splenomegaly, cardiomegaly, hirsutism, lymphadenopathy, hypertrophy of the external genitalia, varicose veins, and (in the congenital forms) muscle hypertrophy. Mental retardation is common and renal disease may develop. A "diabetogenic" peptide has been found in the urine, but its role is not clear. The term *lipoatrophic diabetes* is synonymous with total lipodystrophy. All patients have elevated plasma insulin levels. Resistance may be due to decreased number of receptors, diminished affinity of the receptor for insulin, or a postreceptor defect.

The *pineal hypertrophy syndrome* is characterized by insulin resistance, early dentition with malformed teeth, dry skin, thick nails, hirsutism, and a peculiar sexual precocity with enlargement of the external genitalia. The latter may reach near adult size by age 3 or 4. The insulin resistance is severe and ketoacidosis may occur despite high endogenous insulin levels. The *Alström syndrome* is a rare autosomal recessive disease characterized by childhood blindness due to retinal degeneration, nerve deafness, vasopressin-resistant diabetes insipidus, and, in males, hypogonadism with high plasma gonadotropin levels. The patients thus appear to have multiple end organ resistance to hormones. Other features include baldness, hyperuricemia, hypertriglyceridemia, and amino aciduria. Superficially the patients may resemble subjects with the Lawrence-Moon-Biedl syndrome but can be differentiated on initial exam by the absence of polydactyly and mental deficiency. Insulin resistance in the Alström syndrome is mild. *Ataxia-telangiectasia* is characterized by cerebellar ataxia, telangiectasia, and a variety of abnormalities in the immune system in addition to insulin resistance. Not listed in Table 114-9 is insulin resistance due to hormone excess (acromegaly, Cushing's syndrome), myotonic dystrophy, and leprechaunism. The insulin resistance in these conditions is usually not clinically significant.

INSULIN ALLERGY Insulin allergy is due to IgE antibodies to insulin. Manifestations include immediate reactions with local stinging or itching, delayed local reactions with brawny swelling lasting up to 30 h, and generalized urticaria or frank anaphylaxis. Systemic reactions are usually seen in patients who have stopped insulin therapy for one reason or another and have then resumed treatment. The allergic reaction may occur as early as the second injection on resumption of therapy. Mild reactions can be treated with antihistamines. If the problem is severe, desensitization procedures are required. A 1-day insulin desensitization procedure is shown in Table 114-10. Once the patient is desensitized, insulin therapy should not be interrupted.

Miscellaneous abnormalities Diabetes affects almost every system in the body. Space limitations preclude discussion of all associated features, but several deserve comment. *Infections* in diabetics may not occur more frequently than in normal subjects but they tend to be more severe. This may be due to impaired leukocyte function, a frequent accompaniment of poor control. In addition to common infections of the skin, urinary tract, lungs, and bloodstream, three unusual conditions appear to have specific relationship with diabetes. *Malignant external otitis,* usually due to *Pseudomonas aeruginosa,* tends to occur in older patients and is characterized by severe pain in the ear, drainage, fever, and leukocytosis. Soft tissues around the ear are swollen and tender. A mound of granulation tissue is characteristically present internally at the junction of the osseous and cartilaginous portions of the ear. The facial nerve becomes paralyzed in half the cases, and other cranial nerves may also be involved. Facial nerve paralysis is a poor prognostic sign with mortality reaching 50 percent in this subset of patients. A 6-week course of ticarcillin or carbenicillin together with tobramycin is the treatment of choice. Surgical debridement is often necessary. *Rhinocerebral mucormycosis* is a rare fungal infection which usually develops in patients during or following an episode of diabetic ketoacidosis. Organisms are from the genera *Mucor, Rhizopus,* and *Absidia.* Onset is sudden with periorbital and perinasal swelling, pain, bloody nasal discharge, and increased lacrimation. The nasal mucosa and underlying tissues become black and necrotic. Cranial nerve palsies are not uncommon. There may be thrombosis of the internal jugular vein or sinuses of the brain. Proptosis, chemosis, and retinal vein engorgement indicate cavernous sinus thrombosis. Untreated, death usually occurs in a week to 10 days. Amphotericin B coupled with aggressive debridement is the indicated therapy. *Emphysematous cholecystitis* is a variant of gallbladder disease that tends to affect diabetic men (in contrast to ordinary cholecystitis, a disease predominantly present in women). Gangrene of the gallbladder is 30 times more frequent than in the usual forms, accounting for high rates of perforation and a mortality rate 3 to 10 times higher than in ordinary cholecystitis. Diagnosis is made when gas is seen in the gallbladder wall on plain films of the abdomen. Clostridial species are frequently cultured from bile, but other organisms may be present. Treatment is cholecystectomy coupled with

TABLE 114-10
Insulin desensitization*

Time, h	*Dose, units*	*Route*
0	0.001	Intradermal
0.5	0.002	Intradermal
1	0.004	Subcutaneous
1.5	0.01	Subcutaneous
2	0.02	Subcutaneous
2.5	0.04	Subcutaneous
3	0.1	Subcutaneous
3.5	0.2	Subcutaneous
4	0.5	Subcutaneous
4.5	1	Subcutaneous
5	2	Subcutaneous
5.5	4	Subcutaneous
6	8	Subcutaneous

* *Following desensitization, use 2 to 10 units of regular insulin every 4 to 6 h for 24 to 36 h after the 6-h injection before switching to intermediate-acting insulin.*
SOURCE: *Schedule of JA Galloway. For detailed information see JA Galloway, R Bressler, Med Clin North Amer 62:663, 1978.*

broad-spectrum antibiotics. Clindamycin and an aminoglycoside are adequate coverage until cultures are returned.

Hypertriglyceridemia is common in diabetes, and in the majority of cases is due to insulin deficiency. Both overproduction of very low density lipoproteins in the liver and a disposal defect in the periphery appear to be operative. The latter is a consequence of lipoprotein lipase deficiency, an insulin-dependent enzyme. A number of diabetics continue to exhibit hyperlipemia even when diabetic control is adequate and family studies have suggested that these patients have a primary familial hyperlipoproteinemia which is independent of diabetes. Clofibrate appears to be the drug of choice for treatment in subjects unresponsive to diet and insulin therapy.

Some diabetics have been found to have *recurrent hyperkalemia* in association with hyperglycemia. Hyperkalemia can occur in the absence of potassium loads and serum potassium concentrations may rise acutely in response to oral glucose in contrast to normals where glucose ingestion produces a fall in potassium levels. The presumption is that potassium shifts from intracellular to extracellular water under these circumstances. Traditionally these patients have been considered to have hyporeninemic hypoaldosteronism although basal renin and aldosterone concentrations may be normal. Since the capacity to increase aldosterone production in response to stimulatory signals is impaired even when basal levels are normal, it is likely that functional hypoaldosteronism plays a central role in the syndrome. With a deficiency of aldosterone, renal secretion of potassium is impaired and disposal of a potassium load is dependent on insulin-mediated transport of the cation into the intracellular space. Administration of potassium salts or triamterene to such patients may be dangerous. Whether potassium transport is directly regulated by insulin or is secondary to glucose movement is not clear.

A variety of skin lesions occur in diabetes. *Necrobiosis lipoidica diabeticorum* is a plaque-like lesion with a central yellowish area surrounded by a brownish border. It is usually found over the anterior surfaces of the legs. Ulceration may occur. *Diabetic dermopathy* is also usually located over the anterior tibial surface. The lesions are small rounded plaques with a raised border which may crust at the edges and ulcerate centrally. Several plaques may be arranged in linear fashion. Pigmentation is not prominent early, but as the lesion heals a depressed scar occurs with diffuse brown discoloration. A rarer abnormality is *bullosis diabeticorum.* The bullae may be superficial with clear serum or may be mildly hemorrhagic. The cause is unknown. *Infestations of the skin* with *Candida* and dermatophytes are common, and bacterial infections of a variety of types occur. In women *vaginal moniliasis* may be troublesome during hyperglycemic-glycosuric periods. While the symptoms respond to nystatin, recurrence is inevitable unless glycosuria is reversed. In difficult cases intravaginal gentian violet therapy may be required. *Atrophy of adipose tissue* may occur at the site of insulin injections. The lipoatrophy is said to respond to injection of purified pork insulin into the atrophic area.

Hyperviscosity occurs in diabetes and *platelets aggregate abnormally.* The latter may be caused by increased prostaglandin synthesis. *Wound healing* is impaired in experimental diabetes but probably is not a major factor clinically. An interesting accompaniment of insulin-dependent diabetes is the presence of *joint contractures* coupled with *tight, waxy skin* over the dorsum of the hands. The cause of the tendon contractures is unknown although alterations of cross-linking in collagen has been proposed. Patients with the joint contracture–waxy skin syndrome appear to have accelerated development of diabetic complications.

THE EMOTIONAL RESPONSE TO DIABETES Acceptance of the fact that a person has a chronic disease which requires a complete change in life-style is always difficult. This is particularly true in the case of diabetes since patients generally are aware that they are vulnerable to late complications and that statistically their life expectancy is shortened. It is not surprising that the emotional response to diabetes often hampers treatment. On the one hand the primary reaction may be denial with an accompanying refusal to cooperate. At the other extreme is excessive preoccupation with the illness. The physician should make every effort to define a middle ground wherein the patient acknowledges his or her disease and responds to it prudently without becoming obsessed by it. The goal is to live with diabetes not for it. Diabetics are no different from other patients in that they may attempt to use their disease manipulatively with both family and physician. The problems are particularly acute with children and adolescents. While the psychiatric aspects of diabetes are not discussed here, most problems can be anticipated and handled if common sense is coupled with sympathy and firmness.

REFERENCES

Diabetes mellitus

Brownlee M, Cahill GF Jr: Diabetic control and vascular complications, in *Atherosclerosis Reviews,* R Paoletti, AM Gotto Jr (eds). New York, Raven Press, 1979, vol 4, p 29

Bunn HF: Evaluation of glycosylated hemoglobin in diabetic patients. Diabetes 30:613, 1981

Cahill GF Jr, McDevitt HO: Insulin-dependent mellitus: the initial lesion. N Engl J Med 304:1454, 1981

Ellenberg M: Diabetic neuropathy: Clinical aspects. Metabolism 25:1627, 1976

Foster DW: Insulin deficiency and hyperosmolar coma. Adv Int Med 19:159, 1974

———: Diabetes mellitus, in *The Metabolic Basis of Inherited Disease,* 5th ed, JB Stanbury et al (eds). New York, McGraw-Hill, 1983

Friedman JM, Fialkow PJ: The genetics of diabetes, in *Progress in Medical Genetics IV,* AG Steinberg et al (eds). Philadelphia, Saunders, 1980, p 199

Galloway JA: Insulin treatment for the early 80s: Facts and questions about old and new insulins and their usage. Diabetes Care 3:615, 1980

Genuth SM et al: Community screening for diabetes by blood glucose measurement. Results of a five-year experience. Diabetes 25:1110, 1976

Given BD et al: Diabetes due to secretion of an abnormal insulin. N Engl J Med 302:129, 1980

Green DA et al: Comparison of clinical course and sequential electrophysiological tests in diabetics with symptomatic polyneuropathy and its implications for clinical trials. Diabetes 30:139, 1981

Knowles HB Jr: Joint contractures, waxy skin, and control of diabetes. N Engl J Med 305:217, 1981

Kreisberg RA: Diabetic ketoacidosis: New concepts and trends in pathogenesis and treatment. Ann Int Med 88:681, 1978

Lernmark A, Baekkeskov S: Islet cell antibodies—Theoretical and practical implications. Diabetologia 21:431, 1981

Lestradet H et al: Long-term study of mortality and vascular complications in juvenile-onset (type 1) diabetes. Diabetes 30:175, 1981

Liang JC, Goldberg MF: Treatment of diabetic retinopathy. Diabetes 29:841, 1980

McGarry JD, Foster DW: Regulation of hepatic fatty acid oxidation and ketone body production. Ann Rev Biochem 49:395, 1980

Miles JM et al: Effects of acute insulin deficiency on glucose and ketone body turnover in man. Evidence for the primacy of overproduction of glucose and ketone bodies in the genesis of diabetic ketoacidosis. Diabetes 29:926, 1980

NATIONAL DIABETES DATA GROUP: Classification and diagnosis of diabetes mellitus and other categories of glucose intolerance. Diabetes 28:1039, 1979

PADILLA AJ, LOEB JN: "Low-dose" versus "high-dose" insulin regimens in the management of uncontrolled diabetes. A survey. Am J Med 63:843, 1977

PUTNAM WS et al: Selective potentiation of insulin-mediated glucose disposal in normal dogs by the sulfonylurea glipizide. J Clin Invest 67:1016, 1981

ROTWEIN P et al: Polymorphism in the 5′-flanking region of the human insulin gene and its possible relation to type 2 diabetes. Science 213:1117, 1981

ROY B et al: Time-action characteristics of regular and NPH insulin in insulin-treated diabetics. J Clin Endocrinol Metab 50:475, 1980

SCHIFFRIN A, BELMONTE MM: Comparison between subcutaneous insulin infusion and multiple injections of insulin: A one year prospective study. Diabetes 31:255, 1982

SUNDERLIN FS et al: The renin-angiotensin-aldosterone system in diabetic patients with hyperkalemia. Diabetes 30:335, 1981

UNGER RH, ORCI L: Glucagon and the A cell. Physiology and pathophysiology. N Engl J Med 304:1518, 1575, 1981

WHEAT LJ: Infection and diabetes mellitus. Diabetes Care 3:187, 1980

WINTER RJ: Profiles of metabolic control in diabetic children—frequency of asymptomatic nocturnal hypoglycemia. Metabolism 30:666, 1981

YOON J-W et al: Virus-induced diabetes mellitus. N Engl J Med 300:1173, 1979

Insulin resistance

BAR RS et al: Extreme insulin resistance in ataxia telangiectasia. Defect in affinity of insulin receptors. N Engl J Med 298:1164, 1978

DAVIDSON JK, DEBRA DW: Immunologic insulin resistance. Diabetes 27:307, 1978

EPSTEIN CJ et al: Werner's syndrome. A review of its symptomatology, natural history, pathologic features, genetics and relationship to the aging process. Medicine 45:177, 1966

FLIER JS et al: Receptors, antireceptor antibodies and mechanisms of insulin resistance. N Engl J Med 300:413, 1979

GOLDSTEIN JL, FIALKOW PJ: The Alström syndrome. Medicine 52:53, 1973

KAHN CR: Role of insulin receptors in insulin-resistant states. Metabolism 29:455, 1980

SEIP M: Generalized lipodystrophy. Ergeb Inn Med Kinderheilkd 31:59, 1971

SHIPP JC et al: Insulin resistance: Clinical features, natural course and effects of adrenal steroid treatment. Medicine 44:165, 1965

VAN OBBERGHEN-SCHILLING EG et al: Receptors for insulinlike growth factor I are defective in fibroblasts cultured from a patient with leprechaunism. J Clin Invest 68:1356, 1981

WEST RJ et al: Familial insulin resistant diabetes, multiple somatic anomalies and pineal hyperplasia. Arch Dis Child 50:703, 1975

115 LACTIC ACIDOSIS

DANIEL W. FOSTER

Lactic acidosis is a common problem. This follows from the fact that lactic acid is produced at accelerated rates in skeletal muscle and other tissues whenever oxygenation is inadequate to supply energy needs. Thus lactic acidosis represents a kind of final common pathway for any disease resulting in circulatory collapse or hypoxia. Lactic acidosis can also occur under circumstances in which tissue hypoxia is not apparent. In most cases an etiology can be established, but in some the lactic acidosis is "idiopathic."

BIOCHEMICAL BACKGROUND In the narrowest sense biological life can be defined as the capacity to generate high-energy phosphate bonds within the cell. Adenosine triphosphate (ATP) is the most important high-energy compound, but other nucleotides, such as guanosine triphosphate, also play important roles. Structure and function of every tissue in the body is directly or indirectly dependent on ATP or equivalent high-energy nucleotides. During tissue hypoxia ATP cannot be generated in adequate amounts, and lactic acidosis results. The acidosis is the metabolic consequence of activation of a back-up system for the generation of ATP when the primary energy-forming pathway is impaired. The normal mechanism of ATP generation under aerobic conditions is shown in Fig. 115-1. When substrates such as free fatty acids or glucose are oxidized to acetyl CoA, the constituent hydrogen atoms are transferred to nicotinamide adenine dinucleotide (NAD), producing the reduced form of the pyridine nucleotide (NADH). Oxidation of acetyl CoA to CO_2 in the Krebs cycle generates additional NADH. The bulk of NADH is formed intramitochondrially, where fatty acid oxidizing and tricarboxylic acid cycle enzymes are located; cytosolic NADH must be transported into the mitochondria by "shuttle" systems because NADH cannot directly penetrate the inner mitochondrial membrane. In the presence of oxygen, NADH is oxidized by the electron transport chain, the end product being water ("metabolic water"). For each mole of NADH passing through the cytochrome sequence 2 to 3 mol ATP is formed. When oxygen content of tissues is normal and ATP stores are high, rates of glycogen breakdown and glucose oxidation are low (the *Pasteur effect*). It is believed that control of glycolysis is primarily vested in the enzyme phosphofructokinase (PFK). As shown in Fig. 115-2, this enzyme catalyzes the conversion of fructose 6-phosphate to fructose 1,6-diphosphate. Its activity is accelerated under conditions of tissue hypoxia. Regulatory mechanisms for

FIGURE 115-1
Schematic view of aerobic metabolism. Subcellular compartments are not indicated. Glycolysis occurs in the cytosol while enzymes of fatty acid oxidation and the Krebs cycle are located intramitochondrially. The dotted line indicates that glycogenolysis and glycolysis are inactive in the presence of oxygen. (See text.)

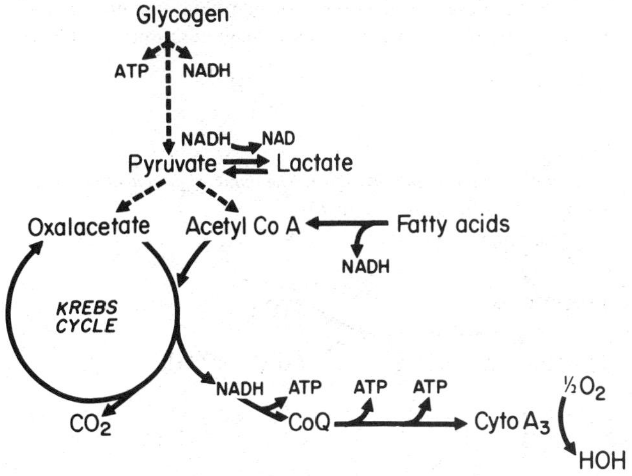

PFK are complicated and a number of allosteric modulators are known. ATP is likely the primary physiological inhibitor, while ADP, AMP, inorganic phosphate, and fructose 1,6-diphosphate all have activating capacity. Other modulators (e.g., citrate, creatine phosphate, NH_4^+, H^+, fructose diphosphatase) probably play secondary roles. In liver, fructose 2,6-diphosphate is the preeminent activator of PFK, its concentration changing reciprocally with glycolytic flux. While PFK in muscle is also activated by fructose 2,6-diphosphate, its role in accelerating glycolysis during the initiation of lactic acidosis has not yet been explored.

The sequence of events occurring during tissue hypoxia is schematically shown in Fig. 115-3. If blood flow to peripheral tissues is diminished such that oxygen delivery is insufficient to meet metabolic demands, electron flow through the transport chain is impaired or blocked (all cytochromes become reduced). Because of the block, NADH, which for a finite period continues to be generated, cannot be oxidized, resulting in high NADH/NAD ratios in both mitochondrial and cytosolic compartments. As a result all near-equilibrium reactions utilizing NADH as cofactor shift to the reduced side (e.g., oxaloacetate → malate, pyruvate → lactate), slowing substrate flux at a number of critical sites. In addition, ATP cannot be generated and tissue ATP concentrations fall. There is a reciprocal rise in ADP and AMP. As a result, phosphofructokinase is activated, with rapid glycogen breakdown and glucose oxidation. Accelerated glycolysis leads to overproduction of pyruvic acid, which, because of the elevated NADH content of the cell, is reduced to lactic acid. Put simply, the acidosis of tissue hypoxia is due to the conversion of neutral substrate, glycogen-glucose, to a strong acid, pyruvate. It is a lactic acidosis because the high NADH/NAD ratio drives the lactic dehydrogenase reaction to the right. These points are shown schematically in Fig. 115-4.

Lactate is produced in significant quantities even in the fully oxygenated subject by a variety of tissues. This lactate passes to the liver, where it enters the gluconeogenic pathway for conversion to glucose (*Cori cycle*). Since the intact organism can rapidly dispose of large lactate loads, impairment of lactate uptake by the liver may be critical for the development of lactic acidosis. Diminished lactate uptake undoubtedly plays a significant role in pathogenesis (especially in patients with vascular collapse, severe hepatocellular disease, or enzymic defects in the gluconeogenic pathway), but significant acidosis probably never occurs in the absence of peripheral overproduction. Whether lactate overproduction in lactic acidosis is generalized or limited to specific tissues such as muscle and intestine is not resolved.

The accelerated glycolysis of hypoxia, as noted above, serves as an alternative system for the generation of ATP when the normal mitochondrial mechanism is impaired. The glycolytic system is not efficient, however. A mole of glucose derived from glycogen and oxidized completely through the Krebs cycle generates about 37 mol ATP, while the yield from glycogen to pyruvate is only 3 mol. Nevertheless, over the short run, this ATP may be life-saving.

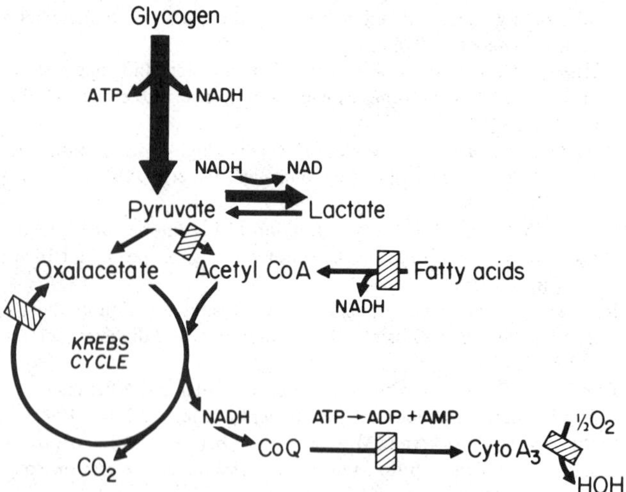

FIGURE 115-3
Schematic view of anaerobic metabolism. Diagonally striped boxes indicate metabolic blocks secondary to failure of delivery of oxygen to tissues and high NADH/NAD ratios. Heavy arrows indicate accelerated glycogenolysis, glycolysis, and lactate production. Glycolysis is permitted to continue in the face of high NADH/NAD ratios in the cytosol because one molecule of NAD (required in the glyceraldehyde 3-phosphate dehydrogenase reaction) is produced for each molecule of lactate formed.

CLINICAL PICTURE Lactic acidosis is usually heralded by the onset of nausea, vomiting, restlessness, and driven respiration of the Kussmaul type. Stupor or coma is sometimes seen. Huckabee, who in 1961 brought the problem of lactic acidosis to the attention of clinicians, recognized that there were two major groups of patients with elevated lactate concentrations in the blood. The first had proportionate increases of lactate and pyruvate and were not considered to be hypoxic. The second group had lactate levels disproportionately elevated when compared with the simultaneously measured pyruvate concentration. Huckabee coined the term "excess lactate" for any increase in lactate that could not be accounted for by a rise in pyruvate concentration and interpreted its presence to mean tissue hypoxia (a high NADH/NAD ratio). The relationship of the lactate/pyruvate concentration to the NADH/NAD ratio is obvious when the lactate dehydrogenase reaction is rearranged:

FIGURE 115-2
Phosphofructokinase and glycolysis. The minus sign indicates inhibition; the plus sign, activation. (See text.)

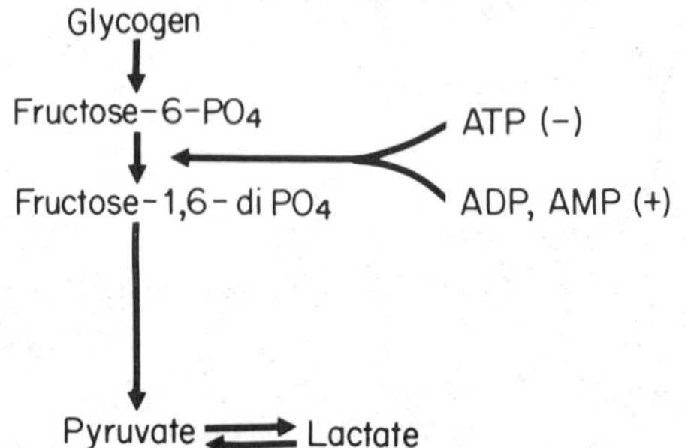

FIGURE 115-4
Summary of biochemical mechanisms in lactic acidosis.

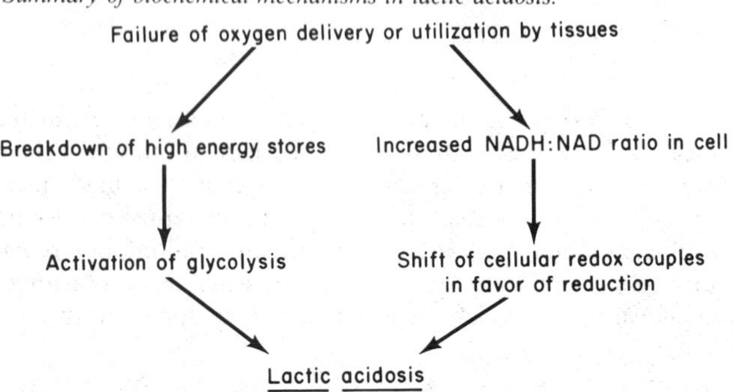

$$\text{Pyruvate} + \text{NADH} + \text{H}^+ \rightleftharpoons \text{lactate} + \text{NAD}^+ \quad (1)$$

$$K \times \frac{[\text{NADH}][\text{H}^+]}{[\text{NAD}^+]} = \frac{[\text{lactate}]}{[\text{pyruvate}]} \quad (2)$$

A sample calculation of "excess lactate" is given in Fig. 115-5.

The mean level of lactate in venous blood normally is about 1 m*M* (range 0.6 to 1.5 m*M*), while the pyruvate concentration is about 0.1 m*M* (range 0.05 to 0.15 m*M*).[1] Accurately determined lactate/pyruvate ratios above 10 to 15 usually mean some degree of hypoxia. In practice pyruvate measurements are often not done because instability and low concentrations make assays difficult. As a consequence, excess lactate is now rarely quantitated. The concept was seminal, however, in providing the insight that led to understanding of the pathophysiology of lactic acidosis.

Cohen and Woods have suggested a classification of lactic acidosis based on clinical findings rather than the lactate/pyruvate ratio (Table 115-1). Type A lactic acidosis is associated with poor tissue perfusion or oxygenation. Most patients with lactic acidosis fall into this category. Vascular collapse is the most common cause, and any condition leading to shock (e.g., myocardial infarction, pulmonary embolism, hemorrhage, septicemia, poisoning) can produce the illness. Hypoxia does not have to be present. Importantly, diminished tissue perfusion may occur in the absence of a measurable fall in the blood pressure. Lactic acidosis occurs physiologically whenever muscular exercise is sufficient to contract an oxygen debt. The pathologic counterpart is lactic acidosis produced by convulsions or hypothermia with prolonged shivering. All type A patients have "excess lactate" in the Huckabee terminology.

Type B patients have elevated blood lactate concentrations without evidence of diminished tissue perfusion. Acidosis may be absent, mild, or severe. Proportionate elevations of pyruvate and lactate may be seen, but high lactate/pyruvate ratios are present when acidosis is severe. Systemic clinical disorders associated with elevations of blood lactate include uncontrolled diabetes mellitus, severe liver disease, leukemia, thiamine deficiency, and metabolic or respiratory alkalosis. Lactic acidosis has been commonly reported with biguanide therapy of diabetes, and because of this, phenformin was removed from clinical use in the United States by the Food and Drug Administration. The syndrome has also been seen with nitroprusside therapy of hypertension, with epinephrine overdosage and in isolated instances with other drug intoxications. Most of the latter are doubtless associated with hypoxia or shock and rightfully belong in the type A category. Ethanol is often listed as a cause of lactic acidosis but in fact rarely induces the syndrome. The oxidation of ethanol by the liver results in the generation of high NADH/NAD ratios in the cell and presumably blocks the recycling of lactate (and alanine) to glucose. Infants with enzyme defects in the glycolytic-gluconeogenic-tricarboxylic acid pathway appear to be peculiarly vulnerable to lactic acidosis, and early death is common. Chronic lactic acidosis also occurs in certain primary myopathies of unknown etiology. If no primary cause can be found, a diagnosis of idiopathic lactic acidosis has to be made.

The pathophysiology of lactate accumulation in type B disease is varied and often incompletely understood. The enzyme defects and alcohol may have diminished hepatic uptake of lactate as a primary mechanism. In other cases, particularly those labeled idiopathic and those with myopathy, subtle mitochondrial disease resulting in functional tissue hypoxia is likely operative. Drugs may also act by the latter mechanism. Hormones such as glucagon and epinephrine raise lactate by stimulating glycolysis. Leukemia probably acts both by direct overproduction of lactate in the white cell mass and through increased blood viscosity that diminishes capillary perfusion. It is likely that most chronic type B conditions cause only mild to moderate hyperlactatemia in themselves and that an additional insult is required for acidosis to develop. The latter might include infection, dehydration, volume depletion, starvation, or unusual exertion. The effect of such an insult would be to add a mild inadequacy of tissue perfusion (insufficient to qualify as type A disease) to the primary abnormality and in combination to cause frank acidosis.

[1] *Measurement of lactate and pyruvate requires precautions. The sample should be iced, and red blood cells (which produce lactate) should be separated immediately.*

FIGURE 115-5

The concept of excess lactate. The symbols L_t and P_t indicate plasma concentrations of lactate and pyruvate, respectively, in the patient. L_n and P_n refer to mean values in normal subjects.

$$XL = (L_t - L_n) - (P_t - P_n) \cdot \frac{Ln}{Pn}$$

	Pyruvate	Lactate
Normal	0.1 mM	1.0 mM
Patient	0.3 mM	11.0 mM

$$XL = (11-1) - (0.3-0.1)\,\frac{1.0}{0.1} = 8\text{mM}$$

DIAGNOSIS The diagnosis of lactic acidosis requires that a significant metabolic acidosis be present and that the measured lactate concentration be sufficient to account for the bulk of the decrease in plasma bicarbonate content. In general the arterial pH is less than 7.2, and the plasma lactate concentration is greater than 12 m*M*. Unfortunately, in many case reports of "lactic acidosis," plasma lactate concentrations are only modestly elevated (3 to 6 m*M*), and pH values are near normal. There are many causes of elevated plasma lactate levels, but

TABLE 115-1

Some causes of hyperlactatemia

A Hyperlactatemia with hypoxia
- *1* Strenuous muscle exercise (convulsions, hypothermia)
- *2* Inadequate tissue perfusion or oxygenation of any cause*

B Hyperlactatemia without apparent hypoxia
- *1* Systemic clinical disorders
  - *a* Alkalosis (respiratory or metabolic)
  - *b* Uncontrolled diabetes mellitus
  - *c* Leukemia, lymphoma, other cancers
  - *d* Severe liver disease
  - *e* Thiamine deficiency
- *2* Drugs, hormones, toxins
  - *a* Phenformin and other biguanides
  - *b* Salicylates
  - *c* Sodium nitroprusside
  - *d* Ethanol
  - *e* Epinephrine, glucagon
  - *f* Fructose, sorbitol
- *3* Enzyme defects
  - *a* Glucose 6-phosphatase
  - *b* Fructose 1,6-diphosphatase
  - *c* Pyruvate carboxylase
  - *d* Pyruvate dehydrogenase
  - *e* Unclassified tricarboxylic acid defect
- *4* Certain primary myopathies
- *5* Idiopathic

* *The most common causes of perfusion-oxygenation defects are myocardial infarction, sepsis, hemorrhage, volume depletion, pulmonary embolism, and heart failure. Hypoxia due to severe pulmonary disease, chronic anemia, carbon monoxide inhalation, and cyanide poisoning are much less frequent.*

SOURCE: *After Cohen and Woods.*

the term *lactic acidosis* should be reserved for situations in which acidosis actually exists. Confusion also occurs when severe acidosis is present but lactate concentrations do not account for the decrement of bicarbonate (i.e., a mixed acidosis is present). In diabetic ketoacidosis, for example, lactate concentrations of 3 to 6 m*M* are frequently seen, but acetoacetate and β-hydroxybutyrate are primarily responsible for the low pH.

Lactic acidosis should be suspected whenever a metabolic acidosis is associated with an "anion gap" in the absence of an explanation for the unmeasured anions. The anion gap can be calculated in several ways, the simplest of which is $[Na^+] - ([Cl^-] + [HCO_3^-])$. The normal range is 8 to 16 m*M* per liter, with the mean about 12. The four most common causes of metabolic acidosis with anion gap are diabetic or alcoholic ketoacidosis, uremic acidosis, lactic acidosis, and acidosis associated with toxin ingestion (salicylates, methanol, ethylene glycol, paraldehyde). Thus if ketoacidosis and uremia are not present and there is nothing to suggest a poisoning, the chances are good that a metabolic acidosis with significant anion gap is due to lactic acid.

TREATMENT If lactic acidosis is caused by shock or hypoxia, reversal of the primary condition cures the secondary acidosis. Persistent acidosis requires that large amounts of sodium bicarbonate be infused intravenously. Bicarbonate should be given in quantities sufficient to raise the pH to about 7.2. This often necessitates the rapid infusion of several hundred to a thousand millimoles over only a few hours. Full restoration of pH is not desirable since a rebound alkalosis will occur when production of lactic acid ceases and circulating lactate is metabolized to bicarbonate. In view of the large quantities required, straight bicarbonate infusions should be used. A near isotonic solution can be prepared by adding three 50-ml vials of bicarbonate (1 mmol/ml) to 850 ml sterile distilled water. Hypertonic (5%) solutions are also commercially available and may be required in certain cases.

Because large volumes of bicarbonate are required in the treatment of lactic acidosis, the problem of fluid overload often arises, especially in elderly patients and subjects with impaired renal function. Diuretics should be routinely given with vigorous alkali therapy after it is clear that any volume deficits have been repaired. Occasionally peritoneal dialysis or hemodialysis with hypertonic solutions may be required to prevent pulmonary edema. Dialysis is not indicated as a treatment of lactic acidosis per se.

Other forms of therapy such as the administration of glucose and insulin or redox dyes have been tried but are of little use. An experimental drug, dichloroacetate, appears to be helpful in some nonhypoxic forms of lactic acidosis in animals. Dichloroacetate causes polyneuropathy, testicular damage, irreversible cataracts, and disturbances of oxalate metabolism when given chronically, probably precluding its use even in acute cases in humans. Another drug, 2-chloropropionate, appears to have similar actions to dichloroacetate but less toxicity. Both act to increase pyruvate dehydrogenase activity and presumably lower lactate by increasing pyruvate oxidation. They do not work in type A lactic acidosis due to hypoxia. Their clinical effectiveness in type B disease has not been adequately tested.

REFERENCES

Cohen RD, Woods HF: *Clinical and Biochemical Aspects of Lactic Acidosis.* Oxford, Blackwell, 1976

Gabow PA et al: Diagnostic importance of an increased anion gap. N Engl J Med 303:854, 1980

Huckabee WE: Abnormal resting blood lactate. Am J Med 30:833, 840, 1961

Kreisberg RA: Lactate homeostasis and lactic acidosis. Ann Intern Med 92:227, 1980

Park R, Arieff AI: Lactic acidosis. Adv Int Med 25:33, 1980

Woods HF et al: The role of altered lactate kinetics in the pathogenesis of type B lactic acidosis, in *Metabolic Acidosis, Ciba Foundation Symposium 87.* London, Putnam, 1982

116 HYPOGLYCEMIA, INSULINOMA, AND OTHER HORMONE-SECRETING TUMORS OF THE PANCREAS

DANIEL W. FOSTER
ARTHUR H. RUBENSTEIN

Maintenance of the plasma glucose concentration within relatively narrow bounds is a fundamental characteristic of the intact organism. Hypoglycemia represents a high-risk metabolic abnormality (in the short run a greater danger than hyperglycemia) because glucose is the primary energy substrate of the brain. Its absence, like that of oxygen, produces deranged function, tissue damage, or even death if the deficit is prolonged. The peculiar vulnerability of the brain to hypoglycemia is due to the fact that it cannot utilize circulating free fatty acids as an energy source in contrast to almost every other tissue of the body. Short-chain derivatives of the free fatty acids, acetoacetic and β-hydroxybutyric acids (the "ketone bodies"), are efficiently oxidized and can protect the central nervous system from damage by hypoglycemia when present at moderate concentrations in plasma. However, development of ketosis requires a number of hours in humans. Accelerated ketogenesis is not, therefore, an effective protective mechanism against hypoglycemia occurring acutely over minutes or even several hours. Preservation of central nervous system function in the early phases of fasting or during hypoglycemia thus requires a prompt increase in the production of glucose by the liver. At the same time glucose utilization in other tissues must be diminished by provision of free fatty acids as alternative substrate. These adaptive mechanisms (Chap. 89) are hormonally controlled and, under ordinary circumstances, are extremely effective. Occasionally, however, the system breaks down or is overwhelmed, resulting in the clinical syndrome of hypoglycemia. In the past, hypoglycemia (apart from insulin reactions in the diabetic) was not a common problem in the practice of medicine. In recent years, however, the diagnosis of postprandial hypoglycemia has been made with great frequency, making it necessary for physicians to be familiar with hypoglycemic syndromes and their differential diagnosis.

SYMPTOMATOLOGY OF HYPOGLYCEMIA Symptoms of hypoglycemia fall into two main categories: those induced by an *excessive secretion of epinephrine* and those due to *dysfunction of the central nervous system.* When plasma glucose concentrations approach the hypoglycemic range, "counterregulatory" hormones are released which cause glycogen breakdown, initiate gluconeogenesis, mobilize free fatty acids, and induce ketogenesis. The four hormones involved are epinephrine, glucagon, cortisol, and growth hormone. It seems probable that only epinephrine produces recognizable symptoms. Rapid epinephrine release causes sweating, tremor, tachycardia, anxiety, and hunger. Central nervous system symptoms include dizziness, headache, clouding of vision, blunted mental acuity, confusion, abnormal behavior, convulsions, and loss of consciousness. When the onset of hypoglycemia is gradual, as in most forms of organic disease, central nervous system symptoms predominate, and the epinephrine phase may not be recognizable. With more rapid drops in plasma glucose (as in insulin reactions), adrenergic symptoms are the prominent complaint. In the diabetic adrenergic symptoms may not be manifest if severe neuropathy is present.

CLASSIFICATION It has been traditional to classify hypoglycemia as either *postprandial* (reactive) or *fasting*. Pathologically low plasma glucose concentrations occur in the former only in response to meals, while in the latter fasting for a few to many hours is necessary to demonstrate the abnormality. Patients with fasting hypoglycemia (particularly insulinomas) may rarely exhibit a reactive component, but reactive patients do not have symptoms when food is withdrawn. Fasting hypoglycemia usually means that an identifiable disease process is associated with the lowered plasma glucose, but symptoms suggestive of postprandial hypoglycemia are often found in the absence of recognizable disease.

CAUSES OF HYPOGLYCEMIA **Postprandial hypoglycemia** Some causes of postprandial hypoglycemia are shown in Table 116-1. The most common category is alimentary. Patients who have undergone gastrectomy, gastrojejunostomy, pyloroplasty, or vagotomy are subject to hypoglycemia following meals, presumably because of rapid gastric emptying with brisk absorption of glucose and excessive insulin release. Glucose concentrations fall more rapidly than insulin under these circumstances, and the resulting insulin-glucose imbalance leads to hypoglycemia. True alimentary hypoglycemia may apparently occur in the absence of gastrointestinal surgery, but this is rare. Ingestion of fructose or galactose induces hypoglycemia in children with fructose intolerance (Chap. 102) and galactosemia (Chap. 101), respectively. Leucine intake has been reported to cause the syndrome in susceptible infants in the absence of insulinoma, but the phenomenon is extremely rare. Diabetes mellitus in its early phase is almost always listed as a cause of reactive hypoglycemia. In our experience symptomatic hypoglycemia as a premonitory symptom of diabetes is uncommon if it occurs at all. Prediabetics, who by definition have normal glucose tolerance, may have a late fall in plasma glucose after oral glucose tolerance testing, but this does not mean hypoglycemia. In fact, this pattern is similar to that frequently present in asymptomatic, healthy individuals (see below).

The fifth cause, idiopathic, has in the past been broken down into two categories, *true hypoglycemia* and *nonhypoglycemia.* The former represents a condition in which adrenergic symptoms appear postprandially and are accompanied by a measurably low plasma glucose at the time the symptoms appear spontaneously during everyday life. Such patients are extraordinarily rare. The mechanism is unknown, although subtle (nonanatomic) dysfunction of the gastrointestinal tract might be operative. *Nonhypoglycemia* is a term coined to describe a large number of patients who reproducibly develop adrenergic symptoms suggestive of hypoglycemia 2 to 5 h after a meal but who do not have measurably low plasma glucose concentrations when symptoms appear spontaneously in everyday life. The condition is often self-diagnosed by those who have read the extensive lay-oriented literature that describes hypoglycemia as a common cause of ill health (as well as a cause of some of the corporate ills of society). Further, in almost every community there are physicians who specialize in "hypoglycemia" and make the diagnosis frequently. The diagnosis is usually made by doing a 5-h glucose tolerance test and demonstrating a lower than "normal" plasma glucose between 2 and 5 h.

Two questions have to be asked about nonhypoglycemia. First, what are the symptoms (which may be incapacitating) due to? Second, is there any validity to a diagnosis of hypoglycemia made by glucose tolerance test? The symptoms of nervousness, weakness, tremor, tachycardia, dizziness, and sweating reported by these patients are probably due to epinephrine release. Many otherwise normal persons have experienced such symptoms at sometime in their lives and may even have gained relief by eating. Patients with nonhypoglycemia, on the other hand, develop the symptoms regularly and repetitively. In one study 80 consecutive subjects with reproducible postprandial symptoms by history were studied by 5-h glucose tolerance testing. Hypoglycemia was considered to be present if (1) the plasma glucose fell below 60 mg/dl during the test, (2) symptoms or signs compatible with hypoglycemia were present, and (3) at least a doubling of plasma cortisol occurred 39 to 90 min after the nadir of plasma glucose (suggesting hypoglycemia sufficient to activate the hypothalamic-pituitary-adrenal axis). Only 18 of the 80 (23 percent) who by history were candidates for postprandial hypoglycemia fulfilled these criteria. Twenty-five percent of asymptomatic matched normal controls also met all three criteria. When the patients and controls were tested after a mixed meal, no subject in either group had a plasma glucose below 60 mg/dl, yet 14 of the 18 patients (78 percent) had symptoms typical of those occurring spontaneously and after glucose tolerance testing. Thus, the syndrome termed *nonhypoglycemia* has been correctly named since the symptoms occur in the absence of chemical hypoglycemia after mixed meals. Most of these patients doubtless have stress and/or anxiety as the primary disorder, and epinephrine is released in consequence thereof. However, it is conceivable that some persons discharge epinephrine abnormally in response to meals to account for the syndrome. Sucrose or glucose overfeeding can cause stimulation of the sympathetic nervous system, but in normal subjects it is norepinephrine and not epinephrine that is released. The possibility that these patients might release epinephrine as well has not been tested. For the present it is suggested that the terms *idiopathic postabsorptive hypoglycemia* and *nonhypoglycemia* be abandoned and the designation *idiopathic postprandial syndrome* be substituted to avoid confusion with true hypoglycemic disorders.

TABLE 116-1
Causes of postprandial (reactive) hypoglycemia

I Alimentary hyperinsulinism
II Hereditary fructose intolerance
III Galactosemia
IV Leucine sensitivity
V Idiopathic

Fasting hypoglycemia The causes of fasting hypoglycemia are many, but in all instances there is an imbalance between the production of glucose by the liver and its utilization in peripheral tissues. In some, hypoglycemia appears to be due primarily to a defect in glucose production ("supply-side" hypoglycemia), while in others the problem is due to excess glucose utilization ("demand-side" hypoglycemia). Clinically the two forms can be distinguished by the amount of glucose required to prevent hypoglycemia during a 24-h period. If more than 200 g, it can be assumed that overutilization is present. This follows from the fact that hepatic glucose output in normal fasting humans is between 100 and 200 g per day and is sufficient to prevent hypoglycemia in the absence of food.[1] The demonstration of overutilization is important since it narrows the diagnostic possibilities. The diseases that can cause accelerated glucose utilization usually also have an element of underproduction (relative or absolute), and in some cases the latter may predominate. Mechanisms by which the hepatic response to increased glucose demand is impaired in conditions of glucose overutilization are probably multiple, but persistent release of insulin or insulin-like growth factors sufficient to blunt the effect of glucagon in the liver is likely of key importance. Other factors include inadequate release of amino acids from muscle (substrate for gluconeogenesis) and/or impairment of fatty acid delivery or oxidation (necessary for maximal rates of gluconeogenesis).

To summarize, if glucose demand is more than 200 g per day, increased glucose flux into peripheral tissues is present. If less than 200 g per day prevents hypoglycemia, no diagnostic implications can be drawn. A classification of fasting hypoglycemia based on underproduction or overutilization of glucose is given in Table 116-2. Hypoglycemia occurs in other conditions in isolated fashion. Only the major types of defects are listed here.

UNDERPRODUCTION OF GLUCOSE As discussed in Chap. 89, the production of glucose by the liver initially involves the breakdown of stored glycogen and subsequently depends on gluconeogenesis, the synthesis of glucose from precursors delivered to the liver from peripheral tissues. The causes of inadequate production of glucose during fasting can be grouped into five general categories: (1) hormone deficiencies, (2) specific defects in glycogenolytic or gluconeogenic enzymes, (3) inadequate substrate delivery, (4) acquired liver disease, and (5) drugs. Hypopituitarism and adrenal insufficiency are the most common of the hormone deficiency states causing hypoglycemia. Defects in catecholamine or glucagon release are rare. Enzymic abnormalities causing hypoglycemia are generally seen in children and not adults. Glucose 6-phosphatase deficiency is the classic example of a defect in glycogen breakdown, but hypoglycemia may occur in young children with deficiencies of hepatic glycogen phosphorylase and in other forms of glycogen storage disease (Chap. 100). The inability to make glycogen because of inadequate glycogen synthetase activity also renders the infant susceptible to fasting hypoglycemia. In addition to glucose 6-phosphatase, three other enzymes are specifically involved in gluconeogenesis: pyruvate carboxylase, phosphoenolpyruvate carboxykinase, and fructose 1,6-diphosphatase (Fig. 116-1). Hypoglycemia has been reported in association with decreased activities of each of these enzymes, often in association with lactic acidosis. Substrate deficiency appears to be one of the mechanisms operative in ketotic hypoglycemia of infancy, since alanine turnover in such patients is low. Inadequate substrate supply may also contribute to the rare instances of hypoglycemia in malnutrition, muscle-wasting states, chronic renal failure, and late pregnancy. Acquired liver disease can cause serious glucopenia. Hepatic congestion due to right-sided heart failure appears to be particularly troublesome, but severe viral hepatitis or cirrhosis may also cause symptomatic hypoglycemia.

[1] *Much more than 200 g glucose can be disposed of by normal humans without developing hyperglycemia. Therefore, the rule is valid only if large quantities of glucose are required to avoid hypoglycemia, i.e., if plasma glucose falls below fasting levels and continues at a low concentration despite the infusion of 200 g glucose per day.*

TABLE 116-2
Major causes of fasting hypoglycemia

I Conditions primarily due to underproduction of glucose
- *A* Hormone deficiencies
  - *1* Hypopituitarism
  - *2* Adrenal insufficiency
  - *3* Catecholamine deficiency
  - *4* Glucagon deficiency
- *B* Enzyme defects
  - *1* Glucose 6-phosphatase
  - *2* Liver phosphorylase
  - *3* Pyruvate carboxylase
  - *4* Phosphoenolpyruvate carboxykinase
  - *5* Fructose 1,6-diphosphatase
  - *6* Glycogen synthetase
- *C* Substrate deficiency
  - *1* Ketotic hypoglycemia of infancy
  - *2* Severe malnutrition, muscle wasting(?)
  - *3* Late pregnancy(?)
- *D* Acquired liver disease
  - *1* Hepatic congestion
  - *2* Severe hepatitis
  - *3* Cirrhosis
- *E* Drugs
  - *1* Alcohol
  - *2* Propranolol
  - *3* Salicylates

II Conditions primarily due to overutilization of glucose
- *A* Hyperinsulinism
  - *1* Insulinoma
  - *2* Exogenous insulin
  - *3* Sulfonylureas
  - *4* Immune disease with insulin antibodies
- *B* Appropriate insulin levels
  - *1* Extrapancreatic tumors
  - *2* Systemic carnitine deficiency
  - *3* Cachexia with fat depletion

A number of drugs cause hypoglycemia. By far the most common, apart from insulin and sulfonylureas, is alcohol. Alcohol only induces hypoglycemia after a period of fasting sufficient to deplete liver glycogen stores. In this circumstance hepatic glucose production is dependent on gluconeogenesis. The oxidation of ethanol in the liver is accompanied by generation of high concentrations of NADH in the cytosol of the cell. The increased NADH/NAD ratio diverts oxaloacetate into malate formation, diminishing its availability to the gluconeogenic sequence via the action of phosphoenolpyruvate carboxykinase

FIGURE 116-1
Simplified scheme of hepatic carbohydrate metabolism. Only the sequence for gluconeogenesis, glycogen synthesis, and glycogenolysis is shown.

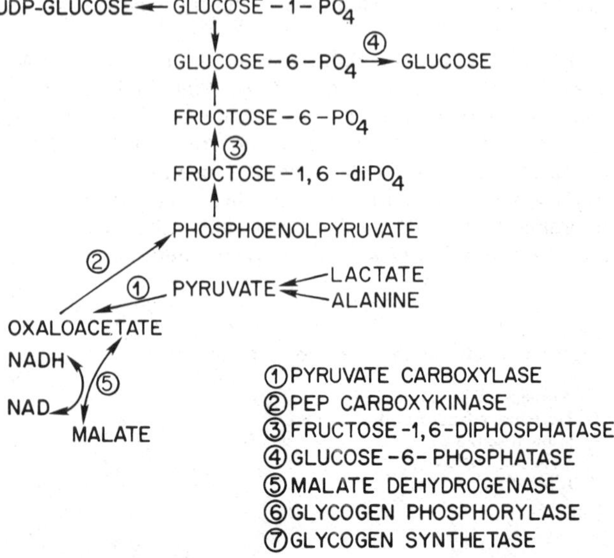

(Fig. 116-1). The normal pathway of gluconeogenesis from pyruvate is thus blocked, leading to a drop in hepatic glucose output and hypoglycemia. Large amounts of ethanol are not required to produce this syndrome, and plasma alcohol concentrations may be as low as 25 mg/dl at the time symptoms occur. Ethanol-induced hypoglycemia usually occurs in adults but is also seen in children who drink alcohol unknowingly. Salicylates (in children) and propranolol are the next most frequently involved drugs. Propranolol presumably causes difficulty in fasting patients or insulin-requiring diabetics by impairing the glycogenolytic response. In diabetes the drug may also prevent recognition of impending hypoglycemia by blunting the symptomatic response to epinephrine release. Other drugs have been reported to cause hypoglycemia in isolated cases, but the relationship is often unproved.

OVERUTILIZATION OF GLUCOSE Overutilization of glucose occurs in two settings. In the first, hyperinsulinism is present, while in the second plasma insulin concentrations are low. There are basically four causes of hyperinsulinemic hypoglycemia: insulinoma, exogenous insulin administration, sulfonylureas, and a peculiar form of insulin autoimmunity. Hypoglycemia in a diabetic taking prescribed insulin or oral agents is not a diagnostic problem. The difficulty comes when a patient induces hypoglycemia deliberately and surreptitiously for psychiatric reasons, raising the possibility of an insulin-producing tumor. The differential diagnosis between insulinoma and factitious hypoglycemia is considered below. Rarely hypoglycemia with hyperinsulinism occurs in autoimmune disease with antibodies to endogenous insulin. Mechanisms are not well understood, although dissociation of free insulin from hormone-antibody complexes at inappropriate times may play a role. By binding insulin, antibodies may also induce insulin release from the beta cell.

Hypoglycemia in the context of glucose overutilization and appropriately low plasma insulin concentrations occurs in two situations. The first is in association with solid extrapancreatic tumors, usually of large size. The most common are of mesothelial origin and include a variety of fibromas and sarcomas. The syndrome can also be seen with hepatomas, carcinomas of the gastrointestinal tract, and adrenal cancers. The mechanism of the hypoglycemia is not clear, although high levels of insulin-like growth factors ("nonsuppressible insulin-like activity") may play a role in some.

Symptomatic hypoglycemia due to overutilization may also occur in situations where free fatty acids are not available for oxidation in muscle and other tissues. A majority of patients with *systemic carnitine deficiency* have hypoglycemia, often very severe. In this condition carnitine, which is necessary to transport fatty acids into mitochondria for oxidation, is low in plasma, muscle, liver, and other tissues. As a consequence, peripheral tissues cannot utilize fatty acids for energy production, and the liver cannot make ketone bodies as alternative substrate. The result is that all tissues become glucose-dependent, exceeding the capacity of the liver to meet the demand. Other features of sytemic carnitine deficiency include nausea, vomiting, hyperammonemia, and hepatic encephalopathy. The illness thus constitutes one form of Reye's syndrome. (In *myopathic carnitine deficiency* only muscle is involved, and a polymyositis-like syndrome without hypoglycemia is produced.) Hypoglycemia is rarely seen with deficiency of *carnitine palmitoyltransferase,* the enzyme that transesterifies fatty acyl CoA to carnitine for oxidation. Presumably the defect is not complete in most patients, allowing some fatty acid oxidation to occur so that the tendency to hypoglycemia is minimized. The clinical picture is that of an exercise-induced myopathy with myoglobinuria. The authors have also seen several cases of hypoglycemia in patients with cachexia due to advanced cancer. At autopsy no recognizable triglyceride stores were present in

adipose tissue, suggesting free fatty acid deficiency as the primary mechanism.

DIAGNOSIS Fasting hypoglycemia If a nondiabetic presents with symptoms suggestive of hypoglycemia—particularly if confusion, loss of consciousness, or convulsions are present—the most important rule is to draw blood for simultaneous determinations of plasma glucose and insulin before intravenous glucose is administered, since the critical diagnostic issue will be the presence or absence of hyperinsulinism. Plasma cortisol should be determined at the same time. Once the patient has become alert, it is important to take a detailed history and carry out a thorough physical examination. Special emphasis should be placed on food intake in the preceding 24 h and the possibility of drug ingestion. Signs of heart failure and hepatic congestion should be sought, and the presence and thickness of the adipose tissue mass should be noted. Pigmentation of the skin may suggest Addison's disease. Workup includes liver function studies and CT scanning or abdominal sonography (to look for solid tumors in the retroperitoneal space or abdominal cavity). Patients with enzyme defects and rare hormonal deficiencies (epinephrine, glucagon) usually require evaluation in referral centers, since definitive assays for these hormones and enzymes are not routinely available. For reasons cited above it is important to quantitate the amount of glucose required to prevent recurrent hypoglycemia during acute phase therapy.

If the patient has a history compatible with hypoglycemia but does not have symptoms at the time of examination, hospitalization for fasting is generally required. The fast should be carried out for at least 72 h unless symptoms develop. Plasma glucose, insulin, and cortisol should be measured every 6 h. Occasionally quantitation of plasma free fatty acids, glucagon, and total ketones is helpful. Two points are at issue. First, does the patient have fasting hypoglycemia? And second, is the hypoglycemia associated with hyperinsulinism? Neither question is easy to answer. There is no definitive lower limit of plasma glucose that unequivocally defines pathologic hypoglycemia. The mean minimal level of glucose attained during a 72-h fast in one study is shown in Table 116-3. It is clear that women develop lower levels than men. Another series reported mean minimal levels of 62 mg/dl in men and 52 mg/dl in women during a 72-h fast. However, values as low as 22 mg/dl have been found in normal women without symptoms. On balance, a presumptive diagnosis of hypoglycemia is probably justified if the plasma glucose falls below 50 mg/dl in men and 40 mg/dl in women at any time during the fast, provided typical symptoms are induced. If symptoms are not produced, the diagnosis should be made with caution.

In interpreting plasma insulin concentrations it is important to remember that absolute values are not very helpful. In normal subjects when glucose concentrations rise, insulin levels also increase and when plasma glucose concentrations fall, insulin release is inhibited. This means that plasma insulin concentrations must be interpreted in the light of the simultaneously determined glucose value. Thus, a "normal" absolute insulin level may be abnormal in the face of hypoglycemia, while high absolute levels may be appropriate if the glucose concentration is elevated. In an attempt to relate the two parameters the concept of the insulin/glucose ratio

$$\frac{\text{Plasma insulin } (\mu\text{U/ml})}{\text{Plasma glucose (mg/dl)}}$$

was developed. In normal persons the ratio is always less than

0.4, while most (but not all) patients with insulinoma have ratios greater than 0.4—often above 1.0. Patients with insulinoma may secrete insulin episodically; the ratio may, therefore, be normal on one occasion and abnormal on another. Multiple sampling is required. A helpful observation is that the insulin/glucose ratio tends to fall during fasting in normal individuals but increases in patients with insulinoma.

Pancreatic insulin release ceases in in vitro studies when the glucose concentration is decreased much below 90 mg/dl, and it is likely that the same holds in vivo. Adam, King, and Schwartz infused glucose at different rates into normal subjects and measured the plasma insulin concentration when a steady state had been reached. Using their data, a plot of the plasma insulin versus the plasma glucose concentration gives a straight line with the relationship expressed by the following equation:

$$y = 0.41x - 34$$

where y is the plasma insulin in microunits per milliliter and x is the plasma glucose in milligrams per deciliter. The intercept on the x axis is 83 mg/dl, indicating that plasma insulin concentration should be functionally zero (background for the assay) at this level of plasma glucose. While other studies have shown lower cutoff points, it is probable that any significant insulin concentration (> 5 to 6 μU/ml) should be considered suspicious if the plasma glucose is below 50 mg/dl in men or 40 mg/dl in women, regardless of the value of the insulin/glucose ratio. This conclusion was also reached in a study of 60 patients with insulinoma at the Mayo Clinic. If hyperinsulinism is not demonstrated, one of the other causes of fasting hypoglycemia must be sought.

Should hypoglycemia not develop during fasting, an insulinoma or other hypoglycemia-producing organic disease is unlikely, although one insulinoma responsive only to glucose loading has been reported. Some authors recommend provocative tests with tolubutamide, glucagon, or leucine in suspected islet cell tumors, but overlap between normals and patients with insulinoma is so great as to render the tests of little value in a given individual.

Postprandial hypoglycemia In patients presumed to have postprandial hypoglycemia the most widely used test has been a 5-h oral glucose tolerance examination. Since normal persons may have chemical hypoglycemia without symptoms in the glucose tolerance test while subjects with idiopathic postprandial syndrome have symptoms in the absence of hypoglycemia following meal testing, the 5-h glucose tolerance test should be abandoned as a tool for diagnosis. The only unequivocal diagnostic test for true idiopathic postprandial hypoglycemia is the demonstration of a low plasma glucose concentration (less than 50 mg/dl) during spontaneously developed symptoms. Patients with idiopathic postprandial syndrome (anxiety) usually have slightly elevated glucose concentrations during spontaneous attacks because of the hyperglycemic actions of epinephrine and cortisol, the stress hormones that induce the symptoms.

TABLE 116-4
Differential diagnosis of insulinoma and factitious hyperinsulinism

Test	*Insulinoma*	*Exogenous insulin*	*Sulfonylurea*
Plasma insulin	High	Very high*	High
Insulin/glucose ratio	High	Very high	High
Proinsulin	Increased	Normal or low	Normal
C peptide	Increased	Normal or low†	Increased
Insulin antibodies	Absent	± Present‡	Absent
Plasma or urine sulfonylurea	Absent	Absent	Present

* *Total plasma insulin in patients with insulinoma is rarely above 200 μU/ml in the basal state and often much lower. Values greater than 1000 μU/ml are highly suggestive of exogenous insulin injection.*

† *C peptide may be normal in absolute terms, but low in relation to the increased insulin value.*

‡ *Insulin antibodies may not be present if only a few injections have been given, especially with purified insulins.*

Insulinoma versus factitious hypoglycemia The self-induction of hypoglycemia by the injection of insulin or the ingestion of sulfonylureas is so common as to equal or exceed the incidence of insulinoma. The demonstration of hyperinsulinism during hypoglycemia cannot, therefore, be taken as definitive evidence of the presence of an islet-cell tumor. Factitious disease should always be suspected when hypoglycemic symptoms appear in medical personnel or families of diabetics. Several additional tests are helpful in making this distinction once hyperinsulinism has been diagnosed. Patients with insulinoma tend to have high concentrations of proinsulin in plasma (> 20 percent of total insulin). Plasma proinsulin is not elevated by the administration of commercial insulin preparations or sulfonylureas. Measurement of the insulin connecting peptide (C peptide) will indicate whether the insulin circulating in plasma is of endogenous or exogenous origin. When insulin is cleaved from its precursor proinsulin molecule, C peptide is released into the portal vein in a 1:1 ratio with insulin. Thus, patients with insulinoma should have high C-peptide concentrations which parallel the plasma insulin values. The characteristic pattern in factitious hypoglycemia due to insulin injection would be a high circulating level of insulin with relatively suppressed C-peptide values. Exogenous insulin suppresses endogenous insulin release, both directly and by inducing hypoglycemia. Animal and human insulins can be distinguished by specific antibodies, but the differentiating immunoassays are not routinely available. Antibodies to insulin are helpful if present since they usually indicate chronic insulin injection. Unfortunately sulfonylureas also elevate both the C-peptide and insulin concentrations in plasma. Therefore, factitious hypoglycemia due to oral agents can only be diagnosed by a high index of suspicion coupled with assay of the drug in plasma or urine.

TABLE 116-3
Plasma glucose and insulin during fasting

		Hours of fast				
Test	*Subjects*	*0**	*24*	*36*	*48*	*72*
Glucose, mg/dl	Men	85 ± 1.5	83 ± 3.6	78 ± 3.4	78 ± 3.3	71 ± 2.4
	Women	83 ± 1.3	63 ± 1.6	50 ± 1.7	46 ± 1.7	48 ± 1.4
Insulin, μU/ml	Men	14 ± 0.9	9 ± 0.8	8 ± 1.1	8 ± 0.9	6 ± 0.7
	Women	12 ± 0.8	6 ± 0.4	4 ± 0.5	3 ± 0.4	4 ± 0.5

* *Zero values obtained after overnight fast. Results represent means ± SEM for 20 normal men and 60 normal women.*
SOURCE: *TJ Merimee, JE Tyson, Diabetes 26:161, 1977.*

The differential characteristics of insulinoma and the two types of factitious hypoglycemia are shown in Table 116-4.

TREATMENT The initial treatment of serious hypoglycemia (producing confusion or coma) is the intravenous administration of a bolus of 25 or 50 g glucose as a 50% solution followed by constant infusion of glucose until the patient is able to eat a meal. The importance of the meal resides in the fact that hepatic glycogen repletion is not effective with small quantities of intravenous glucose. Patients in the overutilization category may require large quantities of intravenous glucose to maintain consciousness, and rates of delivery sufficient to cause mild glycosuria should be given. It is not enough to infuse 5% dextrose at a rate of 1 to 2 ml/min and assume the patient is protected (20 to 30% dextrose solutions may be required in some cases). Frequent measurement of capillary glucose concentrations should be carried out using glucose-sensitive reagent strips to assess effectiveness of glucose infusion rates. Intravenous glucose can usually be stopped once the patient has eaten, but this can only be determined by trial. Adrenergic reactions without central nervous system abnormalities can be treated with oral carbohydrate and do not require parenteral therapy.

It is important to note that hypoglycemia from sulfonylureas may last for prolonged periods (days), particularly with chlorpropamide (Fig. 116-2). It is common experience to have a patient lapse back into coma if glucose infusions are stopped too soon. The reason for the prolonged effect is not always clear, though drug interactions, hepatic disease, and renal failure may play a role in some cases.

Surgery is the treatment of choice for insulinoma. Arteriography (celiac or superior mesenteric) should be done prior to exploration in an attempt to localize the lesion. In some centers preoperative or operative sampling of insulin concentrations by selective pancreatic vein catheterization has been performed but appears to be of minimal benefit even if a rapid insulin assay is available. If the tumor cannot be palpated in the pancreas or located in an extrapancreatic site at the time of surgery, stepwise pancreatectomy (from tail to head) should be carried out with frozen sections made of sequential slices. Frequent plasma samples should be drawn for immediate measurement of glucose and subsequent assay for insulin. A sudden rise in plasma glucose may indicate removal of the tumor. In general resection is stopped with an 85 percent pancreatectomy, even if the tumor is not found, to avoid malabsorptive complications. Evaluation of 1012 cases of insulinoma cited in the literature indicated the following outcomes from surgery: operative mortality, 11 percent; cure, 63 percent; postoperative diabetes, 10 percent; and persistent hypoglycemia, 16 percent. Postoperative complications included acute pancreatitis, peritonitis, fistulas, and pseudocyst formation.

Medical treatment is indicated in insulinoma only in preparation for surgery or after failure to find the tumor at operation. The drug of choice is diazoxide, which can be given intravenously or orally in doses of 300 to 1200 mg per day. Because of its salt-retaining properties a diuretic must always be added when diazoxide is administered. Treatment of metastatic insulin-producing carcinomas is unsatisfactory. Streptozotocin, mithramycin, and doxorubicin have been tried, but the results are dismal.

Therapy of other forms of recurrent hypoglycemia, apart from hormone replacement in pituitary or adrenal insufficiency, is dietary. In most cases avoidance of fasting is all that is required. A high-protein, low-carbohydrate diet is frequently prescribed for patients with the idiopathic postprandial syndrome and often relieves symptoms. With true alimentary hypoglycemia it is probably important to keep the size of the individual meals small. The practice of giving massive amounts of vitamin E, crude adrenocortical extract, and varieties of trace metals to patients with the idiopathic postprandial syndrome is useless even if harmless (which has not been proved).

OTHER HORMONE-SECRETING TUMORS OF THE PANCREAS Tumors of the pancreatic islets can synthesize a variety of hormones other than insulin. Almost all benign tumors are thought to be hormone-secreting, but a fifth or more of islet carcinomas produce no clinically detectable product. Histologically the tumors may be of a single-cell type or of mixed derivation. Despite the capacity of mixed tumors to produce several hormones, one usually predominates such that distinct syndromes result. Tumors are generally named after the primary hormone released. If multiple hormones are produced and none dominates the clinical picture, the tumor is simply classified as "multiple hormone producing." It is critical to remember that pancreatic tumors may be part of the multiple endocrine neoplasia syndrome (Chap. 123). This is particularly

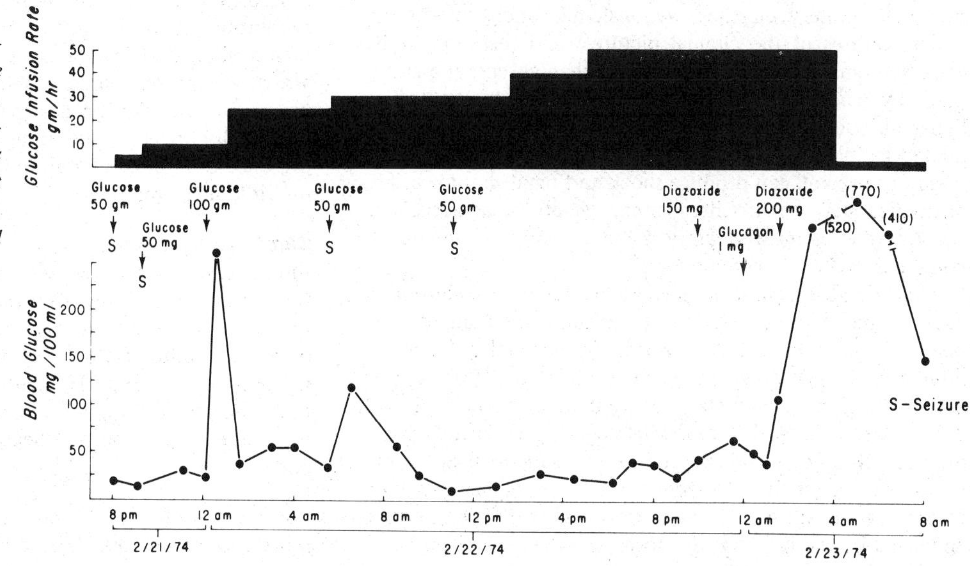

FIGURE 116-2
Prolonged and refractive hypoglycemia in factitious hypoglycemia due to chlorpropamide in an alcoholic. Note continued hypoglycemia despite the infusion of glucose at rates up to 50 g/h. (From RM Jordan et al, Arch Intern Med 137:390, 1977. Copyright 1977, American Medical Association. Used by permission.)

true of the ulcerogenic islet-cell tumor which is now considered to be a typical manifestation of the multiple endocrine neoplasia type I picture. This association is so strong that the designation *multiple endocrine neoplasia–peptic ulcer syndrome* is preferred. In addition to insulin, islet-cell tumors have been associated with the production of gastrin, secretin, vasoactive intestinal polypeptide, human pancreatic polypeptide, gastric inhibitory polypeptide, glucagon, ACTH, melanocyte stimulatory hormone, serotonin, neurotensin, enkephalin, and calcitonin. Chorionic gonadotropin and its β subunit may also be elevated in the plasma; the latter has been suggested to be a specific marker of malignancy in functioning tumors.

Ulcerogenic islet-cell tumor (Zollinger-Ellison syndrome, gastrinoma) This is likely the most common of the non-insulin-secreting tumors. The clinical picture is that of intractable ulcer symptoms, hypersecretion of gastric acid, and diarrhea, which may be watery or due to steatorrhea. Complications such as perforation and hemorrhage occur commonly. X-ray frequently shows the stomach to be filled with fluid, and giant gastric rugae are seen. Often the ulcer is atypically located in the second or third portion of the duodenum. Development of ulcer disease in the very young or very old should always raise suspicion of the Zollinger-Ellison syndrome. Associated endocrine abnormalities are present in half the patients and in a high percentage of first-degree relatives. Hypercalcemia due to parathyroid adenoma is the most common accompanying abnormality. A careful family history designed to elicit evidence of hypoglycemia, renal stones, multiple lipomas, and pituitary adenomas is imperative. All first-degree relatives of patients with gastrinomas should be examined by the physician. Multiple lipomas can be a clue to the presence of multiple endocrine neoplasia. Minimal screening should probably include x-rays of the sella turcica and measurement of serum gastrin, cortisol, prolactin, growth hormone, calcium, and phosphorus. If hypercalcemia is present, workup for hyperparathyroidism can be completed. Evaluation for insulinoma is not indicated in the absence of symptoms suggesting hypoglycemia. Details of diagnosis and treatment for the Zollinger-Ellison syndrome are discussed in Chap. 306.

Diarrheogenic islet-cell tumor The syndrome produced by these tumors has been called pancreatic cholera, the watery diarrhea syndrome, and the WDHA syndrome. The acronym stands for *w*atery *d*iarrhea, *h*ypokalemia, and *a*chlorhydria, major features of the clinical picture. Acid secretion in the basal state may actually be low rather than absent, and stimulation by histamine is intact. About two-thirds of patients have hypercalcemia, and approximately half are hyperglycemic. A dilated gallbladder is characteristic. The secretory diarrhea is often profuse and can produce shock and renal shutdown. Hypokalemia may be life-threatening. Metabolic acidosis, presumably due to bicarbonate loss but possibly also related to volume depletion, is common.

Considerable confusion has existed about the hormonal cause of the syndrome. Originally secretin was thought to be involved, but subsequently vasoactive intestinal polypeptide, human pancreatic polypeptide, gastric inhibitory polypeptide, and prostaglandins were all reported to be associated with diarrheogenic islet-cell tumors. While it is theoretically possible that multiple hormones produce the same clinical picture, it is now thought that vasoactive intestinal polypeptide is the mediator in most cases. The attractiveness of this possibility is enhanced by the fact that the hormone is known to cause hyperglycemia and hypercalcemia in addition to secretory diarrhea. Thus the entire syndrome can be accounted for by one hormone without the need to postulate multiple hormone production. Hypercalcemia usually disappears after removal of the pancreatic neoplasm and in most cases is probably not due to concomitant hyperparathyroidism.

Treatment is surgical removal of the tumor after fluid and electrolyte balance have been restored. Steroids ameliorate the diarrhea in some cases but should be used only if the patient is at risk for life despite conservative management preparatory to surgery. The diarrheogenic tumors tend to be larger than other islet adenomas and may be more easily localized by angiography. Diarrhea disappears, and gastric acid secretion and potassium concentration rapidly normalize if the tumor can be completely removed.

Glucagonoma Glucagonomas, a high percentage of which appear to be malignant and metastasizing, cause a clinical syndrome characterized by a distinctive skin lesion (necrolytic migratory erythema) on the face, lower abdomen, perineum, buttocks, or distal extremities. The characteristic picture is of multiple crusts, scaly macules and papules, occasional pustules, flaccid bullae, and generalized erythema. Glossitis, stomatitis, and angular cheilosis are common. Spontaneous exacerbations and remissions occur, and hyperpigmentation follows healing. Systemically, weight loss and normochromic, normocytic anemia are common. Elevated fasting blood glucose concentrations or abnormal glucose tolerance tests are demonstrable in most patients. Plasma amino acid levels are depressed, and hypocholesterolemia may be present. Plasma ketones may be mildly elevated despite normal plasma free fatty acid concentrations. Glucagon levels in plasma are high and show abnormal responses to a number of provocative tests. It is of interest that four asymptomatic first-degree relatives of one patient with a proved glucagonoma had persistently elevated glucagon concentrations with abnormal responses to glucose suppression and arginine stimulation. Transmission appeared to follow an autosomal dominant pattern. Whether the asymptomatic subjects had small (undetectable) adenomas or whether the alpha cells were functionally abnormal but not neoplastic is not known. Glucagonomas have also been reported in a family with multiple endocrine neoplasia type I.

Treatment of glucagonoma is surgical removal. Chemotherapy of metastatic disease is unsatisfactory.

Somatostatinoma A number of patients have now been reported in whom islet-cell tumors contained somatostatin. The presenting picture includes diarrhea, weight loss, cholelithiasis with a dilated gallbladder, anemia, and hypochlorhydria. Steatorrhea is present in some patients. Abdominal pain may be prominent. In addition to a pancreatic mass, liver metastases are usually present at the time of diagnosis. In one patient the presence of immunoglobulin Gκ-type M led to confusion with multiple myeloma.

Cushing's syndrome ACTH production by pancreatic islet tumors causes less severe clinical manifestations than in other forms of ectopic Cushing's syndrome. Mixed hormone production (insulin, gastrin, serotonin) is common in these tumors in contrast to other islet neoplasms. The problem of differentiating between a single islet tumor producing multiple hormones and the multiple endocrine neoplasia syndrome where two or more adenomas each produce a single hormone may be difficult.

Carcinoid syndrome Serotonin may be synthesized in islet tumors and lead to diarrhea, flushing, and tachycardia. Asthma is not present. It is conceivable that these patients actually have a diarrheogenic tumor with symptoms primarily due to vasoactive intestinal polypeptide and that serotonin production represents a second hormone synthesized by a mixed adenoma (see Chap. 131).

REFERENCES

Hypoglycemia and insulinoma

ADAM PAJ et al: Model for the investigation of intractable hypoglycemia: Insulin-glucose interrelationships during steady state infusions. Pediatrics 41:91, 1968

BAUMAN WA, YALOW RS: Differential diagnosis between endogenous and exogenous insulin-induced refractory hypoglycemia in a nondiabetic patient. N Engl J Med 303:198, 1980

CHARLES MA et al: Comparison of oral glucose tolerance tests and mixed meals in patients with apparent idiopathic postabsorptive hypoglycemia. Absence of hypoglycemia after meals. Diabetes 30:465, 1981

CRYER PE: Glucose counterregulation in man. Diabetes 30:261, 1981

GOLDMAN J et al: Characterization of circulating insulin and pro-insulin-binding antibodies in autoimmune hypoglycemia. J Clin Invest 63:1050, 1979

JORDAN RM et al: Sulfonylurea-induced factitious hypoglycemia. A growing problem. Arch Intern Med 137:390, 1977

MCGARRY JD, FOSTER DW: Systemic carnitine deficiency. N Engl J Med 303:413, 1980

MERIMEE TJ, TYSON JE: Hypoglycemia in man. Pathologic and physiologic variants. Diabetes 26:161, 1977

RIZZA RA et al: Pathogenesis of hypoglycemia in insulinoma patients. Suppression of hepatic glucose production by insulin. Diabetes 30:377, 1981

SCARLETT JA et al: Factitious hypoglycemia. Diagnosis by measurement of serum C-peptide immunoreactivity and insulin-binding antibodies. N Engl J Med 297:1029, 1977

SERVICE FJ et al: Insulinoma. Clinical and diagnostic features of 60 consecutive cases. Mayo Clin Proc 51:417, 1976

STEFANINI P: Beta-islet cell tumors of the pancreas: Results of a study on 1067 cases. Surgery 75:597, 1974

Other hormone-secreting islet-cell tumors

BINNICK AN et al: Glucagonoma syndrome. Report of two cases and literature review. Arch Dermatol 113:749, 1977

CREUTZFELDT W: Endocrine tumors of the pancreas: Clinical, chemical and morphological findings in, *The Pancreas,* PJ Fitzgerald, AB Morrison (eds). Baltimore, Williams & Wilkins, 1980, pp 185–207

JASPAN JB et al: Clinical features and diagnosis of islet cell tumors in, *Tumors of the Pancreas,* AR Moosa (ed). Baltimore, Williams & Wilkins, 1980, pp 469–504

LAMERS CB et al: Prevalence of endocrine abnormalities in patients with the Zollinger-Ellison syndrome and in their families. Am J Med 64:607, 1978

117
DISORDERS OF THE TESTIS

JAMES E. GRIFFIN
JEAN D. WILSON

The testis produces sperm and the steroid hormones that regulate male sexual life. Both of these functions are under complex feedback control by the hypothalamic-pituitary system so that the testis has biosynthetic and regulatory features similar to those of the ovary and the adrenal. Testicular hormones are also responsible for the formation of the basic male phenotype during embryogenesis. The function of the embryonic testis and the disorders that result from abnormalities of testicular function or androgen action during embryogenesis are described in Chap. 120.

PHYSIOLOGY AND REGULATION OF TESTICULAR FUNCTION

The testis consists of two components—a system of spermatogenic tubules for the production and transport of sperm and clusters of interstitial or Leydig cells that lie between the tubules and produce androgenic steroids.

THE LEYDIG CELL **Testosterone synthesis** The biochemical pathway by which the 27-carbon sterol cholesterol is converted to androgens and estrogens is depicted in Fig. 117-1. Cholesterol can either be synthesized de novo in the Leydig cell or derived from plasma lipoproteins. Five enzymes or enzyme complexes are required for the conversion of cholesterol to testosterone. In this process the side chain of cholesterol is cleaved in two steps to reduce the size from 27 to 19 carbons, and the A ring of the steroid is converted to the Δ^4-3-keto configuration. The five enzymes are the 20,22-desmolase, the 3β-hydroxysteroid dehydrogenase-$\Delta^{4,5}$-isomerase complex, 17α-hydroxylase, 17,20-desmolase, and 17β-hydroxysteroid dehydrogenase. The first four enzymes are also present in the adrenal.

The rate-limiting reaction in testosterone synthesis is the conversion of cholesterol to pregnenolone by the 20,22-desmolase; luteinizing hormone (LH) from the pituitary acts at this step to regulate the rate of testosterone formation. Several other steroids including estradiol are synthesized within the

FIGURE 117-1
Pathways of androgen formation in the testis and the conversion of androgens to other active hormones in peripheral tissues.

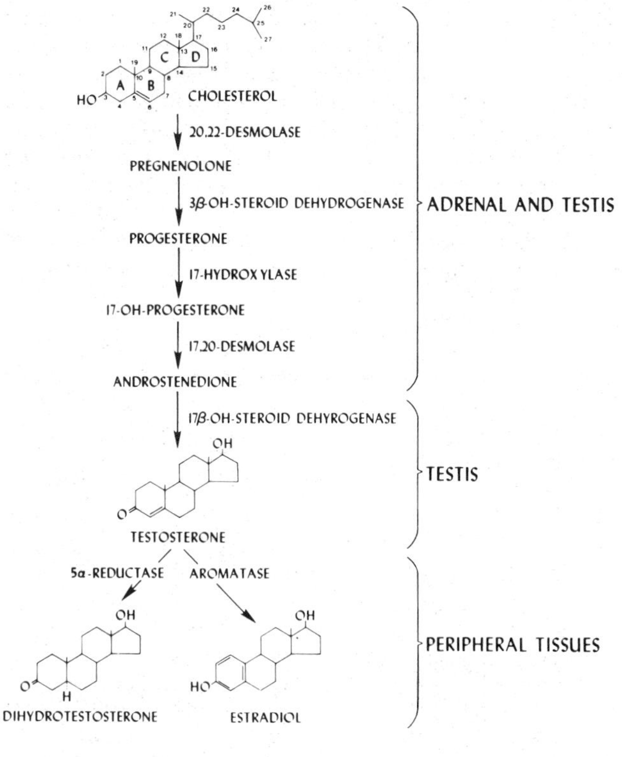

CHOLESTEROL
20,22-DESMOLASE
PREGNENOLONE
3β-OH-STEROID DEHYDROGENASE
PROGESTERONE
17-HYDROXYLASE
17-OH-PROGESTERONE
17,20-DESMOLASE
ANDROSTENEDIONE
ADRENAL AND TESTIS
17β-OH-STEROID DEHYROGENASE
TESTOSTERONE
TESTIS
5α-REDUCTASE
AROMATASE
DIHYDROTESTOSTERONE
ESTRADIOL
PERIPHERAL TISSUES

Leydig cell, but the significance of these in the normal man is thought to be minor.

Testosterone secretion and transport Only about 0.02 mg of testosterone is stored in the normal testes so that the total hormone content turns over about 200 times each day to provide the average of 5 to 6 mg that is secreted into plasma in normal young men (Fig. 117-2). As is true for other steroid hormones, testosterone is transported in plasma bound to protein, largely to albumin and to a specific steroid hormone transport protein, testosterone-binding globulin (TeBG). The bound and unbound fractions in plasma are in dynamic equilibrium, only about 1 to 3 percent being present in the free fraction.

Peripheral metabolism of androgens A special feature of testosterone metabolism is that it serves as a circulating precursor (or prohormone) for the formation of two other types of active metabolites which mediate many of the physiological processes involved in androgen action (Fig. 117-1). On the one hand, testosterone can be converted by 5α-reduction to dihydrotestosterone, which is believed to perform many of the differentiative, growth-promoting, and functional actions involved in male sexual differentiation and virilization. On the other hand, circulating androgens in both sexes can be converted to estrogens in the peripheral tissues. In men estrogens act in some instances in concert with androgens but can also have effects independent of or opposite to those of androgens. Thus, the physiological effects of testosterone are the result of the combined effects of testosterone itself plus those of the active androgen and estrogen metabolites of the parent molecule. (In normal men small amounts of estradiol and dihydrotestosterone are also derived by direct secretion from the testis and indirectly from the weak adrenal androgen androstenedione.)

The quantitative relation between circulating androgens and the formation of estrogen in normal young men is illustrated diagrammatically in Fig. 117-2. The production rates of testosterone and androstenedione average about 6 and 3 mg, respectively, per day. All of estrone production (averaging about 60 μg per day) can be accounted for by formation from circulating precursors. The mean estradiol production rate is about 45 μg per day; about 35 percent of this amount is derived from circulating testosterone, 50 percent is derived from the weak estrogen estrone, and 15 percent is secreted directly into the circulation by the testes. When gonadotropin levels are elevated the amount of estradiol secretion by the testis is increased.

The 5α-reduced and estrogenic metabolites can exert local actions in the tissues in which they are formed or enter the circulation and act as hormones at other sites. Circulating dihydrotestosterone is formed principally in the androgen target tissues, whereas estrogen formation takes place in many peripheral tissues, the most significant site being adipose tissue. The overall rate of peripheral estrogen formation increases with increasing amounts of adipose tissue and with age.

Plasma testosterone and its active metabolites are converted to inactive metabolites in the liver and excreted predominantly in the urine; approximately half of the daily turnover is excreted in the form of urinary 17-ketosteroids (primarily androsterone and etiocholanolone), and the remainder is excreted as a series of polar compounds (diols, triols, and conjugates).

Gonadotropin regulation and testosterone secretion Testosterone secretion is regulated by pituitary LH (Fig. 117-3). (For the details of pituitary function, see Chap. 109.) Follicle-stimulating hormone (FSH) may also augment testosterone secretion, possibly by regulating the number of LH receptors on the plasma membrane of the Leydig cell. Testosterone feeds back on the pituitary to alter the sensitivity of the gland to the hypothalamic-releasing factor luteinizing hormone–releasing hormone (LHRH). Although the pituitary can convert testosterone to dihydrotestosterone and to estrogens, testosterone itself is the primary regulator of gonadotropin secretion. Whether testosterone also acts in the central nervous system to regulate the rate of LHRH formation or secretion is not known. Under ordinary circumstances, LH secretion is exquisitely sensitive to the feedback effects of testosterone, with complete suppression following the administration of amounts of exogenous androgen that approximate the normal daily secretory rate of testosterone (about 6 mg). However, prolonged elevation of plasma LH (as in testicular deficiency) renders the pituitary less sensitive to negative feedback control by exogenously administered androgens.

Neither the plasma concentration of testosterone nor that of LH is constant, each showing fluctuations of a pulsatile nature that reflect changes in secretory rates (Fig. 117-4). In the pubertal male major sleep-related surges in the pulsatile secretion of both LH and testosterone signal the initiation of pu-

FIGURE 117-2
Androgen and estrogen production in normal young men.

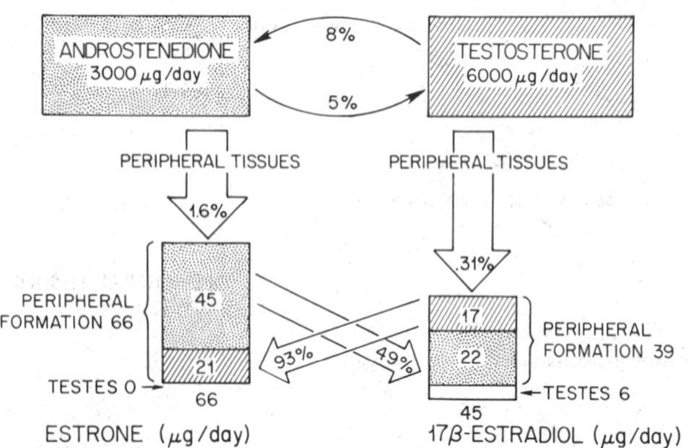

FIGURE 117-3
Regulation of testosterone and sperm production by LH and FSH. (C, cholesterol; T, testosterone.)

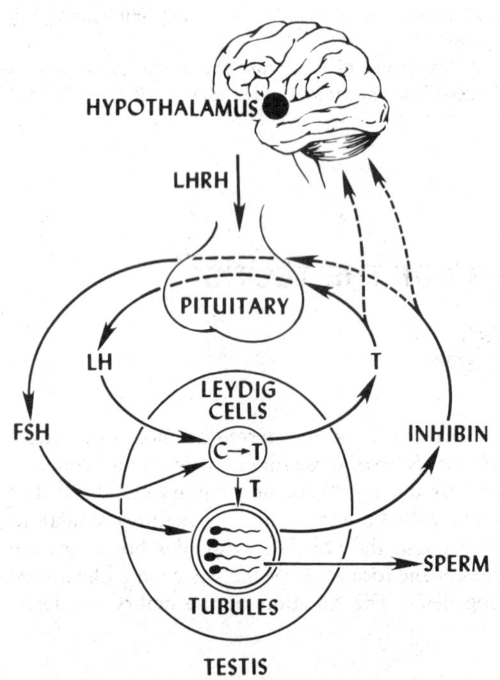

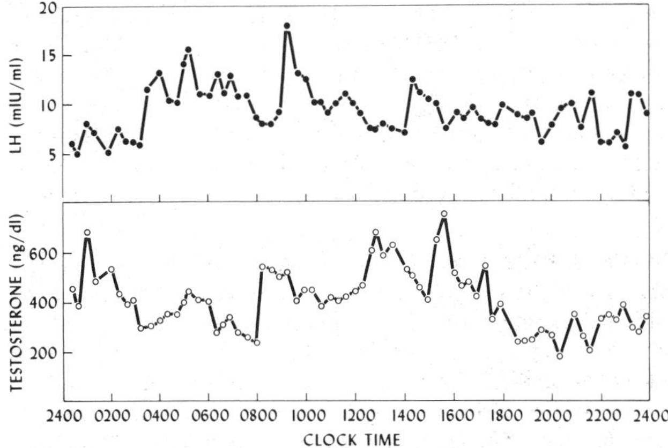

FIGURE 117-4
Twenty-four-hour pattern of plasma LH and testosterone in a normal man sampled every 20 min. (Reprinted from Griffin and Wilson, 1980.)

berty. In the adult the diurnal variation in the magnitude of this episodic secretion of LH and testosterone is minor with peak levels in the morning only about 10 to 15 percent higher than during the rest of the day.

Androgen action The major functions of androgen are the regulation of gonadotropin secretion, the initiation and maintenance of spermatogenesis, the formation of the male phenotype during sexual differentiation, and the induction of sexual maturation and function following puberty. The cellular mechanisms by which androgens perform these functions are summarized schematically in Fig. 117-5. Testosterone (T) enters the cell by passive diffusion. Inside the cell T can be converted to dihydrotestosterone (D) by the 5α-reductase enzyme. T or D is then bound to the androgen receptor protein in the cytosol (R). The hormone-receptor complex (TR or DR) is translocated to the nucleus where it attaches to specific chromosomal sites; as a result, new messenger RNA is transcribed, and ultimately new protein appears within the cytoplasm of the cell.

Although testosterone and dihydrotestosterone bind to the same receptor their physiological roles differ. The testosterone-receptor complex regulates gonadotropin secretion and is responsible for spermatogenesis and for the Wolffian stimulation phase of sexual differentiation (see Chap. 120) whereas the dihydrotestosterone-receptor complex is responsible for external virilization during embryogenesis and the major portion of androgen action during sexual maturation and adult sexual life. The mechanism by which testosterone and dihydrotestosterone mediate these different functions is not known. The mechanisms by which estrogens act to augment or block androgen effects are also not known. It is presumed that estradiol acts by a mechanism similar to that of androgens but involving its own receptor protein (see Chap. 118).

FIGURE 117-5
Current concepts of androgen action. (T, testosterone; D, dihydrostestosterone; R, receptor protein.)

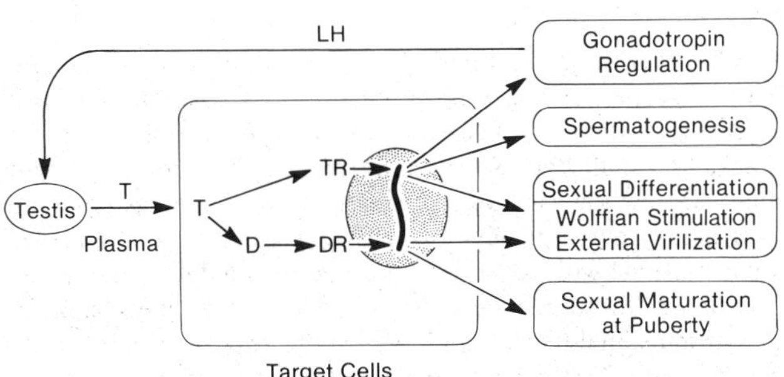

THE SEMINIFEROUS TUBULE AND SPERMATOGENESIS Normal function of the seminiferous tubule is dependent both on the pituitary and on normal function of the adjacent Leydig cells, both FSH and testosterone being essential for spermatogenesis (Fig. 117-3). The major site of FSH action is the Sertoli cell component of the seminiferous tubules. The seminiferous tubule is also a target for testosterone and contains specific androgen receptors. Testosterone appears to be essential for the initial phase of spermatogenesis, whereas FSH is required for the terminal phases of spermatid development. In the normal adult male this machinery produces more than 100 million sperm per day.

The Sertoli cell cannot synthesize steroid hormones de novo and is dependent on testosterone that diffuses in from adjacent Leydig cells. Isolated Sertoli cells (as well as Leydig cells) can convert testoserone to estradiol and to dihydrotestosterone. The role of these various metabolites in spermatogenesis is unclear.

The seminiferous tubules also produce the hormone inhibin that regulates the secretion of FSH by the hypothalamic-pituitary axis (Fig. 117-3). This hormone is a peptide that is formed during the late phase of spermatogenesis. Whether the hormone acts primarily at the level of the pituitary or hypothalamus to regulate FSH secretion is unknown.

The interlocking system in which two pituitary hormones regulate testicular function provides a precise dual-control mechanism by which plasma testosterone and sperm production feed back upon the hypothalamic-pituitary system to regulate their own rates of production (Fig. 117-3).

ASSESSMENT OF TESTICULAR FUNCTION

LEYDIG CELL FUNCTION The presence of male secondary sex characteristics clearly indicates that testosterone levels have been normal at least in the past, and normal libido and normal ejaculate indicate that testosterone levels are currently normal. However, the degree of virilization—for example, beard growth—among men with similar plasma testosterone levels is extremely variable. In addition, sexual function is influenced by many nonendocrine factors. Consequently, the laboratory assessment of Leydig cell function is frequently useful in separating endocrine from nonendocrine causes of male sexual dysfunction and in following the response to replacement therapy in patients with endocrine disorders.

Plasma testosterone and dihydrotestosterone levels Plasma testosterone is measured by a specific radioimmunoassay. Testosterone is secreted into plasma in a pulsatile fashion every 20 to 30 min (Fig. 117-4); a single random sample provides a result within ±20 percent of the true mean value only two-thirds of the time while three equally spaced samples 6 to 18 min apart provide a more accurate assessment. The samples do not need to be assayed separately, and aliquots of the three samples can be pooled for a single determination. The range of plasma testosterone in normal adult men is 300 to 1000 ng/dl. In adult men the plasma values vary slightly throughout the day and at different times of the year, but these variations are not as great as those for plasma cortisol and are not significant in routine clinical assessment. Plasma levels of testosterone correlate in general with testosterone secretory rates as measured by isotope infusion.

The plasma testosterone value in normal prepubertal children is statistically higher in boys than girls, the range in both being 5 to 20 ng/dl. The major change of plasma testosterone at the beginning of puberty occurs as a result of sleep-related nocturnal gonadotropin surges so that during the initial phases plasma testosterone and LH are higher at night than during the day. The random daytime levels of plasma testosterone increase gradually as puberty progresses and reach adult levels at about age 17.

Dihydrotestosterone can also be measured by radioimmunoassay. In normal young men the plasma dihydrotestosterone level is about a tenth that of the testosterone value and averages around 50 ng/dl. In older men with benign prostatic hyperplasia, plasma dihydrotestosterone levels are higher and average about 90 ng/dl.

Urinary 17-ketosteroids The measurement of urinary 17-ketosteroids is not a valid way to assess testicular function. Urinary 17-ketosteroids are mainly weak adrenal androgens or their metabolites, and testosterone contributes only about 40 percent of daily 17-ketosteroid production in men.

Plasma LH Plasma LH is measured by specific radioimmunoassay. LH is also secreted in a pulsatile fashion and fluctuates more widely than does plasma testosterone so that in adult men an isolated random plasma LH is likely to be within ±20 percent of true mean value only a third of the time. Again, assay of a pool of plasma comprised of equal portions of three samples drawn 6 to 18 min apart as described above provides a value approaching the true mean. In early puberty plasma LH secretion increases only during sleep, but the pulsatile secretion in the adult is of similar magnitude during sleep and waking periods. The normal plasma LH values should be established for a given laboratory. The usual normal range in adult men is 26 ±18 ng/ml SD (5 to 20 mIU/ml). A low plasma testosterone concentration can be interpreted correctly only if plasma LH is also measured simultaneously, and likewise the "appropriateness" of a given plasma LH must be interpreted in relation to the plasma testosterone. For example, a low plasma testosterone coupled with a low LH implies pituitary disease, whereas the finding of a low plasma testosterone and a high LH suggests primary testicular insufficiency (see Chap. 108).

Response to gonadotropin stimulation Leydig cell function is difficult to assess prior to puberty when both LH and testosterone levels are low, and it is common to measure response of plasma testosterone to gonadotropin stimulation as an index of Leydig cell capacity. A standard test is to administer human chorionic gonadotropin (HCG) 2000 IU intramuscularly daily for 4 days and to measure plasma testosterone before the first dose and 24 h after the fourth dose. Normal prepubertal boys respond by an increase in plasma testosterone to about 300 ng/dl.

Response to luteinizing hormone–releasing hormone The response of plasma LH (and/or FSH) to the administration of luteinizing hormone–releasing hormone (LHRH) is utilized in some centers to assess the functional integrity of the pituitary-testicular axis. The rationale for this test is discussed in detail in Chap. 109. In normal men LHRH, when given intravenously in a 100-μg bolus, leads to a four- to eightfold increase in plasma LH and a one- to twofold increase in the plasma FSH. Three base-line samples should be obtained in the half hour preceding the injection and again at 30 and 45 min after the injection to allow determination of the peak vlaues of both the LH and FSH. Plasma testosterone does not change significantly after a single bolus of LHRH. However, continuous infusions of 10 μg of LHRH over a 1- to 2-h period result in an increase of plasma testosterone of approximately 20 percent above base line. LHRH is not available for routine use, and in most clinical situations assessment of response to LHRH is not necessary since basal gonadotropin levels correlate adequately with the stimulated response.

SEMINIFEROUS TUBULE FUNCTION Examination of the testes Evaluation of the testes is an essential portion of the physical examination. The seminiferous tubules account for about 95 percent of testicular volume. The prepubertal testis measures about 2 cm in length and 2 ml in volume and increases in size during puberty to reach the adult proportions by age 16. When damage to the seminiferous tubules occurs prior to puberty the testes are small and firm, whereas the testes are usually small and soft following postpubertal damage (the capsule, once enlarged, does not contract to its previous size). Testes average 4.6 cm in length (range, 3.5 to 5.5 cm), corresponding to a volume of 12 to 25 ml in normal adults. Advanced age alone does not influence testicular size, so that the significance of small testes is the same at all ages in the adult.

Semen analysis Seminal fluid analysis is performed after 24- to 36-h abstinence on samples obtained by masturbation into a glass container. Analysis should be performed within an hour. The normal ejaculate volume is greater than 2 ml. Immediately after ejaculation, coagulation of the seminal fluid occurs, followed within 15 to 30 min by liquefaction. Estimation of motility should be made on undiluted seminal fluid; more than 60 percent of the sperm should be motile and of normal morphology. The normal range for sperm density is generally considered to be 20 to 100 million per milliliter with a total count per ejaculate of more than 60 million, but a major difficulty in the interpretation of a semen analysis is the definition of the minimally adequate ejaculate. Some men documented to have low sperm counts are nevertheless fertile. This uncertainty as to the lower level of sperm density, percent motility, and percent normal forms in fertile semen stems from two issues. First, many factors produce temporary aberrations in sperm count, and in men who present with semen of equivocal quality it may be necessary to examine three or more ejaculates to determine whether abnormal findings are permanent or temporary. Second, at present fertilizing capacity can only be assessed by indirect means. A valid in vitro test of the capacity of human spermatozoa to fertilize ova is needed. Until such a test is available, the best functional assessment of spermatozoa is obtained from the cervical mucus penetration test (see Chap. 118), which is sometimes helpful in the evaluation of infertile couples when the routine semen analysis is normal.

Plasma FSH Plasma FSH as measured by specific radioimmunoassay usually correlates inversely with spermatogenesis. In normal adult men, the range of plasma FSH is 102 ±55 ng/ml SD (5 to 20 mIU/ml). Men with intact hypothalamic-pituitary axes have elevations of FSH when damage to the germinal epithelium is severe.

Testicular biopsy Testicular biospy is useful in some patients with oligospermia and azoospermia both as an aid in diagnosis and as an indication of feasibility of treatment. For example, a normal testicular biopsy and a normal FSH in an azoospermic man suggest the diagnosis of obstruction of the vas deferens, which may be surgically correctible. Tissue culture of the biopsy material with subsequent karyotypic analysis is necessary to identify those instances of Klinefelter syndrome secondary to chromosomal mosaicism in which the abnormality is limited to the testes. Testicular biopsy is often followed by a transient decrease in sperm counts, but no permanent adverse effects are usually encountered.

ESTRADIOL Plasma estradiol is measured by radioimmunoassay and in normal men ranges from 20 to 42 pg/ml. As discussed above most estradiol produced in normal men is formed by extraglandular formation from circulating androgens. Elevated estradiol production and elevated plasma levels can be due to elevations in plasma precursors (liver disease), to increases in peripheral aromatization (obesity), or to increased production by the testes (androgen resistance syndromes). The level of plasma estradiol is not always a good index of estradiol production rate in men. One reason is technical difficulty in accurately measuring the low levels normally present in men. Another cause for the poor correlation may be episodic secretion in some men with enhanced estradiol production.

PHASES OF MALE SEXUAL FUNCTION

It is useful to consider the phases of male sexual life in terms of the plasma testosterone value (Fig. 117-6). In the male embryo the production of testosterone by the testis commences at about 7 weeks of gestation. Shortly thereafter plasma testosterone attains a high value that is maintained until late in gestation when it falls so that at the time of birth plasma testosterone is only slightly higher in males than in females. Shortly after birth, plasma testosterone again begins to rise in the male infant and remains elevated for approximately 3 months, falling to low levels by age 1 year. The concentration then remains low (but slightly higher in boys than girls) until the onset of puberty, when it begins to rise in boys, reaching adult levels by age 17 or thereabouts. The mean plasma level remains more or less constant in the adult until late middle age and then declines slowly during the later decades of life. It is only during the third or adult phase of male sexual life that sperm production becomes sufficient to allow reproduction to take place. The physiological events that take place during these various phases differ, as do the pathological consequences of derangements in testicular function at different stages of life. Male sexual differentiation during embryogenesis is considered in Chap. 120. The role of the neonatal surge of testosterone formation during the first year of life is unknown. The focus of this chapter is on testicular pathophysiology during puberty, mature sexual life, and old age.

ABNORMALITIES OF TESTICULAR FUNCTION

PUBERTY The factors that ultimately determine the onset of puberty are poorly understood and may reside in the hypothalamic-pituitary system, the testis, or the adrenal. Prior to the

FIGURE 117-6
Phases of male sexual life. (Reprinted from Griffin and Wilson, 1980.)

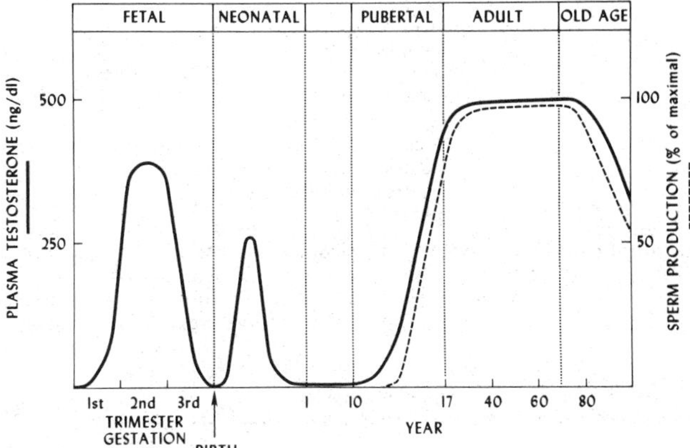

onset of puberty, gonadotropin secretion by the pituitary is low but appears to be under regulatory control by the testis, as prepubertal castration results in a rise in plasma gonadotropin levels. This suggests that prior to puberty the negative feedback control of gonadotropin secretion is exquisitely sensitive to the small amount of circulating testosterone. The onset of puberty is heralded by sleep-associated surges in gonadotropin secretion. Later in puberty the rises in LH and FSH persist throughout the day. Thus, with maturation the hypothalamic-pituitary system becomes less sensitive to negative feedback control, and the consequences are a higher mean plasma testosterone, maturation of the testes, and the onset of spermatogenesis. The remaining anatomical and functional changes at the time of puberty are secondary to the rise in plasma testosterone. Maturation of the accessory organs of male reproduction (the penis, the prostate, the seminal vesicles, and the epididymides) accounts for about a fourth of androgen-mediated nitrogen retention during puberty. Growth of muscle and connective tissue accounts for the remainder. The principal androgen-sensitive muscles are those of the pectoral region and the shoulder. These various androgen-mediated growth and maturation processes reach some limiting value so that once puberty is completed the administration of pharmacological doses of androgen has no further effect. The entire process begins at age 11 to 12 and is usually completed within 5 years, although some aspects of virilization, such as growth of the chest hair, may continue over a decade or more.

The events of normal male puberty are variable in onset, duration, and sequence. The central issue in dealing with disorders of puberty is separating instances of true absence or precocity from subjects at the extremes of normal variation. The use of staging criteria that correlate developmental and anatomical landmarks with chronological age is useful in making this distinction. (See Marshall and Tanner.)

Sexual precocity Sexual development in a boy before the age of 10 should be considered abnormal. Development of feminizing signs in a boy prior to the expected onset of puberty (so-called heterosexual precocity) is usually the manifestation of estrogen secretion by a testicular or adrenal tumor. Virilization in a boy prior to age 10 (isosexual precocity) can be due either to aberrant androgen production by tumors or to true precocious puberty in which both spermatogenesis and virilization are present. True precocious puberty may be idiopathic, the result of a central nervous system tumor that causes enhanced gonadotropin secretion, or due to congenital adrenal hyperplasia (deficiency of 21- or 11-hydroxylase enzyme), in which the increase in adrenal androgen production occasionally triggers elevated plasma gonadotropin levels, as well (see Chaps. 112 and 120). Tumors such as hepatoblastomas that produce gonadotropins may also rarely cause isosexual precocity.

Patients with idiopathic precocious puberty pass through an early but otherwise typical sexual development including a prepubertal growth spurt followed by premature closure of the epiphyses and a short stature. Affected subjects can ejaculate and may produce sperm, and there are rare reports of fatherhood at an early age. Since normal puberty is poorly understood, it is not surprising that the pathogenesis of idiopathic precocious puberty is also poorly defined. Some type of premature activation of the hypothalamic-pituitary-gonadal axis must take place since these individuals have normal pubertal patterns of sleep-associated and LHRH-induced LH release. In evaluating such patients it is necessary to exclude structural lesions of the central nervous system and pituitary tumors as well as disorders of the adrenal and testis. Since the diagnosis is one of exclusion, some "idiopathic" cases later prove to have been misclassified and to be only the first manifestation of lesions of the central nervous system. With improved means of diagnosing CNS lesions (such as CT scanning) such delays in diagnosis should be less frequent.

Management of idiopathic precocious puberty is generally unsatisfactory. Therapy is usually directed toward lowering plasma gonadotropins with the use of medroxyprogesterone acetate, but such treatment usually does not prevent premature closure of the epiphyses. In patients with congenital adrenal hyperplasia or organic CNS lesions therapy is directed toward the primary disease.

Absent puberty The separation of true failure of puberty from variants of normal is one of the most difficult problems in endocrinology. Some patients fail to show the normal spurt of growth and sexual development at the usual time but eventually commence puberty by age 16 or older. Adolescence may then either progress rapidly, or there may be a slow development and growth that continues until age 20 to 22. Many men with delayed onset of puberty attain heights within the normal adult range. At times the history reveals that a parent or sibling has shown a similar pattern of development. The major problem is to separate this group of patients with delayed puberty from patients with organic disorders that impair puberty. Panhypopituitarism and hypothyroidism can cause pubertal failure in males (see Chaps. 109 and 111). Absent puberty can also result from primary disease of the testis including defects in testicular development; this diagnosis is suspected on the basis of low plasma testosterone and elevated FSH and LH. Hereditary androgen resistance (in which plasma testosterone and LH are both high) usually results in hereditary male pseudohermaphroditism, but in milder cases may be manifested by absent puberty (see Chap. 120).

The most frequent finding in boys with absent puberty is both low plasma testosterone and low gonadotropin levels; in these patients it is necessary to distinguish those with delayed puberty from those with hypogonadotropic hypogonadism (the Kallman syndrome). Hypogonadotropic hypogonadism is characterized by eunuchoidal features and testes of prepubertal size. Anosmia or hyposmia and cryptorchidism are common. Histological examination of the testis reveals undifferentiated Leydig cells and immature germinal epithelium similar to a normal prepubertal testis. The disorder appears to be inherited as an X-linked recessive trait or an autosomal dominant trait with variable expressivity. Serum FSH and LH levels are below the normal male range, and plasma testosterone levels are in the female range. The secretion of other pituitary hormones is usually normal. The defect appears to be in the synthesis or release of LHRH, and the administration of synthetic LHRH for a sufficient period corrects the endocrine abnormalities and initiates spermatogenesis. If untreated, these patients usually remain in the prepubertal state indefinitely. A prepubertal manifestation of this disorder is microphallus, in which the size of the penis is below the fifth percentile for the age. Indeed, in a fourth or more of prepubertal patients with isolated microphallus the underlying etiology is hypogonadotropic hypogonadism. Distinction between this disorder and delayed puberty is particularly difficult in patients of early or midpubertal age; the presence of microphallus, anosmia, or a family history of hypogonadotropic hypogonadism may make it possible to establish the diagnosis. In the absence of such evidence, differentiation of the two states may become clear only after several years of observation.

A less severe form of hypogonadotropic hypogonadism is the so-called fertile eunuch syndrome in which spermatogenesis is present despite deficient androgen production. Plasma FSH levels are within the normal adult male range, whereas plasma testosterone and plasma LH levels are low. However, LHRH administration to such patients causes an increase in plasma LH as well as FSH. This implies that the defect in this disorder, as in the Kallman syndrome, is defective LH release.

A few men have been described with isolated FSH deficiency in whom virilization, plasma LH, and plasma testosterone were normal but plasma FSH was persistently low; testicular biopsy in one individual revealed a maturation arrest at the spermatid stage. In some, FSH levels increased following administration of LHRH.

ADULT ABNORMALITIES OF TESTICULAR FUNCTION At the time of the completion of puberty, plasma testosterone levels reach the adult level of 300 to 1000 ng/dl throughout the day, plasma gonadotropins are 5 to 20 mIU/ml each for LH and FSH, and sperm production is sufficient to allow reproduction. The adult set of the complex regulatory system described in Fig. 117-3 is sustained in the normal man for more than 40 years. However, the system is subject to a variety of influences, both at the level of the testis and of the hypothalamic-pituitary system. Spermatogenesis is exquisitely sensitive to alterations in temperature, and brief increases either in systemic or local temperature (as in a hot bath) can be followed by temporary decreases in sperm production. The system is likewise subject

TABLE 117-1
Classification of abnormalities of testicular function in the adult

Site of defect	Presentation: Underandrogenization and infertility	Presentation: Infertility
Hypothalamic-pituitary	Panhypopituitarism	
	Hypogonadotropic hypogonadism	Isolated FSH deficiency
	Cushing syndrome	Congenital adrenal hyperplasia
	Hyperprolactinemia	Hyperprolactinemia
	Hemochromatosis	
Testicular	Developmental and structural defects:	
	Klinefelter syndrome*	Germinal cell aplasia
	XX male	Cryptorchidism
		Varicocele
	Acquired defects:	
	Viral orchitis*	
	Trauma	
	Radiation	Radiation
	Drugs (spironolactone, alcohol, marijuana)	Drugs (cyclophosphamide)
	Autoimmunity (polyglandular endocrine failure)	Autoimmunity
	Granulomatous disease	
	Associated with systemic diseases:	
	Liver disease	Febrile illness
	Renal failure	
	Sickle cell disease	
	Neurological diseases (myotonic dystrophy and paraplegia)	Neurological disease (paraplegia)
Posttesticular	Androgen resistance	Androgen resistance
		Absence or obstruction of the vas deferens (cystic fibrosis)

* *The common testicular causes of underandrogenization and infertility in adults—Klinefelter syndrome and viral orchitis—are associated with small testes.*

to influence by diet, drugs, alcohol, environmental agents, and psychological stress, all of which may cause temporary decreases in sperm count.

Persistent abnormalities of testicular function after the time of normal puberty can be due to pituitary abnormalities (see Chap. 109), testicular defects, or to posttesticular lesions. Certain of these conditions tend to affect Leydig cell function or spermatogenesis selectively, but most influence both aspects of testicular function and cause both underandrogenization and infertility (Table 117-1). The interlocking of defective Leydig cell function with infertility is a consequence of the dependence of spermatogenesis on androgen formation. Even partial decreases in testosterone production can cause infertility. Certain disorders (radiation, androgen resistance, hyperprolactinemia) can cause either isolated infertility or a combined defect in testicular function in different patients.

Hypothalamic-pituitary disorders Disorders of the hypothalamus and pituitary can impair secretion of gonadotropins (and cause as a consequence decreased androgen production and defective spermatogenesis) either as an isolated defect (hypogonadotropic hypogonadism) or as a portion of more complex endocrine and systemic manifestations (see Chap. 109). Alternatively, gonadotropin secretion can be altered by factors other than hypothalamic pituitary pathology. For example, hypercortisolism in the Cushing syndrome can depress LH secretion independent of a space-occupying lesion of the pituitary. Some patients with congenital adrenal hyperplasia have early activation of gonadotropin secretion and true precocious puberty, while other patients have suppressed gonadotropin secretion and consequent infertility. Hyperprolactinemia (either as the consequence of pituitary adenomas or of drugs such as phenothiazines) has been associated with combined Leydig cell and seminiferous tubule dysfunction, presumably the consequence of inhibition of LH and FSH secretion by prolactin. Occasionally, impaired fertility in hyperprolactinemia is associated with normal gonadotropin and androgen levels and is presumed to result from direct inhibition of spermatogenesis by prolactin. Hemochromatosis impairs testicular function most commonly as the result of effects on the gonadotrophs, less often it affects the testis directly.

Testicular defects Abnormalities of testicular function that present in the adult can be grouped into several categories: developmental and structural defects of the testes, acquired testicular defects, and those abnormalities secondary to system and/or neurological disease.

DEVELOPMENTAL ABNORMALITIES The *Klinefelter syndrome* (both the classical and mosaic forms) and the *XX male syndrome* are usually not recognized until after the time of expected puberty (see Chap. 120). Some developmental defects cause infertility in the presence of normal androgen production. These include varicocele, germinal cell aplasia, and cryptorchidism. *Varicocele* is probably the most common treatable cause of male infertility and may be of etiologic importance in as much as a third of all male infertility. It is caused by retrograde flow of blood into the internal spermatic vein that eventuates in progressive, often palpable dilatation of the peritesticular pampiniform plexus of veins. The incidence of varicocele is about 10 to 15 percent in the general population and 20 to 40 percent in men with infertility. It is thought to result from incompetence of the valve between the internal spermatic vein and the renal vein and is more common on the left (85 percent). Unilateral varicocele increases the blood flow and the temperature of both testes as a result of the extensive anastomoses of the venous systems. The findings on semen analysis are usually nonspecific with all parameters showing some abnormality. The increased scrotal (and testicular) temperature is believed to be the cause of the poor-quality semen and infertility (the testes do not have the usual 2°C lower temperature than that of the abdominal cavity). In a number of studies, varicocelectomy caused improved fertility, with the best results (70 percent pregnancy rate) obtained in men whose preoperative sperm counts were over 10 million per milliliter.

Some patients with *germinal-cell aplasia* (the Sertoli cell–only syndrome) have a positive family history and may constitute a specific entity in which the germinal epithelium is missing with resulting azoospermia; plasma testosterone and LH values are normal, and plasma FSH levels are elevated. Other patients with identical histological and clinical findings have androgen resistance or a history of viral orchitis or cryptorchidism. Consequently a variety of conditions are commonly lumped under this term. The syndrome accounts for less than 10 percent of patients with azoospermia.

Unilateral *cryptorchidism*, even when corrected prior to puberty, is associated with abnormal semen in many individuals. This suggests that even in unilateral cryptorchidism the testicular abnormality is usually bilateral.

ACQUIRED TESTICULAR DEFECTS Most acquired testicular failure in the adult results from *viral orchitis*. Mumps is the virus most frequently responsible, although other agents are known to act in a similar fashion, including echovirus, lymphocytic choriomeningitis virus, and group B arboviruses. The orchitis is due to actual infection of the tissue by virus rather than indirect effects of the infection. Orchitis is the most common complication of mumps in adult men. In about two-thirds of the cases it is unilateral, and in the remainder it is bilateral. It usually develops within a few days after the onset of parotitis but occasionally precedes it. The testis may return to normal size and function or undergo atrophy. Atrophy is believed to be due both to direct effects of the virus on the seminiferous tubules and to ischemia secondary to pressure and edema within the taut tunica albuginea. Atrophy is usually perceptible within 1 to 6 months after the orchitis subsides, and the degree of atrophy is not necessarily proportional to the severity of the acute orchitis. Unilateral atrophy occurs in approximately a third of cases of mumps orchitis, and bilateral atrophy occurs in about a tenth.

Trauma is second to viral orchitis as a cause of secondary atrophy of the testes. The exposed position of the testis in the scrotum renders it uniquely susceptible to both thermal and physical trauma—particularly in individuals with harzardous occupations.

Both the seminiferous tubules and the Leydig cells are sensitive to *radiation damage.* Doses higher than 200 mGy (20 rads) almost uniformly cause increases in plasma FSH and LH levels and damage to the spermatogonia. With doses of about 800 mGy (80 rads) extreme oligospermia or azoospermia develops. Higher doses may result in virtual obliteration of the germinal epithelium except for occasional stem and Sertoli cells. Still higher doses [6000 mGy (600 rad)] can cause an increase in the number of Leydig cells. Complete recovery to preirradiation sperm density may require as long as 5 years. Permanent infertility can apparently occur after amounts of radiation used for therapy of malignant lymphoma in spite of shielding the testes. Permanent androgen deficiency rarely results from doses of radiation in the therapeutic range.

In general, *drugs* interfere with testicular function in one of four ways—inhibition of testosterone synthesis, blockade of the peripheral action of androgen, enhancement of estrogen levels, or direct inhibition of spermatogenesis. Certain drugs have multiple effects, and agents such as propanol and guanethidine that block the sympathetic nervous system can impair normal sexual drive and potency in men whose pituitary-testicular axis is normal.

Spironolactone in high doses blocks the synthesis of androgen by interfering with the late reactions in androgen biosynthesis. Spironolactone and cimetidine also compete with androgen for the cytoplasmic receptor protein and thus interfere with androgen action in the target cell. Testosterone levels may be low and estradiol levels may be elevated in patients taking large amounts of marijuana, heroin, or methadone, although the exact reasons are unclear. Alcohol, when consumed in excess for prolonged periods, causes decreased plama testosterone, independent of liver disease or malnutrition. Elevated plasma estradiol levels and decreased plasma testosterone levels have been reported in men taking digitalis.

A number of cancer chemotherapeutic agents interfere with spermatogenesis and rarely with Leydig cell function; the most important is cyclophosphamide which causes azoospermia or extreme oligospermia within a few weeks after the initiation of therapy. Cessation of drug therapy is followed by a return of spermatogenesis within 3 years in about half of patients. Any agent that interferes with testosterone synthesis or action can also result in decreased sperm production.

Testicular failure has been described as a part of a generalized disorder of *autoimmunity* in which multiple primary endocrine deficiencies coexist (Schmidt syndrome) and in which circulating antibodies to the basement membrane of the testes are present (see Chap. 123). Sperm antibodies are a rare cause of isolated male infertility (less than 1 percent of cases). In some instances such antibodies appear to be secondary phenomena resulting from duct obstruction or vasectomy. *Granulomatous diseases* can also destroy the testes, the most common such disorder being leprosy. Testicular atrophy occurs in 10 to 20 percent of men with lepromatous leprosy, the result of direct invasion of the tissue by the mycobacteria. The tubules are involved initially, followed by endarteritis and destruction of Leydig cells.

TESTICULAR ABNORMALITIES ASSOCIATED WITH SYSTEMIC DISEASE The common systemic diseases that cause combined underandrogenization and infertility are liver disease and renal failure. In chronic *liver disease* a combined testicular and pituitary lesion leads to decreased testosterone production. Although plasma LH is elevated, the level may be below the expected range given the degree of androgen deficiency. This is most likely the result of inhibition of LH secretion by the higher estrogen concentrations found in patients with chronic liver disease. Increased estrogen production results from impaired hepatic extraction of adrenal androstenedione and subsequent increased peripheral conversion to estrone and estradiol. In effect there is shunting of estrogen precursors to aromatization sites in peripheral tissues. Testicular atrophy and gynecomastia are present in about half of men with cirrhosis.

In chronic *renal failure* decreased androgen synthesis and diminution of sperm production develop in the setting of elevated plasma gonadotropins. The elevated LH is due to increased production as well as reduced clearance but is incapable of effecting normal testosterone production. In addition, about half of men with chronic renal failure have hyperprolactinemia. The role of the hyperprolactinemia in decreasing testosterone production is unclear. Only slight improvement in testosterone production occurs with hemodialysis, but successful transplantation may lead to return of testicular function to normal.

Men with *sickle cell anemia* often have depressed testosterone levels with elevated gonadotropins, implying a defect at the testicular level. The temporary decrease in sperm density that occurs following *acute febrile illness* usually occurs in the absence of any changes in testosterone production. The major *neurological diseases* associated with altered testicular function are myotonic dystrophy and paraplegia. In myotonic dystrophy small testes may be associated with abnormalities of both spermatogenesis and Leydig cell function. Spinal cord lesions resulting in paraplegia lead to a temporary decrease in testosterone levels that tend to return to normal but persistent defects in spermatogenesis; some patients retain the capacity to obtain erection and to ejaculate.

Posttesticular A posttesticular defect can also result in combined underandrogenization and infertility. Defects of the androgen receptor cause resistance to the action of androgen usually associated with defective male phenotypic development as well as infertility and underandrogenization (see Chap. 120). However, some men with familial Reifenstein syndrome have a less complete androgen resistance with no abnormalities of phenotypic development except for azoospermia but with endocrine and tissue culture evidence of a defective androgen receptor. An even less severe form of androgen resistance is associated with infertility due to oligo- or azoospermia in otherwise phenotypically normal men; this form of androgen resistance may be the etiology in 40 percent of men with infertility previously classified as having idiopathic azoospermia.

A posttesticular disorder that causes about 3 percent of infertility without underandrogenization is absence or obstruction of the vas deferens. The disorder was more common in the past when tuberculosis and gonorrhea often resulted in obstruction to the vas. Congenital defects of the vas deferens can occur as an isolated abnormality associated with absence of the seminal vesicles (and consequently absence of fructose in the ejaculate), in patients with cystic fibrosis, or as a consequence of diethylstilbestrol administration to women during pregnancy.

About 25 percent of infertile men apparently have infertility of unknown etiology; none of the above conditions is found on careful search. The therapy in these patients, as in all infertile men except those with surgically correctable varicocele, vas deferens obstruction, or treatable endocrinopathy, is unsatisfactory. Empirical therapy with androgens or gonadotropins probably has no significant effect on fertility. Although the semen quality may improve with such treatment, the pregnancy rate is usually no greater than in infertile men given no therapy (25 percent fertility in patients followed for a year). This latter fact should be kept in mind, namely that spontaneous resolution may occur in a fourth of patients with idiopathic infertility followed with no treatment.

Fertility control in the male Although a variety of approaches to fertility control in men have been tried, including radiation and drug therapy, the most practical means is ligation of the vas deferens, a procedure that can be performed on an outpatient basis and that has been utilized successfully in large numbers of men. The time required for azoospermia to occur following the operation depends upon the number of sperm in the terminal vas deferens and ejaculatory ducts at the time of surgery but is usually less than 40 days. Azoospermia should be documented in each case to prove effectiveness. No deleterious effects on either testosterone production or the hypothalamic-pituitary axis have been documented. The subsequent infertility is not always reversible. Vasovasostomy for reanastomosis of the vas has a success rate of about 90 percent as judged by return of sperm to the ejaculate, but only about 50 percent subsequently achieve fertility. This discrepancy is possibly due to the development of antisperm antibodies consequent to vasectomy.

OLD AGE Beginning at about age 70 mean plasma testosterone concentrations decline. This decrease occurs despite an elevation in TeBG so that the level of free testosterone decreases even more than the total. Though statistically lower than average, both total and free concentrations of testosterone usually remain within the normal range. There is, however, an associated rise in plasma LH and an increase in the rate of conversion of androgen to estrogen in peripheral tissues so that the effective ratio of androgen to estrogen decreases. These endocrine changes in the aging man are believed to be critical for the development of prostatic hyperplasia and probably for development of gynecomastia in aging men (see Chap. 119), but there is no convincing evidence that such changes have any direct bearing on sexual activity in the elderly.

Prostatic hyperplasia The development of benign prostatic hyperplasia is an almost universal phenomenon in aging men. The prostate weighs only a few grams at birth; at puberty it undergoes androgen-induced growth and reaches the adult size of approximately 20 g by about age 20. It remains stable in weight and histological characteristics for about 25 years. In the fifth decade a second growth spurt starts in the majority of men. Unlike the early growth, which involves the gland diffusely, this second growth phase begins in the periurethral area of the gland as a localized proliferation; it may progress to compress the remaining normal gland, result in a major increase in gland size, and cause urinary and/or rectal obstruction. This growth, like that at puberty, requires a functioning testis. Although the concentration of testosterone in normal and hyperplastic prostates is similar, there is a fivefold increase in the concentration of dihydrotestosterone in hyperplastic as compared to normal glands. The administration to the castrate dog of dihydrotestosterone results in prostatic enlargement comparable to that seen in the naturally occurring disorder. Estradiol acts synergistically with dihydrotestosterone to induce canine prostatic hyperplasia by enhancing the amount of high-affinity androgen receptor protein in the tissue. Since estradiol production is known to increase with age in men and since the human prostate contains a high-affinity estradiol receptor, this finding provides a potential explanation of the occurrence of prostatic hyperplasia with advancing age. Both androgen and estrogen are probably involved in the pathogenesis; its occurrence in elderly men can be explained if dihydrotestosterone is the actual mediator of the hyperplasia and estradiol augments dihydrotestosterone action in the face of declining androgen production. The mechanism by which accumulation of dihydrotestosterone leads to pathological growth remains to be determined. Whatever the etiology, the only treatment at present is surgical.

Cancer of the prostate See Chap. 127.

DISORDERS OF ALL AGES **Testicular tumors** Testicular tumors occur with an incidence of 2 to 2.5 per 100,000 men per year in the United States and account for less than 1 percent of cancer deaths in men. The incidence shows a trimodal curve with peaks in childhood, young adult life, and old age. Testicular maldescent is a predisposing factor for tumor development. About one in five tumors that occur in patients with unilateral cryptorchidism develops in the contralateral descended testis. If boys undergo surgical correction of cryptorchidism before puberty, tumors are rare. Tumors originating from germ cells are more common than those derived from the stroma.

GERMINAL-CELL TUMORS There are four types of germinal-cell tumors: seminomas, embryonal carcinomas, choriocarcinomas, and teratomas; 40 percent of germinal-cell tumors contain two or more cell types.

Seminomas can be divided into spermatocytic and anaplastic types and are characterized by large cells with clear cytoplasm. They account for at least half of testicular neoplasms. Spermatocytic seminomas in older men are associated with a 90 to 95 percent 5-year survival. Embryonal carcinomas are the most frequent testicular tumors in childhood and have 5-year survivals of 70 percent in infants and 20 to 30 percent in adults. Choriocarcinomas contain syncytiotrophoblastic cells, occur primarily in the second and third decades, and carry a poor prognosis. Teratomas contain cells derived from at least two germ layers and may be benign or malignant. They comprise only 9 percent of adult tumors but are the second most common tumor of the testis in childhood. Of the mixed tumors of germ-cell origin, perhaps the most distinctive is the gonadoblastoma which is characterized by the presence of germ cells, sex-cord cells, and usually Leydig cells. These tumors commonly originate from dysgenetic testes containing a Y chromosome and usually produce androgen.

STROMAL-CELL TUMORS The most common stromal-cell malignancies are Leydig cell and Sertoli cell tumors. They are rare in children and are usually benign. Leydig (interstitial) cell tumors may result in masculinization or feminization or both, or they may have no hormonal effect. Sertoli cell tumors (androblastomas) contain cells that are arranged in tubule-like fashion and may also result in feminization or (rarely) virilization.

ENDOCRINE MANIFESTATION OF TESTICULAR TUMORS Chorionic gonadotropin is present in normal testes, and it is therefore not surprising that plasma gonadotropins are elevated in testicular tumors. Indeed, an elevated plasma level of the beta subunit of human chorionic gonadotropins (HCG-β) serves as a sensitive and specific marker of tumor activity in a fourth of cases. Plasma levels of the beta subunit are elevated in all patients with choriocarcinoma, in a third of embryonal carcinomas and teratocarcinomas, and rarely in seminomas. There is a good correlation between change in HCG-β levels and response to therapy.

Elevated estradiol and testosterone production in patients with testicular tumors can arise by at least two mechanisms. In trophoblastic tumors and in tumors of Leydig and Sertoli cells production of both hormones occurs autonomously in the tumor tissue itself; in these instances plasma gonadotropin levels and hormone production by the uninvolved portions of the testes are depressed, and azoospermia is common. However, when gonadotropins are secreted by the tumor, the gonadotropin acts to increase estradiol and testosterone production in the unaffected areas of the testes, and azoospermia is uncommon. When potent estrogens and androgens are formed (directly or indirectly) by the tumors, feminization, virilization, or no obvious change may result, depending on the pattern of hormones produced and the age of the patients involved. Other cellular markers of testicular tumor activity have been described in individual cases, including alpha fetoprotein.

Gynecomastia See Chap. 119.

HORMONAL THERAPY

ANDROGENS **Pharmacologic preparations** Effective androgen therapy requires the use of chemically modified analogues of testosterone. When testosterone itself is administered by mouth it is absorbed into the portal blood and degraded promptly by the liver so that insignificant amounts reach the systemic circulation; when injected parenterally testosterone is rapidly absorbed from the injection vehicle so that it is difficult to sustain effective levels in the plasma. Therefore, it is necessary to modify the molecule so as to retard the rate of absorption or catabolism in order to sustain effective blood levels or to enhance the androgenic potency of each molecule so that full androgenic effects can be achieved at a lower blood level of the drug. Three types of modification of the molecule have received widespread clinical application (Fig. 117-7), namely esterification of the 17β-hydroxyl group, alkylation at the 17α position, and modification of the ring structure, particularly substitutions at the 2, 9, and 11 positions. Esterification serves to decrease the polarity of the molecule. Consequently, the steroid is more soluble in the fat vehicles used for injection, and release of the steroid into the circulation is slowed. Esters cannot be administered by mouth and must be injected parenterally. The more carbon molecules in the acid esterified, the more prolonged the action. Currently available esters such as testosterone cypionate and testosterone enanthate can be injected every 1 to 3 weeks. Because the esters are hydrolyzed before the hormones act, the effectiveness of therapy can be monitored by assaying the plasma level of testosterone with time following administration.

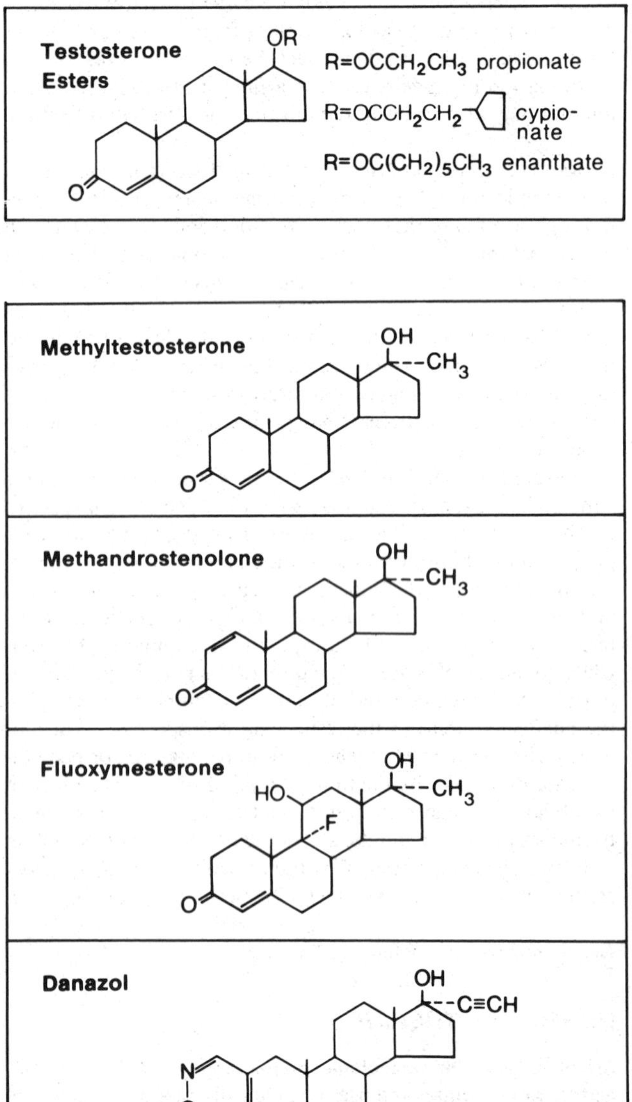

The effectiveness of 17α-alkylated androgens (such as methyltestosterone and methandrostenolone) when given by mouth is due to slower hepatic catabolism than occurs with testosterone itself so that the alkylated derivatives escape degradation by the liver and reach the systemic circulation. For this reason 17α-methyl or -ethyl substitution is a common feature of most orally active androgens. Unfortunately, all 17α-alkylated steroids may cause abnormalities of liver function, and for this reason they have a limited role in medicine.

A variety of other alterations of the ring structure of the androgen molecule have been adopted empirically; in some instances the modification slows the rate of inactivation, in others it enhances the potency of a given molecule, and in still others it alters the conversion to other active metabolites. For example, the potency of fluoxymesterone may be due to the fact that, unlike most androgens, it is a poor precursor for conversion to estrogens in peripheral tissues.

Side effects of androgens All androgens carry the risk of inducing virilization in women. Among the early manifestations are acne, coarsening of the voice, and development of hirsutism. Menstrual irregularities are common. If treatment is discontinued as soon as these effects develop, the manifestations may slowly subside. With prolonged treatment, male-pattern baldness, worsening of the hirsutism and voice changes, and hypertrophy of the clitoris develop and are largely irreversible. There is considerable variation in the frequency and the degree to which these signs develop in women. The variation in response probably results from several factors including individual differences in susceptibility, variability in steady-state blood levels among individuals, and variable duration of therapy. In general, the younger the patient, the more striking the virilizing signs; nevertheless, florid virilization can also occur in adult women.

Some degree of sodium retention is an inevitable consequence of androgen therapy, but usually the amount of retained sodium is limited. However, in patients with underlying heart disease or renal failure, or when androgens are administered in enormous amounts, as in some patients with carcinoma of the breast, the degree of sodium retention may be sufficient to produce edema. Although androgens do not cause malignancy, they may promote growth of and intensify pain from carcinoma of the prostate and from breast carcinoma in men.

Feminizing side effects of androgen therapy in men are poorly understood. Testosterone itself can be converted (aromatized) in peripheral tissues to estradiol. In contrast, 5α-reduction of the molecule precludes estrogen formation. The commonest manifestation of feminization is development of gynecomastia. Such breast enlargement is common in children given androgens and correlates with an increase in urinary estrogens, possibly because of a greater capacity to convert androgens to estrogens in childhood. The administration of testosterone esters to men results in an increase in plasma estrogen levels. In men with normal liver function, gynecomastia usually develops only after high doses of androgens.

All 17α-alkylated androgens produce sodium sulfobromophthalein [Bromsulphalein (BSP)] retention and frequently cause elevation of plasma alkaline phosphatase and conjugated bilirubin. The incidence of clinically manifest liver disease probably depends upon the previous integrity of the liver, but jaundice may occur even in the absence of preexisting liver disease. 17α-Alkylated drugs also cause an increase in a variety of plasma proteins that are synthesized in the liver. The most serious complications of oral androgen therapy are the development of peliosis hepatis (blood-filled cysts in the liver) and

FIGURE 117-7
Some of the androgen preparations available for pharmacologic use.

Testosterone Esters
R=OCCH$_2$CH$_3$ propionate
R=OCCH$_2$CH$_2$- cypionate
R=OC(CH$_2$)$_5$CH$_3$ enanthate

Methyltestosterone

Methandrostenolone

Fluoxymesterone

Danazol

hepatoma. These disorders were initially described in patients with aplastic anemia, many of whom have Fanconi anemia, itself a predisposing factor for the development of malignancy. However, both lesions have also been reported in patients who received oral androgens for a variety of other causes, including use by athletes. There may be a similar increased incidence of hepatocellular neoplasms in women taking oral contraceptives. Although in some individuals these tumors regress and follow a benign course after discontinuation of the drugs, in others the course is rapidly fatal.

One indication for the use of 17α-alkylated androgens is in hereditary angioneurotic edema; in this disorder the desired therapeutic benefit (increase in the level of the inhibitor of the first component of complement) may actually be a side effect of the 17-alkylated steroid rather than an effect of the parent androgen itself. As a consequence, weak androgens such as danazol are effective in this disorder (Fig. 117-6). Another indication for danazol is in the management of endometriosis (see Chap. 45).

Replacement therapy The aim of androgen therapy in hypogonadal men is to restore or bring to normal male secondary sexual characteristics (beard, body hair, external genitalia) and male sexual behavior and to mimic the hormonal effects on somatic development (hemoglobin, muscle mass, nitrogen balance, and epiphyseal closure). Since an assay for plasma testosterone is available for monitoring therapy, the treatment of androgen deficiency is almost universally successful. The parenteral administration of a long-acting testosterone ester such as 100 to 200 mg testosterone enanthate at 1- to 3-week intervals results in a sustained increase in plasma testosterone to the normal male range. Such esters act only through the release of testosterone itself into the circulation. If the hypogonadism is primary and of long duration (as in the Klinefelter syndrome) suppression of plasma LH to the normal range may not occur for many weeks, if at all. Considerable variability exists in the relation between plasma testosterone and male sexual behavior, but in postpubertal testicular failure (even of many years duration) resumption of normal sexual activity is usual following adequate replacement. Androgen does not restore spermatogenesis in hypogonadal states, but the volume of the ejaculate (derived largely from the prostate and seminal vesicles) and male secondary sex characteristics return to normal. The effects of endogenous androgen on hemoglobin, nitrogen retention, and skeletal development are also reproduced.

In patients of all ages in whom hypogonadism developed prior to expected puberty (such as patients with hypogonadotropic hypogonadism) it is appropriate to bring plasma testosterone into the adult range slowly. When therapy is commenced at the time of expected puberty in such patients, the normal events of male puberty proceed in the usual fashion. If therapy is delayed until long after the time of usual puberty the degree to which normal virilization will occur is variable, but many patients undergo a relatively complete anatomic and functional maturation. Intermittent low-dose androgen therapy is indicated in prepubertal hypogonadal boys with microphallus to bring the external genitalia into the normal range. If such patients are monitored closely and given androgens only for short periods such therapy usually has no adverse effects on somatic growth.

In boys of pubertal age with either isolated hypogonadotropic hypogonadism or primary testicular deficiency, the usual practice is to institute androgen therapy between the ages of 12 and 14 years, depending on the subjective need for sexual development. No androgen therapy should be instituted until a diagnosis of either primary or secondary hypogonadism is established and the possibility is excluded that apparent hypogonadism is actually the result only of a delayed puberty. The initial administration of small doses of testosterone esters followed by a gradual increase to 100 to 150 mg/m^2 every 1 to 3 weeks should result in a normal pubertal growth spurt. The time from the start of treatment to the appearance of secondary sex characteristics is variable. Penile development, deepening of the voice, and other secondary sexual characteristics usually commence during the first year of treatment. In normal boys puberty extends over several years, and treatment designed to replicate normal development does not shorten the process greatly.

Testosterone exerts its full action only in the presence of a balanced hormonal environment and, particularly, in the presence of adequate levels of growth hormone. Consequently, prepubertal patients who have coexisting growth hormone deficiency exhibit a diminished response to androgens both in regard to growth and to the development of secondary sex characteristics unless sufficient growth hormone is given simultaneously.

Pharmacologic uses Androgens have been used for a variety of disorders unassociated with hypogonadism, in the hope that potential benefits from the nonvirilizing actions of the agents (such as increase in nitrogen retention and muscle mass, increased hemoglobin, etc.) would outweigh any deleterious actions of the drugs. The most common nonreplacement uses of androgen have been attempts to improve nitrogen balance in catabolic states, self-administration by athletes in the belief that muscle mass and/or athletic performance will be improved, attempts to enhance erythropoiesis in refactory anemias including the anemia of renal failure, adjuvant therapy in carcinoma of the breast, treatment of hereditary angioneurotic edema and endometriosis, and management of growth retardation of various etiologies. Most expectations of beneficial effects in these disorders have been illusory for two reasons. First, pharmacologic doses of androgens do little if anything in men beyond the normal testicular androgen, and in women the virilizing side effects of all agents are formidable. Second, no androgen has been devised that exhibits only the nonvirilizing effects of the hormone. This is not surprising in view of the fact that all known action of androgens are mediated by a single high-affinity receptor protein in the cytoplasm (Fig. 117-5).

Of the current forms of androgen abuse, the most pervasive is the use by male athletes in the expectation that muscle development and athletic performance will be improved. Whether such improvement does result is dubious; if so, it may be the consequence of sodium retention and expansion of the blood volume rather than of a direct effect on muscle development or strength. Under no circumstances do putative benefits outweigh the risks associated with the use of oral androgens, a practice that cannot be condemned too harshly. At present, the only established indications for androgen therapy outside of male hypogonadism are in selected patients with anemia due to bone marrow failure and in patients with hereditary angioneurotic edema or endometriosis.

Parenteral administration of testosterone esters to normal men results in little effects of any kind, except for the suppression of gonadotropin secretion by the hypothalamic-pituitary system and a consequent decrease in the production of sperm. There is no real contraindication to their administration to men with those disorders (such as short stature) where their use has been advocated but the efficacy is not yet established. However, the virilizing side effects in women of androgens in usual dosages preclude their use in all except life-threatening situations. Even in potentially fatal diseases in women such as bone marrow failure and carcinoma of the breast great care must be exercised in androgen use. Administration of small amounts of testosterone cypionate (25 mg every 3 weeks) to women with primary adrenal insufficiency and/or hypopituitarism may be useful in restoring diminished libido that persists despite otherwise adequate replacement therapy; the potential of virilizing side effects exists even with these small dosages (see Chap. 112).

GONADOTROPINS Treatment with gonadotropins is utilized to establish or restore fertility in patients with gonadotropin deficiency of all causes. There are two gonadotropin preparations now available: human menopausal gonadotropins (HMG) (purified from the urine of postmenopausal women) and human chorionic gonadotropin (HCG) (purified from the urine of pregnant women). HMG (Pergonal) contains 75 IU FSH and 75 IU LH per vial. HCG (available from several sources in vials of 5000 to 20,000 IU) has little FSH activity and resembles LH in its ability to stimulate testosterone production by Leydig cells. Because of the expense of HMG, treatment is usually begun with HCG alone, and HMG is added later to stimulate the FSH-dependent stages of spermatid development. Comparison of various combinations of these two preparations in induction of spermatogenesis in prepubertal patients indicates that a high ratio of LH to FSH activity and a long duration of treatment (3 to 6 months) are necessary to bring about the maturation of the prepubertal testis. Once spermatogenesis has been restored in hypophysectomized patients or initiated in hypogonadotropic hypogonadal men by combined therapy, spermatogenesis can usually be maintained with HCG alone.

Men with oligospermia of unknown etiology have been treated with human gonadotropins; the incidence of fertility in patients so treated is probably no greater than would occur in similar groups of untreated controls.

The dosage of HCG required to maintain a normal testosterone level is variable, ranging from 1000 to 5000 IU weekly. A variety of treatment regimens have been utilized to induce maturation of spermatogenesis. Most involve starting with 2000 IU HCG three or more times a week until most of the clinical parameters, including plasma testosterone, indicate normal adult male development. HMG (usually one ampul) is then added three times a week to complete the development of spermatogenesis. After regression of spermatogenesis has occurred the length of therapy required to bring about restoration of spermatogenesis is variable and may be as long as 12 months.

LUTEINIZING HORMONE–RELEASING HORMONE In view of the finding that repeated LHRH injections lead to normal gonadotropin responses in hypogonadotropic hypogonadism, LHRH itself or any of several LHRH analogues has been utilized as the sole form of therapy in some patients with this disorder. Such preparations are not yet available for routine clinical use, and their advantages over gonadotropin therapy are not clear at present.

REFERENCES

AIMAN J, GRIFFIN JE: The frequency of androgen receptor deficiency in infertile men. J Clin Endocrinol Metab 54:725, 1982

AMELAR RD et al: *Male Infertility*. Philadelphia, Saunders, 1977, p 258

BAKER HWG et al: Testicular control of follicle-stimulating hormone secretion, in *Recent Progress in Hormone Research,* RO Greep (ed). New York, Academic, 1976, vol 32, pp 429–476

CROWLEY WF JR et al: The biologic activity of a potent analogue of gonadotropin releasing hormone in normal and hypogonadotropic men. N Engl J Med 302:1052, 1980

DAVIS JE: Male sterilization. Clin Obstet Gynaecol 6:97, 1979

DE KRETSER DM: The effects of systemic disease on the function of the testis. Clin Endocrinol Metabol 8:487, 1979

GOLDZIEHER JW et al: Improving the diagnostic reliability of rapidly fluctuating plasma hormone levels by optimized multiple-sampling techniques. J Clin Endocrinol Metab 43:824, 1976

GRIFFIN JE, WILSON JD: The testis, in *Metabolic Control and Disease,* 8th ed, PK Bondy, LE Rosenberg (eds). Philadelphia, Saunders, 1980, p 1535

LIPSETT MB: Physiology and pathology of the Leydig cell. N Engl J Med 303:682, 1980

MACDONALD PC et al: Origin of estrogen in normal men and in women with testicular feminization. J Clin Endocrinol Metab 49:905, 1979

MARSHALL WA, TANNER JM: Variation in the pattern of pubertal changes in boys. Arch Dis Child 45:13, 1970

MEANS AR et al: Follicle-stimulating hormone, the Sertoli cell, and spermatogenesis, in *Recent Progress in Hormone Research,* RO Greep (ed). New York, Academic, 1976, vol 32, pp 477–527

OAKBERG EF: Effects of radiation on the testis, in *Handbook of Physiology,* sec 7: *Endocrinology,* vol V: *Male Reproductive System,* RO Greep, EB Astwood (eds). Washington, DC, American Physiological Society, 1975, pp 233–243

ODELL WD, SWERDLOFF RS: Male hypogonadism. West J Med 124:446, 1976

PECKHAM MJ, MCELWAIN TJ: Testicular tumors. Clin Endocrinol Metab 4:665, 1975

ROSENBERG E: Gonadotropin therapy of male infertility, in *Human Semen and Fertility Regulation in Men,* ESE Hafez (ed). St Louis, Mosby, 1976, pp 464–475

SHERINS RJ et al: Longitudinal analysis of semen of fertile and infertile men, in *The Testis in Normal and Infertile Men,* P Troen, HR Nankin (eds). New York, Raven Press, 1977, pp 473–488

SNYDER PF, LAWRENCE DA: Treatment of male hypogonadism with testosterone enanthate. J Clin Endocrinol Metab 51:1335, 1980

WILSON JD: Metabolism of testicular androgens, in *Handbook of Physiology,* sec 7: *Endocrinology,* vol V: *Male Reproductive System,* RO Greep, EB Astwood (eds). Washington, DC, American Physiological Society, 1975, pp 491–508

———, GRIFFIN JE: The use and misuse of androgens. Metabolism 29:1278, 1980

118
DISORDERS OF THE OVARY AND FEMALE REPRODUCTIVE TRACT

BRUCE R. CARR
JEAN D. WILSON

The ovary is the source of ova for reproduction and of the steroidal and nonsteroidal hormones that regulate female sexual life. The ovary undergoes striking changes in anatomical structure, response to hormonal stimuli, and secretory capacity at different periods of life. This chapter will review normal ovarian physiology as a background for an understanding of the abnormalities in development, structure, and function of the ovary and related tissues of the female reproductive tract.

DEVELOPMENT, STRUCTURE, AND FUNCTION OF THE OVARY

EMBRYOLOGY During the third week of gestation the primordial germ cells arise from the endoderm lining the yolk sac at the caudal end of the embryo. The germ cells migrate to the genital ridge adjacent to the mesonephric kidney by the fifth week of gestation and undergo mitotic divisions. The gonads exist in an undifferentiated state until the seventh week of fetal life, at which time the primitive ovary can be differentiated from the testis (see Chap. 120). Estrogen formation in the ovary commences between weeks 8 and 10, and by 10 to 11 weeks of gestation some oogonia in the developing ovarian cortex commence development into primary oocytes. The ovary contains a finite number of germ cells, the maximal number of about 7 million oogonia being reached by the fifth to sixth month of gestation. Afterward, the germ cells begin to decrease in number through a process of atresia such that only 1 million remain at birth, 400,000 are present at the time of menarche, and only a few remain at menopause. Two X chromosomes are required for normal development of the ovary; in individuals with a 45,X karyotype ovarian development occurs, but the rate of atresia is accelerated so that only a fibrous streak remains at the time of birth (see Chap. 120).

After the oogonia cease to proliferate meiosis commences, proceeds until the diplotene stage of the first meiotic division is completed, and then change very little until the time of onset of ovulation at puberty. During the fifth month of fetal life, the primordial follicle is formed, consisting of the primary oocyte arrested in meiosis, a single layer of granulosa cells, and a basement membrane that separates the primordial follicle from surrounding stromal (interstitial) tissues.

PUBERTAL MATURATION Final maturation of ovarian follicles commences during puberty. The two major hormones that regulate follicular development are the pituitary gonadotropins—follicle-stimulating hormone (FSH) and luteinizing hormone (LH). As depicted in Fig. 118-1, plasma levels of FSH and LH change throughout life. During the second trimester of fetal development the plasma gonadotropins rise to levels equivalent to those at menopause. This peak in gonadotropin levels may be causally related to the simultaneous peak in replication of oocytes. The hypothalamic-pituitary axis (the so-called gonadostat) undergoes maturation after the second trimester and becomes sensitive to negative feedback by circulating steroid hormones, particularly estrogen and progesterone produced in the placenta. The circulating gonadotropins decrease thereafter and become almost undetectable at the time of birth. In the neonate, concomitant with the decrease in estrogen and progesterone levels due to separation from the placenta at birth, there is a rebound increase in gonadotropin secretion that persists for the first few months of life. With continued maturation of the hypothalamic-pituitary centers the gonadostat becomes sensitive to negative feedback control by the low levels of circulating steroid hormones, and plasma gonadotropins again decrease.

FIGURE 118-1

Pattern of gonadotropin secretion during different stages of life in women. FSH (follicle-stimulating hormone), LH (luteinizing hormone). The secretory patterns of LH during the waking hours (clear area) and night (stippled area) for each stage are indicated in the upper insets. [Adapted in part from C Faiman et al, from SSC Yen, and from L Speroff in P Felig et al (eds).]

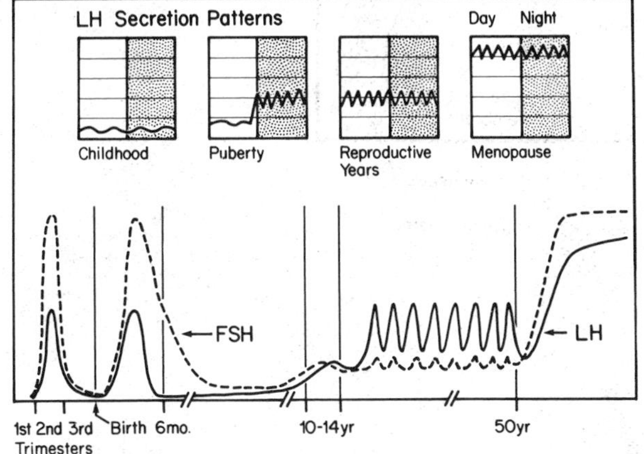

As the time of puberty nears, a decrease in the sensitivity of the gonadostat allows for increased secretion of FSH and LH, possibly secondary to increased production of luteinizing hormone–releasing hormone (LHRH) by the hypothalamus (see Chap. 109). A sleep-induced, pulsatile pattern of LH secretion then occurs, the first step in the development of a cyclic pattern of gonadotropin secretion (Fig. 118-1). The increase in estrogen secretion subsequently exerts a positive feedback which leads to an exaggeration of the pulsatile release of LH and eventually to ovulation and the menarche, after which mean plasma gonadotropin concentrations achieve adult values that are similar during the entire 24 h. After the menopause plasma gonadotropin levels rise, plateau 5 to 10 years later, and remain fairly constant until the eighth to ninth decade of life when the levels of gonadotropins may fall. Although ovarian function is regulated primarily by LH and FSH, specific ovarian receptors have also been identified for prolactin and LHRH, and both hormones inhibit steroidogenesis in in vitro preparations of human ovary, raising the possibility that they play a role in ovarian pathophysiology.

With the pubertal development of decreased sensitivity of the hypothalamic-pituitary centers to circulating steroid hormones, LHRH release by the hypothalamus increases, gonadotropin secretion by the pituitary is enhanced, ovarian estrogen secretion increases, and the anatomical changes of puberty ensue. At approximately 10 to 11 years of age the first signs of secondary sexual characteristics begin to appear in girls, namely development of the breast buds (thelarche), followed by the development of pubic hair (pubarche) and later by the development of axillary hair (adrenarche). The appearance of pubic and axillary hair is believed to be the result of an increase in adrenal androgens which begin to rise at approximately 6 to 8 years of age. A growth spurt then ensues, and a peak growth rate is attained at a mean age of 12 years.

The culmination of female puberty is the onset of predictable, cyclic menses. The average time between the beginning of breast development and the onset of menses (menarche) is 2 years. The age of menarche is variable and is determined in part by socioeconomic as well as by genetic factors and general health. In the United States the mean age of menarche is believed to have decreased at a rate of 3 to 4 months per decade over the last 100 years and is now around 13 years, a decrease believed to be due to an improvement in nutrition in the population at large. A critical body weight of around 48 kg or a critical combination of weight and body fat is associated with development of hypothalamic insensitivity to circulating steroids that leads to increased secretion of gonadotropins and finally to menarche. Obese girls with a body weight 20 to 30 percent above ideal have earlier menarche than do girls with normal weights. In contrast, malnutrition and chronic debilitating disease commonly cause delayed menarche.

MATURE OVARY Morphology The anatomical components and function of the adult ovary are illustrated schematically in Fig. 118-2. Under the influence of gonadotropins, a group of primary follicles is recruited, and by day 6 to 8 of the menstrual cycle one follicle becomes mature or "dominant," a process characterized by accelerated growth of granulosa cells and enlargement of the fluid-filled antrum. The remaining recruited follicles not destined to ovulate begin to undergo degeneration, similar to the atresia observed in other follicles beginning at around 20 weeks gestation. Just prior to ovulation, meiosis again ensues in the ova of the dominant follicle, and the first meiotic division is completed with formation of the first polar body. Rapid enlargement of the antrum (up to 10 to 15 mm in size) occurs with an associated increase in follicular fluid, followed by a thinning of the follicular surface and formation of a conical stigma. Ovulation from the dominant follicle occurs some 16 to 24 h after the LH peak as the result of rupture of the follicular wall at the area of the stigma, followed by expulsion of the ovum together with a mass of surrounding granulosa cells called cumulus cells. The final rupture is believed to result from the action of hydrolyzing enzymes on the surface of the follicle, possibly under the control of prostaglandins. The second meiotic division begins only after the egg is fertilized by a sperm, and a second polar body is then extruded. Following ovulation, the formation of the corpus luteum begins in the retained remnant of the ovulated follicle; the remaining granulosa and theca cells increase in size and accumulate lipids and a yellow pigment, lutein, to become "luteinized." The basement membrane that originally separated the granulosa cells from the stroma and blood vessels breaks, and capillaries, fibroblasts, and lymphatics from the theca invade the granulosa cells and reach the central cavity, thereby filling it with blood. After a period of 14 $\pm$ 2 days (the functional life of the corpus luteum) regression of vessels and fatty degeneration or atrophy of the corpus luteum commence and eventuate in replacement of the corpus luteum by a fibrous scar, the corpus albicans. The factors that limit the lifespan of the corpus luteum in the human ovary have not been identified. However, if pregnancy occurs the corpus luteum persists under the influence of placental or chorionic gonadotropins, and the production of progesterone by the corpus luteum for the support of early pregnancy is maintained.

Hormone formation STEROID HORMONES Like other steroid hormones, ovarian steroids are derived from cholesterol; the predominant pathway by which these hormones are synthesized is illustrated in Fig. 118-3. The ovary can synthesize cholesterol de novo from 2-carbon precursors and can also utilize cholesterol from circulating low-density lipoproteins (LDL) as substrate for steroid hormone formation (Fig. 118-4). Virtually all types of ovarian cells are believed to possess the complete enzymatic complement required for the conversion of cholesterol to estradiol (Fig. 118-3); however, different cell types within the ovary contain different amounts of these enzymes so that the predominant steroids produced differ in the various

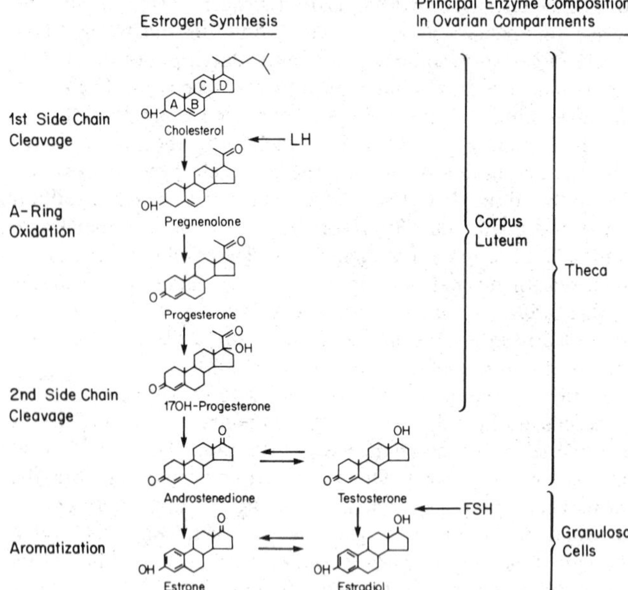

FIGURE 118-3
The principal pathway of steroid hormone biosynthesis in the ovary. Although every ovarian cell probably contains the complete enzyme complement required for the formation of estradiol from cholesterol, the amounts of the various enzymes and consequently the predominant hormones formed differ among the various cell types. The major enzyme complements for the corpus luteum, stroma, and granulosa cells are shown by the brackets; as a consequence these cells produce predominantly progesterone and 17-OH progesterone, androgen, and estrogen, respectively. The major sites of action of LH and FSH in mediating this pathway are shown in the horizontal arrows.

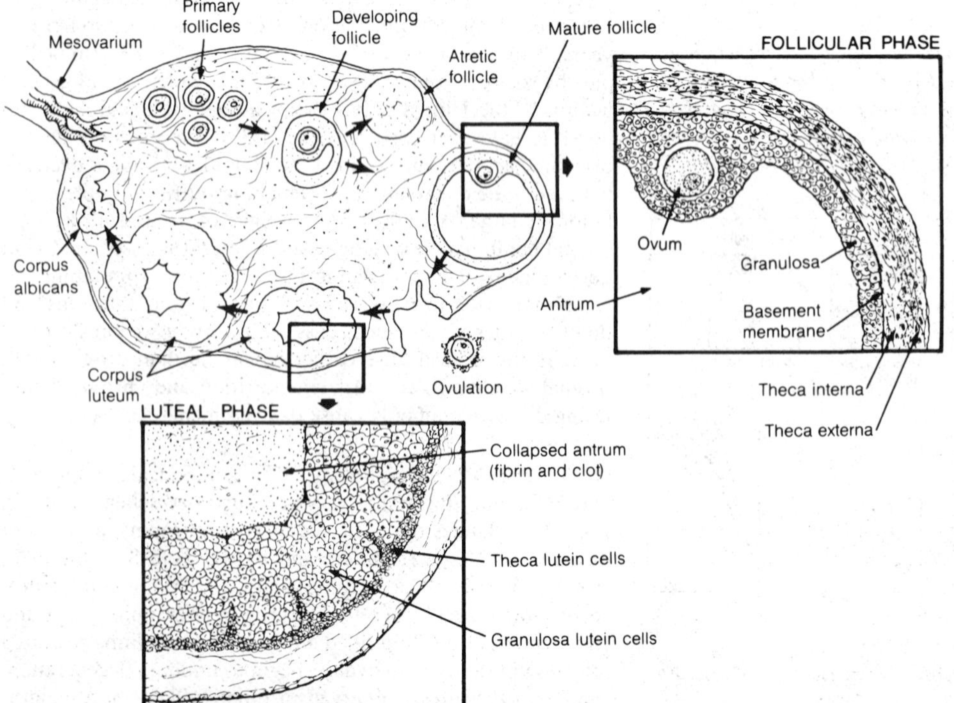

FIGURE 118-2
Developmental changes in the adult ovary during a complete 28-day cycle.

cellular compartments. For example, the corpus luteum forms progesterone and 17-hydroxyprogesterone predominantly, whereas theca and stromal cells convert cholesterol to the androgens androstenedione and testosterone. Granulosa cells are particularly rich in the aromatase activity responsible for conversion of androgens to estrogen and utilize as substrates for this process androgens synthesized within the granulosa cells as well as androgens synthesized by adjacent theca cells.

The principal sites of action of the gonadotropic hormones LH and FSH are also illustrated in Figs. 118-3 and 118-4. LH acts primarily to regulate the first step in steroid hormone biosynthesis, namely the conversion of cholesterol to pregnenolone. FSH acts to regulate the final process by which androgens are aromatized to estrogens. As a consequence LH acts in the absence of FSH to enhance substrate flow and the formation of androgens and/or progesterone, whereas FSH action is impeded in the absence of LH because of diminished substrate for aromatization.

Estrogens. Naturally occurring estrogens are 18-carbon steroids characterized by an aromatic A ring, a phenolic hydroxyl group at C-3, and either a hydroxyl group (estradiol) or a ketone (estrone) at C-17 (Fig. 118-3). (For the numbering of the steroid ring see Fig. 117-1.) The principal estrogen secreted by the ovary and the most potent naturally occurring estrogen is estradiol. Estrone is also secreted by the ovary, but the principal source of estrone is from extraglandular conversion of androstenedione in peripheral tissues. Estriol (16-hydroxyestradiol) is the most abundant estrogen in urine and is believed to arise from the 16-hydroxylation of estrone and estradiol. Catechol estrogens are formed by hydroxylation of estrogens at the C-2 or C-4 position and may act as the intracellular mediators of some estrogen action. Estrogens promote development of the secondary sexual characteristics in women and cause uterine growth, thickening of the vaginal mucosa, thinning of the cervical mucus, and development of the ductular system of the breasts. The mechanism of estrogen action in target tissues is similar to that for other steroid hormones (including progesterone and androgen) and involves the binding of estrogen to a specific cytosolic receptor protein, subsequent conformational change and translocation of the hormone-receptor complex to the nucleus, and attachment of the complex to DNA and initiation of the transcription of messenger RNA, which in turn causes increased protein synthesis in the cell cytoplasm (see Chap. 108).

FIGURE 118-4

Cellular interactions in the ovary during the follicular phase (top) and luteal phase (bottom); LDL (low-density lipoprotein), FSH (follicle-stimulating hormone), and LH (luteinizing hormone). (From BR Carr et al, 1982. Reproduced with permission.)

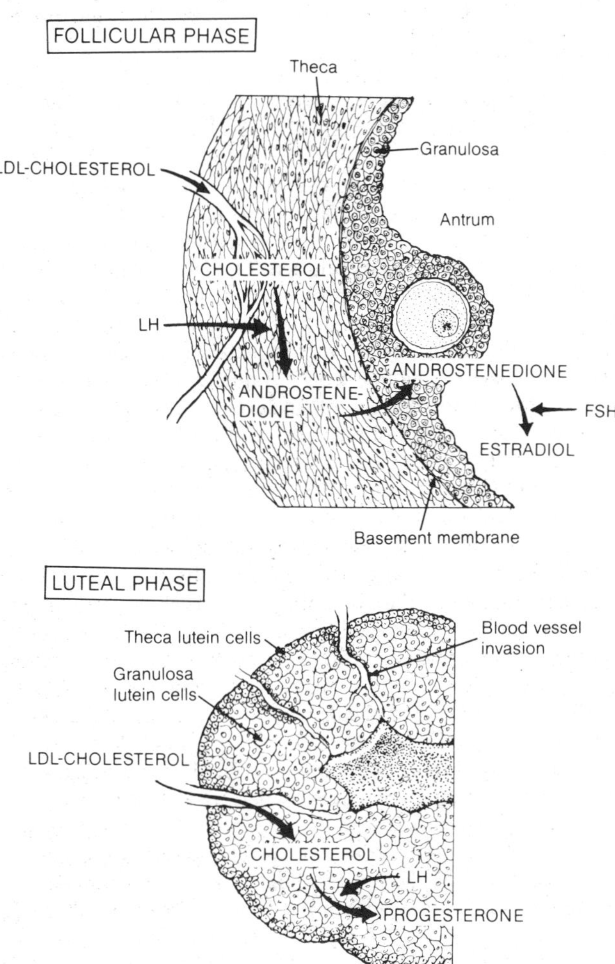

Progesterone. Progesterone, a 21-carbon steroid (Fig. 118-3), is the principal hormone secreted by the corpus luteum and is responsible for progestational effects, namely induction of secretory activity in the endometrium of the estrogen-primed uterus in preparation for implantation of the fertilized egg. Progesterone also induces a decidual reaction in endometrium. Other effects include inhibition of uterine contractions, increased viscosity of cervical mucus, glandular development of the breasts, and increase in basal body temperature (thermogenic effect).

Androgens. The ovary synthesizes a variety of 19-carbon steroids including dehydroepiandrosterone, androstenedione, testosterone, and dihydrotestosterone, principally in stromal and thecal cells. The major ovarian 19-carbon steroid is androstenedione (Fig. 118-3), part of which is secreted into plasma and the remainder of which is converted to estrogen in granulosa cells or to testosterone in the interstitia. In peripheral tissues androstenedione can also be converted to testosterone and to estrogens. Only testosterone and dihydrotestosterone are true androgens with the capacity of interacting with the androgen receptor and thus inducing virilizing signs in women (see Chaps. 48 and 117).

OTHER HORMONES A variety of other ovarian hormones have been identified but play an uncertain role in human physiology. *Relaxin* is a polypeptide hormone produced by the human corpus luteum as well as by the decidua; it causes softening of the cervix and loosening of the symphysis pubis in preparation for parturition in animals. *Follicular inhibin* or *folliculostatin* (the equivalent of testicular inhibin) is secreted by the follicular apparatus and is believed to regulate the release of FSH by the hypothalamic-pituitary unit; this hormone has been recovered and partially characterized in bovine follicular fluid but not in human fluid. *Gonadocrinins,* peptides purified from rat follicular fluid, stimulate the release of both FSH and LH from the pituitary in vitro and in vivo. In addition, in the gonads of both sexes a *meiosis-inducing substance* (MIS) triggers the onset of meiosis, an event that occurs earlier in ovarian than in testicular development. In contrast, male fetal testes secrete predominantly a *meiosis-preventing substance* (MPS) that prevents meiosis until the onset of puberty at which time MIS is formed predominantly.

The normal menstrual cycle A diagrammatic representation of the changes in circulating hormones, the sequence of ovarian and endometrial development, and the pattern of basal body temperature during the normal menstrual cycle is illustrated in Fig. 118-5. The menstrual cycle is usually divided into a follicular or proliferative phase and a luteal or secretory phase. The secretion of FSH and LH is fundamentally under inhibitory control via negative feedback mechanism by ovarian steroids (particularly estradiol) and probably by inhibin, but the response of gonadotropins to different levels of estradiol varies. FSH secretion is inhibited progressively as estrogen levels increase—a typical negative feedback mechanism. In contrast, LH secretion is suppressed maximally by estrogen in low amounts and is enhanced in response to a rising and sustained elevation of estradiol—so-called positive feedback control. Negative feedback of estrogen involves both the hypothalamus and pituitary, whereas positive feedback appears to operate primarily at the level of the pituitary.

The length of the normal menstrual cycle is defined as the time from the onset of one menstrual bleeding episode to the onset of the next. In women of reproductive age the menstrual cycle averages 28 $\pm$ 3 days, and the mean duration of flow is 4 $\pm$ 2 days. Longer menstrual cycles occur both at menarche and prior to menopause. At the end of one menstrual cycle and in the face of a waning corpus luteum, plasma levels of estrogen and progesterone fall. Concomitant increases in circulating levels of FSH are demonstrable at the end of the menstrual cycle. Under the influence of increasing levels of FSH, follicular recruitment is initiated to effect development of the follicle that will be dominant during the next cycle.

After the onset of menses, follicular development continues, but FSH levels decrease during the follicular phase. Approximately 8 to 10 days prior to the midcycle LH surge, plasma estradiol levels begin to rise as the result of secretion of estradiol by the granulosa cells of the enlarging dominant follicle. During the second half of the follicular phase, LH levels also begin to rise (positive feedback). Just prior to ovulation, estradiol secretion reaches a peak and then falls. Immediately thereafter, a further rise in the plasma level of LH occurs, and LH mediates the final maturation of the follicle, followed by follicular rupture and ovulation 16 to 24 h after the LH peak. Concomitant with the rise in LH there is a smaller increase in the level of plasma FSH, the physiologic significance of which is not understood. Plasma progesterone also begins to rise at midcycle.

FIGURE 118-5
The hormonal, ovarian, endometrial, and basal body temperature changes and relationship throughout the normal menstrual cycle.

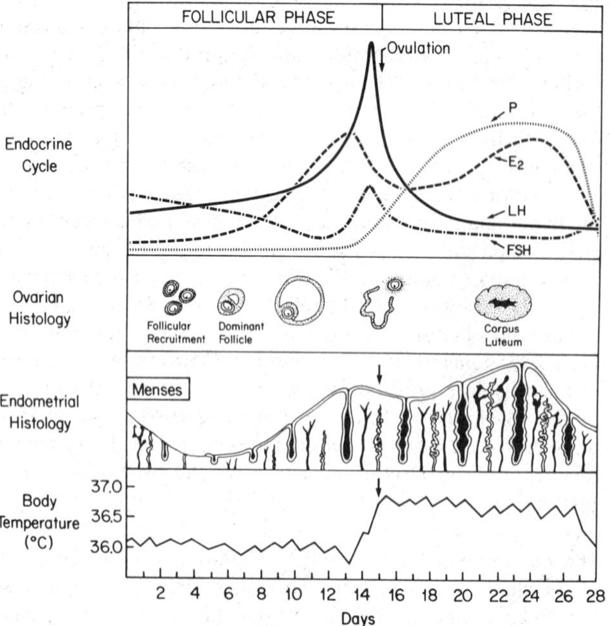

At the onset of the luteal phase plasma gonadotropins decrease, and plasma progesterone increases. A secondary rise in estrogens causes further gonadotropin suppression. Near the end of the luteal phase progesterone and estrogen levels fall, and FSH levels begin to rise again to initiate the development of the next follicle and the next menstrual cycle.

The endometrium lining the uterine cavity undergoes marked alterations in response to the changing plasma levels of ovarian hormones (Fig. 118-5). Concomitant with the decrease in plasma estrogen and progesterone as corpus luteum function declines in the late luteal phase, intense vasospasm occurs in the spiral arterioles supplying blood to the endometrium, followed by an ischemic necrosis, endometrial desquamation, and bleeding. This vasospasm appears to be caused by locally synthesized prostaglandins. The onset of bleeding marks the first day of the menstrual cycle. By the fourth to fifth day of the cycle the endometrium is thin. During the proliferative phase there is an estrogen-mediated increase in glandular growth of the endometrium. After ovulation increased progesterone leads to further thickening of the endometrium, but the rapid growth seen during the proliferative phase slows. The endometrium then enters the secretory phase characterized by tortuosity of the glands, curling of the spiral arterioles, and active glandular secretion. In the absence of conception corpus luteum function begins to wane, and the sequence of events leading to menstruation is again set into action.

Biphasic changes in basal body temperature are characteristic of the ovulatory cycle and are mediated by alterations in progesterone secretion (Fig. 118-5). An increase in basal body temperature of 0.3 to 0.5°C begins after ovulation, persists during the luteal phase, and returns to the normal base line (36.2 to 36.4°C) after the onset of the subsequent menses (see Chap. 9).

Cellular interactions in the ovary during the normal cycle As shown schematically in Figs. 118-3 and 118-4, LH stimulates thecal cells surrounding the follicle to form androgens, and androstenedione diffuses across the basement membrane of the follicle into granulosa cells where it is aromatized to estrogen.

The increase of FSH late in the preceding menstrual cycle stimulates growth and recruitment of the primary follicles by enhancing granulosa-cell proliferation, leading ultimately to the formation of the dominant follicle. FSH also stimulates activity of aromatizing enzymes in the granulosa cells that convert androstenedione to estrogen. Enhanced secretion of estradiol results in at least two other developments, an increase in the number of estradiol receptors and further proliferation of granulosa cells. In the late follicular phase FSH, acting in concert with estradiol, causes induction of LH receptors on the granulosa cells. LH acting via these receptors in turn may be responsible for the increase of progesterone secretion at midcycle. The amount of progesterone formed by the follicle is presumably limited by the availability of LDL-cholesterol to serve as substrate for steroidogenesis and by the fact that most of the progesterone formed is further metabolized to androstenedione by thecal cells. Prior to ovulation the granulosa cells of the follicle are bathed in follicular fluid but have limited access to circulating blood and consequently to plasma LDL. As depicted in Fig. 118-4, the granulosa cells become vascularized after ovulation, and consequently plasma LDL-cholesterol becomes available to serve as the major substrate for progesterone synthesis by the corpus luteum. Thus, increased progesterone synthesis by the corpus luteum is the consequence of increased substrate availability. The peak in progesterone secretion by the corpus luteum is attained 8 days after ovulation and corresponds in time to the maximal vascularization of the granulosa cells.

MENOPAUSE In strict terms, the menopause is defined as the final episode of menstrual bleeding in women. However, the term is used commonly to refer to the period of the female climacteric that encompasses the transitional period between the reproductive years up to and beyond the last episode of menstrual bleeding. During this period there is a gradual but progressive loss of ovarian function and a variety of endocrine, somatic, and psychological changes.

The median age of women at the time of cessation of menstrual bleeding is 50 to 51 years. Since the life expectancy in women is now close to 80 years, approximately a third of life occurs after cessation of reproductive function. Preceding the menopause, the pattern of menstrual cycles is variable, but generally the interval between menses becomes shorter due to a decrease in the length of the follicular phase of the cycle. In addition, there is an increase in the mean levels of plasma FSH and LH, despite the continuation of ovulatory cycles. Thus, the ovary appears to become less responsive to gonadotropins prior to the menopause.

The menopause is the consequence of the exhaustion of ovarian follicles. The decrease in the number of ova begins in intrauterine life; by the time of the menopause few ova remain, and these appear to be nonfunctional. Only a small number of ova are lost as the result of ovulation during reproductive life, the majority of follicles and associated ova being lost by atresia. The cessation of follicular development results in a drop in the production of estradiol and other hormones, which in turn causes a loss of negative feedback on the hypothalamic-pituitary centers. In turn, the levels of plasma gonadotropins increase with FSH levels rising earlier and to a greater extent than those of LH (Figs. 118-1 and 118-6). The higher concentration of FSH than LH in postmenopausal women may result from the decrease in inhibin secretion by the ovary, from the fact that FSH is cleared from plasma less rapidly than LH due to its higher sialic acid content, and possibly from the loss of positive feedback on LH production by estradiol. Intravenous administration of LHRH to menopausal women results in a pronounced increase in the secretion of both FSH and LH, consistent with the enhanced hypothalamic-pituitary secretory activity that occurs in other forms of primary ovarian failure.

The ovaries of postmenopausal women are small, and the residual cells are predominantly stromal in type. Estrogen and androgen levels in plasma are reduced significantly but do not disappear from the circulation (Fig. 118-6). Prior to the menopause, plasma androstenedione is derived almost equally from the adrenals and the ovaries; after menopause the ovarian contribution ceases so that the plasma levels of androstenedione fall by 50 percent (Fig. 118-6). However, the menopausal ovary continues to secrete testosterone, presumably formed in stromal cells.

FIGURE 118-6
Differences in hormone concentration in women during the reproductive years and in women during the menopause. FSH (follicle-stimulating hormone), LH (luteinizing hormone), E_2 (estradiol-17β), E_1 (estrone), Δ^4-A (androstenedione), T (testosterone). [Adapted in part from SSC Yen and RB Jaffe, and from DR Mishell Jr and V Davajan (eds).]

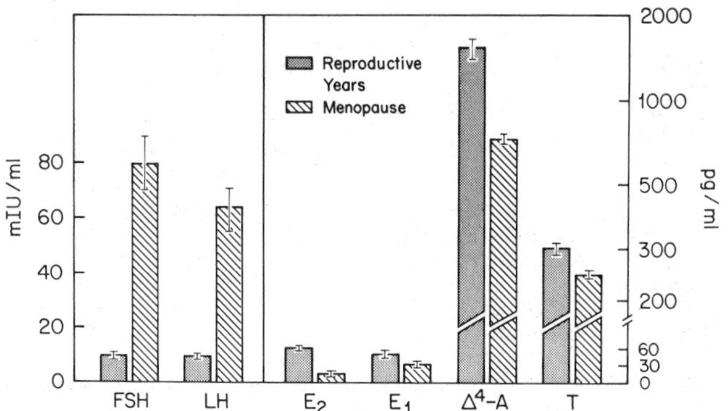

Estrogen production by the menopausal ovary is minimal, and subsequent oophorectomy is not followed by any further decrease in estrogen levels. Plasma levels of estradiol, the principal estrogen secreted by the follicle, are lower in postmenopausal women than are the levels of estrone. Circulating estrogens in the ovulating woman are derived from two sources. Sixty percent of mean estrogen formation during the menstrual cycle is in the form of estradiol formed primarily by ovaries, and the remainder is estrone formed mainly in extraglandular tissues from androstenedione. After menopause, extraglandular estrogen formation becomes the major pathway for estrogen synthesis. The rate of peripheral formation of estrone increases somewhat so that estrone production is usually only slightly less than prior to the menopause, despite the fall in plasma androstenedione. Because a major site of extraglandular estrogen production is adipose tissue, peripheral estrogen formation may actually be enhanced in obese postmenopausal women, so that estrogen production rates may be as great or greater than in premenopausal women. The predominant estrogen formed of course is estrone rather than estradiol.

The most common menopausal symptoms are those of vasomotor instability (hot flash), atrophy of the urogenital epithelium and skin, decreased size of the breasts, and osteoporosis. Approximately 40 percent of women in the postmenopausal period develop symptoms serious enough to seek medical assistance.

The pathogenesis of the hot flash is uncertain. There is a close temporal relationship between the onset of the hot flash and pulses of LH secretion. Alterations in catecholamine or prostaglandin metabolism in conjunction with low estrogen production may also play a role in this phenomenon. Other symptoms commonly associated with the hot flash, including nervousness, anxiety, irritability, and depression, may or may not be due to estrogen deficiency.

The decrease in size of the organs of the female reproductive tract and breasts during the menopause is the consequence of estrogen deficiency. The endometrium becomes thin and atrophic in most (although cystic hyperplasia may occur in about 20 percent of postmenopausal women), and the vaginal mucosa and urethra also become thin and atrophic.

The relationship between estrogen deprivation and the development of osteoporosis is not clear. Osteoporosis is one of the dread afflictions of aging. Approximately a fourth of aging women and a tenth of elderly men sustain a vertebral or hip fracture between the ages of 60 and 90, and the incidence appears to be greatest in elderly white women. Such fractures are a major cause of death as well as morbidity, and the fracture-related mortality increases from less than 10 percent in the 60- to 64-year age group to 30 percent or more in patients over 80. Many factors affect the development of osteoporosis including diet, activity, and general health. Early work suggested that estrogen deprivation plays an important role in the development of osteoporosis; however, subsequent evidence indicates that other factors are the primary causes of the increased bone fragility in elderly women: the decline in bone density commences prior to the menopause, the rate of decline in bone density actually decreases with advancing age, and the loss of bone density occurs at approximately the same rate in men and women. Thus, the loss of mineral content appears to be predominantly the result of aging itself rather than hormone deprivation. The major reason that white postmenopausal women are predisposed to osteoporosis and its consequences is that bone density in such subjects is lower prior to menopause so that loss in bone density has more severe consequences in the group. Despite the evidence that osteoporosis is usually not a disease of estrogen deprivation primarily, premature menopause in women (due either to natural causes or surgical castration) is associated with increased prevalence and symptoms of osteoporosis.

LABORATORY AND CLINICAL ASSESSMENT OF HORMONAL STATUS

A clinical assessment of the hormonal status of women can usually be obtained by taking a thorough history and completing a physical examination. In general, presence of secondary sexual characteristics such as normal female breast development indicates adequate estrogen secretion in the past, and the presence of regular, predictable, cyclic menses implies that ovulation and the production of gonadotropins, estrogen, progesterone, and androgens continue to be adequate and that the outflow tract is intact. Such a history may be more valuable than laboratory tests in evaluating ovarian hormone status. However, certain tests provide valuable ancillary information in the diagnostic workup of patients with endocrine dysfunction or infertility.

PITUITARY GONADOTROPINS Plasma gonadotropins are assessed by radioimmunoassay. Because both FSH and LH are secreted in pulsatile manner, the results obtained from a single serum sample may be difficult to interpret. Consequently, multiple samples at 20-min intervals for 2 h may be pooled to obtain a mean value. Serum gonadotropin levels are of most use in evaluating subjects with suspected ovarian failure and may also be of help in establishing the diagnosis of polycystic ovarian disease and hypogonadotropic hypogonadism. The normal ranges for serum LH and FSH in ovulating women are 5 to 25 mIU/ml and 5 to 30 mIU/ml, respectively. A persistent FSH above 40 mIU/ml is diagnostic of ovarian failure, and an LH value of less than 5 mIU/ml is suggestive of hypogonadotropic hypogonadism. In practice, however, gonadotropin values may be equivocal and must be interpreted in light of the remainder of the clinical findings.

OVARIAN HORMONES The mean plasma concentrations, production rates, and metabolic clearance rates of the principal steroid hormones secreted by the ovary are presented in Table 118-1. The metabolic clearance rate of a hormone is that amount of plasma that is cleared of hormone per unit of time and is inversely proportional to the degree of binding to plasma proteins. Thus, testosterone, which is tightly bound to testosterone-binding globulin (TeBG) (also known as sex hormone–binding globulin or SHBG) has a low metabolic clearance rate. Steroids such as androstenedione that are not tightly bound to carrier proteins have higher metabolic clearance rates. The production rate of a hormone is the sum of the amount of hormone produced by direct glandular secretion and by extraglandular conversion of prohormones and can be estimated by multiplying the concentration of hormone in plasma times the metabolic clearance rate of that hormone.

Estrogen Normal secondary sexual characteristics imply that estrogen production has been adequate (at least in the past), and indication of the current estrogen status can be obtained by pelvic examination. The presence of a moist, rugated vagina with copious, clear, thin cervical mucus that can be stretched and in which arborization or ferning can be demonstrated when spread on a slide is excellent evidence of adequate estrogen production. Demonstration by cytology of a high degree of maturation of vaginal epithelial cells and of abundant cornified squamous epithelial cells with small pyknotic nuclei confirms the presence of adequate estrogen levels.

A frequently used functional assessment of estrogen status is the progesterone withdrawal test. If menses appear within a week after concluding a trial of medroxyprogesterone acetate (10 mg by mouth once or twice a day for 5 days) or the administration of a single intramuscular injection of progesterone (100 mg), then prior estrogen priming was adequate to allow withdrawal bleeding.

Due to its variable level in plasma during the normal cycle and the difficulty of estimating the day of the cycle in women with abnormal cycles, the determination of estrogen levels in plasma or urine by radioimmunoassay is of little use in the routine assessment of estrogen status; plasma estradiol should be measured during attempts to induce ovulation with human menopausal gonadotropins to prevent the development of the ovarian hyperstimulation syndrome.

Progesterone Cyclic, predictable menses also imply that adequate progesterone is secreted during the luteal phase of the menstrual cycle. The indications for specific assay of progesterone are in the evaluation of infertile women to document ovulation or evaluate the adequacy of the luteal phase, and in the separation of subjects with müllerian agenesis from those with the testicular feminization syndrome. Several functional assays of progesterone secretion can be utilized. The least expensive and most useful assay is the daily measurement of basal body temperature throughout a cycle. Due to the thermogenic properties of progesterone, documentation of the monthly biphasic curve with an elevated temperature for approximately 2 weeks after ovulation is a valid indication of normal progesterone secretion during the luteal phase (Fig. 118-5). Presence of viscous cervical mucus that does not stretch or fern and documentation of predominant intermediate cells on vaginal cytology provide additional evidence of progesterone secretion. An endometrial biopsy during the luteal phase on days 20 to 22 of the cycle may also demonstrate a secretory epithelium characteristic of progesterone secretion. Measurement of serum pro-

TABLE 118-1
Concentrations, metabolic clearance rates, and production rates of the major ovarian steroid hormones in blood of ovulatory women

Steroid	*Binding*	*Phase of menstrual cycle*	*Plasma concentration, ng/ml*	*MCR, liters/day*	*Production rate, mg/day*
Estradiol	TeBG and albumin	Follicular	0.06–0.7	1400	0.08–1.0
		Luteal	0.2		0.25
Estrone	Albumin	Follicular	0.05–0.3	2200	0.1–0.7
		Luteal	0.1		0.24
Progesterone	CBG and albumin	Follicular	1.0	2200	2
		Luteal	3–25		25
Androstenedione	Albumin	—	1.6	2000	3
Testosterone	TeBG and albumin	—	0.4	700	0.25

NOTE: *TeBG, testosterone-binding globulin; CBG, cortisol-binding globulin; MCR, metabolic clearance rate.*
SOURCE: *Derived in part from MB Lipsett, in Reproductive Endocrinology, SSC Yen, RB Jaffe (eds). Philadelphia, Saunders, 1978.*

gesterone by radioimmunoassay can also be used to establish progesterone secretion by the corpus luteum. The serum progesterone assay has replaced the older determination of 24-h urinary excretion of pregnanediol, the main urinary metabolite of progesterone.

Androgen Under normal conditions the ovary secretes androstenedione and testosterone as well as small amounts of dehydroepiandrosterone. In conditions of androgen excess, hirsutism and/or virilization are common. The laboratory evaluation of androgen excess is discussed in Chap. 48.

DIAGNOSIS OF PREGNANCY Pregnancy is usually suspected and diagnosed on the basis of the history and findings on physical examination. Namely, a woman with previous cyclic, predictable menses develops amenorrhea accompanied by breast tenderness, malaise, lassitude, and nausea, and on physical examination a softening and enlargement of the uterus is found.

Laboratory assays of placental products excreted in urine facilitate the diagnosis of pregnancy. Human chorionic gonadotropin (HCG) is secreted by the trophoblastic cells of the placenta into the maternal plasma and excreted in the urine. Assays of urinary HCG make it feasible to detect the presence of functioning trophoblasts earlier than can be recognized by clinical assessments. Three types of assay are in current use: (1) the hemagglutination inhibition test, (2) the complement fixation test, and (3) the radioimmunoassay or radioreceptor assay. The most commonly utilized of these tests is the latex slide agglutination-inhibition test, which can be performed in about 2 min; there are occasional false-positive and false-negative results. Radioimmunoassay of the β subunit of HCG in serum or urine makes it possible to differentiate between excess LH and HCG, an important distinction in evaluating women with trophoblastic disease such as hydatidiform mole or choriocarcinoma.

DISORDERS OF OVARIAN FUNCTION

PREPUBERTAL YEARS Puberty in girls is said to be precocious if the onset of breast budding occurs before the age of 8 or if menarche commences before the age of 9. Those disorders in which the developing sexual characteristics are appropriate for the genetic and gonadal sex, i.e., feminization in girls or virilization in boys, are termed *isosexual precocity*, whereas *heterosexual precocity* occurs when sexual characters are not in accord with the genetic sex, namely virilization in girls or feminization in boys. Pubertal disorders of boys are described in Chap. 117.

Isosexual precocious puberty Isosexual precocious puberty in girls can be divided into three major categories (Table 118-2).

TRUE PRECOCIOUS PUBERTY True precocious puberty is characterized by an early but otherwise normal sequence of pubertal development, including ovulatory menstrual cycles. Constitutional or idiopathic precocious puberty comprises 90 percent of all cases. In these individuals no cause for the premature maturation of the central nervous system–hypothalamic-pituitary axis can be identified, and the diagnosis is one of exclusion. As many as half of these individuals have abnormal electroencephalograms. Premature development of secondary sexual characteristics and the appearance of ovulatory cycles with the accompanying risk of fertility may result in significant emotional disturbances. Therefore, prompt initiation of therapy is imperative. The usual treatment is medroxyprogesterone acetate in doses of 100 to 200 mg given intramuscularly every 2 to 4 weeks to suppress gonadotropin secretion. Such a regimen is usually effective in inhibiting ovarian estrogen production and ovulation but does not consistently control bone growth or prevent premature epiphyseal closure and the resultant short stature. More recently, danazol has been used but is apparently no more effective than medroxyprogesterone acetate.

About 10 percent of true precocious puberty is due to any of several organic brain diseases, including brain tumors (hypothalamic gliomas, astrocytomas, ependymomas, germinomas, and hamartomas), encephalitis, meningitis, hydrocephalus, head injury, tuberous sclerosis, and neurofibromatosis. It is essential to separate this group of patients from those with the idiopathic disorder, and occasional patients designated as idiopathic eventually prove to have brain tumors. Fortunately, most patients with organic lesions serious enough to cause precocious puberty have obvious neurological signs and symptoms. Evaluation of all patients with precocious puberty should include, at a minimum, skull films and CT scans of the brain. The success of treatment depends upon the nature of the lesion, but surgical and radiation treatment of well-localized tumors is occasionally successful.

A rare cause of isosexual precocity is virilizing congenital adrenal hyperplasia due to 21-hydroxylase deficiency in girls in whom treatment is delayed until 4 to 8 years of age. After initiation of glucocorticoid replacement, such individuals may undergo true isosexual precocious puberty (see Chap. 112).

PRECOCIOUS PSEUDOPUBERTY Precocious pseudopuberty occurs when girls feminize but do not ovulate or develop cyclic menses. Enhanced estrogen formation in the absence of ovulation can be due to several causes. Ovarian tumors that secrete estrogen (granulosa-theca-cell tumors) are the most frequent cause of precocious pseudopuberty. Granulosa-theca-cell tumors associated with intestinal polyps and pigmentation of the mucous membranes occur in the Peutz-Jeghers syndrome. Other ovarian tumors that secrete estrogens (or androgens that can be converted to estrogens at extraglandular sites) include dysgerminomas, teratomas, cystadenomas, and ovarian carcinomas. Ovarian tumors can usually be detected by rectoabdominal examination, and sonography and/or laparoscopy may also be of help. Ovarian teratomas and choriocarcinomas and other carcinomas that secrete HCG do not cause precocious puberty in girls unless there is concomitant secretion of estrogen by the tumor (HCG or LH in the absence of FSH does not induce ovarian estrogen production.) Rarely, feminizing tumors of the adrenal cause isosexual precocious puberty,

TABLE 118-2
Differential diagnosis of sexual precocity

- *I* Isosexual precocity
  - *A* True precocious puberty
    - *1* Constitutional
    - *2* Organic brain disease
    - *3* Congenital adrenal hyperplasia
  - *B* Precocious pseudopuberty
    - *1* Ovarian tumors
    - *2* Adrenal tumors
    - *3* McCune-Albright syndrome
    - *4* Hypothyroidism
    - *5* Silver syndrome
    - *6* Estrogen-containing medications
  - *C* Incomplete sexual precocity
    - *1* Premature thelarche
    - *2* Premature adrenarche
    - *3* Premature pubarche
- *II* Heterosexual precocity
  - *A* Ovarian tumors
  - *B* Adrenal tumors
  - *C* Congenital adrenal hyperplasia

either by formation of estrogens directly or by secretion of weak androgens to serve as estrogenic precursors in extraglandular tissues.

Other causes of precocious pseudopuberty include the following: (1) The McCune-Albright syndrome (polyostotic fibrous dysplasia), characterized by café au lait spots, cystic fibrous dysplasia of bones, and sexual precocity. In these individuals there is increased gonadotropin secretion, but the first sign of estrogen production is often anovulatory vaginal bleeding that occurs prior to breast budding. Occasionally, this disorder leads to true precocious puberty (see Chap. 123). (2) Primary hypothyroidism in which secretion of thyrotropin-releasing hormone (TRH) as well as the secretion of other hypothalamic hormones is enhanced, leading to increased FSH levels and ovarian estrogen secretion, frequently with galactorrhea. (3) The Silver syndrome, or congenital asymmetry associated with short stature and precocious feminization. (4) Estrogen-containing medications including use of estrogen-containing creams for diaper rash or the ingestion of any estrogen by mouth.

INCOMPLETE ISOSEXUAL PRECOCITY This term is used to describe the premature development of a single clinical pubertal event and encompasses several entities. The appearance of breast budding prior to the age of 8 (premature thelarche) without other evidence of estrogen secretion and without premature bone maturation is believed to be due to a transient increase in estrogen secretion or a temporary increase in sensitivity to the small amounts of circulating estrogens formed prior to puberty. Usually the disorder is self-limited and resolves spontaneously. Occasionally axillary hair and/or pubic hair (so-called *premature adrenarche* and *pubarche*) appear without any other secondary sexual development. The phenomenon is associated with adrenal androgen secretion in the range of normal puberty and can be distinguished from syndromes of virilization by the absence of clitoromegaly. It requires no treatment, and patients enter puberty at about the average time.

Heterosexual precocity Virilization in a prepubertal female is usually due to congenital adrenal hyperplasia or to androgen secretion by an ovarian or adrenal tumor. The manifestations of virilization are described in Chap. 48. Virilization in girls with congenital adrenal hyperplasia usually takes place in a background of variable sexual ambiguity (see Chap. 120).

Evaluation of sexual precocity The evaluation of sexual precocity involves a careful history and physical examination including rectoabdominal examination, abdominal sonography, determination of bone age, and measurement of gonadotropins (and androgen levels when appropriate). Skull films and further diagnostic tests are indicated if a neurological disorder is suspected and no evidence of ovarian or adrenal tumor is found.

REPRODUCTIVE YEARS Disorders of the menstrual cycle

ABNORMAL UTERINE BLEEDING Between menarche and the menopause, almost every woman experiences one or more episodes of abnormal uterine bleeding, here defined as any bleeding pattern that differs in frequency, duration, or amount from the pattern observed during a normal menstrual cycle. A variety of descriptive terms (such as *menorrhagia, metrorrhagia,* and *menometrorrhagia*) have been used to characterize patterns of abnormal uterine bleeding. A more logical approach is to divide abnormal uterine bleeding into those patterns associated with ovulatory cycles and those associated with anovulatory cycles.

Ovulatory cycles. Normal menstrual bleeding with ovulatory cycles is spontaneous, regular, cyclic, and predictable and frequently associated with discomfort (dysmenorrhea). When there are deviations from this pattern but the cycles are still regular and predictable the cause is most often organic disease of the outflow tract. For example, regular but prolonged and excessive bleeding episodes unassociated with bleeding dyscrasias (hypermenorrhea or menorrhagia) are usually due to abnormalities of the uterus such as submucous leiomyomas, adenomyosis, or endometrial polyps. Regular, cyclical, predictable menstruation characterized by spotting or light bleeding is termed *hypomenorrhea* and is due to obstruction of the outflow tract as from intrauterine synechiae or scarring of the cervix. Intermenstrual bleeding occurring between episodes of regular, ovulatory menstruation is also often due to cervical or endometrial lesions. An exception to the association between organic disease of the uterus and abnormal uterine bleeding associated with ovulatory cycles is the occurrence of episodes of regular bleeding more frequently than 21 days apart (polymenorrhea). These cycles may be a normal variant.

Anovulatory cycles. Uterine bleeding that is totally unpredictable with respect to amount, onset, and duration and is usually painless is described as *dysfunctional uterine bleeding.* This disorder is not due to abnormalities of the uterus but rather to chronic anovulation and occurs when there is interruption of the normal progressive sequence of follicular and luteal phases under the influence of a dominant follicle and its resulting corpus luteum. As discussed above normal uterine bleeding in ovulatory cycles is actually due to progesterone withdrawal and requires that the endometrium first be primed with estrogen (when castrates or postmenopausal women are given progesterone withdrawal bleeding usually does not occur).

Dysfunctional uterine bleeding can occur in women who have a transient disruption of the synchronous hypothalamic-pituitary-ovarian patterns necessary for regular ovulatory cycles, most often at the extremes of the reproductive life, namely in the early menarche and in the perimenopausal period, but also as the secondary consequence of a variety of temporary stresses and intercurrent illnesses.

On the other hand, primary *dysfunctional uterine bleeding* can result from at least three pathophysiological mechanisms.

1 *Estrogen withdrawal bleeding* occurs when estrogen is given to a castrate or postmenopausal woman and then withdrawn. As in other types of dysfunctional uterine bleeding, this form of menstrual bleeding is usually painless.
2 *Estrogen breakthrough bleeding* occurs when there is prolonged continuous estrogen stimulation of the endometrium not interrupted by cyclic progesterone secretion and withdrawal. This is the most common type of dysfunctional uterine bleeding and is usually due to anovulation associated with chronic acyclic estrogen production as in women with polycystic ovarian disease. Such women may have histories of irregular, unpredictable menses, oligomenorrhea, or amenorrhea (see below). Alternatively, estrogen breakthrough bleeding can occur in hypogonadal patients given estrogens chronically rather than intermittently or in women with estrogen-secreting tumors of the ovary. Estrogen breakthrough bleeding is unpredictable with respect to duration, amount of flow, and time of occurrence and may be associated with profuse hemorrhage. The endometrium is typically thin because its repair between episodes of bleeding is incomplete.
3 *Progesterone breakthrough bleeding* occurs in the presence of abnormally high ratios of progesterone to estrogen, for example, in women on continuous low-dose oral contraceptives.

The approach to a patient with dysfunctional uterine bleeding in the reproductive years begins with a careful history of menstrual patterns and prior hormonal therapy. Since not all bleeding from the urogenital tract is from the uterus, rectal, bladder, and vaginal or cervical sources must be excluded by physical examination. If the bleeding is from the uterus a pregnancy-related disorder such as abortion or ectopic pregnancy must also be excluded. Once the diagnosis of dysfunctional uterine bleeding is established a rational approach to management is as follows. During a first episode of dysfunctional bleeding the patient can simply be observed, provided the bleeding is not copious and no evidence of bleeding dyscrasia is present. If bleeding is moderately severe, control can be achieved with relatively high dose estrogen oral contraceptives for 3 weeks. Alternatively, a regimen of three or four low-dose oral contraceptive pills per day for 1 week followed by tapering to the usual dosage for up to 3 weeks is also effective. If uterine bleeding is more severe hospitalization, bed rest, and intramuscular injections of estradiol valerate (10 mg) and 17α-hydroxyprogesterone caproate (500 mg) usually control the bleeding. After initial treatment, iron replacement should be instituted, and recurrence can be prevented by cyclic oral contraceptives for 2 to 3 months (or more if pregnancy is not desired). Alternatively, menses should be induced every 2 to 3 months with medroxyprogesterone acetate 10 mg by mouth once or twice a day for 5 days. If hormone therapy fails to control uterine bleeding an endometrial biopsy or dilatation and curettage may be required for diagnosis and therapy. Indeed, uterine sampling may be indicated prior to hormone therapy in women at risk for endometrial cancer (i.e., in women approaching the age of menopause or in massively obese women); endometrial cancer is rare in ovulatory women of reproductive age.

AMENORRHEA An acceptable definition of amenorrhea is failure of menarche by age 16, irrespective of the presence or absence of secondary sexual characteristics, or the absence of menstruation for 6 months in a woman with previous periodic menses. However, women who do not fulfill these criteria should be evaluated if (1) the subject and/or her family are greatly concerned, (2) no breast development has occurred by age 14, or (3) any sexual ambiguity or virilization is present (Chap. 120). Amenorrhea is usually categorized as either primary (in a woman who has never menstruated) or secondary (in a woman in whom menstruation is present for a variable time and then ceases). However, some disorders can cause either primary or secondary amenorrhea. For example, most women with gonadal dysgenesis have primary amenorrhea, but occasional such patients have some follicles and ovulate for short periods so that pregnancies may rarely occur. Furthermore, patients with chronic anovulation (polycystic ovarian disease) most often have secondary amenorrhea but occasionally present with primary amenorrhea. For these reasons, categorization of amenorrhea into primary and secondary types is less helpful in the differential diagnosis than a classification based upon the major underlying physiological derangements: (1) anatomical defects, (2) ovarian failure, and (3) chronic anovulation with or without estrogen present.

Anatomical defects. A variety of anatomical or structural defects of the female genital tract can preclude menstrual bleeding. Starting from the caudal end of the female genital tract, labial agglutination or fusion is often associated with disorders of sexual development, particularly female pseudohermaphroditism (congenital adrenal hyperplasia or exposure to maternal androgens in utero). (See Chap. 120.) Congenital defects of the vagina, imperforate hymen, and transverse vaginal septae can also cause amenorrhea. These women frequently have accumulation of menstrual blood behind the obstruction and may have cyclic, predictable episodes of abdominal pain.

More severe müllerian anomalies include müllerian agenesis (the Mayer-Rokitansky-Küster-Hauser syndrome) (see Chap. 120), second in frequency only to gonadal dysgenesis as a cause of primary amenorrhea. Women with this syndrome have a 46,XX karyotype, female secondary sex characteristics, and normal ovarian function, including cyclical ovulation, but have absence or severe hypoplasia of the vagina. The uterus usually consists of only rudimentary bicornuate cords, but if the uterus contains endometrium, cyclic abdominal pain and accumulation of blood may occur as in other forms of outlet obstruction. A third of patients have abnormalities of the urogenital tract, and a tenth have skeletal anomalies, usually involving the spine. The major diagnostic problem is separating müllerian agenesis from complete testicular feminization in which 46,XY genetic males with testes differentiate as phenotypic women with a blind vaginal pouch and an absent uterus. Women with testicular feminization have feminized breasts but a paucity of pubic and axillary hair. The disorder is due to a defect in the intracellular cytoplasmic androgen-receptor protein that results in profound resistance to the action of testosterone (see Chap. 120). Testicular feminization can be diagnosed by demonstrating a male level of serum testosterone or a 46,XY karyotype, whereas the diagnosis of müllerian agenesis is established by demonstrating a 46,XX karyotype, biphasic basal body temperatures characteristic of ovulating women, and elevated levels of progesterone during the luteal phase.

A rare cause of absence of uterus can occur in 46,XY phenotypic women who are sexually infantile, so-called testicular regression syndrome or testicular agenesis (see Chap. 120).

Other abnormalities of the uterus that cause amenorrhea include obstruction due to scarring or stenosis of the cervix, often resulting from surgery, electrocautery, or cryosurgery. Destruction of the endometrium (Asherman syndrome) may follow vigorous curettage, usually in association with postpartum hemorrhage or therapeutic abortion complicated by infection. This diagnosis is confirmed by hysterosalpingography or by direct vision of the endometrial scarring or synechiae using a hysteroscope.

Treatment of disorders of the outflow tract is surgical. Repair of vaginal agenesis results in normal menstruation and potential fertility only if an intact uterus is present.

Ovarian failure. Primary ovarian failure is uniformly associated with elevated plasma gonadotropins and can result from several causes.

The most frequent cause of ovarian failure is *gonadal dysgenesis,* in which the germ cells are lacking and the ovary is replaced by a fibrous streak. (Also see Chaps. 61 and 120.) Individuals with gonadal dysgenesis may present with a variety of clinical features and can be divided into two broad groups on the basis of karyotype. The most common type is due to deletion of genetic material in the X chromosomes and accounts for about two-thirds of gonadal dysgenesis. A 45,X karyotype is found in about half, and most have associated somatic defects including short stature, webbed neck, shield chest, and cardiovascular defects, collectively termed the Turner phenotype. The remainder of patients with identifiable abnormalities of the X chromosome have chromosomal mosaicism with or without associated structural abnormalities of the X chromosome. The most common form of mosaicism is 45,X/46,XX. Gonadal tumors are rare in 45,X patients, but gonadal malignancies have been reported in several women with chromosomal mosaicism involving the Y chromosome. Therefore, a chromosomal analysis should be obtained in all cases of amenorrhea associated with ovarian failure, and the streak gonad should be removed if a Y chromosome is present. Approximately 90 percent of individuals with gonadal dysgenesis associated with deletion of genetic material in the X chromosome never have menstrual bleeding, and the remaining 10 percent have sufficient residual follicles to experience menses and, rarely, fertility; the menstrual and reproductive lives of such individuals are invariably brief.

A tenth of subjects with bilateral streak gonads have a normal 46,XX or 46,XY karyotype and are said to have *pure gonadal dysgenesis.* These individuals have either normal or above-average stature due to failure of estrogen-mediated epiphyseal closure in the presence of a normal chromosomal constitution. Pure gonadal dysgenesis does not constitute a phenotypic or chromosomally homogenous disorder. Some are the result of X-linked or autosomal gene defects. Other possible causes include chromosomal mosaicism limited to gonadal tissue and destruction of germinal tissue in utero by environmental or infectious processes. Approximately a tenth of such individuals with a 46,XY karyotype develop signs of virilization including clitoromegaly and have an increased incidence of tumors in the gonadal streaks; as a consequence gonadal streaks should be removed prophylactically as previously discussed when a Y chromosome is present. Approximately two-thirds of individuals with 46,XX karyotype experience no menses while the remainder have one or more menstrual episodes and are occasionally fertile.

Other causes of ovarian failure and amenorrhea include 17α-hydroxylase deficiency, premature ovarian failure, and the resistant-ovary syndrome. *17α-hydroxylase deficiency* is characterized by primary amenorrhea, sexual infantilism, and hypertension that is due to increased production of desoxycorticosterone (DOC) (see Chaps. 112 and 120). The diagnosis of *premature ovarian failure* or *premature menopause* is applied to women who cease menstruating prior to the age of 40. The ovaries are structurally similar to the ovaries of postmenopausal women, namely paucity or absence of follicles as the result of accelerated follicular atresia. Premature ovarian failure due to ovarian antibodies may be one component of polyglandular failure together with adrenal insufficiency, hypothyroidism, and other autoimmune disorders (see Chap. 123).

A rare form of ovarian failure is the *resistant-ovary syndrome* in which the ovaries contain many follicles arrested in development prior to the antral stage, possibly because of resistance to the action of FSH in the ovary. To differentiate this disorder from the 46,XX variety of pure gonadal dysgenesis, both of which are associated with sexual immaturity, it would be necessary to perform ovarian biopsy. However, such a distinction is not clinically useful since the treatment of infertility in both conditions is usually unsuccessful.

Chronic anovulation. At least 80 percent or more of gynecological endocrine problems result from chronic anovulation. Chronic anovulation is a disorder in which women fail to ovulate spontaneously but may ovulate with appropriate therapy. The ovaries of women with chronic anovulation do not secrete estrogen in a normal cyclic pattern; it is clinically useful to attempt to separate these women into those who produce sufficient estrogen to have withdrawal bleeding after progesterone therapy and those who fail to produce enough estrogen to have progesterone withdrawal bleeding and who often have hypothalamic-pituitary dysfunction.

Chronic anovulation with estrogen present. Women with chronic anovulation who experience withdrawal bleeding after progesterone administration are said to be in a state of "estrus" due to the acyclic production of estrogen, largely estrone, by extraglandular aromatization of circulating androstenedione. The most common term for this disorder is *polycystic ovarian disease* (PCOD), a syndrome characterized by infertility, hirsutism, obesity, and amenorrhea or oligomenorrhea. When spontaneous uterine bleeding occurs in subjects with PCOD, it is unpredictable with respect to time of onset, duration, and amount, and on occasion the bleeding can be severe. The dysfunctional uterine bleeding in this disorder is usually due to estrogen breakthrough (see above).

The disorder, which may be transmitted as an autosomal dominant or X-linked trait, was originally described by Stein and Leventhal as characterized by enlarged, polycystic ovaries, but in fact the syndrome and its accompanying endocrine abnormalities are now known to be associated with a variety of pathological findings in the ovaries, only some of which result in enlargement of the ovaries and none of which are pathognomonic for the disorder. The most common finding is a white, smooth, sclerotic ovary with a thickened capsule, multiple follicular cysts in various stages of atresia, and a hyperplastic theca and stroma with rare or absent corpora albicans. Other ovaries have the pattern of hyperthecosis in which the ovarian stroma is hyperplastic and may contain lipid-laden luteal cells. Thus, the diagnosis of PCOD is a clinical one, based upon the coexistence of chronic anovulation and varying degrees of androgen excess.

In most women with PCOD menarche occurs at the expected time, but further uterine bleeding is usually unpredictable in onset, duration, and amount. Amenorrhea then follows after a variable time, although in some women the disorder causes primary amenorrhea. Signs of androgen excess (hirsutism) usually become evident around the time of menarche. One theory shown schematically in Fig. 118-7 suggests that this disorder originates as an exaggerated adrenarche in obese girls. It is envisioned that the combination of elevated adrenal androgens and obesity results in an increased formation of extraglandular estrogen and leads to an acyclic positive feedback of LH secretion and negative feedback of FSH secretion so that the LH/FSH ratios in plasma are characteristically greater than 2. The increased LH levels could then lead to hyperplasia of the ovarian stroma and theca cells and increased androgen production, which in turn would provide more substrate for peripheral aromatization and perpetuate the chronic anovulation. In the advanced state of the disesae the ovary is the major site of androgen production, but the adrenal may continue to secrete excess androgen as well. The greater the obesity, the more this cycle would be perpetuated because fat stromal cells aromatize androgens to estrogens, which in turn exaggerates inappropriate LH release by positive feedback.

Thus, the fundamental defect in PCOD is viewed as one of inappropriate signals to the hypothalamus and pituitary. In fact, the hypothalamic-pituitary axis responds appropriately to high levels of estrogen, and ovulation can be induced with antiestrogens such as clomiphene citrate. The concept that the fundamental defect is one of inappropriate signals is supported by the findings in the ovary itself. Ovarian follicles from women with PCOD have low aromatase activity, but normal aromatase can be induced when the follicles are treated in vitro with FSH. In short, the anovulation is not the consequence of an intrinsic abnormality in the ovary itself but rather the result of FSH deficiency and LH excess. Recently, an association between PCOD or hyperthecosis, acanthosis nigricans, and diabetes mellitus due to insulin resistance has been reported. The meaning of this association is not clear.

Treatment of PCOD is directed toward interrupting this self-perpetuating cycle and can be accomplished in several ways, including decreasing ovarian androgen secretion (wedge resection or birth control pills), decreasing peripheral estrogen formation (weight reduction), or enhancing FSH secretion [administration of clomiphene citrate or human menopausal gonadotropin (HMG)]. The choice of therapy depends on the clinical findings and the needs of the individual patient. Attempt at weight reduction is appropriate in all who are obese. If the woman is not hirsute and does not desire pregnancy, periodic withdrawal menses can be induced with medroxyprogesterone acetate every 2 to 3 months; such treatment prevents development of endometrial hyperplasia. If the woman is hirsute but does not desire pregnancy, the ovarian (and possibly the adrenal) component of androgen production can be suppressed with the use of combined estrogen-progestin oral contraceptive agents. Combined oral contraceptives are also indicated if prolonged or excessive menstrual bleeding is present. Once androgen excess is controlled, treatment of previously existing hair growth by shaving, depilatories, or electrolysis may be indicated (see Chap. 48). If the woman wants to become pregnant, induction of ovulation is necessary. The drug of choice for this purpose is clomiphene citrate, which promotes ovulation in three-fourths of cases, and treatment with HMG or wedge resection of the ovaries may be successful in the remainder.

Chronic anovulation with estrogen present may also occur with tumors of the ovary. These include granulosa-theca-cell tumors, Brenner tumors, cystic teratomas, mucous cystadenomas, and Krukenberg tumors. These tumors can either secrete excess estrogen themselves or produce androgens which can then be aromatized in extraglandular sites. As a result chronic anovulation and the clinical features of PCOD are produced. Occasionally areas of the ovary not involved with tumors show the characteristic histological changes of PCOD. Other causes of chronic anovulation with estrogen present include adrenal production of excess androgen and various thyroid disorders.

Chronic anovulation with estrogen absent. Women with chronic anovulation who have low or absent estrogen production and do not experience withdrawal bleeding after progestin treatment usually have hypogonadotropic hypogonadism due either to pituitary disease or to any of several organic or functional disorders of the central nervous system.

Hypogonadotropic hypogonadism associated with defects of smell (olfactory bulb defects) is known as the Kallman syndrome (see Chaps. 109 and 117). Affected women are sexually infantile with a eunuchoid habitus and appear to have a defect in either the synthesis or release of LHRH. A variety of rare hypothalamic lesions can also impair LHRH production and lead to the development of hypogonadotropic hypogonadism; these include craniopharyngioma, germinoma (pinealoma), glioma, Hand-Schüller-Christian disease, teratomas, endodermal-sinus tumors, tuberculosis, sarcoidosis, and metastatic tumors that cause suppression or destruction of the hypothalamus. Central nervous system trauma and radiation can also cause hypothalamic amenorrhea and deficiencies in secretion of growth hormone, ACTH, and thyroid hormone.

More commonly, gonadotropin deficiency leading to chronic anovulation is believed to arise from functional disorders of the hypothalamus or higher centers. A history of a stressful event in a young woman is frequent. For example, chronic anovulation can begin suddenly in a woman who leaves home for the first time or experiences the death of a loved one. Gonadotropin and estrogen levels are in the low to low-normal range as compared to normal women in the early follicular phase of the cycle. In addition, rigorous exercise such as jogging or ballet and diets that result in excessive weight loss may lead to the development of chronic anovulation. The amenorrhea in these women does not appear to be due to weight loss alone but rather to a combination of a decrease in the percentage of body fat and chronic stress. An extreme form of weight loss with chronic anovulation is seen in anorexia nervosa. In this condition, the hypothalamic dysfunction is severe and may involve other pituitary hormones as well. Anorexia nervosa is characterized by the development in a young woman of amenorrhea with associated severe weight loss, distorted attitudes toward eating and weight gain, self-induced vomiting, extreme emaciation, and distorted body image. Amenorrhea in anorexia nervosa can precede, follow, or appear coincidently with the loss in body weight (see Chap. 80). During successful therapy gonadotropin changes recapitulate those observed during normal puberty (Fig. 118-1).

In addition, chronic debilitating diseases such as end-stage kidney disease, malignancy, or the malabsorption syndrome are believed to lead to development of hypogonadotropic hypogonadism via a hypothalamic mechanism.

Treatment of chronic anovulation due to hypothalamic disorders includes reversal of the stressful situation or correction of weight loss if appropriate. Estrogen replacement therapy to induce and maintain normal secondary sexual characteristics is recommended in those women with the Kallman syndrome who do not desire pregnancy, and exogenous gonadotropin therapy is indicated when pregnancy is desired (see therapy section). In other instances therapy is directed at the primary disease of the hypothalamus.

Disorders of the pituitary can lead to the estrogen-deficient form of chronic anovulation by at least two mechanisms—direct interference with gonadotropin secretion by lesions that either obliterate or interfere with the gonadotrope cells (chromophobe adenomas, Sheehan syndrome) or inhibition of gonadotropin secretion in association with excess prolactin (prolactinoma). *Pituitary tumors* comprise approximately 10 percent of all intracranial tumors and may secrete no hormone, one hormone, or more than one hormone (see Chap. 109). In the past most pituitary tumors were assumed to be nonfunctional chromophobe adenomas, but it is now known that prolactin levels are elevated in 50 to 70 percent of cases, as a result of prolactin secretion by the tumor (prolactinomas) or of interfer-

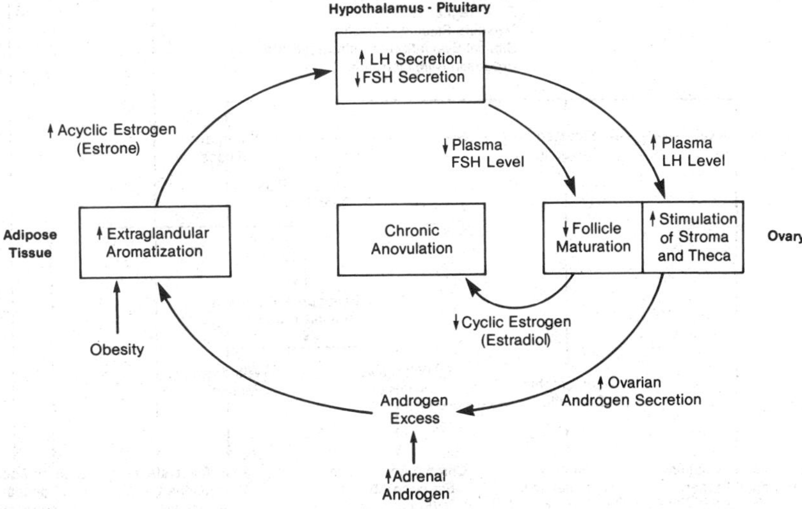

FIGURE 118-7
Proposed mechanism for the initiation and perpetuation of chronic anovulation in polycystic ovarian disease (PCOD). This cycle may be entered or initiated via adrenal androgen excess or obesity, both of which result in enhanced extraglandular formation of estrogens. The therapy of PCOD involves interruption of the cycle at various sites. [Adapted in part from SSC Yen and RB Jaffe, and from U Goebelsmann in DR Mishell and V Davajan (eds).]

ence by tumor mass with the normal inhibitory influence of the hypothalamus on prolactin secretion.

Prolactinomas can be divided into microadenomas (less than 10 mm in diameter) and macroadenomas (greater than 10 mm). Prolactin excess is associated with low levels of LH and FSH and constitutes a specific subgroup of hypogonadotropic hypogonadism. A tenth or more of amenorrheic women have increased levels of serum prolactin, and more than half of women with both galactorrhea and amenorrhea have elevated prolactin levels. The amenorrhea in this disorder is most often associated with decreased or absent estrogen production, but prolactin-secreting tumors may on occasion be associated with normal ovulatory menses or chronic anovulation with estrogen present. Most prolactin-secreting adenomas grow slowly, and some cease growth after attainment of a certain size. The increased frequency of diagnosis of prolactin-secreting adenomas is probably due to several factors, including increased awareness, improved radiographic detection methods, development of radioimmunoassays for prolactin, and possibly to the widespread use of oral contraceptives which are known to increase prolactin levels. However, since in older autopsy series a 9 to 23 percent prevalence of pituitary adenomas was observed in asymptomatic women, the clinical and prognostic significance of small microadenomas remains to be established. When tumors of any size are associated with symptoms of amenorrhea or galactorrhea, however, therapy should be considered, and when visual field defects or severe headaches are present neurosurgical evaluation is mandatory. The evaluation, differential diagnosis, and management of hyperprolactinemia is described in Chap. 109. In the latter half of pregnancy, prolactin-secreting pituitary tumors may expand, leading to headaches, compression of the optic chiasm, and blindness. Therefore, prior to induction of ovulation for the purposes of achieving pregnancy, it is mandatory to exclude the presence of a pituitary tumor.

Large pituitary tumors such as chromophobe adenomas—whether or not hyperprolactinemia is present—are likely to be associated with deficiency of hormones in addition to gonadotropins (Chap. 109).

Craniopharyngiomas, thought to arise from remnants of Rathke's pouch, account for 3 percent of intracranial neoplasms, occur most frequently in the second decade of life, and may extend into the suprasellar region. A large percentage of these tumors calcify and can be diagnosed by conventional skull films. Patients often present with sexual infantilism, delayed puberty, and amenorrhea due to gonadotropin deficiency. Craniopharyngioma may also result in impaired secretion of TSH, ACTH, growth hormone, and vasopressin.

Panhypopituitarism may occur spontaneously, result from surgical or radiation treatment of pituitary adenomas, or develop after postpartum hemorrhage (Sheehan syndrome). The latter patients exhibit characteristic clinical manifestations including failure to lactate or ovulate, loss of sexual and axillary hair, hypothyroidism, and adrenal insufficiency (see Chap. 109).

Evaluation of amenorrhea. A general schema for the evaluation of women with amenorrhea is given in Fig. 118-8. In the initial physical examination, special attention should be given to three features: (1) degree of maturation of the breasts, the pubic and axillary hair, and the external genitalia; (2) the current estrogen status; and (3) the presence or absence of a uterus. All women with amenorrhea should be assumed to be pregnant until proven otherwise. Even when history and physical examination are not suggestive it is prudent to exclude pregnancy by measuring urinary HCG. Once this is done, the cause of amenorrhea can frequently be diagnosed on the basis of the history and physical examination. For example, the Asherman syndrome is suggested by a history of prior curettage in a woman who previously menstruated; in women with clear-cut primary amenorrhea and sexual infantilism the essential differential diagnosis is between gonadal dysgenesis and hypopituitarism, and, in addition, the diagnosis of gonadal dysgenesis (Turner syndrome) or of anatomical defects of the outflow tract (müllerian agenesis, testicular feminization, and cervical stenosis) is frequently suggested on the basis of physical findings. When a specific cause is suspected it is appropriate to proceed directly to confirm the diagnosis (such as obtaining a chromosomal karyotype or measurement of plasma gonadotropins). It is also useful to measure serum prolactin level during the initial evaluation.

Estrogen status is evaluated by determining if the vaginal mucosa is moist and rugated and if the cervical mucus can be stretched and shown to fern upon drying. If these criteria are indeterminate a progestational challenge is indicated, most often administration of 10 mg of medroxyprogesterone acetate by mouth once or twice daily for 5 days or 100 mg of progesterone in oil intramuscularly. (It should be emphasized that progestin should never be administered until pregnancy is ex-

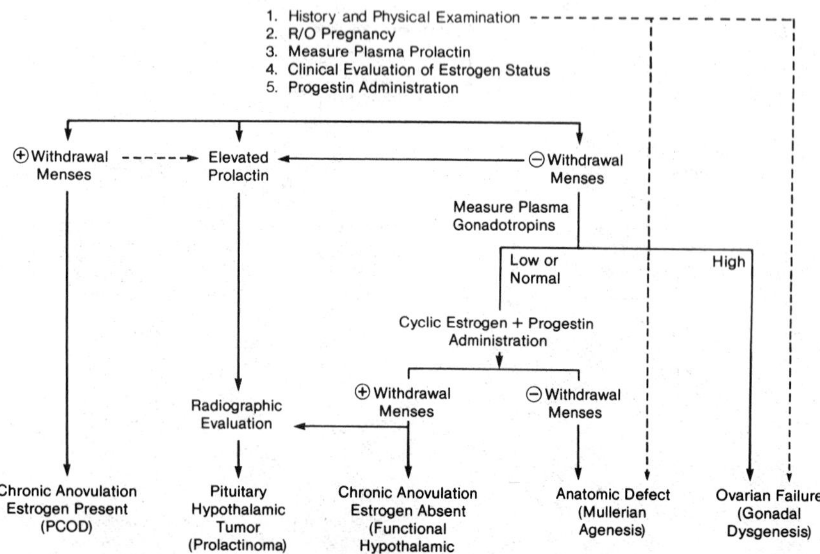

FIGURE 118-8
Flow diagram for the evaluation of women with amenorrhea. The most common diagnosis for each category is shown in parenthesis.

cluded.) If estrogen levels are adequate (and the outflow tract is intact) menstrual bleeding should occur within 1 week of ending the progestin treatment. If withdrawal bleeding occurs the diagnosis is chronic anovulation with estrogen present, usually polycystic ovarian disease.

If no withdrawal bleeding occurs, the nature of the subsequent workup is dependent on the results of the initial prolactin assay. If plasma prolactin is elevated or if galactorrhea is present, radiography of the pituitary should be undertaken.

When the plasma prolactin is normal in the woman who does not develop withdrawal bleeding after progestin administration, the measurement of plasma gonadotropins is required. If the gonadotropin levels are elevated in these women the diagnosis is ovarian failure. If the gonadotropins are in the low or normal range, the diagnosis is either hypothalmic-pituitary disorder or anatomical defect. As indicated previously, the diagnosis of anatomical defects of the outflow tract is usually suspected or established on the basis of the history and physical findings. When the physical findings are not clear-cut, it is useful to administer cyclic estrogen plus progestin [1.25 mg of oral conjugated estrogens per day for 3 weeks with 10 mg of Provera (medroxyprogesterone acetate) added for the last 5 to 7 days of estrogen treatment] followed by 10 days of observation. If no bleeding occurs, the diagnosis of Asherman syndrome or other anatomical defect of the outflow tract is suggested and is confirmed by hysterosalipingography or hysteroscopy. If withdrawal bleeding occurs following the estrogen-progestin combination, the diagnosis of chronic anovulation with estrogen absent (functional hypothalamic amenorrhea) is suggested. Radiologic evaluations of the pituitary-hypothalamic areas should be performed in the latter cases—irrespective of the prolactin level—because of the danger of overlooking a pituitary-hypothalamic tumor and because the diagnosis of functional hypothalamic amenorrhea is one of exclusion (see Chap. 109).

Infertility Infertility, the failure to become pregnant after 1 year of unprotected intercourse, affects approximately 10 to 15 percent of couples and is one of the common complaints for which women seek gynecological assistance. Male factors account for 40 percent of infertility problems (see Chaps. 46 and 117). In women, failure of ovulation accounts for 30 percent, pelvic factors such as tubal disease and endometriosis account for half, and a cervical factor is implicated in about a tenth of infertility evaluations. In approximately 10 to 20 percent of infertile women no obvious reason for infertility is found. An immunological cause may explain a large fraction of infertility in these couples. Finally, infertility in women is rarely due to *luteal phase dysfunction* in which ovulation is assumed to occur but progesterone formation is insufficient to allow preparation of the endometrium for implantation; the disorder is believed to be due to inadequate FSH secretion or action and consequent inadequate estrogen formation by the dominant follicle during the follicular phase.

The first diagnostic step in evaluation of the infertile couple is to determine whether the man or woman is the infertile partner, ordinarily by first obtaining a semen analysis in the man (see Chap. 117) and documentation of presumed ovulation in the woman. Documentation of ovulatory cycles is obtained by daily measurement of basal body temperatures throughout the month. Occasionally, accurate basal body temperature records are not obtained, and demonstration of elevated serum progesterone levels during the luteal phase may be used as evidence of ovulation. Dating of endometrium by histological exam of a biopsy sample is also useful for establishing ovulation or luteal phase dysfunction.

If the infertility is associated with amenorrhea, then the workup is that described in Fig. 118-8. If anovulation due to polycystic ovarian disease is the basis for infertility, ovulation can be induced utilizing clomiphene citrate, human menopausal gonadotropins, or, on occasion, wedge resection of the ovaries. Bromocryptine is used to induce ovulation in cases of hyperprolactinemia in the absence of demonstrable tumors. In the presence of macroadenomas of the pituitary, surgical resection should be performed prior to induction of ovulation (see Chap. 109).

Hysterosalpingograms may be obtained to evaluate the fallopian tubes and uterine cavity. Further evaluation of tubal and ovarian disease is obtained by diagnostic laparoscopy and the demonstration of dye spillage from the fimbria after transcervical injection of dye during laparoscopy. Microsurgical repair of damaged or previously ligated fallopian tubes has resulted in an apparent increase in pregnancy rates. Removal of peritubular and fimbrial adhesions utilizing laser beam surgery is another treatment mode. Endometriosis can be diagnosed by laparoscopy, and treatment of endometriosis associated with infertility includes surgical resection of the endometrial implants or temporary gonadotropin suppression utilizing danazol (400 to 800 mg orally in divided doses for 4 to 6 months) or continuous low-dose oral contraceptive pills to promote regression of the implants.

The cervical factor in infertility is evaluated by study of cervical mucus at an appropriate time after coitus. The test is preferably performed just prior to ovulation (day 12 to 13) when cervical mucus is thin and stretches and provides information as to the penetration and survival of the sperm in the female genital tract. Treatment of infertility due to such abnormality is often unsuccessful.

Since 1978 there have been several reports of successful in vitro fertilization and transfer of embryos to the mother's uterus with subsequent successful deliveries of live-born infants in women with severe tubal disease or obstruction or incompatibility of cervical mucus. The general applicability of such an approach is not established.

Medical aspects of pregnancy The possibility of pregnancy should be considered in all women of reproductive age who are evaluated for medical illness or considered for surgery. Procedures and drugs such as x-ray exposure and anesthetics may be harmful or teratogenic to the developing fetus, and a variety of medical problems may worsen during pregnancy, including hypertension; diseases of the heart, lungs, kidney, and liver; and a number of metabolic and endocrine disorders. Indeed, all women who present with abnormal vaginal bleeding or amenorrhea during the reproductive years should be assumed to have a complication of pregnancy, such as incomplete abortion, ectopic pregnancy, or trophoblastic disease (hydatidiform mole or choriocarcinoma). Women who present with these complications of pregnancy often have histories of abdominal pain and vaginal bleeding and may have evidence of intraabdominal hemorrhage.

Choriocarcinoma is a particular problem because of its protean manifestations. Half of these malignancies follow pregnancies complicated by hydatidiform mole, and the remainder occur after spontaneous abortion, ectopic pregnancy, or normal deliveries. Patients may present with intraabdominal bleeding due to rupture of the uterus, liver, or ovary, with pulmonary manifestations (cough, hemoptysis, pleuritic pain, dyspnea, and respiratory failure), or with gastrointestinal symptoms, usually chronic blood loss or melena. In addition, the tumors can present with symptoms that result from cerebral metastases, or from renal involvement. The diagnosis can be established by demonstrating an elevated level of the β subunit of HCG in plasma. Treatment and cure are possible with chemotherapeutic agents (actinomycin D and/or methotrexate). (For manifestations of choriocarcinoma in men see Chap. 117.)

Ovarian tumors Because of the wide variety of ovarian neoplasms numerous classification systems have been devised. A widely utilized classification based on histogenesis of the ovary is summarized in Table 118-3. About two-thirds of ovarian neoplasms are derived from coelomic epithelium, a fifth are of germ-cell origin, a tenth originate in ovarian stroma, and the remainder are due to metastatic tumors to the ovary. Tumors derived from each of these cell types—whether hormone secreting or not—may either be benign or malignant. Therefore, since the diagnosis is usually only made after a pelvic mass is palpable, each such mass must be considered potentially malignant. This problem is aggravated since ovarian tumors may either be asymptomatic or cause only minimal symptoms such as constipation, pelvic discomfort, or a feeling of heaviness.

Most hormone-secreting tumors of the ovary are derived from the specialized gonadal stroma and cause feminizing or masculinizing signs. The clinical picture depends on the age of the patient. Feminizing tumors in childhood cause isosexual precocious pseudopuberty with symptoms of breast development and uterine bleeding; during the reproductive years symptoms may include the development of amenorrhea or dysfunctional uterine bleeding, and in the menopausal years postmenopausal bleeding due to increased estrogen production may occur. Masculinizing tumors, regardless of the age group affected, can produce hirsutism and progressive virilization (see Chap. 48). Ovarian tumors may feminize due to direct secretion of estradiol by the tumor (as in granulosa-theca-cell tumors) or due to the increased production of androstenedione by ovarian stroma cells adjacent to neoplastic tissue; the androstenedione can then be converted by extraglandular tissues to estrogen. The latter occurs in such tumors as thecomas, teratomas, Brenner tumors, cystadenomas, and cystadenocarcinomas. Ovarian tumors that secrete potent androgens such as testosterone include the Sertoli-Leydig cell tumors (arrhenoblastoma), lipoid-cell tumors, hilar-cell tumors, adrenal-rest tumors, and gynandroblastomas.

Other clinical syndromes associated with ovarian tumors include the Meigs syndrome (ascites and hydrothorax) in association with ovarian fibroma, hyperthyroidism in association with thyroid hormone secretion by struma ovarii tissue in teratomas, and carcinoid syndrome due to serotonin formation by teratomas.

TABLE 118-3
Ovarian neoplasms

I Neoplasms derived from coelomic epithelium
- *A* Serous tumor
- *B* Mucinous tumor
- *C* Endometrioid tumor
- *D* Mesonephroid (clear-cell) tumor
- *E* Brenner tumor
- *F* Undifferentiated carcinoma
- *G* Carcinosarcoma and mixed mesodermal tumor

II Neoplasms derived from germ cells
- *A* Teratoma
  - *1* Mature teratoma
    - *a* Solid adult teratoma
    - *b* Dermoid cyst
    - *c* Struma ovarii
    - *d* Malignant neoplasms secondarily arising from mature cystic teratoma
  - *2* Immature teratoma (partially differentiated teratoma)
- *B* Dysgerminoma
- *C* Embryonal carcinoma (endodermal sinus tumor)
- *D* Choriocarcinoma
- *E* Gonadoblastoma

III Neoplasms derived from specialized gonadal stroma
- *A* Granulosa-theca tumors
  - *1* Granulosa tumor
  - *2* Thecoma
- *B* Sertoli-Leydig tumors
  - *1* Arrhenoblastoma
  - *2* Sertoli tumor
- *C* Gynandroblastoma
- *D* Lipid-cell tumors

IV Neoplasms derived from nonspecific mesenchyme
- *A* Fibroma, hemangioma, leiomyoma, lipoma, etc.
- *B* Lymphoma
- *C* Sarcoma

V Neoplasms metastatic to the ovary
- *A* GI tract (Krukenberg)
- *B* Breast
- *C* Endometrium
- *D* Lymphoma

TREATMENT

PROGESTINS The major use of progestin is in conjunction with estrogen therapy to ensure the full maturation of the endometrium, both in combination birth control pills and in the therapy of hypogonadal states. In certain circumstances, however, progestin therapy is appropriate by itself; this is generally for one of four therapeutic aims—to induce a progestational effect on the estrogen-primed endometrium (diagnostic tests for the evaluation of amenorrhea), to inhibit pituitary gonadotropins (precocious puberty in girls, and the progestin-only birth control pill), for prophylaxis to prevent hyperplasia in PCOD, and for palliation in endometrial and breast carcinoma or treatment of endometriosis. Even when a direct progestational effect is desired the currently available oral drugs substitute a synthetic derivative for the naturally occurring hormone. Oral progestins include medroxyprogesterone acetate, megestrol acetate, norethindrone, and norgestrel. Available parenteral agents include progesterone in oil, medroxyprogesterone acetate suspension, and 17-hydroxyprogesterone caproate.

The most uniform undesirable side effect is breakthrough bleeding, which is common when progestins are used continuously. Other complications include nausea, vomiting, and occasional systemic problems including hirsutism. Abnormal liver function is a side effect of those derivatives with alkyl substitution in the 17α position. Progestins are contraindicated if pregnancy is known or suspected because of a greater risk of birth defects.

ESTROGENS Estrogenic drugs are used for three purposes—the treatment of gonadal failure, control of fertility, and in the management of dysfunctional uterine bleeding and carcinoma of the breast. (The use of estrogens in management of carcinoma of the breast is discussed in Chap. 126). However, none of the presently available orally active or parenteral hormones replaces the pattern or concentration of estradiol characteristic of the normally cycling, premenopausal woman (Fig. 118-5). Estrogens that can be given by mouth are either nonsteroidal agents (such as stilbestrol) that mimic the action of estradiol, estrogen conjugates that must be hydrolyzed before they become active (estrogen sulfates, predominantly estrone sulfate from pregnant mare's urine), or estrogen analogues that cannot be metabolized to estradiol (mestranol, quinestrol) (Fig. 118-9). Even when micronized estradiol itself is given orally, it is rapidly converted in the body to estrone. Consequently, oral therapy neither replaces nor mimics the daily secretory pattern of the lost hormone; in short such therapy is a pharmacological substitution rather than a physiological replacement. Likewise, the use of parenteral estrogens rarely mimics the physiological situation. Parenteral preparations of conjugated estrogens, like the oral derivatives, are poor precursors of estradiol, and estradiol esters (estradiol benzoate and valerate) rarely cause plasma estradiol levels that mimic the normal monthly secretory pattern of the hormone. Furthermore, the side effects of estrogen substitution differ at various times of life.

Gonadal failure In women with early gonadal failure whether due to disease of the ovaries (gonadal dysgenesis) or to pituitary disease (panhypopituitarism) treatment with cyclic estrogens should be instituted at the time of expected puberty for development and maintenance of female secondary sexual characteristics. The most commonly used medications are conjugated estrogens (0.625 to 1.25 mg per day by mouth) or ethinyl estradiol or its precursors (0.02 to 0.05 mg by mouth). The addition of medroxyprogesterone acetate (5 to 10 mg daily) is recommended by most physicians during the last several days of monthly estrogen treatment to prevent development of endometrial hyperplasia in instances where long-term estrogen treatment is planned. Abnormal bleeding in individuals receiving estrogen replacement requires histological evaluation of the endometrium. Such substitution therapy or the use of oral contraceptives (see below) may also be used for the purpose of suppressing pituitary gonadotropins, as in women with PCOD in whom the major therapeutic aim is suppression of ovarian androgen production prior to the time when fertility is desired.

Temporary administration of estrogens in larger quantities (up to two times the usual adult maintenance dose) may be necessary to induce full development of secondary sexual characteristics in girls and for the control of menopausal symptoms in women following surgical removal of the ovaries. Even larger doses of parenteral estrogens (10 mg of estradiol valerate) in conjunction with progestin may be required in some instances of dysfunctional uterine bleeding. In addition to the potential long-term side effects of all estrogens (see below), these dosages may cause specific problems including nausea, vomiting, and edema.

Fertility control Estrogen therapy is only one facet of fertility control in women. Since the use of all contraceptive methods is associated with diverse side effects, an understanding of the use, methods of actions, and consequences of these agents is important to all physicians. Furthermore, since pregnancy may aggravate a variety of chronic illnesses, fertility control should be recommended in many patients.

To be effective all methods of fertility control require patient acceptance and compliance. Presently, the most widely utilized methods for fertility control include (1) rhythm and withdrawal techniques; (2) barrier methods including the condom, jellies, foam, suppositories, and diaphragms; (3) intrauterine devices (IUD); (4) oral steroid contraceptives or birth control pills; (5) sterilization; and (6) abortion.

The rhythm and withdrawal technique and the barrier methods are effective if used correctly and consistently but in actual practice result in high failure rates because of imperfect compliance. Nevertheless, since these methods carry the lowest incidence of side effects and since the side effects, when produced, are minor except for local allergic reactions, their use should be recommended in instances in which there is a relative or absolute contraindication to the use of other therapy.

The most widely utilized nonsurgical methods of contraception are the IUD and birth control pills. Both are effective but are associated with significant side effects.

FIGURE 118-9
The circulating forms of administered estrogenic drugs.

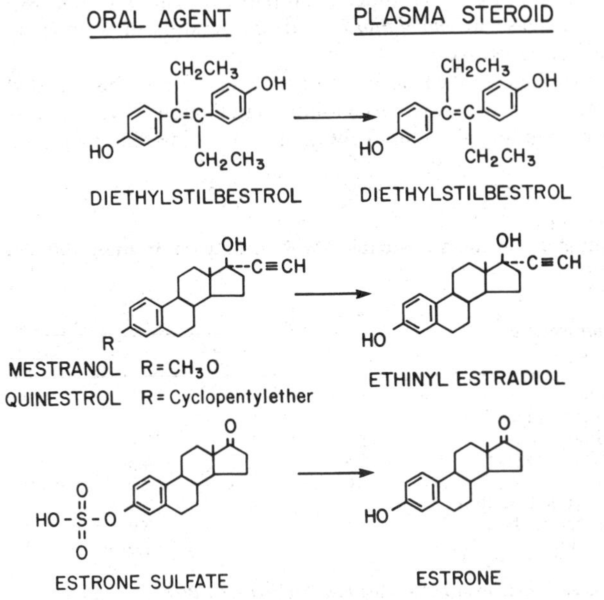

ORAL AGENT — PLASMA STEROID

DIETHYLSTILBESTROL → DIETHYLSTILBESTROL

MESTRANOL R = CH_3O
QUINESTROL R = Cyclopentylether → ETHINYL ESTRADIOL

ESTRONE SULFATE → ESTRONE

IUD The success rates of most IUDs are 95 to 98 percent. These devices are available in a variety of shapes and sizes, but the 7- or T-shaped devices cause minimal pain at insertion and are associated with low expulsion rates. Some IUDs contain copper, which enhances their effectiveness, and some contain slow-release progestational drugs, which makes replacement necessary at 1- to 3-year intervals. The IUD is believed to prevent pregnancy by the induction of a chronic inflammatory reaction in the endometrium, resulting in an unfavorable environment for the implantation of the blastocyst.

Once the IUD is inserted, it is necessary to check occasionally to be certain that the device is still in place. Both minor and serious side effects can occur. Intermenstrual spotting and increased bleeding and pain or cramps at the time of menses are frequent causes of discontinuation of the IUD. In addition, the device may be expelled spontaneously during a menstrual period without the subject being aware of its loss. The most serious side effect is pelvic infection, occasionally leading to the development of tuboovarian abscess and subsequent infertility. For this reason, use in nulligravida women is not advocated by many gynecologists. In addition, pregnancy with an IUD in place is more likely to be ectopic since intrauterine but not extrauterine pregnancies are inhibited. Because of the increased incidence of spontaneous and septic abortions when IUDs are in place, removal of the device is advised if pregnancy is detected. Any user who develops persistent, severe bleeding, abdominal pain, or discharge should have the IUD removed.

ORAL CONTRACEPTIVES Oral contraceptive pills have been used by over 200 million women worldwide and by 1 out of 4 women in the United States under the age of 45. These agents are popular because of ease of administration, low pregnancy rate (less than 1 percent), and a relatively low incidence of side effects.

The most widely utilized oral contraceptive pills are either combination tablets or progestin-only pills. A list of oral contraceptives marketed in the United States is given in Table 118-4. Combination oral contraceptive pills contain one of two synthetic estrogens (mestranol or ethinyl estradiol) and one of five synthetic progestins (norethindrone, norethindrone acetate, norethynodrel, norgestrel, or ethynodiol diacetate). The combination pills are taken for 21 consecutive days followed by 7 days' rest. Progestin-only pills are taken continuously on a daily basis. Presumably, the ideal contraceptive contains the lowest amount of steroid to minimize side effects but at the same time sufficient to prevent pregnancy or breakthrough bleeding. Combination pills containing 30 μg of estrogen and a progestin come closest to this goal.

Oral contraceptives inhibit ovulation by suppressing FSH and LH secretion. As a consequence, the secretion of all ovarian steroids is also suppressed, including estrogen, progesterone, and androgen (Fig. 118-10). In addition, these agents exert minor direct inhibitory effects on the reproductive tract, altering the cervical mucus and thereby decreasing sperm penetration and migration and altering the motility and secretions of the fallopian tube and uterus.

The death rates associated with oral contraceptives and other forms of birth control are summarized in Table 118-5. Up to age 40 the mortality rates in women using oral contraceptives and IUDs are lower than in women using no form of contraception (this difference is because of the increased risk of death associated with pregnancy). The decrease in death rate below age 40 is even more striking in nonsmokers than in smokers using contraceptives, but in all age groups the death rates from IUDs are lower than those associated with oral contraceptives. The increased death rates in women using rhythm or barrier techniques probably results from the higher failure rate and the consequent risk of pregnancy in such women. Oral contraceptive agents are not recommended for women after age 40 or in women of any age who are at increased risk for myocardial infarction (hypercholesterolemia, hypertension, diabetes mellitus, and smoking).

Despite the overall safety of these agents, users are at risk for several serious side effects. In most retrospective and prospective studies an increased risk has been found for *deep-vein thrombosis* and *pulmonary embolism.* The relative increased risk varies from two- to twelvefold and is greater for women taking pills containing more than 50 μg estrogen. The use of oral contraceptives is also associated with an increased risk of thromboembolism after surgery, and for this reason these agents should be discontinued at least 1 month prior to elective surgery.

There is a 3- to 9-times increased risk for *thromboembolic stroke* and a twofold greater risk for *hemorrhagic stroke* in users of oral contraceptives. Therefore, the drugs should be discontinued in women who experience visual complaints or severe headaches. Smoking increases the risk for stroke as well as the frequency of death from complications of deep venous thrombosis, pulmonary emboli, and myocardial infarction.

A small rise in blood pressure while taking oral contraceptives is common, but about 5 percent of women develop significant *hypertension* (blood pressure greater than 140/90) after 5 years of continuous use. Estrogens induce the synthesis of a variety of proteins by the liver including the renin substrate angiotensinogen. The consequent increased formation of angiotensin is believed to be involved in the development of hypertension. In most cases, blood pressure returns to normal when oral contraceptives are discontinued.

Serum lipids and lipoproteins are altered in women on oral contraceptives, the nature of the change depending on the specific components of the oral contraceptives. In general, estrogens increase serum high-density (HDL) and very low density lipoproteins (VLDL). Progestins may either depress or elevate the concentration of HDL.

Some women taking oral contraceptives develop *impairment of glucose tolerance* as manifested by abnormal glucose levels and elevated plasma insulin after an oral glucose load, both of which usually return to normal after discontinuing the agents. Consequently, oral contraceptives are contraindicated in women with adult-onset diabetes. Because juvenile-onset diabetes may cause an increased incidence of myocardial infarction, it is also preferable to utilize other forms of contraception in these individuals.

Oral contraceptive pills should not be used by women with abnormal liver function tests or in women with known acute or chronic liver disease. A rare complication linked to the long-term use of oral contraceptive pills is the development of peliosis hepatitis, which can cause death due to sudden rupture and hemorrhage of the liver. Cholestatic jaundice may occur in those women predisposed to the development of the syndrome of recurrent jaundice of pregnancy.

Oral contraceptives cause an increased concentration of cholesterol in the bile, which is probably the cause for the twofold increase in *cholelithiasis* and cholecystitis in women on oral contraceptives.

Estrogens induce elevation of a variety of proteins secreted by the liver including cortisol-binding globulin (CBG), testosterone-binding globulin (TeBG), and thyroxine-binding globu-

TABLE 118-4
Composition of oral contraceptives

Name	*Estrogen*	*μg*	*Progestin*	*mg*
COMBINATION-TYPE				
Enovid 10	Mestranol	150	Norethynodrel	9.85
Enovid E	Mestranol	100	Norethynodrel	2.5
Enovid 5	Mestranol	75	Norethynodrel	5.0
Ovulen	Mestranol	100	Ethynodiol diacetate	1.0
Norinyl 10	Mestranol	60	Norethindrone	10.0
Norinyl 2	Mestranol	100	Norethindrone	2.0
Norinyl 1/80	Mestranol	80	Norethindrone	1.0
Norinyl 1/50	Mestranol	50	Norethindrone	1.0
Ortho-Novum 10	Mestranol	60	Norethindrone	10.0
Ortho-Novum 2	Mestranol	100	Norethindrone	2.0
Ortho-Novum 1/80	Mestranol	80	Norethindrone	1.0
Ortho-Novum 1/50	Mestranol	50	Norethindrone	1.0
Ortho-Novum 1/35	Ethinyl estradiol	35	Norethindrone	1.0
Modicon	Ethinyl estradiol	35	Norethindrone	0.5
Brevicon	Ethinyl estradiol	35	Norethindrone	0.5
Ovcon 50	Ethinyl estradiol	50	Norethindrone	1.0
Ovcon 35	Ethinyl estradiol	35	Norethindrone	0.4
Ovral	Ethinyl estradiol	50	Norgestrel	0.5
Lo-Ovral	Ethinyl estradiol	30	Norgestrel	0.3
Demulen	Ethinyl estradiol	50	Ethynodiol diacetate	1.0
Norlestrin 2.5	Ethinyl estradiol	50	Norethindrone acetate	2.5
Norlestrin 1/50	Ethinyl estradiol	50	Norethindrone acetate	1.0
Loestrin 1.5/30	Ethinyl estradiol	30	Norethindrone acetate	1.5
Loestrin 1/20	Ethinyl estradiol	20	Norethindrone acetate	1.0
PROGESTIN ONLY				
Micronor	None		Norethindrone	0.35
Nor Q.D.	None		Norethindrone	0.35
Ovrette	None		Norgestrel	0.075

TABLE 118-5
Annual death rates associated with fertility control per 100,000 women

Contraceptive techniques	*Age group* 15–29	30–34	35–39	40–44
None	6.4	13.9	20.8	22.6
Oral contraceptives:				
Smokers	1.6	10.8	13.4	58.9
Nonsmokers	1.4	2.2	4.5	7.1
IUD	1.0	1.4	2.0	1.9
Traditional rhythm or barrier methods	1.5	3.6	5.0	4.2
Abortion	1.5	1.7	1.9	1.2

SOURCE: *Derived from Tietze, Fam Plan Perspect 9:74, 1977.*

lin (TBG). Consequently, various laboratory tests of adrenal and thyroid function may be altered and must be interpreted with caution (see Chap. 108). Oral contraceptives also lower morning plasma ACTH levels, possibly due to an inhibitory effect on ACTH secretion or cortisol catabolism. Finally, serum prolactin levels are elevated in women on oral contraceptives, but whether such treatment leads to the development of pituitary prolactinomas is unknown.

Other effects of oral contraceptive pills include minor dyspepsia, breast discomfort, and weight gain. Other side effects include development of pigmentation of the face (chloasma), which is augmented by exposure to the sun, and a variety of psychological effects, mainly leading to depression and changes in libido. There is no convincing evidence that oral contraceptives are associated with an increased incidence of cancer of the uterus, cervix, or breast.

The absolute contraindications to the use of oral contraceptive pills include previous thromboembolic disorders, cerebral vascular or coronary artery disease, known or suspected carcinoma of the breast or estrogen-dependent neoplasia, undiagnosed abnormal genital bleeding, or known or suspected pregnancy. Further relative contraindications must be weighed against the risk/benefit ratio of the oral contraceptive pills and include hypertension, migraine headaches, diabetes mellitus, uterine leiomyomas, sickle cell anemia, or elective surgery.

OTHER STEROID CONTRACEPTIVES Other types of steroid contraception other than the conventional oral contraceptives include (1) postcoital contraception and (2) injectable steroids. Use of high-dose estrogen for 5 days during the fertile part of the cycle (the morning-after pill) is an effective method of contraception, but this therapy is associated with significant side

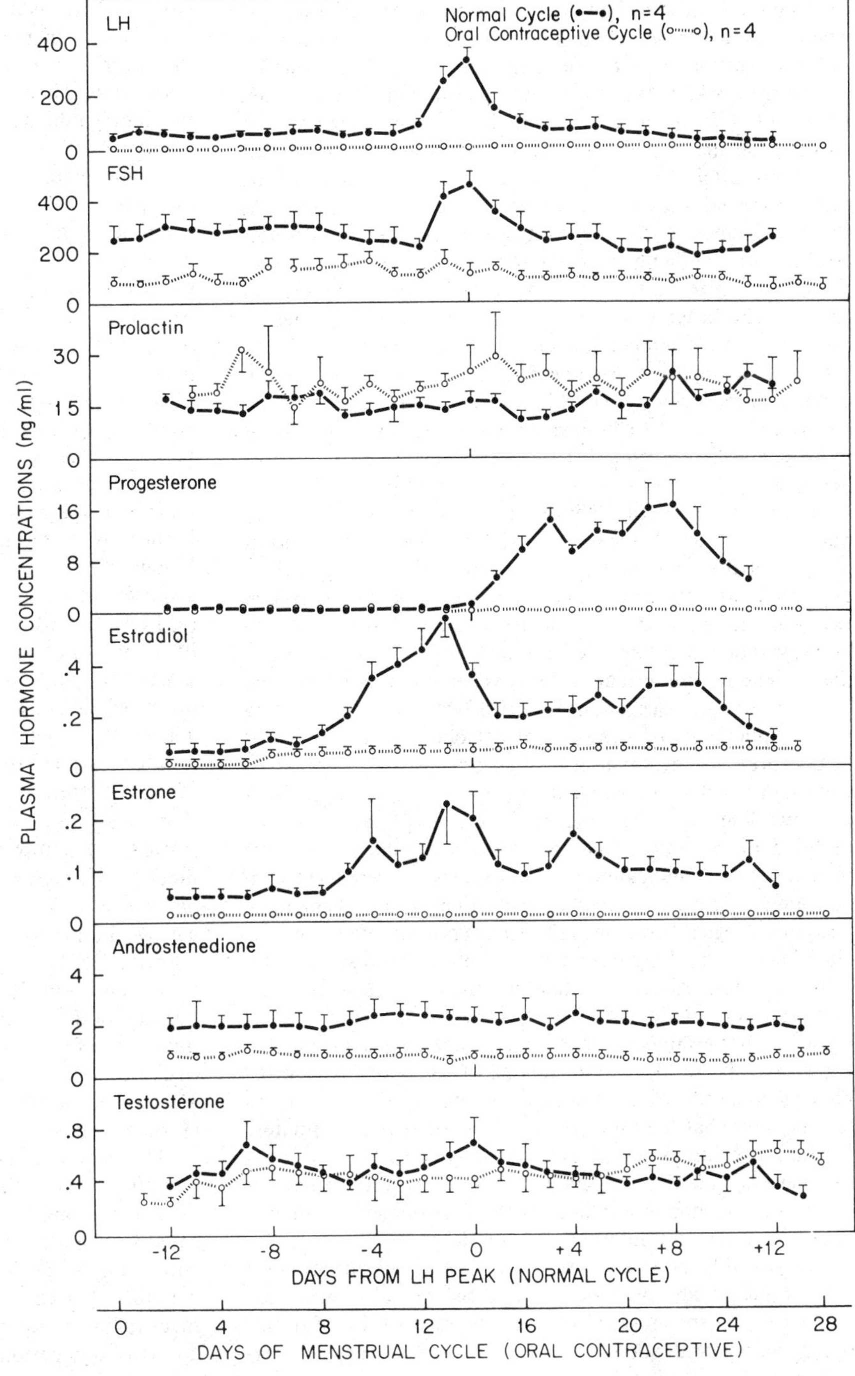

FIGURE 118-10
The mechanism of action of the birth control pill. Mean daily plasma hormone concentrations during the ovarian cycle are shown for four ovulating women and four women treated with combination-type oral contraceptives. Data for the normal ovarian cycle are presented in relationship to the day of the LH peak; day 1 of the contraceptive cycle corresponds to the first day of uterine bleeding. The values are the mean ± SE obtained from four women. (Adapted in part from BR Carr et al, 1979.)

effects, particularly nausea. Administration of depoprogestins by injection is used infrequently in the United States.

Estrogen treatment of the menopause The use of estrogens in postmenopausal women with osteoporosis began in the early 1940s, and there has subsequently been an increase in estrogen use with the widespread belief that such therapy could relieve many of the disorders of the menopause and indeed of aging itself. In some parts of the United States by the mid-1970s as many as half of women in the menopausal age group used one or more forms of estrogen replacement for a median period of 5 years, accounting for more than 30 million prescriptions per year. In the recent past, this practice has come into question because of doubts about the long-term benefits and because the possibility has been raised that serious side effects may result from the routine use of estrogens.

The menopause is not associated with a simple state of estrogen deprivation since some estrogens continue to be produced but is instead a state of altered estrogen metabolism; the predominant estrogen becomes estrone formed by extraglandular conversion of prehormone rather than estradiol secreted by the ovary. As is true for all estrogen therapy, the estrogen treatment of the menopause is actually a pharmacological substitution of one or another estrogen analogue for the physiological estradiol rather than a physiological replacement of the missing steroid. Presently, estrogens available for replacement therapy include conjugated estrogens, estrogen substitutes (stilbestrol), synthetic estrogen (ethinyl estradiol or derivatives), micronized estradiol, and estrogen-containing vaginal creams. The latter can result in significant levels of plasma estrogen, a fact often overlooked when such therapy is utilized for atrophic vaginitis. Regimens associated with low risk of complications include (1) cyclic estrogen therapy in the lowest effective dose for 21 to 25 days per month, (2) cyclic estrogens plus the addition of progestin during the last 10 days of estrogen therapy.

The most clear-cut benefit of estrogen therapy in the menopause is the relief of vasomotor instability (hot flashes) and of atrophy of the urogenital epithelium and skin. Estrogen therapy ameliorates these symptoms in the majority of cases. When estrogen therapy is designed to treat hot flashes alone, such therapy should be continued for only a few years since hot flashes tend to diminish after 3 to 4 years in untreated women.

Whether routine estrogen therapy is beneficial in preventing the complications of menopausal osteoporosis is not established. Ordinary menopausal osteoporosis is due to a variety of causes, of which endocrine factors are not predominant. However, two lines of evidence support the concept that it may be useful. First, in women undergoing premature menopause the incidence and complication rates of osteoporosis are increased, and long-term estrogen replacement appears to be beneficial. Second, estrogen therapy has short-term positive effects on calcium balance and long-term beneficial effects on bone density. Third, in women given combination estrogen and calcium therapy, the incidence of vertebral fractures is decreased. Thus, while it is not established that estrogen itself is responsible for decreasing the serious complications of osteoporosis in ordinary menopausal women (namely hip and vertebral fractures) it is possible that the improved bone densities may ultimately be translated into a diminished morbidity.

There are no clear-cut data that low-dose estrogen treatment in the menopause influences the development of atherosclerosis, myocardial infarction, or stroke.

Of the side effects of estrogen therapy in menopausal women, the possibility of an increased risk of endometrial carcinoma is perhaps most worrisome. The relative risk of developing endometrial adenocarcinoma in estrogen users is between 6 and 8. The risk is increased with duration and dosage of estrogen but may be decreased in women given combination estrogen-progestin therapy.

Depsite the large body of evidence linking endometrial carcinoma and estrogen use, two types of doubt have been raised about the clinical significance of the association. First, some epidemiologists have argued that the increased risk associated with estrogens has been exaggerated because of problems inherent in obtaining adequate controls in retrospective analyses. Second, in spite of an increased incidence of endometrial carcinoma in the United States, there was no concomitant increased mortality from this disease. Indeed the increased incidence apparently involves low-grade malignancies which in fact may be difficult to distinguish histologically from various forms of hyperplasia. These forms of malignancy have little effect on life expectancy.

Most of the apprehension concerning worsening of hypertension and thromboembolic disease is due to reports of the effects of estrogen-progesterone oral contraceptive pills during the reproductive years and not to estrogen use in menopausal women. There is no documented evidence that low-dose estrogen therapy in the menopause enhances the development or the severity of thromboembolic disease, breast cancer, or hypertension. There is a slightly increased risk for the development of gallbladder disease with estrogen use in the menopause.

A reasonable approach to the use of estrogens in the menopause is as follows. (1) For long-term use, estrogens should be given in the minimal effective doses (0.3 to 0.6 mg conjugated estrogen or 0.01 to 0.02 mg ethinyl estradiol per day). Except when hot flashes preclude intermittent use, the agents should be prescribed only for 21 to 25 days each month followed by a rest period. (For women with an intact uterus it is the practice in some clinics to give estrogens alone for 3 weeks and estrogen plus a daily progestin during the third week.) (2) Such replacement therapy is indicated routinely in women undergoing premature menopause (surgically induced or spontaneous) at least until the age of normal menopause. (3) Estrogen therapy is also indicated routinely in women of all ages who have severe hot flashes or symptomatic atrophy of the urogenital epithelium. Hot flashes rarely persist for longer than 4 years, so that if given for this purpose the duration of therapy can be limited. (4) In women who have had prior hysterectomy potential benefits of treatment appear to outweigh the dangers. Whether estrogens should be given routinely to women with intact uteri is unsettled. The complications do not appear to be as serious as was once thought; amelioration of osteoporosis, though not established, may be real. (5) Each woman receiving estrogens must be monitored indefinitely and frequently.

DRUGS TO INDUCE OVULATION The most common treatment for ovulation induction in women with PCOD is *clomiphene citrate.* This agent is an antiestrogen and is believed to act by binding to estrogen receptors in the hypothalamus and allowing FSH to rise to stimulate follicular development and ultimately result in ovulation. Clomiphene therapy is usually begun in a dose of 50 mg by mouth daily for 5 days commencing on the fifth day of progestin-induced uterine bleeding. If ovulation does not occur, the dose may be increased to 100 or 150 mg per day. Such treatment results in ovulatory cycles in 60 percent of women with PCOD.

The most commonly used gonadotropins for induction of ovulation are *human menopausal gonadotropins* (Pergonal) and *human chorionic gonadotropin* (HCG). These agents are indicated in women who fail to ovulate on clomid and in women with hypogonadotropic hypogonadism. One ampul of Pergonal contains 75 units of FSH and 75 units of LH. The usual treatment regimen requires 1 to 3 ampuls of Pergonal per day over a 8 to 12 day period to achieve adequate follicular stimulation and growth, followed by a single injection of 10,000 units of HCG 12 to 24 h after the last injection of Pergonal. Ovulation is successful in 90 percent of women, and pregnancy rates exceed 50 to 60 percent. Measurement of daily estrogen levels and frequent evaluation of ovarian size are indicated to prevent ovarian hyperstimulation. Ovarian hyperstimulation syndrome results from excessive stimulation of ovarian follicles by human menopausal gonadotropins and HCG treatment with resultant enlargement of the ovaries and may progress to the development of ascites, hypotension, and shock.

Bromocryptine (Parlodel) is a dopamine agonist that is effective in inducing ovulation in women with elevated prolactin levels in the absence of demonstrable pituitary tumor. Treatment is instituted (after pituitary tumors are excluded) at a usual dosage of 2.5 mg by mouth two or three times a day. Treatment should be discontinued as soon as pregnancy is diagnosed. The management of prolactin-secreting pituitary tumors is discussed in Chap. 109.

OTHER DISORDERS OF THE FEMALE REPRODUCTIVE TRACT

VULVA Most disorders of the vulva during the reproductive years are due to venereal disease, most commonly syphilis (painless chancre), condyloma acuminata (venereal warts), and herpes vulvitis (painful ulcers) (see Chap. 143). All other lesions of the vulva, particularly in older women, must be biopsied. Early biopsy of cancer of the vulva is mandatory, because when it becomes symptomatic (pruritus and bleeding) it has often progressed to an advanced stage.

VAGINA Infections of the vagina usually present as vaginal discharge and pruritis. The most frequent organisms are *Trichomonas, Candida albicans,* and *Hemophilus vaginalis* (also see Chap. 143). The diagnosis is made by microscopic examination of the discharge, and appropriate therapy can be instituted utilizing vaginal or oral antibiotics.

Abnormalities of the vagina and cervix in female offspring of women given diethylstilbestrol (DES) during pregnancy include adenosis of the vagina as well as structural abnormalities of the vagina, cervix, and uterus; the risk of developing a rare form of vaginal cancer (adenocarcinoma, clear-cell type) is increased (2 per 10,000 exposed women). Periodic examination of women at risk should commence at age 12 to 14, and reevaluation should be undertaken after any episode of abnormal bleeding.

CERVIX Preinvasive lesions of the cervix (also known as cervical intraepithelial neoplasia) as well as invasive carcinoma of the cervix can be detected reliably by obtaining a Papanicolaou smear (Pap smear). Current recommendations by the American Cancer Society are that a Pap smear be obtained every 3 years after 2 negative Pap smears were obtained at yearly intervals in all women between the ages of 20 to 65 and in sexually active women less than 20. However, many gynecologists recommend yearly Pap smears especially in patients with more than one sexual partner.

UTERUS Only 40 percent of endometrial adenocarcinoma is detected by Pap smears. In women at high risk for developing endometrial carcinoma (obesity, history of chronic anovulatory cycles, diabetes, hypertension, estrogen treatment) yearly endometrial sampling should be performed. Low-dose oral estrogen therapy rarely causes breakthrough or withdrawal bleeding in menopausal women. Therefore, irrespective of whether the patient is on estrogen therapy, any occurrence of postmenopausal bleeding makes it mandatory to obtain a tissue diagnosis to exclude endometrial cancer either by endometrial sampling or by curettage.

One of the most common disorders of the uterus and the most frequent tumor of women (1 of 4 women affected) is the uterine leiomyoma, or fibroid tumor. Three-fourths of women with leiomyoma are asymptomatic, and the diagnosis is made on routine pelvic examination. When associated with excessive menstrual blood loss, excessive size or rapid growth, or significant pelvic pain (see Chap. 45), the preferred treatment is surgical removal by hysterectomy if there is no desire for further childbearing. In young women myomectomy may on occasion be indicated when infertility or repeated fetal wastage is a manifestation or where future childbearing is desired.

FALLOPIAN TUBES AND OVARIES Infectious pelvic inflammatory disease is a common disorder of the fallopian tubes and usually becomes symptomatic after a menstrual period; the symptoms include fever, chills, abdominal pain, and vaginal discharge, and pelvic tenderness on physical examination is common. The initiating organism is often *Neisseria gonorrhoeae,* but tuboovarian abscess and sterility are probably caused by mixed aerobic and anaerobic superinfections that complicate *Neisseria* lesions and require wide-spectrum antibiotic treatment (see Chap. 144).

Endometriosis is a benign disorder characterized by the presence and proliferation of endometrial tissue (stroma and glands) outside the endometrial cavity. The clinical manifestations are variable. Endometriosis occurs most commonly between the ages of 30 to 40 and is found incidentally at the time of surgery in approximately a fifth of all gynecological operations. The fertility rate is significantly reduced in affected women. The disorder usually involves the posterior cul-de-sac or the ovaries and can give rise to ovarian enlargement (endometriomas), although it may also involve sites distant to the pelvis (lung, umbilicus). The most significant symptom is pelvic pain, characteristically dysmenorrhea (see Chap. 45). However, the frequency and degree of pelvic symptomatology correlate poorly with the extent of disease. Other symptoms include dyspareunia, pain with defecation, and infertility. The characteristic physical findings are multiple tender nodules palpable along the uterosacral ligament at the time of rectal-vaginal examination, a posteriorly fixed uterus, or enlarged cystic ovaries. The diagnosis can only be confirmed by direct visualization, usually at diagnostic laparoscopy. Treatment depends on the degree of involvement and the desires of the patient and includes observation for mild disease with no associated infertility or pain, hormonal suppressive therapy (see infertility), conservative surgery if fertility is desired, or removal of the uterus, tubes, and ovaries in severe disease. Endometriosis is rarely found after the menopause.

Any adnexal mass that persists for more than 6 weeks or is larger than 6 cm must be evaluated. Although ovarian cysts and neoplasms comprise the largest group of pelvic adnexal masses (see above), tumors of the fallopian tubes, uterus, gastrointestinal tract or urinary tract should also be considered. Sonography or radiographic evaluation is often helpful in identifying the nature of the adnexal mass prior to surgical exploration.

REFERENCES

CARR BR et al: Plasma lipoprotein regulation of progesterone biosynthesis by human corpus luteum tissue in organ culture. J Clin Endocrinol Metab 52:875, 1981

——— et al: Plasma levels of adenocorticotropin and cortisol in women receiving oral contraceptive steroid treatment. J Clin Endocrinol Metab 49:346, 1979

——— et al: The role of lipoproteins in the regulation of progesterone secretion by human corpus luteum. Fertil Steril, 1982 (in press)
DIZEREGA GS, HODGEN GD: Folliculogenesis in the primate ovarian cycle. Endocrinol Rev 2:27, 1981
DMOWSKI WP: Endocrine properties and clinical applications of danazol. Fertil Steril 31:237, 1979
ERICKSON GF et al: Functional studies of aromatase activity in human granulosa cells from normal and polycystic ovaries. J Clin Endocrinol Metab 49:514, 1979
FAIMAN C et al: Patterns of gonadotropins and gonadal steroids throughout life. Clin Obstet Gynaecol 3:467, 1976
FRASIER SD: *Pediatric Endocrinology.* New York, Grune & Stratton, 1980
GEMZELL C, WANG CF: Outcome of pregnancy in women with pituitary adenoma. Fertil Steril 31:363, 1979
GLUCKMAN PD et al: The human fetal hypothalamus and pituitary gland, in *Maternal-Fetal Endocrinology,* D Tulchinsky, KJ Ryan (eds). Philadelphia, Saunders, 1980
GOLD JJ et al: *Gynecologic Endocrinology.* Hagerstown, Harper & Row, 1980
GOLDZIEHER JW: Polycystic ovarian disease. Fertil Steril 35:371, 1981
GRUMBACH MM et al: Hypothalamic-pituitary regulation of puberty in man: Evidence and concepts derived from clinical research, in *Control of the Onset of Puberty,* MM Grumbach et al (eds). New York, Wiley, 1974, p 115
HAMMOND MG, TALBERT LM: *Infertility.* Chapel Hill, Health Sciences Consortium, 1981
HATCHER RA et al: *Contraceptive Technology 1980–1981.* New York, Irvington Publishers, 1980
KAPLAN NM: Complications of the birth control pill, in *Update I: Harrison's Principles of Internal Medicine,* KJ Isselbacher et al (eds). New York, McGraw-Hill, 1981, p 57
MISHELL DR, DAVAJAN V: *Reproductive Endocrinology, Infertility, and Contraception.* Philadelphia, Davis, 1979
PIEPER DR et al: Ovarian gonadotropin-releasing hormone (GnRH) receptors: Characterization, distribution, and induction by GnRH. Endocrinology 108:1148, 1981
PRITCHARD JA, MACDONALD PC: *Williams Obstetrics.* New York, Appleton-Century-Crofts, 1980
RIGGS BL et al: Effect of the fluoride/calcium regimen on vertebral fracture occurrence in postmenopausal osteoporosis. N Engl J Med 306:446, 1982
ROMNEY SL et al: *Gynecology and Obstetrics: The Health Care of Women.* New York, McGraw-Hill, 1980
SCULLY RE: Ovarian tumors: A review. Am J Pathol 87:686, 1977
SITTERI PK, MACDONALD PC: Role of extraglandular estrogen in human endocrinology, in *Handbook of Physiology,* sec 7: *Endocrinology,* SR Geiger et al (eds). Washington, DC, American Physiological Society, 1973, p 615
SPEROFF L et al: *Clinical Gynecologic Endocrinology and Infertility,* 2d ed. Baltimore, Williams & Wilkins, 1978
———: The ovary, in *Endocrinology and Metabolism,* P Felig et al (eds). New York, McGraw-Hill, 1981, p 669
UTIAN WH: *Menopause in Modern Perspective.* New York, Appleton-Century-Crofts, 1980
WALLACH EE, KEMPERS RD: *Modern Trends in Infertility and Conception Control.* Baltimore, Williams & Wilkins, 1979
WILSON JD: The use of estrogens in the menopause, in *Update II: Harrison's Principals of Internal Medicine,* KJ Isselbacher et al (eds). New York, McGraw-Hill, 1981, p 197
YEN SSC: Neuroendocrine regulation of the menstrual cycle. Hosp Prac 14:84, 1979
———, JAFFE RB: *Reproductive Endocrinology.* Philadelphia, Saunders, 1978
YING SY et al: Gonadocrinins: Peptides in ovarian follicular fluid stimulating the secretion of pituitary gonadotropins. Endocrinology 108:1206, 1981

119 ENDOCRINE DISORDERS OF THE BREAST

JEAN D. WILSON

Because the breasts are one of the commonest sites of fatal and preventable disease in women and because they frequently provide clues to underlying systemic disease in both men and women, examination of the breasts is an important part of the physical examination. The internist frequently does not examine the male breast and in the evaluation of women is apt to refer this task to a gynecologist. It is the duty of every physician to distinguish the abnormal from the normal at the earliest possible stage and to call for assistance if there is any doubt. (For cancer of the breast see Chap. 126.)

ENDOCRINE CONTROL OF THE BREAST There is no histological or functional difference in the breasts of boys and girls prior to the onset of puberty, but a profound sexual dimorphism in breast development ensues at the time of puberty. The endocrine control of breast development in the female is illustrated in Fig. 119-1. The development of the normal nonlactating female breast is dependent primarily upon the action of estradiol, which induces the growth, division, and elongation of the tubular duct system and maturation of the nipples. In men the administration of estrogen is equally effective in this regard. To produce true alveolar development at the ends of the ducts, however, the synergistic action of progesterone is required, a ratio of estrogen to progesterone of 1:20 to 1:100 being optimal. Once the anatomical development of the ducts and alveoli is complete, continued action of estrogen and progesterone does not appear to be required for lactation itself.

The formation of milk by the differentiated breast is one of the most complex of endocrinological phenomena, requiring specific lactogenic hormone in addition to appropriate priming of the breast by estrogen and progesterone and the permissive action of glucocorticoid, growth hormone, insulin, and thyroxine. Two lactogenic hormones participate in normal lactation. One is human placental lactogen (HPL or chorionic somatomammotropin), which is secreted in large amounts by the placenta during the latter phases of gestation and plays a role in preparing the breast for milk production. It disappears from the fetal (and maternal) circulation shortly after termination of pregnancy. The second lactogenic hormone is prolactin, a peptide of approximately 20,000 mol wt, which is synthesized in the pituitary and which usually plays the critical role in the initiation and maintenance of normal as well as inappropriate lactation. The plasma level of prolactin rises during pregnancy, and during late pregnancy and lactation 60 to 80 percent of the mass of the anterior pituitary may consist of prolactin-secreting cells.

Unlike most pituitary hormones, the predominant regulation of prolactin secretion is negative, i.e., under ordinary basal condition the hypothalamus secretes an inhibitory peptide hormone, prolactin inhibitory factor (PIF), which is delivered to the pituitary via the portal system and inhibits the release of prolactin into the blood. Many, if not most, factors that influence prolactin release are thought to do so by affecting the synthesis or release of PIF. Basal prolactin levels fall following delivery, but prolactin secretion is enhanced by stimulation of the breasts such as the act of nursing (the so-called sucking reflex), a phenomenon that is believed to be mediated by the reflex release of oxytocin. In the postgestational state the normal woman is capable of forming about a liter of milk per day containing 38 g fat, 70 g lactose, and 12 g protein. Normal lactation can be suppressed either by the administration of estrogens or diethylstilbestrol, which inhibit milk production by direct effects on the breast, or by the administration of bromocryptine mesylate, which inhibits prolactin secretion.

GALACTORRHEA Exactly what constitutes nonpuerperal or inappropriate lactation is not always clearly defined in the literature. According to the studies of Friedman and Goldfien, it is not possible to demonstrate any breast secretion whatsoever in normal, regularly menstruating nulligravid women, but breast secretions can be demonstrated in as many as a fourth of normal women who have been pregnant in the past and may be of no clinical significance in these instances. Spontaneous leakage of milk from the breasts is usually of more concern to the patient than milk that must be expressed. A second problem is related to the composition of the breast secretions. When the breast secretion is milky or white, it is safe to assume that it contains casein and lactose and is in fact milk; however, when the secretion is brown or greenish in color it rarely contains normal milk constituents and consequently may not result from an underlying endocrinopathy. Furthermore, upon repeated sampling the composition of milk carbohydrates and proteins may increase in a given individual from low, colostrum-like values to those typical of milk. Milky discharges must also be distinguished from dark or bloody secretions that may be present with neoplasms of the breast (see Chap. 126).

With these problems in mind galactorrhea can be defined as any inappropriate production of milk that is persistent or worrisome to the patient, recognizing that in some instances no underlying pathology will be demonstrated.

Since the action of a lactogenic hormone is a necessary requirement for the initiation of milk production, it is logical to consider galactorrhea as a manifestation of deranged prolactin physiology. However, as indicated above a complex endocrinological milieu is necessary for lactation, and in many or most instances in which prolactin is elevated in women who have not been appropriately primed or in men no production of milk takes place. As a consequence hyperprolactinemia is more common than galactorrhea. Furthermore, although enhanced prolactin secretion is necessary for the initiation of milk formation, production can be maintained in the presence of minimally elevated or intermittently elevated prolactin levels so that increased basal plasma prolactin levels are not always demonstrated in patients with galactorrhea. For example, repeated stimulation of the nipples of women who have previously been pregnant can cause galactorrhea with minimal elevations of basal prolactin similar to that found in the normal nursing mother. Perhaps the strongest evidence that prolactin is always involved in galactorrhea has been the demonstration that administration of bromocryptine mesylate, which suppresses plasma prolactin levels, causes a disappearance of the galactorrhea even when the initial plasma prolactin levels are within normal limits.

TABLE 119-1
A physiological classification of galactorrhea

- *I* Failure of normal hypothalamic inhibition of prolactin release
  - *A* Pituitary stalk section
  - *B* Drugs
  - *C* Central nervous system disease
- *II* Enhanced prolactin-releasing factor
  - Hypothyroidism
- *III* Autonomous prolactin release
  - *A* Pituitary tumors
    - *1* Prolactin-secreting tumors (Forbes-Albright syndrome)
    - *2* Mixed growth hormone and prolactin-secreting tumors
    - *3* Chromophobe adenomas
  - *B* Ectopic production of human placental lactogen and/or prolactin
    - *1* Hydatidiform moles and chorionephitheliomas
    - *2* Others (bronchogenic carcinoma and hypernephroma)
- *IV* Idiopathic (with or without amenorrhea)

Differential diagnosis It is thus appropriate to consider galactorrhea in terms of deranged prolactin physiology as the result of failure of normal hypothalamic inhibition of prolactin release, of enhanced prolactin-releasing factor, or of autonomous prolactin secretion by tumors (Table 119-1). Pituitary stalk section in humans results in a striking increase in prolactin secretion, as the result of inhibition of delivery of PIF to the pituitary. Likewise, many drugs that influence the central nervous system (including virtually all psychotropic agents, α-methyldopa, reserpine, and antiemetics) result in enhanced prolactin release, presumably by inhibiting PIF synthesis or release. Estrogens enhance prolactin levels by an uncertain mechanism. Extrapituitary central nervous system diseases cause galactorrhea, presumably by interfering with PIF delivery (CNS sarcoidosis, craniopharyngioma, pinealoma, encephalitis, meningitis, hydrocephalus, hypothalamic tumors).

The existence of a physiological prolactin-releasing factor is still a matter of controversy, but in at least one pathological state, primary hypothyroidism, galactorrhea is thought to result from enhanced prolactin-releasing activity. Thyrotropin-releasing hormone (TRH) stimulates prolactin release, and thyroid hormone replacement cures the galactorrhea, suggesting that the galactorrhea of hypothyroidism is due to enhanced TRH secretion.

FIGURE 119-1
Endocrine control of female breast development and function at various stages of life.

STAGE	DUCT SYSTEM	MAJOR HORMONES	PERMISSIVE HORMONES
Prepubertal		None	Unknown
Adult	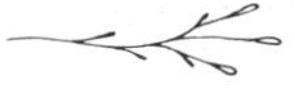	Estrogen (Progesterone)	Thyroxine Glucocorticoids Growth Hormone
Pregnancy	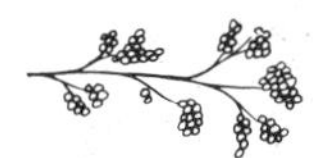	Estrogen Progesterone Prolactin Human Placental Lactogen	
Lactation	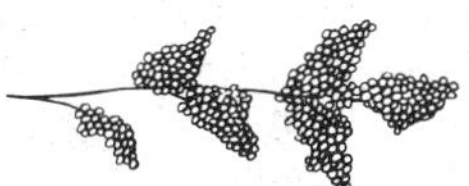	Prolactin Oxytocin	

Enhanced prolactin release can also occur from pituitary or nonpituitary tumors. Three types of pituitary tumors (see Chap. 109) may be associated with galactorrhea—pure prolactin-secreting tumors (micro- or macroadenomas), mixed tumors that secrete both growth hormone and prolactin and result in acromegaly with galactorrhea, and some chromophobe adenomas. The latter may actually either secrete prolactin or interfere with the delivery of PIF to the pituitary. Prolactin can also be secreted on occasion by other malignancies such as bronchogenic carcinoma, and secretion of placental lactogen has been reported in hydatidiform moles and in choriocarcinomas.

All the known etiologies account for only part of the cases of galactorrhea. In four published series totaling more than 500 carefully studied patients, a pituitary tumor was identified in about a fourth of patients, other known causes could be identified in another fourth or fifth, and the remaining half fall into the unknown category. Many of these patients may prove ultimately to have prolactin-secreting pituitary tumors, some probably have subtle disorders of hypothalamic function, and in others a drug-related cause may have been missed, but the fact remains that no satisfactory diagnosis is reached in half or more of patients. It is of note that when normal menses and galactorrhea are both present, the likelihood of establishing a diagnosis is poor.

Galactorrhea is unusual in men, even in the presence of profound elevations of plasma prolactin; when it does occur it is usually upon the background of a feminizing state (see below).

Diagnostic evaluation If hyperprolactinemia is present, the workup is fundamentally that of a pituitary tumor once drug causes and hypothyroidism are excluded (Chap. 109). Even when a specific cause cannot be identified and a diagnosis of idiopathic galactorrhea is made by exclusion, it is necessary to remember that pituitary tumors may subsequently become manifest. The higher the prolactin values and the more persistent the galactorrhea, the greater the likelihood of such a development.

Treatment The aim of all treatment is to remove the source of the elevated prolactin, and resection of pituitary tumor, cessation of causative drugs, and correction of hypothyroidism are often followed by disappearance of galactorrhea. Two other forms of therapy may have some usefulness. Breast binders can be effective in some patients with mild galactorrhea of unknown etiology, presumably by preventing stimulation of the nipple and the consequent perpetuation of lactation. Bromocryptine mesylate, which suppresses plasma prolactin, has been used to treat patients with idiopathic hyperprolactinemia as well as some patients with prolactin-secreting tumors of the pituitary. This drug not only suppresses lactation but may also cause resumption of normal menstrual cycles (and even fertility) in patients in whom amenorrhea accompanies galactorrhea.

GYNECOMASTIA A central issue in the evaluation of breast tissue in adult men is the separation of the normal from the abnormal. It has been the usual belief that no breast tissue is palpable in the normal adult man and that the presence of any breast tissue whatsoever on physical examination is an indication for a diagnostic evaluation. However, Nuttall has recently reported that gynecomastia (less than 4 to 5 cm in diameter) may occur in normal men.

Early gynecomastia is characterized by proliferation both of the fibroblastic stroma and of the duct system which elongates, buds, and duplicates. As gynecomastia persists, progressive fibrosis and hyalinization are associated with regression of epithelial proliferation. Eventually there is a decrease in the number of ducts. Resolution occurs by reduction in size and epithelial content with gradual disappearance of the ducts, leaving hyaline bands which eventually disappear.

In all instances growth of the male breast, as in women, is mediated by estrogen and results from disturbance of the normal ratio of active androgen to estrogen in plasma or within the breast itself. As described in Chap. 117 estradiol formation in the normal man occurs principally by the conversion of circulating androgens to estrogens in peripheral tissues; the normal ratio of production of testosterone to estradiol in adult men is approximately 100:1 (6 mg versus 45 μg), and the normal ratio of the two hormones in plasma is about 300:1. Feminization results when there is a significant decrease in this effective ratio, either as a result of diminished testosterone production or action, enhanced estrogen formation, or both processes occurring simultaneously. The predominant manifestation of feminization in men is enlargement of the breasts.

Enlargement of the male breast can occur as a normal physiological phenomena at certain stages of life or as the result of a variety of pathological conditions. A classification of gynecomastia is given in Table 119-2.

Physiological gynecomastia Physiological gynecomastia occurs under at least three circumstances. In the *newborn* transient enlargement of the breast results from the action of maternal and/or placental estrogens. The enlargement ordinarily disappears in a few weeks, although it may rarely persist longer. *Adolescent* gynecomastia occurs in many boys at some time during puberty. The median age of onset is 14; it is often grossly asymmetric, occasionally unilateral for a portion of its course, and frequently tender, and it generally regresses so that by age 20 only a small number of men have palpable vestiges of gynecomastia remaining in one or both breasts. Although the origin of the excess estrogen in the pubertal male has not been identified, the onset of gynecomastia correlates with transient elevations of plasma estradiol prior to the completion of

TABLE 119-2
Differential diagnosis of gynecomastia

PHYSIOLOGICAL GYNECOMASTIA

- Newborn
- Adolescence
- Aging

PATHOLOGICAL GYNECOMASTIA

- Deficient production or action of testosterone:
  - Congenital anorchia
  - Klinefelter syndrome
  - Androgen resistance (testicular feminization and Reifenstein syndrome)
  - Defects in testosterone synthesis
  - Secondary testicular failure (viral orchitis, trauma, castration, neurological and granulomatous diseases, renal failure)
- Increased estrogen production:
  - Estrogen secretion
    - True hermaphroditism
    - Testicular tumors
    - Carcinoma of the lung
  - Increased substrate for peripheral aromatase
    - Adrenal disease
    - Liver disease
    - Starvation
    - Thyrotoxicosis
  - Increase in peripheral aromatase
  - Drugs
    - Estrogens (diethylstilbestrol, birth control pills, digitalis, marijuana, heroin)
    - Gonadotropins
    - Inhibitors of testosterone synthesis and/or action (alkylating agents, spironolactone, cimetidine)
    - Unknown mechanisms (bisulphan, ethionamide, isoniazid, methyldopa, tricyclic antidepressants, D-penicillamine, diazepam)

puberty so that the androgen/estrogen ratio is altered. *Gynecomastia of aging* also occurs in otherwise healthy men. Forty percent or more of aged men have gynecomastia, as the result of true increase in frequency with age. A likely explanation is the elevation in plasma estrogen in aged men as the result of an increase in the peripheral conversion of androgens to estrogens with age. Since no attempt has been made to exclude abnormal liver function or drug therapy as contributing causes to gynecomastia in the elderly, the real significance of this finding in the aging man is uncertain.

Pathological gynecomastia Pathological gynecomastia can result from one of three basic mechanisms: deficiency in testosterone production or action (with or without a secondary increase in estrogen production), increase in estrogen production, or drugs (Table 119-2). Most of the individual disorders that cause primary and secondary testicular failure have been discussed in Chap. 117. The fact that deficiency in testosterone production per se can cause gynecomastia is illustrated by the syndrome of congenital anorchia in which normal (or slightly low) estradiol production for a male in the presence of profoundly decreased testosterone production results in florid gynecomastia. In some instances of testicular failure diminished testosterone production or action leads to elevated plasma LH, which in turn results in elevated estradiol secretion by the testis and causes or worsens the gynecomastia. Such is the case in some patients with Klinefelter syndrome. In the inherited syndromes of androgen resistance, such as testicular feminization, deficient androgen action and increased testicular estrogen production are both present, although diminished androgen action is the more critical in inducing gynecomastia.

A primary increase in estrogen production can result from a variety of causes. Increased testicular estrogen secretion may result from elevations in plasma gonadotropins, for example, in cases of aberrant production of chorionic gonadotropin by testicular tumors or by bronchogenic carcinoma, from the ovarian elements in the gonads of men with true hermaphroditism, or as the result of direct secretion by testicular tumors (particularly interstitial cell and Sertoli cell tumors). Increased conversion of androgens to estrogens in peripheral tissues can either be due to increased availability of substrate for extraglandular estrogen formation or to increased amount of the enzymes of estrogen formation in peripheral tissues. Increased substrate availability for peripheral conversion can result from increased production of androgens such as androstenedione (congenital adrenal hyperplasia, hyperthyroidism, and most feminizing adrenal tumors) or because of diminished catabolism of androstenedione by the usual pathways (liver disease). Increased amount of peripheral aromatase can either occur rarely as the result of hereditary abnormality or in tumors of the liver or adrenal.

The ingestion of drugs may also cause gynecomastia by several mechanisms. Many drugs either act directly as estrogens or cause an increase in plasma estrogen activity, for example, in men receiving diethylstilbestrol therapy for prostatic carcinoma and in transsexuals in preparation for sex-change operations. The gynecomastia of digitalis ingestion is usually attributed to an estrogen-like side effect of the drug, but in the experience of the author it is usually associated with abnormal liver function tests. Abuse of marijuana and heroin also can cause gynecomastia associated with diminished plasma testosterone and an increase in plasma estrogen. A second mechanism by which drugs can induce gynecomastia is illustrated by gonadotropin itself which causes enhanced testicular secretion of estrogen.

Other drugs cause gynecomastia by interfering with testosterone synthesis (alkylating agents) and/or testosterone action, for instance by blocking the binding of androgen to its cytosol receptor protein in target tissues (spironolactone and cimeti-

dine). Finally, many drugs cause gynecomastia by mechanisms that have not been defined. These include busulfan, ethionamide, isoniazid, methyldopa, tricyclic antidepressants, D-penicillamine, and diazepam. In some instances the feminization is due to effects of the drugs on liver function.

Diagnostic evaluation The evaluation of patients with gynecomastia should include the following procedures: (1) a careful drug history; (2) measurement and examination of the testes (if both are small a karyotype is indicated, and if they are asymmetric an evaluation for testicular tumor should be instituted); (3) evaluation of liver function; (4) an endocrine evaluation to include 24-h urinary 17-ketosteroids (usually elevated in feminizing adrenal states), measurement of plasma estradiol (helpful if elevated but usually normal), and measurement of plasma luteinizing hormone (LH) and testosterone. If LH is high and testosterone is low, the diagnosis is usually testicular failure, if LH and testosterone are both low, the diagnosis is most likely increased primary estrogen production (for example, a Sertoli cell tumor of the testis), and if both LH and testosterone are elevated the diagnosis is either an androgen-resistance state or a gonadotropin-secreting tumor.

Using these various tests a satisfactory diagnosis can be made in only half or less of patients referred for gynecomastia. This implies either that the diagnostic techniques are not sufficiently refined to recognize mild disturbances, that many causes of gynecomastia are as yet undefined, that the causes of many instances are transient and difficult to diagnose, or, as suggested by Nuttall, that gynecomastia may in some instances be normal rather than due to a pathological state. Because of the problem of separating the normal from the pathological, gynecomastia should probably be routinely worked up only if the drug history is negative, and if the breast is tender (indicating rapid growth) or if the breast mass is larger than 4 cm in diameter. In other instances a decision to perform an endocrine evaluation depends on the clinical context. For example, all gynecomastia associated with signs of underandrogenization should be evaluated.

Treatment In instances in which the primary cause of the overestrogenization can be identified and corrected, the breast enlargement usually subsides promptly and eventually disappears. However, if the gynecomastia is of long duration (and fibrosis has replaced the original ductal hyperplasia) correction of the primary defect may not be followed by improvement. In such instances and when the primary cause cannot be corrected, surgery is the only effective form of therapy. Indications for surgery include severe psychological and/or cosmetic problems, continued growth, or a suspected malignancy. Although the relative risk of carcinoma of the breast is increased in men with gynecomastia, it is rare nevertheless. Prophylactic radiation of the breasts prior to the institution of diethylstilbestrol therapy is effective in preventing the development of gynecomastia and has a low complication rate in elderly men. In rare patients who have painful gynecomastia and who are not candidates for other therapy, treatment with antiestrogens such as tamoxifen may be indicated.

REFERENCES

Galactorrhea

ADLER RA: The evaluation of galactorrhea. Am J Obstet Gynecol 127:569, 1977

CHOTINER HC: Lactose and casein content of nonpuerperal breast secretion. J Reprod Med 22:267, 1979

DAVAJAN V: The significance of galactorrhea in patients with normal menses, oligomenorrhea, and secondary amenorrhea. Am J Obstet Gynecol 130:894, 1978

FRIEDMAN S et al: Breast secretions in normal women. Am J Obstet Gynecol 104:846, 1969

GOMEZ F et al: Nonpuerperal galactorrhea and hyperprolactinemia. Am J Med 62:648, 1977

KLEINBERG DL et al: Galactorrhea: A study of 235 cases, including 48 with pituitary tumors. N Engl J Med 296:589, 1977

KULSKI JK et al: Changes in the milk composition of nonpuerperal women. Am J Obstet Gynecol 139:597, 1981

PARKES D: Bromocriptine. N Engl J Med 301:873, 1979

TOLIS G: Prolactin: Physiology and pathology. Hosp Prac, February 1980, p 85

TURKSOY RN et al: Diagnostic and therapeutic modalities in women with galactorrhea. Obstet Gynecol 56:323, 1980

Gynecomastia

CARLSON HE: Gynecomastia. N Engl J Med 303:795, 1980

GAGNON JD et al: Pre-estrogen breast irradiation for patients with carcinoma of the prostate: A critical review. J Urol 121:182, 1979

JEFFERYS DB: Painful gynaecomastia treated with tamoxifen. Br Med J, April 1979, p 1119

NUTTALL FQ: Gynecomastia as a physical finding in normal men. J Clin Endocrinol Metab 48:338, 1979

SATIANI B et al: Cancer of the male breast: A thirty-year experience. Am Surg 44:86, 1978

SPENCE RW et al: Gynaecomastia associated with cimetidine. Gut 20:154, 1979

WILSON JD et al: The pathogenesis of gynecomastia, in *Advances in Internal Medicine,* GH Stollerman (ed). Chicago, Year Book, 1980, vol 25, pp. 1–32

120 DISORDERS OF SEXUAL DIFFERENTIATION

JEAN D. WILSON
JAMES E. GRIFFIN

Known causes of abnormalities in sexual development include environmental insults as in the ingestion of a virilizing drug during pregnancy, nonfamilial aberrations of the sex chromosomes as in 45,X gonadal dysgenesis, developmental birth defects of multifactorial etiology as in most cases of hypospadias, and hereditary disorders resulting from single gene mutations as in the testicular feminization syndrome.

These various etiologic factors produce abnormal sexual development by interfering with one or more of the principal processes involved in sexual differentiation. Normally, *chromosomal sex,* which is established at the moment of fertilization, determines *gonadal sex,* and *gonadal sex* in turn causes the development of *phenotypic sex* in which the male or female phenotype is formed (Fig. 120-1). A disturbance during embryogenesis of any step in this developmental process may result in a disorder of sexual differentiation.

FIGURE 120-1
Jost model for determination of sex.

CHROMOSOMAL SEX
↓
GONADAL SEX
↓
PHENOTYPIC SEX

Current limitations of knowledge make it necessary to make some empiric assignments as to the nature of the physiological derangement in certain disorders. Nevertheless, even in extreme instances of ambiguous genitalia, a specific diagnosis can usually be made as the result of combined genetic, phenotypic, and chromosomal assessment. As a consequence appropriate gender assignment can be made, and tailoring of the phenotype can be undertaken when appropriate.

NORMAL SEXUAL DIFFERENTIATION

The first process in sexual differentiation involves the establishment of chromosomal sex, the heterogametic sex (XY) being male and the homogametic sex (XX) female. The embryos of both sexes then develop in an identical fashion until approximately 40 days of gestation. The second phase of sexual differentiation is the conversion of the indifferent gonad into a testis or an ovary. The differentiation of the indifferent gonad into a testis appears to be dependent on a cell surface antigen that is normally present in males, the H-Y antigen. The structural gene that specifies the antigen is probably located on an autosome, and positive and negative regulatory controls are specified by loci on the Y and X chromosomes, respectively. The final process, the translation of gonadal sex into phenotypic sex, is the direct consequence of the type of gonad formed and the endocrine secretions of the fetal gonads. In the development of phenotypic sex indifferent anlage of the reproductive tract are converted to male or female forms.

The internal genitalia are derived from the wolffian and müllerian ducts that exist side by side in early embryos of both sexes (Fig. 120-2*A*). In the male the wolffian ducts give rise to the epididymides, vasa deferentia, and seminal vesicles, and the müllerian ducts disappear. In the female the fallopian tubes, uterus, and upper vagina are derived from the müllerian ducts, and the wolffian ducts regress. In contrast, the external genitalia and urethra in the two sexes develop from common anlage—the urogenital sinus and the genital tubercle, folds, and swellings (Fig. 120-2*B*). The urogenital sinus gives rise to the prostate and prostatic urethra in the male and to the urethra and a portion of the vagina in the female. The genital tubercle is the origin of the glans penis in the male and clitoris in the female. The urogenital swellings become the scrotum or the labia majora, and the genital folds develop into the labia minora or fuse to form the male urethra and the shaft of the penis.

In the absence of the testis, as in the normal female or in the male embryo castrated prior to the onset of phenotypic differentiation, the development of phenotypic sex proceeds along female lines. Thus, masculinization of the fetus is the positive result of action of hormones from the fetal gonad whereas female development does not require the presence of a gonad or the action of the estrogen from the fetal ovary. Under ordinary circumstances development of the sexual phenotype conforms to the chromosomal sex. That is, chromosomal sex determines gonadal sex, and gonadal sex in turn determines phenotypic sex.

Control over the formation of the male phenotype is vested in the action of three hormones. Two of the three—müllerian-inhibiting substance and testosterone—are secretory products of the fetal testis. Müllerian-inhibiting substance is an incompletely characterized product of the embryonic testis, a protein with a molecular weight greater than 15,000. It acts to suppress the müllerian ducts and consequently prevents development of the uterus and fallopian tubes in the male. Testosterone promotes virilization of the urogenital tract in two ways. It acts directly to stimulate differentiation of the wolffian duct derivatives, and it is the precursor for the third fetal hormone, dihydrotestosterone (see Chap. 117). Dihydrotestosterone, which is formed intracellularly from circulating testosterone, acts in the urogenital sinus to induce formation of the male urethra and prostate and in the genital tubercle, swellings, and folds to cause midline fusion, elongation, and enlargement that eventuate in the formation of the penis and scrotum. Thus, the primary function of androgen during fetal life is to induce the formation of the accessory organs of male reproduction. Testosterone and dihydrotestosterone act in embryonic tissues by the same intracellular machinery as described for differentiated tissues in Chap. 117.

The secretion of testosterone by the fetal testis and of estradiol by the fetal ovary approaches a maximum by the eighth to

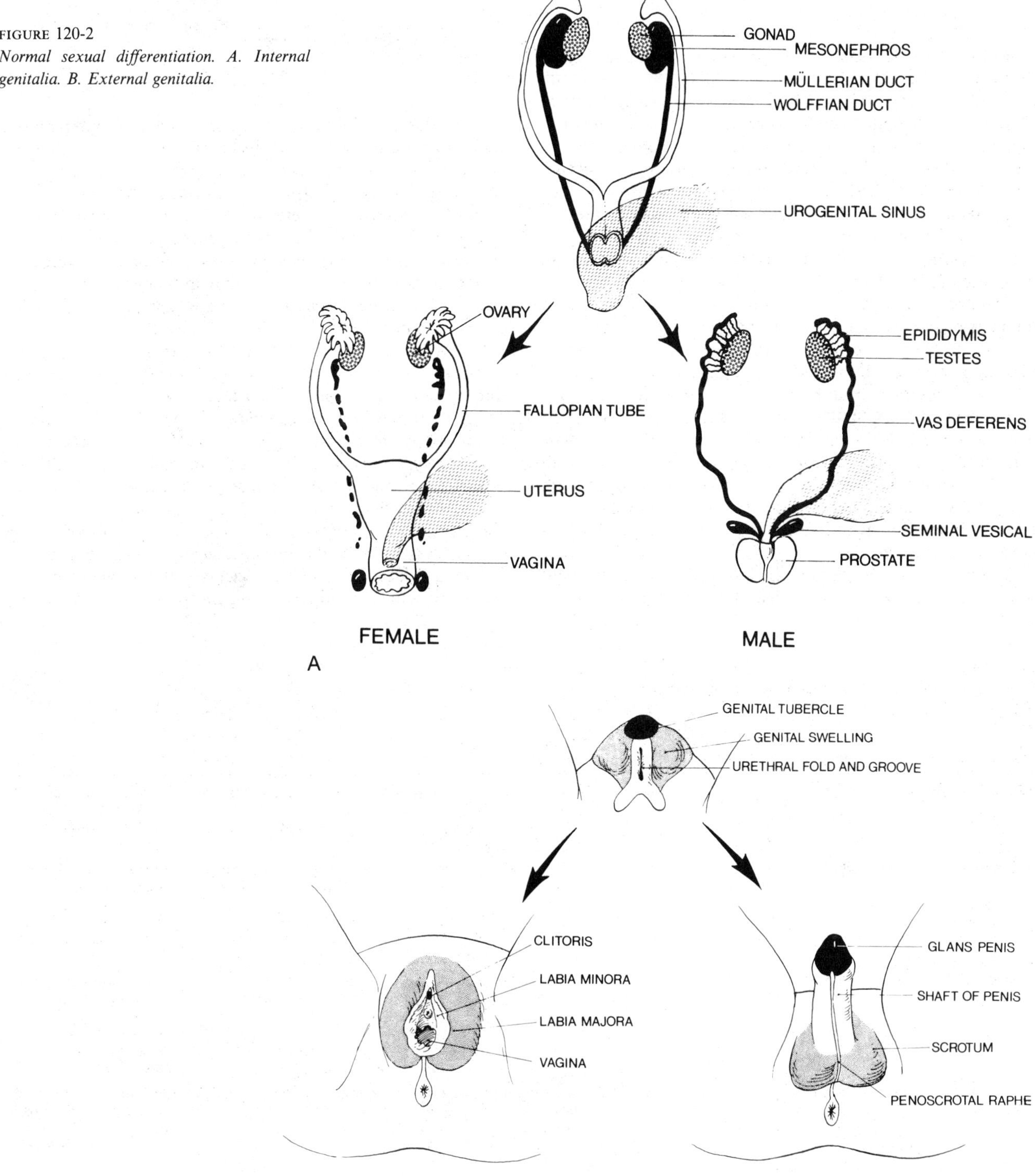

FIGURE 120-2
Normal sexual differentiation. A. Internal genitalia. B. External genitalia.

tenth week of gestation, and both the male and female phenotypes are largely completed by the end of the first trimester. During the latter phases of gestation ovarian follicular development and maturation of the vagina occur in the female, and descent of the testes and growth of the external genitalia take place in the male.

DISORDERS OF CHROMOSOMAL SEX

Disorders of chromosomal sex (Table 120-1) occur when the number or structure of the X or Y chromosomes is abnormal (see Chap. 61).

KLINEFELTER SYNDROME Clinical features Klinefelter syndrome is a disorder in phenotypic men characterized by small, firm testes, azoospermia, gynecomastia, and elevated levels of plasma gonadotropins. The fundamental defect is the presence in a male of two or more X chromosomes. The common karyotype is either a 47,XXY chromosomal pattern (the classic form) or 46,XY/47,XXY (the mosaic form). The disorder is the most frequent major abnormality of sexual differentiation; studies of the buccal smear in the newborn male population and screening studies of young adult men both indicate an incidence of around 1 in 500 men.

Prepubertally, patients have small testes with decreased numbers of spermatogonia but otherwise appear normal. After puberty the disorder becomes manifest as infertility, gynecomastia, or occasionally underandrogenization. The frequency of the various clinical features is given in Table 120-2. Damage to the seminiferous tubules and azoospermia are consistent features of the 47,XXY variety. The small, firm testes are characteristically less than 2.0 cm and always less than 3.5 cm in length (corresponding to 2 and 12 ml volume, respectively). Typical histological changes in the testes include hyalinization of the tubules, absence of spermatogenesis, and apparent increase in Leydig cells.

The increased mean body height in the disorder is the result of an increased lower body segment. Gynecomastia ordinarily appears during adolescence, is generally bilateral and painless, and may progress to become disfiguring (see Chap. 119). Obesity and varicose veins occur in a third to a half, and mild mental deficiency, social maladjustment, subtle abnormalities of thyroid function, diabetes mellitus, and pulmonary disease may be more common than in the general population. The risk of breast cancer is 20 times that of normal men, although the incidence is only about a fifth that in women. Most have a male psychosexual orientation and are capable of functioning sexually as normal men.

The variant with 46,XY/47,XXY mosaicism comprises about 10 percent of the patients, as estimated by chromosomal karyotypes on peripheral blood leukocytes. The frequency of this variant may be underestimated since chromosomal mosaicism may be present only in the testes. Thus, peripheral leukocyte karotype may be normal, and the patient may still have Klinefelter syndrome. As summarized in Table 120-2, the mosaic form is usually not as severe as the 47,XXY variety, and the testes may be normal in size. The endocrine abnormalities are also less severe, and gynecomastia and azoospermia are less common. Indeed, occasional patients with mosaicism may be fertile. In some individuals the diagnosis may not even be sus-

TABLE 120-2
Characteristics of patients with classic versus mosaic Klinefelter syndrome*

	47,XXY, %	*46,XY/47,XXY,* %
Abnormal testicular histology	100	94†
Decreased length of testis	99	73†
Azoospermia	93	50†
Decreased testosterone	79	33
Decreased facial hair	77	64
Increased gonadotropins	75	33†
Decreased sexual function	68	56
Gynecomastia	55	33†
Decreased axillary hair	49	46
Decreased length of penis	41	21

* *Table based on 519 XXY patients and 51 XY/XXY patients.*
† *Significantly different at $p < 0.05$ or better.*
SOURCE: *After Gordon et al.*

TABLE 120-1
Clinical features of the disorders of chromosomal sex

Disorder	*Common chromosomal complement*	*Gonadal development*	*External genitalia*	*Internal genitalia*	*Breast development*	*Comment*
Klinefelter syndrome	47,XXY *or* 46,XY/47,XXY	Hyalinized testes	Normal male	Normal male	Gynecomastia	Most common disorder of sexual differentiation; tall stature.
XX male	46,XX	Hyalinized testes	Normal male	Normal male	Gynecomastia	Shorter than normal men; increased incidence of hypospadias. Similar to Klinefelter syndrome. May be familial.
Gonadal dysgenesis (Turner syndrome)	45,X *or* 46,XX/45,X	Streak gonads	Immature female	Hypoplastic female	Immature female	Short stature and multiple somatic abnormalities. May be 46,XX with structurally abnormal X chromosome.
Mixed gonadal dysgenesis	46,XY/45,X *or* 46,XY	Testis and streak gonad	Variable but almost always ambiguous; 60% reared as female	Uterus, vagina, and one fallopian tube	Usually male	Second most common cause of ambiguous genitalia in the newborn; tumors common.
True hermaphroditism	46,XX *or* 46,XY*or* mosaics	Testis and ovary or ovotestis	Variable but usually ambiguous; 60% reared as males	Usually a uterus and urogenital sinus; ducts correspond to gonad	Gynecomastia in 75%	May be familial.

pected because of the minor degree of the physical abnormalities.

Approximately 30 additional karyotypic varieties of Klinefelter syndrome have been described, including those with uniform cell lines (such as XXYY, XXXY, and XXXXY) and a variety of mosaicisms of the X chromosome with or without associated structural abnormalities of the X. In general, the greater the degree of chromosomal abnormality (and in mosaic forms the more cell lines that are abnormal), the more severe the manifestations.

Pathophysiology The classic form of Klinefelter syndrome is due to meiotic nondisjunction of the chromosomes during gametogenesis (Fig. 120-3). About 40 percent of the responsible meiotic nondisjunctions occur during spermatogenesis, and 60 percent occur during oogenesis. Advanced maternal age is a predisposing factor in the cases in which the defect occurs during oogenesis. The mosaic form of the disorder, in contrast, is thought to result from chromosomal mitotic nondisjunction after fertilization of the zygote and can take place either in a 46,XY zygote (Fig. 120-3) or a 47,XXY zygote. The latter defect or double nondisjunction (meiotic and mitotic) may be the usual cause of the mosaic form and thus explain why the mosaic form is less common than the classic disorder.

Endocrine changes in the pituitary-testicular axis are characteristic. Plasma follicle-stimulating hormone (FSH) and luteinizing hormone (LH) are usually high; FSH shows the best discrimination, and little overlap occurs with normals, a consequence of the consistent damage to the seminiferous tubules. The plasma testosterone averages half normal, but the range of values is broad and overlaps the normal range. Mean plasma estradiol levels are elevated, the cause of which is not entirely clear. Early in the course, the testes may secrete increased amounts of estradiol in response to the elevated plasma LH, but later in the course the testicular secretion of estradiol (and testosterone) declines. Elevated plasma estradiol in this circumstance is probably due to a combination of a decreased metabolic clearance rate and an increased rate of conversion of testosterone to estradiol in extraglandular tissues. The net result both early and late is a variable degree of insufficient androgenization and enhanced feminization. This feminization, including the development of gynecomastia, is thought to depend on the ratio of circulating estrogen to androgen (relative or absolute), and it follows that subjects with the lower plasma testosterone and higher plasma estradiol levels are more likely to develop gynecomastia (see Chap. 119). The increase in plasma gonadotropins after the administration of LHRH is exaggerated after the age of expected puberty, and the normal feedback inhibition of testosterone on pituitary LH secretion is diminished.

Management No method is available for reversing the infertility, and surgical removal is the only available means for effective treatment of the gynecomastia. Some underandrogenized patients benefit from supplemental androgen, but such treatment may paradoxically worsen the gynecomastia, presumably by providing increased androgen substrate for the conversion to estrogens in the peripheral tissues. Following the administration of testosterone, plasma LH returns to normal only after several months, if at all.

XX MALE SYNDROME The incidence of a 46,XX karyotype in phenotypic males is approximately 1 in 20,000 to 24,000 male births. Affected individuals have absence of all female internal genitalia and male psychosexual identification. Indeed, the findings resemble those in the Klinefelter syndrome: the testes are small and firm (generally less than 2 cm), gynecomastia is frequent, the penis is normal to small in size, azoospermia and hyalinization of the seminiferous tubules are usual, mean plasma testosterone is low, plasma estradiol is elevated, and plasma gonadotropin levels are high. Affected individuals differ from typical Klinefelter patients only in that average height is less than in normal men, the incidence of mental deficiency is not increased, and the incidence of hypospadias is increased.

Four theories have been proposed to explain the pathogenesis of this disorder: (1) translocation of all or a portion of a Y chromosome to an autosome, (2) chromosomal mosaicism in which the line containing Y chromosomes exists only in the testes, (3) mutation of an autosomal gene, or (4) deletion of genetic material on X chromosome that controls negative regulation of the H-Y antigen. If either of the first two theories is correct, the disorder is actually a variant of Klinefelter syndrome, and a few XX males have been described in whom translocation of the Y chromosome was identified. Since testicular determinants are located in a circumscribed region of the Y chromosome near the centromere, translocation of small fragments of the Y chromosome that are difficult to detect could be the cause of additional instances. The presence of the H-Y antigen in 46,XX males could be explained either by un-

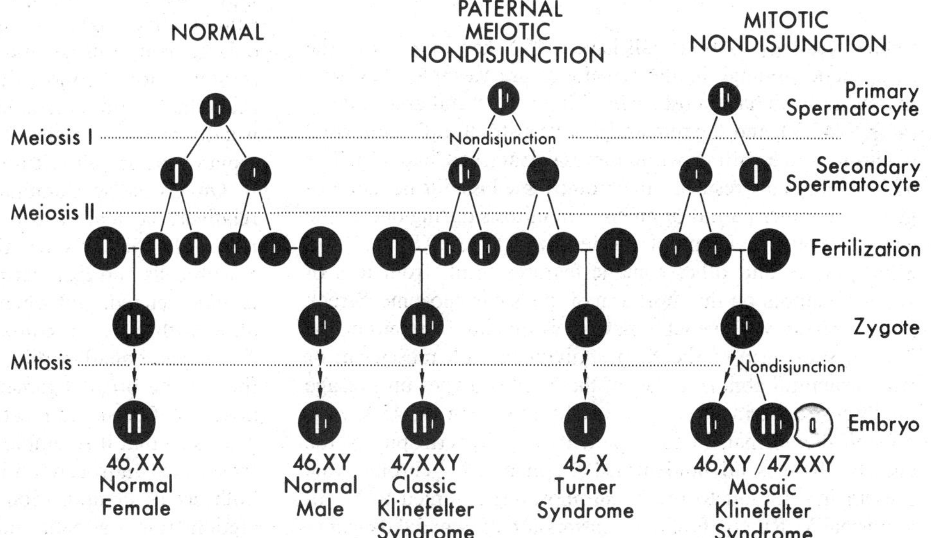

FIGURE 120-3
Schema for normal spermatogenesis and fertilization showing effects of meiotic and mitotic nondisjunction leading to classic Klinefelter syndrome, Turner syndrome, and mosaic Klinefelter. The schema would be similar if the abnormal events took place during oogenesis.

documented translocation or mosaicism of the Y chromosome or by either of the other proposed mechanisms.

GONADAL DYSGENESIS (TURNER SYNDROME) Clinical features Gonadal dysgenesis is characterized by primary amenorrhea, sexual infantilism, short stature, multiple congenital anomalies, and bilateral streak gonads in phenotypic women with any of several defects of the X chromosome. This condition should be distinguished from three similar disorders: (1) mixed gonadal dysgenesis in which a unilateral testis and a contralateral streak gonad are present; (2) pure gonadal dysgenesis in which bilateral streak gonads are associated with a normal 46,XX or 46,XY karyotype, normal stature, and primary amenorrhea; and (3) the Noonan syndrome, an autosomal dominant disorder characterized by the presence of webbed neck, short stature, congenital heart disease, cubitus valgus, and other congenital defects in both males and females with normal karyotypes and normal gonads (see Chap. 107).

The incidence of gonadal dysgenesis is estimated at 1 in 2500 newborn females. The diagnosis is either made at birth because of the associated anomalies or more frequently at puberty when amenorrhea and failure of sexual development are noted in conjunction with the associated anomalies. The external genitalia are unambiguously female but remain immature, and there is no breast development unless the patient is treated with exogenous estrogen. The internal genitalia consist of small but otherwise normal fallopian tubes and uterus, and bilateral streak gonads located in the broad ligaments. Primordial germ cells are present transiently during embryogenesis but disappear as the result of an accelerated rate of atresia (see Chap. 118). After the age of expected puberty these streaks contain fibrous tissue that is indistinguishable from normal ovarian stroma but lack identifiable follicles and ova.

The associated somatic anomalies primarily affect tissues of mesodermal origin, i.e., the skeleton and connective tissue. Lymphedema of the hands and feet, webbing of the neck, low hair line, redundant skin folds on the back of the neck, a shield-like chest with widely spaced nipples, and a low birth weight are features that suggest the diagnosis in infancy. In addition, the facies may be distinctive characterized by micrognathia, epicanthal folds, prominent low-set or deformed ears, a fishlike mouth, and ptosis. Short fourth metacarpals are present in half, and 10 to 20 percent have coarctation of the aorta. In adults the average height rarely exceeds 150 cm. Associated conditions include renal malformations, pigmented nevi, hypoplastic nails, tendency to keloid formation, perceptive hearing loss, and hypertension.

Pathophysiology About half have a 45,X karyotype, and the cytogenetic findings in the remainder are variable. Approximately a fourth have mosaicism with no structural abnormality (46,XX/45,X), and the remainder have a structurally abnormal X chromosome with or without mosaicism (see Chap. 61). The 45,X variety may result from chromosome loss during gametogenesis in either parent or an error in mitosis during one of the early cleavage divisions of the fertilized zygote (Fig. 120-3). Short stature and other somatic features result from loss of genetic material on the short arm of the X chromosome. Streak gonads result when genetic material is missing from either the long or short arm of the X. In individuals with mosaicism or with structural abnormalities of the X, phenotypes on average are intermediate in severity between that seen in the 45,X variety and the normal. In some patients with hypertrophy of the clitoris, there is an unidentified fragment of a chromosome present in addition to the X chromosome, assumed to be an abnormal Y. Rarely, familial transmission of gonadal dysgenesis can be the result of a balanced X-autosome translocation (see Chap. 61).

Assessment of sex chromatin was previously utilized as a means of screening for abnormalities of the X chromosome. Normal sex chromatin (the Barr body) is the result of inactivation of one of two X chromosomes, and women with a 45,X chromosome composition like normal men are said to be chromatin-negative. However, only about half of patients with gonadal dysgenesis (those with 45,X and those with the most extreme mosaicism and structural abnormalities) are chromatin-negative, and karyotypic analysis is necessary both to establish the diagnosis and to identify the fraction with Y chromosomal elements and a high chance of developing malignancy in the streak gonads.

Although sparse pubic and axillary hair develop at the time of expected puberty, the breasts remain infantile, and no menses occur. Serum FSH is usually elevated in infancy, falls during midchildhood to the normal range, and increases to castrate levels at the age of 9 or 10. At this time, serum LH is also elevated, and plasma estradiol levels are low (<10 pg/ml). Approximately 2 percent of 45,X subjects and 12 percent of mosaic subjects have sufficient residual follicles to allow some menstruation. Indeed, occasional pregnancy has been reported in minimally affected individuals; the reproductive life in such individuals is brief.

Management At the anticipated time of puberty replacement therapy with estrogen should be instituted to induce maturation of the breasts, labia, vagina, uterus, and fallopian tubes (see Chap. 118). Linear growth and bone maturation rates are approximately doubled during the first year of treatment with estradiol, but the eventual height of patients rarely approaches the predicted height. Treatment with growth hormone has not been helpful.

Gonadal tumors are rare in 45,X patients. However, gonadal malignancies have occurred in several patients with mosaicism involving the Y chromosome, and, consequently, streak gonads should be removed in any patient with evidence of virilization or a Y-containing cell line.

MIXED GONADAL DYSGENESIS Clinical features Mixed gonadal dysgenesis is an entity in which phenotypic males or females have a testis on one side and streak gonad on the other. Most have 45,X/46,XY mosaicism, but the clinical entity is by no means confined to that chromosomal pattern. The true incidence is unknown, but in most hospitals it is the second most common cause of ambiguous genitalia in the neonate after congenital adrenal hyperplasia.

About two-thirds are reared as females, and most phenotypic males are incompletely virilized at birth. The majority exhibit some degree of ambiguous genitalia, including phallic enlargement, a urogenital sinus, and varying degrees of labioscrotal fusion. In most the testis is located intraabdominally; individuals with a testis in the inguinal or scrotal position are usually reared as males. A uterus, vagina, and at least one fallopian tube are almost invariably present.

On histologic examination, the prepubertal testis appears relatively normal. The postpubertal testis contains abundant mature Leydig cells, but the seminiferous tubules contain only Sertoli cells and lack germinal elements. Frequently, the testis is undescended, and when descended it may present in association with a hernia containing the uterus and fallopian tube. The streak gonad, a thin, pale, elongated structure located either in the broad ligament or along the pelvic wall, is composed of fibrous connective tissue that is often arranged in whorls so that it resembles ovarian stroma. At puberty the testis secretes androgen, and virilization and phallic enlargement both occur. Feminization is rare; when it occurs, estrogen secretion from a gonadal tumor should be suspected.

Approximately a third exhibit the somatic stigmata of 45,X gonadal dysgenesis, i.e., low posterior hairline, shield chest, multiple pigmented nevi, cubitus valgus, webbing of the neck, and short stature (height less than 148 cm).

Virtually all are chromatin-negative. In one series, two-thirds had the 45,X/46,XY karyotype, and in the remainder a 46,XY karyotpe was present but mosaicism might have gone undetected or been limited to certain cell lines. The origin of 45,X/46,XY mosaicism is best explained by the loss of a Y chromosome during an early mitotic division of an XY zygote similar to the postulated loss of the X chromosome in the 46,XY/47,XXY mosaicism shown in Fig. 120-3.

Pathophysiology It has been assumed that the 46,XY cell line stimulates testicular differentiation whereas the 45,X stem leads to the development of the contralateral streak gonad, but actual comparisons between karyotype and phenotypic expression have failed to substantiate such a relationship; furthermore, no clear correlation has been found between the percentage of cells cultured from blood or skin containing 45,X or 46,XY and the degree of gonadal development or of somatic anomalies.

Both masculinization and müllerian duct regression in utero are incomplete. Since Leydig cell function is normal at puberty, it has been suggested that the inadequate virilization in utero is the result of delay in the development of a testis that is ultimately capable of normal Leydig cell function. The capacity of the internal duct structures, the urogenital sinus, and the external genitalia to virilize completely in response to androgen is limited to a critical period between 7 and 14 weeks of gestation, and consequently a delayed but otherwise normal onset of endocrine function in the fetal testis might allow incomplete masculinization of the external genitalia and explain persistence of müllerian ducts. Alternatively, the fetal testis may simply be incapable of synthesizing adequate amounts of müllerian-inhibiting substance and androgen.

Management Several important factors must be considered in the management of patients with mixed gonadal dysgenesis. For the older child or adult in whom gender is fixed prior to diagnosis, the central issue is the possibility of tumor development in the gonads. The overall incidence of gonadal tumors in patients with mixed gonadal dysgenesis is about 25 percent. Seminomas occur more frequently than gonadoblastomas, and the tumors may occur prior to puberty. The tumors occur most frequently in patients with a female phenotype who lack the somatic features typical of 45,X gonadal dysgenesis and are more common in intraabdominal testes than in the streak gonad. When the diagnosis is established in phenotypic females, early exploratory laparotomy and prophylactic gonadectomy are advisable for two reasons; gonadal tumors may occur in childhood, and the testis secretes androgen at puberty and thus causes virilization. Such subjects, like those with gonadal dysgenesis, are then given estrogen to induce and maintain feminization.

When the diagnosis is established in phenotypic males during late childhood or in adults the management is more complicated. Phenotypic males with mixed gonadal dysgenesis are infertile (no germinal elements are present in the testes) and also have a high risk of developing gonadal tumors. Which testes can be safely conserved? In general the following observations apply: (1) tumors develop in scrotal streak gonads but not in scrotal testes, (2) tumors that develop in intraabdominal testes are always associated with ipsilateral müllerian duct structures, and (3) tumors in streak gonads are always associated with tumors in the contralateral abdominal testis. Based on these observations, it is recommended that (1) all streak gonads should be removed, (2) scrotal testes should be preserved, and (3) intraabdominal testes should be excised unless they can be relocated in the scrotum and are not associated with ipsilateral müllerian duct structures. Decisions as to reconstructive surgery of the phallus depend upon the nature of the defect.

When the diagnosis is established in early infancy and the genitalia are ambiguous, the choice of gender for rearing is one of the most complicated issues in gender assignment. Because infertility is inevitable, because the multiple procedures required for construction of the external genitalia often result in a limited ultimate success, because the affected individuals are frequently short in stature, and because of the high risk of developing testicular tumors, gender assignment is usually female. Resection of the enlarged phallus and gonadectomy can then be accomplished in infancy, usually in one procedure. If the decision is for male gender assignment, the same criteria apply as to which testes should be removed in infants as in older males.

TRUE HERMAPHRODITISM **Clinical features** True hermaphroditism is a condition in which both an ovary and a testis or a gonad with histologic features of both (ovotestis) is present. The incidence is unknown, but more than 400 cases have been reported. To justify the diagnosis there must be histologic documentation of both types of gonadal epithelium, the presence of ovarian stroma without oocytes not being sufficient. Three categories are recognized: (1) a fifth are bilateral—testicular and ovarian tissue (ovotestes) on each side, (2) two-fifths are unilateral—an ovotestis on one side and an ovary or a testis on the other, and (3) the remainder are lateral—a testis on one side and an ovary on the other.

The external genitalia display all gradations of the male-to-female spectrum. Two-thirds are sufficiently masculinized to be reared as males. However, less than a tenth have normal male external genitalia; most have hypospadias, and more than half have incomplete labioscrotal fusion. Two-thirds of phenotypic females have an enlarged clitoris, and most have a urogenital sinus. Commonly, differentiation of the internal ducts corresponds to the adjacent gonad. Although an epididymis usually develops adjacent to a testis, development of the vas deferens is complete in only a third. Of the patients with an ovotestis, three-fourths have an epididymis, two-thirds have a fallopian tube, a tenth have a ves deferens, and a tenth have both a vas deferens and a fallopian tube. A uterus is usually present although it may be hypoplastic or unicornuate. The ovary usually occupies the normal position, but the testis or ovotestis may be found at any level along the route of embryonic testicular descent, frequently associated with an inguinal hernia. Testicular tissue is present in the scrotum or the labioscrotal fold in a third, in the inguinal canal in a third, and in the abdominal area in a third.

At puberty signs of variable feminization and virilization develop; three-fourths develop significant gynecomastia, and about half menstruate. In phenotypic men menstruation presents as cyclic hematuria. Ovulation occurs in approximately a fourth and is more common than spermatogenesis. In phenotypic men ovulation may present as testicular pain. Fertility has been reported in women following removal of an ovotestis and in a man who fathered two children. Congenital malformations of other systems are rare.

Pathophysiology About two-thirds of subjects have a 46,XX karyotype, a tenth have a 46,XY karyotype, and the remainder are chromosomal mosaics. In virtually all instances of mosaicism a Y cell line is present. The mechanism responsible for the gonadal development in true hermaphroditism is unknown.

Even if not demonstrable with conventional karyotyping methods, it is assumed that sufficient genetic material derived from the Y chromosome is present (as the result of translocation, nondisjunction, or mutation) to induce the development of testicular tissue. XX true hermaphrodites are usually H-Y antigen positive. In addition cells from the testicular portion of the ovotestis tend to be positive for H-Y antigen whereas the ovarian areas are H-Y antigen negative. Rare instances have been reported in which multiple sibs with a 46,XX karyotype are affected, suggesting that this form of true hermaphroditism may be determined by an autosomal recessive gene or by a common translocation.

Because corpora lutea are present in the ovaries of more than a fourth of subjects, it can be deduced that a female neuroendocrine axis is present and functions normally in such individuals. Feminization (gynecomastia and menstruation) is the result of secretion of estradiol by the ovarian tissue present. It is presumed that in masculinized patients secretion of androgen predominates over secretion of estrogen, and the fact that some patients produce sperm is in keeping with this view.

Management When the diagnosis is made in a newborn or early infant, gender assignment depends largely upon the anatomical findings. In older children and adults gonads and internal duct structures that are contradictory to the predominant phenotype (and the gender of rearing) should be removed, and when necessary the external genitalia should be modified appropriately. Although gonadal tumors are rare in true hermaphroditism, a gonadoblastoma has been reported in an individual with an XY cell line. Consequently, the possibility of future tumor development in the gonad must be taken into consideration when the decision regarding conservation of gonadal tissue is made.

DISORDERS OF GONADAL SEX

Disorders of gonadal sex result when chromosomal sex is normal, but for one of several reasons differentiation of the gonads is abnormal. Thus, chromosomal sex does not correspond to gonadal and phenotypic sex.

PURE GONADAL DYSGENESIS Clinical features Pure gonadal dysgenesis is a disorder in which phenotypic females with gonads and genitalia identical to those with gonadal dysgenesis (bilateral streaks, infantile uterus and fallopian tubes, and sexual infantilism) have normal height, few if any congenital anomalies, and either a normal 46,XX or 46,XY karyotype. In most series this disorder is only about a tenth as common as gonadal dysgenesis. There is a clear-cut genetic basis for considering this a separate disorder from gonadal dysgenesis, but on clinical grounds it cannot be distinguished from those instances of gonadal dysgenesis associated with minimal somatic abnormalities. The height is normal or greater than normal, some subjects being over 172 cm. Estrogen deficiency is profound in that the primary amenorrhea is accompanied by lack of breast development and immaturity of the vagina. Axillary and pubic hair are scanty, and the internal genitalia consist of müllerian derivatives only.

Development of tumors may occur in the streak gonads, particularly dysgerminoma or gonadoblastoma in the 46,XY disorder. Such tumors are frequently heralded by the development of virilizing signs or a pelvic mass.

Pathophysiology Although a variety of chromosomal mosaicisms have been described under this nosology, the designation as used here is restricted to subjects with uniform 46,XX or 46,XY karyotypes. (Those individuals with mosaicism are actually variants of gonadal dysgenesis or mixed gonadal dysgenesis as described above.) The rationale for this restricted definition is based upon the fact that both the XX and XY varieties can result from different single gene mutations. Several sibships have been reported in which more than one individual is affected with the 46,XX type of the disorder, frequently the result of consanguineous matings, suggesting that the disorder is transmitted in an autosomal recessive pattern. Furthermore, several instances of familial occurrence of the 46,XY variety have been described. In some of these latter families the mutation appears to be inherited in an X-linked recessive pattern while in other families segregation analysis is compatible with a male-limited autosomal recessive inheritance. Thus, there appears to be genetic heterogeneity within the familial 46,XY form of pure gonadal dysgenesis. The finding that some (but not all) 46,XY patients are H-Yantigen positive is further evidence for genetic heterogeneity. In both the 46,XX and the 46,XY forms the mutation prevents differentiation of ovary or testis, respectively, by an uncertain mechanism; the development of the female phenotype is the consequence of the failure of gonadal development. According to the current concepts of sexual differentiation, total absence of the gonads—either male or female—would be expected to result in the development of a female phenotype. As also predicted in individuals with nonfunctional gonads, gonadotropin secretion is elevated and estrogen secretion is low.

Management The management of the estrogen deficiency is identical to that in gonadal dysgenesis, namely appropriate estrogen replacement therapy is initiated at the time of expected puberty and maintained in adult life. Because of the high frequency of gonadal tumors in the 46,XY variety, exploratory surgery and removal of the streak gonads should be undertaken once the diagnosis is made. The development of virilizing signs is indication for immediate surgery. The natural history of the gonadal tumors in this disorder is uncertain, but the prognosis after surgical removal appears to be good.

THE ABSENT TESTES SYNDROME (ANORCHIA, TESTICULAR REGRESSION, GONADAL AGENESIS, AGONADISM) Clinical features A spectrum of phenotypes has been described in 46,XY males with absent or rudimentary testes but in whom unequivocal evidence exists that endocrine function of the testis (e.g., invariable müllerian duct regression and variable testosterone synthesis) was present at some time during embryonic life. This rare disorder can be distinguished from pure gonadal dysgenesis in which no evidence can be inferred for gonadal function during embryonic development. The disorder has been reported under a variety of eponyms and varies in its manifestations from complete failure of virilization through varying degrees of incomplete virilization of the external genitalia to otherwise normal males with bilateral anorchia.

The purest form of the syndrome is represented by 46,XY phenotypic females with absent testes, sexual infantilism, and concomitant absence of müllerian duct derivatives and accessory organs of male reproduction. Such individuals differ from the 46,XY form of pure gonadal dysgenesis in that no gonadal remnant whatsoever can be identified, including no streak gonad, and in the absence of müllerian derivatives. In these women testicular failure must have occurred during the interval between the onset of formation of müllerian-inhibiting substance and the secretion of testosterone; that is, after development of the seminiferous tubules but before the onset of Leydig cell function.

In others the clinical features indicate that testicular failure occurred during later phases of gestation, and some of these individuals constitute problems in gender assignment. In some, failure of müllerian regression occurs to a greater extent than the failure of testosterone secretion, but none exhibit complete müllerian development. In individuals with more extensive virilization the external genitalia are phenotypically male, but rudimentary oviducts and vasa deferentia may coexist internally.

At the final extreme is the syndrome of bilateral anorchia in phenotypic men with absence of müllerian structures and gonads but complete male development of the wolffian system and external genitalia. Microphallus in such subjects implies that failure of androgen-mediated growth occurred during late embryogenesis after anatomic development of the male urethra is complete. Persistent gynecomastia may or may not develop after the time of puberty.

Pathophysiology The pathogenesis of these disorders is not understood. The karyotype is 46,XY by definition. Whether the testicular regression is the result of mutant genes, teratogen, or trauma is unclear. Multiple instances of agonadism in the same family have been reported, and since unilateral and bilateral agonadism can occur within the same family, it is necessary to obtain a careful family history.

The quantitative dynamics of gonadal steroid production have been studied in only a few patients. In two phenotypic females who had primary amenorrhea, sexual infantilism, and no internal genital structures, androgen and estrogen kinetics were similar to those in gonadal dysgenesis. The daily production rates of estrogen were low, and no glandular secretion of testosterone could be documented, confirming the functional as well as anatomic absence of the testes. In one phenotypic male with bilateral anorchia there was no glandular secretion of testosterone; total testosterone and estrogen production was accounted for by peripheral conversion from plasma androstenedione. However, some subjects in whom no testes can be identified at laparotomy have blood testosterone values clearly above the castrate range, presumably derived from remnant testes.

Management The management of the two extremes in this disorder is clear-cut. Sexually infantile, phenotypic females should be treated like patients with gonadal dysgenesis, namely given adequate estrogen to ensure appropriate breast and female somatic development, and any coexisting vaginal agenesis should be treated by either surgical or medical means. Likewise, phenotypic males with anorchia should be given adequate androgen replacement to allow development of normal male secondary sexual development. The cases with incomplete virilization or ambiguous development of the external genitalia are more complex and require individual assessment as to whether surgical means are appropriate for improving male or female phenotypes. In either case, appropriate hormonal therapy is mandatory at the time of expected puberty.

DISORDERS OF PHENOTYPIC SEX

FEMALE PSEUDOHERMAPHRODITISM Congenital adrenal hyperplasia CLINICAL FEATURES The pathways by which glucocorticoids are synthesized in the adrenal gland and androgens are formed in the testis and adrenal are schematically summarized in Fig. 120-4. A variety of syndromes result from hereditary defects in the enzymes of steroid hormone synthesis. Three enzymes are common to the formation of glucocorticoids and androgens (20,22-desmolase, 3β-hydroxysteroid dehydrogenase, and 17α-hydroxylase); deficiency of any of these enzymes results in deficiency of glucocorticoid and androgen synthesis and consequently results in both congenital adrenal hyperplasia (due to enhanced ACTH levels) and defective virilization of the male embryo (male pseudohermpahroditism). Two enzymes are involved exclusively in androgen synthesis (17,20-desmolase and 17β-hydroxysteroid dehydrogenase); deficiency in either results in pure male pseudohermaphroditism with normal glucocorticoid synthesis. Deficiency of either of the terminal two enzymes of glucocorticoid synthesis (21-hydroxylase and 11β-hydroxylase) results in defective formation of hydrocortisone; the compensatory increase in ACTH secretion causes enhanced formation of adrenal steroids proximal to the enzymatic defect and a secondary increase in androgen formation. As a consequence, the latter two disorders result in adrenal hyperplasia and either virilization in the female embryo or precocious masculinization in the male.

The *adrenal insufficiency* in these disorders may produce equally severe and life-threatening problems in both sexes and is described in detail in Chap. 112. The major features of the different forms of congenital adrenal hyperplasia are listed in Table 120-3. From the standpoint of *abnormal sexual development* it is helpful to consider separately those enzyme defects in steroidogenesis that result in female pseudohermaphroditism and those that cause male pseudohermaphroditism. (One disorder, 3β-hydroxysteroid dehydrogenase deficiency, can cause either male or female pseudohermaphroditism, but since the more common genital defect is incomplete virilization of the male it will be discussed as an abnormality of male phenotypic differentiation.)

Congenital adrenal hyperplasia due to 21-hydroxylase deficiency is the most common cause of ambiguous genitalia in the newborn, with an incidence of between 1:5000 and 1:15,000 in Europe and the United States. Virilization is usually apparent at birth in the female and within the first 2 to 3 years of life in the male. At birth there is hypertrophy of the clitoris associ-

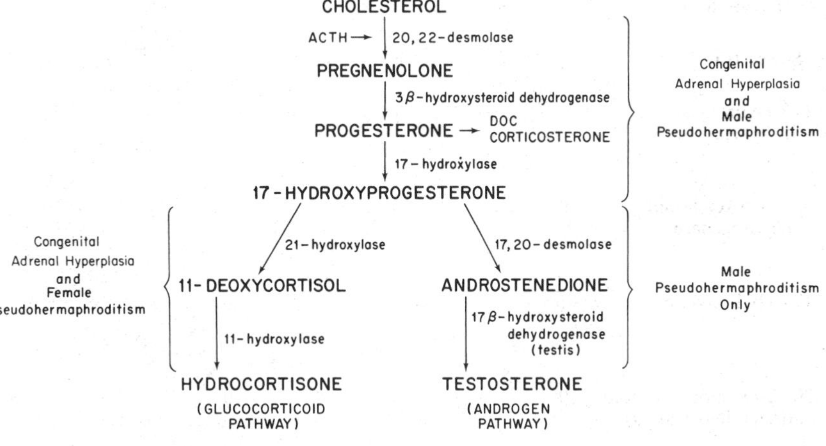

FIGURE 120-4
Pathways of glucocorticoid and androgen synthesis.

ated with ventral binding (chordee), variable fusion of the labioscrotal folds, and differing degrees of virilization of the urethra. The internal female structures and ovaries remain unaltered. The wolffian ducts regress normally, probably because the onset of adrenal function occurs relatively late in embryogenesis. The external appearance of affected females is similar to that of a male with bilateral cryptorchidism and hypospadias. The labioscrotal folds are bulbous and rugated and resemble a scrotum. In a small percentage the virilization is so severe as to result in development of a complete male penile urethra and prostate so that errors in sex assignment may occur at birth. Radiography following the injection of radiopaque dye into the external genital orifice is helpful in defining the internal structure and in particular in demonstrating presence of vagina, uterus, and sometimes even fallopian tubes. In a few cases virilization of the female is slight or absent at birth and becomes evident in later infancy, adolescence, or adulthood, presumably as the result of allelic variation of the mutant genes (the so-called late-onset or adult form of the disorder).

The untreated female grows rapidly during the first year of life and has progressive virilization. At the time of expected puberty there is a failure of normal female sexual development and absence of menstruation. In both sexes rapid somatic maturation results in premature epiphyseal closure and a short adult height. Since male phenotypic differentiation is normal the condition is usually not recognized in the male at birth in the absence of overt adrenal insufficiency. However, there is early growth and maturation of the external genitalia and early appearance of secondary sex characteristics, coarsening of the voice, frequent erections, and excessive muscular development are noticeable in the first few years of life. Virilization in the male can follow either of two patterns. Excessive adrenal androgens can inhibit gonadotropin production so that the testes remain infantile in size despite the acceleration of masculinization. Such untreated adult men are capable of erection and ejaculation but have no spermatogenesis. Alternatively, early adrenal androgen secretion can activate a premature maturation of the hypothalamic-pituitary axis and initiate a true precocious puberty including early maturation of spermatogenesis (see Chap. 117). The untreated male is also subject to the development of ACTH-dependent "tumors" of the testis composed of adrenal rest cells.

In 21-hydroxylase deficiency, which accounts for about 95 percent of congenital adrenal hyperplasia, there is a reduced activity of the 21-hydroxylase enzyme which leads to decreased production of hydrocortisone and consequently to increased release of ACTH, enlargement of the adrenal glands, and partial or complete compensation of the defect in the secretion of hydrocortisone. In about half the enzyme defect appears to be partial, and cortisol secretion is normal. This form is termed "simple virilizing" or "compensated." In the remainder there seems to be a more complete deficiency of the enzyme; the enlarged adrenal fails to produce adequate amounts of cortisol and aldosterone leading to severe salt wastage with anorexia, vomiting, volume depletion, and collapse within the first few weeks of life, the so-called salt-losing form of 21-hydroxylase deficiency. In all untreated patients overproduction of the cortisol precursors prior to the 21-hydroxylase step occurs, leading to increase in plasma progesterone and 17-hydroxyprogesterone. These act as weak aldosterone antagonists at the receptor level and in the compensated form result in greater than normal aldosterone production to maintain normal sodium balance.

A rare form of congenital adrenal hyperplasia associated with female pseudohermaphroditism is 11β-hydroxylase deficiency. In this disorder a block in hydroxylation at the 11 carbon results in the accumulation of 11-deoxycortisol and deoxycorticosterone (DOC), a potent salt-retaining hormone that causes hypertension rather than salt loss. The clinical features that stem from glucocorticoid deficiency and androgen excess are similar to those in 21-hydroxylase deficiency.

PATHOPHYSIOLOGY The reported pedigrees are consistent with an autosomal recessive pattern of inheritance for both disorders. The carrier frequency for 21-hydroxylase deficiency is about 1 in 50. At least three forms of 21-hydroxylase deficiency have been identified, all involving mutations of a gene on the sixth chromosome close to the HLA-B locus: the common type, which acts like an ordinary autosomal recessive enzyme mutation; a cryptic allele, which is clinically silent in homozygous form but which causes typical disease when present as a genetic compound with the common variety; and a late-onset variant. Although no specific HLA markers are pres-

TABLE 120-3
Forms of congenital adrenal hyperplasia

Deficiency	*Cortisol*	*Aldosterone*	*Degree of virilization of females*	*Failure of virilization in males*	*Dominant steroid secreted*	*Comment*
21-Hydroxylase, partial (simple virilizing or compensated)	Normal	↑	++++	0	17-Hydroxyprogesterone	Most common type (~95% of total); from one- to two-thirds salt losers
Severe (salt-losing)	↓	↓	++++	0	17-Hydroxyprogesterone	
11β-Hydroxylase (hypertension)	↓	↓	++++	0	11-Deoxycortisol and 11-deoxycorticosterone	Hypertension
3β-Hydroxysteroid dehydrogenase	0	0	+	++++	Δ^5-3β-OH compounds (dehydroepiandrosterone)	Probably second most common, usually salt loss
17α-Hydroxylase	↓	↓	0	++++	Corticosterone and 11-deoxycorticosterone	No feminization of female, hypertension
20,22-Desmolase (lipoid adrenal hyperplasia)	0	0	0	++++	Cholesterol(?)	Rare, usually salt loss

ent in increased frequency in patients with 21-hydroxylase deficiency, carriers of the disorder (as well as homozygotes) within a given family can be identified on the basis of the HLA haplotype. In 11β-hydroxylase deficiency there is no known linkage of the mutation to the HLA system.

For discussion of the endocrine pathology see Chap. 112. In brief, excretion of ketosteroids is elevated, as is the excretion of the major metabolites that accumulate proximal to the enzymatic blocks. In 21-hydroxylase deficiency, 17-hydroxyprogesterone accumulates in blood and is excreted predominantly as pregnanetriol. In 11-hydroxylase deficiency 11-deoxycortisol accumulates in blood and is excreted predominantly as tetrahydrocortexolone. Plasma ACTH is also elevated in untreated patients.

MANAGEMENT Insofar as is possible, gender assignment should correspond to the chromosomal and gonadal sex, and appropriate surgical correction of the external genitalia should be undertaken promptly. This is of particular importance because appropriately treated men and women are capable of fertility. However, if the correct diagnosis is made late (after 3 years of age) gender assignment should be changed only after careful consideration of the psychosexual background.

Medical treatment with appropriate glucocorticoids prevents the consequences of hydrocortisone deficiency, arrests the rapid virilization, and prevents premature somatic advancement and epiphyseal maturation. The suppression of the abnormal steroid secretion results in cure of the hypertension in patients with 11β-hydroxylase deficiency and allows normal onset of menses and development of female secondary sex characteristics in both disorders. In males glucocorticoid therapy suppresses adrenal androgens and results in normal gonadotropin secretion, testicular development, and spermatogenesis. Measurement of plasma 17-hydroxyprogesterone, androstenedione, ACTH, and renin have all been used to assess adequacy of replacement therapy. In severe forms of 21-hydroxylase deficiency associated with salt loss or with elevated plasma renin activity treatment with mineralocorticoids is also indicated. In such patients the monitoring of plasma renin activity is useful for determining the adequacy of mineralocorticoid replacement.

Nonadrenal female pseudohermaphroditism At present nonadrenal causes of female pseudohermaphroditism are rare. In the past, the administration to pregnant women of progestational agents with androgenic side effects (such as 17α-ethinyl-19-nor-testosterone) to prevent abortion resulted in masculinization of female fetuses. Such infants usually virilize less severely than those with congenital adrenal hyperplasia. Female pseudohermaphroditism may also occur in babies born to mothers who have virilizing tumors (e.g., arrhenoblastomas or luteomas of pregnancy) and, rarely, under circumstances in which no etiology can be determined.

Developmental disorders of müllerian ducts (congenital absence of the vagina, müllerian agenesis) CLINICAL FEATURES Congenital absence of the vagina in combination with some form of abnormal or absent uterus (the Mayer-Rokitansky-Kuster-Hauser syndrome) is second only to gonadal dysgenesis as a cause of primary amenorrhea. Most patients are ascertained after the time of expected puberty because of failure to menstruate and are found to have absence or hypoplasia of the vagina. The height and intelligence are normal, and the breasts, axillary and pubic hair, and habitus are feminine in character. The uterus may vary from almost normal, lacking only a conduit to the introitus, to the more characteristic rudimentary bicornuate cords with or without a lumen. In some patients cyclical abdominal pain indicates that sufficient functional endometrium is present to result in retrograde menstruation and/or hematometra.

Renal, skeletal, and other congenital anomalies are common. About a third have abnormal kidneys, most commonly agenesis or ectopy. Fused kidneys of the horseshoe type and solitary ectopic kidneys located in the pelvis also occur. Skeletal abnormalities are present in a tenth; two-thirds of these involve the spine, and limb and rib abnormalities account for most of the remainder. Specific bone abnormalities include wedge vertebrae, fusions, rudimentary or asymmetric vertebral bodies, and supernumerary vertebrae. The Klippel-Feil syndrome (congenital fusion of the cervical spine, short neck, low posterior hairline, and painless limitation of cervical movement) is a frequent association.

PATHOPHYSIOLOGY The karyotype is 46,XX. Most are believed to be sporadic in nature, but several instances of familial occurrence have been described. It is not known whether the sporadic cases represent new mutations of the type responsible for the familial disorder or are multifactorial in etiology. In the familial cases variable expressivity of the defect is common; some affected family members have skeletal or renal abnormalities only, while others have other abnormalities of müllerian derivatives such as a double uterus. Bilateral renal aplasia in stillborn infants is also commonly associated with absence of the uterus and vagina. Thus, the family histories should be probed for instances of isolated skeletal and renal abnormalities and for stillbirths that might result from congenital absence of both kidneys.

Documentation of ovulatory peaks of plasma LH and biphasic temperature curves during the cycle suggest that ovarian function is normal, and successful pregnancies have been reported following corrective vaginal surgery in patients who have normal uteri.

MANAGEMENT Vaginal agenesis can be treated by surgical or nonsurgical means. Surgical repair generally utilizes a split-thickness skin graft around a solid rubber mold for the creation of an artificial vagina. Medical treatment consists of the repeated application of pressure against the vaginal dimple with a simple dilator to cause development of adequate vaginal depth. In view of the overall complication rate of around 5 to 10 percent in surgical series, medical treatment should be tried in most, and surgery should be reserved for patients in whom a well-formed uterus is present and the possibility of fertility exists. Continued coitus or instrumental dilatation is probably essential for maintaining the neovagina formed either by the nonoperative technique or by the surgical method.

MALE PSEUDOHERMAPHRODITISM Defective virilization of the male embryo (male pseudohermaphroditism) can result from defects in androgen synthesis, defects in androgen action, defects in müllerian duct regression, and uncertain causes. Defects in androgen action are the cause in more than 80 percent.

Abnormalities in androgen synthesis CLINICAL FEATURES Five enzymatic defects have been described that result in defective testosterone synthesis (Fig. 120-4) and consequent incomplete virilization of the male embryo during embryogenesis (Tables 120-3 and 120-4). Each of the enzymes catalyzes a critical biochemical step in the conversion of cholesterol to testosterone. Three (20,22-desmolase, 3β-hydroxysteroid dehydrogenase, and 17α-hydroxylase) are common to the synthesis of other adrenal hormones as well; consequently, their deficiency results in congenital adrenal hyperplasia (Table 120-3) as well as male pseudohermaphroditism. The other two (17,20-desmolase, and 17β-hydroxysteroid dehydrogenase) are unique to the pathway of androgen synthesis, and their deficiency results only in male pseudohermaphroditism. Since 19-carbon androgens are obligatory precursors of estrogens, it likewise follows that in all but the terminal defect (17β-hydroxysteroid dehydrogenase deficiency) synthesis of estrogen is also low in affected individuals of both sexes.

The problems inherent in the adrenal hyperplasia of the three relevant disorders are described in Chap. 112, and the present discussion concerns the abnormal sexual development. In 46,XY subjects there is usually no trace of uterus or fallopian tubes, indicating that the müllerian-inhibiting function of the testis takes place normally during embryogenesis. However, the masculinization of the wolffian ducts, urogenital sinus, and urogenital tubercle and the degree of virilization at puberty vary from almost normal to absent. Therefore, the clinical picture spans the range from phenotypic men with mild hypospadias to phenotypic women who prior to puberty resemble patients with the complete testicular feminization syndrome. This extreme variability is presumed to be the consequence of the varying severity of the enzymatic defects in different patients and of varying effects of the steroids that accumulate proximal to the metabolic blocks in the different disorders. In patients with partial defects and in whom plasma testosterone is normal the diagnosis can only be made by measuring the steroids that accumulate proximal to the metabolic block in question.

20,22-Desmolase deficiency (lipoid adrenal hyperplasia) is a form of congenital adrenal hyperplasia in which virtually no urinary steroids (either 17-ketosteroids or 17-hydroxycorticoids) can be detected and in which the enzyme deficiency is prior to the formation of pregnenolone. The abnormality is assumed to involve one or more of the enzymes of the 20,22-desmolase complex responsible for cleavage of the side chain of cholesterol to form pregnenolone. The syndrome is associated with salt wasting and profound adrenal insufficiency, and most affected individuals die during infancy. At autopsy the adrenals and testes are enlarged and infiltrated with lipid. Affected males are incompletely masculinized whereas affected female infants have normal genital development.

3β-Hydroxysteroid dehydrogenase deficiency is the second most common cause of congenital adrenal hyperplasia. In male infants it causes varying degrees of hypospadias or complete failure of masculinization associated with presence of a vagina. Female infants may be modestly virilized at birth due to the weak androgenic potency of dehydroepiandrosterone, the major steroid secreted. If the enzyme is absent in both the adrenal and testis, no urinary steroids contain a Δ^4-3-keto configuration, whereas in patients in whom the defect is partial or affects only the testis, the urine may contain normal or even elevated levels of Δ^4-3-ketosteroids. Most patients have marked salt wasting and profound adrenal insufficiency, and long-term survival in untreated cases occurs only in states of partial deficiency. Several affected males have been reported who experienced otherwise normal male puberty except for pathological gynecomastia. In these individuals the blood testosterone level is in the low-normal range but is accompanied by elevated Δ^5 precursors. The enzyme in different tissues must be under complex genetic and regulatory control since deficiency of the enzyme in the testis may be less severe than that in the adrenal and since enzyme activity in the liver may be normal in the face of profound deficiency in the adrenal and testis. Individuals with normal liver enzymes can be mistakenly identified as having 21-hydroxylase deficiency if urinary Δ^5-pregnenetriol is not documented to be greater than urinary pregnanetriol.

17α-Hydroxylase deficiency characteristically results in hypogonadism, absence of secondary sex characteristics, hypokalemic alkalosis, hypertension, and virtually undetectable hydrocortisone secretion in phenotypic women. The secretion of both corticosterone and desoxycorticosterone (DOC) by the adrenal is elevated, and urinary 17-ketosteroids are low. Aldo-

TABLE 120-4
Anatomic, genetic, and endocrine profile of hereditary male pseudohermaphroditism

		Phenotype				
Disorder	*Inheritance*	*Müllerian ducts*	*Wolffian ducts*	*Spermatogeneses*	*Urogenital sinus*	*External genitalia*
DEFECTS IN TESTOSTERONE SYNTHESIS						
Five enzyme deficiencies	Autosomal or X-linked recessive	Absent	Variable development	Normal or decreased	Variable from male to female	Generally female
DEFECTS IN ANDROGEN ACTION						
5α-Reductase deficiency	Autosomal recessive	Absent	Male	Normal or decreased	Female	Clitoromegaly
Receptor disorders:						
Complete testicular feminization	X-linked recessive	Absent	Absent	Absent	Female	Female
Incomplete testicular feminization	X-linked recessive	Absent	Male	Absent	Female	Clitoromegaly and posterior fusion
Reifenstein syndrome	X-linked	Absent	Variable development	Absent	Variable from male to female	Incomplete male development
Infertile male syndrome	Probably X-linked recessive	Absent	Male	Absent or decreased	Male	Male
Receptor-positive resistance	Uncertain	Absent	Variable	Absent or decreased	Variable	Female to male
DEFECTS IN MÜLLERIAN REGRESSION						
Persistent müllerian duct syndrome	Autosomal or X-linked recessive	Rudimentary uterus and fallopian tubes	Male	Normal	Male	Male

sterone secretion is low, presumably as the result of high plasma DOC and depressed angiotensin levels, and returns to normal after suppressive doses of hydrocortisone are administered. In 46,XX subjects amenorrhea, absent sexual hair, and hypertension are common, but, since gonadal steroids are not required for female development during embryogenesis, the phenotype is that of a normal prepubertal woman. In males, however, the enzyme deficiency results in defective virilization that varies from complete male pseudohermaphroditism to ambiguous genitalia with perineoscrotal hypospadias. In males with presumed partial enzyme deficiency pathological gynecomastia may develop at puberty. Subjects with this disorder do not develop adrenal insufficiency, since the secretion of both corticosterone (a weak glucocorticoid) and DOC (a mineralocorticoid) is elevated. The hypertension and hypokalemia that are prominent features of the disorder (even in the neonatal period) remit after suppression of the DOC secretion by adequate glucocorticoid replacement.

17,20-Desmolase deficiency has been described in two families in which affected individuals had a 46,XY chromosome pattern, normal adrenocortical function, and a variable pattern of male pseudohermaphroditism. Only trace quantities of 19-carbon steroids are formed.

17β-Hydroxysteroid dehydrogenase deficiency involves the final step in androgen biosynthesis, reduction of the 17-keto group of androstenedione to form testosterone. This disorder is the most common enzymatic defect in testosterone synthesis that causes male pseudohermaphroditism. Affected 46,XY males usually have a female phenotype with a blind-ending vagina and absence of müllerian derivatives, but inguinal or abdominal testes and virilized wolffian duct structures are present. At the time of expected puberty, both virilization (with phallic enlargement and development of facial and body hair) and a variable degree of female breast development take place. Androgen and estrogen dynamics have not been elucidated in detail, but the 17-keto reduction of estrone to estradiol by the gonads is also low. 17β-Hydroxysteroid dehydrogenase is normally present in many tissues besides the gonads, and only the gonadal enzyme appears to be defective in this disorder. Plasma testosterone may be in the low-normal range, making it essential to document a significant elevation in plasma androstenedione to make the diagnosis.

PATHOPHYSIOLOGY The available data for the 17α-hydroxylase and 3β-hydroxysteroid dehydrogenase defects are compatible with autosomal recessive inheritance. The limited family data for 17,20-desmolase deficiency and 17β-hydroxysteroid dehydrogenase deficiency are compatible either with autosomal recessive or X-linked recessive mutations, and insufficient data are available for the 20,22-desmolase defect to warrant any conclusions as to the pattern of inheritance.

The pattern of steroid secretion and excretion depends on the site of the various metabolic blocks (Fig. 120-4). In general, gonadotropin secretion is high, and as a consequence many individuals with incomplete defects are able to compensate so that the steady-state concentration of end products such as testosterone may be normal or almost normal.

Instances of male pseudohermaphroditism have been described in which testosterone formation is deficient for reasons other than a single enzyme defect in androgen synthesis. These include disorders in which Leydig cell agenesis (possibly due to absence of the LH receptor) or the secretion of a biologically inactive LH molecule has been thought to be the primary defect. In addition, as described above, a spectrum of defects in testicular development has been characterized, including familial XY gonadal dysgenesis, sporadic dysgenetic testes, and the absent testis syndrome in which deficient testosterone production is secondary to the underlying disorder of gonadal development.

MANAGEMENT Replacement therapy with glucocorticoids and in some instances mineralocorticoids is indicated in those disorders causing adrenal insufficiency. The decision as to the management of the genital abnormalities depends upon the individual case. Fertility has not been reported, and its consideration does not enter into the decision of sex assignment. In genetic females there is no problem (except in diagnosis) in that affected individuals are raised appropriately as females, and suitable estrogen replacement is indicated at the time of expected puberty to promote development of normal female secondary sex characteristics. The decision as to whether affected newborn males with ambiguous genitalia should be raised as males or females depends upon the anatomic defect; in general the more severely affected should be raised as females, and corrective surgery of the genitalia and removal of the testes should be undertaken as early as possible. In subjects raised as females estrogen therapy is also indicated at the appropriate age to allow development of normal female secondary sex characteristics. In individuals raised as males, corrective surgery is indicated for any coexisting hypospadias, and careful monitoring of plasma androgens and estrogens should be undertaken at the time of expected puberty to determine whether long-term supplemental testosterone therapy is appropriate.

Abnormalities in androgen action Several disorders of male phenotypic development result from abnormalities of andro-

	Endocrine profile relative to normal male		
Breast	Testosterone production	Estrogen production	LH
Usually male	Normal to decreased	Variable	High
Male	Normal	Normal	Normal or increased
Female	High	High	High
Female	High	High	High
Female	High	High	High
Usually male	Normal or high	Normal or high	Normal or high
Variable	Normal or high	Normal or high	Normal or high
Male	Normal	Normal	Normal

gen action. The spectrum of phenotypes is illustrated in Fig. 120-5 and described in Table 120-4.

5α-REDUCTASE DEFICIENCY (FAMILIAL INCOMPLETE MALE PSEUDOHERMAPHRODITISM, TYPE 2; PSEUDOVAGINAL PERINEOSCROTAL HYPOSPADIAS) This form of male pseudohermaphroditism is inherited in an autosomal recessive fashion and is characterized by (1) severe perineoscrotal hypospadias with a hooded prepuce, a ventral urethral groove, and opening of the urethra at the base of the phallus; (2) a blind vaginal pouch of variable size opening either into the urogenital sinus or more frequently onto the urethra immediately behind the urethral orifice; (3) well-developed and histologically differentiated testes with normal epididymides, vasa deferentia, and seminal vesicles, and termination of the ejaculatory ducts into the blind-ending vagina; (4) a female habitus without female breast development but with normal axillary and pubic hair; (5) the absence of female internal genitalia; and (6) normal male plasma testosterone and masculinization to a variable degree at the time of puberty.

The fact that the defective virilization during embryogenesis is limited to the urogenital sinus and the anlage of the external genitalia provided insight into the nature of the fundamental abnormality. Testosterone, the androgen secreted by the fetal testis, is the intracellular mediator for differentiation of the wolffian duct into the epididymis, the vas deferens, and the seminal vesicle, whereas dihydrotestosterone is the functional intracellular hormone for virilization of the urogenital sinus and the anlage of the external genitalia. Consequently, in a male embryo with normal testosterone synthesis and normal androgen receptors a failure of dihydrotestosterone formation would be expected to result in the phenotype observed in this disorder, namely normal male wolffian duct derivatives with defective masculinization of the structures originating from the urogenital sinus, genital tubercle, and genital swellings. Since testosterone itself is the hormone that regulates LH secretion (see Chap. 117), plasma LH is usually only minimally elevated. As a result testosterone and estrogen production rates are those of normal men, and gynecomastia does not develop.

The fact that the 5α-reductase enzyme is deficient in this disorder was suspected on phenotypic and endocrine grounds and was established by direct enzymatic assay in biopsied tissues and fibroblasts cultured from affected individuals. There is considerable genetic heterogeneity; in most subjects the 5α-reductase is either profoundly deficient or functionally absent, and in others the enzyme protein is synthesized at a normal rate but is structurally abnormal. It is not clear why virilization at puberty appears to be more normal than the virilization that takes place during sexual differentiation.

RECEPTOR DISORDERS Disorders of the androgen receptor may result in several distinct phenotypes. Despite differences in clinical presentation and molecular pathology these disorders are similar in regard to endocrinology, genetics, and basic pathophysiology. The major clinical features of the disorders will be considered first and followed by a discussion of the similar endocrinology and pathophysiology.

Clinical features. Complete testicular feminization is the most common form of male pseudohermaphroditism; estimates of frequency vary from 1 in 20,000 to 1 in 64,000 male births. It is the third most common cause of primary amenorrhea in phenotypic women after gonadal dysgenesis and congenital absence of the vagina. The clinical features are characteristic. Namely, a phenotypic female is seen by the physician either because of inguinal hernia (prepubertal) or primary amenorrhea (postpubertal). The development of the breasts after puberty, the general habitus, and the distribution of body fat are female in character so that many patients have a truly feminine appearance. Axillary and pubic hair are absent or scanty, but slight vulval hair is usually present. Scalp hair is that of a normal woman, and facial hair is absent. The external genitalia are unambiguously female, and the clitoris is normal or small. The vagina is short and blind-ending and may be absent or rudimentary. All internal genitalia are absent except for gonads that have histologic features of undescended testes (normal or increased Leydig cells and seminiferous tubules without spermatogenesis).

The testes may be located in the abdomen, along the course of the inguinal canal, or in the labia majora. Occasionally, remnants of müllerian or wolffian duct origin can be identified in the paratesticular fascia or in fibrous bands extending from the

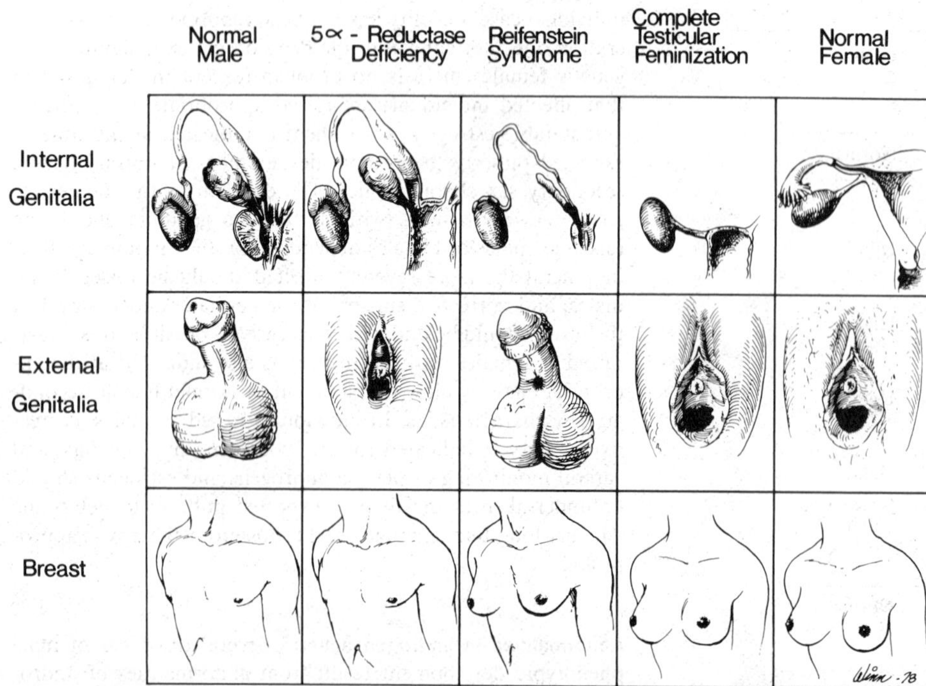

FIGURE 120-5
Schema of the different appearance of the internal and external genitalia and breast development in androgen-resistance syndromes.

testis. Patients tend to be rather tall, bone age is normal, and intelligence is normal. The psychosexual development is unmistakably female in regard to behavior, outlook, and maternal instincts.

The major complication of undescended testes in this disorder as in other forms of cryptorchidism (Chap. 117) is the development of tumors. Since affected individuals undergo a normal pubertal growth spurt and feminize successfully at the time of expected puberty, and since testicular tumors rarely develop until after puberty in patients with intraabdominal testes, it is usual to delay castration until after the time of expected puberty. Surgical intervention is indicated prepubertally if the testes are present in the inguinal region or the labia majora and result in discomfort or hernia formation. (If hernia repair is indicated prepubertally most physicians prefer to remove the testes at the same time so as to limit the number of operative procedures.) If the testes are removed prepubertally, estrogen therapy is required at the appropriate age to ensure normal growth and breast development. When castration is performed postpubertally menopausal symptoms and other evidences of estrogen withdrawal supervene, and suitable estrogen replacement is indicated.

Incomplete testicular feminization is about a tenth as frequent as the complete form. The disorders are similar except that in the incomplete disorder there is a minor virilization of the external genitalia (partial fusion of the labioscrotal folds and some degree of clitoromegaly), normal pubic hair, and some virilization as well as feminization at the time of expected puberty. The vagina is short and blind-ending. In contrast to the complete form, the wolffian duct derivatives are often partially developed. The family history is usually uninformative, but in several instances multiple family members are affected in a pattern compatible with X-linkage.

The management of patients with the complete and incomplete forms of testicular feminization differs. Since patients with the incomplete disorder virilize at the time of expected puberty, gonadectomy should be performed in prepubertal patients with clitoromegaly or posterior labial fusion before the expected time of puberty.

Reifenstein syndrome is the term now applied to a variety of forms of incomplete male pseudohermaphroditism initially described by a number of eponyms (Reifenstein syndrome, Gilbert-Dreyfus syndrome, Lubs syndrome, and familial incomplete male pseudohermaphroditism, type 1). Each of these phenotypes was originally assumed to be a distinct entity. Since several families have now been described in which affected members exhibit variable manifestations that span the phenotypes described under these terms, these syndromes probably constitute variable manifestations of a single mutation. The most common phenotype is a man with perineoscrotal hypospadias and gynecomastia, but the spectrum of defective virilization in such families ranges from men with gynecomastia and azoospermia to phenotypic women with pseudovaginas. Axillary and pubic hair are normal, but chest and facial hair are minimal. Cryptorchidism is common, the testes are usually small, and spermatogenesis is usually incomplete. Some have defects in wolffian duct derivatives such as absence or hypoplasia of the vas deferens.

Since the psychological development in most is unequivocally male, the hypospadias and cryptorchidism should be corrected surgically. The only successful form of treatment of the gynecomastia is surgical removal.

The *infertile male syndrome* is the most common disorder of the androgen receptor and in contrast to the other disorders is not actually a form of male pseudohermaphroditism. Some such individuals are minimally affected subjects in families with Reifenstein syndrome with only azoospermia as a manifestation of the receptor abnormality. More commonly, the individuals present with male infertility and have negative family histories. Evaluation of such men with normal external genitalia, apparently normal wolffian duct structures, and infertility due to azoospermia or severe oligospermia has shown that a disorder of the androgen receptor may be present in a fifth or more of men with idiopathic azoospermia. There is no treatment for the infertility in any of these disorders.

Pathophysiology. The karyotype is 46,XY, and the mutant gene is believed to be located on the X chromosome. The frequency of a positive family history varies from about two-thirds of patients with testicular feminization and Reifenstein syndrome to only occasional patients with the infertile male syndrome. It is assumed that the patients with a negative family history are the result of new mutations.

Hormone dynamics have been best characterized in complete testicular feminization but are similar in all disorders of the androgen receptor. Plasma testosterone levels and rates of testosterone production by the testes are normal or higher than normal. The elevated rate of testosterone production is caused by the high mean plasma level of LH, which in turn is due to defective feedback regulation caused by resistance to the action of androgen at the hypothalamic-pituitary level. Elevated LH concentration is probably responsible also for the increased estrogen production by the testes (see Chap. 117). (In normal men most estrogen is derived from peripheral formation from circulating androgens, but when plasma LH is elevated the testes secrete significant amounts of estrogen into the circulation.) Thus, resistance to the feedback regulation of LH secretion by circulating androgen results in elevated plasma LH levels, and this in turn results in the enhanced secretion of both testosterone and estradiol by the testes. Gonadotropin levels rise even higher (and menopausal symptoms may develop) when the testes are removed, indicating that gonadotropin secretion is under partial regulatory control. Presumably, in the steady state and in the absence of an androgen effect, estrogen alone regulates LH secretion, a control that is purchased at the expense of an elevated plasma estrogen concentrations for a male.

Feminization in these disorders is the result of two interlocking phenomena. First, androgens and estrogens have antagonistic effects at the peripheral level, and normal virilization occurs in normal men when the ratio of androgen to estrogen is 100 to 1 or greater; in the absence of androgen action the cellular effect of estrogen is unopposed. Second, the production of estradiol is greater than that of the normal male (although less than that of the normal female). Variable degrees of androgen resistance coupled with variably enhanced estradiol production result in different degrees of defective virilization and enhanced feminization in the four clinical syndromes. In complete testicular feminization the defective virilization is most severe, and the full feminizing effect of the increased estrogen is expressed. Estrogen production in Reifenstein syndrome is increased to a similar or greater extent to that in testicular feminization, but a less severe androgen resistance results in a predominantly male phenotype and less pronounced feminization. Only a few men with the infertile male syndrome have had evaluation of androgen-estrogen dynamics. The hormonal changes seem to be similar to those in the other receptor disorders but less marked. Some men with this syndrome do not have an elevation of plasma LH or plasma testosterone.

Each of these four syndromes is the result of an abnormality of the androgen receptor. Initially fibroblasts cultured from the skin of some subjects with complete testicular feminization were shown to have a near absence of high-affinity dihydrotestosterone binding. Subsequently, other individuals with complete testicular feminization as well as subjects with incomplete testicular feminization, Reifenstein syndrome, and the infertile male syndrome have been found to have either a decreased amount of an apparently normal receptor or a qualitatively abnormal androgen receptor. Absent or near-absent binding appears to be associated primarily with complete testicular feminization, and decreased amount of an apparently qualitatively normal receptor appears to be most common in the two syndromes with predominant male phenotypes. However, a qualitatively abnormal receptor has been detected in families with each of the four clinical phenotypes. Except for the absent binding in complete testicular feminization there is no consistent correlation between the receptor abnormality as demonstrated in cultured fibroblasts and the clinical severity of the androgen resistance in individual patients.

Receptor-positive resistance. A category of androgen resistance that does not appear to involve either the 5α-reductase or the androgen receptor was first identified in a family with the syndrome of testicular feminization. Subsequent patients have been described with a variety of phenotypes ranging from incomplete testicular feminization to findings similar to those in the Reifenstein syndrome. The hormonal profile is similar to that seen in the receptor disorders. The site of the molecular abnormality in these patients is unclear. It could be due to defects of the androgen receptor too subtle to be detected by the usual assay. If the defect is truly distal to the receptor, there could be failure of generation of specific messenger RNA or an abnormality of RNA processing. Indeed, it is not established that a uniform defect is present, and the disorder may represent a heterogeneous group of molecular abnormalities. Studies designed to detect subtle qualitative abnormalities of the receptor are likely to decrease the number of patients in this category. At present they appear to amount to less than a fifth of patients with androgen resistance. Management depends on the phenotype.

Persistent müllerian duct syndrome Men with this disorder have normal penile development but have in addition bilateral fallopian tubes, a uterus, and an upper vagina, and variable development of the vas deferens. The subjects commonly present with inguinal hernias which contain the uterus, and cryptorchidism is common. Most have uninformative family histories, but several pairs of siblings have been described in whom the condition must be inherited either as an autosomal recessive or an X-linked recessive mutation. Because the external genitalia are well developed and the patients masculinize normally at puberty, it is assumed that during the critical stage of embryonic sexual differentiation the fetal testes produced a normal amount of androgen. However, müllerian regression does not occur for one of three possible reasons: failure of the fetal testis to produce müllerian-inhibiting substance, poor timing of the release of müllerian-inhibiting substance, or failure of the tissues to respond to this hormone.

The preservation of external male appearance and the maintenance of virilization are essential. A primary or staged orchiopexy should be performed. None of the reported cases has developed a malignancy in the uterus or vagina, and because the vasa deferentia are closely associated with the broad ligaments, the uterus and vagina should be left in place to avoid disruption of the vasa deferentia during removal and consequently to preserve possible fertility.

Developmental defects of the male genitalia HYPOSPADIAS Hypospadias is a congenital anomaly in which the urethra terminates in an abnormal position along the midline of the ventral surface of the penis at some site between the normal urethral meatus and the perineum. This malformation is often associated with some degree of ventral contraction and bowing of the penis (chordee). The disorder occurs in 0.5 to 0.8 percent of male births in the United States. Although few authors use the same classification, it is common to categorize hypospadias as glandular (involving the glans penis), penile, or perineoscrotal. Since penile development is mediated by androgens it is assumed that hypospadias results from some defect in earlier androgen formation or androgen action during embryogenesis. Indeed hypospadias occurs in most disorders of male sexual differentiation. A rare cause of hypospadias is maternal ingestion of progestational agents early in pregnancy. However, the known causes (single gene defects, chromosomal abnormalities, and maternal drug ingestion) at best can account for only about a fourth of cases, and the etiology of most remains unknown. The management is surgical.

CRYPTORCHIDISM The normal descent of the testis is perhaps the most poorly understood portion of male sexual differentiation, both in regard to the nature of the forces that result in the movement and to the hormonal factors that regulate the process. In anatomic terms testicular descent can be divided into three phases: (1) transabdominal movement of the testis from its site of origin above the kidney to the inguinal ring, (2) formation of the opening in the inguinal canal (processus vaginalis) through which the testis exits the abdominal cavity, and (3) actual movement of the testis through the inguinal canal to its permanent site in the scrotum. This entire process occurs over a 6- to 7-month period during gestation, beginning at about the sixth week and not completed in some normal individuals until after birth. Whatever its involvement, androgen is probably not the sole hormone responsible for normal descent. Failure of any of the above anatomic events can be responsible for the failure of descent of one or both testes that occurs in 3 percent of full-term males and 30 percent of premature male infants. Cryptorchidism can be classified as intraabdominal, rectractile (intermittently in the groin), obstructed (permanently in the groin), and high scrotal. Most are retractile and descend permanently by 6 weeks to 3 months of age so that the incidence of failure of descent in late teenagers is only 0.6 to 0.7 percent. It is this latter category that requires intervention.

The cryptorchid testis functions poorly after puberty, but the extent to which maldescent is the result of an abnormality of the testis or the cause of abnormal function is unknown. Two general theories have been advanced as to the etiology—inadequate intraabdominal pressure and deficient endocrine function of the testis either because of deficient testosterone synthesis or inadequate formation of müllerian-inhibiting substance. Indeed, hereditary defects that result in inadequate development of intraabdominal pressure or inadequate development of the testes themselves can cause cryptorchidism. As is true for hypospadias, however, the known causes of cryptorchidism constitute only a small fraction of the cases, and the etiology in most remains to be identified. Two complications of cryptorchidism are important; spermatogenesis cannot occur at the temperature of the abdominal cavity, and it is therefore necessary to correct the process as early as possible to allow possible fertility. However, the fact that infertility is common in men who have been treated for unilateral as well as bilateral cryptorchidism suggests that maldescent is usually the consequence rather than the cause of the testicular malfunction. There is also a greater frequency of malignancy in undescended testis, and all should be surgically corrected for this reason (see Chap. 117).

REFERENCES

AIMAN J, GRIFFIN JE: The frequency of androgen receptor deficiency in infertile men. J Clin Endocrinol Metab 54:725, 1982

De La Chapelle A: The etiology of maleness in XX men. Hum Genet 58:105, 1981
Donahoe PK et al: Mixed gonadal dysgenesis, pathogenesis and management. J Pediatr Surg 14:287, 1979
Edman CD et al: Embryonic testicular regression: A clinical spectrum of XY agonadal individuals. Obstet Gynecol 49:208, 1977
George FW, Wilson JD: Sexual differentiation, in *Fetal Physiology and Medicine,* RW Beard, PW Nathanielsz (eds). New York, Marcel Dekker, 1983
Gordon DL et al: Pathologic testicular findings in Klinefelter's syndrome. 47,XXY vs 46,XY/47,XXY. Arch Intern Med 130:726, 1972
Griffin JE et al: Congenital absence of the vagina. The Mayer-Rokitansky-Kuster-Hauser syndrome. Ann Intern Med 85:224, 1976
———, Wilson JD: The syndromes of androgen resistance. N Engl J Med 302:198, 1980
———, Durrant JL: Quantitative receptor defects in families with androgen resistance. J Clin Endocrinol Metab 55:465, 1982
New M, Levene LS: Congenital adrenal hyperplasia and related conditions, in *Metabolic Basis of Inherited Disease,* 5th ed, JB Stanbury et al (eds). New York, McGraw-Hill, 1983, chap 47
Peterson RE et al: Male pseudohermaphroditism due to steroid 5α-reductase deficiency. Am J Med 62:170, 1977
Siiteri PK, Wilson JD: Testosterone formation and metabolism during male sexual differentiation in the human embryo. J Clin Endocrinol Metab 38:113, 1974
Simpson JL: *Disorders of Sexual Differentiation.* New York, Academic, 1976, p 466
Simpson, JL et al: XY gonadal dysgenesis: genetic heterogeneity based upon clinical observations, H-Y antigen status and segregation analysis. Hum Genet 58:91, 1981
Van Niekerk WA, Retief AE: The gonads of human true hermaphrodites. Hum Genet 58:117, 1981
Wilson JD: Sexual differentiation. Ann Rev Physiol 40:249, 1978
———, Goldstein JL: Classification of hereditary disorders of sexual development, in *Birth defects: Original Article Series,* vol XI, no 4: *Genetic Forms of Hypogonadism,* D Bergsma (ed). New York, Grune & Stratton, 1975, pp 1–16
———, Walsh PC: Disorders of sexual differentiation, in *Campbell's Urology,* 4th ed, JH Harrison et al (eds). Philadelphia, Saunders, 1979, vol 2, pp 1484–1532
———, et al: The androgen resistance syndromes: 5α-Reductase deficiency, testicular feminization and related disorders, in *The Metabolic Basis of Inherited Disease,* 5th ed, JB Stanbury et al (eds). New York, McGraw-Hill, 1983, chap 48
Zah W et al: Mixed gonadal dysgenesis. A case report and review of the world literature. Acta Endocrinol Suppl 197:3, 1975

121 DISEASES OF THE PINEAL GLAND

RICHARD J. WURTMAN

Since the discovery of melatonin in 1958, compelling evidence has accumulated that the mammalian pineal functions as a neuroendocrine transducer. It receives sympathetic nervous "information" which is suppressed when the retina responds to light. In response to this input, the pineal secretes a hormone, melatonin, into the bloodstream, much as the adrenal medulla releases epinephrine in response to cholinergic stimulation. The synthesis and secretion of melatonin vary with a 24-h periodicity, thereby providing the body with a circulating "clock" apparatus. Until recently, no assay was available to permit measurement of melatonin in human blood or urine. Largely as a consequence, human pineal physiology remained conjectural. Now melatonin in blood and urine can be measured by bioassay and radioimmunoassay, and it is apparent that the same factors that control the synthesis and secretion of this hormone in experimental animals also do so in humans.

ANATOMY AND BIOCHEMISTRY OF THE PINEAL The pineal is a flattened, conical organ which lies beneath the posterior border of the corpus callosum and between the superior colliculi. It originates embryologically as an evagination of the ependyma which lines the roof of the third ventricle and remains connected to this region by the pineal stalk. The adult gland weighs about 120 mg; its dimensions are 5 to 9 mm in length, 3 to 6 mm in width, and 3 to 5 mm in thickness. Most of the pineal is enveloped by pia mater, from which blood vessels, unmyelinated nerve fibers, and septa of connective tissue penetrate the gland, thereby dividing it into lobules. The glandular or parenchymal cells on the periphery of the lobule are elongated; those in the central zone are ovoid. They contain numerous granular bodies and give rise to processes that terminate adjacent to the capillary endothelium.

The primary innervation of the mammalian pineal originates not within the brain but rather from sympathetic cell bodies in the superior cervical ganglia. The sympathetic nerve endings terminate directly on pineal parenchymal cells in an anatomic relationship that resembles the synapse.

The pineal gland contains melatonin (5-methoxy-*N*-acetyltryptamine) (Fig. 121-1), a factor that causes lightening of amphibian skin by promoting aggregation of dermal melanophores around the cell nuclei. It remains to be shown whether melatonin has any effect on the melanocytes in humans.

Melatonin is a derivative of serotonin (Fig. 121-1), a widely distributed indole stored in large quantities in mammalian pineals. Melatonin differs from all indoles previously identified in mammalian tissues in that it contains a methoxy group. The enzyme that catalyzes this methoxylation reaction (hydroxyindole *O*-methyl transferase, HIOMT) is present in high concentrations in the pineal gland in mammals.

PHYSIOLOGY OF THE MAMMALIAN PINEAL Environmental lighting conditions exert several important effects on the mammalian neuroendocrine apparatus. Light acts as an "inducer" that modifies the rate of sexual maturation: girls who have been blind from birth may show early pubescence. The sequence of day and night also acts to generate some 24-h biologic rhythms and to synchronize the circadian rhythms produced by signals arising from within the body. (Circadian behavioral rhythms in eating and drinking cause chemicals to be introduced into the body intermittently; this produces secondary rhythms in plasma levels of amino acids, choline, insulin, and a variety of additional constituents.) One function of the mammalian pineal is to mediate some of these endocrine and metabolic effects of light. The "information" about light travels to the pineal by a route which involves (1) the accessory optic tracts, (2) centers in the brain and spinal cord that regulate the sympathetic nervous system, and (3) the sympathetic nerves to the pineal that originate in the superior cervical ganglia. When mammals are exposed to light, the resulting increase in optic nerve traffic causes a *decrease* in pineal sympathetic outflow and suppresses the synthesis and secretion of melatonin. The light intensity needed to produce this effect in humans is well below that present out-of-doors on even the cloudiest day but two or three times as great as that available in most offices and hospitals. Pineals of patients with depression may be more responsive to light than those of normal subjects.

The diurnal variation in melatonin secretion from the human pineal causes plasma melatonin levels to peak during the hours of darkness and provides the body with a circulating "clock" under the direct control of the lighting environment (Fig. 121-2). Little is known about which systems take temporal cues from this pineal "clock." It seems likely that melatonin exerts physiologic inhibitory effects on gonadal function (especially in animals with seasonal breeding cycles) and also modifies behavior, electroencephalographic activity, and thyroid function. When tiny amounts of melatonin are implanted in the median eminence of the hypothalamus or the midbrain reticular formation, the increase in pituitary luteinizing hormone (LH) content which normally follows castration is blocked. Melatonin placed in the cerebrospinal fluid suppresses the secretion of pituitary LH and enhances the secretion of prolactin. Melatonin administration also changes the levels of serotonin in the brain.

The mammalian pineal also synthesizes and secretes 5-methoxytryptophol, like melatonin a gonad-inhibiting methoxyindole whose levels exhibit similar daily rhythms. Some (but not all) investigators believe that the pineal also makes a specific octapeptide hormone, arginine vasotocin, similar in structure to oxytocin and vasopressin.

PINEAL PATHOLOGY Two pineal lesions are of interest to the clinician: pineal calcification, which is a universal autopsy finding, and pineal tumors, which are best known for their endocrine sequelae. In rare instances, the pineal gland is the site of cancer metastases, gummas, tuberculous granulomas, or ectopic segments of skeletal muscle.

Pineal calcification often becomes visible on skull roentgenograms around the time of puberty, and it has been suggested that the gland degenerates at this time of life, and then becomes calcified. However, if pineals are examined by appropriate microscopic techniques, evidence of calcification often is seen in patients who die before the age of puberty. A ground substance believed to serve as the matrix for calcification was seen in 8 of 28 pineals from children under a year of age. Moreover, studies of pineal function have failed to show any differences between heavily calcified glands taken from aged subjects and pineals from young subjects without gross calcification. The functional significance of pineal calcification remains entirely unexplained. The calcified material appears to be hydroxyapatite; crystals taken from human pineals are similar to those prepared from bone or tooth.

Pineal tumors may be divided into several categories by their microscopic appearance. More than half are classified as true pinealomas. These tumors contain clusters of two distinct types of cells: large spheroidal epithelial cells and small dark-staining cells with little cytoplasm and an ultrastructure indistinguishable from that of the lymphocyte. About 10 to 15 percent of pineal tumors are teratomas; these may contain mucus-secreting columnar epithelial cells, adenocarcinoma tissue, and areas resembling thyroid, muscle, cartilage, bone, and nerve. Like other midline teratomas, they are often malignant. The remainder of pineal tumors are of vascular or glial origin.

Confirmation of pineal origin of the large pinealoma cells has been hampered by the lack of specific pineal function which could be measured (such as the uptake of ^{131}I by thyroid cells in follicular adenomas). However, the melatonin-forming enzyme HIOMT may provide such a "marker." Two pineal tumors containing this enzyme have been described; one was a metastasis from a parenchymal pinealoma, and the other was a specimen from an ectopic pinealoma. Both had the characteristic histologic appearance of the parenchymal pinealoma. Few data are available on blood or urinary melatonin levels in subjects with pineal tumors.

The natural history of a pineal tumor is related to its size and its histologic appearance. Tumors that originate within the pineal gland usually become clinically manifest because of symptoms which arise from their location (e.g., internal hydrocephalus, elevated cerebrospinal fluid pressure, and oculomotor signs such as paralysis of upward gaze or Parinaud's syndrome); less frequently, the tumors cause precocious puberty. About a third of boys below the normal age of sexual maturation who have pineal tumors develop precocious puberty (see Chap. 117). This neoplasm accounts for about 10 to 15 percent of all precocious sexual development in males. For unexplained reasons, pineal tumors in girls are less common and are not associated with precocious menarche. Some investigators have suggested that the precocious sexual development is a nonspecific consequence of the pressure that these tumors exert on surrounding brain tissue. Kitay and others have summarized the evidence against this "pressure hypothesis": (1) Pineal tumors may produce precocious puberty, no gonadal signs, or even delayed pubescence. The endocrine effects of a particular tumor appear to be unrelated to its size. (2) Most cases of precocious puberty develop in patients with nonparenchymal tumors (frequently teratomas). Occasional parenchymal tumors lead to gonadal enlargement but they are more commonly associated with delayed pubescence or with second-

FIGURE 121-1

Synthesis of melatonin in the pineal gland. The pineal takes up tryptophan from the circulation; the amino acid is hydroxylated to form 5-hydroxytryptophan; this is then converted to the amine serotonin (5-hydroxytryptamine) by the enzyme aromatic L*-amino acid decarboxylase. Some of the serotonin synthesized in the pineal is destroyed by oxidative deamination, forming 5-hydroxyindole acetic acid and 5-hydroxytryptophol; the remainder is N-acetylated and O-methylated to form the hormone melatonin.*

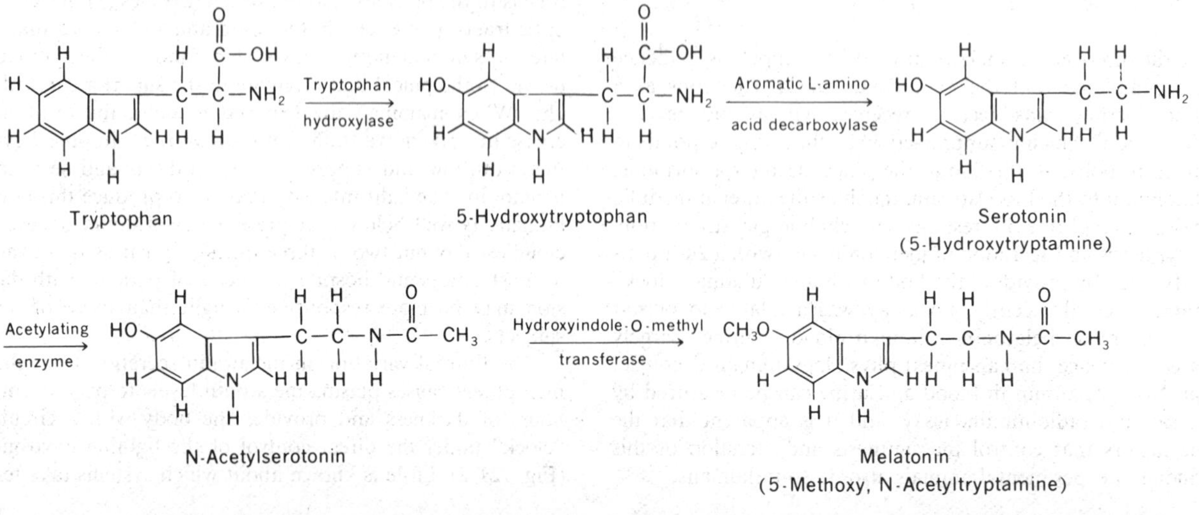

Tryptophan → (Tryptophan hydroxylase) → 5-Hydroxytryptophan → (Aromatic L-amino acid decarboxylase) → Serotonin (5-Hydroxytryptamine)

→ (Acetylating enzyme) → N-Acetylserotonin → (Hydroxyindole-O-methyl transferase) → Melatonin (5-Methoxy, N-Acetyltryptamine)

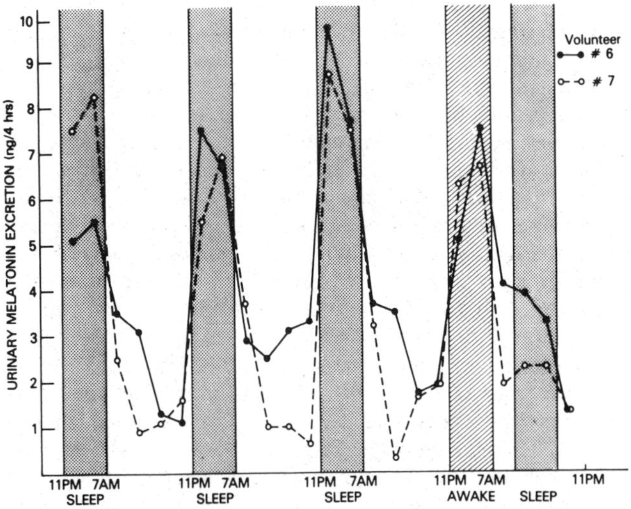

FIGURE 121-2
Effect of diurnal phase reversal on urinary melatonin rhythm. Urinary melatonin was assayed (by radioimmunoassay) in consecutive 4-h urine samples collected from two subjects. After 3 days, the time of onset of the dark period was delayed for 12 h, from 11 P.M. to 11 A.M. Before this time, both subjects had exhibited characteristic daily rhythms in urinary melatonin levels, with high nighttime and low daytime values. On the day that the light period was extended by 12 h, both subjects continued to excrete large amounts of melatonin at the time that they had previously been exposed to darkness (11 P.M. to 11 A.M.). Most subjects require 3 to 4 days to reentrain their rhythms in melatonin secretion to changes in the time of onset of the daily light or dark periods. (From DC Jimerson et al, Life Sci 20:1501, 1977.)

ary gonadal failure. (3) Gonadal abnormalities may occur in patients whose tumors had neither produced signs of a chronic elevation in cerebrospinal fluid pressure nor invaded other brain areas. The demonstration that melatonin influences normal sexual maturation in rats supports the hypothesis that precocious puberty develops in pinealoma patients because the damaged pineal fails to release this or another inhibitory hormone. Both patients described above whose tumors contained melatonin-forming activity showed evidence of depressed sexual function.

Parenchymal pinealomas frequently show a good, if temporary, clinical remission following irradiation. Patients generally receive 30,000 to 50,000 mGy (3000 to 5000 rads); radiation is administered over a wide portal because pinealomas may metastasize throughout the ventricles and the subdural space. Japanese surgeons have reported encouraging results following the surgical extirpation of pinealomas; however, this method is complicated by the relative inaccessibility of the pineal and consequently is used rarely in the United States. A patient with metastatic parenchymal pinealoma has been repeatedly treated during a 10-year period with x-ray and chemotherapeutic agents; each time an objective decrease in tumor mass occurred. In another case, described more recently, repeated courses of daunorubicin (Adriamycin), vincristine, and bleomycin following irradiation have suppressed tumor recurrence for limited periods.

A small number of tumors with histologic appearance of pinealomas originate elsewhere in the brain at some distance from the normal pineal gland. These "ectopic pinealomas" generally arise in the hypothalamus in the region of the infundibulum. Hence, patients usually present a picture similar to that seen with craniopharyngioma with a clinical triad of bitemporal hemianopsia, hypopituitarism, and diabetes insipidus. Most ectopic pinealomas show a good clinical response to irradiation.

REFERENCES

De Tribolet N, Barrelet L: Successful chemotherapy of pinealoma. Lancet 2:1228, 1977

Lynch HJ et al: Daily rhythm in human urinary melatonin. Science 187:169, 1975

Ramsey HJ: Ultrastructure of a pineal tumor. Cancer 18:1014, 1965

Wolstenholme GEW, Knight J (eds): *The Pineal Gland*, Edinburgh, Churchill Livingstone, 1971, p 401

Wurtman RJ, Cardinali DP: The pineal organ, in *Textbook of Endocrinology*, RH Williams (ed). Philadelphia, Saunders, 1974, p 832

Wurtman RJ, Moskowitz MA: Medical progress: The pineal organ. N Engl J Med 296:1329, 1383, 1977

122

ENDOCRINE MANIFESTATIONS OF NONENDOCRINE DISEASE

LOUIS M. SHERWOOD

Hormone production in nonendocrine disease, particularly in patients with malignant disorders, has been recognized with increasing frequency. Advances in our understanding of the biosynthesis, chemistry, and secretion of polypeptide hormones and the development of highly sensitive and specific radioimmunoassays have facilitated this process. Because of an emphasis on earlier diagnosis and modern management of cancer (see Chaps. 124 and 125), many patients with abnormal hormone production associated with tumors have been identified, even in the absence of clinical manifestations of hormone excess. In addition, other nonendocrine "paraneoplastic disorders" have been described. In some, the disorders are associated with production of specific polypeptides or antigens by the tumor; in others, the relation between tumor and clinical manifestations is poorly understood. Although this chapter will focus on the production of hormones by tumors, it should be appreciated that many clinical manifestations of malignancy such as fever, anorexia, weight loss, neurologic syndromes, coagulation and vascular disorders, connective tissue problems, dermatoses, and nephrotic syndrome could be caused by specific proteins produced by the tumors.

DEFINITION The term *ectopic hormone syndrome* refers to the production of hormones by tissues (both nonendocrine and endocrine) other than the primary tissue(s) known to produce the hormone. In the majority of instances the site of aberrant production is a tumor, and the hormone is peptide in nature. Whether the hormone is truly ectopic depends on one's concepts of pathogenesis.

PATHOGENESIS Considerable progress has been made in identifying these disorders, even in the absence of clinical syndromes, but the pathogenesis of ectopic hormone production is poorly understood. Current concepts may be summarized as follows:

1 Production of hormone by nonendocrine tumors may represent dedifferentiation to an embryonic state in which proteins not normally synthesized by a differentiated cell are produced. Since every somatic cell contains the same complement of DNA, any cell could theoretically produce any hormone. That the process is not random is demonstrated

TABLE 122-1
Relationship of tumor type to hormone production

Hormone	*Tumor type*
ACTH and lipotropin (β-MSH, endorphin, and enkephalin)	Oat-cell carcinoma of lung Thymoma Islet-cell tumor Bronchial carcinoid Also ovarian tumors, pheochromocytoma, gastrointestinal, prostate, neurogenic, and parotid tumors, and medullary thyroid carcinoma Inactive "big" ACTH in a wide variety of tumors
Growth hormone	Adenocarcinoma of the lung; bronchial carcinoid
Human placental lactogen	Undifferentiated carcinoma of the lung Hepatoma Lymphoma Pheochromocytoma
Prolactin	Renal-cell carcinoma Undifferentiated carcinoma of the lung Breast carcinoma
Thyrotropin	Choriocarcinoma, hydatidiform mole Epidermoid carcinoma of the lung Mesothelioma
Gonadotropin	Hepatoblastoma, pancreatic, other gastrointestinal tumors Adenocarcinoma and other carcinomas of the lung Choriocarcinoma of male and female, other testicular tumors Islet-cell tumors (malignant) Breast carcinoma Melanoma
HCG β subunit	Adenocarcinoma of the pancreas Islet-cell tumors (malignant)
HCG α subunit	Carcinoid Islet-cell tumors (malignant)
Vasopressin	Oat-cell carcinoma of lung Pancreatic adenocarcinoma
Parathyroid hormone	Epidermoid carcinoma of lung Renal-cell carcinoma Hepatoma, pancreatic, and gastrointestinal carcinoma Other epidermoid tumors
Prostaglandin E_2	Renal-cell carcinoma Lung tumors
Osteoclast-activating factor	Multiple myeloma Burkitt's and other lymphomas
Calcitonin	Oat-cell carcinoma of the lung Breast, pancreatic, and other carcinomas
Somatomedin (NSILA)	Mesodermal and mesenchymal tumors Adrenal carcinoma
Glucagon	Non-beta islet-cell tumors Undifferentiated lung cancer
Gastrin	Non-beta islet-cell tumor Duodenal wall carcinoma Ovarian carcinoma
Vasoactive intestinal peptide	Non-beta islet-cell tumor Carcinoma of lung Pheochromocytoma and ganglio-neuroblastoma
Erythropoietin	Renal-cell carcinoma Cerebellar hemangioblastoma Pheochromocytoma Hepatoma Uterine fibroids
Renin	Juxtaglomerular tumor Wilms's tumor Renal-cell carcinoma
Serotonin and 5-hydroxytryptophan	Non-beta islet-cell tumor Oat-cell carcinoma of the lung Carcinoid (also growth hormone–releasing activity) Pancreatic adenocarcinoma

by the comparison of specific histology with particular clinical syndromes (see Table 122-1).

2 Alternatively, the capacity of different tissues to generate the same peptide hormones may be due to derivation of the tissues from some common embryologic precursor. A specific type of cell that has specific histochemical and biochemical characteristics and is commonly found in some hormone-secreting tumors has been named amine precursor uptake and decarboxylation (APUD) cells. Amines like DOPA and 5-hydroxytryptophan are taken up, decarboxylated, and converted to biogenic amines, which in turn may mediate secretion of other hormones or be used to synthesize more complex polypeptides. The hypothesis of a common embryologic origin of these cells could explain production of hormones by tumors such as medullary thyroid carcinoma, oat-cell carcinoma of the lung, carcinoid tumors, thymoma, islet-cell tumors, pheochromocytoma, neuroblastoma, and possibly others. Tumors containing APUD cells are characterized by similar histologic features and dense neurosecretory-type granules. Because of their clinical features, defined genetic relationships, and characteristic hormones, some consider the multiple endocrine neoplasia syndromes to involve APUD cells (see Chap. 123). The hypothesis does not explain all ectopic hormone-producing tumors, particularly mesodermal tumors that may produce parathyroid hormone (PTH), erythropoietin, gonadotropins, placental lactogen (HPL), nonsuppressible insulin-like activity (NSILA), or renin.

3 Specific information on the biochemical nature of hormones produced by ectopic tumors is limited, particularly their amino acid sequence. The derepression hypothesis would imply that tumors make the same hormones produced by endocrine cells and not abnormal peptide hormones with similar biologic activity. This concept is complicated, however, by the fact that many polypeptide hormones are made from higher-molecular-weight precursors. The first synthetic product in the endocrine cell is a prehormone which contains a "signal" sequence of 15 to 30 amino acids that is necessary to move the polypeptide into the subcellular transport system. The signal peptide is cleaved as the hormone crosses the membrane of the endoplasmic reticulum. For some hormones such as PTH and insulin, there is an additional prohormone precursor (e.g., proPTH and proinsulin) which is converted to mature hormone in the Golgi region of the cell. Some tumors that produce hormones release a precursor form of the hormone rather than the hormone itself [e.g. "big" ACTH or proopiomelanocortin (POMC)]. Since the precursor may be immunologically or biologically different from the usual mature or final hormone, a critical factor in determining whether a clinical or biochemical state of hormone excess results may be the presence of converting enzyme(s) for formation of the final hormone rather than the presence of hormone precursor alone.

Extensive application of radioimmunoassay to tumor extracts and serum of patients has shown that polypeptide hormone synthesis in tumors is more prevalent than previously believed (particularly for ACTH, chorionic gonadotropin and its subunits, vasopressin, and calcitonin). Some have even suggested that hormones may be produced in small amounts by all malignant tumors and by many normal tissues as well. Under such circumstances, it might be suggested that the malignant process enhances the basal capacity of normal cells to produce hormones. It is difficult at present to reconcile the widespread appearance of hormone in tumor tissues with the rather infrequent development of manifest hormone excess, but these associations may be a result of both quantitative and qualitative factors of hormone production. These new findings raise questions both about the definition and the pathogenesis of ectopic hormone syndromes. Resolution of these questions will provide new insights into clinical medicine and basic cell biology.

GENERAL CHARACTERISTICS OF ECTOPIC HORMONE PRODUCTION The common feature involved in documentation of ectopic hormone syndromes is summarized in Table 122-2. These syndromes are being recognized with greater frequency, in part because hormone measurements are carried out both for diagnostic purposes ("tumor markers") and for assessment of tumor recurrence. Since radioimmunoassay techniques are sensitive, the finding of elevated hormone levels in plasma may indicate the presence of malignant cells that are not clinically or radiographically apparent. In such instances, it is critical to differentiate the presence of a hormone-producing malignancy from a coexisting endocrine disorder (e.g., hypercalcemia in a patient with breast cancer could be due to the primary disease or to a concurrent parathyroid adenoma). Occasionally, hormone-induced metabolic disorders such as hyponatremia, hypoglycemia, or hypercalcemia may be a more immediate threat to life than the malignancy itself. When confusion exists as to whether the hormone comes from a nonendocrine tumor or a coexisting endocrine disorder, selective venous catheterization with radioimmunoassay of hormone in effluent veins may be useful in localizing the tissue of origin.

CUSHING'S SYNDROME AND RELATED DISORDERS The first ectopic syndrome recognized was that due to production of ACTH. Several hundred reports of ectopic ACTH production have subsequently appeared, usually in patients with tumors of the lung (oat-cell carcinoma, 60 percent; bronchial adenoma, 4 percent; thymus, 15 percent; or pancreatic islet, 10 percent). Other causes include medullary carcinoma of the thyroid, bronchial carcinoid, and pheochromocytoma. While patients with the above tumors often have clinical Cushing's syndrome, ACTH immunoreactivity has also been noted in other tumors, usually a big form of ACTH that is a precursor with minimal biologic activity. It is now known that ACTH is synthesized through a precursor molecule called POMC which includes the amino acid sequences of ACTH, lipotropin (the latter peptide having melanocyte-stimulating activity), and the opioid peptides (endorphins and enkephalins). In the normal pituitary, POMC is processed to ACTH and the lipotropin peptides. When Cushing's syndrome occurs from ectopic tumors, it is the result primarily of production of biologically active ACTH, a 39-amino acid peptide. However, the majority of tumors that make ACTH precursor do not convert the precursor glycoprotein to mature hormone. Futhermore, the quantity of ACTH in extracts of tumors from patients without Cushing's syndrome is less than in those with clinical manifestations. In a few instances, elevated levels of precursor ACTH have been found in plasma prior to the clinical appearance of a tumor (e.g., in patients with chronic bronchitis).

Ectopic ACTH production due to bronchogenic carcinoma is the most common cause of Cushing's syndrome in men, but the clinical manifestations are usually different than those of typical Cushing's syndrome (see Chap. 112). Weight loss, muscle weakness, hyperpigmentation, hypertension, peripheral edema, and hirsutism are common clinical abnormalities in the ectopic syndrome, while weight gain, centripetal obesity, and striae are rare. In general, the altered manifestations are the result of mineralocorticoid effects. Other possible factors produced by the tumor, debilitation due to malignancy, and rapidity of the course may also contribute to the altered manifestations.

The clinical syndrome is associated with extremely high plasma levels of ACTH and correspondingly increased levels of plasma and urinary steroids. Severe hypokalemic alkalosis in the absence of diuretics, glucose intolerance, and increased urinary 5-hydroxyindoleacetic acid may be present. Autonomy of ACTH secretion is not uniformly present, and in some patients, steroid output is altered by metyrapone and (very rarely) dexamethasone (Chap. 112). The tumors may contain corticotropin-releasing factors in addition to ACTH, a finding that could explain variable autonomy of ACTH production. Selective venous catheterization may be necessary at times to differentiate those with ACTH-producing tumors from patients with hypothalamic-pituitary disease.

Hyperpigmentation is a common manifestation of ectopic ACTH production and is ascribed to the production of lipotropin which contains the melanocyte-stimulating hormone (MSH) sequence. MSH extracted from tumors and plasma is probably artifactual since the activity in vivo is contained in the larger peptide (see Chap. 109).

Therapy should be directed at the primary tumor whenever possible, although oat-cell carcinoma is often metastatic to bone when first diagnosed. The prognosis has been improved with combination chemotherapy but is still poor (median survival about one year). Correction of the hypokalemic alkalosis and hyperglycemia is important. Combined adrenal blockade with metyrapone (11β-hydroxylase inhibitor) and aminogluethimide (which blocks the conversion of cholesterol to pregnenolone), with or without the cytolytic agent mitotane (*o,p'*-DDD), may be useful.

SYNDROMES DUE TO OVERPRODUCTION OF GROWTH HORMONE AND PROLACTIN Ectopic production of growth hormone occurs rarely in bronchogenic and gastric carcinoma. Growth hormone has been extracted from and shown to be synthesized in vitro by such tumors. Since growth hormone secretion in normal subjects varies widely in response to exercise, sleep, and diet, it is critical to differentiate normal physiologic changes in plasma growth hormone from production by tumors. Hypertrophic osteoarthropathy in patients with lung tumors differs from the classical clinical and radiologic manifestations of growth hormone excess noted in acromegaly. Although dramatic reversal of osteoarthropathy may be found following removal of tumors, it has not been demonstrated

TABLE 122-2
Documentation of ectopic hormone production

1 Presence of a clinical endocrine disorder or abnormal level of polypeptide hormone or metabolite in a patient with malignancy. (The presence of a coexisting endocrine disorder, in particular common endocrinopathies such as primary hyperparathyroidism in a patient with a malignant tumor and hypercalcemia must be excluded.)
2 Disappearance or remission of the disorder or biochemical abnormality following surgical removal, radiation therapy, or chemotherapy of the tumor.
3 Recurrence of the disorder or metabolic abnormality when metastases or reappearance of the tumor occurs.
4 Abnormal hormone concentrations in blood or urine or failure of normal hormone suppression or stimulation.
5 Presence of hormone in tumor extracts in amounts greater than in adjacent normal tissue, as determined by bioassay, radioimmunoassay, or radioreceptor assay.
6 Qualitative abnormalities in the hormone in serum or tumor extracts are common (e.g., changes in molecular weight, immunologic activity, biologic activity, or biochemical properties).
7 Increase in hormone concentration from the arterial to venous side of the tumor (e.g., renal artery to vein for hypernephroma).
8 Biosynthesis of polypeptide hormone following incubation of tumor explants in vitro with radioactive amino acids (flask incubation or tissue culture).
9 Cell-free synthesis of ectopic hormone or hybridization of complementary DNA with messenger RNA in tumor extract.

that this is related to elimination of growth hormone or growth hormone-like proteins. More recent reports indicate an association between growth hormone-releasing activity and carcinoid tumors of the lung and pancreatic islet, leading to a clinical picture of acromegaly (see Chap. 109). The production of growth hormone-releasing activity by these tumors leads to enlargement of the pituitary gland and a clinical picture resembling a primary pituitary tumor. Removal of the nonpituitary tumor causes dramatic regression of soft-tissue enlargement and return of plasma growth hormone to normal.

Ectopic production of prolactin is rare, and only one patient with hyperprolactinemia due to renal-cell carcinoma has had galactorrhea. In contrast to patients with primary pituitary tumors that produce prolactin, the sella turcica is normal in ectopic prolactin production. Normal human placenta produces a protein called human placental lactogen (HPL or human chorionic somatomammotropin), a peptide hormone closely related to growth hormone in its biologic and immunologic properties as well as amino acid sequence. Ectopic production of HPL has been described with a number of nontrophoblastic tumors, particularly of the lung, although the concentrations of hormone in blood are quite low. A rare male patient with ectopic HPL production has gynecomastia, but the latter is probably not produced unless there is simultaneous production of gonadotropin or estrogen by the tumor. Identification of HPL in serum may be useful as a tumor marker, and some tumors that produce it also produce chorionic gonadotropin (HCG) as well as the placental form of alkaline phosphatase.

SYNDROMES ASSOCIATED WITH GONADOTROPIN PRODUCTION Clinical syndromes associated with ectopic gonadotropin production have been noted principally in men with choriocarcinoma and, less commonly, with other testicular and lung tumors. In men, the association of gynecomastia with gonadotropin production is well documented (see Chap. 119). Increased estrogen production that is responsible for the gynecomastia is usually the result of HCG-mediated secretion of estradiol by the testis, although estrogen can be formed on occasion directly by aromatization of circulating androgens by the tumor. In the latter instance, HCG may or may not be elevated. A syndrome of precocious puberty has been documented in boys with HCG-producing hepatoblastomas. Gynecomastia due to tumors must be differentiated from other known causes (see Chap. 119). Women usually have no symptoms from tumor-mediated gonadotropin release.

Follicle-stimulating hormone (FSH), luteinizing hormone (LH), thyrotropin (TSH), and HCG each consist of two noncovalently linked subunits. The alpha subunits of the pituitary hormones are identical and are immunologically indistinguishable from the HCG alpha subunit which has a minor structural difference. The beta subunits are biochemically unique and confer biologic and immunologic specificity. The isolated subunits are biologically inactive but may be combined in vitro to produce biologically active hormone. Sensitive radioimmunoassay and radioreceptor assays have been developed for the common alpha and the specific beta subunits. Widespread application of these assays to the serum and tumors of patients with malignancy has revealed the common presence of HCG and its subunits. Isolated beta-subunit production has been useful as an early tumor marker, whereas free alpha subunits are less specific and may be released by the normal pituitary gland (particularly in primary hypothyroidism and in postmenopausal women). In patients with islet-cell tumors of the pancreas, HCG beta subunits in serum provide a strong indication of malignancy. In addition to carcinoma of the lung and liver, tumors of the breast, bladder, adrenal, mediastinum, gonads, melanocytes, and gastrointestinal tract have been reported to produce HCG. Normal tissue such as liver and colon may also produce HCG-like material that contains the polypeptide backbone devoid of normal carbohydrate content.

HYPERTHYROIDISM Nonpituitary production of thyrotropin-like factors is associated principally with trophoblastic tumors (choriocarcinoma of the placenta and testis) and hydatidiform mole, although there are scattered reports of a hyperthyroid syndrome with other tumors. Patients typically have mild hyperthyroidism with smooth skin, increased pulse pressure, tachycardia, tremor, and a small goiter. Thyroid function tests are characteristic of mild hyperthyroidism, but thyroid-stimulating immunoglobulins are not present in plasma. The hormone responsible is probably not TSH but HCG, which has demonstrable thyrotropic activity when present in concentrations as high as those found in the plasma of such patients. Therapy of the hyperthyroidism is not a major problem as the prognosis of the tumor determines the patient's course. These patients must be differentiated from those with ordinary forms of hyperthyroidism (see Chap. 111).

HYPONATREMIC SYNDROMES Ectopic production of vasopressin or antidiuretic hormone (ADH) has been documented both by extraction of ADH from tumors and by demonstration of hormone synthesis in tumor explants. Tumor production of ADH combined with generous fluid intake may produce the syndrome of inappropriate secretion of ADH (SIADH) and cause moderate to severe hyponatremia (see Chap. 110). Other known causes of the SIADH in patients with malignancy include cerebral metastases, mediastinal, or pulmonary infections, renal tubular defects, central nervous system infection, cerebrovascular disease, excessive smoking, pain, trauma, emotional stress, and administration of drugs such as chlorpropamide and vincristine. These must be considered in the differential diagnosis of the hyponatremia. The diagnosis is confirmed by the presence of a low serum sodium and normal to low BUN in the face of a urine osmolality greater than that of serum. The patients usually have no edema. Production of ADH by tumors occurs principally with small-cell carcinoma of the lung and tumors of the pancreas or upper gastrointestinal tract. ADH may be increased in patients with carcinoma of the lung, both with and without SIADH, but the levels tend to be higher in patients with hyponatremia. Some tumors also appear to make the protein neurophysin which binds vasopressin, but this is not associated with clinical abnormalities.

Common clinical characteristics of SIADH, regardless of cause, include nausea, vomiting, headaches, anorexia, confusion, and coma (see Chap. 110). The syndrome is treated with fluid restriction; demeclocycline and lithium carbonate have also been useful in some patients. Symptomatic hyponatremia may require intravenous hypertonic saline.

HYPERCALCEMIC SYNDROMES Hypercalcemia and its associated clinical symptoms are frequent in patients with malignant disease. Both the degree of elevation and the rapidity of change of the plasma calcium are important factors in determining whether symptoms develop. The predominant manifestations of hypercalcemia are in the central nervous system, heart, kidney, and gastrointestinal tract. The signs, symptoms, and differential diagnosis are described in Chap. 339. A number of mechanisms may be responsible for hypercalcemia in patients with malignancy:

1 Direct invasion of bone by tumors; this is particularly true of cancers that metastasize commonly to bone (lung, breast, kidney, and thyroid). Prostatic carcinoma is frequently metastatic to bone but causes osteoblastic metastases that may cause hypocalcemia but do not result in hypercalcemia.

2 Production of parathyroid hormone (PTH) or a PTH-like substance.
3 Production of other calcium-mobilizing substances such as prostaglandin E_2, osteoclast-activating factor, a cyclic AMP–stimulating factor that mimics PTH, or 1,25-dihydroxyvitamin D.
4 Coexistence of the tumor with primary hyperparathyroidism.
5 Coexistence of the tumor with another cause of hypercalcemia such as hyperthyroidism, sarcoidosis, hypervitaminosis D, immobilization, or adrenal insufficiency.
6 Administration of estrogen or androgen to women with carcinoma of the breast that has metastasized to bone.

The differential diagnosis of hypercalcemia can usually be accomplished on clinical grounds plus the radioimmunoassay for PTH. The major difficulty is in separating primary hyperparathyroidism from malignant disorders. An important consideration is to exclude the presence of bony metastases. Bone marrow biopsy and scans are more helpful than routine radiographs (which detect only metastases larger than 1 cm). Demonstration of metastases to bone does not exclude coexisting primary hyperparathyroidism or even the production by the tumor of a calcium-mobilizing substance, but a definitive workup may not be appropriate if the metastatic disease is widespread.

Ectopic production of PTH by tumors has been documented by extraction of PTH-like material from tumors, by an increase in the arteriovenous hormone gradient across the tumor and by demonstration of biosynthesis in tumor explants in vitro. Many patients have had correction of hypercalcemia after removal of the primary tumor, but in only a small number has a fall in PTH been documented. Since PTH levels in serum are usually low or undetectable in the face of tumor-associated hypercalcemia, it follows that other calcium-mobilizing factors produced by neoplasms more often lead to hypercalcemia. One such agent is prostaglandin E_2 (see Chap. 87). Both increased concentrations of circulating prostaglandin E_2 and increased urinary excretion of PGE_m (the major urinary metabolite of E_2) have been demonstrated. Remission of hypercalcemia has occasionally been noted with aspirin or indomethacin, but the clinical response to these inhibitors of prostaglandin synthesis is variable. A third tumor substance that causes hypercalcemia is osteoclast-activating factor (OAF). This low-molecular-weight polypeptide was first identified in the tissue culture supernatant of human lymphocytes stimulated with phytohemagglutinin. OAF induces osteoclastic bone resorption and appears to be the major cause of hypercalcemia in patients with multiple myeloma, Burkitt's lymphoma, and possibly other lymphoid tumors. The biologic activity of OAF can be distinguished experimentally from that of PTH, prostaglandins, or vitamin D metabolites. Its action is inhibited by corticosteroids, partially explaining the successful use of this agent in the hypercalcemia of multiple myeloma. A fourth and very important cause of hypercalcemia is a poorly characterized factor that causes marked hypercalcemia and stimulates nephrogenous cyclic AMP. This substance, which mimics in part PTH activity, is not associated with increased PTH immunologic activity in serum. Unlike PTH, it also causes increased rather than decreased fractional calcium excretion and is associated with low rather than high levels of 1,25-$(OH)_2D_3$ in plasma. Recent studies suggest that this new substance may be the most common cause of the ectopic hypercalcemia syndrome. Bone biopsy shows marked osteoclastic activity and a dissociation between bone formation and resorption. Further studies to characterize the chemical nature of this new physiologic regulator are in process. In patients with ectopic hypercalcemia, a judicious trial of indomethacin together with hydration and diuretics is indicated. If response to indomethacin does not occur, the usual methods for treating hypercalcemia should be instituted (see Chap. 339). These measures include vigorous saline hydration, furosemide, mobilization, oral phosphates, and corticosteroids where indicated. Intermittent treatment with mithramycin (20 to 25 μg/kg) has proved useful, and calcitonin may occasionally be helpful.

Calcitonin is a hormone produced by medullary carcinoma of the thyroid, a tumor of neural crest origin (see Chap. 123). Extrathyroidal production of calcitonin has been reported in many patients with tumors of the bronchus (small-cell), breast, and pancreas. Since calcitonin inhibits mobilization of calcium and phosphate from bone (see Chap. 338), high concentrations should theoretically produce hypocalcemia, but this metabolic abnormality is rare. Since the hormone is clinically silent, demonstration of its presence in serum is useful primarily as a "tumor marker."

METABOLIC BONE DISORDERS Severe osteomalacia, marked hypophosphatemia, and phosphaturia have been described in patients with mesenchymomas, pleomorphic sarcomas, neurofibromas, and sclerosing or cavernous hemangiomas. The etiology of the phosphaturia and metabolic bone disease is unclear, but dramatic remission of the osteomalacia has occurred after tumor removal. This bone disease must be differentiated from the multiple other causes of osteomalacia (see Chap. 341). The tumor may interfere with the conversion of vitamin D to its active form through an action on renal 1α-hydroxylase, but this hypothesis has not been proved and does not adequately explain the phosphaturia.

HYPOGLYCEMIC SYNDROMES The association of symptomatic hypoglycemia with excessive production of insulin by islet-cell tumors has been well described (see Chap. 116). The etiology of hypoglycemia associated with nonendocrine tumors such as sarcomas of the abdomen and thorax, hepatocellular carcinoma, adrenal tumors, lymphomas, and other malignancies is more obscure. More than 200 cases have now been reported. Insulin is usually not found in tumor extracts or tissue sections, and plasma insulin is not elevated. Some patients with this syndrome have increased levels of circulating nonsuppressible insulin-like activity (NSILA-s). NSILA-s consists of two small peptides with a molecular weight of 7500 known as insulin-like growth factors I and II. These are somatomedins, peptides that are normally synthesized by the liver in response to growth hormone and that have insulin-like activity in vitro. Their structure resembles that of proinsulin. Other postulated mechanisms of hypoglycemia include production of metabolites that interfere with gluconeogenesis, induction of an acquired form of glycogen storage disease (as in hepatoma), malnutrition, release of substances that enhance insulin secretion, and depressed normal counterregulatory mechanisms.

Insulin-secreting islet-cell tumors may be differentiated from extrapancreatic neoplasms by inappropriately elevated levels of plasma insulin in the face of hypoglycemia. Proinsulin secretion may also be increased. Plasma free fatty acids and lactate tend to be increased in patients with nonpancreatic tumors and decreased in those with hyperinsulinemia. Prognosis is dependent on tumor type. Although retroperitoneal mesenchymal tumors may grow to extraordinarily large size, they tend to be slow-growing and of relatively low malignancy. Partial or complete resection may ameliorate hypoglycemia. During hypoglycemic attacks, continuous oral or intravenous glucose is required. Diazoxide, which may be useful in treating islet-cell tumors, is not helpful. High doses of glucocorticoids or glucagon infusions are of occasional benefit.

DIARRHEAL SYNDROMES Many hormones are produced in the gastrointestinal tract, including peptides with recognized physiologic function such as secretin, gastrin, and cholecystokinin-pancreozymin, as well as others whose role is not completely clear such as vasoactive intestinal peptide (VIP), gastric inhibitory peptide (GIP), pancreatic polypeptide (PP), and motilin. The pancreatic islet produces several hormones including insulin, glucagon, gastrin, somatostatin, VIP, PP, and prostaglandins. Whether hormone production by pancreatic tumors is truly ectopic is problematic, since these cells normally produce them (see Chap. 116). Tumors outside the islet or gastrointestinal tract also make these hormones, and in such instances they can be more properly defined as ectopic. Aspects of islet-cell tumors that relate to the multiple endocrine neoplasia syndrome are described in Chap. 123.

A well-defined clinical entity known as pancreatic cholera has been associated with non-beta islet-cell tumors. This syndrome classically includes watery diarrhea, hypokalemia, and hypochlorhydria. Agents implicated include secretin, kinins, glucagon, gastrin, calcitonin, GIP, PP, prostaglandins, and VIP. The latter is generally considered to be the primary etiologic agent. Elevations of plasma VIP may be found not only in patients with islet-cell tumors but also in those with bronchogenic carcinoma and neurogenic tumors. VIP is a 28-amino acid peptide with structural similarities to glucagon, secretin, and GIP. Its actions include inhibition of gastric acid secretion and stimulation of myocardial contractility, glycogenolysis, lipolysis, insulin secretion, pancreatic juice, and intestinal cyclic AMP. PP is a 36-amino acid polypeptide with poorly defined function that is found in normal pancreatic islets and in some tumors associated with diarrhea. Indomethacin may ameliorate some cases of watery diarrhea, implicating prostaglandins as a cause. In other patients, the treatment is symptomatic. Regardless of cause, the diagnosis rests on identifying a pancreatic tumor in association with diarrheal states. New diagnostic approaches including ultrasound and computerized tomography, in addition to celiac angiography, may be helpful.

Islet-cell tumors producing somatostatin have recently been identified. This hormone, originally identified as an inhibitor of growth hormone secretion, is widely distributed, particularly in the gastrointestinal tract. In pharmacological doses, somatostatin inhibits gastric acid production, duodenal motility, pancreatic secretion, gallbladder contraction, and the release of gastrin, secretin, insulin, and glucagon. Clinical manifestation of somatostatin excess include abdominal pain, diarrhea, weight loss, hyperglycemia, and gallbladder disease.

A syndrome in which hyperglycemia is associated with a reversible bullous necrotic skin eruption has been described in patients with pancreatic glucagonomas. Weight loss, anemia, and stomatitis are also characteristic of the syndrome. Release of a larger-than-normal form of glucagon may be present. The cause of the reversible rash is unknown but may be due to amino acid deficiencies.

POLYCYTHEMIA The normal source of the hormone that controls erythropoiesis is the kidney. Both benign and malignant disorders of the kidney are associated with increased production of erythropoietin, but extrarenal tumors may also synthesize erythropoietin and cause polycythemia. These include cerebellar hemangioblastomas, uterine fibroids, occasional adrenal, ovarian, and hepatic carcinomas, and pheochromocytoma. Between 2 and 5 percent of patients with renal tumors have polycythemia. Although the clinical syndrome is recognized principally by association of tumor and polycythemia and a fall in hematocrit following surgery, demonstration of elevation of plasma erythropoietin makes possible recognition in the absence of polycythemia. Tumors associated with leukocytosis and thrombocytosis presumably produce leukopoietins and thrombopoietins, respectively.

HYPERTENSIVE SYNDROMES Production of renin by tumors may cause hypertension. This is principally seen with tumors of the kidney, especially of the juxtaglomerular apparatus, Wilms's tumor, and hypernephroma. Clinical manifestations vary from absence of symptoms to severe hypertension; secondary hyperaldosteronism and hypokalemia may or may not be present. Arteriography and selective venous studies for renin are helpful. In some cases, a high-molecular-weight form of renin is released.

ECTOPIC PRODUCTION OF OTHER HORMONES, ENZYMES, AND ANTIGENS WITHOUT SYMPTOMS It is possible that all peptide hormones are produced ectopically, but documentation for some is incomplete. Tumors also produce and release enzymes, antigens, and other proteins. Such enzymes are not detected unless specific screening studies are performed. For example, alkaline phosphatase has been identified in many tumors (primarily lung) and appears to be identical to the heat-stable enzyme produced by the placenta. There has also been considerable interest in clinical syndromes related to antigen production by tumors. Renal disorders varying from minimal change nephropathy to immune-complex glomerulonephritis have been associated with carcinoma and Hodgkin's disease. In some cases, evidence of specific immune-complexes has been found. Some neurologic disorders associated with malignancy (such as myasthenia gravis, dermatomyositis and the Guillain-Barré syndrome) may have an immune basis. It is apparent that tumors may produce a variety of proteins, some of which are responsible for humoral, immunologic, and other pathologic phenomena. In many instances, a sensitive immunoassay may detect hormone or other protein production by the tumor, without the specific protein leading to clinical abnormalities. It is hoped that such measurements may be useful in earlier tumor diagnosis or in following the course of malignancy.

Tumors may also produce more than one ectopic hormone. Those tumors of apparent neural crest origin (producing ACTH, lipotropin, biogenic amines, insulin, calcitonin, glucagon, and secretin) appear to do this more frequently. The production of multiple hormones may not be concurrent, with episodic hormone production of various types being present.

REFERENCES

Baylin SB, Mendelsohn G: Ectopic hormone production by tumors: Mechanisms involved and the biological and clinical implications. Endocrinol Rev 1:45, 1980

Blackman MR et al: Ectopic hormones. Adv Int Med 23:85, 1978

Eipper EA, Mains RE: Structure and biosynthesis of proadrenocorticotropin/endorphin and related peptides. Endocrinol Rev 1:1, 1980

Megyesi K et al: Hypoglycemia in association with extrapancreatic tumors: Demonstration of elevated NSILA-s by a new radioreceptor assay. J Clin Endocrinol Metab 36:931, 1974

Odell WD, Wolfsen AR: Humoral syndromes associated with cancer, in *Annual Review of Medicine,* WT Cregar (ed). Palo Alto, Annual Reviews, 1978, p 379

Sherwood LM: Ectopic hormone syndromes, in *Contemporary Endocrinology,* SH Ingbar (ed). New York, Plenum, 1979, p 341

———, Gould VE: Ectopic hormone syndromes and multiple endocrine neoplasia, in *Metabolic Basis of Endocrinology,* LJ deGroot (ed). New York, Grune & Stratton, 1979, p 1749

———: The multiple causes of hypercalcemia in malignant disease. N Engl J Med 303:1412, 1980

Vaitukaitis JL: Peptide hormones as tumor markers. Cancer 37:567, 1976

Wolfsen AR, Odell WD: ProACTH: Use for early detection of lung cancer. Am J Med 66:765, 1979

123 DISORDERS AFFECTING MULTIPLE ENDOCRINE SYSTEMS

R. NEIL SCHIMKE

This chapter is addressed to those disorders in which multiple endocrine gland hyper- or hypofunction results from mechanisms other than a primary abnormality in the hypothalamic-pituitary axis. Congenital anomalies, vascular lesions, metabolic errors, infiltrative and storage disorders, granulomatous diseases, and primary and secondary neoplastic processes can produce multitropic hormone deficiency by interfering with the central control of pituitary hormone secretion, and such conditions must be excluded before a diagnosis of multiple endocrine system disorder can be made. While not common, many of the conditions that affect multiple endocrine systems are inherited and from the viewpoint of preventive medicine have significance out of proportion to their frequency.

SYNDROMES WITH MULTISYSTEM HYPERFUNCTION

The best known conditions involving a number of endocrine glands are the three multiple endocrine neoplasia syndromes, each of which is inherited as an autosomal dominant trait.

MULTIPLE ENDOCRINE NEOPLASIA, TYPE I (MEN I) This disorder, also termed the *Wermer syndrome,* comprises tumors or hyperplasia of the parathyroids, pancreatic islet cells, pituitary, adrenal cortex, and thyroid. The clinical presentation is variable, depending on which of the potentially affected glands is hyperfunctioning at the time of diagnosis. About two-thirds of patients have adenomas of two or more endocrine systems, and a fifth develop tumors of three or more systems.

The majority of affected subjects present with one of the following problems: (1) peptic ulcer and its complications, (2) hypoglycemia, (3) hypercalcemia and/or nephrocalcinosis, (4) complaints referable to pituitary dysfunction such as headaches, visual field defects, and secondary amenorrhea, and (5) multiple lipomas of the skin. A minority (probably < 10 percent) come to medical attention with acromegaly, Cushing's syndrome, nonfunctional thyroid adenomas, hyperthyroidism, hepatomegaly (due to metastatic liver disease), or flushing.

Parathyroid involvement in MEN I may be asymptomatic for prolonged periods, although most patients eventually show some signs of hyperparathyroidism. Tumors of the islet cells may elaborate excessive insulin or gastrin. Insulinomas cause hypoglycemia (Chap. 116), whereas excess gastrin secretion causes the Zollinger-Ellison syndrome with its multifocal or atypically located ulcers and massive hypersecretion of gastric acid. Symptoms may be identical with those of ordinary peptic ulcer, but there is a higher incidence of complications, including perforation, bleeding, and obstruction. Diarrhea is frequent, often with steatorrhea. Radiographic findings include giant gastric rugae, duodenal nodularity, ectopic ulcers in the esophagus, lower duodenum, and jejunum, and intestinal hyperperistalsis. Associated endocrine abnormalities consistent with the MEN syndrome are present in over half of patients with the Zollinger-Ellison syndrome and in half of the first-degree relatives of such patients. For this reason the Zollinger-Ellison syndrome is now widely regarded as a component of the MEN I syndrome even when no other endocrine abnormalities are apparent.

Islet-cell tumors may also produce glucagon, vasoactive inhibitory polypeptide (VIP), prostaglandins, adrenocorticotropic hormone (ACTH), parathyroid hormone, antidiuretic hormone (ADH), and serotonin. Glucagonomas cause hyperglycemia, weight loss, stomatitis, and a peculiar skin rash called *necrotizing migratory erythema.* VIP and prostaglandins have been implicated in the watery diarrhea (pancreatic cholera) syndrome sometimes seen in MEN I. Cushing's syndrome may be due to an adrenal adenoma or may occur as a consequence of ACTH production by an islet tumor. Some adrenal adenomas produce aldosterone or adrenal androgens. Involvement of the thyroid gland is uncommon in MEN I, and, when it does occur, the lesion is not specific since goiter, simple adenoma, and thyroiditis have all been reported. Other features of MEN I include small-intestinal and bronchial carcinoid tumors, schwannomas, thymomas, multiple lipomas, inclusion cysts, and cutaneous leiomyomas.

Patients with MEN I may develop symptoms at any age, but the condition is rare in childhood and after the age of 60. Affected individuals may demonstrate multiple endocrine system involvement simultaneously, or months or years may elapse between the discovery of one adenoma and the appearance of the next. Once the diagnosis is established, the patient must be surveyed at yearly intervals for appearance of new facets of the syndrome. By the same token, all first-degree relatives should be studied. A reasonable approach for screening relatives at risk is as follows: (1) review history for symptoms of peptic ulcer disease, hypoglycemia, renal calculi, lipomas, or hypopituitarism; (2) examine for multiple lipomas; (3) assay serum calcium, phosphorus, and gastrin; and (4) x-ray the sella turcica. Upper gastrointestinal series have proved of no value as a screening test.

The fundamental lesion in MEN I is unknown. Some have considered the basic abnormality to be in the islet cells with their extensive capability for hormone synthesis, attributing changes in the other glands to secondary effects of islet hormone hypersecretion. Others have classified MEN I as a neurocrestopathy implicating faulty differentiation or regulation of the embryonic neural crest, which is the anlagen of at least part of the endocrine system. The endocrine components of the neural crest have been classified by Pearse and coworkers into a subsystem of APUD cells, so named because of their capacity for amine precursor uptake and decarboxylation. The evidence supporting the contention that all APUD cells are derived from neural crest is not strong; indeed, it is more likely that these are of diverse origin but have developed similar characteristics; i.e., they represent a structural-functional convergence.

The pituitary and parathyroid tumors in MEN I are usually benign, but pancreatic and adrenal cortical tumors are frequently malignant. Surgical removal of the affected gland is the usual therapy, although standard irradiation techniques may be employed for the pituitary tumors. Hyperparathyroidism may be due to a single adenoma, but diffuse hyperplasia of more than one gland is more common. Selective venous catheterization with measurement of serum parathyroid hormone levels can be used to differentiate between those possibilities in some centers. Since new adenomas may arise in normal glands left after removal of an adenoma (and since second operations are difficult because of scar formation), some have advocated removal of all the parathyroid glands with transplantation of extirpated fragments into the thigh or forearm, where they can be easily removed should hyperparathyroidism recur. Successful transplantation obviates the need for long-term therapy of hypoparathyroidism. In hypergastrinemia due to islet-cell lesions, total gastrectomy has been used to prevent recurrent peptic ulcers, and in rare cases distant metastases have regressed after this procedure. H_2-receptor antagonists are efficacious in controlling the hyperacidity and diarrhea seen with hypergastrinemia, but this class of drugs is not known to have any intrinsic chemotherapeutic effect.

MULTIPLE ENDOCRINE NEOPLASIA, TYPE II (MEN II OR IIA) Also known as the *Sipple syndrome,* MEN II consists of pheochromocytoma (frequently bilateral and occasionally extraadrenal), medullary thyroid carcinoma (MTC), and, in about half of the reported cases, parathyroid hyperplasia. MEN II can be related more directly to abnormal neural crest development than can MEN I, since both the adrenal medulla and the parafollicular or C cells of the thyroid originate in neural crest. However, there is no evidence that the parathyroid glands are so derived. The parafollicular cell elaborates calcitonin, the primary marker of medullary carcinoma of the thyroid. MTC is not common, comprising only about 7 to 10 percent of all thyroid malignancies. At least 10 percent of the cases are familial, usually appearing as a component of MEN II or MEN III (see below). Medullary carcinoma may also occur in families without other associated endocrine dysfunction; this form is also transmitted as an autosomal dominant trait. MTC may present as a thyroidal mass or be clinically silent and undetectable by palpation or radioiodine scanning. The diagnosis is usually established by immunoassay of serum calcitonin, provided ectopic sites of calcitonin production can be excluded, e.g., breast, lung, and pancreatic islet-cell tumors. Occasionally, basal serum calcitonin levels are borderline in at-risk individuals, and measurement of plasma levels after calcium-pentagastrin infusion can be used to establish the diagnosis. MTC may on occasion secrete substances other than calcitonin, including ACTH, prolactin, serotonin, VIP, histamine, and various prostaglandins, resulting in a confusing array of symptoms.

The pheochromocytoma of MEN II may produce the classic signs of catecholamine excess as described in Chap. 113 or be asymptomatic. Approximately 7 percent of patients who present with pheochromocytomas also have MTC. Symptoms of hyperparathyroidism rarely bring the patient with MEN II to initial clinical attention.

Examination of cells from both the MTC and the pheochromocytoma components of MEN II using X-linked gene markers has led to the conclusion that the inherited defect in the syndrome produces multiple clones of abnormal cells; tumors then develop from a second mutation in the abnormal clone, accounting for the appearance of varying clinical patterns of tumor formation. Other tumors in MEN II include gliomas, glioblastomas, and meningiomas, all of which may be derived from the neural crest.

The age of the patient at the time of detection of the disorder is variable, ranging in one series from 2 to 67 years. C-cell hyperplasia of the thyroid may precede development of frank malignancy by many years, making early screening studies for calcitonin elevation mandatory in all family members at risk. The only effective therapy for MTC is surgical removal of the entire thyroid, as the tumor is probably always multifocal in origin. Limited node dissection is often indicated since the cancer may progress slowly despite an aggressive histological appearance, and prolonged survival is seen in patients with known metastatic disease. Serum calcitonin levels can be used to assess completeness of surgical removal of the tumor and in concert with selective venous catheterization may be utilized to locate distant metastases that are surgically accessible. Neither radioiodine nor x-ray therapy is helpful in disseminated medullary thyroid cancer, and chemotherapy has been of limited value (see Chap. 111). There are rare reports of thyroxine-induced regression of MTC, but these are of questionable significance. The pheochromocytomas are usually benign and are also treated surgically. Unresectable malignant pheochromocytoma requires long-term sympathetic blockade.

MULTIPLE ENDOCRINE NEOPLASIA, TYPE III (MEN III OR IIB) The third endocrine neoplasia syndrome also consists of medullary thyroid carcinoma and pheochromocytoma, but affected individuals have striking dysmorphic features such as neuromas of the conjunctival, labial, and buccal mucosa, the tongue, the larynx, and the gastrointestinal tract; hence the alternate designation of the condition as the *mucosal neuroma syndrome.* Other physical findings include enlarged corneal nerves, "blubbery" lips, soft-tissue prognathism, and a habitus resembling that seen in the Marfan syndrome with hypotonia, lax joints, kyphoscoliosis, genu valgus, and pes cavus. The patients may have café au lait spots or a diffuse lentiginous type of skin pigmentation along with cutaneous neuromas or neurofibromas. Megacolon may occur.

Despite the resemblance of MEN III to MEN II, the syndromes appear to be distinct. For example, both parathyroid hyperplasia and production of hormones other than calcitonin by MTC are rare in MEN III. The mean survival of patients with MEN III is around 30 years compared with 60 years for those with MEN II, suggesting a more malignant course in the former disorder, although histologically the thyroid tumors appear to be identical. As with MEN II treatment of the medullary carcinoma is surgical. The unusual physical features of MEN III should immediately suggest the diagnosis of underlying thyroid malignancy. MTC has been documented in asymptomatic children with MEN III, and C-cell hyperplasia has been found at operation as early as 15 months of age. Clinically, the associated pheochromocytomas behave as expected (Chap. 113).

McCUNE-ALBRIGHT SYNDROME This condition is characterized by the triad of polyostotic fibrous dysplasia, café au lait spots, and isosexual precocity, the latter occurring predominantly but not exclusively in females. The isosexual precocity is usually hypothalamic in origin, but a primary gonadal abnormality has been implicated in some cases (see Chap. 118). Cushing's syndrome and gigantism or acromegaly may also occur in affected patients. The Cushing's syndrome may result from abnormal ACTH production or adrenal adenomas. Nodular toxic goiter and pheochromocytoma have also been reported. The bone lesion resembles that seen in hyperparathyroidism, and parathyroid hyperplasia has been described histologically, although clinical hyperparathyroidism has not been documented. The condition is sporadic, and its cause is unknown (see Chap. 343).

SYNDROMES WITH MULTISYSTEM HYPOFUNCTION

A number of rather diverse conditions can be grouped under this heading. The combination of endocrine hypofunction and immunologic abnormalities occurs in several of the conditions.

POLYGLANDULAR DEFICIENCY SYNDROME (SCHMIDT SYNDROME) (See also Chaps. 111 and 112) The prototype of a polyglandular deficiency state is the Schmidt syndrome, originally described as the presence of both Addison's disease and lymphocytic thyroiditis in a single patient. This syndrome has subsequently been expanded to include failure of any combination of endocrine organs including adrenal insufficiency, lymphocytic thyroiditis, hypoparathyroidism, and gonadal failure. Diabetes mellitus is a frequent accompaniment. The manifestations may be so extensive as to simulate panhypopituitarism; rarely, true pituitary deficiency has been described. The first evidence of endocrinopathy generally appears in adult life. The most significant laboratory feature, in addition to the low levels of circulating hormones, is the presence of antibodies to one or more endocrine glands. The antibodies may be directed against a clinically normal gland, but with time hypofunction usually supervenes. Additional evidence for an immune pathogenesis is provided by the increased frequency of antibodies to parietal cells, with or without overt achlorhydria or pernicious anemia, and the presence of other disorders felt to have an autoimmune basis such as sprue, vitiligo, myasthenia gravis, pure red cell aplasia, and antibody-mediated IgA deficiency. Hyperthyroidism may complicate the clinical picture.

The majority of affected individuals are female, and most cases are sporadic. A few reports have noted multiple affected family members, indicating that the disorder may occur on a genetic basis. Members of these families who show no endocrine disability frequently have serologic abnormalities indicative of a disturbance in immune function. Many of the component endocrine disorders seen in this syndrome have been shown to be associated with the presence of certain HLA antigens, notably HLA-B8 and -Dw3 (in white populations). Other racial groups show different associations, e.g., hyperthyroidism with HLA-Bw35 in the Japanese. The genes coding for these antigens are inherited as autosomal codominant alleles, and it has been speculated that in certain families some abnormality related to specific HLA antigens predisposes selected individuals to autoimmune disease. Since the HLA region in humans may be linked to the so-called immune response (Ir) genes that have been demonstrated in lower animals, it has been postulated that the basic lesion in the Schmidt syndrome resides in a mutational alteration of an inherited immunologic mechanism. For example, a selective immunodeficient state might render an individual unduly susceptible to certain environmental antigens (e.g., viruses) that have a predilection for the endocrine system. Cell lysis or damage could result in release of intracellular contents and lead to development of autoantibodies. Such autoantibodies would not necessarily be pathogenic but could represent epiphenomena whose importance would be as markers of potential clinical disease. Alternatively the defect could reside in a genetically determined defect with inadequate suppression of antibody synthesis by T cells. It is likely that the syndrome is etiologically heterogeneous and that several pathogenetic mechanisms are operative. At present, treatment is confined to providing hormone replacement.

TABLE 123-1
Disorders with common polyglandular manifestations

		Type of endocrine involvement						
Condition	*Clinical feature*	*Hypothalamic-pituitary*	*Thyroid*	*Parathyroid*	*Pancreas*	*Adrenal*	*Gonads*	*Inheritance*
Ataxia-telangiectasia	Early ataxia Oculocutaneous telangiectasia Immunologic deficiency	?Variably decreased pituitary reserve			Diabetes	Cortical hypoplasia	Dysgenetic ovaries; gonadoblastomas later	Autosomal recessive
Pseudohypoparathyroidism	Short stature Short metacarpals and metatarsals Round facies Ectopic calcification	Variable deficiency of all pituitary hormones Prolactin deficiency	Hypo- or hyperthyroidism	Elevated parathyroid hormone levels with either normo- or hypocalcemia	Diabetes		Ovarian failure	Probable X-linked dominant; heterogeneous
Myotonic dystrophy	Muscular dystrophy Premature baldness Mental retardation	Gonadotropin, growth hormone abnormalities, related to central integrative defect (?)	Hypothyroidism		Diabetes		Primary failure	Autosomal dominant
Noonan syndrome	Short stature Ptosis Webbed neck Pulmonary stenosis	Gonadotropin deficiency	Thyroiditis				Primary failure	Autosomal dominant
Fanconi syndrome	Short stature Bone marrow hypoplasia Abnormal skin pigmentation Radius malformations	Panhypopituitarism			Diabetes	Adrenal atrophy	Gonadal atrophy	Autosomal recessive
Werner syndrome	Premature aging of all organ systems Atrophic skin Cataracts Early osteoporosis		Papillary carcinoma		Diabetes		Gonadal atrophy	Autosomal recessive

CANDIDIASIS-ENDOCRINOPATHY SYNDROME An autoimmune pathogenesis has also been invoked in the candidiasis-endocrinopathy syndrome. Features that differentiate this condition from the Schmidt syndrome include the childhood onset of the disease and the extensive mucocutaneous monilial infection that becomes evident shortly after birth. Hypoparathyroidism is common, and adrenal insufficiency may develop acutely. Organ-specific antibodies against a variety of endocrine glands may be evident early, and both pernicious anemia and sprue may be present. Chronic active hepatitis and membranoproliferative glomerulonephritis also have been seen. Defective cellular immunity to *Candida albicans* has been demonstrated in virtually all affected patients; some have more generalized anergy. A cause-and-effect relationship between the monilial infection and the endocrinopathy has not been demonstrated. The disorder has occurred in sibs, occasionally from consanguineous unions, and it is possible that the disease is inherited as an autosomal recessive trait. No association with the HLA system has been demonstrated, but affected individuals have a deficiency of immunoglobulin A and hypergammaglobulinemia. Suppressor T-cell function is defective. The fungal infection is refractory to conventional chemotherapeutic drugs, although partial remission has been reported with a combination of antifungal agents and transfer factor. Amelioration of the candidiasis in no way affects the endocrinopathy, and conventional replacement therapy is required.

LIPODYSTROPHIC SYNDROMES The lipodystrophic syndromes are described in Chap. 105. Insulin-resistant diabetes mellitus is common and may be associated with elevated growth hormone levels and with an increased incidence of polycystic disease of the ovaries, acromegaly, and Cushing's disease.

DIABETES MELLITUS, DIABETES INSIPIDUS, AND OPTIC ATROPHY This clinical triad has been noted in sibs and likely constitutes a rare autosomal recessive defect. Nerve deafness, usually mild, may also occur. The diabetes mellitus is of the early-onset insulin-dependent type. The diabetes insipidus usually appears prior to age 20. The frequency of the syndrome is uncertain. The varying manifestations of the condition are difficult to reconcile from an etiologic point of view, and treatment requires replacement of the missing hormones.

OBESITY-HYPOGONADISM SYNDROMES A number of seemingly discrete entities share obesity, generally with frank diabetes mellitus, and hypogonadism that may be either primary or secondary. The *Biedl-Bardet syndrome* features retinitis pigmentosa, polydactyly, mental retardation, and renal anomalies along with obesity and hypogonadotropic hypogonadism. Diabetes mellitus has been reported in some patients. There is sufficient resemblance between this syndrome and the *Alström syndrome* (retinitis pigmentosa, nerve deafness, diabetes mellitus, and primary gonadal failure) to cause frequent diagnostic confusion. Both are autosomal recessive disorders. However, polydactyly and mental retardation do not occur in the Alström syndrome. A similar condition is the *Biemond syndrome* in which obesity, diabetes mellitus, secondary hypogonadism, and postaxial polydactyly are combined with iris colobomata rather than pigmentary retinopathy. Patients with the *Prader-Willi syndrome* (obesity, hypogonadism, hypotonia, mental retardation) also have diabetes mellitus of the maturity-onset type. In neither the Biemond nor the Prader-Willi syndrome have the genetics been established. A small deletion of chromosome 15 has been found in some patients with the latter disorder.

CHROMOSOMAL DISORDERS WITH ENDOCRINE DEFICIENCY (See also Chaps. 61 and 120) In addition to hypogonadism, patients with Turner syndrome have an increased incidence of diabetes mellitus and of thyroiditis thought to be on an autoimmune basis. In the Klinefelter syndrome an increased frequency of diabetes mellitus may occur in addition to gonadal failure. In the Down syndrome hypogonadism is probably universal in males, and menstrual irregularities and early menopause are common in women; in addition, increased prevalences of Hashimoto's thyroiditis and diabetes mellitus have been reported.

OTHER CONDITIONS WITH MULTISYSTEM MANIFESTATIONS There are a number of other rare conditions in which involvement of more than one endocrine gland has been recorded often enough to constitute a significant facet of the syndrome. Some, like neurofibromatosis (von Recklinghausen's disease) and tuberous sclerosis, may show either hypo- or hyperfunction of endocrine glands because of interference with central regulatory mechanisms caused by the brain tumors characteristic of the diseases. By the same token, pheochromocytomas not surprisingly occur in neurofibromatosis because the adrenal medulla is derived from the same embryonic source.

Table 123-1 lists a few of the conditions in which disorders of multiple endocrine systems have been seen. It is noteworthy that both primary and secondary failures have been reported within the diagnostic confines of the same syndrome. For example, both gonadotropin deficiency and primary testicular atrophy have been documented in patients with the Noonan syndrome (see Chap. 107) even within the same family. It is also apparent that whenever a clinical condition like diabetes mellitus occurs in such distinct entities as myotonic dystrophy and ataxia-telangiectasia, the molecular mechanisms underlying the disease may be heterogeneous. A better understanding of the genetic defect would provide insight into the development and function of the endocrine system.

REFERENCES

ARULANTHAM K et al: Evidence for defective immunoregulation in the syndrome of familial candidiasis endocrinopathy. N Engl J Med 300:164, 1979

EISENBARTH G et al: HLA type and occurrence of disease in familial polyglandular failure. N Engl J Med 298:92, 1978

IRVINE WJ (ed): Autoimmunity in endocrine disease. Clin Endocrinol Metab, vol 4, no 2, 1975

PEARSE AGE, POLAK JM: Neural crest origin of the endocrine polypeptide (APUD) cells of the gastrointestinal tract and pancreas. Gut 12:783, 1971

RIMOIN DL: Genetic syndromes associated with glucose intolerance, in *The Genetics of Diabetes Mellitus,* W Creutzfeldt et al (eds). New York, Springer, 1976

———, SCHIMKE RN: *Genetic Disorders of the Endocrine Glands.* St Louis, Mosby, 1971

SCHIMKE RN: The multiple endocrine adenoma syndromes. Adv Intern Med 21:294, 1975

———: Syndromes with multiple endocrine gland involvement. Prog Med Genet, 3:143, 1979

section 9 | Neoplasia

124
PRINCIPLES OF NEOPLASIA: APPROACH TO DIAGNOSIS AND MANAGEMENT

JOHN E. ULTMANN
HARVEY M. GOLOMB

Physicians practicing internal medicine should be familiar with the various implications of the diagnosis of cancer in their patients. Cancer is not one disease. There are more than 100 clinically distinct forms of cancer, with differing biological behavior and clinical manifestations. The internist should be especially familiar with the natural history and treatment of common forms of malignancy, such as those of the breast, lung, and gastrointestinal tract. These epithelial cancers comprise over 50 percent of the cancers usually encountered. The magnitude of the cancer problem may be appreciated by a few statistics: one of four Americans will develop cancer during his or her lifetime, and over 420,000 Americans will die of cancer in 1983. Not only is cancer a major health problem, but the management and care of cancer patients is often complex.

With the development of medical oncology as a subspecialty of internal medicine, the internist is playing an ever-increasing role in the care of the cancer patient.

The diagnosis and management of cancer require a knowledge of general internal medicine and an understanding of the characteristics of the growth and spread of malignant neoplasms. For example, a nodular lesion in the lung must be evaluated for the possibility of neoplastic as well as granulomatous disease. Intermittent rectal bleeding must be appraised for benign or malignant neoplasms as well as for inflammatory bowel disease. Cushing's syndrome requires evaluation for bilateral adrenal hyperplasia as well as for an oat-cell carcinoma of the lung capable of producing adrenocorticotropic hormone (ACTH).

This chapter presents an overview of the biology and etiology of neoplasia and summarizes an approach to the diagnosis, staging, and treatment of cancer. The pathophysiologic changes occurring as a consequence of the tumor as a local mass, as a result of metastases, or from the elaboration of various substances by tumor are discussed. Details for the management of cancer will be found in Chap. 125 and in the various sections devoted to specific diseases.

BIOLOGY OF NEOPLASIA *Cancer* is a term used to characterize abnormal growth of cells which may result in the invasion of normal tissues or the spread to distant organs, termed *metastasis.* The degree of malignancy of a cancer is based upon the propensity of these cells for invasion and distant spread. A metastasis is a neoplastic lesion arising from another cancer, with which it is no longer in contiguity. Regardless of mechanism, separation of malignant cells from the primary cancer is an essential part of the neoplastic process. The basic concept that metastases arise directly from the constituent cells of primary cancer originates from observations of histologic similarities between the two. The mode of transport of cells from the primary to the presumptive secondary lesions is inferred from the many observations of cancer cells infiltrating tissues and invading blood vessels and lymphatic channels, and the recognition of circulating cancer cells in the blood of patients with cancer. However, many of the presumed circulating cancer cells have been determined to be megakaryocytes. In addition, the possibility that "metastases" could arise from the release of oncogenic viruses from the primary lesion requires further evaluation.

CYTOGENETICS The characteristics of a particular tumor cell are, in general, permanent and stable and are inherited by descendants of that tumor cell. These characteristics may be explained best by structural alterations of the DNA in genes or chromosomes. These genetic structural changes may range from single gene mutations to gross chromosomal changes. These chromosomal changes may involve loss or gain of chromosomes, translocation of chromosomes, and changes in ploidy. Although the DNA and chromosomes of tumor cells may be clearly different from those of normal cells, the changes are not uniform from tumor to tumor, and no abnormality in the genetic material may be detectable in a substantial number of human tumors. Various techniques are available to analyze the DNA of normal and tumor cells, including the methods of nucleic acid hybridization. This technique allows comparison of analogous nucleotide chains from different cells by analyzing the product of each chain when allowed to interact. With use of radioactive RNA or DNA, comparable sequences of nucleotide chains from different cells can be quantified. Reverse transcriptase (RNA-directed DNA polymerase) has been used to synthesize isotope-labeled DNAs. These DNA templates have been used to show homologies between murine leukemia virus and human leukemias and sarcomas, supporting the hypothesis of a viral etiology of human leukemia.

The most widely used technique for gross examination of genetic material is the examination of metaphase chromosomes. A tumor may be characterized by its "modal" karyotype, i.e., the number of chromosomes and the morphologic pattern of the largest percentage of cells. Major advances in cytogenetics have resulted from development of techniques to demonstrate chromosome banding, utilizing fluorescent acridine dyes, or by treatment of chromosomes by heat, alkali, or enzymes prior to staining. This permits accurate identification of individual chromosomes and regions within the chromosome, increasing the sensitivity of chromosome examination.

Only a few neoplastic diseases in humans are associated with a specific and characteristic chromosome abnormality; these include chronic myelogenous leukemia (CML), acute promyelocytic leukemia (APL), some lymphoproliferative disorders, and meningioma. In about 85 percent of the patients with CML, the material comprising approximately half of the long arm of a G22 chromosome is translocated to the end of a C9 chromosome. This abnormality (Philadelphia chromosome, Ph^1) involves all three hematopoietic cell lines, and has been interpreted as an acquired somatic cell mutation in the bone marrow, with preferential survival and proliferation of this clone. In APL, the material from the distal part of the long arm of an E17 chromosome is translocated to the end of a D15 chromosome. This abnormality is present in approximately two-thirds of the patients with APL. In the lymphoproliferative disorders, an 8/14 translocation has been associated with most Burkitt's lymphomas and a marker 14q+ has been found in the tumors of many patients with multiple myeloma, Hodgkin's disease, and non-Hodgkin's lymphomas. The chromosome abnormality associated with meningioma is hypodiploid, in contrast to the examples cited above, and frequently involves the deletion of chromosome G22.

Approximately 50 percent of patients with acute leukemia have detectable cytogenetic abnormalities. Although the abnormalities are not necessarily uniform, they are probably nonrandom. For any given patient they tend to remain characteristic and recur during a clinical relapse. Leukemias induced by radiation, drugs, or both, such as occur in some patients with treated Hodgkin's disease, have a much higher percentage of chromosomal abnormalities. The use of chromosome-banding techniques may result in grouping of patients with common etiologies or prognoses. Cytogenetic studies also may occasionally be useful in the diagnosis of "preleukemia" when abnormal karyotypes are present.

For technical reasons, only a limited number of chromosome studies have been performed in solid tumors. Cytogenetic abnormalities are frequent and major in solid tumors such as melanoma, lung cancer, and colon cancer. Significant aneuploidy is present in almost all tumors. In melanoma the variation from cell to cell is substantial and has been interpreted as evidence for multiple cell lines, cytogenetic instability, and rapid clonal evolution toward more malignant behavior.

ETIOLOGY Although the etiology of cancer in humans cannot yet be explained at the molecular level, it is clear that genetic composition of the host is important in cancer induction. Related immunologic factors may predispose the host to a putative carcinogen. There is some evidence that viruses may play a role in the neoplastic process. In addition, both environmental and therapeutic agents have been identified as carcinogens.

Genetic factors The fact that not all humans exposed to the same dose of carcinogens develop cancer indicates that host factors play an important role in the cancer-inducing process. Certain familial and genetic disorders may increase the risk of cancer. These may be divided into those that have a well-defined hereditary pattern with a high frequency in family members, such as retinoblastoma, and those familial and genetic disorders having an increased risk, such as multiple polyposis of the colon or breast cancer. In addition, there is a group of familial disorders associated with cytogenetic abnormalities that have an increased risk of cancer, such as Bloom's syndrome, Fanconi's anemia, or the immunologic deficiency states.

Only a small proportion of cancers is inherited in a mendelian fashion, which indicates single-gene transmission. Table 124-1 lists some cancers that occur as an inherited trait (hereditary neoplasms) or as a complication of inherited precursor lesions that are clinically recognizable (preneoplastic states).

Polyposis coli consists of numerous adenomatous polyps of the colon and rectum and occurs in about 1 per 8000 live births. Carcinoma develops in virtually all cases with advancing age and is found at the time of initial diagnosis of the polyps in about 40 percent of patients. A penetrance of about 80 percent is reported in patients with polyps detected any time after the age of 10 years.

Neurofibromatosis (von Recklinghausen's disease), which occurs in about 1 per 3000 live births, is characterized by café au lait spots and multiple neurofibromas. The neurofibromas show sarcomatous degeneration in about 10 percent of patients; in addition, there is an increased risk of meningioma, acoustic neuroma, pheochromocytoma, and gliomas of the brain or optic nerve.

In the *Peutz-Jeghers syndrome,* gastrointestinal polyps are signaled by the presence of melanin spots in the buccal mucosa, lips, and digits. Most of the polyps are in the small intestine and very rarely show malignant degeneration. Ovarian neoplasms, however, occur in about 5 percent of women and may be the initial lead to the syndrome.

Bloom's syndrome is a rare autosomal recessive condition with features of dwarfism, characteristic facies, and a photosensitive telangiectatic erythema on the face. In about one out of eight reported cases acute leukemia has developed.

The apparent association between an inherited abnormality and neoplasia also is found in *ataxia-telangiectasia,* an autosomal recessive trait in which telangiectatic lesions appear in the bulbar conjunctiva and in which there is progressive cerebellar ataxia with spinocerebellar atrophy. Cellular immunity is decreased, and abnormal levels of serum immunoglobulin are often present. The individuals who survive the recurrent sinopulmonary infections into adolescence or their twenties often develop lymphoma (see Chap. 64).

The mechanism by which the hereditary conditions lead to cancer or leukemia is not clear. However, there are some clues to possible pathogenetic mechanisms. Among the genodermatoses, which generally show an autosomal recessive pattern, is xeroderma pigmentosa. In this condition, it has been shown that skin fibroblasts fail to repair DNA damage induced by ultraviolet light. In individuals with Bloom's syndrome, cultured fibroblasts from these patients have increased sensitivity to transformation by oncogenic viruses.

The precise mechanisms of familial cancer are unknown, but it has been shown that daughters of women who develop breast cancer have a three to five times greater chance of developing the disease than women without such a family history. Racial factors are also of importance. For example, blacks and other ethnic groups with deeply pigmented skin are protected from melanoma and other skin cancers induced by exposure to sunlight.

TABLE 124-1
Hereditary cancer syndromes in adults

I Hereditary neoplasms
- *A* Nevoid basal-cell carcinoma syndrome
- *B* Trichoepithelioma
- *C* Multiple endocrine adenomatosis
- *D* Chemodectomas
- *E* Polyposis coli
- *F* Gardner's syndrome

II Preneoplastic states
- *A* Hamartomatous syndromes
  - *1* Neurofibromatosis
  - *2* Tuberous sclerosis
  - *3* Von Hippel-Lindau syndrome
  - *4* Multiple exostosis
  - *5* Peutz-Jeghers syndrome
- *B* Genodermatoses
  - *1* Albinism
  - *2* Werner's syndrome
  - *3* Polydysplastic epidermolysis bullosa
- *C* Chromosome breakage disorders
  - *1* Bloom's syndrome
  - *2* Fanconi's syndrome
  - *3* Ataxia-telangiectasia
- *D* Immune deficiency syndromes
  - *1* Late-onset immunologic deficiency

SOURCE: *JF Froumeni, in Holland and Frei.*

Viruses Viruses can cause neoplasia in almost every mammal, as well as in fish, frogs, and other species. Generally, tumor viruses contain either double-stranded DNA or single-stranded RNA with an icosahedral capsid which may or may not be surrounded by a lipid envelope. So-called C-type RNA viruses usually produce leukemia or sarcomas; these viruses and the transformed cells usually contain RNA reverse transcriptase activity; this RNA-directed DNA polymerase may be necessary for malignant transformation by these viruses. The heteroduplex resulting from transcription of DNA from the single-stranded RNA template is probably replicated by DNA-dependent DNA polymerase to produce a double-stranded DNA molecule that is inserted into the host chromosome by an unknown mechanism. This enzyme activity has been detected in blast cells of some patients with acute leukemia. Also, a C-type human virus has been successfully isolated from a patient with acute myelogenous leukemia. C-type RNA viruses and related viral proteins have been identified in tissue culture specimens of lymph node material obtained from patients with Hodgkin's disease and histiocytic lymphoma. These findings, together with nucleic acid hybridization studies, are presumptive evidence for a virus etiology in some cases of acute leukemia and lymphoma in humans.

The strongest candidate for a human tumor virus is the Epstein-Barr virus (EBV), a DNA herpesvirus that causes infectious mononucleosis. Seroepidemiologic data as well as detection of the viral DNA in the lymphoma cells by nucleic acid hybridization have provided evidence that EBV is associated with Burkitt's lymphoma and nasopharyngeal carcinoma. Burkitt's lymphoma occurs mainly in children in central Africa and New Guinea, and sporadically elsewhere. Because of this geographic distribution, it is believed that in addition to the virus that may act as a cocarcinogen, other factors, such as immunosuppression due to malaria, may be involved. Genetic factors may play a role in the development of nasopharyngeal carcinoma, found in the far east, since Chinese who have migrated to the United States continue to have a high incidence of this disease.

Herpes simplex virus (HSV-2) has been associated with cancer of the cervix by the demonstration of HSV-2 genetic information, as well as HSV-specific antigens in tumor cells.

Occupational and environmental carcinogens In eliciting the occupational history and history of exposure to drugs, as well as chemical agents in the home, various substances which constitute a potential carcinogenic hazard will come to light. The first demonstration of an environmental carcinogen was by Potts, who linked the increased incidence of scrotal cancer in chimney sweeps to exposure to soot. Since that time an ever-increasing number of occupational and environmental carcinogens have been reported (Table 124-2). It has been estimated that up to 70 to 80 percent of cancers in humans are related to chemical and environmental factors. As many as 40 percent of all cancers are related directly or in part to cigarette smoking. There is often a long latent period between exposure to a chemical carcinogen and the development of neoplasia, and unless unusual cancers are produced, the possible association between a chemical exposure and the cancer may not be appreciated. This latent period also makes difficult any screening program in animals to determine whether a given chemical or substance is likely to be carcinogenic. Leads to the presence of environmental carcinogens can be provided by careful monitoring of the incidence of various types of cancer in different populations over a period of time. There is, however, a major disparity in susceptibility to cancer from one species to another and among different populations exposed to the same carcinogen. This may be explained in part by hereditary differences in enzyme levels necessary to process chemicals to be *active* carcinogens and in levels of degrading enzymes necessary to deactivate the carcinogens. For example, it has been suggested, but not proved, that elevated levels of aryl hydrocarbon hydroxylase predispose smokers to lung cancer.

Mapping of cancer mortality by county within the United States has revealed patterns of etiologic significance. For example, bladder cancer in males is probably related to industrial contaminants found in areas of high industrialization and around oil-processing areas. Skin cancer is associated with residence in the "sun belt." Epidemiologic studies on a worldwide scale have revealed geographic areas where certain cancers predominate, and attempts to identify the causal agent are in progress. The high prevalence of bladder cancer in Egypt is related to schistosomiasis haematobia (bilharziasis) and apparently its attendant chronic bacterial infection; the hepatomas of Africa are related to exposure to aflatoxins. Other geographic "epidemic" areas have been identified, but the clues to the etiologic agent(s) involved are not clear: cancer of esophagus around the Caspian Sea, cancer of nasopharynx in China, cancer of stomach in Japan. It has been shown that Japanese migrating to Hawaii or to the continental United States have a decreasing risk of cancer of the stomach, emphasizing the importance of environmental factors.

Other clues regarding etiologic factors predisposing to cancer come from changes in incidence of particular cancers with time. For example, the marked decrease in the prevalence of cancer of the stomach in the United States is attributed to the introduction of refrigeration, with decrease in nitrites formed from nitrate food preservatives; in contrast, the increase in cancer of the colon is attributed to a high-fat, low-fiber diet. The role of bile salts as cocarcinogens is under investigation.

Screening suspect chemicals in animal models is time-consuming and expensive. A number of investigators have proposed in vitro bacterial tests to detect mutagenicity which accurately predict carcinogenicity in test animals and humans. Among these tests, the salmonella mutagenicity test to identify chemical carcinogens and mutagens is the most promising. The unique feature of the test is the use of liver microsomes to activate the potential carcinogenic-mutagenic substance. The test detects these chemicals by means of their ability to damage DNA and cause mutations in bacteria. It is about 90 percent accurate in detecting proven carcinogens or mutagens and therefore a very useful tool for screening for potential carcinogens.

More than 15 carcinogens, including hydrocarbons and aromatic amines, have been isolated from tobacco smoke. The incidence of not only lung cancer but also of head and neck, esophageal, and bladder cancers is increased in smokers. In

TABLE 124-2
Occupational and environmental carcinogens

Carcinogen	*Associated neoplasm*
Cigarette smoke	Lung, upper respiratory tract, and other cancers
Asbestos	Mesothelioma, lung
Arsenic	Skin, lung
Cadmium	Prostate, kidney
Chromium	Lung
Nickel	Lung, nasal sinuses
Uranium	Lung
Aflatoxin	Liver
Nitrites	Stomach
Chloromethyl ethers	Lung
Isopropyl oil	Nasal sinuses
Naphthalene dyes (aniline dyes)	Bladder
Vinyl chloride	Liver hemangiosarcoma
Benzene	Acute myelogenous leukemia
Schistosomiasis haematobia	Bladder

addition, asbestos, uranium, and alcohol exposure act synergistically to increase the risk.

The occurrence of lung cancer as a consequence of occupational exposure to asbestos has been confirmed. Approximately 20 percent of all the deaths of asbestos workers have been attributed to lung cancer. This represents a sevenfold increase in incidence of this neoplasm after 20 years from the time of the first exposure. In addition, approximately 7 percent of the deaths of asbestos workers are caused by either pleural or peritoneal mesothelioma, a risk that is 100 to 1000 times that which might be expected in the general population. A threefold increase in gastrointestinal cancer has been reported for the same workers. With few exceptions, a serious risk begins after 20 years from onset of first exposure and continues from that point on.

Exposure to heavy metals such as arsenic, cadmium, chromium, and nickel has been associated with an increased occurrence of certain cancers. An excess incidence of skin cancer has been observed among patients who have been treated with arsenicals and among workers exposed to this compound, and among persons exposed excessively to arsenic in drinking water. Arsenic also appears to be a lung carcinogen with rate ratios of approximately 7, 5, and 2.5 for heavy, medium, and light exposure. The latent time for arsenic-induced lung cancer is long, ranging from 30 to 35 years for heavy exposure to 40 to 45 years for light exposure. Arsenic may also cause liver cancer.

Occupational exposure to cadmium has resulted in an increased incidence of prostatic carcinoma. The excess was twofold for those whose exposure had commenced less than 30 years earlier and threefold for those with a longer interval. A significant association of renal cancer with exposure to cadmium has also been found.

Chromium exposure has been connected with excess mortality from cancers of the respiratory tract, especially with lung cancers and cancers of the nasal cavities. The rate ratios have been reported as high as thirty- to fortyfold over the expected, while the mean latent period in various studies has ranged from 10 to 20 years. Of the lung cancers reported, at least one-half were anaplastic or undifferentiated; only 10 percent were adenocarcinomas.

An excess of both lung cancer and cancer of the nasal sinuses has been found among nickel refinery workers; rate ratios of about tenfold exist for lung cancer, while they are 100-fold or greater for the nasal sinuses. The mean latent period for lung cancer varies between 13 and 30 years, but may be a few years shorter for nasal cancer. The histology of the tumor is usually epidermoid, although 12 to 30 percent can be anaplastic. The exact identity of the carcinogenic agents in nickel refineries is still unknown, but most cancers occur among employees working in the early stages of nickel refining. It has been suggested there may be a synergistic effect between nickel exposure and cigarette smoking.

Hundreds of chemicals used in industry, on farms, in the home, and in foods as additives or preservatives have been implicated as carcinogens. Some of these are listed in Table 124-2. One example of such a toxic substance is vinyl chloride. This industrial product has been shown to be carcinogenic in both experimental animals and humans. Vinyl chloride administered by inhalation has been found to produce angiosarcomas of the liver in rats at concentrations as low as 25 parts per million. Besides liver angiosarcomas in workers in the vinyl chloride–polyvinyl chloride industry, there also seems to be a high incidence of brain tumors, large-cell carcinomas of the lung, lymphomas, and leukemia.

In view of the large number of potential cancer-causing agents, physicians must be prepared to counsel patients regarding the carcinogenic potential of various chemicals and be aware of the risk-benefit ratio of each of these substances. No doubt food additives which prevent botulism and have a small risk of causing cancer must be dealt with differently from cigarette smoking, which confers a major risk upon the user.

Drugs and radiational agents as carcinogens In addition to occupational and environmental carcinogens listed in Table 124-2, radiation in any form and various drugs have been unequivocally shown to be associated with the induction of cancer. The survivors of Hiroshima and Nagasaki showed an increased incidence of acute and chronic granulocytic leukemia that reached a peak approximately 7 years after the exposure. Radiation therapy for enlarged tonsils and thymus and for ankylosing spondylitis has also led to an increased incidence of acute leukemia, after a similar latent period. These studies show a dose-response relationship until a plateau is reached, and increased doses do not increase the incidence. Why only a small percentage of the population exposed will develop acute leukemia is not known. The risk may be a function of genetic makeup as well as age. Infants and pregnant women are at greatest risk to develop radiation-induced neoplasia. An acceptable safe dose of radiation has not yet been determined with certainty. It has also been shown that in addition to an increased risk of leukemia, patients previously treated with radiation therapy for an enlarged thymus or tonsils have a marked increased risk of developing thyroid carcinoma.

An increase in the frequency of breast cancer in women undergoing repeated x-ray or fluoroscopy examinations of the chest in follow-up of their tuberculosis or as part of a mammography screening program has been shown with a dose as low as 170 mGy (17 rads).

Table 124-3 is a partial list of cancers related to radioisotope and drug exposure in humans. Drugs that are capable of interacting with DNA (alkylating agents) as well as immunosuppressive agents and hormones all have the potential for causing neoplasms in humans. The use of alkylating agents in

TABLE 124-3
Cancers related to drug exposures in humans

Drug	*Cancer*
Radioisotopes:	
Phosphorus (^{32}P)	Acute leukemia
Radium, mesothorium	Osteosarcoma and sinus carcinoma
Thorotrast	Hemangioendothelioma of liver
Immunosuppressive agents (for renal transplantation):	
Antilymphocyte serum; Antimetabolites; Alkylating agents; Corticosteroids	Lymphoma, epithelial malignancies of skin and viscera
Cytotoxic drugs:	
Chlornaphazine; Phenylalanine mustard; Cyclophosphamide	Bladder cancer; Acute myelogenous leukemia
Hormones:	
Synthetic estrogens:	
Prenatal	Vaginal and cervical adenocarcinoma (clear-cell type)
Postnatal	Endometrial carcinoma (adenosquamous type)
Androgenic-anabolic steroids	Hepatocellular carcinoma
Others:	
Arsenic	Skin cancer, lung cancer
Phenacetin-containing drugs	Renal pelvis carcinoma
Coal tar ointments	Skin cancer
? Diphenylhydantoin	Lymphoma
? Chloramphenicol	Leukemia
? Amphetamines	Hodgkin's disease

SOURCE: *After R Hoover, JF Froumeni, J Clin Pharmacol 15:16, 1975.*

therapeutic doses and for a sufficiently long time, either alone or in combination with other drugs and/or radiotherapy, has been associated with an increased incidence of acute myelogenous leukemia or its variants in patients with Hodgkin's disease, non-Hodgkin's lymphomas, multiple myeloma, and ovarian cancer. Since these secondary leukemias are relatively refractory to induction of remission with combination chemotherapy, it is fortunate that the incidence of leukemia appears to be relatively low (1 to 5 percent).

The development of acute leukemia during the course of Hodgkin's disease is probably related to either the immunosuppressive or carcinogenic effects of radiation therapy or a combination of the two. In a study of 81 patients with both acute myelocytic leukemia and Hodgkin's disease, these diseases occurred simultaneously in only three cases. Of the remaining 79 patients, 76 had received radiation therapy for Hodgkin's disease, and acute myelocytic leukemia developed 1 to 19 years later, with a mean interval of 6.5 years. Thirty-four of the 76 patients had also received chemotherapy; only 3 had received chemotherapy alone. The possibility that acute leukemia is a part of the natural history of Hodgkin's disease and is occurring with greater frequency because of improved survival in Hodgkin's disease due to aggressive radiation and drug therapy warrants consideration. Radiation therapy and antineoplastic drugs should be used with caution or not at all in nonneoplastic disorders which are not life-threatening.

Hormones While the relationship of hormone administration in the etiology of breast cancer is well established in mice, such a causal connection has not been demonstrated in women. There appears to be epidemiologic evidence that nulliparous women have a higher incidence of breast cancer than women who have had children. The risk is also increased threefold for women whose mothers and other close relatives have had breast cancer. The role of synthetic hormones in increasing the risk of breast cancer is under investigation, but so far no correlation has been demonstrated. Low doses of hormones used in birth control pills do not appear to cause breast cancer. Prenatal exposure to synthetic estrogens has been associated with vaginal adenosis and vaginal and cervical (clear-cell) adenocarcinomas. It is important to identify the daughters of women who received diethylstilbestrol (DES) during pregnancy. The occurrence of vaginal adenocarcinomas in the offspring of mothers treated with DES during pregnancy demonstrates the problem of detecting carcinogenicity of chemicals. This particular relationship was detected because the neoplasm was unusual, despite the low incidence of tumors. Postnatal exposure to estrogens has led to a fivefold risk for endometrial carcinoma. Estrogens as prescribed in birth control pills also cause hepatic adenomas, which have a tendency to bleed, as well as liver cancers. The relationship of hormones to prostatic cancer is even less clear. It is known that androgenic-anabolic steroids predispose both to benign liver tumors and to hepatocellular carcinoma.

IMMUNOLOGIC FACTORS Cancers may be associated with, or lead to, an altered host immune response; however, the cause-and-effect relationship remains to be determined. The effect can be direct, resulting from replacement of normal by malignant lymphocytes, as in chronic lymphocytic leukemia (CLL); indirect, secondary to treatment required for control of the primary tumor; or an associated effect, as exemplified by situations in which blocking factors can be demonstrated.

Many cancer patients show some resistance to the progress of their disease. Spontaneous regression occasionally occurs in neuroblastoma, hypernephroma, choriocarcinoma, and malignant melanoma. The long-term dormancy of multiple metastases seen after removal of the primary mass can be explained

best by host defense mechanisms. Host defenses are geared to eliminate any tissue recognized as "nonself," in much the same way as an allograft is rejected. Presumably malignant tumors can develop in otherwise healthy hosts only if there has been a breakdown of the host's surveillance mechanism. The ability to mount humoral or cell-mediated immune response against a neoplasm depends on both the host's genetic material and other factors, such as previous exposure to radiotherapy or immunosuppressive drugs. The evidence for these concepts comes largely from the study of animal models; in humans, the data are more limited and this remains an area to be explored further.

An increased incidence of malignancy associated with long-term administration of immunosuppressive drugs has been noted in patients with renal transplants. Of 432 recipients who were followed for up to 11 years, 24 developed neoplasms; this incidence of 5.6 percent is 100 times that observed in the general population when matched for age. In another study of 184 organ homograft recipients who developed cancers de novo, 60 percent were under 40 years of age. Both the incidence of lymphomas and of primary central nervous system lymphomas was greatly increased in such patients.

The host immune response can be blunted by blocking factors present in the host's serum. These blocking factors can decrease the cytotoxic effect of the host's immune lymphocytes. They slowly disappear from the serum if the tumor is removed surgically. The precise component of serum that is responsible for the blocking effect on cell-mediated antitumor immunity is not known, but it may be a noncomplement-fixing antitumor antibody, which, though capable of binding to tumor cell surfaces, is capable of inducing tumor cell lysis.

AGE SPECIFICITY Patients of different ages are at risk for different types of cancer. Fifty percent of the cases of acute lymphocytic leukemia occur in patients under 7 years, whereas only 10 percent of patients with acute myelomonocytic leukemia are under 20 years of age. Chronic lymphocytic leukemia is a disease of middle and old age and is practically unknown in childhood; above the age of 60 it is the most common type of leukemia. Solid tumors demonstrate similar differences. Ewing's sarcoma is a highly anaplastic tumor in bone; 90 percent of patients are under 30 and 70 percent under 20 years of age. Although colon cancer may occur in childhood, the incidence is low until age 40, when it rises rapidly; the peak frequency occurs in the sixth decade.

SEX PREDILECTION Knowledge of the predilection of various malignancies for one of the sexes is also important. Although breast cancer does occur in males, its frequency is about 1 percent of that in females. Lung cancer is three times more common in men than in women, whereas the incidence of rectocolonic cancer is approximately equal in men and women. Differences in sex predilection may be due to hormonal factors, differences in exposure to carcinogens, and other factors.

ROLE OF THE PHYSICIAN IN DETECTION OF CANCER

EARLY DETECTION Early detection and prompt treatment can result in cure or longer survival in many types of cancer. To detect cancer at an early stage, the physician must be aware of certain inherited conditions and environmental factors which predispose to malignancy and must undertake a thorough, systematic clinical evaluation. The partnership of the patient is required if this goal is to be achieved. The patient's awareness of the early signs of malignancy as well as his or her acceptance of diagnostic and therapeutic procedures is essential. The following examples illustrate the usefulness of early detection. For cancer of the cervix, early detection by means of the Papanicolaou test of cervical cytology is responsible for the decrease in the incidence of invasive cancer and has resulted in a 50 percent reduction in mortality. For cancer of the lung, a prospective, controlled project of screening a high-risk group of male, heavy smokers, more than 45 years old with serial sputum cytology and chest roentgenograms has been carried out. Approximately 60 percent of tumors found in persons receiving surveillance examinations every 4 months were resectable for cure compared with 25 percent of tumors detected in controls. The cost-benefit ratio for screening for lung cancer remains to be determined.

The "seven warning signals" of early cancer in special sites, which include skin, breast, larynx, lung, and the gastrointestinal tract, are designed to educate people to seek medical help early (Table 124-4). Patients may participate actively in the detection and diagnosis of their cancer. For example, a self-examination of the breast has resulted in the detection of an increased number of malignant lesions at a time when curative surgery might be feasible. Since more than 90 percent of the 70,000 new cases of breast cancer each year are discovered by the patient, education on thorough, frequent self-examination is a necessity.

In order to identify individuals who are at high risk for cancer and who should participate in screening programs, risk profiles for each site should be constructed for each patient, based on genetic, family, occupational, and social history.

TAKING THE HISTORY A patient's history is important when the physician tries to pinpoint the possible presence of malignant disease; symptoms are frequently nonspecific. For example, fever, weight loss, and night sweats are evidence of systemic disease which can be indicative of a malignant tumor as well as an infectious process. Taking an orderly history with a thorough review of systems is the most revealing and rewarding approach. A persistent cough with or without hemoptysis requires evaluation of the tracheobronchial tree. Recent onset of hoarseness requires evaluation of a lesion along the course of the recurrent laryngeal nerve or of the vocal cords directly. Hematemesis, jaundice, melena, increasing constipation, and/or abdominal pain demand an evaluation of the gastrointestinal tract for possible malignant disease. Painless, recurrent hematuria suggests the need for careful evaluation of the entire urinary tract. Specific points in the history which are highly suggestive of possible malignancy include the presence of an enlarging, firm, fixed mass easily palpated by the patient, such as a mass in the breast or in a lymph node; the development of a thyroid nodule; and the sudden onset of intestinal obstruction in a previously asymptomatic patient above 50 years of age. A history of petechiae, ecchymoses, or uncontrolled bleeding and persistent infections should suggest possible replacement of normal bone marrow elements by malignant cells.

TABLE 124-4
Seven warning signals of early cancer

1 Change in bowel or bladder habits
2 A sore that does not heal
3 Unusual bleeding or discharge
4 Thickening or lump in breast or elsewhere
5 Indigestion or difficulty in swallowing
6 Obvious change in wart or mole
7 Nagging cough or hoarseness

SOURCE: *American Cancer Society.*

PHYSICAL EXAMINATION In conducting the physical examination, the physician should be attentive to abnormalities which indicate neoplastic disease in each organ system. Certain physical findings are highly suggestive of malignant disease. The skin can provide clues to the presence of internal cancer. A subcutaneous or dermal metastatic nodule may be the first indication of cancer arising from such organs as the breast, gastrointestinal tract, lung, ovary, or uterus. Pulsatile nodules may be metastatic foci from a hypernephroma or a cancer of the thyroid gland. Erythema multiforme, dermatomyositis, superficial migratory thrombophlebitis, necrotizing vasculitis, and bullous states have been associated with internal malignancies. The symmetric brownish-black hyperpigmentation of "malignant" acanthosis nigricans is found predominantly in the body folds; it is characterized by rapidly extending skin involvement and by its association with malignant neoplasms. Herpes zoster and unusual fungal diseases may be related to impaired immunity in cancer patients. An ulcerated lesion along the tongue or a unilateral enlargement of a tonsil are suggestive of a primary oropharyngeal tumor; inspection and careful palpation of the oropharyngeal cavity is an important part of the physical examination. Swelling of the neck, face, and upper extremities, especially after a night in the recumbent position, in association with dilated veins in the upper half of the body and with downward venous flow, is typical of obstruction of the superior vena cava, which occurs as a presenting symptom in approximately 4 percent of all patients with lung cancer. The findings of Horner's syndrome—ptosis, miosis, and decreased sweating of the face on the affected side—indicate stellate ganglion involvement and are frequent concomitants of superior sulcus tumors of the lung. A hard, circumscribed mass, which does not move freely in the breast and is clearly felt with the flat surface of the fingers, is indicative of cancer. When fixation to skin, nipple retraction, skin edema, or deep fixation is present, the lesion is almost certainly malignant. A firm, enlarged lymph node in the left supraclavicular region (Virchow's node) suggests an abdominal malignancy which has spread along the thoracic duct. The presence of a palpable, firm mass in the umbilicus suggests seeding of the peritoneal cavity with metastatic tumor. Any abdominal mass or enlargement of the liver or spleen requires further evaluation for the presence of malignant disease. An enlarged spleen, if it is a result of a malignancy, is usually due to a primary lymphoid or myeloid process because metastatic carcinoma to the spleen is rare; it occurs, however, in malignant melanoma. Unilateral leg or scrotal edema suggests an obstruction to the flow of lymph. Enlargement of any lymph node requires a careful evaluation; the presence of enlarged femoral lymph nodes, however, should be considered indicative of a malignant process unless proved otherwise. An ulcerating nodule of the anus can represent squamous-cell carcinoma, whereas a broad, irregular luminal mass noted on digital rectal examination indicates the presence of adenocarcinoma of the rectum. The digital rectal examination may also reveal a firm nodule in the prostate, which requires needle or open biopsy to confirm or disprove carcinoma. A hard, indurated mass confined to the testis suggests malignancy after the possibility of epididymitis has been ruled out by lack of response to appropriate antibiotic therapy.

Pelvic examination of women can reveal an adnexal mass. In premenopausal women, if such a mass is less than 6 cm in diameter, it is usually a physiologic cyst rather than a neoplasm. Any adnexal mass in the postmenopausal patient must be investigated further. Vaginal tumors vary from ulcerated lesions of small or extensive size, often firm in consistency, to papillary or nodular excrescences.

The examples cited above serve only as a guide to the most obvious physical findings which suggest the presence of a malignancy.

DIAGNOSIS OF CANCER

Regardless of the difficulty of the procedures involved, histologic proof of malignancy must be obtained before the risks involved in further staging and in therapy of malignant disease are taken. The only exception to this rule might be in the diagnosis of gliomas in critical areas of the brain. Sometimes this proof is easy to obtain, especially when there is a subcutaneous nodule that indicates the presence of metastatic carcinoma or an enlarged lymph node that suggests lymphoma. At other times, when there is a peripheral lesion in the lung which cannot be sampled by transbronchial biopsy, the patient might have to undergo thoracotomy with resection so that the diagnosis of cancer can be established. For most malignant tumors, the slide which proves the presence of cancer will also allow histologic classification of the tumor. An experienced pathologist is an essential member of the oncology team, and if there is any question, the histologic material should be submitted to a tumor pathology consulting panel.

The greater the lack of differentiation of the malignant tissue, the easier the diagnosis of malignancy; however, the tissue of origin may be more difficult to ascertain in poorly differentiated and anaplastic tumors. The degree of differentiation of a tumor, ranging from poorly to well differentiated, often provides a clue to prognosis and a guide to treatment; the less differentiated the tumor, the more aggressive its behavior and the poorer the prognosis. General features of the malignant cell under the microscope include a large and irregular nucleus, with enlarged nucleoli, that may be increased in number. Polyploidy is common, and there is an increase in mitotic figures, especially in rapidly growing tumors, with abnormal mitosis and macronucleated cells. The cytoplasm may be scanty, with an increase in basophilia due to increased RNA content. Obviously, these are general features that may be found in many, but not all, malignant cells.

HISTOPATHOLOGIC CLASSIFICATION A histopathologic classification should be reproducible in the hands of the same person, should be agreed upon and reproducible by different experts, should allow for a common terminology, and should correlate the histopathology with the clinical stage and the prognosis. Such a system exists in Hodgkin's disease, where the lymphocyte-predominant and the nodular sclerosing types of histology have a more favorable prognosis than the mixed-cell type, which in turn is more favorable than the lymphocyte-depleted type. Equally important is the architecture, or the way in which the cells are arranged in the biopsy specimen. In malignant lymphoma, the "nodular" pattern has been shown to convey a more favorable prognosis than the "diffuse" replacement of the normal architecture. The presence or absence of vascular or lymphatic invasion within the particular cytologic and architectural picture is also important.

Besides using routine hematoxylin and eosin–stained sections for diagnosis, other methods for diagnosis and classification should be utilized. One of these is cytochemistry. For example, the peroxidase and Sudan black cytochemical stains are positive in acute myelomonocytic leukemia and negative in acute lymphocytic leukemia and help to differentiate these two forms. One enzyme, tartrate-resistant acid phosphatase, has been used specifically to define "hairy" cell leukemia. This type of leukemia differs significantly from other types because aggressive chemotherapy is not indicated and may even be harmful. Transmission electron microscopy has been helpful in differentiating some of the tumors that appear identical by light microscopy. Desmosomes found in thin sections are consistent with carcinoma; myofibrils can be seen in a rhabdomyosarcoma; and intercellular lumens with microvilli can be seen in some poorly differentiated adenocarcinomas; premelanosomes can be found in melanoma cells, and secretory granules can be visualized in carcinomas. Functional methods have been used for the subclassification of certain types of malignancy. Surface immunoglobulins have been found in most cases of chronic lymphocytic leukemia, suggesting that this is a B-cell disease, although T-cell cases have been reported. In acute lymphocytic leukemia, E rosettes can be demonstrated in approximately 25 percent of the cases, suggesting that the malignant cells are of T-cell derivation; in the other 75 percent, neither surface immunoglobulins nor E rosettes can be demonstrated, but a common acute lymphocytic leukemia antigen (CALLA) on the cell surface can be identified in the majority of these cases.

TISSUE INVASION Evidence of invasion of normal tissues, especially lymphatic channels, lymph nodes, and blood vessels, and extension of tumors through natural barriers such as the capsule of a lymph node, is used in diagnosing malignancy, and the extent of this invasion is part of some histologic staging systems (e.g., in carcinoma of the colon). The factors that allow neoplastic cells to invade tissues are not well understood. Certain experimental tumors produce proteolytic enzymes or collagenases that may allow tumor cells to invade tissues. Soft tissues are usually easily invaded, while tissues such as cartilage, fascia, and ligaments are usually resistant to tumor invasion.

METASTASIS An important characteristic of certain neoplastic cells is their ability to spread to distant sites, that is, to metastasize. Various human cancers differ appreciably, not only in their propensity to metastasize, but also in the location of the metastasis. Knowledge of the pattern of metastatic spread may provide clinical clues to the origin of the primary tumor. Carcinomas are more apt to spread by lymphatic invasion, initially to regional lymph nodes. For example, in breast cancer the degree of spread to the regional lymph nodes is determined at surgery and provides important prognostic information to help the clinician plan adjuvant chemotherapy. Whether the regional lymph nodes provide immunologic and perhaps mechanical barriers to tumor spread has been debated. Often nodes adjacent to a tumor may not contain tumor but show a "hyperplastic reaction," suggesting a host response to the tumor or its products.

Sarcomas characteristically spread via the bloodstream, and distant metastases, to the lungs from osteogenic sarcoma, are common. Venous invasion is more common than arterial invasion, perhaps due to the elasticity of the arterial wall. Venous invasion characteristically consists of clumps of tumor cells that adhere to the vascular endothelium of the postcapillary venule. Fibrin formation is initiated and is followed by multiplication and invasion through the endothelium. Several studies indicate that anticoagulants may decrease metastases in experimental tumors, perhaps by decreasing endothelial "stickiness." In humans, their value in preventing metastases has not been established.

Two other properties of tumor cells probably also contribute to metastatic spread: (1) decreased adhesiveness of tumor cells to each other, with the resultant ability of individual tumor cells or clumps to break off and enter the lymphatics or the bloodstream and to lodge in other tissues, and (2) the elaboration of tissue angiogenesis factor (TAF). The elaboration of TAF, a macromolecule not yet completely characterized, results in local proliferation of blood vessels and permits the necessary "feeding" of the growing tumor cell mass. In fact, the intense vascularity that may result is responsible for the characteristic "tumor blush" of certain tumors when the arterial supply is examined radiographically after administration of contrast media.

TUMOR AS A GROWTH, TUMOR AS A "FACTORY" The neoplastic lesion can be evaluated in two conceptual ways: as a growth and as a "factory." As a growth, the lesion has local and metastatic manifestations. The site of origin of the neoplastic growth also has important clinical implications, because local manifestations as well as the propensity for and the route of spread are frequently organ-related. In many cases, these manifestations are clues to the diagnosis as well as indications for appropriate therapeutic intervention. As a factory, the tumor may elaborate products normally associated with the tissue of origin, but in an increased amount, or it may produce substances normally not synthesized by the tissue of origin.

Tumor within an organ system The organ within which a tumor arises is of great importance. The histologic characteristics of different tumors within a single organ give clues to the developing clinical pattern, and this pattern often determines its management. Cancer of the lung provides an apt example.

There are four types of histology in lung cancer, each of which has a different clinical characteristic. Adenocarcinoma is frequently found as a peripheral nodule and metastasizes early. Squamous-cell carcinoma and large-cell undifferentiated carcinoma are usually perihilar and at first spread by local extension. In marked contrast to these three types is oat-cell carcinoma, which shows evidence of extrathoracic spread at presentation in over 65 percent of the cases and regional involvement in almost all of the remaining cases. Therefore, in most instances, this tumor cannot be cured surgically.

Knowledge of the natural history of the tumor is important for the design of any staging approach. For example, it is important to know that colon and rectal carcinomas usually begin as a mucosal disease, progress through the bowel wall, invade lymph nodes adjacent to the bowel, and subsequently metastasize to the liver. Prostatic carcinoma is locally invasive, but also metastasizes quite early to bone, especially via Batson's plexus. In contrast, cancers of the head and neck are locally and regionally invasive and only rarely lead to distant metastases.

Tumor as a growth The tumor as a single primary growth can cause the following signs or symptoms: mass and pressure, obstruction, perforation, and invasion with replacement. These conditions can be illustrated with examples from several of the major tumor types, such as cancer of the lung, colon, and brain.

As the malignant cells divide within the neoplastic mass, the dimensions of the tumor continue to increase. The first finding of a mass in the chest could come on a routine annual chest x-ray, and the first finding of a colon mass might occur upon abdominal palpation during a routine physical examination. As the size of the mass continues to increase, there is evidence of increased local pressure. In lung cancer, pressure on the adjacent bronchi might result in an intractable cough; in colon cancer, the patient may complain of lower abdominal cramps.

As it grows in the lung or colon, the tumor will begin to encroach on the function of the organ system and produce symptoms of obstruction. Neoplasms of the left colon tend to be more scirrhous and lead to early production of obstructive symptoms in contrast to the larger, fungating, more friable lesions of the right colon, which tend to present with anemia due to bleeding. Obstructive symptoms are also seen with centrally located squamous-cell carcinoma of the lung. As the tumor grows, bronchial obstruction commonly leads to atelectasis and infection distal to the obstruction, with persistent sputum production and abscess formation.

The most dramatic signs of increased pressure in body cavities occur with primary brain tumors in adults. Patients frequently complain of headache and vomiting. Occasionally, papilledema on fundoscopic examination can be appreciated at initial examination. Localizing signs and symptoms as well as changes in the mental status are frequently present when the diagnosis is first made. The rigid skull contains about $1\frac{1}{2}$ liters brain tissue, only 8 to 10 percent of which may be displaced by either venous blood or cerebrospinal fluid. Brain is a thixotropic substance composed of 80 percent water and is not compressible. Therefore, a single small mass may cause profound dysfunction or an increase in intracranial pressure, depending on its location.

Besides the displacement of cerebral tissue by a brain mass, there can be obstruction to the flow of cerebrospinal fluid; the major portion of this fluid is produced by the choroid plexus of the lateral ventricles and passes through the third ventricle and through the aqueduct. A tumor blocking the aqueduct can prevent the flow of the cerebrospinal fluid, result in secondary dilatation of the lateral ventricle, and lead to increased intracranial pressure.

Enlargement of the tumor mass can cause compression or replacement of the normal structures with tissue less suited to the functional stresses. For example, large-bowel perforation can be associated with a progressive mass lesion.

Invasion and replacement of the organ in which the tumor arises can be a manifestation of the tumor as a primary growth. Approximately 10 percent of resected stomach carcinomas are of the scirrhous form. They may be localized or may involve the entire stomach, producing the classic appearance of "leather bottle" or linitis plastica. Symptoms secondary to total replacement include anorexia, early satiety, weight loss, and occasionally diarrhea. Hepatoma is a primary liver-cell cancer which accounts for slightly less than 1 percent of all cancer deaths. Frequently death ensues from liver failure with no extrahepatic extension of the cancer. Tumor invasion rarely extends to adjacent organs, but frequently involves the portal or hepatic veins, causing thrombosis. Symptoms of osteogenic sarcoma, a primary malignant tumor that probably arises from primitive bone-forming mesenchyme and produces neoplastic osteoid or osseous tissue in its evolution, result from progressive growth of the mass with replacement of the normal trabeculae in one of the long bones. Pain, tenderness, and swelling of either the lower femur or possibly the tibia or humerus are usually present. On x-ray, variable degrees of lytic and sclerotic processes are noted, frequently associated with cortical perforation, subperiostal extension, and new bone formation.

Besides causing signs of obstruction, increased pressure, or organ replacement, a primary growth can invade adjacent structures. The superior vena cava syndrome in lung cancer occasionally results from direct tumor invasion of the cava. Eight to ten percent of all patients with bronchogenic carcinoma are hoarse at their initial presentation. This is a manifestation of laryngeal nerve involvement, which causes vocal cord paralysis. Sharp localized chest pain is often due to extension of the tumor to the chest wall. If the lesion is in the upper part of the lung with invasion of the brachial plexus, the Pancoast or superior sulcus syndrome develops. Uterine cervical cancer tends to spread by direct extension into the surrounding tissues, particularly laterally into the cardinal ligaments; metastases occur late, however. The ureters traverse the cardinal ligaments in the paracervical tunnel and lie in the path of lateral spread of cervical cancer. Extension into these areas obstructs the ureters, resulting in hydroureter and hydronephrosis. If this process is not controlled by therapy, uremia ensues.

Cancer can take the form of a disseminated disease. This is most obvious in malignancies of the hematopoietic tissues, in which the bone marrow is frequently replaced by malignant cells. Symptoms of fever and bleeding can usually be correlated with the absence of mature granulocytes and a decrease in platelets, respectively. Bone marrow aspiration in acute myelogenous leukemia frequently reveals no megakaryocyte, granulocyte, or erythroid precursors; the majority of cells are poorly differentiated myeloblasts.

The two major routes by which tumor cells spread and form metastases are vascular and lymphatic. Occasionally, spread occurs along the peritoneal, pleural, or pericardial lining. The most common sites of metastatic disease are the lungs, especially for osteogenic sarcoma and renal carcinoma; the liver, especially for gastric and colon cancers; and the bones, especially for prostate and breast cancers. Because of the frequent recurrence of tumor at sites distant from the primary tumor, without local recurrence, it is generally accepted that malignant cells were present but not detectable in these sites at the time of initial local resection or radiotherapy. Until recently, 70 percent of patients with osteogenic sarcoma had recurrent disease, with extensive pulmonary nodules, within 1 year of complete resection of the primary lesion; death was usually a result of progressive pulmonary involvement and was directly related to the metastatic characteristics of the tumor. This situation has been reversed dramatically with the use of both preoperative and adjuvant chemotherapy. The poor outcome in half the patients with breast cancer is related to the presence of disseminated disease at the time of surgery. It has been shown that the relapse rate 4 years after mastectomy in premenopausal women with positive axillary lymph nodes has been reduced by half with the use of three-drug adjuvant chemotherapy.

Disseminated or metastatic tumor can also cause symptoms due to an increasing mass associated with increasing pressure, obstruction, perforation, and invasion with replacement of normal tissue. The manifestations result in loss of function of the affected organ or organs and subsequent death.

Tumor as a factory Some tumors can manufacture an increased amount of a normal tissue product or a product not usually associated with the cells of origin. Studies with highly sensitive techniques such as radioimmunoassay have shown that many kinds of tumors, from both endocrine and nonendocrine tissues, secrete or synthesize peptide hormones and other proteins not usually made by these tissues. In some circumstances the substances are proteins ordinarily synthesized at or

TABLE 124-5
Tumor cell markers

Marker	*Tumor*
PRODUCED BY DEDIFFERENTIATION	
Carcinoembryonic antigen (CEA)	Gastrointestinal tract, pancreas, breast, lung
α-Fetoprotein	Hepatoma, embryonal carcinoma of testis
Isoenzyme (placental or tumor specific; Regan enzyme)	Various neoplasms
PRODUCED AS A RESULT OF OVERPRODUCTION BY TUMOR CELLS	
Chorionic gonadotropin (β subunit)	Choriocarcinoma, hydatidiform mole, testicular cancer
Acid phosphatase	Prostatic carcinoma
Vitamin B_{12}–binding proteins	Chronic and acute myelogenous leukemia
Lysozyme	Monocytic leukemia
Polyamines	Various neoplasms
Hormones	Produced by specific endocrine-gland neoplasms

around fetal life (Table 124-5) and are useful markers for neoplastic growth; in other circumstances ectopic hormones are produced, resulting in clinical syndromes that are the result of hormone production (Table 124-6) and other syndromes with less-defined etiologies. In addition, specific tumors may produce an increased amount of a substance normally produced by that cell. Tumor markers are discussed in Chap. 125 and with specific tumors.

The ability to detect the presence of a neoplasm by measurement of a cell product is related to the secretory capacity of a particular cell type, the amount of tumor present, as well as to sensitivity of the technique applied. The beta-cell tumor or *insulinoma of the pancreas* is the most commonly recognized neoplasm of functioning islet cells. Only 10 percent of such tumors are metastatic at the time of presentation. The classic symptoms are those of hypoglycemia. This tumor of the endocrine pancreas presents with signs of physiologic imbalance, whereas tumors of the exocrine pancreas usually are associated with signs of a mass and obstruction.

The most common cancer of the small intestine is the carcinoid tumor. Early manifestations may be caused by the space-occupying effects of the primary tumor. The later manifestations may be due to extension or metastases of the tumor, or to the effects of one or more of its metabolites. Unlike insulinoma of the pancreas, metastases seem to be a definite prerequisite for clinically significant manifestations in most patients with carcinoids. Patients with malignant carcinoids develop flushing spells and peculiar cutaneous vascular phenomena. Most patients show elevated levels of urinary 5-hydroxyindoleacetic acid (5-HIAA). The pharmacologically active agents responsible for the carcinoid syndrome and the resultant excretion of 5-HIAA are covered in Chap. 131. The carcinoid tumor does not manifest itself by mass, perforation, obstruction, or replacement, but by formation of a tumor product that generally occurs only in the presence of hepatic metastases.

Tumors of the testicle have been shown to produce certain markers depending on the cell types present. Tumors with a yolk-sac origin have been shown to produce α-fetoprotein, while those with embryonal elements have been shown to produce the β subunit of human chorionic gonadotropin (HCG). Ten percent of testicular tumors with one or both of these histologic elements will produce no markers. Pure seminomas produce neither of the markers.

Multiple myeloma is an example of a tumor with "factory" characteristics that directly reflect the growth characteristics and that are not the result of a hormonally active end product as in insulinoma, or the result of an unusual tumor product as in the carcinoid syndrome. It is a malignant proliferation of plasma cells. An M protein composed of either heavy and light chains (84 percent of cases) or light chains only (15 percent) can be detected in the serum or urine in 99 percent of the cases. Since all the cells in an M protein–secreting plasma-cell tumor appear to produce this M protein, the total number of tumor cells can be estimated from its serum level.

Certain types of tumors may be associated with the production of several substances. Small-cell (oat-cell) carcinoma of the lung is the histologic type of tumor most frequently associated with ectopic Cushing's syndrome and an inappropriate antidiuretic hormone (ADH) response. Also, oat-cell tumor can cause overproduction of serotonin with resultant carcinoid syndrome. Other lung cancers, such as squamous-cell carcinoma, may show increased production of parathyroid hormone (PTH) and also occasionally release some placental trophoblastic peptides.

These tumor "markers" or products of the cancer cell are important for several reasons. They may provide the clinician with a sensitive measure of tumor-cell progression or regression, as is the case with HCG, α-fetoprotein, and carcinoembryonic antigen, and help guide therapy and estimate prognosis. In other circumstances, especially when ectopic hormones are produced, clinical syndromes may result that offer clues to the etiology of the cancer or present difficult problems in management. In general, resolution of these clinical syndromes usually requires effective treatment of the malignancy, although immediate supportive care may be lifesaving when electrolyte imbalances, such as hypercalcemia, occur (see Chap. 125).

CLINICAL AND PATHOLOGIC METHODOLOGY **Staging classifications** A staging classification has to be both reproducible and clinically feasible. In addition, it must have both therapeutic and prognostic consequences. No single staging system is applicable to all cancers. A variety of staging systems is essential, because no two types of cancer have the same natural history. The clinical and pathologic staging classifications have arisen from a detailed knowledge of the pathophysiology of particular tumors. The following are examples which illustrate the use of different staging classifications.

Cancer of the cervix tends to spread by direct extension via the lymphatic system to the regional lymph nodes in the pelvis, and it metastasizes late. The international classification for the staging of individual cases of carcinoma of the cervix from stage 0 to stage IV predicts the general clinical course that cervical carcinoma follows and reflects the prognosis for each case. Stage 0 represents carcinoma in situ; stage I, carcinoma strictly confined to the cervix; stage II, carcinoma extending beyond the cervix but not yet to the pelvic wall; stage III, carcinoma extending to the pelvic wall; and stage IV, carcinoma extending beyond the true pelvis or involving the mucosa of the bladder and rectum.

Cancers of the head and neck are characterized by local extension and invasion, with subsequent cervical lymph node metastases. Regional lymph node involvement generally follows regular patterns according to the location of the primary tumor, although exceptions with bizarre spread occur. The TMN classification system (Table 124-7) utilizes tumor size and node involvement to describe the stage of a tumor at the time of diagnosis. It is a system designed to take into account the volume or size of the primary tumor T, as well as the degree of local spread to the lymph nodes N and the distant spread M.

The size of the primary tumor ranges from T_1 lesions, which have a maximum diameter of 2 cm or less, to T_3 lesions, which are larger than 4 cm. N stands for regional lymph nodes and varies from N_0, where no palpable cervical lymph nodes are present, to N_3, where clinically palpable lymph nodes are fixed and metastases are suspected. M stands for distant metastases which are either absent (M_0) or present by clinical and radio-

TABLE 124-6
Paraneoplastic syndromes

Syndrome	*Hormone*	*Tumor type*
SYNDROMES ASSOCIATED WITH ECTOPIC HORMONE PRODUCTION		
Cushing's syndrome	ACTH	Oat-cell, thymoma, islet-cell tumors of pancreas, bronchial carcinoids of lung, medullary carcinoma of thyroid
Inappropriate ADH	ADH	Oat-cell, other tumors of lung, duodenum, pancreas, thymoma, lymphosarcoma
Gynecomastia	Gonadotropin	Lung carcinoma, rarely tumors of liver, adrenal, dysgerminoma of ovary
Hyperparathyroidism	PTH	Kidney, lung (squamous), pancreatic, and ovarian tumors
Hyperpigmentation	MSH	Oat-cell, lung tumors
Hyperthyroidism	TSH	Choriocarcinoma, hydatidiform mole, embryonal carcinoma of testis
Hypoglycemia	Insulin-like activity	Retroperitoneal and liver tumors
Hypocalcemia	Calcitonin	Medullary carcinoma of thyroid, breast carcinoma, oat-cell
Aplastic anemia (pure red blood cell hypoplasia)	?	Thymomas
Erythrocytosis	Erythropoietin	Cerebellar hemangioma, renal cell, liver, and uterine tumors
OTHER EFFECTS OF NEOPLASMS ON THE HOST		
Muscle and joint disturbances:		
Polyarthritis (usually mild); Polymyositis (over age 40: 20% have occult cancer)		Ovarian, uterine, breast, stomach, lung
Hypertrophic osteoarthropathy		Lung, esophagus, colon
Neuropathies (often seen with myopathies): Central (Cerebellar degeneration, Cerebral demyelination); Peripheral (Pure sensory, lower motor neuron, mixed)		Oat-cell, lung, breast, ovarian, lymphoma
Multiple thromboses		Pancreatic, other types of cancer
Nephrosis (lipoid nephrosis and membranous glomerulitis)		Occult neoplasm in elderly patients
Acanthosis nigricans		Adenocarcinoma, lymphoma
Cachexia, loss of taste		Various types
Disseminated intravascular coagulation		Mucinous adenocarcinomas

TABLE 124-7
The TNM system

PRIMARY TUMOR (T)	
T_0	No evidence of primary tumor
T_{IS}	Carcinoma in situ
T_1, T_2, T_3, T_4	Ascending degrees of increase in tumor size and involvement
REGIONAL LYMPH NODES (N)	
N_0	Regional nodes not demonstrable
N_{1a}, N_{2a}	Demonstrable regional lymph nodes, metastases not suspected
N_{1b}, N_{2b}, N_3	Demonstrable regional lymph nodes; metastases suspected
N_x	Regional lymph nodes cannot be assessed clinically
DISTANT METASTASES (M)	
M_0	No evidence of distant metastases
M_1, M_2, M_3	Ascending degrees of metastatic involvement of the host including distant nodes

logic evidence in areas other than the cervical lymph nodes (M_1). Other factors besides the clinical and pathologic stage influence the prognosis in head and neck cancer: survival figures are better in patients with well-differentiated tumors than in those with anaplastic tumors; patients whose tumors show lymphocytic infiltration have a better prognosis than those lacking this finding.

The major defect of all staging classifications is their poor assessment of tumor volume. Nevertheless, staging classifications guide clinicians in selection of treatment, assure comparability of cases in various institutions, permit communication between treatment centers, and allow assessment of prognosis. The staging classification applicable to each particular cancer is described in detail in the appropriate chapter in this text.

Clinical staging All diagnostic tools should be used in clinical staging, with local systematic analysis applied to each individual tumor. Table 124-8 summarizes the routine and special clinical, radiologic, laboratory, and surgical procedures which should be utilized in the workup of mass lesions of a particular organ system. Laboratory and x-ray methods make it possible to bridge the gap between the physical examination and the final histopathologic determination.

Analyses of blood chemistries may offer important clues. An increase in the serum calcium is frequently seen with multiple myeloma as well as with metastatic breast carcinoma. A decrease in the serum glucose value is commonly observed with islet-cell tumors of the pancreas that are insulin-secreting, and occasionally with retroperitoneal sarcomas or hepatoma. An increase in blood urea nitrogen (BUN) and creatinine is suggestive of an obstruction of the urinary tract. This can be due to local tumor invasion, as is frequently seen in carcinoma of the cervix with ureteral obstruction, or it can be secondary to uric acid or calcium nephrolithiasis which is occasionally seen in patients with acute leukemia and other myeloproliferative or lymphoproliferative diseases. An increase in direct bilirubin or alkaline phosphatase can result from obstruction of the hepatobiliary system at any point proximal to the ampulla of Vater. An increase in the total protein and, more specifically, the serum globulin can be the first suggestion of multiple myeloma. Special laboratory procedures may be useful in certain tumors, including tests for the presence of fetoprotein in hepatoma or malignant teratomas, carcinoembryonic antigen S (CEAS) in colon cancer, serum immunoglobulins in myeloma, and tartrate-inhibited acid phosphatase in prostatic carcinoma.

Radiographic contrast studies (Table 124-8) that are helpful in mapping the location of a pelvic tumor such as cervical carcinoma include an intravenous pyelogram (IVP), which will demonstrate pelvic or retroperitoneal masses causing either deviation or early obstruction. An inferior vena cavagram (IVC) can be done in patients with malignant lymphoma in the search for a retroperitoneal mass in the high lumbar region. Anterior deviation of the superior vena cava suggests the presence of a tumor mass. A lymphangiogram (LAG) in patients with testicular carcinomas serves to localize enlarged pelvic and low lumbar lymph nodes. An upper gastrointestinal examination with barium as well as a small-bowel follow-through and a barium enema are useful in localizing lesions in the gastrointestinal tract. Selective arteriography has been employed for differentiation of a benign cyst from a malignant renal-cell carcinoma.

Computerized tomography (CT) scan of the brain has been demonstrated to be effective in evaluating brain tumors and is associated with less morbidity than arteriograms and pneumoencephalograms. CT scans of a suspected mass lesion are frequently of value in differentiating solid from cystic lesions. Development of the CT scan for definition of chest and abdominal lesions has resulted in a significant addition to the clinical detection of mass lesions in the mediastinum and the lungs as well as in the retroperitoneal area.

Ultrasonography offers an inexpensive noninvasive technique for the study of orbital, cardiac, pericardiac, hepatic, pancreatic, renal, and retroperitoneal areas. Although ultrasound can demonstrate retroperitoneal lymphadenopathy, studies are occasionally obscured by bowel gas; the CT scan does not encounter this problem. Ultrasound guided biopsies of various tumor masses have been performed successfully.

Highly refined radioisotopic methods, which are noninvasive, have become available for the diagnosis of cancer (Table 124-8). Liver and spleen scans have been used to identify an enlarged spleen which may not be palpable and metastatic lesions in the liver which have not yet become clinically significant. Bone scans can detect metastatic lesions before they are radiologically evident. The only malignancy for which the bone scan is less sensitive than the x-ray is multiple myeloma. The many lytic lesions present will be missed by the bone scan because there are few reactive changes surrounding the lesions. It has been shown that approximately 10 percent of women who are by all other criteria eligible to undergo mastectomy have metastatic lesions in bone as shown by scanning, although the concurrent x-rays are negative. Gallium scans, both whole body as well as tomographic cuts of various sections, are sometimes of value in the clinical staging of Hodgkin's disease and malignant lymphoma but are even more specific and sensitive for lung cancer. In addition, metastatic lung cancer lesions can be picked up in most sites with the gallium scan alone, although the CT scan is more sensitive for brain lesions. Because gallium is a soft-tissue-specific isotope, it can be used for a noninvasive contrast study at the time of clinical staging and may be repeated for follow-up without causing patient discomfort or morbidity.

Pathologic staging Staging operations are used only to find the extent or stage of disease so that appropriate definitive treatment can be selected (Table 124-8). Mediastinoscopy is the major preoperative method for pathologic evaluation of regional spread in lung cancer. Approximately 35 percent of all patients examined preoperatively are found to have mediastinal lymph node metastases. Positive tissue obtained at mediastinoscopy is usually a contraindication to thoracotomy. Patients who have negative mediastinoscopy, a negative metastatic workup, and a tumor that is at least 1 cm distal to the

TABLE 124-8
Evaluative and staging procedures for tumors of selected organ systems

Organ system	*Presenting lesion(s)*	*Routine clinical tests*	*"Obtaining tissue"*	*Special procedures*	*Staging procedures*
Lung	Single mass	Chest x-ray Tomography	Sputum cytology Bronchoscopy and biopsy Mediastinoscopy	Pleural biopsy (if effusion is present) Lung biopsy	Mediastinoscopy Gallium scan
	Multiple masses	Intravenous pyelogram (IVP) Mammogram Thyroid scan Upper gastrointestinal–colon series	Mediastinoscopy	Lung biopsy	Metastatic; if nonlung primary proved, requires no further staging
Breast	Single mass	Mammogram Xerogram	Needle aspiration Excisional biopsy	Estrogen receptor Progesterone receptor	Liver scan Bone scan Brain scan
Lymphoid	Adenopathy	Chest x-ray (hilar adenopathy) Abdominal flat plate (splenomegaly)	Excisional biopsy		Ultrasonogram Gallium scan IVP Inferior vena cavagram (IVC) Lymphangiogram (LAG) Liver-spleen scan Computerized tomography (CT scan) Bone scan Bone marrow biopsy Laparoscopy Laparotomy
	Splenomegaly	Blood counts	Bone marrow aspiration Bone marrow biopsy		Proceed as for adenopathy
Gastrointestinal	Esophageal mass or stricture	Chest x-ray Barium swallow	Esophagoscopy with brushing, cytology, and biopsy		Bronchoscopy Mediastinoscopy CT scan
	Gastric mass	Upper gastrointestinal barium series (double contrast)	Gastroscopy with brushing, cytology, and biopsy		Liver scan Chest x-ray
	Pancreatic mass	Ultrasonogram CT scan	Duodenal drainage for cytology; cannulation of ampulla of Vater for cytology	Percutaneous ("skinny needle") cholangiogram Endoscopic retrograde cholangiopancreatogram (ERCP)	Arteriogram Liver scan Laparotomy and biopsy
	Liver mass: single	Liver scan α-Fetoprotein	Percutaneous biopsy	Peritoneoscopy and biopsy	Arteriogram Laparotomy
	Liver: multiple masses	Liver scan Mammogram Upper gastrointestinal series Barium enema (double contrast) Pancreatic ultrasonogram Chest x-ray	Percutaneous biopsy	Peritoneoscopy and biopsy	Laparotomy

carina are eligible for thoracotomy and resection of bronchogenic carcinoma.

A bone core biopsy is used for establishing the presence of malignant tumor in the bone marrow. In approximately 70 percent of patients with malignant lymphoma, poorly differentiated lymphocytic type, nodular or diffuse, it has been shown that bone core biopsies are positive; the bone core biopsy can serve as easy identification of patients with pathologic stage IV malignant lymphoma.

Mastectomy results in cure in two-thirds of patients with breast cancer who have no axillary lymph node involvement, but the cure rate is less than 10 percent in those who have four or more positive lymph nodes at the time of mastectomy. Although the mastectomy is intended to be therapeutic, it also serves as a pathologic staging procedure, since the number of positive lymph nodes in the axillary dissection identifies a group which benefits from adjuvant chemotherapy in the immediate postmastectomy period.

The most striking example of a staging procedure that is performed only for biopsy and not excision of the tumor is the staging laparotomy used in Hodgkin's disease. It is designed to prove the exact extent of the disease so that patients are not undertreated, which might result in early relapse, or overtreated, which might result in excessive morbidity and mortality. The procedure involves a splenectomy, because splenic involvement can be determined only by thorough pathologic sectioning and evaluation. Biopsies of the liver and various retroperitoneal and mesenteric lymph nodes are also obtained.

Staging procedures can lead to identification of sites of disease as well as definition of the extent of disease at a given site, which can aid in the design of suitable therapy. During the staging laparotomy in Hodgkin's disease, areas of lymph node biopsy are marked with metal clips, as are the margins of any

TABLE 124-8 *(continued)*
Evaluative and staging procedures for tumors of selected organ systems

Organ system	*Presenting lesion(s)*	*Routine clinical tests*	*"Obtaining tissue"*	*Special procedures*	*Staging procedures*
	Gallbladder mass; biliary tract mass or stricture	Liver scan Ultrasonogram	Duodenal drainage for cytology	Percutaneous ("skinny needle") cholangiogram ERCP	Laparotomy
	Colon stricture or mass	Proctosigmoidoscopy Barium enema (double contrast)	Colonoscopy or proctoscopy with brushing, cytology, and biopsy	Carcinoembryonic antigen (CEA) IVP	Laparotomy Liver scan Chest x-ray
Genitourinary	Kidney mass	Urinalysis IVP Nephrotomograms	Ureteral catheterization with cytology and/or brush biopsies Percutaneous fluid aspiration for cytology	Nephrosonogram Arteriogram Erythropoietin	Chest x-ray Liver scan Bone scan Retroperitoneal ultrasonogram Inferior vena cavagram Lymphangiogram Excision of tumor Lymphadenectomy
	Bladder mass	IVP Cystoscopy	Urine cytology Biopsy		
	Testicular mass	Chest x-ray	Radical orchiectomy	α-Fetoprotein Human chorionic gonadotropin (β subunit)	Lymphangiogram CT scan
	Prostate	IVP Acid phosphatase	Biopsy	Iliac crest bone marrow for tumor cells and free acid phosphatase	
	Ovarian mass	Chest x-ray Upper gastrointestinal series Barium enema IVP	Laparotomy	Estrogen receptor Progesterone receptor Peritoneal cytology	Laparotomy Bone scan Liver scan
	Uterine mass	Chest x-ray IVP	Papanicolaou Jet wash cytology Fractional dilatation and curettage (D&C) and/or biopsy Laparotomy (if sarcoma)	Estrogen receptor Progesterone receptor Human chorionic gonadotropin (β subunit)	Fractional D&C Bone scan Liver scan Laparotomy
	Cervical lesion	Papanicolaou Colposcopy Chest x-ray IVP	Biopsy		Clinical staging Lymphangiogram Bone scan Liver scan Staging by lymph node biopsy

masses that have been biopsied. The clips subsequently allow the radiotherapist to design appropriate radiotherapy.

PRINCIPLES OF MANAGEMENT

INDICATIONS FOR SURGERY AND RADIOTHERAPY Management of the patient with suspected or proven cancer involves the evaluation of operability and, if possible, curability. When metastatic disease has been documented, surgery is usually indicated only for staging, as in Hodgkin's disease, or for prevention of local problems, as in colon carcinoma (obstruction secondary to the primary tumor mass is a frequent complication). If there is no evidence of metastatic disease and if a primary lesion is suspected or proven, operability has to be measured against the local extent and known history of the disease.

For example, a patient with lung cancer diagnosed by either positive cytology or bronchoscopic biopsy requires a determination of operability. If it is decided that the patient is not medically operable, further evaluation of the extent of disease must be made prior to the decision regarding radiotherapy or chemotherapy. If medical operability is established, a thorough search for metastatic disease should be made. If there is evidence of metastatic disease, the patient is considered inoperable, and treatment for disseminated disease has to be initiated. If there is no evidence of metastatic disease, the surgical criteria for resectability have to be evaluated. A tumor that has invaded the mediastinum is not curable with resection and will require local treatment such as radiotherapy. If the tumor does not involve the mediastinum, but is less than 0.5 cm from the carina, it is technically unresectable, and local radiotherapy should be planned. Approximately 15 percent of patients with lung cancer pass all the decision points and are eligible for curative surgical therapy. A careful assessment of the patient's clinical status, correlated with the extent of the disease, will probably result in fewer surgical procedures; however, a larger number of the resections will result in cure.

Some tumors are inoperable because of the extent of spread at the time of diagnosis. Others, such as glioma of the brainstem, are inoperable, not because of spread, but because of their location and the loss of essential function that would result from surgical removal.

APPROACH TO DISSEMINATED DISEASE If a patient has disseminated cancer, few surgical staging procedures are indicated, although various radiographic and radioisotopic tests are available for the evaluation of the subsequent response to treatment. When disseminated disease is demonstrated, it is important to look for the primary site only if it involves an organ or cell of origin for which available therapy is effective. For example, it has been shown that the search for the primary site is frequently unrewarding for metastatic undifferentiated carcinoma or adenocarcinoma from an unknown primary cancer site. In a study of 264 patients, only 30 patients had the primary site identified antemortem by extensive radiographic search and eventual biopsy. Even in 23 of 130 patients who underwent autopsy, the primary site could not be found. In the patients in whom a primary site could be found, lung cancer was the most frequent primary tumor above the diaphragm, while the pancreas was the most common primary site below the diaphragm. Although pancreatic cancer is present in autopsy series in about 1.5 percent of cases, in a study of patients dying of unknown primaries, it was found in 20 percent of cases. In contrast, prostatic cancer, which is present in 17 percent of men at autopsy, accounted only for 4 percent of the unknown primaries.

In about 5 percent of the cases of cervical lymph node metastases the primary tumor is undetected. Failure to find the primary site after diligent search has been variously ascribed to the small size or spontaneous regression of the primary tumor or its occurrence in the wall of a branchiogenic cyst or lymph node. In such instances, a curative approach appropriate for head and neck cancer should be undertaken.

Specific therapy for metastatic disease utilizes hormonal treatment and chemotherapy. This is discussed in detail in Chap. 125. Assistance in selecting specific drug therapy is becoming available by means of an in vitro tumor colony-forming assay. Initially it was utilized to measure sensitivity of human tumor stem cells to anticancer drugs in patients with multiple myeloma and ovarian cancer. However, a report utilizing this method to study 800 tumors of 36 separate histologic types showed that only 199 of the 800 tumors (25 percent) formed colonies in vitro and had enough cells in the biopsy or fluid specimen to perform drug sensitivity assays. In 123 instances, the drug tested in vitro against the tumor was also used clinically to treat the patient; the probability of a positive prediction from the assay, given that the patient responded beneficially, was 0.88, whereas the probability for a negative prediction of the assay when the patient did not respond was 0.94. Although the human tumor colony-forming assay can provide useful sensitivity information, it does so for only about 25 percent of the general oncology patients.

MULTIMODALITY THERAPEUTIC APPROACH Although the single-modality approach to treatment, consisting of either surgery, radiotherapy, or chemotherapy, is appropriate in some tumors, others require a combination of all three modalities. Partial colectomy is the treatment of choice in patients with carcinoma of the colon; if there is no evidence of spread through the muscularis mucosa and no evidence of lymph node involvement, most patients will be cured. An acceptable treatment for early carcinoma of the cervix is a radium implant, which is as curative as hysterectomy. The initial treatment of adult acute leukemia is chemotherapy alone, as the disease is widely disseminated and cannot be approached either surgically or with radiotherapy.

Combined-modality therapy has resulted in increased rates of complete remission and prolonged survival in some tumors. Osteogenic sarcoma, although apparently completely excised by removal of the involved limb, recurs with pulmonary metastases in approximately 70 percent of the patients within 1 year. By administration of multiple courses of chemotherapy both before and immediately after resection of the primary tumor, development of lung lesions is prevented in many patients. The period of complete remission has been markedly prolonged, and cures may be possible. Adjuvant chemotherapy has been found useful in Ewing's sarcoma, Wilms's tumors of the kidney, and in premenopausal patients with breast cancer.

In most cases, the combined-modality approach to malignant neoplasms involves surgical removal of the bulk of the primary tumor, followed by radiotherapy to eradicate any tumor left in the margins of resection, and followed, in turn, by chemotherapy to eradicate any distant metastases while the tumor burden is low. This combined-modality adjuvant approach to cancer therapy is designed to cure cancer at the initial presentation when the tumor burden is smallest, rather than when diffuse metastatic disease and a large tumor burden are present. This approach is being tested in cancer of the lung, head, and neck, as well as colon and rectum, and continues to be evaluated in breast cancer and sarcomas. Both nonspecific (e.g., bacillus Calmette-Guérin) and specific (e.g., allogenic tumor cells) immunotherapy is being attempted in acute leukemias and in lung, colon, and rectum cancer as well as in melanoma to further enhance induction of remissions and, in particular, to prolong their duration. Benefit from immunotherapy remains to be proved.

COMPLICATIONS OF MALIGNANT DISEASE AND ITS THERAPY Although each cancer has signs and symptoms specifically associated with its location and cell type, there are certain common complications of tumors. These include hypercalcemia, lactic acidosis, hyperuricemia, ectopic hormone production, both local and remote neurologic manifestations, obstruction, effusions, and bleeding diatheses. Frequently simultaneous therapy is required for both the complication and the underlying tumor. These complications and their management are discussed in Chap. 125.

LONGITUDINAL FOLLOW-UP Cancer patients who are presumed cured need careful follow-up for early detection of recurrences, so that further curative therapy can be undertaken if necessary. These patients must be made aware of possible risk from radiation or chemotherapy to their future children as a result of mutations in their reproductive tissues. They also must be apprised of future risks of developing a second cancer, as is seen in patients treated for multiple myeloma or Hodgkin's disease, some of whom subsequently develop acute myelogenous leukemia. Patients who have undergone curative surgery for lung cancer should be alerted to the risk of resuming smoking. Patients resected for cancer of the oral cavity should be encouraged to discontinue the use of tobacco as well as alcohol.

MANAGEMENT OF THE PATIENT AND FAMILY Undertaking the care of a patient with cancer requires total commitment. Attention must be directed to details of staging and treatment with the potential of cure or prolonged control. In addition, such care demands attention to pain, the nutritional status of the patient, and psychological support for patient and family.

The previous sections of this chapter have addressed the management of the tumor. Pain may be one of the main concerns of the patient. Radiotherapy to the site of tumor can frequently alleviate specific local pain. Generalized pain from widely disseminated tumor requires narcotics. Usually mild analgesics and codeine are started initially. Levophanol tartrate (Levo-Dromoran) and, finally, Brompton's mixture, which includes morphine and cocaine, may be required to control the pain. These agents for pain relief can be prescribed for oral administration and use at home. Once the patient can no longer be cared for at home and is hospitalized, liberal use of morphine is indicated. A hospitalized patient with terminal, disseminated cancer should have as little pain as possible. Pain medication should not be ordered on an "as requested" (prn) basis but around the clock.

The hospice concept has been brought to the attention of cancer patients and their families as well as physicians. The hospice is composed of a group of professionals, including psychiatrists, nurses, and social workers, who help patients to live their terminal period with their family. This form of terminal care should be supported because tertiary care facilities are focusing on the care of those patients who still have the possibility to respond to therapy. Patients supported by a hospice are not abandoned, but, in fact, receive very different care from that which a hospital facility can give them, with the hope of achieving a sense of contentment in their remaining days or months.

REFERENCES

CAPIZZI RL: *Seminars in Oncology,* vol 4, no 2: *The Pharmacologic Basis of Cancer Chemotherapy.* New York, Grune & Stratton, 1977

DEVITA VT JR et al: *Cancer: Principles and Practice of Oncology.* Philadelphia, Lippincott, 1981

GILBERT HA, KAGAN R: *Seminars in Oncology,* vol 4, no 1: *Metastases.* New York, Grune & Stratton, 1977

GOEPP CE: *Seminars in Oncology,* vol 5, no 1: *Heredity and Cancer.* New York, Grune & Stratton, 1978

———, HAMMOND W: *Seminars in Oncology,* vol 2, no 4: *Supportive Care of the Cancer Patient.* New York, Grune & Stratton, 1975

GOLDMAN LI: *Seminars in Oncology,* vol 7, no 4: *Decisions in Surgical Oncology.* New York, Grune & Stratton, 1980

HOLLAND JF, FREI E III: *Cancer Medicine.* 2d ed. Philadelphia, Lea & Febiger, 1981

SANDBERG AA: *The Chromosome in Human Cancer and Leukemia.* New York, Elsevier, 1980

YARBRO JE: *Seminars in Oncology,* vol 5, no 2: *Oncologic Emergencies.* New York, Grune & Stratton, 1978

125 PRINCIPLES OF CANCER THERAPY

VINCENT T. DeVITA, JR.

BIOLOGY OF TUMOR CELL GROWTH AS RELATED TO THERAPY

All living things have an inherent capacity to multiply. Unicellular organisms, such as bacteria, multiply until growth is limited by lack of suitable nutrients or until toxic products accumulate in their environment. At more complex levels of cellular organization a cellular "brake" is required to prevent overgrowth for the benefit of the community of cells. The molecular mechanisms for control of cell growth are unknown, and their understanding forms a key scientific question in cellular biology. Clear examples of the temporary, controlled release of the cellular brake exist, as in wound healing and in regeneration of the liver after partial hepatectomy. In neoplasms, cells no longer cease multiplication when they reach a critical mass, and the uncontrolled growth leads to the death of the host. The three general classes of normal tissue, renewing (marrow, germ cells), expanding (liver, kidney, and endocrine glands), and static (neurons and striated muscle), reach a steady state when normal organ size is attained. For static tissues, such as neurons, the cells live for the duration of the life of the host and are normally not replaced if lost. For expanding tissue, mitotic potential is manifest in cells at random only when cell loss takes place (trauma, surgical resection), and then the tissue is replenished. Adult cells of renewing populations

have a finite, usually short, life span, and continued replacement from a clonogenic, or stem-cell pool, normally takes place. As long as cell birth does not exceed cell loss, a neoplastic process is not evident. Regardless of the tissue of origin, growing populations of tumor cells resemble renewing populations of normal tissue. Maturation takes place in some cells. Although they continue to divide for a time, they lose their capacity to establish new colonies. A subset of the population usually retains the capacity to form new colonies. Although early normal growth in the embryo, and early tumor growth, appear to be exponential, exponential growth soon ceases, and the growth characteristics of expanding tumor masses are best described as a gompertzian function. As the mass increases, the time required for the mass to double also increases; exponential growth is matched by exponential retardation of growth. The tumor doubling time (the time required for a given mass to double its volume) is a complex value influenced by the cell cycle time, the fraction of cells in the population undergoing cell division, and the rate of cell loss from the mass. The phases of a cell cycle are illustrated in Fig. 125-1. Cells not in cycle, but viable, and capable of entering cell division under proper circumstances are said to be in a resting phase (G_0). The fraction of cells in cycle in a given population (proliferative pool, growth fraction) determined by incorporation of tritiated thymidine into DNA (labeling index) markedly influence the growth of the tumor. For a given cycle time, a tumor with a high growth fraction will double faster than a tumor with a low growth fraction if cell loss (death, metastases, shedding) is constant. High rates of cell loss account for long doubling times in tumors known to have high growth fractions.

There are considerable data to suggest that in addition to cells remaining quiescent in G_0, some cancer cells, on their own, or under the influence of drugs or x-ray therapy, may be blocked from proceeding through the cell cycle for long periods of time in other phases of the cycle, a fact of some therapeutic importance in scheduling of treatment programs. Although cell cycle times are relatively constant in tumors of a given histological type, considerable species differences exist in cycle times of normal and tumor tissue. Cell loss begins early in growth of a tumor. Even small (1 to 2 mm), apparently localized, tumors can be assumed to shed cells into surrounding tissue (e.g., shedding from the surface of a colon cancer into the lumen of the bowel) or into lymphatics and/or the bloodstream. The fact that some cancers can be cured by local treatment only reaffirms that many shed cells are nonviable (nonclonogenic) or can be destroyed by the host.

CLONAL EVOLUTION OF CANCER The concept that cancer originates from a single transformed cell, or clone, is supported by clinical studies of human neoplasms. The classic example is multiple myeloma, a malignant proliferation of antibody-secreting plasma cells, which is characterized by elevated blood, or urine, levels of a single immunoglobulin molecule. Tumor-specific abnormalities in chromosome structure have been demonstrated in malignant cells; the most consistent example is the Philadelphia chromosome, which occurs in approximately 95 percent of patients with chronic myelogenous leukemia. The abnormal chromosome 22 has been identified in hematopoietic precursor cells in some cases several years prior to the onset of overt leukemia. The clonal evolution of this disease is further supported by studies of X-inactivation mosaicism. Each cell of the female determines at the early stage in embryogenesis whether the paternal- or maternal-derived X chromosome will remain active or suppressed. The X-linked enzyme glucose 6-phosphate dehydrogenase (G6PD) has proved a useful marker for such studies of clonal origin because it is polymorphic in the black population. Women who are heterozygous at the G6PD locus for the common gene Gd^B and the variant Gd^A normally have two distinct cell populations reflected in their enzyme electrophoretic pattern. While the nonleukemic G6PD heterozygotes have both the A and the B enzyme type in white blood cells, patients with chronic myelogenous leukemia demonstrate only one enzyme type in their leukemic granulocytic series, suggesting that the disorder originated from a single cell. Similar methodology has shown that acute myelogenous leukemia, carcinoma of the uterus and cervix, and Burkitt's lymphoma also have demonstrated a clonal pattern of tumor evolution. Patients with Burkitt's lymphoma have a consistent abnormality of chromosome 14. With early relapse after remission of Burkitt's lymphoma, the cells retain the enzyme phenotype of the initial tumor, and the recurrent tumor appears to represent a reemergence of the original malignant line. In several cases of late recurrent Burkitt's tumor, there have been discordant G6PD phenotypes, indicating the probable emergence of newly induced malignant clones. Cells from meningiomas have also demonstrated a consistent deletion of a portion of chromosome 22. Two hereditary tumors, neurofibroma and trichoepithelioma, have demonstrated a double-enzyme phenotype, indicating multicellular origin. These exceptions suggest that the somatic mutation theories of oncogenesis may not be valid for all neoplasms.

DOSE-RESPONSE RELATIONSHIPS AND DEVELOPMENT OF RESISTANCE TO CHEMOTHERAPY The growth and size of a tumor are generally measured in orders of magnitude or logs. A human tumor, when first diagnosed as, for example, a 1.0-cm mass, contains approximately 1 billion cancer cells or 9 logs, whereas 12 logs has been estimated to represent a lethal body burden for some malignancies. The cytotoxic action of anticancer agents is defined by first-order kinetics; they kill a constant fraction of cells rather than a constant number. Thus, a course of therapy with a capacity to kill 3 logs of tumor cells will reduce a tumor with 10^{10} cells to 10^7, or a neoplasm of 10^5 to 10^2 cells. Unfortunately, the majority of available single drugs, and even drug combinations, used for solid tumors have a limited log cell kill potential, and as a result cannot be expected to have a curative effect when used to treat tumors that are large both in terms of physical size and kinetics. In the past, drug therapy had been largely reserved for advanced cases, after surgery and radiation therapy had failed. While most chemotherapy, used in relatively sensitive tumors, was able to reduce cell numbers by 1 to 3 logs, it was capable of producing only minimal palliation in a patient with 10^{12} tumor cells. Total eradication of tumor cells was not possible for all but the most drug-sensitive malignancies. These concepts, derived from studies of cell kinetics, are now being tested in adjuvant chemotherapy trials. Patients are receiving drug treatment after the tumor mass has been initially reduced by surgery and radiation therapy in the hope that the favorable kinetic features in the remaining microscopic disease will serve to increase the effectiveness of chemotherapy.

Conceptually, the tumor can be divided into three distinct kinetic compartments, each with its particular significance in relation to the effectivenesses of chemotherapy (Fig. 125-2). First, there is the growth fraction of tumor that is most vulnerable to chemotherapy. Second, there is a population of cells which are temporarily nondividing but, nevertheless, have the capability of returning to a replicative stage. In terms of cell cycle kinetics, these cells are in an extended G_1 or G_0 phase and are considerably less sensitive to antitumor agents, particularly the cell cycle phase-specific antimetabolites. Lastly, there is a compartment of cells that have permanent loss of proliferative capacity, until they die and are absorbed, but still contribute to the mass of the tumor and are measured either by physical examination or by x-ray.

With increasing tumor size, the percentage of cells in the drug-sensitive growth fraction decreases and the chance that drug-resistant clones have developed increases. These phenomena are considered to represent the limiting factors of successful chemotherapy. Genetically unstable exponentially growing human cancer cells can develop phenotypic resistance to anticancer drugs without prior exposure, and the chance of resistant lines being present in a tumor varies directly with tumor mass. This provides the basis for the invariable inverse relationship between drug curability and cell number independent of tumor-growth kinetics. Since the number and fraction of resistant cells will vary with mass of tumor, it is easy to appre-

FIGURE 125-1

The cell cycle. The gap terminology divides the cell cycle into phases M, G_1, S, and G_2. M is the period of cell division. G_1 is the period of normal cell metabolism but without replicative DNA synthesis; cells that stay in G_1 for long periods are often referred to as being in the G_0 phase. The S, or DNA synthetic, phase is the period of doubling of the DNA content; it is followed by the G_2, or tetraploid, phase which precedes cell division. Normal and cancer cells have similar cycle times, in general: M, 0.5 to 1 h; G_1, 2 h to infinity; S, 6 to 24 h; G_2, 2 to 8 h.

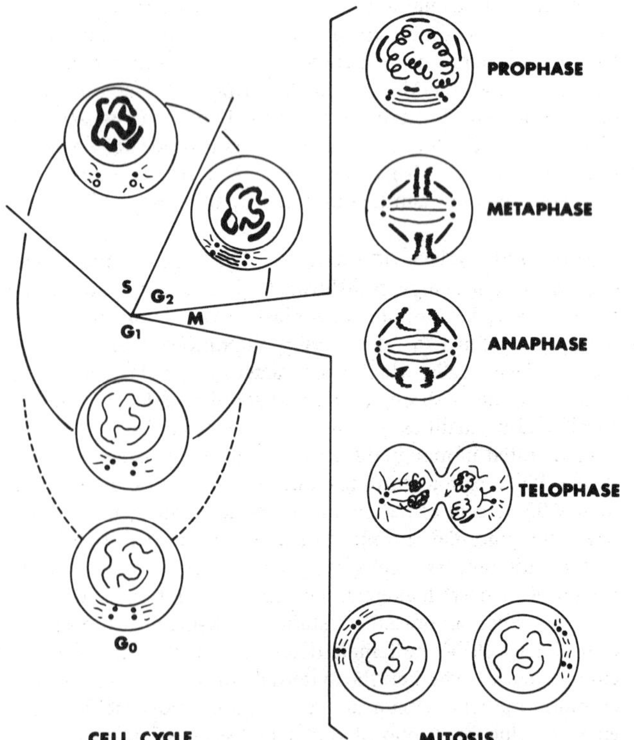

FIGURE 125-2

Various compartments and flow between compartments in a hypothetical tumor mass.

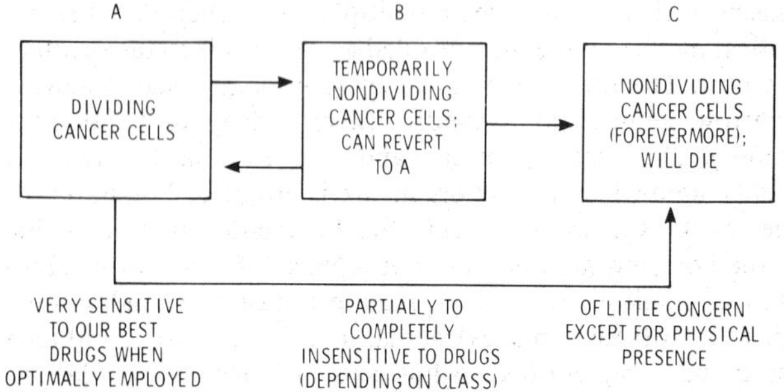

ciate that the possibility of multiple resistant lines is high when patients present with metastatic disease. Such resistance can develop over only 2 logs of growth (about six tumor doublings). For this reason delay in starting drug treatment even in the postoperative period may assume considerable importance. For rapidly growing tumors, such as diffuse histiocytic lymphomas, six doublings could occur in as short a period as 2 to 4 weeks. The data in Fig. 125-3 illustrate the fact that most tumors are in the late stages of their biological growth curves when diagnosed as a 1-cm mass. At this point they have already progressed through approximately 30 doubling times and are only 10 to 15 doublings away from a lethal volume of tumor cells.

The implication of the fractional killing effect is that to eradicate a drug-sensitive tumor population effectively, it is necessary either to increase the dose of drug or drugs within limits tolerated by the host or to start treatment when the number of cells is small enough to allow tumor destruction at reasonably tolerated doses. The killing effect of cancer chemotherapeutic agents has a definite selectivity for cancer cells over normal cells. The clinical counterpart of animal experiments showing a markedly increased sensitivity of tumor cells over normal cells to drugs can, at present, only be inferred from the dramatic antitumor effects noted in some patients with drug-sensitive tumors without permanent damage to their bone marrow or gastrointestinal tract.

DOSE-RESPONSE RELATIONSHIPS AND RADIOTHERAPY A similar effect is seen with x-ray therapy. The radiation dose-response curve is illustrated in Fig. 125-4. The fraction of surviving cells on a log scale is plotted against radiation dose. The slope of the exponential portion of the curve, usually referred to as D_0 (mean lethal dose), is a standard reference point. D_0 is the dose required to place one inactivating event in each pertinent biological entity. The more radiosensitive the cell, the steeper the curve. Owing to the random nature of these energy deposits, some energy will be deposited in a cell which has already been destroyed, while some will escape altogether so that according to the Poisson distribution, instead of destroying all the cells, the D_0 destroys only 63 percent of them. Thus, the dose required to reduce the number of cells in a population to 37 percent of the original number is D_{37}, which is an index of radiosensitivity. For most cells this value lies between 0.80 and 2 Gy (80 and 200 rads). The surviving fraction after two mean lethal doses is 37 times 37 percent or 13.7 percent, and after three mean lethal doses it is 5.1 percent, etc. In practice the logarithmic curve is not exactly a straight line. There is a small shoulder to overcome before the curve is exponential. With a strictly exponential curve D_0 equals D_{37}. The shoulder on the curve reflects doses below which the cell has the ability to repair radiation-induced damage. The dose at the point at which the curve becomes exponential (D_q) is the threshold dose. Repair of radiation-induced damage can take place within 2 h. The identification of D_q, D_0, D_{37} repair time, and mechanisms of repair have important implications in clinical dose fractionation, particularly in studies combining drugs with radiation therapy. For clinical purposes, a dose-response curve can be constructed for specific tumors in which local tumor control is plotted as a function of dose.

TYPES OF IONIZING RADIATION The term *x-ray* or *roentgen ray* is applied to electromagnetic, nonparticulate, ionizing radiations produced by human-made machines, whereas gamma rays emanate from naturally occurring or artificially produced radioactive elements such as radium or cobalt 60. These radiations of very short wavelengths have extremely high penetrating power in materials of low atomic number such as water and tissue but are stopped efficiently in materials of high atomic number such as lead. The ionizing events following irradiation lead to the production of free radicals in the water molecules of the cell microenvironment. Such free radicals and oxidizing agents interact with DNA molecules and produce a large number and variety of DNA breaks and damage. The exact lethal lesion of x-ray irradiation remains undefined, but once alterations in nucleotide sequences occur, a change in transcription, or defective repair, results, leading to cell death.

TYPES OF RADIOTHERAPY EQUIPMENT At one time, the best available apparatus for "deep therapy" operated at 200 to 250 kV, referred to as the *kilovoltage range.* The *supervoltage energy range* is generally taken to be 2 to 10 MeV, and *megavoltage energies* are those above 10 MeV. Radium emits gamma

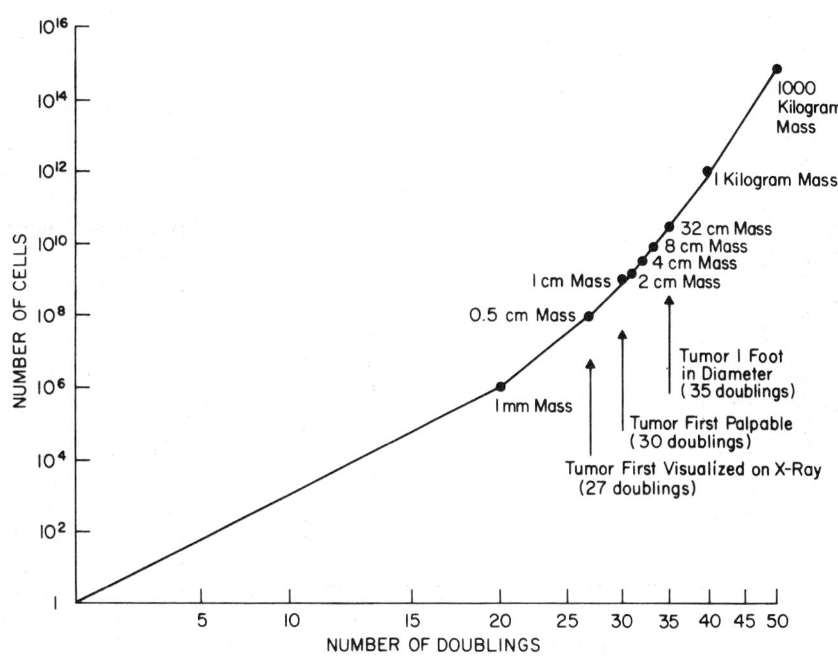

FIGURE 125-3
A schematic representation of the life cycle of a human tumor. Number of cells present in the body is shown on the ordinate with number of population doublings on the abscissa. Clinical phenomena are related to expected size of tumor mass on plotted line. Most tumors have completed at least two-thirds of their growth (32 doublings) at the time of diagnosis of a 1-cm mass.

rays from about 1 MeV, while the artificially produced isotope cobalt 60 (^{60}Co) emits gamma rays of about 1.4 MeV. The mere presence in a unit of a quantity of ^{60}Co does not make it a true supervoltage instrument. The great tissue penetration which characterizes the supervoltage range is obtained only when the radiation source is far removed (preferably 70 cm to 1 m) from the surface of the patient. Since the output of the source decreases inversely as the square of its distance from the patient, units containing very large amounts of ^{60}Co (7.4×10^{13} to 11.1×10^{13} Bq, or 2000 to 3000 Ci) are required to produce adequate intensities and reasonably short treatment times at treatment distances of 1 m or greater. The units which contain smaller amounts of ^{60}Co and are operated at a distance of 50 cm or less should not be thought of as supervoltage devices since the physical distribution of gamma ray beams from these sources is comparable with kilovoltage rays. Linear (electron) accelerators are able to generate high-energy radiations without employing high voltages, and those operating in the range of 4 to 10 MeV are commercially available. A similar device, the betatron, accelerates electrons magnetically in a circular path within a vacuum tube. Commercial units presently available produce electrons and x-rays at a peak energy of 18 to 30 MeV.

Megavoltage radiation equipment has almost completely replaced kilovoltage sources in cancer therapy. Because of reduced skin doses and lesser internal scatter, higher doses of irradiation can be delivered to tumors at any depth in the body by megavoltage irradiation. Linear accelerators in the 4- to 35-MeV range and cobalt sources are the photon generators most widely employed. Linear accelerators deliver radiation with sharper beam margins than cobalt machines. Linear accelerators can also provide electrons, which are particulate and penetrate approximately 0.25 to 0.5 cm per megaelectronvolt of energy with a relatively abrupt falloff in tissues, so that deeper normal tissues are spared from irradiation. The low penetrance of electron beams is proving useful in intraoperative radiotherapy which seeks to avoid radiation to normal tissue moved aside at surgery, and tissues distal to the target organ. Other forms of particulate irradiation are being developed which are more penetrating than electrons and have very favorable physical and biological characteristics for the treatment of cancer. These include fast neutrons, charged particles such as protons or helium ions, and negative pi mesons. These particles cause a more intense deposition of energy per unit path in the tissue [high linear energy transfer (LET)] than does ordinary photon radiation. They also have theoretical advantages of greater relative biological effectiveness (RBE), in part because of lower oxygen-enhancement ratios (OER) which should treat hypoxic fractions of tumors more effectively. Doses of radiation are expressed in units called Grays (Gy). One gray equals 100 rads or 1 rad equals 0.01 Gy. These units indicate the amount of absorbed energy per unit volume of tissue. The biological effects of irradiation are dependent on the time over which the radiation is delivered and the dose per fraction. Usual dose fractionation is about 10 Gy (1000 rads) per week, delivered in 1.5 to 2.5 Gy (150 to 250 rads) fractions. Delivering tumoricidal doses with kilovoltage sources required prolonged periods of time and utilization of many fractions when skin tolerance was the major limiting factor. With megavoltage irradiation, this is no longer the case, and shorter and more intense irradiation dose fractionation is being developed and studied.

FIGURE 125-4
Radiation dose-response curve (see text).

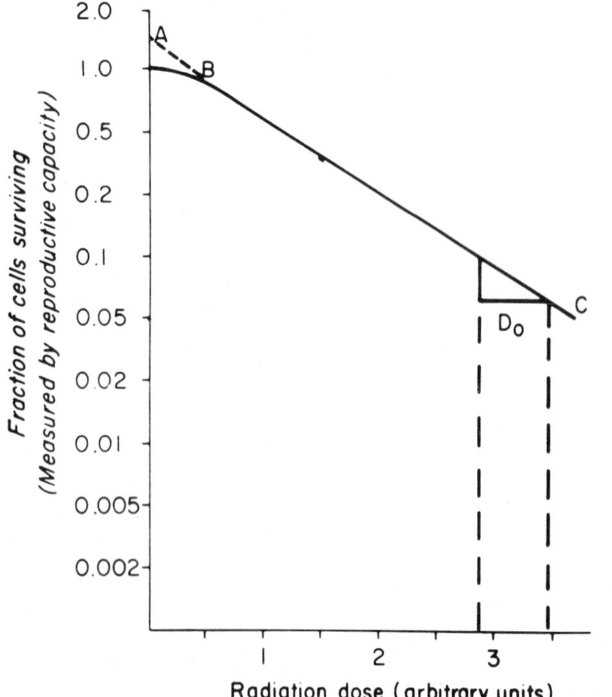

RADIOSENSITIZER DRUGS Tumor masses have been shown to contain significant fractions of hypoxic cells due to the inadequacy of the blood supply in large tumors as the mass increases. Since the free radical state of molecular oxygen interacts with ionization products created by radiation beams, radiation therapy to such tumors is less effective than to fully oxygenated tumors. In experimental tumor systems, the size of the hypoxic fraction has been shown to be directly proportional to the failure rate of local treatment.

Attempts to improve the cell kill of hypoxic cells have involved the use of hyperbaric oxygen, high LET radiation, and hypoxic cell sensitizer drugs. Of the compounds tested as hypoxic cell sensitizers, the nitroimidazoles appear to have the greatest potential because of pharmacological properties that promote distribution of drug to the central portion of tumors in spite of poor blood supply. Among these, metronidazole (Flagyl) and another experimental derivative, misonidazole, have been active in animal model systems and are now in use in several countries. These compounds act by mimicking oxygen in fixing DNA damage caused by radiation. They improve radiosensitivity of hypoxic cells as tested both in vitro and in vivo. They do not sensitize normal oxic cells to radiation and therefore exert a selective effect between tumors and normal tissues. Hypoxic radiosensitizers have the potential of enhancing the usefulness of photon radiotherapy by maximizing the tumor cell kill with doses well within the range tolerated by normal tissue.

DRUGS, HORMONES, AND IMMUNOTHERAPEUTIC AGENTS In 1980, 785,000 patients were diagnosed in the United States as having cancer exclusive of skin cancer. Of these, roughly 505,000 patients presented with disease that appeared localized, and 280,000 presented with visible metastases at the time of first diagnosis. Of the 505,000 with apparently localized tumor, 321,850, or 41 percent of the total with serious cancers (785,000), are expected to remain free of recurrent tumor 5 years later. However, 183,150 patients with operable cancer will develop recurrent tumor because of the presence of micrometastases not noted at the time of surgery or radiation of the primary tumor. For the 280,000 patients who presented with metastatic disease, drug therapy now exists that can prolong useful life in approximately 157,000 patients per year. In fact, of these 157,000 patients, 39,300 have cancers that are now potentially curable with drugs, even though they have widespread metastases at diagnosis. Radiotherapy and surgery offer ways of reducing the tumor mass in specific regions of the body amenable to surgical excision or high doses of radiotherapy. Neither is applicable to the destruction of widely disseminated tumor. In toto, 45 percent of the 785,000 patients with serious cancers are curable in 1980. Of the 321,850 patients with localized cancers in 1980, 219,850 are curable as a result of surgery alone, 90,000 as a result of radiotherapy alone or added to surgery, and 12,000 as a result of chemotherapy added to surgery or radiotherapy for localized tumors. An additional 34,000 patients are curable by chemotherapy used in patients with metastatic disease or as adjuvant therapy in breast, rectal, and testicular and other cancers. Patients with visible metastatic disease or micrometastases require some form of treatment that reaches all the interstices of the body. The stimulus for the development of systemic treatment of cancer can be traced to the success in identifying and using antibiotics for bacterial infections and antiprotozoan drugs for malaria. Drug development for cancer began with the accidental identification of the antitumor activity of nitrogen mustard, a derivative of mustard gases used in World Wars I and II. The initial success in the treatment of Hodgkin's disease and lymphocytic lymphomas with this drug was followed by extraordinary disappointment and skepticism that cancer could be successfully treated by drugs, because all successfully treated patients had relapses of their disease. Further excitement was created with the identification of the effectiveness of the antimetabolite methotrexate, first used successfully against acute childhood leukemia, and then in the treatment of choriocarcinoma in women. In this instance, remissions produced by the drug appeared permanent. The need for a standardized approach to the development of anticancer drugs was recognized in the 1950s. Since then, many synthetic, fermentation, and plant products have been identified as possessing antitumor activity against rodent tumors. These compounds have been selected both by rational synthesis and random screening. Over 40 nonhormone cytotoxic chemicals that possess some anticancer effect in humans with metastatic disease have been identified, and about 30 have been marketed. Six major classes of antitumor agents (alkylating agents, antimetabolites, plant alkaloids, antitumor antibiotics, endocrine agents, and immunologic stimulants) and some miscellaneous drugs are available. The most important agents with their major toxicity, doses, and schedules are described in Table 125-1. The major hormonal agents are described in Table 125-2.

ALKYLATING AGENTS Mechlorethamine (nitrogen mustard) was the first chemical agent used in the treatment of cancer in modern times. It was found to have major antitumor activity against lymphomas. It contains two β-chloroethyl groups which transfer into positively charged ethylenimonium derivatives and combine with negatively charged guanine moieties of complementary DNA strands, resulting in their cross-linking. This leads to miscoding errors or depurination, or, in the case of bifunctional alkylating agents, to cross-linking of adjacent macromolecules, which interferes with mitosis by preventing separation of strands of DNA. Polyfunctional alkylating agents are more cytotoxic than monofunctional alkylators, although the latter may also cause mutagenic and carcinogenic damage that is not lethal to the cell and can, therefore, be reproduced indefinitely as an inherited mutation. Alkylating agents are not cell cycle–specific in their ability to cause cell death. Cell death may occur during the interphase, when many sites, including RNA and protein, are damaged, or it may be delayed until mitosis when separation of the DNA strands is unable to take place. Within a few minutes after administration of mechlorethamine, the drug is no longer detectable in active form and is bound to proteins or intracellular macro-

molecules. Less than 0.01 percent is excreted in the urine. The intracavitary use of mechlorethamine (0.2 to 0.4 mg/kg) after drainage of malignant pleural effusions can be an effective palliative measure. Very dilute solutions (0.25%) can be painted on the skin of patients with generalized mycosis fungoides with good results.

Three major modifications have altered the properties of mechlorethamine. (1) The substitution of electrophilic groups on the nitrogen atom, as in chlorambucil, reduces the reactivity, producing a more stable drug with a longer half-life. (2) An amino acid precursor added to the nitrogen atom as a carrier enhances delivery to sites of greatest tumor activity. Melphalan, for example, is the L-phenylalanine congener. (3) Cyclophosphamide is a derivative in which the activity of the chloroethyl groups is eliminated by the substitution of a ring structure on the nitrogen atom. This drug is activated by enzymatic cleavage of the phosphorus-nitrogen linkage within the ring substitution. In the liver it is activated through conversion to the 4-OH derivative by the drug metabolizing microsomal oxidase system and ultimately broken down to nor-nitrogen mustard. Cyclophosphamide is subject to the influence of other compounds. For example, barbiturates stimulate hepatic enzymes and increase the activation and toxicity of cyclophosphamide, whereas corticosteroids and sex hormones have the opposite effect. After oral administration, maximum plasma levels are achieved in approximately one hour. Disappearance in the plasma is rapid, with a half-life of about four hours; urinary recovery of unchanged drugs is less than 14 percent. Because of its potent immunosuppressive action, cyclophosphamide has been used clinically in Wegener's granulomatosis, rheumatoid arthritis, nephrotic syndrome in children, and other conditions associated with altered immune reactivity. Because gonadal suppression resulting in sterility has been observed and the mutagenic and carcinogenic potential is high, risks and benefits of this drug in patients with reproductive capacity should be weighed carefully. The phenylalanine derivative (melphalan) of nitrogen mustard is particularly useful in multiple myeloma, alone or in combination with other agents. It has the general pharmacological properties of an alkylating agent of intermediate strength, demonstrating activity in the blood for 6 h. The drug can be administered orally. Nausea, vomiting, and alopecia are infrequent. Chlorambucil is the slowest-acting nitrogen mustard derivative in clinical use. In addition to its use in neoplastic disease, good responses have been reported in the treatment of vasculitis following rheumatoid arthritis and in autoimmune hemolytic anemias. The use of busulfan (Myleran) is limited to chronic granulocytic leukemia, polycythemia vera, and myelofibrosis with myeloid metaplasia. Within 3 min, more than 90 percent of the drug disappears from the blood and is excreted in the urine almost entirely as the methane sulfonic acid and other metabolites. The myelosuppressive action of this drug is quite selective, affecting primarily granulocyte production and to some extent platelets.

The *nitrosoureas* are drugs with similar but not identical activity to other alkylating agents. Three of these compounds, 1,3-bis(2-chloroethyl)-1-nitrosourea (BCNU, carmustine), 1-(2-chloroethyl)-3-cyclohexyl-1-nitrosourea (CCNU, lomustine), and 1-(2-chloroethyl)-3,4-methylcyclohexyl-1-nitrosourea (MeCCNU, semustine), have been evaluated clinically and have been shown to have some effect against a variety of tumors; BCNU and CCNU have been used in the treatment of brain tumors and advanced Hodgkin's disease refractory to other agents, and MeCCNU and, in some cases, BCNU have been used in treatment of colon and stomach cancer.

TABLE 125-1
Commonly used anticancer agents

Drugs	*Optimal dose when used alone**	*Route and schedule*	*Marrow suppression*	*Acute toxicity*	*Other toxicity*	*Comments*
ALKYLATING AGENTS						
Mechlorethamine	0.4 mg/kg	IV every 3–4 weeks	4+	Severe nausea and vomiting	Vesicant to skin	Given in tubing of established infusion; used in full doses for intrapleural or intraperitoneal therapy
Cyclophosphamide	40 mg/kg	IV every 3–4 weeks	3+	Nausea and vomiting	Alopecia and cystitis	Causes less severe thrombocytopenia than other alkylators
	3–1 mg/kg	Daily PO continuous	2+	Minimal		
Melphalan	0.2–0.05 mg/kg	Daily PO continuous	3+	Minor nausea and vomiting	Persistent thrombocytopenia after long use	Five-day schedule used for adjuvant treatment of breast cancer
	0.2 mg/kg	qd for 5 days every 4–6 weeks	3+	Minor nausea and vomiting		
Busulfan	0.2–0.05 mg/kg	Daily PO continuous	3+	None	Pigmentation, pulmonary fibrosis	
Chlorambucil	0.2–0.05 mg/kg	Daily PO	3+	None	Pancytopenia with long-term use	
cis-Platinum	60–75 mg/m²	Every 3 weeks	1+	Severe nausea and vomiting	Nephrotoxicity and ototoxicity	Adequate hydration and mannitol therapy used to prevent nephrotoxicity
BCNU	200 mg/m²	IV every 4–6 weeks	4+	Severe nausea and vomiting	Tanning of skin, pulmonary fibrosis, chronic renal failure	Late marrow suppression (4–6 wk)
CCNU	130 mg/m²	PO every 4–6 weeks	4+	Nausea and vomiting	Cumulative marrow suppression, chronic renal failure	
MeCCNU	200 mg/m²	PO every 4–6 weeks	4+	Nausea and vomiting	More pronounced thrombocytopenia, chronic renal failure	
Streptozotocin	500 mg/m²	1-h infusion daily for 5 days every mo	0	Nausea and vomiting, local pain at infusion site	Renal tubular acidosis; renal failure, hepatotoxicity	Dose monitored by presence or absence of proteinuria
Dimethylimidazole carboxamide	250 mg/m²	IV daily for 5 days every 3 weeks	3+	Severe nausea and vomiting, flu-like syndrome	Cumulative marrow toxicity	
ANTIMETABOLITES						
Methotrexate: High dose with citrovorum factor rescue	2–10 g/m²	6-h infusion every 3–4 weeks	±	Nausea and vomiting	Renal failure	These doses lethal without rescue; serum levels should be monitored
Citrovorum factor for rescue	15 mg to 100 mg	Every 3 h for 8 doses, 2 h after methotrexate		None	None	Blood levels of methotrexate must be $< 10^{-8}$ *M* before discontinuing citrovorum factor
Methotrexate doses not requiring rescue	80 mg/m²	IV, IM, or PO weekly	3+	Minimal nausea and vomiting	Fatigue, buccal ulcerations	Used for maintenance treatment of acute leukemia
	20 mg/m²	IV, IM, or PO twice weekly	3+	Minimal nausea and vomiting	Buccal ulcerations	
	15 mg/m²	Intrathecal weekly in Elliot's B solution	0	None	Arachnoiditis, neurotoxicity	Monitor CSF methotrexate levels

TABLE 125-1 *(continued)*
Commonly used anticancer agents

Drugs	Optimal dose when used alone*	Route and schedule	Marrow suppression	Acute toxicity	Other toxicity	Comments
ANTIMETABOLITES *(continued)*						
6-Mercaptopurine	2.5–1 mg/kg	Daily PO continuous	2+	Modest nausea and vomiting	Hepatotoxicity	Reduce dose to 25% with allopurinol
6-Thioguanine	2.0–1 mg/kg	Daily PO continuous	2+	Modest nausea and vomiting		No adjustment of dose required with allopurinol
5-Fluorouracil	12–7.5 mg/kg	IV daily for 5 days, then every other day to toxicity or weekly	3+	Chronic nausea, mucositis, diarrhea	Photophobia, alopecia, cerebellar ataxia	Oral use less effective; intrapleural use effective
Arabinosyl cytosine	200 mg/m^2	IV daily for 5 days every 2–3 weeks	4+	Nausea and vomiting	Alopecia	Can be given subcutaneously
PLANT ALKALOIDS						
Vinblastine	0.3–0.1 mg/kg	IV every 1–2 weeks	3+	Minimal nausea	Minimal paresthesias, jaw pain	
Vincristine	0.033–0.025 mg/kg	IV every week for 6–8 weeks	1+	Minimal nausea, local necrosis at injection site	Paresthesias, motor weakness, alopecia, obstipation	Elderly and immobilized patients have more severe gastrointestinal toxicity
ANTIBIOTICS						
Dactinomycin	15 μg/kg	IV qd for 5 days every month	3+	Nausea and vomiting, mucositis	Alopecia, skin changes	Skin damage severe in irradiated areas
Mithramycin	50 μg/kg	IV every other day to toxicity	3+	Nausea and vomiting	Flushing of skin, hemorrhage	Stop therapy with ↑ lactic dehydrogenase or facial flush
	25 μg/kg	IV every week	0	None	None	Ideal for treatment of hypercalcemia
Daunorubicin	30 mg/m^2	IV qd for 3 days every 2–3 weeks	4+	Nausea and vomiting, mucositis	Myocardiopathy, hepatotoxicity	Not to exceed total dose of 600 mg/m^2
Adriamycin	75 mg/m^2	IV every 3–4 weeks	4+	Nausea and vomiting, mucositis, local reaction at injection site	Myocardiopathy, alopecia	Not to exceed total dose of 550 mg/m^2
Bleomycin	15 units/kg	IV every week	1+	Minimal nausea and vomiting, fever, mucositis	Pulmonary fibrosis, skin changes, alopecia	Not to exceed total dose of 400 units
Mitomycin C	50 μg/kg	IV qd for 5 days every 3–4 weeks	3+	Nausea and vomiting, mucositis	Renal, pulmonary	Extravasation produces local injury
MISCELLANEOUS						
Procarbazine	200–100 mg/m^2 = 100 mg/m^2	Daily PO continuous	3+	Early severe nausea and vomiting subsides with use	Skin rash, side effects of monoamine oxidase inhibitors	CNS toxicity in large doses
L-Asparaginase	200 units/kg	IV daily for 14–28 days	0	Nausea and vomiting	Pancreatitis, CNS toxicity, hypofibrinogenemia	Allergic reactions occur with reusage
o,p'-DDD	2–10 g/day	Daily PO continuous	0	Severe nausea and vomiting	Mental depression, diarrhea, skin eruptions	Nausea and vomiting dose-limiting
Hexamethylmelamine	10–6 mg/kg	Daily PO continuous	1+	Severe nausea and vomiting	Peripheral neuropathy	Limiting toxicity, nausea and vomiting, CNS toxicity at high doses
Hydroxyurea	25 mg/kg	Daily PO continuous	3+	Minimal	None	
	100 mg/kg	IV "push" every 3 days	0	Minimal nausea	None	Used to rapidly decrease blast counts

* *Suggested range of doses from starting to maintenance doses in previously untreated patients. Doses and intervals between doses of all myelosuppressive agents should be continuously adjusted by monitoring white blood cell and platelet counts. Doses differ where used in combinations and are reduced in previously treated patients with compromised bone marrow. Use of milligrams per kilogram of body weight or milligrams per square meter of body surface area is by convention.*

Disappearance of BCNU from the plasma after intravenous administration occurs within 5 min. CCNU and MeCCNU are given orally, and their metabolites have prolonged half-lives (16 to 48 h). Active metabolites, which produce either alkylation or carbamylation, are probably responsible for their cytotoxic actions; entry of these drugs into the cerebrospinal fluid is rapid, and levels 15 to 50 percent of plasma concentrations are achieved. An unusual feature of these agents is the delay in myelosuppressive toxicity which develops 3 to 4 weeks after their administration; dose-related renal toxicity has been reported for these drugs.

Streptozotocin is a naturally occurring nitrosourea which causes diabetes in experimental animals. The sugar moiety attached to a 1-methyl-1-nitrosourea apparently facilitates transport across the membrane of islet cells, an observation which led to its successful use in the treatment of islet-cell carcinoma of the pancreas. The half-life of the drug in plasma is approximately 15 min, and only 10 to 20 percent is excreted unchanged in the urine. Unlike the results with other nitrosoureas, bone marrow toxicity occurs in only 20 percent of cases and is usually mild; nephrotoxicity may be severe and is usually the dose-limiting factor. The presence of albuminuria between doses is used to monitor the administration of the drug. Dimethyltrizenoimidazole carboxamide (DTIC, dacarbazine) has alkylating activity after metabolic activation in the liver and is thought to act by cross-linking DNA. It is not cell cycle phase-specific. After intravenous injection, the plasma half-life is about 35 min, and 43 percent of the drug is excreted intact in the urine in 6 h. It has been reported to be effective in the treatment of malignant melanoma and is now being evaluated as an adjunct to surgical therapy. It is also an integral part of many treatment programs for soft-tissue sarcomas.

ANTIMETABOLITES An antimetabolite is a substance which resembles a normal metabolite so closely that it enters the same metabolic system but differs sufficiently that it interferes

TABLE 125-2
Hormonal agents used in the treatment of cancer

Agents	*Principal route of administration*	*Usual dose*	*Acute side effects*	*Other side effects*	*Indications*
ANDROGENS					
Testosterone proprionate	IM	50–100 mg three times weekly	Fluid retention	Masculinization	Breast cancer: Pre- and postmenopausal women with ER(+) tumors; stimulation of erythropoiesis (6–12 weeks required for effect)
Fluoxymesterone	PO	10–20 mg/day	Fluid retention	Occasional hypercalcemia	
ESTROGENS					
Diethylstilbestrol	PO	1–15 mg/day	Nausea and vomiting, urinary incontinence	Feminization; uterine bleeding; increased mortality from heart disease in males; hypercalcemia	Prostate cancer: Dose not to exceed 1 mg diethylstilbestrol or 0.1 mg ethinyl estradiol per day; 70% respond with prolongation of life
Ethinyl estradiol	PO	0.1–3 mg/day			Breast cancer: Postmenopausal women with ER(+) tumors
ANTIESTROGENS					
Tamoxifen	PO	10–40 mg/day	Mild nausea	Rare thrombocytopenia and leukopenia; hot flashes; mild fluid retention	ER(+) breast cancer
PROGESTINS					
Hydroxyprogesterone	IM	1 g two times weekly			
6-Methylhydroxyprogesterone	PO	100–200 mg/day	Minimal fluid retention	Occasional hypercalcemia; thrombocytosis	Endometrial carcinoma; renal-cell carcinoma; ovarian carcinoma
	IM	200–600 mg two times weekly			
THYROID HORMONES					
Thyroxin	PO	To tolerance	None	Hyperthyroidism; arrhythmias; angina	Papillary adenocarcinoma of thyroid; 70% respond; many remain disease-free > 10 years
ADRENAL CORTICAL COMPOUNDS					
Prednisone	PO	40 mg/m² per day	Hyperglycemia, euphoria; fluid retention	Gastrointestinal bleeding, increased susceptibility to infection; immunosuppression; osteoporosis; hypokalemic alkalosis; hypertension	Lymphomas, leukemias, and multiple myeloma in combination with other drugs; CNS metastases and spinal cord compression to reduce swelling (high-dose dexamethasone)
Dexamethasone	PO	0.5–16 mg/day			
Methylprednisolone sodium succinate	IM or IV	10–125 mg/day			
Hydroxycortisone sodium succinate	IV	100–500 mg/day			

with normal metabolic pathways. Antimetabolites in common use are methotrexate, 6-mercaptopurine, 6-thioguanine, 5-fluorouracil, and arabinosyl cytosine. Antimetabolites act primarily during the DNA synthetic phase of the cell cycle, some exclusively (arabinosyl cytosine) and others (methotrexate) by preventing further entry of cells into the DNA synthetic phase.

Folic acid antagonists Methotrexate was the first important antimetabolite to undergo clinical investigation. Folic acid, an essential dietary factor in humans, is reduced by the enzyme dihydrofolate reductase to dihydrofolic acid and tetrahydrofolic acid. The latter substance accepts single-carbon fragments to form the coenzymes. Several coenzymes exist which differ depending on the oxidation of the carbon fragment. One of these coenzymes, citrovorum factor (N^{10}-formyltetrahydrofolic acid) donates a single-carbon fragment to form deoxythymidine monophosphate, an immediate precursor of DNA. Although synthesis of RNA and protein is also inhibited by lack of tetrahydrofolate coenzymes, the thymidylate block is considered to be the most important site of cytotoxic action leading to "thymineless" cell death. Other "small-molecule" folate antagonists, pyrimethamine and cycloguanil, have been effective against malaria, and trimethoprim has been useful in bacterial infections of the urinary and respiratory tracts. Methotrexate is no longer commonly used orally but is readily absorbed after oral administration. The plasma half-life is approximately 2 h, and about 50 percent of the drug is bound to plasma proteins. Its toxicity may be increased through displacement from plasma albumin by a number of drugs including salicylates, sulfonamides, phenytoin, tetracycline, and chloramphenicol. At usual doses transport across the blood-brain barrier is very poor, and intrathecal administration (10 to 12 mg/m^2) is necessary to obtain high concentrations in the cerebrospinal fluid. The major route of elimination is through the kidney, and 90 percent of the drug is excreted unchanged in the urine. Impaired renal function can produce a marked increase in toxicity. Intravenous or intramuscular doses of 25 to 50 mg can be given once or twice weekly. Constant daily infusions of much higher doses have been administered, but only when the technique of citrovorum "rescue" is used. The rationale for high-dose methotrexate is based on obtaining an excess of unbound intracellular drug and thereby inhibiting DNA synthesis almost completely. In order to achieve this, any deficiency of the active, carrier-mediated, transport system must be overcome by extremely high (10^{-3} to 10^{-4} M) extracellular concentrations of methotrexate. After drug infusions ranging from 6 to 30 h, citrovorum is given as an antidote in order to rescue normal cells and prevent undue toxicity in the host. The use of methotrexate in this fashion can be extremely dangerous. When administered by experienced chemotherapists, however, in laboratories capable of accurately measuring plasma methotrexate concentrations, these investigational regimens are surprisingly free of adverse effects. Since methotrexate precipitates in the renal tubules when the urine is acid, impaired excretion may result in life-threatening toxicity. Accordingly, maintaining a high output of alkaline urine is imperative.

A 7-OH metabolite of methotrexate has been identified as a potential renal toxin after high doses. Because of delayed clearance, high-dose methotrexate may cause extraordinary toxicity in the presence of malignant effusions. Methotrexate is also effective in severe, recalcitrant psoriasis and as an immunosuppressive agent. In addition to bone marrow suppression, it causes ulcerative stomatitis and gastrointestinal toxicity. The adverse reactions can reach serious proportions and even cause death, particularly in the presence of preexisting folate and renal deficiencies. Other complications include dermatitis, alopecia, pulmonary interstitial infiltrates, and hepatic dysfunction, which sometimes eventuates in cirrhosis of the liver.

Purine analogues *6-Mercaptopurine* (6-MP) is a structural analogue of hypoxanthine which is converted to the active nucleotide 6-mercaptopurine ribosphosphate by the enzyme inosinic pyrophosphorylase. The nucleotide interferes with several steps in purine biosynthesis. It decreases the synthesis of 5-phosphoribosylamine, the first step in purine biosynthesis, by pseudofeedback inhibition. It also interferes with the conversion of inosinic monophosphate to xanthine monophosphate and the conversion of inosinic monophosphate to adenosine monophosphate. The drug is well absorbed after oral ingestion, and about 50 percent of the dose is recovered in the urine in 24 h, largely as 6-thiouric acid and inorganic sulfate. Attempts to inhibit this degradation led to the development of allopurinol (Zyloprim), a xanthine oxidase inhibitor capable of blocking the metabolism of 6-MP as well as the formation of uric acid from hypoxanthine and xanthine. Allopurinol has become an important agent in the management of hyperuricemia and gout. Although active as an immunosuppressive agent, 6-MP has been superseded by its imidazolyl derivative azathioprine (Imuran). Cholestatic jaundice has been reported from 6-MP in as many as one-third of adult patients; this is usually reversible upon discontinuation of therapy. Thioguanine (Tabloid) acts in a manner analogous to 6-MP; it is also significantly incorporated into DNA and RNA. After oral administration, peak blood levels are reached in 6 to 8 h, and approximately 40 percent of the dose is excreted in the urine in 24 h, mainly as inorganic sulfate and 2-amino-6-methylthiopurine, instead of 6-thiouric acid. Unlike 6-MP and azathioprine, no reduction in dose of thioguanine is necessary when used together with allopurinol.

Pyrimidine analogues 5-Fluorouracil (5-FU) and fluorodeoxyuridine (FUdR) block thymidylate synthetase, the enzyme involved in transfer of a methyl group from N^5,N^{10}-methylenetetrahydrofolic acid to deoxyuridylic acid (dUMP) in the synthesis of thymidylate and DNA. 5-FU must be converted to its active form 5-fluorodeoxyuridine monophosphate. Inhibition of RNA synthesis and incorporation into RNA also occur and may explain why these compounds are cycle-specific but not phase-specific agents. Clinically, 5-FU is used almost exclusively. Three hours after intravenous injection little 5-FU can be detected in the plasma. Catabolism occurs primarily in the liver. Approximately 15 percent of an injected dose of 5-FU appears intact in the urine, most of it within 1 h. Topical 5-FU as a 2 or 5% solution of propylene glycol or in a hydrophilic cream base, has been successful in eradicating premalignant actinic keratoses, as well as superficial basal-cell carcinomas.

Arabinosyl cytosine is a unique pyrimidine nucleoside analogue, with an alteration in the sugar moiety rather than the base. It interferes with DNA synthesis by inhibiting DNA polymerase. Its effects are exerted strictly during the DNA synthetic phase of the cell cycle. Structurally, it is related to deoxycytidine and is converted to the active nucleotide by the enzyme deoxycytidine kinase. Arabinosyl cytosine is metabolized by deaminase to uracil arabinoside which is excreted in the urine. The drug is incorporated into DNA and RNA. Twenty minutes after intravenous administration, the inactive metabolite uracil arabinoside accounts for 90 percent of the material in the urine. Studies in both animals and humans indicate that the schedule of administration markedly influences the antitumor effect and toxicity of this drug. Arabinosyl cytosine is a potent immunosuppressive agent and, depending on the dosage schedule used, can suppress either humoral or cellular responses or both. The major use of this drug is for treatment of acute myelocytic leukemia.

PLANT ALKALOIDS The alkaloids *vincristine* and *vinblastine* are derived from the periwinkle plant. They are cell cycle–specific and produce metaphase arrest in dividing cells by direct binding to tubulin and interference with the assembly of spindle proteins. Vincristine differs structurally from vinblastine only by replacement of a methyl group with a formyl group. Although they have similar activity, there are some important differences. Vincristine is capable of producing complete remissions in about 70 percent of patients with acute lymphoblastic leukemia, an accomplishment not observed with vinblastine. Vincristine and vinblastine are equally effective in Hodgkin's disease, while vincristine is superior to vinblastine in the lymphocytic and histiocytic lymphomas. Oral absorption of both drugs is unpredictable, and there is poor penetration of the blood-brain barrier by these drugs. Extravasation during intravenous injection may cause considerable irritation and sloughing. The compounds are cleared from the bloodstream in less than 1 h and are excreted primarily through the biliary system. Increased toxicity may be encountered in obstructive jaundice. Vinblastine causes bone marrow suppression and occasional gastrointestinal side effects, but neurological toxicity and alopecia occur less frequently than with vincristine. With vincristine, alopecia occurs in 20 percent of patients. The syndrome of inappropriate antidiuretic hormone secretion has been observed in patients treated with vincristine.

ANTITUMOR ANTIBIOTICS Antibiotics are substances produced by organisms which interfere with the growth of other living cells. The important antitumor antibiotics in clinical use are dactinomycin (actinomycin D), mithramycin, daunorubicin, adriamycin, and bleomycin. Dactinomycin was the first antibiotic used extensively in cancer chemotherapy. The drug forms a complex with DNA which inhibits DNA-dependent RNA synthesis. It is not cell cycle–specific. It has proved to be especially useful in the treatment of childhood malignancies, such as Wilms's tumor, neuroblastoma, rhabdomyosarcoma, and in trophoblastic tumors of women. Because of its immunosuppressive effects, it has been used in renal transplantation. The antitumor activity of *mithramycin* is limited to embryonal cell testicular tumors. The drug can also rapidly reduce serum calcium levels in patients with tumor-related hypercalcemia. This effect appears to be due to inhibition of bone resorption by the drug. Mithramycin inhibits DNA-dependent RNA synthesis, presumably by binding with DNA. The drug causes myelosuppression which results in thrombocytopenia, but additionally produces an acute hemorrhagic diathesis of uncertain etiology which appears to be fatal in about 5 percent of patients receiving the drug in full therapeutic doses. *Daunorubicin* and *adriamycin* are anthracycline antibiotics with activity against a broad spectrum of animal and human tumors. Adriamycin has a broader antitumor spectrum and differs from daunorubicin only by the addition of a hydroxyl group. In animal tumor systems it has twice the therapeutic index of daunorubicin. The anthracycline antibiotics inhibit DNA synthesis and DNA-dependent RNA synthesis by binding with DNA with untwisting of the helix which facilitates intercalation. This distortion impairs the template activity of DNA. Both daunorubicin and doxorubicin (adriamycin) are administered intravenously in large intermittent doses and are rapidly cleared from the plasma. The disappearance curves are biphasic, with a short initial half-life of approximately 1 h and a long secondary half-life of about 17 h. There is rapid uptake of the drugs in the heart, lungs, kidney, spleen, and liver, but they do not cross the blood-brain barrier. Metabolic degradation occurs in the liver by an aldehyde reductase and a microsomal reductive glycosidase. Microsomal enzyme inducers enhance this process, and, conversely, severe toxicity may result if the drugs are administered as standard doses in the presence of impaired liver function. The drugs and their metabolites are primarily excreted in the bile and to a lesser extent in the urine. Patients should be advised that these compounds may impart a red color to the urine for 1 or 2 days after administration. Myelotoxicity is a major complication, and alopecia, stomatitis, and gastrointestinal manifestations are often found. Local vesicant action and tissue necrosis can occur if the drugs extravasate. A peculiar cardiomyopathy has been observed with these agents. Two variants of cardiotoxicity may occur; the first, an acute type characterized by abnormal electrocardiographic changes, includes ST-T wave changes and arrhythmias, which are brief and rarely a serious problem. Cineangiographic data have shown that an acute reversible reduction in ejection fraction occurs 24 h after a single dose. The second variant, chronic cumulative, dose-related toxicity manifested by congestive heart failure, unresponsive to digitalis, is probably a result of repeated acute cardiac insults and has a mortality in excess of 50 percent. Although the frequency of this variant of cardiomyopathy is less than 3 percent at total doses of adriamycin below 500 mg/m^2, it increases markedly in patients receiving total doses greater than 550 mg/m^2. With daunorubicin, the frequency of congestive heart failure is 1 percent at cumulative doses of 600 mg/m^2 but increases rapidly at higher doses. Previous cardiac radiation, cyclophosphamide, or other anthracycline antibiotic exposure increases the risk of cardiotoxicity. There are no reliable tests to predict which patients will develop heart failure, and the onset of heart failure is often delayed, with 50 percent of the cases occurring 6 months from completion of therapy. The mechanism of this cardiomyopathy is unclear. The structural similarities of these agents to the digitalis glycosides and their binding to cardiac DNA, as well as oxidative damage they produce, probably relate to the quinone-hydroquinone moiety which has been shown to liberate free radicals and produce membrane damage. Cardiotoxicity is not too serious in patients with metastatic cancer who achieve only temporary remissions with the drug but should be considered a serious impediment to the use of these drugs in adjuvant therapy. *Bleomycin* is an antibiotic complex consisting of seven polypeptides of similar structure. Sixty percent of the mixture is bleomycin A_2, the most active moiety. Bleomycin inhibits DNA synthesis and reacts with DNA causing strand scission. It is most active against malignancies of the head and neck, skin, and penis, lymphomas, and testicular tumors where its use in combination with vinblastine has produced a remarkably high rate of complete remissions. Total courses exceeding 400 units are associated with pulmonary toxicity and should be given with great caution. Renal excretion is the primary route of elimination, and 20 to 40 percent of the active compound is recovered in the urine. Preferential localization of the drug due to failure of inactivation occurs in the skin and the lung; other tissues inactivate the compound by removing 1 mol ammonia. This probably accounts for the selectivity of therapeutic and toxic effects. Bleomycin alone does not produce significant bone marrow depression. Lung damage is the most serious toxic effect. Although usually age- and dose-related, it occurs more frequently in individuals over 70, and at cumulative doses greater than 400 units. It may be encountered in younger subjects at lower doses, particularly when used in combination with other agents. It begins with a presentation indistinguishable from pneumonitis, and, in 15 to 20 percent of cases, it may progress to pulmonary fibrosis, which has been fatal in about 1 percent of patients. As with the anthracycline antibiotics, the late toxicity appears to be a summation of acute insults to pulmonary tissue, since some patients complain of acute dyspnea with each intravenous dose. Because anaphylactic reactions have been observed in patients with lymphomas, administration of 2 units or less is recommended for the first two doses. *Mitomycin-C* (Mutamycin) appears to cross-link DNA in a manner similar to alkylating agents after intracellular enzymatic reduction. It disappears rapidly from the blood after intravenous administration, with a 50 percent reduction of the blood level within 6 to 7 min. In adults, less than 10 percent is excreted as active drug in the urine and very little in the bile. The currently recommended dose is 50 μg/kg daily for 5 days, repeated for another 5 days, after a 10-day interval. The schedule may be repeated after recovery from hematologic toxicity. Myelosuppression is a major complication, and gastrointestinal, renal, pulmonary, and mucocutaneous toxicity also occur. Extravasation may produce severe local injury.

MISCELLANEOUS AGENTS *Hydroxyurea* is a simple derivative of urea which may be used as an alternative to busulfan in the treatment of chronic myelogenous leukemia. It is also useful for quickly reducing very high white blood cell counts in patients with acute myelogenous leukemia or chronic myelogenous leukemia in blastic crisis who have rapidly proliferating disease. A large dose will significantly reduce myeloblast counts within 24 h with the nadir occurring at 3 days. Hydroxyurea is rapidly absorbed from the gastrointestinal tract, and peak plasma concentrations are reached in 2 h. It is undetectable in the blood within 24 h. About 80 percent is recovered in the urine; the rest is probably metabolized in the liver. *Procarbazine* is a methyl hydrazine derivative. Its major use is for the treatment of patients with Hodgkin's disease, but it has some activity in oat-cell carcinoma of the lung. Procarbazine is not cross-resistant with other antitumor agents in animal tumor systems and is active in patients with Hodgkin's disease resistant to other drugs. Besides inhibiting monoamine oxidase, the drug undergoes autooxidation with formation of hydrogen peroxide leading to denaturization of DNA. In experimental systems, procarbazine causes decreased mitotic activity and chromatin breaks. It is rapidly absorbed from the gastrointestinal tract and readily equilibrates between the plasma and the cerebrospinal fluid. Because of rapid metabolism, primarily in the liver, its half-life in the blood is approximately 7 min, and in 24 h 25 to 40 percent is excreted as a metabolite in the urine. When used alone, the recommended oral daily dose is 50 to 300 mg/m^2. Notable immunosuppressive activity has been reported. Augmentation of sedative effects may accompany the concomitant use of central nervous system depressants. Ethyl alcohol may cause a reaction resembling the acetaldehyde syndrome produced by disulfiram (Antabuse). Since it is a weak monoamine oxidase inhibitor, the use of sympathomimetics, tricyclic antidepressants, and other drugs and foods with high tyramine content, such as bananas and ripe cheese, should be avoided. *Mitotane* (*o,p′*-DDD, Lysodren) is a derivative of the insecticide DDT that causes selective destruction of normal and neoplastic adrenocortical cells. It also modifies the peripheral metabolism of corticosteroids. Approximately 40 percent of the drug is absorbed after oral administration, and about 10 to 25 percent is recovered as a metabolite in the urine. Blood levels are measurable for 6 to 9 weeks after cessation of therapy. The drug is distributed in all tissues; fat is the primary site of storage. The initial daily dose is 8 to 10 g, usually given in three to four portions. Maximum tolerated doses vary from 2 to 16 g per day. Treatment should be continued for at least 3 months. Gastrointestinal disturbances are common. Somnolence, lethargy, vertigo, and dermatitis also occur. Adverse reactions are usually reversible with reduction in dosage and do not contraindicate continuation of therapy. Discontinuation of the drug and administration of exogenous corticosteroids are indicated if shock or trauma supervenes. *L-Asparaginase* is an enzyme which converts L-asparagine to L-aspartic acid, depleting body stores of L-asparagine. Many experimental leukemias and lymphomas require exogenous L-asparagine, whereas normal tissues are able to synthesize the amino acid. Experimentally, a good correlation exists between the absence of L-asparagine synthetase and a requirement for exogenous L-asparagine. Furthermore, tumors which do not respond to L-asparaginase tend to undergo a marked increase in L-asparagine synthetase after exposure to asparaginase. L-Asparaginase interferes with protein synthesis, thereby causing a wide variety of toxic effects. Its major use is in the treatment of acute lymphoblastic leukemia. It causes pancreatitis as well as allergic reactions in some cases. It has been of value occasionally in the treatment of patients with malignant insulinomas, by suppressing the production of insulin, when other more standard agents have failed. *cis-Platinum* (*cis*-diamamine dichloroplatinum, DDP) consists of platinum coordination complexes which are a new class of cytotoxic agents. DDP is not cell cycle– or phase-specific and is capable of cross-linking DNA, although inactivation of DNA also occurs by other mechanisms. After intravenous administration, the initial half-life is 24 to 49 min, and the secondary half-life is 58 to 73 h. More than 90 percent of measured platinum appears to be protein-bound, and there is poor penetration into the central nervous system. During the first 5 days, 27 to 45 percent is excreted in the urine. From 50 to 75 mg/m^2 can be administered once every 3 weeks, or 15 to 20 mg/m^2 daily for 5 days every 3 to 4 weeks. In order to prevent dose-limiting renal toxicity, concomitant administration of intravenous fluids and mannitol, 37.5 to 60 g during a period of 6 to 8 h, with or without 40 mg furosemide, has been recommended. Its major toxic effects are gastrointestinal, renal, and ototoxic. Moderate myelosuppression may occur, and anaphylactic reactions, possibly related to DDP, have been reported.

ENDOCRINE THERAPY (See also Chaps. 126 and 127)

The first demonstration of hormonal control of breast cancer was made in 1896 by Beatson, who induced regression of metastatic tumor by ovariectomy. Since then, it has become obvious that other tumors such as those originating in the prostate and uterine endometrium may respond to hormonal manipulation. The original concept that all hormonal action was mediated by metabolic modification of circulating hormones in the target tissue has been completely superseded since the discovery that receptors which bind with estrogens exist in the cytosol of normal and malignant cells. The mechanism of interaction of hormones and receptors has been carefully studied; apparently hormones bind to receptors in the cytoplasm and sterically alter the shape of the receptor protein itself which, after transport to the cell nucleus, interacts with DNA and is responsible for initiating specific messenger RNA and protein synthesis. Following this interaction, cytoplasmic receptor concentration is restored and the cycle can be repeated. Estrogen receptors (ER) can be quantitated as 8-S and 4-S proteins. Values for estrogen receptor in primary tumors in humans range from 0 to almost 1000 fmol/mg cytosol protein. The adrenal corticosteroids are unique among the steroid hormones because they exert some antitumor effect in tissues not normally considered to be endocrine organs, such as the malignant cells in acute lymphatic leukemia. Receptors for corticosteroids have been identified in the cytosol of leukemic cells which, along with other nonspecific effects of the corticosteroids, probably explains their antitumor action. Receptors are also known to exist for progesterones and androgens.

Although prostate and uterine fundal cancers have been

shown to possess binding proteins for their respective hormones, the correlation between the frequency and quantity of binding proteins and the response to hormonal therapy has not been made. Hormonal agents useful in the management of these diseases are shown in Table 125-2.

ESTROGENS Although estrogens clearly have an antitumor effect, there is a risk of increased mortality from cardiovascular disease which may be related to an increase in production of renin substrate by the liver and subsequent hypertensive cardiovascular disease.

ANTIESTROGENS The discovery that certain estrogen analogues can antagonize estrogen stimulation of target tissue has been applied to the problem of breast cancer. Growth of dimethylbenzanthracene (DMBA) tumors in rodents can be inhibited by clomiphene and tamoxifen (Table 125-2). The ability of tamoxifen to cause regression of DMBA-induced tumors is highly correlated with the presence of estrogen receptors in the tumor. Antiestrogens have been found to bind to the estrogen receptor, translocate with the receptor into the nucleus, and initiate early estrogenic responses. A complete response to the complex apparently does not develop, and the genome remains refractory to the action of estrogens for a time. Some antiestrogens retain the receptor in the nucleus for many days in contrast to several hours for estrogens. Antiestrogens can effect a tumor response in patients who have estrogen-binding proteins in up to 60 percent of patients and have a lower incidence of troublesome side effects than estrogens. Virilization and fluid retention are uncommon with tamoxifen; the most common toxic effects noted are hot flashes, mild nausea, mild fluid retention, and, in a few instances, thrombocytopenia and leukopenia. With doses higher than are normally necessary (100 mg per day), corneal and retinal opacities have been observed.

ANDROGENS In older studies, androgen therapy is most effective in postmenopausal women with breast cancer, particularly those with osseous metastases. The effects of therapy are not seen for several weeks, but 90 percent of those responding will have begun to show a response within 8 weeks. All active androgens have been used with equal success. In comparative studies androgens have not been as effective as estrogens in the postmenopausal period except in patients with osseous metastases.

PROGESTINS Progestins are related to progesterone which is produced by the corpus luteum and placenta. They produce useful responses in 30 percent of women with metastatic endometrial carcinoma. Remissions may last for several years. The best results are seen in older women with well-differentiated tumors who have had a long interval between the appearance of the primary and recurrent disease. Useful responses are also seen in about 10 percent of patients with metastatic renal-cell carcinoma. Studies correlating response rates with the presence or absence of binding proteins for progestins have not been performed.

ADRENAL CORTICOSTEROIDS Prednisone is the adrenal corticosteroid most commonly used for antitumor therapy. It produces complete remission in about 60 percent of patients with lymphoblastic leukemia and partial responses in 70 percent of patients with chronic lymphocytic leukemia. It is also active against lymphomas and myeloma and in about 10 percent of patients with breast carcinoma. Responses in acute leukemia appear related to the presence of a specific corticosteroid-binding protein. In addition, adrenal corticosteroids suppress mitoses and cause lysis of normal and abnormal lymphocytic elements, presumably by inhibiting cellular protein synthesis. Their activity in breast carcinoma is presumed to be due to the suppression of estrogen production by the adrenal cortex.

MEDICAL ADRENALECTOMY An alternate method of ablating adrenal function is the use of aminoglutethamide, a potent inhibitor of the conversion of cholesterol to pregnanelone in the adrenal gland. It is given in a dose of 250 mg four times daily along with corticosteroid replacement. Since aminoglutethamide has been shown to accelerate the metabolism of dexamethasone, hydrocortisone 40 mg per day is the preferred steroid to use. With this approach, the response rate of patients with metastatic breast cancer has been equivalent to that reported after adrenalectomy. This regimen may be particularly useful in markedly debilitated women who have widespread bony metastases, in order to avoid surgical morbidity and mortality. Acute side effects of glutethamide, such as skin rash and lethargy, usually subside spontaneously, without cessation of therapy, and chronic therapy is remarkably free of side effects. Hypothyroidism occurs infrequently and can be managed by replacement therapy.

THYROID HORMONES Death from thyroid cancer occurs in less than 1000 patients per year in the United States, a figure that could easily be exceeded by surgical mortality if indiscriminate surgery for thyroid nodules were performed. Papillary carcinomas, even when metastatic to the neck, are often responsive to suppression of thyroid-stimulating hormone. Suppression of thyroid nodules presumed to be cancer, or suppressive therapy for patients with tumor in the thyroid or surrounding lymph nodes in the neck, is both indicated and effective (see Chap. 111).

IMMUNOTHERAPY AND THE USE OF BIOLOGICALS

Since the host's immunologic system may be involved in the control of malignant process, immunologic approaches to cancer treatment are under investigation. In order to achieve an effect from immunostimulation in rodents, maximum tumor reduction must be accomplished by surgery, radiation, or chemotherapy before immunotherapy is attempted. The host must be immunocompetent, and there may be an optimal, but as yet undefined, time following other treatment before immunotherapy is administered. Most antitumor agents are immunosuppressive, but as patients recover from the effects, their immunologic reactivity may be temporarily enhanced, and this could be the optimal time for immunotherapy. All immunotherapy is predicated on the identification of tumor-associated antigens on the cell surfaces of the tumor which can be used as the specific target for attack by immunocompetent cells or antibodies. Some examples of supposed tumor-specific antigens identified on human tumor tissue are due to the inadvertent measurement of fetal antigens, expressed by benign and malignant human cells grown in tissue culture. There are two main approaches to immunotherapy—passive and active. Passive immunotherapy involves the transfer of immune serum from syngeneic, allogeneic, or xenogeneic hosts into tumor-bearing host. Active nonspecific immunotherapy has been attempted with substances such as bacillus Calmette-Guérin (BCG), the methanol-extractable residue of BCG (MER), and *Corynebacterium parvum.* These substances augment both cellular and humoral immunity. Active specific immunotherapy consists of immunization of the host with tumor cells or cellular extracts. The greatest success has been achieved in animals by using live cells. Preimmunization prevents subsequent tumor transplantation in animals. Since most tumor-associated antigens are weak, attempts have been made to enhance their antigenicity by coupling the antigens with another substance. It has been possible to demonstrate cytotoxic antitumor antibodies in patients immunized in this fashion. The infusion of immune lymphocytes or their extracts into tumor-bearing hosts is known as *adoptive immunotherapy*. This approach has been used successfully in some animal tumors but not in humans.

Local immunotherapy utilizes delayed hypersensitivity reactions at the site of skin tumors. Local injection of BCG has eliminated skin tumors in animals. BCG injection into skin nodules in patients with recurrent breast cancer or melanoma is an effective way of controlling the local disease. The injection of BCG into the pleural space in patients with resectable epidermoid carcinoma of the lung has been shown to prevent or delay recurrence in one small controlled study. A larger clinical trial failed to confirm this observation. Delayed hypersensitivity has been produced in patients by cutaneous application of dinitrochlorobenzene. Subsequent application of this substance in superficial epidermoid and basal-cell carcinomas has a cure rate equal to topical chemotherapy with 5-fluorouracil. The macrophage plays an important role as a sensor cell in the modulation of the immunologic response to antigenic tumors in rodents. The macrophage also regulates other related physiological functions, such as granulocytopoiesis, through production of colony-stimulating factor. Studies aimed at stimulating macrophages are in progress with substances such as glucan, a polysaccharide product from yeast, and levamisole, an antiprotozoan drug that improves depressed lymphocyte function by stimulating macrophages. The early forms of immunotherapy have not produced antitumor responses comparable with other therapeutic modalities in patients with visible metastatic disease. Considerable additional investigation is necessary before the role of immunotherapy in the management of cancer can be defined.

With the development of new techniques such as the formation of hybridoma cells capable of forming highly specific monoclonal antibodies and the identification and purification of numerous lymphokines and thymus hormones, a more specific form of immunotherapy is under investigation. Agents like interferon, now produced by recombinant DNA techniques, and toxins and radioisotopes linked to highly specific antibodies, and purified thymosin fractions are already in clinical trials and showing some promising antitumor effects. These agents are referred to as biological-response modifiers.

PRINCIPLES OF DRUG COMBINATION DESIGN

The potential circumvention of resistance to treatment has been an important factor prompting studies of drug combinations. While phenotypic resistance to anticancer drugs can develop spontaneously, repetitive exposure of tumor cells to chemicals can also accelerate clinical resistance to drugs. This poses two problems—the regrowth of tumor cells between cycles of therapy and reduced tumor cell kill with subsequent cycles of drug treatment because of the evolution of resistant cell lines. Largely on the basis of experimental evidence, various mechanisms for the development of resistance have been proposed (Table 125-3). An effective drug may be required for each distinct line of cells until the number of viable cells can be reduced to zero or "effective zero" (small enough number of cells to be controlled, as with bacteria, by the host's own defense mechanisms). The success of drug treatment programs in rodents depends on the number of resistant lines in the tumor population and the number of available drugs that can be used effectively in combination. Pharmacological influences can be either advantageous or disadvantageous. The action of some drugs can be enhanced by other drugs with no antitumor effect by preventing the metabolic degradation of the active agent. The potential enhancement or depression of cyclophosphamide activity, by drugs that induce or inhibit the oxidative microsomal enzymes which convert the intact inactive parent compound into the 4-OH metabolite, has been recognized. Enhancement of the activity of 6-mercaptopurine by concomitant use of 4-hydroxypyrazolopyrimidine (allopurinol), which prevents its conversion into the inactive thiouric acid, and the prevention of deamination of arabinosyl cytosine and arabinosyl adenine by the ubiquitous deaminases present in serum and tissue by tetrahydrouridine and 2-deoxycorformycin, respectively, are additional examples of such drug interactions.

When drugs are used together in full doses, intermittent treatment at intervals of 2 to 4 weeks rather than continuous daily administration has been employed. Such an approach has two theoretical advantages. The first is that if the treatment programs exert a selective killing effect on tumor tissue over normal bone marrow, an interval of about 2 weeks is usually sufficient to allow recovery of bone marrow to pretreatment levels without allowing regrowth of the tumor population to base-line levels. The second advantage is that intermittent scheduling may permit the recovery of the host's immunologic mechanisms between cycles of chemotherapy.

The most important initial goal of the more intensive drug treatment programs is similar to the goals of surgery and radiation therapy for localized tumor—that is, to erase all clinical evidence of disease (complete remission). The length of time the patient remains free of disease after all therapy is discontinued is used as an indication of the magnitude of the reduction of tumor cell number. These indicators of successful treatment have been valid, and survival has improved commensurate with an increase in the rates and duration of complete remission for many metastatic cancers when drug combinations have been compared with single agents.

TUMOR MARKERS A major obstacle to curative therapy of malignancy is the difficulty of guiding the duration and intensity of further therapy by measuring the small amounts of residual disease presumed to be present, following surgical resection or drug-induced remission. Attempts are being made to identify tumor-specific products in blood and urine that might serve as markers of neoplastic growth. The use of hormones, enzymes, or other proteins as markers requires that their plasma or urine concentration exceed an established upper limit of normal. The so-called oncofetal antigens have the same limitation—they are present in detectable concentrations in

TABLE 125-3
Mechanisms of resistance to commonly used classes of antitumor agents

Mechanisms	*Examples*
Insufficient drug uptake by the neoplastic cell	Methotrexate Anthracyclines Actinomycin D
Insufficient activation of drug	6-Mercaptopurine 5-Fluorouracil Arabinosyl cytosine
Increased inactivation	Arabinosyl cytosine 5-Fluorouracil
Increased concentration of a target enzyme by induction or gene amplification	Methotrexate
Decreased requirement for a specific metabolic product	L-Asparaginase
Increased utilization of an alternative biochemical pathway (salvage)	Antimetabolites
Rapid enzymatic repair of a drug-induced lesion	Alkylating agents

normal adults. In contrast, placental hormones, such as human chorionic gonadotropin (HCG), are not found in the blood of males and nonpregnant females. A measurable level indicates an underlying neoplasm until proved otherwise.

Oncofetal antigens are products of gene expression during fetal tissue differentiation. When full tissue specialization and organization are reached, these genes are normally repressed and remain inoperative in adult life. With neoplastic transformation of a cell, there may be a reactivation of genomes and a reappearance of embryonic antigens. Three such antigens are now in clinical use: carcinoembryonic antigen (CEA), α-fetoprotein (AFP), and pancreatic oncofetal antigen (POA). The CEA is a glycoprotein of 200,000 daltons molecular weight which is secreted onto the glycocalyx surface of the cells that line the normal gastrointestinal tract. When first discovered, CEA was thought to be specific for the digestive organs of the 2- to 5-month-old human fetus and for patients with colorectal cancer. It has, however, been detected in the feces of normal adults as well as the secretions of the colon and pancreaticobiliary systems. Elevated CEA is also found in patients with benign liver disease, such as alcoholic hepatitis or biliary obstruction, as well as alcoholic pancreatitis and inflammatory bowel disease—in this instance, obviating its possible use as a detector of secondary neoplastic transformation. It has also been found in patients with benign rectal polyps and chronic obstructive pulmonary disease. There is no threshold difference in CEA levels that serves to separate benign from malignant conditions. Because of overall lack of specificity and sensitivity, CEA cannot be used as a general diagnostic test for cancer. The principal role of this tumor marker is as a monitor of the response to treatment. Complete surgical resection, or successful radiation or chemotherapy, should bring an elevated plasma level to normal within 1 month following treatment. A persistent elevation, or a progressively increasing titer, is strong, but not definitive, evidence of residual or recurrent tumor. Elevations of plasma CEA above the normal of 2.5 ng/ml in healthy nonsmoking adults have been found in association with a wide variety of malignancies and, in particular, the entodermally derived neoplasms of the gastrointestinal organs and lung in 60 to 90 percent of patients. Approximately 50 percent of women with advanced breast cancer also have an elevation in CEA concentration. The principal factors that influence the incidence of positive tests and the height of the titer include:

1 *The extent of disease.* Eighty to ninety percent of patients with advanced metastatic colon cancer compared with 20 to 40 percent of cases with tumor confined to the colon wall will have positive tests.
2 *The differentiation of the tumor.* A lower incidence of positive tests is associated with anaplastic histology.
3 *The presence of hepatic metastases.* They are frequently associated with an abrupt elevation of CEA resulting from either impaired catabolism or excretion of the glycoprotein.

The *α-fetoprotein* is a 70,000-dalton molecular weight protein with alpha-electrophoretic mobility. It is synthesized by the liver, yolk sac, and gastrointestinal tract of the human fetus, reaching a peak plasma concentration by the twelfth to fifteenth week of gestation. It then gradually decreases to reach a normal adult level by the sixth to twelfth month after birth. Elevations in the plasma concentration of AFP have been found in association with hepatoma, and titers in excess of 40 ng/ml are present in 70 to 90 percent of patients using sensitive radioimmunoassays. Abnormal levels are also detected with teratocarcinoma of the testes and ovary and in extragonadal sites, including the mediastinum and retroperitoneum. In these tumors, AFP is thought to be produced in yolk sac elements. Patients with seminomas and the corresponding dysgerminoma of the ovary have normal blood levels of AFP. Elevated AFP levels have also been detected in a small percentage of patients with pancreatic carcinoma, gastric cancer, and lung cancer. As with CEA, AFP is not a specific marker for malignancy, since abnormal titers are found in association with several benign conditions including viral and alcoholic hepatitis, ataxia telangiectasia, and hereditary tyrosinemia. The clinical application of this test is as a monitor for the effectiveness of anticancer treatment.

The pancreatic oncofetal antigen (POA) is a glycoprotein with a molecular weight of 800,000 daltons found in fetal and malignant pancreatic tissue but not in the normal pancreas. The index substance has, however, been detected in the blood of normal adults and in elevated concentrations in some patients with cancer of the lung, stomach, colon, and breast. The highest titers have been recorded in patients with pancreatic cancer, particularly those with well-differentiated histology.

Several placental proteins including HCG, human placental lactogen, and placental alkaline phosphatase (Reagan isoenzyme) have been demonstrated in cancer patients. Human chorionic gonadotropin is a glycoprotein hormone composed of dissimilar alpha and beta subunits; the alpha subunit is similar in primary structure to the alpha subunit of human luteinizing hormone, but sensitive radioimmunoassays of the beta subunit of HCG permit discrimination between the two hormones. Human chorionic gonadotropin is normally secreted by the trophoblastic epithelium of the placenta, and the presence of a detectable level in a male or a nonpregnant female is indicative of underlying tumor. In addition to the trophoblastic neoplasms of the placenta, the ectopic secretion of HCG has been found in 40 to 60 percent of patients with germ cell tumors, both gonadal or extragonadal, as well as in a smaller percentage of patients with adenocarcinoma of the ovary, pancreas, and stomach, hepatomas, and islet-cell carcinomas. Over 50 percent of patients with malignant insulinomas have elevations of HCG or one of its subunits; the hormone was not detected in association with benign adenomas. In patients with germ cell tumors secreting both HCG and AFP, discordant reduction after treatment suggests that the two markers are synthesized by heterogeneic clones of cells within the tumor.

The placental alkaline phosphatase is an isoenzyme synthesized in the trophoblast and is distinguished from other isoenzymes by heat stability (5 min at 65°C), electrophoretic mobility, and immunochemical specificity. Elevated placental alkaline phosphatase activity has been found in 5 to 15 percent of patients with cancer of the female reproductive organs, breast, and lung.

There are many tumors which, because of increased cellular mass and/or loss of the normal restraints on the rate of secretion, will produce excessive quantities of hormones or proteins that are normally produced by the cell of origin. Typical examples include the hypersecretion of insulin or gastrin by islet-cell neoplasms, the M spike in multiple myeloma, and the elevated serum acid phosphatase found in patients with prostatic carcinoma. There are many other tumors that will secrete index materials which are foreign to the cell or tissue of origin ectopically. In these instances, it is assumed that all somatic cells contain a full and equal genetic complement and that ectopic hormone secretion, after malignant transformation, results from the selected derepression of a previously dormant gene. The abnormally elevated plasma or urine concentration then allows this material to serve as an indirect tumor marker. Examples include the secretion of adrenocorticotropic hormone (ACTH), antidiuretic hormone, and calcitonin by small-cell carcinomas of the lung; ACTH, vasoactive intestinal polypeptide, serotonin, and HCG by islet-cell carcinomas; and ACTH and serotonin by medullary carcinomas of the thyroid. Over the past 10 years it has become apparent that peptide hormones exist in precursor forms that may have little or no bioactivity when compared with the predominant circulating hormones. Examples include increased concentrations of proinsulin in the diagnosis of insulinoma and elevated levels of pro- or "big" ACTH, without clinical Cushing's syndrome, in many patients with lung cancer independent of histology. This phenomenon and related observations had led some investigators to suggest that ectopic hormone protein or hormone secretion is a universal accompaniment of cancer.

TREATMENT OF LOCALIZED OR REGIONAL TUMOR

SURGICAL THERAPY Development of the radical mastectomy by Halsted in 1894 provided the most enduring influence on cancer surgery. Halsted believed that all cancer was unifocal in origin and spread to adjacent structures by direct contiguity; hence he conceived the idea of en bloc resection. Since then, the same surgical principle has been applied to operations for a wide variety of visceral malignancies, and survival has indeed improved. However, for many common cancers, survival, after surgery alone, reached a plateau by 1955. Increasingly radical surgery failed to provide additional benefits because even unifocal malignant tumors constantly shed cells even when tumor mass is below diagnostic levels. Cure after removal of the primary tumor alone, which certainly occurs, may seem inconsistent with persistent showering of tumor cells from all primary lesions. Current data, however, support three explanations for these events. (1) Only a fraction of cells in a tumor mass retain their capacity to create metastases (clonogenic cells); nonclonogenic cells may not continue to grow after they have been shed. (2) There is evidence that the host has the capacity to destroy small numbers of viable shed cells. (3) Tumor mass itself influences the tendency of tumors to metastasize and of the host to deal with residual microscopic metastases, with or without the help of systemic treatment. Surgery (and/or radiotherapy) of localized tumors may be effective because it reduces tumor volume, a source of clonogenic metastases, and in this way removes an adverse influence on the host defense mechanisms.

Surgery is considered the primary treatment for most early cancers (Table 125-4). However, in many patients the disease is not amenable to curative surgery. Many tumors are operable but not fully resectable, and some that appear resectable (control of T and N compartments, see Chap. 124) have micrometastatic disease which will grow to detectable size eventually. This point can best be illustrated using colon and breast carcinoma as examples. Involvement of lymph nodes in breast cancer (stage II) and colon cancer (Duke C) is associated with low 5-year survivals. Treatment failure occurs because of the presence of undetected micrometastases at the time of surgery. Increasingly radical surgery in both these cancers has been unable to provide additional benefit. Unlike surgical approaches to colon cancer, in breast cancer the visible mutilation of the radical mastectomy is significant. There is considerable evidence, however, that lesser surgical procedures, including segmental resection, give results as good as are obtained with radical or modified radical mastectomy, including survival. Most older data on the surgical management of primary breast cancer have been generated in uncontrolled trials. Reports of the controlled trials of the National Surgical Adjuvant Breast Program (NSABP) show that a total (simple) mastectomy is sufficient for patients in clinical stage 1 ($T_1N_0M_0$) and either total mastectomy, or total mastectomy plus radiotherapy, may be sufficient for patients in stage II ($T_1N_1M_0$).

Surgeons also perform procedures for staging purposes only, such as laparotomy in Hodgkin's disease and other lymphomas. Indications for use of these procedures vary with treatment options, and they should never be performed by the surgeon in vacuo, without prior consultation with the physician, or team of physicians, who will eventually be called upon to provide the definitive treatment.

Indications for more mutilating radical surgical procedures such as hemicorporectomy, pelvic exenteration, and radical head and neck surgery vary. They are offered to patients with locally advanced primary tumors or locally recurrent tumors for which no other means of controlling the regional tumor or systemic treatment is available. If the patient fully understands the degree of mutilation involved, a careful search reveals no metastases, the risk of recurrent disease is not unreasonable, and the operation is technically feasible, then the risks of mortality must be weighed against the chance of tumor control. These are very personal decisions shared by the patient, the family, and the physician. Significant advances in reconstructive surgery of the head, neck, and pelvic regions have been made, and greater availability of more acceptable prostheses may make these radical procedures more acceptable.

RADIATION THERAPY Radiation therapy is a regional form of treatment primarily evolved for the control of localized cancers. The ideal in radiation therapy of malignant disease is achieved when the tumor is completely eradicated and the surrounding normal tissues, in the treated volume, show little or no evidence of structural or functional injury. The important factor in successful treatment is the difference in radiosensitivity of neoplastic and normal cells. The difference depends on the capacity for intracellular repair of normal and neoplastic cells and the ability of normal organs to continue to function well if they are only segmentally damaged. If surrounding tissue can tolerate twice the radiation dose of a given tumor, then the tumor is radiosensitive. On the other hand, tumor which extensively involves both lungs, and may be cured by a dose of 30 Gy (3000 rads), cannot be treated effectively with radiation therapy because of the greater radiosensitivity of the surrounding lung tissue. As with normal tissue, however, different tumors have a range of radiosensitivity, some being responsive to as little as a few hundred rads, and others incurable with as much as 100 Gy (10,000 rads), and this variation can even exist within a specific tumor type.

Treatment with radiotherapy instead of surgery, using more sophisticated equipment, has the advantage of less mutilation and, where it provides equivalent results, is the preferred approach (Table 125-4). This choice will depend a great deal on the expertise in a given institution. For example, in the treatment of stage I carcinoma of the cervix, either modality provides equal survival rates. In localized carcinoma of the vocal cords, because radiotherapy has a high cure rate and spares the vocal cords, it is preferred to surgery. In carcinoma of the prostate, with stages A and B, radiotherapy produces survival figures at least equivalent to surgery, with far less risk of impotence, and is the preferred approach. In carcinoma of the rectum below the peritoneal reflection, radiotherapy alone in small, nonulcerated, and superficial lesions is quite effective in controlling the tumors; radiotherapy can improve survival figures when used in conjunction with surgery in patients with rectal cancer with more extensive disease. In patients with localized Hodgkin's disease (stages I and II) radiotherapy is the treatment of choice, with 5- and 10-year disease-free survivals achievable in 80 percent of such patients. In lymphocytic and histiocytic lymphomas cures are possible in the small number of patients with truly localized disease.

In some cases the routine use of radiotherapy as an adjunct to surgery should be avoided. Postoperative treatment of the chest wall and lymph node areas in carcinoma of the breast

TABLE 125-4

Role of available treatment modalities in *localized* and *regional* forms of some visceral and hematologic malignancies

Original cancer	*Surgery**	*Radiotherapy*	*Chemotherapy*	*Immunotherapy*
Breast:				
Stage I	P	Alt	ND	ND
Stage II	P	Alt	P	E
Ovary:				
Stage I	P	Adj,E‡	E	ND
Stage II	P	Adj,E	Adj	E
Uterine fundus	P	Adj	ND	ND
Uterine cervix:				
In situ	P	P	NU	NU
Stage I	P	P	NU	NU
Stage II	P	P	E	ND
Choriocarcinoma	Adj	NU	P	ND
Lung:				
Small (oat) cell	NU	Adj,E	P	E
Epidermoid	P	Adj	E	Adj,E
Adenocarcinoma	P	Adj	E	E
Gastrointestinal:				
Colon	P	NU	E	E
Rectum	P	Alt, Adj	E	E
Stomach	P	Adj	Adj	ND
Pancreas	P	Adj	E	ND
Melanoma:				
Stage I	P	NU	NU	E
Stage II	P	NU	E	E
Other skin cancers	P	P	P	P
Head and neck	P	P	E	E
Thyroid:				
Papillary	P	Adj‡	P§	NU
Follicular	P	Adj‡	P‡	NU
Anaplastic	Adj	P	Adj,E	ND
Testes:				
Seminoma:				
Stage I	P	P	ND	ND
Stage II	Alt	P	ND	ND
Embryonal and teratocarcinoma:				
Stage I	P	Adj,E	ND	ND
Stage II	P	Adj,E	P	ND
Choriocarcinoma	P	NU	P	ND
Prostate	P	Alt	E	ND
Bladder:				
Papillomas	P	Alt	Alt	E
Others	P	Alt	E	E
Kidney	P	Adj	ND	ND
Brain	P	Alt	E	E
Tumors of childhood:				
Wilms's tumor	P	Adj	P	ND
Neuroblastoma	P	Adj	E	E
Ewing's sarcoma	Alt	P	P	E
Rhabdomyosarcoma	P	Alt,E	P	E
Lymphomas:				
Hodgkin's disease:				
Stage I	NU	P	Adj	ND
Stage II	NU	P	Adj	ND
Stage III	NU	Alt	P	ND
Lymphocytic:				
Stage I	NU	P	ND	ND
Stage II	NU	P	E	E
Stage III	NU	Alt	P	E
Histiocytic:				
Stage I	NU	P	Adj	ND
Stage II	NU	P	Alt	ND
Stage III	NU	Alt	P	ND
Mycosis fungoides	NU	P	P	E
Solitary plasmacytomas	Alt	P	Alt	ND

* *For purposes of this table, diagnostic biopsy is not considered treatment when used prior to an alternate method of treatment.*
† *For premenopausal women only.*
‡ *Radioisotopes.*
§ *In the form of thyroid suppression of TSH production.*
NOTE: *P = Considered an integral part of standard primary treatment programs. Alt = An alternate, although less commonly used, method of primary treatment for which data are already available indicating results equivalent to more common approaches. Adj = Use as adjunctive therapy after localized tumor is treated by a primary method; routine use is not considered essential. E = Experimental; role in treatment is under examination in controlled clinical trials. Either a new approach to treatment or an older approach which, in the absence of sufficient data to support its frequent use, is being evaluated in controlled clinical trials. In the latter case, treatment is designated Alt,E. NU = Current information indicates no role in primary treatment program. Control rate of tumor in question may be sufficiently high with other forms of treatment as to preclude testing of this modality. ND = No data available to evaluate this form of treatment.*

after radical mastectomy adds nothing to the results of surgery, does not improve survival, but does cause significant morbidity. Since local recurrences rarely happen in the absence of systemic metastases, and local recurrences can be controlled, when they occur, by radiotherapy or drug treatment, routine postoperative radiotherapy regardless of the location of the primary tumor cannot be recommended in breast cancer. Radiotherapy alone in stage IIB carcinoma of the ovary (limited to the pelvis) should be discouraged since further drug therapy is usually required. Its use as the primary treatment in stage III ovarian cancer (widespread intraabdominal disease) is also contraindicated. Routine radiotherapy in lung cancer has been ineffective, except in rare instances, although it may complement the increasingly effective drug treatment of small-cell carcinoma. The use of routine retroperitoneal radiotherapy after lymphadenectomy for testicular cancer is questionable except in patients with seminomas where even metastatic lesions can be controlled by radiotherapy. Routine preoperative or postoperative therapy of stage I uterine fundal cancer may not offer additional benefit to surgery.

TREATMENT OF ADVANCED CANCER

The most important aspect of cancer chemotherapy trials conducted in the 1960s, and realized in the early 1970s, was the demonstration that drugs could cure patients with advanced cancer. Considering the volume of cancer cells now known to be present in such patients, this presented a formidable challenge. For reasons that are not yet clear, the most effectively treated cancers are those that occur less often and in younger persons.

Cancers can be generally grouped into categories according to the effectiveness of systemic treatment. Table 125-5 lists 12 types of cancer for which current chemotherapeutic programs can render a fraction of patients with metastatic tumor free of disease long enough to be considered cured. Exclusive of skin cancer, which is treated when localized, the numerical impact of therapy on a national mortality ratio from cancer is relatively small since the diseases listed make up only 10 percent of all patients with cancer and 8 percent of all cancer deaths. Successful application of the best available treatment programs, however, can save approximately 15,000 lives per year. Although most of these tumors are not common, they occur at a relatively young age, and their impact in person-years of life or person-years of work lost is larger than their numerical impact suggests. Although in some cases (choriocarcinoma and Burkitt's tumor) excellent results are achievable with highly effective single drugs, in most cases cures are achievable only by drug combinations. The unique feature of the survival curves in these diseases is the long flat tail indicating disease-free survival beyond the high-risk period of recurrence, after therapy is discontinued, as illustrated in advanced diffuse histiocytic lymphoma (reticulum-cell sarcoma, Fig. 125-5). In Hodgkin's disease, acute childhood leukemia, diffuse histiocytic lymphoma, and testicular tumors disease-free survival after cessation of treatment extends to over 10 years. Considering the tumor volume in most of these patients at the time of treatment ($\pm 10^{11}$ cells), these results are quite remarkable. The break in the survival curve varies for each disease. A 2-year disease-free interval from the end of treatment is sufficient to consider patients with such virulent, rapidly growing tumors as choriocarcinoma, Burkitt's lymphoma, and diffuse histiocytic lymphoma cured, while four or more years is necessary to evaluate the results of treatment in Hodgkin's disease, acute childhood leukemia, and testicular cancer. Widespread use of these treatment programs has already resulted in a decrease in national mortality in all patients with Hodgkin's disease, in acute leukemia in children less than 15 years of age, and in renal and bone tumors of children. In ovarian carcinoma, a small fraction of patients with advanced intraabdominal tumor (stage III) remain free of disease over long periods after successful treatment with alkylating agents. Earlier use of chemotherapy holds promise in this disease. Slow but steady progress is being made in the treatment of acute myelocytic leukemia. The complete remission rate attainable with drug combinations is now in excess of 50 percent, and more than 10 percent of treated patients survive, free of disease, without any therapy, beyond 5 years of treatment with minimal risk of recurrence. The improvement in recent years is coincident with the identification of arabinosyl cytosine and adriamycin as active agents in this disease and appreciation of the schedule dependency of arabinosyl cytosine. Retreatment of patients who have been in remission for 2 years (late intensification) holds promise of the control of the cellular phase of the disease.

In Table 125-6, the cancers listed make up 26 percent of all tumors in the United States and an equal percentage of all cancer deaths. In each of the tumor types listed it is possible to achieve sufficient responses to chemotherapy to prolong life of a fraction of these patients and palliate the majority of the rest. In most examples cited, however, the complete remission rate is low, and long disease-free survivals are uncommon when treatment is discontinued. Although drug combinations used in metastatic breast cancer have not yielded long disease-free survivals, for the first time patients treated with many current drug combinations are able to attain complete remissions. Furthermore, these programs have been successfully applied in patients with minimal residual disease (stage II) postoperatively.

Tumors listed in Table 125-7 are frequently thought of as resistant to treatment, but significant palliation can be provided for most patients by the careful use of existing chemotherapeutic agents by an experienced physician. Although studies of large groups of patients with these diseases have not revealed improvement in average survival, a small number of patients with each of these tumors can experience long disease-free survival as a result of the meticulous use of chemotherapy.

FIGURE 125-5

Survival in advanced diffuse histiocytic lymphomas treated with combination chemotherapy. Patients who achieve a complete remission relapse uncommonly. The high-risk period of relapse is the first 2 years after treatment. Patients with partial responses, even if they are associated with greater than 75 percent reduction of tumor volume, rarely survive beyond 2 years.

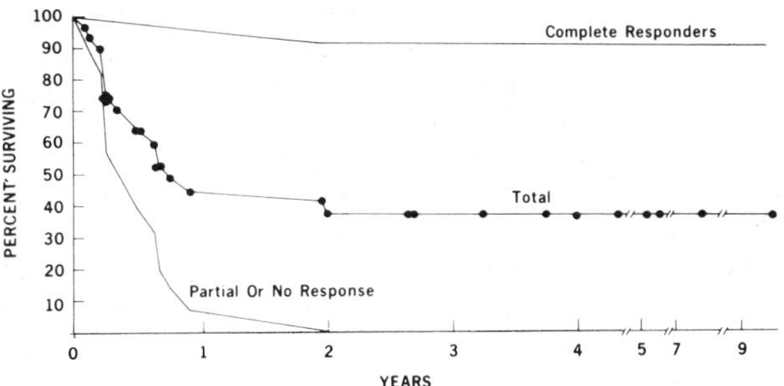

Of particular interest is the identification of the usefulness of methotrexate, bleomycin, and the investigational agent, *cis*-diamine dichloroplatinum, in combination, in patients with cancer of the head and neck. This approach offers particular

TABLE 125-5
Advanced cancers curable by chemotherapy*

Diseases	*Complete remission rates, %*	*Comments*
Acute lymphoblastic leukemia of childhood	90	80% of null-cell and 50% of all patients remain free of disease > 10 years.
Hodgkin's disease, stages III and IV	80	65% of cell complete responders and 90% of asymptomatic patients remain disease-free at 10 years.
Diffuse histiocytic lymphomas, stages III and IV	50	80% of complete responders remain disease-free at 10 years.
Nodular mixed lymphomas	75	80% of complete responders remain disease-free off all therapy beyond 10 years.
Testicular carcinoma (exclusive of seminomas)	75	70% of complete responders remain disease-free beyond 3 years.
Ovarian carcinoma, stages III and IV	35	Half of complete responders remain disease-free as long as 10 years.
Acute myelocytic leukemia	60	20% of complete responders living without recurrences, off therapy, beyond 5 years.
Choriocarcinoma	90	Almost all complete responders remain free of tumor; longest follow-up 20 years.
Burkitt's lymphoma	90	Half of complete responders remain free of recurrences beyond 10 years.
Wilms's tumor		Primary treatment is multimodal. Surgery, radiation, and chemotherapy together now produce 80% cure rate. Latest data indicate surgery and chemotherapy alone can do the same.
Ewing's sarcoma		Primary treatment is multimodal. Use of radiation and chemotherapy produces relapse-free survival in two-thirds of patients at 5 years.
Embryonal rhabdomyosarcoma		Primary therapy is multimodal. Surgery, radiation, and chemotherapy produce disease-free survival in 60% of patients at 5 years.

* *Cancers on this list occurred approximately 53,800 times in 1980. In 39,300 instances, patients had visible metastatic disease. Currently available chemotherapy, mostly given as combinations of drugs, can render one-third to one-half of the patients with metastatic disease free of tumor for periods long enough to consider these patients cured of their tumor. The results listed in this table represent best available data from centers studying these diseases. Because of the availability and effectiveness of systemic treatment in some of the cancers listed, all effective treatments have been integrated into the primary treatment plan (multimodal primary treatment). Skin cancer is not included since it rarely metastasizes. It occurs approximately 300,000 times per year and is highly treatable with topical chemotherapy.*

promise because it may prevent recurrences and allow the use of less radical surgical procedures in this critical area of the body. In colon cancer, controlled studies have demonstrated a doubling of the response rate of patients who have metastatic disease when treated with the combination of 5-FU and MeCCNU when compared with the use of 5-FU alone. The nitrosoureas are a useful adjunct to radiotherapy and surgery in patients with the malignant gliomas, with a doubling of median survival time of patients so treated.

Surgery has an increasingly important role in the treatment of patients with advanced metastatic cancer. Surgery is important to reduce tumor bulk and facilitate the use of drugs or immunotherapy. This may involve removal of a primary tumor when metastases are known to be present (renal-cell carcinoma) or reduction of the bulk of retroperitoneal and mesenteric lymph nodes in testicular and bowel tumors, and mesenteric metastases in ovarian cancer. Not to be overlooked is the surgical attack on metastases in patients who are otherwise doing well. Seemingly solitary brain metastases should be removed surgically, if possible, particularly in young people, since the likelihood of rapid demise without such treatment is high and occasional long-term control is possible. Pulmonary metastases of a variety of sarcomas have been successfully controlled surgically even when multiple nodules are present. Some of these patients have remained free of recurrent disease for periods in excess of 2 years with surgery alone. This has been true particularly in patients whose tumors can be shown to have long doubling times prior to operation. These studies have added significance with the recent development of more effective systemic treatment of sarcomas which can be used following surgery to supplement tumor bulk reduction. Removal of metastases to the lungs is important in patients with testicular tumors because of the histological heterogeneity of this tumor and the likelihood that a metastasis has resulted from growth of a clone of a histological type resistant to the drugs employed.

Surgeons are often asked to provide palliation for patients incurable by any modality. The operative risks are often high and the therapeutic yield, from the surgical point of view, low, but considerations of comfort and ability to return home during the terminal months of illness may make such procedures worthwhile. Palliation should be considered, for example, in intestinal obstruction in ovarian and pancreatic cancer, gastrointestinal bleeding, urinary diversions, and relief of pain through neurosurgical procedures. The primary physician is often in the best position to make the decision as to the feasibility of such palliative procedures.

TABLE 125-6
Malignant diseases which, when widely disseminated, respond sufficiently to systemic treatment that the lives of responding patients are prolonged greater than 1 year*

Carcinoma of the breast
Multiple myeloma
Lymphocytic lymphoma
Prostatic carcinoma
Adrenal cortical carcinoma
Malignant insulinoma
Small-cell (oat-cell) carcinoma of the lung
Sarcoma of soft tissue
Endometrial carcinoma
Malignant carcinoid tumors
Neuroblastoma
Chronic lymphocytic leukemia
Chronic myelocytic leukemia

* *In most examples cited, systemic chemotherapy is able to induce a variable fraction of complete remissions, but eventually most patients who responded completely develop recurrent tumors. Cancers on this list occurred about 120,000 times in the United States in 1980.*

Radiotherapy can also be used to reduce tumor bulk in patients with metastatic disease and decrease the extent of any surgical procedure that might be used in addition. Examples are radiation therapy following lumpectomy in breast cancer and in conjunction with surgery in head and neck, and rectal cancers. In highly radiosensitive tumors, radiotherapy may be used to reduce tumor bulk in patients with advanced metastatic cancers whose primary treatment is with drugs, as in patients with lymphomas. Prophylactic use of radiotherapy to treat the brain and meninges before disease is evident has been successful as an ancillary method to drug treatment and has resulted in prolonged disease-free survival in children with acute leukemia and Ewing's sarcoma and in oat-cell carcinoma of the lung.

Palliative radiotherapy has many applications in patients with metastatic cancer. In emergency situations, it can be used to provide rapid relief of superior mediastinal obstruction in conjunction with drugs or to relieve ureteral obstruction in patients with lymphomas or testicular tumors which are drug-resistant. It can provide frequent and useful relief of bone pain and may prevent fracture if used prophylactically to treat lesions of weight-bearing bones. In these cases the primary treatment is usually with drugs, and radiation fields should be only as large as required to control the lesion in question. For lytic lesions of weight-bearing bones greater than 2.5 cm in diameter, especially those involving the cortex, prophylactic internal fixation, followed by radiation therapy, is the treatment of choice. Radiation of the brain and spinal cord are important examples of palliation which, when used early and effectively, can prevent catastrophic neurological incapacitation in the final months of illness.

MULTIMODAL PRIMARY (ADJUVANT) TREATMENT

A major reduction in national mortality rates from many of the major cancers appears likely only if current drug programs are markedly improved and applied in the postoperative period to the treatment of those patients who develop recurrences after surgery or radiotherapy. Such programs should have the added benefit of stimulating the investigation of less-mutilating surgical approaches. Considerations of biology of tumor growth and the importance of tumor cell number to the dose-response curves of both radiation and chemical treatment serve as the rationale for the use of more than one modality in the perioperative period. The four most important considerations in the development of drug programs for post- or perioperative use are the following: (1) the identification of populations of patients who, even after optimal surgery or radiotherapy for their primary disease, have a high risk of recurrence and death from their cancer (e.g., stage II breast cancer, Duke C colon cancer); (2) the availability of a proven useful systemic form of treatment; (3) the weighing of the potential benefits of treatment against short- and long-term risks of added drug treatment, keeping in mind that a fraction of patients exposed to adjuvant drug treatment would not have developed recurrent tumor; and (4) proper study design. Since the reduction of measurable tumor is not possible during adjuvant studies, few can be accepted unless comparisons of treated groups are made with untreated controls, or the risk of recurrence is known to be very high and is spread over so narrow a time frame as to obviate the need for concurrent controls. In the latter case, historical controls may suffice. An example of a tumor requiring controls in adjuvant studies is stage II ($T_1N_1M_0$) melanoma. Sex, site, level of invasion of the primary, and degree of nodal involvement all affect not only the risk but the time of recurrence, which may be spread over periods of a few months to several years.

The most difficult question is the level of effectiveness required of systemic therapy in patients with advanced metastatic tumor before it is feasible to use it in an adjuvant program. There is uncertainty whether drugs which are apparently inactive against advanced cancer are potentially useful against a small number of cancer cells present in the postoperative period when tumor growth characteristics, sensitivity to chemotherapy, and therefore vulnerability to drugs may be different. Clinical studies have shown that changes in measurements of tumor masses in patients with metastatic disease are sufficiently variable that response rates of 10 percent or less in drug-treated patients should be considered "biological noise." Presently, only single agents or combinations of drugs with response rates of 20 percent or more can be considered acceptable for postoperative drug programs. The attractiveness of a candidate drug program is enhanced considerably if a significant fraction of treated patients attain complete rather than partial responses since complete disappearance of visible tumor indicates a greater log reduction in the number of tumor cells.

In Hodgkin's disease, the fact that radiotherapy for localized tumor and combination chemotherapy for advanced disease have worked so well has led to studies of both used together in patients with regional tumor only (chemotherapy as an adjuvant to radiotherapy) and in advanced tumors to reduce tumor bulk (radiotherapy as an adjuvant to chemotherapy). In localized diffuse histiocytic (reticulum-cell sarcoma) and lymphocytic lymphomas, recurrence of tumor outside the radiation field is common when radiation therapy is used alone. In diffuse histiocytic lymphoma, the fraction of patients with advanced cancer (stages III and IV) achieving long disease-free survivals with drug combinations is often equivalent to that achieved by radiotherapy alone in patients with localized tumor and has led to their combined use in early stages of disease.

Childhood neoplasms are quite responsive to all forms of treatment. Chemotherapy with dactinomycin as an adjuvant to both radiotherapy and surgery has increased the 2-year survival in patients with Wilms's tumor from 43 to 92 percent. Tumor recurrences after this time are unusual. Similar results can be achieved with surgery and chemotherapy only, obviating the need for radiotherapy and avoiding its growth-retarding effect on bones. Similar results have been achieved with embryonal rhabdomyosarcoma. Adjuvant chemotherapy with high-dose methotrexate and citrovorum factor rescue and/or adriamycin in patients with osteogenic sarcoma has reduced the recurrence rate in the first 2 years in this virulent tumor of adolescence.

Many drug combinations have been tried in advanced breast cancer. Several are being tested as a means to prevent metastases in the postoperative period. One combination of cyclophosphamide, methotrexate, and 5-fluorouracil (CMF) has been compared with melphalan in patients with metastatic breast cancer and found to be superior. CMF has been reported to produce a statistically significant 57 percent reduction in recurrence rate when used as adjuvant treatment in premenopausal women with stage II carcinoma of the breast in controlled trials. CMF treatment has also resulted in a significant 20 percent reduction in mortality after 4 years of follow-up. The enhanced capacity of the combination of MeCCNU, 5-FU, and vincristine in inducing remissions in stomach and colon cancer has led to the design of several large studies comparing their effectiveness to untreated or 5-FU–treated controls in patients with operable stomach cancer and Duke C colon cancer. The dramatic increase in the complete remission rates in patients with testicular tumors, treated with bleomycin, *cis*-platinum, and vinblastine, coupled with the precision in detecting residual tumor cells provided by tumor markers in this disease, has led to the routine use of these drugs following surgery in patients with retroperitoneal node disease with highly successful results.

The sequencing of chemotherapy and radiation therapy has varied from site to site with the use of radiotherapy before, during, and after chemotherapy. It is apparent that there has been little or no consistency in the approach, and the limit of tolerance to radiotherapy of normal tissue, not the ability to control tumor, has been used as a guide to therapy. Further research is needed to determine whether combinations of radiation and drugs are additive, synergistic, or inhibitory. Changes in proliferative capacity of tumors after radiation may negatively influence their response to cycle-active drugs. Chemotherapy has been used before radiotherapy in locally inoperable breast cancer with some success. The results of simultaneous chemotherapy and radiotherapy have been difficult to evaluate, and except for glioblastoma multiforme, where some beneficial effect on survival has been observed, this approach is not now standard treatment for any cancer.

COMPLICATIONS OF THERAPY

Acute side effects and other toxicities of chemotherapeutic agents are listed in Table 125-1. Each side effect must be weighed against the potential benefit to be derived. In a highly treatable disease it is rare that nausea, vomiting, and temporary hair loss should be considered significant enough side effects to withhold treatment. Patients must be apprised of all the risks involved both in using therapy and in withholding it. Many chemicals are carcinogenic to some degree, and anticancer drugs and radiotherapy are no exception. The opportunity to identify this risk has only come about following the advent of successful treatment of patients with metastatic cancer as long disease-free intervals provide the necessary follow-up time. Used alone, single drugs or combinations of drugs have not yielded rates of secondary tumors higher than expected following the diagnosis of the primary diseases alone. Radiation treatment is known to be carcinogenic, but the risk when used alone is relatively low in a given treatment field. Combinations of drugs and x-rays, however, may be associated with a higher risk of second malignancies such as acute myelogenous leukemia and other tumors in the radiation field. This has been noted in long-term survivors of Hodgkin's disease who receive both combination chemotherapy (MOPP) and radiation ther-

TABLE 125-7
Malignant diseases which, when widely disseminated, respond to chemotherapy, but, although palliation is often provided, response to drugs in such patients after treatment has not yet been shown to prolong their lives*

Epidermoid carcinomas of the head and neck region
Carcinoma of the colon
Carcinoma of the stomach
Brain tumors
Malignant melanoma
Hypernephromas
Carcinoma of the bladder
Hepatocellular carcinoma
Undifferentiated thyroid cancer
Carcinoma of the cervix uteri
Osteosarcomas
Carcinoma of the penis

* *Complete remissions are uncommon. It should be noted that the treatment programs producing marginal response in these patients, when they have metastatic disease, offer attractive opportunities to test the use of these drugs as adjuvant chemotherapy when the tumor volume is smaller.*

apy. In one study it is estimated that patients treated with both extensive radiation therapy and MOPP chemotherapy may have an incidence of acute myelocytic leukemia between 5 and 10 percent within 10 years. Long-term survivors of patients with Wilms's tumors who receive both radiation and drug therapy have also had a high incidence of secondary malignancies in the radiation treatment field. In addition there is some evidence that long-term exposure to alkylating agents, particularly melphalan, in patients with otherwise normal bone marrows may be associated with late marrow dysplasia which may eventuate in acute myelocytic leukemia. These potential risks are particularly germane to the use of these drugs in adjuvant treatment programs.

The physician should be familiar with normal tissue tolerance for radiation and the acute and late effects. Acute radiation effects are largely on the cell-renewal tissues—skin, oropharyngeal mucosa, small intestine, rectum, bladder mucosa, and vaginal mucosa. Acute radiation effects such as skin reactions, weight loss, nausea and vomiting, mucositis, and blood count depression may appear during or near the end of treatment and usually are reversible. Others, such as pneumonitis, may not appear until several weeks or months later and then resolve. Since the effect on rapid-cell-renewal tissues will be dependent on the balance between cell birth and cell death, it will be crucially affected by the time allowed for repopulation. It will also be dependent on the cell kill per fraction. Therefore, fraction size will be important. The radiotherapist frequently observing the oral mucosa and seeing an excessive reaction knows that a small decrease in fraction size or a small treatment break may allow rapid resolution of the problem since these changes will permit reconstitution of the normal tissue.

Late effects are the dose-limiting effect in radiation therapy, often progress with time, and are usually irreversible. These include necrosis, fibrosis, fistula formation, nonhealing ulceration, and damage to specific organs such as spinal cord transection or blindness. Normal tissues and organs differ in radiosensitivity. The risk of complication increases with dose and, if delivered by megavoltage sources, in the usual fractions, occurs when the dose exceeds the following: both lungs 15 Gy (1500 rads); both kidneys 24 Gy (2400 rads); liver 30 Gy (3000 rads); heart 35 Gy (3500 rads); spinal cord 40 Gy (4000 rads); intestine 55 Gy (5500 rads); brain 60 Gy (6000 rads); bone 75 Gy (7500 rads). While the mechanisms of late toxicity are not clear, they do not appear to depend primarily on the rapid proliferation of a cell-renewal tissue. Clinically they appear to be much more dependent on the total dose of radiation and the size of the radiation fraction. Only if the same fractionation scheme is used with the same normal tissue end point, the same volume irradiated, and the same treatment technique can acute and late effects be correlated. If any of these parameters are varied the acute reactions to radiation may be dissociated from eventual late effects. Rather than serve as a guide, these acute reactions then will be misleading. There are a number of examples in radiation therapy where the total dose has been increased, the fraction size increased or kept the same, but the time has been protracted to minimize acute effects. Such maneuvers have resulted in unacceptable late complications.

There are two hypotheses for the mechanism of late radiation effects. One theory holds that all late effects are due to damage to vasculoconnective tissue stroma. A variation on this hypothesis is that damage to the endothelial cells determines late effects. An alternate hypothesis suggests that both the acute and the late effects of radiation and cytotoxic chemotherapy are due to depletion of the major target cell-renewal tissues. Acute effects depend on the balance between cell killing and compensatory cellular replication of both the stem and proliferative compartments. The development of late effects requires that stem cells have only a limited proliferative capacity. Compensation for extensive or repeated cell killing may exhaust this capacity, resulting in eventual tissue failure.

Chemical and radiation therapy produce sterilization in both sexes which may be reversible but often is not. If reversible at all, the time necessary for reversal may be several years. Anticancer drugs are teratogenic. It should never be assumed that chemotherapy and radiotherapy themselves are sufficient methods of birth control. All patients in the childbearing age treated with radiation or drugs should be fully informed of the risks and advised about contraception. When pregnancy occurs during chemotherapy or exposure to radiotherapy, abortion should be considered if the pregnancy is discovered in the first trimester, because of the high risk of teratogenesis. Treatment of women who develop tumors while pregnant is best withheld until delivery, which may need to be hastened. Chemotherapy can be used safely in the third trimester, but because of the uncertain long-term effects on the fetus, should not be employed unless the situation is critical.

SUPPORTIVE CARE

ANEMIA The first manifestation of malignant disease may be anemia; it is present in 60 percent of patients with disseminated cancer. The peripheral iron profile is similar to that found in chronic infection or inflammation with a low serum iron and iron-binding capacity. Iron stores are normal. The most characteristic anemia is due to both increased destruction of red blood cells and inadequate compensatory erythropoiesis. Other causes of anemia are blood loss, hemolysis, and myelophthisis. Both warm and cold autoimmune hemolytic anemias occur in patients with lymphomas and chronic leukemias, and less frequently in other cancers. Adrenal corticosteroids usually control "warm" autoimmune hemolytic anemia. Splenectomy is often beneficial and should be considered if treatment of the primary disease is ineffective. Radiation of the spleen is simple but rarely effective. Except in cases of blood loss, autoimmune hemolytic anemia, and vitamin deficiencies, there is no specific therapy for the anemia of cancer. Most patients will remain asymptomatic if their hemoglobin is maintained above 8 g/dl with transfusions.

HEMORRHAGE Tumor invasion of blood vessels, thrombocytopenia, and disseminated intravascular coagulation are the major causes of hemorrhage in patients with cancer. Occasional patients with a normal or excessive number of platelets bleed because of defective platelet function. In thrombocytopenic patients, life-threatening hemorrhage is unusual unless the platelet count falls below 20,000 per milliliter or unless additional coagulation defects are present. The routine use of platelet transfusions in severely thrombocytopenic patients has reduced fatal hemorrhage by over 50 percent. Platelets may be obtained by plasmapheresis of normal random donors. Platelets obtained from histocompatible donors, using HLA and mixed lymphocyte culture typing techniques, are more useful when prolonged periods of platelet support are required. Disseminated intravascular coagulation has been described in many patients with several types of cancer. The process is probably initiated by the release of thromboplastic substances from cancer cells as blood passes over poorly endothelialized surfaces of tumors. Most patients with cancer can be shown to have increased levels of fibrin degradation products without evidence of hemorrhage. Patients with acute promyelocytic leukemia often bleed, especially after treatment is initiated, owing to release of thromboplastin-like material. Heparin therapy may be useful before treatment to prevent hemorrhage. Except in this instance, heparin is almost never indicated in cancer patients with intravascular coagulation.

INFECTION Fever occurs in 70 percent of hospitalized patients with cancer and is usually due to infection. Local factors such as obstruction to normal drainage or recent surgery play a prominent role in infections occurring in patients with metastatic carcinoma, particularly those involving the lung. Patients undergoing cancer chemotherapy are especially susceptible to infectious complications because they develop neutropenia and impairment of normal host-defense mechanisms (Chap. 137). Patients with chronic lymphocytic leukemia and multiple myeloma have decreased levels of normal immunoglobulins and respond inadequately to antigenic stimuli. They are particularly susceptible to infections by *Streptococcus pneumoniae*. Patients with generalized Hodgkin's disease characteristically have impaired cellular immunity and are particularly susceptible to infections caused by fungi (*Cryptococcus*) and viruses. Herpes zoster occurs in 10 percent of patients with Hodgkin's disease. The incidence increases to 20 percent if the spleen has been removed during staging. The majority of infections occurring in cancer patients are caused by gram-negative bacilli, especially *Escherichia coli, Klebsiella,* and *Pseudomonas aeruginosa. Bacteroides* infections are sometimes overlooked. However, organisms of low pathogenicity, such as *Bacillus* spp., *Staphylococcus epidermidis,* and *Flavobacterium* spp., may cause fatal infections in some neutropenic patients. Hence, all organisms cultured from the blood or sites of infection should be considered as possible etiologic agents. Sepsis due to encapsulated cocci is increased in lymphoma patients who have undergone splenectomy and received both combination chemotherapy and radiotherapy. Prophylactic treatment with penicillin or vaccination with the pneumococcal vaccine may be useful, especially in patients under 10 years of age. Fungal infections, particularly with *Candida* and *Aspergillus* species, are major problems in patients with hematologic malignancies and are increasing in frequency. Pneumocystis pneumonia has been recognized increasingly in patients with a wide variety of malignant diseases and may occur in small epidemics. It is the most common cause of infectious death in leukemic children while in remission. A peculiar association of infection with cytomegalovirus and immunosuppression leading to a high incidence of Kaposi's sarcoma and death from pneumocystis pneumonia has been described in homosexual men.

Many patients are neutropenic when they develop infection. In these patients infection may be rapidly fatal if not treated promptly. Often, the classic signs and symptoms of infection are absent. Infections due to *Pseudomonas* are the most common cause of death from bacterial infections in cancer hospitals. The best initial antibiotic regimen is carbenicillin or ticarcillin, gentamicin or tobramycin and a penicillinase-resistant penicillin or a cephalosporin. However, the effectiveness of aminoglycoside antibiotics is somewhat reduced in neutropenic patients. Granulocyte transfusions are beneficial for the treatment of infections in neutropenic patients, whose bone marrow function is not expected to return to normal for more than 2 weeks, although adverse reactions to white blood cell transfusions are frequent. Histocompatibility typing of donors and recipients holds promise in increasing their effectiveness and reducing the incidence and severity of the reactions. Granulocytes may be obtained by plasmapheresis of patients with chronic myelogenous leukemia, normal family members, or other donors by use of the special centrifuges developed for blood cell separation or by filtration leukopheresis. A daily dose of 10^{10} white blood cells, at a minimum, is required until the infection clears. Gamma globulin is of little benefit in the prophylaxis or treatment of cancer patients with hypogammaglobulinemia.

NUTRITION IN CANCER A profound state of malnutrition, the cachexia of malignancy, is frequently the most debilitating feature of this disease process. In many instances, it can be attributed to anorexia with an associated distortion of taste sensation or acquired aversions to specific foods, particularly meat. There are, however, patients in whom the extent of the weight loss far exceeds the deficit in quantity and quality of the calories consumed. In addition to the loss of adipose tissue and protein stores, these patients have a marked degree of insulin resistance with abnormal glucose tolerance. It has been demonstrated that malignancies can cause an augmentation of hepatic and renal gluconeogenesis secondary to enhanced Cori cycle activity, as well as an excessive utilization of fatty acids as metabolic fuel, which can theoretically contribute to a net energy loss by normal tissue. Hyperalimentation with total parenteral nutrition (TPN) with solutions based on 50% glucose, mixtures of essential amino acids, and vitamins, containing about 3000 cal per day, is used to restore nutritionally depleted patients who have a chance for tumor control by surgery, chemotherapy, and/or radiotherapy. TPN through a catheter placed in the superior vena cava is also indicated in patients with pain on deglutition, fistulas, or intestinal obstruction. When possible, oral hyperalimentation is preferred and effective. TPN in patients who have lost 10 lb or more body weight is associated with an average weight gain of 6 lb in a mean of 24 days, even when chemotherapy and radiotherapy are given simultaneously. There is no evidence that TPN preferentially enhances tumor growth. Anergic patients receiving TPN recover delayed hypersensitivity, suggesting that anergy may, in many instances, be a metabolic-immunologic abnormality. Catheter-related sepsis occurs in about 2 percent of patients. Hyperosmolar, nonketotic coma can be avoided with gradual increases in the concentration of glucose.

TUMOR HYPOGLYCEMIA Tumor hypoglycemia, unrelated to islet-cell tumors, has been most commonly reported in patients with retroperitoneal or intrathoracic fibrosarcomas, hepatomas, and adrenocortical carcinomas. A variety of mechanisms have been described, including the excessive consumption of glucose, impaired gluconeogenesis, and an acquired glycogen storage disease. Elevated blood and tumor nonsuppressible insulin-like activity has been demonstrated as an important factor in the pathogenesis of this syndrome.

NEUROLOGICAL MANIFESTATIONS OF CANCER Approximately 25 percent of all patients with uncontrolled cancer have intracranial metastases, including intracerebral, meningeal, or dural deposits. Common cancers which lead to intracerebral metastases are melanoma and those arising in the breast and lung. Approximately half of patients with cerebral metastases will present with headache, less than half with motor weakness, and about one-third with changes in mental status. On examination, about three-quarters of these patients will have impaired cognitive functions, two-thirds will have signs of motor system involvement, and only one-fourth will have papilledema. The test most valuable for identifying cerebral metastases is computerized tomography of the brain. Lumbar puncture does not usually provide diagnostic information and may be dangerous. Cerebral metastases are usually multiple, even when thought to be solitary, but on occasion solitary metastases occur and can be removed successfully, and removal may be followed by long periods free of symptoms. The treatment of intracerebral metastases includes dexamethasone 12 to 16 mg per day followed by whole-brain radiation and then tapering of the steroids as tolerated. The usual dose of radiation to palliate these patients is 30 to 40 Gy (3000 to 4000 rads) in 3 to 4 weeks, but high-dose, short-duration radiotherapy has been shown to be equally effective. Meningeal leukemia is a well-recognized complication of acute lymphoblastic leukemia, often occurring in patients in remission following chemotherapy. Meningeal lymphoma and carcinomatosis are also recognized more frequently than in the past. Leukemia patients generally present with cranial neuropathies, increased intracranial pressure, vomiting, and meningeal signs, but these findings may not be present in meningeal carcinomatosis. In the latter case, isolated peripheral neuropathies, back pain, and changes in mental status are more common. Frequent and careful examination of the spinal fluid with search for malignant cells in concentrated samples, obtained by millipore filtration of the cytocentrifuge specimen, is necessary to identify meningeal metastases. Treatment usually includes intrathecal methotrexate and/or whole-brain irradiation. The use of the Ommaya Reservoir for intrathecal chemotherapy improves drug distribution and has been recommended in preference to repeated lumbar punctures. Subdural or epidural metastatic tumors are less common than cerebral metastases and are most frequently associated with overlying skull metastases. These may produce cerebral edema and increased intracranial pressure and/or may interfere with venous drainage, particularly of the sagittal sinus. Radiation therapy is the treatment of choice for these problems, but surgery may be required to establish the diagnosis. Dural tumors are within the systemic circulation and accessible to systemic chemotherapy if effective agents are available for the particular tumor type.

Epidural spinal cord compression is an important complication of metastatic cancer. The most common primary tumors which produce this problem are in the breast, lung, prostate, and kidney. It is also a recognized complication of the lymphomas and multiple myelomas. Local or radicular pain is the most frequent and earliest clinical symptom, with subsequent weakness and bladder and bowel dysfunction; numbness and paresthesias are present in the majority of patients by the time the diagnosis is made. A high index of suspicion is necessary, and the diagnosis is confirmed by demonstrating a lesion by myelography or CT scan. Lumbar spinal taps should be avoided in these patients if the condition is suspected. The spinal tap should be done at the time of the myelogram, and preferably only in consultation with a neurosurgeon, since herniation of the cord into a decompressed region can occur after withdrawal of fluid. The cerebrospinal fluid may be under reduced pressure distal to the compression, and the protein is increased. Malignant cells are usually not found. Radiation therapy is utilized for patients with slowly progressing neurological deficits and radiosensitive tumors. Surgery is usually recommended for patients with rapidly progressing neurological signs, especially if the tumor is relatively radioresistant. Systemic chemotherapy may be of benefit for patients with responsive tumors, and corticosteroids are often used without proven benefit. Neither should be employed to the exclusion of surgery or radiotherapy. Intrathecal chemotherapy is not indicated. In the face of complete motor loss, recovery is rare following radiation or decompressive surgery.

Peripheral nerve or plexus compression and infiltration of the structures by tumor are other neurological complications of metastatic cancer. These problems may result from soft-tissue masses, usually at sites where nerves emerge from neural foramens of the skull or vertebra. Breast and lung cancer are common causes of brachial plexus neuropathy. Lung cancer is the most frequent cause of recurrent laryngeal or phrenic nerve paralysis, and rectal cancer is a common cause of paravertebral nerve compression. However, any tumor may produce these problems, and recognition and differentiation of tumors from metabolic or drug-induced neuropathies are essential if good palliation is to be accomplished. Radiation therapy is usually the most effective treatment but may be unsuccessful if the neurological deficits are marked and long-standing. Chemotherapy, especially for patients with breast cancer and malignant lymphomas, can be beneficial in selected patients.

Neurological and *neuromyopathic* syndromes are associated with malignant disease. Although the histopathology of the tumors producing these syndromes is often well characterized, the causes of the abnormalities are largely unknown. They should always be distinguished from direct effects of neoplasms. Neuromuscular complications are found in 5 to 10 percent of patients with malignant disease. Most often they will be associated with lung cancer, usually of the small-cell (oat-cell) type. Clinical presentation of myositis and dermatomyositis should prompt a search for a hidden malignancy, usually of the gastrointestinal tract. Progressive multifocal leukoencephalopathy is a rare complication in patients with lymphoma and may be due to a papovavirus. Cerebellar degeneration occurs in cancer patients but is also a complication of the use of 5-FU. Carcinomatous myopathy and the characteristic myasthenic syndrome (Eaton-Lambert syndrome) are additional neurological complications.

MALIGNANT EFFUSIONS Peripheral effusions are due to increased fluid formation resulting from tumor on serous surfaces. Central effusions are secondary to decreased fluid resorption due to impaired venous or lymphatic drainage, related to centrally located tumor masses or obstruction of lymphatics by tumor. A combination of peripheral and central causes may occur. A coexisting condition such as an infection or congestive heart failure may be responsible for effusions in patients with cancer. Exudates are usually seen with peripheral effusions; transudates, with central effusions. The presence of true chyle implies central impairment of lymphatic drainage and, in the absence of trauma, is due to tumor or infection. Tetracycline has now been shown to be the drug of choice for the management of pleural effusions due to cancer. Usually, 500 mg is dissolved in 30 ml saline and instilled into the chest, followed by 50 ml saline. A chest tube is required and attached to water-sealed drainage for 6 h. Drainage is continued for 12 h or longer until less than 60 ml fluid is drained per 24 h. Pleural effusions are controlled by this method in 80 percent of all patients. Intrapleural instillation of alkylating agents, 5-FU, and quinacrine is used less frequently. When alkylating agents are used, unpredictable absorption occurs which, in the face of systemic chemotherapy, may further compromise bone marrow function. Malignant pericardial effusions are best managed by external radiation and systemic treatment for the primary cancer. Management of malignant ascites is less successful owing to the large size of the peritoneal cavity.

SUPERIOR VENA CAVA OBSTRUCTION The superior vena cava (SVC) is the major vessel most commonly obstructed by tumor, resulting in facial swelling, distention of the veins of the neck and upper chest wall, loss of venous pulsations, conjunctival injection, headache, and convulsions. Patients often present with these findings as the first sign of malignant disease. The diagnosis is usually based on clinical findings and the presence of a mediastinal mass. While the SVC syndrome is a serious medical problem, it need not be considered a true medical emergency, since patients rarely die from it. There is usually sufficient time to make a histological diagnosis before treatment is instituted, although an occasional patient may require treatment before a tissue diagnosis. Temporizing treatment with corticosteroids and diuretics may be useful while the diagnosis is pursued. More definitive therapy should include systemic treatment for the disease in question, if it is susceptible to drug therapy, and full-dose irradiation therapy to the site of obstruction, in conjunction with corticosteroids. The tumors most commonly associated with superior vena cava syndrome are diffuse histiocytic lymphomas and small-cell carcinoma of the lung.

HYPERCALCEMIA Extensive bone involvement is characteristic of some tumors such as multiple myeloma, breast carcinoma, and prostatic carcinoma and may result in hypercalcemia. A common cause of hypercalcemia is immobilization with or without bony metastases. Some tumors, like epidermoid lung cancer, may produce parathyroid hormone–like substances which cause hypercalcemia. A group of patients with hypercalcemia, normal parathormone levels, and no evidence of bony metastases has been described. Some of these patients with renal-cell carcinoma have elevated tumor levels of prostaglandins and respond to the inhibitor of prostaglandin synthesis, indomethacin. Since prostaglandins cause bone resorption, this may be another mechanism for tumor hypercalcemia in the absence of metastatic disease or identifiable ectopic parathormone production. Myeloma and other lymphoid cell lines are capable of producing, locally, a low-molecular-weight substance known as *osteoclast-activating factor,* which also may be involved in the dissolution of bone. Hypercalcemia requires prompt attention. Chronic hypercalcemia may lead to nephrocalcinosis and irreversible impairment of renal function. The treatment of choice for hypercalcemia associated with malignancy is therapy for the underlying disease. Mithramycin (Table 125-1), proper hydration with isotonic saline solution, and diuretics are the best ancillary methods of controlling hypercalcemia and may lead to control within 2 days. Normal serum calcium levels can be maintained by weekly low doses of mithramycin (25 μg/kg), without risk of marrow suppression or hemorrhage. Adrenal corticosteroids reduce the serum calcium level to normal in 60 percent of patients but may predispose to infection and are no longer the treatment of choice. Sodium sulfate and sodium phosphates facilitate excretion of calcium by the kidney. Phosphates must be used cautiously since they may cause extraosseous calcification.

HYPERURICEMIA AND OTHER CONSEQUENCES OF RAPID CELL LYSIS Hyperuricemia is most common in patients with acute leukemia but occasionally occurs in other malignancies. The high serum uric acid levels are due to the increased formation and destruction of tumor cells and accompanying breakdown of nucleoproteins. Chemotherapy and radiotherapy may cause further elevations in serum uric acid and urinary urate excretion. Uric acid is actively secreted by the kidney, and its solubility is highest in alkaline urine. When the concentration exceeds the solubility, uric acid precipitates in the tubules causing obstruction, decreased glomerular filtration, and eventually anuria. Allopurinol prevents the formation of uric acid from xanthine and hypoxanthine. Prophylactic use of this drug in patients with a large volume of tumor, prior to treatment, in anticipation of a high urate load, should obviate the need to treat uric acid nephropathy. Urate nephropathy can also be prevented by ensuring a water diuresis. Administration of sodium bicarbonate to maintain the urinary pH above 7.0 is helpful. Secondary gout is uncommon except in patients with polycythemia vera. The excessive production of lactate by suboxygenated masses of tumor has been reported to cause lactic acidosis in patients with leukemia and Burkitt's lymphoma. The lactic acidosis can be reversed by cytotoxic chemotherapy directed against the tumor. The elaboration of large quantities of lactic dehydrogenase (LDH) has been observed in these settings. Cytotoxic therapy in highly drug sensitive tumors can cause rapid tumor lysis with release of intracellular phosphates and potassium leading to serious hyperkalemia, hypocalcemia, and potentially fatal cardiotoxicity.

PSYCHOLOGICAL EFFECTS Even the patient whose cancer is treatable faces severe emotional difficulties. There is often readjustment to the home situation, difficult psychosexual readjustment, particularly in women after mastectomy, and difficulties convincing the community that the patient remains a useful member of society. Many such cancer patients are shunned because of unwarranted fears of "catching" cancer. Realization by the patient that he or she has an incurable malignant disease has an even more profound psychological impact, particularly if the disease strikes in youth or middle age. An important aspect of cancer therapy is the hope of improvement it offers to patients. Even experimental chemotherapy which fails to alter the course of the disease significantly may be beneficial and gives some meaning to an otherwise dismal experience, because patients feel they are contributing to the welfare of others even if the drug fails to help them. Suicide is not common in incurable cancer patients, and the prospect of a shortened life is ultimately preferred to death by suicide if a modicum of physical and emotional comfort can be maintained. As the disease progresses, the patient may pass through a variety of mental processes, including denial, hostility, despair, and finally acceptance of the inevitable. The physician should provide hope, encouragement, understanding, sympathy, and support. During this difficult period the physician should also rely upon the nursing staff, clergy, and social workers for assistance in the care of the patient.

Most patients with advanced cancer know they are dying, and attempts at circumventing the truth are usually recognized by them and cause feelings of distrust and hostility toward those the dying patient needs the most, the family, physicians, and nurses. Honesty should be the rule; most patients will surprise their doctors and families by expressing relief at a willingness to discuss what is foremost in their minds, their imminent death.

Uncontrollable pain is uncommon in cancer patients but is a problem more often in those with bony disease. Most hospitalized cancer patients with pain are underdosed usually because of ignorance of the pharmacokinetics of narcotic analgesics. Attending physicians should use narcotics, alcohol, and tranquilizers liberally and often, and in combination in these circumstances, recognizing that the proper dose is whatever is enough to control the patient's discomfort. Fear of addiction is unwarranted. Sufficiently potent narcotics are available to control most types of pain in the cancer patient. Widely spaced doses of narcotics that exceed the half-life of most drugs are inhumane and should not be used. For pain not controllable with narcotics, neurosurgical procedures may be useful.

REFERENCES

Buschke F, Parker RG (eds): Fundamentals of clinical radiation therapy, in *Radiation Therapy in Cancer Management.* New York, Grune & Stratton, 1972

Calabresi P, Parks RE Jr: Chemotherapy of neoplastic diseases, in *Pharmacological Basis of Therapeutics,* LS Goodman, A Gilman (eds). New York, Macmillan, 1980, pp 1249–1313

Chabner BA, Myers CA: Clinical pharmacology of cancer chemotherapy, in *Cancer: Principles and Practice of Oncology,* VT DeVita, S Hellman, SA Rosenberg (eds). Philadelphia, Lippincott, 1981, pp 156–197

DeVita VT Jr: Principles of chemotherapy, in *Cancer: Principles and Practice of Oncology,* VT DeVita, S Hellman, SA Rosenberg (eds). Philadelphia, Lippincott, 1981, pp 132–155

Goldie JH, Coldman AJ: A mathematic model for relating the drug sensitivity of tumors to the spontaneous mutation rate. Cancer Treat Rep 63:1727, 1979

126
BREAST CANCER

JANE E. HENNEY
VINCENT T. DeVITA, JR.

Breast cancer is a major public health problem in the western hemisphere. In 1980 in the United States, 108,000 women and 900 men were diagnosed as having this disease. It is the principal cause of death for women between the ages of 35 and 45.

ETIOLOGY AND EPIDEMIOLOGY Epidemiologic studies indicate that the occurrence of breast cancer varies greatly among different geographic areas and is influenced markedly by migration patterns. For example, oriental women living in eastern countries are at low risk for developing breast cancer. Yet those oriental women whose ancestors migrated to Hawaii or to the continental United States have the higher incidence of breast cancer observed in the populations native to these areas. The incidence also varies among racial groups within the United States; it is highest in Caucasians, intermediate in blacks, and lowest in American Indians in New Mexico and Filipinos in Hawaii.

A woman's age, her menstrual and reproductive history, family history, and prior incidence of benign breast disease all are risk factors in the development of breast cancer. Except for a plateau at age 50, the risk of breast cancer increases with a patient's age. Furthermore, early menstruation, late menopause (after 55), and irregularity of the menstrual cycle all appear to be factors which increase a woman's chances of having this disease. Women who have undergone artificial menopause prior to age 35 have only one-third the risk of developing breast cancer as women who undergo natural menopause. Women who bear their first child before age 18 have one-third the risk of those who bear their first child after age 30. The older primiparas, however, are at slightly higher risk of developing breast cancer than women who are nulliparous. These risk associations pertain even when the women become elderly.

The risk conferred by members of one's family having breast cancer is well known. However, only 10 to 15 percent of patients with breast cancer have a family history of the disease. Women whose mothers or sisters have developed breast cancer are two to three times as likely to develop it as the female population at large. Women whose female relative(s) were premenopausal when they developed breast cancer, particularly if it was bilateral, are at greatest risk. The cause of this familial association is not understood, although a gene that is transmitted in an autosomal dominant manner through both maternal and paternal lines has been described in rare families. This particular gene is felt to have wide distribution but low penetrance. Furthermore, the allele that increases the susceptibility for this penetrance may be linked to the glutamic pyruvate transaminase locus.

A history of benign chronic breast conditions, particularly those associated with epithelial hyperplasia, increases the risk as much as fourfold. It is not clear whether fibrocystic disease is a premalignant state or whether the hormonal determinants in both diseases are similar. Acute conditions such as abscesses and mastitis are not associated with the development of breast cancer.

Dietary content, including high animal fat intake and obesity, may also increase the risk of breast cancer. Although no hypothesis has been firmly established, it is generally thought that dietary factors may act by influencing estrogen metabolism by increasing steroidal estrogen production after menopause, and by affecting the onset of menarche.

The breast is one of the most susceptible organs to the effects of ionizing radiation. Exposure of the breast to ionizing radiation is a major risk enhancer for the development of malignancy. Data which support these observations are derived from studies of survivors of the bombings at Hiroshima and Nagasaki, and women who have undergone radiation therapy, as well as those who have had multiple fluoroscopies during pneumothorax treatment for tuberculosis. The dose-effect relationship appears to be linear with an increased risk present in women who have received as small a dose as 0.5 Gy. There also appears to be an additional risk for those women who are exposed to radiation during adolescence. Fractionated or intermittent dosing does not appear to diminish this risk, nor does time since exposure, even after 45 years. The interval between exposure and the appearance of breast cancer is likely mediated by many factors including the age of the woman and related hormonal factors.

Reserpine has also been implicated in the development of breast cancer, but this is controversial. Hair dyes and other chemicals frequently used by women have been shown to be mutagenic but their role in the etiology of breast cancer has not been demonstrated.

Because of the relatively low incidence of breast cancer in males, its epidemiology and etiology have been largely unexplored. It is known, however, that males with altered estrogen metabolism, gynecomastia, and/or Klinefelter's syndrome are at greatest risk.

NATURAL HISTORY AND PROGNOSTIC FACTORS Breast cancer is a chronic disease in which some patients do not show signs of spread until 15 years after the initial diagnosis. One important tumor characteristic of breast cancer is multicentricity, that is, in approximately 13 percent of patients with breast cancer, microscopic foci of invasive and noninvasive tumor can be detected in quadrants of the breast other than that in which the primary lesion is discovered. Such tumors are regarded as independent cancers. The clinical significance of such lesions is unclear for it is unusual for multiple cancers in a single breast to become clinically overt or for bilateral cancers to occur synchronously. In women over 70 who have died from other causes, the incidence of clinically inapparent intraductal carcinoma is 19 times the reported incidence of breast cancer. Whether these cancers are controlled by the body's immune-defense mechanisms because they represent a low tumor burden or undergo regression for other reasons has not been elucidated. This observation has been central to the debate about the extent of treatment necessary to treat breast cancer with local modalities. Long-term follow-up of the women who are now being treated with segmental mastectomy in a trial conducted by the National Surgical Adjuvant Breast Project (NSABP) should provide an answer to the clinical relevance of multicentricity in breast cancer. This clinical trial is described in the section "Surgical Options."

The size of the primary tumor, a clinical predictor of outcome, can be determined easily by palpation combined with mammography. Tumors less than 2 cm in size are generally associated with the most favorable outcome. Tumor size is also correlated with the likelihood of axillary lymph node involvement, another prognostic indicator. Lesions <1.5 cm are less likely to have nodal metastases (38 percent) in contrast to large lesions (≥ 5.5 cm) which have metastasized to axillary lymph nodes 70 percent of the time. Furthermore, a correlation exists between increased tumor size and those patients who will have four or more positive axillary lymph nodes involved with tumor.

Establishing whether there is nodal involvement and the number of axillary nodes involved is critical (Table 126-1). In those patients with no histologic involvement of axillary nodes, an 83 percent rate of 5-year disease-free survival has been found; those with one to three positive nodes have a 50 percent disease-free, 5-year survival rate. Those patients with four or more positive nodes have a 21 percent disease-free survival at 5 years. Unfortunately, the physical examination of the axillary nodes is an inaccurate predictor of histologic involvement. In approximately 25 percent of cases examined, when axillary nodes are palpable, histologic evidence of disease is not found. Likewise, in 30 percent of cases in which axillary nodes are not palpable, histologic involvement with tumor is discovered. At present, this determination can be made accurately only by surgically removing the nodes.

In addition to the size of the tumor and the number of positive axillary nodes, an important prognostic factor is the presence or absence of the estrogen receptor (ER) protein. The ER protein is capable of binding and transferring the steroid molecule into nuclei to exert specific hormonal functions. The degree of such binding capacity is expressed in femtomoles per milligram of cytosol protein. Values above 10 are positive, 3 to 10 intermediate, and those less than 3 are negative. The degree of positivity is proportional to the degree of cellular differentiation and subtype and is also a measure of potential responsiveness of the tumor to hormonal manipulation. Women who have ER levels in the positive range have a more favorable prognosis than those whose ER is either in the intermediate or negative range. Observations from women who have more advanced disease indicate that approximately 60 percent of patients who are ER-positive respond to hormonal manipulation while fewer than 10 percent of patients who are ER-negative respond to hormonal therapy. Other steroid receptors may be present in the breast cancer cells and generally correlate with the presence of ER and a high likelihood of responsiveness to hormonal manipulation. Perimenopausal women tend to have the lowest levels of ER, premenopausal women an intermediate level, with postmenopausal women the highest levels.

Other factors which are predictive of outcome of breast cancer are the patient's age and menopausal status. The group found to be most likely to have a favorable outcome are those postmenopausal women whose primary cancer is less than 2 cm, positive for ER, and who have no evidence of spread to the axillary lymph nodes.

PATHOLOGY There are four common histologic forms of breast cancer: infiltrating duct–NOS (not otherwise specified), lobular invasive, medullary, and colloid or mucinous tumors. These histologic types are generally seen in their pure form but can appear in combinations. Rare histologic forms of breast cancer include tubular, adenocystic, papillary, and carcinosarcoma. The anatomical units of the female breast are the small, medium, and large ducts. Tumors can arise from any of these structures, but carcinoma of the breast most frequently arises in a large duct. In 70 to 75 percent of cases, no distinctive histologic structure can be distinguished and these infiltrating duct carcinomas are designated NOS (not otherwise specified). In spite of the small size of the primary, these cancers frequently metastasize to axillary lymph nodes and their prognosis is the worst of all breast cancer types. To palpation these lesions are firm and a fibrotic response within the tumor is characteristic.

Lobular carcinoma which makes up approximately 5 percent of breast cancers, arises in the small end ducts, may be either invasive, with tumor extending beyond the duct in which it arises, or noninvasive. In the noninvasive form, carcinoma in situ, the anaplastic cells are contained within the lobules. In the invasive form the tumor extends beyond the lobule or end duct from which it arises.

Medullary carcinoma comprises 5 to 7 percent of all breast cancers. Unlike intraductal carcinomas, these tumors attain large size but are not as likely to infiltrate. Another slow-growing invasive carcinoma that reaches large, bulky proportion is the colloid carcinoma, a mucinous-producing tumor which comprises 3 to 5 percent of breast cancers.

Inflammatory breast carcinoma presents with a unique clinical picture which must be confirmed pathologically. Biopsies of the erythematous areas of the breast as well as normal-appearing skin will reveal undifferentiated cancer cells in the subdermal lymphatics. In Paget's disease, the nipple epithelium contains nests of tumor cells, but the tumor may be either intraductal or of the invasive duct type. Prognosis is related to the histologic type of the tumor. Tumors arising from the large duct that rarely become invasive are the papillary carcinomas. These lesions comprise only 1 percent of all breast cancer. While they do not invade tissue, they grow slowly and often reach considerable size by the time they are diagnosed. Axillary lymph node invasion is a late feature in this type of breast cancer.

Careful staging using both the clinical and surgical staging systems illustrated in Table 126-2 are useful in establishing a patient's prognosis and prescribing an appropriate form of treatment. Frequently, breast cancer metastases to distant sites occur early and metastatic spread follows no predictable pattern. The axillary lymph nodes, liver, bones, skin, and lungs are the most common sites of metastases while the adrenal glands, kidneys, ovaries, spleen, and thyroid are less frequently involved.

SCREENING Because the earlier clinical stages of breast cancer (Table 126-2) have a more favorable outcome, major emphasis has been placed on developing methods for screening large populations for cancer. In approximately 90 percent of cases, the breast mass is found by the patient herself during deliberate or accidental self-examination, with the remaining 10 percent found during examination by health professionals or by mass screening techniques.

The Health Insurance Plan of New York evaluated mammography as a screening tool in 62,000 patients; their screening included physical examination as well. A 9-year follow-up period showed a 30 percent reduction in mortality for women 50 or older who had been screened compared to a control group. The risk/benefit ratio involved in exposing large populations of women to ionizing radiation has been widely debated. In an attempt to resolve this issue, a panel of experts convened by the National Cancer Institute recommended the following guidelines: annual mammograms for women over 50, with annual mammograms of women from 40 to 49 who were considered to be at high risk. This high-risk group was defined as those who had had prior breast cancer or had a mother or sibling with the disease. With current technology, high-quality mammograms can be performed which expose the patient to radiation doses which do not exceed 0.01 Gy. Other screening techniques such as thermography pose a lesser risk to the patient but are not considered sufficiently accurate to be used as the sole screening tool. In addition, ultrasound and computer-

TABLE 126-1
Disease-free survival related to lymph node status

Axillary node status	*Percent surviving disease-free*	
	5-year	*10-year*
Negative	82	76
Positive:	35	24
1–3 nodes	50	35
≥ 4 nodes	21	11

SOURCE: *National Surgical Adjuvant Breast Project.*

ized tomography (CT) are currently being evaluated as screening techniques.

DIAGNOSIS In 70 to 80 percent of cases, the patient presents with a hard, circumscribed mass in the breast. If this mass is fixed to skin or deep muscle, or if there is edema of the skin or retraction of the nipple, cancer is almost a certainty. However, 75 percent of all breast lesions are benign. Breast cancer presents most frequently (in 45 percent of cases) in the upper outer quadrant of the breast; it is present in the central or subareolar portion of the breast in 25 percent of cases, in the upper inner quadrant in 15 percent of cases, and in the lower inner quadrant in only 5 percent of cases. A mobile mass with well-defined margins in a woman under 30 is much more likely to be a fibroadenoma, a benign condition. On rare occasions, infectious mastitis may be mistaken for adenoma.

Two infrequent but nonetheless important clinical presentations of breast cancer are *inflammatory breast carcinoma* and *Paget's disease.* With inflammatory breast disease there is increased local temperature, redness, and a visible erysipeloid margin; the entire breast is often indurated and firm to hard. Patients diagnosed as having inflammatory breast cancer frequently have palpable axillary and supraclavicular lymph nodes as well as evidence of distant metastases, and an extremely poor prognosis. In Paget's disease eczematoid changes in the nipple, including itching, burning, oozing, and bleeding occur over a relatively long period and a mass can be palpated in two-thirds of patients.

Another form of malignancy of the breast, *cystosarcoma phyllodes,* a rare sarcoma, can arise from a fibroadenoma, but usually presents as a warm, tender, cystic mass. In the presence of a breast mass, a bloody discharge from the nipple is a classic sign of cancer. However, *intraductal papilloma,* a benign lesion, is associated with a bloody discharge from the nipple, but without a palpable mass. These tumors are generally exceedingly small but can be located by noting the area which, when palpated, results in bleeding from the nipple. Infrequently, sarcomas, or nonepithelial malignancies, including fibrosarcomas, lymphosarcomas, liposarcomas, and hemangiosarcomas, may be associated with breast masses.

Inflammatory lesions Mammary duct ectasia is a benign condition, usually seen in elderly women with atrophic breats, in which the mammary ducts in or just beneath the nipple become dilated and filled with cellular debris and lipid-containing material. Intermittent pain and local inflammatory changes may be present, and because a discharge, at times bloody, and retraction of the nipple may occur, this condition must be differentiated from carcinoma. Excision of the nipple is usually indicated.

Fat necrosis is a common occurrence following trauma that may be so slight as to have not been noticed. It presents as a painful lump usually associated with some ecchymosis and may be followed by local atrophy and dimpling of the skin, at which stage biopsy must be performed to distinguish it from carcinoma.

Thrombosis of the thoracoepigastric veins and sclerosing subcutaneous phlebitis (Mondor's disease) occur after trauma or for no apparent reason and are manifest by the appearance of long cord-like structures, initially tender, in the outer half of the breast, frequently extending up into the axilla or down toward the epigastrium. They may persist up to a year, but no treatment is indicated.

Sarcoid may very rarely involve the skin of the chest, and secondary amyloidosis may involve the breast tissue itself. Eosinophilic granuloma may occur in the submammary folds.

Fibrocystic disease With each menstrual cycle there is a recurring biphasic stimulation, first of proliferation of breast tissue by estrogens, then of alveolar secretory activity by progesterone, followed by a period of involution. In most women these changes are of such slight degree as to cause few if any clinical symptoms. Not infrequently, however, inflammatory changes may precede each menses, with tenderness, engorgement, and increasing nodularity of the breasts. This is more often seen in nulliparous women and may subside after childbearing and lactation. Suspected cysts in the breast may be aspirated safely in the office with local anesthesia if biopsy is done promptly in any of the following circumstances: (1) no fluid is obtained; (2) the cyst fluid is grossly bloody; (3) the mass does not completely disappear with aspiration; and (4) the fluid reaccumulates during succeeding days. Cytologic examinations of cyst aspirates are of no value.

In the later years of reproductive life the continued recurrent stimulation and involution of the breasts in the course of each menstrual cycle may result in diffuse and nodular fibrosis and the formation of cysts of varying sizes, so-called chronic cystic mastitis. This condition may simulate carcinoma but is usually distinguishable by the fact that it is intermittently painful and may subside to some extent following menstruation. Nevertheless, carcinoma may coexist and be masked by the diffuse nodularity of the cystic disease. Moreover, the incidence of mammary carcinoma is greater in patients with fibrocystic disease of the breasts, and it is unwise to delay biopsy of suspicious areas in the hope that they may subside by the end of the next menstrual cycle.

Once a well-defined breast mass has been detected, a complete history and physical examination should be followed by a biopsy or needle aspiration. A breast mass is an indication for biopsy regardless of the results of mammography. There is no necessity for the biopsy and definitive surgical treatment to be undertaken as a single operative procedure. Prior custom was to perform the initial biopsy while the patient was under general anesthesia, examine a frozen section of the tissue, and proceed with a radical mastectomy if the biopsy was positive. Biopsy can be done using local anesthesia and the interval between diagnostic biopsy and definitive surgery or radiation therapy provides a period during which metastatic disease can be ruled out and the physician can discuss all of the options for further management with the patient. In the workup for metastatic disease, the patient should be questioned and examined thoroughly for signs and symptoms of bone pain, neurologic deficit, or behavioral changes which would indicate the need to search for distant metastases. However, routine scanning of the

TABLE 126-2
Breast cancer clinical stage and prognosis

Stage	American Joint Committee staging	Approximate frequency of stage at presentation, %	Approximate 5-year survival, %
I	Primary tumor <2 cm; nodes, if palpable, not felt to contain metastases; no distant metastases	55–70	80
II	Primary tumor >2 cm and <5 cm; nodes, if palpable, not fixed; no distant metastases evident	20–25	65
III	Tumor >5 cm or fixed to chest wall or skin invasion present; supraclavicular nodes palpable; no distant metastases evident	10	40
IV	Distant metastases	10	10

bones in patients who are asymptomatic has not proved to be cost-effective. Likewise, radioisotopic or CT scans of the liver and brain should be undertaken only in patients with abnormal physical findings or liver function studies.

LOCAL MANAGEMENT OF BREAST CANCER (STAGE I AND STAGE II) Background Until recently, the radical mastectomy, which involves removal of the breast, both the major and minor pectoralis muscles, ipsilateral axillary lymph nodes, and, in the medial lesions, the ipsilateral supraclavicular and mediastinal lymph chains, was considered the sole therapeutic option for breast cancer. This treatment was based on the rationale that breast cancer began as a single focus of disease which, after a considerable period of time, would spread in an orderly fashion from the breast to the axillary nodes and from there into the systemic channels of the blood and lymphatic systems. With this underlying assumption, treatment was targeted at arresting the spread of tumor by removing the primary breast tumor and the surrounding tissue en bloc.

Data from many of the studies discussed in this section have changed the conceptual underpinnings for such radical therapy. Breast cancer is now appreciated to be a disease which is localized for only a brief period and then disseminates into the circulatory and lymphatic channels simultaneously early in its course. The current emphasis in the management of breast cancer is removal of the primary site of tumor with the minimum disfigurement necessary to gain local control and control of the microscopic foci of disease with adjuvant therapy. No single procedure can be recommended as ideal for all patients. Although many investigators favor conservative surgery, some feel that until long-term follow-up studies are available, radical surgery is the most conservative approach.

Surgical options The radical mastectomy described previously not only confers no increased benefit in terms of survival, but often, because of the removal of the pectoralis minor, results in edema of the arm and a shallow, shrunken chest which make fitting a prosthesis difficult. Various other surgical options attain survival outcomes similar to those in patients treated with the radical mastectomy while obtaining a more acceptable cosmetic result.

The modified radical mastectomy is the treatment used in the majority of patients in the United States. However, a prospective clinical trial of the radical mastectomy and the modified mastectomy has never been done. This operation differs from the radical mastectomy in that the pectoralis muscles are spared but an axillary dissection is done en bloc. Reconstructive surgery or fitting of a prosthesis can be accomplished with satisfactory results. Women with little breast tissue often favor complete removal of the breast since the amount of tissue removed in procedures such as the quadrantectomy or even the segmental can result in a distorted-appearing breast.

The total or simple mastectomy is an operation in which the breast is removed, but the pectoralis muscles and the axillary nodes are not routinely excised. To resolve whether this operation would produce survival benefits similar to that of the radical mastectomy, the NSABP conducted such a comparative trial. No significant difference in survival has been found after 8 years of follow-up among three groups of patients: one treated by radical mastectomy, the second by total mastectomy followed by local-regional irradiation, and the third treated with total mastectomy and removal of the axillary nodes only when the nodes became positive. Like the modified radical, a total or simple mastectomy minimizes the disfigurement caused by the radical mastectomy. However, the simple and the total mastectomy are generally not recommended because the axillary nodes are not removed in these procedures and an informed judgment regarding the necessity for further adjuvant therapy cannot be made without this information.

The segmental mastectomy and the tylectomy involve removal of the primary and a minimal amount of surrounding tissue. Both operative procedures are aimed at preserving most of the breast. These procedures are appropriate for women who have small lesions, <2 cm, located in the periphery of the breast, and who have ample breast tissue remaining so that the desired aesthetic effect can be achieved. A prospective trial is in progress to evaluate the benefits of the segmental mastectomy. Patients eligible for a segmental mastectomy are randomized into three groups; one group receives the segmental mastectomy, the second the segmental mastectomy plus radiation of the breast, and the third a total mastectomy. In all patients entered in this trial, an axillary dissection is performed. The group treated with segmental mastectomy alone will have had no treatment to the breast tissue containing multiple foci of microscopic tumor; careful follow-up of this patient population should, therefore, provide an answer about the clinical relevance of multicentricity. To date, 1400 patients have been entered on this important trial.

The quadrantectomy is the removal of the breast quadrant in which the primary occurs with the overlying skin and the fascia of the pectoralis major, and has been evaluated by Veronesi of the Cancer Institute in Milan, Italy. In this study no difference has been observed in the 5-year survival rate of two groups of women with breast cancer, one that had been treated by a radical mastectomy and the other by quadrantectomy plus axillary dissection coupled with radiotherapy. In this trial all 700 women had breast cancers which were smaller than 2 cm. Local control of disease in those treated with the less extensive surgical procedures was not markedly different from those treated with radical mastectomy, and when local recurrences did occur, they could be treated effectively with further surgery or irradiation.

Radiation therapy Other nonsurgical means of achieving local-regional control of tumor, such as radiation therapy, have been under investigation for many years. A study has evaluated a selected group of women with stage I and II breast cancer. The group of women who received local treatment consisting of external beam radiation therapy utilizing tangential and nodal fields to deliver 44 to 50 Gy (2 Gy daily, four to five times per week) plus a booster dose of 10 to 20 Gy from either an external beam or radium implants had basically the same outcome as the group of historical controls that had undergone extensive surgical treatment. While the breast remains intact in those women who receive primary radiation therapy, this procedure can cause fibrosis and hardening of the affected breast and the shrinkage caused by this technique may result in an asymmetrical appearance for the patient with small breasts. This treatment modality also raises the possibility of tumor induction in the irradiated area; data in patients who had received postoperative radiation suggest that this risk is slight. Whether the primary breast cancer is treated with surgery or radiation, sampling of the ipsilateral axillary lymph nodes should be carried out in order to ascertain the number of positive nodes and to determine if further therapy is required.

ADJUVANT THERAPY OF BREAST CANCER Background Because only 80 percent of patients with stage I disease and 65 percent of those with stage II disease (Table 126-2) attained a 5-year survival following surgery, clinicians began to investigate other modalities such as postoperative radiation and hormonal manipulation in an effort to improve these results. Radiation therapy was aimed at achieving survival by increasing local-regional control of tumor, while hormonal manipulation by means of prophylactic castration was designed to reach deposits of tumor that had already undergone systemic dissemination. Neither of these modalities has improved the overall survival of treated patients. Radiation proved ineffective because it could only affect local disease. Hormonal manipulation failed as well, probably because it was not applied selectively to only those patients who were ER-positive, a technology that was not available at the time. Animal experiments with chemotherapeutic agents suggested that these drugs might be effective in patients with breast cancer.

Selected adjuvant chemotherapy trials The NSAPB in 1958 initiated a clinical trial of systemic therapy following surgery. Within the first two postoperative days, one course of triethylenethiophosphoramide (thiotepa) was administered. With even this modest chemotherapeutic regimen, at 10-year follow-up, 35 percent of premenopausal women who had four or more positive nodes had survived as opposed to only 13.5 percent of the control group who had received a placebo—a significant difference. During the 1960s, 10 other groups initiated similar trials of adjuvant chemotherapy but, due to the small patient populations and inadequate controls, few definitive conclusions could be drawn from these studies. One such uncontrolled trial did produce extremely promising results. Seventy-three women with four or more positive nodes were treated with cyclophosphamide, methotrexate, 5-fluorouracil, vincristine, and prednisone. Twenty-seven women received this therapy after postoperative radiotherapy. In the population who received chemotherapy alone, 68 percent were alive 8 years later with no evidence of disease.

With these clinical studies as background, two prospective randomized studies of the efficacy of postoperative chemotherapy were initiated in 1972 and 1973 by the NSABP and the Cancer Institute of Milan, Italy. The first group of investigators studied the agent L-phenylalanine mustard (L-PAM) versus placebo. After 6 years of follow-up, the disease-free survival of those who received treatment is significantly better than those who did not. The Milan group studied the combination of cyclophosphamide, methotrexate, and 5-fluorouracil (CMF). Similar to the findings of the NSABP, after 6 years the treated group has a significantly improved relapse-free survival when compared to controls. Both trials demonstrated that the greatest benefit was achieved in the premenopausal group with low tumor burden, 1 to 3 positive nodes. In the treated NSABP group who were $\leq$ 49 years and who had 1 to 3 positive nodes, after 5 years a 57 percent reduction in treatment failure and a 54 percent reduction in mortality was achieved. The premenopausal women treated in the Milan group with 1 to 3 positive nodes also had a significantly improved disease-free survival.

Investigators at the Cancer Institute of Milan have also suggested that a dose-response effect may be responsible for the less promising results in postmenopausal patients. When they reviewed those patients who had received 85 percent of the planned dose, 77 percent had a relapse-free survival at 5 years. However, the patients who received only 65 percent of the planned dose had only a 48 percent rate of relapse-free survival, a result no different from the controls. These data suggest that adjuvant chemotherapy should be used as aggressively as possible to ensure the best chance of favorable results.

Selecting adjuvant chemotherapy CMF in combination has been studied extensively and is probably the most commonly used combination. Other combinations of drugs have yielded similar results. Although each patient's clinical situation must be considered individually, those generally recommended for adjuvant chemotherapy are stage II (node-positive) premenopausal patients. Adjuvant therapy is not commonly recommended for stage I (node-negative) patients. These patients, however, should be considered candidates for clinical trials. Two studies are currently ongoing in women with stage I (node-negative) disease who are ER-negative. The Southwestern Oncology Group is randomizing such patients to combination chemotherapy consisting of cyclophosphamide, methotrexate, and vincristine or no treatment. The NSABP is randomizing stage I (node-negative) ER-negative patients to either methotrexate and 5-fluorouracil or no further treatment. In addition, they are conducting a study in stage I ER-positive patients employing either tamoxifen or no further therapy.

Side effects of chemotherapy Acute side effects of adjuvant therapy such as malaise, nausea, and vomiting are common. Nausea and vomiting can often be relieved by the administration of phenothiazines prior to and during treatment. Alopecia must be anticipated. It can be minimized by cooling the scalp with a cap specifically designed for this purpose, 30 min prior to, during, and 30 min after the administration of chemotherapy. The long-term side effects of adjuvant therapy have not yet been clearly delineated. Cardiotoxicity from anthracycline-containing combinations and the carcinogenic effects of several of the anticancer drugs should be considered. The acute side effects of each chemotherapeutic agent are presented in greater detail in Chap. 125. Clearly long-term follow-up is required to elucidate the risk/benefit ratio of each adjuvant regimen.

Adjuvant radiotherapy Postoperative radiotherapy, a common practice in the past, has been effective only in decreasing the rate of local-regional recurrence. If a patient has four or more positive nodes, the local-regional recurrence rates range from approximately 15 to 25 percent. If one to three nodes are positive, 5 to 10 percent of patients develop local-regional recurrence. If the nodes are negative, only 2 to 8 percent develop recurrence. Radiation delivered postoperatively can reduce the overall local-regional recurrence rate to less than 5 percent but does not increase overall survival. Patients who have received adjuvant chemotherapy have been reported to have an incidence of local-regional recurrence similar to that observed in women treated with local-regional radiation therapy and have the additional benefit of longer survival. Should a patient who has received adjuvant chemotherapy develop a local-regional recurrence, then radiation therapy can be utilized at that time and is effective in controlling the lesion in 60 to 70 percent of such patients.

Postoperative radiotherapy should only be considered if clinically apparent tumor remains following surgery, if the tumor is >5 cm, or if the histologic type is undifferentiated or inflammatory. These situations are infrequent.

Adjuvant hormone therapy Prior attempts to evaluate hormonal manipulation as an adjuvant therapy were done without the benefit of the assay for the ER protein and were, for the most part, negative. One trial, however, has yielded positive findings. After 10 years of follow-up, Meakin and his coworkers observed an improvement in overall survival for those stage II premenopausal patients whose ovaries were ablated by radiation (20 Gy in five daily fractions) plus prednisone (7.5 mg per day) after surgery and postoperative regional radiation. The survival rate for women in this treatment group was 77 percent, in contrast to a survival rate of 61 percent in women who received only primary surgery and a postoperative regimen of radiation.

MANAGEMENT OF DISSEMINATED BREAST CANCER While fewer than 10 percent of patients present with stage IV breast cancer, approximately one-third to one-half of all breast cancer patients treated with surgery or radiation alone will eventually have recurrence of the disease. Therefore, it is important to document the extent and location, ER status, and rate of progress of the cancer since it is useful in determining a patient's prognosis and in selecting the proper approach to management if metastases appear.

Hormone receptors and hormonal management Conventional forms of hormonal manipulation are aimed at abolishing estrogen or estrogen precursors. In the majority of patients the initial ER determination remains unchanged and the ER values of the primary and metastatic sites are similar. A woman who has changed menopausal status since the original ER determination is the most likely candidate to have changed ER status from negative to positive or vice versa. Although on a statistical basis women who are ER-positive are more likely to respond to estrogen deprivation, in any given patient the absence or presence of ER should not influence the choice of therapy. Certainly patients with absent estrogen receptors may respond to estrogen deprivation therapy, and vice versa. If, at the time of relapse, tissue for ER evaluation is not obtainable, the therapeutic plan should consider the results from earlier evaluation of breast tissue. Even if the ER status of a patient is unknown, a 30 percent response rate of approximately 12 to 18 month's duration has been observed to either additive or ablative hormonal manipulation. In the absence of ER data, clinical parameters which predict a favorable response to hormonal manipulation are postmenopausal status, a disease-free interval longer than 2 years, metastases which are confined to the soft tissue or bones, and a prior positive response to hormone therapy. In general, the response to hormone therapy is not rapid, but 90 percent of those patients who are going to respond do so within an 8-week period.

ANTIESTROGENS These estrogen analogues are the hormonal treatment of choice and bind to the ER and are translocated like estrogens with the receptor into the cell's nucleus. Tamoxifen 10 mg bid is considered the antiestrogen of choice. Sixty percent of patients who are ER-positive respond to antiestrogens, although patients with hepatic metastases are the least likely to respond. Common side effects of tamoxifen are mild nausea, vomiting, and, occasionally, hot flashes. Corneal opacities and retinal degeneration have been observed only rarely at normal dose levels.

CASTRATION Premenopausal females who relapse after having achieved a response to tamoxifen and who have no evidence of hepatic metastases or lymphatic spread to the lungs should be considered as candidates for castration. The response rate to this procedure in ER-positive women is 50 percent, while 20 percent of men respond. The average duration of such a response is 15 to 18 months.

ADRENALECTOMY/HYPOPHYSECTOMY If, after having responded to antiestrogen and/or castration, a premenopausal patient develops recurrent tumor, adrenalectomy or hypophysectomy should be considered. Women who are postmenopausal should also be considered for such therapy to reduce estrogen production further. Approximately 50 percent of patients who were previously hormone sensitive respond to such treatment. Medical adrenalectomy using aminoglutethimide (AG) has become a reasonable alternative to surgical adrenalectomy for ablating adrenal function. The mechanism of action of AG is by its inhibition of adrenal steroid synthesis and the blocking aromatization of adrenal androgens to estrogen. While offering the same response rate as surgical ablation, the drug can be withdrawn should the treatment fail without the patient's being rendered hypoadrenal for the remainder of her life. The recommended dosage of AG is 250 mg every 6 h. Hydrocortisone 40 mg per day is administered to mimic glucocorticoid administration and to prevent the reflex ACTH rise. Hydrocortisone is preferred to replacement doses of dexamethasone because the latter's metabolism is accelerated by AG, thereby reducing availability of the steroid. Side effects of AG include lethargy, rash, transient ataxia, and dizziness; most of these are acute and transient.

ESTROGEN Used primarily in the postmenopausal group, estrogens such as diethylstilbestrol, 15 mg daily, or ethinyl estradiol, 3 mg daily, are frequently effective, particularly in patients with soft-tissue and slowly progressive visceral metastases. Acute side effects include nausea, vomiting, and uterine bleeding, which can be controlled with cyclic administration of progesterone.

ANDROGENS While androgens can be considered for premenopausal patients, their greatest utility is in the postmenopausal patient with bony metastases. Any of the drugs or procedures used to manipulate the hormonal milieu can cause the sudden onset of life-threatening hypercalcemia which occurs in 10 percent of treated patients. Sudden hypercalcemia in a patient who has recently undergone hormonal manipulation may be an indication of an antitumor response to the hormones. Hypercalcemia should be treated with hydration, diuretics, steroids, and mithramycin (see Chap. 339). Hormone therapy need not, in most cases, be discontinued unless the hypercalcemia proves refractory.

Chemotherapy Patients who have failed or exhausted prior hormonal manipulation, or who are ER-negative, and those with visceral disease that is progressing rapidly should be considered for chemotherapy. Single-agent chemotherapy with drugs such as 5-fluorouracil, methotrexate, doxorubicin, or cyclophosphamide is effective in producing partial responses in 20 to 40 percent of patients. While the overall response rates to doxorubicin hydrochloride (Adriamycin) and cyclophosphamide may approach that of some combination programs, the responses are usually only partial. Overall response rates of the more frequently used drug combinations are illustrated in Table 126-3 and range from 50 to 75 percent, with 15 to 20 percent of patients achieving a complete response. Combination chemotherapy has therefore become the treatment of choice in patients with metastatic disease. The "Cooper regimen," CMFVP, was originally reported to attain a response rate of 90 percent with nearly all responses being complete. However, numerous clinical trials using these same drugs in a variety of schedules have attained an overall response rate of 40 percent with 10 to 20 percent of patients achieving a complete response. Clinical studies of other combinations of drugs show similar results. The median duration of response of patients who achieve a complete remission is 1 year, while for those who have partial regression of tumor it is 6 to 9 months. Should the patient initially respond to chemotherapy and then fail, subsequent chemotherapy regimens can produce responses of brief duration in 25 to 40 percent of cases. Following failure of primary or secondary chemotherapy programs, experimental chemotherapy in a protocol setting should be considered.

Clinical predictors of a favorable response to chemotherapy include a disease-free interval of more than 2 years and pre- or perimenopausal status. All sites of metastatic disease are not equally responsive to chemotherapy; metastases to soft tissue, such as skin and lymph modes, are most responsive; visceral sites of metastases show intermediate responsiveness, and bone lesions are least likely to respond to chemotherapy, although pain relief often results.

Selecting an appropriate combination depends primarily on two factors: the patient's prior exposure to drugs in the adjuvant setting, and a medical history which would contraindicate the use of specific drugs in combination. Patients exposed to L-PAM in the adjuvant setting can respond to a non-cross-resistant drug or drug combination such as Adriamycin or CMF if metastases occur. Patients exposed previously to CMF remain responsive to Adriamycin-containing combinations, but are unlikely to respond to single-agent alkylating therapy once combination therapy has failed. Adriamycin-containing regimens should be considered for the patient with a prior history of congestive heart failure only if the patient has failed to respond to non-anthracycline-containing combinations. A maximum total dose of 550 mg per square meter of body surface should be used in all patients who receive Adriamycin (see Chap. 125).

MANAGEMENT OF COMPLICATIONS DUE TO BREAST CANCER **Skeletal system** Painful and destructive lesions of the skeleton often occur in breast cancer patients with advanced disease. Bone scans are the most sensitive test for detecting early signs of metastatic disease, but have not proved to be cost effective in asymptomatic patients. When following a patient, x-rays of sites which become symptomatic are appropriate. Bone-scanning is required only if x-rays are negative.

Limited field irradiation is effective for palliation of pain. The extent of disease, the patient's requirements for narcotics, and overall health status should be carefully evaluated before radiation for pain relief is recommended. Preventing fractures of weight-bearing bones can also be accomplished by limited field irradiation. Total dosage in this instance is generally 20 to 40 Gy over 3 to 4 weeks. If the site of involvement is a weight-bearing bone and if the lesion is approximately 2.5 cm or larger, stabilization by internal fixation or, in some cases, replacement of the femoral head should be considered.

If the patient complains of back pain, a careful neurologic examination should be carried out and, if the findings are equivocal, a CT scan and occasionally a myelogram should be performed to rule out compression of the spinal cord due to pathologic fracture of a vertebra or epidural involvement by tumor. Prevention of paralysis is vastly preferable to treatment after the fact.

Hypercalcemia Markedly elevated levels of calcium occur in breast cancer patients for many reasons. Skeletal metastases which result in destruction of bone can result in hypercalcemia, but the severity of the hypercalcemia does not necessarily correlate with the extent of bone destruction. A response to hormonal therapy, dehydration, and immobilization because of increased bone reabsorption of calcium, as well as use of long-term prednisone can also cause hypercalcemia in breast cancer patients.

The severity of the patient's symptoms dictates the urgency and measures that should be employed to treat the hypercalcemia. In the patient who is relatively asymptomatic and has only mild elevation of calcium, administration of fluids and/or diuretics such as furosemide, as well as increasing the patient's level of activity, may be sufficient. If the hypercalcemia is due to additive hormonal agents, glucocorticoids (40 to 100 mg of prednisone or its equivalent in divided doses) are recommended. In all patients with demonstrated hypercalcemia, substitutes should be found for medications such as thiazide, antacids which contain calcium, and lithium, which also tends to increase the serum calcium level. Dose adjustments should be made in drugs like digoxin which are dependent on calcium for their action. In breast cancer as in other malignancies, treatment of the tumor is the most effective means to control complications such as hypercalcemia. Because effects of such treatment take days to weeks, it may be necessary to administer mithramycin 25 μg/kg as a rapid intravenous infusion to achieve a lowering of calcium levels in the more severe cases. This drug usually acts to lower serum calcium within 48 h of administration and the effect may last for a week or more. If, however, it has not had the desired effect within that period, a similar dose (not to exceed two doses per week) should be given. These dosages of mithramycin rarely result in side effects.

TABLE 126-3
Commonly used combination chemotherapies for the treatment of disseminated breast cancer*

Combination	*Dose and schedule*	*Overall response rate, %*	*Complete response rate, %*
CMFVP:		50–90	10–20
Cyclophosphamide	80 mg/m² P O daily		
Methotrexate	20 mg/m² I V weekly × 8 weeks		
5-Fluorouracil	500 mg/m² IV weekly		
Vincristine	1.0 mg/m² I V weekly × 4–5 weeks		
Prednisone	30 mg/m² P O daily × 15 (then taper)		
CMFP (repeat every 4 weeks):		65	26
Cyclophosphamide	100 mg/m² P O days 1–14		
Methotrexate	60 mg/m² I V days 1 & 8		
5-Fluorouracil	700 mg/m² I V days 1 & 8		
Prednisone	40 mg/m² P O days 1 & 14		
CMF (repeat every 4 weeks):		50	15
Cyclophosphamide	100 mg/m² P O days 1–14		
Methotrexate	30–40 mg/m² I V days 1 & 8		
5-Fluorouracil	600 mg/m² I V days 1 & 8		
CAF (repeat every 4 weeks):		80	18
Cyclophosphamide	100 mg/m² P O days 1–14		
Adriamycin	40 mg/m² I V day 1		
5-Fluorouracil	400 mg/m² I V days 1 & 8		
AC (repeat cycle every 3–4 weeks):		80	12
Adriamycin	40 mg/m² I V day 1		
Cyclophosphamide	200 mg/m² P O days 3–6		

* *Appropriate precautions, as outlined in Chap. 125, should be reviewed prior to prescribing combination chemotherapy.*

Central nervous system Changes in the patient's behavior or evidence of cranial or peripheral neurologic deficit should raise the possibility of brain or spinal involvement. A thorough neurologic examination, CT scan, and lumbar puncture should be undertaken and, if a localized lesion is detected, whole-brain radiotherapy is generally the treatment of choice. Cytologic examination should be carried out on the spinal fluid as well as culture for opportunistic infections. If leptomeningeal metastases are observed, intrathecal administration of methotrexate is recommended.

Eye Breast cancer is the most common cause of retro- or intraorbital metastases. Visual impairment with or without proptosis in the breast cancer patient is an indication for further evaluation. Intraorbital metastases can be revealed by careful fundoscopic examination, but retroorbital metastases require evaluation by CT.

REFERENCES

Bonadonna G et al: Multimodal therapy with CMF in resectable breast cancer with positive axillary nodes: The Milan experience, in *Adjuvant Therapy of Cancer III,* S Salmon et al (eds). New York, Grune & Stratton, 1981, p 435

Fisher B et al: Breast cancer studies of the NSABP: An editorialized overview, in *Adjuvant Therapy of Cancer III,* S Salmon et al (eds). New York, Grune & Stratton, 1981, p 359

Harris J et al: The role of radiation therapy in the primary treatment of carcinoma of the breast. Semin Oncol 5:403, 1978

Hellman S et al: Cancer of the breast, in *Cancer: Principles and Practices on Oncology,* VT DeVita et al (eds). New York, Lippincott, 1982, p 914

Henderson C et al: Cancer of the breast—The past decade. N Engl J Med 302:17, 1980

Miller A et al: The epidemiology and etiology of breast cancer. N Engl J Med 303:1246, 1980

Santen R et al: A randomized trial comparing surgical adrenalectomy with aminoglutethimide plus hydrocortisone in women with advanced breast cancer. N Engl J Med 305:545, 1981

127 CARCINOMA OF THE PROSTATE

ARTHUR I. SAGALOWSKY
JEAN D. WILSON

INCIDENCE Cancer of the prostate is the second most common malignancy in men, and in men older than age 55 it is the third most common cause of cancer death (after carcinomas of the lung and colon). In 1980 there were some 66,000 newly diagnosed cases and 21,500 deaths from the disorder in the United States. The disease is rare before age 50. The incidence increases with advancing age, but only about a third of cases identified at autopsy are manifest clinically.

The frequency varies in different parts of the world. In terms of age-adjusted mortality rates, the United States has 14 deaths per 100,000 men per year compared to 22 for Sweden and 2 for Japan. However, Japanese immigrants to the United States develop prostatic cancer at a frequency similar to the rest of the men in this country, suggesting that an environmental factor is the principal cause for population differences. The incidence among black men is somewhat higher than that in white men in the United States; the reason for this difference is not known.

CLASSIFICATION Some carcinomas of the prostate are slow-growing and may persist for long periods without causing significant symptoms, whereas others behave aggressively. It is not known whether tumors can become more malignant with time. Insight into the natural history of a given tumor is provided by careful histopathological grading of the lesions combined with surgical evaluation of the pelvic lymph nodes.

Histological grading Over 95 percent of prostatic cancers are adenocarcinomas that arise in the prostatic acini. Adenocarcinoma may begin anywhere in the prostate but has a predilection for the periphery. The tumors are frequently multifocal. Variability in cellular size, nuclear and nucleolar shape, glandular differentiation, and acid phosphatase and mucin content may occur within a single specimen, but the most poorly differentiated area of tumor (i.e., the area with the highest histological grade) appears to determine its biological behavior. In one grading scheme the dominant and any other glandular histological patterns are independently assigned numbers from 1 to 5 (best to least differentiated), and these numbers are summed to give a total score of 2 to 10 for each tumor. Such grading is reproducible and correlates with the course of the disease and with patient survival.

The remainder of prostatic cancers are comprised of squamous- and transitional-cell carcinomas that arise in the prostatic ducts, carcinoma of the prostatic utricle (a müllerian-duct remnant), carcinosarcomas that arise in the mesenchymal elements of the gland, and occasional metastatic tumors, usually carcinoma of the lung, melanoma, or lymphoma. These tumors will not be considered further.

Surgical staging Adenocarcinoma of the prostate may spread by three routes: direct extension, the lymphatics, or the bloodstream. The prostatic capsule is a natural boundary against growth of tumor into adjacent structures, but direct extension upward into the seminal vesicles and bladder floor is common. Lymphatic spread can best be assessed by surgical exploration, and the frequency with which it occurs correlates directly with the size and the histological grade of the tumor. Only about a tenth of tumors with a grade of less than 5 have lymph node involvement, while more than 70 percent of tumors with a Gleason grade of 9 or 10 have coexisting lymphatic invasion at the time of diagnosis. The route of lymphatic spread in decreasing order is to obturator, internal iliac, common iliac, presacral, and paraaortic nodes. Hematogenous metastases occur to bone (pelvis > lumbar vertebrae > thoracic vertebrae > ribs) more frequently than to viscera (lung > liver > adrenal). Diffuse pulmonary involvement is infrequent.

The standard staging scheme is that of Whitmore. *Stage A* represents cancer not detectable by rectal exam but found in a surgical specimen obtained during operation for prostatic hyperplasia or at autopsy. Stage A is subdivided into two groups: *stage* A_1, in which tumor is present in only a few transurethral chips from one lobe, and *stage* A_2, in which tumor is more diffuse. *Stage B* disease is palpable but confined to the prostate. *Stage* B_1 disease is a single nodule involving only one lobe, surrounded by tissue normal to palpation, and *stage* B_2 involves the gland more diffusely. In *stage C* palpable tumor extends beyond the prostate, but there are no distant metastases. In *stage D* metastatic disease is present. *Stage* D_1 refers to involvement of pelvic nodes only with no other metastases, whereas in the D_2 category metastatic disease is more widespread. It is generally believed that any of the lower stages (A, B, or C) may progress directly to stage D. Failure to include pelvic lymphadenectomy in the staging process results in marked underestimation of the frequency of lymph node metastases; for example, about a fifth of tumors tentatively classified as A_2 solely on the basis of prostate pathology actually constitute stage D disease when appropriate surgical staging is performed. The frequency with which early hematogenous metastases are missed with the current staging procedures is uncertain.

DIAGNOSIS Symptoms and signs Both early and advanced carcinoma of the prostate may be asymptomatic at the time of diagnosis, but more than 80 percent of patients have stage C or D disease at the time of diagnosis. In symptomatic subjects common presenting complaints (in descending order) include dysuria, difficulty in voiding, increased urinary frequency, complete urinary retention, back or hip pain, and hematuria. A high index of suspicion should be entertained in all men over age 40 with dysuria, frequency, or difficulty in voiding in the absence of mechanical urethral obstruction.

Palpation of the prostate is the best predictor for the diagnosis of all stages of disease other than stage A. Indeed, the importance of the rectal examination in the routine physical examination of men cannot be stressed too strongly. The posterior surfaces of the lateral lobes, where carcinoma begins most often, are easily palpable on digital rectal examination. Carcinoma characteristically is hard, nodular, and irregular, but induration may be due to areas of fibrous benign prostatic hyperplasia, focal infarcts, or calculi as well as tumor. The midline furrow between the lateral lobes may be obscured by either benign or malignant enlargement. Local extraprostatic extension of tumor into the seminal vesicles can also be detected by rectal exam. Scrotal and/or lower-extremity lymphedema secondary to infiltration of pelvic lymph nodes are manifestations of extensive disease.

When a transrectal probe is used for pelvic sonography, carcinoma is manifested by asymmetric densities within the prostate. The procedure is not a sensitive means of establishing a diagnosis but is useful for documenting the degree of extension of the tumor into bladder and seminal vesicles. Computerized tomography (CT) of the prostate may also be helpful in defining the extent of tumor and locating nodes for aspiration needle biopsy.

Biopsy Biopsy of the prostate is essential for establishing the diagnosis. Needle biopsy may be performed transperineally or transrectally with less risk of bacterial contamination with the former and more precise sampling with the latter. Open perineal biopsy is performed infrequently because it carries risk of at least temporary impotence and is a more extensive surgical procedure. Transurethral biopsy is also used infrequently because most early lesions are in the peripheral regions of the gland. Prostate biopsy is indicated when a palpable abnormality is detected or when lower urinary tract symptoms occur in men who have no known cause of obstruction.

Biochemical markers Several biochemical markers provide ancillary information in diagnosing prostatic cancer. Elevated serum *acid phosphatase* occurs in some patients with localized carcinoma and more commonly in patients with bony metastases. However, no technique of assay for the enzyme (including counterimmune electrophoresis and radioimmunoassay) is sufficiently specific or sensitive for use in screening, and the major application of the assay is in following the progress of the disease after the diagnosis is established. Likewise, none of the other plasma markers studied—bone marrow acid phosphatase, carcinoembryonic antigen, lactic dehydrogenase, creatine phosphokinase, hydroxyproline, cholesterol, isoleucine, glycine, aspartic acid, glutamic acid, methionine, or spermidine—has sufficiently high specificity or sensitivity for routine screening.

Assessment of metastatic disease *Bony metastases* from prostatic carcinoma usually contain both osteoblastic and osteolytic components. The bony pelvis and lumbar vertebrae are involved most often, and metastases to thoracic vertebrae, ribs, skull, and long bones also occur. Skeletal survey has a low sensitivity of detection because a significant portion of bone must be involved to permit detection on a routine x-ray. Bone scans using radionuclides such as technetium 99 are more sensitive, but the specificity is not high because positive scans may occur in any metabolically hyperactive bone, including sites of inflammation, healing fractures, osteoarthritis, and Paget's disease. Therefore, although radionuclide scanning is useful as an initial survey for bone metastases, the presence of other lesions must be excluded by conventional radiography of the affected site when a positive scan is obtained. Radionuclide bone scans are also useful for monitoring progression and response to therapy.

Surgical staging is the common modality for assessing *lymph node involvement* and determining therapy. The procedure usually includes removal of the external iliac, internal iliac, and obturator lymph node chains and is performed either by itself or in conjunction with prostatic surgery or implantation of radioactive beads. In some centers the initial procedure is either lymphangiography or pelvic CT scan followed when positive by confirmatory thin-needle biopsy of the affected lymph nodes; when the CT scan or the lymphangiogram is negative, however, operative staging is mandatory.

TREATMENT Surgery Surgical removal is the oldest treatment for carcinoma of the prostate. The radical perineal prostatectomy (total prostatoseminovesiculectomy) and the retropubic procedure, which affords access to the pelvic lymph nodes, are most commonly employed. Both operations almost invariably cause impotence, but in experienced hands the procedures have otherwise low morbidity and low mortality rates ($<$ 1 percent for radical perineal and 1 to 4 percent for radical retropubic prostatectomy).

Radical prostatectomy is not indicated for stage A_1 cancer since this disease is cured definitively by the simple prostatectomy at which the diagnosis is made. The role of radical prostatectomy in stage A_2 is unsettled. However, true stage A_2 disease in which pelvic nodes show no evidence of metastases may behave aggressively and be benefited by radical surgery particularly when the neoplasm is anaplastic. Indeed, 5- and 10-year survivals equivalent to those of age-matched men without prostatic cancer have been reported following such treatment for stage A_2 disease.

Radical prostatectomy has its clearest indication in stage B disease. Nearly all of the apparent surgical cures in this stage are in men who have 1- to 2-cm nodules involving only one lobe of the prostate at presentation (e.g., stage B_1). These data led Walsh and Jewett to suggest that radical prostatectomy be limited to stage B_1 disease, a group comprising only 5 percent of prostatic carcinoma patients. However, subjects with true stage B_2 disease may in fact be appropriate candidates for radical prostatectomy.

The effectiveness of radical prostatectomy for stage C disease is less certain. Morbidity rates from local pelvic symptoms, bladder outlet obstruction, hematuria, and ureteral obstruction may be decreased by radical prostatectomy in stage C disease, but controlled studies comparing morbidity rates after surgery with those of other therapies are lacking. Radical prostatectomy has no place in the treatment of stage D disease, and lymph node removal has no therapeutic benefit. Therefore, other means of therapy should be tried.

Radiation Radiation therapy was developed as a primary treatment in prostatic carcinoma because of a desire to avoid the impotence and occasional incontinence that follows radical prostatectomy. In most series, approximately 6000 to 7000 rads (60,000 to 70,000 mGy) are administered to the prostate over 6 weeks by a variety of delivery patterns. Radiation to the pelvic nodes may or may not be performed. Acute proctitis and urethritis are common side effects but are usually controllable by local measures and adjustments in radiation delivery. Chronic complications after full courses of external beam radiation include impotence in 30 to 60 percent; chronic proctitis in 10 to 15 percent; and occasional rectal stricture, rectal fistula, and rectal bleeding. It is not clear whether external beam radiation actually eradicates prostatic carcinoma, because many patients in whom progression of the tumor is slowed or halted have persistent tumor on rebiopsy, and the biological potential of these persistent tumors is not clear.

The largest series on external beam radiation for prostatic cancer is that of Bagshaw; a variety of delivery techniques and doses were utilized in nearly 1300 patients, many of whom had received prior hormone manipulation. There was about 50 percent 10-year survival in stages A and B and a mean 10-year survival of 30 percent in stage C. The 5-year survival in stage D patients who also received radiation to the pelvis as well was 58 percent. Several smaller studies have reported responses that in the aggregate are similar. The best results are obtained when the tumors are less than 2 cm in size at the time of therapy. There appears to be no consistent correlation between tumor grade and radiosensitivity.

Focal external beam radiation is usually effective as palliation for bone pain due to metastases. The duration of relief is variable. Radiation is less reliable for alleviating ureteral obstruction secondary to metastatic tumor because the time lag for a successful response may take 6 to 8 weeks.

Interstitial radiation involves retropubic implantation of seeds of ^{125}I. This treatment avoids major extirpative surgery and provides a concentrated delivery of radiation to the target tissue. Successful ^{125}I implantation requires a well-defined primary tumor with a diameter less than 5 cm, a tumor volume less than 30 to 40 ml, and uniform distribution of ^{125}I seeds throughout the prostate. In the initial reports, 5-year survival following staging pelvic lymphadenectomy and retropubic implantation of ^{125}I seeds was comparable to survival rates of other forms of treatment. Potency is preserved in more than 90 percent, and early complications are fewer and less severe than after external beam radiation.

In summary, except for impotence following external beam radiation, serious morbidity is infrequent following either form of radiation therapy. Practical considerations make ^{125}I seed implantation most suited to stage B_1 disease. The long-term efficacy of either form of radiation as compared to radical prostatectomy for treatment of localized prostatic carcinoma (pathological stages A_2, B_1, and B_2) is not clear.

Androgen deprivation Since growth of the normal prostate is dependent upon testicular androgens (see Chap. 117) it was logical to try androgen deprivation for treatment of prostatic cancer. On theoretical grounds, there are four ways by which androgen deprivation can be achieved and consequently by which androgen-dependent tumors could be treated: (1) surgical extirpation of the glands that synthesize androgens (castration and adrenalectomy), (2) inhibition of pituitary gonadotropin (and/or ACTH) production (estrogen therapy or hypophysectomy), (3) inhibition of androgen synthesis by the testes and adrenals (aminoglutethimide), and (4) inhibition of androgen binding to its receptor protein (cyproterone acetate or flutamide).

The common techniques to achieve androgen deprivation at the clinical level are castration and estrogen therapy. Since testicular secretion accounts for more than 95 percent of daily testosterone production, bilateral orchiectomy results in a decline of plasma levels from approximately 5 ng/ml to 0.3 to 0.5 ng/ml. Estrogens such as diethylstilbestrol (DES) are potent inhibitors of the release from the pituitary gland of luteinizing hormone, the gonadotropin that regulates testosterone production, and consequently its administration also causes a fall in plasma testosterone to castrate levels. Maximum depression of plasma testosterone is achieved with 3 mg of DES per day. Other estrogens (conjugated estrogens, ethinyl estradiol, diethylstilbestrol diphosphate) are no more effective in lowering plasma testosterone than is DES.

Androgen depletion beyond that achieved by surgical castration or estrogen administration can be accomplished by adrenalectomy. Since adrenal androgen production is under the control of ACTH, the adrenal sources of androgen can also be eliminated by hypophysectomy. The alternative to surgical ablation is the induction of a medical adrenalectomy and/or castration with drugs that inhibit the synthesis and/or binding of androgen to its cytoplasmic receptor protein. While these ancillary surgical and medical means have theoretical benefits for achieving androgen deprivation, their usefulness in treating prostatic cancer is not established.

Androgen deprivation therapy utilizing bilateral orchiectomy, DES therapy, or combined orchiectomy plus DES was a standard form of treatment for carcinoma of the prostate for many years, based largely upon clinical reports comparing treatment groups with historical controls. Subsequently, the role of such therapy was assessed in three controlled prospective studies conducted by the Veterans Administration Cooperative Urological Research Group. These studies failed to establish the effectiveness of high-dose DES or orchiectomy, alone or in combination, in enhancing survival in any stage of prostatic cancer. [Low-dose DES (1 mg per day) may decrease deaths from cancer; since this dosage does not uniformly suppress testosterone levels, the drug may work by means other than or in addition to inhibiting testosterone formation.]

Even when there is no beneficial effect upon survival, androgen deprivation causes a decrease in bone pain in two-thirds of symptomatic stage D patients with carcinoma of the prostate. Whether palliative hormone therapy should be administered early (asymptomatic stage) or late (symptomatic stage) in stage D disease is unsettled.

Chemotherapy The age group at greatest risk for prostatic cancer has poor tolerance for chemotherapy. This feature, coupled with the variable course of the disease, makes it difficult to determine the effectiveness of such therapy. However, several comprehensive trials utilizing chemotherapy have been undertaken in stage D disease following relapse after hormonal treatment, a situation in which mean survival time is only 7 to 8 months. The agents studied most extensively are estramustine phosphate, prednimustine, and *cis*-platinum, and more limited trials have been conducted with 5-fluorouracil, melphalan, and hydroxyurea. Complete response is rare, and only a tenth of stage D patients have an objective partial response. In other trials combinations of chemotherapeutic agents have been tested in stage D disease, most commonly estramustine phosphate plus prednimustine or cyclophosphamide plus another agent. Complete response is again rare, and only a fourth of patients or fewer show any objective improvement. For progressive, symptomatic stage D prostatic cancer, endocrine ablation therapy should be undertaken first, but chemotherapeutic agents may provide some benefit when such patients relapse.

REFERENCES

BAGSHAW MA: External radiation therapy of carcinoma of the prostate. Cancer 45:1912, 1980

BYAR DP, CORLE DK: VACURG randomized trial of radical prostatectomy for Stages I and II prostate cancer. Urology 17(4)(Suppl):7, 1981

CATALONA WJ, SCOTT WW: Carcinoma of the prostate, in *Campbell's Urology*, JH Harrison et al (eds). Philadelphia, Saunders, 1979, p 1085

GUINAN P et al: The accuracy of the rectal examination in the diagnosis of prostatic carcinoma. N Engl J Med 303:499, 1980

HERR HW: Iodine 125 implantation in the management of localized prostatic carcinoma. Urol Clin North Am 7:605, 1980

KLEIN LA: Prostatic carcinoma. N Engl J Med 300:824, 1979

MURPHY GP et al: Current status of classification and staging of prostate cancer. Cancer 45:1889, 1980

SAGALOWSKY AI, WILSON JD: Carcinoma of the prostate: The therapeutic dilemma, in *Update IV: Harrison's Principles of Internal Medicine*, KJ Isselbacher et al (eds). New York, McGraw-Hill, 1982

SCHMIDT JD: Chemotherapy of hormone-resistant stage D prostatic cancer. J Urol 123:797, 1980

STAMEY TA: Cancer of the prostate. An analysis of some important contributions and dilemmas. 1982 Monographs in Urology 3:67, 1982

WALSH PC: Physiologic basis for hormonal therapy in carcinoma of the prostate. Urol Clin N Am 2:125, 1975

——— et al: Radical surgery for prostatic cancer. Cancer 45:1906, 1980

128
THE ACUTE LEUKEMIAS

BAYARD CLARKSON

DEFINITION Leukemia is a disease characterized by neoplastic proliferation of one of the blood-forming cells. The different types of leukemia are classified according to the cell type involved, and as acute or chronic, depending on the duration of the disease. If left untreated, all forms of leukemia are fatal; death is usually due to complications resulting from infiltration of the bone marrow by leukemic cells and replacement of normal hematopoietic cells. The average survival of untreated patients with acute leukemia is about 3 months, but the course of the disease may vary considerably.

This chapter is limited to a discussion of the acute leukemias, i.e., those forms which present de novo with progressive infiltration of the marrow by largely immature cells and which usually have a rapidly fatal course without effective treatment. Chronic myelogenous leukemia and other myeloproliferative disorders, which may terminate by transformation into an acute blastic phase, are discussed in Chaps. 129, 336, and 337.

CLASSIFICATION Because there are significant differences in their age distribution and responsiveness to treatment, the acute leukemias are commonly divided into two major types: *acute lymphoblastic leukemia (ALL)* and *acute nonlymphoblastic leukemia (ANLL)*. These are further divided into several subtypes, which in the case of ANLL are often referred to collectively as *acute myelogenous* or *acute myeloid leukemia (AML)*.

It is important to distinguish between the two major types because the response to chemotherapy is more favorable in ALL than in ANLL and different drugs are used for inducing remission. Conventionally, the diagnosis has been made on the basis of the morphologic appearance of fixed cells on Romanowsky-stained smears, but cytochemical stains, chromosomal analysis, immunological markers, and measurements of selected enzymes are being used increasingly to identify the cell type with greater precision. In ALL, the lymphoblasts characteristically have a high nuclear cytoplasmic ratio; the nuclei are usually not indented or twisted, the number of nucleoli tends to be low (one or two); azurophilic granules are minimal and Auer rods are absent in the cytoplasm; promyelocytes and monocytes are uncommon; and, because they arise from normal precursors, the more mature cells of the granulocytic series appear normal. In contrast to acute myeloid leukemic cells, lymphoblasts do not stain with Sudan black B and the myeloperoxidase reaction is also negative.

The French-American-British (FAB) Co-operative Group has proposed a uniform classification system for the acute leukemias. Lymphoblastic leukemias are subdivided in three groups (L1 to L3) on the basis of cell size, nuclear chromatin pattern, nuclear shape, nucleoli, amount and basophilia of cytoplasm, and extent of cytoplasmic vacuolization. In the L1 type, small cells which are usually homogeneous with respect to the above-listed features predominate; such cases may have a more favorable prognosis than do the L2 types, in which the cells are larger and more heterogeneous. About 25 percent of the L1 and L2 types have T-lymphocyte markers, whereas the rest are "null" or "non-B, non-T" cells, but there are no distinctive morphologic features associated with the minority with T-cell markers. Both T- and null-cell types have elevated terminal deoxynucleotidyl transferase levels; since this enzyme is associated with T-cell differentiation, the null cells are probably pre-T cells. In the L3 (Burkitt) type, the cells are large and homogeneous, frequently have prominent cytoplasmic vacuolization and a high mitotic index, and usually have B-lymphocyte markers.

Leukemic myeloblasts tend to be larger cells, commonly 12 to 20 μm in diameter, although smaller "micromyeloblasts" occur and may be mistaken for lymphoblasts. Myeloblasts usually have ample cytoplasm, which sometimes contains Auer rods. The nucleus has a homogeneous "ground glass" appearance and multiple nucleoli (three to five) are usually present. In the FAB classification, the acute myeloid leukemias are subdivided into six types (M1 to M6), defined according to the direction of differentiation and degree of maturation. M1 to M3 show predominantly granulocytic differentiation and differ from one another in their extent of maturation. In the M1 type (myeloblastic leukemia without maturation) the blasts are nongranular, but 3 percent or more are myeloperoxidase-positive and may contain rare azurophilic granules, Auer rods, or both, but further maturation is not seen. In the M2 type (myeloblastic leukemia with maturation), maturation proceeds to the promyelocyte stage or beyond. More than 50 percent of the cells in the bone marrow are myeloblasts and promyelocytes, and later cells of the granulocytic series may also be found in varying proportions. The latter often demonstrate abnormal features such as the Pelger-Huet anomaly or hypogranulation. In the M3 type (hypergranular promyelocytic leukemia), the majority of cells are abnormal promyelocytes with heavy granulation; this type is often associated with serious coagulation abnormalities.

The M4 type (myelomonocytic leukemia) shows both granulocytic and monocytic differentiation, and the percentages of promonocytes plus monocytes and of myeloblasts plus promyelocytes in the marrow each exceed 20 percent. A chronic form of myelomonocytic leukemia is also described. In the M5 type (monocytic leukemia), there is predominantly monocytic differentiation. Two subtypes are described: (*a*) poorly differentiated (monoblastic) and (*b*) differentiated, in which both monoblasts and more mature cells of the monocytic series are present. The naphthol AS or ASD acetate esterase reaction (NASDA) is strongly positive in monoblasts, promonocytes, and monocytes and is inhibited by sodium fluoride, whereas in granulocytes the positivity of the reaction is unaffected by exposure to sodium fluoride. The serum lysozyme concentration is frequently elevated in the M4 and M5 types with a prominent monocytic component.

In the M6 type (erythroleukemia), the erythropoietic component usually exceeds 50 percent of the nucleated cells in the marrow, and erythroblasts may be present in the blood. The erythroblasts frequently show abnormalities, such as megaloblastosis, distorted nuclear shape, multiple nuclei, nuclear fragmentation, and giant forms. There is an increased percentage of myeloblasts and promyelocytes (30 percent or higher), and abnormal megakaryocytes may also be present. The proportion of erythroblasts varies during the course of the disease, usually decreasing as the disease progresses and eventually becoming replaced by immature cells of the granulocytic series. These findings are characteristic of the acute form of erythroleukemia (acute erythremic myelosis, or Di Guglielmo's syndrome), but a more chronic form of erythroleukemia is also seen and may be related to other dysmyelopoietic syndromes associated with "ineffective erythropoiesis," such as refractory megaloblastic anemia, "smoldering leukemia," and "preleukemia," or with refractory anemia with excess of blasts (RAEB). In the latter condition, the marrow is hypercellular and myeloblasts and promyelocytes may account for 10 to 30 percent of the nucleated cells; a progressive increase toward 50 percent indicates development of acute myeloid leukemia.

Abnormal eosinophils, which are probably derived from the leukemic cell lines, are often present as a minority component in myeloid leukemia, but both acute and chronic forms of eosinophilic leukemia have been described in which eosinophils predominate; the acute form may be associated with cardiac complications. However, the diagnosis should be made with caution, since eosinophilic leukemia is very rare and is often difficult to distinguish from other conditions associated with hypereosinophilia, particularly the hypereosinophilic syndrome (see Chap. 57). Basophilic leukemia and megakaryocytic leukemia seldom, if ever, present as forms of acute leukemia de novo, but may evolve as variants of chronic myelogenous leukemia or other myeloproliferative diseases. Mast-cell leukemia is a rare disease which is associated with urticaria pigmentosa and gastrointestinal symptoms. Plasma-cell leukemia, in which numerous plasma cells appear in the peripheral blood, may occur rarely, either as a terminal event in patients with multiple myeloma or as an initial variant of the disease. When this occurs, in addition to the usual manifestations of myeloma, there may be a prominent involvement of the liver, spleen, and lymph nodes and a marked tendency to bleeding.

In the hands of experienced morphologists, there is usually reasonably close agreement in identifying morphologic subtypes of acute leukemia. The major distinction between ALL and ANLL can be made in about 90 percent of cases by expert morphologists, but in distinguishing between subtypes of ANLL such as acute myelomonocytic leukemia (M4) and acute monocytic leukemia (M5), agreement is less consistent. By means of cell-separation techniques and newer cell markers to identify subpopulations, some acute leukemias have been found to be comprised of mixed subpopulations of lymphoid and myeloid cells (biphenotypic leukemias). Although some cell types have distinctive ultrastructural features, transmission and scanning electron microscopic studies have proved more useful in confirming suspected diagnoses than in providing positive identification in unknown cases. With the use of special staining procedures, myeloperoxidase can sometimes be demonstrated in early myeloblasts which are otherwise indistinguishable from lymphoblasts by light microscopy and conventional cytochemical staining methods.

INCIDENCE AND PREVALENCE The reported mortality from all types of leukemia in the United States increased to about 6.8 per 100,000 persons per year in 1956, and since then the overall rate has remained relatively stable. The mortality rate from leukemia is higher than average in Jews, and has been persistently lower in black than in white Americans, but these differences appear to be diminishing. Leukemia occurs throughout the world; the annual mortality rates in different countries vary from around 3 to 7 per 100,000 population, being highest in the Scandinavian countries and Israel and lowest in Chile and Japan. Still lower death rates are reported in some developing countries, but this may reflect inadequate medical services. Depending on the criteria of classification, about 50 to 60 percent of leukemia deaths in the United States are due to acute leukemia.

All types of leukemia are slightly more common in males than in females. However, male predominance is less marked for acute leukemia (about 3:2) than for chronic lymphocytic leukemia (about 2:1) and the sex incidence is almost the same in very young children. The overall incidence of ALL and ANLL is about equal in the United States, but there are marked age and racial differences in their distribution. Acute leukemia accounts for nearly half of all neoplasms in children. The peak incidence of ALL occurs between the ages of 2 to 4 years; this peak was originally noted only in white children, but a less prominent peak has also been observed in young black and Japanese children. Whereas fewer than 20 percent of cases of acute leukemia in persons under the age of 15 are ANLL, the incidence is reversed in adults; the incidence of ANLL progressively increases with advancing age.

ETIOLOGY AND EPIDEMIOLOGY The etiology of leukemia is still unknown, although there are certain factors which predispose to its development.

Ionizing radiation In doses of 1 Gy (100 rads) or greater, whether from unintentional exposure to nuclear sources or from irradiation therapy, ionizing radiation is clearly associated with an increased incidence of both acute and chronic myelogenous leukemia. It is still controversial whether a threshold dose exists below which there is no attendant increase in the risk of developing leukemia. There is no convincing evidence that doses employed in radiodiagnostic procedures are leukemogenic in adults, unless the exposure is excessive, as it was for pioneer radiologists working without effective protection. Exposure of the fetus to diagnostic radiographic procedures during pregnancy appears to be associated with a slightly increased risk of leukemia later in childhood, but the extent of the increase is controversial. It is also debatable whether any irradiation of the mother prior to conception increases the likelihood of leukemia in children born later.

Chemical agents The leukemias which follow exposure to chemical agents are usually acute or chronic myelogenous leukemia rather than the lymphocytic type. Occupational exposure to benzene and possibly other chemicals is associated with an increased incidence of leukemia. Certain drugs, such as chloramphenicol and phenylbutazone, which are known to cause bone marrow depression, are probably also leukemogenic, although the risk is not great. There are now numerous reports of an increased incidence of acute nonlymphocytic leukemia in patients with Hodgkin's disease, multiple myeloma, chronic lymphocytic leukemia, ovarian cancer, and other types of cancer, as well as in patients with nonneoplastic diseases who have been treated with cytotoxic drugs, especially alkylating agents. Moreover, the risk appears to be greater with combined-modality therapy (irradiation plus chemotherapy). The incidence increases with lengthened survival due to successful treatment of the original disease. Loss of chromosome 5 or 7, or parts of these chromosomes, is common in these secondary leukemias, and they rarely respond satisfactorily to treatment.

Hereditary factors Patients with Down's syndrome, a defect characterized by trisomy of chromosome 21, have approximately a twentyfold higher incidence of acute leukemia than expected in comparable age groups of the general population. The incidence of Down's syndrome increases with advancing maternal age; the incidence of leukemia in otherwise normal children born of older mothers is also slightly higher than average, but not nearly as high as in Down's syndrome. Both ALL and ANLL occur, and the type of leukemia appears to be related to that usually expected at the age of occurrence. All ages have an increased incidence, but the risk is highest in infants. Once diagnosed, with rare exception, leukemia occurring in Down's syndrome runs its usual fatal course if not treated effectively. However, occasional newborns with Down's syndrome have been reported in whom the findings are indistinguishable from those of acute leukemia, but in whom all the abnormalities disappear spontaneously and apparently permanently.

A number of other congenital conditions are also associated with an increased incidence of leukemia, although the risk is less than in Down's syndrome. These include Fanconi's aplastic anemia; Bloom's syndrome; ataxia-telangiectasia; Patau's syndrome, or D trisomy; Wiskott-Aldrich syndrome; congenital sex-linked agammaglobulinemia; and Kostmann's agranulocytosis. Although there is no common specific chromosomal lesion, most of these syndromes are characterized either by chromosomal aneuploidy or by a tendency to chromosomal breakage. Fibroblasts from individuals with Down's syndrome and Fanconi's anemia and from their parents, as well as from one family with no known congenital disease or chromosomal disorder but with multiple cases of AML, have been shown to have increased susceptibility to transformation in vitro by SV40, a simian DNA virus with high oncogenic potential.

Familial leukemia is rare, but a few otherwise normal families have been reported in which multiple cases have occurred during one or more generations. Otherwise normal siblings and fraternal twins of leukemic children have a slightly higher than normal risk of developing leukemia, and although the overall incidence is not increased in twins, if one monozygotic twin develops acute leukemia, the other has about a 20 percent chance of developing it also. Because the majority of concordant leukemias in identical twins occur during the first few years of life and because they are often diagnosed simultaneously or within a short time interval, these cases probably represent only one occurrence of leukemia and not two. Unlike the situation in dizygotic twins, the in utero circulatory systems of monozygotic twins are united by shared placental vessels, and if the initial leukemic transformation occurred in one twin before separation of the placental circulation, the other would almost inevitably be colonized by the progeny of the transformed cell. In confirmation of this hypothesis, an identical karyotypic marker was found in the leukemic cells of both monozygotic twins with near simultaneous development of acute leukemia.

Viruses It is firmly established that viruses may cause leukemia in fowls, rodents, cats, and monkeys. The viruses are leukemogenic when initially inoculated, but infected animals may harbor the virus for their lifetimes, often without themselves developing leukemia. They can pass virus to their offspring through the ovum or shed it in milk or other secretions and thereby transmit it to uninfected animals. There are many environmental and genetic factors which determine whether and what type of leukemia an infected animal will develop. Among the most important are quantity of virus, differences in susceptibility of different strains, age, sex, hormonal and immunologic influences, and exposure to external agents such as irradiation or chemical carcinogens which can release or trigger the virus and cause full expression of the disease. Most of the viruses which are leukemogenic in fowls and mammals are RNA viruses (types C or B); type C viruses have been shown to cause lymphomas or myelogenous leukemia in subhuman primates. Exceptions to this rule are Marek's disease (neural lymphomatosis) in chickens and malignant lymphomas in owl monkeys which are caused by DNA viruses of the herpes group.

Despite clear proof that viruses can cause leukemia in many animal species including primates and an intensive search for human leukemia viruses, there is no conclusive evidence that viruses cause leukemia in humans. There have been numerous reports of electron microscopic demonstration of type C virus particles in plasma pellets or tissues from patients with leukemia, of detection of viruses or virus-related antigens in human leukemic cells by immunologic techniques, and of recovery of virus from human materials in animal or cell culture systems. However, many of these reports have not been substantiated, others have failed to exclude contaminating infections, and none have provided definitive proof that viruses are the etiologic agents of human leukemia.

RNA-directed DNA polymerase (reverse transcriptase) is an enzyme present in type C viruses which permits them to synthesize DNA that can then be inserted into the genome of the infected cell, thereby allowing viral-directed genetic determinants to be passed on indefinitely through the normal process of cell division. Reverse transcriptase with biochemical and immunologic properties similar to those associated with mammalian type C viruses has been reported to be present in some human leukemic cells and also in normal leukocytes of patients with acute leukemia in remission. The enzyme is not present in fresh leukocytes from normal individuals nor in normal lymphocytes transformed to blasts by phytohemagglutinin, but has been detected in some human cell lines in established cultures. The significance of type C RNA tumor virus–related components in human leukemia cells is still disputed.

Several time-space clusters or microepidemics of leukemia have been reported, which might suggest an infectious etiology. However, prospective epidemiologic studies in situations that might reflect an infectious mode of spread have failed to support this suspicion. In a few well-documented instances, leukemic transformation has occurred in the marrow cells obtained from normal donors after transplantation into their siblings who had acute leukemia and who had received intensive chemotherapy and total-body irradiation prior to the marrow transplants. However, this is a rare occurrence, and most instances of recurrent leukemia in patients who have received marrow grafts have been due to regrowth of the recipients' own leukemic cells.

NATURE OF THE DISORDER IN ACUTE LEUKEMIA There is good evidence that acute leukemia usually begins with the transformation of a single hematopoietic stem cell. The nature of the molecular lesion(s) responsible for the transformed cell's neoplastic properties is unclear, but the critical defect is intrinsic and inheritable by the cell's progeny. There have been many attempts to demonstrate qualitative biochemical differences between normal and leukemic cells, but no consistent differences have been found in cells of comparable levels of maturity. In patients who have recognizable karyotypic abnormalities in their leukemic cells prior to treatment and in whom serial cytogenetic studies have been performed, the abnormal metaphases disappear from the marrow or are greatly reduced in number, and normal diploid modes are present during drug-induced remissions. When relapse occurs, the original abnormal leukemic line reappears; in some cases one or more secondary abnormal lines may appear as a result of clonal evolution. Relapse is ordinarily caused by regrowth of residual surviving cells from the original leukemic population rather than as a result of reinduction of a new leukemia.

The leukemogenic transforming event may occur at any stage in the cells' ancestral lineages, but in order for the disease to be fully expressed, it must either take place at an early enough stage so that the cell already has unlimited proliferative capacity, or it must acquire this capacity as a result of becoming transformed. Consequently, if the transformation occurs in a progenitor cell with the capacity to differentiate into both erythrocyte and granulocyte precursors, erythroleukemia will result; whereas if it occurs in a progenitor cell already committed to granulocytic differentiation, the resultant leukemia will be myeloblastic. Biphenotypic leukemias composed of mixed subpopulations of lymphoblasts and myeloblasts or monoblasts have also been described. A critical defect in acute leukemia is defective maturation so that instead of producing equal numbers of committed and stem cells, leukemic stem cells generate an increased proportion of stem cells. In acute leukemia the leukemic population seldom if ever expands exponentially at a maximum rate as do stem cells in uncrowded cultures or transplanted leukemic cells in the mouse during early disease. The kinetic behavior of leukemic cells in human disease can be represented best as intermediate between maximum exponential growth and the steady-state characteristic of normal hematopoiesis. Instead of invariably generating two daughters which both behave as stem cells (which would result in exponential growth) or else one stem cell and one committed cell (as in normal hematopoiesis), there is usually excessive production both of cells with unlimited proliferative potential and of committed cells with finite life spans. However, there must necessarily be a ratio greater than 1:1 of stem cells to committed cells, because otherwise the population would cease to expand. The fraction of leukemic cells with stem-cell capability may vary greatly among different populations, and this variability is partly responsible for differences in the rate of progression of the disease. Other factors influencing rate of progression are the growth fraction, or proportion of actively dividing cells, and the fact that many leukemic populations have a substantial spontaneous death rate. In some leukemic populations, (i.e., RAEB and other dysmyelopoietic states) the majority of the cells may mature to the extent of losing their ability to divide. In such instances their behavior may closely resemble that of normal hematopoietic cells, and the leukemic population may expand only very slowly.

Another important characteristic of the leukemic state is that leukemic cells are relatively unresponsive to normal regulatory mechanisms which maintain the size of the normal hematopoietic compartments within narrow limits. As a result leukemic cells continue to proliferate, albeit sometimes slowly, and commonly reach far higher population densities than do hematopoietic cells in normal individuals. However, the degree of escape from normal control varies widely; some leukemic populations expand to lethal numbers extremely rapidly, whereas others barely exceed normal cell densities in the marrow for long periods, even without treatment.

The normal hematopoietic precursors are generally reduced in advanced leukemia, probably owing to inhibition at the stem-cell level by the leukemic cells. Although the mechanism of inhibition is still unclear, it seems probable that the normal cells recognize the leukemic cells, or their inhibitory products, as "normal," and turn off production in response to excess cell numbers. The cell cycle duration of leukemic cells is no faster, and may be slower, than that of the normal hematopoietic precursors, especially during advanced disease. If chemotherapy reduces the leukemic population sufficiently, the normal stem cells are released from inhibition, and because of their faster proliferative rate, the normal precursors may repopulate the marrow faster than can the surviving leukemic cells. If enough leukemic cells have been destroyed, a remission results.

CLINICAL MANIFESTATIONS The clinical manifestations of acute leukemia are most often related to replacement of the normal hematopoietic cells in the marrow by leukemic cells, and to a lesser extent to infiltration of other organs. Symptoms may appear abruptly with severe prostration, high fever, and bleeding, or the onset may be insidious with progressive weakness, pallor, low-grade fever, minor bleeding tendencies, or recurrent infections. Sometimes there are no antecedent symptoms, and the diagnosis is made while investigating the reason for menorrhagia or excessive bleeding following a dental procedure.

Fever is present in the majority of patients at the time of diagnosis, and some degree of fever occurs almost invariably sometime during attempts at inducing remission owing to further depletion of granulocytes by cytotoxic drugs. High fever is frequently associated with obvious infection, but sometimes no source can be found even on careful search, and there may be no response to antibiotics. It is debatable whether fever can occur in the absence of any infection, but if it can, this phenomenon is certainly less frequent than in the lymphomas or in the blastic phase of chronic myelogenous leukemia. In addition to the usual pathogenic bacteria, microorganisms which are ordinarily relatively avirulent frequently cause serious infections in patients with acute leukemia.

There may be no abnormalities on physical examination, or there may be multiple findings. Enlargement of the tonsils, lymph nodes, and spleen are common, especially in ALL, and splenic infarction, subcapsular hemorrhage, and, rarely, splenic rupture may occur. The liver and kidneys are also frequently enlarged due to leukemic infiltration, but the infiltrates do not ordinarily interfere with the function of these or other organs unless there are associated complications such as infection, hemorrhage, blockage of the ureters or biliary system, or uric acid nephropathy. Leukemic infiltration of the gingivae, skin, and other tissues is especially common in monocytic leukemia. Localized tumor masses which have a greenish appearance sometimes occur in the skin, orbit, or other tissues in granulocytic forms of leukemia. These are called *chloromas,* and the greenish color is due to the presence of myeloperoxidase. Rarely leukemia may present as a localized bony tumor prior to diffuse marrow involvement. Patients with many circulating leukemic cells usually have more rapidly progressive disease, and more extensive infiltration of the marrow and other organs. They may die suddenly from massive intracranial hemorrhage as a result of leukostasis, perivascular infiltration, and weakening of the vessel walls. Bleeding may occur at any site, but the most common sites of fatal hemorrhages are intracranial, gastrointestinal, and pulmonary. Thrombophlebitis and other thromboembolic disorders occur frequently in acute leukemia, even in patients with severe thrombocytopenia.

Local infections are common, especially involving one or more of the body orifices, and can be very serious as in the case of peritonsillar or perirectal abscesses. Leukemic infiltrations often occur at sites of infection and interfere with healing. Leukemic infiltration of the lungs may also occur, but this is frequently difficult to distinguish from pulmonary infections, and often the two are associated. Serous effusions, involving especially the pleural cavities, are also common. Infiltration, intussusception, hemorrhage, infection, or perforation may occur anywhere in the gastrointestinal tract, and local or generalized peritonitis may develop. Sternal tenderness is often present, and there may be severe pain and tenderness of multiple bones and joints due to bone infarcts or subperiosteal infiltrates. Bone and joint pains are especially common in children with ALL and may be misdiagnosed as acute rheumatic fever or rheumatoid arthritis. Anorexia, weight loss, muscle wasting, and contractures sometimes occur, usually as a result of the combined effects of diminished physical activity, hypercatabolism, and nutritional deficiency.

Neurologic findings are unusual at the time of presentation but occur frequently during the course of acute leukemia. There may be infiltration of the peripheral nerves, spinal nerve roots, or cranial nerve palsies, the latter commonly being due to infiltration of the nerve sheaths with compression of the nerves as they pass through their osseous foramens. Severe symptoms due to intracranial hemorrhage and/or infiltration of the leptomeninges may occur, among them being headache, vomiting, seizures, visual disturbance, papilledema, and nuchal rigidity. Leukemic meningitis due to arachnoid infiltration occurs in the majority of patients with ALL sometime during the course of their disease if not prevented by prophylactic intrathecal chemotherapy or cranial irradiation. Arachnoid leukemia also may be seen in ANLL, but less frequently than in ALL. Rarely, leukemic infiltration of the hypothalamus may cause hyperphagia, obesity, and behavioral disturbances. Inappropriate secretion of antidiuretic hormone or true diabetes insipidus is also seen occasionally.

LABORATORY FINDINGS There is usually some degree of anemia which is generally due mostly to decreased erythrocyte production, although hemorrhage can sometimes be an important factor, and a modest decrease in red blood cell survival may also occur. Severe hemolytic anemia is rare, and the direct Coombs test is usually negative. Reticulocytes are reduced, and the erythrocytes are usually normochromic and normocytic. However, in some patients, the red blood cell precursors have prominent megaloblastic features, and macrocytes and erythroblasts may appear in the blood. The megaloblastic changes are not corrected by administration of vitamin B_{12} or other nutritional factors, and it seems likely that the abnormal erythroblasts in such patients are part of the leukemic population.

The platelet count is usually moderately to severely decreased; occasionally it is normal, but it is rarely elevated. Hemorrhagic tendencies are usually correlated with the level of thrombocytopenia, and although occasionally severe hemorrhages occur in patients with more than 100,000 platelets per cubic millimeter, most serious bleeding episodes develop in patients with fewer than 20,000 platelets per cubic millimeter, particularly in the presence of infection. When bleeding occurs in the presence of adequate numbers of platelets, the platelets are often abnormal and function poorly, and may be derived from megakaryocytes which are involved in the leukemic process.

In addition to those attributable to thrombocytopenia, various coagulation abnormalities have been recognized, of which one of the most frequent and serious is disseminated intravascular coagulation (DIC). DIC is most often seen in promyelocytic leukemia but may occur in other types of acute leukemia. When first diagnosed, most patients with acute leukemia have adequate levels of all clotting factors, and indeed fibrinogen and factor VIII are sometimes elevated. However, multiple abnormalities may occur during the course of the disease due to sepsis, hepatic decompensation, nutritional deficiencies, and some of the drugs used in treating leukemia (e.g., L-asparaginase).

Neutropenia is often present. The severity is related to the extent of marrow infiltration by leukemic cells and also to the presence of infection. Various abnormalities of granulocytic function have been described in acute leukemia, but it is uncertain whether the defective granulocytes belong to the leukemic or normal population.

Because most of the manifestations of acute leukemia also may be associated with other diseases, the diagnosis can be made only by careful morphologic examinations of the blood and bone marrow. The number of leukemic cells in the peripheral blood may vary from none to more than 1 million per cubic millimeter; only about 15 percent of patients have leukocyte counts over 100,000 per cubic millimeter. Some patients present with normal erythrocyte and platelet counts, or with pancytopenia, and have only a few (subleukemic) or no (aleukemic) blasts in the blood. In such cases, the peripheral blood leukocytes should be concentrated by centrifugation, and stained smears of the buffy coat prepared. Some leukemic cells will be found in the blood of most patients; moreover, they may be more mature and hence more indicative of the morphologic type of leukemia than those in the marrow. A bone marrow aspiration and differential count should always be performed. Most untreated patients have over 50 percent obviously leukemic cells in the marrow, and a diagnosis of acute leukemia should be made with great caution if the marrow differential count shows less than 30 percent immature cells unless Auer rods are present.

Sometimes even when the marrow is filled with leukemic cells, they cannot be aspirated because they are so adhesive or are enmeshed in reticulin fibers, and in such cases a needle biopsy should always be done. Open surgical biopsy is rarely necessary and should be performed with extreme caution in the presence of severe thrombocytopenia. The pathologist can usually recognize replacement of normal marrow cells by immature cells in hematoxylin-eosin-stained sections, but Wright-stained touch preparations of the biopsy specimen are more useful in identifying the morphologic type of leukemia. A specific granulocyte stain, the naphthol chloroacetate esterase reaction, can be performed on paraffin-embedded tissue sections and aids in identifying the specific cell type in such cases.

Chromosome analysis of dividing leukemic cells in the marrow shows one or more karyotypic abnormalities in about half of patients with acute leukemia, using conventional banding techniques. With high-resolution cytogenetic analysis, the leukemic cells in the majority of patients with ANLL have been reported to have chromosomal abnormalities. Specific abnormalities occur fairly consistently in different types of leukemia. For example, in the acute myeloblastic (M2) type of ANLL, translocation between chromosomes 8 and 21, t(8;21), is especially common, and translocation between chromosomes 15 and 17, t(15;17), occurs in about 40 percent of patients with acute promyelocytic leukemia (M3). Patients with ANLL whose marrow cells are all karyotypically normal by conventional analysis, or who have a mixture of normal and abnormal cells, have a better prognosis than do those with only abnormal cells. ALL patients with hypodiploidy also appear to have a very poor prognosis.

Other laboratory studies are not very useful or specific. Uric acid production is frequently increased in patients with rapidly growing and/or a massive number of leukemic cells. The serum level and urinary excretion of uric acid may rise further after treatment with cytotoxic drugs because of increased cellular breakdown, and gout or precipitation of urate crystals may develop in the renal collecting system. Serum and urinary levels of phosphorus and potassium may also be elevated and rise further after treatment. Hypophosphatemia and hypokalemia may also occur, the latter especially during treatment with amphotericin B, gentamicin, or other nephrotoxic drugs, or in acute monocytic leukemia with lysozymuria. The serum level of lactic acid dehydrogenase (LDH) may be elevated in some types of ANLL and in the L3 type of ALL. Both serum and urinary lysozyme (muramidase) levels are often increased in acute monocytic leukemia. However, both of these enzymes may also be elevated in chronic granulocytic leukemia and other myeloproliferative conditions, and very high LDH levels are sometimes seen in some of the lymphomas. In untreated ALL the muramidase concentration may be subnormal and subsequently rise to normal following successful treatment. The levels of serum vitamin B_{12}-binding protein and serum vitamin B_{12} may be high in acute as well as in chronic granulocytic leukemia.

The cerebrospinal fluid may be under increased pressure, have high concentrations of protein and low glucose, and contain leukemic cells, but sometimes central nervous system involvement may occur without any abnormalities of the cerebrospinal fluid. Conversely, pleocytosis may sometimes be present in the absence of recognizable neurologic signs or symptoms.

DIFFERENTIAL DIAGNOSIS When the blood leukocyte count is elevated, certain infections (e.g., meningococcemia, tuberculosis, abscesses) may be mistaken for acute leukemia, but the majority of leukocytes are more mature in leukemoid reactions than in acute leukemias, and appropriate microbiologic studies should lead to the correct diagnosis. The peripheral blood lymphocytes may be greatly increased in pertussis, infectious mononucleosis, and infectious lymphocytosis, and to a lesser extent in varicella, infectious hepatitis, and several other viral illnesses. However, the bone marrow is less affected, and anemia and thrombocytopenia are either absent or less prominent than in acute leukemia. The lymphocytes are small and mature in pertussis and infectious lymphocytosis and should be readily distinguished from lymphoblasts. Although lymphoblasts indistinguishable from those found in ALL can occur in infectious mononucleosis and sometimes in other viral infections, the abnormal lymphocytes which occur in viral infections are usually more pleomorphic than leukemic lymphoblasts. Other helpful diagnostic tests for infectious mononucleosis are an elevated heterophil antibody titer (Paul-Bunnell test) and rising antibodies to components of the Epstein-Barr (EB) virus; also the circulating lymphocytes in infectious mononucleosis have T-cell markers, whereas this is true in only about 25 percent of cases of ALL. Occasionally, there can be diagnostic confusion when severe anemia and/or thrombocytopenia occurs in infectious mononucleosis or infectious hepatitis as a result of hypersplenism, an autoimmune process, or rarely, aplastic anemia. However, in such cases the bone marrow either shows erythrocytic or megakaryocytic hyperplasia or it is aplastic and is not densely infiltrated with immature cells. Whereas chronic lymphocytic leukemia or hairy-cell leukemia are sometimes misdiagnosed as ALL, with careful morphological examination of the cells and use of appropriate cell markers, the correct diagnosis should be readily apparent.

Usually, there is no difficulty in distinguishing between acute myelocytic leukemia and chronic myelogenous leukemia, but in some patients with chronic myelogenous leukemia the disease has already undergone blastic transformation when they first present; in about 25 percent of cases the blasts have the morphologic appearance of lymphoblasts. The presence of a Philadelphia (Ph′) chromosome is considered by some authorities to be diagnostic of the blastic phase of chronic myelogenous leukemia, whereas others prefer to regard such cases as Ph′+ variants of ALL or ANLL. It is generally agreed such patients have a worse prognosis than the majority of patients with ALL or ANLL.

Some solid tumors which have a tendency to cause myelophthisic anemia are sometimes confused with acute leukemia, especially if there are no extramedullary tumor masses accessible for biopsy, because the tumor cells infiltrating the marrow may resemble leukemic cells. These tumors include neuroblastoma, Ewing's sarcoma, embryonal rhabdomyosarcoma, and small-cell carcinoma of the lung. Infiltration of the marrow and blood occurs frequently in non-Hodgkin's lymphomas, and less commonly in Hodgkin's disease. The neoplastic cells in some diseases diagnosed as lymphomas may, in fact, be indistinguishable from certain types of leukemia, even by surface and biochemical markers. For example, neoplastic cells in the lymphoblastic type of poorly differentiated lymphocytic lymphoma may be "null" or T cells and have a high deoxynucleotidyl transferase content and other properties which are identical with the same cell types found in patients with ALL. Similarly, Burkitt's lymphoma cells are neoplastic B cells which are apparently identical with the L3 type of ALL cells and have the same chromosomal abnormality, t(8;14). Diffuse histiocytic lymphoma (reticulum-cell sarcoma) may be confused with acute monocytic leukemia, since in both diseases the cells may have monocytoid features and a propensity to infiltrate the skin and other tissues. However, elevated lysozyme levels are common in monocytic leukemia, whereas this is not the case in diffuse histiocytic lymphoma, which is usually a B-cell neoplasm. Moreover, gingival infiltrates are common and retroperitoneal node involvement is uncommon in pure monocytic leukemia, whereas the reverse is true in histiocytic lymphoma. When lymphomas clearly originate in lymph nodes or other extramedullary sites and only secondarily involve the marrow, there is little difficulty in diagnosis. However, sometimes lymphomas may be largely confined to the marrow (and perhaps the spleen and liver) at the time of presentation, and there may be no enlarged lymph nodes available for biopsy. Conversely, in rare cases, the first manifestation of monocytic leukemia may be extramedullary infiltration of the bladder, skin, or other organs, and the marrow may not show extensive infiltration until later in the course of the disease. Indeed, with the use of newer cell marker techniques to identify specific cell types more precisely, some diseases previously diagnosed as lymphomas or leukemias are proving to be merely different manifestations of neoplastic proliferations of the same cell type.

When patients with acute leukemia present with few leukemic cells in the blood and reduction of one or more of the normal blood elements, the diagnosis may be confused with several other conditions, including hypersplenism and various neutropenic or thrombocytopenic states. Aplastic anemia, resulting from drugs, chemicals, or unknown causes, can be mistaken for acute leukemia, especially if the marrow is hyperplastic or in a regenerative phase, since numerous blasts and other immature cells may be present. Some patients with aplastic anemia die of infection or bleeding, some recover partially or completely, and still others go on to develop full-blown acute myeloblastic or monocytic leukemia. A rare form of ANLL has been described in which the marrow is hypoplastic even on biopsy, but contains a greatly increased percentage (more than 30 percent) of blasts.

The terms *preleukemia, myelodysplastic syndrome,* and *refractory anemia with excess blasts (RAEB)* are sometimes used to describe such heterogeneous manifestations as anemia, neutropenia, thrombocytopenia, monocytosis, splenomegaly, and various other hematologic abnormalities which precede the development of acute leukemia, but this diagnosis can be made with certainty only in retrospect. If chromosomal abnormalities are present, there is a greater likelihood that acute leukemia will develop.

Erythroleukemia can be particularly difficult to diagnose and may be confused with primary refractory anemia, sideroblastic anemia, and paroxysmal nocturnal hemoglobulinuria (PNH). Since all these conditions may sometimes terminate in myeloblastic or other forms of acute leukemia, it has been suggested that they may represent early or chronic forms of erythroleukemia. The acidified-serum lysis (Ham) test is very useful in diagnosing PNH.

TREATMENT During the last quarter century, a worldwide effort has been mounted to improve the treatment of acute leukemia, and survival has been increased substantially in ALL and to a lesser extent in ANLL. An increasing number of patients remain in complete remission even after discontinuing treatment, but because some patients have had late relapses of leukemia after many years in remission, experienced clinicians are appropriately cautious about predicting curability. Nevertheless, encouraged by the progress that has been made, many therapists are now treating leukemia more aggressively and are directing their efforts toward total eradication of the leukemic cells rather than being content with temporary remissions.

Patients with acute leukemia usually have between 50 billion and 10 trillion (5×10^{10} to 10^{13}) leukemic cells when the disease is diagnosed; the number depends on the patient's size and extent of disease. Assuming that there are 1 trillion (10^{12}) cells, then a 13-decade (log) reduction is necessary to eliminate all of them, but usually only a two- to three-decade reduction (99 to 99.9 percent) is required to cause a complete remission (defined as disappearance of all symptoms and physical abnormalities due to leukemia, and return of blood and marrow cell counts to normal values).

Assuming no cell death, a single leukemic cell will propagate 10^{12} cells after 40 consecutive divisions. If there are 10^{12} cells at diagnosis, and if treatment causes a three-decade reduction, then only 10 doublings are required for the leukemic population to return to its original number. It has not been possible to measure the doubling times of leukemic populations in patients with any precision, and there is undoubtedly considerable variability, but if a doubling time of 5 days is assumed, then after a three-decade reduction, the leukemic cells would return to their original number within 50 days. It is necessary, therefore, to continue treatment to further reduce the leukemic cells long after a complete remission has been achieved. It is not known how long treatment must be continued in order to eliminate all leukemic cells, and the duration undoubtedly varies in different patients and with the intensity of the treatment and types of drugs used. Some drugs, such as alkylating agents and antitumor antibiotics, kill both resting and actively proliferating cells, whereas most of the antimetabolites are lethal only to proliferating cells. Since some leukemic cells can probably remain in a resting state for many months, alkylating drugs and antibiotics would be expected to be more effective in eradicating the last few cells.

Only some of the leukemic cells have unlimited proliferative potential and are capable of reproducing the disease; the rest, which are committed to maturation, will die spontaneously after a limited number of divisions just as committed normal cells do. There are no methods to measure the fraction of clonogenic leukemic cells (i.e., those with stem-cell capability), but this undoubtedly varies greatly in different patients. It is also unknown whether there are host defense mechanisms capable of eliminating small numbers of residual leukemic cells in humans. Since it has been proved in animal leukemias that the number of leukemic cells surviving treatment is inversely related to the duration of remission and that the duration of remission in human leukemia is directly related to lengthened survival, the goal of treatment should be to destroy as many leukemic cells as possible.

The best opportunity to achieve maximum leukemic cell kill is when the disease is first diagnosed, since cells which survive the first round of treatment and later cause relapse of the disease may be relatively resistant to drugs which were highly effective initially. Although prolonged and possibly permanent second remissions have occurred occasionally in ALL, in general, second and later remissions become progressively shorter and are more difficult to maintain. Combinations of effective drugs have produced more frequent and longer remissions than have single agents, but it is difficult to predict how best to use the available or new drugs in the optimal combinations, order, and time sequences to achieve maximum leukemic cell kill with the least toxicity to normal cells. Because there are so many unknown factors, most of the current regimens have been developed empirically. Since none of them has been uniformly successful, no standard treatment schedules have been established, and investigators throughout the world are still trying to improve the results through comparative clinical trials. Exact comparisons between different series are often difficult because of differences in patient selection, age, previous treatment, outcome (whether patients are excluded if they die before receiving an adequate course of treatment), and use of differing criteria for tabulating incidence and duration of remission. In deciding which therapeutic regimen to use, the physician should consider the probability of achieving a durable remission in a disease which kills the average patient within a few months and weigh it against the necessity for prolonged hospitalization and the greater morbidity and disruption of normal life which are associated with some of the more aggressive regimens. Whenever possible, intensive treatment should be carried out under the close supervision of a physician who is experienced in the modern management of acute leukemia; such well-trained specialists are now widely distributed in the United States and in many other countries throughout the world. Because inadequate initial chemotherapy can jeopardize the patient's chance of a long-term response, except in emergency situations *patients with acute leukemia should be referred to the nearest specialist as soon as the diagnosis is made, preferably prior to initiating chemotherapy.* However, death can occur rapidly in acute leukemia, sometimes within days of diagnosis, and if the leukocyte count is very high or if there is evidence of disseminated intravascular coagulation (DIC) or other life-threatening complications, it is mandatory to begin therapy which will reduce the leukemic cell mass immediately.

With the best current treatment regimens, over 90 percent of children and about 85 percent of adults with ALL now achieve complete remissions. All current effective regimens include prednisone (40 to 100 mg per square meter of body surface area per day) and vincristine (1.5 to 2.0 mg/m^2 with a maximum dose of 4 mg every 5 to 7 days) for induction of initial remission because these two agents are highly effective in killing lymphoblasts and are less toxic to normal marrow cells than most of the other drugs. If no further treatment is given after successful induction with prednisone and vincristine, the median duration of remission is only a few months, and it is imperative that the remission be consolidated and maintained with other drugs. Prophylactic intrathecal or intraventricular chemotherapy with or without cranial radiation treatment should also be given because of the high incidence of central nervous system involvement. Cranial irradiation and intrathecal methotrexate are effective in prophylaxis of central nervous system (CNS) leukemia, but there are several reports indicating that this combined modality therapy may result in serious late complications such as leukoencephalopathy and ventricular dilation. On the other hand, if prophylactic intrathecal chemotherapy alone is to be successful in preventing CNS leukemia, it must be given in sufficient dosage and continued for a relatively long period; exactly how long is uncertain, but one successful protocol has continued intrathecal therapy intermittently for 3 years.

The choice of drugs and the sequence of subsequent systemic therapy will depend on the training and preference of the specialist. Several combination drug regimens for ALL which have been shown to produce high rates of remission are listed in the references at the end of the chapter.

The results are less favorable in ANLL. Although remission rates of 60 to 80 percent have been reported with various drug combinations, the median duration of remission has generally been less than a year and, even with the best regimens, only about 10 to 15 percent of patients remain in remission for 5 years or longer. In most, but not all, series the remission rate has been less in older patients, and the age factor should be taken into account when comparing different series. There is no relatively nontoxic drug combination comparable to prednisone and vincristine which will regularly induce remissions in ANLL, and all the effective regimens are moderately to severely toxic to the normal hematopoietic cells and sometimes also to other tissues. This lack of selectivity is one of the major reasons for therapeutic failures. The patient has a high risk of dying during attempted induction of remission from infection or bleeding, because the granulocytes, platelets, and sometimes the immune system are already depressed as a result of the disease and become further depressed after treatment. Patients with ANLL seldom go into remission unless the great majority of morphologically evident leukemic cells in the blood and marrow have been destroyed and the marrow has become markedly hypocellular; the hypoplastic phase usually lasts at least 10 days and may last many weeks before repopulation begins. Repopulation may occur due to regeneration of normal cells, signifying the onset of remission, or from regrowth of leukemic cells, or there may be simultaneous repopulation with both normal and leukemic cells if treatment has been only partially effective.

There is considerable variability in how patients respond to a treatment regimen. This variability is partly explicable on the basis of differences in the kinetic behavior of the various leukemic and normal cell populations, and partly on the basis of differing sensitivities of the various cell populations to the same drugs. Regeneration of normal hematopoietic cells may occur very rapidly after interrupting treatment, especially in younger patients, or may be delayed or fail to occur at all; when this happens, the marrow may remain "empty" for a month or longer before it again becomes repopulated with leukemic cells. The variability in response makes it difficult to design a multiple-drug regimen with a standardized sequence which will be maximally effective in all patients. It is therefore essential to monitor closely the hematologic parameters and to individualize treatment schedules in accordance with the patient's general condition, hematologic status, and therapeutic response.

The hazard of dying during attempted induction is especially great in older patients who have other coexisting diseases, or who have developed serious infections prior to institution of antileukemic treatment. Because older patients often tolerate intensive treatment poorly, or because occasionally they have very slowly progressive disease ("smoldering leukemia") and may survive for a year or more with just supportive treatment, physicians have been understandably reluctant to treat them aggressively with chemotherapy. However, if they are left untreated, the majority of elderly patients die of acute leukemia within a few months just as do younger patients, and it is only the infrequent patient who survives longer than a year. When the diagnosis of smoldering leukemia is suspected, the patient should be observed closely, and as soon as the disease shows evidence of progression, or if the patient becomes incapacitated and unable to function with periodic transfusions, antileukemic treatment should be instituted, preferably before serious complications develop.

The most successful current regimens for ANLL have employed an anthracycline (e.g., daunorubicin or doxorubicin) in combination with arabinosyl cytosine and sometimes also with a purine analogue (e.g., 6-thioguanine or 6-mercaptopurine). In some protocols other drugs are also added in an attempt to increase leukemic cell kill. Several of the most effective regimens which have been reported to give remission rates of 70 percent or higher in ANLL are listed in the references. Any of these regimens can be instituted in emergency situations, since they will all lower the leukemic cell count fairly rapidly in most patients. Daily blood counts should, of course, be obtained to follow the progress of treatment, but the count will usually be brought down to reasonable levels within a few days. If the patient has an extremely high number of circulating blasts or if there are other indications for promptly and drastically reducing the leukemic cell mass, a continuous intravenous infusion of arabinosyl cytosine, 200 mg per square meter of body surface area per 24 h, or of hydroxyurea, 2 to 3 g/m^2 per 24 h, will quickly lower the blast cell count in most patients, and higher doses will do so even more rapidly. Moderately large doses of several other drugs given singly are also usually effective in accomplishing this objective. These include daunorubicin, 45 to 60 mg/m^2 per day by intravenous injection for 2 to 3 days, and cyclophosphamide, 1 to 1.5 g/m^2 per day by intravenous injection for 1 to 2 days. However, the remission rate is lower with single agents than with drug combinations, and whenever possible one of the effective combinations should be employed as primary therapy because previously untreated patients have the best chance of achieving a durable remission.

Massive leukapheresis, using continuous-flow centrifugation or filtration techniques, is effective in lowering the blood leukocyte count rapidly, and up to several kilograms of leukemic cells have been removed in some patients. However, neither massive leukapheresis nor extracorporeal irradiation of the blood have proved useful in the definitive treatment of acute leukemia.

Because some reports are contradictory, and because the morphologic criteria for diagnosis are not necessarily identical, it is not clear whether there are important differences in the response rates of the different types of ANLL. In some series, patients with promyelocytic leukemia, erythroleukemia, or monoblastic leukemia have been reported to have lower than average remission rates, but these differences may reflect differing sensitivities of the cells to specific drugs rather than general unresponsiveness. For example, promyelocytic leukemia appears to be unusually responsive to daunorubicin; in one large series, almost half of patients treated with daunorubicin survived over 3 years.

Good supportive care is essential for patients undergoing intensive chemotherapy for induction of remission, and some of the disparate remission rates in different series of patients treated with the same regimen undoubtedly reflect differences in supportive treatment. Considerable experience and skill are required in anticipating and diagnosing infections and in knowing how best to treat them when they occur, in knowing how and when to use platelet transfusions and other measures to prevent or control bleeding, and in implementing preventive measures to avoid such common complications as perirectal abscesses. These can sometimes be prevented by such simple measures as keeping the stool soft and well lubricated, maintaining good perineal hygiene, and prohibiting the taking of rectal temperatures. Venipunctures should be performed only when absolutely necessary, and meticulous care should be taken to avoid damaging the veins or introducing infections. Unessential subcutaneous or intramuscular injections should be avoided and if prolonged intravenous infusions are planned, it is desirable to place an indwelling catheter. When hyperuricemia is present or is anticipated as a result of drug-induced cell breakdown, allopurinol should be given prophylactically, and sufficient fluids administered to maintain a good urinary output in order to prevent uric acid nephropathy. If 6-mercaptopurine is to be used concomitantly, the dosage must be lowered to about one-quarter of the usual dose because allopurinol interferes with the degradative pathway of this purine analogue and increases its toxicity; this is not true for 6-thioguanine, which may be given in full dosage.

Sometimes leukemic cells form local tumor masses in the central nervous system or elsewhere in the body which cause pressure symptoms, or the cells may infiltrate sites of infection such as perianal abscesses and interfere with healing. In such cases local irradiation may be used as an adjunct to systemic chemotherapy; generally 3 to 6 Gy (300 to 600 rads) will suffice. Irradiation may also be useful in controlling pericardial or other serous effusions due to leukemia. There are conflicting reports about the incidence of CNS leukemia in ANLL; the incidence in the monocytic types (M4 and M5) appears to be higher than in other types of ANLL. It is generally agreed that symptomatic CNS leukemia occurs much less frequently in ANLL than in ALL, but whether this is largely due to the fact that patients with ALL live longer is unsettled, as is the indication for preventive treatment. Most centers do not give prophylactic treatment for CNS leukemia in ANLL but do treat the patient vigorously with cranial irradiation and intrathecal methotrexate and/or arabinosyl cytosine if this complication develops.

Fresh platelets have been shown to be very effective in preventing serious hemorrhagic complications. However, platelet transfusions should be administered judiciously and only when needed, because eventually many patients receiving multiple transfusions from random donors over prolonged periods develop platelet antibodies; subsequent platelet transfusions are then relatively ineffective, perhaps when the need is greatest. If the platelets are obtained from siblings or nonfamily donors who are histocompatible for HLA antigens, the incidence of sensitization is reduced; use of matched donors is essential once refractoriness to random platelets occurs. The level of platelet count at which platelets are required varies greatly. A level of 20,000 per cubic millimeter is commonly taken as the danger threshold, but many patients tolerate platelet counts of 20,000 per cubic millimeter or less without major bleeding, especially if the count has been stable around that level for some time. A rapidly falling platelet count, whether due to progressive disease or drug-induced myelosuppression, is more apt to be associated with serious bleeding, and in these circumstances platelets should be administered prophylactically before the count drops dangerously low.

One unit of concentrated platelets obtained from 500 ml of blood contains about 10^{11} platelets, and 2 to 4 units per square meter of body surface area are usually given; however, the number of units required depends on the clinical situation and the frequency of transfusions. Platelets should preferably be given within a few hours of being obtained, because stored platelets, especially when held beyond 48 h, are clearly less effective. Short-term storage at room temperature is preferable to refrigerated storage. Satisfactory methods have been developed for freezing and long-term storage of frozen platelets, and it can be anticipated that this new technology will become more widely available. The normal platelet life span is about 9 days, but that of transfused platelets in leukemic recipients is always less than this, especially if there is infection, fever, or bleeding, and sometimes platelet transfusions are required daily or more often. Aspirin and other drugs which interfere with platelet function should be avoided in platelet donors and of course also in patients with leukemia.

If bleeding occurs despite an adequate number of normally functioning platelets, other coagulation defects should be looked for. In patients with overt bleeding due to DIC, anticoagulation with heparin should be begun promptly and continued until the leukemic mass has been sufficiently reduced by chemotherapy to arrest the chain of events responsible for the syndrome. Platelets and fresh frozen plasma should also be administered. It is generally assumed that the leukemic cells release proteolytic enzymes or other factors which activate the clotting process. Whether fibrinogenolysis occurs as a primary phenomenon or is secondary to plasmin formation during intravascular coagulation is unclear, but in either case the result is that the fibrinogen falls, fibrinogen and fibrin degradation products appear, and there may also be secondary decreases in other clotting factors, particularly V and VIII. Platelets also decrease and their recovery after an episode of DIC may be prolonged. Heparin should be given prophylactically in acute promyelocytic leukemia, even in the absence of bleeding if there is biochemical evidence of DIC, before starting antileukemic therapy, because massive lysis of leukemic cells will aggravate the process and might precipitate a serious bleeding episode.

Anemia should be corrected by transfusions of packed red cells. The erythrocyte level required to avoid symptoms attributable to anemia varies greatly in different patients, and as in the case of platelet transfusions, red blood cell transfusions should not be overutilized. There is always the danger of serum hepatitis, and if a good remission is obtained, erythropoiesis will resume at a level adequate to maintain normal or near-normal erythrocyte counts. Fresh leukocyte transfusions may be beneficial in treating infections when patients are severely neutropenic, but relatively large quantities must be given repeatedly because of the short life span of granulocytes. Moreover, the necessary facilities for procuring adequate quantities of fresh histocompatible leukocytes are not widely available. Leukocytes should probably not be given if the patient is receiving amphotericin because pulmonary damage may occur. Various measures are being evaluated to try to lower the frequency and severity of infections. These include prophylactic bacterial vaccines, oral nonabsorbable antibiotic regimens for gut sterilization, and placement of patients in laminar airflow rooms or other sterile environments during attempted induction of remission, but their efficacy in increasing the incidence and duration of remissions has not been clearly established.

A diagnosis of acute leukemia can be psychologically devastating to patients and their close relatives, and it is crucial to provide support and sympathetic counseling. Psychiatric consultants and other medical personnel can be very helpful, but patients will rely mainly on the primary therapist to alter the outcome of the disease. The physician must accept this responsibility, which can be very demanding, and be prepared to support patients throughout their course, whatever the outcome. There are no fixed guidelines about how explicitly patients should be informed about their disease, because many factors must be taken into account, such as age, emotional stability, and the patient's general medical condition. In general, however, the wisest course is to be truthful in order to keep the patient's confidence and cooperation; it is essential that there be mutual understanding and consent between the patient and the physician regarding the nature of the disease and the necessity for prolonged treatment with drugs that have many unpleasant and dangerous effects.

Bone marrow transplantation (see Chap. 331) is being used increasingly in acute leukemia, following intensive chemotherapy and total body irradiation to destroy the leukemic population. A histocompatible donor, usually a sibling, must be available. In the two largest reported series, approximately 60 percent of patients with ANLL who received allogenic transplants while in their first remission are surviving without evidence of recurrent leukemia for up to 4 years after transplantation. The major causes of death have been graft-versus-host disease (GVHD) and infections, especially interstitial pneumonia rather than recurrent leukemia. The results in patients transplanted in relapse or while in their second or later remissions have been less favorable, both in ANLL and ALL, and the relapse rate following transplantation has been higher. Because of the relatively good results with chemotherapy in ALL and the high risks associated with allogenic transplantation, relatively few patients with ALL have been transplanted while in their first remission and it is not known if the results will be superior to chemotherapy alone. Since younger patients tolerate the transplant procedure better than older ones, most centers are restricting transplantation to patients under the age of 35 or 40.

There have been many attempts during the last 75 years to treat acute leukemia by immunotherapy. Occasional remissions were noted following administration of various blood constituents, following various infections (either induced or occurring spontaneously), or after immunostimulation by administration of bacterial endotoxins or other substances. However, remissions were infrequent, and attempts to induce remissions by immunotherapeutic maneuvers were largely abandoned after modern chemotherapy was introduced because the results were too inconsistent.

In recent years there have been renewed trials of immunotherapy with the more limited goal of trying to eradicate the relatively small number of leukemic cells remaining after remission has been induced with cytotoxic drugs. Nonspecific immunostimulants have included bacillus Calmette-Guérin (BCG), *Corynebacterium parvum,* mixed bacterial endotoxins, and various other microbial products. Modified autologous or allogenic leukemic cells have also been administered in attempts to increase remission duration. The rationale for these trials is the presumption that leukemic cells have antigenic determinants distinct from those expressed by normal cells against which the host's immune system can be stimulated to react; however, there is as yet no good evidence that human leukemic cells have leukemia-specific antigens. No consistently beneficial effects have been noted from any of these forms of immunotherapy, and the ultimate value of immunotherapy in acute leukemia remains uncertain. A few partial and complete remissions have occurred following administration of large doses of interferon, but they have been of short duration. Interferon cannot be considered a reliable form of treatment, and therapeutic trials should be reserved for patients who have failed conventional chemotherapy.

PROGNOSIS Over 90 percent of children with ALL have complete remissions with modern chemotherapeutic regimens. The average survival for the untreated disease is only a few months; with improved chemotherapy, survival times have increased, and there are several large series in which over 50 percent of children are living after 5 years. Since many of these children have remained free of disease for several years or longer after all treatment has been discontinued, it appears likely that most of them will prove to have been cured. However, a much longer follow-up period will be necessary to ascertain whether they will have a normal life expectancy, because some late relapses have occurred after 5 years, and the incidence of possible delayed adverse effects of intensive treatment is not yet known. Subgroups of children with ALL with differing prognoses are becoming more clearly defined. Favorable risk features include age between 2 and 10 years; relatively low initial white blood cell count; initial hemoglobin level less than 10 g/dl; L1 morphology of leukemic cells with absence of T- or B-cell markers; absence of mediastinal mass and of marked enlargement of liver, spleen, and lymph nodes; absence of central nervous system involvement; and prompt response to chemotherapy with rapid attainment of remission. Children showing these characteristics have a high probability of having lasting remissions with effective treatment regimens, whereas in children with unfavorable risk features, the average duration of remission is usually shorter and there are fewer long-term survivors. No treatment regimens have yet been reported which are highly effective in these poor-risk children. Adults with ALL generally respond less well than children, and most trials have resulted in complete remission rates of 50 percent or less, with a median duration of a year or less. However, in some trials using intensive multidrug combinations, the remission rate has been 80 percent or higher and about 50 percent of patients have remained in remission for over 5 years.

The prognosis remains generally poor in ANLL, both in children and adults. With the best chemotherapeutic regimens and good supportive care, 60 to 80 percent of patients are now attaining complete remissions. In most series the remission rate is higher in younger and lower in older patients, although a few also report good results in elderly patients. Possibly because of lack of uniformity in classifying subtypes, no consistent differences in response have been found among the different types of ANLL according to the FAB classification except that it is generally agreed that patients with the M6 type and those with a preceding history of a myelodysplastic syndrome (e.g., RAEB, preleukemia) usually respond poorly to treatment, and a higher-than-average percentage of patients with the promyelocytic (M3) type become long survivors. Patients developing secondary ANLL following treatment of other diseases rarely achieve lasting remissions.

The survival of nonresponders remains about the same as with no treatment, around 3 months. In patients having remissions, the average duration of remission in most series has been between 6 and 12 months, and the average survival between 1 and 2 years. At best, except for the M3 type, only about 10 to 15 percent of patients with ANLL remain in continuous remission for over 5 years. Recent attempts to increase the proportion of long survivors with combination chemotherapy have been disappointing, and bone marrow transplantation should be considered as a therapeutic option for patients under the age of 40 who have a suitable donor.

REFERENCES

BENNETT JM et al: Proposals for the classification of the acute leukemias. Br J Hematol 33:451, 1976

BERNARD J et al: Treatment of granulocytic leukemias, in *Cancer. Achievements, Challenges, and Prospects for the 1980s,* JH Burchenal, HF Oettgen (eds). New York, Grune & Stratton, 1981, vol 2, pp 271–289

BURCHENAL JH: Leukemia overview, in *Cancer. Achievements, Challenges, and Prospects for the 1980s,* JH Burchenal, HF Oettgen (eds). New York, Grune & Stratton, 1981, vol 2, pp 249–270

CLARKSON B et al: Results of intensive treatment of acute lymphoblastic leukemia in adults, in *Cancer. Achievements, Challenges, and Prospects for the 1980s,* JH Burchenal, HF Oettgen (eds). New York, Grune & Stratton, 1981, vol 2, pp 301–317

GALE RP et al: Intensive chemotherapy for acute myelogenous leukemia. *Ann Intern Med* 94:753, 1981

HAGHBIN M et al: A long-term clinical follow-up of children with acute lymphoblastic leukemia treated with intensive chemotherapy regimens. Cancer 46:241, 1980

LINMAN JW, BAGBY CC JR: The preleukemic syndrome (hemopoietic dysplasia). Cancer 42:854, 1978

MERTELSMANN R et al: Morphological classification, response to therapy and survival in 263 adult patients with acute non-lymphoblastic leukemia. Blood 56:773, 1980

MILLER DR: Childhood leukemias, in *Cancer. Achievements, Challenges, and Prospects for the 1980s,* JH Burchenal, HF Oettgen (eds). New York, Grune & Stratton, 1981, vol 2, pp 319–330.

ROWLEY JD: Chromosome abnormalities in human leukemia. Ann Rev Genet 14:17, 1980

THOMAS ED: Bone marrow transplantation, in *Cancer. Achievements, Challenges, and Prospects for the 1980s,* JH Burchenal, HF Oettgen (eds). New York, Grune & Stratton, 1981, vol 2, pp 625–638

129 THE CHRONIC LEUKEMIAS

GEORGE P. CANELLOS

The term *chronic leukemia* has been applied to those hematologic malignancies in which the predominant leukemic cell is initially well differentiated and can be readily identified as to cell type. They are generally divided into two main categories, lymphocytic and granulocytic. There are less common variants within these groups such as eosinophilic, myelomonocytic, and chronic lymphosarcoma cell leukemias. The term *chronic* also refers to the fact that these disorders have a generally better prognosis than the acute leukemias. Chronic granulocytic leukemia is a variant of the myeloproliferative syndrome (Table 129-1). However, there are some unique cytogenetic and clinical characteristics which distinguish this disease from other disorders in that group.

CHRONIC GRANULOCYTIC LEUKEMIA

CLINICAL AND HEMATOLOGIC FINDINGS Chronic granulocytic leukemia (CGL) can occur at any age, but the majority of patients are between 30 and 50 years old. Although there is no well-defined etiologic factor, an increase in both acute and chronic granulocytic leukemia was noted 5 to 8 years following the atomic bomb explosions in Japan.

The natural history of CGL can be divided into two fairly distinct phases, chronic and blastic. The *chronic phase* of CGL begins as a myeloproliferative disorder in which there is an excessive proliferation and accumulation of granulocytic cells of intermediate maturity as well as polymorphonuclear leukocytes. The median white blood cell count at the time of diagnosis is about 200,000 per cubic millimeter. Myeloblasts usually compose less than 10 percent of cells in the bone marrow and peripheral blood. The bone marrow morphology reflects this hyperproliferation and is usually hypercellular with excessive granulocytic precursors. The cytogenetic and morphologic evidence suggests involvement of all elements derived from the marrow stem cell. Thus, this disease can be considered a "panmyelosis" in the category of the myeloproliferative diseases such as polycythemia vera and myeloid metaplasia (see Chaps. 336 and 337). The predominant cell type in most instances is in the granulocytic series, although rare cases of predominant eosinophilic and basophilic proliferation have been noted. About half the patients will present with a thrombocytosis in excess of 450,000 per cubic millimeter with increased megakaryocytes in the marrow. About 20 percent of cases are diagnosed on the basis of an elevated blood cell count in the absence of symptoms. In the majority, however, the signs and symptoms of the disease are related to the expanded granulocytic mass in the bone marrow, liver, and spleen. *Presenting symptoms* are usually palpable or painful splenomegaly, vague osteoarticular pains, anemia, and hypercatabolic symptoms such as weight loss and fever. Lymphadenopathy is distinctly rare in the chronic phase of CGL. In addition to the above, thrombohemorrhagic complaints such as excessive bleeding either spontaneously or following a surgical or dental procedure may be the first sign of disease. In some instances spontaneous cyclic leukocytosis and thrombocytosis may occur with a periodicity of 50 to 70 days. *Physical examination* will reveal splenomegaly in the majority of patients with the possible exception of those patients who are discovered early in the disease with a leukocytosis of less than 50,000 per cubic millimeter.

The chronic phase of CGL usually can be well controlled by treatment and persists for a median of 36 to 40 months before there is a transformation to the accelerated or blastic phase.

The onset of the *blastic phase* represents an evolution of the leukemic process from hyperplasia of mature elements to a loss of differentiation with increased numbers of blasts and progranulocytes. In approximately half the patients, the blastic phase will be preceded by an intermediate period of 3 to 6 months of myeloproliferative acceleration with progressively increasing leukocytosis, possibly thrombocytosis, and splenomegaly refractory to previously effective chronic phase therapy. In addition, myelofibrosis composed of increased reticulin, basophilia, and abnormalities of erythrocyte and platelet morphology may be seen. In the remainder, the transition can be abrupt, usually within weeks, to a state resembling acute granulocytic leukemia (AGL) (see Chap. 128). The myeloblasts of the acute phase of CGL lack the Auer rods which are often seen in AGL. Rarely the "crisis" of a rising blast cell count is associated with cerebrovascular bleeding secondary to blast cell thrombi in the smaller vessels (leukostasis). A minority of patients will present with or develop extramedullary myeloblastic tumors usually in lymph nodes or skin, or as osteolytic bone lesions. In the past such lymph node masses have been diagnosed as *reticulum-cell sarcoma* because of the very anaplastic appearance of myeloblasts in hematoxylin-eosin tissue sections. Meningeal leukemia is rare and usually occurs in patients whose blastic phase has been in hematologic remission following chemotherapy. The blast-cell morphology can vary and about one-third of cases have some of the characteristics of lymphoblasts. Approximately the same proportion of patients will have the enzyme terminal deoxynucleotidyl transferase, a DNA-synthesizing enzyme, associated with acute lymphoblastic leukemia and normal thymic lymph cells. These cases also demonstrate reactivity with a non-B, non-T, anti-acute lymphoblastic leukemia antiserum. The relationship of these lymphoid characteristics to the presumed myeloid genesis of the disease is unclear. Acute lymphoblastic leukemia in adults has been reported to have the Philadelphia chromosome in a minority of cases. Rarely cytoplasmic IgM has been noted indicating a pre-B phenotype. More often a mixed population of lymphoid and myeloid cells exists with resistance to anti-lymphoblastic chemotherapy characterized by an emerging myeloid or undifferentiated blast-cell population that is terminal-transferase- and ALL-antigen-negative.

The blastic phase of CGL is usually refractory to therapy and has a median duration of about 2 months from onset to death. The fatal complications of this phase are similar to those seen in terminal acute granulocytic leukemia.

CLINICOPATHOLOGIC FINDINGS The chronic phase of CGL is associated with a number of unique biochemical abnormalities. Accompanying the persistent leukocytosis of CGL is a marked elevation of serum vitamin B_{12} levels as well as an increased binding capacity of the serum for the vitamin. This is due to excessive serum content of the vitamin B_{12} transport protein, transcobalamin I, a glycoprotein of alpha globulin electrophoretic mobility. A vitamin B_{12}–binding protein with similar properties has been shown to be produced by mature normal and leukemic granulocytes in vitro. The elevated levels in the serum of CGL are probably derived from the turnover of the increased granulocytic mass. The high levels of vitamin B_{12} as well as the increased serum binding capacity return toward normal with remission of the disease. An enzyme termed *leukocyte alkaline phosphatase* is undetectable biochemically or histochemically in granulocytes of most patients with CGL in relapse. This enzyme has no known function but is often elevated in response to infection, stress, steroid administration, chronic inflammatory diseases, and Hodgkin's disease. Successful therapy of the disease results in normal or elevated levels. It is also known to be increased in polycythemia vera and myeloid metaplasia. The only other hematologic disorder with low or absent leukocyte alkaline phosphatase is paroxysmal nocturnal hemoglobinuria. Rarely, the hyperplastic marrow of CGL may contain glycolipid-laden phagocytic cells which resemble Gaucher's cells. These have also been noted in the spleen. Hyperuricemia related to the increased cell turnover may occur prior to therapy and can be exacerbated by treatment. This problem is also common to other myeloproliferative disorders such as myeloid metaplasia and polycythemia vera. The mature polymorphonuclear leukocyte of CGL is a functionally normal cell with respect to phagocytosis and bactericidal activity. This is especially true in patients with blood counts of less than 90,000 leukocytes per cubic millimeter. The kinetics of the granulocyte in CGL have been studied with isotopic-labeling techniques. There is clear evidence for increased production of mature granulocytes and their prolonged survival in the circulation but only in the presence of leukocytosis.

CYTOGENETICS About 90 percent of cases, which fulfill the hematologic criteria of CGL, have a unique and characteristic chromosome marker in the marrow and peripheral blood cells, the Philadelphia chromosome. It consists of a shortening of the long arms of chromosome G22 due to translocation of genetic material to chromosome 9. The abnormality persists throughout the course of the disease, in remission and relapse, and is generally unaffected by therapy. It is present in granulocytic, megakaryocytic, and erythroid precursors but not in lymphocytes or skin fibroblasts. In addition to the Philadelphia chromosome, the blastic phase of CGL is often associated with other chromosomal abnormalities, such as aneuploidy, which reflect the malignant character of this phase of the disease. Cases of CGL which lack the Philadelphia chromosome usually have a worse prognosis than the chromosome-positive disease.

DIFFERENTIAL DIAGNOSIS CGL must be differentiated from leukemoid reactions associated with infections and neoplasms. In these circumstances the leukocyte alkaline phosphatase is usually markedly elevated, and the Philadelphia chromosome is absent. A closely related myeloproliferative disorder with a similar prognosis is agnogenic myeloid metaplasia. This disease usually presents with marked myelofibrosis and splenomegaly. The white blood cell count and platelet count may be elevated as well. The leukocyte alkaline phosphatase is high, and there is no Philadelphia chromosome. Among the myeloproliferative disorders, the serum vitamin B_{12} level cannot be used as a differential diagnostic test in patients with elevated leukocyte counts. CGL in children is rare. A Philadelphia-chromosome-negative variant referred to as juvenile granulocytic leukemia is characterized by skin rash, splenomegaly, thrombocytopenia, elevated fetal hemoglobin, and poor response to chemotherapy.

TREATMENT The chronic phase of CGL can be controlled by a number of oral alkylating agents such as busulfan, cyclophosphamide, and phenylalanine mustard. Splenic irradiation can be an effective means for systemic control of the disease but in current practice has been replaced by more effective chemotherapy. The most commonly used drug is busulfan. It may be administered on an intermittent schedule or on a continuous daily basis with approximately the same results. The most serious complication of busulfan therapy is prolonged myelosuppression. Occasionally, remission of the disease for periods in excess of 12 months may follow a single course of treatment. The principal side effects include increased skin pigmentation, dryness of skin and mucous membranes, and, rarely, pulmonary fibrosis. An initial daily oral dose of 4 to 8 mg per day will reduce the white blood cell count to less than 20,000 per cubic millimeter in 2 to 3 weeks. It is important to reduce the dose progressively, roughly in proportion to the reduction in white blood cell count. The patient can achieve an excellent hematologic remission with return of blood counts to normal and disappearance of organomegaly. The Philadelphia chromosome will continue to be present in the marrow cells. Thus, a true remission of the disease has not occurred; rather, the proliferating granulocytic mass has been reduced to the point where immature cells disappear from the peripheral blood. Splenectomy has little place in the primary management of CGL but should be reserved for those patients with evidence of hypersplenism, repeated painful splenic infarction, and the rare instance in which prolonged thrombocytopenia has followed a course of busulfan. Splenectomy in the chronic phase of the disease does not appear to abort the occurrence of blastic transformation.

TABLE 129-1
The myeloproliferative syndromes

	Splenomegaly	*RBC count*	*WBC count*	*Platelet count*	*Marrow fibrosis*	*Philadelphia chromosome*	*Leukocyte alkaline phosphatase*
Chronic myelocytic leukemia	Marked	Normal	↑↑↑	↑, Normal	±	+	↓→0
Myeloid metaplasia, myelofibrosis	Marked	↓	↑	Normal, ↑	+	0	↑
Polycythemia vera	Moderate	↑	↑	↑	0	0	↑
Essential thrombocythemia	Moderate	Normal	Normal	↑↑↑	0	0	

Acceleration of the disease is reflected by progressive refractoriness to busulfan with leukocytosis, thrombocytosis, and increasing splenomegaly. In the absence of evidence for frank blastic transformation, the drug hydroxyurea (0.5 to 2.0 g per day by mouth) can effectively control the proliferative aspects of this phase. The blastic phase of CGL is refractory to most drug regimens, but remissions in about 20 percent of cases have been obtained with the use of vincristine and prednisone or other intensive combination chemotherapy programs useful in the treatment of acute leukemia.

The inability to achieve hematologic remission in the blastic phase of CGL may be in some part due to the fact that these patients often have myelofibrosis and/or are totally depleted of a residual stem-cell population capable of producing mature elements. Symptomatic extramedullary myeloblastic tumors, however, can be controlled with local radiation therapy. Recent investigations have demonstrated the eradication of Philadelphia-chromosome-positive cells in the majority of chronic-phase patients treated with intensive radiation and chemotherapy and transplanted with bone marrow from a normal identical twin. Another investigational approach involves the cryopreservation of chronic-phase bone marrow with subsequent autologous transplantation during the blastic phase. Attempts at eradication of the Philadelphia-chromosome-positive cell line during the chronic phase with anti-acute-leukemia-type combination chemotherapy has had only transient effect.

CHRONIC LYMPHOCYTIC LEUKEMIA

CLINICAL AND HEMATOLOGIC FINDINGS Chronic lymphocytic leukemia (CLL) is a hematologic disorder of older people (median age of 60 years) which is characterized by the production and accumulation of functionally inactive but long-lived mature-appearing lymphocytes. Kinetic studies of the small lymphocyte in CLL indicate a turnover time in excess of 12 months.

The signs and symptoms of the disease are related to the infiltration of lymph nodes, bone marrow, liver, and spleen with these cells. As in CGL, the diagnosis can be made on a routine blood count in asymptomatic patients, but the majority of cases will present with lymphadenopathy and moderate splenomegaly. The white blood cell count is usually not as high as in CGL, and only one-third of patients have a count about 100,000 per cubic millimeter. Patients with advanced disease can also present with anemia, granulocytopenia, and thrombocytopenia due to bone marrow involvement. In addition, about 20 percent of patients will develop a Coombs-positive autoimmune hemolytic anemia at some time in the course of the disease. Rarely an idiopathic autoimmune-type thrombocytopenia can occur. As opposed to CGL, infiltrative skin lesions can occur and often precede the systemic manifestations of CLL. Patients with CLL will often have exaggerated cutaneous reactions to insect bites.

The presence of retroperitoneal or mesenteric lymph node enlargement can be associated with gastrointestinal or genitourinary complaints. The prognosis of the disease appears to be related to the extent of organ infiltration at the time of diagnosis. The median survival varies from 24 months for patients with anemia and thrombocytopenia to 8 to 10 years for patients who have only lymphocytosis and lymphadenopathy. The diagnosis can often be made from the peripheral blood film, especially in the presence of generalized lymphadenopathy.

Progression of the disease is associated with anemia, thrombocytopenia, and increased frequency of infection which is the most common cause of death. Splenomegaly and lymph node enlargement can be prominent, but splenic infarction is rare.

LABORATORY FINDINGS The disease is associated with a number of immunologic abnormalities. Almost half the patients with CLL will develop hypogammaglobulinemia which becomes progressively worse during the course of the disease. Antigenic challenge with vaccines has demonstrated a depressed circulating antibody response. Delayed hypersensitivity to antigens such as tuberculin is generally not impaired. The lymphocyte of CLL has a much-delayed transformation in vitro with mitogenic substances such as phytohemagglutinin when compared with normal lymphocytes. Immunofluorescent studies of the malignant lymphocyte of CLL have demonstrated immunoglobulin at the cell surface. Immunofluorescent staining of surface immunoglobulin, usually monoclonal IgM, is characteristically faint. In addition, receptors for immunoglobulin–sheep erythrocyte–complement (EAC) complexes have been noted on these cells. These findings have supported the concept that in most but not all cases of CLL the disease is a malignancy of the bone marrow–derived (B-cell) lymphocyte, but a small number of cases of thymus-derived (T-cell) CLL have been described. These cells form rosettes with sheep red blood cells and possess T-cell surface antigens. Patients with T-cell CLL characteristically have marked hepatosplenomegaly without lymphadenopathy, neutropenia, and skin infiltration. Response to therapy is poor and survival is considerably poorer than in B-cell CLL. There is no characteristic cytogenetic abnormality, and the serum vitamin B_{12} levels are in the normal range.

Several hematologic disorders are related to CLL but can be differentiated on the basis of morphology. Chronic lymphosarcoma-cell leukemia shares most of the features and complications of CLL. The malignant cell is usually a small or intermediate-sized cleaved lymphocyte. Malignant lymphoma with nodes diffusely involved with well-differentiated lymphocytes but without peripheral blood involvement may be associated with autoimmune phenomena and hypogammaglobulinemia and probably represents a lymphomatous expression of CLL.

TREATMENT The course of CLL is quite variable; in general, therapy is reserved for progression of the disease to the point of symptomatic lymphadenopathy, splenomegaly, or interference with normal hematopoiesis.

In the absence of a need for systemic therapy, lymph node enlargement which has become cosmetically or mechanically onerous can be controlled by local radiation therapy. Isolated splenomegaly can be effectively treated by splenic irradiation, often with improvement of the systemic manifestations of the disease including decrease of peripheral lymphocytosis. When systemic therapy is required, the majority of patients can be controlled with the lymphocytotoxic alkylating agents and/or corticosteroids. The drug of choice is either chlorambucil, 0.1 to 0.2 mg/kg per day, or cyclophosphamide, 50 to 150 mg per day. Both are administered on a chronic intermittent schedule. The doses of either alkylating agent usually can be reduced for maintenance therapy, but this requires a degree of individual titration according to disease activity. These agents can reduce lymph node and splenic enlargement and the infiltration of the bone marrow, often resulting in correction of the anemia and thrombocytopenia. Complete remission of CLL following radiation or chemotherapy is rare. Patients should be carefully followed lest the benefits of chemotherapy be canceled by excessive myelosuppression due to the drugs.

Corticosteroids have a marked lymphocytolytic effect and are not myelosuppressive. Thus they are especially useful when given with alkylating agents to patients with extensive marrow involvement. The risk of infection is increased, however, when steroids are given for prolonged periods in patients who are hypogammaglobulinemic and/or granulocytopenic. Corticosteroids are especially useful in the treatment of the autoimmune complications of CLL such as Coombs-positive hemolytic anemia and may be lifesaving in that circumstance. Splenectomy has not been shown to be of benefit in CLL except in some cases where hemolytic anemia and thrombocytopenia are refractory to corticosteroids and are related to excessive peripheral destruction of blood cells in the spleen. Blastic transformation analogous to that seen in CGL does not occur; however, a small number of patients develop lymphomatous transformation with a histologic appearance compatible with diffuse lymphocytic or histiocytic lymphoma.

In addition to the use of chemotherapeutic agents for the systemic treatment of CLL, fractionated total-body irradiation and thymic irradiation have been successful in achieving clinical remission. These radiation techniques are still investigational and are not conventionally employed in the treatment of CLL.

REFERENCES

Chronic granulocytic leukemia

Canellos GP et al: Hematologic and cytogenetic remission of blastic transformation of chronic granulocytic leukemia. Blood 38:671, 1971

———: The treatment of chronic granulocytic leukaemia. Clin Haematol 6:113, 1977

Galton DAG: Chemotherapy of chronic myelocytic leukemia. Semin Hematol 6:323, 1969

Janossy G et al: Comparative analysis of membrane phenotypes in acute lymphoid leukemia and in lymphoid blast crisis of chronic myeloid leukaemia. Leukemia Res 1:289, 1977

Karanas A, Silver RT: Characteristics of the terminal phase of chronic granulocytic leukemia. Blood 32:445, 1968

Koeffler HP, Golde DW: Chronic myelogenous leukemia—New concepts. N Engl J Med 304:1201, 1981

Marks SM et al: Terminal transferase as a predictor of initial responsiveness to vincristine and prednisone in blastic chronic myelogenous leukemia. N Engl J Med 298:812, 1978

Rosenthal R et al: Blast crisis of chronic granulocytic leukemia. Am J Med 63:542, 1977

Rowley JD: A new consistent chromosomal abnormality in chronic myelogenous leukaemia identified by quinacrine fluorescence and Giemsa staining. Nature 243:290, 1973

Whang-Peng J et al: Clinical implications of cytogenetic variants in chronic myelogenous leukemia. Blood 32:755, 1968

Chronic lymphocytic leukemia

Aisenberg AC et al: Cell-surface immunoglobulins in chronic lymphocytic leukemia and allied disorders. Am J Med 55:184, 1973

Brouet J et al: Chronic lymphocytic leukemia of T-cell origin. Immunological and clinical evaluation in eleven patients. Lancet 1:890, 1975

Freymann JG et al: Role of hemolysis in anemia secondary to chronic lymphocytic leukemia and certain malignant lymphomas. N Engl J Med 259:847, 1958

Peterson LC et al: Relationship of clinical staging and lymphocyte morphology to survival in chronic lymphocytic leukemia. Br J Haematol 45:563, 1980

Rai KR et al: Clinical staging of chronic lymphocytic leukemia. Blood 46:219, 1975

Shevach EM et al: Receptors for complement and immunoglobulin on human leukemic cells and human lymphoblastoid cell lines. J Clin Invest 51:1933, 1972

Theml H et al: Kinetics of lymphocytes in chronic lymphocytic leukemia: Studies using continuous H-thymidine infusion in two patients. Blood 42:623, 1973

Wiltshaw E: Chemotherapy in chronic lymphocytic leukaemia. Clin Haematol 6:223, 1977

130 HODGKIN'S DISEASE AND OTHER LYMPHOMAS

JOHN E. ULTMANN
VINCENT T. DeVITA, JR.

DEFINITION The lymphomas are a group of malignant diseases of lymphoreticular origin. Although there are similarities among the various lymphomas, they include a wide spectrum of clinical and pathological pictures.

CELL OF ORIGIN OF THE LYMPHOMAS The lymphomas arise in the lymph nodes or in the lymphoid tissues of parenchymal organs such as the gut, lung, or skin. Ninety percent of cases of Hodgkin's disease originate in lymph nodes; 10 percent are of extranodal origin. In the non-Hodgkin's lymphomas, the tissues of the parenchymal organs are more often involved; 60 percent of these lymphomas originate in the nodes and 40 percent are of extranodal origin. With the availability of information on the subcompartmentalization of the lymphoid system and tests to study human tissue, the lymphomas can be classified by their cells of origin (Table 130-1). Almost all the non-Hodgkin's lymphomas (NHL) appear either to derive from a monoclonal population of B cells or to have no distinctive cell surface markers. Only a few appear to be true derivatives of tissue histiocytes despite the morphological similarity of some malignant lymphomas to these cells.

Normal lymphoid tissue is composed of a mosaic of lymphoid cells within the follicle, and each subpopulation contains different immunoglobulin light chains. This is in sharp contrast to malignant lymphoid tissue. Even those histological types of lymphomas characterized by mixtures of different morphological cell types in the same node (mixed lymphomas of Rappaport, see below) have been shown to derive from a monoclonal B cell line. While identification of immunologically homogeneous clinical pathological entities may have prognostic and therapeutic implications with each major immunologic classification of the lymphomas (T cell, B cell, null cell), great variations in behavior can occur. For example, those B-cell lymphomas which grow in a nodular pattern usually tend to have an indolent natural history with relapses and recurrences spread over 5 to 10 or more years. In contrast, the lymphomas termed diffuse "histiocytic" by Rappaport usually have a more aggressive clinical course, but when responsive to treatment may be more vulnerable to permanent control by drugs. Yet, these lymphomas, like nodular lymphomas, are often monoclonal B-cell neoplasms.

The origin of the Hodgkin's disease (HD) cell may be the dendritic interdigitating cell found in the interfollicular regions of lymph nodes. Cells from the spleens of patients with Hodgkin's disease have now been grown in tissue culture. These cells resemble the Sternberg-Reed cell of Hodgkin's disease. They are aneuploid, a characteristic of malignancy, and have staining characteristics similar to but not identical with macrophages and the dendritic interdigitating cell. When implanted intracerebrally into immune-deprived mice, they produce invasive tumors. They have also been shown to be phagocytic and to possess surface receptors for the Fc fragment of immunoglobulins and complement (C3b). All these findings are more characteristic of cells derived from the monocyte-histiocyte series. Studies employing monoclonal antibodies to Ia antigens have shown that the dendritic interdigitating cell and Reed-Sternberg cells in culture share this antigen, a factor responsible for antigen transfer from macrophage to lymphocyte and a potent stimulus for lymphocyte blastogenesis. All these features point strongly to a monocyte-macrophage lineage of the malignant cell in Hodgkin's disease.

ETIOLOGY There is convincing evidence that viruses are one of the causes of lymphomas in rodents and birds. Such a relationship has been demonstrated in humans with cutaneous T-cell lymphomas by American and Japanese investigators who isolated a unique retrovirus from patients with mycosis fungoides. Clusters of T-cell lymphoma also have been identified independently in China and Japan with isolation of virus as well as demonstration of antibodies to virus. There is also a strong association between the DNA Epstein-Barr virus (EBV) and the rare lymphoma described by Burkitt in East Africa (anti-EBV antibodies appear in serum of patients, and complementary DNA appears in the human genome of Burkitt cells), but the association is less strong in Burkitt lymphomas diagnosed in the United States. In addition, in large series of patients with infectious mononucleosis, a disease caused by the Epstein-Barr virus, a small but consistent increase in the incidence of lymphoma has been noted after long follow-up, compared with controls who did not have infectious mononucleosis. A lymphomatous disease of chickens, Marek's disease, is known to be caused by another herpes-like DNA virus and can now be prevented by vaccines. Cell lines cultured from patients with Hodgkin's disease and some types of diffuse non-Hodgkin's lymphomas have been shown to express type C RNA virus particles and appear to contain viral information such as protein coat antigens and viral reverse transcriptase. All these observations lend credence to a viral etiology of some human lymphomas.

A hereditary influence on the incidence of lymphomas is suggested by their higher incidence in patients with inherited immunologic deficiency diseases and by a small increased incidence in families of patients with immunologic disorders. In one study, a significantly increased incidence of Hodgkin's disease was noted in siblings of the index case, particularly in siblings of the same sex. A slight increase in incidence of lymphomas has been noted in large series of patients with collagen-vascular diseases compared with the general population adjusted for age. This increased incidence approached 10 percent in patients with long-standing Sjögrens syndrome, who tend to develop diffuse lymphomas or immunoblastic sarcomas.

Lymphoma-like syndromes have been found in patients who take phenytoin. Although in most cases the disease regresses when the patients stop taking phenytoin, a significant fraction proceed to develop frank lymphoma of several different varieties, including Hodgkin's disease. Such observations suggest that the drug is acting on patients with an inherited tendency to develop the disease. Patients who are chronically immunosuppressed, particularly those who have received renal transplants, have a higher incidence of diffuse histiocytic lymphoma and immunoblastic sarcomas, often in the brain. Except for the higher incidence of Hodgkin's disease in siblings and the influence of phenytoin on the development of lymphomas, it is difficult to separate the influence of heredity per se from immunosuppression, which may be of etiologic importance without an inherited background.

TABLE 130-1
Immunologic characterization of cells of origin of the lymphomas

LYMPHORETICULAR NEOPLASMS OF B-CELL ORIGIN
Chronic lymphocytic leukemia
Cells in Richter's syndrome*
Diffuse well-differentiated lymphocytic lymphomas
Nodular poorly differentiated lymphocytic lymphomas
Nodular mixed lymphoma
Nodular "histiocytic" lymphomas
Diffuse poorly differentiated lymphocytic lymphomas
Most patients with diffuse "histiocytic" lymphoma
Burkitt lymphoma
5% of children with acute lymphatic leukemia
Poorly differentiated lymphoblastic lymphoma of children
Immunoblastic lymphadenopathy
Immunoblastic sarcomas
LYMPHORETICULAR NEOPLASMS OF T-CELL ORIGIN
Acute lymphatic leukemia of childhood with mediastinal adenopathy and convoluted cells
Sézary syndrome, mycosis fungoides
Chronic lymphatic leukemia—some cases
Diffuse "histiocytic" lymphoma—some cases
LYMPHORETICULAR NEOPLASMS OF HISTIOCYTES
Hodgkin's disease†
<10% of patients with "diffuse histiocytic lymphoma"
Histiocytic medullary reticulosis
Monocytic leukemia
NULL-CELL NEOPLASMS
Most patients with childhood acute lymphatic leukemia, up to 40 percent of patients with diffuse "histiocytic" lymphoma of Rappaport

* *Local overgrowth of lymphoid tumor in patients with chronic lymphatic leukemia; often designated as reticulum-cell sarcoma in past.*
† *See text.*

EPIDEMIOLOGY About 30,000 new cases of lymphoma were diagnosed in 1980; 40 percent of these were Hodgkin's disease. Lymphomas are the seventh commonest cause of death from cancer in the United States; because of the young average age of the population (32 years for Hodgkin's disease and 42 for the other adult lymphomas), the toll in person-years of life lost ranks the lymphomas fourth among cancers in the United States in terms of economic impact. The incidence of lymphomas appears to be increasing each year.

Worldwide, there are differences in the prevalence of lymphomas. In the United States, Hodgkin's disease has a bimodal age-specific incidence rate, one mode occurring at ages 15 to 35 years and the other above age 50. A disproportionate number of patients in the first modal peak have the nodular sclerosing variety of Hodgkin's disease. The first peak is absent in Japan. Hodgkin's disease in children under 10 years is seen much more frequently in underdeveloped countries, and, when it is observed, the histological varieties and stages are characteristic of more advanced disease.

Some of the non-Hodgkin's lymphomas have unique epidemiologic characteristics. The Burkitt lymphoma occurs characteristically in children in central Africa, although a small number of cases with a different clinical presentation has been reported in the United States. Abdominal lymphomas that produce fragments of heavy chains of immunoglobulin occur in the Mediterranean region but are rarely seen in other parts of the world. These observations, and the occasional report of clusters of Hodgkin's disease, suggest environmental and/or genetic influences on the development of these diseases. In the United States following the report of several clusters of Hodgkin's disease, population-based studies using the cancer registries of Connecticut and California indicate that the reported clusters of Hodgkin's disease probably occurred by chance alone. Medical personnel who specialize in the care of patients with lymphoma do not seem to have a higher incidence of these diseases than others. An excellent epidemiological study has made a strong case that Hodgkin's disease may be a rare manifestation of a common infection. Factors that increase the risk of early exposure to infections, such as large families or multiple families per dwelling, decrease the risk of Hodgkin's disease. The data also suggest different risk factors are involved for Hodgkin's disease in the young and in the old. These data may explain several curious epidemiological associations, such as the absent early peak in Japan.

HODGKIN'S DISEASE

NATURAL HISTORY AND CLINICAL MANIFESTATIONS There are two prevalent theories about the origin and spread of Hodgkin's disease. Data from Stanford carefully mapping sites of involvement by tumor suggest the disease is unifocal in origin and spreads initially by involving contiguous lymph node areas. There are two weaknesses in this hypothesis—the high degree of involvement of retroperitoneal lymph nodes without intervening mediastinal involvement and the common involvement of the spleen, which has no afferent lymphatics. Kaplan has proposed that retroperitoneal lymph nodes are involved by retrograde spread through the thoracic duct. This proposal is difficult to accept because almost total occlusion of the duct's flow would be required. Smithers has proposed an alternate hypothesis referred to as the susceptibility hypothesis. He suggests that the malignant cell freely circulates but grows only in preferential sites, giving the appearance of contiguous spread. The ability to cure a multifocal disease with a local form of treatment, irradiation, seems difficult to explain with Smithers's proposal but may be due to destruction of preferential sites of involvement, limiting future growth of the tumor.

Hodgkin's disease usually presents either with asymptomatic, discrete, painless, rubbery enlargement of lymph nodes or with symptoms of fever, night sweats, weight loss, and sometimes pruritus associated with adenopathy. Asymptomatic adenopathy may be noted by the patient or by the doctor on a routine physical examination. Often mediastinal adenopathy is noted on a routine chest x-ray or a film taken because of a persistent, dry, nonproductive cough. These presentations are more common in young people, and such patients often have the nodular sclerosing variety of the disease.

Other, usually older, patients present with fever and night sweats, or both, followed by increasing malaise and weight loss. Whereas superficial adenopathy is present in most such patients at some time in the course of the disease, in some cases the enlarging lymph nodes are located exclusively in the abdomen, and these patients often present to the physician with a differential diagnosis of fever of undetermined origin (see Chap. 9). When diagnosed, they usually have the lymphocyte-depleted variety of Hodgkin's disease.

The fever in Hodgkin's disease is usually remittent. Occasionally, the patient has a cyclical fever pattern, called Pel-Ebstein fever, which is characterized by several days or weeks of fever, alternating with afebrile periods. While fever, night sweats, and weight loss (referred to as B symptoms) have been found to correlate with a poor prognosis in Hodgkin's disease, the prognostic significance of pruritus by itself is unclear. It rarely occurs in the absence of fever and/or night sweats and has been dropped as a staging criterion indicating the presence of more advanced disease. Alcohol-induced pain in Hodgkin's disease is uncommon but has been reported to coincide with heavy eosinophilic infiltration at the sites involved by tumor. If alcohol-associated pain occurs, it may serve to direct the physician's attention to a site of involvement which can be biopsied. Occasionally a patient with Hodgkin's disease will present with obstruction of the superior vena cava as the first symptom. Sudden spinal cord compression can be a presenting complaint in patients with Hodgkin's disease but is usually a complication of progressing disease in a patient with known disease.

Characteristically, asymptomatic patients may have their adenopathy for extended periods of time with waxing and waning of lymph node size. Old x-ray films, in retrospect, may reveal that evidence of mediastinal widening has been present for several years. Slow progression of the disease, usually by extension to contiguous lymph node areas, occurs especially in the nodular sclerosing variety of the disease. With invasion of the hilar lymph nodes, the gateway to the lungs, the tumor mass may invade the pulmonary parenchyma. At some point in the progression of the disease, blood vessel invasion may occur. Vascular invasion can be easily demonstrated in biopsy specimen of lymphoid tissue stained with Weigert's stain, especially in patients with more advanced histological subtypes. Unsuspected involvement of the spleen, an organ which has no afferent lymphatics, suggests that vascular invasion and circulation of the malignant cell may be a common occurrence, even in patients with apparently localized disease. Later, with further progression of disease and clear evidence of vascular invasion, the bone marrow, liver, and other viscera become involved. Symptoms, if they were not present initially, appear as the volume of tumor increases, and if the patient is not successfully treated, cachexia and widespread involvement of visceral organs by tumor occurs, infections complicate the course, and the patient dies.

Patients symptomatic at the outset seem to have disease which progresses more rapidly, have smaller-sized but more widespread lymphadenopathy, and more often have the lymphocyte-depleted or mixed-cellularity varieties of Hodgkin's disease. Bone and visceral involvement occurs earlier in such patients. Bone lesions are often osteoblastic, and the ivory vertebra is characteristic of Hodgkin's disease. Bone pain is common, but pathological fractures are rare.

DIFFERENTIAL DIAGNOSIS The lymphadenopathy of Hodgkin's disease should be distinguished from adenopathy from other causes. Most cervical or axillary adenopathy in young people occurs as a result of infectious diseases with symptoms of fever, headache, and usually pharyngitis, and is often due to infectious mononucleosis, viral syndromes, or infection by *Toxoplasma gondii.* In older patients, adenopathy may occur as a result of local spread of head and neck cancers. A good rule of thumb is that any lymph node 1 cm or greater in diameter, which does not show signs of regression after 6 weeks of observation, should be biopsied.

Mediastinal and hilar adenopathy should be distinguished from sarcoidosis, which is almost always panhilar, erythema nodosum, and primary tuberculosis which, although unilateral like Hodgkin's disease, is almost always accompanied by a resolving pulmonary infection and usually does not cause mediastinal lymph node enlargement. In older patients, the differential diagnosis includes primary tumors of the lung and mediastinum, specifically oat-cell and epidermoid carcinomas. Reactive mediastinitis and hilar adenopathy from histoplasmosis can be confused with lymphoma, particularly in regions where histoplasmosis is endemic, since it occurs in otherwise asymptomatic young people. Histoplasma mediastinitis usually involves the esophagus and should be suspected by obtaining a history of difficulty swallowing; the diagnosis is confirmed by an abnormal esophagogram; occasionally a biopsy may be necessary. Hodgkin's disease presenting as "fever of undetermined origin" may remain undiagnosed despite extensive investigations until an exploratory laparotomy is done. Infrequently, patients present with autoimmune hemolytic anemia or idiopathic thrombocytopenic purpura and are found to have Hodgkin's disease only when splenectomy becomes necessary; on occasion, Hodgkin's disease in the removed spleen has been the only focus of involvement with tumor.

DIAGNOSIS AND PATHOLOGY The diagnosis and classification of a lymphoma can be made only by biopsy and histopathologic examination under a light microscope. Needle aspiration of lymph nodes, while it may suggest the diagnosis, does not yield sufficient tissue to classify lymphomas accurately, and the error rate is high. Even experienced pathologists, using fixed sections of lymph nodes, disagree on subclassification of lymphomas in up to 25 percent of cases and disagree on whether the resected tissue shows evidence of malignancy in as many as 6 percent of cases. Frozen section material should not be used when lymphoma is suspected because slightly crushed normal lymphoid tissue in frozen sections mimics malignancy. Some patients diagnosed by frozen section as having carcinoma of the neck have actually had lymphoma or benign reactive hyperplasia and have undergone neck dissection unnecessarily.

Hodgkin's disease is unique among cancers because the tumor observed by the physician contains largely normal tissue, lymphocytes, plasma cells, and the fibrous stroma of the lymph node and only a scattering of the characteristic malignant cell of Hodgkin's disease, the Sternberg-Reed cell. In the absence of Sternberg-Reed cells the diagnosis of Hodgkin's disease should rarely be made, although the presence of such a cell by itself is not pathognomonic of the disease, since cells simulating Sternberg-Reed cells have been found in patients with infectious mononucleosis and breast cancer. The presence of the mononuclear variety of the Sternberg-Reed cell, which has a large, eosinophilic nucleolus, is sufficient to demonstrate Hodgkin's disease involving the liver or bone marrow in a patient known to have Hodgkin's disease elsewhere; however, the finding of mononuclear Sternberg-Reed cells is not sufficient for the diagnosis of the primary tumor itself.

On the basis of histological classification and knowledge of the rates of spread of tumor, the likelihood that an apparently localized lesion will be disseminated can often be predicted. The histological classification by Lukes and Butler used for Hodgkin's disease is shown in Table 130-2, along with the older Jackson-Parker classification. The original, more complete version of the Lukes and Butler classification was modified at the Rye Conference to include the four major histological subgroups shown in the right column of Table 130-2. Proper classification is important.

TABLE 130-2
Evolution of histopathologic classification of Hodgkin's disease*

Jackson-Parker (1947)	*Lukes-Butler (1966)*	*Rye classification (1966)*
Paragranuloma	Lymphocytic and/or histiocytic *1* Nodular *2* Diffuse	Lymphocytic predominance
	Nodular sclerosis	Nodular sclerosis
Granuloma	Mixed	Mixed cellularity
	Diffuse fibrosis	Lymphocytic depletion
Sarcoma	Reticular	

* *The current classification by Lukes et al. provides greater prognostic information than the old Jackson-Parker classification by virtue of identifying those patients whose tissue shows intense fibrosis in nodules.*

IMMUNOLOGIC ABNORMALITIES In the 1950s, patients with Hodgkin's disease were shown to have a higher incidence of cutaneous anergy to a battery of intradermal skin tests than normal controls. The best clinical predictor of cutaneous anergy is the absolute lymphocyte count. A lymphocyte count less than 1000 per cubic millimeter was significantly associated with cutaneous anergy. The presence or absence of anergy, or the in vitro lymphocyte phytohemagglutinin response, has, however, been shown to have no influence on the prognosis, within a given clinical stage when modern therapy is used. This surprising observation indicates that effective antitumor treatment could eradicate the disease in patients already immunosuppressed by their disease even when the drugs themselves were immunosuppressive.

A functional T-lymphocyte defect can now be detected even in patients with very early stage I Hodgkin's disease, if dose-response curves are done with dinitrochlorobenzene (DNCB) in vivo and the lymphocyte response to phytohemagglutinin (PHA) is measured in vitro. These data suggest that a T-cell defect is always a concomitant of Hodgkin's disease. The T-cell defect in HD appears to be caused by factors external to the cell itself. In normal serum and laboratory media, washed lymphocytes from patients with Hodgkin's disease are able to respond normally to PHA; while circulating immune complexes containing complement that binds to T lymphocytes have been identified in the sera of patients with Hodgkin's disease and cultures of Hodgkin's tissue obtained from resected spleens have been shown to produce high levels of prostaglandin E_2, which may inhibit the lymphocyte PHA response. These factors are not considered the major cause of the T-cell abnormality. A circulating glycoprotein that specifically inhibits T-cell function has been isolated from the sera of patients with Hodgkin's disease.

Following successful treatment with chemotherapy or radiation therapy, a permanent immunologic defect, both in number and function of T lymphocytes, remains, even in patients who have been free of tumor for many years, which does not occur in other lymphoma patients cured with the same treatments.

Antibody production is normal in most patients with Hodgkin's disease, but antibody production can be influenced by therapy. Combined multidrug chemotherapy and radiotherapy have been shown to diminish the primary response to capsular antigens of *Hemophilus influenzae* type B. This therapy combined with splenectomy may lead to a higher incidence of sepsis with *H. influenzae* and other encapsulated pathogens and accounts for the failure of pneumococcal vaccines to prevent infection in treated patients after splenectomy.

HEMATOLOGIC ABNORMALITIES A moderate, normochromic, normocytic anemia associated with low serum iron and low iron-binding capacity, but normal or increased iron stores in the bone marrow, may be present in patients with Hodgkin's disease. Studies have shown the anemia to be due to both increased destruction and decreased production of red blood cells. The iron profile in the peripheral blood is similar to that found in other patients with malignancy. A Coombs-positive hemolytic anemia occurs in less than 1 percent of patients with advanced disease.

The erythrocyte sedimentation rate (ESR) is usually rapid and serves as a useful test to follow disease activity; however, it has limited sensitivity and may return to normal when residual disease is still present. It can be useful in monitoring patients who are in remission to determine the first evidence of recurrence. Extensive radiation therapy may cause the ESR to be elevated for as long as 1 year after treatment without evidence of recurrent tumor. Numerous more complicated, and usually more expensive, laboratory tests of disease activity have not been shown to be superior to the ESR.

A moderate to marked leukemoid reaction is common in Hodgkin's disease, particularly in symptomatic patients. White blood cell count as high as 67,000 per cubic millimeter, a level which can easily be confused with the level found in chronic granulocytic leukemia, may be seen. The leukemoid reaction disappears with successful treatment. Mild peripheral eosinophilia is not uncommon, especially in patients with pruritus. Absolute lymphocytopenia ($<$1000 cells per cubic millimeter) usually occurs in patients with more advanced disease.

A bone marrow examination requires a bone marrow biopsy. Marrow aspiration has not yielded results comparable to those obtained by biopsy, probably because of the fibrosis and granuloma formation in the marrow of patients with Hodgkin's disease. On smear or section, the myeloid/erythroid ratio may be increased, and marrow eosinophilia is common; neither necessarily represents marrow involvement by tumor. Involvement of the marrow by tumor may be demonstrated by finding either classic Sternberg-Reed cells or their mononuclear variant, distributed focally or diffusely throughout the bone marrow. Marrow involvement is often associated with reticular fibrosis, which sometimes obscures the architecture of the marrow. In a patient with known Hodgkin's disease, intense marrow fibrosis, even in the absence of the characteristic malignant cells, is strong evidence of tumor in the bone marrow. Surprisingly, effective treatment by chemotherapy often leads to total resolution of marrow fibrosis in patients who achieve remission.

SELECTED CLINICAL PROBLEMS Infections are common in patients with Hodgkin's disease. Those who have progressive tumor usually die of the complications of bone marrow failure, bacteremia, or disseminated fungal infections. Diffuse pulmonary infiltrates may appear in patients who are in remission between cycles of chemotherapy, radiotherapy, or both; infection with the protozoan *Pneumocystis carinii* then should be suspected. Evidence from rats infected with *P. carinii* suggests that the appearance of this infection between cycles of treatment is related to a rebound inflammatory response to the growing organism. Patients with Hodgkin's disease are prone to develop cryptococcosis, either in the form of meningitis or as a primary pulmonary infiltrate with or without meningitis. Herpes zoster (shingles) occurs in 10 percent of treated Hodgkin's patients and in 20 percent of treated patients who have had a splenectomy. Most patients who develop herpes zoster have a few scattered papules outside the involved dermatone; this minimal evidence of spread usually does not require systemic treatment. Tuberculosis, once thought to "follow Hodgkin's disease like a shadow," is no longer common in these patients.

Cord compression is the most serious acute complication caused by growing tumor masses and is usually seen in patients with progressive tumor who have failed primary treatment. It can be caused by vertebral body involvement with collapse, which is easily seen on x-ray or bone scan, or by invasion of the epidural space from retroperitoneal lymph nodes with compression of the cord or compression of the vascular supply to the cord. Computerized tomograph (CT) scanning can be useful in detecting encroachment on the spinal cord from the retroperitoneal area. Selective electromyography is a useful way to detect regional denervation, but a myelogram is usually needed to confirm the diagnosis. Tumor masses can also obstruct the superior vena cava. This may occur as a presenting syndrome or late in the course of the disease when the diagnosis is obvious.

STAGING The staging classification developed for Hodgkin's disease and used for all lymphomas is shown in Table 130-3. Accurate staging of HD patients is vital for planning long-term management. The primary physician must take a detailed history, do a thorough physical examination, and seek evidence of systemic symptoms such as fever, night sweats, and weight loss. Weight loss of 10 percent or greater, with no attempt at dieting, usually means serious disease in this young population. Soaking night sweats can occur in anxious patients, and a history of sweats preceding knowledge of the diagnosis should be sought carefully. Every lymph node area of the body should be examined carefully, and the presence or absence of enlargement noted for future reference; the size, shape, and consistency should be recorded. Reactive hyperplasia is a cause for lymph node enlargement around lymph nodes involved with tumor, especially in the neck region; the largest lymph nodes in a group should be marked for biopsy. These may be less accessible to the surgeon, who should be urged, nonetheless, to seek them out. Nodes in areas other than the primary site, that might change the patient's stage from local to generalized disease, should be biopsied at the same time. Internists unfortunately are prone to omit examination of the oro- and nasopharynx by indirect laryngoscopy. Such examination is essential to uncovering Waldeyer ring involvement by lymphoma, although this finding is more common in the non-Hodgkin's lymphomas than in Hodgkin's disease. Epitrochlear nodes can also be involved by HD but are also more likely to be present in non-Hodgkin's lymphoma. The size of the liver and spleen should be noted. In HD, palpable splenomegaly is significant because in most cases it indicates more generalized disease. The procedures required for staging patients with Hodgkin's disease under various circumstances are shown in Tables 130-4 to 130-6.

Radiological examination should include a routine chest film. When any evidence of disease is noted on this x-ray, whole-chest tomography is performed to identify the extent of mediastinal or hilar adenopathy or evidence of contiguous invasion of the lung from the hilar nodes. Lower-extremity lymphangiogram should always be done unless medically contraindicated. On occasion, the lymphangiogram will not fill

TABLE 130-3
Staging classification for lymphomas

Stage	*Definition*
I	Involvement of a single lymph node region (I) or of a single extralymphatic organ or site (I_E).
II	Involvement of two or more lymph node regions on the same side of the diaphragm (II) or localized involvement of an extralymphatic organ or site and of one or more lymph node regions on the same side of the diaphragm (II_E).
III	Involvement of lymph node regions on both sides of the diaphragm (III), which may also be accompanied by involvement of the spleen (III_S) or by localized involvement of an extralymphatic organ or site (III_E) or both (III_{SE}).
III_1	Involvement limited to the lymphatic structures in the upper abdomen, that is, spleen, or splenic, celiac, or hepatic portal nodes, or any combination of these.
III_2	Involvement of lower abdominal nodes, that is, paraaortic, iliac, or mesenteric node, with or without involvement of the splenic, celiac, or hepatic portal nodes.
IV	Diffuse or disseminated involvement of one or more extralymphatic organs or tissues, with or without associated lymph node involvement.

NOTE: *E = extralymphatic site; S = splenic involvement. The presence of fever, night sweats, and/or unexplained loss of 10 percent or more of body weight in the 6 months preceding admission is denoted by the suffix letter B. The letter A indicates the absence of these symptoms. Biopsy-documented involvement of stage IV sites is also denoted by letter suffixes: marrow = M+; lung = L+; liver = H+; pleura = P+; bone = 0+; skin and subcutaneous tissue = D+.*

high retroperitoneal lymph nodes. CT scan and ultrasound have been shown to be effective in delineating the status of the retroperitoneal lymph nodes in these upper node regions and should supplement lymphangiography. Bone involvement can be assessed using the lymphangiogram films in most cases. Symptomatic patients should have a separate skeletal survey and/or bone scan. The latter is the more sensitive test for identifying bone lesions.

Routine blood counts, ESR, urinalysis, liver function studies, and renal function studies are all necessary parts of the medical workup but by themselves do not provide information about the extent of Hodgkin's disease or specific organ involvement. Liver function abnormalities, in particular, are poor indicators of Hodgkin's involvement of the liver but are helpful in ruling out the presence of other complicating illnesses. Bone marrow biopsy, not aspiration, should be done in all symptomatic patients with Hodgkin's disease and in those asymptomatic patients with evidence of generalized adenopathy and in patients who undergo staging laparotomy. Asymptomatic patients who have disease clinically localized above the diaphragm, that is, whose lymphangiography, CT scan, and sonogram are found to be negative, rarely have bone marrow involvement, and the biopsy can be omitted in such cases.

In 1968, a group of investigators at Stanford University introduced routine staging laparotomy as a research tool to evaluate the extent of Hodgkin's disease, to define its mode of spread, and to determine the implications of such information for therapy. In one-third of patients with normal-sized spleens, Hodgkin's disease was found in the spleen removed at surgery; conversely, in those patients with clinically enlarged spleens up to 25 percent had no evidence of tumor in the spleen but appeared instead to have reactive hyperplasia. Splenic enlargement due to involvement by HD has been linked to liver involvement. The liver is rarely involved when splenic involvement is not associated with splenomegaly (<0.5 percent). Liver involvement is present in as many as 28 percent of patients with positive lymphangiograms and enlarged spleens. The Stanford data also showed that the lymphangiogram is an accurate test to detect lymph node involvement by tumor. Only 15 percent of patients with positive lymphangiograms are found to have normal lymph node biopsies at surgery. Even in these patients, an explanation may be found in the reactive lymphoid hyperplasia normally found adjacent to tumor.

Retroperitoneal lymph node involvement demonstrated at laparotomy is associated particularly often with low left neck lymph node involvement. This association reinforced the hypothesis that HD spreads from the neck to the retroperitoneum via the thoracic duct. This hypothesis has been invoked to help explain why, in 10 percent of patients with HD, tumor will skip the mediastinal area and involve the retroperitoneal lymph nodes. A more likely explanation is that HD involvement of the retroperitoneal lymph nodes is related to splenic involvement, which is in itself related to dissemination of tumor through the bloodstream.

Staging laparotomy should not be considered a routine concomitant of staging. Knowledge of the type of treatment to be used by the radiotherapist or medical oncologist, for the variety of stages of Hodgkin's disease, should be known in advance of a decision to operate, since general treatment strategy may markedly influence the decision to perform a staging laparotomy. Random biopsy at laparotomy will not often detect lymph node involvement in patients whose retroperitoneal nodes appear normal after examination by lymphangiogram, CT scans, and sonograms. When it is performed, the laparotomy should always be complete and include at least two needle biopsies of each lobe of the liver, a wedge biopsy of the liver edge, biopsies of suspicious areas, splenectomy, and biopsy of selected lymph nodes in the retroperitoneal area, marked on the lymphangiogram prior to the operation. A postoperative film should confirm that the proper lymph nodes were removed. Nodes in the porta hepatis should also be biopsied, and, in female patients in the reproductive period, the ovaries should be moved laterally or centrally to avoid the major part of the radiation ports. If done properly, results from laparotomy will change the stage in as many as 35 percent of patients. In most cases, the change results from evidence that more extensive tumor is present, but in some cases patients are downstaged as well. Laparoscopy has been shown to be a useful alternative approach to laparotomy in staging abdominal disease. Liver involvement can be detected with equal facility by either approach.

The Ann Arbor Conference on staging of Hodgkin's disease recommended that results of staging should be reported using both the clinical stage (CS) (all tests leading up to invasive studies) and the final pathological stage (PS) which includes the results of invasive tests, such as liver biopsy, peritoneoscopy, and laparotomy. This was recommended to ensure that investigators, using different staging approaches, could make comparisons of the results of therapy based on the clinical stage of the patient. When the best diagnostic and therapeutic approaches are used, the change of stage following laparotomy infrequently results in a change in the plan of therapy.

Nationwide, the mortality from staging laparotomy in Hodgkin's disease is 1.5 percent, with a complication rate of approximately 12 percent. However, mortality rates up to 6.6 percent and morbidity rates of greater than 25 percent have been reported from institutions where laparotomies are done infrequently. In some stages of Hodgkin's disease, the operative mortality may exceed the expected death rate at 5 years from the disease itself. It was thought that staging laparotomy would decrease side effects of radiotherapy to the left upper quadrant, but problems from radiating the normal-sized spleen have turned out to be infrequent. Splenectomy itself has not been shown to have a beneficial effect either in the delivery or outcome of radiotherapy or combination chemotherapy.

TABLE 130-4
Staging Hodgkin's disease: Required evaluation procedures

1 Adequate surgical biopsy, reviewed by an experienced hematopathologist
2 A detailed history recording the absence or presence of and duration of fever, unexplained sweating and its severity, unexplained pruritus, and unexplained weight loss
3 A careful and detailed physical examination; special attention to all node-bearing areas, including Waldeyer's ring, and determination of size of liver and spleen
4 Necessary laboratory procedures
- *a* Complete blood count, including an erythrocyte sedimentation rate
- *b* Serum alkaline phosphatase
- *c* Evaluation of renal function
- *d* Evaluation of liver function

5 Radiological studies
- *a* Chest roentgenogram (posteroanterior and lateral)
- *b* Bilateral lower extremity lymphangiogram
- *c* CT scan of abdomen, with or without ultrasonography, if exploratory laparotomy is not performed
- *d* Views of skeletal system to include thoracic and lumbar vertebrae, the pelvis, proximal extremities, and any areas of bone tenderness

TREATMENT Effective treatment of Hodgkin's disease has been developed. Both drugs and radiation therapy eradicate the disease under certain circumstances. As a result of widespread application of these treatment methods, national mortality from Hodgkin's disease has dropped 30 percent in the most recent reporting period. Because of the stringent requirements for shielding and field piecing, the radiotherapy used for Hodgkin's disease is the most difficult treatment a radiation therapist uses. The treatment of Hodgkin's disease by radio-

TABLE 130-5
Staging Hodgkin's disease: Procedures required under certain conditions

1 Whole-chest tomography if any abnormality is noted or suspected on the routine chest roentgenogram
2 Bone marrow biopsy (needle or open) in the presence of:
  a An elevated alkaline phosphatase
  b Unexplained anemia or other blood count depression
  c Other evidence of bone disease (scan or x-ray)
  d Generalized disease of stage III or greater
3 Exploratory laparotomy and splenectomy, if management decisions will depend on the identification of abdominal disease

therapy requires extensive experience with more than a few patients a year and adequate equipment, preferably a 6- to 10-MeV linear accelerator. Kilovoltage equipment is inadequate and should no longer be used. Cobalt 60 equipment can be used effectively, but its use is associated with an increase in side effects from greater scatter of the radiotherapy beam. A linear accelerator is the preferred instrument.

Current drug treatment programs require precise metering of doses using a sliding scale for increases and decreases of doses, based on nadir blood counts and blood counts determined the day a new cycle is to begin. Consistency in delivering chemotherapy safely requires experience with the disease and the drugs and *should not be done by anyone not expert in the field.* Occasional treatment often results in reduced doses, drug omissions, improper sequencing, disrupted schedules, and, ultimately, recurrent tumor.

Treatment of lymphomas is in transition. Clinical trials are in progress to develop and study ways to make both drugs and radiation treatment safer, to further facilitate their general use, and to evaluate the role of each alone and together in various stages and histological subtypes of Hodgkin's disease. Some general principles have, however, emerged. At the present time, the best approach to treatment is to use either radiotherapy or combination chemotherapy alone in the appropriate stage. Studies comparing both types of treatment used together to each used alone have shown that patients who relapse after radiotherapy can be successfully re-treated with combination chemotherapy, with survival results equivalent to those obtained in previously untreated patients of the same stage and histological subtype. This means that patients cured by radiotherapy alone can be spared exposure to drugs, and those patients treated with radiotherapy who relapse have a second chance for cure. The role of radiotherapy as a supplement to drug treatment of stages III and IV disease is still experimental. While adding full-dose radiotherapy to combination chemotherapy has not proved useful in any study so far, some interesting results have been reported using low-dose radiotherapy to organs involved with tumor between cycles of chemotherapy.

The most important parameter to follow after treatment with either radiotherapy or chemotherapy is the initial period of relapse-free survival. Interpretation of current data is somewhat confused by the fact that patients who are inadequately treated with radiotherapy can be salvaged by chemotherapy. Until such time as studies are done to determine the effectiveness of chemotherapy alone in patients with early stages of disease, however, inadequate radiotherapy should not be given intentionally because of the potential for salvage by drugs of patients who fail radiotherapy.

The dose of radiotherapy is important, because the risk of relapse in a treated field is inversely proportional to dose, falling to about 1 percent at 44 Gy (4400 rads). Sharpness of the field edge with minimal scatter is achieved by a linear accelerator. It also allows the large fields required to treat Hodgkin's disease to be given with less toxicity to the bone marrow and less scatter to uninvolved but susceptible essential organs. In spite of shielding and sharp field edges, scatter to the entire lung fields is often in the range of 2 Gy (200 rads), and similar scatter doses are routinely received by the testes if the lower abdomen is radiated, even when extensive shielding is used.

Three types of radiation fields are used. Involved-field (IF) radiotherapy treats only the tumor mass with a minimal margin of normal tissue. Mantle-field irradiation gives radiation treatment to the cervical, axillary, mediastinal, and upper paraaortic nodes, usually as one field; when used in this way, it is referred to as extended-field (EF) radiotherapy. The "inverted Y" field is used to irradiate the retroperitoneal lymph nodes as a single field, and when used with the mantle field is referred to as total nodal irradiation (TNI). Actually TNI is a misnomer since many lymph nodes are outside the usual TNI fields; *total axial lymph node* irradiation (TANI) is a more accurate term. Critical in applying these treatments is to shield the spinal cord in the cervical region and the heart and to avoid overlapping the margins of the mantle and inverted Y fields. Such overlap can result in delivery of sufficient radiotherapy to the spine to cause radiation myelitis.

The four-drug program abbreviated MOPP [nitrogen *m*ustard, vincristine (*O*ncovin), *p*rednisone, and *p*rocarbazine] has emerged as a standard treatment program. Non-cross-resistant drug combinations are now available and are being tested along with MOPP treatment to determine whether alternating cycles of non-cross-resistant drug combinations are superior to combining drug combinations with radiation therapy in patients with advanced disease. Other combinations of old and of new single drugs are also used to salvage those patients who relapse after MOPP-induced remission, or who fail to enter remission. There is little role for single-agent chemotherapy as the primary treatment in patients with advanced disease unless they are medically infirm for reasons other than Hodgkin's disease.

Through use of the MOPP combination program, 80 percent of patients with advanced stages can achieve a complete remission; 63 percent of patients at risk for 10 years have remained free of their disease after remission was induced with only six cycles of treatment. Most patients who relapse do so in the first 4 years of follow-up.

Use of specific treatment approaches INVOLVED-FIELD RADIOTHERAPY Patients with single-node involvement in the high right neck, especially those who have lymphocyte-predominant Hodgkin's disease, do not require a laparotomy, since they rarely have splenic or retroperitoneal lymph node involvement by tumor and can be rendered free of disease for extended periods 95 percent of the time when treated with 35 to 40 Gy (3500 to 4000 rads) to the involved field.

EXTENDED-FIELD RADIOTHERAPY Patients with CS IA and IIA, with nodular sclerosing or mixed cellular Hodgkin's disease, limited to lymph node areas above the diaphragm, can be rendered free of disease more than 90 percent of the time, for periods extending beyond a decade, by EF radiotherapy only,

TABLE 130-6
Staging Hodgkin's disease: Useful ancillary procedures

1 Skeletal scintigrams*
2 Hepatic and spleen scintigrams*
3 Gallium whole-body scans*
4 Serum chemistries to include serum calcium and uric acid for overall management of patient
5 Estimates of the patient's delayed hypersensitivity of the tuberculin type

* *Cannot be used as evidence of Hodgkin's disease without biopsy confirmation.*

without the need for a laparotomy. However, the normal-sized spleen needs to be included in the EF port. Those patients who present with single sites of involvement in the groin should be treated with EF radiotherapy (in this case the inverted Y field) rather than IF radiotherapy. Some assessment of the status of the liver should also be made in such patients either by laparoscopy or laparotomy.

TOTAL AXIAL LYMPH NODE RADIOTHERAPY (TANI) TANI has provided results superior to EF or the mantle field when relapse-free survival is used as the major assay of effectiveness. TANI includes a splenic port and should not be used in the patient with an enlarged spleen. All symptomatic patients with localized disease (CS and PS IB and IIB), if they are to receive radiotherapy alone, should receive TANI, even if a laparotomy revealed no evidence of disease below the diaphragm, since there is no evidence that withholding radiation therapy to retroperitoneal nodes is safe in patients with negative random lymph node biopsies. Laparotomy in most cases is unnecessary. The type of radiotherapy to be given for supradiaphragmatic CS and PS IIA mixed cellularity and lymphocyte-predominant Hodgkin's disease is debatable. Equivalent results are achievable with TANI in clinically staged patients, and EF in patients staged by laparotomy. TANI can be used for patients with stage IIIA Hodgkin's disease, although at least equivalent rates of control have been achieved with MOPP chemotherapy in CS IIIA; results from one study show superiority of radiation in patients with PS IIIA. The choice of treatment for stage IIIA depends in part on the local expertise available.

Chemotherapy with the MOPP program Stage IIIA responds well to MOPP chemotherapy; most studies report nearly a 100 percent remission rate and few relapses over a decade of follow-up. Several studies clearly show that patients with CS and PS IIIB Hodgkin's disease have a better chance of relapse-free survival with MOPP chemotherapy than with TANI, and that the addition of full doses of radiotherapy to chemotherapy does not appear to provide much benefit. An exception may be found in patients with nodular sclerosing stage IIIB Hodgkin's disease, with bulky tumor. These patients may profit by the use of the combination of MOPP and TANI radiotherapy.

All patients with stage IV disease are best treated with MOPP chemotherapy or other drug combinations that have been equally effective in producing relapse-free survivals beyond 5 years with no treatment beyond the initial induction cycles. Therapy rate and duration are not influenced by specific organs involved with tumor. A patient with bone marrow involvement by Hodgkin's disease should receive full doses of chemotherapy and can expect the same frequency and duration of remission as those patients who have liver or lung involvement. Other drug combinations may be useful in patients who fail the MOPP chemotherapy program. One such drug combination using Adriamycin (doxorubicin), bleomycin, vinblastine, and dacarbazine (ABVD) has been shown to produce a significant fraction of durable complete remissions in MOPP treatment failures. When a patient has failed treatment with both MOPP and ABVD the greater side effects produced by combinations of drugs must be weighed against a single drug treatment. Because of the lack of durability of remissions achieved after resistance to the first two drug treatments occurs, cure is usually no longer a reasonable expectation, and under these circumstances it is sometimes helpful to return to the use of single-agent chemotherapy, including drugs used in previous combinations by a different schedule. For example, patients with advancing MOPP-resistant Hodgkin's disease may still respond to daily oral procarbazine or intermittent large doses of alkylating agents.

Many variables influence the outcome of patients within a given stage. These include the presence or absence of symptoms and the various histological subtypes in the treatment groups. Symptoms adversely affect prognosis since they generally indicate a greater volume of tumor as well as rapidity of spread. Volume is a clinical variable that is difficult to assess in current staging classifications; however, a large mediastinal mass, occurrence of more than four splenic nodules, and PS III_2 are poor prognostic factors. Histology is also important. While the nodular sclerosing variety of Hodgkin's disease favorably influences the prognosis of patients treated by radiotherapy alone, the presence of this histological subtype appears to adversely influence the durability of remissions attained with chemotherapy programs. The selection of treatment for patients presenting with a large mediastinal mass, contiguous involvement of the lung (E), more than four splenic nodules, CS III, or PS III_2 is not settled and these patients are often considered for combined modality therapy.

Side effects Acute side effects of radiotherapy are nausea and vomiting, marrow suppression, and gastrointestinal ulceration. All these are troublesome but usually subside shortly after radiation therapy is terminated. Nausea and vomiting are the acute side effects most unpleasant to the patient and are difficult to prevent with antiemetics, although Δ^9-tetrahydrocannabinol and metaclopramide have been shown to be useful in ameliorating nausea and vomiting associated with cancer chemotherapy. After completion of radiotherapy, the more serious side effects of radiation myelitis, pneumonitis, and rarely pericarditis may occur 6 weeks to several months after therapy is completed. Late complications include fibrosis of soft tissue and lungs within the radiation field, coronary artery disease, persistent bone marrow fibrosis, and pancytopenia, as well as an increased incidence of tumors within the treated field.

With chemotherapy, marrow suppression is the most serious acute side effect. It should be monitored carefully, and drug doses adjusted using sliding scales provided in publications reporting the results of treatment. The effective use of drugs requires experience; it is unacceptable to give smaller doses of chemotherapy because of inconvenience or inexperience, both of which adversely affect the efficacy of drug treatment. Sterility, more commonly seen in males, is a consequence of chemotherapy.

In combined treatment with radiation and chemotherapy, particularly in patients with early disease, one of the late complications is an increased incidence of acute myelocytic leukemia. In some series, the incidence has already reached 5 to 7 percent at 10 years after completion of therapy. An increased incidence of non-Hodgkin's lymphoma following combined modality treatment has also been reported. While such a risk may be acceptable in patients who would otherwise have died without treatment, it may not be acceptable in patients who might have been effectively treated with either chemotherapy or radiotherapy alone.

NON-HODGKIN'S LYMPHOMAS (NHL)

This group of diseases, like Hodgkin's disease, has its origin in lymphoreticular tissue and presents clinically in lymph nodes; however, there are differences in the cell of origin, age distribution, presentation, stage at onset, complications, and response to therapy. These diseases are not a single clinical entity and encompass a wide spectrum of disorders, ranging from Burkitt's lymphoma in children in Africa to nodular and diffuse lymphomas in adults. The designation *non-Hodgkin's lymphomas* (NHL) has arisen from common usage. The majority of cases of NHL are monoclonal B-cell neoplasms (see Table 130-1).

CLINICAL FEATURES The NHL usually present as painless, localized or generalized enlargement of lymph nodes with or without hepatosplenomegaly and not infrequently as an abdominal mass. Involvement of Waldeyer's ring is more common in NHL than in HD. A discrete lesion or multiple lesions of the lung, bone, gastrointestinal system, skin, or other parenchymal site may be the presenting feature. The B symptoms described for HD are less common in patients with NHL, but their presence is thought to influence the prognosis negatively. Particularly in the nodular lymphomas, the lymphadenopathy may have been present for a long period of time; often, a previous lymph node biopsy may have been interpreted as "atypical" or "hyperplastic." Review of such material by a hematopathologist at a later time and comparison with a second biopsy often reveals that a lymphoma was present from the start.

DIFFERENTIAL DIAGNOSIS The differential diagnosis of NHL is similar to that of Hodgkin's disease.

DIAGNOSIS AND PATHOLOGY The diagnosis of the NHL is made by histopathologic examination of biopsy material usually obtained from lymph nodes; diagnosis and classification of material obtained from other sites may be more difficult. Selection of therapy depends on the histological type as well as stage of disease. The histological classification proposed by Rappaport is generally employed because it is reproducible and useful in predicting prognosis (Table 130-7); familiarity with this system is important since it has been employed in the majority of clinical trials. In addition to the Rappaport classification, six other classifications have been proposed, leading to considerable confusion. A consortium of hematopathologists developed a "Working Formulation for Clinical Usage"; this classification is shown in square brackets [ ] throughout the text. The Rappaport classification divides lymphomas according to lymph node architecture into (1) the nodular type (N) in which neoplastic cells group in cohesive aggregates which simulate lymphoid follicles (germinal centers) and (2) the diffuse type (D) in which no aggregation occurs and the architecture of the lymph nodes is effaced. The NHL are further classified according to their cytologic characteristics into "histiocytic" (H) and lymphocytic (L) varieties, the latter consisting of poorly differentiated lymphocytic (PDL) and well-differentiated lymphocytic (WDL) types ("histiocytic" is placed in quotation marks to indicate that, except in very rare instances, the tumors so classified are lymphoid in origin). In addition, there is a group of lymphomas of mixed cellularity (MC) which have elements of the "histiocytic" and lymphocytic type.

The presence of a nodular or a diffuse pattern in the nodal architecture is a most influential prognostic factor. The nodular (follicular) lymphomas tend to follow a more indolent course (even when minimally treated) than those with a diffuse pattern, except for the infrequently observed nodular "histiocytic" (NH) variety which, when left untreated or when treated unsuccessfully, evolves rapidly. The diffuse lymphomas are clinically more aggressive than the nodular, except for the diffuse well-differentiated lymphocytic lymphoma (DWDL) [small lymphocytic] which resembles chronic lymphocytic leukemia and follows a chronic course. At the time of initial staging, 40 percent of patients with diffuse "histiocytic" lymphomas appear to have regional disease, but following treatment with radiotherapy alone 30 to 40 percent tend to relapse early, usually in the first 2 years. In contrast, patients with nodular poorly differentiated lymphocytic lymphoma (NPDL) [follicular, predominantly small cleaved cell] show a propensity for widespread dissemination easily demonstrated with routine tests and for a pattern of continuous, late recurrence extending over a period of 5 to 10 years.

Although the Rappaport classification is reproducible and predicts prognosis, the classification is not scientifically accurate because advances in studying lymph node structure and immunologic and cell surface markers of lymphocytes have revealed that each of Rappaport's different cellular types in fact consists of different morphological expressions of B-cell differentiation. For example, Rappaport's category of "histiocytic" lymphoma includes lymphomas mostly derived from transformed B lymphocytes, from large cleaved and noncleaved follicular center cells (FCC), but, only rarely, from T lymphocytes and the true histiocyte (Table 130-9).

Lukes and Collins and others have proposed an alternative pathological classification based on histological findings, surface immunoglobulin markers, lymph node imprints, and results of other immunologic studies. If cases of malignant lymphoma are classified by the system of Lukes and Collins according to the functional designation of B, T, and U cells (undefined cell systems), and histiocytes, it is generally found that 68 to 70 percent of malignant lymphomas are derived from B cells, 18 to 19 percent from T cells, 13 percent from U cells, and a very small fraction from true histiocytes. The U-cell type is a hypothetical classification, which has been proposed for cellular proliferations with primitive morphological features that are not distinctive and in which identifying immunologic or cytochemical markers are not detectable by *presently available* techniques. The classification of Lukes and Collins is shown in Table 130-8, together with the distribution of cases. Table 130-9 shows the relationship of the Rappaport classification to the Lukes and Collins classification.

TABLE 130-7
Classification of non-Hodgkin's lymphomas based on general histology and cell type according to Rappaport*

Type	*Percent of total cases*
NODULAR	
Lymphocytic poorly differentiated (NPDL) [Follicular, predominantly small cleaved cell]	<40
Mixed lymphocytic and "histiocytic" (NMC) [Follicular, mixed, small cleaved and large cell]	>5
"Histiocytic" (NH) [Follicular, predominantly large cell]	<5
DIFFUSE	
Lymphocytic:	
Well-differentiated (DWDL) [Small lymphocytic]	10
Poorly differentiated (DPDL) [Diffuse, small cleaved cell]	>10
Mixed lymphocytic and "histiocytic" (DMC) [Diffuse, mixed, small and large cell]	5
"Histiocytic" (DHL) [Diffuse, large cell] [Diffuse, large cell, immunoblastic]	>25
Lymphoblastic [Lymphoblastic]	
Undifferentiated:	
Burkitt's [Small noncleaved cell]	
Non-Burkitt's (pleomorphic) (DUL) [Small noncleaved cell]	

* *The terminology used in the "Working Formulation for Clinical Usage" is shown in brackets.*

Although the Lukes and Collins immunologic classification of NHL lacks data for extensive clinical and therapeutic correlations and is difficult to reproduce, specific pathological entities are emerging with distinct morphological and immunologic characteristics, recognizable clinical features, and predictable responses to therapy. However, since the majority of available studies showing clinicopathological correlations have used the Rappaport classification system, the subsequent sections of this chapter will discuss the NHL according to the Rappaport schema showing the working formulation designation in brackets and will point out certain specific pathological entities which are emerging from the Lukes and Collins classification.

IMMUNOLOGIC ABNORMALITIES Immune function is less affected in NHL than in HD patients, although a defect in delayed hypersensitivity reactions can be found in patients with DHL [diffuse large-cell lymphoma]. Skin reactivity and phytohemagglutinin response in NPDL [follicular, predominantly small cleaved cell] are sometimes depressed but usually only in association with advanced tumor. A defect in humoral immune function can be demonstrated more frequently in NHL patients than in HD patients. Hypogammaglobulinemia and hypergammaglobulinemia may be present. Monoclonal gammopathy occurs in some patients. Both the primary and the secondary antibody responses may be impaired.

CHROMOSOMES IN NHL In many patients with B-cell lymphomas, additional material at the end of the number 14 chromosome (14q+) can be demonstrated. This abnormality has been reported in adults with lymphomas and multiple myeloma, and in children with African Burkitt's lymphomas. The fact that patients with ataxia-telangiectasia also have abnormalities in chromosome 14 and are subject to an increased incidence of lymphocytic neoplasia suggests that aberrations in chromosome 14 may represent nonrandom chromosomal abnormalities characteristic of lymphocytic neoplasia.

STAGING The staging classification developed for HD (Ann Arbor staging classification, Table 130-3) is often used in NHL; however, the sequence of staging procedures differs because extralymphatic presentations occur more frequently in NHL than in HD. Furthermore, since many approach stage III and stage IV disease in a similar manner, this distinction may be far less relevant in NHL than in HD. The stage of disease must be determined after the confirmation of the histological diagnosis of NHL but prior to treatment. The extent of clinical evaluation must be guided by the type of therapy available and proposed for a particular patient. For patients who, after clinical staging, still appear to have localized disease and are considered eligible for aggressive curative radiotherapy, extensive staging, even employing laparotomy, may be justified. In those whose age or general medical problems limit therapy to local palliation with radiotherapy or systemic treatment with a single drug, few invasive staging procedures are indicated. Surgical staging should not be considered a routine procedure in patients with NHL. The major task of staging is to determine whether the patient has limited nodal or extranodal (E) disease, which is radiocurable (stage I or II), or disseminated disease which requires systemic therapy (stage III or IV).

Because the histological patterns correlate well with specific disease patterns, response to therapy, and prognosis, the histological diagnosis can be used to determine the appropriate staging procedures needed to choose the appropriate treatment strategy for a particular patient. For example, 80 percent of patients with a *nodular* pattern have a histopathologic diagnosis of *lymphocytic* [follicular, predominantly small cleaved cell] or *mixed-cell* [follicular, mixed, small cleaved and large cell] *lymphoma,* and 80 to 90 percent of these patients will be in stages III and IV after clinical staging and simple needle biopsy techniques. Early in the patient's staging evaluation, only diagnostic studies that have a low morbidity and a high probability of disclosing advanced disease should be employed. Lymphangiograms, bone marrow biopsies, and liver biopsy meet these requirements and can usually obviate the need for staging laparotomy.

Approximately 90 percent of patients with nodular lymphocytic and 60 to 70 percent with diffuse lymphocytic lymphomas have positive lymphangiograms. For patients with positive lymphangiograms, the incidence of spleen, liver, and/or bone marrow involvement is high (90 percent); in contrast in patients with negative lymphangiograms, such involvement is 10 percent or less.

Bone marrow aspirates are inadequate for diagnosis, and multiple posterior iliac crest biopsies are recommended. In WDL, PDL, and MC [small lymphocytic; follicular or diffuse, predominantly small cleaved cell; and follicular or diffuse, mixed, small cleaved and large cell, respectively] disease, the incidence of bone marrow involvement is at least 50 to 60 percent even though no evidence in blood count abnormalities is evident.

Search for liver involvement should be pursued if the bone marrow biopsies prove to be negative, and if the therapeutic plan is to treat the patient with less than a systemic approach. Nondirected percutaneous biopsies detect 20 percent of cases with liver involvement, peritoneoscopy-directed multiple biopsies detect an additional 20 to 30 percent of cases, and finally, if no evidence for stage IV disease has been shown after these procedures, liver biopsies at laparotomy detect the remaining 50 percent of cases. Liver involvement with lymphoma occurs in 58 to 65 percent of cases with WDL, PDL, and MC [small lymphocytic; follicular or diffuse, predominantly small cleaved cell; and follicular or diffuse, mixed, small cleaved and large cell, respectively] disease whether the architecture is nodular or diffuse.

In sharp contrast are the findings in patients diagnosed as having "histiocytic" [large cell and large cell, immunoblastic] lymphoma. Only 5 percent will have a nodular pattern. Thirty-five to forty-five percent of patients with DHL [diffuse large cell and diffuse large cell, immunoblastic] or NH [follicular, predominantly large cell] disease appear to be in clinical stages I and II and may be curable with megavoltage radiotherapy alone; in such patients, laparotomy may be advisable to ensure

TABLE 130-8
Distribution of cases of malignant lymphomas by cytologic types of Lukes and Collins

Lymphoma	*No. of cases*	*Percent*
B cell:		
Small lymphocyte (B)	39	9.2
Plasmacytoid lymphocyte	29	6.8
Follicular center cell (FCC)	(193)	(45.4)
Small cleaved	119	28.0
Large cleaved	21	4.9
Small noncleaved	29	6.8
Large noncleaved	24	5.7
Immunoblastic sarcoma (B)	15	3.5
Hairy-cell leukemia	14	3.3
T cell:		
Small lymphocyte (T)	10	2.4
Convoluted lymphocyte	41	9.7
Cerebriform lymphocyte (Sézary, mycosis fungoides)	9	2.1
Immunoblastic sarcoma (T)	15	3.5
Lymphoepithelioid cell	4	1.0
Histiocytes	1	0.2
U cell	55	12.9
Total	425	100.0

accurate staging prior to radiotherapy. Extranodal presentations in Waldeyer's ring and extralymphatic local presentations in bone, brain, testes, or other sites are more frequent in "histiocytic" than in lymphocytic lymphoma. In addition, initial bone marrow involvement is present in only 15 percent or less of cases. Similarly, liver involvement at the time of presentation occurs in less than 20 percent of cases. Bone marrow core biopsies and blind liver biopsy are obviously less rewarding than in the lymphocytic lymphomas. The staging strategy for the "histiocytic" lymphomas [large cell and large cell, immunoblastic] is to seek evidence for stage III disease by lymphangiography or inferior vena cavography or abdominal CT scan.

TYPES OF TUMORS Nodular lymphoma, poorly differentiated lymphocytic type (NPDL) [follicular, predominantly small cleaved cell] This is the most common nodular lymphoma and presents a more uniform clinical picture than the other nodular types. The disease afflicts adults, usually over the age of 40, and is very rare in young adults and children, though instances below the age of 15 are known.

NPDL is usually asymptomatic at the onset and is characterized by painless adenopathy in the cervical, axillary, and inguinofemoral regions. In some patients large abdominal masses of retroperitoneal or mesenteric lymph nodes cause acute gastrointestinal problems, including obstruction, hemorrhage, and intussusception. Some patients have ureteral obstruction with consequent renal failure. Even though the patient may notice only one or several enlarged lymph nodes, examination and study with lymphography or other tests may reveal widespread, often symmetrical, lymphadenopathy. In some patients, the lymph node enlargement may have been present for several years but is so gradual or fluctuating that patients were not concerned enough to seek medical attention. The spleen is often enlarged but rarely produces symptoms at the onset of the disease. Later in the course of the disease, it may become considerably larger and result in local symptoms and significant hypersplenism. Involvement of the lymphoid tissue in Waldeyer's ring is not a common clinical problem.

Nodular lymphomas do not often produce symptoms in nonlymphatic organs or in tissues such as the lung, liver, bones, and skin. Paravertebral lymphoid masses may result in chylous pleural effusions and/or ascites presumably because of lymphatic obstruction. It is extremely rare for the central nervous system to become involved, though peripheral nerve compression and epidural tumor masses may develop.

The peripheral blood picture is usually normal at the onset of the disease, but careful examination of the blood smear may reveal typical notched or cleft, so-called buttock, cells thought to be characteristic, but not diagnostic, of nodular lymphomas. Ordinary bone marrow aspirations are usually normal. However, study of the bone marrow by the needle or open biopsy technique will reveal focal bone marrow involvement in up to 85 percent of patients with NPDL even at the onset of the disease.

Some patients who present an otherwise typical clinical picture of chronic lymphatic leukemia, with white blood cell counts as high as 100,000 per cubic millimeter, will show a nodular lymphoma in lymph nodes. Conversely, a small proportion of patients with nodular lymphoma will develop marked lymphocytosis during the course of the disease. It remains to be determined whether these patients differ significantly from those with typical chronic lymphatic leukemia in whom the lymph nodes show the histological picture of diffuse lymphoma of the well-differentiated lymphocytic type (DWDL) [small lymphocytic].

The clinical course of nodular lymphoma is variable. In some it is indolent, and lymphadenopathy may have been present for years prior to the diagnosis and may be well tolerated for 5 years or more after the diagnosis is established. The disease is malignant, however, and though there may be spontaneous regression of lymphadenopathy, clinical problems gradually appear. In other patients the tempo of the disease is accelerated from the start, and such patients may experience difficulties within months of the diagnosis.

After months or years of being well tolerated, the disease almost always becomes much more aggressive. Lymph node masses grow rapidly, often in localized or asymmetric locations. They cause serious local problems and are less responsive to treatment which was previously effective. Fever, night sweats, and weight loss may appear. Involvement of nonlymphoid organs and tissues occurs, and the prognosis becomes very poor. If biopsy is performed at this time, the histological picture may be unchanged; or a change in histological appearance to a diffuse pattern, often with a larger cell type corresponding to the diffuse "histiocytic" lymphoma of Rappaport, may be seen.

Nodular lymphoma, mixed-cell type (NMC) [follicular, mixed, small cleaved and large cell] There are many similarities between NPDL and the less frequently occurring NMC. The NMC differs in overall prognosis, frequency of initial bone marrow involvement, and type and location of lymph node enlargement: bone marrow involvement at the onset is less common, and unusual large abdominal masses may be seen more often. In contrast to NPDL, combination chemotherapy has been found to yield a significant percentage of complete remissions with long-term disease-free intervals suggesting cure.

Nodular "histiocytic" (NH) lymphomas [follicular, predominantly large cell] This group of lymphomas generally is considered together with the diffuse "histiocytic" lymphomas since the course and prognosis are unlike those of the other nodular lymphomas.

Diffuse lymphomas (DWDL, DPDL, DMC, DHL) The diffuse NHLs consist of a number of diseases with variable presentation and clinical evolution. *Diffuse well-differentiated lymphocytic lymphoma (DWDL)* [small lymphocytic] is generally consid-

TABLE 130-9
Comparisons of classifications

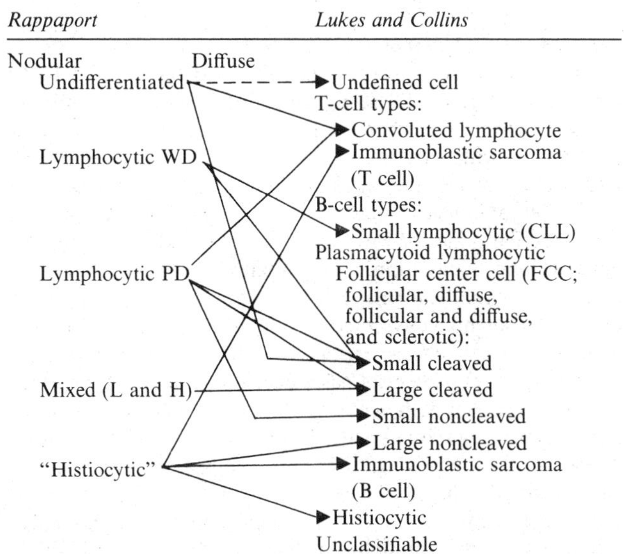

ered the most indolent NHL and in its outcome is usually indistinguishable from chronic lymphocytic leukemia. The *diffuse poorly differentiated lymphocytic lymphomas (DPDL)* [diffuse, small cleaved cell] *and diffuse mixed-cell lymphomas (DMC)* [diffuse, mixed, small and large cell] present much like the nodular lymphomas but spread much more rapidly. When the patient is first seen, the disease usually is disseminated to all lymph node areas, the liver, spleen, and bone marrow. The incidence of bone marrow and liver involvement is over 50 percent. Although response to combination chemotherapy is good and leads to complete remissions in up to 60 percent of cases, disease-free survival has not improved. In contrast, the *diffuse "histiocytic" lymphoma (DHL)* [diffuse, large cell, and diffuse, large cell, immunoblastic] (formerly called *reticulum-cell sarcoma*) and nodular "histiocytic" lymphoma (NH) [follicular, predominantly large cell] often present with localized lymph node enlargement, or local extralymphatic manifestation. The lymph nodes are most prominently located in the neck; presentations in the gastrointestinal tract, bone, thyroid, testes, brain, and the lymph node tissue of Waldeyer's ring, occur frequently. In 25 to 35 percent of the patients, even after extensive diagnostic efforts, the disease is found to be relatively localized. The bone marrow is involved initially in less than 10 percent of the patients and is not commonly involved even late in the course of the disease.

"Histiocytic" lymphoma is highly invasive, and involvement of peripheral nerves, epidural tumors, compression of the vena cava or airways, and destruction of osseous tissue occur during the course of the disease. The skin, liver, kidneys, lung, and even the brain may be involved. Occasionally bone marrow invasion results in the appearance of large, undifferentiated cells in the peripheral blood.

Localized DHL may be curable by megavoltage radiotherapy. In some studies, over 70 percent 5-year actuarial disease-free survival has been obtained. Since 1974, disseminated DHL has been shown to be responsive to combination chemotherapy, and complete remissions can be obtained in 60 percent of cases of whom the majority have a 5-year actuarial disease-free survival. Analysis of DHL responses according to histopathologic subclassification supports the Lukes and Collins hypotheses that DHL is derived most often from follicular center cells for which potentially curative therapy exists.

The diffuse lymphomas that occur in children, adolescents, and young adults must be separated from those that occur in the older age groups because of differences in clinical patterns and in response to therapy. Several unique clinical pathological entities have been recognized.

Lymphoblastic lymphomas [lymphoblastic] These tumors comprise about 30 percent of all childhood NHL and 5 to 10 percent of NHL in adolescents and adults. Males predominate in this group. The characteristic presentation is supradiaphragmatic with cervical, supraclavicular, or axillary lymph nodes and, in half the cases, a massive anterior mediastinal mass. Pleural effusions may occur. Some patients may present with inguinal nodes or with disease in extranodal sites (breast, gonads, long bones, skin, etc.). Initially, the blood and bone marrow may not be involved. The tumors may be composed of convoluted or nonconvoluted lymphocytes, but all are associated with T-cell characteristics. Following a 2- to 3-month period, 30 to 50 percent of cases develop acute leukemia cytologically identical with acute lymphoblastic leukemia of childhood. Central nervous system involvement occurs frequently. These T-cell tumors of children and young adults are cytologically distinct from the B-cell Burkitt's and non-Burkitt's lymphomas. Patients identified by clinical and histopathological criteria as having lymphoblastic lymphoma require only minimal staging procedures. Combination chemotherapy, employing regimens used in acute lymphocytic leukemia together with central nervous system prophylaxis, should be given because of the systemic nature of the process. Overall survival is poor.

Burkitt's lymphoma Burkitt first described this diffuse lymphoma of follicular center B cells in children in Africa. It has unique clinical and epidemiologic features. Although found worldwide, Burkitt's lymphoma appears virtually epidemic in certain areas of east Africa and New Guinea. In epidemic regions, serologic evidence of infection with herpes-like Epstein-Barr virus (EBV) has been documented repeatedly.

The disease appears to predominate in males (male/female ratio in Africa is 8:5; in America it is 2:1). The median age at onset of African children is 7 years, whereas in America it is 11 years. In its *typical African form,* the disease presents primarily as an extralymphatic tumor arising in the bones of the jaw. In addition, there appears to be a predilection for spread to the abdominal viscera, particularly the ovaries, as well as to the breasts and meninges. Bone marrow involvement occurs but is not common; leukemia is seen infrequently. In *American children,* bony tumors of the jaw are less frequent, and abdominal or pelvic sites, particularly the gastrointestinal tract, are involved with tumor at the time of presentation. Bone marrow and/or cerebrospinal fluid involvement occurs eventually in one-third of patients.

The diagnosis is made by recognition of the clinical picture and the characteristic histological and cytochemical findings. The tumor is very responsive to chemotherapy with single drugs, particularly alkylating agents, and long-term complete remissions without maintenance therapy have been reported.

TREATMENT Treatment approaches to NHL have undergone considerable change in the past decade. Although various treatments, including regional radiotherapy, total lymphoid irradiation, single-drug chemotherapy, combination chemotherapy, and combinations of both modalities, have been tested, the results have been difficult to interpret because differing staging and histological classifications were used. By consistent use of the Ann Arbor staging and the Rappaport histopathologic classifications, treatment strategies based on clinical and pathological stages and histology have been developed.

Involved-field (IF) radiotherapy The principles of delivery of effective radiotherapy described for HD are the same for NHL when irradiation is selected as the primary and potentially curative treatment.

Patients with stage I and II NHL should be treated with involved-field (IF) radiation therapy only, since treatment with extended-field (EF) or total nodal irradiation does not appear to improve the results. The effectiveness of regional radiotherapy depends in part on the histological type of lymphoma. For nodular lymphomas following treatment with 44 Gy (4400 rads), the local recurrence rate in the treated field is close to zero; for diffuse lymphocytic and diffuse mixed-cell lymphomas, it is approximately 15 percent. The local recurrence rate (21 to 37 percent) for patients with diffuse histiocytic lymphoma does not appear to be dose-related for doses between 25 and 65 Gy (2500 and 6500 rads), in contrast to the experience with dose-dependent control of HD. Local control with radiotherapy translates into long-term disease-free survival in 60 to 80 percent of patients with pathological stage I and 30 percent with pathological stage II NHL; paradoxically, DHL, the histologically most malignant tumor, has the best disease-free survival rate (70 percent at 5 years) if it is truly localized. However, for all the lymphomas, the main problem remains disease in viscera outside treatment fields.

Chemotherapy The treatment of choice for stages III and IV NHL is chemotherapy. For the nodular variety of the lymphomas, three treatment options are available: no initial treatment, treatment with a single drug, or treatment with combinations of drugs. For NPDL [follicular, predominantly small cleaved cell], the commonest variety of the nodular lymphomas, selected patients may be followed for periods of time with no treatment. Current evidence suggests, however, that even when patients with indolent disease are carefully selected, most will require drug treatment within 12 to 24 months.

When chemotherapy first became available for the treatment of cancer, the most responsive tumors were the lymphomas, and single-agent chemotherapy evolved initially as the treatment of choice. With the availability of many drugs, acting by different mechanisms, and evidence in animals that therapeutic synergism was possible, combination chemotherapy was tested in humans and appeared to provide superior results. Other studies, however, have suggested that single-agent chemotherapy may still produce results equivalent to those obtained with combination chemotherapy in patients with advanced NPDL. Since comparative clinical trials in NHL are relatively new, two well-established facts dictate the use of combination chemotherapy as the first treatment for patients with advanced NHL, if treatment is required. First, combination chemotherapy, using vinca alkaloids, alkylating agents, and prednisone, with or without the anthracycline antitumor antibiotics, induces a greater fraction of complete remissions in the first year of treatment than single-agent chemotherapy (68 vs. 40 percent). Second, patients who attain a complete remission survive longer than those patients who achieve partial responses; therefore, the therapy that induces the greatest fraction of complete remissions is always the best choice, provided toxicity is not too severe. Long-term comparisons of the use of single agents with drug combinations have also shown a slightly larger percentage of patients rendered free of disease with the use of combinations. Surprisingly, combination chemotherapy, in most cases, does not cause significantly greater toxicity than single-agent chemotherapy. Chlorambucil, the single agent most often used, is frequently associated with bone marrow aplasia within 2 years of continuous treatment, a side effect which is not noted when intermittent cyclical combination chemotherapy is used.

As is the case with radiotherapy, once chemotherapy of patients with NPDL is discontinued, the rate of relapse is constant, even in patients who have attained a complete remission. Ten to fifteen percent of patients can be expected to relapse per year over a 6-year period. Maintenance drug treatment of patients with NPDL prolongs the duration of the initial remission, and generally is recommended, but has not been shown to prolong survival when compared with intermittent reinduction of remission.

The situation is clearly different for patients with the nodular mixed lymphomas (NMC) [follicular, mixed, small cleaved and large cell]. Here studies have shown that combination chemotherapy is more effective than single agents. In one study, patients with NMC achieved remission in 76 percent of cases treated with a variety of MOPP which substitutes cyclophosphamide for nitrogen mustard (C-MOPP). In contrast to patients with NPDL, those with NMC who were treated with a combination of drugs and who achieved remission remained in complete remission for periods up to 10 years after therapy was discontinued; the relapse rate diminishes after 2 years. Patients with NH are treated in a fashion similar to those with DHL described below.

Results of treatment in patients who have diffuse lymphomas depend in a major way on the histological characteristics of the tumor. Patients with DWDL [small lymphocytic], even in the absence of nodularity, have a long, indolent course that waxes and wanes in a manner similar to the course of patients with chronic lymphocytic leukemia, regardless of the aggressiveness of the initial therapy. Conservative single-agent treatment, usually with chlorambucil, employed only when disease progression dictates its use, is the treatment of choice. For patients with advanced stages of DPLD, DMC, DHL [diffuse, small cleaved cell; diffuse, mixed, small and large cell; diffuse, large cell and diffuse, large cell, immunoblastic, respectively], and diffuse undifferentiated lymphoma (DUL) [small noncleaved cell], the treatment of choice is one of the several four-drug combinations that produce a significant fraction of complete remissions. In these lymphomas, the dedifferentiation of the cellular component that leads to the more aggressive clinical behavior apparently makes the tumor cells more vulnerable to the killing effects of chemotherapy. Complete remissions in patients with these poorly differentiated diffuse lymphomas are possible in 40 to 80 percent of treated patients. Failure to achieve a complete remission in these patients is associated with an extremely short survival time, usually less than 6 months. Almost all patients who fail to achieve complete remission, even those who have dramatic partial responses, die within 2 years. In contrast, if complete remission is attained, long disease-free survivals are now possible. In some studies, relapse-free survival has been reported to extend for more than 10 years beyond the end of a drug treatment. Patients with the diffuse lymphomas who achieve a complete remission do not benefit from maintenance therapy.

Combined modality treatment of NHL In view of the success of chemotherapeutic regimens in controlling advanced NHL and the apparent irreducible failure rate of radiotherapy alone for stages I and II, programs employing radiotherapy *and* chemotherapy are being explored. In one study, IF radiotherapy with chemotherapy (RT + CT) proved superior to radiotherapy (RT) alone. The 3-year relapse rate was 29 percent for RT + CT but 55 percent for RT alone; the impact of combined treatment was most striking for patients with DPDL, DMC, DHL, and NH histologies, whereas there appeared no significant difference in relapse rates for patients with DWDL, NPDL, and NMC histologies.

Whole-body radiotherapy (WBR) This modality has been employed for the management of patients with lymphocytic types of NHL in stages III and IV. The 56 percent complete remission rate achieved was similar to that obtained in parallel studies using various drug regimens. Nodular histological subtypes had better response than the diffuse types. This approach is prone to complications. Moreover, the difficulty in re-treatment of relapse with drugs dictates the use of WBR only when other treatments have failed.

Immunotherapy of NHL For the past decade studies have been carried out to determine the role of immunotherapy in the management of NHL. Controlled studies show that combination chemotherapy plus bacillus Calmette-Guérin (BCG) vaccination had a slightly better response than combination chemotherapy alone; there is a small difference in survival between patients maintained on BCG and those receiving no immunotherapy or chemotherapy as maintenance.

COMPLICATIONS OF HODGKIN'S DISEASE AND NHL

The complications of lymphoma may be due to progressive enlargement of lymph nodes, involvement of parenchymal organs, and hematologic, metabolic, or immunologic abnormalities. Complications may also result from therapy.

Progressive lymph node enlargement causes compression or obstruction of surrounding structures such as vascular structures (superior vena cava syndrome), airway, esophagus, the urinary tract, or the gastrointestinal tract. Serious complications may ensue depending on the site affected.

Direct infiltration of the lymphoma from involved mediastinal lymph nodes into the parenchyma of the lung, pleura, pericardium, and heart may occur. Infiltration from retroperitoneal lymph nodes through lymphatic channels leads to involvement of the gastrointestinal tract and may result in ulceration, perforation, hemorrhage, intussusception, or malabsorption.

Jaundice may be caused by obstruction of the biliary duct by portal lymph nodes or by infiltration of the liver secondary to hematogenous spread. The liver is often involved in the diffuse lymphocytic lymphomas (DPDL, DWDL, DMC) but less often in "histiocytic" lymphoma. Usually splenomegaly and/or retroperitoneal lymphadenopathy are demonstrable. In Hodgkin's disease, liver involvement is most commonly seen in patients with mixed cellularity or lymphocytic depletion type, who have splenomegaly and B symptoms. The differential diagnosis of jaundice must include hemolytic anemia and drug toxicity.

Central nervous system involvement may occur by direct extension of tumor from the mediastinum or retroperitoneum to the spinal canal. Symptoms of cord compression which are produced in this way occur more frequently in Hodgkin's disease than in NHL and in the latter, most often in DHL. Cranial nerves and brain may be affected by HD and NHL. Occasionally, lymphomatous meningitis may occur, and lymphoma cells, high protein, and low glucose appear in the spinal fluid. In DHL with demonstrated bone marrow involvement, meningitis occurs with such high frequency that prophylactic intrathecal therapy is recommended. More rarely, bizarre neurological manifestations may occur without demonstrable direct involvement by lymphoma. Progressive multifocal leukoencephalopathy, subacute cerebellar degeneration, myelopathy, and neuropathy have been described. Occasionally, polymyositis may occur. The differential diagnosis of these central and peripheral nervous system complications includes bacterial and viral meningitis, herpes zoster, and drug toxicity, particularly with the vinca alkaloids.

The lung may be involved by direct extension from mediastinal–hilar lymph nodes or by hematogenous spread. In the lymphocyte-predominant type of HD and in the nodular NHL the lungs are rarely involved; in contrast, nodular sclerosis–type HD frequently involves the lungs. Pleural involvement by lymphoma with malignant effusion may occur with or without lymphoma of the lung. Pneumonia is a frequent complication of treatment and constitutes the major differential diagnostic problem. Bleomycin, methotrexate, and other drugs may cause pulmonary manifestations and must be considered in the differential diagnosis of lung disease.

Skin involvement occurs as part of hematogenous dissemination of the lymphoma. A number of nonspecific skin lesions occur in lymphoma including excoriations secondary to pruritus, urticaria, erythema multiforme, erythema nodosum, exfoliative dermatitis, and dermatomyositis.

Bone marrow involvement occurs most frequently with DWDL and PDL (nodular or diffuse) (50 to 60 percent) but less frequently with DHL (10 percent). In HD, initial bone marrow involvement is rare; it is seen most often in patients with symptoms (B categories) and in patients with the lymphocyte-depleted subtype. Anemia, neutropenia, and thrombocytopenia are the consequences of bone marrow replacement; however, these conditions may also be caused by hypersplenism, immunologic mechanisms, blood loss, or complications of therapy.

Hematologic complications occur frequently. Anemia may be caused by blood loss secondary to gastrointestinal infiltration and ulceration or nonspecific lesions, malabsorption of iron or folate, bone marrow infiltration by lymphoma, or hemolysis. Coombs' test–positive hemolytic anemia is seen most often with DWDL and DPDL; it occurs less frequently with DMC, DHL, or in the nodular lymphomas and Hodgkin's disease. Chronic illness and radiotherapy or chemotherapy result in diminished or ineffective erythropoiesis. Changes in white blood cell counts are frequent. The leukemic phase of lymphoma is seen most frequently in the lymphocytic lymphomas; rarely, in "histiocytic" lymphoma. Leukopenia in an untreated patient suggests bone marrow infiltration or hypersplenism. In the patient undergoing therapy, leukopenia is usually due to the therapy. Thrombocytosis occurs occasionally in Hodgkin's disease and NHL. Frequently following staging splenectomy, the platelet count rises briefly. More often, thrombocytopenia occurs because of bone marrow replacement by lymphoma, hypersplenism, or therapy.

Metabolic abnormalities may occur as a consequence of the lymphoma or of therapy. Hyperuricemia is seen in patients with large volume of lymphoma. Effective therapy with rapid reduction of the tissue mass may exacerbate the hyperuricemia and lead to a decrease in renal function and infrequently to gouty arthritis. Hydration and administration of allopurinol can prevent these complications.

Hypercalcemia occurs in less than 10 percent of cases and is usually related to bone destruction. It is seen most frequently in DHL and Hodgkin's disease of the lymphocytic-depletion and mixed-cellularity varieties. Occasionally, the hypercalcemia may be due to release of a parathyroid-like substance. Hypercalcemia requires prompt and appropriate treatment to lower the serum calcium level and specific therapy appropriate for the management of the lymphoma.

Serum protein abnormalities occur frequently. Particularly in Hodgkin's disease, but also in NHL, the $alpha_1$, $alpha_2$, and beta fractions of globulins may be increased. The $alpha_2$ increase in Hodgkin's disease has been shown to be due to increases in haptoglobin and ceruloplasmin. Polyclonal gamma globulin elevation is seen in 40 percent of patients with HD; it is less frequent in NHL. Paraproteinemia may occur in NHL, especially in DWDL, and occasionally in HD. Hypogammaglobulinemia may precede the onset of DWDL or PDL, occurs eventually in 60 percent of these patients, but is seen less frequently in advanced Hodgkin's disease. Antibody production is usually decreased both in response to primary and recall challenge.

Complications of treatment include radiation damage associated with therapy of specific sites, toxicity due to chemotherapeutic agents (see Chap. 125), sterility, and second malignancies.

Chemotherapy with four-drug regimens leads to some decrease in ovarian or testicular function in most patients. Amenorrhea, inability to conceive, or hypo- or aspermia may result; however, in those patients who have achieved a complete remission and are off all chemotherapy, these functions may return.

Second malignancies, particularly nonlymphocytic acute leukemias, have been reported to occur in patients with HD and NHL treated with radiation alone, combination chemotherapy alone, or with both modalities. The incidence is estimated to be 1 to 8 percent of cases, with time of onset 1.2 to 19 years and a mean interval of 7 years following initial therapy. Hypoplastic or aplastic bone marrow often antedates the occurrence of frank leukemia. In the preleukemic phase chromosome analysis employing chromosome banding techniques has demonstrated a high incidence of abnormalities in chromosomes 5, 8, and 7.

ANGIOIMMUNOBLASTIC LYMPHADENOPATHY WITH DYSPROTEINEMIA (AILD)

Immunoblastic lymphadenopathy is a lymphoma-like, systemic disorder characterized by acute onset, generalized lymphadenopathy, hepatomegaly, splenomegaly, and severe constitutional symptoms including fever, sweats, and weight loss. Pruritus and skin rashes may be present. These clinical features closely mimic many of the presenting signs and symptoms of advanced Hodgkin's disease and of the other lymphomas.

The disorder occurs in adults (age 28 to 92, median 62). In half the patients a generalized, pruritic maculopapular rash precedes the onset of the other signs and symptoms by weeks or a few months. In some patients, ingestion of drugs, including penicillin or other antibiotics, phenytoin, sulfonamide, halothane, methyldopa, and aspirin, antedates the onset of the disease.

AILD is not considered a histologically malignant disease but rather an extreme form of a hypersensitivity (hyperimmune) reaction. Some have considered this a clinical example of a graft-vs.-host reaction. A proliferation of B cells and a profound deficiency of T cells have been demonstrated.

The laboratory data show anemia, which in one-quarter of the cases is due to a Coombs' test–positive hemolytic anemia. A majority of the patients have a polyclonal hypergammaglobulinemia. Leukocytosis and eosinophilia may be present.

Characteristic lesions are found in biopsy specimens of lymph nodes and consist of alterations of nodal architecture or complete effacement with a pleomorphic cellular proliferation in which immunoblasts, lymphocytes, and plasma cells predominate. In addition, vascular proliferation and prominent eosinophilic interstitial material are seen. The changes in the liver, spleen, and bone marrow do not have the diagnostic specificity of the lesions seen in the lymph nodes.

The course of AILD may be benign or fulminant. Some patients (approximately 25 percent) appear to have a long survival (20 to 45 months) with or without small doses of corticosteroids and do not require intensive chemotherapy. Others (25 percent), although requiring intensive cytotoxic chemotherapy, nevertheless have a long survival (28 to 67 months). A third group of patients (50 percent of cases) have a rapid course (1 to 20 months) terminating in death regardless of the therapeutic approach employed. Many patients die of overwhelming infections, often with pneumonia due to *Pseudomonas* and other gram-negative organisms, *Pneumocystis carinii,* cytomegalovirus, or mycoses. Acute hepatic failure or acute renal failure have also been reported to occur as terminal events.

The correct treatment of AILD has not been devised. Treatment should be initiated with corticosteroids. If there is no response, a combination chemotherapy regimen effective in lymphoma has been advocated. Radiotherapy may be employed for control of local problems. In view of the high failure rate of cytotoxic drugs, brief use of corticosteroids has been recommended to diminish the hyperimmune response along with Levamisole to stimulate T-cell function.

REFERENCES

BERARD CW et al: Malignant lymphomas as tumors of the immune system. Br J Cancer 42:1, 1980

CARBONE PP et al: Report of the committee on Hodgkin's disease staging classification. Cancer Res 31:1860, 1971

CHABNER BA et al: Sequential non-surgical and surgical staging of non-Hodgkin's lymphoma. Ann Intern Med 85:149, 1976

Contemporary issues in Hodgkin's disease: Biology, staging and treatment. Cancer Trmnt Repts, vol 66, no 4, April 1982

DEVITA VT et al: Advanced diffuse histiocytic lymphoma, potentially curable disease. Lancet 1:248, 1975

———: Curability of advanced Hodgkin's disease with chemotherapy: Long-term follow-up of MOPP-treated patients at the National Cancer Institute. Ann Intern Med 92:587, 1980

FIELD R, BODEY GP: Infections in patients with malignant lymphoma treated with combination chemotherapy. Cancer 39:1018, 1977

FISHER RI et al: Factors predicting long-term survival in diffuse mixed, histiocytic or undifferentiated lymphoma. Blood 58:45, 1981

FRIZZERA G et al: Angio-immunoblastic lymphadenopathy with dysproteinemia. Lancet 1:1070, 1974

GLATSTEIN E: Radiotherapy in Hodgkin's disease: Past achievements and future progress. Cancer 39:837, 1977

HELLMAN S et al: The place of radiation therapy in the treatment of non-Hodgkin's lymphoma. Cancer 39:843, 1977

———, DEVITA VT JR: Hodgkin's disease and the non-Hodgkin's lymphomas, in *Cancer: Principles and Practice of Oncology,* VT DeVita Jr et al (eds). Philadelphia, Lippincott, 1982, pp 1331–1392

KAPLAN HS: *Hodgkin's Disease,* 2d ed. Cambridge, Harvard University Press, 1980

LUKES RJ et al: Immunologic approach to non-Hodgkin's lymphomas and related leukemias. Analysis of the results of multiparameter studies of 425 cases. Semin Hematol 15:322, 1978

———, TINDLE BH: Immunoblastic lymphadenopathy: A hyperimmune entity resembling Hodgkin's disease. N Engl J Med 292:1, 1975

MILLER JB et al: Diffuse histiocytic lymphoma with sclerosis: A clinicopathologic entity frequently causing superior venacaval obstruction. Cancer 47:748, 1981

RAPPAPORT H: Tumors of the hematopoietic system, in *Atlas of Tumor Pathology.* Washington, DC, Armed Forces Institute of Pathology, 1966, sec 3, fasc 8

Report of the Writing Committee: National Cancer Institute sponsored study of classifications of non-Hodgkin's lymphomas: Summary and description of a working formulation for clinical usage. Cancer 49(10):2112, 1982

ROWLEY JD: Chromosomes in leukemia and lymphoma. Semin Hematol 15:301, 1978

STEIN RS et al: Anatomic substages of stage III-A Hodgkin's disease: A collaborative study. Ann Intern Med 92:159, 1980

SWEET DL JR et al: Hodgkin's disease: Problems of staging. Cancer 42:957, 1978

——— et al: Survival of patients with localized diffuse histiocytic lymphoma. Blood 58:1218, 1981

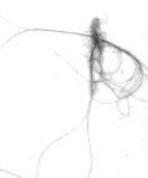

131 CARCINOID SYNDROME

JOHN A. OATES

The association of carcinoid tumors with cutaneous flushes, telangiectasia, diarrhea, cardiac valvular lesions, and bronchial constriction eluded recognition until 1953. Once this connection was established by Thorson, Biörk, Björkman, and Waldenström, and independently by Isler and Hedinger, it was clear that the syndrome was mediated by release of one or more biologically active agents by the tumor. Serotonin was the first such agent to be discovered, and overproduction of this amine is the most consistent biochemical indicator of the carcinoid syndrome. Serotonin, however, is not the sole mediator of the symptoms. These tumors vary in their synthesis of indoles and may elaborate chemically unrelated agents such as bradykinin, histamine, and adrenocorticotropic hormone (ACTH). Furthermore, unidentified substances may participate in the production of flushing. Within the broad classification of carcinoid tumors there is great diversity in the production of biologically active substances and in the mechanisms for their storage and release. Accordingly, there is a varied spectrum of clinical manifestations.

THE TUMOR Carcinoid tumors are slowly growing neoplasms of enterochromaffin cells. The metastatic tumors associated with carcinoid syndrome usually arise from small primary tumors in the ileum. The syndrome is also produced by neoplasms arising from the remainder of the small intestine, from organs derived from the embryonic foregut (e.g., bronchus, stomach, pancreas, and thyroid), and from ovarian or testicular teratomas.

Carcinoid tumors have an unusual proclivity for metastasis to the liver and may involve this organ extensively, with minimal metastatic disease elsewhere. Extrahepatic metastases occur in bone, where they are often osteoblastic, and in lung, pancreas, spleen, ovaries, adrenals, and other organs.

Primary carcinoid tumors of the appendix are common, but they rarely metastasize. Those from the large intestine may metastasize but almost never exhibit endocrine effects.

The usual carcinoid tumor arising from the ileum has the histological pattern of dense nests of cells with uniform size and nuclear appearance. Histochemically, they typically exhibit an argentaffin reaction in which the cells convert a silver salt to metallic silver. A positive argentaffin reaction is not required for the diagnosis, however, and carcinoid tumors arising from organs of the embryonic foregut usually contain few if any argentaffin cells. Tumors from these organs also have a broad histological spectrum, which in the lung ranges from typical bronchial carcinoid to a form indistinguishable from oat-cell carcinoma. Ultrastructural examination of carcinoid tumors reveals electron-dense secretion granules.

CLINICAL FEATURES Unlike most metastatic neoplasms, carcinoid tumors have an unusually slow rate of growth; many patients survive for 5 to 10 years after the disease is recognized. For much of the duration of the illness, morbidity may result largely from the endocrine function of the tumor. Death results from cardiac or hepatic failure and from complications associated with tumor growth.

Vasomotor paroxysms The most common clinical feature is cutaneous *flushing.* The typical flush is erythematous and involves the head and neck (blush area). Some patients exhibit vivid color changes from red to violaceous to pallor during its course. Prolonged flushing attacks may be associated with lacrimation and periorbital edema. The systemic effects of the flush are variable. It may be accompanied by tachycardia, and the blood pressure usually falls or does not change. A rise in blood pressure during flushing is rare, and carcinoid syndrome is not a cause of sustained hypertension.

Flushing may be provoked by excitement, exertion, eating, and ethanol ingestion. In addition, the administration of pentagastrin and beta-adrenoceptor agonists such as epinephrine can trigger episodes of vasodilatation; as the hemodynamic changes associated with such pharmacologically induced attacks may be severe, these drugs should be administered with great caution.

Telangiectasia In addition to paroxysms of cutaneous vasodilatation, some patients also develop purple telangiectasia, primarily on the face and neck and most marked in the malar area.

Gastrointestinal symptoms Intestinal hypermotility with borborygmi, cramping, and explosive diarrhea may accompany the episodic flushes. Chronic diarrhea is more common and may have a secretory component. When this is severe, malabsorption may occur.

Cardiac manifestations There is a unique deposition of fibrous tissue on the endocardium of the valvular cusps and cardiac chambers. It occurs primarily in the right side of the heart but may involve the left side to a minimal degree. The placque-like thickening of the endocardium is composed of smooth-muscle cells embedded in a stroma rich in mucopolysaccharides, collagen, and microfibrils and does not penetrate the internal elastic membrane. Distortion of the valve cusps, chordae tendineae, and papillary muscles interferes with valvular function in the right side of the heart and may lead to regurgitation, stenosis, or combined functional lesions. There is, however, a tendency for the fibrosing process to produce incompetence at the tricuspid valve and stenosis of the smaller pulmonary orifice, a deleterious hemodynamic combination. A high cardiac output, with its attendant imposition on cardiac function, may be found in some patients with carcinoid syndrome; this is due either to a continuing release of a vasodilator or to excessive flow in the metastatic tumors.

Pulmonary symptoms Bronchoconstriction is a less common feature of the syndrome, but it may be severe. It is usually most pronounced during flushing attacks.

General In addition to the endocrine effects, the tumors themselves may cause intestinal obstruction or bleeding. Necrosis of intestinal or hepatic tumor masses may produce abdominal pain, tenderness, fever, and leukocytosis. Hepatomegaly from the metastatic disease is usually present with the syndrome. Extensive metastatic involvement of the liver by these slowly growing tumors may occur before the liver function test results become abnormal. Rarely, a tumor-associated myasthenia accompanies the carcinoid syndrome.

ENDOCRINE FUNCTION OF THE TUMORS Serotonin The most constant biochemical characteristic of carcinoid tumors is the presence of tryptophan hydroxylase, which catalyzes the formation of 5-hydroxytryptophan (5-HTP) from tryptophan (Fig. 131-1). Most tumors also contain the enzyme aromatic L-amino acid decarboxylase, which catalyzes the formation of 5-hydroxytryptamine (serotonin). Carcinoids from the stomach and from other organs derived from the embryonic foregut, however, are frequently deficient in this decarboxylase and release 5-HTP from the tumor.

Following its release from the tumor, serotonin is inactivated primarily by the enzyme monoamine oxidase; uptake into platelets also contributes to removal of free serotonin from blood. Monoamine oxidase oxidizes serotonin to 5-hydroxyindoleacetaldehyde, which is rapidly converted to 5-hydroxyindoleacetic acid (5-HIAA) by aldehyde dehydrogenase. This acid is rapidly excreted in the urine, and almost all circulating serotonin can be accounted for as urinary 5-HIAA.

Carcinoid tumors vary widely in their capacity to store serotonin, with concentrations of the amine in tumors ranging from a few micrograms per gram to 3 mg/g. The concentration in the tumor appears unrelated to the rate of synthesis of serotonin as reflected by urinary 5-HIAA. Generally, tumors from the ileum have a much higher storage capacity for serotonin than do tumors from organs of the embryonic foregut.

Substance P An undecapeptide, substance P is found in enterochromaffin cells, carcinoid tumors, and in the plasma of patients with carcinoid syndrome. It is a vasodilator and promotes intestinal hypermotility.

Bradykinin A vasodilator peptide, bradykinin is released during flushes in some, but not all, cases of carcinoid syndrome. Bradykinin and related kinins are formed by the action of a group of enzymes (kallikreins) which split these peptides from kininogen, a plasma globulin. It is thought that bradykinin formation is initiated either by release of kallikrein from the tumor or by a sequence that leads to activation of the kallikrein normally present in plasma.

Other biologically active substances Some carcinoid tumors, particularly those of gastric origin, produce and release excessive amounts of histamine. This can be detected by an increased excretion of this amine in the urine. In such patients, the release of histamine from the tumors is responsible for the episodic vasodilatation with flushing, tachycardia, and hypotension.

Carcinoid syndrome has been associated with hyperadrenocorticism in a number of instances. This results from ectopic production of adrenocorticotropic hormone or of a corticotropin-releasing factor by the tumors, which usually originate from sites other than the ileum (bronchus, pancreas, ovary, and stomach). (See Chap. 122.)

In a few cases, "multiple endocrine adenomas" have been seen in conjunction with carcinoids arising from organs of the embryonic foregut. The associated tumors have included parathyroid adenomas and pancreatic tumors, producing Zollinger-Ellison syndrome. (See Chap. 123.)

Neoplasms of foregut origin with histological features resembling carcinoids may produce excessive amounts of polypeptide hormones such as gastrin, insulin, calcitonin, glucagon, corticotropin, growth hormone, a growth-hormone releasing factor, and vasoactive intestinal polypeptide without exhibiting the usual features of carcinoid syndrome. These carcinoid tumors probably share a common embryologic origin with those producing carcinoid syndrome.

PATHOPHYSIOLOGY Serotonin contributes to those aspects of the syndrome related to intestinal hypermotility, and there is evidence that the fibrous deposits on the endocardium also result from increased levels of circulating serotonin.

A secondary effect of serotonin overproduction occurs when a large fraction of dietary tryptophan is shunted into the hydroxylation pathway, leaving less tryptophan available for the formation of nicotinic acid and protein. When urinary excretion of 5-HIAA exceeds 200 to 300 mg daily, low levels of plasma tryptophan and evidence of nicotinamide deficiency are seen. (See Chap. 83.)

Mechanism of the flush Although the flushes of patients with gastric carcinoids that secrete histamine can be attributed to this amine, the mechanism of the flush in the more typical carcinoid syndrome has not yet been elucidated. Current evidence suggests that serotonin is not the mediator of the flush, and many patients flush without release of bradykinin. The relation of substance P to the flushing attacks remains to be explored.

Release of the flush-provoking substance(s) can be triggered by catecholamines, and this probably accounts for the association of flushing with excitement and emotional stimuli. For experimental induction of flushing, injection of isoproterenol in amounts of as little as 0.5 μg may be effective. Pentagastrin in doses as small as 0.25 μg also can trigger flushing, an action that may explain the provocation of flushes by eating in some patients. Flushing episodes can be blocked by somatostatin, probably by inhibition of the release of the vasodilator substance(s).

DIAGNOSIS With its full constellation of clinical features, carcinoid syndrome is easily recognized. The diagnosis also must be considered when any one of its features is present.

The diagnostic hallmark of carcinoid syndrome is *overproduction of 5-hydroxyindoles* with *increased urinary excretion of 5-hydroxyindoleacetic acid.* Normally, excretion of 5-HIAA does not exceed 9 mg daily. Ingestion of foods containing serotonin may complicate the biochemical diagnosis of carcinoid syndrome; both walnuts and bananas contain enough serotonin to produce abnormally elevated urinary excretion of 5-HIAA after their ingestion. Some drugs also interfere with the analysis of urinary 5-HIAA; cough syrups containing guaiacolate cause falsely elevated values, and phenothiazines interfere with the colorimetric test. When dietary 5-hydroxyindoles are excluded, a urinary excretion of more than 25 mg 5-HIAA daily is diagnostic of carcinoid. Elevations in the range of 9 to

FIGURE 131-1
Metabolic pathway of serotonin.

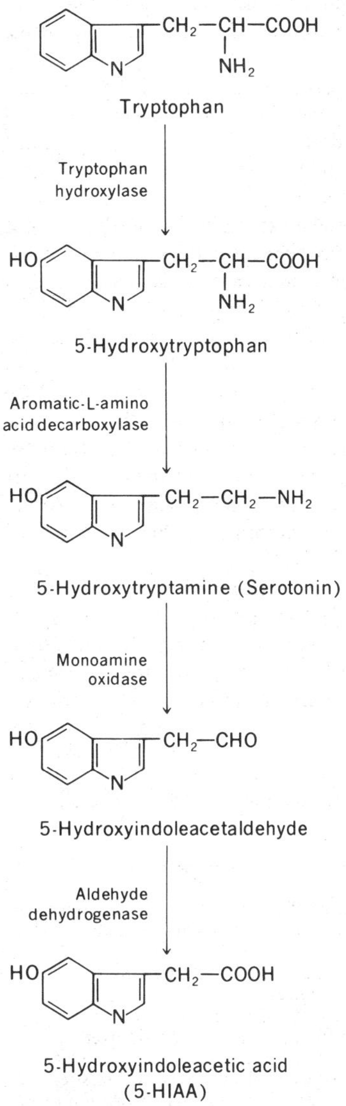

Tryptophan ($-CH_2-CH(NH_2)-COOH$)

↓ Tryptophan hydroxylase

5-Hydroxytryptophan (HO, $-CH_2-CH(NH_2)-COOH$)

↓ Aromatic-L-amino acid decarboxylase

5-Hydroxytryptamine (Serotonin) (HO, $-CH_2-CH_2-NH_2$)

↓ Monoamine oxidase

5-Hydroxyindoleacetaldehyde (HO, $-CH_2-CHO$)

↓ Aldehyde dehydrogenase

5-Hydroxyindoleacetic acid (5-HIAA) (HO, $-CH_2-COOH$)

25 mg may be seen with carcinoid syndrome, nontropical sprue, or acute intestinal obstruction.

Measurement of *serotonin in blood or platelets* is of interest but has less diagnostic value than assay of the major metabolite of serotonin in the urine.

Measurement of an increased concentration of *serotonin in tumor tissue* is a useful and sometimes necessary supplement to histological examination. A portion of suspected tumor should always be frozen for serotonin analysis (see Table 131-1).

Differential diagnosis Attacks of flushing in a patient with normal urinary excretion of 5-HIAA raises other diagnostic possibilities. Systemic mastocytosis produces flushing, hypotension, and even syncope and is the principal consideration when 5-HIAA excretion is not elevated. Flushing also occurs in the postmenopausal state and in conjunction with other tumors, particularly medullary carcinoma of the thyroid.

VARIANTS OF THE SYNDROME: RELATION TO SITE OF TUMOR ORIGIN The origin of the tumor influences the biologically active substances produced and their storage and release. Carcinoid tumors arising from organs derived from the embryonic foregut (bronchus, stomach, and pancreas) tend to differ from those arising distal to the midduodenum (midgut). The typical carcinoid syndrome usually results from tumors of midgut origin, which almost invariably secrete serotonin with little or no 5-HTP. Tumor serotonin content is likely to be high, and the tumor usually contains dense nests of argentaffin-positive cells.

In contrast, tumors arising from the embryonic foregut contain fewer argentaffin cells, have lower serotonin content, and may secrete 5-HTP. Hyperadrenocorticism and multiple endocrine adenomas are more likely to be associated with this group.

In addition to the general characteristics of the foregut group, certain clinical and biochemical features have been associated with gastric and bronchial carcinoids. Patients with gastric carcinoids frequently exhibit unique flushing which begins as a bright red patchy erythema with sharply delineated serpentine borders; these patches tend to coalesce as the blush heightens. Food ingestion is especially likely to produce flushes. The tumors usually are deficient in decarboxylase enzyme and secrete 5-HTP; histamine secretion is also common, as is a high incidence of peptic ulceration. Diarrhea and heart lesions are not prominent features in the patients who secrete largely 5-HTP from the tumor without much preformed serotonin.

When the carcinoid tumor arises from the bronchus, attacks of flushing tend to be prolonged and severe and may be associated with periorbital edema, excessive lacrimation and salivation, hypotension, tachycardia, anxiety, and tremulousness. Nausea, vomiting, explosive diarrhea, and bronchoconstriction may progress to a severe degree. This group is therapeutically unique in that the severe flushes often can be prevented by corticosteroids, and chlorpromazine may be helpful in relieving the symptoms.

TABLE 131-1
Outline of diagnostic approach to a patient with suspected carcinoid syndrome

1 Quantitative determination of 24-h urinary excretion of 5-HIAA (5-hydroxyindoleacetic acid).
2 When elevated 5-HIAA confirms clinical evidence for carcinoid syndrome, curable ovarian, testicular, or bronchial primary tumors should be sought.
3 Consideration of possible treatment of the syndrome by surgical resection of hepatic metastases requires:
  a Assessment of the location and character of hepatic metastases with arteriography and scintillation scanning of the liver.
  b Evaluation of hepatic and cardiac function.
  c A search for extrahepatic metastases in bone and other sites.
4 In patients with substantial diarrhea, possible malabsorption of nutrients should be investigated.

TREATMENT Recognition of the carcinoid syndrome has led to complete surgical cure of a few patients with tumors arising in ovarian or testicular teratomas or in the bronchus; by releasing their secretions directly into the systemic circulation, tumors from these locations can produce the syndrome before metastatic disease occurs. As the humoral substances released by tumors draining into the portal circulation are largely metabolized by the liver, tumors arising in this location produce the syndrome only after metastasis, usually to the liver. Because of the relatively slow growth of carcinoid tumors, palliative resection of hepatic metastases is beneficial in selected cases. Resection of large isolated hepatic metastases has led to relief of the symptoms of carcinoid syndrome and marked reductions in urinary 5-HIAA excretion for periods of several years. In some cases with multiple metastases, removal of as much as a hepatic lobe may be considered when the metastases are located primarily in the portion of the liver to be resected, as determined by arteriography, radionuclide scanning of the liver, ultrasonography, and computerized tomography, and inspection of the hepatic surface at surgical exploration.

There is no universally effective antitumor regimen, and none will eradicate carcinoid tumors. Palliation has been achieved in some patients with 5-fluorouracil, cyclophosphamide, streptozotocin, and doxorubicin (Adriamycin) used alone or in combinations. For the fortunate patient who is responsive to 5-fluorouracil, long-term remission may be maintained with single weekly treatments. Initial doses of chemotherapeutic agents should be reduced in patients with 5-HIAA over 150 mg per day or florid manifestations of the carcinoid syndrome. Troublesome local metastases (e.g., in bone) can be eradicated with radiation therapy.

Pharmacological therapy directed at the humoral mediators of the syndrome is useful in some cases. When the flush is associated with release of histamine, as may be the case with gastric carcinoids, combined treatment with an H_1 antagonist (e.g., diphenhydramine) and an H_2 antagonist (cimetidine) will block the vasodilator action of histamine. Diarrhea should be treated symptomatically if possible, e.g., with loperamide. Methysergide, a serotonin antagonist, improves diarrhea, but prolonged therapy with this agent can produce retroperitoneal fibrosis. Blockade of serotonin synthesis with the tryptophan hydroxylase inhibitor *p*-chlorophenylalanine (an experimental drug) also ameliorates the diarrhea. Somatostatin, an experimental agent, decreases flushing, diarrhea, and bronchoconstriction and may contribute to the management of episodes with massive mediator release or "carcinoid crisis." The prevention of severe flushing by corticosteroids and amelioration of the syndrome by phenothiazines are limited largely to patients with tumors arising from the bronchus and other organs derived from the embryonic foregut.

Nicotinamide should be given to those patients who shunt a large fraction of dietary tryptophan into the hydroxyindole pathway.

Hypotensive episodes should not be treated with catecholamines; by stimulating the release of vasoactive substances from the tumor, norepinephrine, epinephrine, and other agents with adrenergic activity can exaggerate and prolong the circulatory disturbance. If hypotension requires therapy, volume expansion or methoxamine infusion is the preferred approach.

REFERENCES

MOERTEL CG, HANLEY JA: Combination chemotherapy trials in metastatic carcinoid tumor and malignant carcinoid syndrome. Cancer Clin Trials 2:327, 1979

OATES JA, BUTLER TC: Pharmacologic and endocrine aspects of carcinoid syndrome. Adv Pharmacol 5:109, 1967

SJOERDSMA A et al: A clinical, physiologic and biochemical study of patients with malignant carcinoid. Am J Med 20:520, 1956

SKRABANEK P et al: Substance P in ovarian carcinoid. J Clin Pathol 33:160, 1980

132 CUTANEOUS MANIFESTATIONS OF INTERNAL MALIGNANCY

HARLEY A. HAYNES
THOMAS B. FITZPATRICK

One of the most satisfying aspects of dermatologic diagnosis is the detection of previously unknown malignant disease in a treatable stage by recognition of an apparently irrelevant alteration of the skin as a clue to the presence of the neoplasm. Although less satisfying, the recognition of the probability of a neoplastic disease may be of great assistance in clarifying a difficult diagnostic problem, even if the neoplasm should be untreatable when discovered. Sometimes these skin changes are induced directly by infiltration of the neoplasm into the skin, but more often they are induced indirectly by a variety of mechanisms.

This chapter is an attempt to classify the wide range of skin signs of internal malignancy in a logical fashion (Table 132-1). Since the types of skin alterations and the number of neoplasms are extremely large, grouping of the alterations by pathogenetic mechanisms was selected. There remains a substantial idiopathic category; the entities therein will be grouped by pathogenesis when this becomes understood. The skin alterations induced by neoplasms of the endocrine organs are not included here as they generally are the alterations one would expect from excess or deficiency of the hormone in question and are mentioned in the appropriate chapters.

SKIN INFILTRATION BY AN INTERNAL MALIGNANCY

METASTASES FROM CARCINOMA Cutaneous metastases of malignant lesions occur in 3 to 5 percent of patients with metastatic disease. These lesions may provide the first indication of recurrence in a patient with a known primary tumor or may be the presenting lesions of a hitherto unsuspected tumor. Typical skin metastases are dermal nodules, varying from skin color to purple, which are more easily felt than seen, and are very firm to the touch; they ulcerate rarely. Metastases from renal and thyroid carcinomas may be pulsatile and have a bruit. Breast carcinomas may produce an erysipelas-like appearance on the chest. The location of skin metastases may give a clue to the origin of the primary tumor. The abdominal wall is the most common site in both sexes for lesions initially presenting as metastases. In this situation, the primary sites are usually the lung, stomach, or kidney in men, and the ovary in women. In women with metastases on the chest wall, the most likely primary site is the breast. Other skin areas that tend to be involved by metastases are the scalp, from lung, kidney, or breast; the chest, in men, from lung; the back, from lung or breast; the extremities, from malignant melanomas; and the face, from oropharyngeal carcinomas. Histological examination of a skin metastasis may reveal the identity of the primary tumor.

METASTASES FROM LEUKEMIA Leukemic deposits in skin are more common in myelomonocytic leukemia than in lymphocytic or granulocytic leukemias (Chap. 128). Firm papules or nodules ranging in color from pink to purple are the usual lesions, although ulcerations may develop. If thrombocytopenia is present, purpura often occurs in the nodules. Leukemic infiltrates may develop in recent scars, in traumatized areas, and in lesions of herpes zoster and herpes simplex. Cytological

TABLE 132-1
Classification of skin signs of internal malignancy

- *I* Skin infiltration by an internal malignancy
  - *A* Metastatic, lymphatic, hematogenous, or by surgical implantation
    - *1* Carcinoma
    - *2* Leukemia
  - *B* Metastatic, intraepidermal
    - *1* Paget's disease of the breast
    - *2* Extramammary Paget's disease
  - *C* Autochthonous or metastatic (?)
    - *1* Lymphoma
    - *2* Malignant histiocytosis
- *II* Skin changes due to exposure to a carcinogen that also induces internal malignancy
  - *A* Arsenical keratoses
  - *B* Bowen's disease
- *III* Skin malignancies associated with increased risk of separate primary internal malignancy
  - *A* Bowen's disease
  - *B* Kaposi's sarcoma
  - *C* Any skin malignancy (??)
- *IV* Skin changes due to metabolic products of malignancies
  - *A* Malignant carcinoid syndrome
  - *B* Addisonian hyperpigmentation with Cushing's syndrome, from carcinomas producing MSH- and ACTH-like peptides
  - *C* Generalized dermal melanosis (slate gray), from malignant melanoma
  - *D* Nodular fat necrosis, due to lipases from pancreatic carcinoma
  - *E* Raynaud's syndrome with cryoproteinemia, from multiple myeloma
  - *F* Amyloidosis, from multiple myeloma
  - *G* Necrolytic migrating erythema, from functioning glucagonoma
  - *H* Porphyria cutanea tarda secondary to primary hepatoma
- *V* Skin changes due to functional disturbances in other systems induced by nonendocrine malignancies
  - *A* Jaundice, obstructive
  - *B* Addisonian hyperpigmentation from adrenal infiltration by a tumor
  - *C* Purpura, thrombocytopenic
  - *D* Pallor, from anemia
  - *E* Herpes zoster
  - *F* Herpes simplex, severe, protracted, recurrent
  - *G* Pyoderma, recurrent
  - *H* Delayed hypersensitivity, exaggerated to mosquito bites
- *VI* Skin changes, idiopathic
  - *A* Changes frequently related to internal malignancy
    - *1* Dermatomyositis, adult-onset
    - *2* Acanthosis nigricans
    - *3* Thrombophlebitis, migratory
    - *4* Ichthyosis, adult-onset
    - *5* Alopecia mucinosa, adult
    - *6* Pachydermoperiostosis, acquired
    - *7* Hypertrichosis lanugosa, acquired ("malignant down")
    - *8* Erythema gyratum repens
  - *B* Changes occasionally related to internal malignancy
    - *1* Pruritus, without causative skin lesions
    - *2* Clubbing, with and without hypertrophic osteoarthropathy
    - *3* Erythroderma
    - *4* Normolipemic xanthomatosis
    - *5* Erythema multiforme
    - *6* Urticaria and erythema perstans
    - *7* Pyoderma gangrenosum, atypical and acute febrile neutrophilic dermatosis
    - *8* Bullous disease (bullous pemphigoid and dermatitis herpetiformis)
    - *9* Seborrheic keratoses, multiple, sudden onset (sign of Leser-Trelat)
    - *10* Dermatoses, bizarre
- *VII* Heritable diseases with skin manifestations and the propensity to develop internal malignancy (see Table 132-2)

examination of "touch" preparations from the cut surface of a nodule more readily identifies the cell type than examination of histological sections. The only clinically pathognomonic lesion of any of the leukemias is chloroma, named for its green color, which is due to myeloperoxidase in the cells of acute granulocytic leukemia. In addition to specific leukemic cell infiltrates, a variety of lesions occur that are nonspecific on biopsy.

INTRAEPIDERMAL METASTASES: PAGET'S DISEASE *Paget's disease of the nipple* and areola is an uncommon but well-known skin sign of underlying intraductal carcinoma of the breast. The primary ductal carcinoma extends upward within the epithelium of the mammary ducts and into the epidermis, where it causes the skin lesion. The clinical appearance is that of an eczematous, weeping, crusted, or scaly lesion resembling atopic eczema or contact dermatitis. Paget's disease is unaffected by topical corticosteroids, in contrast to the responsiveness of eczema. Therefore, any such "eczematous" lesions that fail to respond to treatment must be biopsied. The histopathologic appearance of Paget's disease is diagnostic; the presence in the epidermis of clear cells containing mucopolysaccharides is apparent.

Extramammary Paget's disease is a similar eczematous-appearing lesion occurring on the pubis, perineum, thighs, or genitalia, related usually to underlying apocrine or eccrine sweat gland carcinoma, but occasionally to rectal or urethral adenocarcinoma. Occasionally, a primary malignant origin cannot be found. The histopathologic appearance of extramammary Paget's disease of apocrine gland origin is identical to that of Paget's disease of the breast, which is an apocrine gland. Special staining of the mucopolysaccharides will permit differentiation between Paget's disease of cloacogenic and apocrine gland origin.

LYMPHOMA Lymphomatous deposits in the skin secondary to an internal lymphoma are seen most often in histiocytic lymphoma and lymphoblastic lymphoma. Such cutaneous deposits are rare in Hodgkin's disease. Mycosis fungoides, the most frequent lymphomatous skin disorder, is discussed in Chap. 133. Lymphoma lesions in the skin are dermal or subcutaneous nodules that typically have a purple or red-brown color. The lesions usually are covered by relatively normal intact epidermis. Skin infiltrates may be the initial manifestations or may appear at any time in the course of the disease. Biopsy of these lesions is necessary to establish the correct diagnosis. The nonspecific skin changes in lymphoma are discussed below.

MALIGNANT HISTIOCYTOSIS In the Letterer-Siwe, Schüller-Christian disease complex a variety of skin lesions may occur: (1) scaly papules or vesicles with or without purpura on trunk or scalp; (2) pruritic seborrheic or eczematous lesions in intertriginous areas that do not respond to local treatment for the benign conditions; (3) petechiae due to perivascular infiltrates, thrombocytopenia, or both; (4) scaly or exudative eruptions of the scalp; and (5) xanthomas, usually late in the course. When there is lack of response to local therapy, directed at presumptive diaper dermatitis, seborrheic dermatitis, moniliasis, or intertrigo, early biopsy of these various lesions should be done and is usually diagnostic if histiocytosis is present. Skin lesions may be the presenting sign and may lead to the correct diagnosis, or they may appear late in the course of the disease if it is not controlled.

SKIN CHANGES DUE TO EXPOSURE TO A CARCINOGEN THAT ALSO INDUCES INTERNAL MALIGNANCY

ARSENICAL KERATOSES Inorganic arsenicals are the only well-recognized carcinogens which cause both skin and visceral malignancies. These salts were widely used in medicine a few decades ago for the treatment of a large variety of disorders, such as arthritis, asthma, and psoriasis, and were also used as herbicides in agriculture. Arsenic contamination of drinking water occurs in many parts of the world. Exposure may therefore be intentional and known or accidental and wholly unsuspected. Multiple, discrete, hard hyperkeratotic wartlike lesions, termed *arsenical keratoses,* on the palms and soles occur characteristically in patients a decade or more after exposure to arsenic. These lesions are similar to actinic or solar keratoses in that they are premalignant lesions, but they have a very low incidence of malignancy. The histopathologic changes produced by these two types of keratosis also are similar.

BOWEN'S DISEASE Squamous-cell carcinoma of the skin in situ is known as Bowen's disease. The lesions are single or multiple sharply defined plaques that are slightly thickened and brownish red and have a varying amount of scale. At times the lesions of Bowen's disease resemble eczema or psoriasis but fail to respond to local therapy. Such lesions must be biopsied. Arsenical exposure is definitely the cause of many cases of Bowen's disease and may be the cause of nearly all. The lesions are easily treated by surgical excision or by various methods of local destruction. Although about 5 percent become invasive, less than 2 percent metastasize. More important is the recognition of the fact that the patient is at significant risk of developing carcinomas of the respiratory, genitourinary, and gastrointestinal systems. This risk is especially high in patients in whom Bowen's disease develops on skin that is not usually exposed to sunlight. Thorough examinations to detect visceral neoplasia must be performed at intervals, as the average latent period between the onset of Bowen's disease and the development of visceral neoplasia is more than 8 years. Even without a history or stigmata of arsenical exposure, there is an increased risk of visceral neoplasms in patients with this condition.

SKIN MALIGNANCIES ASSOCIATED WITH INCREASED RISK OF SEPARATE PRIMARY INTERNAL MALIGNANCY

BOWEN'S DISEASE See preceding section.

KAPOSI'S SARCOMA Initially Kaposi's sarcoma may be a multiple, autochthonous, reactive, lymphoreticular and endothelial cell proliferation rather than a neoplasm. It usually behaves in an indolent fashion, although frank, aggressive, sarcomatous change develops in a small percentage of patients. The lesions begin on the feet or ankles, then may progress proximally and also be found on the hands and arms. Extracutaneous lesions are most frequently seen in the gastrointestinal tract, where bleeding is the major complication. The respiratory tract is the second most frequently involved extracutaneous site. Generally these extracutaneous lesions are not clinically significant, unless frankly sarcomatous. There is a marked genetic predisposition to the disease among Jews, Italians, and the Bantus in the Congo. A pronounced male predominance of 9:1 has been noted. The skin lesions of Kaposi's sarcoma are rather distinctive dark blue or purple-brown nodules or plaques, primarily located on the distal extremities. The color is due to the vascular nature of the lesions and the chronic extravasation of erythrocytes, resulting in hemosiderin deposition. Almost invariably, chronic lymphedema is associated with, and at times precedes, the lesions. Lymphoma and leukemia are associated in about 10 percent of cases in the western hemisphere, but not in the eastern. The histopathologic picture is sufficiently characteristic for confirmation of the clinical diagnosis. For the average case, very conservative therapy, such as elastic support hose to reduce edema and low-dose x-ray treatment of symptomatic skin lesions, is all that is required. Chemotherapy should be considered only in the presence of clinically significant visceral lesions or aggressive sarcomatous behavior.

In recent years Kaposi's sarcoma has been described with increasing frequency in homosexual males. This type of sarcoma is quite aggressive and occurs in association with suppressor T-cell–induced immunological suppression and cytomegalovirus infection. An increased incidence of *Pneumocystis carinii* is also seen.

ANY SKIN MALIGNANCY Neoplasia of the skin of any type may be an indication of increased risk of visceral neoplasia, but the exact relationship is difficult to ascertain because of the high incidence of skin malignancies.

SKIN CHANGES DUE TO METABOLIC PRODUCTS ASSOCIATED WITH MALIGNANCIES

MALIGNANT CARCINOID SYNDROME The hallmark of the syndrome (Chap. 131) is the sudden onset of bright red flushing of the skin, especially of the face, neck, and upper part of the chest.

ADDISONIAN HYPERPIGMENTATION WITH CUSHING'S SYNDROME (See Chap. 112) Some nonendocrine tumors, particularly oat-cell carcinoma of the lung, secrete polypeptide hormones. The most commonly observed syndrome is Addisonian hyperpigmentation with Cushing's syndrome. Intense hyperpigmentation combined with proximal muscle weakness, hypertension, diabetes mellitus, edema, and confusion are typical features. Hypokalemic alkalosis and elevated serum cortisol levels are more frequent findings than are the usual physical signs of Cushing's disease. The syndrome is caused by the production of adrenocorticotropic hormone and β-melanocyte-stimulating hormone by the tumor.

GENERALIZED DERMAL MELANOSIS (SLATE GRAY) In some patients with widespread metastases from malignant melanoma, metabolic precursors of melanin enter the circulation and are deposited in all tissues, where they become oxidized to melanin. Excretion of these intermediates results in urine that turns black upon exposure to air. Inasmuch as most of the visible melanin in this type of melanosis is in the dermis, the Tyndall effect causes the skin to look gray or blue-black rather than brown.

NODULAR FAT NECROSIS The syndrome of tender subcutaneous nodules, fever, eosinophilia, and polyarthritis of the small joints is produced by pancreatic adenocarcinoma as well as by pancreatitis. In this syndrome, the subcutaneous nodules are various shades of red and may undergo central necrosis with discharge of oil material. The increased circulating levels of lipase and other pancreatic enzymes are probably responsible for the syndrome. The histopathologic picture of the nodules usually permits the diagnosis of pancreatic fat necrosis, but does not permit differentiation of benign from malignant etiology.

RAYNAUD'S PHENOMENON (See Chap. 269) The production of cryoglobulins in patients with myeloma may cause Raynaud's phenomena. Such an etiology should be especially suspected when the syndrome is atypical, appears in men, or begins in individuals over 50 years of age.

SYSTEMIC AMYLOIDOSIS From 10 to 20 percent of patients with multiple myeloma develop amyloidosis (Chap. 66). The characteristic presentation resembles "primary" amyloidosis and includes macroglossia, extraordinarily easy bruising, and, occasionally, yellowish papules or plaques visible in the skin. All organs may be affected. The purpura appears to result from vascular fragility as a consequence of deposition of amyloid. Purpura may often be induced by gentle stroking or pinching of apparently normal skin, particularly the eyelids and body folds. When the skin lesions of amyloidosis are isolated rather than scattered diffusely, the etiology is unlikely to be systemic. Such local skin amyloidosis is not rare and must be differentiated from systemic amyloidosis.

NECROLYTIC MIGRATING ERYTHEMA The glucagonoma syndrome includes a characteristic dermatitis, somewhat resembling chronic mucocutaneous candidiasis and acrodermatitis enteropathica. The skin lesions are often most severe on the lower abdomen, groin, perineum, and about the mouth. Their morphology consists of vesicles or bullae with a migrating erythematous, scaly margin. There is a tendency to heal centrally. A red, smooth, painful tongue is common (see Chap. 116).

PORPHYRIA CUTANEA TARDA The cutaneous manifestations of porphyria cutanea tarda include hyperpigmentation (especially on the dorsum of the hands in sun-exposed areas), blisters, erosions, superficial scars with milia as a result of minimal trauma; periorbital erythema; hypertrichosis; and occasionally sclerodermoid changes in exposed skin. Patients do not generally note photosensitivity. Most patients with porphyria cutanea tarda have hepatic dysfunction; a few cases have been reported secondary to primary hepatoma.

SKIN CHANGES DUE TO FUNCTIONAL DISTURBANCES IN OTHER SYSTEMS INDUCED BY NONENDOCRINE MALIGNANCIES

See Table 132-1.

IDIOPATHIC SKIN SIGNS OF INTERNAL MALIGNANCY

SIGNS FREQUENTLY RELATED TO INTERNAL MALIGNANCY
Dermatomyositis (see Chap. 370) Adults with dermatomyositis have an associated malignancy in at least 15 percent of cases, the association being slightly higher in men than in women. The skin changes may be either subtle and transient initially or widespread, persistent, and rapid in onset. Transient, blotchy, red or violaceous areas, with or without fine scaling, may be incorrectly diagnosed as contact dermatitis, eczema, or seborrheic dermatitis. When the initial lesions are sudden in onset and marked on the face, neck, and other sun-exposed areas, a photosensitivity dermatitis or contact dermatitis may be simulated. Indeed, photosensitivity is frequently noted in dermatomyositis. Later, telangiectasia develops in the lesions, and often edema and telangiectasia of the malar area or the eyelids may result in the violaceous (heliotrope) color. Linear telangiectasia adjacent to the cuticles on the nail folds

within areas of periungual erythema are usually seen, as in systemic lupus erythematosus. Accentuation of cutaneous lesions over the joints on the dorsum of the hands, as well as over large joints, is often noted.

Acanthosis nigricans This skin sign is a highly significant marker of probable malignant disease when it develops in adults. The clinical problem is to differentiate between the different types of acanthosis nigricans, all of which look the same clinically and histopathologically. The lesions typically involve the axilla, groin, umbilicus, and nipples, but more extensive lesions may occur. The epidermis shows brown-to-black hyperpigmentation in areas of multiple confluent papillomas, resulting in a velvety elevation of the surface of the epidermis. Pruritus is sometimes present. The histopathologic appearance of the lesions confirms the diagnosis of acanthosis nigricans but does not permit differentiation between the various types. It is the history, the family history, and the physical examination which provide the most helpful data in classifying the type of acanthosis nigricans. Lesions present at birth or developing in childhood or at puberty are genetically determined and not related to malignancy. Obese individuals may develop intertriginous acanthosis nigricans without underlying disease. Various endocrinopathies, particularly Cushing's syndrome, acromegaly, and Stein-Leventhal syndrome, may be associated with acanthosis nigricans. When these conditions are absent and acanthosis nigricans develops in an adult, an underlying malignancy will be associated in most of the cases. Adenocarcinomas are the usual type of malignancy, and 60 percent of these are gastric (Chap. 307). Occasionally an undifferentiated or squamous-cell carcinoma or a lymphoma is the associated neoplasm. Though the course of the acanthosis nigricans in two-thirds of cases tends to parallel the course of the neoplasm, including remission with cure, intervals as long as 6 years between the skin lesion and the onset of the malignancy have been observed. If no benign explanation can be found for acanthosis nigricans in an adult, periodic efforts to locate a neoplasm are mandatory.

Migratory thrombophlebitis Superficial and multiple deep venous thromboses, not readily explained by the usual causes, are likely to be associated with a malignancy, usually pancreatic carcinoma (Chap. 325). Involvement of atypical sites, such as upper extremities, should also alert the physician to this possible association. An involved area may resolve in a few days. Pulmonary embolism is not a frequent complication. The migratory thrombophlebitis may precede detection of the neoplasm by several months. Unfortunately, the neoplasms associated with recurrent phlebitis tend to be inoperable.

Ichthyosis The development of ichthyosis in adults having no personal or family history of the disorder is very likely to be associated with lymphoma (usually Hodgkin's disease), although occasionally other types of malignancy have been reported. The skin appears dry, and the stratum corneum cracks to produce rhomboidal scales with flaky edges. Hyperkeratosis of the palms and soles may occur as well. The histopathologic changes are epidermal atrophy and hyperkeratosis, but they do not distinguish ichthyosis as a manifestation of malignancy from certain hereditary types. Although the association of this ichthyosiform alteration with lymphoma is strong, only a small number of cases have been reported.

Alopecia mucinosa Dermal papules, often with follicular accentuation and usually with hair loss in affected areas, are the typical findings. Usually this disorder is benign and self-limited, especially in patients under 40 and with a small number of lesions. In patients over 40 and when there are multiple infiltrated plaques with alopecia, the lesions are likely to represent a lymphoma with associated follicular mucinosis. However, alopecia mucinosa may develop before the lymphoma can be diagnosed in a certain number of patients.

Pachydermoperiostosis This term describes hypertrophic osteoarthropathy combined with acromegaloid features (Chap. 109). Thickening of the skin of the hands, forearms, and legs, as well as marked accentuation of facial folds, is typical. When the scalp is involved, the skin is reduplicated and furrowed (cutis verticis gyrata). A familial form of the disorder occurs and is unrelated to malignant disease. The acquired form usually occurs in men over 40 years of age who have bronchogenic carcinoma. Some acquired cases are associated with pulmonary infections, congenital heart disease, and hepatic disease.

Hypertrichosis lanugosa This sign is quite rare but so striking in its appearance and in its association with internal malignancy that it deserves discussion. A congenital form, often familiarly known as "dog face" or "monkey face," is inherited as an autosomal dominant trait and has no association with malignancy. Acquired hypertrichosis of lanugo hair type in adults has been associated with malignant disease. The associated neoplasms have been carcinomas of the breast, urinary bladder, lung, gallbladder, colon, and rectum. The hypertrichosis in this condition is composed of extremely fine, silky, and lightly pigmented hairs of the lanugo type. This hair growth is most apparent on the face and ears, but may occur on the trunk and extremities. Care must be taken to differentiate this lanugo hair growth from adult-type hair growth in women with disorders of androgen excess and in either sex with porphyria cutanea tarda, erythropoietic porphyria (Chap. 53), and phenytoin administration.

Erythema gyratum repens See "Urticaria" below.

SIGNS OCCASIONALLY RELATED TO INTERNAL MALIGNANCY **Pruritus** Since pruritus is one of the major symptoms expressed in the skin (Chap. 51), obviously most causes of pruritus are not related to malignant disease. Yet pruritus may be a significant symptom in up to 30 percent of patients with Hodgkin's disease. Other lymphomas are less frequently associated with pruritus, excepting mycosis fungoides, in which pruritus is almost universal. Occasionally carcinomas of the lung, stomach, colon, breast, or prostate are associated with pruritus. In such patients the pruritus usually is not limited to a small discrete area. An association with malignancy should be considered in any patient in whom pruritus cannot be explained by the finding of a metabolic cause (Chap. 51) or a local skin disease, aside from excoriations, which could explain it. Hodgkin's disease is the most likely malignancy in patients in their teens through the thirties. In the elderly, xerosis (dry skin) is common and presents a tempting explanation of pruritus. However, if decreased frequency of bathing and the use of emollients do not eliminate the pruritus, then a malignant disease must be considered. The pruritus of malignant disease will cease upon successful therapy of the malignancy.

Clubbing This alteration of the fingers and toes may sometimes be a manifestation of tumors arising either intrathoracically or metastatic to the thorax (Chap. 284).

Erythroderma This dramatic reaction of the skin is a response to a variety of stimuli (Chap. 50). Approximately 8 percent of persons with generalized erythroderma are patients with lymphoma, particularly mycosis fungoides, or leukemia. Only occasionally is erythroderma a manifestation of a carcinoma. In patients with erythroderma due to mycosis fungoides, atypical cells are present in the skin, and a skin biopsy will often be diagnostic. In erythroderma related to other types of lymphoma, leukemia, or carcinoma, there is not usually a definable infiltration of the skin by the atypical cells, and the diagnosis must be made from the blood smear, the bone marrow, involved lymph nodes, or other such tissue. In such cases, this erythroderma syndrome may represent an expression of a hypersensitivity reaction to tumor products. The course of the erythroderma parallels the response of the malignant disease to therapy, but it may precede the detection of the malignancy by a year or more, making repeated diagnostic investigations necessary.

Normolipemic xanthomatosis Malignant diseases of the reticuloendothelial system have been reported in approximately one-half the reported cases of normolipemic plane xanthomatosis. Multiple myeloma is the most frequent type of associated malignant process, but several cases of lymphoma and malignant histiocytosis have been reported. Lesions are yellow to yellow-brown, flat or slightly elevated plaques. There is marked variation in size, and the lesions may be sharply demarcated or may have indistinct borders. The eyelids, sides of the neck, and upper trunk are favored sites, but lesions may appear on any portion of the body. The histopathologic appearance of these xanthomas does not differ from that of clinically similar lesions not associated with malignant disease.

Erythema multiforme (see Chap. 50) This skin reaction occasionally occurs days to weeks after deep radiation therapy of internal malignant disease, perhaps representing a hypersensitivity reaction to components of tumor tissue. Erythema multiforme is also occasionally reported as an apparent manifestation of a lymphoma, leukemia, or carcinoma, in the absence of radiation therapy. The number of cases which are related to malignant disease is a very small fraction of the total number. The skin reaction tends to resolve spontaneously even in the presence of persistent malignant disease.

Urticaria (see Chap. 50) This frequent skin reaction is an uncommon manifestation of malignant disease. A cause-effect relationship is difficult to establish unless a clear effect on the urticaria results from therapy of the associated condition. In a few patients with chronic urticaria in whom investigation disclosed a malignant disease, removal of the malignant process was associated with remission of the urticaria. Variants of urticaria present with wheal-like lesions that persist for days to months in the same site, possibly slowly changing position to form annular, arcuate, polycyclic, concentric, or other patterns. This reaction pattern is often classified under the heading of *erythema perstans.* One clinically spectacular but rare syndrome is known as *erythema gyratum repens,* in which concentric, arcuate lesions look like the grain of a soft wood. Only a few cases have been reported, but all were associated with a malignant disease, and in several the skin reaction cleared after successful treatment of the malignancy. These urticarial cutaneous vascular reactions are presumed to represent a hypersensitivity reaction to some component of the malignant disease.

Pyoderma gangrenosum, atypical Various myeloproliferative disorders have been found in association with pyoderma gangrenosum. Myelogenous and myeloblastic leukemia, myeloma, myeloid metaplasia, monoclonal gammopathy, and polycythemia have been so described. The lesions begin as papules, nodules, or bullae and progress rapidly to central necrosis and ulceration with an epithelial rim of violaceous hue, undermined edge, and occasionally peripheral bulla formation. The lesions are quite often tender. Bacterial cultures and skin biopsy should be done to evaluate possible sepsis, vasculitis, or leukemia cutis. In pyoderma gangrenosum the biopsy is not diagnostic, but there is a neutrophilic dermal infiltrate with varying degrees of tissue necrosis. Another neutrophilic dermatosis with pustules and/or areas resembling cellulitis (Sweet's syndrome) has also been associated with myeloproliferative disease. Both the atypical pyoderma gangrenosum and Sweet's syndrome have occurred simultaneously, suggesting they are related neutrophilic dermatoses.

Bullous disease Blistering disorders of various types may occur as a manifestation of malignant disease. The most common type is the subepidermal bullous disease known as *bullous pemphigoid* (Chap. 50). This disorder usually occurs in the elderly and may affect any of or all the skin and mucosal surfaces. Although there appears not to be an increased incidence of malignant disease in such patients, this point is not proved. Removal of a neoplasm has been associated with remission of the dermatosis in a few cases. Another bullous reaction which should cause the physician to think of the possibility of a malignant disease is *dermatitis herpetiformis.* The disease is characterized by intensely pruritic, grouped vesicles which tend to be symmetrically distributed on the extensor surfaces of the limbs and over the scalp, buttocks, and back. Any patient over 40 or 50 years of age who has a dermatitis herpetiformis-like disorder which is atypical and which does not respond well to sulfone or sulfapyridine therapy should be suspected of having an occult malignant process. This situation is distinctly uncommon.

Seborrheic keratoses, multiple, sudden-onset This cutaneous lesion (sign of Leser-Trelat) is a rare occurrence, while seborrheic keratoses are very common. The suspicion of any paraneoplastic significance should be reserved for the very sudden appearance of unusually large numbers of seborrheic keratoses and/or a rapid increase in their size. This syndrome can occur along with acanthosis nigricans and may be related. No consistent tumor type has been associated with the sign of Leser-Trelat.

Dermatoses, bizarre From time to time patients present very strange skin reactions, difficult to identify, and are discovered to have a malignant process. Some of these patients appear to have a cutaneous vasculitis, but this eventually is recognized to be a lymphoma. The variety of such skin reactions is great and cannot be clearly defined. The major importance of including this category is to alert the physician to the possibility of occult malignancy in a patient who presents an unusual, or atypical, or bizarre skin reaction.

HERITABLE DISORDERS WITH SKIN MANIFESTATIONS AND THE PROPENSITY TO DEVELOP INTERNAL MALIGNANCY

The role of heredity in neoplasia is interesting and complex. At times congenital immunologic deficiency states predispose to malignancy, as does acquired immune deficiency. In other cases the relationship between the hereditary condition and neoplasia is unclear. Both types are listed here to increase the awareness of the association. The list is not complete but has been selected to include the most significant syndromes. The manifestations in the skin and other organ systems, as well as the predominant type of malignancy, are presented in Table 132-2. The reader should refer to specific discussion of these entities for more complete information.

TABLE 132-2
Heritable diseases with skin manifestations and propensity to develop internal malignancy

Disorder	*Skin signs*	*Alterations of other systems*	*Predominant malignancy*
DOMINANT INHERITANCE			
Multiple hamartoma syndrome (Cowden's disease)	Acral verrucous papules, trichilemmomas of face, fibromas of oral mucosa	Multiple hamartomas: Lipomas, hemangiomas, fibrocystic disease of breast, thyroid adenomas, neuromas	Thyroid carcinoma, breast carcinoma
Gardner's syndrome	Epidermal cysts, sebaceous cysts, dermoid tumors, lipomas, fibromas	Polyposis of colon, osteomas	Colonic adenocarcinomas (very high incidence, unless colectomy done)
Multiple mucosal neuromas	Neuromas on eyelids, lips, tongue, nasal or laryngeal mucosae	Parathyroid adenomas, hypertension	Pheochromocytoma, medullary carcinoma of thyroid (high incidence)
Neurofibromatosis (Recklinghausen's)	Neurofibromas, café au lait spots, axillary "freckles," giant nevi	Acoustic and spinal neuromas, meningiomas, osseous fibrous dysplasia	Malignant neurilemmoma (5% incidence), pheochromocytoma (uncommon), astrocytoma, glioma (uncommon)
Nevoid basal-cell carcinoma syndrome	Multiple basal-cell carcinomas, epidermoid cysts, "pits" on palms and soles	Jaw cysts, rib and vertebral abnormalities, short metacarpals, ovarian fibromas, hypertelorism	Medulloblastoma, fibrosarcoma of jaw (low incidence)
Palmar-plantar hyperkeratosis (tylosis)	Hyperkeratosis of palms and soles (usually onset after age 10)	None	Esophageal carcinoma (95% incidence)
Peutz-Jeghers syndrome	Pigmented macules on lips, oral mucosa, digits	Intestinal polyposis (predominantly small intestine)	Gastric, duodenal, and colonic adenocarcinomas (low incidence)
Tuberous sclerosis	Hypopigmented macules, shagreen patches, adenoma sebaceum, subungual fibromas	Epilepsy, mental retardation, hamartomas in brain, kidneys, heart	Astrocytomas, glioblastomas (low incidence)
AUTOSOMAL RECESSIVE			
Ataxia-telangiectasia	Telangiectasia: neck, malar, antecubital fossae, popliteal fossae, ears	Cerebellar ataxia, sinopulmonary infections, IgA deficiency, ± IgE deficiency	Lymphoma, leukemia (10% incidence)
Bloom's syndrome	Telangiectasia of sun-exposed skin, photosensitivity	Short stature, fine features, dolichocephaly	Leukemia (high incidence)
Chédiak-Higashi syndrome	Dilution of skin and hair color, recurrent pyoderma, giant melanosomes	Recurrent infections, azurophilic leukocytic inclusions, nystagmus, iris translucence, photophobia, pancytopenia	Lymphoma (high incidence)
Fanconi's anemia	Patchy hyperpigmentation	Bone anomalies, chromosomal aberrations	Leukemia (high incidence)
Werner's syndrome (adult progeria)	Premature aging, scleroderma-like changes, graying hair and baldness, leg ulcers	Arteriosclerosis, cataracts	Sarcoma, meningiomas (10% incidence)
SEX-LINKED RECESSIVE			
Bruton's sex-linked agammaglobulinemia	Recurrent infections	Recurrent infections, agammaglobulinemia	Leukemia, lymphoma (5% incidence)
Dyskeratosis congenita	Reticulate hyperpigmentation, leukoplakia of mucosae, loss of nails, hyperkeratosis of palms and soles, atrophy of skin of extensor surfaces	Pancytopenia	Carcinomas (high incidence), leukemia (occasional)
Wiscott-Aldrich syndrome	Eczematous dermatitis, petechiae-purpura, recurrent pyoderma	Decreased IgM, thrombocytopenia	Leukemia, lymphoma (10% incidence)

REFERENCES

BARNES BE: Dermatomyositis and malignancy: A review of the literature. Ann Intern Med 84:68, 1976

BROWNSTEIN MH, HELWIG EB: Metastatic tumors of the skin. Cancer 29:1298, 1972

CALLEN JP: Skin signs of internal malignancy, in *Cutaneous Aspects of Internal Disease,* JP Callen (ed). Chicago, Year Book, 1981, pp 207–222.

———, HEADINGTON J: Bowen's and non-Bowen's squamous intraepidermal neoplasia of the skin. Relationship to internal malignancy. Arch Dermatol 116:422, 1980

CAUGHMAN W et al: Neutrophilic dermatoses of myeloproliferative disorders. JAMA (in press)

CROCKER AC: The histiocytosis syndromes, in *Dermatology in General Medicine,* 2d ed, TB Fitzpatrick et al (eds). New York, McGraw-Hill, 1979

DIGIOVANNA JJ, SAFAI B: Kaposi's sarcoma: Retrospective study of 90 cases with particular emphasis on the familial occurrence, ethnic background, and prevalence of other diseases. Am J Med 71:779, 1981

DURACK DT: Opportunistic infections and Kaposi's sarcoma in homosexual men. N Engl J Med 305:1465, 1981

HAYNES HA, CURTH HO: Cutaneous manifestations associated with malignant internal disease in *Dermatology in General Medicine,* 2d ed, TB Fitzpatrick et al (eds). New York, McGraw-Hill, 1979

KAHAN RS et al: Necrolytic migratory erythema. Distinctive dermatosis of the glucagonoma syndrome. Arch Dermatol 113:792, 1977

LEWIS SJ et al: Atypical pyoderma gangrenosum with leukemia. JAMA 239:935, 1978

MINNA JD, BUNN PA JR: Paraneoplastic syndromes, in *Cancer, Principles and Practice of Oncology,* VT DeVita Jr, et al (ed). Philadelphia, Lippincott, 1982, pp 1500–1505

RIGEL DS, JACOBS MI: Malignant acanthosis nigricans: A review. J Dermatol Surg Oncol 6:923, 1980
SAMSON MK et al: Acquired hypertrichosis lanuginosa: Report of two new cases and a review of the literature. Cancer 36:1519, 1975
STONE SP, SCHROETER AL: Bullous pemphigoid and associated malignant neoplasms. Arch Dermatol 111:991, 1975

133 PRIMARY CANCER OF THE SKIN

HARLEY A. HAYNES

Carcinoma of the skin is the most common carcinoma occurring in Caucasoid individuals. Inasmuch as the lesions can be seen with the naked eye when they are in an early stage, the potential for cure is well over 90 percent. Although not responsible for all carcinomas of the skin, chronic exposure to ultraviolet radiation of the sunburn wavelengths (290 to 320 nm) in individuals not protected by intense melanin pigmentation is the most important single etiologic factor (Chap. 53). Hence, most of these cancers occur on areas of the skin that remain uncovered when the individual is fully clothed. As discussed in Chap. 53, genetic factors markedly mediate this tendency for carcinogenesis. Heritable diseases such as albinism, xeroderma pigmentosum, and the nevoid–basal-cell carcinoma syndrome are less common conditions associated with a greater risk of skin cancer. The routine local use of effective sun-screen preparations by individuals at risk can undoubtedly reduce tumor incidence. Chemical carcinogens, especially inorganic arsenicals and certain organic hydrocarbons, are separate and additional causes of skin cancers, particularly of the squamous-cell variety. Chemical and ultraviolet (UV) carcinogenesis may share some mechanisms as UV radiation is both an initiator and a promotor of carcinoma of the skin. Ionizing radiation, including x-rays, grenz rays, and gamma rays, is also carcinogenic. As with other organ systems, the skin is predisposed to the development of malignant lesions in immunologic deficiency states, such as those associated with lymphoma or immunosuppressive therapy. In fact, there is increasing evidence that UV radiation of the skin is in itself immunosuppressive by several mechanisms: (1) destruction of lymphocyte-activating Ia antigens on the surface of lymphoid cells, (2) impairment of antigen-processing function, (3) induction of suppressor lymphocytes that prevent the rejection of UV-induced tumors in mice, and (4) depletion from the epidermis of the Langerhans cells, the bone-marrow–derived dendritic cells which serve as the sentinel cells for contact dermatitis and other types of delayed hypersensitivity. Although any of the cell types in the skin may give rise to malignant neoplasms, the most common are basal-cell and squamous-cell carcinomas.

BASAL-CELL CARCINOMA Basal-cell carcinoma accounts for over 75 percent of all skin cancers. These carcinomas arise from the epidermis, cytologically resemble the normal basal cells, and show little tendency to undergo the usual differentiation into squamous cells which produce keratin. Although these tumors very rarely metastasize, they are locally invasive and, if neglected, may invade widely and deeply into underlying structures, including nerves, bone, and brain. Like most cancers these tumors are remarkably painless in their course. This lack of symptoms often leads to prolonged neglect of a lesion. The typical basal-cell carcinoma is a noninflamed, smooth, waxy nodule that appears translucent, usually has numerous telangiectatic vessels visible near the surface, and may have variable amounts of melanin pigment in the form of small dots. Such nodules often ulcerate and form a crust. This ulceration may reepithelialize, causing the patient to assume that the nodule is resolving. Basal-cell carcinomas may take many other forms, including subtle infiltrating lesions that do not produce elevated nodules. Biopsy for confirmation of the diagnosis should be routine. The patient with one basal-cell carcinoma is likely to have others, either at the same time or in following years. Some patients come to the physician with a dozen or more concurrent primary basal-cell carcinomas. Although there is no visible premalignant lesion that precedes a basal-call carcinoma, the lesion is usually seen in patients who manifest the stigmata of skin damage from sunlight (or x-rays). Treatment is selected according to the size, depth, type, and location of the lesion, as well as the particular abilities of the physician. If a simple excision will suffice, there is no other procedure that can equal the cosmetic result. Curettage and electrodesiccation for small lesions give a cure rate of more than 95 percent in experienced hands, as does x-ray treatment. Cryosurgery with liquid nitrogen seems to give cure rates similar to curettage and electrodesiccation and often brings a better cosmetic result. The specialized technique of microscopically controlled serial shave excision (Mohs' technique) gives the highest cure rate known (about 99 percent) and is recommended for difficult or recurrent lesions not manageable by the usual forms of therapy. Local chemotherapy with 5-fluorouracil is not recommended as routine treatment of basal-cell carcinomas, but may have a role in the treatment of multiple superficial lesions. Immunotherapy is investigational.

SQUAMOUS-CELL CARCINOMA Squamous-cell carcinoma also arises from the epidermis but shows significant squamous differentiation and usually keratin production. These tumors have a variable tendency to metastasize, depending upon their size, extent of invasion, location, and whether they arise from a premalignant lesion, a burn scar, a chronic inflammatory condition, or from apparently normal skin. The typical squamous-cell carcinoma is a painless, firm, red nodule or plaque with visible scales on the surface. Ulceration and crusting may occur. Relatively undifferentiated lesions that do not produce much keratin may fail to show noticeable scaling on the surface. In contrast to the basal-cell variety, squamous-cell carcinomas most commonly arise from preexisting *actinic* or *solar keratoses.* These premalignant keratoses are scaly, rough, red plaques that occur in chronically sun-damaged skin. Although very few of these keratoses progress to carcinoma, most squamous-cell carcinomas on exposed skin do arise from such keratoses. This type of squamous-cell carcinoma has the lowest frequency of metastasis (under 2 percent). However, because of the potential of malignant change in solar keratoses, which though small is real, it seems prudent to remove them, especially in younger patients. At present, the local application of 5-fluorouracil (1 to 5%) in cream or lotion seems to be the most effective method and one that generally produces no scarring. Squamous-cell carcinomas arising from mucous membranes, mucocutaneous junctions, burn scars, chronic ulcers, or sinus tracts or from apparently normal skin have a much higher tendency to metastasize. An in situ stage of cutaneous squamous-cell carcinoma is known as Bowen's disease (Chap. 132). Although some of these in situ lesions are the result of chronic sun damage, a significant proportion occurs in patients who had received inorganic arsenic preparations either accidentally or for medicinal purposes a decade or more before. In these patients there is also an increased risk of carcinomas of the respiratory, genitourinary, and gastrointestinal systems.

Patients with squamous-cell carcinoma must be examined carefully for the presence of metastases so that therapy may be appropriate. In the absence of metastases, therapy of the local lesion may generally be as indicated for basal-cell carcinoma, with preference for surgical excision or x-irradiation in view of the potential for metastasis. Extensive local or metastatic lesions may benefit from systemic chemotherapy, sometimes via local perfusion.

MYCOSIS FUNGOIDES LYMPHOMA *Lymphoma of the skin* may be a primary or secondary manifestation of various types of lymphoma. Histiocytic lymphoma and lymphoblastic lymphoma may occasionally begin with only skin lesions, but Hodgkin's disease rarely does so. The most common lymphoma of the skin is *mycosis fungoides,* which always begins with cutaneous lesions, usually with no evidence of visceral infiltration for several years. The initial lesions may be clinically confused with eczema, contact dermatitis, or psoriasis, and the biopsy may not be diagnostic. Later, more typical patches of infiltrated skin develop, often with a tendency for central clearing or an arciform or polycyclic arrangement. At this point, the biopsy may be diagnostic. In some patients, diffuse exfoliative erythroderma develops, and there may be circulating mycosis fungoides cells in the blood, at times causing diagnostic confusion with chronic lymphocytic leukemia. The skin biopsy may resolve the confusion if it is sufficiently characteristic, as may electron microscopy of the atypical cells, which are quite distinct in mycosis fungoides. The atypical cells found in the skin appear to be the same cells found in the blood or in visceral infiltrates. These cells have been identified as thymus-dependent lymphocytes and are usually of the helper/inducer type as determined by the monoclonal antibody technique. In blood smears these cells resemble large lymphocytes with scant cytoplasm and folded nuclei. In routine tissue sections these cells sometimes look like lymphocytes and sometimes like reticulum cells with the characteristic infolded nucleus. Electron-microscopic examination shows the nucleus of this cell to be highly irregular, convoluted, lobulated, and drawn into narrow threads and ribbons. At some point in time, most patients develop larger tumors as well. Although any of the viscera may be affected, disability from internal involvement usually does not occur until quite late in the course of the disease. For a patient with the early stage of the disease, the prognosis is for survival for several decades. Once the histologic diagnosis of mycosis fungoides is confirmed, the median survival for all patients is 5 years. Patients with skin tumors, ulceration, or lymphatic involvement have a median survival of 30 months.

Treatment is best planned so as to not restrict unnecessarily the future options of therapy. Topical applications of dilute, nonvesicant concentrations of mechlorethamine are often very effective for months or even years. Photochemotherapy with psoralens and long-wave UV light is often helpful. Selected lesions can be treated with grenz rays. Whole-skin electron-beam treatment may be given without hematologic suppression, since the voltage is regulated to control the depth of penetration of electrons. The use of orthovoltage x-irradiation of multiple sites should be carefully restricted, so as not to compromise the marrow or complicate further therapy with electron beam. Electron beam followed by topical mechlorethamine is probably the most effective therapy for disease limited to cutaneous plaques. Systemic chemotherapy with agents such as methotrexate, cyclophosphamide, vinca alkaloids, procarbazine, chlorambucil, and steroids often can cause dramatic objective regression of disease, but has not yet been proved to prolong life expectancy. Even though most patients at necropsy are found to have infiltrates in various viscera, early systemic chemotherapy has not been found advantageous, as a rule, perhaps because of the adverse effect of such therapy on the clinically very apparent resistance of the host to this lymphoma. In fact, this lymphoma was the first human malignancy to regularly show regression of lesions that were challenged locally with delayed hypersensitivity reactions.

REFERENCES

ANDRADE R et al (eds): *Cancer of the Skin: Biology-Diagnosis-Management.* Philadelphia, Saunders, 1976

BURN PA JR et al: Prospective staging evaluation of patients with cutaneous T-cell lymphomas: Demonstration of a high frequency of extracutaneous dissemination. Ann Intern Med 93:223, 1980

EDELSON RL (ed): Special issue: Cutaneous T-cell lymphoma. J Dermatol Surg Oncol 6:358, 1980

FITZPATRICK TB et al (eds): Neoplasms of the dermis, in *Dermatology in General Medicine,* 2d ed. New York, McGraw-Hill, 1979

GILCHREST BA et al: Oral photochemotherapy of mycosis fungoides. Cancer 38:683, 1976

HAYNES HA, VANSCOTT EJ: Lymphomas, in *Dermatology in General Medicine,* 2d ed, TB Fitzpatrick et al (eds). New York, McGraw-Hill, 1979

——— et al: Phenotypic characterization of cutaneous T-cell lymphoma: Use of monoclonal antibodies to compare with other malignant T-cells. N Engl J Med 304:1219, 1981

LEVENE MB et al: Cancers of the skin, in *Cancer, Principles and Practice of Oncology,* VT DeVita Jr, et al (eds). Philadelphia, Lippincott, 1982

McDONALD CJ, BERTINO JR: Treatment of mycosis fungoides lymphoma—effectiveness of infusions of methotrexate followed by oral citrovorum factor. Cancer Treatment Rep 62:1009, 1978

TOEWS GB, et al: Langerhans cells: Sentinels of skin-associated lymphoid tissue. J Invest Dermatol 75:78, 1980

VONDERHEID EC et al: Topical chemotherapy and immunotherapy of mycosis fungoides. Arch Dermatol 113:454, 1977

ZACARIAN SA (ed): *Cryosurgical Advances in Dermatology and Tumors of the Head and Neck.* Springfield, Ill., Charles C Thomas, 1977

134
MALIGNANT MELANOMA OF THE SKIN

THOMAS B. FITZPATRICK
ARTHUR J. SOBER
MARTIN C. MIHM, JR.
CALVIN L. DAY, JR.

Primary malignant melanoma of the skin is the leading cause of death from all diseases arising in the skin, and the detection of early lesions must be the task of every physician, regardless of specialty. At every occasion when the entire cutaneous surface can be viewed, a careful search for suspicious pigmented lesions should be made.

Pigmented moles are among the most common growths on the skin, and yet cancer involving pigment cells (i.e., malignant melanoma) is relatively uncommon, constituting about 1 percent of all cancers. There has been a disturbing increase in the incidence of primary melanoma of the skin. The rate has doubled in the past 10 years, possibly due to increased "weekend" exposure to sunlight, especially among persons in professional and managerial positions. Primary cutaneous malignant melanoma, moreover, does not respond or responds only poorly to chemotherapy or radiation therapy, and, so far, hope for survival has been based on surgical excision during the very early primary stages before deep invasion occurs. The problem for the physician, therefore, is to recognize early primary malignant melanoma and also those precancerous lesions that will develop into malignant melanoma among the large number of pigmented lesions that occur on the skin.

Primary malignant melanoma of the skin, even in the early stages, is now considered relatively easy to detect by clinical examination alone. In the past, the clinical description of primary cutaneous malignant melanoma was presented incompletely. Physicians and patients were told to have concern only for those pigmented lesions that showed changes in growth pattern or color or were bleeding or ulcerated—criteria indicating deep invasion in the skin and, usually, a poor prognosis.

Follow-up study of more than 1100 patients with primary melanoma has provided evidence indicating that a primary cutaneous melanoma may exist in a "silent," intraepidermal, preinvasive form for several years. These early "silent" primary malignant melanomas, even when 3 to 4 mm in size, can be recognized by certain simple criteria, which are delineated below.

Two criteria, *variegation of color* and *irregular border* often with a "notch," are so characteristic of primary cutaneous malignant melanoma that histologic examination is advised when they are present. The important colors that are signs of primary malignant melanoma *include shades of red, white, or blue* and the shades resulting from their mixture with brown or black. Furthermore, a lesion may be uniformly colored, e.g., *bluish black or bluish red.*

The diagnostic significance of various shades of brown or black, or both, in pigmented primary cutaneous malignant melanoma has been stressed in the past. It is, however, the diagnostic significance of the various shades of red, white, or blue, or all three mixed with brown or black, that requires emphasis. Of the colors present in pigmented primary cutaneous malignant melanomas, shades of blue (bluish red, bluish gray, and bluish black) are the most significant in the diagnosis. *Examination with a magnifying lens and bright lighting* may assist greatly in recognizing the diagnostic feature of melanoma (Table 134-1).

Before 1967, malignant melanoma was considered a single morphological entity with a uniformly grave prognosis. Later histopathologic investigations, especially by Clark, McGovern, Mihm, and colleagues, have permitted a new approach to the classification of primary human cutaneous malignant melanomas, based on the correlation of the clinical and histologic features with prognosis. Four types of primary malignant melanoma have been delineated (Table 134-2) and have been subdivided by the presence or absence of an adjacent intraepidermal component around the tumor nodule:

Malignant melanoma with adjacent intraepidermal component:

1 Superficial spreading melanoma
2 Malignant melanoma, lentigo maligna
3 Acral lentiginous melanoma

TABLE 134-1
Indications for excision or diagnostic biopsy of pigmented lesions

I History
  A Change in size or color, bleeding
  B Symptoms
    1 Itching (25%)
    2 Tenderness
  C Congenital, raised pigmented lesions
II Lesion characteristics
  A Color
    1 Uniform blue or gray
    2 Variegated: blue, gray, white, red, mixed with brown or black
  B Border: irregular, often with a notch
  C Surface: irregular

Malignant melanoma without an adjacent intraepidermal component:

4 Nodular melanoma

It should be emphasized that lentigo maligna melanoma and superficial spreading melanoma may exist for several years in the preinvasive stage. Hence, early diagnosis of malignant melanoma of the skin makes excision of the identified lesions possible before deep invasion has occurred. The survival rate of malignant melanoma is related to the level of invasion of the tumor or the thickness of the primary tumor expressed in millimeters. These levels of invasion have been classified on the basis of anatomic structure as follows:

Level 1: Intraepidermal melanocytic atypism, a level recognized for purposes of research. Patients with this finding are not at present labeled with the diagnosis of melanoma.
Level 2: Tumor invading the papillary layer but not extending to the reticular layer.
Level 3: Tumor filling and expanding the papillary layer but not invading the reticular layer.
Level 4: Tumor penetrating into the reticular layer of the dermis.
Level 5: Tumor invading the subcutaneous fat.

(See Table 134-3 for survival by level of invasion.)

When thickness of the primary tumor is determined by measuring the vertical thickness with a light microscope fitted with an ocular micrometer, tumors measuring less than 0.85 mm in thickness have a uniformly favorable outcome, while patients with tumors greater than 3.60 mm are at high risk for recurrent diseases and death. At the present time, the determination of prognosis by thickness is the most practical (see Table 134-3 for survival by thickness).

Suspicious lesions require biopsy, which will confirm the benign or malignant nature of the lesion. Simple excisional biopsy with narrow margins is the procedure of choice, but trephine (punch) or incisional biopsies are also acceptable depending on the situation and the experience of the physician performing the procedure. Table 134-1 lists the indications for biopsy of cutaneous lesions.

Treatment of malignant melanoma at the present is primarily by surgical excision of the primary lesion; there is no agreement as to whether prophylactic lymph node dissection affects the course of the disease. Data of Breslow and Macht suggest that limited excision may be effective for thin (0.75 mm) lesions. The more advanced primary lesions ($>$ 0.75 mm) should be treated by wide local excision down to the deep fascia, followed by skin grafting if necessary; radical lymph node dissection when the tumor drains to only one lymph node group also is still advocated by many surgeons for primary tumors thicker than 1.5 mm or 2.0 mm. Surgery for lentigo maligna melanoma is less aggressive; the recommendation is for surgical margins of 1 cm and lymph node dissection only if therapeutically indicated.

In the past few years, considerable interest has been directed toward the factors that influence both the development of primary malignant melanomas of the skin and also the rate and degree of dissemination of the tumor. The possibility that there is a population with a high risk for the development of these melanomas is being studied. It is suspected that persons, both male and female, who have poor tolerance to sunlight and who develop sunburn on short exposures and who tan poorly have a higher incidence of malignant melanoma (Table 134-3).

TABLE 134-2
Clinical features of malignant melanoma

Type	*Site*	*Average age at diagnosis, years*	*Duration of known existence, years*	*Color*
Lentigo maligna melanoma	Exposed surfaces usually, and particularly malar region of cheek and temple; on unexposed surfaces sometimes	70	5–20* or longer	In flat portions, shades of brown and black predominant, but whitish gray occasionally present; in nodules, shades of reddish brown, bluish gray, bluish black
Superficial spreading melanoma	Any site (more common on upper back and in women on lower legs)	40–50	1–7	Shades of brown and black mixed with bluish red (violaceous), bluish black, reddish brown, and often whitish pink, and the border of lesion is at least in part visibly and/or palpably elevated
Nodular melanoma	Any site	40–50	Months to less than 5 years	Reddish blue (purple) or bluish black, either uniform in color or mixed with brown or black
Acral lentiginous	Palm, sole, nailbed, mucous membrane	50	1–10	In flat portions, dark brown predominantly; in raised lesions (plaques), brown-black or blue-black color predominantly

* *During much of this time, the precursor stage, lentigo maligna is actively confined to the epidermis.*

It has recently been demonstrated that within countries an inverse relationship exists between melanoma incidence and latitude. For example, incidence rates of 9 per 100,000 per year in Connecticut can be contrasted to rates greater than 20 per 100,000 per year in the Caucasian population of the southwestern United States.

Families have been studied in the members of which malignant melanomas have aggregated. Many of these family members appear to have a type of nevus which resembles clinically miniature early superficial spreading melanomas. These lesions, termed *dysplastic nevi,* may be a genetically determined precursor lesion for malignant melanomas. Patients with large congenital melanocytic nevi are also at recognized higher risk for melanoma development in these lesions.

Only a few factors are presently known to influence the dissemination of melanoma. There is a higher incidence of melanoma in women, but the death rate is higher among men. When multifactorial analyses are performed, the primary tumor site appears to be important in outcome. Torso lesions have a worse prognosis than lower extremity lesions. The most common site for melanoma in males is the torso. The immune status of the patient is another factor under investigation. The possibility that immunologic factors are involved in the course of malignant melanoma is suggested by the high rate of spontaneous regressions of melanoma, by the long periods of freedom from the time of excision of the primary lesion to the development of metastases, and by the improved prognosis of those lesions in which on histologic examination a marked lymphocytic response is found. Both cellular and hormonal immunities to melanoma cells have been demonstrated by in vitro techniques.

TABLE 134-3
Summary data on malignant melanoma of skin

I Incidence: 1% of all cancers (excluding nonmelanoma skin cancer)
- *A* Overall annual crude incidence rates (United States)
  - *1* Caucasians: 4.5/10^5/year (men, 4.4; women, 4.5/10^5/year)
  - *2* Blacks: 0.6/10^5/year (men, 0.7; women, 0.6/10^5/year)
- *B* Increasing with time (Connecticut Registry)
  - *1* 1935–1939: 1.2/10^5/year
  - *2* 1965–1969: 4.8/10^5/year
  - *3* 1976–1977: 7.2/10^5/year
  - *4* 1979–1980: 9/10^5/year
- *C* Latitude-dependent crude incidence rates:
  - *1* Northern United States (Detroit): 3.1/10^5/year
  - *2* Southern United States (Dallas): 7.2/10^5/year

II Frequency for type of melanoma
- *A* Superficial spreading: 70%
- *B* Nodular: 16%
- *C* Lentigo maligna melanoma: 5%
- *D* Unclassified (includes acral lentiginous type): 10%

III Five-year (except where otherwise specified) survival
- *A* Stage III (distant metastases): $<$10%
- *B* Stage II (regional lymph nodes clinically enlarged): 30%
- *C* Stage I (clinically localized disease): 80%
  - *1* Based on level of invasion
    - *a* Level 2: 99%
    - *b* Level 3: 92%
    - *c* Level 4: 68%
    - *d* Level 5: 29%
  - *2* Based on thickness of primary tumor (8-year survival rate)
    - *a* $<$0.85 mm: 99%
    - *b* 0.85–1.69 mm: 93%
    - *c* 1.70–3.60 mm: 69%
    - *d* $\geq$3.65 mm: 38%

The physician examining a patient with many pigmented lesions should recognize the features that are highly suggestive of primary melanoma of the skin and necessarily indicate that the lesion must be removed, or, if it is very large, at least biopsied (see Table 134-1). If these early lesions can be detected and excised, the 5-year survival rate of patients with malignant melanoma should approach 99 percent. The most important clues in the detection of primary malignant melanoma are the areas of bluish gray, bluish red, bluish black, and whitish gray.

REFERENCES

BALCH CM et al: Tumor thickness as a guide to surgical management of clinical stage I melanoma patients. Cancer 43:883–888, 1979

BRESLOW A, MACHT SD: Optimum size of resection margin for thin cutaneous melanoma. Surg Gynecol Obstet 145:691, 1977

CLARK WH JR et al: Human Malignant Melanoma. Grune & Stratton, New York, 1979

DAY CL JR et al: The natural breakpoints for primary tumor thickness in clinical stage I melanoma. N Engl J Med 305:1155, 1981

———: Prognostic factors for melanoma patients with lesions 0.76 through 1.69 mm in thickness: An appraisal of thin level IV lesions. Ann Surg 195:30, 1982

KOPF A et al: *Malignant Melanoma.* Masson, New York, 1979

MIHM MC JR et al: Early detection of primary cutaneous malignant melanoma: Color atlas. N Engl J Med 289:989, 1973

REIMER RR et al: Precursor lesions in familial melanoma. JAMA 239:744, 1978

SOBER AJ et al: Early recognition of cutaneous melanoma. JAMA 242:2795, 1979

———: Primary melanoma of the skin: Recognition and management. J Am Acad Dermatol 2:179, 1980

———: Primary melanoma of the skin: Recognition of precursor lesions and estimation of prognosis in stage I, in *Update: Dermatology in General Medicine,* TB Fitzpatrick et al (eds). McGraw-Hill, New York, 1983

VERONESI U et al: Inefficacy of immediate node dissection in stage I melanoma of the limbs. N Engl J Med 297:627, 1977

PART FOUR | DISORDERS CAUSED BY BIOLOGICAL AND ENVIRONMENTAL AGENTS

section 1 | Important considerations in infectious diseases

135 AN APPROACH TO INFECTIOUS DISEASES

ROBERT G. PETERSDORF

THE SCOPE OF INFECTIOUS DISEASES The vast majority of human and animal diseases of known etiology are produced by biologic agents: viruses, rickettsias, bacteria, mycoplasma, *Chlamydia,* fungi, protozoa, or nematodes. No small part of the past and present importance of infectious diseases in medical practice is attributable to their enormous frequency and the public health implications of their contagiousness. However, developments in sanitary engineering, vector control, immunization, and specific chemotherapy have modified the situation favorably. Although important exceptions remain, infectious diseases as a class are more easily prevented and more easily cured than any other major group of disorders. Despite the elimination of some infectious diseases such as smallpox and the profound reduction in the morbidity and mortality rates of many, humans are by no means free of infection. In fact, the total human load of disease produced by microbial parasites has decreased only modestly, primarily through smallpox and malaria control and better health care in developing countries. As certain specific microbial infections have been controlled, others have emerged as troublesome therapeutic and epidemiologic problems. With the introduction of cytotoxic drugs, massive irradiation in the treatment of malignant diseases, and immunosuppressive agents to control the rejection of transplanted organs, the insertion of prosthetic devices into the bloodstream, and the progressive longevity of people with chronic degenerative diseases, infections due to organisms previously considered saprophytic or commensal have increased. These infections have also been termed *opportunistic.* As Dubos has pointed out, microbial infections appear to form an inherent part of human life.

Because of better environmental sanitation and other measures that now prevent contact with many microbial agents, and the development of acquired immunity early in childhood, certain infections have been seen more frequently in adults. For example, as contact with poliomyelitis virus in childhood declined in many countries, paralytic poliomyelitis became more common in young adults. *Hemophilus influenzae* meningitis and pneumonia is being reported more frequently in adults than heretofore, and decreasing infection with the tubercle bacillus raises questions about the status of antituberculous immunity in adults. For reasons that are not clear, hepatitis A is predominantly a disease of young adults, while non-A, non-B hepatitis tends to occur in individuals over 35 years of age.

As antimicrobial agents reduce the mortality associated with certain common infections, other microbes emerge as important causes of human disease. If an infection occurs during or immediately following a course of chemotherapy, it is often caused by a microorganism that is resistant to the drug that was given; such an infection is termed a *superinfection.* While it is relatively unusual nowadays for patients to die of uncomplicated pneumococcal pneumonia, a disease readily handled with available antimicrobials, it is common to see serious disease produced by microorganisms which are much more resistant even though they are often part of the normal microbial flora in humans. These include staphylococci, gram-negative enteric bacilli, and a variety of anaerobes and fungi. One important mechanism by which resistance is conferred on gram-negative enteric bacteria is the action of R factors (see Chap. 138).

Agents not previously known as causes of human disease are being identified rapidly. *Legionella pneumophila* (see Chap. 162) was first described in 1976 and in the ensuing 6 years much of the epidemiology, microbiology, pathogenesis, clinical course, prognosis, and treatment have been worked out. Since the original description of *L. pneumophila* less virulent but related microorganisms that cause pneumonia have been described (see Chap. 163). However, in contrast to *L. pneumophila,* these organisms turned out not to be new pathogens. Rather, they had been described in the past and given different names and the discovery of *L. pneumophila* placed them into the proper taxonomic and clinical framework. A different manifestation of an old organism is the relationship between *Staphylococcus aureus* and the toxic-shock syndrome (see Chap. 147). In this situation a well-known organism appears to be elaborating a toxin that causes a severe systemic illness. The precise mechanism whereby this toxin produces disease is not known. Yet another relatively new entity that was presumed to be of infectious etiology, Lyme arthritis (see Chap. 350), has been found to be caused by a spirochete. These brief descriptions of new diseases are cited to illustrate the ever-changing array of infectious diseases. Perhaps even more striking than the discovery of new microorganisms that cause infections is the change in the spectrum of infections found in male homosexuals (see Chap. 64), who have been found to be the victims of multiple infections with viruses [cytomegalovirus (CMV) and herpes simplex virus], bacteria (*Mycobacterium tuberculosis, M. avium-intracellulare*), parasites (*Pneumocystis carinii* and *Toxoplasma gondii*), and fungi (*Cryptococcus neoformans* and *Candida albicans*), and some of whom subsequently have developed Kaposi's sarcoma. The relationship of these individuals' heredity, environment, and immune defenses, and the microorganisms involved is by no means clear. No wonder one-quarter of people that seek medical attention, even in developed countries, do so for infections, and the number is much higher in the developing world. It should also come as no surprise that, in the United States, 25 percent of prescriptions that are written consist of antibiotics.

In this and the subsequent chapters, principles of host-parasite interaction, the usefulness of diagnostic procedures, important epidemiologic issues, principles of chemotherapy, major infectious syndromes not associated with specific organ systems (which are found under diseases of these organ systems), and approaches to preventing infections are stressed. In subsequent chapters of this section, diseases caused by specific etiologic agents are described. Together, the syndromic as well as etiologic approach provides a thorough compendium to the study of infectious diseases.

THE PARASITE AND THE HOST The interaction between microorganism and humans that results in infection and disease is complex. Much has been learned about the way in which microbes enter the body, the ways in which they produce tissue injury, the influence of specific immunity and "nonspecific" resistance of the host, and the mechanisms of recovery. It is not yet possible to transfer in any specific way much of the information that has been acquired to the individual patient with an infection. However, considerable progress is being made. Examples are the sexual transmission of hepatitis A virus; the major role that *Chlamydia* are found to play in the causation of pelvic inflammatory disease (see Chap. 144); the role of Norwalk and rotaviruses in infectious diarrheas (see Chap. 142); and advances in antimicrobial therapy in containing heretofore difficult-to-treat bacteria (see Chap. 141).

INFECTION AND CLINICAL DISEASE It is well known that microorganisms of different species or different strains of the same species vary widely in their capacity to produce disease and that human beings are not equally susceptible to the disease caused by a given bacterium or virus. Furthermore, while a specific infectious disease will not occur in the absence of the causative organism, the mere presence of the organism in the body does not lead invariably to clinical illness. Indeed, the production of symptoms in humans by many parasites is the exception rather than the rule, and the *subclinical infection* or the "carrier state" is the usual host-parasite relationship. *Disease* in a clinical sense is not synonymous with the presence of the organism or *infection* in a microbiological sense. In fact, for most organisms the number of subclinical infections far exceeds that of clinical disease.

MECHANISMS OF INJURY It is customary to refer to bacteria or other microorganisms that are capable of producing disease as *pathogenic. Virulence,* the *degree* of pathogenicity, should be distinguished from *invasiveness,* the ability to spread and disseminate in the body. For example, *Clostridium tetani* is pathogenic and, by virtue of its exotoxin, highly virulent, but it is almost completely lacking in invasiveness. Moreover, in certain circumstances and in certain anatomic locations, mildly "pathogenic" organisms can produce fatal disease, or highly "pathogenic" species can multiply without producing any harmful effect.

A few microorganisms produce *toxins* that account for the tissue damage and physiological alterations of infection. *Hypersensitivity* to components of the organism is demonstrable in several infections to account for the manifestations of disease. For many pathogenic agents, an explanation of their damaging effects upon the host is incomplete or wholly lacking. Generally, therefore, the aim of therapy is to stop multiplication or to kill the microorganisms with appropriate drugs; in diseases caused by toxin-producing organisms, the use of antitoxin (as in tetanus or diphtheria) is the definitive procedure, and chemotherapy is of secondary importance. A relatively new example of a toxin-mediated infection is the toxic shock syndrome, in which the toxin is elaborated by *S. aureus.* In this situation, this ordinarily invasive organism does not usually invade local tissues.

The tendency of certain pathogenic organisms to *localize in certain cells or organs* and to produce disease in a specific anatomic site or evoke a combination of symptoms referable to certain organs often suggests the identity of the causative organism. For example, the pneumococcus usually causes infection in the lung but almost never in the kidney, and *H. influenzae* infections are confined almost solely to the respiratory tract and meninges. Similarly, in the presence of disease known to be caused by a given agent, involvement of other tissues can be anticipated or predicted. Examples include the multiple lung abscesses which are so characteristic of hematogenously disseminated staphylococcal disease and the metastatic skin lesions which complicate *Pseudomonas* bacteremia.

Frequently, the proper management of infectious disease involves the use of techniques completely unrelated to microbiology or chemotherapy, in an effort to support the function of damaged organs. Survival in varicella pneumonia usually depends upon treatment of respiratory failure; in the management of endocarditis, valve replacement is often more difficult than the eradication of the causative organism; in cholera the repletion of the volume deficit and in Weil's disease the treatment of acute renal failure with peritoneal or hemodialysis are the important therapeutic objectives.

RESISTANCE AND SUSCEPTIBILITY Many so-called host factors are known to influence the likelihood that disease will occur if organisms enter the tissues, or to play a determining role in the outcome once the infection has become established. These include natural or acquired antibodies, interferon, properdin, phagocytic activity, and the level of the inflammatory response, which is generally manifested by cellular activity such as chemotaxis, phagocytosis, and release of lysozomal enzymes.

In experimental animals, sex, microbial strain, age, route of infection, the presence of specific antibody, associated diseases, nutritional state, and the use of such procedures as exposure to ionizing radiation or high environmental temperature or administration of mucin, antimetabolites, adrenal steroids, epinephrine, and metabolic analogues can be shown to exert a profound effect on infection by bacteria, viruses, fungi, and other agents.

In humans, these factors are no less important, although controlled studies are lacking for many. Alcoholism; diabetes; deficiency or absence of immunoglobulins (see Chap. 64); defects in cellular immunity (see Chap. 67); malnutrition; chronic administration of steroid hormones; chronic lymphedema; ischemia; the presence of foreign bodies such as bullets, calculi, or bone fragments; obstruction of a bronchus, the urethra, or any hollow tube; agranulocytosis or congenital defects in bactericidal or virucidal activity; various blood dyscrasias, and many other circumstances influence susceptibility to systemic or local infection. Furthermore, in those instances where the extenuating condition is remediable, the probability of recovery is enhanced. An interesting example is provided by the high incidence of tuberculous and fungal infections in patients undergoing jejunoileal bypass for morbid obesity. In some of these patients, the infection could not be reversed until the bypass was reconstructed.

Racial differences in susceptibility, such as the poor resistance of dark-skinned people to tuberculosis and their predilection for developing disseminated coccidioidomycosis, are well established. Resistance to infection may be determined genetically. The relation of sickle cell trait to malaria is one example. The increased frequency and severity of some infections in children, of others in pregnant women, and still others in the aged are familiar.

Prior contact with an organism or its products, whether by active infection or by artificial immunization, increases resistance to some infections, such as measles, diphtheria, and pertussis, by stimulating antibody production, but seems to have little influence on resistance to others, such as gonorrhea.

Knowledge of the factors involved in human resistance and susceptibility is incomplete. Explanations such as changes in physical or chemical activity of phagocytes; antibacterial substances such as lysozyme, phagocytin, or lysozomal enzymes; qualitative or quantitative alterations in serum proteins; disordered metabolism at the cellular level; "products of tissue injury" that influence vascular permeability; and the effects of tissue pressure remain to a considerable extent in the realm of hypothesis.

The profound influence of host factors upon the infectious process makes it clear, however, that their understanding is essential for the control of infections in predictable fashion. An example is the "acquired immune deficiency syndrome," in which homosexuals, primarily, have developed a number of severe infections often complicated by Kaposi's sarcoma. It seems likely that these individuals have severe abnormalities in their cellular immune defenses. Until this defect is more completely understood, it seems unlikely that this dread infection complex can be contained.

PATHOGENESIS OF INFECTION With relatively minor variations, the development of an infectious disease follows a consistent pattern. The parasites enter the body through the skin, nasopharynx, lung, intestine, urethra, or other portal. A number of microorganisms adhere to their site of primary attack through fimbriae, pili, and surface antigens; the adherence of *Bordetella pertussis* to respiratory epithelium, the gonococcus to urethral epithelium, and possibly some gram-negative urinary pathogens to the epithelium of the renal pelvis are some examples. Once established in the host, the organisms can multiply and, in so doing, establish a local or primary lesion. From this site, there may be local spread along fascial planes or tubular structures, such as a bronchus or ureter. The next step may be systemic spread of the microorganisms via the circulating blood. Bacteria can enter the bloodstream by direct invasion of vessels, a relatively unusual occurrence, or more commonly by traversing peripheral lymph nodes to enter the thoracic duct lymph and thence the venous system. In the bloodstream, they spread to other tissues and can produce distant or secondary lesions. In infections such as tetanus and diphtheria, distant lesions are produced by toxins elaborated at the primary site without systemic spread of the bacteria. The infectious process may terminate in recovery or death at any stage: the local lesion, systemic spread, or distant lesion.

The apparent inconsistency of this pattern in clinical medicine is attributable to the fact that the infection is recognized as a clinical entity only at the stage when symptoms are most likely to appear. For example, pneumococcal pneumonia is a local lesion, and the distant lesion, pneumococcal meningitis, is referred to clinically as a complication. In meningococcal infections, the local lesion, nasopharyngitis, is rarely symptomatic and has no status as a clinical entity, but the stage of spread, meningococcemia, and the commonest distant lesion, meningitis, are clinical entities. A rarer distant lesion, arthritis, is called a complication. In a patient who has osteomyelitis, a clinical entity, a recent furuncle may be referred to as a predisposing factor. In another patient with extensive furunculosis who develops osteomyelitis, the infection in bone may be regarded as a complication of the superficial infection. The stages mentioned are in no way limited to bacterial diseases; the primary lesion of poliomyelitis is intestinal and is usually asymptomatic, viremia may occur without neurological involvement, or a distant lesion manifested by symptomatic involvement of the central nervous system may be established.

Because clinical usage and terminology are based upon the symptomatic illness that leads patients to seek medical aid, the consistency of this general sequence in the pathogenesis of infection is often not recognized. However, the concept is useful and offers some basis for systematizing what may otherwise seem to be a miscellaneous collection of unrelated clinical signs and symptoms.

CLINICAL MANIFESTATIONS OF INFECTIONS So varied are the disorders attributable to infection or infestation of humans by lower organisms that generalizations about them are difficult. The clinical manifestations of infection can duplicate those of diseases of any other etiology. However, certain clinical features are highly suggestive of infection, including abrupt onset, fever, chills, myalgia, photophobia, pharyngitis, acute lymphadenopathy and splenomegaly, gastrointestinal upset, and leukocytosis or leukopenia. It is obvious that the presence of one, several, or all of these features does not constitute proof of the microbial origin of illness in a given patient. Conversely, serious, even fatal, infectious disease may exist in the absence of fever or other signs and symptoms.

Although there is no infallible clinical criterion of infection, it is possible to recognize accurately many specific infectious diseases from information obtained by *history, physical examination, blood count, and urinalysis.* The importance of interrogation about past illness, predisposing factors such as alcoholism, familial disease, exposure to ill persons, contact with animals or insects, ingestion of contaminated food, type and order of onset of symptoms, and recent or remote residence in endemic areas is discussed in the subsequent chapters that deal with specific diseases and etiologic agents. Cardinal physical signs are also described for each entity.

The mechanisms that produce most of the signs and symptoms of human infection are unknown. The pathogenesis of fever is discussed in Chap. 8. The physiological alterations underlying "malaise," "postinfectious asthenia," "toxicity," and other common complaints are completely mysterious. The factors responsible for leukocytosis or leukopenia are only partially understood (see Chap. 57). Why the rash of typhus begins on the trunk while that of another rickettsiosis, Rocky Mountain spotted fever, begins on the extremities is unanswered. Failure to understand these manifestations does not impair their clinical usefulness, although it is probable that understanding them might lead to more accurate diagnosis and better management.

DIAGNOSTIC PROCEDURES The specific procedures for the diagnosis of infectious disease have become sufficiently complex to warrant separate discussion. This is provided in Chap. 136.

Importance of specific diagnosis in infectious diseases The diagnostic procedures employed for infectious diseases are no more absolute than those in other diseases; they cannot be blindly equated with the science of microbiology. The responsibility for interpreting the facts supplied by the bacteriologist, immunologist, and virologist in the total context of a patient's illness remains that of the physician. A positive tuberculin skin test certainly does not indicate that a patient has active tuberculosis. The finding of *Candida albicans* in a stool culture does not necessarily mean that a patient's diarrhea is caused by intestinal candidiasis. The presence of staphylococci in nasal cultures from a patient with headaches does not establish a diagnosis of staphylococcal sinusitis. A throat culture containing group A beta-hemolytic streptococci does not rule out diphtheria, nor does such a culture establish that a febrile illness in a patient with mitral stenosis is a recurrence of acute rheumatic fever rather than bacterial endocarditis. A positive serologic test for syphilis may indicate a treponematosis other than syphilis, syphilis that is active or inactive, or an unrelated disease such as systemic lupus erythematosus.

The etiologic agent From a practical point of view, two important steps are vital to the correct diagnosis of infection: (1) the organ(s) or organ systems involved must be found, and (2) the etiologic agents causing the infections must be identified precisely. Chapter 136 deals with the diagnostic approaches that are available. Most of the remaining chapters in this part take up the specific bacteria, spirochetes, fungi, rickettsias, viruses, *Mycoplasma*, and Protozoa which cause infections. The common syndromes caused by these agents are described either in chapters dealing with specific organisms or in chapters dealing with infections in individual organ systems such as pneumonia (see Chap. 276), bacterial endocarditis (see Chap. 259), urinary tract infections (see Chap. 301), osteomyelitis (see Chap. 344), meningitis (see Chap. 359), and infectious arthritis (see Chap. 350).

When confronted with specific organ involvement, it is important to know the most common pathogens which cause disease in the involved organ. Table 135-1 provides a listing of those pathogens. Used in conjunction with the individual chapters dealing with specific agents and the summary of chemotherapy (see Chap. 141), the table should provide a rational guide to treatment which often must be instituted before the results of antimicrobial sensitivity tests are available.

ANTIMICROBIAL THERAPY The impact of chemotherapy upon mortality and morbidity from infection and upon epidemic disease is a matter of record. These therapeutic agents, however, have in no way lessened the importance of specific diagnosis; indeed, their availability has increased the need for

TABLE 135-1
The syndromic approach to treatable infections

	Etiologic agents		
Type of infection	*Common*	*Relatively common*	*Unusual but important*
Skin and subcutaneous tissue	*Staphylococcus aureus*	*Streptococcus pyogenes, Candida,* and superficial fungi	Gram-negative bacilli (burns, wounds)
Sinusitis	*Streptococcus pneumoniae, S. aureus*	*S. pyogenes, Hemophilus influenzae*	Mucorales
Pharyngitis	Respiratory viruses, *S. pyogenes*	Gonococcus	*Corynebacterium diphtheriae*
Epiglottitis	*H. influenzae*		
Otitis, mastoiditis	*S. pneumoniae, H. influenzae* (children)	*S. aureus, S. pyogenes*	*Pseudomonas, Proteus*
Pneumonitis	*S. pneumoniae, Mycoplasma pneumoniae, Mycobacterium tuberculosis*	*S. aureus, Klebsiella-Enterobacter,* respiratory viruses, *Legionella pneumophilia*	*S. pyogenes,* gram-negative enteric bacilli, psittacosis, systemic fungi, *Pneumocystis, H. influenzae, Pasteurella multocida*
Empyema and lung abscess	*S. aureus,* anaerobic streptococcus, *Bacteroides, Fusobacterium*	*Klebsiella* (abscess)	
Bacterial endocarditis	*Streptococcus viridans, S. aureus,* enterococcus	*S. pneumoniae,* anaerobic streptococci	*Pseudomonas, Candida, Staphylococcus epidermidis, Listeria monocytogenes*
Gastroenteritis	*Salmonella, Shigella,* enteric viruses, *Campylobacter jejuni, Escherichia coli* (enterotoxic)	*S. aureus,* clostridia, *Giardia*	*Pseudomonas, Entamoeba histolytica, Vibrio cholerae, V. parahemolyticus*
Peritonitis, cholangitis, intraabdominal abscess	*E. coli,* enterococcus, *Bacteroides,* anaerobic streptococcus, *Fusobacterium*	*Klebsiella-Enterobacter, Proteus* species	Clostridia, *S. aureus*
Urinary infection (cystitis, pyelonephritis)	*E. coli, Klebsiella-Enterobacter,* paracolon, *Proteus,* enterococcus	*Pseudomonas*	*S. aureus, S. saprophyticus*
Urethritis	Gonococcus, *Chlamydia*	*Treponema pallidum, Mycoplasma*	
Pelvic inflammatory disease	Gonococcus, *E. coli, Bacteroides,* anaerobic streptococci, *Chlamydia*	*Klebsiella-Enterobacter,* enterococcus, *Fusobacterium*	Clostridia, *S. aureus*
Bones (osteomyelitis)	*S. aureus*	*Salmonella*	*S. pyogenes*
Joints	*S. aureus,* gonococcus, *S. pneumoniae, H. influenzae*	*S. pyogenes, Neisseria meningitidis*	
Meninges	*S. pneumoniae, H. influenzae, N. meningitidis*	*E. coli, Klebsiella-Enterobacter, Proteus, Pseudomonas*	*S. pyogenes, M. tuberculosis, Cryptococcus, S. aureus, Listeria monocytogenes*

obtaining exact etiologic information. It requires but a moment's reflection to realize that the substitution of a prescription for a broad-spectrum antibiotic or a quick injection of penicillin for the systematic collection of facts and thoughtful consideration of diagnostic possibilities is a fallacious, unwise, and dangerous practice. Numerous antibiotics with overlapping spectra are now available, dosages for different infections vary widely, the drugs themselves are potentially dangerous, and their administration entails considerable expense. They should never be prescribed as placebos, antipyretics, or substitutes for diagnosis. In the vast majority of instances in which this is done, patients recover just as they would if no "therapy" had been given, and the drugs are wasted. More importantly, an inadequate dosage of a drug or the wrong agent may suppress symptoms temporarily without achieving cure and may make isolation of the etiologic agent difficult, delay recognition of the true nature of an illness, and postpone the institution of curative treatment. Furthermore, antibiotics may select out resistant variants or facilitate the transfer of R factors between pathogenic and commensal enterobacteria. Resistant variants can then replace sensitive strains and pose the additional hazard of spread to others. Finally, to expose a patient to the risk of a drug reaction without proper indication is inexcusable, whether the drug is an antibiotic, a sedative, a laxative, or a narcotic.

EPIDEMIOLOGIC CONSIDERATIONS Just as the decision to administer antibiotics to a patient with a febrile illness of presumed infectious etiology must be made on an individual basis, the selection of cases in which extensive cultural and serologic testing is required is a matter of judgment. The majority of common grippe-like illnesses subside spontaneously, and symptomatic treatment is sufficient. However, because of this tendency toward spontaneous recovery and also because the results of serologic tests may not be available until after recovery has taken place, the effort to determine the specific etiology of illness is often considered an impractical, "academic" procedure. Such an attitude fails to recognize that in addition to the individual patient, the welfare of the community must be considered. For example, a clinical diagnosis of "virus pneumonia" may turn out, following serologic tests, to be psittacosis. Although the "index" patient may have recovered completely, others in the community may be at risk until the pet parakeet which was the source of the illness has been eliminated. Even more pertinent is the tracing of sexual contacts of patients with sexually transmitted infections. There is no way to eradicate the present-day epidemic of sexually transmitted diseases without this essential "shoe-leather epidemiology." Equally important is the tracing of tuberculosis, particularly in the refugees from southeast Asia who are populating many communities in the United States, and in whom the prevalence of the disease is very high.

Pursuing the diagnosis of obscure, often self-limited, illnesses may be academic, but this approach has led to clarification of some important etiologic relations. For example, the syndrome of infectious mononucleosis has been linked with development of antibody to a herpes-like virus, the EB virus (see Chap. 212), which also has a causal relationship to Burkitt's lymphoma and carcinoma of the posterior nasopharynx. Some congenital anomalies have been related to prenatal viral infections; this relationship is well known for rubella (see Chap. 201), but a number of other viruses (CMV, varicella, herpes simplex) have been implicated, although with less certainty. The finding of bacteria-like bodies in the intestinal mucosa of patients with Whipple's disease and the improvement of these patients with tetracycline therapy provides another example of an entity of unknown etiology entering the realm of infectious diseases. The virus etiology of a number of severe fatal demyelinating diseases of the central nervous system has been well established (see Chap. 360). And the development of Kaposi's sarcoma in the acquired immune deficiency syndrome places that tumor in the realm of viral etiology.

Legionnaires' disease is the most striking example demonstrating the importance of identifying the causative organism of an infection definitively by microbiological and serologic means. This has enabled epidemics to be traced to water sources, air-conditioning towers, and such mundane devices as shower heads.

Similar results can be expected from other "academic procedures" which may have little immediate applicability to infection in a particular patient. Yet, just as was the case with Legionnaires' disease, organisms that seem to have little biological significance at present may assume practical importance in the future.

REFERENCES

BURGDORFER W et al: Lyme disease—A tick-borne spirochetosis? Science 216:1317, 1982

CATANZARO A, MOSER RJ: Health status of refugees from Vietnam, Laos, and Cambodia. JAMA 247:1303, 1982

DURACK DT: Opportunistic infections and Kaposi's sarcoma in homosexual men. N Engl J Med 305:1465, 1981

MANDELL GL et al (eds): *Principles and Practice of Infectious Diseases.* New York, Wiley, 1979

MARMOR M et al: Risk factors for Kaposi's sarcoma in homosexual men. Lancet 1:1083, 1982

SHANDS KN: Toxic-shock syndrome, in *Update IV: Harrison's Principles of Internal Medicine,* 9th ed, KJ Isselbacher et al (eds). New York, McGraw-Hill, 1982, pp 1–8

TOBIN JO et al: Legionnaires disease in a transplant unit: Isolation of the causative agent from shower baths. Lancet 2:118, 1980

TUSTIN AW et al: Unusual fungal infections following jejunoileal bypass surgery. Arch Intern Med 140:643, 1980

136 THE DIAGNOSIS OF INFECTIOUS DISEASES

JAMES J. PLORDE

The diagnosis of an infectious disease requires the direct or indirect demonstration of a pathogenic microbe on or within the tissues of the afflicted host. The major ways in which this is accomplished are described in this chapter.

DIRECT MICROSCOPIC EXAMINATION The direct microscopic examination of body fluids, exudates, and tissues is both the simplest and one of the most helpful laboratory procedures available for the diagnosis of infectious diseases. In many situations the examination allows an accurate, highly specific identification of the causative agent. Examples include the recognition of *Borrelia* or *Plasmodium* species in blood smears taken from patients with relapsing fever or malaria. At times only a tentative identification can be made on the basis of microbial morphology. Nevertheless, this is often sufficiently precise to allow the selection of an appropriate chemotherapeutic agent pending the results of more definitive investigations. A variety of techniques are used in direct microscopy. If the agent being sought is sufficiently large or characteristic, the specimen can be prepared as an unstained wet mount and examined by light-field, dark-field, or phase contrast microscopy. More commonly, a dried smear is made; this allows the application of a variety of stains which assist the visualization and identification of the microbe in question.

Wet mounts Dark-field examination of fluid from genital lesions for the spirochete of syphilis is a well-known, but neglected, procedure. More often, wet mounts are used for the diagnosis of fungal and parasitic infections. The examination of hair fragments, skin scrapings, or nail clippings is useful in establishing the presence of superficial mycoses. The specimens are placed in a drop of 10% KOH, a coverslip added, the preparation cleared by heating, and the mount examined under low-power magnification for the presence of hyphae and arthrospores. At times, as for tinea versicolor infections, the fungous elements will be sufficiently characteristic to allow the specific identification of the causative agent. Occasionally a presumptive diagnosis of a systemic fungous infection can also be established with this procedure. Two examples are cryptococcal meningitis by demonstrating the encapsulated organism in an india ink preparation of cerebrospinal fluid, and coccidioidomycosis by finding characteristic spherules in expectorated sputum.

Examination of saline or iodine mounts of stool or duodenal drainage is also the initial first step in establishing the diagnosis of intestinal protozoal infections such as amebiasis and giardiasis. Moreover, it is the definitive procedure diagnosing intestinal helminthic infections including ascariasis, trichuriasis, strongyloidiasis, and hookworm. Finally, filariasis and sleeping sickness can be recognized by demonstrating the characteristic motility of microfilariae and trypanosomes in blood or other body fluids.

Stain-enhanced microscopy Despite many recent technical advances in the field of microbiology, Gram's stain remains, after 90 years of use, the best single technique available for the rapid diagnosis of bacterial infections. It can be applied to virtually all clinical specimens and is of particular value in the examination of exudates, aspirates, body fluids, including cerebrospinal fluid, and urine. Gram's stains should be examined first under the lower-power objective to demonstrate the presence of pink-staining inflammatory cells. The paucity of such cells in the presence of many squamous epithelial cells suggests that the specimen was contaminated during the process of collection and may not be representative of the inflammatory process. After the evaluation under low-power objective, the smear is then examined for the presence of bacteria using the oil immersion lens; bacteria will appear either as dark blue (gram-positive) or pink (gram-negative) bodies. Their color and morphological appearance often make possible a presumptive identification of the genus and occasionally the species with a significant degree of accuracy. The demonstration of pneumococci in the sputum, Enterobacteriaceae in the urine, staphylococci in localized abscesses, gonococci in urethral exudates, clostridia in foul-smelling discharge, and pneumococci, meningococci, or *Hemophilus influenzae* in stained smears of the cerebrospinal fluid permits the initiation of specific chemotherapy with the assurance that the regimen is the proper one. In some immunosuppressed patients *Candida* blastospores and pseudohyphae can be found in blood smears several days before candidemia is demonstrable by culture.

A variety of other stains are available for the demonstration of specific microbes. Mycobacteria have the unique capacity to resist the decolorization by strong mineral acid alcohol solutions once they have been stained with basic carbol-fuchsin or one of the fluorochromes. This allows their immediate recognition in body tissues and fluids. The presence of a large number of acid-fast bacilli in the expectorated sputum establishes the presumptive diagnosis of respiratory tuberculosis and is sufficient evidence for initiating isolation procedures and antituberculosis therapy once additional specimens are collected for culture. Subsequent examination of the sputum with acid-fast stains is an important element in monitoring the success of therapy. The traditional Ziehl-Neelsen and Kinyoun stains are being supplanted by the fluorochromes which allow a much more rapid scanning of smears using relatively low magnification.

Acid-fast smears can also be used to identify pathogenic strains of *Nocardia* if mineral acid rather than acid-alcohol is used for decolorization. When an even weaker decolorizing agent such as organic acid is used, organisms such as *Actinomyces* may also be visualized.

Both Giemsa's and iodine stains may be used to diagnose chlamydial infections involving the eye, urethra, or cervix. When epithelial cells obtained by scraping these areas are stained with Giemsa's stain, a typical semilunar dense inclusion body composed of many blue- or purplish-staining particles is seen adjoining the nucleus of the cell. Iodine stains reveal a similar reddish-brown mass in scrapings from the eye but are not useful in cervical specimens.

A number of stains are available for the definitive identification of parasites. *Pneumocystis carinii* can be recognized in transbronchial brush biopsies using a modified Wright's stain, toluidine blue, or methenamine silver. The latter produces a very distinctive black-stained cyst. Blood and tissue protozoa such as plasmodia and *Leishmania* can be demonstrated best with Romanowsky-type mixtures containing methyline blue and eosin. These render the nuclei red to violet and the cytoplasm blue. The identification of intestinal protozoa, on the other hand, requires the use of stains such as iron hematoxyline or trichome to demonstrate the taxonomically important nuclear detail.

Immune microscopy This method combines the specificity of immunologic procedures with the speed of direct microscopy. In the immunofluorescent technique, smears thought to contain viral, bacterial, fungal, or parasitic organisms are stained with specific antibody preparations labeled with fluorescent compounds and examined with a fluorescent microscope. The most useful application of this technique is the examination of brain tissue for herpes simplex or rabies virus; lung tissue, pleural fluid, and sputum for *Legionella pneumophila;* and cervical, urethral, and conjunctival scrapings for trachoma-inclusion conjunctivitis agent.

Direct fluorescent antibody staining of nasal epithelial cells may also be used for the rapid diagnosis of influenza, parainfluenza, and respiratory syncytial virus infections.

Finally, the direct immunofluorescence technique for detecting antibody-coated bacteria in the urinary sediment has been useful in distinguishing kidney from bladder infection in females.

Unfortunately, the need for expensive fluorescent microscopes, the poor quality of many of the commercially available conjugated antiserums, and the need for well-trained technologists restrict the routine use of these procedures to reference laboratories.

Enzyme-linked immunoabsorbent assay (ELISA) tests are similar to the immunofluorescence test except that the antiserum is reacted with an enzyme-labeled antispecies conjugate. After treatment with an appropriate substrate, a color change can be visualized with the ordinary light microscope, obviating the need for expensive equipment.

Electron microscopy The electron microscopic examination has been useful in the identification of certain viruses which do not produce cytopathic effects in cell cultures. It has been particularly valuable in the detection of rotaviruses in the stool specimens of infants and small children suffering from gastroenteritis. The large number and characteristic appearance of these virus particles allow specific identification to be made on morphological grounds alone. Electron microscopy has also been used in the diagnosis of the so-called winter vomiting disease caused by the Norwalk and Hawaii agents. These agents are morphologically similar to those of the picornavirus group, and specific identification requires aggregation of the virus particles with immune serum. This technique of immune electron microscopy may have wide application in virology and has been used to identify virus-like particles associated with non-A, non-B hepatitis in experimental animals.

DETECTION OF MICROBIAL ANTIGENS AND THEIR BY-PRODUCTS The relative nonspecificity of many direct microscopic methods and the delay inherent in culture procedures have resulted in the introduction of a variety of techniques aimed at the rapid detection of microbial antigens or their by-products.

Counterimmunoelectrophoresis The most widely used of these techniques is counterimmunoelectrophoresis (CIE). In this variation of the agar gel diffusion test, the specimen being tested for antigen is placed in an agar well and specific antiserum in a second apposed well. An electric current is then passed through the agar resulting in rapid confluence of antigen and antibody with the formation of a precipitant within a matter of minutes. CIE has proved most useful for the rapid diagnosis of bacterial meningitis in childhood where the cerebrospinal fluid is checked for the presence of pneumococcal, meningococcal, group B streptococcal, or *H. influenzae* antigens. The technique has approximately the same order of sensitivity as Gram's stain but has the advantage of heightened specificity. CIE has also been used for the detection of the above-mentioned bacterial antigens in serum, pneumococcal capsular antigens in sputum, and the detection of rotavirus and enterovirus in stool.

Latex agglutination This test has been utilized in many of the same situations as CIE. Although greater sensitivity has been claimed for latex agglutination, the test is plagued by false-positive reactions from heat-labile serum components and rheumatoid factor. Perhaps its greatest usefulness has been in the detection of cryptococcal antigen in the spinal fluid of patients with chronic meningoencephalitis.

Radioimmunoassay (RIA) The most spectacular application of this technique is in the detection of hepatitis B surface antigen–associated (HBsAg-associated) infection and in the prevention of such infections by the screening of blood and blood products for the presence of the antigen. This procedure is highly sensitive, and results can be obtained within a few hours with commercially available test kits. In this method HBsAg-labeled ^{125}I competes with antigen in a test serum for a specific antibody in the test mixture. Free and bound antigens are separated by washing. The reactivity of the antigen-antibody complex is then analyzed with a gamma counter. Experimental RIA procedures have also been developed for the detection of circulating antigens in disseminated fungal infections.

Enzyme-linked immunosorbent assays The method, as described above under "Direct Microscopic Examination," can be adapted for the visual or spectrophotometric detection of microbial antigens. Increasingly, it is coming to replace radioimmunoassay techniques in the diagnosis of hepatitis B infections and is now extensively utilized to ascertain the presence of rotavirus in the diarrheal stool of infants. As with RIA, it has been successfully used to detect circulating fungal antigens in candidiasis and aspergillosis.

Gas chromatography This method involves the direct examination of clinical specimens by gas liquid chromatography for the detection of characteristic microbial by-products. It has been thought helpful in differentiating aerobic from anaerobic organisms in pus and blood. It has also been used to differentiate staphylococcal, streptococcal, and gonococcal from traumatic arthritis and to detect *Candida* in the blood of patients with fungemia. Although the role of gas chromatography in the identification of anaerobic bacteria is established, its usefulness in the direct analysis of clinical specimens remains to be determined.

CULTURE Despite the time and complexity, the isolation of the etiologic agent by cultivation in artificial media, tissue cultures, or animals is generally the most definitive procedure available.

The diagnostic value of a culture specimen, however, depends to a large extent on the likelihood that it has been collected free of contamination with the resident microbial flora and transported to the laboratory in a fashion that ensures survival of fastidious organisms.

Specimen collection When specimens from deep closed lesions are collected, the site of percutaneous needle aspiration should be cleansed first by using 70% isopropyl or ethyl alcohol and then disinfected with a 2% tincture of iodine or an appropriate iodophor. The iodine is applied in a concentric fashion beginning at the site of aspiration and allowed to act for 1 to 2 min before the aspiration is performed. The area should not be probed or manipulated unless sterile gloves are worn or the involved fingers have also been disinfected. If the initial attempt at collection fails, subsequent efforts should be carried out with a new needle through a freshly disinfected site. At the completion of the procedure the iodine should be removed with alcohol to avoid the danger of sensitization. If the specimen for culture is drawn through an indwelling cannula, the site of withdrawal must be disinfected in the same fashion.

When specimens are to be collected from the uterus or a draining wound or sinus tract, the orifice must be thoroughly cleansed and disinfected as described above, a sterile intravenous catheter or multilumen tube is introduced as deeply as possible through the orifice, and the specimen aspirated into a sterile syringe. Culture from an open lesion may be collected by biopsy, aspiration from the margin, or by swabbing the surface. In the first two situations the wound is prepared as for a deep closed lesion. For swab cultures, the wound surface is cleansed only with sterile saline to remove debris and saprophytic flora.

Transportation All specimens submitted for microbial culture should be transported to the laboratory as rapidly as possible, preferably within 1 h. Delay beyond this time may result in death of fastidious organisms, overgrowth of contaminants, and/or change in the number of bacteria unless special procedures are employed to overcome these problems. Rapid transportation is particularly important when dealing with blood, body fluid, and exudates which may harbor pathogenic *Neisseria* or anaerobes. The container should be clean, sterile (stool specimens excepted), and appropriately labeled. Respiratory secretions, urine, large pieces of tissue, and large volumes of fluid can be safely transmitted in plastic containers with leak-proof lids. Aspirates are conveniently and safely transported in the same syringe used in the collection procedure, providing all air is expressed from the syringe and the needle is capped with a sterile holder. Alternatively, such fluid may be injected into a sealed gassed-out vial suitable for transport of anaerobic specimens. If such vials are used, it is important that the indicator in the vial be checked to ascertain whether it is still colorless. A pink or blue color indicates the presence of oxygen and suggests that the vial is no longer adequate for the transport of specimens for anaerobic culture. Small pieces of tissue (less than 1 cm^2) are transported best in sterile rubber-stoppered gassed-out tubes. After the anaerobic indicator is checked, the tube is held upright to minimize the loss of the heavy inert gas, the stopper removed, specimen inserted, and the tube recapped.

Swabs submitted for the culture of group A beta-hemolytic streptococci can be transported in dry sterile test tubes. All other swabs should be submitted in one of several commercially available transport media. These prevent both the desiccation of organisms implanted on the swab and the overgrowth of hardy organisms at the expense of more fastidious ones. Although special anaerobic transport materials are available, use of swab cultures for the recovery of such organisms is not encouraged.

Culture of specific specimens UPPER RESPIRATORY TRACT Because the throat and nasopharynx are normally heavily colonized by both saprophytic and potentially pathogenic bacteria, culture of this area is seldom useful except when a particular bacterial pathogen is being sought, e.g., *Streptococcus pyogenes, Bordetella pertussis, Corynebacterium diphtheriae,* meningococci, or gonococci.

Throat cultures. When throat cultures are submitted to the laboratory without specifying the pathogen being sought, the laboratory will generally report only the presence or absence of *S. pyogenes.* Since a single properly obtained throat swab will detect at least 90 percent of patients with streptococcal pharyngitis, a negative culture is very helpful in excluding the possibility of this disease. Similarly, a heavy or predominant growth of group A beta-hemolytic streptococci in patients presenting with the signs and symptoms of streptococcal pharyngitis is highly predictive of an antibody response to streptococcal antigens and, therefore, presumably disease. It is far more difficult to interpret cultures with a light or nonpredominant growth of *S. pyogenes.* A large proportion of these patients do not mount an appreciable immunologic response, suggesting that bacterial growth represents a carrier state.

Throat cultures may not be indicated in adults presenting with sore throat if they lack fever, cervical lymphadenopathy, or recent exposure to another patient with streptococcal pharyngitis since fewer than 5 percent of this population have positive cultures. Conversely, adults with temperatures of 38°C or higher, tender cervical lymphadenopathy, or pharyngeal exudate are so frequently culture positive that immediate antibiotic therapy is more cost effective than waiting for the result of culture.

Mouth cultures. Usually massively mixed flora of aerobic and anaerobic bacteria is present in mouth cultures, and they are not clinically useful except when a careful attempt to avoid contamination with indigenous flora has been made. This is particularly true for the isolation of *Actinomyces israelii.* This organism is part of the normal oropharyngeal flora, and the time and effort required for its isolation is not justified unless an uncontaminated specimen can be provided.

LOWER RESPIRATORY TRACT Although culture of expectorated sputum is the most frequently employed technique for the diagnosis of lower respiratory tract infections, both its sensitivity and specificity are open to question. Studies of patients with bacteremic pneumococcal pneumonia have shown the etiologic agent to be present in the sputum in only 50 to 94 percent of cases. Moreover, expectorated sputum is almost always contaminated with oropharyngeal flora including, in many cases, bacterial species commonly associated with pulmonary infections. Even when a potential pathogen is recovered, its role in the causation of a lower respiratory tract infection is uncertain. Attempts to remove saliva and nasal secretions from the sputum by repeated washing or to differentiate upper and lower tract organisms on the basis of quantitative sputum culture have been ineffective or unacceptably tedious. Some confusion can be avoided if the specimen is collected appropriately and screened carefully for both gross and microscopic characteristics prior to inoculation of the culture. Ideally, sputum specimens should be collected early in the morning under direct supervision of a physician or respiratory therapist. If the patient is unable to produce sputum, coughing may be stimulated by lowering the head of the patient's bed for a few minutes or exposing the patient to an aerosol of warm hypertonic saline.

Because sputum is rarely homogeneous, it should be examined carefully for bits of pus and blood. These should then be used to prepare a Gram's stain smear which is examined for the presence of squamous epithelial cells (SEC) and leukocytes under the low-power objective (10×) of the microscope. If there are fewer than 10 SEC and greater than 25 leukocytes per field, the results of the culture are more likely to represent lower tract flora. This is particularly true if a single or clearly predominant bacterial type grows, or, in the case of chronic obstructive pulmonary disease, if both pneumococci and *H. influenzae* are isolated. If squamous epithelial cells number more than 10 per low-power field, the specimen can be considered heavily contaminated with oropharyngeal flora and should be discarded. In most cases a second carefully collected expectorated sputum will yield a satisfactory specimen.

Direct endotracheal or endobronchial aspiration may be employed when a satisfactory expectorated sputum cannot be produced. However, such specimens are subject to contamination by oropharyngeal flora which is introduced during the passage of the aspiration instrument. Fiberoptic bronchoscopy, which allows the direct visualization and aspiration of bronchial secretions, is a relatively inocuous procedure and may result in a somewhat better specimen. When it is accompanied by a brush biopsy performed through an occluded double-lumen tube, the material obtained is unlikely to be diluted with saliva or topical anesthetics and may be utilized for anaerobic cultures. Alternatively, the specimen may be collected by a technique that totally bypasses the oropharynx. The most widely used is transtracheal aspiration. This method entails a definite risk of hemoptysis, subcutaneous and mediastinal emphysema, vagal discharge, or respiratory embarrassment and is contraindicated in the presence of a bleeding diathesis. It should be used only when results from expectorated sputum are unsatisfactory and the infection is severe enough to merit the attendant risks. The technique produces a more reliable sputum specimen than expectoration and is probably the only other satisfactory method for collecting specimens for anaerobic culture. However, some 20 percent of specimens from patients without clinical evidence of pneumonia yield potential respiratory pathogens. These "false-positive" specimens are primarily from patients who have chronic pulmonary disease, who have recently suffered minor bouts of aspiration, or in whom the tip of the catheter was coughed into the hypopharynx during the collection procedure.

Needle aspiration of a pulmonary infiltrate under fluoroscopic control also produces specimens of excellent quality. The percutaneous method gives both a high yield and accurate results but has at least a 5 percent chance of complications, particularly pneumothorax. The morbidity risk is greater than with transtracheal aspiration biopsy, but the diagnostic yield may be superior.

Whatever technique is used to sample the lower respiratory tract, a concomitant blood culture should always be obtained. If a pleural effusion is present, it should also be aspirated and cultured.

In addition to bacterial pathogens, pneumonia can be caused by viruses, *Rickettsia, Chlamydia, Mycoplasma pneumoniae,* and *Legionella* and related agents. Techniques for the recovery of these agents from the sputum are generally not available in a routine clinical microbiology laboratory, and the diagnosis is most frequently made by clinical and/or serologic methods. *L. pneumophila* can be cultured from lung tissue or empyema fluid. In addition, it can be demonstrated by direct fluorescent antibody staining in both of these specimen types and in transtracheal aspirates. This allows early diagnosis and rapid institution of appropriate therapy. For discussion of the techniques used for the recovery of mycobacteria and fungi from the lower respiratory tract, the chapters devoted to these organisms should be consulted.

URINE CULTURES Voided urine, like expectorated sputum, is usually contaminated with the normal microbial flora, in this case from the urethra and external genitalia. Urine cultures, however, are more reliable than those of expectorated sputum, because the periurethral area can be disinfected and the urethra itself flushed with the first portion of the urine stream before a sample is taken. In addition, quantitation of the bacterial growth is helpful in separating contaminated specimens from true infection. In general, bacterial counts exceeding 100,000 organisms per milliliter of urine indicate true bacteriuria while those less than 10,000 organisms per milliliter reflect contamination with perineal or urethral flora. Before a high bacterial count can be accepted as evidence of infection, however, the following factors need to be considered: (1) the adequacy of the disinfection procedures, (2) the sex of the patient, (3) the interval between specimen collection and plating, and (4) the number of bacterial species isolated. It is important that patients be carefully instructed in the techniques of collecting clean voided specimens or that the collection be supervised by a trained attendant. In brief, the foreskin of males must be retracted and the labia of females separated. The periurethral area is repeatedly cleansed with an appropriate disinfectant and then rinsed with warm sterile water. Following this, the patient voids. After the first 20 to 25 ml is discarded, the specimen is caught directly in a sterile container without interrupting the stream. The cup should be held in a way to avoid contact with the legs or perineal area. When this procedure is followed conscientiously, a single specimen from a male which yields a colony count in excess of 100,000 organisms per milliliter is highly indicative of bacteriuria. In women, the colony count must exceed 100,000 organisms per milliliter in two consecutive urine specimens before infection can be considered to be present. Because urine is a good culture medium, contaminating organisms will multiply to large numbers if the urine is allowed to stand at room temperature for prolonged periods of time. For this reason, specimens which cannot be dispatched to the laboratory within an hour should be refrigerated. They can be held at 4°C for 4 to 6 h without an appreciable change in the bacterial colony count. In most instances, urinary tract infections are caused by a single bacterial species. The isolation of three or more species in a urine culture usually reflects contamination even when the colony count is high. True polymicrobial bacteriuria does occur but is generally restricted to patients with chronic indwelling urethral catheters. In contrast, colony counts of less than 100,000 organisms per milliliter may sometimes represent true bacteriuria. In fact, up to one-third of urinary tract infections are associated with counts less than 100,000 organisms per milliliter. This is particularly true of specimens from male patients or patients receiving antimicrobial therapy, specimens from women with symptomatic lower tract infections, and specimens obtained by ureteral or urethral catheterization and by suprapubic aspiration.

When an adequate clean-voided urine specimen cannot be obtained, or when anaerobic cultures are desired, suprapubic aspiration may be employed. Specimens obtained in this manner are unlikely to be contaminated, and even slight growth may be significant. When an indwelling catheter is in place, a specimen should be collected directly from the catheter by means of a sterile needle and syringe after careful disinfection of the exterior surface. Urine should not be taken from the drainage tube or bag, because these are frequently contaminated. Occasionally Foley catheter tips are submitted to the laboratory for culture when a catheterized patient shows signs or symptoms of urinary tract infection. Statistical analysis has shown this practice to be both futile and potentially misleading.

Examination of a Gram's stain smear of uncentrifuged urine is often helpful in the rapid diagnosis of urinary tract infection. The presence of many squamous epithelial cells and mixed bacterial flora indicates contamination and the need for another specimen. In the absence of the epithelial cells, the presence of one or more bacterial cells per oil immersion field usually indicates true bacteriuria especially when accompanied by one or more leukocytes.

BLOOD CULTURES Cultures should be obtained from all febrile patients who have rigors, are seriously ill, are thought to have endocarditis or intravascular infection, or are immunosuppressed. If viremia, fungemia, brucellosis, tularemia, leptospirosis, or an infection with cell wall–deficient bacteria is suspected, the laboratory should be contacted for special instructions. In general, three blood cultures taken at intervals of no less than 60 min are adequate to document the presence of bacteremia in an adult. In emergent situations, two cultures taken simultaneously from different anatomic sites will usually suffice. In patients who have received antimicrobial agents within the previous 2 weeks or in whom endocarditis is suspected, a total of six cultures taken over a 2-day period may be useful. If the patient is receiving antimicrobial agents, the cultures should be taken immediately prior to the next dose, and the laboratory should be notified to allow the addition of penicillinase, use of an antibiotic removal device, or extensive dilution of the blood specimen. The collection of specimens over and above the number listed above is seldom helpful in detecting occult bacteremia unless the culture procedures, media, or conditions of incubation are altered to allow detection of fastidious organisms.

Specimens are best collected by percutaneous venipuncture. If possible, aspirations from the femoral vein should be avoided since disinfecting the skin of the groin is often difficult. The increasingly common practice of drawing blood for culture through an indwelling intravascular cannula often results in a higher level of contamination without substantially improving the detection of bacteremia. Similarly there is no evidence that arterial blood cultures possess any advantage over venous cultures. Bone marrow cultures may reveal the etiologic agent when it cannot be obtained by other means in occasional patients with disseminated salmonellosis, tuberculosis, and deep mycoses.

To minimize the chance of contamination with skin flora, the site of aspiration should be carefully disinfected as described above. Following aspiration, the blood should be inoculated into both aerobic and anaerobic broths immediately. The dilution ratio of blood to broth should be at least 1:10 to minimize the normal bactericidal activity of serum and the activity of any antimicrobial agents that may be present. If direct inoculation into broth is not feasible, the blood may be drawn into a sterile Vacutainer tube containing sodium polyethanol sulfanate (SPS). This anticoagulant is anticomplementary and inactivates leukocytes and certain aminoglycoside and polypeptide antibiotics. Nevertheless, it will not delay bacterial death indefinitely, and Vacutainer specimens should be sent to the laboratory for dilution in broth within 30 min of the time the blood is drawn. If fungemia is suspected, the laboratory should be notified since the standard techniques described above are less satisfactory for the isolation of fungi.

Gram's stain examination of buffy coat smears is seldom indicated. Although a number of microorganisms, particularly meningococci and staphylococci, can be detected within granulocytes in approximately 4 percent of submitted blood culture specimens, the procedure is time-consuming and seldom of therapeutic value. It may be justified if fungemia is suspected. The toxicity of amphotericin B therapy precludes initiation of treatment without strong evidence of systemic fungal infection. Because these organisms often require 4 to 5 days to grow, a positive buffy coat smear would be of obvious therapeutic importance.

Approximately two-thirds of blood cultures from bacteremic patients are found to be positive within 24 h and 90 percent within 3 days. Despite strict adherence to disinfectant procedures on the ward and sterile technique in the laboratory, contamination occasionally occurs. The following are characteristics of "false-positive" blood cultures: (1) repeat cultures are seldom positive for the same organism, (2) bacterial growth in broth generally occurs after 3 days of incubation, and (3) the organisms are often identified as diphtheroids, *Bacillus*, or *Staphylococcus epidermidis*. However, any of these species can occasionally be responsible for true bacteremia, particularly in immunosuppressed patients.

CEREBROSPINAL FLUID Examination of the CSF from patients suspected of having meningitis represents one of the major emergency procedures faced by the clinical microbiology laboratory. Bacterial meningitis can be rapidly fatal if treatment is delayed or inadequate, and appropriate therapy often requires specific identification of the etiologic agent. Because of the clinical urgency, CSF specimens should be collected as soon as the diagnosis is considered, and the specimen promptly transported to the laboratory. The laboratory should be notified if the specimen has been collected from an abscess within the CNS to ensure that it is cultured both aerobically and anaerobically. If possible, at least 2 ml CSF should be obtained and the specimen sent for glucose, quantitative protein level, and cell count in addition to microbiologic studies. A simultaneous blood sugar also should be drawn for correlation with the CSF glucose level. Fastidious organisms, particularly *Neisseria meningitidis*, may not survive prolonged storage at temperatures below that of the body. If a delay in CSF examination cannot be avoided, specimens should be held at 37°C.

After receipt, the specimen is concentrated by centrifugation or filtration, Gram stained, and cultured. The inflammatory response in the CSF is helpful in distinguishing acute bacterial meningitis from nonbacterial forms of the disease. In bacterial meningitis, polymorphonuclear leukocytes predominate, while in tuberculous, fungal, or protozoal meningitis, the inflammatory cells usually consist of lymphocytes, and the response is less intense. Although polymorphonuclear leukocytes may dominate early in the course of aseptic meningitis, there is usually a clear shift to mononuclear cells within 8 h. Cytologic changes in the CSF may also be seen in patients with brain abscess. However, smears and cultures are generally negative in these cases unless the abscess ruptures into the subarachnoid space or into the ventricles. The Gram's stain smear of the CSF should be examined carefully for stainable organisms, particularly meningococci, pneumococci, *Enterobacteriaceae*, *Listeria*, and staphylococci in patients with atrioventricular shunts. Stainable, but nonviable, organisms occasionally contaminate sterile plastic containers and may result in a "false-positive" Gram's stain. In addition, in cases of partially treated bacterial meningitis there is a tendency for gram-positive organisms to stain gram-negative.

When a large number of organisms are present and specific antiserums are available, the etiologic agent can often be rapidly identified by the quellung reaction or a precipitin test. Counterimmunoelectrophoresis is even more sensitive and may be positive when the Gram's stain is not. Moreover, detection of microbial antigens in the CSF by CIE is often the only method of identification of an infectious agent from a patient with partially treated meningitis. In the presence of a significant number of mononuclear cells without stainable bacteria, encapsulated cryptococci or cryptococcal antigen can be identified with the India ink preparation or latex agglutination tests, respectively.

Regardless of the results of these studies, the CSF must be cultured and any resulting growth identified to the species level. Mycobacterial and fungal cultures should be set up on patients who present with chronic meningitis and a mononuclear inflammatory response in the CSF.

Naegleria fowleri, the cause of amoebic meningoencephalitis, can often be recognized by its amoeboid movements in wet-mount preparations of cerebrospinal fluid. This organism should be looked for in patients who develop hemorrhagic meningoencephalitis during the summer months (see Chap. 217).

GASTROINTESTINAL TRACT Cultures of the mouth, periodontal lesions, or saliva usually yield a mixed flora of aerobic and anaerobic organisms including *A. israelii* and *Candida* spp. The isolation of these organisms is without significance unless the specimen was collected in a way which avoided contamination with indigenous flora. If actinomycosis is suspected, the laboratory should be contacted for special instructions. The diagnosis of oral thrush and Vincent's infection can be made with stained smears from scrapings of the suspected lesion.

Cultures of ileostomy or colostomy stomata, gastrointestinal fistulas, and rectal fissures invariably grow both aerobic and anaerobic intestinal flora. They are seldom helpful, therefore, unless a search is made for specific intestinal pathogens.

Fecal cultures are helpful in determining the etiology of diarrhea and in detecting carrier states. Such specimens are routinely cultured for species of *Salmonella*, *Shigella*, and *Arizona*. Many laboratories are now also looking for *Vibrio parahemolyticus*, *Yersinia enterocolitica*, *Campylobacter jejuni*, and *Clostridium difficile*, the agent of antibiotic-associated pseudomembranous enterocolitis. Cell culture techniques can be used for the direct detection of *C. difficile* toxin in the stool of diarrheal patients. There is at present no convenient and reliable cultural method of identifying enterotoxogenic strains of *E. coli*, the Norwalk-like viruses, or rotaviruses in the clinical laboratory. The laboratory should be alerted as to whether any of these, or any other unusual infection such as candidiasis, clostridial food poisoning, or cholera, are suspected.

Although rectal swabs are adequate for the diagnosis of bacterial diarrhea, they are less satisfactory for the detection of carrier states. If swabs are used, they should show obvious soiling and be sent to the laboratory in appropriate transport media. Whole stool should be collected free of urine, placed in clean waxed cardboard cartons, and promptly dispatched to the laboratory. If delivery cannot be made within 1 h, the stool should be preserved in phosphate-buffered glycerol to prevent death of fastidious organisms such as *Shigella* spp. It is seldom necessary to submit more than three consecutive daily specimens.

GENITAL TRACT Genital specimens are submitted primarily for the diagnosis of venereal disease including gonorrhea, syphilis, chancroid, trichomoniasis, and chlamydial infections. Instructions for the collection of specimens should be sought in the sections of the text dealing with these specific diseases. In addition to the venereal pathogens, a number of organisms may infect the endometrium, tuboovarian tissues, and vagina. Endometrial cultures must be collected through a double or triple lumen tube inserted through a decontaminated cervical os if contamination with vaginal and cervical flora is to be avoided. The specimens should be delivered to the laboratory in either a gassed-out vial or a sealed syringe to ensure recovery of anaerobic organisms. When a patient presents with vaginitis, a specimen is collected by swabbing the vaginal fornix under direct visualization. If trichomoniasis is suspected, the swab should be placed in a small amount of sterile saline and sent to the laboratory immediately. If the swab is received within 10 to 15 min, the organism can be identified without difficulty by its characteristic motility in a wet-mount preparation. Cultural examination should focus on the recovery of agents thought capable of causing vaginitis such as *G. vaginalis*, group B beta-hemolytic streptococci, and *Candida albicans*.

EXUDATES AND BODY FLUIDS Pus from undrained abscesses as well as pericardial, pleural, peritoneal, and synovial fluids is best collected by syringe and needle aspiration through disinfected skin. Prior rinsing of the syringe with a sterile anticoagulant such as heparin or SPS will help prevent formation of clots. Because anaerobic organisms are commonly involved in infection of these areas, the syringe should be sealed and sent immediately to the microbiology laboratory. Alternatively, the aspirate may be injected into a gassed-out anaerobic transport vial. The use of swabs is not encouraged since the sample size is small and fastidious organisms including anaerobes are unusually susceptible to desiccation and oxidation. Deep suppurative lesions which communicate with the surface of the body through fistulas or sinus tracts present a difficult problem in specimen collection. The communicating pathway is generally colonized by a wide variety of bacterial flora which contaminate drainage being ejected through the fistula opening. The degree of contamination can be lessened in many instances by carefully disinfecting the orifice and aspirating material via a sterile plastic catheter inserted deep into the sinus. Even when these precautions are taken, however, sinus tract cultures often fail to correlate well with pathogens isolated from operative specimens. For this reason, a bacteriologic diagnosis of draining suppurative lesions should be based on a culture of currettings or biopsy rather than sinus drainage. If actinomycosis is suspected, the draining sinus tract may be covered with gauze which is left in place until it is thoroughly saturated. The gauze is then submitted to the laboratory where it is carefully examined for the presence of granules which can be picked out and then identified.

SKIN, SOFT TISSUE, AND SUPERFICIAL WOUNDS Specimens collected from these areas are usually heavily contaminated with the normal flora of their respective sites. Swab cultures should be obtained only if gross pus is present or if there is need to confirm the presence or absence of only a single bacterial pathogen, such as *C. diphtheriae;* in this case, the wound should first be cleansed mechanically with saline to remove as much exudate as possible. Material from bullae and areas of cellulitis is best obtained with a syringe. Successful aspiration of an area of cellulitis may require initial injection of a small amount of sterile saline. It is important that this solution not contain a preservative which may affect the viability of some bacteria. Alternatively, a punch biopsy may be obtained of the area after appropriate disinfection. Similarly, cultures from open lesions may be obtained by biopsy or by aspirating from the margins of these lesions using a syringe and needle. Semiquantitative cultures of burn eschars are useful in identifying patients at risk of bacteremia.

Intravenous and intraarterial catheter tips are best collected by disinfecting the area of the skin penetrated by the catheter, carefully withdrawing the catheter, and aseptically cutting off the 5-cm section that had been located just under the skin into a sterile container. This is then delivered to the microbiology laboratory where semiquantitative cultures are done. In general, catheters which are contaminated during removal will have only a few colonies on agar plates, while infected catheters will show heavy growth.

SKIN TESTS Exposure to antigens of certain types, by various routes, and under circumstances not completely understood often results in the development of immediate (anaphylactic, atopic) hypersensitivity or delayed (bacterial, tuberculin) hypersensitivity.

Active infection with some, but not all, bacteria and viruses results in delayed hypersensitivity to the infecting agent in some, but not all, individuals. Clinically, this allergic state is detected by intradermal injection of the organism or one of its components; in a sensitive individual, induration and erythema will appear at the local site within 24 to 48 h. If an individual is highly "sensitive" or if the amount of antigen injected is excessive, there may be extensive local inflammation with necrosis, vesicle formation, edema, regional lymphadenopathy, and even malaise and fever. Antigens prepared in concentrations unlikely to provoke severe reactions are generally available for intradermal testing for tuberculosis, leprosy, mumps, lymphogranuloma venereum, cat-scratch disease, chancroid, brucellosis, tularemia, glanders, toxoplasmosis, blastomycosis, histoplasmosis, coccidioidomycosis, and many other infections. The immune reaction to vaccination is also an example of delayed dermal hypersensitivity.

The reliability, specificity, and usefulness of the individual tests differ and are discussed in the chapters on specific infection.

Intradermal injection of antigens derived from sources other than microorganisms usually produces an immediate *wheal and erythema* reaction which subsides promptly. The greatest clinical usefulness of this type of reaction is in the detection of allergy to foreign serums, pollens, and animal dander (see Chap. 67). The skin tests for demonstrating infestation with helminths (trichinosis, filariasis) produce reactions of the immediate type in allergic individuals, but many of the antigens employed are so nonspecific that they are of little use in diagnosis.

IMMUNOLOGIC METHODS These diagnostic methods are intended to supply evidence of past or present infection by demonstrating antibodies in serum or other body fluids, or indicating changed reactivity of the host (hypersensitivity, allergy) to products of the organism.

Serologic tests The finding on a single occasion that a patient's serum contains antibody which reacts with a certain antigen merely indicates that the patient has had previous contact with the antigen or a closely related substance. For this reason, with rare exceptions, the clinical interpretation of serologic tests depends on serial determinations. If the antibody titer is found to *rise or fall significantly*, the response likely is a result of recent contact with the antigen. In subsequent chapters, the need for serologic testing of acute phase and convalescent serum is emphasized repeatedly. *In any patient with a puzzling illness, a sterile specimen of serum should be preserved in a frozen state so that it can, if necessary, be studied and compared with serum collected at a later date.*

Prior contact with an antigen may be the result of past immunization with vaccines; interpretation of serum agglutinin titers for typhoid bacilli is often made difficult by prior immunization. The so-called anamnestic reaction, a nonspecific stimulation of antibody formation by an acute illness (e.g., a rise in *Brucella* agglutinins in a patient with acute tularemia), occurs only when the two organisms are antigenically related, and rarely presents a serious problem.

Some mention of "nonspecific" serologic changes may serve to emphasize again that clinical laboratory tests have come into use *only because they have been found to correlate reasonably well with clinical findings.* In several diseases it has been found, often accidentally, that serum antibody develops which will react with antigens derived from sources other than the etiologic agent (which may actually be unknown). Common examples are heterophil agglutinins in infectious mononucleosis, cold agglutinins in mycoplasma pneumonia, and the agglutination of certain strains of *Proteus* bacilli by serum of patients with rickettsial diseases. The VDRL test for syphilis and related flocculation tests are performed with antigens derived from sources completely unrelated to *Treponema pallidum.*

The results of serologic tests must be interpreted in the light of other information about the patient, including such factors as previous immunizations and illnesses, the possibility of exposure to chemically but etiologically unrelated antigens, and the importance of a changing titer in serial tests as opposed to a single isolated observation.

VIROLOGIC SPECIMENS The selection of specimens for the diagnosis of viral illness depends on both the stage of the disease and its clinical presentation. If the patient is seen early in the course of illness, frequently it is possible to demonstrate viral antigen in body tissue or fluids and/or to recover the virus by appropriate culture techniques. If the patient is seen later, during the recovery or convalescent stages, the diagnosis is often best established by serologic means. The type of specimen submitted for culture and the method of specimen transport depend to some extent on the nature of the illness. Throat swabs are helpful in the diagnosis of most viral infections. Because respiratory viruses are extremely labile, the swabs are placed in a buffered, high-protein transport medium containing antibiotic agents. If the specimen is to be transported to another institution, the specimen should be stored at −60°C and shipped on dry ice.

Cerebrospinal fluid from patients presenting with meningitis or encephalitis can also be submitted for culture. As with throat swabs, these specimens should be stored at low temperatures and shipped on dry ice. Stool should be collected in patients with respiratory illnesses, meningitis, or encephalitis, if either adenoviruses or enteroviruses are thought to be involved. Since these organisms are hardy, the feces can be collected in any sterile screw-top bottle and dispatched without refrigeration. Urine cultures are seldom helpful except in the diagnosis of cytomegalovirus infections. Vesicular fluid is a rich source of virus and viral antigen in patients presenting with exanthems. Pericardial fluid may be of help in patients with myocarditis or pericarditis. Viral blood cultures are seldom useful except in the diagnosis of arboviral infections. Isolation techniques for these viruses are highly specialized and are not available in most virus laboratories. Buffy coat cultures for cytomegalovirus and herpesvirus may be of help in immunosuppressed patients. Brain biopsy is the best single method for diagnosing herpes simplex encephalitis (see Chap. 210). The biopsy specimen should be placed in a sterile screw-top bottle and stored and dispatched in the frozen state.

REFERENCES

BARRY AL: Clinical specimens for microbiologic examinations, in *Infectious Diseases,* 2d ed, PD Hoeprich (ed). Hagerstown, Md., Harper & Row, 1977

——— et al: Microscopic examinations in infection, in *Infectious Diseases,* 2d ed, PD Hoeprich (ed). Hagerstown, Md., Harper & Row, 1977

BARTLETT RC: Control of cost and medical relevance in clinical microbiology. Am J Clin Pathol 64:518, 1975

DOLAN CT et al: *Proceedings of the 1975 Aspen Conference on Clinical Relevance in Microbiology.* Chicago, College of American Pathologists, 1977

EISENBERG HD et al: Collection, handling and processing of specimens, in *Manual of Clinical Microbiology,* 3d ed, EH Lennette et al (eds). Washington, DC, American Society for Microbiology, 1980

NEU HC: What should the clinic expect from the microbiology laboratory? Ann Intern Med 89:781, 1978

137
INFECTIONS IN THE COMPROMISED HOST

DAVID C. DALE

DEFINITION An individual who is abnormally susceptible to infections is called a *compromised host.* This heightened susceptibility often is attributable to specific abnormalities in host defense mechanisms (e.g., leukocytes, immunoglobulins, complement, mucosal and epithelial barriers, tissue vascular supply), alterations in normal surface bacteria caused by antibiotics, or the insertion of a foreign body (e.g., endotracheal tube, artificial heart valve, shunt, or catheter) (Table 137-1).

HOST DEFENSE MECHANISMS The skin and mucous membranes are the principal barriers which prevent invasion of the body by microorganisms. A variety of bacteria, including *Staphylococcus epidermidis, Streptococcus pyogenes,* and *Corynebacterium acnes,* inhabit the superficial layers of the normal skin. The mucosal surfaces of the upper respiratory tract, the lower gastrointestinal tract, and lower urinary tract are also in constant contact with bacteria, whereas the lower respiratory and upper urinary tracts are normally free of microorganisms. The subcutaneous tissues are protected from infection by the tough stratum corneum and antimicrobial substances derived from the sweat and sebaceous glands. Mucus in the respiratory and gastrointestinal tracts, together with secretory immunoglobulin (IgA), lysozyme, lactoferrin, α-antitrypsin, and bacteriocins produced by the normal bacterial flora serve to prevent colonization of the mucosal surfaces by new organisms. Bacteria and foreign debris are constantly swept toward the body orifices by the ciliated epithelial cells lining the mucosal surfaces. Normally a constant, low-grade exudation of leukocytes to these surfaces provides added protection.

If an organism penetrates a body surface and enters the

TABLE 137-1
Infections in the compromised host

	Disease	*Infection*	*Etiologic agents*
HUMORAL DEFECTS			
Antibody deficiency	Bruton's X-linked agammaglobulinemia, multiple myeloma, chronic lymphocytic leukemia, Waldenström's macroglobulinemia, Wiskott-Aldrich syndrome, ataxia telangiectasia, isolated IgA deficiency, prolonged chemotherapy	Sinusitis, bacterial pneumonia, bacteremia	*S. pneumoniae, H. influenzae, G. lamblia*
Complement deficiency	C3 deficiency, C5 deficiency, other isolated complement factor deficiencies, systemic lupus erythematosus, sickle cell anemia	Otitis, sinusitis, pneumonia, bacteremia	*S. aureus, E. coli, Pseudomonas, N. gonorrhoeae*
PHAGOCYTIC DEFECTS			
Neutropenia	Agranulocytosis, acute leukemia, aplastic anemia, cyclic neutropenia, cytotoxic drug therapy, Chédiak-Higashi syndrome	Cellulitis, pharyngitis, perirectal abscess, pneumonia, bacteremia	*S. aureus, E. coli, Pseudomonas, Candida, Aspergillus*
Chemotactic defects	Chédiak-Higashi syndrome, diabetes mellitus, rheumatoid arthritis, alcoholism, corticosteroid therapy	Cellulitis, abscesses, septic arthritis, skin ulcers	*S. aureus, S. pyogenes*, gram-negative bacilli
Phagocytic defects	Acute leukemia	Pharyngitis, perirectal abscess, pneumonia, bacteremia	*E. coli, Pseudomonas, Candida*
Microbicidal defects	Chronic granulomatous disease of childhood, myeloperoxidase deficiency, Chédiak-Higashi syndrome, lysosomal granule deficiency	Recurrent skin abscesses, lymphadenitis, osteomyelitis, liver abscess, lung abscess, pneumonia	*S. aureus, Salmonella, Serratia*
DEFECTS OF CELLULAR IMMUNITY			
T-cell deficit, with intact B cells	Hodgkin's disease, chronic mucocutaneous candidiasis, thymic dysplasia (Nezelof's syndrome), thymic-parathyroid hypoplasia (Di George's syndrome), sarcoidosis, lepromatous leprosy	Superficial skin infections (especially with *Candida*), hepatitis, tuberculosis, fungal pneumonia, chronic meningitis, meningoencephalitis	*Candida, Cryptococcus, M. tuberculosis, Listeria, Toxoplasma,* herpes zoster
Combined B-cell and T-cell defects	Severe combined immunodeficiency (adenosine deaminase deficiency), ataxia telangiectasia, Wiskott-Aldrich syndrome, cartilage-hair hypoplasia, thymoma with immunodeficiency, intestinal lymphangiectasia secondary to Whipple's disease, Crohn's disease, pericarditis, tricuspid regurgitation, chronic lymphocytic leukemia, corticosteroid and cytotoxic drug therapy, bone marrow transplantation	Disseminated skin infection (especially viral), otitis, sinusitis, bronchitis, pneumonia, bacteremias, abscesses	*S. aureus,* gram-negative bacilli, herpes zoster, herpes simplex, *cytomegalovirus*
OTHER DEFECTS			
Impaired tissue perfusion	Diabetes mellitus, nephrotic syndrome, sickle cell anemia, severe atherosclerosis	Skin ulcers, cellulitis, wet gangrene, osteomyelitis	*S. aureus, E. coli,* and other gram-negative enteric bacilli
Abnormal drainage	Cystic fibrosis, bronchogenic carcinoma, ureteral and urethral obstruction, obstruction tumors at any site	Bronchitis, bronchiectasis, pneumonia with atelectasis, urinary tract infection, ascending cholangitis	*S. aureus, E. coli,* and other gram-negative bacilli
Integumental damage	Burns, eczema, compound fractures	Cellulitis, pneumonia, bacteremia, osteomyelitis	*S. aureus, S. pyogenes, Pseudomonas*
Antibiotics	Superinfection	Pneumonia, bacteremia	*S. aureus,* resistant gram-negative bacilli, especially *Pseudomonas, Serratia, Mima-Herellea, Candida*
Prosthetic devices and foreign bodies		Abscesses, bacteremia, osteomyelitis	*S. aureus, S. epidermidis,* gram-negative enteric bacilli, *Candida*

tissues, a series of host responses occurs. An inflammatory exudate containing immunoglobulins, complement components, and other plasma proteins quickly appears. If the immunoglobulin is specific for the invading organism, it attaches to the bacterial cell wall, opsonizes the organism, and activates the complement system via the classic pathway. If specific immunoglobulin is lacking, the C3 component of complement will serve to opsonize the organism and facilitate phagocytosis. Complement activation also generates chemotactic factors which attract neutrophils, monocytes, and eosinophils to the inflammatory site (see Chap. 57).

Normally within 1 to 3 h, neutrophils have begun to accumulate at a site of inflammation anywhere in the body, and they continue to arrive until the invading microbes are killed and eliminated, or a chronic inflammatory reaction consisting of monocytes, lymphocytes, and macrophages has developed. When infection spreads from the tissues to the blood, the circulating organisms ordinarily are removed by cells of the fixed mononuclear phagocytic system in the lungs, liver, spleen, and bone marrow.

Certain pathogens, such as mycobacteria, DNA viruses, and fungi, which are not readily killed by neutrophils, tend to persist intracellularly; they require a different host response for their containment. This mechanism, commonly referred to as *cellular immunity,* involves the interaction of monocytes and sensitized lymphocytes, the transformation of monocytes to activated macrophages, and the killing of organisms by macrophages and lymphocytes by both intracellular and extracellular mechanisms. The mediators of cellular immunity include migration inhibitory factor, transfer factor, chemotactic factor, and other lymphokines which are produced by T lymphocytes (see Chap. 63).

SPECIFIC DEFECTS IN HOST DEFENSES **Defects in skin and mucous membranes** Burns and extensive trauma which leave patients with raw skin exposed to endogenous and environmental organisms rapidly become infected. *Pseudomonas* infections are frequently encountered in these patients, particularly those who have received antibiotics (see Chap. 152). Atherosclerosis and neuropathy commonly predispose diabetic individuals to cutaneous infections of the lower extremities, particularly with staphylococci. Decubitus ulcers which become secondarily infected occur in severely ill patients who are not repositioned regularly. Burns, inhalation of toxic materials, and viral infections, e.g., influenza, can damage the respiratory tract epithelium predisposing to secondary infection by upper respiratory tract flora, especially pneumococci and staphylococci. Obtundation, intubation, and mechanical ventilation also enhance the risk of pneumonia because these factors interfere with the clearance of debris and bacteria from the lower respiratory tract. Urinary tract catheters, intravenous catheters, and other devices which connect the integument to any internal organ provide a route for microbial invasion from the skin. This problem is compounded by the fact that the porous surfaces of these foreign bodies provide crevices where bacteria can grow protected from the host's phagocytic cells.

Defects in the humoral system Immunoglobulin deficiency due to B-lymphocyte deficiency or dysfunction occurs in agammaglobulinemia (see Chap. 64), multiple myeloma (see Chap. 65), and chronic lymphocytic leukemia (see Chap. 129) and with intensive immunosuppressive therapies. It results in decreased bacterial opsonization and inefficient function of the phagocytic system. Patients with these disorders are prone to infections by encapsulated bacteria, particularly pneumococci and *Hemophilus influenzae.* Patients with reduced or absent immunoglobulins and patients with defects of complement components C1, C2, or C4 are able to utilize the alternate complement pathway to activate C3 and the later complement components, i.e., C5 through C9. Patients with early complement component defects have fewer problems with infections than patients with deficiencies of complement components C3 through C9. These complement-related host defense defects are, in general, quite uncommon (see Chap. 63).

Defects in the phagocytic system The most frequently encountered problem in phagocytic defenses is neutropenia. Blood neutrophil counts below 500 cells per cubic millimeter, and particularly counts below 100 cells per cubic millimeter, are associated with a greatly increased frequency of fever and infections. This is especially true in idiopathic or drug-induced agranulocytosis, leukemia, and aplastic anemia. Far less commonly, patients are encountered with specific defects in the granulocyte bactericidal mechanisms, e.g., chronic granulomatous disease and the Chédiak-Higashi syndrome (see Chap. 57). In some patients with diabetes, uremia, lupus erythematosus, and rheumatoid arthritis, defects in neutrophils have been recognized which are attributed to abnormalities in the environment (excess glucose, uremic toxins, immune complexes) in which the cells function. When these patients' cells are suspended in normal serum or plasma, they generally function normally.

Defects in cell-mediated immunity Patients with Hodgkin's disease, sarcoidosis, lepromatous leprosy, chronic mucocutaneous candidiasis, and certain congenital syndromes, e.g., Nezelof's syndrome, Di George's syndrome, Wiskott-Aldrich syndrome, and combined immunodeficiency, have defective lymphocyte-monocyte function most easily identified by reduced or absent cutaneous, delayed hypersensitivity responses (see Chap. 64). Tuberculosis, candidiasis, and disseminated viral infections, particularly herpes zoster infections, seem to occur with increased frequency in these patients.

Splenectomy The magnitude of the risk of overwhelming infection in the splenectomized patient is related to the underlying disease which called for removal of the spleen. However, even splenectomy for trauma in an otherwise normal individual appears to increase the risk of severe bacteremic infections. There is an impressive predominance of pneumococcal infections in splenectomized individuals; other organisms encountered frequently have included *Neisseria meningitidis, Escherichia coli,* and *Pseudomonas.* Malaria and other intracellular parasitic infections such as *Toxoplasma* and *Babesia* also may occur with increased frequency.

Defects induced by drugs *Antibiotics,* particularly when taken orally, regularly alter the normal host bacterial flora and predispose patients to superinfections, i.e., infections occurring specifically as a consequence of antibiotic treatment. Characteristically, these infections are caused by organisms resistant to the antibiotic being administered. These infections occur more commonly when antimicrobials are given in large doses, when several antimicrobials are administered concurrently, or when broad-spectrum agents are used.

It is often difficult to distinguish between superinfections and simple surface colonization by new organisms. Usually superinfections are identified by the occurrence of new symptoms, e.g., fever, cough, dysuria, or diarrhea, and the finding of resistant organisms in an area of new inflammation during the course of treating a defined infection (see Chap. 145). Most of the time, antimicrobial therapy does not promote superinfection. However, when the concentration of organisms replacing the normal flora is high and when anatomic conditions are favorable, superinfection is likely. Certain circumstances, such as the tendency for *Pseudomonas* to infect patients treated with the cephalosporins and for *Candida* to infect patients treated with broad-spectrum combinations of antibiotics, are well recognized. Superinfections are also common during treatment of pneumonia in patients with severe, chronic, obstructive pulmonary disease where intubation is necessary, and when urinary tract infections are treated in patients with urinary stones or catheters.

Glucocorticosteroid therapy, particularly when given for long periods and in high doses, is thought to increase the risk of infections in humans. Although this risk is well documented in animal experiments, properly controlled human studies have been difficult to conduct. In the laboratory, steroids decrease mobilization of neutrophils to the sites of inflammation, decrease the killing of microbes by monocytes, and interfere with cell-mediated immune responses, possibly by altering the responsiveness of monocytes and macrophages to lymphokines. Because steroids induce such a broad defect in host defense mechanisms, both common and unusual pathogens must be considered in the steroid-treated patient with a presumed infection.

Immunosuppressive drugs, e.g., cyclophosphamide, chlorambucil, methotrexate, and many others, are now widely used for nonmalignant and malignant diseases. Nearly all of these agents cause neutropenia, lymphopenia, and monocytopenia through suppression of cell production. They also impair the rates of cell renewal in other tissues vital for host defenses including the epithelial cells lining the mucosal surfaces. Most of the infectious complications of these agents occur concomitant with the drug-induced neutropenia. Especially when used with corticosteroids in high doses, patients treated with these agents are severely compromised both in their ability to resist new infections and to handle established ones.

Defects with transplantation Immunosuppressive drugs, antilymphocyte globulin, and corticosteroids are generally used to prolong and to prevent rejection of kidney, heart, and other homografts. Because these agents are used in high doses during periods of impending graft rejection and because cellular resistance to infections may be impaired by the graft rejection process itself, at times these patients are inordinately susceptible to infections, particularly to severe fungal and viral infections (see Chaps. 292 and 331).

Bone marrow transplant patients have marked susceptibility to infection at the time of marrow grafting because of neutropenia and bone marrow ablation. After transplantation and marrow engraftment, despite the rise in their neutrophil counts, their host defenses remain severely compromised for 1 to 3 months because of a persisting impairment in cellular immunity. During this period, they frequently develop catastrophic pulmonary infections due to fungi, viruses, and parasites (see Chap. 331).

RECOGNIZING THE COMPROMISED HOST Most disease states associated with increased susceptibility to infections are easily identified. Examples include patients with leukemia, lymphoma, or aplastic anemia; therapy with steroids, immunosuppressive drugs, and broad-spectrum antibiotics; and specific anatomic defects such as bronchiectasis, chronic obstructive lung disease, or obstructive uropathy. Not infrequently the occurrence of fever and infection leads to the diagnosis of certain diseases associated with defects in host defenses. For example, a diabetic may be recognized because of recurrent abscesses or candidiasis in the perineal region. A severely granulocytopenic patient may be recognized because of fever, sore throat, or sepsis. Recurrent pneumococcal meningitis may lead to recognition of a small skull fracture with chronic CSF leakage. Recurrent fever and lymphadenitis usually precede recognition of chronic granulomatous disease.

Several reasonably reliable associations of specific organisms and certain host defense defects have been recognized and may be helpful in identifying or caring for the compromised host. These include *Staphylococcus aureus* with foreign bodies; *S. aureus, Serratia,* and *Salmonella* with chronic granulomatous disease; *Streptococcus pneumoniae* with agammaglobulinemia and splenectomy; mucoid *Pseudomonas* strains with cystic fibrosis; *Salmonella* with sickle cell disease; *Nocardia* with alveolar proteinosis; *Mycobacterium tuberculosis, Cryptococcus,* and herpes zoster with Hodgkin's disease; and *Candida* with hypoparathyroidism.

The evaluation of a patient to identify a defect in host defenses should proceed systematically. After a complete history and physical examination, complete blood cell counts, blood glucose, liver and renal function tests, and chest and other appropriate x-ray examinations are obtained. Serum protein electrophoresis, quantitative immunoglobulins, and isohemagglutinins or selective febrile agglutinins are then measured to evaluate B-lymphocyte function. T-lymphocyte functions are evaluated with a panel of delayed hypersensitivity skin tests, generally including PPD, mumps, *Candida,* trichophytin, and streptokinase-streptodornase. Contact sensitization with dinitrochlorobenzene (DNCB) or keyhole hemocyanin (KLH) may also be performed. Complement defects usually can be recognized by obtaining total hemolytic complement levels (CH_{50}) or C3 assays. The principal screening test for recognizing the various forms of chronic granulomatous disease is the nitroblue tetrazolium (NBT) test. At this point in any patient's evaluation, consultation with an individual engaged in studying host defense defects is usually necessary.

Useful clues for persisting in a patient's evaluation to try to define a specific abnormality are: repetitive episodes of proven bacterial infections with the same organism; infections which do not respond to treatment that is usually considered to be effective or which relapse when therapy is discontinued; and repeated infections caused by unusual organisms.

THERAPEUTIC CONSIDERATIONS Successful treatment of infections in the compromised host depends upon early diagnosis, prompt intervention, and avoidance of certain pitfalls in patient management. Because infections in the compromised host tend to be chronic, long-term care by a concerned physician who understands the patient's host defense deficiency is vitally important. Laboratory facilities for accurate culture and sensitivity testing also are essential. In the febrile compromised host, the clinician must collect blood, body fluids, and exudate for cultures as quickly as possible. When these materials do not yield a diagnosis promptly, aspiration or biopsy of sites of presumed infection is often necessary and should not be delayed.

Often it is necessary to initiate antibiotic treatment before results of cultures and sensitivity tests are available. This is particularly true in patients with shock and presumed bacteremia, patients with fever and severe neutropenia, and those with severe respiratory tract infections where sputum or transtracheal washings are difficult or impossible to obtain. In these instances broad-spectrum coverage with a combination of antibiotics should be used initially (see Chap. 141), but the coverage should be narrowed as quickly as possible to avoid superinfections. Often patients with neutropenia, corticosteroid treatment, and certain specific host defense defects fail to mount an inflammatory response as rapidly as normal individuals. Consequently, when these patients have pneumonia, cellulitis, or abscesses, the diagnosis may not be apparent when the patient is first seen. Repeated careful examinations are the only way to establish the diagnosis.

Although sometimes essential, indwelling catheters should

be avoided in the compromised host whenever possible (see Chap. 138). The prophylactic use of antibiotics in these patients has rarely been successful (see Chap. 145). With time, the patients simply become colonized by microbes resistant to the prophylactic agents chosen. Oral therapy with trimethoprim-sulfamethoxazole is effective for short-term prophylaxis for bacterial infections in highly susceptible neutropenic hosts, but this combination increases the risk of fungal superinfections. Prophylactic neutrophil transfusions for these patients are not recommended. Gamma globulin therapy can be helpful in patients with agammaglobulinemia (see Chap. 64), but is of no benefit to most patients with multiple myeloma or other hypogammaglobulinemic states in which there is low, but detectable, serum IgG. Active immunization against *S. pneumoniae* is recommended for patients with splenectomies and other causes of compromised defense mechanisms (see Chap. 146). Active and passive immunization to prevent other infections is under investigation. Protective isolation with laminar airflow rooms, sterile food, and antibiotic treatment will prevent or delay infection and probably is useful when the duration of maximum susceptibility to the infection is no longer than a few days to a few weeks.

SPECIFIC INFECTIONS Certain organisms are encountered as pathogens almost exclusively in the compromised host, e.g., *Pneumocystis carinii, Phycomyces,* and *Aspergillus.* Others, e.g., *Candida, Histoplasma,* herpes simplex, and cytomegalovirus, are common pathogens for both the normal and compromised host. The following organisms are encountered frequently or present special problems. Separate chapters in the text deal with each of these and their treatment in greater detail.

Staphylococcus In general, staphylococcal infections are not inordinately difficult to manage in the compromised host. Staphylococcal infections related to intravenous catheters present a special problem. Although it is always best to remove the catheter, it may be possible, on occasion, to cure infections caused by antibiotic-sensitive staphylococci at the site of arteriovenous shunts and at the tips of chronic parenteral nutrition catheters (see Chap. 147).

Listeria Bacteremia, peritonitis, and meningitis are encountered particularly in newborns, alcoholics, diabetics, and patients with lymphoreticular malignancies. The diagnosis may be missed initially because relatively few organisms are found in exudate (e.g., peritoneal fluid or cerebrospinal fluid) or the organism is confused with other gram-positive rods, such as diphtheroids, and regarded as a contaminant (see Chap. 164).

Corynebacterium Diphtheroids are among the most common organisms encountered as contaminants of blood cultures. With increasing frequency, however, they are being found as the cause of significant bacteremias, particularly in severely ill patients with intravenous catheters and cerebrospinal fluid reservoirs and shunts.

Gram-negative bacilli *E. coli, Pseudomonas, Proteus,* and other Enterobacteriaceae remain the major pathogens for patients with compromised host defenses. The portal for entry is generally the gastrointestinal tract. Gram-negative bacteremia, pneumonia, and meningitis are well recognized. *Ecthyma gangrenosum* is an important clue to early recognition of *Pseudomonas* sepsis (see Chaps. 151 and 152).

Mycobacterium With the declining frequency of pulmonary tuberculosis in the United States, an increasing proportion of cases involve patients with compromised host defenses who often present with unusual manifestations of the disease. For this reason it is important to know the tuberculin status of every patient with a chronic debilitating disease which may predispose the patient to infections or which may require treatment with corticosteroids or immunosuppressive drugs. The practice of treating all tuberculin-positive patients receiving steroids with isoniazid is becoming less frequent with recognition of the toxicity of the drug and the relatively small risk of activation of latent disease, at least in certain conditions such as asthma and rheumatoid arthritis. However, this approach necessitates careful follow-up of every tuberculin reactor (see Chap. 147).

Candida This organism has emerged as a major cause for superinfection in the compromised host. *Candida* pharyngitis, laryngitis, esophagitis, pneumonia, and candidemia are common in patients with reduced host defenses who are receiving broad-spectrum antibiotics. The diagnosis of disseminated candidiasis often poses considerable difficulty (see Chap. 184).

Histoplasma Disseminated histoplasmosis is becoming an increasingly important problem, particularly among patients with Hodgkin's disease, chronic lymphocytic leukemia, acute lymphocytic leukemia, and those undergoing intensive immunosuppressive therapy. Both reactivation of latent infections and inordinately severe initial infections have been documented. It is important to establish because the infection responds well to amphotericin in many instances (see Chap. 183).

Nocardia See Chap. 182.

Aspergillus See Chap. 184.

Phycomyces See Chap. 184.

Herpes zoster Disseminated herpes zoster infections occur with increased frequency in disorders of cellular immunity, especially Hodgkin's disease and chronic lymphocytic leukemia, and in patients receiving corticosteroids and immunosuppressive drugs (see Chap. 204).

Herpes simplex Disseminated infections with diffuse skin lesions, pneumonitis, encephalitis, and hepatitis have been increasing, especially in renal transplant patients and in others receiving intensive immunosuppression (see Chap. 210).

Cytomegalovirus See Chap. 211.

Toxoplasmosis See Chap. 221.

Pneumocystis See Chap. 222.

REFERENCES

Fauci AS et al: Glucocorticosteroid therapy: Mechanisms of action and clinical considerations. Ann Intern Med 84:304, 1976

Fraser DW, Broome CV: Pneumococcal vaccine: To use or not. JAMA 245:498, 1981

Gurwith MJ et al: Granulocytopenia in hospitalized patients: I. Prognostic factors and etiology of fever. Am J Med 64:121, 1978

——— et al: A prospective controlled investigation of prophylactic trimethoprim/sulfamethoxazole in hospitalized granulocytopenic patients. Am J Med 66:248, 1979

Heier HE: Splenectomy and serious infections. Scand J Haematol 24:5, 1980

Jackson GG: Considerations of antibiotic prophylaxis in nonsurgical high risk patients. Am J Med 70:467, 1981

Meunier-Carpentier F et al: Fungemia in the immunocompromised host. Am J Med 71:363, 1981

NAUSEEF WM, MAKI DG: A study of the value of simple protective isolation in patients with granulocytopenia. N Engl J Med 304:448, 1981

PETERSON PK et al: Fever in renal transplant recipients: Causes, prognostic significance and changing patterns at the University of Minnesota Hospital. Am J Med 71:345, 1981

PIZZO PA: The value of protective isolation in preventing nosocomial infections in high risk patients. Am J Med 70:631, 1981

RUBIN RH et al: Infection in the renal transplant recipient. Am J Med 70:405, 1981

———, YOUNG LS: *The Clinical Approach to Infection in the Immunocompromised Host.* New York, Plenum, 1981

SCHIMPFF SC: Infection prevention during profound granulocytopenia. Ann Intern Med 93:358, 1980

SMITH FG, PALMER DL: Alcoholism, infection and altered host defenses: A review of clinical and experimental observations. J Chron Dis 29:35, 1976

STRAUSS RG: A controlled trial of prophylactic granulocyte transfusions during initial induction chemotherapy for acute myelogenous leukemia. N Engl J Med 305:597, 1981

TULLY JL: Complications of intravenous therapy with steel needles and teflon catheters. Am J Med 70:702, 1981

WINSTON DJ et al: Infectious complications of human bone marrow transplantation. Medicine 58:1, 1979

YOUNG LS: Nosocomial infections in the immunocompromised adult. Am J Med 70:398, 1981

138 HOSPITAL-ACQUIRED INFECTIONS

PIERCE GARDNER
WILLIAM A. CAUSEY

DEFINITIONS Hospital-acquired infections (also called *nosocomial infections*) are significant causes of human morbidity and mortality. They are defined as infections occurring in patients after admission to the hospital that were neither present nor in incubation at the time of admission. Infections acquired in the hospital but not manifest until after the patient is discharged are also included. Although many of these infections can be prevented, some cannot, and the term *hospital-acquired infection* should not be equated with *iatrogenic infection,* which indicates an infection caused by a diagnostic or therapeutic intervention such as the insertion of a urethral or intravenous catheter. *Opportunistic infections* occur in patients with impaired host defenses and are commonly caused by infectious agents that do not ordinarily produce disease in healthy individuals. Many opportunistic infections are caused by organisms in the patient's own flora (*autochthonous infections*) and are often unavoidable because they are related to defects in mucosal barriers or other host defenses rather than preventable environmental risks.

EPIDEMIOLOGY Incidence and cost Hospital-acquired infections occur in from 2 to 12 percent (average, 5 percent) of patients admitted to general hospitals. The highest infection rates are reported from municipal hospitals and tertiary care centers, while the prevalence of these infections is much lower in community hospitals. Hospital-acquired infections have a mortality rate of 1 percent and contribute to death in an additional 3 percent of cases. Estimates for the United States indicate that 1.5 million hospital-acquired infections occur annually, that they cause 15,000 deaths, and that they contribute to mortality in an additional 45,000 patients. The prolongation in hospital stays and additional diagnostic tests, medications, and physicians' fees contribute significantly to the high cost of hospital care.

ETIOLOGY Causative pathogens Gram-negative bacilli dominate the list of nosocomial pathogens, although *Staphylococcus aureus,* the scourge of the 1950s and early 1960s, remains an important pathogen in all sites except the urinary tract (Table 138-1). Multiply antibiotic-resistant strains of *S.*

TABLE 138-1
Rates* and relative frequencies† of selected pathogens causing nosocomial infections, by site of infection, 1978

	Primary bacteremia	*Surgical wound*	*Lower respiratory*	*Urinary tract*	*Cutaneous*	*Other*	*All sites*
Staphylococcus aureus	2.4	15.8	7.3	3.2	8.4	7.0	44.1
	(13.8)	(14.6)	(10.4)	(2.0)	(31.7)	(14.6)	(10.3)
Staphylococcus epidermidis	1.5	4.8	0.4	4.9	1.6	2.2	15.4
	(8.9)	(4.4)	(0.5)	(3.1)	(5.9)	(4.6)	(3.6)
Streptococcus, group D	1.1	10.4	1.0	21.9	1.8	2.4	38.6
	(6.2)	(9.6)	(1.4)	(13.8)	(6.7)	(5.0)	(9.0)
Escherichia coli	2.7	15.7	5.1	51.1	2.2	3.9	80.8
	(15.6)	(14.6)	(7.3)	(32.1)	(8.4)	(8.0)	(18.8)
Klebsiella spp.	1.9	5.4	7.6	14.5	1.2	2.1	32.7
	(10.9)	(5.0)	(10.8)	(9.1)	(4.5)	(4.3)	(7.6)
Enterobacter spp.	0.9	4.3	4.7	6.9	0.9	1.2	18.7
	(5.0)	(3.9)	(6.7)	(4.3)	(3.3)	(2.5)	(4.4)
Proteus-Providencia spp.	0.4	7.5	4.3	15.2	1.3	1.8	30.6
	(2.4)	(7.0)	(6.1)	(9.6)	(5.0)	(3.8)	(7.1)
Pseudomonas aeruginosa	1.0	5.7	6.2	16.1	1.7	2.8	33.5
	(6.0)	(5.3)	(8.8)	(10.1)	(6.2)	(5.9)	(7.8)
Serratia spp.	0.5	1.3	2.3	4.1	0.3	0.6	9.1
	(3.1)	(1.2)	(3.3)	(2.6)	(1.1)	(1.3)	(2.1)
Candida spp.	0.6	1.1	1.6	6.1	0.9	3.5	13.7
	(3.5)	(1.0)	(2.2)	(3.8)	(3.2)	(7.2)	(3.2)
All pathogens ‡	17.3	108.2	70.1	159.0	26.6	48.3	429.5
	(100.0)	(100.0)	(100.0)	(100.0)	(100.0)	(100.0)	(100.0)
Secondary bacteremia	NA	4.2	4.0	4.5	1.4	5.5	19.5
	(−)§	(3.9)	(5.7)	(2.8)	(5.1)	(11.3)	(4.5)

* *Rate is number of isolates reported per 10,000 patients discharged; up to four isolates may be reported per infection.*
† *Relative frequency is expressed as percent of all isolates from each site.*
‡ *Relative rates differ from those in other tables because more than one pathogen may be isolated from a single site.*
§ *Relative frequency is <0.1% of all isolates from that site.*
SOURCE: *Centers for Disease Control, National Nosocomial Infections Study Report, Annual Summary 1978, issued March 1981.*

aureus have become endemic in some hospitals in Europe and North America in recent years and have been responsible for epidemics of infections primarily on surgical services. These strains may be resistant to not only penicillin and ampicillin but also the penicillinase-resistant penicillins (methicillin, oxacillin, nafcillin), cephalosporins, erythromycin, clindamycin, and some aminoglycosides. There is epidemiologic evidence to suggest that resistant *S. epidermidis* strains are an important reservoir of genes mediating multiple resistance and can transfer these genes to *S. aureus.* Bacterial tolerance (organisms are inhibited but not killed by bactericidal drugs) is common among currently isolated strains of *S. aureus* tested against β-lactamase–resistant penicillins, but the clinical significance of this in vitro observation has not been clearly defined in human infections.

Gram-negative bacilli have tended to develop resistance to multiple antibiotics more readily than gram-positive cocci. In large part, resistance among gram-negative bacilli is due to the acquisition of plasmids called *resistance factors* (R factors). R-factor plasmids consist of extrachromosomal circular deoxyribonucleic acid (DNA) which mediates antibiotic resistance by coding for enzymes that inactivate the drug or by conferring properties altering the permeability of the bacterial cell wall or membrane to the drug. Two properties of R factors are of major public health concern: (1) resistance to several antibiotics is often linked on the same R factor, and (2) R-factor transfer can occur across species lines from one gram-negative organism to another with relative ease. Under appropriate selective conditions, often occurring in hospital environments, these properties make possible the rapid dissemination of multiple antibiotic resistance among a wide variety of gram-negative pathogens.

Whatever the mechanism of resistance, the major reason for the emergence of antibiotic-resistant bacteria in the hospital setting is the use of antibiotics. These drugs tend to suppress susceptible bacteria in the patient's flora and in the hospital environment, creating a competitive advantage for antibiotic-resistant organisms. The importance of antibiotics as a selective force is emphasized by the observation that a number of hospital epidemics due to resistant bacteria have been aborted by limiting the use of some of these drugs and by interdicting others altogether.

In recent years the spectrum of microorganisms reported to be associated with nosocomial transmission has broadened considerably. Opportunistic infections have become so frequent that *Candida* spp. appear among the list of most common nosocomial pathogens. Other opportunistic fungi (including *Aspergillus* and the *Mucor* groups of fungi); viruses (including hepatitis B virus, non-A and non-B hepatitis virus, cytomegalovirus, rubella virus, influenza viruses, respiratory syncytial virus, and others); and protozoan parasites (*Pneumocystis carinii* and *Toxoplasma gondii*) have gained increasing recognition as causes of hospital-acquired infection.

Transmission of nosocomial pathogens Even before the recognition of bacteria as causative agents of disease, Ignaz Semmelweis, by simple epidemiologic methods, identified the contaminated hands of physicians and medical students as the major transmitters of puerperal sepsis, the most significant hospital-acquired infection of his day. Although the major sites and pathogens of hospital-acquired infections have changed during the past century, contact with hospital personnel remains the principal means of transmission of nosocomial pathogens. Usually, transmission occurs via the hands of hospital personnel, but other skin surfaces and respiratory droplets may also be important. Inanimate sources of hospital-associated microorganisms include food and drinking water, sinks and bath water, ventilation systems, contaminated horizontal surfaces, and the catheters and equipment needed for life-support systems and diagnostic procedures.

A *common-source* epidemic occurs when a single contaminating source is responsible for multiple infections. In this situation, patients commonly become colonized with hospital-associated bacteria following exposure to a particular procedure or area of the hospital. The epidemiologic steps in the evaluation of a common-source epidemic include recognition of a clustering of infections in both time and place, use of antibiotic susceptibility patterns or other biologic markers to allow more precise definition of the epidemic strain, and analysis of the geographic distribution and diagnostic experiences which are common to the infected patients but absent from the noninfected patients.

Host factors The age and underlying disease of patients, the integrity of their mucosal and integumentary surfaces, and the status of their immunologic defenses are among the major determinants of both the incidence and outcome of hospital-acquired infections (see Chap. 137).

COMMON HOSPITAL-ACQUIRED INFECTIONS **Urinary tract infections** These infections account for approximately 40 percent of hospital-acquired infections and are usually a consequence of instrumentation of the urethra, bladder, or kidneys. The most common predisposing factor is the insertion of an indwelling urethral catheter which bypasses the normal anatomic barriers to ascending infection. Hospital surveys show that 10 to 15 percent of all adult patients have indwelling urinary catheters, many of which appear to be unnecessary. Because the urinary tract is the most common site of infection resulting in gram-negative bacteremia, steps to prevent catheter-related infections merit special emphasis and include:

1 Restrict the use of indwelling catheters except when required for management of bladder outlet obstruction or for close monitoring of fluid and electrolyte balance in severely ill patients.
2 Rigorously adhere to sterile technique during insertion of the catheter.
3 Maintain a system of closed drainage. Good technique can usually keep the urine sterile for 5 to 7 days. After that, the risk of infection increases with time, 5 to 10 percent for each day of catheterization.
4 Keep the collecting tubing and bag unobstructed and in a dependent position.
5 When urine specimens are required, aspirate the specimen from the catheter by use of a sterile syringe rather than by breaking the closed drainage system.
6 Consider intermittent straight catheterization for patients with anticipated short-term needs for bladder drainage in order to avoid using an indwelling catheter altogether.

Wound infections Most surgical wound infections are caused by organisms introduced into the tissues at the time of the operative procedures. Most infecting organisms originate from the resident flora of the patient, and airborne bacteria are of lesser consequence in wound infections. The major factors affecting the incidence of wound infection include the type of operation, its duration, the skill of the surgeon, and the basic health of the patient. Operations involving contaminated sites, such as the bowel or vagina, are more likely to be complicated by infection than operations on sites which were sterile prior to surgery. Operations of long duration, or ones in which devitalized tissue, foreign bodies, or hematomas are left behind, are associated with increased wound infection rates. Other factors predisposing to wound infection include advanced age, poor nutritional status, the presence of distant foci of infection, diabetes mellitus, renal failure, and corticosteroid therapy.

Most wound infections become manifest from 3 to 7 days following surgery. Early postoperative wound infections (those occurring within 24 to 48 h of surgery) are commonly caused by group A *Streptococcus* or *Clostridium* spp. Staphylococcal wound infections characteristically become evident 4 to 6 days after surgery, and those caused by gram-negative bacilli and anaerobic bacteria may not appear for a week or more. If perioperative antibiotics are used, the manifestations of infection may be delayed. Gram-stained smears of wound exudate, together with culture, often provide valuable early clues to the bacterial cause of wound infections.

In addition to emphasis on maintaining sterility in the operating room and insistence on operative techniques that minimize tissue trauma and blood loss, increasing attention is being given to preventing postoperative wound infections with short prophylactic courses of systemic antibiotics during the perioperative period. The principles that should govern the use of antibiotics in this situation include (1) beginning the drug during the immediate preoperative period but not earlier, (2) ensuring adequate tissue levels throughout the surgery, giving intraoperative doses of antibiotics if necessary, and (3) discontinuing antibiotic prophylaxis within 24 to 48 h following surgery. These brief courses of antibiotics do not appear to alter the patient's flora or promote colonization with resistant strains. Prolonged pre- and postoperative courses are unnecessary, expensive, and potentially harmful because of increased risk of drug toxicity and superinfection. Antibiotic prophylaxis administered according to these principles has reduced infectious morbidity in a wide variety of operative procedures that are traditionally associated with major risk of infection including colon surgery and vaginal hysterectomy.

Nonsurgical wounds that are common sites of nosocomial infection include burns, injection sites, decubitus ulcers, and cutaneous ulcers resulting from venous or arterial occlusive disease. In general, the offending pathogens are similar to those found in wound infections, with the exception that burn wound and soft-tissue infections in neutropenic patients are frequently caused by *Pseudomonas aeruginosa.* Bacteremic *Pseudomonas* infections may result in bacterial arteritis and cutaneous infarction manifested by hemorrhagic bullae (ecthyma gangrenosa, see Chap. 152).

Pneumonia Lower respiratory tract infections are the leading cause of mortality among hospital-acquired infections, although they rank third in incidence behind urinary tract infections and wound infections. The major pathogens are the gram-negative bacilli and *S. aureus,* all of which characteristically cause a necrotizing bronchopneumonia. These organisms usually reach the lower respiratory tract by aspiration of upper respiratory organisms rather than by hematogenous spread. This is consistent with the observation that the pharyngeal flora of seriously ill patients contains an increased number of gram-negative bacilli. The three settings in which nosocomial pneumonias most commonly occur are (1) obtunded patients whose gag reflex and cough are ineffective, (2) patients with underlying pulmonary disease or congestive heart failure whose pulmonary clearance mechanisms are impaired, and (3) patients who require respiratory tract instrumentation or ventilatory assistance.

Because antibiotic treatment of nosocomial pneumonia is often ineffective, preventive measures assume special importance. Positioning the patient in a swimmer's or Gatch position is the cornerstone of preventing aspiration of obtunded patients. Treatment of congestive failure will improve the effectiveness of the lung's defenses and will reduce lung edema fluid that serves as an excellent culture medium. Emphasis should be placed on sterile technique when performing tracheal toilet, and the breathing circuits on ventilatory assistance equipment must be properly maintained. The routine use of positive pressure breathing machines in perioperative care is often unnecessary and subjects patients to the infection risk inherent to exposure to ventilatory equipment. Regular monitoring of the respiratory flora, particularly in intubated patients, with Gram-stained smears and cultures provides useful information in choosing appropriate early therapy for pulmonary superinfections, should they occur.

Most patients with pulmonary tuberculosis are now diagnosed and managed in general hospitals. Recognition of active cases of pulmonary tuberculosis, and prompt institution of respiratory isolation and appropriate chemotherapy, are the principal means by which in-hospital spread of the disease can be limited. General hospitals located in communities with an appreciable incidence of tuberculosis should maintain an active surveillance program for their employees.

Hospital transmission of viral respiratory pathogens is common, especially on pediatric services but, except for influenza and respiratory syncytial virus (in infants), rarely results in severe disease. When influenza A is widespread in the community, amantadine prophylaxis, as well as immunization, should be considered for unimmunized hospital patients identified as being at high risk for complications of influenza.

Bacteremia Although bacterial invasion of the bloodstream can occur in any nosocomial infection, infected vascular cannulas are among the most common and also most preventable causes of hospital-acquired bacteremia. Annually in the United States more than 10 million persons (more than one in four hospitalized patients) receive intravenous therapy, and therefore even a low rate of infection assumes major clinical significance. Infected vascular devices account for about 5 percent of all nosocomial infections and 10 percent of all positive blood cultures. The most common isolates from cannula tips are *S. epidermidis, S. aureus,* gram-negative bacilli (especially *Klebsiella, Enterobacter, Serratia*), and enterococci. Although microorganisms can enter a fluid delivery system at any point, contamination most commonly occurs at the site of skin entry during cannula insertion or subsequent manipulation. The connecting points of the administration set to the cannula or the infusion bag are also vulnerable entry points for microorganisms. Intravenous fluids may become contaminated as a result of adding medications, or rarely in the process of manufacture.

The type of cannula, the choice of insertion site, the adequacy of skin preparation, and the length of time during which the cannula is in use determine the risk of septic complications. Stainless steel needles, especially scalp vein needles, are preferable to plastic cannulas which carry greater risks of local phlebitis, contamination, and sepsis. Suppurative phlebitis, the most feared complication of cannula-related infections, is virtually unknown with steel needles. Arms are better insertion sites than legs owing to lower rates of phlebitis and sepsis. The risk of bacteremia increases with time and is unacceptably high when cannulas are left in place longer than 48 to 72 h. Prolonged use of a vascular cannula and failure to remove it at the earliest sign of inflammation or malfunction are common errors. Preventive measures designed to reduce the incidence of intravenous-associated infections are listed in Table 138-2. With meticulous care, catheters used for parenteral hyperalimentation can be maintained free of infection for prolonged periods. However, infectious complications, particularly *Candida* sepsis, are not uncommon in this setting.

TABLE 138-2
Guidelines to reduce the risk of infusion-associated infections

1 Limit use of vascular cannulas to specified clinical circumstances when other routes of administration of fluids or drugs are not feasible.
2 Avoid high-risk injection sites, such as the legs.
3 Use stainless steel needles in preference to plastic catheters when possible.
4 Adequately disinfect skin over the insertion site.
5 Use sterile technique in insertion of cannulas.
6 Securely anchor the cannula to limit to-and-fro motion.
7 Apply sterile dressing over the insertion site (antibiotic ointment optional).
8 Inspect insertion site daily and remove the cannula if inflammation, phlebitis, or cannula malfunction is present.
9 Change peripheral cannulas at frequent (~48 h) intervals.

Transient bacteremia following diagnostic or therapeutic manipulations of the mouth or respiratory, gastrointestinal, or genitourinary tract are usually well tolerated by the normal host. However, the patient with valvular or congenital heart disease or a prosthetic valve may be at risk of developing endocarditis during such episodes and should receive antibiotic prophylaxis when undergoing procedures associated with significant risk of bacteremia. These procedures include dental manipulations, urinary tract instrumentation, abdominal surgery, and other surgery involving infected tissue. For patients with prosthetic heart valves, these recommendations have been extended. Detailed programs of prophylaxis are given in the chapter on infective endocarditis (see Chap. 259).

Hepatitis B The risk of hospital-acquired hepatitis B is significant not only for patients but also for hospital personnel who work with infected patients or handle their blood specimens. Patients at special risk for hepatitis B virus infection include those who receive blood products or undergo hemodialysis. The widespread practice of screening blood products for the presence of hepatitis B surface antigen (HBsAg) has markedly reduced the incidence of posttransfusion hepatitis B, and most posttransfusion hepatitis is now caused by viruses other than hepatitis B (non-A, non-B hepatitis). However, transmission of hepatitis B virus remains an endemic problem on many hemodialysis units and oncology services. For poorly understood reasons, hepatitis B virus infections are often more severe in clinical and laboratory staff than in patients. Meticulous attention to precautions designed to limit spread of pathogens by direct contact or needle accident is the major emphasis in the prevention of transmission of hepatitis B virus in dialysis units. Hepatitis B immune globulin (HBIG) contains high levels of antibodies to hepatitis B (anti-HBs) and is recommended for susceptible personnel directly exposed to HBsAg-positive material by accidental needle stick, mucosal membrane contact, or oral ingestion. Prophylaxis with HBIG for patients and personnel with continuing exposure to hepatitis B virus is not routinely recommended, but may be indicated in epidemic situations.

Active immunization with a vaccine containing hepatitis B surface antigen appears to be safe and effective in preventing hepatitis B in susceptible individuals with continuous or frequent exposure risks. This vaccine will probably play an important role in future preventive strategies.

Considerable concern has been generated about the infectivity of the approximately 1 percent of physicians and dentists who are asymptomatic carriers of HBsAg. Although several instances of transmission of infection from health care workers to patients have been identified, the great majority of HBsAg-positive health care personnel do not appear to present a hazard to their patients. While they should be encouraged to pay particular attention to personal hygiene and hand washing, their patient-related activities need not be restricted.

CONTROL MEASURES Infection control team The goals of those concerned with infection control are (1) to reduce the risk of patients acquiring infections in the hospital, (2) to provide adequate care for patients with a potentially communicable infection, and (3) to minimize the infectious risks of employees, visitors, and community contacts. The functions of the infection control team include (1) development of enforceable policies necessary for appropriate management of patients with communicable infections; (2) development of a surveillance system which identifies patients with communicable infections, quantitates the incidence and prevalence of hospital-acquired infection, and investigates problems that are likely to be remediable; (3) liaison with personnel from nursing, central supply, housekeeping, maintenance, pharmacy, and other hospital services to ensure that an appropriate infection control environment is maintained; (4) education of employees in appropriate techniques to prevent the spread of infectious agents within the hospital; (5) communication with employee health services to ensure adequate immunization of hospital employees and to provide care when personnel are exposed to a potentially communicable disease; and (6) monitoring of antibiotic utilization and susceptibility patterns of common nosocomial pathogens. Most large hospitals employ full-time personnel, nurses or physicians, to lead the multidisciplinary team effort that is necessary to carry out these functions.

Prevention Sir William Osler once remarked, "Soap, water and common sense are the best disinfectants." The basic principles of hand washing between patient contacts, appropriate isolation of patients harboring communicable microorganisms, and application of epidemiologic methods to identify and correct potential sources of infection remain the cornerstones of preventing nosocomial infections.

EMPLOYEE HEALTH SERVICE Preventive medicine applies not only to patients but also to hospital personnel. The employee health service should be encouraged to maintain an employee surveillance program for communicable diseases such as tuberculosis, hepatitis B, and rubella and to immunize personnel who are susceptible to measles, mumps, poliomyelitis, diphtheria, or tetanus. Personnel of both sexes who are likely to come into contact with pregnant women should be tested for rubella antibodies. It has been recommended that such personnel have proof of prior rubella infection or immunization before being allowed to work in areas where contact with pregnant women is likely. Rubella immunization is especially recommended for susceptible female employees of childbearing age who are practicing effective contraception. The availability of improved influenza vaccines makes it rational to recommend annual immunization for all hospital personnel.

Hospital personnel who develop significant infectious diseases should be removed from patient contact during the period of communicability. The dangers of paronychias and other postular lesions due to *S. aureus* or group A streptococci are often underestimated by the staff, and it is commonly forgotten that susceptible contacts may develop chickenpox following exposure to patients or personnel with herpes zoster.

ADMISSION SCREENING A patient scheduled for elective admission who has, or is thought to be incubating, a communicable disease should not be admitted until the period of communicability has passed. Screening on admission for communicable infections is particularly important for patients being admitted to oncology and transplant services where there may be a concentration of immunocompromised patients. Infections usually considered to be of minor importance, such as chickenpox or measles, can be devastating in such patients, and their spread is to be avoided at all costs.

CONTAINMENT Microorganisms can spread from one person to another by several routes: (1) contact, either directly from person to person or indirectly via contaminated equipment such as bed linens; (2) airborne via infected droplet nuclei that produce infectious particles of respirable size; (3) vehicles such as contaminated food, water, injectable drugs, or blood; and (4) vectors, such as insects.

Each pathogen has its characteristic mode(s) of spread, and, on the basis of this knowledge, isolation precautions can be tailored to fit the situation. Isolation procedures are time-consuming and expensive and can hinder essential patient care activities if applied too rigidly. They should be used only when necessary and for the shortest period consistent with good medical practice.

The following types of isolation and precautions are in common use:

1 *Strict isolation,* where both airborne and contact transmission of an organism are possible, e.g., staphylococcal pneumonia
2 *Respiratory isolation,* where the infectious agent is contained in airborne droplets of respirable size, e.g., tuberculosis
3 *Wound and skin precautions,* where direct or indirect contact with infected skin lesions or dressings may transmit the organism, e.g., a staphylococcal wound infection
4 *Enteric precautions,* where transmission usually occurs via the fecal-oral route and where contact with articles contaminated by feces is to be avoided, e.g., hepatitis A
5 *Protective (reverse) isolation,* where the precautions are designed to protect an unusually susceptible patient with impaired host defenses from organisms in the environment, e.g., patients with burns or with significant granulocytopenia
6 *Blood precautions,* where transmission is by accidental inoculation or ingestion of blood or blood products, e.g., hepatitis B
7 *Resistant-organism precautions,* where precautions are designed to reduce the spread of multiply resistant bacteria to other patients and the hospital environment

If preventive measures fail and a communicable infection develops in an inpatient, the following principles of containment should be observed:

1 Prevent further transmission of disease by the index case by either isolating the patient or, if the patient's condition allows, arranging for discharge from the hospital.
2 Identify all contacts of the index case and determine their susceptibility and degree of exposure.
3 If prophylactic measures are available, administer them appropriately to exposed susceptible individuals.
4 Design a plan to prevent the spread of the infectious agent from the exposed susceptibles to other patients and personnel. This plan must recognize the epidemiology of the communicable disease in question, the effectiveness and feasibility of various control measures, and the potential consequences of further disease transmission.

Methods commonly employed to limit the tertiary spread of communicable diseases by exposed susceptibles are (1) early discharge of patients when feasible, (2) arranging personnel assignments to avoid patient contact during the period of communicability, and (3) cohorting exposed susceptible patients and personnel together and treating them as an epidemiologic unit. Although cohorting is cumbersome, it remains a major measure for control of hospital outbreaks of chickenpox and epidemic diarrhea.

PROGNOSIS Most nosocomial infections are diseases of medical progress, and the ever-increasing orientation of modern medicine to technologically sophisticated procedures, both diagnostic and therapeutic, makes it likely that the risk of patients acquiring infections in the hospital will continue to increase. On the other hand, many of the factors that promote infections in the hospital have been identified, and measures for their control have been developed. Influencing hospital personnel to carry out these control measures, such as hand washing, catheter care, and restraint in the use of antibiotics, remains a major challenge.

REFERENCES

AMERICAN COLLEGE OF SURGEONS: *Manual of Control of Infections in Surgical Patients.* Philadelphia, Lippincott, 1976

BENENSON AS (ed): *Control of Communicable Diseases in Man,* 12th ed. Washington, DC, American Public Health Association, 1975

BENNETT JV, BRACHMAN PS: *Nosocomial Infections.* Boston, Little, Brown, 1978

CENTERS FOR DISEASE CONTROL: *Guidelines for Prevention and Control of Nosocomial Infections.* Springfield, Va., National Technical Information Service, 1981

DIXON RE (ed): Symposium on nosocomial infection. Am J Med 70:379, 631, 899, 1981

GOLDMAN DA et al: Guidelines for infection control in intravenous therapy. Ann Intern Med 79:848, 1973

O'BRIEN TF et al: Dissemination of an antibiotic resistance plasmid in hospital patient flora. Antimicrob Agents Chemother 17:537, 1980

SNYDMAN DR et al: Prevention of nosocomial viral hepatitis, type B. Ann Intern Med 83:838, 1975

STAMM WE: Guidelines for prevention of catheter related urinary tract infections. Ann Intern Med 82:386, 1975

TIPPLE MA, GARDNER P: Control of infections in the pediatric hospital, in *Textbook of Pediatric Infectious Diseases,* RD Feigin, JD Cherry (eds). Philadelphia, Saunders, 1981

139
GRAM-NEGATIVE BACTEREMIA AND SEPTIC SHOCK

DAVID C. DALE
ROBERT G. PETERSDORF

DEFINITION Septic shock is characterized by inadequate tissue perfusion, usually following bacteremia with gram-negative enteric bacilli. Hypotension, oliguria, tachycardia, tachypnea, and fever are observed in most patients. The circulatory insufficiency is due to diffuse cell and tissue injury and the pooling of blood in the microcirculation.

ETIOLOGY Septic shock may be associated with gram-positive infections, notably those due to pneumococci and streptococci, although it is more common following gram-negative bacteremia. The most frequently causative organisms are: *Escherichia coli, Klebsiella-Enterobacter, Pseudomonas,* and *Serratia.* Gram-negative anaerobic bacteremia with *Bacteroides* spp. is also a precursor of septic shock, although in this situation the syndrome is less fulminating than with aerobic gram-negative bacilli. In gram-negative bacteremia, the shock syndrome is not due to bloodstream invasion with bacteria per se but is related to release of endotoxin, the lipopolysaccharide moiety of the organisms' cell walls, into the circulation.

EPIDEMIOLOGY Gram-negative bacteremia and septic shock occur primarily in hospitalized patients who usually have underlying diseases which render them susceptible to bloodstream invasion. Predisposing factors include diabetes mellitus; cirrhosis; leukemia, lymphoma, or disseminated carcinoma; transplantation and its associated immunosuppression; childbirth; and a variety of surgical procedures and antecedent infections in the urinary, biliary, or gastrointestinal tracts. Neonates, childbearing women, and elderly men with prostatic obstruction are prone to develop this syndrome. The incidence of gram-negative bacteremic sepsis is increasing, and it is now as high as 12 cases per 1000 admissions in some large urban hospitals. In addition to the predisposing factors mentioned above, the widespread use of antibiotics, immunosuppressive and cytotoxic agents, adrenal steroids, intravenous catheters, humidifiers and other hospital equipment, and the increasing longevity of patients with chronic diseases contribute to this serious problem (see Chaps. 137 and 138).

PATHOGENESIS AND PATHOLOGY Most of the bacteria causing gram-negative sepsis are normal commensals in the gastrointestinal tract. From there they may spread to contiguous structures, as in peritonitis after appendiceal perforation, or they may migrate from the perineum into the urethra or bladder. Gram-negative bacteremia follows infection in a primary focus, usually the genitourinary tract; biliary tree; gastrointestinal tract or lungs; and, less commonly, the skin, bones, and joints. In burn patients and in patients with leukemia, the skin or the lungs are often portals of entry. In many instances, however, notably in patients with debilitating diseases, cirrhosis, and cancer, no primary focus is apparent. When bacteremia is followed by metastatic lesions in distant sites, classic abscess formation occurs. More often, however, the autopsy findings in gram-negative sepsis reflect primarily the infection at the primary locus and show involvement of target organs: pulmonary edema, hemorrhage, and hyaline membrane formation in the lungs; tubular or cortical necrosis in the kidney; patchy necrosis in the myocardium; superficial ulceration in the gastrointestinal tract; and generalized thrombi in the capillaries.

PATHOPHYSIOLOGY **Cellular injury in shock** Exposure of mammalian cells to endotoxin results in cell injury by several mechanisms: (1) direct cell membrane damage by endotoxin, (2) extracellular release of lysosomal enzymes from leukocytes, (3) activation of the complement cascade, and (4) metabolic injury due to tissue anoxia. The toxic component of endotoxin is principally lipid A. When endotoxin is administered to experimental animals, diffuse endothelial cell damage occurs. The cells show vacuolization and other cytoplasmic and nuclear abnormalities. There is diffuse desquamation of the endothelial cells, and the damaged cells often can be seen in the circulating blood. Endotoxin administration also causes an abrupt thrombocytopenia and granulocytopenia. The damaged endothelial cells, leukocytes, and platelets all release substances activating blood coagulation, which leads to fibrin deposition in many tissues. The damaged platelets release the vasoactive substances serotonin, epinephrine, and thromboxanes. Polymorphonuclear leukocyte injury releases a variety of lysosomal enzymes, cytotoxic products of molecular oxygen, and arachidonic acid derivatives, as well as substances activating the complement system; the complement system is also activated directly by endotoxin, chiefly through the alternate complement pathway (see Chap. 63).

Animal studies suggest a number of interactions between the complement system and the changes in platelets and leukocytes. Animals depleted of complement by pretreatment with cobra venom factor, which depletes C3 and later complement components, are less prone to develop thrombocytopenia and granulocytopenia after endotoxin than normal animals. Activation of complement in the circulation by endotoxin, specifically the component C5a, appears to increase granulocyte margination and to enhance the extracellular release of granulocyte enzymes. Diffuse pulmonary injury, the "shock lung," may occur by this mechanism.

Cells in many tissues are also injured by the hypoxia that results from reduced tissue perfusion in endotoxic shock. The tissue injury closely resembles that occurring in hemorrhagic and cardiogenic shock. The result of hypoxia is uncoupling of oxidative phosphorylation and lactic acidosis.

Hemodynamic alterations Endotoxin exerts its major effects on small blood vessels with sympathetic (alpha-receptor) innervation. The toxin causes intense arteriolar and venospasm leading to significant immobilization of blood in the pulmonary, splanchnic, and renal capillaries, and to stagnant anoxia in these tissues. Through the activation of Hageman factor (factor XII), endotoxin activates bradykinin, a potent vasodilator which may be the humoral substance principally responsible for the pooling of blood in the peripheral tissues. It also increases capillary permeability.

An important role for arachidonic acid derivatives and the endorphins in the hemodynamic changes in septic shock is suggested in several recent experiments. Animals deficient in essential fatty acids, the precursors of arachidonic acid, are resistant to the lethal effects of endotoxin. Animals pretreated with the thromboxane synthesis inhibitor, imidazole, which blocks formation of thromboxane A_2, a potent vasoconstrictor, also are protected from endotoxin's lethal effects. Infusion of prostacyclin, a thromboxane A_2 antagonist, after endotoxin has this same benefit. Both imidazole and prostacyclin prevent platelet aggregation, interrupt intravascular coagulation, and normalize blood pressure in experimental endotoxic shock. A role for the endorphins in causing septic shock is suggested from the finding that naloxone, an endorphin antagonist, corrects hypotension and improves survival in endotoxin-treated animals.

Early in the development of shock, blood pools in the capillary bed and plasma proteins leak into the interstitial fluid. This, in turn, results in a sharp decrease in effective circulating blood volume, lowered cardiac output, and systemic arterial hypotension. Further sympathetic activity, vasoconstriction, and selective reduction of blood flow to visceral organs and skin follow. If ineffective perfusion of vital organs is permitted to continue, metabolic acidosis and severe parenchymal damage ensue, and shock is then irreversible. In humans, the kidneys and lungs are the organs particularly susceptible to endotoxin; oliguria as well as tachypnea and, in some instances, pulmonary edema develop early. In general, the heart and brain are spared early in shock, and myocardial failure and coma are late and often terminal manifestations of the shock syndrome. There is also experimental evidence that, after the administration of live gram-negative bacteria, significant arteriovenous shunting occurs around the capillary beds of susceptible organs. This intensifies tissue anoxia. Finally, in some instances the cells seem unable to utilize available oxygen. The net result of defective tissue perfusion is a sharp decrease in arteriovenous (AV) oxygen difference and lactic acidemia.

Early in septic shock, the picture is usually one primarily of vasodilatation with an increase in cardiac output, a decrease in systemic vascular resistance, a decrease in central venous pressure, and an increase in stroke volume. In contrast, later in septic shock, the predominant picture is one of vasoconstriction with an increase in systemic vascular resistance, a decrease in cardiac output, a decrease in central venous pressure, and a decrease in stroke volume. The study of large groups of patients with septic shock has revealed certain patterns of clinical and laboratory abnormalities. These may be summarized as follows:

1 Shock characterized by a normal cardiac output, normal blood volume, normal circulation time, normal or high central venous pressure, normal or high pH, and *reduced* peripheral resistance. These patients have warm, dry skin. While hypotension, oliguria, and lactic acidemia are present, the prognosis is generally good. Shock in this group has been attributed to shunting of blood through arteriovenous communications, making it unavailable for perfusion of vital organs.

2 Patients with low blood volume, low central venous pressure, high hematocrit, increased peripheral resistance, low cardiac output, hypotension, oliguria, but only a moderate elevation of blood lactate and normal or slightly high pH. These patients may be hypovolemic before bacteremia, and their prognosis is reasonably good, provided intravascular volume is restored, bacteremia is treated with appropriate antibiotics, septic foci are removed or drained, and vasoactive drugs are given.

3 Shock characterized by normal blood volume, high central venous pressure, normal or high cardiac output, reduced peripheral resistance but *marked metabolic acidosis,* oliguria, and very high blood lactate, indicating ineffective tissue perfusion or impaired oxygen utilization. Despite the presence of warm, dry extremities in these patients, the prognosis is unfavorable.

4 Shock characterized by low blood volume, low central venous pressure, low cardiac output, marked decompensated metabolic acidosis, and severe lactic acidemia. In these patients the extremities are cool and cyanotic. The prognosis is extremely poor.

These observations suggest that there are various stages of septic shock, from hyperventilation, respiratory alkalosis, vasodilatation, and high or normal cardiac output in early shock, to perfusion failure characterized by high-grade lactic acidemia, metabolic acidosis, low cardiac output, and small AV oxygen difference in irreversible, late shock. Moreover, in some patients there is little correlation between the outcome and the hemodynamic abnormalities.

COMPLICATIONS Coagulation defects In most patients with septic shock there is a deficiency in several clotting factors, due to consumption of these factors, a syndrome termed *disseminated intravascular coagulation* (DIC). The pathogenesis of this syndrome involves the activation of the intrinsic clotting system by factor XII (Hageman factor) followed by deposition of fibrin-platelet aggregates on the capillary thrombi that have formed as a result of the generalized Shwartzman reaction. The fibrin-platelet aggregates are typical of DIC, which is characterized by a decrease in factors II, V, and VIII, fibrinogen, and platelets. There may be some degree of fibrinolysis, with appearance of split products. These clotting abnormalities are present to some degree in most patients with septic shock, but usually there is no clinical bleeding, although hemorrhagic phenomena due to thrombocytopenia or deficiency in clotting factors occur occasionally. A more important effect of further disseminated intravascular coagulation is development of capillary thrombi, particularly in the lung. Unless there is bleeding, the coagulopathy requires no therapy and disappears spontaneously as shock is treated.

Respiratory failure Respiratory failure is the most important cause of death in patients with shock, particularly after the hemodynamic aberrations have been corrected. The respiratory lesion has been called the "shock lung" and is characterized by pulmonary edema, hemorrhage, atelectasis, hyaline membrane formation, and formation of capillary thrombi. The severe pulmonary edema may be a consequence of a marked increase in capillary permeability, resulting in a "pulmonary leak." It may occur in the absence of heart failure. Respiratory failure may develop and progress even as other abnormalities return to normal. Pulmonary surfactant decreases, and pulmonary compliance becomes progressively compromised.

Renal failure Oliguria occurs early in shock and is probably due to low intravascular volume and inadequate renal perfusion. If renal perfusion remains inadequate, acute tubular necrosis develops. In an occasional patient, renal cortical necrosis, as occurs in the generalized Shwartzman reaction, is seen.

Cardiac failure Many patients with septic shock develop myocardial failure even though they were free of heart disease before development of shock. On the basis of experimental data, heart failure has been attributed to a product of lysosomal enzyme activity in the ischemic splanchnic region. This product has been termed myocardial depressant factor (MDF). Functionally, there is left ventricular failure as indicated by an increase in left ventricular end-diastolic pressure.

Other organs Superficial ulcerations of the gastrointestinal tract manifested by hemorrhage are common, as are abnormalities in liver function, characterized by hypoprothrombinemia, hypoalbuminemia, and mild jaundice.

CLINICAL MANIFESTATIONS Usually gram-negative bacteremia begins abruptly with chills, fever, nausea, vomiting, diarrhea, and prostration. When septic shock develops, there are, in addition, tachycardia; tachypnea; hypotension; cool, pale extremities, often with peripheral cyanosis; mental obtundation; and oliguria. When present in its full-blown form, gram-negative shock is detected readily, but occasionally the findings are quite subtle, particularly in old, debilitated patients or in infants. Unexplained hypotension, increasing confusion, and disorientation or hyperventilation may be the only clues to septic shock. Some patients are hypothermic, and in the absence of fever the diagnosis is often missed. Jaundice occurs occasionally and signifies infection in the biliary tree, intravascular hemolysis, or "toxic" hepatitis. As shock progresses, oliguria persists, and heart failure, respiratory insufficiency, and coma supervene. Death usually occurs from pulmonary edema, generalized anoxemia secondary to respiratory insufficiency, cardiac arrhythmias, disseminated intravascular coagulation with bleeding, cerebral anoxia, or a combination of these factors.

LABORATORY FINDINGS The laboratory data in septic shock vary greatly and depend in many instances on the cause of the shock syndrome and on the stage of shock. The hematocrit is often elevated and falls to below normal as the volume deficit is repaired. There usually is *leukocytosis* with a white blood cell count between 15,000 and 30,000 per cubic millimeter with a shift to the left. However, the white blood cell count may be normal, and some patients have leukopenia. The *platelet count* is usually decreased, and the prothrombin time and partial thromboplastin times may be abnormal, reflecting a consumption of *clotting factors.*

The *urinalysis* shows no specific abnormalities. Initially, the specific gravity is high; as oliguria persists, isosthenuria develops. The *blood urea nitrogen* and *creatinine* are elevated, and creatinine clearance is reduced.

Simultaneous measurements of urine and plasma osmolalities are a useful clue to impending renal failure. If the urinary osmolality is greater than 400 mosmol and the ratio of urine to plasma osmolality is greater than 1.5, renal function is preserved and oliguria is probably due to volume depletion. On the other hand, a urine osmolality of less than 400 mosmol and a urine/plasma ratio less than 1.5 signify renal failure. Other useful clues to suggest prerenal azotemia are urine sodium less than 20 meq per liter, a urine creatinine/serum creatinine ratio greater than 40, or a BUN/serum creatinine ratio greater than 20. Electrolyte patterns vary considerably, but there is a tendency to *hyponatremia* and hypochloremia. The serum potassium may be high, low, or normal. The *bicarbonate concentration* is usually low and *blood lactate* is elevated. A low blood pH and high level of blood lactate are the most reliable clues to poor tissue perfusion.

Early in endotoxin shock there is *respiratory alkalosis* manifested by a low P_{CO_2} and high arterial pH, probably because of progressive anoxemia and an attempt to blow off CO_2 to compensate for developing lactic acidemia. As shock progresses, *metabolic acidosis* develops. There often is striking *anoxemia,* and P_{O_2} values below 70 mmHg are common. The *electrocardiogram* generally shows depression of the ST segment, inversion of the T waves, and a variety of arrhythmias, and may mistakenly suggest the diagnosis of myocardial infarction.

In untreated septic shock, the blood cultures should reveal the causative pathogens, but bacteremia may be intermittent and the blood cultures may be negative. Furthermore, many patients will have received antimicrobial agents when they are first seen, masking the bacteriologic diagnosis. *A negative blood culture does not exclude the diagnosis of septic shock.* Culture of the primary septic focus may aid in the diagnosis, but the bacteriology may have been altered by prior chemotherapy. The ability of endotoxin to coagulate the blood of the horseshoe crab *Limulus* is the basis of a test for endotoxemia, but this test is not widely available and is of limited clinical usefulness.

DIAGNOSIS The diagnosis of septic shock is not difficult in the presence of chills, fever, and an overt focus of infection. However, none of the obvious clues may be present. Elderly, debilitated patients, in particular, may have severe infections in the absence of fever. Unexplained confusion and disorientation and hyperventilation without abnormal chest x-rays should call the diagnosis to mind. Pulmonary embolism, myocardial infarction, cardiac tamponade, aortic dissection, and silent hemorrhage are entities often confused with septic shock.

COURSE The rational treatment of septic shock depends upon careful monitoring of patients. A flow sheet for recording clinical data is very helpful. Specifically four parameters need to be followed at the bedside:

1 The status of the *pulmonary circulation* and, to a lesser extent, of left ventricular function should be monitored by insertion of a Swan-Ganz catheter. A pulmonary wedge pressure in excess of 15 to 18 cmH_2O signifies fluid overload. When a Swan-Ganz catheter is not available, the *central venous pressure* (CVP) should be measured. Insertion of a catheter into the great veins or right atrium provides an accurate index of the relation between right ventricular competence and effective blood volume and should be used as a guide to fluid replacement therapy. When the CVP exceeds 12 to 14 cmH_2O, there is some danger of overloading the circulation and precipitating pulmonary edema. It is important to be sure that the flow through the catheter is free and that the catheter is not in the right ventricle. Either a Swan-Ganz catheter or a CVP line should be placed in every patient with septic shock.

2 The *pulse pressure* serves as an estimate of stroke volume.

3 *Cutaneous vasoconstriction* provides a clue to peripheral resistance, although it does not reflect accurately blood flow to kidney, brain, or gut.

4 Hourly *urine output* should be used to monitor splanchnic blood flow and visceral perfusion. Usually this requires placement of an indwelling urethral catheter.

By means of these four measurements the patient with shock can be followed carefully and managed intelligently. Indirect arterial blood pressure does not provide an accurate picture of the hemodynamic situation, and perfusion of vital organs may be adequate in patients with hypotension; conversely, some patients with normal blood pressures may have marked pooling and inadequate visceral blood flow. Direct measurement of arterial pressure is helpful but usually not necessary.

Where possible, these patients should be treated in intensive care units in hospitals that have laboratories available for measurement of arterial pH, blood gases, blood lactate, renal function, and electrolytes.

TREATMENT **Support of respiration** In many patients with septic shock arterial P_{O_2} is markedly depressed. It is essential to establish an airway at the outset and to administer oxygen nasally or by mask. Tracheal intubation usually suffices; tracheostomy is rarely necessary. However, a positive pressure–volume-cycled respirator should be employed early to achieve proper ventilation and to overcome the severe hypoxia.

Volume replacement With the CVP or pulmonary wedge pressure as a guide, blood volume should be replaced with blood (if anemia is present), plasma, or other colloids, especially human serum albumin, and appropriate electrolyte solutions, primarily dextrose-saline and bicarbonate (which is preferable to lactate for treating the acidosis). Bicarbonate should be given to increase the blood pH to about 7.2 to 7.3 but not higher under most circumstances. The quantity of fluid required may be considerably in excess of "normal" blood volume and may amount to 8 to 12 liters in only a few hours. Large quantities may be required even when the cardiac index is normal. *Oliguria in the presence of hypotension is not a contraindication to continued vigorous fluid therapy.* In order to guard against pulmonary edema, diuresis with furosemide should be attempted when the CVP reaches a level of approximately 10 to 12 cmH_2O and the pulmonary artery pressure 16 to 18 cmH_2O.

Antibiotics Blood cultures and cultures of relevant body fluids or exudates should be taken before instituting antimicrobial therapy. Drugs should be given intravenously, and bactericidal agents used when possible. When the results of blood cultures and sensitivities are known, one of the appropriate drugs recommended in the chapters dealing with the specific infections and discussed in Chap. 141 should be given. Usually cultures and sensitivities are not at hand at the onset of shock, and the etiologic diagnosis entails an educated guess based upon culture from the primary focus—urine, bile, pus, or sputum, or on the setting in which the infection occurs. For example, a young woman with dysuria, chills, and flank pain and septic shock is likely to have *Escherichia coli* bacteremia, while gram-negative sepsis in a burn patient is probably caused by *Pseudomonas.* The drugs of choice for gram-negative bacteremia are:

E. coli	Ampicillin or a parenteral cephalosporin
Klebsiella-Enterobacter	Gentamicin or tobramycin
Proteus mirabilis	Ampicillin or a parenteral cephalosporin
P. rettgeri, morganii, or *vulgaris*	Gentamicin, tobramycin, amikacin, and/or carbenicillin
Acinetobacter	Gentamicin, tobramycin, amikacin, and/or carbenicillin
Pseudomonas	Gentamicin, tobramycin, amikacin, and/or carbenicillin

The dosages and routes of administration for these agents are detailed in Chap. 141. A cephalosporin can be substituted for ampicillin in patients with a history of penicillin allergy. Because of their toxic effect on the vestibular portion of the eighth nerve, the aminoglycosides must be given cautiously to oliguric patients.

When the cause of septic shock is unknown, therapy should be initiated with both gentamicin (or tobramycin) and a cephalosporin or a penicillinase-resistant penicillin; many physicians add carbenicillin to this regimen. If *Bacteroides* is suspected, chloramphenicol, 7-chlorlincomycin (clindamycin), or carbenicillin can be added. As soon as culture results become available, the unnecessary drugs can be deleted.

Surgical intervention Many patients with septic shock have an abscess, infarcted or necrotic bowel, inflamed gallbladder, infected uterus, pyonephrosis, or other local situations which lend themselves to surgical drainage or excision. As a rule, successful treatment of shock requires surgical intervention even if the patient is desperately ill. Operations should not be postponed "to get the patient in shape" because these patients' condition will continue to deteriorate unless the septic focus is removed or drained.

Vasoactive drugs Usually, septic shock is accompanied by maximal stimulation of alpha-adrenergic receptors, and pressor agents which act by stimulating these receptors, such as norepinephrine, levarterenol, and metaraminol are generally not indicated. The two groups of drugs which have been of value in septic shock are beta-receptor stimulants (notably isoproterenol and dopamine) and alpha-receptor blocking agents (phenoxybenzamine and phentolamine).

Dopamine hydrochloride is used widely for treatment of shock. Unlike other vasoactive agents, this drug increases renal blood flow and with it glomerular filtration, sodium excretion, and urine flow. This effect is seen at low doses [1 to 2 (μg/kg)/min]. At a dose of 2 to 10 (μg/kg)/min, the beta receptors in the heart are stimulated with a resulting increase in cardiac output but without increase in heart rate or blood pressure. Between 10 and 20 (μg/kg)/min there is some effect on the alpha receptors with a rise in blood pressure. Above 20 (μg/kg)/min, alpha stimulation predominates, and vasoconstriction may reverse the dopaminergic effects on the renal and splanchnic circulations. Treatment should be started at 2 to 5 (μg/kg)/min and the dose increased until urine flow and blood pressure respond. Most patients respond to doses of 20 (μg/kg)/min or less. Side effects include ectopic rhythms, nausea and vomiting, and occasionally tachyarrhythmias. They usually disappear with reduction in dosage.

Isoproterenol (Isuprel) counteracts arteriolar and venous constriction in the microcirculation by its direct vasodilating effect. In addition, the drug exerts a direct inotropic effect on the heart. Cardiac output is increased by stimulation of the myocardium and by reduction of cardiac work as peripheral resistance decreases. The dose of isoproterenol is 2 to 8 μg/min for the average adult. Ventricular arrhythmias may result from this drug, and shock may be made worse if fluid administration does not keep pace with relieved vasoconstriction.

Phenoxybenzamine (Dibenzyline), an adrenolytic agent, effects a central phlebotomy by reducing resistance and increasing intravascular capacity. Hence there is a redistribution of blood. Blood leaves the lungs, relieving pulmonary edema and enhancing gas exchange. Central venous pressure and left ventricular end-diastolic pressure fall, cardiac output rises, and peripheral venous constriction regresses. The recommended dose is 0.2 to 2.0 mg/kg intravenously. Small doses can be injected instantaneously and large doses over a period of 40 to 60 min. Fluids must be given simultaneously to compensate for the increment in venous capacitance; failure to do so aggravates shock. Phenoxybenzamine[1] is not available for general use, and experience with phentolamine has not been great enough to recommend it.

Diuretics and digitalis It is important to maintain urine flow to try to prevent the development of renal tubular necrosis. Once the volume status of the patient is repaired, a diuretic, preferably furosemide, should be given to keep the hourly urine output up to greater than 30 to 40 ml/h. In patients who remain hypotensive despite an elevated CVP or pulmonary wedge pressure, digoxin may be beneficial but should be given cautiously because of the frequent occurrence of acid-base abnormalities, hyperkalemia, and impaired renal function in shock patients.

Glucocorticosteroids Numerous experimental studies provide a rationale for the use of corticosteroid therapy to ameliorate the effects of endotoxemia and septic shock. Steroids appear to protect cell membranes from endotoxin-mediated injury, to prevent transformation of arachidonic acid to its vasoactive derivatives, to decrease platelet aggregation, and to reduce the extracellular release of leukocyte enzymes. Some studies suggest that steroids also may have a direct effect on reducing peripheral vascular resistance. Because of the complexity of the clinical circumstances surrounding the patient with endotoxic shock, it has been difficult to prove that steroid therapy is clearly helpful. One controlled study has demonstrated a substantial benefit for treating patients with methylprednisolone (30 mg/kg) or dexamethasone (3 mg/kg) as soon as shock was recognized. Therapy was repeated in 4 h in the most severely ill patients. This study and experience in many shock centers support the early use of steroids in high doses for relatively brief periods (24 to 48 h), but many experts regard the data as unconvincing.[2] Prolonged steroid therapy substantially increases the problems of hyperglycemia, gastrointestinal bleeding, and other steroid side effects and should be avoided.

Other measures Hemorrhage must be controlled with whole blood, fresh frozen plasma, cryoprecipitate, or platelet transfusion, depending on the clotting abnormality. The use of naloxone, prostaglandin synthesis inhibitors, and prostacyclin is still experimental. Treatment of disseminated intravascular coagulation with heparin remains a controversial and hazardous procedure. Hyperbaric oxygen has been tried in gram-negative bacteremia with indifferent results.

[1] *This drug has not been approved for this purpose by the Food and Drug Administration at the time of publication.*
[2] *This drug is not approved for this purpose by the Food and Drug Administration at the time of publication.*

PROGNOSIS The measures described above usually will resuscitate most patients, at least temporarily. Indicators of a favorable response are:

1 Improved sensorium and general appearance
2 Decreased peripheral cyanosis
3 Warming of the skin over the extremities
4 Urine output of 40 to 50 ml/h
5 Increased pulse pressure
6 Return of CVP and pulmonary artery pressure to normal
7 Increased blood pressure

The ultimate outcome, however, is dependent upon several other factors:

1 Ability to eliminate the source of infection with surgery or antibiotics. The prognosis of urinary tract infections, septic abortions, abdominal abscesses, gastrointestinal or biliary fistulas, and subcutaneous or anorectal abscesses is better than that of primary foci in the skin or lungs. However, extensive abdominal surgery, even if necessary, is associated with a poor prognosis.
2 Previous contact with the organism. Patients with chronic urinary tract infections who develop bacteremia rarely have severe gram-negative shock, perhaps because they have become tolerant to the endotoxin.
3 Underlying disease. Patients with lymphoma or leukemia who develop septic shock while their hematologic disease is out of control rarely recover; conversely, if hematologic remission is achieved, the shock is more likely to respond to therapy. Patients with antecedent heart disease and with diabetes mellitus also have a poor prognosis.
4 Metabolic status. The development of severe metabolic acidosis and lactic acidemia—irrespective of cardiac output—is associated with a poor prognosis.
5 Development of pulmonary insufficiency even after the hemodynamic abnormalities have been corrected is associated with an unfavorable outcome.

The overall mortality rate of septic shock remains 50 percent; however, with better monitoring and more physiologic treatment, the outcome should improve.

PREVENTION The poor results in the treatment of septic shock are not due to lack of potent antibiotics or vasoactive agents. Rather, failure to institute therapy sufficiently early is a major roadblock to success. Septic shock usually is recognized too late, all too often after irreversible changes have taken place. Because 70 percent of patients who are likely to develop septic shock are in the hospital *before* signs and symptoms of shock appear, it is essential to watch patients who are candidates for development of shock assiduously, to treat their infections vigorously and early, and to perform appropriate surgery before catastrophic complications occur. It is particularly important to watch for infected venous and urinary catheters which may act as portals of entry for the organisms that cause gram-negative sepsis and to remove them from all patients as soon as feasible. There is some preliminary evidence that early therapy of septic shock improves the ultimate outcome. Finally, the protective effect of antiserum in experimental animals may, at some time in the future, be applicable to humans.

REFERENCES

FADEN AI, HOLADAY JW: Experimental endotoxin shock: The pathophysiologic function of endorphins and treatment with opiate antagonists. J Infect Dis 142:229, 1980

FEARON DT et al: Activation of properdin pathway of complement in patients with gram-negative bacteremia. N Engl J Med 292:937, 1975

HARDAWAY RM III: Treatment of severe shock with phenoxybenzamine. Surg Gynecol Obstet 151:725, 1980

KRAUSZ MM et al: Prostacyclin reversal of lethal endotoxemia in dogs. J Clin Invest 67:1118, 1981

KREGER BE et al: Gram-negative bacteremia. III. Reassessment of etiology, epidemiology and ecology in 612 patients. Am J Med 68:332, 1980

———: Gram-negative bacteremia. IV. Re-evaluation of clinical features and treatment in 612 patients. Am J Med 68:344, 1980

LOVE LJ et al: Improved prognosis for granulocytopenic patients with gram-negative bacteremia. Am J Med 68:643, 1980

MACLEAN LD et al: Patterns of septic shock in man: A detailed study of 56 patients. Ann Surg 166:543, 1967

MILLER RI et al: Biochemical mechanisms of generation of bradykinin by endotoxin. J Infect Dis 128:S144, 1973

NISHIJIMA H et al: Hemodynamic and metabolic studies in shock associated with gram-negative bacteremia. Medicine 42:287, 1973

PETERS WP et al: Pressor effect of naloxone in septic shock. Lancet 1:529, 1981

ROBINSON JA et al: Endotoxin, prekallikrein, complement and systemic vascular resistance. Am J Med 49:61, 1975

SCHUMER W: Steroids in the treatment of clinical septic shock. Ann Surg 184:333, 1976

SHEAGREN JN: Septic shock and corticosteroids. N Engl J Med 305:456, 1981

SHINE KI et al: Aspects of the management of shock. Ann Intern Med 93:723, 1980

SIBBALD WJ et al: Alveolo-capillary permeability in human septic ARDS: Effect of high-dose corticosteroid therapy. Chest 79:133, 1981.

TARAZI RC: Sympathomimetic agents in the treatment of shock. Ann Intern Med 81:364, 1974

ULEVITCH RJ et al: Role of complement in lethal bacterial lipopolysaccharide-induced hypotensive and coagulative changes. Infect Immun 19:204, 1978

WINSLOW EJ et al: Hemodynamic studies and results of therapy in 50 patients with bacteremic shock. Am J Med 54:421, 1973

WISE WC et al: Protective effects of thromboxane synthetase inhibitors in rats in endotoxic shock. Circ Res 46:854, 1980

140 LOCALIZED INFECTIONS AND ABSCESSES

JAN V. HIRSCHMANN
ROBERT G. PETERSDORF

GENERAL CONSIDERATIONS

In contrast to many bacterial diseases, which can be conveniently described in terms of their specific etiologic pathogens, there are some in which the clinical picture is determined primarily by their location. Examples of such infections include abscesses, soft-tissue infections, bacterial endocarditis (see Chap. 259), pyogenic infections of the central nervous system (see Chap. 359), urinary tract infections (see Chap. 296), lung abscess (see Chap. 276), mediastinitis (see Chap. 285), appendicitis and appendiceal abscess (see Chap. 312), diverticulitis (see Chap. 310), osteomyelitis (see Chap. 344), and infections of the pericardium (see Chap. 265). Infections in these sites can be caused by many pathogens, and although their bacteriologic identification may be time-consuming, knowledge of the usual flora causing infection in certain anatomic loci should permit institution of therapy before the results of cultures are available. Although treatment of these infections is usually surgical, the internist may be the first one to see these patients and may also be the one to prescribe chemotherapy on the basis of the presumed pathogen.

ETIOLOGY Localized pyogenic infection can develop in any region or organ of the body, and may be initiated by *trauma* and secondary bacterial contamination, by some *alteration in local conditions* that renders a tissue susceptible to infection with organisms already present as part of the "normal flora" to which it is ordinarily resistant, by *contiguous spread* from a nearby lesion, or by *metastatic implantation* of microorganisms carried in blood or lymph.

Under appropriate conditions of lowered local host defenses, almost any of the common bacteria can initiate an infectious process. Cultures from open lesions such as those of the skin or from intraabdominal foci arising from perforations of the gastrointestinal tract frequently contain several bacterial species; as might be expected, the organisms found most frequently are the "normal flora" of these regions.

Infection in some areas is more likely to be caused by certain organisms, staphylococci in the skin and coliform bacteria in the urinary tract, and special features of the tissue reaction produced by some bacterial species make it possible to recognize infection by them with considerable accuracy. The *staphylococci* produce rapid necrosis and early suppuration with large amounts of creamy yellow pus (see Chap. 147). Group A beta-hemolytic streptococcal infections (see Chap. 148) tend to spread rapidly through tissues, causing intense edema and erythema but relatively little necrosis and thin, serumlike exudate; anaerobic bacteria (see Chap. 173) produce necrosis and profuse, brownish, foul-smelling pus.

The identification of infecting organisms is important in the choice of local or systemic chemotherapy. However, when infection occurs in certain areas, as in paranasal sinuses or cutaneous ulcers, or shows up in sputum, it is unlikely that cultured specimens can ever be rendered sterile. In these locations, serial cultures during antimicrobial administration must be interpreted in this light, and therapy should be guided largely by the clinical response.

PATHOGENESIS Factors predisposing to the initiation and persistence of infection in a tissue include trauma, obstruction of normal drainage (sweat glands, biliary tract, bronchial tree, urinary tract), ischemia (infarction, gangrene), chemical irritation (by gastric contents, bile, or intramuscularly injected drugs), hematoma formation, accumulation of fluid (lymphatic obstruction, cardiac edema), foreign bodies (bullets, splinters, sutures), and others such as the occurrence of stasis or turbulence in the vascular system.

Infection in soft tissue usually begins as a *cellulitis,* a diffuse acute inflammation with hyperemia, edema, and leukocytic infiltration but little or no necrosis and suppuration. With some organisms, this is followed by necrosis, liquefaction, accumulation of leukocytes and debris, suppuration, loculation of the pus, and formation of one or more *abscesses.* Abscess formation is particularly likely to follow infection in a preexisting space or cavity, examples being the fallopian tubes or lung cysts.

The local spread of infection generally follows the path of least resistance along fascial planes; proper surgical treatment is based upon a knowledge of these routes, which will be described for specific infections later in this chapter. Lymphatic spread may lead to lymphangitis, lymphadenitis, or, if the regional nodes suppurate, to the formation of a *bubo.* Involvement of local venules or large veins may lead to infective thrombophlebitis with resulting bacteremia, septic embolization, and systemic dissemination of infection. Staphylococci, streptococci, and *Bacteroides* are notorious for the frequency with which they produce vascular lesions of this type.

Depending upon the infecting organism and the anatomy of the affected region, a small abscess may subside completely; there may be gradual encapsulation of the accumulated pus and persistence of the focus in a quiescent state; or the lesion may "point" and rupture into adjacent tissues or to the outside surface of the body, as usually happens with furuncles. Spontaneous drainage ordinarily leads to subsidence and healing of a superficially situated suppurative focus. However, if the abscess is deeply situated and well encapsulated, there are often persistence of a fistulous tract and the formation of a chronic, draining sinus. *The development of persistent sinuses over an area of suppuration produced by ordinary pyogenic bacteria should always suggest involvement of underlying bone or the presence of a foreign body.* Fistulas that open onto the skin are, of course, soon colonized by microorganisms from the external environment. Ordinary bacterial cultures of drainage fluid almost invariably show a mixed flora and should not be relied upon for the etiologic diagnosis of the underlying disease. This is particularly important in disorders that characteristically lead to persistent sinus formation: tuberculosis, actinomycosis, blastomycosis, melioidosis and glanders, and, rarely, amebic abscess of the liver or cecum. In these situations, superficial organisms about the opening of the sinus tract may mask the true nature of the lesion by obscuring the real pathogen.

MANIFESTATIONS Secondary infection of wounds and cutaneous ulcers is usually recognizable by inspection. Infections of the skin and subcutaneous tissues almost invariably produce the classic manifestations: *redness, tenderness, heat,* and *swelling.* Reddish streaks extending proximally and associated with tender enlargement of regional lymph nodes indicate lymphangitis. Systemic symptoms may be absent or mild, or there may be fever, malaise, prostration, and leukocytosis.

Infection and suppuration in deeper tissues or in body cavities are often manifested by local pain and tenderness, but the task of locating and determining the exact nature of the lesion may be difficult. The palpation of a tender mass is helpful, but muscle spasm and intervening structures often interfere. Abdominal or pelvic examination under anesthesia is sometimes useful in these circumstances.

Auscultation may reveal a friction rub over an abdominal viscus, the pleura, or the pericardium. The rapid development of an effusion in the pericardium, pleura, abdomen, or a joint should suggest infection. Similarly, fluid detected by transillumination of paranasal sinuses or inspection of the tympanic membrane may be the first sign of infection.

Depending on the location of an abscess, symptoms and signs referable to encroachment upon adjacent structures may dominate the picture. Respiratory obstruction may be the first sign of mediastinal abscess; dysphagia often first calls attention to peritonsillar or retropharyngeal abscesses; and tamponade is sometimes the initial clue to pericardial infection. Localizing signs of dysfunction are especially striking and important with brain and spinal cord abscesses, although brain abscesses may be clinically silent (see Chap. 359). In some patients local pain and tenderness or signs of dysfunction are mild or equivocal, and fever, prostration, and weight loss dominate the picture. The fever may be low-grade but is often hectic, with repeated rigors and drenching night sweats. Fatigue and anemia are frequent, and weight loss may be so rapid as to result in emaciation within a few weeks. A patient with these symptoms and signs may have chronic subphrenic, perinephric, or other abscess in the complete absence of any detectable physical sign pointing to the location of a large accumulation of pus. With the advent of antibiotics some deep-seated abscesses present the picture of a chronic illness manifested by no more than malaise, easy fatigability, low-grade fever, mild anemia, and an elevated sedimentation rate because of prior treatment with antimicrobials.

Fluctuation of a mass on palpation is a reliable sign that it contains fluid, perhaps pus, but failure to detect this sign when deeper structures are examined is no guarantee that suppuration is absent and should not be taken by itself to indicate that the mass is noninfectious in origin or that drainage is not required.

LABORATORY FINDINGS Peripheral polymorphonuclear leukocytosis is frequent with abscesses, and significant unexplained elevation of the white blood cell count in any patient should lead to a search for localized suppuration. Depending on the severity and duration of infection, there may be a chronic normocytic, normochromic anemia. The sedimentation rate is almost always rapid. Mild albuminuria, occasionally noted in febrile patients, has no diagnostic import.

Pus or fluid obtained by needle aspiration or incision of a suspected lesion should *always* be stained and examined directly in addition to being cultured aerobically and anaerobically. Pus is a poor metabolic substrate, and bacteria may fail to grow in cultures from an abscess of long standing. In such instances, the findings on microscopic examination may be the only guide in choosing proper chemotherapy. *Failure to examine exudates with Gram's stain is the single greatest deterrent to appropriate antimicrobial therapy;* it is the responsibility of the internist as well as the surgeon to see that this procedure is performed.

Blood cultures are often positive in intravascular infections such as septic thrombophlebitis and endocarditis and in pyogenic infections in which localized abscesses are metastatic, as in staphylococcal, streptococcal, and *Salmonella* bacteremias. Moreover, manipulation, including surgical incision, of any localized infection may be followed by transient bacteremia.

Noninvasive techniques are often helpful in the diagnosis of abscess. X-ray examinations may be of considerable help in detecting localized collections of pus when they show atypical collections of gas, displacement of organs, and tissue densities in abnormal locations. Radionuclide scans may demonstrate abscesses in brain, liver, spleen, and thyroid. The isotope [^{67}Ga] gallium citrate is selectively concentrated in areas of suppuration, but in noninfectious inflammation and neoplasms as well, and many have found gallium scans of limited value in locating abscesses. Scans using ^{111}In-labeled leukocytes may be more accurate. The technique of diagnostic ultrasound is not only useful in localizing abscess but also may provide clues to the size of the abscess and to the presence of multiple abscesses or loculation. Angiography is useful in detecting abscesses in highly vascular organs such as the spleen. Computerized tomography (CT scan) may be helpful in demonstrating abscesses, especially in the brain and in areas not easily evaluated by other methods, such as the retroperitoneum.

THERAPEUTIC CONSIDERATIONS Recognition of the striking symptomatic improvement that follows spontaneous evacuation of a suppurative focus led long ago to the adoption of *surgical incision* for the treatment of abscesses. The exact reasons for the amelioration of local and constitutional manifestations that results from drainage of pus are unknown, but clinically the benefits of adequate incision and drainage are unequivocal.

Incision of infected tissue before the stage of liquefaction and accumulation of pus is often deleterious and fails to relieve discomfort. Premature incision may even at times facilitate spread of infection. For this reason, it is sometimes necessary to wait until an abscess "ripens," i.e., localizes and "comes to a head." The *application of heat* to an area of inflammation will relieve pain and often speed the subsidence of cellulitis without suppuration. If necrosis of tissue is already under way, hot applications appear to facilitate localization of the process and accumulation of pus, making incision and drainage feasible at an earlier time. Another procedure that aids in reduction of swelling and relief of pain is *elevation of the affected part.*

The availability of specific chemotherapeutic drugs has modified the need for heat, elevation, and incision surprisingly little. The early administration of chemotherapeutics has reduced the incidence of suppurative complications in many disorders, but once suppuration has appeared, antimicrobial drugs become remarkably incapable of eradicating the infecting organisms, although they may mask the classic clinical features of abscess formation.

Some antimicrobials, notably the penicillins, appear to retain their antibacterial activity in the presence of pus, while others, exemplified by the aminoglycosides and the polymyxins, are at least partially inactivated in purulent exudates. However, inability of the drug to penetrate into an area of suppuration is rarely the reason for therapeutic failure. Although this possibility exists in some infections, such as osteomyelitis, it is usually overcome by increasing dosage. Because direct instillation of the antibiotic into an infected area is not, by itself, a curative procedure, other factors are probably more important than faulty diffusion of the agent into the purulent focus.

An established inflammatory exudate is a relatively poor environment for bacterial multiplication. Because the bactericidal action of the penicillins and the cephalosporins is exerted only against multiplying organisms, failure of these antibiotics to eradicate bacteria in an abscess may be related to the organisms' inactive metabolic state. Although the mechanism of their antibacterial action differs from that of the penicillins, bacteriostatic agents such as tetracycline or chloramphenicol also are incapable of eradicating bacteria in the static phase of growth. Furthermore, by definition, these drugs only inhibit multiplication of bacteria and usually exert no direct lethal action; the death of organisms in any infection treated with bacteriostatic agents depends on other mechanisms. For most pyogenic bacteria, phagocytosis is one of the most important of these mechanisms (although there must be others that have not been studied so carefully), and, in the absence of phagocytes or in circumstances which inhibit their activity, bacteriostatic drugs are relatively ineffective. In fluid-filled cavities, particularly in the metabolically unfavorable milieu of an abscess, phagocytosis is greatly reduced. Consequently, despite inhibition of bacterial multiplication, organisms can remain dormant and survive for long periods of time. It is probably a combination of these two circumstances, decreased multiplication of bacteria and decreased phagocytosis, that makes infection in the heart valves, in the kidney, or in the meninges so relatively resistant to antimicrobial therapy. Relatively large doses of bactericidal drugs for long periods are needed to achieve cure.

Antimicrobial drugs may be expected to prevent suppuration if given early or to prevent spread of an existing abscess, but cannot be substituted for surgical drainage. Indeed, their use in the face of a lesion requiring evacuation of pus is one of the most common serious errors in treating pyogenic infections.

In empyema, suppurative pericarditis, or pyarthrosis, excellent therapeutic results are sometimes achieved by aspiration of pus and systemic antimicrobial therapy. The success of this procedure, however, depends as fully on the adequacy of drainage as it does upon the administration of the antibiotic, and if there is loculation or if the exudate becomes too viscid to allow removal, surgical incision and drainage through a large-bore tube become mandatory.

In the presence of infective thrombophlebitis, surgical interruption of the veins by ligation or, in some cases, by total excision of an infected segment is sometimes indicated to prevent seeding of other organs by infected emboli.

CLINICAL FEATURES OF INFECTIONS IN VARIOUS REGIONS

SUPERFICIAL ABSCESSES Skin and subcutaneous tissues *Impetigo* is a superficial infection caused by group A hemolytic streptococci, sometimes combined with *Staphylococcus aureus.* It is primarily a disease of children, common in warm weather, characterized by multiple erythematous lesions which vesiculate and are intensely pruritic. In adults impetigo is most commonly an infectious complication of a chronic dermatitis. Local spread occurs through scratching and release of infected vesicle fluid. Serious complications are metastatic abscesses and hemorrhagic nephritis. Treatment consists of local and general cleansing of the skin, appropriate systemic antibiotics, and therapy of any underlying dermatologic condition present.

Deeper infections of the skin are almost invariably staphylococcal in origin and are described in Chap. 147. Erysipelas, a characteristic dermal lesion produced by group A streptococci, is described in Chap. 148.

Lymphadenitis with or without suppuration may complicate any pyogenic skin lesion and is often striking with superficial streptococcal infections. Specific diseases characterized by suppurative regional lymphadenitis include lymphogranuloma venereum (see Chap. 193), cat-scratch disease (see Chap. 214), tularemia (see Chap. 159), and bubonic plague (see Chap. 160).

Infections of the hand These are almost invariably secondary to trauma and are very common. Because of the rapidity with which infection can spread through the complex fascial spaces of the hand, wrist, and forearm, with the production of irreparable functional damage, *any deep infection in this area should receive expert surgical attention immediately.* The importance of such care has in no way been lessened by the availability of antibiotics.

The ordinary *paronychia,* or "run-around," is a superficial infection of the epithelium lateral to a nail, usually a result of tearing a hangnail and most frequently caused by staphylococcus. Hot applications will lead to subsidence of paronychial cellulitis, but often a superficial blister of pus appears. A small incision or simply separation of the nail fold from the nail will promote adequate drainage. If the infection burrows beneath the nail to form a painful *subungual abscess,* incision and drainage with partial or complete removal of the nail are necessary. Recurrence is common, especially in nail biters, and this seemingly trivial infection can cause painful disability. Chronic paronychial inflammation produced by various fungi occurs in diabetics, and a similar lesion is seen in psoriasis and some types of pemphigus.

What appears to be a small furuncle of the webs of the fingers sometimes produces a *collar-button abscess,* consisting of a superficial and deep compartment connected by a narrow tract. Evacuation of the shallow pocket without emptying the deeper abscess can lead to puzzling persistence of infection. Sometimes a foreign-body granuloma forms in the skin of the digital webs. This is most common in barbers, in whom a hair is the core of the foreign-body granuloma, the "barber's interdigital pilonidal sinus."

Infection of the distal phalanx of a finger, usually acquired by pinprick, thorn prick, etc., may lead to the formation of a *felon,* or *whitlow.* This is a suppurative infection in the tightly enclosed fibrous compartments of the finger pulp, the "anterior closed space," which can compromise the distal blood supply by compression of the digital arteries, with consequent necrosis of bone and the development of osteomyelitis. The manifestations are swelling, extreme pain, and tenderness of the palmar surface of the fingertip. The treatment is immediate incision directly over the lesion, sometimes by the use of a trephine, and cutting all the fibrous septa that radiate from the periosteum to the subcutaneous fascia.

Suppurative tenosynovitis, usually a complication of a puncture wound, is an even more serious infection of the hand from the point of view of functional damage; early diagnosis and treatment are mandatory to prevent permanent disability from destruction of the tendon or its sheath. The three cardinal manifestations of tenosynovitis are (1) exquisite tenderness limited to the course of the sheath, (2) flexion of the fingers, and (3) excruciating pain, most marked at the base of the digit, on extension of the involved finger. *Immediate incision* of the sheath is indicated, not only to prevent damage to the tendon itself but to avoid proximal extension of the process into the major fascial spaces of the hand or forearm. Vigorous antibiotic treatment should accompany surgery. The definitive treatment of any serious infection of the hand is a matter for a skilled surgeon, but the early recognition of the need for surgery often falls to other physicians.

Human bites lead to very important hand infections which, if neglected, almost invariably produce a highly destructive, necrotizing lesion contaminated by a mixture of aerobic and anaerobic organisms. A deliberately inflicted bite on the hand or elsewhere is usually recognized as dangerously contaminated, but wounds on the knuckles produced by striking an opponent's teeth with the fists may not be recognized as potentially dangerous. In general, bite wounds should be cleaned thoroughly and not sutured. Patients should be given prophylaxis for tetanus and antibiotics, preferably both a penicillinase-resistant penicillin and ampicillin.

Chronic cutaneous ulcers A partial list of the causes of chronic ulcers of the skin includes circulatory disturbances, such as varicose veins and obliterative arterial disease, extensive injury from frostbite or burns, trophic changes accompanying many neurological disorders, bedsores or decubiti, systemic diseases such as sickle cell disease and myxedema, neoplasms, and various infections. No matter what the underlying disease, secondary infection is very likely to occur and to interfere with healing, complicate grafting or other restorative procedures, or produce extension of the process.

The management of secondary bacterial infection in skin ulcers associated with obliterative arterial disease, a common problem in diabetics, is especially important, because infection is frequently the factor that precipitates spreading gangrene and makes amputation necessary.

Studies of the microflora of chronic cutaneous ulcers have almost invariably shown bacteria of many species, including staphylococci, aerobic and anaerobic streptococci, coliform bacilli, and members of the *Proteus* and *Pseudomonas* groups. Depending on the patient's environment and on systemically or locally administered antimicrobial drugs, the predominating bacterial species show great variation when lesions are cultured serially. Particularly noteworthy is the replacement of sensitive organisms by resistant strains or species during the course of chemotherapy.

Treatment of chronic dermal ulcers should be directed toward the underlying disorder but should also include *local debridement* and *chemotherapy.* Debridement by surgical excision is often needed, but the local application of wet-to-dry dressings or other forms of "medical debridement" frequently suffice. Intensive systemic administration of antibiotics should be carried out only in conjunction with definitive surgical procedures or when infection can be controlled in no other way. The prevention of infection by "prophylactic" administration of antimicrobial drugs is futile because it results in the development of a flora resistant to the drugs being used. The *local application of antibiotics* is sometimes highly effective, and it is in the management of chronic mixed infections of this type that several potent but toxic antibiotics have great value. An ointment or solution containing neomycin, bacitracin, and polymyxin exerts a bactericidal effect against a wide variety of organisms and will sometimes temporarily sterilize a chronic lesion. Other useful topical medications are furacin and 3 percent acetic acid, which is especially helpful in *Pseudomonas* infections.

Diphtheritic ulcer of the skin is discussed in Chap. 165.

INFECTIONS OF THE HEAD AND NECK Pustules of the nose and upper lip may be particularly dangerous, because they are likely to extend intracranially through the angular vein to the cavernous sinus. These lesions should be treated conservatively, manipulation or incision should be avoided if possible, and systemic antibiotics should be used if local swelling or redness appears.

Suppurative parotitis Typically, suppurative parotitis occurs in elderly and chronically ill patients who have a dry mouth from decreased oral intake, following general anesthesia and surgery, or from medications with atropine-like effects, such as antihistamines or phenothiazines. In most patients, it is an ascending infection due to *S. aureus,* which normally colonizes the opening to Stensen's duct. Occasionally, there is an obstructing calculus. Its onset, usually sudden, is heralded by unilateral local pain and swelling, frequently with fever and chills. Frank pus can often be expressed from the duct and may show gram-positive cocci in clumps. The gland itself is firm and tender and often shows redness and edema of the overlying skin. Treatment consists of systemic antimicrobial therapy with a penicillinase-resistant penicillin or some other agent effective against *S. aureus,* unless another organism is isolated, combined with improved hydration and oral hygiene. Massage of the gland and sialagogues, like lemon drops, help promote drainage through the duct. Surgery is usually unnecessary and should be reserved for patients failing to improve after 4 to 5 days of medical management.

Rare complications include fistula formation, facial nerve palsy, or extension of the infection to involve the mediastinum. The mortality rate is about 20 to 30 percent, probably because this infection occurs in severely debilitated patients.

The use of penicillin and other antibiotics has reduced the incidence of many formerly common suppurative complications of streptococcal pharyngitis. However, as a result of streptococcal sore throat, *Bacteroides* infections of the pharynx, or introduction of infection by trauma to the floor of the mouth or the pharyngeal wall, abscesses of the deep cervical structures still occur. *Suppurative cervical adenitis,* once an all-too-common sequel to streptococcal pharyngitis in children, is now rare. *Peritonsillar abscess* (*quinsy*) is manifested by fever, sore throat, cervical lymphadenopathy, unilateral pain radiating to the ear on swallowing, and enlargement of the tonsil with redness and swelling of the adjacent soft palate. Treatment with penicillin and irrigations of warm saline solution sometimes lead to subsidence of the process, but if digital palpation reveals fluctuation, surgical drainage with or without tonsillectomy is indicated. Organisms associated with peritonsillar abscess include *Streptococcus pyogenes* and oral anaerobic bacteria.

The course of *deep cervical infections* is fully as dependent upon the anatomic arrangement of fascial planes as is that of infections of the hand. Infection in this area is serious and is attended by fever, prostration, and leukocytosis. A tender mass may be palpated, but *surgical evacuation of such an infection should not be delayed because of failure to detect fluctuation,* which is usually absent because of the dense fascial layers.

Infection of the *sublingual* and submandibular spaces, so-called Ludwig's angina, is characterized by brawny induration of the submaxillary region, edema of the floor of the mouth, and elevation of the tongue. It usually originates from apical abscesses of the second and third mandibular molars. There are severe pain, dysphagia, and, within hours, dyspnea from respiratory obstruction. The causative organisms of this and other neck abscesses are mainly streptococci and oral anaerobes. Mortality was formerly about 50 percent. *Treatment* consists of large doses of penicillin and careful observation. With significant airway obstruction, tracheostomy is necessary. Since the infection is largely a cellulitis, incision and drainage are reserved for evidence of fluctuation.

The retropharyngeal space lies between the muscles anterior to the cervical vertebrae and the pharyngeal mucosa. *Retropharyngeal abscess,* formerly common in children, is manifested by dysphagia, progressive stridor, pain, and fever. The bulging mass is easily seen and can completely occlude the airway within hours. Incision and drainage are mandatory; spontaneous rupture may lead to death by aspiration. Esophageal perforation during endoscopy may result in abscess as a late complication. Tuberculous abscess, secondary to spinal disease, occasionally appears in the retropharyngeal space; it is painless, and relief of obstruction follows surgical incision.

Submastoid abscess, or suppuration in the submastoid space, known as *Bezold's abscess,* is usually secondary to otitis and produces nuchal rigidity, which may lead to a mistaken diagnosis of otogenous meningitis. Infection can extend down the carotid sheath to the mediastinum. A suppurative thrombophlebitis of the jugular vein usually accompanies this infection, and the vessel is easily felt as a tender cord. Bacteremia and systemic spread of infection are common, and the involved venous segment may need to be excised. Spontaneous rupture of the carotid artery with rapid death from exsanguination is a rare complication.

Therapy of head and neck abscesses includes surgical incision and drainage, open treatment of infected wounds, and systemic antibiotics, which should include agents active against anaerobic organisms, particularly if there is foul-smelling pus. Penicillin is usually the drug of choice.

DEEP-SEATED INFECTIONS Hepatic abscess These abscesses are usually amebic (see Chap. 217) or bacterial (pyogenic). Bacterial abscesses usually develop by one of five mechanisms: (1) portal vein bacteremia arising from an infected intraabdominal site, such as appendicitis, diverticulitis, or perforated bowel; (2) systemic bacteremia originating from a distant site, in which bacteria reach the liver via the hepatic artery; (3) ascending cholangitis in a biliary tract completely or partially obstructed by stone, malignancy, or stricture; (4) direct extension from a contiguous focus of infection outside the biliary tract, such as a subphrenic abscess; or (5) trauma, either penetrating, with direct introduction of organisms into the liver, or blunt, causing a hematoma that becomes secondarily infected. In most cases the cause is apparent, but in some the pathogenesis of the abscess is unexplained ("cryptogenic"). Most abscesses are single; multiple abscesses are typically microscopic and associated with systemic bacteremia or complete biliary tract obstruction. In these cases, the onset is acute, and the clinical features of the predisposing disease predominate.

Most other cases of hepatic abscess have a subacute onset, and an illness lasting several weeks is the rule. Fever is nearly always present and is accompanied by such nonspecific symptoms as chills, nausea, vomiting, anorexia, weight loss, and weakness. Right upper quadrant abdominal pain or tenderness is present in about one-half of patients, as is hepatomegaly. Some complain of right pleuritic chest pain. Jaundice is usually evident only when there is biliary tract obstruction.

Laboratory findings in most patients include one or more of the following: anemia, leukocytosis, increased erythrocyte sedimentation rate, increased alkaline phosphatase, decreased serum albumin, and usually mildly increased serum bilirubin. The chest roentgenogram is abnormal in about one-half of patients and shows right-sided basilar atelectasis, pneumonia, pleural effusion, or an elevated hemidiaphragm.

The radionuclide liver scan demonstrates filling defects for most abscesses greater than 2 cm in diameter. Ultrasound scans are usually positive and can distinguish fluid-filled from solid masses, helping to discriminate between infectious and neoplastic lesions. Computerized tomography and hepatic arteriography may also demonstrate the abscesses but generally provide no additional useful information.

The bacteriology of liver abscesses depends upon the cause. With systemic bacteremia staphylococci or streptococci are common. Abscesses originating from an intraabdominal infection, however, usually contain aerobic gram-negative rods, especially *Escherichia coli* and *Klebsiella-Enterobacter;* anaerobic bacteria, especially anaerobic gram-positive cocci, *Fusobacterium nucleatum,* and *B. fragilis;* or a mixture of aerobes and anaerobes. Blood cultures are positive in a substantial minority of patients.

Treatment consists of surgical drainage supplemented by appropriate antibiotic therapy. When the bacteriology is unknown, chloramphenicol or a combination of clindamycin and an aminoglycoside should be effective. Antibiotics are usually continued for several weeks following drainage.

Complications of hepatic abscesses include formation of a subphrenic abscess, bleeding into the abscess, and rupture into the lung, pleural cavity, or peritoneum. In correctly diagnosed and treated patients the mortality rate is about 20 to 40 percent, and is higher in those with multiple rather than single abscesses.

In patients with a clinical picture suggesting a liver abscess and an abnormal hepatic radionuclide or ultrasound scan, it is important to distinguish between a bacterial and an amebic abscess, since the latter usually requires no surgical drainage. Features suggesting an amebic etiology are age under 50; single rather than multiple abscesses; a history of diarrhea, especially if bloody; the presence of *Entamoeba histolytica* in the stool; and the absence of a condition predisposing to bacterial liver abscess. The most helpful differential point is that nearly all patients with amebic liver abscesses have a positive serology for *E. histolytica.*

Splenic abscess Most splenic abscesses are multiple, small, and clinically silent lesions found incidentally at autopsy and occurring as a terminal manifestation of uncontrolled infection elsewhere. Clinically important splenic abscesses are generally solitary and arise from (1) systemic bacteremia originating in another site, such as endocarditis or salmonellosis; (2) infection, probably by the hematogenous route, of a spleen damaged by bland infarction (as occurs in hemoglobinopathies, especially sickle cell trait or sickle cell disease), trauma, penetrating or blunt (with superinfection of a subcapsular hematoma), or other diseases (malaria, hydatid cysts); or (3) extension from a contiguous focus of infection, such as a subphrenic abscess. The most common organisms are staphylococci, streptococci, anaerobes, and aerobic gram-negative rods, including *Salmonella.*

The onset is typically subacute, and the major features are fever and left-sided pain which is often pleuritic and located in the upper abdomen, lower chest, or flank. The pain may radiate to the left shoulder. Left upper quadrant abdominal tenderness and splenomegaly are common, but an audible splenic friction rub is rare. Leukocytosis is usually present.

Radiographic findings may include (1) a left upper quadrant soft-tissue abdominal mass, (2) extraintestinal gas from gas-forming organisms in the abscess, (3) displacement of other organs, including the colon, kidney, and stomach, (4) elevation of the left hemidiaphragm, and (5) left pleural effusion. A liver-spleen radionuclide scan is valuable in detecting abscesses larger than 2 or 3 cm. A combined spleen-lung scan may provide clues to perisplenic (or left subdiaphragmatic) abscesses. An ultrasound scan may be positive for macroscopic splenic abscesses. Arteriography, which may reveal an avascular mass and mycotic aneurysms, or CT scan may be helpful when these other tests fail to demonstrate a suspected lesion.

Treatment consists of appropriate systemic antibiotics and splenectomy. Complications of untreated splenic abscesses include hemorrhage into the abscess cavity or rupture into the peritoneum, bowel, bronchus, or pleural space. Splenic abscesses should be considered a possible, although rare, cause of continued bacteremia in acute endocarditis despite appropriate chemotherapy, and splenectomy may be necessary to achieve final eradication of the infection.

Subphrenic abscess Peritoneal infections show a striking tendency to localize in the upper part of the abdomen between the transverse colon and the diaphragm. True subphrenic abscesses form between the liver and diaphragm on the left or right, and many so-called subphrenic infections are, in fact, subhepatic. Most of these infections are related to perforations in the gastrointestinal or biliary tracts, and over half of them follow operations on the gallbladder, duodenum, or stomach. Subphrenic abscesses following perforated appendicitis occur rarely nowadays. Closed blunt trauma is an important cause. A few abscesses occur without predisposing neighborhood infection. The most common organisms are *E. coli,* non-group A streptococci, staphylococci, *Klebsiella-Enterobacter,* and anaerobes, especially *Bacteroides* spp.; mixed infections are common. About 60 percent of abscesses occur on the right, 25 percent on the left, and 15 percent are bilateral. They are more common in males and elderly patients, who often have a debilitating disease such as cancer. *Any patient with persistent fever and a history of a recent abdominal operation or recent intraabdominal sepsis should be suspected of having a subphrenic abscess.*

Manifestations include fever, upper abdominal pain, and tenderness, usually along the costal margin. Shoulder pain, dyspnea, dullness, and rales at the lung base are more common than abdominal signs and symptoms and emphasize the location of a true abscess between the liver and the diaphragm. Foul sputum connotes perforation of the abscess into the lung. The localizing signs are by no means striking in all cases, however. The widespread practice of "covering" postoperative patients with antibiotics prophylactically can attenuate subphrenic infection without eradicating it and may result in an insidiously progressive illness with weight loss, malaise, fatigue, and low-grade fever beginning weeks or months after a laparotomy, a syndrome termed *chronic subphrenic abscess.* Roentgenograms may show gas, sometimes with an air-fluid level beneath the diaphragm. The gas may be from a perforated viscus or the result of bacterial multiplication.

Other radiographic findings include pleural effusion, which is usually sterile, basilar infiltrates, and elevation—but not necessarily fixation—of the diaphragm. Barium meal with the patient in the head-down position may show indentation of the gastric fundus in left subphrenic abscess, a lesion that is often notoriously difficult to localize. Combined lung-liver scintiscan may show a widened subphrenic space. Ultrasound scans are useful in detecting subphrenic abscesses, and CT scan will usually demonstrate extraintestinal gas or fluid.

Treatment includes adequate surgical drainage and appropriate systemic antibiotics. Chloramphenicol or clindamycin and an aminoglycoside are good choices pending culture results. The outlook in subphrenic abscesses is often poor because of delayed diagnosis, the debilitated state of the patient, and failure to attain complete drainage. Even with proper surgery, the mortality rate is about 30 percent.

Retroperitoneal infections Strictly speaking, all perinephric, most pancreatic, and many subphrenic abscesses are located outside the peritoneum, but the term *retroperitoneal abscess* usually refers to infection in the lumbar and iliac regions. Suppuration in these areas is relatively rare, but the importance of recognizing its existence in patients with fever and pain in the lower part of the back is great. In one series, the average duration of illness in 65 patients before diagnosis was approximately 1 month.

Infection in the retroperitoneal space usually reflects extension from posterior perforations of the appendix, small bowel or colon, pancreatic, renal, or spinal infections, and occasionally suppurative lymphadenitis in the iliac area, usually secondary to streptococcal infections of the lower extremities in children. Sometimes, the infection is apparently spread hematogenously.

Lumbar abscess is characterized by tenderness and spasm of the back muscles on the affected side, and a mass is usually palpable in the lumbar region; or there may be a prominent, tender abdominal mass without lumbar pain or spasm. Infection in the wall of the abdominal aneurysm, often with *Salmonella,* may present as a lumbar abscess. Flexion of the hip (psoas sign) occurs in a few cases but is more often present with infections lower in the retroperitoneal area. *Fever, leukocytosis,* and *lumbar spasm* should suggest the diagnosis. The absence of a palpable mass may lead to protracted observation, and it is in these instances that palpation under anesthesia is often helpful.

Psoas (*iliac*) *abscess* is typically attended by abdominal pain in the iliac or inguinal region, and, particularly when the psoas muscle is involved, severe pain may be referred to the hip, thigh, or knee. Careful palpation of the lower part of the abdomen or groin usually reveals a mass, and fullness and tenderness on rectal examination are common. Hip spasm (psoas sign) is often present. Although psoas abscesses characteristically occur in association with tuberculosis of the spine, the acute bacterial form has been reported in association with perforation or fistula formation of the bowel in appendicitis, diverticulitis, colonic carcinoma, Crohn's disease (regional enteritis), and vertebral osteomyelitis. Occasionally, no other focus of infection is present; these primary psoas abscesses are usually staphylococcal. Roentgenograms may delineate the inflammatory mass; pyelography shows displacement of the kidney or ureter in some cases, scoliosis with concavity on the side of the infection, and blurring of the psoas shadow. Barium studies of the small and large bowel may demonstrate an intestinal site of origin. Computerized tomography may be useful in revealing a suspected abscess when other studies are negative. Treatment consists of surgical drainage and appropriate antibiotic therapy.

Pancreatic abscess These abscesses usually occur in a site of pancreatic necrosis following acute pancreatitis. Typically, the patient improves after the attack of pancreatitis, but about 10 to 21 days later fever, abdominal pain and tenderness, nausea, vomiting, and sometimes persistent ileus occur. Less commonly, the abscess develops shortly after the attack begins. In those cases, persistent fever, leukocytosis, and abdominal findings beyond 7 to 10 days should suggest an abscess. A mass is palpable in about half of cases. The serum amylase is irregularly elevated, but leukocytosis is usually present. The serum alkaline phosphatase may be increased and the albumin decreased.

Chest roentgenograms often show a left pleural effusion, basilar atelectasis or pneumonia, or a raised hemidiaphragm. Plain films of the abdomen or barium studies of the intestinal tract may show extraintestinal gas in the pancreatic area from gas-forming organisms in the abscess or may demonstrate displacement of adjacent structures. Ultrasound is very useful in revealing fluid-filled pancreatic masses but may be unable to distinguish infected from uninfected fluid. Similarly, computed tomography (CT) is a sensitive test for abscesses and may show pancreatic gas, peripancreatic fluid collections, or masses, but only pancreatic gas is diagnostic of infection.

Treatment is surgical drainage and appropriate antibiotic therapy. Since the usual organisms are coliforms, staphylococci, streptococci, and anaerobes in varying combinations, chloramphenicol or clindamycin and an aminoglycoside are reasonable choices until culture results return. Complications of undrained abscess include perforation into adjacent structures; erosion of the left gastric, splenic, and gastroduodenal arteries with exsanguination; and the development of further abscesses in the pancreas or peritoneal and retroperitoneal spaces. Even with surgical drainage the mortality rate is about 40 percent, and recurrent abscesses requiring reoperation are common.

Renal abscess Single or multiple abscesses of the renal *cortex* may be the result of metastatic implantation of staphylococci from another focus. There is no relationship to previous renal disease; the infection occurs in younger individuals, is usually unilateral, and occurs on the right side oftener than on the left. Many patients give a history of recent skin infection such as furuncle. Although acute pyelonephritis is a diffuse disease with foci of cellular infiltrates in the interstitium of the renal medulla, these inflammatory foci may coalesce to form single or multiple distinct abscess cavities in the medulla. This situation probably ensues more frequently than is generally appreciated.

The onset of renal abscess is abrupt, with chills and fever, followed by costovertebral pain and tenderness. If the abscess is cortical, the urine contains *no white blood cells;* medullary abscesses are usually accompanied by pyuria. The stained urinary sediment may show myriads of gram-positive cocci in cortical abscesses and gram-negative organisms in medullary abscesses. Transient gross or microscopic hematuria may occur at the onset. The white blood cell count is usually elevated and may exceed 30,000 cells per cubic millimeter. Physical signs are usually localized to the region of the kidney, but abdominal spasm may lead to confusion with appendicitis, cholecystitis, or pancreatitis. Early in the disease, ureteral calculus or acute hydronephrosis may be considered as possible diagnoses. Sudden onset of *fever, leukocytosis, and renal pain in the absence of pyuria* should suggest the diagnosis of a renal cortical abscess, especially in a patient with infection elsewhere. Obstruction of the ureter by pus or cellular debris may also yield a urine sediment sparse in white blood cells and bacteria. Excretory urograms typically reveal an intrarenal mass, and ultrasound scans usually demonstrate the abscess as a fluid-filled defect. *Treatment* consists of appropriate antibiotics, adequate fluids, and relief of pain. An abscess may suddenly discharge into the renal pelvis, with relief of pain and the passage of cloudy urine containing enormous numbers of leukocytes and bacteria. *Complications* include formation of a thick-walled chronic renal "carbuncle," requiring surgical removal, rupture into the perirenal space, and secondary pyelonephritis, usually produced by coliform bacilli. Recovery is ordinarily prompt, and chronic sequelae are rare. Failure to achieve prompt defervescence following treatment suggests an incorrect diagnosis or the necessity of drainage, either by needle aspiration or by surgery.

Perinephric abscess Rupture of a renal parenchymal abscess into the perinephric space can cause a perinephric abscess. Such an abscess may be staphylococcal following hematogenous dissemination from another site, usually the skin, but more commonly it arises from pyelonephritis, especially associated with renal calculus disease. The causative organisms, therefore, are those responsible for acute pyelonephritis: *E. coli, Proteus* sp., and *Klebsiella-Enterobacter.* The main symptoms are fever, chills, and unilateral flank pain. Dysuria is frequently present. Most patients are febrile and have unilateral flank or abdominal tenderness, often with a palpable mass. Leukocytosis, pyuria, and a positive urine culture are typical. Blood cultures are positive in 20 to 40 percent of patients. Perinephric abscess generally can be distinguished clinically from uncomplicated acute pyelonephritis by the longer duration of symptoms before hospitalization (usually more than 5 days) and the failure of patients to become afebrile within 5 days following the institution of antimicrobial therapy.

The chest roentgenograms often show ipsilateral pneumonia or atelectasis, pleural effusion, or a raised hemidiaphragm. An abdominal plain film may reveal the loss of the psoas shadow, a mass, calculi, or extraintestinal gas in the perinephric area secondary to gas-forming organisms. Findings on excretory urogram may include: a nonvisualizing or a poorly visualizing kidney, distorted calyces, anterior displacement of the kidney on lateral views, and unilateral fixation of the kidney that is demonstrated best by fluoroscopy or inspiration-expiration films. Ultrasound and CT scans are very sensitive in detecting perinephric abscesses. Treatment is surgical drainage and relief of any urinary obstruction; occasionally, nephrectomy is necessary. Appropriate systemic antibiotics (not urinary antiseptics) should be administered along with surgical measures.

Rectal abscess Most of these infections are superficial and involve the perirectal region, and many are associated with fistulas. Infection in the apocrine glands (hidradenitis) or folliculitis in the perianal region, extension of cryptitis or obstructions in the "anal glands" which open into the crypts of Morgagni, and contamination of submucosal hematomas, sclerosed hemorrhoids, or anal fissures may lead to abscess formation. In most patients, the cause of infection is not apparent. These are usually painful, easily palpable, often visible on inspection. Treatment is incision and drainage. Antibiotics are rarely necessary unless there is extensive perineal cellulitis.

Difficulties in diagnosis are likely to arise with infections higher in the rectum. Most are in the ischiorectal area, but those above the pelvic diaphragm, the so-called supralevator abscess, are particularly elusive. Patients with this type of infection often have fever, malaise, and leukocytosis for several days or even weeks before any symptoms referable to the rectum develop. There is vague pelvic discomfort, relieved by defecation, and constipation punctuated by short episodes of diarrhea is common. In males, the inflammation often involves the base of the bladder, and urinary urgency or retention may occur, falsely centering attention on the urinary tract as the source of fever and malaise. Eventually, the abscess produces severe pain, chills, and fever; palpation and instrumentation will reveal the swelling in the rectal ampulla. Such an abscess may surround the rectum and produce narrowing that is differentiated from neoplasm by the fact that the mucosa remains intact. A useful sign of deep rectal abscess is severe pain with pressure in the region between the anus and the coccyx. The supralevator space is continuous with the ischiorectal space, with both the gluteal and obturator regions, and with the retroperitoneal space. In neglected cases, the abscess may drain through the skin of the perineum, the groin, or the buttock or may extend as high as the perirenal areas. Rectal abscesses are not uncommon in patients with preexisting anorectal disease, diabetes, alcoholism, and neurological disease; infections in this area are also peculiarly frequent in patients with acute leukemia, especially when neutropenia is present. Because the clinical picture may be that of "fever of unknown origin" for a long period, it is important that thorough digital and endoscopic examination of the rectum be carried out in patients with unexplained fever. Patients with diabetic ketoacidosis should receive a careful rectal examination because a rectal abscess may be the infection responsible for precipitating the ketoacidosis.

A rectal abscess may be a forerunner of both ulcerative colitis and regional enteritis, and may occur months and even years before other overt manifestations of these diseases. For this reason, proctosigmoidoscopy, colonoscopy, barium enema, and, often, upper gastrointestinal roentgenograms are indicated in nonhealing or recurrent rectal lesions.

Treatment of high rectal abscesses consists of incision and drainage, analgesics, and antibiotics directed at *E. coli, Klebsiella-Enterobacter, Bacteroides,* and a variety of streptococci, which constitute the polymicrobial flora of these lesions.

REFERENCES

BALASEGARAM M: Management of hepatic abscess. Curr Probl Surg, May 1981

BARTLETT JG et al: Anaerobic infections of the head and neck. Otolaryngol Clin North Am 9:655, 1976

CHOW AW et al: Orofacial odontogenic infections. Ann Intern Med 88:392, 1978

CHUN CH et al: Splenic abscess. Medicine 59:50, 1980

FEDERLE MP et al: Computed tomography of pancreatic abscesses. Am J Roentgenol 136:879, 1981

FINNERTY RV et al: Primary psoas abscess: Case report and review of literature. J Urol 126:108, 1981

GOLIGHER JC: *Surgery of the Anus, Rectum, and Colon,* 4th ed. New York, Macmillan, 1980

HOVERMAN IV et al: Intrarenal abscess: Report of 14 cases. Arch Intern Med 140:914, 1980

KNOCHEL JQ et al: Diagnosis of abdominal abscesses with computed tomography, ultrasound, and ^{111}In leukocyte scans. Radiology 137:425, 1980

KONVOLINKA CW et al: Subphrenic abscess. Curr Probl Surg, January 1972

LINSCHEID RL et al: Common and uncommon infections of the hand. Orthop Clin North Am 6:1063, 1975

SART MG, ZUIDEMA GD: Splenic abscess—Presentation, diagnosis and treatment. Surgery 92:480, 1982

SPEIRS CF et al: Acute septic parotitis: Incidence, aetiology, and management. Scott Med J 17:62, 1972

THORLEY JD et al: Perinephric abscess. Medicine 53:441, 1974

WARSHAW AL: Inflammatory masses following acute pancreatitis: Phlegmon, pseudocyst, and abscess. Surg Clin North Am 54:621, 1974

141 CHEMOTHERAPY OF INFECTION

WILLIAM M. M. KIRBY
MARVIN TURCK

Modern chemotherapy of infectious diseases dates from the mid-1930s when the sulfonamides were introduced. Penicillin G, the first of the antibiotics to be used systemically, came into widespread use in the early 1940s, and since then several dozen chemotherapeutic agents have appeared that are effective in a wide variety of bacterial, rickettsial, fungal, viral, and parasitic infections. The efficacy of antimicrobial agents is due primarily to their action in inhibiting growth of the parasite rather than to an enhancement of defense mechanisms, and a large number of substances can interfere effectively with multiplication of invading organisms without seriously damaging the cells of the host. Effective new agents continue to appear, both from large-scale screening programs in which samples of organic matter are tested for antimicrobial activity and from chemical modifications of the known chemotherapeutic drugs. Specific recommendations for therapy are made in chapters dealing with individual diseases; this chapter is devoted to general principles of chemotherapy and to a consideration of individual therapeutic agents.

FACTORS INFLUENCING SELECTION OF ANTIMICROBIAL AGENTS AND THE OUTCOME OF THERAPY

SUSCEPTIBILITY OF THE INFECTING MICROORGANISMS No antimicrobial agent is effective against all pathogenic microorganisms; each has its own spectrum of activity against one or a variety of species, within which the majority of strains have been found to be susceptible. There are a few instances, such as the susceptibility of group A streptococci to penicillin G, in which resistant strains occur rarely if at all, and where treatment with penicillin can be given without concern about resistance. With the majority of chemotherapeutic agents, however, a variable percentage of strains of each susceptible species is resistant, i.e., they are not inhibited by concentrations of the drug attainable in the patient's blood and tissues with the recommended dosage schedules. It is customary, therefore, in serious infections to determine the susceptibility of most pathogens to a variety of chemotherapeutic agents. *Dilution methods* of susceptibility testing, considered to be the most accurate, involve making serial dilutions of each agent to be tested in agar or broth, adding a standardized inoculum of the infecting organisms, and determining the smallest amount (the minimal inhibitory concentration, MIC) of the drug that inhibits growth after overnight incubation. *Agar dilution tests* are used routinely in some laboratories with sufficient volume to justify them, and mechanized or preprepared *broth dilution methods* are available. Some of these techniques have been automated. For the majority of laboratories, however, the simple *agar diffusion method,* which is accurate and reliable when properly performed, remains the one usually used. With this technique, zones of inhibition of growth of a standardized inoculum of the infecting organism around filter paper disks impregnated with antibiotics are measured, and the zone sizes are inversely proportional to minimal inhibitory concentrations (MICs) of drug, which are in turn related to the blood levels usually attained. Susceptibility of 8 to 12 chemotherapeutic agents can be tested on a single large agar plate, and a report of *susceptible, intermediate,* or *resistant* can be made. Intermediate sensitivity indicates the organisms' possible susceptibility with increased doses, or in urinary tract infections where high concentrations of drug can be attained in the urine. Disk testing has a number of limitations; it is applicable chiefly to rapidly growing pathogens, and the results are usually not reported until 24 h after the pathogen is isolated.

BACTERICIDAL VERSUS BACTERIOSTATIC AGENTS Although these are relative terms, some chemotherapeutic drugs can be clearly shown to have a killing (bactericidal) action at or near the minimal inhibitory concentration, while others simply inhibit bacterial growth (bacteriostatic). Bactericidal agents include the penicillins, cephalosporins, aminoglycosides, polymyxins, and vancomycin, while examples of bacteriostatic agents are the tetracyclines, sulfonamides, chloramphenicol, erythromycin, and clindamycin. Chloramphenicol is bactericidal in feasible concentrations against *Hemophilus influenzae* and *Streptococcus pneumoniae.* Bactericidal agents give superior results in diseases such as bacterial endocarditis and may be more likely to give a favorable response in life-threatening infections, particularly when there is impairment of the host's defense mechanisms. In mild infections in otherwise healthy individuals, on the other hand, there is little to choose between "-cidal" and "-static" agents. In uncomplicated urinary tract infections, due to *Escherichia coli,* for example, the clinical results are as good with sulfonamides as with broad-spectrum penicillins or cephalosporins.

CLINICAL PHARMACOLOGY Knowledge of the clinical pharmacology of antimicrobial agents is helpful in prescribing therapy that is both safe and effective. Important information includes details of absorption and excretion, blood and urine levels with various routes of administration, protein binding, volume of distribution, renal clearance, half-lives of drugs, stability in solutions and within the body, and the conversion to metabolic breakdown products. With some agents, such as ampicillin, much higher blood levels are obtained with the same doses given parenterally than orally, whereas with others, such as doxycycline, where there is complete absorption from the intestinal tract, the oral and parenteral doses are the same. Because of possible incompatibilities, *it is advisable never to administer more than one agent at a time by the intravenous route.* Absorption from the intestinal tract is impaired by a variety of foods and chemicals, and, in general, antimicrobials should be administered temporally as far removed from food and other drugs, such as antacids, as possible.

Antimicrobials are bound to a varying extent to serum proteins, especially albumin. Although the significance of protein binding is uncertain and controversial, it is clear that the bound antibiotic has no antimicrobial activity, and it is probable that the concentration of free, unbound antibiotic in the tissues, at any one time, is no greater than the peak level of free antibiotic in the blood. All other features being equal, antimicrobials with relatively low binding may be preferable to those with a high degree of binding. In general, this point of view is reflected in the dosages of antimicrobial agents that are commonly recommended.

Renal clearance is one of the most important determinants of antibiotic blood levels. Antibiotics with a high renal clearance such as penicillin G and cephalothin have a large component of tubular secretion, and their blood levels are elevated to a greater degree by probenecid than those of ampicillin and cephaloridine, where the tubular contribution is less important. Plasma half-life, the time required for a blood level to fall by one-half, is also determined primarily by renal clearance mechanisms and is much shorter for those penicillins and cephalosporins that are secreted by the renal tubules than for antibiotics such as the aminoglycosides with little or no tubular component. Protein binding also has an important influence on the half-life of antibiotics, particularly those that are excreted mainly or entirely by glomerular filtration. For example, the plasma half-life of gentamicin, which is not bound significantly by proteins, is 2 h, whereas that of doxycycline, which is over 90 percent protein-bound, is about 16 h. Antibiotics with little or no protein binding have a much larger apparent volume of distribution (AVD) than those with a high degree of binding, i.e., the AVD of gentamicin is 30 percent of body weight compared with 14 percent for cefazolin. Cephalothin has a high plasma clearance with a high rate of nonrenal clearance due to its partial conversion in the body to a less active metabolic breakdown product. These are a few examples of the pharmacologic features of individual antimicrobial agents; others will be mentioned as the individual drugs are considered.

DOSE, ROUTE, AND DURATION OF THERAPY In prescribing dosages of antimicrobial agents, the objective is to deliver a concentration in excess of that needed to inhibit and/or kill the infecting organism at the site of infection. Since it is difficult to measure tissue concentrations, a blood level that exceeds the MIC two- to eightfold is a commonly accepted guideline. This is an arbitrary concentration of drug and obviously does not take into account all the variations in penetration into different tissues, or the role of host defense mechanisms. These variations may be very important because, in many instances, infections have been cured with antibiotics such as the tetracyclines where the concentration of free, active drug in the blood is not much greater than the MIC. The relation between blood levels and MIC does not hold in urinary tract infection, where the concentration of drug cleared by the kidney usually far exceeds the MIC. In this situation, an excess of drug in the urine or renal medulla is important.

The route of administration, as well as the dose, is important in achieving appropriate drug levels. In general, parenteral therapy should usually be given in severe infections to be certain that high, effective blood levels are attained. The *intravenous route* is especially indicated initially in meningitis, endocarditis, and osteomyelitis, where barriers to penetration of the antimicrobial agent can be overcome by high blood levels. Intravenous therapy is also indicated when there is hypotension, and when bleeding diatheses are present. For milder infections, *intramuscular administration* is often an acceptable or preferable alternative, particularly with antibiotics such as procaine penicillin that cause relatively little pain and produce prolonged, effective blood levels. The *oral route* is used chiefly for mild to moderate infections, and for completion of therapy of severe infections after they have been brought under control with parenteral therapy. Absorption from the intestinal tract is variable even in the fasting state, and all oral antibiotics should be taken at least 1 h before and 3 h after food and other medications. This presents difficulties with drugs such as antacids that need to be taken frequently and that are especially likely to interfere with absorption of antimicrobial agents. Parenteral administration is often the only solution to this problem.

The optimal duration of antimicrobial treatment is unknown for many infections, and there is considerable variation from one medical center to another in the length of time antimicrobial therapy is given. In bacterial endocarditis, for example, the usual course of parenteral therapy may vary from 2 to 8 weeks with an average of about 4 weeks. For most acute infections a good general rule is to continue therapy for 2 to 3 days after the temperature has returned to normal and all signs of infection have subsided. However, fever can continue for weeks from sterile effusions complicating pneumonia, and cerebrospinal fluid abnormalities can persist for considerable periods in bacterial meningitis, leading to a continuation of chemotherapy for much longer than is necessary. Empiricism needs to be tempered with reason and experience, and in actual practice the guidelines for duration of therapy must be sufficiently flexible to be appropriate for the patient being treated.

ALLERGY AND TOXICITY The patient's allergic history should always be explored before prescribing antimicrobial agents. In addition to allergic manifestations in general, a report of previous drug allergies is of particular importance, and agents that have caused clear-cut reactions should be avoided. Unfortunately, no reliable test is available to determine the presence of allergy to the penicillins, and they may or may not be well tolerated by patients with a history of a previous reaction. The possibility of a severe anaphylactic reaction can be reliably excluded by skin tests containing major and minor determinant mixtures, but only the major mixture is commercially available. When administration of a penicillin is considered essential, one approach is to begin with a very small dose intravenously and increase the amount every few minutes until it is learned whether the patient can tolerate the antibiotic. However, the number of alternative antibiotics available is large enough that switching to another agent is usually the best course to follow.

Drug toxicity related to renal function is of particular importance. Some antimicrobials, such as the penicillins, cephalosporins, chloramphenicol, erythromycin, and clindamycin, are relatively safe at normal or only slightly reduced dosage in the presence of impaired renal function. Other agents, such as the aminoglycosides, are potentially quite toxic but can be administered safely at reduced dosage if proper guidelines, based on serial determinations of the serum creatinine, are followed, and particularly if blood levels can be monitored. Certain toxic agents should be avoided if at all possible in the presence of renal insufficiency. These include most of the tetracyclines, streptomycin, cephaloridine, the sulfonamides, the nitrofurans, and nalidixic acid. One of the long-acting tetracyclines, doxycycline, has the same half-life in healthy and uremic subjects, and can be administered to patients with impaired renal function either orally or intravenously. Many patients with chronic renal failure are being maintained on dialysis programs and may require antimicrobials for a variety of infections. Table 141-1 summarizes adult dosage schedules for various antibiotics for patients with renal failure, on or off dialysis.

SITE OF INFECTION Soft-tissue infections in sites with a good blood supply and a minimum of tissue necrosis are, in general, easily treated. In meningitis and endocarditis, on the other hand, penetration into the site of the infection presents formidable problems and is not infrequently responsible for treatment failures. Penetration across the blood-brain barrier is a complex phenomenon involving protein binding, lipid solubility, and ionization of the drug being administered. In addition, the permeability of this barrier to drugs depends on the degree of inflammation. Because of their low toxicity the penicillins can be administered in doses large enough to provide therapeutic concentrations in the spinal fluid, whereas more toxic drugs such as the aminoglycosides must be injected intrathecally to be effective clinically in meningitis. On the other hand, agents such as the sulfonamides, chloramphenicol, and the tetracyclines appear in the spinal fluid in amounts adequate for the treatment of some types of meningitis when they are given in doses appropriate for the treatment of systemic infections.

Other examples of problems of penetration, and of the influence of localized physiologic conditions, may be cited. The sulfonamides are excreted in the saliva in amounts adequate to eradicate the meningococcal carrier state, whereas penicillins and tetracyclines other than minocycline are not. However, most of the strains of meningococci encountered at the present time are sulfonamide-resistant. In urinary infections, erythromycin and the aminoglycosides are relatively ineffective at an acid pH, whereas a pH at less than 5.5 is essential for the activity of methenamine mandelate (Mandelamine). Aminoglycosides also are inactive in anaerobic environments. The lack of efficacy of sulfonamides in the presence of pus, due to the competition for binding sites by the large amounts of *p*-aminobenzoic acid present, limits the usefulness of this class of drugs.

Foreign bodies, abscesses, and obstruction to normal pathways of drainage almost always interfere with the response to chemotherapy and usually prevent cure until they are removed, drained, or relieved. Suture materials, prostheses, sequestrations, and calculi are examples of foreign bodies that interfere with drug therapy and usually, but not always, need to be removed. In many abscesses, bacteria tend to be in a metabolically inactive state in which they are not actively synthesizing cell wall and are not susceptible to the damaging effects of some antimicrobial drugs; hence drainage plus chemotherapy is necessary to eradicate the infection. Obstruction to bronchial, biliary, and renal drainage interferes seriously with the response of bacterial infections to antibiotics, and these infections generally cannot be cured with drugs until the obstruc-

TABLE 141-1
Dosages of antimicrobials in renal failure

			Dose interval for degree of renal failure			*Hemodialysis*		*Peritoneal dialysis*		
Drug	*Normal dose*	*Normal dose interval*	*Mild (C_{cr}* 50–80 ml/min)*	*Moderate (C_{cr}* 10–50 ml/min)*	*Severe (C_{cr}* 10 ml/min)*	*Significant dialysis of drug*	*Add at end of each dialysis*	*Significant dialysis of drug*	*Add parenterally during dialysis*	*Alternative, add to dialysate after the regular parenteral loading dose*
Ampicillin	0.5–3 g	6 h	6 h	9 h	12–15 h (1 g)	Yes	0.5–1 g	No		50 μg/ml
Amoxicillin	0.25–1 g PO	8 h	8 h	12 h	16 h (0.5 g)	Yes	0.5 g	No		
Penicillin G	0.25–4 million U	4 h	4 h (2 million U)	4 h (1.5 million U)	6 h (1 million U)	No		No		
Methicillin, oxacillin, nafcillin	1–2 g	4 h	4 h	4 h	8–12 h (1 g)	No		No		
Cloxacillin, dicloxacillin	0.5–1 g PO	6 h	6 h	6 h	6 h	No		No		
Carbenicillin	4–5 g	4 h	4 h	6–8 h (2 g)	12 h (2 g)	Yes	1–2 g	No	1 g every 6 h	200 μg/ml
Cephalexin, cephradine	0.25–1 g	4 h	4 h	6 h	6 h (0.25 g)	Yes	0.25–0.5 g	Yes	0.25 g PO every 6 h	
Cephalothin, cephapirin	1–2 g	4 h	4 h	6 h	8–12 h (1 g)	Yes	1 g	Yes	1 g every 6 h	50 μg/ml
Cefazolin	0.5–1 g	8 h	12 h	12 h (0.5 g)	24 h (0.5 g)	No	0.5 g	No		75 μg/ml
Cefamandole, cefoxitin	0.5–2 g	6 h	8 h	12 h (1 g)	12 h (1 g)	No	0.5 g	No		50 μg/ml
Gentamicin,†,‡ tobramycin	1–1.7 mg/kg	8 h	8–12 h	12–24 h	48–72 h	Yes	1.5 mg/kg	No		8 μg/ml
Amikacin,†,‡ kanamycin	7.5 mg/kg	12 h	24 h	24–72 h	72–96 h	Yes	3.5 mg/kg	No		20 μg/ml
Streptomycin	0.5 g	12 h	24 h	24–72 h	72–96 h	Yes	0.25 g	Yes	?	
Chloramphenicol	0.25–1 g	6 h	6 h	8 h	8 h	No		No		
Erythromcyin	0.25–1 g	6 h	6 h	8 h	8–12 h	?		?		
Clindamycin	0.3–0.6 g	6–8 h	8 h	8 h	12 h (0.3 g)	No		No		
Vancomycin	0.25–0.5 g	6 h	24 h	48–72 h	7 days	No		No		15 μg/ml
Tetracycline	0.25–0.5 g	6 h	8–12 h	Avoid	Avoid	No		No		
Doxycycline	0.1–0.2 g	12–24 h	12–24 h	24 h	24 h	No		No		
Sulfisoxazole	1 g	6 h	6 h	8–12 h	Avoid	Yes	?			

* *C_{cr}=creatinine clearance rate.*
† *Frequency of the dose can be estimated more accurately by multiplying the serum creatinine by 8 (for gentamicin and tobramycin) or by 9 (for amikacin and kanamycin).*
‡ *An alternate method is to give smaller doses at 8- to 12-h intervals by relating the elimination constants of the drugs to the patient's creatinine clearance. A dosing chart applicable to all the aminoglycosides has been described by Sarubbi and Hull.*

tion is relieved. A thorough knowledge of the mechanical, metabolic, and physiologic factors is essential in planning therapy that will bring about optimal results in infections located in different parts of the body.

COMBINATION THERAPY, SYNERGISM, ANTAGONISM Once the etiologic agent is known or can be anticipated, most bacterial infections can be treated successfully with a *single* antimicrobial agent. Combination therapy is used frequently, however, to broaden the antibacterial spectrum while awaiting the results of cultures, and also to cover the possibility that a polymicrobial infection might be present. For example, in a hospitalized patient who suddenly becomes ill with presumed sepsis, a cephalosporin and an aminoglycoside may be given empirically to provide antibacterial activity against a variety of gram-positive and -negative pathogens that might be fatal if therapy were delayed (see Chap. 139). Over 100 fixed-dose combinations were once available commercially in the United States for oral or parenteral therapy, but virtually all have been ordered off the market by the Food and Drug Administration on the grounds that it has not been shown in controlled studies that both agents contribute to the claimed therapeutic effects, that the amounts of each agent present were often not appropriate, and that patients were often being exposed to the potential hazards of two drugs when only one was needed. When combination therapy is indicated, it is most rational to prescribe separately the indicated drugs in doses that take into account the patient's age, weight, and physiologic status.

A clinically significant enhancement of antibacterial activity from exposing microorganisms to two or more drugs is rare. Usually, the drugs have an indifferent effect in vitro; sometimes an additive action is observed, but this is difficult to demonstrate in patients.

True synergism occurs between penicillins and aminoglycosides with a number of gram-positive and gram-negative pathogens. The classic example is enterococcal endocarditis; penicillins (G, V, ampicillin, carbenicillin) disrupt the cell wall, permitting streptomycin to gain access to the ribosomes where their action is lethal. About one-third of enterococci are ribosomally resistant to streptomycin, but few if any strains are resistant to gentamicin, and so this aminoglycoside is replacing streptomycin in treatment of this disease. With viridans streptococci streptomycin is synergistic with penicillins against virtually all strains, and it is probable that, in bacterial endocarditis due to viridans streptococci, there are fewer relapses with combined therapy than with penicillin G alone (see Chap. 259).

Gentamicin, tobramycin, and amikacin are synergistic with carbenicillin or ticarcillin against *Pseudomonas* and some other gram-negative bacilli. Theoretically, it would be possible to reduce doses of the antibiotics, but in severe *Pseudomonas* infections full doses are usually given so as not to risk compromising the therapeutic result.

Trimethoprim-sulfamethoxazole, another synergistic combination, will be described below.

Clinically significant antagonism between antimicrobial agents is also rare, a prime example being a higher mortality rate in pneumococcal meningitis with penicillin and tetracycline than with penicillin alone. The rate of killing by penicillin is presumably slowed by the bacteriostatic agent, tetracycline, and this can alter the outcome when survival depends on rapid killing of the pneumococci.

SUPERINFECTION AND RESISTANCE DURING ANTIMICROBIAL THERAPY A number of microorganisms are genetically resistant to clinically feasible levels of one or more antimicrobials, and they obviously will not be affected by antibiotic therapy. Most antibiotics will alter the host's normal flora by removing those organisms which are sensitive to the drug. In most cases this ecologic change is of little consequence, but occasionally the commensal bacteria of the host set up infection in the same location as the original infection, a state termed *superinfection* (see Chap. 137). The superinfecting organism is resistant to the drug being administered, and determining its susceptibility is helpful in selecting the most appropriate antimicrobial drug. Some superinfecting organisms, particularly gram-negatives, acquire resistance to multiple drugs by an episomal transfer mechanism (R factors). For example, multiple-resistant *E. coli* and *Klebsiella-Enterobacter* pose a particular hazard to hospitalized patients.

Comparatively few organisms become resistant to the antibiotic being given during therapy. Some that do develop resistance are *E. coli* to streptomycin and nalidixic acid, occasional strains of staphylococci to erythromycin, and *Pseudomonas* to carbenicillin and ticarcillin. In general, however, sensitive organisms are supplanted by resistant ones rather than acquiring resistance themselves. From a practical point of view, it is important to know which agents are likely to induce resistance, and to look for this phenomenon clinically.

SPECIFIC ANTIMICROBIALS

PENICILLINS Natural penicillins (penicillinase-susceptible) The prototype, *penicillin G* (benzyl penicillin), is still widely used, especially parenterally, when high blood levels are desirable, as in meningitis and endocarditis. Large doses are necessary either continuously or at 3- to 4-h intervals because of problems of penetration into vegetations and across the blood-brain barrier, and also because of its high renal clearance, which is due chiefly to rapid tubular secretion. Blood levels can be doubled by the concomitant administration of probenecid, 0.5 g every 6 h, but since penicillin G is now quite inexpensive and the optimal blood levels are not known precisely, it is customary in most instances simply to give more penicillin. *Procaine penicillin* is well tolerated intramuscularly and is absorbed quite slowly so that injections need to be given only every 12 h for the treatment of many infections due to susceptible bacteria. In dosage of 300,000 to 600,000 units every 12 h, it is the drug of choice for most patients with pneumococcal pneumonia. *Benzathine penicillin* provides a depot in the muscle that releases penicillin so slowly that low blood levels are present for 2 to 3 weeks. These low levels are adequate for the therapy and prevention of streptococcal pharyngitis, for the treatment of some forms of syphilis, and for the prevention of recurrences of rheumatic fever.

Penicillin G given orally in doses of 200,000 units (125 mg) once or twice daily is also effective in preventing streptococcal sore throats, but less so than benzathine penicillin (see Chap. 257). Because of its instability in the presence of acid, however, it is less reliable for therapy than the acid-stable penicillin V (phenoxymethyl penicillin), and attempts to overcome this disadvantage by giving larger amounts of penicillin G are associated with an increased incidence of nausea and diarrhea. This has resulted in the development of a number of penicillin G analogues which continue to have some usefulness because very little resistance has developed to them. An exception are the pneumococci, among which a small number of resistant strains have been isolated in various parts of the world.

Aminopenicillins (extended-spectrum penicillins) *Ampicillin* differs from penicillin G only in the presence of an amino group in the side chain, but this minor chemical difference is responsible for some unique features that have led to the widespread use of this antibiotic. Ampicillin is active in low concentrations against a number of gram-negative bacteria causing respiratory (*H. influenzae*), intestinal (*Shigella, Salmonella*), and urinary (*E. coli, Proteus mirabilis*) infections. When it is given orally, the peak blood level occurs later (2 to 3 h versus $\frac{1}{2}$ to 1 h) and is lower than with penicillin V, and the ampicillin blood level then declines more slowly. This more prolonged blood level, along with its greater in vitro activity, is probably responsible for the greater efficacy of ampicillin, compared with penicillin V, in the oral therapy of gonococcal urethritis.

When given in an intravenous infusion, blood levels are more than 80 percent higher with ampicillin than with penicillin G chiefly because of the much higher rate of renal clearance of penicillin G (390 versus 210 ml/min per 1.73 m^2). When the in vitro activity of the infecting organisms is the same for the two antibiotics, this difference can mean equal efficacy with smaller doses of ampicillin, or higher blood levels with the same dose when maximum serum concentrations are considered necessary. Ampicillin is also more stable in the body, with a serum half-life twice as long as penicillin G, due chiefly to slower breakdown by the liver. Serum protein binding of ampicillin is approximately 20 percent compared with 60 percent for penicillin G and 80 percent for penicillin V; this may mean that with ampicillin there is a higher concentration of free, active antibiotic at the site of infection. Although ampicillin has remained an effective drug against most organisms, increasing resistance has developed among a significant number of strains of *E. coli, Salmonella, Shigella,* and *H. influenzae.*

Hypersensitivity reactions occur with about the same frequency with ampicillin as with penicillin G and V, and with all three are much more frequent and severe when the drug is given parenterally and topically than by the oral route. About 5 to 10 percent of patients develop skin rashes with oral ampicillin, but the incidence is as high as 90 percent when patients with infectious mononucleosis take this drug. This remarkably high incidence, which does not occur with penicillins G and V, does not represent true penicillin allergy, and its exact nature is not known. Maculopapular (as opposed to urticarial) rashes beginning 4 days or more after initiating treatment with ampicillin do not indicate a need to discontinue therapy, or to avoid subsequent courses of the antibiotic. Although acid-stable, ampicillin is not very well absorbed when taken orally, giving peak blood levels only one-sixth as high as dicloxacillin and cephalexin. *Amoxicillin,* a derivative with a hydroxyl group on the benzene ring, is much better absorbed orally, with blood levels and urinary excretion more than twice as great on the average as ampicillin. Blood levels are roughly equivalent to those of ampicillin given intramuscularly, and amoxicillin has a lower incidence of intestinal side effects when given in half the dose orally. Amoxicillin has superseded ampicillin in many situations in which oral therapy is required. The main exception is in the treatment of shigellosis, in which ampicillin is superior to amoxicillin because of better in vitro activity. *Bacampicillin,* a rapidly hydrolyzed ester with much better intestinal absorption, provides peak blood levels and urinary excretion of ampicillin approximately twice as great as does ampicillin alone. *Hetacillin,* a penicillin with a complex side chain, is hydrolyzed rapidly in the body to ampicillin, and for practical therapeutic purposes can be regarded as the same as ampicillin. *Cyclacillin* is the most rapidly absorbed aminopenicillin, with peak serum levels approximately four times higher than those achieved with 500 mg ampicillin. However, it is rapidly cleared, and its antibacterial activity is less on a weight basis than either ampicillin or amoxicillin. Both cyclacillin and amoxicillin appear to cause less gastrointestinal side effects than ampicillin, and good toleration is their primary therapeutic advantage.

Anti-*Pseudomonas* penicillins *Carbenicillin* and *ticarcillin* are broad-spectrum penicillins similar chemically to ampicillin, except that the amino group in the side chain is replaced by a carboxyl group. As a result, these penicillins are active in vitro against *Pseudomonas aeruginosa,* indole-positive *Proteus,* and some strains of *Enterobacter,* in addition to the other gram-negatives that are susceptible to ampicillin. Like ampicillin, they are not active against *Klebsiella.* The MIC for *Pseudomonas* is much higher than that usually considered within the therapeutic range for other antibiotics, i.e., about 75 to 100 μg/ml for most strains and as high as 500 μg/ml for a few. However, extraordinarily high blood levels can be readily attained, in the range of 200 to 400 μg/ml, so that carbenicillin (and its analogues) provides the safety and bactericidal activity of a penicillin for some organisms that have been notably refractory to most other antibiotics. The much higher blood levels that can be readily attained with carbenicillin compared with ampicillin are due chiefly to its much lower renal clearance (100 versus 210 ml/min per 1.73 m^2). In addition, carbenicillin is much more stable in the body, so that blood levels obtained with 30 g a day in patients with normal renal function can be achieved with only 3 or 4 g a day in patients with no renal function. Since many patients with severe gram-negative infections have considerable renal impairment, reduced doses can be administered with the knowledge that full therapeutic blood levels will be achieved. To give 30 g daily for the therapy of severe *Pseudomonas* infections in patients with normal renal function, it is customary to administer 5 g intravenously every 4 h, diluting each dose in 100 to 200 ml fluid and allowing it to drip into the vein within 1 to 2 h. Except for severe *Pseudomonas* infections, 30 g daily is not necessary, and smaller doses, 10 or 15 g daily, are adequate for the therapy of other gram-negative infections, including those caused by indole-positive *Proteus* and *Enterobacter.* Urinary concentrations in excess of 1000 μg/ml are attained with 0.5- or 1.0-g doses intramuscularly, so that doses comparable with those used with ampicillin are appropriate for urinary tract infections, including those due to *Pseudomonas.* An oral form of carbenicillin, the indanyl ester, is available, and one or two 0.5-g tablets (each equivalent to 382 mg carbenicillin) every 6 h produce urinary concentrations well in excess of MICs for susceptible gram-negative bacilli, including *Pseudomonas.* The indanyl ester is *not* indicated for the treatment of infection outside of the urinary tract.

An increase in bacterial resistance has been noted in some patients with severe gram-negative infections treated with carbenicillin, but the frequency and extent of the resistance has varied in different reports. The concomitant administration of aminoglycosides has tended to delay the development of resistance to carbenicillin, and in addition a synergistic action has been found to occur with these two antibiotics against many gram-negative bacilli. It has therefore become customary in severe infections to give both these antibiotics in order to enhance antibacterial activity and to delay the emergence of resistance as well. Since there is inactivation of the aminoglycosides, especially gentamicin and tobramycin, when they are present in the same solution for several hours with carbenicillin or ticarcillin, it is preferable to administer them separately, either intramuscularly or intravenously, and under these circumstances the blood levels of each are the same as if they were being given alone. Amikacin appears to be more stable in the presence of either carbenicillin or ticarcillin. Ticarcillin, a newer semisynthetic penicillin, has pharmacokinetic properties very similar to those of carbenicillin but is two to four times as active in vitro against *Pseudomonas.* A daily dose of 18 g is considered equal to 30 g carbenicillin for *Pseudomonas* infections and provides a lower sodium load (both antibiotics contain about 5.5 meq sodium per gram). Disadvantages of the lower dose are that the greater activity of ticarcillin is found only against *Pseudomonas,* and that 18 g ticarcillin may be more expensive than 30 g carbenicillin. However, because of its greater activity against *P. aeruginosa,* ticarcillin frequently is chosen, especially in immunocompromised hosts.

Piperacillin and *mezlocillin* are two new semisynthetic penicillins. Piperacillin is more active than either carbenicillin or ticarcillin against strains of *P. aeruginosa,* and its pharmacology is similar. It inhibits approximately 90 percent of strains of *Pseudomonas* at concentrations of 12 μg/ml antibiotic or less. However, when tested against a large inoculum size of bacterial cells in vitro, it loses much of its activity. The clinical significance of this finding is unclear. Mezlocillin has a spectrum of activity and pharmacology similar to that of carbenicillin and ticarcillin, but it is much more active against strains of *Klebsiella.* Similar to piperacillin, it is less active when tested against a high inoculum size of bacterial cells.

Penicillinase-resistant penicillins (antistaphylococcal penicillins) The advent of these antibiotics in the early 1960s greatly enhanced the ability to cope with severe staphylococcal infections, because at that time over three-fourths of strains causing infections in hospitals were penicillinase producers, and this high incidence has persisted. Furthermore, the number of strains resistant to these new penicillins has remained small, especially in the United States. This is probably due to the low incidence of naturally occurring methicillin-resistant strains, and the fact that only a small proportion of the cells in a "resistant" culture are actually lacking in susceptibility. In contrast, certain European hospitals now report that over 20 percent of strains of *Staphylococcus aureus* are methicillin-resistant; the reason for the difference is unknown.

Five penicillinase-resistant penicillins are currently marketed in the United States: *methicillin, oxacillin, nafcillin, cloxacillin,* and *dicloxacillin.* The first three are available for parenteral administration. Methicillin is less active when tested in broth cultures than are oxacillin and nafcillin, but this is probably offset by its much lower protein binding, 40 percent compared with 90 percent or more for the other two. Clinical studies do not provide convincing evidence of superiority of any of these three penicillins for the parenteral therapy of severe staphylococcal infections. Methicillin is given in the same dose as, or in twice the dose of, the other two because of its lower in vitro activity, i.e., 1 or 2 g every 4 to 6 h in adults. For intravenous administration, each dose is diluted in 50 to 100 ml fluid, and is infused over a period of 30 min to minimize phlebitis. Intramuscular injections are painful and are poorly tolerated for more than a few days. Methicillin interstitial nephritis, an uncommon but important untoward reaction, has been reported rarely with oxacillin and nafcillin. Nafcillin has been found by many observers to give lower blood levels than equal doses of oxacillin; this appears to be due to sequestration of nafcillin in the liver and possibly in other tissues so that less is available to circulate in the blood. The therapeutic implications of this phenomenon are unknown. In many centers, nafcillin has replaced methicillin in the treatment of severe staphylococcal infection because of concern about interstitial nephritis.

With oral administration, both nafcillin and oxacillin give low blood levels, but cloxacillin gives blood levels twice as high and dicloxacillin four times as high as oxacillin when the same doses are given orally. However, there is also a progressive increase in serum protein binding (92 percent for oxacillin, 94 percent for cloxacillin, and 96 percent for dicloxacillin), so that the differences in free, active antibiotic may offset the blood level differences. In general, cloxacillin or dicloxacillin in doses of 0.25 or 0.5 g four times daily is preferred for oral administration. The efficacy of these antibiotics, either initially in mild to moderate soft-tissue infections, or for completion of therapy following administration of one of the three parenteral preparations described above, is well established.

The chief indication for the penicillinase-resistant penicillins is the therapy of infections caused by penicillinase-producing staphylococci, but they are often administered empirically before the etiologic organism is known. Pneumococci and most streptococci are more susceptible to penicillin G, but blood levels are sufficiently high with the penicillinase-resistant penicillins, especially when given parenterally, so that it is not necessary to give both types of penicillins to provide coverage for these organisms. However, infections caused by enterococci and *Neisseria* cannot be expected to respond to therapy with a penicillinase-resistant penicillin given alone, and if these organisms are suspected, penicillin G or ampicillin should be used.

In addition to the various allergic manifestations mentioned above, less frequent reactions to penicillins include myoclonus, seizures, potassium intoxication, hemolysis, leukopenia, thrombocytopenia, and neuropathy, usually with very high blood levels. Mental disturbances occur in a small percentage of patients following large doses of procaine penicillin.

CEPHALOSPORINS The cephalosporins differ from the penicillins in having a six-membered dihydrothiazine ring, instead of a five-membered thiazolidine ring, fused to the β-lactam ring. As a result of this chemical difference there is no true cross-allergenicity, and most patients who are allergic to penicillins can be treated with cephalosporins without hypersensitivity reactions. The small number in whom this is not possible seem to be highly allergic individuals who react separately to the two groups of antibiotics.

Most bacteria susceptible to the penicillins are also susceptible to the cephalosporins, including group A and viridans streptococci, pneumococci, penicillin G–sensitive and –resistant *S. aureus, Neisseria, Clostridia, Actinomyces,* and *Corynebacterium diphtheriae.* Among the gram-negatives most strains of *E. coli, P. mirabilis, Klebsiella, Shigella, Salmonella,* and many strains of *H. influenzae* are susceptible. The spectrum has been extended by the addition of cefamandole and cefoxitin, and more recently by cefotaxime and other newer agents (see below). The cephalosporins act on the cell wall in a manner similar to the penicillins, and are bactericidal. As with the penicillins, there has been little tendency for susceptible species to become resistant despite widespread use of the cephalosporins.

Twelve cephalosporins are now marketed in the United States, and many more are under investigation. Orally, *cephalexin* and *cephradine* are very similar and can be considered interchangeable. They are well absorbed, a 0.5-g dose giving an average peak blood level in adults of about 18 μg/ml, six times as high as with the same dose of ampicillin. Serum protein binding is low and comparable with that of ampicillin (about 15 percent), and over 90 percent of these drugs are excreted in the urine, without nephrotoxicity. These two antibiotics are less active in vitro against gram-positive bacteria, especially staphylococci, than the injectable cephalosporins, but, because of the high blood levels, clinical results have been good, particularly after initial parenteral therapy. There is considerable variability in the susceptibility of *H. influenzae,* and twice the usual dose is recommended in the official labeling for otitis media. *Cephaloglycin,* a drug that is poorly absorbed orally and that gives low blood levels, has gradually been abandoned in the treatment of urinary infections because of the superior characteristics of the other two compounds.

Two newer oral formulations, *cefaclor* and *cefadroxil,* are also available. Cefaclor has the same basic structure as cephalexin except for the substitution of a chloride for a methyl group. Although peak serum concentrations achieved with cefaclor are lower than those reached with a comparable dose of cephalexin, cefaclor is more active in vitro against many microorganisms, including both β-lactamase-positive and -negative strains of *H. influenzae.* Its main application is in pediatrics. Cefadroxil is the parahydroxy analogue of cephalexin, and it has a comparable spectrum. Cefadroxil achieves more sustained serum and urine levels because of its longer serum half-life. Because of the prolonged excretion of cefadroxil, the drug may be administered only once or twice a day for the treatment of certain infections. Following a single oral dose of 500 mg to 1 g, cefadroxil can be detected in the serum for 12 h and in the urine for even longer.

Parenteral preparations of eight cephalosporins are commercially available. Both for therapy and prophylaxis *cephalothin* has had the longest and most extensive use. It is usually administered intravenously, 1 or 2 g every 4 or 6 h in at least 50 ml fluid to minimize phlebitis. It is partially converted in the body to a metabolic breakdown product, desacetylcephalothin, which is less active, particularly against gram-negative bacteria. This appears to have no clinical significance because of the large amount of the parent compound present. Cephalothin may cause some nephrotoxicity, especially when given in conjunction with aminoglycosides, but establishing this point has been difficult. *Cephapirin* is very similar to cephalothin in its in vitro activity and pharmacological characteristics and may be interchangeable clinically, although fewer reports of its efficacy are available. *Cephaloridine,* another early cephalosporin, has low serum protein binding and is well tolerated intramuscularly, but clearly causes renal tubular damage in large doses and, because of its potential nephrotoxicity, should not be used. Cephradine is available parenterally as well as orally, but published documentation of efficacy with parenteral administration is not extensive.

Cefazolin has had increasing use parenterally because of its high and prolonged blood levels, which are due to high serum protein binding (85 percent) and low renal clearance. Its serum half-life is 1.8 h compared with 0.5 h for cephalothin. Cefazolin 0.5 g is probably equivalent to 1.0 g cephalothin therapeutically, taking into consideration the differences in blood levels and protein binding. Cefazolin is also well tolerated intramuscularly, whereas cephalothin and cephapirin are not. Also cefazolin is inactivated by large inocula of some strains of *S. aureus* while cephalothin is not; whether the inactivation is of any clinical significance has not been established.

Cefamandole is a parenterally administered semisynthetic cephalosporin which is more active than cephalothin in vitro against a number of gram-negative bacilli. Because of its instability, this compound has been formulated as the nafate derivative. After administration, cefamandole nafate is hydrolyzed rapidly to cefamandole. The enhanced in vitro activity against certain gram-negative bacilli, including *H. influenzae,* is partly due to the resistance of cefamandole to β-lactamase enzymes. However, some strains that hydrolyze cefamandole are also susceptible to it in vitro, and it has been postulated that the drug may be able to penetrate the cell envelope of certain gram-negative bacilli more effectively than other cephalosporins. Compared with cephalothin, cefamandole blood levels are higher, whereas serum half-life and protein binding are similar. Cefamandole is excreted in the urine unchanged. The drug is generally well tolerated and has been approved for pediatric as well as for adult use. Cefamandole inhibits most Enterobacteriaceae to an equal or greater degree than cephalothin. However, strains of *Klebsiella* which are resistant to cephalothin usually are also resistant to cefamandole. Isolates of *Enterobacter* species frequently are resistant to cefamandole in vitro when tested against a large inoculum size of bacterial cells. The usual adult dosage of cefamandole is 0.5 to 1.0 g every 6 to 8 h.

Cefoxitin is a member of the cephamycin group of antibiotics and differs chemically from cephalothin primarily by having a methoxy group at position 7 of the 7-aminocephalosporanic acid nucleus. This alteration in structure somewhat diminishes its activity in vitro against common gram-positive cocci but enhances its activity against many gram-negative bacilli, including indole-positive *Proteus* species as well as strains of *Bacteroides fragilis* and *Serratia. Acinetobacter* and *Enterobacter* species generally are resistant. Its enhanced spectrum is explained, in part, by cefoxitin's resistance to hydrolysis by β-lactamases. Pain at the site of intramuscular injection is common with cefoxitin, and for this reason the drug is administered primarily by the intravenous route. The half-life of cefoxitin is approximately 45 min, compared with 25 min for cephalothin, and the drug is excreted unchanged in the urine. The usual adult dosage of cefoxitin is 1.0 to 2.0 g every 6 to 8 h. Because of its activity against a wide variety of aerobic and anaerobic organisms found in abdominal and pelvic infections, cefoxitin appears to be replacing cephalothin and cefazolin as the antibiotic that is widely used in surgery.

Further modifications of the 7-aminocephalosporanic acid nucleus and discovery of the cephamycins have brought about a worldwide interest in the development of extended-spectrum β-lactam agents. Although both cefamandole and cefoxitin have a spectrum somewhat greater than that of the initial cephalosporins, there still are notable gaps in the scope of their antimicrobial activity. A number of modified β-lactam antibiotics, some with unique antimicrobial activity, have been developed and are undergoing extensive evaluation in the laboratory and clinic.

Cefotaxime, the first of the third-generation agents to be released in the United States, is a methoxyimino derivative of 7-aminocephalosporanic acid. This parenteral drug demonstrates marked resistance to β-lactamases of certain gram-negative bacilli. A particularly interesting aspect of the spectrum of cefotaxime is its in vitro activity against some isolates of *P. aeruginosa.* Some investigators have reported that median minimal inhibitory concentrations (MICs) for isolates of *P. aeruginosa* were 8 and 6 μg cefotaxime per milliliter. In some studies, however, a rather marked inoculum effect was noted, which showed that the MIC increased as the inoculum was enlarged. This may modify the clinical usefulness of this drug, and cefotaxime is *not* recommended for the treatment of *Pseudomonas.* Similar observations have been made with strains of *Serratia marcescens* tested with cefotaxime, i.e., the activity demonstrated by the antibiotic was confined to studies done with lower inoculum sizes of bacterial cells.

Although cephalosporins penetrate most body fluids quite well, none can be clearly recommended for parenteral therapy of bacterial meningitis. Some of the investigational compounds are being evaluated for this purpose. Compounds soon to be released include moxalactam, cefoperazone, and ceftizoxime. *Moxalactam* is a novel β-lactam antibiotic for parenteral use which possesses a unique chemical structure, namely, the 1-oxa-β-lactam nucleus substituted by 7-α-methoxy and phenylmalonyl groups. The drug is undergoing extensive in vitro and clinical trials and appears to be more resistant to β-lactamases, including the R-plasmid–mediated and cephalosporinase types, than other extended-spectrum β-lactams. *Cefoperazone* is a semisynthetic cephalosporin that is structurally similar to cefamandole and piperacillin, an extended-spectrum experimental penicillin. In vitro studies in agar demonstrate that cefoperazone may possess activity against *P. aeruginosa* comparable to that of the aminoglycosides and greater than that of carbenicillin or ticarcillin. *Ceftizoxime* is the desacetoxymethyl derivative of cefotaxime. Both of these compounds are available only for parenteral use and demonstrate interesting properties in terms of β-lactamase stability, intrinsic activity, and antibacterial spectrum. Ceftizoxime appears slightly more active in vitro than cefotaxime against some species, including *Klebsiella, Enterobacter,* and *Serratia.*

Most patients who are thought to be allergic to penicillins can tolerate cephalosporins without adverse reactions. There is probably not true cross-reactivity, but a small number of highly allergic individuals do react to both drugs. In patients with previous penicillin anaphylaxis, or with positive immediate-type skin reactions to penicillin, therapy with cephalosporins should be instituted in small doses that are increased gradually. Rashes, urticaria, and anaphylaxis have been reported with cephalosporins, as have neutropenia, hemolytic anemia, thrombocytopenia, positive Coombs' tests, and transient rise in serum glutamic oxaloacetic transaminase and alkaline phosphatase.

AMINOCYCLITOLS (AMINOGLYCOSIDES AND SPECTINOMYCIN) Six aminoglycoside antibiotics currently are available for clinical use in the United States: streptomycin, neomycin, kanamycin, gentamicin, tobramycin, and amikacin. Netilmicin is due to be released and sisomicin is available in Europe. Aminoglycoside antibiotics are compounds that contain two or more amino sugars and aminocyclitol components. Spectinomycin does not contain an amino sugar component and is an aminocyclitol but not an aminoglycoside antibiotic.

Streptomycin, one of the first antibiotics available for systemic administration, was widely used during the late 1940s and the 1950s. For a number of years it was given almost routinely in conjunction with penicillin in surgical cases for the prophylaxis and treatment of postoperative infections. Because of the tendency for highly resistant organisms to appear within 2 or 3 days, and its potential for causing vestibular damage and deafness, streptomycin has been largely supplanted by kanamycin, gentamicin, tobramycin, and amikacin, although it is still in use for certain specific purposes. Tuberculosis is still treated with streptomycin, particularly when triple drug regimens are used for the first few weeks. Streptomycin is also used in conjunction with penicillin to treat *S. viridans* endocarditis and some enterococcal infections and for the treatment of certain less common infections such as brucellosis and tularemia. In addition to vestibular nerve toxicity, other adverse reactions of streptomycin include rashes, fever, contact dermatitis, pancytopenia, anaphylaxis, and renal injury.

Neomycin, another aminoglycoside that appeared in the 1940s, is no longer used parenterally because of its nephro- and neurotoxicity. Respiratory arrest is a serious adverse reaction that has occurred when neomycin and less frequently when other aminoglycosides are instilled topically in the peritoneal cavity in anesthetized patients, and deafness has resulted from the topical application of neomycin soaks injudiciously in burns and wounds. Neomycin is useful and relatively safe when given orally in doses of 4 to 6 g daily to "prepare" the bowel preoperatively, and in patients with hepatic insufficiency where inhibition of bacterial growth in the intestine is necessary to reduce the absorption of nitrogenous substances. However, the amount of neomycin absorbed from the intestine is variable, and toxic levels have been demonstrated in some patients. Neomycin is also used as a spray and an ointment in an attempt to decrease the bacterial count in individuals who are nasal carriers of staphylococci. Neomycin ointment also is available in combination with other antimicrobials, usually polymyxin B and bacitracin, for topical application to skin and mucous membranes.

Kanamycin is similar in structure to neomycin but is less toxic and has been widely used parenterally for infections caused by most commonly encountered gram-negative bacilli except *Pseudomonas. Amikacin,* a semisynthetic derivative of kanamycin, has many similar characteristics except that it is active against *P. aeruginosa* as well as against other gram-negative bacilli resistant to other aminoglycosides, and amikacin

has superseded the use of kanamycin in most institutions. Both are active in vitro against staphylococci but are not used to treat severe staphylococcal infections because much higher blood levels can be attained safely with penicillins and cephalosporins.

These and other aminoglycoside antibiotics are not active against aerobic or anaerobic streptococci including *S. pneumoniae.* They should be administered intramuscularly or by slow intravenous infusion in doses not larger than 7.5 mg/kg every 12 h, with the total dose generally not exceeding 15 g. Excretion is by glomerular filtration, the serum half-life is 2 h, and the drugs are not protein-bound. With the ever-increasing occurrence of infections due to resistant gram-negative bacteria, amikacin is receiving increasing use over other aminoglycoside antibiotics, especially in the treatment of infections in immunocompromised hosts.

Gentamicin and *tobramycin* are widely used aminoglycosides that are very similar except that tobramycin is two to four times more active against most strains of *Pseudomonas.* Gentamicin is more active against strains of *Serratia.* Smaller doses are used than for amikacin (3 to 5 versus 15 mg/kg per day), giving peak blood levels following intramuscular injections of 4 to 5 μg/ml for gentamicin and tobramycin versus about 20 μg/ml for amikacin. However, minimal inhibitory concentrations are also higher with amikacin, and it has not been shown that the higher blood levels are necessarily associated with a better clinical response. Amikacin is more stable than the other antibiotics in the presence of carbenicillin or ticarcillin. Tobramycin appears to have less nephrotoxic potential than gentamicin.

Bacterial resistance, transmitted by plasmids and due to enzymatic transformations related to adenylating, phosphorylating, and acetylating isoenzymes, is a potential threat with the aminoglycosides. This problem is more common in certain hospitals than in others. Since amikacin has the least potential for resistance by the mechanism of enzymatic inactivation, many hospitals have held the drug in reserve. However, the use of amikacin in hospitals has not been associated with an increased frequency of resistant strains. In some hospitals where gentamicin resistance has become a significant problem (more than 10 percent of resistant strains), amikacin is the drug of choice for seriously ill patients requiring an aminoglycoside.

Although various nomograms have been used to estimate the dosage and interval between doses in patients with unstable renal function, serum concentrations must be determined by precise measurement, generally employing a bioassay or radioimmunoassay method.

Spectinomycin is an aminocyclitol antibiotic that is administered in a single 2-g dose intramuscularly for the treatment of uncomplicated genital gonorrhea. It is used as an alternative to penicillin in penicillin-allergic patients and is the drug of choice against penicillinase-producing strains of *Neisseria gonorrhoeae.* Spectinomycin is less effective than standard regimens of either procaine penicillin or oral tetracycline in eradicating pharyngeal carriage of gonorrhea. Side effects are minimal and the drug is well tolerated.

TETRACYCLINES Since they first appeared in the late 1940s, the tetracycline antibiotics have been used widely because of their broad spectrum of activity against many gram-positive and gram-negative bacteria, and also other microorganisms such as *Mycoplasma, Rickettsia,* and *Chlamydia.* They have been effective, although not necessarily the drugs of choice, in the treatment of common venereal diseases including gonorrhea, syphilis, lymphogranuloma venereum, and granuloma inguinale. Their use has become more restricted during the last decade because of the advent of bactericidal antibiotics such as the cephalosporins, the penicillinase-resistant penicillins, and the aminoglycosides, together with an increasing awareness of the limitations of the tetracyclines. These limitations include the appearance of resistant strains among commonly encountered pathogens such as group A streptococci and pneumococci, the primarily bacteriostatic action of the tetracyclines, the occurrence of hepatotoxicity with high blood levels, the relatively high incidence of superinfections, and the common occurrence of side effects such as nausea, diarrhea, and photosensitivity reactions. Despite these limitations, the tetracyclines are still widely used for respiratory, urinary, soft-tissue, and venereal infections.

Chlortetracycline and *oxytetracycline,* the two original compounds, have been largely replaced by *tetracycline,* which is marketed by a number of companies, and competition has led to a marked reduction in its price. The usual adult dose is 1 to 2 g daily in two to four equally divided doses. Intramuscular preparations are not very satisfactory, but the intravenous form is well tolerated and gives relatively high blood levels with doses of 0.5 g every 12 h. Excessive blood levels occur with renal insufficiency unless the dose is decreased, and can cause fatty degeneration of the liver which may be fatal. Tetracycline persists in the body for many days when its normal route of excretion through the kidneys is blocked.

Four long-acting tetracyclines are available: *demeclocycline, methacycline, doxycycline,* and *minocycline.* They have high protein binding (over 90 versus 70 percent for tetracycline) and a prolonged plasma half-life, so that blood levels are well maintained when they are administered orally only every 12 to 24 h. However, the half-life of tetracycline is sufficiently prolonged so that blood levels with administration only every 12 h are similar to those of the smaller doses recommended for the long-acting tetracyclines. The potential advantages for the long-active tetracyclines, i.e., greater convenience from less frequent administration and decreased cost from lower doses, have not been realized fully. Minocycline can be used in the management of meningococcal carriers, but because of the frequent occurrence of vertigo, rifampin 600 mg/kg every 12 h for 2 days for adults and 10 mg/kg every 12 h for 2 days for children is preferred. Doxycycline does not give excessive blood levels in the presence of renal insufficiency following either oral or intravenous administration, and this provides a safety feature when the exact status of the patient's renal function is uncertain or unknown. Doxycycline is also active against the majority of strains of *B. fragilis,* and its efficacy in abdominal and pelvic infections has received considerable attention. Doxycycline is administered in the usual dosage of 100 mg every 12 h, and the intravenous and oral doses are the same.

Untoward effects of the tetracyclines include staining of the teeth in children under 10, photosensitivity, intestinal irritation, increased urinary nitrogen loss, potential nephrotoxicity especially when given with other nephrotoxic drugs or with outdated supplies, vertigo (with minocycline), fatty hepatic changes in pregnancy, and increased intracranial pressure in children.

ERYTHROMYCIN, LINCOMYCIN, CLINDAMYCIN *Erythromycin* is primarily a bacteriostatic antibiotic that is active against the commonly encountered gram-positive bacteria, and is used chiefly for the oral therapy of respiratory and soft-tissue infections, particularly in patients thought to be allergic to penicillin. The susceptibility of *Mycoplasma pneumoniae* and *Legionella pneumophila* to erythromycin enhances its usefulness in respiratory infections. Erythromycin base is absorbed in an erratic manner, but some enteric-coated preparations now available give good and reliable serum concentrations. Erythromycin estolate has been thought to give much higher blood levels than erythromycin stearate, but the difference may be not as great as was once postulated because the estolate needs to be hydrolyzed in the body to the active form, and the hydrolysis is not as complete as during the blood level assay procedure. The estolate salt is associated with a low incidence of cholestatic hepatitis, which is readily reversible and rarely serious. Clinical results with the estolate, stearate, and the enteric-coated preparations appear to be comparable. The usual oral dose is 1 or 2 g daily. Intramuscular preparations are irritating, and intravenous administration is not used widely, partly because the preparations are not entirely satisfactory but chiefly because oral therapy is adequate for most infections treated with erythromycin. The recommended dose of erythromycin for the treatment of Legionnaires' disease is 0.5 to 1.0 g every 6 h.

Lincomycin and *clindamycin* are similar in antibacterial activity and clinical usefulness to erythromycin. Clindamycin gives higher blood levels, is more potent, and may cause less gastrointestinal side effects than lincomycin. The usual oral dose is 150 to 300 mg every 6 h. An excellent parenteral preparation of both is available, and 300 to 600 mg is given every 6 or 8 h. Clindamycin is considerably more active against *B. fragilis,* and intravenous administration of this antibiotic in abdominal and pelvic infections is widely advocated for this reason. However, pseudomembranous colitis has been recognized as a potentially serious side effect which has led to recommendations that these antibiotics be used chiefly for hospitalized patients with significant infections, and that they be discontinued at once if diarrhea occurs. The colitis is primarily due to toxin-producing strains of clostridia that are resistant to clindamycin.

CHLORAMPHENICOL This antibiotic has a broad spectrum of activity similar to the tetracyclines and during the 1950s was used widely. However, the occurrence of aplastic anemia, even though quite uncommon (about 1 in 25,000 persons exposed) has led to a restriction of chloramphenicol to those serious infections in which it is quite clearly the drug of choice. Typhoid fever is the principal example, and there are occasionally other severe gram-negative infections where the etiologic agent is susceptible only to chloramphenicol. With increasing interest in anaerobic infections, it is now realized that *B. fragilis* is one of the most common of the anaerobic pathogens and that the majority of the strains are resistant to the penicillins and tetracyclines. This has led to an increase in the use of chloramphenicol since almost all *Bacteroides* strains are susceptible to it. However, clindamycin is also very active against *B. fragilis,* and it has partially replaced chloramphenicol for the treatment of patients with proven or presumed *Bacteroides* infections. Clindamycin lacks the broad aerobic gram-negative spectrum of chloramphenicol, and for this reason, the latter may be preferred under certain circumstances. In addition, clindamycin's propensity to producing colitis and its failure to penetrate into the central nervous system should restrict its use. Chloramphenicol is also used frequently in bacterial meningitis when the causative organism is not clearly recognizable on Gram's stain of the spinal fluid. It is frequently prescribed along with ampicillin when *H. influenzae* is suspected since an increasing number of strains of *H. influenzae* produce a β-lactamase which inactivates ampicillin. If the isolate is susceptible to ampicillin, chloramphenicol can be discontinued.

Chloramphenicol is well absorbed by the oral route, and the usual adult dose is 0.5 g every 6 h. The parenteral preparation, chloramphenicol succinate, is hydrolyzed in the body to the active form, and this conversion is incomplete so that the blood levels with intravenous administration are not much higher than when the antibiotic is taken by mouth. With intramuscular administration, blood levels are considerably lower than with the oral route, and intramuscular administration is not recommended.

In addition to aplastic anemia, which may be an allergic or "idiosyncratic" reaction that usually occurs with prolonged and repeated administration, chloramphenicol inhibits protein synthesis, especially with doses larger than 2 g a day, an effect that is reversible. Clinically this is manifested by leukopenia, inadequate erythropoiesis (anemia), and thrombocytopenia as well as absence of reticulocytosis, high serum iron, and full saturation of transferrin. These hematologic abnormalities appear to be dose-dependent, reversible, and not related to the much less frequent aplastic anemia that has been reported with chloramphenicol. The gray syndrome, consisting of pallor, listlessness, and often death, occurs in neonates who have inadequately developed hepatic and renal mechanisms for metabolizing chloramphenicol; this can be prevented by restricting the dose to 25 mg/kg per day. A similar syndrome appears to occur in adults who receive chloramphenicol and who develop severe impairment in liver function.

POLYMYXINS Polymyxin B and E (colistin) are polypeptide antibiotics that are active in vitro against most gram-negative bacteria except for the *Proteus* group. They have been of historical importance chiefly because of their action against *P. aeruginosa.* However, their use systemically has decreased markedly since the advent of the aminoglycosides and carbenicillin, which are clearly superior.

Polymyxin B is administered intramuscularly every 8 h, or as a continuous intravenous infusion, in doses no larger than 2.0 mg/kg per day. It is effective in treating urinary infections, but its efficacy in systemic infections is uncertain. Polymyxin B is also administered topically for eye and ear infections, and intrathecally for *Pseudomonas* meningitis. Colistin is available as the sodium salt of colistimethate and is administered in doses of 3.0 to 5.0 mg/kg per day intramuscularly or intravenously as described for polymyxin B. These agents are employed infrequently for the management of infection related to nonfermentative gram-negative bacilli resistant to other drugs.

Polymyxin B and colistimethate both cause perioral paresthesias and other neurotoxic manifestations with excessive blood levels; of these, apnea is the most life-threatening. Renal irritation and azotemia, which are usually reversible, may also occur. It is important to monitor renal function and to decrease the dose in the presence of renal insufficiency.

VANCOMYCIN Vancomycin is a bactericidal antibiotic that warrants special consideration because of its usefulness in treating certain specific infections. Vancomycin is effective against gram-positive bacteria including penicillinase-producing staphylococci and enterococci. It is particularly useful in treating severe staphylococcal infections when penicillins and cephalosporins cannot be given, and in the treatment of *S. viridans* and enterococcal endocarditis under the same circumstances. It can be given only by the intravenous route, and 0.5 g every 6 h for 2 or 3 weeks is the usual dose. Thrombophlebitis is the principal side effect; it can be minimized by diluting each dose in 100 ml fluid and administering it over a period of at least 1 h. Chills, fever, renal irritation, and deafness are other adverse reactions that have been described, and these can be minimized by slow administration and by reduction of the dose if renal function is impaired. Vancomycin has had a considerable revival. One special indication is infections in patients with renal failure requiring dialysis, where a single dose of 1 g every 7 to 10 days gives adequate blood levels. Vancomycin also is employed in the treatment of antibiotic-associated colitis due to *Clostridium difficile* toxin.

SULFONAMIDES AND SULFAMETHOXAZOLE-TRIMETHOPRIM The sulfonamides have been used clinically since 1937 and were the principal drugs administered for systemic antibacterial chemotherapy before penicillin and the other antibiotics became generally available. Their role has declined steadily, and they now occupy an important, although relatively small, place in clinical therapy since they are less active than the antibiotics, they are primarily bacteriostatic, resistant organisms occur frequently, and adverse reactions are common. Uncomplicated urinary tract infections due to *E. coli* are the principal indication for sulfonamides because of their efficacy, relative safety, and low cost. In addition, sulfonamides are the drugs of choice for the therapy of nocardiosis. They are no longer the preferred agents for the treatment of bacillary dysentery, meningococcal infections, and *H. influenzae* meningitis. They still are recommended for meningococcal prophylaxis *if* the strains are known to be *sensitive* to sulfonamides.

Sulfadiazine, once widely used as an all-purpose sulfonamide, tends to produce crystalluria and has been largely replaced by the more soluble *sulfisoxazole* and its close congener, *sulfamethoxazole,* which is also used widely now in a fixed-dose combination with trimethoprim. Mixtures of three sulfonamides (trisulfapyrimidines) are also widely used because they are associated with a low incidence of crystalluria. The sulfonamides are usually administered orally, although very satisfactory intravenous preparations of the sodium salts are available. Orally, an initial dose of 2 to 4 g is followed by 1 g every 4 to 6 h.

Long-acting sulfonamides have also been used widely, and their only advantage is that they can be administered orally only once or twice daily. Examples are sulfamethoxypyridazine and sulfadimethoxine. The primary clinical indication for these long-acting compounds has been urinary tract infections, in instances where the convenience of taking only one dose a day has been considered important. However, it is undesirable to use a drug that leaves the body slowly, because this may prolong adverse reactions. Moreover, certain severe toxic reactions such as erythema multiforme or myocarditis have been reported to occur more commonly with long-acting sulfonamides. It is probably best not to use this class of compounds at all.

There are also some poorly absorbed sulfonamides, succinylsulfathiazole (Sulfasuxidine) and phthalysulfathiazole (Sulfathalidine), that are used principally to decrease the number of bacteria in the colon prior to certain types of abdominal surgery. These agents are of doubtful value. The drug sulfasalazine (Azulfidine) (see Chap. 309) is of value in ulcerative colitis.

Adverse reactions caused by the sulfonamides include erythema multiforme, serum sickness, hemolytic (in patients with glucose 6-phosphate dehydrogenase deficiency) and aplastic anemias, arthralgia, hepatitis, nausea, vertigo, lesions resembling those of polyarteritis nodosa, and kernicterus.

The combination of sulfamethoxazole and trimethoprim inhibits the growth of susceptible bacteria at two different steps of folic acid synthesis. Studies in vitro demonstrate that this combination may prevent emergence of bacterial resistance better than when either agent is used alone. The combination also is synergistic in vitro against many gram-negative organisms. Initially, the fixed-dose combination of sulfamethoxazole-trimethoprim was recommended only for the treatment of patients with recurrent urinary tract infections. However, the combination has been approved both for oral and intravenous use in patients with acute exacerbation of chronic bronchitis due to *H. influenzae* and *S. pneumoniae;* diarrheal disease due to *Shigella flexneri* and *S. sonnei;* upper and lower urinary tract infections due to susceptible strains of *E. coli, Klebsiella, Enterobacter,* and *Proteus* species; acute otitis media in children due to *S. pneumoniae* and *H. influenzae;* and in the treatment of pneumonia caused by *Pneumocystis carinii.* Its use prophylactically in immunocompromised hosts also appears promising in preventing *Pneumocystis* infections. It also may be of particular value in the prevention of recurrent bouts of bladder bacteriuria in women who experience multiple reinfections. The combination intended for intravenous use is available in 5-ml ampuls containing 80 mg trimethoprim and 400 mg sulfamethoxazole. The combination also is available in two sizes of tablets containing 80 or 160 mg trimethoprim and 400 or 800 mg sulfamethoxazole. The potential adverse reactions anticipated with the combination are the same as those experienced with the sulfonamides.

Trimethoprim also is available alone without sulfamethoxazole for the treatment of initial episodes of acute uncomplicated urinary tract infection generally caused by *E. coli.* A dose of 100 mg every 12 h is recommended for 7 to 10 days. Trimethoprim also is used clinically in the treatment of bacterial prostatitis, although it is not approved for this indication.

ANTIFUNGAL AGENTS (See also Chap. 181) *Amphotericin B* is a potentially toxic antibiotic that is effective in the treatment of deep-seated mycotic infections. It produces marked improvement and occasional cures in cryptococcosis, histoplasmosis, blastomycosis, disseminated candidiasis, and coccidioidomycosis, and has a beneficial effect in at least some cases of aspergillosis and mucormycosis. It is administered intravenously in 5% dextrose solution over a period of 5 or 6 h. The safest procedure is to administer 1 mg on the first day, 5 mg on the second, and 10 mg on the third. The dose is then increased by 5 to 10 mg each day until 1 mg/kg is being administered daily. The dose may then be changed to 1.5 mg/kg every other day; treatment is continued for 2 to 4 months, depending on the severity of the infection and upon the patient's response. In patients with severe infections where intensive therapy is considered essential, it may be necessary to assume the risk of administering 15 mg very cautiously as the initial dose, with the addition of antihistamines and/or steroids to help ameliorate the chills and fever, which are quite variable from patient to patient. In some debilitated patients who develop *Candida* infections with oral or esophageal lesions, or bacteremias secondary to intravenous catheters, 10 or 15 mg amphotericin B daily for only 3 or 4 days may be adequate to bring the infection under control.

Some degree of renal impairment invariably occurs when amphotericin B is administered for several weeks; this is manifested during therapy by a rise in the blood urea nitrogen (BUN) and serum creatinine. Renal function may return to normal following therapy if attention is devoted to giving the minimum amount of drug that is compatible with a satisfactory therapeutic response, and if particular care is exercised in lowering the dose and frequency of administration when the creatinine becomes markedly elevated. Many patients have permanent renal damage; this poses special problems when relapses occur and subsequent courses of therapy are needed. Other adverse effects of amphotericin B include anemia, hypokalemia, thrombocytopenia, and hepatitis.

Nystatin (Mycostatin) is another antifungal antibiotic that is less potent than amphotericin B and is too toxic for systemic administration. It is applied topically in ointments, tablets, and suspension. It is used particularly for oral, intestinal, skin, and vaginal lesions due to *Candida,* and the best results are obtained when applications are made several times a day. The individual dose varies from 100,000 to 1 million units, depending on the location of the lesion.

Flucytosine is an oral antifungal agent that is relatively nontoxic and has been used successfully in cryptococcal, *Candida,* and *Torulopsis* infections. The dose is 150 mg/kg per day administered in divided doses at 6-h intervals. Some cases of cryptococcal meningitis and pulmonary disease have seemed to respond as well as to amphotericin B, but flucytosine is, in general, less potent than amphotericin and, because of emergence of resistance occurring during treatment, is not recommended to be used as a sole agent. An appreciable percentage of initial isolates of *Candida* also are resistant to the drug. Adverse effects have consisted chiefly of nausea, vomiting, diarrhea, and rashes, but pancytopenia and abnormal liver function tests have also been reported. The drug is excreted in the urine, and the dose needs to be decreased in uremia.

Flucytosine is not effective in histoplasmosis, blastomycosis, and coccidioidomycosis. It is indicated chiefly in patients with severe cryptococcal, *Candida,* and *Torulopsis* infections in conjunction with amphotericin B. It can also be used alone for *Candida* infections of the bladder and for superficial lesions that do not respond to topical therapy.

Miconazole, a synthetic imidazole derivative, has been used intravenously in systemic cryptococcal, *Candida,* and coccidioides infections with at least moderate effectiveness. It causes little or no nephrotoxicity. Itching and nausea have been significant side effects. It probably has no clear-cut therapeutic advantage over amphotericin B except perhaps for less potential toxicity.

Ketoconazole is an imidazole antifungal which is slightly less active than miconazole in vitro, but which is significantly better absorbed when administered orally. It has been approved for clinical use.

ANTITUBERCULOSIS DRUGS *Isoniazid* remains the most important single agent for the treatment of tuberculosis. After years of being considered virtually free from adverse reactions, hepatotoxicity has been reported on a number of occasions. Individuals receiving this drug should be monitored with liver function tests (see Chap. 174). *Ethambutol* has largely replaced *p*-aminosalicylic acid (PAS) as the usual companion drug for isoniazid because it avoids the necessity of taking large numbers of tablets and also avoids the gastrointestinal side effects associated with PAS. *Rifampin* is another important drug that is comparable to isoniazid in activity against tuberculosis; it should be used in combination with other drugs to prevent the emergence of rifampin-resistant tubercle bacilli. Streptomycin is still used to some extent, particularly for triple drug therapy in seriously ill, hospitalized patients. The secondary drugs, used chiefly in cases that have failed to respond to initial therapy, are cycloserine, pyrazinamide, ethionamide, and viomycin. These drugs are all associated with significant toxic side effects and should be administered and monitored by experts who are familiar with their use. A more detailed consideration of the antituberculosis drugs and the present treatment regimens are given in Chap. 174.

MISCELLANEOUS ANTIBACTERIAL AGENTS *Nitrofurantoin* is an antibacterial agent that is effective in treating urinary tract infections although susceptibility of the *Proteus* group is variable and *Pseudomonas* is resistant. It is usually administered orally in doses of 100 mg four times a day. In addition to treating acute uncomplicated urinary tract infections, it is

TABLE 141-2
Conventional antibiotic regimens for adults with normal renal and hepatic function

Organism	*Disease*	*Drug*	*Dosage*	*Route*	*Duration*
Streptococcus pneumoniae (pneumococcus)	Pneumonia	Penicillin G (procaine)	600,000 U q 12 h	IM	5–10 days[a]
	Meningitis	Penicillin G (aqueous)	20 million U/day	IV	7–10 days
	Arthritis	Penicillin G (aqueous)	20 million U/day	IV	7–10 days
	Endocarditis	Penicillin G (aqueous)	20 million U/day	IV	4–6 weeks[b]
Group A streptococcus	Pharyngitis	Penicillin G (procaine)	600,000 U/day	IM	10 days[c]
	Erysipelas	Penicillin G (procaine)	600,000 U/day	IM	10 days[c]
	Other sites	See pneumococcus			
Coagulase-positive *Staphylococcus*[d]	Furunculosis, cellulitis, abscess	Erythromycin or	500 mg q 6 h	PO	7–10 days
		cloxacillin or	500 mg q 6 h	PO	7–10 days
		cephalexin	500 mg q 6 h	PO	7–10 days
	Pneumonia	Methicillin or Nafcillin or	1.0 g q 4 h	IM, IV	10–14 days
		cloxacillin or	500 mg q 6 h	PO	10–14 days
		dicloxacillin or	250 mg q 6 h	PO	10–14 days
		cephalothin	1.0 g q 4 h	IV	10–14 days
	Arthritis	Methicillin or Nafcillin or	1.0 g q 4 h	IV	10–14 days
		cephalothin	1.0 g q 4 h	IV	10–14 days
	Meningitis, endocarditis	Methicillin or Nafcillin	2.0 g q 4 h	IV	4 weeks
	Enterocolitis	Vancomycin	500 mg q 6 h	PO	Until diarrhea ceases
Streptococcus viridans	Endocarditis	Penicillin G, then	6–12 million U/day	IV	14 days
		penicillin V	500 mg q 4 h	PO	14 days
		Penicillin G plus	6–12 million U/day	IV	14 days
		streptomycin	500 mg q 12 h	IM	14 days
Streptococcus fecalis (enterococcus)	Genitourinary infection	Ampicillin	500 mg q 6 h	PO	10–14 days
	Surgical wound	Ampicillin	1 g q 6 h	IM or IV	7–10 days
	Endocarditis	Ampicillin or	8–12 g/day	IV	4 weeks
		penicillin G plus	20 million U/day	IV	4 weeks
		gentamicin, or	3–5 mg/kg/day	IM, IV	4 weeks
		streptomycin	500 mg q 12 h	IM	4 weeks
Streptococcus bovis	Endocarditis	Penicillin G then	6–12 million U/day	IV	14 days
		penicillin V	500 mg q 4 h	PO	14 days
		Penicillin G plus	6–12 million U/day	IV	14 days
		streptomycin	500 mg q 12 h	IM	14 days
Neisseria meningitidis	Meningitis, meningococcemia	Penicillin G or	20 million U/day	IV	7–10 days
		chloramphenicol	50–100 mg/kg/day given q 6 h	IV	7–10 days
Neisseria gonorrheae	Urethritis	Penicillin G (procaine) plus	4.8 million U/day	IM	1 dose
		probenecid or	1 g	PO	1 dose
		spectinomycin[e]	2 g/day	IM	1 dose
	Arthritis	Penicillin G (aqueous)	6 million U/day	IV	7–10 days
	Disseminated infection	Ampicillin	2 g/day	IM, IV, PO	7–10 days
Hemophilus influenzae	Bronchitis and pneumonia	Ampicillin	500 mg q 4 h	PO, IV, IM	5–7 days
		or cefaclor	500 mg q 6 h	PO	5–7 days
		or cefamandole	500 mg q 6 h	IM, IV	
	Meningitis	Ampicillin plus	8–12 g/day	IV	7–10 days
		chloramphenicol[f]	50–100 mg/kg/day given q 6 h	IV	7–10 days
Brucella	Brucellosis	Tetracycline and	500 mg q 6 h	PO	14 days
		streptomycin	500 mg q 12 h	IM	14 days
Salmonella typhosa	Typhoid fever	Chloramphenicol[g] or	1.0 g q 6 h	IV, PO	14 days
		ampicillin[g]	1.0 g q 6 h	PO, IM, IV	14 days
Salmonella	Abscess, bacteremia	Ampicillin	1.0 g q 4 h	IV	2–4 weeks
Shigella	Shigellosis	Ampicillin	500 mg q 4–6 h	PO, IM, IV	7 days
Klebsiella species	Genitourinary infection	Gentamicin or	3 mg/kg/day given q 8 h	IM, IV	10–14 days
		cephalothin or	500 mg q 6 h	IM, IV	10–14 days
		cefazolin	500 mg q 6 h	IM, IV	10–14 days
Klebsiella pneumoniae	Pneumonia, bacteremia	Cephalothin or	1.0 g q 4 h	IV	7 days
		cefazolin or	1.0 g q 4 h	IV	7 days
		gentamicin	5 mg/kg/day given q 8 h	IM, IV	7 days
Francisella tularensis	Tularemia	Streptomycin	1.0 g q 12 h	IM	10–14 days

[a] *Last 3 to 4 days can be given orally as penicillin V 2 g per day in many cases.*
[b] *Last 2 weeks can be given as penicillin V 4 to 6 g per day orally.*
[c] *Penicillin V 1 to 2 g per day for 10 days, or a single shot of 1.2 × 10^6 units benzathine penicillin is an acceptable alternate.*
[d] *Appropriate doses (see pneumococcus and streptococcus) of penicillin G (parenteral) or penicillin V (oral) if organism is sensitive to penicillin G.*
[e] *For patients allergic to penicillin.*
[f] *One of the antibiotics can be discontinued after sensitivity tests are available.*
[g] *Start with parenteral but switch to oral as soon as possible.*

TABLE 141-2 *(continued)*
Conventional antibiotic regimens for adults with normal renal and hepatic function

Organism	*Disease*	*Drug*	*Dosage*	*Route*	*Duration*
Enterobacter species	Genitourinary infection	Cefamandole or	500 mg q 6 h	IV, IM	7 days
		gentamicin	3 mg/kg/day given q 8 h	IM, IV	7 days
	Bacteremia	Gentamicin and/or	3–5 mg/kg/day given q 8 h	IM, IV	7 days
		carbenicillin	4 g q 4 h	IV	7 days
Escherichia coli	Genitourinary infection	Sulfisoxazole[h] or	1 g q 6 h	PO	7–10 days
		tetracycline or	500 mg q 6 h	PO	7–10 days
		ampicillin or	500 mg q 6 h	PO	7–10 days
		sulfamethoxazole-trimethoprim	1 tablet qid	PO	7–10 days
	Bacteremia, arthritis, peritonitis	Ampicillin or	6–12 g/day	IV	7–10 days
		gentamicin or	3–5 mg/kg/day given q 8 h	IM, IV	7–10 days
		cephalothin	1–2 g q 4 h	IV	7–10 days
	Meningitis	Ampicillin or	8–12 g/day	IV	7–10 days
		chloramphenicol	50–100 mg/kg/day given q 6 h	IV	7–10 days
Proteus mirabilis	Genitourinary infection	Ampicillin or	500 mg q 6 h	PO	10–14 days
		cephalexin	500 mg q 6 h	PO	10–14 days
	Bacteremia	Ampicillin or	6.0 g/day	IV	7–10 days
		cephalothin or	6.0 g/day	IV	7–10 days
		gentamicin	5 mg/kg/day given q 8 h	IM, IV	7–10 days
Indole-positive *Proteus*	Genitourinary infection	Carbenicillin[i] or	2 g q 6 h	IV	10–14 days
		gentamicin	3–5 mg/kg/day given q 8 h	IM, IV	10–14 days
	Bacteremia	Carbenicillin or	4 g q 4 h	IV	7–10 days
		gentamicin or	5 mg/kg/day given q 8 h	IM, IV	7–10 days
		cefoxitin	1 g q 6 h	IV	7–10 days
Pseudomonas	Bacteremia, arthritis	Gentamicin, or tobramycin and	5 mg/kg/day given q 8 h	IM, IV	7 days
		carbenicillin	5–6 g q 4 h	IV	7 days
	Meningitis, brain abscess	Gentamicin or tobramycin plus	5 mg/kg/day given q 8 h	IV, IM	7–14 days
		carbenicillin and	5–6 g q 4 h	IV	7–14 days
		gentamicin or tobramycin	4 mg q 12–18 h	Intrathecally	7 days
	Genitourinary infection	Gentamicin or tobramycin or	3 mg/kg/day given q 8 h	IM, IV	10–14 days
		carbenicillin	2 g q 6 h	IM, IV	10–14 days
Bacteroides fragilis	Abscess, bacteremia	Chloramphenicol or	0.5 g q 4 h	IV, PO	10–14 days
		clindamycin	0.6 g q 6–8 h, then	IV	10–14 days
			0.3 g q 6 h	PO	As long as necessary
	Brain abscess	Chloramphenicol	0.5 g q 4 h	IV, PO	10–14 days
Mycoplasma pneumoniae	Sputum	Erythromycin or	250–500 mg q 6 h	PO	7 days
		tetracycline	500 mg q 6 h	PO	7 days
Legionella pneumophila	Sputum	Erythromycin	1 g q 6 h	IV, PO	As long as necessary

[h] *Uncomplicated infections only.*
[i] *The indanyl ester of carbenicillin 1 g every 6 h may be given orally.*

widely used to suppress symptoms of infection in patients with prostatism and other chronic obstructive uropathies. Nausea is sometimes troublesome, and pulmonary hypersensitivity and peripheral neuropathy may occur. The latter is especially likely to occur with renal insufficiency, and nitrofurantoin should be used very cautiously in the presence of uremia. Also available is a macrocrystal preparation of nitrofurantoin which appears to be tolerated and causes less nausea.

Nalidixic acid is another drug used orally for urinary tract infections. Its principal defect lies in the rapidity with which bacteria become resistant to it. This means that cultures should be made during, as well as following, therapy to be sure that bacteria are being cleared from the urinary tract. The usual dose is 2 to 4 g daily in divided doses for 1 to 2 weeks. Nausea, vomiting, and rashes are the chief adverse reactions. Clinoxacin is similar chemically to nalidixic acid.

Metronidazole has been approved for the treatment of anaerobic bacterial infections in addition to its previous indications for protozoan and other parasitic organisms. It is available for both oral and intravenous use. It is a bactericidal agent with excellent activity against *B. fragilis.*

DRUGS OF CHOICE

It is quite clear from reading about the pharmacology of individual agents, as well as about their indications and uses in individual diseases, that many agents are available for the treatment of these diseases. Table 141-2 presents a summary of drugs, indications, dosage schedules, routes of administration, and duration of therapy. The table presents only a limited number of drugs, and many equally acceptable regimens are available. Moreover, while these treatment programs are appropriate for the present, changes in them should be expected as new drugs come on the market and as more experience with the newer agents is gathered. For example, some of the newer cephalosporins, e.g., cefotaxime, or aminoglycosides, e.g., amikacin, may be preferred as initial therapy in immunocompromised hosts or in certain institutions where a large number of resistant gram-negative organisms can be expected on the basis of epidemiologic information.

REASONS FOR FAILURE OF CHEMOTHERAPY

This chapter as well as others dealing with specific disease entities has documented that there are few organisms not sensitive to some antibiotic. Despite this seemingly salutary observation, a large number of patients develop infections and many continue to die from them. In these patients antibiotics appear to have failed. Often this failure of chemotherapy is more apparent than real and may be attributed to one of several causes.

FAILURE TO ADJUST THE DOSE OF THE ANTIBIOTIC Different doses of antibiotics are required in different locations. For example, 600,000 units penicillin G is more than adequate to cure pneumococcal pneumonia, but as much as 20 million units may be required to cure pneumococcal meningitis. The pneumococcus in each of these locations remains exquisitely sensitive to penicillin, and the penetration of the drug is not inadequate. However, the host's environment is such that higher doses are required to cure the infections in different locations. Failure to appreciate this phenomenon may lead to inadequate doses.

TREATMENT OF NONBACTERIAL INFECTIONS Viral infections do not respond to the generally available antibiotic agents, and these drugs must not be expected to exact a therapeutic effect in these situations. Similarly, antibiotics do not prevent bacterial complications of viral infections.

FAILURE TO DRAIN PURULENT MATERIAL OR TO REMOVE OBSTRUCTION Antimicrobial drugs work well only in an environment free of obstruction. Infections will not respond optimally unless obstructions such as a plug of mucus or an enlarged prostate, or a foreign body such as a suture or splinter, are removed, or unless purulent material is drained. It is particularly important to drain an abscess cavity because antibiotics do not kill bacteria enmeshed in pus.

SUPERINFECTIONS The role of antibiotics in promoting superinfections is discussed in Chaps. 137 and 138. In 2 to 3 percent of patients, seeming failure of antimicrobials is a consequence of superinfection.

DRUG REACTION The development of drug fever without rash or any other manifestation of hypersensitivity may make it appear as if the infection were not responding to therapy, when instead the fever is due to the very drug being given to cure the infection. Drug fever is extremely common with certain antimicrobials, particularly penicillin. The best way to make the diagnosis is simply to discontinue therapy. If fever disappears, the diagnosis is established. A second challenge with the suspected drug is neither necessary nor safe.

INCORRECT DRUG Only rarely does chemotherapy fail because the incorrect drug has been administered. Most drugs have a sufficiently broad spectrum, and combinations of drugs are administered with sufficient frequency, whether indicated or not, to make it highly unlikely that the patient is not given an agent active against the etiologic pathogen. One of the most common errors, when the patient is not responding, is to add more antimicrobials indiscriminately, when the correct course should be to discontinue therapy and to watch the patient.

DEFECTS IN HOST RESISTANCE The type of patient requiring antimicrobial therapy has changed from a young or mid-

dle-aged individual to an elderly one with degenerative and debilitating disease or one whose host defenses have been compromised by neoplastic disease, large doses of antimicrobials, antineoplastic or immunosuppressive drugs, x-ray therapy, major surgical procedures, or transplants. For a variety of reasons, this type of patient does not, and should not be expected to, respond to antimicrobials as does a normal individual. This factor is often ignored in gauging the results of chemotherapy. It does not mean that antibiotics should not be used when indicated; rather, no miraculous results should be expected in patients with severe associated disease of noninfectious origin.

REFERENCES

Appel GB, Neu HC: The nephrotoxicity of antimicrobial agents. N Engl J Med 296:663, 1977

Handbook of Antimicrobial Therapy, rev. ed. New Rochelle, NY, Medical Letter, 1981

Kunin, CM: Dosage schedules of antimicrobial agents: A historical review. Rev Infect Dis 3:4, 1981

Meyer RD: Drugs five years later: Amikacin. Ann Intern Med 95:328, 1981

The choice of antimicrobial drugs. *The Medical Letter* 24:21, 28, 1982

Sanford, JP (ed): *Guide to Antimicrobial Therapy.* PO Box 34456, West Bethesda, MD, 1981

Sarubbi FA, Hull JH: Amikacin serum concentrations. Ann Intern Med 89:612, 1978

142 ACUTE INFECTIOUS DIARRHEAL DISEASE AND BACTERIAL FOOD POISONING

CHARLES C. J. CARPENTER

Acute diarrheal illnesses caused by bacterial, viral, or protozoal pathogens vary from slightly annoying bowel dysfunction to fulminant, life-threatening diseases. Until recent years, a specific etiologic agent could not be isolated from most patients with acute diarrhea. During the past decade, however, largely because of the recognition of enterotoxigenic *Escherichia coli* as a major cause of acute diarrheal disease in adults and the identification of rotavirus as a frequent cause in young children, specific etiologic agents have been isolated from 80 to 85 percent of patients with acute diarrheal illnesses. Those illnesses caused by bacterial pathogens are more often life-threatening, at least among adults, and for that reason they will be addressed first. This chapter is aimed at presenting an overview of these diseases; in most instances, the entities are discussed in more detail in the chapters dealing with the specific etiologic agent.

In considering the bacterial diarrheas, it is useful to divide them into two groups, those caused by invasive and those caused by noninvasive microorganisms. The invasive pathogens, of which *Shigella* (see Chap. 155) may be considered the prototype, generally cause abdominal pain, fever, and other systemic symptoms, often including headache and myalgia. Illness caused by the noninvasive pathogens, of which cholera (see Chap. 166) is the prototype, is generally characterized by the absence of fever and few systemic symptoms (except those directly related to intestinal fluid loss). The invasive pathogens characteristically destroy gut mucosal cells, typically involving the terminal ileum and colon, and so both leukocytes and erythrocytes are present, to a variable degree, in the stool. Inflammatory cells are generally absent from the stool in acute diarrheal disease caused by noninvasive bacterial pathogens.

NONINVASIVE BACTERIAL PATHOGENS

ENTEROTOXIGENIC *ESCHERICHIA COLI* **Etiology and epidemiology** Enterotoxin-producing *E. coli* (ETEC), which have the dual capacity to adhere to small-bowel epithelial cells and to produce one or more diarrheagenic toxins, are now recognized as a major cause of acute diarrheal disease throughout most of the world and are the most common cause of "traveler's diarrhea." Largely because current techniques for demonstrating toxigenicity remain cumbersome, the epidemiology of ETEC diarrhea is poorly understood. ETEC are responsible for the majority of cases of traveler's diarrhea in visitors to the developing nations in South America, Africa, and Asia. ETEC are also one of the two (with rotavirus) leading causes of acute diarrheal illnesses in children throughout the developing world. ETEC have been implicated as a major cause of fulminant, cholera-like diarrheal disease in adult patients in south and southeast Asia but generally cause milder, self-limited diarrhea in adults in other parts of the developing world. There is no satisfactory explanation for the difference in severity in diarrhea caused by ETEC in different geographic areas. ETEC are rarely incriminated in episodic diarrheal illness in children and adults in the United States.

Pathogenesis The ability to cause diarrheal disease is not restricted to any one *E. coli* serotype but appears to be dependent upon the presence of both a plasmid-mediated colonization factor, which allows the *E. coli* to adhere to small-bowel mucosal cells, and one or more plasmids which code for the production of one or both of the two diarrheagenic toxins which may be produced by *E. coli.* The kinetics and mode of action of one of the toxins, which is heat labile (LT) and of relatively high molecular weight (~83,000 daltons), are similar to those of cholera enterotoxin (see Chap. 166); the diarrheagenic effect results from stimulation of adenylate cyclase in the gut epithelial cells. The other toxin, which is heat stable (ST) and of a lower molecular weight (<2000 daltons), has a more rapid onset of action and probably exerts its effect through stimulation of guanylate cyclase in the gut mucosal cells. Either or both toxins may be produced by ETEC. Most isolates from patients with severe diarrheal disease in Bangladesh produce both LT and ST, whereas isolates from patients in other developing nations have shown widely varying capacities for the production of LT, ST, or both. The wide clinical spectrum may be, in part, related to the predominant production of either LT or ST by the culpable microorganisms. The nutritional status of the host may also be a factor in determining the clinical response to ETEC.

Manifestations Both clinical observations and volunteer studies indicate that the incubation period is generally between 24 and 72 h. The illness which follows is quite variable, ranging from the fulminant, cholera-like disease often seen on the Indian subcontinent to the much milder Mexican "turista," in which the symptoms of mild, watery diarrhea, abdominal cramps, and occasional low-grade fever are more troublesome than life-threatening. Vomiting occurs in fewer than half the adults with *E. coli* diarrhea and is seldom responsible for major fluid losses.

In fulminant cases, the severe diarrhea seldom lasts longer than 24 to 36 h, and the response to either oral or intravenous electrolyte repletion is predictable and dramatic. With milder disease, the symptoms subside more gradually, occasionally persisting for a week or longer.

Laboratory findings As with cholera, no erythrocytes and few, if any, polymorphonuclear leukocytes are seen in a stool preparation stained by Loeffler's methylene blue. Because *E. coli* occurs normally among stool flora, and because its ability to produce enterotoxin is not restricted to any specific serotype, there is no rapid and simple means of laboratory diagnosis of enterotoxigenic *E. coli.* Bioassays for LT, based on the ability of *E. coli* isolates to produce fluid in isolated intestinal loops of experimental animals or to stimulate adenylate cyclase in cells in tissue culture, as well as the suckling mouse bioassay for ST, are reliable but of little value in patient management. Newer technology, utilizing DNA probes for rapid identification of the genes responsible for ST and LT production, appears promising and may be adapted for widespread use for epidemiologic purposes in the near future.

Treatment The intestinal fluid losses are qualitatively identical to those in cholera. Therefore, in those patients who develop clinically significant saline depletion, the principles of fluid administration are identical to those described for cholera (see Chap. 166). Oral solutions containing electrolytes plus glucose or sucrose are consistently effective in correcting the saline depletion. Tetracycline, 30 mg/kg per day, given orally at 6-h intervals for 48 h, is effective in decreasing the duration of illness but is not an essential element in therapy. Doxycycline, 100 mg per day, is of highly significant *prophylactic* value in preventing ETEC diarrhea in travelers. Bismuth subsalicylate, 60 ml hourly for four doses, provides symptomatic relief (less frequent stools, less severe abdominal cramps) but has no effect on the total stool volume. Antiperistaltic agents such as anticholinergics or Lomotil are of no demonstrable value in enterotoxigenic *E. coli* diarrhea.

Prognosis With even the more fulminant cases of disease caused by ETEC, the prognosis is excellent with adequate fluid replacement.

Prevention Careful hygienic practices, with special attention to ingestion of clean water and adequately cooked foods when one is living in a generally unsanitary environment, provide the most certain protection against enterotoxigenic *E. coli.* Doxycycline prophylaxis is detailed above and is 60 to 90 percent effective, the effectiveness varying with the tetracycline sensitivity of the ETEC in the geographic area.

CHOLERA See Chap. 166.

OTHER ENTEROTOXIGENIC ENTEROBACTERIACEAE Noninvasive strains of *Klebsiella* and *Enterobacter* occasionally have been implicated in acute diarrheal disease in the developing areas of the world. The clinical illness produced is indistinguishable from the milder cases of diarrhea caused by enterotoxigenic *E. coli,* and treatment is the same.

CLOSTRIDIUM PERFRINGENS (See also Chap. 172) This organism remains a significant cause of diarrheal disease and was, in 1973, implicated in more cases of acute food poisoning in the United States than any other single microorganism. Both the epidemiologic background and the clinical picture of *C. perfringens* diarrhea differ strikingly from those of *E. coli.* *Clostridium perfringens* diarrhea tends to occur in a microepidemic pattern following ingestion of contaminated meat, poultry products, or legumes. The relatively short incubation period of 6 to 12 h is an important diagnostic clue. Typically, two or more patients who have ingested the same meat dish for dinner become ill at roughly the same time during the early morning hours. The production of a specific enterotoxin by the actively sporulating microorganisms in the intestinal tract appears to be responsible for all the symptoms.

The clinical picture of diarrhea caused by *C. perfringens* is different from that caused by enterotoxigenic *E. coli* in one important respect, namely, that moderately severe cramping abdominal pain, which is usually not prominent with *E. coli,* is a major presenting symptom.

Treatment consists of symptomatic therapy with codeine to alleviate the cramping abdominal pain and intravenous fluid therapy in the small proportion of patients in whom there is clinical evidence of saline depletion. The illness is self-limited and rarely lasts for more than 24 h. Because of the relatively short natural course of the illness, antimicrobial therapy is of no value. Because *C. perfringens* normally inhabits mammalian and avian intestinal tracts, prevention is dependent upon adequate cooking and handling of meat and poultry products. The practice of allowing cooked meat products to cool slowly toward room temperature over 12 to 24 h permits germination of contaminating clostridial spores; this practice must be avoided.

STAPHYLOCOCCUS AUREUS (See also Chap. 147) Acute staphylococcal diarrhea, classic "food poisoning," is due entirely to ingestion of preformed enterotoxin, and the causative organisms are often absent from the stool during the acute illness. This form of diarrhea often occurs in institutional outbreaks and is characterized by a short incubation period (2 to 6 h), relatively short duration (usually less than 10 h), and very high attack rates (often greater than 75 percent of the population at risk). In addition to its distinctive epidemiologic features, acute staphylococcal diarrhea differs from other noninvasive bacterial diarrheas by the prominence of vomiting. Vomiting is an almost constant feature and is apparently mediated by a direct effect of the absorbed toxin on the central nervous system.

Treatment is directed toward correction of the saline depletion (intravenous fluids are required in 10 to 20 percent of patients) and, when necessary, toward symptomatic relief of vomiting. Because staphylococcal food poisoning is caused by preformed enterotoxin and is not perpetuated by viable microorganisms, antimicrobials are of no value.

A good example of the explosive nature of staphylococcal food poisoning was provided by an outbreak on a jet liner flying from Anchorage to Copenhagen. In this episode, 57 percent of 343 passengers developed an acute illness characterized by vomiting, diarrhea, and cramping abdominal pain. Of the 200 affected individuals, 30 required intravenous fluids, but none had serious sequelae. The food, contaminated by a pustule on the hand of a food handler, had not been adequately refrigerated aboard the plane, allowing abundant growth of the staphylococcus, with production of enterotoxin. Since staphylococci are ubiquitous, the prevention of massive contamination is dependent largely on control of growth conditions, primarily temperature. *Staphylococcus aureus* can multiply at temperatures from 4 to 46°C, and if contaminated food is allowed to remain at ambient temperatures after cooking, these organisms have ample opportunity to multiply, especially in such items as cream pastries, potato salad, and mayonnaise.

BACILLUS CEREUS *Bacillus cereus* is a cause of acute diarrheal disease which, although uncommon, has been identified with increasing frequency in the past decade, especially in Europe. The illness results from gross contamination of food with this gram-positive rod, which is capable of producing at least two discrete enterotoxins, one having characteristics similar to those of the labile enterotoxin of *E. coli* and the other having effects similar to that of staphylococcal enterotoxin. *Bacillus cereus* may, therefore, cause two distinct clinical syndromes, a diarrheal form resulting from the *E. coli* LT type of enterotoxin and an emetic form caused by the staphylococcal type of enterotoxin. The diarrheal syndrome caused by *B. cereus* is generally similar to that caused by enterotoxin-producing *E. coli,* with the exceptions that abdominal cramps are more common (75 percent of cases) and both the incubation period (6 to 14 h) and median duration of illness (20 h) are shorter. The emetic syndrome is clinically indistinguishable from that caused by staphylococcal enterotoxin, with a short incubation period (median 2 h), short duration (median 9 h), and prominent vomiting (100 percent compared with less than 25 percent in the diarrheal syndrome).

Because both syndromes are self-limited and generally mild, no specific therapy is indicated. When *B. cereus* food poisoning is suspected clinically, the diagnosis can be confirmed by demonstration of 10^5 or more *B. cereus* organisms in epidemiologically incriminated food. *Bacillus cereus* grows readily on simple laboratory media, including blood agar, but will not generally be identified as a pathogen unless such identification is specifically requested. Isolation of *B. cereus* from stool alone does not establish it as the etiologic agent because the organism is frequently found in the fecal flora of normal individuals.

Since *B. cereus* is ubiquitous in soil, as well as in many raw, dried, and processed foods, proper food handling is the only practical means of preventing this form of food poisoning. The emetic form of *B. cereus* food poisoning almost invariably has been associated with ingestion of contaminated fried rice. *Bacillus cereus* is commonly present in uncooked rice, and its spores survive boiling and germinate, with production of the enterotoxin, when boiled rice is left unrefrigerated. Brief rewarming before serving is not adequate to destroy the relatively heat-stable toxin. Prompt refrigeration of boiled rice will prevent transmission of the disease.

INVASIVE ENTERIC PATHOGENS

INTRODUCTION Shigellae characteristically invade the colon and terminal ileum, destroy segments of intestinal mucosa, cause extensive inflammatory changes in the lamina propria, and are the prototype of the invasive enteric bacterial pathogens. Other important invasive bacterial enteric pathogens include *Salmonella, Yersinia enterocolitica, Campylobacter jejuni, Vibrio parahemolyticus,* and invasive *E. coli,* which may have the capacity both to damage intestinal mucosa and to produce an enterotoxin. As opposed to the noninvasive pathogens, the invasive enteric organisms frequently cause systemic symptoms, including headache, myalgias, chills, and fever. As a general rule, antiperistaltic agents such as opiates, diphenoxylate, and atropine are contraindicated in diarrheal disease caused by invasive enteric pathogens because they clearly worsen the clinical course in human shigellosis, as well as in salmonellosis and shigellosis in animal models.

The major therapeutic challenge in invasive bacterial diarrheas is that of distinguishing between (1) shigellosis and yersiniosis, in which antimicrobial therapy decreases the duration and severity of illness and shortens the period of fecal shedding of the pathogen, and (2) infections caused by *Salmonella,* which are characterized primarily by watery diarrhea and few systemic symptoms and in which antimicrobial therapy does not alter the duration of illness and may cause prolonged excretion of the pathogen.

SHIGELLOSIS See Chap. 155.

SALMONELLOSIS See Chap. 154.

YERSINIA ENTEROCOLITICA See Chap. 160.

CAMPYLOBACTER JEJUNI **Etiology and epidemiology** *Campylobacter jejuni* was first implicated in acute diarrheal disease in humans in 1972; by 1979 *C. jejuni* was second only to *Giardia lamblia* among recognized causes of waterborne diarrheal disease outbreaks in the United States. *C. jejuni* occurs in the intestinal flora of many domestic animals and poultry, and can clearly be transmitted to humans by milk and water polluted by such animal carriers. Adequate data are not yet available to determine whether or not this is the most common mode of transmission. What information there is suggests that *C. jejuni* causes from 5 to 10 percent of acute diarrheal illnesses in both the industrialized and the developing areas of the world.

Pathogenesis *C. jejuni* causes patchy destruction of mucosa of both the small intestine, especially the distal ileum, and the colon; the stools, therefore, regularly contain pus cells and are occasionally grossly bloody. *C. jejuni* rarely produces transient bacteremia.

Manifestations An incubation period of 3 to 5 days, longer than that of most bacterial enteric pathogens, is followed by fever, cramping abdominal pain, and diarrhea that is initially watery but later contains blood and mucus. The diarrhea, generally mild but occasionally voluminous, ceases within 48 to 72 h without specific antimicrobial therapy. In adolescents and young adults, the diarrhea may be relatively mild, and the clinical picture may simulate acute appendicitis. (This may also be true in *Yersinia* enterocolitis; see Chap. 160.) In such cases, laparotomy has revealed acutely inflamed mesenteric lymph nodes as well as patchy inflammation of the small bowel.

Laboratory findings Diagnosis depends upon isolating *C. jejuni* from stool. Since this curved, motile bacillus does not compete well with other enteric flora on standard enteric media, it will rarely be isolated from stool unless special techniques are utilized. These include incubation at 42°C on blood agar to which a number of antimicrobials have been added. Serological diagnosis is rarely helpful, as there are many serotypes of *C. jejuni,* and agglutination tests require use of the homologous organism.

Treatment Since *C. jejuni* produces a relatively short, self-limited illness, antimicrobial therapy is not essential to management. Erythromycin, 30 mg/kg per day, does, however, significantly decrease the duration of fecal shedding of *C. jejuni* and may shorten the mean duration of illness. In the occasional patient who develops clinical signs of saline depletion, oral and/or intravenous fluids of the same sort used in cholera are uniformly effective (see Chap. 166).

VIBRIO PARAHEMOLYTICUS **Etiology and epidemiology** *Vibrio parahemolyticus* is a curved, aerobic, nonmotile, gram-negative bacillus. Although present in coastal waters throughout the temperate zone, it has most commonly been associated with acute diarrheal illness in Japan, presumably because of the frequency of ingestion of raw seafood. *V. parahemolyticus* is responsible for a relatively small ($<$ 10 percent) proportion of acute diarrheal illnesses in both adults and children in rural Bangladesh, where an association with seafood is less clearly established. It has been implicated in several outbreaks of acute diarrheal disease in the coastal United States, always as a common-source outbreak related to ingestion of inadequately cooked seafood, usually shrimp. Secondary cases caused by person-to-person transmission occur rarely. Several epidemics of *V. parahemolyticus* infections on cruise ships have been reported.

Pathogenesis Although *V. parahemolyticus* produces a toxin capable of causing intestinal fluid accumulation in experimental animals, the role of this toxin in human disease is not certain. *V. parahemolyticus* causes patchy mucosal damage in both distal ileum and colon; stools usually contain numerous polymorphonuclear leukocytes and are occasionally grossly bloody. The volume of fluid lost with *V. parahemolyticus* infection is relatively small, and intravenous fluids are seldom required. The illness is self-limited, with a median duration of just under 24 h.

Manifestations Within 6 to 48 h after ingestion of raw or inadequately cooked seafood, the patient develops an acute diarrheal illness. The volume of fluid lost is not great, moderately severe abdominal cramps may be a prominent feature, and chills and fever are observed in roughly half the cases. Vomiting is generally not a prominent feature and occurs in no more than one-third of patients. The illness is self-limited, and no deaths have been reported in outbreaks involving over a thousand patients in the United States.

Laboratory findings When a common-source outbreak of acute diarrheal disease occurs in a group exposed to fresh or frozen seafood, the index of suspicion should be high and the diagnosis should be confirmed by plating a rectal swab on thiosulfate–citrate–bile salt–sucrose (TCBS) agar, on which typical colonies of *V. parahemolyticus* appear in 24 h. (This organism grows poorly and is therefore easily overlooked on deoxycholate culture plates.) The stool generally has numerous polymorphonuclear leukocytes and a smaller number of erythrocytes, but these findings are less prominent than in shigellosis.

Treatment No therapy is required by the large majority of patients. Antimicrobial therapy shortens neither the course nor the duration of pathogen excretion. Antiperistaltic agents are not of clear-cut benefit. An occasional patient may lose sufficient quantities of intestinal fluid to require oral or intravenous fluid therapy.

Prognosis The outcome is almost always good. Fatal cases, occasionally reported from Japan, have occurred in rare instances in patients with serious underlying disease.

INVASIVE *ESCHERICHIA COLI* Invasive *E. coli,* which are far less common pathogens than enterotoxigenic *E. coli,* may cause a clinical syndrome quite similar to shigellosis with the exceptions that vomiting seldom occurs with the invasive *E. coli* and the illness is of shorter duration. Diarrhea caused by invasive *E. coli* is rare in the United States but has been a significant cause of short-term disability in eastern Europe and southeast Asia. Since the illness caused by invasive *E. coli* is relatively short-lived, antimicrobial therapy has not been shown to be helpful.

ACUTE VIRAL DIARRHEAS

Acute viral gastroenteritis is discussed in detail in Chap. 205. These illnesses are both more common and more life-threatening in small children than adults. In the United States, rotaviruses account for a large proportion of diarrheal illnesses during the first 2 years of life and usually occur during the winter. They have seldom been implicated in adult illness. In rural Bangladesh, infection with rotavirus accounts for roughly 60 percent of episodes of diarrhea in children from 6 to 24 months of age and for about 5 percent in the 2- to 5-year-old age group; it seldom occurs in adolescents and adults. The illness usually presents with vomiting followed by watery diarrhea and low-grade fever, with little or no associated abdominal pain. Vomiting is a prominent and almost constant early manifestation of rotavirus enteritis but rarely persists beyond the first 24 h. Diarrhea often persists for 4 to 8 days. Although the illness is generally not life-threatening, many patients require fluid and electrolyte repletion. Since the vomiting is usually short-lived, fluid repletion can generally be achieved by the oral route, using the same fluids that are effective in the treatment of cholera (see Chap. 166).

The diagnosis can be confirmed by a variety of tests including demonstration of the virus in stool by electron microscopy, a rise in complement-fixing antibody titers, and radioimmunoassay. The most useful and reliable test for rapid diagnosis under field conditions consists of direct demonstration of the antigen in stool by the enzyme-linked immunosorbent assay (ELISA).

Norwalk and Norwalk-like viruses, now implicated in roughly a third of episodes of epidemic gastroenteritis involving adults in the United States, usually cause relatively mild, short (< 36 h), and self-limited disease, for which neither fluid nor drug therapy is necessary (see Chap. 205).

ACUTE PROTOZOAL DIARRHEAS

Over the past decade, *Giardia lamblia* has emerged as a major cause of acute diarrheal disease (see Chap. 224). Although formerly thought to be a pathogen only in children and later considered to be a significant cause of diarrheal disease only in developing nations, this organism was the pathogen most commonly incriminated in outbreaks of waterborne diarrheal disease in the United States in 1976. In North America, it occurs most commonly in the Rocky Mountain states and more frequently causes disease in visitors than in the indigenous population. The illness characteristically presents with the sudden onset of watery diarrhea and malabsorption, accompanied by mild to moderate abdominal discomfort, bloating, and flatulence, and may occasionally persist for weeks unless appropriate antimicrobials are administered. Prolonged disease with malabsorption occurs from time to time in previously normal individuals but is particularly common in patients with IgA deficiency, who tend to have the most severe form of giardiasis.

The attack rate may be quite high (> 50 percent) in individuals exposed to contaminated water sources. In certain groups of North American travelers returning from Leningrad, where the water supply appears to be heavily contaminated with *Giardia* cysts, up to 60 percent of individuals have developed clinical giardiasis. The usual incubation period is 10 to 20 days. The illness, therefore, frequently develops after a traveler returns home, and the travel history is a critical element in suspecting the diagnosis. Occasionally the disease occurs endemically in individuals who have not traveled. The diagnosis can be confirmed in approximately half the cases by examining the stool for cysts; if the stool examination is negative in a patient with characteristic clinical features, duodenal aspirates or biopsies will usually yield the characteristic trophozoites. Treatment with quinacrine, 100 mg tid for 5 to 7 days, is generally curative; metronidazole, 250 mg tid for 7 days, is an equally effective alternative regimen.

REFERENCES

BARKER WH JR et al: *Vibrio parahemolyticus* outbreak in Covington, Louisiana, in August, 1972. Am J Epidemiol 100:316, 1974

BLACKLOW NR, CUKOR G: Viral gastroenteritis. N Engl J Med 304:397, 1981

BLASER MJ et al: *Campylobacter* enteritis: Clinical and epidimeologic features. Ann Intern Med 91:179, 1979

———, RELLER BL: *Campylobacter* enteritis. N Engl J Med 305:1444, 1981

CARPENTER CCJ, SACK RB: Infectious diarrheal syndromes, in *Update I: Harrison's Principles of Internal Medicine,* KJ Issellbacher et al (eds). New York, McGraw-Hill, 1981, pp 209–229

DUPONT HL et al: Pathogenesis of *Escherichia coli* diarrhea. N Engl J Med 285:1, 1971

——— et al: Symptomatic treatment of diarrhea with bismuth subsalicylate among students attending a Mexican university. Gastroenterology 73:715, 1977

EVANS DG et al: Plasmid-controlled colonization factor associated with virulence in *Escherichia coli* enterotoxigenic for humans. Infect Immun 12:656, 1975

GORBACH SL et al: Traveller's diarrhea and toxigenic *Escherichia coli.* N Engl J Med 292:933, 1975

GRIFFIN MR et al: Foodborne Norwalk virus. Am J Epidemiol 115:178, 1982

GUERRANT RL et al: Role of toxigenic and invasive bacteria in acute diarrhea of childhood. N Engl J Med 293:576, 1974

KAPLAN JE et al: Epidemiology of Norwalk gastroenteritis and the role of Norwalk virus in acute nonbacterial gastroenteritis. Ann Intern Med 96:756, 1982

MERSON MH et al: Traveller's diarrhea in Mexico. A prospective study of physicians and family members attending a Congress. N Engl J Med 294:1299, 1976

SACK DA et al: Oral rehydration in rotavirus diarrhea: A double blind comparison of sucrose with glucose electrolyte solution. Lancet 2:280, 1978

——— et al: Prophylactic doxycycline for traveller's diarrhea. N Engl J Med 298:758, 1978

SACK RB et al: Enterotoxigenic *Escherichia coli* isolated from patients with severe cholera-like disease. J Infect Dis 123:378, 1971

——— et al: Human diarrheal disease caused by enterotoxigenic *Escherichia coli.* Annu Rev Microbiol 29:333, 1975

TERRANOVA W et al: Current concepts: *Bacillus cereus* food poisoning. N Engl J Med 298:143, 1978

ZEN-YOJI H et al: Epidemiology, enteropathogenicity and classification of *Vibrio parahemolyticus.* J Infect Dis 115:436, 1965

143
SEXUALLY TRANSMITTED DISEASES

KING K. HOLMES
H. HUNTER HANDSFIELD

Venereology today encompasses not only the five "venerable" venereal diseases (gonorrhea, syphilis, chancroid, lymphogranuloma venereum, and granuloma inguinale), but also a growing number of other diseases which might be considered the "new generation" of sexually transmitted diseases (STDs). Many of these newer STDs have, like gonorrhea, become epidemic in nearly all countries of the world during the past two decades. With increasing interest in these diseases and improved methods for diagnosis has come awareness of the growing consequences of STD in areas of health and society which extend beyond the traditional sphere of venereology. In particular, major impact of the newer STDs has been noted on maternal and infant morbidity and on human reproduction and infertility.

EPIDEMIOLOGY OF SEXUALLY TRANSMITTED DISEASES One of the major reasons for the current STD epidemic has been the failure of clinicians to ensure that the sexual partners of patients with STDs are examined and treated. Most persons with genital discharges, lesions, or pain cease sexual activity and seek medical care. Accordingly, those who transmit infection usually are among the minority who are asymptomatically infected or have mild symptoms whose implications are not understood. Therefore, they often will not spontaneously seek medical attention, and physicians must see that they are examined and treated. In the United States, local health departments will usually identify and treat contacts for some diseases (e.g., syphilis, gonococcal pelvic inflammatory disease), but for most STDs this responsibility is shared by the patient and the physician.

CLASSIFICATION OF SEXUALLY TRANSMITTED DISEASES These diseases can be classified on the basis of either their etiologies or their clinical manifestations. Table 143-1 gives an etiologic classification of STD. Sexual transmission has been implicated as a major factor in the propagation of each of the pathogens listed in this table. There have been sporadic case reports of sexual transmission of many other pathogenic agents, but the diseases caused by these other agents are not generally considered, since sexual transmission seems to be a minor factor in their propagation. For each of the agents listed in Table 143-1, there are one or more diseases or syndromes known to be caused by the agent, and others (indicated by a question mark) for which a causal association is suspected but not proved.

APPROACH TO SEXUALLY TRANSMITTED DISEASE It is necessary for the clinician to consider the approach to STD syndromes before an etiologic diagnosis is established. Table 143-2 lists some of the most common clinical syndromes and complications caused by sexually transmitted pathogens. Strategies for the management of some of the common syndromes are outlined below.

MALE URETHRITIS Urethritis in the male is classified as gonococcal or nongonococcal. The incidence of gonococcal urethritis has stabilized in many western countries, while that of nongonococcal urethritis (NGU) continues to rise (Fig. 143-1), suggesting that current measures for control of NGU are relatively ineffective. In general, gonorrhea and NGU are equally common among men seen in STD clinics in the United States, whereas NGU is approximately three times as common as gonorrhea among men seen by physicians in private practice and 10 times as common as gonorrhea among college students.

About 40 percent of NGU is caused by *Chlamydia trachomatis.* Herpes simplex virus and *Trichomonas vaginalis* each cause a small additional proportion of NGU cases in the United States, but about 50 percent of cases cannot be attributed to any of these three pathogens. *Ureaplasma urealyticum* has been implicated in case-control studies as a probable cause of many of the *Chlamydia*-negative cases. Since facilities for isolation of *C. trachomatis* are not available everywhere and the role of *U. urealyticum* is not certain, the diagnosis of male

TABLE 143-1
Twenty-three sexually transmitted pathogens and the diseases they cause

Agent	*Disease or syndrome*
BACTERIA	
Neisseria gonorrhoeae	Urethritis, epididymitis, proctitis, cervicitis, endometritis, salpingitis, perihepatitis, bartholinitis, pharyngitis, conjunctivitis, prepubertal vaginitis, ?prostatitis, accessory gland infection, amniotic infection syndrome, disseminated gonococcal infection, chorioamnionitis, premature rupture of membranes, and premature delivery
Chlamydia trachomatis	Urethritis, epididymitis, proctitis, cervicitis, endometritis, salpingitis, perihepatitis, bartholinitis, prepubertal vaginitis, otitis media in infants, ?chorioamnionitis, ?premature rupture of membranes, ?premature delivery, inclusion conjunctivitis, infant pneumonia, trachoma, and lymphogranuloma venereum
Mycoplasma hominis	Postpartum fever, ?salpingitis
Ureaplasma urealyticum	?Nongonococcal urethritis, ?chorioamnionitis, ?premature delivery
Treponema pallidum	Syphilis
Gardnerella vaginalis	*Gardnerella*-associated ("nonspecific") vaginosis
Hemophilus ducreyi	Chancroid
Calymmatobacterium granulomatis	Donovanosis (granuloma inguinale)
Shigella sp.	Shigellosis in homsexual men
Campylobacter sp.	Enteritis, proctocolitis
Group B streptococcus	Neonatal sepsis, neonatal meningitis
VIRUSES	
Herpes simplex virus	Initial and recurrent genital herpes, aseptic meningitis, neonatal herpes, cervical dysplasia and carcinoma, ?carcinoma in situ of the vulva
Hepatitis B virus	Acute hepatitis B, chronic active hepatitis, persistent (unresolved) hepatitis, polyarteritis nodosa, chronic membranous glomerulonephritis, ?mixed cryoglobulinemia, ?polymyalgia rheumatica, hepatocellular carcinoma
Hepatitis A virus	Acute hepatitis A
Cytomegalovirus	Heterophil-negative infectious mononucleosis, congenital infection, gross birth defects and infant mortality, cognitive impairment (e.g., mental retardation, sensorineural deafness), ?cervicitis, protean manifestations in the immunosuppressed host
Genital papilloma virus	Condyloma accuminata, laryngeal papilloma, ?cervical dysplasia
Molluscum contagiosum virus	Genital molluscum contagiosum
PROTOZOA	
Trichomonas vaginalis	Trichomonal vaginitis
Entamoeba histolytica	Amebiasis in homosexual men
Giardia lamblia	Giardiasis in homosexual men
FUNGI	
Candida albicans	Vulvovaginitis, balanitis
ECTOPARASITES	
Phthirius pubis	Pubic lice infestation
Sarcoptes scabiei	Scabies

TABLE 143-2
Selected syndromes and complications with corresponding sexually transmitted etiologic agents*

Syndrome	Agent
MEN	
Urethritis	*N. Gonorrhoeae, C. trachomatis,* herpes simplex virus, *U. urealyticum*
Epididymitis	*C. trachomatis, N. gonorrhoeae*
Intestinal infections:	
Proctitis	*N. gonorrhoeae,* herpes simplex virus, *C. trachomatis*
Proctocolitis or enterocolitis	*Campylobacter* sp., *Shigella* sp., *E. histolytica*
Enteritis	*G. lamblia*
Hepatitis	Hepatitis A and B viruses, cytomegalovirus, *T. pallidum*
Acquired immunodeficiency syndrome	Unknown
WOMEN	
Lower genitourinary tract infection:	
Vulvitis	*C. albicans,* herpes simplex virus
Vaginitis	*T. vaginalis, C. albicans, ?G. vaginalis*
Cervicitis	*N. gonorrhoeae, C. trachomatis,* herpes simplex virus
Urethritis	*N. gonorrhoeae, C. trachomatis,* herpes simplex virus
Pelvic inflammatory disease	*N. gonorrhoeae, C. trachomatis, ?Mycoplasma hominis*
Infertility:	
Postsalpingitis, postobstetric, postabortion	*N. gonorrhoeae, C. trachomatis, ?M. hominis*
Pregnancy morbidity: Chorioamnionitis, amniotic fluid infection, prematurity, premature rupture of membranes, postpartum endometritis, ectopic pregnancy	Several STD agents have been implicated in one or more of these conditions
MEN AND WOMEN	
Neoplasia	
Cervical intraepithelial neoplasia, carcinoma	?Herpes simplex virus, ?human papilloma virus type 6, *?C. trachomatis*
Vulvar carcinoma in situ	?Herpes simplex virus
Anal carcinoma in homosexual men	Unknown
Hepatocellular carcinoma	Hepatitis B
Kaposi's sarcoma	Unknown
Genital ulceration	Herpes simplex virus, *T. pallidum, H. ducreyi, Cal. granulomatis, C. trachomatis* (LGV strains)
Acute arthritis with urogenital or intestinal infection	*N. gonorrhoeae, C. trachomatis, Shigella* sp., *Campylobacter* sp.
Genital warts, molluscum contagiosum	Human papilloma virus, molluscum contagiosum virus
Ectoparasite infestations	*Sarcoptes scabiei, Phthirius pubis*
Heterophil-negative mononucleosis	Cytomegalovirus, ?Epstein-Barr virus
NEONATES AND INFANTS	
TORCHES syndrome†	Cytomegalovirus, herpes simplex virus, *T. pallidum*
Conjunctivitis	*C. trachomatis, N. gonorrhoeae*
Pneumonia	*C. trachomatis, ?U. urealyticum*
Otitis media	*C. trachomatis*
Sepsis, meningitis	Group B streptococcus
Cognitive impairment, deafness	Cytomegalovirus, herpes simplex virus, *T. pallidum*

* *For each of the above syndromes, some cases cannot yet be ascribed to any cause and must currently be considered idiopathic.*
† *TORCHES is an acronym for toxoplasmosis, rubella, cytomegalovirus, herpes, and syphilis. The syndrome consists of various combinations of encephalitis, hepatitis, dermatitis, and disseminated intravascular coagulation.*

urethritis usually does not include cultures for *C. trachomatis* or *U. urealyticum.* The following steps should be taken in evaluating sexually active men with symptoms of urethral discharge and/or dysuria.

1 *Establish the presence of urethritis.* Urethral discharge should be demonstrated. Commonly in NGU, and less often in gonorrhea, discharge can be demonstrated only by milking the urethra after the patient has gone several hours, preferably overnight, without voiding. If no overt discharge is demonstrable, urethral exudate can be demonstrated by inserting a small urethrogenital swab 1 to 2 cm into the urethra and examining the Gram-stained direct smear prepared from this swab for leukocytes. Five or more leukocytes per 1000× field in areas containing cells suggests urethritis. Patients with symptoms who lack objective confirmatory evidence of urethritis on two occasions 1 week apart may have functional problems and generally do not benefit from repeated courses of antibiotics.
2 *Exclude complications or alternative diagnoses.* Epididymitis and systemic complications, such as the gonococcal arthritis-dermatitis syndrome and Reiter's syndrome, should be excluded by brief history and examination. Rectal examination for prostatitis is seldom informative in patients with urethritis, unless concomitant symptoms such as perineal, suprapubic, or rectal discomfort are present. Bacterial prostatitis and cystitis should, of course, be excluded by appropriate tests in men with dysuria who lack signs of urethritis.
3 *Evaluate for gonococcal infection.* The diagnosis of gonorrhea is confirmed by demonstrating typical gram-negative diplococci within neutrophils. The diagnosis of NGU is warranted if gram-negative diplococci are not found. Smears containing only extracellular or atypical gram-negative diplococci are equivocal and should lead to attempts to isolate *N. gonorrhoeae* by culture. Because the predictive value of

FIGURE 143-1
Reported cases of nongonococcal urethritis in the United Kingdom, 1960–1981. (Courtesy of RD Catterall.)

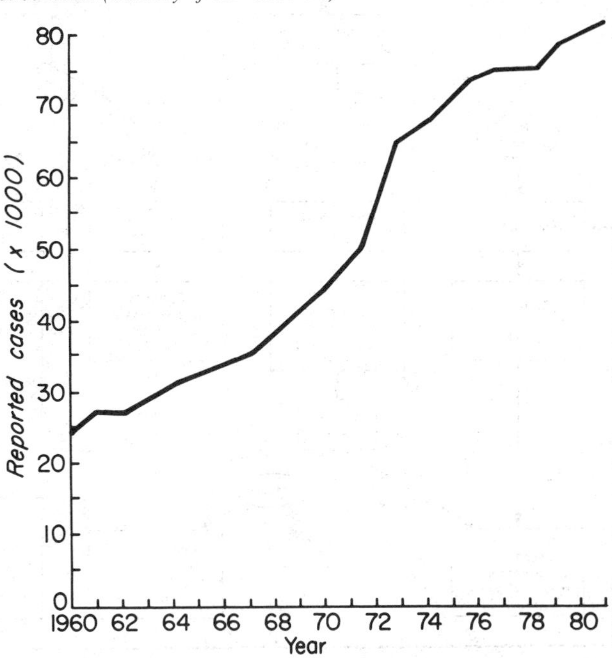

Gram-stained urethral smears is dependent on the experience of the laboratory, most clinicians should routinely culture the urethral exudate for *N. gonorrhoeae.* Treatment should be initiated, however, on the basis of the smear. An approach to the diagnosis of urethritis is illustrated in Fig. 143-2. The treatment of gonorrhea and NGU is discussed in Chaps. 150 and 191, respectively.

EPIDIDYMITIS Acute epididymitis is almost always unilateral and must be differentiated from testicular torsion, tumor, and trauma. Torsion, a surgical emergency, usually occurs in adolescents and young adults and is suggested by sudden onset of pain, elevation of the testicle within the scrotal sac, and absence of blood flow on Doppler examination or ^{99}Tc scan. In sexually active men under age 35, acute epididymitis is usually caused by *C. trachomatis* or by *N. gonorrhoeae* and is usually, but not always, associated with overt or subclinical urethritis. Antimicrobial agents are the mainstay of therapy; optimal treatment for epididymitis due to *C. trachomatis* or penicillinase-negative *N. gonorrhoeae* is doxycycline 100 mg twice daily for 10 days. Bed rest and scrotal elevation may hasten symptomatic relief.

Acute epididymitis in older men is usually caused by urinary pathogens such as coliform bacteria or *Pseudomonas aeruginosa.* Urethritis is usually absent, but bacteriuria is present. Treatment should be initiated with a broad-spectrum, parenteral antibiotic (e.g., tobramycin) and continued with the appropriate antibiotics as determined by sensitivity tests. An algorithm for diagnosis and management of acute epididymitis in sexually active men is presented in Fig. 143-3.

LOWER GENITOURINARY TRACT INFECTION IN WOMEN Infections of the female urinary tract, cervix, vulva, and vagina produce certain overlapping symptoms in women such as dysuria, vulvar irritation, dyspareunia, and altered quality or increased quantity of vaginal discharge. There is insufficient consensus on clinical or laboratory guidelines for differentiating among these various categories on the basis of symptomatology, and they are often referred to in vague terms such as *nonspecific genital infection.* Lack of nosologic precision is attributable not only to overlapping symptomatology, but also to uncertainty about the etiologies of the inflammatory conditions of the urinary tract, vulva, vagina, and cervix in women; to the lack of consistent application of available laboratory testing where the etiology is known; and to the difficulty clinicians and patients experience in differentiating the true inflammatory conditions from functional, psychosomatic genitourinary complaints.

Although the etiology of certain genitourinary inflammatory conditions in women remains uncertain, some data allow improved diagnostic precision, which in turn should lead to improved management. One estimate of the relative frequencies of diagnostic entities that produce lower urogenital symptoms was provided in a study of 821 young women (mean age 24) examined in a primary care clinic. Vaginitis was found to be more than five times as common as bacterial cystitis or urethritis. Two steps are required in the evaluation of lower genitourinary symptoms in women: (1) differentiation among cystitis, urethritis, vaginitis, cervicitis, and cervical ectopy, and (2) exclusion of associated upper tract disease (e.g., pyelonephritis, salpingitis).

Cystitis and urethritis Although dysuria is more common in bacterial urinary tract infection (UTI) than in vaginitis, in

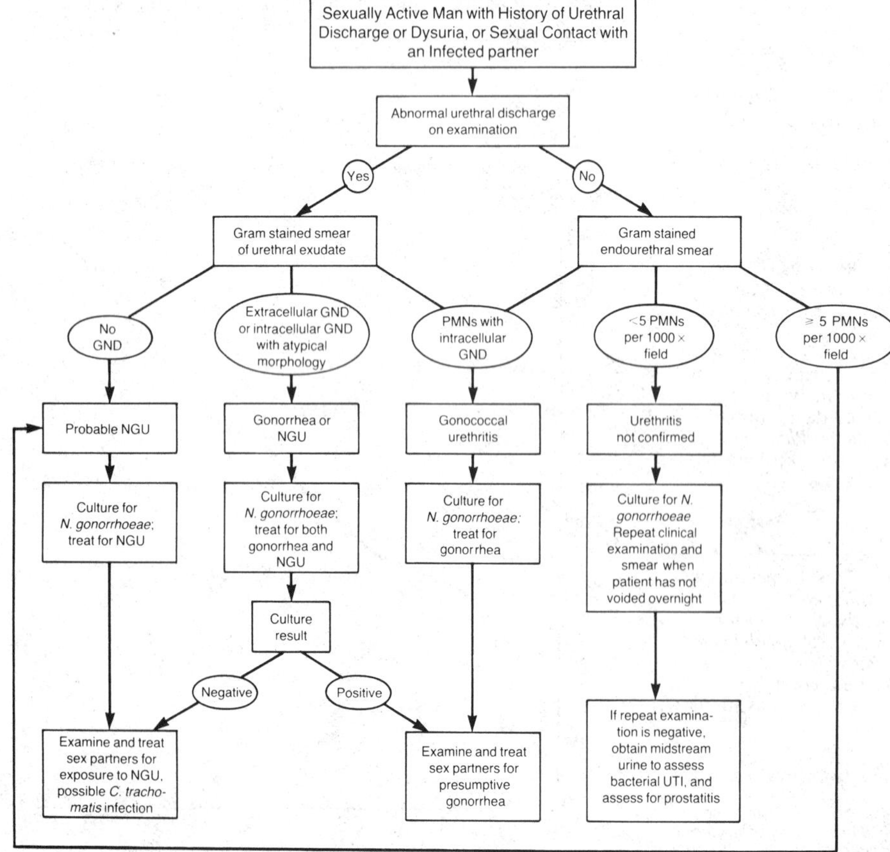

FIGURE 143-2

Evaluation of sexually active men with suspected urethritis. PMN = polymorphonuclear leukocyte; GND = gram-negative diplococci; NGU = nongonococcal urethritis; UTI = urinary tract infection.

young women dysuria is often attributable to vaginitis, because vaginitis is so much more common than UTI. However, when women were asked to localize the dysuria as "internal" (felt inside the body) or "external" (felt on the vaginal labia when the stream of urine passed), "internal" dysuria correlated with UTI and "external" dysuria was associated with vulvovaginitis. In a study of female college students with dysuria, urgency, or frequency without vaginal infection, about half had bacterial cystitis with 10^5 bacteria or more per milliliter of urine, and one-quarter had bacterial cystitis with less than 10^5 bacteria per milliliter (usually between 10^2 and 10^5 per milliliter). About one-quarter had urethral symptoms without bacteriuria—often termed the *urethral syndrome* or *dysuria-frequency syndrome.* In the latter group, about half had pyuria, and most of these were infected with *C. trachomatis,* while most of those without pyuria had no demonstrable infection and improved with placebo therapy alone. In populations whose risk of gonorrhea is higher than that of college students, *N. gonorrhoeae* is also a common cause of the urethral syndrome.

DIAGNOSIS AND THERAPY As outlined in Fig. 143-4, the evaluation of dysuria and frequency in sexually active women involves first the differentiation of cystitis or urethritis from vaginitis by history and examination. Among women without vaginitis, bacterial UTI must then be differentiated from the urethral syndrome. The finding of a conventional urinary pathogen, such as *Escherichia coli* or *Staphylococcus saprophyticus,* in a concentration of $\geq 10^2$ per milliliter in a properly collected midstream urine specimen from a symptomatic woman with pyuria indicates probable bacterial UTI, whereas pyuria with sterile urine on conventional culture suggests the diagnosis of acute urethral syndrome due to *C. trachomatis* or *N. gonorrhoeae.* Gonorrhea should be excluded by appropriate culture of the cervix and urethra. The value of antimicrobial therapy for the urethral syndrome, if gonorrhea is not present, has not been studied in controlled fashion. *C. trachomatis* should be similarly excluded if possible, and treatment with a tetracycline (e.g., tetracycline HCl, 500 mg four times daily for 7 days) should be considered. The sexual partner should also be examined and considered for treatment.

VAGINITIS In self-referred female STD clinic patients, vaginitis is the most common diagnosis. The relative frequencies of candidal vaginitis, trichomoniasis, and *Gardnerella*-associated vaginosis as causes of vulvo-vaginal symptoms vary markedly in different populations.

Vaginitis, without UTI, is characterized by one or more of

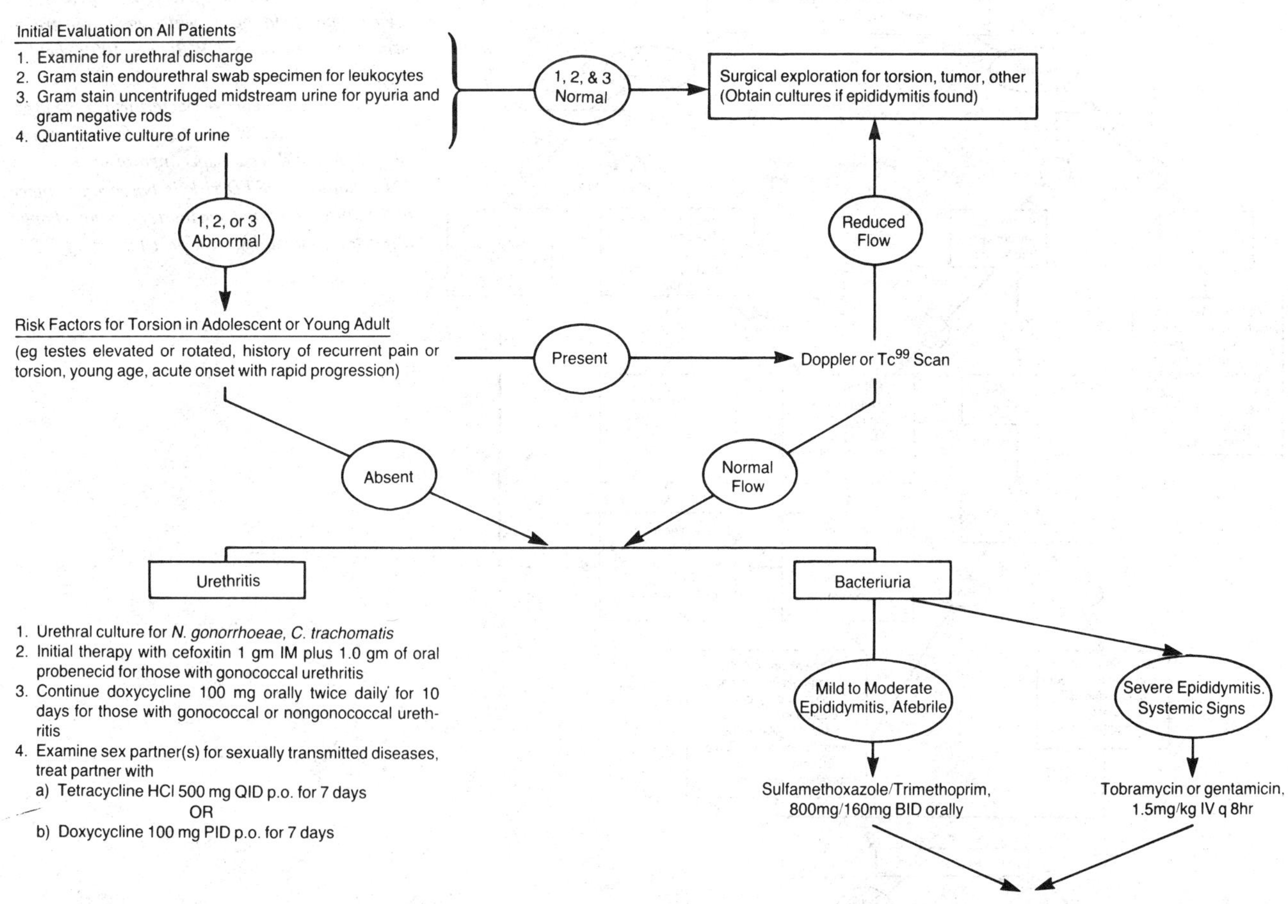

FIGURE 143-3
Evaluation and management of patients with unilateral testicular pain and swelling.

the following symptoms: increased volume of discharge; abnormal yellow or green color of discharge caused by increased concentration of polymorphonuclear leukocytes; vulvar itching, irritation, or burning; introital dyspareunia; and malodor. *Trichomonas vaginalis* usually produces a profuse, yellow, purulent, homogeneous discharge which is often malodorous and may be frothy, presumably because of gas production by vaginal bacteria. The vaginal epithelium is inflamed, and petechial lesions may be present on the cervix. In contrast, the predominant symptom in *Candida albicans* vaginitis is usually vulvar itching, often with signs of vulvitis as well as vaginitis, but without a distinct odor. The discharge in *Candida* vaginitis is typically white and may resemble curds of cottage cheese. The vagina occasionally contains adherent thrush-like plaques of matted mycelia, polymorphonuclear leukocytes, and epithelial cells. *Gardnerella vaginalis* (formerly *Hemophilus vaginalis*) is associated with a condition which has usually been termed *nonspecific vaginitis,* a misnomer since the syndrome is quite specific and is usually noninflammatory. *Gardnerella*-associated vaginosis is characterized by moderately increased malodorous white or gray vaginal discharge which is homogeneous, low in viscosity, contains fewer leukocytes than are usually found in *T. vaginalis* or *C. albicans* infection, and uniformly coats the vaginal walls. Overgrowth of vaginal anaerobes is also associated with this syndrome. *G. vaginalis* is commonly present in low concentrations in the vaginas of normally sexually active women, and the exact pathogenic role of this organism is uncertain. Yeast vaginitis and trichomonal vaginitis can each be demonstrated in 15 to 20 percent of women attending STD clinics, and *Gardnerella*-associated vaginosis can be found in 25 to 30 percent of such patients. These proportions are similar among college women attending students' gynecology clinics, except that trichomonal vaginitis is found in only 1 to 2 percent.

Colposcopy may show abnormally dilated vessels and/or increased density of vessels on the vaginal or cervical wall in *Candida* and *Trichomonas* vaginitis, but not in *Gardnerella*-associated vaginosis. A most important contribution of the clinical evaluation of vaginal discharge is ascertaining by speculum examination whether the discharge emanates from the vagina or cervix and whether the discharge is, in fact, abnormal. Occasionally, increased discharge or other symptoms are not associated with objective signs of vaginitis or cervicitis. Psychological testing is normal in most such cases. The diagnosis and

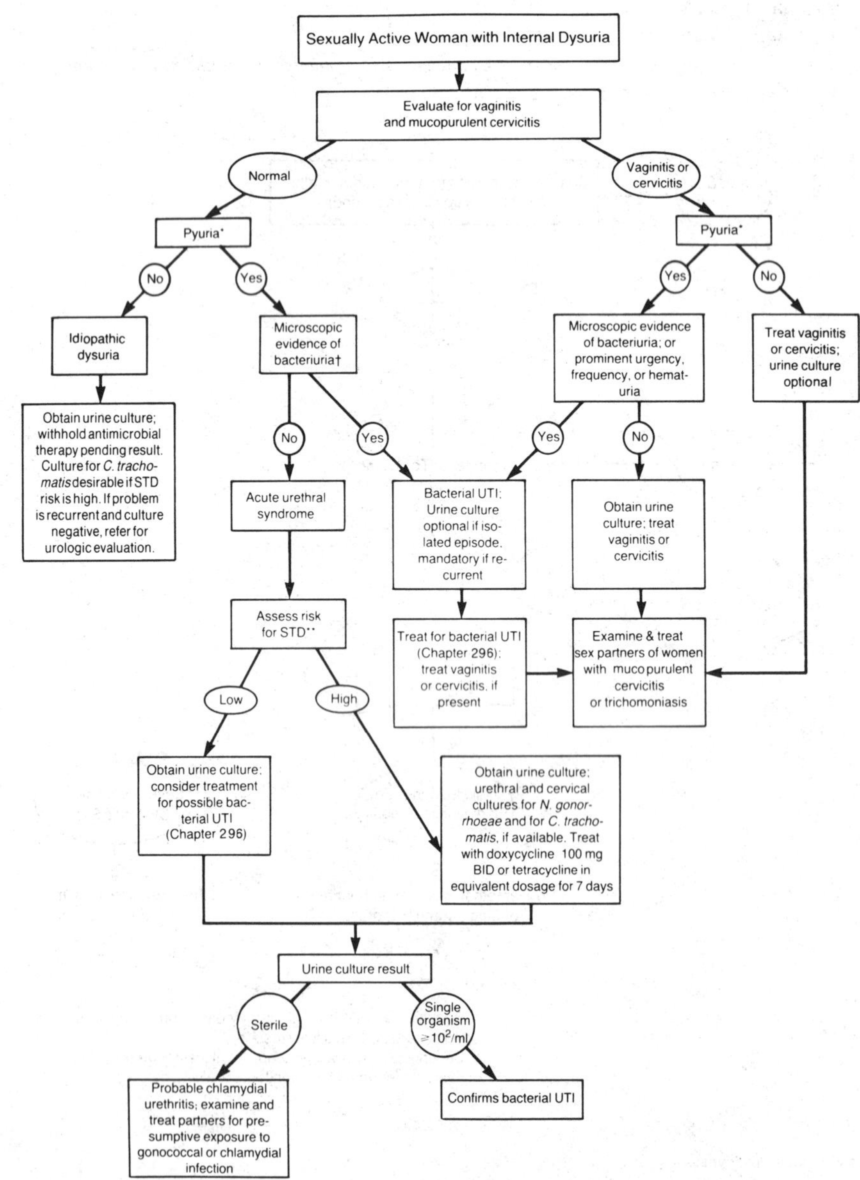

FIGURE 143-4

Evaluation of sexually active women with "internal" dysuria.

**Pyuria is defined as ≥ 20 WBC per 400× microscopic field of a centrifuged midstream urine specimen, or ≥ 1 WBC per 400× field of uncentrifuged urine.*

†Microscopic evidence of bacteriuria is the presence of ≥ 1 bacillus per 400× field of an uncentrifuged midstream specimen of urine.

***Evaluation of STD risk is based on number and nature of sexual partner(s), recent change in partner, marital status, past history of STD.*

therapy of the three major types of vaginal infection are summarized in Table 143-3.

***Trichomonas vaginalis* vaginitis** Sexual transmission of *T. vaginalis* is well established, although the age distribution of trichomoniasis in women is skewed toward the older age group more than for other STDs, suggesting that nonsexual transmission of *T. vaginalis* may be important. Routine sampling indicates that many women and most men with infection are asymptomatic. Among women with asymptomatic infections, however, the potential for development of symptoms is high. Treatment of asymptomatic as well as symptomatic cases is recommended to reduce the reservoir of infection and the risk of transmission, and to prevent the future development of symptoms.

DIAGNOSIS AND THERAPY The diagnosis in women is confirmed by demonstration of motile trichomonads and polymorphonuclear leukocytes in vaginal secretions mixed with normal saline and examined promptly under a low-power or high dry (400×) microscopic field. Wet-mount examination is at least 80 percent as sensitive as culture in symptomatic cases. The diagnosis of *T. vaginalis* infection in men is difficult and requires the use of culture of early morning urethral scrapings obtained before voiding.

The pH of vaginal secretions is usually greater than 5.0 in symptomatic *T. vaginalis* infections, and the addition of 10% potassium hydroxide (KOH) to vaginal secretions may liberate an amine-like fishy odor in trichomonal vaginitis as well as in *Gardnerella*-associated vaginosis.

Nitroimidazoles are the only consistently effective drugs for treating trichomoniasis. Several studies show that a single 2.0-g oral dose is at least 90 percent as effective as more prolonged dosage schedules. Tinidazole, a structurally related nitroimidazole, has a longer half-life than metronidazole but has not been clearly shown to give better results than metronidazole in single-dose therapy of trichomoniasis.

T. vaginalis infection can be demonstrated in one-third to two-thirds of male sex partners of women with trichomonal vaginitis. On the basis of these data, and in view of the difficulty in demonstrating *T. vaginalis* in men, routine treatment of sex partners is advisable to reduce both the risk of reinfection and the reservoir of infection. However, caution is warranted in using nitroimidazoles. It is recommended that metronidazole not be given to women during the first trimester of pregnancy and that alcohol be avoided for 24 h after treatment because of the disulfiram-like effect of the drug. Metronidazole is also mutagenic, and massive doses cause several types of tumors in rodents.

TABLE 143-3
Diagnostic features and management of vaginitis

	Clinical Condition			
	Normal	*Yeast vaginitis*	*Trichomonal vaginitis*	*Gardnerella-associated vaginosis*
Etiology	Uninfected	*Candida albicans* and other yeasts	*Trichomonas vaginalis*	Uncertain; associated with *G. vaginalis* and various anaerobic bacteria
Discharge:				
Amount	Variable; usually scant	Scant to moderate	Profuse	Moderate to profuse
Color*	Clear or white	White	Yellow, green, brownish	Clear or white
Consistency	Nonhomogeneous, flocculant	Clumped; adherent plaques	Homogeneous, low viscosity; occasionally frothy	Homogeneous, low viscosity, uniformly coating vaginal walls; occasionally frothy
Associated inflammatory signs	None	Erythema of vaginal mucosa, introitus; vulvar dermatitis common	Erythema of vaginal mucosa, introitus; occasional cervical petechiae; occasional vulvar dermatitis	None
pH of secretions†	<4.5	<4.5	≥ 5.0	≥ 4.5
Amine ("fishy") odor with 10% KOH‡	None	None	Present	Present
Microscopy	Normal epithelial cells; lactobacilli predominate	Leukocytes, epithelial cells; yeasts or pseudomycelia in 50–80%	Leukocytes; motile trichomonads seen in 80–90% of symptomatic patients	Clue cells; few leukocytes; lactobacilli replaced by profuse mixed flora
Usual treatment	None	Miconazole or clotrimazole intravaginally, each 50–100 mg daily for 7 days Nystatin, 100,000 units intravaginally twice daily for 7–14 days	Metronidazole 2.0 g orally (single dose) Metronidazole 250 mg orally three times daily for 10 days	Metronidazole 500 mg orally twice daily for 7 days
Usual management of sex partners	None	None; topical treatment if candidal dermatitis of penis is present	Examine for STD; treat with metronidazole	Examine for STD; no treatment if normal

* *Color of secretions is determined by examining a swab coated with secretions against a white background.*
† *pH determination is not useful if blood is present.*
‡ *To detect fungal elements, secretions are digested with 10% KOH prior to microscopic examination; to examine for other features, secretions are mixed (1:1) with physiologic saline. Gram's stain also is excellent for detecting yeasts and pseudomycelia and is the only technique useful for distinguishing lactobacilli from other bacteria, but is less sensitive than the saline preparation for detection of* T. vaginalis.

Gardnerella-associated vaginosis Vaginal discharge not associated with *T. vaginalis,* yeast, or cervical infection is usually due to *Gardnerella*-associated vaginosis. The concentration of certain anaerobic bacteria in vaginal washings from women with this syndrome has also been found to be increased. The evidence linking *G. vaginalis* to this syndrome is somewhat similar to that linking *U. urealyticum* to *Chlamydia*-negative nongonococcal urethritis (NGU). That is, *G. vaginalis* is recovered more often and in higher concentrations from women with *Gardnerella*-associated vaginosis than from those with other forms of vaginitis or from normal women, and improvement of clinical signs correlates with eradication of *G. vaginalis.* However, *G. vaginalis* is frequently present in vaginal secretions of asymptomatic women who may or may not have an increased malodorous vaginal discharge. In fact, using selective media, *G. vaginalis* can be isolated from about 40 percent of asymptomatic women with normal vaginal examinations. The factors responsible for the presence or absence of symptoms in women infected by *G. vaginalis* require further study. The prevalence and concentration of anaerobic bacteria, particularly *Bacteroides bivius, B. capillosis, Peptococcus* sp., and *Eubacterium,* also are increased and probably contribute to the pathogenesis of *Gardnerella*-associated vaginosis. *Mycoplasma hominis* and an as yet unspeciated motile, curved, gram-negative or gram-variable rod also may be associated with the syndrome.

DIAGNOSIS AND TREATMENT In a patient with symptoms or signs of abnormal vaginal discharge, the diagnosis of *Gardnerella*-associated vaginosis can be made with reasonable certainty by the following:

1 Exclusion of candidal and trichomonal vaginitis and mucopurulent cervicitis.
2 Demonstration of the presence of "clue cells" by microscopic examination of vaginal secretions diluted 1:1 in normal saline (wet-mount examination) (Fig. 143-5). Clue cells are vaginal epithelial cells coated with coccobacillary forms of *G. vaginalis,* to the extent that the borders of the cells are completely obscured. Several media are available for isolation of *G. vaginalis;* the addition of colistin and nalidixic acid selectively inhibits other organisms, and addition of 5 percent human blood permits rapid detection of beta-hemolytic colonies of *G. vaginalis* on primary isolation.
3 Liberation of an amine-like fishy odor immediately after mixing vaginal secretions with a 10% solution of KOH. Vaginal secretions in *Gardnerella*-associated vaginosis contain several amines, including putrescine, cadaverine, methylamine, isobutylamine, histamine, tyramine, and phenethylamine, and these are volatilized by alkalinization. They also are often present in vaginal secretions of women with *T. vaginalis* infection, but not in secretions from women with candidal vaginitis or normal women.
4 Demonstration of pH of vaginal secretions greater than 4.5. The elevated pH may be partly due to the presence of amines.

FIGURE 143-5

A. Vaginal epithelial "clue cells." Note granular appearance due to adherent H. vaginalis *and indistinct cell margins. 400×. B. Normal vaginal epithelial cells. The cell margins are distinct and lack granularity.*

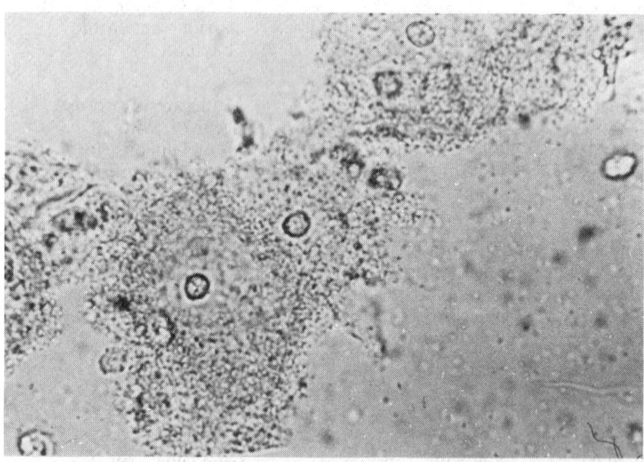
A

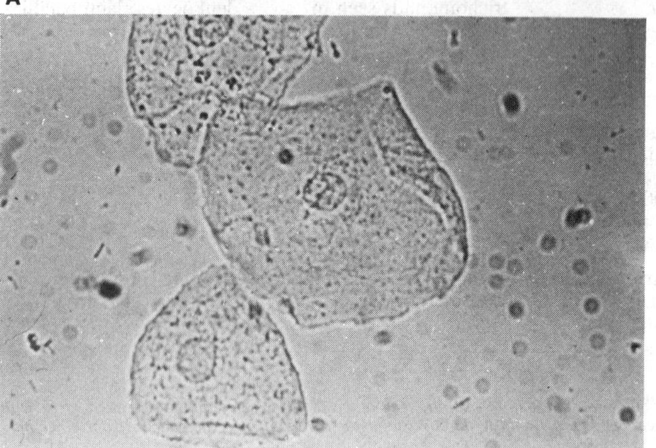
B

Treatment of *Gardnerella*-associated vaginosis generally has been frustrating. Sulfonamide-containing vaginal creams are usually ineffective, probably because sulfonamides are uniformly inactive against both *G. vaginalis* and many vaginal anaerobes. Tetracycline therapy is also usually ineffective, partly because many strains of *G. vaginalis* are resistant to tetracyclines in vitro. Ampicillin, 500 mg four times daily for 7 days, has been effective in about 40 to 50 percent of cases of *Gardnerella*-associated vaginosis. The most consistently effective therapy is metronidazole 500 mg twice daily for 7 days. This observation underscores the role of the anaerobes, which are highly susceptible to metronidazole. The efficacy of this regimen, which is not approved for use for *Gardnerella*-associated vaginosis in the United States, should be weighed against its potential toxicity. Treatment of male partners of women with this syndrome probably does not affect recurrence rates and is not routinely indicated.

Candidal vaginitis *Candida albicans* accounts for about 80 percent of yeasts isolated from the vagina, while *Torulopsis glabrata* and other less commonly encountered *Candida* species are found in the remainder. Pruritus and vulvovaginitis are more common among those with *C. albicans* than among those with *T. glabrata* or other species. Sexual transmission from the male and spread of infection from the anus or urethra may account for some cases of recurrent vaginal yeast infection.

DIAGNOSIS AND THERAPY The diagnosis of *Candida vaginitis* involves demonstration of fungal elements by microscopic examination of vaginal secretions in saline or 10% KOH, or by Gram's stain. Demonstration of pseudohyphae strengthens the diagnosis of *C. albicans* vaginitis. Microscopic examination is less sensitive than culture, but culture has the disadvantage of detecting asymptomatic carriage in women who may not require therapy. The pH of vaginal secretions is usually less than 4.5 in yeast vaginitis, and the vaginal odor is normal. Vulvitis often accompanies vaginitis and may result in excoriations which must be differentiated from genital herpes. Most clinicians recommend therapy for candidal vaginal infection only if the patient is symptomatic. Simultaneous therapy with oral nystatin, with the intent of eradicating colonic colonization with *Candida,* does not reduce the risk of recurrent yeast vaginitis. Treatment of the male sex partner is not routinely indicated, although this has not been rigorously studied.

MUCOPURULENT CERVICITIS Mucopurulent cervicitis in the female can be regarded as the "silent" partner of urethritis in the male, being equally common and caused by the same agents but being more difficult to recognize. It is the most common major STD syndrome in women and can lead to pelvic inflammatory disease. Improved recognition and treatment of mucopurulent cervicitis would greatly improve the control of STD. Although cervicitis may accompany vaginitis due to *C. albicans* or *T. vaginalis,* cervicitis without vaginitis is caused by *N. gonorrhoeae, C. trachomatis,* or herpes simplex virus (Fig. 143-6). The etiologies of mucopurulent cervicitis are similar to those of urethritis in men: in women attending STD clinics, about two-thirds are due to *C. trachomatis, N. gonorrhoeae,* or both; a small percentage is due to herpes simplex virus; and in about one-third the etiology is obscure. *C. trachomatis* is the most common overall cause of this syndrome in industrialized countries.

DIAGNOSIS AND THERAPY The diagnosis of mucopurulent cervicitis is made by demonstrating mucopurulent discharge from the cervical os (analogous to demonstrating purulent exudate in the male urethra) or by demonstrating increased numbers of polymorphonuclear leukocytes on Gram-stained smear of endocervical discharge from women without visible mucopus (analogous to criteria now widely used to diagnose urethritis in men without overt urethral discharge). Cervical ectopy (see below) that is edematous and friable, bleeding readily when swabbed, is also a common sign of mucopurulent cervicitis due to *C. trachomatis.*

The simplest way to demonstrate mucopurulent discharge from the cervix is to observe the color of cervical mucus against the background of a white swab removed from the endocervix. A yellow or green color indicates the presence of mucopus. After the results of this "swab test" are noted, the cervical mucus should be rolled *thinly* on a slide for gram staining. An area of the slide should be identified which contains a monolayer of separated cells, to avoid counting superimposed cells. The presence of ≥ 5 PMN per 1000× microscopic field suggests cervicitis. In studies in STD clinics and student gynecology clinics, the prevalence of *C. trachomatis* infection has been approximately 50 percent among women with mucopurulent cervicitis by the above criteria and <10 percent among women without it.

Mucopurulent cervicitis requires antimicrobial therapy, and nongonococcal endocervicitis should be regarded as being caused by *C. trachomatis* unless infection by that agent can be specifically excluded by culture. The diagnosis of gonococcal cervicitis is made by Gram's stain and culture. If a specimen is properly collected from the endocervical os after first wiping the cervix clean to remove vaginal flora, then the sensitivity of the Gram's stain showing intracellular gram-negative diplococci (in comparison with culture) is about 50 percent, and the specificity approaches 100 percent. The sensitivity of a single endocervical culture for *N. gonorrhoeae* is estimated to be 80 to 90 percent.

Chlamydia trachomatis infection of the cervix can be demonstrated reliably only by isolation of the organism in tissue cell culture, since direct stains of exfoliated cervical cells are insensitive. Pap smears often show atypia of the metaplastic epithelial cells, and cervical biopsy often shows lymphoid germinal centers (follicular cervicitis). If tissue culture isolation capabilities are lacking, and cultures for *N. gonorrhoeae* are negative, tetracycline therapy should be given for nongonococcal mucopurulent cervicitis, as is recommended for NGU in men. The recommended regimens are tetracycline hydrochloride, 500 mg four times per day, or doxycycline, 100 mg twice daily, orally for 1 week. For pregnant women, erythromycin base or stearate can be given in a dose of 500 mg four times daily for 7 days. The male sex partners of women with nongonococcal cervicitis should be examined for NGU and other STD. If cultures for *C. trachomatis* are not available, the partners probably should be treated for NGU, regardless of whether urethritis is documented, although this has not been studied rigorously.

Genital herpes simplex virus (HSV) infection produces ulcerative inflammation of the exocervix, as well as of the endocervix. HSV can be isolated from the cervix in 80 percent of women with an initial attack of genital herpes simplex virus infection, and these patients often have ulcerations of the cervix. In contrast, only about 10 to 20 percent or less of women with recurrent vulvar HSV infection shed the virus from the cervix, and HSV rarely causes overt cervicitis in the absence of external genital herpes lesions. If laboratory facilities for isolation of HSV are not available, HSV can be demonstrated by Papanicolaou smear in about 50 percent of women with HSV cervicitis. In the absence of vaginitis, no infectious cause of cervicitis other than *N. gonorrhoeae, C. trachomatis,* and HSV has been identified.

Cervical ectopy True cervicitis must be differentiated from cervical ectopy, which is often mislabeled "cervical erosion."

FIGURE 143-6
Endocervical exudate in mucopurulent cervicitis. (Courtesy of E Rees, MD.)

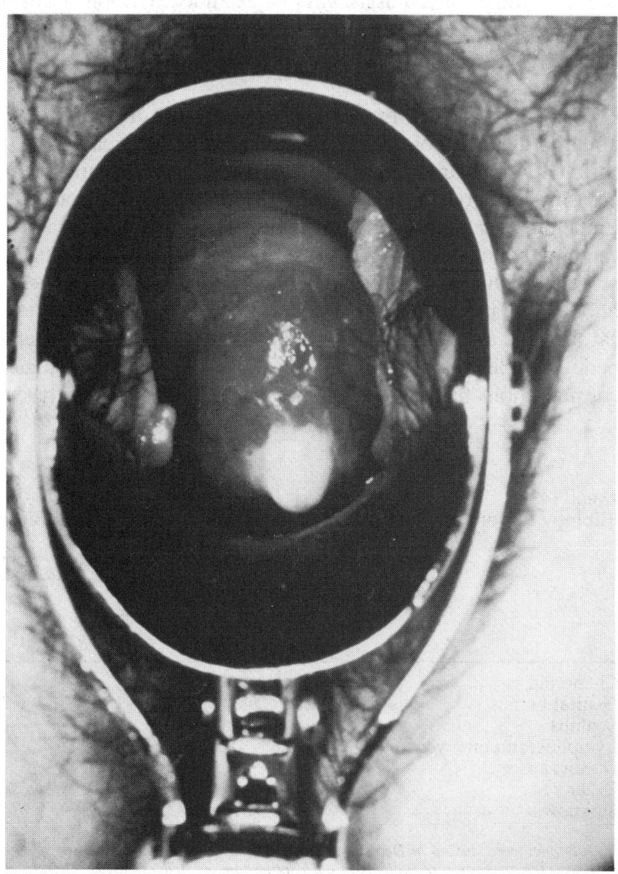

Ectopy represents the presence of the one-cell-thick columnar endocervical epithelium in an exposed visible "ectopic" position on the cervix, where it appears redder than the 20-cell-thick stratified squamous vaginal epithelium. The cervical os may contain clear or slightly cloudy mucous in ectopy, but not mucopus. Colposcopy shows that the epithelium is intact and not ulcerated. Ectopy is normally present during early adolescence and gradually recedes as squamous metaplasia replaces the ectopic columnar epithelium. Oral contraceptive usage or pregnancy favors persistence or reappearance of ectopy. Ectopy may cause increased vaginal discharge which may be symptomatic but which does not require therapy. The use of traumatic cauterizing procedures to eliminate ectopy is no longer recommended. It is speculated that the presence of ectopy makes the cervix more susceptible to infection with *N. gonorrhoeae* or *C. trachomatis.*

ULCERATIVE LESIONS OF THE GENITALIA Genital skin lesions can be classified as ulcerative or nonulcerative. Patients seen in an STD clinic for nonulcerative genital lesions often have a sexually transmitted infection, such as scabies, genital warts, *Candida* balanitis or vulvitis, or genital molluscum contagiosum, but the differential diagnosis involves a broad spectrum of dermatologic conditions.

The incidence and etiology of ulcerative lesions of the genitalia vary greatly in different areas of the world (Table 143-4). In Asia and Africa, genital ulcers are seen as frequently as gonorrhea in some STD clinics, and chancroid is the commonest form of genital ulceration, while genital herpes is relatively uncommon. In the industrialized western countries, genital ulcers are considerably less common than urethritis or vaginitis, and genital herpes simplex virus infection is the commonest form of ulceration, with chancroid being relatively uncommon. Syphilis has been the second commonest form of genital ulcer in most studies and must always be excluded. Lymphogranuloma venereum (LGV) and donovanosis (granuloma inguinale) are rare causes of genital ulceration.

DIAGNOSIS AND THERAPY In industrialized countries, the differential diagnosis of genital ulceration, when trauma and excoriated lesions are excluded, usually rests among genital herpes simplex virus infection, syphilis, and, rarely, chancroid. Epidemiologic factors, such as acquisition of infection in a developing country, or from a prostitute or homosexual contact or an individual of low socioeconomic status, increase the likelihood of chancroid, LGV, or donovanosis. Although the clinical findings are occasionally diagnostic (e.g., presence of herpetic vesicles) and clinical findings plus epidemiologic considerations help dictate the initial therapy pending further studies, many genital ulcerations cannot be diagnosed on clinical grounds. It is axiomatic to exclude syphilis by appropriate serology in all cases. Dark-field examination should also be performed, by experienced technicians when possible, on lesions suggesting primary or secondary syphilis. Chancroid should not be used as a "wastebasket" diagnosis for all ulcerative lesions not attributable to syphilis or genital herpes, since few such lesions are confirmed as chancroid, except in developing nations. Newer selective enrichment media for isolation of *H. ducreyi* should be used for the etiologic evaluation of genital ulcers. However, even when all available diagnostic tests are used by an experienced dermatovenereologist, about 20 to 25 percent of ulcerative genital lesions are still classified as idiopathic.

The following general guidelines are recommended for management of ulcerative genital lesions (Fig. 143-7):

1 *If typical painful herpetic vesicopustules are present.* In this case the clinical diagnosis of herpes is warranted, although a reaginic serologic test for syphilis should be performed. The diagnosis can be confirmed by isolation of herpes simplex virus in 90 percent of patients with intact vesicopustules and by cytology (Papanicolaou) smear in about two-thirds.
2 *If painful nonvesicular ulcer(s) raise the suspicion of herpes or chancroid.* If the lesion(s) or inguinal node(s) are painful or have other features suggestive of herpes or chancroid, attempts to demonstrate herpes simplex virus or *H. ducreyi* are indicated. Culture and cytology for demonstrating herpes virus are somewhat less sensitive in the ulcerative stage than in the vesicular stage. Syphilis should be excluded by dark-field examination and serologic testing, which should be repeated 1 to 2 weeks later if negative initially and if other diagnoses cannot be confirmed.
3 *If painless ulcerative lesions suggest the diagnosis of syphilis.* If lesions are at all suggestive of syphilis, or there are epidemiologic reasons to suspect syphilis, such as recent exposure, then dark-field examination and/or a rapid reagin test should be performed for prompt diagnosis. If these are negative, two more dark-field examinations on successive days are recommended, and a serologic test for syphilis should be repeated 1 week and 6 weeks later.
4 *If chronic painless genital ulceration progresses.* In addition to tests for syphilis and chancroid outlined above, biopsy is required to exclude donovanosis and carcinoma.

Topical antimicrobial therapy is not indicated for undiagnosed ulcerative genital lesions. In settings where genital herpes is much commoner than chancroid, as in the United States, antimicrobial therapy for painful genital ulcers can generally be deferred, pending the results of initial studies. Initial attacks of genital herpes generally begin to improve spontaneously 10 to 14 days after onset, and recurrent episodes 4 to 7 days after

TABLE 143-4
Etiology of genital ulcers in six studies, showing marked difference in populations*

	Percent of patients†					
	Detroit (N=100)	*Seattle (N=82)*	*Nairobi (N=97)*	*Swaziland (N=155)*	*Johannesburg/ Soweto (N=102)*	*Papua New Guinea (N=101)*
Chancroid	2	1	62	44	61	0
Genital herpes	40	55	5	12	17	0
Syphilis	17	12	11	19	9	50
Lymphogranuloma venereum	0	0	0	12	1	23
Donovanosis	0	0	0	1	1	46
Other	12	12	5	0	15	4
Unknown	37	21	24	15		15

* *Only men were studied in Detroit, and only women in Papua New Guinea; the other series included both sexes.*
† *A variable proportion of patients in each series had multiple etiologies; therefore, percentages total >100.*

onset. The value of antimicrobial therapy for idiopathic ulcerative lesions of the genitalia is uncertain, but a course of erythromycin or trimethoprim-sulfamethoxazole, as recommended for chancroid (see Chap. 157), seems reasonable for lesions of recent onset that persist or progress during several days of observation and that cannot be attributed to herpes, chancroid, or syphilis. Trimethoprim-sulfamethoxazole has the advantage of not interfering with the diagnosis of syphilis and is preferred if syphilis has not been reliably excluded and repeated dark-field examinations and serologic tests for syphilis are planned. Antimicrobial therapy should be given promptly when chancroid is probable, especially if regional lymph node suppuration is present or appears imminent. If patients do not improve or worsen during 1 or 2 weeks of observation and the diagnosis remains obscure, attempts to isolate *H. ducreyi* should be made or repeated, and other infectious (e.g., donovanosis) and noninfectious etiologies should be considered.

PROCTITIS, PROCTOCOLITIS OR ENTEROCOLITIS, AND ENTERITIS Anorectal pain and mucopurulent or bloody rectal discharge suggest proctitis or proctocolitis. Proctitis is commonly associated with tenesmus and constipation, whereas proctocolitis is more often associated with diarrhea. In both, anoscopy usually shows the presence of friability and exudate which should be sampled for microbiologic studies and Gram stain. Sigmoidoscopy or colonoscopy, performed if possible without enemas, shows disease limited to the rectum in proctitis, or disease extending at least into the sigmoid colon in proctocolitis.

Most cases of proctitis are due to *N. gonorrhoeae,* HSV, or *C. trachomatis* which are acquired via rectal intercourse. Primary and secondary syphilis can also produce anal or rectal lesions, with or without symptoms. Typically, gonococcal proctitis and proctitis due to non-LGV strains of *C. trachomatis* tend to involve the most distal rectal mucosa and the anal crypts and are clinically mild, without systemic manifestations. In contrast, primary HSV and LGV proctitis usually produce severe anorectal pain and fever. Perianal ulcers and inguinal lymphadenopathy may occur with either but are more common with anorectal herpes. Approximately 50 percent of men with primary anorectal HSV infection have associated neurological symptoms, usually urinary retention or S4–S5 dysesthesias or, less commonly, impotence. Sigmoidoscopy may reveal intact vesicopustular lesions with anorectal herpes but more commonly shows ulcerative proctitis with either herpes or LGV. In herpes, biopsy of the rectal mucosa shows microulcerations and may show intranuclear inclusions or perivascular lymphocytic cuffing. In LGV, biopsy typically shows crypt abscesses, granulomas, and giant cells, mimicking the histopathology of idiopathic inflammatory bowel disease.

Proctocolitis or enterocolitis in homosexual men is most often caused by *Entamoeba histolytica, Campylobacter* sp., and *Shigella* sp., which are presumably acquired by oral-anal contact. These are diagnosed by stool culture and microscopic examination for ova and parasites.

The occurrence of diarrhea and abdominal bloating or cramping pain, without anorectal symptoms, in association with normal anoscopy and sigmoidoscopy, is consistent with inflammation of the small intestine or more proximal colon. In homosexual men, enteritis limited to the small intestine is of-

FIGURE 143-7
Evaluation of sexually active persons with genital ulcer–inguinal lymphadenopathy syndromes.

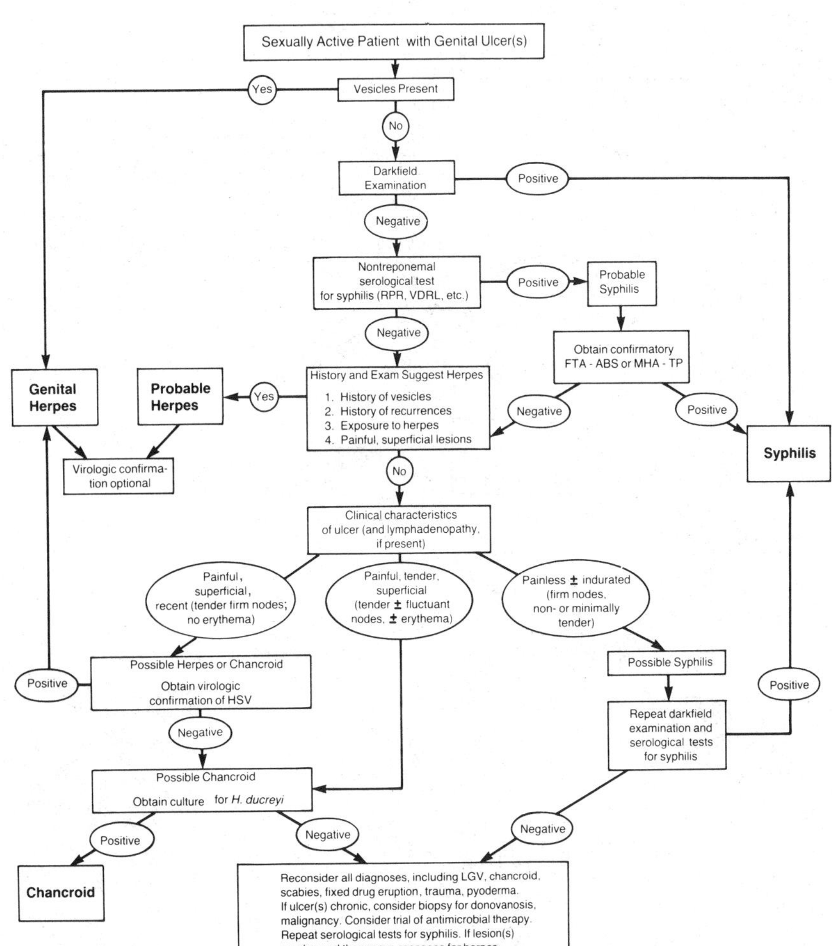

ten attributable to *Giardia lamblia,* while *Campylobacter* sp., *Shigella* sp., and *E. histolytica* can produce enterocolitis with or without lesions involving the distal colon or rectum. *G. lamblia* is presumably also acquired by direct or indirect fecal-oral contact.

The etiologic diagnosis of proctitis, proctocolitis, enterocolitis, and enteritis in homosexual men is confounded by the frequency of mixed infection (e.g., nearly half of those with proctitis who have rectal gonorrhea also have at least one other intestinal or rectal infection). For this reason, the diagnostic evaluation is complicated and potentially expensive. The minimum evaluation should include perianal examination, anoscopy, Gram stain and culture of rectal mucosa (or exudate, if present) for *N. gonorrhoeae,* dark-field examination of any ulcerative lesions, and a serologic test for syphilis. The manner in which a specific etiologic diagnosis should be further pursued is dictated by the syndrome (proctitis, proctocolitis, or enteritis/enterocolitis), by the expense, the results of preliminary microbiologic studies, and the initial response to empiric therapy, if used. One possible approach that takes these factors into account is shown in Fig. 143-8. All the agents discussed above are sexually transmitted, and appropriate treatment of sex partners, to prevent reinfection and reduce community spread of these agents, can be accomplished only if an etiologic diagnosis is established.

ACUTE ARTHRITIS The gonococcal arthritis-dermatitis syndrome is the most common form of acute arthritis in sexually active young adults, and Reiter's syndrome the second commonest. These must be differentiated from each other and from other forms of infective arthritis, various diseases associated with immune-complex deposition, crystal-induced arthropathy, acute rheumatoid arthritis, and other less common rheumatic disorders such as systemic lupus erythematosus. Meningococcemia, *Yersinia* infection, sarcoidosis, and syphilis are other uncommon causes of acute arthritis. In one series of consecutive patients hospitalized because of acute arthritis of 2 weeks or less duration, 52 percent of those aged 15 to 30 had disseminated gonococcal infection (DGI), 13 percent had Reiter's syndrome, and in another 5 percent the arthritis was directly or indirectly related to other sexually transmissible infection.

Demonstration of *N. gonorrhoeae* by culture or specific fluorescent antibody stain in synovial fluid, blood, skin lesions, or cerebrospinal fluid is diagnostic of DGI. Failing this, the diagnosis of gonococcal arthritis is virtually certain if all 3 of the following criteria are met: (1) *N. gonorrhoeae* is recovered from a mucosal site of infection or from the patient's sex partner; (2) pustular, hemorrhagic, or necrotic skin lesions are distributed primarily on the extremities; and (3) a therapeutic antibiotic trial produces defervescence and improvement of the arthritis within 48 h and loss of all objective signs of arthritis within 2 weeks. If only two of the above three criteria are met, the diagnosis of gonococcal arthritis remains highly probable, especially if the other diagnoses listed above are excluded.

DGI due to penicillinase-negative strains of *N. gonorrhoeae* is best treated with intravenous crystalline penicillin G, 10 million units per day until clear-cut clinical improvement occurs,

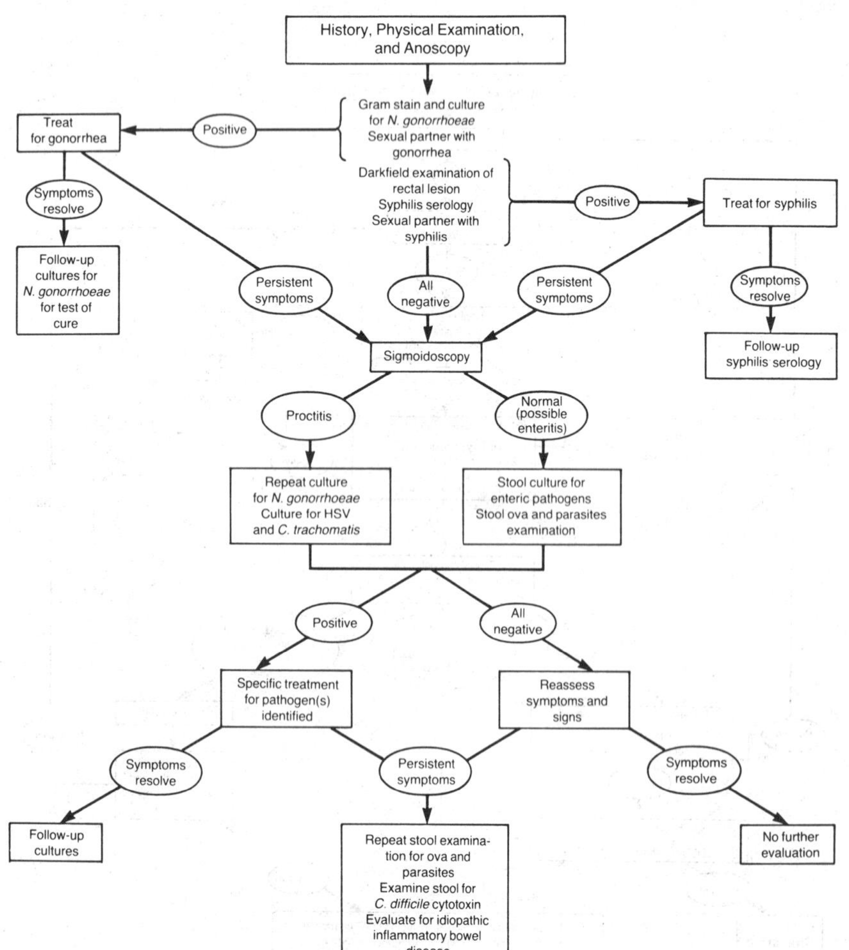

FIGURE 143-8
Evaluation of sexually active patients with symptoms of acute proctitis, proctocolitis, or enteritis. HSV = herpes simplex virus.

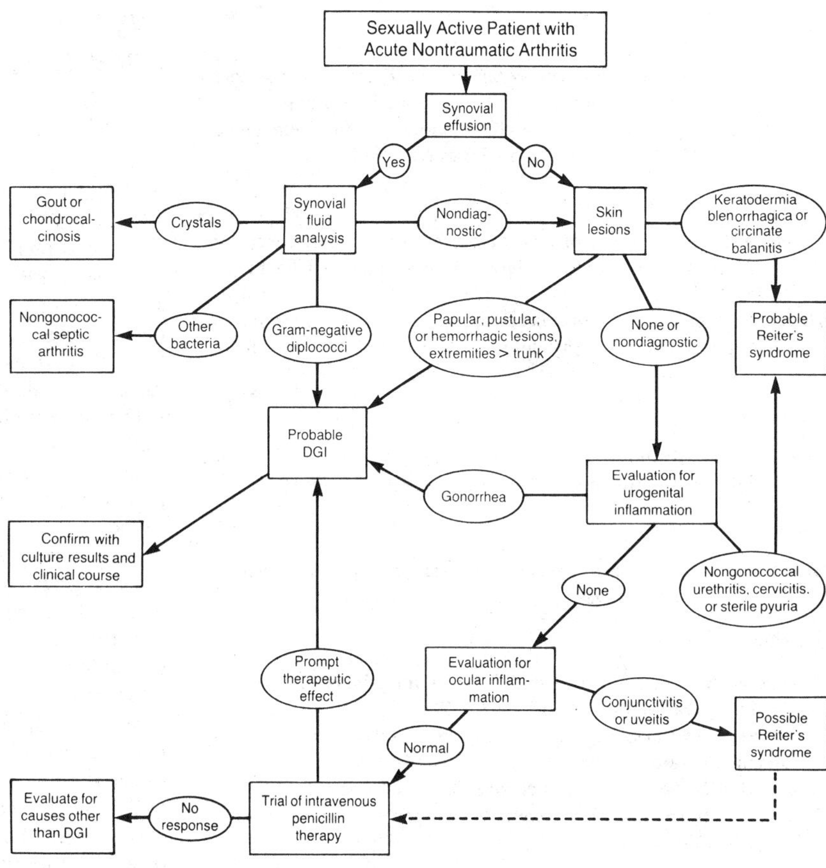

FIGURE 143-9
Evaluation of sexually active patients with acute, nontraumatic arthritis. This algorithm represents the logic used in analyzing the results of the tests or procedures. DGI = disseminated gonococcal infection.

followed by oral ampicillin 500 mg four times daily to complete 7 to 10 days of antibiotic therapy. Patients who are allergic to penicillin may be given cefoxitin or cefotaxime 6 g daily intravenously, or oral tetracycline 500 mg four times daily, for 7 to 10 days. Patients with gonococcal arthritis with highly purulent synovial effusions occasionally have persistent fever and arthritis despite adequate antimicrobial therapy, and they may require repeated closed-point irrigations with saline before improvement occurs.

Reiter's syndrome occurs in a sporadic (apparently sexually transmitted) form and a postdysenteric form, which sometimes occurs in discrete epidemics. It usually involves men, although some series include many women. Approximately 80 percent of patients have the HLA-B27 haplotype, compared with fewer than 10 percent of the general population. The pathogenesis of Reiter's syndrome is not understood, but it is believed that any of several mucosal infections in a predisposed (e.g., HLA-B27 positive) host triggers an abnormal immune response that causes the arthritis and mucocutaneous lesions. *C. trachomatis* is believed to be the most common precipitating infectious agent in the sporadic form and can be isolated from the urethras of up to two-thirds of men with this form of acute Reiter's syndrome. Other implicated infectious agents include *Shigella, Campylobacter, Salmonella,* and *Yersinia* species, and possibly *N. gonorrhoeae.*

The diagnosis of Reiter's syndrome in the male can be made on the basis of urethritis in association with acute, noninfective arthritis that persists at least 1 month, and includes the entities formerly called postgonococcal arthritis, reactive uroarthritis, and others. In women the presence of cervicitis or sterile pyuria may be equivalent to urethritis in the male as a diagnostic criterion for Reiter's syndrome, but this is less well established. One or more of the characteristic mucocutaneous manifestations is present at the time of presentation in half to two-thirds of cases and develops in most of the remainder within a year. The mucocutaneous lesions include acute conjuntivitis or uveitis, painless ulcers of the oral mucosa, circinate balanitis (a characteristic dermatitis of the glans penis), and keratodermia blenorrhagica (a hyperkeratotic papulosquamous eruption that can resemble psoriasis, most prominently involving the palms and soles). Initially, the arthritis usually involves four or fewer joints, distributed asymmetrically. Any joint may be involved and sacroiliac arthritis is common, a differential point compared with DGI. Inflammation often involves tendon insertions (enthesopathy), and fusiform arthritis of the interphalangeal joints produces the characteristic so-called sausage digits. The mainstay of treatment is nonsteroidal anti-inflammatory drugs. The precipitating infection should be treated with an appropriate antibiotic, but there is still no evidence that this affects the course of the arthritis.

Figure 143-9 is an algorithm for the diagnosis of acute arthritis in sexually active young adults, based on synovial fluid analysis, presence or absence of characteristic mucocutaneous lesions, evidence of urogenital inflammation, and therapeutic trials with antibiotics.

REFERENCES

General

HOLMES KK, MARDH PA: *International Perspectives on Neglected Sexually Transmitted Diseases: Impact on Venereology, Infertility and Maternal and Infant Health.* Washington DC, Hemisphere Publishing Corp, 1982

——— et al: *Sexually Transmitted Diseases.* New York, McGraw-Hill, 1983

NIAID STUDY GROUP: *Sexually Transmitted Diseases: 1980 Status Report.* NIH Publication 81-2213. Washington DC, Department of Health and Human Services, 1980

Sexually transmitted diseases treatment guidelines 1982, Morb Mort Week Rep 31:25, 1982

WORLD HEALTH ORGANIZATION: Nongonococcal urethritis and other selected sexually transmitted diseases of public health importance. (Prepared by participants in a WHO Scientific Group Meeting held November 1978.) Technical Report Series 660, 1981

Urethritis in males

BOWIE WR et al: Etiology of nongonococcal urethritis: Evidence for *Chlamydia trachomatis* and *Ureaplasma urealyticum.* J Clin Invest 59:735, 1977

JACOBS NF, KRAUS SF: Gonococcal and nongonococcal urethritis in men: Clinical and laboratory differentiation. Ann Intern Med 82:7, 1975

Epididymitis

BERGER RE et al: Etiology, manifestations and therapy of acute epididymitis: Prospective study of 50 cases. J Urol 121:750, 1979

Urethral syndrome

STAMM WE et al: Causes of the acute urethral syndrome in women. N Engl J Med 303:409, 1980

Vaginitis

KOMAROFF AL et al: Management strategies for urinary and vaginal infection. Arch Intern Med 138:1069, 1978

KRAUS SJ: *Trichomonas vaginalis:* Reevaluation of its clinical presentation and laboratory diagnosis. J Infect Dis 141:137, 1980

ORIEL JD et al: Genital yeast infections. Br Med J 4:761, 1972

SPIEGEL CA et al: Anaerobic bacteria in nonspecific vaginitis. N Engl J Med 303:601, 1980

Cervicitis

REES E et al: *Chlamydia* in relation to cervical infection and pelvic inflammatory disease, in *Nongonococcal Urethritis and Related Infections,* D Hobson, KK Holmes (eds). Washington DC, American Society of Microbiology, 1977, p 67

Genital ulcers

CHAPEL TA et al: The microbiological flora of penile ulceration. J Infect Dis 137:50, 1978

KRAUS SJ: Genital ulcer adenopathy syndrome, in *Sexually Transmitted Diseases,* KK Holmes et al (eds). New York, McGraw-Hill, 1983 (in press)

NSANZE H et al: Genital ulcers in Kenya: Clinical and laboratory study. Br J Vener Dis 57(6):378, 1981

Proctitis, proctocolitis, enterocolitis, enteritis

QUINN TC et al: *Chlamydia trachomatis* proctitis. N Engl J Med 305:195, 1981

——— et al: The etiology of anorectal infections in homsexual men. Am J Med 71:395, 1981

Arthritis

HOLMES KK et al: Disseminated gonococcal infection. Ann Intern Med 74:979, 1971

POLLOCK SM, HANDSFIELD HH: Arthritis, in *Sexually Transmitted Diseases,* KK Holmes et al (eds). New York, McGraw-Hill, 1983 (in press)

144 PELVIC INFLAMMATORY DISEASE

KING K. HOLMES

DEFINITION The term *pelvic inflammatory disease (PID)* usually refers to ascending infection of the uterus, fallopian tubes, and broad ligaments. Intrauterine infection can be caused by invasive intrauterine surgical procedures, such as dilatation and curettage, termination of pregnancy, insertion of an intrauterine device, or hysterosalpingography.

Endometritis or endomyometritis may occur following parturition, particularly following delivery by cesarean section. PID is uncommon during pregnancy itself. There is evidence that the uterotubal junction is closed as early as the seventh week of pregnancy, and the choriamnion becomes approximated to the endocervical os, sealing off the intrauterine cavity, at the twelfth to fifteenth week of gestation. As a consequence, ascending intrauterine infection prior to the twelfth week of gestation may be associated (either as cause or effect) with endometritis and spontaneous abortion, while ascending infection after the twelfth week may be associated with chorioamnionitis.

Rarely, infection may extend secondarily to the pelvic organs from adjacent foci of inflammation, such as appendicitis, regional ileitis, or diverticulitis; as a result of hematogenous dissemination, such as tuberculosis; or as a rare complication of certain tropical diseases, such as schistosomiasis.

However, the great majority of cases of PID arise spontaneously, without predisposing surgical trauma, obstetrical events, other systemic infection, or adjacent intraabdominal disease.

Spontaneously occurring PID can be divided into chronic and acute types. Chronic PID due to tuberculosis has become uncommon in developing countries; other forms of chronic PID, due to chronic infection with *Chlamydia trachomatis* or secondary to IUD usage, have been described but have not been adequately studied.

The term *PID* is most often used today to refer to cases of acute spontaneously occurring infection ascending from the cervix or vagina. The clinical diagnosis of PID is imprecise, since as many as 12 percent of women with suspected acute PID have been found to have other problems, such as acute appendicitis, endometriosis, ectopic pregnancy, or corpus luteum bleeding at laparoscopy, while another 23 percent have had no laparoscopic abnormalities, and only about 65 percent have had laparoscopic evidence of acute salpingitis. However, there is growing awareness of a clinical continuum ranging from cervicitis alone to endometritis, salpingitis, parametritis, and pelvic peritonitis. PID encompasses the latter three conditions, and laparoscopy or laparotomy is necessary to help differentiate between them. In this chapter, the term *PID* is used to refer to the clinical syndrome which includes each of these conditions, and the term *salpingitis* is restricted to patients with visually or histopathologically confirmed inflammation of the fallopian tubes. The distinction between endometritis and salpingitis is important because long-term sequelae are more common after salpingitis. These sequelae include infertility due to bilateral tubal occlusion, ectopic pregnancy due to tubal damage without occlusion, chronic pelvic pain, and recurrent PID.

ETIOLOGY The etiology of PID has seemed to vary greatly in recent studies for reasons that may be more related to patient selection than to methodology. As is summarized in Table 144-1, the agents most often implicated in acute PID include those which are primary causes of cervicitis (*Neisseria gonorrhoeae* and *C. trachomatis*) and those which can be regarded as abnormal components of the vaginal flora.

In the United States, gonococci have been isolated in from 45 to 80 percent of women with acute PID. However, in Scandinavian countries, where gonococcal infection is under better control, endocervical gonococcal infection is found in only 6 to 26 percent of women with acute PID. Conversely, *C. trachomatis* has been isolated from the cervix in only 5 to 20 percent of women with PID in the United States, compared with 22 to 47 percent of women with PID in Scandinavian countries. In general, PID is most often associated with gonorrhea in populations having a high incidence of gonorrhea in developing countries and in indigent, central city urban populations in developed countries.

Acute PID is commonly divided into gonococcal and nongonococcal forms on the basis of isolation of *N. gonorrhoeae* from the endocervix. However, patients with positive endocervical cultures for *N. gonorrhoeae* sometimes have tubal cultures showing gonococci mixed with other organisms or showing only other organisms without gonococci. In several studies, approximately one-third to two-thirds of women with positive endocervical cultures for *N. gonorrhoeae* have had positive peritoneal or tubal cultures for this organism.

C. trachomatis was isolated from the fallopian tubes in 15 and 85 percent of women who had positive cervical cultures for *C. trachomatis* in two Scandinavian studies. This wide disparity might be related to differences in methods used to sample the fallopian tubes. *C. trachomatis* have also been isolated from a high proportion of women with "gonococcal" PID. For example, in one Swedish study, 79 percent of PID patients who had positive cervical cultures for *N. gonorrhoeae* also had positive cervical cultures for *C. trachomatis.*

Anaerobic and facultative anaerobic organisms and genital mycoplasmas have been isolated from the peritoneal fluid or fallopian tubes in a high proportion of women with PID studied in the United States (particularly but not exclusively those with nongonococcal PID), but in only a small portion of women with PID in Scandinavian countries. These differences are not well understood. Much of the evidence for the importance of vaginal organisms in salpingitis is based on cultures obtained by culdocentesis, a procedure in which contamination of the aspirating needle by vaginal flora could occur. However, specimens obtained by laparoscopy in several U.S. studies have also implicated anaerobic and facultative species in many patients with PID. The mixed bacterial species found have generally resembled the organisms associated with the abnormal vaginal flora characteristic of nonspecific vaginitis, except that sometimes *Bacteroides fragilis,* an organism seldom found in the vagina, has been found in the peritoneal fluid from women with PID.

It should be apparent that it is extremely difficult to determine the exact microbial etiology in the individual patient with PID because of the frequency of mixed infection, the difficulty in sampling the fallopian tube itself, and the complexity of microbiologic techniques required to detect the various fastidious pathogens which most often cause this disorder.

In general, first episodes of acute PID are particularly likely to be caused by *N. gonorrhoeae* and/or *C. trachomatis.* Recurrent bouts of acute PID, episodes occurring in IUD users, and episodes precipitated by invasive intrauterine diagnostic or therapeutic procedures tend to be associated with ascending infection caused by the endogenous vaginal flora or by *C. trachomatis.*

EPIDEMIOLOGY It has been estimated that the annual incidence of PID in the United States during the mid-1970s was about 850,000 cases per year, and the direct and indirect costs of PID and its complications (excluding the cost of fetal death due to ectopic pregnancies) totaled an estimated $1.25 billion per year. These cost estimates do not include the growing costs of tubal microsurgery and in vitro fertilization for women rendered infertile because of salpingitis. PID is not a reportable disease in the United States; survey data from the National Drug and Therapeutic Index and the National Ambulatory Medical Care Survey suggest that the incidence of PID increased from 1966 through 1973 and may have decreased since then. However, in England and Wales, and in Sweden, the incidence continued to increase throughout the mid-seventies, even while the incidence of gonorrhea was declining. Furthermore, in the United States, the incidence of one of the major sequelae of salpingitis, ectopic pregnancy, progressively rose each year from 13,200 cases in 1967 to 42,000 cases in 1978. There is some evidence that the percentage of women with involuntary infertility has also increased during the same period.

Acute PID is almost exclusively a disease of sexually active women. The risk appears to be several times greater in sexually active teenagers who are 15 to 16 years old than among women 20 to 24 years of age. Reasons for the higher susceptibility of younger women to PID may include a larger number of sex partners, higher frequency of anovulatory cycles, lower prevalence of immunity to STD pathogens, and possibly delay in securing medical care. Other important risk factors other than young age include a previous history of gonorrhea or of salpingitis, and use of an intrauterine device. The relative risk of PID among IUD users compared with women using no contraception has varied from 1.4 to 7.3 in various studies. In most, but not all, studies, the relative risk of PID among IUD users was higher in nulliparous women than in parous women. On the other hand, women using oral contraceptives appear to be at decreased risk of PID, and for this reason some experts advocate use of oral contraceptives among women at high risk for PID.

PATHOGENESIS The initial step in pathogenesis of gonococcal PID involves passage of the gonococcus from the endocervix, through the lumen of the uterus, into the endosalpinx. Women who have had tubal ligation have a negligible risk of salpingitis. Factors which have been cited as possibly contributing to intracanalicular upward spread include estrogen-dominated (thin) cervical mucus, attachment of gonococci to sperm which migrate upward into the tubes, use of an intrauterine device, and menstruation. The onset of gonococcal PID often occurs during or just after the menstrual cycle. Studies of the interaction between *N. gonorrhoeae* and the mucosal cells in fallopian tube organ cultures in vitro suggest that the gono-

TABLE 144-1
Cervical and vaginal organisms most often implicated in acute PID

	Vaginal flora		
Cervical pathogens	*Anaerobic bacteria*	*Facultative bacteria*	*Mycoplasma*
N. gonorrhoeae *C. trachomatis*	*Bacteroides* sp. *Peptococci* *Peptostreptococci*	*Enterobacteriaceae* *H. influenzae* *G. vaginalis* *Streptococcus,* groups B, D	*M. hominis* *U. urealyticum*

coccus attaches to the surface of secretory columnar cells of the endosalpinx. Gonococcal pili and perhaps other surface proteins are important in this attachment. Gonococci then are taken into the secretory cells by endocytosis. They pass through the cells, and perhaps between cells, and are extruded through the base of the cell into the submucosal connective tissue. Ciliated cells are sloughed from the mucosa during this process—a factor which may render the tubes more susceptible to superinfection by other organisms. It is uncertain whether this loss of ciliated cells is irreversible in vivo. Gonococcal endotoxin is at least partly responsible for these cytotoxic effects.

Gonococci may vary in propensity to cause PID. For example, gonococci which cause disseminated gonococcal infection are significantly more susceptible to penicillin G and more likely to belong to the Arg-Hyx-Ura- auxotype than are strains causing uncomplicated gonorrhea (see Chap. 150), whereas gonococci associated with PID are significantly more resistant to penicillin and less likely to belong to the Arg-Hyx-Ura- auxotype than are strains causing uncomplicated gonorrhea. Also, gonococci isolated from the fallopian tubes reportedly form transparent colonies, whereas paired isolates from the cervix more often form opaque colonies, suggesting that phenotypic changes occur in the protein composition of the gonococcal outer membrane which may be important in the pathogenesis of PID.

C. trachomatis also spreads from the endocervix through the lumen of the uterus to the endosalpinx. *C. trachomatis* has been cultured from the endometrium and tubal mucosa and has been demonstrated by immunofluorescence in both sites. It has been possible to produce chlamydial endometritis and salpingitis in lower primates by direct inoculation of the uterus and fallopian tubes. Among women with chlamydial mucopurulent cervicitis, cervical biopsies show inclusions containing chlamydia within columnar epithelial cells, and submucosal and stromal infiltration by mononuclear cells, forming germinal centers. Endometrial biopsies show plasma cell infiltration. Tubal biopsies from women and from experimental animals with chlamydial salpingitis show destruction of the tubal mucosal epithelium, with predominance of mononuclear cell infiltration.

In fallopian tube organ cultures, *C. trachomatis* is not as cytotoxic as *N. gonorrhoeae,* and it has been speculated that it is the prominent cellular immune response in vivo that is most important in the pathogenesis of mucosal damage in chlamydial salpingitis. Further data supporting this hypothesis might have important therapeutic implications.

The pathogenesis of PID attributable to mycoplasmas or other vaginal anaerobic or facultative organisms is even more speculative. Experimental inoculation of *Mycoplasma hominis* into the fallopian tubes of monkeys produced prominent parametritis as well as salpingitis; however, parametritis has not been especially noteworthy among women with PID when *M. hominis* is isolated from the fallopian tubes or cul-de-sac. Other vaginal organisms implicated in PID are generally believed to cause infection in women whose tubes have already been damaged by a primary STD (sexually transmitted disease) pathogen (e.g., *N gonorrhoeae, C. trachomatis,* or perhaps *M. hominis*). Vaginal organisms are most likely to be found in the upper genital tract in cases of recurrent PID or in neglected cases of PID. PID among IUD users also tends to be associated with polymicrobial infection of the upper genital tract. Since the anaerobic and facultative organisms implicated in PID generally resemble those found in the vagina in nonspecific vaginitis, it is possible that nonspecific vaginitis itself is a predisposing risk factor for PID (in the same manner that poor oral hygiene is a risk factor in aspiration pneumonia). The risk of nonspecific vaginitis is increased fourfold in IUD users, and the IUD may predispose to polymicrobial infection of the uterus not only by providing an access "wick" for ascending infection through the cervix, but also by somehow causing vaginal overgrowth with a more virulent flora.

Certain other iatrogenic factors, such as dilatation and curettage or cesarean section, are known to pose a greater risk of causing PID in women with endocervical gonococcal or chlamydial infection. It remains to be determined whether such procedures are also a greater risk in women with nonspecific vaginitis.

CLINICAL MANIFESTATIONS **Tuberculous salpingitis** Unlike nontuberculous salpingitis, genital tuberculosis often occurs in older women, and about half are postmenopausal. In a large review of cases in Sweden, 38 percent had had previously diagnosed tuberculosis. The commonest presenting symptoms were abnormal vaginal bleeding (41 percent), pain including dysmenorrhea (25 percent), and infertility (13 percent). Most had normal bimanual pelvic examinations, though about one-quarter had adnexal masses. The most common method of diagnosis was endometrial biopsy, showing tuberculous granulomas, associated with a positive culture in many cases.

Nontuberculous salpingitis The sequence of events leading to the first episode of PID caused by *N. gonorrhoeae* or *C. trachomatis* is probably cervicitis→endometritis→salpingitis→peritonitis. The evolution of symptoms classically proceeds from a mucopurulent vaginal discharge caused by cervicitis—possibly associated with dysuria and frequency due to urethritis, or with anorectal pain, tenesmus, rectal discharge, and bleeding due to proctitis—to midline abdominal pain and abnormal vaginal bleeding caused by endometritis, to bilateral lower abdominal and pelvic pain caused by salpingitis, to nausea and vomiting and increased abdominal tenderness caused by peritonitis. Some patients have generalized abdominal pain caused by generalized peritonitis, or pleuritic right upper quadrant pain caused by perihepatitis. The pattern in which symptoms evolve varies from patient to patient and is also related to the etiology of the PID.

The onset of IUD-associated PID is typically gradual, and may be preceded by typical malodorous vaginal discharge characteristic of nonspecific vaginitis. The onset of gonococcal PID is typically more acute than that of chlamydial PID, and is often associated with menses.

The abdominal pain is usually described as dull or aching. In some cases, pain is lacking or is atypical, and active inflammatory changes can be found in the course of an unrelated evaluation or procedure such as a tubal ligation. Metrorrhagia precedes or coincides with the onset of pain in about 40 percent of women with PID. Symptoms of urethritis occurred in 20 percent and of proctitis in 7 percent of patients in one series.

Speculum examination shows evidence of mucopurulent cervicitis in the majority of women with gonococcal or chlamydial PID, but because criteria for the diagnosis of mucopurulent cervicitis have only recently been established, the association of cervicitis with PID has not been systematically studied. Cervical motion tenderness is produced by stretching of the adnexal attachments on the side toward which the cervix is pushed. Bimanual examination reveals uterine fundal tenderness due to endometritis, and abnormal adnexal tenderness due to salpingitis which is usually, but not necessarily, bilateral. A palpable adnexal swelling is found in about one-half of women with acute salpingitis, but evaluation of the adnexae in a patient with marked tenderness is not completely reliable, even by an experienced examiner. An initial temperature $>38°C$ is found in only about one-third of patients with acute salpingitis, and fever is not required for the diagnosis.

Laboratory findings include elevation of the erythrocyte

sedimentation rate (ESR) in 75 percent and elevation of the peripheral white blood cell count in about 60 percent of patients with salpingitis. Microscopic examination of a saline wet mount preparation of vaginal fluid has revealed more than one polymorphonuclear leukocyte per vaginal epithelial cell in nearly all patients with laparoscopically confirmed salpingitis in Swedish studies, and some experts consider the absence of white blood cells in vaginal fluid as incompatible with the diagnosis of acute PID.

Certain clinical manifestations of acute PID have been correlated with etiologic findings. For example, the onset of salpingitis is related to menses in women with gonorrhea but not in women without gonorrhea. Women with gonococcal or chlamydia-associated salpingitis are significantly younger than women with other forms of salpingitis. As is summarized in Table 144-2, women with chlamydia-associated salpingitis tend to have an indolent disease with mild symptoms of significantly longer duration and with less fever when compared to women who have gonococcus-associated salpingitis, but paradoxically, those with chlamydia-associated salpingitis have had significantly higher erythrocyte sedimentation rates and more severe inflammatory reactions seen in laparoscopy. It is suspected that indolent subclinical chlamydial salpingitis may also occur and may be a major cause of infertility in women.

IUD-associated PID also tends to be indolent and is less often associated with fever, but more often with adnexal masses, than is PID not associated with IUD use.

Perihepatitis Symptoms of perihepatitis, including pleuritic upper abdominal pain and tenderness, usually localized to the right upper quadrant, occur in 5 to 10 percent of women with acute PID. The onset of symptoms of perihepatitis occurs during or after onset of symptoms of PID and may overshadow the lower abdominal symptoms, leading to a mistaken diagnosis of cholecystitis. In up to a quarter of all cases of acute salpingitis in some studies, laparoscopy performed early reveals inflammation ranging from edema and erythema of the liver capsule to exudate with fibrinous adhesions between the visceral and parietal peritoneum. When treatment is delayed, and laparoscopy is performed late, dense "violin-string" adhesions are seen over the liver; these cause chronic exertional or positional right upper quadrant pain when traction is placed on these adhesions. Although perihepatitis, also known as the Fitz-Hugh–Curtis syndrome, was for many years attributed to gonococcal PID, it has been recognized that chlamydial salpingitis, and perhaps other types of salpingitis, can lead to perihepatitis.

Physical findings include right upper quadrant tenderness and usually show evidence of adnexal tenderness and cervicitis, even in patients whose symptoms are not suggestive of salpingitis.

Liver function tests may be normal or slightly abnormal. Oral cholecystogram may show nonfunction of the gallbladder, but ultrasonography of the right upper quadrant is normal. The presence of mucopurulent cervicitis and pelvic tenderness in a young woman with subacute pleuritic right upper quadrant pain with normal ultrasonography of the gallbladder points to a diagnosis of perihepatitis.

DIAGNOSIS Early diagnosis and initiation of therapy are essential to minimize tubal scarring. Appropriate treatment must not be withheld from patients who have an equivocal diagnosis. Since delay in therapy may lead to progression of tubal scarring, it is better to err on the side of overdiagnosis and overtreatment. On the other hand, it is essential to differentiate between salpingitis and other pelvic pathology, particularly surgical emergencies such as appendicitis and ectopic pregnancy.

Unfortunately, no clinical or laboratory finding short of laparoscopy is pathognomonic for salpingitis, and there is reluctance to perform laparoscopy in all cases of suspected salpingitis. Weström advocates the following minimum criteria for the clinical diagnosis of salpingitis: (1) lower abdominal pain of <3 weeks' duration; (2) pelvic tenderness on bimanual pelvic examination; and (3) evidence of lower genital tract infection (e.g., white blood cells outnumber all other cells in the vaginal fluid). Approximately 60 percent of such patients have salpingitis at laparoscopy.

The presence of additional findings such as a rectal temperature >38°C, a palpable adnexal mass, and elevation of the ESR >15 mm/h also raised the probability of salpingitis, which was found at laparoscopy in 68 percent of patients with one of these additional findings, 90 percent of patients with two or more, and 96 percent of patients with three or more additional findings. However, only 17 percent of all patients with laparoscopy-confirmed salpingitis had three additional findings.

The meaning of "lower genital tract infection" has not been well defined in any study of PID, and this criterion for the diagnosis of salpingitis has not been widely evaluated. Common sense suggests that it is mucopurulent cervicitis (see Chap. 143) which is responsible for the presence of leukocytes in vaginal fluid in PID, and that mucopurulent cervicitis per se would be the most useful discriminatory sign in differentiating PID from other causes of lower abdominal pain.

Several clinical features other than the presence of cervicitis favor a diagnosis of salpingitis. These include onset with menses, history of recent abnormal menstrual bleeding, presence of an IUD, history of previous salpingitis, and exposure to a male with urethritis. Detection of polymorphonuclear leukocytes in fluid aspirated by culdocentesis supports a diagnosis of suspected salpingitis. Urethritis or proctitis may occur in chlamydial or gonococcal infection but may also represent a urinary tract infection or an intestinal source for the patient's symptoms. Early onset of nausea and vomiting would favor appendicitis or other disorders of the gut. A missed menstrual period dictates evaluation for ectopic pregnancy. The more sensitive assays for human chorionic gonadotropin which are now available are usually, but not always, positive.

Ultrasonography is sometimes useful to differentiate pelvic abscess from an inflammatory mass involving tubes, ovary,

TABLE 144-2
Characteristics of laparoscopically verified salpingitis associated with *C. trachomatis* alone, *N. gonorrhoeae* alone, or neither agent

	Chlamydia-associated, % (N=*68**)	*Gonococcus-associated, %* (N=*19†*)	*Not gonococcus- or chlamydia-associated, %* (N=*64*)
Temperature >38°C	27	74	30
Duration pelvic pain >3 days	85	68	62
ESR >30	65	32	28
Laparoscopic appearance of tubes, moderately severe or severe	78	74	47

* C. trachomatis *isolated from cervix, urethra, rectum, or tubes; or serologic evidence of acute chlamydial infection.*
† N. gonorrhoeae *isolated from cervix, urethra, or tubes; no cultural or serologic evidence of* C. trachomatis *infection.*

bowel, and omentum, but is not sufficiently sensitive to detect salpingitis.

In the hands of an experienced physician, laparoscopy has a low morbidity and is regarded as the most specific method for diagnosis of acute salpingitis. Although it may be normal if inflammation is limited to the endosalpinx or endometrium, patients with suspected PID who have normal laparoscopy have a better prognosis, with few if any sequelae, when compared with patients who have abnormal laparoscopic findings. The primary and uncontested value of laparoscopy in women with lower abdominal pain is exclusion of other surgical problems. Table 144-3 clearly shows that the most common and serious problems that may be confused with salpingitis are usually unilateral. Thus, unilateral pain or pelvic mass, though not incompatible with PID, is a strong indication for laparoscopy unless the clinical picture warrants laparotomy instead. Atypical clinical findings such as the absence of lower genital tract infection, a missed menstrual period, or failure to respond to appropriate therapy are other frequent indications for laparoscopy.

Laparoscopic criteria used for the diagnosis of salpingitis include (1) erythema of the fallopian tube; (2) edema of the fallopian tube; and (3) seropurulent exudate from the fimbriated end or on the serosal surface of a fallopian tube. Laparoscopic findings are further scored as mild, where the above manifestations are mild and the tubes are freely movable and patent; moderate, when the above manifestations are more marked, tubes are not freely movable, and patency is uncertain; and severe, when findings consist of an inflammatory mass.

The etiologic diagnosis of PID can be further studied by cultures or specimens obtained by endocervical swab, endometrial aspiration, or culdocentesis, or by laparoscopy or laparotomy. Endocervical swab specimens should be examined by Gram stain for gram-negative diplococci and by culture for *N. gonorrhoeae.* The sensitivity of Gram stain is about 60 percent and specificity >95 percent, compared with culture. The endocervical swab specimen should also be cultured for *C. trachomatis* whenever possible. Isolation of either *N. gonorrhoeae* or *C. trachomatis* from the cervix does not prove that either agent is also present in the upper genital tract. There is no evidence that isolation of anaerobes or facultative anaerobes from the cervix or vagina correlates with the presence of these organisms in the upper genital tract in acute PID, but this has not been well studied. The value of culture of culdocentesis specimens is disputed because of the risk of contamination of the specimen with vaginal flora. Endometrial aspiration is a relatively easy procedure and is being studied as an alternative to laparoscopy for obtaining upper genital tract cultures from women with PID, but the specimens obtained by this procedure are subject to contamination by cervical flora. When laparoscopy is performed, material can be obtained directly from the cul-de-sac or the fimbriated opening of the tube, or by tubal aspiration if pyosalpinx is present. Such specimens should be cultured for anaerobic and facultative pathogens, as well as for *N. gonorrhoeae* and *C. trachomatis.*

TABLE 144-3
Laparoscopic findings in patients with false-positive or false-negative clinical diagnoses of acute PID

False-positive clinical diagnosis — *Laparoscopic diagnosis*	*Percent*	*False clinical diagnosis, unexpected PID at laparoscopy* — *Clinical diagnosis*	*Percent*
Acute appendicitis	24	Ovarian tumor	20
Endometriosis	16	Acute appendicitis	18
Corpus luteum bleeding	12	Ectopic pregnancy	16
Ectopic pregnancy	11	Chronic salpingitis	6
Pelvic adhesions only	7	Acute peritonitis	6
Benign ovarian tumor	7	Endometriosis	5
Chronic salpingitis	6	Uterine myoma	5
Miscellaneous	15	Atypical pelvic pain	6
		Miscellaneous	6

TREATMENT Hospitalization should be considered in all women with PID. Hospitalization is strongly recommended when (1) the diagnosis is uncertain, (2) surgical emergencies such as appendicitis and ectopic pregnancy must be excluded, (3) a pelvic abscess is suspected, (4) severe illness precludes outpatient management, (5) the patient is pregnant, (6) the patient is assessed as unable to follow or tolerate an outpatient regimen, (7) the patient has failed to respond to outpatient therapy, or (8) clinical follow-up after 48 to 72 h of instituting antibiotic treatment cannot be arranged. The treatment of choice is not established. No single agent is active against the entire spectrum of pathogens (Table 144-4). Several antimicrobial combinations do provide a broad spectrum of activity against the major pathogens in vitro, but many have not been adequately evaluated for clinical efficacy in PID.

Examples of combination regimens with broad activity against major pathogens in PID

1 Doxycycline 100 mg, twice a day, IV, plus cefoxitin 2.0 g, 4 times a day, IV. These drugs should be continued IV for at least 4 days and at least 48 h after the patient defervesces. Doxycycline should be continued in a dose of 100 mg by mouth, twice a day, after discharge from the hospital to complete 10 to 14 days of therapy. This regimen provides excellent coverage for *N. gonorrhoeae,* including penicillinase-producing *N. gonorrhoeae* (PPNG), and *C. trachomatis.* It may not provide optimal treatment for anaerobes, pelvic abscess, or IUD-associated PID.

2 Clindamycin 600 mg, 4 times a day, IV, plus gentamicin or tobramycin 2.0 mg/kg, IV, followed by 1.5 mg/kg, 3 times a day, IV, in patients with normal renal function. These drugs should be continued for at least 4 days and at least 48 h after the patient defervesces. Clindamycin should be continued in a dose of 450 mg, by mouth, 4 times a day, after discharge from the hospital to complete 10 to 14 days of therapy. This regimen provides optimal activity against anaerobes and facultative gram-negative rods but may not provide the best activity against *C. trachomatis* and *N. gonorrhoeae.*

3 Doxycycline 100 mg, twice a day, IV, plus metronidazole, 1.0 g, twice a day, IV. These drugs should be continued IV for at least 4 days and at least 48 h after the patient defervesces. Then both drugs should be continued in the same dosage orally to complete 10 to 14 days of therapy. This regimen provides excellent coverage for anaerobes and *C. trachomatis.* Both drugs can be continued for oral therapy. Activity against some strains of *N. gonorrhoeae,* including PPNG, and against some facultative gram-negative rods, is not optimal.

Patients who are not hospitalized should also receive a combined regimen with broad activity, such as cefoxitin 2.0 g, IM, followed by doxycycline 100 mg, by mouth, twice a day for 10 to 14 days. Although a single loading dose of amoxicillin, ampicillin, or procaine penicillin with probenecid, as recommended for uncomplicated gonorrhea (see Chap. 150), could be used in place of cefoxitin, these regimens are not effective against PPNG and have less activity against anaerobes and facultative gram-negative rods. Tetracycline HCl could also be used in a dose of 500 mg, 4 times a day, in place of doxycycline, but it is less active against certain anaerobes, and requires more frequent dosing; both represent major drawbacks in the treatment of PID.

Management of sexual partners All persons who are sexual partners of patients with PID should be examined for STD and promptly treated with a regimen effective against uncomplicated gonococcal and chlamydial infection.

Follow-up All patients who are treated as outpatients should be clinically reevaluated in 48 to 72 h. Those not responding favorably should be hospitalized. A culture to test whether cure has been achieved should be performed as needed.

Removal of an intrauterine device Although the exact effect of IUD removal on the response of acute salpingitis to antimicrobial therapy and on the risk of recurrent salpingitis is unknown, removal of the IUD is recommended soon after antimicrobial therapy has been initiated. When an IUD is removed, contraceptive counseling is necessary.

Surgery Surgery is necessary only rarely for treatment of salpingitis, except in the face of life-threatening infection such as rupture or threatened rupture of a tuboovarian abscess, or for drainage of an abscess. Ultrasonography is useful for diagnosing and following pelvic abscesses. When surgery is performed, conservative procedures are usually sufficient. Pelvic abscesses can often be drained by posterior colpotomy, and peritoneal lavage can be used if there is generalized peritonitis.

PROGNOSIS Of women treated for PID on an ambulatory basis with ampicillin alone or tetracycline alone, in a recent cooperative trial in the United States, approximately 15 percent treated with either drug failed to improve clinically and required retreatment. Among 900 women who underwent long-term follow-up for a mean period of 8 years after successful treatment of the acute episode with various regimens in Sweden, late sequelae included infertility due to bilateral tubal occlusion, ectopic pregnancy due to tubal scarring without occlusion, chronic pelvic pain, and recurrent salpingitis. Chronic pain lasting longer than 6 months was seen in 18 percent of patients and infertility due to tubal occlusion in 17 percent; 4 percent of pregnancies that did occur were ectopic, representing approximately a sixfold increase over the expected rate of ectopic pregnancies.

The rate of infertility after salpingitis was found to be related to age of the patient, etiology of salpingitis, duration of symptoms when treatment was started, severity of salpingitis by laparoscopy at the time of diagnosis, and number of episodes of salpingitis. The rate of infertility due to tubal occlusion among women exposed to a chance of pregnancy was 14 percent for women 15 to 24 years of age and 26 percent for women 25 to 34 years of age; the risk for women of all ages combined was 11 percent after one episode of salpingitis, 23 percent after two episodes, and 54 percent after three or more episodes. The risk was 6 percent after one episode of *N. gonorrhoeae*-associated salpingitis and 21 percent after one episode of nongonococcal salpingitis.

Although the rate of infertility after *C. trachomatis*-associated salpingitis has not been determined in a similar prospective study, a preliminary analysis of such cases suggests about a 10 percent rate of tubal occlusion after therapy. A striking relationship has also been shown in several countries between infertility due to tubal occlusion and the prevalence and titer of antibody to *C. trachomatis.*

Recurrent salpingitis has been seen in approximately 15 to 25 percent of women treated for salpingitis in various studies.

PREVENTION Prevention of PID depends first on the effective use of current methods for control of gonococcal and chlamydial infection. These methods include providing ready access to modern methods of diagnosis and effective treatment, and treatment of sex partners to control further spread. The decline in popularity of the intrauterine device, particularly in nulliparous women, has undoubtedly helped to reduce the incidence of PID. It is possible, but not proven, that increased use of oral contraceptives might reduce the risk of PID, particularly the risk of recurrent PID among women who have already experienced one episode of PID.

The complications of salpingitis can be minimized by early diagnosis and prompt treatment. It seems logical, but is unproven, that broad-spectrum therapy effective against all of the common causes of PID would offer the best outcome. Similarly, hospitalization to ensure rest and adequate compliance may improve the rather dismal long-term prognosis for tubal function. One placebo-controlled study showed that concurrent anti-inflammatory therapy with prednisolone hastened the reduction of acute inflammatory changes but did not improve the end results as measured by fertility, hysterosalpingographic findings, or chronic pain. However, since the dose of prednisolone used was relatively low, and since the antibiotics used concurrently would not be very effective against chlamydial or anaerobic infection, the potential value of anti-inflammatory therapy has not been adequately evaluated.

REFERENCES

ESCHENBACH DA, HOLMES KK: Acute pelvic inflammatory disease: Current concepts of pathogenesis, etiology and management. Clin Obstet Gynecol 18:35, 1975

———: Pelvic inflammatory disease, in *Update III: Harrison's Principles of Internal Medicine* KJ Isselbacher et al (eds). New York, McGraw-Hill, 1982, pp 67–81

TABLE 144-4
Approximate activity of the antimicrobial agents most commonly used to treat PID against the pathogens most commonly implicated in PID

			Vaginal anaerobes			
	N. gonorrhoeae	*C. trachomatis*	*GPC**	*GNR†*	*Facultative GNR*	*M. hominis*
Ampicillin/penicillin G	4+	1+	4+	2+	2+	0
Tetracycline HCl	3+	4+	4+	2+	2+	4+
Doxycycline	3+	4+	4+	3+	2+	4+
Cefoxitin	4+	0	4+	3+	4+	0
Gentamicin/tobramycin	4+	0	1+	0	4+	3+?
Clindamycin	0	2+	4+	4+	0	3+?
Metronidazole	0	0	4+	4+	0	?

* *GPC = Gram-positive cocci (peptococci, peptostreptococci).*
† *GNR = Gram-negative rods (anaerobic GNR include* Bacteroides; *facultative GNR include Enterobacteriaceae,* H. influenzae*).*
NOTE: *No single antimicrobial agent offers optimal activity against all of these pathogens, but certain combinations (e.g., cefoxitin plus doxycycline, gentamicin plus clindamycin, doxycycline plus metronidazole) have complimentary activity against these pathogens.*

FALK V et al: Genital tuberculosis in women. Am J Obstet Gynecol 138:974, 1980

GJONASS H et al: Pelvic inflammatory disease: Etiologic studies with emphasis on chlamydial infection. Obstet Gynecol 59:550, 1982

HENRY-SUCHET J et al: *Chlamydia trachomatis* associated with chronic inflammation in abdominal specimens from women selected for tuboplasty. Am J Obstet Gynecol 138:1022, 1980

HOLMES KK et al: Salpingitis: Overview of etiology and epidemiology. Am J Obstet Gynecol 138:893, 1980

MÅRDH PA: *Chlamydia trachomatis* infection in patients with acute salpingitis. N Engl J Med 296:1377, 1977

———: An overview of infectious agents of salpingitis, their biology and recent advances in methods of detection. Am J Obstet Gynecol 138:933, 1980

MØLLER BR et al: Pelvic infection after elective abortion associated with *Chlamydia trachomatis*. Obstet Gynecol 59:210, 1982

OSSER S, PERSSON K: Epidemiologic and serodiagnostic aspects of chlamydial salpingitis. Obstet Gynecol 59:206, 1982

ST JOHN RK, BROWN ST (eds): International symposium on pelvic inflammatory disease. Am J Obstet Gynecol 138:845, 1980

WESTRÖM L: Incidence, prevalence and trends of acute pelvic inflammatory disease and its consequences in industrialized countries. Am J Obstet Gynecol 138:880, 1980

WØLNER-HANSSEN P et al: Endometrial infection in women with chlamydial salpingitis. Sex Transm Dis 9:84, 1982

145
PREVENTION OF INFECTION: IMMUNIZATION AND ANTIMICROBIAL PROPHYLAXIS

LAWRENCE COREY
ROBERT G. PETERSDORF

There are three major ways to prevent infections: (1) by reducing exposure, (2) by acquiring or inducing immunity, and (3) by using antimicrobial agents to prevent colonization and infection. Exposure can be reduced by diminishing the prevalence of the infecting agent, by community-wide vaccination programs, and by isolating infected patients in cohorts. On an individual basis, however, the most reliable way to prevent infectious disease is to provide effective immunization or chemoprophylaxis against the causative agent. This chapter summarizes current immunization practices and principles of antimicrobial prophylaxis. Additional details are provided in the chapters dealing with individual diseases.

IMMUNIZATION

Immunity may be defined as the ability of the individual to resist or overcome infection; it may be innate or acquired. For many infectious diseases, immunity is acquired during recovery from an infection or induced by the administration of vaccines prepared from inactivated or live microorganisms of modified disease-producing potential, or from specific antigen(s) derived from these organisms. The purpose of immunization, therefore, is to provoke a specific immunologic response to a selected microbial agent or its antigens with the expectation that this will result in humoral, and/or secretory, and/or cell-mediated immunity. While this protection may diminish over time, future exposures to the same stimulus will result in a rapid return of the immune response because of heightened reactivity of antibody-forming, phagocytic, and other cells that mediate immune mechanisms (see Chap. 63).

Certain infectious diseases present special situations that impede the development of vaccines. For example, *Salmonella* organisms and rhinoviruses consist of several hundred antigenically unique strains, making production of a vaccine unfeasible. Secondly, the portal of entry of an organism and the role of local immunity are important in determining whether a vaccine given parenterally will offer protection from either infection or disease. Finally, even when effective immunizing agents are available, difficulties in delivering them to the susceptible population may preclude their use.

GENERAL PRINCIPLES OF IMMUNIZATION Infections can be prevented or controlled by active and/or passive immunization. Active immunization with live attenuated vaccines generally results in subclinical or mild clinical illness which duplicates, to a limited extent, the disease that is marked for prevention; generally, it provides both local and durable humoral immunity. "Killed" or inactivated vaccines, such as influenza, rabies, typhoid, and cholera vaccines, maintain immunogenicity, without infectivity, but have several disadvantages including the large amount of antigen that must be administered by the parenteral route and the greater time period between administration of the antigen and the appearance of a protective effect. Table 145-1 summarizes active immunizing agents.

The use of any biological substance requires balancing its benefits and risks, and each vaccine must be evaluated accordingly. While some immunizations, such as diphtheria, tetanus, and poliomyelitis, are recommended for all individuals, others should be used only in those who have an increased risk of either acquiring the disease or developing complications. Pneumococcal polysaccharide vaccine, influenza vaccine, hepatitis B vaccine, bacillus Calmette-Guérin (BCG) vaccine, and meningococcal vaccine are some examples.

Inactivated vaccines can be administered simultaneously at separate sites, although vaccines known to be associated with severe side effects should generally be given on separate occasions. Some vaccines contain trace amounts of preservatives or antibiotics to which patients may be sensitive, and, although reactions to them are unusual, reviewing the manufacturers' package insert prior to use of these agents may be helpful. Live virus vaccines prepared by growing viruses in cell culture are usually devoid of potential allergic substances. Many live virus vaccinations can be given simultaneously; measles, mumps, and rubella are some examples. However, when more than one dose of live viral vaccine is required, repeated administration should be separated by at least 1 month.

Contraindications to vaccination Virus replication following administration of live attenuated virus vaccines can be accentuated in immune-deficiency diseases and in patients whose immune responses have been suppressed as in leukemia, lymphoma, or generalized malignancy or following therapy with corticosteroids, alkylating drugs, antimetabolites, and radiation. Such patients should not be given live attenuated virus vaccines. Vaccination of persons with severe febrile disease should be deferred to avoid superimposing the adverse effects of the vaccine on the underlying illness. Occasionally, viral interference, as might occur with concurrent enterovirus infection in the gut, may affect the efficacy of vaccines adversely. Because of a theoretical risk to the developing fetus, live attenuated virus vaccines generally should not be given to pregnant women. For some vaccines, particularly live attenuated rubella vaccine, pregnancy is an absolute contraindication to vaccination. Passively acquired antibody can interfere with the response to live attenuated virus vaccines; therefore, adminis-

TABLE 145-1
Active immunization in adults

	Type of vaccine	*Administration and frequency**	*Comments*
ALL ADULTS			
Tetanus and diphtheria	Adsorbed toxoid	IM at least every 10 years	Usually administered together as Td vaccine
Poliomyelitis	Live attenuated	Oral polio vaccine (OPV)	Preferred for routine use and during epidemics
	Formalin-inactivated	Inactivated polio vaccine (IPV)	Selective use in unimmunized adults
WOMEN OF CHILD-BEARING AGE			
Rubella vaccine	Live attenuated	SC once	Only to women who are antibody (HI) negative and if pregnancy can be prevented for 3 months post-vaccination
POSTPUBERTAL MALES			
Mumps	Live attenuated	SC once	Prevention of orchitis in susceptible seronegative males
PERSONS AT HIGH RISK OF ACQUIRING DISEASE OR DEVELOPING COMPLICATIONS OF DISEASE			
Influenza vaccine	Inactivated	SC yearly	Directed at reducing morbidity and mortality in those at risk of complications of influenza, e.g., chronic heart and lung disease and those over 65 years
Pneumococcal polysaccharide vaccine	Purified tetradecavalent polysaccharide vaccine	SC once	Same population as influenza vaccine, functional or surgical asplenia, agammaglobulinemia, cirrhosis, multiple myeloma, and nephrotic syndrome
Hepatitis B vaccine	Inactivated subunit vaccine	3 doses IM at 0, 1, and 3 months	High-risk groups for acquisition of hepatitis B, including household contacts of hepatitis B patients, patients requiring a large volume of clotting factors, homosexual men, and selected medical and dental personnel
POPULATIONS EXPOSED TO LOCALIZED OUTBREAKS			
Meningococcal vaccine A, C, AC	Purified capsular polysaccharide	SC once	Control of localized epidemics and adjunct to chemoprophylaxis in household contacts
Measles vaccine	Live attenuated	SC once	Control of outbreaks usually among adolescents or young adults
BCG vaccine	Live attenuated	SC or intradermally, once	Used in groups with excessive risk of new infection with tuberculosis or individuals persistently exposed to sputum-positive tuberculosis
Adenovirus vaccine	Live attenuated bivalent (types 4 and 7)	PO once	Used only for military recruits
Typhoid vaccine	Inactivated bacilli	SC in two doses	Household contact of documented *Salmonella typhi* carrier
Rubella vaccine	Live attenuated	SC once	Control of outbreaks among adolescents and young adults (must screen pubertal females with HI test prior to vaccination)
TRAVELERS TO FOREIGN COUNTRIES			
Smallpox	Live vaccinia virus	Intradermally, every 3–5 years	Not recommended except for travel to countries requiring vaccination certificates
Yellow fever	Live attenuated	SC once per 10 years	Administered at yellow fever vaccination centers
Cholera	Phenol-inactivated suspension of *Vibrio cholerae*	SC approximately every 6 months	Only 50% effective and not effective in decreasing transmission of disease
Typhoid	Inactivated bacilli	SC in half doses 4 weeks apart	70–90% efficacy in "normal" exposure
Typhus	Formaldehyde-inactivated *Rickettsia prowazekii*	SC in two doses 4 weeks apart	Only to persons in close contact to those where disease is indigenous
Plague	Formaldehyde-inactivated *Yersinia pestis*	SC in three injections of 0.5 ml at least 1 week apart, booster approximately every 2 years	Agricultural workers who reside in plague-endemic areas
Poliomyelitis	Oral or inactivated polio vaccine	See text	Most adults already immune
Hepatitis A	Immune serum globulin	IM every 3 months	See "Passive Immunization" in this chapter

* *PO, orally; SC, subcutaneously; IM, intramuscularly.*

tration of live vaccine should be postponed until approximately 3 months after passive immunization.

IMMUNIZATION IN ADULTS **Diphtheria** Although the incidence of diphtheria in the United States has declined, localized outbreaks continue to appear. Only 50 to 60 percent of poor urban dwellers in the United States are adequately protected against this infection. The myocardial and peripheral nervous system involvement associated with *Corynebacterium diphtheriae* is due to elaboration of an exotoxin (see Chap. 165). Diphtheria toxoid is a cell-free preparation of diphtheria toxin treated with formaldehyde. The quantity of toxoid varies among products, and the concentration of diphtheria toxoid in adult preparations is lower than in the pediatric formulation. Adverse reactions are thought to be related to dose and age. Extensive worldwide experience has shown that diphtheria toxoid has been associated with a steady reduction in the incidence of diphtheria. Diphtheria immunization reduces both the risk of developing diptheria and the severity of clinical illness. Diphtheria toxoid provides protection against only the toxin and not the somatic components of *C. diphtheriae,* and local infection, either in the respiratory tract or skin, may occur in immune individuals. Nontoxigenic strains also may cause mild, focal infections.

All children less than 7 years of age should receive routine immunization against diphtheria in the form of absorbed diphtheria and tetanus toxoids and pertussis vaccine (DPT). Absorbed toxoids are produced by the addition of aluminum compounds to the formaldehyde-inactivated toxoid and are more antigenic than the fluid (plain) preparation. Children should receive a primary series of three doses of DPT vaccine before they are a year old, a booster at 18 months, and another when they enter school. A preparation without pertussis vaccine is available for primary immunization of children who are unable to tolerate the pertussis vaccine (DT). To avoid the febrile reactions that may accompany repeated exposure to diphtheria toxoid among patients with prior exposure to diphtheria antigens, and because pertussis is less common and less severe in older children and adults, the preparation recommended for use in adults is a combination of tetanus and diphtheria toxoid in which the diphtheria toxoid is reduced to a maximum of two flocculating units per dose. This vaccine (Td) is recommended for primary immunization of adults and children older than 6 years of age and is also routinely used for booster immunization, both for the prevention of tetanus at the time of injury and for diphtheria prophylaxis. For primary immunization in adults, three intramuscular doses of Td should be given, the second dose 1 to 2 months after the first, and the third 6 to 12 months later. Thereafter, boosters at 10-year intervals should be given.

Tetanus (see Chap. 170) Spores of *Clostridium tetani* are ubiquitous. The incidence of tetanus has decreased dramatically with the routine use of tetanus toxoid, a formaldehyde-detoxified bacteria-free filtrate of *Clostridium tetani.* Tetanus occurs almost exclusively in persons who are unimmunized or inadequately immunized. Two doses of the absorbed toxoid or three doses of fluid toxoid usually result in a protective level of antibody, 0.01 unit per milliliter tetanus antitoxin. Tetanus toxoid may be used singly or in combination with diphtheria toxoid (DT or Td), or with both diphtheria toxoid and pertussis vaccine (DPT). When used singly, primary immunization with the fluid toxoid is given in three doses at least 1 month apart with a booster 8 to 12 months later. The absorbed form should be given in two doses, 1 month apart. Primary immunization with tetanus toxoid is highly recommended for all children and adults. Clinical tetanus does not necessarily provide immunity against subsequent tetanus. Boosters after wound infection are recommended at 5-year intervals, routine boosters at 10-year intervals.

Pertussis Endemic pertussis infection is still prevalent throughout the world. Complications and mortality of infection are greatest in children, especially those less than 6 months of age. While recent controversy about the use of pertussis vaccine has occurred, routine use of the vaccine does reduce the morbidity and mortality associated with pertussis infection in the neonate. Pertussis infection in adults and older children is usually mild, while systemic and local side effects from vaccination are increased in older children and adults. Pertussis vaccination is routinely recommended for children 1 year of age. Vaccination is *not* recommended for use in adults or children over 6 years of age. In exceptional cases such as persons with chronic pulmonary disease exposed to children with pertussis, or health care personnel exposed during outbreaks of pertussis, a booster dose of adsorbed pertussis vaccine (0.20 to 0.25 ml) may be useful.

Poliomyelitis (see Chap. 205) While routine polio vaccination of adults residing in the United States is generally not necessary because most are immune and the risk of exposure is small, susceptible adults at increased risk by virtue of travel or exposure to wild or vaccine polio virus should receive primary immunization with either inactivated or wild attenuated polio vaccines. Both a live attenuated oral polio vaccine (OPV) and an inactivated polio vaccine (IPV) are licensed in the United States. OPV has been favored over IPV because it is easier to administer, orally versus injection, confers more resistance in the alimentary tract to reinfection, and interferes with simultaneous infection by wild polioviruses. These properties are of special value during epidemics of poliomyelitis. Vaccination with OPV results in shedding of virus contained in the vaccine, and spread of virus to unvaccinated persons occurs. Rarely, recipients of oral vaccine or people in contact with them have contracted paralytic polio. Between 1969 and 1979, 186 cases of paralytic poliomyelitis were reported in the United States, only 1 percent of whom had had a complete series of polio vaccine; 73 cases (39 percent); were classified as vaccine-associated, 32 percent in recipients of OPV, 53 percent in households, and 15 percent in nonhousehold contacts of vaccinees. The risk of vaccine-associated polio has been estimated to be one case per recipient for every 11.5 million persons vaccinated with OPV, one case in a household contact for every 3.9 million persons vaccinated, and one case in a community contact for every 22.9 million persons vaccinated. The relative risk of paralytic disease is slightly higher in susceptible adults than in children. Such a risk seems acceptable. On the other hand, no serious complications have been reported with IPV. While oral trivalent polio vaccine is the principal vaccine in the United States, use of inactivated polio vaccine may be beneficial in selective circumstances such as primary immunization of susceptible adults.

For infants and children, the primary series of vaccination with OPV consists of three doses. The first two should be given not less than 6 and preferably 8 weeks apart. The third dose should follow 8 to 12 months after the second dose.

A booster dose of trivalent OPV should be given when the child enters kindergarten or first grade. Additional preadolescent immunization (at age 11 to 12) has been recommended to provide additional protection during adulthood. The rationale for this recommendation is twofold: (1) vaccine-associated paralytic disease is rare under age 20; and (2) most vaccine-associated cases have occured in young adults following contact with vaccinated infants.

Inactivated polio vaccine should be considered for persons with heightened susceptibility to infection, including immunodeficient children and their siblings, and immunosuppressed persons and adults undergoing initial vaccination when traveling to areas where the incidence of polio is high or whose household contacts are undergoing OPV vaccination. Live attenuated oral polio vaccine is acceptable for adults who have been vaccinated previously or whose circumstances do not allow adequate time for administration of IVP and who are not in a category in which oral vaccine is contraindicated. Primary immunization with IPV consists of four doses: three at 1- to 2-month intervals and a booster 6 to 12 months after the third. Booster doses at 2- to 3-year intervals either with IPV or with one dose of OPV after primary immunization with IPV will sustain long-lasting immunity.

IMMUNIZATION IN WOMEN OF CHILDBEARING AGE Rubella (see Chap. 201) The purpose of rubella vaccination is to prevent rubella embryopathy in the fetus. The direct approach to this goal would be to immunize all women before they become pregnant. However, the difficulty is being sure that a woman is not pregnant at the time of vaccination, and the increased risk of joint symptoms associated with vaccination in women has rendered this approach impractical. Because children are a major source of spread of rubella to pregnant females, rubella vaccination has been routinely recommended for all children older than 12 months. When given in combination with measles antigen, rubella vaccine should be administered when a child is about 15 months of age to achieve the maximum rate of measles seroconversion.

Since 1969 when rubella vaccine was first licensed, the incidence of rubella has declined steadily, and the lack of a rubella epidemic during the early 1970s suggests that the vaccine is effective in interrupting the 7- to 9-year epidemiologic cycle that has characterized nationwide rubella outbreaks. However, the congenital rubella syndrome still occurs in the United States, and increased emphasis should be placed on vaccinating unimmunized prepubertal girls and susceptible adolescent and adult women who are not pregnant and who agree to prevent pregnancy for 3 months after receiving vaccine. Routine premarital rubella antibody determinations would help identify susceptible females before their first pregnancy. Testing for rubella antibody during the perinatal or antepartum period and vaccination of susceptible women in the immediate postpartum period are warranted. Rubella immunization of medical personnel having frequent contact with pregnant women is also recommended.

Rubella vaccine is prepared in cell cultures and is administered by subcutaneous injection. A single dose induces antibodies in approximately 95 percent of susceptible persons.

Rubella vaccine virus has been demonstrated to cross the placenta and infect the fetus. Infants born to more than 60 susceptible women, who inadvertently received rubella vaccine during early pregnancy and continued their pregnancies to term, did not have any recognizable malformations attributable to rubella. However, fetal infection with vaccine-like rubella virus may produce pathological changes in developing organs. While the risk of teratogenicity is felt to be much lower from the vaccine virus than from the wild virus, if a pregnant woman is inadvertently vaccinated or if she becomes pregnant within 3 months of vaccination, she should be advised of the low (3 percent) but theoretical risk to the fetus.

VACCINATION OF SUSCEPTIBLE POSTPUBERTAL MALES Mumps (see Chap. 206) Mumps is primarily a disease of school-aged children; only about 15 percent of the cases occur in adolescents and adults. Mumps infections are often subclinical and are generally self-limited. Meningoencephalitis associated with mumps is usually uncomplicated and benign, although nerve deafness may occasionally result. Orchitis, usually unilateral, may occur in postpubertal males. While this has been documented to occur as frequently as 20 percent of the time in epidemic mumps, the incidence of subsequent sterility is low. Both a live attenuated mumps vaccine (Jeryl-Lynn strain) grown in chick embryo cell cultures and a killed vaccine have been developed, but only live mumps vaccine has clearly demonstrated safety and efficacy. Mumps vaccination is recommended for all children older than 1 year and especially in children approaching puberty, adolescents, and adults, particularly males, who have not had mumps or who have no serologic evidence of mumps immunity. Skin testing is not a reliable indication of past infection. Persons with prior mumps or who have received vaccine are not at risk from live mumps vaccine. A single dose is given subcutaneously; continuing protection against infection and protective antibodies have both been shown to persist for at least 12 years after vaccination. Parotitis after vaccination has been reported rarely. Patients with severe febrile illness or hypersensitivity to egg products, with malignancy who are receiving immunosuppressive therapy, or who are pregnant should not be vaccinated. Mumps vaccine virus has been shown to infect the placenta, but virus has not been isolated from fetal tissue.

VACCINATION OF PERSONS WITH CHRONIC HEART, PULMONARY, AND METABOLIC DISEASE Influenza (see Chap. 198) Influenza occurs every year in the United States but with variation in incidence and geographic distribution. Epidemics occur periodically; more are caused by influenza A viruses than by influenza B. More importantly, influenza A epidemics are notable for causing mortality in excess of what is usually expected. In the 1957 to 1958 Asian influenza epidemic, nearly 70,000 excess deaths were reported in the United States during the 12-week epidemic period. Most nationwide influenza epidemics have resulted in 10,000 to 20,000 excess deaths. Repeated observations have indicated that during influenza epidemics deaths occur primarily among children and chronically ill adults, especially those over age 65. These high-risk persons should be vaccinated annually. Vaccination of the entire population has not been considered a reasonable public health policy because protection is of limited duration owing both to the antigenic drift of the virus, as well as the short-lived antibody response to the inactivated vaccine, and the low incidence of serious infections in healthy persons.

Influenza vaccines are inactivated products of the prevalent circulating types of influenza virus. The vaccine usually contains influenza A and influenza B prototype antigens. Two types of vaccines are available, whole virus vaccines and "split-product" or subunit vaccines. Generally, whole virus vaccines are more immunogenic but have a slightly higher reaction rate than split-product vaccines. Studies with both preparations indicate a 60 to 95 percent protection rate, depending upon the population group studied and the relationship between the "epidemic" strain and the vaccine strain. In adults either form of vaccine can be used, but because of the high frequency of febrile reactions, children under 12 should receive two doses of split-product vaccine at approximately 3- to 6-week intervals. Vaccine is generally administered during the fall of the year and is given subcutaneously. While intradermal vaccination may elicit a good humoral antibody response, the clinical efficacy of this route of administration has not been well documented. Because even the zonally centrifuged inactivated influenza vaccines contain trace amounts of egg protein, patients who are allergic to egg or egg protein should not receive this vaccine. Severe adverse reactions to influenza vaccine are uncommon. Among recipients of A/New Jersey/76 swine influenza vaccine, an excess risk of Landry-Guillain-Barré syndrome occurs (10 cases for every million vaccinated), an incidence five to six times higher than in unvaccinated persons. Recent (nonswine) influenza vaccines have not been associated with an increased risk of the Landry-Guillain-Barré syndrome.

While influenza vaccine is the preferred form of prophylaxis, because of its low cost, greater efficacy, and slight toxicity, amantadine hydrochloride has been effective in preventing influenza infection especially during interepidemic intervals. Patients at risk of developing the complications of influenza who failed to receive their annual influenza vaccination should be placed on 100 mg amantadine hydrochloride twice daily during the period in which influenza A virus is identified in the community or until adequate protection after receipt of influenza vaccine has occurred.

Pneumococcal vaccine (see Chap. 146) Despite antibiotic therapy, the morbidity and mortality of pneumococcal disease remains a problem. Bacteremic pneumococcal disease appears to be more common in persons with sickle cell anemia, anatomic or functional asplenia, agammaglobulinemia, multiple myeloma, nephrotic syndrome, cirrhosis, alcoholism, diabetes mellitus, and chronic cardiorespiratory disease; in these situations vaccination is generally indicated. Other situations in which pneumococcal vaccine may be of benefit include closed populations in which systemic pneumococcal disease has been identified as an epidemic or endemic problem, or where an antibiotic-resistant strain of pneumococcus has emerged.

The tetradecavalent polysaccharide vaccine licensed for use in the United States is composed of purified capsular material extracted separately from the 14 types of pneumococcal organisms (Danish types 1, 2, 3, 4, 6A, 7F, 8, 9N, 12F, 14, 18C, 19F, 23F, and 25). These 14 types are responsible for about 70 percent of bacteremic pneumococcal disease in the United States. One dose of vaccine contains 50 μg of each polysaccharide. The majority of adults and most children over 2 years of age respond with development of measurable humoral antibody 2 to 3 weeks after vaccination. Immunity exists only against the pneumococcal types contained in the vaccine, although theoretically there may be some degree of cross-protection among immunologically similar types. The duration of protection is unknown, but elevated antibody levels appear to persist for at least 2 years after immunization. Booster doses do not seem to increase the levels of antibody, and children under 2 develop lower levels of antibody than adults. Vaccination reduces the likelihood of acquiring the pneumococcal types in the vaccine in the nasopharynx. There has been no evidence of a relative increase in disease caused by other microbial pathogens among vaccine recipients. In selected populations vaccination has reduced the incidence of pneumococcal pneumonia and bacteremia due to types in the vaccine by 80 percent. These data on effectiveness come primarily from young adults and not the elderly or chronically ill. The vaccine recommendations outlined above are therefore derived from limited data. The vaccine may not be effective in preventing infection in the central nervous system. Local erythema and pain at the injection site occur in approximately half the recipients, but serious adverse reactions are rare, about 5 per 1 million doses given. Local and systemic reactions among adults given second doses within 3 years are of greater intensity and duration; for this reason booster doses are not recommended.

Hepatitis B vaccine Hepatitis B vaccine (HBV) has been approved by the Food and Drug Administration for the prevention of hepatitis B among susceptible persons at high risk of acquiring hepatitis B. The vaccine is a subunit, inactivated preparation containing the hepatitis B surface antigen (HBsAg). It is manufactured by concentration purification and inactivation of the hepatitis B virus from human donors with high titers of hepatitis B surface antigen in their plasma. Hepatitis B vaccine contains 20 μg/ml of HBsAg protein. Three doses of vaccine given 1 and 6 months apart are recommended. Three 10-μg doses are recommended for infants and children from 3 months to 9 years of age. For immunosuppressed patients and patients undergoing hemodialysis three 40-μg doses are recommended. Anti-HBs can be detected in serum of both adults and children in over 96 percent of recipients after a complete vaccination series. The protective efficacy of hepatitis B vaccine for the prevention of clinical hepatitis B has been approximately 95 percent in homosexual men, 90 percent in medical staff of hemodialysis units with endemic hepatitis B, and 75 percent in patients with renal insufficiency undergoing chronic hemodialysis in units with endemic hepatitis B.

Because of the cost and limited availability of vaccine, vaccination strategy is based on selective immunization of high-risk groups. These include susceptible household and sexual contacts of patients with acute and/or chronic hepatitis B, illicit users of injectable drugs, homosexual men, patients requiring blood clotting factor concentrations and large-volume transfusions, and residents and staff of institutions, hemodialysis units, and closed communities where hepatitis B is endemic. Selective vaccination of health care personnel, including laboratory personnel who handle blood and blood products, nursing staff, and medical and dental personnel having frequent contact with groups with hepatitis B or blood products, may also be warranted. These persons should be vaccinated as soon as possible after they begin work in a high-risk environment. Serologic screening of past hepatitis B infection in order to identify susceptibles and those likely to benefit from vaccination is generally useful. The presence of anti-HBs in serum has been associated with protection from clinical hepatitis B. The vaccine appears to have no effect on patients who are carriers of hepatitis B surface antigen and was not associated with either resolution or worsening of chronic hepatitis B infection.

Postexposure immunization with a combination of hepatitis B immune globulin (HBIG) plus hepatitis B vaccine may be useful in some clinical situations, such as immunoprophylaxis of infants born to mothers with acute or chronic hepatitis B and/or sexual contacts of patients with acute or chronic hepatitis B. HBIG does not appear to alter the subsequent development of anti-HBs after hepatitis B vaccine. Clinical studies comparing active and passive immunization with just active immunization are not available.

VACCINES USEFUL IN LOCALIZED OUTBREAKS Meningococcal vaccine (see Chap. 149) Meningococcal disease is endemic in the United States and throughout the world. In recent years meningococcal disease in civilians has occurred primarily in single isolated cases, usually due to groups B or C or, infrequently, in small localized clusters. Secondary cases occur more frequently in household contacts than in the general population, and appropriate antibiotic prophylaxis has been the principal method of reducing the risk for immediate contacts. Vaccines have been used to curtail outbreaks of groups A and C meningococcal disease, and when epidemic meningococcal disease due to groups A or C occurs, the population at risk should be identified and vaccinated. Vaccination also should be considered as an adjunct to antibiotic prophylaxis for household contacts of cases of meningococcal disease. The reason for this is that one-half of the secondary cases in families occurs more than 5 days after the primary case; this is long enough to yield potential benefits from vaccination if antibiotic chemoprophylaxis should not be successful.

Three meningococcal polysaccharide vaccines, monovalent A, monovalent C, and bivalent AC vaccine, are licensed for selective use in the United States. These vaccines are chemically defined antigens consisting of purified capsular polysaccharides and induce specific immunity to the serologic groups. The vaccine is administered parenterally as a single dose. Adverse reactions consist principally of localized erythema lasting 1 to 2 days. The vaccine appears effective in all age groups beyond the first year of life, and there is suggestive evidence of efficacy in children as young as 3 months of age.

Measles (see Chap. 200) Measles vaccine is an attenuated live virus (Schwarz) vaccine derived from passage of the Edmonston strain of measles virus grown in culture of chick embryo cells. This attenuated vaccine is the preferable mode of vaccination over the older Edmonston strain vaccine which was administered with human immune serum globulin.

Measles vaccination is highly effective. Since the introduction of measles vaccine in the late 1960s, a marked reduction in the incidence of measles has ensued. In the late 1970s, localized outbreaks among 10- to 19-year olds were noted, often occurring in children who were vaccinated prior to age 12 months or who received measles vaccine concomitantly with immune serum globulin (ISG). Both of these circumstances may not provide adequate immunity against infection. In 1978, a program to eliminate indigenous measles in the United States was initiated. The program is directed at increasing the incidence of routine measles vaccination for all children, increased emphasis on identifying and vaccinating susceptible adolescents and young adults, efforts to broaden school vaccination requirements, and improved reporting and efficacy of outbreak control measures.

Measles vaccination has been recommended for all children older than 12 months. During measles outbreaks, it is recommended that all susceptible children, as well as adolescents and adults at risk, be immunized. Individuals can be defined as susceptible to measles when they lack a certificate of adequate immunization with live measles vaccine at age of at least 12 months or who lack adequate evidence of having had measles. Persons who should not be considered adequately protected and who should be revaccinated include (1) children vaccinated with live vaccine before they were 12 months old (these children should be revaccinated at 15 months of age or older); (2) children who received live vaccine with immune serum globulin, regardless of their age at vaccination; and (3) persons previously vaccinated with killed measles virus vaccine. Repeat vaccination with live measles vaccine poses no increased risk for individuals who have previously had natural measles or who have been vaccinated.

Up to 15 percent of vaccinated children will have fever between the fifth and twelfth days after vaccination and lasting up to 5 days. Local induration and edema at the injection site may occur in persons who previously received killed measles vaccine.

BCG vaccine Efforts to control tuberculosis in the United States are directed toward the early identification and treatment of active cases and preventive therapy with isoniazid. Use of BCG vaccine should be considered for uninfected persons who are exposed repeatedly to infected cases and who cannot or will not obtain or accept treatment. In selected circumstances, where multiply drug-resistant *Mycobacterium tuberculosis* is the "epidemic" strain, vaccination with BCG may also be useful. In the United States, BCG vaccination should be reserved for persons who are skin test negative to 5 tuberculin units (TU) of tuberculin purified protein derivative (PPD). The protection from BCG vaccine is relative, and neither permanent nor predictable. BCG recipients should have repeat skin tests 2 to 3 months later; if they are negative, vaccination should be repeated. The World Health Organization (WHO) recommends that BCG vaccine be administered by the intradermal route, but vaccine for percutaneous administration is also available. BCG should not be given to persons with impaired immune responses, and although no harmful effects of BCG on the fetus have been observed, it is best to avoid vaccination during pregnancy.

Adenovirus vaccine The epidemiologic syndrome of epidemic acute respiratory disease due to adenovirus 4 or 7 is almost exclusively a problem of military recruits. While an effective oral attenuated adenovirus vaccine has been manufactured, clinical illness caused by these adenoviruses has not been associated with significant morbidity or mortality in the civilian population, and hence use of this vaccine outside the military is not recommended.

Typhoid vaccine Routine typhoid vaccination is no longer recommended in the United States, but selective immunization is indicated for persons who are household contacts of a documented typhoid carrier. Typhoid vaccine is generally not necessary among persons affected by flooding or other natural disasters or for those in rural summer camps. Typhoid vaccine consists of whole typhoid bacilli that have been killed, concentrated, and preserved by various methods. The vaccine should be given in two doses of 0.5 ml subcutaneously or 0.1 ml intradermally, according to the manufacturers' recommendations. Booster doses at intervals of 3 years or more are recommended. Local reactions such as erythema, induration, and moderate fever for about 24 h may occur. Controlled trials indicate a 70 to 90 percent protection rate from clinical typhoid. Immunity may be overcome by exposure to high inocula of *Salmonella,* and localized gastrointestinal infection accompanied by diarrhea may still occur. A newly developed *oral* typhoid vaccine affords protection and is much easier to administer, particularly in endemic areas.

VACCINATION OF TRAVELERS TO FOREIGN COUNTRIES

There are two objectives for immunization of foreign travelers: (1) to satisfy a country's requirements, as modified by international regulations, regarding prevention of the introduction and spread of disease (e.g., yellow fever, cholera, and smallpox), and (2) to protect the traveler.

Smallpox vaccination (see Chap. 203) The success of the WHO smallpox eradication program, the concomitant decrease of worldwide smallpox, and the now low risk of importation of smallpox make the morbidity of smallpox vaccination greater than the risk of exposure to smallpox itself. The complications and contraindications to vaccination are outlined in Chap. 203. In the United States, smallpox vaccination is not recommended for any persons except those who work in high-security laboratories with variola virus or for those traveling to countries that continue to require smallpox vaccination as a condition for entry. In most countries, a written waiver from a physician or health authority indicating that smallpox vaccination is contraindicated for health reasons will be accepted as a substitute for vaccination. Travelers should be aware of the vaccination requirements of each country they visit. Smallpox vaccine should *not* be used for the treatment of warts or prevention of recurrent herpes simplex virus infections.

Yellow fever vaccine Many countries require a current international certificate of vaccination against yellow fever from persons older than 6 months who have been in the countries reporting yellow fever (South America and the African subcontinent) in the preceding 6 days. Because these requirements change and often vary with the length of stay in the country, all travelers to areas where yellow fever is endemic should seek current information from health departments or international airlines before departing. Yellow fever vaccine must be administered at a designated yellow fever center. Vaccination certificates are valid for a period of 10 years, beginning 10 days after vaccination. The only yellow fever vaccine licensed in the United States is a live attenuated vaccine produced in chick embryos which must be administered subcutaneously in 0.5-ml amounts. Fever and malaise occur in 10 percent of recipients, but major reactions such as encephalitis are very rare. While pregnant females should generally not be vaccinated with live attenuated virus, the risk to the fetus is small, and pregnant women who must travel to areas where the risk of yellow fever is high should be vaccinated. Yellow fever virus vaccine should not be given to patients with severe underlying diseases such as leukemia or those receiving immunosuppressive therapy.

Cholera (see Chap. 166) Travelers to the Middle East, Asia, and Africa may require evidence of cholera vaccination. Ideally, travelers to these countries should be vaccinated 1 month prior to their departure. A single primary series or booster dose of vaccine is generally sufficient. The risk of cholera for travelers who use ordinary tourist accommodations is very slight, and currently available cholera vaccines are only about 50 percent effective in reducing the incidence of clinical illness for a period of only 3 to 6 months. They do not prevent transmission of disease.

Typhoid Travelers going to regions where food and water sanitation is poor may wish to receive typhoid vaccine. However, care in selecting food and water is the best protection.

Typhus (see Chap. 189) Vaccination against typhus is not required by any country as a condition for entry, and typhus has not occurred in American travelers in recent years. Typhus vaccination is, therefore, suggested only for persons who work in close contact with the organisms in the laboratory or who live in or visit areas where the disease actually occurs and who will be in close contact with the population in such areas. Typhus vaccine is prepared from formaldehyde-inactivated *Rickettsia prowazekii* grown in embryonated eggs. This vaccine provides protection only against louse-borne (epidemic) typhus, not against murine or scrub typhus. Two subcutaneous injections of the vaccine 4 or more weeks apart are recommended. Boosters at yearly intervals may be necessary.

Plague (see Chap. 160) Immunization against *Yersinia pestis* is recommended only for laboratory workers and for individuals such as Peace Corps volunteers or agricultural advisors who reside in plague-enzootic or plague-epidemic rural areas where avoidance of rodents and fleas is difficult. Travelers to countries or areas reporting endemic plague do not need to receive vaccine.

UNUSUAL OCCUPATIONAL EXPOSURES In general, vaccination of personnel such as laboratory or field workers whose vocation or avocation puts them at particular risk of developing an immunizable disease should receive preexposure immunization. For example, laboratory workers involved with rabies, *Y. pestis,* smallpox, *R. prowazekii, R. rickettsii,* yellow fever virus, or Venezuelan or Eastern equine encephalitis viruses, anthrax bacillus, or tularemia should be vaccinated against the appropriate agent. Occupational exposure requiring vaccination includes preexposure immunization against rabies for veterinarians, spelunkers, and other animal handlers exposed to potentially rabid dogs, cats, skunks, foxes, and bats; *Yersinia* vaccination for field workers in endemic areas; and anthrax vaccination for industrial workers who process hides, hair, bone meal, and wool of potentially infected animals.

PASSIVE IMMUNIZATION (See Table 145-2) Prophylaxis or therapy of infection can also be accomplished in some instances by passive immunization which involves the administration of preformed antibody obtained from humans or other animals who have been actively immunized. Because animal antiserum can induce a hypersensitivity response in the recipient, antiserums from humans are preferable. The duration of immunity provided by passive immunization is brief. Intracellular virus generally is not affected by antibody, and once infection has been initiated, the role of antibody is limited to resisting the spread of the virus.

Hepatitis A (see Chap. 318) Immune serum globulin administered before exposure and during the incubation period of hepatitis A is 80 to 90 percent effective in preventing or modifying the disease. The prophylactic effect of ISG is greatest when given early in the incubation period, and the use of ISG more than 2 weeks after exposure or after onset of clinical illness is not indicated. Immune serum globulin is recommended for household contacts of patients with hepatitis A but not for contacts at school, hospital, or work. In institutional settings where periodic epidemics of hepatitis A are common, the administration of ISG to residents and staff may limit the spread of the disease. The dose of ISG for postexposure prophylaxis is 0.02 ml per kilogram of body weight.

The risk of hepatitis A for residents of the United States traveling abroad is small. Travelers to tropical areas or to developing countries who bypass the usual tourist routes should probably be given ISG. In addition, travelers staying in developing countries or in tropical areas longer than 3 months should receive a single injection of ISG, 0.05 ml per kilogram of body weight. This dose should be repeated every 4 to 6 months.

Hepatitis B (see Chaps. 138 and 318) In selected instances, passive immunization with human globulin containing antibody to the hepatitis B surface antigens may prevent or ameliorate the subsequent development of hepatitis B. Some controversy exists about the relative efficacy and/or cost benefit of ISG-containing antibody to hepatitis B surface antigen (anti-HBs) or hyperimmune globulin containing a high titer of anti-HBs [hepatitis B immunoglobulin (HBIG)]. HBIG is recommended for susceptible health care personnel who are anti-HBs-negative and who have been exposed to needle sticks with blood from documented HBsAg-positive donors. Ideally, HBIG should be administered within 48 h of exposure. Because of its lower cost and more likely potential for preventing non-A, non-B hepatitis, ISG may be used in susceptible persons with needle exposures from unknown sources. HBIG has been shown to be about 75 percent effective in preventing chronic hepatitis B infection in neonates born to mothers with acute or chronic hepatitis B. HBIG should be given to the infant shortly after birth (preferably in the delivery room), and at 3- and 6-month intervals. HBIG has been partially effective in preventing hepatitis B among household contacts of patients with acute hepatitis B. However, in endemic environments, like dialysis units, or among persons continuously exposed to chronic HBsAg carriers, passive immunization may only delay the incubation period of the disease. Passive immunization with ISG and/or HBIG, along with hepatitis B vaccine, may result in improved efficacy in these situations.

Varicella-zoster serum immune globulin (VZIG) If administered within 72 h after exposure, VZIG may prevent or ameliorate varicella-zoster among immunosuppressed susceptible patients. Indications for the use of VZIG are listed in Chap. 204. VZIG is not indicated in established varicella-zoster or in adults with a past history of varicella.

Diphtheria antitoxin (see Chap. 165) Diphtheria antitoxin may be useful in the prophylaxis of asymptomatic unimmunized household contacts along with (1) chemoprophylaxis with either oral erythromycin or intramuscular benzathine penicillin or (2) immunization with diphtheria toxoid. The risk of diphtheria among household contacts, which was approximately 20 percent before the antibiotic era but is negligible now, must be weighed against that of serum sickness from equine antiserum before this product is used.

Tetanus immune globulin (TIG) (see Chap. 170) The product of choice when contaminated wounds are present in persons whose history of previous tetanus immunization is uncertain or inadequate is TIG. The current recommended prophylactic dose of TIG is 250 to 1000 units given intramuscularly. TIG does not interfere with the primary immune response to tetanus toxoid given at the same time but at a different site.

Rabies (see Chap. 207) Postexposure prophylaxis for rabies consists of both passive and active immunization. Although more expensive, human rabies immune globulin is the preferred immunizing agent. The dose is 20 IU per kilogram of body weight given half intramuscularly and half intravenously.

Pertussis (see Chap. 156) Hyperimmune pertussis globulin does not appear effective in preventing disease among unvaccinated susceptible neonates.

Measles (see Chap. 200) Immune serum globulin should not be used to control measles outbreaks. Live measles vaccination can usually prevent development of disease if administered within 2 days of exposure. Immune serum globulin should be reserved for susceptible household contacts of measles patients, particularly for those under 1 year of age, exposed pregnant females, or for persons in whom measles vaccine is contraindicated, such as immune deficient hosts. The usual dose is 10 to 20 ml intramuscularly.

Rubella (see Chap. 201) After exposure to rubella, ISG will not prevent infection or viremia with rubella virus but may modify or suppress symptoms. The routine use of ISG for

TABLE 145-2
Passive immunization

Disease	*Preparation*	*Route and dose**	*Comments*
Hepatitis A	ISG, human	IM (0.02–0.06 ml/kg)	Household contacts
Hepatitis B	Human hepatitis B immunoglobulin ISG, human	IM (0.06 ml/kg; two doses 4 weeks apart) IM (0.05 ml/kg; two doses 4 weeks apart)	HBIG is preferred prophylaxis for direct parenteral exposure (needle stick) or mucous-membrane contact in susceptibles; if unavailable, ISG should be given. HBIG should be administered to neonates born to mothers with hepatitis B.
Vaccinia immunoglobulin	Human VIG	IM (0.3 ml/kg)	Use in eczema vaccinatum, disseminated vaccinia, vaccinia in pregnancy
Herpes zoster	Human varicella-ZIG	IM (125 units per 10 kg, up to 625 units)	Prevention and amelioration of varicella in susceptible immunosuppressed patients
Diphtheria	Diphtheria antitoxin, horse	IM or IV (10,000–100,000 units)	Dose dependent on extent of membrane and degree of toxicity; may also be used in unimmunized household contacts
Tetanus	Human tetanus immunoglobulin (TIG)	IM (250 units)	When given with tetanus toxoid, use separate syringes and sites
Rabies	Human rabies immunoglobulin	One-half locally and one-half IM (20 IU/kg)	Used for postexposure prophylaxis with both tissue culture and duck embryo rabies vaccine
	Equine antirabies globulin	One-half locally and one-half IM (40 IU/kg)	Same as above
Pertussis	Pertussis immunoglobulin, human	IM (1.5 ml, repeat in 5–7 days)	No studies suggest efficacy in susceptible infants
Measles	ISG, human	IM (0.2 ml/kg or 20–30 ml)	Susceptible household contacts less than 1 year old, exposed susceptible pregnant females, or immunodeficient persons
Rubella	ISG, human	IM (20–30 ml)	Exposed susceptible pregnant females who will not consider termination
Botulism (Chap. 171)	Horse serum, trivalent AB	One-half IM and one-half IV (8–32 ml)	Use only therapeutically: greatest efficacy in type E
Snake bite (Chap. 234)	Polyvalent crotaline antivenom (pit vipers)	IV (dose function of severity of bite)	See Chap. 234
Spider bite (Chap. 234)	Equine	IM (2.5 ml)	*Latrodectus* (black widow spider) poisoning

* *IM, intramuscularly; IV, intravenously.*

postexposure prophylaxis of rubella in early pregnancy is not recommended, and infants with congenital rubella have been born to women who were given ISG shortly after exposure.

CHEMOPROPHYLAXIS OF INFECTION

USE OF A SINGLE DRUG Antibiotics have been used prophylactically to (1) prevent the acquisition of an exogenous organism, (2) prevent a resident organism from infecting a normally sterile site, and (3) prevent a dormant pathogenic organism from causing disease. In general, antimicrobial prophylaxis with a single drug, administered over a moderate period of time and directed at a single pathogen, has been successful. Examples of this type of prophylaxis employing low doses of "narrow-spectrum" antimicrobials include the prevention of recurrent episodes of rheumatic fever secondary to group A streptococcal disease with benzathine penicillin, of malaria with chloroquine, and of influenza A with amantadine. Table 145-3 lists some clinical situations where prolonged chemoprophylaxis either to prevent exposure to an exogenous organism or reactivation of a dormant organism in a uniquely susceptible host has been useful.

There are also situations in which the short-term use of antibiotics may prevent bacteremia, as in prophylaxis of bacterial endocarditis in individuals with acquired or congenital heart disease, or may abort localized mucosal infections. Here the use of antibiotics is based on the rationale that brief, low-dose exposure to an antimicrobial, early in the disease before bacterial multiplication has led to established infection, may prevent full-blown disease. Some examples of short-term prophylaxis are given in Table 145-4.

ANTIBIOTIC PROPHYLAXIS IN SURGERY Controlled evaluations of short courses of prophylactic antimicrobials have indicated that the selective use of antibiotics, particularly in operative procedures involving potentially contaminated surgical sites, will lower the rate of postoperative infections. The following principles should be applied in using antimicrobial prophylaxis in surgery (Table 145-5): (1) there must be a high prevalence of postoperative infections that are potentially severe before employing antimicrobial drugs; (2) the prophylactic antimicrobial must be effective against the most frequent postoperative pathogens; (3) the drug should be administered from immediately before and during the operation, and for only a short period thereafter; and (4) where possible, prophylaxis should be carried out with a single drug. In studies of cardiac, colorectal, vaginal, and biliary tract surgery, single-dose antibiotic prophylaxis has been as effective as multiple postoperative administration of antibiotics. Antibiotic prophylaxis is recommended in clean surgical procedures that involve insertion of prostheses where the development of infections can be severe or fatal. Other operations such as those involving clean-contaminated, contaminated, or "dirty" wounds, where the infection rates vary from 10 to 40 percent, also warrant prophylactic antibiotics. This topic is also discussed in Chap. 138. For choice of the appropriate agent, Chap. 141 should be consulted.

ANTIBIOTICS IN SUSCEPTIBLE HOSTS In contrast to short-term antimicrobial prophylaxis with a single drug, which is unlikely to be deleterious, attempts to prevent infection with multiple drugs administered in high doses for relatively prolonged periods are much more likely to be harmful. Adverse effects of "prolonged" antimicrobial prophylaxis include (1) superinfection (defined as an infection with a resistant organism that has developed during antibiotic therapy), (2) increased incidence of toxic or allergic reactions to drugs, (3) increased cost, and last but not least, (4) a sense of false security on the part of many physicians, resulting in less stringent observation of the patient. However, many of the patients who are given antibiotics prophylactically are precisely the ones who are susceptible to complicating infections, and particular care must be taken to watch assiduously for the development

TABLE 145-3
Drugs that may be administered prophylactically for prolonged exposure or for extended periods of time

Disease or organism	*Drug*
Group A streptococcus (rheumatic fever) (Chap. 257)	Penicillin G, sulfonamide
Influenza A infection* (Chap. 198)	Amantadine
Malaria (Chap. 218)	Chloroquine and/or pyrimethamine, sulfadoxine
Tuberculosis contacts (Chap. 174)	Isoniazid
Recurrent urinary tract infection in females (Chap. 296)	Trimethoprim-sulfamethoxazole, nitrofurantoin
Recurrent otitis media (Chap. 283)	Sulfisoxazole or ampicillin
IMMUNOSUPPRESSED PATIENTS	
Pneumocystis carinii in cancer patients receiving cytotoxic agents* (Chaps. 137, 222)	Trimethoprim-sulfamethoxazole
Bacterial infections in granulocytopenic patients (Chap. 137)	Trimethoprim-sulfamethoxazole, liquid nonabsorbable antibiotics (vancomycin, gentamycin, nystatin)
Herpes simplex virus infections in patients receiving cytotoxic agents (Chap. 210)	Acyclovir†
Cytomegalovirus infection in renal transplant patients (Chap. 211)	Leukocyte interferon†

* *May require only short courses.*
† *Neither of these agents has been licensed by the Food and Drug Administration.*

TABLE 145-4
Short-term antimicrobial prophylaxis

Disease	*Antibiotic*
USUALLY EFFECTIVE	
Subacute bacterial endocarditis:	
Streptococcus viridans	Penicillin V or procaine penicillin G plus streptomycin
Enterococcus	Ampicillin or penicillin G plus gentamicin or streptomycin
Neisseria gonorrheae (ophthalmia)	Penicillin, silver nitrate
Neisseria gonorrheae (genital infection)	Tetracycline
Nongonococcal urethritis	Tetracycline
Congenital or incubating syphilis	Penicillin
Toxigenic *Escherichia coli* ("tourista")	Tetracycline
Enteropathogenic *E. coli* diarrhea	Neomycin or kanamycin
Neisseria meningitidis	Sulfonamides (sensitive strains only), rifampin, minocycline
Corynebacterium diphtheriae	Erythromycin, clindamycin, penicillin, benzathine penicillin
SOMETIMES EFFECTIVE	
Shigellosis	Ampicillin, neomycin
Chronic bronchitis*	Ampicillin, tetracycline
Short-term urethral catheterization (<24 h)	Ampicillin, tetracycline, nitrofurantoin, trimethoprim-sulfamethoxazole

* *Prophylaxis may require prolonged administration.*

TABLE 145-5
Systemic antimicrobial prophylaxis in surgery

	Antibiotic
PROPHYLAXIS INDICATED	
Obstetric-gynecologic surgery:	
Vaginal and abdominal hysterectomy	Cephalosporin (cefazolin), metronidazole
Caesarean section after prolonged rupture of membranes	Cefazolin
Colorectal surgery	Neomycin and erythromycin base, doxycycline, cefoxitin, metronidazole, gentamicin plus clindamycin
Appendectomy	Doxycycline, cefoxitin
Cardiac surgery	Cefazolin
Valvular, noncardiac thoracic surgery	Cefazolin
Orthopedic surgery (joint replacement, prosthesis, compound fractures)	A cephalosporin or penicillinase-resistant penicillin
Peripheral artery surgery with graft replacement	A cephalosporin
Contaminated surgical wounds	A cephalosporin
Prostatectomy with preoperative bacteruria	Treat according to bacterial sensitivity tests
PROPHYLAXIS OF VALUE IN SELECTED PATIENTS	
Obstructing duodenal ulcer, achlorhydria, chronic cimetidine therapy, gastric ulcer, malignancy	A cephalosporin
Biliary tract surgery (elderly, obstructed)	A cephalosporin
Microsurgical craniotomy	A cephalosporin
Extensive ear, nose, or throat surgery	A cephalosporin
PROPHYLAXIS UNLIKELY TO BE OF VALUE	
Clean abdominal surgery	
Gynecologic surgery (other than mentioned above)	
Coronary artery bypass surgery	
Genitourinary surgery in persons with sterile urine	

of infection and to treat it promptly when it occurs. Such policy is often superior to the use of antimicrobial prophylaxis.

Prophylactic antibiotics have not been useful in preventing bacterial complications of antecedent viral respiratory illness such as influenza or in preventing colonization of pathogenic organisms in intensive care units. Indeed, in these and many other clinical situations the risk of superinfection with resistant, difficult-to-treat organisms outweighs the unlikely effectiveness of prophylactic antibiotics (Table 145-6). However, in some populations, such as victims of severe burns or patients with severe granulocytopenia, antibiotic prophylaxis may be useful. Infections in granulocytopenic patients are often life-threatening. Most infections develop in persons with prolonged (>14 days) and profound (<100 granulocytes per milliliter) granulocytopenia. Mucosal damage by tumor therapy allows invasion or organisms colonizing the alimentary and respiratory tracts and the oral cavity, resulting in pneumonitis, esophagitis, colitis, and perianal infections. Many infections are due to the patient's indigenous flora, and others are due to organisms acquired from the hospital environment. In selected patients, reduction of indigenous flora and prevention of colonization by microbial suppression using oral nonabsorbable antibiotics such as gentamicin, vancomycin, and nystatin (GVN) with or without laminar airflow rooms or selective suppression of alimentary canal microbial flora with trimethoprim-sulfamethoxazole have been effective. The necessity of maintaining continuous GVN therapy, the difficulty of patient compliance, the emergence of trimethoprim-sulfamethoxazole–resistant organisms, and the existence of localized out-

TABLE 145-6
Antibiotic prophylaxis in susceptible hosts in whom its use is not indicated

OUTPATIENT USE
Viral respiratory disease
Viral exanthems
Preventing acute exacerbations of asthma
HOSPITALIZED PATIENTS
Preventing pneumonia in comatose patients
Preventing tracheal colonization with pathogenic organisms
Preventing infections in patients with congestive heart failure
Prolonged urethral catheterization (>24 h)
Prolonged intravenous catheterization (>48 h)
High-dose steroid therapy
Prematurity
Shock

breaks of unusual organisms indicate that continued evaluation of these prophylactic antibiotic regimens is needed. Similarly, the role of prophylactic antiviral agents such as acyclovir for herpes simplex or interferon for CMV requires clarification.

REFERENCES

Barrett-Conner E: Chemoprophylaxis of malaria for travelers. Ann Intern Med 81:219, 1974

Broome CV: Pneumococcal disease after pneumococcal vaccination. N Engl J Med 303:549, 1980

Dienstag JL: Diagnosis and prevention of viral hepatitis, in *Update IV: Harrison's Principles of Internal Medicine,* 9th ed, KJ Isselbacher et al (eds). New York, McGraw-Hill, 1982, pp 165–196

Goldman PG, Petersdorf RG: Prophylactic antibiotics. Controversies give way to guidelines. Drug Therapy, June 1979, p 539

Hirschmann JV, Inui TS: Antimicrobial prophylaxis: A critique of recent trials. Rev Infect Dis 2:1, 1980

Immunizations and chemoprophylaxis for travelers. Med Lett Drugs Ther 23(25):105, 1981

Kass EH: Assessment of the pneumococcal polysaccharide vaccine. Rev Infect Dis 3(Suppl):S1–197, 1981

Krugman S: Effect of human immune serum globulin on infectivity of hepatitis A virus. J Infect Dis 34:70, 1975

Recommendations of the Immunization Practices Advisory Committee. Diphtheria, tetanus, and pertussis: Guidelines for vaccine prophylaxis and other preventive measures. Morb Mort Week Rep 30:392, 1981 (also Ann Intern Med 95:723, 1981)

———: Inactivated hepatitis B virus vaccine. Morb Mort Week Rep 31:317, 1982

Ruben FL: Antitoxin responses in the elderly to tetanus-diphtheria (Td) immunization. Am J Epidemiol 108:145, 1978

Schimpff SC: Infection prevention during profound granulocytopenia. Ann Intern Med 93:358, 1980

Shasby DM et al: Epidemic measles in a highly vaccinated population. N Engl J Med 296:585, 1977

Willens JS et al: Cost effectiveness of vaccination against pneumococcal pneumonia. N Engl J Med 303:353, 1980

section 2 | Infections caused by gram-positive cocci

146
PNEUMOCOCCAL INFECTIONS

ROBERT AUSTRIAN

ETIOLOGY

The pneumococcus *(Streptococcus pneumoniae)* is a gram-positive encapsulated coccus that usually grows in pairs or short chains. In the diplococcal form, the adjacent margins are rounded and the opposite ends slightly pointed, giving the organisms a lancet shape. In stained preparations of exudate, gram-negative forms are sometimes present. Pneumococcal colonies are surrounded by greenish discoloration on or in blood agar and are confused at times with other alpha-hemolytic streptococci to which they are closely related. Their isolation from respiratory secretions may be facilitated by inclusion of 5 μg gentamicin per milliliter in the medium. Pneumococci can be distinguished by their bile solubility and mouse virulence or by serologic typing. Another method, utilizing inhibition of pneumococci by Optochin-impregnated paper disks, is less cumbersome and very effective, but standard zones of inhibition determined for aerobic cultures cannot be applied to cultures grown in 5% carbon dioxide for the presumptive identification of pneumococcus.

The capsular substances are complex polysaccharides and are the basis for dividing pneumococci into serotypes. Organisms exposed to type-specific antiserum show a positive capsular precipitin reaction, the *Neufeld quellung reaction;* by this means, 84 serotypes have been identified. All are pathogenic for human beings, but types 1, 3, 4, 7, 8, and 12 are encountered most frequently in clinical practice. Types 6, 14, 19, and 23 often cause pneumonia and otitis media in children but are less common in adults.

Specific typing of pneumococci remains of great clinical importance if pneumococcus is to be identified with regularity, but it has largely been abandoned since the introduction of sulfonamides and antibiotics, which are effective against pneumococci of all types. Recognition of pneumococcus has decreased significantly since the abandonment of capsular typing by most clinical laboratories. The detection of pneumococcal capsular polysaccharides in sputum and in other body fluids by counterimmunoelectrophoresis provides an alternative to bacteriologic techniques for the presumptive diagnosis of pneumococcal infection. Because of cross reactions between the polysaccharides of pneumococci and of other bacterial species, immunologic diagnosis is less specific than bacteriologic diagnosis.

PATHOGENESIS

The mechanism by which pneumococci damage the mammalian host is obscure. It is conceivable that toxic substances may be elaborated, but no such toxin has been shown to play a major pathogenic role in pneumococcal infection. The capsular polysaccharides, though nontoxic, are known to be necessary factors in virulence and to protect the organism to a certain extent from engulfment by phagocytes.

Although "pneumococcal pharyngitis" is a doubtful entity, invasion of the tissue of the nasopharynx may occur in the infant and occasionally in the nonimmune adult and be followed by spread to the circulation via the cervical lymphatics. At times, secondary infection of serous cavities in the absence of demonstrable focal infection of the upper or lower respiratory tract may occur. The organisms multiply readily in vivo and may produce acute inflammation of the lungs, serous cavities, and endocardium.

The normal human respiratory tract is provided with a variety of mechanisms which guard the lungs from infection. The lower respiratory tract is protected by the glottis and larynx, and material passing these barriers stimulates the expulsive cough reflex. Removal of small particles impinging on the walls of the trachea and bronchi is facilitated by their mucociliary lining; and growth of bacteria reaching normal alveoli is inhibited by their relative dryness and by the phagocytic activity of alveolar macrophages. Any anatomic or physiologic derangement of these coordinated defenses tends to augment the susceptibility of the lungs to infection. Anesthesia, alcoholic intoxication, convulsions, and disturbed innervation of the larynx depress the cough reflex and may permit aspiration of infected material. Alterations in the tracheobronchial tree leading to anatomic changes in the epithelial lining or to localized obstruction increase the vulnerability of the lungs to infection. Pulmonary edema, local or generalized, resulting from viral infection, inhalation of irritant gases, cardiac failure, or contusion of the chest wall, provides a fluid menstruum in the alveoli for the growth of bacteria and their spread to adjacent areas of the lung. Viral infection of the respiratory epithelium with concomitant disruption of its component cells interferes significantly with the clearance of bacteria from the lungs, an observation in accord with the high incidence of pneumococcal pneumonia during epidemics of viral influenza and its frequent clinical association with sporadic viral respiratory infections.

Pneumonia begins usually in the right lower, right middle, or left lower lobe, those areas to which gravity is most likely to carry upper respiratory secretions aspirated during sleep. Bronchial embolization with infected mucinous secretions during the course of an upper respiratory infection appears to be the initiating factor in many cases of pneumococcal pneumonia. Protected initially from phagocytosis by mucinous material, the bacteria multiply and, in infected alveoli, evoke the outpouring of proteinaceous fluid, which serves both as a nutrient and as a vehicle for spread to adjacent alveoli. Soon thereafter, polymorphonuclear leukocytes migrate from the pulmonary capillaries to phagocytize a part of the pneumococcal population before the appearance of detectable antibody. Delay in the polymorphonuclear leukocytic response occurs during alcoholic intoxication and certain forms of anesthesia, permitting spread of infection. Adrenocortical steroids and their congeners may also interfere with leukocyte migration. Later, as the pneumonic lesion evolves, macrophages appear in the exudate and remove the debris of fibrin and cells. It is probable that antibody to the capsular polysaccharide of the invading pneumococcus makes its appearance locally in the lung before being detectable in the circulation. Such antibody increases the efficiency of phagocytosis approximately twofold and causes agglutination of the organisms and their adherence to alveolar walls, thereby slowing their dissemination in the lung. The outcome of infection depends, therefore, on the rate at which bacteria can multiply in the edema fluid and spread, and on the host's ability to immobilize and destroy them by phagocytosis. Individuals with hypogammaglobulinemia and patients with multiple myeloma incapable of producing anticapsular antibody are liable to recurrent attacks of pneumococcal pneumonia. Repeated infection with the same pneumococcal type should always prompt a search for dysgammaglobulinemia.

Failure of local defense mechanisms in the lung results in lymphatic spread of pneumococci to the hilar lymph nodes. In the sinusoids of these organs, a sequence of events not unlike that in the lung ensues. If infection is not checked in this secondary line of defense, organisms find their way into the thoracic duct and then into the circulation. Although transient bacteremia may occur at the onset of many cases of pneumococcal pneumonia, it is detectable in only 25 to 30 percent of cases. Bacteremia, which reflects the body's inability to localize the pulmonary infection, is a poor prognostic sign and carries with it the danger of metastatic infection. The mortality of treated or untreated bacteremic pneumococcal pneumonia is four times that resulting from comparably managed nonbacteremic infections. Metastatic infection secondary to bacteremia may occur in the meninges, joints, or peritoneum or on the endocardium. Direct spread from the infected lung may give rise to pleural empyema or to pericarditis.

Natural recovery from pneumococcal infection coincides usually, but not invariably, with the appearance of detectable type-specific antibody in the circulation and is often accompanied by a dramatic and abrupt fall in temperature, the so-called crisis. Antibody aids recovery by increasing the efficiency of phagocytosis and by limiting dissemination of the organisms. Bacteriostatic drugs, such as sulfonamides, facilitate control of the infection by limiting the size of the pneumococcal population, but the host's defense mechanisms are still required for the elimination of the bacteria. Bactericidal agents, such as penicillin, cause the death of pneumococci in the lung and are effective when some of the host's defense mechanisms are compromised. With the arrest of infection, the alveolar exudate undergoes liquefaction, the inflammatory debris is removed by expectoration and via the lymphatic channels, and the lung is restored to its normal state. Necrosis of pulmonary tissue as a result of pneumococcal infection is distinctly uncommon. Primary pneumococcal lung abscess is a rare clinical entity, although the diagnosis is mistakenly made at times when pneumococcal infection complicates lung abscess of other origins.

In addition to causing pneumonia and its metastatic sequelae, pneumococcus can extend from the nasopharynx to its adjacent structures, giving rise to otitis media, mastoiditis, paranasal sinusitis, or conjunctivitis. Soft-tissue abscesses are rare but may occur.

PNEUMOCOCCAL PNEUMONIA

Pneumococcal pneumonia is a disease remarkable for its uniformity, in contrast to other infections such as typhoid fever and tuberculosis. The diseases produced by different pneumococcal serotypes show little variation in severity or in clinical manifestations. The prognosis in type 3 pneumococcal pneumonia is usually regarded as poor, probably because type 3 infections occur frequently in the aged and in patients with other debilitating diseases, such as diabetes and congestive heart failure. The usual lesion in adults is segmental or lobar in distribution, but in children and the aged, bronchopneumonia, characterized by patchy involvement, is frequent.

MANIFESTATIONS Pneumonia is often preceded for a few days by coryza or some other form of common respiratory disease. The onset is usually so abrupt that patients frequently can state the exact hour that illness began. There is a sudden *shaking chill* in more than 80 percent of the cases and a rapid rise in temperature, with corresponding tachycardia and an increase in respiratory rate (tachypnea). Most patients with pneumococcal pneumonia have a single rigor unless antipyretic drugs are administered, and repeated chills should suggest another etiologic agent.

About 75 percent of patients develop severe *pleuritic pain* and *cough,* productive of pinkish or "rusty" mucoid sputum within a few hours. The chest pain is agonizing, and respirations become rapid, shallow, and grunting as the patient tries to splint the affected side. Many patients are mildly cyanotic as a result of hypoxia caused by V/Q abnormality or shunt, which accompanies altered respiration, and show dilatation of the alae nasi when first seen. Patients appear acutely ill; but nausea, headache, and malaise are not prominent, and most individuals are alert. Pleuritic pain and dyspnea are the dominent complaints.

In the untreated disease, there are sustained fever of 102.5 to 105°F (39.2 to 40.5°C), continued pleuritic pain, cough, and expectoration; and *abdominal distention* is frequent. *Herpes labialis* is a common complication. After 7 to 10 days, there are diaphoresis, abrupt defervescence, and dramatic improvement in well-being, the "crisis."

In cases which terminate fatally, there is usually extensive pulmonary involvement, and dyspnea, cyanosis, and tachycardia are prominent. Circulatory collapse or a picture resembling heart failure is common. Death in a few patients is associated with empyema or some other suppurative complication such as meningitis or endocarditis.

Physical examination reveals restricted motion of the affected hemithorax. Tactile fremitus may be decreased during the initial day of illness but is usually increased when consolidation is fully established. Deviation of the trachea away from the affected lung suggests pleural effusion or empyema. The percussion note is dull, and if the lesion is in an upper lobe, impaired motion of the diaphragm can be detected on the affected side. Very early in the course of infection, breath sounds are diminished, but as the lesion evolves, they become tubular or bronchial in quality, and bronchophony and whispered pectoriloquy can be elicited. These findings are accompanied by fine crepitant rales.

EFFECT OF SPECIFIC CHEMOTHERAPY Pneumococcal pneumonia usually improves promptly when an appropriate antimicrobial drug is given. Within 12 to 36 h after initiation of treatment with penicillin, temperature, pulse, and respiration begin to fall and may reach normal values, pleuritic pain subsides, and the spread of the inflammatory process is halted. The temperature of approximately half the patients, however, requires 4 days or longer to become normal, and failure of the patient's temperature to reach normal in 24 to 48 h should not prompt a change in antibacterial therapy in the absence of other indications.

COMPLICATIONS The typical course of pneumococcal pneumonia can be modified by the development of one or more local or distant complications:

In the lung ATELECTASIS Atelectasis of all or part of a lobe may occur during the active stage of pneumonia or after treatment has been instituted. The patient may complain of sudden recurrence of pleuritic pain and show rapid respirations. Small areas of atelectasis are often detected by x-ray in the absence of symptoms. These areas usually clear with coughing and deep breathing, but bronchoscopic aspiration is occasionally necessary. If atelectasis is allowed to persist, the affected area becomes fibrotic and functionless.

DELAYED RESOLUTION Return to normal of physical findings in the lung after pneumococcal pneumonia is usually complete within 2 to 4 weeks. X-ray evidence of residual pulmonary consolidation, however, may persist as long as 8 weeks, and other radiologic manifestations of the infection (volume loss, stranding and pleural disease) may persist for up to 18 weeks. The process of resolution may require a longer time in those over 50 years of age and in those with chronic obstructive airway disease or alcoholism.

ABSCESS Lung abscess is a rare sequel to pneumococcal infection, although pneumococcal pneumonia is a not uncommon complication of lung abscess of other origins. It is manifested by continued fever and profuse expectoration of purulent sputum. X-ray shows one or more cavities. This complication is exceedingly rare in patients who receive penicillin therapy and is most likely to follow infection with pneumococcus type 3.

In adjacent structures PLEURAL EFFUSION Pleural effusion occurs in about 5 percent of patients with pneumococcal pneumonia, even with specific therapy. The amount of fluid is usually not sufficient to cause obvious displacement of mediastinal structures. Usually the effusion is sterile and is reabsorbed spontaneously within a week or two. Sometimes, however, the effusion is large and requires aspiration.

EMPYEMA Before the introduction of effective chemotherapy, empyema occurred in 5 to 8 percent of patients with pneumococcal pneumonia; it is now observed in less than 1 percent of treated cases. It is manifested by persistent fever or pleuritic pain, together with signs of pleural effusion. In the early stages, the gross appearance of infected fluid may not differ from that of a sterile pleural effusion; later, there is a profuse outpouring of polymorphonuclear leukocytes and fibrin, resulting in an exudate of thick greenish pus containing large clots of fibrin. The quantity of exudate may become large enough to displace mediastinal structures. In neglected cases, this process leads to extensive pleural scarring, with limitation of thoracic movement. Rupture and drainage through the chest wall *(empyema necessitatis)* occurs, but is rare. Metastatic *brain abscess* is an occasional complication of chronic empyema.

PERICARDITIS A particularly serious complication is spread of infection to the pericardial sac. This lesion is characterized by pain in the precordial region, a friction rub synchronous with the heartbeat, and distention of cervical veins, although one or all of these findings may be absent. The possibility of coexisting purulent pericarditis should be considered whenever a very ill patient with pneumonia develops empyema.

Metastatic infections *Arthritis* occurs more often in children than in adults. The affected joint is swollen, red, and painful, with a purulent effusion. It usually subsides promptly with systemic administration of penicillin, although aspiration and intraarticular injection of penicillin may be necessary in adults.

Acute bacterial endocarditis complicates pneumococcal pneumonia in fewer than 0.5 percent of cases. Its manifestations and treatment are discussed below. *Meningitis,* another complication of pneumococcal pneumonia, is also discussed subsequently.

Paralytic ileus Gaseous abdominal distention is commonly present and in severely ill patients may assume such serious proportions that the term *paralytic ileus* is justified. This complication further impairs respiratory movement by elevation of the diaphragm and constitutes a difficult problem in management. A rarer and more serious gastrointestinal complication is acute gastric dilatation.

Impaired liver function Alterations in hepatic function are common during the course of pneumococcal pneumonia, and mild jaundice is not at all rare. The pathogenesis of the jaundice is not entirely clear, although in some patients it appears to be related to glucose 6-phosphate dehydrogenase deficiency.

LABORATORY FINDINGS *Sputum* should be obtained in the physician's presence before the administration of antimicrobial drugs to ensure its quality. Although resort to transtracheal aspiration or lung puncture may be necessary on occasion to establish the cause of pneumonia, routine use of these invasive techniques is not recommended because of their attendant, albeit infrequent, complications. When stained by Gram's method, the sputum shows polymorphonuclear leukocytes and variable numbers of gram-positive cocci, singly and in pairs. These can be typed directly by the Neufeld quellung or capsular precipitin technique, and this procedure should be followed to facilitate diagnosis whenever possible. The *blood culture* is positive for pneumococci during the first days of untreated illness in 20 to 25 percent of cases. The white blood count usually shows a polymorphonuclear *leukocytosis* ranging from 12,000 to 25,000 cells per cubic millimeter. A normal white count or leukopenia is sometimes observed in patients with overwhelming infection and bacteremia. Occasionally, pneumococci may be seen directly in granulocytes of patients with bacteremia by examining the buffy coat after staining with Wright's stain. These patients often have asplenia. *X-ray of the chest* usually reveals a homogenous density in the affected area of the lung. In well-established cases, the density may occupy one or more entire lobes. Atypical patterns of consolidation may be seen in those with underlying chronic pulmonary disease.

EXTRAPULMONARY PNEUMOCOCCAL INFECTION

PNEUMOCOCCAL MENINGITIS The pneumococcus is second only to the meningococcus as a cause of purulent meningitis in adults; in children, meningitis caused by *Hemophilus influenzae* is also more frequent than pneumococcal infection.

Pneumococcal meningitis can develop as a "primary" disease without preceding signs of infection elsewhere; as a complication of pneumococcal pneumonia; by extension from otitis, mastoiditis, or sinusitis; or following a skull fracture which creates an opening between the subarachnoid space and the nasal cavity or paranasal sinuses. Patients with pneumococcal endocarditis frequently develop meningeal infection. Patients with multiple myeloma and with sickle cell disease seem to be liable to pneumococcal infection of the meninges, just as they are to pneumonia.

The *manifestations* are of those of any acute pyogenic meningitis (see Chap. 359) and include chills, fever, headache, nuchal rigidity, Kernig's and Brudzinski's signs, delirium, and cranial nerve palsies. Evidence of otitis, sinusitis, or pneumonia should be carefully sought by physical and roentgenographic examination in all patients.

The *spinal fluid* is under increased pressure, appears cloudy, often with a greenish tint, and shows a high protein and low glucose content. Stained smears usually reveal gram-positive diplococci and polymorphonuclear leukocytes; in some patients, the number of cells in the spinal fluid is surprisingly small, and much of the cloudiness is produced by the bacterial content. The diagnosis can be established rapidly by identification of pneumococci in the spinal fluid by Gram's stain and by direct typing with the Neufeld quellung reaction.

With appropriate chemotherapy, recovery can be expected in 70 percent of cases; the prognosis is better in children than in infants or in adults. Relapse may occur but is unusual if adequate treatment is carried out. Subarachnoid block, the result of accumulation of large amounts of thick exudate in the meningeal space and at the base of the brain, is now an unusual complication.

PNEUMOCOCCAL ENDOCARDITIS Endocarditis is usually a complication of pneumonia or meningitis. The clinical picture is that of acute bacterial endocarditis (see Chap. 259), with remittent fever, splenomegaly, and metastatic infection of the lungs, meninges, joints, eye, and other tissues. Petechiae are uncommon. The infection can attack normal valves and is particularly likely to occur on the aortic valve. The valvular infection is destructive, and loud murmurs and heart failure develop rapidly. Rupture or perforation of cusps or even rupture of the aorta may occur. The blood culture is consistently positive for the pneumococcus in the absence of treatment with antimicrobial drugs; yet at the same time antibodies to the infecting organism may be demonstrable in the blood, a combination of findings seldom observed except in endocarditis or brucellosis. Although the infection is relatively easy to cure with penicillin, damage to valve leaflets, especially to the cusps of the aortic valve, may be followed by rapidly progressive heart failure. Surgical repair or replacement of damaged valvular structures should be carried out early, before heart failure becomes intractable.

PNEUMOCOCCAL PERITONITIS Pneumococcal peritonitis is a rare disease and is probably the sequel to transient pneumococcal bacteremia, although, because of its somewhat greater frequency in young girls, it has been hypothesized that the organism may gain entry to the peritoneum via the vagina and fallopian tubes. Peritonitis was formerly a common complication of the nephrotic syndrome, particularly in children, but it occurs now with a frequency of approximately 2 percent. In adults, the disease is seen in association with cirrhosis or with carcinoma of the liver. The diagnosis is made by examination of the ascitic fluid; blood cultures are often positive, and a polymorphonuclear leukocytosis is the rule.

TREATMENT

SPECIFIC ANTIMICROBIAL THERAPY Although resistance of pneumococci to antimicrobial drugs has not been regarded as a significant problem in the past, some strains have been found to be resistant to one or the other of the following agents: penicillins, cephalosporins, tetracyclines, chloramphenicol, erythromycin, clindamycin, cotrimoxazole, and aminoglycosides. For this reason sensitivity of the infecting organism to the infecting drug should be determined, particularly in extrapulmonary infection. In the absence of resistance or of hypersensitivity to it, penicillin G (benzyl penicillin) is the drug of choice for all manifestations of pneumococcal infection. Strains of pneumococcus manifesting a modest increase in resistance to penicillin have been recovered infrequently from humans; and although the level of such resistance does not preclude treatment with this antibiotic, awareness of the phenomenon is necessary. The minimum curative dose for *pneumonia* caused by strains of usual sensitivity to penicillin G is less than 60,000 units daily, and a total dose of 600,000 units daily provides a good margin of safety for bacteremic and nonbacteremic pulmonary infection in adults in the absence of an extrapulmonary focus. Treatment may be administered at 12-h intervals in doses of 300,000 units aqueous crystalline penicillin G or procaine penicillin. Therapy should be continued until the patient has been afebrile for 48 to 72 h. The response is usually dramatic, and relapse is extremely uncommon. Pneumococcal pneumonia can be treated adequately with oral penicillin, preferably one of the drugs resistant to gastric acid (see Chap. 141), in dosage of 1.2 to 2.4 million units daily. *Peritonitis* usually responds within 36 to 48 h to 2 to 4 million units of penicillin daily.

Pneumococcal meningitis should be treated with 12 to 20 million units aqueous penicillin G daily intravenously in adults. In many clinics, even larger amounts are used, though care must be taken to avoid neurotoxicity from excessive dosage. Intrathecal administration of penicillin is not necessary. The addition of sulfadiazine to this regimen affords no advantage, and supplementary administration of chlortetracycline (and presumably, of other broad-spectrum drugs) may exert a deleterious effect. In the presence of sinusitis, otitis, or mastoiditis, surgical drainage should be carried out as soon as is feasible. The response of meningitis is usually less dramatic than that of pneumonia; patients often remain febrile and disoriented, and signs of meningeal irritation may persist for several days, but improvement becomes gradually evident with continued treatment.

Moderate doses are required in pneumococcal endocarditis—8 to 12 million units daily by intravenous infusion. Rapidly developing heart failure in these patients and the tendency to form myocardial abscess, however, often lead to a fatal outcome despite large doses of antibiotics. Surgical repair or replacement of damaged heart valves should be considered when cardiac failure develops.

Cephalosporins in parenteral doses of 1 to 2 g daily are effective in pneumococcal pneumonia but must be administered with caution to those hypersensitive to penicillin. These drugs should *not* be used to treat pneumococcal meningitis because of their poor ability to penetrate the blood–cerebrospinal fluid barrier. The *tetracyclines* in doses 1 to 2 g daily, *erythromycin* in doses of 1.6 g daily, or *clindamycin* in doses of 1.2 g daily are effective treatment for pneumococcal pneumonia if it is caused by a sensitive strain, but they are recommended only for patients who have had untoward reactions to penicillins or cephalosporins. Despite its efficacy, *chloramphenicol* should not be used to treat pneumococcal infections other than meningitis in patients hypersensitive to penicillin who are infected with a drug-sensitive strain. For patients with illness caused by multiple drug-resistant pneumococci, *vancomycin* in doses of 2 g daily is the drug of choice. Sulfonamides have little place in the present-day treatment of pneumococcal pneumonia and are useless in endocarditis and meningitis. Aminoglycosides, such as gentamicin, tobramycin, and amikacin, should not be employed to treat pneumococcal infection.

Pneumococcal arthritis responds to systemic penicillin, but aspiration and intraarticular instillation of the drug may be necessary.

Empyema should be detected and treated as early as possible. When an effusion is found, the fluid should be examined for organisms; and if they are present, 50,000 to 200,000 units of penicillin G should be injected intrapleurally. In addition the same antibiotic should be administered systemically in doses of 6 to 8 million units a day. Aspiration of fluid and instillation of penicillin should be carried out at 1- to 2-day intervals until cultures are persistently negative and fever disappears. Fluoroscopic guidance may be needed for aspiration of small empyema pockets. If the exudate is especially thick or viscid, streptokinase-streptodornase (Varidase) may facilitate its withdrawal. When definite improvement is not evident in 4 to 6 days or when the empyema is of long duration, a large-lumen intercostal tube should be placed in the pleural cavity to facilitate drainage. Failure to effect prompt cure of empyema may be followed by pleural fibrosis and necessitate subsequent surgical decortication of the lung to restore pulmonary function.

OTHER MEASURES Oxygen administered through a face mask should be used to treat significant cyanosis, cardiac failure, and delirium. Codeine, 32 to 64 mg every 4 h, will usually control pleuritic pain. When pain is severe, it may require intercostal nerve block with 1 to 2 percent procaine for relief.

PROGNOSIS AND PREVENTION

Although the mortality from pneumococcal pneumonia has diminished significantly since the advent of antimicrobial drugs, available evidence indicates that the incidence of the disease has changed little, if at all. The fatality rate in patients over the age of 12 years with bacteremic pneumococcal pneumonia treated with an antibiotic is 18 percent, and in patients over the age of 50 and in those with underlying systemic illness, it is significantly higher.

Signs of poor prognosis in pneumonia include leukopenia, bacteremia, multilobar involvement, any extrapulmonary focus of pneumococcal infection, presence of preexisting systemic disease, circulatory collapse, and occurrence of the infection in the first year of life or after the age of 55. Infection with pneumococcus type 3 has a higher mortality rate than that caused by other pneumococcal types. Death is most likely to occur in individuals sustaining irreversible physiologic damage early in the course which is unaltered by antimicrobial therapy. Until the nature of the injury produced by pneumococcus is understood and ways devised to repair it, vaccination will remain the only means of protecting those at high risk of a fatal outcome.

A tetradecavalent vaccine containing the capsular polysaccharides of pneumococcal types 1, 2, 3, 4, 6A, 7F, 8, 9N, 12F, 18C, 19F, 23F, and 25, which include the serotypes or groups responsible for 80 percent of bacteremic infections in the United States, is recommended for prevention of pneumococcal infection caused by these types in individuals at high risk of a fatal outcome. Those at higher-than-average risk are individuals over the age of 55 and patients with a variety of chronic systemic illnesses including heart disease, chronic bronchopulmonary disease, hepatic disease, renal insufficiency, diabetes, and a variety of malignancies. Persons of all ages with sickle cell disease have an increased risk of developing pneumococcal infection, and the vaccine is recommended for those with this disorder over the age of 2 years. Since anatomic or functional asplenia is associated with fulminant overwhelming pneumococcal septicemia with disseminated intravascular coagulation, giving rise to a clinical picture resembling the Waterhouse-Friderichsen syndrome, such individuals should also be immunized. However, the vaccine contains a limited number of pneumococcal antigens, and infection caused by other pneumococcal types may occur occasionally in immunized subjects. Reactions to the vaccine are usually absent or mild, although in the occasional individual they may resemble those following immunization with typhoid vaccine: local pain, erythema, and elevation of temperature. The most severe local and systemic reactions to the vaccine appear to be associated with preexisting high levels of antibody to one or more of the antigens in the vaccine. Because of the persistence of pneumococcal antibodies after a single injection of vaccine, reimmunization in less than 5 years after the initial injection is not recommended. The vaccine is 80 to 90 percent effective in immunocompetent adults but may afford little, if any, protection to those with agamma- or dysgammaglobulinemia or to patients who have been subjected recently to intensive antitumor chemotherapy and radiation. In children under 6 years, immunologic responsiveness to different capsular antigens develops at different times as a result of maturational characteristics of the human immune system, and protection may be of shorter duration than in the adults. Further data are needed to define the utility of the vaccine in childhood. If necessary, pneumococcal vaccine may be administered concomitantly with influenza viral vaccine, provided each vaccine is injected from a separate syringe at a separate site.

REFERENCES

AMMANN AJ et al: Polyvalent-polysaccharide immunization of patients with sickle-cell anemia and patients with splenectomy. N Engl J Med 297:897, 1977

AUSTRIAN R, GOLD J: Pneumococcal bacteremia with especial reference to bacteremic pneumococcal pneumonia. Ann Intern Med 60:759, 1964

——— et al: Prevention of pneumococcal pneumonia by vaccination. Trans Assoc Am Phys 89:184, 1976

GOPAL V, BISNO AL: Fulminant pneumococcal infections in "normal" asplenic hosts. Arch Intern Med 137:1526, 1977

HEFFRON R: *Pneumonia with Special Reference to Pneumococcus Lobar Pneumonia.* 2d printing. Cambridge, Harvard, 1979

JACOBS MR et al: Emergence of multiply resistant pneumococci. N Engl J Med 299:735, 1978

KASS EH (ed): Assessment of the pneumococcal polysaccharide vaccine. A workshop. Rev Infect Dis 3, Suppl, March-April 1981

KAUFFMAN CA et al: Purulent pneumococcic pericarditis: Continuing problem in antibiotic era. Am J Med 54:743, 1973

MERRILL CW et al: Rapid identification of pneumococci: Gram stain vs quellung reaction. N Engl J Med 288:510, 1973

SHULMAN JA et al: Errors and hazards in the diagnosis and treatment of bacterial pneumonias. Ann Intern Med 62:41, 1965

STEPHEN JJ et al: The radiographic resolution of *Streptococcus pneumoniae* pneumonia. N Engl J Med 293:798, 1975

TUGWELL P, WILLIAMS AO: Jaundice associated with lobar pneumonia. Q J Med 46:97, 1977

WOOD WB JR: Studies on the cellular immunology of acute infections. Harvey Lect 42:72, 1951–1952

147 STAPHYLOCOCCAL INFECTIONS

MARVIN TURCK
GEORGE W. COUNTS

Staphylococci most commonly produce relatively harmless superficial suppurative infections in human beings. They also produce serious infections of the lungs, pleural space, endocardium, myocardium, long bones, kidneys, and surgical wounds.

The majority of life-threatening staphylococcal infections arise within hospitals, and are among the "diseases of medical progress." Staphylococcal cross infection in hospitals may be less frequent now than it was 10 to 15 years ago, and gram-negative rods are now the most common nosocomial pathogens; nevertheless staphylococci still account for 20 percent of all hospital-acquired infections.

ETIOLOGY *Staphylococcus* and *Micrococcus* are two genera comprised of facultative, aerobic, gram-positive cocci within the family Micrococcaceae. According to current classification, bacteria of the genus *Micrococcus* are of little clinical importance. The name *staphylococcus* derives from the characteristic grapelike clusters of organisms seen in stained smears prepared from colonies on solid media. In material obtained from clinical specimens, smaller clusters, diplococci, and even short chains may be seen. Staphylococci may be separated from micrococci on the basis of anaerobic fermentation of glucose and susceptibility to furoxone. *Staphylococcus aureus,* the most important human pathogen in the genus, is so named because of the golden yellow color of the culture in growth on solid media. All strains producing coagulase are designated as *S. aureus.* Most laboratories label all coagulase-negative strains as *S. epidermidis.* In addition to production of coagulase, two other tests which characterize *S. aureus* and separate isolates from *S. epidermidis* are mannitol fermentation and susceptibility to lysostaphin, a peptidase enzyme active against peptidoglycan in the cell wall. *S. aureus* and *S. epidermidis* differ in the amount of glycine and serine present in the bridging pentapeptides. Other methods to differentiate *S. aureus* from *S. epidermidis* (pigment production, type of hemolysis, and antibiotic susceptibility) are unreliable. In general, *S. aureus* strains exhibit greater expression of biochemical activity (production of coagulase, hemolysins, and toxins) than *S. epidermidis.*

Isolates of coagulase-negative *S. epidermidis* do not represent a homogeneous group. Biochemical testing has identified different subgroups or biotypes within the species. The organism formally called *Micrococcus* biotype 3 (Baird-Parker) and recognized as a frequent cause of urinary tract infection is now tentatively called *S. saprophyticus.* Species names have been proposed for several other biotypes of coagulase-negative staphylococci.

Different strains of *S. aureus* can be recognized by the patterns of lysis produced by staphylococcal bacteriophages. Although it is cumbersome and not performed by most hospital laboratories, phage typing has allowed more precise strain characterization and is commonly used in studies of intrahospital disease and epidemics of staphylococcal infection. It provides no information that is useful clinically in treating an individual patient.

PATHOGENESIS Little is known of the events which allow staphylococci to invade host tissues. Though strains of staphylococci are common skin and mucous membrane inhabitants, an enormous number of bacteria must be used to establish experimental infections in animals or humans, and more than a million organisms are necessary to produce serious infection in most laboratory animals. The inoculum required to produce infection is greatly reduced in the presence of a foreign body. More than 50 percent of serious staphylococcal infections of deep tissues arise from cutaneous foci, and a smaller number originate in the respiratory or genitourinary tract. Direct inoculation of staphylococci into the bloodstream is also an important route of infection in hospitalized patients with intravenous catheters and in drug addicts. The integument and mucous membranes of heroin addicts and insulin-using diabetics appear to have a unique susceptibility to colonization by *S. aureus.*

Staphylococcal disease is more common in patients with *diabetes, liver disease, renal failure,* and severe *debilitation* and/or *malnutrition.* When skin continuity is broken through *abrasions, wounds, insect bites, burns, exfoliative dermatitis,* or *chronic skin diseases,* the areas affected are commonly infected with staphylococci. *Influenza, measles,* and *cystic fibrosis* appear to predispose to primary staphylococcal invasion of the lung. Patients receiving *broad-spectrum antimicrobial therapy* also appear to have a higher incidence of staphylococcal disease.

Staphylococci often invade the integument via hair follicles and sebaceous glands. When skin continuity has been breached, local microbial multiplication is accompanied by inflammation and tissue necrosis at the site of infection. Polymorphonuclear leukocytes rapidly enter the area and ingest large numbers of staphylococci. Thrombosis of surrounding capillaries occurs; fibrin is deposited about the periphery; and, later, fibroblasts create a relatively avascular wall about the area. The fully developed staphylococcal lesion consists of a central core of dead and dying leukocytes and bacteria which gradually liquefies to form characteristic thick, creamy pus, surrounded by a fibroblastic wall.

When host mechanisms fail to contain the cutaneous or subcutaneous infection, staphylococci may enter the bloodstream. Common sites of metastatic seeding are the diaphyseal ends of long bones in children, lungs, kidneys, endocardium, myocardium, liver, spleen, and brain.

Certain biologic properties of staphylococci appear to contribute to pathogenicity. Many *S. aureus* strains elaborate an *exotoxin* (alpha toxin) capable of causing dermal necrosis in animals. Fever, tachycardia, cyanosis, shock, and death ensue when exotoxin is administered to experimental animals, a picture similar to that seen occasionally in certain fulminating cases of staphylococcal bacteremia in human beings. A delta toxin also has been incriminated in the pathogenesis of severe staphylococcal infection. However, the exact role played by both of these toxins remains uncertain. About 40 percent of *S. aureus* lysed by phages in group II produce an exotoxin that causes intraepidermal cleavage and bulla formation.

The high correlation between *coagulase* production and virulence suggests that this substance is important in the pathogenesis of staphylococcal infections. Coagulase has been said to protect staphylococci from phagocytosis by polymorphonuclear leukocytes, to promote abscess formation in humans and in animal species which have coagulable plasmas, or to protect staphylococci from bacteriostatic substances present in normal serum. However, the precise role of coagulase as a determinant of pathogenicity has not been established.

Some *S. aureus* strains produce a *leukocidin* which destroys human and rabbit leukocytes in vitro. Some strains elaborate *hyaluronidase.* Many staphylococci produce an *enterotoxin* which produces nausea, vomiting, and diarrhea in certain experimental animals and in humans.

In vitro and in vivo studies have indicated that pathogenic staphylococci can survive within human leukocytes, whereas nonpathogenic strains do not. Such intracellular survival may be a means of transporting staphylococci and spreading them to distant tissues. This intracellular survival may also account for the relative refractoriness of staphylococcal infection to antibiotic treatment.

Staphylococcus epidermidis strains appear particularly likely to cause infections in the presence of certain foreign bodies: prosthetic heart valves, CSF shunts, and orthopedic prostheses. The unique ability of some *S. epidermidis* strains to adhere to these foreign surfaces seems to at least partly explain this propensity. *S. epidermidis* has also been responsible for an increasing number of bacteremias in immunosuppressed patients. In some centers, this organism is the most frequent isolate recovered from blood cultures. Many of these bacteremias may be related to extensive and prolonged use of indwelling intravascular devices.

IMMUNITY Some degree of resistance to staphylococcal infections develops with age. For example, primary staphylococcal pneumonia is common in infants but rare in adults. Acute staphylococcal osteomyelitis is almost exclusively a disease of children. Both superficial staphylococcal pyoderma and staphylococcal bacteremia are more frequent in infants, while actual abscess formation occurs more often in adults.

Intact polymorphonuclear leukocytes capable of normal chemotaxis, ingestion, and killing appear to be the major protective mechanism against staphylococcal infections. Persons with inherited or acquired defects in any of these leukocyte functions are particularly susceptible to staphylococcal infections (see Chap. 57). Coagulase-positive staphylococci have a characteristic cell wall teichoic acid, which may be antiphagocytic. Certain unusual strains possess a definite mucopolysaccharide capsular structure which impedes phagocytosis, and specific opsonizing antibody is required for the ingestion of these unusual strains. A number of antistaphylococcal antibodies have been shown to pass from mother to fetus, and the incidence of a variety of antibodies rapidly rises with age. Virtually 100 percent of adults possess antibodies to several staphylococcal antigens in their serum. Nevertheless, the role of humoral immunity in modifying or protecting against staphylococcal infection is uncertain. Immunization of animals with alpha toxin, toxoids, coagulase, or whole staphylococci may prolong experimental staphylococcal infection but does not protect against eventual death. There has been no satisfactory demonstration that human staphylococcal disease is followed by immunity or that infection can be modified significantly by vaccination.

EPIDEMIOLOGY *Staphylococcus aureus* transiently colonizes the nasopharynx of 70 to 90 percent of individuals and resides relatively permanently in the anterior nares of 20 to 30 percent. Nasal carriage often leads to skin colonization as well. Hospital patients and personnel have significantly higher staphylococcal carrier rates than the general population.

While staphylococci remain viable for long periods in dust, blankets, or clothing, and viable staphylococci are often demonstrable in the environment by air-sampling techniques, the significance of airborne transmission remains uncertain, and the best evidence suggests that direct person-to-person contact is the most important means of transmission of staphylococci. Most often, staphylococci are carried from patient to patient on the hands of hospital workers who neglect handwashing. Patients or hospital employees with active staphylococcal infections are probably a more serious source of cross infection than the simple carrier state. However, in some circumstances asymptomatic nasal carriers have been the source of staphylococcal infections. The factors which cause some staphylococcal carriers to become dangerous disseminators remain poorly understood. Discontinuation of the use of hexachlorophene in hospital nurseries has been associated with an increase in infection in some hospitals, and it is apparent that continued surveillance is necessary to thwart the development of epidemics of staphylococcal infection.

Certain phage types of staphylococci have been associated with intrahospital infections. Some strains, particularly antibiotic-resistant strains in phage group III, appear to have greater "epidemic virulence" than other staphylococci. In specific hospitals, one phage type often emerges and may cause most of the serious intrahospital infections. Such "epidemic strains" have shifted from time to time and vary from hospital to hospital. In other hospitals, multiple phage types cause infection. The high incidence of active staphylococcal disease in carriers of certain strains (e.g., the 80/81 strains) suggests that some staphylococci may possess higher virulence for humans than others. Some of the decrease in the frequency of staphylococcal infection in hospitals has been attributed to the disappearance of 80/81 strains.

ANTIMICROBIAL RESISTANCE In the past, the introduction of new antibiotics active against staphylococci has generally been followed by the appearance of staphylococci specifically resistant to that agent. When penicillin was first introduced, fewer than 10 percent of staphylococcal strains isolated from patients or carriers were resistant. Now 60 to 90 percent of staphylococci isolated from hospitalized patients throughout the western world are resistant to penicillin G, and the incidence of infection due to penicillinase-producing strains in nonhospitalized individuals is almost as high. The prevalence of resistance to a specific antimicrobial has correlated closely with the frequency of its administration, and the emergence of resistant strains has followed the use of most antibiotics. Vancomycin, first employed in 1958, and the penicillinase-resistant penicillins and the cephalosporins, both introduced in the 1960s, have been exceptions to this rule. In general, these agents have retained a high degree of activity against both penicillin-sensitive and penicillin-resistant staphylococci. However, methicillin-resistant *S. aureus* (MRSA) strains have become increasingly common in Europe and Scandinavia, where up to 25 percent or more of isolates are resistant. In the United States, a marked increase in the number of isolates of MRSA has been noted since 1975. One-third of hospitals surveyed have experienced cases of bacteremia caused by MRSA. The reported frequency of nosocomial bacteremia caused by MRSA doubled between 1975 and 1980. Outbreaks of serious infections (bacteremia, osteomyelitis, pneumonitis, and wound infection) and deaths due to MRSA have been described. The isolates have been resistant to most antibiotics except vancomycin and rifampin. When typable, the isolates have usually belonged to phage group III.

MANIFESTATIONS **Superficial infections** Simple infection of hair follicles manifested by a minute erythematous nodule without involvement of the surrounding skin or deeper tissues is termed *folliculitis.* A more extensive and invasive follicular or sebaceous gland infection with some involvement of subcutaneous tissues is termed a *furuncle,* or *boil.* Itching and mild pain are followed by progressive local swelling and erythema, and the overlying skin becomes exquisitely painful on pressure or motion. Relief of pain occurs promptly after spontaneous or surgical drainage.

Furuncles occur most commonly on the face, neck, axillas, forearms, buttocks, thighs, breast, upper back, and labia. The acne of adolescence is frequently complicated by secondary furunculosis. Staphylococcal infection may involve the sweat glands in the axilla or groin *(hidradenitis suppurativa).* These infections may be deep-seated, slow to localize and drain, and are liable to recurrence and scarring.

Staphylococcal infections within the thick, fibrous, inelastic skin of the back of the neck and upper part of the back lead to formation of a *carbuncle.* The relative thickness and impermeability of the overlying skin lead to lateral extension and loculation, and a large, indurated, painful lesion with multiple ineffective drainage sites results. These extensive lesions appear more frequently among diabetics. Carbuncles produce fever, leukocytosis, extreme pain, and prostration. Bacteremia is common.

Staphylococci frequently colonize impetiginous lesions, but most impetigo in children and adults is due to group A streptococci. However, staphylococcal impetigo does occur, and while it cannot be clearly differentiated from streptococcal impetigo clinically, it tends to produce more localized disease, has a grayish rather than golden yellow crust, and less often produces high fever and lymphadenitis.

One form of impetigo characteristically caused by *S. aureus* is bullous impetigo. This disease represents one of several exfoliative staphylococcal pyodermas. *Staphylococcus aureus* strains lysed by group II phages, usually type 71, cause this group of diseases through production of an exotoxin (exfoliatin), which produces separation of the epidermis at the granular cell layer. Production of this exotoxin is plasmid-mediated.

Several clinical syndromes have been associated with exfoliative toxin-producing strains. Local pyoderma may be followed by a tender, scarlatiniform, finely desquamative rash that can be localized or generalized (staphylococcal scarlet fever). This rash resembles that described as part of the toxic shock syndrome (see below). Bullous impetigo is the more severe form of this disease. Characteristically, local pyoderma precedes the sudden onset of generalized erythema, fever, and leukocytosis. Several days later large flaccid bullae form and then burst, resulting in red, denuded skin resembling a burn. The syndrome may be localized or rarely generalized (toxic epidermal necrolysis, Ritter's syndrome, Lyell's disease, or scalded skin syndrome). In the localized form, staphylococci can usually be recovered from the bullous lesions, while in the generalized form they usually cannot be.

Osteomyelitis Staphylococci are responsible for the majority of cases of *acute osteomyelitis.* This infection occurs most commonly in children under the age of 12, but adults also are susceptible to acute osteomyelitis, especially of the spine. There appears to have been a sharp decrease in the incidence of acute osteomyelitis since the introduction of antibiotics. Approximately 50 percent of patients give a history of a furuncle or superficial staphylococcal infection preceding osteomyelitis. Bone involvement follows hematogenous dissemination of bacteria. In children, the frequent localization in the diaphyseal end of long bones is thought to be due to the endarterial circulation of the diaphysis. Many patients give a history of preceding trauma to the involved area. For example, cases of clavicular osteomyelitis secondary to infected subclavian catheters have been reported.

Once established, infection spreads through the newly formed juxtaepiphyseal bone to the periosteum or along the marrow cavity. If the infection reaches the subperiosteal space, the periosteum is lifted, a subperiosteal abscess forms, and rupture with infection of the subcutaneous tissues may occur. Rarely, the joint capsule is penetrated, producing a pyogenic arthritis. There is death of bone, producing a *sequestrum,* followed by new bone formation, the *involucrum.*

Occasionally indolent staphylococcal infections of bone remain localized within dense granulation tissue about a central necrotic cavity. Such a local infection may persist for years as a so-called Brodie's abscess.

Osteomyelitis in children may present as an acute process beginning abruptly with chills, high fever, nausea, vomiting, and progressive pain at the site of bony involvement. Muscle spasm about the affected bone is a common early sign of osteomyelitis, and the child may refuse to move the affected limb. Leukocytosis is the rule. Blood cultures are positive for staphylococci in 50 to 60 percent of cases early in the disease. The tissues overlying the involved bone become edematous and warm, and the skin becomes erythematous and shiny. Anemia develops during the course of untreated disease. Roentgenograms are usually normal during the first week, but radionucleide scans may be abnormal. Bony rarefaction, local periosteal elevation, and new bone formation can frequently be seen during the second week.

Staphylococcal spinal infection in the adult differs considerably from acute osteomyelitis in the child. The onset is less abrupt, and there is a greater tendency for bony fusion with obliteration of the disk space (see Chap. 344).

DIAGNOSIS Osteomyelitis should be suspected in any child with fever, limb pain, and leukocytosis. Similarly, neck or back pain in an adult, when accompanied by fever, should raise the possibility of acute osteomyelitis or a disk space infection. History of a preceding cutaneous infection, local tenderness over the bone, and the finding of *S. aureus* in blood cultures are confirmatory. In early stages, osteomyelitis must be differentiated from acute rheumatic fever and pyogenic arthritis. Gram-negative bacilli and mycobacteria are relatively more common causes of osteomyelitis in adults compared with children. Procedures such as needle aspiration or biopsy of bone should be performed to obtain a specific etiologic diagnosis prior to initiation of chemotherapy.

PROGNOSIS Before the advent of antimicrobials, the overall mortality was approximately 25 percent. Death was more common in individuals with demonstrable bacteremia. Chronic osteomyelitis with recurrent activation and metastatic foci in other bones was common. However, acute staphylococcal osteomyelitis is declining in incidence, death is rare, and chronic osteomyelitis is also becoming less frequent.

Staphylococcal pneumonia Staphylococci are the cause of approximately 1 percent of bacterial pneumonias acquired outside hospitals. This disease occurs sporadically except during epidemics of influenza, when staphylococcal pneumonia is more common, although even then it is not as frequent as pneumococcal infection.

Primary staphylococcal pneumonia in infants and young children frequently causes pyopneumothorax, and pneumatoceles occur early and should suggest *S. aureus* infection. In older children and healthy adults staphylococcal pneumonia is generally preceded by an influenza-like respiratory infection (influenza, measles, or other viruses). Onset of staphylococcal involvement is abrupt, with chills, high fever, progressive dyspnea, cyanosis, cough, and pleural pain. Early peripheral vascular collapse is common, and examination frequently reveals a patient who seems sicker than the physical findings would suggest. Sputum in the early phases is not characteristic but may be bloody or frankly purulent. Admixture with blood may produce a thick, creamy pink sputum.

Staphylococci are one of the causes of pneumonia occurring in hospitalized patients. These infections usually begin insidiously. Increasing fever, tachycardia, and an elevated respiratory rate may be the only indications of infection. Typical pneumonic symptoms may be absent. The disease is also less abrupt when pulmonary involvement occurs during the course of staphylococcal bacteremia, as may be the case in drug addicts or in patients with endocarditis. Staphylococci generally produce patchy, centrally located areas of pneumonia. Pleural involvement and empyema are common. Many of these patients developing nosocomial staphylococcal pneumonia have chronic lung disease, leukemia, mucoviscidosis, or other debilitating diseases.

Because of the central pulmonary involvement, chest findings are variable. Signs of frank consolidation are rare. Scattered fine to coarse rales and rhonchi may be heard over the involved areas. Empyema produces typical signs of pleural fluid. Signs of abscess may appear late in the course of the disease. Bacteremia is not common in primary staphylococcal pneumonia (less than 20 percent of patients), and *its presence should suggest that the pneumonic involvement is metastatic and secondary to foci of infection elsewhere.*

The course of staphylococcal pneumonia may be stormy despite adequate antimicrobial therapy. Gradual defervescence starting 48 to 72 h after the initiation of therapy is the rule. Pulmonary abscesses or empyema cavities may require surgical treatment.

DIAGNOSIS Staphylococcal pneumonia must be differentiated from other pneumonias. The preceding influenza-like illness, rapid onset of pleural pain, cyanosis, and prostration out of proportion to physical findings should suggest primary staphylococcal pneumonia. The finding of masses of polymorphonuclear leukocytes and gram-positive intraleukocytic cocci strongly suggests the diagnosis. The blood leukocyte count is generally above 15,000 per cubic millimeter. When pneumonia develops suddenly or insidiously, with higher fever, tachycardia, and leukocytosis, in debilitated hospitalized patients receiving antimicrobials, staphylococci should be strongly considered as the etiologic agent.

PROGNOSIS Before 1942, mortality ranged from 50 to 95 percent. The presence of bacteremia was almost invariably associated with a fatal outcome. The prognosis has improved with the use of antimicrobials, but some patients continue to die with staphylococcal pneumonia, especially debilitated individuals acquiring staphylococcal pneumonia in the hospital. Abscess formation and pleural involvement often prolong convalescence.

Staphylococcal bacteremia Staphylococcal bacteremia may arise from any local staphylococcal infection. Infections of the skin (including infections about inlying venous cutdowns or catheters), respiratory tract, bones, or genitourinary tract precede bacteremia. Trauma to local lesions, such as pinching, or surgical drainage before adequate localization may precipitate bacteremia.

Rarely, patients with bacteremia die in 12 to 24 h, with high fever, tachycardia, cyanosis, gastrointestinal symptoms, and vascular collapse. Commonly, the disease progresses more slowly, with hectic fever and metastatic abscess formation in the skin, bones, kidneys, brain, lungs, myocardium, spleen, or other tissues. *Meningitis* is an occasional complication.

Endocarditis (see Chap. 259) may occur in patients with protracted bacteremia. Normal heart valves are frequently involved, the aortic being the most frequent. Typically, staphylococcal endocarditis runs an acute course with high fever, progressive anemia, and metastatic abscesses in the skin and deeper structures. Rupture of the valve leaflets and valve ring abscesses are common. Specific diagnosis of endocardial involvement is difficult; because of its frequency, it should be assumed to be present in patients with staphylococcal bacteremia with demonstrable cutaneous lesions (petechiae or cutaneous pustules) and a significant heart murmur. Echocardiography may facilitate diagnosis if valvular vegetations can be demonstrated. At times, especially among addicts with right-sided valvular lesions, a significant heart murmur may not be audible. In these patients, septic pulmonary emboli often produce chest pain, hemoptysis, and multiple small pulmonary infiltrates. Both *S. aureus* and *S. epidermidis* have been major causes of endocarditis in patients undergoing cardiac surgical procedures, particularly valve replacement. Both coagulase-positive and coagulase-negative staphylococci occasionally produce a subacute endocarditis indistinguishable from that produced by *Streptococcus viridans.* Persistent *Staphylococcus epidermidis* bacteremia has also been common after ventriculoatriostomy.

Staphylococcal bacteremia is generally accompanied by a polymorphonuclear leukocytosis of 12,000 to 20,000 per cubic millimeter, but a normal leukocyte count or leukopenia is occasionally seen. Although a low-yield procedure, diagnosis of bacteremia may be aided by a Gram stain of buffy coat which discloses staphylococci within the cytoplasm of polymorphonuclear cells. Anemia develops rapidly during the course of the illness. Cyanosis and hypoxemia may be seen with staphylococcal bacteremia, even in the absence of significant pulmonary lesions on chest roentgenogram. Demonstration of antibodies to the staphylococcal cell wall component teichoic acid by counterimmunoelectrophoresis or gel diffusion and detection of circulating immune complexes may be of value in identifying patients who have endocarditis or other deep-seated infection.

PROGNOSIS Staphylococcal bacteremia is an extremely serious disease. Before the development of antimicrobials, over 80 percent of individuals died, the majority within 10 days of the onset of illness. The development of endocarditis or meningitis during bacteremia was almost invariably fatal. The sulfonamides produced little alteration in this mortality rate. With the administration of effective antibiotics and appropriate surgical treatment of local sites of infection, 50 to 70 percent of patients survive. With left-sided endocarditis, the fatality/case ratio is 30 percent. The prognosis for drug addicts with right-sided endocarditis appears particularly good; only 10 percent die. However, when staphylococcal endocarditis has occurred on a prosthetic cardiac valve, the outcome has been almost invariably fatal unless reconstructive surgery can be performed. Early surgical intervention is indicated in such cases.

Staphylococcal food poisoning See Chap. 142.

Genitourinary infections *Staphylococcus aureus* rarely causes urinary tract infections by retrograde spread from the bladder. Hence, the isolation of *S. aureus* from a well-collected urine specimen should prompt a search for renal, perinephric, or prostatic abscesses secondary to bacteremic staphylococcal infection elsewhere. Diabetics, drug addicts, and patients with valve prostheses are particularly prone to this complication. One group of coagulase-negative staphylococci has been increasingly recognized as a cause of acute lower urinary tract infection in young women. These strains have the unique characteristic of being novobiocin- and nalidixic acid–resistant and have been given a specific species designation *(S. saprophyticus).*

Toxic shock syndrome Toxic shock syndrome (TSS) is a newly described clinical entity with serious morbidity and mortality affecting primarily menstrual-age women. Clinical features of TSS reflect multisystem involvement with fever, hypotension, a diffuse macular erythematous rash which desquamates, vomiting or diarrhea, myalgia, renal or hepatic insufficiency, thrombocytopenia, disorientation, and mucous membrane inflammation. Approximately 80 percent of cases occur among women under 30 years of age, and only 10 percent of cases are seen in postmenopausal women or in men. Fatality/case ratio has been 10 to 15 percent. The diagnosis of TSS is based on clinical criteria. Differential diagnoses include Rocky Mountain spotted fever, meningococcemia, scarlet fever, erythema multiforme, drug eruption, and leptospirosis. Several similarities exist between TSS and Kawasaki disease (mucocutaneous lymph node syndrome), especially the desquamating rash, fever, and mucosal inflammation. Other features of Kawasaki disease (age less than 5 years, enlarged cervical lymph nodes, and involvement of coronary arteries) are not characteristic of TSS. Up to 30 percent of patients experience more than one episode of TSS, although recurrent episodes have been generally milder in nature.

A strong correlation was found between TSS and the recovery of *S. aureus* from vaginal cultures of affected patients. The organism has been recovered less often from other mucosal sites and only on rare occasions from the bloodstream of TSS patients. The appearance of the rash, the association with *S. aureus,* and the infrequency of bacteremia suggested that a staphylococcal toxin was responsible. New toxins, pyrogenic exotoxin C, and enterotoxin F have been found to be markers for TSS. The toxins are distinct from previously characterized staphylococcal toxins. It is not clear whether these toxins alone are responsible for all the manifestations of TSS. Another strong correlation was menstruation and the onset of TSS. Most patients were previously healthy women who became ill during the first few days of the menstrual cycle. While an association between TSS and tampon use seems likely, it has not been determined how prolonged tampon use might promote vaginal colonization with *S. aureus,* but women with TSS were urged to discontinue or limit tampon use. One brand of tampon, statistically associated with TSS, was withdrawn from the market. In 1981 the number of reported cases decreased dramatically.

Treatment of TSS is directed at the serious manifestations of the illness including the shock, adult respiratory distress syndrome, and renal or hepatic failure. Some patients have developed disseminated intravascular coagulation. Antibiotics are indicated, although it is not certain what role they play in recovery from TSS. The *S. aureus* isolates have been uniformly sensitive to antibiotics with the exception of penicillin and ampicillin. The value of corticosteroids in the treatment of TSS is controversial.

Miscellaneous infections Staphylococci may cause conjunctivitis, otitis, sinusitis, or mastoid infections as well as infection in and around the orbit. Epidemics of staphylococcal pyoderma in newborn infants and maternal breast abscesses are a recurring problem in maternity units.

TREATMENT **Features of staphylococcal infection which influence therapy** While the development of penicillinase-resistant penicillins and cephalosporins has simplified treatment, certain characteristics of staphylococcal disease should be borne in mind in designing therapy.

1 *The host setting in which infection occurs.* Acute staphylococcal infections arising outside the hospital in otherwise healthy adults have a better prognosis than intrahospital infections arising in sick individuals with compromised host defense mechanisms.
2 *The rapid necrosis of tissues produced by staphylococci.* Delays in effective therapy may allow a progressing infection to advance to frank abscess formation. While many antimicrobials reach abscess cavities in adequate concentrations, the physiologic insusceptibility of microorganisms residing in the areas of extensive necrosis or suppuration renders antibiotic therapy quite ineffective in this situation. Surgical drainage of such lesions is often required.
3 *The sluggish response to therapy.* Staphylococci are killed slowly by antimicrobials, and relapses are frequent. Hence antimicrobial therapy must be continued longer than in many bacterial infections.
4 *The problem of antimicrobial resistance.* While treatment must be initiated empirically when serious staphylococcal infection is suspected, rational therapy requires that the antibiotic susceptibility of the infecting strain be known. The recent rise in isolations of staphylococci not inhibited by penicillinase-resistant penicillins further emphasizes the importance of confirming antibiotic susceptibility.

Treatment of serious staphylococcal infections The effectiveness of the penicillinase-resistant penicillins has simplified the approach to life-threatening staphylococcal disease. Since nearly all strains of staphylococci are susceptible to penicillinase-resistant penicillins, and because of the high incidence of penicillinase-producing staphylococci as causes of infection, most authorities initiate treatment with methicillin, oxacillin, or nafcillin alone, shifting to aqueous penicillin G if the strain is subsequently proved to be susceptible to that drug. Because of less interstitial nephritis and fewer other adverse reactions and an identical spectrum of activity, many physicians use nafcillin or oxacillin (1 or 2 g every 4 h) rather than methicillin (2 g every 4 h). For penicillin-sensitive strains, adults should be given aqueous penicillin, 20 million units, by continuous infusion.

Despite differences in structure, the major allergenic properties of the penicillins reside in the 6-aminopenicillanic acid molecule. There is significant cross allergenicity between penicillins, and patients who have had well-established allergic reactions to penicillin G should not receive any type of penicillin antibiotic. Further, there is increasing evidence that a significant number of these individuals may react to the cephalosporin derivatives as well. These agents, which are good antistaphylococcal drugs, have a 7-aminocephalosporanic acid nucleus quite similar to that of penicillins and should be used with caution in patients with prior reactions to penicillin.

Several cephalosporins can be given parenterally for treatment of serious staphylococcal infections. Cephalothin is highly active against both penicillin-sensitive and penicillin-resistant strains; intramuscular or intravenous doses of 1 to 2 g every 4 h are recommended. The usual dose of cefazolin for severe staphylococcal infection is 1 g every 6 h intramuscularly or intravenously, and the dose and route of administration for cephapirin are similar. Nephrotoxicity and an increased susceptibility to penicillinase limit the usefulness of cephaloridine. The newer antibiotics such as cefamandole, cefoxitin, and cefotaxime offer no advantage over older cephalosporins for treatment of stahylococcal infections. Cephalosporins should not be used in the treatment of serious staphylococcal infections caused by methicillin-resistant strains of *S. aureus* or *S. epidermidis.* Such strains are generally resistant to cephalosporins despite disk-diffusion results that may indicate sensitivity.

Vancomycin is uniformly active against most staphylococci regardless of their sensitivity to penicillin. It should be given intravenously in doses of 1 to 1.5 g over a 30- to 40-min period every 12 h.

The development of these new agents has relegated several antibiotics formerly used in treatment to minor or secondary roles. Lincomycin, clindamycin, and erythromycin are still useful in certain circumstances, but are not front-line agents in staphylococcal bacteremia. They are used primarily in patients allergic to penicillin.

Changes in therapy Established staphylococcal infections repond slowly even to the most effective antimicrobial regimens, making it difficult to know when therapy should be considered inadequate. Characteristically, 24 to 48 h elapse before a decline in fever is noted, and recovery is accompanied by slow return of the temperature to normal in 7 to 10 days.

Special therapeutic situations ASYMPTOMATIC NASAL CARRIER STATE The role of asymptomatic carriers in hospital transmission of infection remains controversial. Many hospital personnel carry *S. aureus* in their anterior nares but do not appear to disseminate the strain. However, some persons readily disseminate their strain and are a cause of nosocomial infections. Unfortunately, simple methods for recognition of such "dangerous disseminators" are not available, and they are most often detected when increased numbers of *S. aureus* infections prompt an epidemiologic investigation. It is generally agreed that disseminators must be removed from nursery units, operating theaters, delivery rooms, and surgical floors. Although no method of treatment has been uniformly satisfactory, the following regimens have had limited success in treatment of nasal carriers.

1 Simple removal from the hospital environment for 3 to 4 weeks
2 Frequent baths with germicidal soaps
3 The use of topical antibiotics of low sensitizing potential in a water-soluble base (i.e., bacitracin, neomycin, gentamicin, or a combination of these agents) four to five times daily for 2 weeks

If the carrier state returns, a second course of treatment is indicated. Rifampin has had some success in eradicating methicillin-resistant staphylococci from persons who are persistent asymptomatic carriers.

SUPERFICIAL INFECTIONS Superficial infections frequently do not require the use of antibiotics. There is no adequate therapy for recurrent furunculosis, but if the disease is severe, antimicrobial treatment may be attempted. Antibiotics to which the strain is susceptible should be administered systemically for a minimum of 10 to 14 days. Cloxacillin (2 g per day divided into four doses) or dicloxacillin (2 g per day divided into four doses) can usually be used. Local moist heat, immobilization of the infected part, and incision and drainage should be utilized. The surrounding skin should be protected with a coating of zinc oxide to prevent maceration. Treatment of the nasal carrier state by the local application of topical antibiotics (see above) may be advisable. Careful daily baths with germicidal soaps, attention to personal and family hygiene, and the passage of time appear to be measures most likely to interrupt the process. Attempts to prevent recurrence by autogenous or other vaccines have not been effective.

EMPYEMA Empyema should be treated by aspiration, generally with a large-bore tube since loculation and thick exudate may prevent adequate needle drainage. Intravenous antibiotics as already outlined for serious infections should be given. While the local instillation of proteolytic enzymes may occasionally aid in liquefying the exudate, surgical drainage is generally necessary and should be performed promptly.

OSTEOMYELITIS The initial regimen already outlined for other serious infections is recommended, and treatment should be continued for 14 to 28 days in acute osteomyelitis. Local drainage of abscess cavities in soft tissues or bones should be considered in all patients in whom severe pain persists or when response to antimicrobials is inadequate. If sequestration occurs, devitalized bone should be removed. Lincomycin has been reported to be superior to other agents in the treatment of chronic osteomyelitis, but the evidence for this is not convincing. The optimal duration of treatment in established chronic infection is not known, but frequently several months of antimicrobial therapy are recommended.

BACTEREMIA AND ENDOCARDITIS Most authorities recommend 4 to 6 weeks of parenteral antibiotic therapy in proved or suspected staphylococcal endocarditis. However, shorter courses of therapy may be successful, especially in drug addicts with tricuspid endocarditis. In some centers, gentamicin is given with a penicillinase-resistant penicillin in an attempt to kill staphylococci more rapidly. When staphylococcal bacteremia occurs secondary to a removable focus of localized infection (an abscess or an infected intravenous catheter), 10 to 14 days of parenteral therapy is probably sufficient provided the patient has no clinical evidence of endocarditis and demonstrates prompt clinical improvement.

REFERENCES

BAYER AS, GUZE LB: *Staphylococcus aureus* bacteremic syndromes: Diagnostic and therapeutic update. Dis Mon, June 1979

Conference: The toxic shock syndrome. Ann Intern Med 96 (Part 2):831, 1982

HALEY RW et al: The emergence of methicillin-resistant *Staphylococcus aureus* in United States hospitals. Ann Intern Med 97:297, 1982

LOCKSLEY RM et al: Multiply antibiotic resistant *Staphylococcus aureus:* Introduction, transmission and evolution of nosocomial infection. Ann Intern Med 97:317, 1982

MUSHER DM, MCKENZIE SO: Infections due to *Staphylococcus aureus.* Medicine 56:383, 1977

NOLAN CM, BEATY HN: *S. aureus* bacteremia: Current clinical patterns. Am J Med 60:495, 1976

SHANDS K: Toxic shock syndrome, in *Update IV: Harrison's Principles of Internal Medicine,* KJ Isselbacher et al (eds). New York, McGraw-Hill, 1982, pp 1–8

SORRELL TS et al: Vancomycin therapy for methicillin-resistant *Staphylococcus aureus.* Ann Intern Med 97:344, 1982

TOFTE RW, WILLIAMS DN: Toxic shock syndrome: Clinical and laboratory features in 15 patients. Ann Intern Med 94:149, 1981

148 STREPTOCOCCAL INFECTIONS

ALAN L. BISNO

Streptococci are among the commonest bacterial pathogens of humans. They are responsible for a diverse spectrum of diseases including pharyngitis and tonsillitis, scarlet fever, erysipelas, impetigo, lymphangitis, and perinatal infections of mother and child. Certain representatives of this genus are prominent causes of endocarditis and urinary tract infections. In addition to their role in causing acute pyogenic infections, strains of *Streptococcus pyogenes* are capable of giving rise to the delayed nonsuppurative sequels of acute rheumatic fever and acute glomerulonephritis.

ETIOLOGY AND CLASSIFICATION Streptococci are spherical or ovoid bacterial cells which grow in pairs or chains of varying lengths. Most are facultative anaerobes, although some are strict anaerobes. The organisms are gram-positive, usually nonmotile, non-spore-forming, and catalase-negative. No single system of classification suffices to differentiate this heterogeneous group of organisms. Instead, classification depends upon a combination of features, including patterns of hemolysis observed on blood agar plates, antigenic composition, growth characteristics, and biochemical reactions.

When cultivated on blood agar plates, streptococci may produce one of three different patterns of hemolysis. Alpha-hemolytic colonies are surrounded by a zone of partial hemolysis; in addition, such organisms usually produce a greenish discoloration in the medium due to the presence of an unidentified reductant of hemoglobin. This greening reaction gives rise to the designation "viridans" streptococcus, which is often applied to alpha-hemolytic strains. Strains of *S. pneumoniae* are alpha-hemolytic, as are many other streptococci which normally inhabit the upper respiratory and gastrointestinal tracts. Beta-hemolytic colonies are surrounded by clear colorless zones within which the red blood cells in the medium have been completely lysed. This pattern of complete hemolysis is exhibited by *S. pyogenes* and many of the other streptococci pathogenic for humans. Gamma streptococci are those which fail to produce hemolysis upon blood agar plates.

Although classification of streptococci on the basis of hemolytic reactions is quite useful in certain clinical situations, more precise identification of streptococci is accomplished by differentiation into serogroups, as originally described by Lancefield, on the basis of antigenic differences in cell wall carbohydrates or teichoic acids. These antigens are readily extracted from streptococcal cell walls and identified by precipitin reactions using specific antiserums. Groups A to H and K to T are recognized. The vast majority of beta-hemolytic streptococci isolated from human sources belongs to groups A to D, F, and G. Although the Lancefield grouping system was initially devised for identification of beta-hemolytic streptococci, certain alpha-hemolytic and nonhemolytic strains also contain group-specific antigens. The most important of these are the group D streptococci, including the so-called enterococci, among which many strains fail to show beta hemolysis. There are 21 recognized species of streptococci. Species designation is based upon growth characteristics under varying conditions of temperature, pH, and media composition. Five species do not possess group antigens, and, conversely, a number of serogroups do not encompass any of the recognized species.

Anaerobic and microaerophilic streptococci include members of the family Peptococceae, genus *Peptostreptococcus*; five species are recognized. Hemolytic reactions of these organisms are variable, and no satisfactory method of classifying them has been devised.

GROUP A STREPTOCOCCAL INFECTIONS

Streptococci of Lancefield's group A (*S. pyogenes*) are responsible for the great majority of human streptococcal infections and are uniquely important because of their role as precursors of rheumatic fever and glomerulonephritis.

ETIOLOGY The *group-specific carbohydrate* of group A streptococci is a polymer of rhamnose and *N*-acetylglucosamine. There are approximately 80 recognized and provisionsal group A serotypes. The typing system is based upon antigenic differences in a cell wall constituent known as *M protein,* which is the principal virulence factor of group A organisms. Strains rich in M protein are highly resistant to phagocytosis by polymorphonuclear leukocytes in vitro and are capable of initiating disease in humans and experimental animals. Strains lacking M protein are avirulent. Acquired human immunity to streptococcal infection is based upon development of opsonic antibodies directed against the antiphagocytic moiety of M protein. This immunity is type-specific and lasts for many years, perhaps indefinitely. M protein is a macromolecule which contains, in addition to the type-specific determinant, a variety of non-type-specific antigens which are widely shared by strains of differing serotypes. *T protein* serves as the basis of a subsidiary typing system which has been useful in classifying strains not typable by the M systems; unlike M protein, the T antigen plays no role in virulence. *Lipoteichoic acid,* a substance which has a marked affinity for biological membranes, has been found to play a crucial role in colonization by binding group A streptococci to specific receptor sites on human epithelial cells. The streptococcal *cell membrane* contains a number of antigenic structures, certain of which have been reported to share determinants with constituents of human heart and with basement membrane of the renal glomerulus. Group A streptococci are enveloped in a slimy *hyaluronic acid capsule* which serves to retard phagocytosis and, therefore, represents an accessory virulence factor. Streptococcal hyaluronate is nonantigenic in humans, presumably because it is identical to that found in human connective tissue.

As streptococci grow in vitro or in vivo, they elaborate a number of extracellular products, a few of which require mention. *Erythrogenic toxin (pyrogenic exotoxin),* which is induced by lysogeny with a temperate bacteriophage, is responsible for the rash of scarlet fever. There are three serologically distinct toxins, the effects of which may be neutralized by antibody. Two distinct hemolysins are elaborated. *Streptolysin O* is reversibly inhibited by oxygen (hence exerting its effect primarily on subsurface colonies) and irreversibly inhibited by cholesterol. It is produced by almost all group A strains as well as by many group C and G organisms. Titration of antistreptolysin O (ASO) antibodies in human serums is the most widely used serologic procedure to detect group A streptococcal infection in clinical practice. Hemolysis on the surface of blood agar plates is due primarily to the action of *streptolysin S.* Although streptolysin S differs from streptolysin O in being oxygen-stable and nonantigenic, both hemolysins possess the capacity to damage membranes of polymorphonuclear leukocytes, platelets, and subcellular organelles. A number of other extracellular products exert effects which might serve to facilitate the organisms' survival in vivo by liquefying pus [streptokinase and deoxyribonucleases (DNases) A to D] or by allowing spread through tissue planes (*hyaluronidase* and *proteinase*). The role of these substances in streptococcal virulence remains unproved.

The two most frequent types of group A streptococcal infection are pharyngitis and pyoderma. They differ markedly in their epidemiologic, clinical, and bacteriologic characteristics.

STREPTOCOCCAL PHARYNGITIS Epidemiology The incidence of this ubiquitous infection is highest in children aged 5 to 15 years; males and females are affected equally. The great majority of such infections are due to group A streptococci, but strains of other serogroups, particularly group C or G, are involved occasionally. The organism is ordinarily transmitted directly from person to person, most likely by droplet spread, and crowding markedly facilitates interpersonal transmission. This may account for the increased incidence of streptococcal pharyngitis in northern latitudes during the colder months of the year, as well as for the explosive outbreaks which occur in military recruit camps and other crowded institutional settings. Common-source epidemics of streptococcal sore throat with high attack rates occasionally occur following contamination of a food item with beta-hemolytic streptococci. Environmental reservoirs of streptococci, such as viable organisms in room dust or on blankets, are not important in spread of disease.

Patients with acute streptococcal pharyngitis harbor large numbers of organisms in the anterior nares and throat. If antibiotics are not administered, the organisms may persist in the upper respiratory tract for weeks to months after symptoms have subsided. However, as the length of the carrier state increases, the organisms decrease in number, disappear from the anterior nasal secretions, and lose detectable M protein. Therefore, convalescent carriers are less likely than acutely ill patients to transmit group A streptococci to exposed individuals. Group A pharyngeal carriage rates vary with geographic location, season of the year, and age group. Among school-aged children, rates of 15 to 20 percent have been reported; the carriage rate among adults is considerably lower.

Symptoms The usual incubation period of streptococcal pharyngitis is between 2 and 4 days. The classic syndrome, as observed in older children and adults, is ushered in by the rather abrupt onset of sore throat, manifested particularly by pain on swallowing. Associated symptoms include headache, malaise, feverishness, and anorexia. Chilliness is a frequent symptom, but true rigors are rare. Nausea, vomiting, and abdominal pain are common in children.

Physical signs The patient appears moderately ill with tachycardia and fever which frequently exceeds 38.3°C (101°F). There is diffuse erythema, edema, and lymphoid hyperplasia of the posterior pharynx. The uvula is edematous. The tonsils, if present, are enlarged, reddened, and covered by a punctate or coalescent exudate which may be yellow, gray, or white. Discrete areas of pinhead-size exudate are frequently present on the posterior pharynx but may be concealed by mucopurulent nasal secretions. The anterior cervical lymph nodes at the angles of the jaw are enlarged and tender. Cough and hoarseness, if present, are mild and, in the absence of the signs and symptoms indicated above, do not in themselves suggest the diagnosis of streptococcal pharyngitis. Laryngeal involvement with loss of voice is not a feature of streptococcal infection.

The full-blown clinical syndrome of acute exudative tonsillopharyngitis is seen frequently during explosive epidemics of streptococcal disease, particularly those occurring in institutional settings such as military recruit camps. In endemically occurring infections among civilian populations, however, the illness is frequently much milder. Indeed, in such circumstances, only about half the children with sore throats and positive cultures for group A streptococci will have tonsillar exudate, and a third or less may have fever greater than 38.3°C (101°F) or marked leukocytosis. Patients who have undergone tonsillectomy tend to experience a milder clinical syndrome. In infants, streptococcal upper respiratory infections tend to be less sharply localized to the lymphoid tissue of the faucial and posterior pharyngeal areas. Infections at this age are characterized by rhinorrhea with excoriation of the nares, low-grade fever, anorexia, and a protracted clinical course. Exudative pharyngitis in children less than 3 years of age is rarely streptococcal in etiology.

Course The course of streptococcal pharyngitis is usually brief and self-limited. Fever abates within a week, usually within 3 to 5 days. Constitutional symptoms and sore throat disappear with defervescence or shortly thereafter. Several weeks may be required, however, for the tonsils and lymph nodes to return to normal size.

SCARLET FEVER When streptococcal pharyngitis is due to a lysogenic strain producing erythrogenic toxin, and when the host does not possess neutralizing antibody to the toxin, scarlet fever ensues. The situation may be more complex than was previously thought, because recent studies suggest that a preexisting state of hypersensitivity to streptococcal products may predispose to the development of scarlet fever.

The rash usually appears within 2 days after onset of sore throat, involves first the neck, upper chest, and back, then spreads over the remainder of the trunk and the extremities, and spares the palms and soles. The rash may be difficult to appreciate in black patients. It consists of a diffuse erythema, which blanches on pressure, with numerous 1- to 2-mm punctate elevations that impart a "sandpaper" texture to the skin. Discrete lesions are absent from the face, but there is a generalized facial flush which contrasts with the prominent circumoral pallor. The rash is more intense along skin folds, such as those of the antecubital fossae and axillary folds, and in these locations often produces linear striations of confluent petechiae known as *Pastia's lines.* Increased capillary fragility, which contributes to the formation of Pastia's lines, is confirmed by a positive Rumpel-Leede's test.

The exanthem of scarlet fever is accompanied by an enanthem, consisting of punctate erythema and petechiae on the soft palate. Early in the disease, the tongue is covered with a white coat through which hypertrophied papillae protrude as islands of red (strawberry tongue). By the fourth or fifth day the coating is gone and the entire tongue appears beefy red (raspberry tongue). In rare cases, scarlet fever may be complicated by hepatic involvement with jaundice, pleural effusion, and arthralgia. It is unclear how often arthralgia is a manifestation of scarlet fever or how often it presages the development of rheumatic fever.

The rash usually lasts 4 to 5 days and is followed by extensive desquamation which begins as early as a few days or as late as 3 to 4 weeks after onset of the disease and is often a striking feature of the convalescent phase of scarlet fever.

Although scarlet fever usually follows upper respiratory infection due to group A streptococci, rarely other erythrogenic toxins are produced by streptococci of other groups and by certain strains of staphylococci. Moreover, scarlet fever may follow streptococcal impetigo or secondary streptococcal infection of superficial wounds. The disease must be differentiated from various of the childhood exanthems, toxic shock syndrome, Kawasaki disease, infectious mononucleosis when the latter is associated with rash, and drug eruptions. The management of scarlet fever consists of adequate treatment of the causative infection.

Two tests previously employed in assessment of scarlet fever are no longer in clinical use. The *Dick test* is performed by inoculating erythrogenic toxin intracutaneously. Individuals who are susceptible to the toxin will experience local erythema (positive Dick test), while individuals with antitoxin immunity will have no reaction (negative Dick test). Conversion from a positive to a negative Dick test during the course of a rash illness strongly suggests the diagnosis of scarlet fever. Another test consists of injection of scarlatinal antitoxin into an area of cutaneous rash, which produces blanching if the eruption is due to erythrogenic toxin. This test, previously used for diagnosis of scarlet fever, is known as the Schultz-Charlton reaction.

Complications Streptococcal pharyngitis may give rise to suppurative complications, among which acute otitis media and acute sinusitis are the most frequent. Suppurative cervical lymphadenitis may also occur. Inflammation of the faucial area induced by streptococcal infection may give rise to peritonsillar cellulitis, peritonsillar abscess, or retropharyngeal abscess. The abscesses themselves, however, usually contain a variety of oropharyngeal flora, including anaerobic bacteria, rather than group A streptococci. A variety of other complications, common in the past, are almost never seen in the antibiotic era: (1) extension up the cribriform plate of the ethmoid or via the mastoid, giving rise to meningitis, brain abscess, or thrombosis of cerebral venous sinuses; and (2) bacteremia with metastatic foci of infection such as suppurative arthritis, osteomyelitis, or liver abscess. Much of the intense clinical and investigative interest focused upon streptococcal pharyngitis is due to its association with two delayed nonsuppurative sequels: acute rheumatic fever (ARF) and acute glomerulonephritis (AGN). These are discussed in Chaps. 257 and 294, respectively.

Diagnosis Sore throat due to group A streptococci must be differentiated from that caused by a number of other agents. *Diphtheria* is rare in immunized populations. It is characterized by the presence of an extensive diphtheritic membrane, and in severe cases by respiratory embarrassment due to laryngeal involvement, myocarditis, and cranial nerve palsies. Cultures on Loeffler's medium will be positive for *Corynebacterium diphtheriae.* Gonococcal tonsillopharyngitis should be suggested by a history of homosexuality or fellatio and confirmed by appropriate cultures. *Vincent's angina* is characterized by sore throat and tonsillopharyngeal exudate. Unlike streptococcal sore throat, however, there is an insidious onset without constitutional symptoms, pharyngeal ulcerations are frequent, and the disease is usually unilateral.

The major differential diagnostic confusion is with viral upper respiratory infections, which occur more frequently than does streptococcal infection. In many cases, the viral etiology may be suspected because of the more prominent catarrhal, "common cold–like" quality of these viral infections. *Adenoviruses* may cause an exudative pharyngitis which is virtually indistinguishable clinically from that due to group A streptococci. *Infectious mononucleosis* also produces severe exudative pharyngitis with fever and toxicity and at times is accompanied by a rash which may be confused with scarlet fever. The generalized lymphadenopathy, splenomegaly, prolonged fever, and presence of abnormal lymphocytes and heterophile antibodies in the peripheral blood serve to differentiate this entity. Pharyngitis due to group A coxsackie viruses (*herpangina*) or to primary infection with *herpes simplex* is characterized by formation of vesicles, which rupture and leave shallow ulcers. *Influenza* virus infections frequently occur in epidemics; they are accompanied by severe myalgias, bronchitis is a frequent clinical feature, and all age groups are affected. *Mycoplasma pneumoniae* infections may cause pharyngitis that at times may be exudative. Bullous myringitis, if present, should suggest this diagnosis.

Although use of algorithms incorporating combinations of epidemiologic data, symptoms, and signs may enhance diagnostic accuracy, in many instances it is impossible to differentiate streptococcal from nonstreptococcal sore throat on clinical grounds alone. For this reason, precise diagnosis requires performance of a throat culture. In obtaining the culture, it is important to rub the cotton swab over both tonsils or tonsillar fossae, the oropharynx, and the nasopharynx posterior to the uvula. The swab should be inoculated onto a sheep blood agar plate to allow evaluation of patterns of hemolysis after overnight incubation. If beta-hemolytic streptococci are isolated, they may be presumed to be group A by sensitivity to a low-potency bacitracin disk or may be identified definitively by fluorescent antibody, coagglutination, or precipitin techniques. A number of the positive cultures obtained, particularly those with relatively few organisms on the culture plate, will represent streptococcal carriers rather than cases of acute infection. It is not possible to differentiate cases from carriers confidently on the basis of culture results, but culture does serve to exclude from antimicrobial therapy the bulk of patients with sore throat (approximately 70 percent) who have negative cultures for beta-hemolytic streptococci. Assay of serum antibodies to streptococcal extracellular products (e.g., ASO) provides confirmatory evidence of recent streptococcal infection in patients suspected of having acute rheumatic fever or acute glomerulonephritis, but such tests are of no value in the diagnosis of acute streptococcal infection.

Treatment Therapy of streptococcal pharyngitis is directed primarily toward prevention of ARF and of suppurative sequelae. It is unclear whether treatment of the antecedent streptococcal infection will prevent development of AGN. Prevention of ARF depends upon eradication of the infecting organism from the pharynx, and attainment of this objective requires prolonged antibiotic treatment. Penicillin is the drug of choice because it is inexpensive and nontoxic and because all group A streptococci have remained exquisitely sensitive to this agent. A single intramuscular injection of benzathine penicillin G, 600,000 units for children less than 60 lb and 1.2 million units for all others, ensures a prolonged penicillinemia and is the most effective form of therapy. If oral therapy is elected, penicillin G, 250,000 units, or penicillin V, 250 mg, three or four times daily, is the treatment of choice. Penicillin-allergic individuals may be treated with erythromycin, 20 mg/lb per day (not to exceed 1 g per day). Nearly all group A streptococci in the United States have remained susceptible to erythromycin, but extensive resistance has been reported in certain areas of the world such as Japan. On the other hand, tetracycline-resistant strains are encountered with some frequency in the United States, and this drug is not recommended. Sulfonamides are ineffective in eradication of established streptococcal infection, although they are useful prophylactically in preventing new pharyngeal acquisitions of group A streptococci and in preventing recurrences of ARF (see Chap. 257). All oral regimens are less effective than intramuscular benzathine penicillin G in eradicating the infecting streptococcus, a fact that is due at least in part to the difficulty of ensuring faithful compliance once the acute symptoms have subsided. It is advisable to reculture the throat 48 h after completion of oral therapy. If group A streptococci persist, as they may in 15 percent of cases, retreatment is indicated. Multiple repetitive courses of antibiotics are not of further value and should be avoided.

Appropriate antibiotic therapy is effective in preventing ARF, even when initiated as long as 9 days after the onset of acute pharyngitis. Therefore, in the patient seen early after the course of his illness, the delay in initiating therapy occasioned by obtaining a positive throat culture is not ordinarily a matter of concern. In patients who are severely ill or in whom development of suppurative complications is apparent, therapy may be instituted at the time of the initial visit after a throat culture has been obtained. If oral antibiotic therapy is elected, the throat culture serves as a guide to the necessity of completion of a full 10-day course or, alternatively, of recalling the patient for definitive therapy with an injection of benzathine penicillin G.

Patients with more severe suppurative complications, such as infections involving the mastoid or ethmoids, require larger doses of penicillin than those used for treatment of uncomplicated sore throat. When streptococcal upper respiratory infection is complicated by the development of abscesses associated with suppurative cervical adenitis or in the peritonsillar or retropharyngeal soft tissues, incision and drainage are usually required.

The role of tonsillectomy, if any, in the management of patients with frequent recurrences of acute pharyngitis or in the prevention of ARF remains undefined. Clinical episodes of pharyngitis occur less frequently and tend to be milder following tonsillectomy, but this may possibly make detection and appropriate treatment of immunologically significant streptococcal infections more difficult.

Family contacts of patients with streptococcal sore throat frequently develop symptomatic infections or become asymptomatic pharyngeal carriers. Secondary cases in families should, of course, be treated appropriately. Asymptomatic family contacts should also be cultured in high-risk circumstances. These include the presence of a rheumatic subject in the family, known cases of ARF occurring in the general area, and families in a lower socioeconomic group with a large number of children living in crowded circumstances. In situations where the risk is lower, the decision to culture and treat asymptomatic family contacts must be made for each involved individual and should be based upon factors such as the geographic and socioeconomic setting, and the current prevalence of streptococcal disease and its sequels.

STREPTOCOCCAL SKIN INFECTIONS **Erysipelas** Also known as Saint Anthony's fire, erysipelas is an acute infection of the skin and subcutaneous tissues caused by group A streptococci. Other streptococci, and even staphylococci and pneumococci, have been implicated on rare occasions. The disease most frequently affects infants, young children, and elderly individuals. The commonest site of involvement is the face, where cutaneous infection originates from an upper respiratory source, presumably by way of small or inapparent breaks in the skin. Erysipelas may also result from streptococcal infection of wounds, surgical incisions, or even areas of dermatophytosis, in which case any portion of the body may be involved.

The onset is usually abrupt; initial symptoms include malaise, chilliness, feverishness, headache, and vomiting. The skin lesion may begin with itching and mild discomfort at the site of infection and is followed shortly thereafter by a small area of erythema which enlarges during the ensuing hours. The lesion spreads rapidly, reaching its maximum extent in 3 to 6 days. It is warm, pink to deep red in color, and has an advancing elevated margin which protrudes irregularly into the surrounding areas of normal skin. Vesicles and bullae may appear; these rupture leaving crusts on the surface. While the advancing margin remains inflamed, central clearing may be evident with a return of the skin to normal appearance or with residual pigmentation. The eruption may be less well demarcated in areas where the skin is loose, but edema and erythema are constant features. Facial erysipelas commonly involves the bridge of the nose and one or more cheeks in a "butterfly" distribution (Fig. 148-1).

The disease process may be accompanied by high fever and bacteremia. Recovery is usually apparent by the end of a week, but this varies with the severity of the infection. The substantial mortality attending bacteremic cases of erysipelas in the preantibiotic era has been markedly reduced by penicillin. Fatalities still occur among children within the first few months of life and elderly, debilitated, immunosuppressed individuals. The disease is noted for its propensity to recur, especially in areas of chronic lymphatic obstruction.

The diagnosis of erysipelas is primarily clinical. Group A streptococci may at times be isolated from the respiratory tract or the bloodstream. Culture of edema fluid or of saline injected intracutaneously and then withdrawn from the advancing margin may yield streptococci, but this maneuver is rarely successful.

FIGURE 148-1
This patient with facial erysipelas exhibits the characteristic "butterfly" distribution of the lesion. The picture was obtained after 48 h of penicillin therapy when the acute inflammation and systemic toxicity had abated slightly.

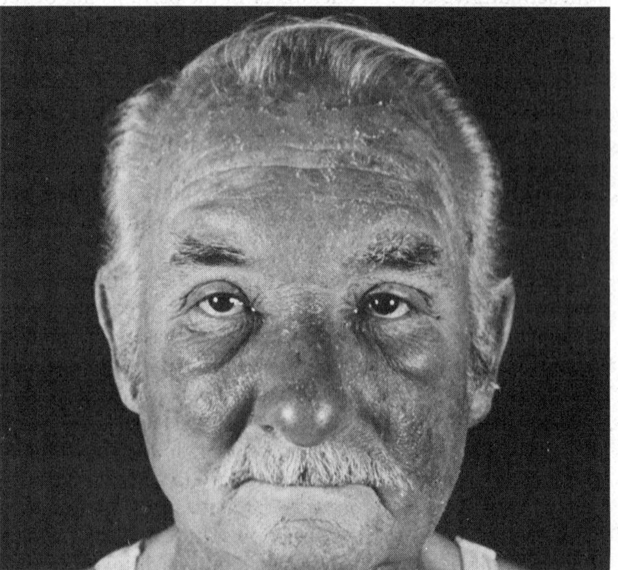

Pyoderma This term is used collectively to denote localized purulent streptococcal skin infections. Some pyoderma lesions represent obvious secondary infections of wounds or burns. For the most part, however, the term is used synonymously with streptococcal impetigo or impetigo contagiosa and refers to discrete purulent lesions which appear to be primary infections of the skin. Streptococcal impetigo differs from streptococcal pharyngitis in a number of particulars (Table 148-1). Epidemiologically, impetigo is more prevalent among underprivileged children residing in warm, humid climates such as the southeastern United States or the tropics. However, the disease may also occur during the summer in northern settings, such as the American Indian reservations of Minnesota. The peak incidence is in young children (2 to 6 years), and there is no definite sex or racial predisposition.

The mode of spread of streptococcal pyoderma is unknown, but personal contact and insect vectors such as *Hippelates* flies are probably both important. "Skin strains" of group A streptococci (i.e., strains of M and T types usually associated with pyoderma) are capable of contaminating unbroken skin, from where they may be inoculated intradermally by local scratches, abrasions, or insect bites. A number of interesting epidemiologic relationships have been observed; they include secondary streptococcal infection in the lesions of scabies and the coexistence of *S. pyogenes* and *Corynebacterium diphtheriae* in impetiginous lesions in Mississippi and Trinidad. Nasal and pharyngeal carriage of skin strains is frequent in children with impetigo, but such carriage does not ordinarily occur until after establishment of cutaneous carriage or overt infection.

The pattern of immunologic responses to streptococcal impetigo differs from that associated with upper respiratory infection. In particular, the ASO response to impetigo is weak, perhaps because streptolysin O is inactivated by lipids present in the skin. Brisk antibody responses to anti-DNAse B and anti-hyaluronidase, as well as to the Streptozyme slide hemag-

TABLE 148-1
Comparative features of pharyngitis and pyoderma due to group A streptococci

	Pharyngitis	*Pyoderma*
Predominant geographic distribution	Temperate	Subtropic-tropic
Season (temperate zone)	Winter-spring	Summer-fall
Peak age group	5–15 years	2–5 years
Mode of spread	Direct contact (droplet)	Unknown (?insects)
Clinical illness	Acute	Indolent
Streptococcal types	Generally lower-numbered M types	Generally higher-numbered M types
ASO responses	Good	Weak
Type-specific antibody responses	Generally good	Variable, often poor
Nonsuppurative sequels	Acute rheumatic fever, acute glomerulonephritis	Acute glomerulonephritis

SOURCE: *After Wannamaker.*

glutination reagent, are observed, however. Type-specific anti-M responses are variable, depending in part upon the antigenicity of the infecting strain, but in general such responses are weaker than in pharyngeal infections. The role of type-specific antibodies in protection against reinfection in pyoderma has not been adequately studied.

Streptococcal impetigo occurs on exposed areas of the body, most frequently on the lower extremities. The lesions remain well-localized but are frequently multiple. They begin as papules but rapidly evolve into vesicles surrounded by an area of erythema. The vesicular lesions are rarely recognized clinically; they give rise to pustules which gradually enlarge, then break down over 4 to 6 days to form characteristic thick crusts. The lesions heal slowly, leaving depigmented areas. A deeply ulcerated form of impetigo is known as *echthyma.* Although regional lymphadenitis often occurs, systemic symptoms are not ordinarily present.

In addition to the indolent, impetiginous skin infections of young children, a more severe and extensive form of pyoderma has been observed in combat troops serving in hot, wet environments such as the jungles of southeast Asia. During the Vietnam conflict, such "jungle sores" became a major medical problem among infantry personnel. In their most common form, they consist of multiple echthymatous ulcers located on the ankle or dorsum of the foot. The ulcers are usually circular, punched-out lesions 0.5 to 3.0 cm in diameter, have borders, and are surrounded by a zone of erythema. They are filled with purulent material and covered with grayish-yellow adherent crusts. Secondary cellulitis or lymphadenitis may be present.

The diagnosis of streptococcal pyoderma is made by bacteriologic culture. Adequate cultures require removal of the surface crusts in order to obtain specimens from the base of the lesions. Although both *S. pyogenes* and *Staphylococcus aureus* may be isolated from the lesions, the former is the major pathogen. Morphologically characteristic lesions respond well to penicillin therapy, even when penicillinase-resistant staphylococci are recovered. These lesions contrast with bullous impetigo, which is ordinarily due to *S. aureus* and not to streptococci. Antibiotic regimens are the same as those for pharyngitis, and benzathine penicillin G, oral penicillin V, or oral erythromycin all result in cure rates in excess of 95 percent. Topical antiseptics and antibiotics are of little, if any, value. Prevention of pyoderma depends primarily upon adherence to good personal hygiene, with special attention to frequent scrubbing with soap and water.

Streptococcal pyoderma does not give rise to ARF. This observation remains unexplained, but may indicate a requirement for infection at the pharyngeal site, with its rich endowment of lymphoid tissue, in order to initiate the immunologic events leading to ARF. On the other hand, studies of populations in which ARF and AGN occur simultaneously indicate that the streptococcal strains responsible for each sequel are distinct and suggest that "pyoderma strains" of group A streptococci may be nonrheumatogenic. When pyoderma is due to a nephritogenic strain of group A streptococcus, AGN may ensue. Indeed, pyoderma is by far the commonest antecedent of poststreptococcal glomerulonephritis in subtropical and tropical regions of the world. Strains of a number of M types (49, 55, 57, and others) have been associated both with sporadic cases and large epidemics of pyoderma-associated nephritis in diverse geographic areas. There are no conclusive data to indicate that treatment of an individual case of pyoderma will prevent the subsequent occurrence of AGN in that patient. Such treatment is important, however, in eradicating nephritogenic streptococci from the environment in epidemiologic settings in which these strains are prevalent.

Cellulitis Streptococcal cellulitis may occur in areas of tissue damage due to trauma, operative wounds, or stasis ulceration. It is an acute inflammation of the skin and subcutaneous tissues marked by pain, tenderness, erythema, fever, and often regional lymphadenopathy. In contrast to erysipelas, the margins of the lesions are neither elevated nor sharply demarcated from the surrounding uninvolved tissue. Rarely such lesions may progress to frank gangrene. Cellulitis of the perianal area may be manifested by painful defecation or by pruritus; asymptomatic anal colonization has been the source of several outbreaks of hospital-acquired streptococcal infection. Vaginal colonization by group A streptococci has a number of features in common with perianal involvement. In both instances there is a close epidemiologic association with streptococcal upper respiratory infection. Anal and vaginal streptococcal infection may be either symptomatic or asymptomatic. At least one outbreak of nosocomial streptococcal infection has been attributed to an asymptomatic vaginal carrier.

LYMPHANGITIS AND PUERPERAL SEPSIS Local trauma, whether or not complicated by frank cellulitis, may give rise to *acute lymphangitis.* This entity is characterized by the appearance of red linear streaks extending from the portal of entry to the draining regional lymph nodes, which are enlarged and tender. Systemic symptoms, including chills, fever, malaise, and headache, are prominent, and the process may be accompanied by demonstrable bacteremia. Streptococcal bacteremia, from whatever cause, may give rise to metastatic foci of infection, such as suppurative arthritis, osteomyelitis, peritonitis, endocarditis, meningitis, or visceral abscesses. The clinical course of streptococcal bacteremia may at times be fulminant and lead rapidly to prostration, shock, purpura fulminans, disseminated intravascular coagulation, and death.

Puerperal sepsis follows abortion or childbirth when streptococci invade the endometrium and surrounding structures and then the lymphatics and bloodstream. The pathological process may be further complicated by pelvic cellulitis, septic pelvic thrombophlebitis, peritonitis, or pelvic abscess. The causative organism may be transmitted to the pregnant woman directly by medical personnel or attendants, as was demonstrated by Semmelweiss in the mid-nineteenth century. In recent years, group B streptococci have supplanted other organisms as the most frequent cause of perinatal streptococcal infections of mother and child (see below). Anaerobic streptococci, along with other anaerobic organisms, have also been implicated.

PNEUMONIA AND EMPYEMA Pneumonia due to group A streptococci is uncommon and usually occurs following viral infections such as influenza, measles, pertussis, or varicella. The illness occurs in epidemic form in military recruit camps and is characterized by abrupt onset of fever, chills, myalgia, dyspnea, cough, pleuritic chest pain, and hemoptysis. Patients are severely ill and often cyanotic. Pathologically and radiologically, this is usually a bronchopneumonia, and lobar consolidation is uncommon. A characteristic feature of streptococcal pneumonia is the early and rapid accumulation of copious amounts of thin, serosanguinous empyema fluid. Bacteremia occurs in 10 to 15 percent of cases. Extension of the pneumonic process to the pericardium may give rise to a purulent pericarditis. Other potential complications include mediastinitis, pneumothorax, and bronchiectasis. Therapy consists of 4 to 6 million units of parenteral penicillin in the form of aqueous procaine penicillin G, given every 6 to 12 h intramuscularly, or intravenous aqueous crystalline penicillin G, and adequate drainage of empyema fluid, which usually requires insertion of a chest tube.

GROUP B STREPTOCOCCAL INFECTIONS

Streptococci belonging to serogroup B have long been of interest to veterinarians because of their association with bovine mastitis, an association which led to their species designation as *S. agalactiae.* The organisms are beta-hemolytic and usually, but not uniformly, resistant to bacitracin. In addition to the presence of group B carbohydrate in their cell walls, *S. agalactiae* may be identified by biochemical means, including their production of hippuricase and so-called CAMP factor. Group B streptococci may be subdivided by means of surface polysaccharides and protein antigens into five serotypes: Ia, Ib, Ic, II, and III.

Human strains of group B streptococci, which appear to be biologically distinct from bovine strains, frequently colonize the female genital tract as well as the throat and rectum. Asymptomatic vaginal carriage rates in postpubertal women generally have ranged between 6 and 25 percent, depending on the bacteriologic methods employed and on the socioeconomic status and geographic residence of the women sampled. The majority of serious group B infections occur as perinatal events. Maternal infections include chorioamnionitis, septic abortion, and puerperal sepsis. *Streptococcus agalactiae* now ranks with *Escherichia coli* as one of the two most frequent causes of neonatal sepsis and meningitis. Neonatal disease takes one of two forms. Early-onset disease, occurring within the first 10 days of life, is usually due to organisms acquired from the maternal genital tract. It involves primarily the lungs, probably as a result of aspiration of infected amniotic fluid, but the organism can be cultured from many sites such as the blood, nasopharynx, skin, and myocardium. Early-onset group B streptococcal infection occurs in approximately two of every thousand live births (the incidence is higher following prolonged or complicated delivery) and is attended by a high mortality rate. Late-onset disease occurs in infants over 10 days old, may be due to nosocomial transmission of group B streptococci, is manifested primarily by meningitis and bacteremia, and has a lower mortality rate than early-onset disease. Although the serotypes involved in early-onset illness are variable, type III organisms predominate as the cause of late-onset meningeal infection. Transplacentally acquired antibodies to type III organisms may protect against late-onset disease: they are reported to be present in serums of most women delivering healthy babies but are usually lacking in serums of mothers whose offspring develop late-onset meningitis due to type III group B streptococci.

Group B streptococci also cause a group of adult infections not associated with the puerperium. These include urinary tract infections in both sexes; the infections in men often occur in elderly individuals, perhaps due to associated prostatism. A second syndrome occurs in patients with adult-onset, insulin-dependent diabetes mellitus, peripheral vascular insufficiency, and suppurative gangrenous lesions, infected with *S. agalactiae.* Bacteremia may accompany this syndrome. Other adult infections due to group B organisms include endocarditis, pneumonia, empyema, meningitis, peritonitis, and terminal bacteremia in patients with malignancy. Although recovered from a small proportion of throat cultures, group B streptococci are rarely, if ever, the cause of clinically significant pharyngitis. All strains are susceptible to penicillin, which is the drug of choice, although group B organisms have slightly higher minimal inhibitory concentrations for penicillin than do group A strains. Only occasional strains are resistant to erythromycin. Tetracyclines should not be used without prior susceptibility testing because resistance to them is quite common.

OTHER STREPTOCOCCAL INFECTIONS

Streptococci of groups C and G are capable of causing exudative pharyngitis, and epidemics of upper respiratory disease due to these organisms have been reported, particularly following ingestion of contaminated food items. Strains of both serogroups produce streptolysin O, and pharyngeal infections with groups C and G elicit rises in ASO titer. However, most reported instances of human disease due to these two serogroups have been skin and wound infections or puerperal infections. Associated bacteremia may result in endocarditis.

Lancefield's group D streptococci consist of enterococcal species (*S. faecalis, S. faecium, S. durans*) and nonenterococci (*S. bovis, S. equinus*). Group D streptococci are frequent causes of urinary tract infection in patients with structural abnormalities of the urinary tract and frequently are associated with bacterial endocarditis. These microorganisms are usually alpha-hemolytic or nonhemolytic but may be beta-hemolytic. The treatment of severe enterococcal infections, particularly bacterial endocarditis, is complicated by the fact that the organisms are resistant to many antibiotics and are relatively resistant to the penicillins. In the therapy of enterococcal endocarditis, a combination of intravenous penicillin G or ampicillin in high doses plus an aminoglycoside antibiotic should be used, because this combination exerts a synergistic effect in the killing of enterococci (see Chap. 259). While formerly streptomycin was the aminoglycoside of choice, high-level resistance (>2000 μg/ml) to streptomycin and kanamycin has been found in a significant number of enterococcal isolates. This is due to a plasmid which is transferable, by conjugation under laboratory conditions, from resistant to sensitive strains. For this reason, aminoglycosides such as gentamicin or tobramycin should be used along with penicillin or ampicillin in treatment of serious enterococcal infections due to organisms which are highly resistant to streptomycin.

In contrast, nonenterococcal group D streptococci, of which *S. bovis* is the major pathogen, remain extremely sensitive to penicillin and are amenable to therapy with this agent alone. Laboratory differentiation of *S. bovis* from enterococci is sometimes difficult. Likewise, *S. mutans,* a penicillin-sensitive viridans streptococcus which is normally found in the mouth and occasionally causes endocarditis, may be confused with group D streptococci. A series of precise biochemical tests is required to identify the various species correctly. In particular, enterococci grow in 6.5% sodium chloride broth, while *S. bovis* and *S. mutans* do not. Treatment of life-threatening enterococcal infections in patients who cannot tolerate penicillin is difficult. Cephalothin and clindamycin are of no value, but vancomycin, often in combination with gentamicin, is likely to be effective.

Streptococci of most groups have been isolated at least occasionally from infected heart valves, soft tissues, or visceral abscesses. Such infections may occur as "opportunists" following surgical manipulation or in patients with malignant disease. Danish and Dutch investigators have reported a number of instances of meningitis and bacteremia in humans due to streptococci of serogroup R, a group of organisms well-known as pathogens of swine. In nearly all human cases there had been a history of contact with pigs.

Viridans streptococci are normal inhabitants of the oropharynx and gastrointestinal tract. They remain the most frequent causative agents of subacute bacterial endocarditis (see Chap. 257). The taxonomy of these organisms is confused, but one classification scheme recognizes five species (in addition to *S. pneumoniae*): *salivarius, mitior, milleri, sanguis,* and *mutans.* Although viridans streptococci are not usually considered to be highly invasive, *S. milleri* is capable of causing serious pyogenic infections such as liver and brain abscesses, peritonitis, and empyema. Cases of endocarditis due to *S. milleri* are more likely to be complicated by abscess formation in peripheral tissues than are similar infections due to other species of viridans streptococci. *Streptococcus milleri* is usually considered "microaerophilic," and its clinical behavior is similar to that of the anaerobic streptococci. All the viridans species, including *S. milleri,* are susceptible to penicillin. Modest increases in the minimal inhibitory concentrations of oral streptococci to penicillin occur following prolonged oral therapy or high-dose intravenous therapy with this antibiotic.

Anaerobic streptococci (see Chap. 173) abound in the mouth, intestinal tract, and vagina. They may be found, either alone or in combination with other anaerobic and aerobic microorganisms, in abscess cavities throughout the body. In the head and neck, anaerobic streptococci may be found in infected paranasal sinuses, brain abscess, dental abscess, infections of the retropharyngeal or lateral pharyngeal spaces, and in cases of Ludwig's angina. In the chest, these organisms occur in lung abscesses and empyema fluids. Abscesses of the liver and other intraabdominal viscera, as well as perirectal abscesses and pelvic abscesses in women, may be due in part to peptostreptococci. Finally, these organisms may thrive in dead or devitalized muscle, skin, or subcutaneous tissue. *Streptococcal myositis* is characterized by marked edema, crepitant myositis, pain, and the presence of chains of gram-positive cocci in a seropurulent exudate. *Progressive synergistic gangrene* usually develops about a surgical incision and consists of an ulcerated lesion surrounded by gangrenous skin. The infection is associated particularly with the use of through-and-through sutures after abdominal surgery, and is thought most often to be due to the synergistic action of *S. aureus* and microaerophilic streptococci. *Chronic burrowing ulcer* is a deep soft-tissue infection caused by microaerophilic streptococci which erodes through subcutaneous tissue to emerge as an ulcer at a distant site. Management of anaerobic streptococcal infections consists of drainage of abscesses, debridement of devitalized tissues, and high-dose intravenous penicillin therapy.

REFERENCES

BAKER CJ, DENNIS KL: Immunological investigation of infants with septicemia and meningitis due to group B streptococcus. J Infect Dis 136:598, 1977

BISNO AL et al: Factors influencing serum antibody responses in streptococcal pyoderma. J Lab Clin Med 81:410, 1973

DUMA RJ et al: Streptococcal infections: A bacteriologic and clinical study of streptococcal bacteremia. Medicine 48:87, 1969

KAPLAN EL et al: Diagnosis of streptococcal pharyngitis: Differentiation of active infection from the carrier state in the symptomatic child. J Infect Dis 123:490, 1971

KROGSTAD DJ: Plasmid-mediated resistance to antibiotic synergism to enterococci. J Clin Invest 61:1645, 1978

LERNER PI et al: Group B streptococcus (*S. agalactiae*) bacteremia in adults: Analysis of 32 cases and review of the literature. Medicine 56:457, 1977

MURRAY HW et al: Serious infections caused by *Streptococcus milleri.* Am J Med 64:759, 1978

STOLLERMAN GH: *Rheumatic Fever and Streptococcal Infection.* New York, Grune & Stratton, 1975

WANNAMAKER LW: Differences between streptococcal infections of the throat and the skin. N Engl J Med 282:23, 1970

section 3 | Diseases caused by gram-negative cocci

149 MENINGOCOCCAL INFECTIONS

HARRY N. BEATY

DEFINITION *Neisseria meningitidis* is the causative organism of a variety of infections, notably meningitis and bacteremia.

ETIOLOGY In stained smears, meningococci are gram-negative and characteristically appear as single cocci or diplococci with flattened adjacent sides. They grow well on solid or semisolid media containing blood, serum, or ascitic fluid, and thrive best at temperatures between 35 and 37°C in an atmosphere reduced in oxygen and containing 5 to 10 percent CO_2. The organism is recovered readily from biological fluids when fresh specimens are inoculated on warm chocolate agar plates which are incubated 18 to 24 h in a candle jar or in a more sophisticated apparatus that provides a suitable environment.

The biochemical reactions of the *Neisseria* are relatively limited, but they contain cytochrome oxidase, which is responsible for the positive "oxidase" test; the clinically significant species usually are differentiated by their ability to produce acid in glucose, maltose, or sucrose. Typically the meningococcus ferments both glucose and maltose, but on occasion maltose-negative strains have been isolated.

Meningococci can be divided into serologic groups on the basis of agglutination reactions with immune serum. The present classification into groups A, B, C, and D was agreed upon in 1950, but since 1960, new groups including 29E, W135, X, Y, and Z have been identified. The major groups are remarkably heterogeneous, but subclassification with additional serologic markers has been possible. Subcapsular antigens, some of which are proteins, have provided the basis for dividing strains of groups A, B, C, and Y into distinct types that are independent of their capsular serogroup.

EPIDEMIOLOGY The natural habitat of meningococci is the nasopharynx of humans, and no other reservoir or vector has been recognized. The principal means of spread is through inhalation of droplets of infected nasopharyngeal secretions. It is unlikely that the disease is spread by contact with contaminated fomites. Meningococci cause either epidemic or sporadic disease, and there is a cyclic variation in the prevalence of meningococcal infection with peaks of increased frequency occurring every 8 to 12 years and lasting 4 to 6 years. The last, quite minor, peak occurred in 1965. Subsequently, the incidence has declined to a fairly constant rate of 1 to 2 cases per 100,000 population per year. The prevalence of meningococcal infection is also subject to seasonal influences; the lowest attack rate occurs in midsummer and the highest in late winter and early spring. The incidence of disease in specific geographic regions varies from year to year and may significantly exceed the national average.

The attack rate of meningococcal disease is highest for children between 6 months and 1 year of age. A second, much lower, peak in incidence occurs among adolescents, and the lowest attack rate occurs in individuals over 25. There is no clear-cut tendency for racial or sexual predominance, but presumably because of an increased opportunity to acquire infection, males develop meningitis and meningococcemia more frequently than females. The attack rate in household contacts of sporadic cases of meningococcal disease is 1000 times the overall endemic rate; in epidemic periods, the attack rate among household contacts may be as much as 15,000 times that of the general population. Experience with group A outbreaks in Alaska and the northwestern part of the United States indicates that alcoholics and Alaska natives are at increased risk of infection. Military recruits also are particularly susceptible to meningococcal disease, although outbreaks that appear to be restricted to the military usually parallel less apparent trends in the civilian population.

Since 1915, most epidemics of meningococcal disease have been caused by group A meningococci, and strains of groups B and C have been associated with sporadic, interepidemic infections. However, in the outbreaks of 1963 and 1964 in the United States a major shift in the pattern of meningococcal infection became apparent as group B meningococci were isolated from the majority of clinical infections in both civilian and military populations. By 1967, over 70 percent of meningococci isolated were group B. Early in 1968, another shift began, and in the epidemic years 1969 through 1972, the majority of meningococcal strains submitted to the Center for Disease Control were group C. More recently, group B has again become the most prevalent serogroup isolated in the United States, and group Y is increasing in importance. This organism is more likely than the others to cause respiratory disease and pneumonia.

Only a small proportion of the meningococci isolated in this country are group A. However, in Alaska and the Pacific Northwest, group A organisms are isolated from 30 to 60 percent of patients with meningococcal disease.

Studies using a serotyping system have allowed identification of a few strains that possess unique epidemic potential. Isolates from group B, C, and Y outbreaks are almost exclusively representatives of two serotypes, with type CII predominating. These observations may have great significance in future vaccine development, because in the case of group B organisms, it has not been possible to develop an effective polysaccharide vaccine.

Coincident with these epidemiologic shifts has been a waxing and waning of the proportion of isolates which are resistant to sulfadiazine. In the early to mid-1960s, the majority of group B meningococci were resistant to sulfadiazine; in 1982 over 90 percent were sensitive. Similarly, when group C emerged as the predominant serogroup, sulfadiazine resistance was the rule, but in the epidemic year 1974, about one-third of group C isolates were sensitive. Sulfadiazine resistance has been recognized among isolates of all major serogroups, and future major shifts may occur.

The potential for the meningococcus to produce serious outbreaks of disease has been reemphasized by events of the last decade in Brazil and Finland. A large urban epidemic was first recognized in São Paulo in 1971, and it increased in intensity over the next several years. In 1974, the predominant strain of meningococcus producing disease there changed abruptly from group C to group A, and the epidemic spread to other major cities in Brazil. In July and August, 1974, about 13,000 cases of meningococcal disease occurred in São Paulo alone. An epidemic of group A meningococcal disease began in Finland early in 1973. It peaked in 1974 when the incidence of infection rose to 15 per 100,000 population. Massive immunization programs curtailed both of these major epidemics.

Carriers Between epidemics, 2 to 15 percent of the individuals in urban centers harbor meningococci in the nasopharynx. When sporadic cases of meningococcal disease occur, the carrier rate in close contacts may rise to 40 percent, and in closed populations or during epidemics, may approach 100 percent. Although some individuals harbor meningococci for years, nasopharyngeal infection is usually transient, and in 75 percent of carriers the organism disappears within a few weeks to a few months. Case-to-case transmission of infection is documented rarely, and carriers, not patients, are the foci from which disease is spread. Even so, the prevalence of meningococcal disease can be attributed to the prevailing carrier rate only in a general way, and the occurrence of clinical disease is most dependent on the immunologic status of the host and other factors that lead to spread of infection beyond the nasopharynx.

Immunity The fact that meningococcal meningitis is primarily a disease of childhood has suggested that natural immunity develops in most individuals within the first two decades of life. There is a correlation between susceptibility to meningococcal disease and absence of bactericidal antibody in the serum, and most adults have antibodies to pathogenic strains of meningococci. Natural immunization appears to result from asymptomatic carriage of meningococci in the nasopharynx. Not only does the carrier state produce antibodies to the infecting strain, but cross-reacting antibodies may develop, even after colonization with nongroupable organisms. Nasopharyngeal carriage of a closely related species, *N. lactamica,* also may play a role in the development of natural immunity to meningococcal disease.

The immunity conferred by meningococcal meningitis or meningococcemia is usually group-specific, and second episodes of meningococcal disease have been encountered. Deficiency of complement components C6, C7, or C8 is a significant risk factor for repeated episodes of bacteremia with the pathogenic *Neisseria.*

PATHOGENESIS The primary focus of meningococcal infection is the nasopharynx. In most instances, this infection is subclinical, but occasionally localized inflammation occurs and mild symptoms develop. Dissemination of meningococci from the nasopharynx occurs via the bloodstream, and generally is followed by clinical manifestations of meningococcal disease. *Purulent meningitis* is a form of metastatic infection and is either associated with signs and symptoms of meningococcemia or constitutes the predominant clinical expression of illness. Organisms in the meninges induce an acute inflammatory reaction, and purulent exudate spreads across the surface of the brain. Rarely, a more extensive inflammatory reaction is responsible for an acute diffuse encephalitis.

Although the mechanisms responsible for the pathologic changes associated with meningococcal infection have not been explained entirely, the tissue injury observed in laboratory animals appears to be caused by an endotoxin which is biochemically and biologically similar to endotoxins of enteric bacilli. It may be responsible for hypotension and vascular collapse observed in fulminant meningococcemia and may also play a role in the pathogenesis of the purpura and visceral hemorrhages associated with meningococcal bacteremia. Thrombosis of dermal venules, adrenal sinusoids, and renal glomerular capillaries is most commonly seen in patients who die of fulminant meningococcemia and is strikingly similar to the pathologic changes observed in the experimental Shwartzman reaction. It is postulated that endotoxin either induces a Shwartzman reaction directly or effects the release of clotting factors which initiate intravascular coagulation and produce these characteristic pathologic changes.

CLINICAL MANIFESTATIONS Ninety to ninety-five percent of patients with meningococcal disease have meningococcemia and/or meningitis.

Meningococcemia Thirty to fifty percent of patients who develop overt disease have meningococcemia without meningitis. The onset of clinical illness may be abrupt, but patients usually have nonspecific prodromal symptoms of cough, headache, and sore throat followed by the sudden development of spiking fever, chills, arthralgia, and muscle pains which may be particularly severe in the lower extremities and back. Patients usually appear acutely ill with an inordinate degree of prostration. In addition to high fever, tachycardia, and tachypnea, mild hypotension may be present. However, clinical shock does not occur unless fulminant meningococcemia supervenes. In the course of meningococcal bacteremia, about three-fourths of the patients develop a characteristic petechial rash. Lesions are frequently sparse, and the axillae, flanks, wrists, and ankles are the most commonly involved sites. Often petechiae are located in the center of lighter-colored macules, and they may become nodular as the disease progresses. The diagnosis of meningococcemia occasionally can be established by demonstrating gram-negative diplococci in scrapings from these nodular lesions. In severe cases, purpuric spots or large ecchymoses develop, and a widespread petechial or purpuric eruption suggests fulminating disease. However, the absence of rash does not necessarily indicate that the illness will be mild.

Fulminant meningococcemia, or the Waterhouse-Friderichsen syndrome, is meningococcemia associated with vasomotor collapse and shock. It occurs in 10 to 20 percent of patients with generalized meningococcal infection, and is associated with a high fatality rate. The onset is abrupt, and profound prostration frequently occurs within a few hours. Petechiae and purpuric lesions enlarge rapidly, and hemorrhage into the skin may be extensive. Early in the preshock stage, there is generalized vasoconstriction; patients are alert and pale, with circumoral cyanosis and cold extremities. Upon entering the shock stage, however, coma develops, the cardiac output decreases, and the blood pressure drops. Unless incipient shock is recognized and appropriate therapy is instituted early, death from cardiac and/or respiratory failure almost invariably occurs. Patients who recover may have extensive sloughing of skin lesions or loss of digits because of gangrene.

Chronic meningococcemia is a rare form of meningococcal infection which lasts for weeks or months and is characterized by fever, rash, and arthritis or arthralgia. Typically, the fever is intermittent, and during afebrile periods, which may last several days, patients appear remarkably well. The usual rash is a maculopapular or polymorphous eruption which waxes and wanes with the fever, but petechial or nodular lesions may be seen. Joint involvement is present in two-thirds of the patients, and splenomegaly is detected in about 20 percent. If the diagnosis is not suspected or treatment is otherwise delayed, complications such as meningitis, carditis, or nephritis may occur.

Meningitis Meningitis is a common form of meningococcal disease which occurs primarily in children over 6 months of age and in adolescents. Fever, vomiting, headache, and confusion or lethargy are the commonest symptoms; in about one-fourth of the patients, symptoms begin abruptly and rapidly increase in severity. The more typical patient, however, has symptoms of an upper respiratory tract infection followed by an illness which progresses over several days. Twenty to forty percent of patients have meningitis without clinical evidence of meningococcemia, and the diagnosis depends upon bacteriologic examination of the cerebrospinal fluid. However, when meningitis occurs in association with a petechial or purpuric rash, a presumptive diagnosis of meningococcal disease is warranted, because this pattern of illness is seen only rarely in other infections.

Rarer manifestations The meningococcus is a rare cause of purulent conjunctivitis or sinusitis. Primary pneumonia previously was considered a rare manifestation of meningococcal infection, but increasing numbers of cases are being reported. In one study of military recruits, 68 cases of clinical pneumonia due to group Y meningococci were reported. Bacterial endocarditis, primary pericarditis, arthritis, and osteomyelitis have also been reported. On rare occasion, meningococci have produced genital infections clinically indistinguishable from gonococcal disease. *N. meningitidis* has been isolated with increasing frequency from the genitourinary tract and anal canal of symptomatic and asymptomatic patients of both sexes.

LABORATORY FINDINGS Aside from bacteriologic data, laboratory studies are of little value in establishing the diagnosis of meningococcal infection. Polymorphonuclear leukocyte counts usually range from 12,000 to 40,000 cells per cubic millimeter, but in meningococcemia, normal or low leukocyte counts may be encountered. Anemia is uncommon, and levels of serum electrolytes and blood urea nitrogen are normal unless shock develops. Patients with prominent hemorrhagic manifestations may have low platelet counts and decreased levels of circulating clotting factors as a result of intravascular coagulation. In meningitis, the cerebrospinal fluid pressure is increased, and the fluid usually contains from 100 to 40,000 polymorphonuclear leukocytes per cubic millimeter. The protein content is increased, and the concentration of glucose is almost always less than 35 mg/dl and often is between 0 and 10 mg/dl.

Meningococci often can be recovered from cultures of blood or spinal fluid, and, on occasion, material aspirated from skin lesions or joints yields the organism. In addition, gram-negative diplococci may be seen in stains of nodular petechiae or the buffy coat of blood from patients with meningococcemia. In meningococcal meningitis, a smear of the spinal fluid is diagnostic in about half the patients but often shows only a few intracellular bacteria which are located with difficulty.

COMPLICATIONS Herpes labialis occurs in 5 to 20 percent of patients with meningococcal disease. Other complications, which result from neurologic damage or secondary foci of infection, are uncommon following appropriate treatment and are often transient. Seizures or deafness occur in 10 to 20 percent of patients during the acute stages of meningitis, but post-meningitic epilepsy is rare, and the frequency of permanent eighth nerve damage is probably less than 5 percent. Peripheral neuropathy, cranial nerve palsies, and hemiplegia are seen occasionally, but usually clear completely within 2 to 4 months. Hydrocephalus and thrombosis of venous sinuses, once frequent sequelae of meningococcal meningitis, are encountered rarely. A number of patients complain of recurrent headache, emotional lability, insomnia, backache, memory loss, and difficulty in concentrating for months after an episode of meningitis. The organic basis for these symptoms is obscure, but they usually disappear a year or two after the infection.

Arthritis is a common metastatic complication of meningococcemia and occurs in 2 to 10 percent of patients. As a rule, multiple joints are involved, and signs and symptoms may not appear until after treatment of meningitis or meningococcemia has been instituted. Joint fluid usually contains many granulocytes, but meningococci are recovered infrequently. Arthritis may be immunologically mediated in those instances when cultures are sterile.

Permanent joint changes are rare. Other purulent complications have become extremely uncommon since antibiotics have gained widespread use. Pneumonia occurs occasionally, but it is uncertain whether it is caused by the meningococcus or coincident infection with other bacteria. Bacterial endocarditis is quite rare, but *a high proportion of patients who die of meningococcal infection have myocarditis.* The etiology of these myocardial changes is uncertain, but cardiac failure may be an important factor in the pathogenesis of the shock syndrome in meningococcemia. A pericardial friction rub or electrocardiographic change of pericarditis is seen in about 5 percent of patients, and rarely purulent pericarditis may develop.

DIAGNOSIS The diagnosis of meningococcal disease depends upon recovering *N. meningitidis* from cultures of blood, spinal fluid, or petechial scrapings from patients with a typical clinical picture. Counterimmunoelectrophoresis of spinal fluid and other materials may help diagnose infections caused by group A or C meningococci, but does not detect antigens of group B organisms or those of the less common serogroups. Recovery of meningococci from the nasopharynx does not, in itself, establish the diagnosis.

Few diseases need to be considered seriously in the differential diagnosis of meningococcal disease. If meningococcal meningitis is not accompanied by manifestations of bacteremia, it is indistinguishable from meningitis caused by other common pathogens. Occasionally, the common viral exanthems, Rocky Mountain spotted fever (see Chap. 189), and vascular purpuras may be confused with meningococcemia, and their differentiation depends upon demonstration of the organism and knowledge of the epidemiology and clinical manifestations of each disease.

TREATMENT Antimicrobial therapy of suspected or documented meningococcal disease should be instituted as early as possible. Penicillin G is the drug of choice, and should be administered intravenously. The dosage for treatment of meningitis in adults is 12 to 24 million units per day, and in the pediatric age group, 16 million units per square meter (day). Meningococcemia alone can be treated with 5 to 10 million units per day, because it is not necessary to achieve high levels of antibiotic in the spinal fluid. If treatment with these doses is continued for a minimum of 7 days, or 4 to 5 days after the patient becomes afebrile, relapse is extremely rare. Ampicillin in doses of 200 to 400 mg/kg per day is as effective as penicillin G. When bacteriologic confirmation of meningococcal disease is available, however, treatment should be switched to penicillin G because it is less costly. Meningococci are susceptible to chloramphenicol, but it should not be used unless a patient is allergic to penicillin. Then chloramphenicol hemisuccinate 4.0 to 6.0 g per day in divided doses (in adults) is an acceptable alternate. Some of the "third-generation" cephalosporins (see Chap. 141) have been used to treat small numbers of patients with meningococcal meningitis, but they should not be employed routinely until more extensive clinical research documents their efficacy. *Because a significant proportion of meningococci isolated are resistant to sulfonamides, these drugs should not be used alone in the treatment of meningococcal infections,* and their use in combination with penicillin offers no advantage.

Patients with meningococcal infections require supportive treatment as well as antimicrobial therapy. Maintenance of fluid and electrolyte balance and prevention of respiratory complications in comatose patients are of primary concern. When shock occurs, visceral perfusion must be improved by maintenance of an adequate intravascular volume, treatment of heart failure, and support of the blood pressure. Vasoactive drugs should be employed according to the pathophysiologic derangement in each individual case. These derangements can be determined best by carefully monitoring the blood pressure, pulse, arterial blood gases, cardiac output, peripheral resistance, pulmonary artery wedge pressures, and arteriovenous oxygen differences. When blood pressure must be raised immediately, norepinephrine may be indicated. However, if improved tissue perfusion is the primary goal, an agent such as dopamine is likely to be more effective. When heart failure is present, diuretics and digitalis should be given. When intravascular coagulation is recognized, treatment with heparin, whole blood, or fibrinogen can be tried, but dramatic results should not be expected. Massive doses of adrenal cortical steroids as used in the treatment of septic shock (see Chap. 139) may be helpful, but lower "replacement" doses are of uncertain value.

PREVENTION With the widespread emergence of sulfonamide-resistant meningococci, alternate methods of preventing meningococcal disease in closed populations were sought. High-molecular-weight polysaccharide antigens from organisms of serogroups A and C have been shown to induce a group-specific bactericidal antibody response after subcutaneous injection. Large-scale field trials with the group C vaccine led to a 90 percent reduction in group C disease among vaccinated recruits. Similar results have been observed with group A vaccine in the Brazilian and Finnish epidemics. An effective group B vaccine has not yet been developed, but a vaccine made from type 2 protein has shown promise in preliminary studies.

For intimate contacts of sporadic cases of meningococcal disease, chemoprophylaxis should be administered. If the organism isolated from the patient is sensitive to sulfonamides, 2 days of prophylaxis with one of these drugs is recommended. When sensitivities are not known or the organism is resistant to sulfonamides, rifampin in dosage of 600 mg a day for 2 days or minocycline in dosage of 100 mg every 12 h for 5 days can be expected to temporarily eradicate the carrier state and minimize spread of meningococci. Because of some reports of a high incidence of vestibular symptoms with minocycline, rifampin is considered by some to be the drug of choice. However, in large populations, rifampin may not be effective because of rapid appearance of rifampin resistance.

With increased availability of group A and C vaccines, their use as adjuncts to chemoprophylaxis for household or other intimate contacts of sporadic cases of group A or C meningococcal disease has been recommended. The rationale behind this recommendation is sound, and this approach to prevention of secondary cases deserves consideration.

PROGNOSIS Before the introduction of antibiotics, meningococcal meningitis and meningococcemia were almost invariably fatal. With prompt and appropriate chemotherapy, the mortality rate of meningitis without fulminant meningococcemia has dropped to less than 10 percent in the United States, and neurologic sequelae are rare. The mortality of fulminant infection remains high primarily because patients are often in irreversible shock when treatment is instituted. Most deaths occur within 24 to 48 h of admission, and the capacity of the meningococcus to kill a perfectly healthy individual within a few hours remains one of the most awesome characteristics of this disease.

REFERENCES

JACOBSON JA et al: Trends in meningococcal disease, 1974. J Infect Dis 132:480, 1975

KOPPES, GM et al: Group Y meningococcal disease in United States Air Force recruits. Am J Med 62:661, 1977

MCCORMICK JB, BENNETT JV: Public health considerations in the management of meningococcal disease. Ann Intern Med 83:883, 1975

MENINGOCOCCAL DISEASE SURVEILLANCE GROUP: Meningococcal disease—Secondary attack rate and chemoprophylaxis in the United States, 1974. JAMA 235:261, 1976

PUBLIC HEALTH SERVICE ADVISORY COMMITTEE ON IMMUNIZATION PRACTICES: Meningococcal polysaccharide vaccines. Ann Intern Med 89:949, 1978

SCHAAD UB: Arthritis due to *Neisseria meningitidis.* Rev Infect Dis 2:880, 1980

150 GONOCOCCAL INFECTIONS

KING K. HOLMES

DEFINITION Gonorrhea, an infection of columnar and transitional epithelium caused by *Neisseria gonorrhoeae,* is the most common reportable communicable disease in the United States. Anatomic sites which can be infected directly by the gonococcus include the urethra, anal canal, conjunctivas, pharynx, and endocervix. Local complications include endometritis, salpingitis, peritonitis, and bartholinitis in the female, and periurethral abscess and epididymitis in the male. Systemic manifestations of gonococcemia include arthritis, dermatitis, endocarditis, and meningitis as well as myopericarditis and hepatitis.

ETIOLOGY *Neisseria gonorrhoeae* is a gram-negative coccus usually found in pairs with flattened adjacent sides. It forms oxidase-positive colonies and is differentiated from other *Neisseria* by its ability to utilize glucose, but not maltose, sucrose, or lactose, or by specific immunological reactions.

At least four morphologically distinct forms of colonies occur when gonococci are passed in vitro. Colony forms T_1 (P^+) and T_2 (P^{++}) retain virulence during repeated selective subculture in vitro and are covered by surface projections called *pili* (Fig. 150-1), which are visible on electron microscopy. Spontaneous transition to colony forms T_3 and T_4 (P^-) results in some loss of virulence, together with disappearance of pili. Gonococcal colonies now are also classified on the basis of colonial opacity, which is not related to pili. Opaque colonies (O^+) have surface proteins (proteins II) which influence the interactions of gonococci with neutrophils and with surface epithelial cells. Transparent (O^-) colonies lack proteins II and have increased serum resistance; most isolates from blood or fallopian tubes form O^- colonies. Gonococcal strains cannot be differentiated by colonial morphology since each strain gives rise to all colony forms. However, gonococcal strains now can be typed on the basis of nutritional requirements (auxotyping) or surface antigenic variation. The predominant protein in the gonococcal outer membrane is termed protein I; gonococci can be divided into three serogroups (WI, WII, and WIII) and into further serological subtypes on the basis of antigenic differences in protein I.

EPIDEMIOLOGY The only natural hosts for *N. gonorrhoeae* are humans. One million cases of gonorrhea were reported in the United States in 1977, and it is estimated that another 2 million cases went unreported. The annual age-specific incidence rates tripled from 1963 to 1976 in the United States and then leveled off. The peak incidence rates occur from ages 18 to 24 (2 cases per 100 population per year); 85 percent of the cases are age 30 or younger. The reported incidence rate in the United States is now three times higher than in England and Wales. The true incidence rate is probably even higher in the United States, since reporting of gonorrhea is far more complete in the United Kingdom, where most patients with gonorrhea are seen in public clinics for sexually transmitted diseases. Suboptimal clinical practice, including use of subcurative therapy and especially failure to trace infected contacts, may contribute to the higher incidence rate in the United States.

Gonorrhea incidence and prevalence rates are known to be related to age, sex, race, socioeconomic status, and marital status—risk factors which influence sexual behavior, illness behavior, and accessibility of health care. Among sexually active individuals, the highest rates occur in teenagers, in non-Caucasians, in the poor, in large cities, and in unmarried persons—particularly those who live alone. The incidence is perceived as highest in men, while the prevalence is perceived as highest in women. The prevalence rate is so high among women in the United States that routine endocervical cultures are advocated for gonorrhea case detection in asymptomatic women age 30 or under who are considered to be at high risk because of sexual behavior or demographic factors cited above. Approximately 2 percent of women tested by private physicians have gonorrhea. However, greater reliance should be placed upon contact tracing, which is far more efficient for control of gonorrhea, than upon routine endocervical culturing, which is expensive and does not focus on those most likely to transmit the infection. The single most important axiom about the epidemiology of this disease is that *gonorrhea is usually spread by carriers who have no symptoms or have ignored symptoms.* Symptomatic patients, male or female, have usually been recently infected by such carriers, who must in turn be

FIGURE 150-1
Diagram of the envelope of N. gonorrhoeae, *showing structures thought to influence pathogenesis, antimicrobial susceptibility, and antigenicity.*

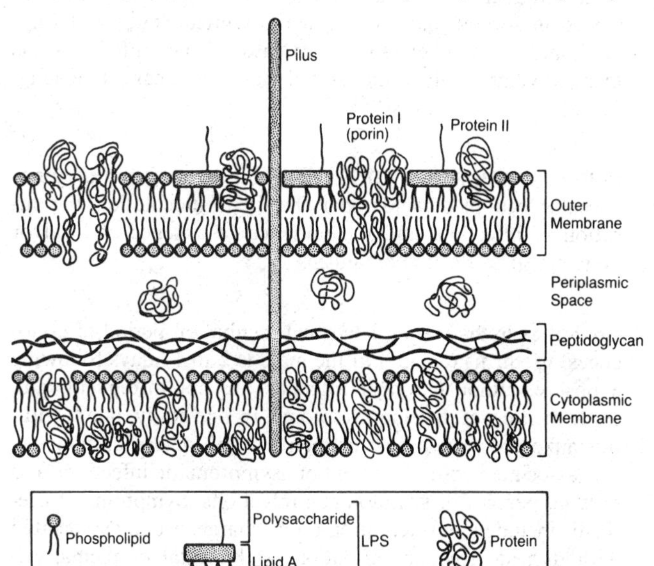

traced and treated to prevent reinfection. *Men and women with symptomatic gonorrhea should always be interviewed to identify their recent sex contacts, who should be examined and treated if infected.*

There are interesting regional differences in the antibiotic resistance of *N. gonorrhoeae.* Resistance is greatest in southeast Asia and Africa where prophylactic or low-dose therapy is common; intermediate in the United States and Australia; and least in Scandinavia, the United Kingdom, and western Europe. Increasing levels of gonococcal resistance to penicillin G and tetracycline were noted during the 1960s in the United States, where subcurative therapy was common and importation of resistant strains occurred during the Vietnam war. From 1970 through 1975, no further increase in resistance to these antibiotics was noted in the United States. However, in 1976, β-lactamase–producing strains of *N. gonorrhoeae* (penicillinase-producing *N. gonorrhoeae,* or PPNG), completely resistant to penicillin and ampicillin, appeared almost simultaneously in two areas of the world: in England, where they had probably been imported from west Africa, and in the United States, where they had clearly been imported from the Philippines. Infections with these penicillin-resistant gonococci are not cured by pencillin therapy. The β-lactamase enzymes produced by these strains are coded on small plasmids which have DNA sequences homologous with the β-lactamase plasmid that first appeared in *Hemophilus influenzae* just 4 years earlier. Such plasmids were not present in gonococci prior to 1976. The African and Asian β-lactamase–producing gonococci show intriguing differences. The β-lactamase plasmid found in most of the African strains has a molecular weight of 3.2 million Daltons and was originally found predominantly in one particular gonococcal auxotype. The Asian plasmid, which can be found in up to 60 percent of gonococci isolated in some cities in the Philippine island of Luzon, and in up to 30 percent of gonococci in other Asian cities, is slightly larger and has entered several different auxotypes and serotypes of gonococci. The Asian β-lactamase more frequently coexists with a larger, conjugative plasmid which is capable of transferring the β-lactamase plasmid to other bacterial cells such as other types of gonococci. This type of molecular epidemiology is instructive—both β-lactamase–producing plasmids apparently enter gonococci and persist in gonococci in areas of the world where prostitution is exceptionally common and where access to subcurative antimicrobial therapy is unrestricted. Although β-lactamase–producing gonococci have not become well established in the industrialized countries, localized outbreaks have occurred in several major cities in the United States and England, and the number of reported cases of such infections has increased alarmingly in the United States since early 1980 (Fig. 150-2).

CLINICAL MANIFESTATIONS The clinical spectrum of gonococcal infections depends upon the site of inoculation, the duration of infection, and the presence or absence of local or systemic spread of the organism.

Gonorrhea in the male The usual incubation period of gonococcal urethritis ("clap") in the male is 2 to 17 days following exposure, although longer intervals are not infrequent, and some men never develop symptoms. In one study, one fastidious auxotype, which has distinctive nutritional requirements, was associated with 96 percent of asymptomatic infections and only 40 percent of symptomatic infections. Symptoms of urethritis include a purulent urethral discharge, usually associated with dysuria, frequent urination, and meatal erythema. Although approximately 90 to 95 percent of men who acquire urethral gonococcal infection develop urethral discharge, most symptomatic men seek treatment and are removed from the infectious pool. The remaining men who never develop symptoms or who ignore their symptoms constitute about two-thirds of the infected men at any point in time, and they serve as the main source of spread of infection to women. Before antibiotic treatment became available, symptoms of urethritis persisted for an average of 8 weeks, and unilateral epididymitis occurred in 5 to 10 percent of untreated men. Epididymitis is now an uncommon complication (see below), and gonococcal prostatitis occurs rarely, if at all. Other local complications of gonococcal urethritis which are now unusual include inguinal lymphadenitis, edema of the penis due to dorsal lymphangitis or thrombophlebitis, submucous inflammatory "soft" infiltration of the urethral wall, periurethral abscess or fistula, unilateral inflammation or abscess of Cowper's gland (which lies between the thumb and forefinger when the forefinger is in the anal canal and the thumb is positioned anteriorly on the perineum), abscess of Tyson's gland(s) (which open on either side of the frenulum), and, rarely, seminal vesiculitis.

In homosexual men, anorectal and pharyngeal gonococcal infection are common. Gonococcal isolates from homosexual men tend to be more resistant to antimicrobials than are isolates from heterosexuals. This may be due to the fact that certain highly susceptible types are rapidly killed by bile salts and fatty acids in feces and rarely occur in homosexual men, while gonococci possessing a gene for multidrug resistance (*mtr*) are resistant to bile salts and fatty acids and occur with increased frequency in homosexual men. Anorectal infection may be asymptomatic from the outset or may produce anorectal pain, pruritus, tenesmus, and a bloody, mucopurulent rectal discharge. Proctoscopy and appropriate laboratory studies are essential to exclude several other conditions which cause similar symptoms (see Chap. 143). These symptoms may subside without treatment, leaving a chronic asymptomatic carrier state. Pharyngeal gonococcal infection occurs in approximately 20 percent of homosexual men or heterosexual women who engage in fellatio with men who have urethral infection, and in a

FIGURE 150-2

Penicillinase-producing N. gonorrhoeae *(PPNG). The number of cases occurring by month in the United States (including outlying areas) from March 1976 to December 1981. (Courtesy of Centers for Disease Control, Atlanta, Ga.)*

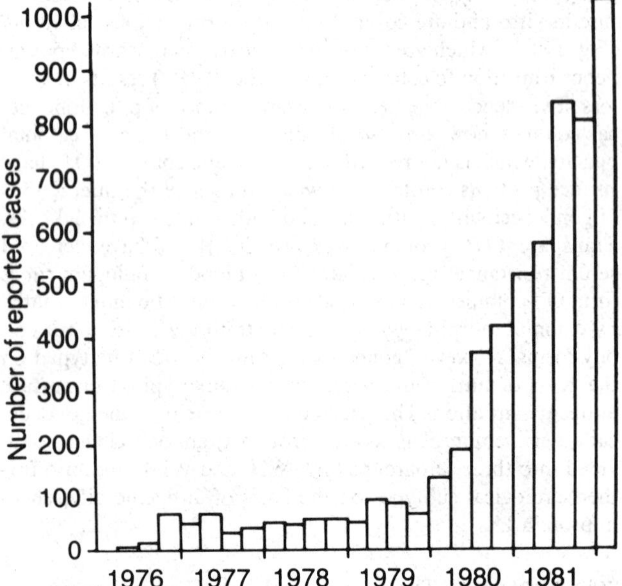

smaller proportion of heterosexual men. Pharyngeal infection may produce exudative tonsillitis but frequently is asymptomatic.

Gonorrhea in the female Acute uncomplicated gonorrhea in the female often causes dysuria, frequent urination, increased vaginal discharge due to exudative endocervicitis, abnormal menstrual bleeding, and anorectal discomfort. While dysuria and frequency in young men arouse the suspicion of gonococcal urethritis, the same symptoms in a young woman are often automatically attributed to "cystitis." Actually, many of those without bacteriuria have gonococcal or chlamydial infection of the urethra. Young women with dysuria should have a thorough pelvic examination. Compression of the urethra through the anterior vaginal wall against the symphysis pubis may express urethral exudate which can be examined by Gram's stain and culture. Symptomatic young women with "sterile pyuria" (i.e., ≥ 10 neutrophils per $100\times$ microscopic field in the centrifuged sediment of clean-catch midstream urine, in whom no uropathogens are isolated from the urine) should be evaluated for gonococcal and chlamydial infection. Acute symptoms of gonococcal urethritis in the female may subside spontaneously or following subcurative therapy with sulfonamides or urinary antiseptics. The proportion of women with gonorrhea who never develop symptoms is undefined.

Asymptomatic gonococcal infection in the female involves the endocervix, urethra, anal canal, and pharynx, in decreasing order of frequency. Extension of infection from the endocervix to the fallopian tubes occurs in at least 15 percent of women with gonorrhea. This tends to occur soon after acquisition of infection or during menstruation and results in acute endometritis, with abnormal menstrual bleeding and midline low abdominal pain and tenderness, followed by *acute salpingitis,* the major complication of gonorrhea. One study suggested one-half of women who became infected after recent exposure to gonorrhea developed signs of salpingitis. Extension of infection to the pelvis may produce signs of pelvic peritonitis, accompanied by nausea and vomiting, and may lead to pelvic abscess. Early antibiotic treatment, before development of adnexal masses, restores normal tubal function and fertility in nearly all cases of salpingitis. However, if prominent adnexal swelling has occurred before treatment is begun, bilateral tubal dysfunction occurs in 15 to 25 percent.

Spread of gonococci into the upper abdomen may cause *gonococcal perihepatitis* (Fitz-Hugh–Curtis syndrome) manifested by right upper quadrant or bilateral upper abdominal pain and tenderness, and occasionally by a hepatic friction rub.

Acute inflammation of Bartholin's gland is usually unilateral and frequently is due to gonococcal infection. The acutely infected duct is surrounded by a red halo and exudes pus at the posterior third of the labium majus. Occlusion of the duct results in formation of a Bartholin's abscess. Chronic Bartholin cysts are rarely caused by active gonococcal infection.

There is suggestive evidence that endocervical gonococcal infection is associated with prematurity and prolonged labor following rupture of membranes, both of which may produce increased perinatal morbidity.

Gonorrhea in children During childbirth, the gonococcus may infect the conjunctivas, pharynx, respiratory tract, or anal canal of the newborn. The risk of contamination increases with prolonged rupture of membranes. Prevention of gonococcal ophthalmia by prophylactic use of 1% silver nitrate eyedrops has led to the emergence of inclusion conjunctivitis caused by *Chlamydia* as a more common form of ophthalmia neonatorum. Since neonates and young infants lack bactericidal IgM antibody against *N. gonorrhoeae,* they may be at increased risk for gonococcal bacteremia. During the first year of life, infection of the infant usually results from accidental contamination of the eye or vagina by an adult. Between 1 year of age and puberty, many cases of gonorrhea involve vulvovaginitis in females who have been molested by a relative, and medicolegal considerations necessitate a complete bacteriologic diagnosis and child welfare consultation.

Disseminated gonococcal infection In some areas of the world, from 1 to 3 percent of adults with gonococcal infection develop gonococcemia. Approximately two-thirds of such patients are women. The majority of men and women with gonococcemia do not have symptoms of urogenital, anorectal, or pharyngeal gonococcal infection. Gonococcemia may occur soon after acquisition of new infection or later, during menstruation. As noted below, serum bactericidal activity, rather than opsonic activity, appears essential for protection against gonococcal bacteremia.

The onset of gonococcemia is characterized by fever, polyarthralgias, and papular, petechial, pustular, hemorrhagic, or necrotic skin lesions. Approximately 3 to 20 such lesions appear, usually on the distal extremities. Gonococci are demonstrable by immunofluorescent staining in about two-thirds of gonococcal skin lesions. The initial joint involvement is characteristically limited to tenosynovitis involving several joints asymmetrically. The wrists, fingers, knees, and ankles are most often involved. Circulating immune complexes have been demonstrated at this stage of infection in some but not all studies. Serum complement levels are normal (except in those with complement deficiency), and the role of immune complexes, if any, is uncertain. Without treatment, the duration of gonococcemia is variable; the systemic manifestations of bacteremia may subside spontaneously within a week. (It is possible that many such cases go undiagnosed and the actual risk of gonococcemia exceeds current estimates.) Alternatively, septic arthritis ensues, often without prior symptoms of bacteremia. Pain and swelling then increase in one or, very occasionally, more joints, with accumulation of purulent synovial fluid, leading to progressive destruction of the joint if treatment is delayed. A continuum exists from the manifestations of bacteremia (polyarthralgias, new skin lesions) to septic arthritis, but the probability of positive blood cultures decreases after 48 h of illness, and the probability of recovery of gonococci from synovial fluid increases with increasing duration of illness. Gonococci are infrequently recovered from early effusions containing less than 20,000 leukocytes per cubic millimeter, but are usually recovered from effusions containing more than 80,000 leukocytes per cubic millimeter. In the individual patient, gonococci are seldom recovered from blood and synovial fluid simultaneously.

Other common manifestations of disseminated gonococcal infection include mild myopericarditis and "toxic" hepatitis. Endocarditis and meningitis are infrequent but severe complications. Endocarditis is suggested by pathological or changing heart murmurs, major embolic phenomena, severe myocarditis, deterioration of renal function, or an unusually large number of skin lesions.

PATHOGENESIS Understanding of the pathogenesis of gonorrhea has developed rapidly. Epidemiologic data suggest that only about one-third of men become infected after a single exposure to gonorrhea, and under experimental conditions an inoculum of 10^3 organisms appears necessary to establish urethral infection in 50 percent of male volunteers. Factors which may confer resistance to infection are undefined. Components of the urethral or vaginal flora, such as *Candida albicans, Staphylococcus epidermidis,* and certain types of lactobacilli, can inhibit *N. gonorrhoeae* in vitro and may provide some natural resistance in vivo. The virulence of gonococcal strains may vary, depending on their ability to remove iron from transferrin in blood or from lactoferrin on mucosal surfaces.

Although it is still not known whether naturally acquired gonorrhea confers immunity to reinfection, there is evidence that one episode of gonococcal salpingitis confers protection against a second attack of salpingitis with the same protein I serotype of gonococcus. Attachment of gonococci to mucosal cells is mediated in part by pili, and local antibody to pili can block attachment. Pili also impede phagocytosis of gonococci by neutrophils, and antibody to pili is opsonic. Antibody to other surface gonococcal antigens might also fix complement (present in low concentration at mucosal surfaces) by the classic or alternate pathway, resulting in opsonization or bactericidal activity. An enzyme produced by the pathogenic *Neisseria,* IgA_1 protease, which inactivates $sIgA_1$, may interfere with the antiadherence activity and with alternate pathway complement activation, resulting in increased attachment and reduced opsonization. However, since 50 percent of sIgA found at mucosal surfaces is present as IgA_2, which is resistant to IgA_1 protease, the role of gonococcal IgA_1 protease is uncertain.

Following attachment to columnar or transitional epithelium, gonococci penetrate through or between cells to reach the subepithelial connective tissue. Gonococci contain lipopolysaccharide which is cytotoxic and also produce proteases, phospholipases, and elastases which may play a role in pathogenesis. Gonococcal strains vary markedly in reactivity with normal serum IgM antibody, which appears to be directed against LPS antigens and results in generation of the chemotactic factor C5a and in the formation of the bactericidal C5–9 attack complex. Normal human serum also appears to contain antibodies, directed against an undefined surface protein antigen present on certain strains of gonococci, which block the bactericidal action of IgM antibody for such strains. These serum-resistant strains, which account for most cases of gonococcal bacteremia and, paradoxically, for most cases of asymptomatic urethral infection in men, are predominantly of the WI serogroup.

Spread of gonococci from the cervix to the endometrium and salpinges appears to be enhanced in women using an intrauterine device and impeded by oral contraceptive usage. Menstruation further increases the risk of intralumenal ascent from the cervix and evidently also predisposes to gonococcal bacteremia. Though natural serum IgM antibody prevents bacteremia by all but the serum-resistant strains of *N. gonorrhoeae,* patients deficient in the terminal complement components C5, C6, C7, or C8 are uniquely susceptible to bacteremia with serum-sensitive strains of gonococci, as well as to meningococcemia. Susceptibility to gonorrhea, to ascending gonococcal pelvic inflammatory disease (PID), and to gonococcemia depends upon a complex interplay of host factors and virulence properties of the organism.

DIFFERENTIAL DIAGNOSIS Gonococcal infection produces several common clinical syndromes which have multiple etiologies or which mimic other conditions. In particular, the epidemiology and clinical manifestations of *Chlamydia trachomatis* infections closely resemble those of gonococcal infections. The differential diagnosis of urethritis, epididymitis, and proctitis in men, vaginitis and cervicitis in women, and of acute arthritis in young adults is discussed in Chap. 143. The differential diagnosis of pelvic inflammatory disease is discussed in Chap. 144.

LABORATORY DIAGNOSIS The Gram's stain of urethral or endocervical exudate is considered diagnostic of gonorrhea when typical gram-negative diplococci are seen within leukocytes, is equivocal if only extracellular or atypical gram-negative diplococci are seen, and is negative if no gram-negative diplococci are seen. When these criteria are employed by experienced microbiologists, the sensitivity and specificity of Gram's stain of the urethral exudate approach 100 percent. Even so, in areas where β-lactamase-positive gonococci are seen, culture should be performed to allow testing of isolates for β-lactamase production. The specificity of Gram's stain of purulent cervical exudate also is high, but the sensitivity is only about 50 percent. Thayer-Martin (TM) medium, which contains antibiotics to inhibit most other organisms selectively, is most useful for recovering the gonococcus from the endocervix, anal canal, and pharynx, which are colonized by a mixed bacterial flora. The concentration of vancomycin should not exceed 3 μg/ml, and even this concentration may inhibit a small proportion of gonococci. Other media have been introduced (e.g., New York City medium) which allow somewhat better growth of gonococcal colonies but are more expensive to prepare. Whatever medium is used, after inoculation, the medium should be placed in an atmosphere containing 3 to 10 percent carbon dioxide to permit growth of the gonococcus. This can be accomplished in a candle jar by generation of carbon dioxide chemically within packets which are sealed after inoculation, or within special CO_2 incubators. Inoculated media should be incubated at 36°C for 48 h, and putative gonococcal colonies should be confirmed by oxidase reaction, Gram's stain, and sugar utilization tests or immunofluorescence using antiserums which are specific for *N. gonorrhoeae.* The latter are especially important for isolates from the pharynx and anal canal and for cultures obtained from populations which have a low prevalence of gonorrhea, such as prenatal patients.

In men with incubating or chronic asymptomatic urethral infection without exudate, or as a test of cure following treatment, a very thin swab or wire bacteriologic loop should be inserted 2 cm into the anterior urethra and used to inoculate TM medium. Cultures of the pharynx and anal canal should be obtained from all homosexual men with suspected gonorrhea.

The most efficient test for gonorrhea in women is the endocervical culture, which is positive on a single examination in approximately 80 to 90 percent of those with gonorrhea. This diagnostic yield can be increased by performing a second endocervical culture and by performing cultures of the rectum, urethra, and pharynx.

Standard blood culture broth medium containing 3 to 10 percent carbon dioxide should be used in culturing blood and is also recommended for culturing synovial fluid. In pus from skin lesions, *N. gonorrhoeae* is more often demonstrable by Gram's stain or immunofluorescent staining than by culture. Techniques designed to detect gonococcal infection by testing of a single serum have been limited thus far by inability to differentiate antibody due to past gonorrhea from antibody due to current infection, and by false-positive tests caused by cross-reactive antibody to *N. meningitidis.* For these reasons, the available serologic tests for gonorrhea have a very low predictive value; for example, only about 10 percent of prenatal patients with a reactive serologic test actually had gonorrhea in one representative study. Gonococcal serology is of no value.

Another diagnostic approach is the detection of gonococcal antigen in urethral or cervical secretion by enzyme-linked immunosorbent assay (ELISA). In men with urethritis, the Gram stain is just as accurate, quicker, and cheaper. In women, the role of such tests remains to be deteremined.

TREATMENT The preferred drugs for gonococcal infection for several years have been penicillin G, ampicillin, or amoxicillin, tetracycline hydrochloride, and spectinomycin. Although long-acting forms of penicillin (such as benzathine penicillin G) are effective in syphilotherapy, they have *no place* in the treatment of gonorrhea. Oral penicillin preparations such as penicillin V and the isoxazolyl penicillins are not recommended for the treatment of gonococcal infection. Since 1979, several important new facts concerning antibiotic sensitivity and resistance of the gonococcus have come to light. The incidence of infections due to penicillinase-producing *N. gonorrhoeae* has increased. Anecdotal reports suggest an emergence of tetracycline-resistant isolates of *N. gonorrhoeae* in certain geographic areas. The relatively high frequency of coexistent chlamydial infection in patients with gonococcal infections has been demonstrated in many populations. The importance of serious complications related to chlamydial infections has been established. Several new and more expensive β-lactam antibiotics which are effective in gonococcal infection have come onto the market. Although uncommon, spectinomycin resistance has been described in several treatment failures from England. The following guidelines for gonococcal infections attempt to consider these new developments, but they do not represent a comprehensive list of all possible treatment regimens. These guidelines are adapted from recommendations made by a CDC advisory committee in 1982. Whenever a specific cephalosporin or cephamycin is recommended, substitution with an equally effective third-generation cephalosporin or related β-lactam antibiotic is acceptable. As is shown in Table 150-1, a regimen combining a single dose of amoxicillin or ampicillin plus probenecid, together with a 7-day course of tetracycline, is recommended for uncomplicated gonococcal infections in heteorsexual adults. Although this combination regimen has not been extensively studied, it can be expected to provide adequate therapy for gonorrhea at any site, including the pharynx, and eliminates coexisting *C. trachomatis* infections. In patients who can not tolerate tetracycline, the single-dose oral ampicillin or amoxicillin/probenecid regimen can be given alone. Patients allergic to the penicillins can be given the 7-day tetracycline course alone. All tetracyclines are ineffective as single-dose therapy. Doxycycline, 100 mg by mouth twice a day for 7 days, may be substituted for tetracycline.

Homosexual men with uncomplicated gonococcal infection should be treated with aqueous procaine penicillin G, 4.8 million units, plus 1.0 g of probenecid. Men allergic to penicillin should receive spectinomycin, 2.0 g, in one intramuscular injection. Either of these regimens will provide adequate treatment for urethral and anorectal gonorrhea. Coexisting chlamydial infection is less common in homosexual men with gonorrhea than in heterosexual men with gonorrhea. With parenteral penicillin G, the risk of anaphylaxis in patients who deny previous penicillin allergy has been about 0.04 percent. The risk of procaine reaction due to transient neurotoxic serum concentrations of procaine is probably between 0.1 and 1 percent with the currently recommended dosage.

All patients with gonorrhea should have a serologic test for syphilis at the time of diagnosis. Patients with incubating seronegative syphilis, without clinical signs of syphilis, are likely to be cured by any of the recommended regimens (except spectinomycin) and need not have later follow-up tests for syphilis. However, patients with gonorrhea who also have syphilis or who are established contacts of someone with syphilis should be given additional treatment appropriate to the stage of syphilis. As a test of cure of gonorrhea, follow-up cervical, anal canal, and other appropriate cultures should be obtained from women, and urethral and other appropriate cultures from men, 3 to 7 days after completion of therapy.

The patient in whom gonorrhea persists after treatment with one of the nonspectinomycin regimens above should be treated with 2.0 g of spectinomycin intramuscularly, because gonococci which demonstrate increased resistance to penicillin G, ampicillin, amoxicillin, or tetracycline show no cross-resistance to spectinomycin. Most recurrent gonococcal infections after treatment with the recommended schedules are due to reinfection and indicate a need for improved contact tracing and patient education. Since infection by PPNG is a cause of treatment failure, posttreatment isolates should be tested for pencillinase production.

Patients with proven PPNG infection or who are likely to have acquired gonorrhea in areas of high PPNG prevalence and their sexual partners should receive spectinomycin, 2.0 g, intramuscularly in a single injection. Tetracycline may be added to treat coexistent chlamydial infection. More recently, certain third-generation cephalosporins have also proved to be highly effective for PPNG infection. Cefotaxime can be used in a single dose of 1 g intramuscularly. Ceftriaxone (not yet commercially available) is the most active of the cephalosporins yet

TABLE 150-1
Recommended treatment for gonococcal infection

Diagnosis	*Treatment of choice*
Uncomplicated gonococcal infection in adults	Amoxicillin 3.0 g or ampicillin 3.5 g single oral dose, given with 1.0 g probenecid by mouth, and followed by tetracycline 0.5 g by mouth four times a day for 7 days (total dose = 14 g) (if penicillin-allergic, give the 7-day tetracycline regimen alone)
Uncomplicated gonococcal infection in homosexual men	Aqueous procaine penicillin G (APPG), 4.8 million units total dose given intramuscularly at two sites, with 1.0 g probenecid by mouth (if penicillin-allergic, give spectinomycin 2.0 g in one intramuscular injection*)
Treatment failures or penicillinase-producing *N. gonorrhoeae*	Spectinomycin 2.0 g single intramuscular dose* *or* cefoxitin 2.0 g single intramuscular injection with 1.0 g probenecid by mouth* *or* cefotaxime 1.0 g single intramuscular injection*
Gonorrhea in pregnancy	Amoxicillin 3.0 g or ampicillin 3.5 g single oral dose, given with 1.0 g probenecid by mouth (if penicillin-allergic, give spectinomycin 2.0 g single intramuscular dose)
Disseminated gonococcal infection	Hospitalization is recommended Aqueous crystalline penicillin G, 10 million units intravenously per day until improvement, followed by ampicillin 0.5 g by mouth four times daily to complete 7 days of antibiotic treatment
Gonococcal PID	Hospitalization is recommended; see Chap. 144 for suggested antimicrobial therapy
Gonococcal epididymitis	See Chap. 143 for recommended therapy
Pediatric gonococcal infection	Children who weigh 100 lb (45 kg) should receive adult regimens; for those who weigh less than 100 lb, see discussion in text

* *Not effective for pharyngeal gonococcal infection (see text).*

tested and has a long half-life which is well suited for single-dose treatment of gonorrhea. A single dose of 250 mg of ceftriaxone intramuscularly cures nearly 100 percent of uncomplicated gonococcal infections, including those caused by PPNG. Cefoxitin, a cephamycin, is effective for PPNG infection in a dose of 2.0 g intramuscularly, together with 1.0 g of probenecid by mouth.

Postgonococcal urethritis (PGU) usually becomes apparent about two to three weeks after treatment of gonorrhea with a penicillin or a cephalosporin. PGU often appears to be caused by *C. trachomatis* which was probably acquired at the same time as gonorrhea but did not become clinically apparent until later because of the longer incubation period of chlamydial infection. When PGU occurs, it can be managed, like nongonococcal urethritis, with tetracycline, 0.5 g four times a day for at least 7 days. Similarly, mucopurulent cervicitis in women often persists or appears after treatment of gonorrhea with a penicillin, is often caused by *C. trachomatis,* and can be treated like PGU with tetracycline 0.5 g four times a day for 7 days. Men and women exposed to gonorrhea should be examined, cultured, and treated with one of the recommended treatment schedules.

All pregnant women should have endocervical cultures for gonococci as an integral part of the prenatal care at the time of the first visit unless epidemiologic data would suggest otherwise. A second culture late in the third trimester should be obtained from women at high risk of gonococcal infection.

Drug regimens of choice in pregnancy are ampicillin or amoxicillin, each with probenecid as described above. Women who are allergic to penicillin or probenecid should be treated with spectinomycin, 2.0 g intramuscularly. Erythromycin in the dosage recommended for chlamydial infection can be added to treat coexistent chlamydial infection. Tetracycline should not be used in pregnant women because of potential toxic effects for mother and fetus.

The management of pelvic inflammatory disease is discussed in Chap. 144. Hospitalization of women with PID is recommended whenever practical. Adequate treatment of women with acute PID must include examination and appropriate treatment of sex partners because of their high prevalence of nonsympatomatic urethral infection. Failure to treat sex partners may lead to recurrent salpingitis.

Treatment of gonococcal arthritis can be accomplished satisfactorily with several regimens. Gonococci recovered from patients with gonococcal arthritis have been significantly less resistant to penicillin or tetracycline than isolates from patients with uncomplicated gonorrhea. However, because of the threat of endocarditis, meningitis, and joint sepsis, all patients with disseminated infection should preferably be hospitalized and treated with aqueous crystalline penicillin G intravenously, 10 million units per day until clinical improvement occurs. Treatment can then be completed on an outpatient basis with ampicillin, 2 g per day orally to complete a 7- to 10-day course of therapy. As summarized in the CDC recommendation, a 3-day course of high-dose intravenous penicillin therapy alone, or treatment with ampicillin, 3.5 g daily orally with 1 g probenecid, followed by 0.5 g four times a day for 7 days, also probably represents adequate therapy for disseminated gonococcal infection. Failure to improve with one of these regimens strongly suggests a diagnosis other than disseminated gonococcal infection. Repeated joint aspiration or closed irrigation of the joint with sterile saline may be required to reduce inflammation in patients with high synovial fluid leukocyte counts. Open drainage is seldom, if ever, required for gonococcal arthritis, except in infants with hip infection. Temporary immobilization of the joint may reduce discomfort for the patient and may be useful during initial ambulation in patients with persistent effusions of the knee or ankle. Antibiotics should not be injected directly into the joint. Once the diagnosis of gonococcal arthritis is proven, then occasional patients may benefit from use of anti-inflammatory agents along with antimicrobial therapy. However, if the diagnosis is suspected, but not proven, then early use of anti-inflammatory drugs will prevent monitoring the response to antimicrobial therapy, which is usually rapid and often of diagnostic importance in gonococcal arthritis.

Meningitis and endocarditis caused by the gonococcus require high-dose intravenous penicillin therapy. In penicillin-allergic patients with endocarditis, cefoxitin 2.0 g or cefotaxime 1.0 g, IV, four times daily for 14 days may be used, but cross-allergenicity with penicillin may occur. Cefotaxime or moxalactam may be used in penicillin-allergic patients with gonococcal meningitis.

Gonococcal conjunctivitis in the adult or newborn should be managed as a medical emergency by irrigation of the conjunctiva with saline, together with penicillin G given intravenously.

Pediatric gonococcal infection The infant born to a mother with gonorrhea is at high risk of infection and requires treatment with a single intravenous or intramuscular injection of aqueous crystalline penicillin G, 50,000 units to the full-term infant or 20,000 units to the low-birth-weight infant. Topical prophylaxis for neonatal ophthalmia is not adequate treatment for infections at other sites. Clinical illness requires additional treatment.

Neonates with gonococcal ophthalmia should be hospitalized and isolated for 24 h after initiation of treatment. Untreated gonococcal ophthalmia is highly contagious and may rapidly lead to blindness. Aqueous crystalline penicillin G, 50,000 units per kilogram per day, in two daily doses intravenously should be administered for 7 days. Irrigation of the eyes with saline or buffered ophthalmic solutions should be performed immediately and then at least at hourly intervals as long as necessary to eliminate discharge. Topical antibiotic preparations alone are not sufficient or required when appropriate systemic antibiotic therapy is given. Both of the parents of a newborn with gonococcal ophthalmia must be treated for gonorrhea.

Neonates with arthritis and bacteremia should be hospitalized and treated with aqueous crystalline penicillin G, 75,000 to 100,000 units per kilogram per day, intravenously in two or three divided doses for 7 days. Meningitis should be treated with aqueous crystalline penicillin G, 100,000 units per kilogram per day, divided into three or four intravenous doses, and continued for at least 10 days.

Uncomplicated gonococcal vulvovaginitis, urethritis, proctitis, or pharyngitis in older children can be treated at a single visit with amoxicillin, 50 mg/kg, orally with probenecid, 25 mg/kg (maximum 1.0 g), or with aqueous procaine penicillin G, 100,000 units/kg, intramuscularly plus probenecid, 25 mg/kg (maximum 1.0 g).

Topical and/or systemic estrogen therapy is of no benefit in gonococcal vulvovaginitis. Long-acting penicillins, such as benzathine penicillin G, are not effective. All patients should have follow-up cultures, and the source of infection should be identified, examined, and treated.

Children who are allergic to penicillins should be treated with spectinomycin, 40 mg/kg, intramuscularly. Children older than 8 years may be treated with tetracycline, 40 mg/kg per day, by mouth, in four divided doses for 5 days. For treatment of complicated disease, the alternative regimens recommended for adults may be used in appropriate pediatric dosages.

PPNG infection in neonates should be treated with cefotaxime or gentamicin in appropriate doses; in children it should be treated with spectinomycin or cefotaxime.

PREVENTION AND CONTROL There is probably no more striking illustration than gonorrhea of the failure of a specific treatment alone to eradicate a communicable disease. Vaccination is not available. Use of the condom can prevent transmission, and the extensive use of condoms for contraception may be responsible for the low rates of gonorrhea in some countries (e.g., Japan). Prophylactic antibiotics (e.g., 200 mg minocycline or doxycycline taken soon after sexual exposure) have been shown to reduce the risk of infection, but are not recommended for general use or for individuals with known exposure to gonorrhea, who should receive one of the regimens recommended for established gonorrhea. The efficacy of local vaginal antiseptic and spermicidal preparations for prevention of venereal disease requires further study.

To try to contain the increasing spread of β-lactamase-producing gonococci, several measures are important: (1) routine use of diagnosis by cultures and testing of isolates for penicillin resistance or β-lactamase production in areas where PPNG is prevalent; (2) routine use of spectinomycin or an appropriate cephalosporin (e.g., cefotaxime) for gonorrhea treatment failures; (3) rapid epidemiologic tracing of contacts of patients with gonorrhea, particularly treatment failures of those known to be infected with PPNG; and (4) routine use of a β-lactamase-resistant antibiotic (e.g., spectinomycin) in areas where PPNG exceeds a certain threshold proportion (e.g., >5 percent) of all gonococcal isolates. The most effective public health measure now available for control of gonorrhea is tracing sexual contacts of infected patients. Experienced interviewers are able to identify and bring to treatment an average of one additional case for every patient interviewed.

REFERENCES

Curran JW et al: Female gonorrhea. Its relations to abnormal uterine bleeding, urinary tract symptoms and cervicitis. Obstet Gynecol 45:195, 1975

Easmon CSF et al: Emergence of resistance after spectinomycin treatment for gonorrhoea due to beta-lactamase-producing strain of *Neisseria gonorrhoeae.* Br Med J 284:1604, 1982

Handsfield HH et al: Asymptomatic gonorrhea in men. Diagnosis, natural course, prevalence and significance. N Engl J Med 290:117, 1974

——— et al: Treatment of the gonococcal arthritis-dermatitis syndrome. Ann Intern Med 84:661, 1976

——— et al: Epidemiology of penicillinase-producing *Neisseria gonorrhoeae* infections: Analysis by auxotyping and serogrouping. N Engl J Med 306:950, 1982

Holmes KK et al: Disseminated gonococcal infection. Ann Intern Med 74:979, 1971

Morse SA: The biology of the gonococcus. CRC Crit Rev Microbiol 7:93, 1978

Petersen BH et al: *Neisseria meningitidis* and *Neisseria gonorrhoeae* bacteremia associated with C6, C7, or C8 deficiency. Ann Intern Med 90:917, 1979

Roberts M et al: Molecular characterization of two beta-lactamase specifying plasmids isolated from *Neisseria gonorrhoeae.* J Bacteriol 131:557, 1977

Roberts RB: *The Gonococcus.* New York, Wiley, 1977

Sparling PF et al: Antibiotic resistance in the gonococcus: Diverse mechanisms of coping with a hostile environment, in *Immunobiology of* Neisseria gonorrhoeae, GF Brooks et al (eds). Washington DC, Am Soc Microbiol, 1978, pp 44–52

St. John RK et al: Gonorrhea therapy—1979. Position papers for the current USPHS recommendations. Sex Transm Dis 6(Suppl):87, 1979

Sexually transmitted diseases treatment guidelines 1982, Morb Mort Week Rep 31:25, 1982

Wiesner PJ, Thompson SE III: Gonococcal disease. Dis Mon 26, 1980

section 4 | Diseases caused by enteric gram-negative bacilli

151 INFECTIONS DUE TO ENTEROBACTERIACEAE

MARVIN TURCK
DENNIS SCHABERG

ESCHERICHIA COLI INFECTIONS

ETIOLOGY *Escherichia coli* is a group of gram-negative nonsporing rods which belong to the family Enterobacteriaceae. They generally ferment lactose, as opposed to the medically significant non-lactose-fermenting organisms, such as *Salmonella, Shigella,* and *Proteus.* The so-called paracolon bacilli are organisms which ferment lactose late, irregularly, or not at all, and on more careful biochemical and antigenic testing are found to belong to one or another of the genera of the Enterobacteriaceae, which comprise *Salmonella, Arizona, Citrobacter, Shigella, Escherichia, Klebsiella, Enterobacter, Hafnia, Serratia, Proteus,* and *Providencia.* All these organisms are readily culturable on ordinary media and are aerobic and facultatively anaerobic. All species ferment glucose, reduce nitrates to nitrites, and are oxidase-negative and catalase-positive. They are differentiated by biochemical and serologic tests, species- or group-specific bacteriophages, DNA relatedness tests, and computerized identification programs. It is important to make this differentiation, not only taxonomically, but also because of epidemiologic and therapeutic implications.

PATHOGENESIS *Escherichia coli* is regarded generally as a normal commensal in the gastrointestinal tract, from which it may spread to infect contiguous structures if normal anatomic barriers are interrupted, as occurs in appendiceal perforation. It is believed that the urinary tract is infected from without via urethral contamination, but direct hematogenous spread may also account for renal infection. Once infection has occurred in a primary focus, further spread to distant organs may occur via the bloodstream. There is experimental and clinical evidence that *E. coli* tends to settle in avascular or necrotic tissue. In more than 50 percent of *E. coli* infections the urinary tract is the portal of entry; infections emanating from the hepatobiliary tree, peritoneal cavity, skin, and lung are not uncommon. A number of patients with *E. coli* bacteremia have no demonstrable portal of entry; they often have neoplastic and hematologic diseases. There may be other defects in host resistance, including diabetes mellitus, cirrhosis, and sickle cell anemia, or recent administration of irradiation, cytotoxic drugs, adrenal steroids, or antibiotics. There also is epidemiologic evidence that *E. coli* and other Enterobacteriaceae tend to colonize the skin and mucous membranes of debilitated patients, possibly accounting for the increased frequency of these infections in patients with advanced illness. Morphologically the lesions produced in various tissues show typical acute inflammation with pus and abscess formation. There is a common misconception that *E. coli* bacterial infections are characterized by a foul-smelling, feculent exudate. Such an odor is caused by anaerobic streptococci or *Bacteroides* species, which are often associated with coliform bacteria in mixed infection. In fact, organisms of the genus *Bacteroides* outnumber *E. coli* as the most prevalent gram-negative flora in the intestine.

EPIDEMIOLOGY Strains of *E. coli* are characterized by their somatic (O), flagellar (H), and capsular (K or B) antigens, and there are hundreds of different serologic varieties. Any of the strains is capable of causing disease. Clinical and epidemiologic studies have demonstrated that certain specific *E. coli* serotypes are more frequently incriminated in diarrheal disease of the infant and newborn. Strains incriminated in infantile diarrhea probably are disseminated within nurseries by symptomatic or asymptomatic infant carriers, mothers, and nurses. Although fecal contamination is the usual mode of spread, airborne contamination and fomite spread may also occur.

Some epidemiologic studies have suggested that *E. coli* 04, 06, and 075 are responsible for most *E. coli* infections other than infantile diarrhea. It is unclear whether these strains actually are more virulent or merely are more prevalent than other somatic types. In fact, virulence factors may be associated more closely with the K than with the somatic antigen and may account for the frequency with which certain strains cause parenchymal infection.

Strains of *E. coli* with K_1 antigen are recovered from an inordinate number of neonates with meningitis. In general, K antigens appear to be highly negatively charged acidic polysaccharides whose effect is to block agglutination by O antiserum. These K antigens have been implicated in promoting adherence to host cells and in resisting phagocytosis.

MANIFESTATIONS Urinary tract infections *Escherichia coli* accounts for well over 75 percent of urinary tract infections, including cystitis, pyelitis, pyelonephritis, and asymptomatic bacteriuria. Strains cultured from patients with acute, uncomplicated urinary tract infections are almost invariably *E. coli,* whereas other Enterobacteriaceae and strains of *Pseudomonas* become prevalent among patients with chronic infection. Urinary tract infections are discussed in Chap. 296.

Peritoneal and biliary infections *Escherichia coli* can usually be cultured from a perforated or inflamed appendix or from abscesses secondary to perforated diverticula, peptic ulcers, subphrenic or lesser sac abscesses, or mesenteric infarction. Often, other organisms, including anaerobic streptococci, clostridia, and *Bacteroides,* are found along with *E. coli.* Acute cholecystitis with gangrene and perforation is often associated with *E. coli* infection. An air-fluid level associated with stones or a circumferential layer of gas in the wall of the gallbladder may be detectable by x-ray and is characteristic of acute emphysematous cholecystitis. From the gallbladder, infection may ascend via the biliary tree to produce cholangitis and multiple liver abscesses. More rarely *E. coli* infection in the peritoneal cavity may produce a septic thrombophlebitis of the portal vein (pylephlebitis), which in turn is followed by liver abscesses.

Bacteremia Invasion of the bloodstream is the most serious manifestation of *E. coli* infection; it is characterized usually by the sudden onset of fever and chills, but sometimes only by mental confusion, dyspnea, or unexplained hypotension. It is most common in patients with urinary tract infection and biliary or intraperitoneal sepsis, and following abortions or pelvic surgery. In some patients no portal of entry is evident. Most cases occur in elderly males, presumably because of the high incidence of urethral instrumentation and catheterization in this group. Fever ranges between 100 and 106°F and is higher in younger patients. Hyperventilation may be an early sign. Hypotension may be present from the onset but usually occurs within 12 to 16 h after bacteremia; if it is persistent, it is accompanied by oliguria and often by mental confusion, stupor, and coma. The skin is warm and dry initially, but most patients develop some evidence of peripheral vasoconstriction characterized by cold and cyanotic extremities. Fortunately hypotension is transient and self-limited in most patients with *E. coli* bacteremia and is absent altogether in some. However, about 25 percent of patients with bacteremia develop more prolonged hypotension, a syndrome known as *gram-negative* or *endotoxin shock,* which is discussed in Chap. 139.

Occasionally *E. coli* bacteremia develops in patients with cirrhosis without an overt portal of entry. This has been variably attributed to portosystemic shunts both in and around the liver, impaired reticuloendothelial function, and diminution in humoral and cellular defense mechanisms.

Other manifestations *Escherichia coli* may produce abscesses anywhere in the body. Subcutaneous infections are found at the site of insulin administration in diabetics, in extremities with ischemic gangrene, or in surgical wounds. Perirectal phlegmons are not uncommon in patients with leukemia. Subcutaneous abscesses are often characterized by formation of gas in tissue, especially among diabetics, which may be detected by crepitation or by x-ray and which must be differentiated from clostridial infection. From 5 to 10 percent of patients with *E. coli* bacteremia develop metastatic infection in bone, brain, liver, and lung. *Escherichia coli* may cause pneumonia de novo; also, *E. coli* are often cultured from sputum in pulmonary superinfections.

Neonatal infection Neonates, particularly premature infants, often develop *E. coli* bacteremia associated with meningitis and bloodborne pyelonephritis. Fecal soiling and absence of maternal gamma-G globulin (IgM) antibody are two of the factors which render this group particularly susceptible to *E. coli* infections.

Gastroenteritis Children under 2 years of age develop gastroenteritis, typified by nausea, vomiting, and diarrhea. Most outbreaks have occurred in nurseries and have been due to specific strains of enteropathogenic *E. coli* (EPEC). These particular strains produce toxins, one of which is heat labile (LT) and similar to the toxin elaborated by *Vibrio cholerae,* while the other is heat stable (ST) (see also Chaps. 142 and 166). Fluorescent antibody techniques have been useful in the rapid identification of organisms with serotypes frequently implicated in this syndrome. Although theoretically any *E. coli* strain might be cultured, since the genetic information coding for toxin production is found on a plasmid and can be transferred between *E. coli* strains, the number of different serotypes involved remains restricted. Although diarrhea is usually mediated through production of enterotoxins, occasionally *E. coli* may be enteroinvasive, involving the mucosa and causing disease akin to *Shigella* dysentery. The rapid dehydration, with its attendant high mortality, demands prompt recognition of this condition, isolation of the infants, and treatment of both patients and contacts with the appropriate antibiotic. *Escherichia coli* is also being recognized as a cause of acute diarrheal disease in adults, especially foreign travelers.

LABORATORY FINDINGS There are no characteristic laboratory abnormalities. The white blood cell count is usually elevated, and there is a preponderance of granulocytes. At times, however, the white count is normal or low. When *E. coli* infection occurs in previously healthy individuals, anemia is absent, but more commonly there is anemia which is usually related to the patient's underlying disease. *Escherichia coli* grows readily in a variety of bacteriologic media and should be cultured from appropriate secretions and blood. In the presence of gram-negative shock, there are often profound metabolic derangements, including azotemia, metabolic acidosis, hypokalemia, and hyperkalemia, as well as a variety of coagulation defects (see Chap. 139).

DIAGNOSIS *Escherichia coli* cannot be differentiated from most other gram-negative bacteria on Gram's stain, and culture followed by appropriate biochemical characterization is necessary to identify the organism precisely. Serologic typing of *E. coli* may be useful in individual patients with recurrent urinary tract infections in order to help differentiate between relapse and reinfection.

TREATMENT As with other infections, drainage of pus and removal of foreign bodies are essential. If *E. coli* is suspected as the etiologic agent in a particular infection, choice of an appropriate antimicrobial will depend upon the site and type of infection as well as upon its severity. Often the outcome of the infection depends upon the status of the associated disease, rather than on eradication of bacteria. For example, in acute, uncomplicated urinary tract infection in females, the disease is frequently self-limited even without antimicrobial therapy, and there is no evidence that antibiotics are superior to sulfonamides. Conversely, *E. coli* bacteremia in a patient with leukemia may not respond to antimicrobials unless a hematologic remission is achieved simultaneously.

In most situations, antibiotics should be selected, when possible, on the basis of their in vitro sensitivity tests. Although no drug is uniformly active against all strains of *E. coli,* a number of agents are effective against the majority of clinical isolates. If average obtainable plasma concentrations become the criteria for in vitro susceptibility, approximately 75 percent of *E. coli* strains are likely to be sensitive to the tetracyclines, 85 to 90 percent to chloramphenicol or ampicillin, and over 90 percent to gentamicin, kanamycin, tobramycin, or amikacin; 75 to 90 percent of *E. coli* will be inhibited by cephalosporin antibiotics. Many strains of *E. coli* are sensitive to high concentrations of penicillin G (50 to 100 μg/ml), and this drug may be used in dosage of 10 to 40 million units intravenously daily, particularly if probenecid is given concomitantly. This regimen has been largely superseded by ampicillin, 2 to 4 g per day intravenously or intramuscularly; for severe infections the dose can be raised to 6 to 12 g per day. The antibacterial spectrum of ampicillin against *E. coli* is probably identical with that achieved with very high concentrations of penicillin G, and with the spectrum covered by the tetracyclines or chloramphenicol. However, the bactericidal properties of ampicillin may be a distinct advantage over these two drugs, particularly in deep-seated infections. Gentamicin and tobramycin have been employed effectively in the initial treatment of severe *E. coli* infections in doses of 5 mg/kg per day in divided doses every 8 h. These drugs have superseded kanamycin in the treatment of many patients, although kanamycin remains effective against most *E. coli* in doses of 15 mg/kg per day given intramuscularly in divided doses every 8 to 12 h. Amikacin, which has been synthetically derived from kanamycin, is very active against isolates which are resistant to the other aminoglycosides. Dose and interval are identical to those recommended for kanamycin. Cephalosporins in concentration of 25 μg/ml or less are effective against many *E. coli* strains. This serum concentration can be obtained only with 1.5- to 2.0-g dosages at 3- to 4-h intervals with cephalothin. Newer cephalosporins have been developed which give slightly higher peak serum concentrations and in some instances have lower MICs for *E. coli* (see Chap. 141). Tetracyclines and chloramphenicol are still widely used in the treatment of *E. coli* infection, but better drugs are now available. Polymyxin B and colistin are also effective in vitro against the majority of *E. coli.* However, it is difficult to obtain adequate tissue and serum concentrations with these agents, and they should probably not be used for treatment of systemic *E. coli* infections. Although combinations of antimicrobials, i.e., streptomycin and tetracycline or streptomycin and chloramphenicol, have been recommended, there is little need to employ more than one agent in most situations. Nitrofurantoin (400 mg) and nalidixic acid (2 to 4 g) are reserved for treating patients with *E. coli* bacteriuria, and should not be employed when infection is suspected outside the urinary tract. Trimethroprim sulfamethoxazole is also useful in urinary tract infections (see Chap. 296).

PREVENTION Isolation and antimicrobial therapy of infants and contacts are essential to abort epidemic infantile diarrhea. In adults, many *E. coli* infections are hospital-associated, and their incidence can be reduced by limiting use of indwelling urinary and intravenous catheters, by careful surgical aseptic technique, by appropriate isolation of infection-prone patients, and by judicious use of antibiotics, steroids, and cytotoxic agents. There is mounting evidence that the promiscuous use of antibiotics may propagate the transfer of resistance factors among intestinal *E. coli.* These organisms may in turn transmit their resistance to other virulent Enterobacteriaceae, such as *Salmonella.*

KLEBSIELLA-ENTEROBACTER-SERRATIA INFECTIONS

ETIOLOGY Next to *E. coli,* strains of *Klebsiella, Enterobacter,* and *Serratia* are the most important enteric organisms infecting humans. In many laboratories *Klebsiella* are, in general, more resistant to antibiotics than *E. coli,* and their isolation from blood, purulent exudates, and urine is of more serious epidemiologic and prognostic significance. The Friedländer bacilli *(K. pneumoniae)* are encapsulated gram-negative bacilli, found among the normal flora of the mouth and intestinal tracts. *Klebsiella pneumoniae* has been considered to be a virulent respiratory pathogen since first described by Friedländer in 1882. *Klebsiella* is closely related to the genera *Enterobacter* and *Serratia* and may be differentiated only by certain amino acid decarboxylase tests. In addition to differentiation by these biochemical tests, which group *Klebsiella, Enterobacter,* and *Serratia,* strains of *Klebsiella* usually are nonmotile and form large mucoid colonies on solid media, whereas the other species are typically motile. Klebsiellas also are usually sensitive to concentrations of older cephalosporin antibiotics, to which *Enterobacter* and *Serratia* are resistant. These characteristics, however, are not invariable enough to differentiate various isolates from clinical sources. Strains of *Klebsiella* can be further distinguished on the basis of type-specific capsular antigens; more than 75 known capsular types have been identified. There is little evidence that certain types are more virulent than others, and the main role of capsular typing of *Klebsiella* is as an epidemiologic tool in nosocomial outbreaks of infection.

Klebsiella rhinoscleromatis is probably the causative agent of rhinoscleroma, and *K. ozenae* has been isolated occasionally from the nose of patients with ozena, a chronic severe rhinitis associated with turbinate atrophy and progressive anosmia. *Klebsiella oxytoca* is the new designation for indole-positive strains of *K. pneumoniae.*

PATHOGENESIS *Klebsiella, Enterobacter,* and *Serratia* are all capable of causing disease in diverse anatomic sites. However, results of clinical and epidemiologic studies suggest that differences in pathogenicity may exist among these genera and that precise taxonomic identification is of value. Although infections of the respiratory tract with *K. pneumoniae* have been emphasized most in the past, the urinary tract presently accounts for the majority of clinical isolates. In this site clinical manifestations and pathogenesis are similar to infections produced by *E. coli,* but klebsiellas are more frequently found in patients with complicated and obstructive urinary tract disease. Infections of the biliary tract, the peritoneal cavity, the middle ear, mastoids, paranasal sinuses, and meninges also are not uncommon. In these locations, *Klebsiella* is more frequent than either *Enterobacter* or *Serratia* and is more likely to produce an illness of greater severity. The apparent increased frequency of infection by *Serratia* represents an increase primarily due to nosocomial spread of this organism. *Enterobacter* species have been incriminated frequently in outbreaks of in-hospital infection attributed to contaminated intravenous solutions.

MANIFESTATIONS Symptoms and signs of common infections caused by *Klebsiella*—namely, those involving the urinary tract, biliary tree, and peritoneal cavity—are indistinguishable from those caused by *E. coli.* These infections commonly occur in diabetics and in the form of superinfections in patients who have received antimicrobials to which these organisms are resistant. *Klebsiella* infection is also an important etiologic factor in septic shock. *Serratia* and *Enterobacter* are almost exclusively nosocomial pathogens. These organisms have been implicated as pathogens in a wide variety of infections, most frequently pneumonia, urinary tract infections and bacteremia.

Pneumonia *Klebsiella* is well recognized as a pulmonary pathogen but probably accounts for less than 1 percent of all cases of bacterial pneumonia. The disease is most common in men over 40 years of age and is most frequently found in alcoholics. Other factors associated with increased susceptibility include diabetes mellitus and chronic bronchopulmonary disease. Aspiration of oropharyngeal secretions containing *Klebsiella* organisms is the likely inciting factor among alcoholic patients. The clinical manifestations are indistinguishable from those of pneumococcal pneumonia (see Chap. 146), with sudden onset of chills, fever, productive cough, and severe pleuritic chest pain. Patients are frequently delirious and prostrated, but this may also occur with pneumococcal infection. A "characteristic" clinical feature, which occurs in only 25 to 50 percent of patients, is the dark-brown or red-currant-jelly sputum which may be so tenacious that the patient has difficulty in expelling it from mouth and lips. The pulmonary lesion is most frequent in the right upper lobe but often rapidly progresses and, if untreated, may spread from lobe to lobe. Cyanosis and dyspnea develop rapidly, and jaundice, vomiting, and diarrhea may be present. Physical findings consist primarily of signs of consolidation unless pleural effusion or necrotizing pneumonitis with rapid cavitation has intervened. The blood leukocyte count may be elevated but is often low, which probably is a reflection of severe infection in an alcoholic patient with poor bone marrow reserve and folate deficiency. Lung abscess and empyema are much more frequent than in pneumococcal pneumonia and are related to the destructive capabilities of this organism. So-called characteristic and radiographic features such as bulging fissures and loss of lung volume occur only occasionally, and also may be found in pneumococcal infection, as well as in necrotizing pneumonia caused by other gram-negative species.

Klebsiella, Serratia, and *Enterobacter* are frequently seen in nosocomial pneumonia. Older patients become colonized with gram-negative bacilli in the oropharynx, and these organisms can then gain access to the respiratory tract and cause pneumonia or purulent bronchitis. Common-source outbreaks, with contamination of a variety of respiratory therapy devices, have been implicated in infections with these pathogens, especially *Serratia.*

Chronic infection of the lung Rarely, infection with *Klebsiella* may progress, often in indolent fashion, to a chronic necrotizing pneumonitis resembling tuberculosis. It may follow acute *Klebsiella* pneumonia but is also seen in patients who give no history of an acute onset. The principal symptoms are productive cough, weakness, and anemia. Hemoptysis, chronic empyema, or sterile serous effusions are also encountered. Cavitation, frequently with thin walls, occurs primarily in the upper lobes.

DIAGNOSIS Diagnosis of community-acquired pneumonia is established by an awareness of the clinical setting in which *Klebsiella* infections occur and by isolation of the organism. A presumptive diagnosis of *Klebsiella* pneumonia should be made on the basis of a Gram stain of the sputum which shows a predominance of short, plump, gram-negative bacilli, frequently surrounded by a clear space because of the capsule. Often these gram-negative organisms occur together with gram-positive cocci, and because the gram-positives are easier to see, the gram-negative bacteria may be ignored and the diagnosis may be missed, which, in turn, may lead to potentially serious delays in instituting therapy. Additional proof of *Klebsiella* infection in the lung is afforded by isolation of the organisms from blood and pleural exudate. In extrapulmonary infections, the organisms are readily seen in, and cultured from, pus or secretions of involved organs.

The diagnosis of nosocomial respiratory infection with these organisms may be more difficult, mainly because colonization has to be distinguished from infection. Careful evaluation of the clinical course is necessary in establishing a diagnosis. Transtracheal aspiration of sputum for culture and Gram's stain may be useful in difficult cases.

TREATMENT *Klebsiella, Enterobacter,* and *Serratia* have variable susceptibility to antimicrobial drugs, and cultures of these organisms need to be tested in vitro. Frequently, however, antimicrobial therapy needs to be insituted before results of antibiotic susceptibility tests become available. In general, the majority of strains of *Klebsiella* is susceptible to the aminoglycosides, the cephalosporins, chloramphenicol, and polymyxin B or colistin. *Klebsiella* isolates do not respond to penicillin and its analogues, although many isolates of *Enterobacter* are inhibited by 25 μg/ml carbenicillin. *Serratia* isolates are frequently resistant to many antimicrobials, and resistance to gentamicin and tobramycin is being encountered with increasing frequency. Amikacin has been used effectively in these drug-resistant infections. The antimicrobial regimen of choice in the treatment of *Klebsiella, Enterobacter,* and *Serratia* infection will vary from one institution to another depending on the resistance patterns as well as upon the degree of clinical severity of infection. In severely ill patients, the combination of an aminoglycoside such as tobramycin or gentamicin (3 to 5 mg/kg per day) or amikacin (15 mg/kg per day) with cephalothin, cephapirin, or cefazolin (4 to 12 g per day) is usually preferred. The newer cephalosporins and/or cephamycins, i.e., cefamandole, cefoxitin, and cefotaxime, also may be active against *Klebsiella, Enterobacter,* and *Serratia.* Occasionally, one or all of these compounds may be more active than the older cephalosporins, and in vitro susceptibility tests will be required to select the most appropriate agent. Because of the relatively poor blood and tissue levels obtained with the polymyxins, they should not be employed as first-line agents in the treatment of severe *Klebsiella* infections despite apparent in vitro susceptibility. Regardless of the antimicrobial regimen employed, treatment should be continued for a minimum of 10 to 14 days and prolonged if there is extensive cavitation. Pleural effusions must be drained; antibiotic therapy alone is not sufficient treatment for closed-space infections of the pleural cavity. At times, rib resection with open drainage may be necessary, and should be considered if effusions recur.

PROGNOSIS Before the introduction of antimicrobials, the fatality rate from these infections varied from 50 to 80 percent, and death within 48 h was not infrequent. Even with antimicrobial treatment the course of these infections is quite variable and the prognosis must be guarded. For the most part, this prognosis reflects the age group involved and the frequent association of *Klebsiella* infections with alcoholism, malnutrition, and severe underlying disease.

PROTEUS INFECTIONS

ETIOLOGY The genus *Proteus* consists of gram-negative bacilli which do not ferment lactose and are characterized by their active motility and spreading growth on solid media. There are four pathogenic species: *P. mirabilis, P. vulgaris, P. morganii,* and *P. rettgeri. P. morganii* has recently been reclassified as *Morganella morganii.* Some biogroups of *P. rettgeri* have been reclassified as *Providencia stuartii* and *Providencia rettgeri. Proteus mirabilis* causes 75 to 90 percent of human infections and is distinguishable from the other three species by its inability to form indole. All four split urea, with production of ammonia. Some strains of *P. vulgaris* share a common antigen with certain rickettsia, accounting for the appearance of antibodies against *Proteus* organisms (Weil-Felix reaction) in typhus, scrub typhus, and Rocky Mountain spotted fever. The *Providencia* group of organisms resembles those of the genus *Proteus* closely except for some differences in biochemical tests.

EPIDEMIOLOGY AND PATHOGENESIS Members of the genus *Proteus* are normally found in soil, water, and sewage and are part of the normal fecal flora. Occasionally, they have been implicated as a cause of epidemic diarrhea in infants, but the evidence for this is inconclusive. The organism is frequently cultured from superficial wounds, draining ears, and sputum, particularly in patients who have received antibiotics, and replaces the more susceptible flora eradicated by these drugs. *Proteus* organisms often localize in already damaged tissues, where they produce a typical exudative inflammatory reaction.

MANIFESTATIONS *Proteus* organisms are rarely primary invaders but produce disease in locations previously infected by other organisms. These locations include the skin, ears and mastoid, sinuses, eyes, peritoneal cavity, bone, urinary tract, meninges, lung, and bloodstream.

Cutaneous infections *Proteus* organisms are frequently isolated from surgical wounds, particularly following antimicrobial therapy, but they do not interfere with normal wound healing provided that the tissues are viable and foreign bodies are not present. Burns, varicose ulcers, and decubiti may become contaminated with *Proteus* organisms, often in company with other gram-negative organisms or staphylococci.

Infections of the ears and mastoid sinuses Otitis media and mastoiditis in which *Proteus* organisms are present can result in extensive destruction of the middle ear and mastoid sinuses. Fetid otorrhea, cholesteatoma, and granulation tissue constitute a chronic focus of infection in the middle and inner ears and mastoid, and deafness ensues. Paralysis of the facial nerve is an occasional complication. The great danger of these infections lies in intracranial extension, leading to thrombosis of the lateral sinus, meningitis, brain abscess, and bacteremia.

Ocular infections *Proteus* infection may cause corneal ulcers, usually following trauma to the eye, which occasionally terminate in panophthalmitis and destruction of the eyeball.

Peritonitis Being part of the normal intestinal flora, *Proteus* organisms may be isolated from the peritoneal cavity following perforation of viscera or mesenteric infarction.

Urinary tract infections *Proteus* organisms are a common cause of urinary tract infections, usually in patients with chronic bacteriuria, many of whom have had obstructive uropathy, a history of instrumentation of the bladder, and repeated courses of chemotherapy. The organism is rarely a pathogen in anatomically normal urinary tracts except occasionally in patients with diabetes mellitus. *Proteus* organisms are also often cultured from bacteriuric patients with renal or bladder calculi. This fact may be related to the urease activity of this organism, which renders the urine alkaline and provides a fertile medium for formation of ammonium-magnesium-phosphate stones.

Bacteremia Bloodstream invasion is the most serious manifestation of infection with this organism. In 75 percent of cases, the urinary tract serves as the portal of entry; in the remainder, the biliary tree, gastrointestinal tract, ears and sinuses, and skin are the primary foci. *Proteus* bacteremia is frequently preceded by cystoscopy, urethral catheterization, transurethral prostatic resection, or other operative procedures. Clinically, the signs, symptoms, and laboratory findings of *Proteus* sepsis—high fever, chills, shock, metastatic abscesses, leukocytosis, and rarely thrombocytopenia—are indistinguishable from those of bloodstream infections with other gram-negative bacteria.

DIAGNOSIS The diagnosis of *Proteus* infection depends on culture of the organism from blood, urine, or exudate and its identification by appropriate biochemical tests. It is especially important to separate *P. mirabilis,* the indole-negative species, from *P. morganii, rettgeri,* and *vulgaris,* which are indole-positive, because only *P. mirabilis* is susceptible to the action of penicillin and many other antibiotics. *Proteus* organisms are often present in mixed infections with other pathogens. Particular care should be exercised in the isolation of other organisms growing in the same medium with members of the genus *Proteus* lest they be masked by its spreading growth. The spreading character of this organism may also make antibiotic sensitivity tests difficult to interpret.

TREATMENT Most strains of *P. mirabilis* are sensitive to penicillin in high concentration (10 units per milliliter or greater), ampicillin, carbenicillin, kanamycin, gentamicin, tobramycin, or amikacin, the cephalosporin antibiotics, and chloramphenicol. *Proteus* bacteriuria can be readily eradicated with any of these drugs during treatment; ampicillin in dosage of 0.5 g every 4 to 6 h is highly effective. In severe infection, therapy should be parenteral: 6 to 12 g ampicillin or 20 million units of penicillin G plus kanamycin or gentamicin in divided doses of 15 mg/kg per day and 5 mg/kg per day, respectively, if renal function is adequate. There is good evidence that an aminoglycoside is synergistic with ampicillin and penicillin G in *Proteus* infections and that chloramphenicol may be ineffective despite the results of in vitro tests. In view of the numerous more effective agents, there is no reason to use chloramphenicol in *Proteus* infections. In general, all strains of *P. mirabilis* are resistant to tetracycline. Most strains other than *P. mirabilis* and *Providencia* bacilli are sensitive only to kanamycin, gentamicin, tobramycin, or amikacin. Gentamicin, tobramycin, and amikacin in particular appear to be effective against indole-positive *Proteus.* In addition, although ampicillin and penicillin G alone are ineffective against indole-positive *Proteus,* a combination of either drug and an aminoglycoside may be synergistic. Carbenicillin and ticarcillin, semisynthetic penicillins, are also effective against the majority of indole-positive *Proteus* species. As with all other gram-negative infections, appropriate attention must be given to drainage of pus, maintenance of fluid and electrolyte status, and treatment of circulatory collapse.

REFERENCES

Enterobacteriaceae: General

MAKI DG: Nosocomial bacteremia: An epidemiologic overview. Am J Med 70:719, 1981

PIERCE AK, SANFORD JP: Aerobic gram-negative bacillary pneumonias. Am Rev Respir Dis 110:647, 1974

SCHABERG DR et al: Epidemics of nosocomial urinary tract infection caused by multiply-resistant gram-negative bacilli: Epidemiology and control. J Infect Dis 133:363, 1976

STAMM WE: Guidelines for prevention of catheter-associated urinary tract infections. Ann Intern Med 82:386, 1975

Escherichia coli infections

CONN HO, FESSEL JM: Spontaneous bacterial peritonitis in cirrhosis. Medicine 50:161, 1971

COOPER R, MILLS J: *Serratia* endocarditis. Arch Intern Med 140:199, 1980

GORBACH SL et al: Travelers' diarrhea and toxigenic *Escherichia coli.* N Engl J Med 292:933, 1975

TULLOCH EF JR et al: Invasive enteropathic *Escherichia coli* dysentery: Outbreak in 28 adults. Ann Intern Med 79:13, 1973

TURCK M et al: Studies on the epidemiology of *Escherichia coli* 1960–1968. J Infect Dis 120:13, 1969

Klebsiella-Enterobacter-Serratia infections

MAKI DG et al: Nosocomial urinary tract infection with *Serratia marcescens:* An epidemiologic study. J Infect Dis 128:579, 1973

MELTZ DJ, GRIECO MH: Characteristics of *Serratia marcescens* pneumonia. Arch Intern Med 132:359, 1973

PRICE DJE, SLEIGH JD: Control of infection due to *Klebsiella* aerogenes in neurosurgical unit by withdrawal of all antibiotics. Lancet 2:213, 1970

RENNIE RP, DUNCAN IBR: Emergence of gentamicin resistant *Klebsiella* in a general hospital. Antimicrob Agents Chemother 11:179, 1978

Proteus infections

JANNINI PB et al: Multidrug resistant *P. rettgeri.* Ann Intern Med 55:161, 1976

LEWIS J, FEKETY FR: *Proteus* bacteremia. Johns Hopkins Med J 124:151, 1969

MUSHER DM et al: Role of urease in pyelonephritis resulting from urinary tract infection with *Proteus.* J Infect Dis 131:177, 1975

152
PSEUDOMONAS, ACINETOBACTER, AND *EIKENELLA* INFECTIONS

MARVIN TURCK
DENNIS SCHABERG

PSEUDOMONAS INFECTIONS

ETIOLOGY *Pseudomonas aeruginosa* is a gram-negative motile rod which generally is not encapsulated and forms no spores. It grows readily in all ordinary culture media, and on agar it forms irregular, soft, iridescent colonies which usually have a fluorescent yellow-green color because of diffusion into the medium of two pigments, pyocyanin and fluorescin. *Pseudomonas* produces acid but no gas in glucose, and it is proteolytic. It is oxidase-positive and produces ammonia from arginine. A number of different strains have been identified by immunofluorescent techniques or bacteriophage typing. There is no evidence that these strains vary in their virulence for humans. Other *Pseudomonas* species (*P. maltophilia, P. cepacia, P. fluorescens, P. testosteroni,* and *P. putida*) also may cause infection in humans. For the most part, these organisms have been associated with common-source nosocomial outbreaks; in addition, they have been incriminated in bacteremia, endocarditis, and osteomyelitis in narcotic addicts.

EPIDEMIOLOGY *Pseudomonas* organisms are present on the skin of some normal persons, particularly in the axilla and anogenital regions. They are uncommon in the stools of adults not receiving antibiotics. In the majority of instances, *Pseudomonas* organisms are cultured as avirulent secondary contaminants in superficial wounds, or from the sputum of patients treated with antibiotics. Ordinarily this is of little consequence because the organisms merely fill the bacteriologic vacuum left by the elimination of more sensitive bacteria. Occasionally, however, infections with *Pseudomonas* organisms occur in the ear, lung, skin, or urinary tract of patients, often when a primary pathogen has been eradicated by antibiotics. Serious infections are almost invariably associated with damage to local tissue or with diminished host resistance. Despite the many potential virulence factors shared by strains of *Pseudomonas,* the organism rarely causes disease in healthy persons. Patients compromised by cystic fibrosis and those with neutropenia appear at particular risk to severe infection with *P. aeruginosa.* Premature infants; children with congenital anomalies and patients with leukemia, usually receiving antibiotics, adrenal steroids, or antineoplastic drugs; patients with burns; and geriatric patients with debilitating diseases are likely to develop *Pseudomonas* infections. Most often these infections occur in the hospital environment and generally are exogenous infections with the organism acquired from sources other than the patient's normal flora. The organisms have been cultured from a variety of sources in hospitals, sharing in common an aqueous environment including such items as sinks, antiseptic solutions, and aqueous medications. The organism is prevalent in urine receptacles and catheters, and on the hands of orderlies, nurses, and physicians; in several outbreaks, *Pseudomonas* urinary tract infections appeared to have been transmitted from patient to patient by human carriers. Similar epidemics have been reported in nurseries among premature infants, and cross infection on burn wards is also common. Although *P. aeruginosa* is found in the gastrointestinal tract of only approximately 5 percent of normal adults, carriage rates increase dramatically in hospitalized patients.

PATHOGENESIS The portal of entry of *Pseudomonas* organisms varies with the patient's age and underlying disease. In infancy and childhood, the skin, umbilical cord, and gastrointestinal tract predominate; in old age, the urinary tract is more often the primary focus. Often the infections remain localized in the skin or subcutaneous tissues. In burns the region below the eschar may become massively infiltrated with bacteria and inflammatory cells, and usually serves as the focus for bacteremia, the single most lethal complication. Hematogenous dissemination is characterized by hemorrhagic nodules in many areas, including the skin, heart, lungs, kidneys, and meninges. The histologic picture is one of necrosis and hemorrhage. Typically the walls of arterioles are heavily infiltrated with bacteria, and the vessels are partially or wholly thrombosed.

The majority of strains of *P. aeruginosa* produce a layer of slime which is rich in carbohydrate and shares heat-stable somatic antigenicity with the cell wall. Antibody against the specific serologic type of slime antigen affords protection to experimental challenge. A majority of isolates also produce a number of exotoxins. Exotoxin A, which shares many properties with diphtheria toxin, is the most potent toxin produced by *P. aeruginosa.* In life-threatening infection with *P. aeruginosa,* high antibody titers against exotoxin A correlate with increased survival.

MANIFESTATIONS *Pseudomonas* infections occur in many locations, including the skin, subcutaneous tissue, bone and joints, eyes, ears, mastoid and paranasal sinuses, meninges, and heart valves. Bacteremia without a detectable primary focus may also occur and should raise the question of contamination of intravenous medications, intravenous solutions, or antiseptics used for preparing the intravenous site, especially when non-*aeruginosa Pseudomonas* species are isolated.

Infections of the skin and subcutaneous tissues *Pseudomonas* organisms are frequently cultured from surgical wounds, varicose and decubitus ulcers, and burns, particularly following antibiotic therapy. Draining tuberculous or osteomyelitic sinuses may become secondarily infected. The mere presence of *Pseudomonas* in these sites is of little significance provided that bacterial multiplication deep in subcutaneous tissues does not occur and bacteremia does not ensue. Cutaneous infections usually heal after removal or slough of devitalized tissue. *Pseudomonas* organisms may be responsible for green nails in persons whose hands are excessively exposed to water, soap, and detergents, who have onychomycosis, or whose hands are subject to mechanical trauma. The organism can usually be cultured from the nail plate.

Pseudomonas has been incriminated in whirlpool-associated dermatitis. One such outbreak caused by *Pseudomonas aeruginosa,* serotype 0:9, occurred in a hockey team in Atlanta in March 1981. The disease is benign and resolves spontaneously.

Osteomyelitis Osteomyelitis is unusual with *Pseudomonas* except as a complication of bacteremia and puncture wounds. If a puncture wound, especially a nail puncture of the foot in children, fails to respond to standard therapy within 3 to 4 days, complicating *Pseudomonas* osteomyelitis must be considered.

Infections of the ear, mastoid, and paranasal sinuses Otitis externa is the most common form of *Pseudomonas* infection which involves the ear. It is particularly troublesome in tropical climates and is characterized by chronic serosanguineous and purulent drainage from the external auditory canal. Otitis media or mastoiditis usually occurs as a superinfection following eradication of pneumococci, streptococci, or staphylococci by antimicrobial agents. Frequently *Pseudomonas* organisms are present in association with other gram-negative or gram-positive organisms.

Infection of the eye Corneal ulceration is the most severe form of ocular *Pseudomonas* infection. It usually follows a traumatic abrasion and may terminate in panophthalmitis and destruction of the globe. Purulent conjunctivitis occurs as a manifestation of *Pseudomonas* infection in premature infants. Contamination of contact lenses or lens fluid may be an important means of infecting the eyes with *Pseudomonas* organisms.

Urinary tract infections *Pseudomonas* organisms are common pathogens in the urinary tract and are usually found in patients with obstructive uropathy who have been subjected to repeated urethral manipulations or to urologic surgery. At times *Pseudomonas* is one of several pathogenic bacteria in the urine, the others being *Escherichia coli, Klebsiella, Proteus,* and enterococci. *Pseudomonas* bacteriuria is in no way unique and cannot be distinguished from infection with other organisms on clinical grounds.

Gastrointestinal tract *Pseudomonas* organisms have been implicated as a cause of epidemic diarrhea of infancy. In addition, a number of infants dying from neonatal sepsis have the classic necrotic, avascular ulcers of *Pseudomonas* bacteremia in the bowel at autopsy. A "typhoidal" form of *Pseudomonas* infection characterized by fever, myalgia, and diarrhea occurs predominantly in the tropics. This illness, also called 13-day fever or Shanghai fever, is self-limited, and the prognosis is good.

Respiratory tract Primary *Pseudomonas* pneumonia is infrequent, and culture of this organism from the sputum usually is indicative of aspiration of oropharyngeal contents with secondary infection or of superinfection following eradication of a more sensitive flora with antibiotics. The normal oropharyngeal flora of hospitalized patients is frequently replaced by gram-negative rods, including *Pseudomonas,* early in hospitalization. A variety of nosocomial events, most notably administration of sedative medications, endotracheal intubation, and intermittent positive pressure breathing treatments, can predispose to respiratory infection with *Pseudomonas.* Pulmonary infection is often associated with microabscesses. The organism is often isolated from the sputum of patients with bronchiectasis, chronic bronchitis, or cystic fibrosis who have lingering infections punctuated by multiple courses of chemotherapy and is recovered frequently from the stomata of tracheostomy sites. *Pseudomonas* bronchitis and bronchiolitis may be the terminal event in cystic fibrosis, and the isolates from these patients often are found to have a characteristic mucoid colonial morphology when cultured on agar.

Meningitis Spontaneous *Pseudomonas* meningitis is most unusual, but the bacilli may be introduced into the subarachnoid space by lumbar puncture, spinal anesthesia, intrathecal medication, or head trauma. Ventriculomastoid or ventriculoatrial shunts performed for hydrocephalus may become contaminated with *Pseudomonas* organisms. Usually revision or removal of the shunt offers the best hope of cure. Meningitis may be a terminal phenomenon in *Pseudomonas* bacteremia and in this instance represents a metastatic infection in the meninges.

Bacteremia Bloodstream invasion tends to occur in debilitated patients, premature infants, children with congenital defects, patients with lymphomas, leukemias, or other malignant tumors, and elderly patients who have undergone surgery or instrumentation of the biliary or urinary tract. *Pseudomonas* bacteremia is an important cause of death in patients with severe burns. In adults, *Pseudomonas* bacteremia is indistinguishable from bloodstream infection with other bacterial species except for two findings: (1) ecthyma gangrenosum, the classic skin lesion, often located in the anogenital or axillary region as a round, indurated, purple-black area about 1 cm in diameter with an ulcerated center and a surrounding zone of erythema; and (2) rarely, the passage of green urine, presumably due to the hemoglobin pigment, verdoglobin. Other features of *Pseudomonas* sepsis include hectic fever, shaking chills, hyperventilation, confusion, delirium, and circulatory collapse. Hypothermia, leukopenia, and thrombocytopenia are more common in *Pseudomonas* bacteremia than in other gram-negative bacteremias but are often related to an underlying blood dyscrasia. In addition to ecthyma gangrenosum, other skin lesions consist of hemorrhagic cellulitis and macular lesions on the trunk similar to "rose spots." Organisms usually can be cultured from cutaneous lesions and may provide an early clue to the diagnosis. *Pseudomonas* organisms may be in the bloodstream concomitantly with other organisms, notably Enterobacteriaceae or staphylococci. More often, however, *Pseudomonas* bacteremia follows staphylococcal sepsis in patients with burns.

Bacterial endocarditis A number of cases of *Pseudomonas* subacute bacterial endocarditis have followed open-heart surgery. Usually the organisms become implanted on a silk suture or a synthetic patch employed for closure of septal defects. Reoperation with removal of the vegetation and foreign bodies offers the best hope of cure. *Pseudomonas* endocarditis has been found on normal heart valves in patients with burns or in drug addicts; it has been postulated that staphylococcal endocarditis develops first and that the vegetation is secondarily infected with *Pseudomonas* organisms. Metastatic abscesses in bone, joints, brain, adrenal glands, and lungs are frequent consequences of *Pseudomonas* endocarditis.

TREATMENT Localized *Pseudomonas* infection can be treated by irrigation with 1% acetic acid or topical therapy with colistin or polymyxin B. Debridement and drainage of purulent material is essential when deeper tissues are involved. For deep-seated tissue infections and life-threatening infection, such as pneumonia or bacteremia, parenteral therapy must be employed. The aminoglycoside antibiotics, tobramycin and gentamicin, inhibit most strains of *Pseudomonas.* In patients with normal renal function, 5 mg/kg per day in divided doses will provide inhibitory levels. Amikacin, a newer aminoglycoside, is also active against *Pseudomonas.* It is especially useful against strains which have developed enzyme-mediated drug resistance to tobramycin and gentamicin. It should be given in doses of 15 mg/kg per day in divided doses. Ticarcillin and carbenicillin are also active against many strains of *Pseudomonas* in doses of 24 to 30 g per day for carbenicillin and 16 to 20 g per day for ticarcillin. The combination of an aminoglycoside active against *Pseudomonas* plus carbenicillin or ticarcillin is frequently employed to delay emergence of resistance during therapy and provides some enhanced activity, especially in the granulocytopenic patient with *Pseudomonas* infection. Asymptomatic bacteriuria, particularly when confined to the bladder, should be treated with the least toxic agent, which at times may be a sulfonamide or tetracycline. The antimicrobial susceptiblity of *Pseudomonas,* other than *P. aeruginosa,* is variable, and many of these isolates may be sensitive to chloramphenicol and resistant to aminoglycoside antibiotics.

PROPHYLAXIS *Pseudomonas* cross infections in hospitals can be reduced by careful attention to aseptic techniques, particularly in nurseries for premature infants, operating rooms, and urologic wards; avoidance of cold sterilization procedures wherever possible; and scrupulous attention to clean plumbing fixtures, humidifying equipment, etc. Judicious use of antibiotics, steroids, and cytotoxic agents should also diminish the incidence of *Pseudomonas* infections. Systemic antibiotic prophylaxis aimed at preventing colonization and infection with *Pseudomonas* organisms has been notoriously unsuccessful and should be interdicted. A polyvalent vaccine for *Pseudomonas* has been developed as well as hyperimmune gamma globulin. The vaccine has proved useful in prophylaxis against *Pseudomonas* infection in patients with thermal injury and may be useful in other selected populations such as those with solid tumors undergoing cancer chemotherapy.

PROGNOSIS The mortality rate in *Pseudomonas* bacteremia is 75 percent and is highest in patients with shock or severe associated disease such as massive third-degree burns, leukemia, or prematurity. When bacteremia originates in the urinary tract and is not accompanied by shock, the prognosis is considerably better. Localized *Pseudomonas* infections do not present a threat to life unless hematogenous dissemination occurs.

ACINETOBACTER INFECTIONS

DEFINITION Organisms of the genus *Acinetobacter* are pleomorphic, gram-negative bacilli which are easily confused with members of the genus *Neisseria.* Severe infections with these organisms, including meningitis, bacterial endocarditis, pneumonia, and bacteremia, have been described with increasing frequency.

ETIOLOGY *Acinetobacter calcoaceticus* var. *lwoffi* was described by DeBord as *Mima polymorpha* in 1939. It is one of two well-characterized varieties of *Acinetobacter,* the other being *Acinetobacter calcoaceticus* var. *anitratus,* formerly called *Herellea vaginicola.* Organisms described as *Bacterium anitratum* and B5W are synonymous with *Acinetobacter.* These organisms are pleomorphic, gram-negative, encapsulated, and nonmotile. They grow well on ordinary media, forming white, convex, smooth colonies. Diplococcal forms predominate in colonies grown on solid media; rods and filamentous forms are more common in liquid media. The species can be differentiated from the Enterobacteriaceae by their negative nitrate reaction and from members of the genus *Neisseria,* which they may resemble morphologically, by their simple growth requirements, their bacillary form in liquid media, and their usually negative oxidase reaction.

EPIDEMIOLOGY AND PATHOGENESIS *Acinetobacter* organisms are ubiquitous and have been cultured from a variety of human sources, including urethral, vaginal, and conjunctival secretions, sputum, pleural fluid, blood, cerebrospinal fluid, feces, cutaneous ulcers, abscesses, chancroid lesions, joint fluid, ascitic fluid, and bone marrow. In addition, these organisms have been found in river water, humidifiers, and oxygen tents. Twenty-five percent of normal subjects are skin carriers of *Acinetobacter.* The striking association of *Acinetobacter* bacteremia with cutdowns or indwelling intravenous catheters favors the skin as a major portal of entry in humans. The increasing incidence of *Acinetobacter* pneumonia, both as a primary infection and as a superinfection, also points to the respiratory tract as an important portal of entry. It appears that *Acinetobacter* organisms are normal human commensals of relatively low virulence with colonization much more frequent than infection. Infections seem to occur in patients subjected to the same epidemiologic pressures encountered with nosocomial, gram-negative bacilli producing serious infections under conditions of decreased host resistance, or in the presence of instrumentation and with prior broad-spectrum antimicrobial therapy. An unexplained predominance of *Acinetobacter* pulmonary infections occurring in late summer has been noted. The role of these organisms as a cause of conjunctivitis, vaginitis, and urethritis requires further documentation.

MANIFESTATIONS Serious infections caused by *Acinetobacter* include (1) meningitis, (2) subacute and acute bacterial endocarditis, (3) pneumonia, (4) urinary tract infections, and (5) bacteremia. Usually, the signs and symptoms associated with infections in these sites are no different from those produced by other pathogens. For example, subacute bacterial endocarditis has usually been reported in patients with congenital or rheumatic heart disease and pursues an indolent course, while urinary tract infections may be manifested by asymptomatic bacteriuria, cystitis, or pyelonephritis. Pneumonia often occurs in the form of a superinfection in patients who have received antibiotics and who have either a tracheostomy or endotracheal intubation. Bronchopneumonia is the most common roentgenographic finding. Occasionally, *Acinetobacter* may be the cause of a fulminating bacteremia, with high fever, vascular collapse, petechiae, and ecchymoses, indistinguishable from fulminant meningococcemia. More often, however, bacteremia is associated with an overt portal of entry, such as infected cutdowns or indwelling intravenous catheters, surgical wounds, or burns, or it may follow urethral or other surgical instrumentation. These patients usually have severe debilitating disease or have undergone surgery. Many times they have received antibiotics, adrenal cortical hormones, irradiation, or tumor chemotherapy and have had infections with other organisms prior to development of sepsis with *Acinetobacter.* The clinical picture presented by these patients is dominated by endotoxemia, and the prognosis is poor.

DIAGNOSIS The diagnosis of *Acinetobacter* infection can be missed because the clinical bacteriology laboratory is unfamiliar with these organisms and reports them incorrectly or because they are considered contaminants. The confusion attending the taxonomic classification of these organisms has not simplified matters. For practical purposes, isolation of *Acinetobacter* or synonyms (*Mimae herelleae, B. anitratum,* B5W, *Diplococcus mucosus,* or *Neisseria winogradskyi*) from blood, spinal fluid, sputum, urine, or pus should be considered significant unless there is no evidence of infection on clinical grounds. Since *Acinetobacter* isolates are resistant to penicillin and members of the genus *Neisseria* are sensitive, differentiation of these organisms is of obvious importance.

TREATMENT Antibiotic sensitivities of *Acinetobacter* strains vary, but most strains are inhibited by kanamycin, gentamicin, tobramycin, colistin, or polymyxin B. Sensitivity to the tetracyclines is unpredictable, and most strains are resistant to penicillin, ampicillin, cephalothin, erythromycin, and chloramphenicol. For serious systemic infections, the appropriate antibiotic, generally an aminoglycoside, should be administered, and since these organisms may produce localized abscesses, surgical drainage may be necessary.

EIKENELLA INFECTIONS

ETIOLOGY *Eikenella corrodens* is a facultatively anaerobic or capnophilic gram-negative rod which is oxidase-positive. As colonies develop on blood agar, characteristic "pitting" or "corroding" of the agar is seen with many strains and generally requires 48 to 72 h of growth to develop.

EPIDEMIOLOGY *Eikenella corrodens* is an inhabitant of the mouth, upper respiratory tract, and gastrointestinal tract of humans. Infections frequently involve bowel or oral contamination. A striking association between *Eikenella* infections and methylphenidate (Ritalin) abuse has been noted, perhaps related to the low redox potential created by "skin popping" of this agent as well as a tendency for needles to become contaminated with oral secretions through needle licking.

MANIFESTATIONS The most common infection caused by *Eikenella* is that of skin or soft tissue. Endocarditis, pneumonia, osteomyelitis, and meningitis are reported but are rare. *Eikenella* infections frequently mimic infections caused by strict anaerobes such as *Bacteroides fragilis* or *Peptostreptococcus.* The infections are indolent, frequently mixed with aerobic gram-positive cocci, and drainage is often foul smelling. Abscess formation is common.

TREATMENT *Eikenella corrodens* is susceptible to penicillin, ampicillin, carbenicillin, and tetracycline. Adequate drainage of purulent material is essential in the management of these infections. Ampicillin or penicillin coupled with surgical drainage generally provides a good response. Of note is the marked resistance of *Eikenella* to clindamycin, making the differentiation of *Eikenella* infections from those caused by mixed anaerobes even more important.

REFERENCES

Acinetobacter infections

Buxton AE et al: Nosocomial respiratory tract infection and colonization with *Acinetobacter calcoaceticus.* Am J Med 65:507, 1978

Glew RH et al: Infections with *Acinetobacter calcoaceticus:* Clinical and laboratory studies. Medicine 56:79, 1977

Retailliau FH et al: *Acinetobacter calcoaceticus:* A nosocomial pathogen with unusual seasonal pattern. J Infect Dis 139:371, 1979

Eikenella infections

Brooks GF et al: *Eikenella corrodens,* a recently recognized pathogen. Medicine 53:325, 1974

Dorff GJ et al: Infections with *Eikenella corrodens.* Ann Intern Med 80:305, 1974

Goldstein EJC et al: Isolation of *Eikenella corrodens* from pulmonary infections. Am Rev Resp Dis 119:55, 1979

Pseudomonas infections

ALEXANDER JW et al: Immunologic control of *Pseudomonas* infection in burn patients: Clinical evaluation. Arch Surg 102:31, 1971

ARTENSTEIN MS, SANFORD JP (eds): Symposium on *Pseudomonas aeruginosa.* J Infect Dis 130:S1, November 1974

DOGGETT RG (ed): *Pseudomonas aeruginosa:* Clinical manifestations of infection and current therapy. Academic, New York, 1979

FLICK MR, CLUFF LE: *Pseudomonas* bacteremia: Review of 108 cases. Am J Med 60:501, 1976

PENNINGTON JE et al: *Pseudomonas* pneumonia: A retrospective study of 36 cases. Am J Med 55:155, 1973

PHILLIPS I et al: Control of respirator-associated infection due to *Pseudomonas aeruginosa.* Lancet 2:871, 1974

153
MELIOIDOSIS AND GLANDERS

JAY P. SANFORD

MELIOIDOSIS Definition Melioidosis is an infection of human beings and animals with a protean clinical spectrum. Melioidosis, which means "a resemblance to distemper of asses," bears a striking resemblance to glanders both clinically and pathologically, but is epidemiologically dissimilar.

Etiology Melioidosis is caused by a gram-negative motile bacillus, *Pseudomonas pseudomallei,* which can be differentiated from *P. mallei* by bacteriologic and serologic means. *P. pseudomallei* (also known as Whitmore's bacillus) is a small, gram-negative, motile, aerobic bacillus. When it is stained with methylene blue, Wayson's, or Wright's stain, marked irregularities with a bipolar "safety pin" pattern are observed. It grows well on standard bacteriologic media, with a characteristic wrinkling of colony surfaces after 48 to 72 h of incubation. Two antigenic types have been distinguished, type I (Asian), found widely, including in Australia, and type II (Australian), found mainly in Australia. Both types are equally pathogenic.

Epidemiology The disease is endemic in Southeast Asia where human and animal cases occur commonly. Disease in humans has been reported from adjacent areas including India, Borneo, the Philippines, Guam, Indonesia, Ceylon, New Guinea, and Australia (North Queensland). Cases in humans or animals have been reported from Madagascar, Chad, Central West Africa (Niger, Upper Volta), Iran, and Turkey. In 1976, *P. pseudomallei* was isolated from animals in the Paris zoo just behind Notre Dame. In Madrid, horses kept for serum died from melioidosis. Human melioidosis has been described only rarely in the western hemisphere (Panama, Ecuador)—a neonatal case in Hawaii, a case in Georgia, and a possible case in Oklahoma. With these exceptions, confirmed melioidosis has occurred in United States or European residents only when they have traveled in endemic areas. As of January 1973, when all American forces had been withdrawn from Vietnam, there had been 343 cases with 36 deaths reported in United States Army personnel who were or had been in Vietnam. The majority of these cases occurred in individuals without intercurrent illness, although patients who sustained burn injuries in Vietnam accounted for a disproportionately high number of the cases.

Pseudomonas pseudomallei is a saprophyte which can be isolated from soil, stagnant streams, ponds, rice paddies, and market produce in endemic areas. Its ubiquitous nature is illustrated by its isolation as a laboratory contaminant. *Pseudomonas pseudomallei* is capable of causing disease in epizootic form among sheep, goats, swine, and horses. Outbreaks have occurred in dolphins in oceanariums in Paris and Hong Kong. Occasional isolates have also been reported from cows, rodents, dogs, and cats. Although animals are susceptible to the disease, they apparently do not represent a reservoir for human disease. A carrier dolphin was identified in Hong Kong. Otherwise, attempts to culture *P. pseudomallei* from the urine and feces of a large variety of healthy animals have been unsuccessful. Arthropod-borne infection does not occur naturally. Human beings contract melioidosis by soil contamination of skin abrasions. Ingestion, nasal instillation, and inhalation are other probable methods of spread. In contrast to glanders, infections have been uncommon, but can occur, in laboratory workers. Person-to-person transmission of melioidosis is rare. Venereal transmission from a patient with chronic prostatitis with *P. pseudomallei* isolated from prostatic secretions to his wife, who had never been in an endemic area and who had a hemagglutination titer of 1:10,240, has been recorded. Also, the development of melioidosis in a 2-day-old newborn in Hawaii and demonstration of a significant antibody titer in a nurse who had never been in an endemic area but who had worked on wards with melioidosis patients raise the question of spread from person-to-person within a hospital.

Pathology In acute infections, the majority of lesions occur in the lungs, with occasional abscesses in other organs. In subacute infections, lung abscesses tend to be more extensive, and lesions are found throughout the body, in the skin, subcutaneous tissue, meninges, brain, eye, heart, liver, kidney, spleen, bone, prostate, synovial membranes, and lymph nodes. The acute abscesses are characterized by an outer border of hemorrhage, a medial zone heavily infiltrated with polymorphonuclear leukocytes, and an inner core of necrotic debris containing large histiocytes with two or three nuclei that have been termed *giant cells.* A striking histological feature has been the marked karyorrhexis. In chronic infections, the lesion consists of a central area of caseation necrosis, mononuclear and plasma cells, and granulation tissue. Calcification does not occur.

Clinical manifestations The clinical manifestations of melioidosis are variable. The illness can present as an acute, subacute, or chronic process. The incubation period has not been defined; however, judging by the lapse of time between injury and the development of infection, it may be as short as 2 days. Following a laboratory accident, an incubation period of 3 days ensued. Clinically inapparent infections may remain latent for a number of years after an individual leaves an endemic area, with an interval of 26 years reported in one patient. Men are more often affected than women, a finding which is thought to represent occupational exposure. Melioidosis may be recognized as inapparent infection, asymptomatic pulmonary infiltration, acute localized suppurative infection, acute pulmonary infection, acute septicemic infection, or chronic suppurative infection.

INAPPARENT INFECTION In Thailand, Vietnam, and Malaysia, 6 to 8 percent of healthy adult men have significant antibody titers against *P. pseudomallei,* with the prevalence reaching 20 percent in a group of Army recruits from the rice-growing states of western Malaysia. Only 1 percent of Thai women had positive reactions. None of the serums from a control group from the United States was positive. The prevalence of significant antibody titers has been reported as 2 percent for Europeans living in Vietnam and 1 to 9 percent in unselected patients in United States Army hospitals and in a group of normal uninjured soldiers who had served in Vietnam. Occasionally, asymptomatic infections have been discovered by routine chest x-ray. Ten percent of serums from inhabitants of a village in Upper Volta were positive, yet melioidosis had never been recognized.

ACUTE LOCALIZED SUPPURATIVE INFECTION Infection by inoculation of a break in the skin usually results in a nodule with an area of acute lymphangitis and regional lymphadenitis. There are usually fever and generalized malaise. This form of infection may rapidly progress to the acute septicemic form.

ACUTE PULMONARY INFECTION The most common form of the disease has been pulmonary infection, which may represent a primary pneumonitis or hematogenous spread. The acute pulmonary infection can vary in severity from a mild bronchitis to overwhelming necrotizing pneumonia. The onset may be abrupt without prodromal symptoms or more gradual, with headache, anorexia, and generalized myalgia. Fever occurs in almost all patients, is often in excess of 38.9°C (102°F), and may be associated with rigors. Dull or pleuritic chest pain is common. Cough, with or without sputum, occurs. There may be mild pharyngitis. Tachypnea may be out of proportion to the fever and findings on physical or x-ray examination. Chest findings may be minimal but usually consist of rales in the area of pneumonitis. In the absence of dissemination, the spleen and liver are not palpable. Laboratory findings include total leukocyte counts ranging from normal to 20,000 cells per cubic millimeter. Mild normochromic, normocytic anemia may appear during the illness. The pneumonia usually involves the upper lobes with the radiographic appearance of consolidation. Thin-walled cavities, usually 2 to 7 cm in diameter, frequently occur. Without specific therapy, the temperature may become normal within a few days; however, the upper lobe cavitation persists, resulting in a radiographic appearance of tuberculosis. While uncommon, pleural effusions and a pleural mass have been reported. Progressive pulmonary spread or hematogenous dissemination with the development of septicemic manifestations may ensue.

ACUTE SEPTICEMIC INFECTION This is the form originally described primarily among narcotic addicts. Subsequent reports, however, have not shown a predilection for debilitated patients. The onset may be abrupt, with the dominant symptoms depending upon site of major involvement. In individuals with bacteremia complicating pneumonitis, symptoms may include disorientation, extreme dyspnea, severe headache, pharyngitis, watery diarrhea, and development of cutaneous pustular lesions on the head, trunk, or extremities. There is high fever, extreme tachypnea, a flushed skin, and cyanosis. Muscle tenderness may be striking. On examination of the chest, signs may be absent, or rales, rhonchi, and pleural rubs may be heard. The liver and spleen may be palpable. Signs of arthritis or meningitis may appear. Patients with the septicemic form usually have a rapidly progressive fatal course, which in some instances may be too fulminant to be altered by therapy. The leukocyte count may be normal or slightly increased. Chest radiographs most commonly show irregular nodular densities 4 to 10 mm in diameter disseminated throughout the lungs. These enlarge, coalesce, and often undergo cavitation as the disease progresses. Pleural effusion is rare. Other radiographic patterns include unilateral irregular mottled densities which become confluent.

CHRONIC SUPPURATIVE INFECTION In some patients secondary abscesses develop which dominate the clinical picture. Organs involved include skin, brain, lung, myocardium, liver, spleen, prostate, bones, joints, lymph nodes, and even the eye. These patients may be afebrile.

RECRUDESCENT INFECTION Activation of inapparent or quiescent infection may present as acute localized suppurative, acute pulmonary, acute septicemic, or chronic suppurative disease remote from the probable time of exposure (up to 26 years having been reported). In reported cases, surgery, trauma, intercurrent illness such as severe influenzal pneumonia, diabetic ketoacidosis, alcoholic debauches, or radiation therapy appeared to act as triggering events.

Diagnosis Melioidosis should be considered in the differential diagnosis of any febrile illness in an individual who has been in an endemic area, especially if the presenting features are those of fulminant respiratory failure, if multiple pustular or necrotic skin or subcutaneous lesions develop, or if there is a radiographic pattern of tuberculosis in a patient from whom tubercle bacilli cannot be isolated.

Microscopic examination of exudates will reveal poorly staining, small, gram-negative bacilli which show the characteristic staining irregularities and "safety pin" bipolar staining with methylene blue. *Pseudomonas pseudomallei* will grow on most laboratory media, including eosinmethylene blue agar (EMB) or MacConkey's agar, in 24 to 48 h. The organisms can be differentiated from *P. mallei* and *P. aeruginosa* by standard bacteriologic procedures, although isolates may pose problems in identification with some commercial medium kits. The characteristic wrinkling of the colonies may require 72 h or longer. The hemagglutination, direct agglutination test, and complement fixation test are aids in diagnosis if a fourfold or greater rise in titer is demonstrated in paired serums. Single low titers are difficult to interpret because of nonspecific responses. The complement fixation test is said to be specific with titers above 1:8 during the acute illness, but may cross-react with *P. mallei.* A negative complement fixation test does not exclude disease. The hemagglutination and agglutination tests show more cross-reactions. Titers of 1:40 or more suggest infection.

Treatment The treatment regimen should vary with the form of the disease. Individuals with low-titer positive serologic tests but with no clinical evidence of infection do not require therapy. The choice of antibiotics in active infection should be based upon sensitivity studies, and therapy should be given for a minimum of 30 days. *Pseudomonas pseudomallei* is usually sensitive in vitro to the tetracyclines, chloramphenicol, novobiocin, kanamycin, sulfadiazine or sulfisoxazole, trimethoprim-sulfamethoxazole, and some of the third-generation cephalosporins (see Chap. 141), and in most instances is resistant to penicillin G, ampicillin, carbenicillin, dicloxacillin, streptomycin, gentamicin, tobramycin, cephalosporins, vancomycin, clindamycin, and rifampin. In patients with pneumonitis who are not too ill, effective therapy has included tetracycline, 2 to 3 g daily (40 mg/kg); chloramphenicol, 3 g daily (40 mg/kg); sulfisoxazole, 4 g daily (70 mg/kg); or trimethoprim-sulfamethoxazole (4 mg/kg trimethoprim, 20 mg/kg sulfamethoxazole) for 60 to 150 days. If the patient is severely ill, two of these antimicrobials in combination have been recommended for 30 days followed by another 30 to 120 days of trimethoprim-sulfamethoxazole alone. The mean interval for sputum cultures to become negative has been 6 weeks. If sputum cultures remain positive for 6 months, surgery with lobectomy should be considered. In patients with extrapulmonary suppurative lesions, therapy should be continued for 6 months to 1 year. The usual principles of surgical drainage should be followed. In desperately ill patients with severe pneumonitis or the septicemic form, multiple antibiotics should be administered by the parenteral route. One such regimen has included the use of chloramphenicol, 12 g per day; novobiocin, 6 g per day; and kanamycin, 4 g per day. In view of the severe potential toxicity of this regimen, its use should be considered only in extremely ill patients, and then only on a short-term basis. Current recommendations for antibiotics in the septicemic form of melioidosis are tetracycline, 4 to 6 g per day (80 mg/kg); chloramphenicol, 4 to 6 g per day (80 mg/kg); and one of the following: trimethoprim-sulfamethoxazole (9 mg/kg trimethoprim, 45 mg/kg sulfamethoxazole), sulfisoxazole (140 mg/kg), kanamycin (30 mg/kg), or novobiocin (60 mg/kg). In vitro studies have revealed antagonism between the following pairs of drugs: chloramphenicol-kanamycin, tetracycline-kanamycin, and sulfadiazine-chloramphenicol. Though the significance of such antagonism in clinical therapy has not been assessed, the data would favor selection of trimethoprim-sulfamethoxazole or novobiocin as the third drug. The dosage should be tapered rapidly as clinical improvement occurs. Experience with the third-generation cephalosporins is extremely limited; however, a combination of ceftriaxone and trimethoprim-sulfamethoxazole may emerge as the recommendation of choice.

Prognosis Prior to antimicrobials, the mortality rate of apparent infection was 95 percent. With better diagnosis and more prolonged appropriate therapy, the mortality rate in all except the septicemic form is low. Even with vigorous appropriate antibiotics and supportive therapy, the mortality rate in patients with melioidosis septicemia is greater than 50 percent. Very few patients have had long-term follow-up, and the incidence of late relapses cannot be predicted but is quite high.

Prevention There is no means of active immunization. In endemic areas, vigorous cleansing of abrasions and lacerations is recommended.

GLANDERS Definition Glanders is a serious infection of equine animals caused by *P. mallei,* which is transmitted occasionally to other domestic animals and to human beings.

Etiology *Pseudomonas mallei* is a small, slender, nonmotile, gram-negative bacillus. When it is stained with methylene blue, marked irregularities in staining are observed. Organisms grow on most common meat infusion media but require glycerol for optimum growth.

Epidemiology Glanders was at one time widespread throughout Europe, but owing to the introduction of control measures, its incidence has decreased steadily in most countries. The disease still occurs in Asia, Africa, and South America, but not in the United States. Glanders has never been common in human beings; the occasional infection, however, may be very serious. There have been no naturally acquired infections in the United States since 1938.

Glanders is primarily a disease of horses, mules, and donkeys, although goats, sheep, cats, and dogs sometimes naturally contract the disease. Pigs and cattle are resistant. In horses, the disease may be systemic, with prominent pulmonary involvement (*glanders*) or may be characterized by subcutaneous ulcerative lesions, and lymphatic thickening with nodules (*farcy*). Inhalation, ingestion, and inoculation through breaks in the skin have been suggested as routes of infection in animals. In human beings, the disease occurs primarily in individuals with close contact with horses, mules, or donkeys through inoculation of or a break in the skin or by exposing the nasal mucosa to contaminated discharges. A number of instances of airborne infection have been reported in laboratory workers.

Pathology The acute lesion is characterized by nodules consisting of polymorphonuclear leukocytes surrounded by a zone of congestion. A characteristic histological feature is a peculiar nuclear degeneration known as *chromatotexis* which occurs early and is extensive. Small foci of deeply staining detritus within the abscess result from this degeneration. In older nodules, the reaction is characterized by epithelioid cells surrounding an area of central necrosis. Giant cells may be present. Virtually any organ may be involved.

Clinical manifestations The manifestations which frequently overlap may be categorized as (1) acute localized suppurative infection, (2) acute pulmonary infection, (3) acute septicemic infection, and (4) chronic suppurative infection. Nearly 60 percent of patients have been between the ages of 20 and 40 years. The disease has been rare in women, probably because of less opportunity for contact.

Infection acquired by inoculation through an abrasion in the skin usually results in a nodule with an area of acute lymphangitis. The incubation period is probably 1 to 5 days. In all types of acute glanders, there are usually fever, generalized malaise, and prostration.

Infection of the mucous membranes may result in a mucopurulent discharge involving the eye, nose, or lips followed by extensive ulcerating granulomatous lesions which may or may not be associated with systemic reactions. With systemic invasion, a generalized papular eruption which may become pustular is frequent. This septicemic form of disease is usually fatal in 7 to 10 days.

Infection by inhalation is followed by an incubation period of 10 to 14 days. The more common symptoms include fever, occasionally associated with rigors, generalized myalgia, fatigue, headache, and pleuritic chest pain. Other symptoms consist of photophobia, lacrimation, and diarrhea. Findings on physical examination are usually normal except for fever and occasional lymphadenopathy, especially in the cervical chain, and splenomegaly. Laboratory findings include mild leukocytosis with 60 to 80 percent neutrophilic leukocytes, but leukopenia with relative lymphocytosis has been recorded. In the acute pulmonary form, chest radiographs characteristically reveal circumscribed densities which suggest early lung abscesses. Other findings may include lobar or bronchopneumonia. In the chronic suppurative form of the disease, the most frequent finding consists of multiple subcutaneous and intramuscular abscesses which most often involve the arms or legs. Approximately one-half the patients will have associated fever, lymphadenopathy, and nasal discharge or ulceration. Visceral involvement including pulmonary or pleural, ocular, skeletal, hepatic, splenic, and meningeal or intracranial involvement occurs in some patients.

Diagnosis Microscopic examination of exudates may reveal small gram-negative bacilli which stain irregularly with methylene blue; however, organisms generally are very scanty. *Pseudomonas mallei* and *P. pseudomallei* cannot be distinguished morphologically. Culturing is often avoided because of the hazard to laboratory personnel; however, if cultures are made, growth occurs on most meat infusion nutrient media. The material is often contaminated with other microorganisms, and incubation with penicillin G (1000 units per milliliter) prior to culturing may be helpful. Subcutaneous inoculation of material into a guinea pig or hamster affords an alternative means of isolation. Blood cultures are usually negative except in the terminal stages of disease. Serologic tests show a rapidly rising agglutination titer, which reaches levels of 1:640 within 2 weeks. Serum from normal persons has been reported to show agglutination titers in dilutions up to 1:320. The complement fixation test is less sensitive but more specific and usually becomes positive during the third week; it is considered positive in dilutions of 1:20 or greater.

Treatment The limited number of recent infections in human beings has precluded evaluation of most of the antibiotic agents. Sulfadiazine has been found to be an effective agent in experimental animals and in humans. The dosage utilized has been approximately 100 mg/kg administered in divided doses. In experimental infections, 3 weeks of therapy gave better results than 1 week. Penicillin is ineffective in vitro and in experimental infections. Streptomycin is bacteriostatic in vitro but was ineffective in experimental infections in hamsters. Antibiotics such as tetracycline, chloramphenicol, the antipseudomonal aminoglycosides, carbenicillin, and trimethoprim have not been evaluated. In the absence of clinical experience and pending in vitro susceptibility studies, it would seem most reasonable to utilize the regimens appropriate for patients with various manifestations of melioidosis. In the acute infections, appropriate supportive measures are essential, and in chronic suppurative infections, the usual principles of surgical drainage should be followed.

Prognosis The prognosis depends upon the type of infection. The acute septicemic form has been uniformly fatal. The localized or chronic forms have a much better prognosis.

Prevention Next to acquisition from diseased horses, the commonest source of natural disease in human beings has been contact with human glanders. Isolation is indicated.

REFERENCES

DODIN A, FERRY R: Recherche epidemiologique du bacille de Whitmore en Afrique. Bull Soc Pathol Exot 67:121, 1974

———, Galimand M: Whitmore's bacillus. Rec Med Vet 152:323, 1976

EICKHOFF TC et al: *Pseudomonas pseudomallei:* Susceptibility to chemotherapeutic agents. J Infect Dis 121:95, 1970

EVERETT ED, NELSON R: Pulmonary melioidosis, observations in 39 cases. Am Rev Resp Dis 112:331, 1975

HOWE C, MILLER WR: Human glanders: Report of six cases. Ann Intern Med 26:93, 1947

——— et al: The pseudomallei: A review. J Infect Dis 124:598, 1971

JACKSON AE et al: Recrudescent melioidosis associated with diabetic ketoacidosis. Arch Intern Med 130:268, 1972

MAYS EE, RICKETS EA: Melioidosis: Recrudescence associated with bronchogenic carcinoma twenty-six years following initial geographic exposure. Chest 68:261, 1975

MCCORMICK JB et al: Human to human transmission of *Pseudomonas pseudomallei.* Ann Intern Med 83:512, 1975

NUSSBAUM JJ et al: *Pseudomonas pseudomallei* in an anophthalmic orbit. Arch Ophthalmol 98:1224, 1980

SANFORD JP: Melioidosis: Another great imitator, in *Infectious Diseases: Current Topics in Diagnosis and Treatment,* DN Gilbert, JP Sanford (eds). New York, Grune & Stratton, 1978

SCHLECH WF III et al: Laboratory-acquired infection with *Pseudomonas pseudomallei* (melioidosis). N Engl J Med 305:1133, 1981

ZAJTCHUK R et al: Surgical treatment of melioidosis. J Thorac Cardiovasc Surg 66:838, 1973

154
SALMONELLA INFECTIONS

RICHARD L. GUERRANT
EDWARD W. HOOK

The genus *Salmonella* consists of three species which include more than 1700 different serologic types. Striking variation in pathogenicity of serotypes occurs, but almost all are pathogenic for animals and humans. Specific host preferences characterize certain serotypes, such as *S. typhi,* which under natural conditions of transmission produces disease only in humans. *Salmonella* infections in humans present a spectrum of clinical syndromes, which sometimes overlap. The syndromes are (1) enteric fever (typhoid or paratyphoid fever), (2) acute gastroenteritis, (3) bacteremia, and (4) localized infection which may occur at almost any site. In addition, *asymptomatic intestinal infections* and *transient convalescent intestinal carrier* states are common. Occasionally, a focus of infection persists in the gallbladder or urinary tract to produce a *chronic carrier* state.

ETIOLOGY Salmonellae are motile gram-negative bacilli that ferment glucose but do not ferment lactose or sucrose. Almost all serotypes produce gas, although *S. typhi* is a notable exception. Salmonellae are divided into three species by biochemical means: *S. typhi, S. cholerae-suis,* and *S. enteritidis.* The species are further subdivided into serotypes, which are identified by highly specific O (somatic) and H (flagellar) antigens. A given serotype will contain a specific combination of multiple O and H antigens. Identification by serotype is accomplished routinely only in major salmonella typing centers, which have the necessary collection of antiserums required for such work. Salmonellae are also divided into groups on the basis of O antigen composition. Most isolates from natural sources fall into five groups, A to E.

The species *S. typhi* and *S. cholerae-suis* consist of only one serotype each (in groups D and C, respectively), whereas the species *S. enteritidis* comprises over 1700 serotypes (in all groups, including C and D). Considerable overlap in antigenic composition is responsible for the cross-reactivity which is commonly seen in serologic tests with salmonellae.

The Salmonella Surveillance Unit of the Centers for Disease Control reports 20,000 to 30,000 isolations of salmonellae annually from human beings in the United States. In descending order, the most frequently isolated serotypes in 1980 were *S. typhimurium, S. heidelberg, S. enteritidis, S. newport, S. infantis, S. agona, S. saint-paul, S. montevideo, S. typhi,* and *S. oranienburg.* The 10 most frequently isolated serotypes account for over 70 percent of the total isolates from humans. *Salmonella typhimurium* perennially accounts for 25 to 35 percent of the isolates. *S. agona,* an organism apparently introduced indirectly via animals fed Peruvian fish meal in 1971, has become established among the 10 most commonly recognized serotypes from humans in the United States. Concern has also arisen over the multiply drug-resistant *S. wein,* which was the most frequent *Salmonella* isolate in France in 1974 and which is now being isolated in the United States; *S. wein* is resistant to chloramphenicol, ampicillin, sulfonamides, and tetracyclines.

In the subsequent section, typhoid fever, the classic example of enteric fever, is considered separately from other *Salmonella* infections because of its historical importance, the host specificity of *S. typhi,* and the extensive clinical experience with the disease.

TYPHOID FEVER

DEFINITION Typhoid fever is an acute systemic disease resulting from infection with *S. typhi.* The disease is unique to humans. It is characterized by malaise, fever, abdominal discomfort, transient rash, splenomegaly, and leukopenia. The most prominent major complications are intestinal hemorrhage and perforation. The disease is the classic example of enteric fever caused by salmonellas. However, enteric fever, similar to typhoid, can also be caused by other *Salmonella* serotypes and is termed *paratyphoid fever*.

EPIDEMIOLOGY *Salmonella typhi* gains access to the body by the oral route in almost all cases as a consequence of the ingestion of contaminated food, water, or milk. Humans are the only true reservoir of *S. typhi* in nature, and persons with typhoid fever, or convalescent or chronic carriers, always serve as the ultimate source of infection. Infected individuals can excrete millions of viable typhoid bacilli in the feces, which are the usual source of contamination of food or drink. Patients with active disease also occasionally have organisms in respiratory secretions, vomitus, or other body fluids. Flies or other insects can carry organisms from feces or other infected material to food or drink and have been implicated in a few outbreaks. The fact that *S. typhi* may survive freezing or drying enhances the possibility of spread by contaminated ice, dust, foods, and sewage. Oysters or other shellfish are contaminated at times in polluted waters and occasionally serve as sources of typhoid.

The incidence of typhoid fever has steadily decreased in the United States during the past century to the present relatively low level of less than 600 cases per year. The decrease in incidence has been coincident with improvement in socioeconomic conditions and is specifically related to development of pure water supplies, effective sewage disposal, pasteurization of milk, and methods to detect and control spread of organisms from persons with active disease or from carriers. Typhoid continues to occur on a large scale in countries where sanitation is suboptimal. About 40 percent of the patients with typhoid fever in the United States appear to have acquired the infection in another area of the world. In the United States 2 to 3 percent of cases appear to be laboratory-acquired.

Typhoid can be eradicated ultimately because the infection is confined to humans and both the disease and the carrier state can be controlled with appropriate drugs. The importance of sewage disposal, a pure water supply, and control of carriers is highlighted repeatedly by the occurrence of outbreaks which develop when defects in sanitation occur during natural disasters such as flood.

The sex distribution of patients with typhoid fever in the United States shows no significant predilection. In recent years, about 75 percent of cases have occurred in persons less than 30 years of age. In contrast, the chronic carrier state is much more common in females than males (the female/male ratio is 3:1) and in older individuals (88 percent are over 50 years of age).

There is no seasonal variation in incidence of typhoid fever in the United States. However, in areas of the world where the disease is endemic, the incidence increases in the summer months.

PATHOGENESIS The outcome of the interaction between the typhoid bacillus and humans is determined during the early hours after ingestion of the organisms. Typhoid bacilli reach the small intestine shortly after ingestion and may multiply there. The organisms may then penetrate the mucosa with minimal epithelial destruction and enter intestinal lymphatics, perhaps via Peyer's patches, to be carried to the bloodstream. This initial early bacteremia apparently occurs within 24 to 72 h after ingestion of organisms and is rarely detected in natural infections because patients are usually asymptomatic at this early stage. The bacteremia is transient and is rapidly terminated as bacilli are phagocytized by cells of the reticuloendothelial system. Nevertheless, viable bacilli are disseminated throughout the body and apparently persist within reticuloendothelial cells. After intracellular multiplication takes place, organisms reenter the bloodstream, producing a continuous bacteremia for days or weeks. The reappearance of bacteremia corresponds with the onset of manifestations of the disease. The intracellular organisms are eventually destroyed as manifestations of disease subside and recovery ensues. Enhanced intracellular killing and recovery appear to be related to the onset of delayed hypersensitivity. Recovery is unrelated to the appearance, even in high titer, of agglutinins against the somatic, flagellar, or Vi antigens of the typhoid bacillus.

The number of organisms ingested is an important determinant of whether typhoid fever results from exposure to *S. typhi.* Studies in volunteers have shown that about 10^7 typhoid bacilli of the Quailes strain must be taken orally to produce typhoid fever in 50 percent of normal volunteers. The number of organisms ingested also influences the incubation period, and short incubation periods, in general, correspond to large doses of organisms. The volunteer studies have also demonstrated that different strains of typhoid bacilli vary considerably in their capacity to produce disease in humans.

The normal flora of the upper intestinal tract is an important protective mechanism against invasion by *S. typhi.* Volunteer studies have demonstrated that antimicrobial therapy a day or so before oral challenge with *S. typhi* markedly decreases the number of viable bacilli required to produce disease. It is possible that certain factors known to be associated with typhoid outbreaks, such as malnutrition, enhance susceptibility to typhoid infection by alterations in the intestinal flora or other host defenses.

During the phase of persistent bacteremia, all organs are repeatedly exposed to typhoid bacilli. Abscess formation may occur but is unusual. However, localization does occur in the gallbladder in almost all cases. Organisms multiply in the bile to high titer, usually without manifestations of cholecystitis, and are excreted with bile into the intestinal tract. Stool cultures, which are usually negative for *S. typhi* during the incubation period and early phases of the disease, become positive in a large proportion of cases during the third or fourth week of the disease, when excretion of organisms in the bile reaches a peak.

The factors responsible for the fever, leukopenia, and other manifestations of typhoid fever have been inadequately defined. Typhoid bacilli contain biologically active lipopolysaccharides or endotoxins which produce fever, leukopenia, thrombocytopenia, and hyperplasia of reticuloendothelial cells when injected into animals or humans. It has been assumed for years that these materials play an important role in the pathogenesis of the signs and symptoms of typhoid fever. However, the evidence regarding the role of endotoxin in the genesis of the manifestations of typhoid is inconclusive. For example, tolerance to the pyrogenic effects of endotoxins can be demonstrated during convalescence from typhoid fever, which suggests release of endotoxins during infection. While laboratory evidence for low-grade, subclinical disseminated intravascular coagulation can often be demonstrated in patients with typhoid fever, endotoxemia is usually not detectable. Other studies show that typhoid fever follows a normal course in volunteers rendered tolerant to endotoxins prior to challenge, indicating that more complex mechanisms than endotoxemia alone are responsible for the sustained fever and toxemia. It has been suggested that endogenous pyrogens released by local inflammatory effects of *S. typhi* endotoxin may sustain the pyrexia in typhoid fever.

PATHOLOGY The most prominent microscopic lesion in typhoid fever is proliferation of large mononuclear cells in many different tissues. Mononuclear hyperplasia leads to lymphadenopathy, splenomegaly, and impressive enlargement of lymphoid tissues in the intestines, especially in the terminal ileum (Peyer's patches). Proliferating mononuclear cells may also be observed in bone marrow, liver, and lung. Studies in volunteers using ^{131}I-tagged aggregated albumin have shown increased phagocytic activity of the reticuloendothelial system by the third to fifth days after onset of symptoms. Necrosis in hyperplastic Peyer's patches may be associated with erosion of blood vessels in the lesions in the intestinal tract, which leads to oozing of blood or massive hemorrhage. Lesions may extend deep into the intestinal wall and cause perforation of the bowel, an event which characteristically occurs late in the disease, most often in the third febrile week. The site of perforation is usually in the distal 24 in of the ileum.

The gallbladder and bile ducts are routinely infected during the disease. As a rule, this biliary infection is asymptomatic, although acute cholecystitis may occur occasionally. Biliary infection terminates spontaneously during convalescence in the vast majority of patients within 12 months, but about 3 percent of adults continue to harbor organisms in the gallbladder and become chronic carriers of the typhoid bacillus.

MANIFESTATIONS The incubation period averages about 10 days but may vary from extremes of 3 to 60 days depending on the infecting dose.

The clinical manifestations and duration of illness vary markedly from one patient to another. Mild forms of the disease, characterized primarily by fever, may last only a week, or illness may be prolonged, lasting 8 weeks or more if untreated.

In a typical patient not treated with antimicrobials, the illness lasts about 4 weeks. The onset is insidious with headache, malaise, anorexia, and fever. Headache may be the first manifestation of disease and is usually generalized and severe. Chilly sensations are common, and frank chills may be observed. The fever is remittent, frequently increasing in a steplike manner from day to day as the illness develops. Abdominal discomfort, bloating, and constipation are common during the early phase of illness. A dry cough is observed in about two-thirds of the patients and occasionally may be so prominent as to direct attention away from the generalized nature of the infectious process. Nosebleeds may occur during the early phase of illness.

The temperature gradually increases for 5 to 7 days and then plateaus as a continuous or mildly remittent fever in the range of 39 to 40°C. The temperature may be sustained at these levels with little variation for 2 or 3 weeks. A relative bradycardia occurs in 30 to 40 percent of the patients. The prolonged persistent fever leads to general debility; patients are weak and anorectic. Mental dullness is common and delirium may occur. Abdominal pain and marked distention are usual. Constipation, relatively common during the early phase of illness, may give way to diarrhea later in the course of the disease.

The characteristic rash (rose spots) is most often observed during the second week of the disease. The lesions are small, 2- to 4-mm, erythematous macules which occur in small numbers on the upper abdomen and anterior thorax. The lesions blanch on pressure and last only 2 to 3 days. Some reports describe rose spots in as many as 90 percent of patients, whereas other reports indicate a frequency of only 10 percent or even less. The evanescent nature of the rash and the difficulties encountered in detecting lesions in highly pigmented individuals probably account for the marked variation in incidence reported in the literature.

The liver and spleen are frequently enlarged and palpable from the end of the first week of illness. The spleen is palpable in about three-quarters of the patients. The liver may be tender, and occasionally a friction rub is audible over the spleen.

Abdominal tenderness is frequent and distention occurs in the majority of cases. Marked abdominal pain with signs of peritonitis should call attention to the possibility of perforation of the bowel.

After the third week, the symptoms slowly abate, and the temperature returns to normal over a period of days.

Jaundice secondary to extensive mononuclear cell infiltration in the liver and hepatic cell necrosis is a rare complication of typhoid. Acute renal failure also is observed rarely; the pathogenesis of this so-called typhoid nephritis has not been adequately defined. Disseminated intravascular coagulation may develop in severe typhoid and lead to additional clinical manifestations secondary to thrombosis or hemorrhage.

Complications Prior to the introduction of chloramphenicol, the prolonged febrile course of typhoid often led to profound debility, weight loss, and multiple nutritional deficiencies. Intestinal hemorrhage and bowel perforation, the most feared complications, were common causes of death. The frequency of complications in typhoid fever has been reduced since the advent of effective chemotherapy.

INTESTINAL HEMORRHAGE Erosion of blood vessels in hyperplastic and necrotic Peyer's patches or in other mononuclear cell accumulations in the wall of the intestine leads to bleeding into the intestinal tract. Occult blood in feces is quite common during the course of the disease, occurring in 20 percent or more of patients. Gross blood is present in feces in about 10 percent of patients, and massive hemorrhage occurs occasionally. Major hemorrhage is usually a late complication, occurring most often during the second or third week of disease. A sudden drop in blood pressure or temperature may be the first manifestation of hemorrhage.

INTESTINAL PERFORATION The pathological process in the lymphoid tissues of the intestine may also involve the muscular and serosal layers of the bowel and lead to perforation. Prior to the advent of chloramphenicol, perforation occurred in about 3 percent of patients with typhoid. The incidence has been reduced by antimicrobial therapy to about 1 percent. Perforation is most common in the distal 60 cm of ileum and is observed most frequently during the third week of the disease. The onset of perforation may be quite unexpected during an otherwise uncomplicated convalescence. Pain in the right lower quadrant of the abdomen is the most frequent initial manifestation, but signs of localized or generalized peritonitis develop rapidly.

OTHER COMPLICATIONS Typhoid bacilli may localize in any tissue in the body with the production of localized suppurative infection. Meningitis, chondritis, periostitis, osteomyelitis, arthritis, and pyelonephritis are examples of localized infections that may be observed occasionally. Pneumonia is not unusual and may be caused by the typhoid bacillus or by a secondary bacterial invader, such as the pneumococcus. Severe deep thrombophlebitis may occur during the febrile period. Late complications also include peripheral neuritis, deafness, and alopecia. Hemolytic anemia may be observed, especially in infected individuals deficient in glucose 6-phosphate dehydrogenase.

Relapse After illness has subsided for a variable period, usually about 2 weeks, all the manifestations which characterized the initial infection may recur. Blood cultures, negative during convalescence, may become positive again. Although relapse may be severe, it is usually milder and of shorter duration than the original illness. The incidence of relapse was about 5 to 10 percent prior to the introduction of effective chemotherapy. Chloramphenicol has not decreased the frequency of relapse; in fact, the relapse rate in chloramphenicol-treated patients is higher than in patients not receiving the drug. Periods of antimicrobial therapy longer than 2 weeks do not seem to alter the incidence of relapse. Relapse cannot be correlated with the titer of agglutinins against the flagellar, somatic, or Vi antigens of the typhoid bacillus.

Chronic carriers Although the vast majority of patients with typhoid fever eradicate the site of infection in the gallbladder during convalescence, about 3 percent of adults do not, and these individuals become chronic typhoid carriers who continue to excrete organisms in feces for years, usually for life. A chronic carrier is defined as a person documented to have been excreting typhoid bacilli in the stool for a period of at least 1 year. In the United States, almost all chronic carriers have a persistent site of infection in the gallbladder from which organisms reach the intestinal tract in bile. Chronic carriers may be detected by follow-up of patients with typhoid fever, but many carriers give no history of typhoid. In these patients, it is assumed that the initial illness was so mild as to go unrecognized or undiagnosed. Once organisms have been demonstrated in the stools for as long as a year, it is quite unlikely that the focus of infection in the gallbladder will terminate spontaneously. The chronic carrier state is rare in children and occurs more commonly with increasing age and is about three times more common in women than men. It is possible that these age and sex characteristics are related to the greater prevalence of gallbladder disease in older women, a factor which would favor persistence of organisms in the biliary tract.

The chronic biliary carrier is usually asymptomatic. Despite millions of organisms entering the intestine in each milliliter of bile, patients show no systemic manifestations. Gallstones and dysfunction of the gallbladder on cholecystogram can be demonstrated in a large proportion of chronic carriers, and carriers occasionally develop acute cholecystitis.

In areas of the world where *Schistosoma haematobium* infections are common, a chronic urinary carrier state results from localization of typhoid bacilli or other *Salmonella* serotypes in the obstructed urinary tract or adjacent lesions resulting from the schistosomiasis. These chronic urinary carriers not only excrete *Salmonella* in the urine but also may have intermittent bacteremic episodes which are not necessarily accompanied by fever.

LABORATORY FINDINGS Leukopenia of 3000 to 4000 cells per cubic millimeter is characteristic of the febrile phase of typhoid fever. A sudden increase in leukocyte count to 10,000 cells per cubic millimeter or higher should suggest the possibility of intestinal perforation, hemorrhage, or a pyogenic complication, but these complications may occur in the absence of leukocytosis. A normocytic normochromic anemia develops during the course of the disease and may be aggravated by blood loss from intestinal lesions. Occult blood and a mononuclear leukocytosis in feces is common from the second week of disease. Urine is usually normal except for transient albuminuria during the febrile period.

The most dependable way to establish a definitive diagnosis of typhoid fever is by blood culture. Organisms can be recovered by culture of blood in 70 to 90 percent of patients during the first week of disease. Bacteremia is continuous and prolonged. Positive blood cultures are obtained in as many as 30 or 40 percent of patients during the third week of disease, but the incidence of bacteremia rapidly decreases after this time. Blood cultures frequently are positive during relapse. Recent evidence in partially treated cases suggests that culture of bone marrow may yield the organism when other cultures are negative, especially after antibiotics have been given.

Only about 10 to 15 percent of patients have positive stool cultures during the first week of disease. However, the frequency of positive stool cultures increases as the disease progresses, reaching a maximum of about 75 percent during the third or fourth week of illness. The frequency of positive cultures then begins to decline so that only about 10 percent of patients have positive stool cultures 8 weeks after onset of illness. Most of these patients' cultures become negative over the next several weeks or months, but about 3 percent of adults continue to excrete organisms even after 1 year. Persistent excretion in these chronic carriers is secondary to infection in the gallbladder and biliary tract.

The incidence of positive urine cultures varies markedly during the course of typhoid fever and parallels the frequency of positive stool cultures. At least some of the positive cultures represent contamination of urine with feces harboring typhoid bacilli.

The majority of patients, but by no means all, develop a fourfold or greater rise in serum agglutinins against the somatic or O antigens of the typhoid bacillus during the course of the disease. Detection of *S. typhi* Vi, D, or d antigens in the urine of patients with typhoid fever may be even more sensitive. A fourfold or greater increase in serum titer in the absence of recent typhoid immunization is compatible with infection with *S. typhi* but is by no means specific. All the group D organisms, one of which is *S. typhi,* as well as organisms in groups A and B, have certain common antigens which can evoke the formation of antibodies reactive with the O antigen used in the Widal test. Agglutinins against flagellar or H antigens also appear, frequently in higher titer than agglutinins against the O antigens. However, the H agglutinins are even more subject to nonspecific variation than O agglutinins and are of no value in diagnosis. Agglutinins begin to appear after about 1 week of illness and reach a peak titer during the fifth or sixth week. Early antimicrobial therapy may dampen the immunologic response in patients with typhoid fever. Relapse bears no relation to agglutinin titer. Rheumatoid factor activity in high titer can be detected in a large proportion of patients with typhoid or paratyphoid fever.

DIFFERENTIAL DIAGNOSIS The clinical features of typhoid fever, while characteristic and suggestive of the diagnosis, are certainly not pathognomonic. Many other diseases give a clinical picture which may be confused with typhoid; these include the rickettsioses, brucellosis, tularemia, leptospirosis, psittacosis, infectious hepatitis, infectious mononucleosis, primary atypical pneumonia, miliary tuberculosis, malaria, lymphoma, and rheumatic fever. Typhoid should be considered in any patient with unexplained fever, especially if there is a history of recent foreign travel to endemic areas.

TREATMENT **Antimicrobial therapy** Chloramphenicol is the antibiotic of choice for the treatment of typhoid fever. Despite the fact that a number of antimicrobial agents show excellent in vitro activity against *S. typhi,* chloramphenicol has consistently been shown to be more effective in terminating the febrile toxic course of the disease in the greatest proportion of patients in the shortest period of time. Nevertheless, the response to chloramphenicol is not dramatic or rapid. Subjective improvement usually occurs within about 48 h after beginning therapy, but the temperature usually does not return to normal for 2 to 5 days after initiating treatment. Bacteremia usually clears within hours after therapy is instituted, but occasionally organisms can be recovered from the blood 24 to 48 h after beginning treatment. The dose of chloramphenicol should be 50 mg per kilogram of body weight per day divided into three or four equal doses given orally at intervals of 6 to 8 h. After the patient has become afebrile, the dose may be reduced to 30 mg/kg per day. Therapy should be continued for 2 weeks. If chloramphenicol cannot be given by the oral route, comparable doses should be given parenterally.

Ampicillin in doses of 80 mg/kg per day or 6 g per day for adults divided into four or six doses given parenterally or a combination of trimethoprim and sulfamethoxazole is effective in the treatment of typhoid, but the response is not as predictable or as prompt as with chloramphenicol. If there is a contraindication to therapy with chloramphenicol, ampicillin, amoxicillin, or trimethoprim-sulfamethoxazole is recommended.

Occasional patients with typhoid without evidence of suppurative complications do not respond clinically even after 4 or 5 days of antimicrobial therapy, even though blood cultures become negative. Delayed responses of this type occur in only about 1 percent of patients treated with chloramphenicol, in contrast to 5 or 10 percent of patients treated with ampicillin.

Chloramphenicol-resistant strains have been reported since 1972 from many areas of the world, predominantly Mexico, southeast Asia, and India. Resistance is due to a transferable R factor which also codes for resistance to sulfonamides, tetracycline, and streptomycin. *Salmonella typhi* resistant to both chloramphenicol and ampicillin have been isolated from a few patients, and the in vivo acquisition of resistance to chloramphenicol, sulfonamide, and trimethoprim in a patient treated with these drugs has been reported. If chloramphenicol resistance is encountered, then ampicillin, amoxicillin, or trimethoprim and sulfamethoxazole should be used.

Adrenal hormones The administration of prednisone or steroids with similar activity can terminate within a matter of hours the severe febrile toxemic state seen in some patients. Because of the lag in time between institution of antimicrobial therapy and evidence of response, patients with life-threatening toxemia should be treated with a brief course of adrenal corticosteroids in addition to chloramphenicol. An appropriate regimen is 60 mg prednisone the first day; no additional steroid therapy should be administered. Hypothermia and hypotension occasionally occur within hours after initiation of steroids.

Supportive treatment Nursing care and attention to nutritional requirements are important. Laxatives and enemas should be avoided despite constipation because of the danger of precipitating hemorrhage or perforation. Salicylates should not be used, because in addition to their effects on blood platelets and irritating action on the bowel, these compounds can induce wide swings in temperature with very uncomfortable chills and sweats. Hypothermia and hypotension occur in some patients after administration of salicylates.

Hemorrhage and perforation Patients should be observed carefully to detect these complications at an early stage. Typing and cross matching should be carried out at the time of initial diagnosis of typhoid, and transfusion is indicated in the event of significant hemorrhage. Patients with typhoid are poor surgical risks. If perforation is suspected, emphasis should be placed on efforts to combat shock and decompress the bowel. Additional antimicrobials may have to be added to control peritonitis. Small perforations may localize and can be managed without surgical intervention. However, if evidence of localization does not develop, surgical intervention may be required.

Relapse The therapy of relapse is identical to that for the primary episode.

Chronic carriers Chronic carriers should be investigated for the presence of gallstones or a nonfunctioning gallbladder. Carriers without evidence of gallstones or gallbladder disease on cholecystogram or with ultrasound usually can be cured with a prolonged course of ampicillin. One program which has been found to be effective consists of 6 g ampicillin divided into four equal oral doses each day with probenecid for a period of 6 weeks. If gallstones or a nonfunctioning gallbladder are demonstrated, antimicrobial therapy is unlikely to be effective in terminating the carrier state. These patients should have cholecystectomy, which cures the chronic carrier state in about 85 percent of patients. Ampicillin may be used in conjunction with cholecystectomy. Therapy should be started a few days prior to the procedure and continued for 2 or 3 weeks. One study has reported success of sulfamethoxazole-trimethoprim and rifampin in the treatment of chronic *Salmonella* carriers.

PREVENTION AND CONTROL Although immunization with typhoid vaccine affords significant protection against typhoid infection, the degree of immunity is not great and can be readily overcome with a large dose of organisms. Nevertheless, immunization is recommended for individuals living or traveling in areas where the disease is endemic and for persons working with the organism in laboratories. Adults should receive 0.5 ml vaccine on two occasions separated by a period of 1 or 2 weeks. A yearly booster is required to maintain immunity. Immunization with typhoid vaccine causes a transient elevation for several months in titer of agglutinins against typhoid O antigens and a persistently elevated titer for H antigens.

All typhoid patients should be reported to local health authorities, and stool specimens should be cultured during convalescence. Three consecutively negative stool cultures obtained at weekly intervals indicate that a carrier state has not developed.

Caution should be observed to prevent spread of infection from persons with active disease or from carriers. Chronic or convalescent carriers should not be allowed to prepare food until clear documentation shows that at least three or more stool cultures are negative for typhoid bacilli. Carriers should be cautioned regarding routine sanitary techniques.

PROGNOSIS The mortality rate of typhoid fever prior to the introduction of chloramphenicol was about 12 percent. Death was associated with toxemia, inanition, pneumonia, bowel perforation, and intestinal hemorrhage. The mortality rate is still 2 or 3 percent; deaths are observed primarily in infants, the aged, or individuals with malnutrition or other underlying diseases.

OTHER *SALMONELLA* INFECTIONS

DEFINITION Bacteria of the genus *Salmonella* may produce asymptomatic infection of the intestinal tract in humans or several different clinical syndromes including acute gastroenteritis (or enterocolitis), bacteremia, paratyphoid fever, or localized infections ranging from osteomyelitis to endocarditis. The clinical syndromes resulting from infection with *Salmonella* cannot always be sharply differentiated and sometimes overlap.

Salmonella infections are among the most prevalent recognized communicable diseases caused by bacteria in the United States today. These infections are transmitted in the vast majority of cases from animals to humans and occasionally from person to person and are usually brief, self-limited, and mild.

EPIDEMIOLOGY Salmonellas can be isolated from the intestinal tracts of humans and many lower animals. The prevalence of asymptomatic excretors of these organisms in the general population is about 0.2 percent, but the most important reservoir of salmonellas is in domestic and wild animal species in which infection rates vary from less than 1 to more than 20 percent. An incomplete list of animals from which *Salmonella* species have been isolated includes chickens, turkeys, ducks, pigs, cows, dogs, cats, rats, parakeets, as well as certain cold-blooded animals and insects. Animals sold as pets, especially baby chicks, ducks, and turtles, may also harbor *Salmonella* and serve as sources of infection.

Salmonella infection is almost always acquired by the oral route, usually by ingestion of contaminated food or drink. Rare exceptions are *Salmonella* infections acquired by intravenous platelet transfusions or contaminated fiberoptic instruments. Any food product is a potential source of human infection. The source of contamination of food or drink may be asymptomatic human carriers or persons with active clinical disease, but the greatest single source of human infection in the United States is the vast reservoir of *Salmonella* in lower animals. The high incidence of infection in domestic animals used as a source of food for humans and present methods of processing foods and food products in bulk result in the availability of foods for human consumption with a potentially high incidence of contamination with *Salmonella.* For example, a significant proportion varying from 1 to more than 50 percent of raw meats purchased in retail markets is contaminated with *Salmonella.* Meat is contaminated by many routes, but the most common are natural infection of the animal used as a source of meat and contamination of the carcass during slaughter and processing. Eggs or egg products, including dried or frozen eggs, are also common sources of *Salmonella* infection. Of the various animal species, domestic fowl, including chickens, turkeys, ducks, and eggs and egg products, constitute the single largest reservoir of infection and the source most often responsible for infection of humans. Adequate cooking of food prior to human consumption serves to decrease the possibility of infection. However, salmonellas may survive cooking at low temperature, or food may be recontaminated after cooking by organisms from kitchen equipment or personnel.

Food or drink may also be contaminated by rats, mice, insects, or other vermin harboring these organisms. Cross infection occurs occasionally by the airborne route from dried foods such as egg whites or dust which contain viable *Salmonella.* *Salmonella* contamination of a large variety of processed foods has also been documented. Some of these foods contain ingredients of animal origin such as eggs, whereas others contain contaminated products of vegetable origin such as coconut or yeast. A variety of pharmaceutical products of animal origin have been shown to be responsible for *Salmonella* infections of humans; these products include carmine dye, pancreatin, bile salts, and extracts of various organs such as thyroid, adrenal, and stomach.

Pet turtles are an important source of *Salmonella* infection in humans, especially in children, accounting for perhaps as many as 10 to 20 percent of reported *Salmonella* infections in certain areas. Turtles are infected on breeding farms and continue to excrete organisms in feces into tank water for long periods of time. Although knowledge of the manner of transmission to humans is incomplete, it is likely that turtle feces or tank water harboring salmonellas contaminate hands of handlers, from which organisms are passed to the mouth or to food or drink.

Salmonella species may also be transmitted directly or via fomites from humans to humans or from animals to humans without the intervention of contaminated food or drink, but this method of spread is not common. However, cross infection of this type has been shown to be responsible for a number of outbreaks of salmonellosis among patients in nurseries and hospitals. Nosocomial salmonellosis poses a particular threat to newborns, immunosuppressed patients, patients in burn units, and those receiving multiple broad-spectrum antibiotics, who may be infected by relatively few organisms. Multiply drug-resistant salmonellas are often found in this setting. Nursery outbreaks have been traced to newborn infants from mothers with recent *Salmonella* infections.

Fish meal, meat meal, bone meal, and other by-products of the meat-packing industry are often contaminated with *Salmonella* organisms. These products are incorporated in animal and poultry feeds and apparently play an important role in the perpetuation of infection among domestic animals that can be spread to humans.

The true incidence of *Salmonella* infection is difficult to determine. The reported isolations of salmonellas from humans in the United States represent about 10 cases per 100,000 population per year. However, reported cases represent only a small proportion of the actual number because bacteriologic studies are usually performed only on patients with severe or protracted diarrhea, and many outbreaks are not investigated. Although *Salmonella* infection occurs throughout the year, the Salmonella Surveillance Unit of the National Communicable Disease Centers has observed a distinct seasonal pattern with the greatest number of isolations reported from July through November for each year.

A close correlation exists between the *Salmonella* serotypes most often responsible for human infection and those isolated from animals in any specific geographic area. The similarities document the importance of nonhuman reservoirs of *Salmonella* in the epidemiology of *Salmonella* infection in humans.

PATHOGENESIS The course of events after salmonellas have gained access to the gastrointestinal tract is determined by the dose, serotype, and invasive potential of the organism, and by the resistance of the host. Different *Salmonella* serotypes show marked variation in invasive potential and capacity to produce disease in humans. For example, *S. anatum* characteristically produces asymptomatic intestinal infection and rarely invades the bloodstream. In contrast, *S. cholerae-suis*, the most invasive serotype, frequently produces bacteremia and metastatic infection. Bloodstream invasion may occur as a complication of gastroenteritis but usually develops without preceding intestinal symptoms. Bacteremia with any serotype may be transient or prolonged, and may be accompanied by recurrent chills and fever or manifestations of paratyphoid fever. Bloodborne bacteria may localize at any site and lead to suppuration in bone, joints, meninges, pleura, or other tissues.

Multiplication of ingested organisms in the intestinal tract may be followed by symptoms of gastroenteritis. The intestinal irritation and inflammation are produced by a true infection deep in the mucosa as evidenced by polymorphonuclear leukocytes typically found in the diarrheal stool. However, studies in animals have shown that mucosal invasion alone is not sufficient to account for the intestinal fluid observed in experimental infections. The secretory effects of certain strains of *S. typhimurium* can be abolished in animals by indomethacin without altering the invasive process. This has led to the hypothesis of a possible enterotoxin-like effect on upper intestinal transport. An enterotoxin-like effect has also been shown with culture filtrates of *Salmonella* in animals and tissue culture models used to study *Escherichia coli* and cholera enterotoxins.

Studies in human volunteers indicate that large numbers of viable organisms must be ingested to produce clinically apparent disease. However, a transient carrier state can be produced with doses 10 or 100 times smaller than those required to evoke symptoms of infection. The minimal infectious dose varies markedly among different serotypes.

Many host factors influence the frequency and nature of *Salmonella* infections. The minimal infectious dose varies considerably among different individual hosts and can be reduced by antacids, antimotility drugs, or antimicrobial agents in experimental animals. Some have reported the precipitation of severe systemic disease following antimotility therapy for mild gastroenteritis.

The bacterial flora of the intestine is important in determining the fate of ingested salmonellas. Administration of certain antibiotics by the oral route to mice results in a 10,000-fold increase in susceptibility to infection with *S. enteritidis.* Somewhat similar observations have been made in experimental typhoid fever in volunteers. In these studies the dose of *S. typhi* required to initiate infection by the oral route in humans can be reduced sharply by giving certain antimicrobials orally prior to challenge. Epidemiologic studies have also shown that prior antimicrobial therapy alters the capacity of the human intestinal tract to eradicate *Salmonella* acquired naturally. The effect of antibiotic therapy may be related to a marked diminution in number of *Bacteroides* or other organisms which produce antimicrobial substances such as short-chain fatty acids that are active against *Salmonella.* Alteration in intestinal flora also has been suggested as a mechanism of the increased susceptibility of patients with previous major gastric surgery, especially gastrectomy and gastroenterostomy, to intestinal infection with salmonellas. However, reduced acidity or rapid emptying time consequent to gastric surgery also appear to play a role by increasing the number of viable organisms reaching the small intestine.

Cell-mediated immune mechanisms appear to be important in host resistance to infection with salmonellas. About one-third of patients who are hospitalized because of salmonellosis have some type of major underlying disease, such as leukemia, lymphoma, lupus erythematosus, or aplastic anemia. This may be coincidence but more often reflects a decrease in resistance to bacterial infection in general. In a few diseases there is evidence to indicate an almost specific predisposition to infection by salmonellas that exceeds susceptibility to other bacterial species. Patients with sickle cell anemia and other hemolytic processes are unusually susceptible to bloodstream invasion by salmonellas. In patients with sickle hemoglobinopathies there is a strong tendency for localization in bone, and salmonellas, not staphylococci, are the most common cause of osteomyelitis in patients with sickle cell diseases. *Salmonella* bacteremia is also an unusually frequent complication of the acute hemolytic phase of bartonellosis (see Chap. 169).

Infants are more susceptible to *Salmonella* infection and remain convalescent carriers for a longer period of time than adults. The mortality rate from the disease is also higher in infants and in the elderly than in young adults.

CLINICAL MANIFESTATIONS **Gastroenteritis** Although gastroenteritis often occurs in large epidemics among individuals who have eaten the same contaminated food, family outbreaks and sporadic cases are even more common. After an incubation period of 8 to 48 h, there is sudden onset of colicky abdominal pain and loose, watery diarrhea, occasionally with mucus or blood. Nausea and vomiting are frequent but are rarely severe or protracted. Fever of 38 to 39°C is common, and there may be an initial chill. Patients usually have mild to moderate abdominal tenderness on palpation, but severe tenderness, even with rebound, occurs in occasional patients. Peristalsis is usually hyperactive. Abdominal findings may be prominent in some patients and lead to confusion with certain intraabdominal emergencies, such as acute appendicitis or acute cholecystitis. Colonic involvement with tenesmus and with mucosal friability and crypt abscess may also occur. Symptoms usually subside promptly within 2 to 5 days and recovery is uneventful. However, the illness is occasionally more protracted, with persistence of diarrhea and low-grade fever for 10 to 14 days. Fatalities rarely exceed 1 percent of the affected population and are limited almost entirely to infants, the aged, and debilitated patients.

The causative organism can often be isolated from the suspected food and from feces during the acute illness. Stool cultures usually become negative for salmonellas within 1 to 4 weeks, but occasional patients continue to excrete organisms for months. Organisms tend to persist in the stools of infants and young children for longer periods than in older children or adults. The blood leukocyte count is usually normal. The blood culture is usually negative.

Enteric or paratyphoid fever Certain species can produce an illness clinically indistinguishable from typhoid fever, with prolonged fever, rose spots, splenomegaly, leukopenia, gastrointestinal symptoms, and positive blood and stool cultures. The organisms most likely to produce this picture are *S. cholerae-suis* and *S. enteritidis,* serotypes *paratyphi A* and *paratyphi B.* Occasionally a typical attack of food poisoning is followed in a few days by manifestations of paratyphoid fever. Generally, paratyphoid fevers tend to be milder than *S. typhi* infections, but differentiation on clinical grounds is not possible in the individual case. Recovery may be followed by continued excretion of the causative organism in the stools for several months, but the chronic carrier state is less frequent than in typhoid fever.

Bacteremia *Salmonella* species may produce a syndrome characterized primarily by prolonged fever and positive blood cultures. Although symptoms of gastroenteritis can precede bacteremia, they are usually lacking, and most cases arise sporadically. In many instances, the only manifestations are prolonged fever, which is usually spiking and is accompanied by repeated rigors, sweats, aching, anorexia, and weight loss. The characteristic features of typhoid and paratyphoid fever, such as rose spots, persistent leukopenia, and sustained fever, are absent. Stool cultures are usually negative. In contrast to the constant bacteremia of typhoid fever, discharge of organisms into the bloodstream is intermittent, and repeated blood cultures may be required to demonstrate the causative organism. At some time in the course of the illness, localizing signs of infection appear in about one-fourth of the cases. Pulmonary infection in the form of bronchopneumonia or abscess, pleurisy, empyema, pericarditis, endocarditis, pyelonephritis, meningitis, osteomyelitis, and arthritis is relatively common. The blood leukocyte count is usually normal, but with the development of focal lesions, polymorphonuclear leukocytosis as high as 20,000 to 25,000 cells per cubic millimeter occurs. *Salmonella* bacteremia can be a very puzzling disorder, especially before localization takes place, and should be considered in cases of fever of unknown origin.

A prolonged febrile illness lasting weeks or months and characterized by weight loss, marked anemia, hepatosplenomegaly, and bacteremia with *Salmonella* has been described in

Brazil and other areas of the world in patients with hepatosplenic schistosomiasis due to *Schistosoma mansoni.* Intermittent bacteremia with *Salmonella* also occurs in patients with *Schistosoma haematobium* infection who are also urinary carriers of *Salmonella.*

Local pyogenic infections *Salmonella* organisms can produce abscesses in almost any anatomic site, and these can occur independently of previous symptoms of gastroenteritis or other systemic illness, or as complications of bacteremias. There is nothing characteristic about the suppurative lesions, and the correct etiologic diagnosis is rarely made on the basis of clinical findings alone. There is a strong tendency for salmonellas to localize in tissues that are the site of preexisting disease. Localization has been described in aneurysms, bone adjacent to aortic aneurysms, hematomas, and many different tumors, including hypernephroma, ovarian cyst, and pheochromocytoma. Meningeal localization of infection is common in newborns and infants, and occasional small outbreaks of *Salmonella* infection in nurseries have consisted almost entirely of meningitis. In addition to suppurative joint disease, a chronic aseptic polyarthritis has been described.

DIAGNOSIS Febrile gastroenteritis produced by presumed viral agents and shigellosis can be distinguished from *Salmonella* gastroenteritis only by appropriate stool cultures, especially in sporadic cases. Polymorphonuclear fecal leukocytes are frequently present in *Salmonella* gastroenteritis and in bacillary dysentery (shigellosis), but not in viral, giardial, or enterotoxin-induced gastroenteritis. Staphylococcal food poisoning usually is not associated with fever, and vomiting is a more prominent feature than in most *Salmonella* infections. Systemic manifestations are usually absent in patients with gastroenteritis caused by enterotoxigenic *E. coli* and *Clostridium perfringens.* Many toxic agents and drugs can produce diarrhea, nausea, and abdominal pain, but fever is rarely a feature of these disorders, and the diagnosis depends upon a history of exposure or ingestion. The diagnosis of paratyphoid fever or *Salmonella* bacteremia depends upon isolation of the causative organism. Agglutination tests with acute and convalescent serums as performed in the usual clinical laboratory are not very helpful. The possibility of an underlying disease should be considered in every patient with a severe *Salmonella* infection.

TREATMENT The treatment of *Salmonella* gastroenteritis is supportive. Dehydration should be corrected by parenteral administration of fluids and electrolytes. Abdominal cramps and diarrhea often are much improved if the patient takes nothing by mouth for 8 to 12 h. Antimicrobial therapy, irrespective of type, does not appear to exert a beneficial effect on the clinical course of *Salmonella* gastroenteritis or decrease the duration of excretion of organisms in the stool. In fact, the period of excretion of *Salmonella* in stools during convalescence is actually longer in patients who have been treated with antimicrobial drugs during the acute illness than in patients who received no antimicrobial therapy. Unless there is documented bacteremia or a protracted febrile course suggesting the diagnosis of enteric fever, antibiotics are *not* indicated in uncomplicated *Salmonella* gastroenteritis.

There appears to be a steady increase in the frequency of antimicrobial resistance due to transferable resistance factors among *Salmonella* isolates from humans. This may be due in part to the widespread use of antibiotics in animals and in humans.

Chloramphenicol in doses of 3 g daily in adults is the antibiotic of choice in systemic infections including *Salmonella* bacteremia, metastatic infection, and paratyphoid fever. The response is characteristically slow, and the temperature rarely returns to normal until 3 to 4 days after beginning therapy. Therapy should be continued for at least 2 weeks, but in certain infections, such as osteomyelitis or meningitis, the duration may have to be extended. Resistance to multiple antibiotics, including chloramphenicol and ampicillin, occurs, particularly in salmonellas acquired outside the United States. Therefore, antibiotic sensitivity of the organism should be tested in cases of bacteremia, metastatic infection, or enteric fever.

Ampicillin is also effective in systemic infections caused by *Salmonella* strains sensitive to the action of this antibiotic. However, a significant proportion of *Salmonella* strains are highly resistant to ampicillin in vitro. For this reason, ampicillin should not be used in therapy of serious infections unless it is known that the causative organism is sensitive. As in cases of typhoid fever, the combination of trimethoprim and sulfamethoxazole holds promise in the therapy of *Salmonella* infection when the organism is resistant to chloramphenicol and ampicillin. The tetracycline derivatives have sometimes appeared to exert a beneficial effect, but streptomycin, polymyxin, neomycin, kanamycin, and the sulfonamides are generally ineffective.

Antimicrobial therapy is usually not indicated in convalescent or asymptomatic transient carriers of *Salmonella* species. The carrier state will cease spontaneously in 1 to 3 months in the vast majority of individuals.

The chronic carrier state with localization of infection in the gallbladder and positive stool cultures for a period of time exceeding 1 year is rarely caused by *Salmonella* serotypes other than *S. typhi* and *S. paratyphi* A and B. Its treatment has been discussed. Surgically accessible suppurative lesions should be drained.

PREVENTION AND CONTROL Continuous surveillance and careful reporting of all *Salmonella* isolates improve awareness of new strains, common sources, antibiotic resistance, and the carrier state. Because of the great number of specific serotypes, surveillance and serotyping have occasionally brought attention to widespread occurrence of relatively rare serotypes traced to single sources. Central surveillance of all reported serotypes led to the discovery of an international outbreak in 1974 of *S. eastbourne,* an otherwise rare serotype that was traced to Canadian chocolates. Adequate cooking of meat and egg products and careful surveillance of poultry products and persons who handle food have been only moderately successful in controlling salmonellosis. Probably most important, besides food surveillance, is personal hygiene, including handwashing. Transient or permanent carriers should be warned to take these precautions and, as much as possible, to avoid food preparation. Minimizing the time that foods are allowed to stand at room temperature (as between cooking and refrigeration) should reduce the chances of bacterial growth to infectious inocula.

Careful obstetrical histories for any diarrheal illness at the time a woman enters for delivery should always be obtained, and mothers and infants so affected should be isolated until cultures rule out *Salmonella* carriage. Finally, because of the increasing antibiotic resistance, the indiscriminate use of unnecessary or "prophylactic" antimicrobial agents should be avoided.

REFERENCES

BAINE WB et al: Institutional salmonellosis. J Infect Dis 128:357, 1973

BENNETT IL JR, HOOK EW: Some aspects of salmonellosis. Ann Rev Med 10:1, 1959

BLASER MJ et al: *Salmonella typhi:* The laboratory as a reservoir of infection. J Infect Dis 142:934, 1980.

BUTLER T et al: Typhoid fever: Studies of blood coagulation, bacteremia and endotoxemia. Arch Intern Med 138:407, 1978

CLARK GM et al: Epidemiology of an international outbreak of *Salmonella agona.* Lancet 2:490, 1973

FELDMAN RE et al: Epidemiology of *Salmonella typhi* infection in a migrant labor camp in Dade County, Florida. J Infect Dis 130:354, 1974

FREERKSEN E et al: Treatment of chronic salmonella carriers. Chemotherapy 23:192, 1977

GIANNELLA RA et al: Pathogenesis of salmonellosis: Studies of fluid secretion, mucosal invasion, and morphologic reaction in the rabbit ileum. J Clin Invest 52:441, 1973

HORNICK RB, GRIESMAN S: On the pathogenesis of typhoid fever. Arch Intern Med 138:357, 1978

KAYE D et al: Treatment of chronic enteric carriers of *Salmonella typhosa* with ampicillin. Ann NY Acad Sci 145:429, 1967

MCHUGH GL et al: *Salmonella typhimurium* resistant to silver nitrate, chloramphenicol, and ampicillin: A new threat to burn units? Lancet 1:235, 1975

MANDAL BK: Typhoid and paratyphoid fever. Clin Gastroent 8:715, 1979

OLARTE J, GALINDO E: *Salmonella typhi* resistant to chloramphenicol, ampicillin, and other antimicrobial agents: Strains isolated during an extensive typhoid fever epidemic in Mexico. Antimicrob Agents Chemother 4:597, 1973

RICE PA et al: *Salmonella typhi* infections in the United States, 1967–1972: Increasing importance of international travelers. Am J Epidemiol 106:160, 1977

RYDER RW et al: Increase in antibiotic resistance among isolates of *Salmonella* in the U.S. J Infect Dis. 142:485, 1980.

SCHROEDER SA et al: Epidemic salmonellosis in hospitals and institutions: A five-year review. N Engl J Med 279:674, 1968

Surveillance summary, human *Salmonella* isolates—United States, 1980. Morb Mort Week Rep 30:377, 1981

TURNBULL PCB: Food poisoning with special reference to *Salmonella*—Its epidemiology, pathogenesis and control. Clin Gastroent 8:663, 1979

155 SHIGELLOSIS

HARRY N. BEATY

DEFINITION Shigellosis is an acute, self-limited infection of the intestinal tract of humans which is characterized by diarrhea, fever, and abdominal pain. The disease is frequently called *bacillary dysentery,* but the term *shigellosis* is preferred.

ETIOLOGY The genus *Shigella* of the family Enterobacteriaceae includes a group of closely related species which are nonmotile, nonencapsulated, slender, gram-negative rods. They are aerobes or facultative anaerobes and grow best at 37°C. Nutritional requirements are relatively simple, and the ability of these organisms to grow in the presence of bile salts is used in devising selective media which facilitate their isolation. *S. dysenteriae* type 1 may be inhibited by these media, however, and growth may not be apparent for several days. Fermentation of carbohydrates differs according to species, but all strains produce acid in glucose and either fail to ferment lactose or do so only slowly. The shigellas are classified into groups A, B, C, or D on the basis of biochemical and antigenic characteristics. The clinically important species within the respective groups are *S. dysenteriae, S. flexneri, S. boydii,* and *S. sonnei.* While these shigellas share antigens among themselves and with other enteric bacilli, serologic classification is not difficult, and with the exception of *S. sonnei* a number of serotypes of each species has been recognized.

The somatic antigen of the shigellas is an endotoxin which is chemically and biologically similar to the endotoxins of other gram-negative bacilli. *Shigella dysenteriae* type 1 (Shiga bacillus) also produces an exotoxin(s) which has cytotoxic, neurotoxic, and enterotoxic properties. The role of this exotoxin in the pathogenesis of shigellosis is unknown, but a biologically and antigenically similar toxin is elaborated by certain strains of *S. flexneri* and *S. sonnei,* and there is increasing speculation that toxin may be a virulence factor.

EPIDEMIOLOGY The principal habitat of the shigellas is the gastrointestinal tract of higher primates. Natural disease occurs in humans, gorillas, and some species of monkey. The convalescent or asymptomatic carrier is the only recognized reservoir. Spread of infection from person to person occurs primarily when organisms on hands and inanimate objects contaminated with infected feces are ingested. In the United States, common source outbreaks usually involve food which has been contaminated by careless handlers. Outbreaks associated with drinking water have been reported, and swimming in contaminated rivers or pools can be a cause of infection. In regions where sanitation is poor, flies which have been in contact with infected human feces may serve as an important vector in the transmission of this disease.

Shigellosis is worldwide in distribution, and is particularly common in countries where effective sanitation is lacking. Around 15,000 cases are reported annually in the United States, but many more undoubtedly occur. *Shigella sonnei* is responsible for about 70 percent of the infections encountered in this country; *S. flexneri* is isolated from all but a small percentage of the rest. *Shigella dysenteriae* type 1, which formerly produced disease predominantly in Asia, has been responsible for large outbreaks of diarrhea in Central America. In the United States, infections with this species occur almost exclusively among foreign travelers or their contacts.

Major epidemics of shigellosis are uncommon in this country, but high-risk groups exist in the inner cities, in mental or penal institutions, and on Indian reservations. Poor sanitation, low standards of personal hygiene, crowded conditions, and a high proportion of children in a population favor spread of the infection. Infected persons may excrete organisms intermittently during convalescence, but the carrier state infrequently persists longer than 3 months.

Humoral antibodies to somatic antigens and toxins frequently develop in response to clinical infection, but there is no evidence that they influence the course of the disease or protect against reinfection. Nevertheless, persons living in endemic areas seem to develop immunity to recurrent episodes of clinical disease, and volunteers infected with a specific strain are resistant to rechallenge with that strain for weeks to months. This immunity may be mediated by coproantibody, which has been identified in the stool of patients with shigellosis, or by cellular defense mechanisms in the wall of the bowel. In any event, it has led to the development of live, attenuated vaccines which, given orally, induce the same degree of immunity as natural infection. Parenteral vaccines are of no value.

PATHOGENESIS AND PATHOLOGY In order to produce disease, viable organisms must first adhere to the mucosal surface and then penetrate the epithelial cell lining. These invasive properties are genetically controlled by at least three separate regions of the chromosome; loss of any one through mutation renders a strain avirulent. Unlike members of the genus *Salmo-*

nella, which require a large inoculum to produce infection, as few as 100 virulent *Shigella* can cause disease. Within 12 h, ingested organisms proliferate in the small intestine to concentrations of 10^7 or more cells per milliliter of luminal contents. This phase of infection is associated with fever and watery diarrhea, but pathological evidence of invasion of the intestine, which appears in the later stages of the illness, is limited to the colon.

Once organisms penetrate the mucosal surface, they multiply within epithelial cells and rarely extend beyond the limits of the intestinal mucous membrane. Although superficial, the inflammatory reaction is severe and usually involves the entire colon. A fibrinous exudate often develops, and necrosis of the mucosa produces shallow ulcers that bleed readily. Microscopic examination shows that the submucosa and muscularis mucosa are infiltrated with bacteria and polymorphonuclear leukocytes. Ulcers are sharply demarcated and are not undermined. Whether toxins are important in the pathogenesis of shigellosis is unsettled. However, there is mounting evidence that species other than *S. dysenteriae* are toxigenic, and the hypothesis has been proposed that toxin produced in the lumen of the jejunum binds to specific receptors on epithelial cells, leading to activation of adenylate cyclase and production of cholera-like diarrhea in the early stages of shigellosis. It has long been proposed that systemic manifestations of this disease are due to absorbed toxins, because bacteremia is extremely rare except when infection is due to the Shiga bacillus.

CLINICAL MANIFESTATIONS *Shigella* infections typically produce a biphasic illness characterized by fever, abdominal pain, and diarrhea. Nonetheless, a significant proportion of infected individuals are asymptomatic or have only mild diarrhea. The initial phase of the illness, which begins after an incubation period of about 24 h, is associated with fever, infrequent, voluminous, watery stools, and colicky abdominal pain. After 24 to 48 h, the frequency of bowel movements increases, but the volume of stools and their water content decreases. Mucus subsequently appears in the stool of half the patients, and gross blood is seen in 40 percent. Fever becomes less impressive, but patients complain more of fecal urgency, tenesmus, and painful defecation during the colitis phase of the illness. Other symptoms seen less consistently include nausea, vomiting, headache, myalgia, respiratory symptoms, and, in children, convulsions. Depending upon the severity of diarrhea and the height of fever, patients may become profoundly dehydrated, and circulatory collapse can occur. Lower abdominal tenderness and hyperactive bowel sounds are common, but there is no peritoneal irritation. Splenomegaly has been reported, but is rare. Sigmoidoscopic examination reveals diffuse mucosal inflammation, often with multiple ulcerations.

LABORATORY FINDINGS Blood leukocyte counts usually range between 5000 and 15,000 per cubic millimeter, but a leukemoid reaction with counts in the range of 30,000 to 50,000 per cubic millimeter is seen occasionally with *S. dysenteriae* infections. Anemia is uncommon. Microscopic examination of stool reveals shreds of mucus and erythrocytes. A methylene blue wet mount preparation shows many polymorphonuclear leukocytes, which correlates with diffuse colitis but does not help establish a specific diagnosis. Stool cultures usually are positive, but blood cultures rarely are. Electrolyte abnormalities depend on the degree of vomiting and diarrhea.

COURSE Shigellosis is generally a self-limited disease, and patients usually become afebrile in about 4 days. Diarrhea and abdominal cramps may continue a few days longer, but within a week most patients have recovered. A significant proportion of untreated patients continue to shed organisms in the stool for 2 or more weeks, however. In about 10 percent of cases a clinical or bacteriologic relapse occurs unless antibiotics are given. In the United States, the overall mortality rate associated with shigellosis is less than 0.1 percent. Among young children and elderly patients, however, the illness is often more severe and the prognosis poorer. *Shigella dysenteriae* type 1 produces particularly severe infections, and mortality rates of 25 to 50 percent have been recorded in epidemics produced by this species.

Complications of *Shigella* infections are encountered infrequently. An uncommon but significant problem is perforation of the colon. Hematogenous dissemination of the shigellas is also rare, but these organisms have been encountered in metastatic foci of infection such as abscesses and meningitis. In some series, bacteremia due to other gram-negative bacilli has been seen in association with shigellosis. Reiter's syndrome has been reported following shigellosis and is particularly likely to occur in patients who have the histocompatibility antigen B27. Likewise, the hemolytic-uremic syndrome has been recognized as an infrequent complication of shigellosis. Conjunctivitis, iritis, and peripheral neuropathy accompany shigellosis on rare occasions.

DIAGNOSIS A definitive diagnosis can be established when pathogenic members of the genus *Shigella* are isolated from cultures. Stool cultures are positive in over 90 percent of cases if they are obtained in the first 3 days of illness; but only about 75 percent are positive if they are obtained more than 1 week after the onset of diarrhea. The organisms survive for only a short time in feces, and fresh stool specimens or rectal swabs should be cultured promptly. Recovery of the shigellas is facilitated if saline suspensions of stool are streaked directly onto selective media such as SS agar or desoxycholate citrate agar. Antibodies can be detected in the serum of the majority of patients with positive cultures and may occasionally be of value in establishing the diagnosis of shigellosis. Immunofluorescent techniques, which allow rapid detection of organisms in the stool, have been developed.

Shigellosis infection should be considered in every febrile illness associated with diarrhea. Occasionally, children with infections such as tonsillitis or otitis have diarrhea, but the major differential diagnosis of shigellosis includes acute ulcerative colitis, viral enteritis, amebic dysentery, clostridial or staphylococcal food poisoning, and bacterial infections caused by enteroinvasive *Escherichia coli, Salmonella* species, *Campylobacter, Yersinia,* and *Vibrio parahemolyticus.* Shigellosis can closely mimic acute ulcerative colitis, and should be excluded with cultures in patients thought to have this disease. In viral infections, fever is uncommon, and the stool usually does not contain gross blood or pus. The onset of amebic colitis is gradual, and the diarrhea is relatively mild. Staphylococcal food poisoning is associated with more nausea and vomiting, and usually is not associated with fever. Bacterial infections can be differentiated with certainty only by microbiologic studies.

TREATMENT Shigellosis is usually a self-limited disease, so supportive therapy is all that is necessary for complete recovery. The role of antibiotics in treatment is controversial. Chemotherapy shortens the course of the illness, but many would reserve their use for the most severely ill patients in order to prevent the development of widespread antibiotic resistance among *Shigella* isolates. Others argue that all patients in the more developed countries should be treated to shorten illness and eradicate organisms from the intestinal tract, the only important reservoir of this infection. Emergence of resistance to antibiotics is not an inconsequential problem; 90 percent of *Shigella* isolates in the United States now are resistant to sulfonamides, and since 1955, epidemics of shigellosis in various parts of the world have been caused by organisms resistant to multiple antibiotics. The molecular basis for multiple resistance involves the episomal transfer (R factor) of drug-resistant determinants between enteric bacilli.

Nonetheless, strains producing shigellosis in the United States are sensitive to a number of antimicrobial agents. Ampicillin for 3 to 5 days, in doses of 50 to 100 mg/kg per day for children and 2 g per day for adults, is effective treatment for susceptible strains. Cotrimoxazole is equally effective, and a single dose of tetracycline (2.5 g) is a simple, effective regimen. Single-dose ampicillin reduces the severity of disease but does not reliably eradicate *Shigella* from the stool.

PREVENTION The most important prophylactic measures are the maintenance of proper sanitation and adequate sewage disposal. The detection and elimination of carriers are difficult and rarely practical. Methods for increasing resistance with oral vaccines may be useful in preventing outbreaks among susceptible populations.

REFERENCES

DuPont HL, Hornick RB: Clinical approach to infectious diarrheas. Medicine 52:265, 1973

———, Pickering LK: Bacillary dysentery, in *Infections of the Gastrointestinal Tract,* HL DuPont, LK Pickering (eds). New York, Plenum, 1980, pp 61–82

Gilman RH et al: Single-dose ampicillin therapy for severe shigellosis in Bangladesh. J Infect Dis 143:164, 1981

Keusch GT, Jacewicz M: Pathogenesis of *Shigella* diarrhea: VII. Evidence for a cell membrane toxin receptor involving β-1,4 linked *N*-acetyl-*d*-glucosamine oligomers. J Exp Med 146:535, 1977

Nelson JD et al: Trimethoprim-sulfamethoxazole therapy for shigellosis. JAMA 235:1239, 1976

156
HEMOPHILUS INFECTIONS

DAVID H. SMITH

Hemophilus influenzae was isolated by Pfeiffer in 1892 from the sputum of individuals afflicted during an influenza pandemic. The requirement of blood for in vitro growth and its presumptive role in the pandemic prompted the designation. Other species have since been classified as members of the *Hemophilus* genus on the basis of morphology and physiology: small, pleomorphic, facultatively aerobic, nonmotile, non-spore-forming, gram-negative bacilli that require enriched media containing blood or certain derivatives and that are strict parasites of humans. Certain of these species are closely related genetically.

H. influenzae and *H. pertussis* are the most important cause of human disease; other pathogenic species include *H. aegypticus, H. aphrophilus, H. ducreyi, H. parapertussis,* and *H. vaginalis. H. hemolyticus, H. parainfluenzae,* and *H. bronchiseptica* infect the upper respiratory tract but rarely cause disease.

HEMOPHILUS INFLUENZAE **Etiology** *H. influenzae* is distinguished by its growth requirement of a heat-labile V factor and a heat-stable X factor found in erythrocytes and its inability to hemolyze erythrocytes during growth. V factor can be replaced by coenzyme I (DPN), coenzyme II (TPN), or nicotinamide

nucleoside, and X factor by hematin. X factor is not required for anaerobic growth. Fermentation reactions and tests of other metabolic activities are variable and not useful in identification but may help in "biotyping" individual isolates.

H. influenzae will grow in any enriched supplemented medium, but optimal growth is realized with media in which erythrocytes are disrupted to release the growth factors, e.g., chocolate or Levinthal agar. "Satellism," growth around colonies of hemolytic *Staphylococcus aureus* which release growth factors, is often used to identify *H. influenzae.* Some strains grow best in 5 to 10 percent carbon dioxide; many laboratories therefore incubate specimens suspected of containing *H. influenzae* in a candle jar or an incubator purged with carbon dioxide. Since viability of this bacterium is lost rapidly on drying or heating, clinical specimens should be inoculated without delay.

The organism exists with or without a polysaccharide capsule. Colonies of nonencapsulated isolates are usually 0.5 to 1.5 mm in diameter and appear granular after overnight incubation on solid agar; those of encapsulated isolates are usually 3 to 4 mm in diameter and initially appear mucoid or glistening. *H. influenzae* grown on enriched media appear microscopically as relatively uniform, small coccobacilli (1×0.3 μm); under less than optimal growth conditions, long filaments or short chains are common. Because *H. influenzae* in clinical specimens often have variable morphology and do not always react with safranin dye, gram-stained smears of infected material are frequently misdiagnosed.

The outer membrane of *H. influenzae,* like that of other gram-negative bacilli, is composed of a lipopolysaccharide (endotoxin)-containing cell wall and a number of proteins, some of which are common to all isolates. Determination of the composition of *H. influenzae* outer membrane proteins has been useful for epidemiologic studies. The antigenic activity of *H. influenzae* endotoxin and these outer membrane proteins has not been defined. Only a small percentage of isolates recovered from the respiratory tract are encapsulated. Six antigenically distinguishable capsular types, designated a to f, have been identified. Each is a complex carbohydrate. Type a, b, and c capsules share antigenic determinants with those of certain pneumococci, while that of type b, polyribose ribitol phosphate (PRP), cross-reacts immunologically with the capsules or cell walls of several species of gram-positive bacteria and enteric bacilli.

Strains with decreased or absent capsular antigen arise spontaneously from encapsulated strains. This variation proceeds: M (fully encapsulated) → S (partially encapsulated) → R (nonencapsulated). The genetic basis of this variation and the natural existence of its converse, i.e., R→S→M, remain undescribed. DNA purified from an M strain can transform an R strain to the serotype of the donor M strain. Transformation of *H. influenzae* in the host has not been studied, but the demonstration of pneumococcal transformation in experimentally infected mice supports the possibility that this occurs. Transformation between *H. aegypticus* and *H. influenzae* and between *H. influenzae* and *H. parainfluenzae* demonstrates the close genetic relation of these species.

The physiologic release by *H. influenzae* b of its capsular antigen (PRP) during growth in vitro and in the host provides the basis for clinically useful immunological detection systems, e.g., countercurrent immunoelectrophoresis or agglutination of latex particles to which antibody is absorbed.

H. influenzae was previously susceptible to many antibiotics, but a significant percentage of strains is now resistant to ampicillin, and resistance to tetracycline has been increasing. Ampicillin-resistant strains are widely but variably distributed and are as pathogenic and transmissible as antibiotic-sensitive strains. Chloramphenicol-resistant and multiple-resistant (chloramphenicol, tetracycline, and/or ampicillin) strains have been isolated infrequently.

Epidemiology *H. influenzae* infects only humans and primarily in the upper respiratory tract. It can be recovered from the nasopharynx of up to 80 percent of healthy individuals with the frequency of infection related inversely to age: greatest with young persons. Asymptomatic nasopharyngeal infection lasts days to a few months, is not eradicated by systemic antibody, and often is not eliminated by antibiotic therapy adequate to cure type b meningitis. Of the isolated strains, up to 25 percent are encapsulated, one-half of which are type b.

H. influenzae diseases occur worldwide and for the most part are endemic. Systemic *H. influenzae* diseases have a marked age relationship: children of 6 to 48 months are highly suspectible; newborns, older children, and adults are uncommonly affected. Systemic type b diseases occur at an attack rate up to 6000 times normal among children of susceptible ages who have intimate contact with primary cases and among persons with certain diseases that increase their susceptibility, e.g., sickle cell disease, splenectomy, agammaglobulinemia, and treated Hodgkin's disease. Alcoholic adults appear to be at modestly increased risk of *H. influenzae* pneumonia. In temperate climates, systemic *H. influenzae* diseases occur most commonly during the late winter and spring.

The incidence of systemic *H. influenzae* b diseases has increased during the past 3 to 4½ decades, and more adults are being affected. The basis for this increased attack rate is not understood, but improved diagnostic laboratories and diminution in the prevalence of type-specific immunity due to excessive use of antibiotics have been suggested as possible mechanisms. Changes in antigenic composition and/or virulence of the organism and the prevalence of cross-reactive antibodies also may be responsible for this change.

Pathogenicity The relatively common asymptomatic nasopharyngeal infection occasionally develops into symptomatic disease which may spread contiguously to involve the sinuses, middle ear, or bronchi, invade local tissues, causing epiglottitis, pneumonia, pericarditis, or facial cellulitis, or enter the bloodstream and produce metastatic disease in the meninges or joints. Nonencapsulated strains produce luminal diseases, while systemic diseases are caused almost entirely by encapsulated *H. influenzae,* of which at least 90 percent are type b.

The pathogenicity of invasive strains is related directly to the inhibition of phagocytosis by the capsule. The basis for the disproportionate virulence of type b strains is under study, as is the role of outer membrane proteins and other constituents. Synergy between *H. influenzae* and certain respiratory viruses has been demonstrated in studies of human disease and experimental models.

Immunity Susceptibility to *H. influenzae* b meningitis was classically correlated inversely to the presence of anticapsular antibody. Continuing research has indicated that immunity results from a composite of antibody activities stimulated by several antigens, including the capsule and certain outer-membrane proteins. The best studied of these antibodies are directed to the capsule (PRP): they promote phagocytosis and bacteriolysis in vitro, protect animals from a lethal concentration of *H. influenzae* b, and were responsible for the efficacy of the anti-*H. influenzae* b serum used in the preantibiotic era. Moreover, field trials with a purified PRP vaccine demonstrated a correlation between protection of young children from systemic diseases and specific antibody activity. Antibody to PRP can be stimulated by infection with bacteria bearing cross-reactive surface antigens and is bacteriolytic in vitro and protective in experimental disease.

Studies of patients recovering from systemic *H. influenzae* b disease and those immunized with PRP have revealed that infants respond infrequently and poorly, younger children have intermediate reactivity, while older children and adults develop marked, nonboostable responses. A few children fail to produce anti-PRP antibody (measured by radioimmunoassay) following systemic disease and subsequently develop a second distinct episode of invasive type b disease. Although these children appear to have been "immunologically nonreactive" for periods up to months, all subsequently raised anti-PRP antibody activity. These observations indicate the need for further study and close follow-up of young children recuperating from invasive *H. influenzae* b disease. Likewise, survivors of intensive therapy for Hodgkin's disease—MOPP, splenectomy, and/or radiation—produce transient, infant-like anti-PRP antibody responses, even following systemic *H. influenzae* b disease.

Clinical manifestations *H. influenzae* can cause local respiratory tract or invasive diseases. Surveys of hospitalized children indicate that *H. influenzae* b is now the most common cause of bacteremic disease and that about one-half of children with *H. influenzae* disease have meningitis, one-sixth pneumonia, about 10 percent bacteremia without a primary focus, facial cellulitis, or epiglottitis, and 1 percent pyarthrosis. Adults may develop *H. influenzae* bacteremia, meningitis, and, less commonly, epiglottitis; however, bronchitis, due to nonencapsulated strains, and pneumonia are more common.

H. influenzae diseases are generally acute with symptoms reflecting the pyogenic process; however, the clinical course of certain of these diseases may be surprisingly prolonged.

MENINGITIS *H. influenzae* is a common cause of bacterial meningitis, primarily affecting children 9 months to 4 years of age. The signs and symptoms depend on the patient's age and the time in the course of the disease when medical care is sought. Young children and those early in the disease generally have a nonspecific clinical picture: preceding upper respiratory tract symptoms, fever, anorexia, lethargy, vomiting, and, with older children and adults, headache. A history of stiff neck or back may be elicited. Mental confusion, paresis of cranial nerves, coma, convulsions, opisthotonus, and shock occur with more prolonged and serious disease. The clinical findings are identical to those of other bacterial causes. Age and certain types of concurrent disease, e.g., cellulitis, pyarthrosis, or epiglottitis, suggest *H. influenzae,* but the diagnosis depends on bacteriologic studies.

PNEUMONIA *H. influenzae* may cause either a broncho- or lobar pneumonia. Approximately one-half of the children with lobar pneumonia have an associated empyema. The pneumonic disease may spread to produce a purulent pericarditis. Lobar disease, particularly with pleural involvement, is most often confused with pneumococcal or *S. aureus* pneumonia, but the course can be prolonged enough to suggest tuberculosis. Elderly patients, particularly those with primary lung disease and/or alcoholism, are being infected increasingly by *H. influenzae.*

BACTEREMIA WITHOUT LOCAL DISEASE Children, particularly those 6 to 24 months of age, may develop bacteremia without evidence of local disease. This condition most often occurs in those with a temperature greater than 102°F and an elevated circulating neutrophil count. Persons with sickle cell disease, previous splenectomy, or chemotherapy for Hodgkin's disease are at increased risk of bacteremia without local disease. Although pneumococci are the most common cause of this syndrome, *H. influenzae* b is the second most common etiologic agent. Fever, chills, anxiety, anorexia, and lethargy dominate the clinical state. Among highly susceptible persons, this disease can progress to shock and death within a few hours.

CELLULITIS *H. influenzae* causes a cellulitis, particularly among children 6 to 24 months of age, which is characterized as a raised, warm, tender area of distinctive reddish-blue hue, usually located on one cheek or, less commonly, the periorbital area. The child is moderately febrile and toxic and has a history of preceding rhinorrhea, fever, and, at times, ipsilateral otitis media. The cellulitis develops and spreads within a few hours. *H. influenzae* cellulitis on the limbs or hands is seen rarely and usually in older children. The distinctive color, location, and clinical course suggest the etiology. A significant percentage of the involved infants develop sepsis and metastatic disease, such as meningitis.

EPIGLOTTITIS *H. influenzae* b is the leading cause of this potentially lethal, septic disease which has a dramatically rapid course. Pre-school-aged children, most often boys, are primarily affected. Acute onset of high fever, dysphagia, and an aura of not feeling well is followed by puddling of oropharyngeal secretions and tachypnea with inspiratory retractions. Increasing airway obstruction is accompanied by increasing hypoxia and anxiety. Over one-half of these patients require hospitalization and airway intubation. The diagnostic examination can provoke further edema of the markedly swollen, inflamed epiglottis and should therefore be conducted only in a locale in which an airway can be inserted.

PYARTHROSIS *H. influenzae* b joint disease occurs during a septic invasion with or without other systemic disease usually in children under 2 years of age. Single, large, weight-bearing joints are usually involved without concomitant osteomyelitis. Response to systemic antibiotics without surgical drainage is dramatic and curative, but long-term follow-up reveals some joint dysfunction in a significant percentage of children.

PERICARDITIS *H. influenzae* b causes purulent pericarditis usually associated with pneumonia. The clinical signs and symptoms are generally similar to those caused by other pyogenic bacteria, but the course is often more prolonged.

OTHER RESPIRATORY TRACT DISEASE *H. influenzae* is the second leading cause of childhood otitis media and often causes sinusitis. Nearly all the etiologic strains are nonencapsulated. These diseases cannot be distinguished clinically from those produced by other microbial agents, nor can the disease caused by encapsulated or nonencapsulated *H. influenzae* be differentiated clinically. Fever, local pain, irritability, and, in sinusitis, foul breath, postnasal drip, and cough predominate. Chronic bronchitis, particularly among adults and those with agammaglobulinemia, is often caused by nonencapsulated *H. influenzae* or mixed bacterial species among which *H. influenzae* predominates. Cough productive of purulent sputum, anorexia, and dyspnea with prolonged expiration dominate this process which is aggravated by smoking and by inhalation of respiratory pollutants.

OTHER DISEASES *H. influenzae* can cause endocarditis and brain abscess, but such cases are rare and are usually associated with a primary underlying disease. *H. influenzae* endophthalmitis, renal disease, and osteomyelitis have been reported. Pharyngitis is only rarely caused by *H. influenzae,* and this organism plays no role in bronchiolitis.

Diagnosis The etiology of many *H. influenzae* diseases, i.e., pyarthrosis in a child under 2 years, facial cellulitis, and epiglottitis, can generally be suspected on the basis of the history and clinical findings. Chemical analysis of infected fluids is consistent with any pyogenic etiology. Leukocytosis is common, and children often have a significant anemia. Gram stains of infected body fluids correlate with culture results in 70 percent of cases. Among the remainder of culture-positive specimens, 15 percent have negative smears, while another 15 percent have misinterpreted smears. Staining such specimens with methylene blue generally does not improve these results. Quellung reactions usually are even less accurate.

PRP can be detected in the serum, CSF, or concentrated urine of up to 90 percent of patients with meningitis by countercurrent electrophoresis. Despite the apparent widespread distribution of immunologically cross-reactive antigens among bacteria in nature, false-positive reactions of this type are unusual. PRP is generally detected in infected pericardial fluid or joint fluid but is found infrequently in the serum of children with epiglottitis, presumably owing to the fulminant course of this disease and the time required for antigen release from invasive bacteria. Detection of antigen in the supernatent of liquid cultures can expedite laboratory diagnosis. Since antigen often persists after antibiotic therapy, its detection is helpful in the diagnosis of patients with systemic *H. influenzae* diseases who have received prior antibiotics.

Positive nasopharyngeal cultures are not meaningful because of the high carriage rate of *H. influenzae* by healthy individuals. Needle aspiration of the edge of the site of cellulitis or of diseased lung markedly increases the rate of bacterial isolation and is recommended, particularly in patients who are critically ill or have a complicated course. Cultures of empyema, pericardial, and joint fluid and an inflamed epiglottis are diagnostic. Blood cultures are positive in up to 80 percent of patients with *H. influenzae* septic arthritis, facial cellulitis, epiglottitis, and meningitis prior to the onset of antibiotic therapy. Even if antibiotic therapy has been initiated, the yield is sufficiently great to recommend that blood cultures be taken. It has been suggested that *H. influenzae* pneumonia, in which 30 percent of persons have a positive blood culture, is underdiagnosed. The role of PRP detection in this diagnosis deserves further evaluation.

Treatment Without treatment, systemic *H. influenzae* disease, particularly meningitis and epiglottitis, has a very high, if not uniform, mortality. Chloramphenicol therapy yields very high concentrations of antibiotic in joint and cerebrospinal fluid relative to serum and produces excellent clinical results. The potential toxicity of chloramphenicol and the excellent results obtained with ampicillin have made this agent the antibiotic of choice for *H. influenzae* diseases. The current prevalence of ampicillin-resistant strains requires that all systemic diseases that might be due to *H. influenzae* should be treated with chloramphenicol, 100 mg/kg per day for children, 4 g per day for adults, given intravenously at 6-h intervals until the etiologic agent is proved to be sensitive to ampicillin. Some, including the American Academy of Pediatrics, recommend that ampicillin also be added to the initial chloramphenicol therapy. If the etiologic strain is sensitive, ampicillin is given intravenously in doses of 200 to 400 mg/kg per day for children and 6 g per day for adults, divided into six infusions given at 4-h intervals.

Chloramphenicol given orally yields higher serum levels of the antibiotic than identical doses given intravenously; administration of chloramphenicol by intramuscular injection yields variable and unpredictable blood levels and is contraindicated. Experience with third-generation penicillins and cephalosporins for systemic *H. influenzae* disease is just beginning to accumulate.

Amoxicillin is recommended for ambulatory therapy of ampicillin-sensitive *H. influenzae* diseases. Tetracycline can be used to treat bronchitis and other respiratory diseases caused by sensitive strains. Cefamandole appears promising for both ampicillin-sensitive and -resistant *H. influenzae* diseases. Trimethoprim-sulfa therapy has been approved for *H. influenzae* upper respiratory tract disease, and on the basis of a good deal of experience in Europe it is also effective in chronic bronchitis.

The duration of chemotherapy for *H. influenzae* disease depends on the disease and the status of the individual patient. All systemic diseases should be treated with intravenous drugs at least until cultures of the infected area are sterile and the patient is afebrile and without clinical and laboratory evidence of active infection for 3 to 5 days. Patients with meningitis are therefore usually treated for 10 to 14 days. Occasionally, ampicillin does not clear the bacteria from the CSF, and relapses follow the cessation of therapy. Most therapeutic failures with ampicillin have been associated with antibiotic courses that are too brief, employ too low a dose, or are given by a route other than intravenously; some result from loculated disease that was not completely eradicated with standard treatment. In treatment failures, re-treatment according to the above guidelines should be undertaken, usually with chloramphenicol.

Patients with endocarditis or pericarditis should receive 3 to 6 weeks of intravenous therapy. Ampicillin and chloramphenicol diffuse well into inflamed joint spaces, and there is no indication for local instillation of antibiotics. Children with otitis media may be treated orally with amoxicillin in dosage of 50 mg/kg per day (adults 2 g per day in four divided doses) until their symptoms are alleviated plus 3 to 4 days; hence, the usually total course is 7 to 10 days. Sinusitis requires therapy of 3 or more weeks; therapy of bronchitis may need to be prolonged even longer.

Only a few *H. influenzae* isolates resistant to chloramphenicol have been recovered in the United States, but their isolation in European centers strongly suggests the need to test invasive strains routinely, particularly when the results of chloramphenicol therapy appear to be less than expected.

Antibiotic therapy is only one facet of the management of the patient with a systemic *H. influenzae* disease. Careful evaluation of the airway, consideration of oxygen therapy and transfusion, vigorous treatment of shock and disseminated intravascular coagulation, conservative fluid replacement, anticonvulsant therapy, and medical management of cerebral edema are often critical. Repeated aspirations of an infected joint or empyema may be needed, but installation of a surgical drain is rarely required. The creation of a pericardial "window" and drainage in patients with pericarditis are preferable to repeated aspirations and are often essential for cure.

Prevention Although secondary cases of invasive *H. influenzae* diseases occur at significantly increased rates among young, intimate contacts of primary cases, no uniformly successful antibiotic prophylaxis exists. Rifampin, in doses of 20 mg/kg given once daily for 4 days, has reduced, but not eliminated, the incidence of such secondary cases. Different regimens of rifampin prophylaxis are much less effective, while other antibiotics are not effective at all. The increased attack rate and the constant mortality (5 to 10 percent) and neurologic morbidity (30 percent) during the past two decades for *H. influenzae* meningitis in children and the prevalence of ampicillin-resistant strains have stimulated an attempt to produce a vaccine to prevent *H. influenzae* diseases. Because of the primacy of the type b capsule in pathogenicity and the efficacy of anticapsular serum, attention was focused initially on a vaccine composed of purified capsular PRP. Such a vaccine has been found to be nontoxic and immunogenic for older children and adults. A single dose protects children older than 18 months from septic diseases for at lease 4 years; however, the vaccine is not immunogenic or protective for younger children. New approaches to develop an effective agent for younger children have therefore been initiated.

Oral ingestion of nonpathogenic species of *Escherichia coli* which have an immunologically cross-reactive capsule may elevate systemic anti-PRP antibody activity. However, the observation in one center of an unusually high incidence of intestinal carriage of such *E. coli* among children with *H. influenzae* b meningitis has precluded further studies. A systemically administered vaccine composed of a native outer membrane protein-PRP complex raises protective antibodies directed against PRP in adults and in children 2 years or older. These antibodies can be boosted by further injections of this vaccine; its immunogenicity for infants is under study. These results suggest that antibodies to PRP can be stimulated provided the polysaccharide has a protein "carrier." Current research is therefore directed to the potential of vaccines in which the polysaccharide antigen is covalently linked to a protein inherently useful as a vaccine, e.g., tetanus toxoid. Other studies are evaluating the role of *H. influenzae* outer membrane proteins as vaccine candidates either as a primary agent or a polysaccharide carrier, with the hope that such a vaccine might be protective against diseases caused by nonencapsulated as well as encapsulated *H. influenzae.*

HEMOPHILUS AEGYPTICUS *H. aegypticus,* also known as the Koch-Weeks bacillus, causes conjunctivitis in humans. Morphologically and biochemically, this organism closely resembles an unencapsulated *H. influenzae.* Moreover, *H. aegypticus* and *H. influenzae* share certain antigens and can be transformed by DNA of the other species.

The conjunctivitis, which primarily affects children, occurs worldwide, often in epidemics, and in some areas seasonally. It must be distinguished from trachoma-inclusion conjunctivitis (TRIC) agents, adenoviruses, and other bacterial agents such as pneumococcus, *S. aureus,* and *N. gonorrhoeae.* Therapy consists of local instillation of antibiotic drops or ointment, such as sulfonamide, polymyxin B, or gentamicin five or six times daily, and moist soaks to keep the eyelids clean.

HEMOPHILUS APHROPHILUS *H. aphrophilus* is an uncommon cause of bacteremia, bacterial endocarditis, acute and chronic sinusitis, pneumonia, and deep tissue abscesses. This organism requires X but not V factor and extra CO_2 for aerobic growth; it grows anaerobically without X factor. Most strains are sensitive to most antibiotics including penicillin, the cephalosporins, aminoglycosides, and chloramphenicol.

HEMOPHILUS DUCREYI *H. ducreyi* causes the localized venereal disease, chancroid (see Chap. 157). The organism requires X but not V factor for growth. In clinical specimens and colonies grown on solid medium, the organism appears as small ovoid rods arranged in pairs, groups, or parallel chains. The disease is characterized by painful, nonindurated ulceration of the genitalia with enlarged, and often suppurative, regional lymph nodes. Chancroid must be distinguished from primary syphilis; not infrequently the two diseases occur simultaneously. Tetracycline or erythromycin therapy cures chancroid.

HEMOPHILUS PARAINFLUENZAE This species differs from *H. influenzae* by requiring V but not X factor for growth. Since *H. influenzae* does not require X factor for anaerobic growth, diagnostic confusion can arise, especially in stabbed cultures. This phenomenon may have played a role in certain systemic infections allegedly caused by *H. parainfluenzae* which, on further testing, were found to be due to *H. influenzae.*

Acute upper respiratory disease, e.g., otitis media, and less commonly meningitis, pneumonia, endocarditis, and brain abscess have been ascribed to *H. parainfluenzae.* A small but significant percentage of *H. parainfluenzae* carries plasmids mediating β-lactamase production and ampicillin resistance.

HEMOPHILUS VAGINALIS *H. vaginalis* (sometimes called *Corynebacterium vaginale*) appears to cause vaginitis and less commonly septic abortion and puerperal fever and asymptomatic urethral infection in men (see Chap. 143). The growth requirements are not precisely defined but include factor V and probably X; incubation in increased CO_2 is important.

Although *H. vaginalis* can be recovered from asymptomatic persons, it has a clear causal etiology to vaginitis; synergy between *H. vaginalis* and anaerobic vaginal flora may exist. The clinical diagnosis is suggested by the presence of "clue" cells—vaginal epithelial cells to which multiple gram-negative bacilli are attached—in a vaginal discharge with a pH of 5.0 which releases an amine-like odor upon alkalinization. *H. vaginalis* is not eradicated by oral tetracycline or ampicillin or by sulfonamide vaginal cream, but oral metronidazole is effective.

HEMOPHILUS PERTUSSIS This bacterium causes an acute bronchitis, primarily in infants and young children, that is characterized by a repetitious, paroxysmal cough and prolonged, inspiratory stridor, "whooping cough."

Etiology *H. Pertussis* is a minute, aerobic nonmotile, nonspore-forming gram-negative coccobacillus that grows slowly even under optimal conditions and is inhibited by many factors present in routine bacteriologic media. The classic medium used for primary culture of *H. pertussis,* Bordet-Gengou, contains blood and starch. The absence of an antigenic relation and with it the ability to transform *H. pertussis* with *H. influenzae* DNA or vice versa suggests that these species are not closely related. *H. pertussis* is closely related, however, to *H. parapertussis,* which can cause a milder, similar disease in humans, and *H. bronchiseptica,* which causes respiratory disease in animals but rarely in humans.

Freshly isolated *H. pertussis* is in phase I, the virulent, morphologically uniform, encapsulated, and piliated form, which also produces several biologically active substances. These include lipopolysaccharide (endotoxin); a heat-labile dermonecrotoxin; a factor that sensitizes animals to histamine and serotonin; a hemagglutinin; and six serologically distinct agglutinogens (K antigens—at least two are present in each isolate). The pili appear to contain the lymphocytosis-promoting activity which is typical of *H. pertussis.* However, neither the capsular substance(s) nor the agglutinogens have been isolated or characterized. With passage in the laboratory, a smooth to rough transition occurs, yielding phase IV cells that are pleomorphic, nonencapsulated, and avirulent. Only phase I *H. pertussis* bacilli are suitable for the preparation of vaccines.

Epidemiology *H. pertussis* exists worldwide and naturally affects only humans, although nonhuman primates and mice can be experimentally infected. Pertussis is one of the most contagious infectious diseases because it is transmitted by aerosolized droplets. (The infectivity of respiratory secretions and contact transmission is not well studied.) Up to 90 percent of exposed, susceptible persons develop the disease. Asymptomatic infection is rare. Although pertussis occurs endemically, it produces epidemics in a susceptible population. The incidence is greatest in the fall in temperate climates.

More than 50 percent of *H. pertussis* disease occurs in infants, presumably owing to deficient maternal immunity and possibly the lack of transplacental transfer of a protective bacteriologic antibody. Although adults were thought to be resistant to pertussis, neither the disease nor active immunization provides lifelong immunity; in fact, pertussis is not an uncommon cause of bronchitis in adults. Hospital personnel also are at increased risk, as evidenced by reports of epidemics involving hospital staff and patients.

About 3000 cases of pertussis are officially reported each year in the United States, but most observers think this number is falsely low because of the difficulty in bacteriologic confirmation. Pertussis remains a very significant health problem in developing countries, particularly in areas of poor nutrition and immunization. The limitation in the rate of immunization to pertussis in Great Britain to 30 percent of children has been accompanied by an epidemic affecting as many persons as in the prevaccine era. Certain adenoviruses can cause a clinical picture identical to that of pertussis, but there can be little doubt that *H. pertussis* is a primary pathogen.

Pathogenesis Inhaled *H. pertussis* attaches to the respiratory epithelium by a pilus; the organisms multiply on the surface of the airway lumen but do not invade the lung or the bloodstream. Acute inflammation results: epithelial cell ciliary action is inhibited and mucous secretions are stimulated. The subsequent necrosis results in patchy ulceration of respiratory epithelium. The bronchi and bronchioles are primarily affected; the trachea, larynx, and nasopharynx may be involved, but less severely. The mucopurulent exudate can compromise the diminutive airway of the infant or small child. Focal atelectasis and emphysema and peribronchial infiltration by inflammatory cells, particularly lymphocytes, are common, but the alveoli are spared in uncomplicated disease. Whatever neurologic symptoms result from the primary action of a bacterial neurotoxin or secondary hypoxia remain undefined.

Clinical manifestations Following an incubation period of 7 to 10 days, sneezing, mild fever, rhinorrhea, anorexia, and a mild cough become evident (catarrhal period) and last 1 to 2 weeks, after which the cough increases in frequency and intensity. Paroxysms of cough are followed, particularly in infants, by a prolonged, often distressing, inspiratory gasp (the whoop). The cough occurs at variable intervals, often every few minutes, for 2 to 3 weeks (paroxysmal period). The disease is much more severe in the infant. The cough inhibits oral intake, and swallowed mucus may provoke vomiting, resulting in significant dehydration and weight loss. The cough can provoke venous congestion with hemoptysis, epistaxis, and small blood vessel hemorrhage. Hypoxia is more common and severe than is usually appreciated clinically. Apprehension is significant among infants; convulsions and subsequent cerebral dysfunction occur rarely. Adults and older children are less ill and have symptoms of a severe, prolonged bronchitis. The paroxysmal period is followed by a recovery period that lasts 1 to 6 weeks, during which the cough decreases in frequency and intensity. Spasms can be provoked during recovery, however, particularly by smoke or irritating inhalants.

Mortality is now less than 5 percent among children hospitalized in the United States, but it is significant in developing countries. Up to 90 percent of deaths occur in children under 1 year of age, up to 70 percent in those of 6 months or younger. Death results primarily from dehydration and electrolyte imbalance, cerebral anoxia or hemorrhage, or secondary bacterial pneumonia. Among survivors, transient atelectasis is frequent, but bronchiectasis, reported commonly a few decades ago, is now uncommon. Permanent cerebral dysfunction is also unusual among children that are treated optimally.

Diagnosis The clinical diagnosis is suggested by a history of contact, the classic cough, and a marked absolute lymphocytosis. The diagnosis depends on the identification of *H. pertussis* in respiratory secretions. Success of isolation is favored by the immediate culture of a deep nasopharyngeal (NP) specimen in a freshly prepared selective medium. Because the characteristic pearl-like colonies cannot be appreciated for 4 to 6 days, inhibitors of normal NP flora, e.g., methicillin, are added to the medium to prevent overgrowth of *H. pertussis.* The recovery rate on "cough plates" is too low to recommend this technique. *H. pertussis* can be isolated from as many as 90 percent of patients during the catarrhal stage of the disease but from no greater than 50 percent during the paroxysmal stage. Fluorescent-labeled antibody can detect *H. pertussis* in NP smears, but false-positive results may be obtained with up to 40 percent of specimens and false-negative tests in 10 to 20 percent. Serologic studies are of little value. Blood cultures are sterile and are not recommended; chest x-rays may show peribronchial thickening but are not diagnostic. Dual infection with adenoviruses occurs, and positive viral cultures do not exclude *H. pertussis* as an etiologic agent.

Pertussis may be distinguished from viral, mycoplasmal, and other bacterial causes of tracheobronchitis by a history of contact, the character and duration of symptoms, and the laboratory findings. The results of cultures are definitive.

Spasmodic coughing may also be associated with bronchiolitis; bacterial, mycoplasmal, and viral pneumonia; tuberculosis; cystic fibrosis; foreign bodies; and disease causing airway compression such as malignancy or chronic obstructive pulmonary disease. These diseases can be distinguished by their clinical and laboratory findings and by the course of the illness.

Treatment General supportive care is critical: careful nursing, avoidance of stimuli that provoke paroxysms, oxygen, suctioning of respiratory secretions, and attention to caloric needs and fluid and electrolyte balance. A single controlled study reporting beneficial effects of steroids deserves attention for severely ill infants.

H. pertussis is sensitive to many antibiotics in vitro. Antibiotics can eliminate infection and, if given in the catarrhal phase, prevent disease. Since the pathologic process has been developed by the time paroxysms occur, antibiotic therapy given thereafter does not affect the clinical course. Erythromycin is preferred and should be used to prevent interpersonal transmission. Tetracycline and chloramphenicol are nearly as effective but are not recommended because of potential toxicity, particularly for infants. Ampicillin appears to be relatively ineffective in eradicating nasopharyngeal infection. Hyperimmune, antibacterial rabbit serum has no effect on bacterial shedding or clinical manifestations and is not recommended.

Prevention Patients suspected of having pertussis should be isolated until the diagnosis is disproved or the infection is eradicated by antibiotics. Exposed susceptibles should be vaccinated to prevent disease (see below) and treated with erythromycin to prevent infection and retransmission.

Prior to the availability of a vaccine, pertussis caused as many deaths in the United States as all other contagious diseases of children *combined!* In order to prevent the disease, a vaccine composed of a chemical extract of bacterial cells was developed. Because of the risk of pertussis to infants, the proposal was made to start immunization as early in life as possible. Unfortunately, pertussis immunization at 7 days of age produced a limited antibody response in only a small percentage of infants and resulted in reduced booster responses at 1 year. This vaccine is now mixed with diphtheria and tetanus toxoids, for convenience and because pertussis enhances the antibody responses to the toxoids, and is given five times during the first 6 years of life, with three doses being given at 2-month intervals starting at 8 weeks of age.

Although the vaccine was 70 to 80 percent effective in preventing disease among intimately exposed children, its effectiveness and toxicity have been questioned. Completely immunized children may develop pertussis, although the disease is milder than among the unimmunized. Furthermore, the protection provided by the vaccine is transient, with minimal resistance being evident a decade or later following the last immunization. Indeed, improved housing, hygiene, and nutrition are cited by some as responsible for the dramatic decline in pertussis during the past several decades. However, available data indicate that the rate of decline in the attack rate of pertussis in the United States has been positively affected by the vaccine. The association of an epidemic of pertussis in Great Britain with a decline in pertussis immunization also strongly supports the efficacy of the vaccine.

Pertussis vaccine provokes local reactions in up to 50 percent of recipients; neurologic complications, including uncontrollable screaming fits, convulsions, and encephalopathy, are a rare but real risk. However, the efficacy of the vaccine far outweighs the risk of significant neurologic complications. Convulsions, alteration of consciousness, shock, screaming, focal neurologic signs, and thrombocytopenic purpura following pertussis vaccination are contraindications to further doses. Because toxic reactions are more common in older persons, the vaccine is rarely given to those over 6 years of age. However, older persons with chronic pulmonary disease and exposed hospital personnel may be candidates for an absorbed pertussis vaccine (0.1 to 0.25 ml).

REFERENCES

Hemophilus aphrophilus

ELSTER SK et al: *Hemophilus aphrophilus* endocarditis: A review of 23 cases. Am J Cardiol 35:72, 1975

SUTTER VL, FINEGOLD SM: *Hemophilus aphrophilus* infections: Clinical and bacteriologic studies. Ann NY Acad Sci 174:468, 1970

Hemophilus influenzae

ALEXANDER HE: Treatment of type B *Hemophilus influenzae* meningitis. J Pediatr 25:517, 1975

BRADSHAW MW et al: Bacterial antigens cross-reactive with the capsular polysaccharide of *Hemophilus influenzae* b. Lancet 1:1095, 1971

LEVIN DC et al: Bacteremic *Hemophilus influenzae* pneumonia in adults: Report of 24 cases and review of the literature. AM J Med 62:219, 1977

LOEB MR, SMITH DH: Outer membrane protein composition in disease isolates of *Haemophilus influenzae:* Pathogenic and epidemiological implications. Infect Immun 30:709, 1980

PELTDA H et al: *Haemophilus influenzae* type b capsular polysaccharide vaccine in children: A double-blind field study of 100,000 vaccines 3 months to 5 years of age in Finland. Pediatrics 60:730, 1977

ROBBINS JB et al: *Haemophilus influenzae* type b: Disease and immunity in humans. Ann Intern Med 78:259, 1973

SMITH DH et al: Responses of children immunized with the capsular polysaccharide of *Hemophilus influenzae* type B. Pediatrics 52:637, 1973

TODD JK, BRUHN FW: Severe *Haemophilus influenzae* infections. Am J Dis Child 129:607, 1975

VANKLINGEREN B et al: Plasmid-mediated chloramphenicol resistance in *Haemophilus influenzae.* Antimicrob Agents Chemother 11:383, 1977

Hemophilus parinfluenzae

CHUNN CJ et al: *Haemophilus parainfluenzae* infective endocarditis. Medicine 56:99, 1977

HABLE KA et al: Three *Hemophilus* species. Am J Dis Child 121:35, 1971

Hemophilus vaginalis

See Chap. 143.

Hemophilus pertussis

BRADFORD WL, SLAVIN B: Nasopharyngeal cultures in pertussis. Proc Soc Exp Biol Med 43:590, 1940

BYERS RK, MOLL FC: Encephalopathies following prophylactic pertussis vaccine. Pediatrics 1:437, 1948

DONALDSON P, WHITACKER J: Diagnoses of pertussis by fluorescent antibody staining of nasopharyngeal smears. Am J Dis Child 99:423, 1960

KOPLAN JW et al: Pertussis vaccine—An analysis of benefits, risks and costs. N Engl J Med 301:906, 1979

KURT TL et al: Spread of pertussis by hospital staff. JAMA 221:264, 1972

MEDICAL RESEARCH COUNCIL INVESTIGATION: The prevention of whooping cough by vaccination. Br Med J i:1463, 1951

NELSON JD: The changing epidemiology of pertussis in young infants: The role of adults as reservoirs of infection. Am J Dis Child 132:371, 1978

Pertussis Surveillance, 1979–1981. Morb Mort Week Rep 31:333, 1982

157 CHANCROID

KING K. HOLMES
ALLAN R. RONALD

DEFINITION Chancroid, or soft chancre (ulcer molle), is an acute sexually transmitted infection characterized by painful genital ulcerations often associated with inflammatory inguinal adenopathy which may progress to suppuration. The diagnosis is established by exclusion of syphilis, genital herpes, and other specific causes of genital ulceration together with isolation of *Hemophilus ducreyi* from the lesion or a suppurative node.

ETIOLOGY The isolation of *H. ducreyi* in mixed cultures from ulcers and rarely in pure cultures from buboes proves the microbial etiology of chancroid. Gram-positive cocci and anaerobic gram-negative rods are often also present, and occasionally spirochetes are seen as well. However, there is no evidence that these organisms play any role as independent pathogens or require specific therapy. In areas where chancroid is common, *H. ducreyi* can be isolated from up to 80 percent of ulcers that clinically appear to be chancroid. The organism is a gram-negative facultative aerobe which requires hemin (X factor) for growth. Some strains also require serum. However, nicotinamide adenine dinucleotide (V factor) is not required. Although no unique biochemical or immunologic characteristics have been demonstrated, the colonial morphology of *H. ducreyi* is unusual in that the yellow-gray colonies can be moved intact across the agar surface. Some strains demonstrate a typical streptobacillary "chaining" appearance on Gram stain, but this feature is too variable and subjective to use as a taxonomic criterion.

EPIDEMIOLOGY The incidence of chancroid is unknown, owing to inaccurate clinical diagnosis and incomplete reporting. It is common in southeast Asia, Africa, and Central America and is probably more prevalent than syphilis in many countries. Less than 1000 cases are reported annually in the United States. However, localized outbreaks of disease do occur (for example, hundreds of cases involving predominantly migrant workers occurred in southern California in 1981 and 1982), and isolates of *H. ducreyi* from sex partners appear identical when restriction enzyme digests of plasmids are compared. The sex ratio of reported cases in the United States is five males to one female. Uncircumcised males are more susceptible to the disease. Prostitution plays a major role in transmission, and among merchant seamen and military troops whose sexual contacts are prostitutes, chancroid is more common than syphilis. The extent of the organism's reservoir and the role of carriers in disease transmission are uncertain.

Many isolates of *H. ducreyi* possess plasmids which have been found to mediate antimicrobial resistance to sulfonamides, tetracycline, chloramphenicol, and/or ampicillin.

CLINICAL MANIFESTATIONS After an incubation period of 3 to 5 days, a small inflammatory papule appears which ulcerates within 2 to 3 days. The classic chancroidal ulcer (Fig. 157-1) is superficial, ranging in size from a few millimeters to several centimeters in diameter. The edge is ragged and undermined. The ulcer base is covered by a necrotic exudate. The ulcers are often multiple and may merge to form giant or serpiginous ulcers. Occasionally, the lesions remain pustular and resemble folliculitis or pyogenic infection. In contrast to syphilis, the chancroidal ulcer in males is painful and not indurated. The most frequent areas of localization are the preputial orifice, the internal surface of the prepuce, and the frenulum in men, and the labia, fourchette, and perianal region in women. The le-

FIGURE 157-1
The classic chancroid.

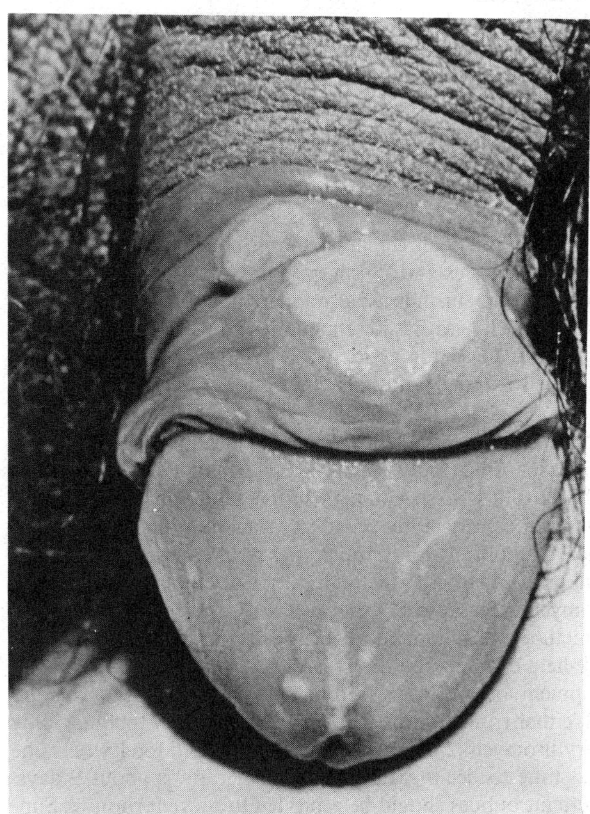

sions in females tend to be more superficial and less painful. Extragenital ulcers are rare.

Acute, painful, tender inflammatory inguinal adenopathy occurs in almost 50 percent of patients and is frequently unilateral. If the patient is untreated, the involved nodes become matted, forming a unilocular suppurative bubo. The overlying skin becomes erythematous and tense and finally ruptures, forming a deep single ulcer.

Diagnosis The morphological diagnosis of genital lesions is fraught with error, and many lesions diagnosed as chancroid in clinical practice may actually be genital herpes, syphilis, or traumatic lesions. In the United States, one study of 100 consecutive men with penile ulceration disclosed genital herpes in 22, syphilis in 17, and traumatic lesions in 8. Classic chancroidal ulcers were noted in 12, only 2 of whom had ulcers that yielded *H. ducreyi* in culture. Most of the remaining ulcers were of uncertain etiology. In contrast, in Kenya, of 97 consecutive men with penile ulceration, 60 were infected with *H. ducreyi,* 11 had syphilis, and only 4 had genital herpes. In a recent U.S. study, a series of patients with suspected granuloma inguinale (donovanosis) were found to have positive cultures from ulcers for *H. ducreyi,* through use of newer microbiologic techniques. These lesions have been termed *pseudogranuloma inguinale chancroid.*

Primary genital infection with herpes simplex virus produces tender inguinal adenopathy in about 50 percent of cases, but primary genital herpes can often be distinguished by the history of onset with vesicular lesions or of recent exposure to herpes. Also, primary genital herpes often produces dysuria, together with systemic symptoms such as fever and myalgia. Chancroid rarely causes systemic symptoms.

The chancre of primary syphilis is indurated, and the associated adenopathy is bilateral, nontender, and nonsuppurative. However, all patients with genital ulcers should have at least two dark-field examinations performed on separate days, together with monthly serologic tests for syphilis for 3 months, to exclude syphilis.

Lymphogranuloma venereum (LGV) differs from chancroid in that the adenopathy develops after the ulcer is healed. It is indolent, often bilateral and nontender, and develops multilocular suppuration and fistulas. LGV can be further excluded by a negative serology and negative *Chlamydia* culture from the lymph node.

The diagnosis of chancroid is confirmed by the isolation of *H. ducreyi* from the ulcer or, less commonly, from the bubo. Exudate should be directly plated onto chocolate agar enriched with 1% Isovitalex and 5% sheep serum, plus 3 μg/ml of vancomycin. The organism is usually apparent within 48 h of incubation in 5% CO_2 with 100% humidity. However, plates should not be discarded for at least 5 days. No serologic tests are available for the diagnosis of chancroid.

TREATMENT Untreated chancroidal ulcers persist for long periods of time and often progress. Small lesions may heal within 2 to 4 weeks. Although sulfonamides and tetracyclines have been considered effective for chancroid, the recent emergence of multiresistant strains has resulted in many failures with both agents. Trimethoprim/sulfamethoxazole and erythromycin are presently the agents of choice for chancroid. Trimethoprim/sulfamethoxazole will not interfere with the dark-field examination for *Treponema pallidum* or with the development of a positive serologic test for syphilis. Therapy with either trimethoprim/sulfamethoxazole 320/1600 mg daily or erythromycin 2 g daily should be continued for 1 week. The usual time to healing after onset of therapy is about 9 days. Fluctuant buboes should be aspirated to prevent rupture. Suppuration may progress despite otherwise effective therapy. Buboes larger than 5 cm in diameter almost always require aspiration.

Sexual contacts of patients with chancroid should be examined for ulcers. Although the epidemiology of chancroid suggests that effective control measures, specifically designed for limited target populations such as prostitutes and known sexual contacts, could halt the spread of this disease, further prospective epidemiologic studies to demonstrate this are required.

REFERENCES

BRUNTON JL et al: Plasmid mediated ampicillin resistance in *Haemophilus ducreyi.* Antimicrob Agents Chemother 15:294, 1979

CHAPEL T et al: How reliable is the morphologic diagnosis of penile ulcers? Sex Trans Dis 4:150, 1977

——— et al: The microbiological flora of penile ulcerations. J Infect Dis 137:50, 1978

HAMMOND GW et al: Antimicrobial susceptibility of *Haemophilus ducreyi.* Antimicrob Agents Chemother 13:608, 1978

——— et al: Comparison of specimen collection and laboratory techniques for isolation of *Haemophilus ducreyi.* J Clin Microbiol 7:39, 1978

——— et al: Determination of the hemin requirement of *Haemophilus ducreyi:* Evaluation of the porphyrin test and media used in the satellite growth test. J Clin Microbiol 7:243, 1978

——— et al: Epidemiologic, clinical, laboratory and therapeutic features of an urban outbreak of chancroid in North America. Rev Infect Dis 2:867, 1980

HANDSFIELD HH et al: Molecular epidemiology of *Haemophilus ducreyi* infection. Ann Intern Med 95:315, 1981

KRAUS SJ et al: Pseudogranuloma inguinale caused by *Haemophilus ducreyi.* Arch Dermatol 118:494, 1982

NSANZE H et al: Genital ulcers in Kenya: A clinical and laboratory study of 97 patients. Br J Vener Dis 57:378, 1981

Sexually transmitted diseases treatment guidelines, 1982. Morb Mort Week Rep 31:25, 1982

TOTTEN PA et al: Characterization of ampicillin-resistance plasmids from *Haemophilus ducreyi.* Antimicrob Agents Chemother 21:662, 1982

158 BRUCELLOSIS

THOMAS M. BUCHANAN
ROBERT G. PETERSDORF

DEFINITION Brucellosis is an infection caused by microorganisms of the genus *Brucella,* which are usually transmitted to humans from lower animals. The illness is characterized by fever, sweats, weakness, malaise, and weight loss, often without localized findings.

ETIOLOGY Human brucellosis is an infection caused by one of three species: *B. melitensis* (goats), *B. suis* (hogs), and *B. abortus* (cattle). *B. canis* (dogs) has caused infections in a few humans, but its incidence may be increasing. Although infections are usually confined to the major animal host, infections of swine with *B. abortus* or of cattle with *B. suis* may occur, and *Brucella* infection has been reported in deer, moose, caribou, horses, cats, and chickens. The species of *Brucella* are separated from one another by biochemical and serological reactions. The organisms are small, nonmotile, non-spore forming, gram-negative rods, which grow best at 37°C in trypticase soy broth or tryptophosphate broth with a pH of 6.6. to 6.8 under increased CO_2 tension.

EPIDEMIOLOGY A natural reservoir of brucellosis is in domestic animals, particularly cattle, swine, goats, and sheep. Animal-to-animal transmission is usually venereal or by ingestion of infected tissue or milk. Human infection most commonly results from ingestion of infected animal tissues or milk products, or directly through the skin.

On the average, approximately 200 cases of brucellosis are reported in the United States every year. On a worldwide basis, the prevalence of the disease correlates closely with the extent of animal brucellosis in a given country. Brucellosis has nearly been eradicated in Scandinavia and Germany, where the incidence of animal brucellosis is also very low. In the United States, areas in which cattle-raising is an important industry generally have a higher incidence of brucellosis.

Brucellosis most frequently occurs in individuals who are exposed to *Brucella*-infected tissues and milk or milk products, including slaughterhouse workers, livestock producers, veterinarians, and individuals who ingest unpasteurized milk products. In most of the instances in which brucellosis has been acquired from unpasteurized dairy products, these products were purchased in other countries, particularly in Mexico and Italy. In the United States, better than half of the reported cases occurred in slaughterhouse workers. Fortunately, isolation of *Brucella* from infected meat decreases following refrigeration, but the high rates of accidental cuts and exposure to blood and lymph of freshly killed animals make abattoir workers particularly susceptible to this infection. In Alaska, a number of cases have been transmitted via raw meat from caribou and moose.

Approximately 2 to 3 percent of cases acquired in this country occur in laboratories, often in veterinarians who are accidentally inoculated with live vaccine.

PATHOGENESIS AND PATHOLOGY *Brucella* invade the body through the skin and, less commonly, through the oropharynx, conjunctivae, or respiratory passages. In the submucosa they interact with polymorphonuclear leukocytes (PMN) and tissue macrophages. Many organisms are phagocytized, but if the inoculum is sufficiently large, they spread via the lymphatics to the regional lymph nodes, most commonly in the axillary, cervical, and supraclavicular regions. If localization does not occur there, the organisms spread via the bloodstream to other reticuloendothelial tissues such as the bone marrow, liver, and spleen, but visceral organs such as kidneys, bones, testes, and endocardium are involved as well.

The usual incubation period between infection and bacteremia with its associated symptoms is 10 to 21 days, depending upon the size of the inoculum. The characteristic but nonspecific reaction of tissues to *Brucella* is the appearance of epithelioid cells, giant cells of the foreign body and Langhans' types, and lymphocytes and plasma cells. Granulomas are formed; usually these are devoid of caseation or necrosis. Although many *Brucella* are killed by PMNs, the macrophage is the ultimate cell that destroys *Brucella.* If the host reaction does not deter granuloma formation, persistent bacteremia with involvement of multiple organs may occur. Although brucellosis is a common cause of abortion in cattle, swine, and goats, there is no evidence that human abortions occur any more frequently with this disease than with other bacteremias.

MANIFESTATIONS The incubation period varies between 7 and 21 days, although many months may elapse between the time of infection and the first appearance of symptoms. The onset is often insidious; patients have a low-grade fever and no localizing findings, and complain only of headache, weakness, insomnia, sweats, constipation, backache, and generalized aches and pains. Most patients are anorectic and lose weight. Cough and arthralgias are present in a minority of patients, along with pain behind the eyes, dizziness, and tinnitus.

The major physical findings are lymphadenopathy, splenomegaly (particularly in the more severe cases), hepatomegaly, and tenderness over the spine. Orchitis occurs after several days of illness and is usually heralded by a chill or chilliness, high fever, and tender, enlarged testes. Painful, swollen joints occur occasionally.

Bacterial endocarditis is a rare but serious complication and is the most common cause of death among patients with brucellosis. It has been reported predominantly in males, follows an indolent course, is accompanied by a high rate of congestive heart failure and arterial embolization, and has required both valve replacement and antibiotic therapy to achieve cure.

Though no complication is very common, among rarer ones described in addition to those already mentioned are pleural effusion, lung abscess, empyema, cholecystitis, suppurative arthritis, osteomyelitis, nephritis, optic neuritis, and meningoencephalitis.

An unusual complication that occurs in veterinarians removing placentas from infected animals consists of a rash which is presumed to be a hypersensitivity reaction to *Brucella* antigens.

The status of chronic brucellosis is difficult to assess. It used to be thought that infection might persist in a relatively small number of individuals for months and years, leaving the patients chronically ill with weakness, fatigue, depression, vague aches and pains, and no abnormal physical findings. Intermittent fever was said to occur. However, in recent series chronic brucellosis has not been found to be a cause of fever of undetermined origin, and there is considerable doubt that the entity exists.

DIAGNOSIS Brucellosis is a relatively rare disease, and there are many more common illnesses that mimic it. Among them are influenza, infectious mononucleosis, toxoplasmosis, viral hepatitis, disseminated gonococcal infection, rheumatic fever, systemic lupus erythematosus, tuberculosis, leptospirosis, and typhoid fever. The clinical suspicion that the patient has brucellosis should be higher in farmers, abattoir workers, and others exposed to infected tissues or animal products.

The definitive evidence of *Brucella* infection consists of isolating the *Brucella* organisms from the patient. However, culturing *Brucella* organisms may be dangerous to laboratory personnel. *All cultures should be clearly marked "possible brucellosis" and should be processed employing sterile techniques in a biohazard hood certified for handling class III infectious agents.* It is recommended that laboratories not having these facilities not undertake *Brucella* cultures.

Blood cultures At least half the patients whose blood is submitted for culture early in the course of infection, and who have not received antibiotics, will have *Brucella* organisms in the blood when a culture is grown in trypticase soy broth for 1 to 3 weeks in the presence of 5 to 10% CO_2. However, many laboratories discard blood cultures after 10 days' incubation. This is another reason for the clinician to communicate any suspicion of brucellosis to the laboratory and to urge the laboratory to hold these cultures for at least 4 weeks. Later in the course of illness, bacteremia is less frequent and organisms may then be isolated from infected lymph nodes or granulomas involving the spleen, liver, and bone. Altogether, only 15 to 20 percent of cases of brucellosis are confirmed by culture. In the majority of instances, the diagnosis is made serologically.

Serology The most reliable serologic test is the standard tube *Brucella* agglutination test which measures antibodies directed primarily at *Brucella* lipopolysaccharide antigens. A fourfold or greater rise in titer of serum specimens drawn 1 to 4 weeks apart is indicative of recent exposure to *Brucella* or *Brucella*-like antigens. The specimen should be tested on the same day, in the same laboratory, under identical conditions. Most patients develop a rise in titer to *Brucella* antigens within 1 to 2 weeks of illness, and within 3 weeks virtually all patients will show seroconversion. False-positive tests may be due to *Brucella* skin tests, cholera vaccination, and infection with *Vibrio cholerae, Francisella tularensis,* or *Yersinia enterocolitica.* These cross-reactive causes of seroconversion are usually readily eliminated.

Significance of serologic findings A titer of 160 or higher is very rare in individuals with no exposure to *Brucella* organisms and is most consistent with past or present exposure to *Brucella* organisms or antigens that cross-react with *Brucella* species. If there is strong clinical suspicion of brucellosis, dilutions as high as 1:1280 should be made, because false-negative tests due to blocking antibodies have been reported in titers as high as 1:640.

Patients develop both IgG- and IgM-agglutinating antibodies in response to infection. When the diagnosis is prompt and is followed by adequate treatment, IgG-agglutinating antibodies rarely persist. However, some patients will maintain elevated IgG *Brucella* agglutinins until diagnosed and treated. These antibodies can be recognized by extraction with 0.5 *M* 2-mercaptoethanol (2-ME). This procedure recognizes only the IgG-agglutinating antibody, and existence of a single elevated titer in the 2-ME *Brucella* agglutination test is good objective evidence of either current or recent infection, and the need for treatment. A titer of 40 to 80 in the 2-ME *Brucella* agglutination test is rarely indicative of recent infection. Many patients maintain elevated IgM-agglutinating antibodies for several years, even after presumed complete cure of their infection. For this reason, a 2-ME *Brucella* agglutination test that measures only IgG-agglutinating antibodies is the most useful indicator of whether the patient has been cured.

Other serologic tests are of no particular value. The *Brucella* skin test is of no more significance than a positive tuberculin test in patients suspected of having tuberculosis. Moreover, the test may interfere with interpretation of serologic tests by causing a rise in titer. For this reason, a skin test should not be performed.

Other laboratory tests An occasional patient will develop anemia. The white blood cell count is normal or low, and the erythrocyte sedimentation rate may be normal or high.

TREATMENT It is generally accepted that the combination of tetracycline 500 mg orally four times daily for 6 weeks plus streptomycin 1 g daily intramuscularly for 2 weeks will result in cure of brucellosis. This regimen has produced lower relapse rates than has treatment with tetracycline alone. The long duration of therapy permits host defenses to be mobilized. With this program, relapses have occurred in only 2 percent of patients, and these have responded to re-treatment.

A variety of other drugs, including gentamicin in lieu of streptomycin, doxycycline instead of tetracycline, or trimethoprim-sulfa or rifampin as supplements have been tried, but none has been found clearly superior to the tetracycline-streptomycin combination. These drugs should be used only when the patient is unable to tolerate either tetracycline or streptomycin.

Febrile patients with either acute or subacute brucellosis characterized by severe anorexia, depression, and generalized debilitation may be given a short course of steroids. Prednisone in an oral dose of 60 mg a day tapered rapidly over a 5- to 7-day period can be administered and may be helpful. However, it is not necessary in most patients.

Therapeutic use of *Brucella* vaccine is of questionable value and is not recommended. Headache, backache, and generalized aches and pains should be treated with analgesics.

PROGNOSIS Even before antimicrobial treatment, the mortality rate of brucellosis was low, and only 15 percent of patients had an illness exceeding 3 months in duration. With chemotherapy, long illnesses have become quite rare, as have complications. When the morbidity exceeds 1 to 2 months, other causes of illness, previously unsuspected underlying disease, or a complication of brucellosis should be considered. The mortality rate of acute brucellosis is less than 2 percent.

The diagnosis of chronic brucellosis, continued active brucellosis, or a complication of brucellosis can best be made by demonstrating a titer of 1:160 or greater in the 2-ME agglutination test. If the titer is less than 1:40 on this test, it is highly unlikely that persistent illness or relapse is due to brucellosis.

Most patients who develop brucellosis in the course of their work can be permitted to return to their place of work. Immunity to reinfection appears to follow the first *Brucella* infection in most cases, and patients who return to work following treatment are less likely to acquire brucellosis than are previously uninfected employees.

PREVENTION Prevention of brucellosis in cattle can be achieved with live attenuated *Brucella* vaccine. No vaccine is available for humans in the United States, although a promising vaccine against *B. abortus* is available in France. The risk of acquiring brucellosis can be reduced by decreasing exposure to freshly killed animal tissue from potentially infected animals and by drinking pasteurized milk and using pasteurized milk products. Slaughterhouse workers, meat inspectors, veterinarians, and others who examine a large number of cattle and hogs can mitigate the risk of infection by wearing protective gloves or goggles and by avoiding hand or arm cuts that would provide a portal of entry for *Brucella.* However, brucellosis will not be eliminated in humans unless it is first eliminated in animals.

REFERENCES

Brown SL et al: Safranin 0-stained antigen microagglutination test for detection of *Brucella* antibodies. J Clin Microbiol 13:398, 1981

Buchanan TM et al: Brucellosis in the United States, 1960–1972: An abattoir-associated disease: I. Clinical features and therapy; II. Diagnostic aspects; III. Epidemiologic evidence for acquired immunity. Medicine 53:403, 415, 427, 1974

———, Faber LC: 2-Mercaptoethanol *Brucella* agglutination test: Usefulness for predicting recovery from brucellosis. J Clin Microbiol 11:691, 1980

Cohen PS et al: Infective endocarditis caused by gram-negative bacteria. Prog Cardiovasc Dis 22:205, 1980

Larbrisseau A et al: The neurological complications of brucellosis. Can J Neurol Sci 5:369, 1978

Llorens-Terol J, Busquets RM: Brucellosis treated with rifampicin. Arch Dis Child 55(6):486, 1980

Medical Staff Conference: Brucellosis. West J Med 122:232, 1975

Pratt DS et al: Successful treatment of *Brucella melitensis* endocarditis. Am J Med 64:898, 1978

Spink WW: *The Nature of Brucellosis.* Minneapolis, University of Minnesota Press, 1956

Young EJ: *Brucella melitensis* hepatitis: The absence of granulomas. Ann Intern Med 91:414, 1978

159 TULAREMIA

THOMAS M. BUCHANAN
EDWARD W. HOOK III

DEFINITION Tularemia is an infectious disease caused by *Francisella tularensis,* a gram-negative bacillus that is usually transmitted to humans from infected animals or insect vectors. It most frequently occurs as an ulcerative lesion at the site of inoculation in association with pronounced regional lymphadenopathy. Tularemia may also present as pneumonia, localized lymphadenopathy, or a febrile illness without localizing findings. Asymptomatic infection with *F. tularensis* also occurs, though its frequency is unknown.

HISTORY *F. tularensis* was first isolated from rodents by McCoy and Chapin in 1912, and from humans in 1914 by Wherry and Lamb. Dr. Edward Francis, for whom the genus *Francisella* is named, contributed much to the early knowledge of the disease including recognition of the role of ticks and deerflies as vectors and the importance of rabbits as animal hosts.

ETIOLOGY *Francisella tularensis* is a small, pleomorphic, nonmotile, poorly staining gram-negative rod. It does not grow well on defined media but may be grown in laboratory animals (mice, rabbits, guinea pigs) or on media containing glucose, cysteine, and serum. Isolation of *F. tularensis* is not attempted by most clinical microbiology laboratories because of its high infectivity and the significant risk of laboratory-acquired infection. The reliability and ease of serologic diagnosis in tularemia obviates the need for isolation of the organism from most suspected cases.

Two types of *F. tularensis* organisms may be distinguished on the basis of geographic distribution, fermentation reactions, and virulence. Jellison type A strains of *F. tularensis* are found only in North America, ferment glycerol, produce citrulline ureidase, and are highly virulent for rabbits and humans. Jellison type B strains have worldwide distribution, are usually avirulent for rabbits, and cause mild disease in humans. Type B organisms lack citrulline ureidase activity and are unable to ferment glycerol.

F. tularensis contains polysaccharide antigen(s), a protein antigen that cross-reacts with *Brucella,* and an endotoxin with biologic activity similar to other gram-negative bacteria.

EPIDEMIOLOGY Tularemia in humans usually results from contact with infected animals or insect vectors, though laboratory-acquired infections occur. In the United States most cases result from contact with infected rabbits or ticks. The organism has been recovered from more than 100 animals, and infections have been documented in squirrels, muskrats, skunks, minks, foxes, coyotes, dogs, cats, chickens, opossums, pheasants, quail, mice, rats, snakes, ticks, lice, mosquitoes, deer, cattle, sheep, and deerflies. In the United States, several species of tick carry the disease (*Dermacentor andersoni,* the Rocky Mountain tick; *D. variabilis,* the western wood tick; *D. occidentalis,* the eastern dog tick; and *Amblyomma americanum,* the Lone Star tick). The infection may persist in ticks through transovarial passage.

Tularemia in the United States has a bimodal prevalence with peaks in May to August and in December and January. In the summer months tick-borne tularemia is greatest, while in the winter months the disease occurs in association with the hunting season and the skinning of infected mammals (primarily rabbits).

In 1981, 268 cases of tularemia were reported in the United States. This figure represents a steady increase in reported cases since 1975 and the greatest number since 1965. Tularemia has been seen in every state. However, the west south central region of the United States (Arkansas, Louisiana, Oklahoma, and Texas) accounts for the greatest number of cases. Although the organism is equally infectious for both sexes, tularemia is more common in men. Individuals at increased risk for development of the disease include hunters, trappers, butchers, agricultural workers, campers, sheepherders, mink farmers, and laboratory technicians.

PATHOGENESIS AND PATHOLOGY The primary route in infection by *F. tularensis* is through the skin. Small cuts or abrasions may be contaminated while a person is skinning an infected animal, or the bite of an infected tick may introduce the organism. Infection may also occur through the conjunctivae, or by inhalation or ingestion of organisms. As few as 10 to 50 organisms are sufficient to cause infection by cutaneous inoculation or by inhalation, though many more bacteria must be ingested to produce the disease. The incubation period averages 3 to 5 days but may be as short as 1 day with a large inoculum or as long as 10 days. Once it has penetrated the skin or epithelial membrane, the organism typically spreads to the regional lymph nodes. These nodes enlarge and, in the ulceroglandular form of the infection (approximately 80 percent or more of cases), the organism may not spread further. If the inoculum is sufficiently large, or the host defenses inadequate, bacteremia occurs with dissemination to phagocytic cells of the reticuloendothelial system. Early in experimental infection foci of necrosis with polymorphonuclear infiltration may be seen in the lymph nodes, spleen, and liver. Subsequently the inflammatory response becomes predominantly mononuclear, and granulomas, with or without giant cells, may form. Coalescence of granulomatous lesions may lead to abscess formation.

Pulmonary tularemia may result following inhalation of organisms or by hematogenous dissemination and histologically appears as foci of edema, alveolar necrosis, and an inflammatory exudate consisting of fibrin and polymorphonuclear leukocytes. As the pneumonia evolves, polymorphonuclear leukocytes are replaced by a predominantly mononuclear infiltrate. Areas of pneumonic involvement may coalesce, but true consolidation or abscess formation is rare. Bilateral patchy infiltrates are most common, though lobar pneumonia and/or pleural effusion may occur.

MANIFESTATIONS Clinical manifestations vary depending upon whether the disease is localized to an entry site and its regional lymph nodes or is more invasive and generalized. Ulceroglandular, oculoglandular, and perhaps true gastrointestinal tularemia are representative of localized disease, and typhoidal and cryptogenic, as well as pulmonary tularemia, are representative of more invasive infection.

Ulceroglandular tularemia is the most common form of disease (75 to 85 percent of reported cases) and consists of a primary cutaneous lesion and pronounced regional lymphadenopathy. At the site of primary inoculation a firm, erythematous papule appears which may be mildly pruritic. It is relatively painless and may be overlooked until ulceration occurs 2 to 3 days later, and even then may not be noticed. The ulcer may require more than 2 weeks to heal and is frequently present when the patient presents to a physician with painful regional lymphadenopathy and fever. Approximately 80 to 90 percent of patients with rabbit-associated tularemia have axillary or epitrochlear adenopathy, presumably reflecting entry of

F. tularensis through broken skin on the hands and arms engendered by skinning infected rabbits. In contrast, 60 to 70 percent of patients with tick-borne tularemia have inguinal or femoral adenopathy, associated with a tick-related ulcer on the lower extremities, buttocks, or perineum. Generalized lymphadenopathy is less common in tick-borne (6 percent) than in rabbit-associated (19 percent) tularemia, perhaps indicating a lower frequency of bacteremia with tick-borne *F. tularensis* infection. Painful lymphadenitis is common in ulceroglandular disease and may be associated with fever as high as 40°C (104°F). The nodes may occasionally suppurate and drain, in which case viable *F. tularensis* can be cultured during the first 3 to 4 weeks of adenopathy.

Ocular inoculation of *F. tularensis* may result in oculoglandular tularemia. This syndrome consists of ocular pain, congestion, photophobia, increased lacrimation, and purulent discharge. Without treatment, corneal ulceration or perforation may occur. Regional adenopathy involving preauricular and submandibular nodes may be striking.

Gastrointestinal tularemia occurs rarely and may follow ingestion of a large number (greater than 10^8) of *F. tularensis.* Patients develop fever, diarrhea, nausea, vomiting, abdominal pain and gastrointestinal bleeding associated with ulcerative intestinal lesions, and marked mesenteric lymphadenopathy.

More invasive tularemia may be associated with high fever, bacteremia, generalized lymphadenopathy, painful hepatomegaly and splenomegaly, headache, myalgias, nausea, prostration, and profound toxicity. The terms *cryptogenic* or *typhoidal tularemia* refer to invasive tularemia in which no obvious site of entry of *F. tularensis* can be demonstrated. Uncommon complications of tularemia include pericarditis, meningitis, endocarditis, peritonitis, appendicitis, perisplenitis, and osteomyelitis.

Pulmonary tularemia may result either from bacteremic spread of *F. tularensis* from a distant site or from inhalation of aerosolized organisms. Pulmonic involvement may be present in 10 to 15 percent of patients with visible ulcers as points of entry and in 30 to 50 percent of patients with cryptogenic or typhoidal tularemia. Nonproductive cough, shortness of breath, and substernal chest discomfort, in addition to fever, chills, malaise, and prostration, are common. Chest x-rays reveal patchy infiltrates that may be bilateral and/or multilobar and that may be associated with hilar lymphadenopathy, pleuritis, pleural effusion, and, rarely, abscesses.

LABORATORY FINDINGS The usual laboratory tests are not distinctive. Leukocytosis is unusual, and the erythrocyte sedimentation rate is also usually normal except in patients with marked systemic toxicity as seen in acute typhoidal tularemia. Although the organism may be isolated from clinical specimens by use of special media, most clinical microbiology laboratories do not attempt isolation because of the high infectivity of even a small number of bacilli. *F. tularensis,* although gram negative, stains poorly and is present in small numbers at sites of infection, making visualization of the organism in clinical specimens (most often sputum or lymph node aspirates) unusual.

Tularemia skin tests are usually positive before diagnostic concentrations of agglutinating antibody are present. Skin tests using whole killed bacilli or purified antigen are usually positive during the first week of illness. The skin test reaction is a delayed hypersensitivity reaction similar to the tuberculin skin test. Skin test reactivity remains positive after tularemia agglutinins are no longer detectable. *The tularemia agglutination test is the method of choice for the diagnosis of suspected tularemia.* Detectable agglutinating antibody to *F. tularensis* usually appears after the second week of illness. Rising antibody levels or a single positive titer of 160 or greater is evidence of infection with *F. tularensis.* In acute tularemia peak agglutination titers of greater than 640 are not unusual, and titers greater than 160 may be present for years following infection. The formalin-fixed *F. tularensis* used for agglutination reactions may cross-react with antibody to *Brucella* or *Proteus* 0-19. However, the elevation in titer to *F. tularensis* is far greater than to cross-reacting antigens, and the specificity for *F. tularensis* may be confirmed by determining agglutination titers to all three antigens.

Aspiration of affected lymph nodes for diagnostic purposes is discouraged because of the risk of handling aspirated fluid, the poor growth of *F. tularensis* on conventional laboratory media, and the ease of diagnosing the infection serologically. Drainage may be required to treat fluctuant buboes but is best delayed until 2 days after initiation of streptomycin therapy or 4 or more weeks after the onset of illness, when the nodes are generally sterile.

DIFFERENTIAL DIAGNOSIS Ulceroglandular tularemia, the most common form of tularemia, should be considered in the differential diagnosis of patients with fever and lymphadenopathy. The disease must be differentiated from melioidosis, glanders, rat-bite fever, sporotrichosis, and lymphangitis secondary to an infected skin lesion. Tularemia has also been reported following cat bite, or presenting as lymphoma. In most of these illnesses lymphadenitis occurs in association with a primary skin lesion, the magnitude of local lymphadenopathy being proportional to the size of the primary skin lesion. As in tularemia, lymphadenopathy in cat-scratch disease and lymphogranuloma venereum may be disproportionately greater than the size of the primary lesion. Extragenital lymphogranuloma venereum is unusual, and in cat-scratch disease clinical illness, if present at all, resolves spontaneously in 6 to 9 days without treatment. Cryptogenic or typhoidal tularemia may be mimicked by infectious mononucleosis, and pneumonic tularemia may resemble atypical pneumonia caused by other organisms. Because of the protean manifestations of *F. tularensis* infection and the rarity of isolation of the organism, a high index of suspicion is critical in order to make the diagnosis. A history of exposure to animal or insect vectors may be an important clue for consideration of the diagnosis, although in some series up to 40 percent of patients will deny exposure to possible vectors.

TREATMENT Streptomycin is the therapy of choice for tularemia. Patients treated early in the course of illness with 1 g daily administered intramuscularly usually experience symptomatic improvement and resolution of fever within 1 to 2 days. Treatment should be continued for 7 to 14 days, and for 5 to 7 days after the patient becomes afebrile. With this regimen, relapses are unusual. When they do occur, it is usually within 2 weeks after therapy is discontinued, and patients then rapidly respond to re-treatment. Patients treated after several weeks of illness may have delayed resolution of fever and incomplete improvement in systemic complaints. Despite improvement of other signs and symptoms of tularemia, the natural history of the primary skin lesion is not changed by treatment, and lymph nodes may continue to enlarge for several days after initiation of therapy. These enlarged local nodes occasionally develop into fluctuant sterile buboes requiring incision and drainage.

Gentamicin and kanamycin are also effective for treatment of tularemia, as are tetracycline and chloramphenicol. However, with tetracycline and chloramphenicol the risk of relapse is increased, particularly when treatment is initiated more than 7 days following the onset of the disease.

PREVENTION Tularemia is transmitted to humans primarily from infected animals and insect vectors. Efforts to avoid and repel ticks, mosquitoes, and deerflies should be made in regions with a high incidence of the disease. Hunters and trappers should wear gloves and proceed cautiously while skinning, dressing, or otherwise handling game, particularly rabbits. Laboratory workers should use caution when working with *F. tularensis* to avoid inhalation of aerosolized organisms or inadvertent inoculation through cutaneous contact.

Killed and live attenuated vaccines have been developed in efforts to prevent tularemia. Live attenuated *F. tularensis* vaccine is more effective than killed vaccine in preventing or mitigating the severity of the disease. The attenuated vaccine induces *F. tularensis* agglutinins and skin test positivity. Protection is long-lived and booster vaccination is not required. In the United States, live attenuated *F. tularensis* vaccine is available through the Centers for Disease Control in Atlanta and is recommended for laboratory workers and others who are at high risk for exposure and development of the disease. Protection from vaccination, like the protection afforded by prior infection, is only partial; patients who acquire tularemia after vaccination usually have mild disease with lower temperatures, less regional lymphadenopathy, and few, if any, systemic manifestations.

In individuals with known exposure to *F. tularensis,* streptomycin treatment will prevent development of clinical illness. Prophylactic treatment with tetracycline or chloramphenicol usually results only in prolongation of the incubation period.

PROGNOSIS The morbidity from tularemia is significant, and fever, anorexia, weight loss, and malaise may persist for months without antibiotic treatment. The overall mortality of untreated infection is less than 6 percent. Significant pulmonic involvement or severe disease increases the likelihood of death to higher than 30 percent without treatment. With early and appropriate antimicrobial therapy, death is rare. Partial immunity to reinfection follows recovery from tularemia.

REFERENCES

BUCHANAN TM et al: The tularemia skin test. 235 skin tests in 210 persons: Serologic correlation and review of the literature. Ann Intern Med 74:336, 1971

BURKE DS: Immunization against tularemia: Analysis of the effectiveness of live *Francisella tularensis* vaccine in the prevention of laboratory-acquired tularemia. J Infect Dis 135:55, 1977

MASON WL et al: Treatment of tularemia, including pulmonary tularemia, with gentamicin. Ann Rev Resp Dis 121:39, 1980

MASSEY ED, MANGIAFICO JA: Microagglutination test for detecting and measuring serum agglutinins of *Francisella tularensis.* Appl Microbiol 27:25, 1974

MCCRUMB FR JR et al: Studies on human infection with *Pasteurella tularensis:* Comparison of streptomycin and chloramphenicol in the prophylaxis of clinical disease. Trans Assoc Am Physicians 70:74, 1957

YOUNG LS et al: Tularemia epidemic: Vermont 1968. Forty-seven cases linked to contact with muskrats. N Engl J Med 280:1253, 1969

160
YERSINIA (PASTEURELLA) INFECTIONS, INCLUDING PLAGUE

JOSEPH E. JOHNSON III

The genus *Yersinia* includes *Yersinia* (fomerly *Pasteurella*) *pestis,* the plague bacillus, *Y. enterocolitica,* recognized increasingly as an important cause of enterocolitis, and *Y. pseudotuberculosis,* an occasional cause of mesenteric adenitis. *Pasteurella multocida* is a cause of human infection, mainly following cat and dog bites. Related species with potential pathogenicity for humans include *P. urae, P. haemolytica,* and *P. pneumotropica.*

PLAGUE Definition Plague is an infectious disease of wild and domestic rodents which is transmitted to humans through the bite of infected ectoparasites (especially the rat flea). Disease in humans is usually characterized by the abrupt onset of high fever, lymphadenopathy with painful enlargement of regional lymph nodes draining the exposure site, bacteremia, and prostration. This clinical form of the disease is known as *bubonic* plague because of the presence of enlarged lymph nodes, or *buboes.* Secondary pneumonia may occur and lead to direct respiratory transmission by infectious aerosols from person to person. This primary *pneumonic* type of human disease is highly fatal.

History Plague was known and feared in ancient times and has been the subject of dread as well as a source of literary stimulation to authors from Dionysius in the third century to Camus in the present. At least three major pandemics have occurred in which large segments of the population were destroyed. The first authentic pandemic was recorded in the sixth century A.D.; the second great pandemic occurred in the fourteenth century and was known as the "Black Death," and the last major pandemic originated in China in 1894, spread eventually to all continents, and was first recognized in the United States in 1900. The disease is now well established in wild rodents in many parts of the world, including the western United States. It is present on every continent except Australia. Human disease is endemic in parts of Asia, Africa, and South America, and sporadic human cases still occur in the United States.

Etiology The causative agent, *Yersinia pestis,* is a gram-negative, nonmotile, and non-spore-forming bacillus which grows both aerobically and anaerobically. It is pleomorphic in exudate or sputum and may appear bacillary, ovoid, or coccal. When stained with Giemsa's or Wayson's stain, it displays a bipolar "safety pin" structure. *Yersinia pestis* grows readily although somewhat slowly on ordinary culture media, forming small, round, transparent colonies which assume a "beaten-copper" appearance after 48 h. At least two types of toxins have been identified, including a soluble exotoxin-like protein and an insoluble endotoxic lipopolysaccharide. The F1 and VW antigens are antiphagocytic. Although readily killed by sunlight, organisms have been shown to survive in sterile soil for 16 months and in nonsterile soil for as long as 7 months, and organisms may be present in rodent burrows in the absence of fleas and rats for long periods.

Epidemiology Plague is firmly entrenched as an enzootic among approximately 200 species of rodents in many parts of the world. While the disease in wild rodents (sylvatic plague) is not usually a direct threat to humans, it nevertheless serves as a vast reservoir for infection of domestic rats (murine or rat plague) which, along with their ectoparasites, live in close association with humans. The endemic reservoir of sylvatic plague includes wild rats, ground squirrels, rock squirrels, mice, marmots, gophers, rabbits, prairie dogs, and chipmunks. Other animal species which are not reservoir hosts are important potential transmitters of the disease. Sick domesticated cats have been implicated in human cases. Dogs are relatively resistant to plague, showing seroconversion following exposure but usually without clinical illness. In the western hemisphere the disease is firmly entrenched in the wild rodent population of California, Oregon, Washington, Utah, Idaho, Nevada, New Mexico, Texas, Arizona, Colorado, Montana, Wyoming, and in wide areas in South America. The principal murine hosts are the domestic rats, *Rattus rattus* and *R. norvegicus,* which are found throughout the world. Although ticks, lice, and bedbugs may occasionally serve as vectors, the principal ectoparasite vectors are the oriental rat fleas, *Xenopsylla cheopis* and *Diamanus montanus.*

Between epidemics the infection persists as a chronic disease of wild rodents which is maintained by the insect vector. Although occasionally acquired through contact with wild rodents and their parasites, in major outbreaks of human disease infection has usually resulted from association with domestic rats and occurs in urban areas in the wake of rat epizootics. When the concentration of people and of rats under circumstances of poor sanitation provides opportunity for the migration of fleas from rats to humans, an outbreak is likely to occur. Because sylvatic plague appears virtually impossible to eradicate, it will continue to pose a constant threat of extension into urban rat populations and thence to humans. Infection of the flea takes place through ingestion of blood of a bacteremic animal. After multiplication in the intestinal tract of the flea, the organisms are regurgitated when the flea attempts to ingest another blood meal. Because rat fleas will attack human beings if rats are not immediately available, the infection is likely to be transmitted as the rat population decreases and the fleas transfer from dead hosts to human beings. Plague can be acquired by direct contact with the tissues of an infected animal, by its bite, or by scratching of infected material into the skin.

The bubonic form of the disease rarely results in transmission from person to person because bacteremia in human disease is rarely of a level sufficient to allow infection of fleas. The principal mode of spread from person to person is by the pulmonary route, which occurs when a patient with bubonic disease develops secondary plague pneumonia and thereafter excretes large quantities of organisms in the sputum. Airborne infection by droplet nuclei is highly contagious, and primary pneumonic plague is common among those attending such a patient. Although asymptomatic oropharyngeal carriers have been identified among healthy family contacts of bubonic plague patients in Vietnam, the role of these carriers in the transmission of the disease has not been determined.

Pathogenesis In the more common bubonic form of disease, *Y. pestis* gains entry into the human host through the bite of an infected flea. Organisms are carried to the local lymphatics, then to the bloodstream and finally are disseminated. The prominent clinical manifestations are usually in the lymphatic system. In bubonic plague, a hemorrhagic zone of edema surrounds an inflamed and suppurating group of regional lymph nodes. The glands are hyperplastic and show multiple areas of necrosis, in which there are swarms of organisms. Metastatic lesions sometimes develop in other lymphatics or in the viscera. Particularly likely is the occurrence of secondary pneumonia, which constitutes a potential source of pneumonic spread. Hemorrhages are numerous, probably as a result of a toxin produced by *Y. pestis,* and it is not unusual for individuals given chemotherapy late in the disease to die of toxemia when plague bacilli can no longer be cultured from any organ. Primary pneumonic spread occurs through the inhalation of infectious aerosols emanating from another case or, rarely, from infected fomites. It is apparent that the tonsils and/or oropharyngeal mucous membranes may occasionally serve as portals of entry resulting in a cervical bubonic-septicemic form of the disease. Rarely a skin papule forms at the site of entry of the bacillus and may develop into a pustule or a carbuncle.

Bacteremia is a constant feature of bubonic and pneumonic plague. The precise mechanisms by which the plague bacillus and its toxic factors produce severe tissue injury are not understood completely.

Manifestations After an incubation period of 1 to 12 days (usually 2 to 4 days), the patient develops an acute and often fulminant illness. In the more common *bubonic* variety, symptoms begin abruptly with chills, a rise in temperature to 38.9 to 40.6°C (102 to 105°F), tachycardia, headache, vomiting, uncertain gait, marked prostration, and delirium. The spleen is sometimes palpable. The fleabite at the portal of entry rarely can be seen; if present, it is marked by a papule or vesicle which ultimately becomes pustular. Pain and tenderness are present in the infected regional lymph nodes. Of the buboes, 60 to 75 percent are in the inguinal or femoral regions because the lower extremities are more commonly the site of the initial fleabite. Less often, especially in children, buboes are found in the axillary or cervical regions. Infection may extend to other superficial or deeply situated groups of glands. The bubo consists of a firm, matted group of glands measuring 2 to 5 cm in diameter and is surrounded by a boggy and frequently hemorrhagic zone of edema. It may occasionally suppurate and drain spontaneously after 1 or 2 weeks, although in some instances there is complete resorption.

There is a marked hemorrhagic tendency, presumably because of the effect of plague toxin on blood vessels, and the development of an intravascular coagulopathy (DIC). Petechiae or ecchymoses occur often. Bleeding may occur into a viscus or a serous cavity, or from the nose and alimentary, respiratory, or urinary tracts.

The course of bubonic plague is marked by an irregular or remittent fever, which often drops at the time of appearance of the bubo, only to rise again. In favorable cases, the temperature falls gradually during the second week concomitant with improvement in the general clinical condition. A rise to hyperpyrexic levels or a precipitous fall to normal or to subnormal frequently heralds approaching death. Most fatalities occur during the first week of illness. Although bubonic plague is usually severe, mild cases called *pestis minor* are sometimes seen during epidemics.

The "primary septicemic" form of plague is actually a variant of bubonic disease. The patient experiences a sudden and overwhelming systemic illness. There is a marked constitutional reaction, with chills, fever, rapid pulse, severe headache, nausea, vomiting, and delirium. Death ensues within a few days, before localizing lesions become clinically apparent.

Plague also may take the form of pneumonia. The initial cases appear in patients with bubonic plague, of whom as many as 5 percent develop secondary lesions in the lungs. These individuals may provide the starting point for a person-to-person epidemiologic cycle of airborne primary pneumonic plague. It is a fulminating infection accompanied by great prostration, cough, dyspnea, and, in the later stages, cyanosis. The sputum is abundant, blood-stained, and teeming with *Y. pestis.* Often there are no clear-cut pulmonary signs, though scattered rales or areas of dullness may be found. In the absence of specific therapy, plague pneumonia invariably ends fatally within 1 to 5 days.

Infection may localize in other regions of the body. Subcutaneous abscesses and cutaneous ulcerations sometimes occur, and occasionally the meninges are involved.

Laboratory findings Laboratory confirmation of plague is relatively simple, although the disease is often misdiagnosed in the United States because of its rarity. Consideration of epidemiologic and clinical features provides highly characteristic leads, and once a suspicion of plague is entertained, it can readily be verified by smear, culture, or animal inoculation of appropriate specimens. The technique of staining a suspected specimen with fluorescent specific antiserum provides an elegant method for rapid identification of *Y. pestis.* If a bubo is present, a small quantity of interstitial fluid should be aspirated from its center. Large numbers of morphologically characteristic bacilli are usually seen in a stained smear. Infected sputum likewise contains many organisms. Bacteremia of varying degrees occurs at some time during the course of the disease in nearly all cases, and blood cultures are essential. Pus and sputum should be cultured on blood agar plates, while blood is inoculated into nutrient broth. Organisms are identified by their morphologic and colonial characteristics, by agglutination with specific antiserum, fluorescent antibody staining, and biochemical reactions. The phage lysis test is relatively simple and helpful in distinguishing *Y. pestis* from other *Yersinia.* Caution should be observed in handling infected materials or animals, because of the great danger of infection to laboratory workers.

Specific antibodies appear in the serum of patients convalescing from the disease and can usually be detected early in the second week by complement fixation, agglutination, passive hemagglutination, or immunoelectrophoretic agar-gel precipitation methods. A passive mouse-protective test serves to indicate the immune status of a convalescent or vaccinated individual.

The white blood cell count is elevated to levels often above 20,000 cells per cubic millimeter, and there is a predominance of polymorphonuclear leukocytes. The red blood cell count usually is normal.

Diagnosis Early in the acute phase of illness, before the appearance of localizing signs, plague may be confused with severe systemic illnesses such as typhoid, typhus, or malaria. The presence of buboes may suggest other forms of infectious lymphadenitis, including tularemia, syphilis, and lymphogranuloma venereum, as well as lymphadenitis of staphylococcal or streptococcal origin. Pneumonic plague must be distinguished from tularemic, pneumococcal, and other gram-negative pneumonias as well as from anthrax, psittacosis, and mycoplasma pneumonia. The consideration of epidemiologic factors, plus bacteriologic studies, will aid in the differentiation. Serologic diagnosis is important for retrospective confirmation. When plague is suspected, it is imperative to begin treatment as soon as adequate specimens have been taken for culture because early institution of therapy is essential to ensure recovery. To delay treatment may risk toxemic death in the face of a bacteriologic cure.

Treatment When antibiotic treatment is instituted early in the course of the disease, the response is usually dramatic and complete. Early treatment in pneumonic and septicemic disease is particularly urgent since irreversible progression may occur within 15 h after onset. Streptomycin and tetracycline are the drugs of choice. Streptomycin is given intramuscularly in doses of 0.5 g every 4 h for 48 h followed by 0.5 g every 6 h for a total of 7 to 10 days or until the patient has been afebrile at least 3 days. Kanamycin is also effective and may be particularly useful if streptomycin resistance increases. Tetracyclines are given in initial doses of 2 to 3 g daily intravenously, and the dose is reduced to 2 g daily orally when improvement occurs. Chloramphenicol is also a potent antiplague agent and should be given in initial doses of 6 to 8 g daily intravenously (100 mg/kg) and the dose reduced to 3 g (50 to 75 mg/kg) daily orally for a total dose of 20 to 25 g. Sulfonamides are less effective, especially in pneumonic plague, and should be used only when the other agents are not available. Trimethoprim-sulfamethoxazole (co-trimoxazole) has been used successfully. Buboes are treated with hot, moist applications. Incision and drainage is not indicated unless the lesion becomes clearly fluctuant and the patient has been treated with antibiotics.

Control Prevention of plague must be directed toward elimination of endemic rodent foci, and in endemic urban areas constant vigilance is required in detecting and combating rodent epizootics. Prevention includes eradication of ectoparasite vectors, extermination of rats, and sometimes the immunization of the human population. The complete elimination of sylvatic plague appears to be impossible in the foreseeable future, and the control program must be aimed at eradicating foci of wild rodent infection around areas of human habitation.

Patients must be disinfested and carefully isolated, while other intimately exposed persons should be quarantined. Chemoprophylaxis with tetracycline or streptomycin is recommended for household and other close contacts.

A formalin-killed vaccine approved for use in the United States has been advised for persons traveling to plague-enzootic areas such as southeast Asia, for those whose vocations bring them into frequent and regular contact with wild rodents in plague enzootic areas, and for laboratory personnel working with *Y. pestis* or with plague-infected rodents. The vaccine appears to reduce the incidence and severity of the disease. Immunity is relative, and protection is not always conferred by the active disease, since a number of reinfections have been described. Although general vaccination may be worthwhile in an area threatened by an epidemic, the results are too slow for immediate prophylaxis. In such epidemic situations, combined use of all available control measures is indicated.

Prognosis The availability of effective antibiotic therapy has improved the prognosis in this formerly highly fatal disease. In the past the mortality rate of bubonic plague varied from 50 to 90 percent, and the pneumonic, septicemic, and meningitic forms were almost invariably fatal. In treated cases the mortality is 5 to 10 percent, and even the gravest infections respond to chemotherapy if treated early enough.

OTHER *YERSINIA* INFECTIONS (*Y. PSEUDOTUBERCULOSIS* AND *Y. ENTEROCOLITICA*) **Etiology** *Y. pseudotuberculosis* is a gram-negative, aerobic, facultatively anaerobic, non-spore-forming bacillus, which is coccobacillary when virulent and bacillary when avirulent. It is easily confused with other non-lactose-fermenting Enterobacteriaceae. It is nonmotile at 37°C (98.6°F) but usually motile at 22°C (71.6°F). *Y. enterocolitica,* a closely related organism, has similar characteristics but is distinguished on the basis of biochemical reactions.

Manifestations *Y. pseudotuberculosis* is a ubiquitous animal pathogen, worldwide in distribution but identified only in the last 20 years as a potentially significant human pathogen. Several hundred cases of human infection have been identified in Europe (especially Scandinavia) and increasingly from Canada and the United States. *Y. enterocolitica,* isolated less frequently from animals in the United States, has been recognized as an important cause of enteritis as well as a potential cause of a variety of human disease syndromes. Both organisms have been associated with diarrheal diseases, both acute and chronic, and also a usually benign and self-limited form of mesenteric adenitis, clinically simulating appendicitis. Cervical adenitis has also been seen. Rarely, potentially fatal typhoidal and septicemic forms of infection have been described, especially in patients with underlying debilitating diseases. Increasingly, polyarthritis with and without associated erythema nodosum has been associated with *Yersinia* infection.

Reported cases have indicated a 3:1 male predominance especially in older children and young adults infected with *Y. pseudotuberculosis,* while equal sex distribution and a greater incidence in young children and infants has been observed with *Y. enterocolitica.* In addition, *Y. enterocolitica* has been incriminated in institutional and multiple-family outbreaks.

Transmission has usually been traced to contact with infected animals or contaminated food or water, although person-to-person, hand-to-mouth transmission appears also to be a significant possibility.

Diagnosis Diagnosis may be confirmed by culture of lymph nodes, occasionally of stools, or by serologic titers. Cross reactions with *Salmonella, Brucella,* and *Escherichia coli* antigens occur, and serums must be cross-absorbed. With use of both agglutination and hemagglutination methods, titers up to 1:10,240 have been found. Titers lower than 1:160 are not considered significant. The highest antibody titers usually occur during the acute phase of illness, rapidly disappearing by the fourth or fifth month of convalescence, probably reflecting the elicitation of IgM-type antibodies.

Although both species are easily grown on standard laboratory media, identification is more difficult, and routine methods for pathogenic Enterobacteriaceae are inadequate.

The variety of clinical syndromes which have been observed in association with *Y. pseudotuberculosis* and *Y. enterocolitica* may also be confusing. Acute or subacute yersinial enteritis may mimic salmonellosis, shigellosis, and other common enteropathogenic syndromes. Fever, diarrhea, and vomiting are the most common findings in infants and younger children. Fecal leukocytosis has been found in yersinial enteritis indicating ulceration of the intestinal mucosa. Acute septicemic yersiniosis may resemble systemic salmonellosis and other "typhoidal" syndromes. Subacute localizing yersiniosis with hepatic or splenic abscesses may resemble amebic hepatitis. Patients with mesenteric adenitis (usually children) may present the clinical picture of acute appendicitis with mid- or right-lower quadrant abdominal pain, fever, and leukocytosis. At laparotomy the appendix is usually normal, but large inflamed mesenteric lymph nodes are found, sometimes with associated terminal ileitis. Histologic examination of inflamed nodes has revealed reticulogranulocytic infiltration with or without small abscess formation. Polyarthritis of varying severity and duration has been observed and most often mimics rheumatic fever or juvenile rheumatoid arthritis. Reiter's syndrome may also be simulated. Erythema nodosum has also been increasingly identified in patients with agglutinin rises to *Yersinia,* with or without associated arthritis. Common features in adults have been abdominal pain and fever, with or without arthritis or erythema nodosum. Possible associations of *Yersinia* infection with glomerulonephritis, thyroid disease, and pulmonary lesions have been reported but need further clarification.

Treatment Antibiotic treatment is indicated in the more severe cases, especially the septicemic and subacute localizing forms of disease. *Y. pseudotuberculosis* is usually susceptible to the aminoglycoside antibiotics (gentamicin, tobramycin, streptomycin, or kanamycin) as well as to tetracycline, chloramphenicol, ampicillin, and the cephalosporins. *Y. enterocolitica* is resistant to penicillin G and only variably sensitive to ampicillin and the cephalosporins. In vitro studies indicate a potential role for trimethoprim-sulfamethoxazole.

***PASTEURELLA MULTOCIDA* INFECTION** *Pasteurella multocida* is a gram-negative nonsporulating bacillus which differs from *Yersinia* organisms in cultural characteristics, antibiotic sensitivity, and pattern of animal parasitism. For example, all strains of *P. multocida* are sensitive to penicillin. *P. multocida* is frequently identified as a commensal in cattle, horses, swine, sheep, fowl, dogs, cats, and rats, and on occasion causes hemorrhagic septicemia, or chronic pulmonary infiltrates, in these species. Human infection with *P. multocida* is uncommon and usually related to animal contact. Related species which have occasionally been identified as human pathogens include *P. urae, P. haemolytica,* and *P. pneumotropica.*

Human disease due to *P. multocida* is usually a consequence of a dog or cat bite and appears as a localized wound infection with cellulitis, suppuration, and adenitis. Osteomyelitis sometimes ensues. Rarely, in patients with bronchiectasis, *P. multocida* is isolated from sputum, and animal handlers are sometimes identified as asymptomatic respiratory carriers. Empyema has occasionally been associated with the organisms. Bacteremia with fever and chills may develop after an animal bite, occasionally without an apparent local lesion. Meningitis, brain abscess, pyogenic arthritis, endocarditis, and pyelonephritis may occasionally complicate the bacteremia. Not all *P. multocida* infections follow documented animal bites or animal contact.

Except for the association with animal (especially cat) bites, local infections with *P. multocida* show no unique characteristics, and may resemble cat-scratch fever, tularemia, or staphylococcal or streptococcal infection. Leukocytosis, uncommon in tularemia and cat-scratch fever, is the rule in *P. multocida* infection. Gram's stain of infected material shows pleomorphic gram-negative bacilli which are usually extracellular. The bacteria may have bipolar staining and may be mistaken for gram-negative diplococci prior to cultural identification.

Penicillin in a dosage of 600,000 to 1.2 million units daily is the preferred antibiotic, but a variety of other antibiotics may be effective.

REFERENCES

Plague

ALSOFROM DJ et al: Radiographic manifestations of plague in New Mexico, 1975–1980. A review of 42 proved cases. Radiology 139:561, 1981

BUTLER T et al: *Yersinia pestis* infection in Vietnam: I. Clinical and hematologic aspects. J Infect Dis 124:5, 1974

CONNOR JD et al: Plague in San Diego. West J Med 129:394, 1978

JOHNSON JE: Plague in the U.S. West J Med 129:421, 1978

KAUFMANN AF et al: Trends in human plague in the United States. J Infect Dis 141:522, 1980

Recommendation of the Immunization Practices Advisory Committee. Plague vaccine. Morb Mort Week Rep 31:301, 1982

VON REYN CF et al: Epidemiologic and clinical features of an outbreak of bubonic plague in New Mexico. J Infect Dis 136:489, 1977

WHITE ME et al: Plague in a neonate. Am J Dis Child 135:418, 1981

P. multocida

FRANCIS DP et al: *Pasteurella multocida:* Infections after domestic animal bites and scratches. JAMA 233:42, 1975

JARVIS WR et al: *Pasteurella multocida.* Osteomyelitis following dog bites. Am J Dis Child 135:625, 1981

OBERHOFER TR: Characteristics and biotypes of *Pasteurella multocida* isolated from humans. J Clin Microbiol 13:566, 1981

FORMAN MB: *Yersinia* arthritis mimicking acute rheumatic fever. S Afr Med J 59:576, 1981

GUTMAN LT et al: An inter-familial outbreak of *Yersinia enterocolitica* enteritis. N Engl J Med 288:1372, 1974

KOHL S: *Yersinia enterocolitica* infections in children. Pediatr Clin North Am 26:433, 1979

LEINO R, KALLIOMAKI JL: Yersiniosis as an internal disease. Ann Intern Med 81:458, 1974

MAKI M et al: Yersiniosis in children. Arch Dis Child 55:861, 1980

SAARI TN, TRIPLETT DA: *Yersinia pseudotuberculosis* mesenteric adenitis. J Pediatr 85:656, 1974

161
RAT-BITE FEVER (*STREPTOBACILLUS MONILIFORMIS* AND *SPIRILLUM MINUS* INFECTIONS)

JAN V. HIRSCHMANN

DEFINITION *Rat-bite fever* refers to infection by either *Streptobacillus moniliformis* or *Spirillum minus.* The latter infection is also known by its Japanese name *sodoku.*

ETIOLOGY AND EPIDEMIOLOGY *Streptobacillus moniliformis* is an aerobic nonmotile gram-negative bacterium that may grow in chains of fusiform bacilli. In blood cultures the typical puffball colonies generally appear in 2 to 7 days. Stable L forms frequently develop spontaneously.

The nasopharynx of rats is the natural reservoir of *S. moniliformis,* which grows from as many as half those studied. Human infection usually follows bites from wild rats, but bites from laboratory rats and occasionally other rodents have caused disease. Infection may also occur from ingestion of contaminated food. An epidemic in Haverhill, Massachusetts, in 1926 involving 86 people and caused by contaminated milk or ice cream has led to the term *Haverhill fever* when infection is food-borne.

Spirillum minus is a short, thick spiral gram-negative organism 2 to 5 μm with two to five curves and terminal flagellae that increase its total length to 6 to 10 μm. On dark-field microscopy the organism has characteristic spasmodic motions of the body and darting movements of the flagella. Although it may be visible on Wright's stains of blood from infected patients or animals, it does not grow on artificial media and requires animal inoculation for isolation from patients.

Carrier rates in wild rats, the natural reservoir, are as high as 25 percent in some locations. In them it may cause interstitial keratitis and conjunctivitis. Human infections with *S. minus* almost always follow rat bites.

CLINICAL MANIFESTATIONS Although up to 22 days may elapse, the incubation period for *S. moniliformis* infection is generally short, typically less than 10 days, usually 1 to 3 days. The onset is sudden, with fever, chills, headache, and myalgias the initial symptoms. The bite site is usually unimpressive; occasionally swelling, ulceration, and regional lymphadenopathy are present. A macular rash develops in about 75 percent of cases, usually 1 to 3 days after the onset of symptoms, and is most prominent on the extremities, where it may involve palms and soles. Sometimes it may be generalized, petechial, purpuric, or pustular. Arthralgias or arthritis occurs in about half the cases within the first week, usually with multiple, asymmetric large joint involvement. Without treatment the course of disease may be prolonged for several weeks with persistent or recurrent fever and arthritis. Complications of *S. moniliformis* infection include endocarditis and localized abscesses in soft tissues or brain.

In *Spirillum minus* infections the incubation period is typically longer, usually 1 to 4 weeks, with a range of 1 to 36 days. Usually the bite site, after initial prompt healing, becomes swollen, painful, and red at the onset of fever and chills. There is often lymphangitis and regional lymphadenopathy as well. The fever is usually relapsing, with febrile periods of 2 to 4 days alternating with afebrile periods of about the same duration. During the fever, headache, photophobia, nausea, and vomiting may occur. Joint complaints are rare. A rash develops in more than half the patients that is usually macular and reddish brown or purple-red and occurs typically on the extremities. When untreated, this relapsing illness may persist for months. Rarely, bacterial endocarditis occurs.

LABORATORY FINDINGS In *S. moniliformis* infections the leukocyte count is typically elevated, with neutrophilia and increased immature forms. The organism can be isolated from blood, joint fluid, or pus. Serologic response can be demonstrated during the second week by agglutination tests.

In *Spirillum minus* infections the leukocyte count may be normal or elevated. The organism may be visible on Wright's stained smears or dark-field examination of the patient's blood. In suspected cases the blood should be injected into the peritoneum of mice or guinea pigs; 5 to 15 days later the organism will be visible on dark-field examination of the animals' blood or peritoneal fluid. In about one-half of patients there are biological false-positive tests for syphilis.

DIFFERENTIAL DIAGNOSIS With a history of a rat bite, the major clinical features distinguishing *S. moniliformis* from *S. minus* infection are the differences in the incubation period, the condition of the bite site, the nature of the fever, and the presence or absence of joint symptoms.

TREATMENT AND PROGNOSIS Before effective chemotherapy was available, the mortality rate from *S. moniliformis* infections was about 10 percent; for *Spirillum minus* it was about 6 percent. The treatment of choice is the same for both organisms: 7 to 10 days of procaine penicillin, 600,000 units twice daily intramuscularly, or oral penicillin V, 2 g daily in four divided doses. For penicillin-allergic patients oral erythromycin or tetracycline, 2 g daily in four divided doses, is an alternative. Patients with endocarditis should receive a 4-week course of intravenous penicillin G in a daily dose of 12 to 16 million units.

REFERENCES

COLE JS et al: Rat-bite fever. Ann Intern Med 71:979, 1969

MCCORMACK RC et al: Endocarditis due to *Streptobacillus moniliformis.* JAMA 200:77, 1967

ROUGHGARDEN JW: Antimicrobial therapy of rat-bite fever: A review. Arch Intern Med 116:39, 1965

section 5 | Other aerobic bacterial infections

162 LEGIONNAIRES' DISEASE

HARRY N. BEATY

DEFINITION Legionnaires' disease is an acute respiratory infection caused by a newly recognized, distinctive gram-negative bacterium that was first isolated from fatal cases of pneumonia among individuals attending an American Legion Convention in Philadelphia.

HISTORY In July of 1976, an explosive outbreak of severe respiratory illness occurred in Philadelphia—chiefly among delegates of an American Legion Convention. Initial investigation failed to document a familiar infective or toxic etiology, and so a comprehensive, coordinated effort was undertaken to define the epidemiology and cause of the outbreak. As the ensuing saga unfolded, it became apparent that at least 220 cases of pneumonia—34 of which were fatal—resulted from a common source of airborne infection that was present for several days inside and in the immediate vicinity outside one of the convention hotels. The infective agent was proved to be a previously unknown gram-negative bacterium.

Using serologic techniques, it has been shown that the same organism, or antigenically related species, has caused other outbreaks of respiratory illness. One occurred in 1965 when 80 patients in a psychiatric hospital in Washington, D.C., developed an unexplained pneumonic illness; 12 of these patients died. Other clusters of cases with additional deaths occurred in Spain (1973) and England (1977). One outbreak of particular significance involved visitors and employees in an office of the county health department in Pontiac, Michigan (1968). Pneumonia was not seen among the 144 persons who developed an influenza-like illness, and there were no deaths. The agent responsible for Legionnaires' disease has been directly linked to this outbreak, because it has been isolated from stored environmental samples and tissues of experimental animals, which were studied unsuccessfully during the initial investigation.

ETIOLOGY The bacterium responsible for Legionnaires' disease is a gram-negative bacillus which is 0.3 to 0.4 μm in width and usually 2 to 3 μm long. However, bacilli from 10 to 50 μm have been seen. Pleomorphism is affected by the medium on which the organism is grown; in tissue, the filamentous forms are not encountered. Electron microscopy reveals a structure typical of gram-negative rods, but gas-liquid chromatography shows a distinctive branched-chain fatty acid profile that is more characteristic of gram-positive bacteria.

With the use of the direct fluorescent-antibody technique, no antigenic cross-reactivity was found with 374 strains including 25 bacterial genera and 59 species. One strain each of *Pseudomonas fluorescens* and *P. alcaligenes* has shown some reaction with anti-Legionnaires' agent conjugate, but numerous other strains of the same species have been tested without additional evidence of cross-reactivity. A search for antigenic cross-reactivity and studies of DNA relatedness also have failed to show that the bacterium responsible for Legionnaires' disease is related to any other organism. As a consequence, it has been named *Legionella pneumophila* and established as the first isolate of a previously unrecognized genus and species.

Legionella pneumophila is fastidious, and either does not grow or grows rather slowly on most artificial media. Mueller-Hinton and charcoal yeast extract agars supplemented with *l*-cystine and ferric salts are best for isolation and growth of the organisms. Inoculated plates should be incubated at 35°C in 5% CO_2 or in candle jars. On clear media, a soluble brown pigment that fluoresces under a Wood's lamp can be seen. The organism is catalase-positive and causes a weakly positive oxidase reaction.

Six distinct serogroups of *L. pneumophila* have been identified; some were first isolated from environmental sources, but all have been associated with human disease. Serologic cross-reactions between groups may be absent or weak, which necessitates the use of multiple diagnostic conjugates to detect all strains of *L. pneumophila.*

Isolation and characterization of *L. pneumophila* paved the way for the discovery of previously unrecognized pathogens with cultural, biological, and ecological characteristics that allow them to be classified in the genus *Legionella.* Other isolates not yet classified are referred to as Legionella-like organisms (LLO) (see Chap. 163).

EPIDEMIOLOGY Knowledge of the distribution of *L. pneumophila* in nature is incomplete, but it has been isolated from soil and water. Several outbreaks of Legionnaires' disease have been linked to contaminated condensates from air-conditioning cooling towers, and drinking water has been implicated as a source of infection in some cases. There is no evidence that ingestion of organisms causes disease, but aerosolization of contaminated water during showering, bathing, etc., undoubtedly leads to inhalation of potentially infectious droplets. The possibility that organisms in soil become airborne during excavation has been considered but not proved to be a source of infection.

Infection appears to be acquired by the respiratory route with a usual incubation period of 2 to 10 days. By use of the direct fluorescent-antibody technique, organisms have been identified in the sputum of patients with Legionnaires' disease, but person-to-person spread has not been documented. Common-source outbreaks have received the greatest public attention, but hundreds of sporadic cases of Legionnaires' disease occur each year. Incidence may increase in the summer and early fall, but the disease occurs year-round.

Although this infection has been reported in children, most patients are middle-aged or older. Cigarette smokers and individuals with serious underlying diseases such as chronic renal failure, malignancy, and immunosuppression have increased susceptibility to infection. The mortality rate of Legionnaires' pneumonia that is serious enough to require hospitalization is around 15 percent; among immunocompromised patients it may exceed 50 percent.

Serologic surveys using the indirect fluorescent-antibody

technique have shown that less than 5 percent of healthy individuals from around the United States have reciprocal antibody titers to *L. pneumophila* of 128 or higher. However, some more geographically restricted surveys have shown that 15 to 25 percent of the population have similar serologic evidence of significant exposure to *L. pneumophila* or antigenically related organisms. This suggests that the infection may be endemic in some regions.

Most cases of Legionnaires' disease are diagnosed by demonstration of at least a fourfold rise in serum antibody titer to *L. pneumophila.* A significant proportion of patients maintain high titers for years. It is not known whether these individuals are immune to reinfection with the same or closely related organisms.

PATHOLOGY AND PATHOGENESIS Pathologic features of Legionnaires' disease are limited to the lungs. Apparent lobar involvement almost always represents confluent bronchopneumonia. Prominent microscopic features include extensive exudation of proteinaceous fluid and inflammatory cells into the alveoli. In most cases, the cellular component of the exudate is a mixture of polymorphonuclear neutrophils and macrophages. Extensive lysis of inflammatory cells, with accumulations of nuclear debris and fibrin, is a distinctive feature of this pneumonia. Alveolar septa usually are edematous and infiltrated with inflammatory cells; hyaline membranes are seen in about half the cases. Terminal bronchioles are routinely involved, but larger bronchioles and bronchi are unaffected. None of these changes is unique to Legionnaires' pneumonia, but the histopathologic alterations are sufficiently distinctive to suggest the diagnosis.

Bacteria usually can be demonstrated in the inflammatory exudate with the Dieterle stain or by direct fluorescent-antibody techniques. Other stains are less reliable. Many bacilli appear to be intracellular, and an increase in the number of organisms is associated with lysis of inflammatory cells.

Little is known about the pathogenesis of Legionnaires' pneumonia. The fact that cigarette smokers are more susceptible to infection than nonsmokers suggests that the defective alveolar macrophage function plays a role in the development of disease. Experimental evidence indicates that *L. pneumophila* can survive and proliferate in normal macrophages and other cells, a characteristic that has important pathogenetic implications. The extensive lysis of inflammatory cells and the edema of the interstitium raise the possibility that a toxin is produced by the Legionnaires' disease bacterium. Such a toxin might be responsible for some of the clinical features seen with this infection.

CLINICAL MANIFESTATIONS The total spectrum of clinical manifestations of Legionnaires' disease is not known. Mild respiratory illness has been recognized, but asymptomatic infection has not been excluded as a possible explanation for elevated antibody titers among healthy individuals. The outbreak in Pontiac, Michigan, was characterized by the acute onset and short duration of a moderately severe influenza-like syndrome of fever, myalgia, and headache.

The more typical patient with Legionnaires' disease has pneumonia that is severe enough to require hospitalization. Some patients have a constellation of symptoms that strongly suggest the diagnosis, particularly in a setting of known Legionnaires' disease activity. These patients have malaise and a slight headache, which precedes a rapidly rising fever by less than a day. Within 24 to 48 h, temperatures reach 40°C in about half the patients, and shaking chills are common. A modest, nonproductive cough frequently is present early; it progresses in severity over the first few days of illness and usually becomes productive of variable amounts of mucoid to mucopurulent sputum. Minimal hemoptysis is seen in about 20 percent of patients. Additional symptoms that occur less frequently include dyspnea, pleuritic chest pain, and myalgia. About 25 percent of patients have various combinations of gastrointestinal symptoms which include nausea and vomiting, diarrhea, and abdominal pain. In a few patients, these manifestations predominate despite the presence of pneumonia. In some individuals, the onset of Legionnaires' disease is more protracted and the clinical expression less distinctive. These cases are likely to be missed unless the epidemiologic setting or subtle clinical clues stimulate physicians to suspect the diagnosis. The findings on physical examination are not specific for Legionnaires' disease, and they are affected by patients' associated diseases. High fever, tachypnea, and tachycardia are common. Patients frequently are flushed, mildly diaphoretic, and appear moderately to severely prostrated. Examination of the chest shows moist rales, but signs of consolidation usually are absent. Chest roentgenograms characteristically show more involvement of the lungs than is suspected on clinical grounds.

During the first 4 to 6 days, the disease becomes progressively worse. An additional 4 to 5 days may pass before definite clinical improvement begins, even though appropriate antimicrobial therapy is given. The average duration of fever in one large series was 13 days. Clearing of pulmonary infiltrates lags significantly behind improvement of other manifestations of infection, and minor residual scarring is not uncommon. Many patients experience weakness and easy fatigability for weeks after the acute stages of the illness.

The major complication of Legionnaires' disease is respiratory failure. Twenty to thirty percent of patients sick enough to require hospitalization have hyperventilation and hypoxemia. In about half of these patients, progression of disease leads to intubation and mechanical ventilation. The mortality rate among patients with respiratory failure is high. Hypotension and shock, with secondary acute renal failure, are additional complications that may be encountered.

LABORATORY FINDINGS Most patients have a modest granulocytosis, but about 20 percent have leukocyte counts in excess of 20,000 per cubic millimeter. The erythrocyte sedimentation rate is elevated, and there is moderate proteinuria. Transient renal insufficiency and mild changes in liver function have been reported, but it is not always possible to attribute these abnormalities to the infection.

Chest roentgenograms show unilateral pulmonary parenchymal infiltrates in about 65 percent of cases early in the illness. By the time of maximal involvement, the pneumonia has progressed to involve both sides in most cases. Nonspecific poorly marginated rounded opacities or diffuse patchy lobar shadows predominate. Small pleural effusions are seen in about a third of cases.

Routine bacteriologic studies including blood and sputum cultures are negative. Lower respiratory tract secretions obtained by transtracheal aspiration or other suitable techniques show many granulocytes and alveolar macrophages but are sterile on Gram's stain and currently available culture media.

DIAGNOSIS In most instances, the diagnosis of Legionnaires' disease is dependent on demonstrating a fourfold or greater rise in serum antibody to a reciprocal titer of at least 128. Despite concerns about its sensitivity and specificity, the indirect fluorescent-antibody technique, using polyvalent antigens, is the most widely used method of serologic testing. Antibody titers rise slowly in some patients, so an acute-phase serum should be obtained as early as possible in the course of the illness and the convalescent-phase sample should be obtained at least 21 days after the onset of symptoms. Even later diagnostic titer rises have been observed in a few patients.

With increasing frequency, the diagnosis of Legionnaires' disease is being made by isolation of *L. pneumophila* from lung tissue, pleural fluid, blood, and sputum. The diagnosis also can be made by demonstrating organisms in tissue with the direct fluorescent-antibody (DFA) technique. A rapid presumptive diagnosis can be made by using DFA to identify organisms in the sputum of patients with pneumonia. Diagnoses made on the basis of sputum cultures or DFA-positive stains should be confirmed with serological tests. A new approach to rapid diagnosis, which involves radioimmunoassays or other techniques to identify antigen in the urine of infected patients, shows great promise. In centers where tests for antigen in urine, DFA stains, and cultures of sputum are being done routinely on all presumptive cases, a highly sensitive and specific diagnosis of Legionnaires' disease can be made within 3 to 4 days.

Legionnaires' disease may be difficult to differentiate from "atypical" pneumonias. When patients have a constellation of findings which include temperature elevations to 40°C, granulocytosis, and sterile lower respiratory tract secretions that contain many granulocytes and alveolar macrophages, Legionnaires' disease should be suspected. Infection with other organisms of the genus *Legionella* can be differentiated from Legionnaires' disease only by serological or microbiological tests. In immunocompromised patients, *Pneumocystis* or fungal infection enters into the differential diagnosis. Rarely, pulmonary embolism can be confused with early Legionnaires' disease.

TREATMENT Although in vitro sensitivity tests indicate that a number of antibiotics might be effective in the treatment of Legionnaires' disease, clinical experience has shown that the lowest case-fatality ratio is achieved with erythromycin in a dose of 0.5 to 1 g every 6 h for adults and 15 mg/kg every 6 h for children. Tetracycline is less effective. Rifampin has shown promise in laboratory testing, but its propensity to induce resistance may limit its potential usefulness.

Although the case-fatality ratio of patients treated with erythromycin is low, response to treatment frequently is not dramatic. If therapy is continued for at least 14 days, relapses are uncommon. When they occur, they usually respond to a second course of erythromycin. Because Legionnaires' disease can cause pneumonia in patients not sick enough to be hospitalized and who are assumed to have either *Mycoplasma* infection or early pneumococcal infection, erythromycin should be considered the drug of choice for the treatment of pneumonia in an ambulatory care setting.

There is more to treatment of Legionnaires' disease than administration of antibiotics. High fever, diaphoresis, and tachypnea produce excessive fluid loss, and volume replacement with intravenous fluids may be needed. Hypoxic patients should receive supplemental oxygen.

PROGNOSIS The overall mortality rate of Legionnaires' disease is unknown. Among patients with pneumonia who are sick enough to require hospitalization, the mortality rate is around 15 percent. The presence of complicating associated illnesses may raise that figure two- or threefold. Individuals who recover from Legionnaires' pneumonia usually have no significant residua. It is not known whether they are immune to reinfection with the same or related organisms.

REFERENCES

BEATY HN et al: Legionnaires' disease in Vermont, May to October 1977. JAMA 240:127, 1978

BLACKMON JA et al: Legionellosis. Am J Pathol 103:429, 1981

CORDES LG, PASCULLE AW: The Legionellae: Newly discovered agents of bacterial pneumonia, in *Update II: Harrison's Principles of Internal Medicine,* KJ Isselbacher et al (eds). New York, McGraw-Hill, 1982, pp 111–130

FRASER DW et al: Legionnaires' disease—description of an epidemic of pneumonia. N Engl J Med 297:1189, 1977

WINN WC et al: The pathology of Legionnaires' disease—fourteen fatal cases from the 1977 outbreak in Vermont. Arch Pathol Lab Med 102:344, 1978

163

PITTSBURGH PNEUMONIA AND OTHER INFECTIONS CAUSED BY RECENTLY DISCOVERED *LEGIONELLA* SPECIES

LESTER G. CORDES
A. WILLIAM PASCULLE

DEFINITION Following the isolation and characterization of *Legionella pneumophila,* six additional species of bacteria belonging to the genus *Legionella* have been discovered. These fastidious gram-negative bacteria resemble *L. pneumophila* in cultural characteristics and ecology but have distinct antigenic and genetic properties. Like *L. pneumophila,* the "newly discovered" legionellae can cause acute respiratory infections in humans and have been isolated from both human tissue and water-associated environments, often during searches for *L. pneumophila* (Table 163-1).

HISTORY ***Legionella micdadei*** This organism was first isolated in 1943 by Tatlock from the blood of two patients with an unusual febrile illness (Fort Bragg fever). Guinea pigs in-

TABLE 163-1
Seven species in the genus *Legionella*

Species	*Original designations (year of isolation)*	*Human isolations*	*Environmental isolations*
L. pneumophila	OLDA (1948) Legionnaires disease bacillus (1977)	Lung tissue Respiratory secretions Pleural fluid Blood	Cooling towers Riparian soil Tap water Shower heads Soil
L. micdadei	TATLOCK (1944) HEBA (1959) Pittsburgh pneumonia agent (1979)	Lung tissue Respiratory secretions Pleural fluid	Cooling towers Shower heads Tap water
L. bozemanii	WIGA (1959) Mi-15 (1979)	Lung tissue	None
L. dumoffii	NY-23 (1978) Tex-KL (1979)	Lung tissue	Cooling towers
L. gormanii	LS-13 (1979)	None	Riparian soil
L. longbeacheae	LB-4 (1981)	Lung tissue Respiratory secretions	None
L. jordanis	BL-540 (1978) ABB-9 (1980)	None	Riparian soil Treated sewage

SOURCE: *Adapted from Cordes and Pasculle.*

oculated with the patients' blood became febrile, and the organism was isolated from the animals' spleens. The bacterium could be propagated in embryonated eggs and guinea pigs but not on artificial media. Testing of paired serums failed to produce serological evidence of infection with this "rickettsia-like" organism, and later studies indicated that *Leptospira autumnalis* was the cause of Fort Bragg fever.

In 1959 Bozeman recovered a similar organism (HEBA) from guinea pigs inoculated with the blood of a patient with suspected pityriasis rosea. Testing of the patient's serum again failed to produce evidence that this organism was responsible for the patient's disease.

In 1978 two clusters of nosocomial pneumonia occurred among immunosuppressed patients in Pittsburgh, Pennsylvania, and Charlottesville, Virginia. Lung biopsy specimens revealed an acute purulent pneumonia caused by gram-negative, weakly acid-fast bacilli. Workers in Pittsburgh subsequently isolated the bacterium and produced serological evidence that this organism, originally termed Pittsburgh pneumonia agent (PPA), was responsible for the outbreaks in Pittsburgh and Charlottesville.

Subsequently, the TATLOCK and HEBA isolates and several isolates of PPA have been grown on media which support the growth of *L. pneumophila.* The isolates are antigenically and genetically similar to each other but distinct from *L. pneumophila* which they resemble culturally. The name *L. micdadei* was given to this group of organisms and honors Joseph McDade who made the first isolation of *L. pneumophila.*

Legionella bozemanii The first known isolate (WIGA) was recovered by Bozeman in 1959 by inoculating postmortem, into guinea pigs, lung tissue from a 38-year-old man who developed fatal pneumonia while scuba diving in Florida.

The second isolate (Mi-15) was recovered in 1979 from ante- and postmortem lung tissue from a 60-year-old man with untreated chronic lymphocytic leukemia who developed pneumonia several weeks following a boating accident in which he was submerged in brackish swampy water. The organism was recovered on charcoal yeast extract agar, in embryonated eggs, and in guinea pigs. The patient's serum demonstrated a rise in antibody titer to both the WIGA and Mi-15 antigens. Genetic and antigenic analysis has shown the two isolates to be similar, and the name *L. bozemanii* was proposed.

Serologic testing of serums originally submitted to the Centers for Disease Control for *L. pneumophila* serology has identified additional patients with community-acquired pneumonia who have developed antibody to *L. bozemanii.* Immunofluorescent studies of autopsy tissues from patients with undiagnosed pneumonias have uncovered two additional cases of *L. bozemanii* infection. One occurred in a patient in Vermont with chronic renal failure and the other in a renal transplant recipient in Boston.

Legionella dumoffii The first isolate (NY-23) was cultured from an air conditioner cooling tower in 1978 during the investigation of an outbreak of Legionnaires' disease in New York City. A second isolate (Tex-KL) was recovered in 1979 from postmortem lung tissue of a patient with pneumonia in Texas who had received steroids and cytotoxic drugs for oat-cell carcinoma. A second case of infection occurred in an 18-year-old woman with systemic lupus erythematosus who had been receiving high-dose steroids and died of overwhelming pneumonia.

The name *L. dumoffii* honors Morris Dumoff who made the first isolation of *L. pneumophila* on artificial media.

Legionella longbeacheae This organism was isolated in 1980 from respiratory specimens from four patients with community-acquired pneumonia in California and Georgia. Two cases were fatal. The name honors the city of Long Beach, California, where the bacterium was first isolated.

Legionella gormanii The only known isolate (LS-13) of this species was found in riparian soil during the investigation of an outbreak of Legionnaires' disease among golfers at an Atlanta country club. The name honors George Gorman of the Centers for Disease Control for his work with the legionellae.

Legionella jordanis This organism was first isolated from water samples taken from the Jordan River in 1978 during the investigation of an outbreak of Legionnaires' disease in Bloomington, Indiana. In 1980, a similar organism was isolated from the effluent of a sewage treatment plant near Atlanta. The name honors the Jordan River where the first strain was isolated.

ETIOLOGY The newly discovered legionellae share several characteristics with *L. pneumophila.* Most notable is their requirement for iron and cysteine in artificial culture media. As a result, they do not grow on common artificial media, and several were initially cultivated only in embryonated eggs and in guinea pigs. All currently recognized species of *Legionella,* however, can be cultivated on buffered or unbuffered charcoal yeast extract agar (BCYE, CYE) from which they appear as gram-negative, non-acid-fast rods 0.3 to 0.4 μm in width and 2 to 3 μm in length.

The legionellae are biochemically inert and cannot be identified by use of standard microbiological tests. The important phenotypic characteristics of the seven species of *Legionella* are listed in Table 163-2. Identification of the legionellae, however, is best made by direct fluorescent antibody (DFA) staining using conjugated antiserums prepared against the known species and serotypes. There are currently six recognized serotypes of *L. pneumophila,* two serotypes of *L. longbeacheae,* and one serotype for each of the remaining species. Since there are few serological cross-reactions between these organisms, identification of an isolate requires the use of a large number of conjugates. In the future, however, the procedure may become simpler as polyvalent antibody pools become available.

DNA relatedness studies allow for the definitive identification of species and the recognition of new species. These studies have shown that the seven species of *Legionella* are not closely related to each other.

EPIDEMIOLOGY Knowledge of the epidemiology of these organisms is incomplete owing to the small number of recognized cases of infection. Approximately 30 cases of culturally proven *L. micdadei* infection have been recognized. In addition to the hospital-associated clusters of infection previously described, sporadic cases have occurred in several other areas of the country. Two-thirds of patients are male, and ages range from 20 to 80 years. Most patients have been immunocompromised either by their underlying disease or by immunosuppressive therapy or both. Many have received high-dose corticosteroid therapy within 3 weeks of the onset of their disease. Twelve were renal transplant recipients, six had leukemia or lymphoma, and the remainder had miscellaneous conditions. Occasional cases also have been community-acquired by relatively healthy persons. Serological studies indicate that infections with the other species of *Legionella* are more common than previously thought. These studies also suggest that infections may be both community- and hospital-acquired, may occur in both healthy and immunosuppressed patients, and may be subclinical.

TABLE 163-2
Phenotypic properties of the various species of *Legionella*

Characteristic	*L. pneumophila*	*L. longbeacheae*	*L. micdadei*	*L. jordanis*	*L. bozemanii*	*L. dumoffii*	*L. gormanii*
Requires iron and cysteine for primary isolation (CYE, BCYE agar)	+	+	+	+	+	+	+
Primary growth on FG agar	V	–	–	–	–	–	–
Brown pigment from tyrosine	+	+	+	+	+	+	NG
Fluorescence	Dull yellow	Dull yellow	Dull yellow	Dull yellow	Blue-white	Blue-white	Blue-white
Catalase	+	+	+	+	+	+	+
Oxidase	+	+	+	+	–	–	–
Gelatinase	+	+	+	+	+	+	+
Hippurate	+	–	–	–	–	–	–
β-lactamase	+	W+,–	–	+	+W	+W	+
Number of serotypes	6	2	1	1	1	1	1

NOTE: *NG = no growth on media used for test, W = most strains give weak reaction, + = most strains give positive reaction, V = variable.*
SOURCE: *Adapted from Cordes and Pasculle.*

The reservoirs and modes of spread of these organisms are not well defined. Preliminary evidence suggests that all the legionellae thrive in moist environments. *L. micdadei* has been isolated from water in ultrasonic nebulizers and cooling towers, and shower head scrapings. However, none of these isolations has been linked conclusively to human infection. The initial isolations of *L. dumoffii, L. gormanii,* and *L. jordanis* from water and riparian soil further suggest that the legionellae thrive in moist environments. *L. bozemannii* and *L. longbeacheae* have not been isolated from the environment.

The mode of transmission is unknown, but it is reasonable to suspect that the bacteria gain entrance to the body via the respiratory tract from a presumed environmental source. The incubation period is probably similar to that of Legionnaires' disease. No evidence of person-to-person spread has been found.

CLINICAL AND LABORATORY FINDINGS Most patients have acute onset of fever accompanied by a pulmonary infiltrate. In some hospitalized patients onset may be insidious, and the infection is first detected on routine chest roentgenogram. Patients usually develop a nonproductive cough which is often accompanied by pleuritic chest pain, dyspnea, tachypnea, and hypoxemia. Because many of the reported patients were immunosuppressed, leukocyte counts have been variable. Leukocytosis or leukopenia may be seen. Abnormal liver function tests have been common; however, too little information is available to determine whether the other multisystem abnormalities often associated with Legionnaires' disease are also characteristic of these infections.

Roentgenographic findings are similar to those of Legionnaires' disease. Pulmonary infiltrates may involve one or several lobes of the lung. The lesions appear radiographically as patchy areas of bronchopneumonia, as well-circumscribed nodular infiltrates, or as segmental or wedge-shaped lesions. Pleural effusions may occur. In several cases lesions have progressed to consolidation of one or more lobes and involvement of the opposite lung field. Occasionally, cavitary abscesses are seen.

Routine blood and urine cultures are usually sterile. Sputum cultures may yield either normal flora or common hospital-acquired organisms. Gram stains of sputum often reveal large numbers of inflammatory cells. Transtracheal aspirates are usually sterile on routine culture although they may contain large numbers of inflammatory cells without readily visible organisms on gram stain.

PATHOLOGY The pathologic findings are similar to those of Legionnaires' disease. Lung biopsy specimens usually reveal an acute purulent bronchopneumonia. The alveolar exudate is composed primarily of polymorphonuclear leukocytes, but later in the disease monocytes begin to appear. The alveolar walls are congested, but the basic architecture of the lung is not destroyed. The pleural surface may be covered by a fibrinopurulent exudate. In the most advanced stages of the disease leukocytoclasis is often present with necrosis of the alveolar walls and frank abscess formation.

The lung tissue usually contains large numbers of organisms which can be visualized by several techniques. The bacilli are generally present within inflammatory cells, but extracellular forms are also seen. *L. micdadei,* like *L. pneumophila,* appear as faintly staining thin gram-negative rods. *L. bozemanii* and *L. dumoffii* are variable in their staining characteristics, appearing either gram-negative or slightly gram-positive. Modified Ziehl-Neelson stains will demonstrate the weak acid-fastness of *L. micdadei. L. bozemanii* and *L. dumoffii* (and *L. pneumophila*) on occasion may also be weakly acid-fast.

All the legionellae stain well with the Dieterle silver stain. This stain will usually demonstrate many more bacilli in tissue than other tissue stains. It is not specific for the legionellae and will identify most other bacteria. The Dieterle stain is best interpreted in conjunction with standard tissue stains, and, when possible, results should be confirmed by culture and immunofluorescent staining.

DIAGNOSIS The diagnosis of infections caused by the newer legionellae can be made by culture and immunofluorescent staining of specimens or by serological testing of patient serums. Materials suitable for culture are lung tissue, transtracheal aspirates, and pleural fluid.

Specimens should be inoculated onto CYE or BCYE agar, as are specimens for the isolation of *L. pneumophila.* Sputum is not a reliable specimen for culture because the media used are not selective and the legionellae are readily overgrown (and possibly inhibited) by other bacteria found in sputum. Selective media used for the isolation of *L. pneumophila* may not be suitable for the isolation of many of the newer legionellae because the media contain cephalosporins which inhibit the growth of many of these bacteria in vitro.

DFA staining is useful for the demonstration of organisms both in fresh and fixed lung tissue and respiratory secretions. Conjugated antiserums are now available for all the currently recognized species and serotypes of *Legionella.* Because the newly recognized legionellae do not appear to share antigens, each specimen must be tested separately with conjugates prepared against each of the species. The sensitivity of DFA testing of respiratory secretions remains to be determined. As with Legionnaires' disease, however, maximal diagnostic yield will occur only if specimens are subjected to both culture and immunofluorescent staining. While the conjugates appear to be highly specific for their respective organisms under laboratory conditions, no data exist concerning possible cross-reactions with organisms in sputum. If sputa are found to be positive by DFA testing, the results should be confirmed by culture and serological testing if possible.

Serological testing using an indirect fluorescent antibody technique is available through reference laboratories. Comprehensive testing requires a large number of antigens, but polyvalent reagents may become available in the future. Most patients with disease caused by one species of *Legionella* have produced antibody only to that species, but a few patients have produced antibody against more than one species or serotype. At least two patients have been seen with culturally documented infection with both *L. pneumophila* and *L. micdadei,* suggesting that some of the previous patients with multiple antibody responses may have had multiple infections. Accurately collected paired serums are essential for diagnosis. An acute-phase specimen should be collected within the first week of illness, and a convalescent specimen about 21 days after disease onset. Most patients with documented infections have demonstrated a fourfold rise in titer of $\geq$ 128 or a standing single titer of at least 256. Additional studies are required to assess the sensitivity and specificity of these criteria.

THERAPY AND PROGNOSIS In vitro susceptibility testing of the newly discovered legionellae has shown susceptibility to a wide range of antibiotics. However, early clinical experience with Pittsburgh pneumonia suggested that penicillins, cephalosporins, and aminoglycosides were ineffective. Erythromycin, to which all species of *Legionella* are susceptible, and rifampin are the current drugs of choice for the treatment of legionellosis. At present, erythromycin, 1 g given orally or intravenously every 6 h, is used to treat patients with Pittsburgh pneumonia. In one series of eight patients, six treated with erythromycin were cured. Two patients with cavitary disease required the addition of rifampin, 600 mg every 12 h, for successful therapy. No good clinical data exist concerning the use of erythromycin for the treatment of pneumonia caused by the other species of *Legionella,* but their in vitro susceptibility and the excellent therapeutic response seen in Legionnaires' disease and Pittsburgh pneumonia make erythromycin the drug of choice.

Therapy should be continued for at least 2 weeks, and patients with cavitary disease should probably be treated until the cavities resolve. Some patients have become afebrile within 24 h, while others have remained febrile for several days. As in Legionnaires' disease, resolution of the infiltrates radiographically has been slow in most cases, and a lack of radiologic response does not imply that therapy has been unsuccessful. Moreover, as has been reported with Legionnaires' disease, organisms may persist in the sputum for several weeks while the patient is receiving adequate therapy and improving clinically. Most patients who have recovered have done so without serious sequelae, although more data on the outcome of the newer forms of legionellosis are needed.

REFERENCES

Cordes LG, Pasculle AW: The *Legionellae:* Newly discovered agents of bacterial pneumonia, in *Update II: Harrison's Principles of Internal Medicine,* KJ Isselbacher et al (eds). New York, McGraw-Hill, 1982, pp 111–130

——— et al: Atypical *Legionella*-like organisms: Fastidious water-associated bacteria pathogenic for man. Lancet 2:927, 1979

Hébert GA et al: The Rickettsia-like organisms TATLOCK (1943) and HEBA (1959): Bacteria phenotypically similar to but genetically distinct from *Legionella pneumophila* and the WIGA bacillus. Ann Intern Med 92:45, 1980

——— et al: A bacterium phenotypically similar to *Legionella pneumophila* and identical to the TATLOCK bacterium. Ann Intern Med 92:53, 1980

Lewallen KR et al: A newly-identified bacterium phenotypically resembling but genetically distinct from *Legionella pneumophila:* An isolate in a case of pneumonia. Ann Intern Med 91:831, 1980

McKinney RM et al: *Legionella longbeacheae* species nova, another etiologic agent of human pneumonia. Ann Intern Med 94:739, 1981

Myerowitz RL et al: Opportunistic lung infection due to "Pittsburgh Pneumonia Agent." N Engl J Med 301:953, 1979

Rogers BH et al: Opportunistic pneumonia: A clinicopathologic study of five cases caused by an unidentified acid-fast bacterium. N Engl J Med 301:959, 1979

164
INFECTIONS CAUSED BY *LISTERIA MONOCYTOGENES* AND *ERYSIPELOTHRIX RHUSIOPATHIAE*

PAUL D. HOEPRICH

LISTERIA MONOCYTOGENES INFECTIONS

DEFINITION Listeriosis, a disease caused by *L. monocytogenes,* consists of many clinical syndromes. Perinatal infection, acquired either transplacentally or during parturition, is the most nearly unique form of listeriosis.

ETIOLOGY *Listeria monocytogenes* are gram-positive, non-acid-fast, microaerophilic, motile bacilli that form smooth colonies but do not produce either capsules or spores. Several serotypes have been defined on the basis of O and H antigens. The epidemiologically essential aid of typing is available from the Centers for Disease Control in Atlanta, Georgia. Types 4b, 1b, and 1a account for more than 90 percent of the cases worldwide. Weakly hemolytic gram-positive bacilli are presumed to be listerias if they are motile (when grown at 20 to 25°C), reduce 2,3,5-triphenyltetrazolium chloride, and display characteristic animal pathogenicity. The Anton test is classic: 3 to 5 days after inoculation into the conjunctival sac of a rabbit or a guinea pig, *L. monocytogenes* causes a keratoconjunctivitis. Also, general listeriosis in the rabbit typically provokes a monocytosis, and focal hepatic necrosis is usual in lethal murine listeriosis.

EPIDEMIOLOGY AND PATHOGENESIS Found on every continent save the Antarctic, *L. monocytogenes* are distinct from the nonhemolytic, nonpathogenic, nonmonocytogenic, and serologically different bacilli (found mainly in soil, decaying matter, and feces) which have been variously assigned either to the genus *Listeria* or to a new genus *Murrayi.* Although typical *L. monocytogenes* have been isolated from silage, other vegetative sources, and 5 to 60 percent of specimens of human feces, listeriosis is uncommon and occurs sporadically; moreover, listeriosis is actually more common in urban than rural dwellers, occurring most frequently in July and August (northern hemisphere). The reservoir from which human beings become infected is frequently occult and the mode of transmission often obscure. Direct transmission from an infected nonhuman animal via contaminated secretions has been documented only rarely. On the other hand, transmission from the infected pregnant female to her offspring is well established as a route of infection.

Transplacental perinatal infection results in disseminated fetal listeriosis. The fetus is usually stillborn or is prematurely ejected, virtually always with lethal listeriosis. Fetal listeriosis acquired during delivery is typically not clinically evident for 1 or 2 weeks postpartum and usually presents as a meningitis.

Listeriosis is preponderantly a disease of persons under 1 year and over 55 years of age.

Persons in apparent good health may develop listeriosis. However, other diseases, particularly those with diminished cell-mediated immunity (listerias are cytophilic), facilitate the occurrence of listeriosis: for example, neoplasms (especially of the lymphoreticular system) and any conditions requiring treatment with pharmacologic doses of glucosteroids, irradiation, or cytotoxic agents; alcoholism; cardiovascular disease; diabetes mellitus; and tuberculosis.

MANIFESTATIONS *Listeriosis of the newborn,* the most nearly unique clinical form of listeriosis, ranges from meningitis that is clinically apparent within 1 month postpartum to diffuse disseminated disease in aborted, premature, stillborn infants, and neonates, who die within minutes to days after birth. If clinical disease is delayed to 1 to 4 weeks postpartum, it is generally localized to the central nervous system, as is the rule when children 1 month to 6 years of age are afflicted.

Infants born alive with listeriosis may or may not have fever; yet these babies are critically ill, with cardiorespiratory distress, vomiting, and diarrhea. Dark-red skin papules are frequent, particularly on the lower extremities. Hepatosplenomegaly may be present. This form of listeriosis is also known as septic or miliary granulomatosis. The findings at necropsy are characteristic and mimic those seen in listeriosis of rodents: widely disseminated abscesses varying in size from grossly visible to microscopic, involving, in order of decreasing frequency, liver, spleen, adrenal glands, lungs, pharynx, gastrointestinal tract, central nervous system, and skin. Typically, the lesions are abscesses, but classic granulomas may be seen, depending principally on the duration of infection before death. Microscopic examination of a Gram-stained smear of meconium from the normal newborn infant does not disclose bacteria; fetal listeriosis results in meconium laden with gram-positive bacilli. For this reason, examination of meconium by Gram's stain and by culture should be carried out whenever there is gross soiling of the amniotic liquid with meconium, prematurity, or unexplained fever in the mother before or at the onset of labor. This is particularly important because listeriosis in the pregnant woman may be asymptomatic or may cause a nonspecific illness. Thus, a week to a month prepartum, there may have been malaise, a chill, diarrhea, pain in the back or flanks, and itching. Even when symptomatic, the disease is benign and self-limited in the mother; however, as symptoms subside, a decrease or cessation of fetal movement may be noted. Infection of the fetus may occur as early as the fifth month of gestation but occurs most often in the third trimester. Following delivery of infants with proved fetal listeriosis, cervical cultures are, or soon become, negative for *L. monocytogenes;* subsequent conception, gestation, and delivery of normal offspring are usual.

Meningitis accounts for about three-fourths of the cases verified by culture and is the predominant clinical form of listeriosis. Meningitis caused by *L. monocytogenes* cannot be distinguished from meningitis caused by other kinds of bacteria.

Nonmeningeal listeriosis of the central nervous system is associated with fever, nausea and vomiting, headache, and listeremia; the cerebrospinal fluid is normal. Localizing neurologic signs may develop (especially if abscess forms), or the picture may be that of an encephalitis.

Listeremia that has no identifiable source and is associated with high fever and severe prostrating illness (typhoidal listeriosis) occurs most often in patients with cancers and immunosuppression. However, primary listeremia may also develop in patients with cirrhosis, alcoholism, pregnancy, and no discernible underlying disease.

Listerial endocarditis is generally a chronic process without singular manifestations. About half of the patients have no known predisposing cardiac disease.

Other rare forms of listeriosis include ocular infections, dermatitis, infections of serous cavities, and abscesses in various organs.

LABORATORY FINDINGS Although *L. monocytogenes* bacilli grow well on the usual culture media, etiologic diagnosis by isolation and identification may be hampered by failure of differentiation from *Corynebacterium* spp., *Erysipelothrix rhusiopathiae,* and *Streptococcus* spp. Recognition of listerial colonies in a mixed culture, as may result with vaginal or cervical specimens, is difficult and may be aided by using selective media and/or enrichment procedures.

Serodiagnosis by assay for agglutinins has not been useful because of the common finding of so-called natural antibodies. Such nonspecific reactions may reflect the known antigenic relationship between *Staphylococcus aureus* and several listerial serotypes. The humoral antibody response to listeriosis in humans is almost exclusively IgM throughout the disease, whereas staphylococci elicit IgG as well as IgM; i.e., treatment of serums with 2-mercaptoethanol may not eliminate nonspecific reactivity.

Monocytosis is not common in human listeriosis. Leukocytosis with neutrophilia, as in any acute bacterial infection, is seen in listerial meningitis, nonmeningeal infection of the central nervous system, primary listeremia, listerial endocarditis, and abscesses in hosts capable of mounting a granulocytic response. The cerebrospinal fluid in meningitis is compatible with that in other purulent meningitides.

DIFFERENTIAL DIAGNOSIS Abortion, premature delivery, stillbirth, and neonatal death are more often due to causes other than listeriosis: Rh incompatibility, syphilis, or toxoplasmosis.

In patients with leptomeningitis, conjunctivitis, endocarditis, bacteremia, or polyserositis, reports of isolation of "diphtheroids" or "nonpathogens" must always be challenged. A statement that *L. monocytogenes* has been excluded should be required.

TREATMENT *Listeria monocytogenes* are susceptible to several antimicrobals in vitro, including penicillin G, ampicillin, erythromycin, rifampin, streptomycin, gentamicin, tobramycin, and the tetracyclines. Tolerance, i.e., inhibition at low concentrations with much higher concentrations needed for killing, is characteristic with the penicillins, erythromycin, rifampin, and streptomycin. Accordingly, combination therapy is necessary for maximally listericidal therapy, e.g., penicillin G [150 to 200 mg (240,000 to 320,000 units) per kilogram of body weight per day, intravenously, as six equal portions every 4 h] plus tobramycin (5 to 6 mg per kilogram of body weight per day, intravenously, as three equal portions every 8 h). Ampicillin and gentamicin (same dosages) may be substituted but offer no advantage. Such treatment is appropriate for listeriosis of the newborn (2 weeks), listeremia in pregnancy (2 weeks), primary listeremia (4 weeks), listerial endocarditis (4 to 6 weeks), and any form of listeriosis outside the central nervous system in immunosuppressed patients (4 to 6 weeks).

As gentamicin and tobramycin do not enter the central nervous system reliably, high-dosage therapy with penicillin G [200 to 300 mg (320,000 to 480,000 units) per kilogram of body weight per day, intravenously, as six equal portions every 4 h] is the primary treatment. Ampicillin may be substituted in the same dose, but the cephalosporins currently available enter the central nervous system too poorly to be useful. In patients who are allergic to the penicillins, tetracycline may be given (15 mg per kilogram of body weight per day, intravenously, as four equal portions every 6 h). Treatment should be continued in full dosage by intravenous injection for at least 7 days after defervescence.

PROGNOSIS Prompt, vigorous antimicrobial treatment of the acute forms of listeriosis, excepting fetal listeriosis, is usually curative. On the basis of agglutinin titers, specific antibody disappears during the months following cure. However, reinfection has not been reported.

ERYSIPELOTHRIX RHUSIOPATHIAE INFECTIONS

DEFINITION Erysipeloid is the commonest and most nearly unique form of infection in humans caused by *Erysipelothrix rhusiopathiae.* Infective endocarditis and arthritis are rare forms of erysipelothricosis in human beings.

ETIOLOGY As gram-positive, microaerophilic bacilli, *E. rhusiopathiae* may be confused with nontoxinogenic *Corynebacterium* spp. and *Listeria monocytogenes.* However, *E. rhusiopathiae* is nonmotile and fails to grow on media selective for *Corynebacterium* spp. Also, unlike *L. monocytogenes, E. rhusiopathiae* only rarely causes conjunctivitis, following conjunctival inoculation, or monocytosis, after intravenous inoculation, in the rabbit. Because alpha hemolysis is commonly evident after 48 h of incubation of *E. rhusiopathiae,* confusion with streptococci may also occur. Isolates of *E. rhusiopathiae* appear to be serologically homogeneous. Although serodifferentiation from other gram-positive bacilli is possible, few laboratories are capable of definitive serodiagnosis.

EPIDEMIOLOGY AND PATHOGENESIS Primarily a saprophyte, *E. rhusiopathiae* is worldwide in distribution. Human beings are virtually always infected by traumatic dermal inoculation; erysipeloid is the usual result. The disease is almost wholly restricted to persons who in their occupations handle edible or nonedible dead animal products. If the bacilli are not successfully confined to the skin, bacteremia may result and may lead to infective endocarditis; in about two-thirds of the reported cases, there was no evidence of preexisting valvular heart disease.

The seasonal incidence of erysipeloid parallels that of swine erysipelas, being highest in summer and early fall. Yet persons who tend pigs, even pigs ill with porcine erysipelas, do not commonly develop erysipeloid.

MANIFESTATIONS Erysipeloid begins 2 to 7 days after injury, often after the initial lesion has healed. An itching, burning, painful irritation may precede and always accompanies the appearance of the maculopapular, nonvesiculated, sharply defined, raised, purplish-red zone surrounding the site of entry. There is local swelling, and when, as is usual, a finger or the hand is involved, nearby joints may become stiff and painful. Centrifugal spread from the site of inoculation is apparent in a day or so. Movement is slow, 1 to 2 cm per 24 h maximally, and more rapid proximally than distally; involvement of the terminal phalanx of a finger is rare, while spread to other fingers and the hand distal to the wrist is common. With extension, the original center subsides without desquamation or suppuration. There are usually no systemic signs or symptoms; regional lymphangitis and lymphadenitis are rare. Untreated, the disease heals within 3 weeks in most patients, although relapse has been observed.

The manifestations of erysipelothrical endocarditis may be either acute or chronic, depending on the virulence of the infecting strain and on the state of resistance of the host. Usually, there are no classic erysipeloid skin lesions to suggest the disease at the time that endocarditis is clinically evident. However, a history of recent erysipeloid may be helpful.

Erysipelothrical arthritis is not clinically characteristic but usually can be related to erysipeloid or erysipelothrical bacteremia. Isolation of *E. rhusiopathiae* from synovial fluid has not been reported.

LABORATORY FINDINGS The usual culture media are adequate for the growth of *E. rhusiopathiae*. However, differentiation from diphtheroids, listerias, and streptococci depends primarily on the clinician's alerting the laboratory to the possibility of erysipelothricosis.

In erysipeloid, *E. rhusiopathiae* are best recovered by incubating, in broth containing glucose, a full-thickness biopsy of skin removed from the advancing edge of a lesion. Culture of an aspirate obtained after injection of sterile, bacteriostat-free 0.9% NaCl solution into the periphery of a lesion is less likely to yield *E. rhusiopathiae.*

With endocarditis and arthritis, the findings are in keeping with the respective clinical syndromes and are in no way characteristic for *E. rhusiopathiae.*

DIFFERENTIAL DIAGNOSIS The appearance and location of erysipeloid, its slow and limited spread, the lack of constitutional reaction, the history of occupation and injury, all serve to identify this disease. The afflicted skin in *erysipelas* is very erythematous, and the face and scalp are affected; there are regional lymphangitis and lymphadenitis, leukocytosis, fever, and malaise. Eczematous lesions may itch, but they display vesicles and little abnormal color. The various erythemas have a different location and do not usually itch or burn; they are more apt to be chronic and nonmigratory.

TREATMENT The penicillins, the cephalosporins, erythromycin, clindamycin, the tetracyclines, and chloramphenicol inhibit *E. rhusiopathiae* in vitro at concentrations practical in therapy. Penicillin G is the agent of choice. Erysipeloid is adequately treated by injection of 1.2 million units of benzathine penicillin G. Erythromycin (15 mg/kg per day in four equal portions taken orally for 5 to 7 days) is an alternative. Cure of erysipelothrical endocarditis has been effected by the daily injection of 2 to 20 million units of penicillin per day for 4 to 6 weeks; the dose should be monitored by determination of the bactericidal activity of serum from the patient against his infecting strain. Intractable cardiac failure may oblige surgical excision of an infected valve and insertion of a prosthesis.

PROGNOSIS Penicillin therapy is highly effective in curing erysipelothrical infections. As with infective endocarditis from any cause, the prognosis is primarily a function of the severity of the valvular damage. Of cases reported since penicillin became available, about 25 percent were fatal; earlier diagnosis, and, perhaps, earlier resort to surgical excision and replacement of infected valves, may improve the outcome.

REFERENCES

BOJSEN-MOLLER J: Human listeriosis. Diagnostic, epidemiological and clinical studies. Acta Pathol Microbiol Scand B 229:13, 1972

HALLIDAY HL, HIRATA T: Perinatal listeriosis—a review of twelve patients. Am J Obstet Gynecol 133:405, 1979

HOEPRICH PD: Listeriosis, in *Infectious Diseases,* 3d ed, PD Hoeprich (ed). Philadelphia, Lippincott-Harper, 1982, chap 51

———: Erysipeloid, in *Infectious Diseases,* 3d ed, PD Hoeprich (ed). Philadelphia, Lippincott-Harper, 1982, chap 103

KAMPELMACHER EH et al: Listeriosis in humans and animals in the Netherlands (1958–1977). Zentralb Bakteriol Hyg (Orig) 246:211, 1980

NELSON E: Five hundred cases of erysipeloid. Rocky Mount Med J 52:40, 1955

NIEMAN RE, LORBER B: Listeriosis in adults: A changing pattern. Report of 8 cases and review of the literature, 1968–1978. Rev Infect Dis 2:207, 1980

RELIER JP: Listeriosis. J Antimicrob Chemother 5(Suppl):51, 1979

SEELIGER HPR: *Listeriosis.* Basel, Karger, 1961

165
DIPHTHERIA

JAMES P. HARNISCH

DEFINITION Diphtheria is an acute infectious disease produced by *Corynebacterium diphtheriae.* It is characterized by a local inflammatory lesion, usually in the upper part of the respiratory tract, and a toxic reaction involving primarily the heart and peripheral nerves.

ETIOLOGY *Corynebacterium diphtheriae* is a gram-positive, nonsporulating, nonmotile rod. There is a characteristic swelling at one end of the bacillus, which gives it a club shape. A Chinese-letter configuration is usually seen in stained smears owing to the alignment of the bacilli at sharp angles with each other. Diphtheria bacilli have been classifed into *mitis, gravis,* and *intermedius* groups on the basis of colonial morphology, appearance on tellurite medium, fermentation reactions, and ability to produce hemolysis. European workers have suggested that there is a significant difference in the clinical manifestations and in the severity of disease related to the strain; gravis and intermedius infections are thought to be accompanied by more severe toxic manifestations and a higher death rate. In the United States, the gravis strain is comparatively uncommon, and less significance is attached to the relationship of the type of organism and the clinical form of the disease.

Corynebacterium diphtheriae produces a protein exotoxin which is responsible for many of the clinical manifestations; as little as 0.0001 mg is lethal for guinea pigs. Strains of diphtheria bacilli which elaborate exotoxin are lysogenic. Absence of lysogeny generally is associated with lack of toxin formation and virulence. However, symptomatic diphtheria may also follow invasion by strains of *C. diphtheriae* that cannot be shown to produce toxin.

EPIDEMIOLOGY Diphtheria occurs primarily in the temperate zone and is still very common in some parts of the world. Since 1966, there has been an irregular increase in the number of cases of diphtheria in the United States. Two outbreaks in Texas early in the 1970s accounted for most of the cases. However, since 1973, more than 75 percent of the cases were reported from the Pacific northwest and the southwest. The western provinces of Canada experienced a similar increase in diphtheria. Until this geographic trend was recognized, the highest frequency had been in children between 1 and 9 years of age. The attack rate for unimmunized children was 70 times higher than the rate for children who had received primary immunization. In the Pacific northwest, isolates have been obtained predominantly from adults with symptomatic skin lesions. Another striking change has been a decrease in the incidence of laryngeal involvement. In general, diphtheria is acquired by droplet transmission from active cases or carriers, but fomites may play a role in the spread of cutaneous infection. Each diphtheria infection must be classifed as either a case or a carrier. A *case* is an individual who is colonized in the respiratory tract with *C. diphtheriae* and is symptomatic. The concomitant presence of other organisms, such as beta-hemolytic streptococci, does not change the definition or prognosis of a diphtheria case. A *carrier* is colonized with *C. diphtheriae* but lacks symptoms. No attempt should be made to classify an instance of cutaneous diphtheria as a case or a carrier.

PATHOGENESIS AND PATHOLOGY The commonest portal of entry for the diphtheria bacillus is the upper respiratory tract. The skin, genitalia, eye, and middle ear may also be sites of invasion. Growth of the organism is superficial in most cases, and there is little tendency to invade the lymphatics or bloodstream except in the terminal stages. The exotoxin elaborated in the local lesion is absorbed and carried by the blood to all parts of the body. The intensity of the toxic effects is greatest when the primary lesion is in the pharynx, less when it is in the larynx, and least when it is on the nasal mucosa or skin. Simultaneous involvement of the pharynx, larynx, trachea, and bronchial tree is associated with most severe intoxication.

The *membrane,* the primary lesion of diphtheria, is thick, leathery, and blue-white and is composed of bacteria, necrotic epithelium, phagocytes, and fibrin. It is surrounded by a narrow zone of inflammation and is firmly adherent to the underlying tissues; bleeding follows its forcible removal. Ulceration is not a regular feature. Regional lymphadenitis is frequent.

The *toxic manifestations* involve primarily the heart, kidneys, and peripheral nerves. The brain is rarely affected. Cardiac enlargement is frequent; this appears to be related to myocarditis rather than hypertrophy. The kidneys may be enlarged and reveal cloudy swelling and interstitial changes. Bronchopneumonia due to *C. diphtheriae* or to secondary invading organisms occurs in some patients, especially those with laryngeal involvement. Membrane is present throughout the bronchial tree when the diphtheria bacillus is responsible for the pulmonary infection. The peripheral nerves may reveal fatty degeneration, disintegration of the medullary sheaths, and involvement of the axis cylinder. Both motor and sensory fibers are affected, but the main impact is on the motor innervation. The anterior horn cells and the posterior columns of the spinal cord may be damaged. Other central nervous system involvement includes cerebral hemorrhage, meningitis, and encephalitis. Petechial and purpuric lesions are occasionally present in the kidneys, skin, or adrenals. Endocarditis due to *C. diphtheriae* is rare.

Death results from respiratory obstruction by membrane or edema, or from the effects of toxin on the heart, nervous system, or other organs.

IMMUNITY Susceptibility to the complications of diphtheria is related to the presence or absence of circulating antibody to exotoxin. The Schick test yields a rough estimate of the quantity of antitoxin in the circulation. This test is carried out in the following manner: 0.1 ml purified diphtheria toxin (one-fiftieth the minimum lethal dose) dissolved in buffered human serum albumin is injected intradermally on the volar surface of the forearm; 0.1 ml purified diphtheria toxoid is injected into the other arm as a control. These areas are examined at 24 and 48 h and between the fourth and seventh days and interpreted in the following way:

1 Positive reaction. The site of injection of toxin begins to redden in 24 h; the reddening increases and reaches a maximum in about a week, at which time the lesion may be as large as 3 cm in diameter and moderately swollen and tender. There is usually a small (1 to 1.5 cm) dark-red central zone which gradually turns brown, desquamates, and leaves a pigmented area. The area of toxoid injection shows no reaction. A positive test indicates little or no circulating antitoxin and no immunity.

2 *Negative reaction.* There is no reaction at the site of injection of either toxoid or toxin. This is consistent with a blood antitoxin level of 1/30 to 1/100 unit and immunity to ordinary exposure.
3 *Pseudoreaction.* Inflammation at both sites of injection within 12 to 14 h, which reaches a maximum in 48 to 72 h and then fades. This usually indicates immunity plus hypersensitivity to the toxin or other materials in the solution.
4 *Combined reaction.* This begins like the pseudoreaction, but the inflammatory response at the toxin site persists after that in the area of toxoid injection has faded. It indicates delayed sensitivity to toxin or other proteins and either low levels or no antitoxin. The incidence of combined reactions increases with age and is highest in unimmunized groups living in areas where diphtheria is prevalent.

Individuals with negative Schick tests occasionally contract diphtheria, and some persons with positive Schick reactions do not develop the disease after exposure. In some parts of the United States fewer than 50 percent of adults have "protective" levels of circulating antitoxin. The Schick test is not used routinely in the United States, and the lack of ability to perform it should not delay the treatment of asymptomatic contacts of diphtheria.

Second attacks of respiratory diphtheria are rare despite the fact that about 10 percent of patients who have had the disease remain Schick-positive. This suggests that factors other than antitoxin may play a role in protection against infection. In general, immunized patients have a milder illness than unimmunized ones when the initial clinical picture and level of circulating antitoxin are the same. Early therapy of diphtheria with antibiotics may lead to recurrence of the disease if exposure to fresh infections occurs shortly after discontinuation of treatment, suggesting that the development of antitoxic immunity is suppressed in these cases. Full immunization with diphtheria toxoid does not prevent nasopharyngeal carriage of the organism but significantly reduces the case fatality ratio. It also ameliorates the symptoms of active disease.

CLINICAL MANIFESTATIONS The incubation period of diphtheria is 1 to 7 days. The local symptoms vary with the site of the primary lesion. A membrane is not always present. The constitutional reaction usually is of only minor to moderate severity in uncomplicated disease. Fever is usually low [37.8 to 38.3°C (100 to 101°F)], unless infection with another organism (often group A *Streptococcus pyogenes*) supervenes. When toxic manifestations are absent, patients feel well except for varying degrees of discomfort at the site of the local lesion. Pallor, listlessness, tachycardia, and weakness are common in more severe cases. Nausea or vomiting is more frequent in young children. Peripheral vascular collapse often develops in the terminal stages of the disease.

Nasal diphtheria Diphtheria is occasionally restricted to the nasal mucosa. It is usually localized to the septum or turbinates in the anterior portion of one side of the nose, does not extend, and may persist for a long time. A foreign body is frequently present. A unilateral serosanguineous discharge is characteristic. When the disease is located in the posterior nasal areas, it commonly extends to the pharynx, from which toxin is absorbed.

Pharyngeal diphtheria The early diphtheritic membrane in the pharynx consists of small areas of soft exudate which wipe off easily and leave no bleeding points. As the disease progresses, the discrete exudate coalesces to form an easily removable thin sheet which spreads to cover tonsils or pharynx, or both. Later, it becomes thicker, bluish white, gray, or black, depending on the degree of hemorrhage, and is so firmly attached to the underlying tissues that attempts to remove it result in bleeding. If infection with group A *Streptococcus pyogenes* is superimposed, the pharynx is diffusely red and edematous. Sore throat is the most common complaint. Pain on swallowing may occur in over 25 percent of the cases and in some patients may be severe. There is a moderate leukocytosis with 15,000 or fewer white blood cells per cubic millimeter.

Local spread of the pharyngeal membrane may occur, and the throat, tonsils, and soft and hard palates become completely covered. Patients with severe disease may develop so-called malignant diphtheria, characterized by marked edema of the submandibular areas and the anterior neck, giving the characteristic "bullneck" appearance. Respiration is noisy, the tongue protrudes, the breath is foul, and the speech thick. The pharyngeal tissues are red and edematous, and the cervical lymph nodes are enlarged. The skin is pale and cool. The patient complains of overwhelming weakness. Purpuric eruptions of the skin, particularly on the neck and anterior chest wall, may appear occasionally. Drowsiness and delirium are common.

Laryngeal diphtheria Involvement of the larynx is usually the result of extension of the diphtheritic membrane from the pharynx. The infection may rarely be limited to the larynx or trachea. This possibility must be considered in the differential diagnosis of all cases of "croup"; it can be ruled out only by direct examination of the airway. The clinical features of this type of disease are described below.

Cutaneous diphtheria Until recently, diphtheria of the skin was a problem primarily in tropical areas where it is responsible for some cases of "jungle sore." However, since 1972, there has been a significant increase in skin diphtheria in the Pacific northwest and the southwest. A high attack rate has occurred in native Americans and in indigent males living in "skid row" areas where crowding and poor personal and community hygiene abound. *Corynebacterium diphtheriae,* being unable to penetrate unbroken skin, invades wounds, burns, or abrasions. Coagulase-positive *Staphylococcus aureus* and/or beta-hemolytic streptococci frequently are recovered concomitantly. Although the lesions develop most often on the extremities, they may appear at any site including the perianal area. In tropical zones, the typical lesion appears as a round, deep, "punched-out" ulcer, 0.5 cm to several centimeters in diameter. In the early stages, it is covered by a gray-yellow or gray-brown membrane which strips off easily to reveal a clean hemorrhagic base that dries quickly and becomes covered by a thin, leathery, dark-brown or black, adherent membrane. In the untreated case, this separates spontaneously 1 to 3 weeks after infection. The margin of the fully developed ulcer is usually slightly undermined, purple, rolled, and sharply defined. When lesions are infected with a toxigenic strain, anesthesia over the lesion develops within a few weeks. In temperate climates, the lesions are not sufficiently specific to permit visual diagnosis. Cutaneous diphtheria should be suspected in any adult with skin lesions, particularly in the proper epidemiologic setting. Antibiotic therapy will change the character of the skin lesions. Twenty percent of patients with cutaneous diphtheria also have infections in the nasopharynx with the same biotype. Myocarditis or neuropathy occurs in about 3 to 5 percent of patients with cutaneous diphtheria. The Landry-Guillain-Barré syndrome develops occasionally.

Diphtheritic lesions in other areas Diphtheria may involve the uterine cervix, vagina, vulva, bladder, urethra, or penis (after circumcision). Toxic manifestations are common. The tongue, buccal mucous membrane, gums, and esophagus may also be affected. Infection of the conjunctiva occurs rarely. Otitis media may occur as an isolated syndrome or secondary to diphtheria in the upper part of the respiratory tract; the aural infection may become chronic; virulent organisms may be isolated from the discharge for many months.

COMPLICATIONS OF DIPHTHERIA The complications of diphtheria are of two types: (1) those that result from spread of the membrane in the respiratory tract, and (2) those due to the effects of the toxin.

Extension and spread of membrane The membrane of diphtheria may spread from the fauces over the posterior pharyngeal wall into the larynx, trachea, and, uncommonly, the bronchial tree, leading to severe illness and a high incidence of toxic manifestations. Occlusion of the airway is manifested by tachypnea and, as obstruction increases, restlessness, use of accessory muscles of respiration, cyanosis, and finally death. In some cases, the membrane extends diffusely into the bronchial tree and produces clinical manifestations of pneumonia. Hoarseness and a crouplike cough are seen with laryngeal involvement. Bronchopulmonary diphtheria is very serious, not only because of obstruction but also because of the large surface from which toxin can be absorbed; the death rate is very high. When the pulmonary lesion regresses, pieces of membrane may break off and produce sudden occlusion of the airway; a cast of the bronchial tree may be coughed up. Occasionally, pharyngeal membrane has extended into the esophagus and cardia of the stomach.

Toxic complications of diphtheria Diphtheria toxin is produced only by isolates of *C. diphtheriae* lysogenic for corynephages that carry the tox structural gene. Nontoxigenic strains can be converted to toxin-producing organisms through transference of this phage. The bacterial host regulates expression of the tox structural gene. The toxin is a single polypeptide chain composed of two fragments. Fragment B recognizes specific surface receptors on sensitive cell membranes, and fragment A crosses the plasma membrane. In the cytoplasm, protein synthesis is inhibited by fragment A through the inactivation of the eukaryotic translocating enzyme, elongation factor 2. A cofactor, nicotinamide adenine dinucleotide, is required for activity of the toxin. The effects of the toxin on the myocardium are thought to result from its ability to decrease the rate of oxidation of long-chain fatty acids by interfering with the metabolism of carnitine. Because of this action, triglycerides accumulate in the myocardium and cause fatty degeneration of muscle.

Myocarditis develops in about two-thirds of patients with diphtheria. However, it is clinically evident in only about 10 percent of cases; alterations in the intensity of the heart sounds, systolic murmurs, bundle branch block, incomplete or complete heart block, atrial fibrillation, and ventricular premature beats or tachycardia, or both, are common. Ventricular fibrillation is a constant threat and is frequently responsible for sudden death. Ninety percent of patients with atrial fibrillation, ventricular tachycardia, or complete heart block die. Overt congestive cardiac failure is uncommon. Evidence of decompensation of the right side of the heart usually develops first; the most common symptom is pain in the right upper quadrant of the abdomen due to rapid engorgement of the liver. Failure of the left side of the heart may appear later. Diphtheritic heart disease is not necessarily "benign" in survivors of the disease; permanent cardiac damage may occur. Fibrosis of the myocardium has been observed in patients who have expired several weeks after "mild" myocarditis was detected electrocardiographically. The degree and extent of fibrotic change have often been greater than could have been predicted on the basis of the type of abnormality present in the ECG.

Peripheral neuritis may occur in the course of diphtheria. Paralysis of the soft palate and posterior pharyngeal wall occasionally appears very early in the disease (2 to 3 days). A more common neuritis (10 percent of cases) usually develops 2 to 6 weeks after onset of the disease. It is characterized by cranial nerve dysfunction; the IIId, VIth, VIIth, IXth, and Xth cranial nerves are most commonly involved. Loss of accommodation, nasal voice, and difficulty in swallowing are the most frequent manifestations. However, any of the peripheral nerves may be affected, with resulting paralysis of the extremities, diaphragm, or intercostal muscles; death may occur from failure of respiration. The peripheral neuritides which appear in the second to the sixth weeks of the disease are characterized primarily by motor loss; sensory changes are uncommon and, when present, are minor. Demyelination is the usual pathologic change. Nerve conduction studies show a marked dissociation between the time course of clinical features and electrophysiologic abnormalities: peripheral nerve conduction velocities are minimally affected early in the disease despite profound weakness. During clinical recovery the electrophysiological abnormalities are most apparent. Peripheral neuritis may not appear until 2 to 3 months after the onset of diphtheria. In these cases, the clinical picture and course resemble infectious polyneuritis. The outstanding findings are loss of sensation in the "glove-and-stocking" distribution and albuminocytological dissociation in the cerebrospinal fluid identical with that observed in the Landry-Guillain-Barré syndrome. Motor weakness and areflexia may develop with progression of involvement. Facial diplegia may accompany the other neurological manifestations. A fatal, rapidly ascending paralysis of the Landry type may develop rarely. Complete recovery is the rule in this late peripheral neuritis, although it may require as long as a year. Encephalitis is a rare toxic complication of diphtheria.

Shock, which develops suddenly and without warning, is an occasional cause of sudden death in this disease. In some instances, this may be a consequence of myocarditis; in others, no cause can be discovered.

Other complications Cerebral infarction with hemiplegia occurs rarely; it is probably due to embolization from atrial thrombi in patients with myocarditis and cardiac dilatation. Superinfection of the lungs is a risk in all patients with diphtheria who are given antimicrobial agents. Purpuric skin eruptions may be seen in severe, malignant cases; thrombocytopenia occurs rarely. A mild morbilliform rash may be present during the early stage of diphtheria. Secondary invasion of the pharynx by group A *S. pyogenes* may take place in patients who have not received an antibiotic. Serum sickness occasionally follows the use of antitoxin. Relapses of diphtheria may occur when patients given antimicrobial agents are exposed to fresh cases soon after therapy has been discontinued. Bacteremia, endocarditis, and meningitis are rare complications.

COURSE AND PROGNOSIS The diphtheritic membrane may be present for only 3 to 4 days in mild cases, even when no antitoxin is given; it usually lasts for about a week in cases of moderate severity. Commonly, the pharyngeal lesion increases in extent and thickness during the first 24 h after the administration of antitoxin. As the disease begins to recede, the exudate softens, wipes off easily, leaving no bleeding areas, becomes patchy so that it resembles the picture of "follicular" tonsillitis, and finally disappears, leaving normal underlying mucous membrane.

The fatality rate of diphtheria prior to the use of specific antitoxin was about 35 percent in average cases and 90 percent in those with laryngeal involvement. Since specific serotherapy has been employed, this rate has been reduced to a range of 3.5 to 22 percent, but it is still highest when the larynx is affected. The overall death rate in the United States is about 10 percent. Death is most frequent in the very young and the old. Immunization is a factor of great importance in prognosis. The fatality rate in immunized individuals is one-tenth that in the unimmunized population. Paralysis is 5 times and "malignant" disease 15 times less common in immune than in nonimmune individuals. As a rule, the longer the delay in the administration of antitoxin, the greater the incidence of complications and death. However, antitoxin is ineffective in reducing risks of complications and death if it is given much later than 48 h after diphtheria begins.

A white blood cell count higher than 25,000 per cubic millimeter is associated with a higher risk of complications and death.

DIAGNOSIS The clinical features of the fully developed diphtheritic membrane, especially in the pharynx, are sufficiently characteristic to suggest the possibility of the disease in most instances. However, the appearance of the pharyngeal exudate alone does not clinch the diagnosis. There are a number of other infections in which pseudomembranes resembling those of diphtheria are present; among those are infectious mononucleosis, streptococcal pharyngitis, viral exudative pharyngitis, fusospirochetal infection, and acute pharyngeal candidiasis.

The specific diagnosis of diphtheria depends completely on demonstration of the organism in stained smears and their recovery by culture. Methylene blue–stained preparations are positive, in experienced hands, in 75 to 85 percent of cases. Diphtheria bacilli can be recovered by culture on Loeffler's medium in 8 to 12 h if patients have not been receiving antimicrobial agents. *Corynebacterium diphtheriae* also multiplies, but more slowly, on ordinary blood agar. If an antibiotic, especially penicillin or erythromycin, has been administered prior to obtaining cultures, the organisms may not grow for as long as 5 days or may fail to grow at all.

Staining of suspected material with fluorescein-labeled diphtheria antitoxin may allow rapid diagnosis. Toxigenicity of *C. diphtheriae* isolates should be determined by passive agar diffusion (Elek plate method), guinea pig inoculation, or counterimmunoelectrophoresis. Biotype determination will help characterize the epidemiology of an outbreak.

TREATMENT Patients with diphtheria should be isolated and kept at strict bed rest; physical effort should be reduced during the early convalescent stages. Local therapy of the diphtheritic pharyngeal lesion is useless. The only specific treatment for diphtheria is antitoxin. Antiserum must never be given until the patient's sensitivity to horse serum, using the eye and skin tests, has been determined. There are several regimens for the administration of antitoxin, and the amount given is often based on an empiric decision. In general, the more severe the disease or the more extensive the membrane formation, the greater the amount of antitoxin required. Mildly symptomatic cases may be treated with 10,000 to 20,000 units. Moderately severe cases, such as those with a pharyngeal membrane, should be given 20,000 to 40,000 units. Severe diphtheria, as with laryngeal involvement, requires 50,000 to 100,000 units. The total dose should be given at one time rather than in split doses over a long period. For doses less than 20,000 units, the intramuscular route is convenient. When this method is used, only one-half the dose should be given intramuscularly and the remainder intravenously in order to expedite delivery of the antitoxin. Alternatively, after appropriate testing for sensitivity, the entire amount of antitoxin may be given intravenously in 100 to 200 ml isotonic saline over a 30-min period. Desensitization should be attempted if the initial skin or eye test is positive. A rare patient may be sensitive to such a high degree that the antiserum cannot be administered without the risk of death.

Antitoxin should be given as early in the course of diphtheria as possible. It is capable of binding or inactivating only the toxin present in blood or extracellular fluid. Once the toxin has entered the cell, the effect cannot be reversed or prevented. Antitoxin must be given when diphtheria is suspected clinically; laboratory confirmation prior to administration of the antitoxin is not necessary. Since mortality increases directly with delay in use of antitoxin, it is better to treat clinically suspect but culture-negative cases than to withhold specific therapy.

A history of military service is not reliable proof of adequate immunization. From World War II until 1956, immunization for diphtheria in the United States military was inconsistent. Since 1957, all branches of the armed forces have routinely immunized their pesonnel. When the immunization history is not clear, it is best to provide antitoxin promptly. Antimicrobial agents do not alter the course, incidence of complications, or outcome of diphtheria.

Patients with laryngeal obstruction should be watched very carefully. In mild cases, inhalation of warm or cool steam may be beneficial. If advancing signs of airway obstruction develop, intubation or tracheostomy is indicated. These procedures must never be delayed until cyanosis appears, because, at this point, stimulation of the pharynx or trachea may produce cardiac standstill and death. Sedative or hypnotic agents should never be given because they may obscure increasing respiratory difficulty.

The pulse and blood pressure should be measured frequently. Little can be done to alter the course of the myocarditis. Quinidine has been tried to prevent and treat arrhythmias but appears to be of no value; there is some suspicion that it may produce deleterious effect. The use of procainamide when ventricular premature beats or tachycardia supervene has been suggested, but no documented observations of its effect have been recorded. The administration of digitalis for cardiac failure in diphtheria is controversial. Some consider this drug to be completely contraindicated; others feel, however, that, used carefully, digitalis may be given safely and with beneficial effects. Shock should be treated according to its etiology (see Chaps. 29 and 139). There is no evidence that corticosteroids and corticotropin are of any value in the treatment of diphtheria or any of its complications. Antibiotics should be used to treat symptomatic cases only after antitoxin is administered. Circulating exotoxin is not affected by antibiotics, and their prompt use may give a sense of false assurance. Patients with diphtheria should be quarantined until two successive cultures of the nose, throat, or other infected areas, taken at 24-h intervals, are negative. If antibiotics have been given, cultures should not be taken until at least 24 h after cessation of therapy.

Treatment of carriers *Corynebacterium diphtheriae* usually disappears from the upper part of the respiratory tract after 2 to 4 weeks in patients who do not receive antimicrobial drugs; in a small number of individuals the organism may persist for a long time or even permanently. The most effective treatment of the acute and chronic carrier state is erythromycin. A dose of 2 g per day orally in divided doses for 7 days appears to be adequate. The enteric-coated base, estolate, and ethyl succinate forms of erythromycin are preferred to ensure adequate serum concentrations without regard to food intake. Alternative antimicrobials include procaine penicillin G, 600,000 units intramuscularly every 12 h for 10 days; clindamycin, 150 mg four times a day orally for 7 days; and rifampin, 600 mg as a single oral dose for 7 days. Tetracyclines, semisynthetic penicillins, aminoglycosides, and oral cephalosporins are inadequate for the eradication of *C. diphtheriae.* Parenteral cephalosporins such as cephalothin or cefamandole are effective. In two areas of North America endemic for cutaneous diphtheria, resistance of *C. diphtheriae* to erythromycin has been recognized. The origin of the plasmid in erythromycin-resistant strains is not clear; fortunately such isolates are uncommon. Initial observations indicate that plasmids are not usually detectable in respiratory isolates of *C. diphtheriae* and are rare in skin isolates. Re-treatment is indicated for carriers whose organisms do not disappear on the first trial. This is preferable to tonsillectomy, which may be considered a last resort should the carrier state persist despite repeated courses of antibiotic. Persistence of the organism after appropriate antimicrobial therapy may represent a lack of compliance rather than drug resistance.

PREVENTION Diphtheria is, for the most part, a preventable disease. Immunization at the age of 3 months should be routine. Diphtheria toxoid is best given together with tetanus toxoid and pertussis vaccine (DPT), because antibody titers are higher with combined immunization than with either agent alone. Booster doses should be administered at the age of 1 year and again just before a child goes to school. Although it has been suggested that Schick testing is not necessary in those who have been immunized, some physicians still carry this out to determine the status of antitoxic immunity. A Schick test acts as a booster. A negative reaction does not indicate absolute protection. The development of highly purified toxoid has made it possible to protect adults with little or no risk of untoward sequelae. In this situation, a combination of adult tetanus-diphtheria (Td) toxoid containing 1 to 2 flocculation (Lf) units per milliliter should be used. With this preparation, severe reactions can be avoided. The Moloney test need not be carried out. Adults should receive booster doses at least every 10 years. Unfortunately, reimmunized adults are the exception, and many elderly patients have low and nonprotective levels of circulating antitoxin. They constitute a high-risk group during any diphtheria outbreak.

Treatment of unimmunized persons exposed to an active case of diphtheria remains controversial. One approach has been to administer 3000 units of equine antitoxin intramuscularly, after appropriate skin and eye tests. In some countries (not in the United States) human diphtheria antitoxin is available. The concentration achieved with this product is sufficient only for passive protection of the asymptomatic, unimmunized contact but is not high enough for treatment of symptomatic disease. If human diphtheria immunoglobulin is used, active immunization must be delayed for 6 weeks. Alternatively, cultures of *C. diphtheriae* can be taken, and a primary series of immunizations initiated. The exposed individual then can be observed closely for signs of active disease. If symptoms occur, antitoxin can be given immediately. In those who have been previously immunized, a booster dose of toxoid is usually sufficient. Cultures from the nasopharynx or open wounds should be obtained from close contacts or family members of a diphtheria case or carrier.

REFERENCES

BELSEY MA, LEBLANC DR: Skin infections and the epidemiology of diphtheria; acquisition and persistence of *C. diphtheriae* infections. Am J Epidemiol 102:179, 1975

BROOKS GR et al: Diphtheria in the United States 1959–1970. J Infect Dis 129:172, 1974

GOOD I: Myocardial changes in fatal diphtheria: A summary of observations in 221 cases. Am J Med Sci 219:257, 1948

GOOR RS, PAPPENHEIMER AM JR: Studies on the mode of action of diphtheria toxin. J Exp Med 126:899, 913, 923, 1967

IPSEN J: Circulating antitoxin at the onset of diphtheria in 425 patients. J Immunol 54:325, 1946

———: Immunization of adults against diphtheria and tetanus. N Engl J Med 251:459, 1954

KURDI A, ABDUL-KADER M: Clinical and electrophysiological studies of diphtheritic neuritis in Jordan. J Neurol Sci 42:243, 1979

MCCLOSKEY RV et al: The 1970 epidemic of diphtheria in San Antonio. Ann Intern Med 75:495, 1971

NAIDITCH MJ, BOWER AG: Diphtheria: A study of 1,433 cases observed during a ten-year period at the Los Angeles County Hospital. Am J Med 17:229, 1954

PAPPENHEIMER AM JR: Diphtheria toxin. Annu Rev Biochem 46:69, 1977

SCHEID W: Diphtherial paralysis: An analysis of 2,292 cases of diphtheria in adults which include 174 cases of polyneuritis. J Nerv Ment Dis 116:1095, 1952

SCHILLER J et al: Plasmids in *Corynebacterium diphtheriae* and diphtheroids mediating erythromycin resistance. Antimicrob Agents Chemother 18:814, 1980

THOMPSON NL, ELLNER PD: Rapid determination of *Corynebacterium diphtheriae* toxigenicity by counterimmunoelectrophoresis. J Clin Microbiol 7:493, 1978

WITTELS B, BRESSLER R: Biochemical lesion of diphtheria toxin on the heart. J Clin Invest 43:630, 1964

166 CHOLERA

CHARLES C. J. CARPENTER

DEFINITION Cholera is an acute illness which results from colonization of the small intestine by *Vibrio cholerae.* The disease is characterized by its epidemic occurrence and the production in the more severe cases of massive diarrhea with rapid depletion of extracellular fluid and electrolytes.

ETIOLOGY AND EPIDEMIOLOGY *Vibrio cholerae* is a curved, aerobic, gram-negative bacillus with a single polar flagellum. It is rapidly motile and possesses both O and H antigens. Serologic identification is based on differences in the polysaccharide O antigens.

Cholera has been endemic for a century and a half in the Gangetic Delta of West Bengal and Bangladesh and is often epidemic throughout south and southeast Asia. The seventh and most recent pandemic spread of this disease, from 1961 to 1981, has extended from the Celebes northward to Korea and westward to the whole of Africa and southern Europe. The last major epidemic of cholera in the western hemisphere occurred from 1866 to 1867. However, in August and September 1978, at least 11 persons developed cholera, serotype Inaba, after ingestion of inadequately cooked crabs caught in lakes or coastal waters of Louisiana.

The majority of epidemics have clearly been waterborne, but direct contamination of food by infected feces probably contributes to spread during major outbreaks. Poor sanitation appears to be primarily responsible for the continuing presence of cholera, but host factors, such as relative or absolute achlorhydria, also play an important role in the susceptibility of the individual to infection. In endemic areas, cholera is predominantly a disease of children; in rural Bangladesh, attack rates are 10 times greater in the 1- to 5-year-old age group than in those above 14 years of age. However, when the disease spreads to previously uninvolved areas, the attack rates are initially at least as high in adults as in children.

A chronic gallbladder carrier state has been observed in a small percentage of elderly convalescent cholera patients. These chronic *V. cholerae* carriers may provide a vehicle for spread outside endemic areas. The basis for the annual cholera epidemics throughout the Gangetic Delta, for the periodic outbreaks throughout the remainder of south and southeast Asia, and for the occasional global pandemics has, however, not been clearly delineated.

PATHOGENESIS *Vibrio cholerae* produces a protein enterotoxin which appears to be responsible for all known pathophysiologic aberrations in cholera. This enterotoxin, which has a molecular weight of 84,000, stimulates adenylate cyclase in the intestine epithelial cells, and the resultant increase in intracellular cyclic adenosine 3′,5′-monophosphate leads to secretion of isotonic fluid by all segments of the small intestine. The enterotoxin-induced electrolyte secretion occurs in the absence of any demonstrable histologic damage to intestine epithelial cells or to the capillary endothelial cells of the lamina propria. Precise studies have demonstrated that the stool of the adult cholera patient is nearly isotonic, with sodium and chloride concentrations slightly less than those of plasma, a bicarbonate concentration approximately twice that of plasma, and a potassium concentration three to five times that of plasma. Disease caused by all known strains of *V. cholerae* results in the same stool electrolyte pattern. The pathophysiologic defect in cholera is extracellular fluid depletion with resultant hypovolemic shock, base-deficit acidosis, and progressive potassium depletion. There is no evidence that the cholera vibrio invades any tissue, nor has the enterotoxin been shown, in human disease, to have any direct effect on any organ other than the small intestine.

MANIFESTATIONS The incubation period generally lasts from 12 to 48 h. This is followed by the abrupt onset of watery, generally painless diarrhea. In the more severe cases, the initial diarrheal stool may be in excess of 1000 ml, and several liters of isotonic fluid may be lost within hours, leading rapidly to profound shock. Vomiting generally follows, but occasionally precedes, the onset of diarrhea; the vomiting is characteristically effortless and not preceded by nausea. As saline depletion progresses, severe muscle cramps, commonly involving the calves, occur.

When first seen, the typical severely ill cholera patient is cyanotic, with pinched facies, scaphoid abdomen, poor skin turgor, and thready or absent peripheral pulses. The voice is faint, high-pitched, and often inaudible, and there are tachycardia, hypotension, and varying degrees of tachypnea. In all epidemics there are many subclinical or mild cases in which gastrointestinal fluid loss is not severe enough to require hospitalization. With the *el tor* strain of *V. cholerae,* which has been responsible for the most recent pandemic, the ratio of subclinical infections to clinical cholera cases is greater than 10:1.

The disease runs its course in 2 to 7 days, and subsequent manifestations depend on the adequacy of electrolyte repletion therapy. With prompt fluid and electrolyte repletion, physiologic recovery is remarkably rapid, and mortality exceptionally rare. The important causes of death, in inadequately treated patients, are hypovolemic shock, metabolic acidosis, and uremia resulting from acute tubular necrosis.

LABORATORY FINDINGS In epidemics or in endemic areas, the clinical picture should arouse strong suspicion immediately. The most reliable technique for identification of *V. cholerae* consists of direct plating of a sample of cholera stool on bile salt, gelatin-tellurite-taurocholate (GTT), or thiosulfate–citrate–bile salt–sucrose (TCBS) agar. On bile salt or GTT agar the organisms appear as typical translucent colonies within 24 h. On TCBS agar, *V. cholerae* appear at 24 h as distinct, large, flat yellow colonies. Further classification requires agglutination with type-specific antiserums. In mild or convalescent cases, recovery of vibrios may be enhanced by initial enrichment for 6 h in alkaline peptone water followed by subculture on bile salt, GTT, or TCBS agar. Rapid presumptive diagnosis is possible either by directly observing immobilization of vibrios by type-specific antiserums, using dark-field or phase microscopy, or by identifying the organisms with immunofluorescent methods.

TREATMENT Successful therapy requires only prompt and adequate replacement of gastrointestinal losses of saline and alkali. A uniformly satisfactory solution for intravenous fluid therapy can be simply prepared by the addition of 5 g sodium chloride, 4 g sodium bicarbonate, and 1 g potassium chloride to 1 liter of pyrogen-free distilled water. If commercially prepared fluids are available, lactated Ringer's solution is generally satisfactory. The intravenous fluids are initially infused at 50 to 100 ml/min, until a strong pulse has been restored. The same fluids should subsequently be infused in quantities equal to the gastrointestinal losses. If losses cannot be measured accurately, intravenous fluids should be given at a rate sufficient to maintain a normal radial pulse and normal skin turgor. Overhydration can be avoided by careful observation of neck venous filling and auscultation of the lungs. Close observation is mandatory during the acute phase of the illness, because the cholera patient can lose as much as 1 liter of isotonic fluid per hour during the first 24 h of the disease. Inadequate or delayed restoration of fecal fluid losses may result in a high incidence of acute renal failure. Serious hypokalemic symptoms are rare in adults, and potassium repletion can be carried out orally if potassium-containing intravenous fluids are not available. Hypokalemia contributes significantly, however, to the morbidity in inadequately treated pediatric cholera, and potassium, 10 to 13 meq per liter, should be included in the intravenous fluids administered to pediatric patients.

Although adequate intravenous saline and alkali repletion alone results in rapid recovery of virtually all cholera patients, a dramatic reduction in the duration and volume of the diarrhea and early eradication of vibrios from the stool may be effected by antibiotic therapy. Oral tetracycline, 500 mg every 6 h for the first 48 h of treatment, has been most successful. Other antibiotics, including chloramphenicol and furazolidone, are also of value, but both appear to be slightly less effective than tetracycline.

Oral therapy Since the cholera enterotoxin does not alter glucose-facilitated sodium absorption, fluid repletion can be effected by the oral administration of glucose-containing electrolyte solutions. Since the limiting factor in treatment of cholera in both epidemic and endemic situations is often the lack of adequate quantities of intravenous fluids, the availability of an oral treatment regimen has greatly reduced the mortality from cholera outbreaks during the most recent pandemic spread of this disease. A solution containing glucose 20 g per liter (or sucrose 40 g per liter), sodium bicarbonate 2.5 g per liter, sodium chloride 3.5 g per liter, and potassium chloride 1.5 g per liter can be readily prepared and should be satisfactory for treatment of all age groups. This solution, administered orally at a rate equal to the stool losses, can be given to patients with milder cholera throughout the course of illness and is also satisfactory in the more severe cases, once the hypovolemic shock has been corrected by intravenous fluid therapy. Oral therapy does not decrease the rate of intestinal fluid loss but provides an electrolyte solution which can be absorbed at a rate sufficient, in most cases, to counterbalance the continuing fluid losses. Therefore, successful management of the cholera patient with oral therapy requires just as close supervision, with careful monitoring of pulse volume, skin turgor, and neck veins, as does management with intravenous solutions. Supplemental intravenous fluids must be administered whenever clinical signs of saline depletion recur.

PROGNOSIS Under ideal conditions and with prompt and adequate fluid replacement, mortality approaches zero, and significant sequelae are rare. Unfortunately, death rates as high as 60 percent still occur, especially during the initial phases of certain outbreaks. This high mortality reflects lack of pyrogen-free intravenous fluids in remote areas, the difficulties of initiating treatment promptly when large numbers of cases are occurring in poverty-striken populations, and the compromises which may have to be made under emergency conditions.

PREVENTION Immunization by standard commercial vaccine, containing 10 billion killed organisms per milliliter, provides only limited (40 to 60 percent) protection for a relatively short (4- to 6-month) period in endemic areas. Vaccination, therefore, is not recommended for Americans who are traveling abroad. Careful hygiene provides the only sure protection against cholera.

REFERENCES

CARPENTER CCJ et al: Clinical studies in Asiatic cholera, I–VI. Bull Johns Hopkins Hosp 118:165, 1966

Cholera, 1981. Morb Mort Week Rep 31:481, 1982

FISHMAN PH: Mechanism of action of cholera toxin: Events on the cell surface, in *Secretory Diarrhea,* M Field, JS Fordtran, SG Schultz (eds). Bethesda, American Physiological Society, 1980, pp 85–106

GANGAROSA EF et al: The nature of the gastrointestinal lesion in Asiatic cholera and its relation to pathogenesis: A biopsy study. Am J Trop Med Hyg 9:125, 1960

HIRSCHHORN N et al: The treatment of cholera, in *Cholera,* D Barua, W Burrows (eds). Philadelphia, Saunders, 1974, p 235

MAHALANOBIS D et al: Oral fluid therapy of cholera among Bangladesh refugees. Johns Hopkins Med J 132:197, 1973

MORRIS JG JR et al: Nm-O group 1 *Vibrio cholerai* gastroenteritis in the United States: Clinical, epidemiologic, and laboratory characteristics of sporadic cases. Ann Intern Med 94:656, 1981

WALLACE CK et al: Optimal antibiotic therapy in cholera. Bull WHO 39:239, 1968

167 ANTHRAX

ROBERT G. PETERSDORF

DEFINITION Anthrax is a disease of wild and domesticated animals that is transmitted to humans by contact with infected animals or their products, by insect vectors which act as mechanical carriers of the etiologic organism, or, rarely, in some developing parts of the world by direct contact, such as use of common household articles. The characteristic lesion of human anthrax is a necrotic cutaneous ulcer. The disease also may be associated with disseminated infection, which is characterized by mediastinitis or meningitis with or without a cutaneous ulcer.

ETIOLOGY The classic studies of Robert Koch established that *Bacillus anthracis* was the cause of anthrax. This was the first demonstration of a single organism causing a single disease. *B. anthracis* is a large, encapsulated, gram-positive, aerobic, spore-forming microorganism that grows well in most nutrient media. Its pathogenicity for laboratory animals, including mice and guinea pigs, differentiates it from *B. subtilis* and *B. cereus,* which it closely resembles. The spores are killed by boiling for 10 min but can survive for many years in soil and animal products, an important factor in the persistence and spread of the disease. Uncultivated soil is more favorable to sporulation, and dry climates also favor the persistence of organisms. Under some conditions, spores may survive for 20 years. The anthrax bacillus possesses a capsule of glutamyl polypeptide, which interferes with phagocytosis of the microorganism. In addition, it contains an anticomplementary substance and elaborates a "protective" antigen and a toxin which is probably of importance in determining virulence.

EPIDEMIOLOGY Anthrax is worldwide; repeated outbreaks have occurred in southern Europe, notably Greece, the Middle East (particularly Iran), Africa (Zimbabwe and Gambia), Australia and New Zealand, and on both American continents.

Cattle, horses, sheep, goats, and swine are most commonly infected. There have been outbreaks of anthrax among animals in the United States, centering mostly in South Dakota, Nebraska, Arkansas, Mississippi, Louisiana, Texas, Washington, and California. The disease tends to occur in animals in late summer and early fall. An outbreak of anthrax, acquired from goatskin bongo drum heads and goatskin rugs, occurred in Haiti and was imported into the United States.

The disease in humans is acquired by butchering, skinning, or dissecting infected carcasses or by handling contaminated hides, wool, hair, or other materials. The majority of cases of human anthrax involve workers handling imported and unprocessed wool, hair, or hides, or bone meal used as fertilizer. Shepherds may be infected during shearing in the dry season, and workers spinning or weaving infected wool develop lesions on the lips. Gardeners have been infected accidentally by inhaling bone meal fertilizers, and inhalation anthrax has been reported following exposure to exhausts of a tanning plant. The disease usually follows inoculation of bacilli or spores into the skin, often through a wound or abrasion. Intestinal infection has followed ingestion of contaminated meat. In Africa outbreaks of anthrax have been attributed to flies which carry the organism from infected carcasses or to biting flies which may carry the bacillus in their blood. This may account for the absence of lesions on the fingers and hands. In Gambia, under crowded conditions, human-to-human transmission has been implicated through the use of common palm-brushes (loofahs).

PATHOGENESIS Germination of spores occurs within hours of inoculation. The spores germinate by polar rupture and form capsules. The malignant pustule which follows cutaneous inoculation of anthrax organisms is characterized by vesiculation, neutrophilic infiltration, gelatinous edema, and necrosis. Suppuration is rare in the absence of secondary pyogenic infection; hence, the term *malignant pustule,* which is often used to describe cutaneous anthrax, is inappropriate. Spread of the bacilli to the regional lymph nodes may be followed by systemic dissemination. Examination of tissues from fatal human cases reveals masses of the bacteria in blood vessels, lymph nodes, and the parenchyma of various organs. There is scanty or no cellular exudation at these foci, but hemorrhage and edema are widespread. In inhalation anthrax the spores are phagocytosed by alveolar macrophages, and germination occurs in mediastinal lymph nodes.

Meningeal anthrax is disseminated via the bloodstream either from a primary cutaneous lesion or without an overt portal of entry.

The rare form of intestinal anthrax presumably occurs by ingestion of infected, poorly cooked animal meat.

The blood of fatally infected experimental animals contains a lethal toxin, which can be neutralized by specific antiserum. This toxin has been isolated in vitro and is important in the pathogenesis of some of the manifestations of the disease.

MANIFESTATIONS **Cutaneous anthrax** Human anthrax usually begins on an exposed body surface as a painless pruritic, erythematous papule which vesiculates and ulcerates to form a black eschar. Tiny satellite vesicles are frequent. The ulcer may be surrounded by extensive edematous swelling which is nontender, nonpitting, and so characteristic of anthrax that it is a valuable diagnostic sign. After about 5 days the ulcer begins to subside, but edema may persist for several weeks. Mild tenderness and enlargement of regional lymph nodes are frequently present. Constitutional symptoms are often absent despite extensive local changes, but there may be mild fever, headache, and malaise.

Septicemic anthrax In 10 to 20 percent of untreated anthrax, the infection spreads from the hemorrhagic regional lymph nodes to the bloodstream. In disseminated anthrax, high fever, prostration, and a rapidly fatal course are seen. These cases usually involve the meninges and the mediastinum.

Inhalation anthrax Also termed *woolsorter's disease,* this is a highly fatal disseminated infection characterized by cyanosis, dyspnea, mediastinitis, and hemoptysis and is probably dependent on the pulmonary route of inoculation. The illness is biphasic and initially consists of an insidious onset of mild fever, malaise, fatigue, myalgia, nonproductive cough, and a feeling of substernal oppression. This phase lasts several days, and there may be some improvement before the acute onset of a second stage consisting of dyspnea, cyanosis, stridor, and shock. Pleural effusions and mediastinal widening are characteristic. Most patients die within 24 h despite treatment. It has been postulated that underlying lung disease, such as sarcoid, may predispose to inhalation anthrax.

Meningeal anthrax This rare complication of anthrax is characterized by the sudden onset of confusion, loss of consciousness, coma, and lateralizing neurological signs. There is often rapid dilation of the pupils followed by death. The cerebrospinal fluid is hemorrhagic, purulent, or both.

Intestinal anthrax Human infection may occur from ingestion of poorly cooked meat of infected animals. Clinically, it resembles an acute abdomen; massive diarrhea similar to cholera may be present. The disease usually has been fatal, although a few patients have been cured by resection of the involved bowel.

LABORATORY DIAGNOSIS The fluid from the cutaneous lesion frequently contains many bacilli, demonstrable by Gram's stain and culture, but when patients have been given topical or systemic antibiotics, cultures and smears may be unreliable. Blood cultures are usually positive in disseminated anthrax, but only 10 percent of patients with cutaneous ulcers have bacteremia. The blood leukocyte count is normal in mild cases, but there is polymorphonuclear leukocytosis in most patients with disseminated disease. Patients with meningeal involvement show bloody spinal fluid, in which the organisms are easily found by direct examination or culture.

A 24-h culture on blood agar shows a characteristic "Medusa's head" on the surface. Inoculation of a suspected colony of *B. anthracis* will kill guinea pigs in 24 h, and the organism can be recovered from the left ventricle. Insertion of a needle contaminated with *B. anthracis* into gelatin gives a characteristic "fir tree" appearance.

The indirect microhemagglutination test (IMH test) has detected antibodies in 93 percent of patients, 98 percent of vaccinees, and none of the controls. It is useful in confirming the diagnosis.

TREATMENT Many antibiotics are effective in the treatment of human anthrax, including penicillin, chloramphenicol, tetracycline, erythromycin, and streptomycin. For cutaneous anthrax, 600,000 units of aqueous procaine penicillin should be given every 6 h until the local edema subsides. The eschar goes through its natural evolution in spite of treatment, and lymph node enlargement may persist for several days. *Bacillus anthracis* cannot be recovered from the skin lesion after 24 to 48 h of penicillin therapy, but it may persist for a longer period when chloramphenicol or tetracycline is used. For inhalation anthrax, 20 million units of penicillin should be given intravenously, but it is doubtful that the drug acts sufficiently rapidly to reverse the process. In meningeal anthrax, similar large doses of penicillin plus 300 to 400 mg hydrocortisone should be given. It is not clear whether the addition of steroids affects the outcome favorably.

PREVENTION Infection of personnel in industrial plants where contaminated animal products are handled still occurs. An outbreak of inhalation anthrax with a high mortality rate was reported in a goat hair processing mill in the United States in the late 1950s. Sterilization of all raw wool, mohair, etc., would probably remove the hazard but has had only limited use. A vaccine prepared from the "protective" antigen of *B. anthracis* is available and is effective in reducing the incidence of infection in an exposed population. Spore vaccines of various types are used with good effect in domestic animals in endemic areas but are not suitable for use in humans.

PROGNOSIS The cutaneous disease was fatal in 20 percent of cases before antimicrobial drugs were available. The mortality rate of cutaneous anthrax now is less than 1 percent with proper treatment. In the rare cases of inhalational, meningeal, and intestinal anthrax the prognosis is poor despite antibiotic therapy.

REFERENCES

Brachman PS: Inhalation anthrax. Ann NY Acad Sci 353:83, 1980

LaForce FM: Woolsorters' disease in England. Bull NY Acad Med 54:956, 1978

Manios S, Kavaliotis I: Anthrax in children: A long forgotten, potentially fatal infection. Scand J Infect Dis 11:203, 1979

Nalin DR et al: Survival of a patient with intestinal anthrax. Am J Med 62:130, 1977

Taaffe A: Anthrax—A review. J Ir Med Assoc 72:437, 1979

168 DONOVANOSIS (GRANULOMA INGUINALE)

KING K. HOLMES

DEFINITION Donovanosis (granuloma inguinale) is a mildly contagious, chronic, indolent, progressive, autoinoculable, ulcerative disease involving the skin and lymphatics of the genital or perianal areas. The disease may be sexually transmitted and is associated with the presence in affected tissues of an intracellular microorganism, identified morphologically as the Donovan body.

ETIOLOGY Donovanosis was described by McLeod in India in 1882, and in 1905 Donovan described the intracellular bodies which are thought to cause the disease. Encapsulated bacteria resembling Donovan bodies have been recovered from lesions and pseudobuboes of granuloma inguinale by inoculation of chick embryo yolk sacs or yolk-agar medium. These bacteria, which are known as *Calymmatobacterium granulomatis,* are antigenically related to *Klebsiella* species but do not reproduce the disease when inoculated intradermally in humans. It is uncertain whether these isolates are responsible for the disease. Electron microscopic studies of Donovan bodies confirm their morphological resemblance to gram-negative bacteria.

EPIDEMIOLOGY Donovanosis is endemic in the tropics, particularly in New Guinea and among Hindus in India. In the United States the disease is rare. Most cases occur in the southeastern states and involve male homosexuals. In reported cases the sex ratio of males to females is nearly 10:1. The disease is uncommon in Caucasians. The reported frequency of donovanosis in conjugal partners of chronically infected patients ranges from 1 to 64 percent. Evidence for sexual transmission includes the age-specific incidence, which corresponds to that of other sexually transmitted diseases, the frequent concomitant presence of syphilis, and the predilection for genital involvement in heterosexuals and for anorectal infection in homosexually active men.

CLINICAL MANIFESTATIONS The incubation period ranges from 8 days to 12 weeks, but most lesions appear within 30 days after sexual exposure.

Donovanosis begins as a papule, which ulcerates and develops into a painless elevated zone of clean, beefy-red, friable granulation tissue. The edges are irregular and spread by continuity or by autoinoculation of approximated skin surfaces. Secondary anaerobic infection may produce pain and a foul-smelling exudate. Less common complications of the disease include deep ulcerations, chronic cicatricial lesions, phimosis, lymphedema, and exuberant epithelial proliferation which grossly resembles carcinoma. In men, the lesions are usually located on the glans, prepuce, or shaft of the penis (Fig. 168-1*A*) or the perianal area, while infection of the labia is most common in women. Lesions in women often arise at the fourchette and progress anteriorly in a V shape along the vulva. Extragenital lesions may occur, involving the face, neck, mouth, and other sites. The chronicity of the disease is of diagnostic importance, since several months often elapse before patients seek treatment. Extension to the inguinal region by autoinoculation, by continuity, or via the lymphatics results in diffuse intradermal and subcutaneous swelling or suppuration, known as "pseudobubo," because involvement of the underlying lymph nodes is minimal. Locally destructive lesions and secondary infection may produce severe morbidity or death. Fatal disseminated disease, involving the bones, joints, or liver, has been reported after several years of chronic local infection. The relationship of donovanosis to subsequent carcinoma of the genitalia is uncertain.

DIAGNOSIS Early donovanosis may be mistaken for the primary chancre or condyloma latum of syphilis. Epithelial proliferation resembling carcinoma in the genital or perianal region in a young subject should always raise the suspicion of donovanosis if unnecessary destructive surgery is to be avoided. Chronic ulcerative or cicatricial changes may resemble lymphogranuloma venereum.

Amebiasis can produce penile lesions resembling donovanosis. In the United States, *Hemophilus ducreyi* has frequently been isolated from lesions resembling donovanosis; this has been termed *pseudogranuloma inguinale-chancroid.* Histological studies in donovanosis reveal marked acanthosis and pseudoepitheliomatous hyperplasia. The dermis contains an inflam-

FIGURE 168-1

A. Extensive granuloma inguinale, extending along the scrotum and involving both inguinal areas, with elevated, clean, exuberant granulation tissue. B. Same patient, following treatment. (Courtesy of A Brathwaite.)

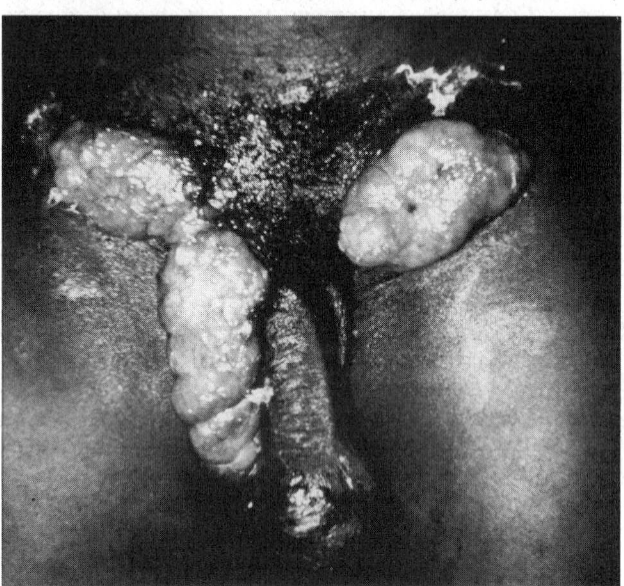

A

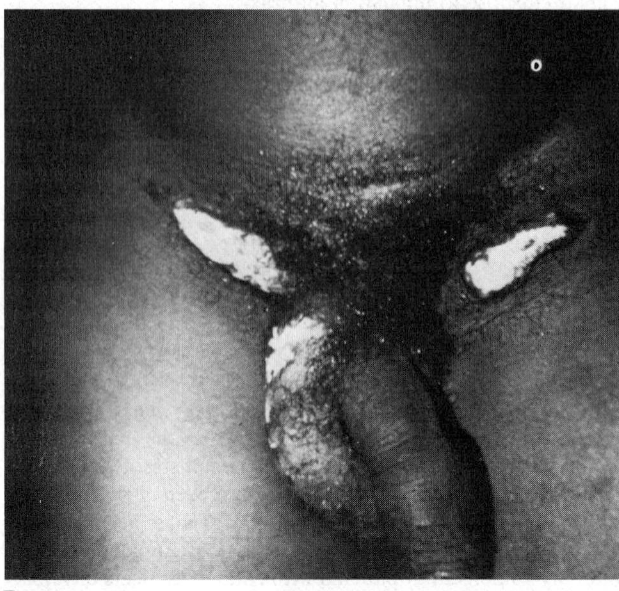

B

matory infiltrate consisting mainly of plasma cells and histiocytes. Because Donovan bodies are seldom detectable in sections stained with hematoxylin and eosin, these changes may lead to an erroneous diagnosis of carcinoma and to unnecessary, destructive surgery. Although silver impregnation techniques are useful for demonstration of Donovan bodies in sections, the diagnosis is best made by examination of impression smears prepared from specimens obtained by punch biopsy of granulation tissue from the periphery of a lesion; the deep portion of the specimen is removed, crushed between two slides which are air-dried and fixed in methanol, and stained with Wright-Giemsa stain. With this method, Donovan bodies appear as very rounded coccobacilli, 1 by 2 μm in size, which lie within cystic spaces in the cytoplasm of large mononuclear cells (Fig. 168-2). The capsule stains as a dense acidophilic zone surrounding the bipolar basophilic bacterium, which resembles a closed safety pin. The pathognomonic mononuclear cell is 25 to 90 μm in diameter and has many cystic areas containing Donovan bodies.

Perianal donovanosis may resemble condylomata lata of secondary syphilis. Other venereal diseases, particularly syphilis, very frequently coexist with donovanosis. Repeated darkfield examinations of lesions before treatment and a serologic test for syphilis should therefore be performed. In countries where donovanosis is endemic, the persistence of suspected condylomata lata after appropriate penicillin therapy for syphilis is highly suggestive of donovanosis.

TREATMENT The treatment of choice is tetracycline, 2 g daily, continued for at least 10 days. The risk of relapse is reduced if treatment is continued until healing is complete. Healing is usually apparent within 3 weeks, as the lesions become pale and flatter and develop peripheral reepithelialization (Fig. 168-1*B*). Donovan bodies disappear from lesions within a few days after onset of therapy. If tetracycline cannot be given, streptomycin may be used in a dose of 1 g intramuscularly every 12 h for 10 to 15 days. In New Guinea, chloramphenicol, 500 mg every 8 h orally, or gentamicin, 1 mg/kg twice daily, is used for cases which appear resistant to tetracycline. Co-trimoxazole (trimethoprim 160 mg, sulfamethoxazole 800 mg) twice daily for 10 days is also reported to be effective.

FIGURE 168-2

Biopsy from granuloma inguinale ulcer, showing mononuclear cells containing Donovan bodies. Wright-Giemsa stain.

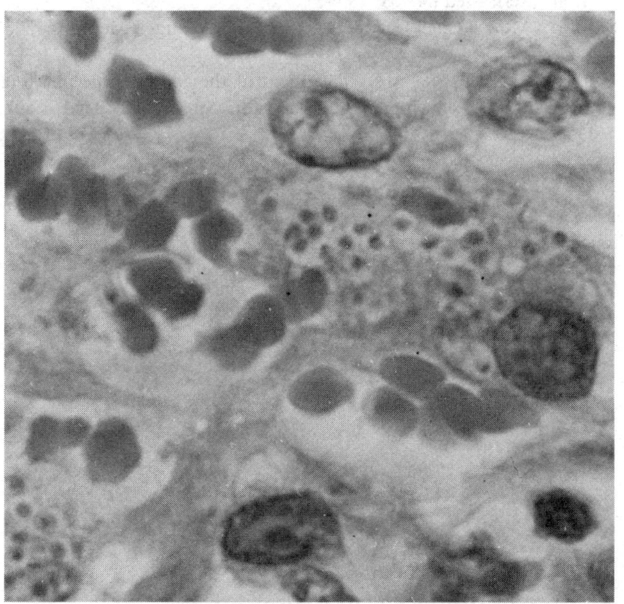

In pregnant women, erythromycin, 500 mg every 6 h, may be effective.

REFERENCES

Davis CM: Granuloma inguinale. A clinical, histological, and ultrastructural study. JAMA 211:632, 1970

Dodson RF et al: Donovanosis: A morphologic study. J Invest Dermatol 62:611, 1974

Garg BR et al: Efficacy of cotrimoxazole in donovanosis. Br J Vener Dis 54:348, 1978

Hart G: Chancroid, donovanosis, lymphogranuloma venerum. US Department of Health, Education, and Welfare Publication (CDC) 75-8302, 1975

Jofre ME et al: Granuloma inguinale simulating advanced pelvic cancer. Med J Aust 2:869, 1976

Kraus SJ et al: Pseudogranuloma inguinale caused by *Haemophilus ducreyi.* Arch Derm 118:494, 1982

Kuberski T: Granuloma inguinale (donovanosis). Sex Transm Dis 7:29, 1980

——— et al: Ultrastructure of *Calymmatobacterium granulomatis* in lesions of granuloma inguinale. J Infect Dis 142:744, 1980

Lal S: Continued efficacy of streptomycin in the treatment of granuloma inguinale. Br J Vener Dis 47:454, 1971

———, Nicholas C: Epidemiological and clinical features in 165 cases of granuloma inguinale. Br J Vener Dis 46:461, 1970

Sowmini CN: Donovanosis, in *International Perspectives on Neglected Sexually Transmitted Diseases: Impact on Venereology, Infertility, and Maternal and Infant Health,* KK Holmes, PA Mardh (eds). Washington, DC, Hemisphere Publishing, 1982, pp 205–217

169 BARTONELLOSIS

JAMES J. PLORDE

DEFINITION Bartonellosis (Carrión's disease) is an infection with *Bartonella bacilliformis.* Two well-defined clinical stages occur: an acute febrile anemia of rapid onset and high mortality, designated *Oroya fever,* and a benign eruptive form with chronic cutaneous lesions, called *verruga peruana.* Either of these types may be mild, and asymptomatic cases constitute the greatest epidemiologic hazard.

ETIOLOGY *Bartonella bacilliformis* is a small, motile, aerobic, pleomorphic, gram-negative bacillus which stains reddish violet with Giemsa's stain. It can be cultured on enriched media and does not produce a hemolysin. The organisms are sensitive to several antibiotics in vitro.

EPIDEMIOLOGY The disease is limited to certain valleys in the Andes Mountains comprising parts of Peru, Ecuador, and Colombia. It occurs in regions between the altitudes of 2400 and 8000 ft where the sandfly vector, *Phlebotomus,* propagates. Although only *P. verrucarum* has been shown to transmit the disease, other species are undoubtedly involved. Asymptomatic cases and convalescent carriers are the only known reservoir of infection. A low-grade bacteremia may persist for years following resolution of symptoms, and *B. bacilliformis* can be recovered from the blood of 5 to 10 percent of the apparently normal population in an endemic area. Epidemics often coincide with immigration of workers from uninfected areas.

PATHOLOGY AND PATHOGENESIS The manifestations of the disease are thought to reflect the immune status of the host. In nonimmune individuals Oroya fever develops. Large numbers of the *Bartonella* bacteria enter the bloodstream, adhere to erythrocytes, and invade the endothelial cells of the capillaries and lymphatics. The presence of the organisms on the surface of the red blood cell results in their phagocytosis and destruction by the liver and spleen. The red blood cell life span is greatly shortened, and anemia develops. This is accentuated by a defective erythropoietic response early in the course of infection. The pathogenesis of the hemolytic anemia remains unknown. Agglutinins and hemolysins have not been found, and tests for mechanical fragility of red blood cells have given variable results. Invasion and swelling of capillary endothelial cells may lead to vascular occlusion and tissue infarcts. It is possible that an impairment of reticuloendothelial function secondary to massive phagocytosis of red blood cells is responsible for the frequency with which *Salmonella* and other coliform bacteremias are seen in Oroya fever.

With developing immunity, the bacteria nearly disappear from the peripheral blood and capillary endothelium. After a latent period they reappear in the skin and subcutaneous tissue where they are apparently responsible for the development of the hemangioid lesions of verruga peruana. Second attacks of Carrión's disease are unusual. When they occur, they almost invariably present as verruga.

CLINICAL MANIFESTATIONS The incubation period is approximately 3 weeks but may be longer. The initial symptoms are fever and pains in the bones, joints, and muscles. At this point the disease often resembles influenza or malaria, but blood cultures are positive. After these prodromes, the patient usually develops one of the two classic forms of the infection.

Oroya fever This form is characterized by sudden onset of high fever, extreme pallor, weakness, and a precipitous drop in the number of red blood cells. The count may fall from normal to 1 million per cubic millimeter within 4 or 5 days. The anemia is characterized by normochromic macrocytes in the peripheral blood, striking polychromasia and polychromatophilia, nucleated red blood cells, Howell-Jolly bodies, Cabot rings, and basophilic stippling. There may also be a mild leukocytosis with a shift to the left. Organisms are numerous in the blood, and stained smears may show 90 percent of the erythrocytes heavily invaded. Salmonellosis, malaria, amebiasis, tuberculosis, and other intercurrent infections may occur and are an important factor in fatal cases.

Muscle and joint pain and headache are severe, and insomnia, delirium, and coma are the terminal manifestations. In untreated patients, the mortality rate may exceed 50 percent; death occurs within 10 days to 4 weeks. With treatment, or sometimes spontaneously, recovery results if the organisms decrease and fever abates. The red blood cell count stabilizes and approaches normal values in about 6 weeks, when convalescence begins.

Verruga peruana This form of the disease, characterized by a profuse skin eruption, may follow the anemic form or may occur in patients without previous symptoms. The verrugas vary in color from red to purple. They may be miliary, nodular, or eroding, and they range in size from 2 to 10 mm up to 3 or 4 cm in diameter. The three types of verruga may occur together; since eruption takes place in successive crops, verrugas of all types and in all stages of development may be found on the same patient. The chief sites involved are the limbs and face, and less frequently the genitalia, scalp, and mucosa of the mouth and pharynx. They may persist for 1 month to 2 years. The eruption is accompanied by pain, fever, and moderate anemia. Bartonellas may be demonstrated in the lesions and cultured from the blood.

DIAGNOSIS A clinical diagnosis can be made with accuracy in endemic areas. During Oroya fever the organism is easily seen on peripheral blood smears. It may be recovered from blood cultures in all stages of the disease.

TREATMENT Oroya fever responds dramatically to a number of antibiotics including tetracycline and chloramphenicol. The latter in a dose of 2 g per day for 7 days is often preferred because of the frequency with which *Salmonella* infections complicate this disease. Fever disappears within 48 h, and the patient recovers rapidly. Transfusions may be required when the anemia is severe. Antibiotic therapy of the verrugal stage may hasten the involution of these lesions. The use of DDT in both the interior and exterior of human dwellings is highly effective in controlling the night-biting sandflies. Insect repellents and bed netting afford personal protection.

REFERENCES

Caudra MC: Salmonellosis complication in human bartonellosis. Tex Rep Biol Med 14:97, 1956

Dooley JR: Haemotropic bacteria in man. Lancet 2:1237, 1980

Kaye D et al: Factors influencing host resistance to *Salmonella* infections: The effects of hemolysis and erythrophagocytosis. Am J Med Sci 254:205, 1967

Ricketts WE: Clinical manifestations of Carrión's disease. AMA Arch Intern Med 84:751, 1949

Schultz MG: Daniel Carrión's experiment. N Engl J Med 278:1323, 1968

Ureteaga OB, Payne EH: Treatment of the acute febrile phase of Carrión's disease with chloramphenicol. Am J Trop Med 4:507, 1955

section 6 | Diseases caused by anaerobic bacteria

170 TETANUS

HARRY N. BEATY

DEFINITION Tetanus is an acute, often fatal, disease caused by an exotoxin produced in a wound by *Clostridium tetani.* It is characterized by generalized increased rigidity and convulsive spasms of skeletal muscles.

ETIOLOGY *C. tetani* is a strictly anaerobic, gram-positive rod which is motile and readily forms endospores. In stained preparations, organisms may occur singly, in pairs, or in long chains. Spore-bearing bacilli usually contain a single, spheric, terminal endospore which swells the end of the organism and produces a characteristic "clubbed" appearance.

The organism grows well on blood agar at 37°C under anaerobic conditions. Slight hemolysis is usually apparent, but isolated colonies are rare because the organism tends to swarm. *C. tetani* is relatively inert biochemically, with no proteolytic activity and no fermentation of carbohydrates. Vegetative forms of the tetanus bacillus are no more resistant to adverse conditions than other bacteria are, but spores are highly resistant to antiseptics and moderately resistant to heat.

Ten distinct types of *C. tetani* can be distinguished on the basis of flagellar antigens. All these types have one or more common somatic antigens and are capable of producing at least two exotoxins. One, a hemolysin, is relatively unimportant clinically. The other, tetanospasmin, generally referred to as tetanus toxin, is a protein with a molecular weight of approximately 145,000 in its dimer form and is responsible for the clinical manifestations of tetanus. The tetanospasmins produced by the various types of *C. tetani* are nearly identical antigenically, and only one antitoxin is needed to neutralize the tetanus toxins produced by all strains.

EPIDEMIOLOGY The tetanus bacillus is found in the superficial layers of soil and as a saprophyte in the intestinal tract of humans and certain animals. It is most frequently encountered in densely populated regions in hot, damp climates and in soil rich in organic matter. This explains, in part, why the disease is rare in the polar regions and relatively uncommon in the U.S.S.R., North America, and most of Europe. Urbanization, mechanization of agriculture, and socioeconomic factors such as poverty and lack of availability of health services also significantly influence the occurrence of this disease.

Worldwide, there are probably 300,000 to 500,000 cases of tetanus each year, with a mortality rate of roughly 45 percent. There is no racial predilection, but the male-to-female ratio is 2.5:1, even among neonates, in which the opportunity for infection is presumably equal. In the United States, there are about 100 reported cases each year, and these occur almost exclusively in nonimmunized or only partially immunized individuals. The incidence of disease is high among nonwhites in the southern states, and in the last decade, about two-thirds of patients have been 50 years of age or older. However, spores of *C. tetani* are distributed widely throughout urban centers and rural areas of the entire country, and are found commonly on clothing and in house dust, placing the nonimmune individual at risk after relatively minor household injuries. Tetanus has been known to follow surgery and innocuous procedures such as skin testing or intramuscular injection of medication. The disease is inordinately common in narcotic addicts, perhaps because heroin is frequently "cut" with quinine, which drastically lowers the redox potential at the site of injection and favors the growth of *C. tetani.*

Tetanus neonatorum is a major cause of infant mortality in developing countries and is directly related to poor obstetric conditions and lack of maternal immunization programs.

PATHOGENESIS AND PATHOLOGY *C. tetani* is a noninvasive organism. Therefore, tetanus can occur only after spores or vegetative bacteria gain access to tissues and produce toxin locally. The usual mode of entry is through a puncture wound or laceration on the hand, foot, or leg. However, tetanus may follow elective surgery, burn wounds, chronic skin ulcers, otitis media, dental infection, abortion, and pregnancy. Neonatal tetanus usually follows infection of the umbilical stump. The disease not infrequently follows injuries too trivial to be seen by a physician, and in 10 to 20 percent of cases there is neither a history of injury nor a detectable lesion.

Wounds are undoubtedly contaminated frequently with spores of *C. tetani,* but tetanus develops rarely because germination of spores occurs only when the oxygen tension is much lower than that of normal tissue. Spores may survive in the body for months to years and finally produce disease at some later date after minor trauma which alters local conditions. Toxin production in wounds is favored by necrotic tissue, foreign bodies, calcium salts, and associated infections which establish low oxidation-reduction potentials. Infection caused by the tetanus bacillus remains strictly localized, but the toxin produced is transported to the central nervous system via neural pathways. Toxin entering the circulation persists for days, and probably must enter peripheral nerves to spread centrally and cause disease.

The typical clinical manifestations of tetanus are caused by the effect of tetanospasmin on the central nervous system. The toxin attacks synaptic functions to produce disinhibition of both the alpha and gamma motor systems. Generalized muscle rigidity arises from uninhibited afferent stimuli entering the central nervous system from the periphery. When the stimuli become more vigorous, spasms occur. Emotional and, to a lesser extent, visual stimuli can also cause muscle spasm. Tetanus toxin also has other effects. Peripherally it produces neuromuscular blockade similar to that of botulinum toxin, and it acts directly on muscle to produce contraction which is unaccompanied by an action potential in nerves. Certain clinical observations have raised the possibility that tetanus toxin also has an effect on the sympathetic nervous system.

All the effects of tetanus toxin appear to be self-limited and completely reversible, because patients who recover from the disease have no residual defect. Although there are no distinguishable pathologic changes which are characteristic of tetanus, brainstem lesions have been reported in patients dying from tetanus, and toxic myocarditis has been recognized.

CLINICAL MANIFESTATIONS The *incubation period* of tetanus, i.e., the time between injury and the appearance of unmistakable symptoms, ranges from 2 to 56 days. However, over 80 percent of patients become symptomatic within 14 days. A short incubation period indicates severe disease, and when symptoms occur within 2 or 3 days of injury, the mortality rate approaches 100 percent.

Nonspecific premonitory symptoms such as restlessness, irritability, and headache are encountered occasionally, but the commonest presenting complaints are pain and stiffness in the jaw, abdomen, or back and difficulty swallowing. As the disease progresses, stiffness gives way to rigidity, and patients often complain of difficulty opening their mouths. In fact, trismus is the commonest manifestation of tetanus and is responsible for the familiar descriptive name of *lockjaw.* As more muscles are involved, rigidity becomes generalized, and sustained contractions of facial muscles produce a characteristic expression called *risus sardonicus.* The intensity and sequence of muscle involvement is quite variable. In a small proportion of patients, only local signs and symptoms develop in the region of the injury. In the vast majority, however, most muscles are involved to some degree, and the signs and symptoms encountered depend upon the major muscle groups affected.

Reflex spasms usually occur within 24 to 72 h of the first symptoms, an interval referred to as the *onset time.* As in the case of the incubation period, a short onset time is associated with a poor prognosis. Spasms are caused by sudden intensification of afferent stimuli arising in the periphery, which increases rigidity and causes simultaneous and excessive contraction of muscles and their antagonists. Spasms may be both painful and dangerous. As the disease progresses, minimal or inapparent stimuli produce more intense and longer-lasting spasms with increasing frequency. Respiration may be impaired by laryngospasm or tonic contraction of respiratory muscles which prevents adequate ventilation. Hypoxia may then lead to irreversible central nervous system damage and death.

Patients are almost invariably conscious and mentally alert at the time of admission. Low-grade fever, profuse sweating, and tachycardia are common. Deep tendon reflexes are hyperactive, and there may be labile hypertension. The physical examination should be undertaken with care, because reflex convulsive spasms may be precipitated easily. The wound through which *C. tetani* was introduced should be evaluated, and the examination should determine the extent of rigidity; the severity of trismus; the presence or absence of dysphagia and respiratory embarrassment; the frequency, intensity, and duration of convulsive spasms; and the presence of complications such as respiratory infection.

Characteristically, the manifestations of tetanus increase in severity for about 3 days after the first sign and then remain stable for the next 5 to 7 days. After about 10 days, spasms begin to occur less frequently, and by the end of 2 weeks, they disappear altogether. Although residual stiffness may persist for a prolonged period, most survivors recover completely in 4 weeks.

Tetanus neonatorum is a severe form of the disease which usually occurs within 10 days of birth. Early signs include difficulty in sucking, irritability, and excessive crying, associated with peculiar grimacing. Intense rigidity characteristically produces opisthotonus, flexion of the arms, clenched fists, extension of the legs, and plantar flexion of the toes. Typical spasms occur with minimal stimuli.

Complications Complications contribute significantly to the morbidity and mortality of tetanus. Some result from overly vigorous therapy and prolonged bed rest, while others are attributed to the action of tetanus toxin. Inadequate ventilation, either from laryngospasm or spasm of respiratory muscles, is a constant threat. In addition to hypoxia, atelectasis is a common consequence of impaired respiration. Difficulty in swallowing leads to aspiration of secretions, which may also cause atelectasis and initiate pulmonary infection. Thrombophlebitis is occasionally encountered, but bland venous thrombosis is more common and may lead to pulmonary embolization. Cardiovascular complications thought to be due to hyperactivity of the sympathetic nervous system include vasomotor instability, hypertension, tachycardia, arrhythmias, and severe vasoconstriction. Pulmonary edema and hypotension may occur as a consequence of myocarditis. High fever usually signifies secondary infection. Pneumonia is a common late complication of tetanus and is found in 50 to 70 percent of autopsied cases. Other frequent sites of secondary infections include the original wound, decubitus ulcers, and the urinary tract of patients with indwelling bladder catheters. Fractures of midthoracic vertebrae are probably due to severe spasms and are particularly common among children and adolescents. Gastrointestinal complications include acute peptic ulceration, paralytic ileus, and constipation. Hemolysis is seen in a small proportion of patients.

Pneumonia is a major cause of death. Other autopsy findings in early deaths include intense congestion of viscera and, occasionally, intracranial hemorrhage or thrombosis. In about 20 percent of cases, no obvious pathology is identified, and death is attributed to the direct effects of tetanus toxin.

LABORATORY FINDINGS There are no laboratory findings characteristic of tetanus. Granulocytosis is seen in about one-third of patients, but anemia is rare. Blood chemistries are almost always normal initially, but various fluid and electrolyte disturbances may arise in the course of the disease. The electrocardiogram usually shows only sinus tachycardia, but occasionally T-wave inversion is seen. Roentgenograms are not helpful except in the evaluation of complications.

The diagnosis of tetanus is entirely clinical and does not depend upon bacteriologic confirmation. *C. tetani* is recovered from the wound in only 30 percent of cases, and not infrequently it is isolated from patients who do not have tetanus. Laboratory identification depends on cultural and morphologic characteristics, absence of fermentative activity, and, most importantly, demonstration of toxin production in mice.

DIFFERENTIAL DIAGNOSIS No disease resembles fully developed tetanus. However, strychnine poisoning and dystonic reactions due to phenothiazines and metoclopramide produce a syndrome that has been referred to as pseudotetanus. These rare reactions usually follow brief exposure to drugs and subside 24 to 48 h after their administration is discontinued. Early in the course of true tetanus, exclusion of local causes of jaw pain may be difficult, and the combination of neck stiffness and fever may suggest meningitis. However, this can be excluded by lumbar puncture, because in tetanus the spinal fluid is normal. When there is doubt about the diagnosis, clinical observation usually settles the issue within a matter of hours.

TREATMENT In order to formulate a rational plan of therapy, it is useful to assess the severity of tetanus. *Mild tetanus* is characterized by an incubation period of at least 14 days and an onset time of more than 6 days. Trismus is usually present, but dysphagia is absent, and generalized spasms are brief and mild. *Moderately severe tetanus* has a somewhat shorter incubation period and onset time; trismus is marked, dysphagia and generalized rigidity are present, but ventilation remains adequate even during spasms. The criteria for *severe tetanus* include a short incubation time, an onset time of 72 h or less, severe trismus, dysphagia and rigidity, and frequent, prolonged, generalized convulsive spasms. Because of the poor prognosis of tetanus in older individuals, the disease should be considered moderate to severe in all patients over 50.

General measures Patients should be hospitalized in an intensive care unit. After initial evaluation, necrotic tissue and foreign bodies should be removed from the infected wound, and abscesses should be drained. Patients should be placed in a quiet room and observed closely for development of complications or unexpected changes in the course of the disease. While it is a good general principle to disturb patients as little as possible, vital signs must be monitored and aspiration must be averted by positioning the patient carefully and by aspirating nasopharyngeal secretions frequently. Care must be taken to prevent development of decubitus ulcers or contractures, but many routine nursing procedures should be omitted because they may precipitate uncomfortable or dangerous spasms. Initially, nutrition is not a major consideration, and fluid and electrolyte balance should be maintained over the first several days by administration of appropriate solutions intravenously, accompanied by careful recording of intake and output. Patients with severe tetanus are in an intense catabolic state, and may have tremendous fluid losses. Early consideration should be given to intravenous hyperalimentation as a means of meeting the nutritional requirements of these patients.

Antiserum Antiserum does not neutralize tetanus toxin fixed in the central nervous system and does little to ameliorate symptoms already present at the time of admission. However, the case/fatality ratio in mild to moderately severe disease is reduced significantly when antiserum is administered early. Human tetanus immune globulin (TIG) is generally available in the United States, and is far superior to equine antiserum. Because its half-life is about 25 days, only one dose of 3000 to 10,000 units intramuscularly is recommended, even though as little as 500 units may be equally effective. Local infiltration at the site of the wound is of no proven value, but intrathecal injections may prove to be effective after more careful study. Hypersensitivity reactions do not occur with TIG, obviating the need for pretreatment testing.

If human antitoxin is not available, a single dose of equine antiserum should be given after the patient has been tested for hypersensitivity to horse serum. Although the dosage of heterologous antitoxin often recommended for adults is 100,000 to 200,000 units, 10,000 units is probably optimal. Anaphylaxis can occur despite negative sensitivity tests, and patients must be observed carefully to institute treatment at the first sign of an anaphylactic reaction. Up to 25 percent of patients develop delayed reactions including serum sickness after equine antitoxin. Occasionally, serious neurologic complications accompany other manifestations of serum sickness.

Active immunization of patients with tetanus is necessary, because the disease does not confer natural immunity. However, there is no need to begin primary immunization until the patient has recovered.

Management of muscle spasms Muscle relaxation is the key to therapy, but mild sedation is desirable also because it reduces the effect of sensory stimuli. Ideally, this should be accomplished without significantly affecting respiration. Although a variety of agents have been used in the treatment of tetanus, none has achieved universal acceptance. Among the barbiturates, phenobarbital, in adult doses of 50 to 100 mg every 3 to 6 h, produces adequate sedation which may suffice in the management of mild tetanus. When rapid action is required, amylbarbital or pentobarbital, 50 to 200 mg intravenously, may be used. Frequent and severe spasms cannot be managed with barbiturates alone, because the dosage required for control leads to unconsciousness and suppressed respiration. For this reason, muscle relaxants usually are used, either alone or in combination with barbiturates, in the treatment of moderate or severe tetanus. Electromyographic studies have shown that the phenothiazines effectively produce relaxation while sparing the sensorium and respirations. Chlorpromazine, in doses of 200 to 300 mg a day, minimizes rigidity and decreases the frequency of spasms. Diazepam, in adult doses of 40 to 120 mg a day, is very effective in the treatment of tetanus; it acts quickly, relieves rigidity, and has significant sedative effect without depressing respiration. Given alone to patients with moderately severe disease, diazepam has been shown to lower oxygen consumption from levels that are three to five times normal to near normal. In combination with other drugs, diazepam may significantly reduce mortality in nonneonates with severe tetanus. Other drugs which have been employed extensively include mephenesin, meprobamate, paraldehyde, and chloral hydrate.

Another approach to the management of muscle spasms involves the use of neuromuscular blocking agents such as tubocurare or pancuronium. This method can be used only where facilities and personnel are available to provide controlled mechanical ventilation for the paralyzed patient. It should be reserved for treatment of severe tetanus that is not adequately controlled by other measures. In centers with a team experienced in handling these patients, this approach, in conjunction with meticulous attention to other details of care, has produced encouraging results.

Tracheostomy Tracheostomy has an important role in the management of tetanus. It protects against suffocation due to laryngospasm, reduces the risk of aspiration, and facilitates mechanical assistance of ventilation. While most patients with mild tetanus and some with more severe disease can be managed without it, all patients should be considered candidates for tracheostomy, and the necessary equipment should be at the bedside. Where secretions are copious or respiration has been compromised, the need for tracheostomy should be recognized early, and whenever possible it should be performed electively rather than as an emergency.

Other measures Although antibiotics are frequently prescribed to treat the infected wound and prevent toxin production, there is no indication that they influence the disease favorably. If antibiotics are used, penicillin G is the drug of choice because it is highly effective against the tetanus bacillus, and its limited spectrum is less likely to predispose patients to superinfections. Appropriate cultures to detect complicating infections should be obtained periodically throughout the course of the disease, and specific antibiotics prescribed when indicated. Adrenocortical steroids have been used empirically in the treatment of tetanus, but there is no experimental or clinical evidence to support their effectiveness. Likewise, beneficial results have been claimed for hyperbaric oxygen, but insufficient information is available to evaluate its potential.

PREVENTION *C. tetani* is so ubiquitous in nature that the only hope for prevention of tetanus lies in massive immunization programs. Effective active immunization is possible, and if applied universally, according to recommendations, tetanus could be virtually eliminated. Even tetanus neonatorum could be prevented, because infants are protected by antibody which passes the placental barrier. Two types of tetanus toxoids are available for immunization, a fluid and an adsorbed form. The adsorbed toxoid is preferred because it produces higher antitoxin titers and longer-lasting immunity. Immunization failures are exceedingly rare.

According to current recommendations, children 2 months to 6 years of age should be immunized with diphtheria and tetanus toxoids and pertussis vaccine (DPT). Ideally, the first dose should be administered within 2 or 3 months of birth, the second and third should follow at 4- to 8-week intervals, and the fourth dose should be given 1 year after the third. Schoolchildren and adults should be immunized with three doses of adult-type tetanus and diphtheria toxoids (Td). The second dose should be given 4 to 8 weeks after the first, and the third 6 months to 1 year after the second. A booster of DPT is recommended for children at the time of entrance into kindergarten or elementary school. Thereafter and for everyone else who has received a primary immunization series, routine boosters of Td should be given every 10 years. Side effects are uncommon after the primary series, but occur more frequently in persons who have received an excessive number of booster injections. Reactions usually take the form of local swelling, erythema, lymphadenopathy, and fever, but on rare occasions more severe hypersensitivity reactions occur.

In the management of wounds, the question of prophylaxis against tetanus frequently arises. Because active immunization is so effective, a reliable immunization history can greatly simplify the problem. If a patient has received three or more doses of toxoid, antiserum need not be given, and a toxoid booster is required only if more than 5 to 10 years has elapsed since the last dose. The shorter interval pertains for all but clean, minor wounds. In all other instances, the decision must be made on an individual basis, taking into consideration the characteristics of the wound, the conditions under which it was incurred, its age, and the patient's previous active immunization against tetanus. Table 170-1 provides guidelines which may be useful in making appropriate decisions about tetanus prophylaxis. For patients who have received fewer than two doses of toxoid, the primary immunization series should be completed in the succeeding weeks to months.

When passive immunization is contemplated, TIG is preferred to horse serum because it offers longer protection and freedom from serious reactions. The currently recommended prophylactic dose for adults is 250 units intramuscularly, which ensures a protective level of antitoxin in the plasma ($>$ 0.01 unit per milliliter) for as long as 4 weeks. If TIG is not available, equine antitoxin in doses of 3000 to 6000 units should be administered after careful screening for sensitivity to horse serum. When both toxoid and antitoxin are indicated, they can be given simultaneously, but separate syringes and separate injection sites should be used. The adsorbed toxin is the preparation of choice in this situation.

TABLE 170-1
Guidelines for tetanus prophylaxis

Active immunization	*Toxoid*	*Antitoxin*	
		*Minor wound**	*Other wounds*
Uncertain	Yes	No	Yes
None	Yes	No	Yes
$<$ 3 doses	Yes	No	Yes‡
$\geq$ 3 doses	No†	No	No

* *Fresh, clean, minor wounds incurred in a setting unlikely to cause tetanus.*
† *Unless more than 10 years since last dose; 5 years if the wound is other than minor.*
‡ *Except in patients who have received at least two previous doses of toxoid and have fresh non-tetanus-prone wounds.*

Prompt and adequate care of wounds is also important in preventing tetanus. They should be cleaned carefully, and foreign bodies or necrotic, devitalized tissue should be removed. Administration of tetracycline or penicillin is advocated by some to prevent multiplication of *C. tetani,* but tetanus may occur in spite of prophylactic antibiotics, and their role in the prevention of tetanus has not been established. However, severe wounds should be examined regularly and treated promptly with antimicrobials if infection develops.

PROGNOSIS The overall case fatality ratio of tetanus is variable, but in the United States it ranges between 40 and 60 percent. This reflects the fact that the incidence of tetanus is 8 to 10 times greater among people over 60 compared with people 10 to 20 years of age, and the mortality rate is 25 to 50 times greater in the elderly. Neonatal tetanus is uncommon in this country but is fatal in more than 60 percent of cases. The shorter the incubation period and onset time, the poorer the prognosis in tetanus. Three-fourths of the deaths occur within the first week, primarily from pulmonary infection, aspiration, or pulmonary embolization. Survivors recover completely, but remain susceptible to the disease unless actively immunized with tetanus toxoid.

REFERENCES

Blake PA et al: Serologic therapy of tetanus in the United States. JAMA 235:42, 1976

Centers for Disease Control: Diphtheria, tetanus, and pertussis: Guidelines for vaccine prophylaxis and other preventive measures. Morb Mort Week Rep 30:392, 1981

Cochlin DL: Dystonic reactions due to metoclopramide and phenothiazines resembling tetanus. Br J Clin Pract 28:201, 1974

Dasta JF et al: Diazepam infusion in tetanus: Correlation of drug levels with effect. South Med J 74:278, 1981

Furste W: Four keys to 100 percent success in tetanus prophylaxis. Am J Surg 128:616, 1974

———, Wheeler W: Tetanus: A team disease, in *Current Problems in Surgery.* Chicago, Year Book, 1972

Gupta PS et al: Intrathecal human tetanus immunoglobulin in early tetanus. Lancet 2:439, 1980

Tsueda K et al: Cardiovascular manifestations of tetanus. Anesthesiology 40:588, 1974

171 BOTULISM

HARRY N. BEATY

DEFINITION Botulism is an acute form of poisoning which results from ingestion of a toxin produced by *Clostridium botulinum.* The illness is characterized by progressive descending muscle paralysis and is often fatal.

HISTORY AND EPIDEMIOLOGY The disease was first recognized over 200 years ago by south German physicians who adopted the term *botulismus* for the often fatal syndrome which sometimes followed the consumption of spoiled sausage (*botulus* is Latin for sausage). Botulism was rare in the United

States before World War I. Subsequent growth of commercial and home canning led to a great increase in cases. A series of studies by K. F. Meyer and his associates in the early 1920s defined the habitat of *C. botulinum*, the foods often incriminated, and the conditions necessary for the destruction of *C. botulinum* spores. This knowledge led to the virtual elimination of botulism from the commercial canning industry, and most cases of clinical botulism now follow consumption of improperly canned, home-preserved foods. However, the need for constant surveillance is emphasized by periodic outbreaks of botulism caused by commercially processed foods. For example, in 1977, 59 people developed botulism after eating home-canned peppers in a restaurant in Pontiac, Michigan; and in 1978, 32 people manifested the disease after dining at a country club in Clovis, New Mexico. These are the largest outbreaks ever reported in the United States, and contrast sharply with the usual situation in which fewer than three individuals are affected after eating home-canned foods.

ETIOLOGY *C. botulinum* is a strictly anaerobic, spore-forming, gram-positive rod which elaborates a potent exotoxin during growth and autolysis. Morphologically and culturally similar strains are differentiated into types A through G on the basis of antigenic characteristics of the toxin each produces. Type A, B, and E toxins have been implicated most frequently in human disease in the United States. Only two outbreaks of type F botulism have been reported. Types C and D produce disease almost exclusively in animals, including wild waterfowl, cattle, horses, and mink. Type G had been isolated from soil only twice since its discovery in 1969, but in 1977 and 1978 the organism and its toxin were recovered at autopsy from five patients in Switzerland who died suddenly and unexpectedly.

Type A and B spores are widely distributed in soil throughout the world. Type A spores are most common in the United States, especially along the Pacific Coast and the Rocky Mountain states. Type B spores have been found more frequently in the eastern states and in Europe. Type E spores have been demonstrated in lakeshore mud, coastal sand, and sea-bottom silt in northern latitudes. Fish apparently contaminate their intestinal tracts with these spores, which accounts for the high incidence of type E strains in fish-borne botulism. Type F spores have been found in marine sediments collected off the coast of California and Oregon and in salmon taken from the Columbia River.

Botulinus toxins are the most potent poisons known. They have been purified and identified as simple proteins. Although they differ in terms of antigenicity, molecular size, electrophoretic mobility, and amino acid content, they appear to have a similar effect on neuromuscular transmission. Pharmacologic differences are manifested by the variable susceptibility of specific animal species to the different toxins.

Spores of *C. botulinum* can withstand 100°C for several hours. Moist heat at 120°C for 30 min will destroy spores of all types, but the toxins are considerably more heat-labile. All varieties of toxin are destroyed by boiling for 10 min, or by temperatures of 80°C for 30 min.

PATHOGENESIS For years, botulism was considered a disease that occurred almost exclusively after ingestion of preformed toxin. With the recognition that infant botulism may follow ingestion of *C. botulinum* spores which germinate, proliferate, and produce toxin in the intestinal tract, this concept has been modified. The Centers for Disease Control now report human cases of botulism in four categories: food-borne botulism, infant botulism, wound botulism, and unclassified. The latter includes a small number of adult cases each year for which no ingestion of contaminated food can be documented. Classifying them separately acknowledges that the pathogenesis of their disease may be more like that of the infant syndrome than classic food-borne botulism.

Food-borne botulism can occur when the following conditions are met: (1) a food product is contaminated with viable *C. botulinum* bacilli or spores; (2) proper conditions for germination of the spores exist; (3) time and conditions permit production of toxin before eating; (4) the food is not heated or is heated insufficiently to destroy botulinus toxin; and (5) the toxin-containing food is ingested by a susceptible host. Though a relatively anaerobic environment and temperatures above 30°C (86°F) are optimal for toxin production, strict anaerobic conditions are not necessary, and toxin production by some type E strains has been observed at temperatures as low as 6°C (42.8°F).

Although a variety of home-processed foods have been sources of botulism in the United States, certain foods seem to be safer than others. This may be because low pH (acidity) inhibits germination of spores and, therefore, toxin production. Commercially processed smoked fish, tuna, peppers, and soup (vichyssoise) have been implicated in outbreaks of botulism. Contaminated foods may appear putrefied, but frequently look and taste perfectly normal, regardless of toxin type.

Botulinus toxins are absorbed primarily in the stomach and upper part of the small intestine. The toxins are large protein molecules which are absorbed after they have been reduced in size by proteolytic enzymes which do not destroy activity. In fact, the toxicity of type E and G toxins is enhanced by tryptic digestion. Either absorption is incomplete or toxins are inactivated partially by digestion, because the amount of toxin which appears in the bloodstream is variable, and in animals the lethal dose orally is 1000 times greater than the lethal dose intravenously. Toxin which reaches the lower part of the small intestine and colon may be absorbed slowly, which probably accounts for the delayed onset and the prolonged symptoms observed in many patients.

It is not clear why infant botulism occurs in some babies who ingest *C. botulinum* spores and not in others. Age certainly is an important factor; 98 percent of recognized cases have occurred in children between 1 and 6 months of age, and in certain animal models the syndrome can only be reproduced during a few days of early life. It has been documented that the intestinal tract of infants with botulism is colonized with *C. botulinum*, and it is assumed that the manifestations of the syndrome are slowly progressive because toxin is absorbed as it is produced rather than all at once, as is the case in food-borne botulism. Limited studies comparing the fecal flora of infants who have botulism with that of controls suggest that colonization of the intestine with *C. botulinum* may occur because of a delay in establishment of the normal fecal flora, the presence of other organisms that promote colonization, the absence of organisms that inhibit *C. botulinum*, or a change in intestinal function that favors germination and growth of ingested spores. Diet is an important factor in the development of infant botulism. Honey has been proved to be the source of *C. botulinum* spores in a number of cases, and the current recommendation is that honey not be fed to children less than 12 months of age. Honey has not been shown to contain botulinus toxin, so it is a safe food for older children and adults. Breast-feeding may provide relative protection against infant botulism. Supplementary iron may increase a baby's susceptibility to the fulminant form of the disease. Spores can be ingested from a variety of environmental sources, and it deserves emphasis that for the majority of cases no source of *C. botulinum* is identified.

Botulinus toxins exert their major effect by blocking neuromuscular transmission in cholinergic nerve fibers. They either inhibit the release of acetylcholine or bind with it at or near its site of release within presynaptic clefts. Muscle reactivity to acetylcholine applied directly to the motor end plate is unimpaired. Central nervous system cholinergic pathways do not appear to be affected significantly in human beings.

CLINICAL MANIFESTATIONS Botulism may vary from a mild illness for which patients seek no medical advice to a fulminant disease which ends in death within 24 h. Symptoms usually begin 12 to 36 h after ingestion of toxin, although the extremes of 3 h to 14 days are recorded. In general, the earlier symptoms appear, the more serious the disease.

The commonest symptoms are ocular; diplopia, blurred vision, and photophobia are frequently the first to appear. Bulbar weakness is manifested by dysphonia, dysarthria, dysphagia, and weakness of the tongue. Symmetric paralysis of the extremities appears and may progress rapidly in a descending or ascending manner. Weakness of the respiratory muscles may occur early, but this is often asymptomatic until function is moderately impaired.

Impairment of cholinergic autonomic transmission may result in constipation, urinary retention, and reduced salivation and lacrimation. Nausea and vomiting are early symptoms in half the patients, but the absence of these symptoms does not rule out botulism. Gastrointestinal symptoms are more common in type B and E disease than in type A. Some patients with type B disease may have minimal weakness but marked constipation and decreased secretions.

On examination patients are usually alert, oriented, and afebrile, even with severe disease. Ocular signs include ptosis, weakness of extraocular motion, and in some patients failure of accommodation. The pupils are normal in many patients, but in some cases may react sluggishly or may be dilated and unreactive to light. Widespread neuromuscular block results in symmetric flaccid weakness of the palate, tongue, larynx, respiratory muscles, and extremities. Severe paralytic ileus and bladder distention may be present. Deep-tendon reflexes are intact in milder cases, but if significant paralysis is present they are reduced or absent. No pathologic reflexes are detectable. Findings on sensory examination are always entirely normal. Some patients have apparent gait disturbances and incoordination, but this is due to generalized weakness.

Once symptoms are noted, the disease may progress rapidly over several days, with significant changes in status occurring at hourly intervals. A period of stabilization is then followed by gradual recovery over a period of days to months, depending on the severity of intoxication. The mechanism of recovery is not well understood. In wound botulism the patient may be febrile, but the clinical manifestations are otherwise similar. A 10- to 14-day incubation period is common from the time of infection to the onset of toxic symptoms. The clinical spectrum of infant botulism ranges from asymptomatic carriage of *C. botulinum* to a fatal illness indistinguishable from the sudden infant death syndrome. Constipation, poor feeding, and "failure to thrive," alone or in combination, may be the only signs of the illness, but these manifestations may be followed by progressive weakness of skeletal muscles, cranial nerve palsies, "floppiness" of the head, and impaired respiration.

LABORATORY FINDINGS Routine laboratory studies do not aid in diagnosing botulism. When botulism is suspected, public health authorities should be consulted to assist in special studies to confirm the diagnosis. Specimens of blood, feces, and gastric contents, as well as suspected foods and their containers, should be obtained. Because of the extreme potency of botulinus toxin, careful collection and laboratory precautions should be used. The food, stool, and serum should be studied for the presence of toxin by injecting extracts intraperitoneally into mice. If toxin is present, the animals will develop botulism and die within 24 h. Mice protected by specific antiserum will survive. The food and stool should be submitted for special anaerobic culture. This battery of tests will result in an overall case recognition rate of about 85 percent. Immunofluorescent techniques are useful for the early recognition of the organisms. If wound botulism is suspected, the exudate should be submitted for culture and toxin analysis.

The spinal fluid is always normal. Electrocardiographic abnormalities, including minor disturbances in conduction, nonspecific T-wave and ST-segment changes, and various disorders of rhythm, have been described. Electrodiagnostic studies have been shown to be of value in differentiating botulism from other paralytic diseases. The evoked motor action potential may be of low voltage but will facilitate with tetanic stimulation in a manner similar to the myasthenic syndrome (Eaton-Lambert syndrome). Electromyography may show small, short-duration, overly abundant motor units. In severe cases, denervation can occur, resulting in fibrillation activity after several weeks.

DIFFERENTIAL DIAGNOSIS Botulism must be differentiated from other conditions that produce generalized paralysis. In the Guillain-Barré syndrome, mild sensory abnormalities are nearly always present, and the spinal fluid protein is often elevated. The variant of the Guillain-Barré syndrome with ophthalmoplegia, areflexia, and ataxia (Fisher's syndrome) may prove particularly confusing. The course of myasthenia gravis is seldom so acute, and the deep tendon reflexes and pupils are normal. Some patients with botulism may show mild improvement after injection of edrophonium (Tensilon), but this improvement is not of the magnitude seen in myasthenia gravis. In tick paralysis the weakness is generally of an ascending pattern, patients may have paresthesias, and a tick is found. In diphtheria, palatal weakness is frequently the first symptom, and a history of prior pharyngitis may be obtained. Cutaneous diphtheria can be differentiated from wound botulism by appropriate cultures. In poliomyelitis the spinal fluid is abnormal and the weakness is often asymmetric and spares the ocular muscles. Vascular accidents of the brainstem can be recognized by associated neurologic signs. Belladonna poisoning presents with markedly dilated pupils and delirium. In organophosphate poisoning the pupils are markedly miotic. Shellfish poisoning, aminoglycoside antibiotic paralysis, and familial periodic paralysis might also prove confusing.

Patients with marked dry mouth may develop a picture simulating pharyngitis. Patients with gastrointestinal complaints and ileus may appear to have other forms of food poisoning or intestinal obstruction.

TREATMENT The most immediate threat to the survival of patients with botulism is respiratory failure. Patients with symptoms or known exposure should be hospitalized. Close observation is essential, and vital capacity should be measured frequently. If respiratory insufficiency develops, the patient may require assisted ventilation with a respirator. Respiratory difficulties may develop rapidly; elective tracheostomy should be performed before onset of respiratory failure, and may be needed to manage secretions even if ventilation is otherwise adequate. Some milder cases may be managed with endotracheal intubation.

If there is no ileus, cathartics and enemas should be given to remove unabsorbed toxin from the intestine, but magnesium citrate and magnesium sulfate should not be given, as the magnesium may potentiate the neuromuscular block produced by botulinus toxin. Nasogastric suction and intravenous hyperalimentation may be needed if ileus is severe. If the bladder is atonic, a catheter will be required. Meticulous nursing care and physical therapy are essential to prevent complications.

As soon as the diagnosis of botulism is suspected, the patient should be tested for hypersensitivity to horse serum and treated with trivalent ABE antitoxin (Connaught), which is available from public health authorities. Type-specific antitoxin has been shown to be of benefit in several outbreaks of type E intoxication, but the value in type A and B outbreaks is less certain, particularly when paralysis has already occurred. Nonfatal hypersensitivity reactions occur in 15 to 20 percent of patients receiving the equine antitoxin, and those that react to a test dose must be desensitized prior to further treatment. Antibiotics should be reserved for specific infectious complications. In infant botulism, where multiplication of ingested organisms may be a factor, antibiotics have been ineffective in eradicating the organism, though this eventually may occur spontaneously. The value of antibiotic therapy in wound botulism has not been determined.

It is essential that public health officials be notified so that toxin-containing foods can be confiscated and so that those with possible exposure can be notified.

A number of reports have appeared since 1967 describing the use of guanidine hydrochloride in the treatment of botulism. This drug presumably acts by enhancing the release of acetylcholine from terminal nerve fibers. About two-thirds of the reported cases have shown some improvement with oral doses of 15 to 50 mg/kg per day, but the drug seems ineffective in those patients with severe respiratory impairment, and probably has no effect on mortality rate. Dose-related side effects include gastrointestinal upset, paresthesias, and fasciculations. Idiosyncratic reactions include cardiac arrhythmias and blood dyscrasias.

PROGNOSIS The current mortality rate of food-borne botulism in the United States is about 10 percent, with type A outbreaks having somewhat higher mortality than types B and E. The case/fatality ratio of hospitalized cases of infant botulism is about 2 percent. Death from botulism is due to complications such as respiratory failure and pneumonia. With rapid diagnosis and aggressive supportive care, even severely involved patients can recover fully. Some patients may have mild residual weakness due to denervation atrophy. Artificial respiratory support may be required for many months, and clinical weakness and autonomic symptoms may be noted for as long as 1 year after the onset of disease.

REFERENCES

Arnon SS: Infant botulism. Annu Rev Med 31:541, 1980

Black RE, Arnon SS: Botulism in the United States, 1976. J Infect Dis 135:829, 1977

Centers for Disease Control: *Botulism in the United States, 1899–1977. Handbook for Epidemiologists, Clinicians, and Laboratory Workers.* 1979

———: Botulism—United States, 1979–1980. Morb Mort Week Rep 30:121, 1981

Cherington M: Botulism: Ten-year experience. Arch Neurol 30:432, 1974

Dowell VR et al: Coproexamination for botulinal toxin and *Clostridium botulinum:* A new procedure for laboratory diagnosis of botulism. JAMA 238:1829, 1977

Faich GA et al: Failure of guanidine therapy in botulism A. N Engl J Med 285:773, 1971

Merson MH, Dowell VR: Epidemiologic, clinical and laboratory aspects of wound botulism. N Engl J Med 289:1005, 1973

Werner SB, Chin J: Botulism—diagnosis, management and public health considerations. Calif Med 118:84, 1973

172
OTHER CLOSTRIDIAL INFECTIONS

MERLE A. SANDE
EDWARD W. HOOK

Bacteria of the genus *Clostridium* are normal inhabitants of soil and of the gastrointestinal tracts of humans and animals. Most of the species that have been described are saprophytic, but some are pathogenic for humans and animals, usually under conditions of lowered host and tissue resistance. Infections with these organisms are often associated with profound systemic manifestations, and all pathogenic clostridia, except *C. tetani* and *C. botulinum,* are capable of causing extensive tissue destruction. Diseases caused by these other clostridia are gas gangrene, cellulitis, postabortal and puerperal sepsis, and, on occasion, pneumonia, empyema, peritonitis, meningitis, endocarditis, osteomyelitis, and arthritis. Ingestion of food contaminated with *C. perfringens* type A is a common cause of enterocolitis, and *C. difficile* has been implicated in antibiotic-induced pseudomembranous colitis.

ETIOLOGY Wounds complicated by gas gangrene may contain a mixture of pathogenic and saprophytic clostridia, often including *C. tetani,* as well as a variety of other bacteria. *Clostridium perfringens* is the most common organism cultured from cases of gas gangrene and clostridial cellulitis, followed in frequency by *C. novyi* or *C. septicum. C. perfringens* causes virtually all clostridial infections of the uterus. *Clostridium bifermentans, C. histolyticum,* and *C. fallax* are less virulent organisms that occasionally cause gas gangrene but are more commonly associated with localized cellulitis. Proliferation of *C. botulinum* in wounds occasionally leads to clinical manifestations of botulism (see Chap. 171).

The clostridia of gas gangrene and related infections are anaerobic or microaerophilic gram-positive bacilli that produce abundant gas in artificial media and form subterminal endospores. *Clostridium perfringens* is encapsulated and nonmotile, rarely sporulates in artificial media, and produces spores that can usually be destroyed by boiling.

Clostridium difficile has been isolated in large numbers from stools of patients with antibiotic-associated pseudomembranous colitis. This organism produces a toxin that is destructive to the intestinal mucosa and is usually resistant to clindamycin, the antibiotic most commonly implicated in enterocolitis.

EPIDEMIOLOGY AND PATHOGENESIS Clostridia can be cultured from one-third to two-thirds of severe traumatic wounds, but gas gangrene develops in only an occasional case. The most important prerequisite for the conversion of clostridial contamination of a wound to a progressive infection is an environment with low oxidation-reduction potential, which permits spore germination and anaerobic growth. Local oxidation-reduction potential can be reduced by failure of the blood supply to a contaminated area, by the presence of foreign bodies such as clothing, soil, or fragments of metal or wood, or by the multiplication of other bacteria in the wound. Once multiplication and toxin production are established, rapid invasion and destruction of healthy tissue follow.

The pathogenicity of clostridia is related to the capacity of these organisms to form exotoxins which destroy tissue cells. The nature and amount of toxins vary considerably for different species and strains. For example, at least 12 different extracellular *toxins* are produced by *C. perfringens.* Alpha toxin, a lecithinase, is the most important and is the principal tissue-destroying, hemolytic, and lethal toxin. Other *C. perfringens* products include collagenase, hyaluronidase, hemolytic theta toxin, leukocidin, deoxyribonuclease, and fibrinolysin.

Gas gangrene is characterized by marked systemic symptoms and a local reaction with extensive necrotizing myositis, edema, thrombosis of small vessels, interstitial gas bubbles, and minimal infiltration by leukocytes. The local reaction in infected tissue can be explained by the action of clostridial toxins, especially alpha toxin, but the factors responsible for the systemic reaction are unknown. Alpha toxin, or other clostridial toxins, have not been demonstrated in circulating blood during the course of severe clostridial myonecrosis.

The toxin responsible for antibiotic-associated pseudomembranous colitis has not been completely characterized. It is found in high titer in cell-free filtrates of feces from patients with this disease. The toxin is produced by *C. difficile,* which is usually resistant to clindamycin and proliferates in the colon when the antibiotic-sensitive flora is suppressed. The toxin is heat labile and cytopathic for certain cells in culture, and it produces an increase in vascular permeability and hemorrhage after injection intradermally in rabbits. Pseudomembranous colitis can be produced by introducing the toxin or the organism into the cecum of hamsters or by treating hamsters with clindamycin. The toxic effects can be blocked by either gas-gangrene equine antitoxin or *C. sordellii* antitoxin; the latter has been shown to cross-react with toxin produced by *C. difficile.*

CLINICAL MANIFESTATIONS **Clostridial myonecrosis (gas gangrene, clostridial myositis)** Gas gangrene develops in anoxic devitalized tissues in which the arterial circulation has been compromised by trauma, constricting tourniquets or casts, or obliterative arterial disease. Infection is most frequent after extensive injury to skeletal muscle, particularly of the thigh and buttock, and is more common in wounds complicated by compound fractures or lodgment of foreign bodies. It may also follow surgical procedures, especially those involving the large bowel and rectum; amputation of ischemic limbs; and reconstructive surgery of the hip. Gas gangrene has also been described following intramuscular injections, especially injection of epinephrine. Minor trauma may occasionally activate clostridial spores dormant in scar tissue and leads to development of myonecrosis years after the original injury. Once infection is established, it rapidly spreads to involve healthy muscle undamaged by previous trauma or ischemia.

The incubation period is usually 1 to 4 days but may vary from 3 h to 6 weeks or longer. The earliest symptom is sudden, severe pain in the injured part, which may develop an intense "woody hard" edema. The distal portion of an involved limb becomes cold and edematous within a few hours, and eventually pulseless and gangrenous. The wound drains a watery, brown, or hemorrhagic material which may have a peculiar sweet odor. The appearance of the wound is usually not that of a pyogenic inflammatory lesion. Depending on the duration of the process, the surrounding skin may be normal, white, and tense, or dusky brown and reddish. Vesicles or hemorrhagic bullae may develop, particularly in *C. septicum* infections. Gas is usually not detectable in the tissues by palpation except in advanced lesions, although it may be visible easily by x-ray. Occasionally, tiny bubbles may be seen in the discharge from the wound; rarely, crepitation can be detected at an early stage by auscultation. The involved muscle appears dark red or black, may herniate through the wound, and is noncontractile when stimulated.

Systemic manifestations developing shortly after onset of severe pain and swelling of an injured extremity strongly suggest gas gangrene. The patient is prostrated, pale, and motionless but is usually well oriented, alert, and extremely apprehensive. The temperature usually does not exceed 38.3°C (101°F) and may be normal. As the illness progresses, there may be anorexia, vomiting, profuse watery or bloody diarrhea, and eventually circulatory collapse. The pulse rate usually exceeds 120 beats per minute and is elevated out of proportion to the temperature. Massive intravascular hemolysis is rare in patients with clostridial myositis. Pericardial effusion is sometimes noted. Delirium and coma may precede death, but more commonly the patient dies suddenly several days after onset of illness, often during surgery or anesthesia. Acute renal failure is occasionally a late complication.

Gas gangrene must be differentiated from nonclostridial infections of gangrenous limbs caused by anaerobic streptococci, aerobic gas-forming coliform bacilli (most commonly *Escherichia coli*), *Bacteroides* species, and group A streptococci (see Chap. 173).

Clostridial cellulitis This is a relatively benign infection of skin and subcutaneous tissues that occurs in a small proportion of wounds contaminated with pathogenic clostridia. The disease is characterized by spreading necrosis of superficial tissues and a profuse, foul-smelling, brown, seropurulent exudate. Gas, which crepitates on palpation, invariably forms in the subcutaneous tissues and may involve an entire limb or form a localized gas pocket. In clostridial cellulitis, the underlying skeletal muscle is not involved, pain is not severe, and the only systemic manifestations are slight fever and moderate tachycardia. It can usually be differentiated from group A streptococcal cellulitis by the presence of subcutaneous gas and the absence of erythema.

Postabortal and puerperal sepsis Uterine infections with *C. perfringens* usually occur after incomplete abortions induced under unsterile conditions and occasionally after spontaneous abortions, prolonged labor at term, ruptured membranes, or operative interference with pregnancy. The organisms presumably invade the damaged endometrium through the retained products of conception. The earliest symptoms may be related to instrumentation and consist of metrorrhagia, suprapubic and back pain, chills, and fever. Fever of 37.8 to 39.4°C (100 to 103°F), often with chills, usually recurs several days after abortion, but the incubation period can be as short as 6 h. Vaginal bleeding is almost invariably present, and there is often a brown, foul-smelling, vaginal discharge containing necrotic tissue. The cervix is soft and patulous, and the uterus and adnexa are usually very tender. The lower abdominal wall is often tense, or signs of generalized peritonitis may be present, secondary to perforation of the uterus or parametrial extension of infection. Nausea, vomiting, and profuse diarrhea are often prominent.

Systemic manifestations may appear with dramatic suddenness. Massive intravascular hemolysis, accompanied by hemoglobinemia, hemoglobinuria, and jaundice, may be the most striking feature of the disease. Icterus may appear within hours after onset of illness. As in gas gangrene, the clinical picture may be dominated by circulatory collapse with hypotension, extreme tachycardia, cyanosis, hyperpnea, and pulmonary edema. Despite severe prostration, the patient is frequently well oriented, alert, and apprehensive. Acute renal failure secondary to shock, dehydration, or hemolysis occurs frequently. The mortality rate in postabortal or puerperal sepsis caused by *C. perfringens* and associated with intense hemolysis is 40 to 70 percent. Death may occur a few hours after onset or may be delayed for days.

Unusual local complications of uterine infection are gas gangrene of the vagina and rectum and clostridial cellulitis of the anterior abdominal wall following cesarean section or hysterectomy. At times, the infectious process is confined to the endometrium and myometrium with intrauterine gas formation (physometra).

Septic abortion with *C. perfringens* bacteremia without overt hemolysis is a more common occurrence than bacteremia with gross hemolysis, as described above. Death is unusual in the absence of hemolysis.

Diseases to be considered in the *differential diagnosis* include perforated uterus, ruptured ectopic pregnancy, ingestion of toxic abortifacients, septic endometritis caused by aerobic or anaerobic streptococci, enteric bacilli or other microorganisms, pelvic thrombophlebitis with septic pulmonary emboli, acute hepatic necrosis of pregnancy, and sickle cell crisis.

Clostridium perfringens food poisoning Meat and meat products contaminated with *C. perfringens* type A are frequently responsible for outbreaks of acute gastroenteritis. In 1976 in the United States, *C. perfringens* accounted for 14.2 percent of cases in reported food-borne outbreaks.

Most outbreaks of *C. perfringens* food poisoning have been associated with the ingestion of meat or poultry dishes. Most market meats and poultry are heavily contaminated, and the organism can be isolated with ease from soil, water, air, and human or animal feces. The usual story is that the food has been prepared and cooked 24 h or more before consumption, allowed to cool slowly at room temperature, and then served either cold or warmed. During this period of incubation, contaminating spores which have survived cooking germinate, and clostridia grow to large numbers sufficient to constitute an infectious inoculum. *Clostridium perfringens* food poisoning can be reproduced experimentally in humans by feeding the actively growing organisms which apparently multiply and sporulate in the small intestine. Sporulation is associated with the production of an enterotoxin in situ.

Typical symptoms of diarrhea with abdominal pain and cramps develop 6 to 24 h after ingestion of meat (especially beef and poultry), stew, or soup which has been stored at a warm temperature for several hours after cooking. Nausea occurs occasionally, but vomiting is rare. Systemic manifestations are usually absent, and recovery is uneventful after 12 to 24 h.

A severe form of clostridial infection termed *enteritis necrotans* was observed in Germany after World War II. This disease was characterized by hemorrhagic necrosis of the small intestine, bloody diarrhea, severe dehydration, shock, and death. A similar infection termed *necrotizing jejunitis* has been described in natives of New Guinea who had eaten inadequately cooked pork.

ANTIBIOTIC-ASSOCIATED COLITIS Diarrhea has been reported in up to 20 percent of patients receiving clindamycin. In one study up to one-half of these patients were found to have evidence of pseudomembranous colitis on proctoscopic examination. *Clostridium difficile* has been implicated as the etiologic agent. Symptoms of cramping, lower abdominal pain, fever, and diarrhea are common. Fever and cramps precede or coincide with the onset of diarrhea which usually develops between the fourth and ninth days of antibiotic therapy, although onset of symptoms has been reported up to 4 weeks after discontinuation of the drug. The diarrhea is usually watery but rarely bloody. Patients may occasionally have abdominal tenderness with rebound and associated leukocytosis. The symptoms usually subside within a week after discontinuation of antibiotics; however, the diarrhea may become protracted, lasting up to 2 to 4 weeks. Severe protracted diarrhea may lead to electrolyte imbalance, protein loss, and death, especially in patients with significant underlying disease. Toxic megacolon is a rare complication. Although clindamycin has received the most attention, other antibiotics such as lincomycin, ampicillin, cephalosporins, tetracyclines, penicillin, trimethoprim-sulfamethoxazole, and chloramphenicol also produce diarrhea and have been implicated as causes of pseudomembranous colitis. Pseudomembranous colitis with *C. difficile* toxin production has been demonstrated in occasional patients who had received no antibiotic therapy.

Miscellaneous clostridial infections Clostridia can be isolated from bile obtained at elective cholecystectomy in patients without symptoms of clostridial infection. Clostridial cellulitis or myonecrosis may occasionally follow surgical procedures, particularly surgery on the gastrointestinal tract or gallbladder. Pathogenic clostridia are occasionally introduced into the abdomen, thoracic cavity, or cranium through penetrating wounds. Primary pneumonia in the absence of a penetrating wound or distant focus has been described. Clostridial pleurisy may involve the underlying lung but is usually an indolent localized infection with minimal systemic manifestations. Meningitis is usually secondary to a puncture wound of the skull and is often associated with a necrotizing cerebritis. Clostridial peritonitis may ocur spontaneously but typically follows perforation of the gallbladder, appendix, or other viscus and is usually rapidly fatal.

Clostridial septicemia, particularly with *C. septicum,* also develops occasionally in patients with aplastic anemia or far-advanced neoplastic disease, including leukemias, lymphomas, and metastatic solid tumors. Over two-thirds of these patients had been receiving antineoplastic chemotherapy or radiation therapy. The primary site of invasion is usually the gastrointestinal tract (the distal ileum or colon) which is frequently extensively involved by the neoplastic process. Abdominal surgical procedures, endoscopy, small-bowel series, and paracentesis have been reported to predispose to sepsis in these patients. The course of the disease is rapid, death often occurring within 24 h after onset of recognizable infection. Mortality rates approach 70 percent. Hypotension, hyperpyrexia, and dyspnea are the most common clinical manifestations. Jaundice and hemolysis occur occasionally. Cellulitis, with or without crepitation, may appear in the flanks and should suggest the diagnosis, especially in patients with leukemia or lymphoma. Conversely, clostridial bacteremia may be seen occasionally in hospitalized patients with unrelated underlying diseases and no clinical evidence of sepsis.

Cystitis with pneumaturia, gaseous cholecystitis, endocarditis, osteomyelitis, arthritis, and bursitis after needle aspiration are other examples of rare clostridial infections.

LABORATORY FINDINGS The diagnosis of gas gangrene, clostridial cellulitis, postabortal sepsis, or other clostridial infections is based primarily on clinical criteria. Smears of wound exudate, uterine scrapings, or cervical discharge may show abundant large gram-positive rods, as well as other organisms. Spores are rarely observed in smears of exudates, and leukocytes are sparse. Thioglycolate broth, deep meat broth, and blood agar plates incubated in an anaerobic jar should be inoculated for definitive identification of specific clostridia. However, interpretation of positive wound cultures is difficult because clostridia are frequent contaminants. *Clostridium perfringens* bacteremia is common in postabortal infections but rare in gas gangrene.

Polymorphonuclear leukocytosis occurs frequently in gas gangrene and invariably in postabortal sepsis; total blood leukocyte counts range from 15,000 to 40,000 cells per cubic millimeter and occasionally exceed 60,000 cells per cubic millimeter. Marked thrombocytopenia develops in about 50 percent of patients with clostridial sepsis. The urine frequently contains protein and casts. Renal insufficiency may lead to severe uremia.

X-ray examination sometimes provides the first clue leading to the correct diagnosis by revealing the presence of gas in muscle, subcutaneous tissue, or uterus; however, demonstration of gas in tissues is not diagnostic of clostridial infection. Other bacteria, especially *Enterobacter, Escherichia,* and anaerobes other than clostridia, may be responsible for gas production. Occasionally air is sucked into a wound at the time of penetrating injury.

Profound alterations of circulating erythrocytes are common in postabortal sepsis but are much less frequent in other clostridial infection. Hemolytic anemia may develop with almost unbelievable rapidity; the red blood cell count occasionally decreases by 2 million cells per cubic millimeter in less than 24 h and is associated with hemoglobinemia, hemoglobinuria, and elevated levels of serum bilirubin. Spherocytosis, increased osmotic and mechanical red blood fragility, erythrophagocytosis, and methemoglobinemia have also been described. Abnormalities of the clotting mechanism characteristic of intravascular coagulation may be observed in patients with severe clostridial infections.

The diagnosis of antibiotic-associated pseudomembranous colitis is established by proctoscopy, which shows raised yellow-whitish plaques that cover an erythematous edematous base. The membrane is composed of mucus, fibrin, desquamated epithelial cells, and polymorphonuclear leukocytes. The classic radiographic findings on plain films of the abdomen are of thickened and distorted haustra, generalized thickening of the colonic wall, "thumbprinting," small marginal irregularities (representing the pseudomembranous plaque), and total colonic involvement. Proctoscopic and x-ray abnormalities are not universally present. The small bowel is usually not involved. Barium enema is not recommended in patients suspected to have colitis because of the possible association with toxic megacolon. The fecal filtrate from a patient with pseudomembranous colitis due to *C. difficile* toxin will demonstrate a typical cytopathic effect in tissue culture. This effect is neutralized by antitoxin to *C. sordellii.* Demonstration of toxin is quite specific and establishes the diagnosis in a patient with a compatible clinical picture.

TREATMENT The traditional therapeutic approach to serious clostridial infection, such as diffuse, spreading myositis, is immediate surgical intervention with wide radical debridement followed by open drainage without closure or open amputation when necessary. Early surgery not only aids diagnosis, but permits decompression of fascial compartments and excision of devitalized muscle and may obviate amputation. Some authorities feel that hyperbaric oxygen therapy has modified this traditional approach to gas gangrene by assuming priority over radical surgical debridement. Proponents report that hyperbaric oxygenation produces impressive, almost immediate improvement in patients with gas gangrene, with rapid disappearance of systemic toxicity and prompt arrest of local spread of the gangrenous infection. Since hyperbaric oxygen facilities are usually not readily available, surgical debridement should not be delayed while vital hours are wasted in transporting patients. If clostridial myonecrosis is suspected, debridement remains the most widely recommended approach.

Curettage of the uterus should be performed for diagnosis and treatment of postabortal clostridial infections. In the absence of hemolysis, standard therapy for septic abortion with antibiotics and uterine curettage usually produces rapid improvement, even in patients with bacteremia. The mortality rate in patients with abortion, *C. perfringens* bacteremia, and intense hemolysis is high regardless of the therapeutic approach. The role of hysterectomy is controversial and ill-defined; some surgeons strongly advocate hysterectomy, whereas others feel that the potential benefits of the procedure do not outweigh the risks. Heparinization, exchange transfusion, and hyperbaric oxygen have been utilized but are not of established benefit.

Simple incision and adequate drainage usually suffice for treating clostridial cellulitis.

Penicillin is the antibiotic of choice for most clostridial infections and should be administered in doses of 20 million units a day by continuous intravenous infusion. Chloramphenicol is also active against most strains of *Clostridium* and may be used as an alternative to penicillin in patients with hypersensitivity. Clostridial myonecrosis has developed while patients were receiving cephalothin (2 to 6 g intravenously daily) for prophylaxis. Cefoxitin in high doses provides good coverage for *C. perfringens* and most other clostridial strains. Clostridia are also generally, but not universally, susceptible in vitro to carbenicillin, clindamycin, metronidazole, doxycycline, minocycline, and tetracycline.

The efficacy of polyvalent gas gangrene antitoxin is controversial. Most centers have discontinued the use of antitoxin in the management of patients with suspected gas gangrene or clostridial postabortal sepsis because of questionable efficacy and the risk of hypersensitivity reactions. At the present time this antitoxin is not being produced in the United States.

Intravenous infusions of blood, plasma volume expanders, fluids, and electrolytes are required to combat shock, anemia, and dehydration. Renal insufficiency should be treated in the same manner as acute tubular necrosis from other causes.

The most reliable protection against gas gangrene is early and adequate wound debridement. Antitoxin is ineffective as a prophylactic agent. The use of clostridial toxoids for prophylactic immunization of individuals in hazardous occupations awaits evaluation.

Therapy of antibiotic-associated pseudomembranous colitis includes immediate discontinuation of the antibiotic and intravenous fluid to maintain an adequate intravascular volume and electrolyte balance. Vancomycin by the oral route has been effective in eradicating the experimental infection in hamsters. Its effectiveness in pseudomembranous colitis in humans has been established in a number of clinical trials. Treatment consists of vancomycin 500 mg orally every 6 h for 10 days. Toxin production persists in 5 to 10 percent of treated patients. Relapses are reported in up to 20 percent of patients, but usually patients respond to a second course of oral vancomycin. Oral bacitracin administration 25,000 units every 6 h for 7 to 10 days has also been effective.

REFERENCES

BARTLETT JG et al: Antibiotic-associated pseudomembranous colitis due to toxin-producing clostridia. N Engl J Med 298:531, 1978

CHANG T-W et al: Bacitracin treatment of antibiotic-associated colitis and diarrhea caused by *Clostridium difficile* toxin. Gastroenterology 78:1584, 1980

DARKE SG et al: Gas gangrene and related infection. Br J Surg 64:104, 1977

DELLINGER EP: Severe necrotizing soft-tissue infections. JAMA 246:1717, 1981

FEKETY R: Antibiotic-associated colitis, in *Update II: Harrison's Principles of Internal Medicine,* KJ Isselbacher et al (eds). New York, McGraw-Hill, 1982, pp 15–23

GEORGE WL: Antimicrobial agent-associated colitis and diarrhea (medical progress). West J Med 133:115, 1980

——— et al: Relapse of pseudomembranous colitis after vancomycin therapy. N Engl J Med 301:414, 1979

HOLLAND JA et al: Experimental and clinical experience with hyperbaric oxygen in the treatment of clostridial myonecrosis. Surgery 77:75, 1975

MacLennan JD: The histotoxic clostridial infections of man. Bacteriol Rev 26:177, 1962

Mahn E, Dantuono LM: Postabortal septicotoxemia due to *Clostridium welchii:* Seventy-five cases from the maternity hospital, Santiago, Chile. 1948–1952. Am J Obstet Gynecol 70:604, 1955

Murrel TGC et al: Pig-bel: Enteritis necroticans: A study in diagnosis and management. Lancet 1:217, 1966

Nakamura M, Schulze JA: *Clostridium perfringens* food poisoning. Annu Rev Microbiol 24:359, 1970

Pritchard JA, Whalley PJ: Abortion complicated by *Clostridium perfringens* infection. Am J Obstet Gynecol 111:484, 1971

Rifkin GD et al: Antibiotic-induced colitis: Implication of a toxin neutralized by *Clostridium sordellii* antitoxin. Lancet 2:1103, 1977

Tedesco RJ: Clindamycin and colitis: A review. J Infect Dis 135S:S95, 1977

Weinstein L, Barza MA: Gas gangrene. N Engl J Med 289:1129, 1973

Wyne JW, Armstrong D: Clostridial septicemia. Cancer 29:215, 1972

173 INFECTIONS DUE TO MIXED ANAEROBIC ORGANISMS

LAWRENCE L. PELLETIER, JR.

Anaerobic bacteria require conditions of reduced oxygen tension and low redox potential for growth. Anaerobes constitute the predominant normal flora on the skin and mucous membranes of humans and outnumber aerobic bacteria 1000 to 1 in the colon and 10 to 1 on the skin, mouth, and vagina. On body surfaces, anaerobic bacteria often coexist with other anaerobic species and aerobic and facultative organisms in poorly understood symbiotic relationships. Any site in the body is susceptible to infection by these endogenous organisms when skin and mucous membrane barriers are compromised by surgery, trauma, or tumor, and when local tissue redox potentials are reduced by ischemia, necrosis, or infection. Multiple species of anaerobic, facultative, or aerobic organisms are often present in infection, and their synergistic interaction is required for pathogenicity. Mixed anaerobic infections frequently cause dental abscess, chronic otitis media and sinusitis, brain abscess, subdural empyema, otogenic meningitis, necrotizing gingivitis, Ludwig's angina, aspiration pneumonia, lung abscess, thoracic empyema, liver abscess, pylephlebitis, peritonitis, intraabdominal abscesses, endometritis, tuboovarian abscess, pelvic cellulitis, gangrene, postsurgical wound infection, perirectal abscess, and human bite infections.

Botulism (Chap. 171), tetanus (Chap. 170), clostridial myonecrosis (Chap. 172), and actinomycosis (Chap. 182) are discussed elsewhere.

ETIOLOGY Because most mixed anaerobic infections develop from normal host flora associated with adjacent mucosal membranes, knowledge of the predominant bacteria at different sites and the pathogenicity of these organisms may permit the selection of appropriate therapy before the results of cultures are available. Advances in culture techniques and methods of microbial identification have clarified the taxonomic classification of anaerobic organisms and the relative pathogenicity of some species in mixed anaerobic infection, but the relative importance of many organisms that participate in mixed infections needs to be established. Certain organisms such as *Vibrio* spp., spirochetes, anaerobic gram-negative cocci, or very oxygen-labile anaerobes that may be seen in stains of clinical material or isolated from culture are not virulent in experimental infections. Formerly, many mixed anaerobic infections of the pharynx, lung, and genital tract were classified as fusospirochetal infections because fusobacteria and spirochetes were seen on stains of material from the lesions. Since spirochetes are not pathogenic and many other species of anaerobes and aerobes have been isolated from infected sites, it is more appropriate to term these infections as mixed anaerobic infections.

Normal anaerobic flora plays a critical role in protecting against both colonization and infection with pathogenic microorganisms and overgrowth of potentially pathogenic endogenous organisms. Administration of clindamycin or other antimicrobials that suppress the majority of anaerobic colon bacteria may be complicated by the overgrowth of clindamycin-resistant *Clostridium difficile,* which produces toxins that may damage colonic mucosa and cause pseudomembranous colitis (see Chap. 172). Likewise, antibiotic suppression of normal flora may predispose to oropharyngeal or perianal symptomatic *Candida* spp. infection (thrush) (see Chap. 184) or prolonged carriage of *Salmonella* spp. in the gut.

The functions of anaerobic gastrointestinal flora in health and disease are poorly understood, but it is known that vitamin K synthesis by *Escherichia coli* and *Bacteroides fragilis* in the gut represent important sources of this essential vitamin. *B. fragilis* and other organisms deconjugate bile acids in the intestine, permitting their reabsorption in the distal ileum and maintenance of the bile acid pool. Alterations in the microbial flora in relation to diet may predispose to the development of carcinoma of the colon and to altered metabolism of dietary chemicals and orally administered drugs. Because of both the complexity of the flora and problems in sampling it, knowledge of this area of normal bacterial physiology is scanty, and it is a fertile area for future investigation.

The major anaerobic pathogens from clinical material include (1) gram-negative bacilli (*B. fragilis, B. melaninogenicus, B. asaccharolyticus, Fusobacterium nucleatum, F. varium, F. necrophorum,* and *F. mortiferum*), (2) gram-positive cocci (*Peptostreptococcus* spp., *Peptococcus* spp., microaerophilic cocci, and streptococci), (3) gram-positive spore-forming bacilli (*Clostridia* spp.), and (4) gram-positive nonsporulating bacilli (*Actinomyces* spp., *Arachina* spp., *Eubacterium* spp., and *Bifidobacterium eriksonii*).

Anaerobic gram-negative bacilli and anaerobic gram-positive cocci are the most commonly isolated anaerobes from clinical infections; *B. fragilis* is the most frequently isolated species. Microaerophilic cocci and streptococci that require reduced oxygen tension and the presence of carbon dioxide for growth are facultative rather than true anaerobic bacteria. *Clostridia* spp. or *Actinomyces* spp. may produce disease as single pathogens or as one organism among many in mixed infections. Anaerobes should be considered significant pathogens when isolated from body fluids or tissues that are normally sterile, or from infected sites where they are repeatedly isolated in high concentrations when measures have been taken to reduce or eliminate contamination by normal flora.

Table 173-1 lists aerobic and anaerobic organisms constituting normal skin and mucosal flora that are potential pathogens. Normal skin flora include anaerobic *Propionibacterium acnes,* a common blood culture contaminant that produces significant infections only in association with a foreign body such as a prosthetic heart valve or cerebral spinal fluid shunts. Anaerobic gram-negative bacilli, e.g., *C. perfringens,* and other anaerobes may be transient skin flora of the perineum and lower extremities and may cause mixed anaerobic infection of decubitus, ischemic, or diabetic ulcers.

Organisms in the oropharynx may play a role in local disease or be involved in pleuropulmonary infections following aspiration of oropharyngeal secretions. Hospitalized patients have a higher frequency of colonization with aerobic coliform bacilli or *S. aureus,* and anaerobes play a greater role in aspiration pneumonias occurring outside the hospital.

Multiple aerobic and anaerobic pathogens are encountered in infections of the abdomen and female genital tract. All potential pathogens isolated from abdominal and genital tract infections should be considered significant including enterococci encountered in abscesses and soft tissue infections.

EPIDEMIOLOGY Mixed anaerobic infections are frequently encountered in hospitals with active surgical, trauma, and obstetrics and gynecologic services. No reliable data are available to establish the true incidence and prevalence of mixed anaerobic infections. The lack of appropriate cultures, the submission of cultures contaminated by anaerobes from normal flora, and the lack, until recently, of reliable culture techniques have made accurate sampling of infectious anaerobes impossible. Anaerobic bacteria, predominately *B. fragilis* and anaerobic cocci, constitute 8 to 20 percent of blood culture isolates in many centers, and anaerobes are isolated in 10 to 54 percent of clinical cultures.

PATHOGENESIS Anaerobes generally are not highly invasive; infection is usually secondary to an underlying disease, surgical procedure, or therapy which impairs the normal defenses of the host. These organisms utilize substances other than oxygen as the final electron acceptor in reactions which generate energy, and will grow only in an environment with a low redox potential. Healthy, well-vascularized tissue has a relatively high redox potential and will not support growth of anaerobes. Conditions that significantly lower redox potential, such as impairment of blood supply, tissue necrosis, or growth of aerobic bacteria, are necessary to create an environment conducive to proliferation of anaerobes. Infections, therefore, frequently occur secondary to vascular disease, trauma, surgery, a perforated viscus, shock, aspiration, intramuscular epinephrine injections, or malignancy.

TABLE 173-1
Potential pathogens that constitute normal flora at different body sites

	Anaerobes	*Aerobes*
Skin	Gram-positive cocci *Eubacterium* spp.	*S. epidermidis* *S. aureus* *C. albicans* *S. pyogenes*
Pharynx	*B. melaninogenicus* *B. asaccharolyticus* *Fusobacterium* spp. Gram-positive cocci *Actinomyces* spp. *Bifidobacterium* spp. *Eubacterium* spp.	*Pneumococcus* *S. aureus* *S. pyogenes* *H. influenzae* *S. viridans* *K. pneumoniae* *Meningococcus* Gram-negative coliform bacilli *C. albicans*
Colon	*B. fragilis* *B. melaninogenicus* *B. asaccharolyticus* Gram-positive cocci *Clostridium* spp. *Bifidobacterium* spp. *Eubacterium* spp. *Fusobacterium* spp.	Gram-negative coliform bacilli *Achromobacter* spp. *Enterococcus* *P. aeruginosa* *S. viridans* *S. aureus*
Vagina	*B. fragilis* *B. asaccharolyticus* *B. melaninogenicus* Gram-positive cocci *Bifidobacterium* spp. *Clostridium* spp. *Eubacterium* spp. *Fusobacterium* spp.	Gram-negative coliform bacilli *Enterococcus* spp. *C. vaginalis* *Mycoplasma* spp. *C. albicans* *S. viridans*

Obligate anaerobes that possess catalase or superoxide dismutase enzymes to protect them from peroxides that form in oxygenated surroundings are more tolerant to exposure to oxygen. However, if the redox potential is low, many species lacking these enzymes can exist in sites that are well oxygenated, such as the mouth. Pathogenic anaerobic species tend to be more resistant to oxygen exposure than nonpathogenic strains.

Anaerobes involved in local infections originating from mucosal surfaces in the mouth, intestinal tract, or vagina may form pseudomembranes on mucosal surfaces, spreading gangrene from a site of trauma or a localized abscess. The characteristic foul odor of anaerobic lesions is caused by certain metabolic end products of bacterial origin, primarily short-chain fatty acids and volatile amines. Many species of anaerobes produce collagenases and proteinases that account for the propensity for abscess formation. *B. fragilis* and strains of *B. melaninogenicus* possesses beta lactamases that inactivate penicillin and cephalothin. Some *Bacteroides* species produce a heparinase which may frequently lead to localized septic thrombophlebitis seen adjacent to areas of infection. Many strains of *B. fragilis* possess a capsule that interferes with phagocytosis by granulocytes, promotes the development of abscesses, and may protect against the nonspecific bactericidal activity of serum. Infection characteristically remains localized, but bloodstream invasion or direct extension to other areas may occur. Localization of blood-borne organisms at distant sites is not unusual and may result in abscess formation in brain, lung, liver, joints, kidneys, or other organs. Disseminated intravascular coagulation complicating *B. fragilis* bacteremia is rare and may relate to the absence of lipid A in the lipopolysaccharide of the cell wall of *B. fragilis.*

CLINICAL MANIFESTATIONS Anaerobic infection should be suspected when a foul odor emanates from lesions or pus; when infection is situated near a mucosal surface; when necrotic tissue or neoplasm is present; when a spreading gangrene involves skin, subcutaneous tissue, fascia, or muscle; when pseudomembranes or abscesses are formed; when gas in tissues is indicated by roentgenogram or crepitance; when septic thrombophlebitis or pulmonary embolus occurs following intraabdominal or pelvic infections; or when infection progresses despite aminoglycoside therapy.

Dental–periodontal infections Root canal infection caused by mixed anaerobic and aerobic oral flora may result from dental caries and produce dental pulp necrosis with periapical destruction of bone. Without drainage of the root canal, mandibular osteomyelitis or extension of the infection into the maxillary sinus, buccal tissues, and submandibular or submental spaces may occur depending upon the teeth involved. Periodontitis with purulent gingival pockets or abscesses may result in spreading anaerobic infection that involves adjacent bone or soft tissues. Secondary pulmonary anaerobic infection may occur from aspiration of purulent material. Mandibular osteomyelitis may also result from infection complicating tooth extraction, from open fractures, or in association with debilitation, diabetes mellitus, radiation therapy, and malnutrition. Most oral infections respond rapidly to penicillin and drainage. Penicillin treatment failures are rare but may be due to β-lactamase–producing *B. fragilis.*

Acute necrotizing ulcerative gingivitis (trench mouth, Vincent's stomatitis) The onset of disease is usually sudden and is associated with tender, bleeding gums, fetid breath, and a bad taste. The gingival mucosa, especially the papillae between the teeth, becomes ulcerated and may be covered by a gray exudate which is removable with gentle pressure. Although involvement of the gums is usually patchy, the process may extend to most of the gingival tissue. If the ulceration is extensive, fever, cervical lymphadenopathy, and leukocytosis are present. The disease may spread to involve other tissues of the oropharynx; it may become less severe and chronic; or it may subside spontaneously. Recurrent ulceration has been described. Most patients who develop ulcerative gingivitis are young adults with poor oral hygiene. Tartar deposits and eruption or extraction of teeth may damage the gums and allow bacterial invasion. Edentulous persons develop the disease infrequently. Ulcerative gingivitis is prevalent in wartime when nutritional deficiency, crowding, and emotional upsets are common. The role of these factors in its pathogenesis is not known. A new genus of facultatively anaerobic bacteria called *Caprocytophaga* has been found to cause periodontal disease and oral ulcerations with bacteremia in granulocytopenic cancer patients.

Acute necrotizing ulcerative mucositis (cancrum oris, noma) Occasionally, ulcerative gingivitis spreads to the buccal mucosa, the cheek, and the mandible or maxilla, resulting in widespread destruction of bone and soft tissue. The first indication of cancrum oris is usually slight inflammation of the skin of the cheek. The destruction of tissue proceeds very rapidly. The teeth may fall out, and large areas of bone, even the whole mandible, may be sloughed. A strong, putrid odor is present. The lesions are not usually painful. The gangrenous lesions eventually heal, but large disfiguring defects are left. Cancrum oris is seen most commonly following a debilitating illness in severely malnourished children in underdeveloped areas of the world. Cancrum oris may complicate acute leukemia or develop in individuals with a genetic deficiency of catalase.

Gangrenous pharyngitis (Vincent's angina) Necrotizing infections of the pharynx may occur alone or in association with ulcerative gingivitis. The main complaints are an extremely sore throat, foul breath, bad taste in the mouth, sensation of choking, and fever. The pharynx in the area of the tonsillar pillars is swollen, red, and ulcerated and is covered with a grayish membrane that peels easily. Lymphadenopathy and leukocytosis are common. The disease may last for only a few days or may persist for weeks if not treated. The lesion begins unilaterally but may spread to the other side of the pharynx or to the larynx. Aspiration of infected material may result in lung abscess.

Sinusitis Acute sinusitis is seldom caused by anaerobic organisms unless it is associated with a dental abscess. However, gram-positive anaerobic cocci and bacteroides are isolated from about one-half of patients undergoing surgery for chronic or recurrent maxillary sinusitis. Anaerobic organisms are also associated with chronic otitis media and mastoiditis. Chronic anaerobic sinusitis, otitis, or mastoiditis may lead to subdural or extradural empyemas, brain abscess, or anaerobic meningitis (see Chap. 359).

Ludwig's angina Mandibular dental or periodontal infections, particularly of the third molar, may produce submandibular cellulitis that results in marked local swelling of tissues with pain, trismus, and superior-posterior displacement of the tongue. Submandibular swelling of the neck also develops. Inability to swallow and respiratory obstruction may result; tracheostomy may be lifesaving. Anaerobes and aerobes originating from oral flora have been implicated in this dramatic clinical syndrome.

Brain abscess Anaerobic bacteria, particularly bacteroides and microaerophilic and anaerobic streptococci, have been isolated from 30 to 89 percent of brain abscesses in adults. In one study, 16 of 18 nontraumatic brain abscesses contained anaerobes, and half of these were bacteroides, including both *B. fragilis* and *B. melaninogenicus.* These lesions may result from either direct extension of suppurative infection involving the sinuses, middle ear, or mastoids, or from hematogenous dissemination from infections elsewhere, particularly the lungs. There is an increased incidence of brain abscess in patients with cyanotic heart disease. Signs and symptoms are mainly those of a space-occupying intracranial lesion with headache followed by changes in mentation, focal neurologic signs, and papilledema. The course may be indolent, and fever is frequently absent. Cerebrospinal fluid findings are variable but may mimic those of purulent or aseptic meningitis.

Computerized tomography (CT) with contrast enhancement permits the accurate location of brain abscesses even at an early stage of cerebritis before a capsule has formed. Serial CT scans detect life-threatening complications such as threatened herniation or hydrocephalus that require emergency surgery, determine the time when surgery is most likely to be successful, and measure response to therapy. CT scan is more sensitive than the radionuclide brain scan for detecting smaller lesions, multiple abscesses, and the presence of satellite lesions. Antimicrobial agents that penetrate the blood-brain barrier (high doses of penicillin G, nafcillin, chloramphenicol, or metronidazole) may be sufficient therapy for cerebritis or small, inaccessible lesions. However, once a capsule has formed, most patients require aspiration or excision of the abscess in combination with prolonged antimicrobial therapy. Patients with multiple abscesses, deep-seated lesions at inaccessible sites, associated meningitis and ependymitis, or hydrocephalus have a worse prognosis. Corticosteroid therapy may be required to decrease life-threatening brain swelling but should not be administered unless absolutely necessary because it may interfere with antimicrobial penetration into the abscess and retard capsule formation.

Pleuropulmonary infection Aspiration of oral secretions leads to production of mixed anaerobic infection of the lungs and pleura. The likelihood of anaerobic pulmonary infection is increased in the presence of poor dental hygiene, periodontal disease, and gingivitis. Bacteroides, fusobacteria, and anaerobic streptococci are isolated alone or in combination in a majority of cases of lung abscess and necrotizing pneumonia. Pneumonitis without necrosis or abscess formation may also occur. These anaerobes are second only to the pneumococcus as a cause of acute bacterial infection of the lungs. *B. melaninogenicus* and *B. asaccharolyticus* are the most frequent *Bacteroides* species isolated in anaerobic pulmonary infections. *B. fragilis* is found in only 5 percent of cases. These infections occur primarily in patients with conditions that predispose to aspiration, such as oral surgical procedures, esophageal dysfunction, and altered consciousness due to alcoholism, major motor seizures, general anesthesia, and drug abuse. Anaerobes may also produce infection distal to obstructive lesions of the bronchus. These infections are characterized by tissue necrosis, abscess formation, and the production of foul-smelling and foul-tasting sputum. Empyema is not an unusual complication of lung abscess or necrotizing pneumonia. Empyema with anaerobes may also occur as an extension from subdiaphragmatic infection. Septic pulmonary emboli may originate from abdominal or female genital tract infections. The bacterial flora of bronchiectatic cavities frequently includes bacteroides and other anaerobes.

Abdominal infection Intraabdominal abscesses and generalized peritonitis almost always contain anaerobes, especially when they are secondary to perforation or leakage from the gastrointestinal tract. These infections are uniformly polymicrobial, with an average of five anaerobic and aerobic pathogens that originate from bowel flora. Symptoms include fever with chills, localized or generalized abdominal pain with peritoneal signs, nausea, and vomiting. The abscess cavity will rarely be large enough to be palpable on abdominal or pelvic examination. *B. fragilis* is isolated from approximately 50 percent of abdominal surgical wounds after trauma involving perforation of the gut and in greater than 50 percent of wound infections following elective colon resection. Anaerobic wound infections may occur following appendectomy or after surgery on the small bowel, stomach, gallbladder, and biliary tract. Polymicrobial bacteremia may complicate local infection and frequently is due to facultative gram-negative bacilli or *B. fragilis.* Abdominal ultrasound, combined liver-spleen scans, and gallium or indium-labeled neutrophil scans may be helpful in localizing intraabdominal abscesses, but often surgical exploration may be necessary to establish the site of intraabdominal infection.

Intrahepatic infection Anaerobic bacteria have rarely been implicated in infections of the gallbladder, but they may produce ascending cholangitis complicating common duct obstruction due to surgery, stones, or neoplasm, and are isolated from half of pyogenic intrahepatic abscesses. *B. fragilis,* peptostreptococcus, *Fusobacterium* sp., and microaerophilic streptococci are the predominant anaerobic pathogens isolated from liver abscesses. Anaerobes gain access to the liver by direct extension from an adjacent intraabdominal focus of infection, embolization through the portal vein, ascent via the common duct, or least often as a result of systemic bacteremia. Anaerobic liver abscess often occurs in elderly males with biliary disease, abdominal trauma, or tumor and is characterized by fever, chills, abdominal pain (particularly in the right upper quadrant), hepatomegaly, and liver tenderness. However, pain and hepatic enlargement may be absent, and fever, malaise, anorexia, and weight loss may be the only symptoms. Over 90 percent of patients with liver abscess have a leukocytosis and elevation of the serum alkaline phosphatase and aspartate transaminase; 50 percent have associated anemia, hypoalbuminemia, and elevation of the serum bilirubin. A basilar pulmonary infiltrate, pleural effusion, and/or elevated hemidiaphragm frequently appears on chest x-ray. One-third of patients with liver abscess have bacteremia. Jaundice and marked elevation of the serum alkaline phosphatase usually indicate multiple abscesses. Hepatic abscesses may be detected by ultrasonography, radionuclide scan of the liver, or CT scan. Open surgical drainage is indicated when an abscess is associated with other lesions requiring surgical therapy; otherwise percutaneous drainage using ultrasonography or CT scan to situate the catheter may be combined with antimicrobial therapy.

Pelvic infection The predominant organisms isolated in greater than 75 percent of nongonococcal gynecologic infections are anaerobic species found in normal vaginal flora. Anaerobic species are the major cause of Bartholin's abscess, endometritis, parametritis, parametrial abscess, pelvic peritonitis, and nongonococcal tuboovarial abscesses. These infections often complicate malignancy or recent surgery and commonly develop within necrotic tissue or products of conception. They are characterized by drainage of foul-smelling pus or blood from the uterus, generalized uterine or localized pelvic tenderness, and continued fever and chills. Suppurative thrombophlebitis of the pelvic veins may complicate these infections and lead to repeated episodes of small septic pulmonary emboli. Anaerobes combined with *Gardnerella vaginalis* produce a nonspecific vaginitis that may be diagnosed by use of gas-liquid chromatography to detect volatile fatty acid anaerobic metabolites and that responds to metronidazole.

Nonclostridial anaerobes, principally bacteroides and anaerobic streptococci, are also the major invasive pathogens in septic abortions. Bacteremia is often transient, frequently polymicrobic, and can be demonstrated in 50 to 60 percent of these patients.

Cutaneous infections Following operation or injury associated with contamination of the subcutaneous tissues, an *anaerobic cellulitis* may develop consisting of a spreading necrosis of skin and subcutaneous tissues with associated subcutaneous gas. This infection is frequently due to a mixed infection from which clostridia, anaerobic gram-positive cocci and gram-negative bacilli, and facultative coliform bacilli, streptococci, and staphylococci are isolated. The onset of anaerobic cellulitis is usually gradual, with erythema, tenderness, and edema of involved tissues followed by the development of necrosis, crepitation, pus, and foul odor over a 2- to 5-day period. Local pain is not marked, and the deep fascia and muscle are spared. Once established, the infection may be associated with high fever, toxemia, and positive blood cultures. In diabetics, an identical syndrome may be produced by gas forming facultative coliform bacilli or *Staphylococcus aureus.* On occasion, intraabdominal abscesses may present as an anaerobic cellulitis or abscess of the thigh. Areas of involvement should be opened surgically with debridement of necrotic tissue and drainage of pus and gas. At surgery, the status of the underlying fascia and muscle should be ascertained.

Necrotizing fascitis caused mainly by group A streptococci, *S. aureus,* or facultative gram-negative rods is associated with separation of the skin from necrotic fascia. A surgical probe may be passed without obstruction in a plane superficial to the deep fascia into areas of undermined skin. Gas gangrene caused by clostridia is usually associated with a more rapid onset and progression than anaerobic cellulitis, with severe pain in the involved areas, tense white overlying skin, and severe systemic toxicity. At surgical exploration, the involved muscle is nonviable.

Bacterial synergistic gangrene occurs 1 to 2 weeks after abdominal or thoracic surgery and is caused by microaerophilic or anaerobic streptococci combined with *S. aureus* or aerobic coliform bacilli. The margin of the surgical wound becomes red, swollen, and tender; central necrosis of skin and subcutaneous tissues occurs; and the margin slowly expands to involve adjacent skin. Systemic toxicity is usually minimal, and treatment consists of local debridement and systemic antibiotics. *Meleney's chronic undermining ulcer* is also a slowly progressive gangrene that occurs following surgery without marked systemic toxicity. It differs from bacterial synergistic gangrene because cutaneous fissures and sinus tracts form and are separated from the leading margin of the ulcer by undermined but intact skin. Anaerobic and microaerophilic streptococci are the usual causative organisms.

Fournier's gangrene is an anaerobic cellulitis involving the scrotum, perineum, and anterior abdominal wall in which mixed anaerobic organisms spread along deep external fascial planes and cause extensive loss of skin. Diabetics are susceptible to a necrotizing infection of skin and subcutaneous tissues that also may involve fascia and muscle. These infections have a foul discharge, marked local pain, gas in tissues, and severe systemic toxemia; they are caused by mixed anaerobic and aerobic organisms, and are associated with bacteremia in one-third of patients.

Mixed anaerobic infection may complicate decubitus ulcers, diabetic ulcers, pilonidal cysts, hidradenitis suppurativa, and vascular gangrene.

Other local infections Anaerobic urinary tract infections are rare and are usually the result of invasion from adjacent foci of infection or from bacteremia. Usually, osteomyelitis also results from adjacent ischemic or diabetic ulcers or abscess, but an increasing number of hematogenous bone and joint infections are being reported. Gangrenous lesions resulting from human bites commonly contain mixed oral anaerobic flora. Gangrenous balanitis and ulcers and gangrene of the vulva have been associated with a mixed anaerobic flora.

Bacteremia Invasion of the bloodstream by anaerobes is usually secondary to local infection, particularly those involving the abdominal cavity and pelvis. The initial manifestations are determined by the portal of entry and may be those of endometritis, appendicitis, intraabdominal abscess, or others. When bloodstream invasion occurs, the patient may become extremely ill with chills and hectic fevers ranging from 101 to 106°F. Shock and disseminated intravascular coagulation may develop. The clinical picture may be quite similar to that seen in sepsis with gram-negative bacilli (see Chap. 139), except for the occasional association of thrombophlebitis. When bacteremia complicates facial or oral infection, the internal jugular vein may be the site of suppurative thrombophlebitis; and in pelvic infections, the iliac and femoral veins may be involved. Palpation along the course of the involved veins may disclose a firm, tender cord, indicating the presence of a thrombus. Emboli may be dislodged from peripheral sites of thrombophlebitis, resulting in multiple septic pulmonary infarcts. The pulmonary abscesses or empyema then become the main focus of clinical attention rather than the initial site of infection.

Transient anaerobic bacteremias may occur following dental manipulation, extraction, periodontal procedures, nasotracheal intubation, percutaneous liver biopsy, barium enema, gastrointestinal surgery, and urinary tract catheterization but usually are not symptomatic. From 8 to 20 percent of clinically significant bacteremias are caused by anaerobes, most commonly by *B. fragilis* originating in abdominal or female genital tract infections. Anaerobic streptococcal bacteremias usually originate from the female genital tract, and fusobacteria from the oropharynx. Anaerobes cause less than 10 percent of infective endocarditis and are predominantly microaerophilic or anaerobic streptococci. *Bacteroides fragilis* is a rare cause of endocarditis. Routine anaerobic cultures should be performed in all cases of suspected bacteremia.

DIAGNOSIS Correct specimen collection and transport are critical for the isolation of anaerobic organisms. Even brief exposure to oxygen may kill the pathogens in clinical specimens. Abscess cavities should be aspirated directly with a syringe, the air expelled, and the needle capped with a sterile rubber stopper. The specimen can then be injected into a carrier bottle containing a reduced environment or transported immediately for direct culture on anaerobic media. Such a technique is preferred over the use of cotton swabs. If swabs must be used, then a swab from a gassed-out container should be placed in a reduced semisolid carrying medium before transport to the laboratory. Delays in transport may lead to failure to isolate anaerobes due to exposure to oxygen or overgrowth with facultative organisms which may eliminate or obscure the anaerobes that are present.

Only certain specimens should be cultured for anaerobic bacteria. Since all mucosal surfaces contain anaerobes, culturing them is of no value, and, in fact, may lead to erroneous conclusions about the etiology of an infection. The following culture specimens are "contaminated" with mucosal bacteria: expectorated sputum, nasotracheal aspirates, bronchoscopic aspirates, feces, voided urine, and cervical or vaginal secretions. Acceptable materials for culture include blood, pleural fluid, transtracheal aspirates, pus obtained by direct aspiration from abscess cavity, culdocentesis, suprapubic bladder aspirates, bronchoscopy, and uterine swab or brush cultures using a double-catheter technique, and other tissues or fluids that are sterile under normal conditions.

All clinical specimens from suspected anaerobic infections should be Gram-stained and examined diligently for organisms with characteristic morphology. Organisms may be seen on Gram's stain that are not isolated in culture. Purulent materials that are "sterile" or that demonstrate organisms on Gram's stain but do not grow on culture should be viewed with suspicion, and the method of collection, transport, and handling in the laboratory reviewed to assure that all reasonable precautions have been taken to permit isolation of fastidious anaerobes. Repeat cultures with immediate inoculation of freshly prepared media and prolonged anaerobic incubation may be required in special circumstances. New techniques for rapid anaerobic diagnosis include fluorescent antibody staining of clinical materials with species-specific antiserums and direct gas-liquid chromatographic analysis of clinical specimens. However, definitive diagnosis depends upon the isolation and identification of pathogenic organisms.

TREATMENT Due to the association of anaerobic infections with abscess formation and tissue necrosis and compression, appropriate surgical management is often essential for the control and elimination of infection. Drainage of abscess cavities should be carried out as soon as fluctuation and localization occur; perforations must be closed promptly; devitalized tissues or foreign bodies removed; closed space infections drained; tissue compartments decompressed; and an adequate blood supply established. Drainage of local suppurative lesions may be all that is required for cure in many cases. However, antimicrobial therapy is indicated in infections involving vital organs; to check the spread of infection into healthy tissues; or when bacteremia or systemic manifestations are present. Surgery also may be indicated to obtain appropriate material for culture by biopsy or excision. Thrombophlebitis not controlled by anticoagulation or recurrent septic pulmonary emboli may require surgical removal of thrombi or vein ligation.

It is often necessary to begin antimicrobial treatment of anaerobic infections before culture and susceptibility data are available. The type and location of infection combined with Gram's stain findings should suggest the likelihood of certain bacterial species and serve as a guide to antibiotic therapy. Chloramphenicol, clindamycin, or metronidazole plus penicillin G is equally effective in therapy for seriously ill patients with suspected anaerobic infection before culture and susceptibility data are available. Generally, anaerobic infections above the diaphragm caused by oral or upper respiratory tract flora are susceptible to penicillin G. However, if *B. fragilis* is isolated, treatment with clindamycin, metronidazole, or chloramphenicol is usually indicated. Mixed abdominal or pelvic infections necessitate multiple drug therapy due to the likelihood of penicillin-resistant strains of *B. fragilis,* or aerobic gram-negative rods and enterococci. A regimen for serious intraabdominal infection includes penicillin G, 24 to 30 million units a day, combined with chloramphenicol, 4 g per day, or combined with clindamycin, 300 to 600 mg every 6 h, or combined with metronidazole, 7.5 mg/kg every 6 h, plus gentamicin, 1.6 to 2.0 mg/kg every 8 h. Chloramphenicol is the drug of choice for central nervous system anaerobic infections as well, although penicillin G and metronidazole also pass the blood-brain barrier. Bactericidal agents such as penicillin G, ampicillin, carbenicillin, cefoxitin, and metronidazole have a definite advantage over bacteriostatic agents only in the presence of endocarditis or in patients with profound neutropenia.

Penicillin G and ampicillin have a wide range of activity against anaerobic bacteria. However, over 90 percent of *B. fragilis* strains, and some strains of fusobacteria, non-*C. perfringens* clostridia, and *B. melaninogenicus*, are resistant. Carbenicillin (25 to 30 g per day) or ticarcillin combine the antimicrobial spectrum of penicillin G with activity against 95 percent of *B. fragilis* strains and may be selected for mixed infections associated with resistant aerobic or facultative gram-negative rods such as *Pseudomonas aeruginosa* or *Proteus* organisms. Semisynthetic penicillinase-resistant penicillins are not active against anaerobes. Many anaerobes are susceptible to cephalothin or cephapirin, but *B. fragilis* is resistant to the cephalosporins. Cefoxitin has widespread activity against anaerobes, due in part to resistance to inactivation by the beta lactamase produced by *B. fragilis*. Clinically cefoxitin is as effective as clindamycin, but 10 percent of *B. fragilis* and one-third of non-*C. perfringens* clostridia are resistant. The new third-generation cephalosporins have activity against anaerobes and a wide range of gram-negative rods, and may ultimately be shown to be effective in single-drug therapy of mixed infections.

Chloramphenicol and clindamycin have been the drugs of choice for *B. fragilis* infections. Both drugs should be reserved for serious infections and should be administered intravenously. Chloramphenicol produces fatal aplastic anemia in 1 of 40,000 to 100,000 patients who receive the drug. The development of aplastic anemia is independent of a dose-related bone marrow suppression that is common with prolonged high dose regimens. Clindamycin produces pseudomembranous colitis in 0.1 to 10 percent of patients and diarrhea in as many as 20 percent of patients. Since diarrhea may precede pseudomembranous colitis, the administration of drug should be stopped if diarrhea develops during therapy. Resistance to chloramphenicol is rare. Clindamycin resistance is common for clostridia other than *C. perfringens* (10 to 20 percent) and peptococci (10 percent); it is rare for *B. fragilis* (1 percent).

Metronidazole has bactericidal activity against most obligate anaerobes and is clinically effective in *B. fragilis* infections. However, actinomyces, eubacteria, and microaerophilic streptococci are resistant to this agent. Metronidazole is now available in a parenteral form and is approved for use in anaerobic infections. As clinical experience with this drug increases, it may replace clindamycin, chloramphenicol, and cefoxitin in the treatment of *B. fragilis* infections.

Tetracycline and doxycycline are not reliable due to widespread resistance among anaerobes. Erythromycin may be used in minor soft-tissue infections above the diaphragm or in bowel preparation for colon surgery, but is less effective than clindamycin. Anaerobes are almost uniformly resistant to the aminoglycosides. Vancomycin is active against most gram-positive anaerobes and is administered orally to treat clostridia-induced pseudomembranous colitis.

Anaerobic lesions that fail to respond to treatment or relapse after responding initially should be recultured, and the need for surgical drainage or debridement should be reassessed. Superinfection with resistant gram-negative facultative or aerobic bacteria may necessitate changes in antimicrobial therapy. During treatment with broad-spectrum antibiotics, superinfection with *Candida* or *Torulopsis* may lead to systemic fungemia.

Additional supportive measures in the management of anaerobic infections include careful attention to fluid and electrolyte balance since extensive local edema formation may lead to hypovolemia; immobilization of infected extremities; therapy for septic shock (see Chap. 139); maintenance of adequate nutrition during chronic infections by enteral or parenteral hyperalimentation if oral intake is inadequate; relief of pain; and anticoagulation with heparin for thrombophlebitis. Hyperbaric oxygen therapy is of no value.

OUTCOME Mortality rates are substantial for serious anaerobic infections and approach 30 percent for necrotizing pneumonia, 25 percent for liver abscess, and 16 to 43 percent for *B. fragilis* sepsis.

PREVENTION Preventive measures include proper therapy of localized infection to prevent metastatic disease; effective debridement, cleansing, removal of foreign bodies, reestablishment of circulation, and early antimicrobial therapy of open traumatic wounds; early exploration and antibiotic therapy for penetrating abdominal wounds associated with bowel perforation; good dental and periodontal hygiene; prophylactic antibiotics for amputation of ischemic lower extremities, vaginal hysterectomy, radical pelvic surgery, and cesarean section with ruptured membranes; measures to prevent pulmonary aspiration; and neomycin-erythromycin bowel preparation for colon surgery.

REFERENCES

Balows A et al: *Anaerobic Bacteria: Role in Disease*. Springfield, Thomas, 1974

Bartlett JG, Finegold SM: Anaerobic pleuropulmonary infections. Medicine 51:413, 1972

——— et al: Percutaneous transtracheal aspiration in the diagnosis of anaerobic pulmonary infection. Ann Intern Med 79:535, 1973

Chow AW et al: Orofacial odontogenic infections. Ann Intern Med 88:392, 1978

———, Guze LB: Bacteroidaceae bacteremia: Clinical experience with 112 patients. Medicine 53:93, 1974

Finegold SM: *Anaerobic Bacteria in Human Disease*. New York, Academic, 1977

Gall SA et al: Intravenous metronidazole or clindamycin with tobramycin for therapy of pelvic infections. Obstet Gynecol 57:51, 1981

Gorbach SL, Bartlett JG: Anaerobic infections. N Engl J Med 290:1177, 1237, 1289, 1974

Harding GKM et al: Prospective randomized comparative study of clindamycin, chloramphenicol, and ticarcillin, each in combination with gentamicin, in therapy for intraabdominal and female genital tract sepsis. J Infec Dis 142:384, 1980

Kasper DL, Finegold SM (ed): Virulence factors of anaerobic bacteria. Rev Inf Dis 1:246, 1979

Ledger WJ: *Infection in the Female*. Philadelphia, Lea & Febiger, 1977

Lennette EH et al: *Manual of Clinical Microbiology*, 3d ed. Washington, D.C., American Society for Microbiology, 1980

Perera MR et al: Presentation, diagnosis and management of liver abscess. Lancet 2:629, 1980

Smith LDS: *The Pathogenic Anaerobic Bacteria*. Springfield, Ill., Charles C. Thomas, 1974

Sutter VL et al: *Wadsworth Anaerobic Bacteriology Manual*, 3d ed. St. Louis, Mosby, 1980

174
TUBERCULOSIS

WILLIAM W. STEAD
JOSEPH H. BATES

DEFINITION Tuberculosis is a necrotizing bacterial infection with protean manifestations and wide distribution. The lungs are most commonly affected, but lesions may occur also in the kidneys, bones, lymph nodes, or meninges or be disseminated throughout the body. The infection may cause clinical disease either (1) shortly after inoculation (sometimes called "primary" tuberculosis) or (2) after a period of months or decades of dormancy (still sometimes erroneously referred to as "reinfection" tuberculosis). In the western world, where bovine tuberculosis has been controlled, the portal of entry in humans is almost exclusively the lung.

ETIOLOGY *Mycobacterium tuberculosis* is a rod 2 to 4 μm in length and 0.3 μm in thickness. Its distinguishing staining property, i.e., resistance to decolorization by acid alcohol when stained with basic fuchsin, is related to the waxy component of the cell wall. This "acid fastness" is dependent in some way upon the structural integrity of the bacillus; it is lost when the organisms are damaged by grinding but is not affected by prolonged extraction with fat solvents.

Tubercle bacilli are strict aerobes and thrive best at a P_{O_2} of about 140 mmHg. The organs most commonly affected by tuberculosis are those with relatively high oxygen tension; metastatic foci are most common in the apexes of the lungs where the P_{O_2} is in the range of 120 to 130 mmHg in the upright position, followed by the kidney and the growing ends of bones, where P_{O_2} approaches 100 mmHg. The liver and spleen, where the P_{O_2} is quite low, are rarely affected, except in overwhelming disseminated infection.

Two species of tubercle bacilli affect humans: *M. tuberculosis* and *M. bovis.* By far the greatest number of cases in the United States are caused by the former strain. Programs for eradication of bovine tuberculosis have been so effective that the disease now appears only sporadically in this country.

Several other species of mycobacteria have been noted to cause chronic pulmonary infection (see Chap. 176). The most common are *M. avium-intracellulare* and *M. kansasii.* Clinical infection due to other atypical mycobacteria is rare. These mycobacteria appear not to be transmissible, and the epidemiology of the infections they cause remains obscure. They tend to infect lungs that have been damaged by silicosis or chronic obstructive lung disease. *M. kansasii* responds well to antituberculous drugs, but *M. avium-intracellulare* is resistant to nearly all drugs presently in use, and a favorable clinical response is less common.

TRANSMISSION Communicable tuberculosis among adults may result from progression of a recent infection or much later from recrudescence of dormant infection with no recent exposure. In either case, liquid caseum from a cavity abounds in tubercle bacilli which are excreted in aerosolized droplets during coughing, sneezing, and speaking. When inhaled, droplets larger than 10 μm are usually caught on the mucociliary blanket and cleared from the lung without harm, but droplets of smaller size may reach the respiratory bronchiole and deposit bacilli beyond the protective mucous blanket. There, in a susceptible host, the organisms may invade tissue and establish an infection. Persons who have been infected previously are largely protected from reinfection by specific immunity, which is mediated by T lymphocytes. Teachers, school bus drivers, and nursery workers with infectious tuberculosis are of particular epidemiologic significance because of the great susceptibility of children.

Infection in a susceptible host is caused by inhalation of tubercle bacilli in *fresh* droplet nuclei expelled by a person with cavitary tuberculosis. Transmission can be blocked effectively by irradiation of the upper air of the room with ultraviolet light and adequate ventilation and by chemotherapy of the infectious case. Even though tubercle bacilli can be cultured from dust in a room of a tuberculous person, they constitute no hazard to others in this state because the irregular shape and electrostatic charge of the attached dust particles prevent them from being carried beyond the mucociliary protective mechanism. Early in the course of tuberculous infection, persons are rarely infectious because they expel very few organisms. Tuberculosis cannot be spread on hands, dishes, glasses, utensils, or fomites.

For patients with smear-positive pulmonary tuberculosis, a regimen containing isoniazid (INH) and rifampin decimates the number of viable organisms in the sputum within 48 h. A further tenfold decrease occurs during the next 7 to 10 days. For clinical purposes patients can be considered noninfectious after receiving effective chemotherapy for 2 weeks, despite the continued presence of a few organisms in the sputum at that time. Patients with smear-negative pulmonary tuberculosis or extrapulmonary tuberculosis rarely infect others even without chemotherapy.

PREVALENCE AND INCIDENCE There has been a great fall in prevalence of tuberculosis in the United States since 1900. Early in this century over 80 percent of the population was infected *before* the age of 20 years. In an autopsy study in 1946, there was evidence of tuberculosis in 80 percent of the persons over the age of 50. In 1980, only 2 to 5 percent of young adults reacted to tuberculin (except in some urban areas), whereas about 15 percent of persons over the age of 50 reacted. The decline in incidence of the infection is most apparent among children and young adults and is due to a reduction in the number of infectious cases, which in turn is attributable to an improved standard of living, reduced risk of late progression of infection, and more prompt recognition and treatment of infectious cases.

The great majority of persons who harbor tubercle bacilli have latent or dormant ("healed") tuberculosis. Apical scars containing viable organisms may remain dormant for many years and then reactivate and produce clinical tuberculosis. Other sites in which tubercle bacilli may lie dormant for years and then recrudesce include the kidney (from which bacilli may spread to the genital tract in the male), spine, long bones, fallopian tubes, brain, and lymph nodes in the hilum and in the neck.

In 1980 there were about 28,000 new cases of clinical tuberculosis in the United States, an incidence of 12 per 100,000. This total represents an increase of 80 cases from 1979. Although there had been a steady decrease of reported cases over the previous 26 years, there is an indication that since 1979 the downward trend has been leveling off. On average, in the past quarter century the number of new cases has decreased about 5 percent per year. In 1979 the decline in new cases was only 3 percent; in 1980 the number of new cases increased by 0.3 percent. Preliminary reports indicate that the number of new cases in 1981 will exceed that for 1980. The substantial number of Indochinese refugees coming to the United States in recent years has contributed to the increase in new cases.

Of new tuberculous infections revealed by conversion of tuberculin reaction from negative to positive, 5 to 15 percent progress to serious disease within 5 years if left untreated. The risk of direct progression varies with age: it is greatest when infection begins in the first years of life and next in adolescence and again when acquired in old age. Among those remaining well for 2 years, a further 3 to 5 percent may develop late recrudescence at some time during life. Thus, the total morbidity rate in persons infected with *M. tuberculosis* is 8 to 20 percent. Both the early and late appearance of tuberculosis can be prevented in 80 percent of individuals if prompt treatment with INH is given when tuberculin "conversion" is discovered.

Mortality has fallen steadily over the past 70 years. Tuberculosis has ceased being the leading cause of death, with over 200 deaths per 100,000 in 1906 but only about 1.5 per 100,000 in 1980. This figure may be somewhat low, because residual pulmonary scarring may lead to cor pulmonale and cause death secondarily.

IMMUNITY Natural resistance The Caucasian and Mongolian races have a distinct natural resistance to tuberculosis consisting of an ability to develop an immune response to the infection which permits spontaneous recovery from initial infection. However, late recrudescence may result in chronic disease characterized by cavitation and scarring. Africans, Asians, American Indians, and Eskimos appear to have decreased ability to develop an effective immune response to new infection, and in them the infection tends to be more rapidly progressive.

The decreased immunity among racial and ethnic groups who have experienced a relatively recent exposure to the tubercle bacillus may be explained, in part, on the basis of selection. Caucasians in Great Britain, Europe, and North America during the seventeenth and eighteenth centuries were the first people to have lived during an epidemic of tuberculosis in which almost everyone was infected and as many as 1300 per 100,000 per year died of the disease. The present population of these areas consists of the descendents of the infected who survived to propagate generation after generation. The selection process continues today in Asia, Africa, and South America, although the severity of the selection process has been modified by such measures as chemotherapy, bacillus Calmette-Guérin (BCG) vaccination, and preventive treatment before development of disease.

Specific (acquired) immunity The alveolar macrophage and circulating monocyte are the key cells in tuberculosis immunity. A network of interactions among the T lymphocyte, B lymphocyte, and macrophage modulates the host defense. When a tubercle bacillus passes into the distal air spaces of the lung of a previously uninfected person, it is engulfed by a macrophage and enclosed within a phagocytic vacuole (phagosome). The phagosome may fuse with a lysosome, causing the tubercle bacillus to be killed by proteolytic enzymes. With or without intracellular killing the macrophage "presents" mycobacterial antigens to T and B lymphocytes and secretes substances which result in lasting changes in lymphocytes. Activated T lymphocytes produce several mediators, including macrophage-activating, chemotactic, migration inhibitory, and blastogenic factors. The ability of activated macrophages to kill tubercle bacilli is greatly increased. Some of the macrophages change into epithelioid or multinucleated giant cells, which are capable of killing ingested tubercle bacilli. Proteolytic enzymes released by the macrophages, epithelioid cells, and giant cells produce a type of tissue necrosis referred to as *caseation.* In the presence of a large number of bacilli the necrotic tissue may liquefy, enabling the infection to spread to other parts of the lung.

Apparently tubercle bacilli may survive within activated macrophages for prolonged periods ("persisters") where they divide only occasionally. There is evidence that sulfatides elaborated by tubercle bacilli render the lysosomes incompetent for fusion with phagosomes containing tubercle bacilli, protecting them from the harmful action of the lysosomal enzymes.

Anergy to PPD in tuberculosis is associated with a marked T lymphocytopenia induced by substances elaborated by antigen-specific suppressor monocytes. Prednisone, in doses greater than 0.3 mg per kilogram of body weight per day, may cause tuberculin anergy, since steroid in this amount causes a marked depletion of circulating T lymphocytes.

Tuberculin hypersensitivity The most readily obtained evidence of a past or present infection with tubercle bacilli is the finding of hypersensitivity to tuberculin, a protein derivative of the broth in which tubercle bacilli have been grown. Epidemiologic evidence strongly suggests that tuberculin hypersensitivity indicates the presence of living tubercle bacilli. The larger the skin reaction, the greater the chance that the infection is of clinical significance.

PATHOGENESIS AND PATHOLOGIC ANATOMY Initial infection ("primary" tuberculosis) In the nonimmune subject tubercle bacilli can gain entrance to the body by several routes: lung, gastrointestinal tract, and direct cutaneous or percutaneous inoculation (as in an accident at the autopsy table). For practical purposes, the only route that is of importance in the United States is the lung. The majority of lesions in the early phase of infection are in the lower two-thirds of the lungs, where ventilation is best and deposition of droplet nuclei more likely. After phagocytosis in the nonimmune host, the bacilli may remain viable or multiply occasionally within macrophages for an extended period. The organisms reach regional (hilar) nodes and even the bloodstream before their progress is inhibited by the gradual development of specific immunity over a period of several weeks. At this time, the characteristic tissue reaction develops, with epithelioid cell granulomas and caseation necrosis in the pulmonary lesion, regional lymph nodes, and any site to which the bacilli have spread. The number of bacilli drops drastically with the appearance of caseation necrosis, indicating that caseation is associated with the release of lymphokines from T lymphocytes and enzymes from macrophages which destroy host tissues as well as tubercle bacilli. Thereafter, the infection in the primary site usually heals by a combination of resolution, fibrosis, and calcification. Occasionally defenses fail, and the infection may overwhelm the host or proceed directly to a chronic stage.

Silent dissemination Early in the course of a new infection tubercle bacilli reach the general circulation in varying numbers. This event is marked only by fever and mild symptoms and is recognized as tuberculosis only when a patient is being observed closely because of recent exposure to tuberculosis. This stage is important in the pathogenesis of tuberculosis, because it is the time when bacilli reach distant sites to establish metastatic foci of infection that are the seeds from which clinical tuberculosis may develop much later.

While bacilli presumably reach all organs during this silent bacillemia, they establish lesions with frequency in only a limited number of sites, which have one feature in common: high tissue oxygen tension. Despite a paucity of ventilation, the apexes of the lungs in the upright position have the highest oxygen tension in the body (130 mmHg) due to a high ventilation-perfusion ratio. Probably for this reason they are the most frequent sites in which viable bacilli persist in a dormant state in metastatic (Simon's) foci and produce clinical disease at a later time.

Latent (dormant) infection When a tuberculous lesion regresses and heals, the infection enters a latent phase in which it may persist without producing illness. Though the infection may remain dormant for life, it may develop into clinical tuberculosis at any time if the persisting intracellular organisms begin to multiply rapidly.

Clinical tuberculosis Fibrocaseous tuberculosis may develop from either direct progression of the initial infection or recrudescence of a dormant lesion, most commonly in the apical portion of the lung. An old caseous hilar lymph node occasionally liquefies and spills its contents into a bronchus, to produce a segmental or lobar tuberculous pneumonia. Massive bloodstream invasion (miliary tuberculosis) may also occur at any stage. Tuberculosis is characterized by localized nodular infiltrations, fibrosis, and cavitation.

MANIFESTATIONS Recent infection Initial tuberculous infection usually produces no clinical illness. A mild illness with fever and malaise may develop about the fourth week after inoculation, but it is usually self-limited. Occasionally, however, the infection progresses, either in the lung or by dissemination through the bloodstream. This turn of events can be extremely serious unless detected promptly and treated adequately.

Massive hematogenous dissemination is most likely to occur in a recently infected child of 3 years or younger. In older children infection usually passes unnoticed. Occasionally it produces pleurisy with effusion, cervical lymphadenitis, miliary tuberculosis, or meningitis.

In the United States, 94 to 99 percent of young adults have never been infected with tuberculosis. There have been several "epidemics" of tuberculosis among such susceptible young persons. For example, when infectious tuberculosis develops aboard ship or in prison, many persons may be infected and some secondary cases may develop. Persons working in the Peace Corps, armed forces, or State Department who are assigned to countries where the prevalence of tuberculosis is high may be heavily exposed to the disease. As in children, recent tuberculous infection usually produces only mild and nonspecific symptoms but may progress to clinical tuberculosis in 5 to 10 percent. There may be an area of pneumonitis in any portion of the lung, but obvious hilar adenopathy is not common. When a young adult has a pleural effusion or a parenchymal infiltrate in the lung, a tuberculin test should be performed. If the skin test is positive, the possibility of tuberculosis should be considered strongly. The source of infection is usually an adult with cavitary tuberculosis.

An epidemic of tuberculosis among elderly residents of a nursing home has been described. One elderly patient who had been infected 2 years earlier developed infectious pulmonary tuberculosis and in the course of a year infected 50 other residents and 22 employees, producing disease in a total of 10 persons. All cases were in persons known to be tuberculin negative, and no case developed in the tuberculin reactors who were exposed to an equal extent. Usually it is a person with a dormant infection which undergoes recrudescence to produce cavitary disease who initiates such an epidemic, but newly infected contacts may become secondary spreaders of the infection. It is this fact that accounts for a rise in PPD reactors from 10 to 15 percent among persons entering nursing homes to 20 to 50 percent in the course of residence.

Pulmonary tuberculosis Pulmonary tuberculosis may follow the initial infection directly or after a short or long period of dormancy. Progressive disease has been observed to develop after 60 years of clinical dormancy. The most striking features of recrudescent tuberculosis are (1) absence of recent exposure to tuberculosis, (2) tendency to chronicity and cavitation, and (3) production of fibrous tissue. The last two phenomena are characteristic of the responses in persons sensitized to tubercle bacilli. While the solid caseation necrosis of the initial stage contains few bacilli, the *liquid* caseum in a tuberculous cavity contains abundant bacilli and may spread infection via bronchi to other portions of the lungs and into the environment.

SYMPTOMS In most instances, the onset of pulmonary tuberculosis is insidious, and the symptoms are quite nonspecific. Many cases are discovered because a routine roentgenogram is taken upon admission of an elderly person to a hospital for some other illness or when a sputum is examined for tubercle bacilli in an elderly person thought to have bacterial pneumonia or chronic bronchitis.

The earliest symptoms are constitutional and probably result from substances secreted by macrophages and leukocytes which have been activated by contact with antigens from the tubercle bacillus. Abdominal symptoms may dominate the clinical picture. It is common for a patient with tuberculosis to be unaware of a fever as high as 40°C. General malaise may be present, but often there is nothing more than irritability, depression, and excessive fatigue at the end of the day. Defervescence during sleep may give rise to profuse sweating which soaks the patient's pajamas (night sweat).

Weight loss is common but is often passed off as being due to overwork or to voluntary caloric restriction, although the weight may be maintained until late in the course of the illness. When abdominal symptoms predominate, loss of weight may be rapid.

Headache may be noted occasionally, especially in the evening. Palpitation may occur during mild exertion. Menstruation is usually not disturbed until the disease is advanced, when amenorrhea may develop.

Cough is frequent but not invariable and is often passed off as a "cigarette cough." When sputum is produced, it is usually odorless, green or yellow in color, and raised principally upon arising in the morning. Hemoptysis may accompany the cough and usually consists of streaking of the sputum with small amounts of blood. In some patients the onset of pulmonary tuberculosis is relatively sudden, with fever, productive cough, or pleuritic pain suggestive of bacterial pneumonia.

PHYSICAL AND ROENTGEN EXAMINATIONS Early asymptomatic infiltrations due to tuberculosis are usually undetectable by physical examination, even though obvious by x-ray. Longstanding tuberculosis with extensive fibrosis causes contraction and distortion of pulmonary tissue and bronchi. In such instances, a wide variety of physical signs may be present, such as apical dullness and bronchial breath sounds, inspiratory crackles, deviation of the trachea, and diminished mobility of one hemithorax.

Because findings on examination of the lungs in the early stages may be unremarkable, the importance of the chest roentgenogram in the diagnosis of tuberculosis cannot be overemphasized. Comparison of abnormal films with those taken in previous examinations makes it possible to detect and treat tuberculosis before liquefaction has occurred with spread of bacilli to other portions of the lungs or to other persons.

COMPLICATIONS OF PULMONARY TUBERCULOSIS *Cavitation.* When defense mechanisms fail, tuberculosis produces extensive tissue necrosis and liquefaction associated with cytotoxicity and enzymatic digestion produced by host lymphocytes and macrophages. Liquefaction of lung tissue results in the formation of a cavity where tubercle bacilli abound, making the disease highly infectious.

Hemoptysis. In the majority of instances of bleeding from the lungs, the blood arises from ulceration of the bronchial mucosa and presents as streaks of bright red in the sputum. On occasion the hemoptysis may be massive and life-threatening.

Pleurisy with effusion. A superficial tuberculous lesion in the lung may involve the overlying pleura and give rise to "dry" pleurisy, attended by localized pleuritic pain on deep inspiration. Or a small, caseous pulmonary focus may actually erode through the visceral pleura and extrude a small amount of liquid caseum. The immune response to such pleural contamination is a vigorous inflammatory reaction with formation of considerable pleural exudate. Although a pleural effusion may develop at any stage of tuberculosis, it is most common within a few months of the initial infection, particularly in young adults (age 15 to 35 years). The fluid is usually clear and light yellow. Its exudative nature is identified by a high protein content ($>$ 3 g per 100 ml), an elevated lactic dehydrogenase (LDH) level, a lymphocytic-cell response, and pH $<$ 7.20.

The importance of recognizing the tuberculous nature of such a pleural exudate in a young adult is reinforced by the finding that 65 percent of untreated patients sooner or later develop active tuberculosis. The diagnosis must often be clinical, because smears of the pleural fluid rarely reveal tubercle bacilli, and even the culture is positive in only 20 to 25 percent of cases. Percutaneous needle biopsy may reveal granulomatous pleuritis, but organisms are often not demonstrable. In most instances, proof of tuberculosis is lacking at the time the antituberculous treatment must be given if development of manifest tuberculosis is to be prevented. Fortunately, the intermediate tuberculin skin test is so regularly negative in healthy young adults that a positive reaction in a patient with a lymphocytic pleural exudate constitutes adequate evidence of tuberculous etiology to warrant initiation of two-drug therapy. However, it is not uncommon for the intermediate-strength purified protein derivative (PPD) test to be negative in patients with large tuberculous effusions, but second-strength PPD will almost always be positive if the effusion is of tuberculous etiology.

Tuberculous pneumonia. The onset of tuberculosis occasionally is quite acute, resembling that of bacterial pneumonia. This picture is seen most often in blacks, persons with diabetes, children with overwhelming infection, and elderly persons whose lungs are flooded with bacilli discharged from an area of liquid necrosis in the lung or hilar nodes. Chills, fever, productive cough, pleuritic chest pain, and leukocytosis may be noted. A stained smear of the sputum usually reveals numerous tubercle bacilli.

Bronchopleural fistula and empyema. Though minimal pleural contamination from a small superficial caseous focus produces only a clear exudate, massive contamination from rupture of a large caseous lesion produces pneumothorax (bronchopleural fistula) and tuberculous empyema. This is one of the most dreaded complications of pulmonary tuberculosis. Tubercle bacilli are usually easily found in the purulent exudate. Management is largely surgical and consists of establishing adequate drainage, in combination with the administration of effective antituberculosis drugs.

Tuberculosis of bronchi, trachea, and larynx. These organs are all protected from implantation of inhaled *M. tuberculosis* by a covering of secreted mucus but may become involved in patients with advanced cavitary pulmonary tuberculosis who excrete numerous tubercle bacilli. Bronchial ulceration may result in hemoptysis and a localized wheeze during respiration. The bronchial lumen also may be compromised by pressure of enlarged hilar lymph nodes early in the course of infection.

In a patient with cavitary pulmonary tuberculosis, hoarseness and pain in the throat accentuated by swallowing suggest tuberculous laryngitis. The diagnosis can be confirmed by indirect laryngoscopy. It is important to exclude cavitary tuberculosis before a laryngectomy is performed for carcinoma of the larynx, because tuberculous laryngitis is occasionally mistaken for carcinoma, even on histologic examination. Antituberculous chemotherapy is highly effective for tuberculosis of the mucous membranes.

Bronchi which lie within tuberculous lesions are regularly weakened by the inflammatory process and dilated by contraction of fibrous tissue in healing. In the upper lobes this is rarely clinically significant, but in portions of the lung which are dependent when the patient is upright, it may lead to secondary infection, producing chronic productive cough and sporadic hemoptysis (see "Bronchiectasis" below).

Gastrointestinal tuberculosis. The normal gastrointestinal tract is resistant to penetration by tubercle bacilli, but in cavitary pulmonary tuberculosis associated with excretion of large numbers of bacilli, the mucosa may be penetrated in the ileocecal region. The symptoms consist chiefly of intermittent abdominal pain, cramping, and diarrhea. Occasionally the infection spreads through the wall of the intestine, to produce tuberculous peritonitis (see "Peritoneum" below).

DIFFERENTIAL DIAGNOSIS The clinical picture presented by pulmonary tuberculosis varies widely and may simulate a great number of other diseases.

Carcinoma of the lung (see Chap. 284). Tuberculosis is commonly confused with carcinoma of the lung because the highest incidence of both diseases is in the upper lobes and in older men. Both cause loss of weight, chronic cough, blood-streaked sputum, and mild fever. In addition to bacteriologic studies for tubercle bacilli, sputum cytology, bronchial brushing, and bronchoscopy should be employed to aid in the differentiation. Comparison of prior roentgenograms may be of considerable help, but in many instances nothing short of a diagnostic thoracotomy will serve to make the distinction. When tuberculosis is considered among the diagnostic possibilities, therapy with two antituberculous drugs should be instituted a few days before thoracotomy in order to minimize complications in the event the lesion is tuberculous.

Mycotic infections (see Chaps. 183, 184). When tubercle bacilli cannot be isolated from a patient suspected of having tuberculosis, appropriate tests should be made for the various fungus infections which may present with a clinical picture indistinguishable from pulmonary tuberculosis. Helpful skin and/or serologic tests are available for coccidioidomycosis, histoplasmosis, and aspergillosis, but blastomycosis, mucormycosis, cryptococcosis, and sporotrichosis can be diagnosed only by demonstrating the organisms in a biopsy specimen or on culture.

Sarcoidosis (see Chap. 235). The typical patient with sarcoidosis is afebrile and has a negative tuberculin test and a roentgen picture of diffuse pulmonary infiltrations and hilar adenopathy, but the disease is protean in its manifestations and may mimic tuberculosis. Mediastinoscopy with biopsy of lymph nodes or lung biopsy is of greatest value in establishing this diagnosis. On occasion tuberculosis may present with a picture which is clinically and pathologically suggestive of sarcoidosis, the correct diagnosis being made only by culture of the tubercle bacillus from biopsied tissue.

Actinomycosis and nocardiosis (see Chap. 182).

Aspiration pneumonia, lung abscess (see Chap. 276). Pulmonary infection which is introduced by the drainage of contaminated saliva during sleep from a focus of pyorrhea occurs predominantly in the upper and midposterior portions of the lung and can mimic tuberculosis. Usually the distinction can be made eventually, but much valuable time can be lost while the patient is treated for the wrong disease. The presence of putrid sputum, hemoptysis, fever, and leukocytosis in a patient who has pyorrhea and has recently undergone surgery or who drinks alcohol to excess strongly suggests a pyogenic abscess. If the differentiation cannot be made readily, it may be advisable to treat with antimicrobials in addition to antituberculosis medications.

Other forms of pneumonia. Bacterial or mycoplasma infection (see Chap. 190) may present with clinical and roentgen appearances which at first may be indistinguishable from pulmonary tuberculosis. Cultures, cold agglutinins, precipitin, and complement fixation tests often establish the correct diagnosis. Cavitation is rare, and sputum examination does not yield tubercle bacilli. Early in the course of infection, tuberculosis may present with a localized infiltrate in the lung and slowly subside spontaneously or coincidentally with tetracycline therapy, similar to mycoplasma pneumonia. If clearing is incomplete, tuberculosis should be strongly considered. A tuberculin skin test should be performed in all patients with "viral pneumonia," particularly if a significant pleural effusion is present, since this is rare in viral pneumonia. A positive tuberculin skin test in an adolescent or young adult with pneumonitis should strongly suggest the possibility of tuberculosis.

Pneumoconiosis. Pulmonary infiltrations associated with exposure to silica dust, asbestos, ferrous oxide, and beryllium as well as hypersensitivity reactions to various organic inhalants may present a roentgenographic appearance suggestive of tuberculosis (see Chap. 274). Silicosis may present great difficulty in diagnosis because it may produce conglomerate masses and even cavitation that mimic tuberculosis. Silicosis impairs the pulmonary defense against tubercle bacilli. When the tuberculin skin test is positive in a patient with silicosis, smoldering tuberculosis is so likely that two-drug therapy is indicated if activity is suggested by x-ray, and prophylaxis with isoniazid is justified if there is no evidence of activity.

Bronchiectasis (see Chap. 277). A productive cough due to chronic infection in dilated bronchi occurs much less frequently than formerly because of more effective antibiotic therapy for necrotizing pneumonias of childhood and the reduction in the number of children whose bronchi have been damaged by tuberculosis. The lower and middle lobes (or lingula on the left) are most often involved, and a bronchogram effectively demonstrates the pathologic condition. If the tuberculin skin test is positive, isoniazid should be administered prophylactically to prevent late progression of tuberculosis from coexistent foci in apexes, whether or not they are visible radiographically.

Confusion caused by systemic effects of tuberculous infection. Because of the insidious nature of tuberculosis, the clinical picture may be mistaken for that produced by several other disorders. Malaise, easy fatigability, inability to concentrate, anorexia, and loss of weight may be mistaken for psychoneurosis. The symptoms may suggest hyperthyroidism or diabetes mellitus, but with a little care the distinction can be made. Tuberculosis should always be considered in the differential diagnosis of fever of unknown origin (see Chap. 9). If the roentgenogram reveals a pulmonary infiltrate, the possibility of tuberculosis is increased, but in cases of disseminated or extrapulmonary tuberculosis, the chest roentgenogram may be normal. In these cases biopsy of an enlarged lymph node, bone marrow, or liver may be of help. Formerly, tuberculosis was overdiagnosed in patients presenting with general systemic symptoms. Today, however, because of a lessening awareness of tuberculosis, the principal danger is that tuberculosis will be overlooked. Furthermore, tuberculosis may appear by recrudescence without recent reexposure.

Tuberculosis of other organs Localized tuberculous infection may occur in a number of other organs, notably, the lymph nodes, kidney, long bones, genital tract, brain, and meninges. Organisms reach these sites during the silent bacillemia which often occurs early in the infection.

LYMPH NODES The most common involvement of lymph nodes occurs in the hilus draining the pulmonary site of initial infection. The enlargement is usually modest but may be massive and give rise to obstruction and even ulceration of a major bronchus. The prognosis is good with proper chemotherapy, but the nodes may continue to enlarge for a few weeks after therapy is started and then resolve slowly.

CERVICAL ADENITIS (SCROFULA) This disease has become uncommon in the United States as a result of the elimination of tuberculous cattle and pasteurization of milk, but it occasionally occurs early in the course of infection. Cervical lymphadenitis may also appear as a late manifestation, especially in blacks. The nodes may be large (several centimeters in diameter) and matted together in a mass with an area of soft fluctuation. Signs of acute inflammation are rarely present. Swelling begins insidiously without systemic symptoms. Spontaneous rupture may occur, with drainage of caseous material. In some cases the offending organism is *M. scrofulaceum, M. kansasii,* or *M. avium-intracellulare,* and for this reason culture of the pus is necessary for accurate diagnosis.

KIDNEY Second to the upper lobes of the lungs, the kidney is the most common site for the late appearance of localized tuberculous infection. The mechanism of implantation is the same as that in the pulmonary apexes, namely, by hematogenous spread early in the infection. The oxygen tension in the cortical portion of the kidney approaches that in arterial blood, which enhances the growth and persistence of tubercle bacilli. As in the lungs, foci of tuberculosis may remain dormant for many years and produce clinical disease late in life. The pathologic process is the same as in the lung: inflammation, followed by caseation, liquefaction, and discharge of contaminated material into the collecting system and down the ureter to the bladder and, in men, to the genital tract.

Symptoms of renal tuberculosis are usually insidious and may be overlooked completely until the appearance of cystitis or epididymitis. Gross or microscopic hematuria and pyuria with a "sterile" urine on culture for bacteria should always call tuberculosis to mind and lead to the performance of a tuberculin skin test and culture of urine for tubercle bacilli. Intravenous pyelography may reveal a cortical cavity communicating with the calyceal system. Symptoms usually subside promptly with chemotherapy. Resection of residual areas of destruction is only rarely necessary.

MALE GENITALS Infection of the genital tract in the male is secondary to renal tuberculosis. Bacilli discharged from a caseous lesion in the kidney may reach the seminal vesicles, prostate gland, and epididymis through their connections with the excretory tract. Symptoms begin insidiously, most commonly with scrotal pain due to inflammation of the epididymis and vas deferens. Tenderness and swelling may be found in the vas, seminal vesicles, and/or the prostate gland.

FEMALE GENITALS When tuberculosis infection occurs after puberty, tuberculosis occasionally spreads hematogenously to the highly vascular fallopian tube. Infection may then spread into the uterus and give rise to endometritis. Symptoms are usually mild and of insidious onset, with abdominal pain, white vaginal discharge, metromenorrhagia, and dyspareunia. Systemic symptoms and signs are uncommon, probably because the infection is indolent and localized. The most common manifestation is sterility, but tubal scarring may cause pregnancy to be ectopic. Tuberculosis of the fallopian tube may also spread to the peritoneum and produce either a tuberculous pelvic abscess or generalized peritonitis.

OSSEOUS TUBERCULOSIS Hematogenous spread of tuberculosis to the long bones and vertebrae is most common when infection occurs in childhood, because of the high P_{O_2} associated with the vascularity at the epiphyseal plates during active bone growth. It usually occurs within 3 years of infection, but dormant lesions may be reactivated by trauma years later. Infection begins in the ends of the long bones but becomes obvious when it involves the adjacent joint: hip, knee, elbow, or wrist. Tenosynovitis is most common at the wrist.

TUBERCULOUS SPONDYLITIS (POTT'S DISEASE) This disease may result from hematogenous seeding or from spread of infection from paravertebral lymph nodes draining a tuberculous pleurisy. Spondylitis may develop in childhood or be delayed until later in life. Localized pain in the back may be present for months before x-rays reveal an abnormality. Though infection begins in the body of a vertebra, the first radiographic sign is usually destruction and narrowing of an intervertebral disk. A paravertebral abscess may be seen as a fusiform density extending the length of several vertebrae and occasionally dissects downward to the inguinal area. Therapy with two bactericidal drugs is the keystone of management, although some patients may require surgical drainage. Extensive orthopedic procedures are no longer necessary.

PERITONEUM The peritoneum may be implanted with tubercle bacilli when they spread by any of at least four routes: (1) through the wall of infected intestine, (2) from a mesenteric lymph node, (3) from an infected fallopian tube, or (4) from hematogenous seeding in the course of disseminated tuberculosis. Symptoms are insidious, with increasing abdominal girth, but ultimately the patient has fever, night sweats, weakness, diarrhea, and abdominal pain. As with other forms of tuberculosis, there is an increased frequency among alcoholics. Tuberculosis should be strongly considered whenever ascitic fluid contains protein in excess of 3 g/dl, when LDH is elevated, and when the white blood cells are mostly lymphocytes. Diagnosis may be made by isolation of *M. tuberculosis* from ascitic fluid or by its demonstration in histologic studies of the peritoneal tissue obtained by peritoneoscopy and biopsy.

PERICARDIUM Tuberculous infection may spread from the mediastinal lymph nodes or contiguous segments of lung to the pericardium in the same manner as to the pleura. The pathologic process is the same as in tuberculous pleurisy, with outpouring of a clear exudate, formation of granulomas, and subsequent fibrosis. The clinical picture may be that of chronic pericardial tamponade, with hepatomegaly, edema, friction rub, and enlargement of the cardiac shadow during the active phase, and constriction during the phase of fibrosis. When such an illness is acccompanied by afternoon fever or night sweats and a positive tuberculin reaction, tuberculosis should be strongly considered. The diagnosis is made best by open pericardial biopsy. A tuberculous pericardial effusion contains more than 3 g protein per deciliter, an elevated LDH, and lymphocytes. Early in the disease, multiple-drug chemotherapy accompanied by corticosteroids is usually sufficient, but surgical resection of the pericardium is occasionally necessary when the process is well established before therapy is begun.

If tuberculous pericarditis has undergone spontaneous healing, the patient may present years later with a picture of constrictive pericarditis (see Chap. 265). Pericardiectomy at this stage may improve cardiac function but may be technically difficult because of extensive calcification extending into the myocardium. The procedure may be complicated by marked impairment of cardiac output postoperatively due to cardiac dilatation and myocardial atrophy.

ADRENALS Occasionally hematogenous tuberculosis localizes in the adrenal glands and may result in their total destruction, giving rise to adrenal cortical insufficiency (Addison's disease, see Chap. 112). This must be differentiated from adrenal cortical atrophy, which is more common, and from other causes of adrenal destruction, such as histoplasmosis. Therapy consists of administration of antituberculosis agents plus physiologic doses of adrenal steroids.

MENINGES Tuberculosis may involve the meninges, either as a part of miliary tuberculosis or as extension of infection from a focus within the brain. In areas with a high incidence of tuberculosis, tuberculous meningitis is seen most commonly in young children during the first year of infection. In areas of low incidence such as the United States, meningitis is more common among older adults as a result of late reactivation of dormant infection. Pathologically, the meninges contain small tubercles and a fibrinous exudate over the base of the brain.

Symptoms consist of headache, restlessness, and irritability, usually accompanied by fever, malaise, night sweats, and loss of weight. Nausea and vomiting may be prominent. Stiffness of the neck and Brudzinski's sign are usually present. Spinal puncture usually reveals increased pressure, clear fluid containing an increased amount of protein, reduced glucose (less than half the blood glucose), and 100 to 1000 white blood cells per milliliter, 80 to 95 percent of which are lymphocytes.

The differential diagnosis includes partially treated pyogenic meningitis, fungal meningitis, carcinomatosis or sarcoidosis of the meninges, and subarachnoid hemorrhage. There is considerable urgency in establishing the correct diagnosis because specific therapy is most effective when instituted early in the course of the illness. Irreversible brain damage may result from waiting 6 to 8 weeks for cultural proof of diagnosis. Frequently it is necessary to begin therapy for tuberculosis on the basis of a presumptive clinical diagnosis while awaiting results of bacteriologic studies. Therapy should include isoniazid and rifampin, both of which cross the blood-brain barrier. Steroids are indicated only when there is an impending subarachnoid block or cerebral edema. Intrathecal therapy is not indicated.

INAPPROPRIATE SECRETION OF ANTIDIURETIC HORMONE (ADH) Older persons with tuberculous meningitis or overwhelming pulmonary tuberculosis occasionally present with somnolence or coma associated with a very low serum sodium concentration (110 to 125 meq per liter), because of inappropriate secretion of ADH. This must be distinguished from adrenal insufficiency, in which the sodium serum concentration is also depressed in concert with an elevated serum potassium level. In addition to antituberculosis agents, adequate sodium chloride should be administered and water intake restricted.

Disseminated tuberculosis SILENT BACILLEMIA Hematogenous dissemination of a small number of tubercle bacilli is common early in the course of infection but usually produces little clinical illness. The principal importance of the event is the seeding of bacilli in sites far removed from the pulmonary site of inoculation.

MASSIVE DISSEMINATION (MILIARY TUBERCULOSIS) When a liquid caseous focus empties its contents into a vein, there is a massive dissemination of tubercle bacilli throughout the body. Defense mechanisms are overwhelmed, and tubercles become established in all organs of the body. Without specific therapy, death is almost a certainty.

Miliary tuberculosis is the most dreaded manifestation of tuberculosis. It may arise shortly after infection or from recrudescence of a dormant focus years or decades later. Because the resistance of the body is overwhelmed, lesions are not limited to those organs with an elevated P_{O_2} but are often found in the liver, spleen, bone marrow, and meninges. The best way to make the diagnosis of miliary tuberculosis is to perform a biopsy of the liver, lymph node, or bone marrow in search of caseating granulomas and tubercle bacilli.

Symptoms are usually nonspecific and consist of weight loss, weakness, gastrointestinal disturbance, fever, and sweats. The patient has usually had a course of penicillin or broad-spectrum antibiotics without control of the fever before the diagnosis comes to mind. Cough is not a prominent feature, but dyspnea may be. The correct diagnosis may not be suspected until the typical "miliary" pattern is noted on the chest roentgenogram. The white cell count may be normal or low, or may show a leukemoid pattern suggesting leukemia. There may be a monocytosis. An identical clinical picture can be presented by histoplasmosis, coccidioidomycosis, blastomycosis, cryptococcosis, and other chronic infections. Therefore, it is imperative to obtain any material possible by biopsy or aspiration to establish a correct diagnosis on which to base therapy.

SUBACUTE AND CHRONIC DISSEMINATION Instead of a single massive invasion of the bloodstream, smaller numbers of tubercle bacilli may escape into the circulation intermittently and give rise to a variety of clinical manifestations, including myelophthisic anemia, low-grade fever, lymphadenopathy, effusion into pleural and peritoneal cavities, and splenomegaly. There may be destructive lesions of bones, kidneys, subcutaneous tissue, or skin. Such a clinical picture is most common in elderly persons with recrudescent infection.

The protean manifestations and bizarre clinical picture caused by subacute and chronic forms of hematogenous tuberculosis provide a tremendous diagnostic challenge. To add to the confusion, the tuberculin reaction is often suppressed in persons with overwhelming infection. The intermediate-strength tuberculin test is often negative, and the PPD no. 2 (see "Diagnosis" below) occasionally so. The solution to the clinical problem most commonly comes when the possibility of tuberculosis is belatedly considered. Confirmation must be sought from appropriate histologic and bacteriologic studies. The prognosis is uniformly bad without treatment but good with appropriate chemotherapy.

DIAGNOSIS Tuberculin skin test Tuberculin is a protein fraction of tubercle bacilli. When introduced into the skin of a person with tuberculous infection, whether clinically apparent or dormant, it triggers release of several lymphokines which over the next 24 to 72 h cause a localized thickening of the skin due to edema and accumulation of sensitized lymphocytes. Although there are several methods for testing healthy populations with tuberculin for evidence of unsuspected infection, the method preferred in clinical practice is to inject 0.1 ml of a solution containing the equivalent of 5 tuberculin units (TU) of purified protein derivative stabilized with Tween 80 (PPD-T) into the skin of the volar aspect of the forearm with a small needle—an "intermediate-strength tuberculin test." The test is read 48 to 72 h later and is considered positive if the diameter of skin thickening measures 10 mm or more, doubtful if it is 5 to 10 mm, and negative if it is less than 5 mm.

Intermediate-strength PPD produces a positive reaction in the majority of persons infected with tubercle bacilli. However, it is a biologic test which is dependent upon the presence of an adequate number of circulating effector T lymphocytes. False-negative results may occur in 15 to 20 percent of persons with clinical tuberculosis, as in persons who are clinically ill, febrile, or have a large pleural effusion. If the intermediate PPD is negative in a patient in whom tuberculosis is suspected, the test should be repeated using "second-strength" PPD (100 or 250 TU). If this is also negative, tuberculosis can be dismissed with considerable certainty, although persons who are moribund from tuberculosis may fail to react even to PPD no. 2.

A positive reaction to intermediate-strength PPD indicates the presence of a tuberculous infection, but it does not help in distinguishing clinical from dormant infection. This distinction must be made on clinical, bacteriologic, and radiographic grounds. A positive reaction which is elicited only by PPD no. 2 in a patient who is clinically ill means that active tuberculosis cannot be dismissed as a diagnostic possibility. In healthy persons, however, it usually signifies only healed tuberculosis or infection with mycobacteria other than *M. tuberculosis.*

Radiography While never providing an etiologic diagnosis, x-rays of the chest provide extremely valuable information. The abnormality which is most suggestive of tuberculosis is a multinodular infiltrate with cavitation in one or both of the upper lobes of the lung. Because of the propensity of tuberculosis to spread via bronchi to other parts of the lungs, the basilar areas may be involved also. Occasionally, especially in the elderly, the lesions are limited to the lower lobe(s). Multiple infiltrates, especially if bilateral, are most suggestive of tuberculosis, because pyogenic pneumonia and primary carcinoma are much more likely to produce single lesions. Carcinoma usually produces a solid lesion, in contrast to the multinodular infiltrate of tuberculosis. Planigrams (laminagrams) are particularly valuable in making such distinctions and in detecting cavitation. Lateral, lordotic, and oblique films are also of value in defining the location and character of lesions. Initially tuberculous infection is not usually apical in location but may involve any other segment of the lungs. Hilar adenopathy is common early in the course of infection in children, but may not be obvious by x-ray in adults. Large pleural effusions are easily detected, but for small or infrapulmonary effusion it may be necessary to place the patient on the *involved* side to permit the fluid to be seen along the lateral chest wall (lateral decubitus film).

Bacteriologic diagnosis The only absolute proof of tuberculosis is the cultural identification of *M. tuberculosis* from tissue or body fluid: sputum, gastric washing, urine, cerebrospinal fluid (CSF), serous effusion, or pus from an abscess or sinus. A useful preliminary examination, however, is to make a smear of the material and stain it for standard microscopy or to apply the auromine-rhodamine stain for easier, though less definitive, detection by fluorescence microscopy. The smear is not a very sensitive method, but it has the virtue of quickly identifying the patient who is discharging great numbers of organisms into the environment. For positive identification, cultures must be made either on solid egg medium (Löwenstein-Jensen) or Middlebrook 7H-11 medium using 20 to 40 mmHg CO_2 in the incubator.

The most commonly examined material is sputum. When it can be produced spontaneously (usually in the early morning), it makes the most satisfactory material for both smear and culture. If none can be produced spontaneously, the patient may be asked to inhale aerosolized heated saline to stimulate production of bronchial secretions. Bacteriologic specimens may also be collected by bronchial washing, bronchial brushing, or tracheal aspiration. Sputum should never be collected over a 24-h period because this increases the frequency of contamination.

When no sputum can be collected, as in young children or senile or psychotic persons, fasting morning gastric contents may be aspirated and cultured. Diagnosis by smear of this material is less reliable than examination of sputum because of the frequency of saprophytic acid-fast bacteria in the stomach, but the presence of large numbers of acid-fast bacilli strongly suggests that they are significant.

Multiple specimens (five or more) may be needed before the organisms are recovered. This is particularly true early in the course of tuberculous infection, tuberculous pleurisy with effusion, and when the pulmonary lesions are small and noncavitary. Patients with old chronic tuberculous lesions may shed organisms only intermittently.

Hematology The white blood cell count is usually not significantly elevated, except in tuberculous pneumonia (when it may suggest a pyogenic infection) and in miliary tuberculosis (when a leukemoid reaction may be mistaken for leukemia). Hemoglobin and hematocrit are usually normal unless a prolonged period of illness has produced anemia of infection.

Urinalysis There are no specific changes except when a urinary tract lesion is present. Renal tuberculosis is not rare in older persons; it most often presents with microscopic hematuria and pyuria with negative cultures for pyogens. Two or three early morning specimens should be submitted for culture. About 10 percent of persons with pulmonary tuberculosis excrete bacilli in their urine, even though the urinalysis is normal and there are no detectable urinary tract lesions.

Other tests Despite great efforts to develop one, there is no specific serologic test to distinguish clinical from dormant tuberculosis. Biopsy of the liver, bone marrow, or lymph node can be of great aid in reaching a presumptive diagnosis of disseminated tuberculosis by revealing caseating granulomas containing acid-fast bacilli. Such a finding may be lifesaving by permitting initiation of specific therapy without allowing the disease to progress while awaiting culture confirmation.

TREATMENT Treatment of tuberculosis is based upon intensive and prolonged exposure of the organisms to bacterial antagonists. With proper management, tuberculosis can be cured in 95 percent of patients, even though return to health may be limited by an associated disease. Heretofore conventional therapy has required 18 to 24 months, but by using a regimen of two bactericidal drugs treatment can be completed in 9 months. Either form of therapy can be accomplished while the patient is ambulatory and even at work.

Principles of chemotherapy To be effective in therapy, a drug must interfere with a vital function of the tubercle bacillus without harming the host. The choice of therapy should be guided by several well-established principles:

1 Drugs should be chosen to which the bacilli are likely to be susceptible. Fortunately, in the United States this presents little difficulty in most newly discovered cases because most strains are susceptible to the major drugs. If a patient has been treated previously or contracted the infection in an area where drug resistance is common (e.g., southeast Asia, Philippines, Mexico), it must be assumed that the bacilli will be resistant to isoniazid (INH) and streptomycin (SM); therefore the regimen should include at least two other drugs until the results of susceptibility studies are known.

2 Even in a generally susceptible population of bacilli, a naturally resistant mutant occurs about once in 10^5 to 10^6 organisms. For this reason at least two effective drugs should always be given to patients with clinical tuberculosis to avoid multiplication of drug-resistant mutants.

3 Bactericidal drugs are always preferred. Both rifampin and isoniazid are bactericidal for both extra- and intracellular bacilli. Isoniazid is superior to rifampin in producing an early bactericidal effect on actively metabolizing bacteria, but rifampin is superior for sterilizing lesions which contain dormant bacilli that show only rare and short bursts of metabolic activity. For this reason these two drugs are effective both for immediate reduction in the large extracellular population of bacilli and for ultimate eradication of the smaller intracellular population.

4 When treatment appears to be failing (bacteriology fails to become negative within 3 to 4 months), the addition of a single drug is an invitation to disaster. Therapy should always be changed to an entirely new regimen of at least two new drugs, and great care should be taken to ensure that the patient takes the medication regularly.

5 Therapy must be continued long enough to eradicate the bacilli from the body. When two bactericidal drugs are used, this can be accomplished in 9 months, but when one of the drugs is bacteriostatic, a treatment period of 18 to 24 months is required.

6 All medications should be given before breakfast and in a single dose, if possible, in order to achieve a single combined peak concentration for maximum effect on the bacilli.

MAJOR DRUGS *Isoniazid (INH).* Isoniazid interferes with DNA synthesis and intermediary metabolism of the tubercle bacillus. It is the keystone of antituberculous chemotherapy. It is acetylated in the liver and excreted by the kidney. The usual dose for adults is 5 mg/kg per day, usually 300 mg, given in a single dose. In children the dosage is higher because of more rapid excretion: 10 to 15 mg/kg per day. It is a safe drug for use in pregnancy, although elective chemoprophylaxis should be deferred until after delivery. Although some persons acetylate INH more rapidly than others, this has proved to be of little clinical significance unless the interval between doses is 5 days or more. When used in "pulse" therapy, the dose is about 15 mg/kg given twice weekly or 10 mg/kg given three times per week. In renal failure the dose must be reduced moderately (to 200 mg per day) in patients on chronic dialysis. Although not common, three types of toxicity from INH occur: (1) Direct toxicity consists of peripheral neuropathy and anemia due to competition of INH with pyridoxine. Pyridoxine in a dose of 30 to 50 mg per day effectively combats this problem, which is most common when a large dose is used and in alcoholics whose nutrition is impaired. With intentional or accidental overdose, pyridoxine, in an equivalent dose to the amount of isoniazid ingested, should be administered in a single, intravenous infusion. (2) Allergic reactions consist of skin rash, swelling of the tongue, arthralgia, and fever and may require withdrawal of the drug. (3) Hepatocellular toxicity is the most serious toxic effect of INH. Contrary to earlier thought, hepatitis is not due to allergy but may be due to a reaction to a metabolic product of INH degradation in the liver. Symptoms consist of malaise and anorexia followed by nausea, vomiting, fever, and finally, jaundice. The best way to detect INH hepatitis is to acquaint each patient with the symptoms for which to be alert (anorexia, nausea, vomiting) with the request that they be reported without delay. No more than a 1-month supply of INH should be given, and inquiry about symptoms should be made each time the patient is seen. A suspected reaction must be confirmed by the following procedure: discontinue INH at once and draw blood for determination of SGOT, alkaline phosphatase, and serum bilirubin. If these tests are normal or SGOT is only mildly elevated, INH therapy may be reinstituted cautiously. If any of the tests show a threefold elevation, INH hepatitis is very likely and the drug should not be given. For minor elevations, one should repeat the studies; if they are normal, restart treatment with INH, beginning with 50 mg (one-sixth of a 300-mg tablet), and recheck the laboratory results. If symptoms recur and the SGOT shows a sharp rise, INH toxicity exists and the drug should be discontinued. The only therapy required is the withdrawal of the drug, but if INH is continued in the face of symptoms of hepatitis, it may prove fatal.

Rifampin (RIF). Rifampin acts by inhibition of RNA polymerase of both extra- and intracellular bacilli. The dose is about 10 mg/kg per day, or 450 to 600 mg per day, for adults and about 15 mg/kg per day for children. Although RIF has not been used extensively during pregnancy, experience to date has produced no evidence of teratogenicity, and its use with isoniazid is an acceptable combination for treatment of tuberculosis in pregnancy. Toxicity consists of jaundice (about 1 percent), gastrointestinal symptoms, and fever. Hypersensitivity reactions such as "flu syndrome," renal failure, and thrombocytopenia may occur when a large dose (900 to 1200 mg) is administered intermittently, but are uncommon when smaller doses (450 to 600 mg) are administered two or three times per week. Hypersensitivity reactions may occur when RIF is resumed after a longer interruption. While there is some laboratory evidence of suppression of immunity, there is no significant clinical effect. Rifampin accelerates the hepatic clearance rates of quinidine, warfarin, corticosteroids, and oral contraceptives, which may require the upward adjustment of the dose of these drugs when they are given concurrently with rifampin.

Streptomycin (SM) and capreomycin (CM). These drugs inhibit protein synthesis and are bactericidal for extracellular bacilli. They are ineffective against intracellular organisms. Dosage for each is 1 g per day for adults, reduced to 0.5 g per day in persons over age 60, of small stature, or with renal impairment. Dosage in children is 20 mg/kg per day. Actually, daily medication can be given 5 days per week with no apparent loss of effectiveness, which facilitates administration of medication by visiting nurses. Toxicity may be allergic in type with fever, rash, malaise, etc., or related to the eighth cranial nerve or the renal tubule. The latter two are total-dose related; therefore, medication is best given daily (five times per week) for only about 2 months and then two or three times per week for an additional 4 to 6 weeks to minimize the total amount of the drug used. Streptomycin may exert a toxic effect upon the eighth cranial nerve of the fetus in late pregnancy and for this reason should not be used when isoniazid and rifampin or ethambutol can be given instead. Slight dizziness and circumoral paresthesias are common immediately after injections, but are generally harmless.

Pyrazinamide (PZA). A very effective drug whose mode of action remains obscure, PZA is bactericidal in the acid intracellular milieu. When used with SM or CM, a very effective bactericidal combination results against organisms located both intra- and extracellularly. Dosage is 30 mg/kg per day given in a single daily dose. PZA can also be given twice a week in a dose of 50 mg/kg. It regularly causes a striking increase in serum uric acid, due to interference with renal excretion of uric acid, but this is harmless except in persons with gout. Toxicity consists of jaundice (rare), fever, or rash.

Ethambutol (EMB). Ethambutol inhibits RNA synthesis and is bacteriostatic against extracellular tubercle bacilli. Its principal value is inhibition of the growth of mutants which are resistant to INH or RIF. It was the second most commonly used drug in the United States until it was realized that the combination of RIF and INH makes it possible to administer two bactericidal drugs and thus reduce the total duration of therapy. Its principal use now is as a substitute drug used when toxicity precludes the use of a more effective one. EMB is well tolerated in a dose of 15 mg/kg per day with only rare instances of ocular toxicity (optic neuritis). In the more effective dose of 25 mg/kg per day which is necessary as a substitute drug, the incidence of optic neuritis approaches 1 percent and requires careful surveillance. It can be used safely during pregnancy but must be used with caution in children who are too young to cooperate in the testing of vision. In addition to periodic examination of visual acuity, color vision, and visual fields, patients should be asked to report any reduction in acuity noted in reading newsprint with their usual glasses. This drug can be used in supervised twice weekly treatment for which the dosage is 50 mg/kg.

OTHER DRUGS *Ethionamide (ETA).* Ethionamide inhibits protein synthesis and is of value in re-treatment of patients who harbor organisms that show multiple drug resistance. Dosage is 750 to 1000 mg per day for adults. Because gastric irritation is so common, this drug must be given in divided doses after meals.

Cycloserine (CS). This drug inhibits cell wall synthesis and is of use in re-treatment cases. Dosage is 750 to 1500 mg per day for adults, divided into two doses, each accompanied by pyridoxine, 100 mg. CS should not be used in epileptics or persons with a history of psychosis.

p-Aminosalicylic acid (PAS). p-Aminosalicylic acid interferes with intermediary metabolism and is bacteriostatic for the tubercle bacillus. Because of a high incidence of gastrointestinal intolerance, it is infrequently used today. It should not be used with RIF because PAS interferes with its absorption. Dosage is 200 mg/kg per day in divided doses.

Kanamycin. An aminoglycoside, kanamycin interferes with protein synthesis and can be used in re-treatment of resistant cases. Eighth nerve toxicity is common when large doses are given over a prolonged period of time, and so the patient should have audiometric tests at least once a month during therapy.

Thiacetazone and isoxyl. These are inexpensive drugs in use in developing countries. They are not available for clinical use in the United States, however, because of a high incidence of toxic side effects.

Choice of therapy for clinical tuberculosis The immediate goal of chemotherapy is to kill the organisms without permitting the selection of resistant mutants. It is very important to adhere to the principles of therapy outlined above in choosing and carrying out a therapeutic regimen. Chemotherapy of tuberculosis is so effective that such modalities as bed rest, collapse therapy, surgical resection, etc., need no longer be discussed.

INITIAL TREATMENT Therapy for tuberculosis, regardless of the organ involved, can be completed in 9 months *provided two bactericidal drugs are given together for the full period.* If the regimen consists of only one bactericidal drug and one bacteriostatic drug, therapy must be given for 18 to 24 months to achieve comparable success.

PREFERRED REGIMENS When there is no reason to suspect resistance to INH (see the first principle of therapy), the regimen should consist of INH and RIF from the start, and usually no other drug is needed. Where the possibility of INH and/or SM resistance is recognized, additional drugs should be given to ensure that at least two effective agents are included pending the report of drug susceptibilities.

Several safe and effective short-course regimens of therapy for tuberculosis have been described. INH 300 mg and RIF 600 mg daily for 9 months is curative in 95 percent of cases with a relapse rate of less than 2 percent. INH and RIF can be given daily for 4 to 6 weeks, after which RIF is given in the same dose of 600 mg, but the INH dose is increased to 15 mg/kg (usually 900 mg for adults) twice a week (e.g., on Tuesdays and Fridays) for the remainder of the 9 months. Advantages of this regimen are that it lends itself to total supervision of drug ingestion when necessary to ensure compliance, and less drug in total is required to achieve results equal to those obtained with therapy given daily for the 9-month period.

The regimen used in Great Britain consists of RIF 600 mg (450 mg for persons of small stature) and INH 300 mg for 9 months with the addition of either SM 0.75 g or EMB 25 mg/kg daily for the first 2 months. The third drug adds little if the organisms are sensitive to INH, but can be good insurance against failure if the organisms should be resistant to INH.

Four bactericidal drugs have been given at the outset to reduce the population of organisms as quickly as possible in an effort to shorten therapy still further. For the moment, this regimen appears to have little advantage to offset the disadvantage of increased drug toxicity, except when drug resistance is known or suspected or when the patient is unlikely to remain cooperative long enough to take therapy for 9 months. Four-drug therapy achieves a culture-negative state in about 85 percent of smear-positive patients after 2 months and a relapse rate of less than 2 percent after only 6 months of therapy.

About 4 to 6 percent of patients are unable to take RIF and INH because of toxicity, forcing the discontinuance of the offending drug(s) and substitution of others (e.g., SM, PZA, EMB). Hepatic toxicity is uncommon, i.e., less than 2 percent in our experience. Whenever the advantage of giving two bactericidal drugs together is lost, therapy then must be prolonged to 18 to 24 months to achieve success.

Prior to the introduction of the bactericidal therapy described above, the most widely used regimen was a combination of INH 300 mg per day combined with EMB in a dose of 15 to 25 mg/kg per day. When a large population of organisms was indicated by a positive sputum smear, it was common practice to add SM 1 g per day for the first 2 months in order to reduce further the risk of selection of INH-resistant mutants. The total period of therapy with this regimen must be 18 to 24 months in order to ensure lasting success. This form of therapy is used principally when toxicity secondary to a bactericidal drug forces substitution of a bacteriostatic one.

With the bactericidal combination of RIF and INH, conversion of cultures to negative is quite prompt, i.e., 89 percent in 2 months and 96 percent in 3 months. This is appreciably better than what could be achieved with earlier regimens. Relapse after successful therapy with RIF and INH has been less than 2 percent, largely within the first 6 months following completion of 9 months of therapy. If the full course of 18 to 24 months of the formerly used regimen is followed, relapses should be uncommon (about 3 to 4 percent), but this is often difficult to achieve. When relapse occurs following treatment with RIF and INH, the organisms almost always remain sensitive to both drugs and further treatment with the same regimen given for a longer period of time is usually successful. When relapse occurs following other forms of therapy, the chance of INH-resistant organisms is greater and a multiple-drug retreatment regimen is often necessary to achieve ultimate success.

The two most important tasks during treatment are (1) careful bacteriologic monitoring to be certain of the effectiveness of the medications and to provide samples of the bacilli to test for susceptibility in the event of failure and (2) careful monitoring for the toxic side effects of the drugs being given. To achieve both these ends, the patient should be seen no less frequently than every week or two at the outset and then at monthly intervals when the patient appears stable and recovery is going smoothly. To detect the occasional relapse, sputum specimens should be collected at monthly intervals for the first 6 months after completion of therapy and then every 3 months for an additional year.

When the patient's clinical condition requires hospitalization, it should be brief. Effective chemotherapy reduces infectiousness promptly even while the sputum smear is still positive for tubercle bacilli. For home therapy to be successful, the patient must comprehend enough of the nature of the disease and chemotherapy to ensure cooperation. Irregularity of medication or premature discontinuation are the major causes of failure and relapse. The booklet *Understanding Tuberculosis Today* by W. W. Stead (Central Press, Milwaukee, 1980) explains tuberculosis and its therapy in terms most patients can comprehend and is helpful in achieving compliance.

RE-TREATMENT OF "RESISTANT CASES" Need for a regimen for re-treatment may arise from inadequate use of drugs at the outset, from premature discontinuation of medication, or from relapse after apparently successful therapy. The skill required to manage a re-treatment case is greater than for initial therapy, and advice should be sought from a physician experienced in this field. Re-treatment must always involve a completely *new regimen of drugs.* When the patient has received several drugs in the past, it is usually desirable to await results of susceptibility tests before selecting therapy. When INH resistance is suspected but not yet proven, an excellent regimen is SM, PZA, RIF, and INH. The drugs should be given daily for 6 to 8 weeks or until drug susceptibilities are known. CM may be substituted if SM resistance is suspected. If the bacilli are later found to be susceptible to RIF and INH, daily or twice weekly therapy with only these medications for another 7 months is adequate. If INH resistance is confirmed, RIF, SM, and PZA should be continued either daily or twice weekly for a total of 9 months. For poorly compliant patients whose ingestion of medication must be supervised, the twice weekly regimen is preferable. When EMB must be substituted for any of the drugs, therapy must be continued for at least 12 to 15 months *after conversion* of sputum to negative.

CORTICOSTEROIDS The use of cortisone and its derivatives has been shown to increase the chance of recrudescence of dormant tuberculosis. Despite this, in patients who are very seriously ill with tuberculosis, these agents may be lifesaving. They should be used only when there is an immediate threat to life, such as hypotension, debilitating fever, dyspnea, or an impending blockage of the subarachnoid space in tuberculous meningitis. Prednisone may be used in a dosage of 40 mg per day for 1 to 2 weeks, then 20 mg for another 8 weeks, and then gradually withdrawn over a period of 3 to 4 weeks in order to prevent a "steroid rebound." The effect upon the temperature and the general well-being of the patient may be dramatic, but there is no decrease in residual fibrosis. In general, the frequency of side effects makes the routine use of steroids in conjunction with chemotherapy unwise. Rifampin, due to its effect on increasing hepatic clearance of corticosteroids, has been noted to induce a state of adrenal insufficiency in the rare patient who, prior to rifampin ingestion, had been able to produce endogenously only marginal quantities of cortisone.

PREVENTION Chemoprophylaxis Clinically inapparent tuberculous infection can be prevented from developing into tuberculosis by judicious use of isoniazid therapy both in recently infected persons and in those with a dormant infection.

Recently infected persons Close contacts of an infectious case of tuberculosis should be tested with tuberculin. Hospital and nursing home personnel should be tested at the time of employment and then annually. Any reactor with detectable disease or symptoms should be examined bacteriologically and given treatment with two drugs as outlined earlier. Newly infected persons with normal chest x-rays should be given preventive treatment with isoniazid. The risk of development of clinical tuberculosis in such persons is appreciable (see "Prevalence and Incidence" above) and greatly exceeds the risk of toxicity from isoniazid.

Close contacts of an infectious case who are under the age of 4 years are at special risk and should be started on therapy even though the tuberculin test is negative and they appear well. If in 3 months the skin test is still negative, therapy may be discontinued; if positive, treatment should be given for a full year.

Hospital and nursing home employees and other individuals such as nursing home residents and prison inmates should be screened initially with tuberculin skin tests, and reactors should be given chest x-rays. Some of these persons may show a weak or doubtful reaction to intermediate-strength PPD initially, but if tested a second time within 1 to 2 weeks a larger reaction may be elicited. This prompt enhancement ("boosting") of a weakly reacting tuberculin reaction is due to an immunologic recall and not a new infection. Its importance turns on the fact that if the second skin test is given after several months or a year, the "boosted reaction" would be erroneously interpreted as a tuberculin conversion. Such a true conversion is an indication that a new infection has occurred, for which preventive therapy is strongly indicated. To circumvent such confusion from the booster effect, it is recommended that all persons in whom the occurrence of new infection is to be monitored by serial tuberculin tests be retested within 2 weeks if the initial skin test shows a negative (< 10 mm) reaction. The reaction to the second test is taken as the base-line reading, and subsequent surveillance is based upon this reading. Then, any later positive reaction can be relied upon as an indication for preventive chemotherapy with isoniazid regardless of the age of the individual.

Persons with dormant infections Dormant tuberculous infection may be prevented from developing into clinical disease by treatment with isoniazid. Treatment is generally recommended for reactors under the age of 35 years but especially for those under 25. Over the age of 35 the risk of hepatitis from isoniazid increases somewhat, and preventive therapy is recommended for reactors of unknown duration only if one of the following factors that increases the risk of tuberculosis is present: (1) radiographically detectable apical scars (Simon's foci) suggestive of healed tuberculosis, (2) diabetes mellitus, (3) prolonged steroid therapy, (4) history of gastrectomy, (5) silicosis, or (6) any chronic malignancy, such as Hodgkin's disease.

Preventive therapy consists of isoniazid, 300 mg for adults and 5 to 10 mg/kg for children given in a single daily dose for 9 to 12 months. Preventive therapy reduces the risk of clinical tuberculosis by about 80 percent, and protection appears to be lasting. When the apparent source case excretes tubercle bacilli which are resistant to isoniazid, rifampin should be given for a year as prophylaxis.

Toxic reactions to isoniazid are uncommon below age 35, but thereafter may be as high as 2 to 3 percent. They need not be serious if early symptoms are heeded and the medication stopped promptly, as outlined earlier. The booklet *Understanding Tuberculosis Today,* mentioned above, can help patients understand the risk of tuberculosis and the rationale for prophylactic chemotherapy.

Biologic prophylaxis BCG VACCINE BCG, or bacillus Calmette-Guérin, is a live, attenuated strain of bovine tubercle bacilli which has been used widely in many countries to induce specific immunity against tuberculosis. Although it does not reduce the chance of natural infection, it does prevent the development of serious forms of tuberculosis when natural infection occurs. There has been controversy on the effectiveness of BCG. Data obtained from trials in Great Britain and Europe show that it affords about 80 percent protection against the development of clinical tuberculosis. Similar trials conducted in the southeastern United States and in India show a much lower level of protection, perhaps due to the presence of infection with mycobacteria of low virulence in these areas. In the United States vaccination is indicated only for nonreactors who cannot avoid exposure, as when assigned to countries of high prevalence in the Peace Corps, State Department, armed forces, etc.

Eradication of tuberculosis The decline in mortality rates from tuberculosis early in the century led some to predict the eradication of the disease in the United States by 1945. This prediction was based on the idea that infection with tubercle bacilli was harmless and that only reinfections were dangerous. It was reasoned that tuberculosis would disappear when reinfections could be prevented by isolating all infectious cases. It is now clear, however, that clinical tuberculosis develops largely from reactivation of dormant infections. Therefore, eradication must await the natural disappearance of tubercle bacilli from the population. It is hoped that this process can be accelerated by the judicious use of INH as prophylactic therapy, but clinical tuberculosis will continue to occur for many years.

Implications of a positive tuberculin reaction In the United States, the chance of a tuberculin reactor developing clinical tuberculosis from a dormant infection is greater than that of a nonreactor acquiring an infection. Therefore, it is preferable to be tuberculin-negative, unless the positive reaction is induced by vaccination. On the other hand, living in a country of high prevalence, a nonreactor would be more likely to become infected than a healthy reactor. Under these circumstances, it would be preferable to be tuberculin-positive and to have the immunologic protection against acquiring a new infection.

REFERENCES

BATES JA: Diagnosis of tuberculosis. Chest (Suppl) 76:757, 1979

———, STEAD WW: Effect of chemotherapy on infectiousness of tuberculosis. N Engl J Med 290:459, 1974

GOREN MB et al: Prevention of phagosome-lysosome fusion in cultured macrophages by sulfatides of *Mycobacterium tuberculosis.* Proc Natl Acad Sci USA 73:2510, 1976

GROSSET J: Bacteriologic basis of short-course chemotherapy for tuberculosis, in *Clinics in Chest Medicine,* WW Stead, AK Dutt (eds). Philadelphia, Saunders, 1980, vol 1, pp 231–241

HADLOCK FP et al: Unusual radiographic findings in adult pulmonary tuberculosis. Am J Roentgenol 134:1015, 1980

JINDANI A et al: The early bactericidal activity of drugs in patients with pulmonary tuberculosis. Am Rev Resp Dis 121:939, 1980

Drugs for tuberculosis. The Medical Letter 24:17, 1982

SNIDER OE et al: Treatment of tuberculosis during pregnancy. Am Rev Resp Dis 122:65, 1980

STEAD WW: Tuberculosis among elderly persons: An outbreak in a nursing home. Ann Intern Med 94:606, 1981

———: Pathogenesis of the sporadic case of tuberculosis. N Engl J Med 277:1008, 1967

———, Dutt AK: Chemotherapy for tuberculosis today. Am Rev Resp Dis 125:94, 1982

———, ———: The changing treatment of tuberculosis, in *Update III: Harrison's Principles of Internal Medicine,* K J Isselbacher et al (eds). New York, McGraw-Hill, 1982, pp 53–65

Thompson NJ et al: The booster phenomenon in serial tuberculin testing. Am Rev Resp Dis 119:487, 1979

175 LEPROSY

CHARLES C. SHEPARD

DEFINITION Leprosy (Hansen's disease) is a chronic granulomatous infection of humans, which, in its various clinical forms, attacks superficial tissues, especially the skin, peripheral nerves, and nasal mucosa. The two major clinical types are *lepromatous* and *tuberculoid;* when the disease has features of both these types, it is called *borderline.* In addition, an early indeterminate form is seen, which may later develop into one of the three types mentioned.

ETIOLOGY *Mycobacterium leprae,* or Hansen's bacillus, is the causal agent of leprosy. It is an acid-fast rod, found in enormous numbers in lepromatous lesions. Although it has not been cultivated in artificial media, nor convincingly in tissue cultures, it can be propagated in cooler tissues of small rodents, very consistently in the foot pads of mice. The bacillus will also produce heavy systemic infections in a proportion of nine-banded armadillos; armadillos have a lower body temperature. The bacillus multiplies very slowly, so mouse experiments take 6 to 12 months and armadillo experiments take several years. The mouse model has been used much for the study of antileprosy drugs, and the high bacterial yield from armadillos is making many immunologic studies possible. Estimates of bacillary viability can be made microscopically by determination of the "solid ratio" or "morphologic index"; only viable bacilli are thought to stain solidly.

Lepromin is a suspension of killed *M. leprae* prepared from the tissues of lepromatous patients. Intradermal injection elicits, somewhat irregularly, a tuberculin-like reaction at 48 h (Fernandez' reaction) and more consistently, a papular reaction at 4 weeks (Mitsuda's reaction). The Mitsuda reaction is usually positive in tuberculoid patients and negative in lepromatous patients and is therefore an aid in clinical classification. However, because it is also positive in nearly all normal adults, it has no diagnostic value.

EPIDEMIOLOGY There are probably 10 to 20 million persons affected with leprosy in the world. The disease is more common in tropical countries, in many of which 1 to 2 percent or more of the population is affected. It is also common in certain regions with cooler climates, such as Korea, China, and central Mexico. In the United States the chief leprosy areas are Texas, California, Hawaii, Louisiana, Florida, and New York. Some of the cases are acquired domestically, most are acquired abroad. The number of new cases of leprosy reported in the United States has increased in recent years with the changing immigration pattern. Most immigrants now come from leprosy-endemic countries.

Leprosy is frequently a family infection. Many patients give a history of prolonged exposure, and in close family contacts (spouse-spouse) of untreated lepromatous patients the attack rate is 5 to 10 percent. Among young children of untreated lepromatous parents, 30 to 50 percent develop a mild, single-lesion type of leprosy which heals spontaneously. After the index case is under treatment, spread within the family does not occur. Transmission from patients with tuberculoid leprosy is uncommon. The portal of entry is a matter of conjecture, but is probably either the skin or the nasal mucosa. The chief portal of exit is thought to be the nasal mucosa of lepromatous patients.

The incubation period is frequently 3 to 5 years, but it has been reported to range from 6 months to several decades.

CLINICOPATHOLOGIC CLASSIFICATION As is true of other chronic infections, such as syphilis and tuberculosis, the manifestations of leprosy are many and variable. The classification now in general use is based on clinical findings, histopathologic changes, and the lepromin test.

Lepromatous leprosy is one of the polar forms. The involvement is extensive, diffuse, and bilaterally symmetrical. Histologically, there is a diffuse granulomatous reaction with macrophages, large foam (Virchow's) cells, and many intracellular bacilli, frequently in spheroidal masses (globi). The lepromin reaction is negative.

Tuberculoid leprosy is the other polar type. Skin lesions are single or few and are sharply demarcated. Neurologic involvement is relatively pronounced and may be severe. The histologic picture consists of lymphocytes, epithelioid cells, and perhaps giant cells; bacilli are few and sometimes difficult to demonstrate. The lepromin reaction is usually positive.

Borderline, or *dimorphous,* leprosy is a form in which the clinical features and histologic changes are a combination of the two polar types. The disease may shift toward the lepromatous form in the untreated patient or toward the tuberculoid form in the treated patient. Change of either polar type to the other is exceedingly rare.

In all forms of leprosy peripheral nerve involvement is a constant feature. In any histologic section involvement of nerves will tend to be more severe than involvement of other tissues, and in some sections the nerves may be the only tissues involved.

PATHOGENESIS *Mycobacterium leprae* probably enters the body through the skin or nasal mucosa. The early stages of infection have not been described accurately. In lepromatous leprosy bacillemia is frequent and often so profuse that the organisms can be seen in stained smears of peripheral blood. Even in the most advanced lepromatous cases, destructive lesions are limited to the skin, peripheral nerves, anterior portion of the eye, upper respiratory passages above the larynx, testes, and structures of the hands and feet. The probable reason for the predilection of the disease for these tissues is that they are all usually several degrees cooler than 37°C. Two sites of preferential involvement are the ulnar nerves near the elbow and the peroneal nerves where they pass around the head of the fibula; above and below these levels where these nerves take deeper courses, they are much less severely involved. In mice that have been experimentally infected in the foot pads, bacillary multiplication is maximal when the mice are kept at air temperatures at which the foot pad tissues are about 30°C; this is also the usual temperature of the most severely involved tissues of human beings. In patients with lepromatous leprosy, collections of bacilli are also found in the liver, spleen, and bone marrow, but these are probably scavenged from the blood.

A profound lack of cellular immunity for *M. leprae* in lepromatous leprosy is indicated by the histology and by the negative lepromin reaction. Further evidence comes from observations that lepromatous patients' lymphocytes fail to react in vitro to *M. leprae* antigens. Under the same in vitro conditions the lymphocytes of tuberculoid patients react positively.

Moreover, many normal persons exposed to leprosy give positive reactions, indicating the presence of subclinical infections. In addition to this depressed specific cellular immunity for *M. leprae,* untreated lepromatous patients frequently have a partial depression of cellular immunity in general. They have been shown to be deficient in the ability to develop delayed hypersensitivity, their lymphocyte transformation response to T-cell mitogens may be weak, and the paracortical areas of their lymph nodes are deficient in lymphocytes. Furthermore, mice that have been rendered T-cell deficient by thymectomy and irradiation followed by bone marrow replacement respond to inoculations of *M. leprae* by developing heavier infections. For these reasons, lepromatous leprosy is thought to be the result of a poor immune response, and tuberculoid leprosy the result of a stronger immune response, but whether these differences in immune state precede the infection or are caused by it is not clear.

CLINICAL MANIFESTATIONS **Early leprosy** The first signs of leprosy are usually cutaneous. One or more hypopigmented or hyperpigmented macules or plaques may be seen. Often an anesthetic or paresthetic patch is the first symptom noted by the patient, but on careful examination skin involvement can also be found. When contacts are being examined, a single skin lesion is often noted, especially in children; usually, this is a hypesthetic macule that may clear in a year or two without treatment, but specific treatment is usually recommended.

Tuberculoid leprosy Early tuberculoid leprosy is frequently manifested by a hypopigmented macule, sharply demarcated and hypesthetic. Later the lesions are larger, and the margins are elevated and circinate or gyrate. There is peripheral spread and central healing. The lesions appear singly or are few in number and are not symmetrical. Nerve involvement occurs early, and the nerves leading from the lesions may be enlarged. The larger peripheral nerves may be palpably and visibly enlarged, especially the ulnar, peroneal, and greater auricular nerves. There may be severe neuritic pain. Neural involvement leads to muscle atrophy, especially of the small muscles of the hand. Contractures of the hand and foot are frequent. Trauma, especially from burns and splinters and from excessive pressure, leads to secondary infection of the hands and to plantar ulcers. Later, resorption and loss of phalanges is frequent. When the facial nerves are involved, there may be lagophthalmos, exposure keratitis, and corneal ulceration leading to blindness.

Lepromatous leprosy The skin lesions are macules, nodules, or papules. The macules are often hypopigmented. The borders of the lesions are not sharp, and the centers of raised lesions are convex (rather than concave as in tuberculoid disease). There is also diffuse infiltration between the lesions. The sites of predilection are the face (cheeks, nose, brows), ears, wrists, elbows, buttocks, and knees. Involvement with infiltration and little or no nodulation may progress so subtly that the disease goes unnoticed. Loss of the eyebrows, especially the lateral portions, is common. Much later the skin of the face and forehead becomes thickened and corrugated (leonine facies), and the earlobes become pendulous.

Nasal symptoms (nasal "stuffiness," epistaxis, and obstructed breathing) are common early symptoms. Complete nasal obstruction, then laryngitis and hoarseness, are also frequent. Septal perforation and nasal collapse lead to saddle-nose.

In adult males infiltration and scarring of the testes lead to sterility. Gynecomastia is common. Invasion of the anterior portion of the eye leads to keratitis and iridocyclitis. Painless inguinal and axillary lymphadenopathy occurs.

Neurologic involvement, of the same type as that seen in tuberculoid disease, is less prominent in the lepromatous form. A diffuse hypesthesia involving the peripheral portions of the extremities is common in advanced lepromatous disease.

Reactional states The general course of leprosy is indolent, but it may be interrupted by two types of reaction, which tend to complicate chemotherapy.

Erythema nodosum leprosum (ENL) occurs in lepromatous patients, most frequently toward the end of the first year of treatment. Tender, inflamed subcutaneous nodules develop, usually in crops. Each nodule lasts a week or two, but more develop. ENL may last only a week or two, or it may continue for long periods. Low-grade fever accompanies severe ENL, and lymphadenopathy and arthralgias may appear. Even in untreated patients with ENL the bacilli have greatly reduced viability, as indicated by low infectivity for mice and by low "solid ratios." Histologically, ENL is characterized by polymorphonuclear infiltration and deposits of IgG and complement; hence, it resembles an Arthus reaction.

Borderline reaction is seen in borderline patients, more often during treatment. Existing skin lesions develop erythema and swelling, and new lesions may appear. An early influx of lymphocytes is followed by edema and a shift toward tuberculoid histology. Cellular immunity increases. Borderline reactions can be differentiated from frank progression, such as occurs when drug-resistant bacilli appear, by mouse inoculations to test bacillary viability and by histologic studies.

The *Lucio phenomenon* is limited to patients with a diffuse nonnodular lepromatous disease; it is seen more often in Mexico and Central America. Arteritis leads to ulceration of the skin, in a characteristic angular shape, and subsequently to angular thin scars.

COMPLICATIONS The crippling that follows involvement of the peripheral nerves has been mentioned. Leprosy is probably the most frequent cause of crippling of the hand in the world. Blindness also is common.

Amyloidosis is a complication of severe lepromatous disease in the United States but is less common in many other countries.

Patients with leprosy are said to be likely to develop other chronic infections. Tuberculosis was the chief cause of death in many leprosariums.

DIAGNOSIS The demonstration of acid-fast bacilli in the skin smears made by the scraped-incision method is strong evidence for leprosy, but in tuberculoid disease bacilli may be too few for demonstration. Wherever possible, a skin biopsy specimen confined to the affected area should be sent to a pathologist knowledgeable in leprosy. The histologic involvement of peripheral nerves is pathognomonic.

The lepromin reaction has no diagnostic value. No diagnostic blood changes occur. Lepromatous patients frequently have mild anemia, elevated erythrocyte sedimentation rate, and hyperglobulinemia. From 10 to 40 percent of lepromatous patients have false-positive serologic tests for syphilis.

The combination of a chronic skin disease and peripheral nerve involvement should always lead to the consideration of leprosy.

The differential diagnosis includes conditions such as lupus erythematosus, lupus vulgaris, sarcoidosis, yaws, dermal leishmaniasis, and a host of banal skin diseases. The skin lesions of leprosy, especially of tuberculoid disease, are characterized by hypesthesia, however, and peripheral nerve involvement can always be demonstrated. Peripheral neuropathy from other causes and syringomyelia may be confused with leprosy.

TREATMENT The treatment of leprosy is largely in the hands of specialists, and hospitalization is advantageous for the first few months while the treatment is being established.

Specific chemotherapy Dapsone (4,4′-diaminodiphenylsulfone, DDS, diaphenylsulfone) is the principal drug. The daily dosage is 50 to 100 mg in adults, often raised gradually to that level during the first few weeks. In a few months in lepromatous disease enough bacilli are killed to render mouse inoculations negative and to reduce infectiousness more than 99 percent. However, in this form of the disease nonviable bacilli disappear slowly and may be found in the tissues for 5 to 10 years. Moreover, a few viable bacilli (persisters) may persist in the tissues for many years and may cause a relapse if treatment is discontinued. Consequently in lepromatous disease, treatment should be continued at least 6 to 10 years after bacilli are no longer demonstrable in skin smears, or perhaps for life.

Sulfone resistance occurs in some patients. After 5 to 20 or more years, during which the response is favorable, such a patient will develop clinical and bacteriologic relapse in spite of regular therapy, and sulfone resistance can be proved on isolates in mice. The frequency of this secondary resistance has been 2 to 30 percent in different countries, depending on the sulfone used and regularity of administration. Occasionally, primary resistance in previously untreated patients has been described.

Because of the problems of drug-resistant bacilli and of persister bacilli, multiple-drug therapy is now recommended for lepromatous disease. The additional drugs most commonly used are clofazimine (B663) and rifampin (rifampicin). Because clofazimine results in cutaneous pigmentation, light-skinned patients often object to the drug. It is also moderately expensive. As rifampin is even more expensive, regimens combining two or three of these drugs in various schedules are under study. In infections with dapsone-resistant *M. leprae,* clofazimine and rifampin are given in combination. Rifampin-resistant *M. leprae* has been demonstrated in patients relapsing after treatment with this drug alone. Other drugs such as prothionamide, ethionamide, thiambutosine, and thiacetazone, thought to be unsuitable for single-drug therapy, are now being studied in combination with dapsone.

Other sulfones, such as sulfoxone or Sulphetrone, are not used much. Acedapsone (DADDS), a repository sulfone, which releases dapsone slowly and is given only five times a year, is under extensive study; in lepromatous leprosy, it has been found necessary to add a 90-day course of rifampin to the continued acedapsone.

In tuberculoid and indeterminate leprosy, persistent and drug-resistant bacilli have not been a problem, and treatment with dapsone or acedapsone alone has been sufficient. Treatment is continued until all signs of activity have been absent for 3 years. The treatment of borderline leprosy depends upon the severity of the disease.

The clinical response to adequate therapy may be confused by the reactional conditions, but the disease stops progressing and the skin lesions gradually improve. Recovery from neurological impairment is limited.

Treatment of reactional states Moderate ENL is managed by antipyretics and analgesics. If severe, it can be treated with corticosteroids; the dosage is adjusted to alleviate severe distress but not to eliminate all signs of reaction. Sulfone therapy should be continued, if necessary, in reduced dosage. In the past some leprologists have discontinued sulfone therapy at the first signs of ENL, but most now feel that such action is not warranted because it allows bacillary multiplication. Corticosteroid therapy promotes the viability of *M. leprae* in mice not given antileprosy drugs. Thalidomide is the most effective drug and in appropriate dosage can completely suppress ENL. Because of its teratogenicity, however, its use is severely restricted, and it can be used only when its administration can be strictly controlled.

Borderline reactions, if severe, can be controlled with corticosteroids. They do not respond to thalidomide.

Other measures Many of the deformities and disabilities of leprosy are preventable through proper attention from the beginning of treatment. Plantar ulcers, which are very common, may be prevented by rigid-soled footwear or walking plaster casts, and contractures of the hand may be prevented by physical therapy and application of casts. Reconstructive surgery is sometimes helpful. Nerve and tendon transplants and release of contractures can give patients more functional ability. Vocational retraining is often necessary for those with permanent disability. Plastic repair of facial deformities assists acceptance of patients in society. The psychologic trauma which results from prolonged segregation is now minimized by permitting patients to continue therapy at home as soon as possible.

CONTROL Case finding and chemotherapy form the present basis of control because infectiousness is quickly suppressed, as is the development of deformity. Early detection of cases is especially important. In endemic countries this means the establishment of clinics or traveling teams. Family and other close contacts need examinations for leprosy. In the United States patients are eligible for treatment by the Public Health Service, and special clinics or hospitals are located in several areas. Chemoprophylaxis with lowered dosages of dapsone or with acedapsone is effective. Field trials of BCG vaccination in endemic areas have given conflicting results. A heat-killed vaccine, prepared from *M. leprae* grown in armadillos, is effective in mice and is under study in humans. Removal of patients from their families and normal environment is generally not necessary.

REFERENCES

Cochrane RG, Davey TF (eds): *Leprosy in Theory and Practice,* 2d ed. Baltimore, Williams & Wilkins, 1964

Enna CD et al: Leprosy in the United States, 1967–1976. Public Health Reports 93:468, 1978

Fasal P: A primer in leprosy. Cutis 7:525, 1971

Godal T: Immunologic aspects of leprosy—Present status. Prog Allergy 25:211, 1978

Levis WR et al: An epidemiologic evaluation of leprosy in New York City. JAMA 247:3221, 1982

Maugh TH II: Leprosy vaccine trials to begin soon. Science 215:1083, 1982

Ridley DS: Histological classification and the immunological spectrum in leprosy. Bull WHO 51:451, 1974

Shepard CC: Immunology and animal experimentation. Cutis 18:80, 1976

WHO Expert Committee on Leprosy: Fifth Report. WHO Technical Report Series 607, 1977

176
OTHER MYCOBACTERIAL INFECTIONS

CHARLES C. SHEPARD

The two most important human mycobacterial pathogens are *Mycobacterium tuberculosis* and *M. leprae,* but morphologically similar acid-fast bacteria are widely distributed in nature as saprophytes and as pathogens of lower animals. In addition, a number of other mycobacteria are known to cause human disease, chiefly chronic cutaneous disease, pulmonary disease, or lymphadenitis. Sometimes in the past, these other human mycobacterial pathogens have been called "atypical mycobacteria" or other confusing terms. An early, tentative classification by Runyon was an important step. In it the slowly growing cultures were placed in three groups: group I, photochromogens; group II, scotochromogens; and group III, nonchromogens. Rapidly growing cultures formed a group IV. As numerical taxonomic studies have now allowed identification of the several pathogenic and nonpathogenic species contained in the groups, the species names should be used. As is the case with other microbial pathogens, individual species cause particular diseases and sometimes several species cause very similar diseases (Table 176-1).

SKIN INFECTIONS ***Mycobacterium marinum* (*M. balnei*, "swimming pool" or "fishtank" bacillus)** This acid-fast organism inhabits swimming pools, aquaria (saltwater and freshwater), and natural bodies of water that are usually brackish or saline. From contaminated swimming pools, it gains entry through human epidermis through cutaneous abrasions from rough concrete; from aquaria, through cuts; and from fish, through cuts and wounds. A few weeks later nodules develop at the site; they may become verrucous, or they may ulcerate and enlarge to form superficial granulation tissue. The involved area is usually not extensive. In another form, new lesions form centrally from the initial site. The lesions usually remain minor and regress after a year or two, but they may last for years. *Mycobacterium marinum* grows optimally at 25 to 35°C and poorly, if at all, at 37°C. This temperature range probably accounts for the lack of systemic spread; regional lymph nodes remain uninvolved unless secondary pyogenic infection occurs.

The diagnosis is made by culturing the organism, usually from biopsy material, at appropriate temperatures. Although it grows slowly on primary isolation, on transfer it grows more rapidly. Histologically, a chronic granuloma with epithelioid and giant cells and sometimes with caseous necrosis is seen. Acid-fast bacteria may be difficult to observe. Many, but not all, patients become tuberculin-positive.

If chemotherapy is needed, ethambutol and rifampin are indicated. Tests for antibiotic sensitivity are helpful.

Prevention of swimming pool outbreaks requires disinfection of the pool. The pool may need to be reconstructed to eliminate rough concrete surfaces.

Mycobacterium ulcerans The ulcers caused by the organism are known by several local names, such as Bairnsdale, Kaferiku, and Buruli, but they are best designated by the name of the organism, since local differences are trivial. The characteristic disease is extensive granulomatous ulceration that destroys subcutaneous tissue down to the muscle or fascia and extends peripherally under an undermined edge. The extensor surfaces of arms or legs are most often affected, but the trunk may be involved. Histologically, necrosis is prominent, and epithelialization extends under the overhanging margins. Systemic invasion does not occur, although new lesions may develop at distant sites. In its natural course, the lesion starts as a local swelling which then ulcerates; it may heal spontaneously or persist for many years with extensive ulceration and contractures. Originally observed in southern Australia, the disease has since been described in central Africa, southeast Asia, and tropical America. While a soil habitat is the suspected source, the organism has not been isolated from soil.

M. ulcerans grows optimally at 30 to 33°C and poorly, if at all, at 37°C. It grows very slowly even at optimal temperature, and colonies require 7 weeks to grow. Inoculation of mouse foot pads may be helpful in isolation.

Treatment is best carried out with surgical extirpation of necrotic tissue and overlapping margins of the ulcer, followed by skin grafting. Although experimental results indicate that clofazimine and rifampin are active against the organism, chemotherapy seems not to be beneficial in human disease.

Other mycobacteria Mycobacterial skin infection caused by an unidentified mycobacterium occurs in a geographically limited area centered on Minnesota and southern Manitoba. A single red raised area enlarges over a period of weeks to a papule, which often breaks down in 1 to 2 months with some drainage. Most patients have enlarged regional lymph nodes. Recovery is prompt after surgery or chemotherapy. Most infections occur in fall or winter and involve people of all ages. Only a few cases have been described in adult males.

M. avium-intracellulare, M. scrofulaceum, M. kansasii, and *M. fortuitum* occasionally cause infections that involve skin.

PULMONARY INFECTIONS Several mycobacterial species other than *M. tuberculosis* can cause chronic progressive pulmonary disease with cavitation and fibrosis closely resembling pulmonary tuberculosis.

Etiology The species are listed in Table 176-1. *M. avium* and *M. intracellulare* are closely related organisms, sometimes difficult to differentiate, and best spoken of as a complex. Cultures have been isolated from soil and from animals, especially chickens, but the source of infection is not established. Cultures of *M. kansasii* have been isolated from the environment. *M. xenopi* was first isolated from a toad. All cultures of *M. szulgai* have originated from human disease. *M. scrofulaceum*

TABLE 176-1
Human mycobacterial pathogens other than *M. tuberculosis* and *M. leprae*

Mycobacterium	*Pigmentation of culture**	*Usual site of disease*	*Usual source of infection*	*Response to drugs*
M. marinum	P	Skin	Swimming pools, aquaria, fish	Good
M. ulcerans	N	Skin	Tropical environment	Variable
M. avium-intracellulare	N	Lungs	Environment, animals?	Poor
M. kansasii	P	Lungs	Environment?	Good
M. xenopi	S	Lungs	Water, animals?	Variable
M. szulgai	S†	Lungs	?	Good
M. scrofulaceum	S	Lungs, lymph nodes	Water, soil	Poor
M. fortuitum	N	Skin (abscesses), lungs	Soil, dirt	Poor
M. chelonei	N	Skin (abscesses), lungs	Soil, dirt	Poor

* *P = photochromogenic (develops yellow-orange pigment only when exposed to light); N = nonpigmented; S = scotochromogenic (develops yellow-orange pigment in dark light).*
† *Scotochromogenic at 37°C, photochromogenic at 25°C.*

needs to be differentiated from *M. gordonae,* also scotochromogenic and commonly found in soil and water. *M. fortuitum* and *M. chelonei,* which are rapidly growing cultures, are best referred to as a complex.

Since similar species may be isolated from normal sputum and the identification of the several species is often carried out in reference laboratories, the etiologic diagnosis may be delayed. However, isolation of the suspect culture from repeated specimens and the presence of multiple (more than 10) colonies in the primary cultures are strong evidence that the organism has an etiologic role. Colonization of the respiratory tract without tissue invasion can occur and gives repeatedly positive culture results with few colonies.

Epidemiology The mode of transmission of all these pulmonary infections is unsettled. There is cross-sensitization between antigens of the tubercle bacillus and other mycobacteria, but sensitization to the etiologic organism is greater. Comparative tests with antigens from *M. avium-intracellulare* and tuberculin indicate that many healthy individuals in the southeastern United States have been infected by organisms of this group, and in this area, chronic pulmonary disease that is not caused by *M. tuberculosis* is often caused by *M. avium-intracellulare.* In Texas, Oklahoma, and Chicago *M. kansasii* is a more frequent causative agent than *M. avium-intracellulare.* The proportion of new cases caused by mycobacteria other than *M. tuberculosis* varies from 2 to 15 percent and is expected to increase as the number of infections due to *M. tuberculosis* decreases. In contrast to tuberculosis, multiple cases in the same family are very rare, and isolation of the patient is not necessary. In terms of frequency *M. avium-intracellulare* and *M. kansasii* are much the most important, followed by *M. scrofulaceum.* Infections with other species are rare.

Manifestations The symptoms and signs are those of pulmonary tuberculosis (Chap. 174), although there is some tendency for most of the infections to be more indolent. Infections with *M. avium-intracellulare* are more frequent in older adults and in men. Underlying chronic obstructive pulmonary disease is often present in infections due to *M. avium-intracellulare, M. scrofulaceum,* and *M. fortuitum-chelonei,* and is sometimes present with the other mycobacteria. Extrapulmonary lesions are rare.

Treatment Rational chemotherapy depends upon identification of the etiologic mycobacterium and determination of its drug sensitivity. *M. kansasii* infections usually respond well to intensive triple-drug therapy with rifampin and a pair selected from isoniazid, ethambutol, and streptomycin. *M. avium-intracellulare* infections are often resistant to chemotherapy. Treatment with four drugs chosen from isoniazid, rifampin, ethambutol, ethionamide, and streptomycin (or capreomycin or kanamycin) is recommended, along with appropriate surgery. Infections with *M. scrofulaceum* also are often resistant to drugs, and therapy is the same as for *M. avium-intracellulare.* Infections with *M. szulgai* have responded well to chemotherapy, but the others have been difficult to treat.

OTHER INFECTIONS *M. avium-intracellulare* and *M. scrofulaceum* cause lymphadenitis in children, especially of the nodes draining the buccal mucous membrane. Excision of the node before it has ruptured or drained is the treatment of choice. *M. fortuitum* and *M. chelonei* cause local abscesses, particularly from injections given with contaminated needles or syringes; cervical lymphadenitis and cellulitis also occur, with the site of entry probably the mouth. *M. chelonei* has caused two outbreaks of infection of sternal incisions after cardiac surgery (coronary bypass and valve replacement). The source of the organism could not be determined. In addition, contamination of porcine cardiac valve prostheses by *M. chelonei* has been detected occasionally, but infection following the implantation of the contaminated valves has been rare. *M. kansasii* and *M. scrofulaceum* can cause disease of bones and joints. Widely disseminated, usually fatal infections with any of these mycobacteria can occur, especially in immunosuppressed patients.

REFERENCES

BARKER DJP: Epidemiology of *Mycobacterium ulcerans* infections. Trans R Soc Trop Med Hyg 67:43, 1973

FELDMAN RA, HERSHFIELD E: Mycobacterial skin infection by an unidentified species. A report of 29 patients. Ann Intern Med 80:445, 1974

JOLLY HW JR, SEABURY JH: Infections with *Mycobacterium marinum.* Arch Dermatol 106:32, 1972

KUBICA GP: Differential identification of mycobacteria. VII. Key features for identification of clinically significant mycobacteria. Am Rev Respir Dis 107:9, 1973

WOLINSKY E: Nontuberculous mycobacterial and associated diseases. Am Rev Resp Dis 119:107, 1979

section 8 | Spirochetal diseases

177
SYPHILIS

KING K. HOLMES

The great ailment of modern syphilological practice is a lack of comprehension of the why and wherefore, rather than the what to do.

J. H. Stokes

DEFINITION Syphilis is a chronic systemic infection caused by *Treponema pallidum,* is usually sexually transmitted, and is characterized by an incubation period averaging 3 weeks, followed by a primary lesion associated with regional lymphadenopathy; a secondary bacteremic stage associated with generalized mucocutaneous lesions and generalized lymphadenopathy; a latent period of subclinical infection lasting many years; and, in about one-third of untreated cases, a tertiary stage characterized by progressive destructive mucocutaneous musculoskeletal or parenchymal lesions, aortitis, or central nervous system disease.

ETIOLOGY The discovery of *Treponema pallidum* in syphilitic material was made by Schaudinn and Hoffman in 1905. *Trepo-*

nema pallidum is one of the many spiral-shaped microorganisms which propel themselves by spinning around their longitudinal axis. The spiral organisms of medical significance, the Treponemataceae, include three groups which are pathogenic for humans and for a variety of other animals: the *Leptospira,* which cause human leptospirosis; the *Borrelia,* including *B. recurrentis* and *B. vincentii,* which cause relapsing fever and Vincent's angina, respectively; and the *Treponema,* responsible for the diseases known as treponematoses. The *Treponema* include *T. pallidum; T. pertenue,* and *T. carateum,* the organisms which cause yaws and pinta (see Chap. 178); and *T. paraluis cuniculi,* the cause of rabbit syphilis. Other treponema include nonpathogenic species found in the human mouth and several species of anaerobic saprophytic genital treponemes of low pathogenicity which often coexist with anaerobic gram-negative rods in ulcerative genital lesions (so-called fusospirochetal infections). These can also be confused with *T. pallidum* on dark-field examination by inexperienced individuals.

Treponema pallidum is a thin, delicate organism with 6 to 14 spirals and tapered ends, measuring 6 to 15 μm in total length and 0.2 μm in width. The cytoplasm is surrounded by a trilaminar cytoplasmic membrane, which in turn is surrounded by a delicate inner mucopeptide layer, the periplast, thought to be composed of alternating molecules of *N*-acetyl glucosamine and *N*-acetyl muramic acid, and which provides some structural rigidity, while an outer lipoprotein membrane is selectively permeable and osmotically sensitive. The unique spiral structure of *T. pallidum* is maintained by six fibrils, three arising at each end of the organism, which wind around the cell body in a groove between the inner cell wall and the outer cell membrane, and may be the contractile elements responsible for motility. None of the four pathogenic treponemes has yet been cultured in vitro in quantities sufficient to permit detailed comparisons of the organisms, and no convincing morphological, serologic, or metabolic differences between them have been discerned. They are distinguished primarily according to the clinical syndrome they produce. Limited animal inoculation studies also indicate some differences in host range and virulence, even among different strains of *T. pallidum.* The only known natural host for *T. pallidum* is the human. Most mammals can be infected with *T. pallidum,* but only humans, higher apes, and a few laboratory animals regularly develop syphilitic lesions. Virulent strains of *T. pallidum* are maintained in rabbits.

HISTORY The first clear descriptions of syphilis were recorded at the end of the fifteenth century, when a pandemic known as the great pox, as distinguished from smallpox, swept over Europe and Asia. Severe morbidity or death often occurred during the secondary stage, indicating an unexplained virulence then which is almost unknown today, except in congenital syphilis. The source of the European pandemic 500 years ago is controversial. It has been proposed that the European pandemic actually reflected increased reporting of a long-standing problem, newly publicized because of the development of the printing process in the fifteenth century. The problem of differentiating increased incidence from increased reporting continues to plague epidemiologists today.

The sexual mode of transmission of syphilis was recognized early during the European pandemic, and description of the primary and secondary stages of the disease followed. The major cardiovascular and neurological complications of late syphilis were recognized during the eighteenth and nineteenth centuries. However, the erroneous concept that gonorrhea, chancroid, and syphilis were the same disease was strengthened by John Hunter, who developed syphilis following self-inoculation with gonorrheal pus in 1767. These three diseases were finally distinguished in the mid-1800s, although their etiologies were not established until the turn of this century. Gummas were not recognized as being syphilitic in origin until this century.

A rapid series of important advances began in 1903 with the successful inoculation of syphilis into primates by Metchnikoff and Rowe. The discovery of *Treponema pallidum* in serum from secondary lesions was made by Schaudinn in 1905 and was confirmed by Landsteiner in 1906. In 1910, Wasserman introduced the complement fixation test for the diagnosis of syphilis, and in the same year, Ehrlich and Hata introduced an arsenic derivative, arsphenamine (Compound 606, Salvarsan), which was effective in treatment.

EPIDEMIOLOGY Nearly all cases of syphilis are now acquired by sexual contact with infectious lesions (i.e., the chancre, mucous patch, or condyloma latum). Uncommon modes of transmission include nonsexual personal contact, contact with contaminated fomites, or infection in utero or following blood transfusions.

In the United States, infant deaths due to syphilis, and new admissions of patients with syphilitic psychoses, have fallen by 99 percent since 1940. The total reported number of cases of late and late latent syphilis has fallen almost every year since 1943. The 9.3 cases per 100,000 population reported in 1980 represent a decrease of over 90 percent since 1943. Only 277 cases of congenital syphilis were reported in 1980, a decrease of 98 percent since 1941. The number of new cases of infectious syphilis reached a peak in 1947, then fell steadily to about 6000 in 1957, but then began to increase again.

In 1980, there were 27,204 cases of primary and secondary syphilis and 20,297 cases of early latent syphilis reported, and the number of unreported cases was estimated to be greater. Comparison of reported case rates of primary and secondary syphilis in the United States with those in England for 1975 shows that the rates per 100,000 persons between ages 20 and 24 were 3.6 times higher for males and 6.1 times higher for females in the United States than in England. The actual difference in case rates between the United States and England is undoubtedly greater, because most cases of syphilis in England are treated by venereologists and reported, whereas many cases in the United States are seen by physicians in private practice and many of these are not reported. The higher case rates in the United States may be partly attributable to inadequate tracing of sexual contacts of unreported cases.

Although the reported incidence of syphilis appears higher in nonwhites than in whites, and is higher in urban than in rural areas, these differences partly reflect the fact that indigent urban racial groups are treated at public clinics, where case reporting is complete. The case rates of early syphilis are highest in the south and southwest, and in those states with large urban populations. The peak incidence of syphilis occurs in the age group 20 to 24. In the United States, the male/female ratio of reported early cases ($<$1 year) has increased from 0.8:1 in 1950 to over 3.2:1 in 1980. In England the ratio is 6:1.

Of all men with primary, secondary, or early latent syphilis interviewed in the United States during 1980, one-half were homosexual or bisexual. Primary syphilis is usually not diagnosed in women or in homosexual men. For example, during 1974 in the United States, 42 percent of cases of early syphilis in heterosexual men were detected in the primary stage, whereas only 23 percent of early cases in homosexual men and 11 percent of early cases in women were detected in the primary stage. Anorectal chancres make up over 50 percent of primary syphilis among homosexuals examined in venereology clinics in the United Kingdom, but only 15 percent of primary syphilis among homosexuals examined in the United States.

This remarkable difference suggests either a greater reticence of physicians in the United States to examine the anal canal or failure to consider syphilis in the evaluation of anal lesions in men.

Interviews of patients with early syphilis disclose an average of 2.8 sexual contacts at risk per patient, and "cluster" tracing of additional associates of the patient or his or her contacts discloses an average of 0.7 others who are also at risk. Approximately one of two individuals named as contacts of infectious syphilis becomes infected. Many contacts will have already developed manifestations of syphilis when they are first seen, and about 30 percent of apparently uninfected contacts of infectious syphilis who are examined within 30 days of exposure will actually be in the incubation stage and will themselves develop infectious syphilis if not treated. Because of this, the identification and "epidemiologic" treatment of all recently exposed contacts has become an important aspect of syphilis control. Also important is the identification of syphilitics by serologic testing of pregnant women, hospital admissions, military inductees, and persons undergoing examination in physicians' offices. Of 45 million blood specimens examined during 1980 in the United States, 1.4 million tests were reactive, representing untreated syphilis, previously treated syphilis, or false-positive tests. Of all reported early syphilis cases of less than 1 year's duration in 1980, 46 percent were detected as a direct result of either contact tracing or serologic testing. More controversial are laws and regulations requiring routine premarital serologic testing for syphilis. This program, which drains approximately 10 percent of all public funds for control of sexually transmitted diseases, yields very few cases of early syphilis. Syphilis is under control in some states in which new cases are limited to sporadic outbreaks which tend to involve homosexual men and are contained by aggressive contact tracing.

NATURAL COURSE AND PATHOGENESIS OF UNTREATED SYPHILIS *Treponema pallidum* can rapidly penetrate intact mucous membranes or abraded skin and within a few hours enters the lymphatics and blood to produce systemic infection and metastatic foci long before and after the appearance of a primary lesion. Blood *from a patient with incubating syphilis is infectious.* The generation time of *T. pallidum* in humans is 30 to 33 h, and the incubation period of syphilis is inversely proportional to the number of organisms inoculated. The concentration of treponemes generally reaches at least 10^7 per gram of tissue before the appearance of a clinical lesion. In experimental infection in rabbits or humans, a single treponeme can initiate infection which leads to a discernible lesion only after 6 weeks, although histopathologic changes are evident earlier, while intradermal injection of 10^7 organisms usually produces a lesion within 72 h. The number of organisms which initiated infection in 50 percent of humans (the infectious dose 50, ID_{50}) was 57. The median incubation period in humans is about 21 days. Although the incubation period is traditionally stated as ranging from 9 to 90 days, experimental inoculations of humans and rabbits show that the period from inoculation until the primary lesion is discernible rarely exceeds 6 weeks. Subcurative therapy during the incubation period may delay the onset of the primary lesion but does not seem to prevent ultimate development of symptomatic disease.

The primary lesion appears at the site of inoculation, persists for 2 to 6 weeks, and then heals spontaneously. Histopathology of primary lesions shows perivascular infiltration, chiefly by plasma cells and histiocytes, capillary endothelial proliferation, and eventually obliteration of small blood vessels. At this time *T. pallidum* is demonstrable in the chancre in spaces between epithelial cells as well as within invaginations or phagosomes of epithelial cells, fibroblasts, plasma cells, and the endothelial cells of small capillaries, within lymphatic channels, and in the regional lymph nodes. Macrophages and polymorphonuclear leukocytes can be seen taking up treponemes into phagocytic vacuoles where the organisms are destroyed.

The generalized parenchymal, constitutional, and mucocutaneous manifestations of secondary syphilis usually appear about 6 weeks after healing of the chancre, although secondary lesions may appear while the chancre is still present, or only several months after the chancre has healed, and some patients enter the latent stage without ever developing secondary lesions. Secondary maculopapular skin lesions show histopathologic features of hyperkeratosis of the epidermis, capillary proliferation with endothelial swelling in the superficial corium, and dermal papillae with transmigration of polymorphonuclear leukocytes, and in the deeper corium, perivascular infiltration by plasma cells. Treponemes are found in many tissues including the aqueous humor of the eye and the cerebrospinal fluid. Cerebrospinal fluid abnormalities are detected in as many as 17 to 33 percent of patients during the secondary stage. Immune complex–induced glomerulonephritis occurs. Generalized lymphadenopathy is present and is characterized by marked follicular hyperplasia, with histiocytic infiltration and lymphocyte depletion of the paracortical areas, where treponema are present in greatest numbers. The reason for the paradoxical appearance of secondary manifestations in the face of high titers of humoral antibody (including immobilizing antibody) to *T. pallidum* is unknown. The secondary lesions subside within 2 to 6 weeks, and the patient enters the latent stage, which is detectable only by serologic testing. In the preantibiotic era, up to 25 percent of untreated patients experienced one or more subsequent generalized or localized mucocutaneous relapses at some time during the first 2 to 4 years after infection. Since 90 percent of such infectious relapses occur during the first year, identification and examination of sexual contacts are most important for patients with syphilis of less than 1 year's duration.

The World Health Organization now arbitrarily divides latent syphilis into early latent (less than 1 year's duration) and late latent (over 1 year's duration) stages. However, because infectious relapse can occur during the first 2 years, and because the risk of congenital syphilis is highest during the first 2 years after acquisition of infection, the International Classification of Diseases definition of early latent syphilis as less than 2 years' duration and late latent as over 2 years' duration is more firmly based on biological (in contrast to epidemiological) criteria. About one-third of patients with untreated latent syphilis develop clinically apparent tertiary disease. In the past, the most common type of tertiary disease was the gumma, a usually benign granulomatous lesion. Today, gummas are very uncommon, perhaps because they respond to very low doses of antitreponemal drugs. The remaining tertiary lesions are caused by obliterative small-vessel endarteritis which usually involves the vasa vasorum of the ascending aorta and less often the central nervous system. Factors which determine development of tertiary disease are unknown.

The course of untreated syphilis has been studied retrospectively in a group of nearly 2000 patients with primary or secondary syphilis diagnosed clinically, before the dark-field and Wasserman tests came into use (the *Oslo Study,* 1891–1951); prospectively in 431 Negro men with seropositive latent syphilis of 3 or more years' duration (the *Tuskegee Study,* 1932–1972); and retrospectively in a review of 198 autopsies of patients with untreated syphilis.

In the Oslo Study, 24 percent of the patients developed relapsing secondary lesions within 4 years, and 28 percent eventually developed one or more manifestations of late syphilis.

Cardiovascular syphilis, including aortitis, was detected in 10.4 percent, with no cases occurring in those infected before age 15; symptomatic neurosyphilis occurred in 6.5 percent, and 16 percent developed benign tertiary syphilis (gumma of the skin, mucous membranes, and skeleton). Syphilis was the primary cause of death in 15.1 percent of males and 8.3 percent of the females. However, many patients alive when the Oslo Study was completed remained at risk for developing complications, while tuberculosis and other infections prematurely eliminated others before complications of syphilis occurred, so the Oslo figures probably represent minimum estimates of the risk of late complications. Cardiovascular syphilis was found in 35 percent of men and 22 percent of women who eventually underwent autopsy. In general, serious late complications were nearly twice as common in men as in women.

The Tuskegee Study showed that the death rate of untreated syphilitic black men, 25 to 50 years of age, was 17 percent greater than in nonsyphilitics, and 30 percent of all deaths were attributable to cardiovascular or central nervous system syphilis. The ethical issues raised by this study, begun in the preantibiotic era but continuing into the early 1970s, had a major influence on development of current guidelines for human medical experimentation. By far the most important factor in increased mortality was cardiovascular syphilis. Anatomic evidence of aortitis was found in 40 to 60 percent of autopsied syphilitics (versus 15 percent of controls), while central nervous system lues was found in only 4 percent. Hypertension was also increased in the syphilitics. The incidence of cardiovascular syphilis was higher and central nervous system syphilis lower in the prospective Tuskegee Study, as compared with the Oslo Study. These studies each show that about one-third of patients with untreated syphilis develop clinical or pathological evidence of tertiary syphilis; about one-fourth die as a direct result of tertiary syphilis; and additional excess mortality not directly attributable to tertiary syphilis is also seen. Untreated syphilis may make people more susceptible to other diseases, or individuals who get syphilis coincidentally may be more susceptible to other diseases, perhaps because of socioeconomic factors.

MANIFESTATIONS **Primary syphilis** The typical primary chancre usually begins as a single painless papule which rapidly becomes eroded and usually, but not always, is indurated, with a characteristic cartilaginous consistency on palpation of the edge and base of the ulcer. Histological examination of the ulcer shows mononuclear and histiocytic infiltrates with obliterative endarteritis and periarteritis of small vessels. *Treponema pallidum* is seen by electron microscopy to lie in interstitial perivascular spaces and within invaginations or phagosomes of neutrophils, macrophages, endothelial cells, and plasma cells.

In heterosexual men, the chancre is usually located on the penis. In homosexual men, the chancre is often found in the anal canal, usually within view if the buttocks are spread, within the mouth, or on the external genitalia. It may occur on any site of the body. In women, primary sites which are commonly overlooked include the cervix and labia. Regional lymphadenopathy accompanies the primary lesion, appearing within 1 week of the onset of the lesion. The nodes are firm, nonsuppurative, and painless. Inguinal lymphadenopathy is bilateral and may occur with anal as well as with genital chancres, since lymphatic drainage of the anus involves inguinal nodes. The chancre heals within 4 to 6 weeks (range 2 to 12 weeks), but the lymphadenopathy may persist for months.

Atypical primary lesions are common. The clinical appearance depends upon the number of treponemes inoculated and upon the preinfection immune status of the patient. A large inoculum produces a dark-field positive ulcerative lesion in nonimmune human volunteers, but in individuals with a previous history of syphilis produces either a small dark-field negative papule, an asymptomatic but seropositive latent infection, or no response at all. A small inoculum usually produces only a papular lesion, even in nonimmune humans. Therefore, syphilis should be considered even in the evaluation of trivial or atypical, dark-field negative, genital lesions. The most common genital lesions which must be differentiated from primary syphilis include traumatic, superinfected lesions, genital herpes simplex virus infection (see Chap. 210), and chancroid (see Chap. 157). *Primary genital herpes* may produce inguinal adenopathy but the nodes are tender and associated with multiple painful vesicles which later ulcerate, and with systemic symptoms including fever; *recurrent genital herpes* typically begins with a cluster of painful vesicles, usually without associated adenopathy. *Chancroid* produces painful, superficial exudative, nonindurated, usually multiple ulcers; adenopathy is either unilateral or bilateral, is tender, and may suppurate.

Secondary syphilis The manifestations of the secondary stage are protean but usually include localized or diffuse symmetrical mucocutaneous lesions and generalized nontender lymphadenopathy. The remnant of the healing primary chancre is still present in many cases. The skin rash consists of macular, papular, papulosquamous, and occasionally pustular syphilides, often with one or more forms present simultaneously. Initial lesions are bilaterally symmetrical, pale red or pink, nonpruritic, discrete, round macules, 5 to 10 mm in diameter, distributed on the trunk and proximal extremities. After 1 to 2 months, red, papular lesions 3 to 10 mm in diameter also appear. These may progress to necrotic lesions (resembling pustules) in association with increasing endarteritis and perivascular mononuclear infiltration. These lesions are distributed widely and may occur on the palms, soles, face, and scalp. Tiny papular *follicular syphilides* involving hair follicles may result in patchy alopecia and loss of eyebrows or beard. Progressive endarteritis obliterans and ischemia result in superficial scaling of papules (*papulosquamous syphilides*) and eventually may lead to central necrosis (*pustular syphilide*). In warm, moist, intertriginous areas, including the perianal area, vulva, scrotum, and inner thighs, axillas, and the skin under pendulous breasts, papules enlarge and become eroded, to produce broad, moist, pink or gray-white highly infectious lesions called *condyloma lata.* Superficial mucosal erosions, called *mucous patches,* occur in about a third of patients and may involve lips, oral mucosa, tongue, palate, pharynx, vulva and vagina, glans penis, or inner prepuce. The typical mucous patch is a silver-gray erosion surrounded by a red periphery and is usually painless.

During relapses of secondary syphilis, condyloma lata are particularly common, and skin lesions tend to be asymmetrically distributed and more infiltrated, resembling skin lesions of late syphilis, perhaps reflecting increasing cellular immunity.

Constitutional symptoms which may accompany secondary syphilis include fever, weight loss, malaise, and anorexia. Headache and meningismus are common. *Acute meningitis* occurs in only 1 to 2 percent of patients, but increased cells and protein have been found in the cerebrospinal fluid in 30 percent or more. *Treponema pallidum* has also been recovered by rabbit inoculation from cerebrospinal fluid during secondary syphilis even in the absence of other cerebrospinal fluid abnormalities.

Gastrointestinal involvement has been found with surprising frequency during secondary syphilis when a systematic search is made. Hypertrophic syphilitic gastritis may present a picture suggestive of linitis plastica or lymphosarcoma of the stomach.

Rectosigmoid involvement may produce patchy proctitis or an ulcerative or mass lesion resembling a neoplasm.

Other less common complications described in secondary syphilis include hepatitis, nephropathy, arthritis and periostitis, and iridocyclitis. Ocular findings which suggest secondary syphilis include otherwise unexplained pupillary abnormalities, optic neuritis, and a retinitis pigmentosa syndrome, as well as the classic iritis (especially granulomatous iritis) or posterior uveitis that do not respond to steroids. *Syphilitic hepatitis* is distinguished by an unusually high serum alkaline phosphatase and by a nonspecific histological appearance which is unlike viral hepatitis and includes moderate inflammation with polymorphonuclear leukocytes and lymphocytes, some hepatocellular damage, and no cholestasis. The *renal involvement* is associated with proteinuria, an acute nephrotic syndrome, or rarely with hemorrhagic glomerulonephritis and is characterized by subepithelial electron-dense deposits and glomerular immune complexes, suggesting that this complication is a form of immune complex glomerulonephritis. Anterior uveitis has been reported in 5 to 10 percent of patients with secondary syphilis, and *T. pallidum* can be demonstrated in the aqueous humor in such cases. Posterior uveitis occurs rarely.

Latent syphilis A diagnosis of latent syphilis is established by the finding of a positive specific treponemal antibody test for syphilis, together with a normal cerebrospinal fluid examination, the absence of clinical manifestations of syphilis on physical examination and chest films, and a history of primary or secondary lesions, history of exposure to syphilis, or delivery of an infant with congenital syphilis. *Early latent* syphilis encompasses the first 2 years after infection, during which relapse of mucocutaneous lesions may occur, while *late latent* syphilis, beginning 2 years after infection, in the untreated patient, is associated with immunity to infectious relapse and with resistance to reinfection. *Treponema pallidum* may still intermittently seed the bloodstream during this stage, pregnant women with latent syphilis may infect the fetus in utero, and transfusion syphilis has been transmitted from patients with latent syphilis of many years' duration. Until recently it was thought that untreated late latent syphilis had three possible outcomes: (1) it could persist throughout the life of the infected individual; (2) it could end in development of late syphilis; or (3) it could end with spontaneous cure of infection, with reversion of serologic tests to negative. It is now apparent, however, that the more sensitive treponemal antibody tests rarely if ever become negative. Fifty to seventy percent of untreated patients with latent syphilis never develop clinically evident late syphilis, but the occurrence of spontaneous cure is in doubt.

Late syphilis The onset of slowly progressive inflammatory disease of the aorta or central nervous system begins early during latent syphilis. Evidence of early syphilitic aortitis is present soon after the secondary lesions subside, while asymptomatic neurosyphilis can be detected readily during life by cerebrospinal fluid (CSF) examination.

ASYMPTOMATIC NEUROSYPHILIS In patients with untreated latent syphilis, if the CSF is normal 2 years or more after infection, there is probably no future risk of subsequent development of neurosyphilis, except for the purely vascular type. The diagnosis of asymptomatic neurosyphilis is made in patients with no clinical manifestations of neurosyphilis who have cerebrospinal fluid abnormalities, including pleocytosis, elevated protein, or positive cerebrospinal fluid Wasserman or Venereal Disease Research Laboratory (VDRL) test. One or more of these findings are present in 20 to 30 percent of patients with untreated syphilis after 2 years. The risk of progression to symptomatic neurosyphilis is two or three times greater in whites than in blacks and is twice as common in men as in women. The risk of parenchymal neurosyphilis (tabes dorsalis or general paresis) is five times greater in men than in women. In patients with untreated asymptomatic neurosyphilis, the overall cumulative probability of progression to clinical neurosyphilis is about 20 percent in the first 10 years, but increases with passing time, and is highest in those who show the greatest degree of pleocytosis or protein elevation. The fluorescent treponemal antibody (FTA) test on undiluted cerebrospinal fluid has been found to be reactive far more often than the VDRL test in cases of latent syphilis. The prognosis of patients with a positive CSF-FTA test without other cerebrospinal fluid abnormalities is not known, but very likely this finding merely represents passive transfer of serum antibody into the CSF, not asymptomatic neurosyphilis, and most specialists do not recommend performing an FTA test on spinal fluid. Similarly, the finding of a positive CSF-FTA test without other cerebrospinal fluid abnormalities in patients with a positive serum FTA-ABS (fluorescent treponemal antibody-absorption) associated with nonspecific neurological findings does not necessarily prove a diagnosis of "atypical" neurosyphilis. However, a therapeutic trial of penicillin in doses adequate for neurosyphilis is warranted in any patient with a positive serum treponemal antibody test who also has unexplained neurological findings.

SYMPTOMATIC NEUROSYPHILIS Although mixed features are common, the major clinical categories of symptomatic neurosyphilis include meningovascular and parenchymatous syphilis. The latter category includes general paresis and tabes dorsalis. The average interval from infection to onset of symptoms is 5 to 10 years for meningovascular syphilis, 20 years for general paresis, and 25 to 30 years for tabes dorsalis. However, many patients with symptomatic neurosyphilis do not present a classic picture, but have mixed or incomplete syndromes. *Meningovascular syphilis* is associated with inflammation of the pia and arachnoid, together with evidence of focal or widespread cerebrovascular disease or often only with pupillary or reflex changes. The manifestations of *general paresis* reflect widespread parenchymal damage and include abnormalities corresponding to the mnemonic *paresis* [*p*ersonality, *a*ffect, *re*flexes (hyperactive), *e*ye (e.g., Argyll Robertson pupils), *s*ensorium (illusions, delusions, hallucinations), *i*ntellect (decreased recent memory orientation, calculations, judgment, insight), and *s*peech]. *Tabes dorsalis* presents symptoms and signs of demyelinization of the posterior columns, dorsal roots, and dorsal root ganglia. Symptoms include ataxic, wide-based gait and footslap, paresthesias, bladder disturbances, impotence, areflexia, and loss of position, deep pain, and temperature sensation. Trophic joint degeneration (Charcot's joints) and perforating ulceration of the feet may result from loss of pain sensation. The Argyll Robertson pupil, seen in both tabes dorsalis and paresis, is a small, irregular pupil which reacts to accommodation but not to light. *Optic atrophy* also occurs frequently in association with tabes.

CARDIOVASCULAR SYPHILIS Cardiovascular manifestations are limited to the large vessels in which the blood supply is provided by vasa vasorum. Endarteritis obliterans of the vasa vasorum produces medial necrosis with destruction of elastic tissue, particularly in the ascending and transverse segments of the aortic arch, resulting in uncomplicated aortitis, aortic regurgitation, saccular aneurysm, or coronary ostial stenosis. Until recently, these complications had not been described following congenital syphilis or syphilis acquired before age 14, suggesting some unexplained resistance of the large blood vessels in youth to invasion by *T. pallidum.* The onset of symptoms occurs from 10 to 40 years after infection. Cardiovascular complications are commoner and occur at an earlier age in men than in women, and in blacks than in whites. The incidence of symptomatic cardiovascular complications in late untreated syphilis is approximately 10 percent, with aortic regurgitation being two to four times as common as aneurysm. However, syphilitic aortitis can be demonstrated at autopsy in about one-half of black males with untreated syphilis.

Asymptomatic syphilitic aortitis may be suspected in life if linear calcification of the ascending aorta is demonstrated on chest x-ray films, since arteriosclerotic disease seldom produces this sign. Aortic dilatation and a tambour quality of the sound of aortic closure are unreliable signs of aortitis. Syphilitic aneurysms are usually saccular, occasionally fusiform, and do not lead to dissection. Approximately 1 in 10 aortic aneurysms of syphilitic origin may involve the abdominal aorta, but tend to occur above the renal arteries, whereas arteriosclerotic abdominal aneurysms usually are found below the renal arteries. With increasing age, the nervous system is also affected in up to 40 percent of patients with cardiovascular syphilis.

LATE LESIONS OF THE EYES Iritis associated with pain, photophobia, and dimness of vision or chorioretinitis occurs not only during secondary syphilis, but also as a relatively common manifestation of late syphilis. Adhesions of the iris to the anterior lens may produce a fixed pupil, not to be confused with Argyll Robertson pupil.

LATE BENIGN SYPHILIS (GUMMA) Gummas may be multiple or diffuse, but are usually solitary lesions which range from microscopic size to several centimeters in diameter, and histologically consist of nonspecific granulomatous inflammation with central necrosis surrounded by mononuclear, epithelioid, and fibroblastic cells, occasional giant cells, and perivasculitis. Although *T. pallidum* is rarely demonstrated microscopically, it can be recovered from the lesions by rabbit inoculation. The most commonly involved sites are the skin and skeletal systems, mouth and upper respiratory tract, larynx, liver, and stomach. Virtually any organ may be involved. Gummas of skin produce painless nodular, papulosquamous, or ulcerative lesions, which are indurated, and form characteristic circles or arcs, with peripheral hyperpigmentation. The lesions are usually indolent, and may heal spontaneously with scarring, but may also be explosive in onset and are often destructive. These lesions may resemble many other chronic granulomatous conditions, including *tuberculosis* and *sarcoidosis*, leprosy, and *deep fungal infections*. Skeletal gummas involve long bones of the legs with greatest frequency, although any bone may be affected. Trauma may predispose to involvement of a specific site. Presenting symptoms usually include focal pain and tenderness. When sufficiently advanced to produce radiographic abnormalities, the findings may include periostitis or destructive or sclerosing osteitis. Gummas of the upper respiratory tract can lead to perforation of the nasal septum or palate. Gummatous hepatitis may produce epigastric pain and tenderness and low-grade fever, and may be associated with splenomegaly and anemia.

The histopathology and extensive tissue necrosis associated with gummas suggest that delayed hypersensitivity to *T. pallidum* produces these lesions. Certain individuals appear to develop an exaggerated delayed hypersensitivity response to *T. pallidum*, presumably mediated by sensitized T lymphocytes and macrophages. In areas where syphilis is endemic in childhood, reinfection may result in gummas; when one member of a household acquires a fresh infection, other members of the household who then become reinfected develop gummas. Experimental inoculation of *T. pallidum* into individuals with latent or late syphilis also sometimes results in gumma formation at the site of inoculation.

Since the histological changes may be suggestive but are nonspecific, the diagnosis of late benign syphilis is confirmed by serologic testing and by therapeutic trial. Treatment with penicillin results in rapid healing of active gummatous lesions.

Congenital syphilis Transmission of *T. pallidum* from a syphilitic mother to her fetus across the placenta may occur at any stage of pregnancy, but the lesions of congenital syphilis develop only after the fourth month of gestation, when immunologic competence begins to develop. This suggests that the pathogenesis of congenital syphilis may depend upon the immune response of the host rather than upon a direct toxic effect of *T. pallidum*. The risk of infection of the fetus during untreated early maternal syphilis is estimated to be 80 to 95 percent, decreases to about 70 percent at 4 years, and is still lower during late latent maternal syphilis. Adequate treatment of the mother before the sixteenth week of pregnancy should prevent fetal damage. During the past decade, the number of reported cases of congenital syphilis in the United States has remained steady at about 5 cases per 100 reported cases of primary and secondary syphilis in women. A study of cases reported in 1972 showed that 37 percent of the mothers of infected children had not sought prenatal examination, while 44 percent had had a nonreactive serologic test during the first trimester, presumably due either to false-negative first trimester tests or to acquisition of syphilis during pregnancy. Syphilis acquired during pregnancy is likely to remain subclinical in the mother while nearly always causing serious fetal infection. Untreated early maternal infection may result in up to 40 percent fetal loss (stillbirth is more common than abortion, because of the late onset of fetal infection), prematurity, neonatal death, or nonfatal congenital syphilis. Therefore, routine serologic testing in early pregnancy as well as at delivery and repeat serologic testing of "high risk" pregnant women in the third trimester are fully justified.

Only fulminant cases of congenital syphilis are clinically apparent in live infants at birth, and these babies have a very poor prognosis. The most common clinical problem is the healthy appearing baby born to a mother who has a positive serologic test.

The manifestations of congenital syphilis can be divided into (1) early manifestations, which appear within the first 2 years of life, often between 2 and 10 weeks of age, are infectious, and resemble severe secondary syphilis in the adult; (2) late manifestations, which appear after 2 years, and are noninfectious; and (3) the residual stigmata of congenital syphilis. Only about 25 percent of cases of congenital syphilis are diagnosed during the first year of life.

The earliest sign of congenital syphilis is usually rhinitis ("snuffles") soon followed by other mucocutaneous lesions. These may include bullae (syphilitic pemphigus), vesicles, superficial desquamation, petechial, and later, papulosquamous lesions, mucous patches, and condyloma latum. The most common early manifestations are osteochondritis and osteitis, particularly involving the metaphyses of long bones, progressing in severity during the first 6 months of life, then spontaneously subsiding; and periostitis, which continues to progress after the first 6 months. Hepatosplenomegaly, lymphadenopathy, anemia, jaundice, thrombocytopenia, and leukocytosis are common. The anemia is usually hypoproliferative but may be hemolytic (paroxysmal cold hemoglobinuria). The nephrotic syndrome in early congenital syphilis, as in adult secondary syphilis, represents an immune complex–induced glomerulonephritis.

Neonatal congenital syphilis must be differentiated from

other generalized congenital infections, including rubella, cytomegalovirus or herpes simplex virus infection, and toxoplasmosis, and also from erythroblastosis fetalis. Neonatal death is usually due to pulmonary hemorrhage, secondary bacterial infection, or severe hepatitis. Pathological findings include interstitial and perivascular inflammation followed by variable fibroblastic proliferation, involving skin, bones, liver, kidneys, pancreas, spleen, lungs, and intestines, and by extramedullary hematopoiesis.

Late congenital syphilis is defined as congenital syphilis which remains untreated after 2 years of age. In perhaps 60 percent of cases, the infection remains latent, while the clinical spectrum in the remainder differs in certain respects from that of acquired late syphilis in the adult. For example, cardiovascular syphilis rarely develops in late congenital syphilis, whereas interstitial keratitis is much more common and occurs between ages 5 and 25. The onset is acute with photophobia, pain, and circumcorneal injection, followed by superficial and deep vascularization of the cornea, which progresses despite antibiotic therapy, and eventually becomes bilateral. The symptoms and signs may be suppressed with corticosteroid therapy. Although treponemes have occasionally been demonstrated in aqueous humor in interstitial keratitis, the pathogenesis is obscure and is ascribed to "hypersensitivity." Other manifestations associated with interstitial keratitis are eighth-nerve deafness and recurrent arthropathy. Bilateral knee effusions are known as *Clutton's joints.* Examination of CSF discloses asymptomatic neurosyphilis in about one-third of untreated patients without other late clinical manifestations, and clinical neurosyphilis occurs in a quarter of untreated individuals with congenital syphilis over 6 years of age. The clinical manifestations of congenital neurosyphilis correspond to those seen in adult neurosyphilis. Gummatous periostitis occurs between ages 5 and 20 and, as in endemic nonvenereal childhood syphilis, tends to cause destructive lesions of the palate and nasal septum.

Characteristic stigmata include Hutchinson's teeth, the centrally notched, widely spaced, peg-shaped upper central incisors, and "mulberry" molars, sixth-year molars which have multiple, poorly developed cusps, rather than the usual four. The abnormal facies, which includes frontal bossing, saddlenose, and poorly developed maxilla, may also be seen in congenital ectodermal dysplasia. Saber shins, or anterior tibial bowing, are rare but were probably more common in the past when syphilitic periostitis of the anterior tibia was associated with vitamin D deficiency. *Rhagades* are linear scars at the angles of the mouth and nose caused by secondary bacterial infection of the early facial eruption. Other stigmata include unexplained nerve deafness, old chorioretinitis, optic atrophy, and corneal opacities due to past interstitial keratitis.

LABORATORY EXAMINATIONS **Dark-field examination technique** Dark-field examination is essential in evaluating cutaneous lesions, such as the chancre of primary syphilis, or condyloma lata of secondary syphilis. Although it is often difficult to demonstrate *T. pallidum* in dry maculopapular lesions in secondary syphilis by dark-field examination, the organism may be demonstrated by saline aspiration of lymph nodes during this stage. The surface of the suspected ulcerated lesion should be cleaned with saline and gauze, then gently abraded further with dry gauze, without production of bleeding. The lesion is then squeezed to express a serous transudate, and a drop of the transudate is picked up on the surface of a glass slide. A drop of saline (without bacteriostatic additives) may be mixed with the transudate if necessary, and this is then covered with a coverslip and examined immediately for *T. pallidum* with a dark-field or phase contrast microscope by an experienced individual. A single negative examination does not exclude syphilis, since at least 10^4 treponemes per milliliter transudate must be present to be detected, and prior use of topical antiseptic or cleansing by the patient may obfuscate the examination. Cleansing or use of topical medication should, therefore, be avoided, and the dark-field examination should be repeated on three successive days before being considered negative.

Demonstration of T. pallidum in tissue It is often necessary to demonstrate *T. pallidum* in tissue when clinical or histopathological features suggest the diagnosis of syphilis. Although the organism can be found in tissue by appropriate silver stains, these should be interpreted with caution, because artifacts resembling *T. pallidum* are often seen. Treponemes can be demonstrated more reliably in tissue by immunofluorescence, using specific antibody against *T. pallidum.*

Serologic tests for syphilis The profusion of serologic tests for syphilis causes much unnecessary confusion. Syphilitic infection produces two types of antibodies, the *nonspecific reaginic antibody* and *specific antitreponemal* antibody.

The term *reagin* is unfortunate, since the unrelated gamma-E globulin (IgE) antibody involved in certain allergic phenomena is also known as *reagin.* The nontreponemal reaginic antibodies produced in syphilis contain both IgG and IgM immunoglobulins directed against a lipoidal antigen that results from the interaction of *T. pallidum* with host tissues, and possibly against a lipoidal antigen of *T. pallidum* itself. The cardiolipin antigens initially used in the detection of reaginic antibody are relatively crude extracts of beef heart, and it is not surprising that false-positive reactions were extremely common in many conditions other than syphilis. The cardiolipin-cholesterol-lecithin antigen now in use in a variety of tests for reaginic antibody (Table 177-1) is more purified and gives fewer false-positive reactions than did earlier antigens. The tests for treponemal antibody employ antigens derived from *T. pallidum,* rather than from tissues, and detect antibody related to past or present treponemal infections.

The most widely used reagin antibody tests are the sensitive rapid plasma reagin (RPR) tests, which can be automated and are used to screen large numbers of serums, and the VDRL slide flocculation test, which is used to determine quantitatively the exact titer of serum reagin antibody. The reagin titer reflects the activity of the disease: false-positive VDRL titers usually do not exceed 1:8; a fourfold or greater rise in titer may be seen during the evolution of primary syphilis; VDRL titers usually reach 1:32 or higher in secondary syphilis; a persistent fall in titer following treatment of early syphilis provides essential evidence of an adequate response to therapy.

The standard antitreponemal antibody test is the FTA-ABS test. The patient's serum is first absorbed with a nonpathogenic treponemal antigen (sorbent) to remove group-specific antibody which may be produced against saprophytic oral and

TABLE 177-1
Common serologic tests for syphilis

NONSPECIFIC (REAGIN) ANTIBODY TESTS

Flocculation: VDRL
Complement fixation: Kolmer
Agglutination: rapid plasma reagin (RPR)

SPECIFIC TREPONEMAL ANTIBODY TESTS

Immunofluorescence: fluorescent treponemal antibody-absorption (FTA-ABS)
Immobilization: *Treponema pallidum* immobilization (TPI)
Hemagglutination: *T. pallidum* hemagglutination assay (MHA-TP, TPHA)

genital treponemes. The patient's absorbed serum is then placed on a slide which contains dried *T. pallidum.* If specific antibody to *T. pallidum* remains in the patient's serum after the absorption step, it is fixed to the dried treponemes, and then is detected by the addition of fluorescein-labeled antihuman gamma-globulin and subsequent examination of the slide by fluorescence microscopy. The *T. pallidum* immobilization (TPI) test, in which immobilization of live *T. pallidum* is produced by immune serum plus complement, is more laborious and in the United States is available only in research laboratories. The *T. pallidum* hemagglutination tests (MHA-TP and TPHA) are convenient tests for treponemal antibody but less sensitive than the FTA-ABS test for detection of early primary syphilis. Both the MHA-TP and FTA-ABS tests are very specific and, when used for confirmation of positive reaginic antibody tests, have a very high positive predictive value for the diagnosis of syphilis. However, even these tests give false-positive rates as high as 1 to 2 percent when used for screening normal populations. The relative sensitivities of the VDRL, FTA-ABS, TPI, and MHA-TP tests in the various stages of syphilis are shown in Table 177-2.

The VDRL is negative in nearly one-third of patients with primary or late syphilis. Obtaining a reagin antibody test alone is not sufficient in evaluating late symptomatic syphilis; the more sensitive FTA-ABS test should be routinely obtained in suspected late syphilis. In early primary syphilis, the detection of antibody can be maximized either by performing an FTA-ABS test or simply by repeating a VDRL test after 1 to 2 weeks if the initial VDRL was negative. However, both tests are always positive during secondary syphilis, and a negative VDRL or FTA-ABS virtually excludes syphilis in a patient with otherwise compatible mucocutaneous lesions. (An estimated 1 percent of patients with secondary syphilis have a negative VDRL test with undiluted serum which becomes positive in higher dilutions—the *prozone* phenomenon.)

False-positive serologic tests for syphilis An estimated 20 to 40 percent of all positive reagin tests are false-positive tests, but the percentages vary widely depending upon the population being examined. False-positive reagin tests are classified as acute if they become negative within 6 months. Acute false-positive reagin tests occur during mycoplasma pneumonia, malaria, and various acute bacterial or viral infections, and following certain immunizations. Chronic reactions, which persist 6 months or longer, occur in addiction, autoimmune diseases, and aging (the three A's). False-positive reagin tests occur in 25 percent of narcotics addicts, and in 10 to 20 percent of patients with active systemic lupus erythematosus. Other antibodies which have been found with great frequency in serums from chronic false-positive reactors include antinuclear, antithyroid, and antimitochondrial antibodies, as well as rheumatoid factor and cryoglobulins. The Donath-Landsteiner antibody responsible for paroxysmal cold hemoglobinuria is a hemolysin which appears in syphilis. The autoimmune nature of the false-positive reagin test is further suggested by the occurrence of systemic lupus erythematosus or other connective tissue diseases in 15 to 45 percent of chronic false-positive reactors. The prevalence of false-positive reagin tests increases with advancing age, and 10 percent of people over 70 years of age have false-positive reactions. Other diseases associated with hyperglobulinemia, such as leprosy, may also produce chronic false-positive reactions.

TABLE 177-2
Reactivity of serodiagnostic tests in untreated syphilis

Test	*Stage of disease,* % positive*			
	Primary	*Secondary*	*Latent*	*Tertiary*
VDRL	72	100	73	77
FTA-ABS	91	100	97	100
TPI	46	98	95	95
MHA-TP	69	100	98	100

* *Percentage figures provided should not be interpreted as absolute values because there are small numbers in certain categories and test results vary from study to study.*
SOURCE: *Data compiled by the Centers for Disease Control.*

In the patient with a false-positive reagin test, syphilis is excluded by obtaining a negative FTA-ABS or MHA-TP test. The results of the FTA-ABS test are reported as negative, borderline, or positive. *Borderline* results are more common in patients who are pregnant or have diseases associated with abnormal or increased globulins, and are frequently not associated with either clinical, historical, or other serologic evidence of syphilis. Borderline results should, therefore, always be repeated in questionable cases and interpreted with caution. A typical "positive" FTA-ABS occurs infrequently in conditions other than syphilis. Although false-positive FTA-ABS tests have been reported in 15 percent of patients with active systemic lupus erythematosus, the fluorescent staining is "borderline" or has an atypical "beaded" appearance in most cases (thought to be due to attachment of antinuclear antibody to treponemal DNA or nucleoprotein leaked through breaks in the outer treponemal membranes). However, because of the occasional occurrence of false-positive FTA-ABS tests, only a positive TPI provides conclusive proof of past or present treponemal infection. Both the FTA-ABS and TPI tests are positive in patients who have had yaws or pinta, and the reagin antibody tests are positive during active yaws or pinta.

For practical purposes, most clinicians need to be familiar with the three uses of serologic tests for syphilis: (1) for screening large numbers of serums for reaginic antibody (e.g., RPR); (2) for quantitative measurement of reaginic antibody titer in order to assess the clinical activity of syphilis, and to follow the reagin titer in response to therapy (e.g., VDRL); and (3) to confirm the diagnosis of syphilis in a patient with a positive reagin antibody test or with a suspected clinical diagnosis of syphilis (e.g., FTA-ABS).

IgM-FTA-ABS test for active congenital syphilis in the newborn All newborn infants of mothers with reactive VDRL or FTA-ABS tests will themselves have reactive tests whether or not they have become infected, because of passive transplacental transfer of maternal IgG immunoglobulins which are reactive in these tests. However, if IgM antitreponemal antibody is present in the infant's serum, it reflects fetal antibody production in response to intrauterine infection, particularly if there is a rise in titer, since maternal IgM antibody does not cross the intact placental barrier. Neonatal IgM antibody is detected in cord or neonatal serums in a modified FTA-ABS test, employing fluorescein-labeled antihuman IgM to detect antitreponemal IgM antibody. Similar tests have been developed for detection of congenital toxoplasmosis, rubella, and cytomegalovirus infections. The IgM-FTA-ABS test is sensitive and is positive in infants with active congenital syphilis. When the mother and fetus become infected very late during pregnancy, this test may be negative in the neonatal period. However, the specificity of this test is in doubt because of evidence that infants with a variety of congenital infections may produce IgM antibody to maternal allotypes of IgG. IgM antibody detected in the IgM-FTA-ABS test may be directed against maternal IgG antibody bound specifically to *T. pallidum,* rather than against *T. pallidum* itself. Such neonatal IgM "rheumatoid factor" antibody could be absorbed onto IgG-coated latex particles to improve specificity of the tests.

TREATMENT AND FOLLOW-UP MANAGEMENT Penicillin G is the drug of choice for all stages of syphilis. *Treponema pallidum* is killed by very low concentrations of penicillin G, although a long period of exposure to penicillin is required for treatment because of the unusually slow rate of multiplication of the organism. The efficacy of penicillin for syphilis remains undiminished after 30 years of use. Other antibiotics which are effective in syphilis include the tetracyclines, erythromycin, and the cephalosporins. Aminoglycosides inhibit *T. pallidum* only in very large doses, and the sulfonamides are inactive. The optimal dose and duration of therapy have not been established for any antimicrobial for any stage of syphilis. The U.S. Public Health Service recommendations are based on limited therapeutic trials and should be interpreted in light of the considerations noted below.

Recurrence rates for a given regimen increase as infection progresses from incubating syphilis to seronegative primary to seropositive primary to secondary to late syphilis. Therefore it is probable, but unproved, that a longer duration of therapy is required to effect cure as the lesion progresses. For these reasons some authorities use more prolonged penicillin therapy than that recommended by the U.S. Public Health Service when treating secondary, latent, or late syphilis.

The optimal dose and duration of therapy have not been carefully evaluated in well-controlled studies. A variety of data suggests that it is necessary to achieve serum levels of penicillin G of 0.03 μg/ml or more for at least 7 days to cure early syphilis. Other tentative conclusions which can be gleaned from published studies include the following: (1) extending therapy with aqueous procaine penicillin G beyond 2 weeks does not improve cure rates for primary or secondary syphilis; (2) studies of experimental syphilis show that *T. pallidum* begins to regenerate if penicillinemia is allowed to fall to subinhibitory levels for periods of 18 to 24 h; (3) in humans, increases in the dosage of crystalline penicillin G administered over 9 h from 0.03 to 0.6 mg/kg progressively increased the rate of disappearance of *T. pallidum* from chancres, but further increases in dosage did not further speed the disappearance of treponemes; and (4) the serum concentration of penicillin G achieved after one injection of 2.4 million units of benzathine penicillin G probably does not kill *T. pallidum* at the maximum rate.

The treatment regimens currently recommended for syphilis by the Centers for Disease Control are summarized in Table 177-3 and described below.

Early syphilis In very early incubating syphilis, treatment of concurrently acquired gonorrhea with 4.8 million units of procaine penicillin G (plus 1.0 g probenecid) aborts the syphilis. The ampicillin-probenecid and tetracycline regimens recommended for gonorrhea are probably also effective against incubating syphilis, although proof is not available. Follow-up serologic testing for syphilis is considered unnecessary in patients treated for gonorrhea with the recommended dose of procaine penicillin G, ampicillin, or tetracycline. Preventive (abortive, "epidemiologic") treatment is recommended for seronegative individuals without signs of syphilis who were exposed to syphilis when the contact was infectious and the exposure occurred within the previous 6 weeks. Before treatment is given, every effort should be made to establish a diagnosis by examination and serologic testing. *The regimens recommended for preventive treatment are the same as those recommended for early syphilis.*

Benzathine penicillin G is the most widely used form of treatment for early syphilis, although it is more painful on injection than procaine penicillin G. A single dose of 2.4 million units cures over 95 percent of cases of primary syphilis. Because efficacy for secondary syphilis may be slightly lower, some physicians administer a second dose of 2.4 million units 1 week after the initial dose for secondary syphilis.

Pregnant patients with early syphilis should receive penicillin in the same doses used for nonpregnant patients. Because of the risk of Jarisch-Herxheimer reaction, women with syphi-

TABLE 177-3
Recommended therapy for syphilis

Stage of syphilis	*Patients without penicillin allergy*	*Patients with penicillin allergy*
Primary, secondary, or early latent	Benzathine penicillin G, 2.4 million units single dose (1.2 million units in each hip) *or* aqueous procaine penicillin G, 600,000 units daily for 8 days	Erythromycin base or stearate, 2 g daily for 15 days *or* tetracycline hydrochloride, 2 g daily for 15 days
Late latent or latent or uncertain duration	*CSF normal:* Benzathine penicillin G, 2.4 million units weekly for 3 weeks *CSF abnormal:* Treat as neurosyphilis	Lumbar puncture *CSF normal:* Treat as neurosyphilis *CSF abnormal:* Treat as neurosyphilis
Late neurosyphilis* (asymptomatic or symptomatic)	Aqueous procaine penicillin G, 600,000 units daily for 15 days *or* aqueous penicillin G, 12 to 24 million units per day intravenously for at least 10 days	Erythromycin base or stearate, 2 g daily for 30 days *or* tetracycline hydrochloride, 2 g daily for 30 days
Late cardiovascular or benign tertiary	Benzathine penicillin G, 2.4 million units weekly for 3 weeks *or* aqueous procaine penicillin G, 600,000 units daily for 15 days	Treat as for neurosyphilis
Congenital (treat *all* neonates with either proved *or* suspected congenital syphilis)	Aqueous procaine penicillin G, 50,000 units/kg per day for at least 10 days *or* aqueous crystalline penicillin G, 50,000 units/kg per day in two divided daily doses for at least 10 days *or, only if CSF normal:* Benzathine penicillin G, 50,000 units/kg in a single dose	Antibiotics other than penicillin should not be used
Syphilis in pregnancy	See text	

* *Benzathine penicillin G has given inferior results for treatment of symptomatic neurosyphilis. Although only erythromycin or tetracycline was recommended by the CDC Syphilis Therapy Advisory Committee for CNS Syphilis in penicillin-allergic patients, there is minimal experience with these drugs (which do not achieve high CSF levels) in CNS syphilis. Many patients who give a history of penicillin allergy prove negative when skin-tested for immediate hypersensitivity to penicillin and could be given aqueous crystalline penicillin G for CNS syphilis under close supervision in the hospital. Certain third-generation cephalosporins (e.g., moxalactam, cefotaxime) have some promise for penicillin-allergic patients with CNS syphilis but require further evaluation.*
SOURCE: *From CDC recommendations, revised 1976.*

lis who are several months pregnant should be hospitalized for treatment, to permit early administration of toxolytic therapy if premature labor should occur during the reaction. If they have well-documented penicillin allergy, and this is confirmed by demonstration of an immediate wheal-and-flare response to skin testing with penicilloyl polylysine or penicillin G minor determinant mixture, no satisfactory alternative is available. Erythromycin, the leading alternative in penicillin-allergic nonpregnant patients, crosses the placenta poorly, with fetal blood levels varying from 0 to 20 percent of maternal levels. Erythromycin estolate is associated with frequent liver toxicity in pregnancy. Doxycycline 100 mg twice daily for 15 days, or a cephalosporin, may be preferable alternatives, although doxycycline has potential toxicity in pregnancy and cephalosporins may be cross-allergenic in penicillin-allergic patients, and therefore should probably be avoided in those with a clear history of penicillin-induced anaphylaxis or with immediate hypersensitivity on penicillin testing. After treatment, a quantitative reagin test should be repeated monthly throughout pregnancy, and if a fourfold rise in titer occurs, treatment should be repeated.

If adequate treatment of the mother is accomplished during pregnancy, the risk of congenital syphilis in the newborn is minimal; the child should then be examined monthly after delivery until his or her reaginic antibody test becomes negative. However, if the seropositive mother received inadequate penicillin treatment or treatment other than penicillin, or her treatment status is unknown, or if the infant may be difficult to follow, treatment should be given promptly. It is unwise to require proof of diagnosis before treatment in such cases. Similarly, every infant with suspected or proved congenital syphilis should be treated promptly. The CSF should be examined as a base line before treatment of such infants. The calculation of penicillin dosage for treatment of late congenital syphilis is the same as for that used in the infant, until dosage based upon body weight reaches that used for adult neurosyphilis.

The response of early syphilis to treatment should be determined by following the quantitative VDRL titer 1, 3, 6, and 12 months after treatment. Because the FTA-ABS and TPHA tests remain positive after 2 years in nearly all patients treated for seropositive early syphilis, this test is not useful in following the response to therapy. After successful treatment of seropositive primary or secondary syphilis, the VDRL titer progressively declines, becoming negative within 3 to 12 months in about 75 percent of seropositive primary cases and 40 percent of secondary cases. After 2 years, nearly all patients with primary syphilis have a negative VDRL, although 25 percent of secondary cases and a higher proportion of those treated for early latent syphilis maintain low titers of reagin. If the VDRL becomes negative or reaches a fixed low titer within 1 or 2 years, performing a lumbar puncture is unnecessary at that time, since the spinal fluid examination is invariably normal and there is no risk of subsequent neurosyphilis. However, if a VDRL titer of 1:8 or more fails to fall at least fourfold within 12 months, the VDRL titer rises fourfold, or clinical symptoms persist or recur, re-treatment is indicated. Every effort should be made to differentiate treatment failure from reinfection. If signs of secondary syphilis recur, the CSF should be examined. Suspected treatment failures, especially those with abnormal CSF, should be treated as described for neurosyphilis. If the patient remains seropositive but asymptomatic after such re-treatment, no further therapy is necessary.

Asymptomatic neurosyphilis The activity of asymptomatic neurosyphilis correlates best with the degree of cerebrospinal fluid pleocytosis. Changes in the cerebrospinal fluid cell count, and to a lesser extent, in cerebrospinal fluid protein concentration, provide the most sensitive index of response to treatment. Spinal fluid examination should be performed every 3 to 6 months for 3 years after treatment of asymptomatic neurosyphilis. An elevated cerebrospinal fluid cell count falls to 10 or less per cubic millimeter within 3 to 12 months in 95 percent of adequately treated cases, and becomes normal in all cases within 2 to 4 years. Elevated levels of cerebrospinal fluid protein fall more slowly, and the cerebrospinal fluid reagin titer declines slowly over a period of several years. Since benzathine penicillin G given in single doses of 2.4 million units to adults or 50,000 units per kilogram to infants does not produce detectable concentrations of penicillin G in cerebrospinal fluid, this form of penicillin is unreliable for the treatment of neurosyphilis in the adult, or for congenital syphilis, and asymptomatic neurosyphilis has been found to relapse in up to one-quarter of patients treated with 2.4 million units of benzathine penicillin. Symptomatic neurosyphilis has rarely, if ever, occurred in patients who received a total dose of 6 million units or more of other forms of penicillin G for asymptomatic neurosyphilis.

Late syphilis Lumbar puncture should be performed even in the evaluation of late complications other than symptomatic neurosyphilis, since asymptomatic neurosyphilis may coexist with other late complications, and abnormal cerebrospinal fluid findings can then be followed serially as a guide to therapy. No studies of benzathine penicillin G for cardiovascular syphilis have ever been reported, and the efficacy of penicillin therapy in any form for cardiovascular syphilis has not been proved. The response of cardiovascular syphilis to penicillin is seldom dramatic because aortic aneurysm and aortic regurgitation cannot be reversed by antibiotic treatment, although further progression of these lesions may be arrested by treatment.

In contrast, the response of benign tertiary syphilis and of meningovascular syphilis to penicillin G is usually impressive. The response of parenchymal neurosyphilis has been variable. In a cooperative study of the treatment of 1086 general paretics with penicillin, the frequency of clinical improvement or termination of progression ranged from 38 percent of those with severe involvement to 81 percent of those with mild involvement. All patients who relapsed following initial improvement in cerebrospinal fluid pleocytosis had received less than 6 million units of penicillin, and all had improvement of CSF pleocytosis with subsequent therapy. Tabes dorsalis or optic atrophy responds less often. In general, treatment of inactive neurosyphilis in which permanent neurological damage has already occurred may not produce any clinical change, and re-treatment of such cases is not warranted. However, persistence of cerebrospinal fluid pleocytosis, or recurrence of pleocytosis following initial response to treatment, indicates continuing active infection, which should respond to additional treatment. The optimal dose and duration of penicillin for neurosyphilis has not been determined, but administration of 600,000 to 900,000 units of procaine penicillin G daily for 10 days has been about 90 percent effective. Some physicians advocate administration of intravenous penicillin G in doses of 12 million units per day or more for 10 days or longer, to ensure maximally treponemacidal concentrations of penicillin G in cerebrospinal fluid. Such therapy has occasionally cured patients who failed to respond to conventional therapy. There are no data to support the use of antibiotics other than penicillin G for the treatment of neurosyphilis. Therefore follow-up for at least 3 years, with reexamination of spinal fluid every 3 to 6 months, is especially important if antibiotics other than penicillin were used.

Jarisch-Herxheimer reaction A dramatic reaction consisting of fever (average temperature elevation, 1.5°C), chills, myalgias, headache, tachycardia, increased respiratory rate, increased circulating neutrophil count (average total white blood cell count, 12,500 per cubic millimeter), and vasodilatation with mild hypotension, may occur following initiation of treatment of syphilis. This reaction occurs in approximately 50 percent of patients with primary syphilis, 90 percent with secondary, and 25 percent with early latent syphilis. The onset occurs within 2 h of treatment, the peak temperature occurs at about 7 h, and defervescence takes place within 12 to 24 h. The reaction is more delayed in neurosyphilis, with peak fever occurring after 12 to 14 h. In patients with secondary syphilis, an increase in erythema and edema of the mucocutaneous lesions occurs; occasionally subclinical or early mucocutaneous lesions may first become apparent during the reaction. The pathogenesis of this reaction is controversial. Patients should be warned to expect such symptoms, which can be managed by bed rest and aspirin. The Jarisch-Herxheimer reaction in neurosyphilis or cardiovascular syphilis has, on very rare occasions, been associated with acute progression of irreversible organ damage.

Persistence of treponemal forms The persistence of *T. pallidum* in the aqueous humor, cerebrospinal fluid, lymph nodes, brain, inflamed temporal arteries, and other tissues following "adequate" penicillin treatment of latent or late syphilis has been suggested by dark-field microscopy and by immunofluorescent antibody and silver staining techniques. Treponemal forms have also been demonstrated in patients with various clinical findings suggestive of syphilis, but in whom serologic tests, including the FTA-ABS test, were negative. Although many of these findings could be explained by artifact or by the coincidental presence of nonpathogenic treponemes, in a few cases the persistence of pathogenic *T. pallidum* after antibiotic treatment was proved by rabbit inoculation experiments. The question has been raised as to whether the lifelong persistence of antitreponemal antibody measured in the TPI and FTA-ABS tests following treatment of latent or late syphilis represents prolonged immunologic memory or continued antigenic stimulation by persisting treponemes in lymph nodes and other tissues.

It is not surprising that *T. pallidum* might persist in the aqueous humor or cerebrospinal fluid despite penicillin treatment, because of poor penetration of the antibiotic, but persistence in lymph nodes and other sites remains unexplained. Limited evidence indicates no increase in resistance to penicillin of such persistent treponemes. Since the data on persisting treponemes are scanty, no modification of the treatment recommendations for latent or late syphilis seems warranted.

IMMUNITY AND PREVENTION OF SYPHILIS Only about 50 percent of the named contacts of primary and secondary syphilis become infected. The actual risk of infection from a single exposure is probably much lower. The relative importance of variations in sexual and hygienic practices, inoculum size, body and environmental temperature, and other local and systemic factors affecting transmissibility of syphilis remains undefined. There is some interest in the possible efficacy of intravaginal contraceptive gels as prophylactics against venereal diseases including syphilis, since many available preparations have bacteriostatic as well as spermicidal properties.

Humans have no natural resistance to infection by pathogenic treponemes. The rate of development of acquired resistance to *T. pallidum* following natural or experimental infection is quantitatively related to the amount of the antigenic stimulus, which depends upon both the size of the infecting inoculum and the duration of infection prior to treatment.

Partial resistance to rechallenge with *T. pallidum* is evident in rabbits as early as 11 days after initial infection. Resistance to a challenge dose of 10^3 organisms is complete by 1 month postinfection. In all cases, the degree of demonstrable resistance is dependent upon the challenge dose, and the rate of development of resistance depends upon the size of the immunizing inoculum. Resistance of human beings to reinfection by intradermal inoculation of *T. pallidum* was studied in volunteers. Those who had previously been treated for *early* syphilis developed a primary lesion and a serologic response, while the majority of those who had previously been treated for *late latent* syphilis and all those with *untreated latent* syphilis developed neither primary lesions nor serologic response following inoculation. Two patients treated for late latent or late congenital syphilis developed gummas at the site of inoculation.

The role of serum antibody in conferring immunity to syphilis remains controversial. Reagin antibody is not protective. Passively administered antibody from rabbits recovering from experimental syphilis prevents or delays appearance of clinical manifestations of syphilis; it does not prevent infection. Evidence for the importance of cellular immunity includes histopathologic studies in experimental rabbit syphilis, which demonstrates clearance of treponemes from primary lesions soon after peak infiltration of the lesion by T lymphocytes and macrophages. Prevention of cellular infiltration by cortisone results in delayed treponemal clearance, despite normal antibody levels. Delayed hypersensitivity to *T. pallidum* has been demonstrated by skin test in late syphilis in humans, and lymphocytes from patients with syphilis have been demonstrated to undergo blast transformation when exposed to treponemal or cardiolipin antigen. The histopathology of gummas suggests that the cellular immune response is somehow involved in the pathogenesis of these lesions.

Inability to cultivate pathogenic treponemes in vitro has hindered analysis, purification, and concentration of treponemal antigens, and attempts to induce immunity to syphilis by vaccination have shown limited promise. Injection of rabbits with gamma-irradiated motile strains has conferred immunity to a rechallenge with 10^5 organisms, but many injections over long periods of time were required. Attempts to provide cross-resistance by immunization of rabbits with cultivated nonpathogenic treponemas have been unsuccessful. Experiments in humans have shown that varying degrees of cross-immunity exist in patients infected with *T. pallidum, T. pertenue,* and *T. carateum,* but chimpanzees with experimental pinta have not developed cross-resistance to syphilis. These findings indicate that the prospects for a syphilis vaccine remain remote, and that the prevention of syphilis depends upon use of mechanical or antiseptic prophylactic agents, and upon detection and treatment of infectious cases.

REFERENCES

BRYCESON ADM: Clinical pathology of the Jarisch-Herxheimer reaction. J Infect Dis 133:696, 1976

CAMPISI D, WHITCOMB C: Liver disease in early syphilis. Arch Intern Med 139:365, 1979

CLARK EG, DANBOLT N: The Oslo study of the natural course of untreated syphilis. Med Clin North Am 48:613, 1964

FISCHER A et al: Tertiary syphilis in Denmark 1961–1970, a description of 105 cases not previously diagnosed or specifically treated. Acta Derm-Venereol 56:485, 1976

FIUMARA NJ: Treatment of primary and secondary syphilis: Serologic response. JAMA 243:2500, 1980

GREENE BM et al: Failure of penicillin G benzathine in the treatment of neurosyphilis. Arch Intern Med 140:1117, 1980

IDSOE O et al: Penicillin in the treatment of syphilis. Bull WHO 47(Suppl):1, 1972

JAFFE HW: The laboratory diagnosis of syphilis: New concepts. Ann Intern Med 83:846, 1975

JOHNSON RC (ed): *The Biology of the Parasitic Spirochetes.* New York, Academic, 1976

LUKEHART SA et al: Characterization of lymphocyte responsiveness in early experimental syphilis: II. Nature of cellular infiltration and *Treponema pallidum* distribution in testicular infection. J Immunol 124:461, 1980

LUGER A et al: Diagnosis of neurosyphilis by examination of the cerebrospinal fluid. Br J Vener Dis 57:232, 1981

MERRITT HH et al (eds): *Neurosyphilis.* New York, Oxford, 1946

MOHR JA et al: Neurosyphilis and penicillin levels in cerebrospinal fluid. JAMA 236:2208, 1976

QUINN TC et al: Rectal mass caused by *Treponema pallidum:* Confirmation by immunofluorescent staining. Gastroenterology 82:135, 1982

REIMER CB et al: The specificity of fetal IgM: Antibody or anti-antibody? NY Acad Sci 254:77, 1975

ROSAHN PD: *Autopsy Studies in Syphilis.* CDC Publication 433, US Department of Health, Education, and Welfare, 1960

ROSS WH, SUTTON HFS: Acquired syphilitic uveitis. Arch Ophthalmol 98:496, 1980

SACHAR DB et al: Erosive syphilitic gastritis. Ann Intern Med 50:512, 1974

Sexually transmitted diseases treatment guidelines 1982. Morb Mort Week Rep 31:25, 1982

Treponematosis research: Report of a WHO scientific group. WHO Tech Rep Ser 455, 1970

TURNER DR, WRIGHT DJM: Lymphadenopathy in early syphilis. J Pathol 110:305, 1973

ZOLLER M et al: Detection of syphilitic hearing loss. Arch Otolaryngol 104:63, 1978

178
NONVENEREAL TREPONEMATOSES: YAWS, PINTA, AND ENDEMIC SYPHILIS

KING K. HOLMES
PETER L. PERINE

GENERAL CONSIDERATIONS Nonvenereal treponematoses occur in remote, impoverished areas of the world. Yaws, pinta, and endemic syphilis are distinguished from venereal syphilis solely by clinical and epidemiologic features. Yaws and pinta are caused by treponemes which are conventionally designated as unique species (*Treponema pertenue* causes yaws, and *T. carateum* pinta), but no convincing morphologic or antigenic differences have yet been demonstrated among *T. pertenue, T. carateum,* and *T. pallidum.* The etiologic agent of endemic syphilis is generally held to be identical with *T. pallidum* and is sometimes designated as *T. pallidum endemicum.* Pinta involves the skin alone; yaws affects skin and bones; and endemic syphilis involves the skin, bone, and mucous membranes. Each disease tends to progress by stages, but these are neither as distinct nor as predictable as in syphilis. Congenital infections and cardiovascular and central nervous system involvement occur rarely, if ever, in the nonvenereal treponematoses but are common in syphilis. It remains unclear whether the clinical and epidemiologic differences among yaws, pinta, endemic syphilis, and venereal syphilis are solely determined by environmental and host factors or are attributable to undefined biological differences among the causal treponemes. The relationship of the treponematoses is summarized in Table 178-1.

EPIDEMIOLOGY Treponemal antibodies are demonstrable in a high proportion of nonhuman primates in regions of Africa where human yaws and endemic syphilis are common, and pathogenic treponemes have been found in skin lesions and lymph nodes of seropositive animals. These treponemes have produced yaws-like lesions in susceptible monkeys and hamsters. Treponemes related to or identical with *T. pertenue* thus may antedate *Homo sapiens.*

Yaws and endemic syphilis are diseases of young children. Yaws occurs throughout the world between the tropics of Cancer and Capricorn, in humid, warm environments. Transmission of yaws among children is favored by scanty clothing, poor hygiene, and frequent skin trauma. Spread occurs by direct contact with infected lesions and perhaps by passive transfer of treponemes by insects. Endemic syphilis occurs in arid subtropical or temperate climates in Africa, the eastern Mediterranean, the Arabian peninsula, and central Asia. It is not observed in the western hemisphere. Skin-to-skin transmission is less important than in yaws; instead, infection of mucous membranes results from direct mouth-to-mouth contact or from contaminated fomites, such as shared drinking or eating utensils. Venereal syphilis can spread by nonvenereal contact among children and cause household outbreaks in modern cities when crowding and poverty favor transmission of *T. pallidum.*

TABLE 178-1
Etiology, epidemiology, and clinical manifestations of the treponematoses

	Venereal syphilis	*Endemic syphilis*	*Yaws*	*Pinta*
Organism	*T. pallidum*	*T. pallidum endemicum*	*T. pertenue*	*T. carateum*
Transmission	Sexual, transplacental*	Household contacts: mouth-to-mouth or via drinking, eating utensils	Skin-to-skin ? Insect vector	Skin-to-skin ? Insect vector
Usual age	Adult	Early childhood	Early childhood	Adolescent
Primary lesion	Cutaneous ulcer (chancre)	Rarely seen	Framboise (raspberry), or "mother yaw"	Nonulcerating papule with satellites
Secondary lesion	Mucocutaneous; occasional periostitis	Florid mucocutaneous lesions (mucous patch, split papule, condyloma latum); osteoperiostitis	Cutaneous papulosquamous lesions	Pintides
Tertiary	Gumma, cardiovascular, and CNS lues	Destructive cutaneous osteoarticular gummas	Destructive cutaneous osteoarticular gummas	Dyschromic, achromic macules

* *Since the nonvenereal treponematoses are usually acquired in childhood and treponemal bacteremia ceases with time, only in adult-onset venereal syphilis is there any likelihood of a mother giving birth to an infected child.*

Although cutaneous pigmentary changes resembling late stages of pinta occur in yaws or endemic syphilis, pinta is a separate, more benign disease which occurs only in the western hemisphere. The onset is typically later than in yaws or endemic syphilis, usually when the person is between 10 and 20 years of age. Pinta is not very contagious, and its mode of transmission is not well defined.

The WHO/UNICEF-assisted mass campaign for eradication of endemic nonvenereal treponematosis from 1948 to 1965 was an unusually successful public health campaign. Over 160 million people were examined in 46 countries, and approximately 50 million cases, contacts, and latent infections were treated. The impact of this program was remarkable. The prevalence of active yaws lesions was reduced from over 20 percent to less than 1 percent in many rural areas. In Bosnia, Yugoslavia, endemic syphilis was eradicated—the only example of eradication of an endemic treponematosis.

Relaxation of active surveillance activities after the mass campaigns has led to a resurgence of yaws, particularly in Africa. Yaws has not been eradicated in any large area. For example, in Ghana reported cases of yaws increased fivefold from 1970 to 1978, and recrudescences have been reported in Senegal, the Congo, Togo, and the Ivory Coast. Among pygmies in Cameroon and Zaire surveyed from 1969 to 1978, the prevalence of clinical yaws was 10 percent, and the prevalence of FTA-ABS antibody ranged from 75 percent for children under 5 years to 90 percent or more for those over 20. Similarly, WHO surveys during the early 1970s showed that the prevalence of active endemic syphilis, though lower than before the eradication program, ranged from 1 to 5 percent in rural poor populations of Senegal, Mauritania, Mali, Chad, Niger, Upper Volta, Kenya, Ethiopia, and Somalia. A new yaws campaign was initiated in Ghana in 1980, and other national campaigns are planned to control resurgent yaws and endemic syphilis in Africa.

Antitreponemal and reaginic seroreactivity has been detected in a small percentage of children without clinical disease born after the mass campaigns in some areas (e.g., Nigeria, New Guinea, and Bosnia). This may represent asymptomatic infection or may simply reflect the decreased predictive value of serologic tests (probability that disease is present if the test is positive) when the prevalence of disease is sharply reduced.

In the Americas, foci of yaws persist in Haiti; Dominica, St. Lucia, and St. Vincent; Peru, Colombia, and Ecuador; a few areas of Brazil; and Guyana and Surinam. Pinta is confined to Central America and northern South America, where it appears to have regressed to remote Indian villages. Its prevalence today is probably less than 1 percent of that found 20 years ago.

BIOLOGICAL RELATIONSHIPS Specific humoral antibodies to *T. pallidum* are produced in individuals with yaws, pinta, or endemic syphilis, but the time of appearance of antibodies after onset of infections is variable. The fluorescent treponemal antibody absorption (FTA-ABS) test, the *T. pallidum* hemagglutination test (TPHA), and the *T. pallidum* immobilization (TPI) test cannot differentiate among the treponematoses.

In addition to the clinical and epidemiologic differences among the treponematoses in humans, the range of susceptible animal hosts and some manifestations of experimental infection are also different. In particular, *T. carateum* has produced an infection in chimpanzees which resembles pinta, but attempts to infect other experimental animals have usually been unsuccessful. Differences between *T. pallidum* and *T. pertenue* have been reported for infections produced in the rabbit and golden hamster, and experimental rabbit infection with one species conferred greater immunity to reinfection with the homologous species than with the heterologous species. However, these interspecies differences in superinfection immunity are no greater than intraspecies differences among different strains of *T. pallidum.* Individuals who have had yaws or pinta are considered relatively immune to syphilis, and persons with active pinta or syphilis cannot be superinfected with *T. pertenue* by experimental inoculation.

CLINICAL MANIFESTATIONS Yaws Also known as pian, framboesia, buba, or bouba, yaws is a chronic infectious disease of childhood caused by *T. pertenue.* The disease is characterized by an initial skin lesion(s) followed by relapsing, nondestructive, secondary lesions of skin and bone. In the late stages, destructive lesions of skin, bone, and joints occur.

The incubation period following experimental inoculation of susceptible human beings is 3 to 4 weeks. Disruption of the skin by insect bites, abrasions, or injuries promotes acquisition of natural infection from infected contacts, most likely by fingers contaminated directly or indirectly with material from early yaws lesions. The initial early lesion is a single papule which is usually located on a leg. The lesion enlarges and becomes papillomatous. This lesion is known as a framboesioma (raspberry) or "mother yaw." It becomes superficially eroded and covered by a thin yellow crust of serous exudate containing *T. pertenue.* Erythema and induration do not occur. The lesion is mildly pruritic, and regional lymphadenopathy occurs. The initial lesion usually heals in 6 months. As a result of treponemal bacteremia and autoinoculation, a generalized secondary eruption of similar lesions appears either before or after the initial lesion has healed and is most extensive on the exposed surfaces of the body. These early cutaneous lesions of yaws have a variety of forms, including desquamative macular and papular as well as papillomatous types (Fig. 178-1). Painful papillomata on the soles of the feet result in a crablike gait referred to as *crab yaws.* Early lesions are infectious and heal slowly; they may result in scarring, hyperpigmentation, or depigmentation, resembling the pigmentary changes seen in pinta. Histological findings are mononuclear-cell infiltration, acanthosis (Fig. 178-2), hyperkeratosis, and the presence of many treponemes. Other manifestations of early yaws include lymphadenopathy and nocturnal bone pain and polydactylitis due to periostitis. Fever and other constitutional symptoms are rare, however, unless lesions become secondarily infected. Infectious cutaneous relapses are characteristic during the first 5 years after infection. Late yaws lesions occur in about 10 percent of cases, starting 5 years or more after infection, and differ histologically from early lesions in showing endarteritis. Late lesions include gummas of the skin and long bones, particularly of the legs, hyperkeratoses of the soles and palms, osteitis, periostitis, juxtaarticular fibromatous nodes, and hydrarthrosis.

Late lesions of yaws are characteristically extensive and usually destructive. Destruction of the nose, maxilla, palate, and pharynx, termed *gangosa,* or *rhinopharyngitis mutilans,* occurs in late yaws, as well as in leprosy and leishmaniasis. Hypertrophic paranasal maxillary osteitis produces distinctive facies known as *goundou.*

The clinical features of yaws have become less reliable for diagnosis as the prevalence of yaws has decreased, necessitating the use of easily performed serologic tests, such as the rapid plasma reagin (RPR) card test, by paramedical field workers engaged in the consolidation phase of yaws surveillance.

T. pertenue can be demonstrated by dark-field examination in early cutaneous lesions but should not be confused with other spirochetes found in tropical ulcers. The serum reagin antibody tests become positive after 1 month, and the FTA-ABS test is also positive.

Endemic syphilis Synonyms for endemic syphilis are Bejel, Siti, Dichuchwa, Njovera, Belesh, and Skerljevo. It is a chronic nonvenereal, treponemal infection of childhood, characterized by early mucous membrane or mucocutaneous lesions, a latent period of indeterminate duration, and late complications including gummas of bone and skin. The causative organism is indistinguishable from *T. pallidum.* Endemic syphilis differs from congenital syphilis in that dental changes, interstitial keratitis, and neurosyphilis rarely, if ever, occur. Cardiovascular complications are considered rare in both endemic and congenital syphilis.

Primary cutaneous lesions are infrequent and when present are extragenital. The earliest manifestation of endemic syphilis is usually an intraoral mucous patch or mucocutaneous lesion resembling the split papules or condylomata of secondary syphilis. Periostitis is common. Regional lymphadenopathy occurs, but generalized lymphadenopathy is unusual. Treponemes are abundant in the moist early lesions and in aspirates from regional lymph nodes. After a variable latent period, late lesions may develop and are the most frequent clinical manifestations. These resemble the lesions of late benign syphilis and include osseous or cutaneous gummas. Destructive gummas, osteitis, and periostitis of nasopharyngeal structures are more common than in late yaws. Gummas occur on the nipples of mothers who have themselves previously had endemic syphilis who breastfeed infants with oral lesions. Both early and late forms of endemic syphilis thus may coexist in the same family. The tertiary lesions of endemic syphilis sometimes may be a consequence of repeated reexposure of a previously sensitized host to reinfection.

Pinta Also known as mal del pinto, carate, azul, or purupuru, pinta is an infectious disease of the skin caused by *T. carateum.* This disease has three cutaneous stages characterized by marked changes in the skin color, does not involve osseous tissue or viscera, and causes no disability other than that associated with cosmetic disfigurement.

The initial lesion is a small papule which appears 7 to 30 days after exposure and is located most often on the extremities, face, neck, or buttocks. It increases in size slowly by peripheral extension and by coalescing with smaller satellite papules. Regional lymphadenopathy occurs. A secondary eruption not associated with generalized lymphadenopathy appears 1 month to 1 year after the appearance of the initial lesion. The secondary lesions are termed *pintides,* may be numerous, and evolve into a psoriatic or circinate configuration. Pintides are initially red but become deeply pigmented, reaching a slate-blue color after a period of time which is related to exposure to sun. Pigmentation occurs most rapidly on the exposed parts of the body. These pigmented lesions are known as dyschromic macules and contain treponemes which are located principally in the epidermis in older lesions. Histologically there is deposition of pigment in the dermis with decreased melanin pigment in the basal-cell layer. Within 3 months to a year, most of the pintides show varying degrees of depigmentation, becoming brown and finally white and giving the skin a mottled appearance. The porcelain-white achromic lesions rep-

FIGURE 178-1
Early papillomatous yaws lesions of the left arm with subcutaneous juxta-articular nodules.

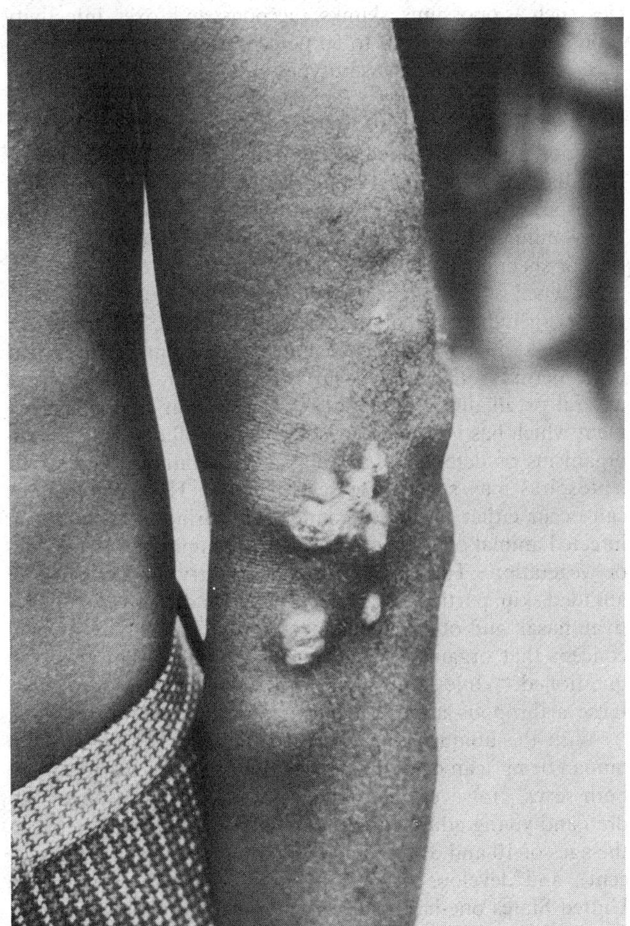

FIGURE 178-2
Secondary yaws ulceropapillomata on the right leg.

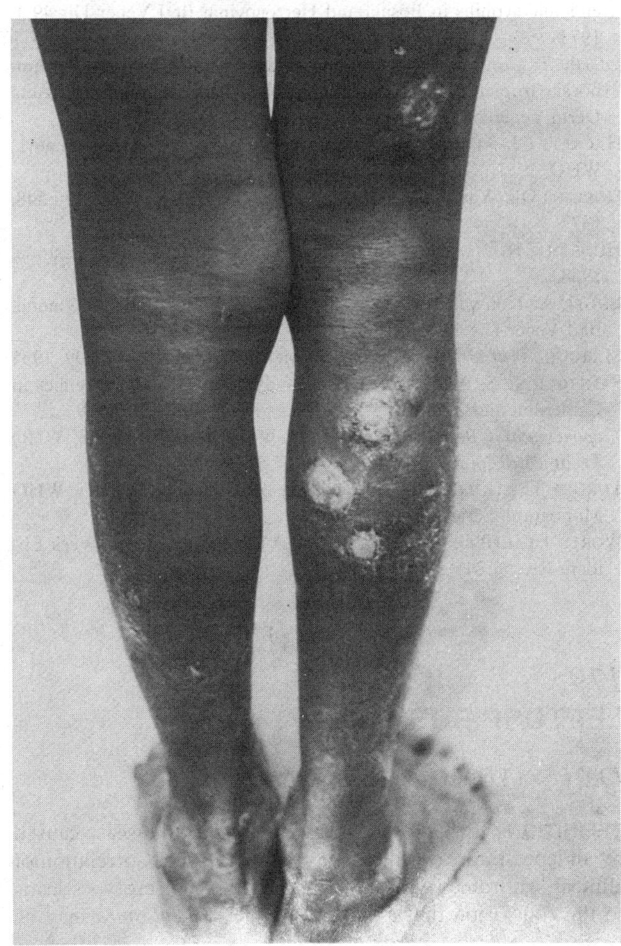

resent the "late" stage of the disease in which the epidermis is atrophic and melanocytes and melanin are absent. *T. carateum* can be demonstrated in transudates from initial, early secondary, or dyschromic lesions. Serologic reaginic and antitreponemal antibody tests are positive, but may take four times longer to become positive in pinta than in venereal syphilis.

TREATMENT Treatment is similar for all the treponematoses. Intramuscular injection of 2.4 million units of benzathine penicillin G in adults and half this dose in children results in rapid resolution of lesions and prevents recurrence. Procaine penicillin G in oil and 2% aluminum monostearate (PAM) has been used extensively. In persons who are allergic to penicillin, tetracycline hydrochloride in a dose similar to that used for infectious syphilis (see Chap. 177) is effective. In areas where less than 5 percent of the population has active disease, cases are managed on an individual basis, and all contacts of infected persons are treated with antibiotics.

PREVENTION Although the nonvenereal treponematoses are less amenable to eradication than smallpox, the resurgence of yaws has led some authorities to suggest that the application of *selective epidemiologic control* as used in smallpox eradication be applied to yaws control. This strategy would emphasize ongoing active surveillance, investigation of outbreaks, and treatment of active cases and their contacts rather than mass treatment.

REFERENCES

Bibliography on Yaws 1905–1962. Geneva, WHO, 1963

Editorial: Yaws again. Br Med J 2:1090, 1980

Grin EI, Guthe T: Evaluation of a previous mass campaign against endemic syphilis in Bosnia and Herzogovina. Br J Vener Dis 49:1, 1973

Guthe T: Clinical, serological and epidemiological features of framboesia tropica (yaws) and its control in rural communities. Acta Derm Venereol 49:343, 1969

Hackett CJ: An international nomenclature of yaws lesions. Geneva, WHO, 1957

Hopkins DR: Yaws in the Americas, 1950–1975. J Infect Dis 136:548, 1977

Hudson EH: *Nonvenereal Syphilis.* Edinburgh, E & S Livingstone, 1958

Luger A: Non-venereally transmitted "endemic" syphilis in Vienna. Br J Vener Dis 48:356, 1972

Marquez F et al: Mal del pinto in Mexico. Bull WHO 13:299, 1955

Pampiglione S, Wilkinson AE: A study of yaws among pygmies in Cameroon and Zaire. Br J Vener Dis 51:165, 1975

Treponematoses Research: Report of a WHO Scientific Group, WHO Technical Report Series 455, 1970

Turner TB, Hollander DH: *Biology of the Treponematoses,* WHO Monograph Series 35, 1957

World Health Organization: Endemic treponematoses. Week Epidem Rec 56:241, 1981

179
LEPTOSPIROSIS

JAY P. SANFORD

DEFINITION *Leptospirosis* is a term applied to disease caused by all leptospiras regardless of specific serotype. Correlation of clinical syndromes with infection by differing serotypes leads to the conclusion that a single serotype of *Leptospira* may be responsible for a variety of clinical features; conversely, a single syndrome, e.g., aseptic meningitis, may be caused by multiple serotypes. Hence there is a preference for the general term leptospirosis rather than the synonyms such as Weil's disease and canicola fever.

ETIOLOGY The genus *Leptospira* contains only one species, *L. interrogans,* which may be subdivided into two complexes, interrogans and biflexa. The interrogans complex includes the pathogenic strains, while the biflexa complex includes saprophytic strains. Within each complex the organisms show antigenic variations that are stable and allow them to be classed as serotypes (serovars). Serotypes with common antigens are arranged in serogroups. Despite contrary common usage, an example of the correct designation of *Leptospira* is as follows: Pomona serogroup of *L. interrogans* or *L. interrogans* serovar pomona, not *L. pomona.* The interrogans complex now contains about 170 serotypes arranged in 18 serogroups (the number in parentheses refers to number of serotypes within the serogroup): Icterohemorrhagiae (18), Hebdomadis (30), Autumnalis (17), Canicola (12), Australis (12), Tarassovi (17), Pyrogenes (12), Bataviae (10), Javanica (8), Pomona (8), Ballum (3), Cynopteri (3), Celledoni (3), Grippotyphosa (5), Panama (2), Shermani (1), Ranarum (2), and Bufonis (1). At least 27 serotypes of *Leptospira* occur naturally in the United States.

EPIDEMIOLOGY Although leptospirosis is not a common disease, it has been reported from all regions of the United States. Between 1970 and 1979, approximately 50 to 150 cases were reported annually. Occasional upswings in number of cases have been the result of common-source outbreaks. Infection in human beings is an incidental occurrence and is not essential to the maintenance of leptospirosis. The disease occurs in a wide range of domestic and wild animal hosts. In many species, such as opossums, skunks, raccoons, and foxes, infectivity ratios in the range of 10 to 50 percent are not unusual. Interspecies spread of specific serotypes of leptospiras between animal hosts is frequent, e.g., Pomona, a serotype principally associated with livestock, has been demonstrated in dogs. Infection in animals may vary from inapparent illness to severe fatal disease. The carrier state, in which the host may shed leptospiras in its urine for months to years, may develop in many animals. Immunization of dogs may not prevent the carrier, or shedder, state.

Survival of pathogenic leptospiras in nature is governed by factors including pH of the urine of the host, pH of soil or water into which they are shed, and ambient temperature. Acid urine permits only limited survival; however, if the urine is neutral or alkaline and is shed into a similar moist environment which has low salinity, is not badly polluted with microorganisms or detergents, and has a temperature above 22°C, leptospiras may survive for several weeks. Human infections can occur either by direct contact with urine or tissue of an infected animal or indirectly through contaminated water, soil, or vegetation. The usual portals of entry in humans are abraded skin, particularly about the feet, and exposed conjunctival, nasal, and oral mucous membranes. The previously held concept that organisms could penetrate intact skin has been questioned. While leptospiras have been isolated from ticks, these arthropods appear to be unimportant in transmission.

With the ubiquitous infection of animals, leptospirosis in human beings can occur in all age groups, at all seasons, and in both sexes. However, it is primarily a disease of teenage children and young adults (about one-half of patients are between the ages of 10 and 39), occurs predominantly in males (80 percent), and develops most frequently in hot weather (in the United States one-half of infections occur from July to October). The wide spectrum of animal hosts results in both urban and rural human disease. Leptospirosis has been considered an occupational disease; however, improved methods of rat control and better standards of hygiene have reduced the incidence among occupational groups such as coal miners and people who work in sewers. Currently less than 20 percent of patients have direct contact with animals; they are mostly farmers, trappers, or abattoir workers. In the majority of patients exposure is incidental; two-thirds of cases occur in children, students, or housewives. Swimming or partial immersion in contaminated water, e.g., riding motorcycles through contaminated pools of water, has been implicated in one-fifth of patients and has accounted for most of the recognized common-source outbreaks.

PATHOLOGY In patients who have died with either hepatic involvement (Weil's syndrome), renal involvement, or both, the significant gross changes include hemorrhages and bile staining of tissues. The hemorrhages, which vary from petechial to ecchymotic, are widespread and are most prominent in skeletal muscle, kidneys, adrenals, liver, stomach, spleen, and lungs.

In skeletal muscle, focal, necrotic, and necrobiotic changes thought to be typical of leptospirosis occur. Biopsies early in the illness demonstrate swelling and vacuolation. Leptospiral antigen has been demonstrated in these lesions by the fluorescent antibody technique. Healing ensues by the formation of new myofibrils with minimal fibrosis. The renal lesions in the acute phase involve predominantly the tubules and vary from simple dilatation of distal convoluted tubules to degeneration, necrosis, and basement membrane rupture. Interstitial edema and cellular infiltrates consisting of lymphocytes, neutrophilic leukocytes, histiocytes, and plasma cells are uniformly present. Glomerular lesions either are absent or consist of mesangial hyperplasia and focal foot process fusion which are interpreted as representing nonspecific changes associated with acute inflammation and protein filtration. Microscopic alterations in the liver are not diagnostic and correlate poorly with the degree of functional impairment. The changes include cloudy swelling of parenchymal cells, disruption of liver cords, enlargement of Kupffer cells, and bile stasis in biliary canaliculi. The changes in the brain and meninges are also minimal and are not diagnostic. Microscopic evidence of myocarditis has been recorded. Pulmonary findings consist of a patchy, localized hemorrhagic pneumonitis. Special staining techniques utilizing silver impregnation methods have demonstrated organisms in the lumina of renal tubules but rarely in other organs.

CLINICAL MANIFESTATIONS **General features** The incubation period following immersion or accidental laboratory exposure has shown extremes of 2 to 26 days, the usual range being 7 to 13 days and the average 10 days.

Leptospirosis is a typically biphasic illness. *During the leptospiremic* or *first phase,* leptospiras are present in the blood and cerebrospinal fluid. The onset is typically abrupt, and initial symptoms include headache, which is usually frontal, less often retroorbital, but occasionally may be bitemporal or occipital. Severe muscle aching occurs in most patients, the muscles of the thighs and lumbar areas being most prominently involved, and often is accompanied by severe pain on palpation. The myalgia may be accompanied by extreme cutaneous hyperesthesia (causalgia). Chills followed by a rapidly rising temperature are prominent. Following the abrupt onset, the leptospiremic phase typically lasts 4 to 9 days. Features during this interval include recurrent chills, high spiking temperatures [usually 38.9°C (102°F) or greater], headache, and continued severe myalgia. Anorexia, nausea, and vomiting are encountered in one-half or more of the patients. Occasional patients have diarrhea. Pulmonary manifestations, usually either cough or chest pain, have varied in frequency of occurrence from less than 25 percent to 86 percent. Hemoptysis occurs but is rare. Adult respiratory distress syndrome has been reported. Examination during this phase reveals an acutely ill, febrile patient, with a relative bradycardia and normal blood pressure, although European authors comment on early hypotension. Disturbances in sensorium may be encountered in up to 25 percent of patients. The most characteristic physical sign is conjunctival suffusion, which usually first appears on the third or fourth day. It may be lacking in some patients but more often is overlooked. This may be associated with photophobia, but serous or purulent secretion is unusual. Less common findings may include pharyngeal injection, cutaneous hemorrhages, and skin rashes that are usually macular, maculopapular, or urticarial and usually occur on the trunk. Uncommon findings are splenomegaly, hepatomegaly, lymphadenopathy, or jaundice. The first phase terminates after 4 to 9 days, usually with defervescence and improvement in symptoms. This coincides with the disappearance of leptospiras from the blood and cerebrospinal fluid.

The second phase has been characterized as the "immune" phase and correlates with the appearance of circulating IgM antibodies. The concentration of C3 in serum has remained within normal range during this phase. The clinical manifestations of this phase show greater variability than those during the first phase. After a relatively asymptomatic period of 1 to 3 days, the fever and earlier symptoms recur and meningismus may develop. The fever rarely exceeds 38.9°C (102°F) and is usually of 1 to 3 days' duration. It is not uncommon for fever to be absent or quite transient. Even when symptoms or signs of meningeal irritation are absent, routine examination of cerebrospinal fluid after the seventh day has revealed pleocytosis in 50 to 90 percent of patients. Less common features include iridocyclitis, optic neuritis, and other nervous system manifestations, including encephalitis, myelitis, and peripheral neuropathy.

Some clinicians recognize a third or convalescent phase, usually between the second and fourth weeks, when both fever and aching may recur. The pathogenesis of this stage is not understood.

Leptospirosis during pregnancy may be associated with an increased risk of fetal loss.

Specific features WEIL'S SYNDROME Weil's syndrome, which may be due to serotypes other than Icterohemorrhagiae, is defined as severe leptospirosis with jaundice, usually accompanied by azotemia, hemorrhages, anemia, disturbances in consciousness, and continued fever. There is uncertainty as to the pathogenesis of the syndrome, i.e., whether it represents direct toxic damage due to leptospiras or whether it is the consequence of immune response to leptospiral antigens. The consensus favors toxic damage.

The onset and first stage are identical with the less severe forms of leptospirosis. The distinctive features of Weil's syndrome appear from the third to the sixth days but do not reach their peak until well into the second stage. As in milder forms of leptospirosis, there is a tendency for defervescence about the seventh day; however, with recurrence, fever is marked and may persist for several weeks. Either renal or hepatic manifestations may predominate. Hepatic disturbances include tenderness in the right upper quadrant and hepatic enlargement, both of which are common when jaundice is present. Serum glutamic oxaloacetic transaminase (SGOT) values are rarely increased more than fivefold regardless of the degree of hyperbilirubinemia, which is predominantly conjugated (direct): e.g., serum bilirubin, 40 mg/dl; SGOT, 170 IU. The predominant mechanism appears to be an intracellular block to bilirubin excretion.

Renal manifestations consist primarily of proteinuria, pyuria, hematuria, and azotemia. Dysuria is rare. Serious renal damage usually occurs in the form of acute tubular necrosis associated with oliguria. The peak elevation of blood urea nitrogen usually is seen on the fifth to seventh day. Hemorrhagic manifestations are most prevalent in this group of patients and include epistaxis, hemoptysis, gastrointestinal bleeding, hemorrhage into the adrenal glands, hemorrhagic pneumonitis, and subarachnoid hemorrhage. These have been explained on the basis of diffuse vasculitis with capillary injury. In addition, in some patients hypoprothrombinemia and thrombocytopenia have been observed.

ASEPTIC MENINGITIS A leptospiral etiology has been incriminated in 5 to 13 percent of sporadic cases of aseptic meningitis. The pleocytosis is not present before the immune phase, when it develops rapidly. There are usually tens to hundreds of leukocytes, occasionally 1000, per cubic milliliter, among which neutrophils or mononuclear cells may predominate. The cerebrospinal fluid glucose concentration is almost always normal, but occasional instances of lowered glucose levels (hypoglycorrhachia) have been recorded. In contrast to the observations with many viral causes of aseptic meningitis, with leptospirosis the cerebrospinal fluid protein may exceed 100 mg/dl early in the course. Xanthochromic cerebrospinal fluid has been observed in the presence of jaundice. Each of the serotypes of leptospiras that are pathogenic for human beings is probably capable of causing aseptic meningitis. The most prevalent serotypes have been Canicola, Icterohemorrhagiae, and Pomona.

PRETIBIAL (FORT BRAGG) FEVER An illness was observed in the summer of 1942 that had an onset identical with that of the first phase of leptospirosis. The most distinctive feature was the development on about the fourth day of a rash, characterized by 2- to 5-cm, slightly raised, erythematous lesions that were usually symmetrically distributed over the pretibial areas. In contrast to other leptospiral syndromes, splenomegaly occurred in 95 percent of these patients. This outbreak was shown to be due to the Autumnalis serogroup. Subsequently, Pomona has been observed in association with rashes, which are usually truncal but which have also been pretibial.

MYOCARDITIS Cardiac arrhythmias including paroxysmal atrial fibrillation, atrial flutter, ventricular tachycardia, and premature ventricular contractions have been described but are usually of little clinical significance. However, on rare occasions definite cardiac dilatation with acute left ventricular failure has been observed. Associated manifestations have included jaundice, pulmonary infiltrates, arthritis, and skin rashes. The serotypes thus far incriminated have included Icterohemorrhagiae, Pomona, and Grippotyphosa.

CHILDREN Several clinical features occur in children which are not seen or are very rare in adults: hypertension, acalculous cholecystitis (five of nine children in one series), pancreatitis, abdominal causalgia, and peripheral desquamation of a rash which may be associated with gangrene and cardiopulmonary arrest. The features of desquamation, myocardial involvement, and hydrops of the gallbladder suggest Kawasaki syndrome [mucocutaneous lymph node syndrome (see Chap. 199)].

LABORATORY FEATURES Leukocyte counts vary from leukopenic levels to mild elevations in the anicteric patients. In patients with jaundice, leukocytosis as high as 70,000 cells per cubic millimeter may be present. However, regardless of the total leukocyte count, neutrophilia of greater than 70 percent is very frequently encountered during the first stage.

Hemolytic substances have been demonstrated in cultures of pathogenic leptospiras. In contrast to many hemolysins of bacterial origin which are not hemolytic in vivo, the leptospiral hemolysins appear to be active in vivo. In patients with jaundice, anemia may be severe and is most characteristically due to intravascular hemolysis. Other mechanisms of anemia include azotemia and blood loss secondary to hemorrhage. Anemia due to leptospirosis is unusual in anicteric patients.

Rarely thrombocytopenia sufficient to be associated with bleeding is encountered. Additional hematologic abnormalities include elevation of the erythrocyte sedimentation rate in over one-half of patients, but it is usually less than 50 mm/h.

Urinalysis during the leptospiremic phase reveals mild proteinuria, casts, and an increase in cellular elements. In anicteric infections, these abnormalities rapidly disappear after the first week. Proteinuria and abnormalities in the urine sediment usually are not associated with elevations in blood urea nitrogen. Since the anicteric form of the disease often has gone undiagnosed, estimates of the frequency of azotemia and jaundice are probably high. Azotemia has been reported in approximately one-fourth of patients. In three-fourths of these patients, the blood urea nitrogen is less than 100 mg/dl. Azotemia is usually associated with jaundice. The serum bilirubin levels may reach 65 mg/dl; however, in two-thirds of patients the levels are less than 20 mg/dl. During the first phase, one-half of the patients have increased serum creatine phosphokinase (CPK) levels, with mean values of five times normal. Such increases are not seen in viral hepatitis, and a slight increase in transaminase with a definite increase in CPK suggests leptospirosis rather than viral hepatitis.

DIAGNOSIS Diagnosis is based upon culture of the organism or serologic proof of its existence. The most common initial diagnostic impressions in patients with leptospirosis are meningitis, hepatitis, nephritis, fever of undetermined origin (FUO), influenza, Kawasaki syndrome, toxic shock syndrome, and Legionnaires' disease. Leptospiras may be isolated quite readily during the first phase from blood and cerebrospinal fluid or during the second phase from the urine. Leptospiras may be excreted in the urine for up to 11 months after the onset of illness and may persist despite antimicrobial therapy. Whole blood should be inoculated immediately into tubes containing semisolid medium, such as Fletcher's medium. If culture medium is not available, leptospiras reportedly will remain viable up to 11 days in blood to which anticoagulants, preferably sodium oxalate, have been added. Prepared concentrated leptospire medium is now available commercially. Animal inoculation (preferably either suckling hamsters or guinea pigs) may be used and is of particular value if specimens are contaminated. Direct examination of blood or urine by darkfield methods has been employed; *however, this method so frequently results in failure or misdiagnosis that it should not be employed.* Serologic methods are applicable during the second phase; antibodies appear from the sixth to the twelfth days of illness. Two serologic methods are commonly used: a macroscopic or slide agglutination test which is easy to perform but lacks specificity and sensitivity, and hence is suitable for screening only, and the microscopic agglutination test which is more complicated but also more specific. Serologic criteria for diagnosis include a fourfold or greater rise in titer during the course of illness. Cross-agglutination reactions between various serotypes commonly occur so that the infection serotype often cannot be determined with certainty without isolation of leptospiras.

PROGNOSIS The prognosis is dependent upon both the virulence of the organism and the general condition of the patient. In 1978, there were five deaths (4.5 percent) in the 110 patients reported in the United States. Age is the most significant host factor related to increased mortality. In a representative series, the mortality rose from 10 percent in men less than 50 years of age to 56 percent in those over 51 years of age. The virulence of the infecting leptospiras correlates best with the development of jaundice. In anicteric patients, mortality does not occur, but with the development of jaundice, mortality in various series has ranged from 15 to 40 percent. The long-term prognosis following the acute renal lesion of leptospirosis is good. Glomerular filtration rates have returned to normal; however, a few patients show residual tubular dysfunction such as a defect in renal concentrating capacity.

TREATMENT A variety of antimicrobial drugs, including penicillin, streptomycin, the tetracycline congeners, chloramphenicol, and erythromycin, have been effective in vitro and in experimental leptospiral infections. Data concerning the efficacy of antibiotics in human beings are conflicting. If antimicrobial drugs are to have any beneficial effect, they must be administered within 4 days, and preferably within 2 days, of the onset of illness. Large doses of penicillin G (usually 600,000 units intramuscularly every 4 h) are considered the preferred treatment, although the tetracyclines are also effective. Within 4 to 6 h after initiation of penicillin G therapy, a Jarisch-Herxheimer type of reaction, which suggests antileptospiral activity, may occur. There is general agreement that antimicrobials administered after the fifth day of illness have no beneficial effect. There exists the clinical impression that early bedrest may minimize subsequent morbidity. Azotemia and jaundice require meticulous attention to fluid and electrolyte therapy. Since the renal damage is reversible, patients with azotemia should be considered for peritoneal dialysis or hemodialysis. From case reports exchange transfusion has been suggested to be beneficial in the management of patients with extreme hyperbilirubinemia.

REFERENCES

ALSTON JM, BROOM JC: *Leptospirosis in Man and Animals.* Edinburgh, E & S Livingstone, 1958

CENTERS FOR DISEASE CONTROL: *Leptospirosis Surveillance: Annual Summary 1978.* August 1979

EDWARDS GA, DOMM M: Human leptospirosis. Medicine 39:117, 1960

FEIGIN RD, ANDERSON DC: Human leptospirosis. CRC Crit Rev Clin Lab Sci 5:413, 1975

HEATH CW JR, ALEXANDER AD: Leptospirosis in the United States: Analysis of 483 cases in man, 1949–1961. N Engl J Med 273:857, 915, 1965

JOHNSON WD JR et al: Serum creatine phosphokinase in leptospirosis. JAMA 233:981, 1975

JOHNSON RC: *The Biology of Parasitic Spirochetes.* New York, Academic, 1976

TURNER LH: Leptospirosis. Br Med J 1:537, 1973

WONG ML et al: Leptospirosis: A childhood disease. J Pediatr 90:532, 1977

ZALTZMAN M et al: Adult respiratory distress syndrome in *Leptospira canicola* infection. Br Med J 283:519, 1981

180 RELAPSING FEVER

JAMES J. PLORDE

DEFINITION Relapsing fever refers to a group of acute infectious diseases that are characterized clinically by cyclic periods of fever and apyrexia. They are caused by spirochetes of the genus *Borrelia* and occur in two epidemiologic varieties, louse-borne and tick-borne.

ETIOLOGY Borreliae are slender helical organisms which measure 10 to 20 μm in length. They have 3 to 10 irregular coils, move in a corkscrew fashion, and divide by transverse fission. Unlike other spirochetes, they readily stain with aniline dyes. *Borrelia recurrentis* is the causative agent of louse-borne relapsing fever. Many strains of *Borrelia* have been found in tick-borne disease; *B. turicatae, B. parkeri,* and *B. hermsii* are responsible for the disease seen in this country. The organisms grow poorly on artificial media and readily in developing chick embryos.

EPIDEMIOLOGY Louse-borne relapsing fever is transmitted from person to person by the human body louse. Spirochetes that are ingested by the vector during feeding penetrate the wall of the intestine and multiply in the body cavity. Human infection occurs when the louse is crushed against an abrasion or wound. There is no known animal reservoir. The disease persists in endemic focuses in Ethiopia, the Sudan, South America, and the far east. Like typhus, it occurs in epidemic form during war and famine. Major epidemics involving millions of people occurred in Europe and Africa after both the First and Second World Wars. A third, much smaller, outbreak was seen at the time of the Korean conflict. An occasional case of louse-borne relapsing fever has been imported into the United States.

The tick vectors of relapsing fever belong to several species of the genus *Ornithodoros.* These soft ticks are reclusive night feeders whose bites are quick and painless. They then detach themselves, leaving their host with a 2- to 3-mm pruritic eschar. Like lice, they ingest the borreliae during feeding. The organisms may remain viable in the ticks for several years and can be passed transovarily to the next generation, making the tick a major reservoir of the disease. It is likely that rodents and other small animals act as vertebrate reservoirs in some locales. Human beings are involved when they come into contact with an infected tick in its natural habitat. Transmission occurs if the tick's saliva or coxal fluid contaminates the feeding site. The tick-borne disease is found in localized areas throughout the world. In the United States it occurs primarily in western mountain states, from Texas in the south to Washington, Montana, and Idaho in the northwest. Outbreaks have occurred among boy scouts in northeastern Washington and tourists visiting the north rim of the Grand Canyon. In both outbreaks, the patients contracted the disease while sleeping overnight in tick-infested cabins. The disease has also been carried to other parts of the country, where it usually does not occur, by western travelers.

PATHOGENESIS AND PATHOLOGY After inoculation into a human, the borreliae reach the bloodstream, producing spirochetemia and a febrile illness. After several days, immobilizing and borrelicidal antibodies appear, the organisms are cleared from the peripheral blood, and the fever resolves. Following a latent period of approximately 1 week, during which the spirochetes are sequestered in the body, a new antigenic variant of the organism arises. There is reinvasion of the bloodstream, causing a second paroxysm of fever and eventually, with the formation of specific antibodies, a second defervescence by crisis. The continued sequential production of new antigenic variants and specific antibodies results in the characteristic relapsing febrile course. In louse-borne disease the fever appears to be produced by a heat-stable, nonendotoxic particulate pyrogen of the spirochete.

At autopsy follicular splenic abscesses, histiocytic interstitial myocarditis, intracranial hemorrhage, and hepatitis with focal necrosis may be seen. Spontaneous splenic rupture and hemorrhagic gastrointestinal lesions have been noted occasionally. Petechiae, the result of a marked thrombocytopenia, are frequent. Borreliae have been recovered from the brain, heart, spleen, liver, and skin.

MANIFESTATIONS Clinical manifestations vary from outbreak to outbreak and between the tick- and louse-borne varieties of the disease. Generally, patients with louse-borne relapsing fever are more seriously ill but have fewer relapses than those with tick-borne illnesses. After an incubation period of 4 to 18 days, the disease begins abruptly with rigors, headache, anorexia, nausea, vomiting, photophobia, and pain in the muscles and joints. The temperature rises rapidly, reaching 39 to 40°C (102.2 to 104°F), where it remains until the time of the crisis. The patient appears dull, apathetic, and is uncomplaining. He or she may have conjunctival suffusion and a macular or petechial rash. Cough, tachypnea, and rhonchi are common. A gallop rhythm and premature ventricular beats may occur in the louse-borne variety. Cardiac enlargement and heart failure are more uncommon. Upper abdominal tenderness is frequent. The liver and spleen are palpable and tender in 20 to 80 percent of cases, and may enlarge 6 to 10 cm during the course of fever. Jaundice secondary to hepatocellular destruction is present in 7 to 36 percent of patients. It is usually seen in louse-borne disease, occurs relatively late in the illness, and if severe, is often associated with purpura.

Bleeding is common in louse-borne relapsing fever. Petechiae develop in the skin and serous membranes, apparently as a result of damage to the capillary endothelium by clumps of spirochetes. Mild epistaxes and microscopic hematuria are present in many patients early in the disease. Later, with the development of liver disease, severe prolonged epistaxes and widespread ecchymoses occur. Infrequently, there may be massive gastrointestinal, urinary, or intracranial hemorrhage. Disseminated intravascular coagulation has been described. Neck stiffness, confusion, and transient focal neurologic signs may be seen even without intracranial bleeding. Patients with tick-borne disease with repeated relapses may develop iritis or iridocyclitis with permanent visual impairment. Pregnant women with relapsing fever often abort.

Three to six days after the onset of illness, the attack ends in a crisis. Clinically this is characterized by a chill and an abrupt but transient rise in temperature, heart rate, respiratory rate, and arterial blood pressure. As the spirochetes disappear, the patient becomes flushed, diaphoretic, and hypotensive. Occasionally, cardiovascular collapse and death may occur at this point. More frequently the blood pressure and temperature return to normal over several hours, leaving the patient comfortable but exhausted. After 7 to 10 afebrile days, a relapse occurs which mimics the original illness. In the louse-borne disease there is usually only a single relapse, but in tick-borne relapsing fever there may be several, each somewhat briefer and milder than the preceding one.

LABORATORY FINDINGS A moderate anemia is common. The leukocyte count is usually normal or slightly elevated. During the crisis, a marked leukopenia occurs which may be followed by a transient rebound leukocytosis. A consumptive thrombocytopenia is seen in most cases, and the prothrombin and partial thromboplastin times may be prolonged. Fibrinogen levels are increased. Liver function tests reveal disturbed hepatocellular function. In severe cases, the total serum bilirubin level may reach 16 mg/dl. Azotemia unrelated to extracellular fluid depletion is common among jaundiced patients. Electrocardiogram abnormalities, including a prolonged QTc interval and ST-T wave changes, may occur. Reagin tests for syphilis are positive in 5 to 10 percent of cases, and experimental data suggest that false-positive FTA-ABS tests may also occur. Patients with louse-borne relapsing fever frequently develop agglutinins to *Proteus* OXK antigens.

The definitive diagnosis is made by demonstrating borreliae in the peripheral blood during a febrile episode. This is most easily accomplished by examining thick and thin films stained with Giemsa's and Wright's stains. Repeated examinations may be required, especially in tick-borne disease. Blood spun in a microhematocrit tube and examined microscopically may reveal organisms when thin and thick smears are negative. Spirochetes may also be seen in wet mounts with phase-contrast microscopy. When the direct methods are negative, blood may be injected into mice or rats and their blood examined frequently for the presence of borreliae.

DIFFERENTIAL DIAGNOSIS Many acute febrile illnesses, including malaria, salmonellosis, typhus, dengue, rat-bite fever, and Weil's disease, must be considered. Practically, there is seldom confusion if blood films are examined carefully.

TREATMENT The peripheral blood is quickly cleared of spirochetes by a variety of drugs, including penicillin, tetracycline, and chloramphenicol. Treatment with these antimicrobial agents, however, is accompanied by a Jarisch-Herxheimer–like reaction which contributes to the morbidity, and perhaps mortality, of the disease. The reaction appears both clinically and pathophysiologically to be an exaggeration of the spontaneously occurring crisis. Its mechanism is unknown, but it may be related to an accelerated release of endotoxin liberated during destruction of spirochetes. It is certainly related temporally to disappearance of spirochetes from the blood, and its severity appears to depend upon the speed with which they are removed.

In louse-borne relapsing fever, where the spirochetemia is often intense and the Jarisch-Herxheimer reaction severe, the drug of choice is a repository penicillin such as penicillin aluminum monostearate (PAM). Unlike tetracycline, this drug achieves a very gradual clearing of the spirochetes and a correspondingly mild reaction. The drug is given intramuscularly in a dose of 600,000 units. If the shorter-acting procaine penicillin is used, the dose should be repeated in 12 to 24 h to prevent relapse. In epidemics, a single 0.5-g oral dose of tetracycline, erythromycin, or chloramphenicol can be used with good results.

In tick-borne disease where penicillin is not effective in terminating relapses, tetracycline is most rapidly borrelicidal. This drug should be given in a dose of 0.5 g four times a day for 5 to 10 days. Doxycycline, 100 mg twice daily, is also effective. The Jarisch-Herxheimer reaction tends to be less severe in this form of the disease.

PROGNOSIS When epidemics strike a nonimmune population, the high mortality rate due to the louse-borne disease shows the potential menace of this disease. Most patients, however, recover quickly and completely; relapses do not occur if antibiotic therapy is adequate. Adverse signs are deep jaundice, uncontrolled bleeding, and a grossly prolonged QTc interval.

Typhus and enteric fever may occur simultaneously with louse-borne relapsing fever, and they probably contribute to the mortality rate, particularly during epidemics.

REFERENCES

AHMED MAM et al: Louse-borne relapsing fever in the Sudan. A historical review and a chemico-pathological study. Trop Geogr Med 32:106, 1980

BOYER KM et al: Tick-borne relapsing fever: An interstate outbreak originating at Grand Canyon National Park. Am J Epidemiol 105:469, 1977

BRYCESON ADM et al: Louse-borne relapsing fever: A clinical and laboratory study of 62 cases in Ethiopia and a reconsideration of the literature. Q J Med 39:139, 1970

BUTLER T et al: *Borrelia recurrentis* infection: Single dose antibiotic regimens and management of the Jarisch-Herxheimer reaction. J Infect Dis 137:573, 1978

———: Infection with *Borrelia recurrentis:* Pathogenesis of fever and petechiae. J Infect Dis 140:665, 1979

JUDGE DM et al: Louse-borne relapsing fever in man. Arch Pathol 97:136, 1974

section 9 | Infections caused by higher bacteria and fungi

181
APPROACH TO THE DIAGNOSIS AND TREATMENT OF FUNGAL INFECTIONS

JOHN E. BENNETT

Actinomycetes and fungi are being considered together in this section, but this should not obscure profound differences between these two groups of organisms. The agents of actinomycosis, nocardiosis, and actinomycetoma are actinomycetes. These organisms are gram-positive higher bacteria which branch but have the diameter, antibiotic susceptibility, and ability to induce a neutrophilic inflammatory response in common with other bacteria. Actinomycetes resemble fungi in causing infections which may be extremely chronic and which are poorly transmissible from person to person. Few other similarities exist between fungi and actinomycetes. The remainder of this introductory section will concern mycoses and will not necessarily apply to actinomycete infections.

The diagnosis of a mycosis requires demonstration of the pathogenic fungus in appropriate patient specimens. Visualization of the fungus by smear or histology is a less precise and less sensitive diagnostic method than culture but is more rapid. Culture allows definitive identification of the pathogen and can detect a small number of organisms. False-positives occur with both methods. Artifacts may be mistaken for fungi in smears or histological sections. *Candida albicans* can be isolated from the mouth, vagina, sputum, urine, or stool in the absence of candidiasis. *Aspergillus* and, occasionally, *Cryptococcus neoformans* appear in sputum of patients without a mycosis. Histology has the uniquely valuable potential of demonstrating the fungus within the area of inflammation. Only this method can show whether *Aspergillus* in the lung or paranasal sinus tissue exists as a pathogen or merely as a saprophyte growing in pooled secretions. Demonstration of fungi in tissue section usually requires special stains, such as methenamine silver.

Skin testing with fungal antigens has little diagnostic value in active infection. Serologic testing is very helpful in diagnosing coccidioidomycosis and cryptococcosis, as well as in following response to therapy of these mycoses. In histoplasmosis, and paracoccidioidomycosis, serologic tests are useful in adding some support to the clinical diagnosis. A positive serology may provide the impetus for more aggressive diagnostic maneuvers. Serologic results differ enough between laboratories that the physician must know the individual laboratory's experience and expertise.

Topical therapy of a mycosis can be very effective if the fungus is confined to the epidermis or squamous mucosa. Ringworm, tinea versicolor, and candidiasis of the skin and mucosa often respond to topical therapy, whereas infection of the skin's deeper layers, such as occurs in sporotrichosis, chromomycosis, mycetoma, and blastomycosis, fails to improve with topical drugs.

Systemic antifungal therapy is limited to a few drugs. Most of the oral drugs have a limited spectrum of activity. *Griseofulvin* is effective in many forms of ringworm but in none of the deep mycoses. *Iodide* is helpful in lymphocutaneous sporotrichosis. *Flucytosine* used with low-dose intravenous amphotericin is active against candidiasis, cryptococcosis, and chromomycosis. *Ketoconazole* is a recently marketed, oral antifungal drug that is effective in chronic mucocutaneous candidiasis and, although not approved as yet for this purpose, is helpful in griseofulvin-resistant ringworm. Early studies with ketoconazole have shown improvement in many cases of disseminated coccidioidomycosis and in some cases of blastomycosis and histoplasmosis. The dose, duration, and indications for ketoconazole therapy are not fully established. *Amphotericin B* and *miconazole* are available as topical preparations for candidiasis, but intravenous administration is required for a systemic effect. Intravenous miconazole has little toxicity and little efficacy. It is being eclipsed by the closely related oral drug, ketoconazole. Intravenous amphotericin B is a notoriously toxic drug that, nevertheless, remains the single most effective agent for a wide variety of systemic mycoses, including aspergillosis, blastomycosis, candidiasis, coccidioidomycosis, cryptococcosis, histoplasmosis, mucormycosis, and extraneous sporotrichosis.

A few details about administration and toxicity of the major systemic drugs may help put them into perspective. The first dose of intravenous amphotericin B causes fever, often chills, and sometimes dyspnea. After a 1-mg test dose to assess this reaction, the rapidity of dose escalation will depend on the severity of the reaction and the rapidity with which the infection is progressing. Hydrocortisone hemisuccinate 25 to 50 mg can be added to the infusion to decrease febrile reactions. A therapeutic dose for most mycoses is 0.5 to 0.6 mg/kg every day or 1.0 to 1.2 mg/kg every other day. Azotemia, nausea, anemia, phlebitis, and hypokalemia are usual. Maintenance amphotericin B dosage is 0.3 mg/kg every day when the drug is used with flucytosine. Toxic reactions due to amphotericin B are less severe because of the lower dose, but flucytosine may cause leukopenia, thrombocytopenia, enterocolitis, hepatitis, or rash. Appropriate reductions in flucytosine dosage as amphotericin B–induced azotemia supervenes will decrease bone marrow toxicity. As a rough rule of thumb, the usual flucytosine dosage of 150 mg/kg per day, given in four equal doses, should be reduced in proportion to the rise in serum creatinine; i.e., the dose should be reduced by half for a doubling of the serum creatinine. Azotemia does not influence the metabolism of amphotericin B. Ketoconazole dosage is similarly uninfluenced by renal function. Approved doses are currently 200 to 400 mg per day, though higher doses are being explored. Toxic reactions have been mild and uncommon, consisting of nausea, pruritus, rash, and abnormal liver function.

Intrathecal therapy is necessary in coccidioidal meningitis and occasionally is employed in other mycotic meningitides. Intracisternal, intraventricular, and lumbar intrathecal routes can all be used, but none is free from potential morbidity. Amphotericin B is preferred over miconazole because of inadequate data on the latter. Triweekly doses are increased from 0.05 to 0.5 mg, which is then given two or three times a week. As therapy progresses, injection frequency is reduced. Addition of hydrocortisone 15 mg to the intrathecal injection decreases the severity of adverse reactions.

REFERENCES

BENNETT JE: Treatment of cryptococcal, candidal and coccidioidal meningitis, in *Current Clinical Topics in Infectious Diseases,* JS Remington, M Swartz (eds). New York, McGraw-Hill, 1980, vol 2, pp 54–67

Drugs for treatment of systemic fungal infections. The Medical Letter 24:35, 1982

EMMONS CW: *Medical Mycology.* Philadelphia, Lea & Febiger, 1977

FETTER BF et al: *Mycoses of the Central Nervous System.* Baltimore, Williams & Wilkins, 1967

MCNAIR AL et al: Hepatitis and ketoconazole therapy. Brit Med J 283:1058, 1981

MEDOFF G, KOBAYASHI GS: Strategies in the treatment of systemic fungal infections. N Engl J Med 302:145, 1980

182
ACTINOMYCOSIS AND NOCARDIOSIS

JOHN E. BENNETT

ACTINOMYCOSIS

DEFINITION Actinomycosis is an indolent suppurative infection caused by certain anaerobic actinomycetes. The microorganisms grow within the tissue as grossly visible tightly knit clusters, called *grains.*

ETIOLOGY *Actinomyces israelii* is the usual causative agent, but *A. naeslundii* and *Arachnia propionica* are occasional causes. These gram-positive branching, anaerobic or microaerophilic organisms are the same width as bacteria. When they are cultured on blood agar, small colonies appear after 2 to 4 days of incubation at 37°C under anaerobic conditions. Catalase and other biochemical tests distinguish these organisms from the common skin contaminant *Propionibacterium acnes.* Final identification is best left to a reference laboratory.

PATHOLOGY AND PATHOGENESIS All agents of actinomycosis are commensals in the mouth and gastrointestinal tract of humans. The portal of entry appears to be either a break in the integrity of the mucosa or aspiration into the lung. Poor dental hygiene and dental abscess predispose to oral lesions. Within the gastrointestinal tract, the appendiceal area is the most common site. Infection presents as a chronic suppurative inflammation, usually in the cervicofacial, thoracic, or abdominal area. In histopathologic section, each grain is typically surrounded by polymorphonuclear neutrophils. Adjacent tissue shows subacute or chronic inflammation with extensive fibrosis and formation of sinus tracts. Giant cells are infrequent. The grain stains variably with hematoxylin and eosin. Grains may have an eosinophilic coating composed of human proteins. Hyphal filaments cannot be seen on hematoxylin and eosin stain but may be demonstrated in the periphery of the grain by tissue Gram's stain (such as Brown and Brenn) or by a heavily stained Gomori methenamine silver. These stains may be useful if there is chance for confusion with the grains of eumycetoma or staphylococcal botryomycosis. Grains are a few millimeters in diameter, making them difficult to miss if they are present in the histological section being examined. Several sections may have to be searched to find a grain. Grains may be observed grossly in pus or on bandages covering draining sinuses. These pale yellow, cheese-like particles can be crushed on a microscope slide, and the gram-positive branching filaments demonstrated on Gram's stain.

Infection spreads by direct extension and hematogenously. Direct extension through the skin causes one or more chronic draining sinuses to appear in the abdomen, chest, or cervicofacial area. Hematogenous foci may appear in bone, brain, liver, or other organs.

CLINICAL MANIFESTATIONS *Cervicofacial actinomycosis* presents as a red or purplish firmly indurated subcutaneous mass, typically in the submandibular area or in the anterior cervical triangle near the angle of the mandible. One or more draining sinuses may be present. Tenderness is slight or absent. Lethargy, weight loss, variable low-grade fever, anemia, and leukocytosis are infrequent in cervicofacial actinomycosis but common in *thoracic* and *abdominal actinomycosis.* Localizing findings in the latter forms include draining sinuses and, in thoracic actinomycosis, cough and purulent sputum. Pain or a palpable mass may appear in abdominal actinomycosis. *Pelvic actinomycosis,* once rare, is now being seen in women with an implanted intrauterine device for contraception. The indolent onset, variable low-grade fever, abdominal pain, and adnexal mass may lead to an erroneous diagnosis of pelvic inflammatory disease or tumor. In all forms of actinomycosis, disease typically has been present for weeks or months at time of diagnosis.

Chest x-ray may reveal an area of dense pneumonitis. Fibrosis, empyema, or cavitation may be seen. Periappendiceal abscess may appear as an extrinsic mass on barium enema.

DIAGNOSIS Laboratory tests other than culture or histological section are not helpful. Blood cultures are rarely positive. Isolation of *Actinomyces* or *Arachnia* species from the mouth, sputum, stool, or feculent draining sinuses is not diagnostic. Demonstration of a grain in pus or deep tissue is diagnostic, if botryomycosis and mycetoma can be excluded. Nocardiosis can be distinguished by the absence of grains, identification of the organism in culture, and, usually, by the weak acid-fast staining of *Nocardia.*

TREATMENT Milder cases of actinomycosis, including most cervicofacial infections, respond well to oral tetracycline or penicillin V, an adult dose being 500 mg qid of either drug. Oral erythromycin would be second choice. More severe cases, including many thoracic and abdominal infections, should receive parenteral penicillin G for roughly 6 weeks (in adults 2 to 5 million units per day) followed by prolonged therapy with oral penicillin V or tetracycline. The likelihood of relapse is reduced if the total duration of therapy is 2 to 4 months in mild cases and up to 6 to 12 months in severe forms. Drug resistance has not been encountered in relapses. Curettage of bone lesions, surgical resection of necrotic tissues, and drainage of empyema, brain abscess, or other large collections of pus facilitate recovery but are usually not curative by themselves.

It is common in actinomycosis to isolate microbes other than actinomycetes from pus. In general, the antibiotic susceptibility of these secondary organisms does not have to be considered in the selection of therapeutic agents.

NOCARDIOSIS

DEFINITION Nocardiosis is an acute, subacute, or chronic infection, most often beginning in the lung.

ETIOLOGY *Nocardia asteroides, N. brasiliensis,* and *N. caviae* are the etiologic agents of two different diseases, nocardiosis and mycetoma. In the latter infection, the organism enters the skin by trauma, forms grains within tissue, and spreads slowly to contiguous tissue (see Chap. 186). In nocardiosis, the organism usually enters via the lung, does not form grains, and is prone to hematogenous spread. Even though the etiologic agents of these diseases do overlap, *N. asteroides* causes most cases of nocardiosis and *N. brasiliensis* is the species usually isolated from mycetoma. *Nocardia caviae* is a rare cause of either disease. *Nocardia brasiliensis* can also cause a lymphocutaneous disease closely resembling sporotrichosis; this infection differs from mycetoma by its lymphangitic spread and by the absence of grains.

Nocardia species are aerobic actinomycetes with branching hyphae the same width as bacteria. Hyphae are weakly gram-positive and weakly acid-fast. Growth appears in 2 to 5 days on blood agar, Sabouraud's agar, or other simple media. Incorporation of antibiotics into the media to inhibit bacterial growth usually inhibits *Nocardia* as well. Colonies become rough and chalky with an orange or yellow hue. Identification of *Nocardia* species, including distinction between *Streptomyces, Actinomadura,* and *Nocardia,* is difficult and best assigned to a reference laboratory.

PATHOGENESIS AND PATHOLOGY *Nocardia* is a soil saprophyte widely distributed throughout the world. Infection is acquired from sites in nature, never from infected persons or animals. Males are infected two to three times more commonly than females. No age or exposure is known to predispose to nocardiosis. Many patients have serious preexisting conditions, such as adrenal corticosteroid therapy, cancer, pulmonary alveolar proteinosis, or chronic granulomatous disease of childhood.

Lesions of nocardiosis show suppuration, necrosis, and abscess formation. Neutrophils are the predominant inflammatory cell. Hyphae are scattered throughout the lesion without formation of grains. Tissue Gram's stain or overstained methenamine silver best demonstrates the hyphae. A modified Fite-Faraco stain of histological sections can be used to demonstrate acid-fastness, but this property is not always demonstrable.

CLINICAL MANIFESTATIONS *Nocardia* pneumonia presents with fever and productive cough of several days' or up to several months' duration. The initial illness may resemble a bacterial pneumonia, but slow radiologic progression continues despite antibiotic therapy often with cavitation of radiodense central areas. Hematogenous dissemination to brain and subcutaneous tissue is frequent in nocardiosis. A pulmonary portal is usually but not always detectable clinically. Brain lesions are typically multiple abscesses. Purulent meningitis may result from rupture of an abscess into the ventricle. The subcutaneous lesion typically consists of one or a few indolent abscesses. Hematogenous dissemination to other organs occurs but is rarely detectable clinically.

DIAGNOSIS *Nocardia* is difficult enough to detect in sputum culture, Gram's stain, or histological section so that the diagnosis is readily missed. A progressive pneumonia with purulent sputum should suggest the diagnosis, particularly if cavitation or spread to brain or subcutaneous tissue occurs. Sputum, pus, bronchial brushing, or bronchial washing specimens should be examined by Gram's stain and modified acid-fast stain. On Gram's stain the hyphae are usually branching, beaded, and refractile. They are not strongly gram-positive but take the red counterstain even less well. Conventional acid-fast staining procedures such as Ziehl-Neelsen or a fluorochrome do not stain *Nocardia.* Identification of branching, weakly acid-fast organisms in histological section or smear of pus or sputum is sufficient to establish the diagnosis of nocardiosis. Cultural confirmation is highly desirable, but isolation of *Nocardia* from heavily contaminated specimens is difficult. Isolation of *Nocardia* from otherwise sterile pus is readily accomplished. *Nocardia* is rarely isolated from blood, but diphasic culture media are said to facilitate isolation.

When *Nocardia* is isolated from sputum, the diagnosis of nocardiosis should be suspected, but occasionally no disease can be detected. Rarely, *Nocardia* is an airborne contaminant.

TREATMENT Surgical drainage of empyema and abscesses in brain or subcutaneous tissue is helpful but not sufficient therapy. Virtually all patients should receive prolonged chemotherapy. The treatment of choice is a sulfonamide, given in sufficient dose to maintain a blood concentration of 10 to 15 mg/dl. Sulfadiazine is preferred because of its penetration into the cerebrospinal fluid and other tissues. Also, more experience is available with sulfadiazine than other sulfonamides. The danger of crystalluria and oliguria requires copious fluid intake and urine alkalinization during high-dose sulfadiazine. A reasonable starting regimen is sulfadiazine 100 mg/kg per day and sodium bicarbonate 50 mg/kg per day, both in four divided doses. Patients who show progressive improvement may be changed to sulfisoxazole or trisulfapyrimidines, 60 mg/kg per day after 4 to 6 weeks. Therapy is continued for a total of 12 to 18 months. Relapse may occur up to many months after therapy.

Sulfisoxazole is a reasonable starting drug when fluid loading and urine alkalinization are difficult. Trimethoprim-sulfamethoxazole has been used successfully in a few cases, but the contribution of trimethoprim is unclear. Addition of other antibiotics to sulfa drugs may be indicated in patients who show continued deterioration. Ampicillin 150 mg/kg per day is preferred. High doses of minocycline or erythromycin also have been advocated. Parsimonious use of other drugs during sulfa therapy of nocardiosis minimizes the probability that a drug allergy will necessitate discontinuance of sulfa. Antimicrobial susceptibility tests are used to guide therapy of patients with serious allergic reactions to sulfa drugs, but such regimens are not of proven efficacy.

Survival has been reported in 92 percent of cases with isolated pulmonary nocardiosis compared to 52 percent in cases with brain abscess. Continued use of immunosuppressive therapy seems to impair therapeutic response in nocardiosis.

REFERENCES

Actinomycosis

BARTELS LJ, VRABEC DP: Cervicofacial actinomycosis—A variable disorder. Arch Otolaryngol 104:705, 1978

DAVIES M, KEDDIE NC: Abdominal actinomycosis. Br J Surg 60:18, 1973

FRADIS M et al: Actinomycosis of the face and neck. Arch Otolaryngol 102:87, 1976

HAGER W, MAJMUDAR B: Pelvic actinomycosis in women using intrauterine contraceptive devices. Am J Obstet Gynecol 133:60, 1979

LOMAX CW et al: Actinomycosis of the female genital tract. Obstet Gynecol 48:341, 1976

SLADE PR et al: Thoracic actinomycosis. Thorax 28:73, 1973

Nocardiosis

FRAZIER AR et al: Nocardiosis. A review of 25 cases occurring during 24 months. Mayo Clin Proc 50:657, 1975

GEISELER PJ, ANDERSEN BR: Results of therapy in nocardiosis. Am J Med Sci 278:188, 1979

KRICK JA et al: Nocardia infection in heart transplant patients. Ann Intern Med 82:18, 1975

ZECLER E et al: Lymphocutaneous nocardiosis due to *Nocardia brasiliensis.* Arch Dermatol 113:642, 1977

183

THE DEEP MYCOSES

Cryptococcosis, blastomycosis, histoplasmosis, and coccidioidomycosis

JOHN E. BENNETT

CRYPTOCOCCOSIS

ETIOLOGY Cryptcoccosis is an infection caused by the yeast-like fungus *Cryptococcus neoformans. C. neoformans* reproduces by budding and forms round, yeast-like cells 4 to 6 μm in diameter. Within the host and on certain culture media, a large polysaccharide capsule surrounds each yeast cell. The fungus grows well as smooth, creamy white colonies on Sabouraud's or other simple media at 20 to 37°C. Certain culture media for ringworm contain cycloheximide, which inhibits *C. neoformans.* Identification is based on gross and microscopic appearance, biochemical tests, and growth at 37°C. The fungus has four capsular serotypes, designated A, B, C, and D, and a perfect state called *Filobasidiella neoformans.*

PATHOGENESIS AND PATHOLOGY Infection is thought to be acquired by inhalation of fungus into the lungs. Pulmonary infection has a tendency toward spontaneous resolution and is frequently asymptomatic. Silent hematogenous spread to the brain leads to clusters of cryptococci in the perivascular areas of cortical gray matter, basal ganglia, and, to a lesser extent, other areas of the central nervous system. Inflammatory response around these foci is usually scant. In the more chronic cases, a dense basilar arachnoiditis occurs. Lung lesions show an intense granulomatous inflammation. Cryptococci are best seen in tissue by staining with methenamine silver or periodic acid Schiff. A strongly positive mucicarmine stain of the organism in tissue is diagnostic, but staining varies from intense to absent.

Cryptococcus neoformans has been isolated from several sites in nature, particularly weathered pigeon droppings. Patients are usually unaware of any unusual exposure to pigeon droppings. No significant case clustering, highly endemic areas, or racial or occupational predisposition is known. Infection before puberty is uncommon. The male/female ratio is about 2:1. Approximately half the patients have a predisposing condition, such as lymphoma or sarcoidosis, or are receiving supraphysiological doses of adrenal corticosteroids. Neither neutropenia nor hypogammaglobulinemia seems to increase susceptibility to cryptococcosis. Cryptococcosis occurs in animals, especially the cat family. Transmission from animals to humans or from person to person has never been documented.

CLINICAL MANIFESTATIONS The majority of patients have *meningoencephalitis* at time of diagnosis. This form of the infection is invariably fatal without appropriate therapy, and death occurs anywhere from 2 weeks to several years from onset of symptoms. Early manifestations include headache, nausea, staggering gait, dementia, irritability, confusion, and blurred vision. Both fever and nuchal rigidity are often mild or absent. Papilledema is present in one-third of the patients at time of diagnosis. Cranial nerve palsies, typically asymmetric, occur in about one-fourth of the patients. Other lateralizing signs are rare. With progression of the infection, deepening coma and signs of brainstem compression appear. Autopsy often reveals cerebral edema in the more acute cases or hydrocephalus in more chronic cases.

Pulmonary cryptococcosis causes chest pain in about 40 percent of patients and cough in 20 percent. Chest x-ray shows one or more dense infiltrates, which are often well circumscribed. Cavitation, pleural effusions, or hilar adenopathy are infrequent. Calcification is not present, and fibrotic stranding is rarely noticeable.

Skin lesions are present in 10 percent of patients with cryptococcosis. These appear to be hematogenously disseminated because the vast majority of patients will be found to have disseminated infection. One or a few asymptomatic tiny papular lesions appear, slowly enlarge, and tend to show central softening leading to ulceration. Osteolytic bone lesions occur in 4 percent of patients and usually present as a cold abscess. Rare manifestations of cryptococcosis include prostatitis, endophthalmitis, hepatitis, pericarditis, endocarditis, and renal abscess.

DIAGNOSIS Cryptococcal meningoencephalitis must be distinguished from tuberculosis, neoplasm, coccidioidomycosis, histoplasmosis, candidiasis, viral aseptic meningitis, and sarcoidosis. Focal lesions are virtually never demonstrable in cryptococcosis by technetium brain scan, cerebral angiography, or electroencephalogram. Computerized tomography (CT) scan will occasionally show one or two sharply demarcated radiodense masses with a central area of lesser density. Lumbar puncture is the single most useful test. An India ink smear of centrifuged spinal fluid sediment reveals encapsulated yeast in one-half the cases, but artifacts resembling cryptococci may cause confusion. Cerebrospinal fluid glucose is reduced in half the cases, protein concentration is usually increased, and 20 to 600 leukocytes per cubic millimeter are typically present and consist predominantly of lymphocytes. Approximately 90 percent of patients with cryptococcal meningoencephalitis, including all those with a positive cerebrospinal fluid smear, will have capsular antigen detectable in cerebrospinal fluid or serum by latex agglutination. False-positive tests occur occasionally, making culture the definitive diagnostic test. *C. neoformans* is often present in urine in patients with meningoencephalitis. Fungemia occurs in only 10 percent of patients and portends a lethal outcome.

Pulmonary cryptococcosis mimics malignancy by x-ray and symptoms. Sputum culture is positive in only 10 percent, and serum antigen tests are positive in only a third. Occasionally, *C. neoformans* appears in one or multiple sputum specimens as an endobronchial saprophyte. Biopsy is usually required for diagnosis of pulmonary cryptococcosis. Cutaneous cryptococcosis may be mistaken for a comedone, basal-cell carcinoma, or sarcoidosis. Biopsy reveals a myriad of cryptococci. Osseous cryptococcosis resembles tuberculosis.

TREATMENT Cryptococcal meningoencephalitis may be treated either with the regimen of flucytosine plus low-dose amphotericin B, outlined in Chap. 181, or with full-dose amphotericin B. Lesser nephrotoxicity and more rapid culture conversion with the combination have led to its general acceptance. With either regimen, approximately 50 to 70 percent of patients can be cured. Treatment with either regimen is continued for at least 6 weeks and until at least four weekly cultures of 2 to 4 ml cerebrospinal fluid are sterile. Intrathecal amphotericin B is usually reserved for treatment of severely azotemic patients not receiving dialysis or for patients who have relapsed. Permanent sequelae include dementia, personality change, hydrocephalus, and blindness.

Patients with extraneural cryptococcosis most often require intravenous amphotericin B, with or without flucytosine. Observation or excision of lesions may suffice for some patients who are previously normal, who have a single focus in lung, skin, or bone, and who have no cryptococci in the cerebrospinal fluid, urine, or blood. All too often, however, patients who present with a presumed single focus of extracranial cryptococcosis are discovered to have early asymptomatic meningoencephalitis or dissemination to other organs.

BLASTOMYCOSIS

ETIOLOGY *Blastomyces dermatitidis* is a dimorphic fungus, growing at room temperature as a white or tan mold but growing within the host or at 37°C as budding, round yeast-like cells. The fungus is identified by its appearance, its dimorphism, and by the appearance of small spores borne on hyphae of the mold form. When isolates of the two opposite mating types are grown closely together on specialized culture media, sporulating structures appear which characterize the perfect form, *Ajellomyces dermatitidis*.

PATHOGENESIS AND PATHOLOGY The infection is restricted by geography and age. Blastomycosis is uncommon in any locality, but the majority of cases have occurred in the southeast, central and midatlantic areas of the United States, with occasional cases in other localities in the United States and Canada. Cases have also been encountered in Africa, Mexico, Central America, and, rarely, South America. Eighty-seven percent of patients are between 20 and 69 years old. The male/female ratio is about 10:1. There is no occupational predisposition.

Infection appears to be acquired by inhalation of the fungus from nature, but the reservoir remains unknown. To date, the fungus has been isolated only from infected humans or animals. No carrier state or transmission from animal to human or from person to person has been observed. The initial pulmonary infection may heal spontaneously or become chronic. Spread to other portions of the lung, cavitation, or endobronchial lesions may appear in chronic cases. Whether or not the lung lesion resolves spontaneously, infection commonly spreads hematogenously to skin, subcutaneous tissue, bone, prostate, epididymis, or mucosa of the nose, mouth, or larynx. Less commonly, infection spreads to the brain, meninges, liver, lymph nodes, or spleen. Dissemination may not be evident for weeks or years after the appearance of the lung lesion. Progressive infection is only rarely attributable to an underlying disease or immunosuppressive treatment. The inflammatory response includes lymphocytes, giant cells, and neutrophils. Pseudoepitheliomatous hyperplasia may be striking and lead to a mistaken diagnosis of squamous-cell carcinoma.

CLINICAL MANIFESTATIONS A small number of patients have been documented to have an acute, self-limited pneumonia. Fever, productive cough, myalgia, and malaise usually have resolved within a month. Pulmonary infiltrates have cleared slowly as *B. dermatitidis* disappeared from the sputum. Laboratory exposure or case clusters in certain geographic sites have suggested the diagnosis in many of these cases. In one such case cluster, the incubation period appeared to be 4 weeks. In none of these case clusters has the exact activity leading to exposure been identified.

The vast majority of patients with blastomycosis have an indolent onset and a chronically progressive course. Fever, cough, weight loss, lassitude, skin lesions, and chest ache are common symptoms. Skin lesions favor exposed areas and enlarge over many weeks from a pimple to a well-circumscribed, verrucous, crusted, or ulcerated lesion. Pain and regional lymphadenopathy are minimal. Large chronic lesions may show central healing with scarring and contracture. Mucous membrane lesions resemble squamous-cell carcinoma. Chest x-ray is abnormal in two-thirds of cases, with one or more pneumonic or nodular infiltrates. Calcification, hilar adenopathy, and large pleural effusions are rare. Osteolytic lesions may occur in nearly any bone and present as cold abscess or a draining sinus. Extension to a contiguous joint may cause indolent swelling, pain, and restricted motion. Prostatic and epididymal lesions resemble tuberculosis clinically.

DIAGNOSIS The diagnosis is made best by demonstrating the fungus in culture of sputum, pus, or urine. In experienced hands, diagnosis by appearance of the organism in wet smear or histopathologic section is adequate. The fungus may be visible in a sputum cytology smear but is easily overlooked. Skin tests and serologic tests lack sufficient sensitivity and specificity to be useful.

TREATMENT A few patients have been observed with transitory lung lesions, but no guidelines are known to distinguish these patients from those who will progress locally or disseminate. Therefore, every patient should receive intravenous amphotericin B. Skin and noncavitary lung lesions should be treated for about 8 to 10 weeks. Recommended total dose for an adult is about 2.0 g. Cavitary lung disease or infection beyond the lung and skin should be treated for about 10 to 12 weeks with 2.5 g or more. Hydroxystilbamidine is less effective and rarely indicated. Iodide therapy is ineffective. The mortality rate in appropriately treated cases is 15 percent or less.

HISTOPLASMOSIS

ETIOLOGY *Histoplasma capsulatum* is a dimorphic fungus that grows in nature or on Sabouraud's agar at room temperature as a mold. Hyphae bear both large and small spores that are used for identification. *H. capsulatum* grows as a small budding yeast in host tissue and on enriched agar, such as blood cysteine glucose, at 37°C. Despite the name, the fungus is unencapsulated. When two isolates of the opposite mating type, both in mold form, are grown closely together on an appropriate culture medium, specialized spore-bearing structures are formed which characterize the perfect state, *Emmonsiella capsulata.*

PATHOGENESIS AND PATHOLOGY Infection with *H. capsulatum* has been encountered in many areas of the world but is much more frequent in certain areas. Within the United States infection is more common in the southeastern, midatlantic, and central states than in other areas. Endemic areas are probably determined by the availability of proper conditions in nature for growth of the fungus. *H. capsulatum* prefers moist surface soil, particularly when it is enriched by droppings of certain birds and bats. The fungus has not only been isolated repeatedly from such sites but many case clusters have occurred 5 to 18 days after groups were exposed to such dust, for example, by raking, cleaning dirt-floored chicken coops, bulldozing, or cave exploring. In many endemic areas, 80 percent or more of residents over age 16 have been exposed, judging by skin test reactivity.

Microconidia, or small spores, of *H. capsulatum* are small enough to reach the alveoli on inhalation and are transformed to budding forms. With time, an intense granulomatous reaction occurs. Caseation necrosis or calcification may mimic tuberculosis. The primary infection in children usually heals completely but may leave spotty calcification in the hilar nodes or lung. Transient dissemination may leave calcified granulomas in the spleen. In adults, a rounded mass of scar tissue, with or without central calcification, may remain in the lung. This has been called a *histoplasmoma.* Previous exposure is thought to confer some protection against reinfection, but infection of persons with prior positive skin tests clearly has occurred.

In a small proportion of patients, histoplasmosis becomes a progressive, potentially fatal infection. The disease occurs either as chronic fibrocavitary pneumonia or, less commonly, as disseminated infection. Patients with either form lack a history of acute primary pulmonary histoplasmosis. Chronic pulmonary infection favors otherwise healthy males over the age of 40 years. A history of cigarette use can be elicited from nearly all patients with chronic progressive pulmonary histoplasmosis. An acute, rapidly fatal course is most likely to be encountered in young children and immunosuppressed patients. A more chronic but equally lethal disseminated infection is more common in previously healthy adults.

CLINICAL MANIFESTATIONS The vast majority of infections are either asymptomatic or mild, and the diagnosis is elusive. Cough, fever, malaise, and chest x-ray findings of hilar adenopathy with or without one or more areas of pneumonitis occur. Erythema nodosum and erythema multiforme have been reported in a few outbreaks. Hilar adenopathy may cause temporary compression of the right middle lobe bronchus in children and young adults. Subacute pericarditis may occur, probably by extension from contiguous lymph nodes. Rarely, many hilar nodes undergo a caseous, granulomatous reaction with perinodal fibrosis. Mediastinal structures become encased by progressive fibrosis, and, over many years, compression of the pulmonary veins, superior vena cava, pulmonary arteries, and esophagus may occur. Late in mediastinal disease only rare nonviable histoplasma can be found in caseous residua of lymph nodes.

Patients with chronic pulmonary histoplasmosis have a gradual onset over weeks or months of increasing productive cough, weight loss, and sometimes nightsweats. Chest x-ray reveals uni- or bilateral fibronodular apical infiltrates. Approximately one-third of cases will stabilize or improve spontaneously early in the course. The remainder have insidious progression. Retraction and cavitation of the upper lobes occur with spread to the apex of the lower lobes and other areas of the lung. Emphysema and bullae formation further compromise pulmonary function. Death from cor pulmonale, bacterial pneumonia, or histoplasmosis occurs after months or years.

Acute disseminated histoplasmosis may be mistaken for miliary tuberculosis (see Chap. 174). Common findings include fever, emaciation, hepatosplenomegaly, lymphadenopathy, jaundice, anemia, leukopenia, and thrombocytopenia. All these features may occur in chronic dissemination, but the disease tends to be more localized. Indurated ulcers of the mouth, tongue, nose, or larynx occur in about a fourth of patients. Other focal findings include granulomatous hepatitis, Addison's disease, gastrointestinal ulceration, endocarditis, and chronic meningitis. Chest x-ray abnormalities occur in half the cases and show discrete nodules or a miliary pattern.

The presumed ocular histoplasmosis syndrome is a distinct clinical form of uveitis. Although a positive histoplasmin skin test is a requisite for diagnosis, none of these patients has had active histoplasmosis.

DIAGNOSIS Histoplasmosis may be suspected by serologic tests and clinical manifestations, but definitive diagnosis requires demonstration of the organism by culture or histology. Serologic tests are performed with either histoplasmin, a culture filtrate, or whole yeast form cells. The results are interchangeable. Complement fixation is quantifiable and is the best test. Agar gel diffusion with histoplasmin is a useful but not quantifiable test. Frequent false-negatives and false-positives limit all current serologic tests. Serologic conversion is helpful but occurs rarely except in acute pulmonary histoplasmosis. Higher complement fixation titers, such as 1:32 or greater, are most suggestive of the diagnosis, but no titer is diagnostic. Cross-reactions with serologic tests for blastomycosis are very common. A 5-mm or more diameter area of induration 24 to 48 h after skin testing with histoplasmin has been very helpful in identifying prior exposure to histoplasma, but false negatives and false positives are so frequent that skin testing has little value in the study of ill patients. Further, approximately one-fifth of normal volunteers with a positive skin test will convert their histoplasmin serology from negative to positive after skin testing.

Culture of *H. capsulatum* from sputum is difficult but is the procedure of choice in chronic pulmonary histoplasmosis. Digestion by proteolytic enzymes and centrifugation of sputum are helpful. In disseminated histoplasmosis, cultures of bone marrow, blood, centrifuged urine sediment, and biopsy specimens are most often positive. Cultures should be performed on agar surfaces of enriched media at room temperature. Growth occurs in 2 to 6 weeks. Histological sections of bone marrow, liver, lymph node, lung, and mucosal lesions may yield the diagnosis.

TREATMENT Acute pulmonary histoplasmosis requires no therapy. Mediastinal fibrosis may benefit by surgery, but the ultimate progress is poor. All patients with disseminated or chronic fibronodular pulmonary histoplasmosis should receive intravenous amphotericin B. Rapid culture conversion and a cure rate in excess of 50 percent can be achieved in both forms, but a formidable relapse rate after short courses has led to use of a 10- to 12-week course of 0.4 to 0.6 mg/kg per day. In chronic pulmonary histoplasmosis, chest x-ray abnormalities improve somewhat, but pulmonary function improves very little. Successful therapy prevents progression. Addisonian crisis is a preventable cause of death in disseminated histoplasmosis.

AFRICAN HISTOPLASMOSIS Patients have been encountered in Africa who seem to be infected with *H. capsulatum* except that the yeast form is larger. Clinical manifestations resemble blastomycosis more than histoplasmosis because skin and bone lesions are very common.

COCCIDIOIDOMYCOSIS

ETIOLOGY *Coccidioides immitis* has two forms, growing as a white fluffy mold on most culture media but as a nonbudding spherical form, a spherule, in host tissue or under specialized conditions. Reproduction in the host tissue is by formation of small endospores within mature spherules. After rupture of the spherule, the released endospores enlarge, become spherules, and repeat the cycle. The fungus is identified by its appearance and by formation of thick-walled, barrel-shaped spores, called *arthrospores,* in the hyphae of the mold form.

PATHOGENESIS AND PATHOLOGY *C. immitis* is a soil saprophyte in certain arid regions of the United States, Mexico, Central America, and South America. Within the United States, most cases are acquired in California, Arizona, West Texas, and New Mexico. A few cases are acquired in bordering areas and by exposure to fomites from endemic areas, such as cotton bales.

Infection in humans and animals results from inhalation of wind-borne arthrospores arising from soil sites. This primary pulmonary infection is symptomatic in only 40 percent of individuals, with symptoms ranging from a mild, influenza-like illness to severe pneumonia. Mild, self-limited infections may come to medical attention because of case clusters or hypersensitivity reactions: erythema nodosum, erythema multiforme, toxic erythema, arthralgia, arthritis, conjunctivitis, or episcleritis. Case clusters occur 10 to 14 days after a group of susceptible individuals is exposed to dust in an endemic area through such activities as unearthing Indian relics, rock hunting, military maneuvers, or construction. Wind storms can carry spores to adjacent nonendemic areas and cause case clusters. The usual course of primary pulmonary infection is complete healing, though an area of pneumonitis on x-ray may heal by forming a coin-like lesion, or coccidioidoma. Less commonly, a single thin-walled cavity remains as a chronic sequela in the area of consolidation. Also, the consolidation may persist as a chronic pneumonia or progress to fibronodular, cavitary disease.

Pleural effusion may be the only manifestation of primary infection. Self-healing of this form is common.

An uncommon but dreaded complication of coccidioidomycosis is dissemination beyond the lung and hilar lymph nodes. Dissemination is more frequent in blacks, Filipinos, native Americans, Mexican-Americans, and pregnant or immunosuppressed patients.

C. immitis incites a chronic granulomatous reaction in host tissue, often with caseation necrosis. Lung and hilar node lesions may show calcification. Both IgM and IgG antibodies against *C. immitis* are induced by infection but neither appears protective. The amount of specific IgG antibody is a rough measure of the antigenic mass, i.e., of the amount of infection, making a high titer a poor prognostic sign. Appearance of delayed hypersensitivity to antigens of *C. immitis* is most common in those clinical forms of disease with a good prognosis, such as self-limited primary pulmonary disease. Negative skin tests to *Coccidioides* antigens occur in roughly half the patients with disseminated disease and portend a poor prognosis.

CLINICAL MANIFESTATIONS Symptomatic primary pulmonary infection is manifested by fever, cough, chest pain, malaise, and sometimes hypersensitivity reactions. Chest x-ray may show an infiltrate, hilar adenopathy, or pleural effusion. Peripheral blood may show a mild eosinophilia. Spontaneous improvement begins after several days to 2 weeks of illness and usually culminates in complete recovery.

The symptoms of a chronic thin-walled cavity include cough or hemoptysis in half the cases; the other patients are asymptomatic. Chronic progressive pulmonary coccidioidomycosis produces cough, sputum, variable degrees of fever, and weight loss. The first indications of dissemination usually appear during the primary infection. Reactivation with dissemination in later years occurs occasionally, especially if Hodgkin's disease, non-Hodgkin's lymphoma, renal transplantation, or other immunosuppression has supervened. Dissemination should be suspected when fever, malaise, hilar or paratracheal lymphadenopathy, and elevated sedimentation rate show abnormal persistence in patients with primary pulmonary coccidioidomycosis. High complement fixation titers support this concern. With time, lesions appear in the bone, skin, subcutaneous tissue, meninges, joints, and other sites. Without therapy, dissemination may progress rapidly to death or wax and wane for years.

DIAGNOSIS When coccidioidomycosis is suspected, sputum, urine, and pus should be examined for *C. immitis* by wet smear and culture. *The laboratory request should indicate clearly that coccidioidomycosis is suspected because the mold form must be handled with extreme care to prevent infection of laboratory personnel.* On biopsy, smaller spherules must be distinguished from nonbudding forms of *Blastomyces* and *Cryptococcus,* but appearance of the mature spherule is diagnostic.

Serologic tests are very helpful in coccidioidomycosis. Latex agglutination and agar gel diffusion tests are useful in screening serums for antibody to coccidioides. The complement fixation test is used on cerebrospinal fluid and to confirm and quantitate serum antibody detected by screening tests. The number of cases with a positive complement fixation test will depend upon the severity of disease and upon the laboratory performing the test. Positive tests are least common in patients with solitary pulmonary cavities or primary pulmonary infection, while serums from patients with multiorgan disseminated disease are nearly all positive. Seroconversion is helpful in primary pulmonary coccidioidomycosis but may not occur for up to 8 weeks after onset. A positive complement fixation test in unconcentrated cerebrospinal fluid is diagnostic of meningitis.

Conversion of the skin test from negative to positive (≥ 5 mm induration at 24 or 48 h) with either coccidioidin or spherulin, the two commercially available antigens, may be observed between the third and twenty-first days of symptoms in primary pulmonary coccidioidomycosis. Skin testing can also be helpful in epidemiologic studies, such as investigation of case clusters or definition of endemic areas. The utility of skin testing as a diagnostic tool is limited by the presence of persistent positive tests resulting from remote exposures to coccidioides and by the frequency of negative skin tests in many patients with either thin-walled cavities or disseminated coccidioidomycosis.

TREATMENT Primary pulmonary coccidioidomycosis usually resolves spontaneously. Some physicians give a few weeks of intravenous amphotericin B when patients show an unusually severe or protracted primary infection, hoping to abort disseminated or chronic pulmonary disease. There is no solid evidence to support this practice, but the stronger the suspicion of dissemination becomes in any given patient, the more logical this approach appears. Once evidence for dissemination becomes incontrovertible, amphotericin B may be palliative rather than curative. Incomplete recovery and relapse after apparent cure with amphotericin B have been distressingly common in both disseminated and chronic progressive pulmonary infection. The low toxicity and possibility of long-term oral therapy with ketoconazole have encouraged study of this drug in nonmeningeal coccidioidomycosis. Doses of 200 to 400 mg per day have improved many patients with skin, bone, and lung coccidioidomycosis, but occurrences of slow, incomplete responses as well as relapses are now prompting courses of 12 months or longer. Higher doses are being explored. As yet, there is reluctance to treat a seriously ill or rapidly deteriorating patient with this new drug. Such patients are given intravenous amphotericin B 0.5 to 0.7 mg/kg daily or double dose on alternate days until infection appears relatively quiescent, often 10 or 12 weeks. More prolonged courses may be changed to 1.0 mg/kg three times a week. Surgical debridement of bone lesions and drainage of abscesses contribute to cure. Resection of chronic progressive pulmonary lesions is a helpful adjunct to chemotherapy when infection is confined to the lung and in one lobe. A single thin-walled cavity tends to close spontaneously, and ordinarily is not resected. Such a cavity responds poorly to chemotherapy. Coccidioidal meningitis is treated with long-term intrathecal amphotericin B. Hydrocephalus, a frequent complication, renders this therapy less effective. The prognosis in all forms of chronic progressive coccidioidomycosis must be guarded.

REFERENCES

Blastomycosis

BLASTOMYCOSIS COOPERATIVE STUDY OF THE VETERANS ADMINISTRATION: Blastomycosis: I. A review of 198 collected cases in Veterans Administration Hospitals. Am Rev Resp Dis 89:659, 1964

CUSH R et al: Clinical and roentgenographic manifestations of acute and chronic blastomycosis. Chest 69:345, 1976

SAROSI GA, DAVIES SF: Blastomycosis. Am Rev Resp Dis 120:911, 1979

WITORSCH P, UTZ JP: North American blastomycosis: A study of 40 patients. Medicine 47:169, 1968

Coccidioidomycosis

BOUZA E et al: Coccidioidal meningitis. An analysis of thirty-one cases and review of the literature. Medicine 60:139, 1980

DERESINSKI SC, STEVENS DA: Coccidioidomycosis in compromised hosts. Medicine 54:377, 1974

DRUTZ DJ, CATANZARO A: Coccidioidomycosis. Am Rev Resp Dis 117:559, 727, 1978

SALOMON NW et al: Surgical manifestations and results of treatment of pulmonary coccidioidomycosis. Ann Thorac Surg 30:433, 1980

STEVENS DA (ed): *Coccidioidomycosis: A Primer for the Clinician.* New York, Plenum, 1980

Cryptococcosis

BENNETT JE et al: A comparison of amphotericin B alone and combined with flucytosine in treatment of cryptococcal meningitis. N Engl J Med 301:126, 1979

DIAMOND RD, BENNETT JE: Prognostic factors in cryptococcal meningitis. Ann Intern Med 80:176, 1974

KERKERING TW et al: The evolution of pulmonary cryptococcosis. Ann Intern Med 94:611, 1981

Histoplasmosis

GOODWIN RA et al: Chronic pulmonary histoplasmosis. Medicine 55:413, 1976

——— et al: Disseminated histoplasmosis: Clinical and pathological correlations. Medicine 59:1, 1980

——— et al: Histoplasmosis in normal hosts. Medicine 60:231, 1981

KAUFFMAN CA et al: Histoplasmosis in immunosuppressed patients. Am J Med 64:923, 1978

PARKER JD et al: Treatment of chronic pulmonary histoplasmosis. N Engl J Med 283:225, 1970

184 THE OPPORTUNISTIC DEEP MYCOSES

Candidiasis, aspergillosis, and mucormycosis

JOHN E. BENNETT

CANDIDIASIS

ETIOLOGY *Candida albicans* is the most common cause of candidiasis, but *C. tropicalis, C. parapsilosis, C. guilliermondii, C. krusei,* and a few other species can cause candidiasis and may even be fatal. *C. parapsilosis* is particularly notable for its ability to cause endocarditis. All *Candida* species pathogenic for humans are also encountered as commensals of humans, particularly in the mouth, stool, and vagina. These species grow rapidly at 25 to 37°C on simple media as oval budding cells. In specialized agar media, hyphae or elongated branching structures called *pseudohyphae* are formed. *C. albicans* can be identified presumptively by its ability to form germ tubes in serum or by the formation of thick-walled large spores, called *chlamydospores.* Final identification of all species requires biochemical tests.

PATHOGENESIS AND PATHOLOGY Either local or systemic factors may lead to tissue invasion by *Candida.* Chronic maceration predisposes to cutaneous candidiasis, as in diaper rash, intertrigo in obese patients, or paronychia in bartenders or cannery workers. Age is important because neonatal colonization often leads to oral candidiasis (thrush). Women in the third trimester of pregnancy are prone to vulvovaginal thrush. Patients with diabetes mellitus or hematologic malignancy, or who are receiving broad-spectrum antibiotics or supraphysiologic doses of adrenal corticosteroids, are especially susceptible to candidiasis. Breaks in the integrity of the skin or mucous membranes may provide access to deeper tissues. Examples include perforation of the gastrointestinal tract by trauma, surgery, and peptic ulceration; indwelling catheters for intravenous alimentation, peritoneal dialysis, and urinary tract drainage; severe burns and intravenous drug abuse.

Candida grows within tissues in both yeast and pseudohyphal forms. Rarely, only one form is present. Visceral lesions are characterized by necrosis and a neutrophilic inflammatory response. Neutrophils kill *Candida* yeast cells and damage segments of pseudohyphae in vitro, suggesting a major role for the neutrophil in host defense against this fungus. Visceral lesions show a preference for kidney, brain, spleen, heart, and liver.

CLINICAL MANIFESTATIONS *Oral thrush* presents as discrete and confluent adherent white plaques on the oral and pharyngeal mucosa, particularly in the mouth and tongue. These lesions are usually painless, but fissuring at the corners of the mouth can be painful. *Cutaneous candidiasis* presents as red, macerated intertriginous areas, paronychia, balanitis, or pruritus ani. Candidiasis of the perineal and scrotal skin may be accompanied by discrete pustular lesions on the inner aspects of the thighs. *Chronic mucocutaneous candidiasis* or *Candida* granuloma typically presents as circumscribed hyperkeratotic skin lesions, crumbling dystrophic nails, partial alopecia in areas of scalp lesions, and both oral and vaginal thrush. Systemic infection is very rare, but disfigurement of the face and hands can be severe. Other findings may include chronic epidermophytosis, dental dysplasia, and hypofunction of the parathyroid, adrenal, or thyroid glands. A variety of defects in T-cell function have been described in these patients. Vulvovaginal thrush causes pruritus, discharge, and sometimes pain on intercourse or urination. Speculum examination reveals an inflamed mucosa and a thin exudate, often with white curds.

From one to multiple small shallow ulcerations due to *Candida* may appear in the esophagus or gastrointestinal tract. Esophageal lesions favor the distal third and may cause dysphagia or substernal pain. Other such lesions tend to be asymptomatic but assume importance in the leukemic patient as a portal for disseminated candidiasis. Within the urinary tract, the most common lesions are either hematogenously disseminated renal abscesses, which can cause azotemia, or bladder thrush. Bladder invasion usually follows catheterization or instrumentation of a patient with diabetes mellitus or who is receiving broad-spectrum antibiotics. This lesion generally is asymptomatic and benign. Rarely, retrograde invasion of the renal pelvis leads to renal papillary necrosis.

Hematogenous dissemination of Candida presents with fever and toxicity but with few localizing findings. One or more retinal abscesses may appear and extend slowly into the vitreous humor. The patient may note orbital pain, blurred vision, scotoma, or opacities floating across the visual field. Pulmonary candidiasis is almost always hematogenous and is visible on chest x-ray only when the abscesses are numerous enough to cause a diffuse, vaguely nodular infiltrate. Candidiasis of the endocardium or around intracardiac prostheses resembles bacterial infection of these sites. Chronic *Candida* meningitis or arthritis may occur, from either disseminated disease or insertion of a plastic prosthesis in the case of arthritis. Rare focal manifestations of disseminated disease include osteomyelitis, pustular skin lesions, myositis, and brain abscess.

DIAGNOSIS Demonstration of pseudohyphae on wet smear with confirmation by culture is the procedure of choice for diagnosing superficial candidiasis. Scrapings for the smear may be obtained from skin, nails, and oral and vaginal mucosa. Culture alone is not diagnostic.

Deeper lesions of *Candida* may be diagnosed by histological section of biopsy specimens or by culture of cerebrospinal fluid, blood, joint fluid, or surgical specimens. Blood culture in vented bottles is very useful in *Candida* endocarditis but is positive less often in other forms of disseminated disease. The utility of serodiagnosis remains controversial.

TREATMENT Cutaneous candidiasis of macerated areas responds to measures which reduce moisture and chafing plus a topically applied antifungal agent in a nonocclusive base. Nystatin, clotrimazole, miconazole, and amphotericin B appear roughly equivalent. The first three of these are available also for vaginal application. Oral candidiasis should be treated with nystatin suspension. Swallowing nystatin suspension or sucking on the tablets compounded for vaginal use may improve symptoms of esophageal candidiasis. When esophageal symptoms are pronounced, a 5- to 10-day course of intravenous amphotericin B, 0.3 mg/kg per day, may be beneficial. Bladder thrush responds to bladder irrigations with amphotericin B, 50 μg/ml for 5 days. In all forms of skin and mucosal candidiasis, relapse after successful treatment is common.

Intravenous amphotericin B is the drug of choice in disseminated candidiasis. The drug is usually given as 0.4 to 0.5 mg/kg every day or as a double dose on alternate days for several weeks. In patients with no contraindication to the use of flucytosine, administration of that drug in dosage of 100 to 150 mg/kg per day plus amphotericin B, 0.3 mg/kg per day, is an effective alternative. Ketoconazole in an adult dose of 200 mg daily is probably the drug of choice for chronic mucocutaneous candidiasis. The efficacy of the drug in systemic candidiasis is unknown.

Candida isolated from a properly obtained blood culture should be considered significant, for true false positives are rare. Whether a patient with candidiasis should receive antifungal therapy will depend on the degree of illness and the likelihood of spontaneous recovery. For example, a febrile, severely immunosuppressed patient with one positive blood culture should receive prompt therapy because a rapidly fatal course is common. A nonimmunosuppressed patient acquiring candidiasis from an indwelling intravenous plastic catheter may recover spontaneously if the catheter is removed promptly. The species of *Candida* is irrelevant to this decision. Patients with candidiasis in whom antifungal therapy is withheld should be observed carefully for the development of endophthalmitis, endocarditis, arthritis, osteomyelitis, or other visceral lesions that require therapy.

ASPERGILLOSIS

ETIOLOGY *Aspergillus fumigatus* is the most common pathogen, but *A. flavus, A. niger,* and several other species can cause disease. *Aspergillus* is a mold with septate hyphae about 4 μm in diameter. Sporulating structures, called *conidial heads,* may be seen when the fungus is growing in nature, on an artificial medium, or within air-containing spaces of the body. The appearance of the colonies and of conidial heads is used for identification.

PATHOGENESIS AND PATHOLOGY All the common species of *Aspergillus* which cause disease in humans are ubiquitous in the environment, growing on dead leaves, stored grain, compost piles, hay, and other decaying vegetation. Inhalation of *Aspergillus* spores must be extremely common, but disease is rare. Invasion of lung tissue is almost entirely confined to immunosuppressed patients. Roughly 90 percent will have two of these three conditions: less than 500 granulocytes per cubic millimeter of peripheral blood, supraphysiological doses of adrenal corticosteroids, and a history of taking cytotoxic drugs such as azathioprine. Infection in such patients is characterized by hyphal invasion of blood vessels, thrombosis, necrosis, and hemorrhagic infarction. Chronic granulomatous disease of childhood also predisposes to invasive pulmonary aspergillosis, but here the inflammatory response is granulomatous. Blood vessel invasion is rare.

Massive inhalation of *Aspergillus* spores by normal persons can lead to an acute, diffuse, self-limited pneumonitis. Epithelioid granulomas with giant cells and central pyogenic areas containing hyphae are seen. Spontaneous recovery taking several weeks is the usual course.

Aspergillus can colonize the damaged bronchial tree, pulmonary cysts, or cavities of patients with underlying lung disease. Balls of hyphae within cysts or cavities may reach several centimeters in diameter and be visible on chest x-ray. Tissue invasion does not occur. The term *allergic bronchial aspergillosis* denotes the condition of patients with preexisting asthma who have eosinophilia, IgE antibody to *Aspergillus*, and fleeting pulmonary infiltrates from bronchial plugging. Some of these asthmatic patients also have endobronchial colonization with *Aspergillus*. It is not clear what role *Aspergillus* plays in noninvasive lung disease. Plugs of hyphae may obstruct bronchi. Perhaps allergic or toxic reactions to *Aspergillus* antigens cause bronchial constriction and damage.

CLINICAL MANIFESTATIONS *Endobronchial pulmonary aspergillosis* presents as chronic productive cough and often hemoptysis in a patient with prior chronic lung disease, such as tuberculosis, sarcoidosis, bronchiectasis, or histoplasmosis. *Aspergilloma* refers to a ball of hyphae within a lung cyst or cavity, usually in the upper lobe. *Aspergillus* may be spread from its endocavitary or endobronchial site to the pleura during the course of bacterial lung abscess or surgery.

Invasive aspergillosis in the immunosuppressed host presents as an acute pneumonia. Infection progresses by hematogenous spread as well as extension to surrounding lung and other contiguous structures. Occasionally the portal of infection in the immunosuppressed host is the paranasal sinus, gastrointestinal tract, skin, or palate.

Aspergillus sinusitis in nonimmunosuppressed patients may take two forms. A ball of hyphae may form in a chronically obstructed paranasal sinus, without tissue invasion. Much less commonly, a chronic, fibrosing granulomatous inflammation with scanty *Aspergillus* hyphae within tissue may begin in the sinus and spread slowly to the orbit and brain.

Growth of *Aspergillus* on cerumen and detritus within the external auditory canal is termed *otomycosis*. Trauma to the cornea may cause chronic *Aspergillus* keratitis. Endophthalmitis follows introduction of *Aspergillus* into the globe by trauma or surgery. *Aspergillus* may infect intracardiac or intravascular prostheses.

DIAGNOSIS Culture of *Aspergillus* from sputum usually has no diagnostic significance. Repeated isolation of *Aspergillus* from sputum or demonstration of hyphae in the sputum smear suggests endobronchial colonization. Fungus ball of the lung is usually detectable by chest x-ray. Antibody of the IgG class to *Aspergillus* antigens is demonstrable in the serum of many colonized patients and of virtually all patients with fungus ball.

Biopsy is usually required to diagnose invasive aspergillosis of the lung, paranasal sinus, or sites of dissemination. Blood cultures are rarely positive, even in patients with infected cardiac prosthetic valves. *Aspergillus* hyphae can be identified presumptively by histology, but culture is required for confirmation and determination of species. Serologic and skin tests have not proved helpful in invasive aspergillosis.

TREATMENT Patients with severe hemoptysis due to fungus ball of the lung may benefit by lobectomy. Poor pulmonary function in residual lung and dense pleural adhesions around the lesion can complicate the resection. Systemic chemotherapy is of no value in endobronchial or endocavitary aspergillosis.

Intravenous amphotericin B has resulted in arrest or cure of invasive aspergillosis when immunosuppression is not severe. Combined flucytosine–amphotericin B may be useful in nonneutropenic patients with invasive aspergillosis.

MUCORMYCOSIS (ZYGOMYCOSIS, PHYCOMYCOSIS)

ETIOLOGY *Rhizopus* and *Mucor* species are the principal pathogens, though *Cunninghamella* and *Absidia* species are occasionally encountered. These molds have broad, rarely septate hyphae of uneven diameter, ranging from 6 to 50 μm. The fungus is inexplicably difficult to grow from infected tissue. When it occurs, growth is rapid and profuse on most media at room temperature. Identification is based upon gross and microscopic appearance of the mold.

PATHOGENESIS AND PATHOLOGY *Rhizopus* and *Mucor* species are ubiquitous, appearing on decaying vegetation, dung, and foods of high sugar content. Infection is uncommon and largely confined to patients with serious preexisting diseases. Mucormycosis originating in the paranasal sinuses and nose occurs predominantly in patients with poorly controlled diabetes mellitus. Mucormycosis in patients with hematologic malignancy or organ transplantation more often originates in the lung than in the nose and paranasal sinuses. Gastrointestinal mucormycosis occurs in a variety of conditions, including uremia, severe malnutrition, and diarrheal diseases. Infection is acquired from nature, with no person-to-person spread. Elastic bandages contaminated with Rhizopus species have caused several skin and subcutaneous infections.

In all forms of mucormycosis, vascular invasion by hyphae is prominent. Ischemic or hemorrhagic necrosis is the predominant histological finding.

CLINICAL MANIFESTATIONS Mucormycosis originating in the nose and paranasal sinuses produces a characteristic clinical picture. Low-grade fever, dull sinus pain, and sometimes nasal congestion or a thin, bloody nasal discharge are followed in a few days by double vision, increasing fever, and obtundation. Examination reveals a unilateral generalized reduction of ocular motion, chemosis, and proptosis. The nasal turbinates on the involved side may be dusky red or necrotic. A sharply delineated area of necrosis, strictly respecting the midline, may appear in the hard palate. The skin of the cheek may become inflamed. Fungal invasion of the globe or ophthalmic artery leads to blindness. Opacification of one or more sinuses is found on x-ray. Carotid arteriogram may show invasion or obstruction of the carotid siphon. Coma is due to direct invasion of the frontal lobe. Early symptoms mimic bacterial sinusitis. Clouding of the sensorium may be attributed to diabetic acidosis. Cavernous sinus thrombosis may be considered when orbital invasion occurs. Without treatment, death may occur in a few days to a few weeks.

Pulmonary mucormycosis is a progressive severe pneumonia, accompanied by high fever and toxicity. The necrotic center of large infiltrates may cavitate. Hematogenous spread to other areas of the lung, as well as to brain and other organs, is common. Survival beyond 2 weeks is unusual. Gastrointestinal invasion presents as one or more ulcers which tend to perforate. Hematogenous dissemination can originate from the gastrointestinal tract, lung, or paranasal sinuses. Sometimes no portal of entry can be found.

DIAGNOSIS Lesions of the lung and craniofacial structures are best diagnosed by biopsy and histological section. Cultural confirmation should be attempted. Wet smear of crushed tissue can provide rapid diagnosis. Cultures of blood and cerebrospinal fluid are negative. Smear and culture of sputum may be positive during cavitation of a lung lesion. Serologic tests are of little assistance.

TREATMENT Regulation of diabetes mellitus and decreasing immunosuppressive drugs aid in the treatment. Extensive debridement of craniofacial lesions appears to be very important. Orbital exenteration may be required. Intravenous amphotericin B is clearly of value in craniofacial mucormycosis and should be employed in the other forms of mucormycosis as well. Maximum tolerated doses are given until progression is halted. The drug is continued for a total of 10 to 12 weeks. Appropriate management results in cure of about half of the craniofacial infections. Survival of patients with pulmonary, gastrointestinal, or disseminated mucormycosis is rare.

REFERENCES

Aspergillosis

FAULKNER SL et al: Hemoptysis and pulmonary aspergilloma: Operative versus nonoperative treatment. Ann Thorac Surg 25:389, 1978

GREEN WF et al: Aspergillosis of the orbit. Arch Ophthalmol 82:302, 1969

MEYER RD et al: Aspergillosis complicating neoplastic disease. Am J Med 54:6, 1973

WANG JLF et al: The management of allergic bronchopulmonary aspergillosis. Am Rev Resp Dis 120:87, 1979

YOUNG RC et al: Aspergillosis: Spectrum of the disease in 98 patients. Medicine 49:149, 1970

Candidiasis

EDWARDS JE et al: Ocular manifestations of Candida septicemia. Review of 76 cases of haematogenous candida endophthalmitis. Medicine 53:47, 1974

———: Severe candidal infections. Clinical perspective, immune defense mechanisms, and current concepts of therapy. Ann Intern Med 88:91, 1978

GAINES JD, REMINGTON JS: Disseminated candidiasis in the surgical patient. Surgery 72:730, 1972

ROSE HD, SHETH NK: Pulmonary candidiasis. A clinical and pathological correlation. Arch Intern Med 138:964, 1978

YOUNG RC et al: Fungemia with compromised host resistance. Ann Intern Med 80:605, 1974

Mucormycosis

ADDLESTONE RB, BAYLIN CJ: Rhinocerebral mucormycosis. Radiology 115:113, 1975

BARTRUM RJ et al: Roentgenographic findings in pulmonary mucormycosis. Am J Roentgenol 117:810, 1973

LEHRER RI et al: Mucormycosis. Ann Intern Med 93:93, 1980

MEYERS BR et al: Rhinocerebral mucormycosis. Premortem diagnosis and therapy. Arch Intern Med 139:557, 1979

185 SPOROTRICHOSIS

JOHN E. BENNETT

ETIOLOGY *Sporothrix schenckii* lives as a saprophyte on plants in many areas of the world. In nature and on culture at room temperature the fungus grows as a mold, but within host tissue or at 37°C on enriched media it grows as a budding yeast. Identification is by appearance of the fungus in mold and yeast forms. Small spores with a hair-like attachment to hyphae give the fungus the name, *Sporothrix*.

PATHOGENESIS AND PATHOLOGY Infection results when minor trauma inoculates the fungus into subcutaneous tissue. Nursery workers, florists, and gardeners acquire the illness from roses, sphagnum moss, and other plants. Infection may be limited to the site of inoculation (plaque sporotrichosis) or extend along proximal lymphatic channels (lymphangitic sporotrichosis). Spread on an extremity, the usual site, even as far as inguinal or axillary nodes is rare, and hematogenous dissemination from the skin remains unproven. The portal for osteoarticular, pulmonary, and other extracutaneous forms of sporotrichosis is unknown but is likely the lung.

Untreated sporotrichosis shows little evidence of self-healing and is capable of extreme chronicity. The inflammatory response contains both clusters of neutrophils and a marked granulomatous response with epithelioid cells and giant cells.

CLINICAL MANIFESTATIONS Lymphangitic sporotrichosis, by far the most common manifestation, forms a nearly painless red papule at the site of inoculation. Over the next several weeks, similar nodules form along proximal lymphatic channels. Nodules intermittently discharge small amounts of pus. Ulceration may occur. The proximal extension of these lesions, often with skip areas, is quite distinctive but may be mimicked by lesions of *Nocardia brasiliensis, Mycobacterium marinum,* or, on rare occasions, by *Leishmania brasiliensis* or *M. kansasii.*

Plaque sporotrichosis is a nontender red maculopapular granuloma confined to the site of inoculation. Osteoarticular sporotrichosis presents as mono- or polyarticular arthritis of indolent onset and progression over months or years, involving the elbows, knees, wrists, ankles, and, rarely, smaller joints of the extremities. Periarticular bone gradually appears "moth-eaten," and draining sinuses may appear over joints and bursas. Hematogenous spread to the skin may be observed during polyarticular disease, but none of the skin lesions shows lymphangitic spread. Immunosuppression predisposes to such spread. Pulmonary sporotrichosis usually presents as a single chronic cavitary upper-lobe lung lesion.

DIAGNOSIS Culture of pus, joint fluid, sputum, or skin biopsy specimen is the preferred method of diagnosis. Appearance of *S. schenckii* in tissue is quite variable. In skin lesions, organisms are hard to find.

TREATMENT Cutaneous sporotrichosis can be cured with oral administration of a saturated solution of potassium iodide, given in increasing divided daily doses up to 9 to 12 ml per day for adults. Gastrointestinal disturbance or acneform rash over the cape area and face are common, but therapy should be continued for 1 month after resolution of all lesions. Patients with serious allergic reactions to iodides may respond to local heat, particularly when plaque sporotrichosis is the only form of disease. Extracutaneous sporotrichosis rarely responds to iodides, but cures have been obtained in over half such patients with prolonged courses of intravenous amphotericin B.

REFERENCES

BULLPITT P, WEEDON D: Sporotrichosis: A review of 39 cases. Pathology 10:249, 1978

CROUT JE et al: Sporotrichosis arthritis. Clinical features of seven patients. Ann Intern Med 86:294, 1977

LYNCH PJ et al: Systemic sporotrichosis. Ann Intern Med 73:23, 1970

ORR ER, RILEY HD: Sporotrichosis in childhood, report of ten cases. J Pediatr 78:951, 1971

RARER DEEP MYCOSES

Paracoccidioidomycosis, petriellidiosis, torulopsosis, mycetoma, and chromomycosis

JOHN E. BENNETT

PARACOCCIDIOIDOMYCOSIS

ETIOLOGY Formerly called *South American blastomycosis,* this is the mycosis caused by *Paracoccidioides brasiliensis.* A dimorphic fungus, *P. brasiliensis* grows as a budding yeast but may be grown as either yeast or mold on a culture medium. Identification is by gross and microscopic appearance. A superficial resemblance to *Blastomyces dermatitidis* may cause misdiagnosis.

PATHOGENESIS AND PATHOLOGY Infection is thought to be acquired by inhalation of spores from environmental sources, but the reservoir in nature remains obscure. Pulmonary infection produces few symptoms initially. Hematogenous spread to the mucous membranes of the mouth and nose, the lymph nodes, and other sites brings the patient to medical attention. Fatal cases show spread to the adrenal, the gastrointestinal tract, and many other viscera.

CLINICAL MANIFESTATIONS Common symptoms include indurated ulcers of the mouth, oropharynx, larynx, and nose, enlarged and draining lymph nodes, lesions of the skin and genitalia, productive cough, weight loss, dyspnea, and sometimes fever. Acquisition of infection is restricted to South America, Central America, and Mexico, but the extreme indolence of this infection may lead to recognition many years after the patient has left the endemic area. Chest x-ray most often shows a bilateral patchy pneumonia.

DIAGNOSIS Cultures of sputum, pus, and mucosal lesions are often diagnostic. The diagnosis can be made by smear or histological section, though confirmation by culture is preferable. Serologic tests are useful in suggesting the diagnosis and monitoring therapy.

TREATMENT Milder cases may be cured by several years of treatment with oral sulfonamide therapy. More advanced cases are given intravenous amphotericin B, followed by prolonged oral sulfa drugs. Recent evidence suggests that ketoconazole is useful in paracoccidioidomycosis.

PETRIELLIDIOSIS

ETIOLOGY Also called *Allescheria boydii, Petriellidium boydii* is a mold frequently found in soil. When the fungus is isolated in the imperfect state, it is called *Monosporium apiospermum.*

PATHOGENESIS AND PATHOLOGY Wind-borne spores of *P. boydii,* arising in soil, are the presumed source of infection. The fungus grows as a mold within tissue, causing necrosis and abscess formation.

CLINICAL MANIFESTATIONS *P. boydii* resembles *Aspergillus* in its ability to colonize the endobronchial tree, to form fungus balls in the lung or paranasal sinuses, to invade the cornea or globe following trauma or surgery, and by its propensity to invade the immunosuppressed host. Hyphae of *P. boydii* in tissue may be difficult to distinguish from *Aspergillus.* Infection with *P. boydii* is much less common than with *Aspergillus. P. boydii* is the single most common cause in the United States of mycetoma. Intravascular hyphae, a hallmark of invasive aspergillosis, also can be found in petriellidiosis. Occasional normal patients have developed necrotizing pneumonia or abscesses in brain or other organs due to *P. boydii.*

DIAGNOSIS Demonstration of hyphae in tissue and culture confirmation are required for diagnosis.

TREATMENT Intravenous miconazole has been recommended, but therapeutic response to all drugs has been poor.

TORULOPSOSIS

ETIOLOGY *Torulopsis glabrata* is a small yeast-like fungus, the same size as the yeast form of *Histoplasma capsulatum. T. glabrata* does not form hyphae or pseudohyphae. Identification is by biochemical tests.

PATHOGENESIS AND PATHOLOGY *T. glabrata* is a normal inhabitant of the human gastrointestinal tract and vagina. Within tissue, *T. glabrata* causes abscess formation with a neutrophilic inflammatory response. In immunosuppressed patients, a scanty or mononuclear inflammatory response may be seen.

CLINICAL MANIFESTATIONS Torulopsosis mimics many of the manifestations of candidiasis, but infection is less common and often less severe. Clinical entities include intravenous catheter–induced sepsis or endocarditis, gastrointestinal and disseminated infection in immunosuppressed patients, and retrograde infection of the urinary tract.

DIAGNOSIS *Torulopsis* may be difficult to distinguish from yeast cells of *Candida* in histological section. Culture is the most reliable diagnostic tool.

TREATMENT Therapeutic measures used in candidiasis appear appropriate for torulopsosis.

MYCETOMA

ETIOLOGY *Actinomycetoma* refers to infection by actinomycetes of the genus *Nocardia, Streptomyces,* and *Actinomadura. Eumycetoma* is caused by true fungi of many different genera. The most common agent varies with the locality.

PATHOGENESIS AND PATHOLOGY The pathogens live in the soil and enter the skin through minor trauma. The most common site of infection is the foot. Infection runs a relentless course over many years, with destruction of contiguous bone and fascia. Grains are found in purulent foci, surrounded by fibrosis and a mononuclear cell inflammatory response.

CLINICAL MANIFESTATIONS *Mycetoma* is a chronic suppurative infection originating in subcutaneous tissue and characterized by the presence of grains, which are tightly clumped colonies of the causative agent. The infected site shows painless swelling, woody induration, and sinus tracts which discharge pus intermittently. Systemic symptoms and spread to distant sites in the body are not seen.

DIAGNOSIS The clinical picture is characteristic, but confusion with chronic osteomyelitis or botryomycosis may occur. The diagnosis requires demonstration of grains in pus from the draining sinus or in biopsy sections. Many histological sections may need to be examined to locate a grain.

TREATMENT Actinomycetoma may respond to prolonged therapy with sulfonamides, trimethoprim-sulfamethoxazole, or other antibacterial agents. Eumycetoma does not respond reliably to any drug. Amputation may be required.

CHROMOMYCOSIS

ETIOLOGY The five species of fungi currently recognized as causing this syndrome have received a bewildering number of different names. Using Emmons' classification, these fungi are called *Phialophora verrucosa, P. pedrosoi, P. compacta, P. dermatitidis,* and *Cladosporium carrionii.*

PATHOGENESIS AND PATHOLOGY Infection occurs in tropical and subtropical areas where workers acquire many small puncture wounds from thorns or splinters. Histopathologic section of the skin lesion shows pseudoepitheliomatous hyperplasia and a granulomatous dermal infiltrate. Microabscesses with neutrophils also occur. Clumps of the pathogenic organism are found in these abscesses or elsewhere in the dermis as rounded, thick-walled brown cells. The epidermis and superficial crusts may contain branching brown hyphae.

CLINICAL MANIFESTATIONS *Chromomycosis* is characterized by chronic verrucoid, ulcerated, or crusted skin lesions. The site of the lesion depends upon the area of trauma but is usually the foot or leg. The lesion begins as a pimple, pustule, or ulcer with slow progression over many years. Lesions may remain flat or become pedunculated. Pain is minimal, but itching is common. Infection usually remains confined to the same extremity, but a few cases have spread hematogenously to cause brain abscess.

DIAGNOSIS Demonstration of the characteristic organisms in histological sections of skin biopsy is the best diagnostic method. Positive cultures are obtained readily, but accurate identification may require the service of a reference laboratory.

TREATMENT Prolonged therapy with oral flucytosine appears helpful. Relapse with secondary drug resistance has been encountered with sufficient frequency to make flucytosine plus low-dose intravenous amphotericin B appear preferable.

REFERENCES

Chromomycosis

LOPES CF: Recent developments in the therapy of chromoblastomycosis. Bull Pan Am Health Organ 15:58, 1981

MAUCERI AA et al: Flucytosine. An effective oral treatment for chromomycosis. Arch Dermatol 109:873, 1974

Mycetoma

GREEN WO, ADAMS TE: Mycetoma in the United States. Am J Clin Pathol 42:75, 1964

MAHGOUB ES: Medical management of mycetoma. Bull World Health Organ 54:303, 1976

TARALAKSHMI VV et al: Mycetomas caused by *Streptomyces pelletieri* in Madras, India. Arch Dermatol 114:204, 1978

Paracoccidioidomycosis

LONDERO AT, RAMOS CD: Paracoccidioidomycosis. A clinical and mycologic study of forty-one cases observed in Santa Maria, RS, Brazil. Am J Med 52:771, 1972

MURRAY HW et al: Disseminated paracoccidioidomycosis (South American blastomycosis) in the United States. Am J Med 56:209, 1974

RESTREPO A et al: Paracoccidioidomycosis (South American blastomycosis). A study of 39 cases observed in Medellin, Columbia. Am J Trop Med Hyg 19:68, 1970

——— et al: Ketoconazole in paracoccidioidomycosis: Efficacy of prolonged therapy. Mycopathologia 72:35, 1980

Petriellidiosis

ARNETT JC, HATCH HB: Pulmonary allescheriasis. Report of a case and review of the literature. Arch Intern Med 135:1250, 1975

LUTWICK LI et al: Visceral fungal infections due to *Petrillidium boydii (Allescheria boydii).* Am J Med 61:632, 1976

WINSTON DJ et al: *Allescheria boydii* infections in the immunosuppressed host. Am J Med 63:830, 1977

Torulopsosis

KAUFFMAN CA, TAN JS: *Torulopsis glabrata* renal infection. Am J Med 57:217, 1974

VALDIVIESO M et al: Fungemia due to *Torulopsis glabrata* in the compromised host. Cancer 38:1750, 1976

187
DERMATOPHYTOSIS

JOHN E. BENNETT

DEFINITION Dermatophytosis, also known as ringworm or tinea, is a chronic fungal infection of the skin, hair, or nails.

ETIOLOGY Species of *Trichophyton, Microsporum,* and *Epidermophyton* are called *dermatophytes.* They grow in and remain confined to the keratinous structures of the body. Other mycoses can show fungal invasion of keratinous structures, such as candidiasis, pityriasis versicolor, and tinea nigra, but are traditionally not termed *dermatophytoses.*

PATHOLOGY AND PATHOGENESIS Dermatophyte species are called anthropophilic, zoophilic, or geophilic, depending on whether their usual reservoir within nature appears to be humans, animals, or soil. Infectivity of all those sources is low, and group outbreaks are largely confined to an occasional case clustering of scalp infections in children. Acquisition of a dermatophytosis appears to be favored by minor trauma, maceration, and poor hygiene of the skin. Infection does not seem to confer solid immunity. Repeated infection with the same species is commonplace, particularly with anthropophilic species. Infrequency of scalp infection in adults has been attributed to local factors rather than immunity.

Invasion of the stratum corneum by dermatophytes may cause little inflammation, or, particularly with zoophilic fungi, inflammation can be intense. Shedding of the stratum corneum is increased by inflammation. To the extent that fungal growth cannot keep up with shedding, inflammation may help terminate infection. Conversely, infection is probably favored when shedding is reduced by corticosteroids and cytotoxic drugs. Antifungal drugs interfere with the ability of fungal growth to keep up with shedding.

CLINICAL MANIFESTATIONS The disease varies with the site of infection and fungal species. Foot infection (athlete's foot, tinea pedis) may present as fissuring of the toe webs, scaling of the plantar surfaces, or vesicles around the toe webs and soles. Interdigital lesions may be pruritic or, when bacterial superinfection occurs, may be painful. Hand infection is less common but resembles foot infection. Scalp dermatophytosis (tinea capitis) is characterized by areas of alopecia and scaling. In so-called endothrix infection, the hair shaft breaks off at the skin surface, leaving the hairs visible as black dots in the scalp. With some forms of scalp infection an intense boggy suppuration occurs, called a *kerion*. Dermatophytosis of the glabrious skin (tinea corporis) presents as circumscribed lesions with a wide variety of appearances. Scales, vesicles, or pustules may appear. Inflammation may be minimal or intense. Central healing of less inflamed lesions may be seen. The serpiginous border of inflammation is the source of the name *ringworm*. Dermatophytosis of the bearded area (tinea barbae) appears as a pustular folliculitis. Onychomycosis (tinea unguium) presents as white discolored nails or thickened, chalky crumbling nails. Peeling and fissuring of the perinychia or keratotic debris under the nail edge may also be seen.

DIAGNOSIS Discolored hairs, scales, and keratotic debris under infected nails should be collected for KOH smear and culture. In the scraping of skin lesions, a drop of water on the skin site may keep the removed scales from flying off and aid in their collection. Culture is important in distinguishing dermatophytes from *Candida* and fungal saprophytes growing in keratinaceous debris.

TREATMENT Skin lesions should be treated topically if the lesions are few and small or located on the feet. Miconazole or clotrimazole cream should be applied twice daily until the lesion disappears and smears are negative. Undecylenic acid, haloprogin, or tolnaftate can also be used. Extensive skin lesions and infection of hair or nails should be treated with oral griseofulvin. The recommended dose for adults is 500 mg bid. Treatment must be continued until all infected keratin is gone. Cutting of infected hair, epilating nails, and cleansing interdigital webs can expedite cure. Secondary bacterial infection of the foot may require soaks or antibacterial agents. Relapse of dermatophyte foot infections may be decreased by measures to keep the feet clean and dry. Griseofulvin-resistant cases may respond to oral ketoconazole, 200 to 400 mg daily.

REFERENCES

ROBERTSON MH et al: Oral therapy with ketoconazole for dermatophyte infections unresponsive to griseofulvin. Rev Infect Dis 2:578, 1980

section 10 | Rickettsial infections

188
APPROACH TO THE DIAGNOSIS AND TREATMENT OF RICKETTSIAL INFECTIONS

THEODORE E. WOODWARD

The rickettsial diseases of humans consist of a variety of clinical entities caused by microorganisms of the family Rickettsiaceae. The rickettsias are obligate intracellular parasites about the size of bacteria and are usually seen microscopically as pleomorphic coccobacilli. Each of the rickettsias pathogenic for humans is capable of multiplying in one or more species of arthropod as well as in animals and humans. Indeed, the majority of the rickettsias are maintained in nature by a cycle which involves an insect vector and an animal reservoir, and infection of humans is unimportant in the cycle. Epidemic typhus presents a number of points of dissimilarity to most of the other rickettsioses, because the natural cycle of the infection involves only humans and the louse.

A compendium of information of the rickettsial diseases is given in Table 188-1. Because each of the rickettsioses responds therapeutically to tetracyclines or chloramphenicol, the table mentions no therapy. Procedures for diagnostic isolation of the rickettsias are omitted because they generally are less useful than serologic methods, and the techniques which they require are highly specialized and hazardous. Information on isolation may be found in textbooks devoted to viral and rickettsial diseases.

Of all the afflictions of the human race the rickettsial diseases, particularly epidemic typhus, rank among the foremost as a cause of suffering and death. The record of deaths from epidemic typhus in this century in the Balkan countries and in Poland and Russia reached astounding figures. Typhus ravaged Russia and eastern Poland from 1915 to 1922, infecting 30 million of the inhabitants and causing an estimated 3 million deaths.

The past two decades have seen the development of excellent methods for the prevention and treatment of rickettsioses. In fact, these measures have been so successful that the rickettsioses have become of minor importance in the United States and in many other countries. Although conquered, the rickettsioses have not been eliminated, and they could again become rampant if the will to control them, the present high standards of sanitation, and the necessary industrial capacities for production of effective insecticides and therapeutic agents should be decreased through war or disaster.

PATHOGENESIS Rickettsial diseases develop after infection through the skin or the respiratory tract. Agents of the typhus and spotted fever group are introduced through the bite of the infected arthropod vector. Ticks and mites, which transmit the agents of spotted fever and scrub typhus, inoculate the rickettsias directly into the dermis during feeding. The louse and flea, which transmit epidemic and murine typhus, respectively, deposit infected feces on the skin; infection occurs when organisms are rubbed into the puncture wound made by the arthropod. The rickettsias of Q fever gain entry through the respiratory tract when infected dust is inhaled; moreover, the respiratory route is occasionally implicated in epidemic typhus when infection results from inhalation of dried infected louse feces.

Although organisms probably multiply at the original site of entry in all instances, local lesions appear with regularity only in certain diseases, namely, the initial cutaneous lesions of scrub typhus, rickettsialpox, and boutonneuse fever, and the pneumonitis which develops in about half the persons infected with Q fever.

Volunteers infected with either scrub typhus or Q fever develop rickettsemia late in the incubation period, often some hours before the onset of fever. Similar events probably occur in all the rickettsial diseases; circulating rickettsias can be detected during the early febrile period in practically all patients. Little is known about the pathogenesis of infection during the midportion of the incubation period. However, it is reasonable to assume that during this time, in patients with typhus or spotted fever, a transient low-grade rickettsemia results from release of organisms multiplying at the initial site of infection and that this seeds infection in the endothelial cells of the vascular tree. Vascular lesions developing at such sites account for the pathologic changes, including the rash.

Rickettsias apparently invade and proliferate in the endothelial cells of small blood vessels. Endothelial cell destruction occurs from the proliferation of organisms and eventual disruption. Rickettsias may exert a cytotoxic effect on endothelial cells; in mice the rickettsial toxin causes remarkable increase in capillary permeability, independent of proliferation. Later manifestations in rickettsial diseases may result from immunopathologic mechanisms, since humoral antibodies are present during the second febrile week, when increases in capillary permeability and vascular thrombosis and ecchymoses are greatest. Also, a delayed type of hypersensitivity occurs during infection.

The underlying cause of the toxic-febrile state which characterizes the rickettsial diseases remains unknown. Several rickettsial species contain type-specific toxins which are lethal for mice; these may play a role.

PATHOLOGIC PHYSIOLOGY Peripheral vascular collapse results in death in fulminating cases during the first week, with capillary dilatation and pooling of blood without increased capillary permeability or loss of fluid into extravascular spaces. As proliferative and thrombotic lesions develop in small vessels, anoxia occurs in the areas supplied, resulting in necrosis and increased capillary permeability, with loss of water, electrolytes, proteins, and erythrocytes. This in turn results in a

TABLE 188-1
Rickettsial diseases

Disease: Type	Disease: Agent	Geographic distribution	Natural cycle: Arthropod	Natural cycle: Mammal	Principal means of transmission to humans	Serologic diagnosis: Weil-Felix reaction	Serologic diagnosis: CF, MA, and IFA reactions*
SPOTTED FEVER GROUP							
Rocky Mountain spotted fever	*R. rickettsii*	Western hemisphere	Ticks	Wild rodents; dogs	Tick bite	Positive OX-19 OX-2	Positive group- and type-specific
Boutonneuse fever	*R. conorii*	Africa, Europe, Middle East, India					
Queensland tick typhus	*R. australis*	Australia		Marsupials, wild rodents			
North Asian tick-borne rickettsiosis	*R. sibirica*	Siberia, Mongolia		Wild rodents			
Rickettsial-pox	*R. akari*	United States, Russia, Africa(?)	Blood-sucking mite	House mouse, other rodents	Mite bite	Negative	
TYPHUS GROUP							
Endemic (murine)	*R. mooseri*	Worldwide	Flea	Small rodents	Infected flea feces into broken skin	Positive OX-19	Positive group- and type-specific
Epidemic	*R. prowazekii*	Worldwide	Body louse	Humans	Infected louse feces into broken skin	Positive OX-19	
	R. Canada	North America	Ticks	?Flying squirrels		Positive OX-19	
Brill-Zinsser disease	*R. prowazekii*	Worldwide	Recurrence years after original attack of epidemic typhus			Usually negative	
Scrub	*R. tsutsugamushi*	Asia, Australia, Pacific islands	Trombiculid mites	Wild rodents	Mite bite	Positive OX-K	Positive in about 50% of patients
OTHER RICKETTSIAL DISEASES							
Q fever	*R. burnetii*	Worldwide	Ticks	Small mammals, cattle, sheep, goats	Inhalation of dried infected material	Negative	Positive
Trench fever	*R. quintana*†	Europe, Africa, North America	Body louse	Humans	Infected louse feces into broken skin	Negative	None available

* *CF = complement fixation; MA = microscopic agglutination; IFA = immunofluorescent antibody.*
† *Some authorities no longer place the agent in the genus Rickettsia because it can be cultured on artificial media.*

decrease in blood volume, together with an increase in extravascular space and clinical edema. Edema, anoxia of the myocardium, and histologic evidence of myocarditis are disclosed by electrocardiographic abnormalities, including serious arrhythmias. Liver function is impaired. The azotemia which develops in seriously ill patients appears to be prerenal. Clinical manifestations resulting from the peripheral vascular collapse are oliguria and anuria, azotemia, anemia, hypoproteinemia, hyponatremia, edema, and coma. In spotted fever and typhus patients with hemorrhagic skin lesions, consumptive coagulopathy is present. All these alterations are absent or minimal in mild cases or in those who are given specific treatment early.

PATHOLOGY The basic changes in the spotted and typhus fever groups are vascular, with resultant widespread lesions in adjacent parenchymatous tissues throughout the body. They are most common in the skin, muscles, heart, lung, and brain. The most conspicuous and diverse are found in Rocky Mountain spotted fever. Here swelling, proliferation, and degeneration of the endothelial cells occur, frequently with thrombus formation which partially or completely occludes the lumen. The muscle cells of the arterioles undergo swelling and fibrinoid changes. The adventitial tissues are infiltrated with mononuclear leukocytes, lymphocytes, and plasma cells. The vascular damage is scattered along the arteries, veins, and capillaries, with normal architecture prevailing throughout most of the vascular bed. The changes in murine, epidemic, and scrub typhus fevers resemble those in Rocky Mountain spotted fever, but thrombosis is uncommon and involvement of the musculature is rare.

Interstitial myocarditis occurs in each of these diseases but is usually most extensive in Rocky Mountain spotted fever and in scrub typhus. In the brain glial nodules are found in all members of the group, but microinfarcts in the brain tissue or in the myocardium are most often observed in spotted fever.

A rickettsial pneumonitis occurs, at least to some extent, in many patients with spotted or typhus fever and is the characteristic pathologic change in patients with Q fever. The process is patchy and consists microscopically of areas of congestion and edema. Within the consolidated areas the alveoli are filled with compact fibrinocellular exudate containing lymphocytes, plasma cells, large mononuclear cells, and erythrocytes but few, if any, polymorphonuclear leukocytes.

Rickettsias can occasionally be observed microscopically in sections of tissue. Failure to demonstrate them is of no diagnostic significance.

LABORATORY DIAGNOSIS Diagnostic procedures which depend on isolation of the etiologic agent from blood or other clinical material are expensive, time-consuming, and hazardous to laboratory personnel. Primary isolation of rickettsias by inoculation in the yolk sac of the chick embryo or tissue cells usually fails because of the small number of organisms in the patient's blood. Rickettsias have been identified in stained cultured monocytes of infected monkeys and by direct or indirect immunofluorescence of tissues of animals infected with *R. rickettsii*. Except in unusual circumstances, however, currently available serologic tests are adequate for laboratory confirmation of the clinical diagnosis in each of the rickettsial diseases. The demonstration of a rise in titer of specific antibody during convalescence is of prime importance in establishing the laboratory confirmation. Table 188-2 summarizes the serologic results usually encountered in persons who have rickettsial diseases in the United States. The Weil-Felix test employing *Proteus* strains OX-19 and OX-2 gives positive results in patients with spotted fever and murine typhus and negative results in those with rickettsialpox and Q fever. It is useful as a screening procedure but cannot be relied upon to differentiate spotted fever from murine typhus. In patients with Brill-Zinsser disease the *Proteus* OX-19 reaction is usually negative or low in titer.

Serologic tests employing group-specific rickettsial antigens provide data which clearly differentiate the most common infections, i.e., murine typhus, Rocky Mountain spotted fever, and Q fever. Moreover, if type-specific rickettsial antigens are employed, it is generally possible to distinguish rickettsialpox from spotted fever and Brill-Zinsser disease from murine typhus.

Utilizing better antigens, other serologic procedures for rickettsial diseases not only distinguish between specific rickettsioses but help to determine the type of immunoglobulin in acute (IgM) and late or recurrent (IgG) illness, such as in recrudescent typhus (Brill-Zinsser disease). The Weil-Felix and complement fixation tests are useful for routine diagnosis; microscopic agglutination, immunofluorescent antibody, and hemagglutination reactions are valuable for specific identification.

Specific antibiotic therapy has little effect on the time of appearance of antibodies or on their ultimate titer, provided treatment is instituted some days after onset of the illness. However, if the illness is cut short by early and vigorous treatment, antibody production may be delayed for a week or so, and also the maximal titers attained may be below those illustrated in Table 188-2. Under these circumstances a sample of blood taken 4 to 6 weeks after onset of illness should also be tested.

The immunofluorescent antibody test is a very useful procedure for detecting rickettsia in the tissues of patients with the typhus group of rickettsioses, the spotted fevers, and Q fever. Identifiable rickettsias have been visualized in skin lesions of patients with Rocky Mountain spotted fever as early as the fourth day of illness and as late as the tenth day. The technique also visualizes rickettsias in ticks and the tissues of animals. This test is useful with paraffin-fixed tissues.

Normochromic anemia occurs in patients severely ill with rickettsial diseases. The white blood cell count in Rocky Mountain spotted fever, rickettsialpox, murine and epidemic typhus, Brill-Zinsser disease, Q fever, and other rickettsial diseases is usually within the normal range; 6000 to 10,000 cells per cubic millimeter. Leukopenia is occasionally observed, and in the presence of complications, such as superimposed infections and extensive vascular lesions, moderate leukocytosis occurs. The differential blood cell count is usually normal.

Thrombocytopenia occurs in severely ill spotted and scrub typhus fever patients with extensive vascular lesions; hypofibrinogenemia, prolonged prothrombin and partial thromboplastin times, and other clotting abnormalties occur. In primates showing peripheral gangrenous ecchymoses caused by *R. rickettsii* there are decreases in complement fractions C2 and C3.

TREATMENT Certain physiochemical changes occurring in the patient seriously ill with one of the diseases of the typhus–spotted fever group should be understood before a therapeutic regimen is outlined. These changes are circulatory collapse, coma, oliguria and anuria, azotemia, anemia, hypoproteinemia, hypochloremia and hyponatremia, and edema. These alterations are often absent in the mildly ill, and in them management is much less complicated. The therapeutic principles necessary for treatment of all rickettsioses are (1) specific chemotherapy and (2) supportive care. Attention to both is mandatory for the seriously ill patient first recognized late in the disease. During the first week in the moderately ill patient, supportive therapy may be less energetic, because specific che-

TABLE 188-2
Serologic diagnosis of rickettsial diseases of the United States

Group	Disease	Weil-Felix reaction: Proteus	Illustrative titer: 10th day	Illustrative titer: 20th day	Cases with diagnostic titer	Complement fixation tests with type-specific antigen: Rickettsial antigen	Illustrative titer: 10th day	Illustrative titer: 20th day	Illustrative titer: 30th day	Cases with diagnostic titer
Spotted fever	Rocky Mountain spotted fever	OX-19 OX-2	40 20	320 160	Most	*R. rickettsii*	20	160	80	Most
	Rickettsialpox	OX-19 OX-2	0 0	0 0	None	*R. akari*	0	64	128	Most
Typhus	Murine typhus	OX-19 OX-2	160 10	640 40	Most	*R. mooseri*	0	160	160	Most
	Brill-Zinsser disease	OX-19 OX-2	160 0	20 0	Infrequent	*R. prowazekii*	1280	640	320	Most
	Q fever	OX-19 OX-2	0 0	0 0	None	*R. burnetii*	10	80	160	Most

motherapy usually suffices. The early mild case may be successfully treated at home; later in the course of the disease patients should receive hospital care.

Therapeutic measures advisable for all the rickettsioses will be described in detail. Variations of this regimen which apply to the individual rickettsioses are described in subsections in the following chapter.

Specific therapy Specific therapy is most effective when initiated during the early stages of disease coincident with the appearance of the rash. When therapy is delayed until the rash has become hemorrhagic and widespread, the response is less dramatic. The antibiotics of choice are chloramphenicol and the tetracyclines, which are effective because of their rickettsiostatic properties. They are not rickettsiocidal.

The following antibiotic regimen is considered optimal: for chloramphenicol, an initial dose of 50 mg per kilogram of body weight, and for tetracycline, 25 mg/kg. Subsequent daily doses are the same as the initial loading dose, with the requirement divided equally and given at 6- to 8-h intervals. Antibiotic treatment is continued until the patient has improved and has been afebrile approximately 24 h. In patients too ill to take oral medication, an intravenous preparation of one of the antimicrobials should be employed.

Adrenal cortical hormones may need to be utilized for their antitoxemic effects, in patients first observed late in the course of severe illness. Large doses for brief periods of about 3 days, in combination with specific antibiotics, are recommended in critically ill patients.

Therapy with antibiotics is continued until the toxemia has abated, the general condition has markedly improved, and the temperature has remained at normal levels for 24 h. In uncomplicated cases of spotted fever, there is symptomatic improvement within 24 h and the temperature becomes normal in 60 to 72 h.

Supportive care Frequent turning of the patient relieves pressure from prominent bony parts and also militates against the development of aspiration pneumonia. Proper mouth care, with frequent swabbing of the oral cavity, may avert the development of parotitis and gingivitis. Sucking of the juice of a lemon or the oral use of glycerin or mineral oil is helpful.

A generous intake of protein should be provided by frequent feedings as soon as the disease is suspected, in order to avoid subsequent protein deficiency. Usually food is well tolerated by patients with rickettsial disease, and the daily diet should provide 3 g protein per kilogram of normal body weight, with adequate carbohydrate and fat to make it palatable. When the patient is uncooperative, the diet may be supplemented by hourly liquid protein feedings via stomach tube, provided that there is no abdominal distention.

At the critical stage, when hypoproteinemia is present and changes in capillary permeability lead to edema and vascular embarrassment, careful attention must be given to parenteral hyperalimentation with high concentration of glucose and amino acids. When indicated by hematologic studies, whole-blood transfusions given slowly are helpful. The judicious administration of one of the plasma expanders at this stage may have a definite favorable effect upon impending circulatory collapse. If the patient is anuric and azotemia is pronounced, overloading the circulation with fluids should be governed by clinical judgment and very careful laboratory studies. Frequent determinations of hemoglobin, hematocrit, electrolytes, and protein, sometimes at intervals of a few hours during crucial periods, are necessary in order to ascertain abnormalities and to permit institution of corrective measures. Dialysis is indicated when there is clear-cut evidence of acute tubular necrosis.

REFERENCES

See Chap. 189.

189
THE RICKETTSIOSES

THEODORE E. WOODWARD

ROCKY MOUNTAIN SPOTTED FEVER

DEFINITION Rocky Montain spotted fever is an acute febrile illness caused by *Rickettsia rickettsii.* It is transmitted to humans by ticks. The disease is characterized by sudden onset with headache and chills and by fever which persists for 2 to 3 weeks. A characteristic exanthem appears on the extremities and trunk about the fourth day of illness. Delerium, shock, and renal failure occur in the severely ill.

ETIOLOGY AND EPIDEMIOLOGY The causative microbe *R. rickettsii* is the prototype for the rickettsial group of agents. The minute organisms are purple when stained by Giemsa's method or red by Macchiavello's technique; most of them are gram-negative. These organisms often occur in pairs and possess a cell wall similar in structure and chemical composition to that of gram-negative bacteria; there are a cell membrane, cytoplasmic granules corresponding to ribosomes, and prokaryotic organization of nuclear material. The cell membrane is selectively permeable; the cell wall is the focus of important antigens and an endotoxin-like substance.

The rickettsias grow in the nucleus and the cytoplasm of infected cells of ticks, mammals, and embryonated eggs; the intranuclear situation of the organisms is shared by the other members of the spotted fever group, but not by rickettsias of the typhus group. *Rickettsia rickettsii* is readily distinguishable from the agents of the typhus fevers by cross-immunity tests in guinea pigs and by complement fixation tests employing antigens prepared from infected yolk sac tissues. The differentiation of *R. rickettsii* from closely related members of the spotted fever group frequently requires elaborate procedures. Strains of the agent of Rocky Mountain spotted fever vary considerably in their virulence for humans and animals.

The first reports of spotted fever in Idaho and Montana during the final decade of the last century led to the name Rocky Mountain spotted fever. However, the disease has been reported from almost all states, as well as from Canada, Mexico, Colombia, and Brazil. Although related diseases are found on other continents, this particular infection is limited to the western hemisphere. In the years 1977, 1978, 1979, and 1980 there were 1115, 1011, 1070, and 1136 cases reported, respectively. The mortality rate was about 20 percent in the days before specific therapy but has decreased to about 7 percent. More than half the cases occur in the south Atlantic and south central states, with the greatest number of these in North Carolina, Virginia, Georgia, Maryland, Tennessee, and Oklahoma.

A number of species of ticks are found infected with *R. rickettsii* in nature, but only two are important in transmitting spotted fever to humans. These are *Dermacentor andersoni,* the wood tick, which is the principal vector in the west, and *D. variabilis,* the dog tick, which assumes this role in the east. Infected female ticks transmit the agent transovarially to at least some of their offspring. Ticks which become infected, either through the egg or at one of the stages during their development cycle by feeding on an infected mammal, harbor the rickettsias throughout their lifetime, which may be several years. Thus, the tick serves as a reservoir in addition to being a vector. Small wild mammals are suspected of playing an important role in spreading the rickettsias in nature by infecting ticks which feed on them during rickettsemia.

Disease in humans is generally acquired from the bite of an infected tick. Transmission is unlikely unless the tick remains attached for a number of hours. Infection may also be acquired through abrasions in the skin which become contaminated with infected tick feces or tissue juices; hence, the hazard associated with crushing ticks between the fingers when removing them from persons or animals. The agent of Rocky Mountain spotted fever has been transmitted accidentally to humans by transfusion of blood taken from a donor just before onset of illness.

There are seasonal variations in the incidence of cases of spotted fever, as well as differences in age and sex distribution of cases. In each instance these differences are related to exposure to ticks. Most cases are seen during the period of maximal tick activity, i.e., late spring and early summer, and 60 percent of cases occur in individuals under 20 years of age. This age distribution is undoubtedly influenced by propinquity to the wood and dog ticks. The mortality rate increases with the age of the patient.

Rocky Mountain spotted fever has been acquired by laboratory workers via aerosol transmission, and special precautions are necessary when the agent is handled in the laboratory.

CLINICAL MANIFESTATIONS **Incubation period and prodromata** A history of tick bite is elicited in approximately 80 percent of patients. The incubation period varies between 3 and 12 days with a mean of 7 days. A short incubation period usually indicates a more serious infection.

Onset In nonvaccinated persons, the onset is usually abrupt, with severe headache, a sudden shaking rigor, prostration, generalized myalgia, especially in the back and leg muscles, nausea with occasional vomiting, and fever which reaches 103 to 104°F within the first 2 days. Pain in the abdominal muscles may be severe, and arthralgia is not uncommon. Deep muscle palpation often elicits tenderness. Occasionally the debut of illness in children and adults is mild, accompanied by lethargy, anorexia, headache, and low-grade fever. These symptoms are similar to those of many acute infectious diseases, making specific diagnosis difficult during the first few days.

Pyrexia Fever continues for approximately 15 to 20 days in untreated cases. The febrile course in children may be shorter. Hyperthermia of 105°F or greater is of unfavorable prognostic significance, although fatalities may occur when the patient is hypothermic, with concurrent vasomotor collapse. Fever generally terminates by lysis over a period of several days, but rarely does so by crisis. Recurrent fever is uncommon except in the presence of secondary pyogenic complications.

The *headache* is generalized and excruciating, and frequently more intense over frontal area. It persists throughout the first and second weeks of illness in untreated cases. Occasionally headache is mild. Malaise continues for the first week; irritability is notable, and the patient shuns distractions such as questioning and examination.

Cutaneous manifestations The rash which is present in practically all cases is the most characteristic and helpful diagnostic sign. It usually appears on the fourth febrile day; the range is 2 to 6 days. The initial lesions are on the wrists, ankles, palms, soles, and forearms. The first lesions are macular, nonfixed, pink, irregularly defined, and measure 2 to 6 mm. A warm compress applied to the extremity accentuates the rash in the early stages. The exanthem is most prominent when the temperature is elevated. After 6 to 12 h, the rash extends centripetally to the axilla, buttocks, trunk, neck, and face. (This is in contrast to the eruption of typhus fever, which begins on the trunk and spreads centrifugally, rarely involving the face, palms, or soles.) The rash becomes maculopapular after 2 to 3 days (it may be felt by light palpation) and assumes a deeper red hue. By about the fourth day it is petechial and fails to fade on pressure. Not uncommonly, the hemorrhagic lesions coalesce to form large ecchymotic blemishes; these lesions tend to form over bony prominences and may ultimately slough to form indolent, slow-healing ulcers. Patients who have had the typical rash show brownish discolorations at the site for several weeks during convalescence. In milder cases, the rash does not become purpuric and may disappear within a few days. Antibiotic therapy may abort the early exanthem; the later fixed lesion fades less rapidly with specific therapy. Occasionally, a rash does not occur or is unnoticed, particularly in dark-skinned patients.

The application of tourniquets for several minutes, or the occasional taking of the blood pressure may provoke additional petechiae (Rumpel-Leede phenomenon), further evidence of capillary abnormalities.

Cardiovascular and respiratory features During the early stages, the pulse is full and regular and is accelerated in proportion to the height of the temperature, and the blood pressure is well sustained. During the peak of illness in seriously ill patients, the pulse is rapid and feeble, and hypotension of 90 mmHg is common. If circulatory failure is sustained, the resultant hypoxia and shock lead to agitation and delirium and contribute to the formation of ecchymoses and gangrene of fingers, toes, genitalia, buttocks, earlobes, and nose. Cyanosis of the peripheral parts of the body is common. Venous pressure determinations show no elevation. A reduction of the total blood volume is occasionally found, as is myocardial impairment as shown by low voltage of ventricular complexes, minor ST-segment deflections, and occasionally delay in atrioventricular conduction on the electrocardiogram. These changes are transient and nonspecific. Severely ill patients have a puffy appearance of the face, hands, ankles, feet, and lower parts of the sacrum. Occasionally a severe arrhythmia associated with myocarditis results in sudden death.

Respirations are either normal or slightly accelerated. Cough may be harassing and nonproductive, and localized pneumonitis may occur, but pulmonary consolidation is extremely rare. Pulmonary edema may develop after injudicious use of intravenous fluids.

Hepatic and renal manifestations In the majority of patients, there is little alteration in renal or hepatic function. The liver may be enlarged, but jaundice is unusual. Oliguria commonly occurs in the seriously ill, and anuria may mark the critically ill patient. Azotemia is common; when marked, it is a very unfavorable sign. Abnormalities in liver function are probably responsible for the hypoproteinemia, with reduction in the albumin fraction.

Neurologic manifestations The principal neurologic manifestations are headache, restlessness, and varying degrees of insomnia. Stiffness of the back is common. The cerebrospinal fluid is clear, with normal dynamics and normal chemical constituents. Coma and muscular rigidity may occur. Athetoid movements, convulsive seizures, and hemiplegia are grave manifestations. Deafness during the active stages of the disease is not uncommon. As a rule, all neurologic signs abate without residua. Findings based upon follow-up examinations and electroencephalograms may be interpreted as indicative of minor residual brain damage for a year or more following recovery of certain patients from Rocky Mountain spotted fever.

Other physical manifestations Patients become dehydrated, with extreme dryness of lips, gums, tongue, and pharynx. The skin is hot and dry, the conjunctivas are frequently injected, and the eyes suffused. Photophobia is common in the early stages of illness. Petechial hemorrhages may be noted in the conjunctivas or in the retina. The spleen is enlarged in approximately one-half the cases and is firm and nontender. Abdominal distention is frequent, and occasionally some degree of intestinal ileus is observed. Constipation is usual.

COURSE In patients with mild and moderately severe cases who are given no specific antibiotic therapy, the disease abates within 2 weeks, and convalescence is rapid. In fatal cases death usually occurs during the latter part of the second week as a result of toxemia, vasomotor collapse and shock, or renal failure. In a few patients, the course is fulminant with death occurring as early as the sixth day of illness.

In vaccinated individuals who contract the disease, the illness is mild, with a short febrile course and an atypical rash.

PROGNOSIS If the serious manifestations of spotted fever mentioned above are regarded as intrinsic parts of the disease, then complications are uncommon and consist mainly of secondary bacterial infections, namely, bronchopneumonia, otitis media, and parotitis. Thrombosis of major blood vessels may result in gangrene of a portion of an extremity. Hemiplegia and peripheral neuritis are rare sequelae.

The overall mortality rate for spotted fever was formerly about 20 percent. Death occurred in more than half of persons over 40 years of age, but the mortality rate was much lower in children and young adults. Since the introduction of the broad-spectrum antibiotics and the development of more precise knowledge regarding correction of the physiologic abnormalities which develop during the disease, fewer deaths occur from this infection. Some of the fatalities can be attributed to failure to consider spotted fever in the differential diagnosis.

DIFFERENTIAL DIAGNOSIS During the early stages of infection before the rash has appeared, differentiation from other acute infections is difficult. History of tick bite while living or traveling in a highly endemic area is helpful. The rash of meningococcemia (see Chap. 149) resembles Rocky Mountain spotted fever in certain aspects, because it is macular, maculopapular, or petechial in the chronic form, and petechial, confluent, or ecchymotic in the fulminant type. The meningococcal skin lesion is tender and develops with extreme rapidity in the fulminant form, whereas the rickettsial rash occurs on about the fourth day of disease and gradually becomes petechial. *Spotted fever is often confused with measles.* The exanthem of rubeola rapidly becomes confluent, while that of rubella *usually remains discrete.*

Murine typhus is a milder disease than Rocky Mountain spotted fever; the rash is less extensive, nonpurpuric, and nonconfluent, and renal and vascular complications are uncommon. Not infrequently differentiation of these two rickettsial infections must await the results of specific serologic tests. Epidemic typhus fever is capable of causing all the pronounced clinical, physiologic, and anatomic alterations seen in patients with Rocky Mountain spotted fever, i.e., hypotension, peripheral vascular collapse, cyanosis, skin necrosis and gangrene of digits, renal failure and azotemia, and neurologic manifestations. However, the rash of classic typhus is noted initially in the axillary folds of the trunk and later extends peripherally, rarely involving the palms, soles, or face. The serologic patterns in these two diseases are distinctive when specific rickettsial antigens are employed. Moreover, louse-borne typhus is not recognized in the United States except in the form of Brill-Zinsser disease (recurrent typhus fever). Rickettsialpox, although caused by a member of the spotted fever group of organisms, is usually readily differentiated from Rocky Mountain spotted fever by the initial lesion, the relative mildness of the illness, and the early vesiculation of the maculopapular rash. The Weil-Felix reaction is positive in Rocky Mountain spotted fever and in murine and epidemic typhus, but is negative in rickettsialpox. Agglutinins against *Proteus* OX-19 and OX-2 appear in the serum of patients with spotted fever, but only those against OX-19 are generally found in murine and epidemic typhus.

TREATMENT See Chap. 188.

COMPLICATIONS *Pyogenic complications,* including otitis media and parotitis, are encountered in patients severely ill with Rocky Mountain spotted fever and other rickettsioses. These localized infections respond to therapy with appropriate antibiotics combined with surgical measures.

Pneumonitis usually develops as a result of specific rickettsial action. The sputum is scant but should be examined to determine whether superimposed bacterial infection is present. Specific therapy is guided by the results of these laboratory studies. The pneumonitis generally responds to the antibiotic therapy the patient is receiving, but if staphylococcal pneumonia is suspected, a penicillinase-resistant penicillin should be added to the broad-spectrum drug.

Circulatory failure of peripheral or central origin is combated by careful administration of plasma expanders and fluids. Heart failure may develop from the disease or as a result of overzealous intravenous therapy and is recognized by rapid pulse, gallop rhythm, and increase in venous pressure. When the clinical signs reveal unmistakable evidence of cardiac failure, digitalis and diuretics should be employed. Oxygen therapy improves the cardiac and circulatory status and is helpful in hypoxemic patients with involvement of the central nervous system.

PREVENTION Prevention is attained primarily by avoidance of tick-infested areas. When this is impractical, prophylactic measures include (1) spraying the ground with dieldrin or chlordane for area control of ticks (though there are environmental objections to the use of residual insecticides in area control of ticks, under special conditions such procedures may be warranted); (2) application of repellents such as diethyltoluamide or dimethylphthalate to clothing and exposed parts of the body, or in very heavily infested areas the wearing of clothing which interferes with the attachment of ticks, i.e., boots and a one-piece outer garment, preferably impregnated with repellent; and (3) daily inspection of the entire body, including the hairy parts, to detect and remove attached ticks. In removing attached ticks great care should be taken to avoid crushing the arthropod with resultant contamination of the bite wound; touching the tick with gasoline or whisky encourages detachment but gentle traction with tweezers applied close to the mouth parts may be necessary; the skin area should be disinfected with soap and water or other antiseptics. Similarly, precautions should be employed in removing engorged ticks from dogs and other animals, because infection through minor abrasions on the hands is possible. Improved vaccines containing inactivated *R. rickettsii* are under development and should be available commercially for those at great risk, namely, persons frequenting highly endemic areas and laboratory workers exposed to the agent. Because the broad-spectrum antibiotics are such excellent therapeutic agents in spotted fever, there has been less impetus for vaccination of persons who run only a minor risk of infection.

After tick bite in a known endemic area an exposed person should be observed for signs of fever, headache, prostration, and rash; therapy is very effective early in the infection.

MURINE (ENDEMIC) TYPHUS FEVER

DEFINITION Murine typhus fever is an acute febrile disease caused by *Rickettsia mooseri* and transmitted to humans by fleas. The clinical illness is characterized by fever of 9 to 14 days, headache, a maculopapular rash appearing on the third to fifth day, and myalgia.

ETIOLOGY AND EPIDEMIOLOGY *R. mooseri* resembles other rickettsias in morphologic properties, staining characteristics, and intracellular parasitism. Under the electron microscope *R. mooseri* is seen to contain dense masses of nuclear material in a less dense homogeneous protoplasmic substance, the whole of which is surrounded by a limiting membrane. It differs from *R. rickettsii* in that it always multiplies within the cytoplasm of cells, in contrast to the intranuclear and cytoplasmic positions of spotted fever rickettsias.

Invasion of the body by *R. mooseri* provokes specific and nonspecific immunologic responses. Utilizing highly purified antigens, specific antibodies may be demonstrated readily by complement fixation, microscopic agglutination, and immunofluorescent antibody reactions. The positive Weil-Felix reaction which occurs in this disease is nonspecific, because it is attributable to the presence of a common carbohydrate antigen in *Proteus* OX-19 and *R. mooseri* and because the reaction is also positive in epidemic typhus and spotted fever. Group-specific rickettsial antigens are common to both *R. mooseri and R. prowazekii.* Furthermore, both murine and epidemic rickettsias possess toxic factors which are lethal to mice and rats and can be neutralized by convalescent serum from humans or lower animals.

The common vector of *R. mooseri* for rats and humans is the rat flea (*Xenopsylla cheopis*). In nature, the rat louse (*Polypax spinulosis*) may transmit the agent among rodents. Customarily, rat fleas become infected on ingestion of blood from diseased rats; the rickettsias multiply within the intestinal cells of the arthropod and are excreted in the feces. Infection in humans occurs after the flea bite and contamination of the broken skin by rickettsia-laden feces. Dried flea feces may also infect via the conjunctivas or the upper part of the respiratory tract.

Rats and mice are naturally infected with murine typhus, and although the rodent disease is nonfatal, viable rickettsias persist in the brain for variable periods.

Murine typhus is one of the most benign and widespread of the rickettsioses in the United States. Prevalent in the southeastern and Gulf Coast states, it has been identified in most of the other states and in harbor centers throughout the world wherever rats and fleas abound. Through control of rats and their fleas a sharp decline in incidence has occurred. In urban areas the disease is more prevalent during the summer and fall months and occurs predominantly among persons working in proximity to granaries or food depots. There has been an extension to certain rural areas when changing agricultural practices have provided rats with ready access to adequate food supplies. Endemic typhus has been reported in laboratory workers. This emphasizes the importance of taking special precautions when working with rickettsial organisms in the laboratory.

CLINICAL MANIFESTATIONS **Incubation period and prodromata** The incubation period ranges from 8 to 16 days, with a mean of 10 days. Common prodromata are headache, backache, arthralgia, and chilly sensations. Nausea, malaise, and transient temperature rises may precede the true onset of disease.

Onset and general symptoms A frank shaking chill and repeated rigors are present at the onset, associated with a severe frontal headache and fever. This triad of headache, chill, and pyrexia is usually followed within a few hours by nausea and vomiting. Prostration, malaise, and weakness are sufficient to enforce cessation of activity in adults, in contrast to children, whose illness is less severe. Occasionally, mild symptoms make it difficult to define the actual onset.

Pyrexia The usual febrile course in murine typhus lasts for about 12 days in adults; the temperature ranges from 102 to 104°F but may reach 105 to 106°F in children. The temperature may reach high levels abruptly after onset or ascend in a stepwise manner during the first few days. With the appearance of the rash, fever is usually sustained, with partial daily remissions which occasionally reach normal levels in the morning. Defervescence is generally by lysis over several days but sometimes occurs by crisis. Transient mild fever of 100°F is not uncommon during early convalescence. A few patients experience only low-grade fever throughout, but this does not necessarily connote a mild illness.

Cutaneous manifestations The early lesions, which are sparse and discrete, are hidden in the axillae and inner surface of the arm. Most patients then develop with surprising suddenness a generalized, dull red macular rash of the upper part of the abdomen, shoulders, chest, arms, and thighs. The individual lesions are discrete and pea size, with an ill-defined border, and fade on pressure during the first 24 h. They later become maculopapular, in contrast to the exanthem of epidemic typhus, which is persistently macular. The distribution over the trunk with sparse involvement of the extremities, palms, soles, and face differs from the peripheral distribution and facial involvement of Rocky Mountain spotted fever. The murine rash generally appears initially on the fifth febrile day, but rarely it is seen concurrently with the onset of fever or develops as late as the seventh day.

Eighty percent of patients develop a rash which persists for 4 to 8 days and fades before defervescence. The cutaneous manifestations vary greatly in intensity and duration and may be fleeting. They are readily overlooked in dark-skinned patients, in whom they should be sought by light palpation and indirect lighting.

Cardiovascular and respiratory features An irritating, nonproductive cough is frequent and is occasionally associated with moderate hemoptysis. Early in the second week, rales may be detected in the basilar lung areas. These changes are generally rickettsial rather than bacterial in origin and respond to the broad-spectrum antibiotics. Pulmonary congestion occurs in extremely ill and elderly patients.

Accelerated pulse, hypotension, and general circulatory weakness occur in this disease, although less frequently than in patients with epidemic typhus or Rocky Mountain spotted fever.

Neurologic manifestations Headache is the most common neurologic manifestation of murine typhus and may dominate the clinical picture. It is frontal and continues into the second week of illness. Stupor and prostration may occur in the second week, and in severe cases, there may be muttering delirium, extreme agitation, or coma. Coma in elderly patients after 2 weeks of illness presages death. Nuchal rigidity and general spasticity often suggest meningitis, although the spinal fluid is normal except for slight increases in pressure and lymphocytes (5 to 30 per cubic millimeter). Transient partial deafness occurs occasionally, but rarely is there localized neuritis or hemiplegia. Neurologic sequelae are unusual. Children experience minimal neurologic changes.

Other physical manifestations During the first 2 days of illness the patient may be nauseated and vomit, but vomiting later in the illness should arouse suspicion of an intercurrent complication. Abdominal pain is bothersome; when associated with diarrhea, it responds to intravenous alimentation. Hepatomegaly and jaundice are unusual. There is splenomegaly in approximately 25 percent of patients.

Photophobia, retroocular pain, suffusion of the eyes, and congestion of the conjunctivas are common but are less severe than in the other typhus and spotted fevers.

Renal function is usually unaltered except in elderly patients with prolonged hypotension. Under these circumstances, azotemia may develop to the degree observed in epidemic typhus. In severe murine typhus, as in the epidemic typhus, hyponatremia and hypoalbuminemia are encountered.

COURSE After defervescence, murine typhus patients recover rapidly. Fatalities occur between the ninth and twelfth days in elderly or debilitated patients, usually as a result of circulatory and renal failure or intercurrent bacterial infection.

PROGNOSIS The mortality rate in murine typhus was low even before the introduction of modern specific therapy. Only 1 death occurred in 114 cases studied by Maxcy and none in the 180 reported by Stuart and Pullen.

DIFFERENTIAL DIAGNOSIS Because murine typhus and Rocky Mountain spotted fever occur in many of the same states, the problem of differential diagnosis often arises. Flea-borne murine typhus, which is predominantly an urban disease, is more likely to occur in late summer and autumn. In contrast, spotted fever is a rural and suburban disease in which exposure to ticks is important. Most cases occur in the spring and summer.

TREATMENT AND PREVENTION Both chloramphenicol and the tetracycline antibiotics have controlled the disease (see Chap. 188).

Prevention of murine typhus in humans is attained by reducing the natural reservoir and vector by applying measures for eliminating rodents and employing appropriate insecticides in rat-infested areas to control fleas. Spraying of rat burrows with DDT effectively reduces the population of the vector.

EPIDEMIC (LOUSE-BORNE) TYPHUS FEVER

DEFINITION The classic epidemic form of typhus is a severe, febrile disease caused by *R. prowazekii* and transmitted to humans by the body louse. Intense headache, continuous pyrexia of about 2 weeks, a macular skin eruption appearing on about the fifth febrile day, malaise, and vascular and neurologic disturbances represent the principal clinical features. Confirmation of the diagnosis is made by demonstration of *Proteus* OX-19 agglutinins and of specific complement-fixing antibodies in convalescence. The broad-spectrum antibiotics are specific therapeutic agents.

ETIOLOGY AND EPIDEMIOLOGY The causative microbe, *R. prowazekii,* is closely related to *R. mooseri,* which causes murine typhus; indeed, the two have a number of common antigens.

Human beings generally are infected when rickettsia-laden louse feces are rubbed into the broken skin; scratching the louse bite facilitates this process. *Pediculus humanus corporis,* which is peculiarly adapted to humans, is the only important vector of epidemic typhus. It dies of its infection and fails to transmit rickettsias to its offspring. *R. prowazekii* has been isolated from flying squirrels, and the organism probably infests their ectoparasites. Generally, however, the organism is maintained by a cycle involving human-louse-human. New epidemics apparently originate from patients with Brill-Zinsser disease (recurrent epidemic typhus). Pathogenic rickettsias reside for long periods in patients with epidemic typhus as well as Rocky Mountain spotted fever and scrub typhus. Lice readily become infected when fed on patients with recurrent typhus. Inhalation of dust containing dried louse feces may cause infection. An established nonhuman reservoir would pose a serious threat.

Epidemic typhus, if uncontrolled, behaves as a cyclic disease in a susceptible population, extending over a 3-year period. During the first year there is a gradual seeding of cases throughout the group; during the second there is epidemic spread; and during the third the epidemic tapers off, because the majority of persons have become immune. Outbreaks of epidemic typhus last occurred in the United States in the nineteenth century, and its presence is now recognized only in the form of Brill-Zinsser disease.

CLINICAL MANIFESTATIONS Epidemic typhus resembles murine typhus but is more severe. After an incubation period of about 7 days an abrupt onset of headache, chill, and rapidly mounting fever ushers in the illness. Headache, malaise, and prostration continue unabated until the rash appears on the fifth febrile day. It is initially macular in the axillary folds but ultimately invades the trunk and extremities as a pink, irregular macular lesion, which becomes fixed, petechial, and confluent in the later stages.

Neurologic features range from headache and general spasticity to extreme agitation, stupor, and coma. Circulatory disturbances consisting of tachycardia, hypotension, and cyanosis are more profound than those observed in murine typhus and are almost as severe as in Rocky Mountain spotted fever. Ultimately, in untreated cases azotemia often reaches high levels as a result of vascular and renal failure, and death occurs late in the second week of illness. Furthermore, thrombosis of major blood vessels and cutaneous gangrene develop in a manner similar to that seen in the virulent form of Rocky Mountain spotted fever.

The complications and sequelae of epidemic typhus are more severe than those in murine typhus, but not as severe as those in Rocky Mountain spotted fever. However, during certain outbreaks, epidemic typhus was fatal in 60 percent of those infected, and convalescence in survivors was prolonged. Broad-spectrum antibiotics have almost eradicated mortality in this dread disease, provided therapy is instituted before irreversible changes have been established in the tissues.

DIFFERENTIAL DIAGNOSIS Differentiation of epidemic typhus from the various rickettsioses and other diseases with which it may be confused was described above. The disease in epidemic form never occurs in the absence of lousiness in the general population. Under the conditions in which typhus epidemics are likely to occur, other diseases which may cause confusion include malaria, relapsing fever, pneumonia, and tuberculosis. Classic typhus contracted by a previously vaccinated person is usually mild and may be clinically indistinguishable from murine typhus except by serologic methods. An illness simulating Rocky Mountain spotted fever is caused by *R. canada,* a member of the typhus group.

TREATMENT AND PREVENTION Both chloramphenicol and the tetracycline antibiotics have been found to be highly efficient therapeutic agents in epidemic typhus. Usually the patient becomes afebrile after 2 days of treatment. Under field conditions, 100 mg doxycycline in a single oral dose resulted in abatement of clinical manifestations and defervescence in epidemic typhus.

The most effective measures for controlling epidemic typhus are those which eliminate lousiness. DDT or lindane powder when dusted into clothing is suitable for this purpose. If resistant lice are found, malathion or carbaryl may prove effective.

A commercially available vaccine prepared from formalin-treated suspensions of infected yolk sac tissue is an effective immunizing agent. A viable vaccine utilizing an attenuated strain of *R. prowazekii* is under development.

BRILL-ZINSSER DISEASE (RECRUDESCENT TYPHUS)

Brill-Zinsser disease is a recrudescent episode of epidemic typhus fever which occurs years after the initial attack, in persons who had recovered from the epidemic disease acquired while residing in countries where it was prevalent. *R. prowazekii* have been isolated from lice fed on patients during the active stages of illness.

The clinical entity, not always mild, resembles epidemic typhus in the character of the rash, circulatory disturbances, and hepatic, renal, and nervous system changes. Recovery is the rule. The Weil-Felix reaction with the various *Proteus* antigens is usually negative, or positive in very low titer. The specific complement fixation, microscopic agglutination, and immunofluorescent antibody reactions are valuable in establishing the diagnosis. In Brill-Zinsser disease the specific complement-fixing antibodies appear as early as the fourth day after the onset of illness; the peak response is attained by the eighth to tenth days. Specific antibody titers in the primary attack of epidemic typhus begin later, about the eighth to twelfth day, with maximum titers on about the sixteenth day after onset. Treatment is the same as for other rickettsial infections.

SCRUB TYPHUS

DEFINITION Scrub typhus is limited to eastern and southeastern Asia, India, northern Australia, and the adjacent islands. It is caused by *R. tsutsugamushi* and characterized by a primary lesion at the site of the bite of an infected mite, a fever of about 2 weeks' duration, a cutaneous rash which develops about the fifth day, and the appearance late in the second week of agglutinins against the OX-K strain of *Proteus* bacillus. The broad-spectrum antibiotics are specific therapeutic agents.

ETIOLOGY The agent of scrub typhus resembles other rickettsias in its physical properties but differs from them in antigenic structure, vector, and reservoir. The disease is transmitted by larvae of several species of mites, especially *Leptotrobidium (Trombicula) akamushi* and *L. deliense.* These tiny chiggers attach themselves to the skin and during the process of obtaining a meal of tissue juice may acquire infection from the host or transmit rickettsias to the vertebrate. The infection is maintained in nature by a cycle involving mites and small rodents and by transovarial transmission in mites; human infection represents an accident attributable to propinquity.

CLINICAL MANIFESTATIONS About 10 to 12 days after infection, illness begins abruptly with chilliness, severe headache, fever, conjunctival injection, and moderate generalized lymphadenopathy, which is most prominent in the nodes draining the area of the primary lesion. The initial lesion at the beginning of fever is evidenced by an erythematous indurated area 1 cm in diameter, surmounted by a multiloculated vesicle; within a few days the vesicle ulcerates and becomes covered with a black crust.

Fever increases progressively during the first week, generally reaching 104 to 105°F, but the pulse remains relatively slow, 70 to 100 beats per minute. The red macular rash, which begins on the trunk about the fifth day and spreads to the extremities, sometimes becomes maculopapular but usually fades in a few days. The course of the disease and the complications resemble those of endemic and epidemic typhus; however, interstitial myocarditis is more prominent than in the other typhus fevers.

PROGNOSIS Before the introduction of the broad-spectrum antibiotics the mortality rate varied from 1 to 60 percent, depending on the geographic area and the virulence of the local strains of *R. tsutsugamushi,* and convalescence was prolonged. With modern therapeutic methods, deaths are rare and convalescence is short.

DIFFERENTIAL DIAGNOSIS Scrub typhus is to be differentiated from the other members of the typhus and the spotted fever group of diseases as well as from measles, typhoid fever, and the meningococcal infections. The geographic localization of scrub typhus, the primary lesion, and the occurrence of OX-K agglutinins are especially useful in establishing the diagnosis.

TREATMENT AND PREVENTION Chloramphenicol and the tetracycline antibiotics are extremely effective in scrub typhus. Scrub typhus is more amenable to drugs than are the other rickettsial infections, and patients with this disease regularly become afebrile and are decidedly improved within 24 to 36 h after beginning treatment, irrespective of the stage of disease. Antibiotic treatment may be discontinued after several afebrile days.

Relapse of clinical illness is unusual unless specific treatment is initiated early, such as before the fifth febrile day. Under these circumstances, recrudescence is obviated by giving the antibiotic for several days and resuming treatment about 5 days after cessation of the initial course of therapy.

Prevention of disease in the individual is accomplished by the application of miticidal chemicals (dibutyl phthalate, benzyl benzoate, diethyltoluamide, and others) to clothing and the skin. There is no satisfactory vaccine.

TRENCH FEVER

DEFINITION Trench fever is a febrile disease transmitted between humans by the body louse, *Pediculus humanus corporis.* It is characterized by a sudden onset with headache and severe pain in the muscles, bones, and joints. In most cases, the fever and other symptoms assume a relapsing character. Fatalities are rare. The disease is also known as shin bone fever, Volhynia fever, His-Werner disease, and quintan fever.

ETIOLOGY AND EPIDEMIOLOGY *R. quintana,* the etiologic agent, grows extracellularly in the louse gut, in contrast to other pathogenic rickettsias which can multiply only within cells. A European strain of *R. quintana* has been cultivated on blood agar, and typical trench fever has been induced in volunteers.

Humans are the only known reservoir of infection. The louse does not transmit the organism transovarially but acquires its infection by ingesting the blood of a person with rickettsemia. The organisms multiply extracellularly in the louse gut, without injury to this host, and are excreted in large numbers with the feces. Humans become infected by the inoculation of the contaminated feces into abraded skin or conjunctivas. *R. quintana* may be recovered periodically from human blood for several years after convalescence from an acute attack. Trench fever is known to exist in Mexico, Tunisia, Eritrea, Poland, the U.S.S.R., and possibly China, and there is serologic evidence for its occurrence in Bolivia, Burundi, and Ethiopia.

PATHOLOGY Since there have been no recorded fatalities, histologic examination has been confined to excised macules of the skin, which have shown nonspecific perivascular infiltrates without the involvement of the vessel walls that is seen in typhus fever.

CLINICAL MANIFESTATIONS A variety of clinical manifestations is displayed in trench fever, ranging from a mild afebrile disease to a debilitating illness with a protracted clinical course involving numerous relapses. Following an incubation period of 10 to 30 days the onset may be insidious or dramatically abrupt. The acute disease is characterized by malaise, headache, fever, and bone and body pain, especially severe in the shins. In some cases only one fever peak occurs; in others the fever continues for 5 to 7 days; and in others there is an initial febrile episode lasting 1 to 3 days followed by relapses which characteristically occur at 4- to 5-day intervals. In some cases the fever and symptoms are continuous for 2 or 3 weeks. Enlargement of the spleen and a red macular rash occur in 70 to 80 percent of the cases. Pain and soreness in the muscles usually recur with each febrile relapse.

The disease is marked by a persistent rickettsemia, which is present during the initial attack and which continues during the relapses, throughout the asymptomatic periods between relapses, and for months or even years after cessation of physical symptoms. A relapse has been reported 10 years after the original attack.

PROGNOSIS The disease causes no known deaths, but its duration is variable. About 85 percent of patients are able to return to work within 2 months of onset, but about 5 percent of all cases become chronic. Recovery is even more delayed in the aged and debilitated.

DIFFERENTIAL DIAGNOSIS During epidemics, typical cases are easily diagnosed on the basis of symptoms. The disease may be differentiated from influenza, typhoid, typhus, dengue, and relapsing fever by the specific laboratory tests available for the diagnosis of each of these diseases.

TREATMENT AND PREVENTION *R. quintana* is highly sensitive in vitro to the broad-spectrum antibiotics, but no reliable information has been obtained about the value of these drugs in treating trench fever. The treatment is symptomatic. Aspirin is used to control pain and discomfort, but codeine may be necessary. Patients should remain in bed for a week or more after complete cessation of subjective and objective evidence of infection. They should be kept under observation for several months and returned to bed at the first sign of relapse.

The methods employed to control epidemic typhus should be equally efficacious in controlling trench fever. These are based on the elimination of lousiness and the improvement of living conditions with provision for frequent bathing and washing of clothing. DDT or lindane powder should be applied by hand or power duster at appropriate intervals to clothes and persons of populations living under conditions favoring lousiness. If resistant lice are found, malathion or other effective lousicides may be substituted as a dusting powder.

RICKETTSIALPOX

DEFINITION Rickettsialpox is a mild, nonfatal self-limited, febrile illness caused by *R. akari,* which is transmitted from mouse to humans by mites. It is characterized by an initial skin lesion at the site of the mite bite, a week's febrile course, and a papulovesicular rash.

ETIOLOGY AND EPIDEMIOLOGY Rickettsialpox was first recognized in New York City in 1946, and about 180 cases were reported annually for several years thereafter. It has been diagnosed in several other areas of the United States, and outbreaks have been reported in European Russia. The vector is a small, colorless mite, *Allodermanyssus sanguineus* (Hirst), which infests small mice and rodents. House mice serve as the reservoir of infection.

R. akari is morphologically and biologically similar to other rickettsias and is antigenically related to, but distinct from, *R. rickettsii,* the cause of Rocky Mountain spotted fever. Mice, guinea pigs, and fertile hen eggs are susceptible to experimental infection. Diagnostic antigens prepared from infected yolk sacs and tissue culture cells are used in serologic reactions.

CLINICAL MANIFESTATIONS The initial skin lesion appears about 7 to 10 days after the mite bite as a firm red papule 1 to 1.5 cm in diameter. In a few days, the center vesiculates, and the papule is surrounded by an area of erythema. The regional lymph glands are moderately enlarged. The primary lesion, which is never painful, becomes covered with a black scab; it heals slowly, and a small scar is visible on separation of the crust.

The febrile phase begins 3 to 7 days after the initial lesion, and exanthem may accompany the fever or begin several days later. The onset of fever is sudden, with chilly sensations or frank chills, headache, sweats, myalgia, anorexia, and photophobia. The pyrexia ranges from 103 to 104°F and continues for about a week, occasionally with morning remisssions.

The exanthem is maculopapular-vesicular, generalized in distribution, and may be abundant or scant. The lesions may involve the oral cavity but not the palms or soles. In a week, the vesicles dry and form scabs which eventually scale but leave no scar.

The constitutional symptoms are generally mild, and the course of illness is uncomplicated. No fatal cases have been reported.

The disease may be confused with chickenpox, which is different because it occurs usually in childhood and has no initial lesion and the papular cutaneous lesion is entirely transformed into a vesicle. Variola (smallpox) is accompanied by a more severe constitutional reaction, and the vesicles become pustules. The skin lesions of the other rickettsioses differ in their lack of vesiculation. The Weil-Felix reaction is usually negative in this rickettsial disease, but specific complement fixation, microscopic agglutination, and immunofluorescent antibody reactions are useful diagnostic aids even though there is considerable crossing with materials from Rocky Mountain spotted fever.

TREATMENT AND PREVENTION Chloramphenicol and the tetracycline antibiotics are all effective for treating patients with rickettsialpox. The temperature reaches normal levels in about 2 days, and recovery is rapid.

Control measures should be directed toward elimination of house mice and the vector mites responsible for transmitting the disease.

OTHER TICK-BORNE RICKETTSIAL DISEASES

DEFINITION Boutonneuse fever, North Asian tick-borne rickettsiosis, and Queensland tick typhus, three diseases occurring in the eastern hemisphere, are caused by rickettsias closely related to one another and to the agent of Rocky Mountain spotted fever. Each is transmitted by the bite of an ixodid tick. These mild to moderately severe illnesses are characterized by an initial lesion (called *tache noire* in boutonneuse fever), a fever of several days to 2 weeks, and a generalized maculopapular erythematous rash which appears on about the fifth day and usually involves the palms and soles. Specific complement-fixing antibodies appear in the patients' serums during convalescence, but agglutinins to *Proteus* OX-19 (Weil-Felix reaction) are frequently found only in low titer.

ETIOLOGY AND EPIDEMIOLOGY The etiologic agents of these three diseases are all members of the spotted fever group of rickettsias. Together with *R. rickettsii* and *R. akari* they possess common group antigens which are readily demonstrated by agglutination, complement fixation, microscopic agglutination, and immunofluorescent antibody reactions.

Boutonneuse fever, which may be regarded as the prototype of the three, is caused by *R. conorii*. Modern serologic methods employing specific rickettsial antigens have shown this rickettsia to be the causative agent for a single widely disseminated disease known by various local names. Information on the distribution and etiology of the various tick-borne rickettsial diseases is contained in Table 188-1.

In general, the epidemiology of these tick-borne rickettsioses resembles that of spotted fever in the western hemisphere. Ixodid ticks and small wild animals maintain the rickettsias in nature; if humans intrude accidentally into the cycle, they become a dead end in the transmission chain. In certain areas, the cycle of boutonneuse fever involves domiciliary environments, with the brown dog tick *Rhipicephalus sanguineus* as the dominant vector.

CLINICAL MANIFESTATIONS These three tick-borne rickettsioses, which occur in different parts of the eastern hemisphere, resemble one another closely. The clinical course is usually milder than that of spotted fever, with a shorter febrile period and fewer severe complications; fatalities are rare and generally limited to the aged and debilitated. The initial lesion, which is present in most cases at the onset of fever, heals slowly; the regional lymph nodes are enlarged. The rash usually remains papular and only in severe cases becomes hemorrhagic.

The clinical picture (including the primary lesion), the geographic location, and epidemiologic considerations are helpful in establishing the diagnosis. The typhus fevers, meningococcal infections, and measles must be considered in the differential diagnosis; the serologic reactions, i.e., Weil-Felix and complement fixation tests, are of value here.

TREATMENT AND PREVENTION Chloramphenicol and the tetracyclines are effective therapeutic agents for boutonneuse fever. Patients generally become afebrile after 2 to 3 days of treatment, and recovery is rapid. Presumably these measures are also applicable to North Asian tick-borne rickettsiosis and Queensland tick typhus.

The major effective methods of control are concerned with avoidance of tick bites; these include application of new repellents and prompt removal of attached ticks. Effective vaccines are not available commercially.

Q FEVER

DEFINITION Q fever is an acute infectious disease caused by *Coxiella burnetii* and characterized by a sudden onset of fever, malaise, headache, weakness, anorexia, and interstitial pneumonitis.Rickettsemia occurs during the febrile period, and specific complement-fixing antibodies are present during convalescence. In contrast to the other rickettsioses, the disease is not associated with a cutaneous exanthem or agglutinins for the *Proteus* bacteria (Weil-Felix reaction).

ETIOLOGY AND EPIDEMIOLOGY *C. burnetii* possesses the general properties of other rickettsias but is somewhat more resistant to inactivation in unfavorable environments and more pleomorphic than the others. Its infectivity after drying under natural conditions is of importance in the spread of infection to humans. *C. burnetii* has a wide host range in nature, but guinea pigs and embryonated eggs are the common laboratory hosts employed for its propagation.

Human cases of Q fever are contracted by inhalation of infected dusts, by handling infected materials, possibly by drinking milk contaminated with *C. burnetii* and, in one instance, by blood transfusion. The disease in Australia is enzootic in animals, especially bandicoots, and is transmitted in nature by ticks. Rickettsia-laden tick feces may contaminate cattle hides, and inhalation of this material has caused infection in humans. In the United States, a number of species of ticks are naturally infected, among them *Dermacentor andersoni* and *Amblyomma americanum,* and in North Africa transovarial transmission of the agent in indigenous ticks has been demonstrated. Sheep, goats, and cows have been found to be naturally infected in North America and in Europe, and *C. burnetii* has been recovered from the milk of such animals. Milk, as well as infected excretions from livestock, probably accounts for certain outbreaks of human disease following inhalation by cows of infected dust from barns and pens. The airborne route of dried contaminated material is the most likely method of spread. A number of epidemics have occurred among laboratory workers engaged in studies on *C. burnetii.* The disease is not transmitted between humans.

CLINICAL MANIFESTATIONS After incubation of approximately 19 days (the range is 14 to 26 days), the disease begins with headache, chilly sensations, fever, malaise, myalgia, and anorexia. For several days, the temperature ranges from 101 to 104°F; the entire course rarely exceeds 2 weeks and usually ranges from 3 to 6 days. There may be wide fluctuations in the fever. Respiratory and gastrointestinal symptoms are not conspicuous in the early stages. Headache and fever predominate. A dry cough and chest pain occur after about 5 days, when rales are usually audible. Roentgenographic findings indistinguishable from those of primary atypical pneumonia are present usually by the third to fourth day of disease, first as patchy areas of consolidation involving a portion of one lobe, giving a homogeneous ground-glass appearance. These manifestations persist beyond the febrile period and may appear in patients who are unaware of pulmonary involvement. Complications are rare, and coincident with defervescence the appetite begins to return. Convalescence progresses slowly for several weeks, during which time the principal disability is weakness. It is not uncommon for patients to lose 15 to 20 lb during the active stages of disease. The disease may be protracted in approximately 20 percent of cases, with fever persisting for longer than 4 weeks, particularly in elderly patients. Occasionally relapse occurs, especially in patients treated with antibiotics during the first several days of disease.

Hepatitis, with the development of clinically detectable icterus, occurs in approximately one-third of patients with the protracted form. This form of Q fever is characterized by fever, malaise, absence of headache or respiratory signs, and hepatomegaly with right upper quadrant pain. Liver biopsy specimens show diffuse granulomatous changes with multinucleated giant cells and scattered infiltrations of polymorphonuclear leukocytes, lymphocytes, and macrophages. *C. burnetii* may be demonstrated in such specimens with the fluorescent antibody technique. Therefore, Q fever must be included in the differential diagnosis of liver granulomas such as tuberculosis, sarcoidosis, histoplasmosis, brucellosis, tularemia, syphilis, and others.

Endocarditis also has been reported, and *C. burnetii* has been identified by smear and isolation in vegetations on the heart valves obtained at operation or autopsy. The aortic valve is most commonly involved, often with large vegetations. It is important, therefore, to suspect the possibility of Q fever in cases of apparent subacute bacterial endocarditis with persistently negative blood cultures. Operative intervention with replacement of damaged valves is usually necessary for recovery because the available antibiotics are not rickettsicidal.

A high complement-fixing antibody titer to phase I antigen is present in patients with endocarditis and granulomatous hepatitis.

PROGNOSIS Few fatalities have been recorded and, except for the patient with protracted illness and hepatic involvement or endocarditis, the course of disease is generally uncomplicated and benign.

TREATMENT AND CONTROL The tetracycline antibiotics and chloramphenicol are effective in the treatment of patients with Q fever. Most patients, when treated early in the course of disease, respond promptly and recover without relapses. The therapeutic procedures are comparable to those used in spotted fever.

Control of Q fever depends primarily on immunization of susceptible persons with specific vaccines. Vaccines made from phase I rickettsias are potent and afford considerable protection to slaughterhouse and dairy workers, herders, rendering-plant workers, woolsorters, tanners, laboratory workers, and others at risk. Measures should be taken to avoid exposure to infected aerosols; milk from infected domestic livestock must be pasteurized or boiled.

REFERENCES

Andrew R et al: Tick typhus in North Queensland. Med J Aust 2:253, 1946

Bozeman FM et al: Serologic evidence of *Rickettsia canada* infection in man. J Infect Dis 121:367, 1970

——— et al: Epidemic typhus rickettsiae isolated from flying squirrels. Nature 255:545, 1975

Derrick EH: The epidemiology of Q fever: A review. Med J Aust 1:245, 1953

DeShazo RD et al: Early diagnosis of Rocky Mountain spotted fever. Use of primary monocyte culture technique. JAMA 235:1353, 1976

Ferguson IC et al: Clinical, virological and pathological findings in a fatal case of Q fever endocarditis. Br J Clin Pathol 15:235, 1962

Gambrill MR, Wisseman CL Jr: Mechanisms of immunity in typhus infections. Infect Immun 8:519, 1973

Harrell GT: Rickettsial involvement of the nervous system. Med Clin North Am 37:395, 1953

Hattwick MAW et al: Rocky Mountain spotted fever: Epidemiology of an increasing problem. Ann Intern Med 84:732, 1976

Hazard GW et al: Rocky Mountain spotted fever in the Eastern United States. N Engl J Med 280:57, 1969

Marmion BP, Stoker MGP: The epidemiology of Q fever in Great Britain: An analysis of the findings and some conclusions. Br Med J 2:809, 1958

McKiel JA et al: *Rickettsia canada:* A new member of the typhus group of rickettsiae isolated from *Haemaphysalis leporis-palustris* ticks in Canada. J Microbiol 12:503, 1967

Mohr CO, Smith WW: Eradication of murine typhus fever in a rural area. Bull WHO 16:255, 1957

Moulton FR (ed): *The Rickettsial Diseases of Man.* Washington, DC, American Association for the Advancement of Science, 1948

Murray ES et al: Brill's disease: I. Clinical and laboratory diagnosis. JAMA 142:1059, 1950

———, Snyder JC: Brill's disease: II. Etiology. Am J Hyg 53:22, 1951

Ormsbee RA et al: The influence of phase on the protective potency of Q fever vaccine. J Immunol 92:404, 1964

——— et al: Serologic diagnosis of epidemic typhus fever. Am J Epidemiol 105:261, 1977

Oster CN et al: Laboratory acquired Rocky Mountain spotted fever: The hazard of aerosol transmission. N Engl J Med 297:859, 1977

Pedersen CE et al: Demonstration of *Rickettsia rickettsii* in Rhesus monkeys by immune fluorescence microscopy. J Clin Microbiol 2:121, 1975

Philip RN et al: A comparison of serologic methods for diagnosis of Rocky Mountain spotted fever. Am J Epidemiol 105:56, 1977

PRATT HD: The changing picture of murine typhus in the United States. Ann NY Acad Sci 70:516, 1958

ROSE HM: The clinical manifestations and laboratory diagnosis of rickettsialpox. Ann Intern Med 31:871, 1949

SCHACHTER J et al: Potential danger of Q fever in a university hospital environment. J Infect Dis 123:301, 1971

SCHAFFNER W, KOENIG MG: Thrombocytopenic Rocky Mountain spotted fever. Arch Intern Med 116:857, 1965

SMADEL JE: Influence of antibiotics on immunologic responses in scrub typhus. Am J Med 17:246, 1954

——— (ed): *Symposium on Q Fever,* Medical Science Publication 6. Washington, DC, Walter Reed Army Institute of Research, 1959

———, JACKSON EB: Rickettsial infections, in *Diagnostic Procedures of Viral and Rickettsial Diseases*, 3d ed. New York, American Public Health Association, 1964, p 743

SOMENSHINE DE et al: Epizootiology of epidemic typhus (*Rickettsia prowazekii*) in flying squirrels. Am J Trop Med Hyg 27:339, 1978

VINSON JW: Etiology of trench fever in Mexico, in *Industry and Tropical Health,* vol V. Boston, Harvard School of Public Health, 1964, p 109

WALKER DH, CAIN BG: A method for specific diagnosis of Rocky Mountain spotted fever on fixed, paraffin-embedded tissue by immunofluorescence. J Infect Dis 137:206, 1978

WOODWARD TE: Rickettsial diseases in the United States. Med Clin North Am 43:1507, 1959

———: A historical account of the rickettsial diseases with a discussion of unsolved problems. J Infect Dis 127:583, 1973

———: Identification of *Rickettsia* in skin tissues. J Infect Dis 134:297, 1976

section 11 | Mycoplasma and chlamydial infections

190 MYCOPLASMA PNEUMONIAE INFECTIONS

VERNON KNIGHT

The mycoplasmas, formerly called pleuropneumonia-like organisms (PPLO) after the organism that caused a highly contagious form of bovine pneumonia and pleurisy in Europe in the eighteenth century, are now designated class Mollicutes, family Mycoplasmataceae, genus *Mycoplasma.*

The only mycoplasma of importance in respiratory disease is *M. pneumoniae. M. pneumoniae* grows on peptone-enriched beef-heart infusion broth as small round colonies partially buried in the agar without the "fried egg" periphery characteristic of growth of other mycoplasmas. *M. pneumoniae* grows aerobically and anaerobically.

M. pneumoniae is resistant to penicillin and antibiotics known to interfere with polymerization of cell wall precursors, and it does not retain the dye-iodine complex of Gram's stain. It is inhibited by tetracyclines, erythromycin, chloramphenicol, and some other antibiotics. Like bacteria, it grows outside the cell, possesses ribonucleic and deoxyribonucleic acids, reproduces by fission, and generates metabolic energy.

DEFINITION Pneumonia caused by *M. pneumoniae* is characterized by fever, pharyngitis, cough, and pulmonary infiltration, often multilobular, in which roentgenographic signs are more extensive than indicated by physical examination. Synonyms are primary atypical pneumonia, Eaton's agent pneumonia, cold agglutinin-positive pneumonia, and "virus" pneumonia. This organism also causes upper respiratory illness without pneumonia and asymptomatic infection.

ETIOLOGY *M. pneumoniae* is distinguished from other mycoplasmas by rapid hemolysis of guinea pig erythrocytes and utilization of glucose and other sugars. It also hemolyzes human and rat erythrocytes and may be distinguished from other mycoplasmas by fluorescent antibody, complement fixation, growth inhibition, and indirect hemagglutination tests, all of which are useful for serologic diagnosis of human infection. In addition to growing on agar, the organism grows on the surface of cells of embryonated eggs and monkey kidney cell culture with little evidence of cytopathic effect. In human cell cultures, however, there is intracellular growth with cytopathic effects.

EPIDEMIOLOGY In the general population *M. pneumoniae* infection is characterized by intrafamily spread. In most cases the infection is introduced into the family by a schoolchild. Once it is introduced, most family members become infected. In family outbreaks, pneumonia occurs with greatest frequency among school-age children, with a predominance in males. The disease is rare above age 40. *M. pneumoniae* pneumonia occurs throughout the year, although prolonged wintertime outbreaks may occur in college groups or communities. The total incidence of *M. pneumoniae* pneumonia in a study in Seattle was 1.3 per 1000 per year, which constituted about 15 to 20 percent of pneumonia from all causes. At intervals of several years, epidemics of *M. pneumoniae* pneumonia may occur with about double the usual incidence of disease.

In the military, *M. pneumoniae* infections account for a small proportion of upper respiratory illness in recruits—in one study, 6.3 percent. However, it accounted for almost one-half of cases of pneumonia in the same military population. No more than 10 percent of infected military personnel develop pneumonia; the rest are asymptomatic. The disease appears to be endemic at military bases.

M. pneumoniae is probably spread by means of infected respiratory secretions. The organisms can be cultured from sputum of naturally occurring cases and from volunteers inoculated artificially. Primary atypical pneumonia has been induced in volunteers both by nasopharyngeal inoculation and by inhalation of a small-particle aerosol containing the agent. In volunteers naturally acquired antibody is associated with a high degree of resistance to infection.

CLINICAL MANIFESTATIONS The incubation period is from 9 to 12 days, but the interval between cases in families is approximately 3 weeks. Illness usually begins with symptoms of upper respiratory infection, which in some patients progresses to bronchitis and pneumonia. Four syndromes of respiratory disease have been identified: pneumonia, tracheobronchitis, pharyngitis, and bullous myringitis. About one-third of cases in family members will develop pneumonia, up to one-half will have tracheobronchitis, 10 percent exhibit only pharyngitis, and 10 percent will be asymptomatic. Children 5 to 10 years old, especially boys, have the greatest incidence of disease. Ear involvement consisting of congestion of the tympanic membrane and of bullous and, rarely, hemorrhagic myringitis may occur in as many as 10 percent of cases of pneumonia, most often in children. Cough is almost universal in pneumonia and is frequent in cases without pulmonary involvement. Blood-flecked sputum may occur in the more severe cases, but gross hemoptysis is rare. A variety of other respiratory and systemic complaints may occur. Fever, nasal congestion, and sore throat are common. In pneumonia, harsh or diminished sounds are frequent but bronchial breathing is uncommon. Fine inspiratory rales are found in most patients but are not impressive. Pleural rubs and pleural effusion are infrequent. Studies on the distribution of pneumonia in one large series showed that more than one-half of cases were multilobular and slightly less than one-half were bilateral. Lower-lobe pneumonia was appreciably more frequent than upper-lobe pneumonia. Pulmonary infiltrates may occur as an isolated area in the lung periphery but more often spread from the hilum.

The disease is variable in severity, but high fever may persist for 1 to 2 weeks in untreated cases. X-ray changes last for as long as 3 weeks in untreated cases, but for 7 to 10 days in treated cases. Even in untreated cases, complications are rare and consist of occasional purulent sinusitis, persistent cough, and, rarely, pleurisy. Prolonged weakness and malaise follow the untreated illness in adults.

Rare complications include meningoencephalitis, polyneuritis, monoarticular arthritis, Stevens-Johnson syndrome, pericarditis, myocarditis, hepatitis, diffuse intravascular coagulation, and hemolytic anemia.

LABORATORY FINDINGS During acute illness leukocytosis in the range of 10,000 to 15,000 leukocytes per cubic millimeter occurs in about 25 percent of cases. Increase in sedimentation rate above 40 mm/h occurs in at least two-thirds of cases. Urinalysis, electrocardiograms, and fluid and electrolyte and liver function studies show no characteristic changes. The complement fixation, fluorescent antibody, indirect hemagglutination, and growth inhibition tests all yield highly specific diagnostic information. The simplicity of the complement fixation test recommends it for general use. Fourfold rises in titer often occur within 2 weeks, and maximum rise is achieved in 4 weeks. A nonspecific test for *M. pneumoniae* infection in use for many years is the detection of cold agglutinins. The end point is the dilution of the patient's serum, which agglutinates human type O red blood cells at 4°C. The test depends on the presence of a macroglobulin antibody to phase I antigen of red blood cells. In *M. pneumoniae* infection, cold agglutinins appear at the end of the first week of illness and disappear in a week or so. The test is positive in a majority of patients, more commonly in those who are severely ill. The cold agglutinin reaction is nonspecific, however, and occurs with other red blood cell antigens in infectious mononucleosis, lymphoproliferative diseases, and in several respiratory infections, particularly in children.

DIFFERENTIAL DIAGNOSIS Pneumonia due to *M. pneumoniae* needs to be distinguished from pneumonia of all other types. It is usually less severe, is associated with less dense pulmonary infiltration than pneumococcal and other bacterial pneumonias, and occurs throughout the year. Pulmonary infiltrate in the absence of symptoms or physical signs may initially suggest acute pulmonary tuberculosis. In military populations adenoviral pneumonia must be excluded. Pneumonic involvement as a direct result of influenza viral infection or its complication by pneumococcal, streptococcal, staphylococcal, or *H. influenzae* infection may cause difficulty in diagnosis. Q fever, psittacosis, and tularemia are less frequent causes of pneumonia that may be difficult to distinguish from *M. pneumoniae* infection. In children, especially young infants, pneumonia due to respiratory syncytial, parainfluenza, adenovirus, and influenza viruses may resemble *M. pneumoniae* infection. Legionnaires' disease (see Chap. 162) resembles severe cases of *M. pneumoniae* pneumonia.

TREATMENT Tetracycline derivatives and erythromycin are effective in treatment of pneumonia due to *M. pneumoniae.* Demethylchlortetracycline may be given to adults in daily doses of 0.9 g; tetracycline, 1.5 g; erythromycin stearate, 1.5 g. Response to treatment is characterized by prompt defervescence, rapid clearing of x-ray signs of pneumonia, and disappearance of malaise and weakness. Persistent cough, despite treatment, is a relatively common finding, especially in women.

Treatment temporarily reduces the frequency of positive cultures from the respiratory tract, but shedding may continue for several weeks after treatment, a finding similar to that in psittacosis pneumonia. Relapse of *M. pneumoniae* pneumonia occurs occasionally, but such cases respond to re-treatment. In cases in which there is doubt between the diagnosis of *M. pneumoniae* and pneumococcal infection, erythromycin should be used in preference to a tetracycline. No vaccines are available.

REFERENCES

CHERRY JD et al: *Mycoplasma pneumoniae* infections and exanthems. J Pediatr 87:369, 1975

COUCH RB: *Mycoplasma pneumoniae,* in *Viral and Mycoplasmal Infections of the Respiratory Tract,* V Knight (ed). Philadelphia, Lea & Febiger, 1973

FOY HM et al: Viral and mycoplasmal pneumonia in a prepaid medical care group during an eight year period. Am J Epidemiol 97:93, 1973

MCDADE JE et al: Legionnaires' disease. Isolation of a bacterium and demonstration of its role in other respiratory disease. N Engl J Med 297:1197, 1978

191

APPROACH TO THE DIAGNOSIS AND TREATMENT OF CHLAMYDIAL INFECTIONS

WALTER E. STAMM
KING K. HOLMES

DIAGNOSIS OF CHLAMYDIAL INFECTION Many infections caused by *Chlamydia trachomatis* produce no symptoms, and, even when symptoms are produced, these are nonspecific and hence not diagnostic of chlamydial infection. For this reason all diseases caused by *C. trachomatis,* except classic trachoma, require laboratory confirmation for diagnosis. The laboratory procedures available include direct microscopic examination of tissue scrapings for typical intracytoplasmic inclusions or specific antigen, isolation of the organism, and detection of antibody in the serum or in local secretions. Direct microscopic examination of Giemsa-stained cell scrapings is inefficient and has a low yield except in neonatal inclusion conjunctivitis. Nevertheless, it may be the only laboratory method available in many areas of the world. Unfortunately, false-positive interpretations by inexperienced observers are common. Direct fluorescent antibody staining of scrapings is more sensitive, particularly with fluorescein-labeled *C. trachomatis*-specific monoclonal antibodies, but experience with such reagents is too limited to permit their assessment in the diagnosis of chlamydial infection by direct staining of scrapings. Cell culture techniques have replaced the yolk sac of embryonated eggs for isolation of *C. trachomatis.* The cell cultures are much more convenient and are more sensitive, particularly for strains from the genital tract. While lymphogranuloma venereum (LGV) strains grow well in many cell lines, the other *C. trachomatis* trachoma strains are much more difficult to culture. The most common cell lines used are McCoy cells and HeLa 229 cells. Both cell lines require special pretreatment and centrifugation of the inoculum onto the monolayer for efficient isolation of genital or ocular trachoma strains. Positive cultures are determined by identifying typical intracytoplasmic inclusions stained by Giemsa's iodine, or immunofluorescent techniques. Isolates may be immunotyped in the microimmunofluorescent (micro-IF) test.

A complement fixation (CF) test with the heat-stable group-reactive antigen has been used to diagnose psittacosis and LGV with limited success. It is too insensitive to be useful with non-LGV *C. trachomatis* (trachoma organisms) infections. The micro-IF test with *C. trachomatis* antigens is sensitive and strain-specific. While it has been greatly simplified for diagnostic purposes, it remains available only in research laboratories. The test measures antibodies by immunotype specificity and by immunoglobulin class (IgM, IgG, IgA, secretory IgA) in both serum and local secretions.

Table 191-1 summarizes the diagnostic tests of choice for patients with suspected chlamydial infection. With few exceptions, the most suitable method for diagnosis is isolation of the agent in tissue-cell culture. Since *C. trachomatis* is an intracellular pathogen, adequate specimens for chlamydial culture must include desquamated cells. Cultures of pus result in fewer isolations of the organism. In urethritis, a thin-shafted urogenital swab should be inserted at least 2 cm into the urethra to obtain an appropriate specimen. When a cervical culture is taken, the external os should first be cleaned of debris and purulent material, and a plastic-shafted swab then inserted into the cervix, rotated slowly for 10 s, and withdrawn. When conjunctival specimens are sought, scrapings rather than purulent material must be obtained. All specimens for chlamydial isolation should be placed immediately into a transport medium and then either refrigerated if they will reach the laboratory within 12 to 18 h or frozen at −70°C if longer storage is anticipated.

As seen in Table 191-1, culture confirmation of infection should be sought in all chlamydial infections. In neonatal conjunctivitis, scrapings of the conjunctiva can be directly stained and examined for rapid diagnosis. Serodiagnosis is not useful in most chlamydial infections for several reasons. First, the test

TABLE 191-1
Diagnostic tests in *C. Trachomatis* infection

Infection	*Suggestive signs/symptoms*	*Presumptive diagnosis**	*Confirmatory test of choice*
ADULT MALES			
Nongonococcal urethritis, postgonococcal urethritis	Discharge, dysuria	Gram stain with more than four polymorphonuclear (PMN) leukocytes per oil immersion field, no gonococci	Urethral culture for *C. trachomatis*
Epididymitis	Unilateral swelling, pain, tenderness; fever; nongonococcal urethritis	Gram stain with more than four PMN leukocytes per oil immersion field, no gonococci	Urethral culture for *C. trachomatis;* micro-IF antibody to *C. trachomatis*—fourfold rise or IgM
Reiter's syndrome	Nongonococcal urethritis, arthritis, conjunctivitis, typical skin lesions	Gram stain with more than four PMN leukocytes per oil immersion field, no gonococci	Urethral culture for *C. trachomatis*
Proctitis	Rectal pain, discharge, diarrhea, blood; homosexual	Negative gonococcal culture and gram stain; PMN leukocytes in stool	Rectal culture for *C. trachomatis*
ADULT FEMALES			
Cervicitis	Mucopurulent cervical discharge, hypertrophic ectopy, friability	Negative culture and gram stain for gonococci	Cervical culture for *C. trachomatis*
Salpingitis	Evidence of pelvic inflammatory disease on examination	*C. trachomatis* should always be suspected in salpingitis	Cervical culture for *C. trachomatis;* micro-IF anibody to *C. trachomatis*—fourfold rise or IgM (especially with associated perihepatitis)
Urethritis	Dysuria and frequency without urgency or hematuria	Mucopurulent cervicitis, sterile pyuria	Urethral and cervical cultures for *C. trachomatis*
NEONATES			
Conjunctivitis	Purulent conjunctival discharge 6 to 18 days postdelivery	Negative cultures and gram stains for gonococci, *Hemophilus* sp., pneumococci, staphylococci	Conjunctival culture for *C. trachomatis;* Giemsa-stained scraping of conjunctival material can provide more rapid diagnosis but is less sensitive than culture
Infant pneumonia	Afebrile, staccato cough, diffuse rales, bilateral hyperinflation, interstitial infiltrates	None	Chlamydial culture of sputum, pharynx, eye, rectum; micro-IF antibody to *C. trachomatis*—fourfold change in IgG or IgM antibody

* *Although a presumptive diagnosis of chlamydial infection is often made in the syndromes listed when gonococci are not found, a positive test for Neisseria gonorrhoeae does not exclude C. trachomatis, which is very often also present in patients with gonorrhea.*

is exacting and time-consuming. More importantly, many chlamydial infections produce few or no symptoms, and hence patients do not seek care until it is too late to demonstrate rising or falling IgG or IgM antibodies. In addition, the prevalence of antichlamydial antibody in sexually active populations often exceeds 60 percent. These factors make it difficult to differentiate current from past infection using serologic techniques alone. However, serologic diagnosis may be useful in several specific instances. In infant pneumonia, a high antibody titer is nearly always produced and, since a definite clinical syndrome may bring the infant to the physician early in the course of disease, high-titer IgM antibody and/or fourfold titer rises can often be demonstrated. For similar reasons, serodiagnosis may be useful in women with chlamydial salpingitis, especially with Fitz-Hugh–Curtis syndrome. In lymphogranuloma venereum the micro-IF antibody titer against *C. trachomatis* is high ($\geq$1:512) and usually has a characteristic pattern of broad reactivity against all immunotypes of *C. trachomatis* (since LGV strains induce broadly reactive antibody).

ANTIBIOTIC SUSCEPTIBILITY *Chlamydia,* like other bacteria, are susceptible to certain antibiotics. In laboratory tests, death of inoculated mice and chick embryos, as well as growth in cell cultures, is prevented or inhibited by tetracyclines, erythromycin, chloramphenicol, and rifampin; sulfonamides and cycloserine are active against *C. trachomatis* but not *C. psittaci;* bacitracin and polymyxin B are less effective; penicillin and ampicillin suppress *Chlamydia* multiplication but do not eradicate the organisms in vitro. The cephalosporins also appear relatively ineffective against *C. trachomatis.* Streptomycin, gentamicin, neomycin, kanamycin, vancomycin, ristocetin, spectinomycin, and nystatin are not effective at concentrations inhibitory for most bacteria and fungi. For treatment of human infection, the tetracyclines, erythromycin, and sulfonamides are most useful.

TREATMENT In general, chlamydial infections cannot be eradicated by single-dose or short-term antimicrobial regimens. In most situations, at least 7 days and sometimes 2 to 3 weeks of antibiotic should be given. Treatment failure after treatment of genital infections with a tetracycline usually indicates inadequate therapy, poor compliance, or reinfection. Tetracycline-resistant strains of *C. trachomatis* have not been described.

Therapy of *C. trachomatis* urethritis is more effective than therapy of other forms of nongonococcal urethritis (NGU). *Chlamydia trachomatis* is eradicated from the urethra by treatment with tetracycline hydrochloride, 500 mg four times daily for 7 days. Alternative regimens which are also effective include erythromycin, 500 mg four times daily for 14 days, and sulfisoxazole, 500 mg four times daily for 10 days. However, sulfonamides are not effective for *Chlamydia*-negative NGU. Minocycline and doxycycline are more active than tetracycline against *C. trachomatis* in vitro and are effective clinically in a dose of 100 mg daily for 7 days.

Eradication of *C. trachomatis* from the cervix has been demonstrated with similar doses of tetracycline and erythromycin. Erythromycin base, 500 mg four times daily for 7 to 10 days, is the regimen of choice for pregnant women with *C. trachomatis* infection. Tetracycline hydrochloride, 500 mg four times daily for 10 days, produces clinical and microbiological cure of epididymitis or salpingitis associated with *C. trachomatis* infection.

Treatment of sex partners The increase in genital *C. trachomatis* infections is related in part to changes in sexual behavior but probably is also due to failure of clinicians to diagnose and treat *C. trachomatis* infections in symptomatic patients or their sexual partners. Cases of NGU, epididymitis, Reiter's syndrome, and mucopurulent endocervicitis are frequently not treated with antimicrobials, and sex partners are treated even less often. Furthermore, even though 20 percent of men and 30 to 50 percent of women with gonorrhea have concurrent *C. trachomatis* infection, only one of the four treatment regimens recommended by the Centers for Disease Control for gonorrhea (tetracycline, but not single-dose procaine penicillin G, ampicillin, or spectinomycin) eradicates *C. trachomatis. Chlamydia trachomatis* urethral or cervical infection has been well documented in the sex partners of patients with NGU, epididymitis, Reiter's syndrome, salpingitis, or endocervicitis. This is analogous to the problem of asymptomatic gonococcal infection in sex partners of patients with gonorrhea. In the absence of facilities for specific diagnosis of *C. trachomatis* infection, sex partners of patients with symptoms that are attributable to *C. trachomatis* should be examined and counseled. Those partners who themselves have clinical evidence of *C. trachomatis* infection clearly should be treated with an effective antimicrobial. Even those without evidence of clinical disease who have been recently exposed to possible chlamydial infection (for example, NGU) should probably also be offered therapy.

In neonates with conjunctivitis or infants with pneumonia, erythromycin estolate can be given orally in a dose of 50 mg/kg per day, preferably as 12.5 mg/kg four times daily, for 2 weeks. Careful attention must be given to compliance with therapy—a frequent problem. Relapses of eye infection are common following treatment with topical erythromycin or tetracycline ophthalmic ointment and may occur after oral erythromycin therapy also, so that follow-up cultures should be obtained after treatment. Both parents should be examined for *C. trachomatis* infection and, if cultures are not readily available, should also be treated with a tetracycline.

REFERENCES

Bowie WR et al: Therapy for nongonococcal urethritis: Double-blind randomized comparison of two doses and two durations of minocycline. Ann Intern Med 95:306, 1981

Brunham RC et al: Treatment of concomitant *Neisseria gonorrhoeae* and *Chlamydia trachomatis* infection in women: Comparison of trimethoprim-sulfamethoxazole vs. ampicillin-probenecid. Rev Infect Dis 4:491, 1982

——— et al: Therapy of cervical chlamydial infection. Ann Intern Med 97:216, 1982

Schachter J et al: Medical progress. Chlamydial infection. N Engl J Med 298:428, 490, 540, 1973

Sexually transmitted diseases treatment guidelines 1982. Morb Mort Week Rep 31:25, 1982

Stamm WE et al: Laboratory diagnosis of nongonococcal urethritis. Lab Med 13(3):147, 1982

Stevens RS et al: Monoclonal antibodies to *Chlamydia trachomatis:* Antibody specificities and antigen characterization. J Immunol 128:1083, 1982

Wang SP et al: Serodiagnosis of *Chlamydia trachomatis* infection with the microimmunofluorescence test, in *Nongonococcal Urethritis and Related Infections,* D Hobson, K Holmes (eds). Washington, DC, American Society for Microbiology, 1977, pp 237–248

World Health Organization: Guide to the laboratory diagnosis of trachoma. Prepared by the participants in a WHO symposium held July 1974, Geneva, 1975

———: Nongonococcal urethritis and other selected sexually transmitted diseases of public health importance. Prepared by participants in a WHO Scientific Group Meeting held November 1978. Technical Report Series 660, 1981.

192
TRACHOMA AND INCLUSION CONJUNCTIVITIS

J. THOMAS GRAYSTON
CHANDLER R. DAWSON

DEFINITION Trachoma is a chronic conjunctivitis. It is still a most important cause of preventable visual loss, having produced an estimated 20 million cases of blindness throughout the world. Inclusion conjunctivitis is an acute ocular inflammation caused by sexually transmitted chlamydial agents in adults exposed to infected genital secretions and in their newborn offspring.

EPIDEMIOLOGY Epidemiologically, two types of eye disease are caused by trachoma biotype strains of *Chlamydia trachomatis*. In trachoma-endemic areas where the classic eye disease is seen, transmission is from eye to eye, via hands, towels, flies, etc. In nonendemic areas, the organisms are transmitted from the genital tract to the eye, usually causing only the inclusion conjunctivitis syndrome with or without keratitis. Rarely the eye disease progresses with the development of pannus and scars similar to endemic trachoma. These cases may be referred to as *paratrachoma* to differentiate them from eye-to-eye transmitted endemic trachoma.

The worldwide incidence and severity of trachoma have decreased dramatically during the past 30 years in areas with improving hygienic and economic conditions. Endemic trachoma is still the major cause of preventable blindness in north Africa, sub-Saharan Africa, the Middle East, and parts of Asia. Transmission of the endemic disease occurs primarily through close personal contact, particularly among young children in the affected rural communities. In endemic areas, trachoma is associated with repeated exposure, but the infection can also be latent. In the United States a mild form of endemic trachoma still occurs in American Indians and in Mexican Americans as well as in immigrants from areas where trachoma is endemic. Acute relapse of old trachoma may be seen occasionally following treatment with cortisone eye ointment or in very old persons exposed in their youth.

C. trachomatis eye infection in nonendemic areas is a complication of what is now recognized as one of the most common venereal infections. Adult inclusion conjunctivitis and paratrachoma are uncommon complications of genital infections, usually in sexually promiscuous young adults. These sporadic, infrequent eye infections occur following transfer of infected genital discharges to the eye, either on the fingers or by orogenital sexual activities. Newborns become infected by exposure in the infected birth canal of their mothers during delivery.

CLINICAL MANIFESTATIONS Both endemic trachoma and adult inclusion conjunctivitis present initially as a conjunctivitis characterized by small lymphoid follicles in the conjunctiva. In regions with hyperendemic classic blinding trachoma, the disease usually starts insidiously before the age of 2 years. Reinfection is common. The cornea becomes involved with inflammatory leukocytic infiltration and superficial vascularization (pannus formation). As the inflammation continues, there is conjunctival scarring that eventually distorts the eyelids, causing them to turn inward so that the inturned lashes constantly abrade the eyeball (trichiasis and entropion); eventually the corneal epithelium is abraded and may then develop a bacterial corneal ulcer with subsequent corneal scarring and blindness. Destruction of the conjunctival goblet cells, lacrimal ducts, and lacrimal gland may produce a "dry-eye" syndrome with resultant corneal opacity due to drying (xerosis) or secondary bacterial corneal ulcers. Communities with blinding trachoma often experience seasonal epidemics of bacterial conjunctivitis with *Hemophilus influenzae* (biotype III or the Koch-Weeks bacillus) and rarely with *Neisseria gonorrhoeae*, which contribute to the intensity of the inflammatory process. In such areas the active infectious process usually resolves spontaneously in affected persons between 10 and 15 years of age, but the conjunctival scars continue to shrink, producing trichiasis and entropion and subsequent corneal scarring in adult life. In areas with milder and less prevalent disease the process may be much slower, with active disease continuing into adulthood; blindness is rare in these cases.

Eye infection with genital *C. trachomatis* strains, usually in sexually active young adults, presents with acute onset of unilateral follicular conjunctivitis and preauricular lymphadenopathy similar to acute adenovirus or herpes virus conjunctivitis. If untreated, the disease may persist for 6 weeks to 2 years. It is frequently associated with corneal inflammation in the form of discrete opacities ("infiltrates"), punctate epithelial erosions, and minor degrees of superficial corneal vascularization. Very rarely conjunctival scarring and eyelid distortion occur, particularly in patients treated for many months with topical corticosteroids. Recurrent eye infections occur most often in patients whose sexual consorts are not treated with antibiotics.

DIAGNOSIS The clinical diagnosis of classic trachoma can be made if two of the following signs are present:

1 Lymphoid follicles on the upper tarsal conjunctiva
2 Typical conjunctival scarring
3 Vascular pannus
4 Limbal follicles or their sequelae, Herbert's pits

For public health purposes, it is necessary to determine whether a substantial proportion of the population has these minimal signs. Public health intervention will depend on the intensity of active inflammatory disease and on the prevalence of blinding or potentially blinding sequelae. In endemic trachoma, laboratory tests to support the clinical diagnosis should be obtained from children with more marked degrees of inflammation. Intracytoplasmic chlamydial inclusions occur in 10 to 60 percent of Giemsa-stained conjunctival smears in such populations, but isolation in cell cultures is more sensitive. Follicular conjunctivitis in adult Europeans or Americans living in trachomatous regions is rarely trachoma.

Sporadic cases of adult inclusion conjunctivitis must be differentiated from adenovirus and herpes simplex virus keratoconjunctivitis during the first 15 days after onset, and later from other forms of chronic follicular conjunctivitis. Laboratory demonstration of chlamydial infection by Giemsa- or immunofluorescent-stained smears or by isolation in cell cultures constitutes definitive evidence of infection, but only a few laboratories carry out these procedures. Serologic demonstration of antibody in serum cannot be taken as evidence of eye infection with chlamydial agents, since so many sexually active young adults have serum antibody titers. A practical diagnostic procedure in cases with chronic follicular conjunctivitis is treatment for 6 days with an oral tetracycline or erythromycin; a marked symptomatic response within 3 to 4 days is highly suggestive of inclusion conjunctivitis, and treatment should be continued for at least 3 weeks.

DIFFERENTIAL DIAGNOSIS Several viral eye infections should be considered in the differential diagnosis of trachoma and inclusion conjunctivitis. The eye and its adnexa may be infected during the course of many cutaneous and systemic viral diseases. Sometimes these ocular infections produce minor manifestations, such as the transient loss of accommodation of dengue and the milder forms of conjunctivitis in systemic adenovirus infections. Other virus infections, however, such as herpes simplex (see Chap. 210), herpes zoster (see Chap. 204), measles (see Chap. 200), and vaccinia or smallpox (see Chap. 203), occasionally produce serious and permanent visual loss. In addition, congenital viral infections are an important cause of blindness, particularly rubella, which leads to cataracts, microphthalmus, and cytomegalic inclusion disease with retinal involvement.

Among the viral infections limited to the outer eye and manifested as a follicular conjunctivitis are epidemic keratoconjunctivitis, herpes simplex keratoconjunctivitis, Newcastle disease virus (NDV) conjunctivitis, and acute hemorrhagic conjunctivitis.

Epidemic keratoconjunctivitis (EKC) Adenovirus types 8 and 19 are the usual cause of epidemics of EKC, although milder cases may be associated with other adenovirus types. The most common method for transmission of adenovirus type 8 is through manipulation of the eye by medical personnel, e.g., for foreign-body removal in industrial dispensaries (thus the name "shipyard eye") or during an ophthalmologic examination. The virus, which is unusually resistant to inactivation, is transmitted on the fingers, by instruments, or in solutions. Medical personnel not infrequently contract the disease and may act as a source of infection for patients. One of the rarer causes of EKC, due to adenovirus type 19, appears to be transmitted person-to-person during small community outbreaks.

Following an incubation period of 5 to 12 days, EKC presents a moderate to very severe follicular conjunctivitis with preauricular lymphadenopathy that is usually unilateral at onset. Severe cases may have subconjunctival hemorrhages and conjunctival membrane formation with subsequent conjunctival scarring. In adults, the associated systemic manifestations are minimal with little if any fever, headache, or malaise, but in children adenovirus type 8 infections may present as febrile upper respiratory disease, or otitis media, with only a minor conjunctivitis; such children may be a source of infection for adults. In EKC, the usual onset of focal corneal involvement is 7 days after onset of conjunctivitis when there is a severe foreign-body sensation, photophobia, and lacrimation. As the conjunctivitis subsides during the second week of the disease, subepithelial corneal opacities 1 to 2 mm in diameter appear, and these opacities may persist for 2 years or longer.

There is no specific treatment for the acute stage of EKC, but the late opacities can be suppressed temporarily with topical corticosteroids if vision is impaired. Explosive epidemics in industrial dispensaries and ophthalmologists' offices can be prevented or controlled by scrupulous hand washing, adequate cleansing of instruments, and replacement of eye drops to break the chain of infection. Medical personnel with conjunctivitis should not come into contact with patients.

Herpes simplex virus (HSV) keratoconjunctivitis Occasionally HSV produces an acute follicular conjunctivitis that is usually accompanied by one or multiple herpetic skin vesicles on the eyelids. In children this may be the primary herpetic infection, but in adults the conjunctivitis is often a recurrent herpetic infection at a new site. The skin lesions may be inconspicuous, misdiagnosed as a sty, or even not present, so that the disease is indistinguishable from early EKC. The cornea may have focal epithelial lesions, a typical linear, branching (dendritic) ulcer, or no involvement at all. The conjunctivitis usually resolves in 2 weeks. If definite herpetic lid lesions are present or if HSV is isolated, treatment with a topical antiviral (idoxuridine, adenine arabinoside, or trifluorothymidine) should be given three to four times daily to prevent corneal involvement. Overt dendritic ulcerations or other corneal involvement should be treated more vigorously as described in Chap. 210. Topical corticosteroids should not be used in acute HSV and other presumed viral infections of the eye except in rare instances and then under frequent supervision by an ophthalmologist.

Newcastle disease virus conjunctivitis Human infection with this avian virus, which is related to influenza, occurs mainly in poultry workers, veterinarians, and virologists. In humans, accidental introduction of contaminated material from naturally infected animals or from live virus (e.g., vaccines) is followed in 24 to 72 h by conjunctivitis, edema of the lids, and tearing. Systemic symptoms occur very rarely, and recovery is complete in 10 to 14 days. The diagnosis may be confirmed by virus isolation in embryonated eggs.

Acute hemorrhagic conjunctivitis (AHC) This disease was first described in 1969 in epidemics in Africa and Asia. It presents as an acute conjunctivitis with numerous punctate hemorrhages on the bulbar conjunctiva which become confluent within 24 h. There is also minor involvement of the cornea. The inflammation subsides in 4 to 5 days, but the hemorrhages do not resolve for 7 to 10 days. The only reported complication has been the rare occurrence of lumbar radiculomyelitis with resultant flaccid paralysis like poliomyelitis. Enterovirus 70 (a member of the picornavirus group) has been identified as the etiologic agent in most epidemics, but some outbreaks have been caused by coxsackievirus A24, another picornavirus. Epidemics of AHC have occurred in the crowded urban populations of developing countries, affecting all age groups and social classes. Occasional outbreaks in Europe have been centered around eye clinics. Community-wide epidemics of AHC have occurred in the United States and Central America.

TREATMENT *C. trachomatis* strains are susceptible to the sulfonamides, tetracyclines, and erythromycin. Public health control programs for endemic trachoma consist of the mass application of tetracycline or erythromycin ointment to the eyes of all children in affected communities for 21 to 60 days or on an intermittent schedule. These programs also include surgical correction of inturned eyelids by a mobile surgical team that visits each locality. Oral erythromycin, but not oral tetracyclines, offers a useful alternative method of mass antibiotic treatment for trachoma of young children and pregnant women.

Adult inclusion conjunctivitis responds well to treatment with full doses of systemic tetracycline or erythromycin for 3 weeks. Treating all sexual consorts of the patient simultaneously is also necessary to prevent ocular reinfection and to avoid the genital diseases due to chlamydial infection. Topical antibiotic treatment is not required in patients treated with systemic antibiotics.

PREVENTION Efforts to develop a practical trachoma vaccine have not been successful. General hygienic measures associated with improved living standards are effective in the elimination of endemic trachoma. Adequate water supply for personal cleanliness may be a key factor. In some areas the reduction of flies in the household is important.

REFERENCES

DAWSON CR, TOGNI B: Herpes simplex eye infections: Clinical manifestations, pathogenesis and management. Surv Ophthalmol 21:121, 1976

HALES RH, OSTLER HB: Newcastle disease conjunctivitis with subepithelial infiltrates. Br J Ophthalmol 57(9):694, 1973

O'DAY DM et al: Clinical and laboratory evaluation of epidemic keratoconjunctivitis due to adenovirus types 8 and 19. Am J Ophthalmol 81(2):207, 1976

SCHACHTER J, DAWSON CR: *Human Chlamydial Infections.* Littleton, Mass., PSG Medical Books, 1978

WHITCHER JP et al: Acute hemorrhagic conjunctivitis in Tunisia: Report of viral isolations. Arch Ophthalmol January 94:51, 1976

193
LYMPHOGRANULOMA VENEREUM

KING K. HOLMES

DEFINITION Lymphogranuloma venereum (LGV) is a sexually transmitted infection caused by *Chlamydia trachomatis.* The acute disease in heterosexual men is characterized by a transient primary genital lesion followed by multilocular suppurative regional lymphadenopathy. Women, homosexual men, and occasionally, heterosexual men may develop hemorrhagic proctitis with regional lymphadenitis. Acute LGV is almost always associated with nonspecific systemic symptoms, usually with fever and leukocytosis, and rarely with systemic complications such as meningoencephalitis. After a latent period of years, late complications include genital elephantiasis, strictures, and fistulas of the penis, urethra, and rectum.

ETIOLOGY Only three immunotypes of *C. trachomatis,* designated L_1, L_2, and L_3, cause LGV, with L_2 being most common. LGV immunotypes also have other distinguishing biological characteristics: they are more invasive than the other immunotypes of *C. trachomatis,* cause disease primarily in lymphatic tissue, grow more readily in tissue culture and in macrophages, and are pathogenic when inoculated intracerebrally into mice and monkeys.

EPIDEMIOLOGY Lymphogranuloma venereum usually is sexually transmitted, but occasional transmission by nonsexual personal contact, fomites, or laboratory accidents has been documented. Laboratory work involving creation of aerosols of this organism (e.g., sonication, homogenization) must be conducted in protective biological chambers. The peak incidence corresponds to the age of greatest sexual activity, the second and third decades of life. The worldwide incidence of LGV is falling, for unexplained reasons, but the disease is still endemic and a major cause of morbidity in certain countries of Asia, Africa, and South America.

Prevalence studies of LGV are difficult to interpret. Most have employed the Frei skin test or LGV complement fixation (CF) serologic test. Since the antigens used in these tests cross-react with other strains of *C. trachomatis* which are much more widely prevalent in developed countries than the three LGV strains, the specificity of the Frei and LGV CF tests is open to question. For example, 18 percent of patients attending a STD clinic had positive skin tests and 2 percent had high LGV titers, but only 1 percent had signs of LGV.

The frequency of infection following exposure is believed to be much less than that associated with gonorrhea and syphilis. Early manifestations are recognized far more often in men than in women, who usually present with late complications. In the United States, where the reported sex ratio is 3.4 males to 1 female, most cases involve homosexually active men; travelers, seamen, and military personnel returning from abroad; and individuals of low socioeconomic status living in areas of low endemicity in the southeast. The main reservoir of infection in the United States is presumed to be asymptomatically infected individuals, but attempts to isolate and identify LGV strains from the urethra or cervix of sexually active persons without clinical LGV have been impeded by the technical difficulties associated with serotyping of chlamydial isolates. The development of monoclonal antibody with apparent specificity for the L_2 immunotype should permit more extensive studies of the epidemiology of LGV.

CLINICAL MANIFESTATIONS In heterosexuals, a *primary genital lesion* occurs from 3 days to 3 weeks after exposure. It is a small, painless vesicle or nonindurated ulcer or papule located on the penis in men or on the labia, posterior vagina, or fourchette in women. The primary lesion is noticed by less than one-third of men with LGV and only rarely by women. It heals in a few days without scarring and even when noticed is usually not recognized as LGV except in retrospect when it is followed by or merges with lymphadenitis. LGV strains of *C. trachomatis* have occasionally been recovered from genital ulcers, and also from the urethra of men and the endocervix of women who present with inguinal adenopathy, suggesting that these areas may be the primary site of infection in some cases.

In women and homosexual men, *primary anal or rectal infection* occurs following rectal intercourse. In women, rectal infection with LGV or non-LGV strains of *C. trachomatis* presumably can also arise either via contiguous spread of infected secretions along the perineum (as with rectal gonococcal infection in women) or perhaps by spread to the rectum via the pelvic lymphatics. During an incubation period of unknown length, multiplication occurs in the rectum (probably within the mucosal epithelium, as well as within histiocytes, although the range of host cells infected within the mucosa and submu-

FIGURE 193-1
Lymphogranuloma venereum. Bilateral inguinal buboes, with the "sign of the groove," caused by adenopathy above and below Poupart's ligament. (Courtesy of A Brathwaite.)

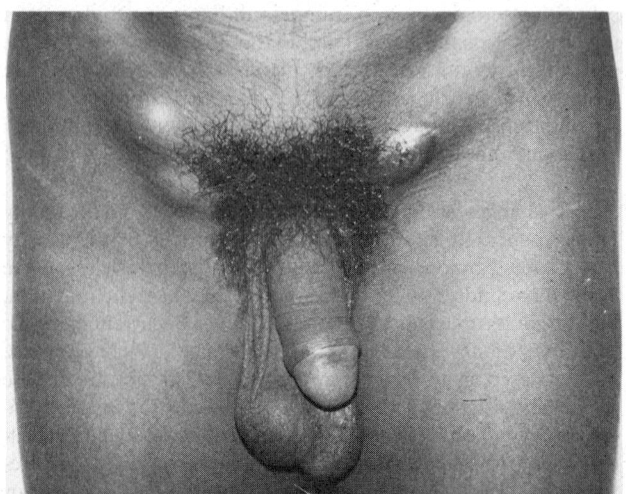

cosa is not well defined), eventually causing symptoms of proctitis.

From the site of the primary urethral, genital, anal, or rectal infection, the organism spreads via the regional lymphatics. Penile, vulvar, and anal infection can lead to inguinal and femoral lymphadenitis. Rectal infection produces hypogastric and deep iliac lymphadenitis. Upper vaginal or cervical infection results in enlargement of the obturator and iliac nodes. The most common presenting picture in heterosexual men is the *inguinal syndrome,* which is characterized by painful inguinal lymphadenopathy beginning 2 to 6 weeks after presumed exposure; rarely the onset occurs after a few months. The inguinal adenopathy is unilateral in two-thirds of cases, and palpable enlargement of the iliac and femoral nodes is often present on the same side as the enlarged inguinal nodes. The nodes are initially discrete, but progressive periadenitis results in a matted mass of nodes which become fluctuant and suppurative. The overlying skin becomes fixed, inflamed, and thinned and finally develops multiple draining fistulas. Extensive enlargement of chains of inguinal nodes above and below the inguinal ligament ("the sign of the groove") is characteristic but is present in only a minority of cases (Fig. 193-1). Histological involvement of nodes initially shows characteristic small stellate abscesses surrounded by histiocytes. These abscesses coalesce to cause large, necrotic, suppurative foci. Spontaneous healing usually occurs after several months, leaving inguinal scars or granulomatous masses of varying size which persist for life. Massive pelvic lymphadenopathy in women or homosexual men may lead to exploratory laparotomy.

As cultures and serology for *C. trachomatis* are being used more often, an increasing number of cases of LGV proctitis is recognized in homosexual men. Such patients present after an unknown incubation period with anorectal pain and mucopurulent, bloody rectal discharge. Although patients may complain of diarrhea, this often actually represents frequent, painful unsuccessful attempts at defecation (tenesmus). Sigmoidoscopy reveals ulcerative proctitis, exudate, and friability, with disease limited to the distal rectum. Since the LGV agent is an obligate intracellular pathogen, the histopathologic findings in the rectal mucosa include granulomas with giant cells, along with crypt abscesses and extensive inflammation. These clinical, sigmoidoscopic, and histopathologic findings may closely resemble Crohn's disease of the rectum (Fig. 193-2).

Constitutional symptoms are common during the state of regional lymphadenopathy and, in the presence of proctitis, include fever, chills, headache, meningismus, anorexia, myalgias, and arthralgias. These findings in the presence of lymphadenopathy are sometimes mistaken for malignant lymphoma. Other systemic complications are infrequent but include arthritis with sterile effusion, aseptic meningitis, meningoencephalitis, conjunctivitis, hepatitis, and erythema nodosum. Chlamydiae have been recovered from the cerebrospinal fluid, and in one case from the blood in a patient with severe constitutional symptoms, indicating the occurrence of disseminated infection. Laboratory infections due to suspected inhalation of aerosols have been associated with mediastinal lymphadenitis.

Associated laboratory findings during the acute stage of infection include leukocytosis and mild elevation of the sedimentation rate. Abnormal liver function tests, hyperglobulinemia, mixed cryoglobulinemia, rheumatoid factor activity, and elevated IgG, IgA, and IgM have been reported in subacute and chronic LGV. False-positive serologic tests for syphilis are rare, and syphilis should be suspected if these tests are positive, as is often the case.

Complications of untreated anorectal infection include perirectal abscess, fistula in ano, and rectovaginal, rectovesical, and ischiorectal fistulas. Secondary bacterial infection probably contributes to these complications. Rectal stricture is a late complication of anorectal infection and usually occurs 2 to 6 cm from the anal orifice, within reach on digital rectal examination. The stricture may extend proximally for several centimeters, leading to a mistaken clinical and radiographic diagnosis of carcinoma.

A small percentage of cases of LGV in men presents with chronic progressive infiltrative, ulcerative, or fistular lesions of the penis, urethra, or scrotum. Urethral stricture may occur and usually involves the posterior urethra, causing incontinence or difficulty with micturition.

An uncommon late complication of LGV is *genital elephantiasis,* a chronic induration and edema of the penis or vulva caused by lymphatic obstruction. Polypoid swelling of the skin and large stellate hyperplastic keloidal scars of the genitalia may be associated with vulvar induration or lymphedema and are difficult to distinguish clinically from granuloma inguinale and genital tuberculosis. Chronic ulcerations of the vulva (esthiomene) and smooth pedunculated perianal growths (lymphorrhoids) also occur. The significance of reports of malignant changes associated with chronic anorectal or genital LGV is uncertain.

DIAGNOSIS Although LGV is uncommon, it frequently enters the differential diagnosis of common conditions such as

FIGURE 193-2
Histopathologic findings in LGV proctitis in a homosexually active man. Note granulomatous changes, with giant cells, and crypt abscess with adjacent giant cell (insert). These changes resemble those seen in Crohn's disease of the rectum. (From Quinn.)

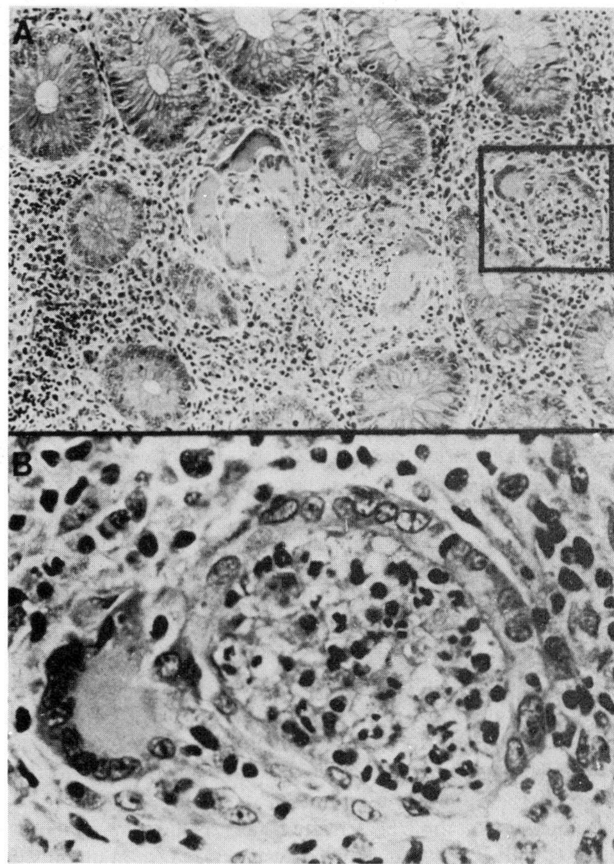

inguinal lymphadenopathy; vesicular, papular, or ulcerative genital lesions; and perirectal abscess, fistula in ano, or proctitis.

The most reliable method of diagnosis is isolation of an LGV strain of *Chlamydia* from aspirated bubo pus from the rectum or from the urethra, endocervix, or other infected tissue. Isolation has been possible from bubo pus in about 30 percent of cases with inguinal lymphadenopathy and from the rectum in most homosexual men who have proctitis. The methods needed for isolation in tissue cell culture are increasingly available. The most widely used immunodiagnostic tests have been the LGV complement fixation test and the Frei skin tests. An LGV CF titer $\geq$1:64 is suggestive of LGV and can be found in most patients after the bubo has appeared. The titer may not increase in paired serums since most patients have already been infected for several weeks when first seen. The LGV CF test can also become positive during infections with non-LGV strains of *C. trachomatis,* and high titers of CF antibody can be seen in patients who have had severe infections with such non-LGV strains. The Frei skin test is less sensitive than the LGV complement fixation test and is no longer available.

The microimmunofluorescent antibody test detects antibody to *C. trachomatis* in nearly all patients with culture-proven LGV. Serum microimmunofluorescent antibody titers from patients with LGV are usually $\geq$1:512, exceeding the highest titers that occur in chlamydial NGU and can usually be shown to have a characteristic broad pattern of reactivity against many immunotypes of *C. trachomatis,* since LGV strains produce broadly reactive antibody. The histopathology of excised nodes or of rectal biopsy specimens is seldom definitive, but suggestive findings may raise the question of LGV and lead to more specific tests. Fluorescein-conjugated monoclonal antibodies against *C. trachomatis,* and against the L_2 strain of *C. trachomatis,* may prove useful for identification of the agent in properly fixed specimens from lymph nodes or other tissue.

TREATMENT The LGV and non-LGV strains of *C. trachomatis* have similar antimicrobial susceptibilities. Antimicrobial therapy does not have a dramatic effect on the duration and healing of inguinal buboes, but acute constitutional symptoms are often terminated abruptly, and LGV proctitis improves rapidly after antimicrobial therapy has been instituted. Antibiotics are usually not helpful in improving late complications such as rectal stricture or genital elephantiasis unless secondary infection is also present. Genital elephantiasis and rectal, penile, and urethral strictures and fistulas usually require surgical correction, although sometimes urethral and even rectal strictures can be managed by repeated mechanical dilation.

The recommended treatment regimen is tetracycline hydrochloride, 0.5 g four times a day for 3 weeks. A sulfonamide preparation, 4 g per day for 3 weeks, can also be used, but occasional isolates have been resistant to sulfonamides in vitro. Fluctuant buboes should be aspirated through normal skin with a syringe and 18-gauge needle as often as necessary to prevent spontaneous rupture. It is not unusual for buboes to increase in size or to develop at another site after initiation of treatment. Although these seldom progress to fistula formation, they should be aspirated if fluctuant. A fourfold or greater fall in complement fixation titer or microimmunofluorescent antibody titer eventually occurs over several months in most treated patients, and LGV *Chlamydia* cannot be isolated from lesions after the initiation of antibiotic treatment.

REFERENCES

ABRAMS AJ: Lymphogranuloma venereum. JAMA 205:199, 1968

CALDWELL HD, KUO CC: Serologic diagnosis of lymphogranuloma venereum by counterimmunoelectrophoresis with a *Chlamydia trachomatis* antigen. J Immunol 118:442, 1977

GREAVES AB: The frequency of lymphogranuloma venereum in persons with perirectal abscesses, fistula-in-ano, or both. Bull WHO 29:797, 1963

HOPSU-HAVU VK, SONCK CE: Infiltrative, ulcerative, and fistular lesions of the penis due to lymphogranuloma venereum. Br J Vener Dis 49:193, 1972

PERINE PL et al: Diagnosis and treatment of lymphogranuloma venereum in Ethiopia. From 11th ICC and 19th ICAAC Proceedings. Curr Chemo Infect Dis, p 1280, 1980

QUINN TC et al: *Chlamydia trachomatis* proctitis. N Engl J Med 305:195, 1981

Sexually transmitted diseases treatment guidelines 1982. Morb Mort Week Rep 31:25, 1982

194 PSITTACOSIS

VERNON KNIGHT

DEFINITION Psittacosis is an infectious disease of birds caused by an organism that has a number of properties in common with gram-negative bacteria. Transmission of infection from birds to humans results in a febrile illness characterized by pneumonitis and systemic manifestations. Inapparent infections or mild influenza-like illnesses may also occur. The term *ornithosis* is sometimes applied to infections contracted from birds other than parrots or parakeets, but *psittacosis* is the preferred generic term for all forms of the disease.

ETIOLOGY The causative agent *Chlamydia psittaci* is a gram-negative obligate intracellular bacterium. Chlamydiae synthesize ribonucleic acid (RNA) and deoxyribonucleic acid (DNA), reproduce by binary fission, and are susceptible to antimicrobial drugs. In contrast to rickettsias, the chlamydias are dependent on their hosts for metabolic energy. Slight but definite homology of the DNA of members of the *Chlamydia* genus with the DNA of *Neisseria meningitidis* has been shown. The psittacosis agent is the prototype of a biologically and antigenically homogeneous class of microorganisms that includes the causative agents of lymphogranuloma venereum, trachoma, and 30 or more mammalian parasites which rarely produce human disease.

EPIDEMIOLOGY Psittacosis is widely distributed throughout the world, and almost any avian species can harbor the agent. Psittacine birds are most commonly infected, but human cases have been traced to contact with pigeons, ducks, turkeys, chickens, and many other birds. Psittacosis may be considered an occupational disease of pet-shop owners, poultry raisers, pigeon fanciers, taxidermists, and zoo attendants. The incidence of human infection in the United States rose steadily from 1930, owing in large measure to the increasing popularity of parrots and parakeets as pets and, as subsequently recognized, transmission of infection by barnyard fowl and pigeons. The number of reported cases reached a peak in 1956 and gradually declined thereafter. By 1963, with acceptance of control measures such as incorporation of tetracyclines in poultry feed, the disease had again become relatively uncommon. However, in recent years the disease has increased with cases occurring primarily among employees of poultry processing plants. In 1976 a plant in Nebraska experienced an outbreak involving 28 of 98 employees, whose disease was contracted from turkeys shipped from Texas. Other outbreaks of this type have occurred. In 1975 and 1976, 58 and 80 cases of psittacosis, respectively, were reported to the Centers for Disease Control, and in 1978 there were 146 cases. The disease appears to be more common in England, where budgerigars are common household pets and where restrictions on the importation of these birds have been eased.

The agent is present in nasal secretions, excreta, tissues, and feathers of infected birds. Although the disease can be fatal, infected birds frequently show only minor evidence of illness, such as ruffled feathers, lethargy, and anorexia. Asymptomatic avian carriers are common, and complete recovery may be followed by continued shedding of the organism for many months.

Psittacosis is almost always transmitted to humans by the respiratory route, and one-half or more of patients infected in fowl-processing plants may have pneumonia indicative of aerosol transmission of the infection. On rare occasions the disease may be acquired from the bite of a pet bird. Intimate and prolonged contact is not essential for transmission of the disease; a few minutes spent in an environment previously occupied by an infected bird has resulted in human infection. The severity of the disease in humans bears no apparent relationship to closeness or duration of contact, although sick birds are more likely to transmit infection than healthy ones. Transmission of a psittacosis-like agent between humans has occurred among hospital personnel, with severe and sometimes fatal infections. There is evidence that these "human" strains are more virulent than native avian organisms. There is no record of infection acquired by eating poultry products.

PATHOGENESIS The psittacosis agent gains entrance to the body through the upper part of the respiratory tract and eventually localizes in the pulmonary alveoli and in the reticuloendothelial cells of the spleen and liver. Invasion of the lung probably takes place by way of the bloodstream rather than by direct extension from the upper air passages. A lymphocytic inflammatory response occurs on both the interstitial and respiratory surfaces of the alveoli as well as in the perivascular spaces. The alveolar walls and interstitial tissues of the lung are thickened, edematous, necrotic, and occasionally hemorrhagic. Histologically, the affected areas show alveolar spaces filled with fluid, erythrocytes, and lymphocytes. The picture is not pathognomonic of psittacosis unless macrophages containing characteristic cytoplasmic inclusion bodies (LCL bodies) can be identified. The respiratory epithelium of the bronchi and bronchioles usually remains intact.

MANIFESTATIONS The clinical manifestations and course of psittacosis are extremely variable. After an incubation period of 7 to 14 days, or longer, the disease may start abruptly with shaking chills and fever ranging as high as 105°F, but the onset is often gradual with increasing fever over a 3- to 4-day period. Headache is almost always a prominent symptom; it is usually diffuse and excruciating and often the patient's chief complaint.

Many patients present with a dry hacking cough which is usually nonproductive, but small amounts of mucoid or bloody sputum may be raised as the disease progresses. Cough may appear early in the course of the disease or as late as 5 days after the onset of fever. Chest pain, pleurisy with effusion, or a friction rub may all occur but are rare. Pericarditis and myocarditis have been reported. Most patients have a normal or slightly increased respiratory rate; marked dyspnea with cyanosis occurs only in severe psittacosis with extensive pulmonary involvement. In psittacosis, as in most nonbacterial pneumonias, the physical signs of pneumonitis tend to be less prominent than symptoms and x-ray findings would suggest. The initial examination may reveal fine, sibilant rales, or clinical evidence of pneumonia may be completely lacking. Rales usually become audible and more numerous as the illness progresses. Signs of frank pulmonary consolidation are usually absent. Symptoms of upper respiratory tract infection are not prominent, although mild sore throat, pharyngeal infection, and cervical adenopathy are often present; on occasion they may be the only manifestations of illness. Epistaxis is encountered early in the course of nearly one-fourth of the cases. Photophobia is also a common complaint.

There is commonly a complaint of generalized myalgia, and spasm and stiffness of the muscles of the back and neck may lead to an erroneous diagnosis of meningitis. Lethargy, mental depression, agitation, insomnia, and disorientation have been prominent features of the illness in some epidemics, but not in others; delirium and stupor occur near the end of the first week in severe cases. Occasional patients are comatose when first seen, and the diagnosis of psittacosis may be missed. Gastrointestinal complaints such as abdominal pain, nausea, vomiting, or diarrhea are present in some cases; constipation and abdominal distention sometimes occur as late complications. Icterus, the result of severe hepatic involvement, is a rare and ominous finding. A faint, macular rash (Horder's spots) simulating the rose spots of typhoid fever has been described.

Patients without cough or other clinical evidence of respiratory involvement come to the physician with fever of unknown origin. The pulse rate is slow in relation to the fever. When splenomegaly is present in a patient with acute pneumonitis, psittacosis should be considered; the reported incidence of splenomegaly ranges from 10 to 70 percent. Nontender hepatic enlargement also occurs, but jaundice is rare. Thrombophlebitis is not unusual during convalescence; indeed, pulmonary infarction is sometimes a late complication and may be fatal.

In untreated cases of psittacosis, sustained or mildly remittent fever persists for 10 days to 3 weeks, or occasionally as long as 3 months. Defervescence is by lysis and is accompanied by abatement of respiratory manifestations. Psittacosis contracted from parrots or parakeets is more likely to be a severe, prolonged illness than infections acquired from pigeons or barnyard fowl. Relapses occur but are rare. Secondary bacterial infections are uncommon. Immunity to reinfection is probably permanent.

LABORATORY FINDINGS The x-ray of the lungs in psittacosis mimics that in a great variety of pulmonary diseases. The pneumonic lesions are usually patchy in appearance but can be hazy, diffuse, homogeneous, lobar, atelectatic, wedge-shaped, nodular, or miliary. The white blood cell count is normal or moderately decreased in the acute phase of the disease but may rise in convalescence. The erythrocyte sedimentation rate is frequently not elevated. Transient proteinuria is common. The cerebrospinal fluid sometimes contains a few mononuclear cells but is otherwise normal.

The diagnosis can be confirmed only by isolation of the causative microorganism or serologic studies. The agent is present in the blood during the acute phase of the disease and in the bronchial secretions for weeks or sometimes years after infection, but it is difficult to isolate. Psittacosis is most readily diagnosed by the demonstration of a rising titer of complement-fixing antibody in the patient's blood. An acute and convalescent specimen should always be tested. Even a low titer of antibody during the acute febrile phase constitutes presumptive evidence of psittacosis. The prompt initiation of treatment with tetracycline has been shown to delay antibody rise in convalescence for several weeks or months. Interpretation of a single complement fixation test may sometimes be difficult because of the antigenic cross reaction between the agent of psittacosis and that of lymphogranuloma venereum.

DIFFERENTIAL DIAGNOSIS A history of exposure to birds may be the only clinical basis for differentiating psittacosis from a great variety of infectious and noninfectious febrile disorders. A partial list of pneumonic disease that may be confused with psittacosis includes *Mycoplasma* pneumonia, Q fever, coccidioidomycosis, tuberculosis, carcinoma of the lung with bronchial obstruction, and bacterial pneumonias. In the early stages, before pneumonitis appears, psittacosis may be mistaken for influenza, typhoid fever, miliary tuberculosis, and infectious mononucleosis. Legionnaires' disease (see Chap. 162), caused by a gram-negative bacillus, causes pneumonia similar to psittacosis.

TREATMENT The tetracyclines are consistently effective in the treatment of psittacosis. Defervescence and alleviation of symptoms usually occur in 24 to 48 h after instituting therapy with 2 g daily in four divided doses. To avoid relapse, treatment should probably be continued for at least 7 days after defervescence. In severe cases, oxygen and other supportive measures are indicated.

REFERENCES

CENTERS FOR DISEASE CONTROL: Morb Mort Week Rep 25:301, 1976
———: Morb Mort Week Rep 29:505, 1980
———: *Psittacosis Annual Summary, 1974,* June 1975.

195
SEXUALLY TRANSMITTED AND PERINATAL CHLAMYDIAL INFECTIONS

WALTER E. STAMM
KING K. HOLMES

GENITAL INFECTIONS

SPECTRUM OF *C. TRACHOMATIS* GENITAL INFECTIONS In adults the clinical spectrum of sexually transmitted *Chlamydia trachomatis* infections is easily understood because it parallels closely the spectrum of gonococcal infections (Table 195-1). Both agents have been associated with urethritis in both sexes, with epididymitis, mucopurulent cervicitis, acute salpingitis, bartholinitis, proctitis, and the Fitz-Hugh–Curtis syndrome (perihepatitis), and both can be associated with systemic complications, particularly with arthritis. The etiologic significance of *C. trachomatis* infection in certain of these syndromes, such as the Fitz-Hugh–Curtis syndrome and Reiter's syndrome, requires further study.

EPIDEMIOLOGY Genital infections other than lymphogranuloma venereum (LGV) are caused by *C. trachomatis* immunotypes D through K. Although data are lacking, the incidence of genital *C. trachomatis* infection is probably increasing, since the incidence of nongonococcal urethritis (NGU) has risen dramatically over the last two decades, and *C. trachomatis* has consistently been isolated from 30 to 50 percent of men with NGU. The peak age incidence of genital *C. trachomatis* infections is in the late teens and early twenties, resembling other sexually transmitted infections. Further evidence for sexual transmission is the rising prevalence of serum antibody to *C. trachomatis* in proportion to an increasing number of sex partners of infected individuals. The prevalence of chlamydial urethral infection in young men ranges from 3 to 5 percent of men seen in general medical settings, to over 10 percent of asymptomatic soldiers undergoing routine physical examination, to 15 to 20 percent of men seen in sexually transmitted disease (STD) clinics. Among homosexual men, urethral infection appears less common (4 to 5 percent of homosexual men in STD clinics) than in heterosexual men, but rectal infections occur with a prevalence of 4 to 7 percent in homosexual male STD clinic patients. Cervical infection in women has ranged from 5 percent or more of asymptomatic college students or prenatal patients in the United States, to over 10 percent of women seen in a family planning clinic, to over 20 percent of women seen in STD clinics. In the United States, the prevalence of *C. trachomatis* in the cervix of pregnant women is 5 to 10 times higher than that of *N. gonorrhoeae.* The prevalence of genital infection with either agent is highest in individuals who are indigent, nonwhite, unmarried, and between ages 18 and 24. The ratio of chlamydial to gonococcal urethritis is highest for heterosexual men and those with high socioeconomic status, and lowest for homosexual men and indigent populations. The ratio of symptomatic to asymptomatic infections appears to be lower for *C. trachomatis* than for *N. gonorrhoeae,* as does the clinical severity of symptomatic infections. However, because the total number of *C. trachomatis* infections exceeds that of *N. gonorrhoeae* infections in industrialized countries, the total morbidity caused by *C. trachomatis* genital infections is comparable with that caused by *N. gonorrhoeae.* The prevalence of *C. trachomatis* is higher than that of *N. gonorrhoeae* in industrialized countries, in part because measures such as treatment of sex partners and routine cultures for case detection in asymptomatic individuals are being applied much more effectively for gonorrhea control than for control of *C. trachomatis* infection.

CLINICAL MANIFESTATIONS **Nongonococcal and postgonococcal urethritis** Nongonococcal urethritis is a diagnosis of exclusion that is applied to men with symptoms and/or signs of urethritis who do not have gonorrhea. Postgonococcal urethritis (PGU) refers to nongonococcal urethritis which develops 2 to 3 weeks after treatment of gonococcal urethritis in men. *Chlamydia trachomatis* causes 30 to 50 percent of the cases of NGU and PGU in heterosexual men but is uncommonly isolated from homosexual men with these syndromes. The cause of the remainder is uncertain, although considerable evidence suggests that *Ureaplasma urealyticum* causes some of these infections.

Since *Chlamydia* cultures are not widely available, current practice is to diagnose NGU by documentation of a leukocytic urethral exudate and by exclusion of gonorrhea by Gram's stain or culture. *Chlamydia trachomatis* urethritis is generally less severe than gonococcal urethritis, although in an individual patient these two forms of urethritis cannot be differentiated solely on clinical grounds. Symptoms include urethral discharge, dysuria, and urethral itching, and examination shows meatal erythema and tenderness and a urethral exudate which is often demonstrable only by stripping the urethra in the morning before voiding. About one-third of male STD patients who have *C. trachomatis* urethral infection have no demonstrable signs or symptoms of urethritis. Such patients frequently have first-glass pyuria (15 leukocytes per 400× microscopic field in the sediment of first-voided early morning urine) in the three-glass test or an increased number of leukocytes on gram-stained smear prepared from a urogenital swab inserted 1 to 2 cm into the anterior urethra. The smear is first scanned at low power to identify areas of the slide containing the highest concentration of leukocytes. These areas are then examined under oil immersion (1000×). An average of four leukocytes in five 1000× (oil immersion) fields is indicative of urethritis and correlates with recovery of *C. trachomatis.* To differentiate between true urethritis and functional symptoms among symptomatic patients, or to make a presumptive diagnosis of *C. trachomatis* infection in asymptomatic men (e.g., male patients in STD clinics, sex partners of women with nongonococcal salpingitis or mucopurulent cervicitis, fathers of children with inclusion conjunctivitis), the examination of an endourethral specimen for increased leukocytes is useful if cultures are not available.

Epididymitis *Chlamydia trachomatis* is also a cause of epididymitis in sexually active males. In one study, *C. trachomatis* infection was found by cultures of the urethra, urine, semen, or epididymal aspirate or by serology in 17 of 34 men under 35 years of age who presented with epididymitis, while 7 had gonorrhea; of 16 men over 35 with epididymitis, only 1 had chlamydial infection, and none had gonorrhea. Coliform bacteria and *Pseudomonas aeruginosa* are the most common causes of epididymitis in men over 35. The presence of a urethral discharge in association with unilateral scrotal pain, swelling, and tenderness suggests the diagnosis of chlamydial or gonococcal epididymitis, whereas the presence of midstream pyuria and bacteriuria in an older patient without urethral discharge suggests coliform or *Pseudomonas* infection. Testicular torsion should be promptly excluded by surgical exploration in a teenager or young adult who presents with acute unilateral testicular pain without urethritis. Testicular tumor or chronic infection (e.g., tuberculosis) should be excluded in the patient with unilateral intrascrotal pain and swelling who does not respond to appropriate antimicrobial therapy.

Reiter's syndrome *C. trachomatis* has been recovered from the urethra from up to 70 percent of men with untreated Reiter's syndrome who have associated urethritis. This striking association is unexplained.

Proctitis *C. trachomatis* of either the genital immunotypes D–K or the LGV immunotype L_2 causes proctitis in homosexual men and heterosexual women who practice anal intercourse. LGV strains produce a more severe ulcerative proctitis which histologically resembles Crohn's disease in that giant-cell formation and granulomas are seen (see Chap. 309). Either asymptomatic infection or mild proctitis not unlike gonococcal proctitis results from infection with immunotypes D–K. Clinically, these patients present with rectal pain, bleeding, mucus discharge, and tenesmus. Most have polymorphonuclear leukocytes in their stool. In chlamydial (non-LGV) proctitis usually sigmoidoscopy reveals mild, patchy mucosal friability, and exudate is limited to the distal rectum. The differential diagnosis of proctitis limited to the distal rectum in homosexual men includes gonococcal or herpes simplex virus infection, in addition to *C. trachomatis* infection.

Cervicitis *C. trachomatis* has been isolated from the cervix of 30 to 60 percent of women with gonorrhea or a history of contact with gonorrhea, from 30 to 70 percent of women whose male partners have nongonococcal urethritis, and from 10 to 20 percent of women attending STD clinics who do not have a history of contact with a partner with urethritis. Women who have cervical ectopy or who use oral contraceptives appear to have an increased prevalence of cervical infection with *C. trachomatis.*

Although many women with *C. trachomatis* cervical infection have a normal cervix, there is a significant correlation of this infection with endocervicitis, manifested by mucopurulent exudate in the cervical os. Endocervicitis appears to be nearly as common in women as is urethritis in men, yet it is detected far less often; this is partly because cervicitis is less often symptomatic than urethritis and the symptoms (i.e., vaginal discharge) are less specific, and partly because clinicians have not been taught how to recognize the signs of cervicitis. However, a very simple screening test for endocervical mucopus involves demonstration of a yellow or green color on a swab after it has been inserted into the endocervix and then withdrawn. The swab should then be used to prepare a *thin* smear for gram staining; demonstration of an average of ≥ 5 polymorphonuclear leukocytes per oil immersion (1000×) field on the smear of secretions from women who do not have visible yellow mucopus (on the swab) appeared to be correlated with an increased rate of isolation of *C. trachomatis* from the cervix in one recent study. These findings, though less sensitive and less specific than culture, are quite analogous to the criteria used for presumptive diagnosis of chlamydial urethritis in men. A distinctive pattern of hypertrophic (edematous and congested) cervical ectopic (red) epithelium and increased friability also may be seen. Herpes simplex virus causes inflammation and ulceration of the exocervix, rather than of the endocervix alone, but can be confused with gonococcal or chlamydial cervicitis. The presence of mucopurulent endocervicitis suggests the presence of *C. trachomatis* or *N. gonorrhoeae* infection. If tests for gonorrhea are negative, nongonococcal endocervicitis should be treated with tetracycline, just as nongonococcal urethritis is treated, and male sex partners should be examined for NGU. There is some evidence that chlamydial cervicitis is associated with cytologic atypia, including reactive and metaplastic atypia and changes suggestive of dysplasia.

Urethral syndrome in women *C. trachomatis* has been found to be the most common pathogen isolated from women with dysuria and frequency among college women who have "sterile pyuria" (e.g., absence of uropathogens such as coliforms or *Staphylococcus saprophyticus* in *any* concentration in clean-catch midstream urine specimens, together with the presence of pyuria) (see Chap. 296). *Chlamydia* can also be isolated from the urethra of women without symptoms of urethritis, and up to 25 percent of female STD clinic patients with urethral or cervical infection have had positive cultures from the urethra only.

TABLE 195-1
Clinical parallels between sexually transmitted infections due to *Neisseria gonorrhoeae* and *Chlamydia trachomatis*

	Resulting clinical syndrome	
Site of infection	*N. gonorrhoeae*	*C. trachomatis*
MEN		
Urethra	Urethritis	NGU, PGU
Epididymis	Epididymitis	Epididymitis
Rectum	Proctitis	Proctitis
Conjunctiva	Conjunctivitis	Conjunctivitis
Systemic	Disseminated gonococcal infection (DGI)	Reiter's syndrome
WOMEN		
Urethra	Acute urethral syndrome	Acute urethral syndrome
Bartholin's gland	Bartholinitis	Bartholinitis
Cervix	Cervicitis	Cervicitis, cervical dysplasia
Fallopian tube	Salpingitis	Salpingitis
Conjunctiva	Conjunctivitis	Conjunctivitis
Liver capsule	Perihepatitis	Perihepatitis
Systemic	DGI	Arthritis-dermatitis (sexually-active reactive arthritis)

Salpingitis and perihepatitis *Chlamydia trachomatis* has been implicated as a cause of acute salpingitis. In one Swedish study, it was isolated from the cervix of 19 of 53 women with acute salpingitis verified by laparoscopy, and it was recovered from the fallopian tube in the absence of other pathogens from six of seven who had *C. trachomatis* in the cervix. *C. trachomatis* was isolated from approximately one-third of consecutive Swedish women with salpingitis; another one-third had negative cultures but had serologic evidence suggestive of chlamydial infection. In the United States, limited studies suggest that a small proportion (perhaps one-third) of women with salpingitis have culture or serologic evidence of *C. trachomatis* infection.

A related development is the demonstration of serologic evidence suggestive of recent *C. trachomatis* infection in 20 of 23 women with acute peritonitis and/or perihepatitis (Fitz-Hugh–Curtis syndrome). *C. trachomatis* has been isolated from the surface of the liver in perihepatitis. Infertility due to bilateral tubal occlusion is more common after gonococcal salpingitis than after nongonococcal salpingitis, and it is not surprising that this form of infertility has been strongly correlated with the prevalence and titer of serum antibody to *C. trachomatis.*

***Chlamydia trachomatis* infection in pregnancy** *C. trachomatis* infection in pregnant women entails a risk of transmitting infection to the neonate. *Chlamydia trachomatis* in pregnancy also has been associated with fetal wastage and with a high risk of postpartum endometritis. Whether these complications are attributable to *C. trachomatis* remains to be determined. If so, detection and treatment of *C. trachomatis* in the mother and father early during pregnancy may be particularly important.

PERINATAL INFECTIONS: INCLUSION CONJUNCTIVITIS AND PNEUMONIA

EPIDEMIOLOGY Several studies in the United States have found *C. trachomatis* infections of the cervix in from 5 to 20 percent or more of pregnant women. In these studies, from approximately one-half to two-thirds of the children who were exposed during birth eventually showed laboratory evidence of *C. trachomatis* infection. Roughly half of the infants who developed laboratory evidence of infection (or 25 percent of the group exposed) developed clinical inclusion conjunctivitis. In addition to eye infection, the *C. trachomatis* organisms were isolated frequently and persistently from the nasopharynx and even the rectum. Pneumonia has also been shown to result in about 10 percent of these birth canal infections, and otitis media may in some cases result from perinatally acquired chlamydial infection.

INCLUSION CONJUNCTIVITIS OF THE NEWBORN (NEONATAL CHLAMYDIAL CONJUNCTIVITIS) In the newborn, chlamydial conjunctivitis generally has a longer incubation period than gonococcal conjunctivitis (5 to 14 days vs. 1 to 3 days), but this is not reliable in the individual patient. The other common causes of conjunctivitis in newborns include *Staphylococcus aureus, Hemophilus influenzae, H. parainfluenzae, Streptococcus pneumoniae,* and herpes simplex virus. Neonatal chlamydial conjunctivitis has an acute onset and often produces a profuse mucopurulent discharge, sometimes with membrane formation. However, it is impossible to differentiate *Chlamydia* conjunctivitis from other forms of neonatal bacterial conjunctivitis clinically, and laboratory diagnosis is required. Inclusions within epithelial cells often can be demonstrated in Giemsa-stained conjunctival smears, but smears are less sensitive than cultures. Similarly, gram-stained smears may show gonococci, or occasional small gram-negative coccobacilli in *Hemophilus* conjunctivitis, but smears should be accompanied by cultures for these agents. Very rarely a trachoma-like eye disease with chlamydial infection occurs in children living in nonendemic areas and probably is the late result of neonatally acquired infection. If neonatal chlamydial conjunctivitis is not treated appropriately with oral antimicrobials, it may be followed by chlamydial pneumonia.

INFANT PNEUMONIA There is a distinctive pneumonia syndrome in infants infected with *C. trachomatis,* which appears to occur in two to six cases per 1000 live births. The diagnosis of *C. trachomatis* pneumonia has been confirmed by isolation of the organism from lung biopsy and by development of high titers of specific IgM antibody to *C. trachomatis.* This pneumonia has been found in infants from 1 to 4 months of age. The onset is gradual and the course protracted, but the child is usually afebrile. There is diffuse interstitial involvement of the lungs. Most of the infants have a distinctive cough (a series of closely spaced staccato coughs, each separated by a brief inspiration), tachypnea, rales, hyperinflation, slight eosinophilia, and elevated serum immunoglobulins. Clinical illness lasts several weeks, while inspiratory rales and radiological signs may persist for months. About half of the infants with pneumonia also have conjunctivitis. While many infants with pneumonia have recovered without therapy, a few in whom the illness has been associated with apnea have been severely ill.

NONGENITAL INFECTIONS DUE TO *C. TRACHOMATIS* IN ADULTS *C. trachomatis* has been reported as an infrequent cause of subacute endocarditis and may cause respiratory infections in older children and adults. Serologic evidence supporting a role for *Chlamydia* in community-acquired pneumonia has been gathered, but as yet the agent has not been isolated from such cases. Immunosuppressed patients with pneumonia have had, in some cases, either serologic or cultural evidence of *C. trachomatis* infection, but more data are necessary to define the role of *Chlamydia* in these patients.

REFERENCES

Beem MO, Saxon EM: Respiratory tract colonization and a distinctive pneumonia syndrome in infants infected with *Chlamydia trachomatis.* N Engl J Med 296:306, 1977

Berger RE et al: Etiology, manifestations and therapy of acute epididymitis: Prospective study of 50 cases. J Urol 121:750, 1979

Bowie WR et al: Etiology of nongonococcal urethritis: Evidence for *Chlamydia trachomatis* and *Ureaplasma urealyticum.* J Clin Invest 59:735, 1977

Harrison JR et al: *C. trachomatis* pneumonitis: Comparison with matched infant controls and other pneumonitis. N Engl J Med 298:702, 1978

Holmes KK et al: Etiology of nongonococcal urethritis. N Engl J Med 292:1199, 1975

Kousa M et al: Frequent association of chlamydial infection with Reiter's syndrome. Sex Transm Dis 5:57, 1978

Mardh PA et al: *Chlamydia trachomatis* infection in patients with acute salpingitis. N Engl J Med 296:1377, 1977

Martin DH et al: Prematurity and perinatal mortality in pregnancies complicated by maternal *Chlamydia trachomatis* infections. JAMA 247:1585, 1982

Punnonen R et al: Chlamydial serology in infertile women, by immunofluorescence. Fertil Steril 31:656, 1979

Quinn TC et al: *Chlamydia trachomatis* proctitis. N Engl J Med 305:195, 1981

Rees E et al: Chlamydia in relation to cervical infection and pelvic inflammatory disease, in *Nongonococcal Urethritis and Related Infections,* D Hobson, KK Holmes (eds). Washington, DC, American Society for Microbiology, 1977, pp 67–76.

Stagno S et al: Infant pneumonitis with cytomegalovirus, chlamydia, pneumocystis and ureaplasma: A prospective study. Pediatrics 68(3):322, 1981

Stamm WE et al: Treatment of the acute urethral syndrome. N Engl J Med 304:956, 1981

Wager GP et al: Puerperal infections morbidity: Relationship to route of delivery and to antepartum *Chlamydia trachomatis* infection. Am J Obstet Gynecol 138:1028, 1980

Wang SP et al: *Chlamydia trachomatis* infections in Fitz-Hugh–Curtis syndrome. Am J Obstet Gynecol 138:1034, 1980

section 12 | Viral diseases

196
AN OVERVIEW OF VIRUS INFECTIONS

A. MARTIN LERNER

Knowledge of the clinical syndromes associated with specific viruses, understanding of appropriate diagnostic tests, and utilization of available means for prevention and therapy are now required of all internists. Common virus infections vary from inapparent to life threatening. Rapid progress in understanding of the acute and longer-term consequences of virus infections continues. Of particular note have been (1) further definitions of immunopathologic mechanisms of hepatitis viruses and (2) understanding of the interferon system in immunoregulation, control of cell growth, and virus infection. Both of these advances are likely to have important effects on the care of patients with virus infections.

GENERAL PROPERTIES AND CLASSIFICATION OF VIRUSES

Viruses are grouped according to their biophysical characteristics: (1) presence of nucleic acid, (2) size, (3) sensitivity to ether, (4) presence of an envelope, and (5) symmetry (cubic or helical). They contain macromolecular cores of ribonucleic acid (RNA) or deoxyribonucleic acid (DNA), but not both. (On the other hand, chlamydiae, *Mycoplasma,* and Rickettsiae contain both RNA and DNA.) Viruses have marked species and organ specificities, and on the whole, viruses infecting plants, insects, rickettsiae, bacteria, and other animals are distinct from their human counterparts.

Human viruses range in size from 17 nm (picornavirus) to 300 nm (poxvirus). They may be naked and contain only nucleic acid (genome) which is protected by a closed shell or tubing, the capsid. Other viruses have, in addition, a lipid envelope, acquired during maturation as virus evaginates from the nucleus (herpes simplex virus) or cytoplasm (influenza, herpes simplex virus). The lipid coat of these viruses surrounds the capsid. The capsid consists of protein and is composed of repeating subunits, capsomeres. The lipid envelope of some viruses is interrupted by spikelike projections. The capsomeres and spikes, of course, represent separate antigenic sites necessary for virus attachment to susceptible cells. Mature virus particles are called *virions.*

The nucleic acid contains all the genetic material necessary to reproduce itself (transcription) and code for structural proteins and enzymes (translation) important in synthesis and attachment to susceptible cells. The nucleic acid core plus the capsid is known as the *nucleocapsid.* When the virion is stripped of its capsid, nucleic acid may enter a host of foreign species and produce a single cycle of mature virus (e.g., poliovirus in mouse renal cells). Species and organ specificities of virus-cell union are functions first of complementary physical characteristics and then of covalent union between proteins of the virus and susceptible cell membranes. For instance, molecules of neuraminic acid act as receptors on human red blood cells, allowing hemagglutination by influenza virus. Within several hours after virus adsorption, neuraminidase, one of the proteins of the influenza capsid, digests the neuraminic acid. Elution of influenza virus from red blood cells follows. Cells which allow virus multiplication are termed *permissive,* while those which do not are termed *nonpermissive.* The membrane fit may be HLA dependent and change with aging of the host. Some virus-cell unions may be permissive at one temperature (37°C) but not at the lower temperatures of the upper respiratory tract (~30°C).

There are nine known families of RNA viruses and five families of DNA viruses (Table 196-1). The classifications of the DNA-containing hepatitis B virus; hepatitis non-A, non-B virus; and the short, highly resistant RNA strands called "viroids," which are likely the cause of the degenerative spongioform encephalopathies of Jakob-Creutzfeldt disease, remain incomplete.

VIRUS MULTIPLICATION Virus adsorption is a specific physical and then chemical reaction. After absorption, virus enters the cell by pinocytosis and is uncoated; i.e., nucleic acid is stripped from the capsid. With DNA viruses, specific virus DNA strands are transcribed into specific messenger RNA (mRNA) which is then translated to synthesize virus-specific proteins and enzymes necessary for biosynthesis of virus DNA. In the case of virus RNA, single-stranded RNA serves as its own messenger. The mRNA is translated, resulting in the formation of an RNA polymerase. Some of the viral proteins are structural parts of the capsid and others are virus-specified enzymes. The complexity of human viruses varies greatly. For instance, there are 4 structural proteins in coxsackieviruses but about 30 structural proteins in herpes simplex virus (HSV) type 1. The DNA genome of that virus is, however, large enough to code for about 100 proteins.

Virus infection suppresses synthesis of host cell protein and nucleic acid to variable degrees. Assembly of protein subunits around virus DNA results in formation of complete virions which may be released by cell lysis or budding from the cytoplasm. Virions of RNA animal tumor viruses contain an enzyme which is capable of catalyzing synthesis of DNA. The product consists of small fragments of DNA, most of which are complementary in base sequence to 70-S RNA of the virion. Information can travel not only from DNA to RNA but also, at least in certain cases, in the reverse direction.

Virus multiplication may lead to a cytolytic infection with

TABLE 196-1
Major families of viruses infecting humans and some associated diseases

Family name, nucleic acid, and prototype virus(es)	*Size, nm*	*Ether sensitive*	*Envelope*	*Symmetry*	*No. of capsomeres*	*Other*	*Characteristic diseases*
Picornaviridae (enteroviruses, RNA) Coxsackieviruses A and B; echo-, rhino-, and polioviruses; "hepatitis A virus"	17–30	No	No	Cubic	20–30	Capsids assembled in cytoplasm Four major polypeptides One minor polypeptide	Rashes, aseptic meningitis, myocarditis, pleurodynia Common cold syndrome Poliomyelitis Hepatitis A
Reoviridae (RNA) Reoviruses; orbivirus; rotavirus	60–80	No	No	Cubic	92 (reovirus) 32 (orbivirus, rotavirus)	RNA (double-stranded and in segments)	Reovirus (uncertain role in human disease) Orbivirus (Colorado tick fever) Rotavirus (nonbacterial infantile diarrhea)
Togaviridae (RNA) Alphaviruses (group A arboviruses) Flaviviruses (group B arboviruses) Rubivirus (non-arbo togavirus)	40–70	Yes	Yes	Cubic			Alphaviruses (Venezuelan, eastern, western equine encephalitis) Flaviviruses (yellow fever, dengue, Japanese encephalitis, St. Louis encephalitis, Omsk hemorrhagic fever, Russian spring-summer encephalitis) Rubivirus (rubella)
Orthomyxoviridae (RNA) Influenzavirus, types A, B, and C	80–120	Yes	Yes	Helical		Spikes at surface are the glycosylated proteins, the hemagglutinin (H), and neuraminadase (N)	Influenza A, B, or C
Paramyxoviridae (RNA) Paramyxovirus (parainfluenza viruses, mumps virus) Morbillivirus (measles virus) Pneumovirus (respiratory syncitial virus)	~ 150	Yes	Yes	Helical		Paramyxoviruses contain H plus N Morbillivirus contains H only Pneumovirus contains neither H nor N	Infantile croup, bronchitis, mumps, measles Infantile pneumonia, bronchitis
Rhabdoviridae (RNA) Lyssavirus (rabies virus, Duvenhage virus, Mokola virus) Vesiculovirus (Chandipura virus) Marburg virus is rhabdovirus-like	60	Yes	Yes	Helical			Rabies Marburg disease
Arenaviridae (RNA) Lymphocytic choriomeningitis virus, Lassa virus, Tacaribe complex (Junin, Machupo viruses of South American hemorrhagic fevers)	50–300	Yes	Yes				Lymphocytic choriomeningitis, Lassa fever, hemorrhagic fevers
Coronaviridae (RNA) Coronavirus	80–130	Yes	Yes				Common cold syndrome
Bunyaviridae (RNA) Bunyavirus (Bunyamwera group)	100	Yes	Yes				California encephalitis, Crimean hemorrhagic fever
Parvoviridae (DNA) Adenosatellovirus, Norwalk agent (The hepatitis B core antigen resembles a parvovirus)	18–26	No	No	Cubic	32	DNA (single-stranded)	Nonbacterial diarrhea
Papovaviridae (DNA) Wart virus, JC virus, BK virus	45–55	No	No	Cubic	72	Unusually heat stable	Warts, progressive multifocal leukoencephalopathy
Adenoviridae (DNA) Adenovirus	70–90	No	No	Cubic	252		Conjunctivitis, pharyngitis, pneumonia

TABLE 196-1 (*continued*)
Major families of viruses infecting humans and some associated diseases

Family name, nucleic acid, and prototype virus(es)	*Size, nm*	*Ether sensitive*	*Envelope*	*Symmetry*	*No. of capsomeres*	*Other*	*Characteristic diseases*
Herpetoviridae (DNA) Herpes simplex virus, types 1 and 2, monkey B virus, varicella-zoster virus, cytomegalovirus, Epstein-Barr virus	100	Yes	Yes	Cubic	162	Establish persistent or latent infections	Herpes labialis and genitalis, herpes encephalitis, chickenpox, mental retardation (cytomegalovirus), congenital deafness (cytomegalovirus), pneumonia in the immunosuppressed patient (cytomegalovirus), infectious mononucleosis
Poxviridae (DNA) Variola virus, vaccinia virus, molluscum contagiosum, orf	~ 300	No		Complex	230		Smallpox, cowpox, milker's nodule
Classifications incomplete:							
Hepatitis non-A, non-B							Acute hepatitis, chronic "active" and chronic "persistent" hepatitis
Hepatitis B (DNA)	42						
"Viroids" (short strand of RNA, molecular weight ~ 75,000)							Jakob-Creutzfeldt disease

release of virus with necrosis of the infected cell, but other infections are persistent or latent and may reactivate at a later time. In turn, the virus nucleic acid may become incorporated into the genome of the cell leading to malignant transformation. Virus infection may also lead to fusion of cellular membranes (giant cells) or demyelinization.

PATHOGENESIS OF VIRUS INFECTIONS The primary site of virus multiplication depends upon the route of acquisition and the special receptor-site complementarity of the host (Table 196-2). The modes of transmission of human virus infections are: respiratory, alimentary, contact (skin or mucosal), bite, injection (transfusion), or transplacental. Respiratory viruses are also exchanged by kissing or by the hands. The hands are also vital in fecal virus transfers.

Virus-specific structures (inclusion bodies) may be present within the cytoplasm (variola), nucleus (herpes simplex virus, varicella-zoster, adenovirus), or both (measles) of infected cells. Viremia may or may not occur. The transit of viruses within the blood is often associated with the cellular components (herpes simplex virus, cytomegalovirus, coxsackieviruses). Buffy coat cultures for attempts at virus isolation are always worthwhile. In many virus infections, in distinct contrast to bacteremias, viremia occurs during the incubation period when the patient is well. Viremia is usual with the exanthems of enteroviruses, rubeola, and varicella-zoster. Herpesviruses may multiply within lymphocytes sequestered from antibodies and phagocytes when there is no viremia. During coxsackievirus B3 viremia in mice, virus is present in the plasma, but erythrocytes, polymorphonuclear leukocytes, and platelets do not contain virus. On the third day of this plasma viremia infectious T and B lymphocyte-virus complexes circulate. Secondary sites of infection may be heart, liver, pancreas, kidneys, or brain.

RESPONSES OF THE HOST At sites of virus multiplication extracellular virus often abounds. Macrophages and a few polymorphonuclear leukocytes migrate to the area producing inflammation. Interferons (see below) are produced locally, and B, T, and null lymphocytes appear. Macrophages attach to antigen markedly augmenting the efficiency of virus inactivation by specific neutralizing antibodies or sensitized T lymphocytes. During the first days of many virus infections there is a circulating lymphopenia of both B and T cells. Lymphocytes migrate to sites of infection and to the liver, spleen, or other organs of the mononuclear phagocytic system.

Interferon Viruses, certain bacteria (pneumococci, streptococci, staphylococci), endotoxin, certain parasites, and double-stranded RNA synthetic polyribonucleotide complexes such as polyinosinic polycytidilic ribonucleic acid (poly rI:rC) stimulate the interferon system to produce antiviral proteins known as α- (leukocyte, Le); β- (fibroblast, epithelial); and γ- (lymphoblastoid) interferon (IFN). The three types of IFN are antigenically distinct, and their mRNAs have been isolated. Through use of techniques of genetic transfer, *Escherichia coli* is being used to produce large quantities of purified IFN for controlled clinical trials in human virus infection and in anticancer treatments. Purified α-IFN with an activity of 10^8 IU/mg has been prepared. α-IFN is produced by unstimulated T cells and monocytes. β-IFN is produced by stimulated epithelial cells in infected organs and by fibroblasts in tissue cultures. γ- (Immune) IFN is produced by sensitized T cells. The molecular weights of the glycoproteins of α- and β-IFN are ~ 20,000, while that of the lipoprotein of γ-IFN is ~ 50,000. About 20 human genes have been found capable of coding for IFNs, and chromosomes 2, 5, and 9 have, so far, been specifically identified as IFN genes.

The appearance of two new enzymes has been associated temporally with the production of IFN, namely, 2′,5′-oligoadenylate polymerase and fatty acid cyclooxygenase. Assays for the former enzyme are far more sensitive than are the usual bioassays for IFN in tissue cultures surveying its antiviral activity versus vesicular stomatitis virus. The initial action of IFN, like that of hormones, resides at the cellular membrane where binding to a specific ganglioside (G_{M1}) and glycoprotein occurs. Anti-ACTH, anti-melanotropin, and anti-gamma-endorphin antiserums neutralize human α-(Le) IFN activity, but not β-(F) IFN activity.

IFNs are regulatory proteins controlling virus biosynthesis, mitogen-induced protein synthesis, and cell growth. Interferon is an immunoregulatory protein as well, with a stimulatory function early and a suppressive one later in the immune responses.

Within several hours after onset of virus infection, and days before humoral antibodies can be measured by ordinary methods, IFN is found in tissues where virus is synthesized and in the blood. IFN is probably most effective as an antiviral substance early in infection when viral titers are low. Later, IFN's effect on virus in tissues is small. IFN also has an important function as an immunoregulatory substance, either stimulator or depressor, depending on the time during infection.

A delay in the appearance of IFN in vesicular fluid has been associated with viremic dissemination in herpes zoster. Likewise, decreased in vitro responsiveness of the patient's lymphocytes after stimulation by herpes simplex virus in the production of IFN has been correlated with recurrences of herpes labialis. Severe repetitive and exhausting exercise in mice infected with coxsackievirus B3 results in a delay in the appearance of circulating IFN and, later, in both a delay and a depression in the quantity of type-specific neutralizing antibody in serum. A marked increase in the quantity of myocardial virus and mortality follows. Exercise augmentation of coxsackievirus B3 virulence is also associated with thymic atrophy. Rest may be a very important factor in recovery from virus infections.

Both α- and β-IFN are acid stable (pH 2), trypsin sensitive, nondialyzable, and nonsedimentable by ultracentrifugal forces sufficient to pellet viruses. γ-IFN is more acid stable, is inactivated at 60°C for 120 min, and is similarly sensitive to treatment with the disulfide-splitting agent, 2-mercaptoethanol. Most cells tested produce IFN, but those of the reticuloendothelial system (especially the spleen) and lymphocytes are particularly important.

IFNs have no effect upon extracellular virus. Following entry of virus nucleic acid into a susceptible cell, the cell nucleus is stimulated to produce IFN. IFN is released through the cytoplasm of the infected cell. Synthesis of virus-directed coat proteins and enzymes is prevented. New virus is not formed.

IFNs are not virus specific and are active against a wide variety of viruses. However, IFN is an effective antiviral substance only in cells of the same species in which it is produced. For instance, anti-influenza A IFN produced in hamster tissue cultures is effective against influenza in hamsters but not in humans. Likewise, IFN produced in human leukocytes or human tissue cultures is effective in humans.

Viruses vary greatly in their sensitivity to IFN. Myxoviruses are quite sensitive, while herpesviruses are more resistant. The importance of IFN in recovery from virus infection probably varies. With coxsackievirus B3, IFN titers in tissues actually parallel virus titers. In animal models, IFN has been shown to have a prophylactic effect in a number of virus infections, but once the titers of virus are high, IFN is ineffective.

TABLE 196-2
Modes of transmission of human viruses

*Mode of transmission**	*Symptoms/ other*	*Viruses*
Respiratory (droplets or droplet-nuclei in air, bites, salivary transfer, mouth to hand or object)	Local	Adenoviruses (many serotypes) Rhinoviruses (many serotypes) Influenza viruses A, B, C Parainfluenza viruses (several serotypes) Coronaviruses (many serotypes)
	General	Varicella-zoster; Epstein-Barr (EB) virus Variola (smallpox) Rubella Mumps; rubeola (measles) Lymphocytic choriomeningitis; Lassa virus
Alimentary	Local	Adenoviruses (a few serotypes) Enteroviruses (a few serotypes) Parvoviruses (Norwalk agent) Reoviruses, orbiviruses, rotaviruses
	General	Enteroviruses (many serotypes, including polioviruses) Hepatitis A virus
Contact (skin, mucous membranes)		Wart virus Herpesviruses [herpes simplex viruses, type 1 (oral) and 2 (genital)]; EB virus Hepatitis B Cytomegalovirus (CMV) Molluscum contagiosum; cowpox; milker's nodules
Arthropod bite	General	California encephalitis virus Western equine encephalitis virus Venezuelan equine encephalitis virus St. Louis encephalitis virus Colorado tick fever virus (reovirus-like orbivirus)
Animal bite	General	B virus Rabies virus
Infection by transfusion	General	Hepatitis B, hepatitis non-A, non-B, CMV EB virus
Transplacental	General	CMV Rubella
Instruments	Tonometer (examination for glaucoma)	Adenoviruses
	Corneal transplants	Jakob-Creutzfeldt "viroid"
	Neurosurgical or ophthalmologic procedures	
	Electrodes (electroencephalograms)	

* *Prevention and isolation/control are specifically directed by understanding the mode of transmission.*

Antibodies Proteins of the virus capsid stimulate B lymphocytes (immunoglobulin-bearing, bone marrow–derived) to synthesize humoral antibodies (IgM, IgG, IgA, IgD) and secretory antibodies (IgA). Cell-associated antibodies (IgE) are also produced. Immunoglobulins are synthesized in local lymph nodes, at body surfaces (saliva, respiratory secretions, colostrum), and in inflammatory exudates within organs (kidney, brain, cervix). During the first 3 to 10 days after an initial exposure to a virus, IgM antibodies predominate. Later, IgG antibodies prevail. Immunoglobulin M is important in clearing viremias remaining within vascular spaces; IgG antibodies also enter interstitial spaces. On surfaces, IgA antibodies contain an added secretory piece, allowing their functional integrity in the presence of hydrolytic enzymes of the secretions. Many molecules of antibody combine with a single virion. Covering a critical number of essential sites on the virion renders an antigen-antibody complex noninfectious. Antigen-antibody complexes attract components of complement which are the mediators for chemotaxis of polymorphonuclear leukocytes. Immune complexes may be fixed in tissues, circulate, or precipitate in the glomerulus, in the synovia of joints, or in the skin.

Secretory IgA antibodies in respiratory secretions are vital to the body's defenses against respiratory viruses. During viral respiratory infections viremia does not occur regularly. Humoral antibodies persist only for months. Immunity is transient and reinfections with the same virus occur. On the other hand, after systemic infections, humoral antibodies and immunity persist. After administration of killed virus vaccines immunity is also briefer than that which follows attenuated virus vaccines.

Circulating neutralizing antibody is effective protection against viremia, except possibly against very large inocula or in the presence of low antibody titers. Some viruses multiply and spread from cell to cell even in the presence of neutralizing antibodies. Herpes simplex virus, type 1, and rubeola in nervous tissues are examples. Cell-mediated immunity is the most important means of defense against enveloped viruses such as herpesviruses, while antibody is vital to recovery from enteroviruses. In some cases antibodies or T lymphocytes (cytotoxic "killer" cells) may be important in continuing the pathogenic process. Cytolytic T cells may be directed against neoantigens induced by, but antigenically distinct from, any structural component of the virus. This appears to be the pathogenetic mechanism in murine coxsackievirus B3 heart disease.

Antibodies to viruses are measured by neutralization of their cytopathic effects in tissue cultures, or by protection tests using embryonated eggs or animals. Complement fixation, precipitin, indirect hemagglutination, fluorescent antibody, immune hemadsorption, enzyme-linked immunosorbent (ELISA) and radioimmunoassays are among the techniques used to measure viral antibodies. Early after infection, certain viruses such as herpes simplex virus, type 1, and cytomegalovirus induce complement-requiring neutralizing antibodies. Myxoviruses, some enteroviruses, and reoviruses hemagglutinate several species of red blood cells. In these cases antibodies can be measured by inhibition of hemagglutination. Virus capsids of nonhemagglutinating viruses may be absorbed to the surface of tanned sheep red blood cells. Antibodies are then assayed by indirect hemagglutination. Kinetics of rises and falls of the several antibodies suggest that different assays may test separate immunoglobulin responses to distinct proteins of the virus capsid.

Cell-mediated immunity Thymic-derived T lymphocytes are responsible for cellular immune functions. In most virus infections, both T and B lymphocytes participate in the containment of virus replication. After a latent period, usually lasting 3 to 4 days, stimulated T lymphocytes transform to lymphoblasts. They release a number of nonspecific, nondialyzable effector molecules which migrate with albumin on electrophoresis. Among these effector molecules are lymphocyte-transforming factor, migration-inhibitory factor, cytotoxin factor, and γ (immune) IFN. Components of complement react with the surface of sensitized lymphocytes, releasing a chemotactic factor to monocytes, which are the most important phagocytes in cellular immunity. After stimulation by an antigen, evoking a potent T-lymphocyte response, macrophages are "activated," becoming more efficient phagocytes. This increased phagocytic ability of activated macrophages is not limited to the stimulating virus.

There are at least three subpopulations of T lymphocytes: T_o (cytolytic cells, antigen specific, without receptors for the F_c portion of immunoglobulin molecules); T_m (helper cells with F_c receptors on their surface for IgM); and T_g (suppressor cells with F_c receptors on their surface for IgG). T_m cells are necessary for a sustained IgG response.

EPIDEMIOLOGY OF VIRUS INFECTIONS Virus infection occurs with disease, or it may be asymptomatic. Clinical illness is the rule with measles (rubeola virus), but inapparent infection is common with enteroviruses. The severity of disease may also be age-related. In adults, chickenpox and mumps are often severe with complications (varicella pneumonia, mumps orchitis, or encephalitis) which are rare during childhood.

The *incidence* of infection is the number of new cases of a disease occurring in a unit of time, while the *incidence rate* is the number of new cases occurring divided by the number of persons in the total population at risk in the area being studied. The incidence rate is usually calculated as the ratio of the number of new clinical cases divided by the population under surveillance in a given year. Incidence rates may also be calculated by measuring virus excretion or rises in antibody titers using acute and convalescent phase serums.

The *prevalence* is the number of cases of a disease existing at one time, while the *prevalence rate* is the number of cases of a given disease at one time divided by the population at risk. The *point prevalence* or *period prevalence* may be calculated.

Unlike most bacterial infections, isolation of virus from an ill patient and even demonstration of a fourfold rise in specific antibodies to that virus in temporally related acute and convalescent serums does not always prove a causative relation to the illness in question. Epidemiologic support is often required for firm etiologic associations. Age-matched, sex-matched, and time- and place-matched controls (compeer groups) must be studied in the same manner as the patients in question. The families of patients are an excellent group to examine. Inapparent simultaneous infection must be sought. Patients within the hospital as well as persons living in the immediate neighborhood of the patient are also often studied. Virus isolation and/or antibody rises in a patient group in significant excess over controls are strong evidence for an etiologic association. *Serologic epidemiology* is the systematic testing of blood specimens from a defined sample of a healthy population for the presence of antigens, antibodies, or other components.

Virus infections often occur in clusters of cases determined by the presence of the virus in the community and the susceptibility (antibody titers to the virus) of the population. An *epidemic* or outbreak is present when the number of cases is in excess of the expected number at that locality based upon past experience. For instance, an increased incidence of a mix of viral respiratory infections and pneumonias is expected each winter, but influenza epidemics occur over 4- to 6-week intervals only every several years. On the other hand, the occurrence of only a dozen cases of St. Louis encephalitis in Michigan during the late summer would constitute an epidemic.

Influenza A epidemics often affect several continents at the same time. When this occurs, *pandemic* influenza is present. Epidemic influenza B is rarely pandemic.

When an epidemic of echovirus type 9 aseptic meningitis occurs in the summer months, most cases of meningitis (often with rash) during mid- to late summer are due to this agent. However, each case must be studied individually so that discovery of the occasional case of bacterial meningitis or herpes simplex virus encephalitis is certain to be made.

The greater the number of persons immune to a given virus among the population of an area, the less is the likelihood of disease due to that agent among that population at that time. "Population immunity," or *herd immunity*, is usually measured by the presence of neutralizing or other protective antibodies. Susceptibles in the population are protected because of the high number of persons in the group who are immune.

The *incubation period* is the time period from first exposure to first symptom. With short incubation periods of 2 to 4 days (e.g., enteroviruses), multiple cases of illness occur at the same time. With longer incubation periods (e.g., several weeks as with chickenpox), illnesses occur sequentially. If common exposure to several persons occurs, illness may be simultaneous irrespective of the length of the incubation period.

An appropriate environment is necessary for the spread of human disease. Mosquito-borne St. Louis encephalitis ends with effective mosquito control or after the first frost. Respiratory contagion is facilitated by rebreathed air laden with aerosolized virus from coughs, sneezes, or speech. Droplets of water over 10 μm in size containing virus travel short distances through air, while droplet nuclei, minus moisture and less than 10 μm in size, waft over greater distances. Successful primary infection in a susceptible host depends upon (1) the number of virions circulating per cubic foot of air, and (2) the time of exposure which, in turn, determine the total size of the inoculum. For instance, if an aerosol contains four virions per liter of air and 30 virions are required for infection, then persons breathing this air will inspire an infectious dose within a half-hour. The smaller number of respiratory infections during summer may be due to the multiple exchanges of air that result from open windows. In hospitals, walls reaching to the ceilings and closed doors are required for adequate respiratory isolation.

DIAGNOSIS OF VIRUS INFECTIONS **Isolation or recognition of viruses** Materials for virus isolation must be obtained as early during illness as possible. The earlier the specimen is taken, the higher is the titer of virus usually present, and the more likely that the specimen will be positive. Generally, specimens are collected in sterile screw-capped vials containing a balanced salt solution with antibiotics. Depending upon the pathogenesis of the particular infection, throat swab (or spu-

TABLE 196-3
Appropriate specimens for virus isolation (or recognition)

		Specimens					
Clinical syndrome	*Viruses*	*Throat/ sputum**	*Stool/ rectal swab**	*CSF**	*Urine**	*Vesicular fluid**	*Other*
Meningitis-encephalitis	Mumps	+	−	+	+	None	Usually none
	Enteroviruses:						
	Coxsackieviruses, group A or B	+	+	+	−†	+‡	Blood and buffy coat, brain, skeletal muscle, heart, pericardial fluid, testicle
	Echoviruses	+	+	+	−†	+‡	
	Polioviruses	+	+	−	−	None	Brain, spinal cord
	Herpes simplex:						
	Type 1	+	−	−	−†	+	Brain, buffy coat of blood
	Type 2	+	−	+	−	+	
	Arboviruses	−	−	+	−	None	Brain
Respiratory diseases	Influenza/parainfluenza viruses	+§	−	−	−	None	Lung, blood, heart
	Rhinoviruses	+	−	−	−	None	Usually none
	Adenoviruses	+	+	−	+	None	Conjunctiva
	Enteroviruses (see above)						
Exanthems	Rubeola (measles)	+	−	−	+	None	Brain
	Rubella	+	−	−	+	None	Brain
	Variola	+	−	−	−	+	
	Vaccinia	−	−	−	−	+	
	Varicella-zoster	−	−	−	−	+	Lung, heart
	Herpes simplex (see above)						
	Enteroviruses (see above)						
Myopericarditis	Enteroviruses (see above)						
Hepatitis	Hepatitis A and non-A, non-B	−	¶	−	−	None	
	Hepatitis B	−	−	−	−	None	Blood ¶
Virus diarrheas	Rotaviruses	−	¶	−	−	None	
	Parvoviruses	−	¶	−	−	None	
Other	Cytomegalovirus	−	−	−	+	None	Buffy coat of blood
	Progressive multifocal leukoencephalopathy	−	−	−	+	None	Brain
	Jakob-Creutzfeldt disease	−	−	?	−	None	Brain, eye

* *+, present; −, absent.*
† *These viruses have occasionally been isolated from urine.*
‡ *Vesicles are only occasionally present during coxsackievirus or echovirus infections.*
§ *These viral antigens can also be promptly recognized in these specimens by immunofluorescent methods.*
¶ *Hepatitis A has been recognized by immune electron microscopy in feces. Hepatitis A, hepatitis B, and hepatitis non-A, non-B viruses have not yet been isolated in tissue cultures. Hepatitis B has been recognized by electron microscopy in blood and liver. Diagnosis is usually made by immunochemical studies of blood (see Table 196-4). HBs, HBe, HBc antibody, and DNA polymerase also identify this virus infection. Rotaviruses and parvoviruses have been recognized in feces of patients by immune electron microscopy, radioimmunoassay for virus antigen, and ELISA for virus antigen.*

tum), stool (or rectal swab), cerebrospinal fluid (CSF), urine, vesicular fluid, or tissues (biopsy or autopsy) should be obtained for inoculation into susceptible tissue cultures (or mice), prepared for electron microscopy, immunofluorescent radioimmunoassay, or enzyme-linked immunosorbent assay (ELISA). These procedures can recognize viral antigens. If the specimen cannot be processed immediately, it should be frozen promptly to −70°C.

Vesicles should be opened and fluids or scrapings inoculated for virus. Scrapings and impression smears should be stained with Tzanck, Wright, and Gram's stains. Instructions relating to collection of specimens for various clinical syndromes are listed in Table 196-3.

Serologic tests At the initial visit with a patient suspected of a viral illness a sample of 10 ml blood should be taken and allowed to clot. The serum should be separated to prevent hemolysis which can interfere with diagnostic tests. A second sample of blood should be obtained 2 to 3 weeks later. Both serums should be sent simultaneously to the virus diagnostic laboratory. Changes in antibody titers are most meaningful when paired serums are tested concomitantly.

Neutralization, complement fixation, hemagglutination inhibition, indirect hemagglutination, immunofluorescence, immune adherence hemagglutination, radioimmunoassay, and ELISA are procedures used to measure viral antibodies. After systemic viral infections neutralizing antibodies confer long-lasting immunity. Complement-fixing antibodies, on the other hand, often fall (or disappear) with convalescence. Particular tests are most appropriate for certain viruses (Table 196-4).

Isolation of virus coupled with a fourfold or greater rise in antibody titers between acute and convalescent-phase specimens is diagnostic of recent infection but is not necessarily diagnostic of the clinical syndrome in question. The most striking example of the possible disparity in isolation of virus and its etiologic relationship is herpes simplex virus (HSV), type 2, the cause of herpes labialis and HSV encephalitis. Biopsy of the brain is required for definitive diagnosis of HSV encephalitis. Rises in complement-fixing antibodies to HSV occur with herpes labialis which may accompany pneumococcal meningitis. Nevertheless, in most virus infections fourfold rises in specific antibodies strongly suggest the proper diagnosis. Cross-reactive antibodies among enteroviruses and among herpesviruses are possible and can be confusing. Isolation of virus from diseased tissues is definitive.

Group-specific antibody tests (e.g., group B arboviruses, influenza A, influenza B) often employ the complement-fixation method and are helpful, lessening the number of diagnostic antigens which must be available. If an initial serum is taken later in the illness, a high single titer or high constant titers in both acute and convalescent serums may be found. Single high titers are probably diagnostic if the disease is rare in the area, if the antibody is short-lived (e.g., complement fixing), or if the antibody is IgM. A fourfold fall in antibody titers is also suggestive. Similar paired serums may be tested from other members of the patient's family for they may be in different stages of apparent or inapparent infection with the same virus.

Nucleic acid hybridization using tumors may recognize viral nucleic acids implicating these viruses in the case of cancers. Through use of nucleic acid probes, herpes simplex virus, type 2, has been linked to cervical cancer and Epstein-Barr virus with Burkitt's lymphoma and nasopharyngeal carcinoma.

PREVENTION OF VIRUS DISEASES Prevention of virus disease has been achieved largely through the development of viral vaccines, either live attenuated and "killed" or inactivated. Inactivated vaccines are generally available for influenza A, influenza B, rabies, and polioviruses, and on a limited and/or experimental basis inactivated viral vaccines have been developed for adenovirus, Japanese-B, equine, and Russian spring-summer encephalitis. Vaccines derived from attenuated tissue cultures are available for rubella, mumps, measles, poliomyelitis, and yellow fever. Indications for use of these vaccines are discussed in Chap. 145.

Passive immunization with pooled human immune serum globulins or globulins with high titers to specific agents such as rabies, hepatitis B, or varicella has also been used in the prophylaxis of virus infections. These preparations generally are most useful when given early during the incubation period in order to prevent clinical illness. In selected instances, use of

TABLE 196-4
Serologic tests employed in virus infections

Virus	*Complement fixation*	*Neutralization*	*Hemagglutination inhibition*	*Indirect hemagglutination*	*Immunofluorescence*	*Immune adherence hemagglutination*	*Radioimmunoassay*	*ELISA*	*Immune electron microscopy*
Mumps	+							+	
Enteroviruses		+							
Herpes simplex viruses	+			+	+	+		+	
Arboviruses	+		+						
Influenza/parainfluenza	+		+		+				
Rhinoviruses	+	+							
Adenoviruses	+								
Rubeola (measles)	+				+				
Rubella			+						
Variola	+				+				
Vaccinia	+				+				
Varicella-zoster	+			+		+			
Hepatitis A	+					+			
Hepatitis B							+		
Cytomegalovirus	+			+					
Rotavirus	+				+		+	+	+
Parvovirus	+				+		+	+	+

hyperimmune globulins may be useful in ameliorating illness once symptoms have developed. Lassa fever is an example. Specific indications for the use of passive immunization in the treatment and prevention of viral infections are discussed in Chap. 145.

Patients with slow virus infections of the central nervous system (Jakob-Creutzfeldt disease) undergoing neurosurgical or ophthalmologic procedures are contagious by means of contaminated surgical equipment. Prolonged autoclaving (121°C, 15 psi, 60 min) and 5% hypochlorite or iodine soaks for 60 min will inactivate large infective doses of this unusual virus. Chemoprophylaxis against smallpox with oral *N*-methylisatin β-thiosemicarbazone (Marboran) is effective as is amantadine hydrochloride (Symmetrel) taken by mouth throughout the period of exposure to influenza A. Amantadine is not effective against strains of influenza B.

TREATMENT OF VIRUS INFECTIONS Amantadine is of some value particularly in the prevention, but also in the symptomatic management, of respiratory tract illness caused by influenza A virus strains (see Chap. 198). The topical preparations idoxuridine, adenine arabinoside, and triflurothymidine are effective, approved, and available therapeutic agents for herpes simplex virus keratitis. Intravenous adenine arabinoside (ara-A) is also an effective therapeutic agent for the treatment of herpes simplex virus encephalitis. This agent has its maximal effect when it is begun before the onset of paralysis or coma. Ara-A (IV) is also effective in promoting healing and in limiting dissemination of herpes zoster in immunosuppressed patients. These drugs have minimal toxicity and are available for general use (see Chap. 210).

Experimental testing of ara-A in other herpesvirus infections as well as in chronic active hepatitis (HBe positive) is under way, and preliminary results are encouraging. HBs, HBe, and DNA polymerase activity has disappeared after IV ara-A with or without exogenous IFN. Exogenous megaunit human interferon will also suppress HBs antigenemia in chronic active hepatitis. Controlled clinical trials have also proved that pharmacological megaunits of leukocytic-derived human interferon are effective therapy for disseminated herpes zoster in immunocompromised patients. Clinical trials with human IFN are under way with IFN (α or β) produced by methods of genetic engineering or produced, in turn, in tissue cultures. The latter method, using a transformed lymphoblastoid cell line, produces large quantities of α-IFN following stimulation by Newcastle disease virus of chickens. Corticosteroids suppress leukocyte chemotaxis and T and B lymphocytes; they may be harmful and should not be given during the period of active virus multiplication. Acycloguanasine (acyclovir, ACV) and BVDU (E-5-[2-bromovinyl]-2′ deoxyuridine) are among the most promising of the newer prospective antiherpes drugs. Both depend for intracellular uptake upon the virus-induced enzyme thymidine kinase and specifically inhibit the virus polymerase. Their therapeutic margin of safety may prove to be greater than that of adenine arabinoside.

REFERENCES

BRAUDE AI: *Medical Microbiology and Infectious Diseases.* Philadelphia, Saunders, 1981

EVANS AS: *Viral Infections of Humans. Epidemiology and Control.* New York, Plenum, 1976

VICEK J et al: *Regulatory Functions of Interferons.* New York Academy of Sciences, 1980

Respiratory viruses

197
COMMON VIRAL RESPIRATORY INFECTIONS

VERNON KNIGHT

GENERAL CONSIDERATIONS

The viral respiratory diseases as a group are responsible for one-half or more of all acute illnesses, and although influenza virus is the only agent among them which causes significant mortality in adults, several different viruses contribute to the 20 percent of childhood mortality due to respiratory disease. Respiratory disease morbidity, due primarily to virus infections, causes 30 to 50 percent of time lost from work by adults, and from 60 to 80 percent of time lost from school by children.

Viral respiratory diseases are associated with a spectrum of host responses ranging from asymptomatic carrier states to severe and sometimes fatal pneumonias. There is a recurring pattern of severe illness in infants and young children and of milder disease with increasing age. A few clinical and epidemiologic entities can be recognized without laboratory aids, such as acute respiratory disease (ARD) in military recruits, caused by adenovirus type 4 and rhinovirus coryza in adults. The causative agent in a large proportion of cases, however, cannot be identified with virologic study.

EPIDEMIOLOGY More than 150 serotypes, representing 12 groups of viruses, have been or may be associated with the majority of acute respiratory illness in humans. With the capacity to isolate this large group of agents and with the recognition of the role of *Mycoplasma pneumoniae* (see Chap. 190) it is possible to define the cause of many respiratory illnesses. The recent identification of coronaviruses as a cause of respiratory illness increases the potential for diagnosis. Though some of the inability to identify agents is caused by lack of efficient application of known diagnostic methods, it is probable that additional viral and possibly other causes of respiratory illness remain to be discovered.

Frequency and severity Since 1957 the National Health Survey has made annual estimates from selected population samples of the incidence of acute respiratory illness in the United States. Since these estimates are designed to measure the socioeconomic impact of illness, cases are reported only if they caused restriction of daily activity or required medical care. There are in excess of 250 million cases of acute respiratory illness in the United States annually, an average of 1.4 illnesses per person per year. Loss of time from work or school averaged 4.2 days for the 80 percent of cases in which some restriction of activity was reported, and about 50 percent of individuals with respiratory disease sought medical attention. Analysis of these data indicates that two-thirds to three-fourths of the cases are caused by viruses; the remainder are divided principally among infections with *M. pneumoniae,* streptococcal sore throat, bacterial pneumonia, and sinusitis.

Acute respiratory disease is a special problem in relation to older persons who have chronic bronchitis. It is a familiar finding that those with chronic pulmonary disease often undergo exacerbations of their disease as a consequence of acute respiratory infections. The question also arises whether individuals with chronic pulmonary disease experience more frequent acute respiratory illness than those without such involvement. Monto and Ross have shown that adults with mild or intermittent chronic cough and sputum production and diminished pulmonary function experience more frequent respiratory illness than those who are asymptomatic. The finding was present at different levels of smoking frequency, apparently excluding the role of smoking in the occurrences. There was no unusual concentration of cases among any of the several etiologic agents studied. The higher frequency of infection, the prolonged morbidity due to exacerbations of chronic bronchitis, and the large and increasing numbers of such patients in our aging population identify a major health problem for which there is no present solution.

Age, sex, and seasonal variation Infants and young children have the greatest number of viral respiratory infections; children under 6 may have twice as many illnesses per year as the average for the entire population. Females have more illness than males. This difference is most marked in adults, where the excess is 25 percent. In children respiratory viral infections appear to affect the sexes about equally, but boys have more lower respiratory tract disease with respiratory syncytial virus infection than girls.

There are prominent seasonal differences in the frequency of acute respiratory illnesses; the rates are highest in winter, with about 30 cases per 100 persons per quarter. Illness is least frequent during the summer—about one-third of the maximum. Epidemics of influenza cause pronounced increases in wintertime frequency of respiratory illness and are the most significant cause of mortality among the respiratory viruses. In pandemic years influenza may begin in summer or fall.

ETIOLOGY The known viral causes of acute respiratory disease and their estimated relative frequency in adults and older children in relation to their common patterns of illness are shown in Table 197-1. In younger or older persons the same agents may cause disease, but the distribution of cases by etiology will vary.

Nearly one-half of respiratory viral illnesses are due to one of the rhinoviruses. The principal nonviral causes of respiratory illness are *M. pneumoniae* and hemolytic streptococci.

The relatively nonspecific response of the respiratory tract to virus infection probably indicates that the target cells of the respiratory tract (i.e., the respiratory epithelium), when damaged by infection, have a limited variability of pathologic response. Classification of viruses will certainly assume greater importance, however, as new chemotherapeutic agents are developed, since many of them will act on specialized viral functions unique to single or related groups of viruses.

CLINICAL MANIFESTATIONS The descriptive term "common cold" was coined to describe the coryzal syndrome before its diverse causes were known. It refers to illness characterized by nasal obstruction and discharge, sneezing, moderate sore throat, and mild constitutional reaction, usually without fever. Patterns of illness shown in Table 197-1 demonstrate that most respiratory viral infections may produce this picture. However, in adults and older children, syndromes more or less restricted to these manifestations are caused by infection with rhinoviruses, respiratory syncytial virus, and coronaviruses. These three groups of viruses may account for as much as two-thirds of cases of acute respiratory viral disease. Herpesvirus causes disease usually localized to the pharynx and tonsils in this age group. The other agents listed, while causing coryzal syndrome, also cause varying degrees of involvement of the lower part of the respiratory tract, with additional symptoms.

This chapter considers six of the seven groups of viruses chiefly responsible for respiratory disease, i.e., rhinoviruses, herpesviruses, parainfluenza viruses, coronaviruses, respiratory syncytial virus, and adenoviruses. Included also is a description of the small contribution to respiratory illness of the enteroviruses, coxsackieviruses A and B, and echoviruses, which are discussed in detail in Chap. 205. Influenza is described in Chap. 198. Respiratory diseases cased by *M. pneumoniae* and the psittacosis agent, both of which resemble viral respiratory diseases, are considered in Chaps. 190 and 194.

RHINOVIRUS INFECTIONS

ETIOLOGY More than 100 types of rhinovirus are known, and others are certain to be found. They resemble the other picornaviruses in being small (15 to 30 nm), non-lipid-enveloped, relatively stable agents. Rhinoviruses can be distinguished from enteroviruses, the other subgroup of picornaviruses, by their loss of infectivity when exposed to an acid medium for 1 to 3 h.

TABLE 197-1
Patterns of illness with respiratory viruses in older children and adults

Agent	*Relative frequency per 100 cases*	*Manifestation*				
		Rhinitis	*Pharyngitis*	*Tracheo-bronchitis*	*Pneumonia*	*Constitutional*
Rhinovirus	40	++	±	+	Rare	± (usually afebrile)
Herpesvirus*	10	+	++	Rare	Rare	+
Influenza A and B viruses	10	+	+	++	Severe when present	++ (high fever common)
Parainfluenza viruses†	8	+	++	++	Rare except in infants	+
Coronaviruses	8	+	+	+	In infants, also bronchiolitis	+
Respiratory syncytial virus	6	++	+	+	As above	+
Adenoviruses	1	+	++	++	Infants and recruits	++ (high fever)
Coxsackievirus and echoviruses	<1	±	+	+	No	++ (fever, visceral, and CNS complications)
Other	13+	?	?	?	?	?

* *College students; lower socioeconomic groups have primary infection earlier.*
† *Laryngeal involvement common.*
NOTE: *++ = severe; + = moderately severe; ± = mild; ? = unknown or uncommon.*

EPIDEMIOLOGY Rhinovirus infection is the cause of approximately 40 percent of respiratory illness in children and adults. While it occurs throughout the year, there are peaks of high incidence in spring and fall. Infection with rhinoviruses, as with other respiratory viruses, is much more frequent in infants and children than was previously thought. Children may develop second episodes of rhinovirus infection and illness with different serotypes within a few weeks. The disease is also more severe in children, especially those under 2 years of age. In the young, fever, cough, croup, and occasionally pneumonia occur.

Family infections are most often initiated by children, and up to three-fourths of family outbreaks may be introduced by children of preschool age; however, at all ages spread is much greater from ill than from well primary cases. Large families have more episodes of infection than small families. Family secondary attack rates are high at all ages, but highest in infants, of whom almost two-thirds of susceptibles may become infected. Infection occurs in about two-thirds or more of exposed persons without antibody, and about 60 percent of these develop illness. In persons with preexisting homotypic antibody, rates of infection and illness are about half that of those without antibody. However, studies in volunteers indicate that high titers of homotypic antibody are uniformly protective. Before 1970 a majority of infections were caused by lower-numbered serotypes; since then the proportion of infections caused by higher-numbered (and also more recently identified) serotypes has increased. Virus is shed in a high percentage of patients from the day before to 6 days after onset of illness. In general, about one-half of individuals whose infection is associated with virus shedding develop a significant serologic response.

CLINICAL MANIFESTATIONS The incubation period for rhinovirus infections is 1 to 2 days. The first signs of disease are scratchy throat, nasal congestion and discharge, malaise, and mild headache. There is usually no fever. Nasal secretions increase sharply between days 1 and 2 and then as promptly return to preillness values. Recovery is rapid and complete. Virus shedding begins a few hours after inoculation and continues for a week or more.

Table 197-2 summarizes clinical experience with naturally occurring rhinovirus infections in adults and children and artificial infection in volunteers. Most adults have only a common cold syndrome, with a rare case of bronchitis the only other form of illness. In contrast, more than one-half of children develop bronchitis, bronchiolitis, or bronchopneumonia. Although these findings resemble those of respiratory syncytial (RS) virus infection, rhinovirus disease is generally milder than that due to RS virus.

TABLE 197-2
Illness associated with rhinovirus infection

Diagnosis	*Adults (n = 61)*	*Children (n = 32)*	*Adult volunteers with nasopharyngeal inoculation (n = 31)*
Common cold	58 (92)*	14 (44)	26 (84)
Croup		1 (3)	
Bronchitis	1 (2)	7 (23)	2 (6)
Bronchiolitis		3 (9)	
Bronchopneumonia		3 (9)	
No disease	2 (3)	4 (12)	3 (10)

* *Values in parentheses are given as percentages.*
SOURCES: *Hamparian et al, Proc Soc Exp Biol Med 117:469, 1964; and Cate et al, J Clin Invest 43:56, 1964.*

LABORATORY FINDINGS In illness with rhinovirus there is usually slight neutrophilia. About one-third of volunteers develop moderate elevations in sedimentation rate.

COMPLICATIONS No serious complications have been reported with rhinovirus infections.

DIFFERENTIAL DIAGNOSIS Among the respiratory viruses, rhinovirus infection most consistently causes coryzal illness. In any one case, however, the illness cannot be distinguished from coryza due to other agents. Except for rare confusion with an atypical case of streptococcal sore throat, only respiratory viral diseases and *Mycoplasma pneumoniae* infection need be considered in differential diagnosis.

TREATMENT AND PREVENTION There is no specific treatment, and no vaccines are currently available for rhinovirus infections. Analgesics, antihistamines, and nose drops may be beneficial.

HERPESVIRUS INFECTIONS

The purpose of this section is to consider the role of herpesviruses in acute respiratory disease. Other aspects of herpesvirus infection are discussed in Chap. 210.

EPIDEMIOLOGY Several studies have shown that about 10 percent of acute respiratory illness in college populations is due to herpesvirus hominis infection. The disease consists almost uniformly of acute ulcerative pharyngitis and tonsillitis, and illness is associated with a significant rise in herpesvirus-neutralizing and complement-fixing antibody, usually from initially immeasurable levels. In one study the early antibody response was predominantly in the IgM fraction, supporting the concept that the disease resulted from a primary infection. Moreover, lesions in the anterior mouth or on the lips were uncommon, suggesting that a superficial recurrent herpetic infection (fever blisters) did not mask disease of another etiology in the pharynx.

The high prevalence of primary disease does not occur at college age in low socioeconomic groups, probably because members of this group experience their primary herpesvirus infections at a much younger age.

The disease occurs predominantly in the fall and winter. The route of transmission is not known, but virus can be readily isolated from respiratory secretions of patients with pharyngitis, or from vesicle fluid of fever blisters, and is occasionally present in the saliva of asymptomatic persons.

CLINICAL MANIFESTATIONS Herpesvirus infections are characterized by pharyngitis similar to that caused by beta-hemolytic streptococci. There are shallow ulcers on the tonsils and posterior pharynx, and in about one-half of patients there is a grayish pharyngeal exudate. Streptococcal infections produce a creamy exudate. Anterior cervical or submandibular glands are enlarged, and tender lymph nodes occur in about one-half of cases. Fever rarely exceeds 102°F and disappears in a day or so. Recovery is rapid without complications.

LABORATORY FINDINGS Leukocyte counts are normal. Herpesvirus can usually be isolated from throat swabs taken early in infection, and neutralizing-antibody titers rise from unmeasurable levels to 1:16 to 1:64 in convalescence. Complement-fixing antibody also shows significant rises in titer.

COMPLICATIONS No significant sequelae have been observed.

DIFFERENTIAL DIAGNOSIS The disease most resembles acute β-hemolytic streptococcal pharyngitis. However, the systemic response is less severe and acute. Adenovirus pharyngitis is similar to herpesvirus pharyngitis. Pharyngitis that accompanies other respiratory viral and *Mycoplasma pneumoniae* infections is usually less severe and does not show ulcerations.

PREVENTION AND TREATMENT The disease does not appear to be highly contagious, but isolation of patients acutely ill with pharyngitis and tonsillitis is probably indicated.

No specific treatment is recommended for this relatively benign, self-limited disease, although potent chemotherapeutic agents are used for other forms of herpesvirus infection. Analgesics are recommended for pain and discomfort, and hot saline gargles may decrease throat symptoms.

PARAINFLUENZA VIRUS INFECTIONS

ETIOLOGY On the basis of antigenic differences, parainfluenza viruses are divided into four types, of which type 4 is divided into two subtypes. They agglutinate avian and mammalian erythrocytes and grow slowly in tissue culture; only type 2 produces readily visible cytopathic effects. Growth of these agents in tissue cultures is detected by addition of guinea pig erythrocytes, which absorb on the surface of infected cells to form rosettes, a process known as hemadsorption. Parainfluenza viruses have antigens common to Newcastle disease and mumps viruses, but influenza virus does not share these. Parainfluenza serotypes are distinguished in complement fixation, hemagglutination inhibition, or tissue culture neutralization tests. The serotypes can also be identified and differentiated from one another by immunofluorescence.

Parainfluenza virus can be isolated in primary monkey or primary embryonic kidney cell cultures, but grows slowly or not at all in embryonated eggs.

EPIDEMIOLOGY The first three types of parainfluenza viruses have been found in many parts of the world; type 4 has so far been isolated only in the United States. Infection with parainfluenza viruses occurs early in life. By the age of 8 years, a majority of children show antibody to types 1 to 3, and it appears that most adults have antibody to all four types.

In children, illness with parainfluenza viruses occurs throughout the year, with seasonal increases in different years in the fall, winter, or spring. Type 3 virus spreads more rapidly than types 1 and 2 and may occur endemically throughout the year. Heterotypic antibody rises are frequent, with antibody to type 3 developing in half the cases with type 1 infection. In both children and adults, reinfection is frequent. In one outbreak, 96 percent of children without antibody, 67 percent with low levels, and 33 percent with high levels of antibody became infected. In adults, the disease is almost invariably a reinfection and is milder than in children.

The total contribution of parainfluenza infections to respiratory illness is variable; its frequency is increasing in institutions in which general health status is lower than average and levels of sanitation and personal hygiene are less than optimum. In studies in the United States parainfluenza infections accounted for 4.3 to 22 percent of respiratory illness in children. The milder illness of adults constituted less than 5 percent of respiratory illnesses.

CLINICAL MANIFESTATIONS In all age groups, the incubation period appears to be 5 to 6 days. The disease is most serious in infants and children, and fever is a constant feature of the disease. The characteristic syndrome with type 1 parainfluenza is laryngotracheobronchitis or croup. Type 2 disease is less frequent but resembles that caused by type 1. Type 3 parainfluenza infections are about equally distributed as causes of croup, tracheobronchitis, bronchiolitis, and bronchopneumonia in infants and children. In older children, the disease is less serious, usually without evidence of pulmonary involvement, and in adults the virus produces a common cold syndrome with hoarseness and cough. Occasionally, adults may experience severe tracheobronchitis with fever with parainfluenza infection. Physical findings are not distinctive.

LABORATORY FINDINGS In adult volunteers given type 2 virus, leukocyte counts were not abnormal. In children there is a considerable variation in leukocyte counts early in illness, making it difficult to distinguish this disease from pneumococcal and other bacterial infections. No characteristic alterations have been reported in other laboratory indexes such as liver or renal function tests, electrocardiograms, and urinalyses.

COURSE AND COMPLICATIONS In children, *otitis media* has occurred as a complication more often with parainfluenza than with the other respiratory viral infections. It is often caused by pneumococci, streptococci, or *Hemophilus influenzae.*

Parainfluenza virus infection is characterized by slow resolution of pulmonary involvement and long persistence of cough and other symptoms. In very young or debilitated children, the outcome can be fatal. In adults, bacterial sinusitis may occur, and in persons with chronic bronchitis, emphysema, or bronchiectasis, the possibility of pulmonary bacterial superinfections should be considered.

TREATMENT There is no specific treatment and no vaccines are available. Therapy is limited to symptomatic measures and efforts aimed at early detection and treatment of bacterial complications such as otitis media or pneumonia. Nursing care is important in pediatric cases, especially children with croup. In adults, analgesics, antihistamines, and small doses of codeine for cough are generally sufficient.

CORONAVIRUS INFECTIONS

ETIOLOGY The disease in humans is caused by an antigenically heterogeneous group of lipid-enveloped RNA viruses sharing morphologic and other properties with mouse hepatitis virus (MHV) and avian infectious bronchitis virus (IBV). A few serotypes of human coronaviruses recovered in tracheal organ culture share antigens with the murine agent.

EPIDEMIOLOGY The disease, characteristically a common cold syndrome, occurs in winter and spring outbreaks that vary from year to year, with greatest incidence in the 15- to 19-year-old age group, but it may involve adults of 40 years of age and older. The incubation period is 3 to 5 days. One study showed lower respiratory tract disease in young children probably caused by coronaviruses ranking in frequency only behind respiratory syncytial virus and parainfluenza 3 infection.

CLINICAL FEATURES The disease resembles rhinovirus common cold with profuse watery and later mucopurulent nasal discharge, sore throat, moderate cough, and mild constitutional symptoms. It is of short duration. In young children, pneumonia and bronchiolitis with coronavirus infection is clinically like that with other respiratory viruses. About one-half of infants may require oxygen because of respiratory distress. Diagnosis is based on isolation of the agent in organ culture or human embryo kidney culture or by antibody rise. The neutralizing antibody test is more sensitive than the complement fixation test, and rises in titer persist for a longer time. Both tests, however, will provide adequate diagnostic information. No treatment is available.

RESPIRATORY SYNCYTIAL VIRUS INFECTION

ETIOLOGY Respiratory syncytial (RS) virus is classified as a subgroup of the myxoviruses. In tissue culture, it causes formation of giant cells, or syncytia, from which its name was derived. It grows well in several human primary and continuous cell lines and in primary rhesus monkey kidney culture. There is a soluble complement-fixing antigen which, with the neutralization test, permits virus identification and serologic studies. Viral antigen can also be detected by immunofluorescence of exudates from infected patients or in infected cell cultures. Respiratory syncytial virus contrasts with other myxoviruses because it does not grow in mice, guinea pigs, rabbits, or chick embryos and does not cause hemagglutination or hemadsorption.

EPIDEMIOLOGY Epidemiologic studies have delineated a very substantial role of this agent in acute respiratory disease in children. Illness in young children occurs most commonly in epidemics in the late winter and early spring. Attack rates are nearly 100 percent among susceptibles, who are mostly children under 4 years of age, but the peak occurrence of bronchiolitis and bronchopneumonia is observed at 2 to 3 months of age. In older children and adults, the disease appears in nonepidemic patterns. The limitation of epidemic disease to the younger age group is also evidence for unchanging antigenicity of the agent, in contrast to the situation with influenza virus, in which antigenic shifts are associated with recurrent epidemics in persons of all ages.

Although antibody is widespread in adult populations, significant illness with RS virus infection, often with lower respiratory tract involvement, has occurred in the elderly and in hospital personnel caring for children with the disease.

RS virus infection is probably transmitted primarily by close contact (fingers, fomites) or by coarse sprays from coughing. Infection is easily initiated by virus deposited in the anterior nares or in the conjunctival sac. The incubation period seems to be 4 to 6 days. Virus shedding occurs for 2 weeks or longer in children and for shorter periods in adults.

CLINICAL MANIFESTATIONS During the first 5 years of life about three-fourths of children will become infected with RS virus and one-third of those will become ill; one-third of the latter, especially during their first year of life, will develop lower respiratory tract disease. The disease also affects children less than 1 month of age, particularly premature infants, but the disease may be mild or atypical, probably owing to a protective effect of maternal antibody. Fever occurs in about 90 percent of ill children, with an average elevation to 102°F. Cough is almost invariably present, and severe malaise is frequent.

Infants with lower respiratory tract involvement often show reduced arterial oxygen saturation which correlates with the duration of virus shedding, occurrence of apnea, and young age. Reduced arterial oxygen saturation may persist for many weeks into convalescence. Fatalities occasionally occur.

In adults the more severe forms of the disease are associated with rhinitis, fever, cough, and prostration. Virus shedding commonly occurs. Respiratory function studies in adults have shown slightly increased respiratory resistance during acute illness and for several weeks thereafter.

LABORATORY FINDINGS In children, leukocytosis with a shift to the left occurs with some frequency.

COMPLICATIONS The prolonged course of these infections in children and adults suggests a role in the development of chronic pulmonary disease in later years. No other complications are known to occur regularly.

DIFFERENTIAL DIAGNOSIS The resemblance of this disease in children to influenza has been suggested. In adults, the differential diagnosis should include rhinovirus and parainfluenza infection and, less often, other respiratory viral diseases and *M. pneumoniae* infection.

TREATMENT As with other respiratory viral diseases, treatment should include rest and palliative medications such as aspirin, nose drops, and medication for sleep when restlessness occurs. Infants may require hospital admission for respiratory therapy.

PREVENTION A formalin-inactivated RS vaccine elicited a high frequency of antibody, but a few months later vaccinated children experienced more severe illness than nonvaccinated children in the same population. This paradoxical effect of vaccination is a major contraindication to further attempts to develop a vaccine. The infection spreads rapidly among children in institutions and poses a threat to debilitated or very young children.

ADENOVIRUS INFECTIONS

ETIOLOGY The adenovirus group contains 31 human and 17 animal serotypes. Strains of types 3, 7, 11, 12, 14, 16, 18, 21, and 31 have been shown to cause sarcomas when injected into newborn hamsters.

Adenoviruses share a common antigenic determinant on a surface structure of the virus called a hexon, designated α. This antigen is the basis for an adenovirus group-diagnostic complement fixation test. It is not exposed on the intact virus and is not associated with immunity. A type-specific antigen ε, exposed on the hexon of the intact virus, gives rise to neutralizing antibody and is associated with immunity. An antigen γ, exposed on the fiber portion of a surface structure called the penton, is type-specific and elicits neutralizing and hemagglutination inhibiting antibody. Serotypes 12 and 18 do not hemagglutinate. An immunofluorescent test is also available that uses antihexon antibody to detect adenoviral group antigen present in exudates from patients or in infected cell cultures. Human adenoviruses grow well in continuous cell lines of epithelial origin.

EPIDEMIOLOGY Adenoviruses are most prevalent in infants and children; they are found in the throat and rectum of both sick and well children. Adenovirus-associated illness occurs throughout the year and accounts for about 2 to 10 percent of all respiratory illness in infants and children, but the highest frequency is in the period from the fall through the spring. Isolations of virus from well children show a similar pattern of seasonal prevalence but a lower frequency of occurrence. Adenovirus types most commonly associated with illness in children are 1, 2, 3, and 5.

The second most frequent occurrence of adenovirus disease is among military recruits. In the general adult population the disease is sporadic. An appreciable prevalence of infection with many adenovirus serotypes is suggested by serologic surveys, but definite virus-associated illness is limited to about 10. These serotypes produce five major patterns of illness, all of which occur in epidemics. A summary of these is presented in Table 197-3.

Acute respiratory disease (ARD) is a respiratory illness of military recruits caused principally by adenoviruses types 4 and 7 that occur in winter and spring outbreaks. Adenoviruses account for 15 to 50 percent of ARD in military groups, but only for about 2 percent of respiratory illness in civilian adults.

Febrile pharyngitis due to adenoviruses usually occurs sporadically or in small outbreaks in children. Its manifestations are summarized in Table 197-3. *Pharyngoconjunctival fever* is febrile pharyngitis associated with acute follicular conjunctivitis. This disease occurs as summer epidemics, frequently among children in relation to exposure in swimming pools. Although it is not limited to swimming pool exposure, it is believed that eye irritation from water, sun, or chlorine may be a factor in its initiation. Conjunctivitis may occur without pharyngitis.

Pneumonia due to adenovirus infection is rare in civilian adults but occurs in military recruits, usually as an extension of ARD. In infants and children, sporadic and epidemic occurrence of highly fatal adenoviral pneumonia has been described in several parts of the world. Such outbreaks have been principally caused by types 3 and 7. The severity of disease in this young age group may reflect the lack of prior experience with these agents, but other factors such as size and route of inoculation, general health, or greater susceptibility due to immaturity may be important.

Acute hemorrhagic cystitis and *pertussis syndrome* are summarized in Table 197-3.

Incubation period The period of incubation for pharyngoconjunctival fever and ARD is 5 to 10 days and is probably similar for other syndromes, since induced disease in volunteers has a similar period of incubation.

PATHOGENESIS When the conjunctival sac is swabbed with suspensions of adenovirus, conjunctivitis occurs and there is sometimes respiratory involvement. The initiation of illness appears to require a significant degree of conjunctival irritation. Administration of virus aerosol by inhalation also produces illness. Volunteers inoculated in this way have developed ARD and mild pneumonia.

These observations suggest the existence of at least two routes of inoculation for naturally occurring respiratory illness with adenoviruses: (1) ocular inoculation associated with eye irritation such as may occur in outbreaks around swimming pools, with the development of *pharyngoconjunctival fever*; (2) inoculation through inhalation of infectious aerosol generated by sneezing and coughing of ill recruits under the crowded circumstances incidental to recruit training. The route of inoculation of infants is less likely to be limited to aerosolized virus, and whatever the route of inoculation, the occurrence of pneumonia may represent primarily a lack of resistance in this young age group.

Nasopharyngeal inoculation in volunteers often produces virus infection without illness, suggesting that the high frequency of antibody to many serotypes in the population may result from asymptomatic infections. Antibody may also result from intragroup cross reactions among serotypes in the three broad immunologic groups of adenovirus.

CLINICAL MANIFESTATIONS *Acute respiratory disease* is an acute febrile illness lasting about 1 week and characterized by fever, cough, hoarseness, and sore throat. Fever has gradual onset and reaches a maximum of 103 to 104°F on the second or third day. There are associated malaise and often headache. Pharyngitis, the most prominent localized manifestation of the disease, reaches maximum severity after about 3 days. There may also be regional lymphadenopathy, pharyngeal injection, some edema, frequent lymphoid follicular hyperplasia, but little or no faucial exudate. Nasal obstruction and discharge occur in almost one-half of cases, but these abnormalities are not usually conspicuous. Cough is almost always present, and hoarseness is frequent.

Pharyngoconjunctival fever is usually a milder respiratory illness than ARD, although fever may be high for 5 or 6 days. Nontender submandibular lymphadenopathy is common even in the absence of sore throat. Lower respiratory tract involvement has not been described. Conjunctivitis is mild to moderate but may last longer than respiratory symptoms. It is an acute, nonpurulent, follicular conjunctivitis. In some cases, unilateral preauricular lymphadenopathy occurs. There is usually no involvement of the cornea or uveal tract.

Febrile pharyngitis without conjunctivitis resembles the foregoing illness, except for the absence of conjunctivitis.

Adenoviral pneumonia in children occurs as a primary illness and is associated with as much as 15 percent mortality. Pediatric texts should be consulted for further details.

For further details about *hemorrhagic cystitis* and *pertussis-like syndrome,* pediatric texts should be consulted.

DIFFERENTIAL DIAGNOSIS The differential diagnosis of ARD should include the respiratory viral diseases described in the present chapter and influenza (see Chap. 198), nonpneumonic forms of *M. pneumoniae* infection (see Chap. 190), streptococcal sore throat, and purulent sinusitis. Pharyngitis and upper respiratory illness may also accompany the onset of infectious hepatitis and infectious mononucleosis.

Differential diagnosis of *pharyngoconjunctival fever,* when conjunctivitis is prominent, includes leptospirosis, influenza, measles, herpangina, and the nonpurulent conjunctivitides, such as inclusion conjunctivitis and physical or chemical trauma to the eye.

TREATMENT There is no specific treatment for adenovirus infection. Treatment is limited to alleviation of general discomfort, headache, and coughing, with analgesics, cough syrup containing terpin hydrate, codeine, antihistamines, or other antitussives.

PREVENTION The communicability of adenovirus infection probably extends from a day or so before onset of illness to recovery, and conventional precautions against respiratory spread should be employed during acute illness for patients in the hospital and to the extent reasonably possible in care of patients at home. Avoidance of swimming pools during outbreaks of pharyngoconjunctival fever is recommended.

Formalin-treated vaccines against types 3, 4, and 7 afford significant protection against infection and illness, but these vaccines were withdrawn from civilian use when it was discovered that some serotypes of adenoviruses produced tumors in hamsters. A live adenovirus vaccine given orally in enteric-coated capsules is effective in preventing infection with adenovirus types 3, 4, and 7 in military recruits. More recently, a vaccine prepared from hexons and the fiber portion of penton demonstrated significant protection against experimental infections in volunteers. No vaccine is now marketed for civilian use.

TABLE 197-3
Illness associated with adenovirus infection

Disease	Occurrence	Order of association (serotypes)		Respiratory tract involvement			
		Common	Less common	Common cold	Pharyngitis	Bronchitis	Pneumonia
Acute respiratory disease (ARD)	Epidemic in winter and spring in military recruits	4, 7	3, 14, 21	Often present	Most frequent	Frequent, usually with fever and laryngitis	Infrequent complication of ARD
Pharyngoconjunctival fever	Summer epidemics in civilians, often in school-age children, related to swimming pools	3, 7	4, 14	Often present	Most frequent, usually with fever	Uncommon	Rare
Febrile pharyngitis	Sporadic or epidemic, resembles ARD, often in children	3, 7	1, 2, 5	Often present	Most frequent, usually with fever	Frequent, especially in older children	Infrequent but severe complication
Pneumonia in children	Severe illness in infants	3, 7		Sometimes present	Very frequent	Very frequent	Primary, with acidophilic necrosis of trachea and bronchi
Keratoconjunctivitis (EKC)	Epidemic disease; sometimes from infected eye solutions	8	11	Unusual	Uncommon	Not reported	Not reported
Acute hemorrhagic cystitis	Year-round sporadic disease	11	21	No respiratory disease syndrome; acute hematuria with dysuria, frequency, bladder pain, more common in boys			
Pertussis syndrome	Infrequent sporadic disease	1, 2, 3, 5		Uncommon	Uncommon	Tracheobronchitis common	Bronchiolitis and bronchopneumonia

COXSACKIEVIRUS AND ECHOVIRUS INFECTIONS

Diseases produced by these agents are described in Chap. 205.

REFERENCES

General considerations

KNIGHT V: *Viral and Mycoplasmal Infections of the Respiratory Tract.* Philadelphia, Lea & Febiger, 1973

MONTO AS, ROSS HW: The Tecumseh study of respiratory illness: X. Relation of acute infections to smoking, lung function and chronic symptoms. Am J Epidemiol 107:47, 1978

Adenoviruses

BRANDT CD et al: Infections in 18,000 infants and children in a study of respiratory disease: II. Variation in adenovirus infections by year and seasons. Am J Epidemiol 95:218, 1972

KASEL JA: Adenoviruses, in *Diagnostic Procedures for Viral, Rickettsiae and Chlamydiae Infections,* 5th ed, EH Lennette, NJ Schmidt (eds). New York, American Public Health Association, 1978

KNIGHT V, KASEL JA: Adenoviruses, in *Viral and Mycoplasmal Infections of the Respiratory Tract,* V Knight (ed). Philadelphia, Lea & Febiger, 1973

MUFSON MB, BELSHO RB: A review of adenoviruses in the etiology of acute hemorrhagic cystitis. J Urol 115:191, 1976

Coronaviruses

CAVALLARO JJ, MONTO AS: Community-wide outbreak of infection with 229E-like coronavirus in Tecumseh, Michigan. J Infect Dis 122:27, 1970

KNIGHT V, MAYOR HD: Coronaviruses, in *Viral and Mycoplasmal Infections of the Respiratory Tract,* V Knight (ed). Philadelphia, Lea & Febiger, 1973

MCINTOSH K et al: Coronavirus infection in lower respiratory tract disease of infants. J Infect Dis 130:502, 1974

WENZEL RP et al: Coronavirus infections in military recruits. Am Rev Resp Dis 109:621, 1974

Herpesviruses

EVANS AS, DICK FC: Acute pharyngitis and tonsillitis in University of Wisconsin students. JAMA 190:699, 1964

GLEZEN WP et al: Acute respiratory disease of university students with special reference to the etiologic role of *Herpesvirus hominis.* Am J Epidemiol 101:111, 1975

MOGABGAB WJ: Acute respiratory illness in university (1962–1966), military and industrial (1962–1963) populations. Am Rev Respir Dis 98:359, 1968

Parainfluenza virus

GLEZEN WP et al: The parainfluenza viruses, in *Viral Infections of Humans,* AS Evans (ed). New York, Plenum, 1976, chap 15

MONTO AS: The Tecumseh study: V. Patterns of infection with respiratory disease. N Engl J Med 258:207, 1978

Respiratory syncytial virus

GLEZEN WP et al: Risk of respiratory syncytial virus infection for infants from low-income families in relationship to age, sex, ethnic group, and maternal antibody level. J Pediatr 98:708, 1981

HALL CB et al: Clinical and physiologic manifestations of bronchiolitis and pneumonia. Outcome of respiratory syncytial virus. Am J Dis Child 133:798, 1979

HALL WJ et al: Respiratory syncytial virus infection in adults. Clinical, virologic, and serial pulmonary function studies. Ann Intern Med 88:203, 1978

Rhinoviruses

CATE TR: Rhinoviruses, in *Viral and Mycoplasmal Infections of the Respiratory Tract,* V Knight (ed). Philadelphia, Lea & Febiger, 1973

FOX JP et al: The Seattle virus watch: V. Epidemiologic observations of rhinovirus infections, 1965–1969, in families with young children. Am J Epidemiol 101:122, 1975

Constitutional reaction	Other
Headache, malaise, often high fever for several days	Usually no other involvement
Headache, malaise, high fever for several days	Acute follicular conjunctivitis, usually unilateral
High fever, malaise, headache	Nausea, vomiting, and diarrhea may occur
High fever, prostration	Conjunctivitis, skin rash, diarrhea, intussusception, and CNS invasion
Usually afebrile	Usually unilateral conjunctivitis followed by corneal subepithelial keratosis
Slight	
Prostration, vomiting with coughing spells	

198
INFLUENZA

VERNON KNIGHT

DEFINITION Influenza is an acute respiratory infection of specific viral etiology characterized by sudden onset of headache, myalgia, fever, and prostration. The terms *influenza* and "flu" should be restricted to those cases with clear-cut epidemiologic or laboratory evidence of infection with influenza viruses.

HISTORY According to the best available records, influenza was uncommon in Europe during the nineteenth century until the pandemic of 1889. Subsequently, the frequency and severity of epidemics increased, culminating in the disastrous pandemic of 1918, which caused an estimated 20 to 40 million deaths. The mortality rate from the disease has decreased progressively since 1918 owing in part to the introduction of antibiotics and also to such factors as possible change in virulence of the virus and improved living standards.

ETIOLOGY There are three distinct antigenic types of influenza virus, designated A, B, and C. Infection with one type confers no immunity to the other two. On the basis of intrinsic properties, the three types are grouped in a virus family named Orthomyxoviridae. The influenza viruses contain a single, segmented, negative-strand RNA genome. They are spherical or filamentous enveloped particles, 80 to 120 nm in diameter, with glycoprotein structures termed *hemagglutinin (H)* and *neuraminidase (N),* which protrude from the envelope. The former are responsible for attachment of virus to cell receptors; the latter enzymatically degrades the active receptor substance, frees virus from attachment sites if cell penetration is unsuccessful, and functions in the release of infectious virus from cells during the replication cycle. The H and N are antigenic and elicit antibodies which correlate with the prevention of infection and disease. Antihemagglutinin antibodies are more potent than those elicited by the N antigen.

The three types of influenza viruses are biologically related by their infectivity for chick embryos, capacity to agglutinate erythrocytes in vitro, and affinity for respiratory epithelium of various mammals.

EPIDEMIOLOGY **Influenza A** Influenza A viruses are the cause of outbreaks of disease almost annually and reach epidemic proportions every 2 or 3 years. Pandemics occur every decade or so.

Influenza, especially type A infection, is a recurring disease, because the virus undergoes continuous antigenic variation with time, involving the surface antigens H and N. This progressive, but not necessarily regular, change produces viruses to which segments of the population become susceptible in numbers somewhat in proportion to the extent of antigenic variation. Thus the annual interepidemic outbreaks are not as severe nor as extensive as the less frequent epidemics. The origin of pandemic viruses is unknown, but they appear to arise by a different mechanism. The segmented genome of type A influenza virus exhibits a high recombination frequency. Consequently, a recombinational event between human and nonhuman type A influenza viruses, or between two human type A viruses in the same host, could possibly give rise to antigenically different subtypes. Table 198-1 shows subtypes of influenza that have appeared in this century.

The characteristics of the 1918 virus are inferred from retrospective serologic analyses. The H antigen is the most important, and each new subtype has had a different H antigen (Hsw, H0, H1, H2, H3). The less mobile N antigen has changed only once, N1 to N2 in 1957.

Pandemics accompanied the introduction of three new subtypes, and the absence of pandemics in 1933 and 1947 is probably due to a limited antigenic relationship that existed among the 1918, 1933, and 1947 subtypes, so that individuals who were ill with swine virus influenza (see below) in 1918 had some resistance to the 1933 subtype, and similarly, individuals ill in 1933 had some resistance to the 1947 agent.

It was also noted that many older people did not become ill during the 1968 epidemic, and it was found that many of them possessed antibody to this subtype that was probably acquired in the period 1889 to 1890, when the subtype then prevalent shared antigenic properties with the 1968 subtype. There is also evidence that the 1957 virus shared antigens with the subtype that was prevalent before 1890, although owing to the time lapse there were too few older people with antibody to have a measurable effect on the pandemic.

Variants within subtypes are identified by the site of first isolation of the new strain and the year of its isolation. The sequence of strains of influenza viruses that have prevailed in the United States since the 1968 pandemic are shown in Table 198-2. Differentiation among variants is important because vaccines to one variant show a progressive loss of protective effect against later emerging variants, so that after about 3 years the vaccine will have little effect.

TABLE 198-1
Subtypes of influenza A and associated disease occurrences in the twentieth century

Pandemic 1918	A/Swine/1931 (HswN1)-like
Epidemic 1933	A/Puerto Rico/1934 (H0N1)
Epidemic 1947	A/FM1/1947 (H1N1)
Pandemic 1957	A/Japan/1957 (H2N2)
Pandemic 1968	A/Hong Kong/1968 (H3N2)

The occurrence of a sequence of H3N2 strains undergoing antigenic drift after 1968 was expected, as was the interruption every few years by epidemics of influenza B disease. Not anticipated was the reappearance in 1978 and 1981 of substantial amounts of illness caused by H1N1 strains that had last been seen before 1957. As might be anticipated, the H1N1 disease occurred almost exclusively in persons 25 years of age or less who had not been exposed to the virus before 1957. It is also recalled that a localized epidemic of H1N1 disease, presumably of swine origin, which occurred in soldiers at Fort Dix, New Jersey, in 1976, was the basis for a national immunization effort. One consequence of the effort was an increased incidence of Guillain-Barré syndrome in persons receiving the vaccine. More recently used vaccines have not shown such an association. The cocirculation of H3N2 and H1N1 viruses may be a new phenomenon; not predicted, it renders even more uncertain prognostication of future changes in influenza occurrence.

Influenza A viruses infect pigs, horses, and fowl, especially ducks and turkeys. H and N antigens of some of these viruses are related to H and N antigens of human influenza A viruses. The internal matrix protein of the virus is an antigen common to all influenza A viruses. The name *swine influenza* was given to the agent that caused the 1918 pandemic because an epidemic of influenza that occurred among swine at that time was thought possibly to have spread to swine from infected people. The swine agent has continued to infect swine populations since that time. The pandemic A (H3N2) strain of 1968 shared antigens with an agent isolated from horses in 1963. Despite these findings and considerable experimentation with induction of infection across species lines, there is no solid evidence that lower animals are involved in the natural history of human influenza.

Influenza A epidemics start abruptly, reach a peak in 2 to 3 months, and subside almost as rapidly. The attack rate is variable but was noted in 1957 to exceed 50 percent in urban populations. An additional 25 percent of individuals may show serologic evidence of infection without clinical manifestations. Experiences in 1957 proved conclusively that crowding, even in summer months or in tropical countries, is a major factor predisposing to epidemics. Schoolchildren, in particular, appear to be the primary focus and disseminators of infection in the United States. If the general immunity of a population is at low levels, community-wide epidemics may occur within a short period after the introduction of new strains of virus. If, however, immune individuals predominate, the case rate will rise slowly and may not reach epidemic proportions.

The mortality rate from all causes always increases markedly during epidemics of influenza. In the fall and winter of 1957 to 1958 it was estimated that 40 million persons in the United States became ill with influenza, and the total number of influenza-associated deaths was reported to be in excess of 8000. In addition, approximately 60,000 more deaths from various causes occurred during this period than would be expected under normal conditions. The greatest incidence of excessive mortality occurred among infants under 1 year of age and adults over 60 years of age. Data from a small series of cases clearly indicate that influenza is frequently fatal in individuals with preexisting pulmonary or cardiac disease, regardless of age. Chronic rheumatic heart disease with mitral stenosis, in particular, appears to predispose to fatal influenzal pneumonia.

TABLE 198-2
Influenza viruses prevalent in the United States since 1968

Year	*H3N2*	*H1N1*	*B*
1968	Hong Kong		
1973	England		
1974	Port Chalmers		
1976	Victoria		
1977			Hong Kong
1978	Texas, Victoria	U.S.S.R.	
1979		Brazil	
1980			Singapore
1981	Bangkok	Brazil	

Influenza B and C Influenza B virus infection occurs sporadically or in localized outbreaks, particularly in schools and military camps and every 4 to 6 years causes more discrete epidemics than influenza A. Although influenza B virus possesses H and N coat proteins, it undergoes less variation than influenza A viruses, and it is not now the practice to designate the virus by these antigens. Illness with influenza B infection is less serious than that caused by influenza A viruses. The most serious problem with influenza B infections is a complication, Reye's syndrome, characterized by encephalopathy and fatty changes in the liver and other organs (see "Complications" below). Illness with influenza C is rarely detected, although antibody surveys indicate a wide prevalence of the infection.

PATHOGENESIS Influenza is primarily an infection of the respiratory epithelium that is produced by inoculation with virus from respiratory secretions of infected persons. Experimental studies show that a small number of virus particles inhaled in a small-particle aerosol or severalfold larger doses in liquid suspension dropped in the nose will produce the disease. Infection thus could result from transfer of infected secretions by personal contact or fomites or, probably much more frequently, by inhalation of aerosols generated by sneezes, coughs, and other expiratory discharges of infected individuals.

After inoculation, the virus multiplies to maximum titers in a few days. Cells lining the respiratory tract, including ciliated epithelium, alveolar cells, mucous gland cells, and macrophages may become infected. Neutrophil leukocytes and endothelial cells do not appear to become infected. Evidence of virus infection by specific immunofluorescence is most conspicuous in cells that show fewest morphologic changes. Infected ciliated cells undergo degeneration after a day or so and are characterized by swelling of nuclei with shift from a longitudinal to a transverse position in the cell. Cytoplasmic changes are granulation, vacuolation, and swelling. Ultimately cells become necrotic and slough, in some areas to be replaced by flattened and metaplastic epithelial regrowth.

In addition to nasopharyngeal infection, tracheobronchitis is also common. The finding of abnormal pulmonary function in apparently uncomplicated cases suggests that viral infection may ordinarily penetrate more deeply into the lung than earlier supposed. When pulmonary involvement is clinically detectable, high titers of virus are recoverable from sputum and tracheal aspirates and autopsy studies show large areas of pulmonary virus infection.

Despite often severe systemic symptoms, direct evidence of influenza infection beyond the respiratory tract is uncommon. It is possible that rare cases of encephalitis with influenza may be associated with viral infection of the central nervous system. One report describes the isolation of influenza virus A from the feces of children ill with the disease.

MANIFESTATIONS The disease assumes its typical form during major epidemics of influenza A, but clinical differentiation between influenza A and B is not possible in localized outbreaks. Sporadic infections with either influenza A or B are likely to result in relatively minor illnesses, with predominantly respiratory symptoms, similar to those of common respiratory disease. Influenza C is particularly difficult to recognize because of its mildness. The clinical description that follows is a composite picture of epidemic influenza A of the past three decades.

The *incubation period* is usually 18 to 36 h but may be as long as 3 days. Mild prodromal symptoms of cough, malaise, and chilliness are sometimes present, but sudden onset is often such a characteristic feature that many patients can recall its exact time. The most common initial symptom is severe generalized or frontal *headache,* frequently accompanied by stabbing retroorbital pain that is accentuated by lateral or upward gaze. Diffuse *myalgia,* particularly marked in the legs and over the lumbosacral area, occurs in more than half the cases. Pain and spasm of the abdominal muscles may simulate acute peritonitis, and incapacitating periarticular pains are sometimes confused with acute arthritis. *Feverishness* and *chilliness,* or occasionally true rigors, may be the first manifestations, but more often they are preceded by headache and myalgia. The temperature rises abruptly to a maximum of 100 to 103°F several hours after onset; rarely it may reach 106°F. Thereafter, the fever and pain usually subside over a 2- to 3-day period but may persist for as long as a week. A common variant in the temperature course is rapid defervescence after the initial peak, with a secondary rise to the original level on the following day. In general, severity of illness parallels the height and duration of the fever. The pulse rate is usually slow in relation to the fever, but marked tachycardia may occur in severely ill patients.

Respiratory symptoms may be present at the onset but become most prominent when the systemic manifestations and fever begin to subside. They are frequently less pronounced than in common respiratory disease and may be entirely absent. Sneezing, watery nasal discharge, and stuffy nose occur in most cases; hoarseness and epistaxis are less frequent. Conjunctival suffusion and burning, with tearing eyes, are often noted. The throat may feel dry, and the pharynx often appears slightly injected. *Cough* develops during the course of the illness in more than three-fourths of the cases, and in about a third of these it is productive of small amounts of tenacious, mucoid sputum. *Chest pain,* usually substernal in location and accentuated by coughing but not by breathing, is present in almost half the patients. Pleurisy and pleural effusion are uncommon. Slight hyperpnea is often noted, but the most ominous, although infrequent, signs are dyspnea and cyanosis, which signal bronchiolar or pneumonic involvement. Findings on physical examination of the lungs are often negative in uncomplicated influenza, but scattered rhonchi, wheezes, and showers of moist rales have been reported in 5 to 40 percent of cases in different epidemics. These changes may persist for several days after apparent recovery. Patients with uncomplicated influenza may have restrictive ventilatory defects and increased alveolar-capillary oxygen tension gradients, suggesting the regular occurrence of lower pulmonary tract involvement. Influenzal bronchiolitis should be suspected if rales persist in the absence of x-ray evidence of pneumonitis and if the patient raises mucopurulent or blood-tinged sputum.

Prostration of some degree is almost invariable and is often the most prominent and alarming manifestation. The face is flushed, and the skin is hot and dry; however, profuse sweating and cold, mottled extremities are sometimes noted. Anorexia, nausea, and constipation are frequent secondary symptoms, but vomiting is rare. Diarrhea occurs with some frequency in children but is rare in adults. Meningoencephalitis, polyneuritis, cranial nerve palsies, transient nerve deafness, aphasia, hemiplegia, psychoses, and other neurologic disorders have been described in association with influenza but are very unusual. Hypotension, heart block, peripheral vasoconstriction, and fatal myocarditis have also been reported in a few cases.

COMPLICATIONS The chief complication of influenza is pneumonia, which occurs as a primary infection with influenza virus or as influenza virus pneumonia with superimposed bacterial pneumonia. In recent years, about 20 percent of pneumonic complications have resulted from primary viral infection. In patients whose pneumonia is complicated by bacterial infection, *Staphylococcus aureus* and pneumococci are the most frequent etiologic agents. Less frequent bacterial etiologies are *Hemophilus influenzae,* hemolytic streptococcus, and various gram-negative bacilli. Staphylococci and gram-negative bacilli are often resistant to some antibiotics, and these resistant strains may have been selected by prior treatment with these drugs. In addition, the incidence of bacterial pneumonias without an apparent viral concomitant is greatly increased during influenza epidemics.

Primary influenza virus pneumonia typically has its onset about 1 week after the onset of influenza, often following a period of apparent improvement. The disease is characterized by severe dyspnea and cyanosis, scanty sputum containing gross blood, leukopenia, few physical signs, and perihilar infiltrates by x-ray. The disease has a rapid course and fatality, when it occurs, results from acute respiratory failure.

Pathologic findings in fatal cases of primary viral pneumonia consist of large areas of inflammatory reaction within alveolar septa, with little exudate in alveolar spaces. Involved septa are edematous and infiltrated with lymphocytes, macrophages, and occasionally plasma cells. Some neutrophils may be present. In severe cases, fibrin thrombi may obstruct alveolar capillaries and cause necrosis and hemorrhage. An eosinophilic hyaline membrane may be found lining alveoli and alveolar ducts, presumably resulting from transudation of fibrin through affected alveolar septa. The pleura is not usually involved. This picture is not specific for influenza virus infection and must be differentiated from *Mycoplasma pneumoniae* pneumonia and from the common respiratory viruses that cause pneumonia, predominantly in children.

Secondary bacterial pneumonia is usually detected by onset of production of purulent sputum, fever, and other signs of bacterial pneumonia after the initial episode of influenzal illness. It may occur at variable intervals in relation to the associated viral pneumonia. The pathologic findings vary with the bacterial etiology. In general, the changes associated with pyogenic infection will obscure the less conspicuous viral lesions.

Staphylococcus aureus causes a necrotizing tracheobronchitis and/or bronchiolitis associated with a neutrophil leukocytosis, tissue necrosis, masses of staphylococci in necrotic areas, thromboses of small blood vessels, and hemorrhage. Purulent exudate plugs the respiratory passages. This process may extend into the lung parenchyma and cause bronchopneumonia associated with large and small abscesses surrounded by areas of hemorrhage, capillary thrombosis, edema, and fibrin deposition.

Pneumococcal pneumonia shows its characteristic fibrinous leukocytic exudate within alveolar air spaces. Necrotizing inflammation as with staphylococcal infection is rare, and the alveolar architecture is preserved. As with staphylococcal infection, the pneumococcal infection may obscure the lesions of viral infection. *Hemophilus influenzae* and gram-negative bacilli produce necrotizing tracheobronchobronchiolitis with lobular pneumonia and sometimes abscess formation. Bacterial pneumonia occurring during influenza epidemics that is not associated with influenza virus pneumonia is a more benign disease with pathologic findings typical of the particular infection.

Many studies have shown that pneumonic complications are most frequent and severe in the aged; in patients with rheumatic valvular or other heart disease, chronic lung disease, and serious systemic illness; and in pregnant women.

Sinusitis and otitis media caused by the usual common pathogens sometimes complicate influenza.

A complication of influenza B and, less frequently, of influenza A and other viral infections that has been identified increasingly is a syndrome of encephalopathy with acute cerebral edema and fatty infiltration of the liver called *Reye's syndrome.* Reduced activity of one or two mitochondrial hepatic enzymes of the urea cycle is noted in these patients. The mortality rate is high. Treatment has consisted of dexamethasone administration under continuous monitoring to maintain intracranial pressure at tolerable levels. Peritoneal dialysis is also used to remove excess blood ammonia commonly present in these patients. Because Reye's syndrome has been associated with the use of salicylates, these drugs should not be used in patients with influenza.

Recovery from uncomplicated influenza is often complete in a week, but convalescence may be prolonged by "postinfectious asthenia" and depression particularly in elderly persons. Minor relapses with fever may occur but are uncommon.

LABORATORY FINDINGS Virus is isolated most readily during the acute phase of the disease by inoculation of throat swab or nasopharyngeal washes into the amniotic cavity of chick embryos or into tissue culture. Influenza virus types A, B, and C may be identified in complement fixation tests. These tests depend on the nucleocapsid antigen found in the viral core and in soluble form in infected cells. Antiserum to whole virions readily detects the same or closely related strains by immunofluorescence in infected cell culture and, on occasion, directly in exudates from patients with infection. This methodology is useful in rapid diagnosis. Serologic diagnosis can be made most reliably by the hemagglutination inhibition test, using paired serum samples obtained in both the acute and convalescent phases. Type-specific antibody against soluble complement-fixing antigens of influenza A virus also appears in the circulation of patients during the acute illness.

In uncomplicated influenza the lungs usually appear normal by x-ray, but pulmonary involvement with viral infection is often marked by increased vascular markings, basilar streaking, small areas of patchy infiltration, atelectasis, or nodular densities. The blood leukocyte count may be low 2 to 4 days after onset of illness, but may be normal or slightly elevated. Leukocytosis with counts above 15,000 cells per cubic millimeter indicates secondary bacterial infection, but leukopenia may occur in severe pneumonia. The reticulocyte count may also be reduced to subnormal levels. Slight proteinuria is common during the height of the febrile illness.

DIFFERENTIAL DIAGNOSIS Many bacterial and viral infections simulate influenza at their onset, but few febrile diseases have such a self-limited course. Noninfluenzal respiratory diseases are generally characterized by more gradual onset; milder systemic manifestations; and predominant symptoms of coryza, rhinorrhea, pharyngitis, and conjunctivitis.

TREATMENT Antibiotics do not affect the course of uncomplicated influenza, nor is there any evidence that they prevent complications. Antibiotics should be reserved for secondary bacterial infections. Clinical trials have shown effectiveness of amantadine, a symmetric amine that inhibits an early step in replication of influenza virus, as a therapeutic agent. The recommended dose for adults is 100 mg twice daily (200 mg per day). There have been few side effects with this dose. Codeine affords relief from incapacitating cough and is more effective than salicylates for symptomatic treatment of headache and myalgia; salicylates often increase discomfort by causing drenching sweats and chills. Bed rest during illness and gradual return to full activity are advisable.

PROPHYLAXIS Formalinized egg vaccines purified by zonal ultracentrifugation or other methods and containing a mixture of influenza A and B viruses in whole or split forms are available commercially in the United States. Current vaccines can be expected to be effective when given in suitable dosage at an interval of several weeks to several months before exposure, and when the antigens of the vaccine are still closely related to the epidemic strain.

The U.S. Public Health Service recommends routine yearly immunization with polyvalent influenza vaccine for high-risk groups, including persons of all ages who suffer from chronic rheumatic heart disease, other cardiovascular diseases, chronic bronchopulmonary diseases, diabetes mellitus, or Addison's disease, and persons 65 years of age or older, regardless of their previous state of health. Pregnant women should be immunized only if they fall into one of the high-risk categories. For initial immunization of adults it is advisable to administer the vaccine subcutaneously in two doses of 0.5 ml each, the first injection in September and the second 4 to 8 weeks later. A single subcutaneous dose of 0.5 ml given each autumn is satisfactory as a yearly booster. Intradermal injection of vaccine is far less satisfactory because a sufficient antigenic mass cannot be administered.

Influenza vaccination is generally safe but not completely innocuous. Fatal anaphylactic reactions and purpura have been reported in individuals sensitive to egg proteins, and inactivated virus itself is pyrogenic and can sometimes produce an illness similar to active influenza. Infants and children have experienced severe febrile convulsions following vaccination, and vaccine should be avoided in children with a history of this syndrome. A decision to vaccinate children, especially the very young, should be made on an individual basis. The subject of influenza prevention is also discussed in Chap. 145.

REFERENCES

CENTERS FOR DISEASE CONTROL: Morb Mort Week Rep 30:279, 1981

GLEZEN WP, COUCH RB: Interpandemic influenza in the Houston area, 1974–1976. N Engl J Med 298:587, 1978

——— et al: Influenza in children: Relationship to other respiratory agents. JAMA 243:1345, 1980

HOCHBERG FH et al: Influenza type B–related encephalopathy, the 1971 outbreak of Reye's syndrome in Chicago. JAMA 231:817, 1975

PRICE DA et al: Influenza virus A2 infections presenting with febrile convulsions and gastrointestinal symptoms in young children. Clin Pediatr 15:361, 1976

WALDMAN RJ et al: Aspirin as a risk factor in Reye's syndrome. JAMA 247:3089, 1982

Exanthems and enanthems

199
APPROACH TO THE PATIENT WITH RASH AND FEVER

LAWRENCE COREY

Because many infectious and noninfectious diseases produce cutaneous lesions, specific diagnosis of an acutely ill febrile patient with a rash is a clinical skill with important therapeutic implications. The cutaneous manifestations of an infectious disease may result from direct inoculation of the organism into skin or indirectly from lymphogenous, hematogenous, or contiguous spread of the pathogen. Exanthems are cutaneous eruptions due to systemic or contiguous spread of an organism. These eruptions may be due to multiplication of the etiologic agent in the skin or dermal vasculature or to the host's immune responses to the organism. The cutaneous manifestations of infections may involve the epidermis or the vascular or extravascular structures of the dermis. Some exanthems are unique to a particular pathogen; others are common to numerous etiologic agents. Classification of exanthematous illness into (1) maculopapular, (2) vesicular, and (3) petechial eruptions is useful in determining the etiology and in understanding the pathogenesis of an exanthem.

PATHOGENESIS The pathogenesis of an exanthem may be caused by (1) multiplication of the pathogen in the skin, (2) carriage of the agent in plasma or in infected hematopoietic cells (leukocytes and/or lymphocytes) into integumentary blood vessels, and (3) antigen-antibody or delayed hypersensitivity reactions to antigens derived from the infecting microorganism. For example, in many viral diseases, such as rubella, rubeola, and the enterovirus infections, initial viral replication occurs in the infected mucosal surface and regional lymphatic tissue. Primary viremia then ensues, and "seeding" of the virus into target organs, such as liver, muscle, central nervous system, or heart, may occur. Continued viral replication and a secondary viremia with hematogenous spread of the virus to the skin may then follow. In this model, regional multiplication of the virus, primary viremia, and visceral dissemination of virus occur prior to the development of the exanthem and explain why the initial clinical manifestations of many viral illnesses occur prior to the development of the rash. Humoral and cellular immune responses which prevent or ameliorate secondary viremia may prevent the development of a rash. This may explain why exanthems associated with enteroviruses occur more frequently in younger children than adolescents or adults: young children do not possess cross-reacting antibodies or cannot mount an anamnestic immune response to the infecting agent.

While some maculopapular exanthems appear to be related to direct viral or bacterial invasion of the skin, other exanthems result from local or systemic immune responses to the microorganism. Rubella virus can be recovered from rubella maculopapules as well as from areas of the body not involved by the exanthem. Administration of pooled immune serum globulin after exposure to rubella may not eliminate rubella viremia but does prevent rash. Similarly, the exanthem of rubeola may be a manifestation of an Arthus reaction produced by the deposition of viral antigen in the endothelium of dermal capillaries. Local factors such as exposure to light or local irritation of the skin have also been shown to modify the distribution of some exanthems.

Vesicular exanthems are usually associated with active viral invasion of the infected area. Characteristically, herpes simplex virus, varicella-zoster virus, or poxviruses can be demonstrated in vesicular fluid by viral culture or by immunologic techniques. Local host and immune responses are important in the progression of varicella lesions, and their duration has been correlated with both α and γ interferon production.

Petechial eruptions may arise from direct invasion of the cutaneous vasculature by a microorganism, as occurs with septic emboli, or may result from immunologic injury to the vascular endothelium. In Rocky Mountain spotted fever, *Rickettsia rickettsiae* can be demonstrated in the smooth-muscle wall of arterioles. Vascular damage, microinfarction, and extravasation of red blood cells produce the characteristic petechial exanthem. Occasionally, a petechial eruption may complicate previous maculopapular or vesicular exanthems, usually coinciding with the development of diffuse intravascular coagulation. This may be seen in hemorrhagic dengue, measles, or varicella. In some petechial eruptions, direct evidence of viral or bacterial invasion can be obtained by direct aspiration and culture of the lesion, by demonstration of the agent with Gram's stain, or by immunofluorescent stain to detect microbial agents.

CLINICAL DIAGNOSIS OF MACULOPAPULAR ERUPTIONS Table 199-1 lists the numerous viral, bacterial, rickettsial, and noninfectious agents that may be associated with maculopapular exanthems. One helpful approach to the physical examination of viral maculopapular (*not* vesicular) rashes is that these eruptions *relatively* spare the palms and soles in contrast to eruptions associated with drug reactions, bacteria, mycoplasma, and rickettsial and/or immunologic diseases. In the latter entities, a prominent palmar or plantar distribution is often present.

While some exanthematous diseases produce characteristic cutaneous patterns, e.g., measles or erythema infectiosum, overlap in the cutaneous manifestations of viral induced maculopapular exanthems is the rule. Therefore, the presence of associated signs or symptoms as well as the epidemiologic characteristics of the disease such as the season of the year, the patient's age, and history of exposure and previous immunization are useful in formulating a diagnostic impression. Because viral maculopapular exanthems are manifestations of the agent's systemic spread, evidence of mucosal viral replication in the form of an enanthem is often a valuable aid in determining the etiology of a viral rash. Koplik spots in rubeola, ulcerative lesions on the hard and soft palate with herpangina due to coxsackievirus A, and palatal petechiae in early infectious mononucleosis are all helpful clinical signs. Associated clinical findings such as coryza, conjunctivitis, and cough with rubeola, mild fever and posterior auricular lymphadenopathy in rubella, or localized mastitis or furunculosis in staphylococcal

TABLE 199-1
Differential diagnosis of patients with rash and fever

Macules or papules	*Vesicles*	*Petechiae-purpura*
VIRAL		
Rubeola Rubella Enteroviruses Cytomegalovirus Hepatitis B Erythema infectiosum Exanthem subitum Adenoviruses Arboviruses Rhabdovirus group Reoviruses Live virus vaccines (measles, rubella)	Herpes simplex Varicella-zoster Vaccinia Enteroviruses (herpangina) Hand-foot-and-mouth disease (A16) Orf Molluscum contagiosum Vesicular stomatitis virus	Enteroviruses (echovirus) Viral hemorrhagic fevers Dengue Adenoviruses Yellow fever Atypical measles
BACTERIAL		
Group A streptococci: Scarlet fever Erysipelas Erythema marginatum Staphylococcal scalded-skin syndrome Staphylococcal toxic shock syndrome Subacute bacterial endocarditis Secondary syphilis Typhoid fever *Erysipelothrix* *Mycobacterium leprae* Rat bite fever Leptospirosis Chronic meningococcemia *Pseudomonas* sepsis	Staphylococcal scalded-skin syndrome Bullous impetigo	Severe sepsis with diffuse intravascular coagulation Meningococcemia Gonococcemia *Hemophilus influenzae* (type B) *Pseudomonas* sepsis Subacute bacterial endocarditis *Listeria monocytogenes*
RICKETTSIAL		
Rocky Mountain spotted fever (early) Murine typhus	Rickettsialpox	Rocky Mountain spotted fever Epidemic (louse-borne) typhus
FUNGAL		
Candidiasis Sporotrichosis Cryptococcosis		
CHLAMYDIAL		
Psittacosis		
PROTOZOAL		
Toxoplasmosis Trichinosis		Trichinosis Plasmodia (blackwater fever)
UNKNOWN		
Mucocutaneous lymph node syndrome		
IMMUNOLOGIC		
Erythema multiforme Erythema nodosum	Stevens-Johnson syndrome Pemphigoid Behçet's syndrome Inflammatory bowel disease	Henoch-Schönlein purpura
DRUGS		
Drug eruptions	Drug eruptions	Drug eruptions

scalded-skin syndrome should be looked for. Concomitant arthritis, renal disease, and/or heart disease generally suggests immunologically mediated entities such as acute rheumatic fever, subacute bacterial endocarditis, serum sickness, or collagen vascular disease.

The distribution of the rash provides important information. Erythema infectiosum presents with a diffuse erythema of the cheeks ("slapped cheeks"). In addition, central clearing of the eruption on the extremities results in a lace-like appearance of the exanthem. Erythema marginatum occurs in 10 percent of patients with acute rheumatic fever and is characterized by a ringed eruption which rapidly spreads to the trunk and extremities. Scarlet fever due to erythrogenic toxin elaborated by a group A streptococcus produces a rash that starts on the neck and spreads to the trunk and extremities within 36 h. The rash consists of numerous punctate papular lesions at the site of hair follicles and feels like rough sandpaper. Circumoral pallor, large red fungiform papillae (strawberry tongue), extension of the rash into body folds including the antecubital fossae, concomitant tonsillitis and cervical lymphadenopathy, and the subsequent desquamation of the rash, especially on the palms and soles, confirm the clinical diagnosis. Erysipelas due to group A (uncommonly group G) streptococci and staphylococci is characterized by an edematous indurated superficial cellulitis. Characteristically, the rash is shiny with a sharply demarcated edge. Occasionally streptococci can be demonstrated on Gram's stain and culture of material aspirated from the advancing edge of the lesion.

Some strains of *Staphylococcus aureus* (phage group 2) can elaborate a toxin which produces a diffuse erythema of the skin (staphylococcal scalded-skin syndrome). The development of bullae resulting in the easy separation of the epidermis (Nikolsky's sign) may occur but is not specific for this entity.

In 1978 Todd described a syndrome, since termed staphylococcal *toxic shock syndrome,* that is characterized by the acute onset of fever, hypotension, vomiting, diarrhea, vaginal discharge, and the development of a diffuse scarlatiniform rash with subsequent desquamation (see Chap. 147). This syndrome was reported with increasing frequency in the United States between 1978 and 1980, especially in young menstruating women using tampons. *Staphyloccus aureus,* often in pure culture, was isolated in a very high percentage of these patients not receiving antimicrobials. Relapses of disease, which are usually milder, are occasionally seen. The staphylococcal strains isolated from these patients appear to elaborate newly described toxin(s).

The course of the eruption is also helpful in differentiating the etiology of viral exanthems. Rubeola usually starts in the hairline area and spreads downward until the involved areas coalesce into a diffuse morbilliform eruption. In contrast, the eruption of rubella tends to disappear from its original sites of involvement as it spreads.

The rash of Rocky Mountain spotted fever usually starts on the extremities and spreads centripetally to the trunk. In contrast, the rash of roseola subitum starts on the trunk and spreads centrifugally to the arms and legs. Pityriasis rosea is characterized by the development of papular lesions along the lines of cleavage of the trunk ("fir tree" effect). The development of the earlier appearing "herald patch" and the lack of fever characterize this exanthem.

While papular lesions may be a manifestation of viral disease, systemic bacterial and/or fungal disease may also produce these lesions. Chronic meningococcemia may be associated with pale rose colored maculopapular lesions that may be mistaken for erythema nodosum when located on the lower extremities. The cutaneous lesions tend to wax and wane with fever. Organisms usually are not demonstrated in Gram's stain or cultures of these lesions. However, blood cultures taken during febrile periods may be positive. The development of discrete papules on the trunk in a patient with a previous history of diarrhea should suggest the possibility of typhoid fever. These "rose spots" are 1- to 3-mm papules which disappear in 3 to 4 days. In the untreated patient new lesions will emerge over the next 2 to 3 weeks. Pseudomonas bacteremia can also produce small painless papules on the trunk. The papulosquamous lesions of secondary syphilis often involve the trunk, palms, soles, and mucous membranes and may be present for days to several weeks. The serology (VDRL) is invariably positive in secondary syphilis.

Papulonodular lesions can be identified in 10 to 15 percent of patients with disseminated candidiasis. The appearance of these lesions in febrile immunosuppressed patients who fail to respond to antimicrobials should suggest the possibility of disseminated candidiasis. Biopsy and culture of the lesions should demonstrate the blastospores and pseudohyphae of *Candida* species.

In all infectious diseases, knowledge of the epidemiologic milieu of the patient is of great aid in arriving at a presumptive diagnosis of a patient with fever and a maculopapular eruption. Erysipeloid should be considered in persons with exposure to swine or saltwater fish; rat bite fever in those with a history of rodent exposure; sporotrichosis in those with contact with roses or sphagnum; leptospirosis in those patients who have contact with potentially infected animals and who also have hepatitis, conjunctivitis, and/or meningitis; and Rocky Mountain spotted fever in individuals who live in areas endemic for tick bites.

Mucocutaneous lymph node syndrome (Kawasaki's disease) Mucocutaneous lymph node syndrome is a multisystem disease of children.

This entity was first described in Japan in the 1960s, but it is now frequently recognized in the United States. It affects children from 2 months to 9 years of age, with 50 percent of cases occurring in children under 2 years of age. Characteristically, the patient presents with a fever between 38.3 and 40°C (101 and 104°F) of 1 to 2 weeks' duration which is unresponsive to antimicrobials. Bilateral conjunctivitis; dryness, redness, and fissuring of the lips; diffuse erythema of the oral and pharyngeal mucosa; "strawberry tongue," and cervical adenopathy may be present. On the third to fifth day of illness, a macular erythematous eruption, usually starting on the extremities, appears. Pronounced reddening of the palms and soles is present, and the child's hands and feet may swell due to an indurative edema. Characteristically during the second week of the illness desquamation of the rash starts at the junction of the nails and skin of the fingers and toes. Myocardial involvement is common, with abnormal ECG findings in over 50 percent of patients. Coronary angiography may reveal aneurysms and pathological changes in the vessels similar to infantile periarteritis nodosa. In severe cases, myocardial infarction due to coronary thrombosis may occur. Laboratory abnormalities include an elevated sedimentation rate, normal antistreptolysin O (ASO) titers, elevated C-reactive protein, and peripheral leukocytosis and thrombocytosis. Urethritis, arthritis, aseptic meningitis, myopericarditis, hepatitis, and hydrops of the gallbladder have also been reported. The prognosis is usually good; death occurs in 1 to 2 percent of patients and is usually due to coronary thrombosis. In the United States, cases have been clustered geographically and temporally. The etiology of this entity is unknown. Aspirin in doses to produce serum salicylate levels of 15 to 25 mg/dl is used during the acute stage of illness. When fever is controlled, the aspirin may be lowered and given in antithrombotic dosages (10 mg/kg per day).

CLINICAL DIAGNOSIS OF VESICULAR ERUPTIONS The distribution of the eruption is often helpful in determining a clinical and etiologic diagnosis of a vesicular exanthem. Varicella begins on the trunk, spreads centrifugally, and demonstrates lesions in all stages of healing, i.e., vesicles, ulcers, and crusts. Variola usually begins on the extremities, spreads centripetally, and is characterized by lesions in similar stages of development. The vesicular ulcerative pharyngeal lesions of herpangina are present only on the palate, whereas primary herpes simplex gingivostomatitis also involves the anterior gingival area and/or the lips. Hand-foot-and-mouth disease due to coxsackievirus A16 presents as multiple linear vesicles or pustules on the palms and soles; this is an unusual distribution for either herpes simplex or varicella-zoster virus.

Primary herpes simplex virus (HSV) infection is clinically distinct from recrudescent disease. Initial oral or genital HSV infection is often accompanied by constitutional symptoms such as fever, malaise, and myalgias; numerous vesicles, bilateral, tender regional lymphadenopathy, and a 2- to 3-week course between the onset of lesions and their complete reepitheliazation are the rule. Contiguous spread of virus as evidenced by the appearance of new vesicles after onset of the initial lesions is common, and inoculation at distant sites such as the fingers, thighs, eyes, and buttocks may be seen in 10 to 20 percent of patients with primary herpes simplex. In contrast, patients with recurrent HSV are usually afebrile and have only a few clustered unilateral lesions which last from 5 to 12 days. Patients will often complain of a "prodrome," a tingling sensation near or at the eventual site of lesion, from 2 to 48 h prior to the appearance of vesicles. Occasionally, HSV infection will present in a dermatomal distribution that is usually characteristic of herpes zoster. Because cytological techniques do not differentiate between these two agents, viral cultures or use of specific techniques such as immunofluorescence must be employed in order to differentiate these two viruses.

The appearance of the vesicles may be helpful. Herpes simplex and varicella lesions have a surrounding zone of erythema and a thin vesicular roof, and they are tender when irritated. The lesions of molluscum contagiosum are umbilicated, contain an expressible white core, and are usually not tender when scraped gently. The lack of surrounding erythema, the large size of the bullae, and the presence of Nikolsky's sign are helpful in differentiating pemphigus or toxic epidermal necrolysis from viral vesicular eruptions. The vesicular-ulcerative lesions associated with Behçet's syndrome or inflammatory bowel disease tend to be present for longer periods than those associated with herpes virus infection. The unremitting course, tendency of the lesions to produce a deep ulcer, and the prevalence of associated clinical findings such as colitis, urethritis, arthritis, and neurological disease in Behçet's syndrome should suggest this entity.

PETECHIAL ERUPTIONS Many hematologic and immunologic entities produce thrombocytopenia as a result of defects in the production, maturation, sequestration, or destruction of platelets. A consequence is the development of petechiae. However, the physician who is presented with an acutely ill patient with a petechial exanthem must be concerned with systemic bacterial or rickettsial disease. The common microorganisms associated with petechial exanthems are listed in Table 199-1. However, any microorganism that is capable of initiating the cascade of hematologic events termed *disseminated intravascular coagulation* may produce a petechial exanthem.

Petechiae due to septic embolization are characteristic of subacute bacterial endocarditis. Lesions may occur anywhere on the skin and/or mucous membranes but are most common over the upper anterior trunk. Splinter hemorrhages under the nails are difficult to differentiate from traumatic lesions and may be seen in hematologic, malignant, and other infective disorders.

Petechial lesions associated with meningococcemia are small, irregularly shaped slightly raised pale grayish lesions with a vesicular-pustular center. The lesions are usually asymmetric and are seen most often on the trunk and extremities, although the conjunctivas and mucous membranes may also be affected. Fulminant meningococcal infection will produce coalescence of the petechiae into grossly ecchymotic areas (purpura fulminans).

Gonococcal infection usually produces lesions on the distal extremities, often over joints. The presence of these pustular, hemorrhagic skin lesions in a patient with asymmetric tenosynovitis or polyarthritis, involving the wrists, fingers, knees, or ankles, should suggest the gonococcal arthritis-dermatitis syndrome. The majority of patients with disseminated gonococcal infection do not have symptoms of urogenital, anorectal, or pharyngeal gonococcal disease.

The metastatic lesions of staphylococcal bacteremia include pustules, subcutaneous abscesses, and purulent petechiae. Aspiration of material from the purulent center of the lesion will often reveal gram-positive cocci in clumps. *Pseudomonas* septicemia may produce ecthyma gangrenosum, a round, indurated, painless, necrotic eschar usually located in the anogenital or axillary area. In addition, hemorrhagic lesions with surrounding erythema resembling erythema multiforme may be associated with *Pseudomonas* sepsis.

Rickettsial disease may produce an arteriolar vasculitis that results in a petechial exanthem. The rash of Rocky Mountain spotted fever generally starts as a blanching maculopapular exanthem on the extremities, and after 2 to 4 days petechiae appear in the involved areas. The lesions no longer fade, and decreased capillary fragility, manifested by a positive Rumpel-Leede test, is often present. These cutaneous findings in a patient with the abrupt onset of fever, chills, headache, myalgias, and arthralgias should suggest this diagnosis. If the patient comes from an endemic area, and a tick bite or tick exposure is present, appropriate therapy should be instituted.

Summer febrile illness due to enteroviruses, especially the echovirus group, may occasionally produce a petechial eruption. While involvement of the face is common, the distribution of the exanthem is usually not distinctive, and because fever, headache, and meningismus may also be present, the clinical differentiation between *Neisseria meningitidis* infection and viral aseptic meningitis may be difficult.

Atypical measles is another viral exanthem that produces a petechial eruption. It begins on the arms and legs and spreads to the trunk and face. The rash differs from typical measles because it has features of raised papules, blisters, and pinpoint hemorrhages into the skin. Koplik's spots are not present, while high fever, cough, bilateral interstitial pulmonary infiltrates, and eosinophils usually are. Patients with this syndrome have a history of previous immunization with inactivated (killed) measles vaccine or of receiving live measles vaccine within 3 months after killed vaccine. The history of previous antigenic exposure to measles virus plus eosinophilia suggests a "hypersensitivity" reaction. A fourfold rise in measles complement fixation antibody titer between acute and convalescent specimens may be demonstrated.

Allergic vasculitis (Henoch-Schönlein purpura) is found most frequently in children less than 16 years of age. The presence of symmetrical red papules ("palpable purpura"), commonly occurring on the lower extremities, accompanied by abdominal pain, gastrointestinal bleeding and renal involvement (edema, hypoproteinemia, hematuria), and arthalgias characterizes this entity.

Petechial eruptions and profuse mucosal bleeding are often major manifestations of the viral hemorrhagic fevers. This syndrome is associated with a number of the arenaviruses (Lassa, Junin), arthropod-borne viruses (dengue), and rhabdoviruses (Ebola, Marburg). Recent travel to endemic or epidemic areas, involvement of the liver, spleen, heart, kidneys, and lungs, and evidence of diffuse intravascular coagulation are usually present.

LABORATORY DIAGNOSIS The laboratory studies most useful in determining the etiology of an exanthem in an acutely febrile patient are directed at demonstrating the microorganism at the cutaneous site. Gram's stain and culture of the lesions, dark-field microscopy of putative spirochetal lesions, and the use of immunofluorescent miscroscopy of skin scrapings or skin biopsy specimens for the detection of microbial antigens should be employed. Because exanthems are generally manifestations of a systemic illness, blood cultures should be taken prior to antimicrobial therapy. The agent should also be isolated from other extravascular sites such as stool specimens in the case of *Salmonella* or enteroviruses or the throat or urethra in the case of gonococci. Histological identification of organisms from skin biopsies of lesions may be of great help, especially with slowly growing agents such as fungi or mycobacteria.

Because local viral invasion is characteristic of vesicular exanthems, isolation of the agent from these lesions provides the diagnosis. The development of rapid viral diagnostic testing has been especially useful to the clinician in the differential diagnosis of vesicular lesions. Biopsies or scrapings of exfoliated cells from vesicular lesions of herpes group viruses (varicella-zoster, herpes simplex virus) contain multinucleated giant cells and/or intranuclear inclusions. However, because the Tzanck smear is only 40 to 70 percent as sensitive as viral isolation, the absence of giant cells does not rule out herpes infection. Herpes simplex and zoster can be differentiated by viral isolation as well as antigen detection techniques such as fluorescent microscopy or enzyme-linked immunoabsorbent assays (ELISA). Immunofluorescence may also be useful in confirming the diagnosis of immunologically related diseases such as pemphigus vulgaris.

Electron microscopy is useful in differentiating the distinct morphology of poxviruses, vaccinia, variola, and molluscum from herpes viruses. In addition, molluscum bodies can be demonstrated by light microscopy with use of a 10% KOH preparation.

In viral exanthems, demonstration of local viral replication in throat secretions or rectal swabs provides presumptive evidence of the etiology of the exanthem; an example is the demonstration of coxsackievirus A16 in throat secretions of patients with hand-foot-and-mouth syndrome. In Behçet's syndrome or in collagen vascular disease, the absence of viruses in an early vesicular or active ulcerative lesion is useful in relating these mucosal lesions to the underlying multisystem illness.

Serologic determinations of acute phase serums are helpful in the diagnosis of syphilis, leptospirosis, streptococcal disease, Epstein-Barr virus infection, hepatitis B, toxoplasmosis, typhoid fever, and occasionally rickettsial disease. Evidence of autoantibody fixation may be useful in diagnosing some collagen vascular diseases. Demonstration of a fourfold or greater rise in antibody titer between acute and convalescent serums will confirm the diagnosis in rubella, rubeola, cytomegalovirus, rickettsial, or chlamydial infection.

REFERENCES

Fulginiti VA et al: Altered reactivity to measles virus. JAMA 202:105, 1967

Gilchest B, Barden HP: Photodistribution of viral exanthems. Pediatrics 54:136, 1974

Heggin AD: Pathogenesis of rubella exanthems. J Infect Dis 137:74, 1978

Kawasaki T et al: A new infantile acute febrile mucocutaneous lymph node syndrome (MLNS) prevailing in Japan. Pediatrics 54:271, 1974

Kimura A et al: Measles rash, light and electron microscopic study of measles skin eruptions. Arch Virol 47:295, 1975

Melish ME: Kawasaki syndrome: A new infectious disease? J Infect Dis 143:317, 1981

Mims CA: Pathogenesis of rashes in virus diseases. Bacteriol Rev 30:739, 1966

Shands KN: Toxic shock syndrome in menstruating women: Its association with tampon use and *Staphylococcus aureus* and the clinical features of 52 cases. N Engl J Med 303:1436, 1980

———: Toxic-shock syndrome, in *Update IV: Harrison's Principles of Internal Medicine,* KJ Isselbacher et al (eds). New York, McGraw-Hill, 1982, pp 1–8

Todd J et al: Toxic-shock syndrome associated with phage-group-I staphylococci. Lancet 2:1116, 1978

200
MEASLES (RUBEOLA)

C. GEORGE RAY

DEFINITION Measles, or rubeola, is an acute febrile eruption which has been one of the most common diseases of civilization. With the development of effective prophylactic measures it is becoming a rarity.

ETIOLOGY The measles virion is composed of a central core of ribonucleic acid with a helically arranged protein coat surrounded by a lipoprotein envelope with small, spike-like structures. The virion is 120 to 250 nm in diameter and is classified as a paramyxovirus.

The measles virus is isolated most easily from infected persons in the first 4 or 5 days of illness, by utilizing primary cell cultures of monkey or human kidney, although primary isolations have been accomplished by using cells from human amnion or chorion or dog kidney. After several passages, the virus can be propagated on a number of types of cell cultures, including chick embryo cells, upon which many of the vaccine strains are grown.

Measles virus infection of cells in culture results in the formation of multinucleated giant cells, many with eosinophilic intranuclear and intracytoplasmic inclusions.

EPIDEMIOLOGY Measles occurs naturally only in human beings, although infection with the virus can be demonstrated in laboratory colonies of monkeys exposed to infected individuals. Before active immunization was available, epidemics of measles occurred in 2- to 3-year cycles, usually during the spring months, and about 95 percent of town and city dwellers developed the disease before the age of 15 years. The virus is transmitted by transfer of nasopharyngeal secretions, either directly or in airborne droplets, to the respiratory mucous membranes or conjunctivas of susceptible individuals. Persons infected with the virus may transmit the disease during a period which extends from 5 days after exposure until 5 days after skin lesions have appeared. The virus is highly contagious, with secondary attack rates among susceptible household contacts usually exceeding 90 percent; asymptomatic primary infections are rare. Measles is typically a disease of childhood in populous areas, but may occur at any age in remote isolated communities if the disease is introduced. In recent years in the United States, there has been a distinct shift in age-specific attack rates, with outbreaks frequently occurring among teenagers and young adults. Infants are uncommonly affected under the age of 6 to 8 months, presumably because of the persistence of maternal antibody acquired by transplacental transmission. With increasingly effective attempts at control, the incidence of measles for 1979, 1980, and 1981 has decreased sharply. However, sporadic outbreaks still occur in the military and in some instances have been transmitted to the civilian sector.

PATHOGENESIS AND PATHOLOGY It is probable that, after infection, measles virus multiplies in the epithelium of the respiratory tract and is disseminated by way of the blood to distant sites. For a few days before the rash appears, and for 1 or 2 days after, the virus can be isolated from blood or washed white blood cells, conjunctiva, lymphoid tissue, and respiratory mucous membranes and secretions. The virus can be obtained from urine for as long as 4 days after the onset of the eruptions.

The mucous membrane lesions (Koplik's spots) consist of vesicle formation and epithelial necrosis. Histology of the Koplik's spots reveals cytoplasmic and intranuclear inclusions, giant cells, and intercellular edema. Electron microscopy of the Koplik's spots and skin lesions has demonstrated microtubular aggregates which are thought to be the measles virus, and suggests that both the exanthem and enanthem are associated with local viral replication. Large multinucleated epithelial giant cells can be found during the prodrome and acute stages of illness in the buccal mucosa, pharynx, tracheobronchial mucosa, and occasionally in the urine. In addition, reticuloendothelial giant cells (Warthin-Finkeldey cells) are found in hyperplastic lymphoid tissues, including lymph nodes, tonsils, spleen, and thymus. An unusually high number of white blood cells from patients with the disease contain broken chromosomes. The epithelium of the respiratory passages may become necrotic and slough, leading to secondary bacterial infection; in addition, interstitial pneumonia with giant-cell infiltration may be observed. Changes in the brain of patients with encephalitis resemble those seen in other postviral encephalitides and consist of focal hemorrhage, congestion, and perivenous demyelination.

MANIFESTATIONS The time from exposure to the development of the first symptoms of measles infection is usually 9 to 11 days, and from exposure to the appearance of rash is about 2 weeks. The initial manifestations of the disease are malaise, irritability, fever as high as 105°F, conjunctivitis with excessive lacrimation, edema of the eyelids and photophobia, moderately severe hacking cough, and nasal discharge. The prodromal period usually lasts 3 to 4 days, with a range of 1 to 8 days before the onset of a rash. Koplik's spots—small, red, irregular lesions with blue-white centers—appear 1 or 2 days before the onset of the rash on the mucous membranes of the mouth and occasionally on the conjunctiva or intestinal mucosa. The findings of the prodromal illness subside or disappear within 1 or 2 days after the appearance of skin lesions, although the cough may persist throughout the course of the disease.

The red maculopapular rash of measles breaks out first on the forehead, spreads downward over the face, neck, and trunk, and appears on the feet on the third day. The density of lesions is greatest on the forehead, face, and shoulders, where coalescence of individual spots usually occurs. The lesions in each area persist for about 3 days and disappear in the same order in which they appeared, resulting in total duration of rash of about 6 days. As the maculopapules fade, a brown discoloration of the skin may be noticed, and finely granular desquamation may occur. In adults the duration of fever may be longer, the rash more prominent, and the incidence of complications higher.

The course of measles can be altered by the administration of gamma globulin soon after exposure. The incubation period may be prolonged for as long as 20 days. The prodromal period of the modified disease may be shorter, the fever, respiratory symptoms, and conjunctivitis milder, and the rash less marked; Koplik's spots may not be present. An atypical, severe form of measles is seen in some persons who received inactivated measles vaccine several years before exposure. The prodromal period with prominent fever, headache, myalgias, and abdominal pain lasts for 1 or 2 days and is followed by an eruption which may be urticarial, maculopapular, hemorrhagic, and/or vesicular. In contrast to natural measles, the rash begins on the hands and feet and progresses toward the head. The rash is especially prominent on the legs and in the body creases. Peripheral edema and pneumonia have been prevalent in this form of atypical measles. The pneumonia is lobar or segmental; hilar lymphadenopathy and pleural effusion are frequent. Ill-defined nodular shadows may persist at the periphery of the lung for as long as 1 to 2 years.

COMPLICATIONS Measles, usually a benign self-limited disease, may be associated with a number of complicating illnesses. Viral involvement of the respiratory tract may lead to croup, bronchitis, bronchiolitis, or rarely to *interstitial giant-cell pneumonia,* which is seen most often in children suffering from severe systemic disease such as leukemia, congenital immunodeficiency, or severe malnutrition, and which is characterized by severe respiratory symptoms, pulmonary infiltrations, and the presence in the lungs of multinucleated giant cells. It may occur in the absence of the typical measles exanthem. *Conjunctivitis,* which is seen regularly in the course of uncomplicated measles, may occasionally progress to corneal ulceration, keratitis, and blindness. *Myocarditis,* characterized by transient changes in the electrocardiogram, occurs in about 20 percent of patients with measles, but clinical evidence of cardiac dysfunction is rare. Viral involvement of the mesenteric lymph nodes and appendix may result in abdominal pain and signs of peritoneal inflammation so severe that surgical exploration is considered. The situation is especially confusing if the evidence of appendiceal involvement becomes manifest during the preeruptive phase of the disease. *Hepatitis,* usually without clinical signs, also frequently occurs. It is usually detected by the presence of a transient elevation of SGOT or SGPT values during the acute phase of illness. Measles infection of pregnant women results in death of the fetus in about 20 percent of the cases; however, a teratogenic effect such as that observed in rubella has not been demonstrated.

Superimposed bacterial pneumonia caused by streptococci, pneumococci, staphylococci, or *Hemophilus influenzae* is considerably more common than giant-cell pneumonia and occasionally may progress to formation of empyema or lung abscess. Bacterial otitis media is a frequent sequel of measles infection in children. In tropical areas, stomatitis, probably of bacterial origin, progressing to cancrum oris may be encountered during the course of the disease.

In addition to conditions associated with the viral infection and the complications resulting from superimposed bacterial infection, several situations may arise after measles infection which are of uncertain pathogenesis. Clinically apparent *encephalomyelitis* occurs in 1 of 1000 patients with measles. It usually begins 4 to 7 days after the appearance of the eruption, but may precede the rash by 10 days or follow it by 24 days. It is characterized by high fever, headache, drowsiness, and coma, and in some patients by focal brain or spinal cord involvement. Death occurs in about 10 percent of affected individuals, and persistent signs of central nervous system damage, including mental changes, epilepsy, and paralysis, are encountered. Electroencephalographic abnormalities without other signs of central nervous system dysfunction may be demonstrated in 50 percent of patients with otherwise uncomplicated measles. Though it is generally postulated that the encephalomyelitis is "postinfectious" or allergic in origin, a report of isolation of the virus from the brain of a patient with a fatal case suggests direct viral invasion of the central nervous system. A progressive, fatal encephalitis has been described in children with lymphatic malignancies treated with immunosuppressive drugs, with onset 1 to 6 months after an episode of measles. Other, more unusual neurologic complications include transverse myelitis and ascending myelitis. An extremely rare condition, *subacute sclerosing panencephalitis* (see Chap. 360), is now thought to be a late complication of measles. *Thrombocytopenia* may occur 3 to 15 days after the onset of symptoms and results in purpura as well as bleeding from mouth, intestine, and genitourinary tract. Measles is also associated with transient suppression of delayed hypersensitivity to tuberculin, exacerbation of existing tuberculosis, and an increased incidence of new tuberculous infections.

LABORATORY FINDINGS Leukopenia is frequent in the prodromal phase of measles, and the appearance of leukocytosis suggests bacterial superinfection or another complication. Extreme lymphopenia (less than 2000 lymphocytes per cubic millimeter) is considered to be a poor prognostic sign. During the prodrome and in the early eruptive phase, multinucleated giant cells can be identified in stained preparations of sputum, nasal secretions, or urine, and the measles virus can be isolated by inoculation of the same materials into appropriate cell cultures. Measles antigen can often be detected quickly by direct fluorescent antibody staining of infected respiratory or urinary epithelial cells. Complement fixation, neutralization and hemagglutination inhibition tests are available for serologic confirmation of measles. Spinal fluid protein of patients with encephalomyelitis ranges from 48 to 240 mg/dl, and lymphocyte counts are usually in a range of 5 to 99 per cubic millimeter, although counts as high as 1000 per cubic millimeter have been reported. Bacterial infection can be identified by appropriate cultures.

DIFFERENTIAL DIAGNOSIS Measles, with its prodrome, Koplik's spots, and characteristic rash, is infrequently confused with other diseases. Rubella is a milder disease of shorter duration with mild respiratory complaints or none at all. Infectious mononucleosis and toxoplasmosis can be identified by the presence of atypical lymphocytes and by serologic tests. Secondary syphilis may display skin lesions similar to the measles rash. Other infections which can sometimes mimic measles include those caused by adenoviruses, enteroviruses, *Mycoplasma pneumoniae,* and *Streptococcus pyogenes,* e.g., scarlet fever. Drug reactions, particularly those associated with ampicillin and Dilantin, can also produce a morbilliform rash. The atypical form of measles in patients previously immunized with inactivated vaccine may suggest Rocky Mountain spotted fever, varicella, scarlet fever, or meningococcemia.

PROPHYLAXIS Measles can be prevented by the administration of 0.25 ml/kg gamma globulin within 5 days of exposure. Passive immunization should be considered for any susceptible person exposed to the disease, but is especially important for children under 3 years of age, for pregnant women, for patients with tuberculosis, and for those patients in whom immune mechanisms are impaired. A modified, less severe form of the disease which results in some degree of active immunity may be observed if 0.04 ml/kg gamma globulin is given within 5 days of exposure (see "Manifestations" above). Prophylactic administration of antibiotics does not decrease the frequency or severity of bacterial superinfections.

Active immunity can be induced by the use of live, attenuated measles virus without spread to contacts of vaccinated individuals. Further attenuated vaccine strains (Schwarz, Attenuvax) derived from additional chick cell culture passages of the original Edmonston B strains are currently recommended and are associated with few local or systemic reactions. Vaccination with these preparations induces antibody formation in more than 95 percent of susceptible individuals. The vaccine can induce protection if given before, or within 2 days after, exposure. After this time, active immunization is less predictable in its ability to confer protection to the already exposed individual, although no ill effects have been noted when vaccination followed exposure by more than 2 days. Vaccination results in protection for at least 10 years, but the total duration of immunity is not known. Live measles vaccine should not be given to pregnant women, to patients with untreated tuberculosis, to patients with leukemia or lymphoma, or to those whose immune responsiveness is depressed. Hypersensitivity reactions have not been associated with the vaccine even among egg-sensitive individuals; however, the vaccine should not be given to persons known to be hypersensitive to vaccine components, such as trace amounts of antibiotics. Except in unusual circumstances, vaccination should not be given in the first 13 months of life. However, if epidemiologic circumstances suggest a risk to infants in the 6- to 13-month age group, the vaccine may be used, and a second dose administered at 15 to 18 months of age to ensure adequate seroconversion. The vaccine seems equally effective when administered alone or simultaneously in combination with rubella and mumps vaccines. Measles vaccination has been very effective in decreasing the incidence of measles in the United States without producing serious side effects. Measles occurs most commonly among the unvaccinated, who, for the most part, are members of low socioeconomic groups. The disease rarely occurs in those who have been vaccinated, although there have been vaccine failures. These failures are related, in part, to early vaccination of infants who still have maternal neutralizing antibody or to the use of improperly stored vaccine.

There is no indication for the use of *inactivated* vaccine because of severe atypical measles which has been observed in persons immunized with it (see "Manifestations" above).

TREATMENT No therapy is indicated for uncomplicated measles. Gamma globulin, although effective in prophylaxis, is of no value once symptoms are evident. Patients should be monitored for the development of bacterial superinfections, which should be treated with appropriate antibiotics on the basis of clinical and bacteriologic findings.

REFERENCES

Aicardi J et al: Acute measles encephalitis in children with immunosuppression. Pediatrics 59:232, 1977

Coovadia HM et al: Immunoparesis and outcome in measles. Lancet 1:619, 1977

Fulginiti VA, Helfer RE: Atypical measles in adolescent siblings 16 years after killed measles virus vaccine. JAMA 244:804, 1980

Hall WJ, Hall CB: Atypical measles in adolescents: Evaluation of clinical and pulmonary function. Ann Intern Med 90:882, 1979

Hinman AR et al: The opportunity and obligation to eliminate measles from the United States. JAMA 242:1157, 1979

Krause PH et al: Epidemic measles in young adults. Ann Intern Med 90:873, 1979

Krugman S: Present status of measles and rubella immunization in the United States: A medical progress report. J Pediatr 90:1, 1977

Meulen V et al: Isolation of infectious measles virus in measles encephalitis. Lancet 2:1172, 1972

Nickell MD et al: Subclinical hepatitis in rubeola infections in young adults. Ann Intern Med 90:354, 1979

Ruuskanen O et al: Measles vaccination after exposure to natural measles. J Pediatr 93:43, 1978

201 RUBELLA ("GERMAN MEASLES")

C. GEORGE RAY

DEFINITION Rubella ("German measles," "3-day measles") is usually a benign febrile exanthem, but when it occurs in pregnant women, it may lead to serious chronic fetal infection and malformations.

ETIOLOGY In the late 1930s and 1940s rubella was transmitted to humans and monkeys, and in 1962 a viral agent was recovered in cell cultures inoculated with nasopharyngeal secretions of infected persons. Human primary amnion cells infected with rubella virus display rounding, clumping of nuclear chromatin, and eosinophilic intranuclear inclusions. Rabbit kidney and some other cell lines also display cytopathic effects. Rubella virus can be detected indirectly in African green monkey kidney cells by the interference or exclusion method. In this system, cells infected with rubella appear normal but are resistant to superinfection with viruses such as echovirus 11 or coxsackievirus A9 that ordinarily produce a cytopathic effect in these cells. Complement-fixing antigen and a hemagglutinin have been identified.

The rubella virion, 50 to 85 nm in diameter, is a somewhat spheroidal RNA virus which has been classified in the togavirus family.

PATHOGENESIS AND PATHOLOGY Rubella can be induced in susceptible persons by the instillation of virus into the nasopharynx, and natural infection is probably induced in the same way. Virus is present in blood, throat washings, and occasionally feces for several days before the exanthem becomes apparent. It can be detected in blood for 1 to 2 days, and in throat washings for as long as 7 days before appearance of rash, to 2 weeks after onset. Lymph nodes show edema and hyperplasia.

Congenital rubella results from transplacental transmission of virus to the fetus from an infected mother, and may be associated with growth retardation, infiltration of liver and spleen by hematopoietic tissue, interstitial pneumonia, a decreased number of megakaryocytes in the bone marrow, and various structural malformations of the cardiovascular and central nervous systems. The virus can persist in the fetus during intrauterine life and may be excreted for 6 to 31 months after birth.

EPIDEMIOLOGY Rubella is not as contagious as measles, and immunity to the disease is not so widespread. Estimates of susceptibility to rubella among women of childbearing age range from 10 to 25 percent. Before the routine introduction of vaccine in 1969, epidemics occurred at 6- to 9-year intervals; however, this cyclical pattern is no longer seen. In 1964 more than 1.8 million cases of rubella were reported in the United States; in 1978, 18,269 cases; and in 1979, 11,795 cases, an all-time low, were reported. Rubella was once most frequent among children 5 to 9 years of age, but with the advent of immunization programs often directed primarily at this age group as well as at preschoolers, a greater proportion of cases is now being reported among older schoolchildren (15 to 19 years) and young adults (20 to 24 years). Over 70 percent of the reported cases in 1979 occurred in persons 15 years of age or older.

MANIFESTATIONS The time from exposure to the appearance of the rash of rubella is 14 to 21 days, usually about 18 days. In adults there may be a prodromal illness preceding the exanthem by 1 to 7 days. The prodrome consists of malaise, headache, fever, mild conjunctivitis, and lymphadenopathy. In children the rash may be the first manifestation of disease. It is apparent from serologic studies that rubella infection may be associated with no signs or symptoms, or may result in lymph node enlargement without skin lesions; however, rash without lymphadenopathy is uncommon. Respiratory symptoms are mild or absent. Small, red lesions (Forchheimer's spots) occasionally may be seen on the soft palate but are not pathognomonic of the disease.

The rash begins on the forehead and face and spreads downward to the trunk and extremities. The small maculopapular lesions, of lighter hue than those of measles, are usually discrete but may coalesce to form a diffuse erythema suggestive of scarlet fever. The rash may last from 1 to 5 days, but is most commonly present for 3 days. Enlarged, tender lymph nodes appear before the rash, are most impressive during the early eruptive phase, and may persist several days after the rash has disappeared. Splenomegaly or generalized lymphadenopathy may occur, but the postauricular and suboccipital nodes are most strikingly involved. Arthralgias and slight joint swellings may be a complication of rubella, especially in young women. The pain and swelling, involving wrists, fingers, and knees, are most marked during the period of rash and may persist for 1 to 14 days after other manifestations of rubella have disappeared. Recurring joint symptoms for a year or more have also been reported. Purpura with or without thrombocytopenia may occur and may be associated with hemorrhage. Encephalomyelitis following rubella resembles other postinfectious encephalitides and is much less common than encephalitis following measles. Testicular pain is also occasionally reported in young adults.

Congenital rubella The syndrome of congenital rubella has conventionally been thought to consist of heart malformations—patent ductus arteriosus, interventricular septal defect, or pulmonic stenosis; eye lesions—corneal clouding, cataracts, chorioretinitis, and microphthalmia; microcephaly, mental retardation, and deafness. In the American epidemic of 1964, thrombocytopenic purpura, hepatosplenomegaly, intrauterine growth retardation, interstitial pneumonia, myocarditis or myocardial necrosis, and metaphyseal bone lesions were encountered frequently in association with the previously recognized manifestations, leading to the term *expanded rubella syndrome.* Some infants have also been found to have significant humoral and/or cellular immunodeficiency, which generally resolves as chronic viral excretion diminishes and eventually ceases. Any combination of lesions may be seen in an individual infant, and the severity is highly variable.

Later complications include an apparent higher risk of subsequent development of diabetes mellitus. In addition, there are reports of patients with congenital rubella who develop a progressive, subacute panencephalitis, with onset in the second decade of life. This is characterized by intellectual deterioration, ataxia, seizures, and spasticity.

Congenital rubella is usually the result of maternal infection during the first trimester of pregnancy, although well-documented cases have resulted from infection several days before conception; deafness may occur as a result of infection in the fourth month. In the 1964 epidemic, about 10 percent of women with clinically recognized rubella during the first trimester gave birth to infants with the rubella syndrome. Serologically identified, asymptomatic maternal rubella can also result in severe fetal disease. It is therefore desirable to ascertain the immune status of every woman, either before conception or as early in the pregnancy as possible, by history of previous immunization or by serologic testing. If rubella antibodies are present before or within 10 days after exposure, the patient is considered immune, and the risk of fetal damage is virtually nil. If antibodies are not detectable and exposure has occurred, acute and convalescent antibody titers should be determined simultaneously on serums obtained 2 to 4 weeks apart, depending upon the time after exposure when the acute sample was drawn.

DIAGNOSIS Rubella is frequently confused with other diseases associated with maculopapular exanthems such as those described in Chaps. 199 and 202, and with infectious mononucleosis (Chap. 212), as well as with drug eruptions and scarlet fever. *A certain diagnosis of rubella can be made only by virus isolation and identification, or by changes in antibody titers.* Rubella hemagglutination-inhibiting antibodies may be present by the second day of rash and increase in quantity over the next 10 to 21 days. Other serologic tests which are frequently used for diagnosis or determination of immunity include complement fixation (CF), enzyme-linked immunosorbent assay (ELISA), radioimmunoassay (RIA), single radial hemolysis (SRH), and IgM-specific antibody tests. Antibodies detected by ELISA and RIA tend to parallel the hemagglutination-inhibiting antibodies, while the appearance of CF antibody lags behind the others by a period of 3 to 7 days and often does not disappear until 1 or 2 years after infection. The presence of IgM-specific antibodies suggests recent rubella infection (within 2 months); however, they have been known to persist as long as 1 year in some cases. The SRH is primarily used as an alternative to hemagglutination inhibition, ELISA, or RIA for semiquantitative screening of serums for the presence of antibody. There are no other laboratory findings helpful in the diagnosis of rubella, although lymphocytosis with atypical lymphocytes may occur.

Patients with the congenital rubella syndrome may lose hemagglutination-inhibiting antibodies at age 3 or 4 years. Therefore a negative serologic test in a child over 3 years does not exclude the possibility of congenital rubella. Congenital rubella should be differentiated by appropriate serologic tests from congenital syphilis (see Chap. 177), toxoplasmosis (see Chap. 221), and cytomegalic inclusion virus disease (see Chap. 211). IgM-specific antibodies are sometimes found early in the first year of life in infants with congenital rubella, but virus isolation is the most reliable way to confirm the diagnosis.

PREVENTION In adults and children rubella is usually a mild disease with infrequent complications. However, the severity of congenital infection has prompted efforts to prevent the disease. Administration of gamma globulin to exposed persons can abort the clinical disease, but seroconversion and transmission of the disease from mother to fetus may occur despite the administration of large amounts of gamma globulin soon after exposure.

Active immunization with live attenuated rubella vaccines prepared in duck, dog, rabbit, or human diploid fibroblast cells has been practiced in this country since 1969, especially among young children. The aim has been to decrease the frequency of the infection in the population, thus decreasing the chance that susceptible pregnant women will be exposed. Because of concern for a possibly enlarging pool of susceptible adolescents and adults, there has been increasing enthusiasm for serologic screening of pubertal females with no history of immunization, followed by selective immunization of those who are seronegative. Such immunization must of course be done with appropriate precautions, as noted below. Persons working in hospitals or clinics who might contract rubella from infected patients or who, if infected, might transmit the infection to pregnant patients should be required to have proof of immunity (either documented immunization or presence of serum antibody).

The attenuated virus can be detected in the respiratory secretions of vaccines for as long as 4 weeks after immunization, but transmission to other susceptible individuals rarely, if ever, occurs, even in households where susceptible pregnant women are in contact with children who are being vaccinated. The vaccine induces antibodies in about 95 percent of recipients, but the degree and duration of protection are still being evaluated. After heavy exposure in closed populations, vaccinated individuals sometimes develop subclinical infections (diagnosed by antibody rises and virus isolation). However, viremia has not been demonstrated in immunized persons, which suggests that previously vaccinated pregnant women will not infect their fetuses even if they acquire subclinical rubella.

Side effects of fever, rash, lymphadenopathy, polyneuropathy, or arthralgias occur very seldom in vaccinated children, but joint pain and swelling or paresthesias were seen in more than 25 percent of women who were immunized with the earlier vaccines. The risk has been reduced to less than 2 percent with the advent of vaccines prepared in human embryonic fibroblast cell cultures (RA 27/3 vaccine). The joint symptoms usually begin 2 to 10 weeks after vaccination, and they may be confused with other forms of arthritis. *Rubella vaccine must never be given to pregnant women or to those who may become pregnant within 3 months of immunization.* This precaution is necessary because the vaccine virus has the theoretical potential to damage the fetus of susceptible women.

REFERENCES

Academy Committee on Infectious Diseases: Revised recommendations on rubella vaccine. Pediatrics 65:1182, 1980

Balfour HH et al: RA 27/3 rubella vaccine. Am J Dis Child 134:350, 1980

Bernstein DI, Ogra PL: Fetomaternal aspects of immunization with RA 27/3 live attenuated rubella virus vaccine during pregnancy. J Pediatr 97:467, 1980

Best JM et al: Rubella immunity by four different techniques: Results of challenge studies. J Med Virol 5:239, 1980

Fox JP et al: Rubella vaccine in postpubertal women. JAMA 236:837, 1976

Hayden JF et al: Subclinical congenital rubella infection associated with maternal rubella vaccination in early pregnancy. J Pediatr 96:869, 1980

Horstmann D: Problems in measles and rubella. Disease-a-month, vol 24, no 6, 1978

Lerman SJ et al: Clinical and serologic evaluation of measles, mumps, and rubella (HPV-77:DE-5 and RA 27/3) virus vaccines, singly and in combination. Pediatrics 68:18, 1981

Mann JM et al: Assessing risks of rubella infection during pregnancy. JAMA 245:1647, 1981

Rubella prevention. Morb Mort Week Rep 30:37, 1981

Sever JL et al: Rubella epidemic, 1964: Effect on 6,000 pregnancies. Am J Dis Child 110:395, 1965

Townsend JJ et al: Progressive rubella panencephalitis: Late onset after congenital rubella. N Engl J Med 292:990, 1975

202 OTHER VIRAL EXANTHEMATOUS DISEASES

C. GEORGE RAY

In addition to the diseases such as measles, rubella, and chickenpox, which historically have been associated with prominent skin lesions, there are other virus infections in which skin manifestations may occur. Table 202-1 and Chap. 199 list the other most commonly recognized causes of maculopapular eruptions. Some of them, particularly the enteroviruses, can also occasionally cause papulovesicular or petechial rashes; others are capable of provoking erythema multiforme-like eruptions. One helpful aspect of the physical examination is the observation that viral-caused maculopapular (not vesicular) exanthems usually *relatively* spare the palms and soles. This is in contrast to eruptions associated with drug reactions, bacteria, *Mycoplasma,* and *Rickettsia,* in which a prominent palmar or plantar eruption is often noted.

EXANTHEM SUBITUM (ROSEOLA INFANTUM) Exanthem subitum is a benign disease of infants 6 to 24 months of age that is characterized by a high fever and rash. The disease can be transmitted to humans and monkeys by the transfer of blood obtained from a patient during the first few days of illness. The infectious agent is probably a virus, although it has not been isolated. The first manifestations of disease, after an estimated incubation period of 5 to 15 days, are the abrupt onset of irritability and fever, which lasts for 3 to 5 days; the temperature may be as high as 105°F. There may be mild pharyngitis and slight lymph node enlargement; convulsions may occur during the height of the fever. On the fourth to fifth day of illness, there is a sudden drop in temperature to normal or below normal; several hours before or after defervescence the rash suddenly and surprisingly appears. It is characterized by faint 2- to 3-mm macules or maculopapules over the neck and trunk and may extend to the thighs and buttocks; it may last for only a few hours or may be present for a day or two. Leukopenia is frequently noted later in the febrile period. The disease is benign and not associated with complications, although rarely an infant may show sequelae as a result of febrile convulsions. In the early, preeruptive phase, the disease may be difficult to differentiate from an acute, occult bacteremia, particularly from one associated with *Streptococcus pneumoniae.* Though a leukocytosis with an increase in band forms is often seen in occult bacteremias presenting in this fashion, blood cultures are necessary to make the diagnosis.

ERYTHEMA INFECTIOSUM (FIFTH DISEASE) Erythema infectiosum is a mild febrile exanthematous disease with little or no prodrome. The incubation period is probably 5 to 10 days. The

TABLE 202-1
Causes of maculopapular eruptions

Viral	*Other*
Measles	*Mycoplasma pneumoniae*
Rubella	Syphilis
Exanthem subitum	Typhoid fever
Erythema infectiosum	Bacterial toxins:
Enteroviruses: coxsackievirus, echovirus	streptococci and staphylococci
Infectious mononucleosis	Rat-bite fever
Adenoviruses	*Rickettsia*
Reoviruses	Live-virus vaccines
Arboviruses	Drug eruptions

first manifestations are low-grade fever and the appearance of indurated, confluent erythema over the cheeks, giving a "slapped face" appearance. A day or so later, a bilaterally symmetric eruption is seen on the arms, legs, and trunk, but rarely on the palms or soles. The lesions are maculopapular and tend to be confluent, forming slightly raised blotchy areas and reticular or lacy patterns. The rash usually lasts about a week, and during this time it may disappear, only to reappear in the same areas a few hours later. The waxing and waning eruption may occasionally persist for several weeks, and can be brought on by fever, heat, exercise, sunlight exposure, or emotional stress. Mild joint pain and swelling have been observed in a large proportion of adults with the disease. Erythema infectiosum affects all ages but is most common in children of school age and may occur in epidemic form. The mode of transmission of the disease is not known, and an infectious agent has not been recovered. A clinical diagnosis of this disease must sometimes be made with caution, since rubella and some enteroviruses have also been shown at times to cause a nearly identical syndrome.

ENTEROVIRAL EXANTHEMS Many individual enteroviruses have been associated with rash. Of these, polioviruses are rarely implicated. More commonly, echovirus serotypes 1 through 7, 9, 11, 12, 14, 16, 18, 19, 20, 25, and 30, coxsackievirus serotypes A4, A5, A6, A9, A10, A16, and B2, B3, and B5 have all been implicated. With the exception of hand-foot-and-mouth disease, usually associated with coxsackievirus A16 or enterovirus 71 infection (see Chap. 205), there is no set of clinical or epidemiologic features that aids in differentiating the specific enteroviral agent involved in a specific case. All are capable of producing maculopapular rashes which vary in intensity and duration, and can also occasionally produce petechial or papulovesicular exanthems and enanthems. In community and household outbreaks, younger children and infants are usually more likely to manifest exanthems, while other features of enteroviral infection, such as fever, myalgia, and aseptic meningitis, are more prominent among older children and young adults. Two enterovirus infections which have been frequently associated with rashes and have been studied extensively are described here as examples of epidemic enteroviral infections.

Boston exanthem (infections with echovirus 16) Echovirus 16 infection was described first and most extensively during an epidemic in Boston in 1951. Children who were infected usually had a disease characterized by exanthem and low-grade fever, while adult family contacts often developed high fever, prostration, and signs of aseptic meningitis with absent or fleeting rash. The first manifestation of the disease in children was fever of 101 to 102°F, lasting for a day or two, pharyngitis with small ulcerated lesions resembling herpangina, and slight enlargement of the cervical and postauricular lymph nodes. The rash appeared during fever or after defervescence and consisted of small pink maculopapules on the face, upper part of the chest, and occasionally on the whole body, including the palms and soles. The rash lasted for 1 to 5 days, and there were no important complications or sequelae. The disease resembled exanthem subitum but occurred in children of all ages and in adults.

Infection with echovirus 9 Infection with this virus in children and adults has been characterized by a febrile illness with a high incidence of aseptic meningitis. The incubation period is 5 to 8 days. About 30 percent of patients have a rash, which may occur with or without meningitis. It is usually maculopapular, developing at the onset of fever. The exanthem appears first on the face and neck, spreads to the trunk and extremities, may involve the palms and soles, although slightly, and persists for 3 to 5 days. Petechiae with or without maculopapules have been recognized; when they are seen in association with meningitis, there may be confusion with meningococcal meningitis. This can be a point of some concern, since concurrent outbreaks of echovirus 9 and meningococcal disease have been observed. A vesicular eruption with crusting lesions has been seen occasionally. An exanthem on the buccal mucosa and soft palate occurs in about 30 percent of patients and consists of small red areas with white centers which resemble Koplik's spots. The disease is usually benign but rarely has been associated with permanent central nervous system damage. Acute rhabdomyolysis with myoglobinuria has also been associated with echovirus 9 infection, and can be severe.

REFERENCES

BALFOUR HH: Erythema infectiosum: Clinical description of 91 cases seen in an epidemic. Clin Pediatr 8:721, 1969

——— et al: Erythema infectiosum: Recovery of rubella virus and echovirus 12. Pediatrics 50:285, 1972

CHONMAITREE T et al: Enterovirus 71 infection: Report of an outbreak with two cases of paralysis and a review of the literature. Pediatrics 67:489, 1981

HALL CB et al: The return of Boston exanthem. Echovirus 16 infections in 1974. Am J Dis Child 131:323, 1977

JOSSELSON J et al: Acute rhabdomyolysis associated with an echovirus 9 infection. Arch Intern Med 140:1671, 1980

LAUER BA et al: Erythema infectiosum. Am J Dis Child 130:252, 1976

NEVA FA et al: Clinical epidemiological features of unusual epidemic exanthem. JAMA 155:544, 1954

WENNER HA: Virus diseases associated with cutaneous eruptions. Prog Med Virol 16:269, 1973

203 SMALLPOX, VACCINIA, AND COWPOX

C. GEORGE RAY

Poxviruses are a group of large (200 to 320 nm), brick-shaped DNA-containing viruses that possess a common antigen and have a predilection for skin. Many of the poxviruses, such as myxoma and fowl pox agents, cause disease mainly in lower animals. Smallpox (variola major), alastrim (variola minor), vaccinia, and cowpox agents are closely related members of the poxvirus group that cause human disease. All these viruses grow and produce pox on the chorioallantoic membrane of chick embryos and can be cultivated in cells from various mammalian tissues with formation of intracytoplasmic inclusions, rounding fusion and heaping up of cells, and eventual degeneration of the infected area. The poxviruses responsible for human disease may be distinguished from one another by minor antigenic differences and by the type and severity of lesions they induce in experimental animals and humans. Smallpox and alastrim viruses produce smaller pox on the chorioallantoic membrane than vaccinia, and there are differences in incubation temperatures at which poxviruses produce lesions.

SMALLPOX (VARIOLA)

DEFINITION Smallpox is a severe, contagious, febrile disease characterized by a vesicular and pustular eruption. Alastrim is a similar but milder illness, with a lower mortality rate. Though the difference in severity between these diseases is apparent, the agents of variola major and variola minor are biologically and immunologically indistinguishable from each other in the laboratory.

At this time, smallpox (both variola major and variola minor) is considered to no longer exist in nature. In 1967, the World Health Organization launched an ambitious program aimed at total eradication of smallpox. Two important epidemiologic factors which suggested that this was possible were the absence of nonhuman reservoirs of the virus and the apparent nonexistence of completely asymptomatic human carriers. As a result of this astonishing effort, the last recorded case of naturally acquired smallpox occurred in Somalia in 1977. After 2 more years of worldwide surveillance with no further infections, global eradication of smallpox was confirmed in 1979 and accepted by the World Health Organization in May 1980. This was followed by destruction of laboratory stocks of virus, with the exception of six laboratories in various parts of the world. Surveillance continues, including studies of poxviruses of animals which are antigenically somewhat similar to smallpox. Some virologists remain legitimately concerned that an animal poxvirus (e.g., monkeypox, whitepox) could undergo mutation and become virulent for humans, although the chance of such an occurrence seems remote. Also, the possibility of "escape" of virus from a laboratory, although unlikely, must be considered.

Because the disease appears to be eradicated, the following description may be more of historical than practical interest. However, the disease might reappear unexpectedly, and a discussion of its features and prevention is still warranted.

PATHOGENESIS AND PATHOLOGY The virus gains access to the body by the respiratory tract and multiplies in unidentified sites, probably in lymph nodes or liver. After several days, during which there is no evidence of infection, viremia ensues, with swelling of the endothelium of blood vessels in the corium and perivascular inflammation. Loculated vesicles are the result of cellular destruction and exudation of serum. The infected epithelial cells are swollen and contain intracytoplasmic inclusions surrounded by a halo (Guarnieri bodies). The extent of skin involvement is greater in smallpox than in chickenpox and reaches into the corium. Pitting, most commonly seen on the face, is said to result from destruction of sebaceous glands, which are abundant in this area. The liver, spleen, and lymph nodes may be enlarged and may show focal accumulations of large mononuclear cells.

EPIDEMIOLOGY Smallpox is not as contagious as measles or influenza, and ordinarily face-to-face contact with an infected person is required to transmit the disease; however, airborne dissemination from contaminated fomites has also been shown to occur. A patient with smallpox is infectious from a day before the rash appears until all lesions have healed and the scabs have fallen off. During the early phase of the illness, the virus is transmitted in nasopharyngeal secretions; when the eruption is fully formed, the lesions themselves are a major source of infectious material. Variola virus may contaminate clothing, bedding, dust, or other inanimate objects and remain infectious for months, necessitating disinfection of articles in the patient's environment.

MANIFESTATIONS The incubation period of smallpox, from the time of exposure to the onset of the prodrome, is about 12 days, with extremes of 4 to 17 days. The disease can be divided into a prodrome, an early eruptive phase, and a period of vesiculation and pustule formation. The prodrome is characterized by a temperature of 102 to 106°F, headache, myalgia especially in the back, abdominal pain, vomiting, and in some patients by a transient, blotchy, erythematous eruption. After 3 or 4 days the fever subsides, the symptoms decrease, and the patient seems to recover. It is at this time, when the patient is afebrile, that the focal eruption begins. Early manifestations are painful ulcers on the buccal mucosa and macules which appear first on the face and forearms, and rapidly become firm, shotty papules. The papules increase in number and spread from the face and distal extremities to involve the trunk. The individual lesions may remain discrete and scattered, or they may become confluent and involve most of the body. They are most concentrated on the face and distal extremities, including the palms and soles, and are relatively sparse in the axilla. On the third or fourth day after the appearance of the focal rash, the papules progress to vesicles containing clear fluid, which, over the next few days, becomes cloudy because of infiltration by pus cells and desquamated epithelial cells; hemorrhage into the vesicles and surrounding skin may also be seen. During the course of smallpox, the lesions at any one time, in one area, are all at the same stage of evolution. At the time the vesicles become pustular, there is recurrence of fever, which may persist until healing occurs. The pustules umbilicate and form crusts and scabs which usually fall off 3 weeks after the beginning of illness, leaving small scars or deep pits.

The above description applies to disease of moderate severity. A milder illness may occur in previously immunized persons or in some who have no history of vaccination. It is characterized by the usual incubation period and prodrome, but is followed either by focal eruption of fewer than 100 papules, or by a rash resembling chickenpox. Smallpox with prodrome but with no eruption of any kind has been recognized (variola sine eruptione). The disease may also occur in a rapidly fulminating form ("sledgehammer" smallpox). After the usual incubation period, the patient develops an initial illness characterized by severe prostration, fever, bone marrow depression, hemorrhagic skin lesions, and bleeding. The disease progresses from inception to death within 3 or 4 days without evidence of the typical focal skin lesions.

Alastrim is similar to mild and moderate forms of variola major in that it has the same incubation period and prodromal illness, but the skin eruption is less extensive, and fatalities are rare and usually related to secondary bacterial infections.

COMPLICATIONS Bacterial superinfections of the lesions, usually with *Staphylococcus aureus,* may occur in the late pustular stage. Bacterial pneumonia and sepsis may be seen in severe forms of smallpox. Mild conjunctivitis is quite common, and iritis and keratitis have been recognized. Encephalomyelitis may occur in the late stage of the disease and is similar to other postinfectious encephalitides. Osteomyelitis and joint effusions may complicate the disease, and orchitis has also been reported.

LABORATORY FINDINGS Leukopenia is present during the prodromal illness, and there is usually leukocytosis during the pustular stage. Rapid diagnosis of poxvirus infection can be made by the finding of characteristic brick-shaped particles in preparations of vesicle fluid examined by electron microscopy. Specific precipitation in agar by use of antigen prepared from lesions and antivariola or antivaccinia immune serum may also allow detection of poxvirus within a few hours. These tests do not distinguish variola from vaccinia or other poxviruses but do allow rapid differentiation from herpes simplex and varicella-zoster viruses. For definitive identification the virus must be grown in cell culture or on the chorioallantoic membrane and neutralized with specific antiserum.

DIFFERENTIAL DIAGNOSIS The major problem in differential diagnosis is in distinguishing smallpox from chickenpox. Smallpox is preceded by a longer prodrome than chickenpox, and the eruption vesiculates over a period of days instead of hours. The smallpox lesions are all characteristically in the same stage of development, whereas those of chickenpox may, in one area, display all stages of evolution. Electron microscopy and agar precipitation techniques (see above) are especially useful in distinguishing between smallpox and chickenpox. Cytologic examination of scrapings of the base of a vesicle can also be helpful in the differential diagnosis. The presence of multinucleated giant cells and/or intranuclear inclusions strongly suggests a herpes group infection (varicella-zoster or herpes simplex); such findings are not seen with poxvirus infections.

Other conditions which are sometimes confused with smallpox include eczema vaccinatum, eczema herpeticum, rickettsialpox, drug eruptions, some cases of contact dermatitis, and Stevens-Johnson syndrome. The fulminant, hemorrhagic smallpox may closely resemble meningococcemia, typhus, and hemorrhagic fevers.

PREVENTION Smallpox may be prevented among the patient's contacts by vaccination. Because this procedure is most successful if carried out during the early part of the incubation period, all exposed persons, regardless of previous immunization, should be vaccinated immediately upon recognition of exposure. Large, controlled, clinical trials have demonstrated that oral administration of *N*-methylisatin 3-thiosemicarbazone (methisazone), a drug which interferes with poxvirus multiplication, can prevent smallpox and alastrim in patients exposed to the diseases. The use of a drug together with prompt vaccination results in greater chance of protection than either measure alone. A drawback to the use of methisazone is its tendency to induce vomiting. The combined use of vaccination and parenteral administration of vaccinia immune globulin early in the incubation period is also effective in the prevention of smallpox in exposed individuals.

TREATMENT There is no specific therapy for smallpox. Thiosemicarbazone, although effective in prophylaxis, has not been shown to be of value in the treatment of established cases. Fluid deficits should be replaced by the administration of appropriate solutions. During the vesicular and pustular phases of the disease, an attempt should be made to prevent bacterial infection by the use of sterile sheets and aseptic nursing procedures. Antihistamines may be helpful in decreasing pruritus. Application of lotions or ointment should be avoided. Later in the course of the illness, when desquamation has begun, showers or baths may be helpful in removing desquamating tissue. If bacterial infection develops, an antibiotic active against the infecting organism should be given by the parenteral route. Topical antibiotics should be avoided.

VACCINIA

Vaccinia is a virus disease of the skin which is induced by inoculation for the prevention of smallpox. The exact origin of the vaccinia virus is obscure. The material first used by Jenner in 1796 was derived from cowpox lesions, and the infectious agent was propagated for many years by successive passage from person to person through use of exudate from fresh skin lesions. The original agent possibly became contaminated with variola virus during the period when transfer was being carried out without strict controls. It has been suggested that vaccinia virus is a hybrid of cowpox and variola agents, a contention supported by the finding that laboratory-induced hybrids of variola and cowpox viruses have many of the characteristics associated with vaccinia.

VACCINATION Use of vaccinia virus is now indicated *only* for a few laboratory workers directly involved with smallpox or closely related animal poxviruses, such as monkeypox. A few countries in Asia and Africa still require an up-to-date certification of smallpox vaccination as a condition of entry, even though there is no medical reason to do so. It has been suggested that travelers to these areas obtain smallpox vaccination–waiver letters indicating that vaccination is contraindicated for health reasons, rather than undergo the risk of complications from the vaccine.

In the past, vaccinia virus has also been occasionally used for the treatment of diseases such as recurrent herpes simplex infection or warts. There is *no* evidence of therapeutic efficacy in these situations, and the use of the virus for these purposes is strictly contraindicated. Live, lyophilized vaccinia virus prepared from vesicle fluid of infected calves maintains potency for 18 months at 46°F. It is dissolved in a diluent solution just prior to use. The usual method for vaccination is to apply a small drop of vaccine to the skin over the deltoid muscle and to press a sterile needle through the vaccine several times in such a way that only the superficial layer of skin is entered, or by simultaneous puncture utilizing a plastic tine device. Vaccination should always induce some form of skin reaction; complete absence of any kind of lesion indicates that the vaccine was not viable or was not administered properly. The reaction which occurs in nonimmune individuals is characterized by a red papule at the site of inoculation 3 to 5 days after vaccination. The papule becomes vesicular on about the fifth or sixth day and pustular by the ninth or eleventh day after inoculation. The vesicle and pustule may be surrounded by a large area of erythema. About 2 weeks after vaccination, the pustule dries and develops a crust which falls off by the end of the third week, leaving a scar. Fever, malaise, and irritability are common in children during the vesicular and pustular phases, and axillary lymphadenopathy may develop and persist for several months. In the partially immune person, a modified reaction develops without fever or constitutional symptoms. A papule appears on the skin within 3 days, vesiculates in 5 to 7 days, and heals without much scarring. The so-called immune reaction described by some, where a papule and/or erythema appears in a few days, then recedes without vesiculation, is an "equivocal" reaction, and may simply represent allergy to the components of an inadvertently inactivated vaccine. A successful vaccination is defined as the presence of a Jennerian vesicle (vesicular, pustular, or crusted) 7 days after inoculation. If the criterion is not met, the patient should be revaccinated, preferably with vaccine from a different lot.

Revaccination every 3 years is required to ensure protection. *Absolute contraindications* to vaccination include individuals with congenital or acquired immune deficiencies, lymphoma, leukemia or other blood dyscrasias, patients being treated with steroids, antimetabolites, alkylating agents, or ionizing irradiation, and individuals with a history of vaccinia encephalitis. *Relative contraindications* include patients or household contacts with eczema or a history of eczema, severe acne, or other similar dermatologic problems, pregnancy, and infants under 12 months of age. If the necessity to vaccinate any individual in this latter group is great, simultaneous administration of vaccinia immune globulin (VIG), 0.3 ml/kg, is suggested, to be given at a separate site intramuscularly at the time of immunization.

COMPLICATIONS Healing of the primary vaccinal lesion may not occur, and some patients go on to develop slowly progressive necrosis with destruction of large areas of skin, subcutaneous tissue, and underlying structures *(vaccinia gangrenosum).* In addition to the local destruction, there may be metastatic lesions on other parts of the skin surface and in bone and viscera. Vaccinia gangrenosum occurs most frequently in persons with disorders of immunity and, if untreated, is nearly always fatal. *Eczema vaccinatum* is a serious complication that is seen in persons with eczema or other types of chronic skin conditions. Widespread infection in the previously affected areas, as well as in normal skin, may result from direct vaccination of an eczematous patient or from exposure to a recently vaccinated individual. *Generalized vaccinia* in patients without preexisting skin disease is characterized by a few satellite lesions surrounding the inoculation site or by widely disseminated pox resembling the primary vaccination lesion. This condition is usually mild with generally complete recovery. Vaccinia virus may be transferred from the primary inoculation site to the eye or other sites by scratching. *Postvaccinal encephalomyelitis* appears from 2 to 25 days after vaccination. The patient suddenly becomes severely ill with nuchal rigidity, drowsiness, vomiting, convulsions, coma, and signs suggesting disease of the spinal cord. The period of coma lasts for a few days, and in those who recover there are usually no permanent sequelae. Death occurs in about 30 to 40 percent of the patients with encephalomyelitis. *Erythema multiforme bullosum,* or *diffuse blotchy erythema,* may occur in vaccinated patients 7 to 10 days after vaccination, and is thought to be an allergic reaction to the virus or other components of the vaccine.

The rates of adverse effects per million primarily vaccinated persons were vaccinia gangrenosum, 0.9; eczema vaccinatum, 10.4; generalized vaccinia, 23.4; vaccinal lesions resulting from accidental implantation of virus, 25.4; postvaccinal encephalitis, 2.9; other complications, 11.8; the death rate was 1 per million.

Active treatment of vaccinia complications, aside from control of bacterial superinfection and treatment of any underlying defects, is limited. VIG is of possible value in accidental inoculation into secondary sites such as the eye, vaccinia gangrenosum, eczema vaccinatum, and generalized vaccinia. Dosage is usually 0.6 ml/kg intramuscularly, although much larger doses are sometimes used in severe cases. VIG is of no use in erythema multiforme or postvaccinal encephalitis. Thiosemicarbazone has apparently been of benefit in some cases of progressive vaccinia gangrenosum. 5-Iodo-2′-deoxyuridine, while not yet proved to be effective, is suggested for topical treatment of vaccinial keratitis and conjunctivitis.

COWPOX

Cowpox is primarily a disease of the teats and udders of cows. Humans are almost always infected by milking, but occasional spread to contacts may occur from an infected person. The human disease is characterized by low-grade fever and by small papules on the fingers and hand, which go through vesicular and pustular stages resembling the course of vaccinia infection. The lesions may be ruptured by trauma and spread to immediately adjacent areas on the hand and continue to ulcerate for several weeks. Edema, lymphangitis, and axillary lymph node enlargement are common. Very rare cases of post-cowpox encephalitis and serious infections of eczematous persons have been reported. In general, the disease is benign, heals without scarring, and is usually uncomplicated.

PARAVACCINIA (MILKERS' NODULES)

Paravaccinia is a poxvirus which is antigenically unrelated to cowpox, but produces similar lesions in humans. It is primarily a disease of calves and milk cows, producing lesions on the teats of the cows and oral lesions in the suckling calf. Humans acquire infection through the skin by direct contact. The lesion is usually solitary, beginning as a macule on the finger, hand, or wrist, and progressing to a firm nodule, 1 to 2 cm in diameter, in 10 days. It then crusts and heals without scarring in 2 to 3 weeks. Occasionally, there is associated lymphadenitis. The lesion and its evolution are closely similar to ecthyma contagiosum (orf), a poxvirus of sheep, which can also infect humans by direct inoculation.

REFERENCES

Adverse reactions to smallpox vaccination. Morb Mort Week Rep 28:265, 1979

Bedson HS, Dumbell K: Smallpox and vaccinia. Br Med Bull 23:119, 1967

Breman JG, Arita I: The confirmation and maintenance of smallpox eradication. N Engl J Med 303:1263, 1980

Dixon CW: *Smallpox.* London, Churchill, 1962

Goldstein JA et al: Smallpox vaccination reactions, prophylaxis, and therapy of complications. Pediatrics 55:342, 1975

Laboratory-associated smallpox—England. Morb Mort Week Rep 27:319, 1978

Rennie AGR et al: Ocular vaccinia. Lancet 2:273, 1974

Smallpox vaccine. Morb Mort Week Rep 29:417, 1980

204
CHICKENPOX (VARICELLA) AND HERPES ZOSTER

C. GEORGE RAY

DEFINITION Chickenpox is a contagious disease characterized by fever and a disseminated vesicular eruption. Herpes zoster, or shingles, is characterized by segmental inflammation of the spinal or cranial nerves and their ganglia, and by a painful localized vesicular eruption of the skin along the distribution of the involved nerve. Chickenpox and herpes zoster are different manifestations of infection with the same viral agent.

ETIOLOGY In 1953 a virus was recovered from patients with chickenpox and herpes zoster that produced intranuclear, eosinophilic inclusions and multinucleated giant cells in lines of cells derived from various monkey and human tissues. The infectivity of varicella-zoster virus in culture is closely cell-associated, and ordinarily can be passed to other tissue cultures only by transfer of infected, intact cells. The structure of the varicella-zoster virion resembles that of herpes simplex and the other viruses of the herpes group.

PATHOGENESIS AND PATHOLOGY Varicella is presumably transmitted by the respiratory route, although the virus has only rarely been isolated from nasopharyngeal secretions of infected persons. Virus multiplication occurs at some unidentified site and probably results in intermittent viremia, as suggested by the successive crops of widely spaced lesions. Focal viral infection of blood vessels in the corium with intranuclear inclusions in endothelial cells results in degeneration of the epidermis and formation of vesicles containing serum, polymorphonuclear leukocytes, and multinucleated giant cells. Virus can be isolated from vesicle fluid, but not usually from crusting lesions or scabs, for 3 to 4 days after eruption. In patients with varicella pneumonia, the tracheobronchial mucosa, the alveolar septa, and the interstitial areas of the lungs are edematous and contain monocytic inflammatory cells, cells with intranuclear inclusions and giant cells. The nodular areas of pneumonia may eventually become calcified. The changes in the central nervous system in patients with postinfectious varicella encephalomyelitis resemble those seen in measles. Rarely, encephalomyelitis with inclusion bodies resembling herpes simplex infection may occur, and varicella-zoster virus can be recovered from the central nervous system. In infants and children, acute encephalopathy with fatty infiltration of the viscera (Reye's syndrome) sometimes follows the acute phase of varicella; in this condition, only cerebral edema is found on pathologic examination of the brain.

The pathogenesis of herpes zoster is not clear (see "Epidemiology" below), but the tissue changes are well documented. The dorsal root ganglion of the affected nerve is swollen and hemorrhagic; the edema spreads along the peripheral nerve and may reach the spinal cord. The nerve tissue shows hemorrhagic infarction, inflammation, and necrosis of many of the ganglion cells, some of which contain intranuclear inclusions. The microscopic appearance of zoster skin lesions is almost identical with that described for chickenpox vesicles. Virus can be cultured from the lesions for as long as 8 days after onset.

EPIDEMIOLOGY Chickenpox is a highly contagious disease with attack rates of 80 percent or more among susceptible household contacts of an index case. The infectious period extends from a day or two before the rash until as long as 6 days after the appearance of new skin lesions, or until all vesicles have crusted over. Patients with herpes zoster may be the source of an outbreak of chickenpox among susceptible contacts. Children from 5 to 9 years of age comprise 65 percent of reported cases, but younger children, including newborn infants, and adults may develop chickenpox; approximately 5 percent of cases occur in persons over the age of 15 years. Serologic surveys are limited, but indicate that as many as 9 percent of parturient women are susceptible to chickenpox. In the United States the disease is endemic, with superimposed epidemics every 2 to 5 years, usually in the winter or spring.

Herpes zoster is mainly a disease of adults who have previously had chickenpox. The epidemiologic evidence strongly suggests that herpes zoster results from reactivation of virus that has remained dormant in spinal ganglia since an episode of chickenpox. Exogenous acquisition of infection directly resulting in herpes zoster rarely, if ever, occurs. Most patients with zoster have had no recent exposure to patients with zoster or varicella, and the incidence of the disease does not increase during seasonal chickenpox epidemics.

Zoster occurs commonly in patients with neoplasms, most frequently in those with Hodgkin's disease, where the incidence may be as high as 25 percent. Advanced disease, cutaneous anergy, recent x-ray therapy to affected nodes, and possibly splenectomy predispose patients with Hodgkin's disease to zoster. The most significant common factor responsible for the development of zoster in these patients appears to be depressed cell-mediated immunity; there is no clear correlation with humoral immune status.

Recurrent herpes zoster is estimated to occur in 2 percent or less of all cases. If such a recurrence is documented, it should raise the suspicion of an underlying malignancy or immunodeficiency. When episodes of so-called recurrent zoster in healthy individuals have been carefully studied, herpes simplex virus has usually been found to be the causative agent. Like varicella-zoster virus, herpes simplex can cause zoster-like disease, but can also cause recurrent lesions. Recurrent chickenpox is exceedingly rare but has been reported in a few patients who were receiving high-dose immunosuppressive therapy.

MANIFESTATIONS **Chickenpox** The incubation period from the time of exposure to the appearance of varicella rash is 10 to 21 days, most often 14 to 17 days. There may be a 1- to 2-day prodrome with fever and malaise, but these symptoms usually begin when the rash appears. The first skin manifestations are pruritic maculopapules that evolve in a few hours to thin-walled vesicles which contain clear fluid and are surrounded by a red border. During the next day the erythema diminishes and the vesicles collapse in the center, forming annular or umbilicated lesions which dry further and form scabs that fall off, after several days, without scarring. New maculopapules continue to erupt during the first 3 or 4 days of illness and go through a similar evolution. The finding at one time, in one area, of skin lesions in all stages of development—maculopapules, vesicles, umbilicated lesions, and scabs—is characteristic of chickenpox. The rash is most concentrated on the trunk, but pox are frequently seen on the face and scalp, occasionally on the mucosal surface of the mouth or conjunctiva, and rarely on the palms and soles.

Chickenpox in adults is often more severe than in children, with more profuse rash, higher fever, and a greater incidence of pneumonia.

Herpes zoster Herpes zoster is a disease of nerves of the skin and other tissues that they supply. It most commonly affects the thoracic (55 percent of cases), cervical (20 percent), and lumbar and sacral nerves (15 percent), and the ophthalmic division of the trigeminal nerve.

Fever and pain that is localized to the areas served by the affected nerves may begin 4 or 5 days before or be concomitant with the appearance of the skin eruption. Rarely, characteristic pain and serologic evidence of zoster occur with no clinical involvement of the skin (zoster sine eruptione). The discomfort is mild to severe and can be sharp, burning, or dull. In addition to disorders of sensation, herpes zoster is occasionally associated with motor paralysis of arms, legs, intercostal muscles, or muscles innervated by cranial nerves. The skin lesion starts with local redness followed by red papules that progress over the next 2 weeks through vesicular, pustular, and crusting stages that resemble the evolution of individual pox of varicella. The lesions are arranged unilaterally in characteristic bandlike clusters which follow radicular lines. They may run transversely along the hemithorax or vertically over the arm or leg.

Disease of the individual cranial nerves leads to characteristic groups of symptoms. If the trigeminal (Gasserian) ganglion is affected, there will usually be pain in the distribution of the nerve, headache, weakness of the eyelid muscles, and occasionally Argyll Robertson pupil. Lesions appear on the face, in the mouth, on the tongue, and frequently on the cornea. Iridocyclitis, anesthesia of the cornea, and scarring may result. If the geniculate ganglion is involved, there may be Bell's palsy, disorders of hearing, and vertigo, with unilateral herpetic lesions of the external ear and canal and of the anterior portion of the tongue. Central nervous system inflammation is prominent when herpes zoster attacks the cranial nerves, and meningeal signs and symptoms are frequent.

COMPLICATIONS Hemorrhage into vesicles and surrounding skin may be seen in adults with severe chickenpox or in children receiving adrenal steroids. Infection of the varicella lesions by bacteria, most commonly *Staphylococcus aureus*, results in delayed healing and scarring of skin, and occasionally in bacteremia.

Of adults with chickenpox, 15 percent develop primary *varicella pneumonia.* Pneumonia is invariably associated with skin lesions and appears 1 to 6 days after onset of rash. The degree of pulmonary involvement correlates to some extent with the severity of the rash; patients may be virtually asymptomatic or may develop serious, life-threatening disease. Tachypnea, dyspnea, cough, and fever, with a temperature of 102°F or more, are present in most patients with symptomatic pneumonia; cyanosis, pleuritic chest pain, and hemoptysis each occur in 20 to 40 percent of the recorded cases. The physical examination may disclose no abnormalities, or there may be intercostal retractions, a few rhonchi, wheezes, scattered rales, and rarely, evidence of pleural effusion. In contrast to the paucity of physical signs, roentgenograms demonstrate widespread nodular infiltration of both lungs, most prominent at the hila and least evident at the apexes. Vital capacity is decreased, arterial oxygen saturation is diminished, and the airways may be blocked by tenacious bronchopulmonary secretions. Most patients with varicella pneumonia show symptomatic improvement when the rash begins to wane; however, seriously ill patients may remain febrile and dyspneic for as long as 2 weeks. Roentgenographic evidence of disease diminishes at the time of clinical improvement, but may persist for several weeks, followed in some cases by persistent miliary calcifications. Persistent abnormalities of pulmonary gas diffusion have been demonstrated several months after apparent recovery.

Central nervous system complications occur most frequently in children, with estimated rates as high as 1 in 200 cases. The most common manifestation is acute cerebellar ataxia, which usually begins 3 to 21 days after onset of rash and is usually benign. Other less common manifestations include acute encephalomyelitis, polyneuritis, ascending or transverse myelitis, optic neuritis, and Reye's syndrome.

Patients who contract *varicella while receiving steroids* may have recurrent crops of new skin lesions for as long as 3 weeks. They have a higher incidence of hemorrhagic and progressive gangrenous lesions and occasionally develop a fatal disseminated disease with viral infection in all the viscera. The fatal form of the disease has been encountered most frequently in children being treated with steroids for leukemia or other disease of the hematopoietic system, but it has also been seen in those receiving therapy for rheumatic fever and allergic disorders. Children with the rare syndrome of cartilage-hair hypoplasia may suffer from unusually severe and occasionally fatal chickenpox. *Other complications of chickenpox* such as myocarditis, corneal lesions, iritis, nephritis, nephrosis, monoarticular arthritis or polyarthritis, thrombocytopenic purpura, purpura fulminans, orchitis, and appendicitis have been recognized but are rare. Hepatic involvement, without evidence of Reye's syndrome, is common in chickenpox. This is most often subclinical and can be detected by elevations in SGOT (up to 920 IU per liter) and/or SGPT (up to 1160 IU per liter) levels. The usually apparent clinical symptoms consist of nausea and vomiting. Like measles, chickenpox can transiently produce anergy to tuberculin, and occasionally there may be reactivation of latent tuberculosis. Congenital infection with varicella can occur, and infants born of mothers with chickenpox may display the typical skin lesions. Congenital malformations as a result of infection in early pregnancy have been reported but are rare. The greatest mortality risk to the newborn infant appears to occur when onset of the maternal rash occurs in the 4-day period immediately before delivery or 48 h after delivery.

Postherpetic neuralgia may last for several months or years and become the most troublesome part of the disease. In nearly all patients with zoster, healing with loss of scab is complete within 2 to 3 weeks. In the young, pain persists for only a week or two after healing and then usually disappears, although hypo- or hyperesthesia may remain. However, in patients over 60 years of age, moderate to severe pain persists for more than 2 months in as many as 70 percent, even though the skin lesions have healed normally.

Zoster skin lesions do not always remain localized. *Generalized zoster* occurs in 5 percent of zoster patients with no underlying disease, and in as many as 70 percent of those with Hodgkin's disease, or in immunosuppressed organ transplant recipients. It is characterized by dissemination to all parts of the skin, producing a picture similar to that of chickenpox. The scattered lesions last 6 to 9 days in normal hosts, but they may persist for 3 to 24 weeks in those with serious underlying disease. In these patients dissemination may also involve the visceral organs (including the lungs) and occasionally results in death.

Atypical generalized zoster is a rare manifestation of infection, characterized by high fever, diffuse lymphadenopathy, and a maculopapular rash over the extremities. The vesicular skin lesions may not appear until 6 weeks after onset of fever.

LABORATORY FINDINGS Multinucleated giant cells and epithelial cells with eosinophilic intranuclear inclusions can be identified in material scraped from the base of a vesicular lesion or in sputum from patients with varicella pneumonia. For specific diagnosis, virus can be isolated from vesicular fluid, and antigens can be demonstrated in vesicular fluid and in crusts of lesions by the use of gel-precipitin or counterimmunoelectrophoresis techniques. Direct immunofluorescent staining of vesicle cells or other infected tissues can also be used to detect the viral antigens. Serologic confirmation is also possible, utilizing complement fixation or the more sensitive immune adherence hemagglutination or indirect immunofluorescent antibody tests. The white blood cell count in patients with uncomplicated chickenpox or zoster is normal. Mononuclear pleocytosis is present in the cerebrospinal fluid of patients with herpes zoster, especially those with involvement of the cranial nerves. The spinal fluid in varicella-zoster encephalomyelitis often contains increased protein, and cell counts may range from zero to 3000 lymphocytes per cubic millimeter.

DIFFERENTIAL DIAGNOSIS Chickenpox can usually be diagnosed by the history of recent exposure and the character of the rash. In situations where smallpox is a possibility, differentiation from chickenpox can be attempted by noting the distribution and evolution of the rash and by examining the cells from vesicles, but definitive diagnosis can be made only by identification of the virus or by serologic methods. Disseminated vaccinia lesions similar to chickenpox lesions may occur in patients, especially those with immune deficiency diseases or eczema, who have recently been vaccinated or exposed to a vaccinated person. Herpes simplex infection in patients with chronic eczema or neurodermatitis may present as a varicelliform eruption confined to previously involved areas of skin. The diagnosis can be confirmed by virus isolation. Rickettsialpox can be differentiated from chickenpox by the presence of an eschar in the area of mite bite, prominent headache, and specific complement-fixing antibodies to *Rickettsia akari.* Rarely, coxsackieviruses can produce a similar eruption in young children, although the lesions all tend to be in the same stage of development in one area. Stevens-Johnson syndrome has also been occasionally confused with chickenpox.

In the preeruptive stage, the diagnosis of herpes zoster is difficult, and the disease is usually confused with other causes of pain, such as pleurisy, appendicitis, pleurodynia, or collapsed intervertebral disk. After the unilateral eruption appears, the clinical features are so characteristic that the diagnosis is usually simple. Occasionally, localized herpes simplex along the distribution of a segmental nerve may simulate zoster, including the localized pain and tenderness. The diagnosis of herpes simplex infection can be confirmed in the laboratory by virus isolation. Atypical generalized zoster most closely mimics a lymphoma; early diagnosis may require electron microscopic and immunofluorescent studies of lymph node biopsies.

PROPHYLAXIS Chickenpox can often be prevented or significantly modified by the administration of specific zoster immune globulin (ZIG) derived from the serum of patients recovering from herpes zoster, varicella-zoster immune globulin (VZIG) prepared from pooled plasma containing high titers of varicella antibody, or intravenous zoster immune plasma (ZIP). Both ZIG and VZIG should be given within 96 h of exposure to be effective, and limited data suggest some usefulness of ZIP if given within 6 days of exposure, in doses ranging from 3 to 14 ml/kg. Table 204-1 lists the current Center for Disease Control criteria which should be fulfilled before the use of VZIG in prophylaxis of chickenpox, and these also generally apply for ZIG and ZIP. Because supplies of VZIG are limited, the following recommendations have also been made: (1) Immunodeficient patients, especially children, with a negative or unknown history of chickenpox should be screened for antibody to varicella-zoster virus prior to any exposure. If antibody is present, there is no need for VZIG prophylaxis. (2) VZIG is not indicated for prophylactic use at any age when there is a past history of chickenpox, unless the patient subsequently received a bone marrow transplant. (3) The use of VZIG in susceptible persons over 15 years of age with serious underlying disease should be evaluated on an individual basis rather than by routine application of the criteria outlined in Table 204-1. (4) VZIG is not recommended for susceptible, otherwise healthy, pregnant women; furthermore, there is no evidence that administration of VZIG in pregnancy is effective in preventing fetal infection. Large doses of pooled human gamma globulin have also been shown to modify the disease if given shortly after exposure, but the quantity required to do so is so great (0.6 to 1.2 ml/kg) that this form of treatment is not generally recommended. There is no evidence that any of these preparations have any value in the prevention of herpes zoster or in the treatment of established infection of either type. There are also data that subcutaneous administration of transfer factor, derived from lymphocytes of patients convalescing from chickenpox, may confer long-term (12 to 30 months) protection on subsequent exposure to chickenpox in susceptible leukemic children.

Live, attenuated varicella-zoster virus vaccines have been tried as immunizing agents in high-risk children in Japan, but larger trials elsewhere have not yet been reported. Such vaccines are not available in the United States, except for limited, controlled trials.

TABLE 204-1
Recommended criteria for the use of varicella-zoster immune globulin for prophylaxis of varicella

1 One of the following underlying illnesses or conditions
  a Leukemia or lymphoma
  b Congenital or acquired immunodeficiency
  c Under immunosuppressive medication
  d Newborn of mother who had onset of chickenpox <5 days before delivery or within 48 h after delivery
2 One of the following types of exposure to varicella or zoster patient(s)
  a Household contact
  b Playmate contact (more than 1 h play indoors)
  c Hospital contact (in same two- to four-bed room or adjacent beds in a large ward)
  d Newborn contact (newborn whose mother had onset of chickenpox* <5 days before delivery or within 48 h after delivery)
3 Negative or unknown prior disease history (see text)
4 Age less than 15 years, with administration to older patients on an individual basis (see text)
5 Time elapsed after exposure is such that VZIG can be administered within 96 h

* *Maternal zoster does not pose a significantly high risk to the neonate and is not a criterion for VZIG administration.*

TREATMENT The patient with uncomplicated chickenpox seems to benefit most from cool, wet compresses or tepid water baths, rather than drying lotions, for the relief of itching. Secondary bacterial infections should be treated with appropriate antibacterial agents. Patients with varicella pneumonia require skillful nursing care, removal of excessive bronchial secretions, administration of oxygen, and on occasion assisted ventilation. Adrenal corticosteroids have been considered by some to be beneficial in the treatment of varicella pneumonia, but convincing evidence of their efficacy in this condition is not available. Patients suspected of having varicella-zoster infection of the eye should be promptly treated by an ophthalmologist. The therapy consists of analgesics for severe pain and the use of atropine to prevent synechiae. Some ophthalmologists recommend the use of steroids if uveitis is present. Topical 5-iodo-2′-deoxyuridine is of possible value for corneal or conjunctival ulcerative lesions.

Intravenous adenine arabinoside or acycloguanosine has been used in cases of severe zoster in patients on immunosuppressive therapy who are at high risk of dissemination, with encouraging results. Other studies, utilizing high doses of intramuscular human leukocyte interferon in similar patients, have also shown promise, but this form of treatment may be limited by the restricted availability of human interferon. However, further data are necessary before the treatment of choice can be recommended. It is also desirable to attempt to reduce the dose of immunosuppressive agents such as azathioprine and antithymocyte globulin as much as possible at the time of onset of zoster lesions.

It has been claimed that in older patients with herpes zoster and no underlying disease, the administration of a short course of adrenal steroids by mouth during the early eruptive phase of the disease reduces the incidence and duration of postherpetic neuralgia without inducing dissemination or other complications. Steroids should *not* be used for this purpose in patients with neoplasms or other underlying disease. More recently, it has been claimed that oral levodopa with benserazide (a peripheral decarboxylase inhibitor) will significantly reduce acute and postzoster pain. The mechanism of this effect is not understood.

REFERENCES

EAGLESTEIN WH et al: The effects of early corticosteroid therapy on the skin eruption and pain of herpes zoster. JAMA 211:1681, 1970

EY JL et al: Varicella hepatitis without neurologic symptoms or findings. Pediatrics 67:285, 1981

FELDHOFF CM et al: Varicella in children with renal transplants. J Pediatr 98:25, 1981

GALLAGHER JG, MERIGAN TC: Prolonged herpes-zoster infection associated with immunosuppressive therapy. Ann Intern Med 91:842, 1979

GERSHON AA et al: Antibody to varicella-zoster virus in parturient women and their offspring during the first year of life. Pediatrics 58:692, 1976

——— et al: Varicella-zoster-associated encephalitis: Detection of specific antibody in cerebrospinal fluid. J Clin Microbiol 12:764, 1981

GROTH KE et al: Evaluation of zoster immune plasma. JAMA 239:1877, 1978

HA K et al: Application of live varicella vaccine to children with acute
HA K et al: Application of live varicella vaccine to children with acute leukemia or other malignancies without suspension of anticancer therapy. Pediatrics 65:346, 1980
KERNBAUM S, HAUCHECORNE J: Administration of levodopa for relief of herpes zoster pain. JAMA 246:132, 1981
KREBS RA, BURVANT MU: Nephrotic syndrome in association with varicella. JAMA 222:325, 1972
MERIGAN RC et al: Interferon for the treatment of herpes zoster in patients with cancer. N Engl J Med 298:981, 1978
MORENS DM et al: An outbreak of varicella-zoster virus infection among cancer patients. Ann Intern Med 93:414, 1980
PATTERSON SD et al: Atypical generalized zoster with lymphadenitis mimicking lymphoma. N Engl J Med 302:844, 1980
RUCKDESCHEL JC et al: Herpes zoster and impaired cell-associated immunity to the V-Z virus in patients with Hodgkin's disease. Am J Med 62:77, 1977
SELBY PJ et al: Parenteral acyclovir therapy for herpesvirus infections in man. Lancet 2:1267, 1979
STEELE RW et al: Transfer factor for the prevention of varicella-zoster infection in childhood leukemia. N Engl J Med 303:355, 1980
TRIEBWASSER JH et al: Varicella pneumonia in adults: Report of seven cases and a review of literature. Medicine 46:409, 1967
Varicella-zoster immune globulin. Morb Mort Week Rep 30:15, 1981
Varicella-zoster immune globulin. Medical Letter 24:51, 1982
WHITLEY RJ et al: Adenine arabinoside therapy of herpes zoster in the immunosuppressed. N Engl J Med 294:1193, 1976

Central nervous system viruses

205
ENTERIC VIRUSES
Coxsackieviruses, echoviruses, polioviruses, reoviruses, parvoviruses, and rotaviruses

A. MARTIN LERNER

GENERAL CONSIDERATIONS

It has been almost 40 years since Dalldorf and Sickles isolated the first coxsackieviruses by inoculating suspensions of feces from two children with signs of clinical paralytic poliomyelitis into suckling mice. Subsequently, some 71 enteroviruses, including polioviruses and coxsackieviruses, and echoviruses, have been shown to multiply at various times in the gastrointestinal tracts of human beings. These viruses include four newly recognized members of the group which have been termed enterovirus, types 68 to 71 (Table 205-1). Enteroviruses have been recovered wherever attempts have been made; their distribution is global. With notable exceptions such as coxsackievirus, type A21, and echovirus 28, which are predominantly respiratory pathogens and are only incidentally isolated from feces, enteroviruses, like *Salmonella,* periodically multiply within the human alimentary canal, predominantly within the oropharynx and small bowel, and sometimes concomitantly produce disease. There is no normal enteric virus flora. In addition to enteroviruses, adenoviruses, reoviruses, and hepatitis A, non-A non-B, parvoviruses, and rotaviruses are commonly recovered from stools. The latter two agents are causes of viral gastroenteritis.

TABLE 205-1
Classification of human enteroviruses

I Enteroviruses
  A Polioviruses (3 types)*
  B Coxsackievirus A (24 types)
  C Coxsackievirus B (6 types)
  D Echoviruses (34 types)†
II Newly recognized enterovirus types
  A Enterovirus, type 68
  B Enterovirus, type 69
  C Enterovirus, type 70
  D Enterovirus, type 71

* *Typing is by neutralization of infectivity with immune serums either in suitable tissue cultures or in suckling mice.*
† *Echovirus, type 10, has been reclassified as belonging to another taxonomic group, now known as reoviruses.*

Coxsackieviruses are named for their site of origin, the village of Coxsackie on the banks of the Hudson River in the state of New York. Echoviruses were descriptively named: *E,* for their *enteric* residence; *C,* the filtrable agents produce *cytopathic* effects in tissue cultures of rhesus kidney; *H, human*; *O, orphan,* indicating that their relationship to disease remained to be established. They were viruses "in search of a disease." It is increasingly evident that a wide but definite variety of human illnesses may result from enterovirus infections. As observations continue to accumulate, these illnesses (Table 205-2) are continually being defined. Associations are now being made with some important chronic human diseases such as insulin-dependent diabetes mellitus and certain forms of "idiopathic" heart disease. Etiologic proof will require well-designed prospective matched case-control epidemiologic studies.

Etiologic associations are difficult to establish and usually require virologic, serologic, epidemiologic, and, when ethically possible, volunteer studies. These are especially useful if viruses are isolated only from the pharynx or anus, where they often multiply without causing significant injury to tissues. More meaningful are isolations from blood, vesicular fluids of patients with rashes, urine, cerebrospinal fluid, or from tissues at biopsy or autopsy. Coxsackieviruses and echoviruses have been recovered from lung, heart, pericardial fluid, liver, spleen, testicle, kidney, muscle, and brain. Dual virus infections and possible bacterial-virus synergisms occur. Until enteroviruses had been repeatedly documented in infants by isolations from pneumonic lungs, the prevalent opinion was that they did not produce pneumonias. The same healthy skepticism exists concerning etiologic associations of enterovirus infections and chronic myocardiopathies, and certain congenital malformations. Firm evidence for an enterovirus cause of chronic coxsackievirus B3 dilated-type cardiomyopathy and coxsackievirus B4 transmural myocardial infarction (sometimes with ventricular aneurysms), at least in a murine model, has now been established. Tissue histocompatibility as well as the age of the host (human or experimental animal model) is apparently critical to the expression of enterovirus disease.

CHARACTERISTICS OF ENTEROVIRUSES The enterovirus group is icosahedral-shaped, with a particle diameter of 17 to 30 nm and a ribonucleic acid core surrounded by a capsid of protein. Enteroviruses share about 20 percent of their nucleotide sequences, while within a grouping such as coxsackievirus B, there is 30 to 50 percent homology among types. The subunit structure of the outer protein capsid (capsomere) determines species, tissue, and age specificities for infection, as well as antigenicity. The RNA of the virus within infected cells transcribes and translates its own genetic information independent of the DNA (deoxyribonucleic acid) of the host. Enteroviruses are quite stable in acid and lipid solvents. They can be protected from thermal inactivation by certain cations.

When inoculated into suckling mice, group A coxsackieviruses induce primarily inflammation and necrosis of skeletal muscle, whereas group B viruses cause lesions of the central nervous system and other viscera, but only focal muscular involvement. Coxsackieviruses B and echoviruses are cytopathogenic for cultures of monkey kidney cells, but this is not the case for coxsackieviruses of group A. These distinctions are not without exception. Some strains of echoviruses, types 6 and 9, have been adapted to produce lesions in baby mice, the former in viscera and the latter in skeletal muscles. Some strains agglutinate human erythrocytes obtained from adults or umbilical cords at the time of delivery. None of the coxsackieviruses or echoviruses has been adapted to grow in embryonated eggs.

EPIDEMIOLOGY Fecal-oral contact is the usual method of transmission. Personal hygiene (particularly hand washing) inhibits the infectious cycle. Toddlers often bring enteroviruses into a household. Insects, including flies and mosquitoes, may act as passive vectors. Echovirus, type 6, may multiply in the gastrointestinal tracts of dogs. This has not been noted with other coxsackieviruses or echoviruses, and with echovirus 6 canine-to-human transmission has not been demonstrated. Respiratory transmission by droplets or their nuclei also occurs.

The incubation period is 2 to 5 days. Multiple concurrent infections within a family are not unusual. Clinical manifestations of infection vary within the family and community. For example, a 2- to 3-year-old child may have a mild fever with rash, while an older sibling may have pleurodynia, myocarditis, or one of a number of syndromes heralding involvement of the central nervous system (Table 205-2). The mechanism of the varied expression of enterovirus disease is not well understood but may relate in part to developmental changes in the number or availability of specific receptors on the surfaces of susceptible cells.

Enterovirus infections are most common during the summer. During infection 10 to 300 million TCD_{50}[1] of virus may be excreted daily into the stool. Following infection, even an asymptomatic person may excrete fecal virus for 3 to 4 weeks. Prevalence is mirrored by virus isolations from samples of sewage. Serotypes present in a community vary from year to year.

[1] *Mean tissue culture dose.*

TABLE 205-2
Illnesses (or syndromes) associated with coxsackievirus, echovirus, or enterovirus infections

	Coxsackievirus types			
	Group A	*Group B*	*Echovirus types*	*New enterovirus types*
I No illness (probably 75% of cases)	1–24	1–6	1–8,* 11–34	69
II Mild or moderate illness				
A Undifferentiated mild febrile illness (nonspecific)	1–24	1–6	1–8, 11–34	
B Upper respiratory syndromes (rhinitis, pharyngitis, including herpangina and lymphonodular pharyngitis, conjunctivitis)	1–10, 16, 21, 22, 24†	1–5	1, 3, 6, 9, 11, 16, 19, 20, 28	70
C Laryngotracheitis	9	5	11	
D Exanthems (various)	5, 9, 16	3, 5	2, 4, 5, 6, 9, 11, 16	
E Lymphadenitis, with or without splenomegaly	5, 6, 9	5	4, 9, 16, 20	
F Pleurodynia (sometimes with pleural effusion)	4, 6, 10	1–5	1, 6, 9	
G Orchitis		1–5	9	
H Gastroenteritis	9	3, 4	2, 3, 6–9, 11–14, 18, 19, 22–24	
I Acute myositis, rhabdomyolysis, myoglobinuria			2, 9	
III Severe or life-threatening illness				
A Hepatitis	4, 9	5	4, 9	
B Hemolytic-uremic syndrome	4	4		
C Pneumonia	9	1, 4	3, 8, 9, 19, 20	68
D Diabetes mellitus‡		4		
E Cardiac				
1 Myocarditis/pericarditis	1, 2, 4, 5, 7, 8, 9, 16	1–6	1, 4, 6, 7, 9, 11, 14, 16, 19, 22, 25, 30	
2 Chronic myocardiopathy		2, 4, 5		
3 Subendocardial fibroelastosis‡		3		
4 Endocardial deformities		4		
5 Constrictive pericarditis		1, 2		
6 Congenital malformations‡	9	3, 4		
F Neurologic				
1 Aseptic meningitis/encephalitis including variants such as hemichorea	7, 9, 16	1–5	1–9, 11–23, 25, 30–32	71
2 Acute cerebellar ataxia	3, 4			
3 Benign intracranial hypertension				
4 Transverse myelitis				
5 Postencephalitic parkinsonism				
6 Guillain-Barré syndrome‡				

* *Asymptomatic infection is common with echovirus, type 9. Variation in attack rates among types (and strains of a single type) occurs.*
† *Coxsackievirus A, type 21, is also known as Coe virus.*
‡ *Suggested (and probable), but cause not established.*

The level of immunity of a population as reflected by the prevalence of type-specific neutralizing antibodies in serums apparently determines the likelihood of infection by a particular enterovirus. In an individual usually one enterovirus multiplies within the intestine at any one time. Vaccination with attenuated polioviruses has virtually eliminated these interfering agents, and there may be a real increase in infections due to coxsackieviruses or echoviruses. Improved hygiene and urbanization have led to an "epidemiologic shift" from infants to adults. On the basis of intrahousehold spread, infectivity of coxsackieviruses is fairly high (76 percent of exposed susceptibles and 25 percent of immunes). For echoviruses, apparent infectivity is substantially lower (43 percent of susceptibles) and immune contacts are rarely infected. At least 49 percent of coxsackievirus and 55 percent of echovirus infections are subclinical.

An interesting correlate has been a seasonal incidence of new cases of insulin-dependent diabetes mellitus in patients under 30 years old. This autumn peak has been correlated with an annual prevalence for coxsackievirus B4, but does not relate to other virus infections. Recent epidemiologic studies show that there is no family history of diabetes mellitus in cases of juvenile onset. These cases show a predilection for certain HLA types, and pathologically, lymphocytes are found in their destroyed pancreatic islets. These data are consistent with, but do not prove, an infectious cause for juvenile diabetes. Coxsackievirus B4 has been isolated at autopsy from the pancreas of a previously well 10-year-old boy admitted to the hospital in diabetic ketoacidosis within 3 days of onset of symptoms of a flu-like illness. Adult-onset diabetes mellitus has a strong familial clustering and appears to be inherited.

VIRUS ISOLATION Primary multiplication occurs in epithelial and paraepithelial lymphatic cells of the pharynx. During this early period of infection the patient may be asymptomatic or have mild malaise, sore throat, or low-grade fever. Slightly later virus multiplies in the intestine. If a critical virus concentration within the pharynx results, viremia follows. During the viremic phase the patient is asymptomatic. Secondary foci of virus multiplication may occur in various tissues (skin, muscle, heart, nervous system, etc.). Major illness of moderate to serious severity sometimes results (Table 205-2). Occasionally (especially during infancy) aspiration of pharyngeal virus leads to lower respiratory infection.

Virus may be isolated from the throat during the minor illness and for as long as a week thereafter. Virus shedding may persist in feces for weeks. Viremia can be documented during the incubation period until type-specific neutralizing antibodies appear.

PROTECTIVE RESPONSES AND SEROLOGIC DIAGNOSIS Intracellular virus multiplication immediately stimulates the interferon system to produce both α (Le, leukocyte) interferon (IFN) and β (fibroblast, epithelial) IFN from within the infected cells (see Chap. 196). About 3 days after the onset of infection specific antibodies appear in saliva and serum. These immunoglobulins combine with extracellular virus to limit spread of virus. Virus-antibody complexes are eliminated by phagocytosis.

Secretory immunoglobulins which are uniquely resistant to the natural proteases in saliva and succus entericus are in the IgA class, while the earliest antibodies to appear in serum are IgM. Both species of macromolecules have complement-fixing and neutralizing qualities. Within 3 to 4 weeks complement-fixing antibodies reach their peak and decline. Neutralizing antibodies of higher avidity (IgG) replace the IgM molecule about 2 weeks after the onset of infection. IgG antibodies persist and provide permanent type-specific immunity.

This information is important in diagnosis, because IgM molecules, recognizable immunologically by specific immunofluorescent or ELISA techniques, are susceptible to reduction and resultant biologic inactivation with sulfhydryl active compounds such as 2-mercaptoethanol (2-ME). IgG immunoglobulins are resistant to 2-ME.

IgG antibodies to coxsackieviruses and echoviruses traverse the placenta freely. IgM immunoglobulins do not. IgA antibodies in colostrum and milk are not absorbed, but apparently provide some local protection in the intestines of nursing babies. Passively acquired type-specific antibodies in serums protect the newborn from viremia and disseminated infection such as disseminated perinatal infection with various coxsackieviruses, belonging to group B, and with echovirus, type 11, for 3 to 6 months. Since the half-life of IgG immunoglobulins is about 3 weeks, duration of firm neonatal immunity depends upon initial titers of the transferred antibodies. Passively acquired antibodies inhibit active synthesis of immunoglobulins, and also may not protect the respiratory tract. Active synthesis of secretory antibody in saliva and nasal secretions is required for local protection. The role of cellular immunity in enterovirus infections remains to be fully defined, but there are examples like coxsackievirus B3 murine cardiomyopathy in which neutralizing antibodies inhibit virus replication. Cytotoxic T lymphocytes responding to a virus-induced, but nonvirion, neomyocardial antigen augment the pathologic changes.

A fourfold rise in neutralizing antibodies or an IgM titer which is similarly diminished by 2-ME indicates recent infection. When applicable, hemagglutination inhibition tests are simpler, and the results parallel those obtained in more cumbersome neutralization tests. Specific IgM, IgA, and IgG ELISA tests are now being more widely applied in the diagnosis of enterovirus infections. Complement-fixing antibodies to enteroviruses are not type-specific. Many cross-reactions render these tests less useful.

The neutralizing antibody response is highly type-specific in primary or initial enterovirus infections. In subsequent infections heterotypic responses occur with increasing frequency; they presumably arise from a booster effect of the current infecting virus on the level of antibodies to other types with which the individual has previously been infected. Levels of heterotypic antibody frequently exceed the level of homotypic antibody. Neutralizing antibodies to group B coxsackievirus, types 1 to 5, are frequently found in titers of 1:64 to 1:512 in patients without evidence of current coxsackievirus infections (Table 196-4).

OTHER LABORATORY FINDINGS Enterovirus infections are usually acute processes, and persistent or chronic infections are unusual [e.g., chronic myopathy (coxsackievirus A9) or chronic coxsackievirus B3 heart disease. In congenital agammaglobulinemias, chronic aseptic meningitis with persistence of enteroviruses in CSF for months occurs]. Hence, changes in concentrations of hemoglobin, albumin, or globulins are unusual. Occasionally hemolysis occurs (see "Group A Coxsackievirus Infections" and "Echovirus Infections," further on in this chapter). White blood cell counts and the erythrocyte sedimentation rates are only mildly elevated. If there is necrosis (e.g., liver, lung), a neutrophilic leukemoid reaction may be noted. Hyperbilirubinemia and elevated transaminase and alkaline phosphatase levels may be seen in cases of hepatitis. Albuminuria often occurs transiently, but hematuria is rare.

PROPHYLAXIS AND TREATMENT Antiviral chemotherapy is not available. The 71 antigenic varieties of coxsackieviruses and echoviruses make prophylaxis with a single vaccine impractical. Pooled human globulin contains enterovirus antibodies, but during serious infections administration usually is not helpful because immunoglobulin production is not impaired. However, in agammaglobulinemic syndromes, passive administration of plasma containing high titers of type-specific neutralizing antibodies has limited virus shedding. Most human enterovirus infections are mild, and globulin prophylaxis is not often warranted. As with poliomyelitis, tonsillectomy and other inoculations are probably best delayed during an outbreak of enterovirus disease. In a murine model of coxsackievirus B3 myocarditis, virus was isolated in higher titer from hearts of mice vigorously exercised daily by swimming, and a benign myocarditis was transformed into a lethal infection. Rest is the cornerstone of symptomatic therapy.

It has been repeatedly shown in experimental animals that during the acute phase of infection administration of steroids appreciably increases the quantity of virus in tissues and the degree of ensuing injury. Corticosteroids also depress cell-mediated immune functions, interferon and antibody synthesis, and leukocyte migration to the area of injury. Therefore at least during the acute phase of enterovirus infections, steroids are contraindicated. Pregnancy may be associated with enhanced susceptibility to these and other infections. Alcohol, cold temperature, and chronic undernutrition are also associated with an increased virulence of coxsackievirus and perhaps other virus infections. Alcohol depresses phagocytic function. Malnutrition suppresses T and B lymphocytes, early mononuclear cell migration, and interferon production.

GROUP A COXSACKIEVIRUS INFECTIONS

Group A coxsackieviruses cause herpangina, lymphonodular pharyngitis, upper and lower respiratory disease, cutaneous eruptions, hepatitis, aseptic meningitis, paralytic disease, including acute infantile hemiplegia and unilateral oculomotor palsy, myopericarditis, and some sudden unexpected deaths in infancy. A chronic myopathy in an 11-year-old girl has been associated with coxsackievirus A9. Picornavirus-like particles were seen on electron microscopy, and virus was isolated from the diaphragm at autopsy. Pharyngeal multiplication may induce infection of superficial vessels or diffuse moderate erythema. Purulent exudate is not seen. More characteristic is *herpangina,* a common febrile illness characterized by small papular, vesicular, or ulcerative lesions on the anterior pillars, soft palate, tonsils, pharyngeal mucous membrane, and posterior part of the buccal mucosa. Herpangina has been seen during infections with coxsackieviruses, group A, types 1 to 10, 16, and 22. Vesicular lesions of herpangina have also been described in patients with illnesses due to coxsackieviruses, group B, types 1 to 5, and echoviruses, types 9, 11, and 17. Coxsackievirus A10 may induce *acute lymphonodular pharyngitis.* Lesions here are raised, discrete, white to yellow 3- to 6-mm papules surrounded by a zone of erythema. All the papules appear at the same time; they do not ulcerate, and they occur on the uvula, anterior pillars, and posterior pharynx. Large outbreaks of mild to severe conjunctivitis have been caused by coxsackievirus A24. Typically, rapid onset of swelling of the eyelids, lacrimation, preauricular adenopathy and, in some cases, a mucopurulent discharge occur.

Coxsackievirus A21 (Coe virus) is predominantly a respiratory pathogen, being regularly isolated from the throat and occasionally from feces. It has been associated with several outbreaks of an illness resembling the common cold in military recruits.

The first enterovirus etiologically implicated in pneumonia was coxsackievirus A9. Subsequently, a number of other enteroviruses have been implicated (Table 205-2). Fatal cases have occurred in infants or young children. Hyperpnea, cyanosis, hyperpyrexia, leukocytosis (or leukemoid reactions), and subsequently coma have been characteristic. Interstitial diffuse polylobed bronchopneumonia with alternate areas of atelectasis and emphysema have been found. Microscopically mixed alveolar septal infiltration without necrosis or formation of giant cells is seen.

A striking cutaneous vesicular eruption, *hand-foot-and-mouth disease,* has repeatedly been associated with infections due to coxsackievirus, group A, type 16. Infants and children with coxsackievirus, group A, type 4 (also coxsackievirus B14) infections have been described with respiratory or gastrointestinal symptoms, acute renal disease, thrombocytopenia, and hemolytic anemia. Reticulocytosis, albuminuria, and hematuria accompany this constellation of findings, which has been described as the *hemolytic-uremic syndrome.* Aseptic meningitis with occasional paralytic disease (especially with A7) also occurs. Acute myopericarditis has been associated with infections with coxsackievirus A, types 1, 2, 5, 8, 9, and 16; there are firmer etiologic data for coxsackievirus, types 4 and 16. One estimate suggests that 23 percent of acute virus myocarditis may be caused by coxsackievirus A. A significantly greater incidence of infection with coxsackievirus, group A, type 9, has been reported in mothers of infants with congenital heart disease.

GROUP B COXSACKIEVIRUS INFECTIONS

Infections with group B coxsackieviruses cause a number of upper respiratory syndromes, exanthems, diarrheas, pleurodynia, orchitis (with subsequent atrophy), pneumonia, hemolytic-uremic syndrome, and cardiac and central nervous system disease. Pleurodynia and cardiac disease due to enteroviruses were first associated with this group of enteroviruses (Table 205-2). In 1965 the Public Health Service (Britain) reported 1160 coxsackievirus B5 infections. Gastroenteritis (90 percent), aseptic meningitis (31 percent), myalgia and Bornholm's disease (23 percent), respiratory disorders (15 percent), and cardiomyopathies (5 percent) were included. There were 41 patients with pericarditis and 5 with myocarditis. Of 6 deaths, 2 each were due to neurologic, respiratory, or cardiac cause. During infancy, the mortality rate of patients with acute infectious myocarditis approaches 50 percent. Many of these infections are perinatal and are associated with mild or asymptomatic infection of the mother at about term. The mode of spread from mother to neonate has not been established, but enteroviruses have been recovered from the mother's vagina at these times. A number of epidemic perinatal echovirus 11 infections have been prevalent recently (some of them with infant death).

PLEURODYNIA (EPIDEMIC MYALGIA, BORNHOLM'S DISEASE, DEVIL'S GRIP) Prodromal symptoms of malaise, sore throat, and anorexia are interrupted by increasing debility, fever, and sudden onset of muscle, pleuritic, and abdominal pain. Pain is sharp, severe, and paroxysmal over the lower ribs or substernal area. It is accentuated by moving, breathing, coughing, sneezing, and hiccuping, and may be referred to the shoulders, neck, or scapulae. Pain and spasm of anterior abdominal muscles occur in about half the cases, often in combination with chest pain. Muscle tenderness is usually not prominent, but some patients complain of intense cutaneous hyperesthesia and paresthesia over the affected area. The illness usually lasts 3 to 7 days, but relapses may occur. Among differential diagnoses are myocardial infarction and acute surgical conditions of the abdomen. Coxsackieviruses B have been isolated from striated muscles of patients with pleurodynia during epidemics. Occasionally pleuritis is accompanied by effusion, and virus has been isolated from pleural fluid. Bornholm's disease may occur at any age but is most common in children and young adults.

Early in the course of illness, meningitis, myocarditis, or hepatitis may ensue. Liver biopsy in patients with complicating jaundice shows subacute portal triaditis and intense cloudy swelling of central-zone hepatocytes. A late complication is orchitis, occurring in 3 to 5 percent of patients with pleurodynia during relapse.

CARDIAC DISEASE Acute myocarditis may be caused by coxsackieviruses of groups A and B as well as echoviruses. Infections with strains of coxsackievirus, group B, have been both most frequent and severe. When congenital or neonatal infection occurs, the course is often rapidly fatal, with concomitant myocarditis, encephalitis, hepatitis, and sometimes adrenal necrosis. Later in childhood or in adult life the heart and pericardium more frequently are involved as the single site of disease. Cardiac inflammation varies in intensity and degree of muscle necrosis. Pericarditis may dominate the clinical presentation, with myalgia, fever, precordial pain, friction rub, and even cardiac tamponade. There may be prominent signs of myocarditis with focal areas of transmural myocardial necrosis or patchy diffuse nontransmural lesions. There may be acute myocardial failure or arrhythmias. Illnesses may be self-limited and recovery complete. However, of 22 episodes of acute virus myocarditis associated with infections due to coxsackieviruses, group B, 12 patients developed chronic heart disease. Strict bed rest until all electrocardiographic changes have reverted to normal (or are stationary) is indicated. This may require 4 to 6 weeks. Since steroids increase virulence of coxsackievirus B myocarditis in mice, they are contraindicated. Some infections may heal with significant myocardial scarring.

Coxsackievirus particles have been localized along tubules of the sarcoplasmic reticulum in infected mice with myocarditis. There is epidemiologic evidence associating coxsackievirus B, types 3 and 4, with congenital heart disease. Most of such infections in pregnant mothers have been subclinical and occur in the first trimester. Transplacental enterovirus viremia has been documented. Suggestive evidence indicates that the following conditions may be caused by infections with coxsackieviruses belonging to group B: chronic continuing cardiomyopathies (B2, B4, B5); congenital calcific pancarditis (B3); and constrictive pericarditis (B1 and B2), with or without superior or inferior vena caval obstruction.

The possible courses and pathogenesis of coxsackievirus acute and chronic heart disease has been extensively studied in mice. It is likely that the similarity to humans is great. Coxsackieviruses affect the myocardium and pericardium, but there is no conclusive evidence to support the occurrence of a murine virus valvulitis. Coxsackievirus A9 induces an interstitial myocarditis in adult mice healing without scar. On the other hand, coxsackievirus B1 and B4 produce transmural necrotizing myocarditis in baby mice. Ventricular aneurysms have followed. There is suggestive but not definitive serologic evidence in humans that some "myocardial infarctions" may be, in reality, a transmural myocarditis. Careful prospective matched case control studies in humans are needed to establish or negate this important question. In weanling mice coxsackievirus B3 causes an immunopathic, cytolytic, T-lymphocyte–induced necrotizing myocarditis leading, over the course of months, to chronic heart disease resembling the dilated type of primary myocardial disease in humans. In coxsackievirus B3 chronic heart disease, extensive fibrosis at the atrioventricular node, enlarged atria with thrombi within, suggest that atrial arrythmias had been present. In these murine animal models the coronary arteries are normal. Constrictive pericarditis with or without superior or inferior vena caval obstruction, endocardial fibroelastosis, and congestive heart failure are other sequelae. The frequency of these illnesses in humans remains a major epidemiologic problem requiring resolution.

ECHOVIRUS INFECTIONS

Echovirus-like coxsackievirus infections may be asymptomatic or mild, moderate, or life-threatening (Table 205-2). Mild to moderate are undifferentiated fevers, upper respiratory infections, various rashes, pleurodynia, and diarrheas. Pneumonia, myopericarditis, hemolytic-uremic syndromes, perinatal infections, and neurologic involvement may be quite serious. They do not differ from similar illnesses caused by coxsackieviruses.

Enterovirus 70 is the most widespread of the enterovirus types. It causes highly contagious infections which became pandemic in 1969 to 1971. After a 24-h incubation period, enterovirus 70 causes acute subconjunctional hemorrhagic conjunctivitis. The lesion may be discrete petechial to large and blotchy and covers the bulbar conjunctiva. Corneal involvement may occur but is transient. In certain parts of the world, notably southeast Asia and India, but not the United States, the conjunctivitis caused by enterovirus 70 has been followed by a neurological syndrome characterized by acute hypotonic, areflexic, asymmetrical proximal paralysis of the legs and, less commonly, isolated cranial nerves and arms. The diagnosis may be difficult, particularly if the conjunctivitis and paralysis are widely separated in time, and requires a rise in neutralization test titers.

ASEPTIC MENINGITIS (See Chap. 360) There may be a mild prodromal malaise, but major illness usually begins with fever, headache, and stiff neck. Papilledema and Kernig's and Brudzinski's signs may be present. Localizing sensory or motor deficits are unusual. Confusion and delirium are common. These acute findings may persist for 4 to 7 days. Cerebrospinal pleocytosis is usually less than 500 cells per cubic millimeter. Early, there may be as many as 90 percent polymorphonuclear leukocytes, but within 48 h the cellular response becomes completely mononuclear. Persistence of polymorphonuclear leukocytes in the cerebrospinal fluid suggests pyogenic meningitis or intracerebral, subdural, or epidural abscess. Gram's stain and appropriate spinal fluid cultures must be done to exclude bacterial meningitis, tuberculosis, or mycotic meningitis. Protein concentration in the cerebrospinal fluid is moderately elevated, but glucose is normal. Early in the illness echoviruses may be isolated from spinal fluid. It usually takes several weeks before the cerebrospinal fluid reverts to normal. In hypo- or agammaglobulinemic syndromes echoviruses have persisted in CSF for weeks to months.

For attempts at virus isolation, throat and rectal swabs, serum, and cerebrospinal fluid should be collected as early in the course as possible (Table 196-3). Acute and convalescent serums should be studied for rises in type-specific neutralizing or ELISA antibodies.

It is not possible to distinguish clinically between aseptic meningitis due to various enteroviruses and mumps. Localizing findings, hemiplegia, prolonged fevers, oculogyric crises, coma, and bloody spinal fluid favor the diagnosis of herpes simplex virus encephalitis (see Chap. 210). Although echovirus aseptic meningitis most often is self-limited and recovery in persons afflicted after the first year of life complete, about 10 percent of patients have more serious involvement of the central nervous system. Minor muscle weakness with reflex changes may persist for weeks to months, but over 90 percent of patients recover completely within a year. Occasionally, choreiform movements, ataxia, nystagmus, transverse myelitis, Guillain-

Barré syndrome, coma, bulbar involvement, and death result.

As with coxsackieviruses, intact B lymphocytes are required for eradication of echovirus infections. Persistent echovirus infection of the central nervous system has been documented by the presence of echoviruses types 5, 30, 19, 9, and 33, which have been recovered for from 2 months to 3 years in five patients with congenital agammaglobulinemias. Additionally, three of the patients had a dermatitis-like syndrome.

POLIOVIRUS INFECTIONS

Enteric infection with the enteroviruses, poliovirus types 1, 2, or 3, is entirely analogous to other similar infections with coxsackieviruses or echoviruses. The unique aspect of poliomyelitis is the predilection of these three viruses for the anterior horn cells of the spinal cord and motor nuclei of the cranial nerves. Nervous tissues necessary for sensation are uninvolved.

ETIOLOGY Three distinct antigenic types have been defined: type 1 (Brunhilde), type 2 (Lansing), and type 3 (Leon). Natural infection leads to type-specific immunity with long-lasting neutralizing antibodies which can be measured in serum.

EPIDEMIOLOGY AND PATHOGENESIS The occurrence, distribution, and pathogenesis (including incubation period) of polioviruses are similar to those of coxsackieviruses and echoviruses. Prior to vaccine prophylaxis with oral attenuated viruses, these were extraordinarily common agents with peaks in prevalence from July through September. Live attenuated vaccine eliminates polioviruses from feces and sewage, but the formalinized killed vaccine, which prevents viremia and neurologic illness, does not limit asymptomatic enteric infection. In countries with poor sanitation, infection and occasional disease occur early in life leading to the designation "infantile paralysis." Physical exertion increases the risk of clinically apparent or paralytic poliomyelitis.

VIRUS ISOLATION AND PROTECTIVE RESPONSES (See Chap. 196) Like coxsackieviruses and echoviruses, polioviruses can be recovered from the throat or feces during the first week of infection. The blood is also positive for virus during the incubation period. In fatal cases polioviruses are easily recovered from affected brain or spinal cord. In aseptic meningitis (nonparalytic poliomyelitis) caused by polioviruses, virus is rarely recovered from cerebrospinal fluid (CSF). This is in contradistinction to the aseptic meningitis syndrome caused by coxsackieviruses or echoviruses in which these viruses are easily recovered from CSF. Long-lasting immunity is mirrored by the presence of serum-neutralizing antibody, which also follows natural infection with wild viruses.

CLINICAL MANIFESTATIONS Infections with polioviruses types 1, 2, or 3 may induce inapparent infection (95 percent of cases), undifferentiated febrile illness (minor illness), aseptic meningitis, or paralytic disease. Recovery is complete except in paralytic disease.

Necrosis and loss of motor nerve cells in any area of the spinal cord, brain, or cranial nerves causes various muscle paralyses. The precentral gyrus, reticular formation of the medulla, the cerebellum, Auerbach's and Meissner's plexuses, and sympathetic ganglia are frequently affected. Bulbospinal poliomyelitis is very serious.

Disease begins with fever and "minor illness." Classically, after several days, symptoms disappear. In 5 to 10 days fever recurs, and signs of meningeal irritation and paralysis ensue. Cramping muscle pain and spasm as well as coarse twitching in affected parts follows. In children younger than 5 years, paralysis of one leg is most common. In patients 5 to 15 years of age, weakness of one arm or paraplegia is most frequent, while in adults quadriplegia is common. Urinary bladder and respiratory muscle dysfunction are also frequent in adults. Inoculations of vaccines are associated with involvement of the muscles around the site of injection.

Tendon reflexes are diminished or absent. Sensation is intact, separating poliomyelitis from the Guillain-Barré syndrome. Paralysis due to heavy metal poisoning, on the other hand, may be more difficult to distinguish clinically from poliomyelitis.

Among paralytic cases, 6 to 25 percent may be bulbar. Tonsilloadenoidectomies should not be done during epidemics of poliomyelitis for 85 percent of patients under these circumstances develop bulbar disease. Myocarditis, hypertension, pulmonary edema, shock, nosocomial gram-negative or staphylococcal pneumonias, urinary tract infections, and emotional problems are among the complications of severe paralytic disease. Treatment is supportive. About 2 to 5 percent of children and 15 to 30 percent of adults with paralyzing infection die. Initially paralyzed muscles usually recover some function, gradually improving over 1 to 2 years.

PREVENTION Poliovirus vaccines, used widely since the introduction of inactivated polio vaccine (IPV), have dramatically reduced the incidence of poliomyelitis in the United States. In 1954 there were more than 18,000 new cases, but there were only 8 in 1976. The risk of poliomyelitis is generally very small in the United States today, but epidemics are certain to recur if the population's immunity is not sustained. Thirty-eight percent of 1- to 4-year-old children have not had primary vaccination against poliomyelitis! In disadvantaged urban and rural areas vaccination rates are even lower. It is essential to immunize all children beginning in infancy.

A Canadian product, inactivated poliovirus vaccine (IPV), is being marketed in the United States. It produces immunity in more than 90 percent of recipients. The vaccine is given by injection and can be administered simultaneously with diphtheria, tetanus, and pertussis antigens. Children or adults with immunodeficiency diseases or altered immune states who are at risk of exposure to poliomyelitis should receive IPV. An antibody response cannot be assured in these immunodepressed persons, but some protection probably results. Four doses are given, the first three at 1- to 2-month intervals and the fourth 6 to 12 months after the third injection. If adults are traveling to areas where poliomyelitis is present, or if they are exposed to vaccine virus following routine immunization of their children, IPV may be given. Except for the possibility of hypersensitivity reactions to the trace amounts of streptomycin and neomycin in IPV, there are no associated risks.

Trivalent oral poliovaccine (TOPV) combines all three strains of polioviruses. Full primary vaccination produces immunity in more than 90 percent of recipients. It is the preferred poliovirus vaccine in the United States. In rare instances oral polio vaccine has been associated temporally with paralytic diseases in vaccine recipients or their close contacts. Of 193 million doses of TOPV, 55 "vaccine associated" cases have been reported. Primary immunization for infants (6 to 12 weeks old), children, and adolescents through age 18 is three doses, the first followed in 6 to 8 weeks by the second, and the third 8 to 12 months later. Routine polio vaccination for adults living in this country is not necessary. A susceptible adult at increased risk of exposure to infection because of travel to an area where poliomyelitis is common should receive complete primary immunization with IPV or TOPV. Supplementary single doses of TOPV should be given to children upon entering school and at the age of 11 or 12. There is no evidence that a pregnant woman or her fetus is at greater risk from TOPV than other persons. Persons with immunodeficiency or altered immune states should not receive TOPV because of the increased risk of vaccine-associated paralysis. These conditions include combined immunodeficiency, hypogammaglobulinemia, agammaglobulinemia, leukemia, lymphoma, generalized malignancy, or lowered resistance from therapy with corticosteroids, alkylating or antimetabolic drugs, or radiation.

REOVIRUS INFECTIONS

Reoviruses were discovered inadvertently in studies of the intestinal viral flora of healthy children and adults. They were initially classified as echovirus, type 10, but were later reclassified. They were named to emphasize their (1) *respiratory* or (2) *enteric* human origins, and their (3) *orphan* status.

Reoviruses are quite different from picornaviruses (Table 205-1). They are about $2\frac{1}{2}$ times larger (70 nm in diameter) and show icosahedral symmetry. Their RNA is unique in that it consists of 10 discrete double-stranded segments, each of which is in essence a distinct gene and is resistant to ribonuclease. The protein capsid consists of an inner core and 92 outer shell capsomeres. The capsid is composed of seven species of polypeptides. Unlike those of enteroviruses, reovirus cytopathic effects are nonlytic. Reoviruses multiply in primate and nonprimate tissue cultures. The particles hemagglutinate human or avian erythrocytes. The hemagglutinin encoded in the S1 gene has been shown to be a virulence factor. On the basis of tests of hemagglutination inhibition antibodies (HIA) with type-specific serums, there are three serotypes.

Human infections with reoviruses are common, and their distribution is worldwide. Like coxsackieviruses and echoviruses, reoviruses spread by enteric and respiratory routes. Fifty to eighty percent of adults in the western hemisphere have had reovirus infections, as measured by the presence of persisting neutralizing or hemagglutinating antibodies. Infections are more frequent in winter but occur in every season. Reoviruses have been isolated from human nasal secretions, posterior pharyngeal and rectal swabs, spinal fluid, brain, and lung. In addition, reovirus isolations or serologic data indicate that natural infections occur in cattle, dogs, cats, mice, horses, swine, birds, and monkeys. Although animal-to-human transmission has never been demonstrated, its possibility is likely.

Widespread evidence of infection and few associations with disease indicate that most infections with reoviruses are asymptomatic. Isolations of virus and fourfold rises in HIA in individual patients with common colds, nonspecific febrile illness, exanthem, and diarrhea suggest an etiologic role in some instances. Provocative data came from three thoroughly studied fatal cases of encephalitis, myocarditis, hepatitis, or interstitial pneumonia. In these patients reoviruses and no other bacterial or viral pathogens have been isolated.

VIRAL GASTROENTERITIS

Within the past decade, with the use of electron microscopic examination of diarrheal specimens of feces and the institution of specific radioimmunoassays, fluorescent antibody and ELISA IgM, IgG, and IgA tests for antibodies in serum, viral gastroenteritis in its epidemic and endemic forms has been effectively studied.

Viral gastroenteritis is the second leading cause of illness in the United States. In the chronically malnourished, the elderly, and in debilitated persons, death may result. Immune electron microscopic examination of virus particles isolated from fecal specimens has uncovered two major virus groups, rotaviruses and parvoviruses (see Table 196-1), which cause viral gastroenteritis.

Parvoviruses and rotaviruses (also called human reovirus-like agents, HRLA) multiply in the small bowel to titers of 10^8 organisms per gram of feces. The viruses can be seen on electron microscopy or recognized by counterimmunoelectrophoresis of fecal filtrates. Neither human rotaviruses nor parvoviruses are easily grown in tissue cultures, and related animal viruses sharing serologic specificity are used in tests for antibodies in serum for rotaviruses. Purified virus preparations from infected human feces are used to prepare parvovirus antigens. The Nebraska calf diarrhea virus can be used as an antigen for tests of rotavirus antibody rises. Clearly, however, the presence of IgG antibodies in serum does not confer immunity for the bowel.

It has been shown that in addition to local inflammation of epithelial cells of the small bowel and subsequent diarrhea, enteric viruses may rapidly enter the systemic circulation during the very early stages of infection before local symptoms occur. Early in experimental reovirus type 1 infection in mice, for instance, striking enlargement of Peyer's patches is noted along with rapid appearance of infectious virus in mesenteric lymph nodes. The M cells, a population of specialized epithelial cells that overlie Peyer's patches, are implicated in this transport of enteric viruses. Initial studies of immunoglobulin isotypes following rotavirus-induced diarrhea in humans indicate that fourfold diagnostic rises in ELISA-IgG antibodies in serums were observed by day 21 after infection, but similar rises in IgA serum antibody were present only after 42 days.

Rotaviruses are responsible for worldwide sporadic and epidemic outbreaks of gastroenteritis, usually occurring in the fall or winter in infants and young children 6 to 24 months old. By the time children in the United States are 2 years old, 50 to 90 percent of them have antibodies to HRLA. Rotaviruses are easily recognized in duodenal biopsies by electron microscopy and are seen as 70-nm particles with double-shelled capsids similar to those of reoviruses. On biopsy, the proximal small intestine shows shortened villi, and crypts are hyperplastic. Polymorphonuclear leukocytes and mononuclear cells infiltrate the lamina propria. Normally, columnar surface cells are vacuolated and cuboidal. During acute illness, a transient peripheral lymphopenia involving all lymphocyte subpopulations ensues.

In several outbreaks of traveler's diarrhea in adults, which is usually caused by enterotoxigenic *Escherichia coli* (see Chap. 142), rotaviruses have been implicated in about one-fourth of the cases.

Parvoviruses are primarily responsible for disease in adults and older children, while reovirus-like agents cause diarrhea in infants and young children. The attack rates for both infections may reach 50 percent, and the incubation period is about 48 h, so that explosive outbreaks are common. Diarrhea may persist for 5 to 8 days and be followed by steatorrhea. A malabsorption syndrome with abnormal xylose and lactose absorption follows for another week. Other viruses (e.g., echoviruses, types 1 or 18, or coronaviruses) may from time to time be involved in sporadic outbreaks of gastroenteritis, but their overall importance seems minor.

The Norwalk, Hawaii, and Montgomery County agents are parvoviruses named after the sites of their original epidemics, and are distinctive in that immunity to one of the agents does not confer protection against the others. Contaminated shellfish (oysters) and person-to-person spread have been implicated in explosive outbreaks associated with festive dinners on cruise ships. Delays in gastric emptying of liquids as well as small bowel peristaltic hyperfunction occur in parvoviral diarrhea. Although the number, weight, or water content of stools, and the extent and magnitude of viral excretion, are not altered, bismuth subsalicylate therapy was beneficial in a randomized double-blind study of 59 volunteers who received Norwalk agent orally because the severity and duration of abdominal cramps and median duration of gastrointestinal symptoms were shortened.

REFERENCES

General

GELFAND HM: Occurrence in nature of coxsackie and ECHO viruses. Prog Med Virol 3:193, 1961

KOGON A et al: The virus watch program: A continuing surveillance of viral infections in metropolitan New York families: VII. Observations on viral excretion, seroimmunity, intrafamilial spread and illness association in Coxsackie and echovirus infections. Am J Epidemiol 89:51, 1969

MELNICK JL: Enterovirus, in *Viral Infections of Humans, Epidemiology and Control,* AS Evans (ed). New York, Plenum, 1976, p 163

MORENS DM et al: Non-polio enterovirus disease in the United States, 1971–1975. Int J Epidemiol 8:49, 1979

Coxsackievirus A infection

CHALHUB EG et al: Coxsackie A9 focal encephalitis associated with acute infantile hemiplegia and porencephaly. Neurology 27:574, 1977

HUEBNER RJ et al: Herpangina: Etiological studies of a specific infectious disease. JAMA 145:628, 1951

LERNER AM et al: Infections due to coxsackievirus, group A, type 9, in Boston, 1959, with special reference to exanthems and pneumonia. N Engl J Med 163:1265, 1960

TANG TT et al: Chronic myopathy associated with coxsackievirus A9. A combined electron microscopical and viral isolation study. N Engl J Med 292:608, 1975

TANS DS et al: An outbreak of acute conjunctivitis caused by coxsackievirus A24 in Kuala Lumpur, Malaysia, 1978. Southeast Asian J Trop Med Public Health 11:24, 1980

Coxsackievirus B infection

BAIN HW et al: Epidemic pleurodynia (Bornholm's disease) due to coxsackie B 5 virus: The interrelationship of pleurodynia, benign pericarditis and aseptic meningitis. Pediatrics 27:889, 1961

EL-KHATIB MR et al: Coxsackievirus B4 myocarditis in mice: Valvular changes in virus infected and control animals. J Infect Dis 137:410, 1978

JOHNSON RT et al: Acute benign pericarditis: Virologic study of 34 patients. Arch Intern Med 108:828, 1961

KATZE MG, CROWELL RL: Indirect enzyme-linked immunosorbent assay (ELISA) for the detection of coxsackie-virus group B antibodies. J Gen Virol 48:225, 1980

KIBRICK S: Viral infections of the fetus and newborn. Perspect Virol Symp NY 2:140, 1961

LERNER AM: Myocarditis and pericarditis, in *Principles and Practice of Infectious Diseases,* GL Mandel et al (eds). New York, Wiley, 1979, chaps 55, 56

SAINANI GS et al: Adult heart disease due to Coxsackievirus B infection. Medicine 47:133, 1968

WOODRUFF J: Viral myocarditis: A review. Am J Pathol 101:425, 1980

YOON JW et al: Isolation of a virus from the pancreas of a child with diabetic ketoacidosis. N Engl J Med 300:1173, 1979

Echovirus and poliovirus infection

Neurovirulence of enterovirus 70 (Editorial). Lancet, Feb 13, 1982, p 373

HENDERSON DA et al: Paralytic disease associated with oral polio vaccines. JAMA 190:41, 1964

HORSTMANN DM, YAMADA N: Enterovirus infection of the central nervous system. Res Publ Assoc Res Nerv Ment Dis 44:236, 1968

JEHN UW, FINK MK: Myositis, myoglobinemia, and myoglobinuria associated with enterovirus echo 9 infection. Arch Neurol 37:457, 1980

JOSSELSON J et al: Acute rhabdomyolysis associated with an echovirus infection. Arch Intern Med 140:1671, 1980

MEASE PJ et al: Successful treatment of echovirus meningoencephalitis and myositis-fascitis with intravenous immune globulin therapy in a patient with x-linked agammaglobulinemia. N Engl J Med 304:1278, 1981

MODLIN JF: Fatal echovirus 11 disease in premature neonates. Pediatrics 66:775, 1980

PETERS AC et al: Echo 24 focal encephalitis and subacute hemichorea. Neurology 29:676, 1979

Poliomyelitis prevention. Recommendation of the Public Health Service Advisory Committee on Immunization Practices. Morb Mort Week Rep 26:329, 335, 1977

WEINSTEIN L: Diagnosis and treatment of poliomyelitis. Med Clin North Am 32:1377, 1948

Reovirus infection

EL-EAI FM, EVANS AS: Reovirus infections in children and young adults. Arch Environ Health 7:700, 1963

JOKLIK WK: The molecular biology of reovirus. J Cell Physiol 76:289, 1970

TILLOTSON JR, LERNER AM: Reovirus, type 3, associated with fatal pneumonia. N Engl J Med 276:1060, 1967

WEINER HL et al: Absolute linkage of virulence and central nervous system cell tropism of reoviruses to viral hemagglutinin. J Infect Dis 141:609, 1980

Viral gastroenteritis

BLACKLOW NR, CUKOR G: Viral gastroenteritis. N Engl J Med 304:397, 1981

GUNN RA et al: Norwalk virus gastroenteritis aboard a cruise ship: An outbreak on five consecutive cruises. Am J Epidemiol 112:820, 1980

LINCO SJ, GROHMANN GS: The Darwin outbreak of oyster-associated viral gastroenteritis. Med J Aust 1:211, 1980

MEEROFF JC et al: Abnormal gastric motor function in viral gastroenteritis. Ann Intern Med 9:370, 1980

MURPHY AM et al: An Australia-wide outbreak of gastroenteritis from oysters caused by Norwalk virus. Med J Aust 2:329, 1979

SHERIDAN JF et al: Traveler's diarrhea associated with rotavirus infection: Analysis of virus-specific immunoglobulin classes. Infect Immun 31:419, 1981

STEINHOFF MC: Bismuth subsalicylate therapy of viral gastroenteritis. Gastroenterology 78:1495, 1980

Viruses from shellfish (Editorial). Lancet 2:1224, 1979

WOLF JL et al: Intestinal M cells: A pathway for entry of reovirus into the host. Science 212:471, 1981

206 MUMPS

C. GEORGE RAY

DEFINITION Mumps is an acute communicable disease of viral origin characterized by painful enlargement of the salivary glands and sometimes by involvement of the gonads, meninges, pancreas, and other organs.

ETIOLOGY The causative agent of mumps is a paramyxovirus of intermediate size (90 to 250 nm in diameter). It has a tight helical inner core (RNA) enclosed in an outer envelope of lipid and protein. The virus of mumps causes in vitro agglutination of erythrocytes of fowl, human beings, and some other species, produces hemolysis, and has two components capable of fixing complement. These are the soluble, or S, antigens derived from the nucleocapsid, and the V antigen derived from the surface hemagglutinin. It elicits a delayed allergic reaction when used as an antigen in persons who have had mumps infection. The virus can be cultivated in chick embryos and in a variety of mammalian cell cultures, including HeLa, monkey kidney and human pancreatic beta cells.

EPIDEMIOLOGY Human beings are the only natural host for mumps. The disease is worldwide and is endemic in urban communities. Epidemics are relatively infrequent and are confined to closely associated groups who live in orphanages, army camps, or schools. The disease is most frequent in the spring, particularly during April and May. Although mumps is generally considered less "contagious" than measles and chickenpox, this difference may be more apparent than real because many mumps infections (at least 25 percent) tend to be inapparent clinically. In some surveys, 80 to 90 percent of an adult population had serologic evidence of previous infection with mumps. The incidence of mumps in the United States has reached its lowest point since reporting began in 1922; in 1977 there were 44.3 percent fewer cases than in 1976, in 1978 there were 21.5 percent fewer cases than in 1977, and in 1979 there were 16.6 percent fewer than in 1978.

Infections are rare before the age of 2 years and then increase rapidly in frequency, reaching a peak at ages 5 to 9. Clinical mumps may be more common in males than in females. In North American cities, most infections are contracted from schoolmates and infected family members. The virus is transmitted in infected salivary secretions, although its isolation from urine suggests that the virus may also spread via this route. Mumps virus is rarely isolated from stools. The saliva is infectious for approximately 6 days prior to the onset of parotitis, and virus has been recovered from this site for as long as 2 weeks after onset of parotid swelling. Viruria also persists for 2 to 3 weeks in some patients. Despite this prolonged secretion of virus, the peak of infectivity occurs a day or two before onset of parotitis and subsides rapidly after the appearance of glandular enlargement.

One attack of clinical or subclinical mumps confers lasting immunity, and second attacks are most unusual. Unilateral parotitis affords protection just as effectively as does bilateral disease.

PATHOGENESIS The virus enters via the respiratory route; during the incubation period of 15 to 21 days it presumably replicates in the upper respiratory tract and cervical lymph nodes, from which it is disseminated via the bloodstream to other organs, including the meninges, gonads, pancreas, breasts, thyroid, heart, liver, kidneys, and cranial nerves. The salivary adenitis is thought by many to be secondary to viremia, but primary spread from the respiratory tract has not been ruled out as an alternative mechanism.

MANIFESTATIONS Salivary adenitis The onset of typical parotitis is usually sudden, although it may be preceded by a prodromal period of malaise, anorexia, chilly sensations, feverishness, sore throat, and tenderness at the angle of the jaw. In many cases, however, parotid swelling is the first indication of illness. The glands enlarge progressively over a period of 1 to 3 days, and the swelling resolves within a week after maximal enlargement. The swollen gland extends from the ear to the lower portion of the mandibular ramus and to the inferior portion of the zygomatic arch, often displacing the ear upward and outward. The skin over the gland is usually not warm or erythematous, in contrast to what happens in bacterial parotitis. There may be reddening and pouting of the orifice of Stensen's duct. Usually, pain and tenderness are marked, although at times they are absent. The edema of mumps has been described as "gelatinous," and when the involved gland is tweaked, it rolls like jelly. Swelling may involve only the submaxillary and sublingual glands and may extend over the anterior part of the chest, producing *presternal edema.* Involvement of submaxillary glands alone can cause difficulty in distinguishing mumps from acute cervical adenitis. Swelling of the glottis occurs rarely but may require tracheostomy. Parotitis is bilateral in two-thirds of cases and remains confined to one side in the remainder. The second gland tends to swell as the first is subsiding, usually 4 to 5 days after onset. In general, parotitis is accompanied by a temperature of 100 to 103°F, malaise, headache, and anorexia, but systemic symptoms may be virtually absent, particularly in children. In most patients, the chief complaints refer to difficulty in eating, swallowing, and talking.

Epididymoorchitis Mumps is complicated by orchitis in 20 to 35 percent of postpubertal males. Testicular involvement usually appears 7 to 10 days after onset of parotitis, although it may precede it or appear simultaneously. Occasionally, orchitis occurs in the absence of parotitis. Gonadal involvement is bilateral in 3 to 17 percent of patients. Orchitis is heralded by recrudescence of malaise and appearance of chilly sensations, headache, nausea, and vomiting. Shaking chills and high fevers, with temperatures between 103 and 106°F, are frequent. The testicle becomes greatly swollen and acutely painful. The epididymis is often palpable as a swollen tender cord. Occasionally there may be epididymitis without orchitis. Swelling, pain, and tenderness persist for 3 to 7 days and gradually subside; lysis of fever usually parallels abatement of swelling. Occasionally, the temperature falls by crisis. Mumps orchitis is followed by progressive atrophy of the testicle in one-half the cases. Even after bilateral orchitis, sterility is unusual, provided no significant atrophy has taken place. However, if bilateral testicular atrophy occurs after mumps, sterility or subnormal sperm counts are quite common. Plasma testosterone levels are depressed during acute orchitis but return to normal with recovery. *Pulmonary infarction* has been noted to follow mumps orchitis. This may be the result of thrombosis of the veins in the prostatic and pelvic plexuses in association with the testicular inflammation. Priapism is a rare but painful complication of mumps orchitis.

Pancreatitis Pancreatic involvement is a potentially serious manifestation of mumps, which may rarely be complicated by shock or pseudocyst formation. It should be suspected in patients with abdominal pain and tenderness together with clinical or epidemiologic evidence of mumps. It is difficult to document, since hyperamylasemia, the hallmark of pancreatitis, is also often present in parotitis. Many times the symptoms resemble those of gastroenteritis, and it is conceivable that the high incidence of gastrointestinal symptoms seen in association with the mumps epidemic in Great Britain in 1961 was due to involvement of the pancreas. Although diabetes or pancreatic insufficiency rarely follows mumps pancreatitis, several children have developed "brittle" diabetes a few weeks after mumps.

Central nervous system involvement Nearly half the patients with mumps have an increased number of cells, usually lymphocytes, in the cerebrospinal fluid (CSF), although symptoms of meningitis, stiff neck, headache, and drowsiness are less common. In typical cases, the onset of overt central nervous system signs and symptoms occurs 3 to 10 days after the onset of parotitis; however, the onset has also been noted to develop prior to the parotitis or 2 to 3 weeks later. In approximately 30 to 40 percent of laboratory-proven cases, there is *no* associated salivary gland involvement at any time in the course of illness. The CSF protein is moderately elevated, and CSF glucose tends to be normal, although in as many as 10 percent of patients low CSF glucose concentrations, in the range of 20 to 50 mg/dl, may be seen. True encephalitis is unusual, although it is responsible for most of the central nervous system sequelae, including behavioral disturbances, headaches, seizures, deafness (usually unilateral), and visual disturbances. At least seven cases of aqueductal stenosis and hydrocephalus have been reported as possible late sequelae to mumps encephalitis, but the association remains unproven. Mumps should also be recognized as capable of presenting a picture of mild paralytic poliomyelitis; definition of the cause depends on isolation of virus or serologic confirmation of mumps in the absence of changing antibody titers to poliomyelitis viruses. Rarely, mumps may produce a transverse myelitis, cerebellar ataxia, or the Guillain-Barré syndrome. Mumps meningitis, without clinical encephalitis, is generally thought to be benign.

Other manifestations Mumps virus tends to involve glandular tissues; inflammation of the lacrimal glands, thymus, thyroid, breasts, and ovaries occurs occasionally. *Oophoritis* may be recognized by persistence of pain in the lower part of the abdomen and fever. It does not result in sterility. Mumps virus has been implicated in the causation of subacute thyroiditis; the diagnosis can be made serologically, and occasionally the virus can be isolated from the thyroid gland. Myxedema following mumps thyroiditis has been reported. Ocular manifestations of mumps include dacryadenitis, optic neuritis, keratitis, iritis, conjunctivitis, and episcleritis. Although these conditions may transiently interfere with vision, complete resolution is the rule. Mumps *myocarditis,* evidenced primarily by transient abnormalities in the electrocardiogram, is relatively common. On rare occasions it can be fatal but it does not usually produce symptomatic disease or impair cardiac function. Similarly, *hepatic* involvement may be manifested by mild abnormalities in liver function, but icterus and other clinical signs of hepatic damage are extremely rare. *Thrombocytopenic purpura* as a complication of mumps has been described, and an occasional patient has a leukemoid reaction involving predominantly lymphocytes. Tracheobronchitis and interstitial pneumonia have also been associated with mumps infection, particularly among young children.

A rare but interesting manifestation of mumps is *polyarthritis* which is often migratory. It is most common in males between the ages of 20 and 30. Joint symptoms begin 1 to 2 weeks after subsidence of parotitis; usually the large joints are involved. The illness lasts 1 to 6 weeks, and complete recovery is the rule. It is not clear whether arthritis is due to viremia or whether it is a "hypersensitivity reaction."

Acute hemorrhagic glomerulonephritis in the absence of streptococcosis has been reported after mumps. The relationship of these two diseases is not clear.

Late complications With the exception of the rare central nervous system sequelae, the most serious of which is nerve deafness, which follow mumps encephalitis, and the occasional patient who is sterile following bilateral testicular involvement, mumps leaves no sequelae. There is no firm evidence that stillbirths and offspring with congenital defects are more common among mothers who have mumps during pregnancy. Likewise, the causal relationship between intrauterine mumps infection and endocardial fibroelastosis has not been clearly established.

LABORATORY FINDINGS In uncomplicated parotitis, the blood leukocyte count is normal, although there may be mild leukopenia with relative lymphocytosis. Patients with mumps orchitis, however, may have a marked leukocytosis with a shift to the left. In meningoencephalitis, the white blood cell count is usually within normal limits. The erythrocyte sedimentation rate is usually normal but may rise with testicular or pancreatic involvement. The serum amylase level is elevated both in pancreatitis and in salivary adenitis. It may also be elevated in some patients in whom the sole evidence of mumps is meningoencephalitis, and probably reflects subclinical involvement of the salivary glands. In contrast to the amylase, the serum lipase level is elevated only in pancreatitis, in which hyperglycemia and glucosuria also may occur. The cerebrospinal fluid contains 0 to 2000 cells per cubic millimeter, almost all mononuclear, although occasionally polymorphonuclear cells will predominate in the early stages. The pleocytosis in mumps meningitis tends to be greater than in aseptic meningitides caused by the poliomyelitis, coxsackie-, and echoviruses. There is no relationship between the cell count and the severity of central nervous system involvement. Transient hematuria and mild reversible abnormalities in renal function, including inability to concentrate the urine maximally and to clear creatinine, occur in association with the viruria of mumps.

DIAGNOSIS The definitive diagnosis of mumps depends on isolation of the virus from blood, throat swabs, secretions from Stensen's duct, cerebrospinal fluid, or urine. Immunofluorescence methods can detect positive cell cultures in 2 to 3 days rather than the 6 days required with standard methods. However, even with the simplification of viral isolation by means of tissue culture techniques, culture of the virus is rarely necessary in the typical case with associated parotitis. When an etiologic diagnosis is needed, as in aseptic meningitis or in atypical cases of parotitis, the complement fixation test is most commonly employed. Antibodies to the S antigen develop rather rapidly, often reaching a peak within 1 week after the onset of symptoms, and usually disappearing in 6 to 12 months. Complement-fixing antibodies to the V antigen follow a more typical pattern, reaching a peak titer within 2 to 3 weeks after onset, remaining elevated for at least 6 weeks, then persisting at lower levels for years afterward. Paired serums obtained 2 to 3 weeks apart are recommended. A fourfold increase in titer confirms recent infection. In cases where an acute serum is not obtained until later in the course of illness, an elevation of antibodies to the S antigen which exceeds the V antibody titer also suggests recent infection. The hemagglutination inhibition reaction is demonstrable somewhat later and persists for several months. The serum neutralization test is the most sensitive indicator of previous mumps infection, although it is more complicated to perform. However, it is a much better indicator of previous mumps infection than the skin test, and individuals with detectable specific neutralizing antibody are highly unlikely to contract mumps. The *skin test* consists of intradermal injection of killed mumps virus; previous exposure will result in a delayed reaction of the tuberculin type and an anamnestic antibody titer rise to mumps. The skin test is unreliable when used alone in determining the immune status of an individual, is useless in the diagnosis of acute mumps, and is no longer commercially available in the United States.

The diagnosis of mumps during an epidemic is usually obvious. Sporadic cases, however, must be distinguished from other causes of parotid enlargement. Parotitis may be caused by other viruses, notably parainfluenza, influenza, and coxsackieviruses. *Bacterial parotitis* usually occurs in debilitated patients with severe underlying diseases, such as uncontrolled diabetes mellitus, cerebrovascular accidents, or uremia. It may also follow surgical operations. The parotid glands are swollen, warm, and tender, and pus can be expressed from the orifices of Stensen's ducts. Marked polymorphonuclear leukocytosis is present. The disease is usually acquired in the hospital, and *Staphylococcus aureus* is the usual causative organism. Dehydration followed by inspissation of secretions in the salivary ducts is an important predisposing factor. *Calculus* in a salivary duct is usually detectable by palpation or by injection of radiopaque media into Stensen's duct. *Drug reactions* may produce tender swelling of the parotid and other salivary glands. "Iodine mumps" is the commonest type; it may follow such procedures as intravenous urography. Mercurialism and the antihypertensive agent guanethidine may also cause parotid enlargement and tenderness. A careful history usually serves to clarify the cause of these reactions. *Cervical adenitis* caused by streptococci, "bullneck" diphtheria, infectious mononucleosis, cat-scratch disease, sublingual cellulitis (Ludwig's angina), and cellulitis of the external auditory canal are usually easy to distinguish from mumps by careful examination. Parotid tumors and chronic infections such as actinomycosis tend to follow a more indolent course, with slowly progressive swelling. The common "mixed tumor" of the parotid is well circumscribed, nontender, and very firm, almost cartilaginous on palpation. Parotid swelling and fever, often accompanied by lacrimal adenitis and uveitis (Mikulicz's syndrome), may occur in tuberculosis, leukemia, Hodgkin's disease, and lupus erythematosus. The onset may be sudden, but the process is usually painless and of long duration. "Uveoparotid fever" of similar type may be the first manifestation of sarcoidosis; in this disease parotid swelling is frequently accompanied by single or multiple palsies of cranial nerves, particularly the facial nerve, and is referred to as Heerfordt's syndrome. Presternal edema may also be a manifestation of malignant lymphoma involving retrosternal lymph nodes. Bilateral painless parotid swelling unassociated with fever is found in patients with Laennec's cirrhosis, chronic alcoholism, malnutrition, diabetes mellitus, pregnancy and lactation, and hypertriglyceridemia.

Sjögren's syndrome (see Chap. 346) is a chronic inflammation of the parotid and other salivary glands which is often associated with atrophy of the lacrimal glands and occurs most commonly in women past the menopause. With cessation of lacrimal and salivary function, there may be striking dryness of the conjunctiva and the cornea (keratoconjunctivitis sicca) and of the mouth (xerostomia). These patients may also have a variety of systemic manifestations, including arthritis of the rheumatoid type, splenomegaly, leukopenia, and hemolytic anemia. The chronicity of the process and its occurrence in elderly women make confusion with mumps unlikely. Finally, benign hypertrophy of both masseter muscles, presumably due to habitual clenching and grinding of teeth, may be confused with painless parotid swelling.

The causes of aseptic meningitis are discussed in Chap. 360.

Orchitis occurring in the absence of parotitis is likely to remain undiagnosed. Serologic testing may later confirm the diagnosis of mumps. Orchitis may occur in association with acute bacterial prostatitis and seminal vesiculitis. It is a rare complication of gonorrhea. Occasionally testicular inflammation accompanies pleurodynia, leptospirosis, melioidosis, relapsing fever, chickenpox, brucellosis, and lymphocytic choriomeningitis.

TREATMENT There is no specific treatment for infections with the mumps virus. Patients with parotitis should receive mouth care, analgesics, and a bland diet. Bed rest is advisable only as long as the patient is febrile; contrary to popular belief, physical activity has no influence on the development of orchitis or other complications. Patients with epididymoorchitis may be acutely ill and in great pain. Many forms of treatment, including surgical decompression of the testicle, infiltration of the spermatic cord with local anesthetics, estrogens, convalescent serum, and broad-spectrum antibiotics, have not been regularly effective. Despite failure to document their effectiveness in controlled studies, adrenal steroids have been of considerable benefit in diminishing fever, as well as testicular pain and swelling, and in restoring the sense of well-being in a number of patients. It is important to give a large initial daily dose corresponding to 300 mg cortisone or 60 mg prednisone. Subsequently, administration of the hormone can be tapered off over 7 to 10 days. Adrenal steroids have not exerted an adverse effect on concomitant pancreatitis or meningitis, although they have not benefited patients with meningeal involvement, and their withdrawal has usually been accompanied by a recrudescence of symptoms. Adrenal steroids have not prevented the appearance of parotid involvement on the contralateral side. Mumps arthritis is usually mild and requires no treatment. Mumps thyroiditis may subside spontaneously, but excellent relief has been obtained with adrenal hormones.

PREVENTION A live attenuated mumps virus vaccine (Jeryl Lynn strain) has been highly effective in producing significant rises in mumps antibody in individuals who are seronegative prior to vaccination, and has afforded 95 percent protection to individuals subsequently exposed to mumps. The vaccine also has boosted antibody levels in vaccinated individuals who are seropositive. The vaccine produces an inapparent, noncommunicable infection. Parotitis after vaccination has been reported only rarely, and central nervous system dysfunction has not been proved to be a complication. It has conferred excellent protection for at least 12 years and has not interfered with vaccines against measles, rubella, and poliomyelitis or with smallpox vaccination given simultaneously. Protection has been demonstrated in both children and adults.

Live mumps vaccine can be administered at any time after 1 year of age, and should be particularly considered for children approaching puberty, adolescents, and adult males who have not had clinical mumps or live mumps vaccine in the past. Individuals living in groups or in institutions should be vaccinated, particularly because it has been shown that physical isolation of mumps patients does not effectively prevent transmission of the infection.

Vaccination is contraindicated in babies under the age of 1 year because of the interfering effect of maternal antibody; in individuals with a history of hypersensitivity to vaccine components; in patients with febrile illnesses, leukemia, lymphoma, or generalized malignancies; in those receiving steroids, alkylating drugs, antimetabolites, or irradiation; and during pregnancy.

It is not known whether the vaccine will prevent infection when administered after exposure, but no contraindication to its use in this situation exists. Neither mumps immune globulin nor ordinary gamma globulin has been shown to be efficacious in postexposure prophylaxis, and therefore neither is recommended.

REFERENCES

Beard CM et al: The incidence and outcome of mumps orchitis in Rochester Minnesota 1935 to 1974. Mayo Clin Proc 52:3, 1977

Brunnell PA et al: Ineffectiveness of isolation of patients as a method of preventing the spread of mumps. N Engl J Med 279:1357, 1968

Caranasos GH, Felker JR: Mumps arthritis. Arch Intern Med 119:394, 1967

FREEMAN R, HAMBLING MG: Serological studies on 40 cases of mumps virus infection. J Clin Pathol 33:28, 1980

KALTREIDER HA, TALAL N: Bilateral parotid gland enlargement and hyperlipoproteinemia. JAMA 210:2067, 1969

LEVITT LP et al: Central nervous system mumps: A review of 64 cases. Neurology 20:829, 1970

Mumps vaccine. Morb Mort Week Rep 29:87, 1980

ST GEME JW JR et al: Immunologic significance of the mumps virus skin test in infants, children and adults. Am J Epidemiol 101:253, 1975

THOMPSON JA: Mumps: A cause of acquired aqueductal stenosis. J Pediatr 94:923, 1979

UTZ JP et al: Studies of mumps: IV. Viruria and abnormal renal function. N Engl J Med 270:1283, 1964

WILFERT CM: Mumps meningoencephalitis with low cerebrospinal fluid glucose, prolonged pleocytosis and elevation of protein. N Engl J Med 280:855, 1969

207
RABIES AND OTHER RHABDOVIRUSES

LAWRENCE COREY

RABIES

DEFINITION Rabies is an acute viral disease of the central nervous system that affects all mammals and that is transmitted by infected secretions, usually saliva. Most exposures to rabies are through the bite of an infected animal, but on occasion a virus aerosol or the ingestion or transplantation of infected tissues may initiate the disease process.

ETIOLOGY The rabies virus is a bullet-shaped, enveloped, single-stranded ribonucleic acid (RNA) virus belonging to the rhabdovirus group. It has a diameter of 750 to 800 Å and varies in length. Excrescenses, 60 to 70 Å long, each with a knoblike structure at the distal end, cover the surface of the virion. These surface structures elicit neutralizing and hemagglutination-inhibiting antibodies, while a nucleocapsid antigen induces a complement-fixing antibody. Neutralizing antibodies to the surface glycoproteins appear to be protective. Antirabies antibodies used in diagnostic immunofluorescent assays are generally directed against the nucleocapsid antigens. Isolates of rabies virus from different animal species and locales may exhibit different biologic properties. Antigenic variations in strains have also been documented. What relevance these strain variations have to the pathogenesis of the infection and the response to immunization or postexposure prophylaxis is unclear. Interferon is induced by rabies virus, particularly in those tissues with high virus concentrations, and may play some role in retarding progressive infection.

EPIDEMIOLOGY Rabies exists in two epidemiologic forms: *urban,* propagated chiefly by unimmunized domestic dogs and/or cats, and *sylvatic,* propagated by skunks, foxes, raccoons, mongooses, wolves, and bats. Infection in domestic animals usually represents a "spillover" from sylvatic reservoirs of infection, and human beings can be infected by either. Hence, human infection tends to occur in locales where rabies is enzootic or epizootic, where there is a large population of unimmunized domestic animals, and where human contact with the outdoors is common. While only about 800 rabies deaths are reported to the World Health Organization (WHO) each year, "guestimates" of the worldwide incidence of rabies is approximated at 15,000 cases per year. Southeast Asia, the Philippines, Africa, and the Indian subcontinent are areas where the disease is especially common. Imported rabies combined with the epizootic of fox rabies in western Europe has increased the importance of this disease in Europe. In the United States human rabies is exceedingly rare, with 0 to 5 cases reported yearly.

In most areas of the world, the dog is the important vector of rabies virus for humans. However, the wolf (eastern Europe, arctic regions), the mongoose (South Africa, the Caribbean), the fox (western Europe), and the vampire bat (Latin America) may also be prominent vectors of the disease. Rodents and lagomorphs are rarely infected with rabies. In the United States the most important recent sources of human disease have been skunks and bats. In the United States, rabies in wildlife accounts for over 75 percent of the reported animal rabies, with dogs and cats comprising only about 4 and 3 percent, respectively, of reported animal rabies. However, most of the reported cases of postexposure prophylaxis are associated with dog bites.

Several cases of human-to-human transmission of rabies through corneal transplantation have been documented.

PATHOGENESIS The first event is the introduction of live virus through the epidermis or onto a mucous membrane. Initial viral replication appears to occur within striated muscle cells at the site of inoculation. The peripheral nervous system is exposed at the neuromuscular and/or neurotendinal spindles. The virus then spreads centripetally up the nerve to the central nervous system, probably via peripheral nerve axoplasm. Experimentally, viremia has been shown to occur, but is not thought to play a role in naturally acquired disease. Once the virus reaches the central nervous system, it replicates almost exclusively within the gray matter and then passes centrifugally along autonomic nerves to reach other tissue—the salivary glands, adrenal medulla, kidney, lung, liver, skeletal muscle, skin, and heart. Passage into the salivary glands facilitates further transmission of the disease via infected saliva. The incubation period of rabies is exceedingly variable, ranging from 10 days to over 1 year (mean 1 to 2 months). The time period appears to depend upon the amount of virus introduced, the amount of tissue involved, host defense mechanisms, and the actual distance that the virus has to travel from the site of inoculation to the central nervous system. Studies in animals have shown that host immune responses and viral strains may also influence disease expression. Attenuated strains of rabies virus produce high cytotoxic responses compared with wild "street virus." Animals which develop paralytic rabies (dumb rabies) appear to have a more marked immune response to infection than those which develop fulminant encephalitis.

The neuropathology of rabies resembles other viral diseases of the central nervous system: hyperemia, varying degrees of chromatolysis, nuclear pyknosis, and neuronophagia of the nerve cells; infiltration by lymphocytes and plasma cells of the Virchow-Robin space; microglial infiltration, and parenchymal areas of nerve cell destruction. The pathognomonic lesion of rabies is the Negri body. This eosinophilic mass, approximately 10 nm in size, is made up of a finely fibrillar matrix and rabies virus particles. Negri bodies are distributed throughout the brain, particularly in Ammon's horn, the cerebral cortex, the brainstem, the Purkinje cells of the cerebellum, and the dorsal spinal ganglia. Negri bodies are not demonstrated in at least 20 percent of rabies, and their absence in brain material does not rule out the diagnosis.

MANIFESTATIONS The clinical manifestations of rabies can be divided into four stages: (1) a nonspecific prodrome, (2) an acute encephalitis similar to other viral encephalitides, (3) a profound dysfunction of brainstem centers which produces the classic features of rabies encephalitis, and (4) rarely, recovery.

The prodromal period usually persists for 1 to 4 days and is marked by fever, headache, malaise, myalgias, increased fatigability, anorexia, nausea and vomiting, sore throat, and a nonproductive cough. The prodromal symptom suggestive of rabies is the complaint of parasthesias and/or fasciculations at or about the site of inoculation of virus. This symptom is present in 50 to 80 percent of patients.

The encephalitic phase is usually ushered in by periods of excessive motor activity, excitation, and agitation. Quickly, confusion, hallucinations, combativeness, bizarre aberrations of thought, muscle spasms, meningismus, opisthotonic posturing, seizures, and focal paralysis appear. Characteristically, the periods of mental aberration are interspersed with completely lucid periods, but as the disease progresses, the lucid periods get shorter until the patient lapses into coma. Hyperesthesia, with excessive sensitivity to bright light, loud noise, touch, and even gentle breezes, is very common. On physical examination the temperature may be found to be as high as 40.6°C (105°F). Abnormalities of the autonomic nervous system include dilated, irregular pupils, increased lacrimation, salivation, perspiration, and postural hypotension. Evidence of upper motor neuron paralysis with weakness, increased deep tendon reflexes, and extensor plantar responses is the rule. Paralysis of the vocal cords is common.

The manifestations of brainstem dysfunction begin shortly after the onset of the encephalitic phase. Cranial nerve involvement causes diplopia, facial palsies, optic neuritis, and the characteristic difficulty with deglutition. The combination of excessive salivation and difficulty in swallowing produces the traditional picture of "foaming at the mouth." Hydrophobia, the painful, violent involuntary contraction of the diaphragm, accessory respiratory, pharyngeal, and laryngeal muscles initiated by swallowing liquids, is seen in about 50 percent of cases. Involvement of the amygdaloid nucleus may result in priapism and spontaneous ejaculation. The patient lapses into coma, and involvement of the respiratory center produces an apneic death. The prominence of early brainstem dysfunction distinguishes rabies from other viral encephalitides and accounts for the rapid downhill course. The median survival after the onset of symptoms is 4 days, with a maximum of 20, unless artificial supporting measures are instituted.

If intensive respiratory support is used, a number of late complications may appear and include inappropriate secretion of antidiuretic hormone, diabetes insipidus, cardiac arrythmias, vascular instability, adult respiratory distress syndrome, gastrointestinal bleeding, thrombocytopenia, and paralytic ileus. Recovery is very rare and when it occurs has been gradual. There have been only three well-documented nonfatal cases of rabies in humans. Two of these survivors received partial postexposure prophylaxis and the third, a case of laboratory-associated rabies, probably from an aerosol exposure, had received preexposure prophylaxis.

Occasionally, rabies may present as an ascending paralysis resembling the Landry-Guillain-Barré syndrome (dumb rabies, *rage tranquile*). This clinical pattern occurs most frequently in those bitten by vampire bats or who have received postexposure rabies prophylaxis.

The difficulty of suspecting rabies when it is associated with ascending paralysis is illustrated by the documentation of person-to-person transmission of the virus by tissue transplantation. Corneal transplants from donors who died of presumed Landry-Guillain-Barré syndrome have produced clinical rabies and death in the recipient. Retrospective pathologic examinations of the brains of both patients demonstrated Negri bodies, and rabies virus was subsequently isolated from each donor's frozen eye.

LABORATORY FINDINGS Early in the disease the hemoglobin and routine blood chemistries are normal, but abnormalities occur as hypothalamic dysfunction, gastrointestinal bleeding, and other complications ensue. The peripheral white blood cell count is usually slightly elevated (12,000 to 17,000 per cubic millimeter) but may be normal or as high as 30,000 per cubic millimeter.

As in any viral infection, the specific diagnosis of rabies depends upon (1) the isolation of virus from infected secretions [saliva, rarely cerebrospinal fluid (CSF), or tissue (brain)], (2) the serologic demonstration of acute infection, or (3) the demonstration of viral antigen in infected tissue, e.g., corneal impression smears, skin biopsies, or brain. Samples of brain obtained either on postmortem examination or from brain biopsy should be subjected to (1) mouse inoculation studies for virus isolation, (2) fluorescent-antibody (FA) staining for viral antigen, and (3) histologic and/or electron microscopic examination for Negri bodies. While the mouse inoculation studies for virus isolation and direct FA staining for viral antigen are quite reliable and sensitive, if the patient's life has been prolonged and high levels of neutralizing antibody are present in serum and CSF, "autosterilization" may occur, and these tests may be negative. The use of FA staining of skin biopsies, corneal impression smears, and saliva for evidence of rabies antigen has been helpful in diagnosing rabies during life. Confirmation of these findings either serologically or by demonstration of virus in brain should be sought.

If the patient has not received antirabies immunization, then a fourfold rise in neutralizing antibody to rabies virus in serial serum samples is diagnostic. If the patient has received rabies vaccination, then a clue to the diagnosis may be obtained from the absolute titers of serum-neutralizing antibody and the presence of neutralizing antibody to rabies in CSF. Postexposure rabies prophylaxis rarely produces CSF-neutralizing antibody to rabies. If present, it is usually in low titer, e.g., less than 1:64, whereas CSF titers in human rabies may vary from 1:200 to 1:160,000.

DIFFERENTIAL DIAGNOSIS There is little to distinguish rabies from other viral encephalitides, and the most helpful point in diagnosis is the history of exposure. Other problems to be considered include hysterical reactions to animal bites (pseudohydrophobia), Landry-Guillain-Barré syndrome, poliomyelitis, and allergic encephalomyelitis to rabies vaccine. The latter occurs most commonly after use of nerve tissue–derived vaccine and usually begins 1 to 4 weeks after vaccination.

PREVENTION AND TREATMENT Each year more than 1 million Americans are bitten by animals. In each instance, a decision must be made whether to initiate postexposure rabies prophylaxis. When deciding whether to institute rabies prophylaxis, the following considerations apply: (1) whether the individual came into physical contact with saliva or another substance likely to contain rabies virus; (2) whether rabies is known or suspected in the species and area associated with the exposure (e.g., all persons within the continental United States bitten by a bat that then escapes should receive postexposure prophylaxis); (3) the circumstances surrounding the exposure; and (4) the treatment alternative and complications. A guide for postexposure rabies prophylaxis is illustrated in Fig. 207-1.

If rabies is known to be present or suspected to be present in the animal species involved in a human exposure, the animal should be captured, if possible. Captured wild animals or any ill, unvaccinated, or stray domestic animal involved in a rabies exposure, particularly any animal involved in an unprovoked bite, exhibiting abnormal behavior, or suspected of being rabid, should be captured and killed, and the head should be sent immediately to an appropriate laboratory for rabies FA examination. If examination of the brain by the FA technique is negative for rabies, it can be assumed that the saliva contains no virus, and the exposed person need not be treated. Persons exposed to escaped wild animals capable of carrying rabies (bats, skunks, coyotes, foxes, raccoons, etc.) in an area where rabies is known or suspected to be present should receive both passive and active immunization against rabies.

If a healthy vaccinated dog or cat bites a person, the animal should be captured, confined, and observed for 10 days. If any illness or abnormal behavior develops in the animal during the observation period, it should be killed for FA examination.

Postexposure prophylaxis Once a decision regarding the necessity to initiate postexposure rabies prophylaxis has been made, the general principle of postexposure therapy is to minimize the amount of virus at the site of inoculation with local treatment of the wound and to establish an early and long-lasting neutralizing antibody titer to rabies virus. The following therapeutic regimen is recommended:

1 *Local wound therapy* with generous scrubbing with soap and then flushing the wound with water is recommended. Both mechanical and chemical cleansing are important. Quaternary ammonium compounds such as 1 to 4% benzalkonium chloride (Zephiran) or 1% cetrimonium bromide (Cetavlon) are also useful. However, 0.1% Zephiran solutions are less effective than 20% soap solutions. Usually tetanus toxoid and antibiotics (generally penicillin) should be administered.
2 *Passive immunization with antirabies antiserum* of either equine or human origin. The latter is preferred because of the high incidence of serum sickness (20 to 40 percent) with the equine product. Fifty percent of the total dose of 20 units/kg for human rabies immune globulin (RIG) and 40 units per kilogram for the equine antiserum is given by local infiltration of the wound, and the rest is administered intramuscularly. When RIG and DEV are used for postexposure prophylaxis, up to 20 percent of recipients do not develop significant levels of neutralizing antibody [$>$ 1:5 by mouse inoculation or equivalent or 1:15 in the rapid fluorescent focus inhibition test (RFFIT)]. For this reason, a neutralizing antibody determination should be obtained after completion of therapy. "Nonresponders" should be given a booster injection with HDCV (see below). When RIG and HDCV are used for postexposure prophylaxis, follow-up antibody titers are *not* routinely needed.
3 *Active immunization with antirabies vaccine.* Two rabies vaccines, human diploid cell vaccine (HDCV) and duck embryo vaccine (DEV), are currently licensed in the United States. Both are "killed virus" vaccines, prepared from laboratory strains of rabies virus grown in either human diploid cell cultures [(WI-38) for HDCV] or embryonated duck eggs, and inactivated with beta-propinolactone or tri-*n*-butyl phosphate. HDCV is more immunogenic than DEV, requires fewer doses, appears to be associated with fewer adverse reactions, and to date has not been associated with vaccine failure, i.e., development of disease after postexposure prophylaxis. For these reasons, HDCV is the preferred rabies vaccine.

FIGURE 207-1
Postexposure rabies prophylaxis algorithm.

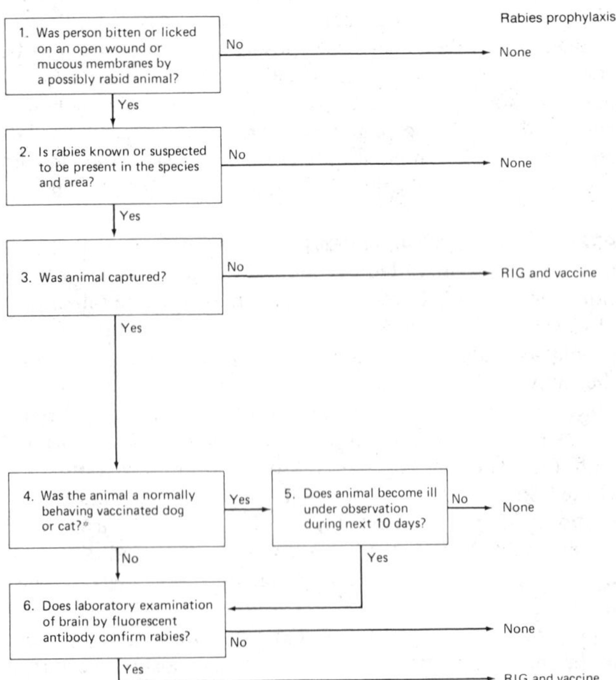

*Livestock exposure should be considered individually and local and state public health officials should be consulted.

Severe reactions to HDCV are uncommon. Immediate hypersensitivity responses such as urticaria have been reported in approximately 1 in 650 recipients. Systemic reactions such as fever, headache, and nausea are generally mild and are reported in 1 to 4 percent of recipients. Local reactions such as swelling, erythema, and induration at the injection site occur in 15 to 20 percent of vaccinees.

Five 1-ml doses of HDCV are given intramuscularly (IM) as soon as possible after exposure. The first dose (day 0) should also be accompanied by antirabies serum (RIG) given in the opposite arm. Subsequent doses of HDCV are given on days 3, 7, 14, and 28.

When DEV has been used in postexposure prophylaxis, local reactions such as pain (100 percent), erythema (97 percent), and pruritus (13 percent) at the site of inoculation are common, and systemic symptoms such as fever, malaise, or myalgia occur in about 33 percent of postexposure recipients. Anaphylaxis is seen in less than 1 percent of DEV recipients and usually occurs during administration of the first five doses. A history of hypersensitivity to avian products should be ruled out before initial therapy.

Preexposure prophylaxis Individuals with a high risk of contact with rabies virus—veterinarians, spelunkers, laboratory workers, and animal handlers—should have preexposure prophylaxis with rabies vaccine. With HDCV, 3 IM injections on days 0, 7, and 21 to 28 should be administered. If DEV is used, two 1-ml subcutaneous injections given 1 month apart, followed by a 1-ml booster 7 months later, should be administered. A neutralizing antibody titer should be checked after vaccination and at approximately 2-year intervals to see that an adequate titer is maintained. Postexposure prophylaxis in individuals previously given preexposure therapy consists of antirabies vaccines only (two doses of HDCV on days 0 and 3 are usually adequate).

MARBURG VIRUS DISEASE

DEFINITION Marburg virus causes an acute systemic febrile illness characterized by the abrupt onset of headache, myalgias, pharyngitis, rash, and hemorrhagic manifestations. It was recognized first in 1967 when it caused simultaneous outbreaks in the Federal Republic of Germany and Yugoslavia among laboratory workers exposed to imported African green monkeys (*Cercopithecus aethiops*). The clinical manifestations are similar to other hemorrhagic fevers of the arenavirus class or flavovirus group (Argentina and Bolivian hemorrhagic fever, Chap. 209). The high case fatality rate and demonstrated ability for nosocomial spread has made recognition of this rare agent an important worldwide public health concern.

ETIOLOGY The Marburg virus has been isolated in guinea pig and various cell culture systems such as vervet monkey kidney. The virus particle contains lipid and RNA, and under the electron microscope the virus appears as an 80- to 100-nm elongated filamentous particle with occasional "blister-like excrescences." While the Marburg virus exhibits some morphologic relationship to other members of the rhabdoviruses (rabies, Ebola, and Mokola viruses), it appears antigenically distinct.

EPIDEMIOLOGY The initial outbreaks affected 31 patients in Marburg and Frankfurt, Germany, and Belgrade, Yugoslavia, and was epidemiologically linked to monkeys imported from the same source in Uganda. Virus was isolated from the blood and tissue of these monkeys. Of the 25 primary infections, there were seven deaths. Six secondary cases, involving two physicians, one nurse, a postmortem attendant, and the wife of a veterinarian, occurred. Person-to-person transmission was felt to take place via accidental needle sticks or abrasions, although respiratory and conjunctival infection could not be ruled out. The wife of one patient developed Marburg virus disease. Marburg virus was demonstrated in semen of the original patient, despite the presence of circulating antibody, and this secondary case is believed to have been acquired through sexual intercourse. The natural reservoir of Marburg virus is unknown. Serologic examination of a large number of primates in Uganda suggests that monkeys appear to be susceptible but incidental hosts.

PATHOLOGY Marburg virus appears "pantropic" and produces lesions in almost all organs including lymphoid tissue, liver, spleen, pancreas, adrenals, thyroid, kidney, testes, skin, and brain. In lymphoid tissue focal necrosis with degeneration of lymphoid tissue is apparent. In the liver, eosinophilic cytoplasmic bodies resembling the Councilman bodies of yellow fever have been noted. The lungs may show interstitial pneumonitis, as well as vascular lesions in small arterioles indicative of endarteritis. Neuropathologic changes consist of multiple small hemorrhagic infarcts with glial proliferation.

CLINICAL MANIFESTATIONS After an incubation period of 3 to 9 days, patients develop the abrupt onset of frontal and temporal headache, malaise, myalgias, especially in the lumbar area, nausea, and vomiting. Fever of 39.4 to 40°C (103 to 104°F) is characteristic, and about half the patients have conjunctivitis. Between 1 and 3 days after onset, watery diarrhea, which is often severe, lethargy, and a change in mentation are noted. An enanthem of the palate and tonsils, and cervical lymphadenopathy, may also be noted during the first week of illness. The most reliable clinical feature is the appearance of nonpruritic maculopapular rash which begins on the fifth to seventh day on the face and neck and spreads centrifugally to involve the extremities. A fine desquamation of the affected skin, especially the palms and soles, appears 4 to 5 days later. Hemorrhagic manifestations, including gastrointestinal, renal, vaginal, and/or conjunctival hemorrhages, generally develop between days 5 and 7 of disease.

During the first week, the temperature continues in the vicinity of 40°C (104°F), falling by lysis during the second week, to increase again between the twelfth and fourteenth days. Other clinical signs apparent in the second week of disease include splenomegaly, hepatomegaly, facial edema, and scrotal or labial reddening. Complications include orchitis, which may lead to testicular atrophy, myocarditis with irregular pulse and electrocardiographic abnormalities, and pancreatitis. The overall case fatality rate has been about 25 percent, with death usually occurring during the eighth to sixteenth days of illness. Recovery is often protracted over a 3- to 4-week period, and during this period loss of hair, intermittent abdominal pain, poor appetite, and prolonged psychotic disturbances have been noted. Late sequelae including transverse myelitis and uveitis have been reported. Marburg virus has been isolated from the anterior eye chamber and semen nearly 3 months after onset of disease.

LABORATORY FINDINGS Abnormalities in granulocyte function are found, and leukopenia is detected as early as the first day, with leukocyte counts as low as 1000 per cubic millimeter and a neutrophilia by the fourth day. Subsequently, atypical lymphocytes, as well as neutrophils exhibiting the characteristic of the Pelger-Huet anomaly, may appear. Thrombocytopenia appears early and is most marked, often less than 10,000 cells per cubic millimeter, between the sixth and twelfth days. In fatal cases, evidence of disseminated intravascular coagulation can be demonstrated. Hypoproteinemia, proteinuria, and azotemia may occur. Elevations in serum glutamic oxaloacetic transaminase (SGOT) and alanine aminotransferase (SGPT) are usual. Lumbar puncture may be normal or reveal a minimal pleocytosis. The erythrocyte sedimentation rate is usually low.

DIAGNOSIS The characteristic clinical course and epidemiologic features are the basis of the diagnosis. Specific diagnosis requires isolation of the virus or serologic evidence of infection in paired serum samples. Viremia coincides with the febrile state of disease, and virus has been isolated from tissue as well as urine, semen, throat, and rectal swabs. Attempts to isolate virus must be carried out only in *specialized high-security laboratories.* All patients should be kept in strict isolation, and all specimens should be handled and shipped according to World Health Organization guidelines.

TREATMENT Patients have received a multiplicity of drugs without apparent influence on the course of the illness. Convalescent serum was administered to four patients, whose subsequent disease followed a mild course. However, similarly benign outcomes were observed in patients who did not receive serum.

EBOLA VIRUS

Between July and November 1976 simultaneous outbreaks of an acute febrile hemorrhagic disease occurred in southern Sudan and northern Zaire. "Secondary and tertiary" spread of infection, particularly among hospital staff, was noted. In the Sudan over 300 cases with 151 deaths and in Zaire 237 cases with 211 fatalities were reported. In one Sudanese hospital, 76 members of a staff of 230 were infected and 41 died. The virus isolated from patients in the Sudan and Zaire was morphologically similar to the Marburg agent but was antigenically distinct. The name Ebola virus, after the river in Zaire located near the epidemic, has been proposed. Sporadic cases of disease also appear to occur, and a recent serosurvey revealed a prevalence rate of 7 percent for antibodies to Ebola virus in endemic areas.

Ebola virus has been propagated in tissue culture (Vero cells) and in suckling mice and guinea pigs. The source of the outbreak in both the Sudan and Zaire is unknown; however, as with other viral hemorrhagic fevers, peridomestic rodents are suspected as being a reservoir of the infection, and serologic evidence of Ebola virus infection was detected in a domestic guinea pig trapped in Zaire. Once established, nosocomial as well as community-acquired cases occur, especially among close and prolonged contact. Parenteral exposure to the virus through disinfected rather than sterilized needles may have played a role in transmission. Barrier nursing and strict isolation precautions using protective clothing appeared to decrease the number of nosocomial cases.

CLINICAL MANIFESTATIONS Clinically, the disease is similar to Marburg virus disease. The incubation period ranges from 4 to 6 days (mean is 7 days). Patients usually present on the fifth day of illness with a history of abrupt onset of headache, malaise, myalgias, high fever, diarrhea, abdominal pain, dehydration, and lethargy. Pleuritic chest pain, a dry hacking cough, and a pronounced pharyngitis were also noted. A maculopapular eruption develops between days 5 to 7 of illness. On black skins the rash is often faint and not recognized until desquamation occurs. Hematemesis, melena, and bleeding from the nose, gums, and vagina are common. Abortion and massive metrorrhagia was a frequent complication among pregnant women. Death usually occurs in the second week of illness and is preceded by severe blood loss and shock.

TREATMENT Patients should be isolated until virological studies indicate they are free of virus, usually 21 days from onset of illness. Malaria parasites were frequently found in blood films of patients with Ebola virus infection in the Sudan indicating that the presence of parasitemia does not rule out concomitant viral illness. Treatment with plasma containing Ebola virus specific antibodies has resulted in diminished levels of viremia; however, further tests are required to establish the effectiveness of this form of therapy. Requests for viral isolation as well as convalescent plasma should be addressed to WHO Regional Centers in Atlanta or Geneva.

MOKOLA VIRUS

Mokola virus was first isolated from wild shrews captured in Nigeria and subsequently was shown to be related morphologically and serologically to rabies. However, neither of the two reported cases of human disease (both children) demonstrated classic clinical features of rabies. One patient had a nonfatal illness characterized by fever, pharyngitis, and convulsions. Mokola virus was recovered from her cerebrospinal fluid. The second patient initially had fever, cough, and vomiting, followed in several days by drowsiness, confusion, and generalized flaccid weakness. Her cerebrospinal fluid was normal. She progressed to deep coma and died within 10 days of onset. Mokola virus was isolated from her brain, and histopathologic sections revealed finely granular cytoplasmic inclusions that were distinguishable from Negri bodies in many neurons.

VESICULAR STOMATITIS VIRUS

Vesicular stomatitis is a viral illness of animals which can occasionally infect humans. It presents as an acute self-limited influenza-like disease. The disease in animals is found in the United States and South America and affects chiefly domestic cattle, horses, swine, and wild deer, raccoons, skunks, and bobcats.

In animals, vesicular stomatitis is characterized by the development of vesicles on the oral mucosa, particularly the tongue, udders, and heels. The mode of spread is probably by direct contact; however, epidemics tend to occur in warm weather, and the virus has been isolated from *Phlebotumus* sandflies in Panama and *Äedes* species in New Mexico, suggesting these as possible vectors. Two distinct serotypes, New Jersey and Indiana, have been recognized, and most of the outbreaks in North America have been attributed to the New Jersey strain. The disease is most common in laboratory workers, and in one report three-fourths of laboratory personnel handling experimentally infected animals or manipulating the virus developed neutralizing antibodies. The disease is transmissible, however, under natural conditions among workers having direct contact with infected animals, especially cattle. The incubation period ranges from 1 to 6 days. This is followed by the sudden onset of fever, up to 40°C (104°F), chills, profuse sweating, myalgias, malaise, headache, and pain on ocular movement. One-third to one-half of patients have sore throat and cervical and/or submandibular adenopathy. Small raised vesicular lesions may appear on the buccal mucosa. Conjunctivitis and coryza are present in about 20 percent of cases. Occasionally, small subcorneal, intraepithelial vesicles may appear on the fingers, usually associated with direct inoculation of the virus. Symptoms generally last 3 to 4 days, but occasionally a diphasic course may occur. Inapparent infection is common, and among laboratory workers with serologic evidence of infection, only about one-half reported clinical symptoms. In some areas of Panama, 17 to 35 percent of the population have neutralizing antibodies against vesicular stomatitis virus.

The differential diagnosis includes hand-foot-and-mouth disease, herpangina, primary herpetic pharyngitis and other mucocutaneous syndromes, and influenza. Viral isolation from patients is not common; however, a rise in complement fixation and/or neutralizing antibodies to vesicular stomatitis virus between acute and convalescent serums will help to confirm the diagnosis. Treatment is nonspecific.

REFERENCES

Marburg virus

GEAR JSS et al: Outbreak of Marburg virus disease in Johannesburg. Br Med J 4:489, 1975

JOHNSON KM: Ebola virus and hemorrhagic fever. Ann Intern Med 91:117, 1979

MARTIN GA, SEIGERT R (eds): *Marburg Virus Disease.* New York, Springer-Verlag, 1971

SIMPSON DIH: Marburg and ebola virus infections: A guide for their diagnosis, management and control. WHO Offset Publication no 36, Geneva, 1977

Mokola virus

FAMILUSI JB: Fatal human infection with Mokola virus. Am J Trop Med Hyg 21:959, 1972

Rabies

ANDERSON LJ et al: Post exposure trial of a human diploid cell strain rabies vaccine. J Infect Dis 142:133, 1980

BAER GM: *The Natural History of Rabies.* New York, Academic, 1975

BAHMANYAR M: Successful protection of humans exposed to rabies: Post exposure treatment with the new human diploid cell rabies vaccine and antirabies serum. JAMA 236:2751, 1976

COREY L, HATTWICK MA: Treatment of persons exposed to rabies. JAMA 232:272, 1975

HATTWICK MA et al: Recovery from rabies: A case report. Ann Intern Med 76:931, 1972

HOUGH SA et al: Human-to-human transmission of rabies virus by a corneal transplant. N Engl J Med 300:603, 1979

PLOTKIN SA: Rabies vaccine prepared in human cell culture: Progress and perspectives. Rev Infect Dis 2:433, 1980

RUBIN RH et al: Adverse reactions to duck embryo vaccine. Ann Intern Med 78:643, 1973

208
ARBOVIRUS INFECTIONS

JAY P. SANFORD

Most viral infections in humans are either asymptomatic or present as undifferentiated illnesses characterized by fever, malaise, headache, and generalized myalgia. The similarities in clinical features between infections caused by viruses as dissimilar as the myxoviruses (e.g., influenza), the enteroviruses (e.g., poliovirus, coxsackievirus, echovirus), some of the herpesviruses (e.g., cytomegalovirus), and the arboviruses usually preclude an etiologic diagnosis based entirely on clinical manifestations without ancillary information regarding epidemiologic features and serologic findings. The purpose of this chapter is to direct attention to the ever-expanding list of viruses which produce febrile disease in humans. Because the number of agents is large, mention will be made of those which have been best documented, have demonstrated unusual features, or seem to be of greatest potential significance.

DEFINITION AND CLASSIFICATION It has not always been easy to determine that an agent is an arbovirus; hence with further characterization some agents which were initially registered as arboviruses have been reclassified; e.g., the zoonotic agents which have unique morphology on electron microscopy have been classified as arenaviruses (see Chap. 209). Similarly, vesicular stomatitis virus, Mokola, and Lagos bat virus, provisionally registered as arboviruses, were found to be related to rabies virus and are now classified as rhabdoviruses (see Chap. 207). The currently accepted definition of an arthropod-borne virus was published in 1967 by the World Health Organization:

Arboviruses are viruses which are maintained in nature principally, or to an important extent, through biological transmission between susceptible vertebrate hosts by hematophagous arthropods; they multiply and produce viremia in the vertebrates, multiply in the tissues of arthropods, and are passed on to new vertebrates by the bites of arthropods after a period of extrinsic incubation.

From this definition it can be appreciated that the term *arbovirus* is used in the ecological sense. Transmission by vectors is not correlated with virus architecture, which forms an important basis for current classification. The broad category arbovirus is being subdivided, and structurally related non-arthropod-borne agents may be classified with agents designated as arboviruses. Casal's serologic groups A and B arboviruses have been shown to be enveloped RNA agents with a spherical nucleocapsid forming the viral core, probably of icosohedral symmetry. Agents with these characteristics are now classified as togaviruses, with group A designated as alphaviruses and group B as flaviviruses. Other members of the togavirus group which are not transmitted by arthropods include rubella virus, equine arteritis virus, European swine fever/hog cholera virus, and viral disease of cattle agent.

There are more than 250 distinct arboviruses, which have been grouped into three families with some agents yet remaining unclassified. Within each family, the agents have been subdivided on the basis of antigenic differences (Table 208-1). The characteristics of individual members of this large group of

TABLE 208-1
Classification of arboviruses

Family	*Group*	*Specific agent**	
Togaviridae	A (alpha viruses)	Bebaru, Chikungunya†, Eastern equine†, Mayaro/Semliki, Forest (Uruma)†, O'nyong-nyong†	Ross River†, Sindbis†, Venezuelan equine†, Western equine†
	B (flaviviruses)	Banzi, Bat salivary gland†, Bussuquara, Central European encephalitis, Dengue 1-4†, Hypr, Ilheus, Japanese (B)†, Kunjin, Koutango, Kyasanur Forest†, Louping ill, Modoc, Murray Valley	Nataya, Negishi, Omsk hemorrhagic†, Powassan, Rio Bravo, Rocio, Russian spring-summer, Spondwenii, St. Louis†, Uganda S, Usutu, Wesselbron, West Nile†, Yellow fever†, Zika†
Bunyaviridae	C	Apeu†, Caraparu†, Itaqui†, Madrid†, Marituba†	Murutucui†, Oriboca†, Ossa†, Restan†
	Bunyamwera	Bunyamwera, Germiston, Guaroa	Ilesha, Wycomyia
	Bwamba	Bwamba	
	California	California, LaCrosse†	Tahyna
	Ganjam	Dugbe	Ganjam
	Guama	Bimiti, Catu	Guama
	Quaranfil	Quaranfil	
	Sandfly fever (*Phlebotomus*)	Candiru†, Chagres†, Naples type†	Punta Toro†, Rift Valley fever*, Sicilian type†
	Simbu	Shuni	Oropouche
	Thogoto	Thogoto	
	Ungrouped	Congo/Crimean hemorrhagic†, Nairobi sheep disease	Tataguine, Zinga
Reoviridae	Orbivirus	Changuinola, Kemerovo, (?) Hantaan (Korean hemorrhagic fever)	Tribec
	Ungrouped	Colorado tick fever†	
Not classified		Nyando	

* *List of specific agents includes those which have caused human infection, natural or laboratory acquired.*
† *Discussed in the text.*

viruses are not uniform; those in group A are 40 to 60 nm in diameter, and those in the Bunyamwera group are about 100 nm in diameter. The majority of agents contain single-stranded RNA, although some, such as Colorado tick fever, contain double-stranded RNA.

Arboviruses are of importance in both temperate and tropical zones. Representative viruses have been isolated in almost every geographic area outside the polar region.

Arbovirus infection of vertebrates is usually asymptomatic. The viremia stimulates an immune response which sharply limits the duration of the viremia. In arbovirus infections other than urban yellow fever, phlebotomus fever, chikungunya, o'nyong-nyong, mayaro, oropouche, and dengue, infection of humans represents an incidental occurrence which is tangential to the basic maintenance cycle of the virus. Hence, the isolation of virus from arthropod vectors or the detection of infection in the natural vertebrate host may provide a means for early detection and enable control of epizootic infection before significant spread to humans occurs.

As determined by serologic evidence of host responses, at least 80 immunologically distinct arboviruses are capable of infecting humans, while somewhat fewer have been incriminated as causing clinical disease. The spectrum of clinical illness produced by the arboviruses is varied both in predominant features and in severity. Five broad, often overlapping, and somewhat arbitrary clinical syndromes may be delineated (Table 208-2).

ARBOVIRUS INFECTIONS PRESENTING CHIEFLY WITH FEVER, MALAISE, HEADACHE, AND MYALGIA **Phlebotomus fever** Phlebotomus (sandfly, pappataci, or 3-day) fever is an acute, relatively mild, self-limited infection caused by at least five immunologically distinct arboviruses (Naples, Sicilian, Punta Toro, Chagres, and Candiru). Serologic evidence of human infection has been demonstrated for four additional agents (Bujaru, Cacao, Karimabad, and Salehabad). Humans, the only known host, probably serve as a dead-end host. Voles are suspected of being an endemic host in the Middle East.

PREVALENCE The disease occurs throughout the Mediterranean Basin, the Balkans, the Near and Middle East, the eastern part of Africa, the Soviet republics of Central Asia, Pakistan, and possibly certain parts of southern China. Recently, sandfly fever has been recognized in Panama and Brazil. In the Middle East and Central Asia native populations acquire the disease at an early age and develop and maintain high levels of immunity. Cases in Panama and Brazil are sporadic, occurring mainly in persons entering the forest. The apparent absence of phlebotomus fever in indigenous adult populations residing in areas where sandflies are abundant may present a deceptive picture of the actual risk to susceptible persons.

EPIDEMIOLOGY In the Middle East and Central Asia, the disease occurs during the hot, dry season (summer or autumn months) and is transmitted to human beings by the bite of infected sandflies (*Phlebotomus papatasi*), which are small (2 to 3 mm) urban flies that can penetrate ordinary house screens. Only the female bites and usually does so during the night. In persons who are not sensitive, there is neither pain nor local irritation after the bite; hence only about 1 percent of patients will remember having been bitten. In contrast, most of the human-biting sandflies of tropical America are sylvan in their habits. Approximately 7 days after feeding on an infected individual, the fly acquires the capacity to transmit infection and remains infectious for its life span. Transovarial transmission of the virus to the next generation has been demonstrated and offers the best explanation for the mechanism of overwinter survival of the virus. In humans, the incubation period averages 3 to 5 days. Viremia is present for at least 24 h before the onset of fever, but is not detectable for more than 2 days after the onset of illness.

CLINICAL MANIFESTATIONS The onset of symptoms is abrupt in over 90 percent of patients, with the temperature rapidly rising to its highest point, which may vary from 37.8 to 40.1°C (100 to 105°F). Headache is nearly always present and often is accompanied by pain on moving the eyes and by retroorbital pain. Myalgia is common and may be localized to the chest, resembling pleurodynia, or to the abdomen. Other symptoms may include vomiting, photophobia, giddiness, neck stiffness, alteration or loss of taste, and arthralgia. Conjunctival injection is present in approximately one-third of patients. Small vesicles may be seen on the palate, and macular or urticarial rashes occur. The spleen is rarely palpable, and lymphadenopathy is absent. The pulse rate may be elevated in proportion to the temperature on the first day; thereafter bradycardia is often present. The fever persists 3 days in most patients, with gradual defervescence. Giddiness, weakness, and feelings of depression are frequently encountered during convalescence. Second attacks 2 to 12 weeks after the first occur in 15 percent of cases.

In common with other arbovirus infections, phlebotomus fever may be associated with *aseptic meningitis.* In one series, 12 percent of patients had symptoms and signs sufficient to warrant a lumbar puncture. Findings in these patients included pleocytosis, with an average cell count of 90 per cubic millimeter and a predominance of either polymorphonuclear or mononuclear leukocytes. Spinal fluid protein concentration ranged from 20 to 130 mg/dl. In another series mild papilledema was observed in a few patients with severe illness.

LABORATORY FINDINGS The changes in leukocyte count constitute the only positive laboratory findings. Total leukocyte counts of less than 5000 per cubic millimeter are observed in 90 percent of patients if daily counts are done during the febrile period and convalescence. The leukopenia may not appear until the last day of fever or even after defervescence. The differential leukocyte count will reveal an absolute decrease in lymphocytes on the first day, accompanied by an increase in nonsegmented neutrophils. During the second or third day, the number of lymphocytes begins to return to normal and may constitute 40 to 65 percent of the total count. Concurrently, there is a reversal in proportion of segmented and band neutrophils. The differential count usually returns to normal within 5 to 8 days after defervescence. Erythrocyte values and urinalyses are usually normal.

DIAGNOSIS In the absence of a specific serologic test, the diagnosis must be made on clinical and epidemiologic grounds.

TREATMENT The disease is self-limited, and no specific therapy is available. Symptomatic care, including bed rest, adequate fluid intake, and analgesia with aspirin, is recommended. Convalescence may require a week or longer.

PROGNOSIS No fatalities have been recorded among the tens of thousands of cases.

Colorado tick fever Colorado tick fever is one of the two tick-transmitted virus diseases of human beings recognized in the United States and Canada, Powassan virus being the other. Though "mountain fever" had been described ever since the advent of immigrants to the Rocky Mountain region, Becker in 1930 differentiated it from mild Rocky Mountain spotted fever, established the clinical picture of disease, and renamed it Colorado tick fever.

ETIOLOGY Colorado tick fever virus is grouped as an arbovirus because it replicates in ticks, but it is an RNA virus belonging to the orbivirus genus of the reovirus family.

PREVALENCE The disease has been contracted in Colorado, Idaho, Nevada, Wyoming, Montana, Utah, the eastern portions of Oregon, Washington, California, and northern portions of Arizona and New Mexico, and Alberta and British Columbia. However, the virus of Colorado tick fever has been reported to have been isolated from the dog tick, *Dermacentor variabilis,* obtained from Long Island. This observation has not been confirmed, but suggests the possibility that Colorado tick fever may occur over a wider geographic area. Mild and clinically inapparent forms of the disease occur. Up to 15 percent of perennial campers have neutralizing antibodies. The number of cases of Colorado tick fever reported in Colorado is 20 times greater than that of Rocky Mountain spotted fever. In fact, almost one-half of the patients diagnosed as having Rocky Mountain spotted fever in Utah were subsequently shown to have Colorado tick fever.

EPIDEMIOLOGY Colorado tick fever is transmitted to humans by the adult hard-shelled wood tick, *Dermacentor andersoni.* The virus has been found in as many as 14 percent of this species of ticks collected in endemic areas. Transovarial transmission of the virus in the tick has been established. Illness occurs from late March through September, with most cases in May and June. Virus can be recovered from blood for 2 weeks in most patients, for at least 1 month in nearly one-half, and from spinal fluid during the acute illness. The virus persists within erythrocytes of convalescent patients for as long as 120 days. Virus can be readily isolated from washed erythrocytes 100 days following infection. Transfusion-associated Colorado tick fever has been reported.

CLINICAL MANIFESTATIONS The incubation period is usually 3 to 6 days, and in 90 percent a history of tick contact within 10 days of onset of illness can be obtained. Failure to obtain such

TABLE 208-2
Summary of clinical and epidemiologic features of arboviruses associated with infection in humans in the Western Hemisphere

Syndrome	*Virus*	*Serologic group**	*Vector*	*Known geographic range*
Fever with malaise, *headaches,* and *myalgia*	Apeu	C	Mosquito	Brazil
	Anhembi	C	Mosquito	Brazil
	Candiru	Sandfly fever	Sandfly	Brazil
	Caraparu	C	Mosquito	Brazil, Panama, Trinidad
	Catu	Guama	Mosquito	Brazil, Trinidad
	Chagres	Sandfly fever	Sandfly	Panama
	Colorado tick fever	Ungrouped orbivirus	Tick	Western United States, Alberta, British Columbia
	Guama	Guama	Mosquito	Brazil, Trinidad
	Guaroa	Bunyamwera	Mosquito	Brazil, Colombia
	Itaqui	C	Mosquito	Brazil
	Madrid	C	?	Panama
	Marituba	C	Mosquito?	Brazil
	Mayaro	A	Mosquito	Brazil, Colombia, Central America, Trinidad
	Murutucui	C	Mosquito	Brazil
	Oropouche	Simbu	Mosquito	Brazil, Trinidad
	Ossa	C	?	Panama
	Punta Toro	Sandfly	Sandfly	Panama
	Quaranfil	Quaranfil	Tick	South America
	Restan	C	Mosquito	Trinidad
	Uruma	A	?	Bolivia
	U.S. bat salivary gland	B	?	Southwestern United States
	Venezuelan equine encephalitis	A	Mosquito	Florida, Texas, Louisiana, Mexico, Central America, Ecuador, Peru, Colombia, Venezuela, Brazil, Trinidad, Surinam, Guyana
	Yellow fever	B	Mosquito	Central and South America
Fever with malaise, headaches, myalgia, *arthralgia,* and *rash*	Changuinola	Changuinola	*Phlebotomus*	Panama
	Mayaro	A	Mosquito	Brazil, Colombia, Central America, Trinidad
Fever with malaise, headaches, myalgia, rash, and *lymphadenopathy*	Dengue 1	B	Mosquito	Caribbean
	Dengue 2	B	Mosquito	Circumglobal
	Dengue 3	B	Mosquito	Caribbean
	Dengue 4	B	Mosquito	Caribbean
Fever with *central nervous system* involvement	California encephalitis	California	Mosquito	United States
	Eastern equine encephalitis	A	Mosquito	Eastern Canada, United States, Mexico, Dominican Republic, Jamaica, Panama, Trinidad, Brazil
	Ilheus	B	Mosquito	Northern South America, Trinidad, Central America, Florida
	Medoc		?	United States
	Powassan	B	Tick	Canada, New York
	Rocio	B	?	Brazil
	St. Louis encephalitis	B	Mosquito	United States, Caribbean, Panama, Brazil, Argentina
	Venezuelan equine encephalitis	A	Mosquito	Florida, Texas, Louisiana, Central America, Caribbean, Northern South America, Peru
	Western equine encephalitis	A	Mosquito	Canada, United States, Mexico, Brazil, Argentina
Fever with malaise, headaches, myalgia, and *hemorrhagic signs*	Dengue 1	B	Mosquito	Caribbean, including Puerto Rico
	Dengue 2	B	Mosquito	Caribbean, including Puerto Rico
	Dengue 3	B	Mosquito	Caribbean, including Puerto Rico
	Yellow fever	B	Mosquito	Central and South America

* *Antibody responses to viruses in the same serologic group often show cross-reactions with other members of the group.*

a history militates against the diagnosis. Persons affected usually are those whose occupational or recreational activities bring them in contact with ticks. The disease may occur at any age, although 40 percent in one series were 20 to 29 years of age. The clinical picture is characterized by the sudden onset of severe aching of the muscles of the back and legs, chilliness without true rigors, a rapid increase in temperature, which usually reaches 38.9 to 40°C (102 to 104°F), headache with pain on ocular movement, retroorbital pain, and photophobia. Abdominal pain and vomiting occur in one-fourth of patients; diarrhea is rare. The physical findings are not specific. Tachycardia in proportion to the temperature, flushed facies, and variable conjunctival injection may be present. Occasionally the spleen is palpable. Rash occurs in only 5 percent of patients, but on occasion a petechial rash involving primarily the arms and legs or a maculopapular rash over the entire body may occur. Rarely, punched-out ulcers may form at the site of tick bite. The fever with the associated symptoms lasts about 2 days, then abruptly lyses to normal or subnormal, leaving the patient very weak. After an afebrile period of about 2 days, the fever recurs, may be higher than in the first phase, and may last as long as 3 days. One-half of patients show this saddleback pattern of temperature. Rarely there may be three febrile phases. Convalescence of more than 3 weeks is reported in 70 percent of patients over age 30, while symptoms last less than 1 week in 60 percent of patients under 20. Prolonged convalescence has no relationship to persistent viremia.

Evidence of central nervous system involvement has been recorded in a few patients. The findings are those of either an aseptic meningitis with stiffness of the neck or encephalitis with clouding of the sensorium, delirium, and coma. Single instances of reported complications include epididymoorchitis and patchy pneumonitis.

LABORATORY FINDINGS The most important laboratory feature is moderate to marked leukopenia, although in one-third of confirmed cases leukocyte counts remain about 4500 per cubic millimeter. On the first day of illness, the total leukocyte count may be at normal levels, but usually by the fifth or sixth day there has been a decrease to 2000 to 3000 per cubic millimeter. Characteristically there is a proportionate decrease in lymphocytes and granulocytes. Toxic changes in neutrophils are often conspicuous, and "virocyte" types of lymphocytes are frequently observed. Bone marrow examination reveals "maturation arrest" in the granulocytic series. Erythrocyte values remain normal. Thrombocytopenia has been recorded in an isolated case report. The blood picture returns to normal within a week after the fever subsides.

DIAGNOSIS The diagnosis of Colorado tick fever is suspected on the basis of the epidemiologic history and clinical findings. Because of the infrequency of rash, patients who develop fever and rash after tick bites should be suspected of having Rocky Mountain spotted fever. The usual methods for confirming Colorado tick fever are mouse inoculation and fluorescent antibody (FA) staining of patients' erythrocyte; a combination of the two is best. Special handling of blood is not necessary for the FA test which remains positive during as well as several weeks after clinical illness.

TREATMENT Treatment is entirely symptomatic.

PROGNOSIS The prognosis is excellent.

PREVENTION Only one patient has been reported as having the disease twice. Active immunity with an attenuated virus has been produced, but the immunization itself frequently produced mild disease. Colorado tick fever is best prevented by avoiding contact with the wood tick. Convalescent individuals should be excluded as blood donors for at least 6 months.

Venezuelan equine encephalitis Venezuelan equine encephalitis (VEE) was first noted in equines in Colombia in 1935.

ETIOLOGY Like other alphaviruses, the causative agent of VEE is a relatively small, 40 to 45 nm, RNA virus. On the basis of serologic tests, differing serotypes have been identified, IA to IE, II, III (Mucambo), and IV. Strains ID, IE, II, III, and IV have remained sylvatic in distribution. IA was the original epidemic strain which occurred in Venezuela, and IB, which was recognized in Ecuador in 1963, spread through Central America into Mexico and was responsible for the epidemic in Mexico in 1971 which spread into southern Texas, with the occurrence of at least 76 laboratory-confirmed human cases. In early 1973, almost 4000 cases occurred in Peru.

EPIDEMIOLOGY VEE has been primarily a disease of equines and other mammals, although occasionally the agent has infected humans. Evidence of human infection (virus isolation or specific neutralizing antibodies) has been found in Colombia, Ecuador, Panama, Surinam, Guyana, French Guiana, Mexico, Brazil, Curaçao, Trinidad, Argentina, Peru, Florida, and Texas. The VEE virus complex in nature has been associated with numerous mosquitoes (at least 9 genera and 37 species), including *Aëdes, Mansonia, Psorophora,* and *Culex.* In this respect it differs markedly from other mosquito-borne encephalitogenic arboviruses, which usually are associated with only one to three vector species. VEE apparently has different vectors for its endemic-epizootic and its epidemic-epizootic cycles. The virus has a wide host range in wild mammals, with at least 20 genera, including capuchin monkeys, rats, mice, opossum, jack-rabbit, fox, and bats being naturally infected. Domestic animals other than equines which have been shown to be infected include cattle and pigs in Mexico and goats and sheep in Venezuela. VEE appears to multiply well in mammals with high titers of virus in the blood; e.g., infected horses may have titers of up to $10^{7.5}$ mouse intraperitoneal lethal doses per milliliter of blood. Though 29 species of wild birds have been shown to be naturally infected with VEE (20 percent of which are colonial nestling herons and related species), whether the VEE-viremia levels in birds are high enough to infect vector mosquitoes is not yet known. During the initial 3 days of illness, viremia has been detected in approximately two-thirds of patients. The levels of viremia are sufficiently high that humans could serve as a reservoir. VEE virus also has been isolated by pharyngeal swab in a few patients, suggesting the potential for person-to-person transmission. The available observations make it reasonable to consider that the natural vector is a mosquito, with the primary reservoir being either wild or domestic terrestrial mammals. However, natural infection can probably take place without an arthropod vector. Laboratory infections have occurred and are probably due to inhalation of aerosols.

CLINICAL MANIFESTATIONS In humans, infection with VEE virus usually results in a mild acute febrile illness without neurological complications. No age is spared, and there is no sex preponderance. The incubation period is 2 to 5 days, followed by the abrupt onset of headache, fever often associated with rigors, malaise, and myalgia. Other common symptoms may include nausea, vomiting, diarrhea, and sore throat. Uncommon features include photophobia, seizures, mental confusion, coma, tremors, and diplopia. Lymphadenopathy occurs in one-third of patients. On laboratory examination initial leukocyte counts are normal with 80 percent neutrophils. By the third day leukopenia occurs in two-thirds of patients. The cerebrospinal fluid may reveal pleocytosis with modest increases in protein concentration and normal glucose concentration. Virus may be isolated both from blood and from cerebrospinal fluid. The symptoms usually last 3 to 5 days in mild cases and up to 8 days in more severe cases, although one patient reported from Florida was febrile for 3 weeks. A biphasic course of illness may be encountered, with recrudescence of symptoms at the sixth to the ninth day. In one case report, palatine petechiae were noted and the patient vomited "coffee-grounds" material. In an epidemic in Venezuela in 1962, almost 16,000 cases of acute disease were evaluated; 38 percent were classified as encephalitis, but only 3 to 4 percent had severe neurological abnormalities: convulsions, nystagmus, drowsiness, delirium, or meningitis. The mortality rate was estimated to be less than 0.5 percent, and nearly all deaths occurred in young children.

Rift Valley fever Rift Valley fever is an acute disease principally of livestock, sheep, goats, cattle, and camels which is widespread throughout east and south Africa. It was first described in humans during an extensive epizootic of hepatitis in sheep in the Rift Valley in east Africa. During an epizootic in South Africa in 1950–1951, an estimated 20,000 humans became infected. In 1977 Rift Valley fever was first recognized in Egypt with a major outbreak. Cases have occurred in each subsequent year. An estimated 20,000 to 100,000 cases with 60 to 600 deaths occurred in 1977. At least one case has been reported in a Canadian tourist.

Virus has been found in several species of mosquitoes: *Culex pipiens, Eretmapodites chrysogaster, Aëdes caballus, Aëdes circumluteolus,* and *Culex theileri. Culex pipiens* has been suggested as the vector in Egypt. While antibodies to Rift Valley fever have been found in wild field rats in Uganda, the reservoir is unknown. Although humans presumably can be infected by arthropods, many infections occur as a result of handling infected animal tissues. In addition, laboratory-acquired infections have been common, which suggests a respiratory route.

The incubation period is usually 3 to 6 days. The onset is abrupt, with malaise, chilly sensation or rigors, headache, retroorbital pain, and generalized aching and backache. The temperature rises rapidly to 38.3 to 40°C (101 to 104°F). Later complaints include anorexia, loss of taste, epigastric pain, and photophobia. Findings on examination are usually unremarkable except for flushing of the face and conjunctival injection. The temperature curve is often saddleback in type, with an initial elevation lasting 2 to 3 days, followed by a remission and second febrile period. Convalescence is typically rapid. Prior to the outbreak in Egypt, Rift Valley fever was a benign illness with almost no fatalities. In Egypt, approximately one percent of patients developed severe complications, such as encephalitis, retinopathy, or hemorrhagic manifestations. Encephalitis appeared as the acute infection waned and was severe with serious residua in survivors. Hemorrhagic manifestations appeared as the disease evolved with generalized hemorrhages and icterus. Deaths from massive hepatic necrosis occurred 7 to 10 days after onset of illness. The fatality rate in severely ill patients may exceed 50 percent. Macular exudates, with decreased vision, occur. A characteristic finding is an initial normal total leukocyte count followed by leukopenia with a decrease in neutrophils associated with an increase in band forms. The diagnosis is made by isolating the virus from the blood by inoculation of mice. Three-fourths of patients are viremic (up to 10^8 mouse intraperitoneal lethal doses per milliliter blood) when first seen. Neutralizing antibodies have been demonstrated as early as 4 days after onset. There is no specific treatment. A killed vaccine which had been stockpiled in the United States is being utilized.

Bat salivary gland virus During a survey of rabies infection in bats, a virus related to the St. Louis encephalitis complex was obtained from the salivary glands of Mexican free-tailed bats in Texas. It is not known how the virus is maintained in nature. Five laboratory-acquired infections have been recorded. The illnesses were characterized by fever associated with headache, myalgia, and a mild nonproductive cough. In two patients, there was evidence of central nervous system involvement with encephalitis and aseptic meningitis. One patient had oophoritis, and two developed orchitis. By the sixth to seventh day of illness, leukopenia in the range of 2000 to 3000 leukocytes per cubic millimeter was observed in two individuals.

Zika virus Zika virus was first isolated from a captive rhesus monkey in Uganda and subsequently from wild mosquitoes. On the basis of serologic surveys, it is known to infect humans in Uganda and Nigeria. During investigation in eastern Nigeria of an outbreak of jaundice that was suspected of being yellow fever, physicians isolated Zika virus from one patient and noted that two others had a rise in neutralizing antibodies. The symptoms in these patients included fever, arthralgia, and headache with retroorbital pain. Jaundice was present in one, and bile was demonstrated in the urine of another. Albuminuria was noted in one patient. Prothrombin times were normal. The clinical syndrome appears to simulate mild yellow fever.

Group C arboviruses Currently 11 viruses are classified as Bunyaviruses, group C, of which 9 have been isolated from blood obtained from humans. The geographic distribution includes Brazil (Apeu, Caraparu, Itaqui, Marituba, Murutucui, Oriboca), Trinidad (Caraparu, Restan), and Panama (Madrid, Ossa). Several of these viruses have been isolated from Culicine and Subethine mosquitoes, as well as from several species of rodents. Isolates have been obtained mostly from forest workers and laboratory technicians. Epidemics have not been recognized. The disease begins with headache, fever [with temperature up to 40.6°C (105°F)], and myalgia. Additional symptoms include malaise, photophobia, vertigo, and nausea. Illness is generally mild, lasting 2 to 4 days, and is occasionally followed by a relapse. No fatalities have been reported. Occasionally a prolonged period of convalescence ensues. Leukopenia, with total leukocyte counts as low as 2600 per cubic millimeter, is a common finding. Diagnosis has been established mainly by virus isolation.

Bunyamwera group Representative viruses of this group are found in all inhabited continents except Australia. Only five viruses of the group—Bunyamwera itself, Germiston, Ilesha, Guaroa, and Wycomyia—have been associated with clinical disease. Serologic surveys give evidence of a high prevalence of inapparent infection in some areas. The clinical patterns of infection due to Germiston, Ilesha, and Guaroa viruses seem similar, while infection due to Bunyamwera virus is associated often with arthralgia and sometimes with a rash. The mild clinical illness is characterized by low-grade fever, headache, and myalgia which last several days, and it may be followed by weakness during convalescence.

ARBOVIRUS INFECTIONS PRESENTING CHIEFLY WITH FEVER, MALAISE, ARTHRALGIA, AND RASH **Chikungunya** In 1952 an epidemic of a disease occurred in Tanzania, which was given the name *chikungunya* ("that which bends up") because of the sudden onset of joint pains. A group A arbovirus was isolated in 1956 both from serum of patients ill with the disease and from a pool of *A. aegypti* mosquitoes.

Chikungunya virus is responsible for a dengue-like illness in Africa, India, Southeast Asia, New Guinea, and Guam, as well as for a rather mild form of hemorrhagic fever in Asiatic children. Outbreaks have been associated with high attack rates, with as many as 80 percent of inhabitants in some settlements becoming ill. The only known host is the human. *Aëdes aegypti* is a vector. Because virus has been isolated from *A. africanus* and because antibodies against the virus can be detected in chimpanzees, they may play a role in the natural cycle in Africa.

After an incubation estimated at no less than 9 days, the onset is typically abrupt, with a rapid rise in temperature to 38.9 to 40.6°C (102 to 105°F), often associated with a rigor and headache. Pain in large joints occurs early, incapacitating some individuals within a few minutes of onset. The arthralgia is often associated with objective arthritis. Sites of involvement include knees, ankles, shoulders, wrists, or proximal interphalangeal joints. Myalgia, especially backache, and malaise occur frequently. In 60 to 80 percent of patients a maculopapular eruption, which may appear at any time during the febrile course, is noted on the trunk or on the extensor surfaces of the extremities. Mild lymphadenopathy, predominantly in the axillary or inguinal areas, may be evident. Pharyngitis and conjunctival suffusion may be observed in a few patients. Fever continues for 1 to 6 days, and in some patients an afebrile interval of 1 to 3 days is followed by a secondary rise in temperature. The joint pains may continue after the temperature has returned to normal. In a few individuals joint pains have persisted for up to 4 months. Hematocrit values remain normal. Total leukocyte counts may be less than 5000 per cubic millimeter in some patients, while in others they remain normal. Urinalyses are normal. There is no specific antiviral treatment. Anti-inflammatory agents such as aspirin or indomethacin have been utilized. No second attacks have been recognized, and in the absence of the hemorrhagic fever syndrome, no deaths have been described.

Mayaro virus disease Outbreaks involving a number of persons have occurred in Brazil and Bolivia. Survey for antibodies in serums obtained from residents in Rio de Janeiro showed that almost one-third were positive. Mayaro virus has been isolated from a wild mosquito, *Mansonia venezuelansis,* and can be maintained serially in *A. aegypti* and *Anopheles quadrimaculatus.*

The incubation period has not been cleary defined but is about 1 week. Ages of patients have ranged from 2 to 62 years, with both sexes involved. Illness begins abruptly with fever, chills, severe frontal headache, myalgia, and dizziness. Temperatures usually exceed 40°C (104°F). Arthralgia occurs uniformly and is very prominent, occasionally incapacitating, and in some patients precedes the fever by a few hours. Involvement of the wrists, fingers, ankles, and toes predominates. Other initial symptoms (in less than one-third of patients) include nausea, vomiting, and diarrhea. Initial examination reveals inguinal lymphadenopathy (one-half of cases), swelling of affected joints (one-quarter of cases), and occasional conjunctival congestion. The initial clinical features last 3 to 5 days except the arthralgia, which may persist for 2 months. On about the fifth day a maculopapular rash develops over the chest, back, arms, and legs. Rash appeared in 90 percent of children and in one-half of adults and lasted about 3 days.

Laboratory findings include leukopenia with leukocyte counts as low as 2500 per cubic milliliter during the first week. Urinalysis revealed albuminuria (2+) in one-fourth of patients. Some patients showed slight elevations in serum glutamic-oxaloacetic transaminase levels.

In Brazil, no relapses were observed and no deaths have been recognized. In Bolivia, more severe illness and several fatalities have been reported.

O'nyong-nyong fever O'nyong-nyong fever was first noted as an epidemic illness characterized by joint pains, rash, and lymphadenopathy in the northern province of Uganda in 1959. The agent is a group A arbovirus which shows close antigenic relationships with chikungunya and Semliki Forest viruses. The original outbreak was associated with an explosive epidemic which spread to Tanzania and other areas in east Africa. By 1961, 2 million cases were recorded. In some areas, 91 percent of the population had either clinical disease or inapparent infection. Local outbreaks extended over the entire year. All age groups were affected. The most likely vector is *Anopheles funestus.* The clinical features are similar to those of chikungunya virus infection.

Sindbis virus Sindbis virus infection in humans rarely presents as a clinical disease. Of five cases from Uganda, one patient gave a history of joint pain. In the only well-studied clinical illness, a South African woman had arthritis as a prominent finding. Two days after a headache she noted swelling in her hands and feet. Soon thereafter she developed a confluent macular rash, followed by vesicle formation. The small joints of the hands and feet were swollen at the time of examination. Slight swelling of the fingers was present at 10 weeks, although she had otherwise recovered.

Ross River virus Epidemics of polyarthritis associated with rashes have been observed in Australia since 1928. Outbreaks occur almost entirely in the period December to June. There is a predilection for women, and children are seldom involved (an obvious similarity with rubella, another Togavirus). The onset is characterized by headache, mild catarrh, and occasionally tenderness of the palms and soles. Initially fever may be absent or minimal [highest 38°C (100.4°F)]. In about one-half of patients, arthritis, involving mainly the small joints, wrists, and ankles and sometimes associated with swelling, and paresthesias precede a rash by 1 to 15 days. In the other half, the rash precedes the arthralgia. The rash, which lasts 2 to 10 days, is usually maculopapular, appears on the cheeks and forehead, occasionally spreads to the trunk, or may be restricted to the limbs. The rash may be pruritic. Vesicles occur rarely. Tender lymphadenopathy occurs in one-fifth of the patients. Joint symptoms persist for 3 weeks to 3 months. Patients with this syndrome have shown infection with Ross River virus, although virus has not been isolated from synovial fluid. Serologic evidence of infection is common in New Guinea. An outbreak occurred between April and October 1979 in Fiji and American Samoa, with cases documented in United States travelers.

Other arboviruses Bunyamwera viruses occasionally have been associated with the syndrome of rash and arthralgia.

ARBOVIRUS INFECTIONS PRESENTING CHIEFLY WITH FEVER, MALAISE, LYMPHADENOPATHY, AND RASH **Dengue fever** Dengue is endemic over large areas of the tropics and subtropics, southeast Asia, the South Pacific, and Africa. Outbreaks of dengue have occurred in the Caribbean including Puerto Rico and the U.S. Virgin Islands since 1969. Approximately 3000 cases were reported in Mexico in 1979. Indigenous infection occurred in the United States for the first time in 35 years in the fall of 1980. Eleven cases have been recognized in residents of the Rio Grande valley of Texas. In the summer of 1981, 79,000 cases of dengue-like illness with 31 deaths were reported from Cuba. *Aëdes aegypti,* the vector, has reappeared along the U.S. Gulf Coast; hence, the threat of dengue along the Gulf Coast is real.

ETIOLOGY There are four distinct serogroups of dengue viruses, types 1, 2, 3, and 4, all of which are group B arboviruses. In the Caribbean, type 1 was associated with the 1977–1978 outbreak, type 2 in 1968–1969, type 3 in 1963–1964, and type 4 was documented in the western hemisphere for the first time in 1981.

EPIDEMIOLOGY So far as is known, dengue infections in nature involve only human beings and *Aëdes* mosquitoes. Attempts have been made to implicate lower vertebrates, especially monkeys, as reservoir sylvatic hosts, but the data are inconclusive. *Aëdes aegypti* is the most important worldwide vector species. This species, as well as the less common vector species, is peridomestic, biting humans readily or even preferentially and breeding in small collections of water such as cisterns and backyard litter. Surveys in Texas have revealed containers with water in which *A. aegypti* were breeding in up to 25 percent of premises. They fly during the day. Humans appear to be uniformly susceptible, and susceptibility is not influenced by age, sex, or race. During outbreaks, attack rates may be very high; in Puerto Rico and the U.S. Virgin Islands, the overall rate of clinical illness was 20 percent, with infection rates as determined by serologic survey as high as 79 per 100.

CLINICAL MANIFESTATIONS Dengue viruses frequently produce inapparent infections in humans. When symptoms develop, three broad clinical patterns may be encountered: classic dengue, hemorrhagic fever (see below), and a mild atypical form. Classic dengue (breakbone fever) occurs primarily in nonimmune individuals, specifically nonindigenous adults and children. The usual incubation period is 5 to 8 days. Prodromal symptoms such as mild conjunctivitis or coryza may occur, followed in hours by the abrupt onset of a severe splitting headache, retroorbital pain, backache, especially in the lumbar area, and leg and joint pains. The headache is aggravated by movement. At least three-fourths of patients have ocular soreness, with pain on moving the eyes. A few have mild photophobia. Though true rigors are common during the course, they are usually not present at the onset. Additional symptoms include insomnia, anorexia with loss of taste or bitter taste, and weakness. Mild transient rhinopharyngitis occurs in as many as one-quarter of the individuals. Cough is almost never seen. Epistaxis has been observed. Examination reveals scleral injection (90 percent), tenderness upon pressure on the ocular globe, and nontender posterior cervical, epitrochlear, and inguinal lymphadenopathy. Over one-half of patients have an enanthem characterized initially by pinpoint-sized vesicles over the posterior half of the soft palate. The tongue is often coated. Skin rashes, varying from diffuse flushing to scarlatiniform and morbilliform, are frequently present over the thorax and inner aspects of the arms. These are transient and fade, only to be followed by a more definite maculopapular rash which appears on the trunk on the third to the fifth day and spreads peripherally. The rash may be pruritic and generally terminates with desquamation. Extreme bradycardia is not observed. Within 2 to 3 days after the onset, the temperature may decrease to nearly normal and other symptoms disappear. The remission typically lasts 2 days and is followed by return of fever and the other symptoms, although they are generally less severe than during the initial phase. This "saddleback" diphasic febrile course is considered characteristic, but often is not encountered. The febrile illness usually lasts 5 to 6 days and terminates abruptly. Complaints of fatigue for several weeks after infection are common.

In addition to this "classic" syndrome, an atypically mild illness may occur. Symptoms include fever, anorexia, headache, and myalgia. On examination, evanescent rashes may be seen, but lymphadenopathy is usually absent. The course is usually less than 72 h in duration.

At the onset both in classic and in mild dengue, the leukocyte counts may be low or normal; however, by the third to the fifth day, leukopenia, usually with counts of less than 5000 leukocytes per cubic millimeter, and neutropenia are usually seen. Occasionally albuminuria of moderate degree occurs.

DIAGNOSIS Virus isolation by tissue culture of serum obtained during the first days of illness is definitive. Diagnosis can be made by serologic tests employing paired serums for hemagglutination inhibition tests and complement fixation tests. Specific serologic diagnosis is complicated by cross-reactions with other group B arbovirus antibodies such as those following immunization with yellow fever vaccine.

TREATMENT Treatment is entirely symptomatic.

PROGNOSIS In the absence of the dengue hemorrhagic fever or dengue shock syndrome, mortality is nil.

PREVENTION An attenuated vaccine for dengue type 2 is undergoing early experimental evaluation. Control depends upon mosquito abatement.

West Nile fever West Nile virus is a group B arbovirus distributed from South Africa to southeastern India, but has been shown as a cause of significant disease only in the Near East, where it can produce a clinical picture closely resembling dengue. Outbreaks of disease involving several hundred patients occurred in Israel in 1950 to 1952. In one outbreak, over 60 percent of the population developed overt disease.

EPIDEMIOLOGY The disease is highly endemic in Egypt but goes largely unrecognized. Presumably most of the adult population is immune, and the infection in childhood is an undifferentiated mild febrile illness, whereas in Israel it mainly affects adults. The infection occurs in the summer both in Israel and in Egypt. The transmission cycle in Egypt is believed to be bird-to-mosquito-to-bird, with *Culex univittatus* as the principal vector. Although humans and a variety of other vertebrates are infected by the virus, their involvement is believed to be tangential. In Israel, the most probable vectors are *Culex molestus* and *C. univittatus.*

CLINICAL MANIFESTATIONS Most of the patients in Israel have been young adults, with neither sex predominating. The onset is usually abrupt and without prodromal symptoms. The temperature quickly rises to 38.3 to 40°C (101 to 104°F), with chills occurring in one-third of patients. Symptoms include drowsiness, severe frontal headache, ocular pain, and pain in the abdomen and back. A small number of patients have anorexia, nausea, and dryness of the throat. Cough is uncommon. Signs observed include flushing of the face, conjunctival injection, and coating of the tongue. The prominent finding is general enlargement of lymph nodes, which are of moderate size but are not hard and are only slightly tender. Occipital, axillary, and inguinal nodes are usually involved. The spleen and liver are slightly enlarged in a small proportion of patients. In one-half the patients a rash may appear from the second to the fifth day of illness and may persist for several hours or until defervescence. The rash occurs predominantly over the trunk and consists of pale roseolar maculopapular lesions. The illness is self-limited and lasts 3 to 5 days in 80 percent of patients.

In a few patients, transitory meningeal involvement may be encountered. Spinal fluid examinations may reveal a pleocytosis and some increase in protein concentration.

Leukopenia occurs in the majority of patients, and total leukocyte counts are lower than 4000 per cubic millimeter in one-third. Differential counts vary from a moderate shift to the left to a slight lymphocytosis.

Convalescence is often prolonged, lasting 1 to 2 weeks, with prominent symptoms of fatigue. Enlargement of lymph nodes subsides over several months. Only rarely have complications, sequelae, or fatalities been seen in natural infections, although in one outbreak in a group of elderly patients a high proportion of patients developed meningoencephalitis, and four fatalities ensued.

Accurate diagnosis rests on virus isolation, which can be accomplished because viremia persists for as long as 6 days, or the demonstration of a rising specific antibody titer.

The treatment is symptomatic.

ARBOVIRUS INFECTIONS PRESENTING CHIEFLY WITH CENTRAL NERVOUS SYSTEM INVOLVEMENT Four arboviruses are presently recognized as numerically important causes of central nervous system disease in the United States: St. Louis encephalitis virus, eastern equine encephalitis virus, western equine encephalitis virus, and the California encephalitis group of viruses. The spectrum of infection caused by these agents includes inapparent infection, fever with headache, aseptic meningitis, and encephalitis. Of the 4308 patients reported with encephalitis during 1975, over 2000 cases (49 percent) were due to arboviruses. Widespread epidemics of St. Louis encephalitis were responsible for 86 percent of these cases. For 12 of the 24 years from 1955 to 1978, St. Louis encephalitis virus was the most common cause of arboviral encephalitis in the United States. Since 1966 when California encephalitis virus was generally recognized, 50 to 150 cases have been reported annually.

ETIOLOGY Despite the diversity of specific viral etiologies (see Table 208-2), in individual patients the clinical manifestations of aseptic meningitis and encephalitis are very similar, and preclude an etiologic diagnosis without ancillary information regarding epidemiologic and serologic features (see Table 208-3). The clinical features of aseptic meningitis due to arboviruses are indistinguishable from those due to the more prevalent enteroviruses (see Chap. 205). Since transmission to humans in the United States and Canada involves arthropods, specifically mosquitoes, except for Powassan and Colorado tick fever, indigenously acquired disease occurs at times when mosquitoes are prevalent, such as late spring through early fall. The broad clinical picture of arbovirus encephalitis will be discussed; then the specific epidemiologic and prognostic features which characterize the major types will be presented.

CLINICAL MANIFESTATIONS The clinical features of arbovirus encephalitis differ among age groups. In infants under 1 year of age, the only consistently noted symptoms are sudden onset of fever, which is often accompanied by convulsions. Convulsions may be either generalized or focal. Typically the fever ranges between 38.9 and 40°C (102 and 104°F). Other physical findings may include bulging of the fontanelle, rigidity of the extremities, and abnormalities in reflexes.

In children between 5 and 14 years of age, subjective symptoms are more easily elicited. Headache, fever, and drowsiness of 2 to 3 days' duration before medical attention is sought are common. The symptoms may then subside or become more intense and may be associated with nausea, vomiting, muscular pain, photophobia, and, less frequently, convulsions (less than 10 percent except in California encephalitis). On examination, the child is found to be acutely ill, febrile, and lethargic. Nuchal rigidity and intention tremors are often present, and on occasion muscular weakness can be demonstrated.

In adults, the initial symptoms commonly include the fairly abrupt onset of fever, nausea with vomiting, and severe headache. The headache is most often frontal but may be occipital or diffuse in location. Mental aberrations, represented by confusion and disorientation, usually appear within the subsequent 24 h. Other symptoms may include diffuse myalgia and photophobia. The abnormalities found on physical examination predominantly relate to the neurological examination, although conjunctival suffusion is frequently seen and skin rashes may occur. Disturbances in mentation are among the most outstanding clinical features. These range from coma through severe disorientation to subtle abnormalities detected only by cerebral function tests such as the subtraction of serial 7s. A small proportion of patients show only lethargy, lying quietly, apparently asleep unless stimulated. Tremor is common and is observed more frequently in individuals over 40 years of age. The tremors vary in location and may be continuous or intention in type. Cranial nerve abnormalities resulting in oculomotor muscle paresis and nystagmus, facial weakness, and difficulty in deglutition may occur, and are usually present within the initial several days. Objective sensory changes are unusual. Hemiparesis or monoparesis may occur. Reflex abnormalities are also common; these include exaggerated palmomental reflexes, and suck and snout reflexes. Superficial abdominal and cremasteric reflexes are usually absent. Changes in the tendon reflexes are variable and inconstant.

TABLE 208-3
Features of arboviral encephalitides common in the United States

Etiology	*Geographic predominance in the United States*	*Urban/ rural*	*Age, years*	*Sex*	*Unique clinical features*	*Mortality, %*	*Residua*
California encephalitis	Midwest	Rural	5–10	M	Seizures	2	Seizures (one-fourth who had them in acute phase), behavioral problems (15%)
Eastern equine encephalitis	Eastern seaboard	Both	<5 >55	=	CSF may have >1000 WBC/mm³	50	Children < 10 years have emotional lability, retardation, convulsions
St. Louis encephalitis	Eastern and midwest	Both	>35	=	Dysuria	2–12	Ataxia, speech difficulties (5%)
Western equine encephalitis	Entire	Both	<1 >55	=	None	3	Children <3 months have behavioral problems, convulsions

The plantar response may be extensor and fluctuates almost hourly. Dysdiadochokinesia often exists.

The duration of the fever and neurological symptoms and signs varies from several days to a month but usually ranges from 4 to 14 days. Clinical improvement generally follows the subsidence of the fever within several days unless irreversible anatomic changes have occurred.

LABORATORY FINDINGS Erythrocyte values are usually normal. Total leukocyte counts often reveal both a slight to moderate leukocytosis (occasionally greater than 20,000 leukocytes per cubic millimeter) and neutrophilia. Examination of the cerebrospinal fluid usually reveals several hundred cells per cubic millimeter, but on occasion cloudy cerebrospinal fluid with cells in excess of 1000 per cubic millimeter may be seen. Within the first several days of illness, polymorphonuclear neutrophils may predominate. The initial cerebrospinal fluid protein is usually only slightly elevated but on occasion may exceed 100 mg/dl. The level of spinal fluid sugar is normal; a significant decrease should raise serious consideration of an alternative diagnosis. As the illness progresses, mononuclear cells in the cerebrospinal fluid tend to increase so that they predominate and the protein concentration may increase. Other laboratory studies have been performed only sporadically, but abnormalities may include hyponatremia, often due to the inappropriate secretion of antidiuretic hormone, and elevations in serum creatine phosphokinase.

DIAGNOSIS Specific diagnosis requires the isolation of the virus or detection of antibodies with a rising titer between the acute phase of disease and convalescence. Antibodies can be detected by hemagglutination inhibition, complement fixation, or virus neutralization techniques.

TREATMENT Treatment is entirely supportive and requires meticulous attention in the comatose patient.

California (LaCrosse) encephalitis A previously undescribed virus was isolated in 1943 from mosquitoes in Kern County, California. Since 1963, a large number of agents now designated as the California group of viruses have been isolated. Almost all the isolates have been LaCrosse virus.

Since 1966 in the midwest United States, California (LaCrosse) encephalitis has been incriminated in 5 to 6 percent of cases of acute central nervous system disease, ranking above all agents except the enteroviruses.

EPIDEMIOLOGY Infection has been demonstrated to occur in the midwest, especially in Ohio, Indiana, and Wisconsin, in wooded areas of eastern Texas and Louisiana, and along the eastern seaboard. The principal animal reservoir is the squirrel. The mosquito vectors are primarily woodland mosquitoes belonging to *Aëdes* species, principally *A. triseriatus.* The LaCrosse virus appears to overwinter in eggs of *A. triseriatus.* Transovarial transmission of California group viruses then occurs. California encephalitis occurs during the summer months (June to October), most often involving boys (60 percent) 5 to 10 years of age (60 percent) who live in rural areas.

CLINICAL MANIFESTATIONS Two clinical patterns have been defined. One is a mild form with a 2- to 3-day prodrome of fever, headache, malaise, and gastrointestinal symptoms. About the third day the temperature increases to 40°C (104°F), and the patient becomes lethargic and develops meningeal signs. These findings abate gradually over a 7- to 8-day period without overt sequelae. The second pattern, a severe form which occurs in at least one-half of the patients, begins abruptly with fever, headache, and vomiting, followed shortly by lethargy and disorientation. During the first 2 to 4 days the course is rapidly progressive with the occurrence of seizures (50 to 60 percent), focal neurological signs (20 percent), pathological reflexes (10 percent), and coma (10 percent). Focal neurological signs may include asymmetrical flaccid paralysis. Uncommon findings have included arthralgia and rash. Clinical laboratory features include peripheral leukocyte counts ranging from 7000 to 30,000 per cubic millimeter (median 16,000 per cubic millimeter) with neutrophilia. Cerebrospinal fluid examination reveals 10 to 500 cells per cubic millimeter, usually with a predominance of mononuclear cells, protein concentrations of less than 100 mg/dl, and normal sugar concentrations. Electroencephalograms are abnormal in at least 80 percent of patients, revealing slow deltawave activity. In one-half of the patients the abnormality is asymmetrical, suggesting focal destructive lesions. Brain scans using [^{99}Tc]pertechnetate also may be abnormal, and localized asymmetrical increased uptake has been observed. Beginning about the fourth day and proceeding over the next 3 to 7 days, there is progressive improvement, with almost all patients becoming afebrile, seizure-free, and ready for discharge from the hospital within 2 weeks after onset.

DIAGNOSIS Neutralizing and hemagglutination-inhibition antibodies usually are present a few days after the onset. Complement-fixing antibodies become detectable 10 to 12 days after onset.

TREATMENT Initial seizure activity is frequently prolonged and difficult to control. The most effective anticonvulsant medication has been parenteral diazepam. Patients with the severe form of disease should be discharged on anticonvulsants such as phenobarbital for 6 to 12 months.

PROGNOSIS The case fatality ratio is low (2 percent or less); however, one-third of patients may have abnormal neurological findings at the time of discharge. During the early convalescent period, emotional lability and irritability are common. In one series, recurrent seizures occurred in one-quarter of the patients who had seizures during the acute phase. In this same series EEGs were abnormal in one-third of patients evaluated 1 to 8 years after their acute illness. In another series, 15 percent had sequelae, predominantly personality or behavioral problems.

Eastern equine encephalitis Eastern equine encephalitis, a group A arbovirus, was first isolated in 1933 from the brain tissue of horses during an outbreak of equine illness in New Jersey. The first recognized human outbreak occurred in Massachusetts in 1938.

EPIDEMIOLOGY The virus is distributed along the eastern coast of the Americas from northeastern United States to Argentina. Viral isolations also have been reported in the Philippines, Thailand, Czechoslovakia, Poland, and the U.S.S.R., but the question of type specificity has not been resolved. In the northeastern United States, epidemics occur in the late summer and early fall. Epizootics in horses precede the occurrence of human cases by 1 to 2 weeks. The disease affects mainly infants, children, and adults over 55 years of age. There is no sex preponderance. Inapparent infection occurs in all age groups, suggesting that the decreased likelihood of developing overt infection in the 15- to 54-year age group is not the result of decreased exposure. The ratio of inapparent infection to overt encephalitis approximates 25:1.

The natural reservoir is unknown. Isolations have been

made from numerous species of wild birds and also from amphibians, reptiles, and mammals. The natural vector is the mosquito, including *A. sollicitans* and *Culiseta melanura. Aëdes sollicitans,* a salt-marsh mosquito which is an avid human feeder, has been postulated as the epidemic vector, while *C. melanura* is important in bird-to-bird transmission. Equine animals and human beings are probably "dead ends" in the transmission cycle, and infection in them is accidental.

CLINICAL MANIFESTATIONS Though human infections have been thought usually to result in serious, if not fatal, central nervous system involvement, the detection of inapparent infection as well as relatively mild disease establishes the occurrence of milder forms. In many patients, the cerebrospinal fluid is cloudy and contains in excess of 1000 cells per cubic millimeter.

DIAGNOSIS The hemagglutination-inhibition or neutralization tests are the serologic methods of choice. The complement fixation test may be negative in patients with confirmed infections.

PROGNOSIS The mortality rate in clinical infection exceeds 50 percent. In the most severe cases, death occurs between the third and fifth days. Children under 10 years of age have a greater likelihood of surviving the acute illness, but they also have a greater likelihood of developing severe disabling residuals: mental retardation, convulsions, emotional lability, blindness, deafness, speech disorders, and hemiplegia.

St. Louis encephalitis St. Louis encephalitis (SLE) was first recognized as an entity during a major outbreak in St. Louis, Missouri, and the surrounding area in 1933. Sporadic, unpredictable outbreaks occurred, for example, in Houston, 1964, Dallas, 1966, Memphis, 1974, northern Mississippi and Illinois, 1975. The attack rate in Greenville, Mississippi, in 1975 was the highest which has been encountered, 10 per 10,000 population.

EPIDEMIOLOGY In the United States, epidemics of SLE fall into two epidemiologic patterns. One pattern is found in the west, where mixed outbreaks of western equine encephalitis and SLE have occurred primarily in irrigated rural areas. The vector has been *Culex tarsalis.* The second pattern occurred in the original St. Louis outbreak and the numerous subsequent epidemics in the midwest, Texas, New Jersey, and Florida. These outbreaks have been more urban in location and are characterized by a marked tendency for the development of encephalitis in older persons. In such urban-suburban epidemics, the epidemic vectors have been mosquitoes of the *Culex pipiens-quinquefasciatus* complex with the exception of the Florida epidemic, in which *Culex nigripalpus* was incriminated. The presence of SLE virus outside the United States has been proved by isolations in Trinidad, Panama, Jamaica, Brazil, and Argentina. However, except for Jamaica, SLE has not been reported outside the United States. The basic transmission cycle is that of wild bird-mosquito-wild bird. The virus survives the winter in female mosquitoes which ingested a blood meal from a viremic bird before overwintering. The disease in humans usually appears in midsummer to early fall. There is no sex preponderance. The human represents an accidental host and plays no role in the basic transmission cycle. Serologic studies following most urban epidemics indicate that infection rates are similar in all age groups, and that the increasing age-specific attack rate for clinical encephalitis which is typical of urban St. Louis encephalitis is probably due to age differences in host susceptibility to overt disease rather than to a higher rate of infection.

CLINICAL MANIFESTATIONS Infection with SLE virus most commonly results in an inapparent infection. Of the patients with confirmed disease, approximately three-fourths have clinical encephalitis; the remainder present with aseptic meningitis, febrile headaches, or nonspecific illness. Virtually all patients over 40 years of age have encephalitic manifestations. Urinary frequency and dysuria have been symptoms in approximately 20 percent of patients despite sterile routine aerobic urine cultures. SLE virus antigen has been demonstrated in urine; this may account for the occurrence of urinary tract symptoms.

DIAGNOSIS The occurrence of either encephalitis or aseptic meningitis as manifested by febrile illness with cerebrospinal fluid pleocytosis in the months of June through September in an adult, especially over 35 years of age, should raise the suspicion of St. Louis encephalitis. Because approximately 40 percent of patients with SLE have antibodies detectable by hemagglutination inhibition at the onset of illness, acute serum for serologic studies should be submitted promptly to a competent laboratory.

PROGNOSIS The case fatality ratio in the original St. Louis epidemic was 20 percent. In most subsequent outbreaks the mortality rate has varied from 2 to 12 percent. Subjective nervous complaints, including nervousness, headaches, and easy fatigability and excitability, appear to be the most common residuals. Late organic defects such as speech defects, difficulty in walking, and disturbances in vision were demonstrated in approximately 5 percent of patients 3 years following infection.

Western equine encephalitis Western equine encephalitis (WEE) virus is a group A arbovirus which was isolated in 1930 in California from horses with encephalitis. In 1938 it was recovered from a fatal human infection.

EPIDEMIOLOGY WEE virus has been isolated in the United States, Canada, Brazil, Guyana, and Argentina. Human disease has been diagnosed in the United States, Canada, and Brazil. In the United States, the virus is found in virtually all geographic areas. The central valley of California represents an important endemic area. The disease occurs mainly in early summer and midsummer. Wild birds, which develop viremia of sufficiently high titer to be able to infect mosquitoes that feed on them, are the basic reservoir, although nonavian vertebrate hosts may be important. *Culex tarsalis* is the principal vector in the western United States. In areas east of the Appalachian Mountains, another vector must be operative. The virus has been repeatedly isolated from *Culiseta melanura;* however, the importance of this species has been questioned, since it is not primarily a human-biting mosquito. The ratio of inapparent infection to disease, as evidenced by serologic survey studies, varies from 58:1 in children to 1150:1 in adults. Approximately one-fourth of patients are less than 1 year of age. The highest attack rates occur in persons 50 years or older. In the summer of 1975, following the flooding of the Red River in North Dakota, an increase in equine and human cases of WEE occurred; 41 cases were reported from this region.

PROGNOSIS The fatality rate approximates 3 percent in laboratory-confirmed cases. The incidence and severity of sequelae are related to age. Sequelae among very young infants are frequent (appearing in 61 percent of a group of patients less than 3 months old) and severe; they consist of upper motor neuron impairment, involving the pyramidal tracts, extrapyramidal structures, and cerebellum, and result in behavioral problems and convulsions. Both the incidence and severity of sequelae diminish rapidly after 1 year of age. Adults may complain of nervousness, irritability, easy fatigability, and tremulousness for 6 months or longer after the acute illness. Probably not more than 5 percent of adults have sequelae which are sufficiently severe to be of practical significance. Postencephalitic seizures are rare.

Japanese encephalitis The name Japanese B encephalitis was employed during an epidemic which occurred in 1924 to distinguish it from von Economo's disease, which was designated as type A encephalitis. The designation as Japanese B no longer seems useful, and the term Japanese encephalitis will be employed.

EPIDEMIOLOGY Japanese encephalitis virus infection is known to occur in eastern Siberia, China, Korea, Taiwan, Japan, Malaya, Vietnam, Thailand, Singapore, Guam, and India. In temperate climates, the disease shows a late-summer early-fall seasonal incidence. In tropical climates there is no seasonal variation. The mosquito *Culex tritaeniorhynchus* is the major vector species. It is a rural mosquito which breeds in rich fields and preferentially bites large domestic animals, such as pigs, but also feeds on birds and humans. The human is an accidental host in the transmission cycle. In several outbreaks, a higher incidence of cases has been reported in children than in adults. The ratio of inapparent infection, as evidenced by a serologic survey study of Australian troops in Vietnam, was 210:1.

CLINICAL MANIFESTATIONS The occurrence of severe rigors at the onset has been noted in almost 90 percent of patients. On admission, most patients are alert, but deterioration of mental status occurs in about three-fourths of patients within 3 to 4 days. Localized paresis is found more often than with other arboviral encephalitides, e.g., in 31 percent of cases, with predominantly upper extremity involvement; however, it resolves rapidly with defervescence. Weight loss has been very striking. The failure of the temperature to lyse, appearance of diaphoresis, tachypnea, and the accumulation of bronchial secretions are grave prognostic signs.

PROGNOSIS The immediate mortality rate has varied from 7 to 33 percent or higher. The rate of occurrence of sequelae varies inversely with the fatality rate; in those series with high fatality rates (33 percent), sequelae occurred in 3 to 14 percent. In another series with a fatality rate of 7.4 percent, the sequelae rate was 32 percent. Individuals who had neurologic abnormalities during the acute phase but survived have no more than an 80 percent chance for complete recovery. Sequelae consist of seizures, persistent paralysis, ataxia, mental retardation, and behavioral disorders.

Other arboviruses with central nervous system involvement A large group of additional arboviruses have been associated with encephalitis or aseptic meningitis. Some of these agents are listed in Table 208-2. Though the epidemiologic picture of each of these agents is unique, the general features are sufficiently similar to require laboratory support for their differentiation.

ARBOVIRUS DISEASES PRESENTING CHIEFLY WITH HEMORRHAGIC MANIFESTATIONS For 300 years, yellow fever was the only epidemic viral disease known to be accompanied by grave hemorrhagic manifestations. Since the 1930s diverse viral etiologies of the hemorrhagic fever syndrome have been recognized and are now known to be responsible for the variety of epidemiologic situations in which this syndrome occurs (Table 208-2). Additional agents include Central Asian hemorrhagic fever, Chikungunya, Congo-Crimean hemorrhagic fever, Kyasanur Forest disease, Omsk hemorrhagic fever, Rift Valley fever, and the arenaviruses (see Chap. 209). Despite the diverse viral etiology, there are many similar clinical manifestations. The onset is usually sudden, with headache, backache, generalized myalgia, conjunctivitis, and prostration. From approximately the third day, the initial stage is followed by hypotension, and hemorrhagic manifestations may occur; these are characterized by bleeding gums, epistaxis, hemoptysis, hematemesis, melena, petechiae, ecchymoses, and hemorrhages into most visceral organs. Early mild leukopenia develops, but with the appearance of hemorrhagic manifestations, leukocytosis may occur. The pathophysiology of the cardinal signs is attributable to hematopoietic and capillary damage, with variable localization of lesions. On the basis of limited confirmatory observations, variable degrees of disseminated intravascular coagulation may be in part responsible for the pathophysiology of the hemorrhagic fever syndromes. Death usually occurs in the second week of disease, at which time a high titer of antibody has developed and the patient may have become afebrile. Death is usually associated with coma, which is due not to encephalitis but to an encephalopathy. The pathological changes may be similar despite diverse viral etiologies, with midzonal hepatic necrosis and acidophilic cytoplasmic inclusions similar to the Councilman bodies of yellow fever.

Yellow fever Yellow fever is an acute infectious disease of short duration and extremely variable severity; it is caused by a group B arbovirus and is followed by lifelong immunity. The classic triad of symptoms—jaundice, hemorrhages, and intense albuminuria—is present only in severe infections, which now compose only a small proportion of the total.

PREVALENCE Yellow fever remains the most dramatically serious arbovirus disease of the tropics. For more than 200 years, after the first identifiable outbreak occurred in Yucatan in 1648, it was one of the great plagues of the world. As late as 1905, New Orleans and other southern United States ports experienced at least 5000 cases and 1000 deaths. Because of the existence of the sylvatic form of the disease, protective measures must be maintained against human disease, as demonstrated by outbreaks in Central America in 1948 to 1957. In southern Ethiopia from 1962 to 1964 there were over 100,000 cases with some 30,000 deaths. From 1978 to 1980 there have been outbreaks in Bolivia, Brazil, Colombia, Ecuador, Peru, and Venezuela. In 1979, yellow fever reappeared in Trinidad. During the same time period extensive epidemics were seen in Nigeria, Ghana, Senegal, and Gambia. In Gambia the attack rate was 2.6 to 4.4 percent with a case fatality rate of 19 percent.

EPIDEMIOLOGY Human infection results from two basically different cycles of virus transmission, urban and sylvatic. The urban cycle is human-mosquito-human, i.e., *Aëdes aegypti*–transmitted yellow fever. After a 2-week extrinsic incubation period, mosquitoes can transmit infection. Sylvan yellow fever differs under various ecologic circumstances. In the rain forests of South and Central America, species of treetop *Haemagogus* or *Sabethes* mosquitoes maintain transmission in wild primates. Once infected, the mosquito vector remains infectious for life; hence it may serve as a reservoir as well as a vector. When humans come into proximity with the forest-canopy mosquitoes, sporadic cases or focal outbreaks may occur. With sylvan yellow fever, males predominate. Focal outbreaks may be quite extensive; in Brazil in 1973 at least 21,000 persons out of 1.5 million (1.4 percent) were infected. In east Africa, the mosquito-primate cycle is maintained by the forest-canopy mosquito, *A. africanus,* which seldom feeds on humans. The peridomestic mosquito *A. simpsoni* feeds upon primates entering the village gardens and can then in turn transmit the virus to humans. Once yellow fever is reintroduced into urban areas, the urban cycle can be reinitiated, with the potential for epidemic disease. Why yellow fever has never invaded Asia despite widespread distribution of human-biting *A. aegypti* mosquitoes has never been satisfactorily explained.

PATHOLOGY The diagnosis of yellow fever may be suspected by the presence of necrobiosis and acidophilic necrosis of the parenchymal cells of the liver with the formation of Councilman bodies which occur in a characteristically discontinuous fashion in the midzones of the liver lobules. In the kidney, the virus produces necrosis of the tubular epithelium. Multiple minute hemorrhages occur in the gastrointestinal tract. In the brain, the chief lesion is perivascular hemorrhage, which is most frequently found in the subthalamic and periventricular regions at the level of the mammillary bodies.

CLINICAL MANIFESTATIONS The incubation period is usually 3 to 6 days. In accidental laboratory- or hospital-acquired infections longer incubation periods (10 to 13 days) have been reported. In considering the clinical features, it is advantageous to classify the illness as to severity: inapparent, mild, moderately severe, and malignant. In mild yellow fever the only symptoms may be the abrupt onset of fever and headache. Additional symptoms may include nausea, epistaxis, relative bradycardia known as Faget's sign [e.g., with a temperature of 38.9°C (102°F) the pulse may be only 48 to 52 beats per minute], and slight albuminuria. The mild illness lasts only 1 to 3 days and resembles influenza except that coryzal symptoms are lacking.

Moderately severe and malignant attacks of yellow fever are characterized by three distinct clinical periods: the period of infection, the period of remission, and the period of intoxication. Prodromal symptoms are usually absent. The onset is characteristically sudden, with headache, dizziness, and temperature elevations to 40°C (104°F) without a relative bradycardia. Young children may have febrile convulsions. The headache is followed quickly by pains in the neck, back, and legs. Often there is nausea with vomiting and retching. Examination reveals a flushed face and injection of the conjunctiva. The congestion of the eyes persists until the third day. The tongue characteristically shows bright red margins and tip and a white furred center. Faget's sign appears by the second day. Epistaxis and gingival bleeding are common. On the third day of illness, the fever may fall by crisis and the patient enters remission, or, in the malignant form, copious hemorrhages, anuria, or delirium may occur. The stage of remission lasts from several hours to several days. In the third stage, the "classic" symptoms develop; the fever returns but the pulse remains slow. Jaundice becomes detectable about the third day; however, jaundice often is not prominent even in fatal illnesses. Increased epistaxis, melena, and uterine hemorrhages are common, but gross hematuria is rare. Of the classic signs, "black vomit" is more characteristic than is jaundice. Hematemesis usually does not occur before the fourth day and is often associated with a fatal outcome. Albuminuria, which rarely develops before the third day, occurs in 90 percent of patients and may be quite marked (3 to 20 g albumin per liter). In spite of this massive albuminuria, edema or ascites has not been reported. In malignant infections, coma frequently occurs 2 to 3 days before death. Shortly before death, which usually occurs between the fourth and the sixth days, the patient commonly becomes delirious and wildly agitated. Though the duration of fever in the third stage is usually 5 to 7 days, the period of intoxication is the most variable of the stages and may last up to 2 weeks. Clinical yellow fever is relatively free from complications, suppurative parotitis being the most striking of those which do occur. Clinical relapses are not characteristic of yellow fever.

LABORATORY FINDINGS Early in the disease, progressive leukopenia may occur. By the fifth day, total leukocyte counts of 1500 to 2500 per cubic millimeter often are found, the decrease being due mostly to a decrease in neutrophils. Total leukocyte counts return to normal by the tenth day, and in fatal cases there may be a marked terminal leukocytosis. Hemoglobin values remain normal except terminally, when hemoconcentration or bleeding may occur. Platelet counts are reported to be normal. Detailed coagulation studies have been performed only in rhesus monkeys experimentally infected with yellow fever, and the results are in conflict. In the earlier studies, a coagulation defect was observed. This was characterized by a prolonged one-stage prothrombin time and a prolonged partial thromboplastin time, reflecting measured deficiencies in factors II, V, VII, VIII, IX, X, and XI. Both the euglobulin lysis time and the thrombin time were prolonged, suggesting a depression of plasminogen activation and accumulation of fibrinogen degradation products. At this time platelet counts and measurements of fibrinogen were normal. The disturbances in coagulation occurred during the stage of viremia and existed before the stage of hepatic necrosis in liver biopsy specimens. These data suggested that the hemorrhagic manifestations were primarily caused by a disseminated intravascular coagulation rather than by hepatic failure. Subsequent studies failed to find evidence for disseminated intravascular coagulation but showed marked acute necrosis of B-cell areas of lymphoid tissues. Also, in experimental infections in primates, modest increases in total bilirubin and alkaline phosphatase levels and marked increases in serum glutamic oxalacetic transaminase occur. In Brazil in 1973, 7 of 29 patients with a clinical diagnosis of viral hepatitis had serologies compatible with recent yellow fever and lacked hepatitis B surface antigen. Electrocardiograms may show T-wave changes. Clinical examinations of cerebrospinal fluid have not revealed abnormalities.

DIAGNOSIS There are three established procedures for the laboratory diagnosis of yellow fever:

1 Isolation of the virus from blood. This must be done early, preferably during the first 3 days. Caution must be exercised to avoid autoinoculation.
2 Demonstration of increase in neutralizing antibody.
3 Demonstration of the typical, although not completely specific, histopathologic lesions on liver biopsy.

TREATMENT The management has been symptomatic and supportive and should be based upon assessment and correction of the circulatory abnormalities. If evidence of disseminated intravascular coagulation is present, the administration of heparin should be considered. Close attention to fluids and electrolytes is essential.

PROGNOSIS The overall fatality rate in yellow fever is between 5 and 10 percent of clinical cases; it may be even less since many infections are mild or inapparent.

PREVENTION Effective control measures are available. Immunization has been effective in the prevention of outbreaks. With the occurrence of sylvatic outbreaks, work in the area of epizootic activity should be discontinued and intensive mosquito abatement measures should be instituted. These measures may provide the time necessary for a mass immunization program.

Mosquito-borne hemorrhagic fevers The term *hemorrhagic fever* was first applied to illness in southeast Asia in the Philippines in 1953. Subsequently the hemorrhagic fevers have grown steadily as a disease problem. Initially they were classified on the basis of geography as Philippine, Thai, and southeast Asian hemorrhagic fevers. With further study it appeared more rational to classify the syndromes as hemorrhagic dengue or chikungunya, depending upon the etiology. These diseases are caused by viruses transmitted by *A. aegypti.*

ETIOLOGY At least four (dengue types 1, 2, 3, 4) and possibly six types of dengue and chikungunya virus have been isolated from arthropods and humans during outbreaks of hemorrhagic fever.

PREVALENCE Once regarded as an inevitable but trivial infection, dengue is now both a feared killer and a pathogenetic enigma. The reasons for the apparent sudden "appearance" of the syndrome in the past 30 years are completely obscure. However, during the 1922 epidemic of dengue fever in Louisiana, hemorrhagic manifestations, including epistaxis, bleeding gums, melena, menorrhagia, and even "black vomit," were observed. Hemorrhagic disease with dengue also was seen in Durban in 1927, in Athens in 1928, and in Curaçao in 1968. Yet no deaths were attributed directly to the dengue. During the past 15 years, dengue has resulted in 200,000 hospital admissions with 5 to 10 percent deaths, and involved every country in tropical Asia except Bangladesh. In Asia, hemorrhagic fever is a disease of children, with virtually all cases occurring in children under age 14 years. In 1962 in Bangkok and Thonburi, an estimated 10 to 20 percent of children under age 15 had illness due either to dengue or to chikungunya virus. Approximately 5 percent of children with dengue or chikungunya had hemorrhagic fever. Dengue hemorrhagic fever occurs almost exclusively in indigenous populations; it has been observed only rarely in Caucasians of European descent despite the frequent occurrence of classic dengue in this group. During the 1975 dengue-2 epidemic in Puerto Rico, three patients with hemorrhagic manifestations, but without shock, were reported. Elsewhere in the western hemisphere, since 1967, dengue hemorrhagic fever has occurred in Curaçao, Jamaica, and Cuba.

EPIDEMIOLOGY *Aëdes aegypti* is the vector of both dengue and chikungunya viruses. It is an urban mosquito which breeds in artificial containers and receptacles. Outbreaks are confined to the rainy season, although in areas without marked seasonal rainfall cases may occur throughout the year. Human-mosquito-human transmission of dengue is responsible for urban epidemics. Recent isolates of chikungunya virus from *Culex tritaeniorhynchus* in Thailand where human population densities are low suggest a nonhuman reservoir for this virus.

CLINICAL MANIFESTATIONS The hemorrhagic dengue syndrome is almost exclusively a disease of children. There is no sex predominance. Illness begins abruptly with a minor stage characterized by fever, cough, pharyngitis, headache, anorexia, nausea, vomiting, and abdominal pain which is often severe. This continues for 2 to 4 days. In contrast to classic dengue, myalgia, arthralgia, and bone pain are unusual. Physical signs include fever varying from 38.3 to 40.6°C (101 to 105°F), injection of the tonsils and pharynx, and palpable lymph nodes and liver. The initial state is followed by abrupt deterioration, with the rapid onset of lassitude and weakness (Table 208-4). On examination the child is found to be restless and to have cold clammy extremities with a warm trunk and a pallid face with circumoral cyanosis. Petechiae, most frequently located on the forehead and distal extremities, are seen in half the cases. Occasionally there may be a macular or maculopapular rash. The extremities are frequently cyanotic. Hypotension, with narrowing of the pulse pressure, and tachycardia occur. Pathological reflexes may be observed. Most fatalities occur in the fourth or fifth day of illness, melena, hematemesis, coma, or unresponsive shock being poor prognostic signs. Cyanosis, dyspnea, and convulsions are terminal manifestations. Following this critical period, survivors show steady and quite rapid improvement.

LABORATORY FINDINGS In one study, hemoconcentration was found in one-fifth of the children. The majority had leukocyte counts between 5000 and 10,000 per cubic millimeter, with one-third showing a leukocytosis. Only 10 percent of children had a true leukopenia. The most characteristic findings were thrombocytopenia, rarely with blood platelets under 75,000 per cubic millimeter, positive tourniquet test, and prolonged bleeding time. Prothrombin time and partial thromboplastin times were usually near normal values. Depression of clotting factors V, VII, IX, and X may be present. Bone marrow examination may reveal maturation arrest of megakaryocytes. In Manila or Bangkok, hematuria has been infrequent even with other serious bleeding manifestations; however, in Tahiti, gross hematuria was common. Cerebrospinal fluid examinations are usually normal. Other abnormal laboratory findings may include hyponatremia, acidosis, elevated blood urea nitrogen levels, elevation in serum glutamic oxalacetic transaminase levels, mild hyperbilirubinemia, and hypoproteinemia. Electrocardiograms may reveal diffuse myocardial abnormalities. Two-thirds of patients have radiological evidence of bronchopneumonia, with many showing pleural effusions.

DIAGNOSIS Specific virological diagnosis of dengue virus infection by serologic means often is difficult because broad antibody responses to group B arboviruses occur. Virus isolation may provide the only means of identifying the specific agent. Chikungunya virus diagnosis poses less difficulty, since it can be isolated from acute serum in suckling mice or hamster kidney cells. Serologic responses can also be demonstrated.

PATHOPHYSIOLOGY The pathophysiologic processes that occur in dengue hemorrhagic fever (DHF) and that distinguish it from unmodified dengue fever are increased vascular permeability in which an increased hematocrit is accompanied by a

TABLE 208-4
World Health Organization's clinical classification of dengue hemorrhagic fever

		Grade	Clinical features	Laboratory findings
DHF*		I	Fever, constitutional symptoms, positive tourniquet test	Hemoconcentration Thrombocytopenia
DHF*		II	Grade I plus spontaneous bleeding (e.g., skin, gums, gastrointestinal tract)	Hemoconcentration Thrombocytopenia
DHF*	DSS*	III	Grade II plus circulatory failure, agitation	Hemoconcentration Thrombocytopenia
DHF*	DSS*	IV	Grade II plus profound shock (blood pressure = 0)	Hemoconcentration Thrombocytopenia

* *DHF, dengue hemorrhagic fever; DSS, dengue shock syndrome.*

decrease in serum protein concentration due to selective extravasation of albumin, decreased plasma volume, hypotension, thrombocytopenia, and a hemorrhagic diathesis. The association of DHF with a secondary-type antibody response suggested that primary dengue infection "sensitizes" the host to a severe response accompanying infection with a second type. Complexes formed between dengue virus and IgG antibodies interacted with the complement system to produce C3a anaphylatoxin with increased vascular permeability. Anamnestic antibody responses with high titers of antidengue IgG antibody early in the course of DHF support this concept. Activation of both the classic and alternate complement pathways has been shown in most patients. In dengue shock syndrome (DSS), the blood clotting and fibrinolytic systems are activated, and levels of factor XII (Hageman factor) are depressed. However, this hypothesis does not explain the occasional cases of DSS which occur with initial infections. Moreover, there is a limit to the time period after primary infection in which a second infection can precipitate DSS. Halstead and associates have reported enhanced growth of dengue viruses in peripheral blood leukocytes obtained from immune, compared with nonimmune, donors. Circulating leukocytes capable of supporting replication of dengue virus in vitro disappear within months to a few years. These observations may relate the difference between benign and severe disease to the number of infected cells.

TREATMENT The mainstay is correction of circulatory collapse while avoiding fluid overload. Administration of 5% glucose in 0.5 *N* saline at a rate of 40 ml/kg restored blood pressure within 1 to 2 h in one-half of patients. When stable, the rate of administration of intravenous fluids was slowed to 10 (ml/kg)/h. If improvement did not occur, plasma or a plasma expander (20 ml/kg) was administered. Transfusion of whole blood is not recommended. Glucocorticosteroids have been used, but doses of 25 mg/kg have not resulted in significant improvement. Since the evidence for severe disseminated intravascular coagulation is questionable, use of heparin is not clear-cut, although in a group of Filipino children with type 3 dengue virus, administration of heparin (1 mg sodium heparin per kilogram) was associated with a dramatic rise in number of platelets and level of plasma fibrinogen. Antibiotics are not indicated; sympathomimetic amines and salicylates are contraindicated. Recovery from vascular collapse usually occurs within 24 to 48 h, at which time diuretics and digitalis may be necessary.

PROGNOSIS Mortality has varied from 6 to 23 percent. Deaths have been most common in infants under 1 year of age.

PREVENTION At present, vector control is the only method available to prevent hemorrhagic fever.

Tick-borne hemorrhagic fevers CRIMEAN-CONGO HEMORRHAGIC FEVER At the close of World War II, a new disease entity was recognized in the Crimea region of the U.S.S.R. Retrospective studies demonstrated that an almost identical syndrome had been recognized in the south central Asian republics of the U.S.S.R. for many years. Soviet workers repeatedly isolated virus strains during 1967 to 1969.

The virus of Crimean hemorrhagic fever (CHF) has been shown to be antigenically identical with Congo virus, which has been isolated from patients, cattle, and ticks in Africa (Kenya, Uganda, Congo, and Nigeria). CHF-Congo (CCHF) isolates now have been made from an area extending from Bulgaria, Yugoslavia, southwestern and central U.S.S.R., and the Middle East into Pakistan and across central Africa from Nigeria to Kenya. Indigenous CCHF was recognized in South Africa.

Approximately 30 cases of CCHF have been recorded annually in each of the known areas of occurrence in the U.S.S.R. The cases occur between April and September. The sex distribution of CCHF is equal, and 80 percent of the cases occur in the 20- to 60-year age group, with the majority occurring in milkmaids and agricultural workers. The major arthropod vectors for transmission to humans are ticks which belong to the genus *Hyalomma*. Cattle and wild hares appear to be important reservoirs, and rooks and other birds have been implicated, although the detailed epidemiology has yet to be defined.

The onset is abrupt, with temperatures to 40°C (104°F), dizziness, headache, and diffuse myalgia. The course of fever is occasionally biphasic, with an average duration of 8 days. Physical signs include flushing of the face, conjunctival injection, vomiting, and, on occasion, epigastric pain. Hepatomegaly is found in half the patients. Splenomegaly has been reported in 2 to 25 percent of patients. Respiratory symptoms or signs are unusual. Hemorrhagic manifestations generally begin on the fourth day with petechiae on the oral mucosa and skin, epistaxis, gingival bleeding, hematemesis, and melena. Neurological abnormalities, seen in 10 to 25 percent of patients, include nuchal rigidity, excitation, and coma. Laboratory findings show leukopenia, with the number of white blood cells falling as low as 1000 per cubic millimeter, and thrombocytopenia, which is often severe. Proteinuria and microscopic hematuria are common, but azotemia and oliguria are not. Convalescence may be prolonged. Death is usually attributed to shock or intercurrent infection. Sequelae include transient alopecia and mononeuritis or polyneuritis. Although the clinical disease seen in Africa due to Congo virus generally has not been associated with hemorrhagic manifestations, one fatal case with gastrointestinal bleeding has been reported from Uganda.

The major approach to therapy has been transfusions of blood or plasma. The clinical similarities to other hemorrhagic fever syndromes in which the phenomenon of intravascular coagulation seems to occur are sufficient to suggest that appropriate studies should be done. If evidence of disseminated intravascular coagulation is demonstrated, treatment with heparin should be considered. The reported mortality rate has shown variation between 9 and 50 percent.

OMSK HEMORRHAGIC FEVER OHF is an acute febrile disease which occurs in the Omsk and Novosibirsk oblasts in the U.S.S.R. and is caused by a group B arbovirus of the Russian spring-summer complex. The seasonal occurrence of OHF shows a biphasic pattern with peaks in May and August. OHF is transmitted to humans either by the bite of infected ticks of the genus *Dermacentor* or by the handling of infected muskrats. The natural reservoir includes muskrats, other rodents, and ticks. Epidemics occurred from 1945 to 1948, but recently the disease has been less prevalent.

Following an incubation interval of 3 to 8 days, illness begins abruptly with fever, headache, and hemorrhagic manifestations, which include epistaxis and gastrointestinal and uterine bleeding. Rarely, neurologic abnormalities may occur. Laboratory features include leukopenia. In contrast to many of the other hemorrhagic fevers, OHF has a low case fatality rate (0.5 to 3.0 percent).

KYASANUR FOREST DISEASE Kyasanur Forest disease was first recognized in south India in 1957 as a discrete clinical entity shown to be due to an arbovirus. The virus is a group B arbovirus immunologically related to the Russian spring-summer complex. Kyasanur Forest disease occurs following occupational exposure to *Haemaphysalis spinigera* ticks in the tropical forests of western Mysore in southern India. The silent reservoir cycle which infects the primate- and bird-feeding *Haemaphysalis* ticks is now believed to be *Ixodes* ticks transmitted among small forest mammals, especially the shrew. Laboratory-associated infections have been common.

The major symptoms include abrupt onset of fever, headache, fatigue, myalgia (especially of the lumbar area and calf muscles), and retroorbital pain. Cough and abdominal pain occur in half the patients. Additional symptoms may include photophobia and polyarthralgia. Epistaxis and hematemesis are observed in some patients. On examination, findings include relative bradycardia, conjunctival injection, and generalized lymphadenopathy. Fine and coarse rales are frequently heard. Hepatosplenomegaly has been encountered occasionally. During the initial phase, generalized hyperesthesia of the skin occurs occasionally. The fever usually lasts from 6 to 11 days. After an afebrile period of 9 to 21 days, approximately half the patients may develop a second phase, which lasts from 2 to 12 days. This is manifested by recurrence of fever, severe headache, neck stiffness, mental disturbance, coarse tremors, giddiness, and abnormalities in reflexes, as well as by recurrence of many of the initial symptoms. No sequelae have been observed, but convalescence is often prolonged.

Only limited laboratory studies have been performed. During the initial phase, leukopenia is a constant feature, with a total leukocyte count of fewer than 3000 per cubic millimeter by the fourth to sixth day. The leukopenia is associated with neutropenia. During the second phase there is a mild leukocytosis. Lumbar puncture during the second phase has shown a pattern of aseptic meningitis. Diagnosis is based upon virus isolation from blood; this is readily accomplished, since viremia is prolonged. Serologic tests of paired serums also can be performed. The management is supportive. The mortality rate is approximately 5 percent.

REFERENCES

Arboviruses: Definition and classification

HORZINCK MC: The structure of togaviruses. Prog Med Virol 16:109, 1973

SUBCOMMITTEE ON ARBOVIRUS LABORATORY SAFETY OF THE AMERICAN COMMITTEE ON ARTHROPOD-BORNE VIRUSES: Laboratory safety for arboviruses and certain other viruses of vertebrates. Am J Trop Med 29:1359, 1980

THE SUBCOMMITTEE ON INFORMATION EXCHANGE OF THE AMERICAN COMMITTEE ON ARTHROPOD-BORNE VIRUSES: Catalogue of arthropod-borne and selected vertebrate viruses of the world. Am J Trop Med 20:1018, 1971

WHO SCIENTIFIC GROUP: *Arbovirus and Human Disease,* WHO Tech Rep Ser 369. Geneva, 1967

WHO STUDY GROUP: *Arthropod-borne Viruses,* WHO Tech Rep Ser 219. Geneva, 1961

Arbovirus infections characterized by fever, malaise, headaches, and myalgia

BECKER FE: Tick-borne infections in Colorado. Col Med 27:36, 1930

BOWEN GS et al: Clinical aspects of human Venezuelan equine encephalitis in Texas, 1971. Bull Pan Am Health Org 10:46, 1976

BRICENO ROSSIE AL: Rural epidemic encephalitis in Venezuela caused by a group A arbovirus (VEE). Prog Med Virol 9:176, 1967

CENTERS FOR DISEASE CONTROL: Rift Valley fever with retinopathy—Canada. Morb Mort Week Rep 28:607, 1980

DAUBNEY R et al: Enzootic hepatitis or Rift Valley fever. J Pathol Bacteriol 34:545, 1931

DIASIO JS, RICHARDSON FM: Clinical observation on dengue fever. Milit Surg 94:365, 1944

DIETZ WH JR et al: Ten clinical cases of human infection with Venezuelan equine encephalomyelitis virus, subtype I-D. Am J Trop Med Hyg 28:329, 1979

FLEMING J et al: Sandfly fever. Review of 664 cases. Lancet 1:443, 1947

GOODPASTURE HC et al: Colorado tick fever: Clinical, epidemiologic and laboratory aspects of 228 cases in Colorado in 1973–1974. Ann Intern Med 88:303, 1978

HUGHES LE et al: Persistence of Colorado tick fever virus in red blood cells. Am J Trop Med Hyg 23:530, 1974

LAUGHLIN LW et al: Epidemic Rift Valley fever in Egypt: Observations of the spectrum of human illness. Trans R Soc Trop Med Hyg 73:630, 1979

LENNETTE EH, KOPROWSKI H: Human infection with Venezuelan equine encephalomyelitis virus. JAMA 123:1088, 1943

SABIN AB: Research on dengue during World War II. Am J Trop Med 1:30, 1952

——— et al: Phlebotomus (pappataci or sandfly) fever; disease of military importance: Summary of existing knowledge and preliminary report of original observations. JAMA 125:603, 693, 1944

SCHERER WF et al: Ecologic studies of Venezuelan encephalitis virus in Southeastern Mexico: VII. Infection of man. Am J Trop Med 21:79, 1972

SMITHBURN KC et al: Rift Valley fever. J Immunol 62:213, 1949

SPRUANCE SL, BAILEY A: Colorado tick fever. A review of 115 laboratory confirmed cases. Arch Intern Med 131:288, 1973

SULKIN SE et al: Bat salivary gland virus: Infections of man and monkey. Tex Rep Biol Med 20:113, 1962

TESH RB et al: Antigenic relationships among Phlebotomus fever group arboviruses and their implications for the epidemiology of sandfly fever. Am J Trop Med Hyg 24:135, 1975

Arbovirus infections presenting chiefly with fever, malaise, arthralgia, and rash

CLARK JA et al: Annually recurrent epidemic polyarthritis and Ross River virus activity in a coastal area of New South Wales. I. Occurrence of the disease. Am J Trop Med Hyg 22:543, 1973

DELLER JJ JR, RUSSELL PK: Chikungunya disease. Am J Trop Med 17:107, 1968

DOHERTY RL et al: Studies of epidemic polyarthritis: The significance of three group A arboviruses, isolated from mosquitoes in Queensland. Aust Ann Med 13:322, 1964

MALHERBE H et al: Sindbis virus infection in man. Report of a case with recovery of virus from skin lesions. S Afr Med J 37:547, 1963

PINHEIRO FP et al: An outbreak of Mayaro virus disease in Belterra, Brazil: I. Clinical and virological findings. Am J Trop Med Hyg 30:674, 1981

ROBINSON MC: An epidemic of virus disease in Southern Province, Tanganyika territory in 1952–53: I. Clinical features. Trans R Soc Trop Med Hyg 49:28, 1955

SHORE H: O'nyong-nyong fever: An epidemic virus disease in East Africa: III. Some clinical and epidemiological observations in the Northern Province of Uganda. Trans R Soc Trop Med Hyg 55:361, 1961

Arbovirus infections presenting chiefly with fever, malaise, lymphadenopathy, and rash

CENTERS FOR DISEASE CONTROL: Dengue—United States. Morb Mort Week Rep 29:531, 1980

MARBERG K et al: The natural history of West Nile fever: I. Clinical observations during an epidemic in Israel. Am J Hyg 64:259, 1956

MICKS DW, MOON WB: *Aëdes aegypti* in a Texas coastal county as an index of dengue fever receptivity and control. Am J Trop Med Hyg 29:1382, 1980

PERELMAN A, STERN J: Acute pancreatitis in West Nile fever. Am J Trop Med Hyg 23:1150, 1974

TAYLOR RM et al: A study of the ecology of West Nile virus in Egypt. Am J Trop Med 5:579, 1956

Arbovirus infections presenting chiefly with central nervous system involvement

BALFOUR HH JR et al: California arbovirus (LaCrosse) infections. Pediatrics 52:680, 1973

DICKERSON RB et al: Diagnosis and immediate prognosis of Japanese B encephalitis. Observations based on more than 200 patients with detailed analysis of 65 serologically confirmed cases. Am J Med 12:277, 1952

FEEMSTER RF, HAYMAKER W: Eastern equine encephalitis. Neurology 8:882, 1958

FINLEY KH et al: Western equine and St. Louis encephalitis. Preliminary report of a clinical follow-up study in California. Neurology 5:223, 1955

GRABOW JD et al: The electroencephalogram and clinical sequelae of California arbovirus encephalitis. Neurology 19:394, 1969

HILTY MD et al: California encephalitis in children. Am J Dis Child 124:530, 1972

KETEL WB, OGNIBENE AJ: Japanese B encephalitis in Vietnam. Am J Med Sci 261:271, 1971

LUBY JP et al: The epidemiology of St. Louis encephalitis (SLE): A review. Ann Rev Med 20:329, 1969

———: Antigenemia in St. Louis encephalitis. Am J Trop Med Hyg 29:265, 1980

SCHNEIDER RJ et al: Clinical sequelae after Japanese encephalitis: One year followup study in Thailand. Southeast Asian J Trop Med Public Health 5:560, 1974

WEAVER OM et al: Japanese encephalitis: Sequelae. Neurology 8:887, 1958

Arbovirus diseases presenting primarily with hemorrhagic manifestations

BOKISCH VA et al: The potential pathogenic role of complement in dengue-hemorrhagic fever syndrome. N Engl J Med 289:996, 1973

BURNEY MI et al: Nosocomial outbreak of viral hemorrhagic fever caused by Crimean hemorrhagic fever—Congo virus in Pakistan, January 1976. Am J Trop Med Hyg 29:941, 1980

CASALS J et al: A current appraisal of hemorrhagic fevers in the USSR. Am J Trop Med 15:751, 1966

Dengue. Lancet 2:239, 1976

DENNIS LH et al: The original hemorrhagic fever: Yellow fever. Blood 30:858, 1967

HALSTEAD SB: Mosquito-borne haemorrhagic fevers of South and Southeast Asia. Bull WHO 35:3, 1966

———, O'ROURKE EF: Dengue viruses and mononuclear phagocytes: I. Infection enhancement by non-neutralizing antibody. J Exp Med 146:201, 1977

KIRK R: An epidemic of yellow fever in the Nuba Mountains, Anglo-Egyptian Sudan. Ann Trop Med Parasitol 35:67, 1941

LOPEZ-CORREA RH et al: Dengue fever with hemorrhagic manifestations: A report of three cases from Puerto Rico. Am J Trop Med Hyg 27:1216, 1978

MONATH TP et al: Yellow fever in the Gambia, 1978–1979: Epidemiologic aspects with observations on the occurrence of Orongo virus infections. Am J Trop Med Hyg 29:912, 1980

———: Pathophysiologic correlations in a monkey model of yellow fever with special observations on the acute necrosis of B cell areas of lymphoid tissues. Am J Trop Med Hyg 30:431, 1981

NELSON ER: Hemorrhagic fever in children in Thailand: Report of 69 cases. J Pediatr 56:101, 1960

PINHEIRO FP et al: An epidemic of yellow fever in Central Brazil 1972–1973: I. Epidemiological studies. Am J Trop Med Hyg 27:125, 1978

PONGPANICH B et al: Management of shock associated with dengue hemorrhagic fever based on pathophysiological findings. Southeast Asian J Trop Med Public Health 6:115, 1975

Technical guides for diagnosis, treatment, surveillance, prevention and control of dengue hemorrhagic fever. World Health Organization, Geneva, 1975

209 ARENAVIRUS INFECTIONS

JAY P. SANFORD

DEFINITION AND CLASSIFICATION The term *arenavirus* is the proposed designation for a group of RNA viruses which have unique morphology (Table 209-1). The virions are round, oval, or pleomorphic, with diameters between 60 and 350 nm, and contain an electron-dense membrane with projections and 2 to 10 inclusion-like dense particles (resembling ribosomes) that give the virion an appearance of having been sprinkled with sand (Latin *arenaceus,* "sandy"). A special property of arenaviruses that causes disease in humans, especially Machupo and lymphocytic choriomeningitis, is their capacity to induce persistent infection in their reservoir hosts with no ill effects and in the absence of an immune response.

LYMPHOCYTIC CHORIOMENINGITIS The first-recognized arenavirus was lymphocytic choriomeningitis (LCM) virus, isolated in 1934 from a laboratory monkey in the course of studies of the 1933 St. Louis encephalitis outbreak. It was recognized early that LCM was carried by apparently healthy laboratory mice. Clinically LCM has been considered primarily in the context of aseptic meningitis; however, it is associated with at least two clinical syndromes in humans: central nervous system and influenza-like illness which may be associated with rash, arthritis, or orchitis. LCM virus has provided a valuable model for the study of chronic, persistent, and generally symptomless viral infections in laboratory animals.

Prevalence In the United States, at present, human infection with LCM virus is rare; however, seroepidemiologic studies on specimens obtained in 1935 to 1940 from persons with no history of central nervous system disease from all parts of the United States revealed neutralizing antibodies in 10 to 28 percent. In a study of aseptic meningitis, Meyer and associates

TABLE 209-1
Classification of arenaviruses

Virus	*Clinical disease*	*Reservoir*	*Known geographic range*
Lymphocytic choriomeningitis	Aseptic meningitis, meningoencephalitis, influenzal syndrome, orchitis, arthritis	Mice, hamsters	Worldwide except Australia
Tacaribe		Bats	Trinidad
Junin	Argentinian hemorrhagic fever	*Calomys musculinus*	Argentina
Machupo	Bolivian hemorrhagic fever	*Calomys callosus*	Northeast Bolivia
Amapari			Brazil
Latino			Bolivia
Parana			Paraguay
Pichinde			Colombia
Tamiami			Florida
Lassa	Lassa fever	*Mastomys natalensis*	Nigeria, Liberia, Sierra Leone, Republic of Guinea, Central African Republic
?	Far eastern hemorrhagic fever (Korean, nephropathica epidemica)	*Apodemus agrarius*	U.S.S.R., Manchuria, China, Korea, Scandinavia

incriminated LCM in 8.1 percent. In recent years, the prevalence of infection seems to have decreased markedly.

Epidemiology The virus of LCM is worldwide in distribution. Although infection can be induced in a variety of animals, mice are the major natural reservoir as well as the primary host in which latent, asymptomatic infection occurs. The latency of infection in the mouse depends upon immunologic tolerance. Animals infected in utero or shortly after birth excrete LCM virus for life without overt disease. Human infections are secondary to contact with an infected rodent. The mode of transmission is thought to be via airborne spread or contact with excrement from infected animals. In the past, most cases have arisen in persons living in rodent-infested houses, but lately outbreaks of LCM virus disease in humans have been reported from Germany and from the United States in which the source of infection was traced to laboratory animals and household pets, specifically hamsters which, like mice, can shed LCM virus in urine and stool. LCM occurs throughout the year but has been more frequent in the colder months when "the mice come in from the fields." Person-to-person transmission has not been demonstrated.

Pathogenesis In natural infection, the portal of entry of the LCM virus is probably through the respiratory tract. Virus multiplication occurs initially in the respiratory epithelium, and an influenza-like illness develops. Dissemination of virus to extrapulmonary sites, presumably to reticuloendothelial cells, with multiplication and viremia occurs. LCM virus crosses the blood-brain barrier. In mice, the resulting meningitis is attributed to a cell-mediated immune reaction. Support for this hypothesis derives from observations that disease but not infection can be prevented in experimental animals by neonatal thymectomy, irradiation, or immunodepressant drugs such as cyclophosphamide. Similar pathogenetic mechanisms may operate in humans, although isolation of LCM virus from the CSF of patients with aseptic meningitis is quite common.

Clinical manifestations The exact incubation period is not known. Following experimental inoculation of LCM virus into volunteers, fever occurred in $1\frac{1}{2}$ to 3 days, while an influenza-like constellation of symptoms developed 5 to 10 days after exposure. An influenza-like illness with many features of other arenavirus and arbovirus infections is the commonest clinical pattern. In some patients, up to one-half in some series, the illness may be biphasic with subsequent aseptic meningitis or encephalomyelitis. Fever, usually from 38.3 to 40°C (101 to 104°F), associated with rigors, is uniformly noted. Other symptoms which are encountered in over one-half of patients include malaise, weakness, myalgia (especially lumbar aching), retroorbital headache, photophobia, anorexia, nausea, and light-headedness. Other prominent symptoms which occur in one-fourth to one-half of patients include sore throat, vomiting, and dysesthesias. Later arthralgias, especially in the hands, occur. Less common complaints (up to one-quarter of patients) include aching pain in the chest, associated with pneumonitis; increased hair loss progressing to generalized alopecia of the scalp, 2 or 3 weeks after the onset of illness; testicular pain or frank orchitis, usually unilateral, again 1 to 3 weeks after onset; and parotid pain, which may lead to a misdiagnosis of mumps. Physical findings in the first week of illness are few. Patients often have a relative bradycardia. Pharyngeal injection without exudate is commonly seen (60 percent). Mild nontender cervical or axillary lymphadenopathy may occur. The initial phase lasts from 5 days to 3 weeks followed by improvement. After a remission of 1 to 2 days many patients relapse with recurrent fever and more prominent headache. Physical signs may include skin rashes, swelling of metacarpophalangeal and proximal interphalangeal joints, meningeal signs, orchitis, parotitis, and alopecia of the scalp. Convalescence generally is of 1 to 4 weeks' duration, characterized by easy fatigability, an excessive need for sleep, dysesthesias, and occasional dizziness. Patients with aseptic meningitis almost always recover without sequelae. With encephalitis, 25 to 30 percent of patients have neurological residua.

Laboratory findings Leukopenia and thrombocytopenia are almost uniform during the first week of illness. Although leukocyte counts usually vary between 2000 and 3000 per cubic millimeter, counts as low as 600 per cubic millimeter have been recorded. Differential counts generally show slight relative lymphocytosis. Platelet counts are usually between 50,000 and 100,000 per cubic millimeter. Anemia is not encountered. The erythrocyte sedimentation rate often is normal. Mild elevations of the serum enzymes, serum glutamic oxaloacetic transaminase (SGOT) and lactic dehydrogenase (LDH), may occur. Chest radiographs may suggest basilar pneumonitis. In patients with meningeal signs examination of the cerebrospinal fluid usually reveals several hundred cells per cubic millimeter, although cell counts in excess of 1000 per cubic millimeter are reported in half the patients in some series. Lymphocytes predominate (greater than 80 percent) even early. The initial cerebrospinal fluid protein is usually slightly elevated, but on occasion levels may exceed 150 mg/dl. Although a normal cerebrospinal fluid glucose level is considered the hallmark of viral meningitides, hypoglycorrhachia has been observed in up to 27 percent of patients with LCM, glucose values as low as 15 mg/dl with normal simultaneous blood sugar levels having been reported.

Diagnosis The diagnosis of LCM can be established with certainty by recovery of the virus from blood or spinal fluid. Complement-fixing antibodies are usually detectable 1 to 2 weeks after the onset of infection, peak at 5 to 8 weeks, and are gone by 6 months. Neutralizing antibodies appear after 6 to 8 weeks, increase in titer slowly, and remain high for years. Immunofluorescent studies have detected antibody to LCM virus earlier in the course of illness, and its appearance seems to parallel the development of the neurological phase. The clinical manifestations of LCM cannot be differentiated from those produced by numerous other viruses.

Treatment The management is supportive and symptomatic.

HEMORRHAGIC FEVER WITH RENAL SYNDROME Synonyms for this disease include Korean hemorrhagic fever, far eastern hemorrhagic fever, endemic or epidemic nephrosonephritis, Manchurian epidemic hemorrhagic fever, Songo fever, and Churilov's disease. A similar but milder disease in Scandinavia has been called *nephropathica epidemica* or *epidemic nephritis* (EN).

Epidemic hemorrhagic fever (EHF) is an acute febrile, often fatal, otherwise self-limited illness caused by an agent, designated Hataan virus, that is characterized by severe toxemia, widespread capillary damage, hemorrhagic phenomena, and renal insufficiency. In 1932, the Russians first observed the disease in southeastern Siberia. In April 1951, a previously unknown illness, subsequently recognized as EHF, broke out among the United Nations forces in Korea.

Etiology In 1978, Lee and associates reported the agent in the lungs of the rodent *Apodemus agrarius Coreae.* It reacted with serums from patients convalescing from Korean hemorrhagic fever. Diagnostic increases in immunofluorescent antibodies were demonstrated in 113 of 116 cases of severe EHF. Hataan virus has been passed in *A. agrarius* and propagated on human lung carcinoma cells. It appears morphologically to be an orbivirus containing double-stranded RNA. There is no serological relationship between Hataan and other orbiviruses. The viruses causing EHF and EN are related but not identical.

Prevalence In Korea between April 1951 and January 1953, 2070 cases of EHF were reported among United Nations personnel. The disease usually occurs as an isolated event; hence, overall attack rates have relatively less meaning. With this reservation, attack rates in two United States Army divisions stationed in Korea varied between 1.9 and 2.9 cases per 1000 persons per epidemic season. Approximately 800 cases per year have continued to occur; however, most cases are now seen in Korean civilians and military with less than 10 cases per year in U.S. military personnel. The U.S.S.R. reports 500 to 2000 cases yearly. Cases have been reported from the People's Republic of China and in laboratory workers in Japan.

Epidemiology In Korea the majority of cases occur in May to June and in October to November. These peaks coincide with the dry seasons. Geographically, EHF originally occurred among troops stationed in the vicinity of Seoul north of the 38th parallel. More recently cases have been encountered throughout the Korean peninsula. The epidemiology of EHF observed in Korea remains unknown. No vector is known or suspected although earlier, chiggers, especially *Trombicula pallida,* correlated closely with the epidemiology of EHF in Korea. Since World War II, rather remarkable outbreaks have occurred in northeast Asia between November and January. In these outbreaks, the peak of the epidemic was preceded by a marked increase in forest rodent populations (usually the red-backed vole *Clethrionomys rutilis*), which migrated into the fields, barns, and even houses near the forest. Antigen has been found in the lungs of both the red-backed and bank vole. There may be a very narrow variety of rodent hosts which distribute virus in urine or by eating dead carcasses. Humans are probably an incidental host who may become infected by the aerosol route.

Clinical manifestations The incubation period in EHF is usually 10 to 25 days, with possible extremes of 7 and 36 days. Individuals who contract the disease in an endemic area may easily not develop illness until their return to the United States. Inapparent or mild disease is less common than typical EHF.

The clinical course of EHF may be divided into phases on the basis of the underlying physiological aberrations: febrile, hypotensive, oliguric, diuretic, and convalescent. There is considerable variation among patients in the severity of the illness. In one study two-thirds of the 264 cases studied were classified as mild, while 14 percent were termed severe. The illness in most patients was of comparable severity in each phase.

FEBRILE (INVASIVE) PHASE From 10 to 20 percent of patients describe vague prodromal symptoms resembling mild upper respiratory infections. The onset is then usually abrupt, often initiated by a chill and accompanied by fever, headache, backache, abdominal pain, and generalized myalgia. Anorexia and thirst are almost universal, while nausea and vomiting are common although not constant symptoms. The headache is most commonly frontal or retroorbital. Eye symptoms, especially mild photophobia and pain on movement of the eyes, are characteristic. Diarrhea is not a feature. Fever is present in almost all patients; the temperature ranges from 37.8 to 41.1°C (100 to 106°F), reaches a peak on the third or fourth day after onset, and falls by lysis on the fourth to seventh day. There is a relative bradycardia. Initially the blood pressure is normal. One of the most typical early findings is a diffuse reddening of the skin, most marked over the face and V area of the neck. It may resemble a severe sunburn. The erythema blanches on pressure. Dermographism can be demonstrated in over 90 percent of patients at the same time as the flush. Slight edema of the upper eyelids causes a bleary-eyed appearance. Bulbar and palpebral conjunctivas show injection. Conjunctival petechiae may develop by the third or fifth day of illness. Subconjunctival hemorrhages may be striking. Intense pharyngeal reddening without significant sore throat is typical. The first location for petechiae is usually the palate, where they occur in half the patients. Within 12 to 24 h, petechiae appear at pressure areas such as the axillary folds, lateral chest wall, belt line, hips, and thighs. Retinal hemorrhages occur rarely. Cervical, axillary, and inguinal nodes are moderately enlarged but nontender. Abdominal and costovertebral tenderness is almost a constant finding. Splenomegaly is unusual and in Korea was generally attributable to malaria with which EHF coexisted in about 1 percent of patients. The degree of flush, fever, and conjunctival injection and the number of petechiae correlate quite well with the overall severity of illness.

Laboratory studies during this phase are often not striking. Initial hemoglobin and hematocrit values are usually normal. Prior to the fourth day, leukocyte counts range from 3600 to 6000 per cubic millimeter but are associated with neutrophilia. Early in the course urine specific gravity may be high. Albuminuria, which is an almost universal finding, appears, often abruptly, between the second and fifth days of illness. The urinary sediment reveals microscopic hematuria and hyaline, granular, red blood cell casts, and/or white blood cell casts. Erythrocyte sedimentation rates are normal during the first week. Capillary fragility tests are usually positive at the time of admission and become most abnormal by the ninth day. Electrocardiographic abnormalities may be seen in 15 to 30 percent of patients; these include sinus bradycardia and low or inverted T waves. Lumbar punctures may reveal gross blood in the spinal fluid.

HYPOTENSIVE PHASE On about the fifth day of illness, during the last 24 to 48 h of the febrile phase, hypotension or shock may occur. In mild cases, only a transient fall in blood pressure occurs; among moderately and severely ill patients shock may persist for 1 to 3 days. In 828 patients, 16.5 percent had clinical shock, and another 14 percent had hypotension without shock. Headache often diminishes, but thirst persists. In the beginning of the hypotensive phase, most patients have warm, dry skin and extremities. As the hypotensive phase progresses and the systolic blood pressure decreases and pulse pressure narrows, the skin becomes cool and moist. Tachycardia replaces the relative bradycardia.

At this stage, an increase in hematocrit with no change in total serum protein level is found. This is thought to reflect a loss of plasma through damaged capillaries. On about the fifth day, all patients develop marked proteinuria. The previously normal urine specific gravity begins to fall and in 2 to 3 days is usually around 1.010. Blood urea nitrogen concentrations begin to increase. Other laboratory findings include leukocytosis with white blood cell counts of 10,000 to 56,000 per cubic millimeter with neutrophilia and toxic granulation. The number of platelets often decreases to less than 70,000 per cubic millimeter. In a single patient who became ill 30 days after leaving Korea and who was studied on the fourth day of illness (i.e., in the hypotensive phase), there was marked thrombocytopenia, hypofibrinogenemia, and hypoprothrombinemia with a prolonged thrombin time. The deficiency of multiple blood coagulation factors suggests that the bleeding defect was due to disseminated intravascular coagulation.

OLIGURIC PHASE (HEMORRHAGIC OR TOXIC PHASE) About the eighth day of illness, blood pressure returns to the normal range and in some instances increases to hypertensive levels. While oliguria may have appeared during the shock phase, it now becomes a prominent feature. Oliguria develops even though hypotension was not recognized. Symptomatically patients continue to feel weak and thirsty and have more severe backache. Protracted vomiting and hiccups may ensue.

Blood urea nitrogen levels increase rapidly and are associated with hyperkalemia, hyperphosphatemia, and hypocalcemia. Metabolic acidosis is rarely severe. Although platelets begin to return to normal, hemorrhagic manifestations become more prominent and include petechiae, hematemesis (analogous to "black vomit" in yellow fever), melena, hemoptysis, gross hematuria, and hemorrhages into the central nervous system. The enlarged lymph nodes may now become tender.

With the onset of diuresis on about the seventh day in moderately ill patients and the ninth to eleventh day in severely ill patients, symptoms of fluid and electrolyte abnormalities and central nervous system or pulmonary complications may appear. Central nervous system symptoms include disorientation, extreme restlessness, lethargy, paranoid delusions, and hallucinations. Grand mal seizures, pulmonary edema, and pulmonary infection occur in some patients.

DIURETIC PHASE With the onset of diuresis, progressive improvement is the rule. Most patients begin to eat and regain their strength. In fatal cases the diuretic phase is associated with a daily urine output of less than 4 liters and often less than 2 liters, in contrast to larger volumes in surviving patients.

CONVALESCENT PHASE The convalescent phase lasts 3 to 6 weeks. Weight is regained slowly. Complaints include muscular weakness, intention tremor, and lack of stamina. Hyposthenuria and polyuria are present; however, within 2 months most patients are able to concentrate their urine to a specific gravity of 1.023 or greater after a 12-h period of water deprivation.

Diagnosis Serologic tests are not currently available; hence, diagnosis is based on clinical-epidemiologic features. The following criteria are necessary for diagnosis: the patient must have been in the endemic area within the limits of the incubation period, and there must be a characteristic history, hemorrhagic findings, and evidence of renal involvement. In addition, studies to exclude other forms of the hemorrhagic fever syndrome must be undertaken, particularly in the sporadic cases.

Pathology The most characteristic fundamental alteration is widespread capillary and endothelial damage, with all subsequent manifestations being the result of this damage. This is manifested by dilatation of all small vessels in tissues, congestion, plasma transudation, and multiple small hemorrhages. Three features are prominent and characteristic: hemorrhage, particularly in the renal medulla, right atrium, and gastrointestinal submucosa; a peculiar type of necrosis of the renal pyramids, anterior lobe of the pituitary body, and adrenal gland; and a mononuclear cellular infiltration of the myocardium, spleen, and liver. Moderate to severe retroperitoneal edema was present in three-fourths of patients who died in the hypotensive phase of EHF.

Pathophysiology The physiological changes correlate with the clinical features. During the early febrile phase, the cardiac index is normal. Late in the febrile phase widespread capillary dysfunction becomes evident. This is manifest by loss of protein-rich plasma through damaged capillaries and results in hemoconcentration and a progressive fall in cardiac output. Measured total peripheral resistance is low, a finding compatible with the observed capillary dilatation and refractoriness to *l*-norepinephrine. During the hypotensive phase, the increases in hematocrit values and decreases in plasma volume are accentuated. These findings have the pathological corollary of marked retroperitoneal edema. The hypotensive phase is associated with a reduction in cardiac output and an increase in peripheral vascular resistance. The reduced cardiac output is probably the result of reduction in circulating blood volume, inadequate vasoconstriction, and possibly myocardial damage. Although adrenal hemorrhages can be seen at necropsy, adrenal insufficiency does not seem to be a contributing cause of shock. The initial pathophysiologic changes may result in impairment of circulation through various organs, with the development of functional and morphologic changes secondary to inadequate perfusion with its attendant hypoxemia. The hemorrhagic manifestations appear to be the result of capillary damage, with diapedesis of erythrocytes and the development of disseminated intravascular coagulation.

The plasma loss and arteriolar dysfunction are limited in duration, and, for unknown reasons, the sequestered plasma rather abruptly returns to the vascular system at the time of oliguric phase. During this phase, examination of nail bed capillaries reveals increased vasomotor activity and vasoconstriction. When patients who became hypertensive were divided on the basis of the presence or absence of diuresis, the clinical and hemodynamic differences became more apparent. During the hypertensive phase in anuric or oliguric patients, some individuals presented with full veins, an exaggerated cardiac apical thrust, and wide pulse pressure. In this group the cardiac index was high, and the peripheral resistance and hematocrit were low. Hypertensive patients who had begun to have diuresis had normal cardiac outputs and significantly elevated values for peripheral vascular resistance.

Although diuresis is a harbinger of convalescence, a daily urine output of 3 to 8 liters contributes to further serious fluid and electrolyte imbalances. If fluid output exceeds intake, low cardiac indexes may be seen and shock may ensue. Conversely, if fluid intake exceeds output, hypertension and pulmonary edema may develop.

Treatment Clinical management primarily revolves around meticulous supportive care. Trials with a variety of agents including antibiotics, adrenocortical steroid hormones, antihistamines, and convalescent serum were without significant beneficial effect during the Korean epidemics. The treatment of shock is discussed in Chap. 139 and that of acute tubular necrosis in Chap. 290.

Prognosis The Soviet experience indicates a mortality rate of 3 to 32 percent; in other early reports the mortality has ranged from 10 to 15 percent. Between April 1951 and December 1976 the overall case fatality ratio in Korea was 6.6 percent.

Residua are uncommon. Of 783 surviving patients cared for at the Hemorrhagic Fever Center in Korea between April and December 1952, only 16 were unable to return to duty within a period of 4 months. Fifteen of these individuals still had hyposthenuria. Follow-up studies on former EHF patients 3 to 5 years later showed that they had many more subsequent hospital admissions for urologic problems than did a control group and that the relative frequency correlated with the severity of the acute episode of EHF. Asymptomatic residual renal tubular dysfunction may be more common than has been appreciated.

ARGENTINIAN AND BOLIVIAN HEMORRHAGIC FEVERS The first cases of a new American hemorrhagic disease were seen near the Argentinian town of Junin near Buenos Aires in 1953. A virus was isolated from patients' blood and from local rodents and their mites. In 1959, cases of a disease thought to resemble severe epidemic typhus were noted among rural workers in northeastern Bolivia. The similarity between these syndromes was recognized. In 1963, the causal virus was isolated from patients and rodents and named the Machupo virus. Machupo virus is serologically related to but distinct from Junin virus.

Prevalence Junin virus infections have occurred in epidemic form since 1958 with between 100 and 3500 cases reported annually. The hemorrhagic disease in Bolivia has been particularly severe. Of a total population of 4000 to 6000 in the endemic area, 750 persons were affected between 1959 and 1963.

Epidemiology Argentinian hemorrhagic fever (AHF) occurs in sharply endemic seasonal form (February to August), mostly among male rural workers, especially those exposed to fields at the time of the maize harvest. Virus is transmitted in the urine of rodents with chronic infection and viruria. Humans acquire the virus through contact with items or foodstuffs which have been contaminated with infected rodent urine. The main reservoir is two species of cricetidae, *Calomys laucha* and *C. musculinus.*

Bolivian hemorrhagic fever (BHF) is similarly transmitted by the urine of *C. callosus* (a mouse-like rodent) chronically infected with Machupo virus. Direct person-to-person transmission is possible and may have occurred in the outbreak in Cochabamba. Disease has not occurred in medical personnel attending infected patients.

Clinical features Argentinian hemorrhagic fever presents manifestations of renal, cardiovascular, and hematologic involvement. Inapparent infections are rare. The incubation period is estimated to be 7 to 16 days, followed by a gradual onset of chills, fever, headache, malaise, myalgia, anorexia, nausea, and vomiting. The temperature reaches 38.9 to 40°C (102 to 104°F), facial flushing may be prominent, and there is a painless enanthem of the pharynx. Lymphadenopathy and splenomegaly are not present. From 3 to 5 days after the onset, the signs and symptoms worsen, with the appearance of signs of dehydration, hypotension to 50 to 100 mmHg, oliguria, and relative bradycardia. In the more severe cases, hemorrhagic manifestations, including bleeding from the gums, hematemesis, hematuria, and melena, occur. Progressive oliguria and tremor of the tongue and extremities may develop. Some patients develop psychic manifestations, with agitation, delirium, or stupor. Progressive shock, hypothermia, gallop rhythm, or gastrointestinal bleeding may occur from the seventh to tenth days. In fatal cases, pulmonary edema usually is the cause of death. During convalescence a temporary alopecia has been noted. Erythrocyte counts are normal or elevated. The total leukocyte count drops to 1200 to 3400 blood cells per cubic millimeter. Thrombocytopenia may occur. Disseminated intravascular coagulation does not seem to be the mechanism responsible for the hemorrhagic manifestations. Complement components C2, C3, and C5 are decreased. The urine is dark and may approach the color of mahogany, with intense albuminuria. Blood urea nitrogen levels rise rapidly.

The clinical picture of Bolivian hemorrhagic fever is similar to Argentinian, although epistaxis and hematemesis at the onset is more common.

Diagnosis Complement-fixing antibodies appear in 15 to 30 days in about 75 percent of the clinically diagnosed cases.

Treatment Treatment consists of supportive measures, including peritoneal dialysis to correct both the azotemia and the pulmonary edema. In AHF, a double-blind trial of administration of immune plasma reduced mortality from 16 to 1 percent. However, fever and cerebellar signs occurred in patients treated with immune plasma. Preliminary studies suggest that ribavirin may be effective in experimental BHF in rhesus monkeys.

Prognosis The mortality rate among patients with Argentinian hemorrhagic fever is usually 3 to 15 percent, while that in Bolivian hemorrhagic fever is 5 to 30 percent.

Prevention In Bolivia, rodent control measures directed primarily against *C. callosus* populations in the houses resulted in a prompt and dramatic cessation of human cases.

LASSA FEVER A new virus disease, which is both highly contagious and virulent, occurred in a missionary nurse in Lassa, a town in northeast Nigeria, in 1969.

Epidemiology Since the initial outbreak at Lassa in 1969, during which one of the patients was transferred to New York City, there have been other outbreaks near Jos in northern Nigeria in 1970 (32 suspected cases with 10 deaths), in Zorzor, Liberia, in 1972 (11 cases with 4 deaths), and in the eastern province of Sierra Leone with 63 suspected cases admitted to two hospitals between 1970 and 1972. In Jos and Zorzor, outbreaks apparently resulted from person-to-person nosocomial spread from the index case to hospital workers or other patients. In Sierra Leone, the great majority of cases were acquired outside the hospital, although hospital workers were at high risk. *Mastomys natalensis,* a multimammate rat widespread in Africa, is known to be an animal reservoir of the virus, and primary human cases probably result from contamination of foodstuffs with rodent urine. Human-to-human transmission may occur through contact with urine, feces, vomitus, or saliva through droplets and aerosols, and particularly through wounds contaminated with blood. Intrafamilial outbreaks have occurred around several cases. There are a number of cases which have been acquired through accidental autoinoculation with needles while starting intravenous fluids. At least one laboratory-acquired infection has occurred. In Sierra Leone 6 percent of the population surveyed had complement-fixing antibody against Lassa virus, while only 0.2 percent had recognized disease, suggesting mild disease or inapparent infection. In Liberia 10 percent of hospital personnel had antibodies. Positive serums were also obtained from individuals in Cameroon and Benin (formerly Dahomey).

Clinical features The incubation period is 1 to 24 days, being 10 days following accidental inoculation. Patients have ranged from 5 months to 46 years of age; approximately two-thirds are women. Three of eight women in one series were 22 to 28 weeks pregnant during their illness. The apparent predilection for women may relate to exposure to contaminated food or work in hospitals rather than to differences in susceptibility. The onset of illness was described by most patients as insidious. The most frequent initial symptoms are fever (100 percent), chilliness and true rigors, headache (50 percent), malaise (100 percent), and myalgia (50 percent). Most patients did not seek medical attention for 4 to 9 days after onset. Symptoms of a systemic viral illness then developed with anorexia, nausea, vomiting, myalgia, and pain in the chest, epigastrium, and lumbar area. Headache was usually present. Early examination reveals fever and flushing of the face and V area of the neck. Pharyngitis developed early and became progressively more severe during the first week; examination may reveal raised patches of whitish exudate occurring on the palatine arches which occasionally coalesce into a pseudomembrane. Oral ulcerations have been noted in up to one-half of cases. Generalized nontender lymphadenopathy occurred in one-half of patients. During the second week severe lower abdominal pain and intractable vomiting are common, and facial and neck swelling with conjunctival edema and infection frequently develop. Occasionally patients have tinnitus, epistaxis, bleeding from the gums and venipuncture sites, maculopapular rashes, cough, and dizziness. During the acute stage, systolic blood pressures of less than 90 mmHg with pulse pressures of less than 20 mmHg occurred in 60 to 80 percent of patients. Initially, relative bradycardia was common. During the second week, the patients who recovered defervesced, while the patients who died often developed signs of shock, clouding of the sensorium, rales, signs of pleural effusion, agitation and, on occasion, grand mal seizures. The duration of illness in surviving patients ranged from 7 to 31 days (average 15 days), while that in fatal cases was 7 to 26 days (average 12 days). The mortality rates in Jos and Zorzor were 52 percent and 36 percent, respectively, while in Sierra Leone the rate was 8 percent. During convalescence occasional flurries of rapid involuntary eye movements (oculogyric crises) occurred. Late sequelae include deafness in a number of patients (two of six in one series) and alopecia in one patient.

Laboratory features The hematologic findings include relatively normal hematocrit values and early leukopenia (less than 4000 cells per cubic millimeter in 36 percent) with a relative neutrophilia and immature forms of leukocytes. In two cases in which it was recorded, the erythrocyte sedimentation rate was normal. Urinalyses revealed proteinuria, which was often massive. Chest radiographs may suggest basilar pneumonitis and pleural effusions. Electrocardiographic abnormalities compatible with diffuse myocardial disease have been encountered. Levels of serum enzymes, serum glutamic oxaloacetic transaminase (SGOT), creatinine phosphokinase (CPK), and lactic dehydrogenase (LDH) have been elevated. Lassa virus has been recovered from cerebrospinal fluid in two patients.

Diagnosis Diagnosis may be made quickly by staining conjunctival scrapings with fluorescent-labeled anti-Lassa antiserums. Confirmation involves growth of the virus in tissue culture and a complement fixation test; however, the latter is rarely positive before the fourteenth day of illness.

Treatment The management has been supportive. Infusion of immune plasma from convalescent patients resulted in a dramatic effect in three of four patients. Because of the self-limited nature of the disease, these results cannot be assessed easily. Ribavirin, an experimental antiviral agent, has prevented hemorrhagic manifestations and death in experimentally infected rhesus monkeys. In view of the hospital association and the presence of virus in pharyngeal secretions and urine, strict isolation is required. Known contacts should be kept under medical surveillance for at least 3 weeks.

REFERENCES

Baum SG et al: Epidemic non-meningitic lymphocytic-choriomeningitis virus infection. N Engl J Med 274:934, 1966

Casals J: Arenaviruses. Yale J Biol Med 48:115, 1975

Dennis LH, Conrad ME: Accelerated intravascular coagulation in a patient with Korean hemorrhagic fever. Arch Intern Med 121:499, 1968

Farmer TW, Janeway CA: Infections with the virus of lymphocytic choriomeningitis. Medicine 21:1, 1942

Frame JD et al: Lassa fever, a new virus disease of man from West Africa: I. Clinical description and pathological findings. Am J Trop Med Hyg 19:670, 1970

Johnson KM et al: Hemorrhagic fever of Southeast Asia and South America. A comparative approach. Prog Med Virol 9:105, 1967

Lee HW et al: Isolation of the etiologic agent of Korean hemorrhagic fever. J Infect Dis 137:298, 1978

———, Cho HJ: Electron microscopic appearance of Hataan virus, the causative agent of Korean hemorrhagic fever. Lancet 1:1070, 1981

MacKenzie RB et al: Epidemic hemorrhagic fever in Bolivia: I. A preliminary report of the epidemiologic and clinical findings in a new epidemic area in South America. Am J Trop Med Hyg 13:620, 1964

Maiztegui JI et al: Efficacy of immune plasma in treatment of Argentine hemorrhagic fever and association between treatment and a late neurological syndrome. Lancet 2:1216, 1979

Mertens PE et al: Clinical presentation of Lassa fever cases during the hospital epidemic at Zorzor, Liberia, March–April 1972. Am J Trop Med Hyg 22:780, 1973

Monath TP et al: Lassa fever in the Eastern Province of Sierra Leone, 1970–1972: II. Clinical observations and virological studies on selected hospital cases. Am J Trop Med Hyg 23:1140, 1974

Powell GM: Hemorrhagic fever. A study of 300 cases. Medicine 33:97, 1954

Rubini ME et al: Renal residuals of acute epidemic hemorrhagic fever. Arch Intern Med 106:378, 1960

Sheedy JA et al: The clinical course of epidemic hemorrhagic fever. Am J Med 16:619, 1954

Stephen EL, Jahrling PB: Experimental Lassa fever virus infection successfully treated with ribavirin. Lancet 1:268, 1979

Svedmyr A et al: Antigenic differentiation of the viruses causing Korean hemorrhagic fever and epidemic (endemic) nephropathy of Scandinavia. Lancet 2:315, 1980

VanZee BE et al: Lymphocytic choriomeningitis in University hospital personnel. Clinical features. Am J Med 58:803, 1975

Herpesviruses

210
INFECTIONS WITH HERPES SIMPLEX VIRUS

A. MARTIN LERNER

Herpes simplex virus types 1 and 2 (HSV-1, HSV-2), sometimes known as *herpesvirus hominis,* establishes diverse relations with humans. Acute disseminated primary infection (gingivostomatitis, herpes genitalis), recurrent infection with intermittent virus shedding (herpes labialis or genitalis), and virus latency in neural ganglia between clinical episodes are all commonplace. Although firm data are not available, the best estimate is that 20 to 40 percent of the population of the United States have had HSV infections and that HSV-2 infections are becoming increasingly prevalent. In fact, the presence and titer of neutralizing antibody, at least to HSV-2 after primary human genital infection, may represent a biologic marker for the presence of latent ganglionic infection, with a subsequent increased likelihood of recurrent infection. Virus multiplies in many tissues, including "activated" lymphocytes, and by its intracellular locus is able to escape anti-HSV antibodies. Herpes simplex virus antibody complexes may be infectious, and when this is the case, are called "sensitized virus." It has been shown that Fc-binding receptors for IgG are induced on the surfaces of cells infected by HSV. Interactions with the complement system are important in neutralizing sensitized virus. Since the decline of poliomyelitis with the development of an effective vaccine, herpes simplex virus encephalitis is the most frequent endemic encephalitis in this country. Type 2 herpes simplex virus is the second most frequent sexually transmitted disease (after gonorrhea). It has been associated with an increased risk of carcinoma of the cervix, but the etiologic association has not been proved.

ETIOLOGY The virus particle consists of DNA, protein, lipid, and carbohydrate (Table 196-1). On an average there are 100 parts DNA, 25 parts carbohydrate, and 320 parts phospholipid to 1000 parts protein. Virus DNA is double-stranded with densities of 1.727 (type 1) and 1.729 (type 2). The molecular weight of the virion is about 100×10^6 daltons. By phosphotungstic acid staining on electron microscopy the virion is seen to consist of a roughly spheric central area or "core" of DNA which measures 75 nm in diameter and a stable "capsid" which measures 100 nm in diameter; it appears to be an icosahedron with a 5:3:2 axial symmetry consisting of 162 capsomeres (9 to 10 nm by 12 to 13.5 nm) of which 150 are hexagonal and 12 pentagonal in cross section, and a surrounding envelope derived from host cell membranes, 145 to 200 nm. Particles appear with or without envelopes [enveloped and/or with or without cores ("full" or "empty")].

Although complete virions are more efficient, both "enveloped" and "naked" particles can infect cells. Phagocytosis of virions by susceptible cells, viropexis, precedes the digestion of virus envelopes and proteins. After initiation of infection, virus absorption is complete in 3 h. New virus infectivity rises sharply from the sixth to the ninth hour, when it levels off. Viral DNA enters the nucleus where new virus DNA is synthesized. Virus proteins are synthesized in the cytoplasm and migrate to the nucleus. The complete virion has a triple-layered envelope. The inner envelope is made within the nucleus, while the second and third are formed by evagination processes at the nuclear and cytoplasmic membranes, respectively. Host materials make up major portions of the envelope. An infected cell may produce about 1000 virus particles, but only 5 to 10 percent are infectious.

BIOLOGIC CHARACTERISTICS By means of neutralization kinetics, hyperimmune unitypic serums in conventional neutralization tests, or direct immunofluorescent methods, strains of herpes simplex virus can be readily typed. Type 1 strains are most often recovered from the eye, nasopharynx, skin (other than thigh or buttocks), and brain in cases of postnatal encephalitis. Type 2 strains are usually related to the adult genital tract. Isolates have been recovered from the penis, cervix, endocervix, vagina, vulva, skin (usually, but not always below the waist), and spinal fluid. In infections of the newborn, HSV-2 has been recovered from brain, liver, adrenal, and lung. Of primary first episodes of herpes genitalis, 15 percent may be caused by HSV-1, but recurrent episodes are much more likely to occur if the first episode of genital herpes was with HSV-2. Recurrences also appear to occur more frequently in men than women.

One of the nonstructural proteins of the HSV genome is

FIGURE 210-1
Cowdry type A ("owl-eye") intranuclear inclusions are seen in this hematoxylin-eosin section (600 ×) in the brain of a patient with encephalitis (arrow). [From ESE Hafez et al (eds), The Human Vagina in Health and Disease, Amsterdam, Elsevier/North-Holland, 1978, with permission.]

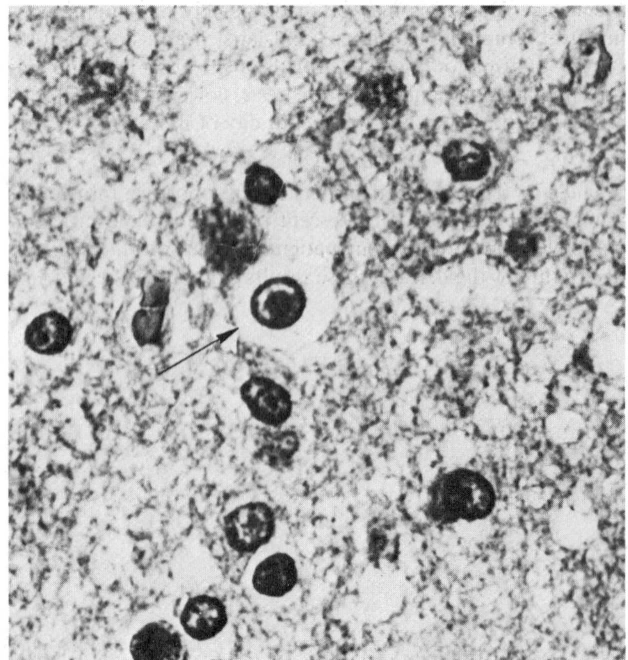

thymidine kinase (TK^+). Thymidine kinase-deficient (TK^-) mutants of HSV grow well in tissue cultures but are much less virulent in animal models than TK^+ strains. The role of TK^- HSV strains in human disease remains to be determined.

Optimal virus isolation occurs in rabbit or baby hamster kidney and human foreskin tissue cultures. Cytopathic effects are usually evident within 72 h after inoculation. However, when isolation of virus by brain biopsy is attempted, trypsinized suspensions of cells, rather than ground tissue suspensions, should be planted, both for primary growth and for co-cultivation with HSV-susceptible tissue cultures. Typical of in vitro and in vivo cytopathic effects is the type A inclusion of Cowdry, an eosinophilic mass surrounded by a halo in a nucleus with marginated chromatin (Fig. 210-1).

In addition to site of recovery, a number of other properties separate type 1 from type 2 herpes simplex virus: HSV-2 produces (1) larger pocks on the chorioallantoic membrane of embryonated eggs, (2) greater virulence in female mice which have been infected by the genital route, and (3) greater tendency toward formation of giant cells in tissue cultures. These strains also exhibit (4) difference in density and base composition of DNA and (5) antigenic distinctiveness. Likewise, (6) minimal inhibitory concentrations (MIC) of idoxuridine (IDU; 5-iodo-2′-deoxyuridine) for type 1 strains are 6.25 μg/ml, while similar values for type 2 herpesviruses are 62.5 μg/ml.

The DNA of HSV isolates can be studied for epidemiological purposes by the molecular technique of restriction endonuclease enzyme analysis. The DNA gel patterns of different HSV strains are each distinctive, but even though viruses have been passaged many times in culture or repeatedly isolated from the same individual, they remain identical. In this manner, when several cases of encephalitis within a short interval of time at a Boston hospital were recognized, it was shown that this cluster of cases was not related to a neurovirulent strain of HSV-1 and that there had not been any transmission of particular strains among these patients. In the same manner, possible nosocomial HSV infections can be proved or disproved.

IMMUNOLOGY Following primary exposure to herpes simplex virus, humoral antibodies appear. Different polypeptides of the virus capsid probably stimulate distinct antibodies which rise and fall, describing separate kinetic curves. In contrast to other antibodies, such as complement-independent neutralizing, complement-fixing, and indirect hemagglutination antibodies (formerly referred to as passive hemagglutinating antibodies), complement-requiring neutralizing antibodies peak during the acute phase of primary infections with HSV-1 and fall during convalescence.

After initial exposure IgM antibodies appear in serum within 1 week. In respiratory secretions IgA antibodies form. In cases of encephalitis, antibodies which are produced locally can be measured in cerebrospinal fluid. Seven days after infection IgG antibodies appear in serum, and antiherpesvirus IgM synthesis decreases. Complement-fixing antibodies appear in 14 days. After an initial exposure, complement-fixing antibodies fall to low levels within several months, while complement-independent neutralizing antibodies persist for many years. Reactivations of infection evoke variable rises in serums of complement-independent neutralizing or complement-fixing IgG antibodies. There are some low-titered cross-reactions when anti-HSV antibodies are measured against varicella-zoster or cytomegalovirus.

Cellular immunity is also stimulated and may be the more important factor in inhibiting virus multiplication and relapse. Chronic persisting clinical herpes labialis and herpes genitalis with virus shedding for several months have been seen in immunosuppressed patients undergoing anticancer chemotherapy.

CLINICAL FINDINGS: HSV-1 Primary infection with HSV-1 causes *acute gingivostomatitis, rhinitis, keratoconjunctivitis, meningoencephalitis, eczema herpeticum* (Kaposi's varicelliform eruption), and *traumatic herpes,* including *herpetic whitlow* and *generalized cutaneous herpes simplex* in burned patients or wrestlers (*herpes gladiatorum*). In immunosuppressed patients initial infection or clinical reactivation may induce esophageal ulceration or interstitial pneumonia.

The incubation period is 2 to 12 days, averaging 6 or 7 days. The route of infection is contact with infected skin or mucosal surfaces. There is little or no evidence to support respiratory contagion by droplets or their dehydrated nuclei. During acute herpetic gingivostomatitis there are fever, irritability, red swollen gums, a vesicular eruption on the mucous membranes of the mouth, oral fetor, and local submaxillary adenopathy. A visit to the dentist may precede an attack. Any portion of the oral mucosa may be affected. Viremia during which the virus is free in plasma or is limited to mononuclear cells may occur. A generalized vesicular eruption may follow and appear in crops. Lesions are generally smaller than those of varicella. In the eczematous infant or adult (Kaposi's varicelliform eruption), large quantities of fluid, electrolytes, and protein may be lost.

Within the tense vesicles is a clear fluid. An impression smear of an opened vesicle demonstrates syncytial giant cells undergoing ballooning degeneration (Fig. 210-2). Intranuclear

FIGURE 210-2

Characteristic intranuclear inclusion bodies of herpes simplex virus infection along with exfoliated multi- and single nucleated cells are shown (high power magnification). Note "ground glass" appearance of nuclear inclusion with peripheral rim of nuclear chromatin (arrow) or scattered polymorphonuclear leukocytes seen in the background. This is a Tzanck impression smear which may be obtained from an opened cutaneous vesicle or from the cervix. (From JW Regan, SF Patten, Cytology of the Female Reproductive Tract, Chicago, American Society of Clinical Pathologists, 1966, with permission.)

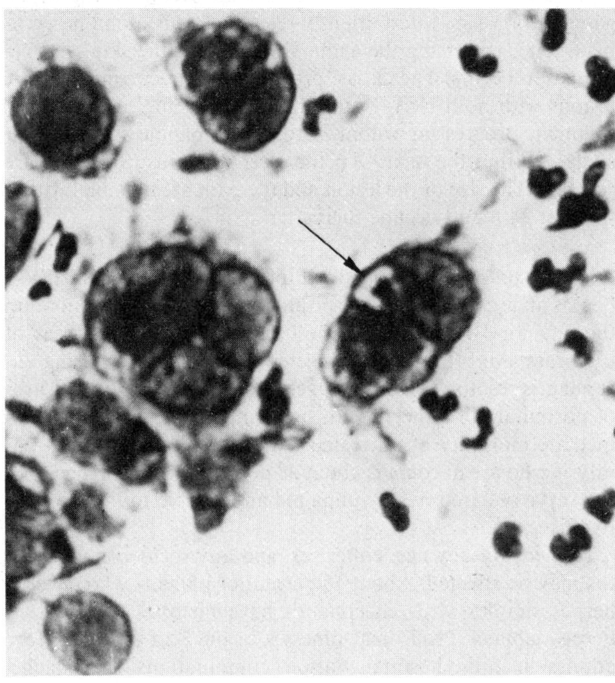

inclusions are seen. Virus is readily isolated from the fluid; no bacteria are seen on Gram's stain, and none may be cultured. Later, vesicles collapse and ulcerate. Sometimes the nose is the site of primary infection. Tiny vesicles surrounding reddened areolae appear in the nostrils. Usually, there is fever and the anterior cervical lymph nodes enlarge.

Patients contaminate their fingers or those of hospital personnel by introducing infected secretions through unnoticed abrasions, producing *herpetic whitlow* in persons without previous experience with HSV. *Herpetic paronychia* may be caused by HSV-1 or HSV-2. Painful deep vesicles appear suddenly and spread locally for about a week. The nail may be separated from its matrix by a lesion at its base. Recrudescent relapses may occur at any time, but the initial infection seems to occur in immunologically "virgin" persons. The importance of wearing rubber gloves when working about the mouth and of handwashing in prevention of infection is obvious.

Follicular conjunctivitis (often unilateral) with chemosis, edema of the lids, and conjunctival ulcers may be seen. The cornea may be involved in primary or recurrent infections; most of these infections are due to HSV-1. When the cornea is affected, a diffuse epitheliolitis develops with superficial punctate erosions which extend into small dendritic ulcers. If untreated, this ulcer increases in size to form a large, anesthetic "geographic" ulcer. Erosions of the cornea recur. *Deeper interstitial keratitis* with secondary bacterial invasion, hypopyon, iridocyclitis, synechia, and opacification of the lens follows.

Others with preexisting complement-independent neutralizing antibodies in serums may suffer *recurrent attacks of herpes labialis,* herpes genitalis, herpes keratitis, herpetic whitlow, or trigeminal neuralgia. Pneumococcal and meningococcal, but not gram-negative infections; menstruation; emotional upset; and other little-understood events seem to trigger recurrent localized episodes. Quiescence and recurrences of herpes labialis may be associated occasionally (about 4 percent of cases) with alternating low and higher titers of virus shedding, but reactivation of latent infection is much more common, with no virus shedding during quiescent intervals. In the prodromal and erythema stages of herpes labialis mean virus titers are $< 10^1$ PFU (plaque-forming unit), but when vesiculation occurs 24 h later, fluids contain about $10^{4.7}$ PFU of HSV. Herpes simplex virus resides in a quiescent state within sacral or trigeminal ganglia for years, intermittently releasing virus along nerve fibers. After traversing the axon, HSV reaches the skin, and vesiculation occurs. The classic progression of recurring herpetic lesions with both HSV-1 and HSV-2 is burning, tingling, and erythema progressing within 24 to 48 h to papule and vesicular stages. Within the next 48 h the ulcer and crusting stages are reached. The size of the lesion and the pain are maximal within the first 24 h and decline thereafter.

Encephalitis Occasionally, and for ill-defined reasons, HSV-1 begins an ascent from the respiratory epithelium of the nose up the olfactory tract to reach the frontal and temporal areas of the brain. An often fatal or severely damaging necrotizing encephalitis results. The data suggest that most (but not all) cases of postnatal HSV encephalitis are primary infections. The immediate mortality of untreated patients with seizures and paralysis who are in coma is about 38 percent, but the majority of the survivors are severely impaired and unable to live productive lives.

Patients of any age, either sex, and any socioeconomic status may be affected. About 15 percent of patients who develop herpes simplex virus encephalitis have histories of recurrent herpes labialis. Prodromal illnesses begin 3 to 4 days before admission to the hospital. Various combinations of headache, rhinorrhea, sore throat, fever, nausea, or vomiting are noted. Less frequently photophobia, vertigo, insomnia, or anorexia occurs. One-third of the patients develop concurrent fever blisters during the course of their illness. Personality changes, lethargy, or seizures necessitate hospitalization, but only a few (3 of 15 brain-biopsy-proven cases) have paralysis or coma at the time of hospitalization. The occurrence of paralysis and coma indicates that irreparable neurologic injury has occurred. In order of frequency, disorientation, personality change, hallucinations, photophobia, ataxia, facial weakness, incontinence of stool or urine, tremors, and amnesia appear. Patients with proven herpes simplex virus encephalitis have been mistaken for inebriates or psychotics. Neurologic signs include stupor, seizures (Jacksonian or generalized), coma, extensor plantar reflexes, nuchal rigidity, motor deficits, cranial nerve palsies, sensory deficits, decorticate and decerebrate posture, abnormal conjugate deviation of eyes, frontal lobe signs (glabella, snout, sucking), asymmetric deep tendon reflexes, and dysphasia. Coma (absence of response to all stimuli) indicates an ominous prognosis.

Leukocyte counts average 13,000 per cubic millimeter with a shift to the left. Cerebrospinal fluid samples are completely normal or contain only a few to several hundred leukocytes which may be predominantly mononuclear or polymorphonuclear. Grossly bloody spinal fluid is an ominous sign of far-advanced disease. Cerebrospinal fluid protein is normal or elevated as high as 250 mg/dl. Glucose in cerebrospinal fluid is usually normal but may be low. In every case electroencephalograms are diffusely abnormal, or show focal lesions in the temporal or frontal regions. The abnormal electroencephalogram is an especially important finding, particularly in cases in which the cerebrospinal fluid is normal. Computerized tomography (CT) scans or carotid angiograms are indicated to rule out an epidural, subdural, or intracerebral hematoma, abscess, or tumor. In a few cases of HSV-1 encephalitis, the focal hemorrhagic necrotic mass deviates carotid vessels, and craniotomy may be necessary for differentiation and diagnosis. Significant rises in HSV antibodies in serum do not determine the diagnosis of encephalitis caused by this virus because rises in these antibodies occur nonspecifically with bacterial pneumonias or bacterial meningitis and in uncomplicated herpes labialis and other conditions. Cowdry type A ("owl-eye") intranuclear inclusions may be demonstrated in the brain (Fig. 210-1). Attempts at isolation of other (e.g., enteroviruses) viruses from throat or rectal swabs, urine, and cerebrospinal fluid as well as, when possible, from brain, spinal cord, and vesicular fluid should be made. Paired serums should be tested for titers of antibody against mumps virus or other agents known to be prevalent at the time of infection.

Isolation of HSV by brain biopsy is at present the only definitive means of diagnosing HSV encephalitis. Brain biopsy must be done as soon after admission to the hospital as possible before the onset of irreversible paralysis or coma, because if intravenous therapy with adenine arabinoside (ara-A) is begun before the onset of coma, full recovery may occur. Efforts toward earlier definitive nonsurgical diagnosis of HSV encephalitis continue. For example, serial concomitant paired serums (S) and cerebrospinal fluids (CSF) were taken from eight patients with biopsy-proven HSV encephalitis. These specimen pairs were compared to 28 others from patients with various neurologic conditions. Both before and after reduction with 2-mercaptoethanol, a ratio of S to CSF antibody titers of ≤ 20 with either the indirect hemagglutinating (IHA) or immune adherence hemagglutinating (IAHA) antibody tests occurred in three patients prior to biopsy of the brain, and in four patients by the tenth day of neurologic disease. Among controls, a ratio of S to CSF titers >20 was observed in all but four patients, each of whom had easily distinguishable neurologic diagnoses (e.g., HSV-2 meningitis, active multiple sclerosis, varicella zoster encephalitis). This work remains promising but must be validated by further experience in several laboratories. The uniform occurrence of S/CSF antibody ratios to HSV-1 equaling ≤ 20 has been corroborated in a rabbit model of HSV encephalitis. It would be better if HSV antigen could be detected in CSF earlier in the course of the disease. Another, perhaps more promising approach, is the early detection of virus-specific glycoproteins in the CSF.

Quantitative HSV and interferon (IFN) titers have been assayed in temporal lobe brain biopsies, various regions of the brain at autopsy, serums, and CSF during courses of HSV encephalitis. Until the tenth day of neurologic disease, IFN (geometric mean titer, 25 μ/ml) was present in each virus-positive brain biopsy. Interferon was not found in virus-negative brain biopsies which have been tested to date. The geometric mean HSV-1 titer at brain biopsy was 328 TCD_{50}/g. On the sixth day of disease, CSF from a single survivor contained 160 μ/ml, but five other samples of CSF contained no detectable IFN. No serums from any of the patients with HSV encephalitis contained IFN. Autopsies performed on the sixth to nineteenth days of neurologic disease showed that 13 to 35 (37 percent) of the regional areas of the brain retained HSV-1, but only a single specimen from a temporal lobe (3 percent of the tested specimens) had measurable IFN.

CLINICAL FINDINGS: HSV-2 Infection with HSV, type 2, is usually sexually transmitted from an individual with active recurrent disease. The chance of infection between relapses is small. In one study seven of eight female contacts of men with penile herpetic infection showed evidence of current HSV genital infection. Similarly, 63 out of 64 HSV isolates from male genitalia and 155 of 162 from the female genital tract were HSV-2. This infection is the most common cause of genital vesicles and/or ulcers found in women, and is second only to primary syphilis as the cause of such lesions in males. Teenagers make up one-fourth to one-half of patients with genital herpetic infections.

In a predominantly white urban study the mean age of acquisition of genital herpes in women was 26.9 years compared with 30.8 years in men. The mean duration of infection for women was 3.9 years, while it was 5.1 years for men. Women usually acquired genital herpes between the ages of 20 to 29 years, while substantial numbers of men continued to experience initial episodes of infection into the next decade. Subjects (especially men) had commonly experienced other sexually transmitted diseases such as gonorrhea or nongonococcal urethritis. Over two-thirds of the subjects with genital herpes experienced over five recurrences every year. The recurrence rate usually remained constant with time.

Neutralizing antibodies to HSV-2 are reported to be present in 35.7 percent of patients who subsequently develop carcinoma in situ of the cervix, and are found in only 7.1 percent of matched controls. However, an etiologic relation between carcinoma of the cervix and infection with HSV-2 is not established.

During primary infections fever, malaise, and inguinal adenopathy may be seen and viremia may follow. A benign aseptic meningitis has resulted. In HSV-2, aseptic meningitis virus can be isolated from CSF. In HSV encephalitis, virus is not found in CSF. In the male there may be tiny vesicles on the glans or shaft of the penis, burning, urgency, frequency, and watery discharge. Herpesvirus is easily cultivated from vesicular fluids.

Antibody surveys suggest that 30 to 100 percent of adults have been infected with one or both of the herpes simplex viruses, with the greatest incidence being among lower socioeconomic groups. Prostitutes have the highest frequency of HSV-2 antibodies. There are roughly 300,000 reported episodes of HSV-2 infection each year, an incidence making it second only to gonorrhea among venereal diseases. Case reporting in other than venereal disease clinics is poor, and herpes may indeed be the most frequent of all the sexually transmitted diseases.

Recurring episodes are probably twice as common as initial attacks. The majority of primary cases occur in young adults between the ages of 19 and 27 (mean 26.5 years). The mean age for recurrences is also 26.5 years. During the acute primary or recurrent attacks of genital herpes, the lesions are painful and sexual contacts are generally avoided. Several days later symptoms abate, but virus may still be present, and this is likely the time of greatest contagion. The attack rate with sexual contact is one in three.

Following recovery from the primary episode of genital herpes (especially due to HSV-1), no further attacks may occur, or recurrences may vary from occasional to frequent. Subclinical primary infection with genital herpes also occurs in some patients with first episodes. The reasons for the variability in the clinical course are unknown. Viremia probably occurs only during initial episodes when serum antibody is absent. Following primary HSV-2 infections, virus follows a retrograde course along sensory nerves to reach spinal dorsal, lumbar, or sacral ganglia. Here the virus remains in a latent stage until lapses in cell-mediated immunity allow retrograde release of virus along nerves to the previously involved sites upon the skin or mucous membrane. Recurrences frequently involve the same locus on skin or mucous membrane.

In women, within several days after sexual relations with an infected partner, paresthesia and burning of the vulva begin, and dyspareunia, dysuria, and tenesmus set in. There may be fever, malaise, headache, neuralgia, and tender inguinal nodes as well.

On examination of patients with primary infection, the skin and mucous membranes of the vulva, genitocrural folds, perianal region, and cervix show crops of 0.5- to 1.5-cm reddened papules which progress to vesicles and then ulcers. The vagina and urethra are affected infrequently. The vesicles (sometimes 20 to 30 of them) ulcerate within several days. Lesions within the vagina consist of mucous patches with collapsed gray, slightly elevated epithelium. Often the mons pubis and vulva are markedly swollen. The cervix is eroded and may appear as a necrotizing mass with a clear profuse or hemorrhagic discharge. Following viremia, similar skin lesions may appear at distant sites. A tender enlarged liver and nuchal rigidity attest to the mild hepatitis and benign aseptic meningitis which may accompany primary HSV-2 infection in the postnatal period.

Over several days systemic signs resolve, but lesions may persist for weeks. Unless secondary bacterial infection follows, ultimately healing is complete without scarring. The subsequent course is variable: (1) some patients remain well and culture negative indefinitely; (2) others have recurring episodes of differing severity at varying intervals; and (3) still others become symptomatic or asymptomatic HSV-2 carriers in their cervical secretions. These patients have an increased incidence of cervical dysplasia.

Approximately two of every three women with primary HSV-2 genital infection suffer relapses. Fever, menstruation, and physical or emotional trauma seem important in induction of some recurrences, but often no obvious inciting cause is recognized. Between clinical episodes the virus remains latent in sensory ganglia. Exogenous reinfection with a new HSV strain has also been documented by restriction endonuclease analysis of viral DNA. The frequency of such reinfection is not known.

During recurrence, the clinical findings are usually milder. Malaise, fever, and adenopathy are often absent and the lesions are localized, less painful, and much less numerous. Pain on urination and defecation is absent, and the entire episode subsides within 7 to 10 days. The milder course reflects a stimulated, but not completely effective, humoral and cellular immune response to latent HSV-2.

The clinical and laboratory findings in initial and recurrent herpes have been studied carefully. The mean number of lesions at first visit for initial (primary) episodes is 6.3, while it is 4.7 in recurrent (secondary) attacks, but patients sought medical advice earlier in relapses (2.5 days in secondary cases versus 4.6 days in primary cases). All attacks were associated with pain (primary, 96 percent; secondary, 89 percent), which lasted longer in primary episodes (13.0 versus 8.6 days). Virus was usually (87 percent) present in cervical secretions in primary episodes but was found rarely during relapses (4 percent). Lesions persisted for 16.6 days in primary attacks opposed to 10.5 days in relapses. During episodes new vesicles appeared for 10.1 days in primary, but for only 4.7 days in secondary, disease. Virus could be recovered from lesions for 8.0 days (primary) versus 4.5 days, (secondary) and from the cervix for 11.4 days (primary) versus 3 days (secondary). For the majority of patients with recurrent attacks of genital herpes, relapses are mild with only a few lesions on the external genitalia that heal within 8 days. The psychologic suffering and social isolation of these patients are often considerably greater. This aspect of genital herpes is now being addressed in clinical investigation.

Cytomegalovirus, varicella-zoster virus, variola virus, Behçet's disease, drug or contact dermatitis, autoimmune disorders, or infections with herpes simplex viruses may cause clusters of vulvovaginal vesicles or ulcers on an erythematous base. Cytologic examinations from open vesicles, the bases of ulcers, or the cervix (Fig. 210-2) and appropriate attempts at isolation or recognition of virus are necessary for the diagnosis. Comparison of antibody titers in paired serums is also useful in establishing the presence of herpes infection. Type-specific neutralizing, immunofluorescent, indirect hemagglutinating (IHA), enzyme-linked immunosorbent (ELISA), IAHA, and several radiolabeled assays are used to measure HSV antibodies. The height of the titers serves as a marker for both neural latency and the number of recurrences.

Tzanck smears are positive in preparations from fresh lesions in two of three cases. Multinucleated giant cells with or without intranuclear inclusions, epithelial cells, and lymphocytes are present. These findings do not differentiate HSV from varicella-zoster virus infection. To perform a Tzanck test, several fresh vesicles are cleansed with alcohol, opened with a no. 22 needle, and a sterile cotton swab or wooden applicator is pressed to the base of the lesion. The swab is smeared onto several clean glass slides. Slides are immersed in 95% alcohol fixed as in Papanicolaou staining. For immunofluorescent staining for HSV-2 antigen, slides are dried in air and fixed with acetone. Hematoxylin-eosin, Giemsa's, Papanicolaou's, Wright's, or Leishman's stains (Tzanck test) may be used.

Herpes simplex virus may be transferred from the vagina or cervix by the hand of patient or attendant to other areas of the skin or to the cornea (herpetic keratitis). Patients must be instructed concerning the importance of hand washing; medical personnel must wear gloves and gowns.

When *genital herpes* occurs in the pregnant mother before the thirty-second week of gestation, the risk of neonatal infection is 10 percent, but when HSV-2 is present at the time of delivery, 40 to 80 percent of the offspring are affected. Pregnant women who have HSV isolated from genital lesions or diagnosed cytologically during the first 20 weeks of gestation have a threefold increase in abortions. After the twentieth week there is a slight increase in prematurity. In every case, effects upon the woman and fetus are most severe when the infection is a primary exposure.

Within 2 to 12 days after delivery, affected newborns may show conjunctivitis, keratitis, papulovesicular rashes, jaundice, cyanosis, seizures, and gastrointestinal bleeding, reflecting disseminated infection to the skin, eye, liver, central nervous system, adrenal glands, lungs, spleen, and bone marrow. Mortality in disseminated infection approaches 67 percent, and another 18 percent of the neonates survive, albeit with significant morbidity. Only 15 percent survive to develop as healthy babies.

Intrauterine transplacental congenital infection has been proved occasionally. The usual outcome is fetal death. However, mental retardation, microcephaly, microphthalmia, intracranial calcification, retinal dysplasia, and vesicles on the skin have been observed at the time of delivery. If HSV-2 infection within 4 weeks of the expected time of delivery is suspected clinically by Papanicolaou smear from the cervix or by culture of HSV-2, delivery by cesarean section prior to rupture of the fetal membranes is indicated.

TREATMENT Neither a killed nor attenuated vaccine has been shown to be effective. When there is a history of recurrent herpetic vulvovaginitis coupled with a clinical exacerbation close to term, delivery by cesarean section is indicated. If primary herpetic vulvovaginitis is documented during gestation, the fetus may be infected during the mother's viremia, and the indication for cesarean section is less clear.

Idoxuridine (5-iodo-2′-deoxyuridine, IDU) and adenine arabinoside (9β-D-arabinofuranosyladenine, vidarabine, ara-A), and trifluorothymidine (trifluridine) are effective topically in herpes simplex virus keratitis. For herpetic keratitis topical IDU is applied in a 0.1% solution every hour during the day and every 2 h during the night. A simpler means of application is a 0.5% ointment four to five times a day. There are no controlled clinical trials to support the clinical efficacy of any local preparation in the treatment of herpes labialis or genital herpes simplex virus infection.

Intravenous ara-A is effective in preventing disseminated perinatal infections and encephalitis if therapy is begun when initial skin vesicles or ulcers are noted on the infant. Therapy with intravenous ara-A (15 mg/kg per day for 7 days) should be instituted if a newborn has cutaneous evidence by positive Tzanck smear from a lesion of HSV infection, because such early treatment often prevents dissemination. Because of the development of resistance of strains of herpes simplex virus to photoactive heterotricyclic dyes (proflavine, neutral red) and the possible induction of malignant transformation by these agents, this treatment is not recommended.

Adenine arabinoside is an established antiherpesvirus agent. It has been effective in varicella-zoster in immunosuppressed patients (Chap. 204), and when given before the onset of coma in biopsy-proven HSV-1 encephalitis, has a good therapeutic index (efficacy/toxicity). Ara-A also inhibits hepatitis B virus multiplication (see Chap. 318). It is active in preventing cytopathic effects in tissue culture of HSV-1, HSV-2, varicella-zoster (VZ) virus, cytomegalovirus, and herpes B and vaccinia viruses. It is much less depressive to the bone marrow than older and now obsolete systemic nucleoside antiviral agents such as idoxuridine or cytosine arabinoside. Ara-A is not an immunosuppressive agent; it is immediately converted within cells by the ubiquitous enzyme adenosine deaminase to hypoxanthine arabinoside (ara-Hx), which, in turn, also has antiviral activity, albeit less than the parent compound. Ara-A specifically inhibits HSV DNA polymerase without major inhibition of similar normal enzymes. The mechanism of action of ara-Hx is unknown, but it may be reaminated to ara-A intracellularly. Experience to date suggests, but does not prove, that ara-A is useful in disseminated cutaneous HSV-1 but is of dubious value in recurrent cutaneous HSV-2 or cytomegalovirus infections.

Ara-A is diluted in 5% dextrose solutions at a ratio of at least 2 ml for each milligram of antiviral compound. Adenine arabinoside is given by slow, continuous intravenous infusions in a dose of 15 mg/kg per day for 10 days for HSV encephalitis (10 mg/kg per day for disseminated varicella-zoster). The National Institute of Allergy and Infectious Diseases Collaborative Antiviral Study Group suggests that in suspected cases of HSV encephalitis ara-A should not be given without a brain biopsy and that treatment should be discontinued after 5 days if brain biopsies are negative for HSV. With ara-A, slight depressions in hemoglobin have been noted, and megaloblasts have been seen in the bone marrow. When patients are receiving other immunosuppressive or cytotoxic treatments or have renal insufficiency, toxicity of ara-A may be greater. A transient reversible akinetic mutism has been observed in several patients. Approximately 40 percent of the daily dose of ara-A is excreted in the urine within 24 h.

Considerable effort is being expended in development of antiviral pharmacokinetics so that antiviral drugs may be used predictively. For instance, ara-A and ara-Hx singly exhibit in vitro anti-HSV inhibitory (MIC) and lethal (MLC) activity at concentrations of drug not inhibiting cellular DNA, RNA, or protein synthesis. This in vitro finding may account for the beneficial therapeutic index in humans. An assay for the combined antiviral activity (AVA) in micrograms per milliliter of ara-A equivalents in human body fluids has been developed which is unaffected by the concomitant presence of anti-HSV antibody or interferon. The combined AVA of ara-A plus ara-Hx (the antiviral drug in vivo) is greater than the predicted values of each drug measured individually by chemical methods. Moreover, sustained AVA in serums (approximately 10 μg/ml) persists throughout the period of treatment. It is clear that the true AVA of ara-A is expressed intracellularly, and concentrations of drug within cells have not yet been measured by microbiologic assay.

Acycloguanosine [9-(2-hydroxyethoxymethyl)guanine, acyclovir, ACV] is an exciting new antiviral agent now under careful clinical evaluation. Like ara-A, ACV selectively inhibits herpesvirus (HSV-1, HSV-2, VZV) DNA polymerases much more actively than similar host cell enzymes. Acycloguanosine in tissue cultures also inhibits infection with Epstein-Barr virus (see Chap. 212) but is not active against vaccinia virus or cytomegalovirus. The active compound (like ara-ATP) is the triphosphate of acycloguanosine (ACG-TP) which binds to the viral polymerase inactivating it. Acyclovir is only minimally metabolized and appears to be excreted largely unchanged in the urine. The drug has the unique property of not being phosphorylated by uninfected cells requiring herpes-specific thymidine kinase for the formation of acycloguanosine-monophosphate. This may account for a unique lack of toxicity which has been demonstrated in phase 1 trials in humans. In human fibroblast tissue cultures, the MIC_{50} for ACV for HSV-1 is 0.09 μg/ml (0.4 μM); for VZV it is 1.0 μg/ml (4 μM). In similar tissue cultures ara-A is one-nineteenth (HSV-1) and one-half (VZV) as active.

Early controlled clinical trials with interferons (α and β) are in progress (see Chap. 196).

REFERENCES

BARZA M, PAUKER SG: The decision to biopsy, treat, or wait in suspected herpes encephalitis. Ann Intern Med 92:641, 1980

CHAMPNEY KJ et al: Anti-herpesvirus activity in human sera and urine after administration of adenine arabinoside (*in vitro* and *in vivo* synergy of adenine arabinoside and arabinosylhypoxanthine in combination). J Clin Invest 62:1142, 1978

COREY L: Chemotherapy of herpes simplex virus infections, in *Update III: Harrison's Principles of Internal Medicine,* KJ Isselbacher et al (eds). New York, McGraw-Hill, 1982, pp 31–52

——— et al: A trial of topical acyclovir in genital herpes simplex virus infections. N Engl J Med 306:1313, 1982

ELION GB et al: Selectivity of action of an antiherpetic agent, 9-(2-hydroxyethoxymethyl) guanine. Proc Natl Acad Sci 74:5716, 1977

GUINAN ME et al: The course of untreated recurrent genital herpes simplex infection in 27 women. N Engl J Med 304:759, 1981

LEGASPI RC et al: Interferon in biopsy and autopsy specimens of brain. Its presence in herpes simplex virus encephalitis. Arch Neurol 37:76, 1980

LEVINE DP et al: Simultaneous serum and CSF antibodies in herpes simplex virus encephalitis. JAMA 240:356, 1978

NAHMIAS AJ, JOSEY WE: Epidemiology of herpes simplex viruses 1 and 2, in *Viral Infections of Humans: Epidemiology and Control,* AS Evans (ed). New York, Plenum, 1976, p 253

——— et al: The human herpesviruses. An interdisciplinary perspective. Elsevier, New York, 1980

PAVAN-LANGSTON D et al: Adenine arabinoside: An antiviral agent. New York, Raven Press, 1975

REEVES WC et al: Risk of recurrence after first episodes of genital herpes. Relation to HSV type and antibody response. N Engl J Med 305:315, 1981

SPRUANCE SL et al: The natural history of recurrent herpes simplex labialis. N Engl J Med 297:69, 1977

WHITLEY RJ et al: Adenine arabinoside therapy of biopsy-proved herpes simplex encephalitis. NIAID Collaborative Antiviral Study. N Engl J Med 294:289, 1976

——— et al: Adenine arabinoside therapy of herpes zoster in the immunosuppressed. NIAID Collaborative Antiviral Study. N Engl J Med 294:1193, 1976

——— et al: The natural history of herpes simplex virus infection of mother and newborn. Pediatrics 66:489, 1980

——— et al: Vidarabine therapy of neonatal herpes simplex virus infection. Pediatrics 66:495, 1980

——— et al: Herpes simplex encephalitis. Vidarabine therapy and diagnostic problems. N Engl J Med 304:313, 1981

———, LERNER AM: Some previously unrecognized features of herpes simplex virus encephalitis. Neurology 28:1193, 1978

211
CYTOMEGALOVIRUS INFECTION (CYTOMEGALIC INCLUSION DISEASE)

JOEL D. MEYERS

DEFINITION Cytomegalovirus is infectious for humans at all ages beginning with gestation. First called *salivary gland virus* after it was found to cause subclinical salivary gland infection as well as a fatal, disseminated illness in newborn infants, it has subsequently been shown to cause a wide spectrum of diseases including severe congenital malformations, a mononucleosis syndrome in adolescents and young adults, and fatal disseminated infection in immunosuppressed patients. The name refers to the characteristic enlargement of infected cells. Similar viruses are found in many animal species, and study of infection in laboratory animals has been important in understanding human disease.

ETIOLOGY Cytomegalovirus (CMV) belongs to the herpesvirus group (herpetoviridae) of double-stranded DNA viruses. It produces large intranuclear (9 to 15 nm) and smaller cytoplasmic (2 to 4 nm) inclusions in infected cells which themselves reach 25 to 40 nm in diameter. The intranuclear inclusion is typically central and surrounded by a clear halo, producing the characteristic "owl's eye" appearance. Inclusion-bearing cells are larger than and usually distinguishable from cells infected with herpes simplex virus and varicella-zoster virus. Though growth in vitro occurs only in human fibroblast cells, infection in vivo may involve virtually any cell type. CMV has been shown to transform hamster cells in vitro and may possess oncogenic potential along with other herpesviruses.

EPIDEMIOLOGY CMV infection occurs throughout the world. The incidence, prevalence, and age at first infection vary depending on cultural and socioeconomic factors. In the United States, about 1 percent of newborns are infected congenitally, while up to 5 percent acquire infection perinatally. Serologic surveys show a gradual increase in seropositivity rates with age with an accelerated rate of infection during adolescence and young adulthood. The virus persists in the host for long periods, perhaps indefinitely, and chronic virus excretion may occur in urine, saliva, semen, cervical secretions, feces, and breast milk. Close and prolonged contact appears necessary for transmission, and the combination of poor hygiene and chronic urinary or salivary excretion is probably responsible for primary infection during childhood, as well as in cultures in which poor hygiene and communal living are more common, including persons in boarding schools and military bases. Evidence that CMV is a sexually transmitted agent is increasing. Such evidence includes the anatomic sites of infection (semen and cervix), the association of CMV infection with other sexually transmitted diseases, the higher prevalence of antibody among persons with other sexually transmitted diseases including homosexual males, the age-specific prevalence of antibody which increases with the onset of sexual activity, and anecdotal reports of transmission of CMV between sexual partners. Primary infection may also occur after exposure to fresh blood or blood products, while reactivation of latent virus occurs among immunosuppressed patients, especially those receiving organ allografts.

PATHOGENESIS CMV infects both the normal host and patients with compromised immunity. Congenital cytomegalic inclusion disease is thought to occur most commonly following primary infection of the pregnant mother, though asymptomatic congenital infections also occur in infants of mothers who were seropositive before pregnancy. The trimester during which maternal infection carries the highest risk and the factors which determine the severity of disease in the fetus are not known. Perinatal infection occurs after exposure to CMV in infected cervical secretions at the time of delivery or after exposure to infected breast milk or other sources early in infancy.

The clinical and laboratory manifestations of primary CMV mononucleosis in older children or adults are similar to those of Epstein-Barr virus–associated infectious mononucleosis (see Chap. 212). The hematologic picture of atypical lymphocytosis is due to the activation of lymphocytes in response to infection, and many of the laboratory manifestations of this disease such as the production of rheumatoid factor are due to a temporarily disordered immune response. Some of the clinical manifestations of CMV infection, such as Guillain-Barré syndrome, may also be mediated immunologically, but others, such as gastrointestinal ulcerations and pneumonia, are due to direct virus invasion of tissue.

The pathogenesis of CMV infection in the compromised host is complex. As in normal persons, primary infection may occur after exposure to exogenous virus in blood products or other sources. However, virus may be transmitted in the organ allograft itself (e.g., kidney, heart, or bone marrow) or may be reactivated from a latent state within the patient. The mechanisms responsible for latency and reactivation are undefined. However, it appears that some form of antigenic stimulation, either host-versus-graft (graft rejection) or graft-versus-host (graft-versus-host disease), is important in virus reactivation. Cytotoxic drugs such as cyclophosphamide and the use of agents that are specific suppressants of cell-mediated immunity such as antithymocyte globulin have also been associated with virus reactivation in both human and animal studies. General suppression of cell-mediated immunity occurs during primary CMV infection and may be responsible for the frequency of combined infections with agents such as *Pneumocystis carinii* (see Chap. 222), fungi, and bacteria in the compromised host. Cell-mediated immunity is important in the predisposition to and outcome of CMV infection, and severe CMV infection usually occurs among patients with suppressed cell-mediated immunity.

PATHOLOGY Enlarged cells with characteristic intranuclear inclusions are the histologic marker of infection. Cytoplasmic inclusions are also seen, though they may be more apparent with Wright-Giemsa or Papanicolaou strains than with hematoxylin-eosin stain. The inflammatory response consists primarily of mononuclear macrophages and lymphocytes, but polymorphonuclear leukocytes may also be present. Either localized or disseminated infection occurs. Localized infection consists most commonly of interstitial pneumonia, hepatitis, or gastrointestinal ulcers. Inclusion bodies are generally not seen in the liver except in disseminated infection; granulomatous hepatitis has been associated with CMV in otherwise normal persons. In disseminated infection virtually every organ may be involved, including the lung, liver, spleen, kidneys, adrenals, pancreas, gastrointestinal tract, and central nervous system. Lung involvement may be diffuse or localized and may include macro- or micronodules (miliary disease) which show focal necrosis. Pulmonary changes may be modified by concomitant infection with a variety of other agents. Similarly, congenital infection may be limited to the salivary glands and kidneys or involve multiple organs. Virus infection of the inner ear has been found in infants with congenital CMV infection and presumably accounts for the hearing loss associated with this disease.

CLINICAL MANIFESTATIONS The manifestations of CMV infection are determined primarily by the age and immune status of the host, but genetic factors of the host and virulence characteristics of the virus about which little is known may play a role. The majority of CMV infections appear to be either very mild or asymptomatic. Because CMV is excreted for many months after the initial infection, association of a specific illness with CMV excretion may be unwarranted if characteristic cytopathology or a specific immune response cannot also be demonstrated.

Congenital CMV infection Approximately 10 percent of newborns with congenital infection have permanent sequelae. Though some develop mild jaundice, respiratory distress, and failure to thrive, others show the full syndrome of cytomegalic inclusion disease including hepatosplenomegaly with hepatitis and cirrhosis, purpura, maculopapular rashes, encephalitis, microcephaly with microgyria, growth retardation, chorioretinitis, pneumonia, hemolytic anemia, and pathologic fractures of the long bones. The differential diagnosis of this syndrome includes congenital syphilis, rubella, enterovirus infection, toxoplasmosis, bacterial sepsis, and neonatal herpes simplex virus infection. Among infants with mild or apparently asymptomatic congenital infection, a substantial proportion develop late sensorineural hearing loss while some also show some degree of mental retardation.

Perinatal or postnatal CMV infection Infants infected at the time of birth or shortly thereafter may excrete virus for months or years but do not show permanent damage similar to that observed after congenital infection. Some infants do have mild illness including poor weight gain, adenopathy, rash, hepatitis, anemia, and atypical lymphocytosis. Pulmonary disease including pharyngitis, bronchitis, and interstitial pneumonia have also been attributed to CMV infection, but concomitant infection with *Chlamydia trachomatis* or *P. carinii* in some of these infants makes the role of CMV less clear.

Infection of normal children and adults A myriad of symptoms and signs have been attributed to primary infection with CMV. Most common is atypical mononucleosis. Transfusion-associated CMV mononucleosis was first described in patients after open-heart surgery and was termed *postperfusion syndrome.* It is now clear that other routes of infection produce the same syndrome. The incubation period after exposure to infected blood is 30 to 60 days, and the illness generally lasts 3 to 6 weeks. The predominant manifestations are fever and both relative and absolute lymphocytosis with atypical lymphocytes. Nonspecific (heterophile) and specific tests for Epstein-Barr virus (EBV) infection are negative. The patient may complain of malaise, myalgias, and a sore throat. However, exudative pharyngitis and tonsillitis are generally mild or absent, and both lymphadenopathy and hepatic involvement are less than those seen with EBV-associated infectious mononucleosis. Rubelliform rashes occur with and without exposure to ampicillin. Other manifestations include interstitial pneumonia, splenomegaly, myocarditis, polyneuritis (Guillain-Barré syndrome), hemolytic anemia, and thrombocytopenic purpura. Even rarer have been encephalitis, jaundice, granulomatous hepatitis, and frank arthritis with effusions. The hematologic profile is identical to infectious mononucleosis, and transient immunologic abnormalities such as the production of rheumatoid factor, cryoglobulins, antinuclear antibodies, and cold agglutinins are observed with both infections. Though most patients recover without residua, some experience fevers and malaise for up to 1 year after onset of the infection.

The differential diagnosis is diverse owing to the multitude of clinical and laboratory manifestations of CMV infection. The primary differential is with EBV-associated infectious mononucleosis. Other diseases to be considered include acquired toxoplasmosis, viral hepatitis, infections with other viruses or mycoplasma, and autoimmune hemolytic anemia or thrombocytopenia. Hematopoietic malignancy may also be an initial concern. These clinical syndromes may occur in the absence of atypical lymphocytosis, and atypical lymphocytosis is generally less common in children than in adults. Rare instances of ulcerative bowel disease and chorioretinitis also have been described in patients who were not apparently immunosuppressed.

CMV infection in the compromised host CMV infection occurs in patients with leukemia or lymphoma, solid tumors, hypogammaglobulinemia, and chronic anemia or renal failure as well as after immunosuppressive or cytotoxic treatment for other illnesses or for organ transplantation. Infection has been most common and most severe among patients receiving organ allografts. The clinical syndromes parallel those in normal persons and are generally thought to be more severe following primary infection than after either reinfection or virus reactivation. A syndrome variably consisting of fever and malaise, hepatitis with or without hepatomegaly, abdominal symptoms including nausea and cramping, arthralgias or arthritis, leukopenia, and lymphocytosis is most common and usually lasts for several weeks. Gastrointestinal disease with focal or diffuse ulcerations in any part of the GI tract occurs with or without other symptomatology. CMV retinitis may occur in one or both eyes and has been observed most commonly after renal or cardiac transplantation. The retinitis has a characteristic appearance that begins with a white granular area of necrosis which spreads centrifugally with sheathing of vessels and subsequent hemorrhage. The differential diagnosis includes herpes simplex virus, varicella-zoster virus, and toxoplasma infections of the retina as well as disseminated candidiasis or cryptococcosis. The diagnosis may be confused by the occurrence of CMV and toxoplasma retinitis in the same individual.

CMV pneumonia may occur in any immunosuppressed patient, though it has been most prominent following allogeneic marrow transplantation for leukemia, occurring in nearly 20 percent of such patients. The roentgenographic appearance is usually that of a diffuse interstitial infiltrate, but localized pneumonia with alveolar infiltrates, nodular or miliary lesions, and cavitary disease has also been seen. The patient has fever and nonproductive cough and is hypoxemic. Though the disease is transient in some, relentless respiratory failure occurs in many and the case fatality rate is high. The differential diagnosis includes *P. carinii,* other viral pneumonias, and a wide spectrum of fungal and bacterial agents as well as noninfectious causes such as pulmonary hemorrhage and radiation or drug toxicity. CMV pneumonia occurs concomitantly with other pulmonary infections, and it is usually not possible to reach a specific diagnosis without open-lung biopsy. In particular, excretion of CMV or a rise in antibody titer is not sufficient to make the diagnosis since CMV infection is common in these patients.

Finally, disseminated CMV infection occurs with involvement of virtually every organ including the central nervous system. CMV infection has also been associated with other serious complications, including a predisposition to bacterial, fungal, or *P. carinii* infections and an increased rate of graft rejection after kidney transplantation.

DIAGNOSIS The diagnosis must include either demonstration of the virus or evidence of an immune response to CMV and cannot be made purely on clinical grounds. However, virus isolation from blood or other sites does not always prove disease since virus excretion persists for some time after infection even in normal persons. Virus isolation may take as little as 3 to 4 days but more commonly takes several weeks; cultures should not be considered negative until they have been observed for 4 to 6 weeks. Virus is most commonly found in the urine, cervical or seminal secretions, throat, or blood. Histologic examination of tissue specimens by standard light microscopy is useful if typical cytopathology can be demonstrated. Detection of cytomegalic cells in the urine of infants with congenital CMV or demonstration of virus in these cells using pseudoreplica electron microscopy has also been useful, but virus cultures are ultimately more sensitive.

CMV infection may also be diagnosed by the demonstration of a rising antibody titer. The complement-fixation antibody test is most widely available, and although it has been shown that CMV strains possess serotypic differences and that the complement-fixation test is relatively insensitive for the detection of low levels of antibody, this test suffices in most instances. Antibody rises may not occur until 4 weeks or more after the initial illness, and study of serially collected serums may therefore be necessary. Other, more sensitive methods for the detection of antibody such as immunofluorescence for both IgG and IgM antibody are also available; in particular, detection of virus-specific IgM antibody by immunofluorescence may be useful for the early diagnosis of infection or for infants with congenital CMV, though false positives may occur in the latter situation owing to circulating rheumatoid factors. These techniques are usually available only in research laboratories and have not been standardized. Other laboratory tests are not specific for the diagnosis of CMV infection.

PREVENTION AND TREATMENT No specific therapy is available. Trials of antiviral drugs such as cytosine arabinoside, adenine arabinoside, and interferon have shown little effect; treatment with adenine arabinoside in high doses (20 mg/kg per day) had a beneficial effect on CMV retinitis in one study. Experience with passive transfusion of specific anti-CMV antibody is limited and would seem to offer no benefit to patients with preexistent antibody. A live, attenuated CMV vaccine is being tested; it seems to be well tolerated and elicits an immune response, but clinical indications and efficacy have yet to be established. The only means presently available for preventing primary CMV infection in seronegative patients who are likely to develop severe disease is to limit exposure to exogenous virus in blood products. In practice this means the elimination of seropositive blood products or the use of frozen deglycerolyzed red blood cells for the transfusion of seronegative patients.

REFERENCES

Dowling P et al: Cytomegalovirus complement fixation antibody in Guillain-Barré syndrome. Neurology 27:1153, 1977

Hanshaw JB: Congenital cytomegalovirus, in *Viral Disease of the Fetus and Newborn,* JB Hanshaw, JA Dudgeon (eds). Philadelphia, Saunders, 1978, pp 97–152

Ho M: *Cytomegalovirus: Biology and Infection.* New York, Plenum, 1982

Jordan MC et al: Spontaneous cytomegalovirus mononucleosis: Clinical and laboratory observations in nine cases. Ann Intern Med 79:153, 1973

Neiman PE et al: A prospective analysis of interstitial pneumonia and opportunistic viral infection among recipients of allogeneic bone marrow grafts. J Infect Dis 136:754, 1977

Pass RF et al: Productive infection with cytomegalovirus and herpes simplex virus in renal transplant recipient: Role of source of kidney. J Infect Dis 137:556, 1978

——— et al: Impaired lymphocyte transformation response to cytomegalovirus and phytohemagglutinin in recipients of renal transplants: Association with antithymocyte globulin. J Infect Dis 143:259, 1981

Phillips CA et al: Cytomegalovirus encephalitis in immunologically normal adults. JAMA 238:2299, 1977

Pollard RB et al: Cytomegalovirus retinitis in immunosuppressed hosts: I. Natural history and effects of treatment with adenine arabinoside. Ann Intern Med 93:655, 1980

Rand KH et al: Increased pulmonary superinfection in cardiac-transplant patients undergoing primary cytomegalovirus infection. N Engl J Med 298:951, 1978

Reynolds DW et al: Congenital cytomegalovirus infection: Relation to auditory and mental deficiency. N Engl J Med 290:291, 1974

Rubin RH et al: Summary of workshop on cytomegalovirus infections during organ transplantation. J Infect Dis 139:728, 1979

Stagno S et al: Congenital cytomegalovirus infection: Occurrence in an immune population. N Engl J Med 296:1254, 1977

Suwansirikul S et al: Primary and secondary cytomegalovirus infection. Arch Intern Med 137:1026, 1977

Winston DJ et al: Cytomegalovirus immune plasma in bone marrow transplant recipients. Ann Intern Med 97:11, 1982

212 EPSTEIN-BARR VIRUS INFECTIONS, INCLUDING INFECTIOUS MONONUCLEOSIS

JAMES C. NIEDERMAN

DEFINITION Epstein-Barr virus (EBV), a lymphotropic herpesvirus, infects all human populations. Primary infection in childhood is usually asymptomatic, but in adolescence or early adulthood clinical manifestations of infectious mononucleosis (IM) develop in approximately 50 percent of infections. The characteristic clinical picture consists of fever, pharyngitis, lymphadenopathy, an increase of peripheral lymphocytes with a high proportion of atypical cells, and the development of transient heterophil and persistent EBV antibody responses.

ETIOLOGY EBV, which has the structural and immunologic characteristics of a member of the herpes group, was discovered by electron microscopic studies of tumor cells from biopsies of Burkitt lymphoma grown in tissue culture. EBV antibodies measured by immunofluorescence techniques, complement fixation, immunodiffusion, enzyme-linked immunosorbent assay (ELISA), and virus neutralization are consistently absent before infectious mononucleosis, regularly develop during the course of the disease, and persist with little change for many years thereafter. In addition to IgG, EBV-specific IgM antibody is present during acute infectious mononucleosis in serums obtained 7 to 10 days after onset and usually persists for several months.

Further evidence of a causative relationship is the presence of EBV in cultures of circulating lymphocytes of patients with acute mononucleosis as well as from subjects with a past history of the disease. The classic heterophil antibody of infectious mononucleosis has been produced experimentally in squirrel monkeys inoculated with EBV-transformed autologous leukocytes. In addition, inadvertent transmission of EBV by transfusion has been reported and in several instances was associated with the development of clinical infectious mononucleosis, including heterophil antibody.

EPIDEMIOLOGY Infectious mononucleosis has been recognized in all parts of the world. Although no yearly or seasonal trends are present in the general population, early fall and spring are periods of high frequency among college students. The most characteristic epidemiologic feature of the disease is its occurrence among young adults, especially in the 15- to 25-year age group.

Seroepidemiologic studies have demonstrated that the absence of EBV antibody correlates with susceptibility to infectious mononucleosis, and its presence indicates immunity. The age at which infection is acquired is related to socioeconomic factors and hygienic environment. Among disadvantaged groups such as children living in certain tropical countries, antibody is acquired early. In contrast, in middle and upper socioeconomic groups, only 50 to 60 percent have detectable antibody during adolescent years and at the time of entry into college. Among these individuals, infectious mononucleosis is a well-recognized disorder. Studies measuring both apparent and inapparent infections suggest a clinical/subclinical ratio of 1:2 to 1:3 in young adults.

When EBV infection develops in early childhood, a mild and nonspecific or an inapparent illness occurs, either of which is associated with the appearance and persistence of specific antibody. If primary infection is delayed until adolescence or young adulthood, the clinical response is frequently typical infectious mononucleosis with the development of both heterophil and EBV antibodies.

Epidemiologic and laboratory evidence has suggested that transmission of EBV occurs through the oropharyngeal route during close personal contact. Table 212-1 indicates that EBV is present in small amounts in throat washings from 1 week to many months after clinical illness; the virus can be cultured from throat washings of 10 to 20 percent of asymptomatic seropositive adults.

This prolonged carrier state following clinical infectious mononucleosis, and presumably also after inapparent EBV infection, may serve as a principal source of transmission. Investigations utilizing the presence of EBV antibody as an index of immunity have confirmed the low contagiousness of both the infection and the disease among susceptible college roommates; secondary attack rates for EBV infection within family units have also been low.

PATHOLOGY Generalized involvement of lymphoid tissue with lymphadenopathy, nasopharyngeal lymphoid hyperplasia, and splenomegaly is the outstanding pathologic feature. Widespread focal and perivascular aggregates of mononuclear cells, including atypical lymphocytes, are found throughout the body. Nonspecific hyperplastic changes in lymph nodes are present without infiltration of the capsule or surrounding tissues. Nonlymphoid organs and tissues, including liver, heart, kidneys, and central nervous system, are also infiltrated, and changes in these organs may be associated with functional disturbances. Marrow specimens are normal or slightly hypercellular, and at times small nonspecific granulomas are present.

MANIFESTATIONS In young adults an incubation period of 30 to 50 days has been suggested on the basis of contact infection studies. Infectious mononucleosis associated with the development of heterophil and EBV antibody has occurred in several patients 5 weeks following blood transfusion. Children appear to have shorter incubation periods, in the range of 10 to 14 days, but there is relatively little information on this point.

During a prodromal period of 3 to 5 days, mild symptoms, including headache, malaise, myalgia, and fatigue, are common. Frank clinical features usually present over the next 7 to 20 days; they are variable in severity, but in over 80 percent of cases include fever, sore throat, and cervical adenopathy. In adults, temperature elevations peaking at 38 to 39°C may persist for 7 to 10 days. In severe cases, daily rise in temperature to 40°C may continue even longer. On the other hand, children often have little or no fever accompanying the infection.

Sore throat occurs in the first week and is the most common feature of infectious mononucleosis. Hyperplasia of pharyngeal lymphoid tissue with inflammation and edema develops. A grayish-white exudative tonsillitis persisting for 7 to 10 days is present in approximately 50 percent of cases. The uvula and palatal arch frequently have a gelatinous appearance. Palatine petechiae, located near the border of the hard and soft palates, are observed in about one-third of patients toward the end of the first week of illness. Although highly suggestive, their presence is not pathognomonic of the disease.

Lymph node enlargement is a hallmark of infectious mononucleosis. The onset is gradual, and anterior and posterior cervical chains are most commonly involved. Generalized adenopathy, including axillary, epitrochlear, and inguinal nodes, may also develop during the course of disease. The nodes are affected singly or in groups and may be small or grape-sized; they are firm, discrete, and moderately tender on palpation.

Splenomegaly occurs in approximately one-half the patients, and enlargement is greatest during the second and third weeks of illness. Although extremely rare, splenic rupture is one of the few potentially fatal complications of the disease.

Percussion tenderness over the liver and hepatomegaly develop in only about 10 percent of patients, but the majority (90 percent) have abnormal liver function test results which persist for several weeks. Jaundice occurs in no more than 4 to 5 percent of cases and is usually mild and uncomplicated.

During the early stages of the disease a transient faint erythematous maculopapular eruption on the trunk and extremities is present in about 10 percent of patients. The rash often resembles rubella but may be urticarial, hemorrhagic, or scarlatiniform in nature. Bilateral supraorbital edema may also be a transient finding early in the course of disease.

A wide variety of neurologic manifestations has been described, but they occur only rarely. Aseptic meningitis, encephalitis, optic neuritis, Bell's palsy, acute cerebellar ataxia, and the Guillain-Barré syndrome may appear at any time during the illness. EBV antibodies have been demonstrated in the cerebrospinal fluid of patients with meningoencephalitis associated with infectious mononucleosis; EBV is cell-associated in cerebrospinal fluid. Most patients experience complete recovery from central nervous system involvement; however, severe paralysis and/or respiratory incapacity occur in rare instances and are potentially fatal complications.

Pneumonia has been described as a rare complication during early infectious mononucleosis. In cases of childhood pneumonia recent observations suggest that EBV may be a primary or secondary pathogen and may be reactivated in the course of pulmonary infections with another agent.

Cardiac complications of significance are infrequent, although a small percentage of patients have electrocardiographic abnormalities during acute illness; cases of associated myocarditis and pericarditis have been reported.

LABORATORY FINDINGS **Blood picture** Essential to the diagnosis of infectious mononucleosis is an increase in relative and absolute numbers of lymphocytes, including at least 10 to 20 percent atypical forms. During EBV infection of B cells early in disease atypical lymphocytosis results from increased numbers of both B and T cells. Later, lymphocytosis is due largely to intense reactive proliferation of T suppressor/cytotoxic cells having a surface phenotype similar to mature thymocytes. The major immunoregulatory T cell consists of activated suppressor cells, defined by monoclonal or heteroantibody techniques. This T5/T8+ Ia^+-positive T cell readily explains the association of infectious mononucleosis with depressed cell-mediated immunity manifested by loss of skin hypersensitivity and lymphocyte hyporesponsiveness to in vitro stimulation by a variety of mitogens and specific antigens.

These studies and others with CMV or toxoplasmosis, for example, show that a virus (or other agent) may activate a specific subset of human T cells which result in immunoregulatory imbalances. In addition, the cell surface phenotype in infectious mononucleosis—a mature activated suppressor cell—readily distinguishes this disorder from acute leukemia and other lymphoproliferative diseases.

The atypical lymphocytes of infectious mononucleosis are

TABLE 212-1
Recovery of EBV in pharyngeal excretions from 25 cases of infectious mononucleosis

Time after onset of symptoms, days	*No. specimens tested*	*No. specimens positive*	*Percent positive*
0–14	16	13	81.3
15–28	12	10	83.3
29–150	11	11	100.0
>150	3	2	66.7
Total	42	36	85.7

SOURCE: *Miller et al.*

large cells with oval, horseshoe-shaped, or indented nuclei and basophilic, vacuolated, foamy cytoplasm. Nuclear chromatin is usually dense and irregular, and nucleoli are rarely seen. During the first week of illness, either the total leukocyte count is normal or there may be a leukopenia due to granulocytopenia. The total count then rises to between 10,000 and 20,000 leukocytes per cubic millimeter by the second or third week of illness; rarely, the number of leukocytes may range as high as 50,000 per cubic millimeter. Characteristic leukocyte changes often persist for 4 to 8 weeks or more. Anemia is rare in infectious mononucleosis, but autoimmune hemolytic anemia has been reported as a complication during the second and third weeks after onset. Cold agglutinins directed against the i antigen are present in about 70 percent of cases. Slight to moderate thrombocytopenia, which is usually symptomless, has been recognized early in the disease. In a few reported cases, the clinical picture has suggested idiopathic thrombocytopenic purpura.

Serologic diagnosis The serum of IM patients characteristically contains heterophil antibodies, i.e., agglutinins against sheep red blood cells, in high titer. Heterophil antibody is associated with the IgM fraction of serum and usually disappears over a period of 3 to 6 months. In general, the higher the titer developed during clinical illness, the longer the antibodies will remain detectable in convalescence. Though a nonspecific serologic response, the heterophil antibody of infectious mononucleosis differs from other antibodies in human serums that also agglutinate sheep red blood cells. The latter are found at low levels in normal human serums and in high titers in serum sickness. Differentiation is based on absorption techniques utilizing guinea pig kidney and beef erythrocytes. The sheep cell agglutinins of infectious mononucleosis are completely absorbed by beef red blood cells but not by guinea pig kidney. Serum sickness agglutinins are absorbed by both, whereas nonspecific Forssman agglutinins are absorbed only by guinea pig kidney. A high order of specificity has been achieved with other qualitative heterophil antibody tests which utilize formalin-treated horse red blood cells, ox red blood cells, and enzyme-treated and -untreated sheep cells.

Usually sheep cell agglutinins are present in the first week of illness, but they may be delayed in appearance. During the first 2 weeks after onset of the illness, 60 percent of young adult patients develop a positive heterophil antibody test. This percentage increases to 80 to 90 percent by the end of 1 month. The height of the titer is not related to severity of the disease or to the degree of lymphocytosis. In the presence of clinical and hematologic findings, a sheep cell agglutinin titer of 1:224 or higher before guinea pig kidney absorption and 1:28 after absorption has diagnostic significance. In the beef cell hemolysin test, a titer of 1:280 or higher may be considered significant; a rising titer in early stages of diseases is the best criterion. The horse red cell test is the most sensitive, and elevated titers may persist over a year after acute illness. An immune adherence test of similar sensitivity has also been developed.

During acute infectious mononucleosis an increase in total serum IgM levels up to 100 percent over control values and an increase of 50 percent in IgG levels has been observed. Other protein alterations associated with the IgM fraction which may be present in the disorder include cold agglutinating antibody and transiently positive serologic tests for syphilis and rheumatoid factor. In IM, the presence of EBV antibody is a regular feature. Prospective clinical studies have shown that the disease occurs only in individuals who lack antibodies to EBV; patients become seropositive in almost all cases by the time acute symptoms appear. As measured by immunofluorescence techniques, levels of 1:80 to 1:320 are often found during early illness, and in only 15 to 20 percent of cases are significant antibody rises demonstrable. Rarely, the appearance of both EBV and heterophil antibodies is delayed several weeks following onset of symptoms. The relationships between clinical features and development and persistence of EBV antibodies in typical heterophil-positive cases are shown in Fig. 212-1. In addition to EB viral capsid antigen (VCA) antibody, which is the most widely used clinically, antibodies to early antigen and EBV-specific IgM occur in 75 to 90 percent of patients with acute mononucleosis. Antibodies to other EBV-associated antigen systems (membrane, nuclear, complement-fixing, neutralizing, and immunoprecipitating) are also absent before infection and appear during the course of disease.

No direct correlation has been found between the levels of EBV and heterophil antibodies, nor between the anti-EBV titer and severity of clinical symptoms or hematologic findings. Heterophil antibody levels are highest during the first 4 to 6 weeks after onset, then decline or disappear after several months. EBV-VCA antibodies also reach peak titers within 3 to 4 weeks but persist at lower levels for many years thereafter, if not for life; titers of 1:20 to 1:40 have been demonstrated in serum collected 45 years after laboratory documentation of heterophil-positive IM.

The appearance of EBV antibody has also been demonstrated in cases which have the clinical and hematologic characteristics of IM but do not develop heterophil antibody. EBV-positive, heterophil-negative cases are apparently frequent in infants and children but rare in adults.

Other laboratory abnormalities These consist primarily of abnormal liver function tests and may include an elevation in alkaline phosphatase level, abnormalities in hepatocellular enzyme levels (serum glutamic oxaloacetic transaminase and serum glutamic pyruvic transaminase), and mild icterus. With recovery, all these values return to normal.

DIAGNOSIS The main diagnostic features of infectious mononucleosis are (1) irregular fever, sore throat, and lymphadenopathy; (2) an absolute increase in lymphocytes and monocytes exceeding 50 percent and including more than 10 percent atypical lymphocytes in the peripheral blood; (3) the transient appearance of sheep cell and horse red blood cell

FIGURE 212-1

Relationships between clinical features, hematologic changes, and antibody levels in a typical case of infectious mononucleosis.

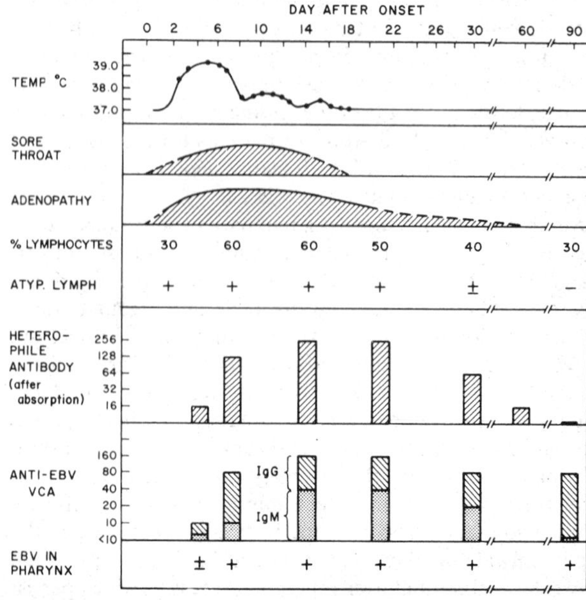

agglutinins and beef cell hemolysins; (4) the development of persistent antibody against Epstein-Barr virus; (5) abnormalities of liver function tests; and (6) appearance of specific suppressor T cells detected by monoclonal antibody techniques, associated with depressed cell-mediated immunity.

Since many of these features are also seen in other diseases, IM may resemble a number of febrile disorders, especially those associated with fever, sore throat, adenopathy, and leukocytosis. In early stages of the disease, it is often difficult to distinguish IM from other forms of febrile exudative pharyngotonsillitis such as *streptococcal infections, exudative tonsillitis of viral etiology, Vincent's angina,* and *diphtheria.* Differentiation depends on results of throat cultures and development of the hematologic and serologic features characteristic of infectious mononucleosis.

Diseases with some similarities in hematologic abnormalities such as *acute leukemia* and other *lymphoproliferative disorders* may be mistaken for IM. Demonstration of very immature leukocytes in blood or bone marrow and the presence of anemia, severe thrombocytopenia, the presence of characteristic suppressor T cells, and a negative heterophil antibody test in IM distinguish these disorders.

Cytomegalovirus (CMV) *mononucleosis* usually involves a slightly older age group, i.e., 20 to 30 years. Splenomegaly, hepatic involvement, and the presence of atypical lymphocytes in blood are common features of this disease, whereas sore throat and cervical adenopathy are usually absent. In transfusion-associated CMV infections, cytomegalovirus is excreted in the urine and a rise in complement-fixing antibody can be demonstrated.

Acute infectious lymphocytosis, a benign disorder of children, should be considered in the differential diagnosis among younger age groups. The majority of these cases are associated with signs of an upper respiratory tract infection; adenopathy is minimal, and splenomegaly is absent. The major feature is leukocytosis consisting of small mature lymphocytes; this abnormal blood picture may persist for 4 to 5 weeks, and occasionally for several months. The heterophil antibody test is negative, and no relationship to EBV antibody has been found.

The prodromal stage of *rubella,* associated with fever, malaise, postauricular and posterior cervical adenopathy, and lymphocytosis, may be indistinguishable from early infectious mononucleosis. A regular feature of the rash of rubella is its invariable presence on the face, while that of IM is prominent on the trunk and usually spares the face; it is rarely as florid as typical rubella. The appearance of large numbers of atypical lymphocytes in the blood and the development of heterophil and/or EB viral antibodies indicate infectious mononucleosis. Isolation of rubella virus from the throat and demonstration of a rising rubella virus antibody titer confirm a diagnosis of rubella.

Acquired *toxoplasmosis* may be associated with fever, generalized adenopathy, splenomegaly, and lymphocytosis. A definitive diagnosis is based on direct isolation of *Toxoplasma gondii* and/or demonstration of the development of specific serologic responses.

Infectious mononucleosis with jaundice can frequently be confused with *infectious hepatitis.* In hepatitis, fever is often lower and disappears when jaundice develops. Similarly, the presence of atypical lymphocytes is usually transitory during the preicteric phase of hepatitis, and the disease is less frequently associated with splenomegaly and leukocytosis. In early illness, hepatocellular enzyme levels are higher in viral hepatitis than in cases of infectious mononucleosis. Severe hepatitis and encephalopathy have been reported in a fatal case of infectious mononucleosis associated with Reye's syndrome in a young child.

A number of fatal lymphoproliferative syndromes associated with primary EBV infection have been described. In one

kindred both lytic and proliferative manifestations have occurred as an X-linked recessive disorder; these include fatal infectious mononucleosis, agammaglobulinemia, and malignant lymphoma. Defects in humoral or cell-mediated immune responses to EBV or in interferon production have been found in the fatal cases.

TREATMENT Therapy is symptomatic. Antibiotics have no effect on uncomplicated infectious mononucleosis. During the febrile period rest in bed is advisable. Salicylates or other analgesics are usually sufficient to control headache and discomfort from sore throat; gargling and irrigation with saline solutions provide symptomatic relief of pharyngitis and stomatitis. As a rule, most patients recover uneventfully on this regimen in 2 to 4 weeks, with gradual return to normal activities. Patients with splenomegaly should be cautioned against heavy lifting and strenuous athletics until splenic enlargement has disappeared.

In patients with severe toxic exudative pharyngotonsillitis associated with extensive pharyngeal edema, corticosteroids are useful to induce a prompt anti-inflammatory effect. A short course of prednisone may be administered, starting with 60 mg the first day and decreasing the dose by 5 to 10 mg daily over the course of a week. Steroids are not necessary in treatment of the usual patient with IM. However, full dosages of steroids should be employed in the management of severe complications, including (1) airway obstruction (intubation or tracheostomy may also be required), (2) neurologic complications, (3) hemolytic anemia and thrombocytopenic purpura, and (4) myocarditis and pericarditis.

Approximately 20 percent of patients with infectious mononucleosis experience concurrent beta-hemolytic streptococcal pharyngotonsillitis and should receive antibiotic treatment; a full 10 days' course of penicillin V 250 mg four times daily, erythromycin 250 mg four times daily, or procaine penicillin G 600,000 units every 12 h should be administered. *Ampicillin should be avoided because of the high frequency of erythematous macular or maculopapular skin rashes associated with the use of this drug in patients with infectious mononucleosis.*

Severe abdominal pain is rare in IM except in association with splenic rupture. This serious complication requires massive transfusions and immediate splenectomy.

REFERENCES

DeWaele M et al: Characterization of immunoregulatory T cells in EBV-induced infectious mononucleosis by monoclonal antibodies. N Engl J Med 304:460, 1981

Epstein MA, Achong BG: Pathogenesis of infectious mononucleosis. Lancet 2:1270, 1977

Henle G et al: Relation of Burkitt's tumor associated herpes-type virus to infectious mononucleosis. Proc Natl Acad Sci USA 59:49, 1968

Ho M: The lymphocyte in infections with Epstein-Barr virus and cytomegalovirus. J Infect Dis 143:857, 1981

Mangi RJ et al: Depression of cell-mediated immunity during acute infectious mononucleosis. N Engl J Med 291:1149, 1974

Miller G et al: Prolonged oropharyngeal excretion of EB virus following infectious mononucleosis. N Engl J Med 288:229, 1973

———: Epstein-Barr herpes virus and infectious mononucleosis. Prog Med Virol 20:84, 1975

Morgan DG et al: Site of Epstein-Barr virus replication in the oropharynx. Lancet 2:1154, 1979

Niederman JC: Infectious mononucleosis: Clinical manifestations in relation to EB virus antibodies. JAMA 203:205, 1968

——— et al: Prevalence, incidence and persistence of EB virus antibody in young adults. N Engl J Med 282:361, 1970

———: Infectious mononucleosis: EB virus shedding in saliva and the oropharynx. N Engl J Med 294:1355, 1976

PURTILO DT et al: Epstein-Barr virus infections in the X-linked recessive lymphoproliferative syndrome. Lancet 1:798, 1978

REINHERZ EL et al: The cellular basis for viral induced immunodeficiency: Analysis by monoclonal antibodies. J Immunol 125:1269, 1980

ROBINSON J et al: Mitotic EBN A positive lymphocytes in peripheral blood during infectious mononucleosis. Nature 287:334, 1980

———: Plasmacytic differentiation of circulating Epstein-Barr virus infected B lymphocytes during acute infectious mononucleosis. J Exp Med 153:235, 1981

ROBINSON JE et al: Diffuse polyclonal B cell lymphoma during primary infection with Epstein-Barr virus. N Engl J Med 302:1293, 1980

Miscellaneous and presumptive viral infections

213 WARTS AND MOLLUSCUM CONTAGIOSUM

LAWRENCE COREY

WARTS Definition Warts are benign neoplasms of the skin and contiguous mucous membranes caused by the human papilloma virus (HPV).

Etiology Warts or papillomata of several different clinical types are caused by the human papovaviruses. Papovaviruses are spherical, small, double-stranded DNA-containing viruses which replicate in the nucleus of the cells. Viruses composing the papovavirus group of agents include (1) the papilloma viruses (human wart virus, Shope papilloma virus of rabbits), (2) the polyoma viruses of mice, and (3) the vacuolating viruses of monkeys (SV_{40}). These agents have been shown to induce the transformation of cells in tissue culture as well as to cause tumors in experimental animals. Human wart virus has been demonstrated by electron microscopy in extracts and thin sections of warts. Studies using restriction endonuclease analysis of HPV DNA indicate that several different subtypes of human papilloma viruses exist and that strain differences vary according to the site from which the viruses are recovered. The nomenclature of this field is still evolving. Plantar or common warts are usually associated with HPV types 1 and 2 and occasionally type 4. Flat or plain warts are associated with HPV-3. While there appear to be some common antigenic determinants among HPV types 1 to 3, HPV-4 appears antigenically distinct from the previous three types. Genital warts are most commonly associated with HPV-6, although some lesions show evidence of containing the genome of HPV types 1 and 2. *Epidermodysplasia verruciformis,* a rare familial disease characterized by flat, wartlike skin lesions that in 25 percent of patients become squamous cell carcinomas, has been associated with HPV types 3 and 5. Further evaluation of the antigenic heterogeneity of the human papovaviruses is likely to increase understanding of the clinical course, complications, and immunology of these infections.

Epidemiology Warts are found in approximately 7 to 20 percent of the population, with the highest frequency in the early teenage years. They occur mainly on the skin areas unprotected by clothing except for the feet. Person-to-person transmission by direct contact with wart tissue and indirectly by virus contamination through contaminated secretions or instruments may occur. Autoinoculation of virus to contiguous or distant sites is frequent. Although warts of several animal species are caused by similar viruses, convincing evidence of interspecies transmission is lacking.

Pathology and pathogenesis Experimentally, cell-free filtrates of human warts will induce the formation of these lesions at the inoculated skin sites of human volunteers. The incubation period varies from 1 to 20 months (mean 3 to 4 months). The skin lesions induced by the wart virus are due to an abnormal proliferation of epidermal cells. In normal epidermis, cell division occurs mainly in the basal layer; however, in the wart, mitotic figures are seen in cells several layers higher. In addition, there is thickening of the cell layers and elongation and broadening of the intrapapillary processes with the development of long, thin papilli containing blood vessels extending high into the wart. These vessels cause bleeding points when the wart is trimmed and, if thrombosed, may appear as small dark spots. Hematoxylin and eosin staining of warty lesions may reveal cells that contain both nuclear and cytoplasmic inclusions. The nuclear inclusions tend to be basophilic and represent aggregates of virus particles, while the cytoplasmic inclusions appear eosinophilic and are felt to represent deranged development of keratohyalin.

Warts are skin colored, can be single or occur in multiple clusters, and are often widely dispersed over the body. While warts may persist and spread within the same person for several years, or may recur in an individual several years after a total remission, most studies indicate that one-third of warts are gone by 6 months and two-thirds of warts will resolve spontaneously within a 2-year period. Whether this is related to a limited life span of infected cells or is due to the host's defenses is unclear. The development of antiwart antibodies has been correlated with clinical regression of the lesions. Resolving warts are associated with histological evidence of a mononuclear cell infiltration in the lower epidermis. As such, cellular immunity has been implicated as an important aspect of the host defenses to human papilloma viruses. During pregnancy warts may increase in size. In immunosuppressed patients, or those with severe combined immunodeficiency, warts may reappear and disseminate during immunosuppressive therapy.

Clinical manifestations Many clinical types of warts exist, and there appears to be a relationship between the clinical manifestations and the antigenic subtype of the virus.

Common warts (verrucae vulgaris) may occur anywhere on the skin but are most common on the hands or around the fingernails. Most lesions appear as solid, rounded tumors with rough, horny projections which may vary considerably in size (1 mm to 2 cm). Lesions occur in both children and adults, either singly or in clusters, may be localized along a scratch (Kobner phenomenon), and are usually asymptomatic.

Plantar warts occur beneath pressure points on the soles of the feet, particularly in children and young adults. The surfaces of the lesions are firm and flat and may occur individually or in mosaic-like clusters. These warts possess a conical shape, probably due to the pressure induced by walking. The lesions are covered by hyperkeratotic epithelial tissue which, upon removal, reveals the papillary structure of the soft whitish core containing thrombosed capillaries that appear as small dark specks. With further paring, capillary bleeding, which is diagnostic of a wart rather than a callous, corn, or scar, can be induced. Local pressure upon the plantar wart usually induces pain, which can be severe upon walking.

Flat warts (verrucae planae) present as skin-colored, smooth, flat or slightly elevated, round or polygonal papules that vary between 1 and 5 mm in diameter. The common sites are the face, neck, chest, dorsum of the hands, and the flexor surfaces of the forearms and shins. The mucous membranes are involved rarely. The surfaces of these lesions show a stippled appearance when examined under a magnifying glass. Flat warts are most frequently confused with the lesions of lichen planus. Multiple lesions on the dorsum of the hands may be mistaken for one of the inherited disorders known as acrokeratosis verruciformis, epidermodysplasia verruciformis, or Darier's disease.

Warts which project fingerlike structures are termed *filiform warts;* when present on the scalp, they are called *digitate warts.* Filiform warts are most frequent in adult males, usually on the bearded area of the face. The lips and eyelids may also be involved. The lesions are either single or multiple, and they grow to considerable size when left unattended. The differential diagnosis includes cutaneous horns and epidermal nevi.

Condylomata acuminata, or venereal warts, generally appear as multiple, polymorphic lesions which may coalesce to large masses in the genital and/or anal area. In men, they are found most frequently in the coronal or frenum area of the penis. Urethral warts usually affect the anterior urinary meatus. In women, warts may occur on the fourchette, on the adjacent labia and/or vulva, the cervix, and the lower and upper one-third of the vagina. In about 20 percent of patients, the lesions spread to the perineum and anal area. Anal warts may, however, appear without concomitant penile or vulvar disease and may extend into the anal canal.

While there are a small number of patients with skin warts who develop flat warts in the genital area due to autoinoculation, most studies indicate that genital warts are sexually transmitted. In one study 60 percent of the patients who had sexual contact with partners having active genital warts subsequently developed disease, usually after an incubation period of 2 to 3 months. Symptomatic flat condyloma of the cervical region, usually not visible to the unaided eye, are noted as white spots with fine punctations on culposcopic examination. Cytologic evidence of flat condylomas (koilocytosis, multinucleated cells, and dyskeratosis) of the lesions has been reported in about 1 percent of patients on routine Papanicoloau screening. In addition, cells suggestive of flat condyloma were noted in one-third of patients with histopathologically proven cervical dysplasia, carcinoma in situ, or invasive cervical carcinoma. Further work on the natural history and characterization of the virus of this entity is needed.

The differential diagnosis of genital warts includes condylomata lata of secondary syphilis (dark-field microscopy for *Treponema pallidum* and serologic testing will differentiate between these two entities), granuloma inguinale in tropical countries, and carcinoma of the penis. Vulvar warts must be differentiated from fibroepitheliomas, molluscum contagiosum, and, in older women, seborrheic keratosis.

Complications Occasionally, a giant condyloma may cause destruction of the affected areas, e.g., the penis in Bushke-Lowenstein tumor. Despite its benign histology, this lesion may cause extensive perforation and destruction of tissue and may simulate a malignant growth. Biopsy is recommended. Vulvar warts may enlarge enough during pregnancy to cause problems in the management of labor and delivery.

Laryngeal papillomatosis of childhood appears related to condyloma acuminatum. These lesions, which are usually multiple, develop within the first 6 months of life, and most mothers of children who develop these multiple lesions have been noted to have genital warts at parturition. This condition appears to be etiologically distinct from the solitary laryngeal papilloma of elderly patients which tends to become malignant. Malignant transformation of warts is rare. An example is *epidermodysplasia verruciformis,* a condition with a familial predisposition that begins with multiple lesions similar to common warts on the dorsum of the hands and feet and soon spreads over the entire body surface.

Treatment There is no specific treatment for warts, although a variety of physical and chemical methods are used for their removal. These methods include electrodesiccation and curettage, surgical excision, x-ray, and cryosurgery by applying liquid nitrogen or dry ice. Repeated paring of warts, followed by the application of caustic agents, such as mono- or trichloracetic acid, calicylic acid, cantharidin, or silver nitrate, is helpful. Topical antimetabolites such as 5-fluorouracil have also been used.

Condylomata acuminata are treated effectively by repeated topical application of a 25 percent podophyllum resin and tincture of benzoin. This preparation is applied to the lesions, washed off after 3 to 4 h, and repeated once or twice a week, while the time of application is lengthened until the lesions have resolved. Large quantities of podophyllum are toxic, however, and may cause hypokalemia and neuropathy. It is also advisable to avoid podophyllum in pregnancy. Radical therapy of warts should be eschewed because most warts will eventually spontaneously disappear without leaving any scars.

MOLLUSCUM CONTAGIOSUM Molluscum contagiosum is an infectious disease of the skin and mucous membranes caused by a member of the poxvirus group. The virus of molluscum contagiosum is the largest of the true viruses to cause human disease, and, because of its size, 240 to 320 nm in diameter, it can be demonstrated in direct touch preparations of lesions using oil-immersion light microscopy. Molluscum contagiosum is a disease of worldwide distribution, occurring in all races and seen most frequently in children. Occasionally, epidemics of the disease are seen in closed populations as in boarding schools among wrestlers. Infection can be transmitted experimentally by injecting material expressed from the lesions. Clinically, infection can be transmitted directly through sexual intercourse or, like other poxviruses, through fomites such as shared towels. The incubation period varies between 2 weeks and 2 months.

Proliferation, hyperplasia, thickening, and degeneration of the epidermis characterize the lesions. Infected epithelial cells become enlarged and develop large intracytoplasmic eosinophilic hyalin inclusion bodies which displace the nucleus to one side.

Molluscum contagiosum is characterized by single or multiple, rounded dome-shaped waxy, pearly white pustules with an umbilical central core. A cheesy material that stains blue with Giemsa's stain can be expressed from the central core. Microscopically, the umbilicated central porous area is composed of horn lamellas, debris, dyskeratotic cells, and molluscum bodies.

These molluscum bodies appear as a mass of viral particles on electron microscopy. The lesions may vary in number and size and range from 1 mm up to 1 to 2 cm in diameter. The principal sites of involvement include the face, especially the eyelids, the trunk, and the anogenital areas. The conjunctiva, lips, and buccal mucosa are involved rarely. Molluscum lesions are frequently traumatized, resulting in autoinoculation. Occasionally, secondary bacterial infection occurs. The lesions are usually present for 6 months to a year but may persist and spread for 3 to 4 years. Spontaneous regression without scarring occurs eventually. In contrast to warts, recurrences are rare. Patients with underlying immunologic defects may develop extensive involvement with an intractable course.

The diagnosis of molluscum contagiosum can usually be made from the characteristic appearance of the lesions. A single lesion may be confused with a keratoacanthoma, basal cell epithelioma, or pyogenic granuloma. The definitive diagnosis can be made histologically from smears of expressed material or by electron microscopy. Treatment by sharp curettage or by expression of the porous material with a curved forceps will help clear up the lesions with little if any scarring.

REFERENCES

EISINGER M et al: Propagation of human wart virus in tissue culture. Nature 256:432, 1975

GISSMAN L et al: Human papilloma viruses (HPV) characterization of four different isolates. Virology 76:569, 1972

ORIEL JD: Genital warts. Sexually Transmitted Dis 8(4):326, 1981

ORTH G et al: Characterization of a new type of human papilloma virus that causes skin warts. J Virol 24:108, 1977

PASS F et al: Identification of an immunologically distinct papilloma virus from lesions of epidermodysplasia verruciformis. J Natl Cancer Inst 59:1107, 1977

ROWSON KEK, MAHY BJW: Human papova virus. Bacteriol Rev 31:110, 1967

SANDERS BB, STRETCHER GS: Warts, diagnosis and treatment. JAMA 235:2859, 1976

SYRJANEN KH et al: Cytologic evidence of the association between condylomatous lesions with dysplastic and neoplastic changes in the uterine cervix. Acta Cytol 25:17, 1981

214
CAT-SCRATCH DISEASE

LAWRENCE COREY

DEFINITION Cat-scratch disease is an infection characterized by indolent, occasionally suppurative, regional lymphadenitis usually occurring following a scratch or a close contact with a cat. A cutaneous lesion at the site of inoculation is often present, and in about 90 percent of the reported cases cat scratches or a history of close contact with cats is elicited. A compatible syndrome has been described following injury due to splinters, thorns, beef-bone fragments, and rabbit, dog, and monkey scratches.

ETIOLOGY A specific etiologic agent has not been identified. Experimental transmission to patients has been reported. Among the agents that have been incriminated are atypical acid-fast bacteria, *Chlamydia*-like organisms, and herpes-like (EB) virus. The evidence for ascribing a causative role to any of these agents is not convincing.

EPIDEMIOLOGY The disease has been reported in numerous geographical areas; it is most common in fall and winter, and 75 percent of cases occur in children. Reactivity to the skin test antigen is seen in 3 to 20 percent of the population. Persons who have frequent contact with cats, such as veterinarians, have a higher prevalence of past infection as detected by a positive reaction to the skin test antigen. Cats appear to act only as vectors of the disease. The animals are usually not ill and have negative skin tests. Familial occurrence of several infections interspersed by months or years suggests that cats are intermittent or long-term carriers.

PATHOLOGY The histopathologic appearance of lymph nodes is not specific. Three stages have been described: (1) early lesions show reticulum-cell hyperplasia; (2) intermediate lesions show granuloma formation; and (3) late lesions show microabscesses. These histologic changes are similar to those seen with atypical mycobacterial infections, lymphogranuloma venereum, toxoplasmosis, sarcoidosis, brucellosis, and even Hodgkin's disease.

MANIFESTATIONS The incubation period ranges from 3 days to several weeks, usually 3 to 10 days. In a typical case, a primary lesion consisting of a raised, slightly tender, nonpruritic papule crowned with a small vesicle or eschar is present. Multiple primary lesions have been described. The lesion is often felt to be an insect bite and usually does not cause the patient to present to the physician. In about 40 percent of cases no primary lesion is present, and in some patients no history of inciting trauma is elicited.

Regional lymphadenopathy becomes evident in a few days or as long as 6 weeks after infection. Adenopathy is usually confined to a single region and is usually unilateral and asymmetric; in most instances only one node is involved. The axillary, cervical, preauricular, submandibular, epitrochlear, femoral, or inguinal nodes (in decreasing order of frequency) on one side become visible swollen and tender, often with redness of the overlying skin. The nodes occasionally suppurate, soften, and drain spontaneously; fistulas heal completely with only slight scarring. Usually the tenderness subsides gradually, and nontender, firm, enlarged nodes remain palpable for some weeks or even months. With rare exceptions, there is no generalized glandular enlargement, and the spleen is not palpable.

Systemic symptoms are usually mild and consist of headache, fever, and malaise, which subside within a few days. Shaking chills and fever with temperatures as high as 104°F can occur but are unusual. Many patients are entirely symptom-free. During the early stages of illness a transient macular or vesicular rash which subsides within 48 h may occur. Erythema nodosum and multiforme and thrombocytopenic purpura have also been reported.

Other clinical forms of this disease include: (1) encephalitis characterized by fever, convulsions, alterations in consciousness, mild cerebrospinal fluid pleocytosis, and elevation in protein (this usually resolves with complete recovery); (2) Parinaud's oculoglandular syndrome characterized by granulomatous conjunctivitis and enlargement of the homolateral preauricular node; (3) mesenteric lymphadenitis; (4) osteolytic bone lesions, which subside spontaneously; and (5) thrombocytopenic and nonthrombocytopenic purpura. In all these syndromes the diagnostic criteria for cat-scratch disease must be present before the illness can be ascribed to this disease.

DIAGNOSIS The following criteria should be fulfilled before a diagnosis of cat-scratch disease is established: (1) history of contact with cats, (2) presence of a primary lesion, (3) regional lymphadenopathy, (4) positive intradermal skin test, (5) biopsy of lymph node with demonstration of histopathologic changes consistent with cat-scratch disease (this may not be necessary if the skin test is positive), and (6) failure to demonstrate other causative agents.

The specific diagnosis is made by means of a skin test. In the United States standardized skin test antigen is not commercially available. Antigen for skin tests is prepared by mixing one part pus aspirated from infected lymph nodes with three parts saline solution and inactivating the mixture by heating or by irradiation. A positive reaction is of the delayed tuberculin type, consisting of 5 mm induration and 10 mm erythema, that appears in 24 to 48 h. Although batches of antigen vary in potency, in general patients reacting to one batch react to another. Skin test material can be preserved by freezing. The test becomes positive within 30 days after infection and may persist for many years. Each batch of antigen must be tested against patients known to have had the disease. False-negative reactions have been reported. Approximately 10 percent of normal individuals will have positive reactions.

Other laboratory abnormalities include mild leukocytosis (up to 15,000 cells per cubic millimeter), occasional mild eosinophilia, and an elevated sedimentation rate.

Patients with cat-scratch disease show significantly depressed lymphocyte transformation responses to phytohemagglutinin and *Candida albicans.* These reactions revert to normal as the disease subsides.

Cat-scratch disease is a benign illness, and the prognosis is uniformly good. Its main clinical importance lies in its possible confusion with other, more serious diseases of the lymphatics. Diseases to be considered are tularemia, lymphatic tuberculosis, sporotrichosis, histoplasmosis, coccidioidomycosis, toxoplasmosis, and bacterial adenitis. Because of the indolent character of the adenopathy, Hodgkin's disease or other lymphomas may be suspected. Cat-scratch disease must be differentiated from tularemia, which occasionally can be transmitted by cats. Neck masses may be confused with thyroglossal duct cysts, cleft cysts, dermoids, cystic hygromas, thryoid and parathyroid adenomas, salivary gland tumors, carotid body tumors, aneurysms, pharyngeal or esophageal diverticula, and mesodermal tumors, as well as lymphomas. Appropriate serologic and cultural tests serve to rule out other infections; biopsy may be needed to exclude tumor. A positive skin test with cat-scratch antigen may obviate the necessity for biopsy.

TREATMENT The disease is self-limited and symptoms resolve spontaneously in 1 to 2 months. Occasionally aspiration of suppurative nodes affords relief of pain. Antibiotics and steroids are ineffective.

REFERENCES

CARITHERS HA et al: Cat-scratch disease; its natural history. JAMA 207:312, 1969

———: Cat-scratch skin test antigen: Purification by heating. Pediatrics 60:928, 1977

EMMONS RW et al: Continuing search for the etiology of cat-scratch disease. J Clin Microbiol 4:112, 1976

FUTRELL JW et al: Unsuspected etiology of lateral neck masses. Arch Otolaryngol 95:277, 1971

LYON LW: Neurologic manifestations of cat-scratch disease. Arch Neurol 25:23, 1971

MARGILETH AM: Cat-scratch disease: Nonbacterial regional lymphadenitis. Study of 145 patients and a review of the literature. Pediatrics 42:803, 1968

SCHULKIND ML, AYOUB EM: Cell-mediated immunity in cat-scratch disease. J Pediatr 95:199, 1974

WARWICK WJ: The cat-scratch syndrome: Many diseases or one disease? Prog Med Virol 9:256, 1967

section 13 | Protozoal and helminthic infections

215 THE DIAGNOSIS AND THERAPY OF PARASITIC DISEASE

JAMES J. PLORDE

Parasitic diseases such as malaria, trypanosomiasis, leishmaniasis, schistosomiasis, and filariasis remain among the major causes of human sickness and death in the world today. A number of technical, social, economic, and political phenomena have combined to produce a dramatic increase in the prevalence of some of these illnesses. This has been most devastating in the case of malaria. Growing resistance of the mosquito vector to insecticides, development of drug-resistant strains of *Plasmodium falciparum,* and cutbacks in many malaria control programs have led to a worldwide resurgence of this disease. At present, over 1 billion people reside in endemic areas; between 125 and 200 million of these are infected at any given time. In Africa, where the intensity of parasite transmission defies current control measures, malaria kills over 1 million children annually. The resurgence of malaria together with an increase in international travel has resulted in an upsurge in the number of infected patients who enter the United States. From 1969 to 1980 civilian malaria cases reported annually to the Centers for Disease Control have increased from 151 to 1864. As only 50 to 60 percent of civilian infections are currently being reported, the total number may be close to 4000, a level similar to that seen during the height of the Vietnam War.

In Africa, from the Sahara in the north to the Kalahari Desert in the south, human strains of *Trypanosoma brucei* cause one of the most lethal of all human diseases, sleeping sickness. Animal strains of this species limit food supply in the same area through their impact on animal husbandry. In South America, a related organism, *T. cruzi,* infects several million people, leaving many with severe heart and gastrointestinal lesions (Chagas' disease).

Leishmaniasis is found in parts of Europe, Asia, Africa, and

South and Central America where it may present as a chronic, highly lethal infection of the reticuloendothelial system (kala azar), a mutilating mucocutaneous infection (espundia), or a self-limiting skin ulcer (oriental sore).

Schistosomiasis is the most serious of the helminthic infections, affecting an estimated 200 million individuals living between the tropics of Cancer and Capricorn. In many it produces bladder, intestinal, and/or liver disease which can eventually result in death. In many countries irrigation schemes have resulted in the dissemination of the disease to previously uninvolved areas, mitigating the economic gains of these development projects. Although not transmitted in the continental United States, exogenously acquired schistosomiasis involves nearly a half million people now residing in this country.

Wuchereria bancrofti and *Brugia malayi*, two closely related filarial worms, obstruct lymphatic circulation and produce grotesque swellings of the legs, arms, and genitals in tropical populations. Onchocerciasis, another filarial infection, affects millions of people in Africa, leaving thousands blind.

Toxoplasmosis, pneumocystosis, giardiasis, and trichomoniasis are four cosmopolitan protozoan infections well known in the United States. The first infects perhaps one-third of the world's population. Although it is usually asymptomatic, congenital toxoplasmosis may result in abortion, stillbirth, prematurity, or severe neurological defects. Even when there are no obvious signs at birth, chorioretinitis with visual impairment may occur years later. Asymptomatic toxoplasma and pneumocystis infections can both result in fatal illness later in life during periods of immunosuppression.

In contrast, giardiasis and trichomoniasis seldom result in severe disability; nevertheless their morbidity can be attested to by millions of otherwise healthy individuals. Both appear to be increasing in incidence, apparently the result of changing American life-styles. Giardiasis is particularly frequent among day-care center attendees, hikers and campers in our western states, and male homosexuals who practice anilingus, while the incidence of trichomoniasis is closely tied to the level of promiscuous heterosexual activity.

DIAGNOSIS Although some of the diseases mentioned above are uncommon in the United States, the continuous arrival of travelers and immigrants from endemic areas of the world makes it necessary to consider them in the differential diagnosis of many illnesses. Typically, neither the clinical manifestations nor the general laboratory findings observed in patients suffering from parasitic infections are sufficiently unique to raise this possibility in the mind of the clinician. Although eosinophilia has long been recognized as a clue to the presence of a hidden parasite, this phenomenon is characteristic only of helminthic infections. Even here its absence does not preclude this diagnosis. The eosinophilia presumably reflects an immunologic response to the complex foreign proteins of the worm and is most marked during the early stages of tissue migration and invasion. Once migration ceases and the worm matures to adulthood, eosinophilia may diminish or disappear.

Unless a careful travel, transfusion, and socioeconomic history is taken, the correct diagnosis may never be entertained. Once considered, however, the presence of a parasitic disease is easily confirmed. Most commonly, this is accomplished by the recovery and morphologic identification of the parasite in the stool, urine, sputum, blood, or tissues of the patient.

In intestinal infections, examination of a wet mount and/or stained smear of the stool is usually adequate. Because many parasites are passed intermittently or in fluctuating numbers, the examination of a single stool specimen may detect only one-third to one-half of involved patients. The testing of three such specimens collected at intervals of 2 or 3 days will improve this yield substantially. Alternatively, a saline cathartic may be administered to evacuate the cecal area where many protozoa are concentrated, and the entire purge examined. The stool must be free of interfering substances such as antidiarrheal or contrast agents, antacids, and antibiotics. If the appropriate specimens cannot be obtained prior to administration of such substances, testing should be performed 1 week or, in the case of antimicrobial agents, 3 weeks after their discontinuation. Occasionally, specimens other than stool must be examined. In small-bowel infections such as giardiasis and strongyloidiasis, the diagnosis, at times, can be established only by sampling the duodenal contents or by performing a jejunal biopsy. Similarly, eggs of *Enterobius* (pinworm) and *Taenia* (tapeworm) are frequently found on the perianal skin when absent from the feces. Recovery of large-bowel parasites such as *E. histolytica* and *Schistosoma mansoni* may require colonic intubation with aspiration or biopsy of suspect lesions. Whenever intestinal aspirates or soft to watery fecal specimens are collected, they should be immediately placed in a preservative such as polyvinyl alcohol (PVA) to prevent rapid disintegration of fragile protozoan trophozoites and allow the preparation of permanently stained smears. Protozoan cysts and helminthic ova found in formed stool will survive for 1 to 2 days at room temperature and indefinitely if placed in 5% formaldehyde.

Direct examination of the blood is useful for the detection of malaria parasites, leishmania, trypanosomes, and microfilaria. Preferably, fresh capillary blood should be used to prepare thin and thick blood smears and, when appropriate, wet mounts. Only specially prepared glass slides should be used as traces of soda lime or potash on uncleaned slides may alter the pH of the stain, making recognition of parasites difficult. If an experienced technologist is not available to assist in the bedside preparation of smears, it is preferable to collect venous blood in an EDTA Vacutainer and send it to the laboratory. As in the case of intestinal parasites, organisms in the peripheral blood may fluctuate, requiring the collection of multiple specimens over a period of several days.

Parasites dwelling within the tissues of the host are more difficult to identify. Some discharge their offspring into the sputum (lung flukes) where they can be found with appropriate concentration procedures. In others, larvae can be recovered with skin (*Onchocerca volvulus*) or muscle (*Trichinella spiralis*) biopsies. In some diseases, however, parasite recovery is uncommon. Reliable immunodiagnostic tests have been developed for a few of these. Unfortunately, serologic tests for parasites often lack the sensitivity and specificity of those developed for viral and bacterial agents. This is particularly true for helminths which are broadly cross-reactive with one another. Table 215-1 lists the serologic tests available through the Centers for Disease Control (CDC). In Table 215-2 the

TABLE 215-1
Parasitic diseases for which serology is available

	Diagnostic usefulness	
Taxonomic group	*High*	*Marginal*
Protozoan	Amebiasis* Babesiosis* Chagas' disease* Leishmaniasis* Toxoplasmosis*	Malaria* Giardiasis Pneumocystosis*
Helminthic	Cysticercosis* Echinococcosis* Paragonimiasis* Toxocariasis* Trichinosis*	Ascariasis* Clonorchiasis* Dracunculiasis* Filariasis* Schistosomiasis* Strongyloidiasis

* *Available at the Centers for Disease Control, Atlanta, Ga.*

diagnostic titer, sensitivity, and specificity of the most frequently requested CDC procedures are given.

TREATMENT Over the past decade, a number of new chemotherapeutic agents have been introduced for the treatment of parasitic diseases. A few, such as praziquantel and nifurtimox, represent the first effective agents available for the treatment of previously refractory diseases (i.e., clonorchiasis, Chagas' disease). Others, such as mebendazole, possess activity against a broad spectrum of helminths, allowing single-drug therapy of multiple intestinal infections. Many of the new agents are better tolerated than the ones they are destined to replace, permitting them to be used in mass therapy programs.

TABLE 215-2
Interpretation of tests frequently performed at the Centers for Disease Control

Disease	*Test**	*Diagnostic titer*	*Sensitivity %†*	*Specificity %†*	*Comments*
Invasive Amebiasis	IHA	≥1:256	70[1], 95[2]	90[3]	*1* Intestinal *2* Extraintestinal *3* Titers may persist for years
Cysticercosis	IHA	≥1:128	50[1], 70[2], 95[3]	83–95[4]	*1* Intracranial calcifications, seizures *2* Meningitis *3* ↑Intracranial pressure *4* Cross-reacts with echinococcosis
Echinococcosis	IHA	≥1:256	10[1], 88[2]	90–95[3,4]	*1* Lung or calcified cyst *2* Liver or peritoneal *3* Cross-reacts with cysticercosis *4* Titer may persist for years
Toxocariasis					
Visceral	ELISA	≥1:32	78	92[1,2]	*1* Cross-reacts with ascariasis but eliminated by preabsorption
Ocular	ELISA	≥1:8	90	91[3]	*2* In children *3* Patients with ocular disease
Trichinosis	BFT	≥1:5	97[1]	90[2]	*1* Detected after third week of illness *2* Titers may persist for years

* *IHA = indirect hemagglutination; ELISA = enzyme-linked immunosorbent assay; BFT = bentonite flocculation.*
† *Superscript numbers refer to comments at right.*
SOURCE: *Adapted from data provided by Kenneth W. Walls, Ph.D., March 1981.*

Despite these gains, however, treatment of parasitic diseases remains unsatisfactory. For a number of infections, including cysticercosis, echinococciasis, and trichinosis, satisfactory anthelmintics are not available. Drug resistance, a phenomenon so common to bacterial pathogens, also threatens the usefulness of some antiparasitic agents. This is particularly serious among the antimalarials. Chloroquine-resistant *P. falciparum,* long present in southeast Asia and Latin America, has now spread to Africa, the continent most devastated by this disease. Some Asian strains of this same organism have now developed resistance to the pyrimethamine-sulfadoxine regimen that has been used so successfully to suppress chloroquine-resistant infections.

Yet another problem relates to the availability of antiparasitic agents in the United States. Many of the drugs recommended in the following chapters have not been approved by the U.S. Food and Drug Administration either for use in this country or for the particular disease indicated. Those available as investigational agents through the Centers for Disease Control are listed in Table 215-3. Others, such as praziquantel, must be obtained directly from the manufacturer. When a clinician prescribes such an agent, the patient should be informed of the drug's investigational status and potential side effects.

Finally, the toxicity of many agents is such that the benefit of treatment must be carefully weighed against its potential side effects. This is particularly true in helminthic infections. Since most worms do not multiply within the body and because disability is usually related to the intensity of infection, treatment is directed primarily at reducing the worm burden of moderately to heavily infected patients. Total eradication is often unnecessary and may be unwise considering the toxicity of many anthelmintics. Light infections should be treated only when (1) small numbers of worms may be dangerous as in the case of strongyloidiasis, (2) the chance of reinfection is slight, and/or (3) the anthelmintic agent in question is without serious side effects. The intensity of many intestinal infections can be determined by enumerating the eggs found in stool (Table

TABLE 215-3
Agents available through the parasitic diseases division, CDC*

Infection	*Therapeutic agent*
Amebiasis	Dehydroemetine Diloxanide furoate
Chagas' disease (*Trypanosoma cruzi*)	Nifurtimox
Dracunculosis	Niridazole
Fascioliasis	Bithionol
Leishmaniasis	Sodium antimony gluconate (stibogluconate sodium) Pentamidine isethionate
Malaria	Parenteral chloroquine hydrochloride Parenteral quinine dehydrochloride
Onchocerciasis	Suramin
Paragonimiasis	Bithionol
Pneumocystosis	Pentamidine isethionate
Schistosomiasis	Metrifonate Niridazole Sodium antimony dimercaptosuccinate
Sleeping sickness (*Trypanosoma brucei*)	Melarsoprol Pentamidine isethionate Suramin
Tapeworms (*Taenia saginata, T. solium, Hymenolepsis nana, H. diminuta, Diphyllobothrium latum, Dipylidium caninum*)	Niclosamide

* *Parasitic Diseases Division, Centers for Disease Control, Atlanta, GA 30333. Day telephone: (404) 329-3670.*

TABLE 215-4
Fecal egg counts associated with illness

Worm	*Approximate egg output per female worm per day*	*Minimum egg output usually associated with illness*
Necator americanus	25,000	>2000/ml
Trichuris trichiura	7500	>3000/g
Schistosoma mansoni	60–300	>200/g

SOURCE: *After DP Stevens, Clin Gastroenterol 7:236, 1978.*

215-4). Multiplying the total seen on direct smear by 750 provides a rough estimate of the number present per gram of feces. The Stoll dilution and the various modifications of the Kato thick-smear technique provide more precise results.

REFERENCES

DOROZYNSKI A: The attack on tropical disease. Nature 262:85, 1976

Drugs for parasitic infections. Med Lett 24:5, 1982

Health Information for International Travel 1981. US Department of Health, Education, and Welfare Publication (CDC) 81-8280. Morb Mort Week Rep vol 30 (Suppl), August 1981

KAGAN IG: Serodiagnosis of parasitic diseases, in *Manual of Clinical Microbiology,* 3d ed, EH Lennette et al (eds). Washington, American Society for Microbiology, 1980, chap 70, pp 724–750

PLORDE JJ: Introduction to pathogenic parasites, in *Medical Microbiology: An Introduction to Infectious Diseases,* JC Sherris (ed). New York, Elsevier North-Holland, 1982

SMITH JW: Perspectives in diagnostic parasitology. Clin Microbiol Newsletter 2:1, 1980

216
THE IMMUNOLOGY OF PARASITES

JOHN R. DAVID

During the past decade interest in parasitic diseases of humans and in new approaches to their control has increased steadily. One reason for this is the enormous scope of the problem. Over a billion people in the world are affected by parasitic diseases. Although accurate statistics are difficult to obtain, it is estimated that over 200 million people have malaria, the most serious protozoan disease of humans, and that more than a million children die of malaria each year in Africa alone. Schistosomiasis, a disease caused by helminths that are transmitted by snails, affects 200 to 300 million persons. Filarial parasites affect an equal number of people, and one of these, *Onchocerca volvulus,* is the second major cause of blindness in the world. *Trypanosoma cruzi,* another protozoan, is the major cause of heart disease in South America, and hookworm infects over 800 million persons.

With the modernization of developing countries, many of these diseases are becoming more prevalent. For example, the pressure to provide energy for industrialization leads to building dams which have brought about profound changes in the local environment; the lake behind the Volta Dam has increased the coastline by 4000 miles, and the snails on its banks infected with schistosomes have increased the prevalence of schistosomiasis in people living on the lake's borders from a few percent to almost 100 percent. Improvement schemes for agriculture often involve extension of irrigation as is necessary for the cultivation of rice. Some of these projects have been associated with increases in transmission of malaria by mosquitoes, which breed in the irrigation ditches. Another example of the unanticipated effects of progress can be seen in the Amazon basin, where the clearing of the forests in order to reclaim the land for industry and agriculture has greatly increased human contact with sandflies which live in these areas and transmit leishmaniasis.

Another reason for the increasing focus on these diseases by scientists and physicians is that the classic control measures are less than adequate. The most telling example of this is malaria. After World War II, there was great optimism that this disease could be eradicated by spraying homes with DDT and by treating the disease in humans with chloroquine. After an extensive eradication program was instituted in the early 1960s in Sri Lanka, only 18 cases of malaria were reported in that country. However, 5 years later there were a million cases. The failure of malaria eradication was due to at least three factors: (1) the surveillance stage of the eradication effort was not maintained; (2) mosquitoes became resistant to DDT; and (3) the parasite became resistant to chloroquine. Moreover, the cost of these control measures proved to be enormous.

The large number of people affected by parasitic diseases, the increasing environmental changes in the developing world, and the failure of classic control programs have stimulated the search for new approaches for the control of these disorders. One of these approaches is immunologic. Currently, immunologists are studying several aspects of parasites' interaction with the host. They are trying to delineate the mechanisms that parasites have evolved to evade the immune response of the host, to define which immune mechanisms they do not escape, and to learn which immune responses are the basis for the pathologic lesions. Immunology is also providing diagnostic tests and ultimately, it is hoped, will provide effective vaccines for some of these diseases. At present, there is not a single vaccine available to protect humans against parasites, despite the availability of several effective vaccines against animal parasitic diseases. For the purposes of this discussion, the most useful way to present the problems of vaccine development in these complex diseases is to give a relatively detailed description of what is being done in one disease, malaria, rather than a cursory summary of many.

MALARIA VACCINE Although investigators are trying to produce vaccines to many parasites, especially intensive work is under way on vaccines for *Plasmodium falciparum,* the most malignant malaria parasite. In order to understand the various approaches that are being pursued, it is necessary to review briefly the life cycle of the malaria parasite (see Chap. 218). When an infected mosquito bites a human, it injects the motile sporozoite, which is in the salivary gland. In less than half an hour, the sporozoite leaves the blood and invades the liver. It then goes through the exoerythrocytic cycle, undergoing asexual division by schizogeny and producing many merozoites. These burst out of the liver cells into the blood and invade erythrocytes. Here, they differentiate into trophozoites, undergo division by schizogony, and burst, liberating more merozoites which reinvade erythrocytes and continue the cycle. Some of the merozoites develop into the sexual stages, the gametocytes. When a mosquito bites an infected person, the gametocytes are taken up in the blood meal and rapidly come out of the erythrocytes. The male microgametes then fertilize the female macrogametes, forming the ookinete and then the oocyst. Further division within the oocyst leads to the infective stage, the sporozoite. Several of these stages can be targeted for immunologic attack by a vaccine.

Sporozoite vaccine Persons can become immune to *P. falciparum* via the sporozoite stage. This has been shown by allowing irradiated infected mosquitoes (containing irradiated sporozoites which cannot divide) to bite humans. Work in animal models has resulted in the characterization of a single sporozoite antigen. Monoclonal antibodies to this antigen can passively transfer resistance to malaria in rodents and monkeys. It is hoped that this antigen can be produced in quantity by recombinant DNA technology. The advantages of a sporozoite vaccine are that it would be effective without an adjuvant and that it may protect against different strains of *P. falciparum.* The disadvantage is that immunity is an all-or-none phenomenon; if a few sporozoites evade the immune response, the person will get malaria.

Merozoite vaccine The host encounters merozoites for short periods, as they leave one erythrocyte and invade another. Erythrocytes infected by parasites develop new antigens, probably of parasite origin, on their surface. Both the merozoite and the infected erythrocyte could be targets for a vaccine. Monoclonal antibodies to merozoites and infected erythrocytes of rodent malaria transferred passively can confer partial protection. These monoclonal antibodies have been used to isolate antigens which can induce protective immunity. This vaccine would have the advantage of acting against stages of the parasite that interact with the host for a longer time period than the sporozoites. The disadvantages are that adjuvants are required for effective protection and that the vaccine may be strain-specific.

Gamete vaccine If an animal is made immune to gametes, a state that does not usually occur in nature because the gamete is isolated from the immune apparatus by the erythrocyte membrane, the antigamete antibodies, when taken up with the gametes in the mosquitoes' blood meal, will neutralize the gametes when they leave the erythrocyte. It appears as if at least two antigens are involved in this process because neutralization will occur when two different monoclonal antigamete antibodies act in concert but not when they act alone. A vaccine aimed at gametes would not protect the vaccinated individual from malaria but might be effective in reducing its transmission. It could be useful, therefore, if it were incorporated into a multivalent vaccine.

IMMUNE EVASION BY PARASITES Parasites have developed a variety of ingenious ways of evading the immune response of the host. Some of these are listed in Table 216-1. The most fascinating mechanism is that of antigenic variation by African trypanosomes, the flagellated protozoa transmitted by the tsetse fly that is the cause of sleeping sickness. The trypanosome has a thick surface coat, which is made up of many molecules of a single antigenic glycoprotein. When cloned organisms, all having the same surface antigen, are injected into certain animals, successive waves of parasitemia ensue similar to those seen when a human is bitten by an infected tsetse fly. Each peak consists of organisms expressing a single variant surface antigen (VSA), and this VSA is different from all other VSAs expressed by organisms in previous peaks of parasitemia in the same animal. A cloned organism can produce waves of parasites with over 100 different VSAs! Each peak of parasitemia induces soluble antibody directed at the major VSA. Presumably the antibody eliminates the organism with that specific VSA, but trypanosomes which can switch to another VSA escape. Analysis of the amino acid sequence of a number of VSAs indicates that they do not differ by only a few substitutions which could be explained by point mutations; on the contrary, the amino acid sequence of each VSA is quite different.

Studies on the genes encoding the VSAs have shown that each VSA is encoded by a distinct gene. Every trypanosome, regardless of the VSA it is expressing, contains a copy of each VSA gene. In addition, the organism expressing a particular VSA gene has an additional, duplicate copy of that gene; this is referred to as the expression-linked copy. Preliminary studies using restriction enzymes indicate that the expression-linked copy is moved to a new site in the trypanosome that is gene-specific for expression. If each gene were visualized as a tape cassette in a library, to express the VSA the cassette is duplicated, the duplicate is removed from the library and inserted into a genetic tape deck, and expressed.

Although it was thought initially that the driving force for antigenic variation was antibody to that antigen, it has been shown that antigenic variation can be triggered in the absence of antibody both in vitro and in vivo.

Some organisms have developed multiple ways of evading the immune response. Schistosomes, for instance, can lose surface antigens after they enter the host, can take up host antigens and masquerade as host tissue, can develop certain intrinsic membrane changes making them resistant to attack even when surface antigens are present, and can shed antigens which may block effector cells and antibodies. A number of parasites, *Toxoplasma* being one example, when engulfed by a macrophage, prevent the fusion of the phagosome with the lysosomes. Others, such as *Leishmania,* do not prevent fusion when engulfed but are resistant to toxic substances in the lysosomes of the macrophage. And still others, such as *Trypanosoma cruzi,* escape from the lysosomes into the cytoplasm.

A number of parasites such as filaria, *Leishmania,* and *Plasmodium* induce strong suppressor mechanisms, including T suppressor cells, which dampen or eliminate the host's effective immune response. Some parasites can destroy mediators of inflammation involved in an effective immune response. For example, *Taenia* destroys complement components, and amoebae produce factors which neutralize chemotactic factors for macrophages. Other parasites such as *Ascaris* appear to have a surface coat which is antigenic and can induce an immune response but is, nevertheless, resistant to its effect. For these parasites, there is no effective protective immune response.

Although some parasites can evade the immune response, they can induce an effective protective immune response to a subsequent infection by the same species. This is called *concomitant immunity* or *premunition.*

EFFECTOR MECHANISMS AGAINST PARASITES Mechanisms that may be effective against parasites include the following: antibodies, cells including cytotoxic T cells, T-cell–induced macrophages, natural killer cells, and a variety of cells that mediate antibody-dependent cell-mediated cytotoxicity. Amplifiers of the immune system such as lymphokines and complement are also involved.

Immunity against several parasites such as malaria, schistosomes, and *Trypanosoma cruzi* can be transferred by antibodies. Nevertheless, evidence obtained in a number of animal models suggests that cell-mediated immunity is also involved

TABLE 216-1
Some mechanisms of immune evasion

Parasite	*Mechanism*
Trypanosoma brucei	Antigenic variation
Toxoplasma	Prevent lysosome-phagosome fusion
Malaria, *Babesia*	Escape into host cells
Schistosomes	Host molecule acquisition
	Loss of surface antigens
	Intrinsic membrane changes
	Immune complex blockade
Filaria, *Leishmania*	Specific T-cell suppression
Taenia, amoeba	Inactivation of mediators of inflammation

against these and other parasites, including the organisms causing malaria, leishmaniasis, toxoplasmosis, schistosomiasis, filariasis, and trichinosis. It is less clear whether immunity develops against amoebae, African trypanosomes, or hookworm. There appears to be no naturally acquired immunity to *Ascaris,* guinea worm, or pinworm.

Two immune mechanisms have been described which appear, so far at least, to be unique for helminths. These involve eosinophils in one case and IgE in the other.

EOSINOPHILS AND ANTIBODY-DEPENDENT CELL-MEDIATED CYTOTOXICITY (ADCC) It has been known for over 100 years that eosinophils are associated with helminth infections, but only in the past few years has it become known that these cells can function as killer cells. Specifically, highly purified preparations of eosinophils, when mixed with antibody-coated schistosomula of *S. mansoni* in vitro, killed the larvae. The antibody formed is of the IgG class, and the eosinophils attach to the Fc portion of the IgG by the cells' Fc receptor. Immune complexes or staphylococcal protein A which can interfere with the binding of esosinophils to the Fc portion of the antibody inhibit the reaction. Incubation at 37°C makes the interaction between eosinophils and antibody-coated schistosomula become irreversible. This is associated with degranulation and the release of major basic protein (MBP), the most abundant protein in the eosinophil granule, over the surface of the schistosomula. MBP, in turn, is toxic to the larvae. Eosinophils can also kill other helminths such as *Trichinella spiralis,* presumably by a similar mechanism.

Eosinophils from patients with eosinophilia exhibit an enhanced ability to kill antibody-coated schistosomula in vitro; they act as if they were activated. Moreover, a number of soluble substances can enhance the killing capacity of eosinophils in vitro. These include eosinophil stimulator promoter (ESP), ECF-A, a soluble substance similar or identical to eosinophil colony stimulating factor, and a soluble mediator produced by blood mononuclear cells in culture.

PROTECTIVE ROLE FOR IgE The observation that IgE levels are elevated in some persons in the tropics, notably those infected with helminths, suggests that IgE may act to protect the host against parasites. The mediators released by triggered mast cells could affect the parasites directly or, by increasing vascular permeability and releasing eosinophil chemotactic factors, they could lead to the accumulation of necessary antibodies (IgG) and cells to attack the parasite. IgE-immune complexes can induce macrophage-mediated cytotoxicity to schistosomula. Rats made specifically IgE-deficient by the repeated injection of antiepsilon chain antibodies show markedly impaired resistance to *Trichinella* infection.

IMMUNOPATHOLOGY Immune mechanisms play a major role in the pathology induced by many parasites. Such mechanisms are the cause of: the granulomatous reaction to eggs of *S. mansoni* which is the basis of the immunopathology of this disease; immune complex renal disease in malaria and visceral leishmaniasis; heart disease due to *T. cruzi;* the obstructive and ocular disease in filariasis and onchocerciasis; the muscle pathology in trichinosis; the allergic reactions to ruptured hydatic cyst fluid; and the pulmonary complications to migrating nematode larvae. Just as suppressor mechanisms are involved in damping protective immunity, they are also involved in modulating the immunopathology. An example of this is the modulation of *S. mansoni* granulomas by T-suppressor cells.

MONOCLONAL AND ANTI-IDIOTYPIC ANTIBODIES Monoclonal antibodies to various stages of malaria parasites have been used to detect antigens that can induce protective immunity. In addition, passive protection has been demonstrated with monoclonal antibodies to the promastigote stage of *Leishmania mexicana* and to schistosomula of *Schistosoma mansoni.* Because of their specificity, monoclonal antibodies can also be used for diagnosis because they can be selected not to show the multiple cross-reactions with other parasites that are frequently found with serums from infected animals. For example, species-specific monoclonal antibodies have been developed which can distinguish between five different species of South American *Leishmania* without cross-reacting with *Trypanosoma cruzi.* Antibodies in the serum of an infected patient will usually cross-react with all these parasites. Diagnostic tests using these antibodies are being developed.

An antibody to an antigen has a specific antigen unique to itself on the immunoglobulin. This antigen is called the *idiotype,* which is the unique amino acid sequence and configuration of the antigen-binding site of that antibody. For instance, it is possible to make an antibody to a particular monoclonal antibody; that antibody will then recognize the idiotype and is called an *anti-idiotypic antibody.* The monoclonal antibody will bind to the anti-idiotype or to the original antigen. If a monoclonal antibody to a parasite were used to induce an anti-idiotypic antibody, it should be possible to induce protective immunity with this anti-idiotype instead of using the antigen. This would have the advantage of bypassing the need to purify antigens and then to produce them in large quantities. This novel strategy for the production of a vaccine is under study.

The rapidly accelerating pace of discovery and definition of the regulatory systems of the immune response, together with the revolution in technology, may soon make it possible to induce stronger protective immunity artificially than that which is acquired naturally, and the prediction that vaccines can be produced against the diseases caused by a number of parasites is based on this assumption.

REFERENCES

BLOOM BR: Games parasites play: How parasites evade immune surveillance. Nature 279:21, 1979

COHEN S, WARREN K (eds): *Immunology of Parasitic Infections,* 2d ed. London, Blackwell Scientific Publications 1982

CROSS GAM: Immunochemical aspects of antigenic variation in trypanosomes. The Third Fleming Lecture. J Gen Microbiol 113:1, 1979

HOMMELL M: Malaria: Immunity and prospects for vaccination. West J Med 135:285, 1981

MAHMOUD AF, AUSTEN KF (eds): *The Eosinophil in Health and Disease.* New York, Grune & Stratton, 1981

MOLLER G (ed): *Immunoparasitology.* Immunological Reviews 161. Copenhagen, Munksgaard, 1982, pp 5–269

217
AMEBIASIS

JAMES J. PLORDE

DEFINITION Amebiasis is an infection of the large intestine produced by *Entamoeba histolytica.* It is an asymptomatic carrier state in most individuals, but diseases ranging from chronic, mild diarrhea to fulminant dysentery may occur. Among extraintestinal complications, the commonest is hepatic abscess, which may rupture into peritoneum, pleura, lung, or pericardium.

ETIOLOGY There are seven species of ameba that naturally parasitize the human mouth and intestine, but of these only *E. histolytica* causes disease. *Entamoeba coli* and *E. hartmanni* are the two species with which it is most likely to be confused in examination of stools.

Entamoeba histolytica exists in two forms: the motile trophozoite and the cyst. The trophozoite is the parasitic form and dwells in the lumen and/or wall of the colon, divides by binary fission, grows best under anaerobic conditions, and requires the presence of either bacteria or tissue substrates to satisfy its nutritional requirements. When diarrhea occurs, the trophozoites are passed unchanged in the liquid stool, where they can be distinguished by their size (10 to 20 μm in diameter), directional motility, sharply demarcated clear ectoplasm with slender finger-like pseudopodia, and finely granular endoplasm. In dysentery, the trophozoites are larger (up to 50 μm in diameter), and often contain ingested erythrocytes. In the absence of diarrhea, the trophozoites usually encyst before leaving the gut. The cysts are highly resistant to environmental changes, chlorine concentrations found in water purification systems, and gastric acid. With rare exception they are responsible for transmission of disease. Young cysts have a single nucleus, a glycogen vacuole, and sausage-shaped chromatoid bodies. As the cyst matures, it absorbs its cytoplasmic vacuoles and becomes quadrinucleate. The cysts of *E. histolytica* can be distinguished from those of *Entamoeba coli* by the presence of one to four nuclei with small centric karyosomes and fine peripheral chromatin and by their thick chromatoid bodies with round ends.

Entamoeba histolytica had been classified into large and small races depending upon whether they form cysts measuring more or less than 10 μm in diameter. Strains of the small race, however, are not pathogenic for human beings and are now considered as a distinct species, *Entamoeba hartmanni.*

Entamoeba histolytica-like amebas are organisms isolated from humans that are morphologically indistinguishable from true *E. histolytica.* However, unlike *E. histolytica* they are nonpathogenic, grow best at 20°C, and can multiply indefinitely in hypotonic solutions.

Entamoeba histolytica can be cultivated in artificial media, a procedure that is essential for the preparation of the purified antigens used in serologic testing. Its diagnostic value remains uncertain.

EPIDEMIOLOGY Although *E. histolytica* can sometimes infect rats, cats, dogs, and primates, humans are the principal host and reservoir. Infection is worldwide. Stool surveys indicate that infection rates as high as 50 percent may occur in areas where the level of sanitation is low. Symptomatic amebiasis is unusual below the age of 10 years in temperate climates, and both intestinal and hepatic lesions predominate in adult males to an extent that is not readily explainable on the basis of different rates of exposure to infection. Reports of amebic liver abscess suggest that invasive amebiasis is concentrated in comparatively few parts of the world, most notably Mexico, western South America, south Asia, and west and southwestern Africa. In the United States, the prevalence of amebiasis is between 1 and 5 percent. Over the past three decades the incidence of invasive disease has decreased sharply, and an increasing proportion of such cases are now acquired outside this country. Patients with dysentery and liver abscess can still be found, however, in institutions for the mentally retarded, Indian reservations, and migrant labor camps.

Because trophozoites die rapidly after leaving the intestine, asymptomatic cyst passers are the source of new infections. The cysts are usually spread directly from person to person under conditions of poor personal hygiene. Oral-anal sexual contact produces high infection rates in male homosexuals. Food- and water-borne transmission may also occur, occasionally in epidemic form. Such outbreaks are never as explosive as those produced by pathogenic intestinal bacteria.

IMMUNITY There are both animal and human data suggesting the presence of protective immunity. However, repeated infections are common, and there is no correlation between the presence of circulating antibodies and immunity to infection. It is likely that immunity is incomplete, serves to limit rather than prevent disease, and is cell mediated.

PATHOGENESIS AND ANATOMIC CHANGES After ingestion, cysts undergo further nuclear division. In the small intestine, the cyst wall disintegrates, and trophozoites are released. The immature amebas are carried to the large intestine, where they live in the lumen of the gut as commensals feeding on bacteria and debris. On occasion the amebas may invade the mucosa, causing ulcerations that are sufficiently extensive to produce symptoms. The factors responsible for this are not completely understood, but the state of the host and the virulence of the infecting organism both play roles. High iron and carbohydrate intake, corticosteroids, and pregnancy all render the host more susceptible. Epidemiologic evidence suggests that amebic strains indigenous to temperate climates are usually avirulent. It has also been shown, however, that invasiveness is not a stable strain characteristic. It can either be lost after continued cultivation in vitro or enhanced by rapid animal passage. The virulence of various strains of *E. histolytica* is dependent upon the association with living bacteria and viruses. Virulent strains are characterized by the presence of the enzyme phosphoglucomutase and the capacity to produce histolysis following direct cell-to-cell contact. Although a cytotoxin-enterotoxin has been described in *E. histolytica,* its presence does not correlate with invasiveness.

Amebic ulceration of the intestinal wall is characteristic. A small mucosal defect overlies a larger, burrowing area of necrosis in the submucosa and muscularis, producing a bottle-shaped lesion. There is little acute inflammatory response, and in contrast to the picture in bacillary dysentery, the mucosa between ulcers is normal. The sites of involvement in order of frequency are cecum and ascending colon, rectum, sigmoid, appendix, and terminal ileum. In the cecum and sigmoid, chronic infection may lead to the formation of large masses of granulation tissue or *amebomas.* Amebas can enter the portal circulation and lodge in venules; liquefaction necrosis of liver tissue leads to the formation of an abscess cavity. Rarely, embolization results in lung, brain, or splenic abscess.

CLINICAL MANIFESTATIONS **Asymptomatic cyst passer** In the majority of patients with this common form of amebiasis, *E. histolytica* probably lives as a commensal in the bowel lumen. Individuals infected in temperate climates are unlikely to develop significant tissue invasion. However, invasion does occur occasionally, and treatment of cyst passers is warranted.

Symptomatic intestinal amebiasis In some patients there is intermittent diarrhea consisting of one to four foul-smelling loose or watery stools daily. The stools sometimes contain mucus and blood. Loose stools alternate with periods of relative normality and may persist for months or years. Flatulence and abnormal cramping are frequent. The only physical findings are occasional tender hepatomegaly and slight pain when the cecum and ascending colon are palpated. Sigmoidoscopy sometimes reveals typical ulcerations with areas of normal mucosa interspersed. The diagnosis depends upon finding the organism in the feces or in ulcers.

Fulminating attacks of amebic dysentery are less common. Waterborne outbreaks may occur, but fulminating dysentery is more likely to occur spontaneously in debilitated individuals. Attacks may be precipitated by pregnancy or corticosteroids. The onset in half the cases is abrupt with high fever, between 40 and 40.6°C (104 and 105°F), severe abdominal cramps, and profuse, bloody diarrhea with tenesmus. There is diffuse abdominal tenderness, often so severe that peritonitis is suspected. Hepatomegaly is very frequent, and sigmoidoscopy almost always demonstrates extensive rectosigmoid ulceration. Trophozoites are numerous in stools and in material obtained directly from the ulcers.

In some cases there may be extensive destruction of the colonic mucosa and submucosa, massive hemorrhage or perforation of the bowel wall, with resultant peritonitis. Repeated severe attacks of intestinal amebiasis can lead to an ulcerative postdysenteric colitis. Amebas can usually not be demonstrated in this condition, but serologic tests are strongly positive. Invasion of the appendix may lead to a clinical picture of *appendicitis.* Penetration of trophozoites through the muscle wall of the bowel may result in the development of large masses of granulation tissue. When the entire circumference of the intestine is involved, there may then be partial obstruction, and a movable, tender, sausage-shaped mass is often palpable. This lesion or ameboma is most frequently seen in the cecum where a palpable mass and radiologic demonstration of a ragged encroachment of the lumen may lead to a mistaken diagnosis of adenocarcinoma.

Hepatic amebiasis The parasites usually reach the liver through the portal vein; rarely, they may traverse the lymphatic vessels. It has been believed for a long time that amebas which lodged in the liver could produce a diffuse hepatitis. Careful postmortem and biopsy studies indicate that the syndrome of tender hepatomegaly, right upper quadrant pain, fever, and leukocytosis in patients with amebic colitis is not a result of amebas in hepatic tissues, is accompanied by nonspecific periportal inflammation, and is rarely, if ever, a prelude to hepatic abscess. It is evident, then, that these manifestations are best regarded as an accompaniment of colitis and do not merit a separate diagnosis of "diffuse amebic hepatitis."

Hepatic abscess may develop insidiously, with fever, sweats, weight loss, and no local signs other than painless or slightly tender hepatomegaly. In other patients, there is abrupt onset, with chills, fever to 40.6°C (105°F), nausea, vomiting, severe upper abdominal pain, and polymorphonuclear leukocytosis. Initially, cholecystitis, perforated ulcer, or acute pancreatitis may be suspected.

Most commonly, the abscess occurs singly and is localized in the posterior portion of the right lobe of the liver, because this lobe receives most of the blood draining the right colon through the "streaming" effect in portal vein flow. This location is responsible for several features that aid in diagnosis. *Point tenderness* in the posterolateral portion of a lower right intercostal space is frequent even in the absence of diffuse liver pain. Most abscesses enlarge upward, producing a bulge in the diaphragmatic dome, obliteration of the costophrenic gutter, small hydrothorax, basilar atelectasis, and pain referred to the right shoulder. Liver function tests may be mildly to moderately disturbed but are of little diagnostic aid. Jaundice is uncommon. Radiologically, unruptured abscesses do not show a fluid level, and calcification of the liver parenchyma is very rare. Isotope liver scan utilizing two, or preferably three, projections is invaluable in confirming both the presence and location of a liver abscess. Ultrasonic scanning and computerized tomography have proved equally effective. Serologic tests are positive in over 90 percent of patients.

Needle puncture results in the withdrawal of "pus" which consists of liquefied, necrotic liver. Typically, it is thick and odorless, resembling "chocolate syrup" or "anchovy paste." It may, however, be thin in consistency and yellow or green in color. The pus contains no polymorphonuclear leukocytes (barring secondary bacterial infection) and, usually, no amebas. The parasites are localized in the cyst wall and may be demonstrated in the terminal portion of the aspirate or, at times, by a Vim-Silverman needle biopsy of the cyst wall following aspiration of the abscess.

Hepatic abscess complicates asymptomatic infection of the colon more often than symptomatic intestinal disease, another factor making recognition difficult. Trophozoites or cysts are demonstrable in the feces of only about one-third of patients with abscess, and fewer than one-half can recall significant diarrheal illness.

Pleuropulmonary amebiasis The right pleural cavity and lung are involved by direct extension from the liver in 10 to 20 percent of patients with liver abscess. Rarely, amebic lung abscess has resulted from embolization rather than direct extension.

Manifestations are those of a consolidating pneumonia or lung abscess. If perforation into a bronchus occurs, patients expectorate large amounts of the typical exudate, some patients even commenting that the sputum "tastes like liver." Cough, pleural pain, fever, and leukocytosis are the rule, and secondary bacterial infection is frequent. Rupture into the free pleural space results in a massive pleural effusion; aspiration of "chocolate" fluid is diagnostic.

Other extraintestinal lesions Extension of an abscess from the left lobe of the liver to the pericardium is the most dangerous complication of hepatic abscess. It may be mistaken for tuberculous pericarditis or congestive cardiomyopathy. Less frequently, rapid cardiac tamponade occurs with ensuing dyspnea, shock, and death. *Peritonitis* is a result of perforation of colonic ulcer or rupture of liver abscess. Painful ulcers or condylomata of the genitalia, perianal skin, or abdominal wall (draining sinuses) are unusual complications which may be mistaken for syphilitic, tuberculous, or neoplastic lesions. They usually result from direct extension of intestinal disease; some are thought to result from sexual transmission. Metastatic brain abscess is rare, and an etiologic diagnosis is seldom made clinically. Splenic abscess has been reported but is very unusual.

DIFFERENTIAL DIAGNOSIS Intestinal amebiasis Patients with nondysenteric amebiasis are often misdiagnosed as having irritable bowel syndrome, diverticulitis, or regional enteritis. Ameboma may mimic colonic carcinoma or granulomatous disease, while the clinical spectrum of amebic dysentery overlaps those of shigellosis, salmonellosis, ulcerative colitis, and, in endemic areas, schistosomiasis. The invasive bacterial infections are usually more acute, severe, and self-limited than amebiasis. Stools from patients with shigellosis, salmonellosis, and ulcerative colitis contain large numbers of polymorphonuclear leukocytes, while those in amebic infection do not. Nevertheless, amebiasis may closely resemble any of the above diseases both clinically and radiologically and must be considered in the differential diagnosis of any chronic diarrhea or dysentery.

The identification of *E. histolytica* in the stool, however, does not eliminate other diagnostic possibilities. Amebic infection is often superimposed on or exacerbated by other colonic disease including cecal carcinoma. For this reason, patients with intestinal amebiasis and abdominal complaints still require stool culture, sigmoidoscopy, and a barium enema.

Hepatic abscess Once a filling defect has been demonstrated by isotope liver scanning, the differential diagnosis includes hepatic neoplasm, hydatid cyst, and pyogenic abscess. Neoplasms can usually be differentiated on the basis of their ultrasonic scanning characteristics, while the lack of constitutional manifestations and presence of an appropriate epidemiologic history is helpful in recognizing echinococcosis. The most difficult problem lies in the exclusion of a pyogenic abscess. An insidious onset in an adult male, a history of chronic diarrhea, significant pleuritic chest pain, and a single right lobe lesion favors the diagnosis of amebiasis. High fever, hyperbilirubinemia, multiple hepatic filling defects, and foul-smelling hepatic aspirate are more suggestive of pyogenic disease. Ultimately, the separation of the two diseases rests upon laboratory procedures.

LABORATORY DIAGNOSIS The diagnosis of intestinal amebiasis depends upon *identification of the organism in the stool or tissues.* Formed stools are examined initially in saline and iodine mounts for amebic cysts; concentration methods such as the formalin-ether technique increase the yield two- to threefold. Liquid or semiformed stools should be examined immediately in saline solution for the presence of motile hematophagous trophozoites. The addition of a supravital stain such as buffered methylene blue to the saline enhances nuclear detail and minimizes the possibility of confusing fecal leukocytes with amebic trophozoites, an error common to inexperienced parasitologists. If there is any delay in examination of the stool, a portion of the specimen may be refrigerated for a few hours at 4°C, or placed in polyvinyl alcohol and 10% formalin. Definitive identification of *E. histolytica* requires the examination of permanently stained slides prepared from the material preserved with polyvinyl alcohol. An ocular micrometer is necessary to separate *E. hartmanni* from its larger relative. Four to six stool specimens may be required for diagnosis. If possible, the stool should be examined before the administration of antimicrobial, antidiarrheal, or antacid preparations, because all these agents may interfere with the recovery of amebas. Likewise, enemas and radiographic procedures utilizing barium sulfate are best postponed until after a thorough search for *E. histolytica* has been made.

Sigmoidoscopy is of value in symptomatic cases. The mucosal lesions should be aspirated and the material examined for trophozoites as described above. Biopsy material obtained from such lesions and stained with periodic acid Schiff solution also will frequently reveal trophozoites.

The diagnosis of extraintestinal amebiasis is difficult. The parasite usually cannot be recovered from stool or tissue. Cultivation of amebas from feces or pus is possible but is not practical in most laboratories. The most important diagnostic procedure in suspected liver abscess is a *therapeutic trial of antiamebic drugs.* The response is often dramatic within 3 days. In the event that demonstrating parasites is difficult, the therapeutic trial should be instituted without hesitation.

Serologic tests employing purified antigens are positive in nearly all patients with proved amebic liver abscess and in a great majority of those with acute amebic dysentery. They are generally negative in asymptomatic cyst passers, suggesting that tissue invasion is required for antibody production. The persistence of significant antibody titers for months to years after complete cure makes serology, particularly in endemic areas, of more value in excluding the diagnosis than in confirming it. Some authors recommend the routine screening of all patients thought to have inflammatory bowel disease for serologic evidence of amebiasis. Steroid therapy could then be withheld in patients with positive tests pending the outcome of parasitological examination. Of the available tests, the indirect hemagglutination and enzyme-linked immunosorbent assays appear to be the most sensitive. Indirect immunofluorescence, countercurrent electrophoresis, and agar gel diffusion are also highly reliable. A number of rapid tests such as latex agglutination and cellulose acetate diffusion have made serologic testing available to most laboratories.

TREATMENT Treatment should be aimed at relief of symptoms, replacement of fluid, electrolyte, and blood losses, and eradication of the organism. Amebas may be found in the lumen of the bowel, in the intestinal wall, or extraintestinally. Most amebicides are not effective at all sites or when used alone, and a combination of drugs is often necessary to achieve cure. The available drugs based on their site of action fall into several different categories, as described below.

Luminal amebicides These oral agents act by direct contact with trophozoites dwelling in the bowel lumen but are ineffective against amebas in tissue. Of the large number of available drugs, diloxanide furoate (Furamide) is one of the most effective and well tolerated but is presently available in the United States only through the Centers for Disease Control. A response rate of 80 to 85 percent has been noted; flatulence appears to be the only major side effect.

Diiodohydroxyquin has been effective in 60 to 70 percent of cases. As with its analogue iodochlorhydroxyquin (Entero-Vioform), myelooptic neuropathy has been reported after long-term use. However, no such case has been noted when the dosage was limited to that given in Table 217-1. The drug should not be used in patients with thyroid disease or preexisting optic neuropathy.

Tissue amebicides *Chloroquine diphosphate* (Aralen) is a systemic amebicide which is useful in hepatic disease because of

TABLE 217-1
Drug therapy of amebiasis

Clinical form and drug	*Dosage*
ASYMPTOMATIC INTESTINAL CARRIER	
Diiodohydroxyquin*	650 mg tid for 20 days
or diloxanide furoate †	500 mg tid for 10 days
MILD TO MODERATE INTESTINAL DISEASE	
Metronidazole	750 mg tid for 5–10 days
plus diiodohydroxyquin	As above
or diloxanide furoate	As above
or tetracycline	500 mg qid for 5 days
SEVERE INTESTINAL DISEASE	
Above regimen	
plus dehydroemetine †	1.0–1.5 mg/kg IM per day (maximum 90 mg per day) for up to 5 days
or emetine	1 mg/kg IM per day (maximum 60 mg per day) for up to 5 days
EXTRAINTESTINAL DISEASE	
Metronidazole	As above
or chloroquine phosphate	1 g per day for 2 days, then 500 mg per day for 4 weeks
plus dehydroemetine †	As above for 10 days
or emetine	As above for 10 days

* *Glenwood Laboratories, Inc., 83 North Summit St., Tenafly, NJ 07670.*
† *Investigational drug available through the Parasitic Drug Service, Centers for Disease Control, Atlanta, Ga., (404) 633-3311, nights and weekends 633-2176.*

its high concentration in the liver. It has little activity elsewhere.

Emetine is an alkaloid derivative of ipecac. When given intramuscularly, it is highly effective in destroying trophozoites in tissue including those in the wall of the intestine. It is ineffective against luminal amebas. Emetine is relatively toxic and may produce vomiting, diarrhea, abdominal cramping, weakness, muscle pain, tachycardia, hypotension, precordial pain, and electrocardiographic abnormalities. The common ECG changes include T-wave inversion and prolongation of the QTc interval. Rarely arrhythmias and prolongation of the QRS complex are seen. A synthetic derivative, dehydroemetine, is thought to be less toxic by virtue of its more rapid excretion and lower concentration in myocardial tissue. It is not free of toxicity, however, and patients treated with either drug should be at bed rest with ECG monitoring. Neither drug should be used in patients with renal, cardiac, or muscle disease, during pregnancy, or in children, unless other drugs fail.

Metronidazole (Flagyl) is unique because it is effective against trophozoites at all sites, intestinally and extraintestinally. It is the drug of choice in most forms of amebiasis. For intestinal amebiasis it is given in dosage of 750 mg three times daily for 5 to 10 days. Smaller doses are effective in hepatic amebiasis. Metronidazole has an Antabuse-like action, and alcohol should be avoided during its administration. The evidence that this drug is carcinogenic and possibly teratogenic in animals when given in large doses is disturbing. The potential risk in human beings must be weighed against the severity of the disease, particularly in pregnant women.

Specific antiprotozoal therapy is outlined in Table 217-1.

In extraintestinal amebiasis including hepatic abscess, metronidazole is the drug of choice. In cases of relapse or in situations where the patient is unable to take oral medication, therapy with dehydroemetine or emetine should be instituted, and oral chloroquine added as soon as possible. Diagnostic trials should employ the chloroquine-emetine regimen because pyogenic liver abscesses may temporarily respond to metronidazole. Most authors prefer to add luminal amebicides to both the metronidazole and chloroquine-emetine programs. Treatment failures have been reported for both emetine-chloroquine and metronidazole. They appear to be unrelated to the organism's resistance.

There is debate over the value of routine aspiration of amebic liver abscesses. Certainly, if there is localized swelling over the liver, marked elevation of the diaphragm, severe localized liver tenderness, and failure to respond to systemic amebicides, it should be done. Adequate drainage can usually be accomplished by needle alone, and surgical drainage is rarely necessary. The greatest hazard in needling an abscess is secondary bacterial infection.

PROGNOSIS Intestinal amebiasis usually responds readily and completely to appropriate drugs. Parasitologic relapses sometimes occur, and posttreatment stools should be checked monthly for 6 months. Repeated relapses, however, are usually a manifestation of reinfection, complicating illness, inadequate therapy, or incorrect diagnosis. The fatality rate is less than 5 percent.

Hepatic and pulmonary amebiasis are still accompanied by an appreciable mortality, but no reliable figures are available.

PREVENTION For the individual, avoidance of contaminated food and water, scalding of vegetables, and the use of iodine-releasing tablets in drinking water (chlorine, in the form of halazone, is ineffective) are important measures. Globaline tablets, containing tetraglycine hydroperiodide, are convenient and effective.

Improvements in general sanitation and the detection of cyst passers and their removal from food-handling duties are general measures in prophylaxis, but such segregation of carriers is rarely practiced. Community control of amebic disease by periodic mass treatment with metronidazole and diloxanide furoate has been successful in some areas. At the present time, however, personal chemoprophylaxis for travelers is not recommended.

PRIMARY AMEBIC MENINGOENCEPHALITIS

Primary amebic meningoencephalitis is caused by free-living amebas of the genus *Naegleria* or *Acanthamoeba.* The former most often affects children and young adults, appears to be acquired by swimming in fresh, warm water, and is almost invariably fatal. *Acanthamoeba* infections involve older immunocompromised individuals, and spontaneous recovery is sometimes seen.

Free-living amebas are ubiquitous in nature where they are commonly found in soil and water. Although generally considered harmless, some varieties are clearly pathogenic for the central nervous system of mammals. In those instances of human meningoencephalitis where the responsible organism has been isolated and cultured, it has, with few exceptions, been identified as an amoeboflagellate, *Naegleria fowleri.*

Over 100 *Naegleria* cases have been reported from different parts of the world including Australia, Czechoslovakia, Great Britain, New Zealand, and the United States. Serologic studies suggest that inapparent infections are much more common. Most of the 35 cases recognized in the United States have occurred in the southeastern states, particularly Florida, Georgia, and Virginia. Characteristically the patients have fallen ill during the summer months approximately 1 week after swimming in fresh or brackish water. The 16 Czechoslovakian cases followed swimming in an indoor pool with chlorinated water maintained at 24°C, and 6 cases have been acquired apparently after bathing in hot mineral water. In sub-Saharan Africa, cases appear to follow inhalation of airborne cysts during the dry, windy harmattan season. Histological evidence suggests that the amebas reach the central nervous system directly via the nasal mucosa at the level of the cribriform plate. Clinically, the illness is rapid in onset, brief in duration, and inexorable in course. The initial symptom is a severe, persistent, frontal headache followed by nausea, vomiting, fever, and nuchal rigidity. Unusual tastes or smells may be noted. Later, drowsiness, confusion, convulsions, and coma appear. Focal neurological findings may occur late in the course of the illness.

A more benign, chronic form of meningoencephalitis is produced by organisms of the genus *Acanthamoeba.* They appear to be disseminated to the brain and other organs from the skin or respiratory tract. Patients with this clinical syndrome are frequently older, are immunocompromised, lack a history of freshwater swimming, and may recover spontaneously. Pathologically, the disease can be distinguished from *Naegleria* infections by the granulomatous nature of the inflammatory reaction and the presence of both trophozoites and cysts in the tissues. Unfortunately, the identification of the responsible organisms remains in some doubt as they have never been recovered by culture techniques. It is possible that the free-living ameba of several species are involved.

A careful examination of the cerebrospinal fluid is the single most helpful diagnostic procedure. In *Naegleria* infections the fluid is usually bloody or sanguinopurulent and demonstrates an intense neutrophilic response. The protein is elevated and the glucose diminished. No organisms are demonstrated on Gram's stain or routine culture. Early examination of a wet preparation of unspun spinal fluid will usually reveal viable trophozoites. They are 10 to 20 μm in diameter, possess a granular cytoplasm, a distinct ectoplasm, and bulbous pseudopodia. If the specimen is allowed to cool, the trophozoites may become immobile and more difficult to recognize. The diagnosis is confirmed with direct fluorescent antibody (DFA) stains. Although the amebas may be easily grown on ordinary culture media which have been seeded with coliform bacteria, this is not helpful in clinical management, so rapidly progressive is the disease. In contrast, the spinal fluid in *Acanthamoeba* infections usually demonstrates a mononuclear response. Trophozoites have been neither cultured nor seen on wet mounts. A positive DFA stain has been seen in a few cases. Treatment with standard antiprotozoal agents seems completely ineffective. *Naegleria,* however, is highly sensitive to amphotericin B, miconazole, tetracycline, and rifampin. To date only four patients have survived a *Naegleria* infection. All were diagnosed early and treated, three with amphotericin B and the other with amphotericin B, miconazole, and rifampin. Intracisternal, as well as intravenous, administration of amphotericin is probably essential to rapidly obtain effective levels in the cerebrospinal fluid. The intraventricular dose is 0.5 to 1 mg for the first few days. The intravenous dose is similar to that for cryptococcal meningitis (see Chap. 183). *Acanthamoeba* are sensitive to sulfanilamides, clotrimazole, 5-FC, and polymyxin B, but no clinical studies have been done.

If the source of the infection can be determined, further *Naegleria* cases might be prevented by closing the area to bathing.

REFERENCES

Amebiasis

ADAMS EB, MACLEOD IN: Invasive amebiasis. Medicine 56:315, 1977

BARBOUR GL, JUNIPER K JR: A clinical comparison of amebic and pyogenic abscess of the liver in sixty-six patients. Am J Med 53:323, 1972

COHEN HG, REYNOLDS TB: Comparison of metronidazole and chloroquine for the treatment of amebic liver abscess. Gastroenterology 69:35, 1975

DOBILER D, MIRELMAN D: Adhesion of *Entamoeba histolytica* trophozoites to monolayers of human cells. J Infect Dis 144:539, 1981

JUNIPER K JR: Amebiasis. Clin Gastroenterol 7:3, 1978

KROGSTAD DJ et al: Amebiasis: Epidemiologic studies in the United States, 1971–1974. Ann Intern Med 88:89, 1978

——— et al: Current concepts in parasitology—Amebiasis. N Engl J Med 298:262, 1978

LUSHBAUGH WB et al: Isolation of a cytotoxin-enterotoxin from *Entamoeba hystolytica.* J Infect Dis 139:9, 1979

SARGEAUNT PG et al: The differentiation of invasive and noninvasive *Entamoeba hystolytica* by isoenzyme electrophoresis. Trans R Soc Trop Med Hyg 72:519, 1978

SCHMERIN MJ et al: Amebiasis—An increasing problem among homosexuals in New York City. JAMA 238:1386, 1977

SUKOV RJ et al: Sonography of hepatic amebic abscess. Am J Radiol 134:911, 1980

Primary amebic meningoencephalitis

CARTER RF: Primary amoebic meningoencephalitis: An appraisal of present knowledge. Trans R Soc Trop Med Hyg 67:193, 1972

DUMA RJ: Meningoencephalitis and brain abscess due to a free-living amoeba. Ann Intern Med 88:468, 1978

HOFFMAN ED et al: A case of primary meningoencephalitis. Am J Trop Med Hyg 27:29, 1978

LAWANDE RV et al: Primary amoebic meningoencephalitis in Nigeria. J Trop Med Hyg 82:84, 1979

SEIDEL JS et al: Successful treatment of primary amebic meningoencephalitis. N Engl J Med 306:346, 1982

218 MALARIA

JAMES J. PLORDE

DEFINITION Malaria is a protozoan disease transmitted to humans by the bite of *Anopheles* mosquitoes. It is characterized by *rigors, fever, splenomegaly, anemia,* and a *chronic relapsing course.* Despite the impressive results of the World Health Organization–sponsored malaria eradication program begun in 1956, technical and socioeconomic difficulties have led to a resurgence of the disease in many areas of the world. Consequently, malaria remains today, as it has been for centuries, one of the most serious infectious disease problems in the world. In the United States and Europe, several thousand imported cases are seen annually in travelers from endemic areas.

ETIOLOGY *The causative organisms are protozoa of the genus Plasmodium.* The four species known to infect human beings are *P. vivax, P. ovale, P. malariae,* and *P. falciparum.* Human infection begins when a female anopheline inoculates plasmodial *sporozoites* into the lymphohematogenous system while feeding. After a brief passage in the peripheral blood, these organisms invade hepatocytes where they initiate the preclinical hepatic (exoerythrocytic) phase of disease. By a process of asexual multiplication referred to as *schizogony,* a single sporozoite eventually produces 2000 to 40,000 hepatic *merozoites.* In 1 to 6 weeks, these daughter cells rupture back into the circulatory system. In *P. falciparum,* and presumably *P. malariae,* infections, the hepatic phase terminates at this point. In the other species, liver forms persist and produce new episodes of bloodstream invasion months to years later.

The erythrocytic or clinical phase of malaria starts with the attachment of a released merozoite to a specific receptor site on the red blood cell surface. This site appears to differ for each species of malaria; in the case of *P. vivax,* it is related to the Duffy blood group antigens (Fy^a or Fy^b). Duffy-negative (FyFy) individuals, who include the majority of people of West African extraction, are resistant to vivax malaria, presumably for this reason. Following attachment, the merozoite invaginates the cell surface and is slowly interiorized. The intracellular parasite first appears as a ring-shaped trophozoite which later enlarges and assumes an irregular or ameboid shape. Its nucleus then divides into several portions to form a multinucleated *schizont.* Eventually, cytoplasm condenses around each daughter nucleus to form a new generation of merozoites. Forty-eight hours after its original invasion (72 h in the case of *P. malariae*) the erythrocyte ruptures, releasing 6 to 24 organisms, each of which is capable of initiating a new red blood cell cycle. With repetition of this cycle, some of the red blood cells become filled with *sexual forms* (gametocytes); these do not induce cell lysis and are unable to undergo further development unless ingested by an appropriate mosquito during a blood meal. In the stomach of the mosquito fertilization occurs, and the resulting *ookinete* encysts on the outer surface of the stomach and releases myriads of *sporozoites.* These migrate to the salivary glands and are inoculated into a human subject at the next feeding.

EPIDEMIOLOGY Malaria survives only in areas of the world where both the anopheline and infected human population remain above certain *critical densities* required for the sustained transmission of disease. Control measures are directed toward reducing both populations to levels that are too low for the infection to survive. Important procedures include drainage or filling of breeding areas, use of residual insecticide sprays, screening, use of skin repellents, effective treatment of cases, and large-scale suppressive drug programs in some human populations.

An active international cooperative program aimed at the eradication of malaria resulted in a significant decline in the incidence of the disease between 1956 and 1968. In over three-quarters of the original malarial areas of the world, the disease was eradicated, or active eradication programs were instituted. Presently, however, malaria still infects between 125 and 200 million inhabitants of 104 countries throughout Africa, Latin America, South America, Asia, and Oceania (Fig. 218-1). Tropical Africa alone harbors 100 million of these afflicted individuals and contributes most of the 1 million deaths that occur annually from this terrible disease. The presence of mobile populations, outdoor-biting mosquitoes, and high levels of disease transmission make successful eradication in these remaining areas unlikely. Furthermore, the emergence of insecticide-resistant mosquitoes as well as a variety of administrative and socioeconomic problems has produced serious setbacks to several previously successful eradication programs, particularly those on the Indian subcontinent. Added to these difficulties has been the continuing spread of drug-resistant *P. falciparum* throughout southern Asia, the western Pacific, Central America, and South America. A limited number of resistant strains have been discovered in Africa, an area previously free of this problem.

Endemic malaria did not disappear from the United States until the 1950s. Imported cases and occasional outbreaks of malaria acquired by mosquito transmission from imported infections (*introduced malaria*) have continued to occur, but until 1966 the total never exceeded 200 cases a year. This number rapidly increased with the return of infected military personnel from southeast Asia, reaching a peak of over 4000 in 1970. Associated with this wave of imported malaria was a smaller increase in the number of infections induced by blood transfusion and intravenous heroin use. Although this epidemic has waned, the incidence of malaria in the civilian population has not (Fig. 218-2). From 1970 to 1979, the number of cases reported annually among tourists, businesspeople, teachers, students, and other civilians rose from 151 to 825; it is estimated that more than 2000 cases occurred in 1980. With rare exceptions, malaria was acquired abroad: approximately 50 percent in Asia, 30 percent in Africa, and 10 percent in the Caribbean or Latin America. Only one-fifth of the recent infections have involved U.S. citizens; most of the remainder have occurred in émigrés from southeast Asia. Surveillance studies suggest that 2 to 5 percent of the latter population are infected at the time of entry to this country. Clinical manifestations usually develop within 6 months of arrival in the United States, but in one-third of the vivax cases they are delayed beyond that point. In 1979, one-fifth of the cases and both of the deaths were caused by the virulent *P. falciparum.* Tragically, most of these cases could have been prevented with appropriate chemoprophylaxis. Until travelers are more fully informed of dangers inherent in traveling unprotected to malarious areas, the number of cases seen in this country each year will continue to increase.

PATHOGENESIS AND PATHOLOGY The invasion, alteration, and destruction of red blood cells by malaria parasites, systemic and local circulatory changes, and immune phenomena are all important in the pathophysiology of malaria.

Red blood cell changes Malaria species differ significantly in their ability to invade red blood cells. *Plasmodium vivax* and *P. ovale* attack only immature erythrocytes; *P. malariae,* only senescent ones. During infection with these species, therefore, no more than 1 or 2 percent of cells are involved at any one time. *Plasmodium falciparum,* although preferring younger erythrocytes, invades red blood cells of all ages and may cause extremely high levels of parasitemia. Only the presence of certain abnormal hemoglobins, notably S, is capable of limiting the intracellular growth and intense parasitemia produced by the

FIGURE 218-1
From Malaria Surveillance: Annual Summary, 1979. Atlanta, Ga., Centers for Disease Control, November 1980.

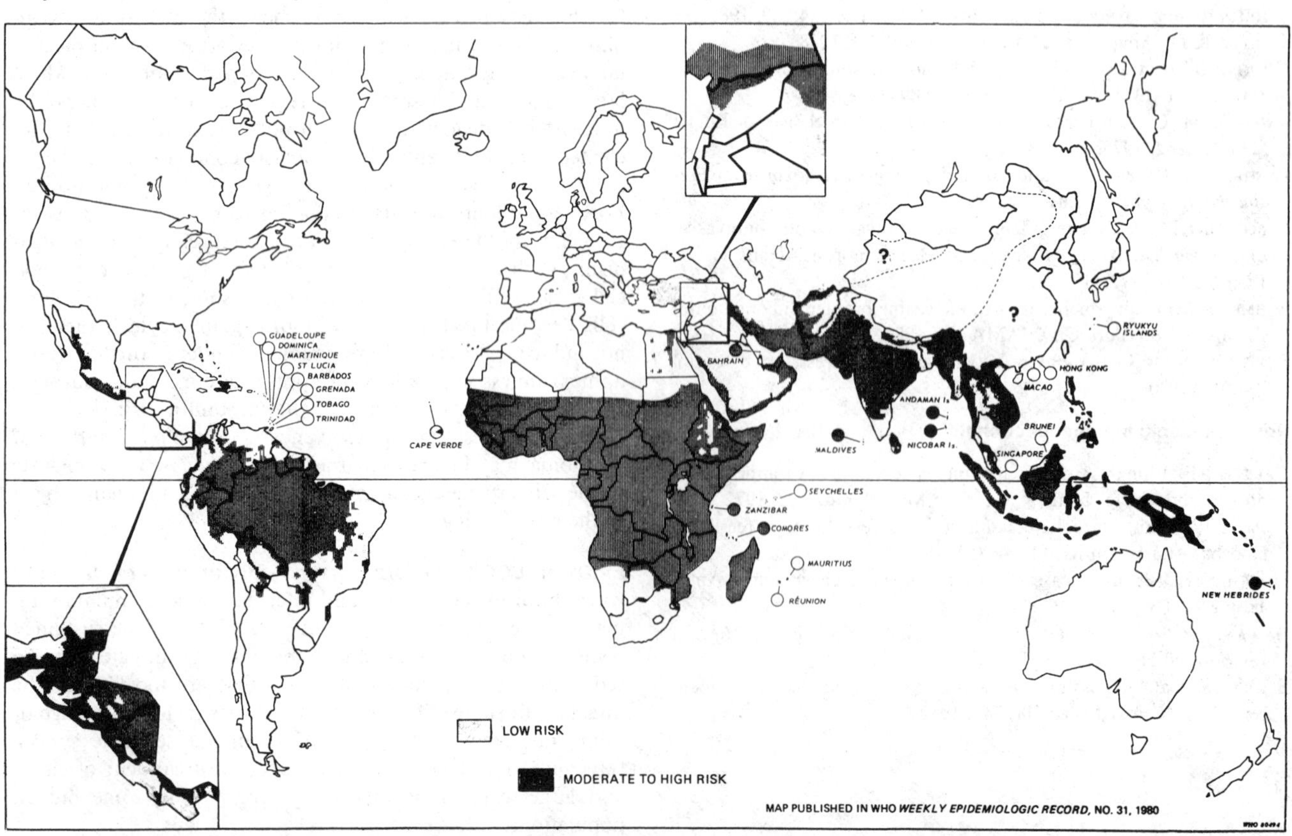

species. The tactoids formed during sickling of *AS* cells may directly damage the parasite and render the deformed erythrocyte more susceptible to phagocytosis. A similar protective effect may be exerted in thalassemia, and glucose 6-phosphate (G6PD) or pyridoxal-kinase deficiency, since these abnormalities are found more commonly in malarious areas. In thalassemia and related hemoglobinopathies, the protection may be related in part to the persistent production of fetal hemoglobin since maturation of *P. falciparum* is retarded in cells containing hemoglobin F and, in part, to the increased susceptibility of such erythrocytes to oxidant damage.

Once parasitized, the cells may be destroyed at the time of sporulation or in the presence of specific opsonizing antibody phagocytosed in the liver or spleen. In the spleen the parasites are also removed from some cells, and the intact erythrocytes are returned into the circulation. However, anemia usually develops and, in the case of falciparum malaria, may be severe. This species also induces physical changes in parasitized cells resulting in intravascular agglutination and sludging.

Although paroxysms of fever coincide with sporulation and the destruction of red blood cells, the cause of the fever remains obscure and may be related to release of an endogenous pyrogen from injured cells.

Circulatory changes The circulatory changes in malaria are characterized by vasoconstriction during the "cold" stage followed by vasodilation during the "hot" stage. In falciparum malaria vasodilation in the skin is accompanied by hypotension, decreased central venous pressure, increased radioiodinated serum albumin space, and increased excretion of aldosterone, suggesting a decrease in effective circulating blood volume due to enhanced vascular permeability and/or capacitance. On the other hand, there may be localized vasospasm, kinin-induced capillary permeability with a resulting increase in blood viscosity, obstruction of capillaries with agglutinated red blood cells, and, occasionally, intravascular coagulation which may compromise perfusion to vital organs such as the kidney, brain, liver, and lung.

Immune phenomena Normal as well as parasitized red blood cells are destroyed in malaria. The explanation for this phenomenon is unknown, although immunologic mechanisms including autoantibody production and adherence of complement-containing immune complexes to uninfected red blood cells have been suggested. The destruction is most profound in blackwater fever where there is massive intravascular hemolysis. More commonly, however, the red blood cells are sequestered and destroyed in the reticuloendothelial system of the liver and spleen. Thrombocytopenia is related to splenic pooling and shortened platelet life span. Both direct parasitic invasion and immune mechanisms may be operative in platelet destruction. Host γ- and β-1C-globulin deposits have been noted along the glomerular capillary basement membrane of patients with the acute transient glomerulonephritis of falciparum malaria and the progressive nephrosis of chronic quartan malaria, establishing these as immune complex nephropathies.

IMMUNITY Recovery from malaria occurs slowly, apparently the function of acquired immunity. In simian malaria, this appears to require the presence of both T and B cell lymphocytes. Although the role of the T cell is known to be vital, its mechanism of action is uncertain. Some authors have suggested that it stimulates effector cells, perhaps macrophages, to release a nonspecific factor capable of inhibiting intraerythrocytic multiplication; others feel it may have a helper effect on antibody formation.

Strain-specific antiplasmodial antibodies do occur early in the course of parasitemia and reach high levels coincident with a fall in the number of circulating organisms. The relative rarity of malaria in young infants has been attributed to transplacental passage of IgG antibodies. It is uncertain whether these are directly lethal, act as opsonizing agents, or block merozoitic invasion of erythrocytes. In simian malaria, antigenic change in the parasite results in cycles of recrudescent parasitemia and production of variant-specific antibodies. It seems probable that similar changes occur in humans, leading to the eventual disappearance of erythrocytic forms. In falciparum malaria, this results in cure. In vivax and ovale infections, the intracellular hepatic forms escape the humoral immune defenses and may later discharge fresh merozoites into the bloodstream to maintain the infection for a period of 3 to 5 years. *Plasmodium malariae* produces chronic disease of extremely long duration, up to 53 years in one case, despite the lack of a persistent exoerythrocytic focus. This effect is presumably due to long-term survival of circulating parasites in concentrations too low to be detected on routine blood films. How these parasites escape immunologic destruction is unknown. In a closely related simian malaria, however, splenectomy rapidly leads to termination of infection, suggesting that suppressor T cells in the spleen may play a protective role.

MANIFESTATIONS General The incubation period between the bite of the mosquito and onset of symptoms is usually 10 to 14 days in vivax and falciparum malaria and 18 days to 6 weeks in malariae infections. This period may be prolonged in persons who have taken antimalarial suppressants. In the United States, the interval between entry into the country and onset of disease exceeds 6 months in one-quarter of the patients developing vivax infections; it exceeds 1 month in a

FIGURE 218-2
Military and civilian cases of malaria, United States, 1970–1979. (From Malaria Surveillance: Annual Summary, 1979. Atlanta, Ga., Centers for Disease Control, 1980.)

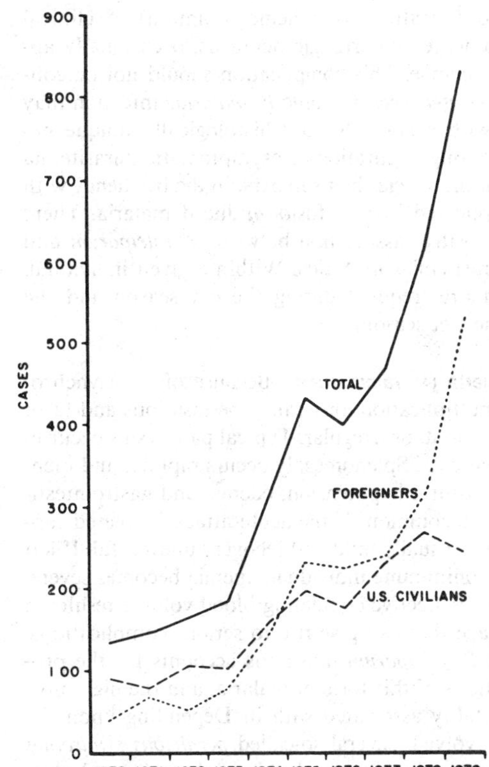

similar proportion of falciparum cases. There is some variation in clinical manifestations produced by the different plasmodia, but in all, chills, fever, headache, muscle pains, splenomegaly, and anemia are common. Herpes labialis is frequent and usually appears after the infection is well established. Hepatomegaly, mild icterus, and edema are often observed, especially in falciparum infections. Urticaria is common in patients with chronic malaria.

The hallmark of the disease is the malarial *paroxysm,* which recurs regularly in all but falciparum infections. The typical paroxysm begins with a rigor that lasts 20 to 60 min—the "cold stage"—followed by a "hot stage" of 3 to 8 h with temperature of 40 to 41.7°C (104 to 107°F). The "wet stage" consists of defervescence with profuse diaphoresis and leaves the patient exhausted.

First attacks are often severe, but repeated episodes become milder, although debilitation may be progressive. In untreated cases, the attacks may persist for weeks. The paroxysms eventually become more irregular and less frequent and finally cease, corresponding with the disappearance of parasites from the blood and marking the end of the primary attack. Relapses occur when exoerythrocytic parasites persisting in the liver reinvade the bloodstream.

Tertian malaria (*P. vivax* or *P. ovale*) This infection is rarely fatal, although relapses are common, and it is the most difficult to cure. A prodrome of myalgia, headache, chilliness, and low-grade fever for 48 to 72 h heralds the onset of the acute illness. Initially, the fever may be irregular because the maturation cycle of the parasite is not synchronized. Synchronization usually occurs toward the end of the first week, and typical paroxysms then occur on alternate days. The spleen becomes palpable at the end of the second week. Infections with *P. ovale* tend to be milder, and primary attacks shorter than those caused by *P. vivax.*

Quartan malaria (*P. malariae*) Paroxysms occur every third day and tend to be regular. The disease is usually more disabling than tertian but responds well to treatment. Edema, albuminuria, and hematuria (*not* hemoglobinuria), a clinical state similar to acute hemorrhagic nephritis, occasionally appear during the course. This complication should not be confused with *blackwater fever.* Chronic *P. malariae* infection may be associated with a clinically and histologically unique nephrosis. The prolonged duration of asymptomatic parasitemia characteristic of the species helps to explain the frequency with which it is implicated in transfusion-induced malaria. There appears to be positive association between *P. falciparum* and *P. malariae* parasitemias in Africa. Within a given individual, the former is more frequent during the dry season and the latter during the wet season.

Falciparum malaria (*P. falciparum*) Because of an asynchronous cycle of multiplication, onset may be insidious and fever continuous, remittent, or irregular. Typical paroxysms occur in a minority of patients. Splenomegaly occurs rapidly, and mental confusion, postural hypotension, edema, and gastrointestinal symptoms are common. If the acute attack is treated rapidly, the disease is usually mild and recovery uneventful. If left untreated in a nonimmune individual, anemia becomes severe, and the decreased effective circulating blood volume results in capillary blockage that can give rise to serious complications. This feature of *P. falciparum* infections accounts for the protean manifestations of this form of malaria, and the high morbidity and mortality associated with it. Depending upon the organ system involved, several so-called *pernicious syndromes* are seen. *Cerebral malaria* can lead to hemiplegia, convulsions, delirium, hyperpyrexia, coma, and rapid death. When the *pulmonary* circulation is involved, there may be cough and blood-streaked sputum, leading to confusion with many other diseases of the lung. Severe pulmonary insufficiency closely resembling the "shock lung" syndrome frequently accompanies cerebral malaria. The splanchnic capillaries can be obstructed, with consequent vomiting, abdominal pain, diarrhea, or melena. Such patients are sometimes thought to have bacillary dysentery or cholera. Fever in these disorders may be low or absent. Indeed, in patients with predominantly gastrointestinal manifestations, there are usually cold, clammy skin, hypotension, profound weakness, and repeated syncopal attacks, so-called *algid malaria.* Tender hepatomegaly, with or without jaundice, and acute renal failure are common. The pernicious syndromes should be anticipated if the intensity of parasitemia exceeds 100,000 organisms per cubic millimeter.

Blackwater fever This is a disorder that occurs in association with malaria, particularly and perhaps only with *P. falciparum* infections. The usual attack begins with a rigor and fever followed by massive intravascular hemolysis, icterus, hemoglobinuria, collapse, and often acute renal failure and uremia. The pathological findings in the kidney are necrosis of tubules and occasionally hemoglobin casts. The mortality is 20 to 30 percent, and survivors are very likely to experience hemolytic episodes with subsequent malarial infections.

Although blackwater fever is often classified as one of the "pernicious" complications of falciparum malaria, its cause is obscure. In many patients, parasitemia is absent at the time hemolysis occurs. Because blackwater fever has usually occurred in patients with chronic falciparum infections who were treated with quinine, it was suggested that the hemolysis results from an autoimmune reaction to the red blood cells that have been altered by the drug, parasite, or both. However, blackwater fever can occur in patients not given drugs. The institution of an appropriate regimen for acute renal failure will reduce the fatality rate considerably.

Complications In addition to the several complications already mentioned, others deserve comment. Rupture of the spleen is relatively rare, but malaria is by far the commonest cause of spontaneous rupture and predisposes to traumatic rupture of this organ. It is most commonly seen in vivax infections.

Chronic malaria or repeated infection in an endemic area leads to anemia, debility, cachexia, and suppression of humoral antibody response to a variety of antigens. These manifestations are particularly severe in children under the age of 3 and in pregnant women. Infection in the latter population is associated with low birth weight of the resulting child and high neonatal mortality. Congenital malaria, although rare, does occur; it is probably most common in the offspring of nonimmune individuals. Secondary bacterial infection is frequent and is often the immediate cause of death. Bacillary dysentery, cholera, and pyogenic pneumonia are common. Tuberculous foci often extend in malarial patients, and miliary tuberculosis is occasionally observed.

Patients living in endemic malarious areas commonly present with chronic hepatosplenomegaly of unknown cause. In some of these, there is infiltration of hepatic sinusoids by lymphocytes, very high levels of serum IgM, and high malaria antibody titers. This condition, which is known as the *tropical splenomegaly syndrome,* is seldom seen before the age of 8. It differs from the ordinary hepatosplenomegaly of malaria in that parasitemia is rare. It has been suggested that the condition results from defective T-cell control of immunoglobulin production, leading to excessive macroglobulin production and immune complex formation. Long-term antimalarial therapy leads to a decrease in spleen size and a disappearance of hepatic sinusoidal lymphocytosis. The epidemiologic evidence implicating malaria as a contributory factor in the etiology of Burkitt's lymphoma has increased. It has been suggested that continuous stimulation of the lymphoid system in chronic malaria makes it more susceptible to neoplastic transformation in the presence of EB virus.

LABORATORY FINDINGS The blood leukocyte count is low or normal. The platelet count is often reduced, especially in falciparum malaria. The erythrocyte sedimentation rate is elevated. Plasmodia are demonstrable in smears of peripheral blood from the vast majority of patients with symptomatic malaria. When the disease is suspected, appropriately stained blood films should be examined diligently. For the inexperienced examiner, a thin smear of fingertip blood on a clean glass slide should be stained with Wright's or Giemsa's stain. Parasitized erythrocytes are most frequent at the edges of a smear; extracellular parasites are not found. Thick smears should be thoroughly dried and stained with diluted Giemsa's or Field stain. This method has the advantage of concentrating the parasites, but artifacts are numerous, and correct interpretations of these preparations require much experience. The value of buffy coat smears in the detection of low-grade parasitemia remains to be determined.

The morphology of the four species of plasmodia that infect humans is specific enough to allow identification in blood smears. The parasitized red blood cells in *P. vivax* infections are enlarged and pale and may contain diffuse bright red dots (Schaffner's dots), and the parasite presents in a wide variety of shapes and sizes; in *P. ovale* infections, the red blood cells containing parasites are oval but otherwise resemble those in *P. vivax;* in *P. malariae* the red blood cells are of normal size and do not contain dots. The parasites often present in "band" forms, and the merozoites are arranged in a rosette around central pigment; in *P. falciparum* infections the rings are very small, may contain two rather than one chromatin dot, and often are found lying flat against the margin of the cell. Only the ring stages of the asexual forms are found in the peripheral smear, and there may be more than one ring in a single red blood cell. The gametocytes are distinctively large and banana-shaped.

There is no advantage of blood over material obtained by splenic or sternal puncture. The administration of epinephrine with the idea of dislodging parasites by producing contraction of the spleen has been advocated, but results are irregular. Serologic tests are used primarily for epidemiologic rather than diagnostic purposes but are also helpful in speciation of the infecting organism and in detection of occult malaria in the bloodstream. The indirect immunofluorescent test seems to be the most sensitive and specific.

DIAGNOSIS The most important diagnostic test is a careful medical history. The diagnosis must be considered in any febrile patient who has resided in or traveled to the Caribbean, Latin America, Asia, or Africa within the previous 12 months. History of previous attacks of malaria, typical malarial paroxysms, or some artificial exposure (blood transfusion, narcotic injections in an addict) should also suggest the disease. Splenomegaly is an almost invariable finding during the second week of illness. Leukocytosis is *not* a feature of malaria. The diagnosis is confirmed by demonstrating the parasites in the peripheral blood. Because the intensity of parasitemia varies greatly from hour to hour, particularly in *P. falciparum* infections, blood smears should be examined every 8 h for 2 or 3 days before the diagnosis is abandoned.

While final cure of malaria may be difficult, particularly in *P. vivax* infections, almost all cases will respond symptomatically to quinine or one of the newer antimalarial drugs, and failure of response to a therapeutic trial argues strongly against the diagnosis.

TREATMENT The use of appropriate chemotherapy can suppress symptoms in individuals exposed in endemic areas or cure malarial infection completely. However, the emergence of drug-resistant falciparum malaria in southeast Asia, including Burma, Indonesia, and the Philippines, in South America, and in adjacent areas of Central America necessitates the use of drug combinations in the treatment of this infection.

Treatment of acute attack Treatment of an acute attack can be accomplished with chloroquine for all types of malaria except drug-resistant falciparum infection (Table 218-1). The drug usually produces complete subsidence of symptoms and destruction of the erythrocytic forms of the parasite. If vomiting is present, chloroquine hydrochloride should be given intramuscularly or, in the case of shock, intravenously. Oral therapy should be resumed as soon as possible. Although side effects are uncommon, this agent may produce epigastric distress, itching, agranulocytosis, and neurotoxicity, including involuntary movements and convulsions.

If patients have transfusion-induced malaria or have contracted the disease in an area known to harbor drug-resistant

TABLE 218-1
Malaria treatment

Purpose	*Drug*	*Dosage*
Cure chloroquine-resistant *P. falciparum* infection	Quinine sulfate*	650 mg PO tid for 10–14 days
	or quinine dihydrochloride*,†	600 mg in 300 ml normal saline IV over 1 h; repeat in 6–8 h; maximum 1800 mg per day
	plus pyrimethamine	25 mg PO bid for 3 days
	plus sulfadiazine	500 mg PO bid for 5 days
	or quinine as above	
	plus tetracycline	250 mg qid for 7 days
Cure *P. malariae* and chloroquine-sensitive *P. falciparum* infection	Chloroquine phosphate	1 g (600 mg base) PO, then 500 mg in 6 h, then 500 mg per day for 2 days
	or chloroquine hydrochloride†	250 mg (200 mg base) IM or IV every 6 h; administer IV dose as for quinine dihydrochloride above; maximum 900 mg per day
Cure *P. vivax* and *P. ovale* infection	Same as for *P. malariae*	
	plus primaquine phosphate	26.3 mg (15 mg base) PO qd for 14 days

* *If quinine is not immediately available, begin with chloroquine and switch when quinine arrives.*
† *For use when patient cannot take oral drug. Switch to oral therapy as soon as possible.*

P. falciparum, they should be treated with a combination of quinine, pyrimethamine, and one of the sulfonamides or sulfones. *Quinine sulfate,* 0.6 g orally three times a day, should be given for 3 days. If nausea and vomiting preclude oral therapy, quinine dihydrochloride diluted in saline solution or glucose can be given very slowly intravenously. During infusion the pulse and blood pressure should be monitored constantly to detect arrhythmia or hypotension. Oral therapy should be instituted as soon as possible. In the presence of renal or hepatic failure, the dose of quinine should be limited to 0.6 g a day. An overdose of quinine produces cinchonism of which tinnitus is an early manifestation. The drug may also cause mild hemolysis, allergic purpura, and drug fever. The appearance of a Coombs-positive hemolytic anemia requires the immediate withdrawal of the drug. Pyrimethamine should be given orally in dosage of 25 mg two times daily for 3 days. This is an antifolate agent and may cause megaloblastic anemia. Sulfisoxazole or sulfadiazine, 2.0 g initially and then 0.5 g every 6 h for 5 days, should be given concurrently with the other two drugs. A variety of other combinations of antifolate agents with sulfonamides or sulfones have also been used with quinine to good effect. Fansidar, a fixed-drug combination containing 25 mg pyrimethamine and 500 mg sulfadoxine, has been particularly effective. The drug was licensed in the United States in January 1982. The combination of tetracycline 250 mg qid for 10 days plus quinine is also an acceptable alternative.

Patients should be followed for 1 month to detect recrudescence of the infection. If there are circulating asexual erythrocytic forms, retreatment with pyrimethamine and a sulfonamide should be instituted. The presence of circulating gametocytes is not, however, an indication for retreatment.

Radical cure *Plasmodium vivax* and *P. ovale* persist in the liver in the exoerythrocytic stage and in this form are not affected by drugs used in the treatment of the acute attack. Unless destroyed, they will eventually reinvade the bloodstream. Primaquine base, 15 mg by mouth daily for 14 days, will effect a radical cure in most cases. If relapse occurs after primaquine therapy, a second course of the drug at twice the dosage should be given. Alternatively, 45 mg primaquine base can be given in combination with 300 mg chloroquine once weekly for 8 weeks. Primaquine may cause hemolysis in patients with G6PD deficiency; this is less likely to occur if the drug is administered once weekly.

Treatment of complications This includes careful attention to fluid and electrolyte balance, prevention of fluid overload in patients with oliguria, and early diagnosis and treatment of renal failure. In severe hemolysis large doses of steroids may be helpful. Transfusions should be given in severe hemolysis, care being taken to match the donor's cells and plasma with those of the recipient. Exchange transfusions are indicated in patients with intense parasitemia. Intravenous low-molecular-weight dextran may be helpful in increasing capillary blood flow in cerebral malaria. Dexamethasone has been used to control cerebral edema, but a controlled study suggests this practice may, in fact, be deleterious. The value of heparin in this syndrome, even when evidence suggestive of intravascular coagulation is present, remains controversial.

PREVENTION General In areas of the world such as Africa where eradication is presently impractical, limited residual insecticides plus chemoprophylaxis for pregnant women and children are recommended. The long-term hope for eradication now depends on the development of new technologies. Two new areas of research hold some promise—biological control of mosquitoes and a malaria vaccine. The latter has been made more feasible by two achievements: the continuous culture of *P. falciparum* in red blood cells and the demonstration that merozoites can serve as effective immunogens. Although merozoite vaccines have been used successfully in test animals, the adjuvants required preclude use in humans. It is hoped that effective human vaccines can be developed within the next decade.

Personal protection In endemic areas, mosquito contact should be minimized through the use of house screens, mosquito netting around beds, insect repellents, and insecticides. In addition, patients traveling to endemic areas should receive chemoprophylaxis.

Chemoprophylaxis (Table 218-2) Although it is not possible to prevent infection with chemotherapeutic agents, it is possible to suppress symptoms while the patient is residing in an endemic area by the administration of chloroquine base in dosage of 300 mg weekly (2 tablets Aralen). Cases of retinopathy have been reported in patients who have taken chloroquine in this dosage over periods of 12 to 20 years (total dose 100 to 1300 g). This, however, is a rare occurrence, and the danger to individuals planning shorter stays in malarious areas is probably nonexistent. Medication should be started at least 1 week prior to entry. Following departure from an endemic area, chloroquine should be continued an additional 6 weeks. This will eradicate *P. malariae* and sensitive strains of *P. falciparum.* The hepatic forms of *P. ovale* and *P. vivax* will not be affected, however, and may produce relapse with clinical manifestations

TABLE 218-2
Malaria chemoprophylaxis

Purpose	*Drug*	*Dosage*
To suppress clinical malaria in areas *without* chloroquine-resistant strains	Chloroquine phosphate	500 mg (300 mg base) PO once weekly, continued 6 weeks after leaving malarious area
	or amodiaquine dehydrochloride	520 mg (400 mg base) PO once weekly, continued 6 weeks after leaving malarious area
To suppress clinical malaria in areas *with* chloroquine-resistant strains	Same as above	
	plus pyrimethamine-sulfadoxine (Fansidar, Hoffmann-LaRoche)	25 mg pyrimethamine and 500 mg sulfadoxine PO once weekly, continued 6 weeks after leaving malarious area
To prevent relapses of *P. vivax* and *P. ovale* infection	Primaquine phosphate*	26.3 mg (15 mg base) PO daily for 14 days or 79 mg (45 mg base) for 8 weeks; start during last 2 weeks of suppressive therapy or immediately upon its completion

**Recommended only for travelers without G6PD deficiency who have had heavy exposure.*

some weeks or months after chloroquine is discontinued. This can be circumvented by administration of primaquine during the final 2 weeks of chloroquine administration.

Chloroquine is not effective in suppressing drug-resistant *P. falciparum.* In areas of the world where this is a problem, pyrimethamine, 25 mg, plus sulfadoxine, 500 mg (Fansidar, one tablet), plus chloroquine, 300 mg base, should be taken orally once weekly. Fansidar is contraindicated in pregnant women, persons allergic to sulfonamides, and children under 2 months. Leukopenia and megaloblastic anemia is a hazard of long-term pyrimethamine therapy, and routine hemograms should be obtained on persons taking this regimen for longer than 6 months.

Transfusions Transfusion malaria continues to occur in the United States; recently *P. falciparum* has been the most common cause. Adherence to recommendations of the American Association of Blood Banking will prevent most of these cases.

REFERENCES

BRUCE-CHWATT LJ: Man against malaria; conquest or defeat. Trans R Soc Trop Med Hyg 73:517, 1979

Chemoprophylaxis of malaria. Morb Mort Week Rep (Suppl) 27(10):81, 1978

DESOWITZ RS, MILLER LH: A perspective on malaria vaccines. Bull WHO 58:897, 1980

Drugs for parasitic infections. Med Lett 24:5, 1982

GALBRAITH RM et al: The human materno-faetal relationship in malaria. Trans R Soc Trop Med Hyg 74:52 and 61, 1980

HURWITZ ES et al: Resistance of plasmodium falciparum malaria to sulfadoxine-pyrimethamine ("Fansidar") in a refugee camp in Thailand. Lancet 1:1068, 1981

LUZZATTO L: Genetics of red cells and susceptibility to malaria. Blood 54:961, 1979

MILLER LH: Hypothesis on the mechanism of erythrocyte invasion by malaria merozoites. Bull WHO 55:157, 1977

MOLINEAUX L, GRAMICCIA G: The Garki project. Research on the epidemiology and control of malaria in the Sudan savanna of west Africa. Geneva, WHO, 1980

NIELSON RL et al: The use of exchange transfusions: A potentially useful adjunct in the treatment of fulminant falciparum malaria. Am J Med Sci 277:325, 1979

PETTERSON T et al: Chloroquine-resistant falciparum malaria from east Africa. Trans R Soc Trop Med Hyg 75:112, 1981

QUINN TC, PLORDE JJ: The resurgence of malaria. Diagnostic and therapeutic dilemmas. Arch Intern Med 141:1123, 1981

Revised recommendations for malaria chemoprophylaxis for travelers to east Africa. Morb Mort Week Rep 31(24):328, 1982

STILMA JS: Chloroquine retinopathy in a rural hospital in Ghana. Trop Geogr Med 32:221, 1980

Tropical splenomegaly syndrome. Lancet 1:1058, 1976

WARRELL DA et al: Dexamethasone proves deleterious in cerebral malaria. A double blind trial in 100 comatose patients. N Engl J Med 306:313, 1982

WERNSDORFER WH, KOUZNETSOV RL: Drug resistant malaria—occurrence, control and surveillance. Bull WHO 58:341, 1980

WOODRUFF AW et al: Cause of anaemia in malaria. Lancet 1:1055, 1979

219 LEISHMANIASIS

RICHARD M. LOCKSLEY
JAMES J. PLORDE

DEFINITION Leishmaniasis designates a disorder produced by flagellated protozoa of the genus *Leishmania.* These parasites of canines and rodents are transmitted from animal to human beings or sometimes from human to human by the bite of phlebotomine sandflies.

ETIOLOGY Four species of *Leishmania* infect humans: *L. donovani* causes visceral leishmaniasis, or kala azar; *L. tropica* and *L. mexicana* produce cutaneous leishmaniasis of the old world and new world types, respectively; and *L. braziliensis* is the agent of mucocutaneous leishmaniasis. Morphologically these organisms appear identical and are generally distinguished by clinical and geographic characteristics. Each contains several subspecies that require sophisticated methods for their separation, including determinations of isoenzyme variants, nuclear and kinetoplast DNA buoyant densities, and data on their vector phlebotomines.

In the sandfly and in culture media, *Leishmania* exist as motile spindle-shaped promastigotes (anterior flagella) which measure 1.5 to 4 μm by 14 to 20 μm. On inoculation into a mammalian host the organisms lose their flagella, enter mononuclear phagocytes, and multiply as small (2 by 5 μm), oval, intracytoplasmic amastigotes known as Leishman-Donovan bodies. In stained preparations a dark, slightly flattened nucleus and rod-shaped kinetoplast may be discerned.

EPIDEMIOLOGY Leishmaniasis is a zoonotic infection which involves the rodents and canines of every continent except Australia. The prevalence varies; 4 to 10 percent of dogs in the Mediterranean littoral and 80 to 95 percent of the gerbils in southern U.S.S.R. are infected, many of them subclinically. The disease is spread when female sandflies of the genus *Phlebotomus* (old world) or *Lutzomyia* (new world) ingest amastigotes while taking a blood meal from an infected mammal. These are transformed to promastigotes within the insect's gut, migrate to the proboscis, and are deposited on the skin of the new host when the insect next engorges. Phlebotomines breed in warm, humid microclimates and are typically found in rodent burrows, termite hills, and rotting vegetation. When humans encroach upon this sylvatic cycle, they may acquire the disease. Establishment of infection in the domestic dog provides an important urban reservoir of leishmaniasis. Human-to-human transmission is infrequent. An exception is the Indian form of kala azar for which there is no known animal reservoir. Rarely, transmission can occur by blood transfusion, contact inoculation, and coitus. It is estimated that over 12 million people are infected with this parasite throughout the world, although human cases are seldom seen in the United States. *Lutzomyia* species capable of transmitting the disease to humans are present in the southern United States.

PATHOGENESIS After inoculation into the skin, promastigotes enter mononuclear phagocytes. Entry is presumed to be rapid, since nonimmune serum, by a mechanism requiring immunoglobulin and complement, is lethal to promastigotes. Neutrophils are able to kill ingested organisms, but in mononuclear phagocytes organisms transform into amastigotes within phagolysosomes and replicate by binary fission. They eventually rupture the cell and invade adjacent mononuclear phagocytes.

The course of the disease from this point is determined by the host's cellular immunity as well as the species of the parasite. In cutaneous leishmaniasis, there is a marked lymphocytic infiltration associated with a reduction in the number of parasites, the development of a delayed skin (leishmanin) reaction, and spontaneous cure. In the mucocutaneous form, the spontaneous disappearance of the primary lesion may be followed by metastatic mucocutaneous lesions at some later date. The destructiveness of the metastatic lesions is attributed to the development of hypersensitivity to parasitic antigens. An interesting exception to the general pattern in cutaneous disease is disseminated cutaneous leishmaniasis in which there is no infiltration of lymphocytes and plasma cells or reduction in the number of parasites, the leishmanin reaction is negative, and the skin lesions become chronic, progressive, and disseminated. The patients appear to have a selective anergy to leishmanial antigens which is mediated at least in part by adherent suppressor cells. In visceral leishmaniasis, the cellular changes are similar, but the parasites spread to reticuloendothelial cells throughout the body. This spread is associated with development of marked hyperglobulinemia. Although antibodies are present, they are nonprotective and may be detrimental when associated with autoimmune hemolytic anemia, immune-complex glomerulonephritis, and amyloidosis. As in disseminated cutaneous disease, the ability of the organism to establish and maintain progressive disease may be related to the development in the host of suppressor T cells. Cure of leishmaniasis confers immunity to the infecting strain.

DIAGNOSIS Establishing a diagnosis of leishmaniasis requires demonstrating the organism by smear or culture of aspirates or tissue. Although Nicolle-Novy-MacNeal (NNN) medium traditionally has been used to culture *Leishmania,* several commercially available liquid media offer improved storage capability and enhanced recovery of organisms. The latter is particularly true with *L. braziliensis,* which grows poorly on NNN medium. Cultures are maintained at 22 to 28°C for 21 days and examined microscopically for the presence of the motile promastigotes. Inoculation of hamsters with infected clinical material results in infection after a period of months.

Antibodies are detectable in all forms of leishmaniasis. The direct agglutination test[1] detects IgM antibody and is more sensitive in acute disease. The test is group-specific, but the titer is generally greatest to the homologous strain. A positive test (>1:32) varies from 97 percent in visceral leishmaniasis to 81 percent in new world cutaneous leishmaniasis. Other serologic tests, including complement fixation, hemagglutination, enzyme-linked immunoabsorbent assays, and indirect immunofluorescence, are less available. Direct agglutination antibodies decline and may disappear with cure.

KALA AZAR Etiology Kala azar touches all continents except Australia. Although the characteristics of the disease are similar throughout the world, certain local peculiarities in its behavior justify the classification of visceral leishmaniasis into at least three main types. These differences are attributed to variations in the strains of *L. donovani* in a given area and, perhaps more important, to the length of time that the disease has been endemic in a population.

African kala azar is found in the eastern half of Africa from the Sahara in the north to the equator in the south. It is a disease of older children and young adults (10 to 25 years) with males being involved more commonly than females. It is endemic in gerbils and other rodents in many areas and is more resistant to therapy with antimony compounds than that found in the rest of the world.

Mediterranean, or *infantile, kala azar* is seen primarily in the Mediterranean area, China, Russia, and Latin America. An outbreak in Kenya and Ethiopia also appears to be of this type. It is a disease of children under the age of 4, but adults, particularly travelers to endemic areas, are not spared. Dogs, jackals, and foxes serve as reservoirs, and human-to-human transmission is thought to be rare. The strains responsible for the Eurasian and American diseases are sometimes referred to as *L. infantum* and *L. chagasi,* respectively.

Indian kala azar has an age and sex distribution similar to African kala azar, and males are involved more commonly than females. The human being is the only known reservoir, and transmission is carried out by anthropophilic species of sandflies.

Manifestations The incubation period is generally about 3 months (3 weeks to 18 months). A primary cutaneous lesion (leishmanioma) is not uncommon in Africa. The onset of disease may be insidious or abrupt; the latter occurs more frequently in individuals from nonendemic areas. Fever, typically nocturnal and occasionally in a double-quotidian pattern, is almost universal and is accompanied by tachycardia without signs of toxemia. Daily fever progresses to recurrent febrile waves. Diarrhea and cough are frequent. Nontender splenomegaly becomes dramatic by the third month. The liver enlarges less conspicuously. Cirrhosis and portal hypertension occur in about 10 percent of patients. Lymphadenopathy accompanies some cases of African kala azar. Atypical forms, including isolated tonsillar infections and cervical adenopathy, have been reported. Asymptomatic or subclinical disease has been suspected.

Pancytopenia is characteristic. Anemia is multifactorial: autoimmune hemolysis, splenomegaly, and gastrointestinal blood loss all contribute. The latter occurs with leishmanial infiltration of the gastrointestinal tract and is exacerbated by thrombocytopenia. Agranulocytosis, cancrum oris, and superinfections complicate untreated cases. Hypoalbuminemia and polyclonal hypergammaglobulinemia are constant features; the latter forms the basis for the nonspecific formol gel test. Proteinuria and microscopic hematuria reflect the development of immune-complex glomerulonephritis. Amyloidosis may occur chronically. Edema, cachexia, and hyperpigmentation (*kala azar* means "black fever") are late manifestations. Without treatment death occurs within 3 to 20 months in 90 to 95 percent of adults and 75 to 85 percent of children, usually due to pulmonary and gastrointestinal superinfections or gastrointestinal hemorrhage.

After successful treatment, 3 percent of African cases and up to 10 percent of Indian cases develop post-kala azar dermal leishmaniasis (PKDL), characterized by a spectrum of lesions ranging from depigmented macules to wart-like nodules over the trunk and face. PKDL appears shortly after symptoms subside in African cases and typically disappears after several weeks. In the Indian disease, PKDL appears after a latent period of 1 to 2 years and may last years, creating a persistent human reservoir.

Diagnosis Buffy coat preparations may demonstrate the parasite, particularly in Indian kala azar (90 percent). Bone marrow aspirate and biopsy are positive in over 85 percent of cases. Although splenic (95 percent) and hepatic (75 percent) samples contain numerous parasites, aspiration of these organs is not recommended because of the risk of fatal hemorrhage. Aspirates or biopsy of enlarged lymph nodes will show parasites in 60 percent of cases. Suspicious skin lesions should be biopsied as well. The direct agglutination test is positive early in the disease. The leishmanin skin test is negative and becomes positive only 6 to 8 weeks after recovery. Other causes of fever in the tropics, including malaria, brucellosis, tubercu-

[1] *The leishmanin skin test (Montenegro test), performed by the intradermal injection of promastigote antigen, is nonstandardized and generally unavailable.*

losis, typhoid, and hepatic abscess can be distinguished by appropriate testing. PKDL must be differentiated from leprosy, syphilis, and yaws.

Treatment Transfusions and treatment of complicating superinfections must supplement specific therapy. Pentavalent antimonials are highly effective against leishmania and relatively nontoxic. Sodium antimony gluconate (Pentostam)[2] is given intravenously or intramuscularly in a single daily dose of 10 mg/kg for adults and 15 mg/kg for children. Treatment should be given for 10 days in Indian kala azar and 30 days in other forms. The cheaper meglumine antimoniate (Glucantime) is available outside the United States. The recommended dose is 50 mg/kg per day for 15 days, although doses twice as high have been used. Resistant cases must be treated with intravenous amphotericin B (0.5 to 1 mg/kg daily or on alternate days) or pentamidine (3 to 4 mg/kg per day for 10 days in three courses). Mortality remains 15 to 25 percent in advanced cases, although the cure rate is over 90 percent when therapy is given early. Relapses can occur up to 2 years after treatment. Both relapses and PKLD should be treated in the same fashion as the initial illness.

Prevention Preventive measures include early treatment of human cases, elimination of diseased dogs, and the use of DDT against sandflies. The cessation of spraying for malaria has resulted in an upsurge in cases of kala azar. Application of insect repellents and the use of fine-mesh netting are important for travelers. There are no useful prophylactic agents.

NEW WORLD CUTANEOUS LEISHMANIASIS Etiology and epidemiology This form of leishmaniasis is produced by several subspecies of *L. mexicana* and *L. braziliensis.* The natural reservoirs of these organisms are the forest rodents of South and Central America. They are transmitted to humans entering the jungle to gather chicle or to clear land for new settlements. Disease is most prevalent in the Amazon basin but occurs in every country of the area except Chile. In some locations 10 to 20 percent of the population is infected. Four autochthonous cases have been reported from southwest Texas.

Disease characteristics There are four clinical varieties of American leishmaniasis: chiclero's ulcer, uta, espundia, and diffuse cutaneous leishmaniasis. All begin with the appearance of a local lesion at the site of infecting sandfly bite after an incubation of 10 days to 3 months. Their course from that point is often sharply different.

Chiclero's ulcer, which is found in Mexico, Guatemala, Belize, and possibly other parts of Central America, is caused by *L. mexicana mexicana.* Chicle gatherers who work in forests during the rainy season when sandflies are abundant develop isolated cutaneous lesions on the hand or head. These show little tendency to ulcerate and generally heal spontaneously within 6 months. Ear lesions, however, persist for years and may cause extensive destruction of the pinna.

Uta, which occurs exclusively on the western slopes of the Peruvian Andes at altitudes of more than 2000 ft, consists of single or multiple skin ulcers of the nose and lips in which parasites are readily demonstrable. Spontaneous healing within 3 months to a year is the rule, and mucosal spread is unusual. The etiologic agent is *L. peruviana,* a member of the *L. braziliensis* group, and the reservoir is the domestic dog. With widespread use of insecticides in Peru, the disease has almost disappeared.

Espundia is caused by *L. braziliensis,* which typically produces one or several lesions on the lower extremities that undergo extensive ulceration; healing occurs with scarring after 3

[2] *Available from the Centers for Disease Control, Atlanta, Ga.*

to 12 months. After months to years, metastatic lesions may appear in the nasopharynx and, less frequently, in the perineum. Nasal obstruction and epistaxis are frequent presenting symptoms. Extensive destruction of soft-tissue structures ensues, with painful mutilating erosions (espundia). In blacks, the lesions are often hypertrophic, and large polypoid masses deform the lips and cheeks. Fever, anemia, and weight loss are common. Death is caused by bacterial infection, inanition, aspiration, and respiratory obstruction.

Diffuse cutaneous leishmaniasis is found in Venezuela and the Dominican Republic. It apparently results from a specific deficiency of cell-mediated immunity to leishmanial antigen. In South America, it is caused by members of the *L. mexicana* complex, usually *L. mexicana amazonensis.* This remarkable disease is characterized by massive dissemination of skin lesions without visceral involvement. The clinical picture often bears a striking resemblance to lepromatous leprosy. The diagnosis is not difficult, because the lesions contain a large number of organisms. In contrast to all other types of cutaneous leishmaniasis, the leishmanin skin test is negative. The disease is progressive and very refractory to treatment.

Diagnosis Skin biopsies are the preferred means of obtaining tissue for stains and culture. Parasites are scanty in most lesions except those of disseminated cutaneous leishmaniasis. In espundia, organisms have been cultured from the blood when the cutaneous sites have been negative; the direct agglutination test and the leishmanin skin test become positive within 4 to 6 weeks. Syphilis, yaws, blastomycosis, sporotrichosis, leprosy, and carcinoma must be considered in the differential diagnosis.

Treatment Uta seldom requires therapy. The antifolate cycloguanil pamoate has been used as a single intramuscular injection for chiclero's ulcer. Espundia is treated with Pentostam as described above for kala azar. Cases that fail to respond to antimalarials should be treated with amphotericin B. Steroids have been used concomitantly with specific therapy to decrease tissue necrosis associated with hypersensitivity, an event that resembles a Jarisch-Herxheimer reaction. Secondary bacterial infection must be treated aggressively. Reconstructive facial prostheses should not be used until the disease has been remittent for at least 1 year without therapy. A rising antibody titer may predict relapse and indicate that further therapy is required. Amphotericin B and pentamidine have been used to produce remissions in disseminated cutaneous infections, but cure is rare.

Prevention Vaccination of forest workers with *L. mexicana* has been successful in establishing immunity and preventing disfiguring ear lesions.

OLD WORLD CUTANEOUS LEISHMANIASIS Etiology and epidemiology This, the least serious form of human leishmaniasis, usually presents as a localized cutaneous ulcer which heals spontaneously. The disease is found throughout the Mediterranean area, Africa, southwest Asia, and India. Three subspecies of *L. tropica* are involved.

Manifestations *L. tropica* causes urban (chronic, dry) cutaneous leishmaniasis, an endemic disease of children and young adults in areas bordering the Mediterranean, the Middle East, southern U.S.S.R., and India. The reservoir is maintained in domestic dogs. The incubation period ranges from 2 to 24 months. Usually the lesion begins as a single, red pruritic papule on the face (oriental sore). The central area ulcerates and slowly enlarges centrifugally, reaching a size of approximately 2 cm. Lymphadenopathy is unusual. Healing occurs over 1 to 2 years and leaves a small depigmented scar. The disease can be complicated by the development of *leishmaniasis recidiva,* a condition marked by persistent facial lesions resembling lupus erythematosus and containing scanty numbers of parasites, and an exaggerated delayed hypersensitivity to parasite antigens. Rarely, the organism may spread to the viscera.

L. tropica major causes rural (acute, moist) cutaneous leishmaniasis, which is endemic to the desert areas of the Middle East, southern U.S.S.R., and Africa. The reservoir is maintained in burrowing rodents. The incubation period ranges from 2 to 6 weeks. The initial lesions are often multiple and located on the lower extremities. Regional lymphadenopathy and satellite lesions are common. Healing with scarring occurs within 3 to 6 months.

L. aethiopica, maintained in rock formations of the Ethiopian and Kenyan highlands, causes cutaneous leishmaniasis which can be complicated by the development of diffuse cutaneous leishmaniasis. This closely resembles the disease of the same name described under "New World Cutaneous Leishmaniasis," above.

Diagnosis Lesions should first be cleansed with alcohol to reduce bacterial contamination, which hinders recovery of the organisms. Aspirates should be obtained from the outer edge of the ulcer. If the aspirated smears are negative, full-thickness skin biopsies from the ulcer margin should be taken for touch smears, histology, and culture. The direct agglutination test and the leishmanin skin test become positive within 4 to 6 weeks, except in diffuse cutaneous leishmaniasis, where the skin test remains negative.

Treatment Secondary bacterial infection must be treated. Specific therapy should be withheld in endemic areas until ulceration takes place, thereby conferring immunity. Exceptions include disfiguring lesions, the presence of lesions for longer than 6 months, and diffuse cutaneous leishmaniasis. Treatment is carried out with sodium antimony gluconate as described above for kala azar. Ulcers should be covered to prevent infection of vectors and other canine and human hosts. *Leishmaniasis recidiva* may require concomitant steroids to abrogate the heightened immune response. Diffuse cutaneous disease often requires multiple courses of therapy with amphotericin or pentamidine. Although *L. tropica major* confers immunity to *L. tropica,* the converse is not true. In Russia and Israel vaccination of children at inconspicuous sites with *L. tropica major* has been extensively practiced.

REFERENCES

HASHEIM-NASAB A, ZADEH-SHIRAZI H: Visceral leishmaniasis in Fars Province, Iran: Study of 130 cases. J Trop Med Hyg 83:119, 1980

HENDRICKS LD et al: Hemoflagellates: Commercially available liquid media for rapid cultivation. Parasitology 76:309, 1978

———, WRIGHT N: Diagnosis of cutaneous leishmaniasis by in vitro cultivation of saline aspirated in Schneider's *Drosophila* medium. Am J Trop Med Hyg 28:962, 1979

MARSDEN PD: Leishmaniasis. N Engl J Med 300:350, 1979

MARU M: Clinical and laboratory features and treatment of visceral leishmaniasis in hospitalized patients in northwestern Ethiopia. Am J Trop Med Hyg 28:15, 1979

PEARSON RD, STEIGBIGEL RT: Mechanism of the lethal effect of serum upon *Leishmania donovani.* J Immunol 125:2195, 1980

PETERSON EA et al: Specific inhibition of lymphocyte-proliferation responses by adherent suppressor cells in diffuse cutaneous leishmaniasis. N Engl J Med 306:387, 1982

SCHUR LF et al: The biochemical and serological taxonomy of visceralizing Leishmania. Ann Trop Med Parasitol 75:131, 1981

SHAW PK et al: Autochthonous dermal leishmaniasis in Texas. Am J Trop Med Hyg 25:788, 1976

ZUCKERMAN A, LAINSON R: Leishmania, in *Parasitic Protozoa,* JP Krier (ed). New York, Academic, 1977, vol 1, pp 58–134

220 TRYPANOSOMIASIS

JAMES J. PLORDE

SLEEPING SICKNESS

DEFINITION African trypanosomiasis, or sleeping sickness, is a disease caused by the hemoflagellate *Trypanosoma brucei,* which is transmitted to human beings by several species of tsetse fly belonging to the genus *Glossina.* Clinically, the untreated disease is characterized by an acute febrile lymphadenopathy followed, after a variable period, by a chronic lethal meningoencephalomyelitis. It occurs in two principal epidemiologic patterns: Gambian, or mid- and west African, sleeping sickness, and Rhodesian, or east African, sleeping sickness.

ETIOLOGY Trypanosomes are fusiform protozoa recognized by an undulating membrane which extends along the length of the cell and terminates in an anterior flagellum. The morphological characteristics of many varieties are so nearly identical that they are distinguishable only by their pathogenicity for certain animals, differences in biochemical requirements, and ability to multiply in insects. *Trypanosoma brucei* strains are polymorphic organisms varying in shape from slender to stumpy and in length from 8 to 30 μm. The slender forms have a long flagellum that in the shorter types is rudimentary or absent. The Gambian and Rhodesian forms of sleeping sickness were previously thought to be caused by two distinct species of trypanosomes, *T. gambiense* and *T. rhodesiense.* It is felt now, however, that they, along with the animal trypanosome responsible for *nagana* in cattle, are all variants of a single species. The individual varieties are referred to as *T. brucei gambiense, T. brucei rhodesiense,* and *T. brucei brucei.*

Trypanosomiasis in animals is a great economic problem in many parts of the world. It is probable that an area of approximately 4 million square miles in Africa is not populated because of the impossibility of keeping animals in sites where tsetse flies are infected with trypanosomes.

EPIDEMIOLOGY Gambian sleeping sickness occurs in tropical, west, and central Africa extending from the Sahara to the Kalahari deserts and east to the Rift Valley. The incidence of disease is particularly high in Zaire. Rhodesian trypanosomiasis is found in tropical east Africa from Ethiopia in the north to Botswana in the south.

Transmission of the trypanosomes of sleeping sickness occurs by what is referred to as the "anterior station." After ingestion by a feeding tsetse, the parasites first develop in the intestine of the fly and then migrate to the salivary glands, where they are discharged when the host is bitten. In some situations it is possible that the trypanosomes can be mechanically transmitted from host to host by the tsetse and other hematophagous arthropods. This may be of importance during epidemics.

The Gambian strains of *T. brucei* are transmitted mainly by *G. palpalis* and *G. tachinoides.* These species live in shaded areas near water. Less than 5 percent of the flies are infected even in the most notorious endemic foci. Although *G. palpalis* and *G. tachinoides* are not exclusively anthropophilic, human beings are thought to be the major reservoir for Gambian sleeping sickness.

Rhodesian sleeping sickness, on the other hand, is primarily a zoonosis. It is transmitted to humans from the bushbuck, a small antelope, by the bite of *G. morsitans*, a savannah tsetse. It is seen typically in individuals who travel away from their villages to hunt or fish. Domestic cattle and sheep may also serve as reservoirs, and transmission from human to fly to human can occur.

PATHOLOGY AND PATHOGENESIS The tsetse fly inoculates the organism into the subcutaneous pool of blood that forms during its feeding. Some of the parasites may reach the bloodstream directly, but most remain at the site of inoculation, where they multiply to produce a local chancre. Following the appearance of this lesion, the trypanosomes spread through tissue spaces and lymphatics, eventually spilling over into the general circulation where they continue to multiply by longitudinal fission. The parasitemia is of low intensity and typically occurs in waves; each wave disappears with the production of antibody to the parasite's glycoprotein surface antigen and reappears in 3 to 8 days as a new antigenic variant arises. A single trypanosomal strain can produce scores of antigenic variants, each apparently encoded by a distinct gene and selected by the host's antibody response. The waves of parasitemia, which are accompanied by fever and mononuclear leukocytosis, tend to become more infrequent and irregular in the later stages of the disease. At some time during this stage of dissemination, trypanosomes localize in the small vessels of the heart and the central nervous system. In the latter it is first manifested as a diffuse leptomeningitis and later by a perivascular cerebritis. If untreated, this parenchymal inflammation gives rise to a demyelinating panencephalitis. Amastigote or short forms have been demonstrated in experimental *T. brucei* infections, suggesting that this organism has an intracellular tissue phase in its developmental cycle. This could be of significance in occult infections.

The mechanism by which the trypanosome elicits tissue damage is unknown. The parasitemia stimulates the production of large quantities of IgM immunoglobulin, perhaps in response to the rapid antigenic variation of the parasite. A small part represents specific protective antibody; the remainder is nonspecific heterophil antibody and rheumatoid factor. High levels correlate well with the presence of circulating immune complexes which may, in turn, produce the vasculitis seen in this disease.

CLINICAL MANIFESTATIONS The Gambian and Rhodesian forms of sleeping sickness differ somewhat in symptoms, severity, and duration. Rhodesian trypanosomiasis is the more acute and severe of the two forms, usually terminating fatally within a year. Fever is higher, emaciation more rapid, and lymphatic involvement less evident. Death from intercurrent infections or myocarditis usually occurs before the typical sleeping sickness syndrome appears. In the Gambian variety there are often successive bouts of clinical activity with intervening latent periods that persist for a number of years. The early stages may be mild, and the disease may go unrecognized until the central nervous system is involved. In both forms of the disease, however, an entry lesion, a febrile period of dissemination, and a stage of central nervous system involvement are found to some degree. The *trypanosomal chancre* appears as an erythematous nodule at the site of inoculation 2 or 3 days after the bite of an infected fly. It may occur anywhere in the body but is most commonly seen on the head or limbs and is accompanied by regional lymphadenopathy. The lesion, which subsides spontaneously, is noted more frequently in Rhodesian sleeping sickness, perhaps because of the acute nature of the disease.

The incubation period is usually about 2 weeks, but in *T. brucei gambiense* infections may be several years. Systemic manifestations generally become apparent during the hematogenous dissemination of the trypanosomes. In the usual case the patient develops a high remittent fever, severe headache, insomnia, and inability to concentrate. In Caucasians a characteristic circinate erythema resembling erythema marginatum is frequent. Transient firm areas of painful subcutaneous edema localized to the hands, feet, and periorbital tissues may appear. All these signs and symptoms may disappear and reappear intermittently over a period of months to years. Tender lymphadenopathy with gradual induration of the nodes and splenomegaly are almost invariably present in Gambian sleeping sickness. The lymph nodes of the posterior cervical triangle are frequently prominent. This is referred to as *Winterbottom's sign.* Eventually the parasites enter the central nervous system. This may occur early in the course of the disease or may be delayed for as long as 8 years. Cerebral trypanosomiasis can be explosive, causing repeated convulsions or deep coma and death within a few days. Most patients show gradual progression to the classic picture of *sleeping sickness.* A vacant expression develops, the eyelids droop, the lower lip hangs loosely, and it becomes more and more difficult to gain the patient's attention or prod him or her to any activity. Patients will eat when offered food, but they never ask for it or engage in spontaneous conversation, and speech gradually becomes blurred and indistinct. Tremors of the hands and tongue, choreiform movements, seizures with transient paralysis, loss of sphincter control, ophthalmoplegia, extensor plantar responses, and finally death in coma, in status epilepticus, or from hyperpyrexia follows inexorably.

Death may also occur from intercurrent infection, of which bacillary and amebic dysentery, malaria, and bacterial (often pneumococcal) pneumonia are the most important.

DIAGNOSIS AND LABORATORY FINDINGS *Anemia* and *hypermacroglobulinemia* are invariably present, and spontaneous clumping of erythrocytes in blood specimens is grossly evident in many cases. The sedimentation rate is rapid, and peripheral monocytosis is frequent. When there has been invasion of the central nervous system, the *cerebrospinal fluid* shows mononuclear pleocytosis and increased protein concentration. The protein concentration is a better index of severity of disease and therapeutic response than the number of cells. The presence of IgM in the spinal fluid is almost pathognomonic of cerebral trypanosomiasis.

The definitive diagnosis depends upon finding the trypanosomes in the blood, aspirate of lymph node, or cerebrospinal fluid. These should be examined first in wet mounts; actively motile organisms are seen easily under high power. For final identification thin and thick blood films should be stained with Wright's or Giemsa's stain. If the direct smears are negative, concentrated specimens are examined. A variety of concentration techniques, including differential centrifugation, microhematocrit buffy coat centrifugation, anion-exchange centrifugation, and membrane filtration, have been used. If these methods are negative, inoculation of rats or mice can be helpful in the diagnosis of Rhodesian disease. A severalfold increase in IgM globulins in the serum is of confirmatory value. Complement fixation, indirect fluorescent antibody, indirect hemagglutination, and ELISA tests utilizing stable antigens are useful in endemic areas.

TREATMENT *Suramin* (Bayer 205, Antrypol) is the most effective agent before central nervous system involvement has occurred. The initial dose should be limited to 0.2 g intravenously because of possible idiosyncrasy. If there is no evidence of sensitivity, a full course of therapy can be instituted the following day. One gram (10 ml fresh 10% solution) is given intravenously on the first, third, seventh, fourteenth, and twenty-first days for a total of 5 g. If red blood cells, casts, or significant amounts of protein occur in the urine, therapy should be discontinued. Pentamidine given in water intramuscularly each day for 10 injections is also effective in early disease. The dose is 3 to 4 mg pentamidine base per kilogram for each injection. When the agent is given too rapidly by the intravenous route, it may cause hypotension.

Lumbar puncture should always be performed in patients who are about to undergo therapy for trypanosomiasis. If the central nervous system is involved, agents that will penetrate the blood-brain barrier must be used; for this purpose the most effective agent is *melarsoprol* (Mel B). This drug, an arsenic derivative of British antilewisite (BAL), is effective at all stages of the disease but is more toxic than suramin. It is given intravenously in a 3.6% solution. The initial dose is 0.5 ml. Each subsequent dose is increased by 0.5 ml until the maximum single dose of 5 ml is reached. The first three doses are given at daily intervals followed by a 7-day rest. This schedule is repeated until a total of 37.5 ml has been given over a period of 1 month. If signs of arsenic toxicity occur, the drug should be discontinued. A reactive encephalopathy, probably due to the release of trypanosomal antigen, may occur early in the course of treatment. Pretreatment with suramin may help avert this complication. A hemorrhagic encephalopathy, a direct arsenic toxic reaction, may also occur and is usually fatal. BAL may be of some use in this situation.

PROGNOSIS The disease is probably always fatal if untreated. If the infection is treated with suramin prior to central nervous system involvement, the cure rate is high and recovery is rapid and complete. When the nervous system becomes involved, the prognosis is less bright, and in far-advanced disease the survivors may suffer neurological damage. Relapses may occur, particularly following treatment with suramin, if the central nervous system was already involved at the time therapy was instituted. Less commonly they may be the result of drug resistance. Examination of the spinal fluid 6 and 12 months after therapy, or earlier if symptoms recur, is helpful in detecting relapse. Such patients must be re-treated with a second therapeutic agent.

PREVENTION Personal protection is best achieved by the use of repellents and protective clothing. A single intramuscular injection of pentamidine in dosage of 3 to 4 mg base per kilogram (maximum 300 mg) will protect against the Gambian form of disease for 6 months or more; its usefulness in Rhodesian trypanosomiasis is controversial. Because of the danger of cryptic infections occurring during chemoprophylaxis, it has been generally restricted to mass prophylactic campaigns. Other methods of disease control include clearing vegetation and the use of insecticides.

CHAGAS' DISEASE

DEFINITION American trypanosomiasis is an infection caused by *T. cruzi* that is characterized by an acute, often asymptomatic illness followed, after a latent period that may span decades, by chronic cardiac and gastrointestinal sequelae.

ETIOLOGY *Trypanosoma cruzi* circulates in the blood as a slender, fusiform trypimastigote measuring 20 μm in length. In stained preparations, its narrow undulating membrane, large kinetoplast, and characteristic C shape are easily recognized. Unlike the trypanosomes of sleeping sickness, it does not multiply within the bloodstream. After invading tissue cells, it loses its undulating membrane and flagellum, assumes its amastigote form, and divides by binary fission. Eventually, new flagellated forms are produced which reenter the general circulation to initiate another cycle.

Strains of *T. cruzi* vary widely in their host preference, geographic distribution, virulence, and tissue tropism. They may be distinguished by specific antiserum, zymotype, and DNA restriction pattern.

EPIDEMIOLOGY This infection is found in scattered foci from Chile and Argentina to Mexico. Within these endemic areas it affects over 12 million people and is the leading cause of heart disease, responsible for one-quarter of all deaths in the 25- to 44-year age group. *Trypanosoma cruzi* has been found in insect vectors and wild animals in several areas of the southern United States, and serologic studies have documented that acquisition of human infection occurs within this country. There are to date, however, only a handful of clinically apparent autochthonous cases reported from Texas.

The disease is transmitted to humans by reduviid ("assassin" or "kissing") bugs, primarily those of the genera *Triatoma, Panstrongylus,* and *Rhodnius.* These winged, hematophagous insects can be found in the burrows of animals and in the cracks and thatches of poorly constructed rural dwellings. The insect attacks human beings at night, usually biting the face at the mucocutaneous junction (most frequently the lip or outer canthus of the eye). The flagellated trypanosomes are ingested by the bug while feeding, and after multiplying and developing in the midgut of the insect for 8 to 10 days, are discharged in the feces; human infection occurs through contamination of the bite wound. This is referred to as transmission by the "posterior station." The reduviid may remain infected as long as 2 years.

Human beings, domestic animals (cats and dogs), and wild animals, especially the opossum and armadillo, may serve as reservoirs for the infection. The close association of human beings, domestic animals, and the vector within human dwellings is of prime epidemiologic importance, but the disease is occasionally transmitted by a blood transfusion and via the placenta to newborn infants. Occasional laboratory infections have also been reported.

PATHOGENESIS AND CLINICAL MANIFESTATIONS Only one-third of newly infected patients have clinical manifestations. In them a local inflammatory reaction, manifested clinically as an erythematous nodule or *chagoma,* appears within 1 to 3 weeks at the site of inoculation of the protozoan. If, as is commonly the case, the portal of entry has been the conjunctiva, the presenting manifestations are a unilateral, painless conjunctivitis, palpebral edema, and preauricular lymphadenopathy (Romaña's sign). This primary complex may persist for ! to 2 months during which parasites can be demonstrated in the lesion.

Following an incubation period of 2 weeks, trypanosomal forms reach the general circulation, producing a parasitemia and initiating the acute phase of the illness. After circulating in the blood for some time, the trypanosomes invade tissue cells of mesenchymal origin, assume the amastigote form, and multiply, producing intracellular pseudocysts. In 4 to 6 days these pseudocysts rupture, releasing both amastigotes and newly formed trypimastigotes. The amastigotes disintegrate, eliciting an intense inflammatory reaction, while the flagellated forms regain the bloodstream to maintain the infection and invade new tissues, particularly the heart, skeletal muscle, smooth muscle, and nervous system. *T. cruzi* antigens can absorb to the surface of both normal and infected cells rendering them susceptible to destruction by the host's hormonal and cellular immune response.

Clinically, the patient experiences a continuous or recurrent fever, generalized lymphadenopathy, hepatosplenomegaly, and in some cases extensive gelatinous edema of the face and trunk. A transient morbilliform or urticarial skin eruption may occur early in the acute phase. Although trypanosomes frequently can be demonstrated in the cerebrospinal fluid at this time, acute meningoencephalitis is relatively rare; newborn infants and young children are affected most commonly. Myocarditis characterized by tachycardia and electrocardiographic changes is very common. In severe cases, there may be conduction disturbances, cardiac dilatation, and heart failure. The duration of the acute illness is variable. In 5 to 10 percent of cases, meningoencephalitis or severe heart disease results in a fatal outcome within a few days or weeks. Most often, the disease, in response to the development of humoral antibody, resolves slowly over a period of several weeks. Parasites become extremely scanty in both the tissues and blood, the patient appears well, and the persistent infection is detectable only by serological means. Rarely, in the face of leukemia or immunosuppression, parasitemia and acute manifestations reappear. In the overwhelming majority of patients, however, the infection remains latent for the remainder of life. In approximately 10 percent, progressive immunologic destruction of mesenchymal tissue eventually leads to the development of chronic organ damage. Most patients presenting with late manifestations deny a history of acute illness, suggesting that subclinical infections often result in chronic disease. It has been suggested that host cell antigens released during the acute phase of the illness initiate an autoimmune inflammatory reaction, and antibodies reactive with endocardium, striated muscle, and vascular tissues have been described. Self-reactive cytotoxic lymphocytes have also been demonstrated in experimental animals, and lymphocytic infiltrates are commonly seen in patients dying of chagasic cardiopathy. Some authors have suggested that the late manifestations of disease are primarily due to neuropathies caused by the destruction of ganglionic nerve cells during this phase of the disease, resulting in the dilatation and malfunction of the affected organs.

The most important late manifestation is heart disease. Symptoms and signs range from precordial pain, arrhythmias, and heart block to chronic congestive heart failure (predominantly right-sided). Thromboembolic phenomena and sudden cardiac arrest are relatively common. Right bundle branch block and left anterior hemiblock, premature ventricular contractions, and inverted T waves are frequently seen on ECG. Echocardiography has been shown to be of value both in screening patients with infection for evidence of cardiac involvement and in following the progress of those with established cardiomyopathy. At autopsy the hearts of patients with Chagas' disease may show a peculiar herniation of the endocardium through the apical muscle bundles. Megacolon and megaesophagus are sequelae seen in southern South America, but they are less common in Central America and in northern South America. Neurological manifestations including mental deficiency and cerebellar symptoms also have been reported in the chronic state of disease.

DIAGNOSIS The diagnosis depends on the demonstration of *T. cruzi* in the patient or upon serologic tests. In the acute phase of the disease the parasite may be seen in the peripheral blood by means of the same direct methods described for African trypanosomiasis. If these are negative, blood may be cultured in a variety of artificial media, or inoculated into rats, mice, or guinea pigs.

Trypanosoma cruzi is easily grown in blood broth and incubated at 28°C; a more sensitive tissue culture method has been described recently. The technique of *xenodiagnosis* is often used in endemic areas; a laboratory-reared vector, known to be parasite-free, is allowed to feed on subjects with suspected cases, and 2 weeks later, the insect's intestinal contents are examined for parasites. Confusion sometimes arises from the finding of trypanosomes in blood. Many children in Venezuela and other South American countries are infected with a harmless species, *T. rangeli,* which produces no symptoms but may be present in the blood for many months. By utilization of both culture and xenodiagnosis repeatedly, organisms can be recovered from most acute cases and from up to 40 percent of chronic ones. Biopsy of an involved lymph node or calf muscle may reveal the organism during the initial illness when the parasites cannot be recovered from the blood. The Machado-Guerreiro test (a complement fixation reaction) is most helpful in the diagnosis of chronic cases and in survey work. Fluorescent antibody and hemagglutination inhibition tests appear more sensitive and less specific. Rapid slide flocculation tests and enzyme-linked immunosorbent assay are being evaluated.

TREATMENT AND PREVENTION There is no satisfactory treatment for Chagas' disease. Although several drugs will clear the blood of trypanosomes, there is some doubt whether any have the capacity to destroy intracellular parasites at tolerable doses. Lampit, a nitrofurazone derivative given in dosage of 10 mg/kg per day for 3 or 4 months, shows the greatest promise. Allopurinol has been shown to have significant antitrypanosomal activity in vitro but its clinical usefulness is unknown. Chronic organ damage, however, is generally thought irreversible. Prevention consists of using residual insecticide sprays—of which benzene hexachloride (BHC) is the most effective—on the walls of houses, the main habitat of the vectors. Reinfestation, however, may occur within a year or two of spraying. Preliminary work on vaccine development is underway. Transfusion infections can be prevented by serologic screening of blood donors in endemic areas and by adding gentian violet to the blood. Leukemic patients from endemic areas should be serologically screened before immunosuppressive therapy is initiated.

REFERENCES

ANDRADE ZA et al: Histopathology of the conducting tissue of the heart in Chagas' myocarditis. Am Heart J 95:316, 1978

COSSIO PM et al: Chagasic cardiomyopathy. Am J Pathol 86:533, 1977

HOFF R et al: *Trypanosoma cruzi* in the cerebrospinal fluid during the acute stage of Chagas' disease. N Engl J Med 298:604, 1978

LAMBERT PH et al: Immune complexes in serum and in cerebrospinal fluid in African trypanosomiasis. J Clin Invest 67:77, 1981

MARTINI-CAMPOS JV, TAFURI WL: Chagas' enteropathy. Gut 14:910, 1973

PUIGBO JJ et al: Diagnosis of Chagas' cardiomyopathy by noninvasive techniques. Postgrad Med J 53:527, 1977

RIBERO DOS SANTOS R, HUDSON L: *Trypanosoma cruzi:* Immunologic consequences of parasite modification of host cells. Clin Exp Immunol 40:36, 1980

SPENCER HC JR et al: Imported African trypanosomiasis in the United States. Ann Intern Med 82:633, 1977

TEIXEIRA ARL: Chagas' disease: Trends in immunological research and prospects for immunoprophylaxis. Bull WHO 57:697, 1979

VICKERMAN K: Antigenic variation in trypanosomes. Nature 273:613, 1978

221 TOXOPLASMOSIS

RIMA McLEOD
JACK S. REMINGTON

DEFINITION The term *toxoplasmosis* refers to disease caused by the obligate intracellular protozoan, *Toxoplasma gondii,* and must be differentiated from the more common asymptomatic infection caused by this organism. The infection and disease in older children and adults are discussed below. The reader is referred to the reference by Remington and Desmonts for information on congenital toxoplasmosis.

ETIOLOGY *Toxoplasma gondii* is classified among the coccidia and exists in three forms: trophozoite, cyst, and oocyst.

Trophozoites Also termed *tachyzoites,* trophozoites are crescent or oval, approximately 3 by 7 μm in size, and stain well with either Wright's stain or Giemsa's stain. Trophozoites invade all mammalian cells except nonnucleated erythrocytes and are found in tissues during the acute stage of infection.

Cysts Tissue cysts are formed within host cells and may contain thousands of organisms. They are 10 to 100 μm in size and stain well with periodic acid Schiff stain; the cyst wall stains with silver stain. Cysts are important in transmission, as they may be present in animal tissues ingested by carnivores. They may persist in virtually every organ, but skeletal and heart muscle and the central nervous system appear to be the most common sites of chronic (latent) infection.

Oocysts Oocysts are oval and 10 to 12 μm in diameter. They are formed only in the mucosal cells of the intestines of members of the cat family and are subsequently excreted in the feces. The cat is the only animal in which the organism has a sexual cycle in the intestine, and cats have systemic infection with *T. gondii* as well. The time of appearance of oocysts in the feces depends on the form of the organism with which the cat becomes infected and varies from 3 to 24 days. Excretion continues for 7 to 20 days, and as many as 10 million oocysts are shed in the feces in a single day. Except under unusual conditions, once a cat has been infected and has excreted oocysts, it will not shed oocysts again. When a cat becomes infected with *Isospora felis,* renewed oocyst excretion has been reported to occur. Sporulation, which occurs from 2 to 3 days (at 24°C) after the oocysts are excreted, is required for the oocysts to become infectious and does not occur below 4°C or above 37°C. Oocysts may remain infectious for more than 1 year under favorable conditions (e.g., in warm, moist soil). This form presumably plays a major role in transmission by the oral route since ingestion of oocysts has been shown to transmit infection.

EPIDEMIOLOGY *Toxoplasma gondii* is ubiquitous and infects herbivorous, omnivorous, and carnivorous animals, including mammals, birds, and reptiles. Prevalence of infection varies with locale; prevalence of positive serologic reaction increases with age. In the United States, approximately 5 to 30 percent of individuals 10 to 19 years old and 10 to 67 percent of individuals over 50 years old have serologic evidence of infection. Generally, less infection occurs in cold regions, in hot and arid areas, and at high elevations. No particular genetic susceptibility has been documented for humans. Epidemics of toxoplasmosis have occurred in humans and in domestic animals.

The natural mechanism of infection is by ingestion of cysts or oocysts or by transplacental transmission. Infection may also be acquired through blood transfusion, leukocyte transfusion, organ transplantation, and laboratory accident. Clinical illness due to reinfection from an exogenous source has not been reported.

Oral transmission Cysts are present in approximately 10 percent of lamb and 25 percent of pork used for human consumption; cysts have been isolated from beef, but their prevalence in beef has not been defined. Direct contact with any material contaminated by infected cat feces may result in ingestion of oocysts, and this form can be transmitted to food by insects. When humans or other animals (including cats) eat infected tissues (from any animal) or mature oocysts (excreted only by cats), the life cycle is completed. Approximately 1 percent of cats have been found to be excreting oocysts in their feces.

Transplacental transmission Accumulated data support the concept that *Toxoplasma* is transmitted to the fetus in utero when the pregnant woman acquires infection during the current pregnancy. Most often, when a mother is infected during pregnancy, the outcome is a normal uninfected infant, but spontaneous abortion, stillbirth, or delivery of a premature or full-term infected infant may result. Congenital infection will occur in approximately one-third of infants born to mothers who acquire their infection during the current pregnancy. In infants born to mothers infected during the first trimester, congenital infection is least common (approximately 17 percent) but disease is most severe; in infants born to mothers infected during the third trimester, congenital infection is most common (approximately 65 percent) but is usually asymptomatic. The fetus is at risk whether or not the infection is symptomatic in the mother.

The following are general guidelines for ascertaining the risk of transmission of the organism to the fetus of a woman who is known to have been infected *prior to the pregnancy in question.* If a woman acquires *Toxoplasma* infection more than 6 months before gestation, she will not deliver an infected infant. When conception occurs less than 6 months after acquisition of *Toxoplasma,* the risk to the fetus is exceedingly low, but transplacental transmission has been documented in this setting. *Toxoplasma* has been isolated on rare occasions from abortuses of women with chronic (latent) infection. At present, the frequency of chronic *Toxoplasma* infection as a cause of abortion has not been defined and is the subject of considerable controversy.

Transmission by blood or leukocyte transfusion or organ transplantation *Toxoplasma* may be transmitted by blood or leukocyte transfusion. The organism has been isolated from leukocytes of individuals without recognized clinical evidence of *Toxoplasma* infection, and parasitemia has been reported to persist in otherwise normal individuals for as long as 1 year after acquisition of infection. The high incidence of isolation of the organism from the blood of patients who have chronic myelogenous leukemia and high antibody titers to *Toxoplasma* is particularly noteworthy. The organism has survived for 50 days in whole citrated blood stored at 4°C. Immunodeficient patients who require multiple blood transfusions may be particularly at risk for transmission of infection by this route. *Toxoplasma* has also been transmitted by transplantation of hearts from acutely infected donors to recipients who were not previously infected with *Toxoplasma.*

PATHOGENESIS Organisms released from cysts or oocysts enter cells of the gastrointestinal tract, multiply, cause cell disruption, and then infect neighboring cells. Extracellular organisms or organisms within leukocytes are transported throughout the body via the lymphatic system and bloodstream and are capable of invading every organ and tissue. Proliferation of trophozoites usually leads to death of invaded cells, resulting in foci of necrosis, surrounded by an intense cellular reaction. The immune response of the host primarily governs the outcome of the acute process. Both humoral and cell-mediated immunity are important. In some apparently normal individuals and in immunodeficient patients, the acute infection may progress with acute necrotizing encephalitis, pneumonitis, or myocarditis which may be fatal. Trophozoites disappear from the tissues with development of the normal immune response.

A unique aspect of the infection is that organisms persist in cysts in many organs during the life span of the host. Either persistence of viable trophozoites within cells of the reticuloendothelial system or disruption of cysts may be the source of the recurrent parasitemias that occur in some asymptomatic individuals with chronic infection. Cysts are the probable origin of the organisms that cause recrudescent disease in immunocompromised patients or chorioretinitis in older children and adults with congenital toxoplasmosis.

PATHOLOGY The histopathologic changes in toxoplasmic lymphadenitis are characteristic and consist of reactive follicular hyperplasia with irregular clusters of epithelioid histiocytes that have vesicular nuclei and abundant eosinophilic cytoplasm and that encroach upon and blur the margins of germinal centers; numerous mitoses in the germinal centers; many necrotic cells and an associated focal distention of subcapsular and trabecular sinuses with monocytoid cells. Trophozoites or cysts are only rarely observed in conventionally stained sections.

Single or multiple foci of necrosis occur as the earliest manifestations of involvement of the eye. Infiltrates are composed largely of lymphocytes, plasma cells, and mononuclear phagocytic cells. There are intra- and extracellular trophozoites and cysts in the retinal lesions. Granulomatous inflammation of the choroid occurs secondary to necrotizing retinitis. Iridocyclitis, glaucoma, and cataracts may be complications of the chorioretinitis.

In cases of acute central nervous system infection, there is a focal or diffuse meningoencephalitis with necrosis and microglial nodules. Margins of areas of necrosis may be infiltrated with monocytes, lymphocytes, and plasma cells. Perivascular mononuclear inflammation frequently is present contiguous to areas of necrosis, and occasionally there is necrosis of vessel walls. Intra- and extracellular trophozoites are usually found at the periphery of areas of necrosis, and these areas of necrosis may mimic mass lesions. Cysts may be present after the first week of infection. The size of lesions and extent and location of central nervous system involvement vary considerably.

In cases of disseminated infection, pathologic changes occur in the heart, lungs, kidney, and multiple other organs. They consist of necrosis and the presence of trophozoites, cysts, and inflammatory cells alone or in combination. Glomerulonephritis with deposits of gamma-M globulin (IgM), fibrinogen, and *Toxoplasma* antigen and antibody has been reported. Involvement of the pancreas has been a prominent finding in infection in immunocompromised patients. Findings in skeletal muscle vary from parasitized fibers without pathologic changes to focal areas of infiltration to widespread myositis with necrosis.

CLINICAL MANIFESTATIONS Lymphadenopathy and other manifestations in the immunocompetent individual Lymphadenopathy is the most commonly recognized clinical manifestation of acute acquired toxoplasmosis. Cervical nodes are involved most frequently. Nodes may be single or multiple, and involvement may be symptomatic or asymptomatic. Asymptomatic lymphadenopathy may mimic lymphoma, and involvement of a pectoral node has been suspected to be carcinoma of the breast when detected on physical examination. Suboccipital, supraclavicular, axillary, inguinal, and mediastinal nodes may be involved. When mesenteric or retroperitoneal nodes are involved, abdominal pain and significant temperature elevation (e.g., up to 40°C) may occur. Involved lymph nodes vary in firmness, may be tender, do not suppurate, and are usually discrete. Confusion, malaise, fever, stiff neck, myalgias, arthralgias, headache, sore throat, maculopapular rash (which spares the palms and soles), urticaria, hepatosplenomegaly, hepatitis, or reactive lymphocytes may occur. In one epidemic, 35 of 37 individuals with serologic evidence of acute acquired *Toxoplasma* infection had signs or symptoms of infection. Although 25 individuals sought medical advice from physicians, only 3 were correctly diagnosed as having toxoplasmosis. Lymphadenopathic toxoplasmosis is self-limited, but malaise and/or lymphadenopathy may persist or recur for months.

Individuals who appear to be normal immunologically rarely may present with any of the following, alone or in combination: pneumonitis, myocarditis, pericarditis, hepatitis, polymyositis, encephalitis, or meningoencephalitis. Signs or symptoms of involvement of these organs are nonspecific. Significant morbidity has occurred, and some of these patients have died of the infection.

Ocular involvement *Toxoplasma* has been estimated to be the cause of approximately 35 percent of cases of chorioretinitis in children and adults. Although chorioretinitis has been estimated to occur in approximately 1 percent of patients with the acute acquired infection, ocular disease is most often a consequence of congenital *Toxoplasma* infection. Blurred vision, scotomas, pain, photophobia, or epiphora may be due to active chorioretinitis. If the macula is involved, impairment or loss of central vision may occur. In children, strabismus may be an early sign of chorioretinitis. Associated signs of systemic infection occur only rarely. Vision improves, but frequently visual acuity recovers only partially as inflammation subsides. Commonly, episodic flares of chorioretinitis cause destruction of irreplaceable retinal tissue. These multiple recurrences may result in glaucoma or loss of vision and ultimately may necessitate enucleation. The acute lesions appear as yellowish white, cotton-like patches that have elevated, indistinct margins surrounded by a zone of hyperemia. Inflammatory exudate in the vitreous may obscure the fundus. Older lesions characteristically appear as atrophic, whitish-gray plaques with distinct borders and black spots of choroidal pigment. Lesions usually are located near the posterior pole of the retina, although they may be peripheral. They may be single but are more commonly multiple, and lesions of varying age may be seen simultaneously. Panuveitis and papillitis with optic atrophy occur less commonly. Isolated anterior uveitis due to *Toxoplasma* infection has never been proved.

Toxoplasmosis in the immunocompromised patient All forms of toxoplasmosis that occur in normal individuals may also occur in immunocompromised individuals. Patients receiving immunosuppressive therapy for lymphoproliferative disorders (especially Hodgkin's disease), for hematologic malignancy, or for prevention of organ graft rejection have the greatest predilection for life-threatening toxoplasmosis. The untreated infection in these patients is frequently fulminant and rapidly fatal. Central nervous system involvement, present in greater than 50 percent of documented cases, is the most characteristic clinical feature of toxoplasmosis in immunocompromised patients. Therefore, the diagnosis of toxoplasmosis must be excluded in any immunosuppressed patient with symptoms or signs referable to the central nervous system. Symptoms and signs are manifestations of diffuse encephalopathy, meningoencephalitis, or cerebral mass lesions and include changes in mental status, headache, focal neurologic deficits, and seizures. Brain involvement has been established by demonstration of trophozoites in material from brain biopsy or in material aspirated from mass lesions that may have the characteristic appearance of a brain abscess on computerized tomography (CT) scan. Typically, the cerebrospinal fluid shows a mononuclear pleocytosis, a moderate elevation in protein, and a normal glucose. Immunocompromised patients also may have other nonspecific manifestations of the infection which are reflections of inflammation and necrosis of the organs involved, particularly the heart and lungs.

Toxoplasmosis and *Toxoplasma* infection in the pregnant woman *Toxoplasma* infection acquired by the mother during pregnancy is symptomatic in only about 10 to 20 percent of cases. See also "Transplacental Transmission" above.

DIAGNOSIS Acute infection with *Toxoplasma* may be diagnosed by isolation of *T. gondii* from body fluids or blood (see qualification under "Isolation Procedures" below), demonstration of trophozoites in histologic sections or in impression smears of tissue or body fluids, demonstration of characteristic lymph node histology, and serologic tests.

Isolation of the organism The organism can be isolated by inoculation of leukocytes, body fluids, or tissue specimens into tissue culture or by subcutaneous or intraperitoneal inoculation into mice. Body fluids should be processed and inoculated immediately, but blood and tissues may be stored at 4°C overnight. Freezing or treatment of specimens with formalin kills the organism. Mice should be examined for the presence of organisms in their peritoneal fluid 6 to 10 days after inoculation, or earlier if they die. Mice that survive 6 weeks should be tested for *Toxoplasma* antibody in their serum. When antibody is present, visualization of *Toxoplasma* cysts in the mouse brain establishes the diagnosis. If cysts are not demonstrable in brains of mice with *Toxoplasma* antibody, portions of brain, liver, and spleen should be inoculated into other mice.

Isolation of *T. gondii* from body fluids reflects the acute stage of infection, as does isolation from blood in most patients. Although persistent parasitemia has been described in asymptomatic individuals with latent infection, this appears to be a rare occurrence, except, perhaps, in patients with chronic myelogenous leukemia. Isolation from tissues (e.g., skeletal muscle, lung, brain, or eye) obtained by biopsy or at autopsy may reflect the presence of tissue cysts and does not prove that infection is acute.

Histologic diagnosis Demonstration of trophozoites in tissue sections or smears (e.g., brain biopsy, bone marrow aspirate) or in body fluids (e.g., cerebrospinal fluid, amniotic fluid) establishes the diagnosis of the acute infection. It is difficult to identify trophozoites by ordinary staining methods; direct and indirect immunofluorescent antibody techniques and a peroxidase-antiperoxidase (PAP) immunohistochemical staining technique have been used successfully for this purpose. Demonstration of tissue cysts does not differentiate between acute or chronic infection. When there are numerous cysts in any organ, infection is usually of recent onset. Characteristic histologic criteria establish toxoplasmic lymphadenitis (see "Pathology" above).

Serologic tests Methods most widely used to establish the diagnosis of acute *Toxoplasma* infection are the Sabin-Feldman dye test, indirect fluorescent antibody (IFA) test, and indirect hemagglutination (IHA) test. Methods that detect antigenemia, although presently experimental, are promising. Measurement of antibodies by enzyme-linked immunosorbent assay (ELISA) or radioimmunoassay is potentially valuable because these techniques may be automated.

The dye test, which measures primarily IgG antibodies, is sensitive and specific. The World Health Organization has recommended that dye test titers be expressed in international units (IU/ml) and will supply a standard reference serum.

The IFA test appears to measure the same antibodies as the dye test and is the most widely available procedure. In both tests, titers tend to be parallel. Dye test and IFA test antibodies usually appear 1 to 2 weeks after infection, reach high titers ($\geq$ 1:1000) in 6 to 8 weeks, and gradually decline over months to years; low titers (e.g., 1:4 to 1:64) commonly persist for life (Fig. 221-1). The magnitude of the antibody titer does not correlate with severity of illness.

The IgM-fluorescent antibody (IgM-IFA) test is useful in establishing the diagnosis of acute infection with *T. gondii* be-

FIGURE 221-1

Antibody response in humans to Toxoplasma *infection. IgM antibodies (— —), detectable by the IgM-IFA test, reach maximum titer within the first few weeks after infection and may decline within a few weeks (----) or persist for months (—— · ——). IgG antibodies (——), detectable by either Sabin-Feldman dye test or conventional IFA test, reach maximum titer within 2 months, plateau for months or years, and then decline, but usually persist at a low titer for life. (After G Desmonts, Feuill Biol 16:61, 1975.)*

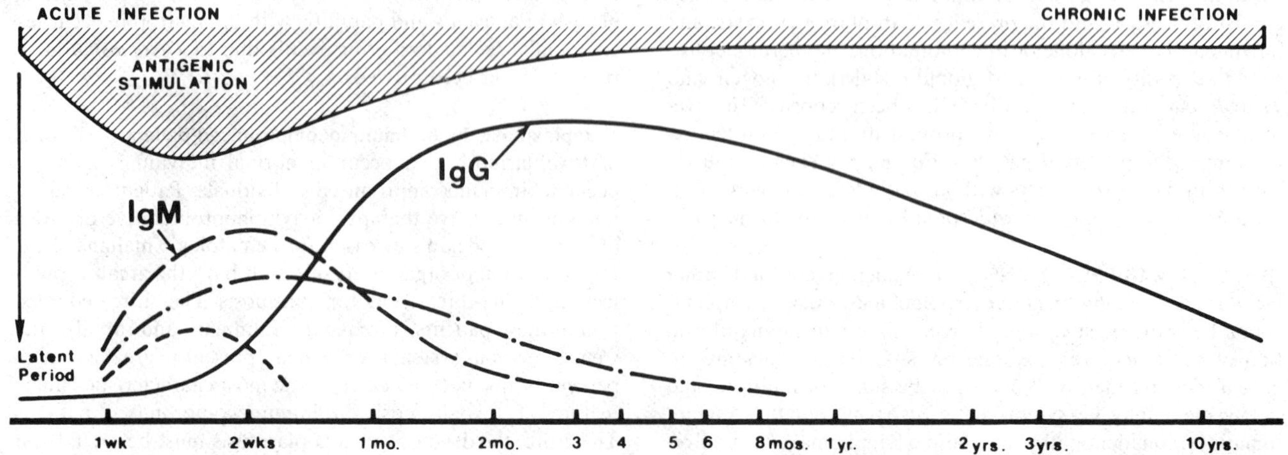

cause IgM antibodies appear early (as early as 5 days after infection) and disappear early as contrasted with gamma-G globulin (IgG) antibodies. In most cases, IgM-IFA test antibodies rise rapidly (to levels of 1:80 to ≥ 1:1000) and fall to low titers (1:10 or 1:20) or disappear within a few weeks or months (Fig. 221-1). However, in some patients they are present at low titer for as long as several years. Some immunodeficient patients with acute toxoplasmosis and most patients with only active ocular toxoplasmosis may not have IgM *Toxoplasma* antibodies. Rheumatoid factor may cause false-positive reactions in the IgM-IFA test. Removal of rheumatoid factor (e.g., by absorption) will eliminate false-positive test results in the IgM-IFA test. Antinuclear antibodies may cause false-positive reactions in both the IFA and IgM-IFA tests.

Detection of IgM antibodies by the double-sandwich ELISA is significantly more sensitive and specific than the IgM-IFA test. Rheumatoid factor and antinuclear antibodies do not cause false-positive test results. As a guideline in the adult, a serum titer of IgM antibodies against *Toxoplasma* of ≥ 1:256 in this test indicates that *Toxoplasma* infection has been acquired within the prior 5 months.

Toxoplasma antigen has been detected in serum of approximately 65 percent of adults tested who had the lymphadenopathic form of toxoplasmosis or other serologic evidence of acute acquired *Toxoplasma* infection. It was not found in serums of uninfected or chronically infected individuals. It was detected in serum, amniotic fluid, and cerebrospinal fluid of the small number of congenitally infected infants tested.

The antibodies measured in the IHA test may persist for years and are different than those measured in the IFA and dye tests. The IHA test may be helpful when titers in the IFA or dye test have stabilized since IHA test titers rise later. However, the rise in titer may occur so late that its demonstration is not helpful in diagnosis of the acute infection at a clinically pertinent time. Because of the frequency of false-negative results, the IHA test should not be used in infants with suspect congenital infection or in screening to determine if the infection has been acquired during pregnancy. Proper standardization of methodology for this and all other serologic tests is needed, as is quality control of commercial kits that are often employed by laboratories inexperienced in performing these serologic tests.

Titers in the complement fixation (CF) test also may appear several weeks later than those measured in the IFA and dye tests and also may persist for years. A negative CF test titer does not exclude acute or chronic infection, and a single positive CF test titer does not prove acute infection. A significant rise in CF test titer (i.e., of two serial dilutions performed at the same time on serums obtained several weeks apart) establishes recent infection.

Local production of antibody in active ocular or central nervous system toxoplasmosis may be demonstrated by comparing the level of *Toxoplasma* antibody in the cerebrospinal fluid or aqueous humor. Application of the following equation may be used to assess local antibody production:

$$C = \frac{\text{antibody titer in body fluid}}{\text{antibody titer in serum}} \times \frac{\text{concentration of gamma globulin in serum}}{\text{concentration of gamma globulin in body fluid}}$$

A significant correlation coefficient *(C)* is ≥ 8 and reflects local antibody production that signifies active central nervous system or ocular infection. It is usually not possible to demonstrate significant local antibody production by application of this formula if the dye test or IFA test serum titer is ≥ 1:1000.

Acute acquired *Toxoplasma* infection in the immunocompetent individual In settings in which acute acquired infection is suspected in an immunocompetent individual, a negative dye test or IFA test virtually excludes the diagnosis. The diagnosis of

TABLE 221-1
Guidelines for interpretation of commonly employed serologic tests in the diagnosis of toxoplasmosis*

	Sabin-Feldman dye test	*Indirect fluorescent antibody (IFA) test*	*Indirect fluorescent antibody test for IgM* Toxoplasma *antibodies (IgM-IFA)*	*Double-sandwich IgM-ELISA*	*Indirect hemagglutination (IHA) test*	*Complement fixation (CF) test*
Positive titer	1:4, undiluted†	1:10‡	1:2 infants‡ 1:10 adults‡	1:64‡	1:16‡	1:4‡
Titer in acute infection	≥1:1000	≥1:1000	≥1:80	≥1:256	≥1:1000	Varies among laboratories
Titer in chronic (latent) infection	1:4–1:2000	1:8–1:2000	Negative to 1:20	≥1:64	1:16–1:256	Negative to 1:8
Duration of elevation of titer	Years	Years	Weeks to months; occasionally years	Months; occasionally years	Years	Years
Special considerations	*1* No known cross-reactions or false-positive results in humans.	*1* Antibody measured is same as that measured in dye test. *2* Antinuclear antibodies may cause false-positive results.	*1* Either antinuclear antibodies or rheumatoid factor (IgM) may cause false-positive results. Rheumatoid factor may be absorbed from serum.	*1* Limited experience with this new test. *2* No cross-reaction with rheumatoid factor or antinuclear antibody if Fab_2 conjugate used.	*1* Not useful for diagnosis of congenital toxoplasmosis. *2* IHA antibodies rise later than in dye test and IFA. May be especially useful if rising IHA titer can be demonstrated.	*1* Antigen preparations have not been standardized. *2* CF antibodies also rise later than dye test and IFA; see special consideration 2 under IHA.

* *These guidelines are useful in the interpretation of test results, but exceptions to these generalizations may occur.*
† *In some cases of eye disease, the dye test may be positive only in undiluted serum.*
‡ *These values are representative, but normal values for each laboratory may differ significantly.*

recent acute acquired infection is confirmed if there is a serial two-tube rise in titer when serums drawn at 3-week intervals are run at the same time or if there is seroconversion from a negative to a positive titer (in the absence of transfer of antibody by transfusion). A single high titer in any test does not prove the presence of active infection.

Guidelines for interpretation of test results are presented below and in Table 221-1. Exceptions to these generalizations may occur.

A dye test or IFA test titer of ≥ 1:1000, a high IgM-IFA test titer (≥ 1:80), or double-sandwich IgM-ELISA titer (≥ 1:256) is probably diagnostic of recent acute infection whether or not symptoms are present. In an individual with a positive titer in the dye test or IFA test, absence of IgM-IFA test or double-sandwich IgM-ELISA antibodies almost always excludes very recent acquisition of infection.

Ocular toxoplasmosis The diagnosis of ocular toxoplasmosis in older children and adults may be difficult because the level of antibody titer in serum does not necessarily correlate with presence of active lesions in the fundus. A patient with active *Toxoplasma* chorioretinitis usually has low serologic test titers (1:4 to 1:64). If a serologic test is negative when performed on undiluted serum, for practical purposes, toxoplasmic chorioretinitis is excluded. If retinal lesions are characteristic and serologic tests are positive (see also "Serologic Tests" above), the diagnosis can be made with a high degree of confidence. If retinal lesions are atypical and serologic tests are positive, the diagnosis of toxoplasmosis is only presumptive; the high prevalence of *Toxoplasma* antibodies in the normal population precludes assumption of a causal relationship.

Active infection in the immunocompromised patient Because antibody formation may be deficient in immunocompromised patients, available serologic methods, including the IgM-IFA test, are at times insufficient for detection of active infection. Serologic tests to screen for *Toxoplasma* infection are useful in asymptomatic immunocompromised individuals in order to identify those patients who are at risk for primary infection or reactivation of latent infection (see also "Prevention" below). Detection of *Toxoplasma* antigen in serum and possibly in cerebrospinal fluid by an ELISA appears to be promising as an adjunct method for establishing the diagnosis of disseminated *Toxoplasma* infection in immunocompromised individuals.

Toxoplasmosis and *Toxoplasma* infection in the pregnant woman It seems advisable to perform serology in any woman considering becoming pregnant to determine whether she has *Toxoplasma* infection prior to pregnancy and to provide essential information when tests are performed during pregnancy (see "Transplacental Transmission" above).

In the absence of a routine screening program in which *Toxoplasma* serology is performed frequently during pregnancy, an IgM-IFA or double-sandwich IgM-ELISA test should be performed if any other serologic test is found to be positive in any titer at any time during gestation. If the IgM-IFA test or double-sandwich IgM-ELISA is not available, a repeat serologic test should be obtained in 3 weeks to determine if the titer is stable or rising. No further evaluation is necessary if the IgM-IFA test or double-sandwich IgM-ELISA is negative and an IFA or dye test titer is stable and < 1:1000 (< 300 IU). If the dye test or IFA test is ≥ 1:1000 (≥ 300 IU) and stable (regardless of titer in the IgM-IFA test), the infection should be considered to have been acquired *at least* 4 weeks earlier and probably more than 8 weeks before the serum was obtained. Thus, for practical purposes, risk to the fetus is very low if the dye test or IFA test titer is ≥ 1:1000 and stable in the first 2 months of pregnancy.

Whereas titers in the dye test or IFA test may have peaked and stabilized by 8 weeks after onset of infection, titers in the CF or IHA test may continue to rise for 4 to 6 months or longer after acquisition of infection. Therefore, rises in these latter two tests may not be helpful in defining when infection occurred relative to the time of conception and should not be used as the sole test for this purpose.

A common problem arises when an asymptomatic woman is tested for *Toxoplasma* antibody late in the first trimester or in the second trimester of pregnancy and her IFA or dye test titer is found to be in the vicinity of 1:2000, her IgM-IFA test or double-sandwich IgM-ELISA titer is found to be negative, and no significant rise in titer in any test is demonstrable. It is not possible to establish whether infection occurred before, at, or after conception in this situation. Detection of *Toxoplasma* antigen in amniotic fluid may become a useful adjunct in determining whether the fetus of a woman who acquired *Toxoplasma* during the current pregnancy is infected. Its use in this setting is experimental at this time, however.

THERAPY Therapy in specific clinical settings The need for and duration of therapy are determined by the clinical severity of illness and by the underlying medical problem.

Most immunologically normal patients with lymphadenopathic toxoplasmosis do not require specific treatment. Indication for treatment in these cases is severe and persistent symptoms. Evidence of serious damage to vital organs is also an indication for therapy. Infections acquired via transfusions or in laboratory accidents may be more severe than naturally acquired infections and probably should be treated.

Patients with active chorioretinitis should be treated with specific therapy. When there is potential for serious visual impairment secondary to macular or optic nerve involvement, corticosteroids are added to the regimen.

Because of the high mortality rate associated with toxoplasmosis in patients whose resistance to infection is compromised by underlying disease or by therapy (e.g., corticosteroids or cytotoxic drugs), toxoplasmosis should be treated in all immunocompromised individuals. In immunocompromised patients, serologic evidence of acute infection (with or without signs and symptoms of infection) or demonstration of trophozoites in tissue (with or without serologic test titers or signs and symptoms) is an indication for therapy. Improvement has been reported to occur in the majority of patients to whom specific therapy was administered. Considering the diagnosis early enough to institute treatment is the major problem.

When a pregnant woman who acquired infection at any time during pregnancy is treated, the chance of congenital infection in her infant is decreased but not eliminated. In separate series reported from France and Germany, treatment decreased the incidence of infection significantly. The drugs employed were spiramycin in the study from France and pyrimethamine plus sulfonamide in the study from Germany. Spiramycin (not available in the United States) has been used safely for treatment in the first trimester. Pyrimethamine is a potential teratogen; therefore, sulfadiazine (which is highly effective in animal models when used alone) should be used alone if a decision is made to treat during the first trimester of pregnancy. When infection occurs during the first trimester, some authorities have recommended therapeutic abortion because of the high probability of severe damage when infection occurs early in fetal life. Other authorities recommend treatment rather than abortion because the risk of transmission of the infection to the fetus is low (approximately 15 percent) in the first trimester and because the incidence of congenital toxoplasmosis can be reduced significantly by intrapartum therapy. They reason that drug therapy would result in saving a significant number of healthy fetuses. The decision about the mode of therapy ultimately must be made by both the well-informed physician and the well-informed patient who must be aware of the risks. Carefully controlled studies are needed to define whether a pregnant woman who has *Toxoplasma* antibody and a history of habitual abortion will benefit from treatment.

Pyrimethamine plus sulfadiazine or trisulfapyrimidines In vivo, pyrimethamine and sulfadiazine act synergistically against *Toxoplasma.* Clinical experience confirms the efficacy of this combination. Comparative tests have shown that sulfapyrazine, sulfamethazine, and sulfamerazine are about as effective as sulfadiazine. In general, other sulfonamides are much less effective.

Pyrimethamine In adults, a loading dose of 100 to 200 mg pyrimethamine is given orally in two divided doses on the first day of treatment. In young children, a loading dose of 2 mg per kilogram of body weight (not to exceed adult loading dose) is given for the first 2 to 3 days of treatment. The maintenance dose is 1 mg per kilogram of body weight (with a maximum of 25 mg) in a single dose. In view of the drug's half-life of 4 to 5 days, administration of the maintenance dose at 3- to 4-day intervals has been suggested. Daily administration is recommended for the patient who is very ill, since there are no data concerning absorption of the drug in this situation. Daily therapy is also recommended for active ocular infection. Pyrimethamine is available only in tablet form.

Pyrimethamine is a folic acid antagonist and produces a dose-related, usually gradual, and reversible depression of the bone marrow. Anemia, leukopenia, and thrombocytopenia may occur. Platelet and peripheral blood cell counts should be evaluated twice weekly in any patient receiving pyrimethamine.

Folinic acid To prevent suppression of the bone marrow, folinic acid (calcium leucovorin) is administered in conjunction with pyrimethamine therapy. Optimal frequency for administration of folinic acid has not been established. A single oral dose of 5 to 10 mg daily is recommended. If folinic acid is not available, bakers' yeast (3 to 4 cakes daily) may be used to prevent toxicity due to pyrimethamine. Neither folinic acid nor bakers' yeast inhibits the action of pyrimethamine on *T. gondii,* whereas folic acid does.

Sulfadiazine and trisulfapyrimidines The loading dose is 50 to 75 mg per kilogram of body weight; thereafter, a total daily dose of 75 to 100 mg per kilogram of body weight is administered in four divided doses at intervals of approximately 6 h. Tablet and liquid oral forms as well as an intravenous form of sulfadiazine are available. The potential toxicities of sulfonamides (e.g., crystalluria, hematuria, and rash) must be carefully monitored.

Other drugs Trimethoprim alone or in combination with a sulfonamide has not been proved to be effective in treatment of toxoplasmosis in humans, but the activity of this combination in vitro and in vivo in animal models warrants carefully designed and controlled clinical trials. This combination is significantly less active than the combination of pyrimethamine with sulfadiazine.

Duration of therapy Optimal duration of specific therapy has not been defined for any form of toxoplasmosis. Specific therapy should be continued for 4 to 6 weeks in a patient who appears to be immunologically normal but who requires treatment for severe and persistent symptoms or evidence of damage to vital organs (e.g., chorioretinitis, myocarditis). Longer treatment may be necessary.

It seems advisable to treat an immunocompromised patient for at least 4 to 6 weeks *beyond* complete resolution of all signs and symptoms of active disease. Careful follow-up of these patients is imperative because relapse may occur and requires prompt reinstitution of therapy. Although therapy may be effective against *T. gondii* trophozoites and may induce a beneficial clinical response, it does not eradicate cysts from the central nervous system.

Desmonts and Couvreur suggest that an acutely infected pregnant woman should be treated with spiramycin and use a total dose of 2 to 3 daily, administered orally in four divided doses. A 3-week course of treatment is alternated with 2 weeks without treatment from the time of diagnosis until term. Another treatment regimen was used in Germany and consisted of a course of sulfonamide and pyrimethamine followed by one or two courses of sulfonamide administered alone or in combination with pyrimethamine. Each course of therapy was given for approximately 2 weeks and was alternated with a 3- to 4-week interval without treatment. Pyrimethamine was not administered during the first trimester of pregnancy.

PREVENTION Measures for prevention of infection involve intervention in the cycle of transmission and are most important for immunodeficient patients and seronegative pregnant women. To kill cysts, meat should be heated to 60°C or frozen at −20°C. (Freezers available commercially do not reach or maintain this temperature reliably.) Hands should be washed after touching uncooked meat, and fruits and vegetables that may be contaminated with oocysts should be washed. Dry heat (66°C) or boiling water renders oocysts noninfectious. Contact with cat feces should be avoided.

There are no definitive data to allow for a firm recommendation regarding the use of whole blood, leukocyte transfusions, or organ transplants when a donor is seropositive for *Toxoplasma* antibodies. It seems reasonable, however, that whenever feasible, blood or blood products donated by an individual with *Toxoplasma* antibody should not be used in an immunosuppressed individual, and an organ transplanted to a seronegative recipient should be from an individual without serologic evidence of *Toxoplasma* infection.

A nontoxic drug that eliminates the organism in the cyst as well as the trophozoite form is needed for prophylaxis against the devastating complications of recrudescent infection in immunocompromised individuals.

See "Therapy in Specific Clinical Settings" above for guidelines concerning prevention of transmission to the fetus.

At present, no effective vaccine to prevent infection with *Toxoplasma* has been developed. Development of a vaccine for use in nonimmune women of childbearing age should be explored since maternal immunity appears to prevent congenital transmission of *T. gondii.* Vaccines that prevent oocyst development in cats could prove valuable by interrupting the life cycle of *T. gondii.*

REFERENCES

Araujo FG, Remington JS: Antigenemia in recently acquired acute toxoplasmosis. J Infect Dis 141:144, 1980

Conley FK, Remington JS: *Toxoplasma gondii* infection of the central nervous system. Use of the PAP method to demonstrate *Toxoplasma* in formalin-fixed paraffin-embedded tissue sections. Hum Pathol 12:690, 1981

Dorfman RF, Remington JS: Value of lymph node biopsy in the diagnosis of acute acquired toxoplasmosis. N Engl J Med 289:878, 1973

Dubey JP et al: Characterization of the new fecal form of *Toxoplasma gondii.* J Parasitol 56:447, 1970

Kimball AC et al: Congenital toxoplasmosis: A prospective study of 4048 obstetric patients. Am J Obstet Gynecol 111:211, 1971

Naot Y et al: Method for avoiding false-positive results occurring in immunoglobulin M enzyme-linked immunosorbent assays due to presence of both rheumatoid factor and antinuclear antibodies. J Clin Microbiol 14:73, 1981

O'Connor GR: Manifestations and management of ocular toxoplasmosis. Bull NY Acad Med 50:192, 1974

Remington JS, Desmonts G: Toxoplasmosis, in *Infectious Diseases of the Fetus and Newborn Infant,* JS Remington, JO Klein (eds). Philadelphia, Saunders, 1982

Ruskin J, Remington JS: Toxoplasmosis in the compromised host. Ann Intern Med 84:193, 1976

Townsend JJ et al: Acquired toxoplasmosis. Arch Neurol 32:335, 1975

222
PNEUMOCYSTIS CARINII PNEUMONIA (PNEUMOCYSTOSIS, INTERSTITIAL PLASMA CELL PNEUMONIA)

JOEL D. MEYERS

DEFINITION *Pneumocystis carinii* pneumonia is a disease of the compromised host which occurs in two settings: as an epidemic illness among premature or debilitated infants and as a sporadic illness among immunosuppressed children or adults. Both forms are often fatal if untreated.

ETIOLOGY *Pneumocystis carinii* is generally accepted as being a protozoan. The organism seen in human beings is morphologically similar to that in animals, but species-specific differences may exist. Maintenance or growth of *P. carinii* in vitro has been accomplished in a number of cell lines, including both human and chick embryonic lung cells, and these studies have expanded knowledge of the life cycle. There are three major forms including 1- to 5-μm trophozoites, 1- to 1.5-μm sporozoites, and cyst forms averaging 5 μm in diameter. Mature cysts are thick-walled and contain up to eight sporozoites. Some cysts are crescent-shaped owing either to incomplete development of the sporozoites or partial collapse of the cyst after excystment of the sporozoites. Following release, the sporozoites develop into mature trophozoites which contain a nucleus, mitochondria, and endoplasmic reticulum, and appear to be eukaryotes. Trophozoites attach to host cells by means of pseudopodal extensions and in this way may obtain nutrients, after which the host cell degenerates. An intracellular form has not been clearly established.

EPIDEMIOLOGY The incidence of *P. carinii* infection is uncertain though serologic studies show that up to 75 percent of children develop detectable antibody by 2 to 4 years of age. This suggests that while disease due to *P. carinii* is rare, *P. carinii* infection may be common. In humans the disease is worldwide and occurs in all age groups either as epidemics in crowded nurseries or as sporadic cases among older children and adults. Most sporadic cases are thought to be due to reactivation of *P. carinii* organisms from latent sites in the lung, but the exact state and site of latency are unknown and cysts are occasionally found in the lungs of patients dying of other causes without evidence of pneumonia. Epidemics in nurseries as well as clustering of cases in cancer wards suggest the possibility of airborne or respiratory spread, as does the presence of high antibody titers among patient care personnel and the isolated reports of intrafamily spread. Virtually all cases in the United States occur among patients with underlying immunodeficiency, though cases are also found among young, debilitated southeast Asian refugees. Intrauterine infection acquired transplacentally has also been reported.

PATHOGENESIS Immunodeficiency is the common denominator for the development of *P. carinii* pneumonia. Disease may be produced in laboratory rats by starvation or by treatment with either corticosteroids or cyclophosphamide. Disease occurring during the first year of life in humans is associated with either protein-calorie malnutrition (epidemic disease) or congenital immunodeficiency of either the cellular or humoral types (sporadic disease). In older children and adults *P. carinii* pneumonia is associated with acquired immunodeficiency, related either to the underlying disease or secondary to cytotoxic or immunosuppressive therapy. The risk of *P. carinii* among children with acute lymphocytic leukemia varies directly with the intensity of chemotherapy, and clinical manifestations in these children commonly occur during periods of remission. In some patients, symptoms begin after steroid withdrawal, and *P. carinii* pneumonia after allogeneic marrow transplantation generally occurs a month or more after initial hematologic recovery. These observations suggest either an obligatory "incubation period" or the need for a partially intact inflammatory response for the production of clinical symptomatology.

The normal immune response to *P. carinii* is unknown. Although *P. carinii* pneumonia is usually associated with dysfunction of the cellular immune system, cases have also been described in children with isolated humoral immunodeficiency as well as in patients without an apparent underlying disease. Recent studies suggest that antibody is important in opsonization and phagocytosis of the organism by macrophages.

The simultaneous occurrence of pneumonia caused by *P. carinii* and other viral, bacterial, and fungal agents is relatively frequent. Combined infection with cytomegalovirus is especially common after organ transplantation, which may be due to either the coincidence of two frequent infections in these patient groups or to an immunosuppressive effect of cytomegalovirus infection itself (see Chap. 211). *P. carinii* infection has been reported in male homosexuals, many of whom were also ingesting, injecting, or inhaling habituating drugs. In a number of instances, infections with other agents including herpes simplex virus, cytomegalovirus, and *Toxoplasma* were present as well. This syndrome, which is associated with *Kaposi's sarcoma* in some patients, is associated with a high mortality. It is discussed in more detail in Chap. 64.

PATHOLOGY Pathologic findings vary depending on whether the pneumonia is of the sporadic or epidemic variety and on the ability of the host to mount an inflammatory response. In the classic epidemic illness there is a foamy honeycombed intraalveolar exudate consisting of masses of cysts and desquamated alveolar cells and an interstitial (septal) infiltrate of plasma cells and lymphocytes. A polymorphonuclear leukocyte alveolar infiltrate is rare in the absence of concomitant bacterial infection. In the sporadic disease, consolidation may be focal rather than diffuse, and the foamy alveolar exudate may be absent. Lymphocytes remain a predominant part of the septal infiltrate, but plasma cells are few or absent. "Atypical" features include interstitial thickening and fibrosis, hyaline membranes, and epithelioid granulomas. Multinucleated giant cells in the absence of other demonstrable organisms, diffuse interstitial infiltrates, and calcification also occur. In latent infections the number of organisms is small and the cellular response sparse. The infection is generally confined to the lung, but organisms have occasionally been found in regional lymph nodes. Pleuritis is characteristically absent, and systemic dissemination of organisms to distant sites is extremely rare. Special stains are needed to demonstrate the organism in tissues or secretions. The cyst form stains best with methanamine silver or toluidine blue O, while the trophozoites stain with polychrome stains such as Gram-Weigert or Giemsa. The organism cannot be detected by Gram's stain or by hematoxylin-eosin stain.

CLINICAL MANIFESTATIONS The sporadic disease in the immunosuppressed child or adult usually has an abrupt onset. Fever, cough, tachypnea, and shortness of breath appear early in the illness, followed by radiologic evidence of pneumonia. Radiologic abnormalities or cough without fever may occasionally precede other signs or symptoms. Fever may be persistent or spiking and as high as 38 to 40°C. Cyanosis is a late sign, though most patients are hypoxemic at the time of diagnosis and develop progressive hypoxemia. The cough is typically nonproductive, but mononuclear cells may be present in scanty expectorated sputum. Auscultatory signs are minimal even in extensive disease. In contrast, the epidemic form is insidious in onset, with nonspecific signs such as restlessness and poor feeding. Symptoms progress over several weeks to tachypnea, dyspnea, intercostal retractions, and cyanosis, but even then fever may be minimal or absent.

The classic early radiologic finding is a hazy perihilar infiltrate spreading to the periphery and appearing predominantly interstitial. The diffuse alveolar nature of the process becomes apparent with time as the infiltrate coalesces and air bronchograms develop. Many variants have been described including segmental infiltrates, localized nodular densities, and asymmetric alveolar infiltrates. The radiologic presentation may be modified by the patient's underlying illness or its treatment (e.g., lung irradiation) or by concomitant infections. Significant pleural effusions and hilar adenopathy are rare and should suggest an alternate diagnosis. Other laboratory studies are unrevealing. The white blood cell count may be normal or slightly elevated, though both lymphopenia and eosinophilia have been reported, the latter usually among children with immunodeficiency syndromes. Elevated cold agglutinin titers have also been observed, but their significance is uncertain.

The differential diagnosis includes other infectious pneumonias, particularly cytomegalovirus, disseminated pulmonary aspergillosis, and occasionally other bacterial and mycotic agents, pulmonary alveolar proteinosis, desquamative interstitial pneumonia, pulmonary hemorrhage, congestive heart failure (with normal heart size), and pulmonary fibrosis, either idiopathic or secondary to radiation or drugs such as bleomycin, methotrexate, busulfan, cyclophosphamide, or nitrofurantoin.

DIAGNOSIS The diagnosis requires the morphologic demonstration of the organism in tissues or secretions. A variety of techniques for obtaining lung tissue have been described as having varying degrees of success. Bronchial brushings, transbronchial needle or forceps biopsy, needle aspiration of the lung, and transthoracic needle biopsy have all been successful, but all include some risk of pneumothorax or bleeding and may be falsely negative. *P. carinii* organisms have also been demonstrated in sputum, gastric aspirates, endotracheal aspirates, and fluid from bronchopulmonary lavage. The most reliable means of diagnosis has been open-lung biopsy, which requires intubation, general anesthesia, and a chest tube but allows visualization and sampling of involved areas of the lung and direct control of intraoperative bleeding. In experienced hands the complication rate with this procedure is low even in seriously ill patients. If the diagnosis cannot be established within 24 to 48 h by alternate procedures, then open-lung biopsy must be considered, and the cooperation of surgeons and pathologists who are familiar with both the patient population and the need for rapid diagnosis will allow the collection of optimal specimens with minimal complications. Examination of touch preparations or frozen sections of tissue obtained at biopsy may provide a diagnosis even before permanent sections are available. Appropriate positive and negative controls should always be included.

Detection of antibody by indirect immunofluorescence has not been useful in the diagnosis of sporadic *P. carinii* infection since both patients and normal persons may have detectable antibody. The presence of antibody may be useful in diagnosing infants at risk of epidemic *P. carinii* infection, however. Circulating *P. carinii* antigen has been detected by counterimmunoelectrophoresis in the serum of patients with proven infection, and antigenemia disappears during successful treatment. However, antigen has also been found in the serum of children without pneumonia and of adults with other types of pneumonia or who have received total-body irradiation. The meaning of these observations is unclear, and the usefulness of detecting pneumocystis antigen remains to be established.

PROGNOSIS There appears to be little direct morbidity attributable to the asymptomatic acquisition of pneumocystis during childhood. The prognosis from sporadic *P. carinii* pneumonia in the compromised host is serious, and mortality rates are 90 to 100 percent without treatment. Even with the availability of effective chemotherapeutic agents, 20 to 40 percent of patients will die, and delays in diagnosis may contribute to this mortality. By comparison, the mortality rate in epidemic infantile disease is lower, although approximately 50 percent die without treatment.

TREATMENT Two drugs are currently available for the treatment of *P. carinii* pneumonia, pentamidine isethionate given intramuscularly and the fixed combination of trimethoprim and sulfamethoxazole given orally. An intravenous preparation of trimethoprim-sulfamethoxazole is available on an investigational basis. The combination of pyrimethamine and sulfadiazine has also been used, but experience with it is limited. All these agents inhibit folate metabolism.

The recommended daily dose of pentamidine is 4 mg/kg given as a single intramuscular injection for 14 days. Nearly half of patients receiving pentamidine develop side effects, including azotemia, changes in liver function, and hypoglycemia as well as local reactions. Immediate side effects such as hypotension and tachycardia occur infrequently. Trimethoprim-sulfamethoxazole is given in doses of 20 mg trimethoprim per kilogram and 100 mg sulfamethoxazole per kilogram of body weight per day, given orally or intravenously in four divided doses for 14 days. Common side effects include rash and nausea. Leukopenia, due either to trimethoprim-sulfamethoxazole or treatment of the underlying illness, has been observed. However, the efficacy of trimethoprim-sulfamethoxazole against *P. carinii* when used concomitantly with folinic acid has not been established and cannot be recommended routinely.

The response rates to pentamidine or trimethoprim-sulfamethoxazole in comparative trials in children were equal at approximately 75 percent, though one-third of patients were changed to the alternative drug after 3 or more days of treatment. Response to treatment is usually slow, with defervescence often occurring in not less than 4 days and radiologic improvement in not less than 10 days. Because of this slow response, early changes in the treatment regimen may be unnecessary for most patients. Serum levels of trimethoprim or sulfamethoxazole should be measured in patients treated with oral trimethoprim-sulfamethoxazole, especially among those who are critically ill and who may have impaired drug absorption. Trimethoprim serum levels of 3 to 5 μg/ml or sulfamethoxazole levels of 100 to 150 μg/ml drawn 2 h after an oral dose are optimal, and if such levels cannot be reached with oral administration, then treatment with either intravenous trimethoprim-sulfamethoxazole or pentamidine should be considered. In animal studies, the use of pentamidine and trimethoprim-sulfamethoxazole together was no more effective than trimethoprim-sulfamethoxazole alone, while treatment with trimethoprim alone was ineffective.

PREVENTION Daily oral administration of low-dose trimethoprim-sulfamethoxazole (5 mg/kg of trimethoprim and 25 mg/kg of sulfamethoxazole per day in two divided doses) will prevent the development of *P. carinii* pneumonia in high-risk patients such as those receiving maintenance chemotherapy with multiple drugs, those who have received marrow transplants, or those who have recovered from *P. carinii* pneumonia. Long-term administration has resulted in few significant adverse effects, though oral candidiasis or leukopenia has occurred in some patients. Prophylaxis is effective only during the period of drug administration, and animal studies have shown that the organism is not eradicated by such treatment. The effectiveness of trimethoprim alone is unknown. Patients being treated for *P. carinii* pneumonia should be in respiratory isolation to prevent possible nosocomial spread of the organism to other compromised patients.

REFERENCES

BURKE BA, GOOD RA: *Pneumocystis carinii* infection. Medicine 57:23, 1973

DOPPMAN JL et al: Atypical radiographic features in *Pneumocystis carinii* pneumonia. Radiology 114:39, 1975

GOTTLIEB MS et al: *Pneumocystis carinii* pneumonia and mucosal candidiasis in previously healthy homosexual men. N Engl J Med 305:1425, 1981

HUGHES WT et al: Successful chemoprophylaxis for *Pneumocystis carinii* pneumonitis. N Engl J Med 297:1419, 1977

——— et al: Comparison of pentamidine isethionate and trimethoprim-sulfamethoxazole in the treatment of *Pneumocystis carinii* pneumonia. J Pediatr 92:285, 1978

MASUR H et al: An outbreak of community-acquired *Pneumocystis carinii* pneumonia. N Engl J Med 305:1431, 1981

MEYERS JD et al: The value of *Pneumocystis carinii* antibody and antigen detection for the diagnosis of *Pneumocystis carinii* pneumonia after marrow transplantation. Am Rev Resp Dis 120:1283, 1979

PIFER LL et al: Propagation of *Pneumocystis carinii in vitro.* Pediatr Res 11:305, 1977

——— et al: *Pneumocystis carinii* infection: Evidence for high prevalence in normal and immunosuppressed children. Pediatrics 61:35, 1978

WEBER WR et al: Lung biopsy in *Pneumocystis carinii* pneumonia. Am J Clin Pathol 67:11, 1977

WINSTON DJ et al: Trimethoprim-sulfamethoxazole for the treatment of *Pneumocystis carinii* pneumonia. Ann Intern Med 92:762, 1980

223

BABESIOSIS

JAMES J. PLORDE

DEFINITION AND HISTORY Known since biblical times, this cosmopolitan infection of domestic and wild animals is caused by protozoa of the genus *Babesia.* These organisms are transmitted by ticks, multiply in red blood cells, and produce an acute febrile hemolytic anemia, the most prominent manifestation of which is hemoglobinuria. The parasite was first described by Babes in 1888 and demonstrated to be tick-borne by Theobald Smith in 1893. This marked the first time a blood-feeding arthropod was implicated in the transmission of a pathogen to a vertebrate host, antedating Ross' description of malaria transmission by 5 years.

EPIDEMIOLOGY AND CLINICAL MANIFESTATIONS The first human infection was described in Yugoslavia by Skrabalo in 1957. This and six other European cases were particularly severe with high fever, hemoglobinuria, jaundice, and renal failure. In both their clinical presentation and in the presence of small intraerythrocytic parasites they closely resembled falciparum malaria with which they were originally confused. All seven occurred in splenectomized patients and five ended fatally. The causative agents were bovine parasites (*B. bovis, B. divergens*). Some 100 cases have now been documented in the United States. Two California cases resembled the European infections and were thought to be caused by equine babesia. The remaining cases have been acquired during the summer months on Cape Cod and the offshore islands lying between New York and Massachusetts, including Long Island, Shelter Island, Nantucket, and Martha's Vineyard. All were caused by a rodent parasite, *B. microti,* and, with few exceptions, occurred in patients with intact spleens. The patients experienced a prolonged illness characterized by the insidious onset of fever, chills, sweating, myalgia, and mild to moderate hemolytic anemia. The physical examination was usually negative except for occasional splenomegaly. Most patients were over 50 years of age and all but one recovered. The carrier state persisted for weeks to months in some patients and in three resulted in subsequent transfusion-induced infections. Two of the three recipients were asplenic; the third was an elderly individual who represents the only fatality in the series. Serologic studies suggest that mild or asymptomatic cases occur with some frequency.

B. microti has been found in field moles and deer mice in New York State, Utah, and California. On the offshore islands of New England, however, the principal reservoir is the white-footed mouse. The northern deer tick, *Ixodes dammini,* serves as a vector. This hard-bodied tick takes a blood meal during each of its three developmental stages: larva, nymph, and adult. Rodents are the principal hosts of the first two stages while deer host the adult ticks. Only the nymphs, which feed from May through September, are capable of transmitting *B. microti* to humans. Since the engorged nymph measures 2 mm in diameter, infested patients may be oblivious to its presence. Transovarial transmission does not occur.

DIAGNOSIS The diagnosis depends on the demonstration of the intraerythrocytic parasite in Giemsa-stained peripheral blood smears. Like malaria parasites, these organisms measure 2 to 3 μm in diameter and demonstrate red-staining nuclear material with blue cytoplasm. In some cases band forms resembling *Plasmodium malariae* may be seen. In contrast to malaria parasites, however, neither gametocytes nor pigment can be demonstrated. Unique basket shapes and tetrads produced by budding are also helpful distinguishing characteristics. In heavy infections, organisms can be seen outside red blood cells. Serologic diagnosis can be made with the indirect fluorescent antibody test. Because the disease is insidious in onset, most infected patients have titers $\geq$1024 at the time they present for medical care. There is no correlation between disease severity and the titer level; cross-reactions with other *Babesia* species and malaria may be seen, but titers with homologous antigens are generally higher. Active infections have been demonstrated in smear-negative, serology-positive infections by inducing infection in experimental animals.

TREATMENT There are no satisfactory drugs available for the treatment of this infection. Mild disease should be managed symptomatically with antipyretics. If significant hemolysis ensues, transfusion may be warranted. In more severe infections specific therapy should be attempted. Although chloroquine provides symptomatic improvement, it appears to have little activity against this parasite. Quinine and clindamycin therapy has been successful in one patient. Antitrypanosomal agents also appear effective, and, in life-threatening infections, pentamidine should be considered. This agent appears to be effective in controlling the clinical manifestations of babesiosis and decreasing parasitemia; it may not eradicate the organism. Exchange transfusions are similarly helpful in fulminant infections.

PREVENTION The prevention of *B. microti* infections in humans is difficult. Individuals summering on the offshore islands of New England should consider the use of insect repellents containing diethyltoluamide and examine themselves daily for the presence of the 2- to 3-m nymphs. A pilot tick control program has been initiated on one of the islands.

REFERENCES

Bredt A et al: Treatment of babesiosis in asplenic patients. JAMA 245:1938, 1981

Chisholm ES et al: *Babesia microti* infection in man: Evaluation of an indirect immunofluorescent antibody test. Am J Med Hyg 27:14, 1978

Dammin GJ et al: Babesiosis, in *Seminars in Infectious Diseases*, L Weinstein, J Fields (eds). New York, Stratton Intercontinental Medical Book, 1978, pp 169–199

———: The rising incidence of clinical *Babesia microti* infections. Hum Pathol 12:398, 1981

Francioli PB et al: Response of babesiosis to pentamidine therapy. Ann Intern Med 94:326, 1981

Jacoby GA et al: Treatment of transfusion-transmitted babesiosis by exchange transfusion. N Engl J Med 303:1098, 1980

Miller LH et al: Failure of chloroquine in human babesiosis (*Babesia microti*). Ann Intern Med 88:200, 1978

Ruebush TK II et al: Development and persistence of antibody in persons with *Babesia microti*. Am J Trop Med Hyg 30:291, 1981

——— et al: Epidemiology of human babesiosis on Nantucket Island. Am J Trop Med Hyg 30:937, 1981

224 GIARDIASIS

JAMES J. PLORDE

ETIOLOGY AND EPIDEMIOLOGY *Giardia lamblia* is a pear-shaped multiflagellar protozoan that parasitizes the human duodenum and jejunum where it multiplies by longitudinal fission. Under a microscope, its two nuclei and central parabasal body give the organism the appearance of a face with two large eyes. It is actively motile but can attach itself to the intestinal mucosa by means of a large ventral sucker. Unattached trophozoites may be carried in the fecal stream to the large bowel. If their passage through the gut is hurried, they will exit unchanged in the liquid stool and perish rapidly. With normal colonic transit times, however, the organisms retract their flagella, envelop themselves in a protective membrane, and undergo nuclear division. The resulting quadrinucleate cysts are infectious and may be transmitted to new hosts by a number of fecal-oral routes. Cysts deposited in cold water can survive for more than 2 months and have been shown to be resistant to chlorine concentrations (0.4 mg per liter) routinely used in community purification systems. The ingestion of water contaminated with as few as 10 cysts is sufficient to establish human infection. Not surprisingly, waterborne outbreaks have been documented repeatedly in the United States during the past two decades. They have involved campers who have drunk from remote surface waters, skiers who have used well water, and ordinary citizens served by chlorinated municipal systems. Contamination of the water supply with raw sewage has been found in several outbreaks. In others, *G. lamblia*-infected beavers were located within the watershed, suggesting that these mammals may serve as alternate reservoirs. Waterborne cysts are also thought to be responsible for the high incidence of giardiasis in travelers returning from third-world countries. Food may also serve as a transmission vehicle in these areas as well.

Direct person-to-person spread occurs with some frequency. This is most dramatically evident among male homosexuals practicing anilingus and groups of ambulatory, non-toilet trained children. It also appears to be responsible for the secondary cases seen in families of infected children.

Giardiasis is a cosmopolitan infection that is particularly common in areas with poor sanitation and among populations unable to maintain adequate levels of hygiene. In the United States, *G. lamblia* is found in 4 percent of stools submitted for parasitologic examination, making it the most frequently identified intestinal parasite. Young children are three times more likely to be involved than adults; the prevalence may be particularly high among toddlers attending day-care centers and the institutionalized retarded where rates exceeding 50 percent have been reported. Giardiasis is also frequent in individuals with immunoglobulin deficiencies and may be a major cause of intestinal abnormalities in this population. It has been suggested that the parasite is able to persist in such patients because of a relative deficiency of secretory IgA.

Among adults, parasitism is common in travelers and campers, but the precise prevalence in these populations is unknown. Achlorhydric individuals may be more susceptible to infection. Several studies have emphasized the association between male homosexuality and intestinal parasitosis; infection rates for *G. lamblia* and/or *E. histolytica* have ranged from 11 to 40 percent. In a New York study, all nontraveled immunocompetent males with giardiasis were, in fact, homosexual.

PATHOLOGY AND PATHOGENESIS Clinical manifestations appear to be caused by an impairment of the absorptive capacity of the gut, particularly for fat and carbohydrates. The mechanism responsible for these changes is unknown. Mechanical blockage of the intestinal mucosa by large numbers of trophozoites, altered jejunal mobility with or without overgrowth of Enterobacteriaceae or yeasts, and organism-induced deconjugation of bile salts have been implicated. None, however, correlates well with disease severity, and eradication of associated microorganisms does not result in clinical improvement. Disaccharidase deficiency with lactose intolerance, altered levels of peptide hydrolyase and enteropeptidase, and decreased vitamin B_{12} absorption indicate that *G. lamblia* produces direct or indirect damage to the microvillar structure of the small bowel. Mechanical irritation to the fuzzy coat by the trophozoite's sucking disk might induce an accelerated turnover of the mucosal epithelium, resulting in functional immaturity of the transport systems. Alternatively, mucosal invasion may provoke a T-cell-mediated insult to the jejunal mucosa. In experimentally infected nude mice immunologic reconstitution with lymphoid cells from previously infected animals results in marked mucosal changes including cellular infiltration and a decreased villus/crypt ratio. Similar pathologic findings have been reported in humans with giardial malabsorption. Both the structural changes and the malabsorption are reversible with specific therapy.

Although reinfection is common, the frequent occurrence of giardiasis in patients with immunologic defects, and the rarity with which it is seen in older adults, suggest that protective immunity, albeit incomplete, does develop with time.

CLINICAL MANIFESTATIONS In endemic situations, over two-thirds of infected patients may be asymptomatic. This ratio is usually reversed in point-source outbreaks. From 1 to 3 weeks after exposure, the patient notes the explosive onset of watery diarrhea. The stool is foul smelling, greasy in appearance, and floats on the toilet water. There is neither blood nor mucus. Abdominal cramping is present and, in contrast to most other causes of diarrhea, is epigastric in location. The formation of large quantities of intestinal gas produces distention, sulfuric eructation, and flatulence. Anorexia, nausea, vomiting, and low-grade fever may be present. Typically, acute symptoms continue for at least 5 to 7 days. In an occasional patient, they may persist for months, leading to significant malabsorption and weight loss. More commonly, the illness resolves spontaneously in 1 to 4 weeks or lapses into a chronic phase characterized by intermittent bouts of flatulence, epigastric pain, and the passage of mushy stools. It is not unusual for patients to present in this fashion without having experienced the more acute manifestations described above. Eventually, both parasites and symptoms disappear. Lactose intolerance, however, may persist, producing a clinical picture easily confused with the parasitologic disease and subjecting the patient to unnecessary therapy.

DIAGNOSIS The diagnosis is made by identifying the cyst in formed feces or the trophozoite in diarrheal stools, duodenal secretions, or jejunal biopsies. In the majority of acute cases, the parasite can be demonstrated easily in a series of stool specimens collected and examined in the manner described for amebiasis (see Chap. 217). Excretion of the organism is often scanty or intermittent in chronic cases, however, making parasitological confirmation more difficult. Purgation does not improve the yield. Many of these patients, however, can be diagnosed by examining specimens collected at weekly intervals for a period of 4 to 5 weeks. Alternatively, the duodenal contents can be sampled with a nylon string (Enterotest) or gastric tube and examined by direct wet-mount preparation. Occasionally, jejunal biopsy is required to establish the diagnosis in patients with typical clinical manifestations. An indirect fluorescent antibody test using axenically cultured *G. lamblia* has been developed. Its diagnostic usefulness remains to be established.

TREATMENT Treatment is usually carried out with quinacrine hydrochloride or metronidazole. Tinadazole, a third highly effective agent, is presently not available in the United States. Quinacrine, 0.1 g given three times daily for 5 days, eliminates the organisms in 70 to 95 percent of cases. Although the drug is usually well tolerated, it may produce gastrointestinal disturbances, exacerbate psoriasis, and, rarely, produce toxic psychosis. Metronidazole appears to be better tolerated and equally effective. However, it is not currently licensed for giardiasis, and there is concern over its mutagenicity. Household contacts and sexual partners of infected patients should be examined; individuals harboring the parasite should be treated even if asymptomatic to prevent the spread to others. Pregnant women, however, should receive therapy only if severely symptomatic and never in the first trimester.

PREVENTION Chemoprophylactic drugs are not effective in preventing the acquisition of giardiasis. Individuals visiting endemic areas should avoid the ingestion of potentially contaminated food and water. The latter may be made potable by boiling or by treating with a suitable halogen disinfectant. Most of the commercially available tablets appear effective when appropriate concentrations and contact times are utilized; they are temperature-dependent, and their dose should be increased when dealing with cold water. Custodial institutions for children should screen new admissions for the presence of *G. lamblia* and treat those found to be positive. Handwashing by children and staff must be emphasized. Community water purification systems should provide for adequate filtration as well as disinfection.

REFERENCES

AMENT ME, RUBIN CE: Relation of giardiasis to abnormal intestinal structure and function in gastrointestinal immunodeficiency syndromes. Gastroenterology 62:216, 1972

BLACK RE et al: Giardiasis in day-care centers—Evidence of person to person transmission. Pediatrics 60:486, 1977

DYKES AC et al: Municipal waterborne giardiasis: An epidemiologic investigation. Ann Intern Med 93:165, 1980

JARROLL EL JR et al: *Giardia* cyst destruction: Effectiveness of six small-quantity water disinfection methods. Am J Trop Med Hyg 29:8, 1980

MEYER EA, JARROLL EL: Giardiasis. Am J Epidemiol 111:1, 1980

OSTERHOLM MT et al: An outbreak of foodborne giardiasis. N Engl J Med 304:24, 1981

PHILLIPS SC et al: Sexual transmission of enteric protozoa and helminths in a venereal-disease-clinic population. N Engl J Med 305:603, 1981

SMITH JW, WOLFE MS: Giardiasis. Ann Rev Med 31:373, 1980

VISVESVARA GS et al: An immunofluorescence test to detect serum antibodies to *Giardia lamblia.* Ann Intern Med 93:802, 1980

225
MINOR PROTOZOAN DISEASES

JAMES J. PLORDE

TRICHOMONIASIS Trichomoniasis is a venereal infection caused by the protozoan *Trichomonas vaginalis.* Of the many members of the genus *Trichomonas,* three are parasites of human beings: *T. hominis* in the intestine, *T. tenax* in the oral cavity, and *T. vaginalis,* the only one capable of producing disease, in the vagina, urethra, and prostate. All three exist only in the trophozoite stage and resemble one another morphologically. *Trichomonas vaginalis* is the largest, however, and confusion in diagnosis is rare because of the anatomic specificity of their habits.

Trichomonas vaginalis is transmitted by sexual intercourse. Although the organism is viable for up to 24 h in urine, semen, and water and may survive on moist washcloths for a few hours, transmission by fomites is probably uncommon. Newborn children of infected mothers have, on occasion, acquired the infection. The parasite is cosmopolitan in its distribution. It is estimated that in the United States 3 million women are infected annually; data on males are lacking. Prevalence correlates directly with the number of sexual contacts; rates as high as 70 percent have been seen in prostitutes, individuals with other venereal disease, and sexual partners of infected patients.

In the female, trichomoniasis usually presents as a persistent vaginitis. In approximately two-thirds a discharge is present and is frequently accompanied by vulvar itching, dysuria, and odor. This acute stage may persist for a week or months, often fluctuating in intensity; it may worsen following menstruation. Eventually the discharge and other symptoms subside and may actually disappear completely, even though the patient still harbors trichomonads. Examination shows inflammation ranging from mild hyperemia of the vaginal vault and endocervix to extensive erosion, petechial hemorrhages, and perianal intertrigo. The finding of a granular, friable, reddened endocervix (strawberry cervix) is a highly characteristic, although uncommon, finding. A discharge, typically thin, yellow, and frothy in nature, is found pooled in the posterior vaginal fornix.

The prostate and urethra are the usual sites of infection in the male. It may present as persistent or recurring nonspecific urethritis, or, more commonly, it may be completely asymptomatic. Acute purulent urethritis occurs rarely.

The diagnosis is made by examining vaginal, prostatic, or urethral secretions for the presence of *Trichomonas.* The organism may also be found in the sedimented urine. A wet mount is highly specific when positive but is often negative in asymptomatic women and in patients who have douched in the previous 24 h. Stained smears provide little additional help. Culture is more sensitive but is not generally available.

Trichomonas is sometimes responsible for confusing changes in the cytologic pattern of exfoliated vaginal cells. Moreover, ordinary Papanicolaou preparations are not well suited to the diagnosis, and when trichomoniasis is suspected, fresh material should be looked at immediately.

Oral metronidazole (Flagyl), given either in dosage of 250 mg three times daily for 7 days or in a single 2-g dose, is an extremely effective therapeutic agent. Concurrent treatment of sexual partners will minimize recurrent infections.

The evidence that metronidazole is carcinogenic in rodents and mutagenic in bacteria has placed the role of this agent in trichomonas infections in doubt. The drug should not be used in pregnancy until further information on its teratogenicity is available. Some authorities suggest that the drug should not be used at all unless patients cannot be rendered asymptomatic by other means. Because of the agent's antabuse-like action, alcohol consumption is contraindicated during therapy and for 24 h following its completion.

COCCIDIOSIS This is an infrequently recognized disease characterized by fever, diarrhea, abdominal pain, and weight loss which results from ingestion of the oocysts of coccidia belonging to the genus *Isospora.* These sporozoan protozoa are widespread in the animal kingdom. *Isospora hominis, I. belli,* and *Cryptosporidium* have been shown to infect humans. Parasitization is much more common in children and is worldwide in distribution, particularly in tropical areas.

Like the related plasmodia, there is both an asexual and sexual stage of multiplication in *I. belli* infections. However, both occur within a single host. Following the ingestion of an oocyst, *sporozoites* are released which invade the epithelial cells of the intestine to become trophozoites. These multiply asexually producing a large number of *merozoites,* which in turn invade other epithelial cells to continue the cycle. In some cells sexual gametocytes are produced. With the fertilization of the female gametocyte, an oocyst is formed which is then passed in the stool. Transmission is by the fecal-oral route. Volunteers develop symptoms about 1 week after the ingestion of viable oocysts. The illness usually has an acute onset with fever, headache, abdominal cramps, and diarrhea. Stools are often fatty and weight loss is common. Coccidiosis may be associated with a malabsorption syndrome and abnormalities of the mucosa in the small bowel. Symptoms, which presumably continue as long as the asexual cycle of multiplication continues, usually subside spontaneously within a few weeks. In some cases, however, they may persist for months or even years, eventually resulting in death.

A peripheral eosinophilia occurs in approximately half of the infected patients. The diagnosis can be made by examination of stool for oocysts. These are often scanty, and concentration techniques such as zinc sulfate flotation or the formol-ether method must usually be employed. Incubation of the stool for 2 days at room temperature improves the recovery rate. Duodenal aspiration and jejunal biopsy are less cumbersome and more reliable. *Isospora belli* infections have been successfully treated with combinations of pyrimethamine-sulfonamide and trimethoprim-sulfamethoxazole.

Isospora hominis is probably identical to *Sarcocystis fusiformis.* Its oocysts are believed to be infectious only for pigs and cattle in which it produces tissue sarcocysts. Humans become infected by eating undercooked pork or beef containing the cysts. These liberate trophozoites which invade intestinal epithelial cells to undergo gametogony with the formation of new oocysts. The disease in humans is usually asymptomatic, but mild self-limited gastrointestinal manifestations have been described. Therapy is not required.

A third intestinal coccidian, *Cryptosporidium,* is a newly defined human pathogen. This parasite, which infects a wide range of vertebrates, differs from the other coccidia in that it is found extracellularly in the brush border of the small bowel. Oocysts are small (4 μm) and scanty; to date, none has been found in human stool. Clinically, cryptosporidiosis presents as a profuse, chronic, watery diarrhea. Its tendency to occur in immunosuppressed hosts, the frequency with which it is associated with other secondary infections, and its resistance to antimicrobials serve to distinguish it from isosporiasis. Three of the six reported human infections have ended in death. Remission in one case followed withdrawal of immunosuppressive agents. Diagnosis requires small-bowel biopsy. The jejunal tissue reveals microvillous distortion, mononuclear inflammatory cells, and the 2- to 4-μm spherical parasite lying on the mucosal surface.

BALANTIDIASIS *Balantidium coli,* the largest protozoon of human beings, inhabits the large intestine. In addition to producing an asymptomatic carrier state, it elicits disease ranging from mild recurrent diarrhea to fulminant ulceration with perforation and death. In many respects the disease is similar to amebiasis in its range of manifestations, exclusive of spread to the liver.

The illness has been reproduced by feeding the organism to volunteers. The diagnosis is made by finding the trophozoite or cyst in the stool, but repeated examinations may be required because shedding of *Balantidium* is intermittent. The disease is more likely to occur in tropical areas, but at least 60 cases have been reported in the United States. Swine and rats are frequent carriers of *B. coli* and may play an important role in the spread of the disease to humans. Outbreaks have been noted in mental institutions where coprophagy implicated direct person-to-person transmission.

The tetracyclines in ordinary doses are highly effective in

treatment, as is diiodohydroxyquin given in the dosage of 650 mg three times daily for 20 days. Metronidazole in the dosage used for amebiasis has also been effective (see Chap. 217).

REFERENCES

Balantidiasis

KNIGHT R: Giardiasis, isosporiasis and balantidiasis. Clin Gastroenterol 7:31, 1978

NICHOLOSON NW: Case report of *Balantidium coli* infection. East Afr Med J 55:133, 1978

WALZER PD et al: Balantidiasis outbreak in Truk Islands. Am J Trop Med Hyg 22:33, 1973

Coccidiosis

TRIER JS: Chronic intestinal coccidiosis in man: Intestinal morphology and response to treatment. Gastroenterology 66:923, 1974

WEINSTEIN L et al: Intestinal cryptosporidiosis complicated by disseminated cytomegalovirus infection. Gastroenterology 81:584, 1981

WESTERMAN EL, CHRISTENSEN RP: Chronic *Isospora belli* infection treated with co-trimoxazole. Ann Intern Med 91:413, 1979

Trichomoniasis

FOUTS AC, KRAUS SF: *Trichomonas vaginalis:* Reevaluation of its clinical presentation and laboratory diagnosis. J Infect Dis 141:137, 1980

KUBERSKI TT: Ankylosing spondylitis associated with *Trichomonas vaginalis* infection. J Clin Microbiol 13:880, 1981

WAITKINS SA, THOMAS DJ: Isolation of *Trichomonas vaginalis* resistant to metronidazole. Lancet 2:590, 1981

226
TRICHINOSIS

JAMES J. PLORDE

DEFINITION Trichinosis is an intestinal and tissue infection of humans and other mammals caused by the nematode *Trichinella spiralis.* The disease is characterized by diarrhea during the development of the adults in the intestine and by myositis, fever, prostration, periorbital edema, eosinophilic leukocytosis, and, occasionally, evidence of myocarditis, pneumonitis, or encephalitis during the stage of larval migration in tissue.

ETIOLOGY Trichinosis in humans is contracted by ingestion of meat containing the encysted larvae of *T. spiralis.* The meat has almost always been pork, but for the past several years about 10 percent of cases reported in this country have been attributed to bear meat. This has been particularly frequent in the northern and western states including Alaska, California, and Idaho. There are no intermediate hosts, and both the adult and larval stages develop in the same animal. Infection has been produced or observed in the bear, wild boar, wolf, coyote, fox, muskrat, horse, cow, dog, cat, rabbit, guinea pig, mouse, and marine mammals, in addition to the rat and the pig. Humans are particularly susceptible; most fowl are resistant. Among pigs, infection is contracted following feeding of the uncooked scraps, less often by eating infected rats. The incidence of infection in pigs has been reduced by laws requiring that garbage be cooked thoroughly before being fed. Rats also feed on uncooked pork scraps and, in addition, maintain a high incidence of infection by their cannibalism.

Soon after ingestion, the larvae are liberated from their cysts by gastric digestion and migrate into the intestinal mucosa, where copulation takes place. The male dies, and within a week, the viviparous female is discharging larvae (100 by 6 μm), which enter vascular channels and are distributed throughout the body. Larviposition continues for about 4 to 16 weeks, each female producing approximately 1500 offspring. The larvae enter skeletal muscle, grow, and begin encysting within 3 weeks; calcification of cysts begins in 6 to 18 months. The life span of the encysted organism has been estimated at 5 to 10 years. The muscles of the diaphragm, tongue, and eye, and the deltoid, pectoral, gastrocnemius, and intercostal muscles are most often affected. Larvae carried to sites other than skeletal muscles do not encyst but disintegrate, often stimulating a granulomatous inflammatory reaction. The life cycle can be carried further only if a new host ingests the encysted larvae.

The description of a fatal case of trichinosis in an immunosuppressed patient emphasizes the importance of the immune response in limiting the intensity of infection. Apparently, it does so by acting directly on circulating larvae, inhibiting the reproduction of the female worms, and accelerating the expulsion of the adult parasites from the intestine. Eosinophils as well as B and T cell lymphocytes are involved in the response. The T cells appear to have a "helper" function in promoting the production of FS antibodies which, in collaboration with eosinophils, induce fracture of the larval cuticle and disintegration of its internal structures. Once safely encysted in striated muscle, the larvae appear resistant to immunologic attack.

EPIDEMIOLOGY Trichinosis is particularly common in Europe and North America, but with the exception of Australia and Asia it is found worldwide. In the United States its prevalence as measured by finding cysts in human diaphragms at autopsy has declined from 16.1 to 4.2 percent over the past 30 years. This decline has been accompanied by a similar reduction of trichinosis in pigs. The prevalence appears highest in the New England states, New Jersey, Louisiana, and Alaska. Currently, it is estimated that 1.5 million Americans carry live trichinae in their musculature and that somewhere between 150,000 and 300,000 acquire new infections annually. The overwhelming majority of these infections are asymptomatic, and many of those that become clinically manifest are never correctly diagnosed. In 1980 only 130 cases and one death were officially reported in the United States. Large outbreaks are usually caused by consumption of ready-to-eat pork sausage prepared in noninspected facilities or at home. The incidence appears highest among Americans of Italian, German, Polish, or Portuguese descent, presumably because of their inclination to make and eat pork sausage over the holiday season. Notable epidemics have followed the ingestion of trichinae-infected wild pig in Hawaii and California and walrus in Alaska. The latter is the first reported outbreak caused by this host in North America. Each year, a few cases are acquired from ground beef, attesting to the frequency with which this meat is adulterated with pork.

PATHOLOGY The most striking lesions are in the skeletal muscles, where there is a severe myositis with basophilic granular degeneration of the invaded muscle fiber. Adjacent fibers exhibit hyalin or hydropic degeneration, and the focus becomes infiltrated with neutrophilic and eosinophilic leukocytes, some lymphocytes, and mononuclear macrophages. Hyperemia, edema, and hemorrhages are constant features.

Larvae do not encyst in cardiac muscle, but an intense myocarditis has been observed in fatal cases.

In cases of central nervous system involvement, there may be granulomatous nodules, and vasculitis involving small arterioles and capillaries of the brain and meninges. Encystment of larvae in the brain is unusual.

CLINICAL MANIFESTATIONS The severity of the clinical manifestations is generally related to the number of larvae disseminated to the tissues of the host; patients with severe disease usually harbor 50 to 100 larvae per gram of muscle, while those with 10 or less are often asymptomatic. The first symptoms usually appear within 1 to 2 days after ingestion of the uncooked or undercooked meat containing encysted larvae. At that time diarrhea, abdominal pain, nausea, and sometimes prostration and fever develop. The next stage, that of muscular invasion, begins about the end of the first week and may last as long as 6 weeks. During this period, patients have fever, periorbital edema, conjunctivitis and subconjunctival hemorrhages, muscle pain and tenderness, and often severe weakness. There may be a maculopapular rash which lasts for several days and subungual "splinter hemorrhages." More serious manifestations accompany lung, heart, or central nervous system invasion. Lung involvement is manifested by hemoptysis and consolidation on chest x-rays. Central nervous system involvement may be evident as polyneuritis, poliomyelitis, myasthenia, meningitis, encephalitis, focal or diffuse pareses, delirium, psychosis, and coma. Despite the severity of central nervous system involvement in some patients, the cerebrospinal fluid remains normal.

Myocarditis is characterized by persistent tachycardia or development of congestive heart failure. There are marked electrocardiographic alterations, including ST-T wave changes and conduction abnormalities in 20 percent of patients. High levels of circulating eosinophils may produce damage to the ventricular endothelium with superimposed thrombosis.

A causal relationship between trichinosis and polyarteritis nodosa has been reported, presumably related to the presence of circulating immune complexes.

LABORATORY FINDINGS The most constant finding, and one of significance early in the course of the disease, is the eosinophilic leukocytosis (over 500 eosinophilic leukocytes per cubic millimeter) which generally appears before the end of the second week. In cases of moderate severity, the proportion of eosinophilic leukocytes ranges between 15 and 50 percent. In severe cases, particularly terminally, the eosinophilic leukocytosis may disappear entirely.

The skin test to larval antigen becomes positive early in the third week of infection and may remain so for up to 20 years. The usual positive response is a wheal of 5 mm or more appearing within 30 min. Unfortunately, the commercially available skin test preparations are not reliable and should not be used.

There are a variety of serologic tests for trichinosis, including the countercurrent electrophoresis test, the complement fixation test, the indirect fluorescent antibody test, and the bentonite flocculation test, which is probably the best. A commercially available latex agglutination test appears as sensitive but is somewhat less specific. These serologic tests all become positive during the third week of the disease and may remain positive for a few years. An enzyme-linked immunosorbent test is able to detect specific antibody earlier in the course of infection. Since each may occasionally be falsely negative, two or more tests should be used. The serologic tests are most valuable if they are negative initially and then in turn positive or if there is a change in titer.

Muscle biopsy when carried out during the third week of infection remains the most useful test for demonstration of larvae or cysts. The deltoid or gastrocnemius muscles are the most useful sites for biopsy. A 1-g portion of the excised muscle should be compressed between glass slides and examined under a low-power microscope for the presence of larvae. Calcified cysts or larvae represent an old infection. The remainder of the biopsy should be submitted for routine processing because myositis is a significant finding even in the absence of larvae or cysts.

In severe trichinosis there may be marked hypoalbuminemia, probably because of protein leakage from damaged capillaries. During the fourth, fifth, and sixth weeks of the disease, concomitant with a rise in antibody, diffuse hypergammaglobulinemia occurs. Elevated levels of circulating IgE have been reported. There may be moderate rises in serum glutamic oxaloacetic transaminase, serum aldolase, and creatine-phosphokinase, probably related to myositis; electromyography may show evidence of altered motor function. Typically the sedimentation rate is slow.

DIFFERENTIAL DIAGNOSIS Trichinosis must be differentiated from diseases which are characterized by eosinophilia (such as Hodgkin's disease, eosinophilic leukemia, and periarteritis nodosa) and from entities which are characterized by myopathy, such as dermatomyositis. When the central nervous system is involved, the diagnosis may be very difficult.

TREATMENT Thiabendazole, in dosage of 25 mg/kg bid for 5 to 7 days, has resulted in apparent improvement in a number of patients, with relief of muscle pain and tenderness and with lysis of fever. The results have not been uniform, however, and the use of this drug in trichinosis has been associated with nausea, vomiting, abdominal discomfort, dermatitis, and drug fever. The usefulness of mebendazole in human disease has not been established.

Patients with "allergic" manifestations of trichinosis, including angioedema and urticaria as well as myocardial or central nervous system involvement, should be treated with prednisone in dosage of 20 to 60 mg per day. Response to steroids usually has been prompt, particularly in central nervous system trichinosis. Not all focal lesions have resolved, however.

Other measures should be directed at relief of pain and maintenance of adequate caloric and fluid intake.

PROGNOSIS The prognosis in trichinosis has improved markedly, and even when the central nervous system is involved, the mortality rate has fallen to under 10 percent. The overall mortality rate is now approximately 1 percent.

PREVENTION The responsibility for control rests with the consumer. Adequate cooking of pork involves heating all portions of the meat to 60°C. Freezing procedures to kill porcine larvae require a temperature of −15°C for 20 days or −18°C for 24 h. Larvae isolated from arctic animals appear much more resistant to freezing. Proper smoking and pickling will also destroy the larvae. Important in control is the cooking of garbage fed to hogs. There is no practical method of inspection which will detect trichinous pork.

REFERENCES

ANDY JJ et al: Trichinosis causing extensive ventricular mural endocarditis with superimposed thrombosis. Evidence that severe eosinophilia damages endocardium. Am J Med 63:824, 1977

BARRETT-CONNER E et al: An epidemic of trichinosis after ingestion of wild pig in Hawaii. J Infect Dis 133:473, 1976

DESPOMMIER D: Immunity to *Trichinella spiralis.* Am J Trop Med Hyg 26:68, 1977

FRAYHA RA: Trichinosis-related polyarteritis nodosa. Am J Med 71:307, 1981

KAZURA JW, AIKAWA M: Host defense mechanisms against *Trichinella spiralis* infection in the mouse: Eosinophil mediated destruction of newborn larvae *in vitro.* J Immunol 124:355, 1980

MARGOLIS HS et al: Trichinosis: Two Alaskan outbreaks from walrus meat. J Infect Dis 139:102, 1979

MCCRACKEN RO, TAYLOR DD: Mebendazole therapy of parenteral trichinosis. Science 207:1220, 1980

METZLER MH et al: Second-degree atrioventricular block in acute trichinosis. Am J Dis Child 124:598, 1972

MOST H: Current concepts in parasitology. Trichinosis—preventable yet still with us. N Engl J Med 298:1178, 1978

227 FILARIASIS

JAMES J. PLORDE

DEFINITION Filariasis is a group of disorders produced by infection with the threadlike nematodes of the superfamily Filarioidea. These worms invade the lymphatics and subcutaneous and deep tissues of humans producing reactions ranging from acute inflammation to chronic scarring. The viviparous female discharges microfilariae into the blood or subcutaneous tissues where they live for weeks or months until taken up by hematophagous arthropods. Within these vectors they are transformed into filariform larvae which then infect a new host when the arthropod takes another blood meal. The clinical pictures produced by various species in this group are more or less specific. The term *lymphatic filariasis* is commonly used to designate the disease produced by *Wuchereria bancrofti* and *Brugia malayi,* the organisms responsible for lymphatic blockade and elephantiasis. *Loa loa* causes loiasis, a disease characterized by transient subcutaneous (Calabar) swellings, and *Onchocerca volvulus* produces the blindness and pruritic skin rash typical of onchocerciasis. *Mansonella ozzardi, Dipetalonema perstans,* and *D. streptocerca* cause infections of questionable clinical significance to humans.

These parasites are identified by the location, periodicity, and morphological characteristics of their microfilariae. Those of *W. bancrofti, B. malayi, L. loa, D. perstans,* and *M. ozzardi* are all found in the blood, and, with the exception of the last, all display nocturnal or diurnal periodicity. *Onchocerca volvulus* and *D. streptocerca* are found in the subcutaneous tissues and are nonperiodic. Morphologically, the microfilariae are distinguished by the presence or absence of a sheath and by the distribution of their deeply staining column of nuclei. The sheath, which is an elongation of the original eggshell, can be seen extending beyond the head and tail only in the microfilariae of *W. bancrofti, B. malayi,* and *L. loa.* The nuclear column extends to the very tip of the microfilariae of *B. malayi, L. loa,* and the two species of *Dipetalonema.*

Skin and serologic tests are group-specific, lack sensitivity, and may be falsely positive in other nematode infections. In the absence of microfilariae and other helminthic infections, however, they may be helpful in establishing a diagnosis in clinically suspect cases.

LYMPHATIC FILARIASIS (BANCROFTIAN AND MALAYAN) Etiology and epidemiology The threadlike adult worms live coiled together in human lymphatics. The male *W. bancrofti* measures 35 mm and the female 80 to 100 mm. The *B. malayi* adults are about one-half as long. Gravid females release microfilariae in large numbers into the lymphatics. These embryos, which are sheathed, measure approximately 200 to 300 μm. They eventually reach the peripheral blood, where further development depends on their ingestion by a proper mosquito vector. Species of *Culex, Aëdes,* and *Anopheles* transmit Bancroftian filariasis; *Mansonia* and *Anopheles* serve as vectors in Malayan disease. After further development in the vector, larvae migrate to the mouthparts. If the mosquito feeds on a human host, they penetrate the puncture site and reach maturity in about a year. In the absence of reinfection, humans harbor microfilariae for 5 to 10 years, the reproductive life of the adult worms. In most *W. bancrofti* and *B. malayi* infections, the microfilariae are found in the blood in greatest numbers between 9 P.M. and 2 A.M. During the day, apparently in response to changes in oxygen tension, they accumulate in the pulmonary vessels and disappear from the peripheral blood. However, in Polynesia and New Caledonia there is an *Aëdes*-transmitted variety of *W. bancrofti* (*W. pacifica*) that displays a diurnal periodicity in which the peak occurs in the early evenings (subperiodic form). Periodicity is of epidemiologic significance because it determines which species of mosquito serves as the vector. Furthermore, several subperiodic forms of *B. malayi* have been found in animals, suggesting the possibility that this disease has an animal reservoir. The human is the only known vertebrate host for *W. bancrofti.*

More than 250 million persons throughout the world are presently infected, and both the prevalence and distribution of the disease seem to be increasing in many parts of Africa and Asia.

Wuchereria bancrofti infection is endemic between latitudes 41°N and 30°S involving primarily Africa, the Pacific Islands, and southeastern Asia from Korea on the north to India in the west. The West Indies, Central America, and the eastern coastal plains of South America are also involved. Distribution is irregular, and there are many peculiar "skip areas" in this geographic pattern, presumably because the endemic disease can be maintained only where human infection and mosquitoes are prevalent. *Brugia malayi* infection is much more restricted in its distribution and occurs in India, Burma, Thailand, Vietnam, China, South Korea, Japan, Malaysia, Indonesia, Borneo, New Guinea, and the Philippines. The parasite has disappeared from Sri Lanka.

Two new types of microfilaria have been described. One, found in Brazil, has been named *W. lewisi,* while the strain from Portuguese Timor is called *Brugia timori.*

There were approximately 15,000 *W. bancrofti* infections among American military personnel in World War II. A small endemic focus of *W. bancrofti* once existed near Charleston, South Carolina, but no new cases have been observed since 1930.

Pathogenesis Pathological changes are caused primarily by the presence of the adult worm in the lymphatics and may be divided into inflammatory and obstructive. The inflammatory response, thought to be due to an immediate-type hypersensitivity reaction to molting larvae, consists of infiltration with lymphocytes, plasma cells, and eosinophils. There are hyperplasia of lymphatic endothelium, acute lymphangitis, and thrombosis. This is followed by a granulomatous reaction to dead or dying adults which may lead to reversible lymphatic obstruction. Repetition of this process over a period of years leads to permanent lymphatic blockade. The tissues become edematous, thickened, and fibrotic. Secondary streptococcal infections are common and may contribute to lymphatic blockade. Dilated lymphatics may rupture into surrounding tissue. Elephantiasis is actually a relatively unusual complication of filarial infections and is actually more common in immigrants to endemic areas. Apparently, exposure to filarial antigens early in life provides some protection against elephantiasis. If repeated reinfections do not occur, the disease is self-limited.

Manifestations The clinical manifestations vary with the geographic area, species of parasite, immune response of the infected patient, and intensity of infection. Light infections may be completely asymptomatic. Symptoms may occur within 3 months of infection, but ordinarily the incubation period is 8 to 12 months. The clinical findings closely reflect the pathological changes, with inflammation early in the disease followed by obstruction later. Inflammatory filariasis consists of a series of brief febrile attacks occurring over a period of weeks. Fever is usually low grade but may reach 40.6°C (105°F) and be accompanied by chills and sweats. Other symptoms include headache, nausea and vomiting, photophobia, and muscle pain. If the involved lymphatics lie close to the surface, the local symptoms dominate the clinical picture. Lymphangitis is very common, involving the legs more frequently than the arms. It often begins as a tender spot in the region of the malleoli or femoral area and spreads centrifugally. The involved vessels are palpably tender and painful. The overlying skin is red and swollen. When abdominal lymphatics are involved, the picture may simulate that of an acute abdomen. In Bancroftian filariasis the vessels of the spermatic cord and testes may be involved, resulting in painful orchitis, epididymitis, or funiculitis. Lymphadenitis almost always accompanies and may sometimes precede lymphangitis. The inguinal, femoral, and epitrochlear nodes are involved. Abscesses which may form about involved lymphatics and lymph nodes may discharge to the surface, resulting in persistently draining sinus tracts. The acute manifestations last only a few days and then subside spontaneously, only to recur at irregular intervals over a period of weeks or months. Recovery finally ensues. With repeated infections, slowly progressive lymphatic obstruction may develop in areas where the inflammatory reactions have occurred previously. Edema, ascites, lymph scrotum, hydrocele, pleural effusion, or joint effusion may appear as a result of interference with lymphatic drainage. Lymphadenopathy persists. The lymphatic vessels become palpably enlarged as tense elastic masses beneath the skin, especially in the femoral, inguinal, and scrotal areas. They may rupture and form draining sinuses. Internal rupture of lymphatics may give rise to chylous ascites or chyluria. In a small percentage of cases elephantiasis develops. This complication is rare below the age of 20 even in natives of heavily infested areas. The chronic obstructive phase of the disease often is punctuated by acute inflammatory episodes.

TROPICAL EOSINOPHILIA Attention has been focused on an aberrant type of filariasis which is characterized by the presence of hypereosinophilia, circulating filarial antibodies, microfilariae in tissue but *not in the blood,* and a chronic, clinical course that can be terminated with specific antifilarial treatment. These amicrofilaremic forms were originally thought to be caused by zoonotic parasites, but it is more likely that they represent an atypical host response to various filariae including *W. bancrofti* and *B. malayi.* The syndrome is most commonly seen in India, Indonesia, Sri Lanka, Pakistan, and southeast Asia, all areas of intense transmission for these organisms. Involved patients lack the IgG-blocking antibodies present in the patients with circulating microfilariae. Animal models suggest that microfilariae are removed from the peripheral circulation and trapped in various tissue sites by an IgG-dependent cell-mediated effector mechanism. Antigens released when the parasites are destroyed initiate an immediate IgE-mediated reaction. The eosinophilic inflammatory reaction, in time, progresses to granuloma formation and fibrosis. Clinically there may be marked enlargement of the lymph nodes and spleen (Meyers-Kouwenaar syndrome) and/or chronic cough, nocturnal bronchospasm, and miliary pulmonary infiltrates (Weingarten syndrome). The former syndrome is most frequently seen in children, and the latter in young male adults. Only one-quarter of the patients with pulmonary manifestations demonstrate obstructive defects on pulmonary function testing. All show restrictive disease, and irreversible pulmonary hypertension has been described in a few. A number of diseases characterized by pulmonary infiltration and eosinophilia (PIE) must be considered in the differential diagnosis of this disease. They include other helminthic infections, Loeffler's syndrome, chronic eosinophilic pneumonia, allergic aspergillosis, vasculitis, idiopathic hypereosinophilia, and drug allergies.

Diagnosis A history of exposure, the long incubation period, the occurrence of typical inflammatory episodes, and the finding of regional lymphadenopathy, thickening of the spermatic cord, or swelling of an extremity should suggest the diagnosis. There is usually eosinophilia during acute episodes. Lymphangiography may reveal dilated afferent and small efferent lymphatics. The definitive diagnosis depends on demonstration of the parasite. Although adult worms can be demonstrated in biopsied lymph nodes, biopsy is not recommended because it may interfere further with lymphatic drainage. Microfilariae are found in the blood during intermediate stages but not early or late in the disease. As they are motile, they can often be seen in a wet mount. Definite identification, however, requires staining with Giemsa. As in malaria, both thin and thick smears should be prepared. Either the Knott concentration, counting chamber, or membrane filtration technique should be employed if the parasite is not found in thick smears. Because the appearance of microfilariae in peripheral blood is periodic, it is essential to obtain blood at appropriate times. When this proves difficult, the oral administration of 100 mg diethylcarbamazine usually produces positive blood specimens within 30 to 60 min. Microfilariae may also be found in lymphatic fluid, hydrocele fluid, ascites, and pleural fluid. Indirect hemagglutination, bentonite flocculation, and soluble antigen fluorescent antibody tests are available and, although not completely reliable, are helpful when microfilariae cannot be demonstrated. An indirect immunofluorescent test utilizing adult *B. malayi* as the source of antigen appears to be both more sensitive and specific than previously developed procedures.

The diagnosis of *tropical eosinophilia* is confirmed by (1) a history of prolonged residence in an endemic area, (2) lack of microfilariae in the peripheral blood despite examination of both day and night specimens by concentration techniques, (3) peripheral eosinophilia in excess of 3000 cells per milliliter, (4) high titers of filarial antibodies, (5) IgE levels of at least 1000 units per milliliter, and (6) response to diethylcarbamazine within 7 to 10 days of initiating therapy. Recovery of microfilariae from the tissues is uncommon, and biopsy is not warranted.

Treatment Diethylcarbamazine (Hetrazan) rapidly eliminates microfilariae from the blood. It probably also kills or injures adult worms, impairing their ability to reproduce, and clears microfilariae permanently from the bloodstream of many patients. The drug is given in doses of 2 mg/kg three times a day for 3 or 4 weeks. Treatment with this agent is often followed by allergic reactions to the dying parasite. These reactions may be quite severe, especially in Malayan filariasis. They can be controlled with aspirin, antihistamines, or corticosteroids. In heavy infections, it may be desirable to begin treatment with antihistamines before administration of Hetrazan.

Reassurance of the patient is very important in this disease. Effective and safe vaccines are presently not available. Pressure bandages and surgery sometimes benefit elephantiasis. The prognosis for life is excellent, particularly if infected individuals leave endemic areas or otherwise avoid reinfections. Disease control is accomplished by combining mass treatment with mosquito control measures.

ONCHOCERCIASIS ("RIVER BLINDNESS") Definition Onchocerciasis is a cutaneous filariasis caused by *Onchocerca volvulus.* It is characterized by subcutaneous nodules, a pruritic skin rash, and ocular lesions.

Etiology and epidemiology The disease is found in focal areas within Mexico, Guatemala, Colombia, Venezuela, Ecuador, Surinam, Brazil, and Yemen, and throughout tropical Africa. It is estimated that at least 50 million individuals are infected and that about 5 percent of these are blind as a result of the disease.

The infection is transmitted by black flies of the genus *Simulium,* which breed along fast-moving streams. An inoculated larva matures into a single male or female in approximately one year. Since larvae do not multiply within the human host, heavy parasite loads are the result of repeated infections. The adult worms are found coiled together in fibrous subcutaneous nodules. The gravid females, which may live as long as 15 years, release thousands of unsheathed microfilariae daily. These migrate in the skin, subcutaneous tissue, and eye for up to 30 months until they either degenerate or are ingested by a feeding *Simulium.*

Pathogenesis and clinical manifestations The subcutaneous nodules which enclose the adult worms are usually 2 to 3 cm in diameter when fully developed. They are firm, nontender, and freely movable, although occasionally they may be adherent to underlying tissue. Their location on the body is related to the biting habits of the vector. In Central America, where the fly bites on the upper part of the body, the nodules are frequently over the head; in Africa they are primarily on the trunk and thighs. They usually number less than 10, but more than 100 have been reported in a single patient.

The important pathological changes occur as a result of a hypersensitivity reaction to the dead or dying microfilariae. Pruritus is often severe and constant. The skin lesion may appear as an erysipelas-like reaction over the face or a papular rash over one extremity. In chronic cases thickening, lichenification, and depigmentation may be present. In Africa microfilariae produce a fibrosing obstructive lymphadenitis, possibly by stimulating the deposition of immune complexes. This lesion is frequently associated with large folds of skin called *hanging groins* and with elephantiasis. Children living in endemic areas may not demonstrate these changes for decades even though microfilariae are present. The most serious complications of onchocerciasis are eye lesions which are usually found in patients repeatedly infected on the upper part of the body. A punctate and later sclerosing keratitis, iridocyclitis, optic atrophy, or chorioretinitis may eventually lead to blindness.

Diagnosis The diagnosis is made by demonstrating microfilariae in a skin snip taken from an involved area. A thin sliver of superficial skin is removed with a razor or punch. Care must be taken to prevent bleeding and possible contamination with blood microfilariae. The skin is weighed and then is placed in saline, teased with a pair of sharp dissecting needles, and observed for emerging microfilariae over the next hour. The results should be expressed in microfilariae per milligram of tissue. Multiple skin snips may be necessary. In patients with eye lesions, microfilariae can sometimes be seen in the anterior chamber with a slit lamp. If organisms cannot be detected by the above methods, the patient may be given 50 mg diethylcarbamazine orally. The occurrence of a pruritic rash within 24 h strongly suggests the presence of cutaneous microfilariae (Mazzotti's test). One of the filarial serologic tests may also be helpful.

Treatment and prevention Diethylcarbamazine is effective in destroying microfilariae but has little effect on the adult worm. The drug must be used with great care as rapid destruction of the parasites may cause a severe allergic reaction. If the eye is involved, this can result in further ocular damage. The initial adult dose is 50 mg orally. It is increased to 50 mg three times daily on the second day, 100 mg three times daily on the third day, and finally 200 mg three times a day for an additional 7 days. Antihistamines, or in rare cases corticosteroids, can be used to control allergic reactions. In ocular reactions, the pupil should be dilated and topical steroids applied.

The adult worms may be eliminated by excision of nodules on the head and neck, a procedure which is useful in preventing ocular complications, or by chemotherapy with suramin. Details of the administration and toxicity of this drug are given in Chap. 220. The dosage is 0.1 g given intravenously to detect drug idiosyncrasy, followed by 1.0 g intravenously once weekly for five to six doses.

Mebendazole may prove to be an effective alternative to these agents. It appears to lower microfilarial counts by interrupting embryogenesis in the female adult.

Chemoprophylaxis is not practical, and personal protection depends upon the use of protective clothing. Insecticides, mass therapy, and nodulectomies have been used but have not been very satisfactory. A massive control project in west Africa utilizing insecticides dropped by airplane and helicopter has been more successful.

LOIASIS This form of filariasis is produced by *Loa loa* and is prevalent in west and central Africa. The infection is transmitted by deer flies of the genus *Chrysops.* The adult worms, which like the other filariae may live for 10 to 15 years, migrate continuously through the subcutaneous tissue. The resulting localized areas of allergic inflammation, *Calabar swellings,* are the hallmark of the disease. Occasionally the adult worms may be seen crossing the eye subconjunctivally. This usually results in intense lacrimation, pain, and anxiety. Infestation may, however, be completely asymptomatic. An association between loiasis and endomyocardial fibrosis has been reported. The diagnosis can be made by finding the adult worm or by demonstrating the distinctive sheathed microfilariae in contents of the Calabar swellings or in the bloodstream during the daytime. Microfilariae are often not found. In these cases, there are usually marked eosinophilia and a positive filarial complement fixation test. Diethylcarbamazine, administered for 2 to 3 weeks in the manner described for onchocerciasis, will kill both adult worms and microfilariae. This drug must be used with great care as it may induce an encephalopathy in this disease. It is taken in a dose of 200 mg twice daily for 3 days each month and is also effective as a chemoprophylactic agent.

DIPETALONEMIASIS *Dipetalonema perstans* (*Acanthocheilonema perstans*) is a filarial parasite of humans and other primates inhabiting the tropical areas of Africa and Latin America. The adult worm lives encysted in the subserosal tissues of the pericardium, pleura, and peritoneum, particularly the mesentery. The unsheathed microfilariae, which can be found in the peripheral blood throughout the day, have four to six nuclei in their tail. They are transmitted from host to host by blood-sucking gnats of the genus *Culicoides.* Most infections are asymptomatic, and their principal significance lies in the fact that they may be confused with other, more serious, forms of filariasis. Nevertheless, some patients complain of fever, pruritus, Calabar swellings, erysipelas-like rashes, and abdominal pain. Peripheral eosinophilia is common, but filarial complement fixation tests are generally negative. The diagnosis is made by finding the characteristic microfilariae in the peripheral blood. Treatment with diethylcarbamazine is of doubtful benefit.

Dipetalonema streptocera is found in equatorial Africa where it inhabits the dermis and subcutaneous tissues of chimpanzees and humans. Like *D. perstans,* it is transmitted by *Culicoides.* The microfilariae inhabit the dermal collagen where they elicit a lymphocytic and eosinophilic inflammatory response, fibrosis, lymphatic dilatation, pruritus, hypopigmented macules, and a papular rash. The diagnosis is made by recovering the nonperiodic microfilariae from skin snips as described for Onchocerciasis above. They are unsheathed and possess a sharply crooked tail with nuclei. Diethylcarbamazine, as described for Bancroftian filariasis above, is effective.

MANSONELLIASIS OZZARDI *Mansonella ozzardi* are found as adult worms in the mesentery and visceral fat of people living in the tropical areas of Latin America and the Caribbean. This species is thought to be transmitted by flies of the genus *Simulium* and gnats of the genus *Culicoides.* The nonperiodic microfilariae are released into the peripheral blood where they can be identified by their lack of a sheath or caudal nuclei. This common infection is thought to be asymptomatic, but reports of patients presenting with fever, lymphadenopathy, and hydroceles have been published. Diethylcarbamazine is ineffective.

DIROFILARIASIS *Dirofilaria immitis* (canine heartworm) is a large, cosmopolitan filaria of dogs which lives in their right ventricle and pulmonary arteries and releases its microfilariae into the peripheral blood. It is transmitted by several types of mosquitoes. Human infections are increasingly reported, particularly from the eastern and southern United States. The worm does not mature in humans, and hence microfilaremia is not present. Although cardiac infections have been noted at autopsy, most human infections present as well-defined pulmonary nodules. The patients are most frequently asymptomatic and are discovered to have a "coin lesion" on pulmonary roentgenography. Less commonly they complain of cough and chest pain or, rarely, of hemoptysis, fever, chills, and myalgia. The diagnosis is usually made by the microscopic examination of excised pulmonary nodules.

Other *Dirofilariae* may rarely invade humans producing subcutaneous eosinophilic granulomas of the eyelid, trunk, or extremities. The nodules, which measure 1 to 2 cm in diameter, may be painful or completely asymptomatic. In the southern United States, the filaria most frequently involved is *D. tenuis,* a parasite of raccoons. The nodules are removed by surgical excision.

REFERENCES

Akisada M, Tani S: Lymphangioadenopathy of filariasis. Trans R Soc Trop Med Hyg 64:885, 1970

Christie RW: *Dirofilaria tenuis* in Vermont. N Engl J Med 297:706, 1977

Connor DH: Onchocerciasis. N Engl J Med 298:379, 1978

Edeson JFB: Filariasis. Br Med Bull 28:60, 1972

Hawking F: The 24-hour periodicity of microfilariae: Biological mechanisms responsible for its production and control. Proc R Soc London Ser B 169:59, 1967

Ive FA et al: Endomyocardial fibrosis and filariasis. Q J Med 36:495, 1967

Merril JR et al: The dog heart worm (*Dirofilaria immitis*) in man. An epidemic pending or in progress. JAMA 243:1066, 1980

Meyers WM et al: Human streptocerciasis. A clinico-pathological study of 40 Africans (Zaireans) including identification of the adult filaria. Am J Trop Med Hyg 21:528, 1972

Nelson GS: Current concepts in parasitology. Filariasis. N Engl J Med 300:1136, 1979

Neva FA, Ottesen EA: Current concepts in parasitology. Tropical (filarial) eosinophilia. N Engl J Med 298:1129, 1978

Onkel TC: Infections with *Dipetalonema perstans* and *Mansonella ozzardi* in the aboriginal Indians of Guyana. Am J Trop Med Hyg 16:628, 1967

Scientific Working Group on Filariasis: The immunology of filariasis. Bull WHO 59:1, 1981

Thylefors B: Ocular onchocerciasis. Bull WHO 56:63, 1978

Weller PF et al: Tourism acquired *Mansonella ozzardi* microfilaria in a regular blood donor. JAMA 240:858, 1978

228 SCHISTOSOMIASIS (BILHARZIASIS)

JAMES J. PLORDE
ELAINE C. JONG

DEFINITION Schistosomiasis (bilharziasis) designates a group of diseases caused by five closely related species of dioecious trematodes belonging to the family Schistosomatidae. *Schistosoma mansoni, S. haematobium,* and *S. japonicum* are the most widespread and important species. *S. mekongi* and *S. intercalatum* are found in limited areas of Asia and Africa, respectively. These blood flukes inhabit the portal system of humans living in tropical and subtropical countries. Here they deposit large numbers of eggs, many of which are retained within the body of the host with the production of inflammatory lesions. The organs and tissues most frequently affected are the colon, urinary bladder, liver, lungs, and central nervous system.

ETIOLOGY AND LIFE CYCLE The adult worms, which grow and mature within the portal venous system of the liver, measure 1 to 2 cm in length. The male has a central trough, the gynecophoral canal, that enfolds the longer, more slender female during most of their 4- to 30-year life span. After copulation the male carries the female against the flow of portal blood to the small mesenteric vessels. *Schistosoma japonicum* and the closely related *S. mekongi* ascend the superior and *S. mansoni* and *S. intercalatum* the inferior mesenteric vein. All eventually reach the submucosal vessels of the intestine. The first two settle in the small intestine and ascending colon; the latter two in the descending colon and rectum. *Schistosoma haematobium* finds its way through the hemorrhoidal anastomoses to the systemic capillaries of the bladder and other pelvic organs. When they can travel no further, the female deposits her eggs in clusters (or one by one in the case of *S. mansoni*), slowly retreating down the vessel in front of them. The daily egg output of each worm pair varies from 300 for *S. mansoni* to over 3000 in *S. japonicum* infections. The eggs, which remain viable for 3 weeks, secrete an enzymatic substance which destroys the surrounding tissue. If the eggs lie close to the mucosal surface, they rupture into the lumen of the gut (or bladder in the case of *S. haematobium*) and are carried to the outside in the urine or feces. On reaching fresh water, the embryonated eggs quickly hatch, liberating ciliated *miracidia.* These miracidia have a life span of 6 to 8 h in which to search out and penetrate the specific snail host appropriate to the species. Within the snail the miracidia are transformed over a 1- to 2-month period into thousands of infective larvae called *cercariae.* These free-swimming cercariae are gradually shed into the water where they can remain infectious for hours to days. If they contact human skin within this time, the cercariae penetrate, discard their tails, and become *schistosomula.* Within 24 to 36 h the schistosomula work their way into the peripheral venules and are carried to the right side of the heart and then to the pulmonary capillaries. After some delay, they enter the systemic circulation. Those parasites that survive the passage through the mesenteric capillary bed finally reach the portal venous system, where they mature into adult flukes in 5 to 12 weeks.

EPIDEMIOLOGY The worldwide distribution and extensive pathologic changes produced by these parasites make schistosomiasis the single most important helminthic infection of humans. Over 200 million people in 71 tropical and subtropical countries are believed to be involved. The continuing presence of this infection requires the disposal of human waste into fresh water, the presence of suitable snail hosts, and the exposure of susceptible individuals to cercariae during play, bathing, work, or the collection and consumption of water. Ironically, in several countries, economic development schemes appear to have substantially increased disease incidence. Construction of dams and irrigation ditches has promoted the spread of the snail host and the migration of infected humans into previously uninvolved areas.

Within an endemic area there are wide variations in both the prevalence and intensity of infection. In general, there is a close correlation between infection rates and the degree of water contact. Typically, an infected patient harbors less than 10 worm pairs and lacks clinical manifestations of disease. Because flukes do not multiply within the body, large worm burdens are the result of repeated infections occurring over a period of years. The intensity of infection peaks during the second decade of life and then decreases with advancing age. This might be explained in part by reduced exposure to contaminated water but also may reflect slowly developing immunity.

IMMUNITY In animal models, protective immunity is directed against the invading larvae or schistosomula. Specific IgG antibodies attach to the parasite and then bind eosinophils to their Fc fragment. The eosinophils degranulate, releasing basic proteins which destroy the schistosomula. Adult worms already present in the body are not affected, a situation referred to as *concomitant immunity*. The adults appear to protect themselves from immunologic attack by shedding larval antigens and incorporating host molecules into their integument as they mature.

PATHOGENESIS AND CLINICAL MANIFESTATIONS Disease manifestations result from the immunopathologic consequences of three events: (1) cercarial penetration of the skin and subsequent migration of the schistosomula to the intrahepatic portal veins, (2) the onset of oviposition and extrusion of eggs, and (3) the retention of the remaining eggs in the tissues of the host. Within hours of penetration many cercariae die, producing a round-cell infiltration of the skin, papular eruption, edema, and pruritus. This is the result of an immediate and delayed hypersensitivity reaction to cercarial antigen and rarely occurs in primary infections. The rash is commonly followed by headache, myalgia, cough, and abdominal pain, manifestations presumably related to the migration of schistosomula. These symptoms may persist for 1 or 2 weeks, terminating with a modest fever.

After reaching maturity 1 or 2 months later, the worms initiate oviposition. The growing egg mass creates a state of relative antigen excess. This leads to the formation of circulating immune complexes and a concomitant serum sickness-like illness. This so-called *Katayama syndrome* is characterized by high spiking fever, cough, arthralgia, urticaria, lymphadenopathy, tender hepatomegaly, diarrhea, and, occasionally, melena. Sigmoidoscopy reveals an inflamed engorged mucosa with small areas of hemorrhage and ulceration. Peripheral eosinophilia is usually marked. The concentration of the circulating immune complexes correlates with both the number of eggs found in the stool and the clinical severity of disease. The illness may last as long as 3 months and, on rare occasion, may result in death. The syndrome is seen in its full intensity only in previously unexposed individuals who suffer massive cercarial exposure. In endemic areas it is usually brief and mild.

The eggs which are extruded into the lumen of the bowel or bladder elicit little damage. Soluble antigens secreted by the retained eggs stimulate an eosinophilic and mononuclear cell infiltration followed by edema, granuloma formation, and vascular obstruction. This has been shown to be T-cell mediated. The intensity of the reaction varies with the stage of disease. Early in infection granulomas may exceed the volume of the inciting egg by a hundredfold; those formed later are smaller and less damaging. Current evidence suggests that antibody blockade and suppressor T-cell activity both play a role in this modulation of host response. The correlation in Egyptian patients between A1 and B5 HLA types and the development of hepatosplenomegaly suggests that the extent of immunoregulation is influenced, at least in part, by the genetic character of the host. Secretion of a fibroblast stimulator by the granuloma eventually leads to deposition of fibrous tissue, scarring, and permanent vascular obstruction. In the bowel and bladder this results in mucosal congestion, thickening, ulceration, and formation of polyps.

Eggs deposited in the larger intestinal veins may be carried back to portal radicles of the liver. Granuloma formation and periportal fibrosis result in hepatic enlargement, presinusoidal portal hypertension, splenomegaly, and esophageal varices. Repeated bouts of esophageal bleeding may occur, but because hepatocellular function is usually well preserved, hepatic encephalopathy is rare.

With the development of portacaval anastomosis, some eggs are carried past the liver to the vessels of the lung where they produce interstitial fibrosis, destruction of pulmonary capillaries, and eventually pulmonary hypertension with cor pulmonale and aneurysms of the pulmonary artery. On roentgenograms the granulomas may resemble miliary tuberculosis.

Occasionally ova are carried to the central nervous system through anastomotic venous channels or are deposited there by ectopic adults.

DIAGNOSIS AND LABORATORY FINDINGS A history of residence or travel in an endemic area is the prerequisite for considering the diagnosis of infection with any of the schistosome species. The adult flukes of all species have a similar morphology and are not easily differentiated. Species diagnosis is usually made by finding characteristic eggs in stool specimens, urine, or biopsied tissue. Stool and urine concentration techniques are often required for detection of ova. Quantitation of the egg output by the Kato thick-smear or membrane filtration method is useful in estimating the severity of infection and in following the response to therapy.

Biopsy of the rectal or bladder mucosa is probably the single most reliable method of diagnosis and is often positive when repeated stool or urine examinations are negative. The mucosal snips are compressed between two glass slides and examined under the low-power lens of a microscope. Eggs, often numbering in the hundreds, are clearly visible. Because dead eggs may persist in tissue for a long time after the death of the adult worms, active infection is confirmed only if the eggs can be shown to be viable. This may be done by observing the eggs for movement under the high-power lens or by hatching them in water.

The absolute eosinophil count in the peripheral blood may be elevated but is a nonspecific finding seen in other tissue-invasive parasitic infections.

Immediate hypersensitivity (IH) skin tests, enzyme-linked immunosorbent assays (ELISA), and radioimmunoassays (RIA) employing antigens from adult worms and eggs are used primarily in research and epidemiologic studies but are not generally available for diagnosis. As immunodiagnostic tests are developed that identify schistosome infections by species and that correlate with activity and intensity of infection as judged by egg counts, they could replace detection and counting of schistosome eggs in urine and stool.

TREATMENT No specific therapy is available for the treatment of schistosomal dermatitis or the acute illness resembling serum sickness seen in the early months of infection. Antihistamines and steroids have been used to control the manifestations of these two symptoms. Because late schistosomiasis is caused by the continued deposition of eggs by the mature worm pairs, the aim of therapy in this stage of the disease is the sterilization and destruction of these parasites. Adult schistosomicides are available for this purpose, but in light of their considerable toxicity, therapy should not be initiated unless the presence of an active infection is first proved by the recovery of *viable eggs* from the stool or rectal mucosa. Moreover, since the severity of disease is related to the intensity of infection, some authorities believe light infections (e.g., fewer than 50 eggs per gram of stool) do not require therapy. In heavier infections therapy will usually reduce egg output by 90 percent or more, and attempts to achieve cure by repeated use of toxic agents are unwise.

Success of treatment is judged by the disappearance of eggs from the stool, reduction in eosinophils, and alleviation of symptoms. Patients should be examined monthly for 6 to 12 months to detect relapses. The decision to re-treat is based on factors such as intensity of egg output, presence of potentially reversible clinical manifestations, and the likelihood of reinfection.

Treatment of the patient with severe hepatic or pulmonary disease is largely symptomatic. There is little enthusiasm for portacaval shunting in the presence of esophageal varices. These patients usually have good hepatocellular function and, if treated carefully, will probably survive longer even with repeated bleeding episodes than with surgery. Additionally, splenectomy makes these patients more susceptible to the recrudescence of chronic malaria.

PREVENTION Prevention of schistosomiasis must be addressed at several levels. Theoretically sound public health measures, including the use of appropriate technology in the development of safe water supplies for endemic areas and in the detection and treatment of infected individuals, often conflict with the realities of political, administrative, and financial constraints.

Large molluscicidal programs to control snail populations have been implemented. Improved designs for irrigation ditches and canals that are inhospitable to snails, and biological snail control techniques, have been developed. In many cases, however, permanent eradication of snails has been limited by ecological factors and the magnitude of the snail problem.

Proper disposal of human excreta depends on acceptance of behavior that may be at variance with local customs and religious practices, despite manipulation of the physical environment.

Mass anthelmintic therapy in endemic areas has been an effective means of curing infections and reducing transmission of schistosomiasis. Drugs such as hycanthone, metrifonate, oxamniquine, and praziquantel have been employed in programs to control schistosomiasis in Africa, South America, and the far east.

Development of a schistosomal vaccine for use in humans is the subject of intense current research. Naturally occurring initial infections do not seem to confer immunity to further infections of the human host, permitting the acquisition of heavy worm burdens in some individuals. The infection rates and intensity of infection both peak in the second decade of life and then decrease with advancing age. This is thought to reflect slowly developing immunity, although decreased water contact may also be a factor. An effective vaccine would significantly increase the efficiency and protectiveness of the immune response. Animal studies suggest that immunity to schistosomiasis depends on the presence of specific antibodies and that parasite toxicity is mediated by eosinophils. An irradiated *S. bovis* cercarial vaccine for cattle has been developed and appears to confer a significant degree of protective immunity against infection in field trials in the Sudan. No vaccine is presently available for human use.

SCHISTOSOMIASIS *MANSONI* (INTESTINAL BILHARZIASIS, SCHISTOSOMAL DYSENTERY) Etiology *Schistosoma mansoni* is distinguished from the two other major species by the structure of its eggs and the adult flukes. The eggs are bluntly oval, have a lateral spine, and measure about 140 by about 60 μm. They are passed in feces and, rarely, in the urine. The intermediate snail hosts belong to the genera *Biomphalaria* and *Tropicorbis*. Humans are thought to be the principal host, but baboons in Kenya have been found to be infected naturally. It is not known whether they constitute an important reservoir of the disease independent of humans.

Epidemiology *S. mansoni* is the most widespread species of schistosomiasis and the only one present in the western hemisphere. It was brought to the Caribbean area and South America by African slaves. It is present in Venezuela, Surinam, Brazil, Puerto Rico, Dominican Republic, St. Lucia, and several other islands in the Caribbean. Owing to a lack of suitable snail hosts, transmission does not occur within the continental United States. However, there may be as many as 400,000 imported cases of infection (*S. mansoni, S. japonicum,* and *S. haematobium*) involving Puerto Ricans and immigrants from the Philippines, Yemen, Saudi Arabia, and southeast Asia. In the eastern hemisphere *S. mansoni* infections are found in the Nile delta, limited areas of east and south Africa, tropical Africa, and the Middle East, including Yemen, Saudi Arabia, and Israel.

Clinical manifestations Schistosomal dermatitis is not commonly noted in residents of endemic areas. The *Katayama syndrome* is, however, frequently observed in patients experiencing a primary infection. It may present in one of two clinical forms. In the first, upper abdominal pain and hepatosplenomegaly are the predominant manifestations. In the second, lower abdominal pain and bloody diarrhea occur. With the development of intestinal lesions, abdominal pain, diarrhea with or without blood, and a mild protein-losing enteropathy may be seen. Intestinal obstruction and rectal prolapse are rare complications. With the development of portal hypertension, the spleen occasionally becomes enormous, producing a visible abdominal mass and the anemia, leukopenia, and thrombocytopenia of hypersplenism. Hepatic enlargement is common but spider nevi, gynecomastia, jaundice, ascites, and other signs of hepatocellular deterioration are uncommon in the absence of other liver disease. Exsanguination from esophageal varices is a common cause of death. Central nervous system involvement usually presents as a transverse myelitis.

There is impressive evidence that circulating antigen antibody complexes may produce an immune-complex nephropathy in schistosomiasis *mansoni.* This has been observed primarily in patients with the chronic hepatosplenic form of the disease and may present as asymptomatic albuminuria, the nephrotic syndrome, or progressive renal failure. There is little information on its incidence or public health significance.

Chronic *Salmonella* and *Escherichia coli* bacteremias have been noted in patients suffering from hepatosplenic schistosomiasis. The chronicity of these infections may be related to the ability of adult parasites to harbor bacteria in their tegument. Antibiotic therapy is unsatisfactory unless the parasites are first eradicated with appropriate antischistosomal treatment.

Diagnosis and laboratory findings *S. mansoni* infections as evidenced by characteristic ova in the stool are sometimes an incidental finding in asymptomatic persons from endemic areas. If an individual has a relevant geographic history, gastrointestinal complaints, and negative stool examinations, a rectal biopsy should be performed.

Treatment *Oxamniquine* (Vansil) is the drug of choice for the treatment of *S. mansoni* infections, in both the acute phase and the chronic phase with hepatosplenic involvement. It is given orally in a total dose of 60 mg/kg divided between two consecutive days for *S. mansoni* acquired in Africa. It is given as a single dose of 15 mg/kg for *S. mansoni* acquired in the western hemisphere. Giving the drug after meals will reduce the most common side effects of transitory dizziness and drowsiness. Few serious side effects are associated with treatment, although treatment is contraindicated in persons with a history of previous seizures. Episodes of fever and an episode of hematemesis with onset 1 to 3 days following treatment of hepatosplenic disease have been reported. The drug is available commercially in the United States.

Niridazole (Ambilhar) is an alternate agent that is given orally in a dose of 25 mg/kg per day in divided doses for 7 days. The side effects of this drug include ECG changes, oligospermia, and a high incidence of neurological abnormalities, including EEG changes. Psychotic episodes or convulsions, which disappear when administration of the drugs is discontinued, have also been reported. Neuropsychiatric side effects are more common in *S. mansoni* infections with hepatic involvement. The drug is contraindicated in patients with a prior history of seizures. It is available in the United States from the Centers for Disease Control (CDC), Atlanta.

Praziquantel (Embay 8440) has a broad spectrum of activity and is active against the three major schistosome species. It has undergone field trials in Africa, South America, and Asia. The drug is given as a single oral dose of 50 mg/kg for *S. mansoni.* The main reported side effects are giddiness, drowsiness, and mild gastrointestinal symptoms. The drug is not presently available in the United States.

Prognosis The prognosis is good. Many patients never develop symptoms, and early states of colonic, hepatic, pulmonary, and central nervous system disease are completely reversible with adequate therapy. In the late fibrotic stage, the prognosis is worse.

SCHISTOSOMIASIS JAPONICA (KATAYAMA DISEASE) Etiology *Schistosoma japonicum* lives in the superior mesenteric venules and frequently migrates to those of the colon for oviposition. Its oval eggs are shorter, wider, and smaller than those of the other two species, measuring about 90 by 70 μm. Mature eggs have a minute hook, or spine, laterally situated and smaller than that of *S. mansoni.* The ova are passed in the feces only. The life cycle is similar to that of *S. mansoni,* except that amphibious snails of the genus *Oncomelania,* which are capable of prolonged existence away from water, are utilized as intermediate hosts. Water buffalo, horses, cattle, pigs, dogs, and cats as well as humans may harbor the adult worms. The nature of the host and presence of nonhuman reservoirs add to the difficulty of disease control.

Epidemiology *S. japonicum* affects 60 million people in the agricultural areas of Japan, China, the Philippines, and the Celebes. An important source of infection is the use of human excreta ("night soil") as a fertilizer in vegetable gardens.

Pathogenesis and clinical manifestations The early manifestations of infection are seen less commonly than in schistosomiasis *mansoni.* However, because *S. japonicum* eggs are deposited in greater number and in closer proximity to the liver than are those of *S. mansoni,* the intermediate and late manifestations of disease are usually both more frequent and more severe.

The allergic manifestations accompanying oviposition are particularly impressive in *japonicum* infections. From 4 to 6 weeks after exposure the patient notes the onset of a high spiking fever, chills, cough, urticaria, generalized lymphadenopathy, tender hepatosplenomegaly, and eosinophilic leukocytosis. The deposition of large numbers of eggs in the intestinal wall results in ulcerations, bloody mucoid stools, and abdominal pain. The acute illness may persist for 1 to 2 months but usually subsides leaving the patient relatively well. Death may occur in severe cases.

With continued oviposition fibrosis of the small bowel and liver develops. These changes are seen earlier than in *mansoni* infections, and as a result the entire disease may run its course in 2 to 5 years, ending in death.

In advanced cases the gross postmortem findings are emaciation and pallor; a large or contracted liver with periportal fibrosis; splenomegaly, with fibrosis of pulp; ascites; fibrotic nodules over the colonic peritoneum; fibrous thickening and rigidity of the colon, with small polyps projecting from the mucosa; and thickening and fibrosis of the omentum.

Clinically, signs of portal obstruction such as engorgement of superficial abdominal veins and ascites appear. Some individuals present marked splenomegaly, a small contracted liver, profound anemia, leukopenia, and thrombocytopenia associated with severe malnutrition and hypoproteinemia. The majority of individuals suffering from schistosomiasis *japonicum* die of cirrhosis and cachexia, massive hemorrhage from rupture of esophageal varices, or intercurrent infections.

Central nervous system lesions occur more frequently in the brain than in the spinal cord, appear clinically as epilepsy on an expanding tumor, and usually result from the presence of ectopic adults.

Diagnosis and laboratory findings The characteristic ova must be found in the stools in order to establish the diagnosis. In established cases, ova are more difficult to demonstrate in the stools or in a rectal biopsy.

Treatment In general, *S. japonicum* infections are more difficult to treat and relapses are more frequent than those of other types of schistosomiasis. *Praziquantel* is potentially the most effective and least toxic of the available drugs. It is being studied as an oral regimen of three doses of 20 mg/kg at intervals of 4 h. The toxicity of this drug has been discussed above.

Niridazole is a drug with limited efficacy against serious *S. japonicum* infections. It is given orally in a dose of 25 mg/kg per day (maximum 1.5 g) for 10 days. The toxicity of this drug has been discussed above.

Antimony sodium dimercaptosuccinate (Astiban) is an alternative drug used in severe cases of *S. japonicum* disease. The drug is prepared in a 10% solution for injection. A total of 6 to 8 mg/kg (maximum 500 mg) is given intravenously in weekly doses for 5 to 7 weeks up to the total adult dose of 35 to 50 mg/kg (maximum 2.5 to 3.0 g). This drug may be obtained from the CDC. Temporary ECG changes are common during therapy; however, arrhythmias, collapse, and sudden death have been reported. Antimonials also may cause hepatitis, acute nephritis, hemolytic anemia, and thrombocytopenic purpura. Heart, renal, or liver disease constitutes a contraindication to therapy with this drug. If a lesion is present in the brain, prompt treatment may forestall the need for surgical intervention.

Prognosis If the condition is not treated early, the prognosis is poor in the majority of cases encountered in endemic communities.

SCHISTOSOMIASIS HAEMATOBIA (GENITOURINARY SCHISTOSOMIASIS, ENDEMIC HEMATURIA) Etiology and life cycle The adult worms live in the hemorrhoidal plexus of veins, some going to the rectum for oviposition but most of them passing on to the vesical plexus. The eggs are compact, elongated spindles, dilated in the middle and measuring about 140 by 50 μm. At one pole they present a short terminal spine. The ova are passed in the urine and occasionally in the feces. The life cycle is similar to that of *S. mansoni.* The intermediate hosts are snails of the genera *Bulinus, Physopsis,* and *Biomphalaria.*

Epidemiology *S. haematobium* is largely confined to Africa and the Middle East where its distribution overlaps that of *S. mansoni.* It is not uncommon for individuals within the endemic areas to harbor both flukes.

Pathogenesis and clinical manifestations Large numbers of ova are deposited in the submucosa of the bladder where they incite an eosinophilic granulomatous reaction. The trigone is involved at first, but soon the entire mucosa is thickened and ulcerated. In chronic infections, the other coats become scarred and the muscularis hypertrophies. Pedunculated papillomas often develop at the trigone and about the urethral orifices. The bladder capacity becomes greatly reduced as the organ loses its contractility. Lesions occur in the distal third of the ureters in many cases, causing vesicoureteral reflux, obstruction, and hydronephrosis. Bacterial pyelonephritis may occur. In about 10 percent of cases, calculi develop in the bladder, renal pelvis, or ureters, and occasionally the entire calcified bladder can be visualized on roentgenograms. Fistulas between the urogenital tract and intestines may develop. The prostate and seminal vesicles in men and the cervix and vagina in women may be affected; lymphatic blockade with elephantiasis of the genitalia occurs rarely. Carcinoma of the bladder is a frequent late complicaton in Egypt but not in other areas. Because the ova are deposited in the vesical plexus, ectopic eggs are carried to the lungs where they produce miliary granulomas. Although in endemic areas the egg output usually decreases in adolescence, the pathological changes continue to progress in untreated infection.

Painful micturition, frequency, and terminal hematuria are the leading symptoms. Secondary bacterial infection of the urinary tract is frequent, and repeated hemorrhages from the bladder produce severe anemia. Chronic *Salmonella* bacteriuria with recurrent bouts of bacteremia has been reported from Egypt. An associated nephrotic syndrome which responds to antibiotic and anthelmintic therapy also occurred. With progressive obstruction, renal failure and uremia ensue.

Diagnosis and laboratory findings As in the other types of schistosomiasis, the diagnosis is made by finding the characteristic ova in the urine, in tissues obtained from vesical mucosa, or, less frequently, in the stools. Eggs are most numerous in the midday urine where they are best detected with membrane filtration techniques. If these are negative, cystoscopy and biopsy of the bladder are usually diagnostic. In long-standing infections, urine culture and intravenous urograms should be obtained.

Treatment Chemotherapy often results in dramatic reversal of symptoms and even obstructive phenomena.

Metrifonate (Bilarcil) is the drug of choice, in a dose of 10 mg/kg once every 2 weeks for three doses. This drug has minimal side effects. Prophylaxis with the drug in a dose of 4 mg/kg weekly along with its lack of significant toxicity and its low cost make it a valuable tool in large-scale efforts to control *S. haematobium* infections in endemic areas. The drug is available from the CDC.

Niridazole can be used in a dose of 25 mg/kg per day orally divided into three doses for 5 to 7 days (maximum 1.5 g). Toxicity of the drug has been discussed previously. Niridazole possesses anti-inflammatory action as well as direct parasite toxicity and is useful in advanced urinary tract disease with obstructive lesions as it promotes resolution of granulomas.

Praziquantel given 50 mg/kg as a single oral dose has been shown to be highly effective for treatment of *S. haematobium* infection. Since this drug is also effective in treatment of *S. mansoni,* it may be particularly useful in patients with mixed infections with both species. Toxicity of the drug has been discussed above.

Hycanthone (Etrenol) is useful in *S. haematobium* infections but has not fared well in mutagenesis studies and is dangerous in patients with hepatosplenic disease or a history of jaundice. The drug is used in endemic areas in a dose of 3 mg/kg as a single IM injection. Common side effects include nausea and vomiting.

Prognosis Provided treatment is started without delay, the prognosis is good in recent infection and fair when damage to the bladder and urinary infection have already occurred. The prognosis is very poor in chronic, late infections. After age 45, the mortality rate increases fourfold. The frequent coexistence of infection with *S. mansoni* aggravates both the prognosis and the clinical picture.

SCHISTOSOMIASIS *MEKONGI* Etiology *S. mekongi* is a newly described species that is closely related to *S. japonicum.* It may be distinguished from the latter by its snail host, distribution, and egg morphology. The intermediate host, *Lithoglyphopsis aperta,* is found in a relatively limited area along the Mekong River and its tributary, the Man River, in Thailand, Cambodia, and Laos. Although resembling those of *S. japonicum, S. mekongi* eggs are rounder and smaller and can be mistaken for ascaris eggs by the inexperienced examiner. Dogs as well as humans may serve as definitive hosts. The adult worms live in the mesenteric venules, and the eggs, like those of *S. japonicum,* are passed in the stool.

Pathogenesis and clinical manifestations *S. mekongi* infections may be asymptomatic. The serious clinical sequelae of *S. mekongi* infections resemble the hepatosplenic disease of *S. mansoni* and *S. japonicum* infections, with the development of hepatosplenomegaly, portal hypertension, and esophageal varices. The pathology of serious disease is presumed similar to that of hepatosplenic disease caused by the other species.

Diagnosis A compatible geographic history is essential in first suspecting the diagnosis. It is confirmed by demonstrating the eggs in the stool. Egg excretion is variable and multiple examinations are often required. Rectal biopsy may be required in light infections.

Treatment Praziquantel may be the drug of choice for this infection.

SCHISTOSOMIASIS *INTERCALATUM* Etiology Although closely resembling *S. haematobium* eggs in morphology, *S. intercalatum* eggs are passed exclusively in the feces. There are two strains of the parasite spread by intermediate snail hosts *Bulinus forskali* in Lower Guinea and *B. africanus* in the Congo.

Pathogenesis and clinical manifestations Many infections are asymptomatic. The symptoms range from minimal gastrointestinal discomfort to severe watery, bloody diarrhea.

Diagnosis Definitive eggs must be found in the stool.

Treatment Praziquantel has shown significant activity against this parasite in laboratory studies.

SCHISTOSOME DERMATITIS Definition and geographic distribution Cercariae of certain nonhuman schistosomes are capable of penetrating human skin but are unable to develop further. The cercariae die just beneath the epidermis, leaving a residue that may serve as a sensitizing agent. Subsequent exposure to cercariae stimulates an allergic response and results in a schistosome dermatitis similar to that seen with the species pathogenic for humans. This condition is known also as *swimmer's itch* or *cercarial dermatitis.* Vertebrate definitive hosts for some common dermatitis-producing schistosomes are migratory birds, muskrats, mice, voles, and deer.

Schistosome dermatitis has been reported from the freshwater areas of the north central and western United States, Alaska, Canada, Central and South America, western Europe (particularly Switzerland), and the far east.

A seawater dermatitis believed to be produced by nonhuman schistosome cercariae has been reported in clam diggers and bathers along the coasts of New York, Rhode Island, California, Hawaii, and Florida.

Clinical manifestations The initial symptom is usually a prickling sensation; occasionally urticaria is noted as the water evaporates from the skin. These manifestations disappear within an hour, leaving only a few macules to mark the site of cercarial penetration. Several hours later an intense itching accompanied by a papular and occasionally a vesicular rash begins. This is most intense on the second or third day and gradually subsides over the next few days. The rash may be easily mistaken for insect bites.

Treatment Local application of antipruritic lotions such as calamine with menthol or phenol is used to allay itching and thereby reduce the likelihood of secondary infection. Treatment with antihistaminic drugs will relieve the pruritus.

Prevention The best prevention is avoidance of water contact in areas where the disease is a problem. Immediate drying of the skin after swimming has been recommended as a prophylactic measure. This will not completely prevent lesions, since some penetration occurs during immersion. In some areas, control has been effected by destruction of snails with molluscicides or with removal of vegetation.

REFERENCES

Bassily S et al: Treatment of complicated schistosomiasis mansoni with oxamniquine. Am J Trop Med Hyg 27:1284, 1978

Davis A, Hegner DHG: Multicentre trials of praziquantel in human schistosomiasis—design and techniques. Bull WHO 57:767, 1979

Heyneman D: Schistosomiasis: Recent developments in immunology and treatment. Medical Staff Conference, University of California, San Francisco. West J Med 133:49, 1980

Hiatt RA et al: Factors in the pathogenesis of acute schistosomiasis mansoni. J Infect Dis 139:659, 1979

Hoeffler DF: "Swimmers' itch" (cercardial dermatitis). Cutis 19:461, 1977

Hofstetter M et al: Infection with *Schistosoma mekongi* in Southeast Asian refugees. J Infect Dis 144:420, 1981

Lehman JS et al: Urinary schistosomiasis in Egypt: Clinical, radiological, bacteriological and parasitological correlations. Trans R Soc Trop Med Hyg 67:384, 1973

Mahmoud AA: Current concepts—Schistosomiasis. N Engl J Med 297:1329, 1977

Warren KS: The pathology, pathobiology and pathogenesis of schistosomiasis. Nature (Parasitol Suppl) 273:609, 1978

———: Schistosomiasis japonicum. Clin Gastroenterol 7:77, 1978

Wright CA et al: What is *Schistosoma intercalatum* Fisher 1934? Trans R Soc Trop Med Hyg 66:28, 1972

229 TISSUE NEMATODES

JAMES J. PLORDE

ANGIOSTRONGYLIASIS CANTONENSIS Definition *Angiostrongylus cantonensis,* the rat lungworm, is the etiologic agent of the common form of *eosinophilic meningitis* found in southeast Asia and the tropical areas of the Pacific.

Etiology The delicate filariform adults (20 mm in length) reside and lay their eggs in the pulmonary arterioles of rats and certain other rodents. After hatching, the larvae break into the alveoli, migrate up the respiratory tract, are swallowed, and pass in the feces. They develop into infective third-stage larvae within snails and slugs, their natural intermediate host. Viable third-stage organisms may also be found in land planarians, crabs, and freshwater prawns. These carriers appear to acquire the larvae by feeding on the tissues of infected mollusks. Humans, like rodents, become parasitized when they ingest raw intermediate or carrier hosts containing the infective stage. In rodents the larvae migrate to the brain where they grow into young adults. After a period of further maturation, the worms travel to the lungs and begin to deposit eggs. The nematode does not complete its life cycle in humans and dies after reaching the central nervous system.

Epidemiology The majority of human infections with *A. cantonensis* have been found in Thailand, Vietnam, Cambodia, Indonesia, the Philippines, Taiwan, Hawaii, and several smaller Pacific islands from Okinawa in the north to New Caledonia and Tahiti in the south. Cases have been described in Cuba, Egypt, and the Ivory Coast. In addition, rodent infections have been found in the islands of East Africa, Sri Lanka, India, and China. The rat lungworm may have been spread from Madagascar to Asia and to the Pacific by the recent dispersal of the giant African land snail, *Achatina fulica.*

Pathology and pathogenesis The nematode can produce extensive tissue damage by moving through the brain when alive and provokes a marked inflammatory reaction when dead. The pathological lesions are characterized by (1) marked lymphocyte and eosinophilic infiltration of the meninges, (2) hemorrhagic and nonhemorrhagic worm tracts through the brainstem and spinal cord, (3) granuloma formation around dead parasites and necrotic debris which sheathes the worm, and (4) engorgement of almost all blood vessels, particularly the veins. Necrosis of vessel walls, aneurysmal dilatation of arteries, and perivascular hemorrhages have been noted. Living worms have been removed from the eyes of patients without central nervous system involvement.

Clinical manifestations The eosinophilic meningitis usually presents as an acute severe headache. Fever is usually mild or absent, and only 15 percent of patients show signs of meningeal irritation. Patients frequently complain of visual impairment and, in a majority of these, visual defects or blurring of the optic disk can be demonstrated. Paresthesias of the trunk and lower extremities are a common complaint, and paralysis of the sixth and seventh nerves is seen in 3 to 7 percent of cases. Paralysis of the limbs, convulsions, and loss of consciousness are rare. Although some patients have experienced significant neurologic residua, the disease usually ends in complete spontaneous recovery. Death is rare. The cerebrospinal fluid contains several hundred cells per cubic millimeter and many eosinophils, and the cerebrospinal fluid protein is elevated. There may or may not be an eosinophilia in the peripheral blood.

The second clinically distinct form of eosinophilic meningitis has been reported from Thailand. This presents as a radiculomyeloencephalitis with limb pain and paresis and is thought to be caused by the nematode *Gnathostoma spinigerum.* The cerebrospinal fluid eosinophilic leukocytosis is less marked than in *angiostrongylus* infections. The fluid is often xanthochromic. Death may occur from cerebral hemorrhage or destruction of vital centers.

Diagnosis The diagnosis is made on the basis of the clinical manifestations in an endemic area. Rarely, the adult worm is found in the cerebrospinal fluid. Angiostrongyliasis must be differentiated from other ectopic worm infections of the central nervous system including strongyloidiasis, filariasis, paragonimiasis, hydatid disease, schistosomiasis japonicum, trichinosis, cysticercosis, toxocariasis, and gnathostomiasis.

Treatment and prevention There is no known effective treatment. Anthelmintic therapy should not be given since the simultaneous death of many worms might produce a severe inflammatory reaction. Steroids may be beneficial in severe cases. Prevention depends upon avoidance or proper cooking of such foods as snails, prawns, and crabs. Raw vegetables should be carefully inspected for the presence of planarians and mollusks before they are eaten. Freezing of crustaceans and mollusks at $-15°C$ for 12 h will destroy infective larvae of *A. cantonensis.*

ANGIOSTRONGYLIASIS COSTARICENSIS *Angiostrongylus costaricensis* is a nematode that dwells in the mesenteric arteries of Central American rats. Larvae pass in the stool and develop in slugs, the intermediate hosts. Rats, and incidentally humans, are infected when they ingest slugs or vegetables contaminated with third-stage larvae deposited in the mucous trail of these mollusks. The larvae mature in the lymphatics and move to the mesenteric radicals of the cecum. Here they may cause arterial thrombosis, ischemic necrosis, ulceration, and eosinophilic granuloma formation. Infected patients present with fever, eosinophilic leukocytosis, abdominal pain, and a right lower quadrant mass. Occasionally perforation of the bowel and generalized peritonitis occur. The fever may persist for up to 2 months. Children are more frequently involved than adults. Neither larvae nor eggs are seen in the stool of the human host. No specific therapy is available.

GNATHOSTOMIASIS Definition Gnathostomiasis is a tissue infection of humans caused by *Gnathostoma spinigerum,* an intestinal nematode of carnivores. Clinically it is manifest as migratory subcutaneous swellings, creeping eruption, or a lethal eosinophilic meningitis.

Etiology and epidemiology The parasite, which is found throughout the far east, lives encysted in the gastric mucosa of dogs, cats, and wild felines. The ova are passed to the external environment via the feces, hatch in water, and are ingested by *Cyclops,* the first intermediate hosts. These in turn are eaten by freshwater fish, frogs, snakes, and eels in whose flesh the infective third-stage larvae develop. Ducks and chickens fed on these second intermediate hosts may also come to harbor infective larvae. Human infections, which are most commonly seen in Thailand and Japan, occur when humans ingest infected uncooked fish (somfak, sashimi), duck, or chicken.

Pathogenesis and manifestations The parasite cannot complete its cycle in humans, and the immature worms migrate through the abdominal and thoracic organs producing localized areas of inflammation and hemorrhage. Clinically, this is manifest as fever, eosinophilic leukocytosis, urticaria, and pain. Typically, the systemic manifestations subside within a month as the worms make their way to the subcutaneous tissues. Here, their continued migration results in the production of transient serpiginous pruritic swellings, subcutaneous tunnels, and abscesses. If the worm invades the epidermis, the resulting lesions closely resemble those of cutanea larva migrans. Rarely the eye may be involved with orbital cellulitis, iritis, or uveitis. Migration into the central nervous system results in a lethal eosinophilic meningitis (see "Angiostrongyliasis cantonensis" above). This presents as a radiculomyeloencephalitis with limb pain and paresis. The cerebrospinal fluid eosinophilic leukocytosis is present but less marked than in *Angiostrongylus* infections. The fluid is often xanthochromic. Death may occur from cerebral hemorrhage or destruction of vital centers.

Diagnosis and treatment Painless, recurrent migratory subcutaneous swellings and eosinophilic leukocytosis occurring in an endemic area make the diagnosis likely. It must be differentiated from cutanea larva migrans, however, and from angiostrongyliasis cantonensis when the central nervous system is involved. Definitive diagnosis depends upon the removal and identification of the worm. Other than excision, there is no specific therapy. The disease can be prevented by the adequate cooking of fish, chicken, and duck in endemic areas.

DRACUNCULIASIS Definition Dracunculiasis is an infection of human connective and subcutaneous tissues by the guinea worm, *Dracuncula medinensis.* The gravid female produces symptoms when she ruptures the skin to discharge her eggs.

Etiology and epidemiology Dracunculiasis affects about 50 million people in west, central, and northeast Africa, the Middle East, Iran, Pakistan, India, northeastern South America, and the Caribbean islands. Humans acquire the parasite when they ingest raw drinking water containing infected copepods (*Cyclops* spp.) which serve as the intermediate host. Shallow ponds, cisterns, and wells are the usual habitat of these crustaceans. In the stomach the copepod is digested and the larvae are released. The larva penetrates the intestinal wall and matures in the connective tissue of the retroperitoneal space. The adult male is small, seldom seen, and presumably dies after mating. In contrast, the female *Dracunculus* is one of the largest nematodes known—1 to 2 mm in diameter and 300 to 800 mm in length. The female reaches gravidity in approximately one year and then migrates to the subcutaneous tissue of the lower extremities. When the anterior end of the worm approaches the skin, a blister forms. This breaks down in a few days, forming a superficial ulcer. When the protruding portion of the worm comes in contact with water, the uterus prolapses through the body and discharges large numbers of motile rhabditiform larvae. Following ingestion by one of several species of *Cyclops,* the larvae undergo further development, becoming infective in 10 to 12 days. Mammals other than humans may be infected, but their importance as a disease reservoir is uncertain.

Pathogenesis and manifestations The infection is asymptomatic until the gravid female appears in the subcutaneous tissues where it may, on occasion, be palpable. A few days before the formation of the blister, the patient frequently has fever, generalized urticaria, periorbital edema, and wheezing. Blister formation is accompanied by intense local pain and pruritus; like the systemic manifestations, this is thought to represent an allergic reaction to prematurely liberated larvae. The local lesion is usually found over the feet and ankles but may occur on the trunk or the upper extremities. Multiple infections are common. With the rupture of the blister and the release of embryos, the systemic manifestations abate, and the worm is slowly extruded over a period of 4 to 5 weeks. Secondary infection and cellulitis are common, particularly if the worm is ruptured during the process of extraction. In Nigeria, guinea worm ulcers are a common portal of entry for the spores of *Clostridium tetani.* The female worm often fails to reach the surface and discharge her larvae. In most of these cases, it dies without producing symptoms. The calcified appearance on roentgenograms is characteristic. Occasionally the worm may invade the deep tissues, causing serious symptoms, and sterile abscesses may follow the release of embryos. Invasion of joint spaces by the adult worm or larvae results in arthritis.

Diagnosis The clinical picture is characteristic. Placing a small amount of water on the worm results in discharge of larvae which can then be examined microscopically. A fluorescent antibody test may permit the diagnosis to be made prior to emergence of the gravid female.

Treatment and prevention If the outline of the worm can be clearly seen or palpated, it may sometimes be completely removed with a single incision. The gradual extraction of the worm can be accomplished by winding a few centimeters onto a stick each day. Administration of niridazole (Ambilhar) results in prompt remission of symptoms. The dose is 25 mg per kilogram of body weight given in three divided doses for 7 days. Thiabendazole in dosage of 25 mg/kg twice daily for 2 days or metronidazole 250 mg three times a day for 7 days is also effective in the relief of symptoms. At present, there is serious question whether any of the above agents hasten worm extrusion or death. Some authorities suggest the rapid symptomatic improvement induced by these agents is secondary to their antiinflammatory rather than anthelmintic properties. Dracunculiasis can be prevented by the chemical treatment of drinking water.

REFERENCES

Loria-Cortes R, Lobo-Sanahuja JF: Clinical abdominal angiostrongylosis. A study of 116 children with intestinal eosinophilic granuloma caused by *Angiostrongylus costaricensis.* Am J Trop Med Hyg 29:538, 1980

Muller R: Guinea worm disease: Epidemiology, control and treatment. Bull WHO 57:683, 1979

Nye SW et al: Lesions of the brain in eosinophilic meningitis. Arch Pathol 89:9, 1970

Pascual JE et al: Eosinophilic meningoencephalitis in Cuba caused by *Angiostrongylus cantonensis.* Am J Trop Med Hyg 30:960, 1981

Punyagupta S et al: Eosinophilic meningitis in Thailand. Am J Trop Med 24:921, 1975

230 INTESTINAL NEMATODES

JAMES J. PLORDE

ENTEROBIASIS Definition Enterobiasis (pinworm, seatworm, or threadworm infection, oxyuriasis) is an intestinal infection of humans caused by *Enterobius vermicularis* and characterized by perianal pruritus. Eggs of this parasite have been found in a 10,000-year-old coprolith, making it the oldest demonstrated infection of humans. It has been estimated that the worm infects 200 million people, 30 to 40 million of them in the United States and Canada.

Etiology The female averages 10 mm in length, the male 3 mm. They live with their heads attached to the mucosa of the cecum, appendix, and adjacent parts of the bowel. The gravid female migrates through the anal canal at night, deposits her 10,000 eggs on the perianal skin, and dies. In female patients the worm may enter the vagina and occasionally gain access to the peritoneal cavity through the fallopian tubes. Each egg contains an embryo which, within a few hours, develops into an infective larva. After the egg has been ingested, the larva is released in the small intestine and migrates down the bowel lumen to the cecum. In less than 1 month from the time of ingestion, newly developed gravid females are again discharging eggs. They are planoconvex and measure approximately 20 by 50 μm. The shell is clear and doubly contoured.

Epidemiology Humans are usually infected by the direct transfer of eggs from the anus to the mouth by way of contaminated fingers. Retroinfection, which is seen primarily in adults, may occasionally take place when eggs hatch in the perianal area and the larvae migrate back into the bowel to mature. The eggs, which are relatively resistant to desiccation, also contaminate nightclothes and bed linen, where they remain viable and infective for 2 to 3 weeks. Airborne transmission is possible, and spread within family and children's groups occurs readily. Enterobiasis is found in all climates and is probably the most common helminthic infection of humans. Its low incidence in some tropical areas, however, is not fully explained.

Clinical manifestations The most common symptom is pruritus ani, which is most troublesome at night, being related to the migration of the gravid female worms. Irritability, insomnia, enuresis, and other minor complaints are probably secondary to the pruritus. Scratching may lead to perianal eczema or pyogenic infection. Vaginal discharge has been reported, and rarely a chronic granulomatous salpingitis or endometritis results from the presence of ectopic adults. An association between enterobiasis and cystitis in young females has been reported. This, it is suggested, results from the transport of enteric bacteria into the bladder by the migrating worm. Other rare ectopic locations include the lung, liver, and peritoneum. Probably the worms can penetrate the bowel wall only if its continuity has been compromised by some other disease.

Laboratory findings Examination for ova of material obtained from the perianal skin by means of a Scotch brand cellophane tape swab is the preferable method for the detection of enterobiasis. The tape is folded sticky-side out over the end of a tongue blade, pressed firmly against the perianal area, and then spread on a glass slide and examined under the lower power of a microscope. The swab should be taken at home by the patient on three to five consecutive mornings prior to bathing and brought to the laboratory for examination. Searching for ova in the feces is rarely helpful, but scrapings from under the nails may reveal ova. The diagnosis is sometimes made by finding adult worms in the perianal area or in the feces following a laxative or an enema. Eosinophilic leukocytosis may occur but is not a typical finding.

Treatment All infected individuals in a family or communal group should be treated simultaneously. The frequently recommended sanitary measures aside from daily bathing and hand washing before meals and after stools are of dubious benefit. It is relatively easy to eradicate the worms, but reinfection is frequent. Retreatment does not appear necessary unless symptoms recur.

Two highly satisfactory drugs are available. Pyrantel pamoate (Banminth) given in a single oral dose of 11 mg/kg (maximum 1.0 g) is probably the drug of choice. Alternatively, a single 100-mg oral dose of mebendazole (Vermox) can be used. This drug is not recommended for infants or pregnant women. Pyrvinium pamoate (Povan) is equally effective but less convenient. It is given orally as a single dose of 5 mg/kg in tablet or liquid form. This compound turns the stool red and may stain bedclothes or undergarments. In heavily contaminated environments, treatment with the above drugs may be repeated after an interval of 2 weeks to eliminate any new infections.

Prevention Methods of preventing autoinfection and dissemination within a group involving children are extremely difficult to enforce. Personal environmental hygiene should be stressed, and anthelmintic and symptomatic treatment of pruritus ani should be instituted. To control infection within a group, simultaneous treatment of all cases is mandatory.

TRICHURIASIS Definition Trichuriasis (whipworm infection, trichocephaliasis) is an intestinal infection of humans caused by *Trichuris trichiura* and is characterized by invasion of the colonic mucosa by the adult trichuris. Five hundred million persons are thought to be infected with this parasite including 2 million in the United States. It may be the most commonly encountered helminthic infection in Americans returning from tropical areas.

Etiology The adult whipworms are found in the large intestine with their anterior ends deeply embedded in the mucosa. They are 30 to 50 mm in length and possess a threadlike anterior two-thirds with a stouter posterior third, giving them a whiplike structure. The female produces about 5000 eggs each day. They are characteristically barrel-shaped (20 to 50 μm), brown, thick-walled, and translucent with knoblike ends. The eggs, like those of *Ascaris,* must incubate at least 3 weeks in soil before they become infective. After ingestion, the eggs hatch in the small intestine and the larvae become embedded in the intestinal villi. After several days they migrate to the large intestine where they mature in about 3 months. The adult worms may live for 4 to 8 years. Occasionally, *T. vulpis,* the whipworm of dogs, may infect humans. The eggs are larger (35 by 75 μm) but otherwise identical to those of the human parasite.

Epidemiology Whipworm is a cosmopolitan parasite but is most commonly found in the tropics where the level of sanitation is low and environmental conditions necessary for the incubation of the eggs are optimal. In the United States, it is found throughout the rural areas of the southeast. Its distribution is similar to that of *Ascaris* and hookworm, but the eggs are less resistant than those of *Ascaris* to sunlight and drying. Because of their general lack of sanitary habits, children and the mentally retarded have the highest incidence of infection. For example, 13 percent of patients confined to hospitals for the mentally subnormal were found to harbor *Trichuris.*

Pathogenesis and clinical manifestations Symptomatic infection generally requires the presence of large numbers of adult whipworms and may be correlated in part with the degree of mucosal involvement. Heavy infections usually occur only in children and may be accompanied by finger clubbing, nausea, abdominal pain, diarrhea, and dysentery. It has been estimated that infected patients lose 0.005 ml blood per worm per day. Infections with more than 800 worms often result in anemia. In heavier infections, the distribution of worms throughout the colon and rectum may result in rectal prolapse while straining at stool. Some investigators also feel that *Trichuris* infections predispose to amebic dysentery and bacterial gastroenteritis.

Laboratory findings In symptomatic infection, large numbers of eggs are present in the feces, and there may be eosinophilic leukocytosis and anemia. In light infections, concentration techniques may be necessary to recover the eggs. Quantitation of egg output is helpful since only counts above 3000 eggs per gram of feces are likely to be associated with symptoms. Stools should be cultured for bacterial pathogens and examined for the presence of *E. histolytica.*

Treatment Treatment is unsatisfactory. Mebendazole in the oral dose of 100 mg twice daily for 3 days is the drug of choice. Its cure rate is 60 to 70 percent, and it achieves a 90 percent reduction in egg burden. The dose may have to be repeated in patients with heavy infections. It is not recommended for children under the age of 2 or pregnant women.

Prognosis Whipworm infection, unless characterized by severe diarrhea, blood loss, and systemic reaction, usually responds well to treatment. Serious infections may require supportive treatment as well as chemotherapy.

Prevention Measures recommended for ascariasis apply also to trichuriasis.

ASCARIASIS Definition Ascariasis is an infection of humans caused by *Ascaris lumbricoides* and characterized by an early pulmonary phase related to larval migration and a later, prolonged intestinal phase. It is estimated that 25 percent of the world's population, including 4 million Americans, are infected with this nematode.

Etiology The adult ascarids are large (15 to 40 cm in length), cylindric worms with blunt ends which maintain themselves in the lumen of the jejunum by virtue of their muscular activity. Despite a life span of only 6 to 18 months, the female releases millions of eggs, both fertile and infertile, into the fecal stream; the daily output is estimated to be 200,000 per worm. Fertilized eggs are elliptic (30 to 40 μm by 50 to 60 μm) with an irregular, dense outer shell and a regular, translucent inner shell. They require a period of soil incubation before they become infective. Under optimum conditions of warmth and moisture this occurs in 2 to 3 weeks. The eggs may then remain viable for up to 6 years in temperate climates. When an infective egg is ingested, the larva is liberated in the small intestine. It migrates through the wall and is carried by the bloodstream or lymphatics to the lung. After about 10 days in the pulmonary capillaries and alveoli, the larvae pass in turn up the bronchioles, bronchi, trachea, and epiglottis, are swallowed, and return to the jejunum. There they develop into mature adult worms within 2 to 3 months of ingestion. *Ascaris suum,* a roundworm of pigs, may occasionally complete a similar life cycle in humans.

Epidemiology Infection follows the ingestion of the embryonated eggs contained in contaminated food, or, more commonly, the introduction of the eggs into the mouth by the hands after contact with contaminated soil. Geophagia may produce massive infections. In endemic areas, the infection is maintained primarily by small children who defecate indiscriminately in the area of the home. In dry, windy climates, eggs may become airborne, get into the mouth, and be swallowed. Since the eggs are relatively resistant to desiccation and wide variations in temperature, the disease is worldwide. In the developing areas of the world where the lack of sanitary facilities exposes populations to the greatest risk, the prevalence of infection may be as high as 80 to 90 percent; children are almost universally infected in these areas. In temperate areas, the infection occurs in family clusters.

Pathogenesis and clinical manifestations Because of the extensive migration of which both the larvae and adults are capable, the manifestations may be diverse. Bronchopneumonia characterized by fever, cough, dyspnea, wheeze, eosinophilic leukocytosis, and migratory pulmonary infiltrates may occur during the passage of the larvae through the lung. This is most commonly seen in communities where *Ascaris* transmission is seasonal. The severity of symptoms is apparently related to both intensity of infection and the degree of sensitization resulting from previous exposures. Significant arterial oxygen desaturation and, rarely, death may occur. Adult worms may produce no symptoms if the infection is light and may be detected accidentally when the adult worm is vomited or passed in the stool. Heavier infections may cause abdominal pain and malabsorption of fat, protein, carbohydrate, and vitamins. In marginally nourished children this may produce growth retardation. Occasionally a bolus of worms may result in volvulus, intussusception, or intestinal obstruction in the iliocecal area. Children are most likely to have these complications because of their anatomically smaller intestine and larger worm loads. Up to 2000 worms have been found in children, although the usual load is less than 50. In the United States where worm loads are usually modest, the incidence of obstruction is 2 per 1000 infected children per year. It often follows a febrile illness or drug therapy which stimulates the worms to increase motility. Rarely, an adult worm will migrate into the appendix, bile ducts, or pancreatic ducts, causing obstruction and inflammation of these organs. Biliary tract obstruction may be associated with bacterial cholangitis and liver abscess. Worms may also penetrate the intestinal wall, particularly at a site of surgical anastomosis, and patients should be dewormed prior to elective surgery. Migration of the worms into the oral pharynx and mouth may lead to acute respiratory distress.

Laboratory findings The diagnosis is usually made by finding the ova in the feces. The fertilized eggs are usually numerous, characteristic, and not easily confused with those of other helminths. The occasional unisexual infection may pose diagnostic problems. The male produces no eggs, and the unfertilized ova produced by a single female may be atypical and difficult to recognize. Occasionally the worms may be seen after a barium meal, either as negative images or after ingesting barium themselves. In biliary ascariasis an intravenous cholangiogram will often demonstrate dilatation of the common duct and/or the negative image of the parasite. Ascaris pneumonia may be diagnosed by finding larvae and eosinophils in the sputum or gastric aspirate. Eggs will usually not be found until after the larvae have matured in the intestine. Eosinophilic leukocytosis is usually noted during larval migration, but diminishes and often disappears during the chronic intestinal phase of infection.

Treatment Only symptomatic treatment can be used during the period of pulmonary involvement by the migrating larvae. For removal of the adult worms from the intestines, either pyrantel pamoate or mebendazole should be used. Pyrantel is given as a single oral dose of 11 mg/kg (maximum 1.0 g). Mebendazole is given as described for trichuriasis and is the preferred agent if both *Ascaris* and *Trichuris* are present. An older agent, piperazine citrate, is highly effective, less expensive, but slightly more toxic than the above two agents. It is given as a flavored syrup administered in a single dose after breakfast on two successive days and will cure the majority of cases. The drug acts by paralyzing the ascarids, which are then passed in the stool. The dose of piperazine is 75 mg/kg with a maximum of 4 g. No particular dietary regulation is necessary. The drug must be administered with caution to patients with renal insufficiency, because impaired elimination may produce neurotoxic signs. In intestinal obstruction, nasogastric suction should be initiated. After vomiting is controlled, piperazine should be given through the nasogastric tube every 12 to 24 h in dosage of 65 mg/kg (maximum 1.0 g) for six doses. Surgery usually is not required.

Prognosis The prognosis in intestinal infection is generally good. When acute or chronic obstruction of ducts or hollow viscera has occurred, the immediate prognosis is determined by the promptness of diagnosis and treatment. The case fatality rate of intestinal obstruction in the United States is 3 percent.

Prevention Ascariasis is primarily a household infection of rural areas. All infections should be treated, personal hygiene stressed, and adequate toilet facilities provided. Mass therapy administered at 6-month intervals may be effective in controlling ascariasis in small communities.

TOXOCARIASIS (VISCERAL LARVA MIGRANS) Definition This is a human infection with *Toxocara canis.* The animal ascarid is usually unable to complete its life cycle in humans, but they may be widely disseminated in the body, producing a variety of clinical manifestations, collectively referred to as *visceral larva migrans.*

Etiology and epidemiology The large adult toxocaral worms live in the intestine of dogs. Their eggs must be passed in the stool and incubate in soil for 2 to 3 weeks before they become infective. If the ova are then ingested by a human, larvae are liberated in the intestine, penetrate the wall, and are carried in the blood to the liver, where most remain, and lung. At the time the larvae reach the pulmonary capillaries, they are still very small (approximately one-half the size of *A. lumbricoides*) and many pass through the lungs to reach the systemic circulation. Larvae penetrate the tissues when their gradually increasing size approaches the diameter of the vessel through which they are traveling. Rarely the organisms break into the alveoli, ascend the respiratory tract, and are swallowed to reach the small intestine where they mature into adult worms. *Toxocara* infections of dogs are common and widespread. Transplacental transmission occurs and accounts for infection rates of 80 percent or more in young puppies; they can shed a large number of ova within 4 weeks of birth. Viable ova were found in 25 percent of soil samples taken from public parks in Great Britain. Although most human infections have been reported from the United States and Europe, it seems likely that the disease is present in other areas of the world as well. Children from the age of 2 to 5 years, because of their sanitary habits and intimate association with domestic pets, are most frequently involved. In Great Britain, 4 percent of children who play in public parks have positive skin tests to *Toxocara* antigens.

Pathogenesis and clinical manifestations The larvae migrate freely in tissues, causing hemorrhage, necrosis, eosinophilic inflammatory reaction, and eventually granuloma formation. The most frequently involved organs are the liver, lungs, brain, eye, heart, and skeletal muscles. Symptoms and signs are related to the number and location of the granulomas as well as sensitization to the parasite antigen. Commonly, only asymptomatic eosinophilia marks the presence of infection. Symptomatic patients most frequently present with fever and tender hepatomegaly. Splenomegaly, skin rash, and recurrent pneumonitis with wheezing respirations may occur in more severe infections. Respiratory failure with death has been reported. Most fatalities, however, result from involvement of the myocardium or central nervous system; the latter may result in convulsions, behavior disorders, or focal neurological defects. There is often a history of dirt eating and contact with puppies. Leukocytosis with eosinophilia to high levels (over 60 percent) and hypergammaglobulinemia with raised levels of IgG, IgM, and IgE are common. These manifestations may persist for months or years. At surgery or autopsy the liver may be studded with small granulomas. A granulomatous endophthalmitis, which may be mistaken for retinoblastoma, may be observed in older children and adults. Typically, this is unilateral and occurs in the absence of other clinical manifestations of visceral larva migrans. Decreased visual acuity or strabismus brings the patient to the attention of the physician.

Diagnosis The diagnosis can usually be made on the basis of clinical findings. Infections with *A. lumbricoides,* hookworm, and *Strongyloides stercoralis,* as well as other nonhuman nematodes, may also on occasion present as visceral larva migrans, making the etiologic diagnosis difficult. Eosinophilic leukemia, trichinosis, trematode infections, and periarteritis nodosa must be ruled out. Isoagglutinin, particularly anti-A, titers of 1:1024 or greater are present in 85 percent of patients with visceral but in very few with ocular disease. Antibodies to *Toxocara* and *Ascaris* antigens may be found, but, as with the isoagglutinins, these tests are neither very sensitive nor specific. The adaption of larval antigens to the enzyme-linked immunoabsorbent assay has, for the first time, provided clinicians with a serologic test of diagnostic value. In one study, the sensitivity and specificity were 78 and 92 percent, respectively. A definitive diagnosis depends on the identification of the larvae in sputum or tissue granuloma. Biopsy of the liver with serial sections of the specimen may reveal eosinophilic granulomas or a *Toxocara* larva.

Treatment No uniformly effective therapy is available. Diethylcarbamazine as used in Bancroftian filariasis (see Chap. 227) is probably the drug of choice. Thiabendazole in dosage of 25 to 50 mg/kg for 7 to 10 days may be helpful. Adrenocortical steroids may be beneficial when respiratory difficulty is pronounced. Control measures are directed toward preventing ingestion of eggs. Removal and repeated worming of infected dogs must be considered. Animals less than 6 months of age should be wormed monthly; older ones every 2 or 3 months.

ANISAKIASIS Ascarids belonging to family Anisakidae infect seals, dolphins, porpoises, whales, and other large sea mammals. Their larval stages are found in the flesh of squid and several marine fish including cod, salmon, and herring. Humans are infected by eating raw, pickled, or slightly salted fish delicacies such as "green herring," sashimi, sunomono, ceviche, and gravlax which contain the third-stage larvae. The infection may be asymptomatic and noted only when the worm is coughed or vomited up. More characteristically, the larvae burrow into the mucosa of the stomach, small intestine, or more rarely the colon. Here they produce eosinophilic granulomatous tumors with edema, thickening, and induration of the bowel wall which may be mistaken for gastric carcinoma or regional enteritis. Occasionally, larvae may penetrate the intestinal wall to involve other abdominal organs. Perforations of the bowel with peritonitis have also been described. The pathological changes are thought to be the result of a hypersensitivity reaction. In the acute gastric syndrome common in Japan, the patient may develop epigastric pain, nausea, and vomiting within a few hours of ingesting infected fish. With a gastroscope 2- to 4-cm larvae can be seen penetrating the mucosa and can sometimes be removed. In Europeans, the small intestine has been the site most frequently involved. The clinical picture may be severe enough to simulate an acute surgical abdomen. More commonly, colicky pain, diffuse abdominal tenderness, fever, and leukocytosis develop a week or more after the ingestion of fish. Peripheral eosinophilia is not always present, and a definitive diagnosis can be made only by the identification of larvae in tissue. Serologic tests are being developed, but are neither highly reliable nor generally available. The disease usually subsides spontaneously with conservative therapy. Occasionally, a chronic illness develops which requires surgical resection of the lesion.

Hundreds of cases have been recognized in the Netherlands and Japan, and several cases have been reported from North America. The disease can be prevented by storing marine fish at $-20°C$ for a single day or by cooking it at normal cooking temperatures.

HOOKWORM DISEASE Definition Hookworm disease is a symptomatic infection caused by *Ancylostoma duodenale* or *Necator americanus.* Asymptomatic infection may be termed simply *hookworm infection,* and the individual with such infection is called a *carrier.*

Etiology *Ancylostoma duodenale,* also known as the "Old World" hookworm, possesses four prominent hooklike teeth in its adult stage. The adults are about 1 cm long and inhabit the upper part of the human small intestine, where they attach to the mucosa by means of the mouth parts and suck blood. Each adult extracts approximately 0.20 ml blood daily. The adults migrate within the small intestine, and each site of attachment persists temporarily as a bleeding point. Following fertilization, the female liberates approximately 20,000 eggs per day.

They measure about 40 by 60 μm and are usually in the two-to-four-celled stage when discharged in the feces.

Necator americanus, the "New World" hookworm, has a buccal capsule containing dorsal and ventral plates rather than teeth. It is slightly smaller, deposits fewer eggs, and causes much less blood loss than *A. duodenale* (0.03 ml per worm daily). *Ancylostoma cylonicum,* a hookworm of cats found in the far east, may occasionally reach maturity in humans.

The life cycles of both hookworms are similar. Under appropriate conditions, the eggs hatch in 24 to 48 h, releasing free-living or rhabditiform larvae. Within a few days, these develop into infective or filariform larvae which may remain viable in the soil for several weeks. These, in turn, penetrate the skin to enter vessels which carry them to the lungs. The larvae leave the alveolar capillaries, enter the alveoli, ascend the respiratory tree, enter the pharynx, and are swallowed. They reach the intestine about 1 week after penetration of the skin and mature within 5 weeks. Larval development of *Ancylostoma* may be arrested or retarded in the human host. This may result in a prolonged latent period between the onset of infection and the appearance of gravid females in the intestine. Adults have been known to survive in the human intestine for as long as 14 years, but *A. duodenale* seldom persists beyond 6 to 8 years, and most *N. americanus* infections are eliminated within 2 to 4 years.

Epidemiology It has been estimated that hookworms infect 700 million people and cause the loss of 7 million liters of blood daily throughout the world from 45°N to 30°S latitude. *Necator americanus* is found predominantly in the tropical areas of Africa, Asia, and the Americas, while *A. duodenale* occurs in the Mediterranean Basin, the Middle East, northern India, China, and Japan. In many areas both species are found. In general, *Ancylostoma* presents a greater public health hazard than *N. americanus,* the species which is most prevalent in the southern United States, because it is more persistent in the environment, more harmful to the host, and less amenable to treatment. Conditions conducive to the development of the hookworm egg into infective filariform larvae are a mean temperature between 23 and 33°C, abundant rainfall, shade, and well-drained sandy soil. Hookworm infection occurs where there is opportunity for direct contact of the skin with soil contaminated by promiscuous defecation. The disease may also be acquired by oral ingestion of infective larvae, particularly those of *A. duodenale.* Lactogenic transmission may also occur with this species; presumably this results from the activation of larvae whose development within the tissues of the host has been arrested or retarded. Probably because of greater exposure, males show a higher incidence of infection than females. Infections are particularly common in closed, heavily populated communities such as coffee or tea plantations.

Repeated infections of hookworm in dogs result in immunity and elimination of the parasite. It seems probable that a similar phenomenon occurs in human infections. When the possibility of reinfection is eliminated, the majority of worms is eliminated spontaneously within 1 or 2 years.

Pathogenesis and clinical manifestations During the invasion of the exposed skin by the larvae, there may be an erythematous maculopapular skin rash and edema with severe pruritus. These manifestations, which may persist for several days, are more marked in *N. americanus* infection. The lesions are most common about the feet, particularly between the toes, and have been termed "ground itch."

During migration through the lungs, cough, pneumonia, and, in severe infections, fever may occur. Usually, however, pulmonary involvement does not give rise to clinical symptoms.

Various gastrointestinal symptoms, ranging from vague epigastric distress and pica to typical ulcer pain, have been reported in association with hookworm infection. Roentgenographic studies may reveal nonspecific changes such as excessive peristalsis and "puddling," particularly in the proximal jejunum. However, gross and microscopic examination of the bowel itself reveals conspicuously little damage. Previous reports of absorptive abnormalities in hookworm infection have not been supported.

The major clinical manifestations of hookworm disease clearly are those of iron-deficiency anemia and hypoalbuminemia consequent to chronic intestinal blood loss. Whether anemia develops and how severe it becomes depends on the balance between iron lost in the gut and iron absorbed from the diet. In many endemic areas, dietary iron is largely of vegetable origin and is absorbed poorly. General dietary deficiency also may lower resistance to parasitic infections. The severity of the disease and the prognosis depend on such factors as the age of the patient, the magnitude of the worm burden, the duration of the disease, and diet. Young children often have extreme anemia, with cardiac insufficiency and anasarca. These conditions may precipitate kwashiorkor. Those who survive to puberty show retarded physical, mental, and sexual development. Milder degrees of the disease, as seen in older children and adults, are characterized by lassitude, dyspnea, palpitation, tachycardia, constipation, and pallor of the skin and mucous membranes.

Asymptomatic infections outnumber symptomatic infections, considering all age groups, 20 to 40 times in endemic areas. The worm burden is small in asymptomatic infections, and the carrier state may be indicative of some degree of acquired host resistance.

Laboratory findings In symptomatic infection, hookworm eggs are usually numerous enough to be detected by microscopic examination of a direct or concentrated fecal smear. A quantitative egg count, using the Stoll or Beaver technique, allows an estimation of the intensity of infection. If a stool specimen is allowed to stand for several hours before examination, the eggs may hatch, releasing larvae which are easily confused with those of *Strongyloides.* The eggs must be differentiated from those of *Trichostrongylus* and *Ternidens diminutus,* which are larger and in a later stage of maturation when observed in a fresh fecal specimen than are those of *Necator* or *Ancylostoma.* Abdominal and pulmonary symptoms appear before the eggs are discharged, although a presumptive diagnosis may be made on the basis of the clinical history and the eosinophilic leukocytosis. The feces seldom contain gross blood in hookworm disease, although tests for occult blood are usually positive.

Generally, the leukocyte count is normal. However, in some early cases, leukocytosis may be marked, with an eosinophilia as high as 70 or 80 percent. The anemia is characteristically hypochromic and microcytic.

The species of hookworm may be determined by the identification of the adult worm passed in the stool following treatment or by culturing the feces and identifying the third-stage larvae. This is seldom important in clinical practice.

Differential diagnosis Since hookworm disease occurs in areas in which beriberi and malaria are also common, these diseases must be differentiated from hookworm disease, or their coexistence must be established.

Treatment Therapy specific for the infection and directed toward the improvement of nutrition and the anemia should be considered simultaneously. In areas where reinfection is likely, administration of anthelmintics to patients with light infections (less than 2000 eggs per milliliter of feces) is probably not beneficial. In most cases requiring specific therapy, anthelmintics may be administered immediately, followed by iron and a high-protein diet. A number of satisfactory anthelmintic agents are available, but two, pyrantel pamoate (see "Ascariasis" above) and mebendazole (see "Trichuriasis" above) are currently favored. Where expense remains a major consideration, the drug of choice is tetrachloroethylene (TCE). It is highly effective, nontoxic, inexpensive, and ideal for mass treatment. (The USP tetrachloroethylene available to veterinarians may be used.) In most instances a single dose of this agent will decrease the worm load substantially. Complete cure may require several courses of treatment but is not necessary in endemic areas; the aim of therapy is reduction of the worm load to an asymptomatic level. Tetrachloroethylene is administered as a single 5-ml oral dose. Children should receive 0.12 ml/kg (to a maximum of 5 ml) by the same route. The night before treatment, the patient is permitted a light fat-free meal. The following morning, breakfast is omitted and the drug is administered. No food is permitted for 4 h and no alcohol for 24 h. Treatment can be repeated in a week if complete cure is desired and has not been accomplished. Bitoscanate (Jonit) in oral dosage of 100 mg every 12 h for three doses is equally effective against *N. americanus* and *A. duodenale.* It is not available in the United States.

The anemia requires iron replacement. When anemia is severe and there is malnutrition with anasarca, blood transfusions and a high-protein diet should be given before drug treatment is begun. Blood should be given in an amount sufficient to raise the hemoglobin level to 10 g/dl. In advanced cases it may be necessary to delay drug treatment for 2 to 3 weeks.

Prognosis The immediate prognosis is good. When opportunity for reinfection persists and nutrition cannot be maintained, a state of chronic debility develops. Maturation of children is impaired, and intercurrent disease is a serious problem in adults.

Prevention Many of the measures required are obvious but difficult to apply on a large scale. Even if facilities for proper disposal of feces are provided, it is no simple matter to educate the population in their use. Soil pollution must be eliminated. Avoidance of direct skin contact with the soil (by wearing shoes) is often not practical in endemic areas. Periodic mass treatment of the population has been used in some hookworm control programs.

CUTANEOUS LARVA MIGRANS (CREEPING ERUPTION) Definition Creeping eruption is an infection of human skin caused by the larvae of the dog and cat hookworm, *A. brasiliense.* The other dog hookworms, *A. caninum* and *Uncinaria stenocephala,* as well as the human parasites, *Strongyloides stercoralis* and *Necator americanus,* may also produce the disease. The larvae of *Gnathostoma spinigerum,* a nematode found in the Orient, and *Gasterophilus,* the horse bat fly, may produce a similar cutaneous infection.

Etiology *Ancylostoma brasiliense* reaches adulthood regularly only in the dog and cat. The larvae emerging from eggs discharged in the feces develop to the filariform stage and then are capable of penetrating the skin. In humans, the larvae usually remain in the skin and migrate, producing an irregular erythematous tunnel visible on the skin surface.

Epidemiology and distribution Transmission to humans requires environmental temperature and humidity appropriate for development of the egg to the infective filariform larva stage. Beaches and other moist, sandy areas are hazardous, because animals choose such areas for defecation, and the *A. brasiliense* eggs develop well in such soil. In the United States infection is found in the southern Atlantic and Gulf states.

Pathogenesis and clinical manifestations The site of penetration of the skin by the larvae becomes apparent in a few hours. The migration of the larvae in the skin is accompanied by severe itching. Scratching may lead to bacterial infection. In the course of 1 week, the initial red papule develops into an irregular, erythematous, linear lesion which may attain a length of 15 to 20 cm. The larvae may persist for weeks to months without treatment.

Loeffler's syndrome has been observed in 26 of 52 cases of creeping eruption. Transient, migratory pulmonary infiltrations associated with an increased number of eosinophils in the blood and sputum were interpreted as an allergic reaction to the helminthic infection.

Laboratory findings Eosinophils occur in the lesion, but eosinophilic leukocytosis is slight, except when Loeffler's syndrome appears. The percentage of eosinophils in the blood may then rise to 50 percent and in the sputum to 90 percent. Only rarely are larvae found on skin biopsy.

Treatment Thiabendazole is the drug of choice; it should be given orally in the dosage suggested for hookworm. It may be repeated if necessary. Alternatively, it may be applied topically as a 10% aqueous suspension. Topical administration avoids systemic toxicity. Superficial bacterial infections are improved by the application of wet dressing and elevation of the extremity. For intense itching, oral antihistaminics may be of aid.

Prognosis Untreated infections last several months. Treatment, which is usually sought because of severe pruritus, is usually successful.

Prevention Dogs and cats should be prevented from contaminating recreation areas and children's sandboxes.

TRICHOSTRONGYLIASIS Definition Trichostrongyliasis is an intestinal infection of herbivorous animals throughout the world. Humans are an intermediate host.

Etiology Almost a dozen species of *Trichostrongylus* are known to have infected humans. The disease is common in Asia, the Middle East, and South America, but few human infections have been reported in the United States. In view of the high frequency of animal infections here, the low incidence of human infections is difficult to understand. The possibility exists that some such infections are mistaken for hookworm infections.

The ova resemble those of the hookworm but are larger, have more pointed ends, and, when observed in a fresh fecal specimen, show a more advanced stage of segmentation (16- to 32-cell stage).

Pathogenesis Infection is acquired by ingestion of green leafy plants contaminated with third-stage larvae. On reaching the small intestine, they attach themselves to the mucosa and develop into adult worms within 4 weeks. The adult at that time sucks blood and maintains residence in the intestine for long periods. Sandground, who infected himself, observed infection to last more than 8 years.

Manifestations Most infections are asymptomatic, but massive infections may result in epigastric distress and anemia. The parasite owes its importance primarily to the resemblance of its ova to those of the hookworms. Moreover, because the trichostrongylidae do not respond to anthelmintics effective in hookworm infection, it may be assumed incorrectly that refractory hookworm infection is present.

Laboratory diagnosis The diagnosis depends on the finding of the ova in the feces. Since they are few, they are usually found only when a concentration method is used. In symptomatic infections, there may be leukocytosis with marked eosinophilia (for example, 80 percent).

Treatment These infections do not respond to tetrachloroethylene. Thiabendazole 25 mg/kg twice daily for 2 or 3 days, or pyrantel pamoate as used in hookworm infections, is effective in symptomatic infections. Both are considered investigational drugs for this condition by the U.S. Food and Drug Administration.

Prevention Leafy vegetables should be cooked before ingestion in endemic areas.

STRONGYLOIDIASIS **Definition** Strongyloidiasis is an intestinal infection of humans caused by *Strongyloides stercoralis* or, on occasion, the primate species, *S. fuelleborni.* Extraintestinal involvement may occur in severe cases.

Etiology The tiny (2 mm in length) adult female resides and lays her eggs in the mucosa of the upper part of the jejunum. In heavy infections, the biliary and pancreatic ducts, the entire small bowel, and the colon may be parasitized. The eggs quickly hatch, releasing rhabditiform larvae which enter the lumen of the bowel and are passed in the feces. On reaching the soil, the larvae develop into the infective filariform stage. There, as in the case of the filariform larvae of hookworm, they penetrate the skin and small blood vessels of humans. They are then carried to the lungs where they leave the alveolar capillaries, ascend the respiratory tree, enter the pharynx, and are swallowed. On reaching the small intestine, they mature and copulate. The fertilized female burrows into the jejunal mucosa, while the male is excreted in the stool. Oviposition (up to 40 eggs per day) begins 17 to 28 days after the initial infection. It is likely that the females also reproduce parthenogenetically. In addition to the *direct* host-soil-host cycle, *Strongyloides* has two alternative cycles. In the first, or *indirect,* cycle, the rhabditiform larvae, after passing from the host, develop into free-living adults which reside and reproduce in the soil, thus creating a reservoir of infection independent of the human host. Under certain environmental conditions, the free-living larvae are capable of transforming back into filariform larvae which initiate a new cycle in humans. In the second, or *autoinfection,* cycle, the rhabditiform larvae develop into filariform larvae before they are passed in the stool. They may then invade the intestinal mucosa or perianal skin of the same host without first going through a soil phase. This may explain the long persistence (20 to 30 years) of strongyloidiasis in patients who have left endemic areas and may also account for the extremely heavy worm loads in some individuals. The early transformation of the filariform larvae is probably also responsible for the frequency with which strongyloidiasis is seen in crowded, unsanitary institutions for the mentally retarded. It appears to occur frequently in patients with achlorhydria, delayed intestinal transit time, and blind loops or diverticula.

Epidemiology The usual mode of infection is the penetration of the skin by larvae. Some infections may result from ingestion of contaminated food and drink, and some are believed to be transmitted by contact. Transmammary passage in humans has been demonstrated for *S. fuelleborni.* This disease is endemic in the tropics, where the warmth, moisture, and lack of sanitation favor its spread. Sporadic cases appear among Puerto Ricans and throughout the rural south of the continental United States. Former British and American soldiers imprisoned in southeast Asia during World War II were examined for the presence of this parasite. Over one-quarter were found infected nearly four decades after exposure; the majority were symptomatic.

Pathogenesis and clinical manifestations The initial cutaneous penetration of the filariform larvae usually produces no symptoms. However, *larva currens,* transitory skin eruptions characterized by blotchy erythema, serpiginous lesions, and urticaria, may be seen. These may recur at irregular intervals thereafter and are particularly common following recovery from an acute febrile illness. In these situations the lesions are generally found over the lower back and buttocks and are related to episodes of autoinfection. Cough, dyspnea, gross hemoptysis, and bronchospasm may accompany migration through the lungs. Chest x-rays may show pulmonary infiltration at this time. The intestinal infestation is usually asymptomatic or productive only of vague abdominal complaints. In heavier infections, epigastric pain and tenderness, nausea, flatulence, vomiting, and diarrhea alternating with constipation may be observed. Peptic ulcer may be simulated, but food often aggravates the pain. The mucosal inflammation may be severe enough to produce subacute obstruction, segmental ileus, and impaired absorption. A severe form of ulcerative colitis, accompanied by intestinal perforation and peritonitis, has been encountered. In debilitated, immunodepressed, or steroid-treated patients massive autoinfection with widespread dissemination of larvae to the extraintestinal organs including the central nervous system may occur. This hyperinfection is often associated with pulmonary manifestations, severe enterocolitis, persistent gram-negative bacteremia, and occasionally gram-negative meningitis. Unrecognized, it usually leads to death. Disseminated strongyloidiasis should be considered in any compromised host with unexplained gram-negative bacteremia, abdominal complaints, and pulmonary infiltrates with or without eosinophilia.

Laboratory findings Although clinical findings may be suggestive, the definitive diagnosis can be made only in the laboratory. Fresh fecal specimens should be examined to avoid confusion with hookworm infection; generally, fresh specimens contain *larvae* in strongyloidiasis infections, while in hookworm infection they contain *eggs.* Since the number of larvae in the stool is small and varies from day to day, several samples should be checked, using concentration and culture techniques. If pulmonary involvement is present, the sputum should be examined for larvae. Microscopic examination of the duodenal aspirates and jejunal biopsies may also establish the diagnosis. Alternatively, a weighted string can be passed into the duodenum, allowed to remain for a short time, and then withdrawn. The bile-stained section of the string is stripped of fluid which is then examined for the presence of larvae. An enzyme-linked immunosorbent assay utilizing *S. stercoralis* larval antigens was shown to be positive in approximately 80 percent of patients and may have some diagnostic utility.

Eosinophilic leukocytosis is common, except in very severe cases. When eosinophilia occurs in association with peptic ulcer symptoms, strongyloidiasis should be suspected.

Treatment All infected patients should be treated to prevent the occurrence of severe invasive disease. The drug of choice is thiabendazole, which should be given orally in dosage of 25 mg/kg twice a day for 2 or 3 days. In disseminated strongyloidiasis, treatment should be continued for 7 days or more. Lightheadedness, nausea, and vomiting are common accompaniments of therapy with this agent. Hypersensitivity reactions may occur but usually respond to treatment with antihistamines. The stools should be rechecked at intervals of 3 months because the parasite is not easily eradicated and retreatment may be necessary. Cambendazole, a new benzimidazole derivative, appears to be superior to thiabendazole but is not yet available in the United States.

Prognosis In the usual case, the prognosis is good. Since the occurrence of hyperinfection is unpredictable, every effort should be made to eradicate the infection in each case. In severe cases with hyperinfection, the prognosis is poor.

Prevention In general, the measures are those for the control of hookworm infection. In addition, it is well to remember that infection may be contracted by ingestion of contaminated food (especially uncooked vegetables) or of contaminated drinking water and by contact. Patients who have a history of residence in an endemic area should be carefully checked for the presence of the parasite prior to the initiation of steroid or immunosuppressive therapy. Because the larvae may not appear in the stool for several weeks after the initiation of such therapy, repeated examinations of stool and upper intestinal aspirates are indicated. Since sputum, vomitus, stool, and body fluids of patients with disseminated disease may contain infective filariform larvae, gloves and gowns should be worn by hospital personnel caring for such patients.

INTESTINAL CAPILLARIASIS Definition Intestinal capillariasis is an infection of humans caused by the roundworm *Capillaria philippinensis.* This species of *Capillaria* was first discovered in 1963 from a fatal human infection occurring in the Philippines. The infection results in intractable diarrhea with a high mortality rate. Clinical studies have shown a severe protein-losing enteropathy and malabsorption of fats and sugars.

Etiology *Capillaria* are nematodes of the family Trichuroidea and are closely related to comembers *Trichuris* and *Trichinella.* Adult *C. philippinensis* are small, measuring 2 to 4 mm in length. The peanut-shaped eggs have flattened bipolar plugs and an average size of 42 by 20 μm. The adults inhabit the mucosa of the small intestine, especially the jejunum. Adults, larval forms, and eggs are found in the stool.

Epidemiology The infection has been found almost exclusively in persons residing along the north and west coastal areas of Luzon, Philippines. Several cases from Thailand have also been reported. Since 1966 the disease has occurred in epidemic form, and more than 1000 cases and 100 deaths have been reported. Males are infected more frequently than females, perhaps because of occupational exposure. Prior to the discovery of an effective chemotherapeutic agent, the mortality rate in untreated cases was about 30 percent. With chemotherapy, the case fatality rate has been reduced to 6 percent.

The mode of transmission and life cycle of the parasite are incompletely understood. First-stage larvae have been found in several species of freshwater fish. When these fish or the larvae are fed to gerbils, they develop to adulthood within their intestinal lumina. These adults rapidly produce new larvae which mature to a second generation of adults. Most of the females from this generation are oviparous, the resulting eggs passing in the gerbil's stool. Some, however, remain larviparous, leading to another generation of intestinal adults. Eggs must presumably embryonate in fresh water before being ingested by the fish host. No naturally infected mammal other than humans has been found. The presence of many adult worms, larviparous females, embryonated eggs, and all larval stages in human intestinal contents suggests that the parasitic cycles in gerbils and humans are the same. The mechanism by which humans originally became infected remains unproven. However, it is known that many of the naturally infected lagoon fish, particularly "bagsit" or *Hypselotris bipartita,* are eaten raw by the people of Luzon.

Pathogenesis and manifestations Adult worms in large numbers invade the small-intestinal mucosa and cause a severe protein-losing enteropathy and malabsorption. Hypokalemia, hypocalcemia, and hypoproteinemia are the rule. Autopsy studies have failed to show extraintestinal spread of the parasite. Initial symptoms of intestinal "gurgling" (borborygmi) and recurrent vague abdominal pain are followed, usually within 2 to 3 weeks, by a voluminous watery diarrhea. Other findings, consistent with the basic pathophysiologic process, are anorexia, vomiting, weight loss, muscle wasting and weakness, hyporeflexia, and edema. Abdominal tenderness and distention may occur. The period between onset of symptoms and death is usually 2 to 3 months. Subclinical infection has not been noted.

Diagnosis The diagnosis is made by finding ova in the stool. The ova of *C. philippinensis* must be differentiated from those of *T. trichiura,* which are similar. Care must be taken that capillaria are not overlooked in patients with *Trichuris* infections because in the endemic area most patients with capillariasis have coexistent *Trichuris* infection.

Treatment Administration of mebendazole combined with fluid and electrolyte replacement leads to dramatic improvement; 400 mg per day in divided dosage should be given for 20 days to prevent relapse.

REFERENCES

AUR RJA et al: Thiabendazole in visceral larva migrans. Am J Dis Child 121:226, 1971

AZIZ MA, SEDDIQUI AR: Morphological and absorption studies of small intestine hookworm disease (ancyclostomiasis) in West Pakistan. Gastroenterology 55:242, 1968

BANWELL JG, SCHAD GA: Hookworm. Clin Gastroenterol 7:129, 1978

BLUMENTHAL DS: Current concepts—intestinal nematodes in the United States. N Engl J Med 297:1437, 1977

CROSS JH et al: Further studies on *Capillaria philippinensis:* Development of the parasite in the Mongolian gerbil. J Parasitol 64:208, 1978

DAVIS CM, ISRAEL RM: Treatment of creeping eruption with topical thiabendazole. Arch Dermatol 97:325, 1968

GROVE DI: Strongyloidiasis in Allied ex-prisoners of war in southeast Asia. Br Med J 280:598, 1980

IGRA-SIEGMAN Y et al: Syndrome of hyperinfection with *Strongyloides stercoralis.* Rev Infect Dis 1:397, 1981

KAMATH KR: Severe infection with *Trichuris trichuria* in Malaysian children. Am J Trop Med Hyg 22:600, 1973

MARKETT EK: Pseudohookworm infection—trichostrongyliasis: Treatment with thiabendazole. N Engl J Med 278:831, 1968

MARSEN JM, TURNER JA: Reinfection of enterobiasis (pinworm infection): Simultaneous treatment of family members. Am J Dis Child 118:576, 1969

MILLER MJ et al: Mebendazole. An effective anthelmintic for trichuriasis and enterobiasis. JAMA 230:1412, 1974

PAWLOWSKI Z: Ascariasis. Clin Gastroenterol 7:157, 1978

PINKUS GS et al: Intestinal anisakiasis. First case report from North America. Am J Med 59:114, 1975

SCHANTZ PM, GLICKMAN LT: Current concepts in parasitology—toxocaral visceral larva migrans. N Engl J Med 298:436, 1978

STEPHENSON LS: The contribution of *Ascaris lumbricoides* to malnutrition in children. Parasitology 81:221, 1980

WOLFE MS: Oxyuris, trichostrongylus and trichiuris. Clin Gastroenterol 7:201, 1978

ZINKHAM WH: Visceral larva migrans—a review and reassessment indicating two forms of clinical expression: visceral and ocular. Am J Dis Child 132:627, 1978

231
OTHER TREMATODES OR FLUKES

JAMES J. PLORDE

The trematodes of humans are long-lived parasites which produce progressive damage to the tissues of their hosts. With the exception of schistosomes, they are similar in morphology and life cycle. The adult flukes are flat, leaflike hermaphrodites that vary in length from a few millimeters to several centimeters. Their digestive tract, unlike that of the nematodes, ends blindly. As their name indicates, they have two "holes" in the form of oral and ventral suckers which are used as organs of attachment and locomotion. The operculated eggs, which are passed in the feces or sputum, hatch in the water to produce a ciliated, free-swimming *miracidium.* The miracidium reaches and penetrates the tissue of an intermediate snail host to undergo a period of development, eventuating in the release of thousands of swarms of free-living *cercariae* from the snail. These thousands of tail-bearing larvae must, in turn, reach a second intermediate host, usually an aquatic animal or vegetation, where they encyst forming *metacercariae.* The definitive host is infected when he or she ingests the parasitized second intermediate host. The distribution of flukes is usually limited by the location of their molluscan intermediate host. With the exception of *Opisthorchis* and *Fasciola,* most hermaphroditic flukes are found only in tropical or subtropical areas.

PARAGONIMIASIS Definition Paragonimiasis (endemic hemoptysis) is a chronic infection of the lung caused by trematodes of the genus *Paragonimus.* Clinically, the disease is characterized by cough and hemoptysis. Ectopic worms may cause a variety of other manifestations. Geographically, it is probably the most widely distributed disease caused by hermaphroditic flukes.

Etiology and epidemiology Although *P. westermani,* which is widely distributed in the far east, is the most common cause of human paragonimiasis, a number of other species, including *P. skrjabini, P. heterotremus* (China), *P. africanus, P. uterobilateralis* (Cameroons, Nigeria, and Zaire), *P. mexicanus, P. peruvianus,* and *P. caliensis* (Central and South America), may cause the disease. Approximately 1 percent of recent Laotian Hmong immigrants to the United States harbor *P. westermani.* The short, plump adults (7 to 12 mm in length, 4 to 6 mm in width) have a life span of 4 to 5 years which they typically spend encysted in the lung parenchyma of the host. Their golden-brown operculated eggs (50 by 90 μm) reach the bronchioles from where they are coughed up and excreted in the sputum or swallowed and passed in the feces. They must embryonate several weeks in fresh water before hatching to release the miracidia.

The infection is acquired by ingestion of cysts in the second intermediate host, a freshwater crab or crayfish. The metacercariae excyst in the duodenum, burrow through the intestinal wall into the peritoneal cavity, and then usually migrate through the diaphragm and into the lung. The worms also may be found in the intestinal wall, liver, pancreas, kidney, mesentery, skeletal muscle, subcutaneous tissues, and central nervous system, particularly the brain. The dog, cat, pig, rat, and wild carnivores are definitive hosts for the parasite in addition to humans. In some of these, very young adults can be found in their striated muscles. Human infection has been reported following the ingestion of this undercooked flesh.

The incidence of paragonimiasis is often affected by food shortages or local customs. The metacercariae survive in vinegar, and lightly pickled or inadequately cooked food usually serves as the source of infection in the far east. Fresh crab juice used for the treatment of measles in Korea and for infertility in the Cameroons may also transmit the parasite. Children may acquire the disease in endemic areas while handling or eating raw crabs during play.

Pathogenesis and clinical manifestations An eosinophilic granuloma forms about the adult worm, eventually leading to the formation of a fibrous cyst. The pulmonary lesions which measure up to 1 cm in diameter frequently communicate with a bronchiole, resulting in secondary bacterial infection. Small, fibrous nodules representing reaction around deposited eggs also occur. Clinically the picture is one of chronic bronchitis and bronchiectasis with production of brownish sputum and hemoptysis. A poorly resolving pulmonary infiltrate, lung abscess, or pleural effusion may be present in heavy infections. The roentgenographic findings vary with the stage of infection. Initially one or more soft infiltrates may be seen anywhere in the lungs excepting the apexes. These are then gradually replaced by round nodules which not infrequently cavitate. Eventually, fibrosis and calcification occur, presenting a picture closely resembling tuberculosis, a disease which often coexists with paragonimiasis.

An abdominal mass, pain, and dysentery characterize intestinal or peritoneal infections. Various types of paralysis and epilepsy occur in cerebral involvement. Homonymous hemianopsia, optic atrophy, and papilledema are common. The cerebrospinal fluid usually shows an eosinophilic leukocytosis and elevated protein. Cerebral calcifications are seen on x-ray in 50 percent of cases. *Paragonimus skrjabini* infections are characterized by migratory subcutaneous nodules that contain adult flukes.

Laboratory findings Eosinophilia is a constant finding. Definitive diagnosis depends upon finding the characteristic operculated ova in the sputum, stool, pleural fluid, or tissue. Eggs may be rare or totally absent from the sputum during the first 3 months of infection but are eventually found in 75 to 85 percent of infected patients. Even later, however, repeated examinations using concentration techniques may be required for their recovery. Ziehl-Neelsen staining, often carried out for suspected tuberculosis, usually will not demonstrate the eggs. In fact, the sputum concentration techniques for tuberculosis may destroy the eggs that are present. Since many patients have concomitant tuberculosis, the diagnosis may be overlooked. Stool examination is frequently helpful in children. A complement fixation test is available, and the results correlate well with active infection. It usually becomes negative within 6 months of successful therapy. The skin test does not distinguish present and past infections and is used primarily for epidemiologic purposes.

Treatment and prevention Praziquantel is the drug of choice. A total of 75 mg/kg is given in three divided doses over a single 24-h period. Alternatively, bithionol may be administered. From 30 to 40 mg/kg in divided doses should be given every other day for a total of 10 to 15 treatment days. The symptoms disappear rapidly, and most infiltrates resolve within 3 months. Side effects are minor and consist of nausea, vomiting, and urticaria. Concomitant bacterial infection must be treated. Prevention of superinfection by the same parasite is important, because the disease is self-limiting.

The most practical control measure is the adequate cooking of all shellfish before they are eaten.

CLONORCHIASIS **Definition** Clonorchiasis is an infection of the biliary passages caused by *Clonorchis sinensis,* the most important liver fluke of humans. Although the infection is usually asymptomatic, heavy worm loads may produce manifestations of biliary obstruction.

Etiology and epidemiology *Clonorchis sinensis* is a small fluke (5 by 15 mm) that lives as long as 50 years in the biliary tree of its host. Here the flukes feed on mucosal secretions and pass operculated eggs into the feces. On reaching fresh water, the eggs are ingested by the intermediate snail host. After multiplication and development within the snail, the cercariae are released and penetrate freshwater fish. Infections result from ingestion of the raw, dried, salted, or pickled flesh of freshwater fish containing encysted metacercariae. The larva is released in the duodenum. It enters the common bile duct and migrates to the second-order bile ducts, where it develops into the adult form in about 1 month. In addition to humans, dogs, cats, pigs, and rats serve as disease reservoirs. The main endemic areas are Korea, Japan, Taiwan, Hong Kong, southern China, and Vietnam where, in previous years, clonorchiasis was perpetuated by the practice of fertilizing fish ponds with manure and human feces. Improvements in the disposal of human feces have dramatically decreased transmission in most areas, but the infection rate has remained high due to the prolonged life span of the adult worm. Twenty-five percent of the population of Hong Kong and a small proportion of Chinese immigrants to this country have been shown to be infected. The disease may also be acquired in the United States by the ingestion of infected, dried, frozen, or pickled fish imported from the far east. Clinically apparent cases are restricted to the adult population in whom the accumulated worm load eventually produces pathological effects.

Pathogenesis and clinical manifestations Light infections are usually asymptomatic, but worm loads of 500 to 1000 flukes often result in clinical manifestations. During the migration of the larvae, the patient may have fever, chills, tender hepatomegaly, mild jaundice, and eosinophilia. The mature worm causes proliferation of the biliary epithelium, increased mucin production, adenoma formation, chronic pericholangitis, and periductal fibrosis. Hepatic parenchymal damage and portal hypertension are not seen in uncomplicated infections. Recurrent attacks of suppurative cholangitis with or without intrahepatic choledocholithiasis may follow biliary obstruction with dead flukes. These occasionally present as hypoglycemic coma. The occurrence of biliary stones in clonorchiasis is associated with an increased incidence of chronic *Salmonella typhi* carriage. Cholangiocarcinoma may occur in patients with severe, long-standing infections. The adult worms may infest the pancreatic ducts, where they can cause squamous metaplasia, periductal fibrosis, and acute pancreatitis.

Laboratory diagnosis Clinical and epidemiologic findings often suggest the diagnosis. There may be elevation of the alkaline phosphatase and hyperbilirubinemia. Eosinophilia is variable. Occasionally, a plain film of the abdomen will demonstrate intrahepatic calcification. Liver scan is usually negative in asymptomatic infections but may show multiple areas of diminished uptake in acute symptomatic disease. Percutaneous transhepatic cholangiography in such patients often reveals dilatation of the peripheral intrahepatic bile ducts. The adult worms appear as round filling defects several millimeters in diameter. Definitive diagnosis depends on the demonstration of the eggs in the feces or the duodenal contents. They measure 29 by 16 μm, possess a conspicuous opercular rim as well as a posterior knob, and can be distinguished from the eggs of *Metagonimus, Heterophyes,* and *Opisthorchis* only with difficulty. An antigen extracted from adult worms can be used in a complement fixation test for the detection of the host's antibody response.

Treatment and prevention The recent introduction of praziquantel has, for the first time, provided an effective chemotherapeutic agent for clonorchiasis. It is administered as described above for paragonimiasis. Thorough cooking of freshwater fish will prevent infection.

OPISTHORCHIASIS Opisthorchiasis is caused by *Opisthorchis felineus* or *O. viverrini* and is characterized by hepatic lesions produced by adult worms in the larger bile ducts. The life cycle resembles that of *C. sinensis.* The geographic distribution differs in that *O. felineus* is endemic in eastern and central Europe and in Siberia and occurs in some parts of Asia, while *O. viverrini* is found in Thailand and Laos. Cats and wild carnivores act as the principal reservoir hosts, and the infection is found most commonly along rivers and lakes which harbor an abundant fish life. Up to 25 percent of inhabitants of northeastern Thailand are purported to carry the parasite. The clinical lesions are similar to those seen in clonorchiasis except that gallstones are rare. Cholangiocarcinoma occurs in approximately 50 percent of infected patients who come to autopsy. The diagnosis usually is based on the finding of the eggs in the feces or duodenal contents. Treatment as recommended for clonorchiasis may be used. Infection can be prevented by eating only well-cooked fish.

FASCIOLIASIS Fascioliasis is caused by *Fasciola hepatica,* which, like *Clonorchis,* inhabits the bile ducts of the definitive host. When fully matured, the adult measures about 3 by 1 cm and discharges large operculate eggs 140 by 70 μm which must embryonate in fresh water before hatching.

Fascioliasis produces so-called liver rot in sheep, the principal definitive host. The disease is most common in sheep- and cattle-raising countries but has been reported from many parts of the world. In North America it occurs in the southern and western United States, Central America, and in the Caribbean Islands.

Infection is contracted by ingestion of the encysted forms of the fluke attached to edible aquatic plants such as watercress. The larvae excyst in the duodenum, migrate through the intestinal wall, pass into the peritoneal cavity, penetrate the liver capsule, and finally reach the bile ducts, where they mature. Occasionally larvae may migrate to and mature in ectopic locations including subcutaneous tissue, chest cavity, or brain.

Early clinical manifestations are related to the migration of the larval form to and within the liver. Epigastric pain, fever, diarrhea, jaundice, urticaria, pruritus, arthralgia, and eosinophilia may be observed during this stage. Fibrosis of the liver similar to that found in clonorchiasis appears only after prolonged residence of many adult worms in the bile ducts. Obstruction of the bile duct occurs frequently and may be the presenting manifestation of disease. A pharyngeal form of the disease, called *halzoun*, can result from eating infected raw liver, the young adults attaching themselves to the pharyngeal mucosa, occasionally interfering with respiration.

The diagnosis usually is based on the finding of the eggs in the feces or in the duodenal contents. It is difficult to distinguish the eggs from those of *Fasciolopsis buski*. Complement fixation, hemagglutination, and precipitin tests have been reported to be helpful. A skin test is also available.

Treatment is as described above for paragonimiasis.

To prevent infection, aquatic plants such as watercress should not be eaten, vegetables grown in fields irrigated with polluted water should be boiled, and safe drinking water should be provided.

FASCIOLOPSIASIS Fasciolopsiasis is caused by the large intestinal fluke *F. buski*, which inhabits the upper part of the intestine of its definitive host. The principal definitive host is the pig. In parts of China, India, and other areas in the far east, infection of humans occurs following ingestion, or peeling with the teeth, of water chestnuts and other edible aquatic plants. The large adults attach themselves to the intestinal mucosa, and these sites may later ulcerate. The infection is usually asymptomatic. In heavy infections, diarrhea, abdominal pain, gastrointestinal hemorrhage, and intestinal obstruction may appear early. Later, asthenia with ascites and anasarca occurs. Diagnosis is based upon the history and the finding of eggs in the feces. The eggs resemble those of *Fasciola hepatica*. The prognosis in untreated heavy infections, especially in children, is poor. Praziquantel as given for paragonimiasis is the treatment of choice. Tetrachloroethylene as given for hookworm infections may also be used.

HETEROPHYIASIS AND METAGONIMIASIS *Heterophyes heterophyes* and *Metagonimus yakagawa* are small intestinal flukes of humans and other fish-eating mammals. They are found in the far east and, in the case of *Heterophyes*, in India, Egypt, and Tunisia. Both are acquired by ingesting the raw or undercooked flesh of metacercarial-infected freshwater fish. The 2- to 3-mm adults attach themselves to the mucosa of the small intestine. If present in sufficient numbers, they may cause abdominal pain and/or diarrhea. Rarely the eggs have been found in sites such as the brain, spinal cord, or heart where they produce granulomatous lesions. Most commonly, they are passed in the stool where they very closely resemble those of *Clonorchis*. Both species can be treated with praziquantel as described for paragonimiasis or tetrachloroethylene as outlined in Chap. 230 for hookworm. As the life span of these trematodes is limited to a year or less, treatment is not indicated unless the patient is symptomatic.

REFERENCES

JONES EA et al: Massive infection with *Fasciola hepatica* in man. Am J Med 63:842, 1977

KOENIGSTEIN RP: Observations on the epidemiology of infections with *Clonorchis sinensis*. Trans R Soc Trop Med Hyg 42:503, 1949

KOOMPIROCHANA C et al: Opisthorchiasis: A clinicopathologic study of 154 autopsy cases. Southeastern Asian J Trop Med 9:60, 1978

MCFADZEAN AJS, YEUNG RTT: Hypoglycemia in suppurative pancholangitis due to Clonorchis sinensis. Trans R Soc Trop Med Hyg 59:179, 1965

MINH V et al: Pleural paragonimiasis in a S.E. Asian refugee. Am Rev Resp Dis 124:186, 1981

PLANT AG et al: A clinical study of *Fasciolopsis buski* in Thailand. Trans R Soc Trop Med Hyg 63:470, 1969

RIM H-J et al: Clinical evaluation of the therapeutic efficacy of praziquantel (Embay 8440) against *Clonorchis sinensis* infection in man. Ann Trop Med Parasitol 75:27, 1981

SADUN EH, BUCK AA: Paragonimiasis in South Korea—Immunodiagnostic, epidemiologic, clinical, roentgenologic and therapeutic studies. Am J Trop Med 9:562, 1960

SEAH SKK: Digenetic trematodes. Clin Gastroenterol 7:87, 1978

YOKOGAWA M: *Paragonimus* and paragonimiasis, in *Advances in Parasitology*, B Dawes (ed). London, Academic, 1969, vol 7, p 375

232 CESTODE (TAPEWORM) INFECTIONS

PAUL G. RAMSEY
JAMES J. PLORDE

The tapeworms, or cestodes, are ribbon-shaped segmented hermaphroditic worms which inhabit the intestinal tract of many vertebrates. Unlike other helminths, they lack a digestive tract but absorb food through their entire surface. Tapeworms have a primitive nervous system, a muscular system, and excretory canals. Attachment to the host's intestinal mucosa is accomplished by sucking cups or grooves located on the head, or *scolex*. In some species, attachment is aided by hooklets located on the scolex. Behind the globular scolex lies a short, narrow neck from which segments or *proglottides* develop to form the chainlike *strobila* of the worm. The proglottides progressively mature as they are displaced further from the neck by new segments. As each section becomes gravid, eggs are released either through a uterine pore, by splitting open, or by simply disintegrating. Because the eggs of many tapeworms appear identical, species identification depends on the morphological characteristics of the scolex or gravid proglottides.

Except for *Hymenolepsis nana* the human tapeworms require one or more intermediate hosts for larval development. After ingestion by a susceptible intermediate host, the eggs develop into larvae or *oncospheres* which are capable of penetrating the intestinal mucosa, migrating in tissues, and developing into encysted forms. If the cyst contains a single scolex, it is called a *cysticercus*, or *cysticercoid* in the case of *H. nana*. A *coenurus* is a cyst which contains several scolices, and a *hydatid* is a structure with daughter cysts each containing several scolices. Ingestion of tissues containing cysts with viable scolices by a definitive host allows development of the larval stage into an adult tapeworm. Cestodes in the *Diphyllobothrium* genus have a more complex life cycle involving two intermediate hosts (see below).

Human tapeworm infections may be divided into two major clinical groups. In the first, humans act as the definitive host and harbor the adult tapeworm in their intestines. The important species in this group include *Taenia saginata, Diphyllobothrium latum, Hymenolepsis* species, and *Dipylidium caninum*. In the second group, humans are intermediate hosts and harbor the larval forms in their tissues. This is exemplified by echinococcosis, sparganosis, and coenurosis. *Taenia solium* is unique because humans may act as both the definitive and intermediate hosts.

TAENIASIS SAGINATA **Definition** Taeniasis saginata is an intestinal infection of humans caused by the beef tapeworm.

Epidemiology Infection with *Taenia saginata* occurs in all countries where raw or undercooked beef is eaten. It is particularly prevalent in Ethiopia, Kenya, Yugoslavia, the Middle East, Mexico and parts of South America, and the U.S.S.R. Taeniasis saginata is uncommon in the United States except in areas where cattle and humans are concentrated such as around feedlots in the southwest.

Etiology and pathogenesis Humans are the only definitive host for the adult stage of *T. saginata* which inhabits the upper jejunum for as long as 25 years. The cestode is 5 to 10 m long and has a small, unarmed scolex with four prominent suckers and between 1000 and 2000 proglottides. The gravid segments are longer than they are wide (5 by 20 mm) and have 15 to 30 lateral uterine branches (*T. solium* has 8 to 12). The eggs, which are passed within the intact proglottid, measure 30 by 40 mm, have a thick brown radially striated shell, and contain a fully developed embryo with three pairs of hooklets. They are indistinguishable from *T. solium* eggs. After the eggs are deposited on soil or vegetation, they are ingested by cattle or other herbivores. The embryo is released in the intestine, invades the intestinal wall, and is carried by vascular channels to striated muscle in the hind limbs, diaphragm, and tongue where it is transformed over a period of 3 to 4 months into an ovoid bladder worm, or cysticercus. This form, which may be viable for 1 to 3 years, measures about 5 by 10 mm and consists of one scolex suspended in a fluid-filled sac. After ingestion of the cyst in raw or undercooked beef by humans, about 2 months is required for the adult worm to develop in the intestine.

Clinical manifestations The majority of patients have minimal or no symptoms. Mild epigastric discomfort, nausea, and hunger sensations are most common, with weight loss, diarrhea, irritability, and an increase in appetite being more unusual. Movements of the worm are sometimes apparent, and occasionally proglottides may crawl through the anus, appearing in the bed linen or underclothing of the distraught host. Rarely segments become impacted in the appendix or cystic or pancreatic duct producing obstruction and inflammation of these organs.

Diagnosis After the adult tapeworm has been established for 2 to 3 months, several proglottides are shed daily in the stool and can be detected with relative ease. Eggs may be distributed in the stool or on the perianal area if a proglottid ruptures during defecation and should be looked for in the absence of segments. The perianal region may be examined as for pinworm infection, using a Scotch brand cellophane tape swab. By this method 85 to 95 percent of infections may be detected, whereas by stool examination only 50 to 75 percent are recognized. Since egg morphology is not diagnostic, examination of either the proglottides or the scolex is necessary to identify the tapeworm species correctly.

Treatment Niclosamide (Yomesan) is a highly effective taenicide which kills the scolex and immature segments of the worm on contact. Four 0.5-g tablets are thoroughly chewed at one time and swallowed with a small amount of water. No preparation or purge is necessary, and few side effects have been reported. As the worm is digested before it is passed in the stool, no attempt should be made to recover the scolex. Stool should be examined at 3 and 6 months for test of cure. Paromomycin (Humatin), 1.0 g orally every 15 min for four doses, is an alternative drug. Quinacrine hydrochloride, for many years the standard medication, has been supplanted by the newer medications because of its inconvenience and side effects. Mebendazole in doses of 300 mg twice daily for 3 days has shown promise in a clinical trial but remains experimental.

Prevention Thorough cooking of beef is the major means of preventing taeniasis saginata. Temperatures as low as 56°C for as little as 5 min will destroy cysticerci. Refrigeration and salting for prolonged periods or freezing at −10°C for 9 days also destroys the cysticercus. General preventive measures include adequate meat inspection and proper disposal of human feces.

TAENIASIS SOLIUM AND CYSTICERCOSIS **Definition** *Taenia solium*, the pork tapeworm, inhabits the intestinal lumen of humans, its only definitive host. The hog is the usual intermediate host, although humans, dogs, cats, and sheep may harbor the larval form. When human tissue is invaded by the larval form, the condition is referred to as *cysticercosis.*

Epidemiology Taeniasis solium is worldwide but is most common in Mexico, Africa, southeast Asia, eastern Europe, and South America. Recently, *T. solium* has been found in swine in Colorado and New Mexico, but autochthonously acquired human disease has not been reported in the United States.

Etiology and pathogenesis The adult worm is about 3 m in length, resides in the upper jejunum, and may live for decades. The globular scolex contains a rostellum with two rows of hooklets. There are usually less than 1000 proglottides. The gravid proglottid is about 6 by 12 mm and contains a uterus with 8 to 12 lateral branchings. The eggs are infective for both human and hog. Infection usually occurs by the fecal-oral route, but humans may be autoinfected when gravid segments are returned to the stomach by reverse peristalsis. In the intermediate host, the embryo is released from the egg, penetrates the intestinal wall, and is carried by vascular channels to all parts of the body. Localization with development over a period of 2 to 3 months to the encysted larval stage ("bladder worm") occurs primarily in striated muscle of the tongue, neck, and trunk. The cysticerci are ovoid, grey-white opalescent structures about 1 cm in diameter. They can survive for 5 years. Humans become infected with the adult stage following ingestion of undercooked pork containing cysticerci.

Clinical manifestations Clinical manifestations of adult worm infestation resemble those with *T. saginata.* When humans serve as the intermediate host (cysticercosis), the clinical picture is entirely different. Cysticerci develop in the subcutaneous tissues, in muscles, in viscera, and, most significantly, in the eye and brain. Only a moderate tissue reaction occurs while the scolex is viable, but the dead larvae invoke a marked tissue response with muscular pains, weakness, fever, and eosinophilia. Brain cysts are usually located in the cerebrum, ventricles, or subarachnoid space. The cerebral cysts are often less than 2 cm in diameter but may rarely be as large as 5 cm. If the cysticerci are widely distributed, the patient has signs and symptoms of meningoencephalitis. Epilepsy, brain tumors, and other types of neurological or psychiatric disorders may also be simulated.

Diagnosis Infection with the adult worm can be detected by finding eggs in perianal scrapings or in the feces. However, to differentiate *T. solium* from *T. saginata,* proglottides or the scolex must be examined. Cysticercosis should be suspected in an individual who has lived in a hyperendemic area and who develops neurological findings. Degenerated cysticerci calcify, and roentgenograms of soft tissue will usually reveal typical calcifications. The encysted larvae may be identified by biopsy of subcutaneous nodules. Brain cysts can be seen by computerized tomography (CT) or radioisotope scan. At present, the indirect hemagglutination is the best serological test available.

Treatment The stage and location of the parasite determine the prognosis and treatment. For removal of the adult worm in the human intestine, niclosamide or paromomycin is given as for taeniasis saginata. However, because these drugs cause maceration of the proglottides with release of ova, cysticercosis could theoretically occur. To prevent this, a saline purge should be administered 1 h after the medication. Drugs or procedures that induce vomiting should be avoided. Treatment of cerebral and ocular cysticercosis should usually be surgical. Mebendazole has shown activity against both the adult and larval stages of *T. solium*, but its value in therapy is not yet defined.

HYMENOLEPIASIS NANA Definition Hymenolepiasis nana is an intestinal infection of humans, rats, and mice by *Hymenolepsis nana*, the dwarf tapeworm. The life cycle is unique in that both the larval and adult phases occur in the same host.

Epidemiology Dwarf tapeworm infection has been reported in temperate and tropical regions around the globe. It is the most common autochthonously acquired tapeworm in the United States, most of the infections occurring in the southern states. The infection is spread by the direct fecal-oral route and is particularly common in children and institutional populations.

Etiology and pathogenesis The adult worm is small, about 2 cm, and lives for only a few weeks in the proximal ileum. Its proglottides are wider than they are long and may number 100 to 200. The gravid segments break apart in the fecal stream releasing spherical eggs. These measure 30 to 44 mm in diameter and have a double membrane enclosing the embryo which has six hooklets. The inner vitelline membrane has four to eight slender filaments arising from each pole. The eggs are immediately infective and when ingested by a new host, the freed oncospheres penetrate the intestinal villi, becoming cysticercoids. Larvae migrate back into the intestinal lumen, attach to the mucosa, and mature into adult worms. The eggs may also hatch before passing in the stool, causing internal autoinfection with gradually increasing numbers of worms in the host.

Clinical manifestations Dwarf tapeworm infection may be asymptomatic even with many adult worms in the intestine. When infection is massive, abdominal cramps and diarrhea occur. Rarely, dizziness or seizures have been seen in children and have been attributed to a neurotoxic product of the worms.

Treatment Niclosamide, 2 g per day, must be given for 5 to 7 consecutive days. The dosage for children must be adjusted for body weight. The longer treatment course is necessary because niclosamide is not effective against the cysticercoid stage, and the encysted larvae continue to release organisms for 4 days. A repeat treatment course may be required in 2 weeks for patients with heavy infections. Paromomycin, 45 mg/kg daily for 5 to 7 days, may also be effective.

Prevention With a single host involved and the eggs being immediately infective, eradication of the disease presents problems similar to those encountered with enterobiasis. Personal hygiene is imperative. In an institution, epidemics can be avoided by proper screening programs.

HYMENOLEPIASIS DIMINUTA *Hymenolepsis diminuta* is a cestode of rats and mice that occasionally infects small children. Larval development occurs in a wide variety of insects including fleas and mealworms. Humans become infected with the adult worm when they ingest uncooked cereal foods contaminated by these insects. Infection is usually asymptomatic, and the diagnosis is made only when characteristic eggs are found in the stool. The eggs resemble those of *H. nana* but are longer and lack polar filaments. Niclosamide, as prescribed for *H. nana*, results in approximately a 90 percent cure rate.

DIPYLIDIASIS *Dipylidium caninum* is the common tapeworm of cats and dogs. The orange-brown proglottid, which resembles a pumpkin seed, is often passed intact in the stool or migrates through the anal canal. This may cause animals harboring the parasite to drag their buttocks across the floor. The characteristic egg packets are then expelled by the proglottides and ingested by fleas to develop into infective larval forms. The definitive host becomes infected by swallowing involved fleas. Human infections occur primarily in small children who ingest fleas while playing with their pets. The diagnosis is made by recovering the characteristic proglottid or egg packet. Treatment is the same as for *T. saginata* described above. Periodic deworming of pets provides the best prevention.

DIPHYLLOBOTHRIASIS Definition *Diphyllobothrium latum* and other *Diphyllobothrium* species, the fish or broad tapeworms, produce an intestinal infection in the definitive host (including humans).

Epidemiology Diphyllobothriasis is common in the Baltic and Scandinavian countries, Japan, U.S.S.R., Switzerland, Italy, Chile, and central Africa. It occurs in the north central United States, Florida, and with increased frequency along the Pacific coast. The prevalence of infection is enhanced by the disposal of raw sewage into freshwater lakes. Anadromous Alaskan salmon have been implicated in an outbreak along the west coast. The growing popularity of raw fish dishes such as Japanese sushi and sashimi may lead to increased prevalence of the disease in the United States.

Etiology and pathogenesis The adult worm lies attached to the mucosa of the ileum and occasionally the jejunum by a pair of sucking grooves located on the scolex. It can live 20 years and achieve a length of more than 10 m. The 3000 to 4000 proglottides are wider than they are long. Unlike *Taenia*, the gravid segments are retained by the worm, and each day a million operculated ova are passed directly in the stool. On reaching water, the egg hatches, releasing a free-swimming embryo. This is eaten by small freshwater crustaceans belonging to the species *Cyclops* or *Diaptomus*, in which it develops into a *procercoid*. When the infected crustacean is swallowed by a fish, the larva migrates into the flesh and grows into a *plerocercoid*, or *sparganum*, larva. Humans acquire disease by ingesting raw infected fish. In 3 to 5 weeks the tapeworm matures in the intestine into an adult capable of discharging eggs. Several *Diphyllobothrium* species can infect humans, and *D. latum* cannot be distinguished from other species by its eggs or proglottides. Species determination requires examination of the scolex.

Clinical manifestations Most infections are asymptomatic or produce slight, transient abdominal discomfort. Rarely, there may be severe cramping abdominal pain, diarrhea or constipation, vomiting, weakness, and loss of weight. Intestinal obstruction has been reported in multiple infections. In 0.1 to 2 percent of infected patients, an anemia develops, and about 40 percent of fish tapeworm carriers will have low serum vitamin B_{12} levels. The anemia appears to result from the ability of the tapeworm to compete successfully with its host for vitamin B_{12} and resembles pernicious anemia including central nervous system involvement. A worm located high in the jejunum may take up 80 to 100 percent of labeled vitamin B_{12} ingested by a patient with anemia. These patients tend to be elderly, have diminished production of intrinsic factor, and have worms located in the proximal small bowel. Folate absorption may also be decreased and contribute to the anemia. Lysolecithin, a product of the tapeworm, may contribute to the severity of the disease. Neurological manifestations are more common than in pernicious anemia and may occur in the absence of hematologic findings. Typically, they include paresthesias, impaired vibration sense, numbness, weakness, and, less commonly, central scotomas secondary to optic atrophy. These findings are reversible with proper treatment.

Diagnosis The characteristic eggs are present in the stool in large numbers, making the diagnosis easy. They measure 55 to 76 by 41 to 56 mm and possess a single shell with an operculum at one end and a knob on the other. Mild eosinophilia may be present.

Treatment Niclosamide or paromomycin as prescribed for taeniasis saginata will cure most infections. In the presence of severe macrocytic anemia, parenteral vitamin B_{12} should be given.

Prevention Fish tapeworm infection can be prevented by cooking to a temperature of at least 56°C for 5 min. Freezing at −10°C for 72 h or placing the fish in a brine solution with appropriate salt concentration and exposure time can also prevent disease. Commercially prepared lox is usually brined appropriately before smoking.

SPARGANOSIS The *sparganum,* or plerocercoid larva, of *Diphyllobothrium*-related tapeworms belonging to the genus *Spirometra* will develop in humans following ingestion (usually in drinking water) of a *Cyclops* bearing the procercoid larva. Sparganosis also follows ingestion of infected frogs or application of infected fresh frog flesh as a poultice. The frog tissues contain the sparganum, which is capable of invading human tissues. The dog and cat are definitive hosts for *Spirometra.* The infection often presents as a painful subcutaneous swelling. The periorbital tissues may be involved with marked palpebral edema and destruction of the globe. A marked eosinophilia is usually present. The location of the larvae determines the prognosis of the infection in humans. Surgery and injection of ethyl alcohol with epinephrine-free procaine to kill worms is the preferred method of treatment.

COENUROSIS This is a rare infection of humans by the larval stage, or coenurus, of the dog tapeworm *Taenia multiceps.* As in cysticercosis, the subcutaneous tissue, eye, and central nervous system may be involved. In tropical areas the brain has often been invaded, and the cases have been fatal. The clinical presentation is that of a slowly growing space-occupying lesion. Diagnosis and treatment both rely on surgical excision of the lesion. Treatment with drugs including mebendazole has not been effective.

ECHINOCOCCIASIS Definition Echinococciasis is a tissue infection of humans caused by the larval stage of *Echinococcus granulosus* or *E. multilocularis.* These species of echinococcus are distinct morphologically and biologically. In humans, *E. granulosus* produces cystic lesions primarily involving the liver and lungs, whereas *E. multilocularis* causes multilocular (alveolar) lesions that are locally invasive. A "sylvatic" form of *E. granulosus* differs significantly in clinical findings from a "pastoral" form.

Epidemiology Canines are the definitive hosts for *E. granulosus.* Sheep, cattle, and, in the Middle East, camels are the common intermediates for the pastoral form. This form of the disease has its highest incidence in countries where sheep and cattle raising is carried out with the help of dogs, particularly in the Middle East, Australia, New Zealand, east and south Africa, South America, and central Europe. Approximately 200 cases per year of echinococciasis are diagnosed in the United States, but most are imported. Autochthonously acquired cases have been reported from 16 states with most coming from well-defined populations, including Basque sheep farmers in California, southwestern Indians, and sheep raisers in Utah.

The sylvatic focus of *E. granulosus* exists primarily in Alaska and western Canada, where wolves act as the definitive host and caribou and moose as the intermediate. A second sylvatic cycle involving deer and coyotes has been reported from California. A survey of deer in California showed that the disease was common in only two of the counties studied. A domestic cycle can be established when humans kill the herbivores and feed their viscera to dogs.

In *E. multilocularis* infections, rodents and deer mice are the natural intermediate hosts, while wolves, foxes, coyotes, and domestic dogs and cats may serve as definitive hosts. An urban cycle involving the cat and common house mouse has been described. Human infection in the United States is most common in Alaska but has also been described in Minnesota. Large series of patients with *E. multilocularis* have been reported from Siberia and Switzerland.

Etiology The adult *E. granulosus* is a small worm measuring 5 mm in length which resides in the jejunum of canines for 5 to 20 months. In addition to the scolex and neck, it has three proglottides, one immature, one mature, and one gravid. The gravid segment splits, either before or after passage in the stool, to release eggs which appear identical to those of *T. saginata.* When ingested by an appropriate intermediate host, the embryos escape from the eggs, penetrate the intestinal mucosa, and enter the portal circulation. Most are filtered out by the liver or lung, but some escape into the general circulation to involve brain, kidney, bones, and other tissues. The larvae that are not phagocytosed and destroyed develop into hydatid cysts which are unilocular and consist of an external laminated cuticula and an inner germinal layer. The laminated membrane in the sylvatic form may be semitranslucent in appearance and more fragile than in the pastoral type. Fluid fills and distends the cyst. Brood capsules and second- or third-generation daughter cysts develop from the germinal layer. "Hydatid sand" found in the cyst consists of scolices liberated from ruptured brood capsules. The cysts grow slowly over a period of years. In the pastoral type cysts often reach a diameter of over 10 cm, while cysts in the sylvatic form are usually only 3 to 5 cm. When the hydatid cyst is ingested by a canine, the cycle is complete.

The life cycle of *E. multilocularis* is similar except that small rodents serve as the natural intermediate host. However, the cyst is quite different. The larval stage of *E. granulosus* develops normally in humans, and the unilocular cyst remains unattached to host tissue. In contrast, humans do not provide optimal conditions for development of *E. multilocularis,* and the larval form remains in the proliferative phase. The hydatid cyst is always multilocular or alveolar in type. Its vesicles progressively invade the host tissue, usually the liver, by extension of processes from the germinal layer. In general, the growth pattern is like a neoplasm, and the lesions may metastasize when growth extends into blood vessels.

Clinical manifestations Echinococciasis is usually acquired in childhood, but a latent period of 5 to 20 years occurs before diagnosis. In one patient the latent period of a hepatic cyst was 75 years. Enlarging cysts usually produce tissue damage by mechanical means. The resulting symptoms depend upon the site, type, and rate of growth of the cystic lesions.

Patients with the sylvatic form of *E. granulosus* are usually asymptomatic at the time of diagnosis. Approximately 60 percent of the cysts are found in the lung and 40 percent in the liver. The cysts are diagnosed as an incidental finding on routine x-ray. Rarely, a patient may present with hemoptysis or a palpable mass in the liver. Morbidity and mortality are almost never seen.

With the pastoral type the ratio of pulmonary to liver cysts is reversed, and the hydatids may reach enormous size. In as many as 20 percent of patients, the pulmonary hydatid may rupture producing cough, chest pain, or hemoptysis. Hepatic lesions often present as abdominal pain or a palpable mass. Rupture through the diaphragm or into the peritoneal cavity can occur. Intrabiliary extrusion of calcified hepatic cysts has been reported in 5 to 15 percent of affected patients and mimics recurrent cholecystitis. Obstruction of the bile duct may result in jaundice. Rupture of a hydatid into the bile duct, peritoneal cavity, lung, pleura, or bronchus may produce fever, pruritus, urticarial rash, or an anaphylactoid reaction which may be fatal. Release of the numerous scolices leads to disseminated infection. Most patients initially have one or more hydatids in a single site, but in about 10 percent other tissues are involved. In bone, the cysts are semisolid, invade the medullary cavity, and slowly erode bone, producing pathological fractures. Central nervous system involvement may produce epilepsy or blindness. Cardiac cysts can lead to conduction blocks, pericarditis, and ventricular rupture. Hydatid antigen has been shown by fluorescent antibody in the glomerulus and has been related to membranous glomerulonephritis. Many other sites can be involved including spleen, ovary, prostate, and thyroid.

The alveolar cyst of *E. multilocularis* usually presents as a slowly growing hepatic tumor, with a minority of patients having metastatic disease to lung, brain, or other tissues. The natural course is one of malignant growth with massive destruction of the liver and extension into vital structures. If untreated, the disease is fatal in 70 percent of cases, but there is considerable individual variation in the course of the disease.

Diagnosis If a hydatid cyst ruptures or leaks fluid, an anaphylactoid reaction associated with eosinophilia and increased IgE levels may suggest the diagnosis. However, the clinical picture is usually not characteristic, and eosinophilia is seen in less than 25 percent of cases. Echinococciasis is most commonly discovered by routine x-ray. Pulmonary lesions usually are round, somewhat irregular masses of uniform density. They do not calcify. In contrast, hepatic cysts of *E. granulosus* show a smooth rim of calcification in about 50 percent of cases. Diffuse radiolucencies (2 to 4 mm) outlined by calcific densities may be seen in the liver with *E. multilocularis.* CT can be useful in demonstrating more details of the hydatid. In some cases of *E. granulosus,* simple, fluid-filled cysts indistinguishable from benign hepatic cysts are seen. In others, the findings of daughter cysts and hydatid sand strongly suggest echinococciasis. Thin eggshell calcification may indicate active disease. With alveolar hydatids, CT reveals indistinct solid masses often with central necrosis, and plaque-like calcification. Ultrasound can also be helpful in distinguishing hydatid structure, and angiography may be necessary prior to surgical therapy.

Specific diagnosis is best accomplished by histological examination. However, diagnostic aspiration should not be attempted because of potential anaphylactoid reactions to leakage of cyst fluid. Occasionally scolices may be found in sputum, stool, or urine and are best shown by Ziehl-Neelsen stain. The skin test (Casoni's test) is sensitive but gives 40 percent false-positive results. Serologic tests including indirect hemagglutination and latex agglutination are more useful if positive, but many cyst carriers will not develop an immune response. Indirect hemagglutination should be positive in 90 percent of patients with hepatic cysts but in only 50 to 60 percent of those with pulmonary hydatids. The presence of "arc 5" in the immunoelectrophoresis test provides the most specific serological diagnosis of hydatid disease, and the adaptation of this technique to an enzyme-linked immunoelectrodiffusion assay may provide a more sensitive, rapid test. Following surgical removal of cysts, serological tests may be helpful in screening for residual or recurrent disease. The Clq assay has also been employed for this purpose.

Treatment Surgical treatment remains the standard therapy. Patients with small calcified hepatic cysts and pulmonary hydatids of the sylvatic type need to be operated on only if the cysts are symptomatic or enlarge dramatically over time. All others should have their cysts excised if possible, or sterilized and drained. With a large cyst, the contents should be sterilized with hypertonic saline before an attempt is made to open it. The entire endocyst should then be removed if possible, and all biliary or bronchial fistulas carefully closed. The residual space must be obliterated to prevent postoperative infection or prolonged drainage. Aspergillomas have been seen in residual cavities of pulmonary cysts.

Medical therapy with "high-dose" mebendazole (40 mg/kg per day) remains experimental. In animal models, mebendazole is larvacidal for *E. granulosus* but not for *E. multilocularis.* In human trials, all forms of echinococciasis appear to respond to the agent, although the experience with *E. multilocularis* is limited. Significant side effects including neutropenia have been reported. Mebendazole may be considered in patients with other medical problems that preclude surgery or in patients with extensive disease that makes surgical cure impossible. In selected patients, it may also be considered in conjunction with definitive surgery to reduce risk of metastatic spread of viable organisms. At present, the agent can be used only with the patient's informed consent. The absorption is erratic and drug levels should be followed. The drug is contraindicated in pregnancy.

Prevention The incidence of echinococciasis can be reduced by appropriate control measures as demonstrated in Iceland. Contact with infected dogs must be avoided, infected carcasses and offal should be burned or buried, and infected dogs should be treated.

REFERENCES

BEARD TC et al: Medical treatment for hydatids. Med J Aust 1:633, 1978

BENGER A et al: A human coenurus infection in Canada. Am J Trop Med Hyg 30:638, 1981

CALAMAI G et al: Hydatid disease of the heart: Report of 5 cases and review of the literature. Thorax 29:451, 1974

GAMBLE WG et al: Alveolar hydatid disease in Minnesota: First human case acquired in the contiguous United States. JAMA 241:904, 1979

GHARBI HA et al: Ultrasound examination of the hydatidic liver. Radiology 139:459, 1981

JONES TC: Cestodes. Clin Gastroenterol 7:105, 1978

JONES WE: Niclosamide as a treatment for *Hymenolepsis diminuta* and *Dipylidium caninum* infection in man. Am J Trop Med Hyg 28:300, 1979

KATZ R et al: Pulmonary echinococcosis: A pediatric disease of the Southwestern United States. Pediatrics 65:1003, 1980

PAWLOWSKI Z, SCHULTZ MG: Taeniasis and cysticercosis *Taenia* (*Taenia saginata*). Adv Parasitol 10:269, 1972

PINON JM et al: Immunological study of hydatidosis. Am J Trop Med Hyg 28:318, 1979

PORAT S, JOSEPH KN: Hydatid disease of bone. Israel J Med Sci 14:223, 1978

TAYLOR RL: Sparganosis in the United States. Report of a case. Am J Clin Pathol 66:560, 1976

TODOROV T, STOJANOV G: Circulating antibodies in human echinococcosis before and after surgical treatment. Bull WHO 57:751, 1979

TURNER JA et al: Diphyllobothriasis associated with salmon—United States. Morb Mort Week Rep 30:331, 1981

VON BONSDORFF B et al: Vitamin B_{12} deficiency in carriers of the fish tapeworm, *Diphyllobothrium lathum*. Acta Haematol 24:15, 1960

WERCZBERGER A et al: Disseminated echinococcosis with repeated anaphylactic shock treated with mebendazole. Chest 76:482, 1979

WILSON JF et al: Cystic hydatid disease in Alaska. Am Rev Resp Dis 98:1, 1968

———, RAUSCH RL: Alveolar hydatid disease. A review of clinical features of 33 indigenous cases of *E. multilocularis* infection in Alaskan Eskimos. Am J Trop Med Hyg 29:1340, 1980

XANTHAKIS D et al: Hydatid disease of the chest. Report of 91 cases surgically treated. Thorax 27:517, 1972

section 14 | Diseases caused by bites and stings

233 SCABIES, CHIGGERS, AND OTHER ECTOPARASITES

JAMES J. PLORDE

SCABIES Scabies is a cosmopolitan skin infection commonly referred to as the "seven-year itch." It is caused by a burrowing mite, *Sarcoptes scabiei,* and is transmitted from person to person by close bodily contact, particularly among bed partners. Although the disease is more common in the poor and unclean, sporadic cases involve individuals of all socioeconomic groups. There has been a worldwide resurgence of this infection over the past 20 years, and in the United States it currently involves 2 to 4 percent of patients seen in dermatologists' offices.

The turtle-shaped female measures 0.4 mm in length and possesses four pairs of legs. With the help of the two anterior pair and her mouth, she burrows into the superficial layer of the epidermis. Here she deposits two or three enormous eggs daily until she dies 30 to 60 days later. The newly hatched larvae mature to adulthood within 2 weeks to continue the cycle of infection. Although an involved person may harbour thousands or occasionally millions of adult mites, the average number of adult females per infection is 11.

Two-thirds of the burrows are found in the upper extremities, particularly on the interdigital spaces of the hands and the flexor surface of the wrists. In heavy infections, other sites are typically involved. These include the dorsal surfaces of the elbows, anterior axillary folds, female breasts, periumbilical area, penis, and buttocks. In bedridden patients, lesions are often concentrated over pressure points. The face, head, palms, and soles are seldom involved in adults. Characteristically, a burrow appears as a short dark wavy line which may end in a small vesicle, the site of the adult female.

Sensitization to the mites and their products begins approximately one month after infection and results in a papular or eczematous reaction at the sites of involvement. Itching is often severe and tends to be more marked at night or after a hot bath. Scratching frequently leads to secondary infection with pustulation; acute glomerulonephritis has followed infection with nephrogenic strains of streptococci. Occasionally, reddish pruritic nodules are seen in the groin and axillary regions. Infected individuals with good personal hygiene usually have few lesions, and burrows may be difficult to identify. In mentally retarded, debilitated, or immunosuppressed patients, a particularly virulent infection known as *Norwegian scabies* is sometimes seen. Millions of mites may be present, producing a highly infectious exfoliative dermatitis; itching is often mild or absent. Scabies usually terminates spontaneously in a few months, but chronic cases do occur.

The diagnosis should be considered in any patient presenting with a pruritic eruption, particularly if it involves several members of a living group. The occurrence of symmetric lesions at the sites of predilection should initiate a search for the characteristic burrows. These should be vigorously scraped with a sterile needle or scalpel blade, and the scrapings transferred to a drop of 10% potassium hydroxide on a glass slide. A cover slip is placed over the top, and the preparation examined for adults, larvae, and eggs. The diagnosis can also be made on histological sections prepared from a punch biopsy. Considering the mode of disease transmission, individuals shown to have scabies should also be checked for venereal disease.

All sexual contacts and household members should be treated simultaneously with the patient to prevent the occurrence of "ping-pong infections." The therapeutic agents are applied topically, covering the skin thinly but completely from the neck down. Although the patient is rendered noninfectious within 24 h, up to 2 months may be required for the clinical manifestations of the disease to disappear completely. Needless retreatment during this period can lead to contact dermatitis.

A number of effective agents are available for use. Gamma benzene hexachloride (Gamene, Kwell) is left on for 12 h and then thoroughly washed off. Care must be taken to keep it away from eyes and mucous membranes. It should not be used in infants or pregnant adults. Benzyl benzoate (25%) is administered in a similar fashion. Crotamiton (Eurax) is massaged into the skin, and a second dose applied 24 h later. Antihistamines or salicylates are helpful in counteracting pruritus. Topical steroids may potentiate the infection and should not be used. Antibiotics are required occasionally when there is a significant bacterial superinfection.

CHIGGER MITES The term *chigger* is used to refer to larvae of harvest mites belonging to the family Trombiculidae. The cosmopolitan adults feed on vegetable matter and deposit their eggs upon the ground. The tiny (0.4 mm) emergent larvae crawl along the ground and upward onto vegetation. Here, they await the passage of a vertebrate host, upon which they must feed before again dropping to the ground and molting. In humans, the chigger usually attaches about the ankles, but some advance along the skin until they are stopped by tight-fitting clothing. It then pierces the skin, releases a digestant to liquefy tissue cells, and feeds for 3 or 4 days. Within a few hours, the chigger's secretions have produced an intensely pruritic papule 0.5 to 2 cm in diameter. This usually vesiculates, resulting in a chickenpox-like lesion. Occasionally, subcutaneous bleeding results in a surrounding area of ecchymosis. The lesion and itching may persist for several weeks. In the United States, most clinical cases are seen during the summer months; in warm climates, the seasonal pattern is missing. Treatment is directed at the relief of itching and the prevention of secondary infections. Insect repellants are highly effective prophylactic agents.

FLEAS Fleas are small wingless laterally compressed ectoparasites of humans and other warm-blooded animals. They tend to be found on the hairy portions of the host where they feed and deposit their eggs. The active larvae which hatch in 3 days can be found on the host, in its nest, or in dust. They eventually pupate and may remain dormant for weeks or months before completing their development to adults.

Medically, fleas serve as both vectors and agents of disease. Rodent fleas of the genus *Xenopsylla* are the most important. They are responsible for the transmission of both plague (*Pasteurella pestis*) and murine typhus (*Rickettsia mooseri*) from animal reservoirs to humans. Humans may also acquire the rat tapeworm *Hymenolepis diminuta* by swallowing fleas containing the cysticeroid. The dog tapeworm *Dipylidium caninum* may be transmitted in a similar fashion. The bites of these and other species of fleas belonging to the family Pulicidae can induce an irritating dermatitis. In addition, the tungidae (*Tunga penetrans*) may burrow into the subcutaneous tissues, producing a painful and debilitating disease.

Flea dermatitis The fleas of humans (*Pulex irritans*), cats and dogs (*Cetenocephalides*), and rodents (*Xenopsylla*) may all induce dermatitis. In many individuals, the bites seem completely innocuous, but in sensitive persons, the saliva induces an erythematous raised pruritic papule. Repeated scratching may result in secondary infection with pustulation or ulceration. The intense pruritus, the ability of the flea to escape capture by virtue of its prodigious jumping ability, and the difficulty involved in crushing their hard chitinous bodies has led to many a frustrating nocturnal safari dedicated to the destruction of this unwanted bed partner. Control is effected by the use of frequent vacuuming to remove eggs, larvae, pupae, and adults from the environment. Insecticide sprays are also of help, but fleas have developed resistance to many of these. Dogs and cats should be washed, flea collars should be applied, and kennels should be dusted or sprayed with DDT or Malathion. If rat runs can be located, they should also be dusted.

Tunga penetrans, sometimes referred to as a *jigger* or *chigoe flea,* is a burrowing flea found in the tropical areas of South America and Africa. These small (1 mm) free-living insects reside in sandy soil. The fertilized female burrows into the skin of the first warm-blooded animal encountered. In humans, they usually embed on the sole of the foot or under a toenail with only their anal pore exposed to the outside. Multiple infections are common. As the female becomes engorged with blood and eggs, a painful and pruritic pea-sized swelling is produced. Eventually, the overlying skin ulcerates, the flea dies, and the eggs are extruded. Secondary bacterial infections including tetanus and gas gangrene occur commonly. Autoamputation of the toes has been reported from Africa. The intact flea can usually be extracted by gently enlarging the entrance hole with a sterile needle and then applying pressure from the side. Alternatively, the lesion can be soaked in Lysol, the flea penetrated with a needle, and the lesion resoaked to kill the eggs and sterilize the wound. Antibiotics may be required to treat secondary bacterial infections.

PEDICULOSIS Lice are obligate human ectoparasites that complete their entire 30- to 40-day life cycle on the body of the host. *Pediculus humanis* var. *capitis* infests the head, *P. humanis* var. *corporis* the body and clothing, and *Phthirius pubis* (crab lice) the genital and occasionally other hairy areas of the body. All three are flattened dorsoventrally and measure 2 to 3 mm in length. The crab louse is broader and flatter than *Pediculus* and possesses powerful claws on its second and third legs with which it clings to the pubic hair. The females lay five or six eggs daily which they firmly attach to the hairs or, in the case of the body louse, the clothing of the host. These clearly visible tiny white nits hatch in 8 to 10 days. The resulting nymph matures to adulthood in an additional 2 weeks. Both the larvae and adults take two blood meals daily, leaving behind a small purpuric puncture site. With repeated exposure, the host develops an inflammatory hypersensitivity reaction manifested as a small red papule at each new feeding site. Pruritus results in scratching, a weeping dermatitis, and secondary infection. Chronic infections of the scalp may result in a fetid mass of matted hair and exudate. On the body and genital areas, the lesions may become pigmented—so-called "vagabond disease." Heavy infections with *P. pubis* may involve the eyebrows and eyelids leading to blepharitis.

Lice can be transferred from person to person by direct contact or via discarded clothing in which the body louse can survive for up to a week. Migration is stimulated by fever, making *P. humanis* var. *corporis* an efficient vector of relapsing fever (*Borrelia recurrentis*), typhus (*R. prowazeki*), and trench fever (*R. quintana*). *Phthirius pubis* is not known to be a vector of human disease.

Pediculosis corporis is typically seen in the poor and transient who are unable to maintain even minimal levels of personal hygiene. In contrast, head and pubic lice are found on patients of all socioeconomic classes and are currently enjoying a resurgence in the United States. *P. capitis* most frequently infests white schoolchildren, blacks being seldom involved. Pubic lice are more common among the sexually active; their presence should stimulate a search for venereal disease.

The diagnosis is suggested by the typical dermatitis and confirmed by finding the adults or nits on the hair or clothing of the patient. Treatment may be carried out with 1% gamma benzene hexachloride (lindane, Kwell) or pyrethrins with piperonyl butoxide (RID). In head infections, the hair should first be shampooed with ordinary soap. Kwell shampoo is then rubbed in at least 4 min (pyrethrins with piperonyl butoxide, 10 min), the hair rinsed, dried, and combed with a fine-tooth comb to remove the nits. The process should be repeated in 7 days. Combs and brushes should be heated in water to 65°C for 5 min or soaked in 2% Lysol. The clothing and bedding of the patient with body lice are heat-sterilized. The patient's body should be lathered for 4 min with Kwell and then rinsed thoroughly. The therapy may be repeated in 7 days. In crab louse infestations, Kwell cream or lotion should be used on the involved areas and left for 24 h. In hirsute individuals, the treatment can be repeated in 1 week. If the eyelashes are involved, 0.25% physostigmine ophthalmic ointment is applied twice daily for 10 days. Lice and nits are carefully removed with a cotton-tipped applicator. Narrow-angle glaucoma should be ruled out before the physostigmine is used.

MYIASIS Infections with maggots or fly larvae are seen worldwide in a variety of animals. Human involvement occurs most frequently where people live in close contact with domestic animals. Many different species of flies are involved. In some, an animal host is required for larval development; in these, the larvae are capable of invading normal tissue or enter the body through the nose, mouth, or ears. Others are opportunists, depositing their eggs or larvae in the open wounds of debilitated patients. The clinical manifestations vary with the species of fly and site of involvement. Four of the more common clinical syndromes are described below.

Localized cutaneous myiasis In tropical America the lesions are produced by *Dermatobia hominis,* the human bot fly. This remarkable forest-dwelling diptera captures a mosquito or other blood-feeding insect on which to deposit its packet of eggs. When this unwilling vector then lands on a warm-blooded animal to feed, the eggs hatch and penetrate the feeding site. Within the skin of the host, the larva develops for 2 or 3 months. Finally, it emerges, drops to the ground, and pupates. The lesions are most frequently seen on unprotected areas of the body including the hands, feet, head, and neck. During the first week of infection, the pruritic lesion closely resembles a mosquito bite. As the larva grows and begins to move, it produces severe pain and itching. Tissue destruction and inflammation results in the development of a furuncle-like lesion. Generally, a central opening is present through which the posterior end of the larva protrudes. A dark serosanguinous discharge containing the feces of the insect may be noted.

In Africa, a similar lesion is produced by *Cordylobia anthropophaga* (Tumbu fly). These flies deposit their eggs on sandy soil or laundry laid out to dry. The larvae hatch and invade the unbroken skin of humans or wild rodents, where they mature in 8 or 9 days. In either case, the larvae can be surgically extracted without difficulty. In Tumbu fly infections, letting the larvae mature and drop off spontaneously may be appropriate. This process can occasionally be hastened by applying mineral oil to the central opening. This results in the suffocation of the larva and stimulates its early exodus.

Cutanea larva migrans This is usually caused by the large (1 to 2 cm) horse bot flies belonging to the genus *Gasterophilus.* When the larvae hatch on the skin, they penetrate to the lower epidermis. Because they do not mature in humans, they may migrate in the skin for several months. Clinically, the infection presents as a pruritic serpiginous band of erythema closely resembling cutanea larva migrans produced by *Ancylostoma braziliense.* The diagnosis can be made by placing a small drop of mineral oil on the skin just in advance of the worm tract. This allows visualization of black backward-directed spines on its body segments. The parasite can be easily removed with a sharp needle. Occasionally, the larvae may penetrate the eye. A similar clinical picture is sometimes produced by the larvae of *Hypoderma* spp. (cattle bot fly). These, however, often penetrate deeply into the subcutaneous tissue and produce more pain and less pruritus than *Gasterophilus* larvae.

Deep-tissue myiasis Screw flies of several genera can deposit large batches of eggs on unbroken skin or in wounds, ears, or the nose. After hatching, the larvae burrow into the tissues and develop for 2 or 3 weeks. The mature 1- to 2-cm larvae then drop to the ground and pupate. At times, they penetrate deep tissues, including the eye, nasal sinuses, and cranium, where they produce destructive foul-smelling lesions. Bacterial superinfection is common. In India and Africa, the flies are usually of genus *Chrysomyia.* In the western hemisphere, *Callitroga* spp. are involved. The occurrence of human cases in the United States often accompanies epizootics of screw worm activity. Flesh flies of the family Sarcophagidae have also been implicated in deep-tissue myiasis both in the United States and elsewhere. In all the above infections, the lesions should be surgically incised and debrided, the larvae removed, and secondary infections treated.

Intestinal myiasis When humans ingest food contaminated with the eggs or larvae of several genera of flies, some survive passage through the stomach and later mature in the intestine before they are extruded in the stool. In the United States, *Tubifera tenax* is the most frequently implicated species. Invasion of the intestinal mucosa may occur with *Sarcophaga* infections.

REFERENCES

ACKERMAN AB: Crabs—The resurgence of *Phthirius pubis.* N Engl J Med 278:950, 1968

HUNTER GW et al: *Tropical Medicine,* 5th ed. Philadelphia, Saunders, 1976

LEIBOWITZ M et al: Keratotic scabies (Norwegian scabies): Case reports and literature review. S Afr Med J 57:363, 1980

MACIAS EG et al: Cutaneous myiasis in South Texas. N Engl J Med 289:1239, 1973

ORKIN M, MAIBACH MI: Current concepts in parasitology. The scabies pandemic. N Engl J Med 298:496, 1978

Sexually transmitted diseases treatment guidelines 1982. Morb Mort Week Rep 31:25, 1982

234
DISORDERS CAUSED BY VENOMS, BITES, AND STINGS

JAMES F. WALLACE

Humans have the propensity to come into contact with a great variety of venomous animals. These contacts occur with many zoologic classes including snakes, lizards, sea animals, spiders, scorpions, and numerous species of insects. In general two types of injuries result: those due to the direct effect of venom on the victim, as exemplified in snakebite, and those due to indirect effects of the poison, of which hypersensitivity reaction to bee stings is an example. Each year in the United States at least 50 persons die as the result of venomous injuries. Three groups of animals—hymenopterous insects, snakes, and spiders—account for over 90 percent of the fatalities. Of even greater public health significance is the loss in economic productivity and human potential resulting from the many serious, nonfatal envenomations which occur annually in otherwise healthy children or working adults.

SNAKE BITE Epidemiology Fewer than one-tenth of the nearly 3500 known species of snakes are venomous. These poisonous varieties belong to five families or subfamilies: Elapidae (cobras, kraits, mambas, and coral snakes) found in all parts of the world except Europe; Viperidae (true vipers) found in all parts of the world except the Americas; Hydrophidae (sea snakes); Crotalidae (pit vipers) found in Asia and the

Americas; and Colubridae (boomslangs, bird snakes) of the African continent. The poisonous varieties of the United States, with the single exception of the coral snake, are pit vipers and include rattlesnakes, the water moccasin, and the copperhead. Although this discussion centers around these species, the therapeutic measures outlined are applicable to snakes in all parts of the world.

The number of individuals bitten by poisonous snakes in the United States is estimated to be about 8000 per year, with a relatively large number occurring in the southeastern and Gulf states, particularly Texas. Deaths are not reported separately but are undoubtedly rare, numbering fewer than 20 per year, and most are due to bites of various species of rattlesnake. In many European countries deaths from snakebite have averaged only one every 3 to 5 years for the last half-century. In contrast, the estimate of annual deaths from snakebite throughout the world is between 30,000 and 40,000 with the largest number occurring in the countries of Burma and Brazil, where 2000 deaths are estimated to occur each year.

Etiology The *coral snake* is found in the southern states from Florida to Arizona. It is usually marked by alternating red and black bands separated by yellow rings; however, black and albino forms exist. Coral snakes are generally nocturnal in their activities, shy and elusive, and rarely bite humans. Their fangs are short and permanently erect; the highly toxic venom is injected into multiple puncture wounds produced by a series of chewing movements.

The *pit vipers* are so named because of a small pit between the eye and the nostril. Large venom glands in the temporal regions give the head a triangular appearance. They are generally aggressive and likely to strike if disturbed. The fangs are long and hinged, folding posteriorly when the mouth is closed. Pit vipers strike suddenly with a forward thrust of the head. The instant that the erect fangs make contact, venom is expressed by sudden muscular contraction.

The *rattlesnakes,* recognized by the horny rattle on the tail, which buzzes when the snake is disturbed, are widely distributed. The diamondbacks (*Crotalus adamanteus* in the southeast and *C. atrox* in the southwest) are the largest and most dangerous snakes in this country. Others include the prairie rattler (*C. confluentus*), the timber rattler (*C. horridus*), and the pigmy rattlers.

The *water moccasin,* or cottonmouth (*Agkistrodon piscivorus*), is found in swampy areas or along the banks of streams. It is a strong swimmer and can bite under water. This snake is notorious for inflicting severe facial bites when disturbed in the branches of small trees. The copperhead, or highland moccasin (*A. mokasen*), is a closely related species. Its bite is painful but rarely fatal.

Pathogenesis SNAKE VENOMS The venoms of most species which have been analyzed have been found to be mixtures of several toxic proteins and enzymes with diversified and complicated pharmacological effects. An an example, the venom of the Indian cobra (*Naja naja*) contains these distinct and separate substances: a neurotoxin, a hemolysin, a cardiotoxin, a cholinesterase, at least three phosphatases, a nucleotidase, and a potent inhibitor of cytochrome oxidase. Several venoms, including those of the pit vipers, contain hyaluronidase and numerous proteolytic enzymes. Although the exact roles of these components in toxicity are incompletely understood, the venom of a given species is usually predominantly neurotoxic or necrotizing and is frequently associated with hemolysis, abnormalities of blood coagulation, changes in cardiac dynamics, and alterations in vascular resistance. The venom of elapids, including the coral snake, is neurotoxic, with death resulting from respiratory paralysis probably caused by damage to brain centers and a curariform interference with transmission at the neuromuscular junction. The venom of crotalid snakes produces local tissue injury, hemorrhage, and hemolysis; death is often preceded by circulatory collapse associated with a marked fall in circulating blood volume resulting from pooling of blood in the microcirculation, and loss of plasma due to increased capillary permeability. Systemic absorption of venom occurs through the lymphatics, and therapeutic measures designed to reduce lymphatic function are helpful in controlling symptoms.

FACTORS AFFECTING SEVERITY OF SNAKE BITE Several factors affect the outcome of snake bite:

1 The age, size, and health of the patient. Envenomation in children is usually serious, and a fatal outcome is more likely, since a relatively large dose of poison is injected into a small victim.
2 Location of bite. Bites on extremities or into adipose tissue are less dangerous than those on the trunk, face, or directly into a blood vessel. A direct strike of the fangs is more dangerous than a scratch, a glancing blow, or one hitting a bone. The discharge orifice of a fang is well above its tip so that the point of the fang can penetrate the skin without envenomation; even a thin layer of clothing may afford great protection. Because of the superficial nature of the wound as many as one-fifth of patients bitten by venomous snakes will have no evidence of envenomation, even though the fangs have penetrated the skin.
3 The size of the snake (a large pit viper can inject over 1000 mg venom, six times a lethal dose for an adult), the extent of its anger or fear (if hurt it may inject a larger amount of venom), the condition of the fangs (broken or recently renewed), and the condition of the venom glands (recently discharged or full). All these factors are important. Contrary to popular belief, the bite of a snake which has recently killed and fed is not necessarily less venomous for humans; the snake usually does not exhaust its venom in a single bite.
4 The presence of various bacteria, particularly clostridia and other anaerobic organisms, in the mouth of the snake or on the skin of the victim. This may lead to serious infection in the necrotic tissues at the local site.
5 Exercise or exertion, such as running, immediately after the bite. This speeds systemic absorption of toxin.

Manifestations Following the bite of a pit viper, severe burning pain develops within a few minutes at the site of the wound. Local swelling rapidly develops and spreads in all directions, accompanied by the appearance of ecchymoses and bullae over the involved area. As the edema spreads, serosanguinous fluid oozes from the puncture wounds. Later gangrene of the skin and subcutaneous tissues may develop. Systemic effects resulting from the absorption of venom and local tissue destruction may include fever, nausea and vomiting, circulatory collapse, bleeding into the skin and from all body orifices, low-grade jaundice, neuropathic muscle cramping, pupillary constriction, disorientation, delirium, and convulsions. Death may occur after 6 to 48 h. Survival may be attended by massive local tissue loss from gangrene or secondary infection, or may be complicated by acute renal failure, secondary to disseminated intravascular clotting and cortical necrosis, or by tubular necrosis following circulatory collapse.

The bite of the coral snake causes little pain and local swelling. There are usually multiple fang marks. Within 10 to 15 min numbness and weakness begin in the region of the bite, followed by ataxia, ptosis, pupillary dilatation, palatal and pharyngeal paralysis, slurring of speech, salivation, and occasionally nausea and vomiting. The patient becomes comatose, develops respiratory paralysis and seizures, and dies within 8 to 72 h.

Cobra bites are painful and are often accompanied by severe hemolysis, local necrosis, and sloughing in addition to their neurotoxic effects. There is little pain and no edema at the site of a sea snake bite. Symptoms of systemic envenomation follow a latent period which may vary from 15 min to 8 h. Although the venom is both myotoxic and neurotoxic, the injury to skeletal muscle is most prominent and is characterized by generalized muscle pain, weakness, and myoglobinuria. Hemorrhagic manifestations predominate following envenomation by colubrids (boomslangs and bird snakes) and many pit vipers including certain species of rattlesnake.

Laboratory abnormalities In severe cases, laboratory abnormalities may include progressive anemia, polymorphonuclear leukocytosis of 20,000 to 30,000 cells per cubic millimeter, thrombocytopenia, hypofibrinogenemia, disordered tests of coagulation, proteinuria, and azotemia.

Treatment An attempt should be made to determine with certainty that the patient has been bitten by a poisonous snake. Absence of distinct fang punctures and failure of local pain, edema, numbness, or weakness to appear within 20 min are strong evidence against snake venom poisoning. If the species of snake is not known, the offending reptile should be killed for the purpose of identification.

FIRST AID This consists of reassuring and calming the victim and instituting measures to retard the absorption of venom and to remove it from the tissues as quickly as possible after the bite. The patient should be promptly placed at rest and the bitten extremity immobilized to reduce the rate of spread of the venom. If anatomically feasible, a wide tourniquet should be placed a few centimeters above the bite and made tight enough to allow one finger to pass beneath with difficulty. The purpose is to impede lymph flow; it is not necessary to obstruct venous return. The tourniquet should be loosened and moved proximally at hourly intervals when local swelling causes it to tighten. Unless the victim can be transported to a hospital within less than 15 min, incision and suction of the wound should be started prior to evacuation. By use of whatever antisepsis is available, 1.0 cm *linear* (not cruciate) incisions about 0.5 cm deep should be carefully made through each fang mark and suction applied. A rubber bulb, breast pump, or heated jar are all preferable to mouth suction, but if other means are not available and no oral lesions are present, this method may be employed. Suction should be continued for at least 1 h following the bite, or until antivenin has been administered. The practice of making multiple incisions along the advancing edge of edema as swelling progresses has not been found to be beneficial and is no longer advised. *Incision and suction are extremely important and should be diligently carried out in every poisonous snake bite.* When begun promptly, they may result in the removal of up to 50 percent of subcutaneously injected venom.

As soon as possible, the patient should be transferred to a hospital. Immobilization of the affected part during transportation is important in controlling lymph flow and is best achieved by splinting. Although ice packs relieve pain and slow lymphatic drainage, they do not neutralize venom, and even a small amount of cooling may result in irreparable damage to already injured tissues by causing ischemia. For this reason, it is recommended that no form of cryotherapy be used.

IMMEDIATE HOSPITAL CARE This should include appropriate treatment for shock and respiratory difficulty, antivenin, measures to combat infection, and general supportive care.

Antivenin is the only specific treatment of snake venom poisoning, and its use in severe bites is vital. In the United States polyvalent crotaline antivenin effective against all American pit vipers and antivenin for North American coral snake poisoning are commercially available. Both products are a lyophylized powder of refined horse serum. Kits are available containing antivenin powder (reconstituted by diluting with water to 10 ml per ampul), syringe, normal horse serum for prior sensitivity testing of the patient, and detailed instructions. Intravenously administered antivenin leads to the most rapid and effective response. It is not advisable to infiltrate antivenin at the local site. The initial dose should depend upon the amount of envenomation; for pit viper bites accompanied by local swelling but no systemic symptoms, 2 to 5 vials (20 to 50 ml) is usually sufficient. When swelling has progressed beyond the site of the bite, and mild systemic symptoms and/or hematologic abnormalities are present, moderate envenomation has occurred, and initial treatment should be 5 to 9 vials (50 to 90 ml). For severe bites, associated with marked local as well as systemic effects and evidence of hemolysis or coagulation abnormalities, 10 to 15 vials (100 to 150 ml) or more should be administered. Larger doses of antivenin should be given to children or small adults to neutralize the relatively higher venom concentrations. When progressive swelling in the bitten part ceases, an adequate dose has generally been achieved; improvement in the victim's clinical signs is often extremely rapid.

If *any* evidence of envenomation appears during the first several hours following a coral snake bite, antivenin should be given without waiting for systemic manifestations to develop. Three vials of antivenin should be given intravenously for bites associated only with minimal swelling and/or local paresthesias. If evidence of a bite is more definitive, particularly if there was initial pain, 5 vials of antivenin should be given as soon as possible.

In the patient with severe envenomation who is allergic to horse serum, the relative risks of death from anaphylaxis rather than from venom poisoning should be carefully weighed before undertaking desensitization with small doses of diluted horse serum.

No antivenin for other snakes is manufactured in the United States, but antiserum for various types is usually kept on hand at large zoos all over the world. A national antivenin index is maintained by the Oklahoma Poison Information Center in cooperation with the Oklahoma City Zoo [(405) 427-6232 and (405) 424-3344], and telephone consultation service for physicians is also available at the Venom Poisoning Unit of the Los Angeles County/University of Southern California Medical Center.

Maintaining *respiration* by mechanical or other means is important. In patients bitten by elapid snakes, respiratory failure is usually reversible. *Tetanus toxoid* or *tetanus immune globulin* of human origin should be given. If wound infections appear, antibiotics should be used with the knowledge that the predominant microorganisms in the mouths of snakes are gram-negative pathogens. Treatment should be preceded by appropriate aerobic and anaerobic cultures. *Fasciotomy* may be necessary to prevent further ischemic injury to a massively swollen limb. *Surgical debridement* of vesicles and superficial necrotic tissue should be instituted near the end of the first week following the bite. *Relief of pain* with salicylates or meperidine, moderate sedation, maintenance of fluid balance, measures to combat shock and hemorrhagic diathesis, and appropriate management of coma or convulsions are all important.

The usefulness of corticosteroids to prevent tissue damage

or systemic intoxication has not been convincingly demonstrated. However, these drugs may be of value in the management of severe shock associated with envenomation and for allergic reactions following the administration of antivenin.

Prevention In snake-infested regions long trousers, high shoes, boots or leggings, and gloves should be worn. Most important of all is to look where one steps or reaches. A sharp knife or lancet, tourniquet, suction bulb, and antiseptic suffice for an emergency kit, and in inaccessible areas, antivenin should also be carried.

POISONOUS LIZARD BITE Of the nearly 3000 species of lizard in the world, only two are venomous: the Gila monster (*Heloderma suspectum*) of the arid southwestern United States and the closely related Mexican beaded lizard (*H. horridum*) which inhabits the lowland forests of western Mexico. These reptiles are not aggressive, and virtually every instance of their attacking a human has involved teasing or handling the animals in captivity. The venom is elaborated in eight glands in the floor of the mouth and secreted directly into the oral cavity, where it bathes the teeth, which are grooved posteriorly. The lizard clings tenaciously and is often dislodged only after considerable effort; envenomation occurs by contamination of the wound. The venom contains a potent neurotoxin which is undoubtedly responsible for its lethal effect on experimental animals. Death in humans following a bite is extremely rare. Most often, human envenomation results in tissue injury, excruciating pain, massive edema, and patchy erythema. Acute systemic symptoms may last for 3 to 4 days and include nausea, vomiting, hematemesis, blurred vision, dyspnea, dysphonia, and profound weakness. Intense hyperesthesia of the bitten extremity may persist for several weeks. There is no antivenin available. Treatment should consist of tourniquet, incision, suction, cooling of the bitten area, measures to prevent or combat infection, including tetanus, and supportive measures. Parenteral meperidine (Demerol) or infiltration of local anesthetic around the bite should be used to relieve pain.

SPIDER BITES The bite of many spiders is locally irritating, and several species can cause severe, even fatal systemic poisoning in humans. In North America, only two types of spiders are of medical importance: the widow spiders (*Latrodectus* species) and the recluse spiders (*Loxosceles* species).

Widow spider bite The most numerous and important of the venomous spiders are members of the genus *Latrodectus,* widely distributed throughout the world. In the United States and Canada, *L. mactans,* the black widow or show-button spider, causes a majority of clinically significant arachnidism. In Florida, *L. bishopi,* the red-legged widow spider, has been reported to produce human poisoning resembling mild black widow bite.

It is the female *L. mactans,* the black widow, that bites humans. She is glossy black with a body 1 cm in diameter, a leg span of 5 cm, and a characteristic red hourglass mark on her abdomen. She spins her web in woodpiles, sheds, basements, or outdoor privies, is very aggressive, and will bite on slight provocation. The venom produces diffuse central and peripheral nervous excitement, autonomic activity, muscle spasm, hypertension, and vasoconstriction.

In the United States, most black widow bites occur between April and October, and many patients are males bitten on the genitalia or buttocks while using a privy. After a momentary sharp pain at the site, there is cramping pain that begins locally within 15 to 60 min and gradually spreads. It may involve all extremities and the trunk. The abdomen is boardlike, and the waves of pain become excruciating, causing the patient to turn, toss, and cry out. Respirations are often labored and grunting. There are also nausea, vomiting, headache, sweating, salivation, hyperactive reflexes, twitching, tremor, paresthesias of the hands and feet, and occasionally, systolic hypertension. A mild polymorphonuclear leukocytosis is usual, and many patients have slight fever. After several hours, the pains subside, although mild recurrences for 2 or 3 days are common. It may be a week before well-being is restored. Deaths due to cardiac or respiratory failure have occurred, mostly in children and the aged.

Because the bite itself is not prominent, patients are often thought to have some abdominal catastrophe such as perforated ulcer, pancreatitis, or volvulus. Renal colic, coronary occlusion, tetanus, strychnine poisoning, tabetic crisis, lead colic, and porphyria are other conditions to be ruled out. The abdomen is not tender to palpation in arachnidism, and pains in the extremities are not typical of most of these other disorders.

Treatment For *Latrodectus* poisoning, treatment consists of measures to relieve pain and administration of antivenin. Initial treatment should include a hot tub bath which affords prompt, although temporary, relief. An ampul (10.0 ml) of 10% calcium gluconate injected intravenously usually produces dramatic, but transient, cessation of cramps. Opiates are sometimes necessary. When symptoms are severe or when the patient is a small child or is at special risk due to other associated medical problems, treatment with *Latrodectus* antivenin is indicated. An intravenous injection of 1 ampul (2.5 ml) is usually quite effective within a few hours and can be repeated if symptoms recur. Since the antivenin is prepared from horse serum, appropriate testing for hypersensitivity should be undertaken prior to its administration.

***Loxosceles* spider bite** During the past 25 years in the United States, there have been increasing numbers of reports of severe necrotizing bites due to *Loxosceles* spiders. Originally thought to be a problem only in the midwestern states and associated only with the brown recluse spider, necrotic arachnidism has now been seen in many of the southern and southwestern states as well as in southern California and has been attributed to at least six species of *Loxosceles* spider. The bite of these spiders may initially produce only a mild stinging discomfort. In severe bites, intense local pain appears within 2 to 8 h, accompanied by bullae formation and erythema at the site of the wound. Subsequently, ischemic necrosis occurs leaving a deep ulcer with a necrotic base. The pathogenetic mechanism for the local reaction is not completely understood but is thought to involve complement-activated tissue damage. Some patients also experience a systemic reaction characterized by fever, myalgias, and a morbilliform rash 24 to 48 h after the bite. Intravascular hemolysis is seen occasionally, and in severe cases hemoglobinuria and acute renal failure may occur. Fatalities have been reported, mostly in children.

Treatment depends upon the severity of the bite. If bullae formation, intense pain, and signs of ischemia do not appear within the first 6 to 8 h, the bite is probably not severe and treatment is unnecessary. When symptoms of more serious local reaction are present, the parenteral use of corticosteroids within the first 24 h following a bite has been advocated to prevent progression of the lesion, but convincing evidence that this is effective is lacking. Other therapeutic measures consist mainly of local wound care, timely surgical debridement, and treatment of secondary infection, if it occurs. The ulcer usually heals spontaneously, although skin grafting may be required on occasion. Renal failure should be treated as advised in Chap. 290.

SCORPION STING Scorpions are eight-legged arthropods. Glands in the terminal segment produce venom, which is injected into the victim by a stinger located on the tip of the tail. Scorpions often enter dwellings. During the day they retreat into crevices; emerging at night, they often get into shoes and clothing and even into bedding. They do not deliberately attack humans, but accidental contact results in a sting.

Of about 650 species, roughly 40 occur in the United States, distributed over three-fourths of the nation. They are most numerous in the south from Florida to California, but the only two lethal species, *Centruroides sculpturatus* and *C. gertschi,* are limited to Arizona and portions of neighboring states. These two species reach a maximal length of about 7 cm. Their sting may be fatal to young children or old people, but seldom to a healthy adult.

Most of the nonlethal species of scorpions in the United States cause only minor reactions, like a beesting. Some in the southwest, however, produce local edema and ecchymosis, with burning pain. In contrast, many species whose venom has potentially dangerous systemic effects, including the Arizona *Centruroides,* evoke little or no visible reaction at the site of the sting. There is an immediate burning sensation followed by local paresthesia ("pins and needles"), hyperesthesia, or numbness. These sensations spread to involve the whole extremity, and within an hour or two, malaise, restlessness, lacrimation, rhinorrhea, salivation, perspiration, nausea, and vomiting appear.

The patient passes from an agitated state with hyperactive reflexes into coma; convulsions follow. In addition to these neurotoxic symptoms, cardiovascular effects due to myocarditis may be seen and include various arrhythmias and intractable heart failure. Death usually occurs within 12 h, but sometimes as late as 2 days after the sting.

Treatment This consists of immediately placing a tourniquet on the extremity just proximal to the sting in order to delay the absorption of venom. If available, ice packs may be applied to the wound and to the affected limb, with care not to create additional tissue injury through freezing. The tourniquet must be removed in 5 to 10 min, but the limb is kept cool for at least 2 h. After this time, if treatment has been applied promptly, no serious effects are experienced following the sting of *C. sculpturatus* or *C. gertschi.* If the sting is on the head, trunk, or genitalia, of course, a tourniquet cannot be used, but the area may be cooled.

Although tourniquet, incision, and suction as in the treatment of snake bite have been recommended, the amount of venom is minute; it produces no local necrotizing effect and is absorbed very rapidly.

Specific antivenin, reconstituted from lyophilized cat serum, is available in some areas and should be employed if the victim develops signs of central nervous system or cardiac involvement. Supportive therapy is directed at combating shock and dehydration. Barbiturates in large doses are useful in reducing restlessness.

Prevention This depends upon alertness in avoiding contact with scorpions in infested areas. Clothing and shoes should be well shaken before being put on in the morning. Towels and bedclothes should be inspected. A house infested with scorpions can in time be rid of them by closing all obvious ways of ingress; picking up debris in the environment, such as piles of brush, logs, stones; introducing a mixture of fuel oil or kerosene, containing a small amount of creosote, between the earth and the house foundation; and spraying with a mixture of 2% chlordane, 10% DDT, and 0.2% pyrethrins in an oil base.

HYMENOPTERA STINGS Each year in the United States, nearly twice as many people die as a result of bites by hymenopterous insects (including bees, wasps, hornets, yellow jackets and fire ants) as from poisonous snake bites. Occasionally, multiple stings in enormous numbers (500 to 1000) are the cause of death. However, the majority of systemic reactions and deaths are due to allergic reactions to the venoms of these insects.

Hymenopteran venoms contain histamine, various kinins, and other vasoactive substances, phospholipases, and hyaluronidase. They are hemolytic and neurotoxic in addition to being effective hypersensitizing agents. The usual reaction to a single wasp sting or bee sting is sharp pain, local wheal and erythema, intense itching, and in loose tissues, such as the eyelid or genitalia, considerable edema which subsides in a few hours. Only in the rare case when a bee is swallowed or inhaled and edema of the laryngopharynx or glottis develops is there danger. A sting directly into a peripheral nerve can destroy its function for a time, much as does an injection of alcohol. Bell's palsy has followed a sting into the trunk of the facial nerve. Unusual reactions such as optic neuritis, generalized polyneuropathy, and myasthenia gravis may follow a sting. The etiology of these reactions is unknown.

In hypersensitive individuals, a single sting may produce serious anaphylaxis with urticaria, nausea, abdominal or uterine cramps, bronchospasm, massive edema of the face and glottis, dyspnea, cyanosis, hypotension, coma, and death. Sensitization is usually the result of previous stings although most fatalities have occurred in individuals who experienced no apparent allergic reaction to the earlier envenomation. Beekeepers who develop allergic rhinitis followed by asthma when near bees or objects that have been in contact with bees are likely to have serious reactions to stings. It has been estimated that nearly 1 percent of the general population in this country has hymenoptera allergy.

Many species of ant can produce stinging bites with local redness and swelling. The most notorious of these are the fire ants (*Solenopsis*), particularly two "imported" South American species (*S. invicta* and *S. richteri*) which were accidentally introduced into the United States in the 1930s. The *invicta* species is now found in more than 150 million acres of land in nine southeastern states and has largely supplanted all others, including several domestic species. In addition to being a major agricultural pest, fire ants, whose bites may result in extensive vesiculation and skin necrosis or cause serious hypersensitivity reactions, have become a significant health hazard to humans. Unlike other hymenopterous venoms, fire ant venom is mostly a simple insoluble alkaloid rather than a complex mixture of proteins. There is limited cross-sensitivity between it and the venoms of bees, wasps, hornets, and yellow jackets.

Treatment The wound site should be examined for a stinger which, if present, should be carefully removed in order to prevent further envenomation from the attached gland. The local reaction to the usual sting is treated by local cool application and antipruritic lotions or oral antihistamines. Fire ant stings, which are frequently multiple, should be thoroughly cleaned with soap and water. Secondary bacterial infection is common and should be anticipated and treated promptly. Epinephrine, 0.3 to 0.5 ml of a 1:1000 aqueous solution subcutaneously repeated every 20 to 30 min, may be lifesaving in patients with an anaphylactic reaction to a sting. A tourniquet to slow the absorption of venom and ice packs to relieve pain may be used. Oxygen, endotracheal intubation, vasopressors, and other supportive measures should be used as needed. In addition, corticosteroids should be employed in severe cases, although their maximum effect is not achieved until several hours after administration.

Prevention Allergic persons should make every effort to avoid contact with these insects, including wearing shoes when outside and not wearing perfumes or bright colors which may attract them. In addition, they should keep epinephrine readily available for immediate use in case of a sting, without waiting for symptoms to develop. Sting kits containing premeasured doses of 1:1000 epinephrine in disposable syringes, tourniquets, and antihistamine tablets are commercially available. Careful instruction in their use should be provided by the person's physician.

Immunotherapy Desensitization by injection of preparations containing venom of the specific insect has long been recommended for any patient who has had a systemic or generalized reaction to hymenopterous insect sting. To date, the only products available for this purpose have been extracts of the crushed whole bodies of the stinging insect. However, skin testing with whole-body extracts was frequently unreliable in identifying persons at risk for systemic reactions, and immunization with these materials did not increase IgG-blocking antibodies to venom proteins, a response felt to be essential for protection against insect allergy. In contrast, purified hymenopterous venoms, which were approved for clinical use in the United States in 1979, have proved to be highly accurate in the diagnosis of sting allergy by skin testing, consistently stimulate production of circulating venom-specific IgG antibodies, and provide much better protection than whole-body extracts. They have not been associated with a greater number of adverse reactions than treatment with whole-body extracts or with desensitization for pollinosis. These purified venom antigens are now the preferred materials for diagnosis and immunotherapy of high-risk patients.

TICK BITE Although ticks may be vectors for such serious diseases as Rocky Mountain spotted fever, Q fever, tularemia, borreliosis, human babesiosis, and Lyme disease, the local reaction to the bite of a tick may be nothing more than an itching papule which subsides within a few days unless there is secondary bacterial infection. However, incomplete removal of a tick, with retention of the mouthparts, may result in the local formation of a nodule which continues to grow and is sometimes annoyingly pruritic. The definitive treatment is surgical excision of the nodule. Histologically, the nodule is a granuloma, but the inflammatory response is sometimes so bizarre and changes in the overlying epithelium are so striking that, in the absence of a history of tick bite, a mistaken diagnosis of malignant tumor may be made.

Removal of a tick by gentle, steady traction is preferable to crushing. Application of a drop of oil, petrolatum, nail polish, or other organic solvent may facilitate removal without leaving embedded remnants. However, touching with a hot object such as a glowing cigarette should be discouraged because of the likelihood of injuring the host.

Tick paralysis A progressive, ascending, flaccid paralysis, acute ataxia, or a combination of both sometimes develops in humans and certain other mammals while a tick is engorging upon them. Human cases have most frequently been reported from the northwestern United States and western Canada, where the wood tick, *Dermacentor andersoni* Stiles, is responsible. The dog tick, *D. variabilis* Say, has been identified in a number of cases occurring in the southeastern states. *Amblyomma americanum,* the Lone Star tick, *A. maculatum,* the Gulf Coast tick, and *Ixodes scapularis,* the black-legged deer tick, have also been incriminated.

This disorder is caused by a neurotoxin secreted in the saliva of the engorging tick which acts upon spinal and bulbar nuclei, slowing motor nerve conduction without affecting neuromuscular transmission. The tick must feed for several days before symptoms develop.

Most human cases occur in children, generally in young girls. The tick is usually attached to the scalp and hidden by the hair, but may be found on any part of the body, especially the ear, axilla, groin, vulva, or popliteal region.

The patient may be irritable or restless for up to 24 h before frank motor involvement appears. Weakness usually is noted first in the distal muscles of the lower extremities, progressing over the next 24 to 48 h to flaccid paralysis, which may extend to involve the trunk, arms, neck, tongue, pharynx, and bulbar centers. Sensory changes are typically absent, and there is little or no fever unless a secondary infection is present. Results of routine laboratory tests including cerebrospinal fluid examination are normal. Nerve conduction studies may reveal decreased velocities and compound action potentials of nerves and their corresponding muscles.

Tick paralysis is apt to be confused with poliomyelitis, the more so because ticks are active in warm weather when poliomyelitis is most prevalent. Among other diseases which might be considered in differential diagnosis are diphtheritic polyneuropathy, transverse myelitis, the Guillain-Barré syndrome, myasthenia gravis, the Eaton-Lambert syndrome, and botulism.

Definitive treatment is removal of the tick, including any mouthparts retained in the skin. After this is done, there is striking improvement of motor function within a few hours and complete recovery within 48 h.

The patient should be observed until the recovery trend is established, because if other ticks or retained mouthparts have been overlooked, the paralysis may progress. When bulbar or respiratory paralysis is present, death may occur if the tick is not removed in time. The mortality rate is 10 percent; nearly all who die are children.

OTHER ARTHROPOD BITES **Flea bite** There are many fleas that attack humans, including *Pulex irritans* and chicken fleas. In sensitive individuals, the salivary secretion of these bloodsuckers produces large, itching papules. It is thought that much of the papular urticaria of children is probably due to flea bites. Treatment is symptomatic only. Elimination of fleas from the environment may be very difficult, but persistent treatment of animals and of premises with appropriate insecticides is usually successful.

Centipede bite Local irritation is the usual reaction to centipede venom, although extensive necrosis and systemic illness have followed severe poisoning by tropical species. Treatment is symptomatic.

Caterpillar sting Contact with hairy caterpillars of many species produces irritation of skin or mucous membranes. The type of venom involved is not known, but severe pain, erythema, urticaria, and even blister formation may come on rapidly after direct contact with caterpillars, after handling cocoons, or on being exposed to windblown fuzz. There are often a regional lymphangitis and transient eosinophilic leukocytosis. The discomfort subsides within 24 h, but local soaks, oral antihistaminics, and oral analgesics are often indicated. When pain is severe, treatment with 10% calcium gluconate, 10.0 ml given intravenously, usually achieves prompt relief of pain.

Bedbug bite Members of the genus *Cimex* inflict bites that leave reactions varying from a simple puncture to large urticarial lesions, apparently depending on the sensitivity of the bitten individual. There is no specific treatment.

Chiggers or redbugs These are tiny mites which are commonly found in foliage, grass, etc., in many parts of the world. In the United States, the larval form of *Eutrobicula alfreddugesi* attacks the skin by secreting a substance which digests tissue, creating a red papule that itches intensely. The tiny reddish larva can be seen in the center of the lesion. Treatment is palliative and consists of antipruritic applications. The use of insect repellents, appropriate protective clothing, and prompt bathing after exposure reduce the risk of infestation considerably.

Bloodsucking-fly bite Many species of flies, particularly the horsefly and the deerfly, viciously attack and feed upon warm-blooded animals, including humans. Occasionally, transmission of diseases such as anthrax, tularemia, loiasis, and trypanosomiasis has been attributed to horseflies and deerflies. More commonly in North America, however, their bites are responsible for painful, intensely pruritic cutaneous lesions which may be followed by delayed localized allergic reactions characterized by erythema, edema, and urticaria. Treatment should include thorough cleaning of the bite sites, topical corticosteroids, and oral antihistaminics for severe itching. Antibiotics may be necessary if the wounds become secondarily infected.

MARINE ANIMAL VENOM DISEASES The venoms of certain marine animals are known to cause illness in humans after injection or inoculation under naturally occurring conditions. Information concerning these toxins is limited; most appear to be composed of proteins and peptides as well as other substances that are pharmacologically active. Although probably less complex than the venoms of reptiles, many marine animal venoms are capable of causing several pathologic effects including neurotoxicity as well as local necrosis.

Portuguese man-of-war and jellyfish stings The burning discomfort induced by contact with sea nettles or jellyfish is familiar to most surf bathers. Contact with the tentacles of the colorful Portuguese man-of-war (*Physalia* species), which is found mainly in or near the Gulf of Mexico, or the more toxic jellyfish (*Chiropsalmus* of the Indian Ocean and *Rhizostoma* of the Atlantic) is followed by burning pain, swelling, and erythema. Severe, generalized muscular cramps, nausea, vomiting, and pulmonary edema may occur. Victims have died as a result of jellyfish stings, sometimes within minutes after contact. In nonfatal cases, systemic symptoms usually subside within several hours.

Treatment consists of removing any tentacles still clinging to the skin after first inactivating the toxins in their nematocysts with local application of alcohol, ammonia, or even dry sand. Analgesics should be used for pain control, and antihistaminics if there is an accompanying pruritic rash. Corticosteroids may be helpful in severe cases.

Sea anemone sting ("sponge diver's disease") Contact with certain sea anemones (especially *Sargatia elegans*) in Mediterranean and African waters produces extensive dermatitis with chronic ulceration. Occasionally, especially during August and September, systemic symptoms of headache, sneezing, nausea, chills, fever, and collapse are noted. Rare fatalities have occurred. No specific therapy is known; symptomatic treatment with topical steroids or oral antihistaminics may provide temporary relief.

Cone shell poisoning The colorful cone shells are highly prized by collectors. However, many species in the Pacific are venomous, a great danger to unwary hobbyists who pick them up. The poison, a neurotoxin, is delivered into a wound inflicted by pointed hollow teeth resembling darts in the long proboscis of the animal. Local manifestations include sudden intense pain, followed by swelling and numbness which may persist for several days. Symptoms of serious poisoning include muscular incoordination and weakness progressing to respiratory paralysis. Death may occur within 3 to 6 h, but recovery within 24 h is the rule. There is no specific therapy; recommended treatment is the use of tourniquet, incision, and suction (as for snake bite), and supportive measures which may include artificial respiration and administration of oxygen.

Sponge dermatitis Direct contact with several species of sponge results in a painful dermatitis, which may persist for several weeks. The lesions appear to be caused by mechanical irritation from the exoskeleton of the sponge as well as by toxins within its tissues. Delayed hypersensitivity reactions may also occur. Antihistaminics provide relief from the pruritus; dilute acetic acid ameliorates local pain strikingly, while alkali will intensify it. The lesions are self-limited.

Sea urchin sting Contact with the spines of some species of sea urchin results in painful erythema and ulceration, occasionally accompanied by neurotoxic symptoms of weakness and frank paralysis of lips, tongue, and face lasting for several hours. Treatment is purely symptomatic and supportive. The toxins isolated from sea urchins have produced paralysis in animals and are notably resistant to heat. Deaths from paralysis and drowning have been reported.

Paralytic and neurotoxic shellfish poisoning Certain dinoflagellates, which compose part of the marine phytoplankton, elaborate a potent neurotoxin. Occasionally, conditions in coastal waters become favorable for the growth of excessive numbers of these organisms, causing the water to develop an amber appearance termed the "red tide" and killing massive numbers of fish by exhausting their oxygen supply. When humans ingest shellfish which have themselves ingested toxic dinoflagellates, an illness occurs characterized by paresthesias of the face and extremities, dysphonia, and generalized muscular weakness, often accompanied by nausea, vomiting, and diarrhea and occasionally by paralysis and respiratory arrest. The more severe syndrome, known as paralytic shellfish poisoning, is encountered along the Pacific northwest and New England coasts. A milder form, not associated with paralysis in humans, is seen along the Gulf and Atlantic coasts of Florida. Treatment should include induced emesis and purgation to remove unabsorbed toxin from the gastointestinal tract and whatever additional supportive measures are necessary. Spontaneous recovery usually takes place within 24 h. There is a standardized mouse bioassay procedure for demonstrating and quantitating toxin in shellfish but no diagnostic test for detecting toxin in clinical specimens.

Venomous fish stings The dorsal fins or spines of bullhead sharks, dogfish, and ratfish and the dorsal and other fins of the lionfish, weeverfish, toadfish, and catfish are grooved, and at their bases are found venom glands. Injury by these spines results in severe pain and swelling and, in some instances, neurotoxic manifestations. Local necrosis with extensive tissue loss is a complication, particularly of lionfish and catfish stings, which may prolong convalescence. Little or nothing is known of the venoms involved. Tetanus toxoid or antitoxin should be given. Narcotics are often required to control the pain. Secondary pyogenic infection is a frequent complication.

Probably the most frequent type of venomous fish injury in the United States is that produced by the lashing tail of the stingray of the California coast (*Urobatis halleri*). The bony spine is encased in a sheath of epithelial cells containing venom which is expressed into the puncture wound. The wound may be several centimeters deep; portions of the bony spine may break off in it, or, more often, the integumentary sheath remains in the wound. The venom is a circulatory depressant in animals, but local injury predominates in humans. There are immediately severe pain and blanching followed by erythema and edema. Symptoms due to systemic absorption of venom are infrequent but may include salivation, muscle cramps and weakness, cardiac arrhythmias, seizures, and death. Treatment consists of application of a tourniquet (the vast majority of these injuries occur on the legs) and copious syringing of the wound with saltwater to remove fragments of sheath followed by immersion in water as hot as the patient can stand for 1 h. The venom is heat-labile, and extensive trials have indicated the usefulness of this last procedure. Tetanus toxoid or antitoxin is indicated; as with other fish stings, pyogenic infection is a frequent complication.

REFERENCES

Hymenoptera stings

HUNT KJ et al: A controlled trial of immunotherapy in insect hypersensitivity. N. Engl J Med 299:158, 1978

GOLDEN DBK et al: Regimens of hymenoptera venom immunotherapy. Ann Intern Med 92:620, 1980

——— et al: Treatment failures with whole-body extract therapy of insect sting allergy. JAMA 246:2460, 1981

LICHTENSTEIN LM et al: Insect allergy: The state of the art. J Allergy Clin Immunol 64:5, 1979

LIGHT WC et al: Unusual reactions following insect stings. J Allergy Clin Immunol 59:391, 1977

RHOADES RB et al: Hypersensitivity to the imported fire ant in Florida: Report of 104 cases. J Fl Med Assoc 64:247, 1977

Marine animal venoms

HALSTEAD BW: *Poisonous and Venomous Marine Animals of the World*, rev. ed. Princeton, N.J., Darwin Press, 1978

HUGHES JM, MERSON MH: Fish and shell fish poisoning. N Engl J Med 295:1117, 1976

SCOGGIN CH: Catfish stings. JAMA 231:176, 1975

STRAUSS MB, ORRIS WL: Injuries to divers by marine animals: A simplified approach to recognition and management. Mil Med 139:129, 1974

Other arthropod bites

FRAZIER CA: *Insect Allergy: Allergic and Toxic Reactions to Insects and Other Arthropods.* St. Louis, Grace, 1969

HANEVELD GT: Centipede bites. Br Med J 2:592, 1952

HILLIER FF, WARM RP: Caterpillar dermatitis. Br Med J 1:346, 1967

HUNT GR: Bites and stings of uncommon arthropods. Postgrad Med 70:91, 1981

Scorpion stings

BARTHOLOMEW C: Acute scorpion pancreatitis in Trinidad. Br Med J 1:666, 1970

HOREN WP: Insect and scorpion sting. JAMA 221:894, 1972

STAHNKE HL: Arizona's lethal scorpion. Ariz Med 29:490, 1972

Snake and lizard bites

MINTON SA JR: *Venom Diseases.* Springfield, Ill. Charles C Thomas, 1974

RUSSELL FE: *Snake Venom Poisoning.* Philadelphia, Lippincott, 1979

———: Snake venom poisoning in the United States. Ann Rev Med 31:247, 1980

SIMON TL, GRACE TG: Envenomation coagulopathy in wounds from pit vipers. N Engl J Med 305:443, 1981

STAHNKE HL et al: Bite of the Gila monster. Rocky Mount Med J 67:25, 1970

Treatment of snakebite in the USA. Med Lett 24:87, 1982

VISSER J, CHAPMAN DS: *Snake and Snakebite.* Capetown, Purnell, 1978

WATT CH JR: Poisonous snakebite treatment in the United States. JAMA 240:654, 1978

Spider bites

HOREN WP: Arachnidism in the United States. JAMA 185:839, 1963

HUNT GR: Bites and stings in uncommon arthropods. Postgrad Med 70:91, 1981

STOCHOSKY BA: Necrotic arachnidism. West J Med 131:143, 1979

Tick bite and tick paralysis

GOTHE R et al: The mechanisms of pathogenicity in the tick paralysis. J Med Entomol 16:357, 1979

SCHMITT N et al: Tick paralysis in British Columbia. Can Med Assoc J 100:417, 1969

SPIELMAN A: How to diagnose and treat tick and mite infestations. Drug Therapy 11:77, 1981

section 15 | Diseases of uncertain etiology

235 SARCOIDOSIS

RICHARD H. WINTERBAUER

DEFINITION Sarcoidosis is a multisystem granulomatous disorder of unknown etiology. The lungs and intrathoracic lymph glands are the most common sites of involvement, producing characteristic bilateral hilar lymphadenopathy and/or pulmonary parenchymal infiltrates on chest roentgenogram. The diagnosis is established by the presence of a compatible clinical illness, histologic demonstration of noncaseating epithelioid-cell granulomas, and, most importantly, a thorough evaluation designed to exclude infectious and neoplastic diseases capable of mimicking sarcoidosis. The clinical course in the majority of patients is benign, with spontaneous resolution within 2 years. However, approximately 10 percent of patients have a progressive syndrome proceeding from granulomatous inflammation to fibrosis.

PATHOLOGY Multiple noncaseating granulomas are the characteristic morphologic feature of sarcoidosis. The sarcoid granuloma consists of a tightly packed central follicle of epithelioid cells surrounded by a perimeter of lymphocytes and fibroblasts. The epithelioid cells are derived from blood monocytes and tissue macrophages. Multinucleated giant cells up to 150 μm in diameter are frequent within the granuloma. The giant cells are most commonly of the Langhans type, with multiple, peripherally located, irregular nuclei. There is no histologic specificity to the sarcoid granuloma. Identical lesions may occur in berylliosis, tuberculosis, leprosy, hypersensitivity pneumonitis, Crohn's disease, primary biliary cirrhosis, fungal disease, and local reactions which occur in lymph nodes that drain neoplastic or chronic inflammatory processes.

The lungs are the primary target of the disease and are involved histologically in all cases. Granulomas are always present in the alveolar septa and usually in the walls of bronchi. The walls of pulmonary arteries and veins are involved in almost one-third of patients. There is increasing evidence that the sarcoid granuloma is preceded by a nonspecific inflammation of the alveolus characterized by the presence of monocytes, macrophages, and lymphocytes. As the granuloma matures, the number of epithelioid cells increases, and inflammatory and immune-effector cells become fewer. In patients with extensive alveolitis, very few granulomas are present; in patients with the greatest density of granuloma, the alveolitis is minimal or absent. Sarcoid granulomas usually involve multiple organs (Table 235-1).

IMMUNOLOGY Although the initial stimulus for the development of sarcoid granulomas is unknown, understanding of the immune mechanisms responsible for their formation and perpetuation is growing (Fig. 235-1). The pulmonary parenchyma in sarcoidosis is rich in active T lymphocytes despite a peripheral T lymphocytopenia. The pulmonary parenchymal T lymphocytes elaborate a monocyte chemotactic factor that attracts blood monocytes. The monocyte changes to assume the appearance of an epithelial cell, developing an extensive rough endoplasmic reticulum, a large Golgi apparatus, and numerous cytoplasmic transport vesicles. These monocytes are in a state of activation with increased numbers of IgG-FC and C3 receptors. Lysozyme and angiotensin-converting enzyme content are also increased. The epithelioid metamorphosis and increased biologic activity are mediated by a second lymphokine called *monocyte activation factor.* The monocyte-macrophages are held at the site of inflammation by a third lymphokine, *macrophage migration inhibition factor.*

Most patients with sarcoidosis demonstrate cutaneous hyporeactivity to common antigens such as trichophyton, mumps virus, streptokinase, and streptodornase. The change in cutaneous reactivity appears soon after the onset of sarcoidosis and disappears as disease activity wanes. The abnormality of cell-mediated immunity is relative. Sarcoid patients with active tuberculosis, for instance, have the same frequency of tuberculin reactivity as do nonsarcoid patients with active tuberculosis. Cultures of circulating lymphocytes show a decreased level of lymphoblastic transformation and mitotic activity after stimulation by phytohemagglutinin M. This impaired response correlates inversely with both activity and extent of disease. The abnormalities of cell-mediated immunity demonstrated in sarcoidosis are not specific for this disease and play little or no role in diagnosis.

The number of B lymphocytes in the peripheral blood of patients with sarcoidosis is normal or high. Antibody production in sarcoidosis is well preserved and may, in certain instances, be hyperactive. Immunization with bacterial vaccines leads to expected levels of circulating antibody. Patients frequently have a polyclonal gammopathy. The serum IgE level may be elevated, and higher than normal antibody titers to common environmental antigens such as the Epstein-Barr virus and *Mycoplasma pneumoniae* are frequent. There is no evidence of an antecedent immunologic abnormality in patients who ultimately develop sarcoidosis. Increased circulating immune complexes have been demonstrated in some patients with sarcoidosis. There has been no demonstrable correlation between presence of immune complexes and stage of disease.

TABLE 235-1
Frequency of clinical involvement of extrapulmonary organs in sarcoidosis

Extrathoracic organs	%
Peripheral lymph nodes	73
Skin	32
Liver	21
Eye	21
Spleen	18
Bone	14
Salivary glands	6
Joints	6
Heart	5
Nervous system	5
Kidneys	4
Nose and mouth	3
Lacrimal glands	3
Skeletal muscle	1
Larynx	1
Stomach and intestine	1
Uterus	1

SOURCE: *From Mayock et al.*

FIGURE 235-1
A schematic representation of the formation and stabilization of a granulomatous inflammatory reaction. After exposure to specific antigens, activated T lymphocytes secrete lymphokines which attract blood monocytes to the site of reaction, activate, and then immobilize the monocyte-macrophage effector cells to form a granuloma. (From AP Fishman, Update I: Pulmonary Diseases and Disorders, New York, McGraw-Hill, 1982.)

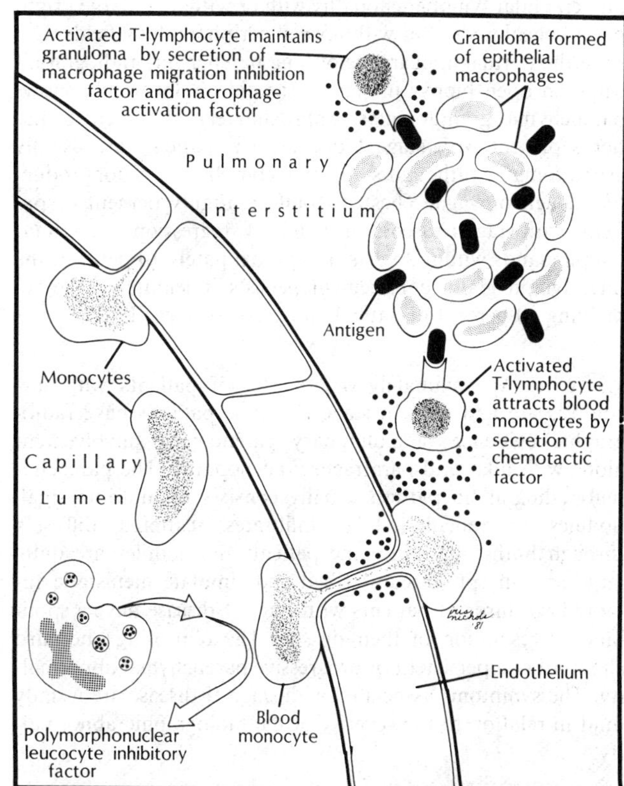

CLINICAL MANIFESTATIONS Sarcoidosis is worldwide in distribution. Women are slightly more often affected than men, and the disease is 10 to 20 times more prevalent among blacks than whites. The black patients in general have more severe disease with more frequent involvement of extrathoracic organs. Approximately two-thirds of patients are under 40 years of age at the time the disease begins.

Sarcoidosis may be either acute, subacute, or chronic in its presentation. An acute onset with erythema nodosum or acute polyarthritis developing in days to weeks is seen in 10 to 15 percent of patients. This presentation is particularly common among Caucasian women. The chest x-ray almost invariably shows bilateral hilar lymphadenopathy. The sudden onset of an infiltrating granulomatous skin rash may also be a presenting feature of acute sarcoidosis. Acute-onset sarcoidosis is usually a benign syndrome with a high incidence of spontaneous resolution.

Chronic and subacute sarcoidosis have been empirically defined as having a disease duration greater or less than 2 years, respectively. Subacute sarcoidosis is often asymptomatic and initially is recognized through periodic health screening or routine chest x-rays. These patients generally have few extrathoracic lesions and usually recover spontaneously. Patients with chronic sarcoidosis are usually older than 30 years and frequently show a progression to pulmonary fibrosis. Extrathoracic involvement is frequent, and most of the 4 percent mortality attributed to sarcoidosis is seen in patients with the chronic form of the disease.

Intrathoracic sarcoidosis Ninety percent of patients with sarcoidosis have roentgenographic evidence of thoracic involvement, either with enlarged intrathoracic lymph glands or parenchymal infiltrates. The current system of classification groups intrathoracic sarcoidosis into three radiographic stages which parallel the progression of the disease.

STAGE I The radiographic appearance of stage I disease is bilateral hilar lymphadenopathy with or without enlarged right paratracheal nodes but with normal peripheral lung fields. Despite the normal appearance of lung parenchyma radiographically, an open biopsy in stage I sarcoidosis invariably shows parenchymal granulomatas. Approximately 50 percent of patients present with stage I disease. The patients are usually asymptomatic, although some may complain of a nonproductive cough or vague chest discomfort. Eighty percent of patients with stage I sarcoidosis will show regression of the hilar lymph glands within 2 years. In approximately 10 percent, the hilar lymph gland enlargement persists indefinitely. The remaining 10 percent of patients progress to stage II.

STAGE II Approximately one-quarter of patients with sarcoidosis are first seen in stage II. These patients have radiographic evidence of pulmonary parenchymal involvement along with hilar and paratracheal adenopathy. The parenchymal radiographic pattern usually consists of multiple small nodules or reticulonodular infiltrates scattered diffusely through both lungs. In some patients the nodules are quite large and sharply circumscribed and simulate metastatic tumor. Two-thirds of patients with stage II disease have a spontaneous resolution of their disease. The remaining one-third show either a persistent or progressive parenchymal abnormality. The symptoms associated with stage II disease are usually mild in relation to the severity of the radiographic abnormality.

STAGE III Approximately 15 percent of patients will have stage III disease at the time of diagnosis. These patients have a diffuse parenchymal abnormality without hilar lymphadenopathy. The chest x-ray frequently suggests fibrosis with small lung volumes, elevated diaphragms, and honeycombing. Cough, dyspnea, and weight loss are common complaints. In the most severely affected, cor pulmonale and respiratory failure may ensue.

Extrathoracic sarcoidosis Approximately 40 percent of patients with sarcoidosis will present with extrapulmonary involvement (Table 235-1).

OCULAR INVOLVEMENT The lesions may be either acute or chronic and include iridocyclitis, chorioretinitis, keratoconjunctivitis, and conjunctival follicles. Patients with acute iritis occurring in association with erythema nodosum or hilar lymphadenopathy tend to have a benign self-limited course. However, patients with chronic uveitis frequently also have cutaneous granulomas, pulmonary fibrosis, and bone cysts. These patients frequently follow a prolonged, complicated course, and some will progress to blindness despite therapy.

PERIPHERAL LYMPHADENOPATHY The most common sites of involvement are cervical, supraclavicular, epitrochlear, axillary, inguinal, and pre- and postauricular nodes. The enlargement may be generalized or localized to a single region. These patients frequently present after accidental discovery of an enlarged gland. There are rarely any symptoms related to the lymphadenopathy. The glands may remain palpable for years and sometimes demonstrate a repetitive cycle of enlargement and regression.

SKIN Skin involvement can be subdivided into specific or nonspecific reactions. The specific lesions consist of noncaseating granulomas and are usually associated with chronic disease. The common nonspecific skin lesion is erythema nodosum. Granulomatous cutaneous lesions appear as discrete 3- to 6-mm-diameter epidermal papules with an erythematous or violaceous hue. A second variety is the deeper, larger plaque-like lesion which occupies the full thickness of the dermis. The most distinctive form of plaque-type sarcoidosis is *lupus pernio,* a disfiguring involvement of the nose, cheeks, or ears. The cutaneous granulomas of sarcoid often occur in scars or in areas of skin chronically damaged by infection, radiation, or mechanical trauma.

HEPATOSPLENOMEGALY The liver and spleen are palpably enlarged at some time in 20 percent of patients with sarcoidosis. Hepatic involvement is usually asymptomatic, and the scattered granulomas resolve leaving no residual. Liver function tests reveal a disproportionate elevation of the alkaline phosphatase with normal or minimally abnormal SGOT, SGPT, and bilirubin. Rarely, there is progressive hepatic dysfunction with jaundice, ascites, and esophageal varices. Enlargement of the spleen is usually asymptomatic. A few patients may have nonspecific abdominal discomfort due to splenic enlargement. There are rare instances of hypersplenism with anemia, leukopenia, and thrombocytopenia.

HEART The clinical manifestations are varied and include sudden death, congestive heart failure, recurrent pericardial effusion, papillary muscle dysfunction, and conduction disturbances. Many patients with cardiac sarcoidosis have little or no evidence of dysfunction in organs other than the heart. The elusive nature of the diagnosis is emphasized by the fact that one-quarter of people with sudden death due to sarcoid cardiomyopathy have no history of prior cardiac symptoms. The duration of symptoms is usually brief, less than 12 months, in patients who ultimately die of cardiac sarcoidosis.

MUSCULOSKELETAL AND JOINT INVOLVEMENT Sarcoidosis begins as an acute polyarthritis in 15 percent of patients. The arthritis typically involves the ankles, knees, wrists, and small joints of the hands. It is frequently associated with erythema nodosum and iridocyclitis. The syndrome usually resolves within 3 months, leaving no chronic deformity. Synovial granulomas have been demonstrated in rare patients with chronic periarticular swelling and tenderness.

Osseous involvement is seen only in chronic sarcoidosis. The lesions are usually asymptomatic and appear on x-ray as small, sharply circumscribed lytic areas. The small bones of the hands and feet are most commonly affected. Less frequently involved areas include the skull, vertebrae, and long bones. Associated infiltrative skin changes are common.

NEUROLOGIC INVOLVEMENT Central nervous system involvement usually occurs in the earlier phases of the disease, while peripheral nervous involvement is characteristically seen in the chronic stages. The cranial nerves, meninges, hypothalamus, and pituitary gland are the most frequently involved regions of the central nervous system. The facial nerve is most commonly affected, with the optic nerve second. The triad of facial palsy, parotid enlargement, and anterior uveitis is known as the *Heerfordt syndrome.* The innervation of the extraocular muscles is rarely involved. Cranial nerve involvement may be sudden in onset and often will show spontaneous resolution.

Encephalopathies due to space-occupying granulomata and granulomatous meningitis with increased intracranial pressure may occur. Focal signs are often absent. The lumbar puncture will demonstrate an increased protein and pleocytosis and, in rare instances, low glucose due to diffuse meningeal infiltration. Seizures occur in 5 to 15 percent of patients with neurologic sarcoidosis. These may be grand mal, focal, psychomotor, or myoclonic. Seizures are associated with a poor prognosis and a high mortality.

Peripheral nerve involvement may present as either mononeuritis or polyneuropathy. Mechanical destruction and segmental demyelination of nerves by granuloma have been demonstrated.

DIAGNOSIS The diagnosis of sarcoidosis requires a compatible clinical picture, the histologic finding of noncaseating epithelioid granulomas, and exclusion of other diseases capable of producing a similar histologic and/or clinical picture. Since the clinical picture is varied and the histology nonspecific, it is important to recognize that sarcoidosis is often a diagnosis of exclusion.

Forty percent of patients with sarcoidosis have distinctive bilateral hilar lymphadenopathy with or without right paratracheal adenopathy on chest x-ray, are asymptomatic, and have negative physical examinations. Such patients have an 80 percent chance of spontaneous resolution within 1 year and do not require specific treatment. This picture is quite specific, and some clinicians who are experienced in dealing with this disease feel that the diagnosis of sarcoidosis may be made without histologic support in these patients. Similarly, the clinical picture of bilateral hilar lymphadenopathy with erythema nodosum, uveitis, and/or arthritis is highly specific for sarcoidosis; again, some people working in the field do not seek tissue confirmation in these "characteristic" cases. On the other hand, a few patients with bilateral hilar adenopathy have subsequently been found to have diseases other than sarcoid. This observation has made some investigators want to biopsy the hilar (or other accessible) nodes on these patients. This controversy remains unresolved.

There are many possible sites for biopsy. Tissue is easily obtained from palpable lymph glands or cutaneous lesions. Random biopsy of the minor salivary glands of the lower lip is positive for granuloma in about 60 percent of patients. Percutaneous liver biopsy gives a 65 to 75 percent frequency of demonstration of granuloma. Transbronchial biopsy of the lung with fiberoptic bronchoscopy has been an effective and safe method for establishing the diagnosis. The accuracy of diagnosis varies with the stage of disease. Approximately 60 percent of patients with stage I sarcoidosis will show parenchymal granulomas on transbronchial biopsy. This figure rises to 80 to 85 percent in patients with stage II and III disease. In contrast, an open-lung biopsy will provide a 100 percent yield of granuloma, even in stage I disease. However, open-lung biopsy is very rarely required to diagnose sarcoidosis. In patients with negative transbronchial biopsy and no extrathoracic biopsy site clinically evident, mediastinoscopy is the procedure of choice. This has a yield of 85 to 90 percent. A reliable Kveim antigen may provide the diagnosis if the antigen is available.

Laboratory studies Hypercalcemia is found in 2 to 10 percent of patients with sarcoidosis. Calcium metabolism in the sarcoid patient is characterized by hypersensitivity to vitamin D with an enhanced intestinal absorption of calcium and hypercalciuria, which is twice as common as hypercalcemia. Vitamin D is converted by the liver to 25-hydroxyvitamin D, which, in turn, undergoes 1α-hydroxylation by the kidney to form 1α,25-dihydroxyvitamin D, the most active metabolite of the vitamin. Patients with sarcoidosis have an increased level of the active metabolite for any given dose of vitamin D. Experimental studies suggest that either abnormal renal production of 1α,25-dihydroxyvitamin D or its decreased degradation are important in the pathogenesis of the hypercalcemia of sarcoidosis. The hypercalcemia is readily reversed by prednisone through its ability to increase the conversion of 1α,25-dihydroxyvitamin D to a biologically inactive metabolite.

Serum angiotensin-converting enzyme (ACE) has been found elevated in 50 to 80 percent of patients with sarcoidosis. In general, the level is highest in untreated patients with active disease and falls toward normal during a spontaneous remission or coincident with corticosteroid therapy. The elevated serum ACE has been shown to come from epithelioid granulomas at multiple sites including lymph nodes, liver, skin lesions, and lung tissue. The secretion of ACE by epithelioid cells appears to be stimulated by active T lymphocytes at the periphery of the granulomas. There is an approximate 15 percent incidence of false-positive elevated ACE levels in patients with diseases mimicking sarcoidosis. Sarcoid granulomas actively take up gallium, and gallium scanning with accumulation of the marker in hilar lymph glands, lung parenchyma, and especially extrapulmonary sites such as the parotid and lacrimal glands has been combined with serum ACE for diagnosis. A positive gallium scan in patients with an elevated ACE has a diagnostic specificity for sarcoidosis of 99 percent.

Lysozyme is a weak proteolytic enzyme found in cells of the monocyte-macrophage system. Serum lysozyme levels reflect the total body pool of such cells. Elevation of the serum lysozyme is not specific for sarcoidosis and may be found in other granulomatous diseases such as tuberculosis, fungal infection, and Wegener's granulomatosis. Elevated lysozyme levels correlate best with extrapulmonary sarcoidosis, especially with splenic involvement. The levels may be used to monitor disease activity as they return to normal with corticosteroid therapy or spontaneous resolution of the disease.

Pulmonary function tests Pulmonary sarcoidosis commonly causes a reduction in vital capacity, reduced diffusing capacity, decreased pulmonary compliance, abnormal gas exchange, and, rarely, abnormal airway function characteristic of an obstructive pulmonary syndrome. The correlation between pulmonary function tests and the severity of roentgenographic abnormality or histologic change is poor. Thirty-five percent of patients with stage II or III sarcoidosis have a normal vital capacity, and approximately one-third have a normal diffusing capacity. There are no known pulmonary function criteria that allow prediction of the natural course of parenchymal sarcoidosis or its response to therapy. Moreover, there is no conclusive evidence that measurements of arterial blood gas tensions or pulmonary compliance add significantly to the sensitivity and specificity of the vital capacity and DLCO (carbon monoxide diffusing capacity) in the management of sarcoidosis. Pulmonary function data should be correlated with roentgenographic and symptomatic information to facilitate clinical decision making. The greatest clinical value of pulmonary function tests is to assess changes in disease severity during its course.

TREATMENT Common indications for corticosteroid therapy in sarcoidosis are (1) progressive pulmonary impairment or respiratory symptoms, (2) ocular involvement, (3) myocardial sarcoidosis, (4) central nervous system sarcoidosis, (5) disfiguring cutaneous lesions, and (6) persistent hypercalcemia or hypercalciuria with renal insufficiency.

The influence of corticosteroid therapy on the natural history of pulmonary sarcoidosis is not precisely defined. The disease is characterized by frequent spontaneous remissions. Therefore, distinguishing between therapeutic effect and the natural course of the disease is difficult. Patients with stage I sarcoidosis, erythema nodosum, and arthritis have an 80 percent or greater chance of spontaneous remission and should be treated symptomatically with anti-inflammatory agents such as aspirin or indomethacin; steroids are not indicated in stage I patients. Patients with stage II or III pulmonary disease present more difficult problems. Spontaneous clearing will be seen in half, but there is no method for predicting accurately the patient in whom the disease will progress or in whom it will improve spontaneously. The clinician must weigh the patient's symptoms, pulmonary function test results, and chest roentgenogram in assessing the need for therapy. Most would agree that patients with significant respiratory symptoms, abnormal pulmonary function tests, and diffuse abnormalities on chest x-ray should receive treatment. Corticosteroids appear to suppress granuloma formation and frequently result in symptomatic and roentgenographic improvement. Patients with stage II or III sarcoidosis who have no symptoms and minimal, if any, measurable abnormality of pulmonary function are managed best by careful follow-up at 2- to 3-month intervals. Treatment may be begun if symptoms, chest x-ray, or pulmonary function tests show evidence that the disease is progressing. There is no conclusive evidence that early treatment with corticosteroids reduces the chance of residual pulmonary dysfunction.

Prednisone is the most commonly used corticosteroid, and an initial dose of approximately 30 mg daily is adequate. Higher doses are rarely required. Symptomatic improvement is usually first evident in 1 to 2 weeks, with maximum improvement in 1 to 2 months. Corticosteroids should be continued for at least 6 to 12 months. Even with prolonged therapy, over half of patients will relapse when therapy is discontinued. Alternate-day therapy is very effective in maintaining improvement and helps to minimize the long-term side effects of corticosteroids. The effect of corticosteroids should be monitored closely through serial chest x-ray and pulmonary function tests. The improving patient frequently will show evidence of radiographic clearing. Seventy-five percent of patients with radiographic improvement will have a coincident increase in vital capacity, and approximately half will increase their diffusing capacity. Half of patients with radiographic stability during treatment will demonstrate an increase in vital capacity and 40 percent an increase in DLCO.

Patients with hypercalcemia usually can be managed by a low calcium diet and elimination of supplemental vitamin D. A few individuals will require corticosteroid therapy for hypercalcemia or hypercalciuria.

Local steroid therapy has been effective in ocular sarcoidosis characterized by anterior uveitis or iritis. Intradermal steroids have been used with some success for disfiguring cutaneous lesions. For chronic skin involvement of either the nodular or plaque-like variety, chloroquine 250 mg daily or hydroxychloroquine 200 mg daily may be useful. Patients must be followed with periodic ocular examinations to monitor the side effects of these drugs.

Despite corticosteroid therapy, the fatality rate of sarcoidosis is approximately 4 percent. Causes of death are respiratory failure, azotemia from renal damage caused by chronic hypercalciuria, myocardial sarcoidosis, and central nervous system involvement.

COMPLICATIONS The development of pulmonary tuberculosis in corticosteroid-treated sarcoid patients has become rare. Nor is there a recognizable increase in bacterial, invasive fungal, or viral infections in patients with sarcoidosis. *Aspergillus* mycetoma may complicate chronic sarcoidosis. Mycetoma formation is related to the presence of parenchymal cysts and is no more frequent among corticosteroid-treated than among untreated patients. Mycetoma may occasionally be responsible for life-threatening hemoptysis; however, bleeding from mycetoma, while often recurrent, is usually self-limited. The mycetoma is medically incurable. Surgical resection of these lesions is often dangerous because of technical difficulties related to resection of stiff, fibrotic lung tissue. Some also feel that there is a high incidence of recurrence in other areas of the lung. For these reasons and because mycetomas almost never progress to invasive aspergillosis, they are best handled medically.

REFERENCES

Bell NH et al: Evidence that increased circulating l-alpha, 25-dihydroxy vitamin D is the probable cause for abnormal calcium metabolism in sarcoidosis. J Clin Invest 64:218, 1979

Crystal RG et al: Pulmonary sarcoidosis: The disease characterized and perpetuated by active lung T-lymphocytes. Ann Intern Med 94:73, 1981

Delaney P: Neurologic manifestations in sarcoidosis: Review of the literature, with a report of 23 cases. Ann Intern Med 87:336, 1977

Fanberg BL: Drug therapy reviews: Treatment of sarcoidosis. Am J Hosp Pharm 36:351, 1979

Gilman MJ et al: Transbronchial lung biopsy in sarcoidosis: An approach to determine the optimal number of biopsies. Am Rev Resp Dis 122:721, 1980

Hanno R et al: Sarcoidosis: A disorder with prominent cutaneous features and their interrelationship with systemic disease. Med Clin North Am 64:847, 1980

Kaplan J et al: Mycetomas and pulmonary sarcoidosis: Nonsurgical management. Johns Hopkins Med J 145:157, 1979

Katz P et al: Serum angiotensin-converting enzyme and lysozyme in granulomatous diseases of unknown cause. Ann Intern Med 94:359, 1981

Lauttman RJ et al: Biopsy of minor salivary glands in the diagnosis of sarcoidosis. N Engl J Med 301:922, 1979

Mayock RL et al: Manifestations of sarcoidosis analysis of 145 patients with a review of nine series selected from the literature. Am J Med 35:67, 1963

NOSAL A et al: Angiotensin-1-converting enzyme in gallium scan in noninvasive evaluation of sarcoidosis. Ann Intern Med 90:328, 1979
OBENAUF CD et al: Sarcoidosis and its ophthalmic manifestations. Am J Ophthalmol 86:648, 1978
ONAL E et al: Nodular pulmonary sarcoidosis: Clinical, roentgenographic, and physiologic course in five patients. Chest 72:296, 1977
ROBERTS WC et al: Sarcoidosis of the heart: A clinical pathologic study of 35 necropsy patients (group 1) and review of 78 previously described necropsy patients (group 2). Am J Med 63:86, 1977
WINTERBAUER RH et al: A clinical interpretation of bilateral hilar adenopathy. Ann Intern Med 78:65, 1973
——— et al: The infectious complications of sarcoidosis: A current perspective. Arch Intern Med 136:1356, 1976
——— et al: The use of pulmonary function tests in the management of sarcoidosis. Chest 78:640, 1980

236 FAMILIAL MEDITERRANEAN FEVER (FAMILIAL PAROXYSMAL POLYSEROSITIS)

SHELDON M. WOLFF

DEFINITION Familial Mediterranean fever (FMF) is an inherited disorder of unknown etiology, characterized by recurrent episodes of fever, peritonitis, and/or pleuritis. Arthritis, skin lesions, and amyloidosis are seen in some patients.

TERMINOLOGY The variety of names given to FMF has led to confusion concerning its clinical features. None of the names, including FMF, is completely satisfactory. Such terms as *periodic disease, periodic peritonitis, la maladie periodique* are inaccurate because the disease often is not cyclical. *Benign paroxysmal peritonitis* is inappropriate because many of the patients have involvement of serosal surfaces other than the peritoneum, and some die of amyloidosis. *Familial paroxysmal polyserositis* is an acceptable alternative for the term *familial Mediterranean fever.*

ETHNOLOGY AND GENETICS FMF occurs predominantly in patients of non-Ashkenazi (Sephardic) Jewish, Armenian, and Arabic ancestry. However, the disease is not restricted to these groups, and has been seen in patients of Italian, Ashkenazi Jewish, and Anglo-Saxon descent as well as others.

The best studies of the genetics of FMF have been done in Israel, where the disease appears to be inherited as an autosomal recessive. Nevertheless, approximately 50 percent of patients give no family history of the disease. Consanguinity among the parents of FMF patients is as high as 20 percent, a figure which may be an underestimate because most patients came from very inbred ethnic groups. Approximately 60 percent of patients are male.

ETIOLOGY Although numerous pathogenetic mechanisms have been suggested, the etiology of FMF is unknown. Fever and inflammation are such prominent signs that frequent attempts have been made to implicate infectious agents and/or their products. However, extensive studies utilizing modern microbiological and serologic techniques have failed to implicate these or any other specific infectious agents.

It has been reported that FMF is due to an allergy or to hypersensitivity, but such hypersensitive states have not been substantiated. There is no firm evidence favoring an autoimmune etiology.

It has been suggested that FMF may be a pathological exaggeration of normal periodic temperature rhythmicity. However, extensive studies of temperature and other circadian rhythms in FMF patients have failed to demonstrate alterations from normal.

Because many FMF patients note that certain emotional or environmental changes may have profound effects on the frequency with which episodes of their disease occur, a psychosomatic basis has been suggested for the illness. There is no question that most patients eventually have transient or even permanent psychological alterations, which probably reflect their reaction to a chronic recurring illness that is forever threatening their social, economic, and personal well-being, but there is no evidence for a functional etiology for FMF.

The demonstration that FMF is inherited as an autosomal recessive disorder has led to the thesis that it is another inborn error of metabolism. Despite extensive studies, no such error has been found. Reported instances of excessive urinary excretion of porphyrins in FMF are probably examples of true porphyria and not FMF.

It has been reported that blood levels of unconjugated etiocholanolone were elevated during fever in six patients with FMF. Subsequent studies, however, showed no correlation between levels of etiocholanolone and fever.

PATHOLOGY Despite the striking clinical manifestations during an acute attack of FMF, no specific pathological alterations have been found. At laparotomy, only acute peritoneal inflammation in which the exudate contains a predominance of polymorphonuclear leukocytes is found to be present. A disproportionately large number of male patients develop gallbladder disease with and without cholelithiasis, but extensive histopathologic examination has failed to reveal any specific pathological changes. Pleural and joint inflammation are also nonspecific.

In the amyloidosis which accompanies FMF, amyloid is deposited in the intima and media of the arterioles, the subendothelial region of venules, the glomeruli, and the spleen. Aside from their vessels, the heart and liver are uninvolved.

MANIFESTATIONS In the majority of patients, the symptoms of FMF begin between the ages of 5 and 15, although attacks sometimes commence during infancy, and onset has occurred as late as age 52. The duration and frequency of attacks vary greatly in the same patient, and there is no set rhythm or periodicity to their occurrence. The usual acute episode lasts 24 to 48 h, but some may be prolonged for 7 to 10 days. The attacks range in frequency from twice weekly to once a year, but 2 to 4 weeks is the commonest interval. Spontaneous remissions lasting years have been seen. In the majority of cases, pregnancy is associated with an absence of acute episodes and many patients note less frequent attacks in the summer than in the winter. There may be a decrease in the severity and frequency of the attacks with age or with development of amyloidosis.

Fever Fever is a cardinal manifestation of FMF and is present during most but not all attacks. Rarely, fever may be present without serositis. The temperature may be preceded by a chill and will peak in 12 to 24 h. Defervescence is often accompanied by diaphoresis. The fever ranges from 38.5 to 40°C but is quite variable.

Abdominal pain Abdominal pain occurs in more than 95 percent of patients, and may vary in severity in the same patient. Minor premonitory discomfort may precede an acute episode by 24 to 48 h. The pain usually starts in one quadrant and then spreads to involve the whole abdomen. The initial site is usually very tender. Tenderness may remain localized with referred pain in other areas, and there may be radiation to the back. There may be splinting of the chest and pain in one or both shoulders, typical of diaphragmatic irritation. Nausea and vomiting sometimes occur. The abdomen is usually distended, and may become rigid with decreased or absent bowel sounds. On x-ray, the wall of the small intestine may appear edematous, transit of barium is slowed, and fluid levels may be seen. Because the manifestations of an acute abdominal attack can simulate those of a perforated viscus so closely, patients should be advised to have an elective appendectomy between attacks so that acute appendicitis will not obfuscate the picture at a later date. An abdominal operation may precipitate an acute attack of FMF which may be confused with other postoperative complications.

Chest pain Most patients with abdominal attacks have referred chest pain at one time or another, and 75 percent also develop acute pleuritic pain with or without abdominal symptoms. In 30 percent, the attacks of pleuritis precede the onset of abdominal attacks by varying periods of time, and a small number of patients never develop abdominal attacks. Chest pain is usually unilateral and is associated with diminished breath sounds, a friction rub, or a transient pleural effusion.

Joint pain In Israel, 75 percent of patients report at least one episode of acute arthritis. Arthritis can be distinct from abdominal or pleural attacks, can be acute or, rarely, chronic, and may involve one or several joints. Effusions are common and the large joints are involved most frequently. Radiologic findings are nonspecific. Despite careful search, frank arthritis rarely has been seen in the United States. Some patients have a history of rheumatic fever-like illness in childhood, but in a large series of patients, including 30 from the Middle East, acute arthritis was not observed. Mild arthralgia is common during acute attacks but is nonspecific.

Skin manifestations Skin involvement is reported by 25 to 35 percent of patients. These lesions consist of painful, erythematous areas of swelling from 5 to 20 cm in diameter, usually located on the lower legs, the medial malleolus, or the dorsum of the foot. They may occur without abdominal or pleural pain and subside within 24 to 48 h.

Other signs and symptoms Involvement of other serosal membranes has been reported, but pericarditis is rare, and it is probable that descriptions of recurrent meningitis have been diseases other than FMF. Hematuria, splenomegaly, and small white dots called *colloid bodies* in the ocular fundus are among the findings of questionable significance. Rarely migraine-like headaches accompany acute abdominal attacks, and some patients have become somewhat irrational or show extreme emotional lability during attacks. Whether these are primary manifestations of FMF or secondary effects of pain and fever is not known.

Complications The most serious complication of FMF in the United States is drug addiction or habituation, and obviously efforts should be made to avoid use of narcotics. Depression and lack of motivation are common, and patients with FMF require considerable encouragement and support. A striking number of patients in one American series have developed gallbladder disease.

Another major complication of FMF is *amyloidosis.* Some investigators believe that few patients in Israel escape this complication and that it is an expression of the same gene that is responsible for the other manifestations of FMF. If the attacks occur first, as they do in over 90 percent of the patients, the patients are classified as being of phenotype I. Amyloidosis also occurs in siblings of FMF patients or precedes the abdominal attacks (phenotype II). The infiltration by amyloid involves the kidneys, and death is often attributable to renal failure.

Amyloidosis has been reported in Israel and North Africa, but there have been only three reported instances of amyloidosis complicating FMF in the United States. These findings are even more striking because there are probably as many known FMF patients in the United States as in Israel. These differences are unexplained and suggest that environmental or nutritional, as well as genetic, factors may play a role in the development of amyloidosis in FMF.

LABORATORY FINDINGS There is no specific diagnostic test. Polymorphonuclear leukocytosis ranging from 15,000 to 30,000 cells per cubic millimeter is almost invariable during acute attacks. The erythrocyte sedimentation rate is elevated during attacks but returns to normal between attacks. Plasma fibrinogen, serum haptoglobin, ceruloplasmin, and C-reactive protein increase during the episodes. Plasma lipids are normal, and there are no consistent abnormalities of hepatic or renal function. When amyloidosis is present, laboratory findings are typical of a nephrotic syndrome followed by renal insufficiency. Electrocardiographic and electroencephalographic changes are inconstant and nonspecific.

DIAGNOSIS When the typical acute attacks of FMF occur in an individual of appropriate ethnic background who has a family history of FMF, the diagnosis is easy. When a patient is seen for the first time, a variety of other febrile illnesses must be excluded by appropriate study or observation. These include acute appendicitis, acute pancreatitis, porphyria, cholecystitis, intestinal obstruction, and other major abdominal catastrophes.

Some of the inherited forms of the hyperlipidemias may mimic the clinical picture of FMF, but measurement of serum cholesterol and triglycerides will eliminate them from consideration. The patient with FMF is not immune to the other diseases, and when an attack differs from the usual pattern or is more prolonged, consideration should be given to other diagnostic possibilities. The pleural form of the disease is sometimes difficult to differentiate from acute pulmonary infection or infarction, but the rapid disappearance of signs and symptoms resolves the problem. The joint manifestations may be more prolonged than other forms of FMF, and differentiation from septic arthritis, gout, and acute rheumatoid disease may be necessary. The erythema is sometimes difficult to differentiate from superficial thrombophlebitis or cellulitis.

Whether or not the patient is of the appropriate ethnic group, the most difficult diagnostic problem in FMF is the patient who presents with fever alone. In this situation, an extensive diagnostic workup for fever of unknown origin may be required. Fortunately, such patients are rare, and all eventually develop serosal involvement. Until specific diagnostic tests for FMF are available, patients with recurrent fever but without signs of inflammation of one of the serosal membranes should not be categorized as having FMF.

PROGNOSIS Despite the severity of the symptoms during some acute attacks, most patients are remarkably free of any debilitation during the intervals between attacks. With encouragement and an understanding of their disease, most FMF patients lead fairly normal lives. The greatest hazard to patients is prolonged periods of hospitalization due to erroneous diagnoses or failure to understand the disease. In the United States, the prognosis of patients with FMF does not seem to be different from that of patients with other chronic nonfatal illnesses. Death usually results from causes unrelated to the underlying disease.

The complication of amyloidosis in Israel, parts of north Africa, Turkey, and other parts of the Middle East makes the prognosis quite different from that in America. Approximately 25 percent of FMF patients in Israel are known to have amyloidosis, and this complication usually leads to death. Because a majority of patients under observation in Israel are under 40 years of age, it has been suggested that fatal amyloidosis may eventually occur in nearly all patients.

TREATMENT Among the therapies tried have been antibiotics, hormones (including estrogens and adrenal corticosteroids), antipyretic drugs, immunotherapy, psychotherapy, elimination and low-fat diets, chloroquine, and phenylbutazone. When carefully studied and followed up, none of these therapies proved effective.

During the past 10 years, the outlook of patients with FMF has been altered dramatically. Goldfinger reported in 1972 that the prophylactic use of colchicine in five patients dramatically reduced the number of attacks. Subsequently, controlled trials in the United States and Israel have shown that chronic administration of colchicine will greatly reduce the number of acute attacks of FMF. It is recommended that 0.6 mg colchicine be taken by mouth three times a day. Patients often develop gastrointestinal side effects with this dose, however, in which case the dose should be reduced to 0.6 mg taken twice a day. Although an occasional patient will respond to 0.6 mg taken only once a day, this amount is less likely to be beneficial. Most but not all FMF patients will respond favorably to colchicine prophylaxis.

Since colchicine is known to result in nondisjunction of chromosomes and in azospermia in some patients, it should not be given to any patient, especially a young one, unless the disease is severe enough to warrant taking the risk. In some patients, intermittent therapy may be beneficial. The patient should take 0.6 mg colchicine by mouth every hour for 4 h, then every 2 h for 4 h, and every 12 h thereafter for 48 h. The colchicine should be given at the first premonitory sign of an attack. If both acute and prophylactic colchicine therapy fail, supportive therapy is all that can be offered. Except for unusual circumstances, narcotics should not be given to FMF patients.

The mechanism of colchicine's action against acute attacks of FMF is unknown. It is postulated that it may work by preventing the normal cellular response to inflammation. Although preliminary, there are suggestions that as colchicine therapy becomes more widespread, the incidence of amyloidosis is decreasing.

REFERENCES

DINARELLO CA et al: Colchicine therapy for familial Mediterranean fever. A double-blind trial. N Engl J Med 291:934, 1974

——— et al: Effect of prophylactic colchicine therapy on leukocyte function in patients with Familial Mediterranean Fever. Arthritis Rheum 19:618, 1976

SCHWABE AD, PETERS RS: Familial Mediterranean fever in Armenians. Analysis of 100 cases. Medicine 53:453, 1974

WRIGHT DG et al: Efficiency of intermittent colchicine therapy in Familial Mediterranean Fever. Ann Intern Med 86:162, 1977

237 WEGENER'S GRANULOMATOSIS AND MIDLINE GRANULOMA

SHELDON M. WOLFF

WEGENER'S GRANULOMATOSIS

DEFINITION Wegener's granulomatosis is characterized by necrotizing vasculitis and granulomatous inflammation which affect primarily the upper and/or lower respiratory tract and the kidneys. However, small vessels anywhere can be involved. Rarely is the disease restricted to the respiratory tract (localized Wegener's granulomatosis). In the vast majority of cases the kidneys are involved and such patients have generalized Wegener's granulomatosis.

ETIOLOGY The cause of Wegener's granulomatosis is unknown, but most studies suggest a hypersensitivity reaction. The vasculitis, glomerulonephritis, the occasional ultrastructural findings of subepithelial glomerular deposits which look like immune complex deposition, and the reported presence of immune complexes in the serums of a few patients strongly implicate immune complex formation as the basis for the pathogenesis of this disease. On the other hand, the granulomas seen in many tissues suggest that cellular immune responses may also be involved. The antigen initiating the response(s) is unknown but may be microbial or tissue in origin and probably has as its site of origin the respiratory tract.

PATHOLOGY In order to make the diagnosis of Wegener's granulomatosis, both granulomas and necrotizing vasculitis must be demonstrated. These lesions can occur anywhere but are most commonly found in the sinus mucosa, lungs, and skin. The necrotizing vasculitis and granulomatous inflammation are in and of themselves not distinctive, but the demonstration of both is required. In the kidney the most common lesion is a focal and segmental glomerulonephritis, although on occasion frank vasculitis or even a granuloma may be observed.

CLINICAL FEATURES Wegener's granulomatosis has been reported as early as the first and as late as the eighth decade of life, but the mean age of onset is approximately 40 years. The disease occurs twice as often in males as in females. The initial signs or symptoms can occur anywhere but usually are seen in the upper or lower respiratory tract. For example, patients may have headache, sinusitis, rhinorrhea, and otitis media with or without hearing loss. Other prominent presenting symptoms can include fever, arthralgias, and anorexia. Cough, pain in the chest, and hemoptysis may predominate in some patients. Associated with the respiratory findings may be signs or symptoms of any of the organ systems involved, and these can include all organ systems. It is rare for a patient to present initially with signs or symptoms of renal failure.

In most patients Wegener's granulomatosis is a generalized disease associated with involvement of multiple organ systems, often with manifestations of acute inflammation. The respiratory tract (upper, lower, or both) is involved in all patients. The sinuses are affected in over 90 percent of patients. Saddle-nose deformities are common, as is mucosal ulceration, but mutilation does not occur. Very often the sinuses become secondarily infected with bacteria, and such infections require aggressive antibiotic therapy and often surgical intervention. Radiographs demonstrate the sinus involvement. The pulmonary manifestations are varied. Signs and symptoms suggestive of a pneumonitis may occur. Pleuritic manifestations are sometimes seen. Occasionally massive hemoptysis or pneumothorax develops. The typical x-ray features are those of nodular and cavitary infiltrates. These lesions can be evanescent and spontaneously disappear even without therapy. Lung biopsy is commonly performed in these patients and often leads to the diagnosis.

Renal involvement is present in over 90 percent of patients with Wegener's granulomatosis and is a prerequisite for a diagnosis of the generalized form of the disease. Prior to the availability of effective therapy, the mean survival of patients with renal involvement was 5 months. The urinary findings are consistent with acute glomerulonephritis, and an active sediment is common. About one-half the patients have glomerulonephritis, and on biopsy a focal glomerulitis is seen. Others also have a picture compatible with the nephrotic syndrome. Approximately 10 percent of patients have rapidly progressive glomerulonephritis and on biopsy have necrotizing and proliferative glomerulonephritis and marked crescent formation. Such patients should be treated as medical emergencies. Deposition of immunoglobulins and possible immune complex deposits have been noted in some patients.

Approximately 50 percent of patients with Wegener's granulomatosis have involvement of the eyes. Iritis, scleritis, and conjunctivitis are common. Proptosis due to retrobulbar granulomatous inflammation is occasionally seen. About one-third of patients have cardiac involvement, ranging from coronary arteritis to pericarditis. In approximately one-quarter of the patients the nervous system is involved. Most commonly, patients have mononeuritis multiplex while others have cranial neuritis.

In addition to serous otitis media, hearing loss is common in Wegener's granulomatosis. Almost one-half of patients have dermatologic manifestations including petechiae, vesicles, and necrotic ulcerations. Although frank arthritis is uncommon, about two-thirds of patients have arthralgias.

LABORATORY FINDINGS There are no specific laboratory abnormalities in Wegener's granulomatosis. A normochromic, normocytic anemia is sometimes present. Leukocytosis is present in some patients but is usually seen when a superimposed bacterial infection has occurred. Thrombocytosis is seen in approximately 10 percent of patients with the generalized form of the disease. The sedimentation rate is increased in almost all patients with active disease and is the most useful parameter with which to follow therapeutic efficacy. About 50 percent of patients have a positive test for rheumatoid factor, and many patients have hyperglobulinemia, particularly IgA. When renal involvement occurs, there are changes in the urine consistent with an active glomerulonephritis, and as the disease progresses, renal insufficiency is reflected in the usual laboratory abnormalities of uremia.

DIFFERENTIAL DIAGNOSIS The diagnosis of Wegener's granulomatosis is made when histological evidence of vasculitis and granulomatous inflammation is present. Vasculitic diseases such as polyarteritis nodosa do not have granulomatous inflammation as a histological hallmark. Conversely, granulomatous diseases such as tuberculosis and sarcoidosis do not show histological evidence of vasculitis. Certain diseases do present problems in differentiation from Wegener's granulomatosis. Occasional patients with Wegener's granulomatosis will present with hemoptysis, pulmonary hemorrhage, and rapidly progressive renal failure, and a clinical diagnosis of Goodpasture's syndrome is suspected. However, appropriate biopsies and immunofluorescent studies should differentiate these two conditions. Midline granuloma is restricted to the head and neck and is not associated with vasculitis. Lymphomatoid granulomatosis can present with a clinical picture indistinguishable from Wegener's granulomatosis. However, biopsy of involved organs (e.g., lung, skin) should demonstrate the characteristic cellular infiltrates. Occasional malignant tumors, particularly malignant lymphomas, will result in granulomatous inflammation and even vasculitis, but histological demonstration of the malignant cells leads to differentiation from Wegener's granulomatosis.

TREATMENT The use of cytotoxic agents in Wegener's granulomatosis has resulted in one of the most striking examples of the way modern chemotherapeutic intervention can alter the course of a hitherto lethal illness. Properly treated, over 95 percent of patients will go into remission, and since some remissions have lasted up to 15 years, it is not inappropriate to talk of cures in this disease.

The treatment of choice is cyclophosphamide, although in many cases azathioprine is equally as effective. Other alkylating agents, such as chlorambucil, may be used. In those patients where the disease is progressing rapidly, intravenous cyclophosphamide therapy may be used, but in general the oral route is preferred. Therapy ordinarily begins with 2 mg/kg cyclophosphamide daily, and this dose is adjusted according to the peripheral white blood cell count. Generally, the dose will decrease with time owing to depression of the white blood cell count. Treatment should be carried on for 1 year after the patient goes into remission. Relapses occur occasionally and should be treated like the initial event. In patients with irreversible renal failure, dialysis may have to be employed, but renal transplantation should be considered in such patients as well. Adrenal corticosteroids are often used as adjunctive therapy in patients whose disease shows active inflammation. The steroid regimen of these patients should be converted to an alternate-day schedule as early as possible.

MIDLINE GRANULOMA

DEFINITION Midline granuloma is an uncommon disease characterized by localized inflammation, destruction, and often mutilation of the tissues of the upper respiratory tract and face. This condition has also been referred to as *lethal midline granuloma, malignant granuloma,* and *granuloma gangrenescens,* none of which is an appropriate term.

ETIOLOGY The etiology of midline granuloma is unknown. In view of the intense granulomatous inflammation, the disease is thought to represent a localized hypersensitivity reaction which leads to tissue destruction and mutilation. However, the responsible antigen(s) is unknown, and there is no immunologic evidence supporting this hypothesis. A variety of microorganisms have been considered as possible causative agents, but detailed microbiologic investigations have failed to detect the consistent presence of pathogenic organisms. In view of the clinical and pathological features of the illness as well as the fact that some upper-airway tumors can elicit a similar intense inflammatory response, some authors have suggested a neoplastic basis for midline granuloma. However, when malignant tissue (usually of a lymphomatous nature) is found in the lesions, the diagnosis of midline granuloma is no longer tenable.

PATHOLOGY The most characteristic pathological finding is acute or chronic inflammation with necrosis. Superimposed pyogenic infection of the involved tissues, including the sinuses, may contribute to nonspecific histological findings. The pathological hallmark, noncaseating granulomas, with or without giant cells, may be obscured by the inflammatory reaction, but when present are strong evidence in favor of the diagnosis. Primary vasculitis is seen rarely, and when it occurs, a search for other causes, most notably Wegener's granulomatosis, should be made. The presence of malignant cells makes the diagnosis of midline granuloma unacceptable. Until an etiology is established, the diagnosis of midline granuloma will rest on the characteristic clinical features outlined below.

CLINICAL FEATURES The disease may occur at any age, but the majority of patients are in the fifth and sixth decades. It is more common in women than men and has been reported in all races. Many patients report recurrent "sinus" problems, and some have histories of allergic rhinitis, although the significance of these features is unknown.

The major symptoms are usually related to the nose. Patients frequently complain of nasal stuffiness and occasionally of discharge. The first symptom in a smaller percentage of patients relates to ulceration of the mucosa of the nose, the buccal mucosa, or the gums. This has led to loosening of the teeth, and dentists are often first consulted by these patients. Rarely, patients will present first with eye findings related to conjunctival inflammation or even ulceration. Although the progression of symptoms in some patients may be slow, all too often the disease steadily, and sometimes rapidly, progresses. The characteristic symptoms of nasal discharge, difficulty in breathing through the nose, and pain over the sinuses, nose, or eye become more prominent with time. Once ulceration begins, the disease often progresses rapidly. The ulcers frequently involve the nasal septum and will lead to the characteristic septal perforation and a saddlenose deformity. The majority of patients develop ulceration and eventually perforations of the soft and hard palates. Untreated, the disease can lead to massive destruction and mutilation of the tissues involved, including the skin of the face and the eyes. Frequently, the necrotic tissue becomes infected, and systemic symptoms such as fever and anorexia appear. The destructive lesions can become very malodorous. The disease extends to involve local tissues and does not progress below the neck; if this happens, other diseases should be considered. As the necrotic process progresses and involves vital organs, patients may lose sight in the affected eye, experience dysphagia, and have difficulty in speech. Although spontaneous temporary remissions have been reported, untreated midline granuloma is fatal. The progression of the disease can be rapidly accelerated by surgical procedures in the affected areas. The patient usually dies from secondary infection, although erosion by the process into a major blood vessel or penetration into the central nervous system with superimposed meningitis can also cause death.

Aside from the granulomatous inflammation, necrosis, and destruction, no other specific clinical or pathological findings are associated with midline granuloma. Occasionally, with superimposed infection, local lymphadenopathy may be noted, but it is not characteristic of the disease per se.

LABORATORY FINDINGS With progression of the disease, a variety of nonspecific abnormalities may be noted. These changes are characteristic of inflammatory processes in general or of secondary infections. For example, mild anemia, leukocytosis, elevated sedimentation rate, and hyperglobulinemia are common in these patients. Radiographic examination reveals pansinusitis, and as the disease advances, destruction of bone in the involved areas is characteristic.

DIFFERENTIAL DIAGNOSIS The diagnosis of midline granuloma is made by finding the characteristic histological lesions in biopsies of the affected tissues. When the specimens show only inflammatory tissue, a presumptive diagnosis of midline granuloma can be made only when the characteristic clinical picture is present and other diseases with similar presentation have been excluded. The diagnosis of Wegener's granulomatosis is ruled out by the absence of vasculitis in the biopsy specimens and the localized nature of midline granuloma (i.e., no pulmonary or renal involvement). In addition, Wegener's granulomatosis rarely, if ever, causes erosion through facial tissues. It is often difficult to differentiate true midline granuloma from neoplasms of the upper airways such as malignant reticulosis and certain lymphomas. These may be clinically similar to midline granuloma and are often associated with granulomatous inflammation. Careful examination of generous biopsy material as well as concomitant workup for disseminated neoplasm often provides the clinicopathological distinction. Other diseases to be excluded by appropriate laboratory techniques are histoplasmosis, blastomycosis, coccidioidomycosis, leprosy, tuberculosis, syphilis, mucocutaneous leishmaniasis, rhinoscleroma, and pseudotumor of the orbit.

TREATMENT The complications of midline granuloma such as superimposed infections can be treated specifically. Although adrenal corticosteroids are often used in the therapy of midline granuloma, they are of no value and probably are contraindicated if infection is present. Sporadic reports of therapy with cytotoxic agents are difficult to interpret, since some of the patients reported clearly had lymphoma or Wegener's granulomatosis, diseases where such agents are of definite value. Surgical removal of the involved tissue has been attempted but is useless and may, in fact, cause rapid progression of the disease.

The treatment of choice is radiotherapy to the local lesion. Although low dosages [10,000 mGy (1000 rads) and below] have been reported to be effective, many patients relapse after such therapy. Radiotherapy should be given in a dose of 50,000 mGy (5000 rads) to the involved areas. Where such a regimen is employed, long-lasting (more than 15 years) remissions and possible cures have been achieved. Following irradiation and after an appropriate period to allow for tissue healing (usually 1 year), reconstructive and plastic surgery, which may be of enormous cosmetic and functional value, can be undertaken.

REFERENCES

Midline granuloma

Fauci AS et al: Radiation therapy of midline granuloma. Ann Intern Med 84:140, 1976

Fechner RE, Lamppin DW: Midline malignant reticulosis. Arch Otolaryngol 95:467, 1972

Wegener's granulomatosis

Fauci AS et al: Wegener's granulomatosis: Studies in eight patients and a review of the literature. Medicine 52:535, 1973

——— et al: Wegener's granulomatosis and related diseases. Dis Mon 23:7, 1977

Wolff SM et al: Wegener's granulomatosis. Ann Intern Med 81:513, 1974

Harrison's

PRINCIPLES OF INTERNAL MEDICINE

Tenth Edition

Harrison's
PRINCIPLES OF INTERNAL MEDICINE

VOLUME 2

PART FIVE
DISEASES DUE TO ENVIRONMENTAL HAZARDS AND PHYSICAL AND CHEMICAL AGENTS

PART SIX
DISEASES OF THE ORGAN SYSTEMS

PART FIVE | DISEASES DUE TO ENVIRONMENTAL HAZARDS AND PHYSICAL AND CHEMICAL AGENTS

238 POISONING AND ITS MANAGEMENT

PAUL A. FRIEDMAN

GENERAL PRINCIPLES

Poisoning by chemical agents is a common and serious medical problem. In the United States accidental poisonings cause about 5000 deaths each year. Suicides by chemical agents annually number more than 6000. Malicious poisoning has become less common since the development of scientific toxicology, but toxic chemicals administered by homicides and abortionists are responsible for more deaths than is generally appreciated. In addition to fatal poisonings there is a much greater number of persons who are made seriously ill by chemical agents but recover after appropriate therapy. Unfortunately, some such victims are left with permanent sequelae of their intoxication. Finally, chemical agents impair the health of very many people by mechanisms not generally thought of as intoxications. Chemical carcinogenesis and mutagenesis, chronic alcoholic liver disease, allergic reactions, and chemical addiction and withdrawal syndromes are the most important examples.

Accidental poisonings may occur in the home or through industrial exposure. The former are far more frequent and usually acute; industrial intoxication is more often the result of chronic exposure. Accidental poisoning results most commonly from ingestion of toxic substances and involves children in the majority of cases. Each year 1 to 2 million American children accidentally swallow toxic materials, and approximately 1 ingestion in 1000 is fatal. Medicines are involved in 50 percent of all ingestions. Cleaning and polishing agents are ingested by 15 percent, while cosmetics, pesticides, petroleum products, and turpentine paints account for 20 percent.

The frequency of accidental poisonings reflects the enormous number of toxic substances found in the American home. Many such accidents could be avoided by simple preventive measures. Physicians can play an effective role in safety education. All toxic substances must be kept out of the reach of small children. Household chemicals and medicines should be kept in the original containers, and all such containers should be labeled. Before taking or administering any medicine, one should check the label carefully.

Despite all precautions, accidental, suicidal, and criminal poisonings will remain an important problem which every physician must be prepared to treat promptly and effectively. Besides their immediate therapeutic responsibilities, physicians have legal obligations in cases of attempted suicide, homicide, criminal abortion, and industrial exposure. The physician should also obtain psychiatric care for any patient who has attempted suicide by poison.

DIAGNOSIS OF CHEMICAL POISONING

Optimal management of the poisoned patient requires a correct diagnosis. Unfortunately, in many such patients poisoning is not considered as a possible cause of the clinical picture. The patient may be unaware of exposure to poison or, as after attempted suicide or abortion, may be unwilling to admit it. Although the toxic effects of some chemical substances are quite characteristic, most poisoning syndromes can simulate other diseases.

Poisoning usually is included in the differential diagnosis of coma, convulsions, acute psychosis, acute hepatic or renal insufficiency, and bone marrow depression. It may not be considered when the major manifestation is a mild psychiatric disturbance or neurological disorder, abdominal pain, bleeding, fever, hypotension, pulmonary congestion, or skin eruption. Chronic, insidious intoxications are more frequent than acute poisonings whose symptoms appear suddenly and may be related immediately to a specific event. Physicians always should remember the variegated manifestations of poisoning and maintain a high index of suspicion.

In every case of poisoning, identification of the toxic agent should be attempted. Specific antidotal therapy is obviously impossible without such identification. In cases of homicide, suicide, or criminal abortion the identity of the poison may be of legal importance. When poisoning results from industrial exposure or therapeutic mishap, accurate knowledge of the responsible agents is essential for future prevention.

In acute accidental poisoning the offending substance may be known to the patient. In many other cases information can be obtained from relatives or acquaintances, by a search for containers at the scene of the poisoning, or by questioning the patient's physician or pharmacist. Frequently such procedures yield only the trade name of a product, which gives no clue to its component chemicals. A number of books which identify the active ingredients of household products, agricultural compounds, proprietary medicines, and poisonous plants are listed in the references to this chapter. A small handbook of this type should be carried in every physician's bag. Poison control centers and manufacturers' representatives are other useful sources of such information. When poisoning is chronic, rapid identification of the toxic agent from the history is often impossible. The lesser therapeutic urgency of such cases usually permits the required painstaking exploration of the patient's habits and environment.

Some poisons can produce clinical features characteristic enough to strongly suggest the diagnosis. Careful examination of the patient may reveal the unmistakable odor of cyanide; the cherry-colored flush of carboxyhemoglobin in skin and mucous membranes; the pupillary constriction, salivation, and gastrointestinal hyperactivity produced by cholinesterase-inhibitor insecticides; or the lead line and extensor paralyses of chronic lead poisoning. Unfortunately, these features are not always present, and in any case telltales are the exception in chemical poisonings.

Chemical analysis of body fluids provides the most definite identification of the intoxicating agent. Some common poisons, such as aspirin and barbiturates, can be identified and even quantitated by relatively simple laboratory procedures. Others require more complex toxicologic techniques, such as gas or high-pressure chromatography, which are performed only in specialized laboratories. Furthermore, the results of toxicologic determinations are rarely available in time to guide the initial treatment of acute poisoning. Nevertheless, specimens of vomitus, gastric aspirate, blood, urine, and feces should be saved for toxicologic study if diagnostic or legal questions are likely to arise. Chemical analyses of body fluids or tissues are of particular value in the diagnosis and evaluation of chronic intoxications. Finally, they are useful in following the success of some forms of therapy.

TABLE 238-1
Treatment of acute chemical poisoning

- *I* Prevention of further absorption of poison
  - *A* Poisoning by ingestion
    - *1* Emptying the stomach
      - *a* Induction of vomiting
      - *b* Gastric lavage
    - *2* Minimizing gastrointestinal absorption
      - *a* Adsorption
      - *b* Catharsis
  - *B* Poisoning by other routes
- *II* Removal of absorbed poisons from body
  - *A* Detoxification—enzyme induction?
  - *B* Biliary excretion—interruption of enterohepatic circulation
  - *C* Urinary excretion
    - *1* Forced diuresis
    - *2* Alteration of urinary pH
  - *D* Dialysis
    - *1* Peritoneal dialysis
    - *2* Hemodialysis
  - *E* Charcoal or resin hemoperfusion
  - *F* Exchange transfusion
  - *G* Chelation and chemical binding
- *III* Supportive therapy
- *IV* Administration of systemic antidotes
  - *A* Chemical agents
  - *B* Pharmacological antagonists

TREATMENT OF CHEMICAL POISONING

Although the physician should always try to identify the poison, such attempts must never delay vital therapeutic measures. Most poisons do not have specific antidotes. Essential supportive care must be given as indicated by the patient's clinical state and does not require knowledge of the toxic agent. Symptomatic treatment of circulatory, respiratory, neurological, and renal function should be administered immediately as to any other seriously ill patient.

Correct treatment of the poisoned patient thus requires knowledge of both the general principles of management and the details of therapy for specific poisons. Treatment involves four steps: (1) prevention of further absorption of the poison, (2) removal of absorbed poison from the body, (3) symptomatic or supportive therapy, and (4) administration of systemic antidotes (Table 238-1). The first three are applicable to most types of poisoning. The fourth is most often used only when the toxic agent is known and a specific antidote is available. However, naloxone is given sometimes if the index of suspicion is high that the patient has had an overdose of an opiate. Success often depends upon speed of treatment, and, when indicated by the clinical situation, several approaches should be used simultaneously.

PREVENTION OF ABSORPTION OF INGESTED POISONS If appreciable amounts of a poison have been ingested, one should attempt to minimize its absorption from the gastrointestinal tract. The success of such endeavors depends upon the time elapsed since ingestion and upon the site and speed of absorption of the poison.

Evacuation of the stomach Attempts to empty the stomach are always worthwhile unless specifically contraindicated. They can be highly successful if made soon after ingestion. Significant amounts of poison still may be recovered from the stomach hours after ingestion because gastric emptying may be delayed by gastric atony or pylorospasm.

Emesis occurs spontaneously after the ingestion of many poisons. In a minority of instances it may be induced in the home by mechanical stimulation of the posterior pharynx. The emetic action of syrup of ipecac (not the 14 times more concentrated fluid extract) in 15- to 30-ml dosage is more effective and is safe enough for home use. Its action has an average latent period of 20 min and depends in part on gastrointestinal absorption, so that concurrent administration of charcoal, to which it adsorbs, is to be avoided. A second dose of ipecac should be given if the patient fails to vomit after 20 min (90 to 95 percent of patients will vomit after two doses). If ipecac is not available at home, every effort should be made to locate some, even if this requires taking the patient to the hospital. Apomorphine, 0.06 mg/kg intramuscularly, acts within 5 min but may cause prolonged vomiting. When given intravenously in doses of 0.01 mg/kg, apomorphine tends to produce almost immediate vomiting which is not followed by any other central nervous system effects. On occasion it is impossible to induce vomiting, and valuable time should not be lost with hopeful waiting. Induction of vomiting should not be attempted in convulsing patients, in patients with severe central nervous system depression, or (because of the danger of gastroesophageal perforation or tracheal aspiration of vomitus) in patients who have ingested strong caustics or liquid hydrocarbons which are potent lung irritants (e.g., kerosene, furniture polish).

In comparison with emesis, *gastric lavage* is more predictably and immediately active but usually no more effective in removing poison from the stomach. It can be employed in unconscious patients, and removal of gastric contents reduces the risk of aspiration of vomitus in such patients. It is, however, contraindicated after the ingestion of strong corrosives because of danger of perforating injured tissues. When properly performed, gastric lavage carries little risk of aspiration of gastric contents into the lungs. The patient should be prone, with head and shoulders lowered. A mouth gag is placed, and a gastric tube of sufficient diameter to permit withdrawal of particulate matter (size 30) is passed into the stomach. If central nervous system function is depressed, if introduction of the tube produces retching, or if pulmonary irritants have been ingested, it is wise to place a *cuffed endotracheal tube* before lavaging. Gastric contents are withdrawn with a large syringe and usually contain most of the poison that will be removed. Thereafter 200 ml (less in children) of warm water or dilute solution alternately is instilled and withdrawn until the aspirate becomes clear.

Interference with gastrointestinal absorption Since neither emesis nor gastric lavage empties the stomach completely, one should attempt to minimize absorption by administering substances which trap ingested poisons. Many poisons are adsorbed by powdered, activated charcoal. A good grade of activated charcoal can adsorb as much as half its weight of many common poisons. A slurry of activated charcoal (20 to 50 g in 100 to 200 ml) should be administered after evacuation of the stomach.

Adsorption by charcoal is reversible, and the effectiveness of adsorption of many poisons varies with the pH. Acidic substances are adsorbed better in acid solutions and therefore may be released in the small intestine. It is desirable to speed the charcoal with its adsorbed poison through the intestine as quickly as possible. This will also decrease intestinal absorption of any unabsorbed poison which has passed beyond the pylorus. In patients with good renal and cardiac function this is best accomplished by oral or gastric administration of an osmotic cathartic such as magnesium or sodium sulfate (10 to 30 g given in solution at a concentration of 10% or less).

PREVENTION OF ABSORPTION OF POISON FROM OTHER SITES Most topically applied poisons can be removed by copious flushing with water. In certain instances weak acids or bases or alcohol plus soap or detergent are more effective, but rapid and voluminous washing with water should always proceed while they are being obtained. Chemical antidotes can be hazardous because tissue injury may result from the heat of the chemical reaction.

The systemic distribution of injected poisons can be slowed by the application of cold to the injection site or by the proximal application of a tourniquet.

Following inhalation of toxic gases, vapors, or dusts, the victim should be moved to clean air and adequate ventilation maintained. If the patient cannot be moved, a protective mask should be applied.

REMOVAL OF ABSORBED POISON FROM THE BODY Unlike prevention or retardation of absorption, measures to speed removal of the toxic agent from the body rarely have much influence on the peak poison concentration. However, they can significantly abbreviate the time during which the concentration of many poisons remains above any given level and may thereby reduce morbidity, avoid complications, and save lives. In judging the need for such measures, one must consider the patient's clinical state, the properties and metabolic fate of the poison, and the amount absorbed as judged by the history and the blood level. Removal of some poisons can be accelerated by several methods; selection depends on the clinical urgency, the amount in the body, and the skills and equipment available.

Biliary excretion Certain organic acids and active drugs are secreted into the bile against large concentration gradients. This process takes time and cannot be accelerated. However, the intestinal resorption of substances already secreted into the bile, such as glutethimide, can be decreased by the administration of charcoal every 6 h. The organochlorine pesticide, chlordecone (kepone), is eliminated slowly from the body (blood half-time 165 days). Cholestyramine (16 g per day) significantly accelerates elimination (blood half-time 80 days).

Urinary excretion Acceleration of renal excretion is applicable to a much larger number of poisons. Renal excretion of toxic substances depends on glomerular filtration, active tubular secretion, and passive tubular resorption. The first two processes should be protected by maintenance of adequate circulation and renal function, but for practical purposes they cannot be accelerated. On the other hand, passive tubular resorption of many poisons plays an important role in the prolongation of their action and can frequently be decreased by readily available methods.

The effectiveness of forced diuresis by administration of large volumes of electrolyte solutions together with intravenous furosemide in increasing renal excretion has been demonstrated for many drugs, such as salicylates and long-acting barbiturates, and potentially is applicable to all ultrafiltered poisons which are reabsorbed passively.

Alteration of the urinary pH can also inhibit passive back-diffusion of some poisons and increase their renal clearance. The renal tubular epithelium is more permeable to uncharged molecules than to ionized solutes. Weak organic acids and bases readily diffuse out of the tubular fluid in their un-ionized form but are trapped in it when ionized. Acidic poisons are ionized only at pHs above their pK_a. Alkalinization of the urine greatly increases the ionization in the tubular fluid of such organic acids as phenobarbital and salicylate. In contrast, the pK_a of pentobarbital (8.1) and secobarbital (8.0) is so high that renal clearance is not increased greatly by raising the urinary pH into the physiological alkaline range. Alkalinization of the urine is achieved by the infusion of sodium bicarbonate at a rate determined by the urinary and blood pH. Excessive systemic alkalosis or electrolyte disturbances must be prevented. A combination of forced diuresis and alkalinization of the urine can raise the renal clearance of some acidic poisons tenfold or more and has been found highly effective in poisoning by salicylate and phenobarbital. Conversely, depression of the urinary pH below its usual range has been shown to augment the clearance of amphetamines and phencyclidines.

Finally, the renal excretion of certain poisons can be increased in a highly specific fashion. An example is the removal of bromide by administration of chloride and chloriuretics. Such methods are discussed with the individual poisons.

Dialysis and hemoperfusion Dialysis has been found effective in the removal of many compounds, including barbiturates, borate, chlorate, ethanol, glycols, methanol, salicylate, sulfonamides, theophylline, and thiocyanate. Theoretically, it should accelerate the removal from the body of any dialyzable toxin which is not bound irreversibly to tissues. Its effectiveness does not extend to large-molecule, nondialyzable poisons and is decreased by a high degree of protein binding or lipid solubility of the toxic substance.

Peritoneal dialysis can be performed easily in any hospital and may be continued for long periods. It is valuable for the removal of poisons only if renal function is impaired, hemodialysis or hemoperfusion is not possible, or forced diuresis cannot be carried out.

Hemodialysis is unquestionably a more effective procedure for removing large amounts of dialyzable poisons. For barbiturates dialysance rates of 50 to 100 ml/min have been achieved, a removal rate 2 to 10 times faster than during peritoneal dialysis or forced diuresis. Perfusion of blood through activated charcoal or exchange resin achieves even higher clearance rates than hemodialysis for most poisons. Extracorporeal dialysis and hemoperfusion are clearly the procedures of choice for the rapid removal of poisons from patients who have absorbed amounts which make survival unlikely even under the best supportive care. Since the required equipment and skilled personnel are not available in every hospital, the possibility of transfer of such patients to an institution with these capabilities should be considered.

Chelation and chemical binding The removal of some poisons is accelerated by chemical interaction with other substances followed by renal excretion. These substances are considered systemic antidotes and are discussed with the individual poisons.

SUPPORTIVE THERAPY Most chemical poisonings are reversible, self-limited disease states. Skillful supportive therapy can keep many seriously poisoned patients alive and their detoxifying and excretory mechanisms functioning until the concentration of poison in the body has fallen to safe levels. Symptomatic measures are especially important when the poison is one of the many compounds for which no specific antidote is known. Even when an antidote is available, disturbances of vital functions must be prevented or controlled by appropriate supportive care.

The poisoned patient may suffer a variety of physiological disturbances. Most of these are not peculiar to chemical intoxications, and their therapeutic management is described elsewhere in this text. Only those aspects of supportive therapy specially relevant to poisonings are discussed briefly here.

Central nervous system depression Specific therapy directed against the depressant effects of poisons on the central nervous system is usually both unnecessary and difficult. Most poisoned patients will emerge from coma as from a prolonged anesthesia. During the period of unconsciousness meticulous nursing care and close observation are essential. If depression of medullary centers results in circulatory or respiratory failure, these vital functions must be immediately and vigorously supported by chemical or mechanical means.

The use of analeptics in the treatment of poison-induced central nervous system depression has been largely abandoned. Certainly these agents should never be employed to restore consciousness, and it is doubtful whether their use to hasten the restoration of spontaneous breathing and active reflexes is ever justified. By contrast, the narcotic antagonist naloxone administered intravenously in adequate doses generally will reverse central nervous system depression secondary to narcotic overdosage.

Convulsions Many poisons (e.g., chlorinated hydrocarbons, insecticides, strychnine) cause convulsions by their specific excitatory effects. Poisoned patients also may have convulsions because of hypoxia, hypoglycemia, cerebral edema, or metabolic disturbances. In such cases these abnormalities should be corrected as far as possible. Regardless of the cause of the convulsions, anticonvulsant drugs often are required. Intravenously administered diazepam, phenobarbital, or phenytoin is usually effective.

Cerebral edema Intracranial hypertension due to cerebral edema is also a characteristic effect of some poisons and a nonspecific result of other chemical intoxications. For example, cerebral edema is seen in poisoning by lead, carbon monoxide, and methanol. Symptomatic treatment consists of use of adrenocortical steroids and, when necessary, the intravenous administration of hypertonic solutions of mannitol or urea.

Hypotension The causes of hypotension and shock in the poisoned patient are legion, and often several of them coexist. Poisons can depress the medullary vasomotor centers, block autonomic ganglia or adrenergic receptors, directly depress the tone of arterial or venous smooth muscle, reduce myocardial contractility, or induce cardiac arrhythmias. Less specifically, the poisoned patient may be in shock because of tissue hypoxia, extensive tissue destruction from corrosives, loss of blood or fluids, or metabolic disturbances. When possible, these abnormalities should be corrected. If the central venous pressure is low, fluid replacement should be the first therapeutic approach. Vasoactive drugs are often helpful and sometimes essential in the hypotensive poisoned patient, particularly in shock resulting from central depression. As in shock from other causes, choice of the most appropriate agent requires an analysis of the hemodynamic disturbance which goes beyond determination of the arterial pressure.

Cardiac arrhythmias Disturbances of cardiac impulse generation or conduction in the poisoned patient arise from the effects of certain poisons on the electrical properties of cardiac fibers or from myocardial hypoxia or metabolic disturbances. The latter should be corrected, and antiarrhythmic agents administered as indicated by the nature of the arrhythmia (Chap. 254).

Pulmonary edema The poisoned patient may develop pulmonary edema because of depressed myocardial contractility or because of alveolar injury from irritant gases or aspirated fluids. The latter type of edema is less responsive to treatment and may be associated with laryngeal edema. Therapeutic measures include suctioning, administration of high concentrations of oxygen under positive pressure, aerosols of surface-active agents, bronchodilators, and adrenocortical steroids.

Hypoxia Poisoning may cause tissue hypoxia by various mechanisms, and several of these may operate in one patient. Inadequate ventilation can result from central respiratory depression, from muscular paralysis, or from airway obstruction by retained secretions, laryngeal edema, or bronchospasm. Alveolar-capillary diffusion may be impaired by pulmonary edema. Anemia, methemoglobinemia, carboxyhemoglobinemia, or shock can interfere with oxygen transport. Cellular oxidation may be inhibited (e.g., cyanide, fluoroacetate, or general protoplasmic poisons). Maintenance of an adequate airway is essential to treatment. The clinical situation and the site of obstruction may indicate frequent suctioning, insertion of an oropharyngeal airway or of an endotracheal tube, or a tracheotomy. If despite a clear airway ventilation remains inadequate, as judged by clinical appearance or by measurement of minute volume or blood gases, artificial ventilation by appropriate mechanical means is imperative. Administration of high concentrations of oxygen is indicated whenever tissue hypoxia occurs. When the central nervous system is severely depressed, oxygen administration often results in apnea and must be combined with artificial ventilation. Hyperbaric oxygen may be helpful in some situations. The treatment of methemoglobinemia, carboxyhemoglobinemia, and inhibition of cellular oxidation is discussed with the specific poisons which produce these changes.

Acute renal insufficiency Renal failure with oliguria or anuria may occur in the poisoned patient because of shock, dehydration, or electrolyte disturbances. More specifically, it may be due to the nephrotoxic potential of some poisons (e.g., mercury, phosphorus, carbon tetrachloride, bromate), many of which are concentrated and excreted by the kidney. Renal damage due to poisons is usually reversible. The management of acute renal insufficiency is outlined in Chap. 290.

Electrolyte and water disturbances Imbalances of fluid and electrolytes are common features of chemical poisoning. They may result from vomiting, diarrhea, renal insufficiency, or therapeutic maneuvers such as catharsis, forced diuresis, or dialysis. These disturbances are corrected or, ideally, prevented by appropriate therapy. Certain poisons produce more specific defects, such as metabolic acidosis (e.g., methanol, phenol, salicylate) or hypocalcemia (e.g., fluoride, oxalate). These abnormalities and any specific treatment are described under the individual poisons.

Acute hepatic insufficiency The primary manifestation of some poisonings (e.g., chlorinated hydrocarbons, phosphorus, cinchophen, certain mushrooms) is acute hepatic failure. Its management is described in Chap. 318.

ADMINISTRATION OF SYSTEMIC ANTIDOTES Specific antidotal therapy is available for only a few poisons. Some systemic antidotes are chemicals which exert their therapeutic effect by reducing the concentration of the toxic substance. They may do this by combining with the poison (e.g., ethylene diaminetetraacetate with lead, dimercaprol with mercury, sulfhydryl-containing reagents with a toxic metabolite of acetaminophen) or by increasing its excretion (e.g., chloride or mercurial diuretics in bromide poisoning). Other systemic antidotes compete with the poison for its receptor site (e.g., atropine with muscarine, naloxone with morphine; physostigmine reverses some of the anticholinergic effects of the tricyclic antidepressants, and those of the antihistamines, belladonna, and other atropinic substances). Specific antidotes are discussed with the individual poisons.

COMMON POISONS

The poisons discussed in this section are some of those encountered by the general population such as commonly used drugs, household products, solvents, pesticides, and poisonous plants. It has been necessary to disregard many uncommon toxic materials as well as products to which exposure occurs only in specialized industrial environments. Details concerning poisoning by such compounds may be found in some of the references to this chapter. Toxic effects of many drugs are considered throughout this text in conjunction with their therapeutic use. Manifestations of hypersensitivity to chemicals are described in Chap. 72. The following discussions of specific poisons stress those details of their action which are pertinent to the recognition or treatment of clinical poisoning.

ACETAMINOPHEN Termed *paracetamol* in the United Kingdom, acetaminophen has become a popular alternative to salicylates as an analgesic and antipyretic. It is a frequent cause of poisoning. While the toxic and lethal doses of acetaminophen may vary from patient to patient, hepatic damage may be expected if an adult has taken more than 8 g as a single dose. A plasma concentration of greater than 200 μg/ml at 4 h after ingestion is also cause for concern. Clinical manifestations of acetaminophen poisoning are nonspecific. In the first few hours after ingestion lethargy, pallor, nausea, vomiting, and diaphoresis may occur; there are no acid-base derangements like those which may accompany aspirin overdose. Hepatic damage, the most important manifestation of acetaminophen toxicity, becomes evident 1 to 2 days after ingestion. While some patients show only elevation of serum transaminase and others show tender hepatomegaly and jaundice, more severe damage can lead to hyperammonemia, asterixis, mental confusion, coma, bleeding, and death from acute liver failure. Acute tubular necrosis, pancreatitis, hypoglycemia, cardiac damage, and hypersensitivity reactions sometimes are seen.

There is good evidence that damage to tissue (especially liver) is caused by metabolites of acetaminophen and not the drug itself. At therapeutic doses acetaminophen is eliminated mainly conjugated to sulfate or glucuronic acid. A small amount of acetaminophen is activated by the cytochrome P_{450} system and conjugated with the sulfhydryl group of glutathione to yield a nontoxic mercapturic acid. After an overdose, the pathways of conjugation to the sulfate and glucuronic acid become saturated, an increasing fraction of the drug is activated by the P_{450} system, glutathione stores are depleted, and the reactive intermediates then become free to bind covalently to liver macromolecules and cause necrosis.

Treatment of acetaminophen poisoning should begin with induction of emesis or gastric lavage followed by administration of activated charcoal. Since endogenous glutathione appears to have a protective effect, the administration of one of several other sulfhydryl compounds has been studied for protection against acetaminophen hepatotoxicity. When administered orally within 10 h of ingestion, either *N*-acetylcysteine (Mucomyst) or cysteamine is effective in decreasing hepatotoxicity. A potentially toxic dose ($>$7.5 g) ingested within the previous 24 h is an indication for *N*-acetylcysteine therapy. Since early treatment is paramount, a patient suspected of having ingested a potentially hepatotoxic dose should be started on sulfhydryl therapy while awaiting the plasma acetaminophen level. A 5% solution of Mucomyst in a cola beverage or fruit juice is given with a loading dose of 140 mg/kg and a maintenance dose of 70 mg/kg every 4 h for 3 days. If sulfhydryl therapy is to be instituted, charcoal and osmotic cathartic administration are contraindicated since both may reduce absorption of the antidote. In a mixed poisoning, charcoal may be removed by lavage prior to administration of the antidote.

ACIDS Corrosive acids are used widely in industry and laboratories. Ingestion is almost always with suicidal intent. Death has occurred after an oral dose of 1 ml of a corrosive acid.

Toxic effects of corrosive acids are due to their direct chemical action. Ingestion of acids may produce irritation, bleeding, and sloughing in the mouth and esophagus with more severe burns occurring in the stomach, particularly in the pylorus. Perforations with peritonitis, though uncommon, may occur. Mouth and pharynx may be brownish black and may have a charred appearance. Yellow staining is seen after ingestion of nitric and picric acids. Severe pain in mouth, pharynx, chest, and abdomen is the rule and soon is followed by hematemesis and bloody diarrhea. Frequently profound shock develops. About half of those who ingest significant amounts of acid die from its immediate effects. Survivors can develop mediastinitis or peritonitis from esophageal or gastric perforation, and delayed perforation of the esophagus or stomach can also occur. Recovery from acid ingestion can be associated with stricture formation which most commonly involves the pylorus.

Ingested acid should be diluted immediately with large amounts of water or milk (when possible, in a hundredfold excess). The danger of perforation contraindicates the use of emesis or gastric lavage. Diagnostic esophagoscopy, if performed, should be done in the first 24 h after ingestion. Following the emergency measures, appropriate supportive therapy is administered for the relief of pain and the treatment of shock, perforation, and infection.

ALKALIES Strong alkalies such as ammonium hydroxide, potassium hydroxide (potash), potassium carbonate, sodium hydroxide (lye, Clinitest tablets), and sodium carbonate (washing soda) are used widely in industry and in cleansers and drain cleaners. Sodium and potassium phosphates find use as water softeners. Strong alkalies form soaps with fats and proteinates with proteins, resulting in penetrating necrosis of tissues. Fatalities have occurred from the ingestion of 5 to 30 g of such compounds.

The toxic effects of alkalies are due to irritation and destruction of local tissues. Ingestion is followed by severe pain in mouth, pharynx, chest, and abdomen. Vomiting of blood and sloughed mucosa and diarrhea are common. Reflex loss of vascular tone frequently leads to profound shock. Perforation of the esophagus or stomach may be immediate or delayed for several days. Mouth and pharynx show erythema and gelatinous necrotic areas. After ingestion of water softeners profound reduction in serum calcium may be seen and lead to tetany and hypotension. Survivors usually suffer from esophageal strictures.

Treatment consists of immediate administration of large amounts of water or milk. Because of the danger of perforation, both induction of emesis and gastric lavage are contraindicated. Esophagoscopy should be done within the first 24 h. In patients with significant esophageal or gastric burns steroids usually are administered for about 3 weeks to decrease the incidence of stricture formation, although definitive evidence of efficacy is lacking. After the ingestion of water softeners (phosphates), calcium gluconate should be administered intravenously as needed. Treatment is otherwise symptomatic and directed at the relief of pain, respiratory obstruction due to edema of the hypopharynx, fluid loss, and shock.

Inhalation of ammonia, which is used as a refrigerant, results in irritation of the upper and lower parts of the respiratory tract. Laryngeal and pulmonary edema may occur and must be treated symptomatically.

ANILINE This substance is used in printing and clothmarking inks, paints, and paint removers. Both aniline and its derivatives, such as toluidine, nitroaniline, and nitrobenzene, are widely used in industrial synthesis. Aniline is absorbed from the gastrointestinal tract and through the lungs or skin. Ingestion of 1 g aniline has been fatal. Methemoglobinemia is the most important manifestation. Headache, dizziness, hypotension, convulsions, and coma may occur. If the acute period is survived, jaundice and anemia may appear. Treatment consists of correction of methemoglobinemia (see Chap. 330) and supportive measures.

ANTIHISTAMINES The common and unprescribed use of antihistamines makes them readily available for accidental overdosage and suicidal attempts. There is wide variation from patient to patient in tolerance to these drugs and in the manifestations of poisoning. A dose of 200 mg diphenhydramine has been fatal in one adult, whereas another tolerated 2 g. Manifestations of poisoning are central nervous system excitement or depression. In adults depressive manifestations with drowsiness, stupor, and coma predominate, but convulsions followed by further depression may occur.

Treatment is supportive and directed toward removal of the unabsorbed drug and maintenance of vital functions. Convulsions may be controlled with phenobarbital or diazepam. Some antihistamines have prominent atropine-like properties. Patients poisoned with these drugs may show manifestations of atropine poisoning and are treated correspondingly.

ANTIMUSCARINIC COMPOUNDS Atropine, related belladonna alkaloids (hyoscyamine and scopolamine), and synthetic substitutes (e.g., benztropine, cyclopentolate, homatropine, methantheline, propantheline) are widely prescribed drugs and occur in many proprietary mixtures.

Individual sensitivity to the toxic effects of belladonna alkaloids varies widely; fatalities have occurred from as little as 10 mg atropine, but doses of 500 mg have been nonfatal. Young children are particularly susceptible to poisoning with belladonna alkaloids. Older persons appear to be more sensitive to the central nervous system effects of these drugs. Since atropine is both hydrolyzed in the liver and excreted unchanged in the urine, insufficiency of hepatic or renal function may lead to poisoning on therapeutic dosage.

The most characteristic manifestations of atropine poisoning are those of parasympathetic blockade: dryness of mucous membranes, thirst, dysphagia, hoarseness, xerophthalmia, dilated pupils, blurring of vision, rise in intraocular tension, flushing, dryness and increased temperature of the skin, fever, tachycardia, hypertension, urinary retention, and abdominal distention. This widespread parasympatholysis is almost diagnostic of belladonna poisoning, but the diagnosis can be strengthened further by the reversal of blockade by physostigmine (2 mg administered intravenously over several minutes).

Central nervous system symptoms are also very common during belladonna intoxication. Atropine and scopolamine produce similar toxic psychoses. Restlessness, excitation, confusion, and incoordination precede mania, hallucinations, and delirium. Patients intoxicated by scopolamine not infrequently show lethargy and somnolence rather than excitement. In severe intoxication with belladonna alkaloids, central nervous system depression and coma are the rule. When death results it is because of circulatory collapse and respiratory failure.

In the treatment of belladonna poisoning, emesis or gastric lavage should be followed by the administration of activated charcoal. Symptomatic treatment is directed at the reduction of body temperature, the moistening of mucous membranes, and, when necessary, urethral catheterization. Excitement or convulsions may require appropriate pharmacotherapy. Patients with deep coma, life-threatening cardiac arrhythmias, severe hallucinations, or severe hypertension have been treated with physostigmine with some reversal of these effects. It has not been established whether physostigmine reduces mortality.

Death occurs in fewer than 1 percent of cases of atropine or scopolamine poisoning. No permanent sequelae have been observed, but manifestations may persist for several days.

BARIUM Poisoning may be due to the ingestion of rodenticides which contain soluble barium salts or of depilatories that contain barium sulfide. A soluble barium salt may be present as a contaminant in the insoluble barium sulfate used as a radiopaque contrast medium. Barium is extremely toxic, producing intense stimulation of muscles of all types. Its action on the gastrointestinal musculature causes vomiting, colic, and diarrhea. Skeletal muscle tremors and spasm are commonly seen. Arteriolar spasm results in marked hypertension. Cardiac arrhythmias may proceed to ventricular fibrillation. Anxiety, weakness, and convulsions may occur. Death is usually due to cardiac arrhythmia or respiratory arrest.

Treatment consists of the oral administration of 250 ml 10% sodium sulfate or 5% magnesium sulfate. This will precipitate and remove any unabsorbed barium in the gastrointestinal tract. A dose of 10 ml of a 10% solution of sodium sulfate should be slowly administered intravenously every 15 min until symptoms subside. Procainamide may be used to reduce the danger of fatal cardiac arrhythmias. Serum potassium may be reduced, in which case oral or intravenous supplementation is indicated. If necessary, pain should be relieved and artificial ventilation with oxygen administered.

BENZENE, TOLUENE These solvents are used in paint removers, dry-cleaning solutions, and rubber or plastic cements. Benzene is also present, to some extent, in most gasolines. Poisoning may result from ingestion or from the breathing of concentrated vapors. Toluene is an ingredient in some cement used by glue sniffers.

Acute poisoning by these compounds causes central nervous system manifestations. With sufficient exposure, symptoms progress from an initial period of restlessness, excitement, euphoria, and dizziness to coma, convulsions, and respiratory failure. Ventricular arrhythmias may occur. Renal tubular acidosis can occur following repeated inhalation of toluene.

Chronic poisoning by benzene or toluene results from repeated exposure to their vapors in low concentration. Central nervous system symptoms include irritability, insomnia, headache, tremors, and paresthesias. Anorexia and nausea are also common. Fatty degeneration of the heart, liver, and kidneys may occur. By far the most important manifestation of chronic exposure to benzene is bone marrow depression, which may progress to aplastic anemia and complete aplasia of the bone marrow. Individual susceptibility to this effect varies greatly and may not become apparent for months after the initial exposure to the poison.

Treatment of both acute and chronic poisoning is symptomatic. Neurological, pulmonary, or cardiovascular problems are treated as in poisoning by petroleum distillates.

BLEACHES Industrial strength bleaching solutions contain 10% or more sodium hypochlorite, while household products (e.g., Clorox, Purex, Sanichlor) contain 3 to 6%. The solution used for chlorinating swimming pools is 20%. Their corrosive action in mouth, pharynx, and esophagus is similar to that of sodium hydroxide. Acid gastric juice releases hypochlorous acid from such solutions. This compound is very irritating to mucous membranes, and inhalation of its fumes causes severe pulmonary irritation and pulmonary edema. However, the systemic toxicity of hypochlorous acid is low. Perforation and stricture formation are rare after the ingestion of household bleaching solutions.

Treatment consists of dilution of the ingested bleach with water or milk. The usual household bleaching solutions do not cause enough corrosive injury to the esophagus to preclude the induction of emesis or gastric lavage, but one should be wary of this possibility if one of the more concentrated solutions has been ingested. Although sodium thiosulfate (100 ml of a 1 to 2.5% solution by lavage), which will reduce hypochlorite to nontoxic products, has been administered routinely to these patients, there is great doubt that it is of any use except very early after ingestion of very large quantities of bleach.

BORIC ACID This compound is a very weak germicide and has been employed widely in powders, lotions, solutions, and ointments. Though not highly toxic, boric acid is not nearly as benign as widely assumed. The lethal dose is approximately 15 g in adults and 5 g in infants. Such amounts can be absorbed through abraded skin, from serous cavities, and after ingestion.

Regardless of the route of administration, the first symptoms of poisoning are nausea, vomiting, and diarrhea. These are followed by headache, weakness, restlessness, and erythroderma which may progress to desquamation of skin and mucous membranes. Renal toxicity and shock are common, and more than 100 fatalities have occurred. Renal excretion of boric acid is slow, and clearance can be increased markedly by dialysis. Boric acid should always be labeled as poison, and since this substance has no therapeutic function which cannot be served equally well by less toxic preparations, it should be removed from home and hospital.

CARBON MONOXIDE Carbon monoxide is a colorless, odorless, tasteless, and nonirritating gas produced by the incomplete combustion of carbonaceous materials. Almost any flame or combustion device emits carbon monoxide. The gas is present in the exhaust of internal combustion engines in a concentration of 3 to 7 percent. Much higher concentrations are present in most illuminating and heating gases, but not in natural gas. Carbon monoxide annually is responsible for about 3500 accidental and suicidal deaths in the United States alone.

The toxic effects of carbon monoxide are the result of tissue hypoxia. Carbon monoxide combines with hemoglobin to form carboxyhemoglobin. Since carbon monoxide and oxygen react with the same group in the hemoglobin molecule, and since the affinity of hemoglobin for carbon monoxide is 200 times greater than for oxygen, carboxyhemoglobin is incapable of carrying oxygen. (At equilibrium 1 part of carbon monoxide in 1500 parts of air will result in 50 percent conversion of hemoglobin to carboxyhemoglobin.) Carboxyhemoglobin also interferes with the release of oxygen from oxyhemoglobin. This further reduces the amount of oxygen available to the tissues and explains why tissue anoxia appears in the carbon monoxide-poisoned person at levels of arterial oxyhemoglobin concentration well tolerated by the anemic patient.

The extent of saturation of hemoglobin with carbon monoxide depends on the concentration of the gas in inspired air and on the time of exposure. The severity of hypoxic symptoms depends further on an individual's state of activity, tissue oxygen needs, and hemoglobin concentration. As a general rule, no symptoms will develop at a concentration of 0.01 percent carbon monoxide in inspired air, since this will not raise blood saturation above 10 percent. Exposure to 0.05 percent for 1 h during light activity will produce a blood concentration of 20 percent carboxyhemoglobin and result in a mild or throbbing headache. Greater activity or longer exposure to the same concentration causes a blood saturation of 30 to 50 percent. At this point headache, irritability, confusion, dizziness, visual disturbances, nausea, vomiting, and fainting on exertion may be observed. After exposure for 1 h to concentrations of 0.1 percent in inspired air, the blood will contain 50 to 80 percent carboxyhemoglobin, which results in coma, convulsions, respiratory failure, and death. On inhalation of high concentrations of carbon monoxide, saturation of the blood proceeds so rapidly that unconsciousness may occur suddenly and without warning. When poisoning is more gradual, the individual may notice decreased exercise tolerance and dyspnea on exertion or even at rest. Excessive sweating, fever, hepatomegaly, skin lesions, leukocytosis, bleeding diathesis, albuminuria, and glycosuria also have been described. Cerebral edema and intracranial hypertension may result from the increased permeability of hypoxic capillaries. Myocardial hypoxia is reflected by electrocardiographic abnormalities.

The most characteristic sign of severe carbon monoxide poisoning is the cherry color of skin and mucous membranes, which results from the bright red carboxyhemoglobin. If the characteristic flush is not present and carbon monoxide poisoning is suspected, 1 ml of the patient's blood can be diluted with 10 ml water; when 1 ml of 5% sodium hydroxide is added to this dilution, an oxyhemoglobin solution will turn brown. If significant amounts of carboxyhemoglobin are present, the solution will turn straw yellow ($<$20% carboxyhemoglobin) or will remain pink ($>$20% carboxyhemoglobin).

Treatment of carbon monoxide poisoning requires effective ventilation in the presence of high oxygen tensions and in the absence of carbon monoxide. If necessary, ventilation should be supported artificially. Pure oxygen should be administered. This will result not only in the replacement of carbon monoxide by oxygen in the hemoglobin molecule but also in the partial relief of tissue hypoxia by oxygen dissolved in the plasma. For the same reasons hyperbaric oxygen is helpful in seriously poisoned patients. Transfusion of blood or packed cells is also of value. In order to reduce tissue needs for oxygen, the patient must be kept absolutely quiet. Induction of hypothermia is not indicated. Cerebral edema should be treated with diuretics and steroids.

During the recovery from carbon monoxide poisoning symptoms regress gradually. If severe tissue hypoxia has obtained too long, neurological symptoms such as tremors, mental deterioration, and psychotic behavior may persist. Histological changes characteristic of hypoxia may be observed in cerebral cortex, medulla, myocardium, and other organs.

CHLORATES Sodium and potassium chlorates are strong oxidizing agents and are found in gargles, mouthwashes, matches, and weed killers. After oral ingestion, 2 g has been fatal for children and 10 g for adults. Chlorate ion acts as a catalyst in the production of methemoglobinemia, and absorption of a small amount can result in a high methemoglobin concentration. The symptoms of chlorate ingestion are those of local mucosal irritation and of methemoglobinemia (see Chap. 330). Intravascular hemolysis and acute renal failure are common. Treatment is directed primarily at the methemoglobinemia. Absorbed chlorate can be removed effectively by dialysis.

CHLORINATED INSECTICIDES These compounds are ingredients of dusts, sprays, and solutions used as insecticides. The great majority of these compounds are chlorinated diphenyls (e.g., DDT, TDE, DFDT, DMC, Neotran) or chlorinated polycyclic compounds (e.g., aldrin, chlordane, dieldrin, endrin, heptachlor). Lindane is a hexachlorobenzene. Their toxicity has led to their greatly diminished use in recent years, and many are banned in certain locales, including the United States. The chlorinated insecticides are soluble in lipid and organic solvents but not in water. They are poorly absorbed unless dissolved in a vehicle such as kerosene, petroleum distillates, or other organic solvents. Under these circumstances they readily enter the body through the skin, lungs, or gastrointestinal tract. These compounds vary considerably in toxicity, and the toxicity of the dissolving vehicle must also be considered. The effects of the solvent may overshadow or modify those of the insecticide.

The initial symptoms of acute poisoning are nausea, vomiting, headache, dizziness, apprehension, excitement, and muscular tremors and weakness. These symptoms progress to generalized central nervous system hyperexcitability and delirium and clonic or tonic convulsions. This stage is in turn followed by progressive depression with paralysis, coma, and death. Except for endrin, which is strongly hepatotoxic, liver toxicity occurs only at extreme dosage levels. Treatment consists of induction of emesis or gastric lavage, activated charcoal administration, catharsis, anticonvulsive therapy, artificial ventilation, and other supportive measures. Sympathomimetic compounds should be avoided, since chlorinated insecticides apparently increase susceptibility to ventricular fibrillation. Cholestyramine accelerates the excretion of the chlorinated hydrocarbon chlordecone (kepone) by preventing reabsorption following biliary excretion, and it may well have a similar effect on the excretion of pesticides such as DTT, dieldrin, chlordane, and heptachlor which remain in the body for prolonged periods.

CHOLINESTERASE INHIBITOR INSECTICIDES Many substances used in agriculture for control of soft-bodied insects are potent inhibitors of cholinesterase. Most of these compounds are organic phosphates (e.g., Parathion, Malathion, Guthion), others are carbamates (e.g., Carbaryl, Mactacil). The toxicity of these compounds varies widely. Usually they are prepared for use by dilution with powders, organic solvents, or water. Formulations containing 1 to 95 percent of the active ingredient are available. The cholinesterase inhibitor insecticides are absorbed rapidly through the intact skin and after inhalation or ingestion.

The toxicity of these agents results from inactivation of acetylcholinesterase which allows accumulation of excessive amounts of acetylcholine at a number of sites: central nervous system, autonomic ganglia, parasympathetic nerve endings, and motor nerve endings. In the central nervous system coma and respiratory depression and less commonly seizures can occur. Toxic muscarinic effects include nausea, vomiting, diarrhea, involuntary defecation and urination, blurring of vision due to miosis, sweating, lacrimation, and salivation. Nicotinic effects include muscle twitching, fasciculations, weakness, and flaccid paralysis. Cardiac arrhythmias and pulmonary edema, as well as EEG abnormalities, also occur.

Management consists of emesis or lavage, charcoal instillation, catharsis, and washing of contaminated skin with soap and water. Atropine should be given immediately to block the parasympathetic and central nervous system effects. Care should be taken to ensure that the patient is receiving adequate oxygen as myocardial infarction has occurred with atropine administration in this setting. A dose of 2 mg is injected intramuscularly and repeated every 10 min until parasympathetic manifestations are controlled and signs of atropinization appear. The same dosage must be repeated frequently to maintain xerostomia and mild tachycardia. Fatal respiratory failure or pulmonary edema may occur quickly upon cessation of atropine therapy, and the drug should be withdrawn judiciously. Atropine is virtually ineffective against the autonomic ganglionic actions of acetycholine and against the peripheral neuromuscular paralysis. Relief of muscle weakness, in particular respiratory paralysis, can be achieved with certain oximes which can reactivate cholinesterase by reversing the phosphate ester bond formed by the organic phosphate at the enzyme active site. Pralidoxime is useful in the treatment of organic phosphate cholinesterase inhibition but should not be used if the inhibition is due to a carbamate. A dose of 1 g pralidoxime in aqueous solution is administered intravenously over a 5-min period, and this dose is repeated up to four times every 8 to 12 h. Supportive therapy includes administration of oxygen with artificial ventilation if necessary, removal of pulmonary secretions by suction, and treatment of convulsions with diazepam and phenobarbital. Energetic therapy with artificial ventilation, atropine, and pralidoxime allows survival after doses of organic phosphate esters vastly exceeding the usual fatal dose.

CYANIDE The cyanide ion is an exceedingly potent and rapid-acting poison, but one for which specific and effective antidotal therapy is available. Cyanide poisoning may result from the inhalation of hydrocyanic acid or from the ingestion of soluble inorganic cyanide salts or cyanide-releasing substances such as cyanamide, cyanogen chloride, and nitroprusside. Parts of many plants also contain substances such as amygdalin which release cyanide on digestion. Among these are the seeds of certain stone fruits (chokecherry, pin cherry, wild black cherry, peach, apricot, bitter almond), cassava roots, the berries of the jet berry bush, the leaves and shoots of elderberry, and all parts of hydrangea. The controversial drug Laetrile, composed in part of an extract of apricot kernels, has been responsible for fatal cyanide poisoning. Cyanides are widely used in industry and for fumigation and may reach the home in photographic chemicals or silver polishes. As little as 300 mg potassium cyanide may cause death.

The extreme toxicity of cyanide is due to its ready reaction with the trivalent iron of cytochrome oxidase. Formation of the cytochrome oxidase-cyanide complex blocks electron transport, thus inhibiting oxygen utilization. This results in cellular dysfunction and death.

Inhalation of hydrogen cyanide may cause death within a minute. Oral doses act more slowly, requiring several minutes for the appearance of symptoms and up to several hours for death. The first effect is an increase in ventilation because of the blockade of oxidative metabolism in the chemoreceptor cells. As more cyanide is absorbed, there are headache, dizziness, nausea, drowsiness, hypotension, profound dyspnea, characteristic electrocardiographic changes, coma, and convulsions.

Cyanide poisoning is a true medical emergency. Treatment is highly effective if given rapidly. The chemical antidotes should be immediately available wherever emergency medical care is dispensed. The diagnosis may be made by the characteristic "bitter almond" odor on the breath of the victim, and physicians should familiarize themselves with this smell. Since the saturation of hemoglobin is not disturbed by cyanide, cyanosis is not seen until respiratory depression supervenes. The objective of treatment is the production of methemoglobin by the administration of nitrite. The trivalent iron of methemoglobin competes with cytochrome oxidase for the cyanide ion. The cytochrome oxidase-cyanide complex dissociates, and enzymatic function and cell respiration are restored. Further detoxification then is achieved by the administration of thiosulfate. The enzyme rhodanese catalyzes the reaction of thiosulfate with cyanide liberated by the dissociation of cyanmethemoglobin; thiocyanate, which is relatively nontoxic, is formed and readily excreted in the urine.

Since speed is of the essence, nitrite should be immediately administered by inhalation of amyl nitrite perles, one every 2 min unless blood pressure is below 80 mmHg. This is followed as soon as possible by the intravenous injection of 10 ml of 3% sodium nitrite over a 3-min period. An intravenous infusion of norepinephrine may be necessary to maintain blood pressure during this injection period. After the administration of sodium nitrite, 50 ml of 25% sodium thiosulfate should be administered intravenously over a 10-min period. Supportive measures, especially artificial respiration with 100% oxygen, should be instituted as soon as possible, but, unless methemoglobinemia is produced promptly, other forms of treatment are of no value. Administration of sodium nitrite and sodium thiosulfate may have to be repeated. Ideally, dosage should be based on methemoglobin determinations, and the methemoglobin should not exceed 40%. If the patient survives 4 h, recovery is likely but residual cerebral symptoms may persist.

DETERGENTS AND SOAPS These substances fall into the three groups of anionic, nonionic, and cationic detergents. The first group contains common soaps and household detergents. They may cause vomiting and diarrhea but have no serious effects, and no treatment is required. However, some laundry compounds contain phosphate water softeners whose ingestion may cause hypocalcemia. The ingestion of nonionic detergents also requires no treatment.

Cationic detergents, such as benzalkonium chloride (Zephiran) and many others, are commonly used for bactericidal purposes in hospitals and homes. These compounds are well absorbed from the gastrointestinal tract and interfere with cellular functions. The fatal oral dose is approximately 3 g. Concentrated preparations ($>$20% detergent) are corrosive to mouth and esophagus. Ingestion produces nausea and vomiting, and shock, coma, convulsions, and death may occur in a few hours. Treatment after ingestion of dilute preparations consists of minimizing gastrointestinal absorption by emesis and gastric lavage with ordinary soap solution, which rapidly inactivates cationic detergents. Emesis and lavage are contraindicated in the presence of esophageal injury which is unlikely to occur except after ingestion of concentrated preparations. Activated charcoal and an osmotic cathartic should be administered. If significant absorption has occurred, intensive supportive therapy may be required.

FLUORIDES Fluoride salts are used in insecticides. The gases fluorine and hydrogen fluoride are used in industry. The latter is a strong corrosive. Fluorine and fluorides are cellular poisons which inhibit a number of enzymatic reactions, probably the most important of which is to block the glycolytic degradation of glucose. Fluorides also form an insoluble precipitate with calcium and cause hypocalcemia. Finally, in an acid medium fluorides form the corrosive hydrofluoric acid. Ingestion of 1 to 2 g sodium fluoride may be fatal.

Inhalation of fluorine or hydrogen fluoride produces coughing and choking. After an asymptomatic period of a day or two, fever, cough, cyanosis, and pulmonary edema may develop. Ingestion of fluoride salts is followed by nausea, vomiting productive of corroded tissues, diarrhea, and abdominal pain. Consequent to the decrease in serum calcium the victim develops muscular hyperirritability, fasciculations, tremors, spasms, and convulsions. Death results from respiratory paralysis or circulatory collapse. If the patient survives the acute period, jaundice and oliguria may appear. Chronic fluoride poisoning (fluorosis) is characterized by weight loss, weakness, anemia, brittle bones, and stiff joints. Mottling of teeth is seen when exposure occurs during enamel formation.

Acute fluoride poisoning is treated by immediate administration of milk, lime water, calcium gluconate, or calcium lactate solution to precipitate calcium fluoride. After lavage or emesis and charcoal instillation, calcium (e.g., calcium gluconate, 10 g) can be given again followed by an osmotic cathartic. Then 10% calcium gluconate or 1% calcium chloride should be slowly injected intravenously and repeated as needed to prevent a positive Chvostek's sign. Symptomatic and supportive therapy is administered as indicated.

FORMALDEHYDE This gas is available as 40% solution (formalin) which is used as a disinfectant, fumigant, or deodorant. Poisoning by formalin may be diagnosed by the characteristic odor of formaldehyde. formaldehyde reacts chemically with cellular constituents, depresses cellular functions, and causes cell death. The fatal dose of formalin is about 60 ml.

Ingestion of formalin immediately causes severe abdominal pain, nausea, vomiting, and diarrhea. This may be followed by collapse, coma, severe metabolic acidosis, and anuria. Death is usually the result of circulatory failure.

Since any organic material can inactivate formaldehyde, milk, bread, soup, etc., should be administered immediately unless activated charcoal is available. Formaldehyde is a corrosive, and emesis and lavage are not recommended.

Parenteral administration of sodium bicarbonate is indicated to combat acidosis. The treatment is otherwise supportive.

GLYCOLS Ethylene glycol and diethylene glycol are used in antifreeze solutions. The more than 50 annual deaths from these compounds usually result from intentional drinking of antifreeze by alcoholics. The fatal dose of ethylene glycol is about 100 g, that of diethylene glycol somewhat lower. Glycols are metabolized by alcohol dehydrogenase to the aldehyde which is ultimately converted to oxalate. It is the metabolites of the glycols (particularly the aldehyde and oxalate) which are most responsible for toxicity after glycol ingestion.

The initial symptoms of acute poisoning by these glycols resemble those of alcoholic intoxication. They may progress to vomiting, stupor, coma with absent reflexes and anisocoria, and convulsions. Tachypnea, bradycardia, and hypothermia are seen commonly, as are metabolic acidosis and hypocalcemia. After massive ingestion death may occur from respiratory failure within a few hours or from pulmonary edema within a day or two. If the patient survives this stage, acute tubular necrosis often develops.

Intravenous infusion of ethanol to maintain a blood level of 100 mg/dl is effective in competing for alcohol dehydrogenase, thus slowing the conversion of glycol to the more toxic aldehyde. Pyridoxine (100 mg daily administered intravenously) and thiamine (100 mg daily administered intravenously) are given to stimulate conversion of glyoxalate, the immediate metabolic precursor of oxalate, to the nontoxic metabolites, glycine and α-hydroxy-β-ketoadipate, respectively. However, the effectiveness of these latter procedures has not been established. Dialysis is highly effective in the removal of ethylene and diethylene glycol from the body. Acidosis and hypocalcemia must be treated vigorously.

HALOGENATED HYDROCARBONS Halogenated hydrocarbons (carbon tetrachloride, ethylene chlorohydrin, ethylene dichloride, methyl halides, trichloroethane, trichloroethylene) find wide industrial use as solvents, refrigerants, fumigants, and in chemical synthesis. They enter the home in household cleaners, floor waxes, fire extinguishers, and rubber or plastic cements. These compounds are highly fat-soluble and produce cell damage either directly or after conversion in the body to other compounds. Individual halogenated hydrocarbons differ considerably in the degree and the exact manifestations of their toxicity, but in sufficient concentration all these compounds are capable of inducing central nervous system depression and varying amounts of hepatic and renal toxicity. Myocardial depression, vascular damage, and pulmonary edema also may occur.

The most important halogenated hydrocarbon is carbon tetrachloride, which still is employed widely as a nonflammable solvent and fire extinguisher fluid but which largely has been replaced in products intended for household use by the less toxic trichloroethane. Poisoning may occur from inhalation of the vapor, ingestion, or, rarely, percutaneous absorption. An oral dose of as little as 4 ml may be fatal. Absorption from the gastrointestinal tract is slow and unpredictable but is increased by the presence of fats and alcohol. Abdominal pain, hematemesis, and hepatic damage are more common and severe after ingestion than when the poison is inhaled. Inhalation may lead to irritation of the upper part of the respiratory tract.

Acute systemic absorption of carbon tetrachloride results in nausea, dizziness, confusion, and headache within a few minutes. Depending upon the quantity absorbed, the symptoms may quickly progress to stupor, coma, convulsions, respiratory failure, hypotension, or ventricular fibrillation. The patient may recover from these immediate manifestations until evidence of hepatic or renal toxicity appears several hours to several days after the exposure. Liver and kidney damage also may occur in the absence of any severe early central nervous system effects. Initially tender hepatomegaly may be present, jaundice may be rapidly progressive, and death due to severe centrilobular necrosis may occur within days. The renal lesion has the characteristics of acute tubular necrosis, and manifests itself by proteinuria, hematuria, oliguria, or anuria. Uremia, acidosis, hypertension, and pulmonary edema may develop as complications of renal failure. Optic neuritis, pancreatitis, and adrenal cortical necrosis are less common manifestations of carbon tetrachloride intoxication.

Chronic poisoning may occur after repeated exposures to low concentrations of carbon tetrachloride and may also lead to liver or kidney damage. Usually it manifests itself by vague symptoms of fatigue, weakness, mental confusion, abdominal pain, anorexia, nausea, blurring of vision, and paresthesias.

Treatment of acute poisoning by halogenated hydrocarbons includes vigorous efforts at minimizing gastrointestinal absorption by lavage or emesis and catharsis. Treatment is otherwise symptomatic. Sympathomimetic drugs should be avoided because of the danger of inducing ventricular arrhythmias in the sensitized myocardium. Acute renal and hepatic failure must be managed carefully. Often, hemodialysis is required and may be lifesaving until kidney function returns three or more weeks after poisoning. Both hemodialysis and hemoperfusion will effectively remove carbon tetrachloride and trichloroethane from the body but are potentially useful in preventing severe toxicity and death only when begun early in the postingestion period.

IODINE The traditional antiseptic iodine tincture is an alcoholic solution of 2% iodine and 2% sodium iodide. Strong iodine solution (Lugol's solution) is an aqueous solution of 5% iodine and 10% potassium iodide. The fatal dose of tincture of iodine is approximately 2 g. Iodides are very much less toxic, and no fatalities have been reported.

The diagnosis of iodine poisoning is suggested by the brown staining of the oral mucous membranes. The effects largely result from the corrosive effects of the compound on the gastrointestinal tract. Burning abdominal pain, nausea, vomiting, and bloody diarrhea may occur soon after ingestion. If the stomach contained starch, the vomitus is blue or black. Tissue trauma from corrosive gastroenteritis and fluid loss by vomiting and diarrhea may result in shock. Severe edema of the glottis, fever, delirium, stupor, and anuria also have been observed.

Treatment consists of the immediate administration of milk, starch, bread, etc., or activated charcoal to provide a source other than human tissue with which the iodine can react. Catharsis should be induced. Sodium thiosulfate will reduce iodine to less toxic iodide; 100 ml of a 5% solution should be given orally followed by an osmotic cathartic. Ten milliliters of a 10% thiosulfate solution also should be given intravenously every 4 h. Induction of emesis and lavage should not be attempted if esophageal injury is suspected. With appropriate treatment most patients poisoned by iodine survive, but esophageal strictures may complicate their recovery.

IRON SALTS Ferrous or ferric salts produce gastrointestinal corrosive damage. Following mucosal damage, large amounts of iron may be absorbed, particularly in children. Toxicity can be seen with as low as 200 mg (calculated as elemental iron in the preparation), and fatalities have been reported at doses as low as 60 mg/kg. Ingestion in the range of 300 mg/kg are those much more likely to be fatal.

The potential toxic effects of iron ingestion can be divided conveniently into five phases: (1) within 30 min to 2 h there may be nausea, vomiting, abdominal pain, bloody diarrhea, lethargy, restlessness; (2) a period of apparent recovery may follow; (3) 2 to 12 h after ingestion the victim may develop shock, refractory acidosis, and fever; (4) 2 to 4 days after ingestion hepatic necrosis may occur; and (5) 2 to 4 weeks after ingestion gastrointestinal obstruction may develop—the end result of the initial corrosive effects of iron.

Treatment is initiated by emesis and lavage with a 5% sodium bicarbonate solution which will precipitate the ferrous ion. A dilution of Fleet's phosphate enema solution also can be used, but excessive lavage can cause hypernatremia, hyperphosphatemia, and hypocalcemia. When possible, at this point an abdominal roentgenogram should be obtained. If radiopaque tablets are still in the stomach, further lavage is indicated, and then an osmotic cathartic should be administered. Optimal management is aided by determination of the presence or absence of free serum iron. If free iron is present, if the total serum iron exceeds 350 μg/dl, or if clinical symptoms are severe (coma, shock), the iron chelator deferoxamine (Desferal) should be infused intravenously at no more than 15 (mg/kg)/h or given intramuscularly at a dose of 20 mg/kg every 4 h (maximum dose of 6 g per 24 h). The iron deferoxamine complex turns the urine pink to orange, and chelator therapy is continued until the urine loses this color. Treatment is otherwise supportive.

ISOPROPYL ALCOHOL This compound is used as a sterilizing agent or as rubbing alcohol. Ingestion produces gastric irritation and raises the danger of vomiting with aspiration. The systemic effects of isopropyl alcohol are similar to those of ethyl alcohol, but it is approximately twice as potent as the latter. Coma is produced readily but rarely lasts longer than 12 h. About 15% of an ingested dose of isopropanol is metabolized to acetone; transient acetonuria is common, but significant acidosis does not occur. Emesis should be induced, or gastric lavage should be performed. Supportive therapy is required only after ingestion of massive amounts, and there are no sequelae other than transient gastritis.

MAGNESIUM Magnesium sulfate is used intravenously as a hypotensive agent and orally as a cathartic. The magnesium ion is a profound depressant of the central nervous system and of neuromuscular transmission. Poisoning after oral or rectal administration is unlikely in the presence of normal renal function, because the kidney removes magnesium more rapidly than it is absorbed by the gastrointestinal tract. In the presence of impaired renal function an oral dose of 30 g may be fatal. Symptoms begin at a serum magnesium level of 4 meq per liter, and concentrations of over 12 meq per liter may be fatal. Oral ingestion of concentrated solutions may cause gastrointestinal irritation. Manifestations of systemic poisoning are depression of reflexes, flaccid paralysis, hypotension, hypothermia, coma, and respiratory failure. Respiratory death usually precedes significant myocardial depression. The actions of magnesium on neurological and neuromuscular function are antagonized by calcium. Treatment of magnesium poisoning therefore includes the intravenous administration of 10 ml of a 10% solution of calcium gluconate, which may be repeated as necessary.

METHYL ALCOHOL This simplest of alcohols, also called wood alcohol or methanol, is used as a solvent, antifreeze, paint remover, and as a denaturant in ethyl alcohol. Denatured ethyl alcohol preparations, such as Sterno or Solox, contain 5 to 15 percent methyl alcohol as well as other denaturants. Methyl alcohol poisoning results almost entirely from its ingestion as a substitute for ethanol or to the drinking of denatured ethyl alcohol. The toxic dose is quite variable: death has occurred after a dose of 20 ml, but 250 ml has been ingested with survival. As little as 15 ml methanol has caused permanent blindness.

Methanol is less inebriating than ethyl alcohol, and inebriation is not a prominent symptom of methyl alcohol intoxication. Methanol is oxidized in the body by alcohol dehydrogenase first to formaldehyde and then to formic acid; these metabolites cause the toxic manifestations of methanol poisoning. The rate of its metabolism is only 15 percent that of ethanol for which alcohol dehydrogenase has a greater affinity and which can inhibit competitively the rate of metabolism of methanol. Formic acid and especially formaldehyde have toxic actions on many cells; the retina and optic nerve are damaged specifically. The toxic metabolites of methyl alcohol are also responsible for the severe acidosis, which is the most prominent feature of methyl alcohol poisoning. This acidosis results partly from the accumulation of formic acid, but formate also appears to exert an inhibitory effect upon enzymes involved in the oxidation of carbohydrate with consequent accumulation of acid intermediates.

Symptoms of methanol poisoning usually do not appear until 12 to 24 h after ingestion, when sufficient toxic metabolites have acccumulated. Manifestations include headache, dizziness, nausea, vomiting, vasomotor disturbances, central nervous system depression, and respiratory failure. Visual disturbance is almost universal and ranges from mild blurring of vision to total blindness. Impairment of vision may be transient, but permanent blindness may follow survival of the acute intoxication. The pupils are dilated and nonreactive, and there is hyperemia of the optic disk and retinal edema. Acidosis is commonly severe.

In the treatment of methyl alcohol intoxication emesis and gastric lavage are of use only within the first 2 h after ingestion. Intravenous administration of large amounts of sodium bicarbonate combats acidosis. Return of acidosis is frequent after initial correction, and additional alkali must be administered as indicated by close observation of the patient and laboratory determinations. It is most useful to obtain a blood methanol level as soon as possible. At any time after ingestion, levels between 20 and 50 mg/dl are associated with acidosis and significant symptomatology and are an indication for intravenous ethanol therapy (1 g ethanol per kilogram of body weight in 5% dextrose in water over 30 min to load, then 7 to 10 g/h in adults to maintain the blood ethanol level at about 100 mg/dl). Severely symptomatic patients should be treated even if a methanol level cannot be obtained. A methanol level exceeding 50 mg/dl is indication for hemodialysis as well as ethanol therapy; dialysis also is indicated in the presence of severe acidosis with lower blood levels.

MUSHROOMS There are many species of poisonous mushrooms, but in the United States most poisoning is due to the *Amanita.* More than 100 deaths result each year from consumption of wild poisonous mushrooms, 90 percent being due to *A. phalloides* (death cap) or closely related species. Fatalities have occurred after ingestion of only part of one mushroom.

A usually less severe poisoning follows ingestion of *A. muscaria* (fly agaric) which contains the parasympathomimetic alkaloid muscarine, as well as variable amounts of a substance active on the central nervous system and a parasympatholytic alkaloid. Symptoms are largely those of parasympathetic stimulation: lacrimation, pupillary constriction, perspiration, salivation, nausea, vomiting, diarrhea, abdominal pain, bronchorrhea, wheezing, dyspnea, bradycardia, and hypotension. Muscular tremors, confusion, excitement, and delirium are common in severe poisoning. Very rarely symptoms of atropine poisoning have predominated. After ingestion of *A. muscaria,* symptoms appear within minutes to 2 h. The patient may die within a few hours, but with appropriate therapy complete recovery in 24 h is the rule.

A. phalloides, A. virosa (destroying angel), some other *Amanita* species, and *Galerina venenata* contain heat-stable cyclopeptide cytotoxins which are rapidly bound to tissues. The principal toxin is α-amanitin which binds to and inhibits specifically the mammalian RNA polymerase responsible for messenger RNA synthesis. Severe cell damage and fatty degeneration may occur in liver, kidneys, striated muscle, and brain. Ingestion of these dangerous mushrooms is followed by a latent period of 6 to 20 h. Manifestations of cytotoxicity then may appear suddenly and consist of severe nausea, violent abdominal pain, bloody vomiting and diarrhea, and cardiovascular collapse. Headache, mental confusion, coma, or convulsions are common. Painful and tender hepatomegaly, jaundice, hypoglycemia, dehydration, and oliguria or anuria frequently appear on the first or second day after ingestion. The victim may die from acute hepatic necrosis (yellow atrophy) within 4 days. About one-half of all poisonings with *A. phalloides* have a fatal outcome in 5 to 8 days. Recovery tends to be slow.

Ingestion of other poisonous mushrooms may cause gastrointestinal symptoms, visual disturbances, ataxia, disorientation, convulsions, coma, fever, hemolysis, and methemoglobinemia.

Treatment of mushroom poisoning depends upon the species ingested. If parasympathomimetic manifestations are prominent, atropine in doses of 1 to 2 mg is given intramuscularly and repeated every 30 min until symptoms are controlled. Poisoning by cytotoxic mushrooms is treated mainly symptomatically. Fluid and electrolyte balance must be carefully maintained. Hypoglycemia should be avoided; large quantities of carbohydrate may exert some protective effect on the liver. Excitement, convulsions, pain, hypotension, and fever may need symptomatic therapy. Early intensive hemoperfusion can remove α-amanitin from the body and probably is indicated in *A. phalloides* poisoning. Both thioctic acid (α-lipoic acid) and cytochrome c have been advocated as antidotes for α-amanitin poisoning, but convincing data as to their efficacy are lacking.

NAPHTHALENE Poisoning by this substance almost always results from ingestion of moth repellents. An oral dose of 2 g has been fatal. Nausea, vomiting, and diarrhea are the initial symptoms. Larger doses may produce hepatic damage with jaundice and renal toxicity which may progress to hematuria, oliguria, or anuria. Depending upon the amount ingested, central nervous system manifestations may range from headache, mental confusion, and excitement to coma and convulsions. In persons with glucose 6-phosphate dehydrogenase–deficient red blood cells the ingestion of naphthalene will produce hemolysis. Treatment consists of emesis or gastric lavage, catharsis, and supportive measures.

NICOTINE This alkaloid is an exceedingly potent and rapidly acting poison. It is a component of many insecticides. Nicotine is absorbed readily from the oral and gastrointestinal mucosa, from the respiratory tract, and through the skin. The lethal dose for an adult is approximately 50 mg, the quantity contained in two cigarettes. However, tobacco is much less toxic than would be anticipated on the basis of its nicotine content. Nicotine is poorly absorbed from ingested tobacco, and on smoking, most of the nicotine is burned. Nicotine acts on chemoreceptors, on synapses in the central nervous system and in autonomic ganglia, on the adrenal medulla, and on neuroeffector junctions. Furthermore, its transient initial stimulant effects are followed by a more persistent depressant phase of action. It is not surprising that the manifestations of nicotine poisoning are highly complex and somewhat unpredictable.

Small doses of nicotine produce nausea, vomiting, diarrhea, headache, dizziness, and neurological stimulation manifested by tachycardia, hypertension, hyperpnea, tachypnea, sweating, and salivation. Larger doses also cause cortical irritability, progressing to convulsions, and myocardial arrhythmias. Finally coma, respiratory depression and arrest, and cardiac arrest or fibrillation may supervene. Severe poisoning may cause death from respiratory failure within a few minutes.

Treatment consists of induction of emesis or gastric lavage, followed by the instillation of activated charcoal and the administration of an osmotic cathartic. Potassium permanganate will oxidize nicotine, and a 1:10,000 solution can be used for lavage. Atropine, 2 mg, and phentolamine, 5 mg, may be given intramuscularly or intravenously and repeated as often as required to control signs and symptoms of parasympathetic or sympathetic hyperactivity. These compounds are ineffective in preventing paralysis of the respiratory muscles and disturbances in cardiac rhythm. Careful attention must be given to artificial ventilation with oxygen and to therapy of catecholamine-induced cardiac tachyarrhythmias. Propranolol is the drug of choice for the latter purpose. Nicotine is rapidly detoxified in the liver, and recovery will be prompt if the patient can be tided over the initial period.

NITRITES Poisoning by the nitrite ion may result from the ingestion of large amounts of drugs such as amyl, butyl, isobutyl, or sodium nitrite. Ingested nitrates may be reduced to nitrite by intestinal bacteria, especially *Escherichia coli.* Except after the ingestion of very large amounts, adults usually absorb all nitrate before this reduction takes place. However, in children nitrite poisoning may result from the ingestion of nitrates or nitrate-containing well water. Fatalities have occurred from the oral ingestion of 2 to 4 g nitrites.

Acute nitrite poisoning may lead to severe headache, flushing, dizziness, hypotension, and syncope. Usually the patient only need be positioned to facilitate venous return to the heart. Pressor agents seldom are required. The most important toxic effect of the nitrite ion is its ability to oxidize hemoglobin to methemoglobin (Chaps. 54 and 330).

OXALIC ACID This acid is found in ink eradicators and stain removers. Ingestion causes irritation and corrosion of mouth, esophagus, and stomach, followed by vomiting and abdominal pain. After absorption it precipitates serum calcium as insoluble calcium oxalate, and the resultant hypocalcemia leads to muscular tremors, tetany, convulsions, and cardiovascular collapse. Ingestion of 5 g may cause death within minutes. Following recovery from the acute episode, there may be renal failure due to blockage of renal tubules by calcium oxalate crystals.

Treatment consists of precipitating oxalate in the gastrointestinal tract by giving calcium orally in any form, such as milk, limewater, chalk, or calcium salts. If tissue corrosion is suspected, neither emesis nor gastric lavage is indicated. A dose of 10 ml of 10% calcium gluconate should be given intravenously and repeated as required to maintain normal serum calcium and prevent tetany. In supportive therapy the maintenance of a high urine output is essential.

PARAQUAT Paraquat is a dipyridilium compound which is used in 5 to 20% aqueous solutions as a herbicide. An oral dose of 5 mg/kg may be fatal. Some victims die within 24 h in respiratory failure, often with refractive pulmonary edema. In others a serious toxic effect is the delayed (3 days to 2 weeks postingestion) development of progressive pulmonary fibrosis. The lungs selectively accumulate paraquat from the blood over several days until a critical concentration is reached, after which pulmonary edema and fibrosis ensue. Progressive respiratory failure is the usual cause of death. The metabolism of paraquat by lung tissue leads to the production of radical intermediates as well as the superoxide radical; the latter appears to be at least partly responsible for the toxicity of the compound.

Prolonged absorption (up to several days) of paraquat from the gastrointestinal tract is common. After gastric emptying, diluted bentonite (fuller's earth) or activated charcoal should be administered followed by an osmotic cathartic twice daily for 48 h. Forced diuresis, hemodialysis, and hemoperfusion significantly augment clearance of paraquat. Oxygen administration to animals experimentally poisoned with paraquat is associated with increased mortality; it would seem prudent to avoid, if possible, oxygen-enriched breathing mixtures in patients poisoned with paraquat. Intravenous administration of superoxide dysmutase has been reported to decrease lung toxicity from paraquat in animals, but no beneficial effect has been demonstrated yet in humans.

PETROLEUM DISTILLATES Petroleum distillates (diesel oil, gasoline, kerosene, paint thinner, solvent distillate) are liquids with a boiling point between 50 and 325°C. They contain variable amounts of branched or straight-chain aliphatic and aromatic hydrocarbons. Kerosene is used widely as a fuel and as a vehicle for cleaning agents, furniture polishes, insecticides, and paint thinners. Not surprisingly, each year petroleum distillates cause about 100 accidental deaths in the United States, 90 percent of these in young children. Furthermore, these products are annually responsible for almost 20,000 hospitalizations. Ingestion of 10 ml kerosene has been fatal, but adults have recovered from as much as 250 ml. Petroleum distillates are central nervous system depressants; they damage cells by dissolving cellular lipids. Pulmonary damage manifested by pulmonary edema or pneumonitis is a common and serious complication.

Inhalation of gasoline or kerosene vapors induces a state resembling alcoholic intoxication. Headache, nausea, tinnitus, and a burning sensation in the chest may also be present. When aliphatic hydrocarbons are inhaled, these symptoms may progress to profound drowsiness or coma with absence of deep reflexes. If the distillate contains a high proportion of aromatic hydrocarbons, the coma is characterized by tremors, muscle jactitations, hyperactive reflexes, and convulsions. Death usually results from respiratory depression, rarely from ventricular fibrillation.

The oral ingestion of petroleum distillates causes irritation of the mucous membranes of the upper part of the intestinal tract. When large amounts have been ingested, the same manifestations as after inhalation may appear. Frequently eructation or vomiting results in aspiration of petroleum distillates into the trachea. Because of their low surface tension, minute amounts of these substances then may spread widely throughout the lungs and produce pulmonary edema and pneumonitis. Pulmonary damage also may arise because of absorption of ingested petroleum distillates from the gastrointestinal tract. However, kerosene is at least one hundred times more toxic by the intratracheal route than when ingested.

In the treatment of poisoning by petroleum distillates extreme care must be used to prevent aspiration. If the patient is coughing when seen, aspiration is likely already to have occurred. When large amounts (>100 ml) have been ingested, gastric emptying is indicated. In the alert patient emesis may be induced; when vomiting occurs, the patient's head should be lower than his or her hips. Otherwise, gastric lavage should be performed but only after insertion of an endotracheal tube with an inflatable cuff. A saline cathartic may be administered. All victims of kerosene poisoning should be hospitalized for at least 24 h for observation. If signs or symptoms of pulmonary irritation appear, oxygen should be given. Steroids do not appear useful in treatment of this pulmonary lesion and may be detrimental. Prophylactic antibiotics are not indicated. Symptomatic therapy for central nervous system depression or treatment of convulsions may be necessary. Sympathomimetic amines should be avoided because of the danger of inducing ventricular fibrillation in the hydrocarbon-sensitized heart.

PHENCYCLIDINE Phencyclidine (PCP, "angel dust") has become a common and dangerous drug of abuse. It is structurally similar to ketamine hydrochloride and is used as a general anesthetic in veterinary medicine, but its powerful psychomimetic properties make it unsuitable for human use. The drug can be inhaled, smoked, swallowed, or injected; at doses as low as 1 to 5 mg euphoria, numbness, and emotional lability result. Higher doses cause disorientation, confusion, restlessness, and psychosis. Doses as high as 1 g have reportedly been taken and have resulted in prolonged comatose states, seizures, spasticity, opisthotonos, hypertension on occasion severe enough to cause intracranial hemorrhage, respiratory depression, and death.

Phencyclidine is metabolized by the liver, and the metabolites as well as some free drug are excreted in the urine. Since the drug is a base, it is trapped in ionized form in the stomach, and treatment begins with emesis or lavage even if the drug was not taken orally. This is followed by charcoal instillation and administration of an osmotic cathartic. The drug's renal clearance can be increased as much as twentyfold by forced diuresis after acidification of the urine (pH<5). Oral ammonium chloride and intravenous ascorbic acid are used to achieve and maintain the urinary pH, and a diuretic is administered. In addition, a significant clearance of phencyclidine is obtained by a continuously draining nasogastric tube. Hypertension occasionally requires treatment, seizures should be controlled with diazepam, and psychosis is best treated with butyrophenones and not phenothiazines.

PHENOL Phenol and related compounds (creosote, cresols, hexachlorophene, hydroquinone, Lysol, resorcinol, tannic acid) are used as antiseptics, caustics, and preservatives. These substances poison all cells by denaturing and precipitating cellular proteins. The approximate fatal oral dose ranges from 2 ml for phenol and cresols to 20 ml for tannic acid.

Ingestion of phenolic compounds produces erosion of mucosa from mouth to stomach. The corroded areas may have a characteristic dead-white appearance. Hematemesis and bloody diarrhea may occur. After an initial phase of hyperpnea due to stimulation of the respiratory center, stupor, coma, convulsions, pulmonary edema, and shock are seen. The initial respiratory alkalosis is soon followed by a profound acidosis which results from the renal excretion of base during the alkalotic stage, from the acidic nature of phenol, and from disturbances in carbohydrate metabolism presumably the result of defects in enzymatic function. If the patient survives the acute stage, acute tubular necrosis may lead to oliguria or anuria and hepatic toxicity to jaundice.

Poisoning by phenolic compounds often may be diagnosed by their characteristic odor. Development of a violet or blue color of the urine after addition of a few drops of ferric chloride indicates the presence of a phenolic compound.

Emesis and lavage are indicated for treatment in the absence of significant corrosive injury to the esophagus. Activated charcoal should be administered. Although definitive proof of efficacy is lacking, olive oil or castor oil, which dissolve phenol and are reputed to retard its absorption, may be given, followed by an osmotic cathartic. Supportive therapy consists of correction of the acidosis, the control of shock and convulsions, and the maintenance of a patent airway in the face of glottal edema by intubation or tracheotomy.

PHOSPHORUS Phosphorus occurs in two forms: a red, nonpoisonous form and a yellow, fat-soluble, highly toxic form. The latter is used in rodent and insect poisons and in fireworks. Yellow phosphorus and phosphides cause fatty degeneration and necrosis of tissues, particularly of the liver. The lethal ingested dose of yellow phosphorus is approximately 50 mg.

Ingestion of yellow phosphorus is followed within 1 h by burning pain in the upper part of the gastrointestinal tract, vomiting, diarrhea, and a garlic odor of the breath and excreta. The patient may die in coma during the first day or two, or symptoms may subside after a few hours. Then, 1 to 2 days later, the victim may develop tender hepatomegaly, jaundice, hypocalcemia, hypotension, and oliguria and may die following convulsions and coma. Death from acute hepatic necrosis may occur in a few days.

Treatment consists of induction of emesis or gastric lavage, instillation of activated charcoal, and administration of an osmotic cathartic. Calcium gluconate is given intravenously to maintain the serum calcium level. Treatment is otherwise supportive.

SALICYLATES Each year 30 million pounds of aspirin is consumed in the United States, and salicylates can probably be found in most American households. Aspirin is found in many compound analgesic tablets. Methyl salicylate (oil of wintergreen) is present in most skin liniments, and salicylic acid is used in ointments and corn plasters. The ingestion of 10 to 30 g aspirin or sodium salicylate may be fatal to adults, but survival has been reported after an oral dose of 130 g aspirin.

Salicylate intoxication may result from the cumulative effect of therapeutic administration of high doses. There is considerable individual variation: toxic symptoms may begin at dosages of 3 g per day or may not appear when 10 g per day is given. Toxic symptoms are also poorly correlated with the serum salicylate concentration, but few patients become intoxicated at levels less than 15 mg/dl and most at levels over 35 mg/dl. Therapeutic salicylate intoxication is usually mild and is called "salicylism." The earliest symptoms are vertigo, tinnitus, and impairment of hearing. Further overdosage causes nausea, vomiting, sweating, diarrhea, fever, drowsiness, headache, dimness of vision, and mental aberrations. The latter may be characterized by confusion, excitement, restlessness, and talkativeness; this "salicylate jag" resembles alcoholic intoxication without the euphoria. The central nervous system effects may progress to hallucinations, convulsions, and coma. Toxic doses of salicylates also have a direct stimulant effect on the respiratory center, resulting in hyperventilation, loss of carbon dioxide, and respiratory alkalosis. Renal excretion of bicarbonate may compensate partially for this.

In acute salicylate poisoning due to accidental or suicidal ingestion of massive amounts, the same manifestations may be seen in more rapid succession. However, they usually are overshadowed by severe disturbances in the acid-base balance which follow a definite sequence. Early in the course of intoxication there may be only hyperpnea, and the seriousness of the poisoning may not be appreciated at that time. The hyperventilation causes a fall in blood P_{CO_2} and an increase in pH. Renal excretion of bicarbonate, sodium, and potassium will bring the pH back toward normal and produce a compensated respiratory alkalosis. At that point the buffering capacity of the extracellular fluid will have been decreased significantly. In young children and after large doses in adults further developments may then produce a combination of respiratory acidosis and metabolic acidosis which stems from a number of factors. High concentrations of salicylate depress the respiratory center and cause CO_2 retention. Renal function becomes impaired because of dehydration and hypotension, and inorganic metabolic acids accumulate. Furthermore, salicylic acid derivatives may displace several milliequivalents of blood bicarbonate. Finally, salicylates impair carbohydrate metabolism and cause accumulation of acetoacetic, lactic, and pyruvic acids. Severe acidosis and disturbances in electrolyte balance are seen most commonly in febrile young children.

Blood salicylate levels are of value in the estimation of the severity of poisoning. Serious poisoning is rare at levels less than 50 mg/dl but usual at levels between 50 and 100 mg/dl. Levels above 100 mg/dl during the first 6 h after poisoning signify severe intoxication and may be fatal. Excretion of salicylates is renal, and in the presence of normal renal function about 50 percent will be excreted in 24 h. Addition of a few drops of ferric chloride solution to 5 ml boiled acidified urine containing salicylate yields a violet color and may aid in diagnosis.

Treatment of salicylate poisoning consists of initially inducing emesis or of gastric lavage after which activated charcoal and then an osmotic cathartic are administered. Disturbances of acid-base or electrolyte balance and hypoglycemia are corrected by the intravenous administration of appropriate solutions. Respiratory depression may require artificial ventilation with oxygen. Convulsions may be treated with diazepam or phenobarbital. The renal clearance of salicylate is enhanced ten- to twentyfold if the pH of the urine can be kept between 7 and 8. In addition to intravenous bicarbonate and a diuretic to raise the pH above 7, it may be necessary to give potassium to prevent paradoxical aciduria. Peritoneal dialysis and hemodialysis are also highly effective in removing salicylate from seriously poisoned patients, but forced alkaline diuresis is so effective in clearing salicylate that these maneuvers most often are not required.

SMOKE Poisoning by smoke is usually due to carbon monoxide inhalation. However, burning material may also release irritant fumes. Many irritant gases combine with water to form corrosive acids or alkalies and cause chemical burns of exposed skin and of the upper part of the respiratory tract. Such gases (and the corrosives formed) are ammonia (ammonium hydroxide), nitrogen oxide (nitric acid), sulfur dioxide (sulfurous acid), and sulfur trioxide (sulfuric acid). These irritating gases as well as hydrogen sulfide also may be present in smog. Another highly toxic gas which may be inhaled by firefighters or victims is phosgene. This compound is formed by the high-temperature decomposition of chlorinated hydrocarbons and is released when carbon tetrachloride from fire extinguishers comes into contact with hot surfaces.

After inhalation of irritant gases the victim may notice burning pain in throat and chest and severe coughing. These symptoms may subside completely, but from several hours to a day after exposure dyspnea and cyanosis may appear and progress rapidly to severe pulmonary edema and death from respiratory and circulatory failure. Treatment consists of administration of oxygen and adrenal steroids and appropriate therapy of pulmonary edema, should that develop.

SULFIDES Hydrogen sulfide is a gas released by the decomposition of organic sulfur compounds and is used widely in industry. Carbon disulfide is an industrial solvent. Other sulfides have industrial uses and release hydrogen sulfide in contact with water or acids. Significant concentrations of hydrogen sulfide may be present in smoke or smog. Inhalation of hydrogen sulfide in concentrations above 50 ppm (50 times the minimum detectable by smell) causes conjunctivitis, headache, nausea, soreness of the upper respiratory passages, pulmonary edema, and drowsiness. Concentrations in excess of 300 ppm may cause coma, respiratory depression, and death. Ingestion of carbon disulfide or soluble sulfides is followed by vomiting, headache, hypotension, respiratory depression, tremors, coma, convulsions, and death. The fatal oral dose of carbon disulfide is approximately 1 g. Treatment of sulfide intoxication is supportive. Administration of sodium nitrite may promote the binding of sulfide in sulfmethemoglobin.

REFERENCES

General

ARENA JM: *Poisoning,* 3d ed. Springfield, Ill., Charles C Thomas, 1974

ARLEFF AL et al: Coma following nonnarcotic drug overdosage—management of 208 adult patients. Am J Med Sci 266:405, 1973

BOURNE PG: *Acute Drug Abuse Emergencies.* New York, Academic, 1976

Casarett and Doull's Toxicology: The Basic Science of Poisons, 2d ed, J Doull, CD Klaasen, MO Amdur (eds). New York, Macmillan, 1980

DREISBACH RH: *Handbook of Poisoning: Diagnosis and Treatment,* 10th ed. Los Altos, Calif., Lange, 1980

EASOM JM, LOVEJOY FH: Efficacy and safety of gastrointestinal decontamination in the treatment of oral poisoning. Pediatr Clin North Am 26:827, 1979

LOOMIS TA: *Essentials of Toxicology,* 3d ed. Philadelphia, Lea & Febiger, 1978

LOVEJOY FH JR: Acute poisoning, in *Current Pediatric Therapy,* 9th ed, SS Gellis, BM Kegan (eds). Philadelphia, Saunders, 1980, pp 654–675

SMITH RP, GOSSELIN RE: Current concepts about the treatment of selected poisonings. Annu Rev Pharmacol Toxicol 16:189, 1976

WINCHESTER JF et al: Dialysis and hemoperfusion of poisons and drugs—update. Trans Am Soc Artif Intern Organs 23:762, 1977

ZENZ C: *Occupational Medicine.* Chicago, Year Book, 1975

Toxic product information

GLEASON MN et al: *Clinical Toxicology of Commercial Products,* 4th ed. Baltimore, Williams & Wilkins, 1976

GOODMAN and GILMAN: *The Pharmacological Basis of Therapeutics,* 6th ed, AG Goodman, LS Goodman (eds). New York, Macmillan, 1980

HAYES WJ: *Toxicology of Pesticides.* Baltimore, Williams & Wilkins, 1975

The Merck Index, 9th ed. Rahway, NJ, Merck & Co, 1976

Poisonous Plants and Fungi. Philadelphia, Rittenhouse, 1976

SCHERZ RG: The history of poison control centers in the United States. Clin Toxicol 12:291, 1978

WILSON CO, JONES TE: *American Drug Index.* Philadelphia, Lippincott, 1981

COMMON POISONS

Acetaminophen

BLACK N: Acetaminophen hepatotoxicity. Gastroenterology 78:382, 1980

PRESCOTT LF et al: Treatment of paracetamol poisoning with *N*-acetylcysteine. Lancet 2:432, 1977

RUMACK BH: Aspirin and acetaminophen. Clin Toxicol 15:313, 1979

Antimuscarinic compounds

GOWDY JM: Stromonium intoxication. JAMA 221:585, 1972

RUMACK BH: Anticholinergic poisoning: Treatment with physostigmine. Pediatrics 52:449, 1973

Barium

GOULD DB et al: Barium sulfide poisoning. Arch Intern Med 132:891, 1973

Benzene, toluene

HAYDEN JW: The clinical toxicology of solvent abuse. Clin Toxicol 9:169, 1976

TAHER SM et al: Renal tubular acidosis associated with toluene "sniffing." N Engl J Med 290:765, 1974

Boric acid

VALDES-DAPENA MA, AREY JB: Boric acid poisoning. J Pediatr 61:531, 1962

WONG LC et al: Boric acid poisoning: Report of 11 cases. Can Med Assoc J 90:1018, 1964

Carbon monoxide

REMICK RA, MILES JE: Carbon monoxide poisoning: Neurologic and psychiatric sequelae. Can Med Assoc J 117:654, 1977

TURINO GM: Effect of carbon monoxide on the cardiorespiratory system. Circulation 63:253A, 1981

WINTER PM, MILLER JN: Carbon monoxide poisoning. JAMA 236:1502, 1976

Castor bean

BENSON S: On the mechanism of protein-synthesis inhibition by abrin and ricin. Eur J Biochem 59:573, 1975

BRUGHSCH HG: The castor bean. N Engl J Med 262:1039, 1960

Caustics

CAMPBELL GS et al: Treatment of corrosive burns of the esophagus. Arch Surg 112:495, 1977

RUMACK BH, BURLINGTON JD: Caustic ingestions: A rational look at diluents. Clin Toxicol 11(1):27, 1977

Chlorate

HELLIWELL M, NUNN J: Mortality in sodium chlorate poisoning. Br Med J 1:1119, 1979

Chlorinated insecticides

BOYLAN JJ et al: Cholestyramine: Use of a new therapeutic approach for chlordecone (Kepone) poisoning. Science 199:893, 1978

STARR GH, CLIFFORD NJ: Acute lindane intoxication. Arch Environ Health 25:374, 1972

TAYLOR JR, CALABRESE VP: Organochlorine and other insecticides. Handbook Clin Neurol 36:391, 1979

Cholinesterase inhibitor insecticides

LUZHNIKOR EA et al: Plasma perfusion through charcoal in methylparathion poisoning. Lancet 1:38, 1977

MILBY TH: Prevention and management of organophosphate poisoning. JAMA 216:2131, 1971

QUINBY GE: Further therapeutic experience with pralidoximes in organic phosphorus poisoning. JAMA 187:202, 1964

WYCKOFF W et al: Diagnostic and therapeutic problems of parathion poisonings. Ann Intern Med 68:875, 1968

Cyanide

BRAICO KT et al: Laetrile intoxication: Report of a fatal case. N Engl J Med 300:238, 1979

BURROWS GE et al: Effect of oxygen on cyanide intoxication. J Pharmacol Exp Ther 184:739, 1973

CHEN KK, ROSE CL: Treatment of acute cyanide poisoning. JAMA 162:1154, 1956

HUMBERT JR et al: Fatal cyanide poisoning: Accidental ingestion of amygdalin. JAMA 238:482, 1977

Detergents

ARENA JM: Poisonings and other health hazards associated with use of detergents. JAMA 190:56, 1964

WILSON, JT, BURR, IM: Benzalkonium chloride poisoning in infant twins. Am J Dis Child 129:1208, 1975

Fluorides

YOLKEN R et al: Acute fluoride poisoning. Pediatrics 58:90, 1976

Glycols

MORIARTY RW, MCDONALD RH: The spectrum of ethylene glycol poisoning. Clin Toxicol 7:583, 1974

PARRY MF, WALLACH R: Ethylene glycol poisoning. Am J Med 57:143, 1974

PETERSON CD et al: Ethylene glycol poisoning. N Engl J Med 304:21, 1981

Halogenated hydrocarbons

BAERG RD, KIMBERG DV: Centrilobular hepatic necrosis and acute renal failure in "solvent sniffers." Ann Intern Med 73:713, 1970

OETTINGEN WF VON: *The Halogenated Hydrocarbons of Industrial and Toxicological Importance.* Amsterdam, Elsevier, 1964

RECHNAGEL RO: Carbon tetrachloride hepatotoxicity. Pharmacol Rev 19:145, 1967

SCHWARZBECK A, KOSTERS W: Extracorporeal hemoperfusion in acute carbon tetrachloride intoxication. Arch Toxicol 35:207, 1976

Iron salts

FISCHER DS et al: Acute iron poisoning in children. JAMA 218:1179, 1971

HADDAD LM: Iron poisoning. J Am Coll Emergency Physicians 5:691, 1976

Isopropyl alcohol

FREIREICH AW et al: Hemodialysis for isopropanol poisoning. N Engl J Med 277:699, 1967

Methyl alcohol

BENNET H JR et al: Acute methyl alcohol poisoning: A review based on experiences in an outbreak of 323 cases. Medicine 32:431, 1953

COOPER JR, KINI MM: Biochemical aspects of methanol poisoning. Biochem Pharmacol 11:405, 1962

KEYVAN-LARIJARNI H, TANNENBERG M: Methanol intoxication: Comparison of peritoneal and hemodialysis. Arch Intern Med 134:293, 1974

Mushrooms

LITTEN W: The most poisonous mushrooms. Sci Am 232(3):90, 1975

PAASO B, HARRISON DC: A new look at an old problem: Mushroom poisoning. Am J Med 58:505, 1975

Naphthalene

HAGGERTY RJ: Naphthalene poisoning. N Engl J Med 255:919, 1956

Nicotine

GEHLBACH SH et al: Nicotine absorption by workers harvesting green tobacco. Lancet 1:478, 1975

TAYLOR WJR et al: Pesticide poisoning in children. Drug Ther 1(11):15, 1971

Nitrites

KEATING JP et al: Infantile methemoglobinemia caused by carrot juice. N Engl J Med 288:824, 1973

Paraquat

FAIRSHTER RD, WILSON RF: Paraquat poisoning: Manifestations and therapy. Am J Med 59:751, 1975

OKONABE S, HOFMANN A: Efficacy of gut lavage, hemodialysis and hemoperfusion in the therapy of paraquat and diquat intoxication. Arch Toxikol 36:45, 1976

Petroleum distillates

BROWN J et al: Experimental kerosene pneumonia: Evaluation of some therapeutic regimens. J Pediatr 84:396, 1974

SHIRKEY H: Treatment of petroleum distillate ingestion. Mod Treat 8:580, 1971

TAUSSIG LN et al: Pulmonary function 8 to 10 years after hydrocarbon pneumonitis. Clin Pediatr 16:57, 1977

Phencyclidine

ARONOW R, DONE AK: Phencyclidine overdose: An emerging concept of management. J Coll Emergency Physicians 7:56, 1978

PEARLSON GD: Psychiatric and medical syndromes associated with phencyclidine (PCP) abuse. Johns Hopkins Med J 1:25, 1981

Phosphorus

SIMON FA, PICKERING LK: Acute yellow phosphorus poisoning. JAMA 235:1343, 1976

TALLEY RC et al: Acute elemental phosphorus poisoning in man: Cardiovascular toxicity. Am Heart J 84:139, 1972

WINEK CL et al: Yellow phosphorus ingestions: Three fatal poisonings. Clin Toxicol 6:541, 1973

Salicylates

ANDERSON RJ et al: Unrecognized adult salicylate intoxication. Ann Intern Med 85:745, 1976

BUSCHANUN N, RABINOWITZ L: Infantile salicylism: A reappraisal. J Pediatr 84:391, 1974

DONE AK, TEMPLE AR: Treatment of salicylate poisoning. Mod Treat 8:528, 1971

HILL JB: Salicylate intoxication. N Engl J Med 288:1110, 1973

PROUDFOOT AT, BROWN SS: Acidaemia and salicylate poisoning in adults. Br Med J 2:537, 1969

SEGAR WE, HOLLIDAY MA: Physiologic abnormalities of salicylate intoxication. N Engl J Med 259:1191, 1958

239 HEAVY METALS

DAVID C. POSKANZER

Three highly effective chemicals, BAL, Versene, and penicillamine, are available for treatment of systemic poisoning with heavy metals by forming nontoxic, stable cyclic compounds with polyvalent metallic ions, thus permitting the offending material to be excreted safely in the urine.

The first to be developed was BAL (British antilewisite, 2,3-dimercaptopropanol, dimercaprol), which was originally intended as an antidote against the arsenical war gas, lewisite. Its tendency to combine with certain metallic ions such as arsenic, mercury, cobalt, nickel, antimony, and gold is so great that it can remove them from combination with the enzymes whose function they impair in the body. By itself BAL is not useful in treating lead poisoning. Because the effectiveness of BAL depends to some extent upon the speed with which its administration is begun, every attempt should be made to avoid delay in its use. For serious systemic intoxications, BAL should be given in doses of 5 mg per kg body weight intramuscularly as a 10% solution in oil and 20% benzyl benzoate. No single dose should exceed 300 mg. This dose should be repeated every 4 h on the first day and every 6 h on the second day. Thereafter, it should be given three times daily for several days; doses should then be tapered and discontinued about 10 days after acute poisoning. When the dose of poison has been relatively small, the schedule of BAL administration may be reduced by one-third. Because BAL is excreted in part by the kidneys, it can accumulate to toxic concentrations in anuric patients. Overdosage results in nervousness, hyperactivity, muscle twitching, and hyperreflexia. Large doses may produce convulsions. The presence of the material in tears sometimes causes blepharospasm. In patients with anuria or oliguria, therefore, BAL should be administered with caution and at a lower dosage than outlined above. If symptoms of overdosage occur, sedatives should be administered.

The second antidote to metal poisons is the chelating agent Versene (ethylenediaminetetraacetate, EDTA), which forms cyclic, stable, soluble, nontoxic compounds with most metals. Because Versene reacts with calcium in the same way as with other metals, it must be given as the calcium salt (Calcium Disodium Versenate; calcium disodiumedetate) to avoid hypocalcemia. The material has been used with notable success in the treatment of lead poisoning. It is given in a dosage of 1.0 g in 250 ml of 5% glucose intravenously every 12 h for 5 days. After a pause to allow for further solution of metal from body stores a second and even a third course may be given.

Penicillamine (Cuprimine, β,β-dimethylcysteine) is an excellent chelating agent for copper, mercury, and lead, promotes their excretion in the urine, and has the additional advantage of being well absorbed from the gastrointestinal tract. It may be given orally, while BAL and Versene require systemic injection. N-Acetyl-*dl*-penicillamine is even more effective than penicillamine in protecting against the effects of mercury, probably because it is more resistant to metabolic degradation, and it has the advantage of being less toxic. Penicillamine is administered orally in a dose of 1 to 4 g daily on an empty stomach to avoid chelation of dietary metals. It has much lower toxicity than BAL, the only other agent which is effective in the treatment of Wilson's disease (hepatolenticular degeneration), in which toxic amounts of copper are deposited in various tissues, but has the disadvantage of acute sensitivity reactions. It has also been shown to be useful in lead poisoning, but the excretion of urinary lead may not be as high after oral penicillamine as after intravenous Calcium Disodium Versenate.

N-Acetyl-*dl*-penicillamine, available as an investigational drug, has been demonstrated to be effective in mercury poisoning and has the advantage of allowing much higher doses with fewer toxic effects. It has less effect on copper levels than penicillamine and is therefore used in the treatment of mercury poisoning when one would wish to maintain copper levels. The administration of 1 to 2 g daily in divided doses for 10 days gives good results.

ANTIMONY Symptoms of poisoning after the ingestion of antimony may occur when an acid food is allowed to stand in cheap enamelware or "graniteware" for a sufficient time to allow solution of antimony, which is used in the manufacture of these products. Certain parasiticidal drugs also contain this metal. The symptoms are similar to those produced by arsenic, except that antimony causes a more rapid onset of gastrointestinal symptoms. Treatment is the same as for arsenic, including use of BAL. Circulatory collapse occurs early and requires vigorous supportive treatment.

ARSENIC Arsenic poisoning is usually the result of accidental or suicidal ingestion of insecticides or rodenticides containing Paris green (copper acetoarsenate) or calcium or lead arsenate. Pesticides containing arsenic are a frequent source of poisoning in rural areas of the United States. Workers at copper-smelting factories are also at risk of arsenic poisoning as arsenic trioxide is a by-product of the smelting process. Some workers have been noted to have abnormal nerve conduction studies in the absence of overt clinical signs of peripheral neuropathy.

The toxic dose of inorganic arsenic varies considerably and seems to depend upon individual susceptibility. Orchardists have been found to ingest as much as 6.8 mg arsenic a day without any signs of intoxication. On the other hand, as little as 30 mg arsenic trioxide has been fatal. Arsenic has a predilection for keratin, and the concentration of arsenic in the hair and nails is higher than that in other tissues. Arsenic reacts with the —SH groups in certain tissue proteins and thus interferes with a number of enzyme systems essential to cellular metabolism. Pathologic changes in fatal inorganic arsenical poisoning are fatty degeneration of the liver, hyperemia and hemorrhages of the intestine, and renal tubular necrosis. The peripheral nerves often show disintegration of axis cylinders (axonal neuropathy) with fragmentation and resorption of myelin.

The symptoms of acute poisoning by the oral route are nausea, vomiting, diarrhea, severe burning of the mouth and throat, and agonizing abdominal pains. The vomitus often contains blood. Circulatory collapse is frequent, and death may ensue within a few hours. With chronic exposure, the first signs of poisoning are usually weakness, prostration, muscular aching, or nervous system involvement; gastrointestinal symptoms are minimal. In patients exposed to arsine gas (hydrogen arsenide), the outstanding features are hemolysis, chills, fever, and hemoglobinuria.

Patients who recover from acute poisoning and those with chronic intoxication usually develop skin and mucosal changes, peripheral neuropathy, and linear pigmentations in the fingernails (see Chap. 368). The *cutaneous manifestations* appear within 1 to 4 weeks and consist of a diffuse, dry, scaly desquamation, occasionally with hyperpigmentation, over the trunk and extremities. Hyperkeratoses of the palms and soles and edema of the face and extremities may also occur. The mucous membranes also show evidence of irritation, with conjunctivitis, photophobia, pharyngitis, or irritating cough. About 5 weeks after exposure to arsenic, a transverse white stria, 1 to 2 mm in width, appears above the lunula of each fingernail (*Mees line*). Patients with more than one exposure to arsenic may show double lines several millimeters apart.

Symptoms of headache, drowsiness, confusion, and convulsions are seen in both acute and chronic intoxication. Evidence of peripheral neuropathy usually appears 1 to 3 weeks after exposure. There are numbness, tingling, and burning of the feet and hands, followed by muscular weakness. The extremities show a decrease in touch, pain, and temperature sensations, in a symmetrical "stocking-glove" distribution, and distal weakness with inability to walk or stand, weakness of grip, and wrist drop. Tendon reflexes are absent or diminished, and atrophy of the affected muscles develops rapidly.

The laboratory findings usually consist of moderate anemia and a leukopenia of 2000 to 5000 white blood cells per mm^3 with mild eosinophilia. There is slight proteinuria, and liver function tests show mild abnormalities. The spinal fluid is normal.

None of the clinical or laboratory manifestations of arsenic poisoning is specific, and the diagnosis depends upon analysis of the urine for arsenic. Because arsenic is found widely in nature, and hence in water and food, its discovery in hair and nails may not be diagnostic. Normal persons have an average concentration of 0.05 mg arsenic per 100 g hair. Concentrations of arsenic greater than 0.1 mg per 100 g hair are considered indicative of poisoning. The minimal level of arsenic in the urine indicating intoxication is difficult to establish. Normal persons have been found to excrete between 0.01 and 0.06 mg arsenic per liter, and a few individuals as much as 0.2 mg per liter. Although there is considerable overlap, most patients with evidence of arsenic intoxication will be found to excrete more than 0.1 mg per liter; soon after acute exposure, many will show levels greater than 1 mg per liter.

The treatment for acute ingestion is gastric lavage (see Chap. 238). Replacement of lost fluids and elevation of blood pressure by vasopressor agents is often indicated. Immediate treatment with BAL should be instituted. Patients with peripheral neuropathy rarely show significant improvement with BAL and continue to have sensory disturbances and weakness for many months. Dramatic responses, however, have been observed with the use of BAL in the treatment of exfoliative dermatitis, bone marrow depression, and encephalopathy caused by the arsphenamines and the organic arsenicals. BAL is of little value in the treatment of the hemolysis caused by inhalation of arsine.

BISMUTH Poisoning by bismuth was formerly almost entirely a complication of antisyphilitic therapy. However, within the past 7 years, a new neurologic disease associated with oral intake of bismuth for chronic digestive disorders has appeared in Australia and France. The illness is characterized by a long prodromal phase with incoordination, depression, and irritability followed by a fairly rapid deterioration with severe confusion, myoclonic jerking, dysarthria, and inability to stand or walk. Osteoarthropathy of the shoulders has occurred in some patients. In France, where over 900 cases have been reported, death has occurred in 72 patients. Recovery invariably follows the withdrawal of bismuth in 2 to 3 weeks. In some patients there may be residual memory loss. Elevations of bismuth blood levels have sometimes been found to reach 2500 μg per liter. Patients who ingested comparable doses of bismuth but did not develop bismuth encephalopathy showed blood levels of less than 50 μg per liter. The mechanism by which bismuth encephalopathy occurs is not known. The development of a bluish stippled line of pigmentation just at the margin of the gums is not dangerous but suggests that oral hygiene should be improved. Bismuth subnitrate occasionally gives rise to methemoglobinemia (Chap. 330).

CADMIUM Cadmium is released into the environment through smelting of zinc and lead ores, coal and oil combustion, and industrial waste disposal. Pigments that contain cadmium are used in the production of plastics, luminous paints, antiseptics, and fungicides. Chronic cadmium poisoning occurs after prolonged inhalation of cadmium fumes or dust; signs of pulmonary dysfunction and renal damage may not appear until many years after the last exposure. Clinically, cadmium nephropathy results from damage caused by accumulation of the metal in the proximal tubular cells of the kidney. Acute poisoning is likely to occur after ingestion of an acid food prepared in a cadmium-lined vessel. The classic example is lemonade served from metal cans. Symptoms of nausea, vomiting, diarrhea, and prostration usually develop within 10 min after ingestion. Treatment is symptomatic, and symptoms ordinarily subside within 24 h. The short length of time after ingestion and the typical circumstances suggest the diagnosis. The use of BAL is not recommended for cadmium intoxication, as the BAL-cadmium complex dissociates in the kidneys and cadmium is nephrotoxic.

COPPER See Chap. 84 for a discussion of disturbances in trace element metabolism, including copper, zinc, cobalt, nickel, silicon, and fluorine.

GOLD Because practically all cases of poisoning by gold are associated with its use in the treatment of arthritis, diagnosis is usually easy. Manifestations are skin rashes of various types, bone marrow depression, icterus, oliguria, nausea, vomiting, and gastrointestinal bleeding. Treatment consists of symptomatic relief of discomfort and the use of BAL, an effective antidote.

LEAD Poisoning results from inhalation of fumes as from burning storage batteries, solder, paint spraying, or processes requiring the remelting of metallic lead. Ingestion of lead-containing materials such as paint, or water which has stood in lead pipes, is less important in adults. Illicit whiskey contaminated by lead solder in the pipes of stills has been responsible for cases of poisoning. Bullets or buckshot containing lead can cause poisoning years after becoming embedded in a serous cavity. The most common form of lead poisoning today is that encountered in children who ingest lead-containing outdoor paint, often used indoors in older houses. It has a sweetish, apparently attractive taste. Absorption is slow by any route, and prolonged exposure is required for the development of symptoms. Lead is a cumulative poison, excreted slowly. Acute poisoning is virtually nonexistent. Symptoms may develop suddenly after chronic exposure. Most of the absorbed lead is deposited in the bones; blood, urine, and feces contain only small amounts.

Manifestations of poisoning are colic, encephalopathy, peripheral neuritis, and anemia.

Lead colic, or painter's cramps, is characterized by agonizing, wandering, poorly localized abdominal pain, often with spasm and rigidity of the musculature of the abdominal wall. There is no fever or leukocytosis. Needless surgery has been carried out in these patients for supposed perforation of peptic ulcer or other catastrophe. Morphine has surprisingly little effect upon the pain; intravenous injection of calcium salts affords relief within a short time, although pain may recur. Attacks of colic seem to be brought on by intercurrent infection or alcoholic overindulgence.

Encephalopathy occurs chiefly in children and is manifested by convulsions, somnolence, mania, delirium, or coma. The mortality rate is high when convulsive seizures and coma occur. In an unexplained acute encephalopathy of childhood, increased intracranial pressure associated with high protein and the absence of cells should suggest the possibility of lead poisoning.

Peripheral neuritis with paralysis, characteristically involving the muscles most used (e.g., wrist drop in painters, etc.), occurs in patients exposed to lead, often in the absence of other symptoms. It is rare in children. (See Chap. 368.)

Mild anemia, probably the result of increased brittleness of the erythrocytes as well as a defect in cell maturation, is common. Pallor is out of proportion to anemia in patients with chronic plumbism and is attributed to spasm of small vessels in the skin. Anemia is almost never severe and is characterized by the presence of large numbers of erythrocytes with basophilic stippling. This is seen in other hematologic disorders, but a smear showing stippling should arouse suspicion of lead poisoning. In patients with poor oral hygiene a "lead line" of black lead sulfide may develop along the gingival margins. This is not seen in edentulous persons and is rare in children.

Patients with lead poisoning excrete increased amounts of coproporphyrin III in the urine (see Chap. 99). This is so consistent that examination of a urine specimen for porphyrin is the best screening test in suspected cases. A few milliliters of urine should be acidified with acetic acid and shaken with an equal volume of ether. Exposure of a specimen prepared in this manner under a Wood's lamp will reveal reddish fluorescence of the ether layer if coproporphyrin is present. A positive test result is strongly in favor of lead intoxication. Urinary lead determinations are of aid in confirming the diagnosis; a level of 0.2 mg per liter or more is usually regarded as significant, although interpretations vary. Diagnosis can be confirmed by promoting lead excretion with three doses of Calcium Disodium Versenate (25 mg per kg) at 8-h intervals. Excretion of over 500 μg in 24 h is indicative of excessive lead burden. A single blood lead level is rarely of help in diagnosis in adults because blood is cleared promptly of circulating lead.

Lead encephalopathy occurs chiefly in children, has a significant mortality rate, and causes severe permanent brain damage in 25 percent of survivors. Encephalopathy in adults is rare and usually results from consumption of lead-contaminated illicit liquor. Once minor symptoms of poisoning are present, acute encephalopathy can develop with unpredictable rapidity. Any child with symptoms suggestive of lead poisoning should be considered to have a medical emergency and should be hospitalized immediately. The onset of encephalopathy is signaled by the development of gross ataxia, persistent vomiting, and intermittent lethargy and stupor. These symptoms are followed by convulsions, confusion, and coma.

The most important single feature of treatment is removal of the patient from further exposure to lead. Once abnormal absorption is terminated, virtually all the lead in the body is shifted into bone. Chelating agents do not remove significant quantities of lead from bone. It takes approximately twice as long to excrete a given burden of lead as it does to accumulate it. As long as significant quantities of lead remain in bone, any intercurrent illness which causes demineralization can cause mobilization of toxic quantities of lead into soft tissues and exacerbate plumbism.

The treatment of lead encephalopathy is begun once adequate urine flow is established. A combination of BAL and Calcium Disodium Versenate is employed, and the Versene therapy continued for 5 to 7 days. If Calcium Disodium Versenate is given alone in the presence of very high tissue concentrations of lead, some of the toxic effects may be intensified. Acute symptoms usually subside within 48 to 72 h after Versene is begun. Within 2 weeks urinary excretion of coproporphyrin ceases, and there is sometimes a dramatic improvement in neuritis.

Symptoms of acute increased intracranial pressure are best treated with repeated doses of mannitol given intravenously. High-potency corticosteroids are also useful in relieving cerebral edema in patients with lead encephalopathy.

Lead-based paint in old, low-income housing is the major source of lead poisoning in children. Although mass screening programs of lead exposure among children in the United States show a sharp decline of severe lead poisoning, asymptomatic lead absorption is still a serious problem. Impairment of neuropsychological and classroom behavior has been demonstrated in children with elevated dentine lead levels. Nonadaptive classroom behavior increases in a dose-related fashion to dentine lead and is not limited to children with the highest lead levels.

In adults, combined therapy with BAL and Calcium Disodium Versenate followed by oral penicillamine is probably indicated whenever blood levels exceed 100 μg lead per 100 g blood, even in the absence of symptoms. Evidence of lead toxicity is usually present at this level, and the risk of symptomatic episodes is considerable. The use of oral penicillamine alone in a dose of 1 to 1.5 g daily for 3 to 5 days in mildly symptomatic cases has been suggested and has the advantage of easy administration and the avoidance of painful injections.

MERCURY Poisoning occurs chiefly as a result of the acute ingestion of a soluble salt, usually mercuric chloride (bichloride of mercury). Toxic symptoms may occur with 0.1 g, and 0.5 g is almost always fatal unless immediate treatment is instituted. The mercuric ion is corrosive and produces severe local inflammation. Oral, pharyngeal, and laryngeal pain are severe; abdominal cramps with nausea and vomiting occur within 15 min. As mercury is absorbed, it is concentrated in the kidneys, where it poisons the tubular cells, producing a tendency to diuresis within the first 2 to 3 h. The combination of vomiting, dehydration, shock, and progressive tubular damage, however, soon leads to anuria and uremia. The poison is also excreted into the colon and produces severe enteritis, with bloody diarrhea and tenesmus. Death is usually from uremia. The chief objectives of treatment are to prevent the shock of dehydration and to remove mercury from the body. Early in treatment, copious quantities of fluid should be infused intravenously to prevent dehydration and to reduce the concentration of mercuric ion in the renal tubules. That the patient is anuric early is often simply the result of dehydration and shock. In such instances, forcing fluids is advisable. However, the gradual development of oliguria and anuria in a hydrated patient indicates renal damage by mercury, and at this stage a regimen for acute renal shutdown should be instituted (Chap. 290).

Chronic poisoning from metallic mercury vapor occurs in persons exposed to large amounts of the metal in laboratories or in industry and occasionally as a result of prolonged therapeutic use, as in vaginal douches. Manifestations may be those of subacute poisoning, with salivation, stomatitis, and diarrhea or primary neurologic signs, including tremors of the extremities, tongue, and lips, ataxia and dysarthria, erethism, a state of easy embarrassment, irritability, apprehension, withdrawal, and depression.

Methylmercuric salts were discovered to have a special effect, mainly on the nervous system. First it was observed that workers exposed in the manufacture of an insecticide containing this compound developed an acute cerebellar ataxia. Later in Minimata, Japan, an effluent from a factory was noted to cause cerebellar ataxia and cortical blindness. In some cases there was involvement of peripheral nerves and impairment of neuromuscular transmission (Rustam et al.). The damage to the central nervous system usually is permanent. Public health measures have been taken to eliminate such compounds from the environment.

Some poison can be removed from the body by gastric lavage, but more important in treatment is the binding of the mercuric ion in a harmless compound by BAL. The therapeutic usefulness of BAL depends on its immediate administration. In chronic mercury poisoning, N-acetyl-*dl*-penicillamine may well be the drug of choice. It can be administered orally and appears to chelate mercury selectively, with considerably less effect on copper, which is essential to many metabolic processes.

SILVER Most poisoning by silver involves silver nitrate, a caustic salt. There are intense nausea, vomiting, and diarrhea after swallowing nitrate (lunar caustic), and death from shock may occur within a few hours. The mouth is usually deeply stained by silver nitrate. Treatment is entirely supportive, with fluid replacement and control of pain.

Chronic exposure (usually to nose drops) produces a peculiar bluish skin discoloration (argyria).

THALLIUM Thallium is a component of certain rodenticides and depilatories, and clinical poisoning is usually a result of accidental ingestion of these materials. The fatal dose is approximately 1.0 g. Manifestations are vomiting, diarrhea, and leg pains, followed by a severe and sometimes fatal sensorimotor polyneuropathy. About 3 weeks after poisoning, the patient's hair falls out, providing a strong diagnostic clue if the cause has not previously been determined. Treatment is symptomatic. The alopecia is temporary if the patient recovers.

REFERENCES

ARENA JM: Treatment of mercury poisoning. Mod Treat 4:734, 1967
BANK WJ et al: Thallium poisoning. Arch Neurol 26:456, 1974
BUGE A et al: Encéphalopathies myocloniques bismuthiques formes évolutives, complications tardives durables ou définitives. A propos de 41 cas. Rev Neurol (Paris) 133:401, 1977
CHISHOLM JJ JR: Poisoning due to heavy metals. Pediatr Clin North Am 17:591, 1970
DOOLAN PD et al: Acute renal insufficiency due to dichloride of mercury: Observations of gastrointestinal hemorrhage and BAL therapy. N Engl J Med 249:273, 1953

Feldman RG et al: Peripheral neuropathy in arsenic smelter workers. Neurology 29:939, 1979

Hamilton A, Hardy HL: *Industrial Toxicology,* 3d ed. Acton, England, Publishing Sciences Group, 1974

Jenkins RB: Inorganic arsenic and the nervous system. Brain 89:479, 1966

Kark RAP et al: Mercury poisoning and its treatment with *N*-acetyl-D,L-penicillamine. N Engl J Med 285:10, 1971

Keusler CJ et al: Arsine poisoning, mode of action and treatment. J Pharmacol Exp Ther 88:99, 1946

Le Quesne PM: Toxic substances and the nervous system: The role of clinical observation. J Neurol Neurosurg Psychiatry 44:1, 1981

Levine WH: Heavy-metal antagonists, in *The Pharmacological Basis of Therapeutics,* 5th ed, LS Goodman, A Gilman (eds). New York, Macmillan, 1975, p 912

Longcope WT, Luetscher JA: The use of BAL (British antilewisite) in the treatment of the injurious effects of arsenic, mercury, and other metallic poisons. Ann Intern Med 31:545, 1949

Murray T et al: Cadmium nephropathy: Monitoring for early evidence of renal dysfunction. Arch Environ Health 36:165, 1981

Needleman HL et al: Deficits in psychologic and classroom performance of children with elevated dentine lead levels. N Engl J Med 300:689, 1979

Rustam H et al: Evidence for neuromuscular disorder in methyl mercury poisoning. Arch Environ Health 30:190, 1975

240
OPIATES AND SYNTHETIC ANALGESICS

MAURICE VICTOR
RAYMOND D. ADAMS

The opiates, strictly speaking, include all the naturally occurring alkaloids in opium, which is prepared from the sap of the poppy *Papaver somniferum.* For clinical purposes, the term refers only to those alkaloids which have a high degree of analgesic activity, i.e., morphine and codeine (3-methoxymorphine). Thebaine, another opium alkaloid which, like morphine, possesses a phenanthrene nucleus, has few or no analgesic properties and is therefore not ordinarily considered an opiate. The terms *opioid* and *narcotic-analgesic* refer to any drug with actions similar to those of morphine. Compounds that are chemical modifications of morphine include heroin or diacetylmorphine (now the most commonly abused opioid), hydromorphone (Dilaudid), codeine dihydrocodeinone (Hycodan), dihydroxycodeinone (Eucodal), oxymorphone (Numorphan), and oxycodone (Percodan). A second class of *purely synthetic analgesics* which lack the phenanthrene nucleus but are classed as opioids includes pethidine or meperidine (Demerol), the meperidine derivatives anileridine and alphaprodine (Nisentil), methadone (Dolophine or amidone), metopon (6-methyldihydromorphinone), racemorphan (Dromoran), levorphanol (*l*-Dromoran), *d*-propoxyphene (Darvon), diphenoxylate (the main component of Lomotil), and phenazocine (Prinadol). The latter drugs are similar to the opiates, both in their pharmacological effects and in the patterns of abuse, the differences being mainly quantitative. In fact, *d*-propoxyphene has such low addictive liabilities that it is not controlled by the federal narcotic laws. The same statement applies to the synthetic analgesic pentazocine (Talwin), and although its overall addictive quality is low, cases of physical dependency do occur.

The opioids will be considered from two points of view: (1) acute poisoning and (2) addiction.

OPIOID POISONING Because of the high incidence of addiction, which leads to irregular and nonmedical usage of opioids, poisoning is not an infrequent accident. This may happen as a result of ingestion with suicidal intent, errors in calculation of dosage, variations in drug potency, or unusual sensitivity. Children may exhibit an increased susceptibility to opioids, so that relatively small doses prove toxic. This is true also of adults with myxedema, Addison's disease, chronic liver disease, or pneumonia. Many cases of acute poisoning occur in addicts who are unaware that tolerance for opioids declines quickly after the withdrawal of the drug: upon resuming the habit a formerly well-tolerated dose can be fatal.

Varying degrees of unresponsiveness, shallow respirations, slow respiratory rate (e.g., two to four per minute), or periodic breathing, miosis, bradycardia, and hypothermia are the well-recognized clinical manifestations of acute poisoning. In the most advanced stage the pupils dilate, the skin and mucous membranes become cyanotic, and the circulation fails. The immediate cause of death is usually respiratory depression, with consequent asphyxia. Patients who have a cardiorespiratory arrest are sometimes left with a residuum of anoxic encephalopathy. Others who recover from coma may occasionally reveal a hemiplegia, presumably due to vascular occlusion. In the stage of mild intoxication, anorexia, nausea, vomiting, constipation, and loss of sexual interest are the only symptoms.

Severe opioid intoxication demands immediate intervention. If respirations are depressed, the patient should be intubated and attached to a respirator. The presence of hypotension requires that an intravenous line be established and fluid replacement begun. Pressor amines may be necessary. Should the patient be comatose, gastric lavage (after oral ingestion) with a cuffed endotracheal tube in place may be beneficial. This procedure may be efficacious many hours after ingestion, since one of the toxic effects of opioids is severe pylorospasm, which may cause much of the drug to be retained in the stomach. If the patient does not respond rapidly to these measures, *naloxone* (Narcan) should be administered. This is a specific antidote to the opiates and also to the synthetic analgesics. It is now preferred to *N*-allylnormorphine (Nalline) because naloxone has no agonistic properties; hence, naloxone will not depress respiration further if the diagnosis of opioid poisoning is mistaken. For such poisoning, the dose of naloxone is 0.7 mg per 70 kg by *slow intravenous* injection repeated once or twice if necessary at 5-min intervals. The cardinal signs of successful opioid antagonism are an increase in respiratory rate and pupillary dilatation. In fact, failure of naloxone to produce such a response should cast doubt on the diagnosis of opioid intoxication. If an adequate respiratory response to naloxone is obtained, the patient should be observed carefully for 24 h, and further doses of naloxone (50 percent higher than previously found effective) may be given *intramuscularly* as often as necessary. Naloxone has little direct effect on impaired consciousness, however, and the patient may remain drowsy for many hours. This is not harmful, provided respiration is well maintained.

Naloxone must be used with caution if the acutely intoxicated individual is thought to be an established addict. Once such a patient regains consciousness, usually in about 8 h, signs of a precipitated opioid abstinence syndrome—lacrimation, rhinorrhea, piloerection, profuse sweating, etc.—may become manifest and necessitate symptomatic treatment. Nausea and severe abdominal pain, due presumably to pancreatitis (from spasm of the sphincter of Oddi), are other troublesome symptoms.

In addition to the toxic effects of the opioid itself, the addict is exposed to a variety of neurological and infectious complications, resulting mainly from the injection of crude adulterants (quinine, lactose, powdered milk, fruit sugars) and various infectious agents (injections often administered by unsterile methods). Amblyopia, due probably to the toxic effects of quinine in the heroin mixtures, has been reported, as well as transverse myelopathy and several types of peripheral neuropathy. The spinal cord disorder expresses itself clinically by the abrupt onset of paraplegia with a sensory level on the trunk. Pathologically, there is an acute necrotizing lesion involving both grey and white matter over a considerable vertical extent of the thoracic cord and occasionally the cervical cord. In some cases the myelopathy has followed the first intravenous injection of heroin after a prolonged period of abstinence. Involvement of single peripheral nerves, particularly of the radial nerve, and painful affection of the brachial plexus, independent of compression and remote from the site of injection, have been observed.

An acute generalized myonecrosis with myoglobinuria and renal failure has been ascribed to the intravenous injection of adulterated heroin. Brawny edema and fibrosing myopathy are the sequelae common to venous obliteration resulting from the administration of heroin and its adulterants by the intramuscular and subcutaneous routes. Occasionally there may be an inexplicable swelling of an extremity (sometimes massive) into which heroin had been injected subcutaneously or intramuscularly. Infection and venous thrombosis appear to be involved in its causation.

The diagnosis of drug addiction or the suspicion of this diagnosis should always encourage surveillance for infectious complications, particularly abscesses and cellulitis at injection sites, septic thrombophlebitis, serum hepatitis, septic arthritis, and periarteritis. Tetanus, endocarditis (due mainly to *Staphylococcus aureus*), spinal epidural abscess, meningitis, brain abscess, and tuberculosis are found less frequently.

OPIOID ADDICTION Fifteen years ago there were some 100,000 persons addicted to narcotic drugs in the United States, not including those who were receiving drugs because of hopeless medical diseases. This represented a relatively small public health problem, in comparison with alcoholism and barbiturate addiction; and the opioid addiction problem was of serious proportions in only a few cities—New York, Chicago, Los Angeles, Washington, and Detroit. In the past 15 years a remarkable increase in opioid (principally heroin) addiction has taken place. The precise number of opioid addicts is not known but was estimated by Dupont, in 1978, to be about 500,000. Some idea of the magnitude of the problem can be obtained from Dupont's statements that there are about 250,000 persons receiving treatment (65 percent of them for heroin dependence) in 3000 drug abuse clinics in the United States, and that the cost to the nation, of heroin abuse alone, is about $6 billion a year.

Etiology and pathogenesis A number of factors, socioeconomic, psychological, and pharmacological, all contribute to the genesis of opioid addiction. In our culture, the most susceptible subjects are young men or delinquent youths living in the economically depressed areas of large cities, but a significant number are now found in the suburbs, in small cities, and in rural areas in southern states. The onset of opioid use is usually in adolescence, with a peak at 17 to 18 years. Fully two-thirds of addicts start using the drug before the age of 21. A disproportionately large number are American Negroes and persons of Puerto Rican or Mexican descent. In the southern states, addicts are predominantly white. Almost 90 percent of addicts engage in criminal activity, often necessary to obtain their daily ration of drug, but most of them have had arrests or convictions prior to addiction. Also, many of them show psychiatric disorders, psychopathy and psychoneurosis being the most common. Monroe et al. examined a group of 837 opioid addicts, using the Lexington Personality Inventory, and found evidence of characterologic disorder (psychopathy or sociopathy) in 42 percent, emotional disturbance in 29 percent, and thinking disorder in 22 percent; only 7 percent were asymptomatic. Nevertheless, the precise "personality" factor which renders certain individuals vulnerable to addiction has not been defined.

Association with addicts is the chief reason for beginning addiction. One addict recruits another person into addiction, and the new recruit does likewise. In this sense opioid addiction is contagious, and as a result of this pattern of opioid abuse, heroin addiction, since the late 1960s, has attained virtually epidemic proportions. A small, almost insignificant, proportion of addicts are introduced to drugs by physicians in the course of an illness.

Opioid addiction evolves in three successive phases: (1) episodic intoxication, (2) pharmacogenic or physical dependence, or addiction, and (3) the propensity to "relapse after cure."

Some of the symptoms of opiate intoxication have already been considered. In persons who are distressed by pain or pain-anticipatory anxiety, the administration of opioid produces a sense of unusual well-being, a state that has been referred to in medical writings as "morphine euphoria." It should be emphasized that only a negligible proportion of such persons continue to use opioids habitually after the pain has subsided. The vast majority of potential addicts are not suffering from painful illnesses at the time they initiate opioid use, and in them the initial effects of the drug are not aptly described as euphoric. The latter persons are mainly teenagers who self-administer opioids (mainly heroin) under the tutelage of their peers and who learn, after several repetitions, to recognize what they refer to as a heroin "high," despite the recurrence of unpleasant symptoms (nausea, vomiting, faintness). The repeated self-administration of drug ("reinforcement," in the language of operant psychology) is the most important factor in the genesis of addiction. Regardless of how one characterizes the state of mind that is produced by episodic reinitiation of the drug, the individual quickly discovers the need to increase the dose in order to obtain the original effect. Although the initial effects may not be fully recaptured, the progressively increasing dose of drug does abate the discomfort which arises as the effects of each injection wear off. In this way a new *pharmacogenically induced need* is developed and the use of opioids becomes self-perpetuating. At the same time a marked degree of tolerance is produced, so that enormous amounts of drugs, e.g., 5000 mg morphine daily, have been administered without the development of toxic symptoms. The mechanism of tolerance is still not understood fully, although it is a subject of much interest and speculation. The various theories related to physical dependence have been discussed fully by Wikler (see "References").

The altered physiological state that develops with continued use of the drug is manifested in another dramatic way at the time of withdrawal. This constitutes a specific illness, termed the *abstinence syndrome.* Strictly speaking, addiction is defined as physical or pharmacological dependence. This definition distinguishes between *addicting drugs* (opiates, alcohol, barbiturates) and *habit-forming drugs* (bromides, cocaine, and marihuana), since no consistent abstinence symptoms follow the discontinuation of the latter group, even after prolonged exposure. Stated in another way, all addicting drugs are habit-forming, but the opposite is not true. The place of amphetamines in this scheme is somewhere between these two groups. Undoubtedly they are habit-forming. Tolerance develops over a period of a few weeks to the euphoric, anorexic, and REM (rapid eye movement)-sleep-suppressant actions of amphetamine, but no tolerance appears to develop to the "stimulant" effects of high doses. Withdrawal of *d*-amphetamine, following prolonged oral or intravenous use, is regularly followed by prolonged sleep (with REM rebound) followed by hyperphagia and depression. The deep sleep can be reversed by administration of *d*-amphetamine.

The intensity of the opioid abstinence syndrome depends mainly on the dose of the drug and duration of addiction, but also on individual factors. In respect to morphine it has been found that the majority of individuals receiving 240 mg daily for 30 days or more will show moderately severe abstinence symptoms following withdrawal, whereas mild abstinence signs can be precipitated by narcotic antagonists in persons who have taken as little as 15 mg morphine, or an equivalent dose of methadone or heroin, three times daily for 3 days.

The abstinence syndrome which occurs in the morphine addict may be taken as the prototype of the opioid group. The first 8 to 16 h of abstinence usually pass asymptomatically. At the end of this period yawning, rhinorrhea, sweating, and lacrimation become manifest. At first mild, these symptoms increase in severity over a period of several hours and then remain constant for several days. The patient may be able to sleep during the early period but is restless, and thereafter insomnia remains a prominent feature. Dilatation of the pupils, recurring waves of gooseflesh, and twitchings of the muscles appear. The patient complains of severe aching in the back, abdomen, and legs and of hot and cold "flashes" so that he or she covers up with blankets. By the end of about 36 h the restlessness becomes more extreme, and nausea, vomiting, and diarrhea usually develop. The temperature, respiration, and blood pressure are slightly elevated. All these symptoms reach their peak intensity 48 to 72 h after withdrawal, and then gradually decline. The opioid abstinence syndrome is rarely fatal. After 7 to 10 days, all clinical signs of abstinence have disappeared, although the patient may complain of insomnia, nervousness, weakness, and muscle aches for several more weeks, and a small deviation of a number of physiological variables can be detected with refined techniques for up to 10 months (protracted abstinence).

Two types of abstinence changes have been recognized: *nonpurposive* and *purposive.* The former comprises the various autonomic and neuromuscular signs and are relatively transient in nature. That these symptoms represent an altered physiological state and are not psychic in origin has been clearly demonstrated experimentally. Signs of physical dependence on morphine and other opioids can be induced in the lower limbs of dogs whose spinal cords have been transected; the flexor and crossed extensor spinal reflexes that are depressed or abolished by the opioid become remarkably exaggerated when the drug is withdrawn. The purposive changes refer to the patient's craving for the drug and the manipulative activity directed toward obtaining it. These symptoms may persist indefinitely and are important in relation to that characteristic of addiction referred to as *habituation, emotional dependence,* or *psychic dependence.* These terms are used interchangeably and refer to the substitution of drug-seeking activities for all other aims and objects in life.

Psychic dependence is regarded as the most important quality of addiction, since it is this feature which governs the initial use of the drug and relapse following apparent cure of addiction. Relapse to the use of the drug may occur long after the nonpurposive abstinence changes seem to have disappeared. The cause of relapse is imperfectly understood. It has been theorized that fragments of the abstinence syndrome may remain as a conditioned response, and that these abstinence signs may be evoked by the appropriate environmental stimuli. Thus, when a "cured" addict finds himself or herself in a situation where narcotic drugs are readily available, or in circumstances that were responsible for the initial use of drugs, the incompletely extinguished drug-seeking behavior reasserts itself.

The characteristics of addiction and of abstinence are qualitatively similar with all the drugs of the opiate group as well as the related synthetic analgesics. The differences are mainly quantitative and are related to the differences in dosage, potency, and length of action. Heroin is two to three times more potent than morphine but otherwise the same; nevertheless, the heroin withdrawal syndrome encountered in hospital practice is usually mild in degree because of the low dosage of this drug in the street product. Dilaudid and metopon are more potent than morphine and have a shorter duration of action; hence the addict requires more doses per day, and the abstinence syndrome comes on and subsides more rapidly. The length of action of racemorphan is somewhat longer than that of morphine, but withdrawal phenomena are similar to those of morphine in temporal course and intensity. Abstinence symptoms from codeine, while very definite, are less than those from morphine. The addiction liabilities of *d*-propoxyphene are even less than those of codeine. Abstinence symptoms from methadone are less intense than those from morphine and do not become evident until 3 to 4 days after withdrawal; furthermore, autonomic signs are less severe in the abstinence period. For these reasons methadone is used in the treatment of morphine and heroin addiction. Meperidine addiction is of particular importance because of the high incidence among physicians and nurses and because there is still a widespread belief that this drug is nonaddicting. Tolerance to the toxic effects of meperidine is not complete, so that the addict may show tremors, twitching of the muscles, confusion, hallucinations, and at times convulsions. Signs of abstinence appear 3 to 4 h after the last dose and reach their maximum intensity between 8 and 12 h, at which time they may be worse than those of morphine abstinence.

Diagnosis of addiction This is usually made on the basis of the patient's statement that he or she is using and needs drugs. Should the patient decide to conceal this fact, one must rely on collateral evidence such as miosis, needle marks, emaciation, or abscess scars. Meperidine addicts are likely to have dilated pupils and twitching muscles. A method for the testing of the urine for opiates is now generally available. The finding of morphine or opiate derivatives (heroin is excreted as morphine) in the urine confirms the suspicion that the patient has taken or has been given a dose of such drugs within 24 h of the test.

Formerly it was necessary to isolate questionable cases and to observe the patient over a period of at least 2 days for signs of abstinence. Through use of the specific morphine antagonist and naloxone (Narcan), a diagnosis of addiction to opiates and related analgesic drugs can be made within an hour. Naloxone should be administered only in the presence of another physician or nurse, with the full understanding and permission of the patient. The drug is given intravenously, slowly, using a syringe containing 1 ampul (0.4 mg). The injection is stopped when pupillary dilatation, increased respiratory rate, lacrimation, rhinorrhea, sweating, and yawning appear. If, after 5 to 10 min, no such signs appear, a second injection may be given in the same way. If again the patient shows no abstinence signs, it may be assumed that he or she is not physically dependent upon opiates. Naloxone may be injected *subcutaneously,* in the same dosage as intravenously. Again, if the patient has taken more than occasional doses of the drug within a week of the test, the administration of naloxone will precipitate symptoms of abstinence. These become evident within 5 min of the first injection, reach their peak intensity in 20 min, begin to decline in 60 min, and disappear after 3 h. Naloxone does not precipitate abstinence symptoms in meperidine addicts unless the patient has been taking more than 1600 mg daily.

Management and avoidance of addiction The ambulatory treatment of addiction never succeeds and should therefore not be undertaken, except in special settings, such as a carefully supervised methadone treatment program (see below). Addicts who are refused opiates may ask for methadone, meperidine, or racemorphine, on the ground that these drugs are synthetic and nonaddicting. These are addicting drugs and have been legally defined as such. Physicians should also be aware that they are breaking both the letter and the spirit of the regulations if they prescribe narcotics for an addict merely for the purpose of preventing abstinence changes. Occasional exceptions may be made in seriously ill addicts who are awaiting treatment in a hospital or methadone program, or in patients who are suffering from incurable, painful disease.

The method that is now used almost exclusively is to substitute methadone for opioid, in the ratio of 1 mg methadone for 3 mg morphine, 1 mg heroin, or 20 mg meperidine. Since methadone is long-acting and effective orally, it need be given only twice daily by mouth—10 to 20 mg per dose being sufficient to suppress abstinence symptoms. After a stabilization period of 3 to 5 days on this dosage of methadone alone, the drug may be reduced rapidly and withdrawn over a similar period of time. Treatment is best carried out in an institution with proper facilities for postwithdrawal rehabilitation in a drug-free environment or where methadone or a morphine antagonist may be administered.

The physician must be constantly alert to the dangers of addiction, particularly in susceptible individuals, i.e., those with psychoneurosis, antisocial personality, or alcoholism. The use of opioids should be limited to cases where pain is the chief problem; they should not be used primarily as sedatives, for the relief of asthma, or even in patients with chronic pain until all other measures have been exhausted. It follows that it is most important to make a precise diagnosis of the cause of pain, since in some cases measures other than opioids will suffice, while in others, such as hysteria and depression, narcotic analgesics are contraindicated.

If narcotics have to be used for the relief of pain, consideration should be given to the choice of the appropriate drug and to the mode of administration. Morphine is still the drug of choice for most patients requiring relief of severe pain for short periods. Meperidine may be useful in patients who cannot tolerate morphine. Patients with chronic pain should be managed with the least potent and smallest dosage of drug that will relieve them; doses should be spaced as far apart as possible and discontinued as soon as the need for pain relief has passed. In general, the opioids should be administered orally whenever possible, and the intravenous route should be avoided, since this method produces maximum "euphoria" and, hence, the greatest danger of addiction. The oral administration of codeine and aspirin is a useful way to begin treatment of the patient with chronic pain. If these drugs fail to control the pain, the parenteral administration of codeine should be tried. If the more potent opioids are needed, methadone and levorphan should be used, because of their effectiveness by the oral route and the relatively slow development of tolerance. Should long-continued injections of morphine or meperidine become necessary, maximum analgesic effect is obtained with 10 mg morphine rather than with 15 mg, as is often prescribed, and with 60 to 70 mg rather than with 100 mg meperidine. In these cases, use of the narcotic antagonist pentazocine (Talwin), ad-

ministered parenterally in doses of 40 to 60 mg, might be considered. The respiratory depression produced by pentazocine, like that due to opioids, can be counteracted by naloxone.

Ambulatory treatment of opioid addiction The most significant development in the treatment of opioid (almost exclusively heroin) addiction has been the establishment and growth of ambulatory methadone maintenance clinics. The scope of this activity, like the incidence of addiction, cannot be stated precisely, but can be judged by the fact that in 1974, 135,000 addicts were participating in such programs nationwide.

The method of treatment consists of the oral administration of methadone, beginning with 40 mg or less once daily and then increasing the dose to an amount sufficient to suppress the craving for heroin and to abolish the euphoria-producing effects of that drug given intravenously (heroin blockade). The daily dosage of methadone required to achieve these effects varies between 60 and 100 mg; some patients can be maintained on as little as 40 mg per day, and with higher dosage they need take the drug only once in 48 h. A longer-acting form of methadone—*l*-alphaacetylmethadol (LAAM)—which can be taken thrice or even twice weekly is now under investigation. In principle, these effects could be achieved by multiple daily injections of heroin or morphine, but the effectiveness of methadone orally, its prolonged duration of action, and the fact that it precludes the desire and need for taking other opioids make methadone far more practical.

Methadone is no longer dispensed in tablet form but only as a liquid (dissolved in fruit juice), which is taken under supervision. The collection of urine samples is also supervised, and these are analyzed for opiates and other drugs, to monitor the patient's adherence to the program. Once this has been established, the patient is allowed to take home a 1- to 3-day supply. These measures are designed to prevent the diversion of methadone into illicit channels. Various forms of individual psychotherapy, group psychotherapy, social service counseling, and vocational guidance are included in most programs. The use of former heroin addicts (who are themselves on methadone treatment) as counselors is considered to be a particularly important adjunct to methadone treatment.

The results of methadone treatment are difficult to assess and vary considerably from one program to another. Even the best programs suffer an attrition rate of about 25 percent after several years. In the patients who remain, heroin use is markedly reduced, and between 75 and 85 percent achieve a high degree of social rehabilitation, i.e., they are gainfully employed and no longer engage in criminal behavior or prostitution. These have been the most notable achievements of the methadone maintenance programs.

Although the effectiveness of methadone treatment in the social rehabilitation of many addicts cannot be doubted, a number of questions about this method remain. The usual practice of methadone programs is to accept only addicts over the age of 16 years, with a history of heroin addiction for at least 1 year. This leaves unanswered the problem of the adolescent addict. Although some individuals have been withdrawn from methadone, this has been accomplished so far in a relatively small number, and their capacity to maintain a drug-free existence appears doubtful. This means that the large majority of addicts now enrolled in methadone programs are committed to an indefinite period of methadone maintenance, and the effects of such a regimen are uncertain.

An alternate method of ambulatory treatment of the opioid addict involves the use of narcotic antagonists. Cyclazocine is the best known of these. After withdrawal of the opiate, cyclazocine is administered orally, in increasing amounts over a period of 2 to 6 weeks, until a dosage of 2 mg per 70 kg is being taken twice daily. The cyclazocine-stabilized individual is highly refractory to the euphoria-producing and pharmacological effects of opiates. The idea of treatment is to continue the administration of cyclazocine until all drug-seeking behavior is extinguished, after which it is withdrawn. Good results have been achieved with this drug, but only in small numbers of highly motivated patients who chose cyclazocine maintenance in preferance to other forms of treatment. More recently, interest has centered on the opiate antagonist naltrexone which is virtually devoid of agonistic activity and twice as potent as naloxone; it has the added advantages of being effective orally and in much smaller doses than naloxone. The value of this kind of "extinction therapy" has not yet been determined, but the results in some patients have been encouraging, and the search for improved methods of using opioid antagonists continues. One such agent, buprenorphine, presently under investigation, shows promise both as an analgesic of low abuse potential and as a maintenance drug in narcotic addiction (Jasinski et al.).

Obviously none of these methods promise lasting success unless combined with reeducation, vocational habilitation, and social adjustment.

REFERENCES

Bourne PD (ed): *Acute Drug Abuse Emergencies: A Treatment Manual.* New York, Academic, 1976

DuPont RL: International challenge of drug abuse: A perspective from the United States, in *The International Challenge of Drug Abuse,* RC Peterson (ed). Washington, Superintendent of Documents, US Government Printing Office, 1979

Hollister LE: Effective use of analgesic drugs. Ann Rev Med 27:431, 1976

Jasinski DR et al: Human pharmacology and abuse potential of the analgesic buprenorphine. Arch Gen Psychiatry 35:501, 1978

Martin WR: Realistic goals for antagonist therapy. Am J Drug Alcohol Abuse 2:353, 1975

——— et al: Naltrexone, an antagonist for the treatment of heroin dependence: Effects in man. Arch Gen Psychiatry 28:782, 1973

Monroe JJ et al: The decline of the addict as "psychopath": Implications for community care. Int J Addictions 6:601, 1971

Opioid Dependence, Mechanisms and Treatment. New York, Plenum, 1980

Richter RW et al: Neurological complications of heroin addiction. Bull NY Acad Med 49:3, 1972

Wikler A: Theories related to physical dependence, in *The Chemical and Biological Aspects of Drug Dependence,* SJ Mule, H Brill (eds). Cleveland, Chemical Rubber Press, 1972, p 359

———: Drug dependence, in *Clinical Neurology,* AB Baker, LH Baker (eds). Hagerstown, Md., Harper & Row, 1975

———: Characteristics of opioid addiction, in *Psychopharmacology in the Practice of Medicine,* ME Jarvik (ed). New York, Appleton-Century-Crofts, 1977, p 417

Zinberg NE: The crisis in methadone maintenance. N Engl J Med 296:1000, 1977

241
COMMONLY ABUSED DRUGS

JACK H. MENDELSON
NANCY K. MELLO

The evanescent decline and recrudescence of heroin and marijuana use, as well as the initiation of new drug abuse fads (e.g., phencyclidine, smoking coca paste), are determined by a complex interaction of the pharmacological properties and relative availability of each drug, the personality and expectancy of the user, and the environmental context in which the drug is used. Neither specific biomedical factors nor a constellation of sociocultural variables has satisfactorily explained the causation of drug abuse. No unique personality profile has been identified which places an individual at high risk for abuse of street drugs or alcohol. Whereas drug abuse was once thought to be most prevalent among the economically disadvantaged, it is now apparent that polydrug abuse is not uncommon among individuals from all socioeconomic strata.

MARIJUANA AND CANNABIS COMPOUNDS *Cannabis sativa* contains over 400 compounds in addition to the psychoactive substance Δ^9-tetrahydrocannabinol (THC). Marijuana cigarettes are prepared from the leaves and flowering tops of the plant, and a typical marijuana cigarette contains 0.5 to 1 g of plant material. Although the usual THC concentration in most cigarettes has varied from 5 to 20 mg, concentrations as high as 100 mg per cigarette have been detected. Hashish is prepared from concentrated resin of *Cannabis sativa* and contains a THC concentration between 8 to 12 percent by weight. "Hash oil," a lipid soluble plant extract, may contain a THC concentration of 25 to 60 percent, and it may be added to marijuana and hashish to enhance their THC concentration. The most common mode of marijuana or hashish self-administration is by smoking. During pyrolysis over 150 compounds in addition to the THC are released in the smoke. Although most of these compounds do not have psychoactive properties, they do have potential physiological effects.

THC is quickly absorbed from the lungs into blood and is then rapidly sequestered into tissues. THC is metabolized chiefly in the liver, where it is converted to 11-hydroxy-THC, a psychoactive compound, and more than 20 other metabolites. Most THC metabolites are excreted through the feces, and their rate of clearance is relatively slow in comparison with most other psychoactive drugs.

Prevalence of use The most recent survey by the National Institute on Drug Abuse (1979) revealed that by the ages of 12 and 13 approximately 8 percent of all youths had used marijuana one or more times. Thirty-two percent of 14- and 15-year-olds and 68 percent of 18- to 25-year-olds reported using marijuana at least once.

An interesting but perhaps not surprising finding was that relatively few of the individuals surveyed perceived marijuana as having "no bad effects." For example, the majority of young adults associated impaired performance in automobile driving with marijuana use. Despite an awareness of potential health hazards, the use of marijuana appears to be steadily increasing among adolescents and young adults in the United States.

Acute and chronic intoxication Marijuana and cannabis compounds produce acute intoxication which is related to both THC dose and route of administration. THC is absorbed more rapidly from marijuana smoking than from orally ingested cannabis compounds. The most frequent form of acute intoxication consists of a subjective perception of relaxation and mild euphoria. This condition is usually accompanied by some impairment in thinking, concentration, and perceptual and psychomotor functions. This acute marijuana intoxication resembles mild to moderate alcohol intoxication. Higher doses of cannabis may produce behavioral effects analogous to severe ethanol intoxication. Although the effects of acute marijuana intoxication are relatively benign in normal users, it may precipitate severe emotional disorders in individuals who have antecedent psychotic or neurotic problems. As with other psychoactive compounds both set (users' expectancy) and setting (environmental context) are important determinants of the type and severity of behavioral intoxication.

The behavioral consequences of *chronic* marijuana use are similar to those observed in chronic abusers of alcohol. Such individuals may lose interest in common socially desirable goals and devote progressively more time to drug acquisition and use. However, it should be emphasized that THC does not cause a specific and unique "amotivational syndrome." The range of symptoms sometimes attributed to marijuana use are difficult to distinguish from mild depression and the maturational dysfunctions often associated with protracted adolescence. Chronic use of marijuana has also been reported to increase the probability of exacerbation of psychotic symptoms in individuals with a past history of schizophrenia.

Physical effects Conjunctival injection and tachycardia are the most frequent immediate physical concomitants of smoking marijuana. Although tolerance for marijuana-induced tachycardia develops rapidly among regular users, angina may be precipitated by marijuana smoking in persons with a history of coronary insufficiency. Exercise-induced angina may be increased following marijuana use to a greater extent than after tobacco cigarette smoking. Patients with cardiac disease should be strongly advised not to smoke marijuana or use cannabis compounds.

Significant decrements in vital capacity have been found in regular daily marijuana smokers. Because marijuana smoking typically involves deep inhalation, with prolonged retention of marijuana smoke, marijuana smokers may develop pulmonary disease such as chronic bronchial irritation. There may be, at present, no evidence that marijuana smoking induces lung cancer, although it should be emphasized that heavy marijuana use among Americans may be of too brief duration for detection of this problem.

Although marijuana has also been associated with adverse effects on a number of other systems, many of these studies await replication and confirmation. For example, the reported correlation between marijuana use and decreased testosterone levels in males has not been confirmed. Decreased sperm count and motility and abnormalities of morphology of spermatozoa following marijuana use have also been reported. Administration of high doses of marijuana to female rhesus monkeys has revealed significant marijuana-induced suppression of pituitary gonadotropins and gonadal steroids. Carefully conducted prospective studies demonstrated a significant correlation between heavy marijuana use by pregnant women and impaired fetal growth and development. Marijuana also has been implicated in derangements of the immune response system, in chromosomal abnormalities, and inhibition of DNA, RNA, and protein synthesis, but these findings have not been confirmed or related to any specific physiological effect of marijuana in humans. One report of cannabis-induced brain atrophy in young adults has not been confirmed in studies of computerized transaxial tomography with young men who had documented histories of heavy marijuana smoking.

Tolerance and physical dependence Habitual marijuana users rapidly develop tolerance to the psychoactive effects of marijuana, then smoke more frequently, and try to secure more potent cannabis compounds. Tolerance for physiological effects of marijuana develops at different rates; e.g., tolerance for marijuana-induced tachycardia develops rapidly, but tolerance for marijuana-induced conjunctival injection develops more slowly. Tolerance to both behavioral and physiological effects of marijuana decreases rapidly upon cessation of marijuana use.

Mild to moderate withdrawal signs and symptoms have been reported in chronic cannabis users. These include tremor, sweating, nausea, vomiting, diarrhea, irritability, anorexia, and sleep disturbances. The severity of symptoms is related to dosage and duration of use. Withdrawal signs and symptoms observed in chronic marijuana users have been relatively mild in comparison with those observed with heavy opiate or alcohol users and rarely require medical or pharmacological intervention. Somewhat more severe and protracted abstinence syndromes may occur after sustained use of high-potency cannabis compounds for long periods.

PHENCYCLIDINE Phencyclidine (PCP), a cyclohexylamine derivative, is widely used in veterinary medicine to immobilize large animals for short periods of time and is sometimes classified as a *dissociative anesthetic.* It is easily synthesized and has become an abused drug, primarily among youth and polydrug users. The true extent of its abuse is unknown, but recently national surveys indicate an increase in frequency of use.

The most common street preparation, "angel dust," is a white, granular powder which contains 50 to 100 percent of the drug. Phencyclidine is taken orally, by smoking, or by intravenous injection. It is also used as an adulterant in illicit sales of THC, lysergic acid diethylamide (LSD), amphetamine, or cocaine. Low doses (5 mg) produce agitation, excitement, impaired motor coordination, dysarthria, and analgesia. Users may have horizontal or vertical nystagmus and also show flushing, diaphoresis, and hyperacusis. Behavioral changes include distortions of body image, disorganization of thinking, and feelings of estrangement. Ingestion of doses of 5 to 10 mg may produce hypersalivation, vomiting, myoclonus, fever, stupor, or coma. Doses of 10 mg or more cause convulsions, opisthotonus, or decerebrate posturing which may be followed by prolonged coma.

The diagnosis of PCP overdose is difficult because the patient's initial symptoms may suggest an acute schizophrenic reaction. Confirmation of PCP use is possible by determination of PCP levels in serum or urine (currently available at most toxicological centers). Large quantities of PCP are present in urine for 1 to 5 days following high-dosage PCP intake.

PCP overdose requires prompt life-support measures including treatment of coma, convulsions, and respiratory depression in a hospital intensive care unit (see Chap. 20). There is no specific antidote or antagonist for PCP. PCP excretion from the body can be enhanced by acidification of urine and gastric lavage (see Chap. 20). Death from PCP overdose may occur as a consequence of some combination of pharyngeal hypersecretion, hyperthermia, respiratory depression, severe hypertension, seizures, hypertensive encephalopathy, and intracerebral hemorrhage.

Acute psychosis associated with PCP use should be considered a psychiatric emergency since patients may be at high risk for suicide or extreme violence toward others. *Phenothiazines should not be used for treatment of acute PCP psychosis because these drugs potentiate PCP's anticholinergic effects.* Haloperidol (5 mg intramuscularly) has been administered on an hourly basis to induce suppression of psychotic behavior. PCP as well as LSD and mescaline produce vasospasm of cerebral arteries at relatively low doses. The use of specific calcium antagonists such as verapamil for the treatment of PCP toxicity is under study. Chronic PCP use has been shown to induce insomnia, anorexia, severe social and behavioral changes, and, in some predisposed individuals, chronic schizophrenia.

COCAINE Cocaine is a stimulant and a local anesthetic with potent vasoconstrictor properties. Leaves of the coca plant (*Erythroxylon coca*) contain 1 to 1.5 percent cocaine. The drug is marketed illicitly in the form of a white crystalline powder, usually adulterated with lactose or glucose to 50 percent purity. Its biological effects are the result of alteration and block of cellular membrane transport, particularly preventing the reuptake of biogenic amines, an effect shared with the tricyclic antidepressants. Frequently cocaine is adulterated with other local anesthetics such as lidocaine, procaine, and tetracaine. Cocaine is very expensive in comparison with other illicit drugs and has attained the reputation of a "status" drug in western industrialized societies. The actual extent of illicit cocaine use is unknown, but the most prevalent pattern of use in America appears to be occasional, sporadic intake of relatively low doses.

The most common mode of drug administration is through inhalation or "snorting." The drug is rapidly absorbed from the nasal mucosa and produces a brief, dose-related stimulation and enhancement of mood. There is also a dose-related increment in cardiac rate and blood pressure. Cocaine is less frequently administered by intravenous injection, but during recent years, smoking of coca paste (a product made by extracting illicit cocaine preparations with flammable solvents) has become increasingly popular.

Although it has been assumed that use of cocaine is relatively safe, death caused by respiratory depression and cardiovascular collapse has been documented after cocaine snorting and after intravenous administration. Severe pulmonary disease has developed in individuals who smoke coca paste and is attributed to both the direct effects of cocaine and residual solvent contaminants in the smoked material. Numerous clinical reports dating from the late nineteenth century strongly suggest that protracted cocaine abuse may induce paranoid ideation and visual and auditory hallucinations, a state which resembles alcoholic hallucinosis. Psychological dependence upon cocaine, as manifested by inability to abstain from frequent compulsive use, has also been reported. Although occurrence of withdrawal syndromes involving psychomotor agitation and autonomic hyperactivity remains controversial, severe depression ("crashing") may be a concomitant of drug withdrawal.

Treatment of cocaine overdose is a medical emergency which involves resuscitation in an intensive care unit. Cocaine toxicity produces hypertension, tachycardia, tonic-clonic seizures, dyspnea, and ventricular arrhythmias. Intravenous diazepam in doses up to 0.5 mg/kg administered over an 8-h period has been shown to be effective for control of seizures. The systemic concomitants of a hypermetabolic state produced by cocaine toxicity with concurrent ventricular arrhythmias have been managed successfully by administration of 0.5 to 1.0 mg of propranolol intravenously. Since many of the reported instances of cocaine-related mortality have also been associated with concomitant use of other illicit drugs (particularly heroin), the physician must be prepared to institute effective emergency treatment for multiple drug toxicity.

POLYDRUG ABUSE Although drug abusers often state a preference for a particular drug, such as alcohol or opiates, the occasional or concurrent use of other drugs is common. Multiple drug use often involves substances which may have different pharmacological effects from the preferred drug. Concurrent use of such dissimilar compounds as stimulants and opiates or stimulants and alcohol is not unusual. The diversity of reported drug use combinations suggests that achieving some perceptible change in state, rather than any particular direction of change (stimulation or sedation), may be the primary reinforcer in polydrug use and abuse.

A practical determinant of polydrug use patterns is the relative availability and cost of the drugs. There are many examples of situationally determined drug use patterns. Soldiers who became dependent on heroin in Viet Nam seldom continued heroin use after separation from military service. However, a significant number of Viet Nam heroin addicts abused alcohol and became alcohol-dependent when they returned to the United States. Alcohol abuse, with its attendant medical complications, is one of the most serious problems encountered in former heroin addicts participating in methadone maintenance programs.

The physician must recognize that perpetuation of polydrug abuse and drug dependence is not necessarily a symptom of an underlying emotional disorder. Neither alleviation of anxiety nor reduction of depression accounts for initiation and perpetuation of polydrug abuse. Severe depression and anxiety are as frequently the consequences of polydrug abuse as they are the antecedents. There is also evidence that some of the most adverse consequences of drug use may be reinforcing and contribute to the continuation of polydrug abuse.

Adequate treatment of polydrug abuse, as well as other forms of drug abuse, requires innovative and eclectic programs of intervention. The first step in successful treatment is detoxification, a process which may be difficult because the patient has abused several drugs with different pharmacological actions (e.g., alcohol, opiates, and cocaine). Since patients may not recall or may deny simultaneous multiple drug use, diagnostic evaluation should always include urinalysis for qualitative detection of psychoactive substances and their metabolites. Treatment of polydrug abuse requires hospitalization or inpatient residential care during detoxification and the initial phases of drug abstinence. When possible, specialized facilities for the care and treatment of chemically dependent persons should be used. Outpatient detoxification of polydrug abuse patients is likely to be ineffective and may be dangerous.

As in the treatment of alcohol abuse, no single therapeutic modality has been shown to be uniquely effective in inducing remission. Polydrug abuse is a chronic disorder with an unpredictable pattern of remission and recrudescence. Therapeutic management of chronic disorders such as cardiac or neoplastic disease should serve as a model for helping the person with polydrug abuse problems. Even temporary remissions with attendant physical, social, and psychological improvement are preferable to the continuation or progressive acceleration of polydrug abuse and its related adverse medical and interpersonal consequences. In polydrug abuse, as in most chronic disorders, definitive "cures" rarely occur. The concerned physician should continue to assist polydrug abuse patients throughout the cyclic oscillations of this complex behavior disorder, recognizing that resumption of drug use may be the rule rather than the exception.

REFERENCES

ALTURA BT, ALTURA BM: Phencyclidine, lysergic acid diethylamide and mescaline: Cerebral artery spasms and hallucinogenic activity. Science 212:1051, 1981

BERNSTEIN JG: Medical consequences of marijuana use, in *Advances in Substance Abuse, Behavioral and Biological Research,* NK Mello (ed). Greenwich, Conn., JAI Press, 1980, vol I, 255–288

DOMINO EF (ed): *PCP (Phencyclidine): Historical and Current Perspectives.* Ann Arbor, Mich., NPP Books, 1981

MENDELSON JH: Chronic effects of cannabis on human brain function and behavior. *WHO/ARF Conference on Adverse Health and Behavioral Consequences of Cannabis Use,* 1981 (in press)

PETERSEN RC, STILLMAN RD (eds): *Phencyclidine (PCP) Abuse: An Appraisal,* NIDA Research Monograph Series no 21, US Department of Health, Education, and Welfare Publication (ADM) 78–728, 1978

VAN DYKE C, BYCK R: Cocaine use in man, in *Advances in Substance Abuse, Behavioral and Biological Research,* NK Mello (ed). Greenwich, Conn., JAI Press, 1982, vol III (in press)

WESSON DR et al (eds): *Polydrug Abuse, the Results of a National Collaborative Study.* New York, Academic, 1978

242 ALCOHOL

MAURICE VICTOR
RAYMOND D. ADAMS

Intemperance in the use of alcohol creates many problems in modern society, the importance of which can be judged by the repeated emphasis it receives in contemporary writings, both literary and scientific. These problems may be divided into three categories—psychological, medical, and sociological. The main psychological problem is why individuals drink excessively, often with full knowledge that such action will result in physical injury to themselves and irreparable harm to their families. The medical problem embraces all aspects of the diseases which result from the abuse of alcohol. The sociological problem comprises the effects of sustained drinking on the patient's work, family, and community.

The various problems raised by excessive drinking cannot be separated from one another, and physicians must, therefore, be conversant with all parts of the subject. They may be asked to help patients conquer their alcoholic tendencies or to diagnose and to treat the numerous diseases to which they are subject; often they must admit or commit patients to a general or mental hospital, according to the nature of the presenting clinical disorder; and, lastly, they may be required to enlist the aid of available social agencies when such services are needed by either patients or their families.

In the most general terms it should be known that over 90 percent of Americans drink alcohol at some time in their lives and that some 30 to 40 percent of young men have problems with alcohol. There is a lifetime risk of alcoholism in 5 to 10 percent of men and 3 to 5 percent of women. Of adults admitted to medical and surgical wards, approximately 15 percent use alcohol in excess. In 1971, the Department of Health, Education, and Welfare estimated that about 9 million men and women (7 percent of the adult population) "manifested the behavior of alcohol abuse and alcoholism." It requires little projection of the imagination to conceive of the havoc wrought by alcohol in terms of decreased productivity, accidents, crime, mental and physical disease, and disruption of family life.

Alcoholism has been defined as both a chronic disease and a disorder of behavior, characterized in either context by drinking of alcohol to an extent that surpasses the social drinking customs of the community and that interferes with the drinker's health, interpersonal relations, or means of earning a livelihood. Reduced to pharmacologic terms, it is addiction to alcohol. Alcoholics are individuals who satisfy these medical, social, and pharmacologic criteria.

The causation of alcoholism is obscure, as one would suspect from the multiplicity of theories that have been proposed (see critical reviews by Roebuck and Kessler and by Schuckit and Haglund). The most significant recent observations are those pointing to a genetic influence in the development of alcoholism. It has been shown that the concordance rate for alcoholism in identical twins is 55 percent or higher and for fraternal twins of the same sex, 28 percent (Kaij). Other studies have indicated that the incidence of alcoholism is four to five times higher in the biologic offspring of alcoholic parents than in the offspring of nonalcoholic parents (Goodwin et al.). The risk of alcoholism is not increased in either group by being raised by an alcoholic parent. Thus it appears that genetic factors are important, in addition to psychological and sociocultural ones.

PHARMACOLOGY AND METABOLISM OF ALCOHOL Ethyl alcohol, or ethanol, is the active ingredient in beer, wine, whiskey, gin, brandy, and other less common alcoholic beverages. In addition, the stronger spirits contain enanthic ethers, which give the flavor but have no important pharmacologic properties, and small amounts of impurities such as amyl alcohol and acetaldehyde, which act like alcohol but are more toxic. Contrary to prevailing opinion, the content of B vitamins in American beer and other liquors is so low as to have little nutritional value.

Alcohol is absorbed unaltered from both the stomach and the small intestine. Its presence may be detected in the blood within 5 min after ingestion, and the maximum concentration is reached in 30 to 90 min. The ingestion of milk and fatty foods impedes the absorption of alcohol, and water facilitates it. The rate of absorption increases after Billroth I and II gastrectomies, and in these individuals maximum blood alcohol concentrations are higher and attained faster than in those with intact stomachs.

After entering the bloodstream, alcohol enters the various organs of the body, as well as the spinal fluid, urine, and pulmonary alveolar air, in concentrations which bear a constant relationship to that in the blood. It is eliminated chiefly by oxidation to carbon dioxide, less than 10 percent being excreted chemically unchanged in the urine, sweat, and breath. The energy liberated by the oxidation of alcohol is equivalent to 7 kcal/g.

The metabolism of alcohol takes place mainly in the liver, where several enzyme systems can independently oxidize alcohol to acetaldehyde. The most important of these systems is alcohol dehydrogenase (ADH) which is found in the cell sap of the hepatocyte and which utilizes nicotinamide adenine dinucleotide (NAD) as a cofactor. A second pathway for oxidation of alcohol utilizes catalase, which is located in the peroxisomes and mitochondria, and a third utilizes the microsomal ethanol oxidizing system (MEOS), located in the microsomes of the endoplasmic reticulum. The MEOS probably does not account for much of the alcohol metabolized in ordinary circumstances but may be responsible for the increased rate of alcohol metabolism observed in chronic alcoholics. Acetaldehyde, in turn, is converted by acetaldehyde dehydrogenase of live mitochondria (a reaction that also requires NAD as a cofactor) to acetyl coenzyme A and acetate, and the latter are metabolized further through well-established pathways to yield carbon dioxide and water.

Acetaldehyde has a number of unique biochemical effects, and this has led to the suggestion that acetaldehyde might be responsible for the manifestations of alcohol intoxication. However, the rate of oxidation of acetaldehyde is very rapid and greatly exceeds the rate of oxidation of ethanol to acetaldehyde (except in the presence of disulfiram and similar acting drugs, such as sulfonylureas, metronidazole, furazolidone; see below). For this reason, acetaldehyde blood levels remain low, even in the face of high blood alcohol levels. It is unlikely that these low blood acetaldehyde concentrations have serious toxic effects, considering the high doses of acetaldehyde required to produce such effects in animals. Also there are no substantive data to support the view that acetaldehyde is the major addicting agent in alcoholism.

For all practical purposes it may be accepted that once absorption is ended and an equilibrium established with the tissues, ethyl alcohol is oxidized at a constant rate, independent of its concentration in the blood (about 150 mg alcohol per kilogram of body weight per hour, or about 1 oz 90-proof whiskey or 10 to 12 oz beer per hour). Actually, more alcohol is burned per hour when the initial concentrations are very high, but this increment is of little clinical significance. On the other hand, the rate of oxidation of acetaldehyde does depend on its concentration in the tissues. This fact is of importance in connection with the drug disulfiram (Antabuse) which raises the tissue concentration necessary for the metabolism of a certain amount of acetaldehyde per unit of time. Patients taking both disulfiram and alcohol will accumulate an inordinate amount of acetaldehyde, resulting in nausea, vomiting, and hypotension, sometimes pronounced in degree. Knowledge of these symptoms may deter an alcoholic on disulfiram from drinking.

Very few factors are capable of increasing the rate of alcohol metabolism. Chronic alcoholics metabolize alcohol somewhat faster than normal individuals. Amino acids (especially alanine), insulin, and fructose also enhance ethanol metabolism, but the clinical usefulness of these agents is limited. On the other hand starvation slows the rate of alcohol metabolism in the liver. Alcohol also reduces the intestinal absorption of nutrients such as glucose, amino acids, calcium, folate, and vitamin B_{12}, which may contribute to the nutritional deficiencies that characterize chronic alcoholism.

PHYSIOLOGIC EFFECTS OF ALCOHOL Chronic intake of alcohol in high doses adversely affects almost all body systems. Medically it is important to recognize this fact for it may explain unexpected findings in unrecognized alcoholic patients, e.g., the elevations of mean corpuscular volume, of uric acid, of gamma glutamyltransferase. The following organs, however, sustain the most severe injury from alcohol abuse.

Liver Alcohol has a number of important effects on liver function. In the area of *lipid metabolism* it can cause hypertriglyceridemia and lead to a fatty liver. It interferes with *carbohydrate metabolism* and can produce hypoglycemia by impairing gluconeogenesis; however, a significant degree of hypoglycemia will occur only if hepatic glycogen stores are depleted. Under certain conditions alcohol can also interfere with the peripheral utilization of glucose and produce hyperglycemia, and a valid glucose tolerance test cannot be obtained in the presence of active heavy drinking. When ethanol is oxidized, there is a simultaneous generation of reduced nicotinamide adenine dinucleotide; as a result pyruvate is converted to lactate. Thus, alcoholism may result in increased levels of serum lactate, occasionally *lactic acidosis,* and also *hyperuricemia,* which is secondary to the inhibitory action of lactic acid on the renal excretion of uric acid.

Renal and endocrine effects Alcohol causes an increased urinary excretion of *phosphate and magnesium,* resulting in low serum levels of these ions and an increased *urinary excretion of ammonium.* In addition to lactic acidosis, other types of metabolic and respiratory acidosis may occur in alcoholics. The metabolic acidosis is presumably due to an accumulation of acid metabolites, especially β-hydroxybutyrate. The respiratory acidosis is attributed to a direct action of alcohol on the respiratory center. As indicated further on, all but the mildest instances of alcohol withdrawal are associated with a respiratory alkalosis.

There are also well-recognized effects of alcohol on water excretion. The ingestion of 4 oz 100-proof bourbon whiskey may result in a diuresis comparable to that which follows the drinking of large amounts of water. This diuresis is most likely due to the transient suppression of the release of antidiuretic hormone (ADH) from the supraopticohypophyseal system. Alcohol does not alter the sensitivity of the kidney tubules to endogenous or exogenous ADH (pitressin) and has no discernible effect on renal hemodynamic function in normal persons. The degree of diuresis seems to be more closely related to the duration of the elevated blood level than to the rate of increase or the absolute level attained if the period of alcohol intoxification is sustained. Diuresis occurs only during the initial phase of alcohol administration and does not persist during prolonged drinking. As a result, the average alcoholic undergoing withdrawal is not likely to be dehydrated and may in fact be overhydrated.

Alcohol also appears to inhibit the hypothalamic and neurohypophyseal release of vasopressin and oxytocin. It has been demonstrated that the administration of alcohol to normal young men for periods up to 4 weeks decreased the rate of production and the plasma concentration of testosterone. These abnormalities in testosterone metabolism were traced to both a central (hypothalamus-pituitary) and gonadal effect of alcohol and were independent of nutritional deficiency and liver disease.

Heart and circulation Alcohol has a direct effect on the excitability and contractility of heart muscle. With intoxicating doses there is a rise in cardiac rate and output and in systolic and pulse pressures, and a cutaneous vasodilatation at the expense of splanchnic constriction. Some of these circulatory effects in response to alcohol are said to be more prominent in Orientals than in Caucasians (Ewing), perhaps accounting for the purportedly low rate of alcoholism in the former. Increased sweating and vasodilatation cause a loss of body heat and a fall in body temperature. It is now generally accepted that prolonged intoxication has a damaging effect on cardiac muscle. There is also some evidence that excessive drinking is associated with an increased vulnerability to cardiac arrhythmias, particularly atrial fibrillation, even in the absence of cardiomyopathy. Some authors have stated that the regular use of alcohol increases the risk of hypertension. Also to be noted is the effect of alcohol on high-density lipoproteins. These are decreased in individuals imbibing small amounts of alcohol each day (40 ml of 80-proof beverage or its equivalent). This results in a lower incidence of myocardial infarction and stroke. Ingestion of larger amounts of alcohol is suspected of causing an increased risk of cardiovascular problems, especially those associated with hypertension and cardiomyopathy.

Gastrointestinal system In low concentrations, by whatever route it is administered, alcohol stimulates the parietal cells of the stomach mucosa to produce acid, apparently by releasing gastrin from the antral region, and possibly by causing the tissues to form or release histamine. With the ingestion of alcohol in concentrations of over 10 to 15 percent, the secretion of mucus is increased, the stomach mucosa becomes congested and hyperemic, and the secretion of acid may then become depressed. This is a state of acute *gastritis,* from which recovery may be relatively rapid. The increase in appetite following ingestion of alcohol is due to the stimulation of the end organs of taste and to a general sense of well-being. Similarly, the reviving effect of alcohol in fatigue states is a cerebral one, not due to a direct stimulating effect on muscle or other organs.

Hematopoietic effects Alcohol has a direct effect upon all cells of the bone marrow. Human volunteers who were given alcohol in doses equaling half their caloric intake for several weeks manifested an increase in vacuolation of red and white blood cell precursors. In addition there was a depression of the platelet count. Serum iron fell, but only during the withdrawal period. All these hematologic defects occurred despite excellent nutrition and concomitant administration of folic acid (Lindenbaum and Lieber). The result is usually a mild macrocytosis either with or without accompanying anemia, a mildly decreased white cell count (except during withdrawal), and a mild decrease in platelets.

Behavioral effects of alcohol and the phenomenon of tolerance The most obvious actions of acute, nonlethal doses of alcohol are those exerted on the nervous system, constituting the characteristic symptoms and signs of alcohol intoxication. It is now accepted that alcohol is not a stimulant of the central nervous system but a depressant. Some of the early effects of alcohol, manifested by garrulousness, aggressiveness, excessive activity, and increased electrical excitability of the cerebral cortex, all of which suggest stimulation, are due probably to the inhibition of certain subcortical structures (probably the high brainstem reticular formation) which ordinarily modulate cerebral cortical activity. Similarly, the initial hyperactivity of tendon reflexes may represent a transitory escape of spinal motor neurons from higher inhibitory centers. With increasing amounts of alcohol, however, the depressant action spreads to involve the cerebral cortical neurons as well as other brainstem and spinal neurons.

The behavioral effects of acute ingestion of alcohol (1 to 6 oz) in the nonaddicted person have been the subject of many studies. They have shown that all manner of motor performance, whether the simple maintenance of a standing posture, the control of speech and eye movements, or highly organized and complex motor skills, is adversely affected by alcohol. The movements involved in these acts are not only made more slowly than normal but also more inaccurately and randomly in character and therefore are less adapted to the accomplishment of specific ends.

Alcohol also impairs the efficiency of mental function by interfering with the learning process, which is slowed and rendered less effective. The facility of forming associations, whether of words or of figures, tends to be hampered, and the power of attention and concentration is reduced. The person is not as versatile as usual in directing thought along new lines appropriate to the problems at hand. Finally, alcohol impairs the faculties of judgment and discrimination and, all in all, the ability to think and reason clearly.

A scale relating the various degrees of clinical intoxication to the blood alcohol levels *in nonhabituated persons* has been constructed by Miles. At blood alcohol levels of 30 mg/dl (30 mg/dl = 0.03 percent) a mild euphoria is detectable, and at 50 mg/dl, a mild incoordination. At 100 mg/dl, ataxia is obvious; at 200 mg/dl, the subjects are drowsy and confused; at 300 mg/dl, they are stuporous; and a level of 400 mg/dl is accompanied by deep anesthesia and may prove fatal. These figures are valid provided that the alcohol content in the blood rises steadily over a 2-h period. Such a scale has little pertinence to the chronic alcoholic patient since it does not take into account the adaptive changes that the organism makes to alcohol, which are an increased rate of alcohol metabolism by the liver and particularly the development of tolerance. These phenomena account for the large amounts of alcohol that can be consumed by the chronic drinker without significant signs of intoxication. In the chronic alcoholic the ingestion of a given amount of alcohol will result in a lower blood alcohol level than in a nonalcoholic individual; furthermore, for a given blood alcohol level one will observe lesser degrees of intoxication.

The organism is capable of adapting to alcohol after a very short exposure. If the alcohol concentration in the blood is raised very slowly, few symptoms appear, even at quite high levels. Contrariwise, the degree of intoxication is severe when the blood alcohol level peaks rapidly. It seems that the important factor in this rapid adaptability is not so much the rate of increment or the height of the blood alcohol level, but the length of time the alcohol had been present in the body. It has also been shown that if the dosage of alcohol which causes blood levels to reach a certain height is held constant, the blood alcohol concentration falls and clinical evidence of intoxication disappears. The cause of this fall in alcohol concentration is not clear. It appears that ethanol has an important effect upon the neuronal membrane, but the nature of this effect or how it contributes to central nervous system (CNS) depression or to the development of tolerance is still an enigma. Removal of alcohol from the habituated CNS results in another disturbance in neuronal function, presumably an overactivity (see below).

CLINICAL EFFECTS OF ALCOHOLISM The possible damaging effects of chronic alcohol ingestion on cardiac and skeletal muscle have already been mentioned. These are considered further on and in Chaps. 263 and 374.

That alcoholics are often anemic and thrombocytopenic is common clinical experience. Until recently these abnormalities were attributed to the malnutrition, infection, and liver disease that complicate severe alcoholism, but increasingly it has become apparent that the chronic ingestion of alcohol has a direct damaging effect upon cells of the bone marrow.

The most frequent and important clinical effects of alcoholism are on the digestive organs and on the nervous system.

Effect on digestive organs Symptoms of disordered gastrointestinal function are particularly common in alcoholics; of these the most distinctive are *morning nausea and vomiting.* Characteristically, patients can suppress these symptoms by taking a drink or two, after which they are able to consume large quantities of alcohol without their recurrence until the following morning. Since sufficient alcohol actually relieves these symptoms, they are probably not due to the local effects of alcohol on the stomach, but have a "central" origin and represent the mildest manifestations of the withdrawal syndrome (see below).

Other complaints referable to the gastrointestinal system are abdominal distention, epigastric distress, belching, typical or atypical ulcer symptoms, and hematemesis. The most common pathological basis for these symptoms is a superficial *gastritis,* which is an almost invariable sequel to prolonged drinking. Most instances of gastritis are benign, and the symptoms subside after a few days of abstinence, but more severe forms are associated with mucosal erosions or ulcerations and may be the source of serious bleeding. The incidence of *peptic ulcer* is exceptionally high in alcoholics. A serious cause of hematemesis is the *Mallory-Weiss syndrome,* which is characterized by lacerations of the mucosa at or just below the gastroesophageal junction. In many of these cases bleeding is preceded by an episode of forceful vomiting or protracted retching. The typical lesions appear to depend upon raising the intragastric pressure to 100 to 150 mmHg, i.e., to the range of pressure attained by normal subjects during a period of induced straining and retching.

Patients admitted to the hospital following a period of prolonged drinking and severe dietary depletion almost invariably show enlargement of the liver because of infiltration of the parenchymal cells with fat (see Chap. 315). Fatty liver is reversible provided that patients remain abstinent and receive a nutritious diet. A form of hepatocellular necrosis or *alcoholic hepatitis* is observed frequently in chronic alcoholics, especially following a severe drinking bout. About 8 percent of patients with severe alcoholism develop a permanent form of liver disease, i.e., *cirrhosis,* in which a diffuse proliferation of fibrous tissue replaces the normal lobular architecture of the organ. The alcoholic forms of liver disease are discussed in Chap. 320.

The excessive use of alcohol is also a significant factor in the causation of *pancreatitis.* The mildest form of this disorder may be attributed to gastritis or may go unnoticed, unless discovered by elevations of the serum amylase level. In more severe form pancreatitis presents as an acute abdominal catastrophe, i.e., with epigastric pain, vomiting, and rigidity of the upper abdominal muscles. In these circumstances the pancreas appears tense and edematous, often with a serosanguineous exudation of fluid on its surface. The most severe abnormality takes the form of hemorrhagic pancreatitis (Chap. 325). Alcoholics may also develop a chronic relapsing form of pancreatitis. This type is often associated with irregular calcification of the pancreas. Steatorrhea is a not infrequent complication and is probably related to abnormalities of pancreatic exocrine function, malnutrition, and interference with intestinal absorption of fat.

[The *management* of the various gastrointestinal complications of alcoholism is considered in the section dealing with these diseases (Chaps. 303 and 307).]

Effect on nervous system A large number of neurological disorders are associated with alcoholism. The factor common to all of them is the abuse of alcohol, but the mechanism by which alcohol produces its effects varies from one group of disorders to another, a feature which serves as the basis for the following classification. For the most part this classification is based on known mechanisms.

1 Alcoholic intoxication—drunkenness, coma, "blackouts," pathological intoxication
2 Abstinence or withdrawal syndrome—tremulousness, hallucinosis, "rum fits," delirium tremens
3 Nutritional diseases of the nervous system secondary to alcoholism
  a Wernicke-Korsakoff syndrome
  b Polyneuropathy
  c Cerebellar degeneration
  d Optic neuropathy ("tobacco-alcohol amblyopia")
  e Pellagra
4 Diseases of uncertain pathogenesis, associated with alcoholism
  a Pontine and extrapontine myelinolysis
  b Marchiafava-Bignami disease
  c Alcoholic deteriorated state (alcoholic dementia)
  d Alcoholic cerebral atrophy
  e Fetal alcohol syndrome
  f "Alcoholic" cardiomyopathy and myopathy
5 Neurological disorders consequent upon Laennec's cirrhosis and portosystemic shunts
  a Hepatic stupor and coma
  b Chronic hepatocerebral degeneration

ALCOHOLIC INTOXICATION Drunkenness is such a common phenomenon that its clinical features require little elaboration. The signs consist of varying degrees of exhilaration and excitement, loss of restraint, impairment of judgment and irregularity of behavior, loquacity, slurred speech, incoordination of movement and gait, irritability, drowsiness, and, in advanced cases, stupor and coma.

On rare occasions, alcohol has an extreme excitatory effect. Following the ingestion of a relatively small amount of alcohol, in an individual who need not be an alcoholic, there occurs an outburst of blind fury with assaultive and destructive behavior. The attack terminates with deep sleep, which occurs either spontaneously or in response to sedation, and on awakening the patient has no memory for the episode. This state is referred to as *pathological intoxication,* and it has been variously ascribed to constitutional differences in susceptibility to alcohol, previous cerebral injury, and "an underlying epileptic predisposition." However, there are no critical data to support any of these contentions. An analogy may be drawn between this state of alcoholic excitement and the paradoxic reaction which occasionally complicates the administration of barbituates. The differential diagnosis of pathological intoxication is from rare instances of temporal lobe epilepsy that take the form of rage and violence, and similar episodes that characterize the behavior of some sociopaths.

"Blackouts," in the language of alcoholics, are transient episodes of amnesia which accompany heavy intoxication. After patients become sober, they cannot recall events that had occurred over a period of several hours, even though the state of consciousness (as observed by others) was not importantly altered during this period. The significance of these episodes is not clear; they do not necessarily indicate progression of alcoholic addiction, as is generally assumed.

In all these forms of intoxication, alcohol acts on nerve cells in a manner akin to the general anesthetics. Unlike the latter, however, the margin between the dose of alcohol that produces surgical anesthesia and that which dangerously depresses respiration is a very narrow one, a fact which adds an element of urgency to the diagnosis and treatment of alcoholic narcosis.

The usual forms of alcohol intoxication are distinctive and present no problem in diagnosis or management. On the other hand, *coma* due to alcohol may present difficulties in differential diagnosis. It should be stressed that the diagnosis of alcoholic coma is made not merely on the basis of a flushed face, stupor, and odor of alcohol, but only after the careful exclusion of all other causes of coma.

Treatment of alcoholic intoxication Mild to moderate degrees of intoxication require no special treatment. Certain time-honored remedies such as a cold shower, strong coffee, or forced activity may be helpful, but there is no evidence that any of these methods influences the rate of disappearance of alcohol from the blood. *Alcoholic stupor* is also a relatively brief, self-limited state, and if the vital signs are normal, no special therapeutic measures are necessary. *Pathological intoxication* may require the use of restraints and the parenteral administration of diazepam (10 mg, repeated in 15 to 20 min if necessary).

Coma due to alcoholic intoxication is a medical emergency. The main object of treatment is to prevent respiratory suppression and the complications which it engenders. The management of the comatose patient is described in Chap. 20. The administration of insulin and glucose or fructose for the purpose of lowering the blood alcohol level is of little practical value. Analeptic drugs such as amphetamine, pentylenetetrazole (Metrazol), and various mixtures of caffeine and picrotoxin are antagonistic to alcohol only insofar as they are powerful cerebrocortical stimulants and overall nervous system excitants; they do not hasten the combustion of alcohol. Hemodialysis should be instituted in patients with extremely high blood alcohol levels (> 500 mg/dl), particularly if accompanied by acidosis and in those who have concurrently ingested methanol, ethylene glycol, or some other dialysable drug.

ABSTINENCE OR WITHDRAWAL SYNDROME A second category of alcoholic neurological disease comprises the tremulous, hallucinatory, epileptic, and delirious states. Although a sustained period of chronic intoxication is the underlying factor in each of these disorders, the symptoms become manifest only *after a period of relative or absolute abstinence* from alcohol—hence the designation *abstinence* or *withdrawal syndrome.* Each of the major manifestations of the withdrawal syndrome may occur in more or less pure form and will be so described; more frequently, however, they occur in various combinations. Only for the most severe form is the term *delirium tremens* justified. Unfortunately physicians often incorrectly apply the term to the minor withdrawal symptoms which are relatively benign. The prototype of the patients afflicted with these symptoms is the spree or periodic drinker, although the steady drinker is not immune if, for some reason, he or she stops drinking.

Tremulousness By far the most common manifestation of the abstinence syndrome is a state of tremulousness, commonly referred to as "the shakes" or "the jitters," combined with general irritability and gastrointestinal symptoms, particularly nausea and vomiting. The symptoms first show themselves after several days of drinking, usually in the morning, after the short period of abstinence that occurs during sleep. Patients then need to "quiet their nerves" with a few drinks. Indeed the symptoms are relieved by alcohol, only to return on successive mornings with increasing severity. The usual spree lasts about 2 weeks, but the duration varies greatly. It is terminated not only because of recurrent tremor and vomiting, but for one or more other reasons such as lack of funds, weakness, self-disgust, injury, illness, or collapse. The symptoms then become greatly augmented, reaching their peak intensity 24 to 36 h after the complete cessation.

At this state the patient presents a distinctive picture. The face is deeply flushed, the conjunctivas are injected, and there is usually tachycardia, anorexia, nausea, and retching. The patient is alert and startles easily and complains of insomnia. He or she is inattentive and disinclined to answer questions, and may respond in a rude or perfunctory manner. There may be a mild temporal disorientation, and memory for events of the last few days of the drinking spree may be poor, but there is usually no serious confusion. The patient is usually aware of the nature of the illness.

Generalized tremor is an outstanding feature of this illness. It is of fast frequency (6 to 8 oscillations per second), slightly irregular, and variable in its severity, tending to diminish in quiet surroundings and to increase with motor activity or emotional stress. The tremors may be so violent that the patient cannot stand without help, speak clearly, or feed himself or herself. Sometimes there is little objective evidence of tremor, the patient complaining only of being "shaky inside."

The flushed facies, anorexia, tachycardia, and tremor subside to a large extent within a few days, but the patient does not regain full composure for a much longer time. The overalertness, tendency to startle easily, and jerkiness of movement may persist for a week or longer; the feeling of uneasiness may not leave the patient completely for 10 to 14 days, and only at the end of this time is the patient able to sleep undisturbed, without sedation. An attempt should be made to keep the patient in the hospital for this length of time.

Hallucinosis Symptoms of disordered perception occur in about one-quarter of the tremulous patients. Patients may complain of "bad dreams"—nightmarish episodes associated with disturbed sleep, which are difficult to separate from real experience. Sounds and shadows may be misinterpreted, or familiar objects may appear distorted and assume unreal forms. Although these are not hallucinations in the strict sense of the term, they represent the most common forms of disordered sense perception in the alcoholic. Hallucinations may be purely visual or auditory in type, mixed visual and auditory, and occasionally tactile or olfactory. There is little evidence to support the popular belief that certain visual hallucinations are specific to alcoholism. They are more commonly animate than inanimate and may comprise various forms of human, animal, or insect life. They may occur singly or in panoramas, appear shrunken or enlarged, and may be natural in appearance or take distorted and hideous forms.

ACUTE AND CHRONIC AUDITORY HALLUCINOSIS A special form of alcoholic psychosis, in which vivid auditory hallucinations are the major abnormality, has been recognized for many years. Kraepelin referred to it as the *hallucinatory insanity of drunkards or alcoholic mania.* The central feature of the illness is the occurrence of auditory hallucinations despite an otherwise clear sensorium; i.e., confusion, disorientation, and obtundation are minimal or absent, and memory is not significantly impaired. The hallucinations may be musical in nature, like a low-pitched hum or chant, or they may take the form of unstructured sounds such as buzzing, ringing, shots, or clicking. Usually vocal hallucinations are associated. When the voices can be identified, they are attributed to the family, friends, or neighbors of patients, rarely to God, radio, or radar. Usually the voices discuss the patient in the third person. In the majority of cases the voices are maligning, reproachful, or threatening in nature and are disturbing to the patient; a significant proportion, however, are not unpleasant and leave the patient undisturbed. The voices are intensely real and vivid, and they tend to be exteriorized; i.e., they come from behind the door, from the corridor, or through the floor. Patients may call on the police for protection or barricade themselves against invaders; they may even attempt suicide to avoid what the voices threaten. The hallucinations are most prominent during the night, and their duration varies greatly—they may last for a few minutes to an hour or two or for days, and they may recur intermittently for days on end and, in exceptional instances, for weeks or months.

Most patients, while hallucinating, have no appreciation of the unreality of their hallucinations. As improvement occurs, the patient begins to doubt their reality, is reluctant to talk about them, and may even question whether he had been sane during the episode. Full recovery is characterized by the realization that the voices were imaginary and by the ability to recall, sometimes with remarkable clarity, the abnormal thought content of the psychotic episode.

A unique feature of this psychosis is the evolution of a chronic auditory hallucinosis in a small proportion of the patients. The chronic disorder begins like the acute one, but after a short period, perhaps a week, the symptoms change. The patient becomes quiet and resigned, even though the hallucinations remain threatening and derogatory. Ideas of reference and influence and other poorly systematized paranoid delusions become prominent. At this stage the illness may be mistaken for schizophrenia. There are important differences between the two disorders, however: the alcoholic illness develops in close relation to a drinking bout, and the past history rarely reveals schizoid personality traits. Alcoholic patients with hallucinosis are not distinguished by a high incidence of schizophrenia within their families. A large number of such patients, whom we studied long after their acute attacks, did not show an increased incidence of schizophrenia. There is some evidence that repeated attacks of acute auditory hallucinosis render the patient more vulnerable to this chronic schizophrenia-like syndrome.

Withdrawal seizures ("rum fits") In this particular setting (i.e., where relative or absolute abstinence follows a period of chronic inebriation) there is a marked tendency to develop convulsive seizures. Over 90 percent of withdrawal seizures occur during the 7- to 48-h period following the cessation of drinking, with a peak incidence between 13 to 24 h. During the period of seizure activity electroencephalograms may be abnormal, but they revert to normal in a matter of days, even though the patient may go on to develop delirium tremens. Also during the period of seizure activity patients are unusually sensitive to stroboscopic stimulation. About half of them respond to this activating procedure with generalized myoclonus (photomyoclonus) or a convulsive seizure (photoconvulsion). In contrast, patients with idiopathic epilepsy show this type of response to photic stimulation infrequently.

Seizures occurring in the abstinence period have a number of other distinctive features. There may be only a single seizure, but, more often, a flurry of two to six seizures occurs over a span of several hours, and an occasional patient develops status epilepticus. The seizures are grand mal in type, i.e., major generalized convulsions with loss of consciousness. A focal seizure or seizures should always suggest the presence of a focal lesion (often traumatic) in addition to the effects of alcohol. Almost 30 percent of patients with generalized seizure activity go on to develop delirium tremens, in which case the seizures invariably precede the delirium. The postictal confusional state may blend imperceptibly with the onset of the delirium, or there may be a clearing of the postictal state, over several hours or even a day or two, before the delirium sets in. Seizures of this type occur in patients who have been drinking for many years, and so they have to be distinguished from other forms of epilepsy beginning in adult life.

It is suggested that the terms "rum fits" and "whiskey fits" be reserved for seizures which possess the attributes described above. These are the terms used by the alcoholic and serve to distinguish seizures that occur only in the immediate abstinence period from those which occur in the interdrinking period, long after withdrawal has been accomplished. Alcohol also has an adverse effect on "idiopathic" or posttraumatic epilepsy. In patients with these latter types of epilepsy, seizures may be precipitated by only a short period of drinking (e.g., a weekend, or even one evening of heavy social drinking); interestingly, in these circumstances, the seizures occur not when patients are intoxicated, but usually the morning after, in the "sobering-up" period.

Electroencephalographic findings in patients with "rum fits" do not support the notion that the seizures merely represent latent epilepsy made manifest by alcohol. Instead, the electroencephalogram (EEG) reflects a sequence of changes induced by alcohol itself—a decrease in the frequency of brain waves during the period of chronic intoxication; a rapid return of the EEG to normal immediately after cessation of drinking; the occurrence of a brief period of dysrhythmia (sharp waves and paroxysmal changes) which coincides with the flurry of convulsive activity; and, again, a rapid return of the EEG to normal. Except for the transient dysrhythmia in the withdrawal period, the incidence of EEG abnormalities in patients who have had "rum fits" is not greater than in the normal population, in sharp contrast to patients who are indeed subject to seizures (see Chap. 355).

Delirium tremens This is the most dramatic and serious form of the alcohol withdrawal syndrome. It is characterized by profound confusion, delusions, vivid hallucinations, tremor, agitation, and sleeplessness, as well as by increased activity of the autonomic nervous system, i.e., dilated pupils, fever, tachycardia, and profuse perspiration. The clinical features of delirium have been presented in detail in Chap. 21.

Delirium tremens develops in one of several settings. The patients, excessive and steady drinkers of many years' duration, may have been admitted to the hospital for an unrelated illness, accident, or operation, and 2 to 4 days later become delirious. Or, following a prolonged spree, they may have already experienced several days of tremulousness and hallucinosis, or one or more seizures, and may even be recovering from these symptoms, when they suddenly develop delirium tremens.

In the majority of cases delirium tremens is benign and short-lived, ending as abruptly as it begins. Consumed by the relentless activity and wakefulness of several days' duration, patients fall into a deep sleep; they awaken lucid, quiet, and exhausted, with virtually no memory for the events of the delirious period. Less commonly, the delirious state subsides gradually; more rarely still, there may be one or more relapses, several episodes of delirium being separated by intervals of relative lucidity, the entire process lasting several days or as long as 4 to 5 weeks. When the delirium occurs as a single episode, the duration is 72 h or less in over 80 percent of the cases.

Approximately 5 percent of cases of delirium tremens, as defined above, end fatally. In many of the fatal cases there is an associated infectious illness or injury, but in a few no complicating illness is discernible. Patients frequently die in a state of hyperthermia or peripheral circulatory collapse; in some, death comes so suddenly that the nature of the terminal events cannot be determined.

Closely related to typical delirium tremens and about as common are *atypical delirious-hallucinatory* or *confusional states,* in which one facet of the delirium tremens complex assumes prominence to the practical exclusion of the other symptoms. Patients may simply exhibit a transient state of quiet confusion, agitation, and peculiar behavior lasting several days or weeks. Other patients present a vivid hallucinatory-delusional state and abnormal behavior, consistent with their false beliefs. Unlike typical delirium tremens, the atypical states always present as a single circumscribed episode without recurrences, are only rarely preceded by epilepsy, and do not end fatally. This may be another way of saying that they are a partial or less severe form of the disease.

Abnormalities of the spinal fluid, blood nonprotein nitrogen, serum sodium, chloride, glucose (both hypoglycemia and hyperglycemia), potassium, calcium, and phosphorus occur unpredictably in the alcohol withdrawal syndrome. Decrease in serum magnesium, rise in arterial pH, and decrease in P_{CO_2} occur in all but the mildest cases and are probably critical in the genesis of alcohol withdrawal syndrome, as discussed below. Electroencephalographic findings have been discussed in relation to alcoholic epilepsy.

Pathologic examination is singularly unrevealing in patients with delirium tremens and other withdrawal syndromes. Edema and brain swelling have been absent in the authors' pathologic material except when there had been shock or hypoxia terminally, and there have not been any significant microscopic changes in the brain.

The *pathogenesis* of the tremulous-hallucinatory-delirious state has been a matter of considerable controversy. The idea that it simply represents the most severe form of alcohol intoxication is not tenable. The symptoms of toxicity, consisting of slurred speech, uninhibited behavior, staggering gait, stupor, and coma, are distinctive and different from the symptom complex of tremor, hallucinations, fits, and delirium. The former symptoms are associated with an elevated blood alcohol level, whereas the latter become evident only when the blood alcohol is reduced. Finally, the toxic symptoms increase in severity as more alcohol is consumed, whereas tremor and hallucinosis and even full-blown delirium tremens may be nullified by the administration of alcohol. Although much discussed in the past, there is no evidence that endocrine abnormality or nutritional deficiency plays a role in the genesis of delirium tremens and related symptoms.

It is evident from observations in both humans and experimental animals that the one indispensable factor in the genesis of delirium tremens and related disorders is the withdrawal of alcohol, following a period of chronic intoxication. The emergence of withdrawal symptoms depends upon a decline in the blood alcohol level from a previously higher level and not necessarily upon the complete disappearance of alcohol from the blood. The mechanism(s) by which the withdrawal of alcohol produces symptoms is only beginning to be understood. The early phase of alcohol withdrawal (beginning 7 to 8 h after cessation of drinking) is regularly attended by a drop in serum magnesium levels and a rise in arterial pH values, on the basis of respiratory alkalosis. Indeed it is possible that the compounded effect of these two factors, both of which are associated with hyperexcitability of the nervous system, might be responsible for seizures and perhaps for other symptoms which characterize the early phase of withdrawal. The elevation in pH and drop in P_{CO_2} are explained as withdrawal release of the neurons of the "respiratory center," which had been rendered insensitive to circulating CO_2 during the period of chronic intoxication. In the "rebound" phase these cells become more sensitive than normal to CO_2, with resultant hyperventilation and respiratory alkalosis. But in the genesis of delirium tremens, hypomagnesemia is probably not important, since the serum magnesium level has frequently been restored to normal before the onset of the delirium.

Treatment of alcoholic withdrawal syndrome The general aspects of management of the delirious and confused patient have been described in Chap. 21. More specifically the treatment of full-blown delirium tremens begins with a careful search, followed by appropriate treatment, for associated injuries (particularly head injury with cerebral lacerations or subdural hematoma), infections (pneumonia or meningitis), gastrointestinal bleeding, pancreatitis, and liver disease. Because of the frequency and seriousness of these complications, skull and chest roentgenograms should be obtained and lumbar puncture should be performed if there are meningeal signs. In severe forms of delirium tremens, the temperature, pulse, and blood pressure should be recorded at 30-min intervals in anticipation of peripheral circulatory collapse and hyperthermia, which, added to the effects of injury and infection, are the usual causes of death in this disease. In the case of shock, one must act quickly, utilizing whole-blooded transfusions, fluids, and vasopressor drugs. The occurrence of hyperthermia demands the use of a cooling mattress in addition to specific treatment for any infection that may be present.

A very important element in treatment is the correction of fluid and electrolyte imbalance. The osmolality of the blood should be checked. Severe degrees of agitation and perspiration may dehydrate the patient. The specific electrolytes and the amounts in which they should be added are governed by the laboratory values for these electrolytes. Occasionally, the withdrawal syndrome is characterized by hypoglycemia, in which case the administration of glucose becomes of prime importance. Rarely, alcoholic patients present with severe ketoacidosis and normal or only slightly elevated blood glucose concentrations; usually such patients recover promptly without the use of insulin.

A special danger attends the use of glucose solutions in alcoholic patients. Usually these persons have subsisted on a diet disproportionately high in carbohydrate (alcohol is metabolized almost entirely as carbohydrate) and low in thiamine, and their reserves of B vitamins may have been further reduced by gastroenteritis and diarrhea. The administration of intravenous glucose may serve to consume the last available stores of thiamine and precipitate Wernicke's disease. For this reason it is good practice to add B vitamins in all cases requiring parenterally administered glucose, even though the alcoholic disorder under treatment, e.g., delirium tremens, is not primarily due to vitamin deficiency.

In respect to the use of drugs, it is important to distinguish between mild withdrawal symptoms, which are essentially benign and responsive to practically all sedative drugs, and delirium tremens, which has a serious mortality and is relatively unresponsive to drugs. In the case of minor withdrawal symptoms, the purpose of medication is to ensure rest and sleep. In delirium tremens, the object of drug therapy is to blunt agitation, prevent exhaustion, and facilitate the administration of parenteral fluid and nursing care; one does not attempt to suppress agitation at all costs, since to accomplish this requires an amount of drug that might seriously depress respiratory function.

In general one can manage most of the milder withdrawal symptoms by giving either chlordiazepoxide (Librium) in doses of 10 to 50 mg orally, repeated every 4 to 6 h, or diazepam (Valium), 10 mg every 4 to 6 h. We have not found it practical to give the patients alcohol in diminishing amounts, especially when in the hospital. For impending or fully developed delirium tremens, Librium should be given parenterally in an initial dose of 50 to 100 mg and repeated every 4 h (up to 300 mg per day) until the agitation is controlled. Some physicians prefer the shorter-acting Valium in intravenous doses of 5 to 10 mg repeated every 30 to 60 min. There is little difference in the therapeutic efficacy of these two drugs, and it is not certain that either can prevent hallucinosis or delirium tremens or shorten the duration of the latter disorder. The advantage of these two drugs, given orally, over paraldehyde has not been proved by controlled studies. Paraldehyde has the additional advantage of being extremely safe, provided it is freshly prepared and kept in brown, tightly stoppered bottles to prevent deterioration and the accumulation of acetaldehyde. If the patient can take medication orally, doses of 8 to 12 ml in orange juice should be given. Paraldehyde may also be administered rectally, but the intramuscular route should be avoided if possible, since it may damage nerves. It should be given intravenously only with great caution because of the danger of respiratory depression; intravenous therapy requires careful monitoring to avoid hypotension and hypoventilation. Adrenocorticotropic hormone and cortisone have no place in the treatment of the withdrawal syndrome. In general, phenothiazine drugs should be avoided unless the patient is psychotic and belligerent because of their tendency to lower the seizure threshold. Chlorpromazine can then be given parenterally in doses of 25 to 50 mg, or haloperidol (Haldol) can be given in doses of 3 to 5 mg and repeated as often as necessary to control the patient.

Treatment of "rum fits" In most cases the seizures that occur in the withdrawal period ("rum fits") do not require the use of anticonvulsant drugs. In this setting there may be only a single seizure or a brief flurry of seizures which usually have ceased by the time that certain medicines, such as phenytoin (Dilantin), become effective. The parenteral administration of sodium phenobarbital or Valium early in the withdrawal period could conceivably prevent "rum fits" in patients with a previous history of this disorder or who might otherwise be expected to develop seizures on withdrawal. Also, the long-term administration of anticonvulsants is not necessary; if patients remain abstinent, they will be free of seizures, and if they resume drinking, they usually abandon their medicines. Rarely withdrawal seizures take the form of status epilepticus and should be managed like status of any other type (see Chap. 355). Alcoholics with a history of idiopathic or posttraumatic epilepsy should be urged to drink only in moderation or not at all, because of the deleterious effects of relatively short periods of drinking on their epilepsy, and they should be maintained on anticonvulsant drugs.

NUTRITIONAL DISEASES OF THE NERVOUS SYSTEM These diseases compose a relatively small but serious group of illnesses in chronic alcoholics. In contrast to alcoholic intoxication and the abstinence syndromes, the role of alcohol in the genesis of nutritional diseases is secondary, serving mainly to displace food in the diet. These illnesses, the role of alcohol in their production, and their treatment are discussed in Chap. 363, "Deficiency Diseases of the Nervous System."

ALCOHOLIC DISEASES OF UNCERTAIN PATHOGENESIS Included under this heading is a group of diseases which have little in common except that they either are confined to or predominate in alcoholics. The relationship to alcohol is not understood in any one of these diseases and is probably not crucial, insofar as some of them also occur in nonalcoholics. There is indirect evidence that some of these disorders are nutritional in origin, but as yet this relationship must be regarded as unproved.

Central pontine myelinolysis (CPM) This term refers to a unique pathological change affecting the center of the basis pontis, in which the medullated fibers are destroyed in a single symmetrical focus of varying size. In contrast, the axis cylinders, nerve cells, and blood vessels are relatively well preserved. Although the lesion is usually confined to the basis pontis, tegmental structures may be involved in advanced cases, and occasionally there are symmetrically placed lesions of similar histologic type in other parts of the brain. The disease may manifest itself clinically by pseudobulbar palsy, quadriplegia, and pseudocoma ("locked-in syndrome"), evolving over a period of several days, but usually the lesion is so small that it causes no symptoms and is found only at postmortem examination. Most cases of CPM have occurred in severely malnourished alcoholics, but the relationship of this condition to nutritional deficiency, alcohol, or other toxic factors is obscure. Recently, attention has been drawn to the frequent occurrence of *hyponatremia* in patients with CPM. In dogs that were made severely hyponatremic (100 to 115 meq/liter) by repeated injections of vasopressin and intraperitoneal infusions of water, a rigid quadriparesis developed, *following* the correction of the hyponatremia by rapid infusion of hypertonic saline (Laureno). At autopsy, these animals showed pontine and extrapontine lesions that were indistinguishable in their distribution and histologic features from those of the human disease.

Marchiafava-Bignami disease (primary degeneration of the corpus callosum) This is a rare complication of alcoholism originally described in Italian men addicted to crude red wine. The symptoms are diverse and include psychic and emotional disorders and intellectual deterioration (mainly of frontal lobe type; see Chap. 24), convulsive seizures, and varying degrees of tremor, rigidity, paralysis, apraxia, aphasia, and sucking and grasping reflexes. The duration is variable, from several weeks to months, and recovery is possible. The pathologic picture is more constant than the clinical one. It consists of symmetrical demyelination in the corpus callosum, particularly of the middle lamina, and less consistently of the anterior commissure and other parts of the white matter. Axis cylinders are better preserved than medullated fibers in these areas, and there are appropriate reactions in the macrophages and astrocytes. Various degrees of recovery may occur if abstinence from alcohol and good nutrition are established and maintained.

ALCOHOLIC DETERIORATED STATE Alcoholic dementia The syndrome designated as alcoholic dementia or deteriorated state has never been delineated satisfactorily, either clinically or pathologically. Purported examples of this state show a remarkably diverse group of symptoms, including jealousy and suspiciousness; blunting of moral fiber and other personality and behavioral disorders; deterioration of work performance, personal care, and living habits; disorientation, impaired judgment, and defects of intellectual function, particularly of memory; and even certain physical manifestations, such as dilatation of facial capillaries, a bloated look, flabby muscles, chronic gastritis, tremors, and recurrent seizures. Recently, Seltzer and Sherwin, on purely clinical grounds, have attempted to sharpen the definition of alcoholic dementia. It is their contention that patients with alcoholic dementia can be distinguished from patients with senile dementia by their stable course and absence of language abnormality, and from patients with Korsakoff's psychosis by their difficulties with constructional tasks and prominent behavioral disturbances in addition to amnesia.

A large variety of cerebral cortical changes have been attributed to the toxic effects of alcohol and have been considered to be the basis of the alcoholic deteriorated state, but some of them (e.g., neuronal pyknosis) are insignificant artifacts, and others, such as opacity of the meninges and moderate dilatation of the lateral ventricles, are nonspecific, being observed in both alcoholics and nonalcoholics as well as in persons who had shown no neurologic or psychiatric abnormalities during life. Some of the cellular changes said to underlie alcoholic dementia may have reflected a state of hepatic failure or terminal anoxia, and others nothing more than the effects of aging or artifacts of tissue fixation and staining. The majority of cases that come to autopsy with the label of "alcoholic dementia" or "deteriorated state" prove to have the lesions of the Wernicke-Korsakoff syndrome. Traumatic lesions of varying degrees of severity are commonly present as well. Other cases show the lesions of anoxic or hepatic encephalopathy, communicating hydrocephalus, Alzheimer's disease, ischemic infarction, or some other disease quite unrelated to alcoholism. Practically always, the clinical state can be accounted for by one or a combination of these disease processes, and there has been no need to invoke a hypothetical diffuse toxic effect of alcohol on the brain.

Alcoholic paranoia and jealousy are outmoded terms that were used in the past to designate what was thought to be a special type of paranoid reaction in chronic alcoholics, in which the patient, usually a male, developed ideas of infidelity on the part of his wife. The morbid jealousy which develops in alcoholics does not merit classification as a distinctive complication of alcoholism because it differs in no major way from that in nonalcoholics. Nevertheless, among individuals with the syndrome of morbid jealousy, chronic alcoholism may be an important associated factor. Among alcoholic patients, the delusions of jealousy may at first be evident only in relation to episodes of acute intoxication, but later they evolve, through a stage of constant suspicion and efforts to detect infidelity, into definite morbid beliefs which persist during periods of sobriety as well.

Alcoholic cerebral atrophy This disorder, like the "alcoholic deteriorated state," does not constitute a clinical-pathologic entity. Usually this diagnosis is made on the basis of radiologic findings. In several pneumoencephalographic studies of chronic alcoholics a symmetrical enlargement of the lateral ventricles was demonstrated in more than half the cases, and a smaller number also showed a widening of the sulci, mainly in the frontal lobes. Similar findings have been reported in chronic alcoholics examined by CT scan.

The clinical correlates of these radiologic findings are quite unclear. In some patients "cerebral atrophy" is associated with an overt complication of alcoholism, but in some alcoholic individuals the finding of large ventricles comes as a surprise, because no symptoms or signs of neurologic disease were found in the course of the usual neurologic and mental status testing.

The term "alcoholic cerebral atrophy" implies that chronic ingestion of alcohol causes an irreversible loss of cerebral tissue, a concept to which there is a serious objection. One cannot assume that dilated ventricles and sulci, observed in a single CT scan, represent a loss of tissue. Such CT changes may in fact be reversible, as has been observed in patients with Cushing's syndrome, anorexia nervosa, and Lennox-Gastaut syndrome (treated with ACTH), as well as in alcoholic patients. This reversibility would suggest that a shift of fluids had occurred in the brain (over many months), rather than a loss of tissue. Until this matter has been studied further, it would be preferable to refer to the asymptomatic ventricular enlargement in alcoholics as such, rather than as cerebral atrophy.

"Alcoholic" myopathy and cardiomyopathy Alcoholics as a group are particularly vulnerable to several disorders of cardiac and skeletal muscle, loosely referred to as *alcoholic cardiomyopathy* and *alcoholic myopathy.* Apart from their high incidence in alcoholics, these myopathies possess no unique features, and the same disorders may be observed in a variety of clinical settings in which alcohol plays no part.

One type of myopathic syndrome occurs acutely in the course of a prolonged bout of heavy drinking and is manifested by severe pain and tenderness and swelling of muscles, accompanied by cramps and muscle weakness. The muscular affection may be generalized or remarkably focal, and an affected limb may give the appearance of a deep phlebothrombosis or lymphatic obstruction. Some of the focal lesions are surely induced by trauma or pressure-ischemic injury during a period of alcoholic coma. Diffuse necrosis of muscle fibers, all in one stage of degeneration (rhabdomyolysis), is the underlying pathologic change and is reflected by myoglobinuria and high serum levels of creatine phosphokinase (CPK). Some patients show a diminished rise in blood lactic acid in response to ischemic exercise, similar to that which occurs in McArdle's disease. In distinction to the latter, however, myophosphorylase levels are not consistently reduced in the alcoholic patients. How these biochemical abnormalities are related to muscle cramps and weakness is a matter of speculation. Most patients with this disorder recover, usually in a matter of weeks; in severe cases, complete restoration of motor power may take several months.

In other cases, a painless and predominantly proximal weakness develops over a period of several days or weeks in the course of a prolonged drinking bout and is associated with a severe degree of hypokalemia. The urinary excretion of potassium is not significantly increased. Often the depletion of potassium is the result of vomiting and diarrhea, which precede the onset of muscular weakness, but sometimes the mechanism of depletion is unclear. In several reported cases with low serum phosphorus levels a bone tumor (e.g., an ossifying angioma) was found, and its removal restored muscle power to normal. The oral administration of phosphates has been beneficial in nontumorous cases. Some of the latter are accompanied by pain and stiffness.

From time to time, one observes in alcoholics the subacute or chronic evolution of painless weakness and atrophy of the proximal muscles of the limbs, especially of the legs, with only minimal signs of polyneuropathy in the distal segments of the limbs. Cases such as these have been referred to as *chronic alcoholic myopathy,* but the data are insufficient to warrant this designation. Muscle biopsies from such patients suggest that it represents a proximal form of polyneuropathy. Treatment is much the same as for alcoholic neuropathy, and complete recovery can be expected if the patient abstains from alcohol and improves his or her nutritional status.

Alcoholic cardiomyopathy is discussed further in Chap. 263.

Fetal alcohol syndrome That maternal heavy alcohol intake may have an adverse effect on the offspring has been a recurrent theme in medical lore, but only in the past decade have the effects of alcohol abuse on the fetus been clearly documented. This congenital disorder has been termed the *fetal alcohol syndrome.* The affected infants are small in length in comparison with weight, and most of them fall below the third percentile for head circumference. They are distinguished also by the presence of short palpebral fissures (probably a reflection of microphthalmia) and epicanthal folds; maxillary hypoplasia, thin vermillion of upper lip, micrognathia, and cleft palate; dislocation of the hips, flexion deformities of the fingers, and limited range of motion of other joints; cardiac anomalies (usually spontaneously closing septal defects); anomalous external genitalia; and capillary hemangiomata. The newborn infants suck and sleep poorly, and many of them are irritable, hyperactive, and tremulous; the latter symptoms resemble those of alcohol withdrawal, except that they persist. In one series of such infants there was a neonatal mortality of 17 percent. Seriously affected infants who survive the neonatal period fail to achieve normal weight, length, and head circumference and remain backward mentally to a varying degree, even under optimal environmental conditions.

The anatomic basis of this syndrome, and the mechanism by which alcohol produces its effects, are not fully understood; the limited evidence to date favors a toxic effect of alcohol or perhaps one of its metabolites or contaminants, rather than a nutritional or genetic factor. The critical degree of maternal alcoholism that is necessary to produce the syndrome and the critical stage in gestation during which it occurs also need to be determined. Cases of fetal alcohol syndrome have occurred only in children born to severely alcoholic mothers who continued to drink heavily (80 ml absolute alcohol per day) throughout their pregnancy. Studies of the effects on the fetus of lesser degrees of maternal alcoholism are in progress.

NEUROLOGICAL DISORDERS CONSEQUENT UPON CIRRHOSIS AND PORTAL-SYSTEMIC SHUNTS *Hepatic coma* refers to an episodic disorder of consciousness which frequently complicates (or terminates) advanced liver disease and/or portal-systemic shunts. This condition and the more chronic type of acquired hepatocerebral degeneration are described in Chaps. 320 and 362.

TREATMENT OF ALCOHOL ADDICTION Following recovery from the acute medical and neurological complication of alcoholism, the underlying problem—that of alcohol dependence—remains. To treat only the medical complications and to leave the management of the drinking problem to patients themselves is indeed shortsighted. Almost always drinking is resumed, with a predictable recurrence of medical illness. For this reason the physician must be prepared to deal with the addiction or at least to initiate treatment.

The problem of excessive drinking is formidable but not necessarily as hopeless as it is made out to be. A common misconception among physicians is that specialized training in psychiatry and an inordinately large amount of time are required to deal with the addictive drinker. Actually, a successful program of treatment can be initiated by any interested physician, using the standard techniques of history taking, establishing rapport with the patient, and seeing him or her frequently, though not necessarily for prolonged periods. A useful point at which to undertake this task is during convalescence from a serious medical or neurologic complication of alcoholism or in relation to loss of employment, arrest, or threatened divorce. Such crises may help convince the patient, better than any argument presented by the family or physician, that the drinking problem has reached serious proportions.

The requisite for successful treatment is total abstinence from alcohol, and for all practical purposes, this represents the only permanent solution. It is generally agreed that any attempt to curb the drinking habit will fail if the patient continues to drink. There are said to be alcoholics who have been able to reduce their intake of alcohol and eventually to drink in moderation, but they must represent a tiny proportion of the addicted population. Also, it is frequently stated that patients must recognize that they are alcoholics, i.e., that their drinking is beyond their control, and they must express willingness to be helped. Undoubtedly there is truth in both these statements, but they should not be interpreted to mean that patients must gain this recognition and willingness entirely on their own initiative and that they will be helped only after they do so. Physicians can do a great deal to help patients understand the nature of their problem and to motivate them to accept treatment. The help of family, employer, courts, and clergy should be enlisted in an attempt to convince them that abstinence is preferable to chronic inebriety. Patients must be made fully aware of the medical and social consequences of continued drinking and must also be made to understand that because of some constitutional peculiarity they are incapable of drinking in moderation. These facts should be presented in much the same ways as one would explain the essential features of any other disease. There is nothing to be gained from adopting a punitive or moralizing attitude; on the other hand, patients should not be given the idea that they are in no way blameworthy for their illness. There appears to be an advantage in making patients feel that they are responsible for doing something about their drinking.

The prevalent belief that alcoholics will not stop drinking under duress also requires qualification. In fact, one of the few careful studies of this matter disclosed that relatively few patients would have sought help unless pressure had been exerted by family or employer; furthermore, in patients who came to the clinic under duress the incidence of sustained abstinence was much the same as in those who came voluntarily.

If earnest and sustained efforts by the physician fail to convince the patient that alcohol is a problem, it is usually impossible to modify the alcoholic tendency. The only way to make such individuals discontinue drinking is to commit them to psychiatric hospitals or special institutions for the management of alcoholism in the hope that with forced abstinence and improvement in their physical state they will gain insight and later accept psychiatric or other forms of therapy.

On the other hand, if patients come to realize that the drinking is beyond their control and that something needs to be done about it, their chances of being helped are raised considerably. Indeed, under these circumstances, many persons stop drinking of their own volition for periods of several months or years. Some of these patients, despite the best of intentions, will relapse. This should not serve as an excuse to abandon treatment; many patients have attained a state of prolonged sobriety after several false starts.

A number of methods have proved valuable in the long-term management of the alcoholic patient. The most important of these are the use of disulfiram (Antabuse), psychotherapy, and the participation in social organizations for combating alcoholism.

Disulfiram interferes with the metabolism of alcohol, so that patients who take both alcohol and disulfiram accumulate on inordinate amount of acetaldehyde in the tissues, resulting in nausea, vomiting, and hypotension, sometimes pronounced in degree. It is no longer considered necessary to demonstrate these effects to patients; it is sufficient to warn them of the severe reactions that may result if they drink while they have the drug in their body. Treatment with disulfiram is instituted only after patients have been sober for several days, preferably longer. It should never be given to patients with cardiac or liver disease. The drug is taken each morning, or at another suitable time daily, in a dosage of 250 mg, preferably under supervision. This form of treatment is of particular value in the spree or periodic drinker, in whom relapse from abstinence usually represents an impulsive rather than a carefully planned or premeditated act. The patient taking disulfiram, aware of the dangers of mixing liquor and the drug, is "protected" against the impulse to drink, and this protection may be renewed every 24 h by the simple expedient of taking a pill. The willingness with which the patient accepts this form of treatment also serves as a rough index of motivation. Compliance can be checked by measuring disulfiram in the blood. Should patients drink when they are taking disulfiram, the ensuing reaction is usually severe enough to require medical attention, and a protracted spree can thus be prevented. Disulfiram may in rare instances lead to a mild polyneuropathy if continued over a period of months or years. It must then be discontinued.

Alcoholics Anonymous (AA), an informal fellowship of former alcoholics, can be helpful in the rehabilitation of alcoholic patients. The philosophy of this organization is embodied in its "twelve steps," a series of propositions about alcohol and alcoholism which guide the patient to recovery. In particular, the AA philosophy stresses the practice of making restitution, the necessity to help other alcoholics, trust in God, the group confessional, and the belief that alcoholics are powerless over alcohol. AA philosophy also embodies the 24-h plan, in which alcoholics strive for just 24 h of abstinence (a concept inspired by the Sermon on the Mount) as a means of facilitating the maintenance of sobriety. Although accurate statistics are lacking, it is stated that about one-third of the members who express more than a passing interest in the program attain a state of long-sustained or permanent sobriety.

The methods used by AA are not suited to every patient; some prefer the more personalized approach offered by special clinics and centers for the treatment of alcoholism. The physician should, therefore, be fully aware of all the community resources which are available for the management of this problem and should be prepared to take advantage of them in appropriate cases.

Alcoholism is frequently associated with psychiatric disease of some other type. There is among alcoholics an increased frequency of schizophrenia, psychoneurosis, sociopathy, and particularly manic-depressive disease. In the latter case, the prevailing mood is far more often one of depression than of mania and is more often encountered in the female who is more apt to drink under these conditions than the male. The presence of concomitant psychiatric disease complicates the management of the alcoholism, and in these circumstances expert psychiatric help should be sought.

REFERENCES

Baekeland F, Lundwall LK, Kissen B: Methods for the treatment of chronic alcoholism: A critical appraisal, in *Research Advances in Alcohol and Drug Problems,* Y Israel (ed). New York, Wiley, 1975, vol 2, pp 247–328

Clarren SK, Smith DW: The fetal alcohol syndrome. N Engl J Med 298:1063, 1978

Epstein PS et al: Alcoholism and cerebral atrophy. Alcoholism. Clin Exp Res 1:61, 1977

Ewing JA et al: Alcohol sensitivity and ethnic background. Am J Psychiatry 131:206, 1974

Gessner PK: Drug therapy of the alcohol withdrawal syndrome, in *Biochemistry and Pharmacology of Ethanol,* E Majchrowicz, EP Noble (eds). New York, Plenum, 1979, vol II

Goodwin DW: *Is Alcoholism Hereditary?* New York, Oxford, 1976

Isselbacher KJ: Metabolic and hepatic effects of alcohol. N Engl J Med 296:612, 1977

Kaij L: *Alcoholism in Twins.* Stockholm, Almqvist & Wiksell, 1960

Laureno R: Experimental pontine and extrapontine myelinolysis. Trans Am Neurol Assoc 105:354, 1980

Lindenbaum J, Lieber CS: Hematologic effects of alcohol in man in the absence of nutritional deficiency. N Engl J Med 281:333, 1969

Mendelson JH, Mello NK: Medical progress: Biologic concomitants of alcoholism. N Engl J Med 301:912, 1979

Miles WR: The comparative concentrations of alcohol in human blood and urine at intervals after ingestion. J Pharmacol Exp Ther 20:265, 1922

Roebuck JB, Kessler RG: *The Etiology of Alcoholism: Constitutional, Pyschological, and Sociological Approaches.* Springfield, Ill., Charles C Thomas, 1972

Rosett HL: A clinical perspective of the fetal alcohol syndrome. Alcoholism. Clin Exp Res 4:119, 1980

Schuckit MA, Haglund RMJ: An overview of the etiological theories on alcoholism, in *Alcoholism: Development, Consequences and Interventions,* NJ Estes, ME Heinemann (eds). St. Louis, Mosby, 1977, pp 15–27

Seltzer B, Sherwin I: Organic brain syndromes: An empirical study and critical review. Am J Psychiatry 135:13, 1978

Thompson WL et al: Diazepam and paraldehyde treatment of severe delirium tremens. A controlled trial. Ann Intern Med 82:175, 1975

Victor M: The pathophysiology of alcoholic epilepsy, in *The Addictive States.* Res Publ, Assoc Res Nerv Ment Dis 46:431, 1968

———, Wolfe SM: Causation and treatment of the alcohol withdrawal syndrome, in *Alcoholism: Progress in Research and Treatment,* PG Bourne, R Fox (eds). New York, Academic, 1973

243 SEDATIVES, STIMULANTS, AND PSYCHOTROPIC DRUGS

MAURICE VICTOR
RAYMOND D. ADAMS

SEDATIVE-HYPNOTIC DRUGS

This class of drugs, also referred to as *depressants,* may be divided into two main groups. The first includes the barbiturates, bromides, chloral hydrate, and paraldehyde. In the past 15 years these drugs have been largely displaced by a second group of sedatives comprising meprobamate and other glycerol derivates, and the benzodiazepines, the most important of which are chlordiazepoxide (Librium) and diazepam (Valium). Indeed, the benzodiazepines are the most commonly prescribed drugs in the world today. According to Hollister, more than 1.4 billion prescriptions for these drugs are filled each year. Their advantages over the older sedatives are their *relatively* low toxicity (hypnotic action) and addictive potential and their minimal interactions with other drugs.

BARBITURATES Despite the steadily diminishing medical use of barbiturates, the high incidence of addiction, suicides, and accidental deaths attributable to the improper use of these drugs is a matter of continuing concern. The production of barbiturates greatly exceeds the amount needed for therapeutic purposes. It is estimated that barbiturates account for 20 percent of acute poisonings admitted to general hospitals and that they are responsible for 6 percent of suicides, figures exceeded by no other single poison. The Domestic Council Drug Abuse Task Force (1975) estimated the total number of regular users of barbiturates who were "in trouble" (suicidal and accidental overdoses as well as medical complications of barbiturate abuse) to be 300,000.

About 50 barbiturates have been marketed for clinical use, but only the following are encountered with any frequency: pentobarbital (Nembutal), secobarbital (Seconal), amobarbital (Amytal), aprobarbital (Alurate), thiopental (Pentothal), barbital (Veronal), and phenobarbital (Luminal). In the United States, pentobarbital, secobarbital, and amobarbital are the most commonly abused barbiturates. All the barbiturates are similar pharmacologically and differ only in their speed of onset and duration of action. The clinical problems posed by the barbiturates vary, however, according to whether the intoxication is acute or chronic.

Acute barbiturate intoxication This results from the ingestion of large amounts of the drug either accidentally or with suicidal intent. The latter is most frequently the act of a depressed person. The hysteric or psychopath may take an overdose as a suicidal gesture and sometimes become seriously intoxicated because of a miscalculation or ignorance of the toxic dosage. The combination of alcohol and barbiturate intoxication is frequent and particularly dangerous, since these drugs have an additive effect.

The symptoms and signs of acute barbiturate intoxication vary with the type and the amount of drug. Pentobarbital and secobarbital produce their effects after a short delay, and recovery is relatively rapid. Phenobarbital induces coma more slowly, and its effects tend to be prolonged. In general, much larger doses of long-acting barbiturates are required to produce a depth of unconsciousness comparable with that produced by the short-acting ones. The ingestion by adults of more than 3.0 g secobarbital, pentobarbital, amobarbital, or diallylbarbituric acid at one time may be fatal unless intensive and skillful treatment is applied promptly; it has been estimated that to produce a comparable effect, the following amounts of long-acting barbiturates would have to be ingested: 6.0 to 9.0 g phenobarbital, 5.0 to 20.0 g barbital, and 15.0 g aprobarbital. Because of the serious complications of prolonged coma, the fatalities are greater with the long-acting than with the short-acting drugs.

Clinically, it is useful to recognize three grades of severity of acute barbiturate intoxication. Mild intoxication follows the ingestion of approximately 0.6 g pentobarbital or its equivalent. The patient is drowsy or asleep but can be readily roused by being called loudly or shaken. The symptoms resemble those of alcohol intoxication, except that the face is not flushed, the conjunctivas are not suffused, and there is no odor of alcohol. The patient thinks slowly, and there may be mild disorientation, lability of mood, impairment of judgment, slurred speech, drunken gait, and nystagmus. Reflex activity and vital signs are not affected.

Moderate intoxication follows the ingestion of 5 to 10 times the oral hypnotic dose. Here the state of consciousness is more severely depressed and is usually accompanied by depressed or absent deep reflexes and slow but not shallow respiration. Corneal reflexes are retained, with occasional exceptions. At times patients can be roused by vigorous manual stimulation; when awakened, they are confused and dysarthric and, after a few moments, drift back into coma. At other times they cannot be roused by any means. In the latter case the depth of coma and seriousness of the respiratory depression may be roughly judged by the response of respiration to the inhalation of 10% carbon dioxide or to painful stimulation. If these stimuli cause an increase in the depth and rate of respiration, the outlook for recovery is good, and only symptomatic treatment is indicated.

Severe intoxication occurs with the ingestion of 15 to 20 times the oral hypnotic dose. Patients cannot be roused by any means. Respiration is slow and shallow or irregular, and pulmonary edema and cyanosis may be present. The deep tendon reflexes are usually but not invariably absent. Most often, patients show no response to plantar stimulation, but in those who do the plantar responses are extensor. In the most advanced cases the corneal and gag reflexes may also be abolished. The pupillary light reflex is retained in severe intoxication and is lost only if the patient is asphyxiated. In the early hours of coma, there may be a phase of rigidity of the limbs, hyperactive reflexes, ankle clonus, extensor plantar signs, and decerebrate posturing; persistence of these signs indicates a severe degree of anoxia. The temperature may be subnormal, the pulse thready and rapid, and the blood pressure at shock levels.

The *diagnosis* of barbiturate intoxication is made from the history and physical findings. One should examine the mouth and gastric contents for any characteristically colored capsules. Acute barbiturate intoxication which presents as a state of coma must be distinguished from other forms of coma by the methods outlined in Chap. 20. Actually there are few other conditions which cause a flaccid coma with reactive pupils, hypothermia, and hypotension. Glutethimide poisoning may produce an identical clinical picture, excepting that the pupils are fixed (a parasympathomimetic action). Laryngeal spasm and sudden apnea also characterize glutethimide intoxication. In the differential diagnosis, hysteria presents the main problem.

The type and amount of barbiturate in the blood can be determined by gas chromatography. The blood level also helps to identify the drug as long- or short-acting, thus giving information as to whether the therapeutic problem will be short or prolonged. A blood barbiturate level of 2 mg/dl in a *comatose* patient is usually due to poisoning with secobarbital or pentobarbital; although the immediate mortality is high in such instances, the therapeutic problem will be short. A level of 11.5 to 12.0 mg/dl is usually due to poisoning with barbital or phenobarbital, and the comatose state will be prolonged. Because of the additive effects of alcohol, a patient who has ingested both drugs may be comatose with relatively low blood barbiturate levels. For this reason, and also because of differences in individual tolerance, the correlation between blood barbiturate levels and depth of coma is not entirely dependable.

The *electroencephalogram* (EEG) may also be useful in diagnosis. In mild intoxication, normal activity is replaced by fast activity, in the range of 20 to 30 Hz, appearing first in the frontal regions and spreading to the parietal and occipital regions as intoxication worsens. In more severe intoxication, the fast waves become less regular and interspersed with 3- to 4-Hz slow activity. In still more advanced cases, there are short periods of suppression of all activity, separated by bursts of slow (delta) waves of variable frequency. In extreme overdosage, all electrical activity ceases. This is one instance in which a "flat" EEG cannot be equated with brain death, and the effects are fully reversible, unless anoxic damage has supervened.

The management of acute barbiturate intoxication depends on its severity. In mild or moderate intoxication, recovery is the rule, and no vigorous treatment is required. If the type and amount of ingested drug cannot be ascertained, it is important to empty the stomach and analyze its contents. In the *responsive* patient, gastric lavage with a large tube is difficult, and a simpler procedure is to induce vomiting with syrup of ipecac. Once this has been accomplished, the patient should be checked at frequent intervals for signs of deepening stupor and coma. If the patient is *unresponsive,* a patent airway should be established by the insertion of an endotracheal tube; suctioning should be used when necessary, and the patient should be turned frequently. Also early on, an intravenous line should be established. Tracheotomy and bronchoscopic suctioning usually become necessary if atelectasis becomes manifest, or if intubation must be maintained for longer than 48 h. Any degree of underventilation requires the use of a positive-pressure respirator. In the unresponsive, intubated patient gastric lavage may be a useful therapeutic as well as a diagnostic measure. It must be performed within several hours of ingestion of the drug, since barbiturates are absorbed rapidly and completely.

Cases of severe respiratory depression, with cyanosis and pupillary dilatation, represent a serious medical emergency. A clear airway should be secured immediately, and some form of assisted respiration begun with an automatic intermittent positive-pressure respirator. If the patient is in shock, the foot of the bed should be elevated, and norepinephrine and whole blood or plasma administered. Catheterization is required to determine the adequacy of urinary output, to obtain samples for laboratory examination, and to prevent distention of the bladder. Since the amount of barbiturate cleared by the kidney is directly proportional to the amount of urine formed, 8 to 10 liters of 5% glucose in saline solution should be given daily. Forced diuresis is also important because toxic amounts of barbiturate have an antidiuretic effect. Coma of any significant duration requires the administration of other electrolytes as well, the amounts being governed by their serum and urinary values. The occurrence of pulmonary and urinary infections calls for the use of appropriate antibiotic treatment.

Hemodialysis has proved to be an effective form of therapy and should be used in all patients with profound coma who fail to respond to the measures outlined above. It is particularly useful in cases of coma due to long-acting barbiturates and is mandatory if anuria or uremia has developed. Alkalinization of the blood by the use of large amounts of bicarbonate solution, as a means of mobilizing the barbiturate and increasing its rate of excretion, seems to be a useful measure, particularly where phenobarbital is the responsible agent.

Occasionally, in the case of a barbiturate addict who has taken an overdose of the drug, recovery from acute intoxication is followed by the development of abstinence symptoms, which have to be managed by the methods outlined below.

Chronic barbiturate intoxication (Barbiturate addiction) Chronic barbiturate intoxication, like other addictions, tends to develop on a background of some psychiatric disorder, most commonly depression or psychoneurosis with symptoms of anxiety and insomnia. As the desired effects of the drug are lost, the patient increases the dose gradually until he or she is taking an amount sufficient to produce symptoms when it is withdrawn. Alcoholics find that barbiturates effectively relieve their nervousness and tremor (cross tolerance); then they may continue to take both alcohol and barbiturates, or the barbiturates may replace the alcohol. Heroin and morphine addicts may turn to barbiturates when they are unable to obtain opiates. As with other addicting drugs, the incidence of barbiturism is particularly high in individuals with ready access to drugs, such as physicians, pharmacists, and nurses.

The manifestations of chronic barbiturism are much like those of mild acute barbiturate or alcohol intoxication. The barbiturate addict thinks slowly, shows an increased emotional lability, and becomes untidy in dress and personal habits. The neurological signs are quite characteristic and include dysarthria, nystagmus, and cerebellar incoordination. Both the mental and neurological signs fluctuate greatly, being more severe if the drug is taken in the fasting state and tending to increase during the day as more of the drug is ingested. If the dosage is elevated rapidly, the signs of moderate or severe intoxication become manifest.

A characteristic feature of chronic barbiturate intoxication is the development of tolerance, sometimes striking in degree. The average addict will ingest about 1.5 g daily of a potent barbiturate and will not develop signs of severe intoxication unless this amount is exceeded. Tolerance to barbiturates does not develop as rapidly as to opiates. Daily doses of 2 g have been reached, but this takes many months. Most persons can ingest 0.4 g daily for as long as 3 months without developing major withdrawal signs (seizures or delirium). With a dosage of 0.8 g daily, the efficiency at all tasks is greatly reduced, and after the daily ingestion of this amount for a period of 2 months, abrupt withdrawal will result in serious symptoms in the majority of patients. Even after 2 weeks at this dosage, some patients will show mild withdrawal symptoms and paroxysmal electroencephalographic changes with photic stimulation. Individuals taking 0.4 to 0.7 g daily fall into an intermediate category; practically all show some mental dulling, and episodes of forgetfulness and occasionally severe withdrawal symptoms may occur.

ABSTINENCE OR WITHDRAWAL SYNDROME Following the withdrawal of barbiturates from chronically intoxicated individuals, a characteristic sequence of symptoms occurs. Over a period of 8 to 12 h the symptoms of intoxication subside and are then replaced by a new group of symptoms, consisting of nervousness, tremor, postural hypotension, weakness, and generalized seizures. With phenobarbital or barbital, the onset of withdrawal symptoms may not occur until 48 to 72 h after the final dose. Seizures usually occur on the second or third day of abstinence, occasionally as long as 6 or 7 days after withdrawal. There may be a single seizure, several, or rarely status epilepticus. The convulsive phase may be followed directly by a delusional-hallucinatory state or a full-blown delirium, indistinguishable from delirium tremens, or a varying degree of improvement may follow the seizures, before the delirium becomes manifest. Death has been reported under these circumstances. The abrupt onset of seizures or an acute psychosis in adult life should always raise the suspicion of addiction to barbiturates or other sedative-hypnotic drugs and withdrawal effects.

The EEG shows a number of changes during chronic barbiturate intoxication and following withdrawal. During chronic intoxication, the predominant pattern is that of fast activity of moderate voltage, interspersed with some 6- to 8-Hz activity chiefly in the frontal and parietal regions. On withdrawal the fast activity diminishes and paroxysmal bursts of mixed spike and slow waves or 4-Hz "spike and dome" paroxysmal discharges may occur, not necessarily associated with seizures. Also, in the withdrawal period, there is a greatly heightened sensitivity to photic stimulation, to which the patient responds with myoclonus or a seizure, accompanied by paroxysmal changes in the EEG. Most of these abnormalities disappear after 4 or 5 days, and the EEG pattern is usually completely normal in 2 weeks.

Treatment of chronic barbiturate intoxication If the diagnosis of addiction is made before signs of abstinence have appeared, the first step in treatment should be the determination of the "stabilization dosage." This is the amount of short-acting barbiturate required to produce mild symptoms of intoxication (nystagmus, slight ataxia, and dysarthria). Usually 0.2 g pentobarbital given orally every 6 h is sufficient for this purpose. The patient is examined 1 h after each dose. If the signs of intoxication are severe, the next scheduled dose is reduced or omitted. If, instead, tremulousness and postural tachycardia appear, an additional 0.1 g pentobarbital is given and the next scheduled dose is increased. This method is preferable to a blind reduction of dosage, since patients frequently underestimate the amount of drug taken. Then a gradual withdrawal of the drug is undertaken, 0.1 g daily. The reduction is stopped for several days if abstinence symptoms appear.

An alternate method of managing barbiturate addiction is to stabilize the patient with phenobarbital rather than pentobarbital. The longer-acting barbiturate permits a withdrawal characterized by fewer fluctuations in blood levels (Wesson and Smith). The initial dosage of phenobarbital is calculated by substituting one sedative dose (30 mg) of phenobarbital for each hypnotic dose (100 mg) of the short-acting barbiturate which the patient had been using. With either of these methods a severely addicted person can achieve abstinence in 14 to 21 days.

If the patient presents with delirium or withdrawal seizures, he or she should be given 0.3 to 0.5 g phenobarbital intramuscularly and then enough to maintain a state of mild intoxication. Most anticonvulsant medicines have been shown to be ineffective against barbiturate withdrawal convulsions. Withdrawal should then be carried out as indicated above. If the abstinence symptoms are not severe, it is not necessary to reintoxicate the patient, but treatment can proceed along the lines laid down for the delirious and confused patient (Chap. 21).

After recovery has taken place, whether from symptoms of chronic intoxication or withdrawal or from acute intoxication due to attempted suicide, the psychiatric problem requires evaluation and an appropriate plan of therapy. Many of the considerations in the management of alcoholism are equally applicable to the patient addicted to barbiturate or nonbarbiturate hypnotic drugs (Chap. 242, "Alcohol").

BROMIDES Bromides are now seldom prescribed by physicians but are contained in certain "nerve tonics" and proprietary remedies (Nervine, Neurosine), so that cases of bromide intoxication are still encountered from time to time. Acute poisoning with bromide is rare because large doses of the drug are irritating to the gastric mucosa, and vomiting prevents the attainment of significant blood levels. Taken in smaller doses, however, bromide tends to accumulate in the body because of its slow excretion by the kidneys, and toxic symptoms may appear in a matter of weeks.

The symptoms of chronic bromide intoxication range from dizziness, drowsiness, irritability, and emotional lability to a quiet confusional state, with impairment of thinking and memory and, in severe cases, to delirium and hyperactivity or stupor and coma. Skin manifestations are often associated, taking the form usually of acne-like eruption and less frequently of proliferative nodular lesions. Headache, mild conjunctivitis, gastric distress, anorexia, and constipation may be associated. Blood bromide levels of 75 mg/dl (9 meq per liter) or more are diagnostic of bromism, if the clinical picture suggests it. However, higher levels are sometimes well tolerated, and symptoms of bromism may persist for some days even after the blood levels have been reduced to normal or near-normal levels.

Treatment consists of removing the source of bromide and administering sodium chloride (at least 6 g daily, in divided doses). Ammonium chloride may be substituted if an accumulation of sodium is to be avoided. Confused or delirious patients require sedation, and anorectic and emaciated patients need careful nursing care and special attention to diet. The administration of a mercurial or thiazide diuretic serves to promote a bromide diuresis. Hemodialysis is an effective means of removing bromide and should be utilized in severe cases.

CHLORAL HYDRATE This is the oldest and one of the safest, most effective, and cheapest of the sedative-hypnotic drugs. After oral administration, chloral hydrate is reduced rapidly to trichloroethanol, which is responsible for the depressant effects on the central nervous system. A significant portion of the trichloroethanol is excreted in the urine as the glucuronide, which may give a false-positive test for glucose.

In large doses, chloral hydrate is toxic to the heart, kidneys, and liver, but only in the presence of preexisting disease in these organs. Chloral hydrate is a strong gastric irritant, so that it requires dilution and should not be taken on an empty stomach. Tolerance and addiction to chloral hydrate develop only rarely, and for these reasons it is an appropriate medication for the management of insomnia, particularly the type which is associated with depression. Poisoning with chloral hydrate is a rare occurrence and resembles acute barbiturate intoxication, except for the finding of miosis, which is said to characterize the former. In combination with alcohol, the well-known "Mickey Finn" or "knockout drops," its effects are additive, leading to a rapid onset of coma. Death from poisoning is due to respiratory depression and hypotension; patients who survive may show signs of liver and kidney disease.

PARALDEHYDE This sedative-hypnotic is also effective and safe, providing that certain precautions are taken in its preparation and administration as indicated in Chap. 242. Paraldehyde is unique in that a significant proportion is excreted unchanged through the lungs, which accounts for its lingering, unpleasant odor and the main objection to its use. It has a wide margin of safety when administered orally (or rectally), and even three or four times the usual dose of 8 to 10 ml causes no more than prolonged sleep or mild stupor. It is particularly effective in suppressing the tremulousness, restlessness, and insomnia that characterize the early phase (6 to 60 h) of the alcohol withdrawal period (see Chap. 242).

BENZODIAZEPINE GROUP As indicated above, the foregoing sedative drugs have been replaced to a large extent by two drugs of the benzodiazepine group, namely, chlordiazepoxide (Librium) and diazepam (Valium). These latter drugs have been used extensively to control anxiety, and they are probably more effective than the barbiturates in this respect. They have also been used to control overactivity and destructive behavior in children and the symptoms of alcohol withdrawal. Diazepam is particularly useful in the treatment of delirious patients who require parenteral medication. The benzodiazepines possess anticonvulsant properties, and the intravenous use of diazepam is an effective means of controlling status epilepticus, as indicated in Chap. 355. In addition, diazepam has been used with moderate success in the treatment of certain extrapyramidal movement disorders and dystonic spasms.

Other widely used benzodiazepine drugs are flurazepam (Dalmane), which is useful in the treatment of insomnia (see Chap. 19), and clonazepam, in the management of seizure disorders.

The benzodiazepine drugs, while comparatively safe in the recommended dosages, are far from ideal. They frequently cause unsteadiness of gait and drowsiness and at times hypotension and syncope, particularly in the elderly. Additional central nervous effects are slurred speech, dysphagia, confusion, and faulty memory. In severely disturbed schizophrenic patients, rage, hostility, uncontrollable excitement, confusion, and depersonalization may develop. Nausea, diminished libido, headache, skin rashes, leukopenia, eosinophilia, agranulocytosis, and enhancement of the effects of alcohol have all been reported but are rare.

CARBONIC ACID DERIVATIVES These drugs have a modest sedative action and can relieve mild degrees of nervousness, anxiety, and muscle tension. Meprobamate (Equanil, Miltown) is the best-known member of this group. With usual doses (400 mg, three or four times a day) the patient is able to function quite effectively; large doses cause ataxia, drowsiness, stupor, coma, and vasomotor collapse. Hypersensitivity reactions and cutaneous petechiae or ecchymoses may also occur, without thrombocytopenia. Diplopia, syncope, menstrual irregularities, peripheral edema, and pancytopenia are other rare complications.

Addiction to meprobamate, though reported infrequently, does occur, and if four or more times the daily recommended dose is taken over a period of weeks to months, withdrawal symptoms (including convulsions) may appear, resembling those which follow chronic barbiturate intoxication. Several other nonbarbiturate sedative drugs, when taken in increasingly large doses, have the same liability. These drugs are glutethimide (Doriden), ethinamate (Valmid), ethchlorvynol (Placidyl), methyprylon (Noludar), chlordiazepoxide (Librium), diazepam (Valium), methaqualone (Quaalude), and perhaps oxazepam (Serax). As with the barbiturates, the toxic effects consist of slurred speech, nystagmus, ataxic gait, drowsiness, confusion, and coma. Abrupt discontinuation of these drugs, after chronic administration of high daily doses, may give rise to abstinence symptoms, which are also like those of the barbiturate and alcohol withdrawal syndromes except for their delayed onset (4 to 8 days after discontinuation of the drugs)—a feature that is probably due to their slow metabolism and excretion. There have been occasional reports of death following the withdrawal of meprobamate, methyprylon, and diazepam in persons who had been taking large doses of these drugs for protracted periods. In view of these observations, physicians must exercise caution in prescribing new sedative drugs which are continually being introduced and which are said to possess no addicting or habit-forming properties.

The management of patients addicted to nonbarbiturate sedatives follows the lines indicated above, under "Barbiturates." If the drug and its dosage can be determined, it should be withdrawn at the rate of one therapeutic dose per day. Should abstinence symptoms appear, the reduction in dosage is stopped for several days. If the offending drug cannot be identified, a barbiturate such as secobarbitol should be administered to the point of mild intoxication and then withdrawn, in the manner indicated above. It should be noted that phenytoin and phenothiazine derivatives are not effective against abstinence convulsions.

ANTIPSYCHOTIC DRUGS

Since the mid-1950s, a large series of pharmacologic agents, loosely referred to as *tranquilizers* (because of their sedative properties), has come into prominent use. They are also referred to as *neuroleptics* because of their ability to increase motor activity in some patients. Mainly these drugs are used for the control of schizophrenia and to a lesser extent for psychotic states associated with organic brain syndromes, and certain instances of manic-depressive disease. The mechanism by which these drugs ameliorate disturbances of thought and affect in these psychotic states is poorly understood but has been attributed to their ability to inhibit or partially block transmission in dopaminergic pathways in the brain. Probably their parkinsonian side effects are attributable to blockade of the dopaminergic striatonigral pathways.

A large number of antipsychotic drugs are on the market (almost 200 have been given generic names). Some have had only an evanescent popularity, and others have yet to prove their value. Chemically these compounds form a heterogeneous group, but six categories are of particular clinical importance: (1) the phenothiazines, (2) the thioxanthines, (3) the butyrophenones, (4) the *Rauwolfia* alkaloids, (5) an indole derivative, molindone (Moban), and (6) a dibenzoxazepine derivative, loxapine (Loxitane). In the management of schizophrenia, molindone and loxapine are about as effective as the phenothiazines, and their side effects are also the same. The main use of the newer antipsychotic drugs is in patients who are not responsive to the older ones or who suffer intolerable side effects from them. A new antipsychotic agent, clozapine (a dibenzodiazepine derivative), is of current interest since it appears to be uniquely free of extrapyramidal side effects. Clozapine, metiapine, and timozide (a diphenylbutylpiperidine) are presently under investigation in the United States.

PHENOTHIAZINES This group comprises some of the most widely used tranquilizers such as chlorpromazine (Thorazine, Largactil), promazine (Sparine), triflupromazine (Vesprin), prochlorperazine (Compazine), perphenazine (Trilafon), fluphenazine (Permitil, Prolixin), thioridazine (Mellaril), and trifluoperazine (Stelazine). In addition to their psychotherapeutic uses, certain members of this group are used as antiemetics (prochlorperazine) and antihistaminics (promethazine).

The phenothiazines have had their widest application in the treatment of the psychoses (schizophrenia and to a lesser extent manic-depressive psychosis). Their use outside psychiatry should be discouraged. Under the influence of these drugs, many patients who would otherwise be hospitalized are able to live at home and even work productively. And the use of these drugs has greatly facilitated the hospital care of hyperactive and combative patients.

Side effects of the phenothiazines are frequent and often serious. All of them may cause a cholestatic type of jaundice, agranulocytosis, convulsive seizures, orthostatic hypotension, skin sensitivity reactions, mental depression, disorientation and hallucinations, and disorders of the extrapyramidal motor system. Jaundice and blood dyscrasias have occurred less often with prochlorperazine, perphenazine, and fluphenazine than with other members of the group, but the extrapyramidal side effects have been relatively more pronounced. Several types of extrapyramidal symptoms have been noted.

1 *A parkinsonian syndrome*—masked facies, tremor, generalized rigidity, shuffling gait, and slowness of movement; these symptoms appear after several weeks of drug therapy.
2 *Muscle spasms and dystonia,* taking the form of involuntary movements of facial muscles and protrusion of the tongue (so-called *buccolingual or oral masticatory syndrome*), dysphagia, torticollis and retrocollis, oculogyric crises, and tonic spasms of a limb (dyskinesias); these complications usually occur early in the course of administration of the drug, sometimes after the initial dose, and can be improved dramatically by the intravenous administration of diphenhydramine hydrochloride (Benadryl).
3 An inability to sit still and an inner restlessness, such that the patient is constantly moving the limbs or pacing the floor (*akathisia*).
4 Lingual-facial-buccal dyskinesia, restlessness, and choreoathetotic and dystonic movements of the trunk and limbs may occur as late and persistent complications (*tardive dyskinesia*) of long-term therapy with phenothiazines or haloperidol.

These extrapyramidal reactions must be recognized at once and the medication discontinued. The purely parkinsonian syndrome and the dystonic spasms usually improve, but tardive dyskinesia may persist for months or years. Administration of antiparkinsonian drugs of the anticholinergic type (trihexyphenidyl, procyclidine, benztropine) may hasten the recovery from some of the symptoms. Oral, lingual, and laryngeal dyskinesias are affected relatively little by any of the antiparkinsonian drugs. Sometimes, however, one such medication has a better effect than another. Amantadine (Symmetrel) in doses of 50 to 100 mg tid has been useful in some cases of postphenothiazine dyskinesia and reserpine in others. No treatment has proved to be uniformly successful. The authors have noted a tendency for some cases of tardive dyskinesia to subside slowly after several years of unsuccessful therapy.

Probably the most threatening side effect, fortunately rare, is the neuroleptic malignant syndrome of hypertonicity, dyskinesia, stupor, hyperthermia, pallor, and pulmonary edema. This has been reported after the use of fluphenazine enanthate alone and with haloperidol. The treatment is immediate discontinuance of the drugs and measures outlined in Chap. 20.

BUTYROPHENONES These drugs (haloperidol, trifluperidol) have much the same antipsychotic effects as the phenothiazines, as well as the same side effects. Unlike the phenothiazines, they have little or no adrenergic blocking action. The butyrophenones are effective substitutes for the phenothiazines in patients who are intolerant to the latter drugs, particularly to their autonomic effects.

RESERPINE This is the prototype of the *Rauwolfia* alkaloids. It was in relation to the sedative effects of these drugs that the term *tranquilization* was used for the first time. These drugs, so effective in controlling hypertension, are no longer recommended for the treatment of mental disorders, except perhaps in patients who cannot tolerate phenothiazines. The *Rauwolfia* alkaloids often provoke a parkinsonian syndrome or a serious depression of mood, which may prove more troublesome than the disorder for which they were prescribed.

Meprobamate, chlordiazepoxide, and diazepam are often referred to as "minor tranquilizers," the implication being that these drugs share the properties of the "major tranquilizers" or antipsychotic drugs. This is not the case. The so-called minor tranquilizers differ from the antipsychotics in both their chemical structure and pharmacologic effects. In fact, the minor tranquilizers more closely resemble the barbiturates in their pharmacologic effects (including the ability to produce tolerance and physical dependence) and are more appropriately referred to as *antianxiety* drugs.

It hardly need be pointed out that the tranquilizing drugs have been much abused. This would be suspected just from the frequency with which they are being prescribed. It is stated that in the decade 1955 to 1965, 50 million patients in the United States received chlorpromazine alone. These powerful medications have specific indications, noted above, and the physician should be certain of the diagnosis before using them. The fact that these drugs can produce tardive dyskinesia in nonpsychotic patients is reason enough not to use them for nervousness, apprehension, anxiety, mild depression, and the many normal psychologic reactions to trying environmental circumstances. These drugs are not curative, but only suppress or partially alleviate symptoms, and they should not serve as a substitute for, or divert the physician from, the use of other measures for the relief of the abnormal mental state.

ANTIDEPRESSION DRUGS

Two classes of drugs—the monoamine oxidase (MAO) inhibitors and dibenzazepine derivatives—are particularly useful in the treatment of depression. The adjective *antidepressant,* referring to their therapeutic effect, is frequently applied to these drugs, but the terms *antidepressive* or *antidepression* would be preferable since *depressant* still has a pharmacologic connotation which does not necessarily equate with the therapeutic effect. For example, barbiturates and chloral hydrate, which may ameliorate the symptoms of depression, are in fact depressants in the pharmacological sense but act as mood elevators or antidepressants in the clinical sense. These terms must not be confused, the one referring to a drug that reduces nervous system excitability and the other to the capacity of the drug to ameliorate the symptoms of mental depression.

MONOAMINE OXIDASE INHIBITORS The observation that iproniazid, an inhibitor of MAO, had a mood-elevating effect in tuberculous patients initiated a great deal of interest in compounds of this type and led quickly to their exploitation in the treatment of depression. Iproniazid (Marsilid) proved exceedingly toxic and was soon taken off the market, as were several subsequently developed MAO inhibitors; but other drugs, much better tolerated, have become available. These include isocarboxizid (Marplan), nialamide (Niamid), phenelzine (Nardil), and tranylcypromine (Parnate), the latter two being the most frequently used. Tranylcypromine, which resembles dextroamphetamine chemically, has proved to be the most potent of these agents, but it has also produced the most serious toxic effects.

The exact mode of action of the MAO inhibitors has not been determined. They have in common the ability to block the oxidative deamination of naturally occurring amines (norepinephrine, dopamine, and serotonin), and it has been suggested that the accumulation of these neurohormonal substances is responsible for the antidepression effect. However, these drugs inhibit many enzymes other than monoamine oxidases and have numerous actions unrelated to enzyme inhibition. Furthermore, many agents with antidepression effects like those of the monoamine oxidase inhibitors do not inhibit this enzyme. At the present time, one cannot assume that the therapeutic effect of these drugs has a direct relation to the property of MAO inhibition.

The MAO inhibitors must be dispensed with great caution and a constant awareness of their potentially serious side effects. They may cause agitation, insomnia, and anxiety, and occasionally mania and convulsions may occur (especially in epileptic patients). Other side effects are increased neuromuscular activity in the form of muscle twitching, urinary retention, skin rashes, tachycardia, jaundice, visual impairment, enhancement of glaucoma, impotence, sweating, muscle spasms, and a variety of paresthesias. Orthostatic hypotension of a serious degree may develop.

Patients taking MAO inhibitors must be warned against the use of dibenzazepine derivatives (see below) and also sympathomimetic amines and tyramine, for they may induce a severe hypertensive episode and cerebral vascular accident, headache, atrial and ventricular arrhythmia, and pulmonary edema. Sympathomimetic amines are contained in some of the commonly used nasal sprays, nose drops, and so-called coryza tablets, and in tyramine-containing foods (cheeses, yogurt, beer, and wine). Phenothiazines and other powerful central nervous system stimulants should not be given with the MAO inhibitors. Exaggerated responses to the usual dose of meperidine (Demerol) and other narcotic drugs have also been observed; respiratory function may be depressed to a serious degree, and hyperpyrexia, agitation, and pronounced hypotension may occur as well, sometimes with fatal issue. Unpredictable side effects may also accompany the simultaneous administration of barbiturates and MAO inhibitors.

DIBENZAZEPINE DERIVATIVES (TRICYCLIC ANTIDEPRESSANTS) Soon after the first successes in the treatment of depression with MAO inhibitors, a new class of tricyclic compounds appeared. The first of this group was imipramine (Tofranil), which was soon followed by amitriptyline (Elavil), and then by desipramine (Norpramin), nortriptyline (Aventyl), protriptyline (Vivactil, Triptil), and doxepin (Sinequan). The first two members of this group have proved to be the most popular (see Chap. 376). Carbamazepine (Tegretol), another dibenzazepine derivative, widely used in the treatment of lancinating pain and seizures, is also occasionally used as an antidepressant.

The exact mode of action of these agents is unknown, but there is evidence that they block the reuptake of amine neurotransmitters released into the synaptic cleft, supporting the hypothesis that exogenous depression is due to a deficiency of noradrenergic or serotonergic transmission. The tricyclic compounds are presently the most effective drugs for the treatment of patients with depressive illnesses, particularly those associated with insomnia (early morning awakening), decreased appetite, weight loss, and decreased libido. Persistence of their pharmacologic effects after the drug is stopped is very short in comparison with the MAO inhibitors, and their side effects are far less frequent and serious.

The tricyclic compounds are potent anticholinergic agents, and their most prominent side effects (orthostatic hypotension, urinary bladder weakness) are due to peripheral anticholinergic action. They may also produce central nervous system excitement, leading to insomnia, agitation, and restlessness, but usually these effects can be controlled readily by the use of phenothiazines or chlordiazepoxide given concurrently or in the evenings. Occasionally they may cause ataxia and blood dyscrasias. The dibenzazepine drugs should never be given with an MAO inhibitor, since serious reactions may occur; hypertensive crises and lethal hyperpyrexia have been reported.

STIMULANTS

Drugs which act primarily as stimulants of the central nervous system have a relatively limited therapeutic use but assume clinical importance for other reasons. Some members of the group, e.g., the amphetamines, are much abused, and others are not infrequent causes of poisoning.

AMPHETAMINE (BENZEDRINE) This drug and its *d*-isomer, dextroamphetamine, are powerful analeptics and in addition have significant hypertensive, respiratory-stimulant, and appetite-depressant effects. These drugs are useful in the management of narcolepsy, but they are much more widely and indiscriminately used for the control of obesity and the abolition of fatigue. Undoubtedly, the initial effect of a moderate oral dose of amphetamine is to reverse fatigue, postpone the need for sleep, and elevate mood, but these effects are not entirely predictable and certainly not indefinite, and the user must pay for the period of wakefulness with even greater fatigue and often with depression. The intravenous use of a high dose of amphetamine produces an immediate ecstasy, "the flash." Because of the popularity of the amphetamines and ease with which they can be procured, instances of acute and chronic intoxication are observed frequently. The toxic signs are essentially an exaggeration of the analeptic effects—restlessness, excessive speech and motor activity, tremor, and insomnia. Occasionally grimacing, tic-like, choreoathetotic, and dystonic movements, similar to those produced by the phenothiazines, may develop as an acute idiosyncratic reaction to amphetamine. The chronic administration of large doses of amphetamine may give rise to hallucinations, delusions, and changes in affect and thought processes, a state that may be indistinguishable from paranoid schizophrenia. The development of tolerance to and physical dependence to drugs is discussed in Chap. 241.

METHYLPHENIDATE (RITALIN) This drug has much the same type of action as amphetamine. It is useful in the treatment of narcolepsy and, paradoxically, like dextroamphetamine, in the management of overactive children.

PICROTOXIN A powerful nervous system excitant, this drug exerts its main effects by producing convulsive seizures and reversing respiratory depression induced by drugs, particularly by barbiturates. It has been shown by Eccles and his colleagues that picrotoxin increases neuronal activity by blocking presynaptic inhibition, i.e., blocking the action of inhibitory fibers that synapse with the presynaptic terminals of excitatory fibers. However, the modern treatment of barbiturate intoxication does not include the use of picrotoxin or other analeptics, because of their epileptogenic properties and because barbiturate intoxication can be managed successfully by other means (see above).

STRYCHNINE The action of this drug is to increase neuronal excitability by interfering with postsynaptic inhibition; the therapeutic value is negligible. In children accidental poisoning may occur from ingestion of AS&B cathartic pills or "rat biscuits." Rarely, strychnine is taken with suicidal intent. After a period of heightened irritability and muscle twitching, tonic seizures occur, characterized by opisthotonus, rigid extension of the legs, facial tetanus, and apnea due to spasm of the muscles of respiration. Death from anoxia may follow several seizures. The immediate need is to control the convulsions. This calls for the intravenous administration of a short-acting barbiturate or the use of inhalation anesthesia; endotracheal intubation is an important safeguard. The patient must then be observed carefully, and if any signs of irritability recur, more sedative should be given. During this period, supportive care is indicated, as for any comatose patient. Morphine, which is principally a medullary depressant, is contraindicated.

PENTYLENETETRAZOL (METRAZOL, CARDIAZOL) This drug is a potent stimulant of all parts of the nervous system. For a number of years it served as the convulsive agent in shock treatment of depression and schizophrenia but was abandoned in favor of less dangerous and more effective forms of convulsive therapy. The use of this drug to activate latent epileptogenic foci or to reproduce convulsions, with the purpose of studying the underlying cerebral mechanisms, has been discontinued.

BEMEGRIDE, NIKETHAMIDE (CORAMINE) These two drugs act much like pentylenetetrazol. For many years common clinical practice was to administer nikethamide as a final therapeutic gesture in patients dying of cardiac and respiratory failure, but there is little evidence that the drug has a significant stimulant effect on either heart or respiration. Poisoning with these drugs, which is usually due to parenteral overdosage, is best treated with barbiturates.

CAFFEINE The therapeutic value of caffeine and other xanthine derivatives stems from their diuretic effects and their ability to stimulate the heart and nervous system. The major use of these agents is to abolish fatigue and maintain wakefulness, and the usual mode of administration is in coffee, a cup of which contains 100 to 150 mg caffeine. Overdosage leads to insomnia, tremulousness, mild delirium, tinnitus, tachycardia, prominent diuresis, and cardiac arrhythmias. The excitatory effects are easily controlled with barbiturates and other sedatives, and fatalities due to caffeine poisoning are extremely rare.

CAMPHOR Formerly a popular stimulant, camphor is now rarely used therapeutically; however, occasional cases of poisoning are still seen as a result of ingestion of liniment (camphorated oil) or moth flakes. The manifestations of poisoning are headache, sensation of warmth, confusion, clonic convulsions, and terminal respiratory depression; the characteristic odor of camphor facilitates the diagnosis. Treatment consists of supportive care and the cautious use of barbiturates to combat convulsions.

REFERENCES

Baldessarini RJ, Tarsy D: In *Psychopharmacology: A Generation of Progress,* MA Lipton et al (eds). New York, Raven, 1978

———: Drugs and the treatment of psychiatric disorders, in *Goodman and Gilman's The Pharmacological Basis of Therapeutics,* 6th ed, AG Gilman, LS Goodman, A Gilman (eds). New York, Macmillan, 1980, pp 391–447

Bloomer HA, Maddock RK Jr: An assessment of diuresis and dialysis for treating acute barbiturate poisoning, in *Acute Barbiturate Poisoning,* H Mathew (ed). Amsterdam, Excerpta Medica, 1971, chap 15

Bourne PG (ed): *Acute Drug Abuse Emergencies. A Treatment Manual.* New York, Academic, 1976

Clemmesen C, Nilsson E: Therapeutic trends in the treatment of barbiturate poisoning: The Scandinavian method. Clin Pharmacol Ther 2:220, 1961

DiMascio A, Shader RI (eds): *Clinical Handbook of Psychopharmacology.* New York, Science House, 1970

DiPalma JR (ed): *Drill's Pharmacology in Medicine.* New York, McGraw-Hill, 1971

Domestic Council Drug Abuse Task Force: *White Paper on Drug Abuse.* Washington, DC, US Government Printing Office, September 1975

Essig C: Chronic abuse of sedative-hypnotic drugs, in *Drug Abuse,* CJD Zarafonetis (ed). Philadelphia, Lea & Febiger, 1972, p 205

Harvey SC: Hypnotics and sedatives, in *Goodman and Gilman's The Pharmacological Basis of Therapeutics,* 6th ed, AG Gilman, LS Goodman, A Gilman (eds). New York, Macmillan, 1980, pp 339–375

Hollister LE: *Clinical Pharmacology of Psychotherapeutic Drugs.* New York, Churchill Livingstone, 1978

Isbell H et al: Chronic barbiturate intoxication: An experimental study. Arch Neurol Psychiatry 64:1, 1950

Iversen SD, Iversen LL: *Behavioral Pharmacology.* New York, Oxford, 1975

Marks J: *The Benzodiazepines: Use, Overuse, Misuse, Abuse.* Baltimore, University Park Press, 1978

Plum F, Swanson AC: Barbiturate poisoning treated by physiological methods. JAMA 163:827, 1957

Snyder SH: Receptors, neurotransmitters and drug responses. N Engl J Med 300:465, 1979

Wesson DR, Smith DE: *Barbiturates: Their Use, Misuse and Abuse.* New York, Human Sciences Press, 1977

Wikler A: Drug dependence, in *Clinical Neurology,* AB Baker, LH Baker (eds). New York, Harper & Row, 1975

244
TOBACCO SMOKING

JOHN H. HOLBROOK

Tobacco smoke is a ubiquitous personal and environmental pollutant. Although tobacco has been used in western culture for more than 400 years, human inhalation of cigarette smoke is a twentieth century phenomenon with major medical and economic consequences. In industrialized nations cigarette smoking is a principal cause of preventable disease and premature death.

Important changes in smoking trends are occurring in the United States. In general, the trend is downward. For example, between 1975 and 1979 per capita cigarette consumption declined at an average annual rate of 1.4 percent, reaching a level of 3900 cigarettes per adult. Between 1965 and 1980 the proportion of adult cigarette smokers in the United States declined from 53 to 37 percent of men and 33 to 29 percent of women (see Table 244-1); however, per capita cigarette consumption of current regular smokers may be increasing. There are 52.4 million current smokers and 33.3 million former smokers in the United States. Except among 17- and 18-year-old females, the percentage of current teenage smokers is also decreasing (Table 244-1). While consumption of cigar and pipe tobacco has decreased, use of chewing tobacco has increased.

CIGARETTE SMOKE Large prospective epidemiologic studies have shown a strong association between cigarette smoking and several diseases. Identification of more than 4000 substances in cigarette smoke provides a framework for understanding these diverse biologic effects.

Cigarette smoke is a heterogeneous aerosol produced by incomplete combustion of the tobacco leaf. It is composed of gases and vapors in which droplets are dispersed. Mainstream smoke emerges from the mouthpiece during puffing. Sidestream smoke is emitted between puffs at the burning cone and from the mouthpiece. The composition of the smoke is influenced by several factors including type of tobacco, temperature of combustion, length of the cigarette, porosity of the paper, additives, and filters. The major tobacco leaf constituents are carbohydrates, nonfatty organic acids, nitrogen-containing compounds, and resins. Cigarette temperatures vary greatly from 30°C at the mouthpiece to 900°C at the burning cone. In the presence of intense heat some tobacco constituents undergo thermic decomposition (pyrolysis). Volatile substances are distilled directly into the smoke. Unstable molecules recombine to generate new compounds (pyrosynthesis). Concentration of smoke constituents occurs as the smoke is filtered by unburnt tobacco and is redistilled by the burning cone. Some substances found in tobacco pass unchanged into cigarette smoke.

TABLE 244-1
Estimated percentage of current, regular cigarette smokers in the United States

Year	Female (Percent smokers 17 years of age and over)	Male
1955	24.5	52.6
1965	33.3	51.1
1970	31.1	43.5
1974	31.9	42.7
1980	28.9	36.7

	Percent teenage smokers by age					
	Ages 12–14		*Ages 15–16*		*Ages 17–18*	
Year	*Female*	*Male*	*Female*	*Male*	*Female*	*Male*
1968	0.6	2.9	9.6	17.0	18.6	30.2
1974	4.9	4.2	20.2	18.1	25.9	31.0
1979	4.4	3.2	11.8	13.5	26.2	19.3

Each cigarette generates approximately 500 mg mainstream smoke of which 92 percent is present in a gas phase and 8 percent is present in a particulate phase. Mainstream smoke contains 2 to 5 billion particles per milliliter, with the particle size ranging from 0.1 to 1.0 μm. Nitrogen, oxygen, and carbon dioxide account for 85 percent of the smoke's weight. The remaining gases, vapors, and particulate matter are the substances of medical importance. (See Table 244-2.)

Because a pack-a-day cigarette smoker puffs more than 50,000 times a year, the membranes of the mouth, nose, pharynx, and tracheobronchial tree are exposed repetitively to tobacco smoke. Some constituents act directly on the membranes, while others are absorbed into the blood or are dissolved in saliva and swallowed.

PHARMACOLOGY Tissue and organ system responses to cigarette smoke inhalation are multiple and complex. Most studies in humans have dealt with exposure to whole smoke or selected constituents which are thought to pose the greatest risk to health, for example, nicotine and carbon monoxide. Relatively little is known about the individual effects and interactions of other potentially toxic smoke constituents that are often present in low concentrations.

Nicotine, the component most characteristic of tobacco, is a highly toxic alkaloid that is both a ganglionic stimulant and depressant. Many of its complex effects are mediated by catecholamine release. Acute cardiovascular responses to nicotine observed in normal smokers include increases in systolic and diastolic blood pressure, heart rate, force of myocardial contraction, myocardial oxygen consumption, coronary artery blood flow, myocardial excitability, and peripheral vasoconstriction. Nicotine has also been shown to increase serum concentrations of glucose, cortisol, free fatty acids, and antidiuretic hormone and to increase platelet aggregation. Nicotine plays an important but not exclusive role in maintaining the smoking habit.

TABLE 244-2
Selected cigarette smoke constituents

Substance	*Effect*
PARTICULATE PHASE	
"Tar"*	Carcinogen
Polynuclear aromatic hydrocarbons	Carcinogen
Nicotine	Ganglionic stimulator and depressor
Phenol	Cocarcinogen and irritant
Cresol	Cocarcinogen and irritant
β-Naphthylamine	Carcinogen
N-Nitrosonornicotine	Carcinogen
Benzo[a]pyrene	Carcinogen
Trace metals (e.g., nickel, polonium 210)	Carcinogen
Indole	Tumor accelerator
Carbazole	Tumor accelerator
GAS PHASE	
Carbon monoxide	Impairs oxygen transport and utilization
Hydrocyanic acid	Ciliotoxin and irritant
Acetaldehyde	Ciliotoxin and irritant
Acrolein	Ciliotoxin and irritant
Ammonia	Ciliotoxin and irritant
Formaldehyde	Ciliotoxin and irritant
Oxides of nitrogen	Ciliotoxin and irritant
Nitrosamines	Carcinogen
Hydrazine	Carcinogen

* *The aggregate of particulate matter in cigarette smoke after subtracting nicotine and moisture.*

Carbon monoxide is a toxic gas which interferes with oxygen transport and utilization. Because cigarette smoke contains 2 to 6 percent carbon monoxide, smokers inhale concentrations as high as 400 parts per million (ppm) and develop elevated carboxyhemoglobin (COHB) levels. While the range of COHB found in smokers is 2 to 15 percent, levels for nonsmokers are near 1 percent. The average COHB level of moderate cigarette smokers is 5 percent. Carbon monoxide produces its adverse effects by reducing the amount of available oxyhemoglobin and myoglobin, and displacing the oxygen-hemoglobin dissociation curve to the left. Chronic, mild elevations of COHB due to smoking are a common cause of polycythemia and may produce subtle impairment of central nervous system function.

Cigarette smoke and its condensate are carcinogenic in several species of animals. The major identified carcinogens in cigarette smoke are polynuclear aromatic hydrocarbons (Table 244-2). Tumor promoters and tumor accelerators present in cigarette smoke, such as catechol, greatly enhance its carcinogenicity. Sister chromatid exchange rates in the lymphocytes of smokers are higher than in nonsmokers. Cigarette smoke condensate is also mutagenic in a microbial test system.

Potent pulmonary irritants and ciliotoxins are found in cigarette smoke (Table 244-2). These substances cause increased bronchial mucus secretion, and they mediate acute and chronic decreases in pulmonary and mucociliary function.

EPIDEMIOLOGY Data from large prospective studies of populations in several countries show that cigarette-smoking men, taken as a whole, have 30 to 80 percent higher death rates than nonsmokers. This excess male mortality is present in all groups over the age of 35, but it is proportionately greatest in the age group 45 to 54. In a study of British physicians it was shown that 40 percent of 35-year-old men who smoked more than 25 cigarettes per day died before the age of 65, compared with 15 percent of nonsmokers in the same category. The excess mortality of female smokers has been somewhat less than that of male smokers, but recent trends suggest it is increasing. Smoking is responsible for an estimated 325,000 premature deaths each year in the United States. Coronary heart disease is the chief contributor to smoking-related excess mortality. In the United States cigarette smokers experience more disability due to chronic illness and report 45 percent more days absent from work than do nonsmokers.

A strong dose-response relationship exists between tobacco exposure and excess mortality, as measured by age at onset of smoking, cigarette consumption, and smoke inhalation. Cessation of smoking is associated with a decrease in the excess mortality. These observations together with clinical, experimental, and pathological studies suggest that smoking, per se, causes the excess mortality.

CHARACTERISTICS OF SMOKERS Demographic, anthropometric, physiological, and laboratory features which distinguish cigarette smokers from nonsmokers are due both to baseline differences between these groups and to the effects of smoking. Smokers drink more alcohol, coffee, and tea than do nonsmokers. Their weight and blood pressure are slightly less and their heart rate is slightly faster than those of nonsmokers. In women the menopause comes earlier in smokers than in nonsmokers. Smokers have impaired maximum exercise performance. A markedly increased number of pulmonary alveolar macrophages is present in smokers, and these cells show abnormal function and metabolism. Serum thiocyanate levels are much higher in smokers. When compared with nonsmokers, smokers show small increases in total white blood cell count and serum cholesterol, as well as small decreases in serum high-density lipoprotein, vitamin C, uric acid, and albumin. Other laboratory findings observed more commonly in smokers than in nonsmokers include proteinuria, increased levels of carcinoembryonic antigen, and an increased frequency of antinuclear autoantibodies.

CLINICAL CORRELATIONS **Cardiovascular disease** Premature coronary heart disease (CHD) is one of the most important consequences of cigarette smoking (see Chap. 260). The risk of fatal or nonfatal CHD is 60 to 70 percent greater in male smokers than nonsmokers. Sudden death may be the first manifestation of CHD, and it is two to three times more likely to occur in 35- to 54-year-old male cigarette smokers than in nonsmokers. Women cigarette smokers are also at greater risk of developing CHD than nonsmokers, and the use of both cigarettes and oral contraceptives increases this risk approximately tenfold. Cigarette smoking acts both independently and synergistically with other factors to increase the risk of developing CHD. Cessation of smoking is associated with decreased CHD mortality, an effect which is measurable within 1 year. Those who continue to smoke after an acute myocardial infarction are more likely to die from CHD than are those who quit smoking. Cigarette smoking produces an imbalance between myocardial oxygen supply and demand, a decrease in the threshold for ventricular fibrillation, and an increase in platelet aggregation; avoidance of these effects may explain the rapid cardiac benefits of quitting smoking. Coronary atherosclerosis and intimal thickening of intramyocardial arteries and arterioles are more frequent in smokers than in nonsmokers.

Cigarette smoking is a major risk factor for arteriosclerosis obliterans (see Chap. 266) and thromboangiitis obliterans (see Chap. 269). It also aggravates peripheral ischemia and may adversely affect peripheral bypass grafts. The mortality rate for atherosclerotic aortic aneurysm is greater in male smokers than nonsmokers. Cigarette smoking is not a risk factor for the development of hypertension; however, hypertensives who smoke appear to be at greater risk to develop malignant hypertension. Subarachnoid hemorrhage is more likely to occur in women smokers than nonsmokers, and the use of both cigarettes and oral contraceptives greatly increases this risk. Because of the association with chronic obstructive lung disease, cigarette smoking is an important factor leading to cor pulmonale.

Cancer In spite of the well-documented cause-and-effect relationship between cigarette smoking and lung cancer, more Americans die from this cancer than from any other tumor (see Chap. 284). In 1981 an estimated 105,000 lung cancer deaths occurred in the United States; approximately 80 percent of these deaths are attributable to cigarette smoking. The risk of developing lung cancer is quantitatively related to cigarette smoke exposure. Men who smoke one pack a day increase their risk tenfold compared with nonsmokers; men who smoke two packs a day may increase their risk more than 25 times compared with nonsmokers. Workers in the asbestos and uranium mining industries who smoke cigarettes are at especially high risk for developing lung cancer. Cigarette consumption by women increased rapidly in the United States during the past 25 years, and lung cancer mortality is currently increasing at a faster rate in women than in men. Projections indicate that by 1984 lung cancer will become the leading cause of cancer death among American women. Because 5-year survival rates for lung cancer are less than 10 percent, emphasis must be placed on prevention. Giving up cigarettes is associated with a gradual decline in the risk of developing lung cancer. After 15 years the ex-smoker's risk approximates that of the nonsmoker. Squamous-cell and oat-cell carcinomas are the histological types of lung cancer most closely associated with cigarette smoking.

Cigarette smoking is causally associated in men and women with cancer of the larynx, oral cavity, and esophagus; alcohol consumption acts synergistically with cigarette smoking to increase the risk for these neoplasms. Carcinoma of the bladder, kidney, and pancreas is also associated with cigarette smoking.

Respiratory disease Cigarette smoking is the most important factor contributing to the development of chronic obstructive pulmonary disease (COPD), that is, chronic bronchitis and emphysema (see Chap. 279). Of the estimated 50,000 deaths from COPD that occurred in the United States in 1980, approximately 70 percent were attributable to smoking, and many of these deaths were preceded by prolonged respiratory disability. Depending upon the extent of smoke exposure, male cigarette smokers experience from 4 to 25 times higher mortality secondary to COPD than do nonsmokers. Although the death rate from COPD among female smokers is somewhat lower than among male smokers, it is increasing much more rapidly in female than in male smokers. Chronic cough, sputum production, and breathlessness are much more common in smokers. Smokers are more likely than nonsmokers to show abnormalities in a number of pulmonary function tests including measurements of elastic recoil, large and small airway obstruction, ventilation-perfusion mismatching, and diffusing capacity. Mild pulmonary function abnormalities may be present even in teenage smokers. When compared with continuing smokers, ex-smokers experience a decrease in mortality from COPD, a decrease in prevalence of pulmonary symptoms, and improved pulmonary function. British studies suggest that regular measurement of the forced expiratory volume in middle age may identify individuals who are at high risk for developing symptomatic COPD. Cessation of smoking would be especially valuable for these patients. Chronic inhalation of pulmonary irritants and ciliotoxins (Table 244-2) may contribute to the development of COPD. Studies of the pathogenesis of emphysema suggest that smoking results in an excess of pulmonary proteases, which may produce pulmonary damage. The major site of obstruction in chronic bronchitis is the bronchiole measuring less than 2 mm in diameter, and cigarette smoking is associated with bronchiolitis and increased stickiness of bronchiolar mucus. For most people in the United States cigarette smoking is a more important cause of COPD than are occupational or environmental factors; however, several factors may act conjointly to increase morbidity and mortality from COPD. In a rare disorder, homozygous α_1-antitrypsin deficiency, smoking accelerates the tendency to panacinar emphysema; smoking may play an additive role in individuals heterozygous for this state.

Cigarette smoking has been associated with an increased incidence of respiratory infections and deaths from pneumonia and influenza. Postoperative respiratory complications and spontaneous pneumothorax are also more common in smokers. Because tobacco smoke may increase airway obstruction, asthmatics should be urged not to smoke. Chronic stomatitis and chronic laryngitis occur more frequently in smokers than in nonsmokers.

Pregnancy Smoking during pregnancy may affect the fetus adversely. Infants whose mothers smoked during pregnancy weigh, on an average, 170 g less than infants whose mothers did not smoke. Maternal smoking during pregnancy is related to an increased risk of spontaneous abortion, fetal death, and neonatal death. This increased risk may be much greater in pregnancies already at high risk due to other factors. Smoking by a woman during pregnancy may also adversely affect the long-term physical growth and intellectual development of the child.

Gastrointestinal disorders Gastric and duodenal ulcer disease is more prevalent in male and female cigarette smokers and causes more deaths in male smokers than in nonsmokers. Smoking impairs healing of peptic ulcers, inhibits pancreatic bicarbonate secretion, and decreases the pressure of esophageal and pyloric sphincters.

Involuntary smoke inhalation Indoor atmospheres and other confined spaces are often contaminated by tobacco smoke which is inhaled involuntarily by both smokers and nonsmokers. Most of the atmospheric pollutants arise from sidestream smoke. It contains greater concentrations of many smoke constituents than does mainstream smoke, but since sidestream smoke is diluted in a large volume of air, the smoke exposure from involuntary inhalation is less than that associated with smoking.

Initially, involuntary or passive smoking was thought to cause primarily an irritation, e.g., ocular burning, nasal congestion. Later, accumulated data documented that patients with symptomatic CHD and COPD may note exacerbation of symptoms when exposed to smoke-contaminated air. Even asymptomatic nonsmokers who are chronically exposed to smoke-contaminated air may develop small-airways dysfunction. Studies from Japan and Greece suggest that passive smoking may increase the risk for lung cancer.

Drug metabolism Tobacco smoke constituents induce hepatic microsomal enzyme systems which are important in the metabolism of many drugs. For example, cigarette smoking appears to increase the metabolism of phenacetin, propoxyphene, and antipyrine. The theophylline half-life is shorter in heavy smokers than in nonsmokers, and consequently smokers may require higher maintenance doses of this drug. With cessation of smoking, adjustment of the dose may be necessary.

TYPES OF SMOKING During the past 20 years the amount of tar and nicotine delivered by cigarettes made in the United States decreased by more than 50 percent. In 1980 the average American cigarette delivered 1 mg nicotine and 14 mg tar. Although there is a paucity of scientific data concerning the relative risks of lower-tar and -nicotine cigarettes compared with higher-tar and -nicotine cigarettes, filter-tipped cigarettes and lower-tar and -nicotine cigarettes now account for more than 90 and 50 percent of sales, respectively. Lung cancer is the only tobacco-related disease for which the use of lower-tar and -nicotine cigarettes has been shown to result in risk reduction, compared with the use of higher-tar and -nicotine cigarettes; however, compared with not smoking or quitting, the benefits are minimal. Consumers who choose lower-tar and -nicotine cigarettes and then smoke a larger number of cigarettes or inhale more frequently or deeply may actually increase their exposure to harmful substances. There is also concern because unidentified flavoring agents are added to these cigarettes to enhance consumer acceptance. Their presence represents an unmeasured risk for the active smoker, passive smoker, and fetus.

Cigar and pipe smokers usually inhale less smoke than cigarette smokers. This is presumably related to the alkaline pH of cigar and pipe tobacco, which is irritating to the respiratory tract. The smoke exposure and overall mortality rates of pipe and cigar smokers in the United States are substantially less than those of cigarette smokers. Death rates of cigarette, cigar, and pipe smokers are approximately equal for carcinoma of the oral cavity, larynx, and esophagus, sites where exposures to cigarette, cigar, and pipe smoke are similar. The mortality rates of most cigar and pipe smokers for cancer at other sites, CHD, and COPD are not greatly elevated above the rates of nonsmokers, but cigar and pipe smokers who inhale consistently may experience adverse health effects comparable with those of cigarette smokers.

CESSATION OF SMOKING Psychosocial forces lead to the onset of smoking, especially among teenagers. Later, drug dependency and psychological factors maintain the smoking habit. It is estimated that more than 30 million people in the United States have stopped smoking. Many long-term smokers quit because of smoking-related health problems. This seems to explain Hammond's observation that the death rate of men smoking more than 20 cigarettes a day was somewhat higher in the months immediately after quitting than that of continuing smokers. Thereafter, a gradual decline in death rates was observed in ex-smokers. Ten or more years after quitting, the death rate of those who had smoked more than 20 cigarettes a day decreased about two-thirds, and the death rate of individuals who had smoked 20 cigarettes a day or less was about the same as that of nonsmokers. Ex-smokers usually experience prompt symptomatic improvement. On the average they also gain less than 5 lb, compared with continuing smokers.

In the United States more than 80 percent of cigarette smokers would like to stop smoking. Many self-care and organized programs are available to assist these individuals. Organized programs employ several techniques including instruction, counseling, withdrawal clinics, behavioral modification, hypnosis, aversive conditioning, self-monitoring, and drug therapy. Even though individual successes result from these programs, their value is uncertain. One-year abstinence rates of 20 to 30 percent are common. Relapse usually occurs during the 3-month interval after quitting. Successful programs emphasize maintenance of the nonsmoking state during this critical period.

All smokers should be encouraged to quit, especially those in high-risk groups with chronic pulmonary disease, coronary artery disease, and pregnancy. Physicians can help their smoking patients in the following manner:

1 Obtain a quantitative smoking history.
2 Explain the health risks in a personally relevant fashion.
3 Emphasize the benefits associated with cessation.
4 Advise and assist the patient to quit smoking.
5 Support the patient in a maintenance program.

Patients who are unable or unwilling to stop cigarette smoking should be assisted to reduce their smoke exposure by smoking lower-tar and -nicotine cigarettes, smoking fewer cigarettes, inhaling less, taking fewer puffs, and leaving a longer stub.

Ultimately, primary smoking prevention in the pediatric and adolescent age groups may be the most effective program. Young people who understand the consequences of smoking to their health and who appreciate the difficulty of quitting are less likely to start smoking.

REFERENCES

Friedman GD et al: Mortality in cigarette smokers and quitters. N Engl J Med 304:1407, 1981

Hammond EC: Smoking in relation to the death rates of one million men and women, in *Epidemiological Approaches to the Study of Cancer and Other Chronic Diseases,* W Haenszel (ed). National Cancer Institute Monograph no 19, 1966, pp 127–204

———, Selikoff IJ: Passive smoking and lung cancer with comments on two new papers. Environ Res 24:444, 1981

Royal College of Physicians: *Smoking or Health.* Tunbridge Wells, Kent, Pitman Medical, 1977

US Department of Health, Education, and Welfare: *Smoking and Health.* PHS Publication no 1103, 1964

———: *Smoking and Health: A Report of the Surgeon General.* DHEW Publication no (PHS) 79-50066, 1979

US Department of Health and Human Services: *The Health Consequences of Smoking for Women: A Report of the Surgeon General,* 1980

———: *The Health Consequences of Smoking—the Changing Cigarette: A Report of the Surgeon General.* DHHS Publication no (PHS) 81-50156, 1981

World Health Organization: *Smoking and Its Effects on Health.* WHO Technical Report Series no 568, 1975

245 ELECTRICAL INJURIES

JAMES F. WALLACE

EPIDEMIOLOGY Electrical injury has become progressively more common since the first human fatality from accidental electrocution was reported in 1879. In the United States, approximately 1000 deaths occur annually from electric current accidents, while another 200 persons die as a result of being struck by lightning. In addition, major electrical burns presently constitute nearly 5 percent of all admissions to burn centers in this country. Electrical injuries occur most commonly among utility pole linemen and construction workers who come into contact with high-tension current, but nearly a third result from accidents in the home or other settings including the hospital with its many electrically powered instruments and appliances.

PATHOGENESIS In understanding the fundamental aspects of electric current injury, it is helpful to consider some electrophysical principles. For an electric current to flow, there must be a closed pathway or circuit, and a difference in potential or voltage must exist between two points in this completed circuit. The flow of current is directly related to the voltage difference and inversely proportional to the electrical resistance between two points in the circuit (Ohm's law). High-resistance paths allow relatively small currents to flow, while low resistances permit large currents to flow. When the voltage is very high, the flow of current will likewise be relatively great, unless the resistance is increased proportionally to the voltage; however, if the potential difference between the two points can be minimized, the current flow can also be minimized regardless of resistance.

Although the end result of passage of an electric current through the human body is unpredictable in the individual case, many factors are known to influence the nature and severity of electrical injuries. Body tissues vary considerably in their *resistance* to the flow of current, with conductivity being roughly proportional to water content. Bone and skin offer relatively high resistance, while blood, muscle, and nerve are good conductors. The resistance of normal skin can be lowered by *moisture,* and this factor alone can convert what might ordinarily be a mild injury to a fatal shock. Of importance at the time of contact is *grounding* which, if effective, can minimize the voltage difference between two points in the electric circuit and lower the intensity of current passing through the body. The *pathway of the current through the body* is also crucial. An accident involving passage of a current between a point of contact on the leg and the ground is less likely to be injurious than one between the head and the foot, in which the heart lies between the two poles of the circuit. Similarly, a small current leak which would be innocuous when applied to the surface of the intact body may result in a fatal arrhythmia when conducted directly to the heart via a low-resistance intracardiac catheter. *Duration of contact* also influences the outcome of electrical injury. Alternating current is much more dangerous than direct current, partly because of its ability to produce tetanic muscular contractions which prevent the victim from being able to release contact with the circuit. This is usually accompanied by sweating, which lowers skin resistance, allowing current of still greater intensity to pass into the body until fatal cardiac arrhythmia results.

While the effects of electricity upon the body are incompletely understood, many pathophysiologic features of severe electrical injury have been described. In general, when sudden death occurs following low-voltage shock, it is due to the direct effect of relatively small amounts of current upon the myocardium resulting in ventricular fibrillation. With high-tension injury (greater than 1000 V) cardiac asystole and respiratory arrest occur probably as a result of injury to the medullary centers of the brain.

In addition, contact with high-intensity current may cause three types of thermal injuries. Current coursing externally to the body from the contact point to the ground may generate temperatures as high as 10,000°C and cause extensive carbonification of skin and immediately underlying tissues termed *arc* or *flash burns.* Such burns often ignite surrounding clothing or nearby objects which result in *flame burns.* Finally, there is injury due to the *direct heating* of tissues by electric current. As it traverses the skin, energy from current is converted into heat which produces coagulation necrosis at the points where it enters and exits from the skin as well as in striated muscle and blood vessels through which it passes. The associated vascular injury results in thromboses, often at sites distant from the body surface, and accounts for the observation that a greater amount of tissue destruction characteristically occurs in an electrical injury than is apparent on first inspection.

PATHOLOGY In patients who die immediately, autopsy findings are limited to burns and generalized petechial hemorrhages. If patients survive for a period of days or longer, postmortem examination reveals focal necrosis of bone, large blood vessels, muscle, peripheral nerves, spinal cord, or brain. Renal tubular necrosis may also be seen when acute renal failure follows extensive tissue destruction.

CLINICAL MANIFESTATIONS Immediately after a severe electrical shock, patients are usually comatose, apneic, and in circulatory collapse from ventricular fibrillation or cardiac standstill. If they survive this stage, they often are disoriented, combative, and frequently may have seizures. Often they will be found to have fractures of bone caused either by convulsive muscular contractions accompanying the shock or from falls at the time of the accident. Hypovolemic shock often appears soon after high-tension electrical injury and is due to the rapid loss of fluid into areas of tissue damage, and from body surface burns. Hypotension, direct injury to the kidneys by the electric current, and renal tubular damage from myoglobin and hemoglobin pigments liberated during massive muscle necrosis and hemolysis may lead to acute renal failure.

Besides the extensive destruction of tissue occurring instantly in electrical burns, additional injury from ischemia produced by swelling of damaged tissues may appear later and is often accompanied by severe metabolic acidosis. Other serious complications which may be seen are gastrointestinal hemorrhage from preexisting or acute ulcers and both anaerobic and aerobic infections originating in inadequately debrided necrotic muscle masses.

Late effects include various neurological disabilities, visual disturbances, and the residual damage left by burns. Nervous system injuries are frequent and include peripheral neuropathies, incomplete transection of the spinal cord, and reflex sympathetic dystrophies, as well as late convulsive disorders and intractable headache. The development of cataracts of one or both eyes has been reported to occur up to 3 years following electrical injury.

LABORATORY FINDINGS Immediately following major electrical injury the hematocrit is elevated and the plasma volume reduced, reflecting sequestration of fluid in the wound. Unless extensive flame burns are also present, serial determinations of either of these parameters provide a good means of monitoring the adequacy of fluid replacement therapy. Myoglobinuria is seen frequently in association with severe shocks, and when it persists following establishment of urine flow, usually indicates massive muscle injury. In many patients arterial blood pH determinations will indicate the presence of metabolic acidosis. Lumbar puncture may show elevated pressure associated with cerebral edema or bloody spinal fluid as a result of intracerebral hemorrhage. The electrocardiogram not infrequently shows tachycardia and minor ST-segment alterations which can persist for several weeks following injury. Unexplained acute hypokalemia leading to respiratory arrest and cardiac arrhythmias has developed in some patients between the second and fourth weeks following injury.

TREATMENT Removal of victims from contact with the current should be accomplished immediately without touching them directly. Rescuers should use a rubber sheet, a leather belt applied as a sling, a wooden pole, or other nonconductive material to detach them, and this should be preceded by cutting off the source of current when possible. If the victim is not breathing, mouth-to-mouth ventilation should be instituted at once. Although most cases who survive develop spontaneous respiration within half an hour, complete recovery after longer periods occurs often enough so that respiratory support should be continued for at least 4 h. If there is no evidence of heartbeat, external cardiac massage should accompany ventilatory resuscitation. Persons struck by lightning frequently have cardiac asystole which responds to a manual blow to the chest, while victims of low-voltage shocks will usually require defibrillation to restore heart action. During cardiopulmonary resuscitation and evacuation to the hospital, attention should be paid to possible broken bones and spinal cord injuries incurred at the time of the accident.

Subsequent hospital management of patients with electrothermal injuries requires considerable specialized care; whenever feasible, they should be referred to an appropriate burn or trauma unit.

Rapid institution of fluid and electrolyte therapy for hypovolemic shock and acidosis is essential, with guidelines being the patient's urine output, hematocrit, osmolality, central venous pressure, and arterial blood gases. Standard burn formulas should not be used to estimate fluid therapy since these are based only upon extent of body surface area injury and do not take into account the extensive damage to muscle which is usually present. Instead, fluid replacement principles used in the treatment of crush injury, which electrical injury closely resembles, should be followed. Large volumes of fluid, preferably lactated Ringer's solution, should be administered in order to maintain urine output greater than 50 ml/h. If myoglobinuria persists after adequate urine flow has been established, the use of furosemide or an osmotic diuretic such as mannitol along with alkalinization of the urine is indicated. Management of the electrical wound should include adequate debridement of necrotic tissue and often will require fasciotomy to prevent further ischemic injury. Anticlostridial prophylaxis, including tetanus toxoid and high doses of penicillin, should be administered to all severely injured patients, while topical antimicrobial chemotherapy with mafenide (Sulfamylon) or silver sulfadiazine may be useful in preventing or delaying infections in extensive surface burns. Survivors of the acute episode often require extensive treatment for infection, cerebral edema, visceral injury, and delayed hemorrhage as devitalized tissues slough. If acute renal failure occurs, it should be managed as described in Chap. 290.

PREVENTION Proper installation of appliances, grounding of telephone lines and radio and television aerials, and the use of rubber gloves and dry shoes when working with electric circuits should be routine. Unused wall sockets should be kept plugged and live extension cords not left unattended, particularly in households where there are young children. During a severe thunderstorm, refuge near hilltops, riverbanks, hedges, telephone poles, and trees should be avoided. The safest shelter is the closed house, while a closed automobile, cave, ditch, or even lying on the ground curled up with hands close together is relatively secure. In hospitalized patients, the hazard of ventricular fibrillation precipitated by minute current leaks conducted directly to the myocardium from monitoring equipment via pacemakers or intravascular manometric catheters should be more widely appreciated. Hospital personnel should be aware that, in addition to medical instruments, patient contact with two or more other power line–operated devices such as television sets, radios, electric razors, lamps, and especially electric beds can also result in electrocution if the heart lies within the current path through the patient. These hazards can be minimized by proper grounding of equipment *before* a patient is connected to the instrument, periodic measurement for leakage of current supplied by each device, and by instruction in the principles of electrical safety for hospital personnel who use the complex and dangerous equipment that is so much a part of modern medical practice.

REFERENCES

Apfelberg DB et al: Pathophysiology and treatment of lightning injuries. J Trauma 14:453, 1974

Artz CP: Changing concepts of electrical injury. Am J Surg 128:600, 1974

McCrady-Kahn VL, Kahn AM: Lightning burns. West J Med 134:215, 1981

Rouse RG, Dimick AR: The treatment of electrical injury compared to burn injury. A review of pathophysiology and comparison of patient management protocols. J Trauma 18:43, 1978

Sances A Jr et al: Electrical injuries. Surg Gynecol Obstet 149:97, 1979

Solem L et al: The natural history of electrical injury. J Trauma 17:487, 1977

Strasser EG et al: Lightning injuries. J Trauma 17:315, 1977

246 DROWNING AND NEAR-DROWNING

JAMES F. WALLACE

EPIDEMIOLOGY In the United States, drowning accounts for approximately 7000 fatalities per year and is one of the three leading causes of accidental death. In addition, although no national statistics are available, it has been estimated that as many as 48,000 persons annually are near-drowning victims: those who live at least temporarily following an immersion incident. Children and young adults are most often the victims, and nearly 80 percent are males. However, with the increasing popularity of boating and water sports in this country nearly half the population is at risk of drowning each year, especially during the summer months.

PATHOPHYSIOLOGY Ten to twenty percent of drowning victims have no evidence of water aspiration in their lungs at autopsy ("dry drowning"). Death is due to asphyxia secondary to reflex laryngospasm and glottic closure. It is probable that a similar number of near-drowning victims also do not aspirate. If ventilation is reestablished before they sustain irreversible anoxic brain damage, prompt and complete recovery can be anticipated.

When aspiration accompanies drowning ("wet drowning"), the clinical situation is further complicated by the amount of surrounding water that is introduced into the respiratory tract as well as by the solutes and solids contained in it. A severe pulmonary injury often occurs, resulting in persistent arterial hypoxemia and metabolic acidosis even after ventilation has been restored.

In the past, an important distinction was made between the pathophysiology of saltwater and freshwater drowning with respect to changes in blood volume, serum electrolyte concentrations, and cardiovascular function. However, it has been established that the most important problem in human near-drowning is hypoxia and that the other disturbances are of considerably less significance in determining survival.

The mechanisms by which hypoxia develops in near-drowning with aspiration are often multiple: laryngospasm, bronchospasm, airway obstruction secondary to aspirated particulate matter, and pulmonary edema following prolonged hypoxia can take place regardless of the composition of the water aspirated, while other types of lung injury causing hypoxemia depend upon the osmolar and chemical characteristics of the immersion fluid. Aspiration of seawater, which is hypertonic compared with blood and chemically irritating to the pulmonary alveolocapillary membrane, causes a rapid shift of plasma proteins and water from the circulation into the alveolar lumen. Continued perfusion of these nonventilated, edema-filled alveoli results in an intrapulmonary right-to-left shunt and arterial hypoxemia. When hypotonic fresh water is aspirated, fluid is rapidly absorbed from the lung into the circulation. Injury to alveolar lining cells takes place, altering or destroying the properties of pulmonary surfactant that maintains surface tension, and leading to alveolar collapse. Ventilation-perfusion ratios change in these atelectatic areas of lung, and hypoxemia is the result. Metabolic acidosis, which is present in as many as 70 percent of near-drowning victims, is a consequence of tissue hypoxia and may be severe.

Although changes in electrolyte concentrations occur, depending upon the type and volume of fluid aspirated, these disturbances are rarely life-threatening. Most persons who aspirate sufficient quantities to produce marked electrolyte abnormalities do not survive the immersion incident. Similarly, profound changes in circulating blood volume are unusual. However, hypovolemia requiring treatment may be seen in massive saltwater aspiration accompanied by shifts of fluid from the vascular space into the lung.

Although rarely of clinical significance, some hemolysis of red blood cells often takes place, especially with freshwater aspiration. Free hemoglobin may be found in the urine and blood, but the abnormality requires no specific therapy. Disseminated intravascular coagulation has been reported as a complication of freshwater near-drowning. It is thought that with extensive pulmonary injury "tissue factor" in lung parenchyma and plasminogen activator from pulmonary endothelium are released, triggering the extrinsic clotting and fibrinolytic systems. Other pathophysiologic events in near-drowning include the development of renal failure secondary to acute tubular necrosis, probably due to the combined effects of hypoxia and hypotension, and neurological deficits secondary to cerebral anoxia. Although the extent of the central nervous system injury tends to correlate with the duration of hypoxia, hypothermia accompanying the incident may be a moderating factor by reducing cerebral oxygen requirements. Complete neurological recovery has been reported in victims submerged as long as 40 min in water temperatures less than 20°C.

CLINICAL MANIFESTATIONS The clinical features in near-drowning are variable and depend upon many factors including the amount and type of water aspirated and the promptness and effectiveness of treatment. Pulmonary and neurological abnormalities usually predominate. Patients may present with mild cough and tachypnea, or with fulminant pulmonary edema. At least a third will require endotracheal intubation and some type of ventilatory therapy for the management of pulmonary injury. Instead of gradual recovery during the first 48 to 72 h of treatment, some patients will develop the adult respiratory distress syndrome, associated with progressive respiratory failure and reduction in lung compliance (see Chap. 287). Other pulmonary complications often include regional atelectasis due to aspirated particulate matter; secondary bacterial pneumonia; lung abscess; empyema; and injuries such as pneumothorax or pneumomediastinum sustained during resuscitation or related to ventilator therapy.

Early neurological manifestations include seizures, especially during resuscitative efforts, and altered mental status, ranging from normal alertness to agitation, combativeness, or coma. Patients may present with speech, motor, or visual abnormalities or with more diffuse organic brain syndromes. Some of these neurological deficits will improve gradually and resolve over several months. However, 5 to 20 percent of patients will have permanent sequelae, many of which prove ultimately fatal. Neurological status usually does not continue to worsen after a near-drowning victim is admitted to the hospital unless there has been a preceding deterioration in pulmonary status. The possibility of unrecognized head trauma coincident with the drowning episode or a subdural hematoma should be considered as well.

Near-drowning victims often require treatment for cardiac as well as respiratory arrest during resuscitation. If this is successfully accomplished, most patients experience few additional cardiovascular problems. Supraventricular arrhythmias are common but usually resolve promptly when acidosis and hypoxia are treated. Heart failure secondary to myocardial ischemia or acutely expanded blood volume is unusual. Instead, pulmonary edema and low cardiac output states are usually due to the pulmonary injury from water aspiration with extravasation of fluid into the lung, resulting in hypovolemia.

Fever, frequently greater than 38°C, is seen in most patients within the first 24 h following significant aspiration. Its appearance later in the hospital course usually indicates a complicating infection. Vomiting is common during and after resuscitation. This often is associated with gastric distention by large quantities of fluid and air swallowed during the near-drowning episode and may result in additional aspiration. Other rare, but clinically important, features which may be encountered include acute renal failure and a severe hemorrhagic diathesis.

LABORATORY FINDINGS Arterial blood gas and pH determinations on admission reveal varying degrees of hypoxia and acidosis; follow-up values are the most reliable indicators of the effectiveness of ventilatory therapy. In 25 percent of near-drowning victims the initial chest x-ray film may be normal; however, this finding does not exclude the possibility that the patient has significant hypoxemia. In the remainder of cases, radiologic findings range from fine, symmetric, perihilar infiltrates with relative sparing of apexes, bases, and lateral lung fields to massive bilateral pulmonary edema with little or no areas of sparing. Marked clearing of these abnormalities usually takes place within 72 to 96 h.

Alterations in serum sodium and potassium may be noted, but these are generally mild and require no corrective treatment. Although leukocytosis up to 40,000 white blood cells per cubic millimeter is common during the first 24 to 48 h following near-drowning, significant changes in hematocrit and hemoglobin are rare, irrespective of the type of fluid aspirated. A *falling* hematocrit should raise the possibility of bleeding, not hemolysis, which, if it has occurred, should be apparent at the time of initial evaluation. Thrombocytopenia, prolonged prothrombin and partial thromboplastin times, hypofibrinogenemia, and elevated fibrin degradation products may be seen if disseminated intravascular coagulation takes place (see Chap. 334).

THERAPY The primary objective of therapy is to correct hypoxemia and acidosis as rapidly as possible. On-the-scene efforts should include immediate institution of mouth-to-mouth breathing and, if necessary, closed-chest cardiac massage. Time should not be wasted with attempts to drain water from the victim's lungs. However, it is important to establish and maintain a clear airway at the onset of resuscitation in order to avoid accidental overdistention of the stomach which might result in regurgitation and aspiration. One hundred percent oxygen should be administered by inhalation as soon as possible, and other necessary resuscitative efforts continued during evacuation to the hospital. Even if spontaneous ventilation returns and the patient seems coherent, high concentrations of oxygen should be continued, since severe hypoxemia and acidosis may be present even in persons who are alert and without cyanosis.

All near-drowning victims should be taken to a hospital for further evaluation. Initial diagnostic studies should include arterial blood gas and pH determinations, hemogram, serum electrolytes, and chest x-ray. Patients who are alert, have normal chest x-rays, and show no evidence of hypoxemia or acidosis usually require no further therapy. Nevertheless they should be observed for several hours for evidence of deterioration in blood gas and acid-base status prior to discharge. Metabolic acidosis should be treated by intravenous administration of sodium bicarbonate ($NaHCO_3$), and hypoxemia with supplemental oxygen. If bronchospasm is present, aerosol inhalation of a bronchodilator may be given. Patients with pulmonary edema or hypoxemia which fails to respond to increasing inspired oxygen tensions up to 40 percent should be intubated endotracheally and have positive end-expiratory pressure (PEEP) applied to the airways. When respiratory failure is present, lung compliance is markedly reduced, or the patient is unable to breathe spontaneously, mechanical ventilatory support should be used in addition to PEEP. Arterial blood gas tensions and pH should be determined frequently to assess the adequacy of respiratory therapy. Treatment with PEEP should be continued long enough for the lung injury to stabilize before it is withdrawn. This may take 48 to 72 h or even longer. Monitoring the magnitude of the intrapulmonary shunt, the pulmonary wedge pressure, and cardiac output by means of a Swan-Ganz intraarterial catheter is often very helpful in weaning patients from PEEP as well as in managing cases complicated by low cardiac output and hypotension.

Intensive therapy, including controlled hyperventilation,

deliberate hypothermia, barbiturate-induced coma, and continuous muscular paralysis, has been recommended for near-drowning victims who are comatose when admitted to the hospital, in order to preserve cerebral function. Although preliminary results suggest that there may be fewer major neurologic sequelae, particularly in children treated in this manner, the need for such aggressive and potentially hazardous therapy requires further study.

Other therapeutic measures are largely supportive. Patients should be observed closely for evidence of pulmonary infection and treated with appropriate antibiotics on the basis of results of cultures of respiratory secretions. Prophylactic use of antibiotics and corticosteroids has been of no benefit in near-drowning victims. Fluid and electrolyte balance should be carefully maintained. If hypovolemia is associated with low urinary output or hypotension, plasma expanders may be required. Transfusion with packed red blood cells or whole blood, depending upon circulating blood volume status, may be used for significant anemia. Acute renal failure should be managed as described in Chap. 290.

PROGNOSIS The prognosis depends largely upon the extent and duration of the hypoxic episode. In addition, such factors as the temperature of the submersion medium, the availability and appropriate application of specific treatment, and coexisting medical illness or trauma are often important in determining the outcome. In general, patients who are alert and have normal chest x-rays upon arrival at the hospital can be expected to recover fully. Those who are obtunded but arousable and have normal respirations have nearly as good a prognosis, while approximately two-thirds of those who present in coma or cardiopulmonary arrest die or are left with significant neurological deficits. Prediction of outcome on the basis of other presenting neurological features or laboratory abnormalities is unreliable. The fact that nearly 90 percent of victims who live long enough to receive definitive hospital care will survive should serve to emphasize that extensive resuscitative efforts are advisable in all cases of near-drowning.

REFERENCES

Aquatic deaths and injuries—United States. Morb Mort Week Rep 31:417, 1982

Conn AW et al: Cerebral salvage in near-drowning following neurological classification by triage. Can Anaesth Soc J 27:201, 1980

Fuller RH: Drowning and the postimmersion syndrome: A clinicopathologic study. Mil Med 128:22, 1963

Giammona ST, Modell JH: Drowning by total immersion: Effects on pulmonary surfactant of distilled water, isotonic saline and seawater. Am J Dis Child 114:612, 1967

Modell JH: Biology of drowning. Annu Rev Med 29:1, 1978

——— et al: Near-drowning: Correlation of level of consciousness and survival. Can Anaesth Soc J 27:211, 1980

Peterson B: Morbidity of childhood near-drowning. Pediatrics 59:364, 1977

Young RSK et al: Neurological outcome in cold water drowning. JAMA 244:1233, 1980

PART SIX | DISEASES OF THE ORGAN SYSTEMS

section 1 | Disorders of the heart

Diagnostic methods

247
APPROACH TO THE PATIENT WITH HEART DISEASE

EUGENE BRAUNWALD

The initial symptoms of the patient with heart disease result most commonly from myocardial ischemia, from disturbance of the contractile activity of the myocardium, or from an abnormal cardiac rhythm or rate. Ischemia is manifest most frequently as chest pain, while reduction of the pumping ability of the heart commonly leads to weakness and fatigability or, when severe, produces cyanosis, hypotension, syncope, and elevated intravascular pressure behind a failing ventricle; the latter results in abnormal fluid accumulation, which in turn leads to dyspnea, orthopnea, and edema. Cardiac arrhythmias often develop suddenly, and the resulting signs and symptoms—palpitation, dyspnea, angina, hypotension, and syncope—generally occur abruptly and may disappear as rapidly as they develop.

A cardinal principle useful in the evaluation of the patient with suspected heart disease is that myocardial or coronary function which may be adequate at rest may be inadequate during exertion. Thus, a history of chest pain and/or dyspnea which appears only during activity is characteristic of heart disease, while the opposite pattern, i.e., the appearance of these symptoms at rest and their remission during exertion, is rarely observed in patients with organic heart disease.

Patients with cardiocirculatory disease may also be entirely asymptomatic, both at rest and during exertion, but may present an abnormal physical finding, such as a heart murmur, elevated systemic arterial pressure, or an abnormality of the electrocardiogram or of the cardiac silhouette on the chest roentgenogram.

Diseases of the heart and circulation are so common and the laity is so well acquainted with the major symptoms resulting from these disorders that patients, and occasionally physicians, erroneously attribute many complaints to organic cardiovascular disease. Furthermore, the combination of the widespread fear of heart disease in the western world with the deep-seated emotional connotations concerning this organ's function results in the frequent development in persons with normal cardiovascular systems of symptoms which mimic those of organic disease. The correct interpretation of symptoms in patients with recognized organic cardiovascular disturbances is occasionally quite difficult. Such persons, in addition to having symptoms resulting from their disease, may also develop functional complaints referable to the cardiovascular system. The unraveling of symptoms and signs due to organic heart disease from those which are not directly related is an important and challenging task in these patients.

It must be recognized that dyspnea, one of the cardinal manifestations of diminished cardiac reserve, is not limited to disease of the heart, but is also characteristic of conditions as diverse as pulmonary disease, marked obesity, and anxiety (Chap. 26). Similarly, chest pain (Chap. 4) may result from a variety of causes other than myocardial ischemia. Whether heart disease is responsible for these symptoms can frequently be determined by carrying out a detailed clinical examination. The electrocardiogram and roentgenogram provide additional helpful information; more specialized examinations are often helpful but only occasionally essential.

In every branch of medicine the establishment of the prognosis and development of a rational plan of management are based on a correct diagnostic appraisal. However, in the case of patients with disorders of the cardiocirculatory system, particular care must be taken to establish not only a correct but also a *complete* diagnosis. As outlined by the New York Heart Association, the elements of a complete cardiac diagnosis include consideration of:

1 *The underlying etiology.* Is the disease congenital, rheumatic, hypertensive, or arteriosclerotic in origin?
2 *The anatomic abnormalities.* Which chambers are enlarged? Which valves are affected? Is there pericardial involvement? Has there been a myocardial infarction?
3 *The physiologic disturbances.* Is an arrhythmia present? Is there evidence of congestive heart failure or of myocardial ischemia?
4 *The extent of functional disability.* How strenuous is the physical activity required to elicit symptoms?

Two simple examples may serve to illustrate the importance of establishing a complete diagnosis. The identification of myocardial ischemia as the cause of exertional chest pain is of great clinical importance. However, this diagnosis is insufficient to develop either a strategy of specific treatment or prognosis until the underlying disease process, e.g., coronary atherosclerosis or aortic stenosis, which is responsible for the myocardial ischemia, is identified and a judgment made as to whether severe anemia, thyrotoxicosis, or supraventricular tachycardia plays a contributory role. Similarly, determining that heart disease is congenital provides an important starting point, but the decision about whether surgical treatment is advisable depends upon the specific anatomic defect present and often upon the nature of the physiologic disturbance and the functional impairment.

The establishment of a correct and complete cardiac diagnosis often requires the use of six different methods of examination: (1) history, (2) physical examination (Chap. 248), (3) electrocardiogram (Chap. 249), (4) chest roentgenogram (Chap. 250), (5) noninvasive graphic examinations (echocardiogram, radionuclide scanning techniques, and other "noninvasive" tests, Chap. 250), and occasionally (6) specialized "invasive" examinations, such as cardiac catheterization or angiocardiography (Chap. 251). In order to be most effective, each of these six approaches should be analyzed independently of one another as well as with the information derived from the other methods clearly in mind. Only in this way can one avoid overlooking a subtle, though extremely significant, finding. For example, an electrocardiogram should be obtained in every patient suspected of having heart disease. It may provide the critical clue in establishing the correct diagnosis, e.g., the finding of an atrioventricular conduction disturbance in a patient with unexplained syncope, even when all other methods of examination reveal no abnormal findings. On the other hand, when combined intelligently with the results of other methods of examination, the electrocardiogram may provide essential confirmatory data. Thus, the knowledge that a patient has an apical diastolic rumbling murmur may direct particular attention to the P waves, and the recognition of left atrial enlargement electrocardiographically would support the suggestion that the murmur is caused by mitral stenosis. Under these circumstances the additional finding of right ventricular hypertrophy suggests that pulmonary hypertension is present.

Although the electrocardiogram is an invaluable aspect of every cardiovascular examination, with the exception of the identification of arrhythmias it rarely permits establishment of a specific diagnosis. In the absence of any other abnormal findings, electrocardiographic changes must not be overinterpreted. The range of normal electrocardiographic findings is wide, and the tracing can be affected significantly by many noncardiac factors, such as age, body habitus, and serum electrolyte concentrations.

In obtaining the history of the patient with known or suspected cardiovascular disease, particular attention should be directed to the family history. Familial clustering is common in many forms of heart disease. Genetic transmission may occur, as in hypertrophic cardiomyopathy (Chap. 263) or Marfan's syndrome (Chap. 106). In patients with essential hypertension or coronary atherosclerosis the genetic component may be less obvious but also of considerable importance. The nature of the response of the myocardium to an increased hemodynamic load, such as hypertension, or a valvular lesion may also be conditioned by hereditary factors. Familial clustering of cardiovascular diseases may not only occur on a genetic basis but may also be related to familial, dietary, or behavior patterns.

When an attempt is made to ascertain the severity of functional impairment in a patient with heart disease, it is essential to determine the precise extent of activity and the rate at which it is performed before symptoms develop. Thus, breathlessness which occurs after running up two long flights of stairs denotes far less functional impairment than similar symptoms occurring after taking a few steps on the level. Also, the degree of customary physical activity at work and during recreation should be considered. The development of two-flight dyspnea by a marathon runner may be more ominous than dyspnea on far less exertion by a previously sedentary person. Similarly, the history must include a detailed consideration of the patient's therapeutic regimen. For example, the persistence or development of edema in a patient whose diet is rigidly restricted in sodium content and who is receiving optimum doses of digitalis and diuretics must be interpreted quite differently from the finding of edema in the absence of these measures.

PITFALLS IN CARDIOVASCULAR MEDICINE Increasing subspecialization in internal medicine and the perfection of advanced diagnostic techniques in cardiology may sometimes be accompanied by several undesirable consequences, which can be summarized as follows:

1 Failure by the noncardiologist to recognize cardiac manifestations of systemic illnesses. The latter include but are by no means limited to (*a*) mongolism (often associated with endocardial cushion defect); (*b*) gonadal dysgenesis, i.e., Turner's syndrome (associated with a variety of congenital defects, particularly coarctation of the aorta); (*c*) bony abnormalities of the upper extremities (associated with atrial septal defect); (*d*) muscular dystrophies (associated with cardiomyopathy); (*e*) hemochromatosis and glycogen storage disease (associated with myocardial infiltration); (*f*) congenital deafness (associated with serious cardiac arrhythmias); (*g*) Raynaud's disease (associated with primary pulmonary hypertension); (*h*) connective tissue disorders, i.e., Marfan's syndrome, Ehlers-Danlos syndrome, Hurler's syndrome, and related disorders of mucopolysaccharide metabolism (aortic dilatation, prolapsed mitral valve, a variety of arterial abnormalities); (*i*) chronic hemolytic anemia (cardiac dilatation); (*j*) Refsum's disease (myocardial failure and conduction defects); (*k*) acromegaly (accelerated coronary atherosclerosis, conduction defects, cardiomyopathy); (*l*) hyperthyroidism (heart failure, atrial fibrillation); (*m*) rheumatoid arthritis (pericarditis, aortic valve disease); (*n*) Whipple's disease (pericarditis and endocarditis); (*o*) scleroderma (cor pulmonale, myocardial fibrosis, pericarditis); (*p*) lupus erythematosus (valvulitis, myocarditis); (*q*) polymyositis (pericarditis, myocarditis); (*r*) sarcoidosis (arrhythmias, cardiomyopathy); (*s*) Fabry's disease (myocardial ischemia, heart failure); (*t*) exfoliative dermatitis (high-output heart failure). In patients in whom these and other systemic disorders in which cardiovascular involvement may occur, a detailed cardiovascular examination should be carried out.

2 Failure by the cardiac specialist to recognize systemic illnesses in patients with cardiac disorders. Patients known or suspected of having heart disease require a detailed general assessment and a search for the frequent noncardiac manifestations of cardiac disorders. Indeed, the cardiovascular abnormality may provide the clue critical to the recognition of these disorders. Closely related is the failure to appreciate the profound effects of stress, such as that resulting from an intercurrent infection, of pregnancy, or from emotional disturbances, on cardiovascular performance and symptoms.

3 Overreliance on and overutilization of laboratory tests, particularly specialized invasive techniques. Catheterization of the right and left sides of the heart, selective angiography, and coronary arteriography (Chap. 251), provide precise diagnostic information under many circumstances. For example, they aid in establishing a specific anatomic diagnosis in patients with congenital heart disease, in patients with chest pain of uncertain etiology in whom coronary artery disease is suspected, and in determining the functional significance of valvular abnormalities in patients with rheumatic heart disease being considered for surgical treatment. Although a great deal of attention has been lavished on the newer specialized laboratory examinations, it should be recognized that they serve to *supplement,* not *supplant,* a careful clinical examination. There is an unfortunate tendency to carry out procedures such as coronary arteriography instead of taking a detailed and thoughtful history; although it may be established whether the coronary arteries are obstructed, the results often do not provide a definite answer to the question of whether a patient's complaint of chest pain is clearly attributable to coronary arteriosclerosis. Similarly, catheterization of the left side of the heart is all too frequently employed to determine whether operative treatment of valvular disease is indicated, even before the patient has had a trial of medical therapy. Despite their enormous value, it must not be overlooked that these specialized examinations entail some risk to the patient, involve discomfort and cost, and place a strain on existing medical facilities. Therefore, *they should be carried out only if there is a specific indication and if the results can be expected to modify or aid in the patient's management.*

REFERENCES

BRAUNWALD E (ed): *Heart Disease,* 2d ed. Philadelphia, Saunders, 1983

FOWLER NO: *Cardiac Diagnosis and Treatment,* 3d ed. Hagerstown, Harper & Row, 1981

HURST JW et al (ed): *The Heart,* 5th ed. New York, McGraw-Hill, 1982

NEW YORK HEART ASSOCIATION, INC, CRITERIA COMMITTEE: *Nomenclature and Criteria for Diagnosis of Diseases of the Heart and Great Vessels,* 8th ed. Boston, Little, Brown, 1981

PERLOFF JK (ed): *Physical Examination of the Heart and Circulation.* Philadelphia, Saunders, 1982

SELZER A: *Principles of Clinical Cardiology: An Analytical Approach.* Philadelphia, Saunders, 1975

248 PHYSICAL EXAMINATION OF THE HEART

ROBERT A. O'ROURKE
EUGENE BRAUNWALD

The general examination of a patient with cardiac disease often provides important information concerning the status of the cardiovascular system. The general physical appearance should first be assessed. The patient may appear tired because of a persistently low cardiac output; the respiratory rate may be increased, indicating pulmonary venous congestion. Central cyanosis, often associated with clubbing of the fingers and toes, indicates right-to-left shunting of blood in the heart or great vessels or inadequate oxygenation of blood by the lungs. Cyanosis in the distal extremities, cool skin, and increased sweating result from vasoconstriction in patients with severe heart failure (Chap 27). Noncardiovascular details can be equally important. For example, the diagnosis of infective endocarditis is highly likely in patients with petechiae, Osler's nodes, and Janeway lesions (Chap. 259).

The blood pressure should be taken in both arms and with the patient supine and upright; the heart rate should be timed for 1 min. Orthostatic hypotension and tachycardia may indicate a reduced blood volume, while resting tachycardia may be a clue to the presence of severe heart failure.

Careful examination of the optic fundi is essential (Chap. 267), and the retinal vessels may show evidence of systemic hypertension, arteriosclerosis, or embolism. The latter may result from atherosclerosis in larger arteries (e.g., carotid) or may represent a complication of valvular heart disease (e.g., endocarditis).

Palpation of the peripheral arterial pulses in the upper and lower extremities is necessary to define the adequacy of systemic blood flow and to detect the presence of occlusive arterial lesions. It is also important to examine both legs for evidence of edema, varicose veins, or thrombophlebitis (Chap. 269). The cardiovascular examination includes careful evaluation of both the carotid arterial and the jugular venous pulses, as well as deliberate precordial palpation and attentive cardiac auscultation. An understanding of the events of the cardiac cycle (Fig. 250-1, page 1331) is vital to carrying out an accurate cardiovascular examination.

ARTERIAL PRESSURE PULSE The normal central aortic pulse wave is characterized by a fairly rapid rise to a somewhat rounded peak (Fig. 248-1). The anacrotic shoulder, present on the ascending limb, occurs at the time of peak rate of aortic flow just before maximum pressure is reached. The less steep descending limb is interrupted by a sharp downward deflection, synchronous with aortic valve closure, called the *incisura.* As the pulse wave is transmitted peripherally, the initial upstroke becomes steeper, the anacrotic shoulder becomes less apparent, and the incisura is replaced by the smoother dicrotic notch. Accordingly, palpation of a peripheral pulse (e.g., the brachial arterial) frequently gives less information than examination of a more central pulse (e.g., the carotid arterial) regarding alterations in left ventricular ejection or aortic valve function. However, certain findings such as the bounding pulses of aortic regurgitation or pulsus alternans are more readily evident in peripheral than in central arteries. The carotid pulse usually is best examined with the sternocleidomastoid muscle relaxed and with the head rotated slightly toward the examiner. In examining the brachial arterial pulse, the examiner can support the subject's relaxed elbow with his or her right arm while compressing the brachial pulse with this thumb. The usual technique for palpating the pulse is to compress the artery with the thumb or forefinger until the maximum pulse is sensed. The examiner should apply varying degrees of pressure while concentrating on the separate phases of the pulse wave. This method, referred to as *trisection,* is useful for assessing the sharpness of the upstroke, systolic peak, and diastolic slope of the arterial pulse. In most normal persons a dicrotic wave is not palpable.

A small weak pulse, *pulsus parvus,* is frequently present in conditions with a diminished left ventricular stroke volume, a

FIGURE 248-1
A. Simultaneous recordings of electrocardiogram, aortic pressure pulse (AOP), phonocardiogram recorded at the apex, and apexcardiogram (ACG). On the phonocardiogram, S_1, S_2, S_3, *and* S_4 *represent the first through fourth heart sounds; OS represents the opening snap of the mitral valve, which occurs coincident with the O point of the apexcardiogram.* S_3 *occurs coincident with the termination of the rapid-filling wave (RFW) of the ACG, while* S_4 *occurs coincident with the a wave of the ACG. B. Simultaneous recording of electrocardiogram, indirect carotid pulse (CP), phonocardiogram along the left sternal border (LSB), and indirect jugular venous pulse (JVP). ES, ejection sound; SC, systolic click.*

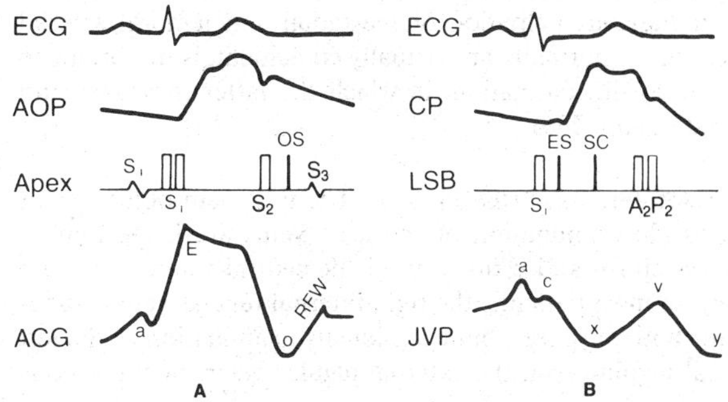

narrow pulse pressure, and increased peripheral vascular resistance. This may be due to hypovolemia, to left ventricular failure secondary to myocardial disease or myocardial infarction, to restrictive pericardial disease, or to mitral valve stenosis. In aortic valve stenosis the delayed systolic peak, *pulsus tardus,* is the result of mechanical obstruction to left ventricular ejection and is often accompanied by the transmission of a coarse systolic thrill. In contrast, a large bounding pulse is usually associated with an increased left ventricular stroke volume, a wide pulse pressure, and a decrease in peripheral vascular resistance. This occurs characteristically in patients with abnormally elevated stroke volumes as in complete heart block, hyperkinetic circulation due to anxiety, anemia, exercise, or fever, or in patients with an abnormally rapid runoff of blood from the arterial system (patent ductus arteriosus, peripheral arteriovenous fistula). Patients with mitral regurgitation or a ventricular septal defect may also have a bounding pulse, since vigorous left ventricular ejection produces a rapid upstroke in the arterial pulse even though the duration of systole and the forward stroke volume may be diminished. In aortic regurgitation the rapidly rising, bounding arterial pulse results from increased left ventricular stroke volume and the associated increased rate of ventricular ejection.

The *bisferiens pulse,* which consists of two systolic peaks, is characteristic of aortic regurgitation (with or without accompanying stenosis) and of hypertrophic obstructive cardiomyopathy (Chap. 263). In the latter the pulse wave upstroke rises rapidly and forcefully, producing the first systolic peak ("percussion wave"). A brief decline in pressure follows, because of the sudden decrease in the rate of left ventricular ejection as severe obstruction develops during midsystole. This pressure trough is followed by a smaller and more slowly rising positive pulse wave ("tidal wave") produced by continued ventricular ejection and by reflected waves from the periphery. The *dicrotic pulse* has two palpable waves, one in systole and one in diastole. It occurs most frequently in patients with a very low stroke volume, particularly in those with diffuse myocardial disease.

Pulsus alternans refers to a pattern in which there is regular alteration of the pressure pulse amplitude, despite a regular rhythm. It is due to alternating left ventricular contractile force, usually denotes severe left ventricular decompensation, and commonly occurs in patients who also have a loud third heart sound. Pulsus alternans may also occur during or following paroxysmal tachycardia or for several beats following a premature beat in patients without heart disease. In *pulsus bigeminus* there is also regular alteration of pressure pulse amplitude, but it is caused by a premature ventricular contraction that follows each regular beat. *Pulsus paradoxus* is an accentuation of the decrease in systolic arterial pressure accompanying the reduced amplitude of the arterial pulse which normally occurs during inspiration. In patients with pericardial tamponade, airway obstruction, or superior vena cava obstruction, the decrease in systolic arterial pressure frequently exceeds the normal of 10 mmHg and the peripheral pulse may disappear completely during inspiration.

Simultaneous palpation of the radial and femoral arterial pulses, which normally are virtually coincident, is important to rule out aortic coarctation, in which the latter is weaker and delayed (Chap. 256).

JUGULAR VENOUS PULSE (JVP) The two main objectives of the bedside examination of the neck veins are inspection of their waveform and estimation of the central venous pressure (CVP). In most patients, the right internal jugular vein is superior for both purposes, but occasionally examination of the left internal jugular vein, the external jugular veins, or the venous pulsations in the supraclavicular fossae may yield more information. In most normal subjects, maximum pulsation of the internal jugular vein is observed when the trunk is inclined by less than 30°. In patients with elevated venous pressure it may be necessary to elevate the trunk further, sometimes to as much as 90°. When the neck muscles are relaxed, shining a beam of light tangentially across the skin overlying the vein exposes the pulsations of the internal jugular vein. Simultaneous palpation of the left carotid artery aids the examiner in deciding which pulsations are venous and in relating the venous pulsations to their timing in the cardiac cycle.

The normal JVP reflects phasic pressure changes in the right atrium and consists of two or sometimes three positive waves and two negative troughs (Fig. 248-1). The positive presystolic *a* wave is produced by venous distention consequent to right atrial contraction and is the dominant wave in the JVP, particularly during inspiration. Large *a* waves indicate that the right atrium is contracting against an increased resistance, such as occurs with obstruction at the tricuspid valve (tricuspid stenosis) or more commonly with increased resistance to right ventricular filling (pulmonary hypertension or pulmonic stenosis). Large *a* waves also occur during dysrhythmias whenever the right atrium contracts while the tricuspid valve is closed by right ventricular systole. Such "cannon" *a* waves may occur regularly (as during junctional rhythm) or irregularly (as in atrioventricular dissociation with ventricular tachycardia or complete heart block). The *a* wave is absent in patients with atrial fibrillation, and there is an increased temporal delay between the *a* wave and the carotid arterial pulse in patients with first-degree atrioventricular (AV) block.

The *c* wave, often but not invariably observed in the JVP, is a positive wave produced by the bulging of the tricuspid valve into the right atrium during right ventricular isovolumetric systole and by the impact of the carotid artery adjacent to the jugular vein. The *x* descent is due to a combination of atrial relaxation and the downward displacement of the tricuspid valve during ventricular systole. In patients with constrictive pericarditis, there is often increased prominence of the *x* descent wave during systole, but this wave is reduced with right ventricular dilatation and may even be reversed in tricuspid regurgitation. The positive, late systolic *v* wave results from the increasing volume of blood in the venae cavae and right atrium during ventricular systole when the tricuspid valve is closed. With mild tricuspid regurgitation the *v* wave becomes more prominent, and when tricuspid regurgitation becomes severe, the prominent *v* wave and the obliteration of the *x* descent result in a single large positive systolic wave ("ventricularization"). After the peak of the *v* wave is reached, the right atrial pressure diminishes because of the decreased bulging of the tricuspid valve into the right atrium as right ventricular pressure declines and the tricuspid valve opens.

Following the summit of the *v* wave there is a negative descending limb, referred to as the *y* descent or "diastolic collapse," which is produced mainly by tricuspid valve opening and the rapid inflow of blood into the right ventricle. A rapid, deep *y* descent in early diastole occurs with severe tricuspid regurgitation. A venous pulse characterized by a sharp *y* descent, a deep *y* trough, and a rapid ascent to the base line is seen in patients with constrictive pericarditis or with severe failure of the right side of the heart and a high venous pressure. A slow *y* descent in the JVP suggests an obstruction to right ventricular filling, as occurs with tricuspid stenosis or right atrial myxoma.

For accurate estimation of the CVP, the right internal jugular vein is best utilized, with the sternal angle as the reference point, since in the average patient the center of the right atrium lies approximately 5 cm below the sternal angle, regardless of body position. The patient is examined at the optimum degree of trunk elevation for visualization of venous pulsations. The vertical distance between the top of the oscillating venous column and the level of the sternal angle is determined and generally found to be less than 3 cm (3 cm + 5 cm = 8 cm blood). The most common cause of an elevated venous pressure is an elevated right ventricular diastolic pressure. In patients suspected of having right ventricular failure who have a normal CVP at rest, the abdominojugular reflux test may be helpful. The palm of the hand is placed over the abdomen and firm pressure is applied for 30 to 60 s. Normally, the jugular venous pressure is not significantly altered, but with impaired function of the right side of the heart the upper level of venous pulsation usually increases. Also, abdominal compression may elicit the typical JVP of tricuspid regurgitation when the resting pulse wave is normal.

PRECORDIAL PALPATION The location, amplitude, duration, and direction of the cardiac impulse can usually be best appreciated by using the fingertips. The normal left ventricular apex impulse is located at or medial to the left midclavicular line in the fourth or fifth intercostal space and is a tapping, early systolic outward thrust localized to a point not more than 2 to 3 cm in diameter. It is due primarily to recoil of the heart as blood is ejected and should be evaluated with the patient supine and in the left lateral decubitus. Left ventricular hypertrophy results in an exaggerated amplitude and duration of the normal left ventricular thrust. The impulse may be displaced laterally and downward into the sixth or seventh interspace, particularly in patients with a left ventricular volume load such as occurs in aortic regurgitation.

Additional abnormal features of the left ventricular apex include marked presystolic distention of the left ventricle, often accompanying a fourth heart sound in patients with an excessive left ventricular pressure load, and a prominent early diastolic rapid-filling wave, often accompanying a third heart sound in patients with left ventricular failure or mitral valve regurgitation (Fig. 248-1). A double systolic impulse is frequently palpable in patients with idiopathic hypertrophic subaortic stenosis.

Right ventricular hypertrophy results in a sustained systolic lift at the lower left parasternal area which starts in early systole and is synchronous with the left ventricular apical impulse. In patients with chronic obstructive pulmonary disease a right ventricular impulse may often be detected by sliding the fingers up under the rib cage just beneath the sternum. The enlarged right ventricle strikes the ends of the fingertips as an inferiorly directed movement.

Abnormal precordial pulsations occur during systole in patients with motion disorders of the left ventricular wall due to coronary artery disease or to diffuse myocardial disease from some other cause. These pulsations often occur in patients with a recent transmural myocardial infarction and may be present in some patients only during episodes of anginal pain. They are most commonly felt in the left midprecordium one or two interspaces above and/or 1 to 2 cm medial to the left ventricular apex. When a systolic bulge occurs in the region of the apex, it is difficult to distinguish it from the impulse of left ventricular hypertrophy.

A left parasternal lift is present frequently in patients with severe mitral regurgitation. This pulsation occurs distinctly later than the left ventricular apical impulse, is synchronous with the *v* wave in the left atrial pressure curve, and is due to anterior displacement of the right ventricle by the large left atrium. A similar impulse occurring to the right of the sternum has been noted in some patients with severe tricuspid regurgitation and a giant right atrium. Pulsation of the right sternoclavicular joint may indicate a right-sided aortic arch or aneurysmal dilatation of the ascending aorta. Pulmonary artery pulsation is often visible and palpable in the second left intercostal space and may be normal in children or thin young adults. However, this pulsation usually denotes pulmonary hypertension, increased pulmonary blood flow, or poststenotic pulmonary artery dilatation.

Thrills are palpable low-frequency vibrations associated with heart murmurs. The diastolic rumble of mitral stenosis and the systolic murmur of mitral regurgitation may be palpated at the cardiac apex. When the palm of the hand is placed over the precordium, the thrill of aortic stenosis crosses the palm of the hand toward the right side of the neck, while the thrill of pulmonic stenosis tends to radiate more often to the left side of the neck. The thrill due to a ventricular septal defect is usually located in the third and fourth intercostal spaces near the left sternal border.

Percussion should be performed in each patient to identify normal or abnormal position of the heart, stomach, and liver. However, in patients with a normal cardiac situs, percussion adds little to careful inspection and palpation in the recognition of cardiac enlargement.

CARDIAC AUSCULTATION To obtain maximal information from cardiac auscultation, the observer should keep in mind several principles: (1) This portion of the examination should be carried out in a quiet room to avoid the distractions caused by the noises of normal activity. (2) In order to hear a faint heart sound or murmur, it is necessary to focus attention on that phase of the cardiac cycle during which the auscultatory event may be expected to occur. (3) The accurate timing of a heart sound or murmur necessarily involves ascertaining its relation to other observable events in the cardiac cycle—the carotid arterial pulse, the JVP, or the apical impulse. (4) To determine the significance of a cardiac sound or murmur, it is often necessary to observe alterations in its timing or intensity during various phases of the respiratory cycle, with changes in position, during and following a premature ventricular depolarization, with handgrip exercise, and during the administration of vasoactive drugs such as amyl nitrite.

HEART SOUNDS The major components of heart sounds are vibrations associated with the abrupt acceleration or deceleration of blood within the cardiovascular system, but there is continuing controversy regarding the relative significance of the vibrations of valves, muscles, vessels, and supporting structures in the production of the heart sounds. Recent studies using simultaneous echocardiographic-phonocardiographic recordings indicate that the first and second heart sounds are produced primarily by the closure of the AV and semilunar valves and the events that accompany these closures. The intensity of the *first heart sound* (S_1) is influenced by (1) the position of the mitral leaflets at the onset of ventricular systole, (2) the rate of rise of the left ventricular pressure pulse, (3) the presence or absence of structural disease of the mitral valve, and (4) the amount of tissue, air, or fluid between the heart and the stethoscope. S_1 is increased in intensity if diastole is shortened because of tachycardia, if atrioventricular flow is increased because of high cardiac output or prolonged because of mitral stenosis, or if atrial contraction precedes ventricular contractions by a short (PR) interval. The loud S_1 in mitral stenosis usually signifies that the valve is pliable and that the valve remains open at the onset of isovolumetric contraction because of the elevated left atrial pressure. A reduction in the intensity of S_1 may be due to poor conduction of sound through the chest wall, a slow rise of the left ventricular pressure pulse, a long PR interval, or imperfect closure due to reduced valve substance, as in mitral regurgitation. S_1 is also soft when the anterior mitral leaflet is immobile because of rigidity and calcification even in the presence of predominant mitral stenosis.

Splitting of the two high-pitched components of S_1 by 10 to 30 ms is a normal phenomenon (Fig. 248-1). The first component of S_1 normally is attributed to mitral valve closure and the second to tricuspid valve closure. A widened split of S_1 is most often due to complete right bundle branch block and the resulting delay in onset of the right ventricular pressure pulse. Reversed splitting of the S_1 with the mitral component following the tricuspid component has occasionally been noted in complete left bundle branch block and frequently is present in patients with severe mitral stenosis or a left atrial myxoma.

Splitting of S_2 into audibly distinct aortic (A_2) and pulmonic (P_2) components occurs normally during inspiration when augmented inflow into the right ventricle increases its stroke volume and ejection period and delays closure of the pulmonic valve. P_2 is coincident with the incisura of the pulmonary artery pressure curve, which is separated from the right ventricular pressure tracing by an interval termed the "hangout time." The absolute value of this interval reflects the resistance to pulmonary blood flow and the impedance characteristics of the pulmonary vascular bed. This interval is prolonged, and physiologic splitting of S_2 is accentuated in conditions associated with right ventricular volume overload and a distensible pulmonary vascular bed. However, in patients with an increase in pulmonary vascular resistance, the "hangout time" is markedly reduced and narrow splitting of S_2 is present. Audible expiratory splitting, heard best at the pulmonic area or left sternal border, is usually abnormal when the patient is in the upright position. Such splitting may be due to delayed activation of the right ventricle (right bundle branch block), to prolongation of right ventricular contraction with an increased right ventricular pressure load (pulmonary embolism or pulmonic stenosis), or to delayed pulmonic valve closure because of an increased right ventricular flow load associated with diminished impedance of the pulmonary vascular bed and a prolonged "hangout time" (atrial septal defect). In pulmonary hypertension, P_2 is increased in intensity and splitting of the second heart sound may be diminished, normal, or accentuated, depending on the cause of the pulmonary hypertension, the pulmonary vascular resistance, and the presence or absence of right ventricular decompensation. Early aortic valve closure, occurring with mitral regurgitation or a ventricular septal defect, may also produce audible expiratory splitting. In patients with large atrial septal defects the proportion of right atrial filling contributed by the left atrium and the venae cavae varies reciprocally during the respiratory cycle so that right atrial inflow remains relatively constant. Therefore, the volume and duration of the right ventricular ejection are not significantly increased by inspiration, and there is little inspiratory exaggeration of the splitting of S_2. This phenomenon, termed "fixed splitting" of the second heart sound, is of considerable diagnostic value.

A delay in aortic valve closure causing P_2 to precede A_2 results in so-called reversed (paradoxic) splitting of S_2. Splitting is then maximal in expiration, and decreases during inspiration with the normal delay of pulmonic valve closure. The commonest causes of reversed splitting of S_2 are left bundle branch block and delayed excitation of the left ventricle from a right ventricular ectopic beat. Mechanical prolongation of left ventricular systole, resulting in reversed splitting of S_2, may be caused by severe aortic outflow obstruction, a large aorta-to-pulmonary artery shunt, systolic hypertension, and ischemic heart disease or cardiomyopathy with left ventricular failure. P_2 is normally softer than A_2 in the second left intercostal space; when P_2 is greater than A_2 in this area, it suggests pulmonary hypertension, except in patients with atrial septal defect.

The *third heart sound* is a low-pitched sound produced in the ventricle 0.14 to 0.16 s after A_2, at the termination of rapid filling. This sound is frequent in normal children and in patients with high cardiac output. However, in patients over 40 years of age, an S_3 usually indicates ventricular decompensation, AV valve regurgitation, or other conditions which increase the rate or volume of ventricular filling. The left-sided S_3 is best heard with the bell piece of the stethoscope at the left ventricular apex during expiration and with the patient in the left lateral position. The right-sided S_3 is best heard at the left sternal border or just beneath the xiphoid and is increased with inspiration. Often it is accompanied by the systolic murmur of functional tricuspid regurgitation. Ventricular third heart sounds often disappear with treatment of heart failure.

An earlier (0.10 to 0.12 s after A_2), higher-pitched third heart sound (pericardial knock) often occurs in patients with constrictive pericarditis; its presence is dependent upon the restrictive effect of the adherent pericardium, which halts diastolic filling abruptly.

The opening snap (OS) is a brief, high-pitched, early diastolic sound which is usually due to stenosis of an AV valve, more commonly the mitral valve. It is usually heard best at the lower left sternal border and radiates well to the base of the heart. The A_2-OS interval during exercise is inversely related to the height of the mean left atrial pressure, and ranges from 0.04 to 0.12 s. At the base an OS is often confused with P_2. However, careful auscultation at the upper left sternal border will reveal both components of the second heart sound, followed by the opening snap. The OS of tricuspid stenosis occurs later in diastole than the mitral OS. Since most patients with tricuspid stenosis also have severe mitral valve disease, the tricuspid OS is often overshadowed by the diastolic rumble and OS originating in the stenotic mitral valve. An OS also may occur when there is increased flow across an AV valve, such as exists with left-to-right intracardiac shunts and mitral or tricuspid regurgitation.

The *fourth heart sound* is a low-pitched, presystolic sound produced in the ventricle during the ventricular filling associated with an effective atrial contraction, and is heard best with the bell piece of the stethoscope. The sound is absent in patients with atrial fibrillation. The S_4 occurs when diminished ventricular compliance increases the resistance to ventricular filling, and it is present frequently in patients with systemic hypertension, aortic stenosis, hypertrophic cardiomyopathy, coronary artery disease, and acute mitral regurgitation. Most patients with an acute myocardial infarction and sinus rhythm have an audible S_4. The fourth heart sound is frequently accompanied by visible and palpable presystolic distention of the left ventricle. It is maximal in intensity at the left ventricular apex with the patient in the left lateral position, and is accentuated by mild supine exercise. The right-sided S_4 is present in patients with right ventricular hypertrophy, secondary to either pulmonary stenosis or pulmonary hypertension, and frequently accompanies a prominent presystolic *a* wave in the JVP.

Audible fourth heart sounds also may be present during increased ventricular filling and normal ventricular compliance such as occurs in patients with severe anemia, thyrotoxicosis, or a peripheral arteriovenous fistula. An S_4 frequently accompanies delayed AV conduction even in the absence of clinically detectable heart disease. The incidence of an audible S_4 increases with increasing age. Whether an audible S_4 in adults without other evidence of cardiac disease is abnormal remains controversial.

The *ejection sound* is a sharp, high-pitched event occurring in early systole closely following the first heart sound. Ejection sounds occur in the presence of semilunar valve stenosis, i.e., opening snaps of the aortic or pulmonic valves, and in conditions associated with dilatation of the aorta or pulmonary artery. The aortic ejection sound is usually heard best at the left ventricular apex and the second right interspace; the pulmonary ejection sound is of maximal intensity at the upper left sternal border. The latter, unlike most other right-sided acoustical events, is heard better during expiration.

Nonejection systolic clicks, occurring with or without a late systolic murmur, often denote mitral valve regurgitation due to prolapse of the posterior leaflet (Chap. 258). They probably result from functional unequal length of the chordae tendineae of the mitral valve and are heard best along the lower left sternal border and at the left ventricular apex. Systolic clicks may be single or multiple, and they may occur at any time in systole but usually later than the systolic ejection sound. Frequently the midsystolic click is misinterpreted as S_2, and the actual second heart sound is called an OS or S_3.

Heart murmurs Cardiac murmurs result from vibrations set up in the bloodstream and the surrounding heart and great vessels as a result of turbulent blood flow, the formation of eddies, and cavitation (bubble formation as a result of sudden decrease in pressure).

The intensity or loudness of murmurs may be graded from I to VI. A grade I murmur is so faint that it can be heard only with special effort, and a grade VI murmur is audible with the stethoscope removed from contact with the chest. The configuration of a murmur may be crescendo, decrescendo, crescendo-decrescendo (diamond-shaped), or plateau. The precise time of onset and time of cessation of a murmur depend on the instant in the cardiac cycle at which an adequate pressure difference between two chambers appears and disappears (Fig. 248-2).

The location on the chest wall where the murmur is best heard and the areas to which it radiates can be helpful in identifying the cardiac structure from which the murmur originates. For example, the murmur of aortic valve stenosis is loudest usually in the second right intercostal space and radiates to the carotid arteries. By contrast, the murmur of mitral regurgitation is most often loudest at the cardiac apex and may radiate to the left sternal border and base of the heart when the posterior mitral leaflet is predominantly involved or to the axilla and back when the anterior leaflet is more severely affected. In the former case, the regurgitant blood is directed toward the posterior left atrial wall.

FIGURE 248-2
Simultaneous recordings of ECG, aortic pressure (AOP), left ventricular pressure (LVP), and left atrial pressure (LAP). HSM is a holosystolic murmur; PSM, a presystolic murmur; MDM, a middiastolic murmur; MSM, a midsystolic murmur; EDM, an early diastolic murmur; LSM, a late systolic murmur; and CM, a continuous murmur.

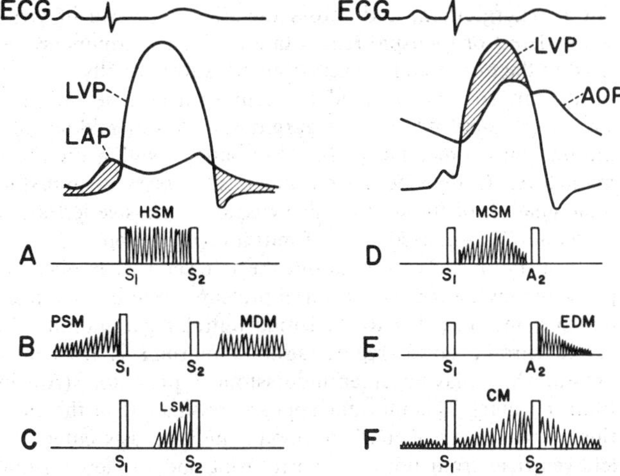

Many times it is difficult to classify with certainty a cardiac murmur based on its timing, configuration, location, radiation, pitch, or intensity. However, by noting changes in the characteristics of the murmur during maneuvers which alter cardiac hemodynamics, the auscultator often can identify its correct origin and significance.

Accentuation of a murmur during inspiration with the augmentation of systemic venous return implies that it originates on the right side of the circulation; expiratory exaggeration has less significance. Prolonged expiratory pressure against a closed glottis, the Valsalva maneuver, reduces intensity of most murmurs by diminishing both right and left ventricular filling. The systolic murmur associated with *obstructive hypertrophic cardiomyopathy* and the late systolic murmur due to a *prolapse of the mitral valve* are exceptions and may be accentuated during the Valsalva maneuver. Murmurs due to flow across a normal or obstructed semilunar valve increase in intensity in the beat following a premature ventricular contraction or a long RR interval in atrial fibrillation. In contrast, murmurs due to AV valve regurgitation or a ventricular septal defect do not change appreciably during the beat following a prolonged diastole. Standing, which decreases heart size, accentuates the murmur of hypertrophic cardiomyopathy and occasionally the murmur due to a prolapse of the mitral valve. Squatting, which increases both venous return and systemic arterial resistance, increases most murmurs, except those due to hypertrophic cardiomyopathy and mitral regurgitation due to a prolapsed mitral valve, which often decrease. Sustained handgrip exercise, which increases the systemic arterial pressure and heart rate, often accentuates the murmurs of mitral regurgitation, aortic regurgitation, and mitral stenosis but usually diminishes those due to aortic or subaortic stenosis.

Holosystolic (pansystolic) murmurs are generated when there is a flow between two chambers which have widely different pressures throughout systole, such as the left ventricle and either the left atrium or the right ventricle. The pressure gradient is established early in contraction and lasts until relaxation is almost complete. Therefore, holosystolic murmurs begin before aortic ejection, and at the area of maximal intensity they begin with S_1 and end after S_2. Holosystolic murmurs accompany mitral or tricuspid regurgitation, ventricular septal defect, and under certain circumstances, aorta-pulmonary shunts. Although the typical high-pitched murmur of mitral regurgitation usually continues throughout systole, the shape of the murmur may vary considerably. The holosystolic murmurs of mitral regurgitation and ventricular septal defect are augmented by raising the arterial pressure with intravenous phenylephrine and are diminished by lowering the left ventricular systolic pressure by inhalation of amyl nitrite. The murmur of tricuspid regurgitation associated with pulmonary hypertension is holosystolic and frequently increases during inspiration, a feature of diagnostic importance. Not all patients with mitral or tricuspid regurgitation or ventricular septal defect have holosystolic murmurs (Chap. 258).

Midsystolic murmurs occur when blood is ejected across the aortic or pulmonic outflow tracts. The murmur starts shortly after S_1 when the ventricular pressure rises sufficiently to open the semilunar valve. Ejection then begins and with it the onset of the murmur; as ejection increases, the murmur is augmented, and as ejection declines, it diminishes. The murmur ends before the ventricular pressure falls enough to permit closure of the aortic or pulmonic leaflets. In the presence of normal semilunar valves and increased flow rate, as may occur in states of elevated cardiac output, ejection into a dilated vessel beyond the valve, or increased transmission of sound through a thin chest wall may be responsible for the production of this murmur. Most benign, functional murmurs are midsystolic and originate from the pulmonary outflow tract. Valvular or subvalvular obstruction to either ventricle may also cause such a midsystolic murmur, the intensity being related to the flow.

The murmur of aortic stenosis is the prototype of the left-sided midsystolic murmur. The location and radiation of this murmur appear to be influenced by the direction of the high-velocity jet within the aortic root. In *valvular aortic stenosis* the murmur is usually maximal in the second right intercostal space, with radiation into the neck. In *supravalvular aortic stenosis* the murmur is occasionally loudest even higher, with disproportionate radiation into the right carotid artery. In obstructive hypertrophic cardiomyopathy, the murmur originates within the left ventricular cavity, and is usually maximal at the lower left sternal edge and apex, with relatively little radiation to the carotids. When the aortic valve is immobile (calcified), the aortic closure sound (A_2) may be soft and inaudible so that the length and configuration of the murmur are difficult to determine. Midsystolic murmurs also occur in patients with mitral regurgitation or, less frequently, tricuspid regurgitation resulting from papillary muscle dysfunction. Murmurs due to mitral regurgitation are often confused with those originating in the aorta, particularly in elderly patients.

The patient's age and the area of maximal intensity aid in determining the significance of midsystolic murmurs. Thus, in a young adult with a thin chest and high velocity of blood flow, a faint or moderate midsystolic murmur heard only in the pulmonic area is usually without clinical significance, while a somewhat louder murmur in the aortic area may indicate congenital aortic stenosis. In elderly patients pulmonary flow murmurs are rare, while aortic systolic murmurs are frequent and may be due to aortic dilatation, to a significant degree of valvular aortic stenosis, or to nonstenotic deformity of the aortic valve. Midsystolic aortic and pulmonic murmurs are intensified by amyl nitrite inhalation and during the cardiac cycle following a premature ventricular contraction, while those due to mitral regurgitation are unchanged or softer. Aortic systolic murmurs are diminished by interventions which increase systemic arterial resistance such as intravenous phenylephrine. Cardiac catheterization may be necessary to separate a prominent and exaggerated functional murmur from one due to congenital semilunar valve stenosis.

Early systolic murmurs begin with the first heart sound and end in midsystole. They may be due to a very small *ventricular septal defect, a large defect with pulmonary hypertension,* or *severe acute mitral* or *tricuspid regurgitation.* In large ventricular septal defects with pulmonary hypertension the shunting at the end of systole may be small or absent, resulting in an early systolic murmur. A similar murmur may occur with very small muscular ventricular septal defects, the shunt being interrupted in late systole. An early systolic murmur is a feature of tricuspid regurgitation occurring in the absence of pulmonary hypertension. This lesion is common in drug addicts with infective endocarditis, in whom a tall regurgitant right atrial *v* wave reaches the level of the normal right ventricular pressure in late systole, confining the murmur to early systole. In patients with acute mitral regurgitation and a large *v* wave in a noncompliant left atrium, a loud early systolic murmur is frequently heard which diminishes as the pressure gradient between left ventricle and left atrium decreases in late systole (Chap. 258).

Late systolic murmurs are faint or moderately loud high-pitched apical murmurs, which start well after ejection and do not mask either heart sound. They are probably related to papillary muscle dysfunction caused by infarction or ischemia of these muscles or to their distortion by left ventricular dilatation. They may appear only during angina but are common in patients with myocardial infarction or diffuse myocardial disease. Late systolic murmurs following midsystolic clicks are associated with late systolic mitral regurgitation caused by prolapse of the mitral valve into the left atrium (Chap. 258).

Early diastolic murmurs begin with or shortly after the second heart sound as soon as the corresponding ventricular pressure falls sufficiently below that in the aorta or pulmonary artery. The high-pitched murmurs of aortic regurgitation or pulmonic regurgitation due to pulmonary hypertension are generally decrescendo, since there is a progressive decline in the volume or rate of regurgitation during diastole. Faint, high-pitched murmurs of aortic regurgitation are difficult to hear unless they are specifically sought by applying firm pressure with the diaphragm over the left midsternal border while the patient sits, leans forward, and holds a breath in full expiration. The diastolic murmur of aortic regurgitation is enhanced by an acute elevation of the arterial pressure such as occurs with handgrip exercise; it diminishes with a decrease in arterial pressure such as occurs during amyl nitrite inhalation. The diastolic murmur of congenital pulmonic regurgitation in the absence of pulmonary hypertension is low to medium pitched. The onset of this murmur is delayed because at the onset of pulmonic valve closure the regurgitant flow is minimal, since the reverse pressure gradient responsible for the regurgitation is negligible at this time.

Middiastolic murmurs usually arise from the AV valves, occur during early ventricular filling, and like most midsystolic murmurs, are due to disproportion between valve orifice size and flow rate. Such murmurs may be loud despite only slight AV valve stenosis when there is normal or increased blood flow. Conversely, the murmur may be soft or even absent despite severe obstruction if the cardiac output is markedly reduced. When stenosis is marked, the diastolic murmur is prolonged and the duration of the murmur is more reliable than its intensity as an index of the degree of valve obstruction.

The low-pitched, middiastolic murmur of mitral stenosis characteristically follows the opening snap. It should be specifically sought by placing the bell of the stethoscope at the site of the left ventricular impulse, which is best localized with the patient on the left side. Frequently the murmur of mitral stenosis is present only at the left ventricular apex, and it may be increased in intensity by mild supine exercise or by inhalation of amyl nitrite. In tricuspid stenosis the middiastolic murmur is localized to a relatively limited area along the left sternal edge and may increase in intensity during inspiration.

Middiastolic murmurs may be generated across the mitral valve in ventricular septal defect, patent ductus arteriosus, or mitral regurgitation, and across the tricuspid valve in atrial septal defect or tricuspid regurgitation. These murmurs are related to the torrential flow across an AV valve, usually follow a third heart sound, and tend to occur with large left-to-right shunts or severe AV valve regurgitation. A soft middiastolic murmur may sometimes be heard in patients with acute rheumatic fever (Carey-Coombs murmur). It has been attributed to inflammation of the mitral valve cusps or excessive left atrial blood flow as a consequence of mitral regurgitation.

In acute aortic regurgitation, the left ventricular diastolic pressure may exceed the left atrial pressure, resulting in a middiastolic murmur due to "diastolic mitral regurgitation." In severe chronic aortic regurgitation a murmur is frequently present which may be either middiastolic or presystolic (Austin Flint murmur). This murmur appears to originate at the anterior mitral valve leaflet when blood simultaneously enters the left ventricle from both the aortic root and the left atrium.

Presystolic murmurs begin during the period of ventricular filling that follows atrial contraction and therefore occur in sinus rhythm. They are usually due to AV valve stenosis and have the same quality as the middiastolic filling rumble but are usually crescendo, reaching peak intensity at the time of a loud S_1. The presystolic murmur corresponds to the AV valve gradient, which may be minimal until the moment of right or left atrial contraction. It is the presystolic rather than the middiastolic murmur which is most characteristic of tricuspid stenosis and sinus rhythm. A right or left *atrial myxoma* may occasionally cause either middiastolic or presystolic murmurs that resemble the murmurs of mitral or tricuspid stenosis.

Continuous murmurs begin in systole and persist through S_2 into all or part of diastole. These murmurs signify continuous flow due to communication between high- and low-pressure areas which persists through the end of systole and the beginning of diastole. A *patent ductus arteriosus* causes a continuous murmur as long as the pressure in the pulmonary artery is much below that in the aorta. The murmur is intensified by elevation of the systemic arterial pressure and is reduced by amyl nitrite inhalation. When pulmonary hypertension is present, the diastolic portion may disappear, leaving the murmur confined to systole. A continuous murmur is uncommon in aortopulmonary septal defects, since this malformation is generally associated with severe pulmonary hypertension. Surgically produced aortopulmonary connections and the subclavian–pulmonary artery anastomosis result in murmurs similar to that of a patent ductus.

Continuous murmurs may result from congenital or acquired *systemic arteriovenous fistula, coronary arteriovenous fistula,* anomalous origin of the left coronary artery from the pulmonary artery, and communications between the *sinus of Valsalva and the right side of the heart.* Continuous murmurs may also occur when high left atrial pressure results in continuous flow across a small defect in the atrial septum. Murmurs associated with *pulmonary arteriovenous fistulas* may be continuous but are usually only systolic. Continuous murmurs may also be due to disturbances of flow pattern in constricted systemic (e.g., renal) or pulmonary arteries when marked pressure differences between the two sides of the narrow segment persist; a continuous murmur in the back may be present in *coarctation of the aorta; pulmonary embolism* may cause continuous murmurs in partially occluded vessels.

In nonconstricted arteries continuous murmurs may be due to rapid flow through a tortuous bed. Such murmurs typically occur within the bronchial arterial collateral circulation in cyanotic patients with severe pulmonary outflow obstruction. The "mammary souffle," an innocent murmur heard during late pregnancy and early postpartum, may be systolic or continuous. The innocent cervical venous hum is a continuous murmur usually heard over the medial aspect of the right supraclavicular fossa with the patient upright. The hum is usually louder during diastole and can be instantaneously abolished by digital compression of the ipsilateral internal jugular vein. Transmission of a loud venous hum to the area below the clavicles may result in a mistaken diagnosis of patent ductus arteriosus.

The *pericardial friction rub,* which may have presystolic, systolic, and early diastolic scratchy components, may be confused with a murmur or extracardiac sound when heard only in systole. It is best appreciated with the patient upright and leaning forward and may be accentuated during inspiration.

REFERENCES

Braunwald E: Physical examination, in *Heart Disease,* 2d ed. E Braunwald. Philadelphia, Saunders, 1983, chap 2

Crawford MH, O'Rourke RA: A systematic approach to the bedside differentiation of cardiac murmurs and abnormal sounds. Curr Probl Cardiol 1(11):1, 1977

Fowler NO: Cardiac auscultation, in *Cardiac Diagnosis and Treatment,* 2d ed, NO Fowler (ed). Hagerstown, Harper & Row, 1980, chap 5, pp 62–76

Leatham A: *Auscultation of the Heart and Phonocardiography,* 2d ed. New York, Churchill Livingstone, 1976

Luisada AA, Portaluppi F: *The Heart Sounds: New Facts and Their Clinical Implications.* New York, Praeger, 1982

Mills P, Craig E: Echophonocardiography. Prog Cardiovasc Dis 20:337, 1978

Perloff JK (ed): *Physical Examination of the Heart and Circulation.* Philadelphia, Saunders, 1982

Schlant RC, Felner JM: The arterial pulse—clinical manifestations. Curr Probl Cardiol 2(5):1, 1977

Shaver JA, O'Toole JD: The second heart sound. New concepts. Mod Concepts Cardiovasc Dis 46:7, 1977

249 ELECTROCARDIOGRAPHY

ROBERT J. MYERBURG

CARDIAC ELECTROPHYSIOLOGY The electrocardiogram (ECG) is a graphic description of the electrical activity of the heart recorded from the body surface by electrodes positioned to reflect activity from a variety of spatial perspectives. The source of cardiac electrical activity resides within the working (contracting) myocardial cells as well as within the automatic and specialized cells. Most cardiac cells maintain a *resting* membrane *polarization* of 90 mV, the inside of the cell negative with respect to the outside (that is, −90 mV); but the cells are electrically active, and a sufficient stimulus is able to initiate a *depolarization.* Cardiac tissue is unique among other electrically active tissues in the magnitude of the time delay between depolarization and the completion of recovery of excitability or *repolarization.* This results in refractory periods—the minimum intervals required for two successive responses—which are relatively long. After repolarization and before the next depolarization, most cells maintain the state of resting polarization; but certain cardiac tissues undergo slow, *spontaneous depolarization.* If this continues to threshold potential, an impulse is initiated. It is this mechanism which permits the sinoatrial (SA) node to function as the pacemaker of the heart and other regions to provide normal backup pacemakers, or to usurp this function abnormally. Recently, another form of depolarization, which drives single cell membranes toward threshold potential, has been observed. This is referred to as *triggered activity* because it can be elicited by premature stimulation or increasing rates of stimulation. In contrast to spontaneous depolarization, which usually spans diastole, triggered depolarization of single cells occurs relatively early in diastole and may establish sustained activity. The clinical significance of this form of activity has not yet been determined although some arrhythmias have now been attributed to triggered activity.

Under resting, steady-state conditions, ionic gradients are maintained across cardiac cell membranes. The extracellular concentration of Na^+ is about 10 to 15 times the intracellular concentration, and the intracellular concentration of K^+ is 30 to 35 times its extracellular concentration. The K^+ gradient is responsible for the resting transmembrane potential. During depolarization of most normal cardiac tissue, on the other hand, specific Na^+ channels in cell membranes open, permitting the rapid influx of Na^+ down its electrochemical gradient and very rapid depolarization, which is paralleled by rapid impulse conduction. Stimulation of partially depolarized tissue causes a slower rate of depolarization and a more slowly conducted impulse. The Na^+ channel is inactivated at membrane potentials less negative than −55 mV. Depolarization initiated at resting potentials less than −55 mV appears to result from ionic currents across a different channel—the so-called slow channel—carried primarily by Ca^{2+} ions. Such impulses are conducted more slowly. At levels of partial depolarization between −90 and −55 mV, slow depolarizations might result from either the partially inactivated fast (Na^+) channel or slow channel impulses.

In addition to the uniquely long delay between depolarization and repolarization in cardiac tissue, there is considerable variability in the electrical properties among the various cardiac tissues, including important variations in refractory periods. The electrically active tissues may be conveniently divided into two general types: (1) ordinary muscle and (2) specialized conducting tissue (SCT). The ordinary muscle of the atria and ventricles accounts for most of the cardiac mass. These tissues conduct impulses at a velocity much lower than the intraventricular SCT (the His-Purkinje system), but considerably faster than the atrioventricular (AV) node. The refractory periods of muscle are shorter in duration than SCT, and the SCT of the heart has a broader range of functional properties than does muscle. The primary function of the SA node is initiation of the cardiac impulse, and the cells are highly specialized for the purpose of impulse formation (automaticity). Spontaneous depolarization is the most prominent feature.

The AV node is a complex structure, in which the electrical activity may be predominantly or entirely dependent upon "slow channel," Ca^{2+}-dependent currents. Impulses propagating from the atria into the AV node undergo an abrupt and progressive decrease in conduction velocity, a phenomenon termed *decremental conduction;* i.e., the amplitude and velocity of the impulse diminish as it is conducted into an area which is less responsive, causing a still weaker response, which acts as a yet weaker stimulus for continued propagation. Should this sequence continue, the impulse eventually would be extinguished. However, at some point within the AV node the process reverses, responses to the weakly conducted impulse becoming stronger and propagating into more responsive tissue. After approximately 90 to 100 ms, propagation across the AV node is complete, and the impulse enters the next area of specialized conducting tissue, the bundle of His.

Propagation through the bundle of His is very rapid as this structure moves through the lower portion of the interatrial septum, giving off fibers which become the left bundle branch (LBB) as they pierce the membranous portion of the interventricular septum below the aortic ring. The rest of the bundle of His continues across the crest of the interventricular septum and courses down the right side of the septum as the right bundle branch (RBB). When the RBB reaches the apex of the right ventricle, it fans out onto the free wall as the Purkinje network.

The main LBB is a relatively short structure which bifurcates into two general collections of fibers on the upper portion of the interventricular septum, forming structures which have been referred to as the anterior (superior) and posterior (inferior) divisions of the LBB. The two divisions are not isolated end structures, there being numerous interconnections between them on the surface of the left ventricular septum. The cells of the RBB and LBB systems are highly specialized and conduct more rapidly than any other within the heart. Specialization for rapid conduction achieves an orderly and appropriately synchronous sequence of activation of the ventricles.

The magnitude and direction of the electrical activity recorded on the body surface is an average of the numerous cell depolarizations or repolarizations occurring at a given instant. Although much of the electrical activity from individual cells is canceled out before reaching the body surface by opposing forces from other cells, the resultant recording is a reasonably reproducible and accurate approximation of net cardiac electrical activity. However, the signals recorded at the body surface lack specificity in regard to site of origin because a given vector at the body surface can be accounted for by innumerable combinations of cellular signals at their source in the heart.

Early in the development of the ECG, Einthoven popularized the concept that the human body represents a large volume conductor having the source of cardiac electrical activity at its center. While this theory is not strictly true, it still provides the clinician with a practical point from which to work. As an extension of this concept, the *net* electrical activity at any instant in the cardiac cycle may be viewed as originating from a polarized point source at a theoretical "electrical center" of the heart. Since this "equivalent dipole" would have direction and magnitude, one might then extend the pattern into a sequence of instantaneous vectors recordable from the body surface. The application of this concept to ECG analysis is discussed below.

LEAD SYSTEMS The ECG lead system is composed of five electrodes, one on each of the four limbs and one placed at various sites on the precordium. Each lead is a continuous recording of the change in electrical potential during the cardiac cycle between two of the electrodes, or between one electrode and a combination of the others. The right-leg electrode is an inactive ground electrode in all leads.

The original lead system developed by Einthoven is based on assumptions of (1) the homogeneity of the body volume conductor, (2) the symmetry of the leads, and (3) a single equivalent dipole at the center of the volume conductor. The *standard limb leads* (I, II, and III) are composed of three permutations of the right arm (RA), left arm (LA), and left leg (LL) electrodes [Fig. 249-1*A* (1)]. Lead I records the potential difference between the LA and the RA, the positive electrode on the LA, and the negative electrode on the RA [Fig. 249-1*A* (2)]. Lead II records the potential difference between the electrodes on the RA and the LL, the positive electrode on the LL. Lead III records the potential difference between the LA and the LL, with the positive electrode on the LL. It is likely that Einthoven arbitrarily selected the relationships between positive and negative electrodes in the three leads in order to have the major deflection of the QRS complex (see below) moving in an upward (positive) direction in most normal individuals.

The central terminal of Wilson (CTW) is constructed by connecting the RA, LA, and LL electrodes through 5000 Ω resistance, in order to cancel out the potentials from these three points. With the forces canceled out, the CTW theoretically remains inactive during the entire cardiac cycle, and an exploring electrode will function as a unipolar lead [Fig. 249-1*B* (1)]. The selection of the positions for the six *unipolar chest leads* [Figs. 249-1*B* (2) and 249-2] was based on the concept that the proximity of the heart to the anterior chest wall resulted in the unipolar chest leads functioning as semidirect leads, being influenced primarily by the tissue immediately beneath the electrode. While this concept does not have the quantitative significance originally assigned to it, and the recordings do reflect the activity of the total heart, there is weighting of the voltages recorded by the tissue closest to the exploring electrode. The six standard chest leads (V_1 to V_6) are recorded by positioning the exploring chest electrode as follows: V_1 in the fourth intercostal space (4ICS) at the right ster-

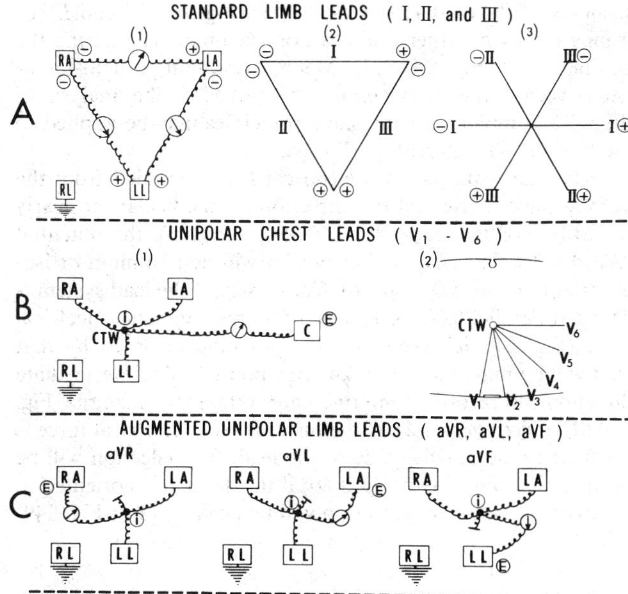

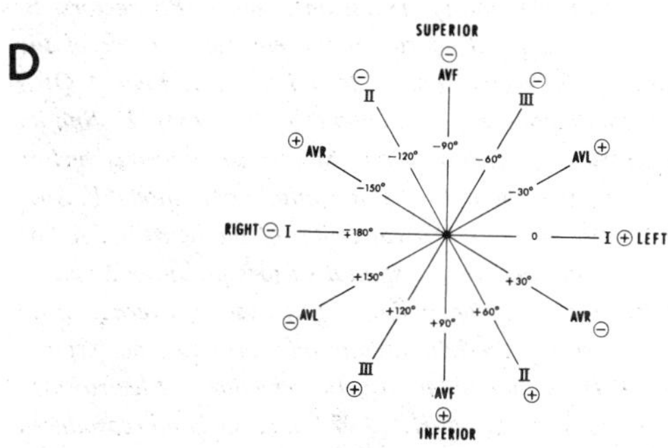

FIGURE 249-1

Lead systems. A. Standard limb leads, showing (1) electrode positions, (2) the equilateral triangle of Einthoven, and (3) the conversion of the triangle to a triaxial reference system with positive (+) and negative (−) polarity. B. The unipolar chest leads, showing (1) the central terminal of Wilson (CTW) (or the indifferent electrode −i) and the chest electrode (C) (or the exploring electrode −E). The 5000 Ω between CTW and each limb electrode is not shown. The relationship between CTW and V_1 to V_6 in the horizontal plane is shown in B (2). C. The augmented unipolar limb leads, using the modified CTW. D. The hexaxial frontal plane reference system. Normal ranges are described in the text, and applications are derived in Figs. 249-5 and 249-6. RA, right arm; LA, left arm; LL, left leg; RL, right leg.

nal border; V_2 in the 4ICS at the left sternal border; V_4 in the 5ICS at the midclavicular line; V_3 midway between V_2 and V_4; V_5 at the left anterior axillary line at the level of V_4 horizontally; and V_6 at the left midaxillary line at the level of V_4 horizontally (Fig. 249-2). The CTW is the indifferent electrode, and the exploring chest electrode is the active electrode.

Unipolar limb leads may be recorded by a system in which the CTW constitutes the indifferent electrode and the exploring is one of the three active limb electrodes. These leads are referred to as VR, VL, and VF. By disconnecting the input to the CTW from the extremity being explored, the voltage of the unipolar limb leads is augmented by as much as 50 percent. This modification is universally used for clinical ECGs, and the leads are labeled aVR, aVL, and aVF (Fig. 249-1*C*).

In recent years, the clinical value of chest wall mapping has been studied by a number of investigators. Multiple electrodes (32 to 192) are used for simultaneous recording, and computer processing for data reduction and display. This procedure

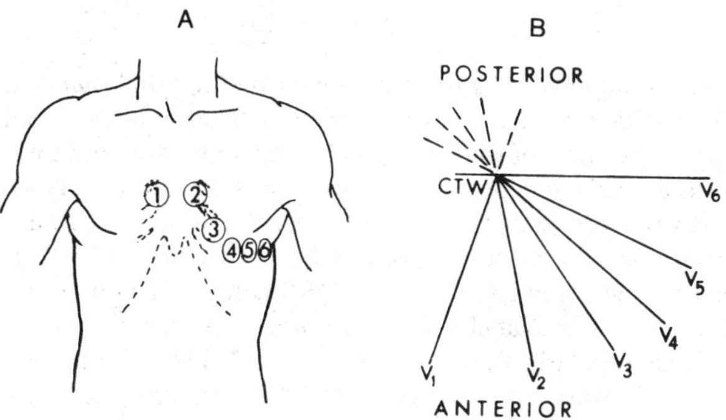

FIGURE 249-2

The unipolar chest leads. A. The position of the chest electrode for V_1 to V_6. B. The relationship between the CTW and the chest electrode (C) in the horizontal plane.

yields information not available from the standard 12-lead ECG. New insights into normal and abnormal depolarization and repolarization patterns are evolving, and the value of sequential changes in ST segments during acute myocardial infarction is being studied.

ELECTROCARDIOGRAPHIC WAVEFORMS, DURATIONS, AND INTERVALS Clinical ECGs are recorded on paper having a graphic background (Fig. 249-3) to permit rapid measurement of standardized time intervals and voltages. Time lines are 1 mm apart, with every fifth line intensified. Standard paper speed is 25 mm/s. Thus, 1 mm = 0.04 s (lighter lines), and 5 mm = 0.20 s (heavier lines). The horizontal lines, 1 mm apart, permit calibration of the voltage deflections of the ECG. Usual standardization is ↑10 mm = +1 mV (Fig. 249-3).

The P wave of atrial depolarization is normally the initial wave of activity during the cardiac cycle (Fig. 249-4). Ventricu-

FIGURE 249-3

Standardization of the ECG. Standard time calibration is 1 mm = 0.04 s or 5 mm = 0.20 s. Standard voltage is 0.1 mV/mm. A repetitive event occurring every 5 mm (A) on time axis (0.20 s) is occurring at 300 per minute. A repetitive event occurring every 10 mm (B) (0.40 s) is occurring at 150 per minute. C, D, and E indicate that repetitive events at 0.60, 0.80, and 1.00 s are occurring at rates of 100, 75, and 60 per minute, respectively.

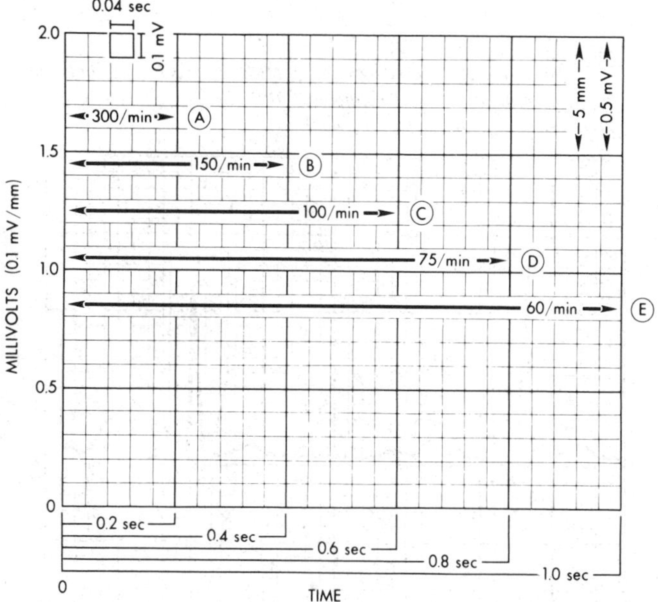

lar muscle depolarization is represented by the *QRS complex.* A Q wave is an initial negative wave; an R wave is an initial positive wave or a positive wave following a Q wave; and an S wave is a negative deflection following an R wave (Fig. 249-4). A QRS complex having a Q wave which returns to the base line but does not produce a positive wave is labeled a QS complex, and the second R wave in a QRS complex having more than one R wave is labeled R′. The T wave represents ventricular muscle repolarization and is sometimes followed by a small wave, the U wave, the mechanism of which remains uncertain. Repolarization of atrial muscle is represented by the T_a (or T_p) wave, which occurs during the PR interval and QRS complex, and is usually difficult to identify. The interval between the end of the QRS complex and the onset of the T wave is the ST segment, representing the period of time between depolarization of the ventricles and the period of rapid repolarization of ventricular muscle.

The interval between the P wave and the QRS complex is the PR (or PQ) interval, measured from the *onset* of atrial depolarization (P) to the *onset* of ventricular depolarization (Q) (Fig. 249-4). The duration is 0.12 to 0.20 s in the adult. Since AV nodal activation begins before the end of depolarization of atrial muscle, the PR interval may be used as a rough approximation of AV conduction time.

The duration of the QRS complex (0.04 to 0.10 s) reflects the time required for depolarization of ventricular muscle. It may be slightly prolonged by regional block in a portion of the intraventricular SCT or by delayed conduction in a region of ventricular muscle. Block in a bundle branch prolongs the QRS to a greater extent. An approximation of the refractory period of the ventricles may be obtained by measuring the QT interval (from the onset of the QRS to the end of the T wave) (Fig. 249-4). The QT interval is rate dependent, and may be altered by numerous pathophysiologic or pharmacologic influences.

THE VECTOR CONCEPT AND ELECTRICAL AXIS The representation of a force by a graphic description of its direction and magnitude is referred to as a *vector.* In specific reference to cardiac electrical activity, a vector may be projected onto a two-dimensional plane as a scalar vector (Fig. 249-5*A* to *D*), or considered in three dimensions as a spatial vector (Fig. 249-5*E* to *H*). It may be used to represent instantaneous forces in the sequence of the cardiac electrical cycle (Fig. 249-5*A* and *E*), or it may represent either the mean or maximum axis during the cardiac cycle (Fig. 249-5*H*). Mean, maximum, and instantaneous vectors are most commonly applied to the analysis of the QRS complex, but the same principles may be applied to the P wave, ST segment, or T wave.

When an instantaneous electrical force recorded from the body surface is oriented in a direction perpendicular (or nearly so) to one of the leads (Fig. 249-5*C,* vector 6), the potential recorded by that lead at that instant will be minimum or isoelectric (Fig. 249-5*D,* point 6). Conversely, if the lead system is oriented parallel to the direction of an instantaneous electrical force (Fig. 249-5*C,* vector 4), the potential recorded by that lead will be maximum (Fig. 249-5*D,* point 4). An intermediate direction will record an intermediate voltage (for example, Fig. 249-5*C* and *D,* vector 2). If the instantaneous electrical force is oriented to the positive side of the lead, the deflection will be positive (4 in Fig. 249-5*C* and *D*); if the direction is oriented to the negative side, the deflection will be negative (1 in Fig. 249-

FIGURE 249-4

The waves of the electrocardiogram—P, QRS, T, and U—are indicated. The measurements of the PR interval, QRS complex, ST segment, and QT interval are identified on the right.

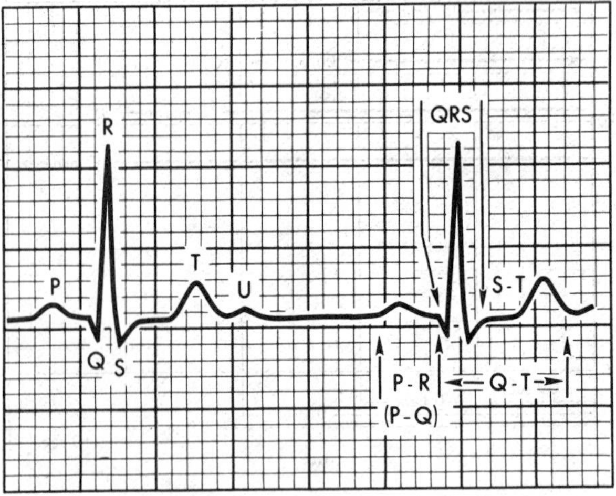

FIGURE 249-5

A. Frontal plane scalar projection of six instantaneous QRS vectors. B. Vectors originating from a point source at the electrical center of the heart. C. Projection of the vectors on the lead I axis. D. Lead I QRS produced by the instantaneous vectors in panel C (see text). E. Spatial representation of ventricular depolarization. Seven instantaneous vectors in the sequence of depolarization indicated in spatial orientations. F. Spatial vectors originating from the electrical center of the heart. G. A line drawn through the terminations of the spatial vectors produces a spatial QRS loop (vector loop). H. The mean spatial QRS vector, average of all the instantaneous vectors—to the left, slightly inferiorly, and posteriorly. (See text.) (From JW Hurst, RJ Myerburg, Introduction to Electrocardiography, 2d ed, New York, McGraw-Hill, 1973; modified and reproduced by permission of the publisher.)

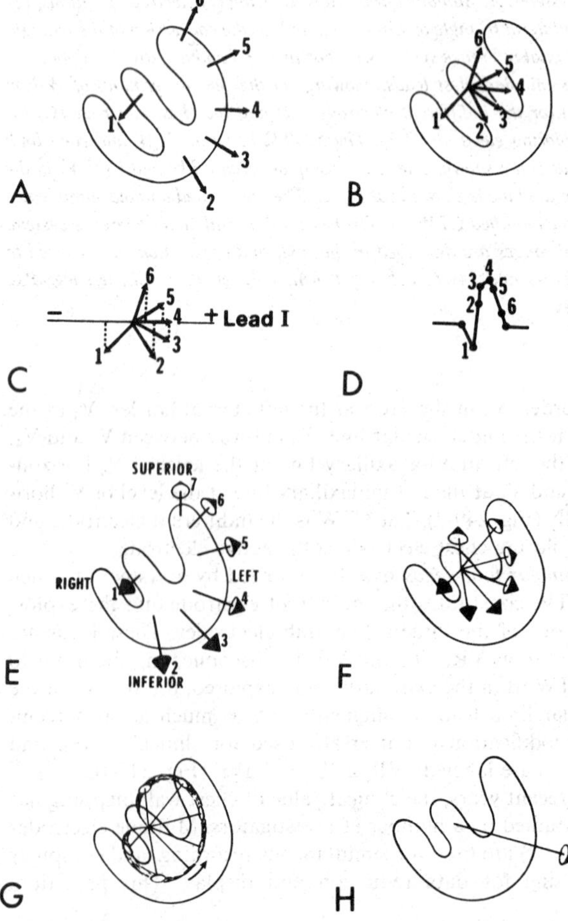

5*C* and *D*). These general considerations may be applied to either instantaneous vectors occurring at any point during the inscription of the QRS complex, or the mean vector produced by total ventricular depolarization (see below).

In Fig. 249-5*E* to *H*, seven instantaneous vectors are represented in three dimensions, indicating the spatial sequence of ventricular depolarization. In panel *E*, the mean spatial QRS vector, representing the net vector of all instantaneous forces, is shown. If the principles described above were applied, the QRS voltage would be large in lead I and small in aVF in the frontal plane (limb leads), and oriented posteriorly in the horizontal plane (chest leads).

When a triaxial system representing the augmented unipolar limb leads is superimposed on the triaxial system of Einthoven, a hexaxial system is obtained which is convenient for estimating the mean QRS axis, or any of the instantaneous vectors, in the frontal plane (Fig. 249-1*D*). When the appropriate positive and negative voltage orientations are assigned to each of the leads, the hexaxial reference system becomes a simple means of scalar vector analysis, requiring a minimum of two leads for estimation of the mean axis. An ECG which reveals a maximum positive QRS deflection in lead I and an isoelectric deflection in aVF would be oriented at 0°. Conversely, if the QRS voltage is positive and maximum in lead II and isoelectric in aVL, it would be oriented at +60°. The mean QRS axis in the frontal plane in normal adults ranges from −30 to +110°. Overlap between normal and abnormal occurs in the range of +90 to +110°. Generally, an axis > +90° is referred to as *right axis deviation,* and more negative than −30° as *abnormal left axis deviation.* The determination of the mean QRS axis in the horizontal plane (Fig. 249-2*B*) is similarly derived, normal orientation being to the left and posteriorly.

Three normal ECGs are shown in Fig. 249-6. Analysis of the mean QRS axis in the *frontal plane* (I, II, III, aVR, aVL, aVF) reveals the axis of *A* to be oriented horizontally, of *C* to be oriented vertically, and of *B* to be oriented in an intermediate range. In *A* the net voltage of the QRS complex is largest in lead I, almost isoelectric in lead III, and low in aVF, placing the mean axis in a direction almost perpendicular to lead III. In *B,* the voltages in lead I and aVF are almost identical, and maximum in lead II and aVR. The mean QRS axis is between lead II (+) and aVR (−). In *C,* net voltage is largest in leads II and aVF and almost isoelectric in lead I, placing the mean QRS axis almost perpendicular to lead I. A similar approach is applied to QRS axis determination in the *horizontal plane.* In *C,* the lead in which the net forces are isoelectric is V_3. Therefore, as shown in the axial representation of the horizontal plane of tracing *C,* the QRS is oriented to the left and posteriorly. If this information is added to that obtained from the frontal plane axis, it is apparent that the mean QRS vector of electrocardiogram *C* is oriented inferiorly, to the left, and posteriorly. Similar principles may be applied to the analysis of the mean T-wave axis, which is normally oriented in the same general direction as the QRS axis. An angle between the QRS and T axes >45° in the frontal plane, or >60° in the horizontal plane, is abnormal.

ELECTRICAL ACTIVITY OF THE ATRIA The mean P-wave vector is normally directed to the left, inferiorly, and slightly anteriorly; the frontal plane P axis is usually oriented between +30 and +60°. Right atrial enlargement causes tall, peaked P waves (≥0.25 mV), most prominent in standard leads II and V_1 (Fig. 249-7). Left atrial enlargement causes broad, notched P waves in lead II, and inverted or biphasic P waves (with the inverted portion of the biphasic P wave broader and deeper than the upright portion) in lead V_1. The upper limit of normal for P-wave duration is 0.11 s, and the broad P wave of left atrial enlargement usually is ≥0.12 s. However, criteria for left atrial enlargement are nonspecific, similar changes occurring in intraatrial conduction disturbances (Fig. 249-7), and the two must be distinguished on clinical grounds.

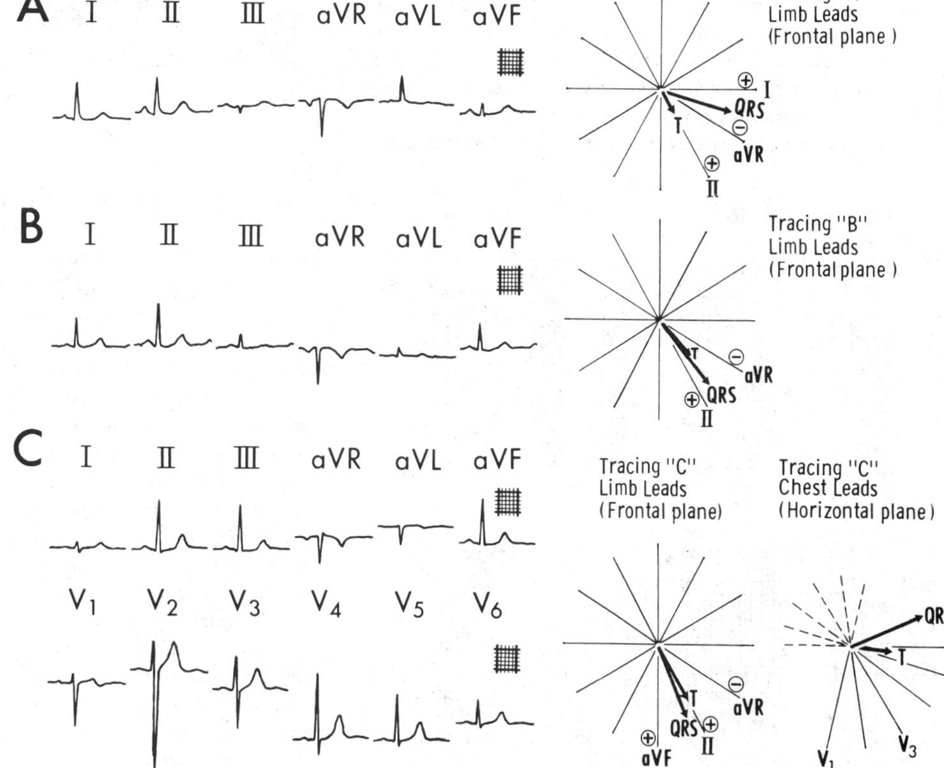

FIGURE 249-6
Three normal ECGs demonstrating: (A) horizontal, (B) intermediate, and (C) vertical mean frontal plane QRS axes constructed on the hexaxial system. In addition, the horizontal plane vector in C is constructed on an axial system and is posteriorly oriented. T-wave vectors are similarly constructed.

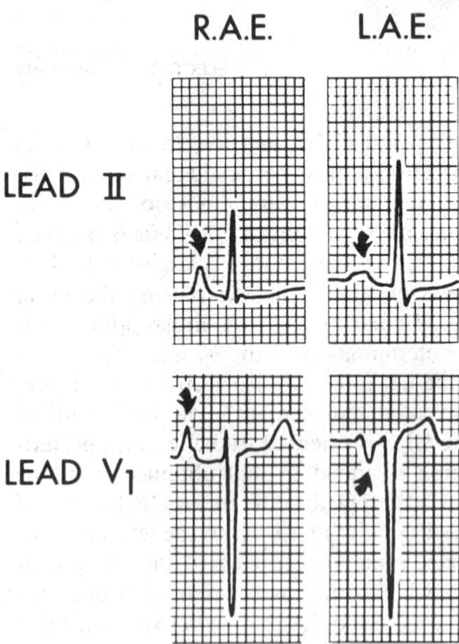

FIGURE 249-7

P waves of right atrial enlargement (RAE) and left atrial enlargement (LAE).

ABNORMALITIES OF VENTRICULAR DEPOLARIZATION: QRS COMPLEX Since the QRS complex is the ECG representation of the sequence, time, and synchronization of total ventricular muscle depolarization, focal or diffuse abnormalities in ventricular muscle or in the SCT may cause changes in QRS form. Abnormalities may be confined to initial depolarization (Fig. 249-8*B*), terminal depolarization (Fig. 249-8*C*), or mid and late depolarization (Fig. 249-8*D*) or may be diffuse (Fig. 249-8*E* to *G*).

The normal earliest site of activation is in the midportion of the left side of the interventricular septum, followed closely by a site on the lower portion of the right side of the interventricular septum and the adjacent free wall endocardium. The dominant wavefront is that one arising on the left septum, which results in a small initial R wave in V_1 (anterior movement), and a small initial Q wave in I, aVL, and/or V_6 (rightward movement). Small initial Q waves in II, III, and aVF may be observed as an indication of a small superior movement of the initial wavefront. Normal septal Q waves are ≤ 0.02 s and of low amplitude. A normal R in V_1 is ≤ 0.4 mV.

After septal depolarization has been initiated, rapid endocardial propagation occurs through both ventricles. In the normal heart, the greater mass of the left ventricle predominates, and the magnitude and direction of the electrical vectors reflect

FIGURE 249-8

QRS complexes. The lead is indicated above each example. A. Normal. B. Prolongation due to initial QRS delay between arrows (1→2) in Wolff-Parkinson-White syndrome (see Chap. 254). C. Prolongation due to terminal delay (1→2) in right bundle branch block. D. Prolongation due to mid (1→2) and late (2→3) delay in left bundle branch block. E. Minor uniform prolongation (1→2) in left ventricular hypertrophy. F. Distortion of total QRS pattern (1→2) in a cardiomyopathy. G. Uniform prolongation (1→2) in an electrolyte abnormality. H. Pathologic Q wave (1→2) in myocardial infarction. Intrinsicoid deflection = 2→3 in D and S→2 in E.

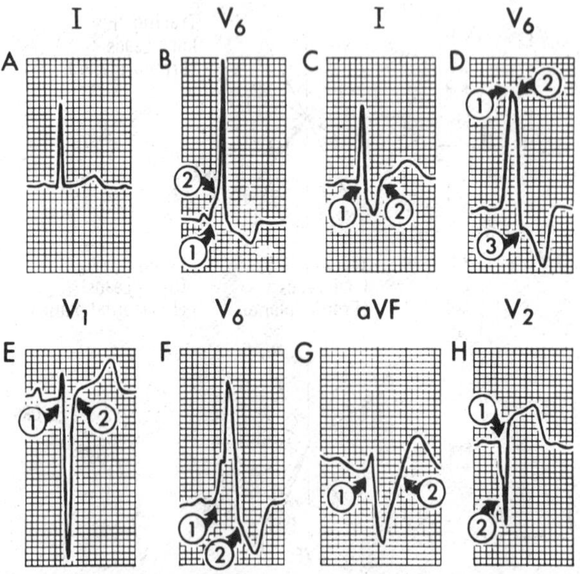

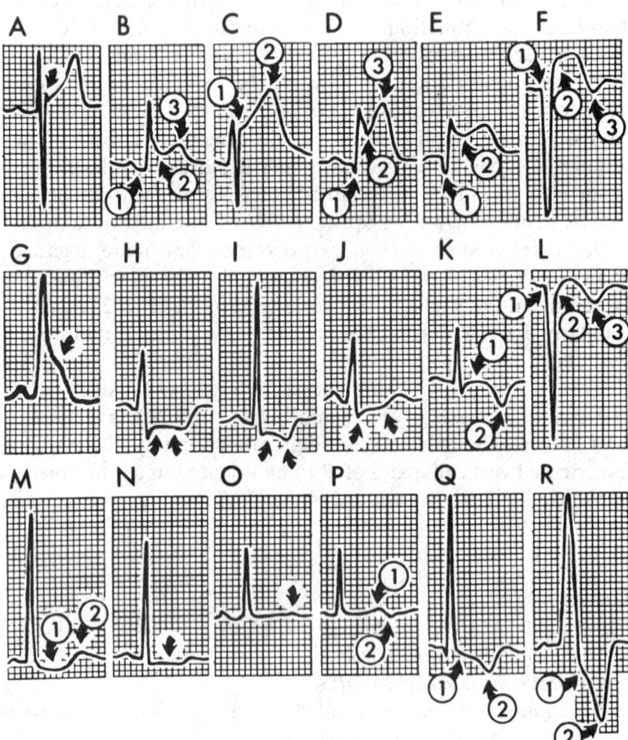

FIGURE 249-9

ST-segment and T-wave changes. Arrows in each panel indicate the major features of each complex. A. Early repolarization (J-point elevation), normal variant. B. Acute pericarditis: (1) depressed T_a; (2) elevated ST; (3) normal T. C. Early acute myocardial infarction (AMI): (1) elevated ST; (2) tall, peaked T wave; steep angle between 1 and 2. D. AMI: (1) small Q wave; (2) elevated ST segment; (3) tall, peaked T wave with steep 2→3 angle. E. AMI: (1) pathologic Q wave; (2) elevated ST segment. F. AMI: (1) Q wave; (2) elevated ST segment; (3) terminal T-wave inversion. G. Angina pectoris (Prinzmetal variant) with ST elevation during pain. H and I. Angina pectoris (usual form) with horizontal or downward sloping ST segment during pain or exercise. J. J-point depression with upsloping ST segment during exercise, normal response. K. Primary T-wave inversion (2) in ischemia or primary muscle disease. L. Myocardial infarction (healed): (1) pathologic Q; (2) ST returning to base line; (3) symmetrically inverted T wave. M. Digitalis effect: (1) downward coving of ST segment, merging into (2) an upright T wave. N to P. Nonspecific ST-segment and T-wave changes often seen in chronic ischemic heart disease. Q. Left ventricular strain pattern with (1) downsloping ST segment and (2) asymmetrically inverted (secondary) T wave. R. Downsloping ST segment merging into a deeply inverted T wave in ventricular conduction abnormality.

this fact (Fig. 249-6). During normal depolarization, the sequence of instantaneous vectors rotates from rightward and anterior to leftward, posterior, and superior, as illustrated in Fig. 249-5*E* to *G*. Most individuals will have maximum QRS duration (i.e., the lead having the longest measurable QRS) of 0.05 to 0.08 s (normal range is 0.04 to 0.10 s). A QRS duration of 0.09 or 0.10 s may be a normal variant or may represent a conduction delay to limited regions of either ventricle. QRS durations $\geq$0.12 s represent left or right bundle branch block or severe degrees of diffuse intraventricular conduction delay (see below).

Abnormal initial Q waves or an abnormal initial R in V_1 usually represents (1) a loss of muscle mass; (2) abnormal sequence of depolarization; or (3) a change in the relative muscle mass in the two ventricles.

The *intrinsicoid deflection* of the QRS complex is the major deflection *returning* to the base line in a left (for example, 2→3 in Fig. 249-8*D*) or a right (S wave→2, Fig. 249-8*E*) precordial lead. Its *onset* does not exceed 0.035 s from the *onset* of the QRS complex in V_1, or 0.055 s from the *onset* of the QRS in V_5 or V_6. Delayed onset of the intrinsicoid deflection may indicate hypertrophy or conduction abnormalities (see below and Fig. 249-8).

ABNORMALITIES OF VENTRICULAR REPOLARIZATION: ST SEGMENT, T WAVE, AND U WAVE In the normal ECG, the ST segment is "isoelectric," resting at the same potential as the interval between the T wave and the next P wave. Deviations of the ST segment from the base line may occur as a result of injury to cardiac muscle, changes in the synchronization of ventricular muscle depolarization, or drug or electrolyte influences. Elevations of the ST segment, in association with an elevation of the takeoff point of the ST segment from the QRS complex (the J point), may occur as a normal variant, especially in young individuals (Fig. 249-9*A*). The most common pathologic causes of ST-segment elevation are acute myocardial infarction and pericarditis (Fig. 249-9*B* to *F*), and the normal variant must be differentiated from these. Horizontal depression or a downsloping ST segment merging into the T wave occurs as a result of ischemia, ventricular strain, changes in the pattern of ventricular depolarization, or drug effects (Fig. 249-9*H, I, M, N, Q,* and *R*).

Since the sequence of ventricular muscle *de*polarization is from endocardium to epicardium, and *re*polarization represents an electrical current opposite in direction to depolarization, the T wave would be in the opposite direction to the QRS complex if the sequence of repolarization were in the same direction as depolarization. However, T waves generally assume the same direction as the major deflection of the QRS complex (see Fig. 249-6). It is assumed, therefore, that the direction of normal repolarization is opposite to the wave of depolarization—from epicardium to endocardium. T waves are generally considered abnormal when they are of low voltage, flat, or inverted in leads in which they are normally upright, or when they are abnormally tall and peaked. T-wave inversions are reflected vectorially by a widening of the angle between the QRS vector and the T vector (Fig. 249-6). Common causes of abnormalities of the T waves include ischemic heart disease, ventricular hypertrophy and strain, primary muscle disease, abnormal sequences of depolarization, electrolyte abnormalities, and drug influences (see Fig. 249-9*C, D, F, I, K, L,* and *N* to *R*). However, T-wave changes are often not specific.

The U wave is usually positive in leads in which the QRS complex is positive. The abnormal U wave is manifested as either an exaggeration of normal U-wave voltage, the appearance of a U wave in leads in which it is not normally seen, or inversion of a U wave. U-wave abnormalities occur in ischemic heart disease, left ventricular strain, and electrolyte disturbances. Unfortunately, the information they provide is usually nonspecific.

ECG MANIFESTATIONS OF VENTRICULAR HYPERTROPHY The normal dominance of the left ventricle on the features of the QRS complex is decreased or reversed in right ventricular hypertrophy (RVH) and exaggerated in left ventricular hypertrophy (LVH) (Fig. 249-10). RVH causes a shift of the net forces of depolarization from the left and posterior toward the right and anteriorly. On the ECG, this produces tall R waves in V_1 ($\geq$0.5 mV), with an abnormal S wave in V_5 or V_6 ($\geq$0.7 mV). In the frontal plane, the mean QRS axis shifts to the right of vertical (usually $>$110°). Less extreme degrees of RVH may result in preservation of a moderately deep S wave in V_1, with an R-wave voltage exceeding the S-wave voltage, or a normal R wave with a shallow S wave and prominent terminal S waves

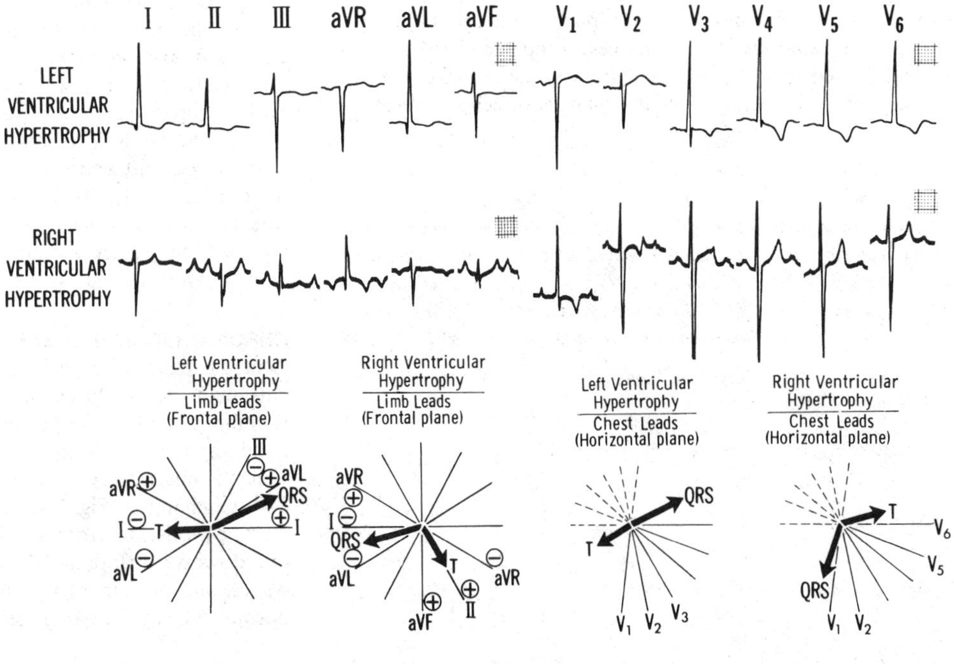

FIGURE 249-10
Ventricular hypertrophy. Left ventricular hypertrophy and strain with R wave $>$2.0 mV in limb leads; R $>$2.5 mV in V_5 and V_6, and S in V_1 $>$2.5 mV. The sum of S-V_1 or S-V_2 and R-V_5 or R-V_6 exceeds 3.5 mV. Strain is indicated by the downsloping ST segments and asymmetrically inverted T waves, especially in the lateral chest leads. The QRS-T vector angle is abnormally wide. Right ventricular hypertrophy is indicated by right axis deviation in the frontal plane and abnormal anterior forces in the horizontal plane. The former is indicated by a small R and deep S wave in lead I, and the latter by tall R waves in V_1 and V_2 with deep S waves in V_5 and V_6. The QRS-T angle is wide (strain).

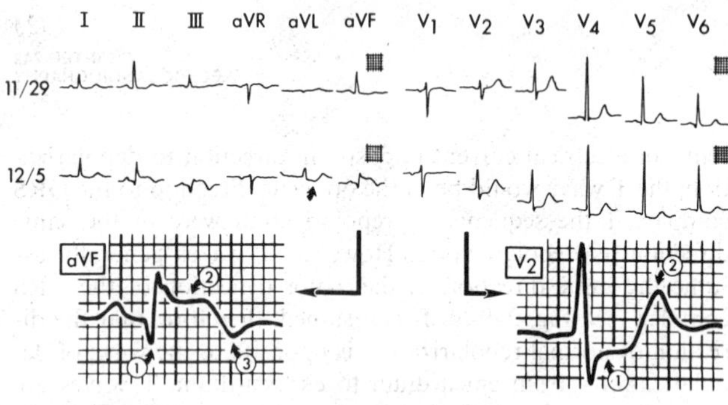

FIGURE 249-11

Acute inferior wall myocardial infarction. The ECG of 11/29 shows minor nonspecific ST-segment and T-wave changes. On 12/5 an acute myocardial infarction occurred. There are pathologic Q waves (1), ST-segment elevation (2), and terminal T-wave inversion (3) in leads II, III, and aVF indicating the location of the infarct on the inferior wall (see text). Reciprocal changes in aVL (small arrow). Increasing R-wave voltage with ST depression and increased voltage of the T wave in V_2 is characteristic of true posterior wall extension of the inferior infarction.

in V_5 and V_6. The primary QRS manifestation of LVH is an increase in voltage in those leads which reflect the electrical activity of the left ventricle. R waves in the standard limb leads may increase beyond the normal limit of 2.0 mV. Concomitantly, there is a tendency for a shift of the frontal plane QRS axis to the left. It is not likely that LVH alone will cause a shift in the QRS axis beyond $-30°$, but it commonly causes a shift in the range of 0 to $-30°$ (Fig. 249-10). LVH causes a deep S wave in lead V_1 or V_2 (>2.5 mV) or an abnormal R wave in lead V_5 or V_6 (>2.5 mV). When T waves are normal, the presence of voltage criteria for LVH must be interpreted in terms of body habitus of an individual. Young, healthy, thin-chested individuals will frequently exceed the QRS voltage criteria for LVH in its absence. However, when the ST-segment and T-wave changes associated with "strain" are present (Figs. 249-9*Q* and 249-10), the diagnosis of LVH is clarified. Similarly, borderline voltage criteria carry more significance when associated with the ST-segment and T-wave changes of left ventricular strain.

ACUTE MYOCARDIAL INFARCTION Three pathophysiologic events occur, either in sequence or simultaneously, in an acute myocardial infarction—ischemia, injury, and infarction. The ECG manifestations of these processes include changes in the T waves (ischemia), ST segments (injury), and QRS complexes (infarction). The earliest T-wave changes of acute myocardial ischemia are tall, peaked T waves ("hyperacute") (Fig. 249-9*C* and *D*), followed later by symmetrically inverted T waves (Fig. 249-9*F* and *K*). When the electrical integrity of the cell membranes is affected, currents of injury develop. The injury pattern on ECG during evolution of a transmural infarction is an elevation of the ST segments in the leads facing the infarcting area (Fig. 249-9*C* and *F*). The combination of ischemia and injury causes elevated ST segments, followed by either tall, peaked T waves (in the very early stages) or inverted T waves (Fig. 249-11). In leads opposite the region of the acute infarction, reciprocal changes occur: depressed ST segments and upright or isoelectric T waves (Figs. 249-11 and 249-12). As the period of active injury resolves, the ST segments return to the base line, but the inverted T waves may persist for months or years (Fig. 249-9*L*). Pathologic Q waves are the QRS manifestation of a transmural myocardial infarction. Q waves are pathologic when they appear in a lead in which Q waves were previously not present, or when the Q waves of normal septal depolarization become exaggerated (>20 ms; >0.2 mV).

FIGURE 249-12

Acute anterior wall myocardial infarction. On 4/11, changes of a very early acute myocardial infarction in leads I, aVL, V_2, and V_3, with reciprocal changes in II, III, and aVF. On 4/12, ST segments remain elevated in the anterior leads, but T waves are inverted. On 4/25, a completed large anterior myocardial infarction is recorded—Q in I, aVL, V_1 to V_4.

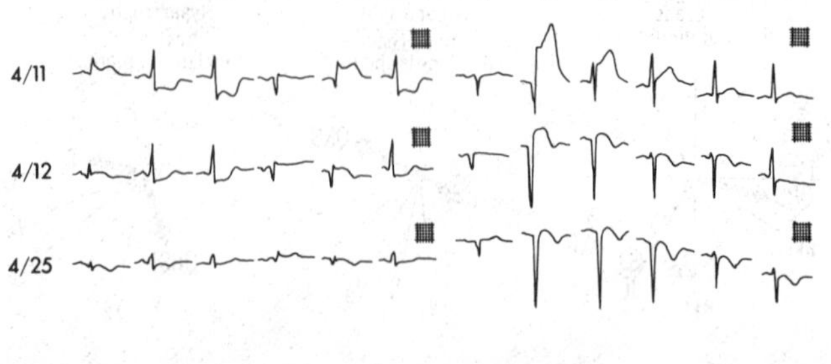

The ECG in an acute inferior wall myocardial infarction is shown in Fig. 249-11. Leads II, III, and aVF, which face the inferior surface of the left ventricle (see Fig. 249-1*D*), demonstrate the direct patterns of infarction (pathologic Q waves), injury (elevated ST segments), and ischemia (inversion of the T waves). Reciprocal changes (depressed ST, tall T) are demonstrated in aVL. The evolution of an acute anterior myocardial infarction is demonstrated in Fig. 249-12. The most obvious direct changes occur in aVL, V_2, and V_3, and reciprocal changes in II, III, and aVF. In the tracing of 4/11, ST elevations (most prominent in aVL, V_2, and V_3) are accompanied by "hyperacute" peaked T waves in V_2 and V_3. On 4/12, deeper Q waves are present in aVL and V_1 to V_3, and T waves have inverted in aVL and V_2 to V_5. ST elevations persist but less prominently. On 4/25, the pattern of a healing infarction—pathologic Q waves and ischemic T waves—is present. Eventually, the T waves might become partially or completely normal, with persistence of the Q waves. An infarction of the true posterior wall of the left ventricle causes ECG changes opposite to those of an anterior infarction. Instead of Q waves, ST elevation, and T-wave inversion in the anterior precordial leads (V_1 and V_2), true posterior infarction is characterized by tall R waves, ST depression, and upright T waves in these leads. These infarctions usually occur in combination with inferior wall infarctions. Right ventricular myocardial infarction may occur infrequently and is almost always associated with inferior and/or posterior infarction of the left ventricle. It has no specific ECG pattern.

A nontransmural (subendocardial or subepicardial) myocardial infarction may cause persistent ST-segment and T-wave changes similar to those seen in transmural infarctions. However, pathologic Q waves do not appear on the QRS complex, although R-wave and/or S-wave voltages may change. The ST-segment depressions and T-wave inversions are common in leads I, II, III, aVL, aVF and/or V_4 to V_6. Similar, but transient, changes may occur during the pain of angina pectoris, in shock, after pulmonary embolism, and secondary to acute central nervous system lesions.

CHRONIC ISCHEMIC HEART DISEASE The ECG in chronic ischemic heart disease is often nonspecific. The patterns of chronic myocardial ischemia are intrinsically variable, and this is compounded by the problem of coexistent ECG changes related to pharmacologic interventions and/or LVH. Chronic ischemic heart disease causes a broad range of ST-segment and T-wave changes (Fig. 249-9*G* to *I*, *K*, *L*, and *N* to *P*). There may be moderate degrees of horizontal ST-segment depression or a downward sloping ST segment, flattening of inversion of T waves, and prominent U waves. It is difficult to define an abnormal ST-segment depression in precise quantiative terms.

However, if the J point is more than 0.5 mm below the isoelectric line, the ST segment is horizontal or downsloping, and there is an associated T-wave abnormality, myocardial ischemia should be considered. The common clinical expression of chronic ischemic heart disease, angina pectoris, may be accompanied by a normal resting ECG or nonspecific ST-segment and T-wave changes. However, during spontaneous or exercise-induced pain, the ECG may demonstrate the horizontal or downward sloping ST-segment depressions shown in Fig. 249-9*H* and *I*, or rarely the variant pattern of spontaneous transient ST elevations (Prinzmetal variant) (Fig. 249-9*G*).

INTRAVENTRICULAR CONDUCTION DISTURBANCES The complex anatomy of the specialized conducting system of the ventricles, in conjunction with the focal nature of most cardiac diseases, is reflected in the multiplicity of ECG patterns which result from disorders of the sequence of activation of the ventricles. Disease of both the SCT and ventricular myocardium plays a role in the various patterns. The universal feature of ventricular conduction disturbances is a prolongation of the time required for depolarization of a portion of a ventricle, an entire ventricle, or both ventricles. Delayed or slow conduction may be diffuse or may be confined to a portion of the QRS complex (Fig. 249-8). Prolongation of the QRS may be modest as in left ventricular hypertrophy or extremely prolonged as in cardiomyopathies or metabolic abnormalities (Fig. 249-8).

The classic bundle branch block patterns are associated with specific lesions in the left or right bundle branch in the majority of cases. Complete right bundle branch block (RBBB) (Fig. 249-13) is characterized by prolongation of the QRS complex ($\geq$0.12 s) with the delayed activation of the right ventricle accounting for a terminal delay on the ECG. Since septal activation from the left bundle branch system normally precedes right ventricular activation, the initial forces of ventricular depolarization are not disturbed in RBBB, and the ability to identify coexistent pathologic Q waves is not hindered. The delayed activation of the right ventricle is reflected by the presence of terminal forces directed anteriorly and to the right.

The rightward direction of the slow terminal forces are indicated by the broad terminal S wave in leads I, aVL, and V_6 (Fig. 249-13). The anterior orientation of these forces is indicated by a large terminal R wave (R′) in V_1. Since initial forces are not disturbed, the normal initial R wave in V_1 persists, followed by an S wave. Incomplete RBBB is present when the

FIGURE 249-13

Intraventricular conduction abnormalities. Illustrated are right bundle branch block (RBBB); left bundle branch block (LBBB); left anterior hemiblock (LAH); right bundle branch block with left anterior hemiblock (RBBB + LAH); and right bundle branch block with left posterior hemiblock (RBBB + LPH) (see text).

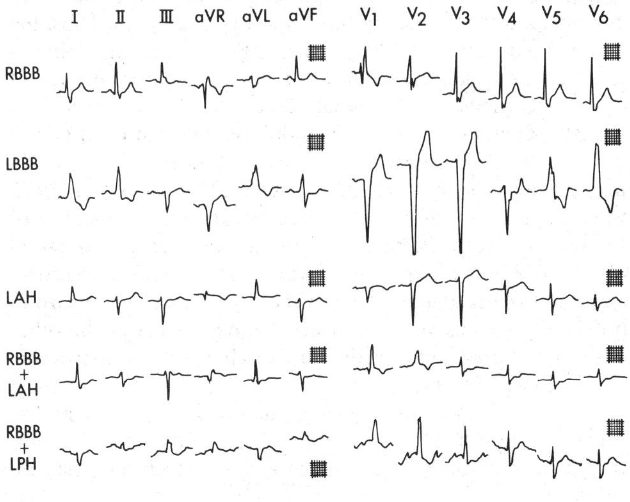

waveform criteria for RBBB (rSR′) are present, but the QRS duration is <0.12 s.

Left bundle branch block (LBBB) is also characterized by a QRS duration $\geq$0.12 s. However, since normal initial ventricular depolarization is dependent upon the LBB to deliver the impulses of initial depolarization to the left septum, the patterns produced by LBBB are more complex. Normal septal depolarization is disturbed, and delay of the normally dominant left ventricular forces produces a more generalized disturbance of QRS morphology. The septal Q wave in standard leads I, aVL, and V_6 is typically lost. In addition, the initial anterior force reflected by the small R wave in lead V_1 may be lost because of a less anterior orientation of the initial forces. The delay in left ventricular activation produces the greatest degree of slowing in the mid and late portion of the QRS complex. This often results in notching at the peak of the upstroke in leads I and V_6 (see Figs. 249-8*D* and 249-14), with a late intrinsicoid deflection (>0.055 s) in V_5 and V_6. Most cases of LBBB produce secondary T-wave abnormalities as demonstrated in Fig. 249-14. Because of the changes in the initial forces, and the secondary ST-segment and T-wave changes, it is usually difficult to evaluate the QRS-complex, ST-segment, and T-wave changes of coexistent ischemic heart disease. When the intrinsicoid deflection is delayed in leads V_5 or V_6, but the QRS duration is <0.12 s, incomplete LBBB may be present. LBBB may be associated with either a normal QRS axis (Fig. 249-13) or left axis deviation.

In recent years a great deal of attention has been given to the ECG patterns referred to as the *left* hemiblocks. As the name implies, *left anterior hemiblock* (LAH) has been proposed to result from disease in the anterior radiation of fibers referred to as the anterior division of the LBB. *Left posterior hemiblock* (LPH) has been assumed to result from disease in the left posterior radiation. The complex nature of the LBB system has thus far defied a determination of whether focal proximal disease or diffuse distal disease in the distribution of these portions of the LBB is the mechanism responsible for the hemiblock patterns, although it is known that the pathologic process tends to be diffuse in those cases studied at autopsy.

LAH results in a moderate delay of activation of the superior portion of the left ventricular free wall, causing a modest prolongation of the QRS complex and shift of the front plane axis to the left. Initial septal depolarization is undisturbed (Fig. 249-13), and the QRS complex rarely exceeds 0.09 to 0.10 s. The differentiation between LAH and left ventricular hypertrophy (LVH) may occasionally be difficult. In general, LVH alone will not produce a left axis shift beyond $-30°$, and LAH will often produce left axis deviation $\geq -60°$. The key QRS features in left anterior hemiblock include small Q waves in leads I and aVL, with small initial R waves and deep S waves in leads II, III, and aVF.

LPH results in a moderate delay of activation of the posterior-inferior portion of the left ventricular free wall. Again, there is a modest prolongation of the QRS complex, but a shift of the frontal plane QRS axis to the *right*. Thus, the initial septal forces, though generally undisturbed, may be oriented more superiorly, producing small initial Q waves in leads II, III, and aVF. Since the specificity of the ECG manifestations of LPH is not very reliable, many clinicians will not make a diagnosis of isolated LPH without demonstrating a right axis shift on serial ECGs, plus definite exclusion of other causes of right axis shift. Of all the intraventricular conduction disturbances, isolated LPH is the most difficult to diagnose.

The hemiblocks frequently coexist with disease in the RBB system. The combination of RBB, plus LAH or LPH, is referred to as *bifascicular block*—the implication being that two fascicles of the trifascicular model of the intraventricular SCT are diseased. This probably represents a pathophysiologic oversimplification, but it is useful for clinical purposes. Since RBBB alone does not produce abnormal axis deviation either to the left or to the right, the coexistence of RBBB with abnormal left axis deviation (Fig. 249-13) is usually interpreted as LAH plus RBBB. Similarly, abnormal right axis deviation in association with RBBB is usually interpreted as the coexistence of LPH with RBBB, when the QRS criteria for LPH are met (Fig. 249-13). As is the case in isolated LPH, the diagnosis of LPH plus RBBB is difficult because a number of clinical settings may cause abnormal right axis deviation in conjunction with RBBB.

Trifascicular block describes abnormal conduction in all three divisions of the intraventricular SCT. The ECG diagnosis can be made only by inference, when a patient has bifascicular block and a prolonged PR interval. Confirmation can be achieved only with His bundle electrocardiography (Chap. 254).

PERICARDITIS, MYOCARDITIS, AND THE CARDIOMYOPATHIES Acute pericarditis causes elevation of the ST segments in many leads without the reciprocal changes seen in acute myocardial infarction (Fig. 249-14*A*). ST-segment elevation may occur in all leads except aVR and rarely involves V_1. After a period of days, the diffuse ST elevations return to the base line, and T-wave inversions may occur. Coexistent ST elevations and T-wave inversions do not occur as often as they do in myocardial infarction (compare Figs. 249-11 and 249-14*A*). T-wave abnormalities may persist for weeks or months after the acute episode of pericarditis. If the pericarditis is accompanied by significant degrees of pericardial effusion, electrical alternans may occur. On alternate beats, ECG voltage shifts in magnitude. There also may be low voltage of the QRS complexes and T waves in all leads. Finally, the T_a waves may be transiently depressed because of atrial involvement by the inflammatory process [see Fig. 249-9*B* (1)].

The ECG changes of myocarditis (Chap. 263 and Fig. 249-14*B*) are often difficult to differentiate from the late phase of pericarditis, in which symmetric T-wave inversions are present. However, myocarditis may occur in many other settings, and an appreciation of the range of the ECG changes is important. Almost all systemic infections may produce minor myocardial involvement. Measles, mumps, influenza, hepatitis, infectious

FIGURE 249-14

A. Acute pericarditis with ST-segment elevations in all leads except III, aVR, and V_1. B. Myocarditis: diffuse ST-segment and T-wave changes, with low-voltage T waves in the limb leads and primary T-wave changes in the chest leads. C. Cardiomyopathy: gross distortion of the QRS complex.

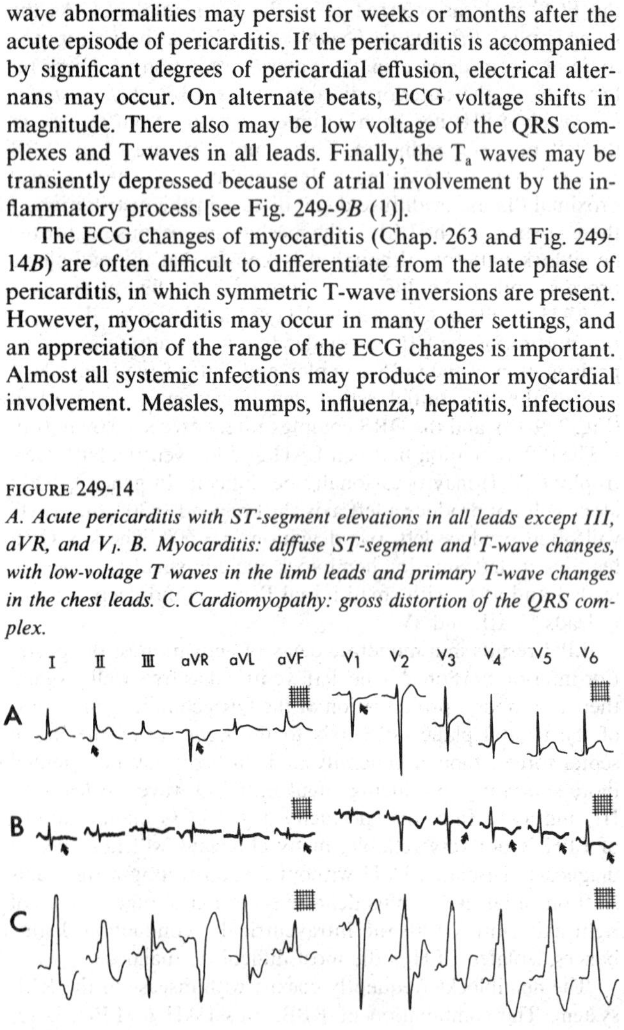

mononucleosis, and scarlet fever, just to name a few diseases, may be associated with ECG abnormalities and with histopathologic evidence of myocardial inflammation. When the myocardial involvement is subclinical, the ECG changes are usually subtle and nonspecific. There are minor T-wave changes, manifested as flattening or perhaps shallow inversion of the T waves in multiple leads (Fig. 249-9*O* and *P*). The conducting system may be involved, and prolongation of the PR interval may be noted.

In clinically evident myocarditis, the ECG demonstrates symmetrically inverted T waves in most of the standard limb leads and in the lateral precordial leads (Fig. 249-14*B*). When the specialized conducting system is involved, bundle branch block or patterns of nonspecific intraventricular conduction defects may occur.

The ECG may be helpful in distinguishing types of cardiomyopathies (Chap. 263). In the hypertrophic cardiomyopathies, the most common ECG pattern is LVH and strain (Fig. 249-10). When asymmetric septal hypertrophy is present, abnormal septal depolarization may be indicated by the presence of deep abnormal Q waves in leads I, aVL, V_5, and/or V_6, and a tall initial R wave in V_1. In the congestive cardiomyopathies, nonspecific intraventricular conduction abnormalities, indicated by broad, notched QRS complexes without a specific bundle branch block pattern, are common (Fig. 249-14*C*). Nonspecific ST-segment and T-wave abnormalities are almost universal in congestive cardiomyopathies. In the restrictive cardiomyopathies, intraventricular conduction defects, low-voltage QRS complexes, or loss of R-wave progression across the precordium may occur.

ECG ABNORMALITIES IN METABOLIC AND ELECTROLYTE DISTURBANCES The electrically active tissues of the heart are particularly sensitive to changes in the extracellular concentration of K^+, and dramatic ECG changes may accompany abrupt changes in K^+. The initial effect of acute *hyper*kalemia is the appearance of tall, peaked T waves (Figs. 249-15 and 43-1). As the severity of hyperkalemia increases, the QRS complex widens and blends into the tall, peaked T waves, P-wave voltage decreases and may disappear entirely, and the PR interval is prolonged. As these changes evolve, there is marked prolongation of the QRS complex (Fig. 249-15) with the evolution of continuity between the S wave and T wave, ultimately producing a sine wave configuration. This pattern is a very late and ominous manifestation of hyperkalemia. Equally dangerous is the occurrence of severe *hypo*kalemia, which also produces characteristic ECG changes. Instead of the tall, peaked T waves of hyperkalemia, hypokalemia produces a flattening or inversion of the T wave, with concomitant prominence of the U wave. In its fully developed state, the ECG gives the appearance of a very long QT interval. Careful analysis reveals that the QT interval is not so prolonged, and the U wave has assumed the appearance of the T wave (Fig. 249-15). Thus, the major prolongation is a "QU" prolongation. This ECG manifestation of hypokalemia may forewarn of the occurrence of serious ventricular arrhythmias, especially in the presence of digitalis. One must be careful to differentiate the ECG effects of hypo*calcemia* from hypo*kalemia.* Whereas hypokalemia may produce the appearance of a long ST segment and late T wave because of flattening of the T wave and prominence of the U wave, hypocalcemia does, in fact, produce prolongation of the ST segment with a late T wave (Fig. 249-15). Hypocalcemia is not as immediately ominous as hypokalemia in regard to potentially serious ventricular arrhythmias. Most of the other electrolyte imbalances produce ECG changes too nonspecific to be clinically useful.

Abnormalities of metabolism, such as hyper- or hypothyroidism, Addison's disease, diabetic ketoacidosis, and the infiltrative diseases such as amyloidosis and hemachromatosis, all may produce ECG abnormalities which may be helpful in the recognition of the disease process but are often nonspecific.

VECTORCARDIOGRAPHY

A vectorcardiogram (VCG) is a continuous loop representing the sequence of instantaneous electrical vectors in a two-dimensional plane (shown diagrammatically in Fig. 249-5*G*). This form of recording, requiring simultaneous voltage information from two leads, is achieved by recording one ECG lead on the vertical axis and replacing time by a second lead on the horizontal axis. The resulting loop is photographed on an oscilloscope screen. Most VCG systems today employ an XYZ lead system in which X is analogous to lead I (left-right), Y is analogous to lead aVF (superoinferior), and Z represents a lead in the anteroposterior orientation, most closely analogous to lead V_2. The XY plane records a vectorial loop in the frontal plane, projected on the hexaxial reference in Fig. 249-1*D*. The XZ plane records the horizontal loop in which the left-right orientation is plotted against the anteroposterior orientation on a reference system similar to that in Fig. 249-2*B*. In the YZ plane, the loop is in the sagittal orientation—the anteroposterior orientation (Z) plotted against the superoinferior orientation (Y). Recording in three planes provides information of spatial vectors, as in Fig. 249-5*F*. The loops are interrupted every 1 to 2.5 ms with intentional distortion of the interrupted display points. The result is a loop consisting of comma-shaped dots, the orientation of the comma indicating the direction of rotation, and the frequency of interruption providing a measurement of time. Closely grouped dots indicate a slow change in the magnitude and direction of the vector, while widely spread dots indicate rapid changes. Vectorial information of P waves, QRS complexes, ST segments, and T waves may be obtained, but the most valuable information is that derived from the QRS complexes.

The greatest value of the VCG today lies in the analysis of Q waves of uncertain significance and of certain intraventricular conduction abnormalities. When normal septal Q waves are absent in lead I or V_6, and no other evidence of septal infarction is present, the VCG may demonstrate either that the normal Q loop in the horizontal plane is absent, indicating a septal infarction or scarring, or conversely that the Q loop in the horizontal plane is morphologically normal but oriented directly anteriorly, accounting for the absence of the initial rightward forces. Similarly, the VCG can be helpful in assessing confusing initial forces or poor R-wave progression in the anterior precordial leads. Small Q waves, QS complexes, or poor R-wave progression may indicate anterior myocardial infarction (see above) but may also occur as a normal variant, as a consequence of chronic lung disease, or due to improperly positioned electrodes. The initial forces of the horizontal loop of the vectorcardiogram may be helpful when the VCG is either definitely normal or definitely abnormal.

The VCG is particularly useful in identifying inferior wall myocardial infarctions. When the ECG is equivocal, the VCG may show the superior displacement of initial forces in the frontal plane and the clockwise rotation that is characteristic of inferior wall myocardial infarction. Furthermore, the difficulty in differentiating inferior wall infarctions from left anterior hemiblock on ECG, or recognizing their coexistence, may be aided by a VCG. In left anterior hemiblock, the initial forces are often normal, but there is superior displacement of the major portion of the frontal plane loop. However, the rotation is counterclockwise, in contrast to the clockwise rotation of inferior wall myocardial infarction. When the combination of inferior wall myocardial infarction and left anterior hemiblock is present, the infarction may be masked on the ECG; but the VCG may show the distinctly abnormal superiorly displaced initial forces of inferior wall myocardial infarction plus the counterclockwise rotation in the frontal plane, characteristic of left anterior hemiblock.

In most other settings, the usefulness of VCG is limited, since much of the information can be obtained from the standard ECG. However, it may be helpful in patients with complex disease processes in which infarction and conduction disturbances are suspected, with chest wall deformities and unusual electrocardiographic patterns, and ECG abnormalities in the absence of clinical suspicion of heart disease.

FIGURE 249-15

Electrolyte disturbances. Hyperkalemia *($K^+ = 6.8$) with tall, peaked T waves. Severe hyperkalemia ($K^+ = 9.1$) with (1) flattening of the P wave, and ↑PR interval (1→2), (2) marked widening of the QRS complex (2→3), and (3) merging of the S wave into the T wave.* Hypokalemia *produces flat or inverted T waves with prominent U waves, causing prolonged "QU" interval, while hypocalcemia produces true prolongation of the ST segment with marked QT prolongation.*

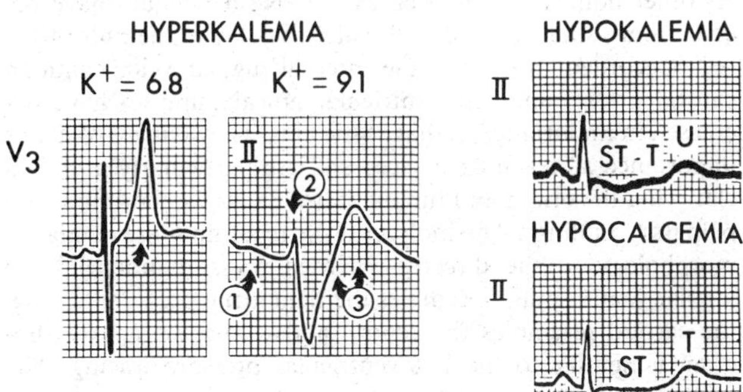

REFERENCES

Berne RM (ed): Electrophysiology of the heart, in *Handbook of Physiology,* sec 2: *The Cardiovascular System,* vol 1: *The Heart.* Washington, DC, American Physiological Society, 1979, pp 187–428

Castellanos A, Myerburg RJ: Electrocardiography, in *The Heart,* 5th ed, JW Hurst et al (eds). New York, McGraw-Hill, 1982

Cooksey JD et al: *Clinical Vectorcardiography and Electrocardiography,* 2d ed. Chicago, Year Book, 1977

Fisch C (ed): *Cardiovascular Clinics,* vol 5, no 3: *Complex Electrocardiography I.* Philadelphia, Davis, 1973

——— (ed): *Cardiovascular Clinics,* vol 6, no 1: *Complex Electrocardiography II.* Philadelphia, Davis, 1974

———: Electrocardiography and vectorcardiography, in *Heart Disease,* 2d ed, E Braunwald (ed). Philadelphia, Saunders, 1983, chap 7

Hoffman BF, Cranefield PF: *Electrophysiology of the Heart.* New York, McGraw-Hill, 1960

Horan L, Flowers NC: Electrocardiography and vectorcardiography, in *Heart Disease,* E Braunwald (ed). Philadelphia, Saunders, 1980, chap 7, pp 198–252

250
NONINVASIVE METHODS OF CARDIAC EXAMINATION

Roentgenography, phonocardiography, echocardiography, and radionuclide techniques

JOSHUA WYNNE
ROBERT A. O'ROURKE
EUGENE BRAUNWALD

ROENTGENOGRAPHY

The *chest roentgenogram* provides two principal forms of information: (1) pathoanatomic information regarding the size and configuration of the heart and great vessels, and (2) pathophysiologic information regarding pulmonary arterial and venous pressures and flow, derived from analysis of the pulmonary vascular pattern. Dilatation of a cardiac chamber is usually readily recognizable on the chest film by a change in cardiac size and contour. Concentric cardiac hypertrophy, on the other hand, often results in thickening of the ventricular wall at the expense of the chamber cavity, and usually produces only slight cardiac enlargement or alteration of the cardiac silhouette. Although standard 6-ft posteroanterior and lateral chest roentgenograms may provide adequate information, overpenetrated frontal, lateral, and oblique views obtained when the esophagus is filled with barium paste are essential for visualization of specific regions of the heart.

The standard chest roentgenogram may be supplemented by image-intensification fluoroscopy to detect areas of calcification within the cardiac valves, coronary arteries, pericardium, or myocardium. It is also useful to define further the size of the pulsations of the cardiac chambers and great vessels.

CARDIAC SILHOUETTE Enlargement of the *right atrium* may be noted on the posteroanterior (PA) and left anterior oblique (LAO) views by a bulging of the cardiac silhouette to the right, along with an increase in curvature of the right cardiac border. However, estimation of right atrial size from the chest film is the least reliable of all the cardiac chambers. The *right ventricle* is best seen in the lateral view, where its anterior wall lies directly behind the lower third of the sternum. The retrosternal space above the right ventricle is composed of lung and is radiolucent. As the right ventricle enlarges, it displaces this lung tissue, and the retrosternal space becomes filled in by the dilated right ventricle. Dilatation of the right ventricle may passively displace other cardiac chambers, particularly the adjacent left ventricle, and it is hazardous to assess left ventricular size when the right ventricle is enlarged.

While enlargement of the left atrial appendage may be suspected when a bulge is noted beneath the pulmonary artery segment in the PA film, dilatation of the body of the *left atrium* is best demonstrated by an indentation of the barium-filled esophagus in the lateral or right anterior oblique (RAO) view. As the left atrium dilates further, it may be seen behind the right atrium, forming a second border or "double density" adjacent to the right atrial wall. As the *left ventricle* enlarges, it moves downward, posteriorly and to the left. A variety of criteria for quantifying left ventricular size have been proposed, but the only widely used measurement is the cardiothoracic ratio, where the maximal diameter of the cardiac silhouette is divided by the maximal internal thoracic diameter. The normal ratio is less than 0.50. The plain chest roentgenogram remains a useful, relatively inexpensive noninvasive procedure, particularly as a screening or initial test, although echocardiography provides a much more precise and comprehensive assessment of the size of individual cardiac chambers.

PULMONARY VASCULATURE Because the size of the pulmonary vessels is proportional to the flow within them, a regional or global reduction of pulmonary blood flow results in a reduction of the caliber of the vessels, and the lung usually appears relatively radiolucent. A focal area of decreased flow in a part of one lung may be seen with a pulmonary embolus, although this is not a sensitive sign, while a diffusely oligemic pattern is characteristic of a right-to-left intracardiac shunt. Increased flow, as seen with left-to-right shunts, results in enlargement and tortuosity of the vessels.

With mild increases in pulmonary venous pressure, perivascular edema formation in the dependent portions of the lung leads to a reduction in flow at the lung bases and an increase in flow at the apex. This results in equalization of vascularity in the upper and lower lung fields. With further increases in venous pressure the lung bases become oligemic, and there is redistribution of flow to the upper-lobe vessels, resulting in their distention. Further increase in venous pressure results in visible accumulation of interstitial edema which collects in the dependent interlobular septa, producing short, horizontal linear shadows oriented perpendicular to the pleural surface (Kerley B lines). Peribronchial cuffing, along with perihilar and peripheral haze, are additional evidence of interstitial edema. A further rise in pulmonary venous pressure, particularly if it occurs rapidly, culminates in alveolar pulmonary edema (Chap. 26). Unfortunately, the chest films may demonstrate a considerable temporal lag behind the actual hemodynamic changes.

Pulmonary artery hypertension produces dilatation of the main pulmonary artery and its central branches. When associated with conditions marked by elevated pulmonary vascular resistance, such as primary pulmonary hypertension, the more peripheral arteries are small, resulting in tapering or "pruning" of the distal vessels with increased radiolucency of the peripheral lung fields.

SPECIALIZED RADIOGRAPHIC METHODS *Digital radiography* is a new technique which uses computer processing to digitize high-resolution fluoroscopic images. By computer comparison of images obtained before and after an intravenous injection of a relatively modest dose of a radiopaque contrast agent, a picture is obtained of vascular structures free of overlapping soft tissues and bony densities. It is particularly useful for assessing left ventricular size and function, although the applications and indications for this technique are yet to be defined completely.

Computed tomography utilizes a finely collimated x-ray beam and a circular array of detectors to obtain a cross-sectional image of excellent spatial resolution. It is possible to obtain images of high temporal resolution as well. Current uses include evaluation of myocardial infarction, aortic dissection, and the patency of coronary artery bypass grafts.

PHONOCARDIOGRAPHY AND SYSTOLIC TIME INTERVALS

As other noninvasive as well as invasive techniques have become more sophisticated and widely available, the pulse tracings (recorded from over the internal jugular vein, common carotid artery, and left ventricular apical impulse) have decreased in importance as diagnostic aids. They remain of major importance as teaching devices and are particularly useful in clarifying the origin and timing of heart sounds, murmurs, and palpatory findings. The indirect pulse recordings are similar in morphology to the directly recorded pressure tracings; the jugular venous pulse resembles the right atrial pressure tracing, the carotid resembles the central aortic, and the apexcardiogram is similar to the left ventricular pressure tracing. The

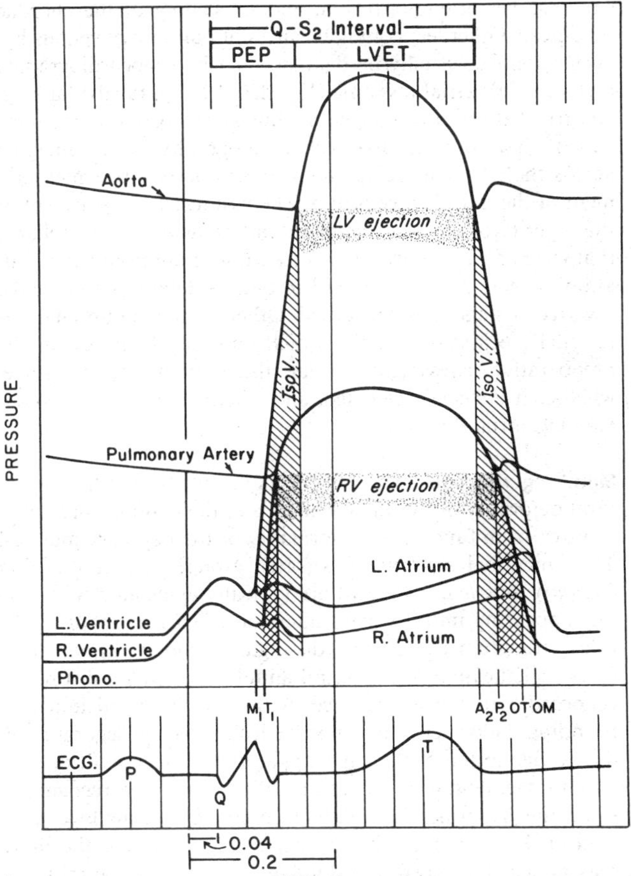

FIGURE 250-1
Diagrammatic representation of pressure tracings recorded within the left and right ventricles correlated with the ECG and the phonocardiogram (Phono). The striped areas labeled IsoV represent the isovolumetric phases of left ventricular contraction and relaxation; isovolumetric right ventricular contraction and relaxation are shown as cross-hatched areas. M_1 and T_1, sounds produced by closure of the mitral and tricuspid valves, respectively; A_2 and P_2, sounds produced by the closure of the aortic and pulmonic valves, respectively; OT and OM, sounds produced by opening of the tricuspid and mitral valves, respectively. The QS_2 interval includes the preejection period (PEP) and the left ventricular ejection time (LVET), the latter being measured noninvasively from the delayed indirect carotid pulse tracing (see text).

phonocardiogram provides a graphic display of heart sounds and murmurs, and through the use of filters permits the selective recording of low- and high-frequency sounds. Although it is useful for determining the configuration and frequency composition of individual cardiac murmurs, its most important application is in the precise timing of cardiac events.

The *carotid pulse morphology*, and the derived *systolic time intervals* (Fig. 250-1), are useful aids in the evaluation of left ventricular function and outflow tract obstruction (both in fixed obstruction, as with valvular aortic stenosis, and in dynamic obstruction, as with obstructive hypertrophic cardiomyopathy). The systolic time intervals consist of electromechanical systole (QS_2) measured from the onset of the QRS complex to the aortic component of S_2; the left ventricular ejection time (LVET), which begins with the upstroke of the carotid arterial pulse and ends with the dicrotic notch; and the preejection period (PEP), the difference between the duration of left ventricular mechanical systole and LVET (PEP = QS_2 − LVET). Systolic time intervals can be corrected for both heart rate and the patient's sex by using regression equations (see Appendix). The ratio of the PEP to the LVET (PEP/LVET) is particularly attractive because it need not be corrected for heart rate or sex (normal = 0.345 ± 0.036 SD). In the presence of left ventricular failure, the PEP lengthens (reflecting primarily a decrease in the rate of ventricular pressure generation) and the LVET diminishes (reflecting a reduced stroke volume), while the total duration of electromechanical systole is unchanged. There is a resultant increase in the PEP/LVET ratio. In fixed-orifice left ventricular outflow obstruction the carotid upstroke is slow, while in dynamic obstruction the flow is unimpeded early, and the upstroke is brisk. In both cases, the duration of ejection (left ventricular ejection time) is prolonged, and in the absence of concomitant heart failure, PEP/LVET is reduced.

ECHOCARDIOGRAPHY

Echocardiography utilizes short pulses of ultrasound in a frequency of approximately 2 to 5 MHz to image the heart and great vessels. The sound waves are generated by a piezoelectric crystal, which has the unique property of transforming electrical energy into mechanical (i.e., sound) energy, and vice versa. A transducer containing the crystal is placed on the chest wall, and it acts as both a transmitter and receiver of short pulses of ultrasound which reflect off surfaces of the heart and return to the crystal for detection. The traditional technique (called M-mode or time-motion echocardiography) transmits and receives ultrasound waves along a single line; the resulting image has been termed an "ice pick" view of the heart (Fig. 250-2). The orientation and position of the transducer must be changed by the operator to view different parts of the heart.

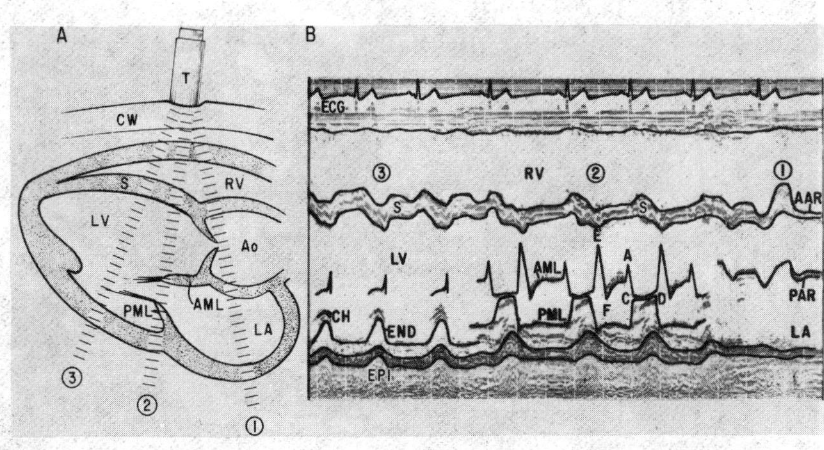

FIGURE 250-2
A schematic presentation of the cardiac structures traversed by three echo beams (A) is shown with a continuous echo "sweep" from a normal subject (B). T, transducer; CW, chest wall; RV, right ventricle; S, interventricular septum; Ao, aorta; LA, left atrium; and LV, left ventricle; AML, anterior mitral leaflet; PML, posterior mitral leaflet; AAR, anterior aortic root; PAR, posterior aortic root; CH, chordae tendineae; END, endocardium; and EPI, epicardium.

Newer echocardiographic machines provide a cross-sectional or two-dimensional view by steering the ultrasound beam through an arc of up to 90°, resulting in a tomographic image of high spatial resolution (Fig. 250-3). By obtaining many such images each second (typically 30 or more images per second), the motion of the heart can be viewed in real time. While two-dimensional echocardiography provides high *spatial* resolution, M-mode echocardiography (with a sampling rate of 1000 Hz) provides high *temporal* resolution; both forms of imaging are usually employed in clinical practice, although for most forms of heart disease, two-dimensional imaging provides a more complete appreciation than M-mode echocardiography of the degree of structural and functional abnormality present.

Doppler echocardiography is a technique for the evaluation of the velocity and turbulence of blood flow within the heart. When ultrasound waves strike moving red blood cells, a frequency change is produced which can be measured and analyzed. While this technique has been quite useful in identifying abnormal blood flow patterns as are produced by valvular regurgitation and cardiac shunts, it has not achieved universal reliability in quantitating flow.

VALVULAR HEART DISEASE (See also Chap. 258) The site of stenotic lesions, be they subvalvular, valvular, or supravalvular, can usually be easily resolved by echocardiography. The severity of valve disease is determined directly, by visualization of the involved valve and, indirectly, by assessing the secondary alterations produced by the valve disease (such as dilatation of the left atrium and ventricle with mitral regurgitation). Although exceptions occur, the presence of an apparently normal valve on two-dimensional echocardiography excludes hemodynamically significant pathology in most forms of valvular heart disease.

Mitral stenosis The echocardiographic appearance (Fig. 250-4*A*) is distinctive and virtually diagnostic, with thickening and restricted diastolic motion of the leaflets, fusion of the commissures, and shortening, fusion, and thickening of the chordae tendineae. Other less common causes of pulmonary venous hypertension can usually be distinguished by echocardiography, including left atrial myxoma (Fig. 250-4*B*), supravalvular ring, cor triatriatum, and congenital mitral stenosis ("parachute" valve). Two-dimensional echocardiography with imaging across the left ventricular minor axis permits direct measurement of the mitral valve orifice. The noninvasive assessment of the severity of *isolated* rheumatic mitral stenosis is so reliable that cardiac catheterization is often not required in the evaluation of these patients, at least insofar as determination of the severity of stenosis is concerned. Other associated findings detected by echocardiography which may be of interest in the preoperative assessment include the mobility of the valve, whether it is heavily calcified, and whether there is an associated left atrial thrombus.

Mitral regurgitation This lesion may result from either structural deformity of the valve leaflets and their supporting apparatus or from functional abnormality of the papillary muscles. The functional abnormalities (often grouped under the term *papillary muscle dysfunction*) are typically associated with normal-appearing mitral valve leaflets on echocardiography. The echocardiogram can usually distinguish among various etiologies; calcification of the mitral annulus presents a distinctive echocardiographic appearance, with a shelf of calcium surrounding the posterior mitral valve leaflet. Mitral regurgitation due to disruption of the valve apparatus (as seen with rupture of chordae tendineae or endocarditis) is easily recognized, since the hypermobile and flail components usually can be identified. In mitral valve prolapse (Fig. 250-4*C*), the valve may appear thickened or redundant on echocardiography due to myxomatous changes in the leaflets. Systolic bulging of one or both leaflets toward the left atrium is found; this abnormal leaflet motion is often associated with a midsystolic click and late systolic murmur on auscultation.

Aortic stenosis Determination of the site of left ventricular outflow tract obstruction is usually easily determined with two-

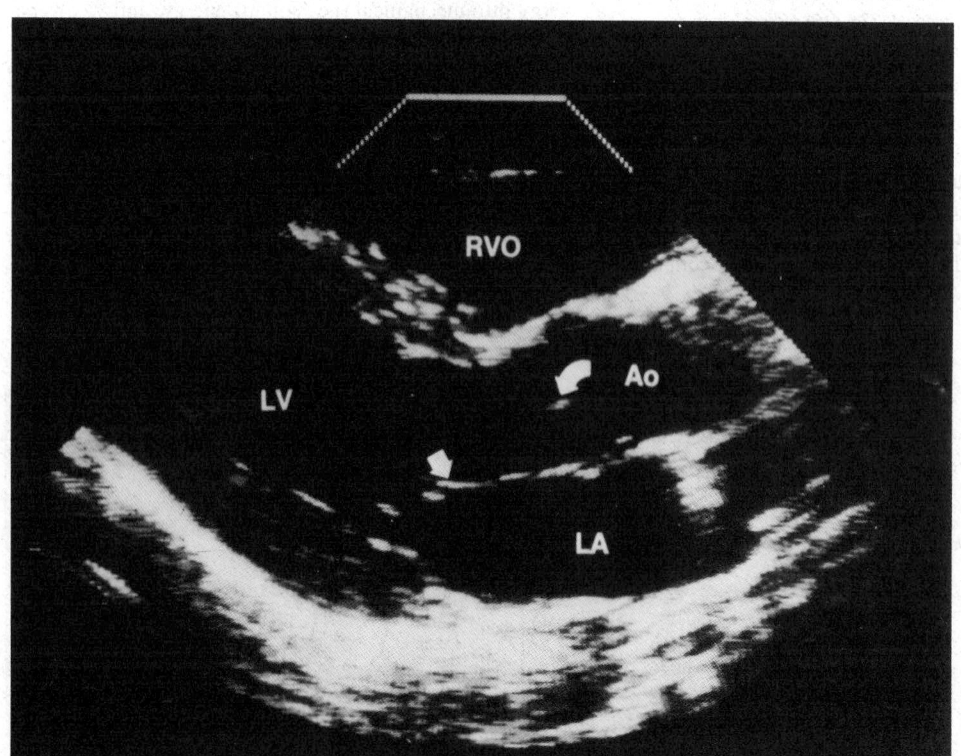

FIGURE 250-3
Two-dimensional echocardiographic scan through the long axis of the left ventricle. The curved arrow indicates the aortic valve, while the straight one points to the anterior mitral valve leaflet. (Ao = aortic root; LA = left atrium; LV = left ventricle; RVO = right ventricular outflow tract.) (Courtesy of Advanced Technology Laboratories, Inc., Bellevue, Wash.)

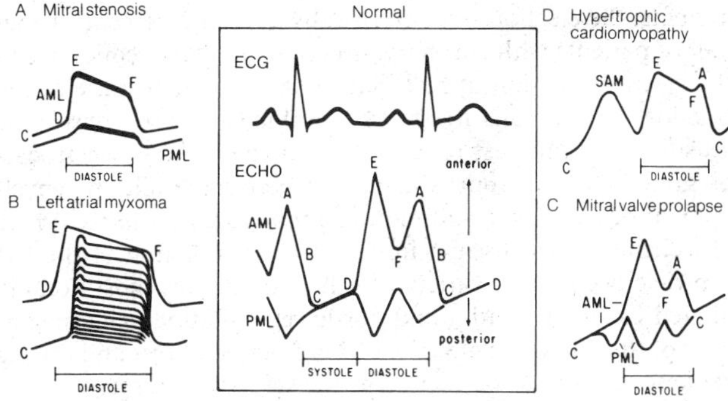

FIGURE 250-4
A schematic presentation of the normal echocardiographic (ECHO) recording of anterior (AML) and posterior mitral leaflet (PML) motion is shown in the center with the simultaneous ECG. Abnormal mitral echocardiograms which occur in (A) mitral stenosis, (B) left atrial myxoma, (C) mitral valve prolapse, and (D) obstructive hypertrophic cardiomyopathy are also depicted. In the ECHO, the A point represents the end of anterior movement resulting from left atrial contraction, the CD segment represents the closed position of both mitral leaflets during ventricular systole, and point E ends the anterior movement as the leaflet opens. The slope EF results from posterior motion of the AML during rapid ventricular filling. In obstructive hypertrophic cardiomyopathy SAM represents systolic anterior movement.

dimensional echocardiography. Dynamic subvalvular stenosis (obstructive hypertrophic cardiomyopathy) is readily recognized by the disproportionate thickening of the ventricular septum in relation to the left ventricular free wall, and the systolic anterior motion (SAM) of the anterior mitral leaflet (Fig. 250-4*D*). Valvular aortic stenosis in the adult, regardless of etiology, is usually associated with calcification of the valve, which is readily recognizable. M-mode echocardiography is of limited value in determining the *severity* of valvular stenosis, but severe obstruction can usually be recognized by the two-dimensional technique. Two-dimensional echocardiography also permits the determination of the severity, location, and type of supravalvular aortic stenosis.

Aortic regurgitation The echocardiogram is helpful in distinguishing between the two principal causes of aortic regurgitation in the adult, i.e., disease of the aortic cusps, and enlargement of the aortic root (due to hypertension, aortic aneurysm, or anuloaortic ectasia) without direct involvement of the cusps themselves. Aortic regurgitation usually results in high-frequency diastolic vibrations of the anterior leaflet of the mitral valve or interventricular septum. Acute, severe aortic regurgitation (usually due to endocarditis) may result in premature closure of the mitral valve as a result of marked elevation of the left ventricular diastolic pressure. While the severity of chronic aortic regurgitation cannot be determined directly, associated echocardiographic findings, such as left ventricular size and function, are moderately useful in providing an estimate.

Vegetations (see also Chap. 259) The vegetations of infective endocarditis are demonstrated by echocardiography in approximately 50 percent of patients with infective endocarditis, and a normal echocardiogram therefore does not exclude endocarditis. Patients with demonstrable vegetations are at higher risk of complication and death than those without vegetations, and more often require cardiac surgery with valve replacement. However, cardiac surgery is not usually required unless there is associated congestive heart failure, uncontrolled sepsis, or embolization. Vegetations may persist on the echocardiogram despite apparent bacteriologic cure and do not indicate treatment failure.

Left ventricle The echocardiogram has been widely used to measure left ventricular size, wall thickness, and function. The degree of fractional shortening of the minor axis of the left ventricle, normally greater than 28 percent, is one useful measure of left ventricular systolic performance. Since the M-mode technique is able to visualize only selected portions of the ventricle, the tracings obtained may not be representative of the function of the entire ventricle. Particularly when regional wall motion abnormalities are present, as with coronary artery disease, M-mode echocardiograms may be misleading as to global left ventricular function, and the two-dimensional technique is required.

Two-dimensional echocardiography has been particularly useful in identifying left ventricular aneurysms, and the mural thrombi which are often associated with them. Increased left ventricular wall thickness is usually due to myocardial hypertrophy, but on occasion myocardial infiltration may present a similar picture. Amyloidosis may be suspected when the thickened myocardium has a distinctive "speckled" appearance. (The echocardiographic findings in dilated, restrictive, and hypertrophic cardiomyopathy are outlined in Table 263-3.)

Pericardial effusion (see also Chap. 265) Echocardiography is the procedure of choice for evaluating pericardial effusions; effusions as small as 15 to 20 ml may be detected. While specific echocardiographic features (such as small chamber size, phasic variation in right and left ventricular dimensions, and gross cardiac oscillation) may suggest tamponade, a conclusion regarding the significance of the fluid is based on clinical and hemodynamic observations.

Congenital heart disease Two-dimensional echocardiography has been of major benefit in the evaluation of congenital cardiac lesions (Chap. 256), since the relationship of atria, ventricles, and great vessels to one another can easily be assessed by the wide field of view. In adults, the most common congenital abnormality (other than valve lesions) is an atrial septal defect (ASD). Perhaps the most sensitive indicator of a hemodynamically significant ASD is right ventricular enlargement, which is easily detectable on M-mode or two-dimensional echocardiography. Further evaluation of a shunt at the atrial level may be aided by the use of contrast echocardiography.

RADIONUCLIDE IMAGING OF THE HEART

There are four principal clinical nuclear medicine procedures in current use: (1) assessment of ventricular function by means of radionuclide ventriculography (Fig. 250-5*A*); (2) identification and quantification of intracardiac shunts by means of radioangiocardiography; (3) study of acute myocardial infarction by means of infarct-avid radionuclides (Fig. 250-5*B*); and (4) assessment of myocardial perfusion by means of ionic tracers, principally thallium 201 (Fig. 250-5*C*).

VENTRICULAR PERFORMANCE Radionuclide ventriculography (RVG) is similar to contrast ventriculography in that an intravascular indicator (in this case radioactive) is used to delineate the chambers of the heart and great vessels. The radionuclide, usually technetium 99m, is often attached to red blood cells to ensure that it remains intravascular. Two principal methods of performing RVGs are used. The *first-pass method* involves the bolus intravenous injection of the radiotracer, and its initial transit through the right heart chambers, lungs, and left heart chambers is recorded by a computer. Upon reaching the systemic circulation, the bolus soon becomes diluted, and its utility for cardiac imaging is lost. In the *equilibrium or gated method* (Fig. 250-5*A*), changes in counts within the ventricle which occur during many (often 400) cardiac cycles are measured and averaged, and changes in volume are inferred because of the proportional relationship between counts and volume. The scintigraphic information in each cardiac cycle is divided by computer into multiple frames (often 30 or more segments of the cardiac cycle) using the QRS complex of the electrocardiogram as a timing reference; this technique is termed *gating.* Since multiple frames are acquired throughout the cardiac cycle, rather than merely at end diastole and end systole, this method has been termed *multiple gated acquisition.* Both right and left ventricular ejection fractions may be calculated, as well as ventricular volumes, and ejection and filling rates. Agreement with standard catheterization methods has been excellent. RVG avoids catheterization, is largely noninvasive, is repeatable, does not alter ventricular performance, and, since analysis is based on changes in counts, is largely independent of ventricular geometry.

RVG DIAGNOSIS OF CORONARY ARTERY DISEASE Assessment of ventricular function is typically performed prior to and during bicycle ergometry. The normal response in patients under 65 years of age is an ejection fraction at least 50 percent at rest with an increase of at least 5 percent (ejection fraction percentage units) without the development of a regional wall motion abnormality; in older (> 65 years), otherwise normal, patients, the ejection fraction rises by at least 2 percent. About half of patients with coronary artery disease have reductions of the ejection fraction at rest, but in about 85 percent, ejection fraction falls or fails to increase normally with exercise. The sensitivity of this test exceeds that of the exercise electrocardiogram, which is approximately 75 percent. While the development of a *regional* wall motion abnormality is characteristic of ischemic heart disease, impaired *global* function of the left ventricle occurs in a variety of other conditions, most notably dilated cardiomyopathy and aortic regurgitation. The magnitude of the fall in the global ejection fraction at rest and during exercise appears to be related to the severity of disease.

Since symptoms of congestive heart failure may be due to a variety of cardiac as well as noncardiac causes, assessment of biventricular function may provide important diagnostic information. It is useful, for example, in the differential diagnosis of dyspnea (Chap. 26), which may be due to pulmonary congestion caused by a damaged left ventricle (decreased left ventricular ejection fraction, normal right ventricular ejection fraction), pulmonary disease (normal left ventricular ejection fraction, normal or depressed right ventricular ejection fraction), or increased stiffness of the left ventricle due to myocardial hypertrophy (normal ejection fraction of both ventricles).

The left ventricular ejection fraction is more depressed in patients with anterior than with inferior infarcts. On the other hand, right ventricular dysfunction, presumably due to infarction, occurs almost exclusively in patients with inferior infarction. In patients in cardiogenic shock, the RVG readily distinguishes between patients with extensive left ventricular

FIGURE 250-5
Examples of the use of three different scintigraphic techniques in patients with ischemic heart disease. Actual scintigrams at top and explanatory diagrams below. (A). A gated blood pool scan in a postinfarction patient with septal and inferior wall akinesis (↑). ED = end-diastolic image and ES = end-systolic image. The posterior wall (far right) moves normally from ED to ES. (B). A technetium pyrophosphate (TcPYP) scan shows a localized region of heavy uptake (↑) in a patient with a recent inferior wall myocardial infarction. R = ribs and S = sternum. (C). Thallium 201 scan immediately after exercise in the left anterior oblique (LAO) view shows an inferior wall perfusion defect (↑). RV = right ventricle and LV = left ventricle. (Courtesy of S Sorenson.)

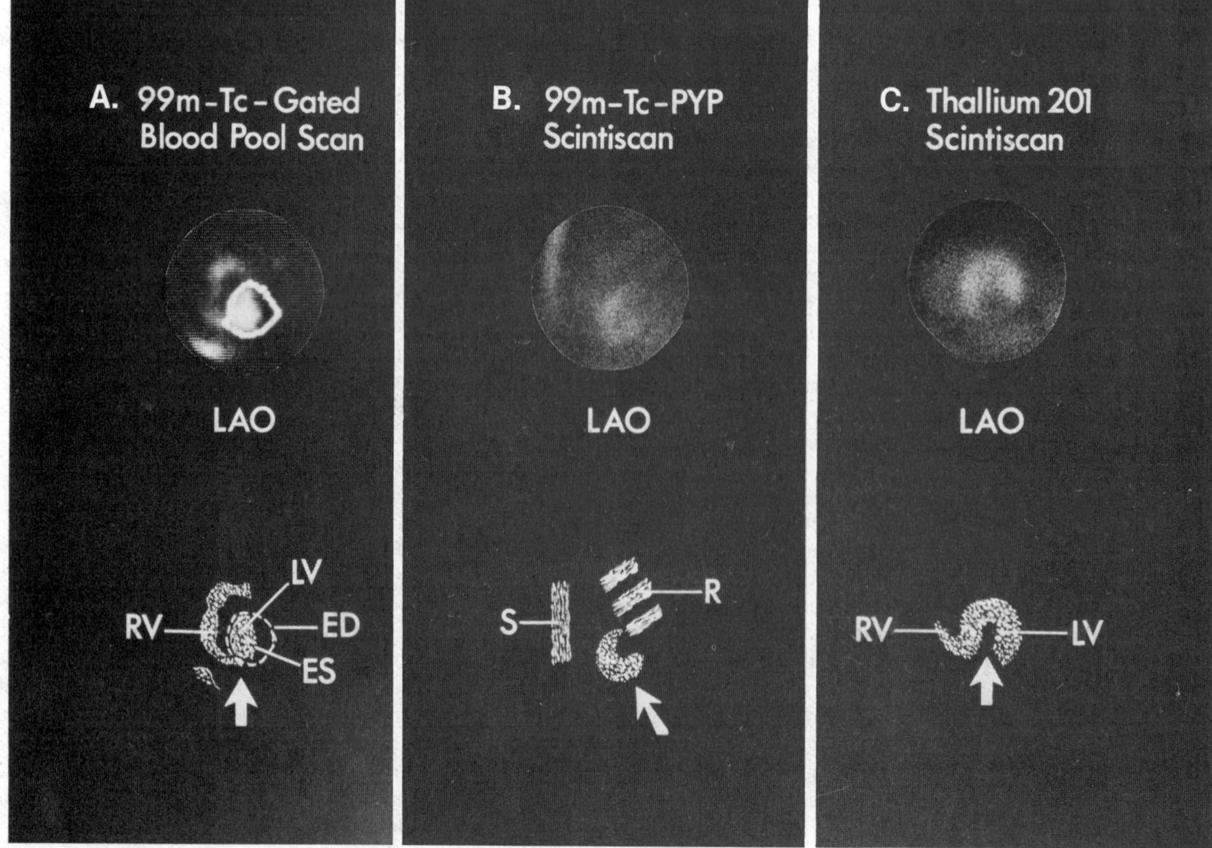

damage and those with predominant right ventricular infarction; therapy is importantly affected by this differentiation. Prognosis after recovery from infarction is closely related to ventricular performance at rest and particularly during exercise. By demonstrating disorders of regional wall motion, the RVG can also distinguish between a discrete left ventricular aneurysm and diffuse myocardial damage.

The RVG is particularly well suited for assessing changes in ventricular function produced by a wide variety of pharmacologic agents, including vasodilators, positive inotropic agents, and cardiac depressants such as doxorubicin and disopyramide.

SHUNT SCINTIGRAPHY Evaluation of left-to-right shunts utilizes a modification of the first-pass RVG, in which a bolus of radiotracer is injected intravenously and its passage through the heart and great vessels is recorded by a gamma camera/computer system. By focusing on a "region of interest" over the lung, a pulmonary time-activity curve is generated. As the bolus passes through the lungs, the normal pulmonary time-activity curve demonstrates a sharp peak, a smooth descent, and a later bump due to recirculation of the radiotracer through the lungs after it has completed its normal circulation through the systemic circuit. In a left-to-right shunt, there is an interruption of the descending limb and/or an early recirculation wave. Computer analysis of the curves permits determination of the ratio of pulmonary to systemic flow and therefore of the size of the left-to-right shunt. Agreement with cardiac catheterization has been excellent. While massive valvular regurgitation or bidirectional shunting may invalidate the results, a normal scan virtually excludes a significant left-to-right shunt.

ACUTE INFARCT SCINTIGRAPHY (See also Chap. 261) Pyrophosphate appears to bind to calcium deposits as well as to organic macromolecules in necrotic myocardium. Technetium m 99m stannous pyrophosphate (^{99m}Tc-PYP), a bone-imaging agent, is concentrated by acutely necrotic, but not by normal, myocardium and yields a scintigraphic image of a "hot spot" of radioactivity (Fig. 250-5*B*). Maximal uptake of ^{99m}Tc-PYP occurs in regions with 30 to 40 percent of normal myocardial blood flow, between 2 and 4 days after infarction. About 90 percent of patients with transmural infarcts have positive scans, while only about 60 percent of scans in nontransmural infarcts will be abnormal. Small infarcts are often not imaged, but a negative scan excludes a large transmural infarct. Scans are usually positive 2 to 5 days postinfarction and then become negative, although persistently positive scans are not uncommon, particularly with formation of a left ventricular aneurysm. Abnormal ^{99m}Tc-PYP scans, especially when there is diffuse uptake in the region of the heart, may be seen in a variety of conditions besides myocardial infarction, including unstable angina pectoris, left ventricular aneurysm, and some forms of cardiomyopathy.

Acute infarct scintigraphy is usually not necessary for an otherwise uncomplicated myocardial infarction. Specific situations where ^{99m}Tc-PYP may be of particular utility include (1) diagnosis of myocardial infarction after cardiac surgery, (2) suspected infarction in patients with left bundle branch block, (3) patients with atypical chest pain and equivocal enzymatic or electrocardiographic changes, and (4) suspected myocardial contusion.

MYOCARDIAL PERFUSION IMAGING (See also Chap. 260) A variety of radioactive monovalent cations have been used as indicators of normally perfused myocardium. Currently, the most widely used ionic tracer is *thallium 201* (half-life 72 h), a potassium congener which is concentrated by viable myocardium. The initial distribution of thallium 201 in the myocardium following an intravenous injection is proportional to the regional myocardial blood flow. Myocardial regions containing acutely infarcted tissue, ischemic tissue, or scar all show a relative decrease in thallium 201 uptake, demonstrating a "cold spot" of decreased radioactivity compared with the normal uptake of tracer by the uninvolved myocardium (Fig. 250-5*C*).

Thallium 201 is typically injected during exercise, and imaging performed immediately thereafter. Imaging is then repeated several hours later and the images are compared. Segments initially demonstrating diminished thallium 201 uptake due to exercise-induced ischemia will concentrate the tracer over the next several hours, at the same time that there is efflux of the tracer from normal regions; there will be a resultant filling in of the initial cold spot, a process termed *redistribution.* In contrast, necrotic myocardium, whether it is due to an acute infarct or chronic scar, is unable to concentrate thallium 201 at any time, so the initial defect will remain unchanged or "fixed."

Thallium 201 imaging at rest and during exercise is more accurate than exercise electrocardiography in the diagnosis of coronary artery disease, particularly in patients unable to achieve an adequate heart rate response during the stress test. Sensitivity and specificity for the detection of coronary artery disease have been reported to be in the 80 and 90 percent range, respectively. Unfortunately, thallium 201 scintigraphy has limitations in predicting the location of coronary artery stenoses and in identifying patients with left main coronary artery stenosis. Thallium 201 imaging at rest may be useful in patients with acute myocardial infarction. While almost all patients imaged soon after an infarction demonstrate defects in the thallium 201 image, only about three-quarters of patients have abnormalities if studied after the first day, presumably because blood is able to perfuse the necrotic zone through the development of collateral vessels. The size of the thallium 201 defect appears to correlate with subsequent prognosis. Patients with unstable angina pectoris and coronary artery spasm demonstrate transient resting thallium 201 cold spots in the absence of infarction.

REFERENCES

BERGER HJ, ZARET BL: Nuclear cardiology. N Engl J Med 305:799 and 305:855, 1981

COHN PF, WYNNE J (eds): *Diagnostic Methods in Clinical Cardiology.* Boston, Little, Brown, 1982

FEIGENBAUM H: *Echocardiography,* 3d ed. Philadelphia, Lea & Febiger, 1981

LUISADA AA, PORTALUPPI F: *The Heart Sounds: New Facts and Their Clinical Implications.* New York, Praeger, 1982

MASON DT et al: *Principles of Noninvasive Cardiac Imaging: Echocardiography and Nuclear Cardiology.* New York, Le Jacq, 1980

POPP RL et al: Echocardiography: M-mode and two-dimensional methods. Ann Intern Med 93:844, 1980

251
CARDIAC CATHETERIZATION AND ANGIOGRAPHY

JOHN ROSS, JR.
KIRK L. PETERSON

The application of techniques for catheterizing both the left and right sides of the heart, and for selective injection of contrast media into the coronary arteries and cardiac chambers during the exposure of high-speed x-ray motion pictures (cineangiography), provides precise information about the dynamic physiology and anatomy of the heart in the normal state and a variety of cardiac disorders (Table 251-1). By permitting accurate anatomic and functional diagnoses of complex cardiac lesions, these procedures have placed the selection of patients for surgical treatment of heart disease on a firm, objective basis.

INDICATIONS

There are several types of problems for which hemodynamic or angiographic investigations commonly are performed, although other specific indications and contraindications may exist in the individual patient. These broad areas may be summarized as follows:

1 In patients with acquired valvular heart disease, hemodynamic assessment and angiographic studies often are required to determine whether the nature and severity of a mechanical valvular defect render it amenable to surgical treatment. In particular, cardiac catheterization studies are indicated when both the mitral and aortic valves are involved, or when associated tricuspid valve disease is suspected to be of significance, and to search for associated coronary artery disease.
2 In patients with congenital heart disease, hemodynamic studies and angiography usually are necessary to characterize the primary defect and to determine whether associated lesions are present.
3 In patients with chest pain of undetermined cause, angiographic visualization of the coronary arteries may be indicated to determine the presence or absence of atherosclerotic coronary disease or coronary artery spasm. In patients with known coronary heart disease such studies may provide information that is useful prognostically and helpful in determining whether operative treatment is feasible.
4 In patients who have undergone cardiac operations, cardiac catheterization studies may be indicated to evaluate the success of the operation, particularly when residual symptoms are present. Such studies may reveal malfunction of a prosthetic valve, loss of patency of a coronary artery bypass graft, inadequate correction of a congenital defect, or residual disease of the ventricular myocardium.
5 In patients with suspected myocardial or pericardial disease, cardiac catheterization may be undertaken in an effort to exclude lesions potentially amenable to surgical treatment, such as mitral regurgitation, coronary heart disease, constrictive pericarditis, and obstructive hypertrophic cardiomyopathy.
6 In patients with evidence of pulmonary hypertension, cardiac catheterization should be performed to search for such lesions as mitral stenosis, left-to-right shunts, multiple pulmonary emboli, or peripheral pulmonic stenosis.
7 In some patients in an intensive care setting (e.g., for hypotension or heart failure following acute myocardial infarction) catheterization of the right side of the heart by means of a balloon-tipped flotation catheter (Swan-Ganz catheter) often is employed to measure the pulmonary artery pressure, the pulmonary artery wedge pressure (as a measure of the left ventricular filling pressure), and the cardiac output. Such studies permit proper diagnosis, and repeated measurements allow accurate assessment of the effects of treatment.

TABLE 251-1
Information that can be obtained by cardiac catheterization and angiography

1 Intracardiac and intravascular pressure measurements and determination of pressure gradients across the cardiac valves
2 Cardiac output, pulmonary vascular resistance, and systemic vascular resistance
3 Radiographic anatomy of the cardiac chambers and great vessels (aorta, pulmonary artery)
4 Radiographic anatomy of the coronary arteries and detection of coronary artery spasm
5 Detection and quantification of intracardiac shunts
6 Intracardiac electrograms, His bundle electrograms, electrical pacing studies, and intracardiac phonocardiograms
7 Acute effects (hemodynamic and electrophysiologic) of cardioactive drugs
8 Quantification of coronary blood flow
9 Histology of myocardium from endomyocardial catheter biopsies

GENERAL METHODS OF USE

CATHETERIZATION OF THE RIGHT SIDE OF THE HEART Catheterization of the right side of the heart is now a safe and well-standardized procedure in the cardiac catheterization laboratory, as well as at the bedside in the intensive care unit. With the patient under local anesthesia, an antecubital or saphenous vein is isolated and a long, flexible radiopaque catheter is introduced. Alternatively, the percutaneous approach is employed, in which a needle is positioned in the vessel, a small, flexible wire passed through the needle, and with a vein dilator, a sheath is then passed over the dilator into the femoral or other vein. The guide wire is removed, leaving the sheath in place, and a catheter is introduced into the vein through it. Under fluoroscopic control, the cardiac catheter is guided into the right atrium, right ventricle, the pulmonary artery, and pulmonary arterial wedge position. At the bedside, when fluoroscopy is not available, a balloon-flotation catheter (often with a thermistor mounted near its tip) may be passed through the sheath, or directly into an exposed vein, and advanced blindly until it is considered to be near the right atrium. Then, while intracardiac pressure is being monitored, the balloon is inflated and the catheter advanced further, whereupon it is usually carried by the bloodstream directly into the right ventricle, the pulmonary artery, and into a third- or fourth-order pulmonary artery branch, from which a pulmonary arterial wedge tracing is obtained. When the balloon is deflated, the pulmonary artery pressure is recorded. Also, with a thermistor-tipped catheter, cardiac output can be measured serially by using the indicator dilution principle discussed subsequently in this chapter.

The course of the catheter alone in the right side of the heart on fluoroscopy or cineangiography may provide a clue to the diagnosis of certain congenital malformations. The catheter may enter an anomalous pulmonary vein or left superior vena cava; it may directly traverse a patent ductus arteriosus or an atrial septal defect; and inability to cross the tricuspid valve may indicate tricuspid atresia.

CATHETERIZATION OF THE LEFT SIDE OF THE HEART Various methods for catheterization of the left side of the heart have been devised, and each has found application under certain circumstances. Currently, the retrograde arterial approach is used most widely for catheterization of the aorta and left ventricle. The catheter usually is inserted via the femoral artery by the percutaneous method, or through a small incision directly into the exposed brachial artery. The transseptal approach often is employed to gain access to the left atrium and left ventricle, particularly when disease of the mitral valve is suspected. With this method, a catheter is inserted via the right saphenous or femoral vein, and its tip is positioned in the right atrium. A long needle, curved at its tip, is introduced through the catheter and employed to puncture the intact interatrial septum in the region of the fossa ovalis. Commonly, the catheter then is advanced over the needle into the left atrium and ventricle. Other methods of catheterization of the left side of the heart are used less commonly; e.g., with the anterior percutaneous approach a needle is introduced directly into the left ventricle in the region of the cardiac apex. This procedure sometimes is useful for measuring the left ventricular pressure in patients with valvular aortic stenosis or in postoperative patients with prosthetic valves in both the aortic and mitral positions.

CARDIAC ANGIOGRAPHY **Right side of heart** Selective injection of radiopaque contrast media at various sites within the right side of the heart also may be performed during cardiac catheterization. Injections into the superior or inferior vena cava are useful for detecting the thickened right atrial wall of constrictive pericarditis and for defining certain congenital lesions such as Ebstein's malformation of the tricuspid valve and tricuspid atresia. Selective right ventriculography is used commonly in the delineation of congenital cardiac lesions such as pulmonic stenosis and tetralogy of Fallot. Injection into the main pulmonary artery permits visualization of pulmonary thromboemboli, congenital pulmonary arterial branch stenosis, and anomalous pulmonary venous connections, and may be useful in the detection of tumor or thrombus within the left atrium.

Left side of heart Selective left ventriculography is employed to define congenital and acquired lesions affecting the mitral valve and the left ventricular outflow tract and to assess the adequacy of left ventricular function. Mitral stenosis may be detected by left ventriculography as thickening and/or calcification of the valve leaflets, shortening of the chordal subvalvular apparatus, and reduced excursion and delayed closure of the leaflets. Mitral regurgitation may be detected and estimated by noting the amount and density of contrast agent which enters the left atrium (Fig. 251-1). In addition, systolic prolapse into the left atrium of one or both of the mitral valve leaflets, secondary to either chordal malfunction or primary myxomatous degeneration and redundancy of the leaflets themselves, may be identified. The site of discrete subvalvular, valvular, or supravalvular aortic stenosis may be visualized, and the abnormal apposition of the ventricular septum and the anterior mitral valve leaflet in hypertrophic cardiomyopathy can be defined.

Both regional as well as global left ventricular function can be determined from analysis of the left ventricular cavity silhouette on the left ventriculogram. Regions of absent contraction (akinesia), reduced contraction (hypokinesia), or paradoxical systolic expansion (dyskinesia), as well as frank aneurysm formation, can thereby be detected and assessed as to severity (Fig. 251-2). Mural thrombi also may be visualized within such areas of wall motion disorder. In addition, by determination of a magnification factor, the area of the left ventricular cavity can be measured accurately, and by assumption of a geometric model of an ellipse, the volume of the chamber at end-diastole and end-systole can be determined (Fig. 251-1), and the total stroke volume can be calculated. The total stroke volume minus the forward stroke volume (calculated by an independent method for determining cardiac output, as discussed below) can then be used to derive the amount of aortic or mitral regurgitation per beat.

Values for end-diastolic volume greater than 90 ml per square meter of body surface area (average normal, plus one standard deviation) generally indicate left ventricular dilatation due to heart failure, or to a volume overload such as occurs in aortic regurgitation. The ejection fraction, the ratio of stroke volume to end-diastolic volume, reflects the percent shortening of the left ventricular myocardium (normal range 0.56 to 0.78). When the ejection fraction is reduced, the presence of depressed left ventricular contractile function is suggested. A further useful index of myocardial function is the mean velocity of circumferential fiber shortening (mean V_{cf}) or the fractional shortening per unit time of the minor axis of the left ventricular chamber (Fig. 251-1). Mean V_{cf} values below 1.2 end-diastolic circumferences per second in the basal state are considered indicative of depressed myocardial contractility. (Other measures of depressed contractility are discussed below under intravascular pressures.)

Selective ascending aortography is used for assessing the severity of aortic regurgitation, for determining the size and location of aortic aneurysms, and for visualizing less common congenital or acquired malformations such as sinus of Valsalva aneurysm, paraaortic sinus tract or aortic valvular vegetation (infective endocarditis), or dissection of the aorta due to cystic medial necrosis. Direct injection of contrast medium into the left atrium has been used to study left atrial function or the

FIGURE 251-1

Cineangiogram with injection of contrast medium into the left ventricle (LV). End-diastole is on the left and end-systole on the right. Study is performed in the right anterior oblique projection in a patient with severe mitral regurgitation in whom the left atrium (LA) is densely opacified simultaneously with the aorta (Ao) during ventricular systole.

Volume of LV is determined by planimetry of chamber area (enclosed by dashed line) and measurement of longest length (solid line between base and apex), using a geometric model of an ellipsoid. Thus, $D = 4A/\pi L$ *and* $V = \pi(D^2L/6)$, *where* D = *calculated diameter,* L = *longest measured length,* A = *area, and* V = *LV volume. Mean velocity of circumferential fiber shortening (mean* V_{cf}, *normalized to per unit circumference) can also be calculated by direct measurement of the minor axis (indicated by line with arrows) perpendicular to the midpoint of the long axis, and determination of the ejection time from cine frame rate and number of frames exposed from the beginning to the end of ejection.*

$$\text{Mean } V_{cf} = \frac{\text{end-diastolic } D - \text{end-systolic } D}{\text{end-diastolic } D \times \text{ejection time}}$$

where D = *minor axis diameter.*

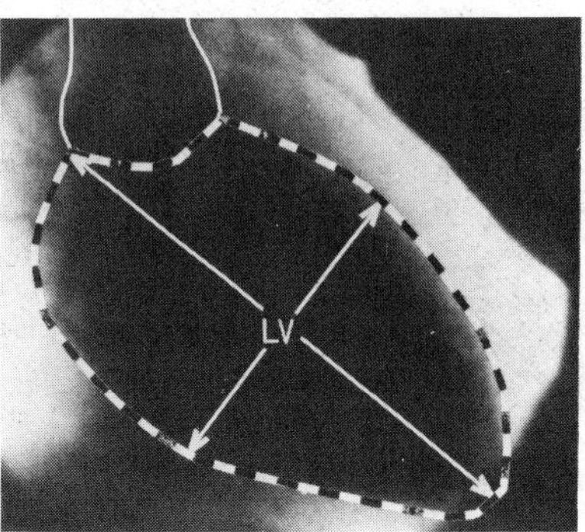

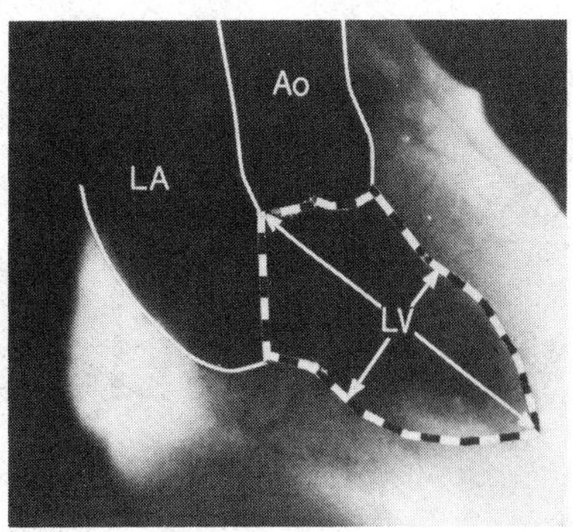

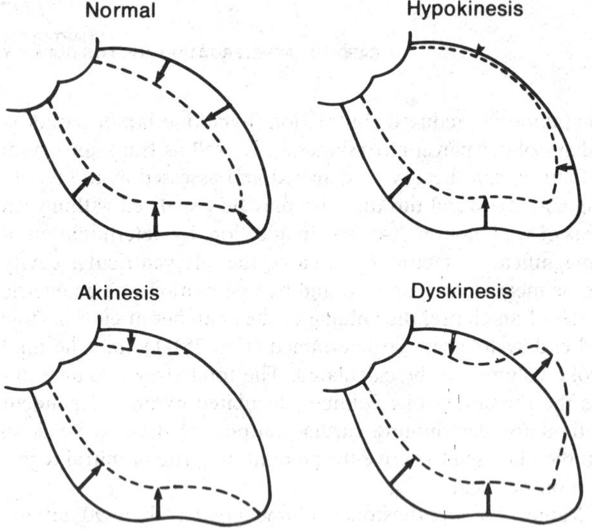

FIGURE 251-2
Diagrammatic representation of end-diastolic (solid line) and end-systolic (dashed line) silhouettes of left ventricular cineangiograms in various forms of localized wall motion disorders in patients with coronary heart disease. Normal patient exhibits relatively symmetrical contraction; patient with hypokinesis exhibits reduced contraction over anterior and apical surfaces; patient with dyskinesis exhibits paradoxic, outward movement over anterior surface during systole.

movement of the mitral valve, and to detect thrombi or tumor (myxoma) within that chamber.

Coronary arteriography Selective angiographic visualization of the coronary arterial tree is one of the most commonly applied diagnostic procedures in the cardiac catheterization laboratory. Accurate visualization of coronary artery atherosclerotic lesions has significantly increased understanding of the pathogenesis and natural history of coronary heart disease. Moreover, this procedure has contributed in large measure to the advent of surgical procedures for bypassing obstructive lesions within the coronary arteries. Visualization of coronary artery anatomy is useful, likewise, for defining congenital abnormalities such as anomalous origin of the coronary arteries, or a coronary arteriovenous fistula. Administration of ergonovine maleate is useful for inducing focal coronary artery spasm, particularly in patients with chest pain at rest in whom this etiology is suspected.

Coronary arteriography is performed by selective injection of 5 to 10 ml of contrast medium directly into each coronary artery orifice with cinefilming in multiple oblique and angulated projections at 30 to 60 frames per second and/or large film or photospot exposures at 4 to 6 per second, thereby obtaining dynamic as well as high-resolution images of the coronary arterial tree (Fig. 251-3). Specially designed catheters are used: one type, which has an open, tapered tip and multiple side holes, is inserted via a brachial arteriotomy (Sones technique); another type is advanced over a guide wire inserted percutaneously via the femoral artery and is preshaped to allow ready access to the right or left coronary artery orifices (Judkins technique). Both techniques provide diagnostic visualization of obstructive lesions within the main branches of the coronary vessels (Fig. 251-4*A* and *B*). In addition, collateral vessels, or new vascular pathways which serve to carry blood around a significant obstruction, can often be seen, and the vessel beyond a complete obstruction thereby visualized (Fig. 251-4*C*). The latter finding has obvious importance in determining the site for implantation of the distal end of a bypass graft.

COMPLICATIONS Catheterization of the right side of the heart is rarely associated with morbidity or mortality when performed under proper laboratory or bedside conditions. However, catheterization and angiography of the left side of the heart are procedures which unavoidably, although uncommonly, can lead to serious complications. Nevertheless, diagnostic cardiac catheterization procedures have been increasingly applied in recent years, primarily in response to the need for precise functional and anatomic information prior to carrying out cardiac operations. In the pediatric age group great attention has been paid to preventing metabolic disorders (hypoxia and acidemia) and pulmonary difficulties, utilization of small amounts of contrast agents, and use of flexible catheters; such precautions have significantly reduced the incidence of major complications and decreased the overall mortality rate in infants markedly. In adults, the advent of coronary artery bypass graft surgery has brought about a marked predominance in the application of coronary arteriography and left ventriculography by retrograde aortic catheterization, compared with other catheterization procedures. A prospective survey in 7553 patients of complications due to coronary arteriography reported in 1979 by the Collaborative Study of Coronary Artery Surgery (CASS) reported an overall mortality rate of 0.2 percent, an incidence of myocardial infarction of 0.025 percent, and an incidence of systemic embolization and vascular injury of 0.09 and 0.74 percent, respectively (all figures apply to 0 to 48 h after completion of the procedure). The brachial artery (Sones) technique increased the risk of death 3.6 times compared with the femoral approach, but this multiple did not apply if a given laboratory performed greater than 80 percent of its procedures by the brachial artery approach.

It seems clear that specialized invasive cardiac procedures in any age group should be performed only in well-equipped laboratories by highly experienced personnel, and the risks of cardiac catheterization and angiography should be weighed carefully in relation to the potential therapeutic benefits to be derived from an accurate anatomic and functional diagnosis.

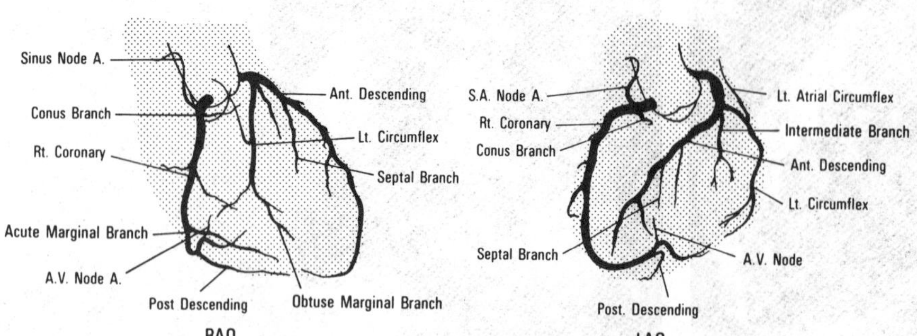

FIGURE 251-3
Diagram of the coronary arterial tree as viewed in two projections commonly used in coronary arteriography, the right anterior oblique (RAO) and left anterior oblique (LAO) projections. A., artery; Ant., anterior; A.V., atrioventricular; Lt., left; Post., posterior; Rt., right; S.A., sinoatrial; post., posterior.

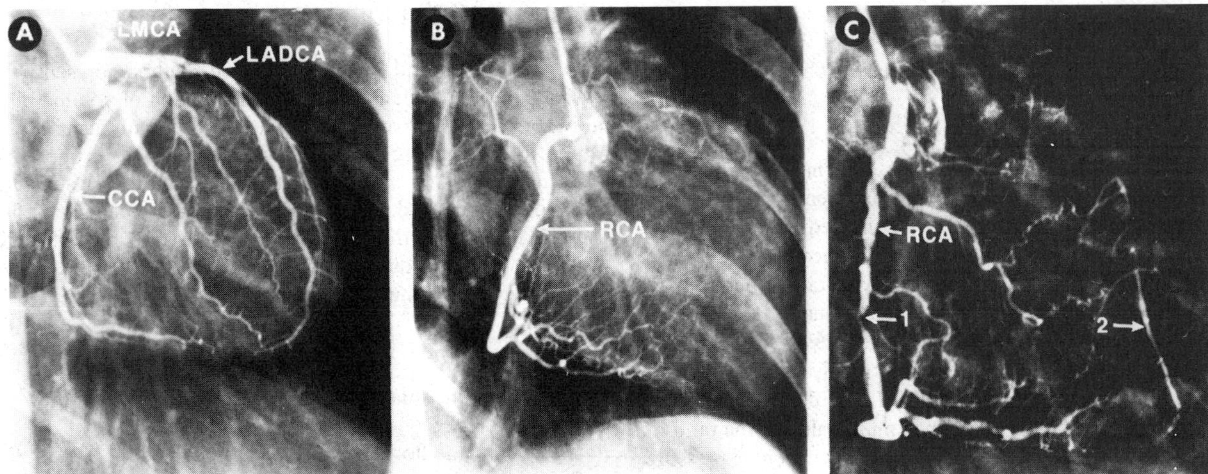

FIGURE 251-4
Selective coronary arteriograms obtained in the right anterior oblique projection. A and B show a normal subject and C a patient with severe stenosis of the right coronary artery. LMCA, left main coronary artery; CCA, circumflex coronary artery; LADCA, left anterior descending coronary artery; RCA, right coronary artery. In C, arrow 1 indicates the area of narrowing in the right coronary artery, and arrow 2 shows retrograde filling of the anterior descending coronary artery via collateral vessels, indicating that a severe obstruction is present in that vessel as well. (Courtesy of MP Judkins.)

MEASUREMENT OF INTRAVASCULAR PRESSURES

The upper limits of normal for intracardiac pressures and certain other hemodynamic variables are shown in Table 251-2. In understanding the contours of the intracardiac pressure pulses, thorough knowledge of the temporal relations between the electrical and mechanical events of the cardiac cycle is important.

The *a* wave in the right atrium normally is larger than the *v* wave, whereas in the left atrium the *v* wave is dominant (Table 251-2). Therefore, when the *v* wave in the right atrial pressure pulse exceeds the *a* wave, abnormal filling of the right atrium during ventricular systole, as occurs in tricuspid regurgitation or atrial septal defect, should be suspected. A characteristic right atrial pressure pulse also may be seen in the presence of tricuspid stenosis, the contour resembling that of mitral stenosis (see below), as well as in constrictive pericarditis, when an early diastolic "dip" and "plateau" elevation of pressure in mid- and late diastole occur. In many patients, the *mean* level of pressure in the left atrium is reflected with reasonable accuracy by the pulmonary artery wedge pressure (also sometimes termed the pulmonary "capillary" pressure), although the excursions of the wedge tracing often do not coincide with those measured directly within the left atrium. The characteristic contours of the left atrial pressure pulse in a normal subject and in patients with several forms of mitral valve disease are shown in Fig. 251-5. In the normal pressure pulse, or in the presence of mitral regurgitation without stenosis, there is a rapid fall in pressure during early diastole (the *y* descent), and a slow rise in pressure occurs during late diastole (diastasis), reflecting equilibration between the atrial and ventricular pressures during this slow phase of ventricular filling (Fig. 251-5*A*). In contrast, in patients with mitral stenosis the *y* descent is slow and prolonged; pressure in the left atrium continues to fall throughout diastole, and evidence of diastasis on the left atrial pressure pulse is absent because of the persistent atrioventricular pressure gradient (Fig. 251-5*B*). When mitral stenosis is present with normal sinus rhythm (Fig. 251-5*C*), the *a* wave is present, and a large pressure gradient accompanies atrial contraction (often associated with a loud presystolic murmur in such patients). In patients with pure mitral regurgitation, the *v* wave is prominent and the descending limb of this wave (the *y* descent) is rapid (Fig. 251-5*D*).

The left ventricular end-diastolic pressure immediately precedes the onset of isometric contraction in the left ventricular pressure pulse. This pressure point therefore follows the *a* wave and precedes the *c* wave, and the coincident pressure point in time in the left atrial tracing is termed the *z* point (Fig. 251-5*A*). The left ventricular end-diastolic pressure may be elevated in several situations: (1) in the presence of myocardial failure, (2) when the ventricle bears a high flow load (as in aortic or mitral regurgitation), (3) when the ventricle is hypertrophied and relatively noncompliant (restrictive myocardial disease), (4) in the presence of constrictive pericarditis, and (5) with cardiac tamponade secondary to a pericardial effusion.

The systolic pressure in the left ventricle exceeds that in the aorta in any of the forms of aortic stenosis which produce significant obstruction to ventricular outflow. In patients with valvular aortic stenosis, the left ventricular pressure pulse resembles that of an isometric contraction, the contour being more symmetric and the pressure peak more delayed than normal (a similar phenomenon is observed in the right ventricle in patients with pulmonic stenosis). The characteristics of the peripheral arterial pressure tracing also may be distinctive in patients with different types of aortic stenosis. Thus, when valvular stenosis is present, a slow and delayed rise of the peripheral arterial pulse wave is seen, while in hypertrophic obstructive cardiomyopathy an initially sharp upstroke is followed first by a rapid decline in pressure and then by a secondary positive

TABLE 251-2
Normal hemodynamic values,* mmHg

	a wave	*v wave*	*Mean*	*S/D*
Right atrium	8	7	6	
Right ventricle				30/7
Left ventricle				145/12
Pulmonary artery			17	30/14
Pulmonary artery wedge or left atrium	10	15	12	

Cardiac index = 2.4–3.8 (liters/min)/m² body surface area.
AV O_2 difference = 3.5–5.0 ml/dl.
Pulmonary vascular resistance = 250 (dyn•s)/cm⁵ (3 resistance units).

* *The figures shown indicate the upper limits of pressure (mmHg) in normal adult subjects. The values for the pressure waves, the mean pressures, and the systolic and diastolic pressures (S/D) are shown; in the ventricles, D = end-diastolic pressure. The ranges for cardiac index and arterial–mixed venous (AV) O_2 differences are shown.*

wave, which reflects the development of the obstruction during systole.

Derivatives of pressure pulses The rate of change, or slope, of the isovolumetric phase of the right or left ventricular pressure pulse, called the first derivative or *dp/dt,* frequently is used in addition to ejection phase measures mentioned above (ejection fraction, mean V_{cf}) to characterize the contractile behavior of the ventricular myocardium. The *dp/dt* may be measured manually by determining the slope of the pressure rise, but it is recorded more accurately by means of an electronic circuit or by computer processing. The peak of this derivative tracing (maximum *dp/dt*) as well as the maximum value of the ratio of *dp/dt* to the corresponding instantaneous ventricular pressure [peak (*dp/dt*)/*p*] provide indexes of the speed of contraction of the ventricle and therefore can help to define the level of the inotropic or contractile state of the heart. These measures tend to be below 1200 mmHg/s and 32 per second, respectively, in the left ventricles of patients with disease of the left ventricular myocardium, and they may be augmented strikingly by agents which improve the contractility of the heart, such as digitalis or catecholamines.

MEASUREMENT OF CARDIAC OUTPUT

The direct Fick and indicator-dilution methods presently are widely used in humans for the determination of volume blood flow, or the cardiac output. In general, the equations used with these techniques are derived from the principle proposed by Adolf Fick, which states that the rate at which a substance distributed in a fluid is delivered to an area by the moving fluid stream is equal to the product of the flow rate and the difference between the concentration of the substance at sites proximal and distal to the area. Thus,

$$q = F(C_a - C_v)$$

where q = the quantity of substance delivered per unit time

F = the flow rate

$C_a - C_v$ = the concentrations of the substance at proximal and distal sampling sites, respectively

(The same equation is applicable to the measurement of the removal rate, or clearance, of a substance.) When flow is the quantity to be derived, the equation is rearranged to

$$F = \frac{q}{C_a - C_v}$$

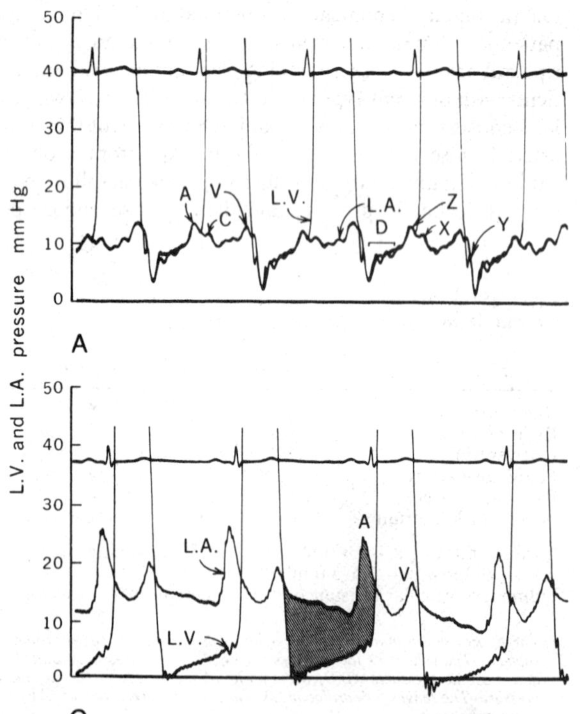

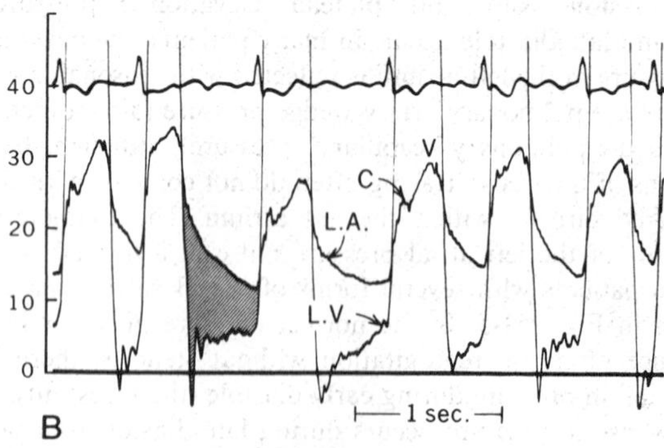

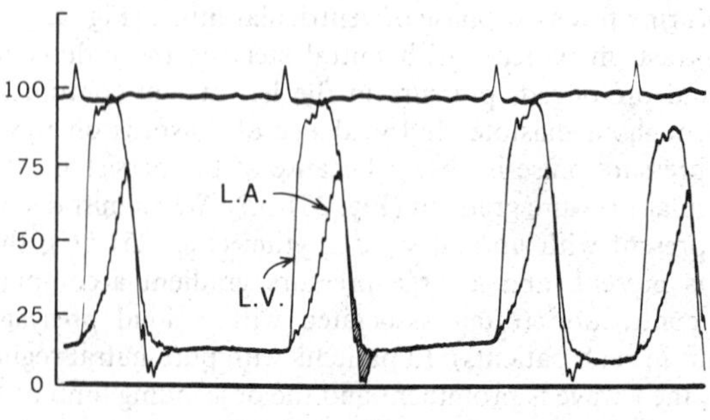

FIGURE 251-5

Simultaneously recorded left ventricular (LV) and left atrial (LA) pressure tracings in a normal subject (A) and in patients with various forms of mitral valve disease (B to D). The tracings are recorded at high sensitivity (0 to 40 mmHg), and therefore the top portion of the left ventricular pressure tracing is cut off. The electrocardiogram is recorded in the upper portion of each panel.

A. In the normal heart, diastole is initiated by a rapid-filling wave, which is followed by a period of slow ventricular filling or diastasis (bracket D), in which atrial and ventricular pressure rise together slowly. This period of diastasis is followed by the atrial contraction wave (a), which precedes the onset of isometric contraction in the ventricle, the end-diastolic pressure. The c wave occurs during the phase of isometric ventricular contraction and is followed by the x descent. The v wave occurs during late systole and the downslope of the v wave, constituting the y descent, occurs immediately after opening of the mitral valve.

B. Tracings obtained in a patient with mitral stenosis and atrial fibrillation. The pressure gradient from left atrium to left ventricle during diastole is indicated by the diagonally shaded area. The a wave is absent, and the c-V wave is prominent, and the y descent is slowed.

C. Tracings from a patient with mitral stenosis and normal sinus rhythm. The pressure gradient is indicated by the diagonally shaded area. A large pressure gradient occurs at the time of atrial contraction. No pressure rise during the period of diastasis is evident in the left atrial pressure tracings of panels B and C.

D. Tracings from a patient with isolated, severe mitral regurgitation and atrial fibrillation. The c wave is not evident, and the giant v wave in the left atrial pressure pulse is nearly 70 mmHg. There is small pressure gradient during the phase of rapid ventricular filling, because of the large volume of antegrade flow across the mitral valve.

DIRECT FICK METHOD In this method for measuring the cardiac output it is assumed that at rest the oxygen uptake in the lungs is equal to that used by the tissues, and systemic flow, i.e., left ventricular output, therefore is equated with blood flow through the lungs. It is essential to this method that a sample of mixed venous blood be obtained, because blood samples in the venae cavae and the coronary sinus have widely differing oxygen concentrations, and therefore the venous blood sample generally is withdrawn from the right ventricular outflow tract or the pulmonary artery. In practice, arterial and venous blood samples ($C_a - C_v$) are obtained during the measurement of oxygen consumption q over a 3-min period by spirometry and subsequent chemical analysis of the expired gas. Flow F, or cardiac output, is then calculated. The subject must be in a steady state throughout the period of measurement to avoid transient changes in systemic blood flow or in the rate of ventilation that can negate the assumption that oxygen uptake in the lungs equals that taken up in the tissues.

INDICATOR-DILUTION METHOD This is a special application of Fick's principle. A variety of relatively nondiffusible indicators have been employed, the indicator substance being injected into the circulation and its concentration measured at a downstream sampling site by a suitable detector. For example, the dye indocyanine green is injected intravenously and blood is withdrawn from an artery at a constant rate through a calibrated densitometer, which provides direct measurement of the dye concentration. Generally, a single bolus of the indicator is injected rapidly and is thoroughly mixed in one of the vascular spaces, such as a ventricular chamber; the concentration versus time curve then provides a measure of the rate at which indicator was washed out of the mixing site. Prior to recirculation of the indicator, the downslope of this curve is exponential, and therefore extrapolation of the curve using semilog paper permits the elimination of recirculated indicator. The mean concentration $\bar{c}$ of the dye is determined from the area of this corrected curve and its duration. The rate of blood flow F then is directly related to the quantity of indicator injected i and is inversely related to the mean concentration of the indicator $\bar{c}$ and the duration of the curve t (in seconds) by the formula $F = 60i/\bar{c}t$. A simple example will serve to illustrate this principle: if 8 mg dye is injected and a mean concentration of 2 mg per liter is recorded, and if the indicator takes 60 s to pass the sampling site, then the flow is 4 liters per minute.

Cold saline is another indicator which is used commonly when a thermodilution catheter is situated in the pulmonary artery. A standard amount of saline is injected at the junction of the superior or inferior vena cava with the right atrium, and the resultant change in temperature (analogous to concentration) is measured in the pulmonary artery by a small thermistor located 2 to 5 cm from the tip of the catheter. The thermodilution technique has demonstrated empirically an excellent correlation with other methods of measuring cardiac output. Cardiac output can also be computed by continuous infusion. Single thermodilution curves provide certain advantages: (1) no arterial entry is required, (2) the indicator is inexpensive, (3) recirculation is minimal, and (4) the analogue signal is well suited to rapid calculation of the cardiac output by computer analysis.

MEASUREMENT OF PULMONARY VASCULAR RESISTANCE The formula for calculating pulmonary vascular resistance in simplified form which omits consideration of vessel length and blood viscosity, states that resistance is directly proportional to the pressure drop across the bed and inversely proportional to the rate of blood flow. This ratio of mean pressure difference to volume flow is expressed in dyne-seconds per cm^5 [(dyn·s)/cm^5], the mean pressure difference across the pulmonary bed being obtained by subtracting the mean left atrial or pulmonary artery wedge pressure from the mean pulmonary artery pressure.[1] The *resistance unit* (i.e., the pressure difference in millimeters of mercury divided by the cardiac output in liters per minute and expressed in arbitrary units) also is commonly employed as an index of arteriolar resistance (Table 251-2). Estimation of the pulmonary vascular resistance, which normally is about 15 percent of that in the systemic vascular bed, is of importance in patients with congenital heart disease and circulatory shunts, as well as in certain forms of acquired cardiac and pulmonary diseases. Its calculation provides a useful means of interpreting the level of pulmonary arterial pressure relative to pulmonary blood flow, high pressure and high flow obviously bearing a different connotation than high pressure and low flow.

VALVE ORIFICE SIZE AND VALVULAR REGURGITATION When the cardiac output is normal, the severity of a stenotic valve lesion may be estimated from the magnitude of the pressure gradient across the valve. When the cardiac output is elevated or reduced, however, reliance on the pressure gradient alone may lead to an erroneous estimate of the degree of mechanical obstruction. In addition, it is of importance to consider the heart rate in assessing the significance of a pressure gradient. When the heart rate is rapid, systole occupies a disproportionate amount of time in each cardiac cycle, diastole filling time is limited, and a large pressure gradient across the atrioventricular valve may exist in the face of relatively mild stenosis. The application of the hydraulic formula devised by Gorlin and Gorlin to the calculation of valve orifice size has proved helpful in analyzing the degree of valve stenosis in these situations. In simplest terms, this formula states that the area of a short-bore orifice is directly proportional to the rate of blood flow across the orifice and inversely proportional to the square root of the pressure gradient. For example, if the flow rate across a narrowed valve orifice of fixed size doubles, as may occur when the cardiac output increases during exertion, the pressure gradient will quadruple. Conversely, when the flow rate is reduced, as in patients with heart failure, a small pressure gradient may exist in the presence of a severe degree of valve stenosis. This relationship differs from the general resistance equation discussed above and reflects the fact that the kinetic energy losses across a stenotic valve are high, a large pressure head being expended in developing a rapid flow velocity across the narrowed orifice.

It should be pointed out that use of the orifice formula is not valid when significant valvular regurgitation is present and forward cardiac output alone is measured, since an unknown volume of blood is regurgitated and recrosses the valve during the subsequent cardiac cycle. Application of the formula under these circumstances leads to an underestimation of the valve orifice area, since forward flow across the valve is underestimated.

DIAGNOSIS OF CIRCULATORY SHUNTS

When a communication exists between the left and the right sides of the heart, and when pulmonary vascular resistance is lower than that in the systemic vascular bed, a left-to-right shunt of oxygenated blood will occur. Conversely, when the resistance in the pulmonary bed is higher than that in the sys-

[1] $$\text{Resistance} = \frac{[P_{PA}\,(\text{mmHg}) - P_{LA}\,(\text{mmHg})] \times 1332\ \text{dyn/cm}^2}{\text{cardiac output (ml/s)}}$$

where P_{PA} and P_{LA} = mean pulmonary artery and left atrial pressures, respectively. 1 mmHg = 1.36 cmH_2O; 1 cmH_2O = 980 dyn/cm^2 force.

temic circulation, or an obstruction such as pulmonic stenosis exists distal to an intracardiac communication, a right-to-left shunt of venous blood may occur. These shunts can be readily visualized and localized by exposure of cineangiograms during selective injections of contrast medium.

Many types of indicators have been employed in the quantification and detection of circulatory shunts. The indicator may be the oxygen in room air, blood samples being withdrawn and analyzed for oxygen manometrically or by an oximeter. Foreign, inert gases such as hydrogen or krypton 85 may be employed; these, like oxygen, are "injected" into the pulmonary circulation by inhalation and sampled from the right side of the heart. They may be measured by a catheter-tip sensor (hydrogen) or by withdrawal of blood samples for analysis. In obtaining indicator-dilution curves, the substance most commonly injected is indocyanine green dye, detected by withdrawing blood through a densitometer.

The techniques used for localizing and quantifying shunts at cardiac catheterization may be divided into two basic categories: (1) Those methods in which an indicator is delivered distal to the site at which blood is sampled (the so-called upstream sampling method), e.g., indicator is injected into the pulmonary artery or is inhaled to enter the pulmonary veins and left side of the heart. Blood samples are then obtained upstream in the right side of the heart and analyzed for concentration of the indicator. (2) Those methods in which an indicator is delivered proximal to the sampling site (the so-called downstream sampling method), in which most frequently an indicator-dilution curve is obtained by intracardiac dye injection with sampling from a peripheral artery. This approach permits detection of right-to-left as well as left-to-right shunts.

UPSTREAM SAMPLING METHOD Blood samples are withdrawn in serial fashion from the pulmonary artery, right ventricle, right atrium, and venae cavae, the indicator being introduced downstream (in the case of oxygen into the lungs). This approach permits localization of the site of a left-to-right shunt. With the oxygen sampling method, a step-up of 2.0 ml/dl from the venae cavae to the right atrium, of 1.0 ml/dl from the right atrium to the right ventricle, or of 0.5 ml/dl from the right ventricle to the pulmonary artery is considered to be evidence of a left-to-right shunt. The use of a foreign gas improves the sensitivity of this approach, even a small left-to-right shunt being readily detected by appropriate sampling within the right side of the heart using a catheter-tip hydrogen electrode, for example.

For determination of the size of a left-to-right shunt, samples of venous blood proximal to the shunt and samples from the pulmonary artery and a systemic artery are obtained in close time sequence. The oxygen uptake at the lungs is measured simultaneously, or estimated, and the pulmonary and systemic blood flow rates (and hence the magnitude of the left-to-right shunt relative to systemic flow) can be calculated using Fick's equations. Generally a pulmonary to systemic flow ratio of 1.5:1 or greater is considered to indicate a left-to-right shunt of substantial magnitude.

DOWNSTREAM SAMPLING METHOD A needle is placed into a systemic artery and a time-concentration curve is recorded following upstream injection of the indicator. This technique is particularly useful for localizing the site of a right-to-left shunt. For example, when a right-to-left shunt exists at the ventricular level, an injection into the right ventricle and at all sites proximal to the right ventricle will result in an early appearance time of dye that has immediately traversed the defect (Fig. 251-6). However, an injection into the pulmonary artery, distal to the right-to-left shunt, shows a normal appearance time. A left-to-right shunt also may be detected, but not localized, by injection of indicator into the right side of the heart using peripheral arterial sampling. The indicator-dilution curve will show a reduced peak concentration of dye and a break on the downslope when compared with a normal indicator-dilution curve (Fig. 251-5). This contour occurs because a portion of the indicator traverses the left-to-right shunt during its initial passage to the left side of the heart, recirculates rapidly through the right side of the heart and lungs, and reappears at the peripheral artery before the downslope of the primary curve has been completely inscribed.

OTHER SPECIAL CARDIAC CATHETERIZATION TECHNIQUES Miniaturization of electronics has permitted the construction and application of cardiac catheters with special measuring devices mounted on, or close to, the tip. For example, a catheter-tip micromanometer permits the measurement of intracardiac pressure free of the artifacts produced by fluid-filled manometer systems and catheter motion. Accurate high-fidelity pressure measurements are of particular utility in the assessment of the contractile and distensibility properties of the left ventricle. Micromanometer-tipped catheters also can be used for highly sensitive recordings of intracardiac sounds, murmurs, and clicks. In fact, an intracardiac phonocardiogram in the right ventricle is perhaps the most reliable method for documenting pulmonic insufficiency as the source of a diastolic, decrescendo murmur along the left sternal border. Other special catheters have been designed to record the intracardiac electrocardiogram and have made it possible to record selective potentials from the right atrium, right ventricle, and along the bundle of His. Recordings from the latter area are useful, for

FIGURE 251-6
Diagrammatic representation of indicator-dilution curves using the downstream sampling method. The time of injection (Inj.) of an indicator, such as cardiogreen dye, is indicated by the arrow and by the square wave response on the recorded tracing. With right atrial (RA) injection and sampling at a peripheral artery, the normal appearance time is about 8 s, and the normal contour of the indicator-dilution curve is represented by the solid line. In a patient with a right-to-left (R-L) shunt at the atrial, ventricular, or pulmonary arterial levels, early appearance time of the dye is indicated by the dashed line. In a patient with a left-to-right (L-R) shunt, the appearance time need not be altered, but there is a reduced peak concentration of dye, and a break on the downslope, indicating early recirculation of the indicator.

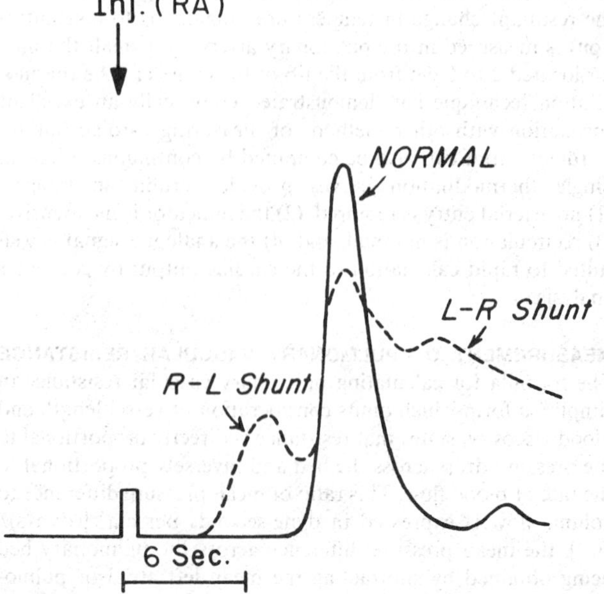

example, in determining whether a conduction delay or block on the surface electrocardiogram is located at or below the atrioventricular junction. His bundle recordings also have improved understanding of the mechanisms underlying paroxysmal atrial tachycardia and the preexcitation syndromes. Electrophysiologic studies with cardiac pacing are now being used in the diagnosis and selection of therapy for refractory cardiac dysrhythmias (Chap. 255). Electromagnetic or ultrasonic catheter-tip velocity probes also are available and have proved useful for study of phasic blood flow patterns in the venae cavae and pulmonary artery in patients with constrictive pericarditis and cardiac tamponade, and for analysis of the pattern and velocity of left ventricular ejection into the ascending aorta in patients with disorders of left ventricular function.

Transvascular intracardiac biopsy of the right and left ventricles by specially designed catheters also has been accomplished safely in a large number of patients. The specimens have proved to have some value from a diagnostic standpoint in uncommon varieties of infiltrative cardiomyopathy, e.g., those due to amyloid, iron, glycogen, granuloma, and neoplasm. Endomyocardial biopsy has also been used to detect early cardiac rejection following cardiac transplantation.

Recently, small balloon-tipped catheters have been developed which can be passed through a preshaped guiding catheter into the coronary arterial tree and used to dilate areas of partial coronary obstruction (transluminal coronary angioplasty). At the present time, this technique is most successfully applied to patients with single-vessel coronary disease involving the proximal left anterior descending artery when the stenosis is concentric, isolated, and noncalcified.

REFERENCES

Barry W, Grossman W: Cardiac catheterization, in *Heart Disease,* 2d ed, E Braunwald (ed). Philadelphia, Saunders, 1983, chap 9

Davis K et al: Complications of coronary arteriography from the Collaborative Study of Coronary Artery Surgery (CASS). Circulation 59:1105, 1979

Grossman W (ed): *Cardiac Catheterization and Angiography,* 2d ed. Philadelphia, Lea & Febiger, 1980

Rackley CE: Quantitative evaluation of left ventricular function by radiographic techniques. Circulation 54:862, 1976

Shabetai R, Adolph RJ: Principles of cardiac catheterization, in *Cardiac Diagnosis and Treatment,* 3d ed, NO Fowler (ed). Hagerstown, Harper & Row, 1980, p 106

Functional abnormalities of the heart

252 DISORDERS OF MYOCARDIAL FUNCTION

EUGENE BRAUNWALD

CELLULAR BASIS OF CARDIAC CONTRACTION

The myocardium is composed of individual striated muscle cells (fibers), normally 10 to 15 μm in diameter and 30 to 60 μm in length. Each fiber contains multiple cross-banded strands (myofibrils), which run the length of the fiber and are composed of a serially repeating structure, the sarcomere. The remainder of the cytoplasm, lying between the myofibrils, contains other cell constituents, such as the single centrally located nucleus, numerous mitochondria, and intracellular membrane systems.

The sarcomere, the structural and functional unit of contraction, is delimited by two adjacent dark lines, the Z lines (Fig. 252-1). The distance between Z lines varies with the degree of contraction or stretch of the muscle and ranges between 1.6 and 2.2 μm. Within the confines of the sarcomere, alternating light and dark bands are seen, giving the myocardial fibers their striated appearance under the light microscope. At the center of the sarcomere is a broad dark band of constant width (1.5 μm), the A band, which is flanked by two lighter bands, the I bands, which are of variable width. The sarcomere of heart muscle, like that of skeletal muscle, is made up of two sets of myofilaments. Thicker filaments, composed principally of the protein myosin, traverse and are limited to the A band. They are about 100 Å in diameter, with tapered ends, and measure 1.5 to 1.6 μm in length. Thinner filaments, composed primarily of actin, course from the Z line through the I band into the A band. They are approximately 50 Å in diameter and 1.0 μm in length. Thus, there is overlapping of thick and thin filaments only within the A band, while the I band contains only thin filaments (Fig. 252-1). On electron-microscopic examination, bridges may be seen to extend between the thick and thin filaments within the A band.

The "sliding" model for muscle rests on the fundamental observation that both the thick and thin filaments are constant in overall length, both at rest and during contraction. With activation of the sarcomere, repetitive interactions take place at the bridges between the actin and myosin filaments, and the actin filaments are propelled further into the A band. In the process, the A band remains constant in width, whereas the I band becomes more narrow and the Z lines move toward one another.

The myosin molecule is a complex, asymmetric fibrous protein with a molecular weight of about 500,000; it has a rod-like portion that is about 1500 Å in length with a globular portion at its end. This globular portion contains the adenosine triphosphatase (ATPase) activity and forms the bridges. In forming the thick myofilament, the rod-like portions of the myosin molecules are laid down in an orderly, polarized manner, leaving the globular portions projecting outward so that they can interact with actin to generate force and shortening. Actin has a molecular weight of 47,000. The thin filament is composed of a double helix of two chains of actin molecules wound about each other, intimately associated with the protein tropomyosin, which appears to form the central core of this filament. Another protein complex, troponin, which can be separated into three components, is located periodically along the actin filament. In contrast to myosin, actin has no intrinsic enzymatic activity, but it has the ability to combine reversibly with myosin in the presence of ATP and Mg^{2+}, which activates the myosin ATPase. In relaxed muscle this interaction is inhibited by one of the components of troponin. During activation, Ca^{2+} becomes attached to another of the components and removes this inhibition. As a result, ATP is split, and linkages between actin and myosin filaments are made and broken cyclically. Mechanical forces are generated by these reactions, with resultant shortening of the sarcomere.

The sarcoplasmic reticulum, a complex network of anastomosing, membrane-lined intracellular channels, which invests the myofibrils, and which is less profuse in cardiac than in skeletal muscle, consists of a series of interconnecting longitudinally disposed membrane tubules closely applied to the surfaces of the individual sarcomeres; it has no direct continuity with the outside of the cell. Closely related, both functionally and structurally, are the transverse tubules or T system,

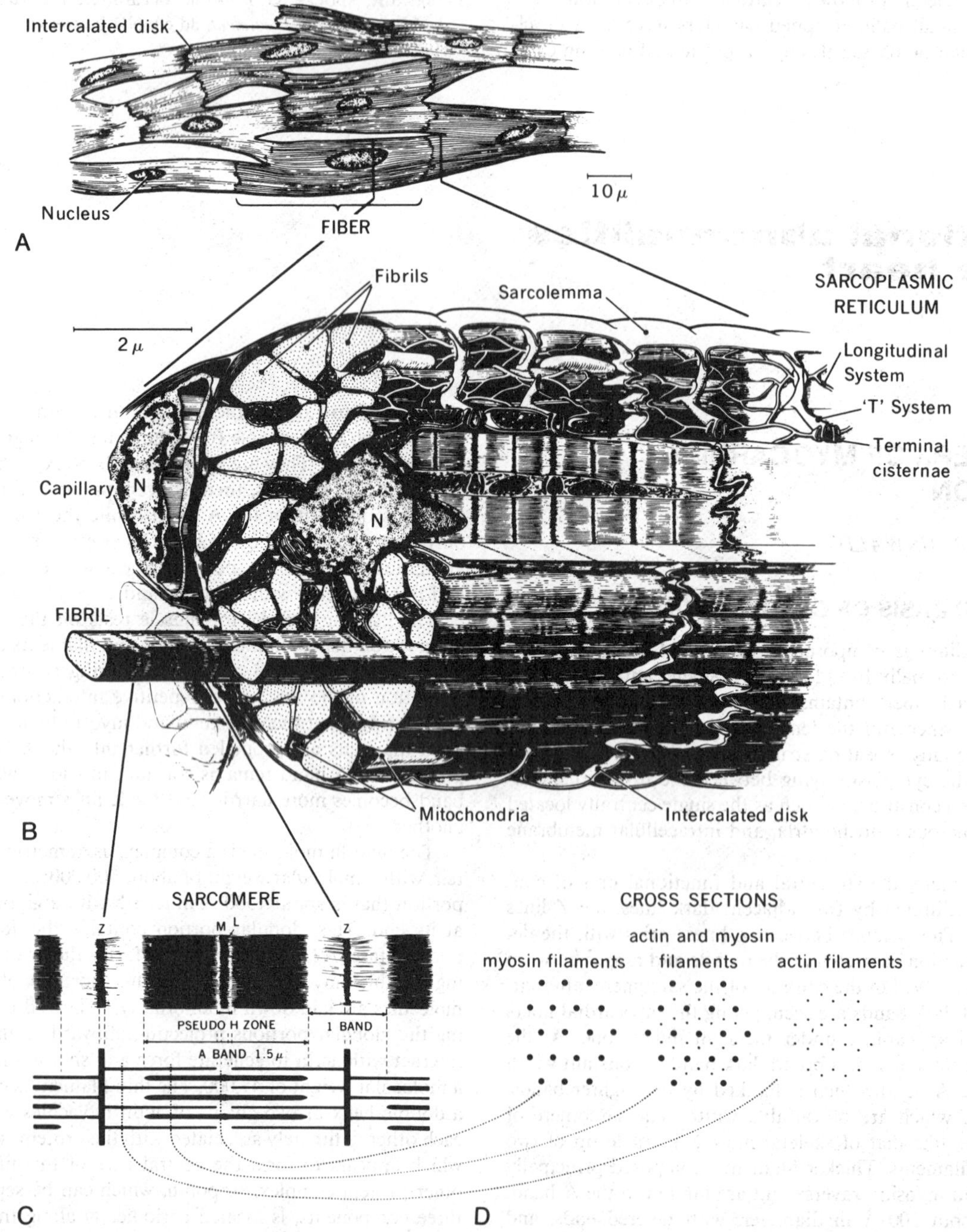

FIGURE 252-1
Microscopic structure of heart muscle. A. Myocardium as seen under the light microscope. Branching of fibers is evident. Each fiber, or cell, contains a centrally located nucleus. B. Myocardial cell, reconstructed from electron micrographs. Each cell is composed of multiple parallel fibrils. Each fibril is composed of serially connected sarcomeres (N, nucleus). C. Sarcomere from a myofibril, with diagrammatic representation of myofilaments. Thick filaments (1.5 μm long, composed of myosin) form the A band, and thin filaments (1 μm long, composed primarily of actin) extend from the Z line through the I band into the A band. The overlapping of thick and thin filaments is seen only in the A band. D. Cross sections of the sarcomere indicate the specific lattice arrangements of the myofilaments. In the center of the sarcomere only the thick, or myosin, filaments arranged in a hexagonal array are seen. In the distal portions of the A band, both thick and thin, or actin, filaments are found, with each thick filament surrounded by six thin filaments. In the I band only thin filaments are present. (From Braunwald et al, 1976.)

formed by tubelike invaginations of the sarcolemma, which extend into the myocardial fiber, along the Z lines, i.e., the ends of the sarcomeres.

At rest, the cardiac cell is polarized; i.e., the interior has a negative charge relative to the outside of the cell, with a transmembrane potential of -80 to -100 mV (Chap. 249). The sarcolemma, which in the resting state is largely impermeable to Na^+ and has a Na^+ - and K^+ -stimulated pump requiring adenosine triphosphate (ATP) which extrudes Na^+ from the cell, plays a critical role in establishing this resting potential. Thus, the inside of the cell has relatively large quantities of K^+ with far less Na^+, while the extracellular milieu is high in $[Na^+]$ and low in $[K^+]$. At the same time, in the resting state, the extracellular $[Ca^{2+}]$ greatly exceeds the free intracellular $[Ca^{2+}]$.

During the plateau of the action potential (phase 2) there is a slow inward current which reflects primarily a movement of Ca^{2+} into the cell. However, the absolute quantity of Ca^{2+} that crosses the surface membrane is relatively small and in and of itself appears to be incapable of bringing about full activation of the contractile apparatus. However, the depolarizing current not only extends across the surface of the cell but penetrates deeply into the cell by way of the ramifying T system. A flux of Ca^{2+} as well as Na^+ into the cell takes place, which may then lead to depolarization of the sarcoplasmic reticulum; this in turn leads to the release of much larger quantities of Ca^{2+} from the sarcoplasmic reticulum.

The Ca^{2+} then diffuses toward the sarcomere, combines with troponin, and, by repressing the inhibitor of contraction, activates the myofilaments to produce contraction, the strength and velocity of which are dependent on the quantity of Ca^{2+} that reaches the contractile sites. The sarcoplasmic reticulum then appears to reaccumulate Ca^{2+}, thereby lowering its concentration in the myofibril to a level that inhibits the actin-myosin interaction which is responsible for contraction, and in this manner leads to relaxation. Thus, the cell membrane, transverse tubules, and the sarcoplasmic reticulum, with their ability to transmit an action potential, to release and then reaccumulate Ca^{2+}, appear to play a fundamental role in the rhythmic contraction and relaxation of heart muscle.

The ATP formed from substrate oxidation is the principal source of energy for almost all of the mechanical work of contraction performed by the myocardial cell. The high-energy phosphate stores in ATP are in equilibrium with those in the form of creatine phosphate.

In all forms of striated muscle, including cardiac muscle, the force of contraction depends on initial muscle length. The sarcomere length associated with the most forceful contraction is 2.2 μm. It is at this length that the two sets of myofilaments of the sarcomere are most ideally situated to provide the greatest area for their interaction. In support of the sliding-filament hypothesis, force development diminishes in direct proportion to the decrease in the overlap between thick and thin filaments, and the resultant decrease in the number of reactive sites. The

FIGURE 252-2

Relation between sarcomere length and band patterns in skeletal muscle (frog sartorius). A. Band patterns as seen electromicroscopically. B. Disposition of the thick and thin filaments that create band patterns. The vertical arrows in both panels denote the ends of the thin filaments that insert at the Z line at the left. Line 3 represents the sarcomere at the apex of the length-tension curve, i.e., at L_{max}. In lines 1 and 2, sarcomere length has been progressively decreased, whereas in 4 and 5 it has been progressively elongated. Throughout, the A band remains constant in width. The placement of filaments to provide for maximum overlap is shown in B (3). Line 1 shows the sarcomere pattern in the contracted muscle; the I band has disappeared, and a secondary dark band has been formed at the center of the sarcomere, termed the C contraction band, which is due to the passage of thin filaments through this area as in B (1). In A (4 and 5), an expanding H zone has appeared, owing to the withdrawal of the thin filaments from the A band, as shown diagrammatically in B (4 and 5). (From Braunwald et al, 1976.)

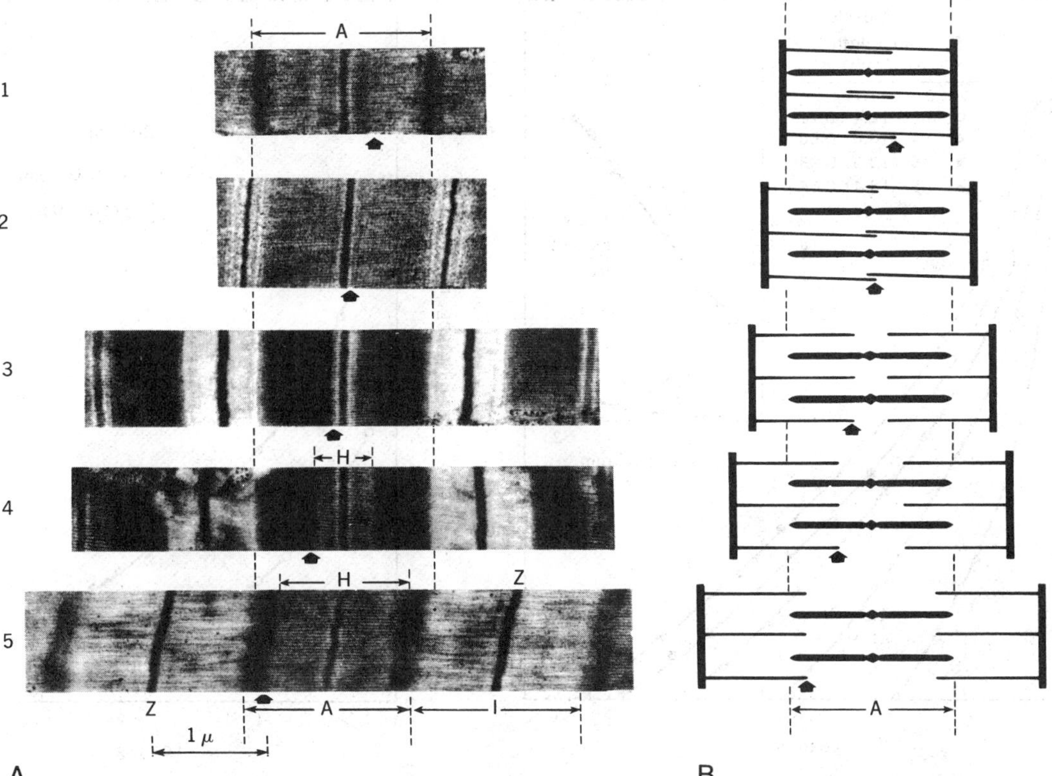

length of the sarcomere also appears to regulate the extent of activation of the contractile system, i.e., its sensitivity to Ca^{2+}, which is greatest at 2.2 μm. When sarcomere length is increased to 3.65 μm, developed tension falls to zero, and it is at this point that the thin filaments are entirely withdrawn from the A band. Similarly, when the sarcomeres are shorter than 2.0 μm, the thin filaments bypass one another, producing a double overlap of the thin filaments (Fig. 252-2), a reduction of sensitivity of the contractile sites to Ca^{2+}, and force also falls.

The relation between the initial length of the muscle fibers and the developed force is of prime importance for the function of heart muscle. This forms the basis of the Frank-Starling relation (Starling's law of the heart), which states that, within limits, an augmentation of initial volume of the ventricle, which is a function of the initial length of the muscle, results in an increase in the force of ventricular contraction. It has been shown for heart muscle that sarcomere length is directly proportional to muscle length along the ascending limb of the length–active tension curve. As muscle length decreases to the point at which developed tension approaches zero and at which sarcomere length approaches 1.5 μm, the I bands at first narrow, then disappear while the A band remains constant in length. At this latter point, the Z lines abut on the edges of the A bands. Thus, the sarcomere length–active tension curve forms the ultrastructural basis of Starling's law of the heart.

MYOCARDIAL MECHANICS

The mechanical activity of all muscle may be expressed externally in only two ways: shortening and the development of tension. Hill showed in skeletal muscle that the velocity of shortening is inversely related to the magnitude of tension development, an expression of the so-called force-velocity relation, now acknowledged to be a fundamental property of muscle. Expressed simply, the greater the load the muscle is called upon to lift, the lower the velocity of shortening and vice versa. More recently, the concept of the force-velocity relation has been extended from skeletal to cardiac muscle. However, in this respect there is a basic difference between skeletal and cardiac muscle. Skeletal muscle has a single, essentially fixed, force-velocity curve; i.e., at any given muscle length, force and velocity are always related to each other in the same manner. The contractile activity of skeletal muscle is increased by the recruitment of additional muscle fibers, i.e., motor units, and by increasing the frequency of nerve impulses, while the contractile properties of each individual fiber remains constant. Although resting length also influences the characteristics of contraction, this variable remains essentially fixed in vivo. In contrast, the number of cardiac cells and within them the myofibrils and sarcomeres which become activated during each contraction is constant. However, the contractile activity of the myocardium may be readily altered under physiological conditions by changes in resting fiber length and by changes in the inotropic state, i.e., the contractility, both of which shift the myocardial force-velocity curve.

Variations in myocardial contractile activity may be expressed as displacements of the force-velocity curve in two fundamental ways. Figure 252-3*A* shows a family of force-velocity curves obtained from an isolated cardiac muscle; each curve was obtained at a different preload, i.e., with a different degree of stretch on the muscle. Note that changing the preload alters the intercept of the force-velocity curve on the horizontal axis; i.e., it increases the isometric force developed by the muscle. However, within limits, these alterations in preload do not ap-

FIGURE 252-3
A. Effects of increasing initial muscle length on the force-velocity relation of the cat papillary muscle. Initial velocity of shortening has been plotted as a function of load for five different muscle lengths. The maximum velocity of shortening is essentially unchanged, whereas the maximum force of contraction is augmented. The insert shows the places along the length-tension curves at which these force-velocity curves were determined. B. Effects of norepinephrine on the force-velocity relation of the cat papillary muscle. Both the maximum velocity of shortening and the force of contraction are increased. (From Braunwald et al, 1976.)

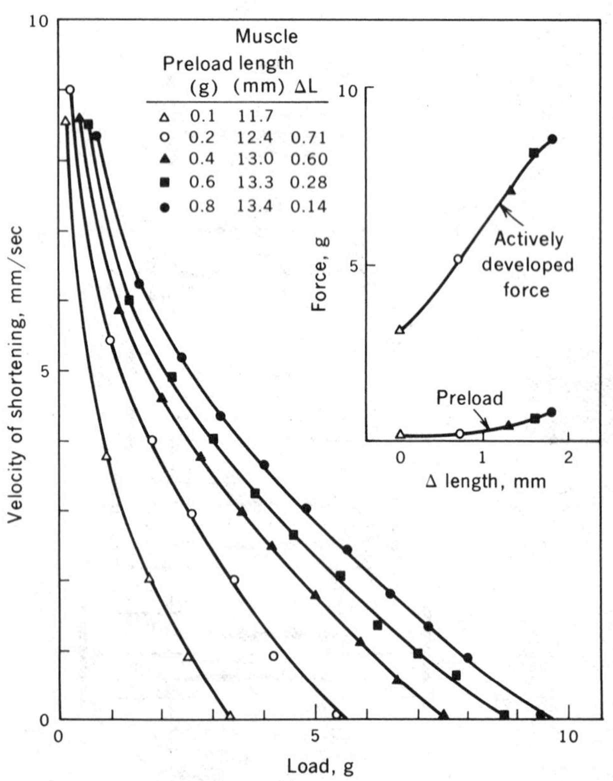

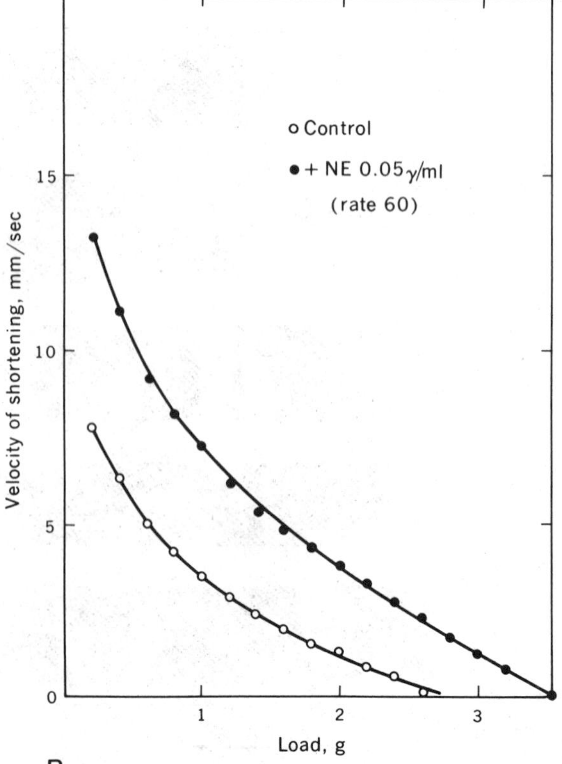

pear to alter the velocity of shortening, since all the curves extrapolate to the same intercept on the vertical axis. Thus, a change in initial length of heart muscle shifts the force-velocity curve primarily by altering the total force which can be developed by the muscle, as illustrated by the isometric length-tension curve, shown in the insert of Fig. 252-3*A*.

This type of shift in the force-velocity curve may be contrasted with that obtained when a positive inotropic agent, such as Ca^{2+}, digitalis, or norepinephrine (which act ultimately, either by increasing the concentration of Ca^{2+} in the vicinity of the myofilaments and/or their sensitivity to Ca^{2+}) is added to the muscle while the initial length is held constant (Fig. 252-3*B*). These agents not only increase the weight which the muscle is capable of lifting, i.e., the intercept of the force-velocity curve on the horizontal axis, therefore shifting the isometric length-tension curve upward, but they also increase the velocity of shortening of the unloaded muscle, i.e., the extrapolated intercept on the vertical axis.

It has been postulated that an increase in initial muscle length up to an optimal length brings about an increase in the number of effective force-generating sites as a consequence of a more advantageous overlap of interdigitating contractile filaments within the sarcomere and in the extent of activation of the contractile sites, i.e., their sensitivity to Ca^{2+}. A change in the inotropic state, characterized by an increase in the velocity of shortening of the unloaded muscle, can also result from an increase in the rate of cyclic force-generating processes at the contractile sites, without a change in the number of these sites, i.e., at a constant muscle length. Increased contractility appears to be related primarily to an increased availability of Ca^{2+} within the cell.

CONTRACTION OF THE INTACT VENTRICLE

Analysis of the heart as a pump has classically centered upon the relation between the filling pressure, or diastolic volume, of the ventricle (length of the muscle fibers) and its stroke volume (the Frank-Starling relation). In the heart-lung preparation the stroke volume is a function of diastolic fiber length, and the failing heart delivers a smaller-than-normal stroke volume from a normal or elevated end-diastolic volume. The relation between the mean atrial or the ventricular end-diastolic pressure and the stroke work of the corresponding ventricle (the

ventricular function curve) provides a useful definition of the level of the contractile, or inotropic, state of the ventricle. Significant increases in the level of ventricular contractility are accompanied by shifts of the ventricular function curve upward and to the left, while depression of contractility is identified by downward and rightward displacement of this relation.

It has been observed that during the adrenergic stimulation of the myocardium accompanying a stress such as exercise, relatively little change in ventricular end-diastolic size occurs, while cardiac output, aortic flow velocity, stroke work, and the rate of ventricular pressure development are all greatly augmented. Thus, reflex and humorally mediated changes in myocardial contractility, heart rate, venous return, and peripheral vascular resistance may be of greater importance in circulatory adaptation than changes in ventricular end-diastolic volume and the operation of the Frank-Starling mechanism.

The important influence of the neurotransmitter substance norepinephrine on the mechanical properties of the myocardium has long been recognized. Direct stimulation of the cardiac sympathetic nerves augments ventricular function as a consequence of the release of norepinephrine from sympathetic nerve endings in the heart. These adrenergic effects are evidenced by tachycardia, a reduction in cardiac dimensions, increased velocity of ejection, and an enhanced rate of tension development.

CONTROL OF CARDIAC PERFORMANCE AND OUTPUT

The extent of shortening of mammalian heart muscle and, therefore, the stroke volume of the intact ventricle are, in the final analysis, determined by three influences: (1) the length of the muscle at the start of contraction, i.e., the preload; (2) the inotropic state of the muscle, i.e., the position of its force-ve-

FIGURE 252-4
Diagram of a Frank-Starling curve, relating ventricular end-diastolic volume (EDV) to ventricular performance (top right) and the major influences that determine the degree of stretching of the myocardium, i.e., the magnitude of the EDV (bottom left). (From Braunwald et al, 1976.)

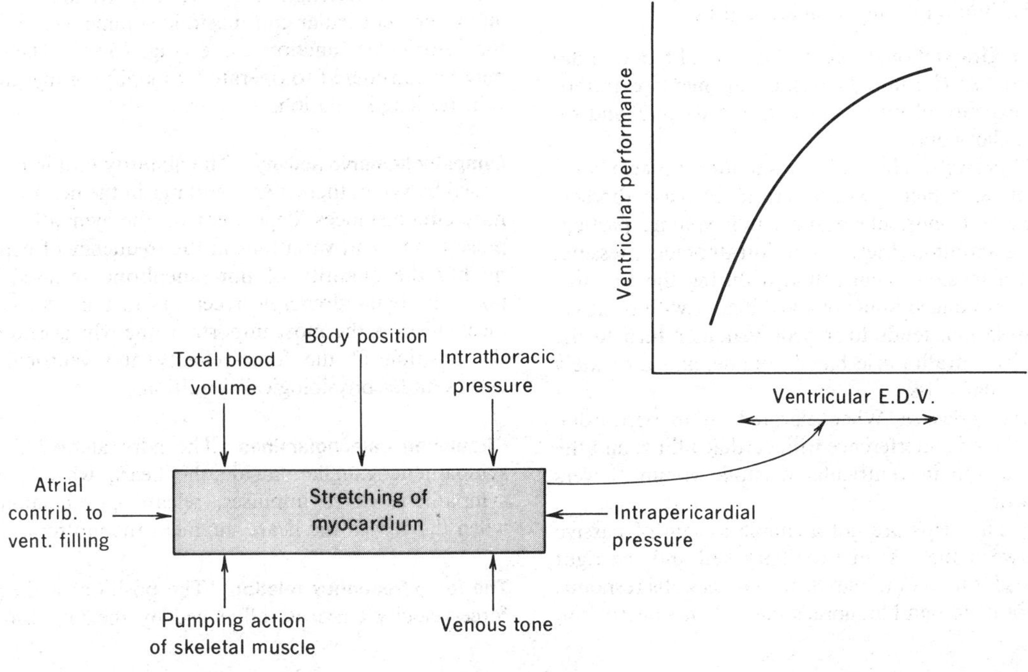

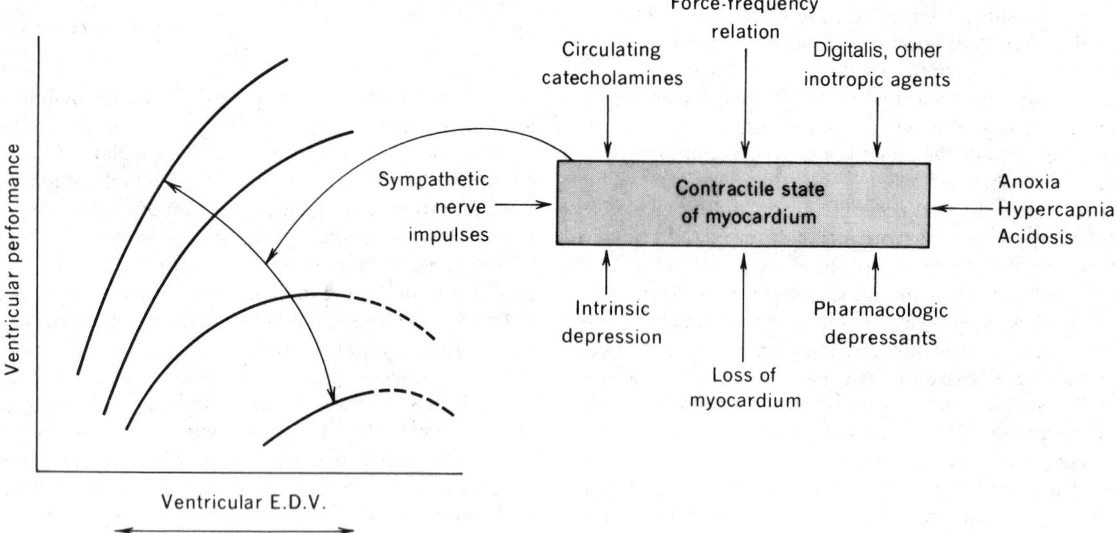

FIGURE 252-5
Diagram showing the major influences that elevate or depress the inotropic state of the myocardium (top right), and the manner in which alterations in the inotropic state of the myocardium affect the level of ventricular performance at any given level of ventricular end-diastolic volume (bottom left). (From Braunwald et al, 1976.)

locity-length relation or function curve; and (3) the tension which the muscle is called upon to develop during contraction, i.e., the afterload. Heart rate determines the cardiac output at any stroke volume as long as ventricular filling is maintained.

VENTRICULAR END-DIASTOLIC VOLUME (PRELOAD) At any level of its inotropic state, the performance of the myocardium is influenced profoundly by ventricular end-diastolic fiber length and therefore by diastolic ventricular volume. The following are the major determinants of ventricular end-diastolic volume in the intact organism (see also Fig. 252-4):

Total blood volume When depleted, as in hemorrhage, venous return to the heart declines and ventricular end-diastolic volume falls, as does ventricular performance, as reflected in ventricular work.

Distribution of blood volume At any given total blood volume, the ventricular end-diastolic volume is influenced by the distribution of blood between the intra- and extrathoracic compartments. This distribution in turn is influenced by:

1 *Body position.* Gravitational forces tend to pool blood in dependent portions. The upright posture augments extrathoracic at the expense of intrathoracic blood volume, and reduces ventricular work.
2 *Intrathoracic pressure.* Normally, mean intrathoracic pressure is negative, a factor which acts to increase thoracic blood volume and ventricular end-diastolic volume, particularly during inspiration. Elevation of intrathoracic pressure, as occurs in a tension pneumothorax, during the Valsalva maneuver, in prolonged bouts of coughing, or with positive-pressure ventilation, tends to impede venous return to the heart, diminish intrathoracic blood volume, and ultimately reduce ventricular work.
3 *Intrapericardial pressure.* When elevated, as in pericardial tamponade, there is interference with cardiac filling, and the resultant reduction in ventricular diastolic volume lowers ventricular work.
4 *Venous tone.* The veins are not a simple system of passive conduits between the systemic capillary bed and the right atrium. Instead, the smooth muscle in venous walls responds to a variety of neural and humoral stimuli. Venoconstriction occurs during muscular exercise, deep respiration, fright, or marked hypotension, tending to diminish extrathoracic and to augment intrathoracic blood volume, venous return to the heart, and ventricular performance.
5 *The pumping action of skeletal muscle.* During exercise the contracting skeletal muscles tend to squeeze blood out of the veins and, with the aid of the venous valves, to displace it centrally, thereby increasing intrathoracic blood volume, ventricular end-diastolic volume, and ventricular work.

Atrial contraction Vigorous, appropriately timed atrial contraction augments ventricular filling and end-diastolic volume. The atrial contribution to ventricular filling is of particular importance in patients with ventricular hypertrophy, in whom the loss of atrial systole (as in atrial fibrillation) tends to reduce ventricular end-diastolic pressure and volume, ultimately lowering myocardial performance.

INOTROPIC STATE (MYOCARDIAL CONTRACTILITY) A number of factors determine the level of ventricular performance at any given ventricular end-diastolic volume, i.e., the position of the ventricular function curve (Fig. 252-5). These influences may be considered to operate by modifying myocardial force-velocity-length relations.

Sympathetic nerve activity The quantity of norepinephrine released by sympathetic nerve endings in the heart is, under ordinary circumstances, dependent on the sympathetic nerve impulse traffic, and variations in the frequency of nerve impulses modify the quantity of norepinephrine released and acting upon the beta-adrenergic receptors in the myocardium. This mechanism is the most important one which acutely modifies the position of the force-velocity and ventricular function curves under physiological conditions.

Circulating catecholamines The adrenal medulla and other sympathetic ganglia outside the heart, when stimulated by sympathetic nerve impulses, release catecholamines, which, when they reach the heart, augment the inotropic state.

The force-frequency relation The position of the myocardial force-velocity curve is influenced by the rate and rhythm of cardiac contraction; e.g., ventricular extrasystoles result in post-extrasystolic potentiation, presumably by increasing the Ca^{2+} which enters the cardiac cell.

Exogenously administered inotropic agents The cardiac glycosides, isoproterenol and other sympathomimetic agents, calcium, caffeine, theophylline, and their derivatives, all improve the myocardial force-velocity relation and therefore may be used therapeutically to augment ventricular performance at any given ventricular end-diastolic volume.

Physiological depressants Included among these are severe myocardial hypoxia, hypercapnea, and acidosis. Acting either singly or in combination, these influences exert a depressant effect on the myocardial force-velocity curve and lower the level of the left ventricular work at any given ventricular end-diastolic volume.

Pharmacological depressants These include quinidine, procainamide, barbiturates, and other local and general anesthetics, as well as many other drugs.

Loss of ventricular substance When a portion of ventricular myocardium becomes nonfunctional or necrotic, as occurs temporarily in bouts of ischemia (Chap. 260), and permanently in myocardial infarction (Chap. 261), total ventricular performance at any given level of end-diastolic volume is depressed, even if the remaining myocardium functions normally.

Intrinsic myocardial depression Although the fundamental mechanisms responsible for depression of myocardial contractility in heart failure still remain to be elucidated, it is now apparent that in this condition the inotropic state of each unit of myocardium is depressed and that the level of ventricular performance at any ventricular end-diastolic volume is thereby lowered.

VENTRICULAR AFTERLOAD The stroke volume is ultimately a function of the extent of ventricular fiber shortening. As in isolated cardiac muscle, the velocity and extent of shortening of ventricular muscle fibers at any given level of diastolic fiber length and myocardial inotropic state are inversely related to the afterload imposed on the muscle. The afterload on the intact heart is dependent on the level of aortic pressure, but it may be defined as the tension or stress developed in the wall of the ventricle during ejection. Therefore, the afterload on the ventricular muscle fibers also is dependent on the size of the heart, according to Laplace's law, which indicates that the tension of the myocardial fiber is a function of the product of the intracavitary ventricular pressure and ventricular radius. Thus, at the same level of aortic pressure, the afterload faced by an enlarged left ventricle is higher than that encountered by a ventricle of normal size. The aortic pressure, in turn, is influenced largely by the peripheral vascular resistance, the physical characteristics of the arterial tree, and the volume of blood it contains at the onset of ejection. At any given ventricular end-diastolic volume and level of the inotropic state, the left ventricular stroke volume is a function of the afterload.

The critical role played by the ventricular afterload in cardiovascular regulation is summarized in Fig. 252-6. As already noted, increases in both preload and contractility increase myocardial fiber shortening, while increases in afterload reduce it. The extent of myocardial fiber shortening and left ventricular size are the determinants of stroke volume. Arterial pressure, in turn, is related to the product of cardiac output and systemic vascular resistance, while afterload is a function of left ventricular size and arterial pressure. An increase in arterial pressure induced by vasoconstriction, for example, augments afterload, which through a negative feedback depresses myocardial fiber shortening, stroke volume, and cardiac output; this in turn tends to restore arterial pressure to its previous level.

When left ventricular function becomes impaired, left ventricular afterload becomes increasingly important in determining cardiac performance. Increases in afterload may result from the influence on the arterial bed of neural, humoral, or structural changes which can occur in response to a fall in cardiac output. This increased afterload may further reduce cardiac output while myocardial oxygen requirements are increased. In this way, alterations in the peripheral vascular bed probably play an important role in the hemodynamic and metabolic events which usually are attributed to progressive impairment of the myocardium.

All of the influences acting on cardiac performance enumerated above interact in a complex fashion to maintain cardiac output at a level appropriate to the requirements of the metabolizing tissues, and in a normal person interference with one of these mechanisms may not influence the cardiac output. For example, a moderate reduction of blood volume or the loss of the atrial contribution to ventricular contraction can ordinarily be sustained without a reduction in the resting cardiac output. Presumably other factors, such as an increase in the frequency of sympathetic nerve impulses to the heart and an increase in heart rate, will, in the normal person, augment contractility and sustain output. Mechanisms are also available which prevent elevation of the cardiac output when there is no physiological demand for augmented flow. For example, augmentation of myocardial contractility by means of cardiac glycosides does not increase the cardiac output in normal humans. Thus, in analyzing the effect of an intervention on

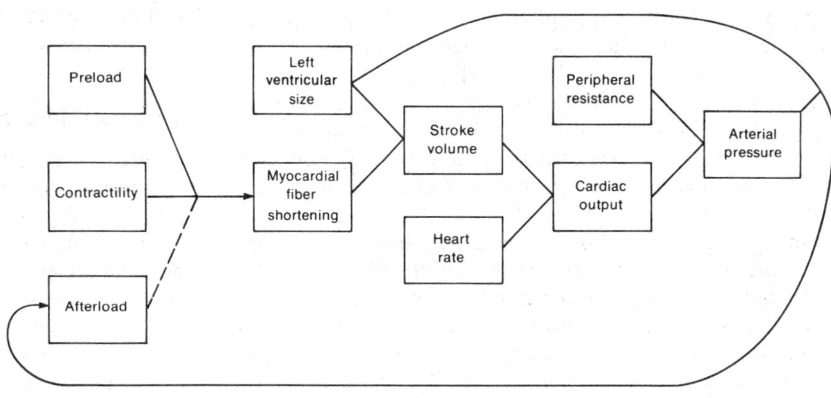

FIGURE 252-6
Scheme of interactions among various components that regulate cardiac activity. Solid lines indicate an augmenting effect; broken line represents an inhibiting effect. (From Braunwald et al, 1976.)

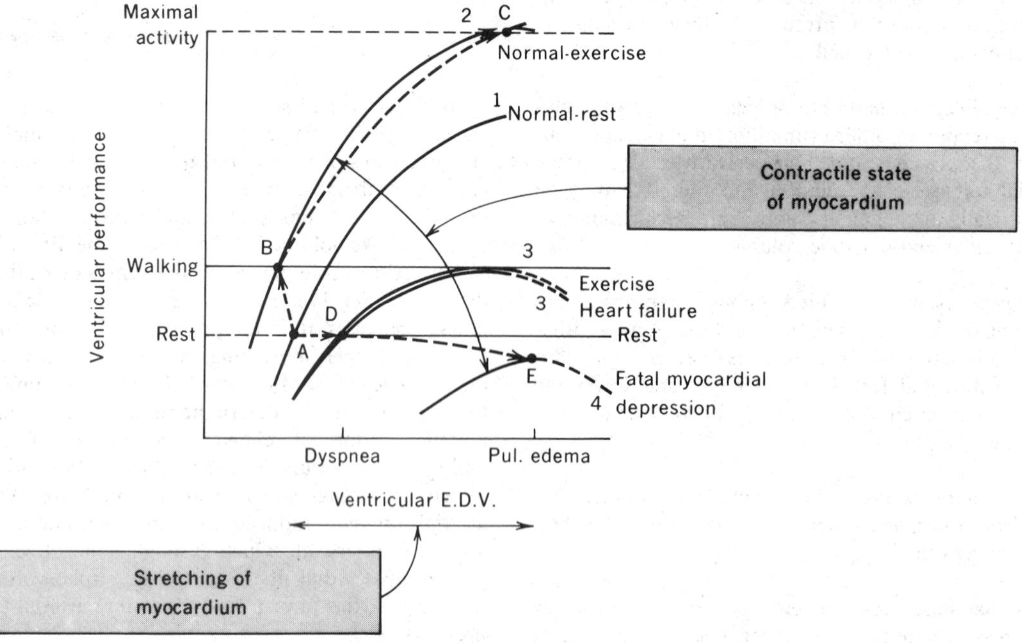

FIGURE 252-7
Diagram showing the interrelations among influences on ventricular end-diastolic volume (EDV) through stretching of the myocardium and the contractile state of the myocardium. Levels of ventricular EDV associated with filling pressures that result in dyspnea and pulmonary edema are shown on the abscissa. Levels of ventricular performance required when the subject is at rest, while walking, and during maximal activity are designated on the ordinate. The dotted lines are the descending limbs of the ventricular-performance curves, which are rarely seen during life but which show the level of ventricular performance if end-diastolic volume could be elevated to very high levels. (From Braunwald et al, 1976.)

cardiac output, it is important to recognize that under normal circumstances it is the preload, which in turn is related to the volume of blood available for filling the heart, rather than the inotropic state of the myocardium or the afterload which limits cardiac output in the normal individual and that an improvement of myocardial contractility by a drug such as digitalis or the reduction of afterload with nitroprusside should not be expected to elevate the output in a normal subject. On the other hand, in the presence of congestive heart failure, the cardiac output usually is limited by the depressed contractile state of the myocardium, and a positive inotropic influence or reduction of afterload would be expected to raise cardiac output, and, indeed, does so.

EXERCISE The hemodynamic changes which normally occur during exercise in the upright position are complex (Fig. 252-7). The hyperventilation, the pumping action of the exercising muscles, and the venoconstriction which occur all tend to augment venous return and hence ventricular filling and preload. Simultaneously, the increase in the sympathetic nerve impulses to the myocardium, the increased concentration of circulating catecholamines, and the tachycardia which occur during exercise all result in an augmentation of the contractile state of the myocardium (Fig. 252-7, curves 1 and 2) and an elevation of stroke volume, with no change or even a decrease of end-diastolic pressure and volume (Fig. 252-7, points A and B). Vasodilatation occurs in the exercising muscles, thus tending to reduce the afterload. This ultimately allows the achievement of a greatly elevated cardiac output during exercise, at an arterial pressure usually only slightly higher than in the resting state.

In heart failure, the fundamental abnormality resides in depressions of the myocardial force-velocity relationship and of the length–active tension curve, reflecting reductions in the contractile state of the myocardium (Fig. 252-7, curves 1 to 3). In many instances, cardiac output and external ventricular performance at rest are within normal limits but are maintained at these levels only by an increased end-diastolic fiber length and an elevated ventricular end-diastolic volume, i.e., through the operation of the Frank-Starling mechanism (Fig. 252-7, points A to D). The elevation of left ventricular preload is associated with similar changes in the pulmonary capillary pressure, contributing to the dyspnea experienced by patients with heart failure. The normal improvement of contractility due to augmented sympathetic activity during exercise is attenuated or even prevented by norepinephrine depletion which occurs in heart failure (Fig. 252-7, curves 3 and 3′). The factors which tend to augment ventricular filling during exercise in the normal subject push the failing myocardium even farther along its flattened length–active tension curve, and although the left ventricle may perform somewhat better, this occurs only as a consequence of an inordinate elevation of ventricular end-diastolic volume and pressure and, therefore, of the pulmonary capillary pressure. The elevation of the latter intensifies dyspnea and therefore plays an important role in limiting the intensity of exercise which the patient can perform. Left ventricular failure becomes fatal when the myocardial length–active tension curve is depressed (Fig. 252-7, curve 4) to the point at which cardiac performance fails to satisfy the requirements of the peripheral tissues even at rest, and/or the left ventricular end-diastolic and pulmonary capillary pressures are elevated to levels which result in pulmonary edema (Fig. 252-7, point E).

THE FAILING HEART

Though heart failure may be readily described as a clinical syndrome, characterized by well-known symptoms and physical signs, a precise physiological or biochemical definition is far more difficult. However, from the clinical point of view, heart failure may be considered to be the condition in which *an abnormality of cardiac function is responsible for the inability of the heart to pump blood at a rate commensurate with the requirements of the metabolizing tissues.* Though a defect in myocardial contraction is characteristic of heart failure, this defect may result from a primary abnormality in the heart muscle, as in cardiomyopathy, or it may be secondary to a chronic excessive work load as in hypertension and valvular heart disease, as well as in many forms of congenital heart disease. In ischemic heart disease heart failure results from a loss in the quantity of normally contracting cells. It is important to distinguish heart failure from (1) states of circulatory insufficiency in which myocardial function is not primarily impaired, such as cardiac tamponade or hemorrhagic shock, (2) conditions in which there is circulatory congestion because of abnormal salt and water retention but in which there is no serious disturbance of the heart's function, and (3) conditions in which a normally contracting myocardium is suddenly presented with a load which exceeds its capacity, e.g., accelerated hypertension or rupture of a valve cusp secondary to infective endocarditis.

Acute heart failure in the intact canine heart, studied in situ or in the heart-lung preparation, is characterized by a depression of ventricular stroke volume or stroke work at any given level of left ventricular end-diastolic volume or filling pressure. Further, as diastolic volume is augmented in the failing heart, an abnormally small increase or no change in stroke volume occurs. Thus, in an effort to maintain stroke volume at a normal level, the heart dilates and the Frank-Starling mechanism therefore might be considered one of the first lines of defense called upon to maintain cardiac output when myocardial contractility declines. An increase in the end-diastolic volume of the ventricle permits the ejection of a larger stroke volume, even when the extent of shortening of individual muscle fibers remains constant. The fact that when end-diastolic volume is augmented in the failing heart, stroke volume shows little change or is actually diminished clearly indicates that the relative degree of muscle fiber shortening must have decreased. Thus, an important mechanical defect which can be delineated in acute heart failure is a decrease in the extent of shortening of cardiac muscle fibers.

The intrinsic contractile state of myocardium removed from normal, hypertrophied, and failing animal hearts has been evaluated, and both ventricular hypertrophy and heart failure were shown to reduce the maximum isometric tension and velocity of shortening to subnormal levels; the changes were more marked in the myocardium of animals in which heart failure had been present than in those with hypertrophy alone. However, ventricular hypertrophy, in the absence of heart failure, also appears to be associated with a depression of the inotropic state per unit of myocardium, although the absolute increase of total muscle mass maintains overall cardiac compensation. Papillary muscles removed from the left ventricles of patients with heart failure have also shown a depression of the maximum degree of active tension which they can develop. Electron-microscopic analysis of failing cat papillary muscles fixed at the apexes of the length–active tension curves revealed sarcomere lengths averaging 2.2 μm. Thus, the abnormalities of contractility do *not* appear to be produced by an alteration in the overlap of filaments within the sarcomere.

The failing ventricle may still eject a normal or nearly normal stroke volume despite considerable depression of function, when its end-diastolic volume increases, i.e., through the operation of the Frank-Starling mechanism. As outlined above, an increase in the initial volume of the ventricle is associated with stretching of the sarcomere, a process which augments the number of sites at which the actin and myosin filaments can interact and/or which increases their sensitivity to Ca^{2+}. Furthermore, the development of ventricular hypertrophy may be considered to provide additional contractile units, and thereby constitutes an important compensatory mechanism when the myocardium's intrinsic inotropic state is depressed.

Several techniques are available for defining impaired ventricular contractility in intact humans. With the patient at rest, the cardiac output and stroke volume may be depressed, but not uncommonly these variables are within normal limits. A more sensitive index is the ejection fraction, i.e., the ratio of stroke volume to end-diastolic volume, which may be estimated by standard radiologic or radionuclide angiography (Chaps. 250 and 251), and which is frequently depressed in heart failure even when the stroke volume itself is normal. An even more sensitive method for detecting impaired ventricular performance is based on the measurement of the circulatory changes occurring during stresses such as exercise or increased afterload. Thus, left ventricular performance may be estimated accurately by measuring the left ventricular end-diastolic pressure, cardiac output, and total body O_2 consumption at rest and during exercise. In normal persons, the cardiac output rises by more than 500 ml/min for each 100-ml increase in minute O_2 consumption. The left ventricular end-diastolic pressure at rest is less than 12 mmHg and rises slightly, remains unchanged, or decreases slightly during exercise, while stroke volume usually rises. The failing left ventricle, on the other hand, is characterized by an elevation of end-diastolic pressure during exercise, which reaches a value exceeding 12 mmHg, accompanied by either no change or a fall in stroke volume and a subnormal increase in cardiac output related to the increase in minute O_2 consumption. Various degrees of impairment intermediate between the normal response and that of the failing left ventricle during the stress of exercise also have been described.

The potential value of stressing the left ventricle is emphasized by the fact that the basal values for left ventricular end-diastolic pressure, cardiac index, and ventricular stroke work may be in the same range in patients with depressed ventricular function as in normal persons. The response to stress may prove useful not only in the detection of the impairment of myocardial function, but also in expressing the severity of this impairment quantitatively.

The performance of the left ventricle in humans may also be characterized by examining the instantaneous myocardial force-velocity relations and the extent of shortening during individual cardiac cycles. Angiocardiographic and echocardiographic studies (Chap. 250) and analyses of the rate of change of intraventricular pressure (*dp/dt*) as a function of the simultaneously recorded pressure during isovolumetric contraction have shown that depressions in the velocity of myocardial fiber shortening and of tension development exist in patients with heart failure. Further evidence for reductions in the velocity of myocardial fiber shortening is provided by the finding of a reduced mean systolic ejection rate in patients with heart failure and a failure of the mean systolic ejection rate to rise normally during muscular exercise. Noninvasive, graphic techniques, particularly echocardiography and radionuclide angiography, are of great value in the clinical assessment of myocardial function (Chap. 250).

CARDIAC METABOLISM IN HEART FAILURE The common forms of low-output heart failure, secondary to arteriosclerosis, hypertension, and certain valvular and congenital lesions, are characterized by an absolute or a relative reduction in the useful external work delivered by the heart. Considerable attention has been directed to the question of whether cardiac failure is due to a defect in the production of energy, its conservation, or its utilization. Only in isolated instances of heart failure, such as those associated with beriberi, are there clear-cut disturbances of myocardial energy production. The major pathway by which pyruvate enters the citric acid cycle and some reactions within the cycle itself are dependent on the presence of adequate concentrations of thiamine (Chap. 85). Thiamine deficiency results in diminished pyruvic acid utilization by heart slices, and in abnormally low pyruvate extraction coefficients in intact dogs and in humans.

The principal defect in the common forms of low-output heart failure does not appear to be in an impairment of energy production by the myocardium through the oxidation of substrate. In the second phase of cardiac metabolism, energy conservation, the energy of substrate oxidation is converted into the terminal-bond energy of creatine phosphate (CP) and of ATP, the immediate source of chemical energy utilized by heart muscle. This process, known as oxidative phosphorylation, occurs in the mitochondria. The effectiveness of the combined energy production-conservation mechanisms may be studied by measuring the stores of ATP and CP existing in the myocardium, while energy conservation may be evaluated by determining (1) the P/O ratio, i.e., the ratio of high-energy phosphate produced to oxygen consumed in the mitochondria, and (2) the degree of coupling between electron transport and the generation of high-energy phosphate compounds. Although lively controversy exists concerning the status of this phase of metabolism in heart failure, it now appears that severe impairment of myocardial performance may occur *without* disturbances of mitochondrial function or reduction of high-energy phosphate stores, although abnormalities in these processes do occur in some forms of experimental heart failure. Thus, there may be an inability of the energy-producing system to keep pace with the increased energy needs of the hypertrophied contractile system.

In the absence of a definitive abnormality of energy liberation or conservation in the failing myocardium, attention has naturally been directed to the possibility that energy *utilization* is abnormal. An abnormality of energy liberation could certainly occur if the contractile proteins themselves were altered. A cardiac myosin isoenzyme characterized by immunological and electrophoretic properties exhibiting a lower Ca^{2+}-dependent ATPase activity has been shown in some forms of experimentally produced heart failure, particularly those produced by mechanical overloading. It is possible that this depression may be responsible for a defect in the breakdown of ATP, the process which leads to contraction. In addition, substantial evidence has been obtained that in heart failure there is an *abnormality of excitation-contraction coupling,* which alters the delivery of Ca^{2+} to the contractile sites, thereby impairing cardiac performance.

THE ADRENERGIC NERVOUS SYSTEM IN HEART FAILURE In view of the importance of the adrenergic nervous system in stimulating the contractility of the normal myocardium, the activity of this system has also been studied intensively in patients with congestive heart failure. An index of the activity of this system, at rest and during exercise, is provided by measurements of the concentration of norepinephrine (NE) in arterial blood. No change or very little increase in the NE concentrations occurs during exercise in normal subjects; much greater increases are seen in patients with congestive heart failure, presumably because of an increased activity of the adrenergic nervous system during exercise in these patients. Marked elevations of a 24-h urinary NE excretion occur in patients with heart failure, indicating that the activity of their adrenergic nervous systems is also augmented at rest.

The importance of the increased activity of the adrenergic nervous system in maintaining ventricular contractility when the function of the myocardium is depressed in congestive heart failure also is shown by the effects of adrenergic blockade in patients with heart failure. Antiadrenergic drugs such as propranolol or guanethidine may cause sodium and water retention, as well as intensify heart failure. The adrenergic nervous system thus plays an important compensatory role in the circulatory adjustments of patients to congestive heart failure, and caution must be exercised in the use of antiadrenergic drugs, particularly beta-adrenergic blocking agents, in the treatment of patients with limited cardiac reserve (Chap. 253).

Both the concentration and content of the NE in atrial and ventricular tissue in patients with heart failure are reduced, sometimes to only 10 percent of normal. This reduction in NE content in the heart is not the result of a simple dilution of sympathetic nerve endings in a hypertrophied muscle mass. The mechanism responsible for the depletion of cardiac NE stores is not entirely clear. A prolonged increase in cardiac sympathetic tone appears to play a critical role and to interfere in some manner with the biosynthesis of NE. Deficiencies in the activities of two of the enzymes involved in biosynthesis—tyrosine hydroxylase and dopamine oxidase—have been incriminated. Also, there is evidence that the beta-adrenergic receptor density is reduced in the chronically failing heart.

In view of the strongly positive inotropic effect exerted by the NE released from these nerves, the adrenergic nervous system may be considered to provide an important potential source of support to the failing myocardium. However, the increments of heart rate and contractile force which occur in animals with experimental heart failure and cardiac NE depletion are abolished or markedly reduced with stimulation of the cardiac sympathetic nerves. Thus, it is likely that when congestive heart failure is accompanied by depletion of cardiac NE stores, the quantity of NE released by the sympathetic nerve endings in the heart is deficient relative to the impulse traffic along these nerves.

Cardiac stores of NE are not fundamentally necessary for maintaining the intrinsic contractile state of the myocardium. However, since the reduction of NE stores in heart failure is associated with a diminished release of neurotransmitter, this depletion of NE may be responsible for loss of the much-needed adrenergic support in the failing heart. In the later stages of heart failure, when the levels of circulating catecholamines are elevated and the cardiac NE stores depleted, the myocardium is largely dependent on a more generalized adrenergic stimulation derived from extracardiac sources, presumably the adrenal medulla; this would explain the deterioration of cardiac performance which may occur in patients with heart failure who are treated with beta-adrenergic blocking drugs. This generalized adrenergic stimulation resulting from circulating catecholamines may, however, also exert undesirable side effects, because it elevates vascular resistance and may present the heart with an afterload which is higher than optimal.

REFERENCES

BRAUNWALD E et al (eds): *Congestive Heart Failure: Current Research and Clinical Applications.* New York, Grune & Stratton, 1982

———, et al: *Mechanisms of Contraction of the Normal and Failing Heart,* 2d ed. Boston, Little, Brown, 1976

———, Ross J: Control of cardiac performance, in *Handbook of Physiology,* sec 2, vol 1, RM Berne (ed). Washington, DC, American Physiological Society, 1979, pp 553–580

———, Sonnenblick EH, Ross J: Contraction of the normal heart, in *Heart Disease,* 2d ed, E Braunwald (ed). Philadelphia, Saunders, 1983, chap 12

FISHMAN AP (ed): *Heart Failure.* Washington, DC, Hemisphere, McGraw-Hill, 1978

FORD LE: Effect of afterload reduction myocardial energetics. Circ Res 46:161, 1980

JAMES TN: Ultrastructure of the myocardium, in *The Heart,* 5th ed, JW Hurst et al (eds). New York, McGraw-Hill, 1982, chap 2, p 57

LOMPRE AM et al: Myosin isoenzyme redistribution in chronic heart overload. Nature 282:105, 1979

SORDAHL LA: Some biochemical lesions in myocardial disease. Tex Rep Biol Med 38:121, 1979

THOMAS JA, MARKS BM: Plasma norepinephrine in congestive heart failure. Am J Cardiol 41:233, 1978

253
HEART FAILURE

EUGENE BRAUNWALD

Heart failure may be defined as the pathophysiologic state in which an abnormality of *cardiac* function is responsible for the failure of the heart to pump blood at a rate commensurate with the requirements of the metabolizing tissues. Heart failure is frequently, but not always, caused by a defect in myocardial contraction, and then the term *myocardial failure* is appropriate. The latter may result from a primary abnormality in the heart muscle, as occurs in the cardiomyopathies (Chap. 263). Myocardial failure may also result from extramyocardial abnormalities, such as coronary atherosclerosis which leads to myocardial ischemia, as well as from abnormalities of the heart valves in which the heart muscle is damaged by the long-standing excessive hemodynamic burden imposed by the valvular abnormality, and/or by the rheumatic process (Chap. 258). In patients with chronic constrictive pericarditis, myocardial damage resulting from infiltration of the heart muscle by pericardial inflammation and calcification is common (Chap. 265).

In other patients with heart failure, however, a similar clinical syndrome is present, but without any detectable abnormality of *myocardial* function. In these patients the normal heart is suddenly presented with a load that exceeds its capacity, such as an acute hypertensive crisis, rupture of an aortic valve cusp, or massive pulmonary embolism. Heart failure, in the presence of normal myocardial function, also occurs in chronic conditions in which there is impairment of filling of the ventricles due to tricuspid and/or mitral stenosis, constrictive pericarditis without myocardial involvement, and endocardial fibrosis.

Heart failure should be distinguished from (1) conditions in which there is circulatory congestion consequent to abnormal salt and water retention but in which there is no disturbance of cardiac function per se (the latter syndrome, termed the *congested state,* may result from the abnormal salt and water retention of renal failure, or from excess parenteral administration of fluids and electrolytes), and (2) from noncardiac causes of inadequate cardiac output, including shock due to hypovolemia and redistribution of blood volume (Chap. 29).

CAUSES OF HEART FAILURE

In evaluating patients with heart failure, it is important to identify not only the *underlying cause* of the heart disease but the *precipitating cause* of heart failure as well. The cardiac abnormality produced by a congenital or acquired lesion may exist for many years and produce no or only trivial disability. Frequently, however, the manifestations of clinical heart failure appear for the first time in the course of some acute disturbance which places an additional load on a myocardium that chronically is excessively burdened, resulting in further deterioration of cardiac function. Identification of such precipitating causes is of critical importance because their prompt alleviation may be lifesaving. However, in the absence of underlying heart disease these acute disturbances do not usually, by themselves, lead to heart failure.

PRECIPITATING CAUSES

1 *Pulmonary embolism.* Patients with low cardiac output, circulatory stasis, and physical inactivity are at increased risk of developing thrombi in the veins of the lower extremities or the pelvis. Pulmonary embolization may result in further elevation of pulmonary arterial pressure, which in turn may produce or intensify failure of the right ventricle. In the presence of pulmonary vascular congestion, such emboli may also cause infarction of the lung (Chap. 282).

2 *Infection.* Patients with pulmonary vascular congestion are also more susceptible to pulmonary infections, but any infection may precipitate heart failure. The resulting fever, tachycardia, hypoxemia, and the increased metabolic demands may place a further burden on the overloaded, but compensated, myocardium of a patient with chronic heart disease.

3 *Anemia.* In the presence of anemia the oxygen needs of the metabolizing tissues can be satisfied only by an increase in the cardiac output (Chap. 54); though such an increase in the cardiac output might be sustained by a normal heart, a diseased, overloaded, but otherwise compensated heart may be unable to augment the volume of blood which it delivers to the periphery.

4 *Thyrotoxicosis and pregnancy.* As in anemia and fever, in these conditions adequate tissue perfusion requires an increased cardiac output. The development or intensification of heart failure may actually be one of the first clinical manifestations of hyperthyroidism in a patient with underlying heart disease (Chap. 111). Similarly, heart failure not infrequently occurs for the first time during pregnancy in women with rheumatic valvular disease in whom cardiac compensation may return following delivery.

5 *Arrhythmias.* These are among the most frequent precipitating causes of heart failure in patients with underlying but compensated heart disease for a variety of reasons: (*a*) tachyarrhythmias reduce the time period available for ventricular filling; (*b*) the dissociation between atrial and ventricular contractions characteristic of many arrhythmias result in the loss of the atrial booster pump mechanism, thereby tending to raise atrial pressures; (*c*) in any arrhythmia associated with abnormal intraventricular conduction, myocardial performance may become further impaired because of the loss of normal synchronicity of ventricular contraction; (*d*) the marked bradycardia associated with complete atrioventricular block requires a greatly elevated stroke volume if a marked reduction in cardiac output is to be prevented.

6 *Rheumatic and other forms of myocarditis.* Acute rheumatic fever and a variety of infectious or inflammatory processes affecting the myocardium may further impair myocardial function in patients with preexisting heart disease (Chaps. 257 and 263).

7 *Infective endocarditis.* The additional valvular damage, anemia, fever, and myocarditis which often occur as a consequence of infective endocarditis may, singly or in concert, precipitate heart failure (Chap. 259).

8 *Physical, dietary, environmental, and emotional excesses.* The augmentation of sodium intake, the discontinuation of medications to treat heart failure, physical overexertion, excessive environmental heat or humidity, and emotional crises may all precipitate cardiac decompensation.

9 *Systemic hypertension.* Rapid elevation of arterial pressure, as may occur in some instances of hypertension of renal origin or upon discontinuation of antihypertensive medica-

tion, may result in cardiac decompensation (Chap. 267).

10 *Myocardial infarction.* In patients with chronic but compensated ischemic heart disease, a fresh infarct, often otherwise silent clinically, may further impair ventricular function and precipitate heart failure (Chap. 261).

A systematic search for these precipitating causes should be made in every patient with heart failure, particularly if it is refractory to the usual methods of therapy. If properly recognized, the precipitating cause of heart failure can usually be treated more effectively than the underlying cause. Therefore, the prognosis in patients with heart failure in whom a precipitating cause can be identified and treated is more favorable than in patients in whom the underlying disease process has advanced to the point of producing heart failure.

FORMS OF HEART FAILURE

Heart failure may be described as *high-output* or *low-output, acute* or *chronic, right-sided* or *left-sided,* and *forward* or *backward.* Although these terms may be useful in a clinical setting, they are descriptive and do not signify fundamentally different disease states.

HIGH-OUTPUT VERSUS LOW-OUTPUT HEART FAILURE With the development of methods for the measurement of cardiac output, it became useful to classify patients with heart failure into those with a low cardiac output, i.e., *low-output heart failure,* and those with an elevated cardiac output, i.e., *high-output heart failure.* The cardiac output is often depressed in patients with heart failure secondary to ischemic heart disease, hypertension, cardiomyopathy and valvular and pericardial disease, but tends to be elevated in patients with heart failure and hyperthyroidism, anemia, arteriovenous fistulas, beriberi, and Paget's disease. In clinical practice, however, it is not always easy to distinguish between low-output and high-output heart failure. The normal range of cardiac output is wide [2.5 to 4.0 (liters/min)/m^2], and in many patients with so-called low-output heart failure the cardiac output may actually be near the lower limits of normal at rest, although it may fail to rise normally during exertion. On the other hand, in patients with so-called high-output heart failure the output may not be excessive but rather may be close to the upper limit of normal, particularly when heart failure is severe. Regardless of the absolute level of the cardiac output, however, cardiac failure may be said to be present when the characteristic clinical manifestations described below are accompanied by a depression of the curve relating ventricular end-diastolic volume to cardiac performance (Fig. 252-5).

An integral part of the heart failure syndrome is evidence that the heart does not deliver the quantity of oxygen required by the metabolizing tissues. In the absence of peripheral shunting of blood, such inadequate delivery of oxygen to the metabolizing tissues is reflected in an abnormal widening of the normal arterial-mixed venous oxygen difference (3.5 to 5.0 ml/dl in the basal state), relative to the total body oxygen consumption. In mild cases, such an abnormality may not be present at rest but become evident only during exertion or other hypermetabolic states. In patients with the high-output cardiac states associated with arteriovenous fistula, beriberi, thyrotoxicosis, Paget's disease, etc., the arterial-mixed venous oxygen difference is often abnormally low, because the mixed venous oxygen saturation is raised by the admixture of blood which has been diverted from the metabolizing tissues, and it may be presumed that even in these patients the delivery of oxygen to the latter is reduced despite the normal or even elevated mixed venous oxygen saturation. When heart failure occurs in such patients, the arterial-mixed venous oxygen difference may be normal or even reduced, but it still exceeds the level which existed prior to the development of heart failure, and therefore the cardiac output, though normal or elevated, is lower than before heart failure occurred.

The mechanisms responsible for the development of heart failure in patients whose cardiac outputs are initially high are complex and depend on the underlying disease process. In most of these conditions the heart is called upon to pump abnormally large quantities of blood in order to deliver the normal quota of oxygen to the metabolizing tissues. The burden placed on the myocardium by the increased flow load resembles that produced by regurgitant valvular lesions. In addition, thyrotoxicosis and beriberi may impair myocardial metabolism directly, and severe anemia may interfere with myocardial function by producing myocardial anoxia.

ACUTE VERSUS CHRONIC HEART FAILURE The prototype of acute heart failure develops in patients with large myocardial infarctions or valve rupture, while chronic heart failure is typically observed in patients with slowly progressive dilated cardiomyopathy or multivalvular heart disease. In acute failure, the sudden reduction in cardiac output often results in systemic hypotension without peripheral edema, while in chronic heart failure, arterial pressure tends to be well maintained, but there is accumulation of edema. Frequently, however, there is no fundamental distinction between acute and chronic failure. For example, intensive efforts to prevent expansion of blood volume by means of dietary sodium restriction and the administration of diuretics will frequently delay the development of exertional dyspnea and edema in patients with chronic valvular heart disease, i.e., it will mask the clinical manifestations of chronic heart failure, until an acute episode, such as an arrhythmia or infection precipitates acute heart failure. Without intensive efforts to restrict blood volume the same patients would have been considered to have been suffering from chronic heart failure, even though their underlying myocardial disease were no further advanced.

RIGHT-SIDED VERSUS LEFT-SIDED HEART FAILURE Many of the clinical manifestations of heart failure result from the accumulation of excess fluid behind one or both ventricles (Chaps. 26 and 28). This fluid usually localizes upstream to the specific cardiac chamber which is initially affected. For example, patients in whom the left ventricle is mechanically overloaded (e.g., aortic stenosis) or weakened (e.g., postmyocardial infarction) develop dyspnea and orthopnea as a result of pulmonary congestion, a condition referred to as *left-sided heart failure.* In contrast, when the underlying abnormality affects the right ventricle primarily, e.g., valvular pulmonic stenosis or pulmonary hypertension secondary to pulmonary thromboembolism, symptoms resulting from pulmonary congestion such as orthopnea or paroxysmal nocturnal dyspnea are less common, and edema, congestive hepatomegaly, and systemic venous distention, i.e., clinical manifestations of *right-sided heart failure,* are more prominent. However, when heart failure has existed for months or years, such localization behind the failing ventricle may no longer exist. For example, patients with long-standing aortic valve disease or systemic hypertension may have ankle edema, congestive hepatomegaly, and systemic venous distention late in the course of their disease, even though the abnormal hemodynamic burden initially was placed on the left ventricle, in part because of the secondary pulmonary hypertension and resultant right-sided heart failure, but also because of the persistent retention of salt and water. It is also useful to recall that the muscle bundles composing both ventricles are continuous and both ventricles share a common wall, the interventricular septum. Also, biochemical changes which occur in heart failure and which may be involved in the impairment of myocardial function, such as norepinephrine depletion and alterations in the activity of myosin ATPase, occur in the myocardium of both ventricles, regardless of the specific chamber on which the abnormal hemodynamic burden is placed.

BACKWARD VERSUS FORWARD HEART FAILURE For many years a controversy has revolved around the question of the mechanism of the clinical manifestations resulting from heart failure. The concept of *backward heart failure,* propounded by James Hope in 1832, contends that when heart failure occurs, one or the other ventricle fails to discharge its contents normally, the end-diastolic volume of the ventricle rises, the pressures and volumes in the atrium and venous system behind the failing ventricle become elevated, and retention of sodium and water occurs as a consequence of the elevation of systemic venous and capillary pressures and the resultant transudation of fluid into the interstitial space (Chap. 28). In contrast, the proponents of the *forward heart failure* hypothesis, expounded by MacKenzie in 1913, maintain that the clinical manifestations of heart failure result directly from an inadequate discharge of blood into the arterial system. Salt and water retention, then, is a consequence of diminished renal perfusion and excessive proximal tubular sodium reabsorption and of excessive distal tubular reabsorption, through activation of the renin-angiotensin-aldosterone system.

A rigid distinction between *backward* and *forward heart failure* is artificial, since both mechanisms appear to operate to varying extents in most patients with heart failure. However, the rate of onset of heart failure often influences the clinical manifestations. For example, when a large portion of the left ventricle is suddenly destroyed, as in myocardial infarction, acute pulmonary edema may develop rapidly, and although stroke volume is reduced, the patient may die of acute pulmonary edema, a manifestation of backward failure, before the reduced cardiac output can be responsible for the renal retention of salt and water. However, if the patient survives the acute insult, clinical manifestations resulting from the abnormal retention of fluid within the systemic vascular bed might develop. Similarly, the right ventricle may dilate and the systemic venous pressure may rise to high levels immediately following acute massive pulmonary embolism, but this state may have to be maintained for some days before sodium and water retention sufficient to produce peripheral edema occurs.

REDISTRIBUTION OF CARDIAC OUTPUT The redistribution of cardiac output also serves as an important compensatory mechanism when flow is reduced. This redistribution is most marked when a patient with heart failure exercises or when an additional burden is imposed, such as fever or anemia, but as heart failure advances, redistribution occurs even in the basal state. Blood flow is redistributed so that the delivery of oxygen to vital organs, such as the brain and myocardium, is maintained at normal or near-normal levels, while flow to less critical areas, such as the cutaneous and muscular beds and splanchnic viscera, is reduced. Vasoconstriction mediated by the sympathetic nervous system is largely responsible for this redistribution, which in turn may be responsible for many of the clinical manifestations of heart failure, such as fluid accumulation (reduction of renal flow), low-grade fever (reduction of cutaneous flow), and fatigue (reduction of muscle flow).

SALT AND WATER RETENTION IN CHRONIC HEART FAILURE (See also Chap. 28)

When the volume of blood pumped by the left ventricle into the systemic vascular bed is chronically reduced, and when one or both of the ventricles fail to expel the normal fraction of their end-diastolic volume, a complex sequence of adjustments occurs which ultimately results in the abnormal accumulation of fluid. Though, on the one hand, many of the clinical manifestations of heart failure are secondary to this excessive retention of fluid, on the other hand, this abnormal fluid accumulation and the expansion of blood volume which accompanies it also constitutes an important compensatory mechanism which tends to maintain cardiac output and therefore perfusion of the vital organs. Except in the terminal stages of heart failure, the ventricle operates on an ascending, albeit depressed and flattened function curve (Fig. 252-7), and the augmented ventricular end-diastolic volume and pressure characteristic of heart failure must be regarded as aiding the maintenance of cardiac output, despite causing pulmonary and systemic venous congestion.

In the presence of heart failure, effective filling of the systemic arterial tree is reduced, a condition which initiates the complex hemodynamic, renal, and hormonal adjustments that interact to promote reduced renal sodium and water excretion. Patients with very severe heart failure often exhibit a reduced capacity to excrete a water load, which may result in dilutional hyponatremia. These abnormalities may be caused, in part, by excess antidiuretic hormone activity and/or factors that prevent sodium reabsorption in the distal tubule, such as avid proximal tubular reabsorption of sodium or the action of a diuretic acting on the distal tubule.

The importance of elevated systemic venous pressure and of the alterations of renal and adrenal function characteristic of heart failure vary in their relative importance in the production of edema in different patients with heart failure. The renin-angiotensin-aldosterone axis is activated most intensely by acute heart failure, and its activity tends to decline as heart failure becomes chronic. In patients with tricuspid valve disease or constrictive pericarditis the elevated venous pressure and the transudation of fluid from systemic capillaries appear to play the dominant role in edema formation. On the other hand, severe edema may be present in patients with ischemic or hypertensive heart disease, in whom systemic venous pressure is within normal limits or is only minimally elevated. In such patients, the fluid retention is probably due primarily to a redistribution of cardiac output and a concomitant reduction in renal perfusion, as well as activation of the renin-angiotensin-aldosterone axis. Regardless of the mechanisms involved in fluid retention, untreated patients with chronic congestive heart failure have elevations of total blood volume, interstitial fluid volume, and body sodium. These abnormalities diminish after clinical compensation has been achieved by treatment.

CLINICAL MANIFESTATIONS OF HEART FAILURE

Dyspnea Respiratory distress which occurs as the result of increased effort in breathing is the most common symptom of heart failure (Chap. 26). Dyspnea is at first observed only during activity, when it may simply represent an aggravation of the breathlessness which normally occurs under these circumstances. As heart failure advances, however, it appears with progressively less strenuous activity. Ultimately, breathlessness is present even when the patient is at rest. Thus, the chief difference between exertional dyspnea in normal persons and in cardiac patients is the degree of activity necessary to induce the symptom. Cardiac dyspnea is observed most frequently in patients with elevations of left atrial, pulmonary venous, and pulmonary capillary pressures. Such patients have engorged pulmonary vessels and interstitial pulmonary edema, which reduces the compliance of the lungs and thereby increases the work of the respiratory muscles required to inflate the lungs.

The activation of receptors in the lungs results in the rapid, shallow breathing of cardiac dyspnea. The oxygen cost of breathing is increased by the excessive work of the respiratory muscles. This is coupled with the diminished delivery of oxygen to these muscles, which occurs as a consequence of the reduced cardiac output and which may contribute to fatigue of the respiratory muscles and the sensation of shortness of breath.

Orthopnea Dyspnea in the recumbent position occurs in part because of the redistribution of fluid from the abdomen and lower extremities into the chest as well as an increase in the average pulmonary capillary hydrostatic pressure. Patients with orthopnea generally elevate their heads on several pillows at night and frequently awaken short of breath if their heads slip off the pillows. The sensation of breathlessness usually is relieved by sitting bolt upright, since this position reduces venous return and pulmonary capillary pressure, and many patients report that they find relief from sitting in front of an open window. As heart failure advances, orthopnea may be so severe that patients cannot lie down at all and must spend the entire night in a sitting position. On the other hand, in other patients with long-standing, severe heart failure, symptoms of pulmonary congestion may actually diminish with time as the function of the right ventricle becomes impaired.

Paroxysmal (nocturnal) dyspnea This term refers to attacks of severe shortness of breath which generally occur at night and usually awaken the patient from sleep. Though simple orthopnea may be relieved by sitting upright at the side of the bed with legs dependent, in the patient with paroxysmal nocturnal dyspnea coughing and wheezing often persist even in this position. The depression of the respiratory center during sleep may reduce ventilation sufficiently to lower arterial oxygen tension, particularly in patients with interstitial lung edema and reduced pulmonary compliance. Also, ventricular function may be further impaired at night because of reduced adrenergic stimulation of myocardial function. Acute pulmonary edema (Chap. 26) is a severe form of cardiac asthma due to further elevation of pulmonary capillary pressure leading to alveolar edema, associated with extreme shortness of breath, rales over both lung fields, and the transudation and expectoration of blood-tinged fluid. If not treated promptly acute pulmonary edema may be fatal.

Cheyne-Stokes respiration Also known as *periodic* or *cyclic respiration,* Cheyne-Stokes respiration is characterized by diminished sensitivity of the respiratory center. There is an apneic phase, during which the arterial P_{O_2} falls and the arterial P_{CO_2} rises. These changes in the arterial blood stimulate the depressed respiratory center, resulting in hyperventilation and hypocapnia, followed in turn by apnea. Cheyne-Stokes respiration occurs most often in patients with cerebral atherosclerosis and other cerebral lesions, but the prolongation of the circulation time from the lung to the brain which occurs in heart failure, particularly in patients with hypertension and coronary artery disease and associated cerebral vascular disease, also appears to precipitate this form of breathing.

Fatigue and weakness These nonspecific but common symptoms of heart failure are related to the reduction of perfusion of skeletal muscle. Anorexia and nausea associated with abdominal pain and fullness are frequent complaints which may be related to the congested liver and portal venous system.

Cerebral symptoms In severe heart failure, particularly in elderly patients with accompanying cerebral arteriosclerosis, arterial hypoxemia, and reduced cerebral perfusion, there may be alterations in the mental state characterized by confusion, difficulty in concentration, and impairment of memory, headache, insomnia, and anxiety.

PHYSICAL FINDINGS In moderate heart failure the patient appears to be in no distress at rest except that he may become uncomfortable if asked to lie flat for more than a few minutes. In more severe heart failure the pulse pressure may be diminished, reflecting a reduction in stroke volume, and occasionally the diastolic arterial pressure may be elevated as a consequence of generalized vasoconstriction. There may be cyanosis of the lips and nail bed and sinus tachycardia. *Systemic venous pressure* is often abnormally elevated in heart failure and may be recognized most readily by observing the extent of distention of the jugular veins. In the early stages of heart failure the venous pressure may be normal at rest but may become abnormally elevated during and immediately after exertion as well as with sustained pressure on the abdomen (positive abdominojugular reflux).

Third and fourth heart sounds (Chap. 248) are often audible but are not specific for heart failure, and *pulsus alternans,* i.e., a regular rhythm in which there is alternation of strong and weak cardiac contractions and therefore alternation in the strength of the peripheral pulses, may be present. Pulsus alternans may be detected by sphygmomanometry and in more severe instances by palpation; it frequently follows an extrasystole and is observed most commonly in patients with cardiomyopathy or with hypertensive or ischemic heart disease. It is caused by a reduction in the number of contractile units during weak contractions and/or by alternation in the ventricular end-diastolic volume.

Basal pulmonary rales Moist, inspiratory, crepitant rales and dullness to percussion over the posterior lung bases are common in patients with heart failure and elevated pulmonary venous and capillary pressures. In patients with pulmonary edema, rales may be heard widely over both lung fields; they are frequently coarse and sibilant and may be accompanied by expiratory wheezing. Rales may, however, be caused by many conditions other than left ventricular failure.

Cardiac edema Cardiac edema is usually dependent, occurring in the legs symmetrically, particularly in the pretibial region and ankles in ambulatory patients, and in the sacral region of individuals at bed rest. Pitting edema of the arms and face occurs rarely and only late in the course of heart failure.

Hydrothorax and ascites Pleural effusion in congestive heart failure results from the elevation of pleural capillary pressure and transudation of fluid into the pleural cavities. Since the pleural veins drain into both the systemic and pulmonary veins, hydrothorax occurs most commonly with marked elevation of pressure in both venous systems, but may also occur with marked elevation of pressure in either venous bed. It is more frequent in the right pleural cavity than the left. *Ascites* also occurs as a consequence of transudation and results from increased pressure in the hepatic veins and the veins draining the peritoneum (Chap. 39). Marked ascites occurs most frequently in patients with tricuspid valve disease and with constrictive pericarditis.

Congestive Hepatomegaly An enlarged, tender, pulsating liver also accompanies systemic venous hypertension and is observed not only in the same conditions in which ascites occurs, but also in milder forms of heart failure from any cause. With prolonged, severe hepatomegaly, enlargement of the spleen may also occur.

Jaundice This is a late finding in congestive heart failure and is associated with elevations of both the direct- and indirect-reacting bilirubin levels; it results from impairment of hepatic function secondary to hepatic congestion and the hepatocellular hypoxia associated with central lobular atrophy. Serum enzyme concentrations, particularly SGOT and SGPT, are frequently elevated. If hepatic congestion occurs acutely, the jaundice may be severe and the enzymes strikingly raised.

Cardiac cachexia With severe chronic heart failure there may be serious weight loss and cachexia because of (1) elevation of the metabolic rate, which results in part from the extra work performed by the respiratory muscles, the increased oxygen needs of the hypertrophied heart, and the discomfort associated with severe heart failure; (2) anorexia, nausea, and vomiting due to central causes, to digitalis intoxication, or to congestive hepatomegaly and abdominal fullness; (3) some impairment of intestinal absorption due to congestion of the intestinal veins; and (4) rarely, in patients with particularly severe failure of the right side of the heart, a protein-losing enteropathy.

Other manifestations With reduction of blood flow the extremities may be cold, pale, and diaphoretic. Urine flow is depressed, and the urine contains protein and has a high specific gravity and a low concentration of sodium. In addition, prerenal azotemia may be present.

ROENTGENOGRAPHIC FINDINGS In addition to the enlargement of the particular chambers characteristic of the lesion responsible for heart failure, vascular changes in the lung fields are common in patients with heart failure and elevated pulmonary vascular pressures (Chap. 250). Also, pleural effusions may be present and associated with interlobar effusions.

CLINICAL MANIFESTATIONS OF HIGH CARDIAC OUTPUT STATES ASSOCIATED WITH HEART FAILURE

THYROTOXICOSIS (Chap. 111) The characteristic clinical features of hyperthyroidism may be so conspicuous even after the development of heart failure that the diagnosis is simple on clinical grounds. In other cases, when eye phenomena and thyroid enlargement are not striking, there is no or little clinical evidence of hyperthyroidism, which should be suspected as a contributing factor in patients with cardiac disease under the following circumstances: tachycardia that persists after prolonged rest and during sleep; any suggestion of heart failure with a high cardiac output in the absence of other recognizable causes; failure of the usual treatment measures to bring about a satisfactory response; attacks of paroxysmal atrial fibrillation or chronic atrial fibrillation in a person without obvious cause such as mitral valve disease and/or left atrial enlargement, particularly when the ventricular rate is resistant to the slowing effect of full doses of digitalis. After treatment has restored the euthyroid state, remarkable improvement in a previously intractable form of heart disease usually follows.

HEART FAILURE SECONDARY TO ANEMIA The clinical picture is that of high-output failure with anemia. One may find cardiac enlargement, occasionally with hypertrophy; systolic murmurs resulting from the combined effects of decreased viscosity, increased flow velocity, or an aortic diastolic blowing murmur, presumably due to dilatation of the aortic ring. The latter may present a confusing problem of diagnosis. Furthermore, when slight fever is also present, infective endocarditis may be mimicked. In patients with sickle cell anemia with fever and joint pains, acute rheumatic fever may be suspected.

HEART FAILURE SECONDARY TO THIAMINE DEFICIENCY (BERIBERI) (See Chaps. 83 and 263) The defect in the peripheral tissues causes peripheral vasodilatation, increased venous return and cardiac output, and, consequently, an increased load on a heart already handicapped by the metabolic defect. The usual clinical picture of beriberi heart disease, as seen in the Orient, is characterized by enlargement of the heart, systemic venous hypertension, bounding arterial pulsations, and the classic phenomena of heart failure with a high cardiac output. The diagnosis depends mostly on securing a good dietary history and on observing the response to treatment. Beriberi heart disease should be suspected when heart failure with a normal or elevated cardiac output is observed in the absence of thyrotoxicosis or anemia. Furthermore, thiamine deficiency may contribute to the development of heart failure in alcoholic cardiomyopathy (Chap. 263).

DIFFERENTIAL DIAGNOSIS The diagnosis of congestive heart failure may be established by observing some combination of the clinical manifestations of heart failure, enumerated above, together with the findings characteristic of one of the etiologic forms of heart disease. Since chronic heart failure is usually associated with an enlarged heart, the diagnosis should be questioned, but is by no means excluded, when all chambers are normal in size. Heart failure may be difficult to distinguish from pulmonary disease, and the differential diagnosis is discussed in Chap. 26. Pulmonary embolism also presents many of the manifestations of heart failure, but fixed splitting of the second heart sound, a right ventricular lift, hemoptysis, pleuritic chest pain, and the characteristic mismatch between ventilation and perfusion on lung scan should point to this diagnosis (Chap. 282).

Ankle edema may be due to varicose veins, cyclic edema, or gravitational effects (Chap. 28), but in these patients there is no generalized systemic venous hypertension at rest, following exertion, or with pressure over the abdomen. Edema secondary to renal disease can usually be recognized by appropriate renal function tests and urinalysis and is rarely associated with elevation of the venous pressure. Enlargement of the liver and ascites occur in patients with hepatic cirrhosis, but may also be distinguished from heart failure by normal jugular venous pressure and absence of a positive abdominojugular reflux.

TREATMENT OF HEART FAILURE

The treatment of heart failure may be divided into three components: (1) removal of the precipitating cause, (2) correction of the underlying cause, and (3) control of the congestive heart failure state. The first two are discussed together in subsequent chapters with each specific disease entity or complication. The third component of the treatment of heart failure may, in turn, be divided into three categories: (1) reduction of cardiac work load, including afterload, (2) enhancement of myocardial contractility, and (3) control of excessive salt and water retention. The vigor with which each of these measures is pursued in any individual patient should depend upon the severity of the heart failure state. Following effective treatment, recurrence of the clinical manifestations of heart failure can often be prevented by continuing those measures that were originally effective.

REDUCTION OF CARDIAC WORK LOAD This consists of reducing physical activity, instituting emotional rest, and reducing afterload. The latter is generally instituted *after* the use of glycides and diuretics. Modest restriction of physical activity in mild cases and rest in bed or in a chair in severe failure remain cornerstones in the treatment of heart failure. Meals should be small in quantity, and every effort should be made to diminish the patient's anxiety. Physical and emotional rest tend to lower arterial pressure, and reduce the load on the myocardium by diminishing the requirements for cardiac output. These influences act in concert to diminish the need for redistribution of the cardiac output, and in many patients, particularly those with mild heart failure, simple bed rest and mild sedation often result in an effective diuresis.

Rest at home or in the hospital should be maintained for 1 to 2 weeks in patients with overt congestive failure and should be continued for several days after the patient's condition has stabilized. The hazards of phlebothrombosis and pulmonary embolism which occur with bed rest may be reduced with anticoagulants, leg exercises, and elastic stockings. In any event, absolute bed rest rarely is required, and the patient should be encouraged to sit in a chair and be given toilet privileges unless heart failure is extreme. Heavy sedation should be avoided, but small doses of barbiturates or tranquilizers may be helpful in calming the emotionally disturbed patient through the first few days of therapy and in permitting much-needed sleep. In patients with chronic, mild heart failure, bed rest on weekends will frequently allow continuation of gainful employment. Following recovery from heart failure, the patient's activities must be carefully assessed, and often his or her professional, family, and/or community responsibilities must be reduced. Intermittent rest during the day and the avoidance of strenuous exertion are often helpful once compensation has been restored. Weight reduction by restriction of caloric intake in the obese patient with heart failure also diminishes cardiac work load and is an essential component of the therapeutic program.

ENHANCEMENT OF MYOCARDIAL CONTRACTILITY—DIGITALIS The improvement of myocardial contractility by means of cardiac glycosides is the second of the cornerstones in the control of heart failure. The basic molecular structure of the digitalis glycosides is a steroid nucleus to which an unsaturated lactone ring is attached at C-17. These two elements together are called *aglycone* or *genin,* and it is this portion of the molecule which is responsible for the cardiotonic activity. The addition of a sugar to this basic structure enhances both the potency and duration of action of the glycoside, probably as a result of increasing solubility.

Pharmacokinetics Although, in the absence of severe malabsorption, digitalis is adequately absorbed from the intestinal tract even in the presence of vascular congestion secondary to heart failure, some glycosides, including ouabain, are poorly absorbed and, therefore, are effective only when administered parenterally; the intravenous route is preferable to the intramuscular, since absorption is erratic with the latter. When they are administered orally, absorption is close to complete within 2 h. The fraction of orally administered glycoside which is absorbed varies. Approximately 40 percent of digitalis powder is absorbed, almost 100 percent of digitoxin, and 65 to 75 percent of digoxin. Considerable variability of bioavailability has been found in different commercial preparations of digoxin. Cholesterol-lowering resins, antidiarrheal agents containing pectin and kaolin, nonabsorbable antacids, and neomycin can reduce the absorption of digoxin and digitoxin. Varying degrees of protein-binding of glycosides occur in the bloodstream (for example, 97 percent for digitoxin and 25 percent for digoxin), and though these differences may account in part for the varying durations of the effect of different glycosides, they are not related to the speed of action of these drugs. The plasma contains only approximately 1 percent of the body stores of digoxin; therefore, digoxin is not effectively removed from the body by dialysis, exchange transfusions, or during cardiopulmonary bypass, presumably because of tissue binding. The major fraction of the glycosides is directly bound by various tissues including the heart, in which the concentration is approximately 30 times that in the plasma for digoxin and 7 times for digitoxin, which is less polar and more lipid-soluble than digoxin.

Digoxin, which has a half-life of 1.6 days, is filtered in the glomeruli, and 85 percent is excreted in the urine, most in unchanged form; only 10 to 15 percent of digoxin is eliminated in the stool through biliary excretion in the presence of normal renal function. The ratio of digoxin clearance to endogenous creatinine clearance is 0.8, and the percentage of the body's total stores of digoxin lost per day can be calculated as $(14 \pm 0.2) \times$ creatinine clearance in milliliters per minute. In patients with normal renal function a plateau concentration in the blood and tissue is reached after 5 days of daily maintenance treatment without a loading dose (Fig. 71-2). Therefore, significant reductions of the glomerular filtration rate reduce the elimination of digoxin (but not of digitoxin) and, therefore, may prolong digoxin's effect, allowing it to accumulate to toxic levels if it is administered as in normal subjects. The administration of most diuretics does not alter the excretion of digoxin significantly, but spironolactone can inhibit tubular secretion of digoxin, resulting in significant accumulation of the drug. Serum levels and pharmacokinetics are essentially unchanged by massive weight loss. *Digitoxin,* with a half-life of approximately 5 days, is metabolized chiefly in the liver; only 15 percent is excreted in the urine unchanged and an equal fraction in the stool. Drugs such as phenobarbital and phenylbutazone that increase activity of hepatic microsomal enzymes accelerate the metabolism of digitoxin. To reach a steady state, digitoxin requires maintenance doses for 3 to 4 weeks. *Ouabain* is very rapid acting, exhibiting an onset of action 5 to 10 min and a peak effect 60 min following intravenous injection. It is poorly absorbed from the gastrointestinal tract and, therefore, is not suitable for oral use; it is excreted by the kidneys, has a half-life of 21 h, and is useful in emergencies.

Mechanism of action The cardiac actions of all digitalis glycosides are alike. The clinical effects result from augmenting contractility and irritability and from slowing heart rate and atrioventricular conduction. In addition, the cardiac glycosides potentiate vagal influences on the heart.

The most important effect of digitalis on cardiac muscle is to shift its force-velocity relation upward (Chap. 252). This positive inotropic effect is exhibited in normal, nonfailing hypertrophied as well as in failing hearts. In the absence of heart failure, however, when cardiac output is not limited by cardiac contractility, the drug does not elevate the output. The finding that digitalis increases the contractility of the nonfailing heart has led to its use (1) in patients with heart disease but without heart failure prior to operation or other stressful situations such as serious infections, and (2) in the presence of a chronically increased load, such as hypertension without heart failure. However, definitive evidence of its efficacy in these circumstances has not been provided.

Excitation-contraction coupling is the membrane and intracellular process most likely involved in producing the positive inotropic effect of digitalis glycosides. These drugs inhibit transmembrane sodium and potassium movement by inhibition of the monovalent cation transport enzyme–coupled Na-K-ATPase. The latter, localized to the sarcolemma, appears to be the receptor for cardioactive glycosides whose action results in an increase in intracellular sodium content, and this in turn increases intracellular calcium concentration through a Na^+-Ca^{2+} exchange carrier mechanism. The increased myocardial uptake of calcium augments calcium released to the myofilaments during excitation and, therefore, invokes a positive inotropic response. There is a correlation between inhibitors of the enzyme and the inotropic potency of the glycoside.

The action of glycosides on the inhibition of the sarcolemmal Na^+- and K^+-stimulated ATPase also produces alteration in the electrical properties of both the contractile cells and the specialized automatic cells. While low concentrations of glycosides produce little effect on the action potential, high concentrations result in a reduction in the resting potential (phase 4) with an augmented rate of diastolic depolarization (Chap. 249). The reduction in the resting potential brings the cell closer to the threshold for depolarization. These two effects lead to increased *rhythmicity* and ectopic impulse activity. With the lowering of the resting potential, the rate of rise of the action potential is reduced, resulting in a slowing of conduction velocity, which is conducive to the development of reentry. Thus, the known electrophysiologic effects of digitalis glycosides are capable of explaining both reentry and ectopic foci and the resultant arrhythmias associated with digitalis intoxication.

The glycosides also prolong the *functional refractory period* of the atrioventricular node, through a direct action, as well as an enhanced vagal effect. Digitalis also shortens the refractory period of the atrial and ventricular muscle. Small action potentials are propagated in a decremental fashion in the atrioventricular junction. Most do not reach the ventricles but leave some of the atrioventricular junctional cells in a refractory state. Together with the action of digitalis to augment vagal activity, this helps to explain the slowing of ventricular rate produced by digitalis glycosides in supraventricular tachycardias. In atrial fibrillation, the slowing of ventricular rate is explained by several factors, in addition to prolongation of the functional refractory period of the atrioventricular node, including increased fibrillation rate (shortened atrial refractory period) and increased concealed conduction with fewer impulses penetrating the atrioventricular junction owing to both direct and vagal effects of glycosides on junctional tissue.

Digitalis exerts a negative chronotropic action, which in part is a vagal effect and in part is due to a direct action on the sinus pacemaker. In heart failure, slowing of the sinus rate following the administration of digitalis results also from withdrawal of sympathetic activity secondary to general improvement in circulatory status due to the positive inotropic effect of the glycoside. In the nonfailing heart the slowing effect is negligible, and digitalis should not be used for the treatment of sinus tachycardia unless heart failure is present. The apparent suppression of pacemaker activity which may take place following large doses of digitalis is probably due not to arrest of the pacemaker but rather to a sinoatrial block related to a depression of conduction.

In addition, the digitalis glycosides also exert an action on the peripheral vasculature, causing venous and arterial constriction in normal individuals and reflex dilatation resulting from withdrawal of sympathetic constrictor activity in patients with congestive heart failure.

Use in heart failure By stimulating the contractile function of the heart, digitalis improves ventricular emptying; i.e., it augments the ejection fraction, increases cardiac output, promotes diuresis, and reduces the elevated diastolic pressure and volume and end-systolic volume of the failing ventricle with consequent reduction of symptoms resulting from pulmonary vascular congestion and elevated systemic venous pressure. It is most beneficial in patients in whom ventricular contractility is impaired secondary to chronic ischemic heart disease, or when hypertensive, valvular, or congenital heart disease imposes an excessive volume or pressure load. It is helpful in slowing the rapid ventricular rate of patients with atrial flutter and fibrillation. It is of relatively little value in most forms of cardiomyopathy, myocarditis, beriberi with heart failure, mitral stenosis, thyrotoxicosis and sinus rhythm, cor pulmonale when the lung disease is not being treated concurrently (Chap. 262), and chronic constrictive pericarditis (Chap. 265). Nonetheless, it is not contraindicated in these disorders and is frequently used since it may exert a beneficial effect, albeit not a striking one.

Digitalis intoxication Although digitalis is one of the cornerstones of the treatment for heart failure, it is a two-edged sword, because intoxication due to digitalis excess is a common, serious, and potentially fatal complication of its use. The therapeutic-to-toxic ratios are identical for all cardiac glycosides. In most patients with heart failure the lethal dose of most glycosides is probably 5 to 10 times the minimal effective dose and only about twice the dose which leads to minor toxic manifestations. In addition, old age, acute myocardial infarction or ischemia, hypoxemia, magnesium depletion, renal insufficiency, hypercalcemia, carotid sinus massage, electrical cardioversion, and hypothyroidism all may reduce the tolerance of the patient to the digitalis glycosides or provoke latent digitalis intoxication. The most common precipitating cause of digitalis intoxication, however, is depletion of potassium stores, which often occurs as a result of diuretic therapy and secondary hyperaldosteronism. Since it is not necessary for a patient to receive a maximally tolerated dose of digitalis to derive a beneficial effect, even small doses provide some therapeutic action; this point should be considered if these drugs are to be used in patients prone to toxicity.

Anorexia, nausea, and vomiting, which are among the earliest signs of digitalis intoxication, are caused by direct stimulation of centers in the medulla and are not of gastrointestinal origin. The most frequent disturbance of cardiac rhythm caused by digitalis is premature ventricular beats, which may take the form of bigeminy because of increased myocardial irritability or facilitation of reentry. Atrioventricular block of varying degrees of severity may occur. Nonparoxysmal atrial tachycardia with variable atrioventricular block is quite characteristic of digitalis intoxication. Finally, sinus arrhythmia, sinoatrial block, sinus arrest, and atrioventricular junctional and multifocal ventricular tachycardia may also occur. These arrhythmias are due to action of the glycoside both on cardiac tissues and on the central nervous system. Chronic digitalis intoxication may be insidious in onset and characterized by exacerbations of heart failure, weight loss, cachexia, neuralgias, gynecomastia, yellow vision, and delirium. Digitalis-toxic cardiac arrhythmias precede extracardiac (gastrointestinal or central nervous system) toxicity in about one-half of cases.

Digitalis intoxication has been reported to occur in as many as 20 percent of hospitalized patients receiving a cardiac glycoside, which emphasizes the importance of the ability to diagnose this condition. The administration of quinidine to patients receiving digoxin raises the serum concentration of the latter and increases the incidence of digitalis intoxication. Therefore, serum digoxin concentrations and electrocardiograms should be followed carefully when quinidine is given to digitalized patients. The radioimmunoassays for digoxin and digitoxin make possible the correlation of serum glycoside levels with the presence of toxicity. In patients receiving standard maintenance doses of digoxin and digitoxin and in whom no sign of intoxication is present, serum concentrations approximate 1 to 1.5 and 20 to 25 ng/ml, respectively. When signs of intoxication are present, serum levels of more than 2 and 30 ng/ml, respectively, of these glycosides are often found. Since many factors other than the serum concentration determine digitalis intoxication, and since there is overlap in serum glycoside concentrations in patients with and without toxicity, it is clear that these levels cannot be used as a sole guide to digitalis dosage. However, when taken together with findings on the clinical examination and electrocardiogram, they add useful information to the clinical evaluations of digitalis intoxication. In addition they will indicate whether a patient for whom the history of digitalis intake is in doubt has, in fact, been receiving the drug.

Treatment of digitalis intoxication When tachyarrhythmias result from digitalis intoxication, withdrawal of the drug and treatment with potassium, phenytoin, propranolol, or lidocaine are indicated. Potassium should be administered cautiously and by the oral route whenever possible if hypokalemia is present, but small doses may also be helpful when serum potassium levels are normal; *potassium must not be employed in the presence of atrioventricular block or hyperkalemia,* when phenytoin is more appropriate. Propranolol should not be used to treat digitalis toxicity in the presence of severe heart failure or atrioventricular block but may be useful otherwise; lidocaine is effective in the treatment of digitalis-induced ventricular tachyarrhythmias in the absence of preceding atrioventricular block. A cardiac pacemaker may be required in digitalis-induced atrioventricular block. Electrical conversion may not only be ineffective in treating these arrhythmias but may induce more serious arrhythmias. However, it may be lifesaving in digitalis-induced ventricular fibrillation. Quinidine and procainamide are not useful in the treatment of digitalis intoxication. Fab fragments of purified, intact digitalis antibodies represent a potentially lifesaving approach to the treatment of severe intoxication.

SYMPATHOMIMETIC AMINES Four sympathomimetic amines which act largely on beta-adrenergic receptors—epinephrine, isoproterenol, dopamine, and dobutamine—improve myocardial contractility in various forms of heart failure. The latter two agents appear to be most effective; they must be administered by constant intravenous infusion and are useful in intractable heart failure, particularly in patients who have undergone cardiac surgery, and in some instances of myocardial infarction and shock or pulmonary edema. While they improve the hemodynamics in that condition, it is not clear that they improve survival. Their administration must be accompanied by careful and continuous monitoring.

Dopamine, the naturally occurring immediate precursor of norepinephrine, has a combination of actions which make it particularly useful in the treatment of a variety of hypotensive states and congestive heart failure. At very low doses, that is, 1 to 2 (μg/kg)/min, it dilates renal and mesenteric blood vessels through stimulation of specific dopaminergic receptors, thereby augmenting renal and mesenteric blood flow and sodium excretion. In the range of 2 to 10 (μg/kg)/min dopamine stimulates myocardial beta receptors but induces little tachycardia, while at higher doses it also stimulates alpha-adrenergic receptors and elevates arterial pressure.

Dobutamine is a synthetic catecholamine which acts primarily on $beta_1$-adrenergic receptors, and stimulates $beta_2$ and alpha receptors only slightly. Consequently, it exerts a potent inotropic action. It has only a modest cardioaccelerating effect and lowers peripheral vascular resistance, but since it raises cardiac output, it has little effect on systemic arterial pressure. Dobutamine, given in continuous infusions of 2.5 to 15 (μg/kg)/min, is useful in the treatment of acute heart failure without hypotension. Like other sympathomimetic amines it may be particularly valuable in the management of patients requiring relatively short-term inotropic support—up to 1 week—in conditions which are reversible, such as the cardiac depression which sometimes follows open-heart surgery, or in patients with acute heart failure who are being prepared for operation. Adverse effects include sinus tachycardia, tachyarrhythmias, and hypertension.

A variety of orally active sympathomimetic amines, such as pirbuterol and salbutamol, as well as the orally active noncatecholamine, nonglycoside, amrinone, are under intensive investigation for the chronic treatment of heart failure.

CONTROL OF EXCESSIVE FLUID RETENTION Many of the clinical manifestations of heart failure are secondary to hypervolemia and expansion of the interstitial fluid volume. When fluid retention due to heart failure first becomes clinically evident, considerable expansion of the extracellular space has already occurred, and heart failure usually is already advanced. Treatment aimed at reducing extracellular fluid volume is dependent primarily on lowering total body sodium stores, while fluid restriction is of less importance. A negative sodium balance can be achieved by reducing the dietary intake and increasing the urinary excretion of this ion with the aid of diuretics. In severe heart failure mechanical removal of extracellular fluid by means of thoracentesis, paracentesis, hemodialysis, or peritoneal dialysis may also be employed.

Diet In patients with mild heart failure, considerable improvement in symptoms may result from the simple reduction of sodium intake, particularly if accompanied by bed rest. In patients with more severe failure the sodium intake must be controlled more rigidly, even when other measures such as cardiac glycosides and diuretics are used, and following recovery from a bout of heart failure, at least moderate sodium restriction should be maintained. The normal diet contains approximately 6 to 10 g sodium chloride; this intake can be reduced by half simply by excluding salt-rich foods and salt which is added at the table. Reduction of the ordinary dietary intake to approximately one-fourth of normal may be achieved if, in addition, all salt is omitted from cooking. In patients with severe heart failure, in whom the daily sodium chloride intake should be reduced to between 500 and 1000 mg, milk, cheese, bread, cereals, canned vegetables and soups, some salted cuts of meat, and some fresh vegetables, including spinach, celery, and beets, must be eliminated. A variety of fresh fruit, green vegetables, specially processed breads and milk, and salt substitutes are permissible, but such diets are difficult to keep palatable. Water intake may be ad libitum in all but the most severe forms of congestive heart failure. However, late in the course of heart failure, dilutional hyponatremia may develop in patients who are unable to excrete a water load, sometimes because of excessive secretion of antidiuretic hormone. In such cases water intake as well as sodium intake must be restricted.

Attention must also be directed to the caloric content of the diet. Substantial improvement can result from caloric restriction in obese patients with heart failure, in whom weight loss will reduce the load placed on the myocardium. On the other hand, in individuals with severe heart failure and cardiac cachexia, an attempt must be made to maintain nutritional intake and to avoid caloric and vitamin deficiencies.

Diuretics A variety of diuretic agents is available, and in patients with mild heart failure almost all are effective. However, in the more severe forms of heart failure, the selection of diuretics is more difficult, and any existing abnormalities in serum electrolytes must be taken into account. Overtreatment must be avoided, since the resultant hypovolemia may reduce cardiac output, interfere with renal function, and produce profound weakness and lethargy.

THIAZIDE DIURETICS These agents are widely used in clinical practice because of their effectiveness when administered orally. In patients with chronic heart failure of mild or moderate severity the continued administration of chlorothiazide or one of its many analogues abolishes or diminishes the need for very rigid dietary sodium restriction, although salty foods and table salt should still be avoided. Thiazides are well absorbed following oral administration; chlorothiazide and hydrochlorothiazide reach their peak action in 4 h, and diuresis persists for approximately 12 h. Thiazide diuretics reduce the reabsorption of sodium and chloride, and water follows the unreabsorbed salt. Thiazides fail to increase free water clearance, and in some instances reduce it, supporting the hypothesis that these drugs inhibit selective sodium chloride reabsorption in the distal cortical diluting segment, at a site where the urine is normally diluted (Chap. 289). This may result in the excretion of a hypertonic urine and may contribute to dilutional hyponatremia. As a consequence of increased delivery of sodium to the distal nephron, sodium-potassium ion exchange is enhanced and kaliuresis results. The weak carbonic anhydrase-inhibiting properties of the thiazides are of limited importance and need not be invoked to account for most of the diuretic action.

Chlorothiazide is administered in doses of up to 500 mg every 6 h. Many derivatives of this compound are available but differ principally in dosage and duration of action and therefore offer few, if any, significant advances over the parent compound, except for chlorthalidone which may be administered once daily. Potassium depletion and metabolic alkalosis (the latter due to increased H^+ secretion as a substitute for the depleted intracellular stores of potassium and increased proximal tubular reabsorption of filtered HCO_3^- when there is relative depletion of the extracellular fluid volume) are the chief adverse effects following prolonged administration of chlorothiazide (and of ethacrynic acid and furosemide), and may seriously enhance the dangers of digitalis intoxication and induce fatigue and lethargy. Hypokalemia may be prevented by the oral supplementation of potassium chloride. However, the solution is not palatable and may be hazardous in patients with renal failure. Therefore, to control potassium depletion, intermittent dosage schedules, e.g., omitting the diuretic every third day, and the addition of a potassium-retaining diuretic, such as a spironolactone or triamterene, may be preferable. Other side effects of thiazides include reduction of the excretion of uric acid, which may lead to hyperuricemia, and a hyperglycemic effect, which rarely may precipitate hyperosmolar coma in the poorly regulated diabetic. Skin rashes, thrombocytopenia, and granulocytopenia have also been reported.

ETHACRYNIC ACID AND FUROSEMIDE These two "loop" diuretics are similar physiologically but differ chemically. Ethacrynic acid is an unsaturated ketone derivative of aryloxyacetic acid, while furosemide differs from the thiazides in that the thiadiasine ring has been replaced by a furfuryl group on the amino nitrogen of the anthranilic acid.

These are extremely powerful diuretics which reversibly inhibit the reabsorption throughout the nephron, but especially inhibit active chloride reabsorption in both the medullary and cortical segments of the thick ascending limb of the loop of Henle. These agents may induce renal cortical vasodilatation and can produce rates of urine formation which may be as high as one-third of the glomerular filtration rate. While other diuretics lose their effectiveness as blood volume is restored to normal levels, ethacrynic acid and furosemide remain effective despite the elimination of excessive extracellular fluid volume. The major side effects of these agents are due to this marked diuretic potency, which may result in circulatory collapse and in reductions in the renal blood flow and glomerular filtration rate. There is an inability to generate a dilute urine; alkalosis is produced by a large increase in the urinary excretion of chloride, hydrogen, and potassium ions. Hypokalemia (see discussion of thiazides, above) and hyponatremia may occur, and hyperuricemia and hyperglycemia are observed occasionally, as with thiazide diuretics.

Both drugs are readily absorbed orally and are excreted in the bile and urine. They are usually effective by mouth, in doses of 25 to 100 mg two or four times daily, and intravenously in doses ranging from 10 to 100 mg. Both can be given intravenously, and furosemide intramuscularly as well. Weakness, nausea, and dizziness may accompany both diuretics; ethacrynic acid has been associated with skin rash and granulocytopenia, as well as with transient or permanent deafness.

These extremely effective diuretics are useful in all forms of heart failure, particularly in otherwise refractory heart failure and pulmonary edema. Both agents have been shown to be effective in patients with hypoalbuminemia, hyponatremia, hypochloremia, hypokalemia, and reductions in the glomerular filtration rate, and to produce a diuresis in patients in whom thiazide diuretics and aldosterone antagonists, alone and in combination, are ineffective.

Ethacrynic acid and furosemide may be potentiated by spironolactone, triamterene, thiazide diuretics, carbonic anhydrase inhibitors, or osmotic diuretics. These latter agents act on the cortical collecting ducts, are relatively weak, and therefore are rarely indicated as sole agents. However, their potassium-sparing properties make them particularly useful in conjunction with the more potent kaliuretic agents, the thiazides and loop diuretics, discussed above. These agents fall into two classes, as noted below.

ALDOSTERONE ANTAGONISTS. The 17-spironolactones resemble aldosterone structurally and act on the distal renal tubule by competitive inhibition of aldosterone, thereby blocking the exchange between sodium and both potassium and hydrogen in the distal tubules and collecting ducts. These agents produce a sodium diuresis, and, in contrast to the thiazides, ethacrynic acid, and furosemide, they result in potassium retention. Although secondary hyperaldosteronism exists in some patients with congestive heart failure, the spironolactones are effective even in patients in whom the serum aldosterone concentration is within normal limits. Aldactone A may be administered in doses of 25 to 100 mg three to four times daily by mouth. The maximal effect of this regimen is not observed for approximately 4 days. Spironolactones are most effective when administered in combination with thiazide diuretics, ethacrynic acid, or furosemide. The opposing action of these drugs on urine and serum potassium makes possible a sodium diuresis without either hyper- or hypokalemia when spironolactone and one of these other agents are administered in combination. Also, since spironolactone (and triamterene) act on the distal tubule, they are particularly effective when used in combination with one of these other diuretics which acts more proximally.

Spironolactone should not be administered alone to patients with hyperkalemia, renal failure, or hyponatremia. Reported complications include nausea, epigastric distress, mental confusion, drowsiness, gynecomastia, and erythematous eruptions.

TRIAMTERENE AND AMILORIDE. These two drugs exert renal effects similar to those of the spironolactones; i.e., they prevent sodium reabsorption and interfere with sodium-potassium exchange in the distal tubules. However, their fundamental mechanism of action differs from those of the spironolactones, since they are active in adrenalectomized animals. The effective dose of triamterene is 100 mg once or twice daily. Side effects include nausea, vomiting, diarrhea, headache, granulocytopenia, eosinophilia, and skin rash. Both triamterene and the chemically unrelated diuretic amiloride, resemble Aldactone A in that their diuretic potency is not great, and they are effective in preventing the hypokalemia characteristic of the administration of thiazides, furosemide, and ethacrynic acid.

ORGANOMERCURIALS Presumably these diuretics act by releasing inorganic mercury within the tubule cell, which then combines with sulfhydryl enzymes essential for active sodium transport in the ascending limb of Henle's loop. Since mercurial diuretics are not particularly effective when given by mouth, they are usually administered intramuscularly in doses of 0.5 or 1.0 ml.

CHOICE OF DIURETICS Orally administered thiazides are the agents of choice in the treatment of chronic cardiac edema of mild to moderate degree in patients without hyperglycemia, hyperuricemia, or hypokalemia. Spironolactones, triamterene, and amiloride are not potent diuretics when used alone, but they potentiate other diuretics, particularly the thiazides, ethacrynic acid, and furosemide. However, in patients with heart failure and severe secondary aldosteronism, spironolactone may be quite effective. Ethacrynic acid or furosemide, given alone or with spironolactone or triamterene, are the agents of choice in patients with severe heart failure refractory to other diuretics. Rarely, in very severe failure the combination of a thiazide, a loop diuretic (ethacrynic acid or furosemide), and a potassium-sparing diuretic (spironolactone, triamterene, or amiloride) are required. Mercurial diuretics are occasionally useful when a rapid diuresis is desired in patients with hyperglycemia or hyperuricemia in whom loop diuretics may be undesirable.

VASODILATOR THERAPY In many patients with heart failure, left ventricular afterload is increased as a consequence of the many neural, humoral, and/or structural changes which constrict the peripheral vascular bed, and as the elevation of ventricular end-diastolic volume compensates for impaired cardiac function as a consequence of the operation of Laplace's law, myocardial wall tension (afterload) rises. The maintenance or even the elevation of arterial pressure is generally considered to be a useful compensatory mechanism that allows blood flow to vital organs to persist in the presence of hypovolemia, despite inadequacy of the total cardiac output. However, in the presence of severely impaired cardiac function, the increase in afterload may reduce cardiac output and elevate myocardial oxygen consumption further.

As shown in Fig. 252-6, afterload is a major determinant of cardiac function. A modest elevation in afterload will not necessarily alter stroke volume when cardiac function is normal, because the resultant small increase in left ventricular end-diastolic volume, i.e., preload, can be tolerated easily. However, when myocardial function is impaired, such an increase in preload evoked by an elevation of afterload may raise ventricular end-diastolic and pulmonary capillary pressures to levels that may produce pulmonary congestion and pulmonary edema. In many patients with heart failure, the ventricle is already operating at the peak, flat portion of its Frank-Starling curve (Fig. 252-7), and any additional increase in afterload will reduce stroke volume (page 1350). Conversely, a reduction of afterload will elevate the stroke volume of the failing ventricle.

The pharmacological reduction of impedance to left ventricular ejection, i.e., of afterload, with vasodilator drugs may be considered to be a form of reduction of cardiac work load and an important adjunct in the management of heart failure. This approach may be particularly helpful in patients with acute heart failure due to myocardial infarction (Chap. 261) and valvular regurgitation. The reduction of afterload by means of a variety of vasodilators, or mechanically by intraaortic balloon counterpulsation, reduces left ventricular end-diastolic pressure and oxygen consumption, while raising stroke volume and cardiac output and causing only modest reductions in aortic pressure.

In patients with both acute and chronic intractable heart failure secondary to coronary artery disease, cardiomyopathy, or valvular regurgitation who are treated with vasodilators, cardiac output increases, the pulmonary wedge pressure falls, the signs and symptoms of heart failure are relieved, and a new steady state is achieved in which cardiac output is higher and afterload lower with only mild reduction of arterial pressure (Fig. 253-1). Furthermore, the reduction of elevated left end-diastolic pressure might improve subendocardial perfusion.

Vasodilator therapy is particularly useful in the treatment of acute pulmonary edema, which, if not precipitated by myocardial infarction, is often associated with hypertension. Also, vasodilator therapy is often helpful in refractory congestive heart failure; when heart failure is acute, the addition of an inotropic agent such as dobutamine may be required.

The several available vasodilators vary in their hemodynamic effects, locus and duration of action, and mode of administration (Table 253-1). Some vasodilators, such as the alpha-adrenergic blocking agents, hydralazine, and captopril, act predominantly on the arterial bed, while others, such as nitroglycerin, act exclusively, or almost so, on the venous side of the circulation. Some agents, such as sodium nitroprusside, must be administered by continuous intravenous infusion, nitroglycerin requires administration in ointment form when a prolonged effect is desired, while isosorbide dinitrate is most effective when it is administered by the sublingual route.

The ideal vasodilator for the treatment of *acute* heart failure should have a rapid onset and brief duration of action when

FIGURE 253-1

Effects of various vasodilators on the relationship between left ventricular end-diastolic pressure (LVEDP) and cardiac index or stroke volume in normal (N) and failing (F) hearts. H represents hydralazine or any other pure arterial dilator. It produces only a minimal increase in cardiac index in the normal subject (A′ → H′) or in the patient with heart failure with normal LVEDP (C′ → H″). In contrast, it elevates output in the patient with heart failure and elevated LVEDP (A → H). P represents a balanced vasodilator, such as sodium nitroprusside or prazosin. It reduces filling pressure in all patients, elevates cardiac output in patients with heart failure and elevated LVEDP (A → P), lowers cardiac output in normal subjects (A′ → P′), and has little effect on cardiac output in heart failure patients with normal filling pressures (C → P″). (Reprinted with permission from E Braunwald (ed), Heart Disease: A Textbook of Cardiovascular Medicine, Philadelphia, Saunders, 1980.)

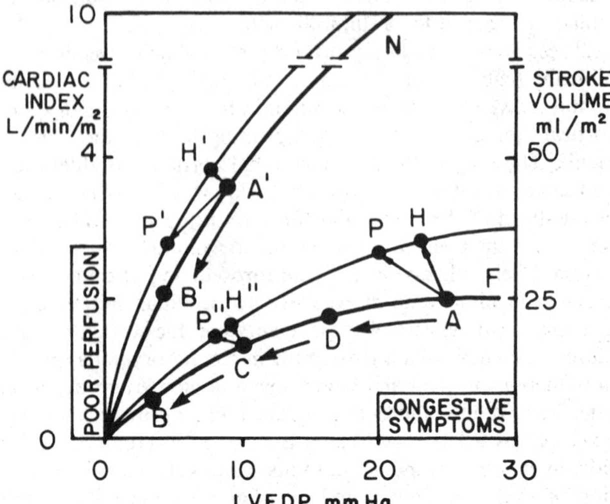

administered by intravenous infusion; sodium nitroprusside qualifies as such a drug, but its use requires careful hemodynamic monitoring. For the treatment of chronic congestive heart failure, the agent should be effective on oral administration, and its action should persist for at least 6 h. Hydralazine, prazosin, and captopril satisfy these requirements. Hydralazine acts on the arterial bed, prazosin dilates both the arterial and venous beds, while captopril is most active on the arterial bed.

In view of the spectrum of actions of available vasodilators, the selection of the specific agent or combinations of agents for any given patient should depend on the pathophysiologic state. For example, when the primary defect is a reduction of cardiac output and/or mitral regurgitation, an arterial vasodilator is the drug of choice; when pulmonary congestion is the principal problem, a venodilator would be preferable. When it is desired both to elevate cardiac output and to reduce pulmonary vascular pressures, an agent which acts both on the arterial and venous beds, such as prazosin or captopril, is indicated.

Vasodilators are ineffective, indeed they may even exert a deleterious action, in patients without heart failure (Fig. 253-1). Arterial dilators may produce postural hypotension with little effect on cardiac output. Venodilators lower arterial pressure and cardiac output in patients with normal cardiac function, and in patients with heart failure whose ventricular filling pressures have previously been restored to normal by diuretic therapy.

REFRACTORY HEART FAILURE When the response to treatment is inadequate, heart failure is considered to be refractory. Before assuming that this state simply reflects advanced, perhaps preterminal, myocardial depression, careful consideration must be given to several possibilities: (1) an underlying and overlooked cause of the heart disease that may be amenable to specific surgical or medical therapy, such as silent aortic or mitral stenosis, constrictive pericarditis, infective endocarditis, hypertension, or thyrotoxicosis; (2) one or a combination of the precipitating causes of heart failure, such as pulmonary or urinary tract infection, recurrent pulmonary emboli, arterial hypoxemia, anemia, or arrhythmia; and (3) complications of overly vigorous therapy, such as digitalis intoxication, hypovolemia, or electrolyte imbalance.

Recognition and proper treatment of the aforementioned complications are likely to make the patient responsive to therapy again. Perhaps the most common complication results from overzealous treatment with diuretics. When they are administered too rapidly, sudden hypovolemia can occur before edema fluid can be mobilized to replace the loss of blood volume, the result being a shocklike state with evidence of systemic hypoperfusion in the presence of edema. The chronically excessively diuresed patient has exchanged the hazards of pulmonary edema and the inconvenience of systemic edema for a persistently depressed cardiac output with its associated weakness, lethargy, prerenal azotemia, and sometimes cardiac cachexia. Temporarily easing up on salt restriction and diuretic administration may overcome this difficulty, but as heart failure worsens, this course of action may lead to increased pulmonary congestion which is equally unacceptable.

Hyponatremia is a late manifestation of refractory heart failure. It, too, may be a complication of overaggressive diuresis leading to reduced glomerular filtration rate and decreased delivery of NaCl to the diluting sites in the distal tubule. Hyponatremia may also result from nonosmotic stimuli for the continued secretion of antidiuretic hormone. Therapy involves improvement of the cardiovascular status, if possible, as well as temporary cessation of diuretic therapy and restriction of oral water intake.

The combination of an intravenously administered vasodilator, such as sodium nitroprusside, along with a potent sympathomimetic amine, such as dopamine or dobutamine, often results in an additive effect, raising cardiac output and lowering filling pressure. Once compensation is established, therapy can be continued with the combination of oral hydralazine or captopril to reduce afterload and one of the experimental orally active nonglycoside inotropic agents, such as amrinone, salbutamol, or pirbuterol.

TABLE 253-1
Spectrum of vasodilators used for the treatment of heart failure*

	Principal site of action	*Mode of administration*	*Duration of action*
Phentolamine	Arterial	Continuous intravenous	Minutes
Phenoxybenzamine	Arterial	Oral	Hours
Hydralazine	Arterial	Oral	Hours
Minoxidil	Arterial	Oral	Hours
Captopril	Arterial and venous	Oral	Hours
Nitroprusside	Arterial and venous	Continuous intravenous	Minutes
Trimethaphan	Arterial and venous	Continuous intravenous	Minutes
Prazosin	Arterial and venous	Oral	Hours
Nitroglycerin	Venous	Intravenous or sublingual	Minutes
		Ointment	Hours
Isosorbide dinitrate	Venous	Sublingual	Minutes to hours

* *Although all these drugs have been demonstrated to be effective vasodilators in the treatment of heart failure, not all have been approved for this use in the United States.*

TREATMENT OF ACUTE PULMONARY EDEMA Pulmonary edema secondary to left ventricular failure or mitral stenosis is described in Chap. 26. It is life-threatening and must be considered a medical emergency. As is the case for the more chronic forms of heart failure, in the treatment of pulmonary edema, attention must be directed to identifying and removing any precipitating causes of decompensation, such as an arrhythmia or infection. However, because of the acute nature of the problem, a number of additional nonspecific measures are necessary. When possible, and if it does not delay treatment unduly, recording pulmonary vascular pressures through a Swan-Ganz catheter and intraarterial pressure directly is advisable.

1 Morphine is administered by the subcutaneous, intramuscular, or intravenous routes in doses from 3 to 20 mg, depending upon the route chosen and the severity of the problem. This drug reduces anxiety, and thereby reduces adrenergic vasoconstrictor stimuli to the arteriolar and venous beds, and thereby helps to break a vicious cycle. Naloxone should be available in case respiratory depression occurs.
2 Because the alveolar fluid interferes with oxygen diffusion, resulting in arterial hypoxemia, 100 percent oxygen should be administered, preferably under positive pressure. The latter increases intraalveolar pressure and therefore reduces transudation of fluid from the alveolar capillaries and impedes venous return to the thorax, reducing pulmonary capillary pressure.
3 The patient should be maintained in the sitting position, with the legs dangling along the side of the bed, if possible, which also tends to reduce venous return to the heart.
4 Rotating tourniquets should be applied to the extremities.
5 Intravenous diuretics, such as furosemide or ethacrynic acid (40 to 100 mg), will, by rapidly establishing a diuresis, re-

duce circulating blood volume and thereby hasten the relief of pulmonary edema. In addition when given intravenously, furosemide also exerts a venodilator action, reduces venous return, and reduces pulmonary edema even before the diuresis commences.

6 Afterload reduction is achieved with intravenous sodium nitroprusside at 20 to 30 μg/min in patients whose systolic arterial pressures exceed 100 mmHg.

7 If digitalis has not been administered previously, three-fourths of a full dose of a rapidly acting glycoside, such as ouabain, digoxin, or lanatoside C, should be administered intravenously.

8 Aminophylline (theophylline ethylenediamine), 240 to 480 mg intravenously, is effective in diminishing bronchoconstriction, increasing renal blood flow and sodium excretion, and augmenting myocardial contractility.

After these emergency therapeutic measures have been instituted, and the precipitating factors treated, the diagnosis of the underlying cardiac disorder responsible for the pulmonary edema must be established if it is not already known. After stabilization of the patient's condition a long-range strategy for prevention of future episodes of pulmonary edema must be established, and this may require surgical treatment.

PROGNOSIS

The prognosis in heart failure depends primarily on the nature of the underlying heart disease and on the presence or absence of a precipitating factor which can be treated. Also, the long-term prognosis for heart failure is most favorable when the underlying forms of heart disease can be treated. When one of the latter can be identified and removed, the outlook for immediate survival is far better than if heart failure occurs without any obvious precipitating cause. The prognosis can also be estimated by observing the response to treatment. When clinical improvement occurs with only modest dietary sodium restriction and/or digitalis without the administration of diuretics, then the outlook is far better than if, in addition to these measures, intensive diuretic therapy and vasodilators are necessary.

REFERENCES

ADER R et al: Immediate and sustained hemodynamic and clinical improvement in chronic heart failure by an oral angiotensin-converting enzyme inhibitor. Circulation 61:931, 1980

ARNOLD SB et al: Long-term digitalis therapy improves left ventricular function in heart failure. N Engl J Med 303:1443, 1980

BARRY WH et al: Drug therapy: Digitalis: how does it work? J Cardiovasc Med 7:217, 1982

BRAUNWALD E et al: Heart failure, in *Mechanisms of Contraction of the Normal and Failing Heart,* 2d ed. Boston, Little, Brown, 1976, chap 11

——— et al (eds): *Congestive Heart Failure: Current Research and Clinical Applications.* New York, Grune & Stratton, 1982

CHERNIACK NS, LONGOBARDO GS: Cheyne-Stokes breathing: An instability in physiologic control. N Engl J Med 288:952, 1973

DZAU VJ et al: Relations of the renin-angiotensin-aldosterone system to clinical state in congestive heart failure. Circulation 63:645, 1981

———: Angiotensin converting enzyme inhibition in the treatment of congestive heart failure and hypertension, in *Update IV: Harrison's Principles of Internal Medicine,* KJ Isselbacher et al (eds). New York, McGraw-Hill, 1982, p 137

GOODMAN LS, GILMAN A (eds): Cardiovascular drugs, in *The Pharmacological Basis of Therapeutics,* 6th ed. New York, Macmillan, 1980, pp 729–760, 892–915

SMITH TW, BRAUNWALD E: Management of heart failure, in *Heart Disease,* 2d ed, E Braunwald (ed). Philadelphia, Saunders, 1983, chap 16

STEIN J, KUNAU R: Mechanisms of action and clinical use of diuretics, in *The Kidney,* 2d ed, BM Brenner, FC Rector (eds). Philadelphia, Saunders, 1980, chap 22

254

BRADYARRHYTHMIA—SINUS NODE DYSFUNCTION AND CONDUCTION DEFECTS

KENNETH M. ROSEN
STEVEN S. SWIRYN

This chapter will focus upon sinus node dysfunction and conduction defects and will cover abnormalities of heart rhythm which relate to interference in impulse generation and/or propagation. As with all arrhythmia, the physician managing the patient with sinus node dysfunction and/or a conduction defect must be cognizant of the exact arrhythmic diagnosis, and also of the presence and extent of underlying heart disease. The natural history of a given arrhythmia, and often its hemodynamic consequences, relates quite clearly to the presence and extent of cardiovascular disease.

THE SICK-SINUS SYNDROME

PHYSIOLOGY AND PATHOPHYSIOLOGY OF THE SINUS NODE

Under normal conditions, the biologic clock responsible for determining heart rate is the sinus node. This structure lies subepicardially at the junction of the superior vena cava and the high right atrium. The blood supply to the sinus node is either a branch of the right coronary artery (approximately 60 percent of the time) or a branch of the left circumflex system (approximately 40 percent of the time). The sinus node is richly supplied with autonomic nerves, both sympathetic and parasympathetic.

The major electrophysiologic property allowing the sinus node to function as the predominant pacemaker is the presence of automaticity, which reflects the presence of spontaneous phase 4 diastolic depolarization of sinus node cells (Fig. 254-1). These cells depolarize spontaneously, reaching a threshold potential which triggers the cell to depolarize and generate an impulse.

FIGURE 254-1

Sinus node action potential. Shown is a schematic diagram of an action potential from a sinus node cell. The y axis represents voltage and the x axis represents time. Note the presence of gradual depolarization during phase 4 (spontaneous phase 4 depolarization) which allows threshold potential to be reached. This results in generation of the cardiac impulse.

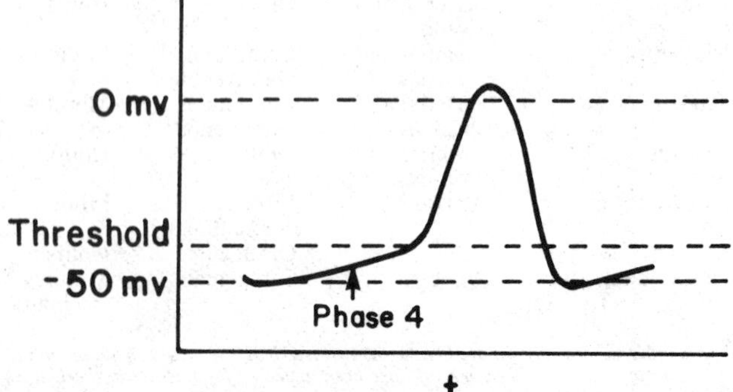

In adults under basal conditions, sinus rates can be expected to vary between 60 and 100 beats per minute. Speeding of heart rate is the normal response to an increase in sympathetic nerve impulses acting on beta-adrenergic receptors and/or withdrawal of parasympathetic (vagal) impulses acting on muscarinic receptors, while slowing results from the opposite. The sinus node can be considered to have an intrinsic heart rate which is then modulated by the autonomic nervous system. This modulation gives the heart the ability to increase rate with stress and to slow during periods of rest. The range of normal rates under all conditions is difficult to define. Rates can slow to 35 or 40 beats per minute during sleep and rise to as fast as 180 to 200 beats per minute during strenuous exercise.

Sinus rates are also a function of age. Heart rate is rapid at birth, somewhat slower during childhood years, and slows progressively during late adulthood. The slowing of heart rate with aging probably reflects both anatomic maturation and, ultimately, aging of the sinus node, as well as changes in autonomic tone. The slowing of sinus rate observed with aging complicates the diagnosis of sinus node dysfunction in the elderly, since the normal rate range in this age group has not been clearly characterized.

The sinus node is not directly represented on the surface electrocardiogram, so that the presence of sinus node dysfunction must be inferred from the behavior of P waves. The sinus node impulse is directly transmitted to the surrounding atrium via perinodal tissue. Activation of atrial muscle generates the P wave on the surface electrocardiogram. Abnormalities both of automaticity and/or conduction from the sinus node manifest themselves clinically as sinus node dysfunction.

The sinus node displays the phenomenon of *overdrive suppression.* Rapid stimulation of any automatic cardiac tissue is followed by suppression of automaticity for a measurable period of time, termed the *recovery time.* Sinus node recovery times are measured after cessation of rapid atrial stimulation as the elapsed time until resumption of sinus node automaticity (see below).

ETIOLOGY OF SINUS NODE DYSFUNCTION Sinus bradycardia (rate $<$ 60 per minute) may be a normal finding in the trained athlete, reflecting the presence of increased vagal tone. In addition, specific disease states may be associated with sinus bradycardia, including hypothyroidism, liver disease with jaundice, hypothermia, typhoid fever, and brucellosis. Paroxysmal decreases in sinus rate may be observed during vasovagal syncope (Chap. 12), acute hypoxia and hypercarbia, acute ischemia, and acute hypertension.

With aging, the sinus node exhibits loss of excitable sinus node cells and an increase in fat, collagen, and elastic tissue. These changes, which are part of the normal aging process, probably play a role in the sinus slowing normally seen with aging, as well as in patients with the sick-sinus syndrome. Sinus node dysfunction has also been postulated to reflect interference in the blood supply of the sinus node and the presence of inflammatory changes in autonomic ganglia located in the atria.

There is a close association between sinus node dysfunction, atrial dysrhythmia, and atrial disease, which can occur in any condition producing atrial stretching, such as elevation of ventricular end-diastolic pressure or disease (stenosis or regurgitation) of an AV valve. The atria and sinus node have a predilection for involvement by senile amyloidosis, a frequent concomitant of aging. Rarely, the atria may become totally inexcitable, reflecting either severe metabolic injury or extensive infiltrative disease. The resultant arrhythmia is known as *atrial standstill* and is seen most commonly with drug intoxication (digitalis, quinidine, etc.), with acute generalized atrial ischemia, and following cardiovascular surgery utilizing the pump oxygenator. Extensive infiltration and degeneration of the atria may be observed complicating several varieties of amyloidosis, sometimes with muscular dystrophy, neoplastic invasion, and occasionally as a selective atrial cardiomyopathy. In most patients with the sick-sinus syndrome, a clear etiology is not established.

ELECTROCARDIOGRAPHIC AND CLINICAL DIAGNOSIS Since the normal range of sinus rates in adults is 60 to 100 beats per minute, sinus bradycardia is defined as a sinus rate slower than 60 beats per minute. It must be recognized that sinus bradycardia occurs normally during sleep and frequently at other times in healthy people. Clinically significant sinus bradycardia is usually slower than 50 beats per minute and often is characterized by lack of response of the sinus node to interventions, such as atropine and exercise, which normally increase sinus rate.

Sinus arrhythmia may be defined as a greater than 10 percent variation in the length of adjacent sinus cycles. Sinus arrhythmia may be respiratory (slowing with inspiration) or independent of respiration. *Sinus pause* is the term used to describe sudden cessation of atrial activity during sinus rhythm (generally greater than two PP intervals). The term *sinoatrial block* refers to interference with impulse conduction between the sinus node and the atrium. Sinoatrial block of one sinus impulse will be characterized by sudden loss of a P wave, with the next sinus P wave occurring when anticipated. This will create a PP interval equal to two sinus cycle lengths. The term *sinus arrest* refers to total cessation of sinus node activity (due to complete sinoatrial block or loss of automaticity) and usually produces a prolonged period of atrial asystole or a change to an ectopic atrial rhythm, generally at a slower rate.

The term *sick-sinus syndrome* refers to a clinical syndrome in which sinus node dysfunction produces symptomatic bradyarrhythmia, including sinus bradycardia, sinoatrial block, and sinus arrest, either singly or in combination. Symptoms referable to bradyarrhythmia include dizziness, confusion, chronic fatigue, recurrent syncope, and congestive heart failure (particularly if there is significant coexistent ventricular disease). Each of these symptoms is nonspecific and can result from many other cardiovascular or noncardiovascular conditions, even in a patient with sinus bradycardia, and each is therefore of limited diagnostic value.

Atrial dysrhythmia is common in patients with the sick-sinus syndrome since this syndrome often occurs in patients with extensive atrial disease. The atrial tachyarrhythmias observed include paroxysmal atrial fibrillation, paroxysmal atrial flutter, and paroxysmal atrial reentrant tachycardia; each of these may produce palpitation, and depending on the ventricular rate, the duration of the tachycardia, and the presence and severity of underlying heart disease, may also cause dizziness, syncope, congestive heart failure, and angina pectoris. The sudden cessation of atrial tachyarrhythmia may produce syncope due to suppression of sinus node automaticity and failure of an escape pacemaker. There is a group of patients with subclinical sinus node dysfunction who present with atrial tachyarrhythmia, in whom treatment with cardiac glycosides, beta-adrenergic blocking drugs, or type I antiarrhythmic agents, such as quinidine, may produce a clinically manifest sick-sinus syndrome.

LABORATORY TESTING The diagnosis of sick-sinus syndrome does not usually require elaborate testing. In some patients, bradyarrhythmia is striking and symptomatology is marked so that a clear-cut relationship of bradyarrhythmia and symptoms is established. However, in many patients the diagnosis is not clear. In such patients symptoms may be sporadic (for example, single syncopal episodes) or mild (slight fatigue). Electrocardiograms may provide a clue if varying degrees of bradyarrhythmia are demonstrated. However, a clear-cut relationship between the bradyarrhythmia and the symptoms is not easily established. In such patients, 24-h ambulatory electrocardiograms may provide more definitive information. The following should be quantified on the 24-h ambulatory electrocardiogram in patients with suspected sinus node dysfunction: average and minimum heart rates and maximum sinus pauses, both while awake and asleep. In evaluating 24-h recordings in patients with suspected sick-sinus syndrome, it must be remembered that rather marked bradycardia is sometimes seen in normal subjects, with sleeping rates as slow as 30 beats per minute and pauses as long as 2.5 s. The diagnosis of the sick-sinus syndrome is best established when it is possible to demonstrate a concordance of severe bradyarrhythmia and symptomatology.

Provocative testing also plays a role in the diagnosis of the sick-sinus syndrome and is most useful when resting electrocardiograms and 24-h ambulatory electrocardiograms do not provide a definitive diagnosis. Treadmill testing can be used to delineate the range of sinus node responses to exercise. The failure of sinus rate to increase with exercise is abnormal, while this lack of response does not establish the sick-sinus syndrome as the cause of symptoms. The response to infusions of atropine and isoproterenol can also be used to evaluate sinus node function, the response to these agents normally being an increase in sinus rate. However, clear ranges of normal dose-response relationships have not been established, making interpretation of pharmacologic response to these agents difficult. Determination of the patient's intrinsic heart rate after autonomic blockade with atropine and propranolol may also be useful in identifying individuals whose bradyarrhythmia is due to abnormal sinus node automaticity rather than autonomic imbalance.

Sinus node function can also be evaluated in the electrophysiology laboratory. Sinus node recovery times can be measured by noting the duration of atrial asystole following cessation of rapid pacing of the atrium. The normal sinus node recovery time is less than 1.6 s. Marked prolongation of sinus node recovery time suggests the likelihood of symptomatic prolonged sinus pauses following spontaneous atrial tachyarrhythmias.

Testing with atrial extra stimuli during sinus rhythm allows calculation of the sinoatrial conduction time, i.e., the time necessary for emergence of the sinus impulse from the sinus node to the atrium. Marked prolongation of sinoatrial conduction time is usually found in patients who have clinically apparent sick-sinus syndrome. However, it may occasionally identify individuals who are prone to the subsequent development of overt sinoatrial exit blocks. In patients with atrial standstill, electrophysiologic study may demonstrate total loss of atrial excitability. Unfortunately, abnormalities of sinus node function as determined in the electrophysiology laboratory are most marked in patients with obvious sick-sinus syndrome. Electrophysiologic testing frequently shows equivocal abnormalities in patients in whom the sick-sinus syndrome is only suspected. Also, it is possible for a patient to have transient severe bradyarrhythmia but normal sinus node function as measured in the electrophysiology laboratory.

TREATMENT Management of the sick-sinus syndrome involves the elimination of significant bradycardia, as well as suppression of any associated atrial tachyarrhythmias. This is most readily done by utilizing some variety of permanent demand pacemaker (see below). If it has been established that AV conduction is intact, this can be achieved with atrial pacing. However, in most patients, the simplest form of therapy is to establish demand ventricular pacing. It is possible to manage patients with milder degrees of bradyarrhythmia and slight symptoms with reassurance, withholding permanent pacing unless and until symptoms become marked. There is little place for vagolytic drugs or beta-adrenergic stimulating drugs, such as sublingual isoproterenol, in the management of sinus node dysfunction. Once pacemaker control is established for management of bradyarrhythmia, atrial tachyarrhythmia may be managed appropriately with type I antiarrhythmic agents, beta-blocking agents, and/or digitalis (see Chap. 255).

CONDUCTION DEFECTS

PHYSIOLOGY AND PATHOPHYSIOLOGY OF CONDUCTION DEFECTS The specialized cardiac conduction system (Fig. 254-2) is designed to deliver the sinus impulse in an organized fashion to the atria and then to the ventricles. The atria and ventricles are separated electrically by fibrous AV rings which are penetrated by the specialized conduction system. Conduction defects may be atrioventricular (interfering with conduction from atrium to ventricle) or intraventricular (interfering with conduction within the ventricles).

Sinus impulses are conducted to the atrium and then to the AV node, which lies at the caudal end of the atrial septum, and which is in continuity with the His bundle, a structure which traverses the fibrous AV rings through the central fibrous

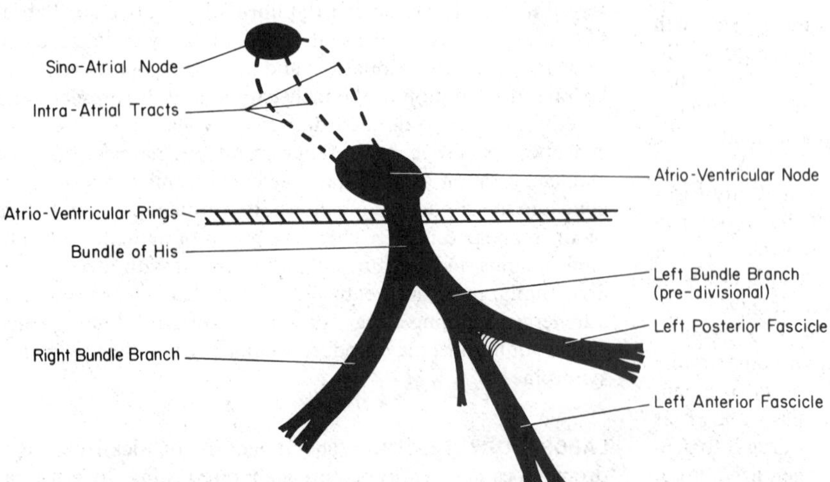

FIGURE 254-2
The specialized conduction system. Shown is a schematic drawing of the specialized conduction system of the heart with the atria above and the ventricles below. See text for discussion.

body. The His bundle, in turn, gives rise to the trifascicular conduction system, consisting of the right bundle branch (delivering the cardiac impulse to the right ventricle) and the two divisions of the left bundle branch (which has a short predivisional section before separating into two fascicles which deliver the cardiac impulse to the left ventricle). The two divisions of the left bundle branch are the anterior superior division and the posterior inferior division. These divisions should be thought of as groups of interconnecting fascicles as opposed to individual, insulated, free-running divisions. The AV node contains slowly conducting cells, while the His bundle and trifascicular conduction system are composed of rapidly conducting His-Purkinje tissue.

Simple catheter techniques have evolved for recording the electrical activity of the bundle of His (the His bundle electrogram). An electrode catheter is passed via a femoral vein to the right side of the heart, with electrodes positioned at the right AV ring. With proper amplification and filtering, a high-frequency electrogram may be recorded from the bundle of His. This high-frequency potential is not detectable on the routine surface electrocardiogram.

In patients with intact AV conduction, recording of the His bundle electrogram allows the division of the PR interval into three subintervals (Fig. 254-3). The PA interval (normally 9 to 45 ms), from the onset of the P wave to the onset of the low septal right atrial electrogram (a site very close to the AV node), is a measure of intraatrial conduction time. The AH interval (54 to 130 ms), from the onset of the low septal right atrial electrogram to the onset of the His bundle electrogram, is a measure of AV nodal conduction time. The HV interval (31 to 55 ms), from the onset of the His bundle electrogram to the onset of the QRS complex, is a measure of His-Purkinje conduction time.

A prolonged PA interval reflects intraatrial conduction delay, while a prolonged AH interval suggests AV nodal dysfunction. Splitting or prolongation of the His bundle electrogram suggests dysfunction of the His bundle. A prolonged HV interval suggests trifascicular disease, since even if only one of the three fascicles is normal, it will cause the onset of the QRS to occur at a normal time. Slow or absent conduction at any of these levels may result in AV block.

Under normal circumstances, the trifascicular conduction system delivers the cardiac impulse to both ventricles simultaneously, resulting in a QRS that is narrow (less than or equal to 0.10 s in duration) with an axis in the frontal plane of 0 to +110° (Chap. 249). Block or marked conduction delay in one or two fascicles (uni- or bifascicular block) results in abnormalities of activation diagnosable from the surface electrocardiogram but does not totally interrupt conduction since the remaining fascicle(s) will activate the ventricles. Block of three fascicles (trifascicular block) results in complete AV block.

The most important determinant of the natural history of AV block is the site of conduction disease. Total interruption of conduction can occur at the atrial approaches to the AV node, at the AV node, within the His bundle, or within the trifascicular conduction system. The His-Purkinje system possesses latent automaticity, allowing protection from the consequences of AV nodal block. Thus, the patient with AV block may be protected from asystole by the occurrence of escape rhythms distal to the site of interruption of conduction. Thomas Lewis proposed a *law of the heart,* in which he noted that rhythmicity and automaticity decrease (in terms of both rate and reliability) as one moves distally within the conduction system. In accord with this law more distal conduction disease is more likely to produce symptomatic bradyarrhythmia.

Complete AV nodal block usually results in a His bundle escape rhythm, characterized by escape rates of approximately 40 to 60 beats per minute. In the absence of additional His-Purkinje disease, this escape rhythm is conducted with a normal (narrow) QRS complex. Proximal His bundle block usually results in emergence of a distal His bundle pacemaker, whose escape rate is somewhat slower than the more proximal His bundle escape rhythms. This rhythm may be conducted with either a wide or narrow QRS complex. For patients with complete trifascicular block, the escape rhythm is idioventricular (arising in the distal intraventricular His-Purkinje system). Idioventricular escape rhythms are quite slow and unreliable. They produce a wide QRS complex since they arise in either the right or left ventricle and must traverse the ventricular septum to activate the other ventricle.

In order to understand conduction defects complicating acute ischemic heart disease, it is necessary to know the blood supply to the conduction system. The AV node is supplied by a branch of the right coronary artery in 90 percent of patients. Thus, in acute diaphragmatic infarction (generally reflecting obstruction of right coronary flow), if conduction defects arise, they are usually AV nodal. The blood supply to the trifascicu-

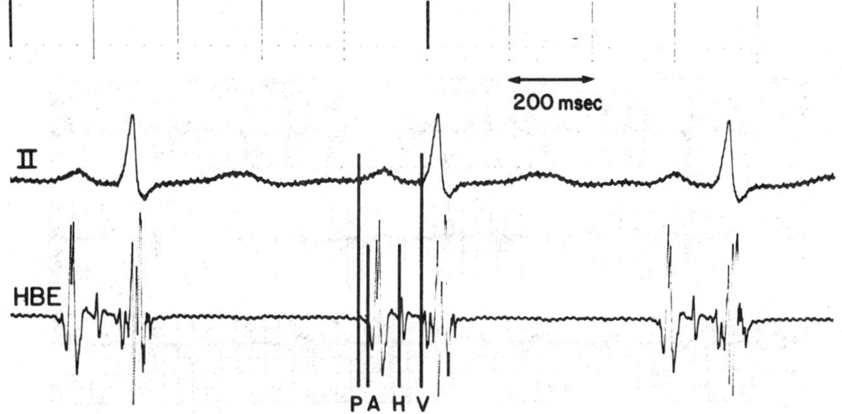

FIGURE 254-3
The His bundle electrogram. Shown is electrocardiographic lead II and the corresponding His bundle lead at 100 mm/s paper speed. See text for discussion.

lar conduction system reflects the blood supply to the ventricular septum, i.e., predominantly branches of the left anterior descending coronary artery. In addition, the posterior septum is supplied by branches of the posterior descending coronary artery, which is usually a branch of the right coronary artery. Unifascicular, bifascicular, and trifascicular block therefore may result from acute anteroseptal infarction (reflecting major disturbances in blood flow to the ventricular septum).

ETIOLOGY OF CONDUCTION DEFECTS The AV node has considerable autonomic supply (both parasympathetic and sympathetic) and is thus sensitive to marked variations in autonomic tone. It is also markedly susceptible to ischemia. Acute AV nodal block may be seen with acute diaphragmatic myocardial infarction, spasm of the right coronary artery, digitalis intoxication, acute myocarditis (typically rheumatic), and cardiovascular surgery. Acute AV nodal block occurs in some patients during episodes of vasovagal syncope. It has also been reported in association with Lyme disease.

Chronic AV nodal dysfunction may be seen as a normal variant in healthy people, in trained athletes, and with almost any disease process involving the heart (arteriosclerotic, hypertensive, valvular, etc.). Most congenital heart block is AV nodal. Specific infiltrative disease processes may selectively involve the AV node. These include amyloidosis, sarcoidosis, and hemochromatosis. The AV node may rarely be involved with primary tumors (mesothelioma) or metastatic disease. Nocturnal AV nodal block may complicate the sleep-apnea syndrome.

Unifascicular, bifascicular, and trifascicular disease have similar etiologies. Trifascicular conduction system disease can be classified as either primary or secondary; primary trifascicular disease is diagnosed when major intraventricular conduction disease is present without apparent complicating heart disease. One variety of trifascicular disease reflects the effects of aging on the cardiac skeleton. There is sclerosis and calcification of the structures making up the mitral and aortic valve rings, the central fibrous body, the pars membranacea of the ventricular septum, and the summit of the ventricular septum. It is possible for calcific lesions to impinge upon one, two, or three fascicles (Lev's disease). In other patients with primary conduction disease, pathologic studies reveal sclerodegenerative changes within the conduction system without involvement of other cardiac structures (Lenegre's disease).

In most patients unifascicular, bifascicular, or trifascicular disease is secondary to readily apparent organic heart disease. The most common cause of trifascicular disease is hypertensive cardiovascular disease, which accelerates aging of the cardiac skeleton, with resultant secondary involvement of the trifascicular conduction system. Calcific aortic stenosis is another common cause of trifascicular conduction disease, since the aortic valve ring is adjacent to the upper portions of the trifascicular conduction system. Trifascicular block may also accompany acute anteroseptal myocardial infarction. If the patient survives the acute infarction, he or she may be left with residual unifascicular, bifascicular, or trifascicular block. Trifascicular disease may also occur in any disease process involving the ventricular myocardium, including all varieties of cardiomyopathy, a number of congenital heart diseases, and, occasionally, the results of trauma due to cardiovascular surgery. There are also hereditary forms of trifascicular block, usually reflecting autosomal dominant inheritance, and manifesting as heart block later in life. There is a specific predilection for trifascicular disease in patients with myotonia dystrophica, Kearns-Sayre syndrome, and polymyositis.

The causes of His bundle block are generally similar to those producing trifascicular block and include hypertensive cardiovascular disease, calcific aortic stenosis, arteriosclerotic heart disease, Lev's disease, trauma, cardiovascular surgery, and sarcoidosis. Acquired idiopathic His bundle block is most commonly seen in females, who appear to have specific predilection to sclerosis and calcification of the cardiac skeleton with resultant interference with His bundle function.

DIAGNOSIS OF AV BLOCK The surface electrocardiogram is the usual tool for diagnosing AV block, which is characterized by disordered relationships of P waves and QRS complexes. First-degree AV block is defined as a prolonged PR interval (greater than 0.20 s in adults) with intact AV conduction. Second-degree AV block is defined as incomplete AV block with blocked P waves. Second-degree block can be further classified into Mobitz type I (Wenckebach), Mobitz type II, and advanced. Type I block is characterized by progressive PR-interval prolongation prior to the blocked P wave (Fig. 254-4*A*). Mobitz type II block is characterized by fixed PR intervals prior to the blocked P wave (Fig. 254-4*B*). Advanced second-degree AV block is defined by the presence of 2:1 or greater degrees of AV block (less than complete) and cannot be categorized as being type I or type II since there are not two consecutive conducted P waves by which to judge the increase or lack of increase in PR interval. Complete heart block (third-degree block) is defined by the total lack of conduction between atria and ventricles (Fig. 254-4*C*). Paroxysmal AV block

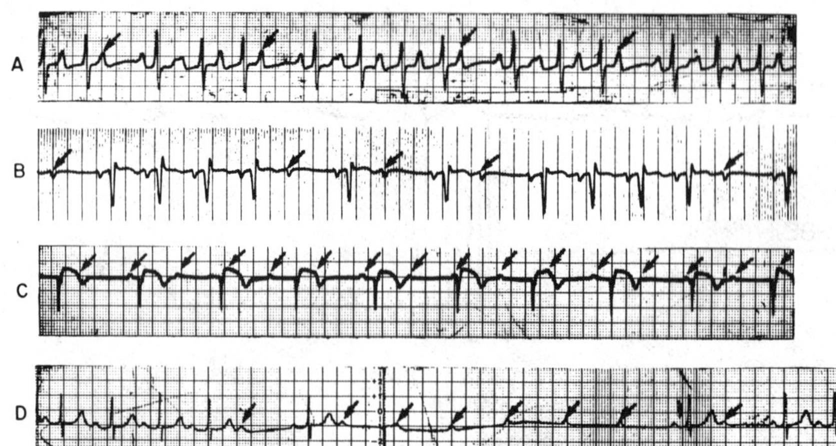

FIGURE 254-4
AV block. All blocked P waves are labeled with arrows. A. Mobitz type I (Wenckebach) second-degree AV block. Note the progressive lengthening of PR interval before the blocked P. B. Mobitz type II second-degree AV block. Note the absence of progressive lengthening of the PR interval before the blocked P wave. This figure also demonstrates periods of 2:1 AV block, which is commonly associated with Mobitz type II block. C. Complete (third-degree) AV block complicating acute diaphragmatic myocardial infarction. Note the fixed PP intervals which are different from the fixed RR intervals, resulting in a changing AV relationship. The atrial rate is faster than the ventricular rate (AV dissociation due to complete AV block). D. Paroxysmal AV block. Intact AV conduction is followed by sudden block of many P waves.

is the sudden onset of complete heart block with prolonged asystole following a period of previously intact AV conduction (Fig. 254-4*D*).

Complete AV block results in complete AV dissociation, usually with an atrial rate faster than the ventricular escape rhythm. Scrutiny of the electrocardiogram in patients with AV dissociation reveals fixed PP intervals which differ from the RR intervals, which are also fixed. Although AV dissociation often reflects AV block, it can also occur when there is an increased rate of a secondary pacemaker, such as with junctional or ventricular tachycardia and when there is a decreased rate of the primary pacemaker such as with sinus bradycardia and a junctional escape rhythm.

ELECTROCARDIOGRAPHIC DIAGNOSIS OF FASCICULAR BLOCKS *Left anterior fascicular block* (block of the anterior superior division of the left bundle branch) is characterized by a narrow QRS complex (less than or equal to 0.10 s) and left axis deviation (a mean frontal plane QRS axis of between −45 and −90°). This results in a qR complex in lead I and rS complexes in leads II and III. Left anterior fascicular block may mask the Q wave of a previous diaphragmatic infarction and sometimes simulate a lateral infarction (because of the qR in lead I). *Left posterior fascicular block* (block of the left bundle branch) is uncommon and is also characterized by a narrow QRS complex but with right axis deviation (QRS axis greater than 110°). This produces a QRS pattern with an rS in lead I and qR in leads II and III. In order to make this electrocardiographic diagnosis, there must be no clinical evidence of right ventricular hypertrophy.

Right bundle branch block is also a variety of unifascicular block. However, in this unifascicular block, impulses are delivered by the left bundle branch and then must cross the septum to activate the right ventricle. This produces QRS widening. Complete right bundle branch block is characterized by a wide QRS complex (0.12 s or greater), and typically an rSR′ pattern in lead V_1. Alternate patterns seen in V_1 with right bundle branch block include a qR and a notched R.

The term *bifascicular block* refers to block of two fascicles of the trifascicular conduction system. The combinations producing bifascicular block are thus left bundle branch block, which may be predivisional or reflect involvement of both divisions of the left bundle branch, right bundle branch block with left anterior fascicular block, and right bundle branch block with left posterior fascicular block. The electrocardiographic diagnosis of left bundle branch block is dependent upon QRS widening (0.12 s or greater) and the presence of a notched or M-shaped R wave in lead V_6. Right bundle branch block with left anterior fascicular block is diagnosed when V_1 demonstrates right bundle branch block and the frontal plane leads demonstrate left axis deviation (Fig. 249-13). Right bundle branch block with left posterior fascicular block is diagnosed when V_1 demonstrates right bundle branch block and the frontal plane leads demonstrate right axis deviation. In such cases, an independent means (such as echocardiography) must be utilized to exclude the presence of right ventricular hypertrophy.

INTRACARDIAC RECORDINGS In patients with manifest AV block, the His bundle recording technique allows delineation of the site of block. In patients with first-degree AV block (with or without additional bifascicular block), conduction delays may be noted in the atrium, AV node, His bundle, or within the trifascicular conduction system. In a patient with bifascicular block a long HV interval suggests the presence of disease in the remaining fascicle and is associated with a relatively increased risk of subsequent complete AV block (although the absolute risk is still low). In patients with second- or third-degree AV block, the exact site of block may be localized as being proximal to the His bundle (AV nodal), within the His bundle (this is frequently manifest by split His bundle potentials, one potential being recorded proximal to an area of His bundle block, and the other recorded distal to such an area), or distal to the His bundle (trifascicular block) (Fig. 254-5). In general, AV nodal blocks do not lead to serious clinical consequences, while His bundle blocks and trifascicular blocks do. Therefore, AV nodal blocks often do not necessitate pacing, while His bundle and trifascicular blocks do (see below).

ADDITIONAL LABORATORY TESTING In patients with conduction defects or AV block, it is often useful to evaluate cardiac structure and function utilizing a host of noninvasive tests. These include echocardiography (both M-mode and two-dimensional), gated or first-pass nuclear angiography, and thallium scintigraphy (Chap. 250). These tests provide information regarding the presence or absence of complicating or-

FIGURE 254-5

Diagnosis of the site of second-degree AV block using intracardiac recording of the His bundle electrogram. Shown in each panel are electrocardiographic lead II and the His bundle electrogram at 50 mm/s paper speed. Atrial electrograms and His bundle electrograms are labeled A and H, respectively. The distal recording of a split His potential is labeled H′. A. Block proximal to H (AV nodal block). Note that the blocked P wave (the fourth in the tracing) occurs with A not followed by H, indicating that conduction was interrupted within the AV node. Note that this is Mobitz type I (Wenckebach) second-degree AV block (characteristic of AV nodal block). B. Block within H (His bundle block). Note that two His bundle electrograms are recorded (split His potentials). The blocked P wave (the third in the tracing) occurs with A followed by H, but not H′, indicating that conduction was interrupted within the bundle of His. C. Block distal to H (trifascicular block). Note that the blocked P waves (the second and the seventh in the tracing) occur with A followed by H, indicating that conduction was interrupted at a site beyond the His bundle recording site. Note that this is Mobitz type II second-degree AV block (characteristic of His-Purkinje block).

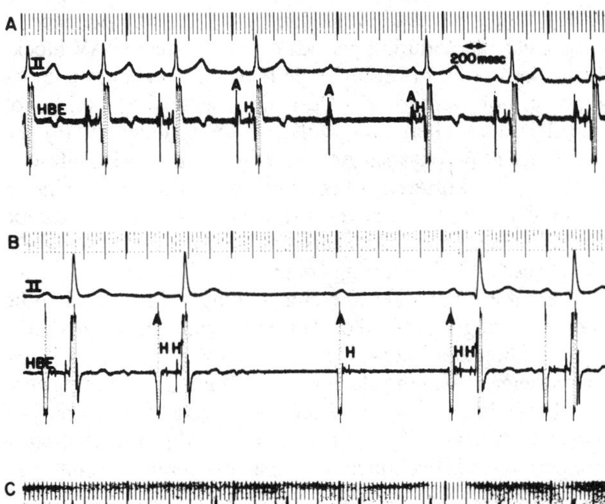

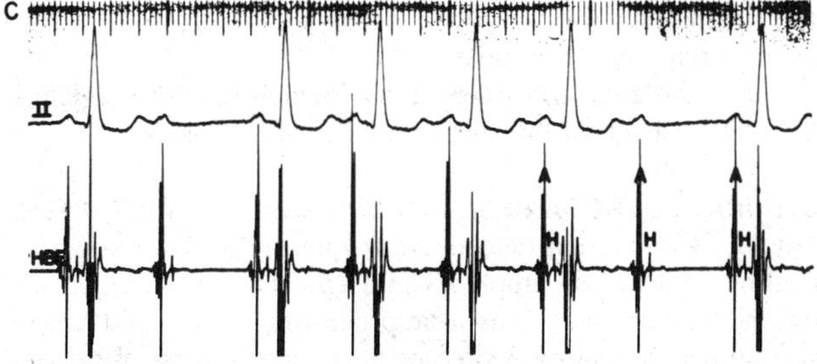

ganic heart disease and the accompanying hemodynamics. *Twenty-four hour ambulatory electrocardiographic monitoring* can be used to enhance the detection of AV block in patients with suspected bradyarrhythmia. Episodes of second-degree, third-degree, or paroxysmal AV block may be detected with this technique. However, it should be noted that normal persons may occasionally manifest second-degree AV nodal block on 24-h ambulatory recording. This is particularly true during nocturnal vagotonic periods.

Treadmill testing may also be utilized in patients with suspected or proven AV block. In patients with bifascicular block, treadmill provocation of complete AV block (a rare event) strongly suggests the occurrence of spontaneous complete block. Treadmill testing in patients with established block may also be of some value in delineating the site of block. AV nodal block is generally improved with exercise, while block within or distal to the His bundle is usually worsened.

DIAGNOSIS OF SITE OF CONDUCTION DISEASE The site of AV block is a major determinant of the clinical course in patients with second- and third-degree AV block. Thus, when evaluating a patient with AV block, it is important to arrive at a clinical decision regarding the probable site of block. Clues to the presence of AV nodal block include: (1) the clinical setting in which AV block is seen (see discussion of etiology of conduction disease above); (2) the occurrence of typical Wenckebach periodicity, which is characteristic (but not absolutely diagnostic) of AV nodal block; (3) the occurrence of conducted beats with narrow QRS complexes in patients with second-degree AV block, or the occurrence of a narrow QRS escape rhythm in patients with complete AV block; (4) improvement in conduction with atropine and/or exercise in patients with second-degree block, or significant increase in escape rates with atropine and/or exercise in patients with established complete block; (5) in patients with complete block, the presence of an escape rhythm more rapid than 50 beats per minute.

Clues to the presence of trifascicular block include: (1) the clinical setting in which AV block is seen (see discussion of etiology above); (2) the presence of preexistent bifascicular block during periods of intact conduction; (3) the presence of bifascicular block during periods of second-degree AV block; (4) the occurrence of Mobitz type II block (this is not pathognomonic, however, for His-Purkinje disease); (5) periods of fixed 2:1 block alternating with 1:1 AV conduction; (6) the occurrence of paroxysmal AV block in a patient with bifascicular block; (7) worsening of conduction with either atropine or treadmill testing (see above); (8) slow idioventricular escape rhythms (rates below 40 beats per minute) with wide QRS complexes ($\geq$ 0.12 s) during complete heart block.

There are times when the clinical diagnosis of His bundle block is strongly suggested. The most common such occurrence is idiopathic block with narrow QRS complexes in elderly women in whom calcification of valve rings and the central fibrous body may be detectable by echocardiography. It frequently is manifest as periods of 1:1 conduction alternating with periods of 2:1 conduction with a near-normal PR interval. Paroxysmal AV block with a narrow QRS complex is also characteristic of His bundle block.

His bundle electrocardiography frequently allows a definitive diagnosis of all the above varieties of AV block.

CLINICAL COURSE AND SIGNIFICANCE OF CONDUCTION DEFECTS Conduction defects are frequently discovered during routine electrocardiography. The diagnosis of isolated left anterior fascicular block has little prognostic import and can be seen either in healthy people or as a complication of organic heart disease. The extent and severity of heart disease are the determining factors in regard to life history of these patients.

The occurrence of acquired left or right bundle branch block is of somewhat greater diagnostic and prognostic importance. Recent data reported from Framingham, Massachusetts, have improved our understanding of bundle branch blocks and their significance. Most patients who develop right or left bundle branch block will have evidence of significant organic heart disease, usually either hypertensive or ischemic. The age-corrected mortality for patients with newly discovered bundle branch block in Framingham is three to five times that of an age-matched control group (reflecting the presence of organic heart disease). However, it should be noted that there are "benign" varieties of bundle branch block. One does encounter young people (and occasionally older people) who have bundle branch block in whom careful evaluation reveals no additional evidence of organic heart disease. Such patients generally do well and need no therapy other than reassurance.

There are a number of complications of bifascicular block. The most common variety of acquired heart block in adults is that within the trifascicular conduction system, and most adults developing trifascicular block have had antecedent bifascicular block. Of patients with chronic bifascicular block, approximately 2 percent per year will develop AV block (approximately half of which is trifascicular and half of which is AV nodal). Progression of conduction disease appears to be independent of age, but it is more common in patients with obvious organic heart disease. In patients with acute anteroseptal myocardial infarction, newly developed bifascicular block carries a risk of trifascicular block of approximately 30 to 80 percent within 2 weeks of the acute infarction.

Syncope is among the most common of the clinical problems encountered in patients with chronic bifascicular block. In patients with chronic bifascicular block, syncope may reflect an intermittent bradyarrhythmia (AV block or sinus node dysfunction), or a variety of other conditions, such as intermittent ventricular or supraventricular tachyarrhythmia, valvular obstruction, and central nervous system disease. Recurrent syncope in a patient with chronic bifascicular block *usually* reflects either recurrent AV block or recurrent ventricular dysrhythmia.

In a patient with second- or third-degree AV block, the significance of the conduction defect relates both to the site of conduction disturbance (see above) and to the extent and severity of complicating organic heart disease. Acute or chronic AV nodal blocks are generally benign in regard to clinical course and are usually not complicated by the development of significant symptomatic bradyarrhythmia. In contrast, His bundle block and trifascicular block are associated with progressive and usually symptomatic bradyarrhythmia, and with a high incidence of Stokes-Adams attacks. Once bradyarrhythmia is appropriately managed with pacemakers in such patients, the natural history will be determined by the extent and severity of the complicating heart disease.

MANAGEMENT OF CONDUCTION DEFECTS The *asymptomatic* patient with bundle branch block or chronic bifascicular block can be followed without prophylactic pacemaker therapy since the risk of symptomatic bradyarrhythmia or sudden death in such patients is relatively low. Prophylactic pacing is not indicated prior to surgery because of the low risk of AV block.

Patients with bifascicular block who develop syncopal episodes should be hospitalized and evaluated by means of clinical examination, serial electrocardiograms, prolonged electrocardiographic monitoring, routine laboratory studies, central nervous system evaluation, noninvasive cardiovascular evaluation, and electrophysiologic testing. The results of His bundle recordings should be evaluated along with additional clinical data. Marked HV prolongation (> 100 ms) and the development of block distal to the His bundle with atrial pacing and intact AV nodal conduction are indications of significant trifascicular disease, and may be indications for permanent pacing. Recurrent syncope in patients with bundle branch block in whom no cause can be delineated may also be an indication for permanent pacing. Our experience suggests that permanent pacing will prevent further episodes in approximately 50 percent of these patients.

The decision to institute permanent pacing in patients with second- or third-degree AV block is largely dependent upon the site of the block and the presence or absence of symptoms secondary to bradyarrhythmia. Thus, asymptomatic patients with second-degree AV nodal or even complete AV nodal block may be followed closely without recourse to pacemaker therapy, while asymptomatic patients with second- or third-degree block within or distal to the His bundle (His bundle or trifascicular block) should have demand pacing instituted prophylactically because of the high risk of Stokes-Adams attacks and the potential risk of sudden cardiac death due to prolonged asystole. Patients whose symptoms can be attributed to the conduction disturbance generally require pacing, regardless of the site.

The management of heart block complicating acute myocardial infarction essentially follows along the lines of management of chronic AV block (Chap. 261). Acute second-degree AV nodal block (most commonly seen complicating diaphragmatic infarction or digitalis intoxication) is generally self-limited. Temporary pacing need be utilized only if severe bradyarrhythmia is encountered. In patients with new bifascicular block complicating acute anteroseptal infarction, temporary prophylactic pacing is indicated because of the high risk of trifascicular block and the adverse hemodynamic consequences of this block, should it occur. In this group of patients, however, the mortality is high, both with and without pacing, since bundle branch block alone is associated with approximately a 50 percent mortality in acute infarction patients, and trifascicular block is associated with almost a 90 percent mortality even with pacing. These high mortalities reflect the extensive myocardial damage required to produce advanced intraventricular conduction defects in the patient with acute myocardial infarction.

The management of patients surviving anteroseptal infarction with trifascicular block is somewhat controversial. If trifascicular block does not resolve, then permanent pacing is indicated. If trifascicular block resolves, and the patient is left with chronic bifascicular block, then permanent pacing is suggested by some workers, based upon data indicating that this will decrease the risk of late sudden death. It is our opinion that further life history data are needed before a firm recommendation can be made regarding the long-term management of such patients.

PACEMAKERS

Cardiac muscle is electrically excitable and capable of propagating a response, a property which allows the use of external energy sources to replace the normal automatic cardiac function responsible for impulse generation. This type of therapy (electrical pacing) is of use when there is either failure of impulse generation or failure of impulse conduction. Pacing the heart depends upon the local delivery of an electrical impulse which is then propagated. Pacing can be either temporary or permanent.

Temporary pacing with catheter electrodes is generally utilized for stabilization of heart rate in acute settings, where bradyarrhythmia is most likely a self-limited event (such as due to acute infarction, acute metabolic derangement, or drug intoxication) or while awaiting institution of permanent pacing. Temporary pacing under special circumstances (Chap. 255) may be utilized for management of tachyarrhythmia.

Permanent pacing is primarily utilized for ensuring the presence of adequate heart rates because of either permanent or intermittent chronic bradyarrhythmia. Indications for permanent pacing include intermittent or established asymptomatic His bundle block and trifascicular block, symptomatic block at any site within the conduction system, and symptomatic bradyarrhythmic sinus node dysfunction. Permanent pacing may also be utilized in patients with bifascicular block and recurrent syncope, and prophylactically following acute anteroseptal infarction which has been complicated by transient trifascicular block. Prophylactic pacing of asymptomatic patients with bifascicular block or patients who have suffered a single syncopal episode without documented cause does not appear indicated at present. Permanent pacing is generally not necessary in patients with chronic second- or third-degree AV nodal block although, if ventricular rates are quite slow, this therapy may become necessary.

Pacemakers may be defined on the basis of the site and type of lead systems utilized. Leads may be endocardial (placed transvenously) or epicardial (implanted via thoracotomy). Leads may be placed in either the atria or the ventricles (or both); they may be unipolar or bipolar, each having advantages and disadvantages regarding ease of stimulation and sensing. Although type of energy sources vary, the most commonly used is the lithium battery, which appears to have a useful life of 7 to 8 years.

Pacemakers are frequently used in a demand mode in which, when spontaneous impulses are sensed, the pacemaker does not deliver competitive impulses. The demand function is a safety feature which protects against initiation of ventricular fibrillation because of competitive pacing during the vulnerable period of the cardiac cycle. *Programmability* is a useful pacemaker function, in which pacemaker parameters can be changed via a source external to the patient. Programmable functions can include rate, stimulus strength and duration (which can be useful for prolonging battery life), and sensing circuitry (changing the ability of the pacemaker to sense spontaneous cardiac depolarization). Programmability increases the utility and safety of pacemakers and will almost certainly soon become routine for all permanent pacemakers.

A new terminology, involving a three-letter code, has been developed for describing the increasingly complex varieties of permanent pacemakers available. In this code, the first letter indicates the chamber paced; the second, the chamber sensed; and the third, the mode of response. The following abbreviations are utilized: I = inhibited, T = triggered, A = atrium, V = ventricle, D = dual-chamber pacing (both chambers), O = neither chamber. Thus, the VVI pacemaker would pace the ventricle, sense the ventricle, and be inhibited by a spontaneous QRS complex. This is the description of a commonly used demand ventricular pacemaker. The value of atrioventricular triggered or synchronous pacing is currently being explored because of the possibility of utilizing the atrial contribution to ventricular filling in a hemodynamically beneficial manner and of allowing the sinus node to control the rate. The place of such "physiological" pacemakers has yet to be accurately defined.

REFERENCES

ALPERT MA et al: Natural history of high-grade atrioventricular block following permanent pacemaker implantation. J Chron Dis 35:341, 1982

BONKE FLM (ed): *The Sinus Node: Structure, Function, and Clinical Relevance.* The Hague, Martinus Nijhoff Medical Division, 1978

DHINGRA RC et al: Incidence and site of A-V block in patients with chronic bifascicular block. Circulation 59:238, 1979

——— et al: Significance of H-V interval in 517 patients with chronic bifascicular block. Circulation 64:1265, 1981

JOSEPHSON ME: The role of programmed stimulation and intracardiac recording in the diagnosis and management of arrhythmias, in *Update IV: Harrison's Principles of Internal Medicine,* KJ Isselbacher et al (eds). New York, McGraw-Hill, p 99

———, Seides SF: *Clinical Cardiac Electrophysiology.* Philadelphia, Lea & Febiger, 1979

SCHNEIDER JF et al: Comparative features of newly acquired left and right bundle branch block in the general population: The Framingham Study. Am J Cardiol 47:931, 1981

STRASBERG B et al: Natural history of chronic second degree A-V nodal block. Circulation 63:1043, 1981

WELLENS HJJ et al (eds): *The Conduction System of the Heart.* Leiden, H. E. Stenfert Kroese B.V., 1976

255
THE TACHYARRHYTHMIAS

KENNETH M. ROSEN
ROBERT A. BAUERNFEIND

ATRIAL FLUTTER, ATRIAL FIBRILLATION, AND ATRIAL PREMATURE BEATS

PHYSIOLOGY AND PATHOPHYSIOLOGY While it has long been established that depolarization of atrial muscle generates the P wave on the surface electrocardiogram (Chap. 249), many aspects of atrial activation are still controversial. Sir Thomas Lewis proposed that activation of the atria takes place via radial spread from the sinoatrial node. James and others, on the other hand, have postulated that atrial activation takes placed via specialized internodal pathways (anterior, middle, and posterior) which connect the sinoatrial and AV nodes (Fig. 254-2).

A number of abnormalities, including atrial stretch, hypoxia, and electrolyte imbalance, serve as the background upon which atrial ectopic activity develops. Considerable evidence suggests that *atrial flutter* reflects the presence of an intraatrial circus movement (see below), but whether the circus movements underlying flutter are microscopic or macroscopic is not clear. It is possible that some cases of flutter result from triggered automaticity (see below) in diseased atrial tissue. *Atrial fibrillation* results from the total disorganization of atrial depolarization, with multiple microreentrant circus movements. In normal atria, electrotonic interactions between neighboring atrial cells maintain the almost simultaneous depolarization of atrial cells in any region, so that fibrillation, should it develop, is self-terminating. However, such normal interactions between adjacent cells are less likely in diseased atria and may account for the perpetuation of atrial fibrillation, once begun.

During either atrial flutter or fibrillation, atrial impulses enter the AV node at a very high frequency (> 250 per minute). Many of these impulses are usually blocked in the AV node, a mechanism which protects the ventricles.

ETIOLOGY OF ATRIAL FLUTTER AND FIBRILLATION Both atrial flutter and fibrillation usually occur in patients with heart disease which is associated with atrial distention so that elevation of either right or left ventricular end-diastolic pressures or obstruction of either AV valve predisposes to these arrhythmias. In addition, any condition associated with infiltrative or inflammatory changes involving the atria may be associated with flutter or fibrillation.

Several disease processes, including pulmonary embolism, thyrotoxicosis, mitral stenosis and/or regurgitation, and mitral valve prolapse, should be specifically searched for in the patient with apparently idiopathic atrial flutter or fibrillation. Atrial fibrillation is a frequent arrhythmia in patients with the sick-sinus syndrome (Chap. 254). It also occurs occasionally in a familial form and is inherited in an autosomal dominant fashion. Atrial fibrillation can also occur in the absence of definable organic heart disease, a condition termed *lone atrial fibrillation.*

ELECTROCARDIOGRAPHIC DIAGNOSIS OF ATRIAL ARRHYTHMIA The electrocardiographic diagnosis of *atrial premature beats* (APBs) depends upon the recognition of P waves that are premature relative to sinus cycle length, and which differ in morphology from sinus P waves (Fig. 255-1*A*). APBs frequently reset the sinus node, producing pauses which are only partially compensatory. Less commonly, APBs are interpolated between two sinus P waves, without pauses. APBs may be blocked in the AV node or conducted to the ventricles and activate them normally, producing a normal QRS complex, or occasionally they may produce an aberrantly conducted beat. Closely coupled (early) APBs are usually either blocked or conducted aberrantly.

The electrocardiographic features characteristic of *atrial flutter* (Fig. 255-1*B*) include the presence of flutter waves which are identical in shape, usually sawtooth in configuration, with the major deflection being negative in leads II, III, and aVF and precisely regular, at rates usually between 250 and 350 per minute. This classification is somewhat arbitrary, in that atrial rhythms identical to flutter sometimes occur with rates as rapid as 400 per minute, particularly in children and in patients with thyrotoxicosis. The atrial rate may be relatively slow, i.e., below 250 per minute following administration of type I antiarrhythmic drugs (quinidine, procainamide, and disopyramide) which reduce automaticity and conduction velocity, but which

FIGURE 255-1
Atrial arrhythmia. Rhythm strips show (A) sinus rhythm with atrial premature beats (third and fifth beats); (B) atrial flutter with variable block; and (C) atrial fibrillation with rapid ventricular response.

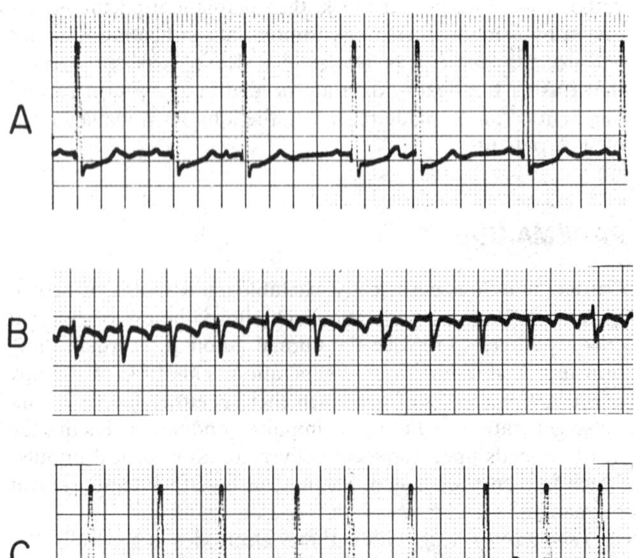

prolong the duration of the action potential and the effective refractory period. *Atrial fibrillation* is characterized by lack of organized atrial activity, with atrial fibrillatory waves, i.e., irregular undulation of the base line visible on the surface electrocardiogram (Fig. 255-1*C*).

The ventricular rate during atrial flutter or fibrillation varies inversely with the refractoriness of the AV node. Atrial flutter is characteristically conducted with a fixed ratio of flutter waves to QRS complexes, most often a 2:1 ratio, so that an atrial rate of approximately 300 per minute is associated with a ventricular rate of 150 per minute. However, flutter may also occur with 3:1, 4:1, or with varying AV conduction, producing an irregular ventricular response. Flutter may be associated with varying degrees of heart block, leading to a slow and sometimes irregular ventricular rate. Atrial flutter with 1:1 AV conduction is rare and usually follows administration of quinidine, which slows the atrial rate and also exerts a vagolytic effect on the AV node, both actions predisposing to 1:1 AV conduction.

The ventricular response in patients with atrial fibrillation is usually totally irregular, reflecting varying penetration of atrial impulses into the AV node, resulting in the passage of impulses to the ventricles in an irregular fashion. In a patient with atrial fibrillation and a normal AV node not under the influence of drugs, the ventricular rate usually exceeds 150 per minute. Atrial fibrillation can also occur with advanced AV block, resulting in an irregular ventricular rate of 60 per minute or less, or with complete heart block, resulting in a regular ventricular rate below 60 per minute.

In patients with atrial flutter or fibrillation, the arrhythmia should be classified as paroxysmal, when it represents a new event or an episode which is self-terminating within 2 weeks of onset, or established, when it represents an episode exceeding 2 weeks in duration.

Carotid massage and laboratory testing Although the electrocardiographic diagnosis of atrial tachyarrhythmias is usually straightforward, it is sometimes difficult, as in atrial fibrillation with a very rapid (and relatively regular) ventricular rate and in atrial flutter with fixed 2:1 block, where alternate flutter waves are obscured by the superimposed QRS complexes and T waves. In both of these circumstances, an increase in AV nodal refractoriness with carotid sinus massage or the administration of edrophonium may simplify the electrocardiographic diagnosis by slowing ventricular rate, thereby allowing visualization of atrial activity on the surface electrocardiogram.

Right atrial electrograms can be recorded from a transvenous catheter inserted into the right atrium, and left atrial electrograms from an esophageal lead, or the coronary sinus. By utilization of these techniques, atrial activity is found to be totally disorganized in atrial fibrillation and regular in atrial flutter.

Echocardiography is frequently of diagnostic value since a number of the conditions which are frequently associated with atrial fibrillation or flutter, such as mitral stenosis, mitral valve prolapse, hypertrophic cardiomyopathy, and atrial septal defect, can often be diagnosed by this technique. Echocardiography is also useful for estimating atrial size, which may correlate with the likelihood of recurrence of the atrial arrhythmia. Ambulatory electrocardiography and treadmill testing are useful in defining the range of ventricular rates in a variety of circumstances in patients with established atrial flutter or fibrillation. These examinations are also of help in defining the adequacy of therapy; an inappropriately rapid ventricular response during activity signifies inadequate treatment.

CLINICAL SIGNIFICANCE OF APBs, ATRIAL FLUTTER, AND FIBRILLATION APBs are common, usually of little importance, and do not produce significant symptoms. They occur frequently during periods of sinus rhythm in patients with paroxysmal atrial fibrillation. Symptoms during atrial flutter or fibrillation relate to the ventricular rate and to the presence and severity of underlying heart disease. In otherwise healthy patients with these arrhythmias, ventricular rates of 70 to 100 per minute at rest usually are not associated with symptoms, whereas more rapid ventricular rates may produce only palpitations (Chap. 4). However, patients with significant ventricular dysfunction, in whom loss of the atrial contribution to ventricular filling may be hemodynamically deleterious, tolerate atrial flutter or fibrillation poorly. In patients with mitral stenosis, atrial flutter or fibrillation can precipitate heart failure or acute pulmonary edema, largely as a consequence of the rapid ventricular rate. Systemic embolism is one of the feared complications of these arrhythmias.

TREATMENT APBs usually do not necessitate therapy. However, if frequent, the ventricular rate may be controlled by increasing AV nodal refractoriness with digitalis or beta blockade, so that some premature beats do not conduct to the ventricles. Type I antiarrhythmic drugs (quinidine, procainamide, and disopyramide) may suppress APBs.

One approach to the management of the patient with paroxysmal, or new onset, atrial flutter or fibrillation is to control the ventricular rate, while waiting for the paroxysm to self-terminate. Cardiac glycosides, beta-adrenergic blockers, and the calcium channel blocker verapamil generally increase AV nodal refractoriness, and thereby slow the ventricular rate. Cardiac glycosides can also shorten atrial refractoriness and thus help to convert atrial flutter to atrial fibrillation, which may then self-terminate. Rapid atrial pacing may sometimes be used to convert atrial flutter (not fibrillation). This modality may be utilized when cardioversion is contraindicated because of cardiac glycoside therapy.

Another approach to the management of these arrhythmias is to attempt their conversion to sinus rhythm usually by direct-current cardioversion (page 1382). Atrial flutter frequently can be terminated with low-energy synchronized cardioversion (less than 100 W·s), whereas atrial fibrillation usually requires higher energy (100 to 400 W·s). Cardioversion is indicated when the arrhythmia is poorly tolerated and/or when one anticipates that sinus rhythm can be maintained, as when atrial flutter or fibrillation has been of short duration, and when either occurs in the absence of marked atrial enlargement, significant mitral stenosis or regurgitation, or right or left ventricular failure. Cardioversion can sometimes produce long-standing sinus rhythm, especially when a reversible cause of the arrhythmia, such as thyrotoxicosis, pulmonary embolism, infections, and surgically correctable valvular or congenital heart disease can be identified and corrected or controlled. Atrial flutter or fibrillation can also be converted to sinus rhythm with type I antiarrhythmic drugs, which exert a direct antifibrillatory effect on the atria. However, these drugs also have the potential for slowing the rate of atrial flutter and for exerting a vagolytic effect on the AV node, facilitating AV nodal conduction and increasing ventricular rate. In addition, these drugs also have the potential for provoking QT prolongation which may predispose to the development of ventricular tachyarrhythmias (page 1382).

Once sinus rhythm is established in a patient with paroxysmal atrial flutter or fibrillation, digitalis and/or beta-blocking drugs can be administered chronically so that the ventricular rate will be controlled should the arrhythmia recur. However, when paroxysms are frequent and not well tolerated, therapy with type I drugs may prevent recurrences of the arrhythmia.

However, this approach to therapy may fail, or there may be adverse effects of chronic therapy with these drugs. When chronic atrial flutter or fibrillation is the only stable rhythm that can be achieved, the goal of therapy is to ensure adequate control of the ventricular rate. Most patients require digitalis, a beta-adrenergic blocking drug, or verapamil to accomplish this.

Chronic anticoagulation is indicated when paroxysmal or established atrial flutter or fibrillation complicates mitral valve disease, and when there is a history of thromboembolic disease. Anticoagulation for 1 to 3 weeks is indicated prior to cardioversion in these circumstances.

PAROXYSMAL SUPRAVENTRICULAR TACHYCARDIA (PSVT)

PATHOPHYSIOLOGY Most paroxysmal tachycardias, supraventricular and ventricular, reflect the occurrence of sustained *reentrance,* i.e., a circus movement, in which an impulse is continually propagated in a circuit of excitable tissue. The wave fronts radiating from the circus movement produce the tachyarrhythmia. Such circuits may exist because of abnormal anatomic structures, such as bypass tracts, or because of functional abnormalities of diseased cardiac tissue and may be either microscopic or macroscopic in size. Such an excitable circuit, shown schematically in Fig. 255-2*A,* consists of two limbs joining common pathways both proximally and distally. If the two limbs have different refractory periods, a critically timed premature beat may be blocked in the first limb but conducted in the second (Fig. 255-2*A*). The impulse can then be conducted retrograde via the first (originally blocked) limb and can reenter the second (originally unblocked) limb (Fig. 255-2*B*). Total unidirectional block in one limb of the circuit predisposes to induction of circus movements, which continue as long as the propagating impulse does not encounter refractory tissue. The rate of a circus movement tachycardia varies inversely with the length of the circuit and directly with the velocity of conduction. Tachycardias due to reentry can be terminated by increasing refractoriness and/or increasing the velocity of conduction, thereby resulting in the propagating impulse encountering refractory tissue (Fig. 255-2*C*).

Electrophysiologic studies have demonstrated that reentrance involving the AV node is the most common mechanism in patients with recurrent PSVT, occurring in 60 to 70 percent of patients with this arrhythmia. Since both the proximal and distal common pathways of the circuit are located within the AV node, the path of the circus movement is microscopic. AV nodal reentrance can occur when the AV node has two pathways with different refractory periods and conduction velocities. The most common type of AV nodal reentrant tachycardia is characterized by antegrade conduction in the slowly conducting AV nodal pathway and retrograde conduction in the rapidly conducting one. This tachycardia is usually induced by a critically timed APB, which is blocked when it traverses the fast pathway in an antegrade direction. Whenever the propagating impulse reaches the distal common pathway, a wave front traverses the His bundle and activates the ventricles; whenever the impulse reaches the proximal common pathway, the atria are activated and a retrograde P wave results. Because of the extensive innervation of the AV node by the autonomic nervous system, both pharmacologic agents (such as edrophonium) and physiologic maneuvers (such as carotid sinus pressure) which have potent autonomic actions can significantly affect the properties of the AV nodal circuit.

The second most common variety of PSVT, occurring in up to 20 percent of patients, results from a circus movement involving a concealed Kent bundle, i.e., an anomalous pathway which connects the atrium directly to the ventricle and which conducts only in a retrograde direction. In contrast to the situation in preexcitation (page 1376), a concealed Kent bundle is undetectable during sinus rhythm because it cannot conduct an impulse in an antegrade direction. However, the presence of a concealed pathway can be demonstrated by means of ventricular pacing, which reveals intact VA conduction with an eccentric sequence of retrograde atrial activation. The reentrant circuits in patients with concealed anomalous pathways are macroscopic in dimension. The wave front travels in an antegrade direction through the AV node and bundle of His; the ventricle constitutes the distal common pathway, and the impulse then traverses the anomalous pathway in a retrograde direction, with the atrium serving as the proximal common pathway. The tachycardia traversing this circuit can be considered "AV reentrant," because the circus movement reenters back and forth between atria and ventricles, and it may be induced by a critically timed atrial or ventricular premature beat.

Other varieties of PSVT are less common. In approximately 10 percent of patients circus movements, usually microscopic in dimension, may exist in and around the sinus node or elsewhere in the atria (sinoatrial reentrance) and are believed to be caused by inhomogeneous refractoriness.

Although enhanced atrial automaticity may also produce tachycardias emanating from ectopic foci within the atria, the specific precipitating events have not been well established. Electrocardiographic features include initiating beats which are identical to subsequent beats (rather than APBs or VPBs), gradual acceleration of frequency at the onset of tachycardia (warm-up phenomenon), and gradual slowing before its termination, in contrast to the sudden onset and termination characteristic of reentrant tachycardias. Experimental studies have also revealed a type of automaticity which has been termed "triggered" and which may occur in injured or digitalis-intoxicated cells which utilize slow, calcium-dependent channels. Premature stimuli, or rapid stimulation, can evoke series of afterpotentials which reach threshold, producing a train of depolarizations. The clinical importance of this mechanism of producing paroxysmal tachycardia has not yet been established.

Organic heart disease, frequently of minor degree, is detectable in about 50 percent of patients with AV nodal reentrance. Concealed anomalous pathways are congenital abnormalities

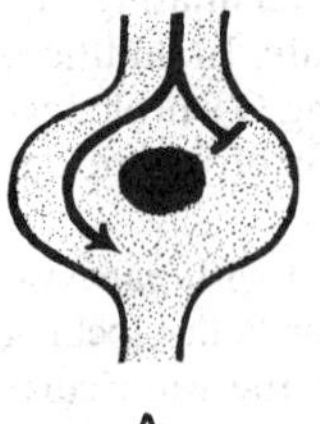

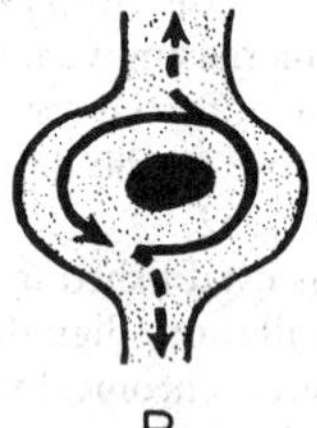

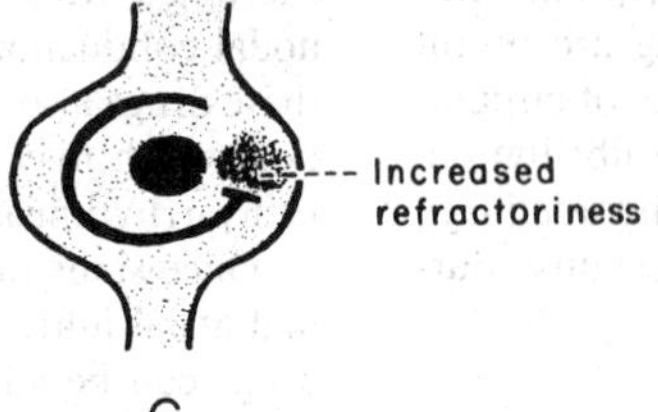

FIGURE 255-2
Schema of reentrant (circus) mechanism causing an arrhythmia. A. An impulse enters both limbs in antegrade direction; it is blocked in one limb (right) but conducts in the other (left). B. The impulse is conducted retrogradely in the originally blocked limb (right), initiating a circus movement. Antegrade and retrograde conduction from the circus movement (broken arrows) depolarize cardiac tissues, resulting in tachycardia. C. The circus movement is broken when the circling impulse encounters refractory tissue and its further conduction is blocked.

which are usually found in patients without demonstrable organic heart disease. Sinoatrial reentrant tachycardia is associated with the sick-sinus syndrome (page 1364), usually occurs in patients with organic heart disease, and probably results from pathologic changes within the atria.

Multifocal atrial tachycardia, an atrial tachycardia characterized by changing P-wave morphology and frequency, with some conducted and some nonconducted P waves, is frequently associated with digitalis intoxication, poorly compensated chronic lung disease, and electrolyte imbalance. *Atrial tachycardia* with block is usually mutifocal but may sometimes be unifocal with ectopic P waves. This arrhythmia is typically associated with digitalis intoxication but may complicate metabolic imbalance and atrial disease. The range of atrial rates is quite broad.

Electrocardiographic diagnosis The following classic electrocardiographic criteria for the diagnosis of PSVT were established prior to the development of electrophysiologic techniques and do not take into consideration the mechanism of the paroxysmal tachycardia: (1) The tachycardia is paroxysmal in onset and offset. (2) The rhythm is precisely regular and remains so for the duration of the paroxysm. (3) Atrial rates usually range between 140 and 220 per minute. Occasionally, they exceed these limits, and P waves may be difficult or impossible to identify on the surface electrocardiogram. (4) The ventricular rate equals the atrial rate (if AV conduction is normal). (5) The QRS complexes are usually narrow ($\leq$ 0.10 s) but may be widened when aberrant conduction is present.

The *mechanism* responsible for the tachycardia may be difficult to identify utilizing surface electrocardiography alone. However, in AV *nodal* reentrant tachycardia, with its microreentry within the AV node, atrial activation usually occurs simultaneously with ventricular activation, so that no P waves are visible and AV block is absent. In AV reentrant tachycardia, with its macroreentry involving an anomalous pathway, retrograde P waves usually follow the QRS complexes, and functional bundle branch block is frequent. Sinoatrial reentrant tachycardia is characterized by relatively slow rates ($\leq$ 150 beats per minute), P waves that may or may not resemble sinus P waves, but which are clearly visible, and the frequent occurrence of AV block during tachycardia.

CAROTID MASSAGE AND LABORATORY EVALUATION Carotid sinus massage is a useful diagnostic, and sometimes therapeutic, maneuver in patients with PSVT. It may have no effect or may accomplish any of the following: (1) conversion to sinus rhythm; (2) slowing of tachycardia without conversion; (3) increasing AV conduction ratio (particularly in cases of sinoatrial reentrant or automatic atrial tachycardia); (4) rarely, conversion to atrial flutter or fibrillation.

It is important to document, if possible, the occurrence of episodes of PSVT in patients with a history of paroxysmal palpitation. Twenty-four hour ambulatory monitoring may not be useful because frequently the arrhythmia is sporadic and may not occur during a given 24-h period. Treadmill testing is also not particularly helpful since most episodes are not provoked by exercise. More useful, however, are the recently developed electrocardiographic transmitting systems which allow patients to transmit their rhythms over the telephone when they develop palpitations; the transmitted signal can then be recorded on an electrocardiograph in the physician's office.

Electrophysiologic study is extremely useful in patients with known or suspected PSVT, when arrhythmia is clinically troublesome because of frequent episodes, severe symptoms, or drug resistance. The techniques utilized include recording of atrial electrograms from multiple sites, obtaining His bundle potentials, and studying the effects of atrial and ventricular extra stimuli as well as of incremental pacing of the atria and ventricles (programmed stimulation). Such studies usually allow replication of PSVT, delineation of its mechanism, and distinction between PSVT and ventricular tachycardia. The effectiveness of various drugs in the prevention of the arrhythmia induced in the electrophysiologic laboratory can also be determined (Fig. 255-3). There is an excellent correlation between a drug's ability to prevent electrically provocable tachy-

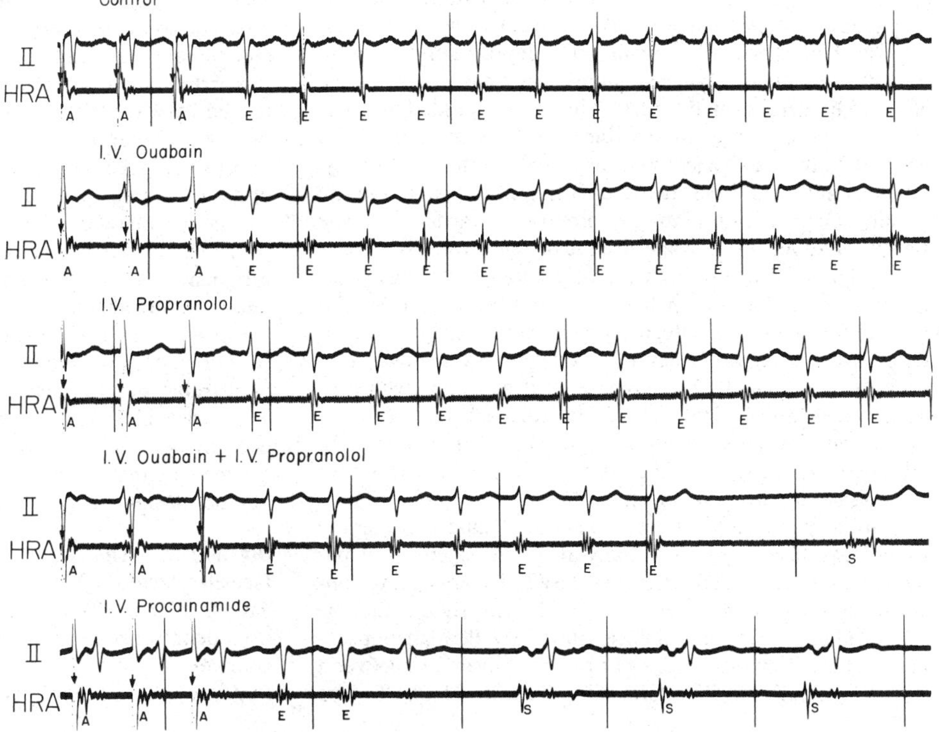

FIGURE 255-3
Electrophysiologic testing of serial IV drugs in a patient with recurrent AV nodal reentrant tachycardia. Each panel shows electrocardiographic lead II and a high right atrial (HRA) recording. Time lines are at 1-s intervals. Sustained tachycardia was induced by atrial pacing (arrows) during control study (top panel) and following administration of ouabain (second panel) or propranolol (third panel). However, following administration of ouabain and propranolol in combination (fourth panel) or procainamide (bottom panel), only brief episodes of nonsustained tachycardia could be induced (A = paced atrial beat; E = atrial echo beat). (Reproduced with modification from RA Bauernfeind et al (with permission of the American Heart Association).

cardia and its subsequent effectiveness in preventing spontaneous recurrences of tachycardia, when given as chronic oral therapy. Thus, electrophysiologic testing can be used to select specific antiarrhythmic therapy, with low morbidity and a high probability of effectiveness.

MANAGEMENT Patients with PSVT have great variability with respect to the frequency, severity, and duration of attacks. The presence and severity of symptoms relate to the ventricular rate, the duration of the attack, and the presence or absence or organic heart disease. Frequent symptoms include palpitation and dizziness, while dyspnea, angina, and syncope are less common. Attacks are often relatively benign in terms of cardiovascular function but frightening to the patient. Treatment of PSVT has two goals—the conversion of acute attacks and the prevention of recurrent attacks. In both instances, the purpose of therapy is to inhibit the ability of one or both limbs of the circus movement to sustain the reentrant arrhythmia. Many episodes of paroxysmal tachycardia, particularly AV nodal reentrant or AV reentrant tachycardia, can be converted by simple vagotonic maneuvers, which increase refractoriness within the AV node. Maneuvers eliciting potent vagotonic responses include carotid massage, ocular pressure (which involves the risk of retinal detachment and is not recommended), evoking a diving reflex by immersion of the face in cold water, and provoking a baroreceptor reflex with a vasopressor.

Drugs that can convert, or potentiate, vagotonic maneuvers in the conversion of acute attacks of PSVT include cardiac glycosides and beta blockers. Intravenous verapamil (5 to 10 mg) is the treatment of choice, since approximately 90 percent of attacks can be converted by this drug with few adverse effects. Attacks of PSVT can also be converted by performing rapid atrial stimulation using an electrode catheter, by dc cardioversion, or by administration of type I antiarrhythmic drugs. The latter methods should be used when conversion does not occur with verapamil or a cardiac glycoside, or when these drugs are contraindicated.

Prophylactic therapy is usually not necessary in patients who have infrequent attacks of relatively short duration. In patients with frequent and/or disabling attacks, an attempt should be made to delineate effective antiarrhythmic therapy. In patients with AV nodal or AV reentrant tachycardia, digitalis, beta blockers, or verapamil may depress conduction in the antegrade limb, while type I antiarrhythmic drugs may be effective by depressing conduction in the retrograde limb. The choice of appropriate antiarrhythmic therapy must take into account both effectiveness and long- and short-term toxicity. Digitalis and beta blockers are usually well tolerated and are usually effective in preventing recurrent tachycardia. The type I antiarrhythmic drugs, while also usually effective, have a relatively high incidence of both short- and long-term adverse effects. While trial and error has been the most frequently used method for delineating effective prophylactic therapy, the random variation in frequency of attacks makes evaluation of drug therapy difficult. Therefore, serial drug testing with programmed electrical stimulation, as described above, is an alternate means for delineating effective prophylactic antiarrhythmic therapy and should be carried out in patients who have drug-resistant paroxysmal tachycardia.

Cardiac pacing and surgery are alternate modes of therapy which have been used successfully in the management of patients with drug-resistant recurrent PSVT. Patients being considered for either of these forms of therapy should first be evaluated in an electrophysiologic laboratory. Permanent pacemakers have been designed which can be activated to deliver a train of stimuli and thus terminate an attack of PSVT. One variety of pacemaker, the radio frequency–triggered model, can be activated by the patient, whereas another can recognize the tachycardia and become activated automatically. Surgical therapy consists of section of an anomalous pathway, or transection of the bundle of His, followed by insertion of a pacemaker. Surgery can be carried out with a cryoprobe which produces a relatively small lesion; it should be reserved for patients in whom the precise mechanism of the tachycardia has been diagnosed and appropriate treatment with drugs and a pacemaker has failed.

PREEXCITATION—THE WOLFF-PARKINSON-WHITE SYNDROME

PATHOPHYSIOLOGY The fibrous AV rings electrically insulate the atria from the ventricles and are normally penetrated only by the specialized AV conduction system (Fig. 254-2). However, in patients with preexcitation an anomalous pathway, the muscular bundle of Kent, connects atrium directly to ventricle. The surface electrocardiogram reveals a short PR interval as a result of bypass of the AV node, while insertion of the anomalous pathway into the ventricle causes abnormal ventricular activation with initial slurring of the QRS complex, the so-called delta wave. The QRS complex reflects fusion of wave fronts which have traversed the normal and anomalous pathways. The presence of preexcitation interferes with the electrocardiographic recognition of ischemia, ventricular hypertrophy, bundle branch block, and infarction.

The Wolff-Parkinson-White (WPW) syndrome consists of preexcitation complicated by recurrent paroxysmal tachycardia, usually AV reentrant tachycardia. Thus, the tachycardia results from antegrade conduction via the normal pathway and retrograde conduction via the anomalous pathway. Patients with preexcitation are also predisposed to attacks of paroxysmal atrial fibrillation. In some patients AV reentrant tachycardia degenerates into atrial fibrillation, while others have organic heart disease with atrial distention which predisposes to atrial fibrillation. The ventricular rate may be very rapid in patients with preexcitation and atrial fibrillation because antegrade conduction takes place over the anomalous pathway with short refractoriness and the AV node, which usually protects the ventricles from the fibrillating atria, is short-circuited. The recognition of paroxysmal atrial fibrillation complicating preexcitation is of great importance, since errors in diagnosis and therapy can lead to serious complications. Superficially, this arrhythmia resembles ventricular tachycardia; it is characterized by wide QRS complexes, reflecting antegrade conduction over the anomalous pathway, but occurring at irregular intervals (Fig. 255-4*C*). The ventricular rate can be very rapid, often in the range of 300 beats per minute.

There is marked variability in the frequency and severity of tachyarrhythmias in patients with preexcitation. Some patients experience no arrhythmias, or episodes which are only a minor nuisance. In others, arrhythmias may be frequent, disabling, life-threatening, and even fatal.

Although most patients with preexcitation do not have demonstrable heart disease, this condition may be associated with Ebstein's anomaly, hypertrophic cardiomyopathy, and possibly with mitral valve prolapse. Thyrotoxicosis may allow a latent anomalous pathway to become manifest. In a small number of patients preexcitation is familial.

DIAGNOSIS The typical features of preexcitation on the surface electrocardiogram (Fig. 255-4*A*) are (1) a short PR interval ($\leq$ 0.12 s); (2) a widened QRS complex ($\geq$ 0.12 s); and (3) a delta wave, i.e., slurring of the initial portion of the QRS complex. When the major deflection in lead V_1 is an R wave (type A preexcitation), the anomalous pathway usually involves the left ventricle, while a dominant S wave in V_1 (type B) results from an anomalous pathway involving the right ventricle.

In the patient with WPW and AV reentrant tachycardia, during the tachycardia antegrade conduction usually occurs across the AV node, and retrograde conduction via the anomalous pathway, producing a PSVT with a normal QRS complex ($\leq$ 0.10 s) (Fig. 255-4*B*). Less commonly, the tachycardia complicating the WPW syndrome exhibits antegrade conduction through the anomalous pathway and retrograde conduction via the AV node; this produces a tachycardia with a wide QRS complex ($\geq$ 0.12 s), resembling ventricular tachycardia, but without AV dissociation.

The *Lown-Ganong-Levine syndrome* refers to a condition with short PR interval ($\leq$ 0.12 s), narrow QRS complexes, and reentrant tachycardia. Patients with this syndrome, unlike those with the WPW syndrome, usually have a propensity to AV nodal reentry.

ELECTROPHYSIOLOGIC STUDY This can establish whether an anomalous pathway is present or absent and allow its localization; the atrial pacing site which results in the shortest stimulus to delta wave interval is usually closest to the atrial insertion of the anomalous pathway. There is a strong correlation between the ability to induce an AV reentrant tachycardia in the laboratory in the patient with WPW and the clinical occurrence of the arrhythmia. Thus, if the tachycardia can be induced, it suggests the diagnosis in a patient whose tachycardia has escaped electrocardiographic documentation. The ability to induce AV reentrant tachycardia and atrial fibrillation with programmed stimulation can also be used to test the efficacy of antiarrhythmic drugs.

TREATMENT The principles for the treatment of PSVT (page 1376) are usually applicable to the treatment of the patient with the WPW syndrome and this arrhythmia. However, the management of the patient with preexcitation, atrial fibrillation, and rapid ventricular rate requires special consideration.

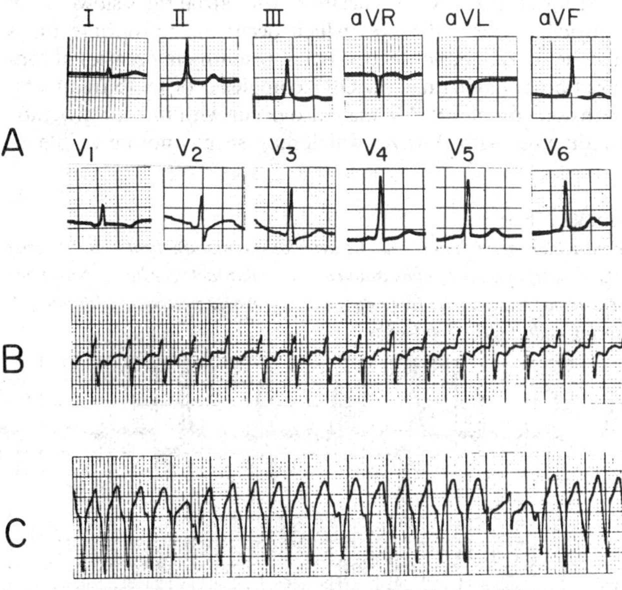

FIGURE 255-4
The Wolff-Parkinson-White syndrome. A. Standard electrocardiographic leads during sinus rhythm in type A preexcitation. Note short PR (0.09 s), widened QRS (0.13 s), and delta waves. B. Paroxysmal supraventricular tachycardia through normal AV pathway resulting in narrow QRS complexes. C. Paroxysmal atrial fibrillation, conducted predominantly over the anomalous pathway, with widened QRS complexes.

Digitalis is contraindicated because it does not increase the refractoriness of the anomalous pathway and therefore does not slow the ventricular rate and because it may predispose the patient with preexcitation and atrial fibrillation to ventricular fibrillation. Verapamil or propranolol also do not increase the refractoriness of the anomalous pathway, but by depressing left ventricular function they may interfere with tolerance of a rapid rate. In some patients, type I antiarrhythmic drugs, particularly disopyramide, may increase the refractoriness of the anomalous pathway, resulting in slower ventricular rates during recurrences of paroxysmal atrial fibrillation, while inhibiting the ability of the atria to sustain atrial fibrillation. The safest therapy for the WPW patient with atrial fibrillation and rapid ventricular rate dc is cardioversion.

Surgical treatment is indicated in patients with the WPW syndrome with drug-refractory recurrent PSVT or atrial fibrillation. Electrophysiologic study in the catheterization laboratory can delineate the arrhythmic mechanism and localize the anomalous pathway. Epicardial mapping in the operating room can further define the location of the anomalous pathway, allowing its transection. Patients with anomalous pathways in the free wall can usually be cured with low morbidity by surgical ablation. Ablation of anomalous pathways in the ventricular septum is more difficult and is associated with risk of transection of the normal as well as the anomalous pathway, resulting in complete AV block.

NONPAROXYSMAL JUNCTIONAL TACHYCARDIA

This arrhythmia is believed to reflect increased automaticity of AV junctional tissue, i.e., of the AV node and bundle of His. The escape rate of the AV junction, as occurs in failure of impulse formation in the sinoatrial node, is normally in the range of 40 to 60 per minute. Nonparoxysmal junctional tachycardia reflects enhanced automaticity of the AV junction, with a rate ranging between 60 and 140 per minute. This arrhythmia may persist for hours or days, and since its onset and termination are usually gradual, it is termed "nonparoxysmal." It is usually a manifestation of digitalis intoxication, acute ischemia (most often acute diaphragmatic infarction), acute myocarditis, or chronic obstructive lung disease with respiratory failure. Nonparoxysmal junctional tachycardia may also occur following cardiac surgery, as a manifestation of electrolyte imbalance, or rarely without apparent cause.

The electrocardiographic diagnosis depends upon recognition of an AV junctional rhythm with a rate between 60 and 140 per minute, usually with narrow, regular QRS complexes. Typically, retrograde conduction is blocked so that there is AV dissociation, with the ventricular rate more rapid than the atrial rate. However, AV dissociation is usually incomplete, so that appropriately timed P waves may capture the ventricles, producing early QRS complexes during the tachycardia. Occasionally, nonparoxysmal junctional tachycardia occurs with exit block, resulting in irregularity of QRS complexes. His bundle electrograms demonstrate that a His bundle potential precedes each QRS, with a normal or prolonged HV interval. Nonparoxysmal junctional tachycardia due to digitalis intoxication should be suspected when the ventricular rate becomes regular in a patient with atrial fibrillation.

The hemodynamic effects of nonparoxysmal junctional tachycardia are usually relatively minor, reflecting the relatively moderate ventricular rates characteristic of this arrhythmia. However, there is loss of the atrial contribution to ventricular filling, which may be deleterious in hemodynamically compromised patients. Digitalis intoxication should be recognized when it is the cause because more serious consequences of digitalis intoxication can occur if cardiac glycosides are continued. When nonparoxysmal junctional tachycardia complicates diaphragmatic myocardial infarction, it is frequently self-limited and disappears within 24 to 48 h.

This arrhythmia generally does not require specific therapy. If due to digitalis intoxication, cardiac glycosides should be discontinued and electrolyte abnormalities or hypoxemia corrected if present.

VENTRICULAR ARRHYTHMIAS (PREMATURE BEATS, VENTRICULAR TACHYCARDIA, FIBRILLATION, AND SUDDEN CARDIAC DEATH)

PATHOPHYSIOLOGY Enhanced automaticity and reentrance are the major mechanisms involved in the occurrence of ventricular premature beats (VPBs) and ventricular tachycardia (VT). The normal His-Purkinje system is characterized by latent automaticity, and injured ventricular muscle cells may also be automatic. Experimentally, automaticity of all these structures can be increased by ischemia, hypoxia, electrolyte abnormalities, catecholamines, and stretch. Ventricular reentry as a mechanism for ventricular arrhythmias appears to occur as a consequence of areas of slow conduction. Microscopic reentry occurs predominantly with ventricular muscle or the distal His-Purkinje system, while macroscopic reentry involves the bundle branches and is less common. In the animal laboratory, reentrant ventricular arrhythmia can be observed in areas of acute ishcemia or chronic myocardial infarction.

The ability to induce sustained VT and to replicate the spontaneous tachycardia by programmed electrical stimulation strongly implicates reentry as the mechanism of the tachycardia. Endocardial recordings, either in the catheterization laboratory or the operating room, frequently demonstrate continuous electrical activity during sustained VT, further suggesting the presence of a continuously propagating circus movement. Endocardial maps usually reveal that VT arises on the endocardial surface in proximity to a ventricular aneurysm. On the other hand, ventricular fibrillation (VF) involves total disorganization of ventricular electrical activity and presumably reflects the occurrence of multiple circus movements in the ventricles. A critical mass of ventricle is necessary for ventricular fibrillation to occur. This arrhythmia can be provoked in the dog by delivering a suprathreshold stimulus during the vulnerable period (during the upstroke of the T wave), and the VF threshold, i.e., the amount of energy required to provoke VF, can thus be measured. The vulnerability to VF varies inversely with the threshold. A number of stimuli, including ischemia, reperfusion of an occluded coronary artery, toxic doses of cardiac glycosides, electrolyte abnormalities, stretch, and unilateral sympathetic nerve stimulation may decrease the threshold, and VPBs which are normally harmless could provoke VF. There has been an association between the occurrence of closely coupled premature beats (R-on-T phenomenon) and the development of VF. An increase of the VF threshold and protection against this arrhythmia may be achieved experimentally by vagal stimulation in the presence of intact sympathetic nerves, or by the administration of drugs, such as lidocaine and bretylium. The healthy nonischemic human heart is not prone to VF unless provoked by specific circumstances such as powerful electric shocks.

ETIOLOGY Ventricular arrhythmias are frequently associated with chronic ischemic heart disease. In general, there is an association between the severity of the arrhythmia and the extent of the ischemic heart disease, i.e., the number of diseased vessels, the presence of previous infarction, and the extent of wall motion abnormality (Chap. 260). Mitral valve prolapse (Chap. 258) and hypertrophic cardiomyopathy (Chap. 263), and congenital or acquired QT prolongation, are also associated with ventricular arrhythmias. The syndrome of arrhythmogenic right ventricular dysplasia is characterized by fatty infiltration of the right ventricle, leading to right ventricular wall motion abnormalities, as well as disturbances of right ventricular repolarization, and is frequently associated with serious ventricular dysrhythmia.

VPBs and VT may also occur in patients without any evidence of organic heart disease, and in them are usually of little prognostic significance.

ELECTROCARDIOGRAPHIC DIAGNOSIS A VPB is characterized by the occurrence of a QRS complex which (1) has a duration $\geq$ 0.12 s; (2) is premature relative to the normally conducted beats; (3) does not follow a P wave; and (4) typically produces a fully compensatory pause, so that the interval between conducted beats bracketed by the VPB equals two basic RR intervals (Fig. 255-5*A*). Occasionally, VPBs are conducted retrogradely and reset the sinus node (producing less than a fully compensatory pause), or are interpolated between two normal beats (producing no compensatory pause). Grading systems emphasize the complexity of VPBs. Characteristic measures of complexity include frequency, multiformity, and occurrence of couplets and salvos and of close coupling intervals. VPBs are frequently coupled by a fixed interval to preceding QRS complex, reflecting a reentry mechanism. *Parasystole* occurs when premature beats happen at a regular interval unrelated to normally conducted beats and is due to the enhanced automaticity of an abnormal focus. Other characteristics of parasystole include a common denominator for interectopic intervals and entrance block, resulting in protection from normally occurring beats, and fusion beats.

VT is defined as the occurrence of three or more consecutive VPBs at a rate $\geq$ 100 beats per minute (Fig. 255-5*B*); ventricular rhythms with rates between 60 and 100 per minute are classified as accelerated idioventricular rhythms. During most VTs there is AV dissociation, with atrial rates slower than ventricular rates; P waves which occur at appropriate times may be conducted to the ventricles, resulting in occasional captured beats having narrow QRS complexes or more frequently in fusion complexes. VT may also occur with intact retrograde conduction, with P waves which may or may not be visible on

FIGURE 255-5

Ventricular arrhythmias. A. Ventricular premature beats. B. A brief (three-beat) episode of nonsustained ventricular tachycardia. C. Sustained ventricular tachycardia (note dissociated P waves preceding fifth and following eighth QRS complexes).

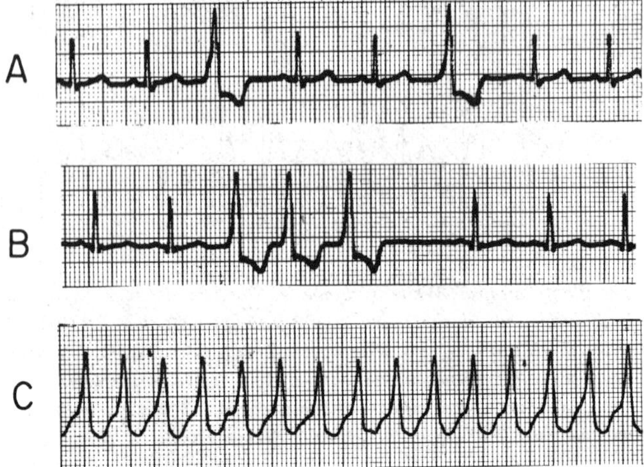

the surface electrocardiogram. Although VT may be confused with supraventricular tachycardia and bundle branch block, the configuration of the QRS complexes tends to be more bizarre in VT than in supraventricular tachycardia with bundle branch block.

By definition nonsustained VT terminates spontaneously (Fig. 255-5*B*), while paroxysmal sustained VT persists until it is terminated by specific interventions, such as drugs or dc conversion (Fig. 255-5*C*). A specific variety of VT known as *torsade de pointes* is associated with QT prolongation (see below).

VF, reflecting total disorganization of ventricular electrical activity, is recognized electrocardiographically by fibrillatory waves and by an absence of regular QRS complexes. It should be differentiated from *cardiac asystole,* which is characterized by a flat base line.

Detection of ventricular arrhythmias Twenty-four hour ambulatory electrocardiographic recordings are useful in the detection of transient ventricular arrhythmias, which may not be present on routine electrocardiograms. VPBs can be classified (R-on-T, multiform) and quantified (number of individual VPBs, couplets, or salvos per hour or day). Treadmill exercise testing is also frequently useful as a means of provoking ventricular arrhythmias.

ELECTROPHYSIOLOGIC STUDY These investigations have proved extremely useful in the diagnosis, understanding, and management of VT. In establishing the diagnosis in the presence of a tachycardia with a wide QRS complex, it is necessary to delineate atrial activity, and when P waves are not apparent on the surface electrocardiogram, either an esophageal electrode or an electrode catheter in the right atrium may be employed. The differentiation between supraventricular and ventricular tachycardia may require the recording of His bundle electrograms; conducted beats of a supraventricular tachycardia, regardless of the duration of the QRS complex, are preceded by His bundle potentials, with normal or prolonged HV intervals. In contrast, VT is characterized by either no His bundle potentials preceding the QRS complexes or a short or negative HV interval.

In most patients with VT, programmed stimulation of the ventricles allows replication of the arrhythmia in the electrophysiologic laboratory with critically coupled impulses which engage reentrant pathways. If sustained VT is induced, catheter mapping of the ventricles can provide information regarding the anatomic origin of the VT, information which may subsequently be useful to the surgeon. This technique also provides an excellent means for delineating effective antiarrhythmic therapy by testing the ability of various drugs to prevent the induction of VT (Fig. 255-6). This arrhythmia may also be induced in the operating room. Both epicardial and endocardial maps delineating the path of the arrhythmia can be made and can be useful for planning the surgical treatment of VT. It should be noted that most patients with VT can be managed medically.

Electrophysiologic testing has also been useful in patients resuscitated from out-of-hospital VF in whom it may be possible to induce a rapid sustained VT in the catheterization laboratory, which is likely to be identical to the spontaneous rhythm which preceded the VF. This approach may be used to develop a suitable antiarrhythmic drug regimen (Chap. 30).

CLINICAL SIGNIFICANCE VPBs are a frequently encountered clinical problem, in patients both with and without organic heart disease; they can be detected in approximately 80 percent of patients with recent myocardial infarction if Holter recording and/or treadmill provocation are utilized. In patients with chronic ischemic heart disease, there is an association between the presence of high-grade ventricular ectopy (repetitive or early VPBs) and the subsequent occurrence of both sudden and non-sudden cardiovascular death. The extent of ventricular arrhythmia is strongly related to the severity of heart disease. Patients with ischemic heart disease and high-grade ventricular ectopy usually have low ejection fractions, multiple wall motion abnormalities, and obstructive disease involving at least two major coronary arteries (Chap. 260). The combination of congestive heart failure and complex ventricu-

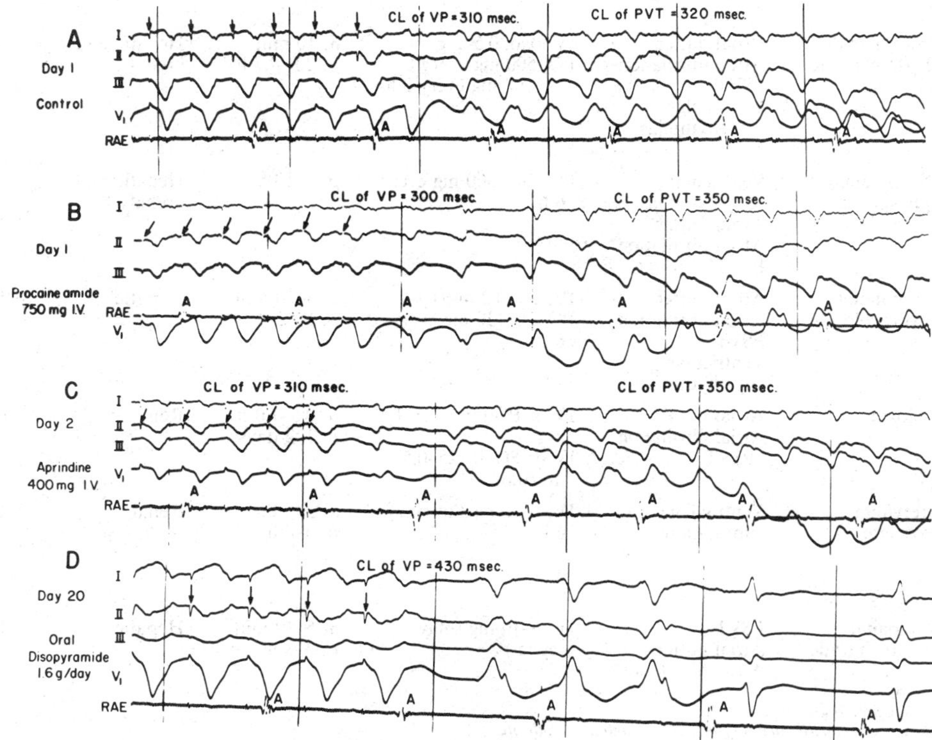

FIGURE 255-6
Electrophysiologic testing of serial drugs in a patient with recurrent sustained paroxysmal ventricular tachycardia. Each panel shows electrocardiographic leads I, II, III, and V_1 as well as a right atrial electrogram (RAE). Sustained tachycardia was induced by ventricular pacing (arrows) during control study (A) and following administration of IV procainamide (B) or IV aprindine (C). However, following administration of oral disopyramide (D), only brief episodes of nonsustained tachycardia could be induced. A = atrial electrogram. (Reproduced from P Denes et al, Chest 77:478, 1980, with permission of the American College of Chest Physicians.)

lar ectopy has been shown to be a powerful predictor of subsequent cardiovascular mortality.

The significance of ventricular ectopy in the patient with acute myocardial infarction (Chap. 261) is somewhat controversial. The previously widely accepted concept that VPBs are warning arrhythmias for the development of VF appears to be an oversimplification, since many patients who develop VF have no warning arrhythmia and many patients with frequent VPBs do not develop VF. Available insurance data suggest that in patients without organic heart disease VPBs are usually benign. Although annoying, they generally have relatively little hemodynamic or prognostic significance.

The clinical significance of VT varies with the frequency of attacks, the rate and duration of the episodes, and the presence or absence of complicating heart disease. VT ranges from a benign insignificant to an incapacitating and/or life-threatening arrhythmia. Transient episodes may be noted during 24-h ambulatory recordings in asymptomatic patients. In others, particularly patients with severe ischemic heart disease, longer bouts of VT may produce significant symptoms, necessitate multiple cardioversions and hospitalizations, or precipitate sudden death.

VF can be classified as being either primary or secondary. If it occurs as a consequence of or in association with a serious illness, cardiovascular or noncardiovascular, it may be considered secondary, and the successful management of the arrhythmia has little effect on the ultimate outcome. In contrast, in primary VF, the major derangement appears to be electrophysiologic. If the latter can be managed, then the prognosis can be significantly improved. Sudden cardiac death is usually due to primary VF (see Chap. 30).

THERAPY OF VENTRICULAR ARRHYTHMIA The major therapeutic decision in patients with VPBs relates to whether therapy is to be attempted and, if so, what the appropriate end point should be. The following principles are useful in reaching this decision: (1) All antiarrhythmic drugs have significant short- and long-term toxicity, some of which may be life-threatening; (2) there is no conclusive evidence that therapy of asymptomatic ventricular arrhythmias in patients with or without organic heart disease results in improved survival; (3) the appropriate end point for measuring the efficacy of therapy for preventing sudden death has not been delineated. Thus, it remains to be determined whether it is necessary to eradicate all or some VPBs or specific categories of VPBs, such as early VPBs or couplets. Since it has not been convincingly demonstrated that the potential benefits of antiarrhythmic therapy outweigh the risks in asymptomatic patients, the authors believe that antiarrhythmic therapy is *not* required in most cases of asymptomatic ventricular arrhythmias, despite the recognition that under certain circumstances VPBs may be harbingers of sudden death.

If and when ventricular ectopy is treated, the treatment should be carried out in a rational manner. Before therapy is attempted, the frequency and complexity of VPBs should be quantified on one or more 24-h ambulatory electrocardio-

TABLE 255-1
Antiarrhythmic drugs

Drugs	*Indication*	*Route/dose*	*Half-life*	*Predominant metabolic route*	*Therapeutic plasma concentration*	*Major side effects*
Lidocaine hydrochloride	Ventricular dysrhythmias	IV load, 50–100 mg (may repeat) Infusion, 2–4 mg/min	α, 5–10 min β, 1.2–2.2 h	Hepatic	1.5–5.0 μg/ml	CNS (convulsions)
Quinidine sulfate	Atrial flutter Atrial fibrillation PSVT Ventricular dysrhythmias	PO, 200–600 mg every 6 h	β, 6–7 h	Hepatic and renal (10–50%)	2.5 μg/ml	Gastrointestinal Cinchonism Purpura Rash Fever Torsade de pointes
Procainamide hydrochloride	Atrial flutter Atrial fibrillation PSVT Ventricular dysrhythmias	IV load, 0.5–2 g PO, 500 mg every 6 h–1500 mg every 3 h	α, 10 min β, 2.5–4.7 h	Hepatic and renal	4–10 μg/ml	+ANA and lupus syndrome Fever Rash Leukopenia Torsade de pointes
Disopyramide phosphate	Ventricular dysrhythmias Atrial flutter* Atrial fibrillation* PSVT*	PO, 100–300 mg every 6 h	β, 4–10 h	Hepatic and renal	2–4 μg/ml	Anticholinergic (vision, urinary) Negative inotropy Torsade de pointes
Propranolol hydrochloride	Atrial flutter Atrial fibrillation PSVT Ventricular dysrhythmias	IV, 0.1–0.2 mg/kg PO, 20–120 mg every 6 h	α, 5–20 min β, IV 2–4 h, PO 3.5–6 h	Hepatic	Uncertain for arrhythmia	Bronchospasm Bradycardia Hypotension Negative inotropy
Digoxin	Atrial flutter Atrial fibrillation PSVT	IV or PO load, 0.5–1.5 mg IV or PO, 0.125–0.5 mg/day	α, 0.5–1.0 h β, 1–2 days	Renal	0.5–2.0 ng/ml	Gastrointestinal Visual disturbances Arrhythmia
Bretylium tosylate	Ventricular fibrillation	IV, 5–10 mg/kg every 6 h	α, 30 min β, 5–8 h	Renal	Unknown	Initial hypertension and ventricular irritability Postural hypotension
Verapamil hydrochloride	PSVT Atrial flutter Atrial fibrillation	IV, 5–10 mg (may repeat)	α, 5–10 min β, 3–8 h	Hepatic	Unknown	Hypotension Negative inotropy Bradycardia

* *Unapproved use.*
NOTES: *α = distribution half-life; β = elimination half-life.*

graphic recordings as well as one or more treadmill tests. Recent literature suggests that because of the large fluctuations in frequency of VPBs, a reduction of greater than 80 percent is required to signify a beneficial effect. The therapy of nonsustained VT also requires determination of the frequency of attacks. If multiple attacks occur during each 24-h period, then it is usually possible to identify an effective response, i.e., suppression of VT. However, if episodes of nonsustained VT are infrequent, it is much more difficult to do so.

Attacks of sustained VT generally necessitate rapid attempts at conversion. If the attack is well tolerated, conversion can be attempted with intravenous lidocaine or procainamide. If the VT is poorly tolerated, or if the above medications fail, then elective or emergent dc cardioversion is indicated. Prevention of recurrent paroxysmal sustained VT is a difficult problem. Since the arrhythmia is sporadic in many patients, a trial-and-error approach is difficult. A type I antiarrhythmic drug may be administered with appropriate monitoring of blood levels, although recent work suggests that previously described levels may be too low (specifically with procainamide) (Table 255-1). If an episode of VT occurs despite an effective blood level, other agents should be tried. Combination drug therapy may be helpful but increases the frequency and severity of adverse effects. In patients who have frequent VPBs or nonsustained VT provoked by exercise, therapy with beta-blocking drugs is usually effective.

VT can usually be reproduced in the catheterization laboratory, and if a specific drug is found to prevent induction of sustained VT, then oral, chronic administration of this drug will generally prevent spontaneous recurrences of sustained tachycardia (Fig. 255-6).

Surgical treatment may be considered in patients with drug-resistant, recurrent sustained VT, most of whom have chronic ischemic heart disease with prior myocardial infarction. The electrophysiologic evaluation includes (1) induction of the VT in the laboratory as well as in the operating room; (2) endocardial mapping to delineate the site of origin of the VT in the laboratory, using electrode catheters; (3) epicardial mapping in the operating room utilizing probe electrodes; (4) endocardial mapping in the operating room through a ventriculotomy. The surgical approaches in these patients include (1) simple aneurysmectomy; (2) aneurysmectomy with resection of residual endocardial scar, since many tachycardias appear to arise from the endocardium on the periphery of ventricular aneurysms; and (3) encircling ventriculotomy, consisting of surgical isolation of the origin of the VT from the remainder of the heart. Although the relative merits of these procedures have yet to be firmly established, aneurysmectomy with endocardial resection, based upon an endocardial map of the VT prior to operation, may prove to be the procedure of choice. In patients with arrhythmogenic right ventricular dysplasia (page 1378) recurrent VT has been cured with surgical ablation of areas of slow conduction in the right ventricular epicardium.

The management of VF is discussed in Chap. 30.

TORSADE DE POINTES

This arrhythmia, also termed *polymorphic ventricular tachycardia,* is a very rapid VT, characterized by a gradually changing QRS morphology (Fig. 255-7*B*). Torsade de pointes is often self-terminating but may degenerate into VF. Most patients with this arrhythmia have prolonged QT intervals during sinus rhythm (Fig. 255-7*A*), and the combination of QT prolongation and torsade de pointes has been designated the QT syndrome. It is important to recognize this arrhythmia, both because of its life-threatening potential and because of the specific modalities of therapy which it requires.

The congenital varieties of the QT syndrome are rare and are usually seen in children but may become manifest for the first time in adulthood. The Jervell and Lange-Nielsen syndrome is characterized by autosomal recessive transmission, nerve deafness, QT prolongation, torsade de pointes, syncope, and sudden death. The Romano-Ward syndrome is similar but is characterized by autosomal dominant transmission and lack of nerve deafness. In the adult, the QT syndrome is usually acquired and most frequently results from drug administration. The most common offending agent is quinidine, torsade de pointes being the mechanism of most cases of quinidine syncope. Other drugs which are responsible include procainamide, disopyramide, several experimental antiarrhythmic drugs, phenothiazines (particularly thioridazine), and tricyclic antidepressant drugs. Other causes of torsade de pointes include electrolyte abnormalities such as hypokalemia, hypomagnesemia, and hypocalcemia, ingestion of the liquid protein diet, acute ischemia, bradycardia, particularly AV block, mitral valve prolapse, central nervous system disease, amyloidosis, and acute myocarditis.

Congenital QT syndromes are generally treated with beta-blocking drugs, although transection of the left stellate ganglion has been used in resistant cases. Since the acquired QT syndromes are usually caused by drugs, they are treated primarily by discontinuing the offending agent and correcting any electrolyte abnormalities. Most patients with acquired QT syndrome can be temporarily managed (torsade de pointes prevented) by ventricular pacing or isoproterenol infusion.

ANTIARRHYTHMIC DRUGS

It is inappropriate to administer antiarrhythmic drugs on the basis of a history of palpitations alone, without documentation of the arrhythmia. However, the latter can be accomplished by standard electrocardiography, 24-h ambulatory recordings, phone transmission of electrocardiograms, treadmill testing, and electrophysiologic study.

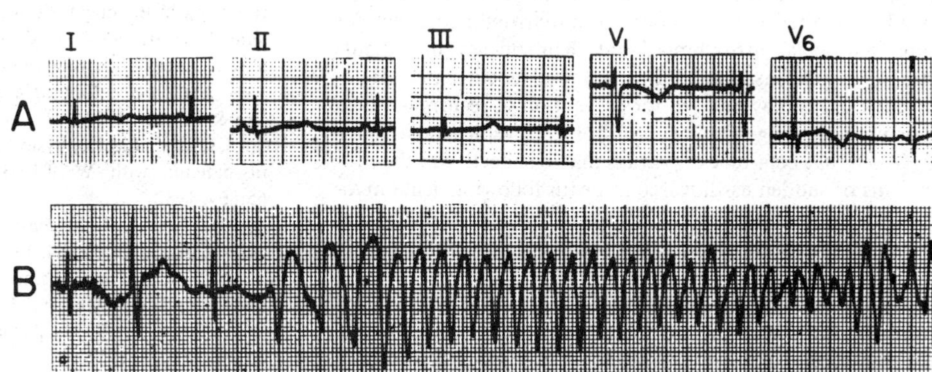

FIGURE 255-7
QT syndrome. A. Five standard electrocardiographic leads during sinus rhythm (note markedly prolonged QT interval of 0.60 s). B. Onset of torsade de pointes.

LIDOCAINE This drug, available only in the parenteral form, is particularly useful in the treatment of ventricular arrhythmias because of its rapid onset of action following intravenous bolus administration (Chap. 71) and its relative lack of significant side effects. There is evidence that a lidocaine infusion (3 to 4 mg/min) has a prophylactic antifibrillatory effect in patients with acute myocardial infarction during the first 48 h, and it is reasonable to administer lidocaine prophylactically to all patients with acute myocardial infarction, unless a specific contraindication exists (Chap. 261). Lidocaine is metabolized primarily by the liver, and higher than expected concentrations can be anticipated with liver disease and in conditions in which hepatic flow is reduced, such as congestive heart failure or cardiogenic shock.

QUINIDINE, PROCAINAMIDE, AND DISOPYRAMIDE PHOSPHATE Individual patients may respond to one or another of these agents in an unpredictable fashion even though these three type I antiarrhythmic drugs have the following similar effects: (1) an antifibrillatory effect on the atria; (2) depression of conduction in the retrograde limb in reentrant PSVT and in anomalous pathways; (3) possible interference with circus movements within the ventricles; and (4) reduction in automaticity of ectopic atrial or ventricular foci.

The toxicities of these three agents differ. Quinidine is associated with a high incidence of gastrointestinal intolerance, and this drug is probably more likely than the other type I drugs to produce torsade de pointes; approximately 2 percent of patients who receive therapeutic doses of quinidine chronically develop quinidine syncope, which is caused by brief episodes of rapid VT. Quinidine can also produce immunologically mediated thrombocytopenic purpura. Serum digoxin levels in patients receiving chronic oral digoxin approximately double with initiation of quinidine therapy.

In patients receiving long-term therapy with procainamide there is a high (50 to 75 percent) incidence of positive antinuclear antibodies, and a lupus erythematous syndrome becomes clinically manifest in a smaller number of patients. This lupus-like syndrome is most common in patients who are slow acetylators of procainamide. Fever and arthralgias are characteristic of this syndrome, while central nervous system and renal involvement are rare. The procainamide-induced lupus syndrome generally disappears when the drug is discontinued.

Administration of disopyramide phosphate is characterized by a high incidence of vagolytic side effects, most notably urinary retention and blurred vision. In addition, disopyramide probably has the most potent negative inotropic action of the three type I drugs and should be used with caution in patients with latent or manifest congestive failure.

BETA-ADRENERGIC BLOCKING AGENTS (See also Chap. 260) These drugs increase AV nodal refractoriness, thus slowing the ventricular response in atrial fibrillation and flutter, and can abolish PSVT when the AV node is in the reentrant pathway. In addition they exert a moderate antiarrhythmic effect for some ventricular arrhythmias, but their efficacy in patients with recurrent, sustained VT is not well documented. Beta-blocking drugs may be used for prevention of recurrent VF in patients with congenital QT syndrome. Several studies have suggested that beta-blocking drugs may be effective in the prophylaxis of sudden cardiovascular death following acute myocardial infarction (Chap. 260). However, because of their negative inotropic effect, these drugs must be used cautiously in patients with latent or overt heart failure.

CARDIAC GLYCOSIDES (See also Chap. 253) These drugs, like propranolol, can be used to (1) increase AV nodal refractoriness and thereby to slow the ventricular rate in atrial fibrillation and flutter; and (2) to break up circus movements responsible for PSVT. Cardiac glycosides are contraindicated in paroxysmal atrial fibrillation complicating the WPW syndrome because of lack of effectiveness and predisposition to occurrence of VF.

BRETYLIUM This drug, which has been reported to have a relatively potent antifibrillatory effect, is currently available only in the parenteral form. The one clear indication for bretylium is the prophylaxis of recurrent VF refractory to lidocaine and procainamide.

VERAPAMIL Intravenous verapamil is probably the drug of choice for conversion of acute attacks of PSVT. The value of oral verapamil for prophylaxis of recurrent paroxysmal tachycardia has not yet been firmly established. In patients with atrial flutter or fibrillation, verapamil usually results in significant slowing of the ventricular response.

DC CARDIOVERSION

Cardioversion is the application of a large direct current to the heart, usually via external paddles. This causes total depolarization of the atria and ventricles, often resulting in instantaneous conversion of tachyarrhythmia to sinus rhythm.

Elective cardioversion is usually synchronized, with the impulse timed to the QRS complex, in order to avoid its delivery during the ventricle's vulnerable period and thereby prevent VF. Synchronized cardioversion can be utilized electively for attempted conversion of atrial flutter, atrial fibrillation, PSVT, and sustained VT. Emergent cardioversion is currently the only effective measure for conversion of VF. Elective cardioversion is performed with the aid of diazepam or with an anesthesiologist in attendance to administer light general anesthesia. The energy necessary for cardioversion relates to the nature of the arrhythmia and usually varies from 10 to 400 W·s. Elective cardioversion should generally be avoided in digitalized patients, because of the hazard of unmasking digitalis toxicity. Prophylactic anticoagulation for 1 to 3 weeks is indicated before cardioversion of atrial fibrillation or flutter in patients with a history of thromboembolic disease and in patients with mitral valve disease.

REFERENCES

BAUERNFEIND RA et al: Serial electrophysiologic testing of multiple drugs in patients with atrioventricular nodal reentrant paroxysmal tachycardia. Circulation 62:1341, 1980

GALLAGHER JJ et al: The preexcitation syndromes. Prog Cardiovasc Dis 20:285, 1978

HARRISON DC et al: Clinical pharmacokinetics of antiarrhythmic drugs. Prog Cardiovasc Dis 20:217, 1977

HOROWITZ LN et al: Ventricular resection guided by epicardial and endocardial mapping for treatment of recurrent ventricular tachycardia. N Engl J Med 302:589, 1980

JOSEPHSON ME: The role of programmed stimulation and intracardiac recording in the diagnosis and management of arryhthmias, in *Update IV: Harrison's Principles of Internal Medicine,* KJ Isselbacher et al (eds). New York, McGraw-Hill, p 99

———, SEIDES SF: *Clinical Cardiac Electrophysiology.* Philadelphia, Lea & Febiger, 1979

KERR CR et al: Electrophysiologic effects of disopyramide phosphate in patients with Wolff-Parkinson-White syndrome. Circulation 65:869, 1982

MARCUS FI et al: Right ventricular dysplasia: A report of 24 adult cases. Circulation 65:384, 1982

MORADY F et al: Diagnosis and treatment five years later: Disopyramide. Ann Intern Med 96:337, 1982

PICK A, DOMIGUEZ P: Nonparoxysmal A-V nodal tachycardia. Circulation 16:1022, 1957

SCLAROVSKY S et al: Polymorphous ventricular tachycardia: Clinical features and treatment. Am J Cardiol 44:339, 1979

WALDO AL (ed): Seminar on surgical therapy for ventricular arrhythmias. Am J Cardiol 49:163, 1982

WU D et al: Clinical, electrocardiographic and electrophysiologic observations in patients with paroxysmal supraventricular tachycardia. Am J Cardiol 41:1045, 1978

ZIPES DP, TROUP PJ: New antiarrhythmic agents: Amiodarone, aprindine, disopyramide, ethmozin, mexiletine, tocainide, verapamil. Am J Cardiol 41:1005, 1978

Specific cardiac diseases

256
CONGENITAL HEART DISEASE

WILLIAM F. FRIEDMAN

GENERAL CONSIDERATIONS

INCIDENCE Approximately 1 percent of all live births are complicated by a cardiovascular malformation. If the problem is recognized early, these anomalies can now be diagnosed accurately, and most of these babies may be salvaged by aggressive medical and surgical management.

Children with congenital heart disease usually show an overall male preponderance. Moreover, specific defects may show a definite sex preponderance; patent ductus arteriosus and atrial septal defect are common in females, whereas valvular aortic stenosis, coarctation of the aorta, tetralogy of Fallot, and transposition of the great arteries are more common in males. Table 256-1 demonstrates the frequency of occurrence of specific cardiovascular malformations in clinical and pathologic studies.

ETIOLOGY Congenital cardiovascular malformations are generally the result of aberrant embryonic development of a normal structure or a failure of such a structure to progress beyond an early stage of embryonic development. Malformations appear to result from a complex interaction between multifactorial genetic and environmental systems that does not allow a single specification of etiology; only rarely may a causal factor be identified. Maternal rubella and chronic maternal alcohol abuse are environmental insults that are known to interfere with normal cardiogenesis in humans. The *rubella syndrome* consists of cataracts, deafness, microcephaly, and, either singly or in combination, patent ductus arteriosus, pulmonary valvular and/or arterial stenosis, and ventricular septal defect (see Chap. 201). The *fetal alcohol syndrome* consists of microcephaly, micrognathia, microphthalmia, fetal growth retardation, developmental delay, and cardiac septal defects. Hypoxia, deficiency or excess of several vitamins, intake of several categories of drugs, and ionizing irradiation are teratogens that are capable of causing cardiac defects in experimental animals, but their precise relation to human malformations requires further definition.

A single gene mutation (Chap. 58) may be incriminated in the familial forms of atrial septal defect, mitral valve prolapse, ventricular septal defect, congenital heart block, situs inversus, the combination of supravalvular aortic stenosis and peripheral pulmonary arterial stenosis, idiopathic hypertrophic subaortic stenosis, and the syndromes of Noonan, Holt-Oram, Ellis–van Creveld, and Kartagener. Table 256-2 provides a partial list of syndromes in which cardiovascular anomalies may be manifestations of the pleiotropic effects of single genes or examples of gross chromosomal defects. Despite the long list presented in Table 256-2, it must be appreciated that recognized chromosomal aberrations and mutations of single genes account for less than 10 percent of all cardiac malformations.

The finding that, with some exceptions, only one of a pair of monozygotic twins is affected by congenital heart disease indicates that the vast majority of cardiovascular malformations are not inherited in a simple manner. Family studies indicate a two- to fivefold increase in the incidence of congenital heart disease in the siblings of affected patients. The malformations are concordant or partially concordant in at least half of such cases. Nonetheless, the incidence of congenital heart disease in the siblings of an index patient is only 2 to 5 percent. With few exceptions, therefore, patients with isolated heart defects have a negative family history for malformations and a normal chromosome pattern, and it is rarely wise to discourage the parents of one affected child from having additional children. The low recurrence rate and the increasing possibilities for effective therapy for nearly all cardiac lesions usually justify a positive approach to family counseling. If, however, two or more members of a family are affected, the recurrence risk may be quite high, and a pedigree should be obtained prior to further counseling. If a dominant or recessive mendelian pattern is established, the mendelian laws apply, and the risk of recurrence in each pregnancy is equal.

PREVENTION The feasibility of preventive programs will depend upon what is learned in the future about the cause of the 90 percent or more of cardiovascular anomalies for which no cause is now known.

TABLE 256-1
Frequency of occurrence of cardiac malformations at birth*

Disease	*Percent*
Ventricular septal defect	30.5
Atrial septal defect	9.8
Patent ductus arteriosus	9.7
Pulmonary stenosis	6.9
Coarctation of the aorta	6.8
Aortic stenosis	6.1
Tetralogy of Fallot	5.8
Complete transposition of the great arteries	4.2
Persistent truncus arteriosus	2.2
Tricuspid atresia	1.3
All others	16.5

* *2310 cases = 100 percent.*

TABLE 256-2
Syndromes with associated cardiovascular involvement

Syndrome	*Major cardiovascular manifestations*	*Major noncardiac abnormalities*
HERITABLE AND POSSIBLY HERITABLE		
Ellis–van Creveld	Single atrium or atrial septal defect	Chondrodystrophic dwarfism, nail dysplasia, polydactyly
TAR (thrombocytopenia-absent radius)	Atrial septal defect, tetralogy of Fallot	Radial aplasia or hypoplasia, thrombocytopenia
Holt-Oram	Atrial septal defect (other defects common)	Skeletal upper limb defect, hypoplasia of clavicles
Kartagener	Dextrocardia	Situs inversus, sinusitis, bronchiectasis
Laurence-Moon-Biedl-Bardot	Variable defects	Retinal pigmentation, obesity, polydactyly
Noonan	Pulmonary valve dysplasia	Webbed neck, pectus excavatum, cryptorchidism
Tuberous sclerosis	Rhabdomyoma, cardiomyopathy	Phacomatosis, bone lesions, hamartomatous skin lesions
Multiple lentigines (leopard) syndrome	Pulmonic stenosis	Basal-cell nevi, broad facies, rib anomalies
Rubenstein-Taybi	Patent ductus arteriosus (others)	Broad thumbs and toes, hypoplastic maxilla, slanted palpebral fissures
Familial deafness	Arrhythmias, sudden death	Sensorineural deafness
Osler-Rendu-Weber	Arteriovenous fistulas (lung, liver, mucous membranes)	Multiple telangiectasia
Apert	Ventricular septal defect	Craniosynostosis, midfacial hypoplasia, syndactyly
Incontinentia pigmenti	Patent ductus arteriosus	Irregular pigmented skin lesions, patchy alopecia, hypodontia
CONNECTIVE TISSUE DISORDERS		
Cutis laxa	Peripheral pulmonic stenosis	Generalized disruption of elastic fibers, diminished skin resilience, hernias
Ehlers-Danlos	Arterial dilatation and rupture, mitral regurgitation	Hyperextensible joints, hyperelastic and friable skin
Marfan	Aortic dilatation, aortic and mitral incompetence	Gracile habitus, arachnodactyly with hyperextensibility, lens subluxation
Osteogenesis imperfecta	Aortic incompetence	Fragile bones, blue sclera
Pseudoxanthoma elasticum	Peripheral and coronary arterial disease	Degeneration of elastic fibers in skin, retinal angioid streaks
INBORN ERRORS OF METABOLISM		
Pompe's disease	Glycogen storage disease of heart	Acid maltase deficiency, muscular weakness
Homocystinuria	Aortic and pulmonary arterial dilatation, intravascular thrombosis	Cystathionine synthetase deficiency, lens subluxation, osteoporosis
Mucopolysaccharidosis:		
Hurler, Hunter	Multivalvular and coronary and great artery disease, cardiomyopathy	Hurler: Deficiency of α-L-iduronidase, corneal clouding, coarse features, growth and mental retardation Hunter: Deficiency of L-iduranosulfate sulfatase, coarse facies, clear cornea, growth and mental retardation
Morquio, Scheie, Morateaux-Lamy	Aortic incompetence	Morquio: Deficiency of *N*-acetylhexosamine sulfate sulfatase, cloudy cornea, normal intelligence, severe bony changes involving vertebrae and epiphyses Scheie: Deficiency of α-L-iduronidase, cloudy cornea, normal intelligence, peculiar facies Morateaux-Lamy: Deficiency of arylsulfatase B, cloudy cornea, osseous changes, normal intelligence
CHROMOSOMAL ABNORMALITIES		
Trisomy 21 (Down's syndrome)	Endocardial cushion defect, atrial or ventricular septal defect, tetralogy of Fallot	Hypotonia, hyperextensible joints, mongoloid facies, mental retardation
Trisomy 13 (D)	Ventricular septal defect, double-outlet right ventricle	Single midline intracerebral ventricle with midfacial defects, polydactyly, nail changes, mental retardation
Trisomy 18 (E)	Ventricular septal defect, patent ductus arteriosus, pulmonic stenosis	Clenched hand, short sternum, low-arch dermal-ridge pattern on fingertips, mental retardation
Cri-du-chat (short-arm deletion-5)	Ventricular septal defect	Cat cry, microcephaly, antimongoloid slant of palpebral fissures, mental retardation
XO (Turner)	Coarctation of aorta	Short female, broad chest, lymphedema, webbed neck
XXXY and XXXXX	Patent ductus arteriosus	XXXY: hypogenitalism, mental retardation, radial-ulnar synostosis XXXXX: small hands, incurving of fifth fingers, mental retardation

An effective rubella vaccine has been developed, and immunization of children with this vaccine may be anticipated to lessen maternal rubella and its cardiac consequences. Strict testing in animals of new drugs that may be teratogenic when taken early in pregnancy may be expected to reduce the chances of another thalidomide tragedy. In this regard, no medications should be taken during pregnancy without prior consultation with a physician. Physicians dealing with pregnant women should be aware of known teratogens, as well as of drugs for which inadequate information exists relative to their teratogenic potential. Similarly, appropriate use of radiologic equipment and techniques for reducing gonadal and fetal radiation exposure may be expected to reduce the potential hazards of this likely cause of birth defects.

The presence of a cardiac malformation as one component of a multiple system involvement that may exist in Down's, Turner's, and the trisomy 13-15 (D_1) and 17-18 (E) syndromes may be anticipated in occasional pregnancies by the detection of abnormal chromosomes in fetal cells obtained from amniotic fluid. Similarly, identification in such cells of the enzyme disorders observed in Hurler's syndrome, homocystinuria, or type II glycogen storage disease may allow one to predict the ultimate presence of cardiac disease.

THE FETAL AND TRANSITIONAL CIRCULATIONS

The fetal circulation is a single circulation in which the pulmonary vasculature exists in parallel, not in series, with the systemic circulation. Prenatal survival is not endangered by extremely severe cardiac anomalies as long as one side of the heart can drive blood from the great veins to the aorta. Inferior vena caval blood is deflected across the foramen ovale into the left atrium. Most of the blood that reaches the right ventricle bypasses the high-resistance, unexpanded lungs and passes through the ductus arteriosus into the descending aorta. In fetal life, pulmonary arteries and arterioles are surrounded by a fluid medium, have relatively thick walls and small lumens, and resemble comparable arteries in the systemic circulation.

Although fetal somatic growth may be unimpaired, the hemodynamic effects in utero of some cardiac malformations may alter the development and structure of the fetal heart and circulation. Thus, premature closure in utero of the foramen ovale may result in hypoplasia of the left ventricle. Moreover, postnatally the caliber of the aortic isthmus may be reduced in the presence of lesions, such as aortic stenosis with ventricular septal defect, that divert a portion of left ventricular output away from the ascending aorta while increasing right ventricular output and ductus arteriosus flow in utero. Similarly, obstruction in utero to right ventricular outflow is associated with an increase in proximal aortic flow and diameter and almost never with aortic coarctation. In these and other examples it is important to recognize that malformations compatible with fetal survival may nonetheless result in abnormal development of the circulation in utero and also affect circulatory adjustments after birth.

Normally the fundamental change which occurs at birth is the division of this single circulation into two separate circulations operating in series. Inflation of the lungs at the first inspiration produces a marked reduction in pulmonary vascular resistance. Fetal pulmonary vessels, heretofore supported by fluid media, are suddenly suspended in air, reducing extravascular pressure. New vessels are opened, and already patent vessels enlarge. Pulmonary arteriolar vasodilatation results from the increase in oxygen tension to which these vessels are exposed. Pulmonary arterial pressure falls, and pulmonary blood flow increases greatly. The systemic vascular resistance rises when clamping the umbilical cord removes the low-resistance placental circulation. Increased pulmonary blood flow increases the return of blood to the left atrium and raises left atrial pressure, which in turn closes the foramen ovale. The shift in oxygen dependence from the placenta to the lungs produces a sudden increase in arterial blood oxygen tension, which, in concert with alterations in the local prostaglandin milieu, initiates constriction of the ductus arteriosus, and total anatomic closure follows within a few days.

PULMONARY HYPERTENSION Pulmonary hypertension frequently complicates congenital heart disease, and the status of the pulmonary vascular bed may be the principal determinant of the clinical picture, its rate of progression, and whether corrective surgical treatment is feasible. Elevation of pulmonary arterial pressure results from elevation of pulmonary blood flow and/or resistance, the latter often reflecting structural alterations in the pulmonary vascular bed. Normally, following the fall in the pulmonary arterial pressure, resistance, and vasomotor tone which occurs shortly after birth, there is a gradual postnatal reduction in the thickness of the media of the pulmonary arterioles and widening of the lumens. Hence, the pulmonary circulation of the normal adult has evolved from a high-pressure, high-resistance, highly reactive vascular bed with relatively small cross-sectional area, to a low-pressure, low-resistance, less reactive bed with a large cross-sectional area.

As in the other vascular beds, the pressure in the pulmonary artery is determined by the product of the volume of blood flow, per unit of time, and the resistance to that flow. Equalization of pressures in the systemic and pulmonary circulations may be expected if a large communication exists between the two great arteries or between the two ventricles in the absence of semilunar valve obstruction. Pulmonary vascular resistance is calculated as the transpulmonary pressure difference per unit of pulmonary blood flow (Chap. 251). When blood flow increases, existing patent vessels are distended and additional vessels are opened, so that calculated vascular resistance diminishes. Therefore, in a normal pulmonary vascular bed, pressure will rise substantially only if flow is very greatly increased. In the vast majority of patients with congenital heart disease and elevated pulmonary vascular resistance, the pulmonary arterioles are the principal locus of this abnormal resistance.

A delay in the normal involution of the pulmonary vascular bed often occurs postnatally in the presence of an intra- or extracardiac communication with a large left-to-right shunt. In patients having high pulmonary arterial pressure from birth, anatomic changes in the pulmonary vessels, in the form of medial thickening and intimal proliferation, usually progress so that in the older child or adult the vascular resistance may ultimately be fixed by obliterative changes in the pulmonary vascular bed. However, if pulmonary arterial hypertension is not present in infancy or childhood, it may never occur or may not develop until the third or fourth decade, or even later.

Because pulmonary vascular obstructive disease may be the factor limiting a decision concerning the advisability of operation, it is important to quantify and compare pulmonary to systemic flows and resistances in patients with severe pulmonary hypertension. Furthermore, the lability of the pulmonary vascular resistance should be evaluated; a marked reduction with the infusion of tolazoline or the inhalation of oxygen suggests that resistance is not fixed and may fall after successful operation. Some defects between the left and right sides of the heart should be closed in order to eliminate a sizable left-to-right shunt, which, in turn, may result in a significant drop in pulmonary arterial pressure because of reduction of pulmonary blood flow. Conversely, little or no benefit and high mortality rates may be expected from the closure of defects that are associated with bidirectional or predominant right-to-left shunts in patients with high-resistance and obstructive pulmonary hypertension. The designation *Eisenmenger's reaction* is applied to this condition in patients who may have a large communication between the two circulations at the aortopulmonary, ventricular, or atrial levels. The actual mechanism for the persistence, delayed reduction, or late onset of elevated pulmonary vascular resistance is not known.

The clinical manifestations of the hyperkinetic form of pulmonary hypertension, i.e., that associated with a large left-to-right shunt, reflect the specific malformation responsible. When a significant right-to-left shunt exists, the patient is cyanotic, and polycythemia and clubbing of the digits may be noted (Chap. 27). A dominant *a* wave in the jugular venous pulse may be seen, reflecting vigorous right atrial contraction due to diminished compliance of the right ventricle; in some instances there are large systolic *c-v* waves, which suggest tricuspid regurgitation. A prominent right ventricular parasternal lift and palpable systolic expansion of the pulmonary artery are present. On auscultation, one often hears a soft pulmonary systolic ejection murmur following a loud ejection sound, marked accentuation of the pulmonic component of the second heart sound, and often, a fourth heart sound. The decrescendo diastolic murmur of pulmonary valvular regurgitation may be heard. The electrocardiogram shows right ventricular hypertrophy. Roentgenologic examination reveals enlargement of the right ventricle, a conspicuously enlarged pulmonary artery, prominent hilar pulmonary vascular markings, and attenuated peripheral vessels. The site of the underlying defect may be localized by means of echocardiography and/or cardiac catheterization and angiocardiography (Chap. 251). Pressures in the right side of the heart are essentially identical to systemic pressures in cyanotic patients if the shunt is at the ventricular or aortopulmonary levels, but they are usually lower than systemic pressure in patients with an interatrial shunt. No specific treatment has proved beneficial for obstructive pulmonary vascular disease.

CIRCULATORY SHUNTS

Although equal quantities of blood flow through the pulmonary and systemic circulations in normal subjects postnatally, the systemic circulation has a flow resistance approximately six times that of the pulmonary circuit, which is reflected in the markedly higher arterial and ventricular systolic pressures in the systemic circulation; the lower compliance of the thicker left ventricle is reflected in higher ventricular end-diastolic and mean atrial pressures on the left side of the heart. Therefore, if an abnormal communication is present, blood will flow from the left to the right side of the heart. The size of the opening and the pressures on either side of it generally determine the direction and magnitude of the shunt flow. A right-to-left shunt usually requires either an obstructive lesion at some point in the right-sided circulation (i.e., tricuspid stenosis or atresia, pulmonary valvular or infundibular stenosis, elevated pulmonary vascular resistance), a mixing of systemic venous and arterialized blood (i.e., total anomalous pulmonary venous drainage, a single atrium or ventricle, or a persistent truncus arteriosus), or some form of obligatory recirculation of systemic venous blood (e.g., transposition of the great arteries). The location, direction, and magnitude of the right-to-left shunt may be determined during hemodynamic study by measuring the admixture of venous and arterial blood at various sites in the central circulation, by indicator-dilution curves, and by angiocardiography, as outlined in Chap. 251.

CLINICAL MANIFESTATIONS OF RIGHT-TO-LEFT SHUNTS

Cyanosis and polycythemia These signs are discussed in Chap. 27.

Clubbing A prominent accompaniment of arterial hypoxemia consists of a widening and thickening of the terminal phalanges of the fingers and toes, accompanied by convex nails. These digits have an increased number of capillaries with increased blood flow through extensive arteriovenous aneurysms, and an increase of connective tissue.

Hypoxic spells and squatting A sudden marked increase in cyanosis due to an abrupt reduction in pulmonary blood flow occurs in younger children with certain types of cyanotic heart disease, particularly tetralogy of Fallot. The spells may lead to convulsions and may even be fatal; they may be precipitated by fluctuations in intravascular volume or in arterial P_{CO_2} and pH, a sudden fall in systemic or increase in pulmonary vascular resistance, or an acute increase in the severity of right ventricular outflow tract obstruction, either by augmented contraction of the hypertrophied muscle in the right ventricular outflow tract or by a decrease in right ventricular cavity volume due to tachycardia. Treatment consists of oxygen administration, placing the child in the knee-chest position, and intravenous administration of fluids and of sodium bicarbonate to correct the accompanying acidosis. Additional medications that may prove of value include morphine, alpha-adrenergic receptor stimulants such as phenylephrine to raise peripheral resistance and to diminish right-to-left shunting, and beta-adrenergic blocking agents, which may increase ventricular volume by reducing heart rate and lessen infundibular obstruction by reducing contractility.

Patients with cyanotic heart disease, especially tetralogy of Fallot, typically assume a squatting posture after exertion to obtain relief from breathlessness. Squatting appears to hasten an increase in the arterial oxygen saturation by increasing systemic vascular resistance and thereby diminishing the right-to-left shunt and by trapping markedly unsaturated blood in the legs. Also, systemic venous return and therefore pulmonary blood flow may rise.

"Paradoxic" embolus and brain abscess In patients with cyanotic congenital heart disease, venous blood bypasses the normal filtering action of the lungs, and emboli arising in systemic veins may pass directly to the systemic circulation. Patients with severe cyanosis or polycythemia have often had previous occlusive microcirculatory damage to the central nervous system. These predisposing factors are primarily responsible for the relatively high incidence (2 to 4 percent) of brain abscess in such patients.

Impaired growth Physical underdevelopment and a delayed onset of adolescence are common features of many types of cyanotic and, to a lesser extent, acyanotic forms of congenital heart disease. Mental development is rarely affected. Various explanations for the mechanisms of growth interference have implicated malnutrition, tissue anoxia, diminished peripheral blood flow, hypermetabolic state, chronic cardiac decompensation, genetic and endocrine factors, and frequency of upper and lower respiratory infections.

SPECIFIC CARDIAC DEFECTS

Various classifications of congenital cardiovascular lesions have been proposed, depending on hemodynamic, anatomic, and radiographic factors. Although there is overlapping between groups, the following arrangement of the more common anomalies is used in this chapter:

1 Communications between the systemic and pulmonary circulation without cyanosis (left-to-right shunts)
2 Obstructing valvular and vascular lesions with or without associated right-to-left shunts
3 Abnormalities in the origins of the great arteries and veins; the transpositions
4 Malpositions of the heart

COMMUNICATIONS BETWEEN SYSTEMIC AND PULMONARY CIRCULATION WITHOUT CYANOSIS (LEFT-TO-RIGHT SHUNTS) **Atrial septal defect** Atrial septal defect, the most commonly recognized congenital cardiac anomaly in adults, occurs more frequently in females than in males. Defects of the *sinus venosus* type occur high in the atrial septum, near the entry of the superior vena cava, and are associated frequently with anomalous connection of pulmonary veins from the right lung to the junction of the superior vena cava and right atrium. Most often, an atrial defect involves the fossa ovalis, is midseptal in location, and is of the *ostium secundum* type. This type of defect should not be confused with a patent foramen ovale. Anatomic obliteration of the foramen ovale ordinarily follows its functional closure soon after birth, but residual "probe patency" is a common normal variation; atrial septal defect denotes a true deficiency of the atrial septum and implies functional as well as anatomic patency. *Ostium primum* anomalies are a form of endocardial cushion defect that lie immediately adjacent to the atrioventricular valves, either of which may be deformed and incompetent, or which may form together a common atrioventricular valve; this defect may also involve the basal portion of the interventricular septum. *Ostium primum defects* occur commonly in patients with *Down's syndrome* (mongolism), although the more complex endocardial cushion anomalies are more characteristic. *Lutembacher's syndrome* is the designation applied to the rare combination of atrial septal defect and mitral stenosis; this component of the malformation almost invariably is the result of acquired rheumatic valvulitis.

The magnitude of the left-to-right shunt through an atrial septal defect depends on the size of the defect, the relative compliance of the ventricles, and the relative resistances in the pulmonary and systemic circulations. The left-to-right shunt causes diastolic overloading of the right ventricle and increased pulmonary blood flow. The pulmonary vascular resistance is usually normal or low in the child and young adult with atrial septal defect, and the volume load is usually well tolerated even though pulmonary blood flow may be three to six times greater than systemic.

Patients with atrial septal defect are usually asymptomatic in early life although there may be some physical underdevelopment and respiratory infections; cardiorespiratory symptoms occur in many of the older patients. Beyond the fourth decade, a significant number of patients develop atrial arrhythmias, pulmonary arterial hypertension, bidirectional and then right-to-left shunting of blood, and cardiac failure. Patients exposed to the chronic environmental hypoxia of high altitude tend to develop pulmonary hypertension at younger ages. Historical features suggesting that the defect is of the endocardial cushion variety include the onset of disability, pulmonary hypertension, and heart failure in infancy or childhood.

Physical examination usually reveals a prominent right ventricular cardiac impulse and palpable pulmonary artery pulsation. The first heart sound is normal or split, with accentuation of the tricuspid valve closure sound. Increased flow across the pulmonic valve is responsible for a midsystolic pulmonary ejection murmur. The second sound is widely split and is relatively fixed in relation to respiration, because of reciprocal changes in the magnitude of the left-to-right shunt and of the systemic venous inflow into the right ventricle during respiration, so that filling of the right ventricle remains constant and the stroke volume of the right ventricle exceeds that of the left throughout the respiratory cycle. With pulmonary hypertension the splitting is still fixed throughout respiration, although the width may be reduced. A middiastolic rumbling murmur at the fourth intercostal space and along the left sternal border reflects increased flow across the tricuspid valve. In patients with ostium primum defects, an apical thrill and holosystolic murmur indicate associated mitral or tricuspid incompetence or a ventricular septal defect.

The *physical findings* are altered when an increase in the pulmonary vascular resistance results in diminution of the left-to-right shunt. Both the pulmonary and tricuspid murmurs decrease in intensity, the pulmonic component of the second heart sound and a systolic ejection sound are accentuated, the two components of the second heart sound may fuse, and a diastolic murmur of pulmonic incompetence appears. Cyanosis and clubbing accompany the development of a right-to-left shunt.

The *electrocardiogram* in patients with an ostium secundum defect usually shows right axis deviation, right ventricular hypertrophy, and a right intraventricular conduction defect. A coronary sinus pacemaker or first-degree heart block is occasionally noted in patients with defects of the sinus venosus type. In patients with an ostium primum defect, the right ventricular conduction defect is characteristically accompanied by left axis deviation and by superior orientation and counterclockwise rotation of the QRS loop in the frontal plane. Varying degrees of right ventricular and right atrial hypertrophy may be seen with each type of defect, depending on the height of the pulmonary artery pressure; prolongation of the PR interval is most common with defects of the ostium primum variety. Chest roentgenograms reveal enlargement of the right atrium and ventricle, dilatation of the pulmonary artery and its branches, and increased pulmonary vascular markings. Left atrial enlargement is extremely uncommon. Echocardiographic features include pulmonary arterial and right ventricular dilatation and anterior systolic (paradoxical) or "flat" interventricular septal motion if significant right ventricular volume overload is present. Mitral valve prolapse may be recognized in 10 to 20 percent of patients with secundum defects. Abnormal "mitral" motion and septal-atrioventricular valve relationships are typically observed in endocardial cushion anomalies.

The diagnosis may be confirmed readily at cardiac catheterization by passage of the catheter across the atrial defect. The site at which the catheter crosses, if high in the cardiac silhouette, may suggest a sinus venosus defect, or, if low, a primum defect. Serial determinations of the oxygen saturation, or indicator-dilution curve techniques, may be used to estimate the magnitude of the shunt. In young patients, pressures in the right side of the heart are often normal despite a large shunt; pulmonary arterial hypertension occurs with greater frequency in the older patients. If an endocardial cushion defect is present, a left ventricular angiogram will frequently demonstrate a "gooseneck" deformity of the left ventricular outflow tract caused by an abnormal anterior mitral valve leaflet; it may also show mitral regurgitation. When a high oxygen saturation is found in the superior vena cava, or when the catheter enters pulmonary veins directly from the right atrium, a sinus venosus defect is likely, and indicator-dilution curves and selective angiography will aid in identifying the number and location of the anomalous veins. *Partial anomalous pulmonary venous con-*

nection, although generally associated with a sinus venosus defect, may occasionally accompany primum and secundum defects, or be unassociated with any defect of the interatrial septum.

Endocardial cushion anomalies more complex than the ostium primum defect are associated with high morbidity and mortality rates in infancy and childhood. Patients with atrial septal defect of the sinus venosus or secundum types rarely die before the fifth decade. During the fifth and sixth decades, the incidence of progressive symptoms, often leading to severe disability, increases substantially. Medical management should include prompt treatment of respiratory tract infections, antiarrhythmic medications for atrial fibrillation or supraventricular tachycardia, and the usual measures for heart failure (Chap. 253) if these complications occur. Although the risk of subacute bacterial endocarditis is low, antibiotics should be administered prophylactically prior to dental procedures (see Chap. 259).

Operative repair, ideally in patients between 3 and 6 years of age, should be advised for all patients with uncomplicated atrial septal defects in whom there is evidence of significant left-to-right shunting, i.e., with pulmonary-to-systemic flow ratios exceeding approximately 1.5:1.0. Excellent results may be anticipated, at low risk, even in patients beyond 40 years of age in the absence of pulmonary hypertension. The defect is closed by suture or with a patch of prosthetic material with the patient on cardiopulmonary bypass. Special attention must be given to the atrioventricular valves in patients with endocardial cushion defects; cleft, deformed, and incompetent valves may require repair or replacement to prevent significant regurgitation and failure in the postoperative period. The operative risk and the incidence of such complications as complete heart block and the persistence of significant mitral regurgitation are significantly higher in patients with endocardial cushion defects. Electrophysiologic mapping of the course of the conduction system during operation may reduce the risk of postsurgical heart block. Operation should not be carried out in patients with small defects and trivial left-to-right shunts, or in those with severe pulmonary vascular disease without a significant left-to-right shunt.

Ventricular septal defect Isolated defects of the ventricular septum are among the commonest cardiac malformations, and they are encountered as one component of a combination of anomalies more often than any other. Most frequently, the opening is single and situated in the membranous portion of the septum. The functional disturbance caused by a ventricular septal defect is dependent primarily on its size and the status of the pulmonary vascular bed, rather than on the location of the defect. A substantial left-to-right ventricular pressure gradient occurs in the presence of a small defect (*maladie de Roger*), and a small shunt, limited by the size of the defect, occurs throughout systole. Larger defects offer less resistance to flow, while in the presence of very large defects both ventricles will function hemodynamically as a single pumping chamber with two outlets, equalizing the pressures in the systemic and pulmonary circulations. In such patients, the magnitude of the left-to-right shunt varies inversely with the ratio of pulmonary-to-systemic vascular resistance. In patients with large defects and large left-to-right shunts, the left ventricle is overloaded and may fail. Survival through infancy in many of these patients is predicated on delayed regression of the fetal pulmonary vascular pattern, the development of an elevated pulmonary vascular resistance, or the secondary development of infundibular hypertrophy and obstruction to right ventricular outflow. Irreversible obliterative changes in the pulmonary vessels with dominant right-to-left shunts and cyanosis become manifest in many patients with large defects after the second decade of life. Spontaneous closure of small and even large ventricular defects occurs in a significant number of patients, especially before the age of 3 years. In some others, the relative size of the interventricular communication may diminish as normal growth of the heart occurs with advancing age. Rarely, incompetence of the aortic valve resulting from insufficient cusp tissue or prolapse of a cusp through the interventricular defect complicates and dominates the clinical course of patients with ventricular septal defect.

The clinical picture varies greatly, depending on the patient's age, the size of the defect, and the level of the pulmonary vascular resistance. Patients with small defects are generally asymptomatic; moderate left-to-right shunts may be associated with effort intolerance and fatigue. Large defects are commonly accompanied by frequent pulmonary infections, growth retardation, and cardiac failure in infancy, but survival past this period is often associated with an amelioration of symptoms until adulthood. In patients with severe pulmonary vascular obstruction, symptoms develop most often in adult life and consist of exertional dyspnea, chest pain, syncope, and hemoptysis. The right-to-left shunt leads to cyanosis, clubbing, and polycythemia.

Patients with moderate-sized defects exhibit cardiomegaly with a forceful left ventricular impulse and a prominent systolic thrill along the lower left sternal border. The second heart sound is normally or closely split, with moderate accentuation of the pulmonic component; a third heart sound and diastolic rumbling murmur, reflecting increased flow across the mitral valve during rapid ventricular filling, are often audible at the cardiac apex. The characteristic holosystolic murmur results from flow across the defect; it is best heard along the third and fourth interspaces to the left of the sternum, and is widely transmitted over the precordium. A basal midsystolic ejection murmur may also be heard, because of increased flow across the pulmonic valve. In patients with pulmonary vascular obstruction and small left-to-right shunts, both the systolic thrill and murmur decrease in intensity and duration and may disappear entirely, to be replaced by a marked right ventricular precordial lift, pulmonary ejection sound and soft systolic ejection murmur, a closely split second heart sound with accentuation of the pulmonic component, and the diastolic murmur of pulmonic incompetence.

The electrocardiographic pattern, the relative size and contour of the two ventricles roentgenographically, and the appearance of the lung fields serve as indicators of the underlying pathophysiologic condition. The electrocardiogram is generally normal in patients with small defects. Left or combined ventricular hypertrophy is seen with large left-to-right shunts; right ventricular hypertrophy occurs with pulmonary vascular obstruction. The roentgenograms may be normal in patients with small defects; large defects are characterized by an enlarged left atrium, biventricular hypertrophy, a prominent pulmonary artery segment, and increased pulmonary vascular markings. Relative diminution and attenuation of the peripheral pulmonary vasculature occur in patients with obstructive pulmonary vascular disease.

In approximately 90 percent of patients with this malformation, the defect occurs in the membranous septum. A shunt from the left ventricle to the right atrium may occur with a defect in the most superior portion of the ventricular septum, since the tricuspid valve is lower than the mitral valve. The clinical, electrocardiographic, and radiologic findings in these patients often do not differ appreciably from those with a simple ventricular septal defect, although right atrial enlargement and evidence of right ventricular volume overload may be present; the diagnosis can be established by left ventriculography. Prolapse of an aortic valve leaflet through a subpulmonary ventricular defect or the combination of subcristal ventricular septal defect and underdevelopment of an aortic valve commissure may produce aortic regurgitation that is frequently progressive and is the most significant hemodynamic lesion. In these patients complete operative repair may necessitate insertion of a prosthetic aortic valve.

The pathophysiology of a single or common ventricle may resemble that of a large ventricular septal defect, although the two lesions are dissimilar embryologically. There is an obligatory admixture of systemic and pulmonary venous return in patients with a single ventricle, but there is occasionally little or no cyanosis if selective streaming and increased pulmonary blood flow occur. Severe pulmonary hypertension is invariably present unless pulmonic stenosis coexists. It is imperative to differentiate a large ventricular septal defect from a single ventricle by echocardiography and angiography, because attempts at corrective operation for single ventricles have met with little success.

The risk of bacterial endocarditis is higher in patients with small or moderate-sized defects than in those with large ones, but appropriate prophylaxis is essential in all. In the small infant with a large left-to-right shunt, congestive failure may be severe and intractable despite intensive medical management; this problem is managed best by primary closure of the defect. Operation is indicated in children and adults when there is a moderate or large left-to-right shunt with a pulmonary to systemic flow ratio which exceeds 1.5:1.0 or 2.0:1.0 regardless of the level of pulmonary artery pressure. Operation is contraindicated in patients with small defects and left-to-right shunts and in patients in whom the pulmonary vascular resistance is elevated to a level which eliminates the net left-to-right shunt and carries an increased risk whenever pulmonary resistance is significantly elevated.

Patent ductus arteriosus The ductus arteriosus is a vessel leading from the bifurcation of the pulmonary artery to the aorta just distal to the left subclavian artery. Normal closure of the ductus immediately after birth may be due to the sudden increase in arterial oxygen tension that accompanies ventilation and abrupt alterations in the disposition of vasoactive substances, particularly prostaglandins. Intimal proliferation and fibrosis proceed more gradually, so that total anatomic obliteration may not occur for several months after birth. Persistent patency of the ductus after birth is a relatively common anomaly, occurring more frequently in females, in the offspring of women whose pregnancies were complicated by first-trimester rubella, in premature infants, and in children born at high altitudes. A distinction should be made between patency of the ductus arteriosus in the preterm infant who lacks the normal mechanisms for postnatal ductal closure because of immaturity and the full-term newborn in whom patency of the ductus is a true congenital malformation related, most likely, to a primary anatomic defect of the elastic tissue within the wall of the vessel. Although the latter anomaly occurs most frequently in the isolated form, it may coexist with other malformations, particularly coarctation of the aorta, ventricular septal defect, pulmonic stenosis, and aortic stenosis. Patency of the ductus may provide the only route for maintaining pulmonary or systemic blood flow in the presence of such lesions as pulmonary atresia or aortic arch interruption, respectively.

The flow across the ductus is determined by the pressure and resistance relationships between the systemic and the pulmonary circulations, and by the cross-sectional area and length of the ductus itself. Most commonly, pulmonary pressures are normal, and a gradient and shunt from aorta to pulmonary artery persists throughout the cardiac cycle. Physical examination reveals a characteristic thrill and a continuous "machinery" murmur, with a late systolic accentuation at the upper left sternal border. The left atrium and ventricle enlarge to accommodate the increased pulmonary venous return, and flow murmurs across the mitral and aortic valves may be detected. With large or moderate-sized left-to-right shunts, the runoff of blood through the ductus causes a widened systemic pulse pressure and bounding peripheral pulses. The hemodynamic abnormality is reflected by left ventricular and, occasionally, left atrial hypertrophy on the electrocardiogram and by left atrial and ventricular enlargement, a prominent ascending aorta and pulmonary artery, and pulmonary vascular engorgement on the chest roentgenogram. Left atrial and ventricular size determined echocardiographically provide an estimate of the magnitude of left-to-right shunting.

The clinical recognition of patent ductus arteriosus may be difficult in infancy and in patients with pulmonary hypertension or heart failure. In these circumstances, the pressure gradient between the aorta and pulmonary artery is reduced or absent, as is the typical continuous murmur, and there may be only a systolic ejection murmur at the base, a diastolic blowing murmur of pulmonary regurgitation (Graham Steell), or no murmur audible at all. When severe pulmonary vascular disease results in reversal of flow through the ductus, unoxygenated blood is shunted to the descending aorta, and the toes, but not the fingers, become cyanotic and clubbed, a finding termed *differential cyanosis.*

Although a large ductus often results in cardiac failure and pulmonary edema in the premature infant, its occurrence in the full-term baby is often compatible with survival until adult life. The symptomatic *preterm* infant may be managed either by pharmacologic inhibition of prostaglandin synthesis with indomethacin to constrict and close the ductus or by surgical ligation. Pharmacologic approaches are ineffective in full-term infants or children in whom patency of the ductus is a true malformation, unrelated to immaturity of the normal mechanism for closure. The leading causes of death in adults with patent ductus are cardiac failure and bacterial endocarditis. In older patients, severe pulmonary vascular obstruction may cause aneurysmal dilatation, calcification, and rupture of the ductus.

In the absence of severe pulmonary vascular disease with predominant right-to-left shunting of blood, the simple presence of a patent ductus is generally considered a sufficient indication for operation, at least in patients over 2 years of age. Ligation or division of the ductus is associated with a low risk (under 2 percent) when it is performed electively in an otherwise healthy person. The operative risk is reduced if cardiac failure can be treated successfully before operation. Operation should be deferred for several months in patients treated successfully for bacterial endarteritis, because the ductus may remain somewhat edematous and friable.

Aortopulmonary septal defect Aortopulmonary window, partial truncus arteriosis, and aortic septal defect are other designations applied to this relatively uncommon anomaly, which consists of a communication between the aorta and the pulmonary artery just above the semilunar valves. Such defects are usually large and are accompanied by varying degrees of obstructive pulmonary vascular disease and severe pulmonary arterial hypertension. The anomaly may be difficult to distinguish from patent ductus arteriosus with which it is often associated. Its presence should be suspected whenever a large shunt into the pulmonary artery is demonstrated at catheterization. Distinction from patent ductus and persistent truncus arteriosus is facilitated by catheter passage across the defect and selective angiocardiography, with the injection of contrast material into the left ventricle and/or the root of the aorta. Operative correction is indicated in patients with large left-to-right shunts; cardiopulmonary bypass is required, and the defect is closed, generally with a prosthetic patch.

Aortic sinus aneurysm and fistula Congenital aneurysm of an aortic sinus of Valsalva, particularly the right coronary sinus, is an uncommon anomaly with a predilection for males; it consists of a separation, or lack of fusion, between the media of the aorta and the annulus fibrosus of the aortic valve. Progressive aneurysmal dilatation of the weakened area develops but may not be recognized until the third or fourth decade of life, when rupture into a cardiac chamber occurs. The receiving chamber of the aorticocardiac fistula is usually the right ventricle, but occasionally the fistula drains into the right atrium.

The unruptured aneurysm generally does not produce symptoms or a hemodynamic abnormality. Rupture is often of abrupt onset, causes chest pain, and creates continuous arteriovenous shunting and volume overloading of both right and left heart chambers, with resultant heart failure. Bacterial endocarditis may originate either on the edges of the aneurysm or on the jet lesions in the right side of the heart. This anomaly should be suspected in a patient with a history of recent onset of chest pain, symptoms of diminished cardiac reserve, bounding pulses, and a loud, superficial, continuous murmur accentuated in diastole when the fistula opens into the right ventricle, as well as a thrill along the right or left lower parasternal area. The diagnosis may be established definitively by retrograde thoracic aortography. Operation is indicated in patients with large left-to-right shunts.

Coronary arteriovenous fistula Coronary arteriovenous fistula is an unusual anomaly that most often consists of a communication between the right coronary artery and the right atrium or ventricle. The shunt is usually of small magnitude, and myocardial blood flow is not usually compromised. Potential complications include bacterial endocarditis, thrombus formation with occlusion or distal embolization, rupture of an aneurysmal fistula, and rarely, pulmonary hypertension and congestive failure. The finding of a loud, superficial, continuous murmur at the lower or midsternal border usually prompts a further evaluation of asymptomatic patients. Retrograde thoracic aortography or coronary arteriography permits identification of the size and anatomic features of the fistulous tract, which may be closed by suture obliteration.

Anomalous pulmonary origin of coronary artery In this rare malformation, the left coronary artery originates from the pulmonary artery. As the elevated pulmonary vascular resistance declines immediately after birth, perfusion of the left coronary artery from the pulmonary artery ceases and the direction of flow in the anomalous vessel reverses. Thus, blood flows from the aorta to the right coronary artery, then through collateral channels to the left coronary artery, and finally to the pulmonary artery. Total myocardial perfusion must pass through the right coronary artery and may be sufficient for normal activity if adequate collateral channels develop between the two coronary circulations. Myocardial infarction and fibrosis commonly develop during the first 6 months of life, leading to death within the first year. From 10 to 20 percent of patients survive to childhood or adolescence without surgical correction. Occasionally, in older children or adults one may find an example of mitral regurgitation which results from dysfunction of ischemic or infarcted papillary muscles. In some instances the coronary anomaly is unsuspected until a previously well adolescent or adult experiences angina, heart failure, or sudden death.

The diagnosis of anomalous origin of the coronary artery is supported by the electrocardiographic findings of an anterolateral myocardial infarction. Chest roentgenograms show moderate to severe enlargement of the left atrium and ventricle. Aortic root or coronary angiography demonstrates the retrograde drainage of the coronary vessel into the pulmonary artery and the presence of a single right coronary artery arising from the aorta.

Ideal operative management of these patients consists of anastomosis of the left coronary artery to the subclavian artery or to the aorta via a graft. The outcome of operation and ultimate prognosis are influenced significantly by the degree of myocardial damage suffered preoperatively.

Persistent truncus arteriosus Persistent truncus arteriosus is a rare but serious anomaly in which a single vessel forms the outlet of both ventricles and gives rise to the systemic, pulmonary, and coronary arteries. It is always accompanied by a ventricular septal defect. The designation "pseudotruncus arteriosus" refers to the condition in which a single vessel arises from the heart but is accompanied by a remnant of atretic pulmonary artery; pseudotruncus arteriosus does not differ from tetralogy of Fallot with pulmonary atresia (see below). In truncus arteriosus pulmonary flow is governed by the size of the pulmonary arteries and the pulmonary vascular resistance. Most often, mild cyanosis coexists with the cardiac findings of a large left-to-right shunt. The most frequent physical findings include cardiomegaly, a systolic ejection sound, a loud, single second heart sound, a harsh systolic murmur accompanied by a thrill, an early diastolic blowing murmur of truncal valve regurgitation, and a low-pitched middiastolic rumbling murmur. The diagnosis should be suspected at catheterization if the catheter fails to enter the central pulmonary arteries from the right ventricle despite evidence of increased pulmonary blood flow; aortography is the diagnostic procedure of choice.

The early fatal course and, in patients surviving infancy, the development of pulmonary vascular obstructive disease are responsible for the poor prognosis associated with persistent truncus arteriosus. Corrective operation employs a valve-containing prosthetic tubular conduit to construct a pulmonary trunk.

VALVULAR AND VASCULAR LESIONS WITH OR WITHOUT RIGHT-TO-LEFT SHUNT **Pulmonary stenosis with intact ventricular septum** Obstruction to right ventricular outflow is relatively common; it may be localized to the supravalvular, valvular, or subvalvular levels or occur at a combination of these sites. Multiple sites of narrowing of the peripheral pulmonary arteries are often a feature of rubella embryopathy and may be associated with both the familial and sporadic forms of supravalvular aortic stenosis. Valvular pulmonic stenosis is the most common form of isolated right ventricular obstruction.

The severity of the obstructing lesion, rather than the site of narrowing, is the most important determinant of the clinical course. In the presence of a normal cardiac output, a peak systolic transvalvular pressure gradient between 50 and 80 mmHg is considered to be moderate stenosis; levels below and above that range are classified as mild and severe, respectively. Patients with mild pulmonic stenosis are generally asymptomatic and demonstrate little or no progression in the severity of obstruction as they grow older. In patients with more significant stenosis, the severity of the obstruction may increase with time. Atresia of the pulmonary valve is commonly associated with a hypoplastic right ventricle and interatrial communications. Symptoms vary according to the degree of obstruction. Infants with pulmonary atresia often die from hypoxia. Fatigue, dyspnea, right ventricular failure, and syncope may limit the activity of older patients, in whom moderate or severe obstruction may prevent an augmentation of pulmonary blood flow with exercise.

In patients with severe obstruction, the systolic pressure in the right ventricle may exceed that in the left ventricle, since the ventricular septum is intact. Right ventricular ejection is prolonged in patients with moderate or severe stenosis, and the sound of pulmonary valve closure is delayed and soft. Right ventricular hypertrophy reduces the compliance of that chamber, and a forceful right atrial contraction is necessary to augment right ventricular filling. A fourth heart sound, prominent *a* waves in the jugular venous pulse, and occasionally, presystolic pulsations of the liver reflect the vigorous atrial contraction. The clinical diagnosis is further supported by the presence of a right parasternal lift and harsh systolic ejection murmur and thrill at the upper left sternal border, typically preceded by a systolic ejection sound if the obstruction is valvular. The systolic murmur becomes louder, and its crescendo occurs later in systole, with more severe degrees of valvular obstruction resulting in a greater prolongation of right ventricular systole. The holosystolic decrescendo murmur of tricuspid regurgitation may accompany severe pulmonic stenosis, especially in the presence of congestive heart failure. Cyanosis usually reflects venoarterial shunting through a patent foramen ovale or atrial septal defect. In patients with supravalvular or peripheral pulmonary arterial stenosis, the murmur is systolic or continuous and is best heard over the area of narrowing, with radiation to the peripheral lung fields.

The electrocardiogram may be helpful in assessing the degree of obstruction to right ventricular output. In mild cases, the electrocardiogram is often normal, whereas moderate and severe stenoses are associated with right axis deviation and right ventricular hypertrophy. A ventricular strain pattern, as well as high-amplitude P waves in leads II and V_1, indicating right atrial enlargement, is associated with severe stenosis. The chest roentgenogram in patients with mild or moderate pulmonic stenosis often shows a heart of normal size and normal vascularity of the lungs. In the presence of valvular stenosis, poststenotic dilatation of the main and left pulmonary arteries may be evident. In patients with severe obstruction and resultant right ventricular failure, right atrial and right ventricular enlargement are generally evident. The pulmonary vascularity may be reduced in patients with severe stenosis, right ventricular failure, and/or a venoarterial shunt at the atrial level.

Cardiac catheterization and angiocardiography with right ventricular injection are necessary to localize the site of obstruction and evaluate its severity and to document the coexistence of additional cardiac malformations. The treatment of moderate and severe degrees of pulmonary valvular and subvalvular stenosis is surgical. Direct surgical relief of the obstruction may usually be accomplished at a low risk. Multiple stenoses of the peripheral pulmonary arteries are usually inoperable, but narrowing of a single branch or at the bifurcation of the main pulmonary trunk may be corrected.

Tetralogy of Fallot The four components of this malformation are (1) ventricular septal defect, (2) obstruction to right ventricular outflow, (3) overriding of the aortic orifice above the ventricular defect, and (4) right ventricular hypertrophy. Systolic pressures are equal in the right ventricle and aorta as a consequence of the first two components. The overall incidence of tetralogy approaches 10 percent of all forms of congenital heart disease, and it is the most common anomaly responsible for cyanosis after the age of 1 year. The ventricular septal defect is usually large, approximating the aortic orifice in size, and located high in the septum beneath the crista supraventricularis and just below the aortic valve. The aortic root may be displaced anteriorly and straddle or override the septal defect. Infundibular stenosis occurs as the only major site of obstruction to right ventricular outflow in about one-half the patients and coexists with valvular obstruction in another 25 percent. Supravalvular and peripheral pulmonary arterial narrowing may be observed. When the main pulmonary artery, pulmonic valve, or right ventricular infundibulum is atretic, the condition may be called *pseudotruncus arteriosus* (see "Persistent Truncus Arteriosus" above). In such cases, the lungs are perfused through enlarged bronchial arteries and/or through the pulmonary arteries via a patent ductus arteriosus. A right-sided aortic knob, arch, and descending aorta occur in approximately 25 percent of patients with tetralogy of Fallot.

The relationship between the resistance to blood flow from the ventricles into the aorta and into the pulmonary vessels plays the major role in determining the hemodynamic and clinical picture. Therefore, it is the severity of obstruction to right ventricular outflow which is of fundamental significance. When right ventricular outflow obstruction is severe, the pulmonary blood flow is markedly reduced and a large volume of unsaturated systemic venous blood is shunted from right to left across the ventricular septal defect, severe cyanosis and polycythemia occur, and symptoms of systemic anoxia are prominent. The term *pink*, or *acyanotic, tetralogy of Fallot* is used often to describe an interventricular communication and a milder degree of obstruction to right ventricular outflow with no appreciable venoarterial shunting. In many patients the obstruction to right ventricular outflow is mild but progressive, so that early in life pulmonary exceeds systemic blood flow and the symptoms resemble those produced by a simple ventricular septal defect.

Most children with tetralogy of Fallot are cyanotic from birth or develop cyanosis before 1 year of age. Dyspnea with exertion, retarded growth and development, clubbing, and polycythemia are common. When resting after exertion, infants with tetralogy characteristically assume a squatting posture. Spells of severe anoxia and cyanosis (see "Hypoxic Spells" above) constitute a major threat to survival.

Physical examination reveals variable degrees of underdevelopment and cyanosis. Clubbing of the terminal digits may be prominent after the first year of life. A right ventricular impulse and systolic thrill may be palpable along the left sternal border; there is no generalized cardiomegaly. The second heart sound is single, and the pulmonic component is rarely audible. A systolic ejection murmur is produced by flow across the narrowed right ventricular outflow tract or pulmonic valve. The intensity and duration of the murmur vary inversely with the severity of obstruction, the opposite of the relation existing in patients with an intact ventricular septum and pulmonary stenosis. Polycythemia, decreased systemic vascular resistance, and increased obstruction to right ventricular outflow may all be responsible for a decrease in the intensity of the murmur. A continuous murmur over the paravertebral area may indicate collateral circulation to the lungs through bronchial arteries.

The electrocardiogram ordinarily shows right ventricular and, less often, right atrial hypertrophy. Radiologic examination characteristically reveals a normal-sized, boot-shaped heart (*coeur en sabot*) with prominence of the right ventricle and a concavity in the region of the pulmonary conus. The pulmonary vascular markings are typically diminished, and the aortic arch and knob may be on the right side. Echocardiography demonstrates discontinuity between the ventricular septum and anterior aortic wall, a thickened anterior wall of right ventricle, an enlarged, anteriorly displaced aorta, and small pulmonary artery. Selective angiocardiography with right ventricular injection is necessary to confirm the diagnosis and to evaluate the architecture of the right ventricular outflow tract, pulmonary valve and annulus, and caliber of the main branches of the pulmonary artery.

Among the factors that may complicate the management of patients with tetralogy are iron-deficiency anemia, infective endocarditis, paradoxic embolism, polycythemia, coagulation defects, and cerebral infarction or abscess. The paroxysmal cyanotic spells may respond quickly to oxygen, placing the child in the knee-chest position, and morphine. If the spell persists, metabolic acidosis will develop from prolonged anaerobic metabolism, and infusion of sodium bicarbonate may be necessary to interrupt the attack. Vasopressors, beta-adrenergic blockade, or general anesthesia may occasionally be necessary.

Total correction is ultimately advisable for almost all patients with tetralogy of Fallot. However, if cyanosis or symptoms are marked in an infant, the risk of primary repair may be high unless performed in a center experienced with this form of intracardiac surgery in infancy, and a palliative operation designed to increase pulmonary blood flow may be recommended. These procedures include aortopulmonary or subclavian-pulmonary arterial anastomosis or transventricular infundibulectomy or valvulotomy. Total correction can then be carried out at a lower risk later in childhood.

Ebstein's anomaly In this rare anomaly there is abnormal morphogenesis of the tricuspid valve, with redundancy of tricuspid valve tissue, and the attachment of portions of the septal and posterior leaflets of the tricuspid valve is lower than normal; the leaflets originate from the right ventricular wall rather than from the atrioventricular ring. Hence, the portion of the right ventricle that lies between the atrioventricular ring and the origin of the valve is continuous with the right atrial chamber. The tricuspid valve is usually incompetent, the foramen ovale is patent, and the right ventricle exhibits varying degrees of hypoplasia. The clinical manifestations of Ebstein's anomaly are variable, depending on the severity of the anatomic changes in the tricuspid valve. Ultimately, however, progressive cyanosis resulting from the right-to-left shunt across the interatrial communication, symptoms resulting from right ventricular dysfunction, and/or paroxysmal arrhythmias develop.

A prominent systolic pulsation of the liver and a large *v* wave in the jugular venous pulse accompany the systolic thrill and murmur of tricuspid regurgitation. Wide splitting of the first and second heart sounds and prominent third and fourth heart sounds may produce a characteristically rhythmic auscultatory cadence. The electrocardiogram shows giant P waves, a prolonged PR interval, and complete or incomplete right bundle branch block. Roentgenography usually demonstrates an enlarged right atrium and a small right ventricle and pulmonary artery, and reduced pulsations; the pulmonary vascularity may be reduced if a large right-to-left shunt is present. The principal echocardiographic findings include a large anterior tricuspid leaflet with delayed tricuspid valve closure with respect to mitral closure. At cardiac catheterization the intracavitary electrocardiogram recorded just proximal to the tricuspid valve shows a right ventricular type of complex, while the pressure recorded is that of the right atrium.

Most patients survive to the third decade at least. In some disabled patients moderate improvement has resulted from anastomosis of the superior vena cava to the right pulmonary artery to divert systemic venous return from the right atrium and to increase pulmonary blood flow. Patients beyond early childhood have occasionally benefited from prosthetic replacement of the tricuspid valve; at all ages, however, patients with Ebstein's anomaly are poor surgical risks.

Tricuspid atresia Atresia of the tricuspid valve, an interatrial communication, and, frequently, hypoplasia of the right ventricle and pulmonary artery exist in this malformation. The clinical picture is usually dominated by severe cyanosis as a result of greatly diminished pulmonary blood flow.

Balloon atrial septostomy and palliative operations consisting of increasing pulmonary blood flow, often by systemic arterial or venous–pulmonary artery anastomosis, may allow many patients to survive to the age of 10 to 20 years; functional correction of the anomaly can then be accomplished in those with normal or low pulmonary arterial pressure by anastomosis of the right atrial appendage to the right ventricle with the aid of a pericardial patch or by insertion of a prosthetic conduit between the right atrium and pulmonary artery and closure of the interatrial communication.

Coarctation of the aorta Narrowing or constriction of the lumen of the aorta may occur anywhere along its length but is most commonly localized just distal to the origin of the left subclavian artery near the insertion of the ligamentum arteriosum. Coarctation is encountered in approximately 7 percent of patients with congenital heart disease and is twice as common in males as in females, although the lesion occurs frequently in patients with gonadal dysgenesis (Turner's syndrome, Chap. 118). Clinical manifestations depend on the site and extent of obstruction and the presence of associated cardiac anomalies, which occur in the majority of patients. These include most commonly bicuspid aortic valve, congenital aortic stenosis, patent ductus arteriosus, ventricular septal defect and mitral regurgitation. When diffuse narrowing of the aorta is located proximal to the ductus arteriosus, right ventricular hypertrophy develops in utero and pulmonary hypertension and congestive heart failure are common in early life. *Differential cyanosis* may result from preferential shunting of unsaturated pulmonary arterial blood through a patent ductus arteriosus to the lower part of the body.

More commonly, the coarctation is localized at or just distal to the attachment of the ductus or ligamentum arteriosus. The majority of children and young adults with isolated juxta- or postductal coarctation are asymptomatic. Headache, epistaxis, cold extremities, and claudication with exercise may be noted, although attention is usually directed to the cardiovascular system when a heart murmur or hypertension in the upper extremities is detected on routine physical examination. In childhood, mechanical factors, rather than those of renal origin, play the primary role in the production of hypertension.

Absence, marked diminution, or delayed pulsations in the femoral arteries and a low or unobtainable arterial pressure in the lower extremities with hypertension in the arms are the basic clues to the diagnosis. In adults, enlarged and pulsatile collateral vessels may be palpated in the intercostal spaces anteriorly, in the axillae, or posteriorly in the interscapular area. Also, the upper extremities and thorax may be preferentially more developed than the lower extremities. A midsystolic murmur over the anterior part of the chest, back, and spinous processes is most frequent, becoming continuous if the lumen is narrowed sufficiently to result in a high-velocity jet across the lesion throughout the cardiac cycle. Additional systolic and continuous murmurs over the lateral thoracic wall may reflect increased flow through dilated and tortuous collateral vessels. The *electrocardiogram* reveals left ventricular hypertrophy of varying degree, depending on the height of the arterial pressure proximal to the obstruction and the patient's age; predominant right or combined ventricular hypertrophy may be seen in infants and children, and usually implies a complicated lesion. *Roentgenograms* may show a dilated left subclavian artery high on the left mediastinal border and a dilated ascending aorta. Indentation of the aorta at the site of coarctation and pre- and poststenotic dilatation (the "3" sign) along the left paramediastinal shadow are almost pathognomonic. Notching of the ribs, an important radiographic sign, is due to erosion by dilated collateral vessels, increases with age, and usually becomes apparent between the sixth and twelfth years of life. Cardiac catheterization and aortography may be indicated to localize accurately the site of obstruction, determine the length of the coarctation, and identify associated malformations.

The *treatment* of uncomplicated coarctation of the aorta is surgical; resection and end-to-end anastomosis or subclavian flap angioplasty can be accomplished with excellent results in most patients, although it is occasionally necessary to use a tubular graft or patch in the repair if the narrowed segment is long. Paradoxic hypertension of short duration is often noted in the immediate postoperative period, and occasionally a necrotizing panarteritis of the small vessels of the gastrointestinal tract of uncertain cause complicates the course of recovery. In those who survive the first 2 years of life complications are uncommon before the second or third decade; operation on asymptomatic patients is advised ideally between the ages of 3 and 6. The chief hazards to patients with coarctation result from severe hypertension and include the development of cerebral aneurysms and hemorrhage, rupture of the aorta, left ventricular failure, and infective endocarditis. Systemic hypertension in the absence of residual coarctation has been observed in resting or exercise-stressed patients postoperatively and appears to be related to the duration of preoperative hypertension, as well as incomplete operative repair; lifelong observation is desirable because of the late onset of hypertension in some postoperative patients.

CONGENITAL AORTIC STENOSIS Malformations that cause obstruction to the ejection of blood from the left ventricle include congenital valvular aortic stenosis, the discrete form of congenital subaortic stenosis, congenital narrowing of the supravalvular ascending aorta, and hypertrophic cardiomyopathy with outflow tract obstruction (Chap. 263).

Valvular aortic stenosis Valvular aortic stenosis occurs in approximately 4 percent of patients with congenital cardiovascular defects and occurs three to four times more often in males than in females. However, the congenital bicuspid aortic valve, which is not necessarily stenotic, may actually be the most common congenital malformation of the heart, although it may go undetected in early life. Because bicuspid valves may become stenotic with time or be the site of infective endocarditis, the lesion may become of clinical significance only in adult life, when it may be difficult to distinguish it anatomically from acquired rheumatic aortic stenosis. Commonly associated anomalies include patent ductus arteriosus and coarctation of the aorta.

The dynamics of blood flow associated with a congenitally deformed, rigid aortic valve commonly lead to thickening of the cusps and, in later life, to calcification. When the obstruction is hemodynamically significant, concentric hypertrophy of the left ventricular wall and dilatation of the ascending aorta occur.

The hemodynamic abnormalities produced by obstruction to left ventricular outflow are discussed in Chap. 258. A peak systolic pressure gradient exceeding 70 mmHg, in association with a normal cardiac output, or an effective aortic orifice less than 0.6 cm^2 per square meter of body surface, is considered to represent critical obstruction to left ventricular outflow. In children and young adults, the resting cardiac output is generally within normal limits, but often fails to rise normally during muscular exercise.

Most children with congenital aortic stenosis are asymptomatic and grow and develop normally. Usually, a murmur is detected on a routine examination. At least moderately severe obstruction should be suspected if there is a definite history of fatigability and exertional dyspnea. In patients with severe obstruction, the inability of the left ventricle to increase its output and to maintain cerebral flow during exercise may result in exertional syncope, while the disparity between the oxygen supply to the left ventricle and myocardial oxygen requirements may be responsible for anginal pain. The symptomatic patient with valvular aortic stenosis generally has critical stenosis, although a lack of symptoms does not preclude the presence of moderately severe obstruction. Sudden death is a distinct threat to patients with critical stenosis. Its precise cause is poorly understood, but ventricular arrhythmias, perhaps initiated by acute myocardial ischemia, may be responsible.

When obstruction is hemodynamically significant, a left ventricular lift is usually palpable and a precordial systolic thrill is felt over the base of the heart, with transmission to the jugular notch and along the carotid arteries. Presystolic expansion is often palpable. A systolic aortic ejection sound, signifying opening of the aortic valve, is typically present at the cardiac apex when the valve is mobile, particularly in patients with mild to moderate stenosis. Delayed closure of the stenotic aortic valve leads to a single or a closely split second heart sound, and paradoxic splitting may be present. A fourth heart sound is generally associated with severe obstruction. The systolic murmur starts after the completion of left ventricular isometric contraction, is rhomboid-shaped, loud, harsh, and best heard at the base of the heart. The murmur, like the thrill, radiates to the jugular notch and carotid vessels, as well as to the apex. In some patients, an early diastolic blowing murmur of aortic regurgitation is present, but unless the valve leaflets have been eroded by infective endocarditis, the regurgitation is usually not hemodynamically significant; occasionally, in patients with a congenital bicuspid valve, aortic regurgitation may be severe and the dominant lesion hemodynamically.

Electrocardiographically, left ventricular hypertrophy tends to vary with the severity of obstruction, although a *normal or near-normal electrocardiogram does not exclude severe aortic stenosis.* The left ventricular "strain pattern" generally indicates that severe aortic stenosis is present.

Roentgenographically, the overall heart size is most often normal or only slightly enlarged. Left atrial enlargement and concentric left ventricular hypertrophy accompany moderate or severe obstruction. Poststenotic dilatation of the ascending aorta is a common finding. Echocardiographic findings include multiple eccentric diastolic closure lines in the aortic lumen, thickening of the left ventricular posterior wall and septum, reduced separation of thickened aortic valve leaflets, and aortic dilatation. Cardiac catheterization is indicated when the clinical diagnosis of aortic stenosis has been established and when the history, clinical examination, roentgenogram, electrocardiogram, or echocardiogram suggests the possibility of severe obstruction. The site and severity of obstruction are established, and any associated malformations are identified. In patients with mild or moderate obstruction repeat left-sided heart catheterization should be carried out every 5 to 10 years because stenosis may progress.

The medical management of congenital valvular aortic stenosis includes prophylaxis against infective endocarditis and, in patients with diminished cardiac reserve, the administration of digitalis and diuretics and sodium restriction while awaiting operation. If severe aortic stenosis is present, avoidance of strenuous physical activity is advised even when the patient is asymptomatic, and participation in competitive sports should probably also be restricted in patients with milder degrees of obstruction. The decision concerning the advisability of operation depends on the severity of obstruction rather than on the symptoms described by the patient. Operation is carried out under direct vision with the aid of cardiopulmonary bypass, and in children without valvular calcification the fused commissures are opened. Commissurotomy may result in aortic regurgitation which can progress to require prosthetic valve replacement. Moreover, since the valves remain deformed after valvulotomy, further degenerative changes, including calcification, may lead to significant stenosis later. The treatment of congenital aortic stenosis in the adult is described in Chap. 258.

Subaortic stenosis The most common form of subaortic stenosis is the *idiopathic hypertrophic* variety, also termed *hypertrophic cardiomyopathy,* which occurs in a congenital form in about one-third of the patients and is discussed in Chap. 263. Both clinically and physiologically, however, it is the *discrete* form of subaortic stenosis which resembles valvular aortic stenosis. The lesion usually consists of a membranous diaphragm or fibrous ring encircling the left ventricular outflow tract just beneath the base of the aortic valve. It is less common than isolated valvular obstruction, but it also occurs more frequently in males than in females. There are no clinical criteria which can be relied upon to distinguish the two forms of obstruction, although a systolic ejection sound is rarely heard in patients with discrete subvalvular aortic stenosis and the diastolic murmur of aortic regurgitation is more common than in patients with valvular aortic stenosis. Valvular calcification is not observed roentgenographically in patients with subaortic stenosis. Echocardiography may demonstrate the subaortic obstruction, and usually reveals an abnormal pattern of motion of the aortic valve leaflets. Definitive differentiation between valvular and subvalvular obstruction is best accomplished at cardiac catheterization by recording pressure tracings as a cardiac catheter is withdrawn across the outflow tract and by left ventricular angiocardiography.

Because of the likelihood of progressive obstruction and aortic regurgitation, the presence of even mild or moderate subaortic stenosis warrants consideration of elective operation. Surgical correction consists of excising the membrane or fibrous ridge.

Occasionally, valvular and subvalvular aortic stenosis coexist in the same patient, producing a tunnel-like narrowing of the left ventricular outflow tract. Associated findings are often a small ascending aorta, hypoplasia of the aortic valve ring, and thickened valve leaflets. It may be recognized by angiography. Operative treatment frequently necessitates prosthetic replacement of the aortic valve, as well as enlarging the aortic annulus, proximal aorta, and left ventricular outflow tract, or the interposition of a valved conduit between the left ventricular apex and the aorta.

Supravalvular aortic stenosis Supravalvular aortic stenosis is a localized or diffuse narrowing of the ascending aorta, originating just above the level of the coronary arteries at the superior margin of the sinuses of Valsalva. In contrast to other forms of aortic stenosis, in the supravalvular variety the coronary arteries are subjected to the elevated pressures that exist within the left ventricle, and are often dilated and tortuous. Adherence of the free edges of the aortic cusps to the sites of supravalvular stenosis may interfere with coronary arterial inflow.

The designation *Williams'* or *supravalvular aortic stenosis syndrome* has been applied to the distinctive clinical picture produced by coexistence of the cardiovascular lesion and a metabolic disorder, idiopathic infantile hypercalcemia, that is probably related to deranged vitamin D metabolism. Other manifestations of this syndrome include mental retardation, a peculiar "elfin facies," craniosynostosis, strabismus, narrowing of peripheral systemic and pulmonary arteries, inguinal hernias, cryptorchidism in males, premature development of secondary sexual characteristics in females, and abnormalities of dental development. Supravalvular aortic stenosis and peripheral pulmonary arterial stenosis are also seen in familial and sporadic forms unassociated with the other features of the syndrome. Genetic studies suggest that when the anomaly is familial it is transmitted as an autosomal dominant trait with variable expression.

The physical findings resemble those in valvular aortic stenosis, except that the sound of aortic valve closure is accentuated, ejection sounds are infrequent, and transmission of the thrill and murmurs into the jugular notch and along the carotid vessels is more prominent; the systolic pressure in the right arm is characteristically higher than in the left. Poststenotic dilatation of the ascending aorta is rarely present.

The electrocardiogram reveals left ventricular hypertrophy. The diagnosis is confirmed by the demonstration at retrograde aortic catheterization of a pressure gradient just above the aortic valve, and a constriction at this level as revealed by aortography.

Surgical treatment consists of widening the lumen of the aorta by the insertion of a fabric prosthesis, and operative treatment is indicated if the obstruction is discrete and severe without generalized hypoplasia of the ascending aorta and arch.

Hypoplastic left heart syndrome This syndrome is a significant cause of neonatal mortality; it may be caused by atresia and/or hypoplasia of the aortic and mitral valves and of the aortic arch, lesions which are presently inoperable.

Malformations obstructing pulmonary venous flow A number of rare malformations at or upstream to the mitral valve may cause obstruction to flow of pulmonary venous blood into the left ventricle. These include pulmonary vein stenosis, the "parachute" deformity of the valve (in which shortened chordae tendineae converge and insert into a single large papillary muscle), and *cor triatriatum,* a correctable malformation in which an abnormal fibromuscular diaphragm divides the left atrium into a posterosuperior chamber, into which the pulmonary veins drain, and an anteroinferior chamber, which communicates with the mitral valve and atrial appendage.

TRANSPOSITION COMPLEXES The term *transposition* identifies a complicated group of malformations that have in common abnormal relationships between the cardiac chambers and the great arteries.

Complete transposition of the great arteries The aorta arises from the right ventricle to the right of and anterior to the pulmonary artery, which emerges from the left ventricle. This results in two separate and parallel circulations, and some communication between the two circulations must exist after birth in order to sustain life. Almost all patients have an interatrial communication, two-thirds have a patent ductus arteriosus, and about one-third have an associated ventricular septal defect. Transposition occurs more frequently in the offspring of diabetic mothers and in more males than females. It is a leading cause of death due to congenital heart disease in the first 2 months of life and accounts for approximately 10 percent of all patients with cyanotic heart disease. Without treatment, about 70 percent of the patients with this malformation die by the age of 6 months. A few survive into childhood, and rarely a patient survives into young adult life. Those who live beyond infancy have, as a general rule, either an isolated large atrial septal defect or a single ventricle or ventricular septal defect and pulmonic stenosis.

The clinical course is determined by the degree of tissue hypoxia, the ability of each ventricle to sustain an increased work load in the presence of reduced coronary arterial oxygenation, the nature of the associated cardiovascular anomalies, and the anatomic and functional status of the pulmonary vascular bed. Severe morphologic alterations develop in the pulmonary vascular bed by the age of 1 to 2 years in almost all patients with this anomaly with an associated large ventricular septal defect or large patent ductus arteriosus in the absence of obstruction to left ventricular outflow.

The usual clinical manifestations are dyspnea and cyanosis from birth, retardation of growth, and congestive heart failure. Murmurs and the electrocardiogram are of little diagnostic help. The roentgenographic findings are often highly suggestive of the diagnosis and consist of (1) progressive cardiac enlargement in early infancy, (2) characteristic oval or egg-shaped cardiac configuration in the anteroposterior view and a narrow vascular pedicle, and (3) increased pulmonary vascular markings. In the absence of dextrocardia, transverse cross-sectional echocardiography may strongly suggest the diagnosis by demonstrating that the anterior great artery (aorta) is to the right of the posterior great artery (pulmonary). Cardiac catheterization shows a lower oxygen saturation in the aorta than in the pulmonary artery. Angiocardiography is diagnostic and demonstrates that the anteriorly placed aorta arises from the right ventricle, and the posteriorly placed pulmonary artery in continuity with the mitral valve arises from the left ventricle.

The creation or enlargement of an interatrial communication is the simplest procedure for providing increased intracardiac mixing of systemic and pulmonary venous blood; it may be achieved surgically or, preferably, by rupturing the valve of the foramen ovale with a balloon catheter during cardiac catheterization (Rashkind's procedure). Pulmonary artery banding should be considered as an adjunct in infants with ventricular septal defect, and high pulmonary arterial pressure. Systemic-pulmonary artery anastomosis may be indicated in the patient with severe obstruction to left ventricular outflow and diminished pulmonary blood flow. Intracardiac repair may be accomplished by rearranging the venous return so that the systemic venous blood is directed to the mitral valve and thence to the left ventricle and pulmonary artery, while the pulmonary venous blood is diverted through the tricuspid valve and right ventricle to the aorta (Mustard or Senning operation). The risk of this corrective operation is lowest in those patients with an intact ventricular septum and no obstruction to pulmonary flow. For those patients with a ventricular septal defect in whom it is necessary to bypass a severely obstructed left ventricular outflow tract, corrective operation employs an intracardiac ventricular baffle and extracardiac prosthetic conduit to replace the pulmonary artery (Rastelli's procedure).

Partial transposition This designation is usually applied to the anomaly referred to as *double-outlet right ventricle* or *origin of both great vessels from the right ventricle.* The aorta is transposed and arises entirely from the right ventricle, while the pulmonary artery takes its usual origin. A ventricular septal defect serves as the sole outlet of the left ventricle. The clinical and physiologic picture is determined by the size of the ventricular septal defect and the presence or absence of pulmonary stenosis. These patients may resemble clinically those with isolated, large ventricular septal defects without cyanosis. However, when there is accompanying pulmonary stenosis, the clinical findings are similar to those of cyanotic tetralogy of Fallot. Diagnosis of these lesions is dependent on echocardiographic and angiocardiographic analysis, and increased preoperative recognition of the partial transposition anomalies may be expected to result in improved operative results. In the *Taussig-Bing* form of partial transposition, the ventricular septal defect is related to a nonstenotic pulmonary orifice. This malformation resembles complete transposition with ventricular septal defect and pulmonary hypertension clinically.

Corrected transposition The two fundamental anatomic derangements composing this malformation are transposition of the ascending aorta and pulmonary trunk and inversion of the ventricles. This arrangement permits functional correction, so that systemic venous blood passes into the pulmonary trunk while arterialized pulmonary venous blood flows into the aorta. The systemic veins drain into the right atrium; venous blood hence flows across an atrioventricular valve, which has the structure of a normal *mitral* valve, into the right-sided "venous ventricle." This chamber, however, has the morphologic characteristics of a normal *left* ventricle, and it ejects blood into the pulmonary trunk, which arises *posterior* to the ascending aorta. Oxygenated blood returns from the lungs to the left atrium, from which it flows into the left-sided "arterial ventricle" across an atrioventricular valve, which has the structure of a normal *tricuspid* valve. The arterial ventricle has the morphologic characteristics of a normal *right* ventricle, and it ejects blood into the aorta, which arises anterior to the pulmonary trunk.

Patients in whom corrected transposition exists as an isolated anomaly present no functional alterations and have no symptoms. Ebstein-type anomalies of the left-sided, tricuspid atrioventricular valve, ventricular septal defect, obstruction to outflow from the venous ventricle, and congenital heart block are those malformations most often associated with corrected transposition. An accentuated, single second heart sound in the second left intercostal space, representing closure of the aortic valve, which lies lateral and anterior to the pulmonic valve is often heard. An abnormal direction of initial (septal) ventricular depolarization is manifested electrocardiographically by a reversal of the precordial Q-wave pattern (Q waves are present in the right precordial leads and absent on the left). The His bundle is elongated, often leading to atrioventricular conduction disturbances. Roentgenographic examination characteristically reveals absence of the normal pulmonary artery segment and a smooth convexity of the left supracardiac border produced by the displaced ascending aorta. The displaced aorta may be visualized by cross-sectional echocardiography and by radionuclide scintillation scans of the central circulation. The diagnosis of corrected transposition can usually be established by selective angiocardiography.

Specific problems have attended operative repair of the lesions associated with corrected transposition, owing primarily to the course of the conduction system and the coronary arterial pattern. The incidence of surgically induced heart block has been reduced by intraoperative electrophysiologic mapping of the course of the conduction system. Occasionally, the inversion of the coronary arterial system may limit and preclude an incision into the venous ventricle, thereby interfering with exposure of intracardiac defects in the usual manner.

Transposition of the pulmonary veins When all the pulmonary veins connect either to the right atrium directly or to the systemic veins or their tributaries, the condition is called total anomalous pulmonary venous connection (TAPVC). Because all venous blood returns to the right atrium, an interatrial communication is an integral part of this malformation. Additional major cardiac malformations occur in about one-third of these patients. The anomalous connection is usually supradiaphragmatic and to the left brachiocephalic vein, right atrium, coronary sinus, or superior vena cava. The distal site of connection may be below the diaphragm, a condition which is hazardous because it is typically associated with marked obstruction to pulmonary venous return.

Most infants with the more usual, unobstructed form of supradiaphragmatic TAPVC fail to thrive, are subject to repeated respiratory infections, and have congestive heart failure by the age of 6 months. Cyanosis is not usually prominent in the absence of congestive failure unless the patient survives long enough to acquire secondary pulmonary vascular changes and a reduction in pulmonary blood flow.

A characteristic physical finding is the presence of multiple heart sounds, consisting of a first sound followed by an ejection click, a fixed, widely split second heart sound with an accentuated pulmonic component, and a third, and often a fourth, heart sound. The electrocardiogram shows right axis deviation, as well as right atrial and ventricular hypertrophy. Roentgenograms of the chest reveal increased pulmonary blood flow; the right atrium and ventricle are dilated and hypertrophied, and the pulmonary artery segment is enlarged. In addition, the specific site of anomalous connection may result in a characteristic appearance of the cardiac silhouette. Thus in patients with TAPVC to the left brachiocephalic vein, the superior vena cava on the right, left brachiocephalic vein superiorly, and left vertical vein on the left produce a cardiac shadow that resembles a "snowman" or figure-of-eight. The upper right cardiac border may be prominent when the anomalous connection is to the right superior vena cava. Echocardiography demonstrates marked enlargement of the right ventricle and, occasionally, the common pulmonary venous chamber behind the left atrium. Selective pulmonary arteriography is especially helpful in determining the drainage pathways of the pulmonary veins.

Balloon atrial septostomy may provide dramatic palliation for the infant in whom the small size of the interatrial communication limits the amount of blood reaching the left side of the heart and systemic circulation. Unless serious pulmonary vascular disease is present, results of operation for TAPVC in patients more than 1 year of age are good. The procedure consists of creating an anastomosis between the common pulmonary venous channel and left atrium and closing the atrial defect and the anomalous venous pathway.

Partial transposition of the pulmonary veins In this condition, one of the pulmonary veins (or more than one) is connected to the right atrium or to one or more of its tributaries. An atrial septal defect, particularly one of the sinus venosus type, usually accompanies partial transposition of the pulmonary veins, and the usual connection involves the veins of the right upper and middle lobes and the superior vena cava. The physiologic disturbance is determined by the number of anomalous veins and their site of connection, the presence and size of an atrial septal defect, the state of the pulmonary vascular bed, and associated anomalies. In the usual case of isolated partial transposition of the pulmonary veins, the hemodynamic state and physical findings are similar to those in atrial septal defect. Occasionally, drainage is into the inferior vena cava. This condition may be associated with pulmonary parenchymal abnormalities, hypoplasia of the right pulmonary artery and lung, and dextroposition of the heart. This complex has been designated the "scimitar syndrome," because of the characteristic roentgenographic finding of a crescent-like shadow in the right lower lung field which is produced by the anomalous venous channel.

MALPOSITIONS OF THE HEART Positional anomalies of the heart refer to conditions in which the cardiac apex is located in the right side of the chest (dextrocardia) or at the midline (mesocardia), or in which there is a normal location of the heart in the left side of the chest but abnormal position of the viscera (isolated levocardia). Knowledge of the position of the abdominal organs is important in diagnosing these malpositions. For example, a mirror-image dextrocardia is usually observed in a patient with complete situs inversus; this condition occurs more frequently in an otherwise normal person than in one with a malformed heart. In contrast, when dextrocardia occurs without situs inversus, associated cardiac malformations are the rule. When the heart occupies its normal position but situs inversus of the viscera is present, the heart is almost always seriously malformed. Moreover, when the visceral situs is indeterminate, there is a striking association of asplenia or polysplenia with complex, multiple cardiac anomalies, which usually include a combination of systemic and pulmonary venous abnormalities, defects in the atrial and ventricular septa, and endocardial cushion defects. In addition, pulmonary arterial obstruction and maldevelopment of the great arteries may occur with both asplenia and polysplenia but are more common in the former. Transposition of the great arteries occurs frequently in cardiac malposition, and double-outlet right ventricle is common in asplenia. It is important to recognize these complex syndromes in order to distinguish them from forms of cyanotic heart disease that are more amenable to corrective surgical therapy. The diagnosis is suggested by a symmetric liver shadow roentgenographically, and by the presence of Howell-Jolly and Heinz bodies in red blood cells demonstrated by blood smear, and confirmed by a negative or abnormal radioactive spleen scan.

REFERENCES

General

Borow, KM, Alpert J, Braunwald E: Congenital heart disease in the adult, in *Heart Disease,* 2d ed, E Braunwald (ed). Philadelphia, Saunders, 1983, chap 30

Friedman WF: Congenital heart disease in infancy and childhood, in *Heart Disease,* 2d ed, E Braunwald (ed). Philadelphia, Saunders, 1983, chap 29

——— et al: *Neonatal Heart Disease.* New York, Grune & Stratton, 1973

Moss AJ et al: *Heart Disease in Infants, Children and Adolescents,* 2d ed. Baltimore, Williams & Wilkins, 1977

Perloff JK: *The Clinical Recognition of Congenital Heart Disease,* 2d ed. Philadelphia, Saunders, 1978

Roberts WC: Congenital heart disease in adults, in *Cardiovascular Clinics,* 10/1, AN Brest (ed). Philadelphia, Davis, 1979

Specific malformations

Allwork SP et al: Congenitally corrected transposition of the great arteries. Am J Cardiol 38:910, 1976

Arciniegas E et al: Management of anomalous left coronary artery from the pulmonary artery. Circulation 62(Suppl):180, 1980

Berger TJ et al: Survival and probability of cure without and with operation in complete atrioventricular canal. Ann Thorac Surg 24:104, 1979

Doty DB et al: Supravalvular aortic stenosis. J Thorac Cardiovasc Surg 74:362, 1977

Friedman WF: The patent ductus arteriosus in the newborn. Clin Perinatol 5:411, 1978

——— et al: Congenital aortic stenosis in adults, in *Congenital Heart Disease in Adults,* A Brest (ed). Philadelphia, Davis, 1979, pp 235–251

Fuster V et al: Long-term evaluation (12–22 years) of open heart surgery for tetralogy of Fallot. Am J Cardiol 46:635, 1980

Gale AW: Fontan procedure for tricuspid atresia. Circulation 62:91, 1980

Garson A Jr et al: The surgical decision in tetralogy of Fallot: Weighing risks and benefits with decision analysis. Am J Cardiol 45:108, 1980

Giuliani ER et al: Special review Ebstein's anomaly. Mayo Clin Proc 54:163, 1979

Gutgesell HP et al: Prognosis for the newborn with transposition of the great arteries. Am J Cardiol 44:96, 1979

HENRY CG et al: Treatment of D-transposition of the great arteries: Management of hypoxemia after balloon atrial septostomy. Am J Cardiol 47:299, 1981

LIBERTSON RR et al: Coarctation of the aorta. Review of 234 patients and clarification of management problems. Am J Cardiol 43:835, 1979

——— et al: Congenital coronary arteriovenous fistula. Circulation 59:849, 1979

———: Right ventricular function in adult atrial septal defect. Preoperative and postoperative assessment and clinical implications. Am J Cardiol 47:56, 1981

MYER J et al: Aneurysm and fistula of the sinus of Valsalva. Clinical considerations and surgical treatment of 45 patients. Ann Thorac Surg 19:170, 1975

NEUGENT EW et al: Clinical course in pulmonary stenosis. Circulation 56:I-38, 1977

NEWFELD EA et al: Pulmonary vascular disease and total anomalous venous drainage. Circulation 61:103, 1980

RICHARDSON JV: The spectrum of anomalies of aortopulmonary septation. J Thorac Cardiovasc Surg 78:21, 1979

SOTO B et al: Classification of ventricular septal defects. Br Heart J 43:332, 1980

SUNG CS et al: Discrete subaortic stenosis in adults. Am J Cardiol 42:283, 1978

TYNAN MJ et al: Nomenclature and classification of congenital heart disease. Br Heart J 41:544, 1979

WHITMER JT et al: Exercise testing in children before and after surgical treatment of aortic stenosis. Circulation 63:254, 1981

257 RHEUMATIC FEVER

GENE H. STOLLERMAN

DEFINITION Rheumatic fever is an inflammatory disease which occurs as a delayed sequel to pharyngeal infection with group A streptococci. It involves principally the heart, joints, central nervous system, skin, and subcutaneous tissues. The usual manifestations in the acute form are migratory polyarthritis, fever, and carditis. Sydenham's chorea, subcutaneous nodules, and erythema marginatum may occur as other typical manifestations. No single symptom, sign, or laboratory test is pathognomonic of rheumatic fever, although several combinations of them are diagnostic. Although the name *acute rheumatic fever* emphasizes involvement of the joints, rheumatic fever owes its importance to the involvement of the heart, which can be fatal during the acute stage of the disease or can lead to rheumatic heart disease, a chronic condition due to scarring and deformity of the heart valves.

ETIOLOGY AND PATHOGENESIS The etiologic relationship of group A streptococci to rheumatic fever can be summarized briefly, as follows. (1) Numerous clinical and epidemiologic studies have shown a close association of group A streptococcal infections and rheumatic fever. (2) Antecedent streptococcal infection can almost always be demonstrated immunologically in the acute stage of rheumatic fever by increased titers of antibodies to streptococcal antigens. Moreover, in long-term prospective follow-up studies, rheumatic fever recurs only as a result of intercurrent streptococcal infections. (3) Both primary and secondary attacks of the disease can be prevented by prompt treatment or prevention of streptococcal infections with antimicrobial therapy. The pharyngeal route of infection is necessary to initiate the rheumatic process. Streptococcal skin infections do not do so. Furthermore, throat infections with some group A strains appear to produce rheumatic fever rarely or not at all.

The mechanism by which the group A streptococcus initiates the disease process remains unknown. A relatively small percentage of persons who suffer from streptococcal sore throats subsequently develops rheumatic fever. The organism is not demonstrable in the lesions when rheumatic fever appears several days or weeks after the acute streptococcal infection. No one product of the streptococcus has been incriminated as a cause of the lesions, either as a direct tissue toxin or as an antigen inducing hypersensitivity. Gamma globulin has been demonstrated by fluorescent antibody methods to be deposited in the sarcolemma of myocardial fibers of patients who have died of rheumatic carditis and in the biopsied auricular appendages of patients operated upon for mitral stenosis. Also streptococcal membrane antigens have been purified which cross-react immunologically with myocardial sarcolemma. Furthermore, patients with rheumatic carditis or chronic rheumatic heart disease often have circulating antibodies to heart tissue. This finding has led to the suggestion that the myocardial lesions of rheumatic fever are the result of some form of autoimmunity induced by streptococcal antigens. The validity of this concept has not been confirmed, however, since the immunologic phenomena might be secondary to cardiac tissue damage rather than a cause of it.

INCIDENCE AND EPIDEMIOLOGY Although rheumatic fever may occur at any age, it is extremely rare in infancy; it appears most commonly between the ages of 5 and 15 years, when streptococcal infection is most frequent and intense. Similarly, the geographic distribution, incidence, and severity of rheumatic fever are, in general, a reflection of the frequency and severity of streptococcal pharyngitis. The attack rate of rheumatic fever following exudative streptococcal pharyngitis in epidemics averages approximately 3 percent. When streptococcal pharyngitis is sporadic and mild or due to strains of lesser rheumatic potential, the attack rate of rheumatic fever may be very much lower. Strains of group A streptococci that cause epidemics of streptococcal pharyngitis are most likely to be rheumatogenic. Following such infections, the attack rate of rheumatic fever is directly correlated with the magnitude of the streptococcal immune response. Analysis of reported epidemics of acute rheumatic fever caused by a variety of serotypes shows some, such as type 5, to be overrepresented, and others, such as type 12, to be conspicuously absent. In some populations, such as in Trinidad, strains responsible for rheumatic fever and acute glomerulonephritis are serotypically distinct.

Environmental, bacterial, and host factors which appear to play a role in the development of rheumatic fever are important primarily as they are related to the incidence and severity of preceding streptococcal infection. Such factors as latitude, altitude, dampness, economic factors, and age all affect the incidence of rheumatic fever because they are related to the incidence of streptococcal infection in general. Crowding is, however, the major environmental factor relating to the occurrence of this disease because, regardless of other variables, it promotes interpersonal spread of the most virulent group A streptococcal strains. Such crowding as occurs in military barracks, closed institutions, large families in small quarters, and those massed in the densely populated core of major urban centers is most likely to be associated with an increase in incidence of rheumatic fever.

The attack rate of rheumatic fever following streptococcal infections in patients who have had previous attacks of rheumatic fever is increased to as high as 5 to 50 percent and is also related to the virulence of the reactivating infection. Furthermore, the frequency of rheumatic recurrences following streptococcal infection is consistently greater in those with rheumatic heart disease than in those who escaped cardiac injury during prior attacks. The tendency to suffer recurrences of rheumatic fever following streptococcal infections declines with the passage of years since the preceding attack. It appears, therefore, that certain host variables, as well as probable qualitative and quantitative differences in the nature of the antecedent streptococcal infection, also influence the development of rheumatic fever. To what extent such variables are genetic or acquired has not been settled. It is common to obtain a family history of rheumatic fever as well as to encounter multiple cases among siblings of a single family. However, the concordance of rheumatic fever in identical twins is approximately 20 percent, which does not exceed that of poliomyelitis or tuberculosis, suggesting only a limited penetrance of genetic predisposition to rheumatic fever. Although investigations of the distribution of haplotypes in rheumatic hosts have been limited in scope and number, there has been so far no consistent association of rheumatic fever, or any of its major manifestations, with any predominant histocompatibility locus antigens.

The mortality of acute rheumatic fever has been declining steadily for the past 30 years. It is still, however, a major cause of death and disability in children and adolescents in socioeconomically depressed areas of the world. The incidence of rheumatic fever has been decreasing for several years in countries where housing and economic conditions have been improving steadily. The rate of decrease may have been accelerated by the wide use of antimicrobial therapy. The decrease also may be due to a change in the prevalence of rheumatogenic streptococcal strains. Rheumatic fever remains, however, a worldwide disease having its greatest incidence wherever poor economic conditions, overcrowding, and substandard housing are most common.

PATHOLOGY The lesions of rheumatic fever are disseminated widely throughout the body, with special predilection for connective tissues. Focal inflammatory lesions occur particularly around small blood vessels.

Cardiovascular lesions The heart is the site of the most characteristic and consequential involvement, and all its layers—endocardium, myocardium, and pericardium—may be involved. This generalized involvement gives rise to the term *rheumatic pancarditis.* The most characteristic and specific pattern of rheumatic inflammation is found in the *myocardial Aschoff body,* a submiliary granuloma. This lesion, when present in its classic form, is generally considered to be pathognomonic of rheumatic fever. In many areas the inflammatory lesion is accompanied by swelling and fragmentation of the collagen fibers and alteration in the staining properties of the ground substances of the connective tissues. This change is described as *fibrinoid degeneration of collagen,* but its chemical basis has not been established. Aschoff bodies with less exudative and more productive changes may persist for many years as the lingering traces of chronic rheumatic inflammation in patients with rheumatic heart disease, long after rheumatic fever has become clinically quiescent. The persistence of such lesions is most common in patients who develop severe mitral stenosis. Eventually the Aschoff body is converted into a spindle-shaped or triangular scar lying between the muscle bundles and surrounding blood vessels.

Rheumatic endocarditis produces the verrucous valvulitis of acute rheumatic fever which leads to the most serious permanent cardiac damage. It may heal with fibrous thickening and adhesion of the valve commissures and chordae tendineae, leading to variable degrees of valvular regurgitation and stenosis. Deformity resulting in functional impairment of the heart occurs most commonly in the mitral and aortic valves, less frequently in the tricuspid, and almost never in the pulmonic valves. *Rheumatic pericarditis* (Chap. 265) produces a serofibrinous effusion, with the deposit of shaggy elements of fibrin on the surface of the heart. The pericardium may become calcified, but pericardial constriction does not occur.

Extracardiac lesions Involvement of the *joints* is characterized by exudative rather than proliferative changes, and healing of these structures occurs without significant scarring or deformity. *Subcutaneous nodules,* seen during the acute phase of the disease, are composed of granulomas with localized areas of "fibrinoid" swelling of subcutaneous collagen bundles, and perivascular collections of large cells with pale nuclei and prominent nucleoli. Synovitis is usually mild and nonspecific. *Pulmonary* and *pleural* lesions are less definite and less characteristic. Fibrinous pleurisy and rheumatic pneumonitis may occur with exudative and proliferative lesions but without definite Aschoff bodies. Patients with active *chorea* rarely die. The pathologic findings which have been reported in the central nervous system are not consistent, and no characteristic lesion has been reported to explain this clinical manifestation. During active chorea the spinal fluid remains normal, being free of cells, with no increase in total protein and no change in the relative concentration of various proteins.

CLINICAL FEATURES The major clinical manifestations by which rheumatic fever can be recognized are polyarthritis, carditis, chorea, erythema marginatum, and subcutaneous nodules.

Arthritis The classic attack of rheumatic fever appears as an acute migratory polyarthritis accompanied by signs and symptoms of an acute febrile illness. The large joints of the extremities are most frequently affected, but no joint is impervious to the inflammatory process; one may find arthritis of the hands and feet but only rarely of the spine or of the sternoclavicular or temporomandibular joints. Joint effusions occur but are not persistent. As pain and swelling subside in one joint, others tend to become involved. Although such "migratory" involvement is characteristic, it is not invariable, and several large joints may be inflamed at one time. To be acceptable as a criterion for the diagnosis of rheumatic fever, the polyarthritis should involve two or more joints, should be associated with at least two minor manifestations such as fever and elevation of sedimentation rate, and should be associated with high titer of anti-streptolysin O or some other streptococcal antibody (Table 257-1). There is nothing distinctive about the arthritis of rheumatic fever, and other causes of migratory polyarthritis that may be associated only fortuitously with high streptococcal antibody levels must, of course, be excluded.

Acute rheumatic carditis Acute rheumatic carditis first manifests itself by the appearance of the heart murmurs of either mitral or aortic regurgitation, the former most frequently. Signs and symptoms of pericarditis and of congestive heart failure may supervene in more severe cases. Death may result from heart failure during the acute stage of the disease, or permanent valvular damage may be sustained which results ultimately in serious disability. Carditis may vary from a fulminating, fatal course to a low-grade, inapparent inflammation. *It is well to bear in mind that the vast majority of patients with carditis do not have symptoms referable to the heart.* The latter occur only in more severe cases when heart failure or pericardial effusions produce characteristic symptoms. For this reason, unless extracardiac manifestations, such as polyarthritis and chorea, are present, patients whose rheumatic fever is manifested only by carditis are frequently not diagnosed and in later life may be discovered to have rheumatic heart disease without a definite history of rheumatic fever.

When carditis is manifest, there is usually tachycardia disproportionate to the degree of fever, gallop rhythms are often heard, and the heart sounds may become fetal or "tic-tac" in quality. Occasionally, arrhythmias and/or a pericardial friction rub may be present. Prolongation of the conduction time may lead to dropped beats with varying degrees of heart block. Prolongation of the PR interval and other changes in the electrocardiogram are very common, but these findings, in the absence of clinical manifestations of carditis, have a benign prognosis. Therefore, changes in the electrocardiogram alone, unassociated with significant murmurs or cardiac enlargement, do not by themselves constitute an acceptable criterion for the diagnosis of rheumatic carditis. Pericarditis may cause precordial pain, and a friction rub may be audible.

A definite clinical diagnosis of carditis can be made if one or more of the following can be demonstrated: (1) the appearance of, or change in the character of, organic heart murmurs; (2) definite increase in heart size demonstrated by radiogram or fluoroscopy; (3) pericardial friction rub or effusion; or (4) signs of congestive heart failure. Rheumatic carditis is almost always associated with a significant murmur.

Subcutaneous nodules These are usually small, pea-sized, painless swellings over bony prominences and therefore frequently go unnoticed by the patient. The skin moves freely over them. Characteristic locations are the extensor tendons of the hands and feet, the elbows, margins of the patellae, the scalp, over the scapulae, and over the spinous processes of the vertebrae.

Chorea (Sydenham's chorea, chorea minor, Saint Vitus' dance) This is a disorder of the central nervous system characterized by sudden, aimless, irregular movements, often accompanied by muscle weakness and emotional instability. Chorea is a delayed manifestation of rheumatic fever, and other manifestations may or may not still be present at the time it appears. Polyarthritis, when part of the same attack, always subsides before chorea appears. Carditis is often discovered for the first time when the presenting feature of rheumatic fever is chorea. Chorea usually appears after a long latent period (up to several months) from the antecedent streptococcal infection and at a time when all other manifestations of rheumatic fever have abated. When no previous rheumatic manifestations are noted, such cases are called *pure chorea.*

The clinical onset of chorea is often gradual. Patients may be unusually nervous and fidgety and may have difficulty in writing, drawing, and handiwork. They may stumble or fall, drop things, and grimace. As symptoms become more severe, spasmodic movements extend to all parts of the body, and muscular weakness may become so marked that patients cannot walk, talk, or sit up. Often the weakness is severe enough to simulate paralysis. The irregular, jerky, spasmodic movements may become so violent that cribs and beds must be padded to prevent injury. Symptoms are exaggerated by excitement, effort, or fatigue but subside during sleep. Emotional instability is almost invariable in patients with chorea. All degrees of speech disturbance are seen. Central nervous stimulants exacerbate and sedatives suppress choreiform activity.

Erythema marginatum This evanescent pink rash is characteristic of rheumatic fever. The erythematous areas often have clear centers and round or serpiginous margins. They vary greatly in size and occur mainly on the trunk and proximal part of the extremities, never on the face. The erythema is transient, migratory, and may be brought out by the application of heat; it is nonpruritic, not indurated, and blanches on pressure.

Minor clinical criteria These are clinical features which occur frequently in rheumatic fever but are also common to many other diseases and are therefore of minor diagnostic value. They include fever, arthralgia, abdominal pain, tachycardia, and epistaxis.

LABORATORY FINDINGS There is no specific laboratory test to indicate the presence of rheumatic fever. The appraisal of rheumatic activity by laboratory findings is, however, of value, since various tests may indicate *continued* rheumatic inflammation when clinical features are not apparent.

Streptococcal antibody tests to disclose preceding streptococcal infection Streptococcal antibody titers differentiate preceding streptococcal from other acute respiratory infections and are increased following asymptomatic as well as symptomatic streptococcal infections. These antibody levels are increased in the early stages of acute rheumatic fever. They may be declining, or low, if the interval between the acute streptococcal infection and the detection of rheumatic fever has been longer than 2 months, a situation which occurs most often in patients whose presenting rheumatic manifestation is chorea. However, patients whose only major manifestation is rheumatic carditis also may have low antibody titers when first seen. Their rheumatic attack may have been in progress several months before becoming symptomatic and recognized. Except in these two instances, *one should be reluctant to make the diagnosis of acute rheumatic fever in the absence of serologic evidence of a recent streptococcal infection.* The anti-streptolysin O test (ASO) is the most widely used and best-standardized streptococcal antibody test. In general, single titers of at least 250 Todd units in adults and at least 333 units in children over 5 years of age are considered to be increased. Depending on the general prevalence of streptococcal infections, a varying percentage of the normal population may show titers of this magnitude.

About 20 percent of patients in the early stages of acute rheumatic fever, and most patients who present with chorea, have a low or borderline ASO titer. In these instances, it is advisable to obtain another streptococcal antibody test. Other streptococcal antibody tests that can be employed include the following: antihyaluronidase (AH), antideoxyribonucleotidase B (anti-DNase B), antinicotinamide-adenine dinucleotidase (anti-NADase), and anti-streptokinase (ASK). The anti-streptozyme test (ASTZ) is a hemagglutination reaction to a concentrate of extracellular streptococcal antigens absorbed to red blood cells. It is a very sensitive indicator of recent streptococcal infection; virtually all patients with acute rheumatic fever have titers greater than 200 units per milliliter. The real value

TABLE 257-1
Jones criteria (revised)

Major manifestations	*Minor manifestations*
Carditis	Fever
Polyarthritis	Arthralgia
Chorea	Previous rheumatic fever or rheumatic heart disease
Erythema marginatum	Elevated ESR or positive CRP
Subcutaneous nodules	Prolonged PR interval

Two major criteria or one major and two minor criteria indicate a high probability of the presence of rheumatic fever with supporting evidence of preceding streptococcal infection: history of recent scarlet fever; positive throat culture for group A streptococcus; increased ASO titer or other streptococcal antibodies.

SOURCE: *American Heart Association, 1965.*

of the ASTZ test is in *ruling out* rheumatic fever when the titer is low in patients with isolated polyarthritis. To date, the specific antigens involved in the ASTZ test remain unidentified and therefore the test has not yet been adequately standardized. A rise in titer of two dilution tubes or more can be demonstrated for at least one of the streptococcal antibodies in almost all recurrent as well as primary attacks of rheumatic fever (Table 257-2). Increased streptococcal antibodies, however, do not reflect rheumatic activity per se, and their rate of decline is independent of the course of the rheumatic attack.

Isolation of group A streptococci Some patients continue to harbor group A streptococci at the onset of acute rheumatic fever, but these organisms are usually present in small numbers and may be difficult to isolate by a single throat culture. The administration of penicillin or other antibodies may also result in failure to isolate the infecting organism. In addition, a significant number of *normal* individuals, particularly children, may harbor group A streptococci in the upper respiratory tract. For these reasons, throat cultures are less satisfactory than antibody tests as supporting evidence of recent streptococcal infection.

Acute phase reactants These tests offer objective but nonspecific confirmation of the presence of an inflammatory process. *The erythrocyte sedimentation rate* (ESR) and the test for *C-reactive protein* (CRP) in serum are used most commonly. Unless the patient has received corticosteroids or salicylates, these reactions are almost always abnormal in patients presenting with polyarthritis or acute carditis, whereas they are often normal in patients with chorea. Other laboratory findings which reflect inflammation include reactions such as leukocytosis, and increases in serum complement, mucoproteins, and alpha$_2$ and gamma globulins. Prolongation of the PR interval of the electrocardiogram, although neither specific for rheumatic fever nor diagnostic of serious cardiac involvement, is frequent in acute rheumatic fever (about 25 percent of all cases), and other nonspecific electrocardiographic changes are also common. Anemia, due to the suppression of erythropoiesis characteristic of chronic inflammatory diseases, is another feature of rheumatic activity.

COURSE AND PROGNOSIS The course of rheumatic fever varies greatly and is impossible to predict at the onset of the disease. In general, however, approximately 75 percent of acute rheumatic attacks subside within 6 weeks, 90 percent within 12 weeks, and less than 5 percent persist more than 6 months. The latter usually consist of severe, intractable forms of rheumatic carditis or stubborn, prolonged attacks of Sydenham's chorea, both of which may persist for as long as several years. Once acute rheumatic fever has subsided and more than 2 months have elapsed after withdrawal of treatment with salicylates or adrenal corticosteroids, rheumatic fever does not recur in the absence of new streptococcal infections. Recurrences are most common within the first 5 years of the initial attack and tend to decline with increasing duration of freedom from rheumatic activity. The frequency of recurrences is dependent upon the frequency and severity of streptococcal infection, the presence or absence of rheumatic heart disease following an attack, and the duration of freedom from the last attack.

Approximately 70 percent of patients who develop carditis do so within the first week of the disease, 85 percent within the first 12 weeks of the disease, and almost all within 6 months from the onset of the acute attack. Thereafter, if significant murmurs have not appeared, the prognosis for a patient in whom recurrences are prevented is excellent.

Chronic rheumatic carditis and the course of rheumatic heart disease The remarkable variability in the course of rheumatic carditis and rheumatic valvular disease stems from several factors: (1) the variability in the duration and severity of the rheumatic inflammation; (2) the amount of scarring of the valves and myocardium following the abatement of the acute inflammation; (3) the location and severity of the hemodynamic lesion due to valvular insufficiency or stenosis; (4) the frequency of recurrent bouts of carditis; and (5) the progression of valvular calcification and sclerosis, which occurs as a secondary phenomenon in a deformed or injured valve without recurrent or persistent rheumatic inflammation (as seen in congenital valvular disease or following healed acute bacterial endocarditis). These factors, and possibly others not yet appreciated, produce striking variations in the clinical syndromes of rheumatic heart disease.

Chronic rheumatic myocarditis In this syndrome, the presenting picture is one of chronic heart failure in a patient with a markedly dilated heart and with physical, roentgenographic, and electrocardiographic findings of mitral regurgitation. The differentiation of this syndrome from other forms of chronic myocarditis may be very difficult, if not impossible, when the associated extracardiac features of rheumatic fever (chorea, polyarthritis, and so forth) are not present (Chap. 263). Although rheumatic fever does not produce *isolated* myocarditis, and is almost invariably a pancarditis, the pericardial inflammation may not be clearly evident, and the mitral valvulitis may not be distinguishable from mitral regurgitation due to dilation of the mitral ring. In such cases one must search diligently for an evanescent friction rub, evidence of pericardial effusion, appearance of a soft aortic regurgitation murmur, and extracardiac clues such as fever responding promptly to salicylates, arthralgias, transient subcutaneous nodules, evanescent erythema marginatum, and subtle signs of chorea.

The course of chronic rheumatic carditis may be intractable and end fatally after months or even several years. Often, however, the patient improves rather suddenly and even recovers cardiac reserve dramatically in association with the disappearance of systemic manifestations of the inflammatory process. The heart may remain large, may decrease somewhat in size, or in occasional instances may return to normal size with varying degrees of residual valvular deformity. Such a course signals the termination of the "toxic" phase of the rheumatic process, and thereafter the course of rheumatic heart disease depends on the variables in healing cited above.

DIFFERENTIAL DIAGNOSIS Early cases of rheumatic fever may be confused with other diseases which begin with acute polyarthritis. It is wise to exclude *bacteremia* by blood cultures, particularly because such infections may be masked by penicillin given for presumed acute rheumatic fever. Polyarthritis due

TABLE 257-2
Serologic results in patients with streptococcal disease

	Percent of patients whose serums were "positive"				
Patient group (no.)	*ASO*	*AH*	*Anti-DNase B*	*At least 1 of 3*	*ASTZ*
Acute rheumatic fever (20)	90	65	85	95	100
Acute glomerulonephritis (22)	50	63	72	91	95
Convalescent pharyngitis (11)	81	54	54	91	91
Convalescent pyoderma (23)	35	35	91	96	91
Total (76)	61	54	79	93	95

SOURCE: *AL Bisno, I Ofek, Am J Dis Child 127:676, 1974.*

to *infective endocarditis* in a patient with preexisting rheumatic heart disease may be mistaken for a recurrence of acute rheumatic fever. If streptococcal antibodies are not increased, polyarthritis should be attributed to some cause other than rheumatic fever. Gonococcal polyarthritis may be distinguished from rheumatic fever by the dramatic response of the former to a therapeutic trial of penicillin. In rheumatoid arthritis, joint involvement will persist and characteristic joint deformities may appear. The latter are not seen in rheumatic fever. The rheumatoid factor so characteristic of rheumatoid arthritis is not present in rheumatic fever. Antibodies against nuclear components and other autoantibodies are absent in rheumatic fever. Rheumatic pericarditis and myocarditis, associated with cardiac enlargement and heart failure, are both almost invariably associated with valvular lesions which produce significant murmurs.

Overdiagnosis of rheumatic fever should be avoided. Unless ill-defined febrile syndromes are clearly associated with a major manifestation of rheumatic fever, the diagnosis of rheumatic fever should not be made. A common error is the premature, vigorous administration of corticosteroids or salicylates before the signs and symptoms of rheumatic fever are unmistakable. In the absence of a curative agent, one should not suppress the signs and symptoms of rheumatic fever until they are clearly expressed.

Particularly confusing in the differential diagnosis of rheumatic fever is the drug sensitivity with fever and polyarthritis which may occur after administration of penicillin for a previous pharyngitis. Urticaria or angioneurotic edema, if present, helps differentiate penicillin sensitivity in such cases. The abdominal pain of rheumatic fever may be mistaken for appendicitis, and the crisis of sickle-cell anemia may also be associated with joint pain, enlargement of the heart, and cardiac murmurs. The rapidity with which the arthritis symptoms of rheumatic fever are controlled with salicylates is characteristic of this disease. Dramatic response to salicylates does not in itself, however, establish a diagnosis of rheumatic fever.

In order to help clarify the diagnosis of rheumatic fever, the American Heart Association has accepted and modified criteria usually referred to as the *Jones criteria* (Table 257-1). They are not to be used as a substitute for good medical judgment but are recommended as a guide for careful study of questionable cases. The finding of two major criteria, or of one major and two minor criteria, indicates a high probability of the presence of rheumatic fever if supported by evidence of a preceding streptococcal infection. The absence of the latter should always make the diagnosis questionable, except in the situation in which rheumatic fever is first discovered after a long latent period from the antecedent infection (Sydenham's chorea or low-grade carditis). Because the prognosis may differ according to the major manifestations, for recording purposes the diagnosis of rheumatic fever should be followed by a list of the major manifestations present, e.g., rheumatic fever manifested by polyarthritis and carditis. An indication of the severity of carditis in terms of presence or absence of congestive heart failure and cardiomegaly is also advisable.

TREATMENT There is no specific cure for rheumatic fever, and no known measures change the course of the attack. Good supportive therapy, however, can reduce the mortality and morbidity of the disease.

Chemotherapy After rheumatic fever is first diagnosed, a course of penicillin should be given to eliminate group A streptococci. This is advisable even if bacteriologic examination yields throat cultures negative for streptococci, since the organisms may be present in areas inaccessible to swabs. It is preferable to administer penicillin parenterally. An effective course is a single injection of 1.2 million units of benzathine penicillin intramuscularly or 600,000 units of procaine penicillin intramuscularly daily for 10 days. Attempts to reduce ultimate heart damage by administering penicillin early in the acute rheumatic attack in larger doses have not been successful. After completion of the therapeutic course of penicillin, continuous protection from reinfection with streptococci should be provided by instituting one of the prophylactic regimens described below.

Suppressive therapy For patients without carditis treatment with adrenal corticosteroids is unnecessary. Acute arthritis can be relieved with codeine or with salicylate, the latter being preferable to reduce fever and joint inflammation. When salicylate is used in the therapy of rheumatic fever, the dosage should be increased until the drug produces either a clinical effect or systemic toxicity characterized by tinnitus, headache, or hyperpnea. A starting dose of 100 to 125 mg/kg per day in children and 6 to 8 g in adults given in four or five divided doses is recommended. Of the various salicylate preparations ordinary aspirin is cheapest and most effective. Gastric intolerance can usually be diminished by administering aspirin after meals or by giving antacids 15 to 30 min after each dose of aspirin.

Many physicians prefer corticosteroids to salicylates for the treatment of carditis, despite the lack of a demonstrated advantage of these adrenal hormones in controlled clinical trials. Corticosteroids are more potent anti-inflammatory agents but are more likely to be followed by posttherapeutic "rebounds," and they have the additional disadvantage of more frequent side effects, particularly acne, hirsutism, and cushingoid changes in facies and habitus. For this reason it is preferable to begin treatment of patients who have carditis with salicylates; if these drugs fail to reduce fever and to ameliorate heart failure, therapy with corticosteroids may be initiated promptly. Prednisone is administered in doses of 60 to 120 mg or higher when necessary in four divided doses daily. After the inflammation has been brought under control by either salicylates or corticosteroids, treatment should be continued until the sedimentation rate approaches near-normal values and should be maintained for several weeks thereafter. To prevent poststeroid rebounds, an "overlap" course of salicylate therapy may be added when steroids are tapered off over a 2-week period. A useful method for tapering steroids is outlined in Chap. 112. Salicylates may then be continued for an additional 2 to 3 weeks. Rebounds of rheumatic activity are usually of short duration and, when mild, are best managed without resuming anti-inflammatory treatment, because a second or even a third rebound may occur when suppressive therapy is discontinued. About 5 percent of rheumatic attacks persist for 6 months or longer, either in the form of spontaneous acute recrudescences or as posttherapeutic rebounds. These "chronic" attacks are most likely to occur in patients with cardiac damage and with previous rheumatic episodes. Weekly tests for C-reactive protein in blood and for erythrocyte sedimentation rate are useful in following the healing process, particularly while treatment with corticosteroids or salicylates is gradually withdrawn.

Treatment of chorea The signs and symptoms of chorea usually do not respond well to treatment with antirheumatic agents. Because the patient with chorea is frequently emotionally unstable and because the manifestations of chorea may be exaggerated by emotional trauma, complete mental and physical rest is essential. Patients with chorea should be kept in a quiet room and cared for by sympathetic attendants. Corticosteroids or salicylates have little or no effect on chorea. Sedatives and tranquilizers, particularly diazepam and chlorpromazine, are useful. If the chorea is severe, large doses of phenobarbital rather than tranquilizers alone are usually necessary to control purposeless movements. Padded sideboards for the bed may be necessary to avoid injury to the patient. In the absence of other evidence of acute rheumatic disease, it is advisable to allow gradual resumption of physical activity when improvement is apparent rather than waiting for all choreiform movements to disappear, which may require many months.

Because of the great variability in the course of chorea, evaluating the effectiveness of various therapeutic measures is difficult. It is well to remember that chorea is a self-limited disease which is usually not followed by significant neurologic sequelae and that good results are almost invariably obtained by patient, attentive nursing care and by conservative medical management.

PREVENTION OF RECURRENCE The most efficient regimen for continuous prophylaxis against group A streptococci is a monthly intramuscular injection of 1.2 million units of benzathine penicillin. The disadvantages and discomfort of this regimen have to be weighed against the individual patient's susceptibility to recurrences. Those with rheumatic heart disease, recent rheumatic fever, and exposure to an environment in which the incidence of streptococcal infection is frequent deserve the most effective protection. As a second choice, prophylaxis may be administered orally with either 1 g sulfadiazine daily in a single dose or 200,000 units of penicillin given twice daily on an empty stomach. The duration of continuous prophylaxis cannot be fixed arbitrarily for all patients, although the safest generalization is that it be continued indefinitely. Certainly, those under the age of 18 years should receive a continuous prophylactic regimen. A minimum period of 5 years is recommended for patients who develop rheumatic fever without carditis over the age of 18 years. The decision to continue prophylaxis beyond this period should take into account a number of variables. Patients with rheumatic heart disease are more susceptible to reactivation of rheumatic fever if they contract a streptococcal infection. Moreover, patients who have had carditis in a previous attack are much more likely to suffer carditis again in a subsequent attack. Climate, age, occupation, household situation, cardiac status, and length of time since the previous attack are all significant variables which influence the risk of recurrence. The decline in recurrence rates with increasing age is due to (1) decreased rate of streptococcal infection and (2) decrease in the rate of rheumatic reactivation following streptococcal infection in older rheumatic subjects. Despite this decreased rate, however, the risk of rheumatic recurrence in adults remains relatively high when the streptococcal disease encountered is severe or epidemic.

PREVENTION OF INITIAL RHEUMATIC ATTACKS Early and adequate treatment of pharyngeal infection due to group A streptococci will prevent initial attacks of rheumatic fever. If clinical streptococcal disease were properly detected by throat cultures and adequately treated, the spread of infection in a given population would be prevented, the epidemiology of streptococcal disease would be modified markedly, and the incidence of rheumatic fever in the community would be diminished. In communities where group A streptococcal disease has been diagnosed early and treated well and where socioeconomic standards are high, the group A organisms cultured frequently from schoolchildren's throats may be of relatively low virulence and may cause rheumatic fever less frequently than do more virulent strains prevalent in many epidemics.

Streptococcal pharyngitis is adequately treated by a single intramuscular injection of 600,000 units of benzathine penicillin in children less than 10 years of age or 1.2 million units in older children and adults. Any alternate plan of parenteral therapy or combined parenteral and oral therapy should provide for treatment over a period of 10 days. If oral penicillin is employed, at least 800,000 units per day in four divided doses must be given for no less than 10 days to achieve results comparable with a single injection of benzathine penicillin. Erythromycin in daily doses of 1 g for 10 days may be substituted in penicillin-sensitive individuals. Tetracycline is not recommended because some strains of group A streptococci have acquired resistance to it. All group A streptococci have so far remained extremely sensitive to penicillin.

REFERENCES

AHA Committee on Rheumatic Fever and Bacterial Endocarditis: Prevention of rheumatic fever. Circulation 55:1, 1977

American Heart Association: Jones criteria (revised) for guidance in the diagnosis of rheumatic fever. Circulation 32:664, 1965

Joint Report of UK-US Cooperative Study: The natural history of rheumatic fever and rheumatic heart disease. 10 year report of a cooperative clinical trial of ACTH, cortisone and aspirin. Circulation 32:457, 1965

Read S, Zabriskie JB (eds): *Streptococcal Diseases and the Immune Response*. New York, Academic, 1980

Stollerman GH: *Rheumatic Fever and Streptococcal Infection*. New York, Grune & Stratton, 1975

———: Global changes in group A streptococcal diseases and strategies for their prevention. *Advances in Internal Medicine* 27:373, 1982, Chicago, Year Book Medical Publishers

Wannamaker LW, Matsen JM (eds): *Streptococci and Streptococcal Diseases*. New York, Academic, 1972

258 VALVULAR HEART DISEASE

EUGENE BRAUNWALD

The role of physical examination in the evaluation of patients with valvular disease is considered in Chap. 248; of echocardiography, phonocardiography, and other indirect graphic techniques in Chap. 250; and of cardiac catheterization and angiography in Chap. 251.

MITRAL STENOSIS

PATHOPHYSIOLOGY In normal adults the mitral valve orifice is 4 to 6 cm^2. In the presence of significant obstruction, i.e., when the orifice is less than one-half of normal, blood can flow from the left atrium to the left ventricle only if propelled by an abnormally elevated left atrioventricular pressure gradient, the hemodynamic hallmark of mitral stenosis. When the mitral valve opening is reduced to 1 cm^2, a left atrial pressure of approximately 25 mmHg is required to maintain a normal cardiac output. The elevated left atrial pressure in turn raises pulmonary venous and capillary pressures, reducing pulmonary compliance and causing exertional dyspnea. The first bouts of dyspnea are usually precipitated by clinical events which increase the rate of blood flow across the mitral orifice, which results in further elevation of the left atrial pressure. In order to assess the severity of obstruction, it is essential to measure both the transvalvular pressure gradient and the flow rate. The latter is dependent not only on the cardiac output but on the heart rate as well. An increase in heart rate shortens diastole proportionately more than systole, and diminishes the time available for flow across the mitral valve. Therefore, at any given level of cardiac output tachycardia augments the transvalvular gradient and elevates further left atrial pressure.

The left ventricular diastolic pressure is normal in isolated mitral stenosis; coexisting mitral regurgitation, aortic valve disease, the residua of damage produced by rheumatic myocarditis, systemic hypertension, or ischemic heart disease may be responsible for elevations which reflect impaired left ventricular function and/or reduced left ventricular compliance. Left ventricular dysfunction, as reflected in reduced ejection fraction and circumferential fiber shortening rate, occurs in about one-fifth of the patients. In pure mitral stenosis and sinus rhythm, the mean left atrial and pulmonary artery wedge pressures are usually elevated and the pressure pulse shows a prominent atrial contraction (*a* wave), and a gradual pressure decline after mitral valve opening (*y* descent). In patients with mild to moderate mitral stenosis without elevation of the pulmonary vascular resistance, the pulmonary arterial pressure may be normal at rest and may rise only with exercise. In severe mitral stenosis and whenever the pulmonary vascular resistance is significantly increased, the pulmonary arterial pressure is elevated even when the patient is at rest, and in extreme cases it may exceed the systemic arterial pressure. Further elevations of left atrial, pulmonary capillary, and pulmonary arterial pressures occur during exercise. When the pulmonary arterial systolic pressure exceeds approximately 50 mmHg in patients with mitral stenosis, or for that matter with any valvular lesion, the increased right ventricular afterload impedes the emptying of this chamber, and right ventricular end-diastolic pressure and volume (preload) usually rise as a compensatory mechanism.

The cardiac output at rest varies considerably in patients with mitral stenosis. Thus, the hemodynamic response to a given degree of mitral obstruction may be characterized by a normal cardiac output and a high left atrioventricular pressure gradient or, at the opposite end of the hemodynamic spectrum, by a reduced cardiac output and low transvalvular pressure gradient. In a small fraction of patients with moderately severe mitral stenosis, the cardiac output is normal at rest and rises normally during exertion; under these circumstances, the high atrioventricular pressure gradient elevates the left atrial and pulmonary capillary pressures markedly, and this elevation is responsible for symptoms of relatively severe pulmonary congestion. In the majority of patients, however, the cardiac output is normal at rest but rises subnormally during exertion. In patients with severe stenosis, particularly those in whom the pulmonary vascular resistance is strikingly elevated, the cardiac output is subnormal at rest and may fail to rise or may even decline during activity. The depressed cardiac output in patients with mitral stenosis is related primarily to the obstruction of the mitral orifice but may also be due to the impairment of the function of either ventricle which can accompany it.

The clinical and hemodynamic features of mitral stenosis are dictated largely by the level of the pulmonary artery pressure. Pulmonary hypertension results from (1) the passive backward transmission of the elevated left atrial pressure, (2) pulmonary arteriolar constriction, which presumably is triggered by left atrial and pulmonary venous hypertension (reactive pulmonary hypertension), and (3) organic obliterative changes in the pulmonary vascular bed. The elevation of pulmonary vascular resistance may be considered to be a complication of long-standing and severe mitral stenosis; in time, the resultant severe pulmonary hypertension results in tricuspid and pulmonary incompetence as well as right-sided heart failure. However, the changes in the pulmonary vascular bed may also be considered to exert a protective effect; the elevated precapillary resistance reduces the likelihood of symptoms of pulmonary congestion by preventing the surge of blood into the pulmonary capillary bed which then dams up behind the stenotic mitral valve. However, this protection occurs at the expense of a decreased cardiac output.

ETIOLOGY AND PATHOLOGY Mitral stenosis is generally rheumatic in origin. Pure or predominant mitral stenosis occurs in approximately 40 percent of all patients with rheumatic heart disease; two-thirds of all patients with mitral stenosis are females. A history of one or more attacks of acute rheumatic fever can be elicited from approximately one-half of patients with predominant or pure mitral stenosis. The valve leaflets are diffusely thickened by fibrous tissue and/or calcific deposits. The mitral commissures fuse, the chordae tendineae fuse and shorten, the valvular cusps become rigid, and these changes in turn lead to narrowing at the apex of the funnel-shaped valve. While the initial insult to the mitral valve is rheumatic, the later changes may be a nonspecific process resulting from trauma to the valve caused by altered flow patterns due to the initial deformity. Calcification of the stenotic mitral valve immobilizes the leaflets and narrows the orifice. Thrombus formation and arterial embolization may arise from the calcific valve itself. Rarely, mitral stenosis is congenital in origin (Chap. 256), most commonly the so-called parachute mitral valve, in which all the chordae insert into a single left ventricular papillary muscle.

SYMPTOMS In temperate climates the latent period between the initial attack of carditis and the development of symptoms due to mitral stenosis is generally on the order of two decades; most patients begin to experience disability in the fourth decade. Once a patient with mitral stenosis becomes seriously symptomatic, continuous progression of the disease to death usually occurs in 2 to 5 years unless the stenosis is relieved by operation. In economically deprived areas, particularly in the Indian subcontinent, Central America, and the Middle East, mitral stenosis tends to progress more rapidly and frequently causes serious symptoms before the age of 20 years. On the other hand, slowly progressive mitral stenosis in the elderly is also being recognized with increasing frequency.

When valvular obstruction is mild, many of the physical signs of mitral stenosis may be present in the absence of any symptoms. However, even in those patients whose mitral orifices are large enough to accommodate a normal blood flow with only mild elevations of left atrial pressure, extreme exertion, excitement, fever, severe anemia, paroxysmal tachycardia, sexual intercourse, pregnancy, and thyrotoxicosis all may precipitate elevations of pulmonary capillary pressure and lead to dyspnea and cough. As stenosis progresses, the stresses that precipitate dyspnea become less severe, and the patient becomes limited in his or her daily activities. Redistribution of blood from the dependent portions of the body to the lungs, which occurs when the recumbent position is assumed, leads to orthopnea and paroxysmal nocturnal dyspnea. *Pulmonary edema* develops when there is a sudden increase in flow rate across a markedly narrowed mitral orifice (Chap. 26). When moderately severe mitral stenosis has existed for several years, *atrial arrhythmias*—premature contractions, paroxysmal tachycardia, flutter, and fibrillation—tend to occur with increasing frequency. The rapid ventricular rate associated with untreated or inadequately treated atrial fibrillation is frequently responsible for acute exacerbations of dyspnea. The development of permanent atrial fibrillation often marks a turning point in the patient's course and is generally associated with acceleration of the rate at which symptoms progress.

Hemoptysis (Chap. 25) results from rupture of pulmonary-bronchial venous connections secondary to pulmonary venous hypertension. It occurs most frequently in patients who have elevated left atrial pressures without markedly elevated pulmonary vascular resistances and is almost never fatal. True hemoptysis must be distinguished from the bloody sputum that occurs with pulmonary edema, pulmonary infarction, and bronchitis, three conditions that occur with increased frequency in the presence of mitral stenosis.

When the pulmonary vascular resistance rises or when tricuspid stenosis or regurgitation develops, symptoms secondary to pulmonary congestion may diminish, and the episodes of acute pulmonary edema and hemoptysis become reduced in frequency and severity. Elevation of pulmonary vascular resistance further increases right ventricular systolic pressure, leading to right ventricular failure, fatigue, weakness, abdominal discomfort due to hepatic congestion, and edema.

Recurrent pulmonary emboli with infarction (Chap. 282) are an important cause of morbidity and mortality late in the course of mitral stenosis, occurring most frequently in patients with right ventricular failure. *Pulmonary infections,* i.e., bronchitis, bronchopneumonia, and lobar pneumonia, commonly complicate untreated mitral stenosis. *Infective endocarditis* (Chap. 259) is rare in pure mitral stenosis but is not uncommon in patients with combined stenosis and regurgitation. *Chest pain* occurs in about 10 percent of patients with severe mitral stenosis; it may be due to pulmonary hypertension, myocardial ischemia secondary to coronary embolization or coronary atherosclerosis; most often the cause cannot be discovered despite careful investigation.

In addition to the aforementioned changes in the pulmonary vascular bed, fibrous thickening of the walls of the alveoli and pulmonary capillaries occurs commonly in mitral stenosis. The vital capacity, total lung capacity, maximal breathing capacity, and oxygen uptake per unit of ventilation are reduced, and in patients with severe stenosis the latter fails to rise normally during exertion. The reduction of pulmonary compliance that occurs generally correlates directly with the severity of the dyspnea and inversely with the left atrial pressure, and these changes are intensified during exercise. In some patients airway resistance is abnormally increased. These changes contribute to an increase in the work of breathing and play an important role in the genesis of dyspnea. These changes in the lungs are due, in part, to increased transudation of fluid from the pulmonary capillaries into the interstitial and alveolar spaces as a consequence of the elevated pulmonary capillary pressure. The distribution of blood flow and ventilation may be uneven; as in other conditions in which left atrial pressure is elevated, pulmonary blood flow in the erect position is displaced from the basal to the superior segments of the lung (Chap. 271). The diffusing capacity may be reduced, particularly during exertion, as a result of structural changes in the diffusing surface and reduction of the pulmonary capillary blood volume. The thickening of the alveolar and capillary walls impedes the transudation of fluid into the alveoli and the development of pulmonary edema at times when the pulmonary capillary pressure exceeds the plasma oncotic pressure. The increased capacity of the pulmonary lymphatic system to drain excess fluid also retards the development of pulmonary edema.

Thrombi may form in the left atria, particularly in the enlarged atrial appendages of patients with mitral stenosis. When they embolize, they do so to the systemic vessels, most commonly the brain, kidneys, spleen, and extremities. This complication occurs much more frequently in patients with atrial fibrillation or unstable rhythms, in older patients, and in those with a reduced cardiac output, but it is also seen in patients with relatively mild as well as severe obstruction. Thus, systemic embolization may be the presenting complaint in otherwise asymptomatic patients with mild mitral stenosis. At operation, thrombi are not found more frequently in the left atria of patients with past history of embolization than in those without this complication, indicating that it is usually the freshly formed clots that dislodge. Patients who have had one or more systemic emboli have the predilection to have further embolic episodes more often than patients with stenosis of comparable severity without previous embolization. Rarely, a large pedunculated thrombus or a free-floating clot may suddenly obstruct the stenotic mitral orifice. Such "ball valve" thrombi produce syncope, angina, and changing auscultatory signs with alterations in position, findings that resemble those produced by a left atrial myxoma (Chap. 264).

PHYSICAL FINDINGS (See also Chap. 248) Peripheral and facial *cyanosis* may occur in patients with extremely severe mitral stenosis. In advanced cases there is a malar flush and the facies appear pinched and blue. The jugular venous pulse reveals prominent *a* waves due to vigorous right atrial systole in patients with sinus rhythm who have associated tricuspid stenosis or severe pulmonary hypertension. When atrial fibrillation is present, the jugular pulse reveals only a single expansion during systole (*c-v* wave). The systemic arterial pressure is usually normal or slightly low. A right ventricular tap is present along the left sternal border, signifying an enlarged right ventricle. The first heart sound may be palpable in patients with pliable valve leaflets. In patients with pulmonary hypertension, the impact of pulmonary valve closure can usually be felt in the second and third left intercostal spaces just left of the sternum; the left ventricle is not palpable in severe, pure mitral stenosis. A diastolic thrill may frequently be felt at the cardiac apex, particularly if the patient is turned into the left lateral recumbent position. The apex cardiogram (Chap. 250) reveals a slow rate of left ventricular filling during early diastole; when a rapid left ventricular filling phase is present, either mitral stenosis is very mild or there is associated mitral or aortic regurgitation.

The first heart sound is generally accentuated and snapping, and since the mitral valve does not close until the left ventricular pressure reaches the level of the elevated left atrial pressure, this sound is often slightly delayed on phonocardiography, particularly in patients with severe stenosis. In patients with pulmonary hypertension, the pulmonary component of the second heart sound is often accentuated, and the two components of the second heart sound are closely split. A pulmonary systolic ejection click is heard commonly in patients with severe pulmonary hypertension and extensive dilatation of the pulmonary artery. The opening snap of the mitral valve is most readily audible in expiration at, or just medial to, the cardiac apex but may also be easily heard along the left sternal edge or at the base of the heart. This sound generally follows the sound of aortic valve closure by 0.06 to 0.12 s, that is, it follows the pulmonic valve closure sound. Since the opening snap of the mitral valve occurs at the instant at which the left ventricular pressure falls below the left atrial pressure, the time interval between aortic closure and the opening snap varies inversely with the severity of the mitral stenosis. It tends to be short, that is, 0.06 to 0.07 s, in patients with severe obstruction and long, that is, 0.10 to 0.12 s, in patients with mild mitral stenosis. The intensities of the opening snap and the first heart sound correlate with the mobility of the anterior mitral leaflet.

The opening snap usually ushers in a low-pitched, rumbling, diastolic murmur, heard best at the apex with the patient in the left lateral recumbent position, and often accentuated by exercise carried out just before auscultation. In general, the duration of this murmur correlates with the severity of the stenosis. In patients with sinus rhythm the murmur often reappears or becomes reaccentuated during atrial systole, as atrial contraction reelevates the rate of blood flow across the narrowed orifice. Soft (grade I or II/VI) systolic murmurs are commonly heard at the apex or along the left sternal border in patients with pure mitral stenosis and do not necessarily signify the presence of mitral regurgitation. Hepatomegaly, ankle edema, ascites, and pleural effusion, particularly in the right pleural cavity, may occur in patients with mitral stenosis and right ventricular failure.

Associated lesions With severe pulmonary hypertension a loud pansystolic murmur produced by functional tricuspid regurgitation may be audible along the left sternal border. This murmur is often accentuated by inspiration, diminishes during forced expiration or during performance of the Valsalva maneuver, may disappear as compensation is restored, and must not be confused with the apical pansystolic murmur of mitral regurgitation, since management is quite different if mitral regurgitation is present.

The recognition of associated mitral regurgitation is of considerable clinical importance in patients with mitral stenosis. A presystolic murmur and an accentuated first heart sound speak against the presence of serious associated mitral regurgitation, but when the first heart sound and/or the opening snap are soft or absent in a patient with mitral valve disease, it is likely that significant mitral regurgitation and/or serious calcification of the deformed mitral valve leaflets are present. A third heart sound at the apex often signifies that the mitral regurgitation is serious; this sound is generally duller and lower pitched and follows the opening snap. Occasionally, in patients with pure mitral stenosis, physical signs may falsely suggest mitral regurgitation. Thus, in the presence of severe pulmonary hypertension and right ventricular failure, a third heart sound may originate from the right ventricle and be audible along the left sternal border. In such patients the enlarged right ventricle may rotate the heart in a clockwise direction and form the cardiac apex, giving the examiner the erroneous impression of left ventricular enlargement. Under these circumstances the rumbling diastolic murmur and the other auscultatory features of mitral stenosis become less prominent or may even disappear. When congestive heart failure is severe in a patient with calcific mitral stenosis, none of the auscultatory findings typical of mitral stenosis may be detectable, but they may reappear again as compensation is restored. Associated tricuspid stenosis also tends to obscure many of the physical signs of mitral stenosis.

The Graham Steell murmur of pulmonary regurgitation, a high-pitched, diastolic, decrescendo blowing murmur along the left sternal border, results from dilatation of the pulmonary valve ring and occurs in patients with mitral valve disease and severe pulmonary hypertension. This murmur may be indistinguishable from the more common murmur produced by mild aortic regurgitation except that it is rarely audible at the second right intercostal space, and may disappear following successful surgical treatment of the mitral stenosis.

Electrocardiogram In mitral stenosis and sinus rhythm the P wave usually suggests left atrial enlargement (Chap. 249). It may become tall and more peaked in lead II and upright in lead V_1 when severe pulmonary hypertension or tricuspid stenosis complicates mitral stenosis and right atrial enlargement occurs. When atrial fibrillation is present in patients with mitral valve disease, the base line usually shows coarser undulations than when this arrhythmia occurs as a consequence of coronary artery disease. The QRS complex may be normal, even in patients with critical mitral stenosis. However, with severe pulmonary hypertension, right axis deviation and right ventricular hypertrophy are usually found. When left ventricular hypertrophy is present in patients with mitral stenosis, it generally indicates that an additional lesion which places a burden on the left ventricle, such as mitral regurgitation, aortic valve disease, or hypertension, is present.

Echocardiogram (see also Chap. 250) The echocardiogram is the most sensitive and specific noninvasive method for diagnosing mitral stenosis. The M-mode tracing reveals that the anterior and posterior mitral leaflets do not separate widely in early diastole (i.e., less than 15 mm) and they maintain a fixed relation to each other throughout diastole. A reduction in the EF slope reflects failure of the anterior leaflet of the mitral valve to float back to midposition in middiastole. In the presence of a mobile valve and normal cardiac output, this slope is related to the severity of the obstruction. Calcification and thickening of the mitral valve are detected as multilayered echoes or a thickening of the echo pattern. Mitral orifice area is best determined with cross-sectional (two-dimensional) imaging systems. The left atrium is usually enlarged.

Roentgenographic features The earliest changes are straightening of the left border of the cardiac silhouette, prominence of the main pulmonary arteries, dilatation of the upper lobe pulmonary veins, and backward displacement of the esophagus by an enlarged left atrium. In patients with mild or moderate stenosis, the overall cardiac size is not grossly enlarged. In severe mitral stenosis, however, all chambers and vessels upstream to the narrowed valve are prominent, including the two atria, the pulmonary arteries and veins, right ventricle, and superior vena cava. Kerley B lines are fine, dense, opaque, horizontal lines which are most prominent in the lower and midlung fields and which result from distention of interlobular septa and lymphatics with edema when the resting mean left atrial pressure reaches approximately 20 mmHg. As the pulmonary arterial pressure rises, the smaller pulmonary arteries become attenuated, at first in the lower, then in the mid-, and finally in the upper lung fields. Deposits of hemosiderin occur in the lungs of patients who have had multiple hemoptyses; the hemosiderin-containing macrophages fill the air spaces, and if they become confluent result in a fine, diffuse nodulation most prominent in the lower lung fields. Ossified nodules are also more common in this region and are produced by true lamellar bone, which tends to develop in areas of chronic interstitial edema.

DIFFERENTIAL DIAGNOSIS Significant mitral regurgitation may be associated with a prominent diastolic murmur at the apex, but this murmur commences slightly later than in patients with stenosis, and there is often clear-cut evidence of left ventricular enlargement on physical examination, roentgenography, and electrocardiography. In addition, a pansystolic murmur of at least grade III/VI intensity as well as a third heart sound should arouse the suspicion of significant associated regurgitation. Similarly, the apical middiastolic murmur associated with aortic regurgitation (Austin Flint murmur) may be mistaken for mitral stenosis. However, in a patient with aortic regurgitation the absence of an opening snap or of presystolic accentuation if sinus rhythm is present points to the absence of mitral stenosis. Tricuspid stenosis, a valvular lesion that occurs very rarely in the absence of mitral stenosis, may mask many of the clinical features of mitral stenosis. The echocardiogram is particularly useful in detecting mitral stenosis in patients who have or are suspected of having other valve lesions.

Exertional dyspnea and recurrent pulmonary infections may be falsely ascribed to pulmonary emphysema in patients with both *chronic lung disease* and mitral stenosis. Careful auscultation, however, will generally reveal the characteristic opening snap and rumbling diastolic murmur. Similarly, the hemoptysis that occurs in many otherwise asymptomatic patients with mitral stenosis may be improperly attributed to bronchiectasis or tuberculosis. Actually, the latter condition is uncommon in patients with significant mitral obstruction.

Primary pulmonary hypertension (Chap. 281) results in a number of the clinical and laboratory features observed in mitral stenosis. It occurs most frequently in young women; however, the opening snap and diastolic rumbling murmur are absent, there is no left atrial enlargement, and the pulmonary artery wedge and left atrial pressures are *normal.*

Atrial septal defect (Chap. 256) may also be mistaken for mitral stenosis; in both conditions there is often clinical, electrocardiographic, and roentgenographic evidence of right ventricular enlargement and accentuation of the pulmonary vascularity. The widely split second heart sound of atrial septal defect may be confused with the mitral opening snap, and the diastolic flow murmur across the tricuspid valve mistaken for the mitral diastolic murmur. However, the absence of left atrial enlargement on the roentgenogram, electrocardiogram, or echocardiogram, the absence of Kerley B lines, and demonstration of fixed splitting of the second heart sound all favor atrial septal defect over mitral stenosis.

Cor triatriatum is an unusual congenital malformation that consists of a fibrous ring within the left atrium (Chap. 256). It results in elevation of the pulmonary venous, capillary, and arterial pressures. This lesion can be recognized most readily by means of left atrial angiography.

A *left atrial myxoma* (Chap. 264) may obstruct left atrial emptying, resulting in dyspnea, a diastolic murmur, and hemodynamic changes that resemble those of mitral stenosis. However, patients with left atrial myxoma often demonstrate findings suggestive of a systemic disease, with weight loss, fever, anemia, systemic emboli and elevated erythrocyte sedimentation rate, and serum gamma-globulin concentration. Usually an opening snap is not audible, there is no clinical evidence of associated aortic valve disease, and the auscultatory findings frequently change with body position. The diagnosis can be established by demonstrating a characteristic echo-producing mass in the left atrium by echocardiography and a lobulated filling defect in the left atrium by angiocardiography.

Specialized techniques Left-side heart catheterization (Chap. 251) is extremely helpful in deciding whether valvulotomy is necessary in patients in whom it is difficult to estimate the severity of obstruction by clinical means alone. When combined with aortography and left ventricular angiocardiography, this procedure serves as the ultimate method for detecting and estimating associated mitral regurgitation and coexisting lesions such as aortic stenosis and regurgitation as well as left ventricular dysfunction. Left atrial thrombi and tumors may be detected or excluded by angiocardiography, particularly when the contrast medium is injected directly into the left atrium. These "invasive" methods are also helpful in the detection of conditions that impair left ventricular function and would thereby contraindicate or reduce the effectiveness of mitral valvulotomy. Left-side heart catheterization and angiography are indicated in most patients who have undergone previous mitral valve operations and who have redeveloped serious symptoms; in such patients clinical assessment may be particularly difficult, and the hemodynamic studies allow determination of the severity of the lesion, intelligent planning of the operative procedure when it is indicated, and a more accurate estimate of the risk.

MANAGEMENT In the asymptomatic adolescent with mitral valve disease, penicillin prophylaxis of beta-hemolytic streptococcal infections (Chap. 257), prophylaxis for infective endocarditis (Chap. 259), and vocational counseling are particularly important; physically strenuous occupations should be avoided so that premature retirement will not be necessary should symptoms develop later. In symptomatic patients some improvement usually occurs with restriction of sodium intake and maintenance doses of oral diuretics. Digitalis glycosides do not alter the hemodynamics and usually do not benefit patients with pure stenosis and sinus rhythm, but they are necessary for slowing the ventricular rate of patients with atrial fibrillation and for reducing the manifestations of right-sided heart failure in the advanced stages of the disease. Small doses of propranolol (10 to 20 mg qid) may be added when cardiac glycosides fail to control ventricular rate in patients with atrial fibrillation or flutter in the absence of ventricular failure. Particular attention should be directed to detecting and treating any accompanying anemia and infections. Hemoptysis is treated by measures designed to diminish pulmonary venous pressure, including bed rest, the sitting position, salt restriction, and diuresis. The administration of anticoagulants for at least 1 year is indicated in patients with mitral stenosis who have suffered systemic and/or pulmonary embolization and those with intermittent atrial fibrillation.

If atrial fibrillation is of relatively recent origin in a patient whose mitral stenosis is not severe enough to warrant surgical treatment, reversion to sinus rhythm, by means of either electrical countershock or quinidine, is indicated. Usually this should be undertaken following 4 weeks of anticoagulant treatment. Conversion to sinus rhythm is rarely helpful in patients with severe mitral stenosis, particularly those in whom the left atrium is especially enlarged or in whom atrial fibrillation has been present for more than 1 year, since it is frequently impossible to maintain sinus rhythm, and reversion to atrial fibrillation is common.

Surgical treatment Unless there is a specific contraindication, operative treatment is indicated in the symptomatic patient with pure mitral stenosis whose effective orifice is less than approximately 1.0 cm^2 per square meter of body surface area. Operation not only usually results in striking symptomatic and hemodynamic improvement but also clearly prolongs survival. In uncomplicated cases, the surgical mortality rate should be less than 2 percent, and comparisons of the natural history of patients with serious symptoms treated by valvulotomy with those who did not receive the benefits of surgical therapy have shown considerable improvement following operation. However, there is no evidence that surgical treatment improves the prognosis of patients with slight or no functional impairment. Therefore, unless recurrent systemic embolization has occurred, valvulotomy is *not* recommended for patients who are entirely asymptomatic, regardless of hemodynamic findings. When there is little symptomatic improvement following valvulotomy, it is likely that the procedure was ineffective, that it induced mitral regurgitation, or that associated valvular or myocardial disease was present. The recurrence of symptoms several years after what appeared to be a satisfactory initial result is usually due to an inadequate valvulotomy, but progression of other valvular lesions, the development of myocardial disease, restenosis of the mitral valve, or some combination of these conditions may also be responsible. In the *pregnant patient* with mitral stenosis operative treatment should be carried out if pulmonary congestion occurs despite intensive medical treatment.

A closed operation (with "pump standby") is usually preferable for patients with pure mitral stenosis who have not been operated upon previously, in whom no valvular or perivalvular calcification is detected on fluoroscopic and/or echocardiographic examination, and in whom there is no suspicion of left atrial thrombosis. Transventricular instrumental dilatation of the mitral valve usually results in more effective relief of stenosis than transatrial finger fracture, and the importance of loosening any existing subvalvular fusion of papillary muscles and chordae tendineae must be appreciated since closed valvulotomy is occasionally ineffective or may result in severe regurgitation. The ready availability of an extracorporeal system is prudent. Operative treatment of patients with extremely severe obstruction, significant associated mitral regurgitation, valvular calcification, left atrial thrombi, or a mitral valve distorted by previous operative manipulation is usually carried out under direct vision, with open-heart techniques. The valve may have to be replaced with a prosthesis or a heterograft in those patients who were severely symptomatic preoperatively and in whom the surgeon does not find it possible to improve valve function significantly. Since the operative mortality rate of replacement of the mitral valve is still approximately 5 to 8 percent and since there is some uncertainty concerning the long-term fate of valve replacements, patients in whom preoperative evaluation suggests the possibility that replacement may be required should be operated on only if they are symptomatic on ordinary activity despite optimal medical therapy.

The results of valve replacement are dependent primarily on (1) the patient's myocardial function and level of pulmonary artery pressure at the time of operation, (2) the technical abilities of the operative team and the quality of the postoperative care, and (3) the durability and long-term functioning of the valve used for replacement. Increased operative mortality is associated with the degree of preoperative functional disability and pulmonary hypertension. Patients who have undergone valve replacement with a prosthesis must be maintained permanently on anticoagulants postoperatively. Late complications of replacement of any valve, which fortunately are declining in incidence, include paravalvular leakage, thromboemboli, bleeding due to anticoagulants, mechanical dysfunction of the prosthesis, and infective endocarditis. The primary advantage of tissue valves over prosthetics is the elimination of thromboembolic complications and the necessity for anticoagulants. However, infective endocarditis and late deterioration of the graft in a few instances have been associated with their use.

The overall 5-year survival following mitral valve replacement approximates 70 percent. Long-term prognosis is worse in subgroups of older patients and those with marked disability and striking depression of the cardiac index preoperatively.

MITRAL REGURGITATION

PATHOPHYSIOLOGY The regurgitant mitral orifice may be considered to be in parallel with the aortic orifice, and therefore the resistance to left ventricular emptying is reduced in patients with mitral regurgitation. As a consequence, the left ventricle decompresses itself into the left atrium early during ejection, and with the reduction in left ventricular size there is a rapid decline in left ventricular tension, allowing a greater proportion of the contractile activity of the left ventricle to be expended in shortening. The initial compensation to mitral regurgitation consists of more complete systolic emptying of the left ventricle. However, a progressive increase in left ventricular end-diastolic volume occurs as the severity of the regurgitation increases and the function of the left ventricle deteriorates. The atrial contraction wave in the left atrial pressure pulse (*a* wave) is usually not as prominent as it is in mitral stenosis, but the *v* wave is often much taller, since it is inscribed during ventricular systole, when the left atrium fills from the pulmonary veins as well as from the left ventricle. During early diastole, as the distended left atrium suddenly empties, there is a particularly rapid *y* descent as long as there is associated mitral stenosis. The left ventricular end-diastolic pressure may be slightly elevated. However, in chronic mitral regurgitation, there is often an increase in left ventricular compliance, so that ventricular volume may be greatly increased with little elevation in end-diastolic pressure. The effective cardiac output usually declines in seriously symptomatic patients. Although a left atrioventricular pressure gradient persisting throughout diastole signifies the presence of significant associated mitral stenosis, a brief, early diastolic gradient may occur in patients with pure regurgitation as a result of the torrential flow of blood across a normal-sized mitral orifice.

The prompt appearance of contrast material in the left atrium following its injection into the left ventricle signifies the presence and can be useful in the diagnosis of mitral regurgitation. The regurgitant volume can be measured by determining the difference between the total left ventricular stroke estimated angiocardiographically, while simultaneously measuring the effective forward stroke volume by the Fick method. The results of such studies suggest that the regurgitant volume may be of the same magnitude as the effective forward stroke volume or may even exceed it in patients with severe regurgitation. Qualitative, but clinically useful, estimates of the severity of regurgitation may be made by observation on cineangiograms of the degree of left atrial opacification following the injection of contrast material into the left ventricle.

Patients with severe mitral regurgitation may be divided into several subgroups, depending on the compliance, i.e., the pressure-volume relationship, of the left atrium and pulmonary venous bed, which appears to be capable of affecting the clinical and hemodynamic picture. Among patients with severe mitral regurgitation, three major groups have been identified:

1. *Normal or reduced compliance.* In this group there is little enlargement of the left atrium, but marked elevation of the mean left atrial pressure, particularly of the *v* wave. In these patients severe mitral regurgitation has usually developed suddenly, as when it follows rupture of chordae tendineae, infarction of one of the heads of a papillary muscle, or tear of a mitral leaflet. Pulmonary vascular resistance is frequently markedly elevated, presumably as a consequence of the left atrial hypertension, and therefore both right-sided heart failure and pulmonary edema are common clinical manifestations; sinus rhythm is usually present.
2. *Marked increase in compliance.* At the opposite end of the spectrum from group 1 are those patients with severe chronic mitral regurgitation, massive enlargement of the left atrium, and normal left atrial pressure. The pulmonary artery pressure and pulmonary vascular resistance are normal or only slightly elevated at rest. Clinically, these patients are usually disabled with fatigue and exhaustion, because of a low cardiac output, while symptoms resulting from pulmonary congestion are less prominent. The mitral regurgitation is long-standing, and atrial fibrillation is almost invariably present. The association of a normal left atrial pressure with a markedly enlarged, thin-walled left atrium indicates that this chamber is far more compliant than normal. Thus, long-standing mitral regurgitation may, in some instances, alter the physical properties of the left atrial wall and thereby displace the atrial pressure-volume curve, allowing a normal pressure to exist in a greatly enlarged left atrium.
3. *Moderate increase in compliance.* By far the most common

group are patients whose clinical and hemodynamic features are between those in the other two groups with variable degrees of enlargement of the left atrium and with significant elevation of the left atrial pressure.

ETIOLOGY In about half the patients mitral regurgitation is caused by chronic *rheumatic heart disease,* but in contrast to mitral stenosis, pure or predominantly rheumatic mitral regurgitation occurs more frequently in males. The rheumatic process produces rigidity, deformity, and retraction of the valve cusps, and commissural fusion, as well as shortening, contraction, and fusion of the chordae tendineae. Mitral regurgitation may also occur as a congenital anomaly (Chap. 256), most commonly as (1) a defect of the endocardial cushions or in association with (2) corrected transposition, (3) endocardial fibroelastosis, and (4) the "parachute" mitral valve deformity. It may follow rupture or fibrosis of a papillary muscle or of one of its heads in ischemic heart disease. Myocardial infarction, fibrosis, or a ventricular aneurysm, at the base of the papillary muscle but not necessarily involving it, may lead to abnormal anchoring of the latter, also resulting in mitral regurgitation. The latter may also occur during transient periods of ischemia involving a papillary muscle or adjacent myocardium and may accompany bouts of angina pectoris. Mitral regurgitation may occur with marked left ventricular dilatation of any cause in which dilatation of the mitral annulus and lateral displacement of the papillary muscles interfere with coaptation of the valve leaflets. In hypertrophic cardiomyopathy the anterior leaflet of the mitral valve is displaced anteriorly during systole, leading to regurgitation (Chap. 263). Systemic lupus erythematosus, rheumatoid arthritis, and ankylosing spondylitis are less common causes. Massive calcification of the mitral annulus of unknown cause, which occurs most commonly in elderly women, can also be responsible for significant mitral regurgitation. Mitral regurgitation may occur acutely in patients with infective endocarditis involving the valve or chordae tendineae, as a consequence of trauma or as a complication of cardiac surgery.

Abnormal elongation of chordae tendineae and/or redundant posterior cusps of the mitral valve with prolapse of the cusps into the left atrium, the so-called floppy valve, leading to the syndrome of midsystolic click and midsystolic murmur, also referred to as the prolapsing mitral valve leaflet syndrome (see below), is another important cause of mitral regurgitation.

Regardless of etiology, significant mitral regurgitation tends to be gradually progressive since enlargement of the left atrium places tension on the posterior mitral leaflet, pulling it away from the mitral orifice, thereby aggravating the valvular dysfunction. Similarly, the dilatation of the left ventricle increases the regurgitation, which in turn further enlarges the left atrium and ventricle, resulting in a vicious cycle; hence the aphorism, "mitral regurgitation begets mitral regurgitation."

SYMPTOMS Only a fraction of patients with chronic mitral regurgitation ever experience any reduction of cardiac reserve, but in those who do become symptomatic, fatigue, exertional dyspnea and orthopnea may be prominent complaints. Symptoms resulting from pulmonary congestion tend to be less episodic in nature in patients with chronic severe mitral regurgitation than mitral stenosis, since fluctuations of the mean pulmonary capillary pressure are less marked. Indeed, acute paroxysmal pulmonary edema is quite rare in patients with chronic mitral regurgitation. Similarly, hemoptysis and systemic embolism occur far less frequently in mitral regurgitation than in stenosis. On the other hand, fatigability, weakness, exhaustion, weight loss, and even cachexia are more prominent and occur most frequently in patients with marked reduction of cardiac output. Right-sided heart failure, with painful hepatic congestion, ankle edema, distended neck veins, ascites, and tricuspid regurgitation, is observed commonly in patients with mitral regurgitation who have associated pulmonary vascular disease. In patients with *acute* severe mitral regurgitation, left ventricular failure with acute pulmonary edema and/or cardiovascular collapse is common. In contrast to patients with mitral stenosis, pure regurgitation rarely leads to hemoptysis, systemic emboli, or chest pain.

PHYSICAL FINDINGS The arterial pressure is usually normal, and the arterial pulse is often characterized by a sharp upstroke. The jugular venous pulse shows abnormally prominent *a* waves in patients with sinus rhythm and marked pulmonary hypertension. A systolic thrill is usually palpable at the cardiac apex, the left ventricle is hyperdynamic with a brisk systolic impulse and a palpable rapid-filling wave, and the apex beat is often displaced laterally. When the left atrium is markedly enlarged, it may extend anteriorly, and its expansion may be palpable along the sternal border late during ventricular systole. The combination of the retraction of the left ventricle and expansion of the left atrium during systole may produce a characteristic rocking motion of the chest with each cardiac cycle. A right ventricular tap and the shock of pulmonary valve closure may be palpable in patients with marked pulmonary hypertension.

The first heart sound is generally absent, soft, or buried in the systolic murmur, and an accentuated mitral closure sound is useful in excluding severe regurgitation. A pulmonary ejection sound is often audible in patients with associated pulmonary hypertension. Splitting of the second heart sound is usually normal, but in patients with severe regurgitation, aortic valve closure may occur early, resulting in wide splitting of the second heart sound. An opening snap indicates associated mitral stenosis but does not exclude predominant regurgitation. A low-pitched third heart sound, occurring 0.12 to 0.17 s after the aortic valve closure sound, at the completion of the rapid-filling phase of the mitral valve, is believed to be caused by the sudden tensing of the papillary muscles, chordae tendineae, and valve leaflets and is an important auscultatory feature of severe mitral regurgitation. The absence of a third heart sound indicates that if mitral regurgitation exists, it may not be severe. The third heart sound may be followed, often after a brief interval, by a short, rumbling, diastolic murmur, even in the absence of mitral stenosis. A fourth heart sound is heard characteristically in patients with acute severe regurgitation in sinus rhythm. A presystolic murmur is not ordinarily heard in patients with pure regurgitation and sinus rhythm but is present when there is significant associated mitral stenosis.

A systolic murmur, grade III/VI in intensity or louder, is the most characteristic auscultatory finding in patients with severe mitral regurgitation. It is usually holosystolic (Chap. 248), but it may be decrescendo because the tall *v* wave in the left atrial pressure pulse results in a reduced late systolic left ventricular-atrial pressure gradient in patients with acute severe mitral regurgitation. Although the systolic murmur usually radiates into the axilla, in a minority of patients, particularly those with ruptured chordae tendineae or primary involvement of the posterior mitral leaflet, the regurgitant jet strikes the left atrial wall adjacent to the aortic root, and the systolic murmur is referred to the base of the heart and therefore may be confused with the murmur of aortic stenosis. In patients with ruptured chordae tendineae the systolic murmur may have a cooing or "sea gull" quality.

Electrocardiogram There is electrocardiographic evidence of left atrial enlargement in patients with sinus rhythm, but right atrial hypertrophy may be present when pulmonary hypertension is extreme. Prolonged, severe mitral regurgitation with left atrial enlargement is generally associated with atrial fibrillation. In many patients there is no clear-cut electrocardiographic evidence of enlargement of either ventricle. In severe regurgitation the signs of left ventricular hypertrophy are often present, although in patients with pulmonary hypertension combined ventricular hypertrophy or rarely pure right ventricular hypertrophy may be present.

Echocardiogram The left atrium is usually enlarged and/or exhibits increased pulsations. The left ventricle is hyperdynamic. With ruptured chordae tendineae or a flail leaflet there is coarse erratic motion of the involved leaflets. The echocardiogram in the syndrome of midsystolic click and midsystolic murmur is described below.

Roentgenographic features The left atrium and left ventricle are the dominant chambers; the latter may be enlarged to aneurysmal proportions and form the right border of the cardiac silhouette. Though both mitral stenosis and regurgitation tend to increase left atrial size, extreme left atrial enlargement usually signifies that regurgitation is the predominant lesion and has existed for years. On fluoroscopy the left ventricle is hyperdynamic and the left atrium exhibits vigorous systolic expansions. Marked calcification of the mitral leaflets occurs commonly in patients with long-standing combined severe regurgitation and stenosis but is uncommon in patients with pure regurgitation. Cineangiography commonly reveals late systolic prolapse of a leaflet (usually the posterior) of the mitral valve into the left atrium in patients with the syndrome of mid-late systolic click and late systolic murmur (see below).

TREATMENT The nonsurgical management of mitral regurgitation is directed toward restricting those physical activities which regularly produce extreme fatigue and dyspnea, reducing sodium intake, and enhancing sodium excretion with the appropriate use of diuretics (Chap. 253). Digitalis glycosides (Chap. 255) augment the output of the overburdened left ventricle even in the presence of sinus rhythm. The same considerations as in patients with mitral stenosis apply to the reversion of atrial fibrillation to sinus rhythm. In the late stages anticoagulants and leg binders are used to diminish the likelihood of venous thrombi and pulmonary emboli. Effective surgical treatment of rheumatic mitral regurgitation generally requires valvular replacement with a suitable prosthesis or tissue valve. Though most patients who survive operation appear to be greatly improved, some degree of myocardial dysfunction may persist.

When surgical treatment is contemplated, right- or left-side heart catheterization and selective left ventricular angiocardiography are indicated. These studies are helpful in confirming the presence of severe regurgitation and aid in the identification of patients with primary myocardial disease and relatively mild, functional mitral regurgitation, who usually do not benefit from operation. Hemodynamic studies are also helpful in detecting and assessing the severity of any associated valve lesions, which may have to be dealt with at the time of operation or which might limit the patient's ultimate improvement if they are left untreated.

In the selection of patients for surgical treatment, the chronic, often slowly progressive nature of the disease must be balanced against the immediate risks and long-term uncertainties attendant upon valve replacement. Patients with mitral regurgitation who are asymptomatic or who are limited only during strenuous exertion are not considered to be ideal candidates for surgical treatment, since they may live for many years with little deterioration. However, surgical treatment should be considered seriously in patients whose limitations do not allow them to work full time or carry out normal household activities despite optimal medical management. The risks of valve replacement rise sharply and the recovery of impaired left ventricular function is incomplete when the patient has developed congestive heart failure which is refractory to medical therapy. In addition, long-term survival of these patients is reduced (approximately 60 percent in 5 years). However, conservative management has little to offer these patients, so that operative treatment may be indicated even at these advanced stages of the disease, and occasionally the clinical and hemodynamic improvement following surgical treatment is dramatic. It is likely that the immediate results of surgical treatment will continue to improve considerably and will lead to recommendations of operative treatment for selected patients with mitral regurgitation before they become severely disabled.

SYSTOLIC CLICK-MURMUR SYNDROME This is also variously termed the *prolapsing mitral valve leaflet syndrome, Barlow's syndrome, floppy-valve syndrome,* and *billowing mitral leaflet syndrome,* a common, but highly variable, clinical syndrome resulting from diverse pathogenic mechanisms of the mitral valve apparatus. Among these are excessive or redundant mitral leaflet tissue, which is commonly involved with myxomatous degeneration and greatly increased concentration of acid mucopolysaccharide. This is a frequent finding in patients who have the typical features of Marfan's syndrome or cystic medial necrosis (Chap. 268), although in most patients myxomatous degeneration is confined to the mitral valve leaflets without other clinical or pathological manifestations of disease; the posterior leaflet is usually more affected than the anterior, and the mitral valve annulus is often greatly enlarged. In other patients, elongated redundant chordae tendineae as well as short attenuated chordae have been identified. In still others, abnormalities of shortening and/or orientation of the papillary muscles, as well as localized or diffuse abnormalities of left ventricular contraction, appear to be responsible. There are probably several subsets of these patients, who differ in regard to the etiology and hemodynamic and clinical sequelae of abnormal mitral valve function. In the majority of patients, the etiology is unknown, but the condition may occur in acute rheumatic fever, chronic rheumatic heart disease, following mitral valvulotomy, ischemic heart disease, and cardiomyopathies, in 20 percent of patients with ostium secundum and atrial septal defect. The resulting syndrome has protean manifestations.

This syndrome is a usually benign abnormality that may progress to a stage involving significant regurgitation and ventricular dilatation in some individuals. In these, prolapse of the valve leads to excessive stress on the papillary muscles, which in turn leads to dysfunction and ischemia of the papillary muscle and subjacent ventricular myocardium. The characteristic ventriculographic deformity (see below), the electrocardiogram showing changes of ischemia, and many of the recurrent arrhythmias appear to result from regional ventricular dysfunction related to abnormalities of the papillary muscles; these abnormalities usually are not manifestations of a diffuse cardiomyopathy, of some general disorder of the coronary circulation, or of myocardial metabolism.

The syndrome is more common in females and occurs in a wide age range but most commonly between the ages of 14 and 30. Echocardiographic surveys have suggested that it may occur in as many as 10 percent of this group. There is an increased familial incidence suggesting an autosomal dominant form of inheritance. In many patients the echocardiographic abnormality is not accompanied by any other clinical manifestation of cardiac disease, and the significance of this finding is uncertain.

Most of the patients are asymptomatic and remain so for

their entire lives, but arrhythmias, most commonly ventricular premature contractions and paroxysmal supraventricular and ventricular tachycardia, have been reported. In patients with supraventricular tachycardia a left-sided atrioventricular bypass tract can often be discerned. Patients with arrhythmias complain of palpitations, light-headedness, and syncope. Sudden death is a very rare complication. Many patients have chest pain which is difficult to evaluate. It is often substernal, prolonged, and poorly related to exertion and rarely resembles typical angina pectoris.

The most common finding on *physical examination* is the mid- or late systolic click, which occurs 0.14 s or more after the first heart sound, and is thought to be generated by the sudden tensing of slack, elongated chordae tendineae or by the prolapsing mitral leaflet when it reaches its maximum posterior excursion; systolic clicks may be multiple and are often followed by a high-pitched late systolic crescendo-decrescendo murmur, occasionally "whooping" or "honking," heard best at the apex with the patient in the left lateral decubitus position. The click and murmur occur earlier with maneuvers such as standing, the Valsalva maneuver, or inhalation of amyl nitrite, all of which decrease left ventricular volume, exaggerating the propensity of mitral leaflet prolapse. Conversely, squatting or isometric exercise, which increases left ventricular end-diastolic volume, diminishes the propensity for the mitral valve leaflets to prolapse, and the click-murmur complex is delayed and may even disappear. Some patients have a midsystolic click without the murmur; others have the murmur without a click. Many patients with this syndrome but without overt features of Marfan's syndrome have certain bony abnormalities such as a high arched palate and deformities of the chest and thoracic spine.

The *electrocardiogram* most commonly shows biphasic or inverted T waves in leads II, III, and aVF. The *echocardiogram* characteristically shows an abrupt posterior displacement of the posterior or sometimes of both mitral valve leaflets in mid- to late systole immediately after the click and during the systolic murmur. *Angiocardiography* generally reveals prolapse of the posterior and sometimes of both mitral valve leaflets and, rarely, severe mitral regurgitation. Many patients have bulging of the posteroinferior wall of the left ventricle into the left ventricular cavity during systole and/or hypokinesis of the anterolateral left ventricular wall.

The *treatment* of patients with mitral valve prolapse is directed toward reassurance of the asymptomatic patient, the prevention of infective endocarditis, and the relief of the atypical chest pain; propranolol has been found to be helpful in this regard, although its use is on an empiric basis. Antiarrhythmic agents are administered if frequent ventricular premature contractions are present at rest or during exercise, and propranolol has been advocated in patients with arrhythmias and prolongation of the QT interval. If mitral regurgitation is severe, mitral valve replacement is indicated.

AORTIC STENOSIS

This lesion occurs in about one-fourth of all patients with chronic valvular heart disease; approximately 80 percent of adult patients with symptomatic valvular aortic stenosis are male.

PATHOPHYSIOLOGY The primary hemodynamic abnormality is obstruction to left ventricular outflow which leads to a pressure gradient between the left ventricle and aorta during systole. When severe obstruction is suddenly produced experimentally, the left ventricle responds by dilatation and reduction of stroke volume. However, in patients the obstruction may be present at birth or it increases gradually over the course of many years, and left ventricular output is maintained by the presence of left ventricular hypertrophy, which serves as a useful compensatory mechanism since it reduces toward normal the systolic stress developed by each segment of myocardium. A large transaortic valvular pressure gradient may exist for many years without a reduction of cardiac output, left ventricular dilatation, or the development of any symptoms. As aortic stenosis progresses in severity, the left ventricular systolic pressure continues to rise, but rarely exceeds 300 mmHg.

A peak systolic pressure gradient exceeding 50 mmHg in the face of a normal cardiac output or an effective aortic orifice less than 0.5 cm^2 per square meter of body surface area, i.e., less than approximately one-third of the normal orifice, is generally considered to represent critical obstruction to left ventricular outflow. The left ventricular pressure pulse exhibits a rounded summit as the contraction of this chamber becomes progressively more isometric, and pulsus alternans in the left ventricle may occur in patients with severe stenosis. The elevated left ventricular end-diastolic pressure observed in many patients with severe aortic stenosis does not necessarily signify the presence of left ventricular failure or dilatation, but may instead reflect diminished compliance of the hypertrophied left ventricular wall.

A large *a* wave in the left atrial pressure pulse is usually present with severe stenosis, because of enhanced atrial contraction and diminished ventricular compliance. Atrial contraction tends to raise left ventricular end-diastolic pressure without producing a similar elevation of mean left atrial pressure. This "booster pump" function of the left atrium prevents the pulmonary venous and capillary pressures from rising to levels which would produce pulmonary congestion, while at the same time maintaining left ventricular end-diastolic pressure at the elevated level necessary for effective left ventricular contraction. Loss of an appropriately timed, vigorous atrial contraction, as occurs in atrial fibrillation or atrioventricular dissociation, may result in a rapid aggravation of symptoms, even when the ventricular rate is not particularly rapid.

Although the cardiac output at rest is within normal limits in the majority of patients with severe aortic stenosis, it may fail to rise normally during exercise. Late in the disease the cardiac output and left ventricular–aortic pressure gradient decline, and the mean left atrial, pulmonary artery wedge, pulmonary arterial, and right ventricular pressures become elevated.

The hypertrophied left ventricular muscle mass elevates myocardial oxygen requirements. In addition, even in the absence of obstructive coronary artery disease, there may be interference with coronary blood flow, because the pressure compressing the coronary arteries exceeds the coronary perfusion pressure. Metabolic evidence of myocardial ischemia, i.e., lactate production, can be demonstrated in patients with aortic stenosis both in the presence and in the absence of coronary arterial narrowing, when myocardial oxygen needs are stimulated by isoproterenol.

A significant fraction of patients with rheumatic aortic stenosis has associated mitral valve disease. Aortic stenosis intensifies the severity of mitral regurgitation by increasing the pressure driving blood from the left ventricle to the left atrium. The dilatation of the left ventricle which occurs late in the course in some patients with aortic stenosis further raises the mitral regurgitant flow.

Etiology Aortic stenosis may be congenital in origin, secondary to rheumatic inflammation of the aortic valve, or due to calcification of the aortic cusps of unknown cause. The *congenitally affected valve* may already be stenotic at birth and may gradually become calcified during the first three decades of life, becoming progressively more stenotic. In others, the valve may also be congenitally bicuspid without serious narrowing of the aortic orifice during childhood; its abnormal architecture makes its leaflets susceptible to otherwise ordinary hemodynamic stresses, which ultimately lead to valvular calcification, increased rigidity, and narrowing of the aortic orifice.

Rheumatic endocarditis of the aortic leaflets produces commissural fusion, resulting, sometimes, in a bicuspid valve. This, in turn, also makes the leaflets more susceptible to trauma, and ultimately leads to calcification and further narrowing. By the time the obstruction to left ventricular outflow causes serious clinical disability, the valve is usually a rigid calcified mass, and careful examination may make it difficult or even impossible to determine whether the underlying process was rheumatic or congenital. Rheumatic aortic stenosis is almost always associated with rheumatic involvement of the mitral valve. A rheumatic etiology is also favored by a history of active rheumatic fever and by associated severe aortic regurgitation. *Idiopathic calcific aortic stenosis* occurs most often in the elderly and is occasionally associated with fibrosis and fusion of the valve cusps; the pathological process is considered to be a degenerative one—a "wear-and-tear" phenomenon. It may produce many of the characteristic physical signs of aortic stenosis. The valvular obstruction is usually relatively mild and of little if any hemodynamic significance; it may, however, on occasion, produce severe obstruction.

OTHER FORMS OF OBSTRUCTION TO LEFT VENTRICULAR OUTFLOW Besides valvular aortic stenosis, three other lesions may be responsible for obstruction to left ventricular outflow.

1 *Hypertrophic cardiomyopathy.* This is the most important of these conditions numerically. It is characterized by marked hypertrophy of the left ventricle, involving in particular the interventricular septum of the left ventricular outflow tract, as described in Chap. 263.
2 *Discrete congenital subvalvular aortic stenosis.* This condition is produced by either a membranous diaphragm or a fibrous ridge just below the aortic valve (Chap. 256).
3 *Supravalvular aortic stenosis.* This uncommon congenital anomaly is produced by narrowing of the ascending aorta or by a fibrous diaphragm with a small opening just above the aortic valve (Chap. 256).

SYMPTOMS Aortic stenosis is rarely of hemodynamic or clinical importance until the valve orifice has narrowed to approximately one-third of normal. In contrast to mitral stenosis, which results in symptoms as soon as the obstruction becomes severe because the chamber just proximal to the narrowed valve, i.e., the left atrium, provides little compensation, severe aortic stenosis may exist for many years without producing any clinical disability because of the ability of the hypertrophied left ventricle to generate the elevated intraventricular pressures and the presence of a competent mitral valve behind the left ventricle.

Most patients with pure or predominant aortic stenosis have gradually increasing obstruction for years but do not become symptomatic until the fourth or fifth decade. Exertional dyspnea, angina pectoris, and syncope are the three cardinal symptoms. Often there is a history of insidious and subtle progression of fatigue and dyspnea associated with gradual curtailment of activities. Dyspnea results primarily from elevation of the pulmonary capillary pressures, which in turn is caused by elevations of left atrial and left ventricular end-diastolic pressures. Angina pectoris usually develops somewhat later and reflects an imbalance between the augmented myocardial oxygen requirements and oxygen availability; the former results from the increased myocardial mass and intraventricular pressure, while the latter may result from accompanying coronary artery disease which is not uncommon in patients with aortic stenosis, as well as compression of the coronary vessels by the hypertrophied myocardium. Therefore, angina may occur in severe aortic stenosis without organic coronary obstruction, but the absence of angina usually signifies that severe coronary obstructive disease is unlikely. Exertional syncope may result from a decline in arterial pressure caused by vasodilatation in the exercising muscles and inadequate vasoconstriction in nonexercising muscles in the face of a fixed cardiac output, or from a sudden fall in cardiac output produced by an arrhythmia (Chap. 12). If prolonged, the syncopal episode may be accompanied by convulsions and loss of sphincteric control.

Since the cardiac output is usually well maintained at rest until the late stage of the disease, marked fatigability, weakness, peripheral cyanosis, and other clinical manifestations of a low cardiac output are usually not prominent until this stage is reached. Orthopnea, paroxysmal nocturnal dyspnea, and pulmonary edema, i.e., symptoms of left ventricular failure, also occur only in the advanced stages of the disease. Severe pulmonary hypertension leading to right ventricular failure and systemic venous hypertension, hepatomegaly, atrial fibrillation, and tricuspid regurgitation are usually preterminal findings.

When aortic stenosis and mitral stenosis coexist, the latter lesion masks many of the clinical findings of aortic stenosis. The reduction of cardiac output induced by mitral stenosis lowers the pressure gradient across the aortic valve, diminishes the frequency of anginal episodes, and retards the development of aortic calcification and severe left ventricular hypertrophy. On the other hand, symptoms considered more characteristic of mitral stenosis, such as pulmonary congestion and hemoptysis, occur more frequently in patients with combined stenotic lesions than in those with isolated aortic stenosis. Physical, electrocardiographic, radiological, and echocardiographic examinations in patients with aortic and mitral stenosis generally reveal more evidence of left ventricular enlargement than in patients with pure mitral stenosis, and catheterization of the left side of the heart is helpful in defining the relative importance of each valvular abnormality.

PHYSICAL FINDINGS AND GRAPHIC TRACINGS The systemic arterial pressure is usually within normal limits. In the late stages, however, when stroke volume declines, the systolic pressure may fall and the pulse pressure narrows. Systemic hypertension is unusual in patients with marked aortic stenosis, and a basal systolic arterial pressure exceeding 200 mmHg practically excludes severe narrowing of this valve. The peripheral arterial pulse, as palpated in the carotid or brachial arteries, rises slowly, to a delayed sustained peak. Indirect recordings of the carotid pulse exhibit a gradually ascending limb, often with a prominent anacrotic notch or shoulder on the upstroke, as well as a delayed peak, with coarse systolic vibrations. The left ventricular ejection period is prolonged, the preejection period is abbreviated, and the ratio of these two, i.e., the preejection period/systolic ejection period, is characteristically reduced (Chap. 250). Late in the course of the disease, in the presence of heart failure, the ratio may be normal. A palpable double systolic wave, the so-called bisferiens pulse, excludes pure or predominant aortic stenosis and signifies dominant or pure aortic regurgitation or obstructive hypertrophic cardiomyopathy (Chap. 263). In the late stages of the disease, when the pulse pressure is reduced, the pulse amplitude is so small that the anacrotic nature of the pulse and the delay in its upstroke may become more difficult to appreciate. The jugular venous pulse may be normal, although in many patients the *a* wave is accentuated. This results from the diminished distensibility of the right ventricular cavity caused by the bulging, hypertrophied, interventricular septum and/or the presence of pulmonary hypertension.

The apex beat is usually active and displaced inferiorly and laterally, reflecting the presence of left ventricular hypertrophy. A double apical impulse may be appreciated, particularly with the patient in the left lateral recumbent position; the first outward expansion occurs during atrial systole and reflects the important contribution made by atrial contraction to ventricular systole, while the second occurs during ventricular systole, usually is forceful and sustained during ejection. The right ventricle is usually palpable only when pulmonary hypertension develops in the late stages of the disease. A systolic thrill is generally present at the base of the heart, in the jugular notch, and along the carotid arteries, but occasionally it is palpable only during expiration and with the patient leaning forward. In patients who do not have marked pulmonary emphysema, a thick chest wall, thoracic deformity, or heart failure, the absence of a systolic thrill suggests that the aortic stenosis is relatively mild.

The rhythm is generally regular until very late in the course; at other times, atrial fibrillation should suggest the possibility of associated mitral valve disease. An early systolic ejection sound, actually the opening snap of the aortic valve, is frequently audible in children and adolescents with noncalcific valvular aortic stenosis. This sound usually disappears when the valve becomes calcified and rigid. The sound of aortic valve closure can also be identified most frequently in patients with aortic stenosis with pliable valves, and calcification tends to diminish the intensity of this sound. As aortic stenosis increases in severity, left ventricular systole may become prolonged so that the aortic valve closure sound no longer precedes the pulmonic valve closure sound, and the two components may become synchronous, or aortic valve closure may even follow pulmonic valve closure. This is called paradoxic splitting of the second heart sound (Chap. 248); in patients with aortic stenosis in the absence of a left intraventricular conduction defect this finding usually signifies severe obstruction to left ventricular outflow. A fourth heart sound is audible at the apex in many patients with severe aortic stenosis, reflects the presence of left ventricular hypertrophy and an elevated left ventricular end-diastolic pressure; a third heart sound generally occurs when the left ventricle dilates and fails.

The murmur of aortic stenosis is characteristically midsystolic; i.e., it commences shortly after the first heart sound, increases in intensity to reach a peak toward the middle of the ejection period, and diminishes progressively thereafter to end just before aortic valve closure (Chaps. 248 and 250). The murmur is usually low-pitched, rough, and rasping in character and is loudest at the base of the heart, most commonly in the second right intercostal space. It is transmitted to the jugular notch and upward along the carotid arteries. In patients with mild degrees of obstruction or in those with severe stenosis with heart failure in whom the stroke volume and therefore the transvalvular flow rate is reduced, the murmur may be relatively soft and brief. However, in almost all patients with significant obstruction, the murmur is at least grade III/VI. Occasionally, the murmur is transmitted downward and to the apex and may be confused with the systolic murmur of mitral regurgitation. However, the latter is usually holosystolic, while that of aortic stenosis is diamond-shaped and of the ejection type (Chap. 248).

Electrocardiogram This reveals left ventricular hypertrophy in the majority of patients with severe aortic stenosis (Chap. 249). In advanced cases, ST-segment depression and T-wave inversion in standard leads I, aVL, and in the left precordial leads are evident. However, there is no close correlation between the electrocardiogram and the hemodynamic severity of obstruction, and the absence of electrocardiographic signs of left ventricular hypertrophy does not exclude severe obstruction. Left bundle branch block or the presence of intraventricular conduction defects suggests diffuse fibrotic involvement of the myocardium. The presence of left atrial enlargement should suggest the possibility of associated mitral valve disease.

Echocardiogram This reveals thickening of the left ventricular wall, and in patients with valvular calcification, multiple, bright, thick, echoes from within the aortic root, without the normal box-like separation of the aortic cusps during systole. While cusp calcification does not necessarily indicate significant valve stenosis, its absence can usually be used to exclude such a diagnosis after the age of 25. Eccentricity of the aortic valve cusps is characteristic of congenitally bicuspid valves (Chap. 250). Left ventricular dilatation and reduced systolic shortening reflecting impairment of left ventricular function can be recognized. Echocardiography is particularly useful for identifying valvular abnormalities such as mitral stenosis and aortic regurgitation which sometimes accompany aortic stenosis, and for differentiating valvular from obstructive hypertrophic cardiomyopathy.

Roentgenographic features The chest roentgenogram may show no or little overall cardiac enlargement for many years, since the development of concentric left ventricular hypertrophy is the initial response to obstruction to left ventricular outflow. Hypertrophy without dilatation may produce some rounding of the cardiac apex in the frontal projection and slight backward displacement in the lateral view; significant aortic stenosis is usually associated with poststenotic dilatation of the ascending aorta. Aortic calcification is usually readily apparent on fluoroscopic examination with an image intensifier or by echocardiography; indeed, *the absence of valvular calcification in an adult suggests that severe valvular aortic stenosis is not present.* In later stages of the disease as the left ventricle dilates, there is progressively more evidence of left ventricular enlargement, and there may also be roentgenologic signs of pulmonary congestion, as well as enlargement of the left atrium, pulmonary artery, right ventricle, and right atrium.

Catheterization and angiocardiography Catheterization of the left side of the heart should be carried out in the majority of patients suspected of having severe aortic stenosis, particularly before a final decision concerning operative treatment is made. The goals are to document (1) the severity of the aortic obstruction, (2) the status of left ventricular function, and (3) the location of left ventricular outflow obstruction. These investigations are especially indicated in:

1 Young, asymptomatic patients with noncalcific aortic stenosis, in order to define the severity of their obstruction to left ventricular outflow, since operation may be indicated in them even in the absence of symptoms if severe aortic stenosis is present.

2 Patients in whom it is suspected that the obstruction to left ventricular outflow may not be at the aortic valve, but rather in the sub- or supravalvular regions.

3 Patients with clinical signs of aortic stenosis and symptoms of myocardial ischemia, in whom associated coronary artery disease is suspected. An effort should be made to determine whether aortic stenosis or coronary atherosclerosis is primarily responsible for the symptoms, and coronary arteriography should be carried out in addition to catheterization of the left side of the heart.

4 Patients with multivalvular disease, in whom the role played by each valvular deformity must be defined before operative treatment is planned.

Angiographic studies with left ventricular injection of contrast material are helpful in defining the size of the left ventricular cavity, the thickness of the wall, the site of obstruction, the degree of deformity and mobility of the aortic valve cusps, the diameter of the ascending aorta, and the presence and degree of accompanying mitral regurgitation. In patients with severe narrowing, a jet of contrast substance passing through the aortic orifice is readily visualized. When contrast substance is injected into the ascending aorta, the aortic valve cusps can also be outlined, and associated aortic regurgitation can be detected and its severity assessed.

NATURAL HISTORY The advanced age at death of patients with severe aortic stenosis is a consistent feature of this disease, and averages 63 years in men. In several studies, based on analysis of data obtained at postmortem examination, the average duration of various symptoms was as follows: angina pectoris, 3 years; syncope, 3 years; dyspnea, 2 years; and congestive heart failure, 1.5 to 2 years. Moreover, in more than 80 percent of these patients who died with aortic stenosis, symptoms had existed for less than 4 years. Congestive heart failure was considered to be the cause of death in one-half to two-thirds of patients.

Among adults dying with valvular aortic stenosis, sudden death, which presumably results from an arrhythmia, occurred in 10 to 20 percent, and at an average age of 60 years (Chap. 30). About one of every six patients dying suddenly has evidence of old or recent myocardial infarction at postmortem examination.

TREATMENT Strenuous physical activity should be avoided even in the asymptomatic stage in patients with *severe* aortic stenosis. Digitalis glycosides, sodium restriction, and diuretics are indicated in the treatment of congestive heart failure. While nitroglycerin is helpful in relieving angina pectoris, vasodilator therapy for heart failure is usually of little value. The most critical decision in the management of aortic stenosis, indeed of any valvular lesion, concerns the advisability of surgical treatment. The indications and results of operation, as well as the techniques, differ considerably, depending on the patient's age and the nature of the valvular deformity.

In children and adolescents with noncalcific aortic stenosis, considerable hemodynamic improvement can be anticipated from simple commissural incision under direct vision (Chap. 256). When carried out by an experienced surgical team, this procedure may be expected to be hemodynamically effective and to be associated with a mortality rate of less than 3 percent. This operation is recommended not only for symptomatic patients but also for asymptomatic children and adolescents with hemodynamic evidence of severe obstruction to left ventricular outflow, with a peak systolic pressure gradient exceeding 50 mmHg when the cardiac output is normal, or a calculated effective orifice less than 0.7 cm^2 per square meter of body surface area. Though this procedure can be expected to result in complete or almost complete relief of obstruction in the majority of patients, the valve cannot be rendered entirely normal anatomically, and it may become deformed, calcified, and stenotic again, entailing the possibility of reoperation, and perhaps valve replacement at some later date.

In the majority of adults with calcific aortic stenosis, satisfactory valve function cannot be restored, even by deliberate sculpturing procedures carried out under direct vision, and replacement of the valve is necessary. In most instances, it is prudent to postpone operation in patients with severe calcific aortic stenosis who are asymptomatic, since their future course is difficult to predict and they may continue to do well for many years. However, they should be followed carefully by clinical examination for the development of symptoms and by the various noninvasive tests, such as echocardiograms and/or radionuclide angiograms (Chap. 250), for evidence of deteriorating left ventricular function. It is likely that as the results of surgical replacement of the aortic valve continue to improve, many of these patients will become candidates for operation before their disease reaches the symptomatic stage. At the present, replacement of the aortic valve should be undertaken in patients with symptoms, even when relatively mild, that are believed to result primarily from aortic stenosis and who have hemodynamic evidence of severe obstruction.

It is clear that when symptoms of angina pectoris, syncope, or left ventricular decompensation develop in adults with valvular aortic stenosis, the outlook, despite medical treatment, is poor and can be improved significantly by replacement of the aortic valve with a prosthesis or tissue valve. Therefore, the risk entailed by operation in this group of patients is considerably lower than the risk involved by nonoperative treatment; moreover, the symptomatic improvement in many survivors of operation has been remarkable.

Operation should, if possible, be carried out before frank left ventricular failure supervenes; at this late stage, the operative risk is high (15 to 25 percent), and evidence of myocardial disease may persist even when the operation is technically successful. Furthermore, long-term postoperative survival correlates inversely with preoperative functional disability. Nonetheless, in view of the very poor prognosis of such patients when they are treated medically, there is usually little choice but to advise immediate surgical treatment. In patients in whom severe aortic stenosis and coronary artery disease coexist, relief of the aortic stenosis and revascularization of the myocardium by means of aortocoronary bypass grafting (Chap. 260) may result in striking clinical and hemodynamic improvement. Since many patients with calcific aortic stenosis are elderly, particular attention must be directed to the adequacy of hepatic, renal, and pulmonary function before valve replacement is recommended. Aortic valve replacement in symptomatic patients with severe obstruction but without heart failure is associated with a higher immediate mortality rate than is aortic commissurotomy in childhood (5 to 10 percent in most centers), and the long-term results and complications associated with the use of the several available prostheses and heterografts show some variation. The mortality rate depends to a substantial extent on the patient's preoperative clinical and hemodynamic state. Accordingly, a more conservative approach to operative treatment is warranted in adults with calcific aortic stenosis than in children with noncalcific stenosis. The 8-year survival rate following aortic valve replacement is approximately 65 percent. Fortunately, there is evidence that regression of left ventricular hypertrophy may occur following relief of obstruction.

AORTIC REGURGITATION

PATHOPHYSIOLOGY The total stroke volume expelled by the left ventricle (i.e., the sum of the effective forward stroke volume and the volume of blood which regurgitates back into the left ventricle) is increased in aortic regurgitation. In patients with free aortic regurgitation the volume of regurgitant flow may be of the same order of magnitude as the effective forward stroke volume. In contrast to mitral regurgitation, in which a fraction of the left ventricular stroke volume is delivered into the low-pressure left atrium, in aortic regurgitation the entire left ventricular stroke volume must be ejected into a high-pressure zone, the aorta. Although the low aortic diastolic pressure facilitates ventricular emptying during early systole, an increase of the left ventricular end-diastolic volume constitutes the major hemodynamic compensation to aortic regurgitation. The dilatation of the left ventricle allows this chamber to expel a larger stroke volume without requiring any increase in the relative shortening of each myofibril. Therefore, severe aortic regurgitation may occur with a normal effective forward stroke volume and a normal ejection fraction [total (forward plus regurgitant) stroke volume/end-diastolic volume], together with an elevated left ventricular end-diastolic pressure and volume. On the other hand, through the operation of Laplace's law (which indicates that myocardial wall tension is the product of intracavitary pressure and left ventricular radius), left ventricular dilatation increases the left ventricular systolic tension required to develop any given level of systolic pressure. As left ventricular function deteriorates, the end-diastolic volume increases without further elevation of the aortic regurgitant volume; the ejection fraction and forward stroke volume decline. Deterioration of left ventricular function often precedes the development of symptoms. Considerable thickening of the left ventricular wall also occurs with chronic aortic regurgitation, and at autopsy the hearts of these patients may be among the largest encountered, occasionally exceeding 1000 g in weight.

The reduction of the aortic diastolic pressure in aortic regurgitation shortens the left ventricular isometric contraction period, which is advantageous since it prolongs the left ventricular ejection period. The reverse pressure gradient from aorta to left ventricle, which is responsible for the aortic regurgitant flow, falls progressively during diastole, accounting for the decrescendo nature of the diastolic murmur. Equilibration between aortic and left ventricular pressures may occur toward the end of diastole, particularly when the heart rate is slow, and the left ventricular end-diastolic pressure may be elevated, occasionally to extremely high levels (>40 mmHg). Rarely, the left ventricular pressure exceeds the left atrial pressure toward the end of diastole, and this reversed pressure gradient closes the mitral valve prematurely, or may cause diastolic mitral regurgitation.

In patients with free aortic regurgitation the effective forward cardiac output usually is normal or only slightly reduced at rest, but often it fails to rise normally during exertion. In advanced stages there may be considerable elevation of the left atrial, pulmonary artery wedge, pulmonary arterial, and right ventricular pressures, and lowering of the effective cardiac output at rest. A qualitative index of the severity of aortic regurgitation may be obtained by determining the intensity of left ventricular opacification and the size of the left ventricle during thoracic aortography. In addition, this technique allows the detection of associated mitral regurgitation. However, quantitative angiographic techniques are required for accurate estimates of aortic regurgitant flow.

Myocardial ischemia occurs in patients with aortic regurgitation because both left ventricular dilatation and the elevated left ventricular systolic pressure tend to augment myocardial oxygen requirements. However, the major portion of coronary blood flow occurs during diastole, when arterial pressure is subnormal, thereby reducing coronary perfusion pressure. The result is a combination of increased oxygen supply and reduced demand.

ETIOLOGY Approximately three-fourths of all patients with pure or predominant regurgitation are males; however, females predominate among patients with aortic regurgitation who have associated mitral valve disease. In approximately 75 percent of patients with aortic regurgitation the disease is rheumatic in origin, resulting in a chronic form of the disorder with thickening, deformation, and shortening of the individual aortic valve cusps, changes which prevent their proper closure during diastole. A rheumatic etiology is less common in patients with isolated aortic regurgitation. Acute aortic regurgitation may also result from infective endocarditis, which may attack a valve previously affected by rheumatic disease, a congenitally deformed valve, or rarely a normal aortic valve, and may result in the perforation or erosion of one or more of the leaflets. Patients with discrete membranous subaortic stenosis may develop thickening of the aortic valve leaflets, which in turn leads to mild or moderate degrees of aortic regurgitation and makes these valves particularly susceptible to endocarditis. Aortic regurgitation may also occur in patients with congenital bicuspid aortic valves. Prolapse of an aortic cusp, resulting in progressive chronic aortic regurgitation, occurs in approximately 15 percent of patients with ventricular septal defect (Chap. 256). Congenital fenestrations of the aortic valve occasionally produce mild aortic regurgitation. Although traumatic rupture of the aortic valve is an uncommon cause of acute aortic regurgitation, it does represent the most frequent serious lesion observed in patients surviving nonpenetrating cardiac injuries. In patients with aortic regurgitation due to primary valvular disease, dilatation of the aortic annulus may occur secondarily and intensify the regurgitation.

Aortic regurgitation, both acute and chronic, may also be due entirely to marked aortic dilatation, without primary involvement of the valve leaflets; widening of the aortic annulus and separation of the aortic leaflets are responsible for the aortic regurgitation. Syphilis and ankylosing rheumatoid spondylitis may be associated with cellular infiltration and scarring of the media of the thoracic aorta, leading to aortic dilatation, aneurysm formation, and severe regurgitation. In syphilis of the aorta (Chap. 266), the involvement of the intima may narrow the coronary ostia, which narrowing in turn may be responsible for coronary insufficiency. Cystic medial necrosis of the ascending aorta, which may or may not be associated with other manifestations of Marfan's syndrome (Chap. 266), idiopathic dilatation of the aorta, and severe hypertension all may also widen the aortic annulus and lead to progressive aortic regurgitation. Occasionally, retrograde dissection of the aorta involving the aortic annulus produces aortic regurgitation.

The coexistence of hemodynamically significant aortic stenosis with aortic regurgitation usually excludes all of the rarer forms of aortic regurgitation because it occurs almost entirely in patients whose aortic regurgitation is on a rheumatic or congenital basis.

HISTORY A family history may frequently be elicited from patients with Marfan's syndrome, and a history of a heart murmur heard early in life may be obtained from patients with congenital aortic regurgitation. Patients with aortic regurgitation of obscure cause should also be questioned in detail about a positive serologic test for syphilis and about prior chest trauma; a history compatible with infective endocarditis may sometimes be elicited from patients with rheumatic or congenital involvement of the aortic valve, and the infection often precipitates or seriously aggravates preexisting symptoms. Ankylosing spondylitis is usually self-evident.

The interval between the first episode of acute rheumatic fever and the development of hemodynamically significant aortic regurgitation averages approximately 7 years, and this period is followed by an asymptomatic interval of approximately 10 to 20 years, during which the severity of the aortic regurgitation usually increases. Thus, severe aortic regurgitation may exist for many years without producing symptoms.

In chronic severe aortic regurgitation, the first complaint is often an uncomfortable awareness of the heartbeat, especially on lying down. Sinus tachycardia occurring during exertion or with emotion, or premature ventricular contractions, may produce particularly uncomfortable palpitations, as well as head pounding. These complaints may persist for many years before the development of exertional dyspnea, usually the first symptom of diminished cardiac reserve. This is followed by orthopnea, paroxysmal nocturnal dyspnea, and excessive diaphoresis. Symptoms of left ventricular failure are more common than symptoms of myocardial ischemia. Chest pain occurs frequently, even in younger patients, and it is not necessary to invoke the presence of coronary artery disease to explain this symptom in patients with aortic regurgitation. It may be due to myocardial ischemia, or it may originate from excessive cardiac pounding on the chest wall. Anginal pain may develop at rest as well as during exertion. Nocturnal angina may be a particularly troublesome symptom and is frequently accompanied by marked diaphoresis. The anginal episodes may be prolonged and often do not respond satisfactorily to sublingual nitroglycerin. Late in the course of the disease, evidence of systemic fluid accumulation, including congestive hepatomegaly, ankle edema, and ascites, may develop. Patients with severe aortic regurgitation tolerate high fevers, infections, or cardiac arrhythmias poorly, and may die in pulmonary edema as a result of one of these complications.

In patients with acute severe aortic regurgitation, as may occur in trauma or infective endocarditis, the left ventricle rapidly exhausts its ability to dilate, and left ventricular diastolic pressure rises rapidly with associated elevations of left atrial and pulmonary capillary pressures.

PHYSICAL FINDINGS The examination should be directed toward the detection of causes predisposing to aortic regurgitation, such as Marfan's syndrome, rheumatoid spondylitis, syphilis, essential hypertension, and ventricular septal defect. Even prior to the examination of the heart of the patient with free aortic regurgitation, the jarring of the entire body and the bobbing motion of the head with each systole can be appreciated, and the abrupt distention and collapse of the larger arteries are easily visible. A rapidly rising "water-hammer" pulse, which collapses suddenly as arterial pressure falls rapidly during late systole and diastole (Corrigan's pulse), and capillary pulsations (Quincke's pulse), an alternate flushing and paling of the skin at the root of the nail while pressure is applied to the tip of the nail, are characteristic of free aortic regurgitation. A booming, "pistol-shot" sound can be heard over the femoral arteries, and a to-and-fro murmur (Duroziez's sign) is audible if the femoral artery is lightly compressed with a stethoscope.

The arterial pulse pressure is widened, with an elevation of the systolic pressure, sometimes to as high as 300 mmHg, and a depression of the diastolic arterial pressure. The measurement of arterial diastolic pressure with a sphygmomanometer may be complicated by the fact that systolic sounds are frequently heard with the cuff completely deflated. However, the level of cuff pressure at the time of muffling of the Korotkoff sounds generally corresponds fairly closely to the true intraarterial diastolic pressure. The severity of aortic regurgitation does not always correlate directly with the arterial pulse pressure, and in many instances severe regurgitation exists in patients with arterial pressures in the range of 140/60. As the disease progresses, and the left ventricular end-diastolic pressure becomes markedly elevated, the arterial diastolic pressure may actually rise since the aortic diastolic pressure cannot fall below the left ventricular end-diastolic pressure.

The apex beat is displaced laterally and inferiorly. The left ventricle is hyperdynamic in patients with free regurgitation, and the systolic expansion and subsequent retraction of the apex are prominent and contrast sharply with the sustained systolic thrust characteristic of severe aortic stenosis. A diastolic thrill is often palpable along the left sternal border, and a prominent systolic thrill may be palpable in the jugular notch and transmitted upward along the carotid arteries. This thrill and the accompanying systolic murmur are due to the markedly increased blood flow across the aortic orifice, and do not necessarily signify the coexistence of aortic stenosis. Palpation, or indirect recording of the carotid arterial pulse, reveals it to be bisferiens, i.e., with two systolic waves separated by a trough, in many patients with pure aortic regurgitation, or with combined stenosis and regurgitation.

In patients with severe regurgitation the aortic valve closure sound is usually diminished or absent, and the indirectly recorded carotid arterial pulse does not usually show a clear-cut incisura. A third heart sound is common, and occasionally a fourth heart sound may also be heard. A loud systolic ejection sound is frequently audible; presumably it results from the sudden dilatation of the aorta by a greatly increased stroke volume.

The murmur of aortic regurgitation is typically a high-pitched, blowing, decrescendo diastolic murmur which is usually heard best in the third left intercostal space. In patients with mild regurgitation this murmur is brief and usually lasts less than one-third of diastole. However, as the severity increases, the murmur generally becomes louder and longer, and in patients with free aortic regurgitation it is usually holodiastolic. When the murmur is soft, it can be heard best with the diaphragm of the stethoscope and with the patient sitting up, leaning forward, and with the breath held in forced expiration. As it increases in intensity it tends to radiate widely, particularly down the lower sternal edge. In patients in whom the regurgitation is caused by primary valvular disease, the diastolic murmur is usually louder along the left than the right sternal border. However, when the decrescendo diastolic murmur is heard best along the right sternal border, it suggests that the aortic regurgitation is caused by dilatation or an aneurysm of the aortic root. "Cooing" or musical diastolic murmurs suggest eversion of an aortic cusp vibrating in the regurgitant stream.

On a purely statistical basis, a diastolic blowing murmur along the left sternal border is much more commonly caused by aortic than by pulmonic regurgitation. Unless it is trivial in magnitude, the aortic regurgitation can also be recognized by peripheral signs such as a widened pulse pressure or a collapsing pulse. On the other hand, the Graham Steell murmur of pulmonary regurgitation is usually accompanied by clinical evidence of severe pulmonary hypertension, including a loud and palpable pulmonary component of the second heart sound. In addition, the phonocardiogram reveals that the murmur of aortic regurgitation begins with the aortic second sound and therefore commences somewhat before the murmur of pulmonary regurgitation.

A systolic ejection murmur is generally heard best at the base of the heart and is transmitted to the jugular notch and along the carotid vessels. This murmur may be as loud as grade V or VI without indicating the presence of organic obstruction; it is often higher pitched, shorter, and less rasping in quality than the ejection systolic murmur heard in patients with predominant aortic stenosis.

A third murmur which is frequently heard in patients with aortic regurgitation is the Austin Flint murmur, a soft, low-pitched, rumbling middiastolic or presystolic bruit. It is probably produced by the displacement of the anterior leaflet of the mitral valve by the aortic regurgitant stream. However, this displacement of the mitral valve does not appear to be associated with hemodynamically significant obstruction to left ventricular filling; earlier onset and longer Austin Flint murmurs correlate with more severe aortic regurgitation. In patients with rheumatic aortic regurgitation it may be difficult to distinguish the Austin Flint murmur from the rumbling diastolic murmur of mitral stenosis. Both are loudest at the apex, but the murmur of mitral stenosis is usually accompanied by a loud first heart sound and immediately follows the opening snap of the mitral valve, while the Austin Flint murmur is often shorter in duration than the murmur of mitral stenosis, and in patients with sinus rhythm the latter more frequently is characterized by presystolic accentuation. The auscultatory features of aortic regurgitation are intensified by isometric exercise such as strenuous handgrip, which augments systemic resistance, and reduced by inhalation of amyl nitrite, which evokes the opposite effect. A blowing holosystolic murmur at the apex, which is transmitted to the axilla, may also be heard in patients with marked left ventricular dilatation and functional mitral regurgitation.

In *acute* severe aortic regurgitation, the elevation of left ventricular end-diastolic pressure may lead to early closure of the mitral valve, an associated middiastolic sound, a soft or absent S_1, a pulse pressure that is not particularly wide, and a soft, short diastolic murmur.

Electrocardiogram In patients with mild aortic regurgitation there may be no electrocardiographic abnormalities, but as the severity of aortic regurgitation increases, so do the electrocardiographic signs of left ventricular hypertrophy (Chap. 249). In addition to the abnormally tall R waves over the left precordium and deep S waves over the right precordium, patients with severe aortic regurgitation frequently exhibit ST-segment depressions and T-wave inversions in leads I, aVL, V_5, and V_6. Electrocardiographic signs of previous myocardial infarction generally indicate associated coronary artery disease. Left axis deviation and/or QRS prolongation denote diffuse myocardial disease, generally associated with patchy fibrosis; these signs usually denote a poor prognosis.

Echocardiogram This reveals increased systolic excursion of the posterior left ventricular wall; the velocity of wall motion is supernormal or normal until myocardial contractility declines. A rapid, high-frequency fluttering of the anterior leaflet of the mitral valve produced by the impact of the aortic regurgitant jet is a characteristic finding. The echocardiogram is also useful in detecting dilatation of the aortic root and of the left atrium in patients with aortic regurgitation.

Roentgenogram Moderate or severe degrees of regurgitation are always associated with varying degrees of left ventricular enlargement. The apex is displaced downward and to the left on the frontal projection, and frequently the cardiac shadow extends below the left diaphragm. Left ventricular enlargement also occurs in the left anterior oblique and lateral projections, in which the left ventricle is displaced posteriorly and encroaches on the spine. In patients in whom primary valvular disease is responsible for the aortic regurgitation, the ascending aorta and aortic knob may be moderately dilated and may extend further to the right than the right atrial shadow in the frontal view. On fluoroscopic examination the aorta and left ventricle pulsate vigorously in opposite directions during systole. When aortic regurgitation is caused by primary disease of the aortic wall, aneurysmal dilatation of the aorta may be seen roentgenographically, and the aorta may fill the retrosternal space in the lateral view.

TREATMENT The left ventricular failure of chronic aortic regurgitation at first usually responds to treatment with digitalis glycosides, salt restriction, and diuretics. Digitalis may also be indicated in patients with severe regurgitation and dilated left ventricles without symptoms of frank left ventricular failure. Cardiac arrhythmias and infections are poorly tolerated in patients with free aortic regurgitation, and must be treated promptly and vigorously. Although nitroglycerin and long-acting nitrites are not as helpful in relieving anginal pain as in patients with coronary artery disease or aortic stenosis, they are worth a trial. Patients with syphilitic aortitis should receive a full course of penicillin therapy (Chap. 177).

In deciding upon the advisability and proper timing of surgical treatment, it should be recognized that patients with chronic aortic regurgitation usually do not become symptomatic until after the development of myocardial dysfunction. Also, surgical treatment often does not restore normal left ventricular function. Therefore, careful clinical follow-up and repeated noninvasive testing, with judicious timing of catheterization of the left side of the heart, are necessary if operation is to be undertaken at the optimal time, i.e., with the onset of left ventricular dysfunction but prior to the development of severe symptoms.

Replacement of the aortic valve with a suitable prosthesis or porcine heterograft is generally necessary in patients with rheumatic aortic regurgitation and in many patients with other forms of regurgitation. Rarely, when a leaflet has been perforated during an episode of infective endocarditis, or torn from its attachments to the aortic annulus, surgical repair may be possible. When aortic regurgitation is due to aneurysmal dilatation of the annulus and ascending aorta, rather than to primary valvular involvement, it may be possible to reduce the regurgitation by narrowing the annulus or by excising a portion of the aorta without operating on the aortic valve itself. More frequently, however, regurgitation can be eliminated only by replacing the aortic valve, excising the aneurysm responsible for the regurgitation, and replacing the latter with a graft. This formidable procedure entails a higher risk than aortic valve replacement alone.

As in patients with aortic stenosis, the operative risks of aortic valve replacement are largely dependent on the stage of the disease. Surgical treatment should be considered in patients who have free aortic regurgitation and cardiomegaly who have become symptomatic on exertion in spite of medical therapy. Late mortality is also dependent on myocardial function at the time of operation; patients with marked cardiac enlargement and prolonged left ventricular dysfunction have a late mortality of approximately 5 percent per year despite a technically satisfactory operation. It is likely, however, that as in the case of aortic stenosis, further reductions of the operative mortality rate and increased confidence in the long-term effects of valvular prostheses and tissue valves will make it possible to extend the recommendation for operative treatment to asymptomatic patients with severe regurgitation and cardiomegaly. In patients with acute, severe aortic regurgitation producing left ventricular failure, early surgical treatment is generally indicated and may be lifesaving. Long-term postoperative survival correlates inversely with the height of the preoperative left ventricular end-diastolic pressure.

TRICUSPID STENOSIS

Tricuspid stenosis, a relatively uncommon valvular lesion, is generally rheumatic in origin and is much more common in women than in men. It does not usually occur as an isolated lesion or in patients with pure mitral regurgitation, but most commonly is observed in association with mitral stenosis, and sometimes with combined mitral and aortic stenosis. Hemodynamically significant tricuspid stenosis occurs in 5 to 10 percent of patients with severe mitral valve disease; rheumatic tricuspid stenosis is commonly associated with some degree of regurgitation.

PATHOPHYSIOLOGY A diastolic pressure gradient between the right atrium and ventricle is characteristic of tricuspid stenosis. This gradient can be recorded most accurately and conveniently with a double-lumen cardiac catheter, by placing the distal opening into the right ventricle and the proximal opening into the right atrium. It is augmented when the transvalvular blood flow increases during inspiration, and reduced when flow declines during expiration. A mean diastolic pressure gradient exceeding 5 mmHg is usually sufficient to elevate the mean right atrial pressure to levels which result in systemic venous congestion and, unless sodium intake has been restricted or diuretics have been given, is associated with ascites and edema. In patients with sinus rhythm, the right atrial *a* wave may be extremely tall and may even approach the level of the right ventricular systolic pressure. The resting cardiac output is usually quite reduced and fails to rise during exercise. The low cardiac output is responsible for the normal or only slightly elevated left atrial, pulmonary arterial, and right ventricular systolic pressures despite the presence of even moderately severe mitral stenosis.

SYMPTOMS Since mitral stenosis generally precedes the development of tricuspid stenosis, many patients initially have symptoms of pulmonary congestion. Amelioration of the symptoms of pulmonary congestion in a patient with mitral stenosis should raise the possibility that tricuspid stenosis may be developing. Characteristically, patients with hemodynamically significant tricuspid stenosis complain of relatively little dyspnea for the degree of hepatomegaly, ascites, and edema which they present. In some patients tricuspid stenosis may be suspected for the first time when symptoms of right ventricular failure persist after an adequate mitral valvulotomy. Weakness secondary to a low cardiac output and discomfort due to refractory edema, ascites, and marked hepatomegaly are common in patients with tricuspid stenosis and/or regurgitation.

PHYSICAL FINDINGS The diagnosis is often missed unless it is specifically considered and searched for. Severe tricuspid stenosis is associated with marked hepatic congestion, often resulting in cirrhosis, jaundice, serious malnutrition, severe edema, and ascites. Congestive hepatomegaly and, in cases of severe tricuspid valve disease, splenomegaly are present. The jugular veins are distended, and in patients with sinus rhythm there may be giant *a* waves. The *v* waves are less conspicuous, and since tricuspid obstruction impedes right atrial emptying during diastole, there is a slow *y* descent. In patients with sinus rhythm there may be prominent presystolic pulsations of the enlarged liver as well.

The right ventricle and the shock of pulmonary valve closure are usually not easily palpable. Indeed, a giant *a* wave in the jugular venous pulse without palpatory evidence of pulmonary hypertension or right ventricular enlargement suggests the possibility of tricuspid stenosis. The pulmonic closure sound is not accentuated on auscultation, and occasionally an opening snap of the tricuspid valve may be heard or recorded phonocardiographically approximately 0.06 s after pulmonary valve closure. The diastolic rumbling murmur of tricuspid stenosis has many of the qualities of the mitral diastolic murmur, and since tricuspid stenosis almost always occurs in the presence of mitral stenosis, the less-common valvular lesion may be missed. However, the tricuspid murmur is generally heard best along the left lower sternal margin and over the xiphoid process and is most prominent during presystole in sinus rhythm. It is augmented during inspiration, when negative intrathoracic pressure increases the velocity of blood flow across the tricuspid orifice, and it is reduced during expiration and particularly during the Valsalva maneuver, when tricuspid blood flow is reduced. This finding (Carvallo's sign) is often most easily elicited when the patient is in the erect position. In patients with sinus rhythm the presystolic component is often loudest. The diastolic murmur is reduced in amplitude as the stethoscope is inched laterally, only to intensify or reappear as the mitral murmur at the apex. In patients with sinus rhythm the presystolic component is often louder at the tricuspid than at the mitral area; the tricuspid presystolic murmur commences before the mitral, and it often is of the crescendo-decrescendo type. As already indicated, severe tricuspid stenosis may obscure many of the physical signs of accompanying mitral stenosis.

Electrocardiogram and roentgenogram The features of right atrial enlargement (Chap. 249) include tall, peaked P waves in lead II, as well as prominent, upright P waves in lead V_1. The absence of electrocardiographic evidence of right ventricular hypertrophy in a patient with right-sided heart failure who is believed to have mitral stenosis should suggest the possibility of associated tricuspid valve disease. The chest roentgenograms in patients with combined tricuspid and mitral stenosis show particular prominence of the right atrium and superior vena cava without much enlargement of the pulmonary artery and with less evidence of pulmonary vascular congestion than occurs in patients with pure mitral valve disease.

TREATMENT Patients with tricuspid stenosis generally exhibit marked systemic venous congestion; intensive salt restriction, digitalization, and diuretic therapy are required during the preoperative period. Such a prolonged preparatory period may diminish hepatic congestion and thereby improve hepatic function sufficiently that the risks of operation are diminished. Surgical treatment of the tricuspid valve is not ordinarily indicated at the time of mitral valve surgery in patients with mild tricuspid stenosis. On the other hand, definitive surgical relief of the tricuspid stenosis should be carried out, preferably at the time of mitral valvulotomy, in patients with moderate or severe tricuspid stenosis who have mean diastolic pressure gradients exceeding 5 mmHg and tricuspid orifices less than 1.5 to 2.0 cm^2. Tricuspid stenosis is almost always accompanied by significant tricuspid regurgitation; simple finger-fracture valvulotomy often does not result in significant hemodynamic improvement, but may merely substitute severe regurgitation for stenosis. However, open operations utilizing cardiopulmonary bypass may permit substantial improvement of tricuspid valve function. If this cannot be accomplished, the tricuspid valve may have to be replaced with a prosthesis.

TRICUSPID REGURGITATION

Tricuspid regurgitation is usually functional and secondary to marked dilatation of the right ventricle and the tricuspid valve ring. Functional tricuspid regurgitation may complicate right ventricular failure of any cause, including inferior wall infarcts that involve the right ventricle, and is commonly seen in the late stages of heart failure due to rheumatic or congenital heart disease with severe pulmonary hypertension, i.e., with systolic pressures exceeding 60 mmHg, as well as ischemic heart disease, cardiomyopathy, and cor pulmonale. It is in part reversible if pulmonary hypertension is relieved. Rheumatic fever may also produce organic tricuspid regurgitation, which is often associated with tricuspid stenosis. Less commonly, regurgitation results from congenitally deformed tricuspid valves, and it occurs with defects of the atrioventricular canal, as well as with Ebstein's malformation of the tricuspid valve (Chap. 256). Carcinoid heart disease, endomyocardial fibrosis, infective endocarditis, trauma, and infarction of right ventricular papillary muscles may also produce tricuspid regurgitation.

As is the case for tricuspid stenosis, the clinical features of tricuspid regurgitation result primarily from systemic venous congestion and reduction of the cardiac output. With the onset of tricuspid regurgitation in patients with pulmonary hypertension, as cardiac output declines, symptoms of pulmonary congestion diminish, but the clinical manifestations of right-sided heart failure become intensified. The neck veins are distended, with prominent *v* waves, and marked hepatomegaly, ascites, pleural effusions, edema, systolic pulsations of the liver, and positive hepatojugular reflux are common. A prominent right ventricular pulsation along the left parasternal region and a blowing holosystolic murmur along the lower left sternal margin which is generally intensified during inspiration and reduced during expiration or the Valsalva maneuver are characteristic findings; atrial fibrillation is usually present.

The electrocardiogram is usually characteristic of the lesion responsible for the enlargement of the right ventricle which leads to this form of valvular dysfunction. In the rare instances of isolated tricuspid regurgitation the electrocardiogram often shows incomplete right bundle branch block. Roentgenographic examination usually reveals enlargement of both the right ventricle and right atrium, and the latter chamber expands during systole. The cardiac output is usually markedly reduced, and the right atrial pressure pulse may exhibit no *x* descent during early systole, but a prominent *c-v* wave, with a rapid *y* descent. The mean right atrial and the right ventricular end-diastolic pressures are often elevated.

Isolated tricuspid regurgitation, without pulmonary hypertension, such as that occurring as a consequence of infective endocarditis or trauma, is usually well tolerated and does not require operation. Indeed, excision of an infected tricuspid valve is often well tolerated. Treatment of the underlying cause of heart failure usually reduces the severity of functional tricuspid regurgitation. In patients with mitral valve disease and tricuspid regurgitation due to pulmonary hypertension and massive right ventricular enlargement, effective surgical correction of the mitral valvular abnormality results in lowering of the pulmonary vascular pressures and gradual reduction or disappearance of the tricuspid regurgitation without direct treatment of the tricuspid valve. However, recovery may be much more rapid in patients with severe secondary tricuspid regurgitation if, at the time of mitral replacement, tricuspid annuloplasty or, if necessary, tricuspid valve replacement is performed. In patients with severe regurgitation secondary to deformity of the tricuspid valve due to rheumatic fever, particularly those without severe pulmonary hypertension, surgical treatment of the tricuspid regurgitation, consisting of either valve replacement or narrowing of the annulus, should be carried out.

PULMONIC VALVE DISEASE

The pulmonic valve is affected by rheumatic fever far less frequently than the other valves and is uncommonly the seat of infective endocarditis. The most common acquired abnormality affecting the pulmonic valve is regurgitation secondary to dilatation of the pulmonary valve ring as a consequence of severe pulmonary hypertension of any cause. This produces the Graham Steell murmur, a high-pitched, decrescendo, diastolic blowing murmur along the left sternal border, which is difficult to differentiate from the far more common murmur produced by aortic regurgitation. It is of little hemodynamic significance; indeed surgical removal or destruction of the pulmonic valve by infective endocarditis does not produce heart failure unless serious pulmonary hypertension is also present.

Congenital pulmonic stenosis is discussed in Chap. 256.

REFERENCES

Braunwald E: Mitral regurgitation: Physiological, clinical and surgical considerations. N Engl J Med 281:425, 1969

———: Acquired valvular heart disease, in *Heart Disease,* 2d ed, E Braunwald (ed). Philadelphia, Saunders, 1983, chap 32

Chizner MA et al: Natural history of aortic stenosis in adults. Am Heart J 99:419, 1980

Cohn LH et al: Five- to eight-year followup of patients undergoing porcine heart valve replacement. N Engl J Med 304:258, 1981

Crawford MH, O'Rourke RA: Mitral valve prolapse syndromes, in *Update I: Harrison's Principles of Internal Medicine,* KJ Isselbacher et al (eds). New York, McGraw-Hill, 1981, pp 91–106

Dalen JA, Alpert JS (eds): *Valvular Heart Disease.* Boston, Little, Brown, 1981

Duran et al: Is tricuspid valve repair necessary? J Thorac Cardiovasc Surg 80:849, 1981

Greenberg BH et al: Arterial dilators in mitral regurgitation: Effects on rest and exercise, hemodynamics and long-term clinical follow-up. Circulation 65:181, 1982

Henry WL et al: Observations on the optimum time for operation interruption for aortic regurgitation. Circulation 61:471, 484, 1980

Lingameni R et al: Tricuspid regurgitation: Clinical and angiographic assessment. Cath Cardiovasc Diag 5:7, 1979

Mahapatra RK et al: Rheumatic tricuspid stenosis. Indian Heart J 30:1381, 1978

Morganroth J et al: Acute severe aortic regurgitation. Ann Intern Med 87:223, 1977

Ross J Jr: Left ventricular function and the timing of surgical treatments in valvular heart disease. Ann Intern Med 94:498, 1981

259 INFECTIVE ENDOCARDITIS

LAWRENCE L. PELLETIER, JR.
ROBERT G. PETERSDORF

DEFINITION Infective endocarditis is a microbial infection of the heart valves or of the endocardium in proximity to congenital or acquired cardiac defects. A similar clinical illness develops when there is infection of arteriovenous fistulas or aneurysms. The infection may develop abruptly or insidiously, may pursue a fulminant or prolonged course, and is fatal unless treated. The infection caused by indigenous microorganisms with low pathogenicity is ordinarily subacute, whereas infection by microorganisms with high pathogenicity is often acute. Fever, cardiac murmurs, splenomegaly, anemia, hematuria, mucocutaneous petechiae, and embolic manifestations are characteristic of the disease. Valve destruction may result in acute mitral or aortic regurgitation requiring urgent surgical intervention. Mycotic aneurysms may develop in the aortic root, cerebral artery bifurcations, or other remote sites.

ETIOLOGY AND EPIDEMIOLOGY Acute infective endocarditis is caused by relatively pathogenic microorganisms, exemplified by *Staphylococcus aureus,* pneumococcus, group A streptococcus, and rarely gonococcus, *Histoplasma capsulatum, Brucella,* and *Listeria.* Endocarditis attributed to these organisms usually follows dissemination from an infected focus, which is often undetectable. Endocarditis caused by staphylococci, coliform bacilli, and *Candida* has been described frequently among intravenous drug users. Infection of the heart due to staphylococci, *Candida, Aspergillus,* or coliform bacilli and resembling endocarditis is a rare but serious complication of surgery in which sutures or prostheses have been placed in the heart or peripheral arteries. Primarily in alcoholics, endocarditis is sometimes observed in association with pneumococcal meningitis and bacteremia (see Chap. 146). Staphylococcal endocarditis can result from bacteremia associated with septic thrombophlebitis due to infected intravenous catheters, hyperalimentation lines, or arteriovenous shunts; or a cutaneous, bone, or pulmonary infection. Group A streptococcal endocarditis is probably never a complication of streptococcal pharyngitis but may follow the bacteremia of streptococcal skin or puerperal infection. Polymicrobial infections may occur occasionally in parenteral drug addicts or after prosthetic valve surgery.

Subacute infective endocarditis usually develops in persons with rheumatic valvular or congenital cardiac lesions. It is most commonly caused by the viridans streptococci, which are part of the normal upper respiratory bacterial flora. *Streptococcus faecalis* (enterococcus), indigenous to the fecal and perineal flora, is an increasingly important cause of subacute infective endocarditis, particularly in elderly men with prostatism or women with genitourinary tract infections. *Streptococcus bovis* endocarditis is associated with an intestinal portal of entry, such as a colon carcinoma. *Staphylococcus aureus* may produce subacute as well as acute infective endocarditis. Suppuration, cellulitis, or other infected foci may precede subacute infective endocarditis but are recognized infrequently. Viridans streptococci are commonly found in the blood immediately after dental manipulation or extraction. Tonsillectomy and rigid bronchoscopy are also occasionally associated with transient bacteremia. Chewing of food or use of a water jet may result in bacteremia in patients with gingival disease or dental infection. Transient bacteremia of this sort is probably an important initiating factor in some cases of subacute infective endocarditis.

PATHOGENESIS Infective endocarditis occurs most frequently in persons with preexisting heart disease. Infection most commonly involves the left side of the heart. The mitral, aortic, tricuspid, and pulmonary valves may be involved, in the order of frequency listed. Valves damaged by rheumatic fever are most commonly involved, but valves damaged by syphilis and arteriosclerosis are also susceptible to infective endocarditis. Enterococcal endocarditis in elderly men is associated with involvement of the aortic valve, and frequently results in marked valvular damage. Infective endocarditis rarely involves interatrial septal defects. Prosthetic heart valves, mitral valve leaflet prolapse, or idiopathic hypertrophic subaortic stenosis may predispose to endocarditis. Infection in patients with interventricular septal defects often involves the endocardium opposite the septal defect in the direction of the shunt. Infection associated with patent ductus arteriosus develops on the pulmonary side of the ductus. Drug addicts frequently develop right-sided endocarditis involving the tricuspid valve. Valvular infection in association with rheumatic heart disease is usually on the valve edge along the line of closure.

Hemodynamic events are important in the pathogenesis of the disease. Alterations in blood flow can cause marked changes in vascular endothelium. It has been demonstrated experimentally that bacteria are deposited on the endothelium in areas of high flow with decreased lateral pressure. These factors are undoubtedly important in determining the situations and location where infective endocarditis develops. Infection in the heart is most often at a site of a structural change or abnormality. Thrombi that develop on endocardial irregularities have been implicated as foci for bacterial implantation, and it seems likely that a sterile vegetation consisting of platelets and fibrin is the nidus on which bacteria become implanted.

Serum antibodies in high titer against the infective microorganisms are often found in patients with infective endocarditis and circulating antigen-antibody complexes are commonly found, sometimes associated with immune complex glomerulonephritis and cutaneous vasculitis. The presence of opsonizing antibodies to bacteria may facilitate localization of organisms on the endocardium during transient bacteremias. Nonspecific complement fixing antibodies probably protect against gram-negative enteric rod endocarditis, explaining the low incidence of this entity in an era of increasing gram-negative rod bacteremia.

Infective endocarditis leads to deposition of fibrin and platelets about the site of infection, producing a vegetation. Highly pathogenic microorganisms often cause rapid valvular destruction and ulceration. Less pathogenic microorganisms usually cause less valvular destruction or ulceration but can lead to development of large polypoid vegetations. The infection may extend from the valve to the surrounding mural endocardium or penetrate the valve ring to produce a mycotic aneurysm, myocardial abscess, or cardiac conduction defects. Involvement of chordae tendineae may lead to rupture and valvular insufficiency. Acute infective endocarditis, particularly when caused by *S. aureus,* often is associated with abscesses in the valve ring. Vascularization of involved valves may increase during endocarditis but rarely extends into the area of infection. Phagocytes are not prominent in the area of microbial growth, which may explain why infection by microorganisms of low pathogenicity progresses uncontrolled without bactericidal antimicrobial therapy. The lack of vascularization of the granulation tissue in the vegetation also may account for ineffectiveness of host defenses and the requirement for intensive treatment.

The microbemia of intravascular infections is ordinarily continuous. For this reason few blood cultures are required to demonstrate the microorganisms. The microorganisms are primarily cleared from the blood by the reticuloendothelial cells of the liver and spleen. There is no obvious reduction in the number of bacteria in the blood during circulation through the extremities. Arterial blood cultures, therefore, are no more likely to show bacteremia than are venous blood cultures.

Embolization is a characteristic feature of infective endocarditis. The friable fibrin vegetations may separate from the site of infection and be propelled as emboli into the systemic or pulmonary circulation, depending on whether the endocarditis involves the left or right side of the heart. Emboli vary in size and most often involve the brain, spleen, kidney, gastrointestinal tract, heart, or extremities. Emboli in fungal endocarditis tend to be large and occlude major vessels. Pulmonary infarction or abscess is common in right-sided endocarditis. Septic infarction is uncommon in subacute bacterial endocarditis caused by microorganisms of low pathogenicity, and suppurative complications are rarely seen at these sites when viridans streptococci are the offending agents. Osteomyelitis has been described, however, as an embolic complication of endocarditis due to viridans streptococci and enterococci. Septic infarction is common in acute infective endocarditis attributable to bacteria of high pathogenicity, as are metastatic abscesses. Involvement of major arteries by emboli produces mycotic aneurysms, which may rupture. Myocardial infarction may develop after coronary embolization. In addition, focal myocarditis is common in subacute infective endocarditis and may be embolic.

The spleen is frequently enlarged, particularly in subacute cases. Three types of renal lesions may be produced. When large emboli find their way into the kidney, infarction may develop. Small emboli may produce a focal glomerulitis. In some instances, there is a diffuse glomerulonephritis that is indistinguishable from other types of immune complex glomerulonephritis. Petechial skin lesions, characterized histologically by acute vasculitis, are probably not embolic and may be immunologic in origin. Other skin lesions associated with pain, tenderness, and cellulitis, however, may be embolic.

MANIFESTATIONS **Subacute infective endocarditis** Patients ordinarily cannot date the onset of the infection. Symptoms begin insidiously, and gradually the illness becomes apparent. In some individuals, however, the onset of infection can be related to a recent dental extraction, urethral instrumentation, tonsillectomy, acute respiratory infection, or abortion.

Weakness, fatigability, weight loss, feverishness, night sweats, anorexia, and arthralgia are the usual symptoms of subacute bacterial endocarditis. Emboli may produce paralysis, chest pain due to myocardial or pulmonary infarction, acute vascular insufficiency with pain in the extremities, hematuria, acute abdominal pain, or sudden blindness. Painful fingers or toes and painful skin lessions may also be important symptoms. Chills are not common. Transient cerebral ischemic attacks, toxic encephalopathy, headache, brain abscess, subarachnoid hemorrhage from rupture of a mycotic aneurysm, or purulent meningitis may develop.

Physical examination may reveal a variety of findings, none of which alone is pathognomonic of subacute infective endocarditis. Physical examination may be normal early in the course of infection. The association of the different manifestations, however, usually provides a characteristic picture of the disease. The patient usually appears chronically ill and pale and has an elevated temperature. The fever is most often remittent, with afternoon or evening peaks. The pulse is usually rapid, and if cardiac failure complicates the infection, it may be greater than expected with the degree of fever.

Mucocutaneous lesions are common and vary in type. Petechiae are most frequent and may be found in the mucosa of the mouth, pharynx, or conjunctivas. These small, red, hemorrhagic-appearing lesions do not blanch on pressure and are not tender or painful. On the mucous membranes or conjunctivas these petechiae may have a pale center. Petechiae may be found anywhere on the skin but are most common over the upper part of the trunk anteriorly. They are frequently difficult to distinguish from angiomas, but they gradually become brownish and disappear. Frequently, petechiae continue to appear, even during convalescence. Linear hemorrhages (splinter hemorrhages) may be found under the nails, but these are difficult to differentiate from traumatic lesions, particularly in manual laborers. These mucocutaneous lesions are not specific for bacterial endocarditis but may be found in patients with other conditions such as profound anemia, leukemia, trichinosis, and sepsis without endocarditis. Erythematous or purple, painful, tender nodules (Osler's nodes) may develop on the palms of the hands, soles of the feet, pulp of the fingers, or other sites. These are probably embolic lesions. Emboli to larger peripheral arteries may result in gangrene of fingers, toes, or larger portions of the extremities.

Clubbing of the fingers is observed in long-standing or prolonged infective endocarditis. Mild jaundice is found occasionally.

Findings in the heart are usually those of underlying heart disease. Major changes in cardiac murmurs, primarily development of a new diastolic murmur, may be attributable to ulceration of a valve, dilatation of the heart or valve ring, rupture of chordae tendineae, or development of a very large vegetation. Minor changes in systolic bruits are usually of little significance. In rare instances, no cardiac murmurs are detected. In this situation, right-sided endocarditis or an infected mural thrombus, or pulmonary, or peripheral arteriovenous fistula should be suspected.

Splenomegaly is common in subacute infective endocarditis. Rarely is the spleen tender, but a friction rub may be heard over it when there is infarction. Hepatomegaly is not characteristic unless heart failure develops.

Arthralgia is relatively common, and arthritis resembling acute rheumatic fever may occur.

Embolic phenomena may precipitate awareness of the infection. Sudden development of hemiplegia, flank pain with hematuria, abdominal pain with melena, pleuritic pain and hemoptysis, left upper abdominal pain with splenic friction rub, blindness, or monoplegia in a patient with fever and cardiac murmurs makes infective endocarditis suspect. Pulmonary emboli in right-sided endocarditis may be confused with pneumonia.

Acute bacterial infective endocarditis Endocarditis caused by highly pathogenic microorganisms usually begins abruptly. Suppurative infection commonly antedates the onset of endocarditis. For example, infection of the heart may develop as a complication of pneumococcal meningitis, septic thrombophlebitis, group A streptococcal cellulitis, or staphylococcal abscesses. The source of cardiovascular infection, therefore, is often evident.

Acute endocarditis often involves the normal heart, in contrast to the subacute infection, which almost invariably involves the abnormal heart. It is particularly common in intravenous drug users and individuals with previously undetected abnormalities of the aortic valve. The acute infection is fulminant and pursues a rapid course. Fever is often greater, may be intermittent, and in certain instances (as in gonococcal endocarditis) may be characterized by a double quotidian temperature curve. Chills are common. Petechiae may be numerous, and embolic phenomena are prominent. Small, occasionally flame-shaped hemorrhages that may have pale centers (Roth spots) are found in the retina. Osler's nodes are uncommon, but the pulp of the fingers may show nontender subcutaneous erythematous maculopapular lesions (Janeway's spots) that may ulcerate. Hematuria is seen with embolic lesions of the kidney, and diffuse glomerulonephritis may occur. Destruction of the cardiac valves can be complicated by rupture of chordae tendineae or perforation of cusps, leading to rapidly progressing cardiac failure. Metastatic abscesses following septic emboli are frequent.

Right-sided endocarditis Tricuspid valve and rarely pulmonary valve endocarditis or pulmonary artery mycotic aneurysm are seen in parenteral drug addicts with skin cellulitis or septic phlebitis. Infected peripheral or central venous catheters or transvenous pacing wires may also result in right-sided infective endocarditis. The infecting organisms originate from the skin (*S. aureus, C. albicans*) or presumably from injected materials (*Pseudomonas aeruginosa, Serratia marcescens*). *S. aureus* is the most frequently isolated organism, and the tricuspid valve the most common site of involvement in parenteral drug addicts. The clinical presentation is that of acute endocarditis with pulmonary infarction and abscess formation. The most frequent symptoms are high fever of several weeks' duration, pleuritic chest pain, hemoptysis and sputum production, dyspnea on exertion, malaise, anorexia, and fatigability. A tricuspid valve regurgitant murmur accentuated by inspiration with pulsatile neck veins and liver may be present, but more often there is no audible murmur at all or the murmur is difficult to detect. Two-dimensional echocardiogram may be required to confirm the presence of endocardial vegetations. Blood cultures are as likely to be positive in right-sided endocarditis as in left-sided lesions. The chest roentgenograph usually shows peripheral wedge-shaped pulmonary infiltrates with cavitation. Due to the absence of emboli to vital organs, acute hemodynamic decompensation secondary to valve destruction, and a generally younger, healthier patient population, and perhaps because of a better response to antimicrobial agents, patients with right-sided endocarditis have a better prognosis. Large (greater than 1 cm diameter) vegetations or infection caused by resistant microorganisms may require valve debridement or excision in conjunction with antimicrobial therapy to eradicate the infection.

Prosthetic valve endocarditis Prosthetic valve infections develop in 1 to 2 percent of patients following prosthetic valve placement. About one-third of these infections develop *within 2 months of surgery* and are probably due to colonization of the prosthesis or suture sites during surgery. *Staphylococcus aureus, S. epidermidis,* coliform bacilli, *Candida* spp., *Aspergillus* spp., and diphtheroid organisms that cause early infections are often resistant to antimicrobial agents; such infections are associated with a high mortality due to septic shock, valve dehiscence, and myocardial invasion. Gram-negative bacteremia in the immediate postoperative period may originate from the urinary tract, wound, pulmonary infections, or septic phlebitis and is often not associated with prosthetic valve infection.

Prosthetic valve infections that occur *more than 2 months after surgery* are frequently caused by viridans streptococci, enterococci, *S. aureus,* or *S. epidermidis.* These infections probably result from colonization of the prosthesis or its site of attachment during transient bacteremias. Patients with prosthetic valves should receive prophylactic antimicrobial agents when undergoing procedures known to produce bacteremia, and minor infections that might produce bacteremia should be treated promptly. Late onset infections caused by streptococci have a better prognosis than early infections and may be controlled with antibiotics alone.

Prosthetic valve infections often produce symptoms and signs indistinguishable from infections on natural valves, but there is a greater frequency of valve ring infection that may involve part or all of the circumference producing valve dehiscence or penetration into the myocardium or surrounding tissues. Myocardial abscess, conduction disturbances, sinus of Valsalva aneurysm, or fistulas into the right side of the heart or pericardium may result. Prolongation of the PR interval, a new left bundle branch block, or right bundle branch block with left anterior hemiblock should suggest involvement of the ventricular septum in aortic valve infections. Extension of infection from the mitral valve annulus may be associated with nonparoxysmal junctional tachycardia, or second- or third-degree heart block with a narrow QRS complex. Prosthetic valve stenosis due to vegetations narrowing the orifice or interfering with valve excursion may be detected by auscultation or echocardiography. A postoperative regurgitant murmur or abnormal position or movement of the valve on fluoroscopic examination or echocardiogram may indicate partial dehiscence of the prosthesis. Prosthetic valve infections complicated by valve stenosis, valve dehiscence with congestive heart failure, recurrent emboli, resistance to antimicrobial therapy, or evidence of myocardial invasion require early surgical intervention. Patients receiving anticoagulants to prevent embolism who develop endocarditis should generally continue to take the medication because the risk of embolization without anticoagulation is high and accept a slightly increased risk of intracranial hemorrhage. Relapse following appropriate antimicrobial treatment or fungous infections also requires early surgical removal of the infected prosthesis.

LABORATORY FINDINGS Leukocytosis with neutrophilia is the rule but is by no means invariable. Macrophages (histiocytes) may be found in the blood, particularly in the first drop obtained from the earlobe. Normocytic, normochromic anemia is almost always found in subacute bacterial endocarditis but may not be present early in acute bacterial endocarditis. The erythrocyte sedimentation rate is rapid. Serum immunoglobulins are increased but return to normal during convalescence. The anti-gamma globulin latex fixation test is commonly positive, and the Rose-Waaler test is negative. Circulating immune complexes are present and titers decline with successful antimicrobial therapy. Mild bilirubinemia is detected occasionally. Proteinuria is common, and microscopic hematuria is frequently present. Serum total hemolytic complement and the third component of complement may be decreased.

An echocardiogram may identify high-risk patients with large vegetations or unsuspected preexisting valvular lesions, or it may provide an indication for early operation in patients with acute aortic insufficiency and severe volume overload of the left ventricle. The echocardiogram does not detect vegetations smaller than 2 mm, nor does it differentiate active from healed lesions. Two-dimensional scanners are more sensitive than M-mode echocardiography but still demonstrate vegetations in only 43 to 80 percent of patients with endocarditis.

Blood cultures are positive in the majority of cases. Three to five cultures of 20 ml of blood, taken at intervals determined by the patient's clinical status, are usually adequate to demonstrate the bacteremia, if it is demonstrable at all. Blood cultures may not become positive for several days, if at all, in patients who have received antibiotics prior to the time when cultures are obtained. Failure to demonstrate bacteremia or delayed growth in blood cultures also may be due to infection by unusual microorganisms such as *Hemophilus parainfluenzae, Cardiobacterium hominis, Corynebacterium* spp., *Histoplasma capsulatum, Brucella, Pasteurella,* or anaerobic streptococci that require special nutrient media or extended (up to 4 weeks) incubation. Thiol-requiring streptococcal variants may require pyridoxine- or cysteine-supplemented broth. Castañeda-type culture bottles assist in the recovery of fungi and *Brucella. Aspergillus* endocarditis is seldom associated with positive blood cultures. *Coxiella burnetii* endocarditis and *Chlamydia psittaci* endocarditis are diagnosed by serologic tests, since blood cultures are always negative. Bone marrow cultures and serologic testing for *Candida, Histoplasma,* and *Brucella* may be helpful in culture-negative endocarditis.

DIFFERENTIAL DIAGNOSIS When several of the manifestations of infective endocarditis occur together, the diagnosis is not difficult. In particular, the presence of fever, petechiae, splenomegaly, microscopic hematuria, and anemia in a patient with cardiac murmurs is most suggestive of infection. When only a few manifestations are present, however, the diagnosis is not simple. Prolonged fever in a patient with rheumatic heart disease is particularly troublesome, but the diagnosis of bacterial endocarditis should be considered in every patient with fever and a heart murmur. The diagnosis becomes even more difficult when blood cultures show no growth.

Acute rheumatic fever with carditis is often difficult to distinguish from infective endocarditis, and in a few instances, active rheumatic fever has been found to coexist with the valvular infection. The diagnosis of rheumatic carditis hinges on a combination of clinical and laboratory criteria (see Chap. 257).

Subacute infective endocarditis is no longer a common cause of "fever of undetermined origin" (see Chap. 9). However, occasionally it may be mistaken for a hidden neoplasm, systemic lupus erythematosus, periarteritis nodosa, poststreptococcal glomerulonephritis, and intracardiac tumors such as myxoma of the atrium. Aortic dissection with acute aortic regurgitation also may mimic bacterial endocarditis. Postoperative endocarditis should be suspected in patients who develop fever, anemia, and leukocytosis after cardiovascular surgery. In these postoperative patients, the various postthoracotomy and postcardiotomy syndromes must also be considered.

PROGNOSIS Recovery from untreated infective endocarditis is rare. With appropriate antibiotic therapy, however, over 70 percent of the patients with infection on endogenous valves and 50 percent with infection on prosthetic valves survive the infection. Intravenous drug users with right-sided staphylococcal endocarditis generally have a good prognosis. Factors that suggest a less favorable outcome are the presence of congestive heart failure, extreme age of the patient, involvement of the aortic valve or multiple heart valves, polymicrobial bacteremia, failure to identify the etiologic agent owing to negative blood cultures, antimicrobial resistance to nontoxic bactericidal drugs, and delay in initiating therapy. Prosthetic-valve, gram-negative bacillus, and fungal endocarditis are associated with the poorest prognosis.

The commonest cause of death in treated endocarditis is congestive heart failure, attributable either to valve destruction or to myocardial damage. Additionally, death may be precipitated by embolization to vital organs, by renal insufficiency, by rupture of a mycotic aneurysm, or by complications following cardiac surgery. Many patients recover completely without apparent worsening of the underlying cardiovascular disease. When recurrent endocarditis develops, it usually involves the same valve and is due to failure to kill microorganisms in an environment of suboptimal host resistance.

Further reduction in the mortality rate of infective endocarditis will depend primarily on the increased use of cardiac surgery in combination with antimicrobial therapy to eliminate refractory infections, and the early replacement of damaged valves in patients with congestive heart failure.

PROPHYLAXIS Patients with suspected congenital or acquired heart disease, prosthetic heart valves, ventriculoseptal patches, or prior history of infective endocarditis should receive antimicrobial prophylaxis for viridans streptococci immediately before any dental manipulation that causes bleeding, oral surgery, and tonsillectomy or adenoidectomy. Likewise, patients with similar cardiac risks undergoing urinary catheterization, cystoscopy, prostatectomy, obstetrical or gynecologic manipulation of infected tissues, or rectal or colon surgery should receive prophylaxis directed against the enterococcus. Patients with mitral valve prolapse, asymmetrical septal hypertrophy, and tricuspid or pulmonary valve lesions are at lower risk of developing endocarditis but should also receive antimicrobial prophylaxis. Prophylaxis is not required for atherosclerotic arterial plaques, coronary artery bypass grafts, isolated atrial septal defects, or transvenous pacemakers. The high-risk patients mentioned above undergoing surgical manipulation of infected tissues at other sites should receive an antimicrobial active against the most likely infecting organism.

The rationale for antimicrobial prophylaxis is that when these patients develop bacteremia, they are more likely to develop endocarditis. The best experimental evidence available holds that for prevention of endocarditis caused by viridans streptococci with penicillin, both a high concentration and relatively prolonged duration of action are necessary. It has been shown that penicillin and streptomycin act synergistically in killing viridans streptococci. These data suggest a regimen consisting of a single dose of 1.2 million units of aqueous procaine penicillin G plus 1.0 g streptomycin administered intramuscularly within 30 min of dental surgery, followed by penicillin V 0.5 g orally at 6-h intervals for four doses, is effective. A loading dose of 2 g penicillin V followed by 0.5 g of the drug at 6-h intervals for 24 h is probably equally effective. Patients who are allergic to penicillin should receive vancomycin, 1.0 g intravenously over 30 min, 1 h before the procedure or erythromycin, 1.0 g orally 1 h before the procedure. Either antibiotic should be followed with erythromycin, 0.5 g orally every 6 h for four doses. The best regimen for preventing enterococcal endocarditis is ampicillin plus gentamicin. Ampicillin, 1 g, plus gentamicin, 1.5 mg/kg (not over 80 mg), should be given intramuscularly or intravenously 30 to 60 min before the procedure, and both agents should be repeated every 8 h for two doses. Penicillin-allergic patients should receive vancomycin, 1.0 g intravenously, and streptomycin, 1.0 g intramuscularly, 30 to 60 min before the procedure; administration of both agents is repeated 12 h later. Although not proved definitively, antistaphylococcal prophylaxis may be indicated during surgery associated with implantation of prosthetic heart valves, intracardiac materials, or vascular prostheses. Cephalothin or cefazolin, 1.0 g intravenously, every 4 to 6 h should be given 30 min prior to surgery and continued no longer than 72 h.

The prophylactic doses of penicillin used to prevent group A streptococcal infection and recurrent rheumatic fever will not prevent bacterial endocarditis. The dose of benzathine penicillin given for rheumatic fever prophylaxis does not predispose to bacterial endocarditis caused by penicillin-resistant microorganisms, whereas oral penicillin V does promote the emergence of penicillin-resistant oral flora. All high-risk patients should be cautioned to maintain a high level of oral hygiene, avoid the use of a water jet in the mouth, and seek prompt treatment of infections that occur at any site.

TREATMENT The best treatment of infective endocarditis is assured when treatment is begun early in the illness, when an effective *bactericidal* antimicrobial agent is selected, and when treatment is continued over a relatively long period of time.

Selection of the most effective antibiotic for treatment of infective endocarditis depends on the sensitivity of the infecting microorganism. When bacteremia is not demonstrated, selection of the therapeutic agent depends on predicting the most probable infecting bacteria and their probable antibiotic sensitivity.

Infective endocarditis in young persons with rheumatic or congenital disease is most often due to the viridans streptococci. These microorganisms are usually very sensitive to penicillin G (minimum inhibitory concentration $\leq 0.1\ \mu g/ml$). Administration of aqueous penicillin G 10 to 20 million units per day intravenously in divided doses at 4-h intervals or 1.2 million units of procaine penicillin intramuscularly at 6- or 12-h intervals to these patients is usually effective in eliminating the infection when therapy is continued for 4 weeks. The penicillin should be given parenterally for 2 weeks but for the second 2 weeks may be given orally (penicillin V if adequate serum levels are assured by a peak serum bactericidal titer of more than 1:8 dilution). There is a synergistic effect of streptomycin with penicillin on viridans streptococci. If streptomycin in a dose of 0.5 g twice a day is administered in addition to penicillin, then therapy of 2 weeks' duration is sufficient.

Infective endocarditis in older men and in women after abortion or endometritis is often due to enterococci (*Streptococcus fecalis, S. faecium, S. durans*). These microorganisms are relatively resistant to penicillin alone. Enterococci should be differentiated from group D nonenterococcal organisms (*S. bovis*) that are susceptible to penicillin alone. The combination of penicillin with gentamicin is synergistic against the enterococcus, and the administration of these two antibiotics together is the treatment of choice in the infection. Penicillin G should be given parenterally in a dose of 15 to 24 million units per day, together with gentamicin in a dose of 3 to 5 mg/kg per day divided into three doses. Ampicillin, in a dosage of 8 to 12 g per day, may be substituted for penicillin G. Streptomycin, 1 g intramuscularly every 12 h for 2 weeks followed by 0.5 g every 12 h for 2 weeks, may be substituted for gentamicin if high-level streptomycin resistance ($\geq$ 2000 μg/ml) is not present. Treatment should be continued for a minimum of 4 weeks. Adjustment of the gentamicin and streptomycin dosage may be necessary in renal insufficiency, or if therapeutic serum levels are not attained.

Penicillin G, 6 to 12 million units a day given parenterally, is satisfactory for treatment of pneumococcal and group A streptococcal endocarditis. Treatment should be continued for 4 weeks. Penicillinase-resistant penicillin analogues should be used in the initial treatment of staphylococcal endocarditis because of the high probability that the infection is due to a penicillin-resistant organism. Nafcillin should be given intravenously in a dose of 12 g per day in divided doses at 4-h intervals in 50-ml volumes injected over 20 to 30 min. Oxacillin, methicillin, cephalothin, cefazolin, 1 to 2 g intravenously every 6 h, or vancomycin, 0.5 g intravenously every 6 h, may be administered in lieu of nafcillin. The addition of gentamicin to a penicillinase-resistant penicillin or cephalosporin results in enhanced staphylococcal killing in vitro and may improve the clinical response in some patients. If the staphylococcus is found to be sensitive to penicillin G, this antibiotic should be given rather than methicillin, in a dose of 16 to 24 million units per day. Treatment should be continued for at least 4 weeks. In staphylococcal endocarditis in particular, attention must be given to possible metastatic abscesses requiring surgical drainage.

Prosthetic valve infections should be treated for 6 to 8 weeks. *Staphylococcus epidermidis* or *Corynebacterium* spp. frequently are sensitive only to vancomycin and should be treated with vancomycin combined with rifampin 300 mg orally every 12 h. Culture-negative prosthetic valve infections should be treated with vancomycin plus streptomycin. This regimen should be effective against most streptococcal, enterococcal, staphylococcal, and corynebacterium infections. Parenteral drug addicts with culture-negative endocarditis should be treated with a semisynthetic penicillinase-resistant penicillin in combination with penicillin G or ampicillin and gentamicin or tobramycin. Patients with culture-negative endocarditis who are neither drug addicts nor prosthetic valve recipients should be treated as though they had enterococcal endocarditis.

In patients allergic to penicillin, the alternative drugs are cephalothin, cefazolin, and vancomycin. Cephalosporins should be administered with caution to patients who have shown severe immediate hypersensitivity reactions to penicillin. Skin testing with major and minor penicillin antigens may be used to guide antimicrobial selection in patients with an unclear or positive past history of penicillin allergy.

In patients allergic to penicillin, the alternative drugs are cephalothin, cefazolin, and vancomycin. Vancomycin and gentamicin should be administered to penicillin-allergic patients with enterococcal endocarditis. If an allergic reaction to penicillin develops during the course of therapy, antihistamines or corticosteroids may be used to alleviate the manifestations of the reaction.

Usually fever begins to disappear within 3 to 7 days after the start of treatment of infective endocarditis. Embolic complications of the disease, heart failure, and infection with resistant microorganisms, however, may delay defervescence. Drug fever or phlebitis may occasionally supervene and complicate the febrile course. Cessation of all therapy for 72 h is not hazardous and may identify such a drug reaction readily. Sterile emboli or late valve rupture occurs occasionally up to 12 months after cessation of therapy.

Many patients with arteriovenous fistulas, valve ring abscess, recurrent embolization, endocarditis produced by resistant organisms, or infected cardiac prostheses require surgical intervention before the infection can be controlled. In addition, early valve replacement should be considered in patients who develop congestive heart failure associated with marked

valvular damage (particularly aortic or mitral regurgitation) as a consequence of bacterial endocarditis. Valve replacement has been lifesaving and must be undertaken before intractable heart failure ensues.

Fungal endocarditis is usually fatal. However, a few survivors have been reported after surgical debridement and replacement of the infected valve combined with amphotericin B therapy.

When infective endocarditis recurs, it usually develops within 4 weeks after treatment is terminated. Reinstitution of antibiotic therapy is required, but the sensitivity of the microorganism to the antibiotic must be reevaluated. Relapse may indicate inadequate or inappropriate therapy, or the need for surgical intervention. Recrudescence of infective endocarditis more than 6 weeks after cessation of treatment usually connotes a new infection.

REFERENCES

DINUBILE MJ: Surgery in active endocarditis. Ann Intern Med 96:650, 1982

DUMA RJ (ed): *Infections of Prosthetic Heart Valves and Vascular Grafts.* Baltimore, University Park Press, 1977

FREEDMAN LR: Endocarditis updated. Dis Mon, vol 26, December 1979

KAPLAN EL et al: Prevention of bacterial endocarditis. Circulation 56:139A, 1977

———, TARANTA AV (eds): *Infective Endocarditis: An American Heart Association Symposium*, Monograph 52. Dallas, American Heart Association, 1977

KARCHMER AW et al: Late prosthetic valve endocarditis. Am J Med 64:199, 1978

KAYE D (ed): *Infective Endocarditis.* Baltimore, University Park Press, 1976

MELVIN ET et al: Noninvasive methods for detection of valve vegetations in infective endocarditis. Am J Cardiol 47:271, 1981

PETERSDORF RG: Prophylaxis of bacterial endocarditis: Prudent caution or microbial overkill. Am J Med 65:220, 1978

ROY P et al: Spectrum of echocardiographic findings in bacterial endocarditis. Circulation 53:474, 1976

SANDE MA, SCHELD WM: Combination therapy of bacterial endocarditis. Ann Intern Med 92:390, 1980

SIPES JN et al: Prophylaxis of infective endocarditis: A re-evaluation. Annu Rev Med 28:371, 1977

VON REYN CF et al: Infective endocarditis: An analysis based on strict case definitions. Ann Intern Med 94:505, 1981

WILSON WR et al: Prosthetic valve endocarditis. Ann Intern Med 82:751, 1975

——— : Short term therapy for streptococcal infective endocarditis. JAMA 245:360, 1981

260
ISCHEMIC HEART DISEASE

EUGENE BRAUNWALD
PETER F. COHN

Ischemia refers to oxygen deprivation resulting from reduced perfusion. The term *ischemic heart disease* defines a disease spectrum of diverse etiology, with the common factor being an imbalance between myocardial oxygen supply and demand. This imbalance is usually related to either an absolute reduction in coronary blood flow or an inability to increase coronary blood flow relative to the needs of the heart, and is most often due to atherosclerotic obstruction of large coronary arteries. The myocardium can be rendered ischemic also by nonatheromatous coronary obstructive lesions, such as embolism, coronary ostial stenosis associated with luetic aortitis, coronary artery spasm, or very uncommonly an arteritis of the coronary vessels. Congenital abnormalities of the coronary circulation, especially anomalous origin of the left coronary artery from the pulmonary trunk, may cause myocardial ischemia in the infant or child and, rarely, in the adult. The imbalance between myocardial oxygen supply and demand is less commonly due to an increase in myocardial oxygen demands exceeding the supply capabilities of a normal coronary circulation, as occurs in severe myocardial hypertrophy especially when aortic stenosis is present. Myocardial ischemia may also occur when the oxygen-carrying capacity of the blood is reduced, as in anemia or the presence of carboxyhemoglobin, or as a consequence of an inadequate perfusion pressure due to hypotension of any cause. Not infrequently, two or more causes of ischemia can be identified in the same patient, i.e., the combination of left ventricular hypertrophy secondary to hypertension or aortic stenosis and reduced myocardial blood flow consequent to coronary atherosclerosis.

The location of atherosclerotic lesions in the coronary circulation and the degree of luminal narrowing they cause determine whether the lesions will bring about significant and clinically evident ischemia. Luminal narrowing is important because flow through a tubular conduit varies with the fourth power of the radius if other conditions are kept constant. Location is important because it relates to the mass of myocardium perfused by the vessel in question. Thus, occlusive disease of the proximal left anterior descending artery jeopardizes the septum and anterior left ventricular free wall, whereas a similar lesion in a distal branch of this vessel compromises the flow of a lesser mass of myocardium. The state of the collateral circulation also helps determine whether ischemic heart disease develops as a consequence of coronary atherosclerosis. Although all the factors responsible for collateral development and their influence on the course of the disease remain uncertain, it appears that the potential for the development of collaterals is present in many and possibly all hearts, but that these channels do not develop sufficiently to be visualized until the stimulus of ischemia is manifest.

Asymptomatic coronary arteriosclerosis develops at an unknown rate and is detected only when death occurs from another cause, such as trauma, or when the coronary vessels are visualized angiographically (Chap. 251); the latter may be carried out in asymptomatic individuals when an exercise electrocardiogram or thallium 201 scan performed for screening purposes shows evidence of "silent" myocardial ischemia. The disease begins early in life, as evidenced by the relatively frequent finding of significant obstructive lesions in the coronary arteries of young men killed in war. The symptomatic phase presents most commonly as angina pectoris, acute myocardial infarction (Chap. 261), or sudden death; the latter presumably is due to ventricular arrhythmia (Chap. 30). Alternatively, patients may present with a symptom complex that shares features of both acute myocardial infarction and angina and is termed *unstable angina* or the *intermediate syndrome* (Chap. 261). A less common presentation is with arrhythmias, generally ventricular electrical instability, of sufficient severity to cause symptoms in the absence of angina or infarction. Frequently, however, these arrhythmias do not result in symptoms, and the tentative diagnosis of ischemic heart disease is suggested only when arrhythmia is discovered on a routine physical examination or exercise testing.

Once in the symptomatic phase, the patient may remain symptomatic with either a stable or progressive course, return to the asymptomatic stage, or die suddenly. The average mortality rate following entry into the symptomatic phase of ischemic heart disease is 4 percent per year irrespective of whether the initial event is the development of angina pectoris or a myocardial infarction from which the patient has recovered.

The two principal prognostic indicators are the *state of function of the left ventricle* and the *extent of coronary artery disease.* Patients with compromised ventricular function are at increased risk. Compromised function may be noted by symptoms of congestive heart failure, roentgenographic evidence of cardiac enlargement, and/or angiographic evidence of altered cardiac performance (reduced ejection fraction, elevated left ventricular end-diastolic volume, and, perhaps most importantly, elevated left ventricular end-systolic volume). The mortality rates in patients with normal left ventricular function and disease in all three or in two of the three major coronary arteries average 11 and 8 percent per year, respectively, as compared with 2 percent per year in patients with single-vessel involvement. In patients with obstruction in the left main coronary artery, mortality averages 15 percent. With any degree of coronary artery obstruction the mortality is correspondingly elevated in patients with impaired left ventricular function. Within each angiographic class, additional prognostic subsets have also been defined. For example, patients with obstructive lesions isolated to a single artery segregate into different mortality groups. Lesions isolated to the proximal left anterior descending coronary artery appear to carry a greater risk than those to the right or left circumflex vessels. Data concerning mortality in patients with specific coronary arterial lesions have generally been obtained from patients with symptomatic disease. Prognosis of asymptomatic individuals with similar anatomic abnormalities is not well established, but preliminary data suggest that it may be better than in symptomatic patients. High-grade ventricular ectopic activity is yet another index of increased risk, especially in patients with impaired left ventricular function (Chap. 30).

It is useful to conceptualize coronary atherosclerosis as a process that destroys myocardial tissue at an unpredictable rate, thus reducing cardiac reserve. The greater the degree of muscle cell death at any point in time, the less the cardiac reserve, the less the ability to tolerate additional myocardial damage, and therefore the higher the expected mortality rate. In this light, the various indexes of increased risk, such as an abnormal electrocardiogram and left ventricular failure, should be taken as evidence of advanced degrees of myocardial cell death.

The pathogenesis of myocardial infarction remains a matter of debate. It is clear that the simplistic concept of thrombosis superimposed on an atheroma or of hemorrhage into an atheromatous lesion is not adequate in patients with subendocardial infarcts. Severe atheromatous disease and thrombosis are usually present in patients with transmural infarcts. Further complicating any simplistic explanation of the pathogenesis of myocardial infarction are recent arteriographic studies documenting normal coronary anatomy in a small percentage of patients with evidence of remote acute myocardial infarction. Many investigators consider these to be examples of a recanalized embolus or a thrombus that has lysed.

Variant (Prinzmetal's) angina (see "Angina Pectoris" below) has been demonstrated to result from spasm of a large coronary artery. Coronary artery spasm may also be an important contributing factor in some instances of typical angina pectoris and myocardial infarction. While the stimulus for such spasm remains unclear, it is most likely related to a combination of neural and chemical factors, including increased platelet aggregation with subsequent release of vasoconstrictor agents, such as thromboxane A_2 (Chap. 88).

PREVENTION

See Chap. 266.

PATHOPHYSIOLOGY

CORONARY CIRCULATION Under basal conditions, the heart extracts a high and relatively fixed percentage of the oxygen from coronary arterial blood. Since increased oxygen extraction is thus not possible, augmented myocardial oxygen demands must be met by increases in coronary blood flow. Blood flow in the coronary bed, as in other vascular beds, is related directly to coronary perfusion pressure and inversely to vascular resistance. Since arterial pressure does not increase sufficiently or at all during a stress, such as exercise, variation in the resistance vessels of the coronary bed is the mechanism by which coronary flow, and thus oxygen supply, are regulated. The immense dilatory reserve of the normal coronary circulation is proved by the observation that patients without coronary disease may tolerate prolonged periods of hypotension or severe anemia without sustaining ischemic myocardial damage.

Coronary vascular resistance is mediated at the level of the coronary arterioles, while the large coronary arteries located on the epicardium serve more of a conduit function. Pathological studies have defined the large conduit vessels as the major sites of atherosclerosis, and arteriographic studies have shown them to be the site of spasm in vasospastic angina. In animal experiments it has been shown that when there is a significant narrowing of the lumen of the conduit vessel (i.e., greater than 80 percent) by the atherosclerotic process, flow through the vessel decreases in the basal state, and a pressure gradient across the obstruction develops. In response to the reduction in pressure distal to the obstruction, resistance vessels at this site dilate in order to maintain flow. In this manner, the dilatory reserve of the resistance coronary vessels is progressively diminished by the advancing atherosclerotic process. As stenotic lesions become critical, the resistance vessels become permanently dilated in order to maintain basal flow, thus explaining the inability of patients with ischemic heart disease to augment coronary flow appropriately in response to stress. The observation that myocardial infarction without coronary occlusion occurs most commonly in the presence of severe coronary artery disease is explained by the lack of dilatory reserve; i.e., if myocardial oxygen demands are augmented in excess of supply capability, infarction will occur in the absence of total obstruction once a persistent discrepancy develops between oxygen supply and demand. In addition, the existence of pressure gradients across stenotic sections of coronary vessels explains the inability of patients with coronary artery disease to tolerate hypotension. In the presence of such obstruction, coronary flow may decline precipitously as perfusion pressure drops, despite dilatation of the resistance vessels.

EFFECTS OF ISCHEMIA The state of inadequate myocardial oxygenation induced by the atherosclerotic process results in abnormalities of the biochemical, electrical, and mechanical function of the heart. One biochemical response to ischemia which is used to evaluate the adequacy of myocardial perfusion relates to the aerobic metabolism of the normal heart; i.e., in the nonischemic heart, glucose and glycogen are oxidized completely to CO_2 and H_2O, and intermediary metabolites of carbohydrate breakdown such as lactate neither accumulate in the myocardium nor appear in coronary sinus blood. Under conditions of impaired oxygenation, anaerobic patterns of metabolism are utilized and lactate is formed and is eventually released into coronary sinus blood. Myocardial lactate production is thus an index of ischemia. Unfortunately, the use of coronary arteriovenous lactate analysis is of limited clinical value, since the blood sample obtained in the coronary sinus represents *mixed* coronary venous blood, and regional increases of lactate in coronary venous blood draining a small ischemic area may thus escape detection.

Ischemia alters the electrical properties of the heart, the most characteristic early changes in the electrocardiogram being those of the repolarization process, as evidenced by inversion of T waves and later by displacement of the ST segment (Chap. 249). ST-segment shifts are usually seen during episodes of angina pectoris and also in the early stages of myocardial infarction. Another important consequence of myocardial ischemia is electrical instability, leading sometimes to ventricular tachycardia and even ventricular fibrillation. Most patients who die suddenly from ischemic heart disease do so from one of these malignant ventricular arrhythmias (Chap. 30).

The contractile function of ischemic myocardium is markedly impaired. Transient ischemia, as occurs with angina pectoris, induces a reversible depression of myocardial function. Prolonged ischemia and the resultant process of infarction create both necrosis and an area of ischemia in tissue adjacent to the necrotic core. The necrosis causes an irreversible loss of contractile function with eventual scar formation, while the impaired contractility of the ischemic zone remains potentially reversible. This ischemic zone may progress to necrosis or revert to a normal state, depending upon the interaction of numerous factors which are as yet only partially defined. The potential for worsening and/or improvement in the ischemic zone explains why abnormalities of contractile function noted in the early phase of acute infarction are not static and may either progress or resolve. In addition to impairing left ventricular systolic function and thereby interfering with the volume of blood ejected, ischemia also interferes with ventricular relaxation and filling, thereby elevating ventricular diastolic pressure, causing a rise in pulmonary capillary pressure and pulmonary congestion.

Coronary atherosclerosis is a regional process which causes nonuniform ischemia. This results in an asymmetric distribution of disordered contractility, which in turn alters the symmetry and synchrony of ventricular contraction and reduces the efficiency of myocardial pump function. When the ischemic process involves the papillary muscles and other segments of myocardium responsible for the normal function of the mitral valve, mitral regurgitation may also occur. The ischemic or infarcted portion of myocardium may bulge outward (myocardial dyskinesis) when the normal portion of the ventricle contracts, further reducing the effectiveness of ventricular systole.

ANGINA PECTORIS

Angina pectoris is a clinical syndrome resulting from transient myocardial ischemia. The various diseases that result in myocardial ischemia as well as the numerous pain syndromes that may be confused with angina are discussed in Chap. 4. Approximately four-fifths of all patients with angina pectoris are men, and an even larger fraction of those younger than 50 years of age are men. The typical patient is in his fifties or early sixties and seeks medical advice because of chest discomfort. The patient commonly declines to apply the word *pain* to his chest symptoms, may have difficulty describing the sensation, and will usually select words such as heaviness, pressure, smothering, tightness, choking, or squeezing. The typical discomfort is substernal in location, but other sites are also commonly involved (see below). The most important diagnostic feature of angina pectoris is its relation to exertion or emotion and its relief by rest. The discomfort comes on during physical or emotional stress, anger, fright, hurrying, or sexual activity.

The threshold for the development of angina varies with the time of day more than from day to day. The typical patient may have to stop at exactly the same spot on his way to work each morning, yet by midday he may be able to cover many times that distance without discomfort. Symptoms which develop soon after arising are common, and the patient may not be able to shave without stopping; yet he may perform moderately heavy manual labor later in the day after he has "warmed up."

Manual chores which have been performed for many years may be well tolerated, whereas unfamiliar tasks requiring comparable effort may cause angina. This pattern is commonly observed in a laborer who is asymptomatic at work but notices chest discomfort with household or recreational activities. Relatively nonstressful activities which require the hands to be held at or above the level of the head (combing hair, shaving) frequently cause symptoms in patients who are asymptomatic while performing more strenuous chores which do not require elevation of the arms. This phenomenon is thought to be related to the increased total body oxygen requirements associated with continuous contraction of the antigravity muscles of the arms and shoulder girdles. The pain may occur during or after eating. Exposure to cold temperature or to wind may accentuate or precipitate the symptoms. Coronary spasm may play a particularly important role in patients in whom the anginal threshold varies considerably.

Variation in the location and character of the discomfort may occur, and so angina pectoris should not be ruled out just because the location of the pain is atypical, especially if there is a strong relation to exertion. Myocardial ischemia may be characterized by pain in the neck, jaw, throat, back, shoulder, abdomen, or arm, with no symptoms in the chest. Radiation to the arms, particularly the ulnar aspect of the left arm, is common in typical angina, and sometimes the only discomfort may be in the arms or wrists, where it is often described as numbness or heaviness. Sharp pains of brief duration and prolonged dull aches localized to the left submammary area are rarely due to myocardial ischemia, but the words *knife-like* and *cutting* are occasionally utilized to describe angina.

The term *angina decubitus* has been applied to the variant of angina pectoris which develops while the patient is in the recumbent position. The patient may report that he is awakened at night by a sensation which is similar to his exertional pain. Angina decubitus may resemble paroxysmal nocturnal dyspnea, and dyspnea actually often accompanies the chest discomfort. It is postulated, but not proved, that the pathophysiology is also similar and that angina decubitus is a form of left ventricular failure precipitated by the expansion of the intrathoracic blood volume which occurs with recumbency and which may increase myocardial oxygen requirements. Elevation of systemic arterial blood pressure has been demonstrated to precede attacks of pain in some instances and may be another precipitating factor; in other patients hypertension follows, and occurs as a consequence of angina. Dreaming has also been implicated in the pathogenesis of angina decubitus. In those instances of angina decubitus in which an increase in myocardial oxygen requirements does not precede angina, coronary spasm is probably the precipitating cause.

Variant angina, or *Prinzmetal's angina,* is characterized by the development of the anginal syndrome, usually at rest, and it may be accompanied by ventricular arrhythmias. Characteristically the electrocardiogram demonstrates ST-segment *elevations* during the episodes of pain, in contrast to the more characteristic ST-segment depression of the typical effort angina syndrome. Variant angina usually causes transmural ischemia, often due to spasm of one of the major epicardial coronary arteries. Varying degrees of atherosclerotic obstruction, usually just proximal to the site of spasm, occur in approximately two-thirds of patients with variant angina.

PHYSICAL EXAMINATION Although patients are often overweight and of mesomorphic habitus, there are many exceptions to this traditionally accepted description. Evidence of atherosclerosis may be present in vessels other than the coronary arteries; the peripheral vessels may be thickened on palpation, there may be bruits over the carotid arteries, and the fundi may show an increased light reflex and arteriovenous nicking. Physical findings are often normal in the patient with angina pectoris between episodes, but transient abnormalities of contractile function induced by the ischemia associated with angina pectoris may result in transient auscultatory and palpatory evidence of ventricular dysfunction which helps to establish the diagnosis. These include third and fourth heart sounds (Chap. 248). Frequently, an asymmetric contraction pattern, localized lack of contraction, or paradoxical contraction (akinesis or dyskinesis) may be palpated as a transient ectopic left ventricular impulse. The third and fourth sounds and aneurysmal lift are best appreciated with the patient in the left lateral decubitus position. Another manifestation of ischemia is dysfunction of the papillary muscles, which may be reflected in a late systolic murmur of mitral regurgitation. The transient arterial hypertension induced by isometric handgrip may cause a previously undetectable murmur of mitral regurgitation associated with papillary muscle dysfunction to become detectable. While this maneuver is useful in the evaluation of patients with stable disease, acute induced hypertension may be hazardous during acute myocardial infarction or during an episode of angina pectoris. In order to determine whether left ventricular outflow tract obstruction plays a role in the etiology of the anginal syndrome, auscultatory evidence of aortic valve disease (Chap. 258) or hypertrophic cardiomyopathy (Chap. 266) should be sought.

Physical examination is also valuable in detecting evidence of a systemic disease, a metabolic state or risk factor which predisposes to coronary atherosclerosis. For example, systemic hypertension is a finding of great significance because it accelerates the atherosclerotic process and is amenable to treatment. Xanthelasma and xanthoma may indicate abnormalities of lipid metabolism which may be associated with an increased incidence of coronary atherosclerosis (Chaps. 103 and 266). Nicotine stains on the fingertips suggest prolonged, excessive smoking.

LABORATORY EXAMINATION The tentative diagnosis of ischemic heart disease may frequently be made by means of the history, but in the absence of a history of documented infarction, the definitive diagnosis requires laboratory confirmation. Laboratory evaluation of all patients with suspected or documented coronary disease should include an electrocardiogram at rest and chest roentgenogram. When a diagnosis cannot be established with these techniques, the indicated procedure is electrocardiographic stress testing, which in certain instances is followed by radionuclide studies (thallium 201 perfusion scans, Chap. 250) and/or coronary arteriography. A positive response to a therapeutic trial of nitroglycerin is also helpful in supporting the diagnosis of angina pectoris.

Electrocardiogram The electrocardiogram may establish the diagnosis of ischemic heart disease if characteristic changes are present. The absence of abnormalities, however, by no means excludes the diagnosis. The 12-lead electrocardiogram recorded at rest and in the absence of pain is normal in approximately one-half of patients with typical angina pectoris and arteriographically demonstrable coronary atherosclerosis. The most definite and diagnostic electrocardiographic changes are those of old myocardial infarction (Chap. 249). The electrocardiographic diagnosis of myocardial infarction can be made with greater certainty when a previously normal electrocardiogram can be used as a reference. In some instances the vectorcardiogram may be helpful as well.

T-wave changes are more difficult to interpret as evidence of ischemic heart disease. Inverted T waves may appear as the only manifestation of ischemic heart disease, but they may also occur in other conditions which may be associated with chest pain, such as pericarditis, myocarditis, and abnormalities of vasoregulation.

Great diagnostic significance can be placed upon ST-segment and T-wave changes which occur *during* attacks of pain and disappear thereafter. The most characteristic change is displacement of the ST segment, with or without T-wave inversion, which is similar in every way to that induced during the course of an exercise test. Long-term monitoring (ambulatory electrocardiography) may be useful in documenting the association of ECG changes and chest pain. The ST segments are usually depressed but rarely may be strikingly elevated, as in the early stages of myocardial infarction, or in variant (Prinzmetal's) angina.

Chest roentgenogram The chest roentgenogram may aid in the diagnosis of ischemic heart disease when a ventricular aneurysm or calcification in a coronary artery is identified. Cardiac enlargement is a nonspecific finding, but in patients with ischemic heart disease it usually reflects the presence of a large quantity of infarcted myocardium.

Stress testing Two general classes of stress test have been defined for the evaluation of cardiac function. One, the measurement of cardiac output and intraventricular pressure, by means of cardiac catheterization or the ejection fraction by radionuclide or radiographic ventriculography, assesses the adequacy and/or reserve of myocardial pump function. Stress tests of this type are of little value in establishing the diagnosis of ischemic heart disease since many forms of heart disease other than ischemic heart disease may impair ventricular function.

The second form measures the capability of the coronary circulation to augment coronary blood flow in response to increased myocardial oxygen demands. Although such evaluation may be occasionally obtained with catheterization techniques (coronary arteriovenous lactate analysis, atrial pacing), the application of invasive testing is obviously limited. The ideal test for application to a large number of patients would employ a form of stress that augments myocardial oxygen demands in a safe and reproducible fashion and in the presence of ischemic heart disease results in an easily observable and specific alteration of cardiovascular function. At the present time electrocardiographic stress testing is the best approximation of this ideal because electrocardiographic ST-segment displacement is a characteristic response to ischemia and occurs during and immediately following an exercise stress. Unfortunately, certain known factors (K^+, digitalis), and many as yet undefined factors, affect ST-segment morphology; therefore ST-segment depression is not specific for ischemia (i.e., false-positive responses may occur). Similarly, false-negative responses are known to occur and may be due to the complex geometry of the heart and the fact that certain areas of the heart are electrically silent. These limitations notwithstanding, the realization that ST-segment depression is a clinically useful, readily available index of ischemia has prompted the development of standardized exercise tests which use ST-segment depression as the end point to define ischemia.

The ischemic ST-segment response is generally defined as a flat depression of the ST segment 0.1 mV below the base line, i.e., the PR segment, lasting more than 0.08 s. The depression is of the "square-wave" or "plateau" type and is flat or slopes downward (unlike the ST-segment depression that slopes upward, which is referred to as a *junctional change* and does not constitute a positive test result unless the slope is shallow). T-wave abnormalities, ventricular arrhythmias, and conduction disturbances may develop with exercise but do not constitute certain evidence of myocardial ischemia. If 0.1 mV or more ST-segment depression is required before the test is considered to be positive, the percentage of false-positive results will be less than 10 percent, and only about 15 percent of patients with severe coronary atherosclerosis will have negative test results; these are usually patients with only single-vessel disease. If the threshold of positivity is set at 0.05 mV, there will be more false-positive tests and fewer false-negative ones.

The duration of exercise, presence of anginal symptoms, heart rate, and blood pressure response are also important in evaluating the results of a stress electrocardiogram. Thus, false-positive results are *least* likely in those patients who demonstrate ST-segment depression *early* in the test, in whom the changes persist for relatively long periods ($>$ 5 min) following cessation of exercise, who experience typical angina during the test, or who have only minimal increases in heart rate and blood pressure (compared with the control values) when the ECG changes occur. It is also important to emphasize that, according to Bayes' theorem, the probability that coronary artery disease exists in the population under study must be considered along with the diagnostic features of the test in the interpretation of a positive or negative exercise test result. For example, on the basis of arteriographic studies, patients with typical angina, who have not had an exercise electrocardiogram, have a high (approximately 90 percent) probability of demonstrating coronary artery disease, patients with atypical angina have a 50 percent probability, patients with chest pain deemed unlikely to be angina about a 10 percent probability, and asymptomatic middle-aged males about a 5 percent probability. A positive exercise result indicates that the likelihood of coronary artery disease is 98 percent in patients with typical angina, 88 percent in patients with atypical pain, 44 percent in patients with nonanginal chest pain, and only 33 percent in asymptomatic persons.

Approximately 10 percent of patients with a positive test will have ST-segment changes only *during* exercise; hence, the sensitivity of the test is improved by monitoring during, in addition to immediately after, exercise. Exercise testing is safer with in-exercise monitoring because ST-segment changes or arrhythmias may develop before pain or other symptoms occur (or even in the absence of symptoms) and the stress can be discontinued before severe ischemia develops. Multiple leads should be recorded, and precordial leads should be included, because one-third of patients with a positive test will have changes only in one lead, most likely V_5 or V_6.

Three formats of stress testing are commonly used; tests with standardized external workloads, tests which are standardized by heart rate response, and tests designed to reach the maximal possible exercise load. The two-step system of exercise developed by Master is an example of the first variety. The second and third varieties employ a treadmill or bicycle and differ only with respect to the method of determining the end point of the exercise. In the *target heart rate* test, exercise is continued until the patient attains 80 to 90 percent of his predicted maximum heart rate, which can be obtained from available tables. In the *maximal exercise* test, exercise is progressively increased until maximal workload is attained. Both tests are discontinued at a lower level of work if the patient develops chest pain, signs of cerebral insufficiency, fall in blood pressure, or significant electrocardiographic changes. The percentage of positive tests in a population of patients with angina and arteriographically proven coronary atherosclerosis is greater with the graded exercise methods (85 to 90 percent) than with the tests standardized on the basis of external workload (double two-step test). A physician must be in attendance throughout the exercise test to observe the patient, to evaluate the in-exercise ECG and in-exercise blood pressure recordings, and to decide whether the testing should continue. The risk of an exercise test is small but real, being estimated at approximately one fatality and two nonfatal complications per 10,000 tests. The test is probably unusually hazardous and hence contraindicated in patients with unstable angina pectoris and patients who have suffered acute myocardial infarction during the preceding few weeks. However, in the latter situation, *modified* exercise tests have been used (for prognostic purposes) with little risk. Combining the exercise test with myocardial perfusion imaging (using thallium 201, for example) has been demonstrated to improve its diagnostic accuracy even further.

Other forms of stress testing have been developed for use in the recumbent subject during the course of cardiac catheterization and angiography. Under these circumstances the heart can be stressed by having the patient perform leg exercise with a bicycle device, or isometric handgrips by squeezing an ergometer. Probably the most widely used form of stress at catheterization is the pacing stress test, in which the heart rate is increased by electrical pacing with a pacing catheter in the right atrium. Pacing-induced tachycardia increases the myocardial oxygen demands and hence produces ischemia in the patient with limited ability to increase myocardial blood flow in proportion to oxygen demands. Ischemia is manifested by the development of angina or ST-segment depressions on the electrocardiogram. One of the advantages of this form of stress is that it can be conducted on a recumbent subject, and therefore hemodynamic measurements can be made during the test.

Other noninvasive procedures Two types of noninvasive *radionuclide studies* discussed in Chap. 250 are helpful in diagnosing ischemic heart disease. The first is myocardial perfusion imaging with thallium 201 in which areas of underperfused myocardium can be identified in the basal state or during stress. The second type of study, the gated radioisotopic angiogram, can provide a measure of ventricular volumes and ejection fraction at rest and during exercise and permits identification of disorders of global left ventricular function and of localized wall motion. *Echocardiography,* particularly two-dimensional (cross-sectional) echocardiographic techniques, can also be used to evaluate regional left ventricular motion.

Coronary arteriography (see also Chap. 251) Coronary arteriography is the only method which can provide unequivocal diagnostic information concerning the presence or absence of coronary atherosclerosis in living patients. It also permits estimation of the severity of obstructive lesions which may be present. Opinion is nearly unanimous that arteriography is indicated in the following specific situations: (1) Patients with either chronic, stable angina pectoris or unstable angina (Chap. 261) who are refractory to medical treatment, and others who, on clinical grounds, are considered to be candidates for coronary bypass surgery, as discussed under "Operation" below. No uniform statement regarding the indications for arteriography in the evaluation and management of the patient with stable but unequivocal coronary disease and in the patient who has recovered from a recent myocardial infarction can be made at present. The uses of arteriography in such patients vary among physicians and among institutions and are predicated upon the local definition of "intractable angina" and the prevailing attitude toward the indications for coronary bypass operations. (2) Patients with a variety of diagnostic problems in which the diagnosis of ischemic heart disease needs to be established or ruled out.

Six groups of patients exemplify the latter situation. (1) Patients with negative exercise tests and a disabling chest pain syndrome. Included in this group are patients with a chest pain syndrome that the physician believes is *probably* not angina but who need unequivocal evidence either for psychological reasons or for personal decisions relating to career planning, family planning, insurability, etc. (2) Patients with frequent hospital admissions with the diagnosis of possible myocardial infarction which has never been substantiated and in which the diagnosis of coronary atherosclerosis has not been established. (3) Commercial and military flight personnel or others with careers in which more than individual safety is concerned and in whom there is a reasonable doubt as to the status of the coronary circulation. (4) Patients with severe aortic valve disease and angina pectoris in whom this symptom could be secondary to the valvular lesions and/or to coronary arteriosclerosis. (5) Young patients (under age 45) with angina or documented myocardial infarction in whom none of the risk factors associated with premature coronary disease can be identified and who may not have extensive coronary atherosclerosis and, hence, a more favorable prognosis. (6) Patients with severe congestive heart failure, postmyocardial infarction suspected to be related to papillary muscle dysfunction, ventricular septal defect, or discrete aneurysm rather than global ventricular dysfunction.

The diversity of opinion concerning the role of arteriography in the evaluation of patients with suspected or documented coronary disease is due to a combination of factors: (1) the continuing controversy over the role of coronary artery bypass surgery in the management of patients with ischemic heart disease, (2) the invasive nature of the test and the attendant small but distinct morbidity and mortality, and (3) the fact that the quality of study and complication rate vary widely. In general, the performance record of laboratories doing less than 100 studies per year, for example, is not comparable with that of more active laboratories.

MANAGEMENT OF ANGINA PECTORIS The term *management* is more appropriate than *treatment* with reference to angina pectoris because far more is required than the prescription of a drug or the recommendation of operation. The patient must be evaluated with particular reference to the interaction between his disease and life pattern. The physical and emotional stresses which precipitate pain and the pleasurable activities prohibited by angina must be identified. The management plan has six parts: (1) reassurance, (2) general measures directed toward preventing progression of ischemic heart disease, (3) definition of a protocol of activity designed to prevent and minimize the attacks of ischemia, (4) elimination of the possibility of coexistent disease capable of exacerbating angina, (5) institution of a program of drug therapy, and (6) definition of end points which will be indications for consideration of coronary bypass surgery.

Reassurance The patient must be made to realize that long, useful life is possible even though he has angina pectoris. A realistic explanation of the pathophysiology of the disease is worthwhile for the intelligent patient and can be used as a basis for the life plan which is to be described. It is usually not advisable to quote statistics, but the recital of case histories of persons in public life may be of great value.

General measures There is no definitive proof in humans that the lesions of coronary atherosclerosis can be made to regress, but extrapolation from animal experiments makes this appear likely. It is clear that certain factors accelerate the progression of these lesions. It seems reasonable, therefore, to make the reduction of these risk factors a keystone of treatment in all patients with coronary atherosclerosis. Ideal weight should be attained and maintained, hypertension treated if present, and cigarette smoking forbidden. It has been demonstrated that the cardiac mortality rate of individuals who have discontinued cigarette smoking for several years is the same as that for those who have never smoked. Thus, the facts do not support the excuse often offered by patients that it is too late to stop. Diabetes and the hyperlipidemias should be treated when they are present (Chap. 266). The patient should be encouraged to engage in steady dynamic exercise, such as walking; isometric exercise may be hazardous. The maintenance of good physical condition enables him to perform physical work more efficiently at a lower pulse rate and, therefore, reduces the frequency of anginal episodes. The patient in good physical condition also may have a better chance of surviving a myocardial infarction.

Activity Specific therapy depends on the elimination of the discrepancy between the demand of the heart muscle for oxygen and the ability of the coronary circulation to meet this demand. Most patients can be made to understand this fundamental concept and utilize it in the rational programming of activity. The patient must be taught that many tasks which usually cause pain may be accomplished without symptoms simply if the speed with which the task is performed is lessened. The patient must appreciate the variation in tolerance with the time of day and reduce activity requirements in the morning and immediately after meals; it is helpful sometimes to alter the eating pattern to one of smaller, more frequent meals. It may be necessary to counsel a change in employment or residence to avoid physical stress, but with the exception of the manual laborer it is usually possible for the patient to continue to function merely by allowing more time for the completion of each task. In some patients, anger and frustration may be the most important precipitating factors of myocardial ischemia. If these cannot be avoided, tranquilizing and sedative drugs should be prescribed. A treadmill exercise test to determine the approximate heart rate at which ischemic electrocardiographic changes or symptoms may occur may be of help in developing a specific exercise program. Ambulatory electrocardiography during daily activities may also be helpful in this regard.

Exacerbating conditions A number of illnesses, not primarily cardiac in nature, may either increase oxygen demand of or decrease oxygen supply to the myocardium and may precipitate or exacerbate angina pectoris. In the former category are hyperthyroidism (iatrogenic or spontaneous), hypertension, and anemia. Frequently, severe angina may be treated successfully by appropriate antihypertensive or antithyroid therapy. Decreased oxygen supply to the myocardium may be due to decreased oxygenation of the blood (intrinsic pulmonary disease, carboxyhemoglobin due to cigarette or cigar smoking) or decreased oxygen-carrying capacity (anemia).

Drug therapy NITRATES The mechanism of action of nitroglycerin, the most valuable drug in the treatment of angina pectoris, is discussed in Chap. 253. The activity of the agent depends upon its absorption, which is most rapid and complete through the mucous membranes. For this reason, nitroglycerin is administered sublingually, in tablets of 0.4 or 0.6 mg. Patients with angina should be instructed to take the medication to relieve an attack and also in anticipation of stress which is likely to induce angina. When the patient develops pain on exertion, he should cease activity and place a tablet under his tongue. The discomfort generally disappears more rapidly with nitroglycerin than would be expected if the drug were not administered. A flight of stairs, a walk up a hill, or sexual intercourse may produce pain consistently, but often the pain can be prevented by the anticipatory use of nitroglycerin. The value of this *prophylactic* use of the drug cannot be overemphasized.

The dose of nitroglycerin should be large enough to relieve pain but not large enough to produce a feeling of pulsating fullness in the head or a frank headache. The latter is the most common side effect of nitroglycerin and fortunately only rarely becomes disturbing at a dose required to relieve angina. Nitroglycerin deteriorates with exposure to air, moisture, and sunlight; therefore, if it produces neither relief of pain nor a headache, nor a slight sensation of burning at the sublingual site of absorption, the preparation may be inactive, and a fresh supply should be obtained. If the patient does not experience relief after the first dose of nitroglycerin, he may take a second, or even a third, but should be instructed not to continue to take the medication if the first few doses prove unsuccessful. If pain continues despite nitroglycerin, the patient should consult his physician, or report promptly to a hospital emergency room for evaluation for the possibility of an acute myocardial infarction (Chap. 261).

A diary or log of the time of occurrence of pains in relation to activity and other precipitating factors and nitroglycerin administration is often helpful to the physician attempting to tailor a management program for a new patient. A log may also be valuable in detecting a change in frequency and severity of pains which may herald an impending myocardial infarction. The stable patient may keep the log only intermittently or discontinue it, especially if the recording of pains focuses attention on the disease and has undesirable psychologic consequences.

Unfortunately, none of the long-acting nitrates is as effective as nitroglycerin in the relief of angina pectoris. However, several of these preparations are useful in prolonging the time interval between attacks and, hence, in reducing the amount of nitroglycerin which has to be taken as therapy for acute attacks. Preparations which are chewed or taken sublingually and therefore depend upon absorption through the mucous membranes are more effective than those that are simply swallowed. If one preparation is ineffective, another should be tried, as many patients find one preparation more effective than others. There is marked variation among patients in the dose required to produce a result, especially in the preparations to be swallowed, just as there is variation in the dose of nitroglycerin required for relief of an acute attack. The dosage of the long-acting agent should be increased gradually until either a therapeutic or a toxic effect is encountered. It may be taken on a regular basis every few hours by patients with frequent anginal attacks, in addition to being taken in anticipation of events known to provoke angina. Nitroglycerin ointment applied to the chest can be utilized as a slow-release preparation which is especially useful in the treatment of angina decubitus. An application of ointment at bedtime may give the patient a night's sleep which had not been possible before.

BETA-ADRENERGIC BLOCKADE The beta-adrenergic blocking agents represent a useful addition to the pharmacological treatment of angina pectoris (Chap. 73). The effects of beta-adrenergic blockade are described best as being the opposite of those of isoproterenol, an agent which stimulates the cardiac beta receptors. Isoproterenol produces an increase in heart rate, myocardial contractility, cardiac output, and myocardial oxygen consumption, associated with a decrease in total peripheral resistance, while the beta-adrenergic blocking agents prevent these changes. The effects of these drugs are most apparent during exercise; there is only a small decrease in cardiac output, heart rate, and arterial pressure at rest, but beta blockade reduces these variables more strikingly during exercise. Beta blockade is useful in angina pectoris because it reduces the myocardial oxygen consumption during exercise, rather than because of any direct effect on the coronary arteries. Thus, the goal of treatment with beta blockade is not only to decrease the resting heart rate but also to blunt the heart rate response to exercise. Propranolol is usually administered in an initial dose of 40 mg per day in four divided doses and is increased as tolerated to doses of 160 to 320 mg per day. Some patients require much higher doses, as much as 640 mg per day to obtain relief, however. A recently approved beta blocker, nadolol, offers the advantage of one-a-day dosage at 40 to 160 mg. If heart failure is present and/or there is cardiomegaly on radiographic examination, prior treatment with digitalis and a lower initial dose of these drugs are in order. Treatment is monitored by observation of the pulse rate and examination for signs of congestive failure: a resting pulse rate below 45 beats per minute and clinical evidence of impairment of left ventricular function are grounds for reduction of the dose or discontinuation of the drug.

CARDIAC GLYCOSIDES AND DIURETICS During an attack of angina pectoris, left ventricular systolic function becomes impaired, leading to an elevation of left ventricular end-diastolic volume; in addition the ischemic myocardium becomes stiffer in diastole, leading in turn to an elevation of ventricular end-diastolic and pulmonary vascular pressures. Agents useful in the treatment of congestive heart failure (Chap. 253) may also be valuable in the management of angina pectoris. A decrease in heart size reduces wall tension and hence myocardial oxygen requirements. However, if the heart is of normal size, the cardiac glycosides may aggravate angina by increasing contractility and hence the oxygen requirements. Oral diuretics are useful in many patients, and are especially valuable in the prevention of attacks of nocturnal angina and of angina at rest.

Newer forms of therapy Two new—and very different—forms of therapy for angina pectoris have recently been introduced. Calcium channel blockers (nifedipine, verapamil, diltiazem), widely used in Europe for several years, have recently been released in the United States. Because of their potent coronary vasodilatory properties, they have proved to be extremely useful in the treatment of Prinzmetal's angina and other forms of angina in which coronary spasm plays a role. In addition calcium channel blockers reduce myocardial oxygen demands by reducing arterial pressure and myocardial contractility and are useful in the treatment of chronic stable angina. They can be used together with beta blockers and nitrates and produce an additive effect. However, when such combination pharmacotherapy is employed, it is important to follow the patient carefully to ensure that hypotension and heart failure do not occur.

Nonoperative dilatation of coronary artery stenoses (percutaneous transluminal angioplasty) was developed in Switzerland by Grüntzig, using a special type of catheter. (This procedure has also been carried out successfully on the renal artery in patients with renovascular hypertension and on arteries in the lower extremities in patients with peripheral vascular disease associated with discrete lesions.) Patients with proximal single-vessel lesions that are soft and noncalcified are the best subjects for the procedure. However, it is estimated that only about 10 percent of candidates for bypass surgery are suitable for coronary artery dilatation.

Operation Numerous surgical procedures have been proposed for the treatment of ischemic heart disease, but the only procedure for which there is enthusiasm at present is the aortocoronary bypass graft. A section of vein, usually the saphenous, is used to form a connection between the aorta and the coronary artery distal to the obstructing lesion. Alternatively, the end of the mammary artery may be anastomosed to a coronary artery distal to the obstructing lesion. The operation is attractive because it represents a simple, direct mechanical attack on the obstructive lesions in the major coronary arteries.

Despite the controversy surrounding the indications for coronary bypass procedures and the problems enumerated above, certain areas of agreement can be identified: (1) The operation is relatively safe, with reported mortality rates as low as 1 percent in elective operations carried out by experienced surgical teams in patients with normal or near-normal left ventricular function. (2) Operative and postoperative mortality increases with left ventricular dysfunction and with surgical inexperience. (3) The graft procedure is surgically feasible, with patency rates of 70 to 85 percent reported at 2 to 3 years. Ultimate patency of the graft correlates with graft flow at the time of operation. The frequency of occlusion of grafts with flow rates exceeding 50 ml/min is very low. (4) Grafts that become occluded usually do so within 1 year. (5) When a bypass operation is performed on a partially occluded vessel, the probability of the partial obstruction in the native circulation proximal to the graft progressing to completion is increased. (6) Angina is abolished or unequivocally reduced in 85 percent of patients, although drug therapy may still be necessary in many. In most instances this relief can be attributed to increased blood flow to the ischemic myocardium, but this is not an adequate explanation in all patients. For example, relief of symptoms in the presence of occluded grafts could be due to infarction of the ischemic or angina-producing segment of the myocardium. The well-known placebo effect of operation is another possible mechanism for symptomatic improvement, but relief due to this mechanism would not be expected to be long-lasting. The fact that symptomatic relief is attributable to increased flow is supported by the arteriographic demonstration that in patients in whom pain has recurred abruptly, a graft is usually found to be occluded. (7) The inability to demonstrate ventriculographic or hemodynamic improvement of global ventricular function at rest after bypass operation in some patients is not surprising when it is recognized that improvement could not be expected in those patients who have normal ventricular function prior to operation or in patients with ventricular function impaired by previous infarction and scar or aneurysm formation. (8) Perioperative and intraoperative myocardial infarction occurs in 5 to 10 percent of patients. In most instances these infarcts are small. (9) The mortality rate of patients with unoperated left main coronary artery lesions is exceedingly high, and it appears that this rate can be reduced by operative intervention. There is also some evidence, although it is less clear-cut, that coronary bypass surgery can improve survival in patients in whom the major portion of residual viable myocardium is perfused by a single, critically narrowed vessel, and in whom heart failure or death might be precipitated by progression to occlusion of this obstructive lesion. (10) The mortality of patients with unoperated single-vessel disease limited either to the circumflex or right coronary arteries is low and does not differ greatly from that of age-matched controls without any disease.

The objectives of surgical treatment include the relief of symptoms and improvement of exercise tolerance, improvement of ventricular function, prevention of myocardial infarction, and improvement of life expectancy. The impressive ability of the procedure to relieve pain in most patients has been discussed above. Available data have not shown unequivocally that the procedure is capable of improving ventricular function at rest for the reasons discussed above, although myocardial function during exercise can be improved in many patients in whom exercise-induced ischemia is abolished. However, dramatic clinical improvement in ventricular function should not be anticipated from bypass surgery unless the surgical procedure includes the correction of some mechanical deficit (i.e., repair of mitral regurgitation or closure of ventricular septal defect or resection of aneurysm).

Major controversy as to indications for bypass graft operations exists because of lack of knowledge of the effect of the operation on the natural history of the disease. The largest group of potential candidates for operation consists of patients with two- or three-vessel disease and some disorder of left ventricular function. The only certain effect of operation in this group is the relief of symptoms. However, recent data from some centers reporting on 3- to 7-year follow-up of surgically treated patients with three-vessel disease using the life table analysis technique *suggest, but do not prove,* that bypass graft surgery favorably affects the natural history of coronary artery disease. This impression is strengthened when patients with similar degrees of angiographically proven disease who have been treated medically are used as controls. Whether the operation can forestall infarction or other complications of coronary artery disease is not known.

The considerable disagreement concerning the indications for, and/or results of, bypass surgery is attributable to a number of factors: (1) Although it is acknowledged that many different subsets of patients with coronary artery disease exist, the morbidity and mortality of patients in each group have not been defined. Therefore, it is difficult to estimate the natural history of patients not treated by operation, and attempts to define a beneficial effect of operation are thereby compromised. (2) Most life table analyses of patients with ischemic heart disease utilize patients in whom the diagnosis was proved by coronary arteriography. As a rule, only symptomatic patients are subjected to arteriography. Thus, the use of life table analyses to document the history of untreated coronary disease may represent a biased approach since untreated, asymptomatic, or mildly symptomatic patients with comparable findings on coronary arteriography are excluded. (3) The indications for surgical treatment and the effectiveness of operation vary among institutions and surgeons, thus rendering interinstitutional comparisons of limited value.

In view of these considerations, the role of this operation in the treatment of ischemic heart disease cannot be defined precisely at this time, and it is, therefore, possible to list indications only in terms of current practice. Three factors are usually considered in arriving at a decision to advise coronary bypass operations: (1) symptomatic status and age of the patient, (2) coronary anatomy as demonstrated by coronary arteriography, and (3) ventricular function as determined by left ventricular angiography and hemodynamics. Most patients advised to undergo operation are symptomatic, although the severity of the symptoms in surgical candidates varies widely among institutions. The ideal candidate has severe (80 percent or greater) obstructive lesions in the proximal portions of at least two of the three major coronary arteries. In some centers, patients with lesions in a single vessel are also considered to be operative candidates, particularly if they are severely symptomatic. This seems justified if the proximal left anterior descending rather than the right or circumflex coronary artery is the vessel involved. Patients with severe lesions in the left main coronary artery are at high risk and should have operative therapy if there are no contraindications. The best results are obtained in patients with normal ventricular function or at most a single area of impaired myocardial contractility.

Major controversy persists as to the indications for operation in the asymptomatic or mildly symptomatic patient with obstructive coronary artery disease. If the studies purporting to demonstrate a beneficial effect of the operation on the natural history of the disease can be confirmed, the indications will obviously be less stringent than if relief of symptoms is the only goal of the procedure. Patients who have definite symptomatology, but in whom significant relief with medical therapy is obtained, present a difficult problem. The definition of a level of symptomatology which indicates the need for operation must represent a joint decision between physician and patient. Older patients, i.e., those over 70 years, are generally treated medically unless the symptoms are truly disabling, whereas in a younger individual less disability is generally required before operation is advised. An important additional factor frequently not discussed relates to the technical skills of the surgical and diagnostic teams, and the quality of care in the early postoperative period. The variation in results of operative therapy from different institutions reflects this factor as well as differing selection criteria for operation. As a general rule, the poorest results are reported from institutions performing the least number of operations, and the advisability of having operation carried out by an experienced surgical team cannot be overemphasized. Operative mortality is also a function of case selection. If only patients with good ventricular function are selected, mortality may be less than 1 percent, but such a policy may exclude many patients who could benefit from the procedure.

MANAGEMENT OF THE PATIENT WITH ASYMPTOMATIC CORONARY ARTERIOSCLEROSIS

The widespread use of exercise testing during routine annual examinations has defined a heretofore unrecognized group of patients with asymptomatic coronary artery disease. Longitudinal studies of young military personnel have demonstrated an increased incidence of coronary events (sudden death, infarction, angina) in asymptomatic patients with positive exercise tests. In addition, patients who are asymptomatic after an infarct are nonetheless at greater risk for a second coronary event than the general population. Although medical therapy (elimination of smoking, antihypertensive medication, diet, etc.) aimed at preventing progression of the disease is indicated, recent surgical data suggesting that bypass surgery improves mortality in coronary patients have led some to advocate routine coronary arteriography to establish a diagnosis and subsequent bypass surgery if anatomically feasible despite the asymptomatic state. While such an approach cannot be condoned on the basis of available data, a number of factors should be considered when faced with this dilemma: (1) the degree of positivity of the exercise test and duration or stage of exercise at which it appears, (2) the ECG leads in which the test is positive (changes in the anterior precordial leads appear to indicate less favorable prognosis than changes in the inferior leads), (3) the age of the patient, and (4) the occupation of the patient. Whereas most would agree that the asymptomatic, 45-year-old, commercial airline pilot with 4-mm ST-segment depression in leads V_1 to V_4 during mild exercise should have arteriograms and the asymptomatic sedentary 75-year-old retiree with 1-mm ST-segment depression in leads II and III during maximal exercise should not, there is no consensus about the appropriate procedure in less extreme situations. There is now evidence that beta-adrenergic blockade, when begun 7 to 35 days following acute myocardial infarction, improves survival. This therapy is recommended, even in the absence of angina pectoris, as long as there are no contraindications (heart failure, bradycardia, heart block, asthma).

REFERENCES

BRAUNWALD E (ed): Coronary artery disease, in *Heart Disease*, 2d ed. Philadelphia, Saunders, 1983, chaps 34–40

CHRISTIE LG et al: Systematic approach to evaluation of angina-like chest pain: Pathophysiology and clinical testing with emphasis on objective documentation of myocardial ischemia. Am Heart J 102:897, 1981

COHN PF (ed): *Diagnosis and Therapy of Coronary Artery Disease*. Boston, Little, Brown, 1979

CORYA BC: Echocardiography in ischemic heart disease. Am J Med 63:10, 1977

FROEHLICH RT et al: Recognizing and treating left ventricular aneurysms. J Cardiovasc Med 6:484, 1981

GRÜNTZIG AR et al: Nonoperative dilatation of coronary-artery stenosis. N Engl J Med 301:61, 1979

GUNTHER S et al: Therapy of coronary vasoconstriction in patients with coronary artery disease. Am J Cardiol 47:157, 1981

HILLIS LD, BRAUNWALD E: Myocardial ischemia. N Engl J Med 296:971, 1034, 1093, 1977

———, ———: Coronary artery spasm. N Engl J Med 299:695, 1978

PROUDFIT WL et al: Natural history of obstructive coronary artery disease: Ten-year study of 601 nonsurgical cases. Prog Cardiovasc Dis 21:53, 1978

RAHIMTOOLA SH: Coronary bypass surgery for chronic angina—1981. A perspective. Circulation 65:225, 1982

261 ACUTE MYOCARDIAL INFARCTION

EUGENE BRAUNWALD
JOSEPH S. ALPERT

Myocardial infarction is one of the commonest diagnoses occurring in hospitalized patients in western countries. In the United States, approximately 1.3 million myocardial infarctions occur each year. Mortality during the first year following infarction is approximately 50 percent, with half of the deaths occurring before the stricken individual reaches the hospital. Risk of excess mortality persists in patients who recover; indeed, the age-corrected risk of death is increased 3.5 times even 10 years after infarction.

CLINICAL PRESENTATION *Pain* is the most common presenting complaint in patients with myocardial infarction. In some instances, the discomfort may be severe enough to be described as the worst pain the patient has ever experienced (Chap. 4). The pain of myocardial infarction is deep and visceral; adjectives commonly used to describe it are *heavy, squeezing*, and *crushing*. It is similar in character to the pain of angina pectoris but is usually more severe and lasts much longer. Typically the pain involves the central portion of the chest and/or epigastrium, and in about 30 percent of cases it radiates to the arms. Less common sites of radiation include the abdomen, back, lower jaw, and neck. The location of the pain beneath the xiphoid may be responsible for the mistaken diagnosis of indigestion. The pain of myocardial infarction does not radiate above the maxilla or below the umbilicus. The pain is often accompanied by weakness, sweating, nausea, vomiting, giddiness, and anxiety. The discomfort usually commences with the patient at rest. However, when it begins during a period of exertion, in contrast to angina pectoris, it does not usually subside with cessation of activity.

Although pain is the most common presenting complaint, it is by no means always present; a minimum of 15 to 20 percent of myocardial infarcts are *painless*. The frequency of such silent infarcts is probably even higher than this estimate because patients without pain may not seek medical attention. The incidence of painless infarcts is greater in patients with diabetes mellitus, and it increases with age. In the elderly, myocardial infarction may present as sudden-onset breathlessness, which may progress to pulmonary edema. Other less common presentations in the absence of pain include sudden loss of consciousness, a confusional state, a sensation of profound weakness, the appearance of an arrhythmia, or merely an unexplained drop in arterial blood pressure.

PHYSICAL FINDINGS In many instances the dominant feature of the patient's presentation is the reaction to the chest pain. Patients are typically anxious and restless, attempting to relieve the pain by moving about in bed, squirming, stretching, belching, or even inducing vomiting. This is in contrast to the pain of angina pectoris which causes the patient to remain relatively immobile for fear of making the pain reappear. Pallor is common and is often associated with perspiration and coolness of the extremities. No alteration of pulse rate is specific for myocardial infarction, with bradycardia, normal sinus rhythm, and sinus tachycardia being observed both early and late in the course of the disease. This is not unexpected in view of the multiplicity of hemodynamic derangements that may occur with infarction.

The precordium is usually quiet, and the apical impulse may be difficult to palpate. In about one-fourth of patients with anterior wall infarction, an abnormal systolic pulsation develops in the periapical area within the first days of the illness and then may resolve. This abnormality is best brought out with the patient in the left lateral decubitus position and represents a transient, palpable systolic bulging of the infarcted ventricle. Other physical signs of ventricular dysfunction that may be present include, in decreasing incidence, fourth (S_4) and third (S_3) heart sounds, decreased intensity of heart sounds, and, rarely, paradoxical splitting of the second sound (Chap. 248). A transient apical systolic murmur, presumably due to mitral regurgitation secondary to papillary muscle dysfunction during acute infarction, may be midsystolic or late systolic in timing. A pericardial friction rub is heard in many patients with transmural myocardial infarction at some time in their course if they are examined frequently. Jugular venous distention occurs in patients with right ventricular infarction. The carotid pulse is often decreased in volume despite a normal upstroke. Temperature elevations in the range of 37 to 38°C, and occasionally as high as 39°C, may be observed during the first week following acute myocardial infarction; however, a temperature exceeding 38°C should prompt a search for other causes. Like the pulse, the arterial pressure is variable; it may be normal, elevated, or low. In most patients with transmural infarction systolic pressure declines approximately 10 to 15 mmHg from the preinfarction state.

LABORATORY DIAGNOSIS The laboratory tests of value in confirming the diagnosis of myocardial infarction may be divided into three groups: (1) nonspecific indices of tissue necrosis and inflammation, (2) the electrocardiogram, and (3) serum enzyme changes.

The *nonspecific reaction* to myocardial injury is associated with polymorphonuclear leukocytosis, which appears within a few hours after the onset of pain, persists for 3 to 7 days, and often reaches levels of 12,000 to 15,000 leukocytes per cubic millimeter. The magnitude of the leukocytosis yields some information about the size of the infarct: higher white blood cell counts are associated with larger infarcts. The erythrocyte sedimentation rate rises more slowly than the white blood cell count, peaking during the first week, and sometimes remaining elevated for 1 or 2 weeks.

The *electrocardiographic manifestations* of acute myocardial infarction are described in Chap. 249. Although electrocardiographic/pathologic correlations are not excellent, transmural infarction is diagnosed if the electrocardiogram demonstrates Q waves or loss of R waves; nontransmural infarction is said to be present if the electrocardiogram shows only persistent ST-segment and T-wave changes. However, these changes are variable and nonspecific and should not form the sole basis for the diagnosis of infarction. A more rational nomenclature for designating electrocardiographic infarction would be *Q-wave* or *ST-T-wave infarction* in place of the terms *transmural* or *nontransmural infarction,* respectively.

SERUM ENZYME STUDIES Enzymes are released in large quantities into the blood from necrotic heart muscle following myocardial infarction. The rate of liberation of specific enzymes differs following infarction, and the temporal pattern of enzyme release is of diagnostic importance. The time course of the serum concentration of the most commonly used enzymes is shown in Fig. 261-1. Levels of two of the enzymes, SGOT and creatinine phosphokinase (CK), rise and fall rapidly, while that of lactic dehydrogenase (LDH) rises later and remains elevated longer. SGOT is widely used but has the disadvantage that it is also present in skeletal muscle, liver, and red blood cells and may be liberated from these extracardiac stores. The MB isoenzyme of CK has an advantage over SGOT in that it is not present in significant concentrations in extracardiac tissue, and therefore it is more specific than SGOT. Since rises in serum concentration of CK and SGOT are short-lived, they may be missed if initial blood samples are obtained more than 72 h after the infarct develops. MBCK isoenzymes are particularly useful when there has been skeletal muscle or brain damage since both tissues contain large amounts of the enzyme but none of the MB isoenzyme. In myocardial infarction, the level of LDH rises during the first day, peaks at 3 to 4 days, and returns to normal in 14 days. Five common LDH isoenzymes may be separated by starch-gel electrophoresis. Tissues differ with respect to the specific isoenzyme patterns; the rapidly migrating isoenzyme which predominates in the heart is referred to as LDH_1, while the slowly migrating components predominate in liver and skeletal muscle. LDH_1 rises before total LDH in patients with myocardial infarction and may rise when there is no change in total LDH. Therefore, increased LDH_1 is a more sensitive indicator of myocardial infarction than total LDH. Its sensitivity exceeds 95 percent.

Of particular importance in the clinical situation is the fact that a two- to threefold elevation of CK may follow an intramuscular injection. This may lead to the erroneous diagnosis of myocardial infarction in a patient who has been given an intramuscular injection of a narcotic for chest pain of noncardiac origin. Other potential sources of total CK elevation worthy of note include: (1) myopathy associated with chronic alcoholism, (2) clofibrate therapy, (3) electrical cardioversion, (4) cardiac catheterization, (5) hypothyroidism, (6) stroke, and (7) surgery. Cardiac surgery and electrical cardioversion often result in elevation of serum levels of MB isoenzyme.

It has long been recognized that the amount of enzyme released correlates with the size of the infarct. It has been demonstrated that the mass of heart muscle infarcted can be estimated from analysis of the concentration-time curve of the enzyme if the kinetics of the release, degradation, disposal, etc., of the enzyme are known. The size of an infarct in terms of grams of infarcted tissue can be estimated from an analysis of the MB CK time curve.

Characteristic rises occur in serum enzyme concentration in more than 95 percent of patients with clinically proven myocardial infarction. CK and SGOT levels generally do not rise in unstable angina (see "Unstable Angina" below), rheumatic carditis, or pericarditis. The list of conditions other than myocardial infarction which may result in elevated SGOT includes (1) right ventricular failure with hepatic congestion, (2) administration of salicylates, opiates, or coumarin-type anticoagulants, (3) primary muscle disease, including muscular dystrophy and surgical trauma, (4) cardiac operations, (5) acute pancreatitis, (6) extensive central nervous system damage, (7) toxemia of pregnancy, (8) hemolytic crisis, (9) crush injuries or burns, (10) infarction of kidney, spleen, or intestine, and (11) hypothyroidism.

Many patients with suspected infarction have base-line enzyme levels which are normal and increase threefold in a pattern consistent with infarction, although the absolute level of enzyme in the blood never exceeds the upper limits of normal. This situation is most commonly observed in patients with small infarctions and, although not diagnostic, is highly suggestive of acute infarction. Isoenzyme studies are particularly helpful in this situation.

Several radionuclide imaging techniques are of value in the diagnosis of or assessment of the patient with acute myocardial infarction (Chap. 250). Acute infarct scintigraphy ("hot-spot" imaging) is carried out with an infarct-avid imaging agent such as ^{99m}Tc stannous pyrophosphate. Scans are usually positive 2 to 5 days after infarction, particularly in patients with transmural infarcts; they aid in localizing infarcts and provide a measure of infarct size (page 1335). Myocardial perfusion imaging with thallium 201, which is taken up and concentrated by viable myocardium, reveals a defect ("cold spot") in most patients during the first few hours after development of a transmural infarct. This localized area of decreased radioactiv-

FIGURE 261-1
The time course of serum enzyme concentration changes following a typical myocardial infarction. CK, creatinine phosphokinase; LDH, lactic dehydrogenase; GOT, glutamic oxaloacetic transaminase.

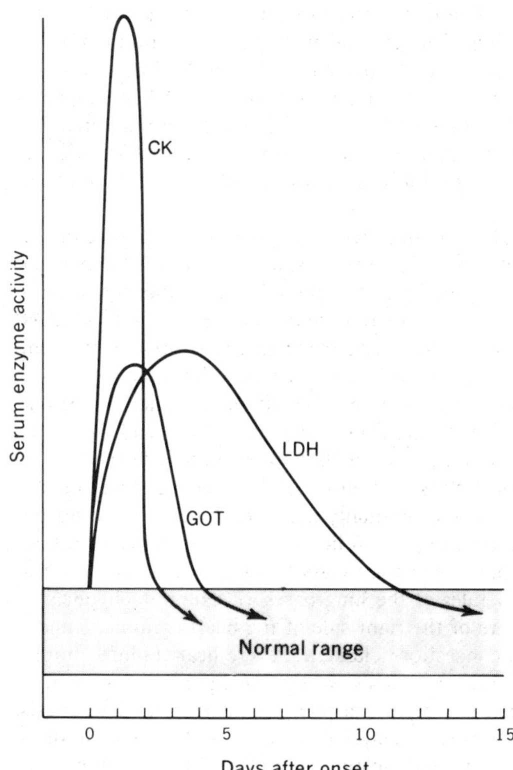

ity may fill in during the following hours (page 1335). However, it is not possible to distinguish acute infarcts from chronic scars. Radionuclide ventriculography, carried out with ^{99m}Tc-labeled red blood cells (page 1335), frequently demonstrates wall motion disorders and reduction in ventricular ejection fraction in patients with acute myocardial infarction. While of value in assessing the hemodynamic consequences of infarction, and in aiding in the diagnosis of right ventricular infarction when the right ventricular ejection fraction is depressed, the technique is quite nonspecific, since many cardiac abnormalities other than myocardial infarction alter the radionuclide ventriculogram.

MANAGEMENT

By virtue of experience in coronary care units and extensive research on acute myocardial infarction during the past decade, the management of this disorder has been substantially altered. Two general classes of complications have been defined: (1) electrical (arrhythmias) and (2) mechanical ("pump failure"). Ventricular fibrillation is the most common form of arrhythmic death in acute myocardial infarction. The observation that ventricular tachycardia or ventricular premature beats were almost uniformly present in patients during the early phases of infarction and appeared to be harbingers of ventricular fibrillation led to a therapeutic plan based upon aggressive suppression of all ventricular ectopic activity. It was realized that the potential for arrhythmic death was greatest during the early phase of infarction; that is, 65 percent of male subjects under 50 years of age who died of myocardial infarction did so within 1 h of the onset of symptoms, and 85 percent died within the first 24 h. Simultaneously, lidocaine was identified as an antiarrhythmic drug of unique effectiveness for the prophylactic treatment of ventricular ectopic activity in acute myocardial infarction. It became apparent that ventricular fibrillation could, in many instances, be prevented by aggressive antiarrhythmic drug therapy, and the focus of coronary care changed from resuscitation to prevention. These developments led to the formulation of the therapeutic tenets which are now the hallmark of care for patients with acute myocardial infarction. Reduction of in-hospital mortality for acute myocardial infarction from 30 to 15 percent is the result of institution of measures such as rapid transfer of patients with acute myocardial infarction to facilities with ECG monitoring capability staffed by personnel (not necessarily physicians) knowledgeable in the recognition and treatment of ventricular arrhythmias.

With sudden and unexpected in-hospital arrhythmic deaths essentially eliminated by the preventive approach to ventricular arrhythmias, attention has turned to the other major complication of acute myocardial infarction, i.e., pump failure. Although advances have been made in the treatment of pump failure, it remains the primary cause of in-hospital death from acute myocardial infarction. The extent of ischemic necrosis correlates well with the degree of pump failure and with mortality, both early, i.e., within 30 days of infarction, and later as well. A clinical classification dependent on the status of cardiac pump function originally proposed by Killip divides patients into four groups as follows: class I, no signs of pulmonary or venous congestion; class II, moderate heart failure as evidenced by rales at the lung bases, S_3 gallop, tachypnea, or signs of failure of the right side of the heart including venous and hepatic congestion; class III, severe heart failure, pulmonary edema; class IV, shock with systolic pressure less than 90 mmHg and evidence of peripheral constriction, diaphoresis, peripheral cyanosis, mental confusion, and decreased urine output. The expected hospital mortality rate of patients in these clinical classes has been established by a number of investigators as follows: class I, 0 to 5 percent; class II, 10 to 20 percent; class III, 35 to 45 percent; and class IV, 85 to 95 percent.

GENERAL CONSIDERATIONS The primary therapeutic objectives of management of the patient with myocardial infarction are to prevent death from arrhythmia and to minimize the mass of infarcted tissue.

Arrhythmias can usually be managed successfully if trained personnel and appropriate equipment are available when this complication develops. Since mortality from arrhythmia is greatest during the first few hours after infarction, it is obvious that the effectiveness of coronary care units relates directly to the speed with which patients come under medical observation. The biggest delay usually is not in transportation to the hospital but rather between the onset of pain and the patient's decision to call for help. One hopes that this delay can be reduced by education of the public concerning the significance of chest pain and the importance of seeking early medical attention.

An occlusive or near-occlusive thrombus overlying or adjacent to an atherosclerotic plaque in a coronary artery appears to be the cause of most transmural infarcts. Therefore, reperfusion of the ischemic zone by the prompt dissolution of the thrombus with a thrombolytic agent (streptokinase or urokinase) is a logical approach to the reduction of infarct size. Pilot studies carried out within the first 4 h following the onset of the clinical event have demonstrated the feasibility of this approach. At the time of this writing, however, the role of this therapeutic maneuver in the management of acute myocardial infarction remains to be established.

The amount of myocardial tissue which becomes necrotic secondary to a vascular occlusion is determined by factors other than just the site of occlusion. Infarct size is now known to be variable with time and affected by a number of therapeutic agents currently in use. The balance between myocardial oxygen supply and demand in areas rendered ischemic determines the ultimate fate of these areas of jeopardized myocardium. While no routine therapeutic approach to reduce infarct size in all patients is currently recommended, the realization that infarct size may be increased by interventions which adversely alter the supply-demand balance has prompted the reevaluation of previously accepted therapeutic maneuvers in the management of patients with acute infarction.

A number of "common sense" rules in the management of acute myocardial infarction deserve particular emphasis. First and foremost, it is mandatory to maintain an optimal balance between myocardial oxygen supply and demand in order to salvage as much as possible of the jeopardized zone of myocardium surrounding the center of the infarct. Therapeutic strategies that help to attain this goal include rest, analgesia, mild sedation, and a quiet atmosphere in order to reduce anxiety and thereby lower heart rate, a major determinant of myocardial oxygen consumption.

If the patient was receiving a beta-adrenergic blocking agent at the time the clinical manifestations of infarction commence, it is reasonable to continue the drug unless a specific contraindication develops, such as left ventricular failure or a bradyarrhythmia. Marked sinus bradycardia (heart rate less than approximately 45 beats per minute) should be treated by leg elevation and atropine or by electrical pacing. However, routine administration of atropine, with resultant increase in heart rate, to patients without serious bradycardia seems unwise. Patients with acute myocardial infarction who have a hyperdynamic state, i.e., tachycardia and elevation of arterial pressure, should be treated with a beta-adrenergic blocking agent. Initially, 0.1 mg/kg propranolol given intravenously in three divided doses is safe, if there are no contraindications, such as heart failure, AV block, or asthma. All forms of tachyarrhythmias require prompt and direct treatment. Drugs that exert a positive inotropic effect, such as digitalis glycosides and cardioactive sympathomimetics, should be administered only if there is evidence of heart failure. They should not be given prophylactically. Of the various sympathomimetic amines available, isoproterenol with its chronotropic and vasodilator effects is the least desirable. Dopamine and Dobutamine, which have less effect on heart rate and systemic vascular resistance, are more desirable when it is necessary to augment cardiac contractility. Obviously, diuretics are indicated in the presence of heart failure and should, in fact, be used prior to cardiac stimulants unless the patient is hypovolemic or hypotensive.

All patients should inhale oxygen-enriched air (see below). Particular attention must be paid to preserving arterial oxygenation in patients with hypoxemia, as occurs in patients with chronic pulmonary disease, pneumonia, or left ventricular failure. Severe anemia, which can also extend the area of ischemic injury, should be corrected by cautious administration of packed red blood cells, sometimes accompanied by a diuretic. Associated conditions, particularly infections with accompanying tachycardia and elevated myocardial oxygen demand, require immediate attention. Systolic arterial pressure should not be allowed to deviate by more than 25 to 30 mmHg from the patient's usual level.

Coronary care units Coronary care units have resulted in improved care of patients with myocardial infarction, reduction in mortality rates, and major increases in knowledge about myocardial infarction. The coronary care unit is a specially designed *nursing unit,* the most important feature of which is a staff of highly trained nursing personnel with authority to take immediate action in emergency situations. The unit should be equipped with systems which permit continuous monitoring of the electrocardiogram of each patient. Defibrillators, respirators, and facilities for introducing pacing catheters and flow-directed balloon-tipped catheters should be available. However, equipment alone does not ensure an effective coronary care unit. Of prime importance is the organization of a highly trained team of nurses who can recognize arrhythmias, adjust the dosage of antiarrhythmic drugs, and perform cardiac resuscitation, including the application of electroshock when necessary. A physician should be available at all times, but many lives have been saved because nurses have treated ventricular tachycardia or fibrillation before the physician's arrival.

The policies and procedures for admission to a coronary care unit should ensure that patients are admitted early in their illness when they may expect to derive maximum benefit from the care provided. In order to accomplish this, the threshold for admission of patients with suspected infarction should be low, and this is best monitored in terms of the fraction of total admissions in whom myocardial infarction is eventually proven. If this fraction exceeds 50 percent, the admission policies may well be too restrictive, and not enough patients are being admitted for suspected myocardial infarction which did not develop. Mortality rates for myocardial infarction treated in coronary care units vary from 10 to 20 percent; this variation can be explained, in part, by variations in admission policies as regard age limitations, the type of population being served (tertiary care center versus community hospital), and other as yet unidentified factors.

TREATMENT OF THE PATIENT WITH AN UNCOMPLICATED INFARCT **Analgesia** Since myocardial infarction usually presents with severe pain, one of the important initial therapeutic objectives is the relief of pain. Morphine, the agent traditionally used for this purpose, is still the most effective and remains the drug of choice. It may lower arterial pressure by reducing sympathetically mediated arteriolar and venous constriction. The resultant venous pooling may produce a reduction in cardiac output. This must be recognized but does not necessarily contraindicate its use. The skin may become cool and moist, and the patient may complain of nausea, but these events usually pass and are replaced by a feeling of well-being associated with the relief of pain. It is important to recognize this syndrome as one attributable to morphine, because the hypotension and signs of peripheral constriction may be incorrectly interpreted as manifestations of the shock syndrome and taken as grounds for the initiation of vasoconstrictor or other therapy which would be inappropriate. Hypotension associated with venous pooling usually responds promptly to elevation of the legs, but in some patients volume expansion with intravenous saline is required. Morphine also has a vagotonic effect and may cause bradycardia or advanced degrees of heart block, particularly in patients with posteroinferior infarction. These side effects of morphine usually respond to atropine, and prophylactic atropine (0.4 mg intravenously) should be administered prior to the injection of morphine if bradycardia or any degree of heart block is present. Because of these potential side effects, it is advisable to select the minimal effective dose of morphine which relieves pain. This can be accomplished by repetitive (every 5 min) intravenous injection of small doses of drug (2 to 4 mg) rather than the administration of a larger quantity by the subcutaneous route, from which site absorption may be unpredictable. Demerol or Dilaudid may be effectively employed in place of morphine. Inhalation of 30 to 50 percent inspired nitrous oxide is effective in relieving both pain and anxiety associated with the discomfort of myocardial ischemia and/or necrosis. Nitrous oxide may be administered in addition to narcotic analgesics with little or no depression of left ventricular function.

Oxygen The routine use of oxygen is supported by the observation that the arterial P_{O_2} is reduced in many patients with myocardial infarction and that oxygen inhalation reduces infarct size in experimental animals. Inhalation of oxygen increases arterial P_{O_2} and hence increases the concentration gradient responsible for the diffusion of oxygen into the ischemic myocardium from adjacent, better-perfused areas. Although oxygen therapy has been associated with theoretically deleterious effects such as elevation of peripheral resistance and slight reduction of cardiac output, the weight of evidence favors its administration. It should be administered by face mask or nasal prongs for the first 2 or 3 days after infarction.

Activity Factors which increase the work of the heart may increase the size of the infarct. Circumstances in which heart size, cardiac output, or myocardial contractility are increased should be avoided. It has been demonstrated that 6 to 8 weeks are required for complete healing, i.e., replacement of the infarcted myocardium by scar tissue. The purpose of reduced physical activity is to provide the most favorable possible circumstances for this healing.

All patients with myocardial infarction should be admitted to a coronary care unit and remain there for 3 or 4 days under constant observation by trained personnel utilizing continuous electrocardiographic monitoring. A catheter should be introduced into a peripheral vein, firmly fixed so that it is not easily dislodged, and kept open by the slow infusion of isotonic glucose solution. This is a route of administration for antiarrhythmic or other drugs which may be necessary. In the absence of heart failure during the first 2 to 3 days, the patient should be in bed most of the day, with one or two periods of 15 to 30 min in a bedside chair. The patient may use a bedside commode and should be bathed by a nurse. Patients may eat unassisted. The bed should be equipped with a footboard, and the patient should push his feet against the footboard firmly 10 times during each waking hour to prevent venous stasis and thromboembolism and to maintain muscle tone in the legs.

The patient with an uncomplicated course may be discharged from the coronary care unit on the third or fourth day. By this time, he or she should be spending at least 30 to 60 min in a chair twice a day. It is advisable at this stage to measure the patient's blood pressure when standing in order to be aware of postural hypotension, which may be a problem when ambulation is begun. Standing and gradual ambulation are usually begun somewhere between the fourth and seventh days postinfarction in patients with uncomplicated myocardial infarction. Initial ambulation is to the bathroom if it is in the patient's room or nearby. Ambulation is progressively increased, eventually including walks about the hospital floor. In many hospitals a cardiac rehabilitation program with progressive exercise is initiated in the hospital and continued after discharge. The total duration of hospitalization in uncomplicated cases is usually 10 to 14 days, but many physicians still hospitalize patients with Q-wave infarction for 3 weeks, while others have reduced the period to as short as 1 week when the opportunities for home convalescence are ideal. Patients in clinical class II or higher may require 3 or more weeks of hospitalization, depending upon the rapidity with which heart failure resolves and the home situation to which the patient is returning. Many physicians perform a limited (heart-rate limited) exercise tolerance test just prior to discharge in selected patients with myocardial infarction. Such testing identifies high-risk patients as those who develop angina, ST-segment change, or serious ventricular ectopic activity during or immediately following exercise. These patients require special attention, including measures such as antiarrhythmic drugs for ectopic activity, and beta-adrenergic blockers, long-acting nitrates and calcium channel blocking agents for evidence of ischemia. These tests also aid in formulating an individualized exercise prescription, which can be much more vigorous in patients who tolerate exercise without any of the above-mentioned adverse signs.

The remainder of the convalescent phase of myocardial infarction may be accomplished at home. Some physicians restrict the patient to one floor until he has completed 5 weeks of convalescence, and then allow only one trip upstairs a day. Other physicians allow patients to make one daily trip up and down a single flight of stairs after discharge from the hospital. From 5 to 8 weeks, the patient should be encouraged to increase activity by walking about the house and outdoors in good weather. Patients should still spend 8 to 10 h in bed each night. Additional rest periods in the morning and afternoon may be advisable for selected patients.

From 8 weeks onward, the physician must regulate the patient's activity on the basis of his or her exercise tolerance. It is during this period of increasing activity that the patient may become aware of profound fatigue. Postural hypotension may still be a problem. Most patients will be able to return to work after 12 weeks. A submaximal exercise test is frequently performed prior to returning to work. A trend toward earlier ambulation, hospital discharge, and resumption of full activity for patients recuperating from acute myocardial infarction has developed in recent years.

Diet During the first 5 days, a low-calorie diet divided into multiple small feedings is preferred. Cardiac output increases following ingestion of food, and therefore the quantity of feedings should be kept down. If heart failure is present, sodium intake should be restricted. Since constipation commonly occurs during convalescence from myocardial infarction, it is reasonable to give average or even increased amounts of bulk in the diet. In addition, the ingestion of potassium-rich foods should be encouraged in patients receiving diuretics. During the second week, increasing amounts of food may be introduced into the diet. At this time, the importance of restriction of calories and saturated fat may be explained to the patient, and he or she can be started on an appropriate diet. Willingness to accept dietary restriction and to discontinue cigarette smoking is usually never greater than it is during this early period of convalescence.

Bowels Bed rest of 3 to 5 days and the effect of the narcotics utilized for the relief of pain often lead to constipation. Most patients are not comfortable using a bedpan, which frequently results in excessive straining at stool. A bedside commode, a diet rich in bulk, and the routine use of a stool softener such as dioctyl sodium sulfosuccinate, 200 mg daily, are recommended. If the patient remains constipated despite these measures and becomes distressed and uncomfortable, a laxative can be safely used. It is safe to perform a gentle rectal examination on patients with acute myocardial infarction.

Sedation Most patients require sedation during hospitalization in order to withstand the period of enforced inactivity with tranquillity. Chlordiazepoxide 10 mg, or diazepam 5 mg, given four times daily is usually effective. Appropriate sleeping medication may be given at night to ensure adequate sleep. Chloral hydrate 0.5 to 1.0 g or flurazepam 15 to 30 mg is usually sufficient to induce sleep. Attention to this problem is especially important during the first few days in the coronary care unit, where the atmosphere of 24-h vigilance may interfere with the patient's sleep. Sedation is no substitute for reassuring, quiet surroundings.

Anticoagulants Few topics are more controversial than the use of anticoagulants in the routine treatment of acute myocardial infarction. The lack of a confirmed, statistically clear-cut demonstration of a lower mortality rate in the first few weeks following myocardial infarction suggests that the benefit of anticoagulant therapy, if any, is small. The use of anticoagulant therapy to retard the process of coronary occlusion during the initial phases of myocardial infarction is not justified. However, there is agreement that anticoagulant therapy does reduce the incidence of both arterial and venous thromboembolic complications. Since the incidence of venous thromboembolic disease is known to be increased in patients with heart failure, shock, and previous venous or thromboembolic disease, the routine, prophylactic use of anticoagulant drugs to prevent pulmonary embolism in the coronary care unit is recommended for those patients at high risk for this complication. Routine anticoagulation as prophylaxis against venous thromboembolism is not recommended in class I patients. Patients in classes III and IV are at greater risk for pulmonary embolism and should routinely receive anticoagulants during the initial 10 to 14 days of hospitalization, or until ambulatory. This is best accomplished initially by the continuous intravenous administration of heparin with a constant infusion pump with measurement of the clotting time or partial thromboplastin time to define the need for increasing or decreasing the infusion rate. Once the patient is out of the intensive care area, oral anticoagulants may be substituted for heparin. Alternatively, small subcutaneous doses of heparin (5000 units every 8 to 12 h) can be employed. Controversy as to the need for anticoagulant therapy in class II patients persists. It would seem appropriate to anticoagulate these patients only if the signs of congestive heart failure persist for more than 3 or 4 days.

The incidence of arterial embolism from clot originating in

the ventricle at the site of infarct is small (i.e., less than 5 percent) but definite. Frequently, arterial embolism presents as a major complication, such as hemiparesis, when the cerebral circulation is involved, or hypertension if the renal circulation is compromised. The low incidence of this complication, contrasted with its severity, renders it impractical to establish firm guidelines for the use of anticoagulant drugs as prophylaxis against arterial embolism in acute myocardial infarction. The likelihood of arterial embolism appears to increase with the extent of infarction and the resultant inflammation and endocardial stasis due to akinesis. Therefore, as is the case with venous thromboembolism, the indication for anticoagulation as prophylaxis against arterial embolism increases with the extent of infarction.

TREATMENT Arrhythmias (see also Chaps. 254 and 255) The improved management of arrhythmias constitutes a most significant advance in the treatment of myocardial infarction.

VENTRICULAR PREMATURE SYSTOLES Infrequent, sporadic ventricular premature systoles occur in almost all patients with infarction and do not require therapy. Indications for suppression of ventricular ectopic beats are generally considered to be the following: (1) the presence of more than five isolated ectopic beats per minute, (2) the occurrence of consecutive or multifocal ventricular extrasystoles, and (3) the occurrence of ectopic ventricular beats early in diastole and hence superimposed on the T wave of the preceding beat (the so-called "R-on-T phenomenon"). Intravenous lidocaine has become the treatment of choice for ventricular premature beats and ventricular arrhythmias, because it acts rapidly and side effects disappear soon (15 to 20 min) after its administration is discontinued. Lidocaine is given initially as a single intravenous injection of 50 to 100 mg to establish adequate blood levels quickly. This initial dose usually eliminates the ectopic activity and is followed by an intravenous infusion of 1 to 4 mg/min. Usually, ventricular premature beats spontaneously disappear after 72 to 96 h. If significant ventricular ectopic activity persists past this time, chronic antiarrhythmic therapy is often initiated.

Procainamide and quinidine are most commonly used for the treatment of persistent ventricular ectopic activity; beta-adrenergic blocking agents and disopyramide are also effective in abolishing ventricular ectopic activity in infarction patients. The latter agent should be used with great care in patients with left ventricular failure since it has a significant negative inotropic action. If the usual doses of these drugs (Chap. 255), singly or in combination, are not effective, blood levels should be measured to ensure that adequate blood concentrations are being obtained. Frequent clinical and electrocardiographic assessment of the patient for signs of drug toxicity are mandatory when higher doses of these agents are employed.

VENTRICULAR TACHYCARDIA AND VENTRICULAR FIBRILLATION Recent studies have demonstrated that ventricular tachycardia and fibrillation often occur without prior warning arrhythmia. The occurrence of such primary arrhythmias can be materially reduced by prophylactic administration of intravenous lidocaine. The use of prophylactic antiarrhythmic drug therapy is particularly well suited to patients who cannot reach a hospital or those treated in hospitals that lack constant physician presence in the coronary care unit. Sustained ventricular tachycardia is treated first with lidocaine, and if it cannot be terminated by one or two 50- to 100-mg doses, electroconversion should be employed (Chap. 255). Electroshock is used immediately in patients with ventricular fibrillation, or when ventricular tachycardia causes hemodynamic deterioration. If fibrillation has persisted for more than a few seconds, the first shock may be unsuccessful, and in this situation it is advisable to administer closed-chest massage, mouth-to-mouth respiration, and intravenous sodium bicarbonate solution (40 to 90 meq) before attempting electroconversion again. Improvement of oxygenation and perfusion and correction of acidosis increase the likelihood of successful defibrillation (see also Chap. 30).

Long-term survival is good in patients with *primary* ventricular fibrillation, i.e., ventricular fibrillation resulting as a primary response to acute ischemia and not associated with predisposing factors such as congestive heart failure, shock, or ventricular aneurysm. In one series, 87 percent of patients with primary ventricular fibrillation left the hospital alive. This prognosis is in sharp contrast to that for patients who develop ventricular fibrillation *secondary* to severe pump failure. A far smaller percentage, 29 percent, of patients in this group was discharged from the hospital alive.

ACCELERATED IDIOVENTRICULAR RHYTHM Accelerated idioventricular rhythm (AIVR, "slow ventricular tachycardia"), a ventricular rhythm with a rate of 60 to 100 beats per minute, occurs in 25 percent of patients with myocardial infarction. It is especially frequent in inferoposterior infarction, where it is usually associated with sinus bradycardia. The rate of AIVR is usually similar to that of the sinus rhythm which precedes and follows it, and this similarity of rate and the relatively minor hemodynamic effects make this rhythm difficult to detect other than by electrocardiographic monitoring. The rhythm comes and goes spontaneously as fluctuation in sinus rate causes the atrial rate to fall below the accelerated escape level. For the most part, this rhythm is benign and does not presage the development of classic ventricular tachycardia. However, a number of cases have been documented wherein AIVR was associated with more dangerous forms of ventricular ectopic activity or where AIVR degenerated into a potentially fatal ventricular arrhythmia. Since one cannot predict when this complication will occur, it may be best to treat AIVR whenever it is identified. This can be done by using a drug which decreases the ventricular escape rate (lidocaine) and/or one that increases the sinus rate (atropine).

SUPRAVENTRICULAR ARRHYTHMIAS The common arrhythmias in this group are junctional rhythm and tachycardia, atrial tachycardia, atrial flutter, and atrial fibrillation. These rhythm disturbances are often secondary to left ventricular failure. The administration of a short-acting glycoside, such as digoxin or ouabain, is the treatment of choice. If the abnormal rhythm persists for more than 2 h with a ventricular rate in excess of 120 beats per minute, or at any time when tachycardia induces heart failure, shock, or ischemia (as manifested by pain or ECG changes), electroshock should be utilized.

Junctional arrhythmias are of diverse etiology, are not indicative of any specific abnormality, and from a therapeutic viewpoint must be considered on an individual basis. Even in the presence of acute myocardial infarction, digitalis excess must be ruled out as a cause of junctional tachycardia. In some patients with severely compromised left ventricular function, the loss of appropriately timed atrial systole results in a marked decrease in cardiac output. Right atrial or coronary sinus pacing is indicated in such instances. The hemodynamic effects of these two modes of pacing are identical, but coronary sinus pacing offers the advantage of better catheter stability.

SINUS BRADYCARDIA The significance of bradycardia as a predisposing factor to ventricular fibrillation in acute myocardial infarction is controversial. While the incidence of ventricular tachycardia in patients with sustained bradycardia is twice that observed in patients with normal heart rates, sinus bradycardia has also been identified in hospitalized patients as an index of a favorable prognosis. Experience with mobile coronary care units indicates that sinus bradycardia occurring within the first hour after infarction is more consistently associated with ventricular ectopic rhythms than that occurring later in the course of the illness. Treatment of sinus bradycardia is indicated if significant ventricular ectopic activity is present or if hemodynamic compromise results from the slow heart rate. It is unclear whether bradycardia need be treated in asymptomatic, normotensive, arrhythmia-free patients. Elevation of the legs and/or the foot of the bed is frequently helpful in the treatment of sinus bradycardia. Atropine is the most useful drug for increasing heart rate and should be given intravenously in doses of 0.4 to 0.6 mg. If the rate remains below 60 beats per minute, additional doses of 0.2 mg, up to a total of 2.0 mg, may be given in divided doses. Persistent bradycardia (< 40 beats per minute) despite atropine may be treated with electrical pacing. Isoproterenol should be avoided, if possible, in the treatment of this condition.

CONDUCTION DISTURBANCES Malfunction of the conduction system in acute myocardial infarction is similar to that seen in other disease states in that block or failure to conduct may develop at three different levels in the conduction system: the atrioventricular (AV) node, the bundle of His, or the more peripheral portions of the conduction system (Chap. 254). If the block occurs in the AV node, the escape rhythm originates in the AV junction and the QRS complexes are of normal duration; but when the block occurs distal to the AV node, the escape site is ventricular and the QRS configuration is abnormal and its duration is prolonged. Rosenbaum has directed attention to disturbances of conduction in the three peripheral branches of the conduction system as being of value in predicting the occurrence of complete heart block (Chap. 249). When block occurs in any two of the three fascicles, bifascicular block is said to exist; trifascicular block, resulting in complete AV block, often develops in such patients. Patients with the combination of right bundle branch block and either left anterior or left posterior hemiblock have a particularly high risk of progression to complete heart block.

The mortality rate of patients with complete AV block in association with anterior infarction (80 to 90 percent) is almost three times that of patients who develop conduction disturbances with inferior infarction (30 percent), and the risk of subsequent death in those who survive to leave the hospital is also increased in the former group. This difference is related to the fact that heart block in inferior infarction is usually caused by AV nodal ischemia. The AV node is a small discrete structure, and thus a small amount of ischemia or necrosis can result in AV nodal dysfunction. In anterior wall infarction, heart block is related to ischemic malfunction of the three fascicles of the conduction system and thus results only from extensive myocardial necrosis.

Electrical pacing provides an effective means of increasing the heart rate of patients with bradycardia due to AV block, but it is not possible to be sure that such acceleration is always beneficial. For example, in patients with anterior wall infarction and complete heart block, the large size of the infarct is the major factor determining the outcome, and correction of the conduction deficit does not clearly improve the poor prognosis in this group. Pacing does appear to be beneficial, however, in patients with inferoposterior infarction who have complete heart block associated with heart failure, hypotension, marked bradycardia, or significant ventricular ectopic activity.

Some cardiologists advocate the placement of a pacing catheter prophylactically in patients with conduction disturbances known to be precursors of complete heart block. Unanimity of opinion does not exist on this point. Pacing may diminish the risk of treating ventricular ectopic beats with antiarrhythmic agents such as procainamide or lidocaine in the presence of heart block or sinus bradycardia. Permanent pacing has been advocated for patients who develop the combination of persistent bifascicular and transient third-degree heart block during the acute phase of myocardial infarction. Retrospective studies in small numbers of such patients suggest that the incidence of sudden death is decreased in those in whom permanent pacing was instituted.

Heart failure Some degree of transient heart failure occurs in over half of patients with myocardial infarction. The most common clinical signs are pulmonary rales and S_3 and S_4 gallop rhythms. Pulmonary congestion is also frequently seen on chest roentgenogram. However, roentgenographic signs of pulmonary congestion often fail to parallel temporally clinical evidence of pulmonary congestion, i.e., the presence of rales. Elevation of left ventricular filling pressure and pulmonary artery pressure are the characteristic hemodynamic findings. The therapy of heart failure in association with myocardial infarction is similar to that of heart failure secondary to other forms of heart disease, with a few exceptions (Chap. 253). The major difference concerns the use of cardiac glycosides. The benefit following the administration of digitalis is less impressive in acute myocardial infarction. This is not surprising in that the agent would not be expected to improve the function of infarcted tissue, and the function of the noninfarcted tissue may be normal. On the other hand, diuretic agents are extremely effective in the treatment of heart failure following myocardial infarction. A fall in left ventricular filling pressure and an improvement in orthopnea and dyspnea follow the intravenous administration of furosemide. This drug should be used with caution, however, as it can result in a massive diuresis with associated decrease in plasma volume, cardiac output, systemic blood pressure, and hence coronary perfusion. The patient with pulmonary edema is treated in the manner described in Chap. 253. Recent studies with agents that reduce cardiac afterload, i.e., nitrates, alpha-blockers, hydralazine, prazosin, and sodium nitroprusside, indicate that the reduction in cardiac work which results from the lowered afterload may significantly improve left ventricular performance with a reduction of ventricular filling pressure and pulmonary congestion concomitant with an elevation of cardiac output.

Hemodynamic monitoring Hemodynamic evidence of abnormal left ventricular function becomes apparent when contraction is seriously impaired in 20 to 25 percent of the left ventricle. Infarction of 40 percent or more of the left ventricle will usually result in the syndrome of cardiogenic shock (see below). Compensatory increases in left ventricular filling pressures occur in patients with myocardial infarction and reduced systolic contractile function. Impaired left ventricular compliance also contributes to elevated left ventricular filling pressures in these individuals.

Pulmonary capillary wedge pressure and pulmonary artery diastolic pressure correlate well with left ventricular diastolic pressure and are therefore often referred to as left ventricular filling pressures. Positioning of a balloon flotation catheter in the pulmonary artery enables the physician to monitor left ventricular filling pressure constantly, a technique which is useful in patients who exhibit clinical evidence of hemodynamic abnormalities or instability. Cardiac output can also be determined with a pulmonary artery catheter. Some patients with acute myocardial infarction have markedly elevated left ventricular filling pressures (> 22 mmHg) and normal cardiac outputs [> 2.6 and < 3.6 (liter/min)/m^2], while others have low filling pressures and reduced cardiac indices. The former usually benefit from diuresis, while the latter respond to volume expansion by means of intravenous administration of colloid-containing solutions.

Cardiogenic shock—power failure With the development of effective methods for treating arrhythmias, shock or "power failure" has become the most important fatal complication of myocardial infarction. It is useful to consider this syndrome as a severe form of left ventricular failure. Cardiogenic shock is characterized by marked hypotension with systolic arterial pressure < 80 mmHg and a marked reduction of cardiac index [< 1.8 (liter/min)/m^2] in the face of elevated left ventricular filling (pulmonary capillary wedge) pressure > 18 mmHg. Shock occurs in about 20 percent of patients with myocardial infarction and accounts for at least 70 percent of the in-hospital deaths, now that the mortality rate due to primary arrhythmias has been reduced. The mortality rate in myocardial infarction with shock (Killip class IV) ranges from 85 to 95 percent.

Hypotension alone is not a basis for the diagnosis of the shock syndrome, because many patients who make an uneventful recovery will have serious hypotension (systolic pressures < 80 mmHg) for several days. Such patients often have low left ventricular filling pressures, and their hypotension usually resolves with intravenous administration of colloid-containing solutions. The shock syndrome is considered to be present when hypotension is accompanied by other clinical signs of circulatory inadequacy. The following criteria for the shock syndrome define a population of patients with a mortality rate of greater than 95 percent: (1) systolic arterial blood pressure less than 90 mmHg which has declined by at least 30 mmHg below the previous level, as recorded by direct intraarterial pressure measurements rather than sphygmomanometry; (2) clinical signs of peripheral circulatory insufficiency, e.g., cold, moist skin and cyanosis; (3) dulled sensorium; (4) oliguria with urine flow of less than 20 ml/h; and (5) failure of improvement following relief of pain and administration of oxygen. Specifically *excluded* are patients with hypotension secondary to vasovagal reaction, arrhythmia, drug reaction, or hypovolemia.

PATHOPHYSIOLOGY OF PUMP FAILURE Marked reduction in the quantity of contracting myocardium is the cause of the shock syndrome in myocardial infarction, although all organ systems are ultimately involved. The function of the heart is impaired by the initial insult; this results in a decrease in arterial pressure and hence in coronary blood flow because of its dependence on aortic perfusion pressure (Fig. 261-2). The reduction in coronary perfusion pressure and myocardial blood flow further impairs myocardial function and may increase the size of the myocardial infarction. Arrhythmias and metabolic acidosis also contribute to this deterioration because they are the result of inadequate perfusion, and both tend to perpetuate the precipitating conditions. It is this positive feedback loop (impaired cardiac function → arterial hypotension → reduced coronary blood flow → impaired cardiac function) which accounts for the high mortality rate associated with the shock syndrome.

Arterial blood pressure is a function of two factors—the cardiac output and total peripheral resistance—and a decrease in either without a compensatory rise in the other will result in a fall in arterial blood pressure. Cardiac output is lower in a population of patients with shock than in those who do not have the shock syndrome, but a low cardiac output is by no means the whole explanation for the development of shock. Many patients with myocardial infarction without shock have cardiac outputs in the same range as those in patients with shock, and therefore it is not possible to characterize these patients on the basis of reductions of cardiac output alone.

Total peripheral resistance, the other factor important in determining blood pressure, may be either normal or increased in myocardial infarction. Here again, a range of values for total peripheral resistance may be seen in patients in the absence of shock. Normally, a fall in cardiac output is accompanied by a compensatory rise in total peripheral resistance, but in patients with shock due to myocardial infarction, the appropriate elevation in peripheral resistance may fail to occur.

It is necessary to return to the heart itself as the site of the fundamental physiological alteration in the shock syndrome. It is axiomatic that if the diagnosis of myocardial infarction is correct, there will be a reduction in myocardial contractile function. Measurement of left ventricular filling pressure has demonstrated that left ventricular function may be impaired in the absence of the usual clinical manifestations of left-sided heart failure, such as pulmonary congestion.

A simple schematic diagram depicting the relationship between left ventricular work and filling pressure is seen in Fig. 261-3. The upper curve represents the familiar Frank-Starling relationship in the normal heart; the lower curve shows the relation which might be expected in the patient with shock secondary to myocardial infarction. It is obvious that at all levels of end-diastolic pressure, the left ventricular work of the patient with myocardial infarction is depressed. At point C, the end-diastolic pressure is elevated, but at point B, it may be normal despite the fact that myocardial work is well below that expected of the normal heart at this diastolic pressure, as indicated by point A.

Treatment of pump failure The physiology of this condition dictates that all patients with shock should, if possible, have continuous monitoring of arterial pressure and left ventricular filling pressure as reflected in the pulmonary capillary wedge pressure measured with a pulmonary artery balloon catheter, as well as frequent determinations of cardiac output. All patients with the shock syndrome should receive 100 percent oxygen continuously to help combat the hypoxemia which is uni-

FIGURE 261-2
Diagram depicting the sequence of events in the vicious cycle in which coronary artery obstruction leads to cardiogenic shock and progressive circulatory deterioration.

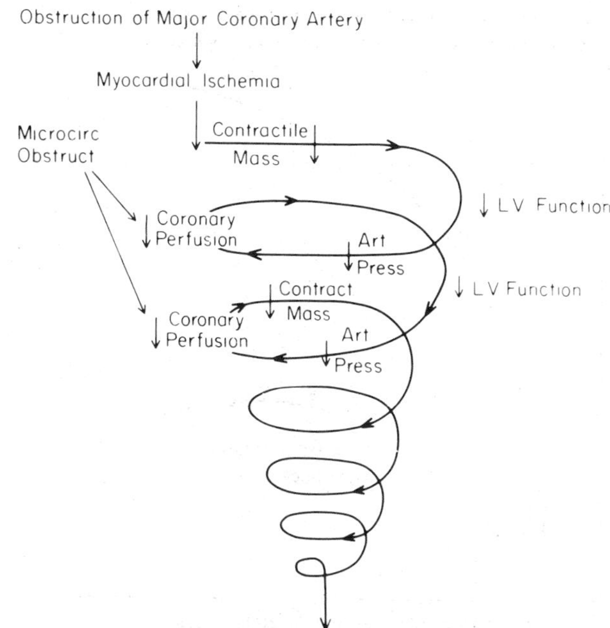

versally present. The relief of pain is important, as some vasodepressor reflex activity may be a response to severe pain. However, narcotics should be used cautiously in view of their propensity to lower arterial pressure.

Treatment is directed at the interruption of the feedback loop (Fig. 261-2), whereby impaired myocardial function leads to a reduction in arterial pressure, decreased coronary blood flow, and further depression of left ventricular function. This objective is approached by attempting to maintain coronary perfusion by raising the arterial blood pressure with vasopressors (see below), intraaortic balloon counterpulsation, and volume replacement to a level that ensures an optimum left ventricular filling pressure (approximately 18 to 20 mmHg).

Hypovolemia This is an easily corrected condition which may contribute to the hypotension and vascular collapse associated with myocardial infarction in some patients. Fluid loss may be secondary to previous diuretic use, to reduced fluid intake during the early stages of the illness, and/or vomiting associated with pain or medications. In addition, a state of relative hypovolemia may exist; i.e., with the acute reduction in contractile function and ventricular compliance resulting from infarction, an increase in vascular volume is needed to maintain cardiac output. Owing to the acute nature of the process, there is insufficient time for compensatory fluid retention to accommodate this need, and relative hypovolemia in a normally hydrated patient results. Consequently, hypovolemia should be identified and corrected in patients with acute myocardial infarction and hypotension before embarking upon more vigorous forms of therapy. If left ventricular filling pressure is in the normal range, fluid should be administered until the left ventricular filling pressure increases to 18 to 20 mmHg. Central venous pressure measurements reflect right rather than left ventricular filling pressure and are inadequate in this situation, since left ventricular function is almost always affected much more adversely than is right ventricular function in acute myocardial infarction.

VASOPRESSORS In cardiogenic shock, the coronary vascular bed distal to an obstructing lesion is maximally dilated, and myocardial blood flow is totally dependent on the perfusion pressure. Agents such as methoxamine, phenylephrine, and angiotensin, which are pure vasoconstrictors, have no place in the treatment of shock due to myocardial infarction, since failure of arterial constriction usually plays only a minor role.

Dopamine is useful in patients with the power failure syndrome. At low dosages [≤ 5 (μg/kg)/min] the drug has positive chronotropic and inotropic effects as a consequence of stimulation of beta receptors. At high doses a vasoconstrictor effect as a result of the stimulation of alpha receptors is noted. Dopamine at lower doses [≤ 2 (μg/kg)/min] also has the unique effect of dilating the renal vascular bed. Experience with this drug in the treatment of pump failure syndromes has been favorable, although it is not clear that it reduces mortality in patients with cardiogenic shock. It appears that dopamine has little effect on myocardial oxygen consumption when employed at low dosages. Intravenous dopamine infusion is started at 2 to 5 (μg/kg)/min with increments in dosage every 2 to 5 min up to a maximum of 20 to 50 (μg/kg)/min. Systolic arterial blood pressure should be maintained at approximately 90 mmHg. *Dobutamine* is a synthetic catecholamine with positive inotropic action and minimal positive chronotropic or peripheral vasoconstrictor activity in the usual dose range, [3 to 10 (μg/kg)/min]. It is unclear whether dobutamine is more effective than dopamine in the treatment of patients with cardiogenic shock and should not be employed when a vasoconstrictor effect is deemed desirable.

Norepinephrine should be administered intravenously through an indwelling catheter to avoid the risk of extravasation, which results in necrosis of subcutaneous tissue. It is desirable to determine the smallest effective dose of norepinephrine by starting with 4 mg dissolved in a liter of 5% glucose solution. The infusion rate should maintain a systolic pressure of around 90 mmHg, which usually provides adequate perfusion of the heart, brain, and kidneys. Increasing the pressure above this level imposes an unnecessary load on the heart and may be undesirable. Should 4 μg/min (1 ml/min) prove inadequate to maintain systolic pressure near 90 mmHg, the concentration of the infused solution should be increased, but if pressure cannot be maintained with a dosage of 15 μg/min, it is unlikely that a further increase in dosage will be beneficial. The lack of response to norepinephrine probably indicates that the remaining functional myocardium is already maximally stimulated by endogenous catecholamines. Renal blood flow is decreased early in the development of circulatory failure, and therefore urine flow constitutes a sensitive indicator of the rate of renal perfusion, which may be considered adequate if a urine flow of 0.5 ml/min is maintained.

Every effort should be made to use the smallest effective dose of positive inotropic agent for the shortest possible time. Weaning the patient from pressors is often difficult and requires close observation and the exercise of considerable clinical judgment. The rate of administration must be reduced cautiously. The systolic arterial pressure may fall to 80 mmHg, but if there are no hemodynamic or clinical signs of circulatory deterioration, i.e., increasing left ventricular filling pressure, cyanosis, clouded sensorium, or cold, moist extremities, it is wise not to reinstitute therapy. Close observation often reveals that arterial pressure rises gradually with passage of time. If, on the other hand, the arterial pressure falls further or clinical signs of circulatory inadequacy appear, therapy should be reinstituted. Pressor amines cause fluid to shift from the intravascular space to the extracellular fluid space, and their prolonged use may result in a depletion of intravascular volume in patients who do not lose weight and who may actually appear edematous. In such instances, blood pressure falls dramatically when pressor amine support is withdrawn. Hypovolemia which results from these internal fluid shifts must be treated in patients who cannot be weaned from pressor amines.

Isoproterenol is a synthetic sympathomimetic amine which

FIGURE 261-3
Schematic representation of the Frank-Starling relationship as applied to patients with the shock syndrome in myocardial infarction.

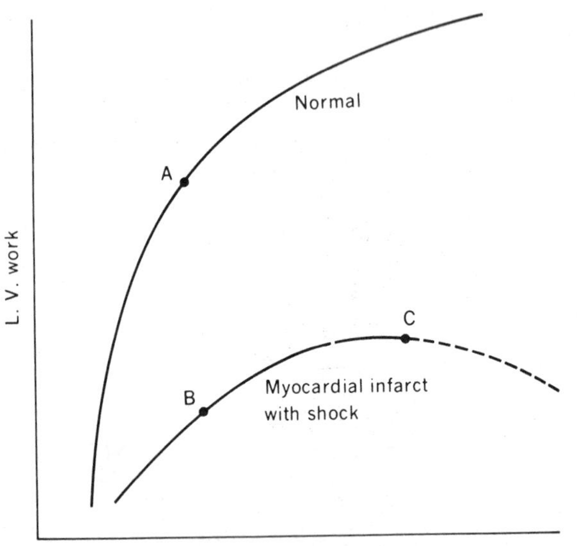

has enjoyed unjustified popularity in the treatment of shock due to myocardial infarction. This agent increases myocardial contractility and, unlike norepinephrine, produces peripheral vasodilatation and increases heart rate. The increase in contractility results in an increase in myocardial oxygen consumption, which may extend the area of ischemic injury. It has also been demonstrated that isoproterenol results in metabolic deterioration, as evidenced by an increase in lactate production by the heart. For all of these reasons, isoproterenol is of little if any value and may actually be detrimental in the treatment of shock due to myocardial infarction.

CARDIAC GLYCOSIDES Consideration of the central role of impaired myocardial function in the shock syndrome leads to the conclusion that cardiac glycosides should be administered to all patients with this condition. Controlled studies, however, have failed to demonstrate significant beneficial effects of glycoside therapy in the early phases (0 to 48 h) of acute myocardial infarction. Hemodynamic improvement has been documented at later times, but this effect is marginal. Since cardiac glycosides cannot improve the function of necrotic myocardium and since pump failure is thought to be related to the total mass of infarcted tissue, digitalis therapy does not result in dramatic improvement in patients with acute myocardial infarction. Nonetheless, it is probably worthwhile to treat patients with signs and symptoms of left ventricular failure with digitalis. It has been demonstrated that when scrupulous attention is paid to the dosage, incidence of arrhythmias and cardiac rupture is no higher in patients with myocardial infarction treated with digitalis than in a control group, and therefore digitalis can be administered with relative safety.

COUNTERPULSATION The basic defect in the shock syndrome is impaired myocardial function; therefore, mechanical assist devices have been developed to supplement the pumping action of the heart. The largest body of clinical experience has been obtained with the intraaortic balloon system of diastolic pressure augmentation. A sausage-shaped balloon at the end of a catheter is introduced into the aorta via the femoral artery, and the balloon is inflated during early diastole, thereby enhancing both coronary blood flow and peripheral perfusion. The balloon collapses in early systole, thereby reducing the afterload against which left ventricular ejection takes place. Improvement in hemodynamic status has been observed with balloon pumping in a large number of patients, but long-term survival following this mode of therapy alone is still disappointing. The balloon counterpulsation system appears to be of greatest use for the support of patients during and after coronary arteriography and bypass surgery.

There is reason to believe that results of therapy of the shock syndrome secondary to myocardial infarction will continue to be disappointing because a large fraction of patients with the syndrome have severe, diffuse coronary atherosclerosis with large areas of infarcted myocardium. Although occasional dramatic results have been reported with emergency revascularization surgery alone, or in combination with infarctectomy, the overall results with this approach have been disappointing.

Other complications MITRAL REGURGITATION Apical systolic murmurs of mitral regurgitation appear in more than one-half of patients during the first 5 days after the onset of a myocardial infarction, but mitral regurgitation is of hemodynamic importance in only a minority of these patients. In most patients the murmur is present during the acute phase of infarction, disappearing with recovery. The most common cause of mitral regurgitation following myocardial infarction is dysfunction of the papillary muscles of the left ventricle, due to ischemia or infarction.

Mitral regurgitation may also be the result of alteration in the size or shape of the ventricle due to impaired contractility or to aneurysm formation. Either papillary muscle may rupture, the posterior one twice as frequently as the anterior. Left ventricular function may deteriorate dramatically with superimposition of mitral regurgitation. The differential diagnosis includes perforation of the ventricular septum (see below), and the differentiation from mitral regurgitation is conveniently made at the bedside with a flow-directed balloon catheter. Large *v* waves may be recorded in the pulmonary capillary wedge position in patients with hemodynamically significant mitral regurgitation, and there is no oxygen "step up" as the catheter is advanced from the right atrium to the right ventricle. Surgical replacement of the mitral valve may be followed by dramatic improvement in patients in whom acute heart failure results primarily from severe mitral regurgitation due to papillary muscle rupture or dysfunction and in whom myocardial function is relatively well maintained.

If aortic systolic pressure is lowered in patients with mitral regurgitation, a greater fraction of the left ventricular output will be ejected antegrade, thus lessening the regurgitant fraction. To this end, both intraaortic balloon counterpulsation, which lowers the aortic systolic pressure mechanically, and the infusion of sodium nitroprusside, 0.5 to 8.0 (μg/kg)/min, which reduces peripheral vascular resistance, have been used with success for the interim management of patients with severe mitral regurgitation in the setting of acute myocardial infarction; the results of definitive operative treatment are better if it can be postponed for 4 to 6 weeks after the infarct. However, if the patient's hemodynamic and/or clinical condition does not improve and stabilize, surgical treatment should be undertaken, even in the acute stage.

VENTRICULAR ANEURYSM The term *ventricular aneurysm* is usually used to describe *dyskinesis* or local expansile paradoxical wall motion. Normally functioning myocardial fibers must shorten more if stroke volume and cardiac output are to be maintained in patients with ventricular aneurysm, and if they are unable to do so, overall ventricular function is impaired.

The complications of left ventricular aneurysm include congestive failure, arterial embolism, and ventricular arrhythmias. Apical aneurysms are the most common and the most easily detected by clinical examination. The physical finding of greatest value is a double, diffuse, or displaced apical impulse. The standard roentgenogram frequently reveals an abnormal bulge distorting the contour of the left heart border, but the roentgenogram may be entirely normal, especially with posterior aneurysms. The electrocardiographic finding of ST-segment elevation at rest is present in precordial leads in 25 percent of patients with either apical or anterior aneurysms. Ventricular aneurysms are readily detectable by two-dimensional echocardiography, which may also reveal a mural thrombus in aneurysms involving the anterior wall and/or apex. Ventricular aneurysms may cause persistent ventricular arrhythmias such as ventricular tachycardia.

RIGHT VENTRICULAR INFARCTION Approximately one-third of patients with inferoposterior infarction demonstrate at least a minor degree of right ventricular myocardial necrosis. An occasional patient with inferoposterior left ventricular infarction also has extensive right ventricular myocardial infarction. These individuals often present with signs of severe right ventricular failure (jugular venous distention, hepatomegaly) with or without hypotension. Catheterization of the right side of the heart often reveals a distinctive hemodynamic pattern resembling cardiac tamponade or constrictive pericarditis (Chap. 265). Intravenous administration of colloid-containing solutions (volume expansion) is often successful in treating low cardiac output and hypotension associated with extensive right ventricular infarction.

THROMBOEMBOLISM Clinically apparent thromboembolism complicates myocardial infarction in approximately 10 percent of cases, but embolic lesions are found in 45 percent of patients in necropsy series, suggesting that thromboembolism is often clinically silent. Thromboembolism is considered to be at least an important contributing cause of death in 25 percent of infarct patients. Arterial emboli originate from left ventricular mural thrombi, but most pulmonary emboli arise in the leg veins. Thromboembolism most commonly occurs in association with large infarcts in the presence of heart failure. The high incidence of thromboembolism constitutes one of the best arguments for the use of systemic anticoagulant therapy in patients with extensive infarction.

CARDIAC RUPTURE Myocardial rupture is a dramatic complication of myocardial infarction most likely to occur during the first week after the onset of symptoms; its frequency increases with the age of the patient. First infarction, female sex, and hypertension are associated with a higher incidence of cardiac rupture. The clinical presentation may often be that of a sudden disappearance of the pulse, blood pressure, and consciousness while the electrocardiogram continues to show sinus rhythm (apparent electromechanical dissociation). The myocardium continues to contract, but forward flow is not maintained as blood escapes into the pericardium. Cardiac tamponade ensues (Chap. 265), and closed-chest massage is ineffective. Although almost universally fatal, there have been a few instances in which cardiac rupture has been recognized and successfully treated by pericardiocentesis and emergency cardiac surgery.

SEPTAL PERFORATION The pathogenesis of perforation of the ventricular septum is similar to that of external rupture of the myocardium, but the therapeutic potential is greater. Patients with ventricular septal rupture present with severe heart failure in association with the sudden appearance of a pansystolic murmur, often accompanied by a parasternal thrill. It is often impossible to differentiate this condition from rupture of a papillary muscle, and a tall *v* wave in the pulmonary capillary wedge pressure further complicates the differentiation between these two conditions. The diagnosis can be established by the demonstration of a left-to-right shunt (i.e., an oxygen step-up at the level of the right ventricle) by limited cardiac catheterization performed at the bedside using a flow-directed balloon catheter. Rupture of the ventricular septum is amenable to immediate surgical treatment, albeit at a high mortality. If the clinical condition permits, however, surgical intervention should be postponed for 6 to 8 weeks, at which time the margins of the defect are composed of firm scar tissue, and surgical closure is easier and more likely to be successful. The physiology of acute mitral regurgitation and acute ventricular septal perforation are similar in that the level of aortic systolic pressure determines in part the regurgitant fraction, the only difference being the chamber into which the regurgitant fraction is ejected. In septal perforation, a fraction of left ventricular output is ejected into the right ventricle. In a manner analogous to mitral regurgitation, lowering of aortic systolic pressure by mechanical (intraaortic balloon counterpulsation) or pharmacological (nitroglycerin or nitroprusside) means can decrease the hemodynamic compromise caused by perforation.

PERICARDITIS (see also Chap. 265) Pericardial friction rubs and/or pericardial pain are frequently encountered in patients with acute transmural myocardial infarction. This complication can usually be managed with aspirin (650 mg qid). It is important to diagnose the chest pain of pericarditis accurately, since failure to appreciate it may lead to the erroneous diagnosis of recurrent ischemic pain and/or infarct extension with resultant inappropriate use of anticoagulants, nitrates, propranolol, or narcotics. No definite cause and effect relationship between anticoagulant administration and pericarditis or tamponade has been proved. Nonetheless, the possibility that anticoagulants can cause tamponade in the presence of acute pericarditis is sufficiently high to contraindicate their use in patients with pericarditis, as manifested by either pain or persistent rub, unless there is a compelling indication.

POSTMYOCARDIAL INFARCTION SYNDROME—DRESSLER'S SYNDROME (see also Chap. 265) This syndrome, characterized by fever and pleuropericardial chest pain, is thought to be due to an autoimmune pericarditis, pleuritis, and pneumonitis. It may begin from a few days to 6 weeks after myocardial infarction. The pain can often be distinguished from that of an extending infarction by its characteristic pericardial pattern: it is substernal, radiates to the neck and shoulders, is relieved by leaning forward, and exacerbated by deep breathing. The syndrome usually responds promptly to therapy with salicylates. On occasion, corticosteroids may be required to relieve discomfort of an unusual, refractory nature. Effusions associated with Dressler's syndrome may become hemorrhagic if anticoagulants are administered.

SHOULDER-HAND SYNDROME A few patients develop pain and stiffness of the left arm and shoulder following myocardial infarction. The syndrome is probably related to immobility during the early period of therapy and is less frequent in patients who have been mobilized at an early stage in convalescence.

UNSTABLE ANGINA The manifestations of ischemic heart disease may be thought of as representing a spectrum ranging from stable angina pectoris at one end to acute myocardial infarction at the other. In angina pectoris, the myocardial blood supply is temporarily inadequate, but there is no death of tissue, whereas myocardial infarction is, by definition, characterized by death of myocardial tissue. Some patients develop manifestations which logically place them at an intermediate position between these two extremes, the syndrome of unstable angina. Included under this heading are syndromes known as acute coronary insufficiency, unstable angina, intermediate syndrome, and preinfarctional angina. Unstable angina may be superimposed upon a background of stable exertional angina pectoris, or it may represent the first manifestation of symptomatic ischemic heart disease.

Unstable angina pectoris may be characterized by discrete episodes of severe ischemic chest discomfort which may come on at *rest.* On occasion, the discomfort begins during exertion and does not disappear with rest. The pain lasts 30 min or more and is of such severity that the diagnosis of myocardial infarction is considered. Although there may be transient electrocardiographic ST-segment and T-wave changes, myocardial infarction is ruled out by the absence of both evolutionary QRS changes in the electrocardiogram and diagnostic elevation of serum enzyme concentrations. Unstable angina may be superimposed upon chronic stable angina pectoris. The patient notes that his pain is precipitated by less severe exertion, comes more frequently, lasts longer, or has changed in pattern. Alternatively, unstable angina, characterized by pain at rest or with minimal exertion, may be the first manifestation of ischemic heart disease.

Coronary arteriography in patients with unstable angina has revealed a spectrum of morphological abnormalities ranging from severe three-vessel involvement to normal coronary anatomy, indicating that the term *unstable angina* does not define a specific clinical entity but rather a pattern of presentation in the spectrum of coronary artery disease. Coronary vasospasm may play an important role in the pathophysiology of unstable angina pectoris, in patients both with and without obstructive coronary artery disease.

Most patients with unstable angina stabilize with intensive medical therapy, i.e., hospitalization, bed rest, oxygen, sedation, and drug therapy with nitrates, beta-blocking agents, and calcium channel blockers. The adequate dose of beta-blocking agent varies from patient to patient, and increasing amounts of drug should be administered until the resting pulse rate is below 60 beats per minute. Patients with unstable angina pectoris should receive continuous electrocardiographic monitoring. Given the high success rate with medical therapy (> 75 percent) and the slightly increased risk of coronary arteriography and coronary artery bypass graft surgery in patients with unstable angina, intensive medical therapy should be the initial approach in these patients. Should such therapy be successful, as defined by the disappearance of rest pain and/or the resumption of previous activity levels, the need for immediate coronary arteriography with a view toward emergency surgery is obviated. The question of coronary arteriography and coronary bypass graft surgery may then be considered on an elective basis as it would be in any patient with chronic stable severe coronary artery disease. On the other hand, if unstable angina persists despite intensive medical therapy, it is advisable to carry out coronary arteriography and, if the anatomy is suitable, revascularization surgery. Often these procedures may be aided by stabilizing the patient with intravenous nitroglycerin infusion and/or intraaortic balloon counterpulsation.

REFERENCES

ALPERT JS: *The Heart Attack Handbook: A Commonsense Guide to Treatment, Recovery, and Prevention.* Boston, Little, Brown, 1978

———, BRAUNWALD E: Pathological and clinical manifestations of acute myocardial infarction, in *Heart Disease,* 2d ed, E Braunwald (ed). Philadelphia, Saunders, 1983, chap 37

COHN JN, FRANCIOSA JA: Pathophysiology of shock in acute myocardial infarction, in *Progress in Cardiology,* PN Yu, JF Goodwin (eds). Philadelphia, Lea & Febiger, 1973, vol 2

FORRESTER JS et al: Medical therapy of acute myocardial infarction by application of hemodynamic subsets. N Engl J Med 295:1356, 1404, 1976

HILLIS LD, BRAUNWALD E: Myocardial ischemia. N Engl J Med 296:971, 1034, 1093, 1977

KARLINER JS, GREGORATOS G: *Coronary Care.* New York, Churchill Livingstone, 1981

MILLER DH et al: Exercise testing early after myocardial infarction. Am J Med 72:427, 1982

PANTRIDGE JF et al: *The Acute Coronary Attack.* New York, Grune & Stratton, 1975

RUDE R, MULLER JE, BRAUNWALD E: Efforts to limit the size of myocardial infarcts. Ann Intern Med 95:736, 1981

SOBEL BE, BRAUNWALD E: Management of acute myocardial infarction, in *Heart Disease,* 2d ed, Philadelphia, Saunders, 1983, chap 38

WENGER NK et al: Physician practice in the management of patients with uncomplicated myocardial infarction: Changes in the past decade. Circulation 65:421, 1982

262 COR PULMONALE

ALFRED P. FISHMAN

Cor pulmonale denotes enlargement of the right ventricle secondary to malfunctioning lungs. Often, but not invariably, hypertrophy and dilatation coexist; in chronic cor pulmonale, hypertrophy is more apt to predominate than in acute cor pulmonale. Moreover, the abnormal performance of the lungs need not be due to intrinsic lung disease: in some instances, an abnormal chest bellows or a depressed ventilatory drive from the respiratory centers (Table 262-1) is the cause. Invariably, if the cause is in the lungs, the disease will be diffuse, bilateral, and extensive, in most cases affecting airways as well as parenchyma.

Pulmonary arterial hypertension invariably precedes cor pulmonale. In practice, cor pulmonale is synonymous with pulmonary hypertensive heart disease, even though hypoxemia and polycythemia, as well as pulmonary hypertension, often contribute to overloading the right ventricle. But before making the diagnosis of cor pulmonale, *primary disease of the left side of the heart* and *congenital heart disease* must be excluded. It is worth emphasizing that the term *cor pulmonale* does not automatically imply heart failure. However, it is understood that if the pulmonary hypertension that led to enlargement of the right ventricle is not relieved, cor pulmonale will become associated with right ventricular failure.

Hypertrophy and/or dilatation of the right ventricle are usually much more difficult to detect and to quantify, both clinically and at autopsy, than are left ventricular hypertrophy and dilatation. Consequently, in interpreting the size of the right ventricle it is helpful to understand the mechanisms that operated during life to impose an abnormal hemodynamic load upon it.

These caveats have several practical implications. By underscoring the critical role of abnormal performance of some component(s) of the respiratory system in the pathogenesis of cor pulmonale, the point is being emphasized that prognosis and treatment of cor pulmonale *depend more on relieving the respiratory disorder than on improving the performance of the right ventricle.* Moreover, by stressing *enlargement* of the right ventricle as the hallmark of cor pulmonale, they indicate that pulmonary hypertension may exist without detectable enlargement of the right ventricle and that right ventricular failure is a complication, rather than an essential feature, of cor pulmonale.

TABLE 262-1
Respiratory disorders predisposing to chronic cor pulmonale*

1 Intrinsic disease of the lungs and intrapulmonary airways
- *a* Chronic obstructive lung disease (COLD)
- *b* Diffuse pulmonary interstitial disease
- *c* Pulmonary vascular disease

2 Upper airways obstruction
- *a* Tracheal stenosis
- *b* Obstructive sleep apnea syndromes
- *c* Congenital anatomic abnormalities of oropharynx

3 Malfunctioning chest bellows
- *a* Kyphoscoliosis
- *b* Neuromuscular incompetence
- *c* Marked obesity ("Pickwickian syndrome")

4 Inadequate ventilatory drive from respiratory centers
- *a* Primary or idiopathic alveolar hypoventilation ("Ondine's curse")
- *b* Chronic mountain sickness
- *c* Central sleep apnea syndromes

* *The term respiratory disorders includes not only the diseases and disorders of the lungs, airways, and chest bellows, but also malfunctioning of the centers that control breathing and the support structures of the oropharynx. In essence, respiratory disorders refers to malfunctioning of any part or parts of the entire respiratory system and of the structures that impinge upon it.*

TYPES OF COR PULMONALE By tradition, the designation "acute" is generally reserved for the dilatation of the right side of the heart which follows acute embolization of the lungs. The designation "chronic" is less specific. Usually chronicity is judged by the type and duration of the respiratory disorder that led to the cardiac enlargement (Table 262-1). Just how long, and to what degree, the heart remains enlarged will depend on fluctuations in the level of pulmonary arterial pressure.

INCIDENCE Reliable estimates of the prevalence of chronic cor pulmonale are sparse. After the age of 50, cor pulmonale is the most common cardiac disorder except for coronary and hypertensive heart disease. However, because obstructive disease of the airways is so prevalent and is so often the precursor of pulmonary hypertension, cor pulmonale is a common type of heart disease. Indeed, in parts of the world where cigarette smoking and air pollution have resulted in a high incidence of chronic bronchitis and emphysema (described in detail in Chap. 279), cor pulmonale may comprise up to one-quarter of all types of heart failure. By virtue of exposure rather than predisposition, men are more often affected than women. Chronic cor pulmonale is also a common sequel to cystic fibrosis (Chap. 278). In contrast, it is an unusual complication of allergic asthma.

Most diffuse pulmonary diseases are either too limited in extent or too circumscribed in their effects on alveolar-capillary gas exchange to set in motion the train of events leading to cor pulmonale. Thus, the bulk of patients with silicosis, emphysema, or diffuse fibrosis suffer from breathlessness for years but fail to develop pulmonary hypertension or cardiomegaly.

PATHOGENESIS

Pulmonary hypertension is a prerequisite for cor pulmonale. Although a high cardiac output, tachycardia, an expanded blood volume, or myocardial damage from hypoxia and acidosis may all contribute to the pulmonary hypertension, the crux in the pathogenetic sequence is an increase in pulmonary vascular resistance to blood flow through small muscular arteries and arterioles. The increase in vascular resistance may be anatomic or vasomotor in origin; often both mechanisms are involved (Table 262-2).

It has been noted above that the increase in the work of the right ventricle imposed by the pulmonary hypertension may cause it to fail. However, even in patients with evidence of depression of right ventricular stroke volume due to pulmonary hypertensive overloading, the myocardium of the right ventricle seems capable of normal contractile behavior.

ANATOMIC INCREASE IN PULMONARY VASCULAR RESISTANCE In the normal resting individual, the pulmonary circulation is a highly distensible, low-resistance circuit, accommodating the same blood flow as the systemic circulation at approximately one-fifth the mean blood pressure; during moderate exercise, tripling the blood flow elicits only slight increments in pulmonary arterial pressure. Even after pneumonectomy, the residual pulmonary vascular bed accepts considerable increments in pulmonary blood flow with only slight increase in pulmonary artery pressure as long as the lung is free of fibrosis, emphysema, or pulmonary vascular change. Similarly, disappearance of a large portion of the pulmonary capillary bed in emphysema generally fails to elicit pulmonary hypertension.

However, when pulmonary vascular reserve has been exhausted by progressive reduction in the extent and distensibility of the pulmonary vascular tree, even the increments in blood flow associated with daily living may suffice to elicit marked pulmonary hypertension. The essential component of this vulnerability is a decrease in the cross-sectional area of the pulmonary resistance vessels. The restricted vascular bed stems from widespread narrowing and obstruction of small pulmonary arteries and arterioles, usually accompanied by a decrease in the distensibility not only of the vessels but also of the adjacent lung.

VASOMOTOR INCREASE IN PULMONARY VASCULAR RESISTANCE (HYPOXIA AND ACIDOSIS) The most potent stimulus for pulmonary vasoconstriction is alveolar hypoxia which acts directly on adjacent small pulmonary arteries and arterioles; systemic arterial hypoxemia supplements the local effects of alveolar hypoxia indirectly by way of the sympathetic nerves to the pulmonary circulation. Experiments in dogs indicate that severe acidosis ($pH < 7.2$) also elicits pulmonary vasoconstriction. In humans, acidosis acts synergistically with hypoxia, whereas alkalosis diminishes the pressor response to hypoxia. The biologic basis for this interplay remains unclear. In chronic hypoxia, the effects of these pulmonary hypertensive

TABLE 262-2
Pathogenetic mechanisms in chronic pulmonary hypertension and cor pulmonale

Pathogenetic mechanism	*Intermediaries*	*Examples*
PRIMARY MECHANISMS		
Anatomic increase in pulmonary vascular resistance	Obliteration, obstruction, reduction, and stiffening of pulmonary vascular tree	*Vascular disease:* Primary pulmonary hypertension; recurrent pulmonary emboli *Extravascular disease:* Diffuse interstitial disease; fibrosing alveolitis; pneumoconiosis
Vasomotor increase in pulmonary vascular resistance	Pulmonary vasoconstriction by hypoxia and acidosis	*General alveolar hypoventilation with normal lungs:* *1* Disorders of chest bellows: neuromuscular; extreme obesity; kyphoscoliosis *2* Diminished ventilatory drive: primary alveolar hypoventilation; sleep; hypercapnia
Combined anatomic restriction and vasomotor	Combination of above	*Net alveolar hypoventilation with abnormal lungs:* Chronic obstructive lung disease: "blue bloater"; cystic fibrosis of pancreas
SECONDARY MECHANISMS		
Increase in cardiac output	Increase in metabolic rate; acute hypoxia	Daily activities; acute respiratory infection
Increase in blood viscosity	Secondary polycythemia	Chronic hypoxia
Tachycardia	Aggravation of hypoxia	Heart failure

stimuli are often intensified by increased viscosity of the blood arising from secondary polycythemia.

HYPERCAPNIA In contrast to the effects of hypoxia and acidosis, the effects of CO_2 on the pulmonary circulation appear to be by way of the acidosis that it generates rather than by a direct action on pulmonary vessels. However, because heart failure in cor pulmonale is often associated with respiratory insufficiency, and because management of the respiratory insufficiency generally determines the prognosis, the noncardiac effects of hypercapnia merit consideration.

Hypercapnia affects mainly the central nervous system, producing cerebral vasodilatation, increased cerebrospinal fluid pressure, and neurologic derangements ranging from weakness, irritability, lassitude, and cloudy sensorium to somnolence, confusion, and coma. These derangements are most apt to occur if hypercapnia is acute in onset and severe, or if chronic hypercapnia is acutely aggravated. In contrast, during chronic hypercapnia, the patient may be virtually free of central nervous system disturbances if respiratory acidosis is fully compensated. When severe hypoxemia and hypercapnia coexist, it may be impossible to distinguish between their neurologic effects because severe hypoxia causes anatomic damage to nervous tissues.

Carbon dioxide retention, with elevated CO_2 tensions in the blood and tissues, is self-perpetuating. On the one hand, hypercapnia from any cause blunts the responsiveness of the respiratory center to the CO_2 stimulus; on the other, hypercapnia promotes retention of bicarbonate by the kidney. Not only the hypercapnia originating in disorders of the lungs or ventilation, but also the hypercapnia of metabolic alkalosis, such as that produced by powerful diuretics, causes ventilatory depression. This is why patients with chronic hypercapnia are particularly vulnerable to the effects of sedatives or oxygen breathing, both of which may cause calamitous increments in the degree of hypercapnia: sedatives by depressing further the respiratory centers in the brain, and oxygen by abolishing the hypoxic peripheral drive to ventilation. A large diuresis in which the loss of chloride is inordinate for the output of chloride may be equally effective in depressing the ventilation. It is usually in the severely hypoxic, hypercapnic patient that right-sided heart failure occurs.

ALVEOLAR HYPOVENTILATION A large disparity commonly exists between the degree of pulmonary hypertension recorded during life and the anatomic changes in the lungs and pulmonary vessels at autopsy. This discrepancy is particularly marked in patients with obstructive disease of the airways, in whom the anatomic changes in the gas-exchanging parts of the lungs consistently appear to be inadequate to explain either the blood-gas abnormalities or the pulmonary arterial pressor response. Similarly, the most extensive emphysema may be associated with normal levels of blood gases and normal pulmonary arterial pressures. Much of this discrepancy disappears when account is taken of alveolar hypoventilation, an important functional disorder which cannot be quantified at autopsy. Recognizing that alveolar hypoventilation is an essential component in the pathogenesis of cor pulmonale is critical for two reasons: (1) elimination of the initiating mechanism (e.g., acute respiratory infection) usually reverses the alveolar hypoventilation, and (2) unless alveolar ventilation is improved, other therapeutic measures are apt to be ineffective.

The importance of alveolar hypoventilation in the pathogenesis of cor pulmonale has been underscored in recent years by observations of its occurrence in patients with sleep apnea syndromes in whom hypoxia is a consequence of inadequate ventilatory drive (central apnea) or of upper airways obstruction (peripheral apnea) whereas the lungs and chest bellows are normal. Dramatic improvements have often followed relief of the initiating mechanism, e.g., hypertrophied tonsils and adenoids, or bypassing an area of obstruction, e.g., tracheostomy for tracheal stenosis.

PULMONARY HYPERTENSION

Two distinct patterns characterize the natural history of cor pulmonale at sea level: (1) The pattern of *episodic* pulmonary hypertension, due to exacerbations of the underlying pulmonary disorder, is more common. Generally, each bout leaves its imprint and predisposes to continuing hypertension even though recovery from the early bouts frequently is associated with the return of pulmonary arterial pressures to normal. (2) The pattern of *progressive,* unremitting pulmonary hypertension and cor pulmonale leading inexorably to right-sided heart failure is generally a consequence either of progressive pulmonary vascular or interstitial disease or of unremitting hypoxia (as in continuing alveolar hypoventilation). Distinction between the two sequences tends to become blurred if intercurrent respiratory infections decrease the intervals between bouts of hypoxia and pulmonary hypertension. Also, each bout of pulmonary hypertension seems to predispose to a subsequent bout of cor pulmonale because of residual hypertrophy of the muscular pulmonary arteries or further curtailment of the extent and distensibility of the pulmonary vascular tree. Consequently, although relief of hypoxia may restore the pulmonary arterial pressure to normal or near-normal levels, with each attack the pulmonary vascular tree seems to lose some of its adaptability and the patient moves a little closer to the verge of persistent pulmonary hypertension and cor pulmonale.

As a general rule, pulmonary hypertension appears in a predisposed individual either when blood flow is increased (exercise, fever) or during a bout of acute hypoxia (bronchopulmonary infection). In time, pulmonary hypertension is present even at rest. The highest pulmonary artery pressures occur in pulmonary vascular and interstitial disease; the levels of pulmonary hypertension are neither as high nor as fixed in chronic obstructive diseases of the airways, even during an acute exacerbation.

The pulmonary hypertension that comes on only during exercise or hypoxia is associated with normal end-diastolic pressure in the right ventricle. However, as pulmonary hypertension becomes persistent and severe, abnormally high filling (end-diastolic) pressure develops in the right ventricle as a result either of incomplete emptying of the ventricle as it dilates or of the decrease in ventricular compliance associated with hypertrophy; cardiac output is still normal at rest and increases normally during exercise (cor pulmonale without heart failure). Finally, the onset of right-sided heart failure is identified by abnormally high end-diastolic pressures in the right ventricle. At this stage, the cardiac output, which may still be normal at rest, fails to increase normally during exercise; the systemic veins are engorged, reflecting the inability of the right ventricle to empty normally.

THE LEFT VENTRICLE IN COR PULMONALE Recent observations on the interplay between the two ventricles ("interdependence") have served as a reminder that both ventricles not only are encased in common muscle bundles and pericardium but also have one wall in common, i.e., the ventricular septum. Increasing pressures in the right ventricle displace the septum into the left ventricle, thereby encroaching upon its lumen and modifying left ventricular pressures as well as volumes. However, the clinical significance of these changes is uncertain.

Except in the case of the few severely hypoxemic high-altitude dwellers who develop mountain sickness, the left ventricle does not seem to share in the cardiomegaly of high altitude. Consequently, *tolerable* levels of hypoxia do not exert serious noxious effects on the myocardium; nor are they associated with an inordinate hemodynamic load on the left ventricle. Conversely, severe, intolerable levels of hypoxia and arterial hypoxemia at altitude may impair myocardial function of both ventricles as well as produce right ventricular overload. The left ventricle then enlarges and fails, primarily because of inadequate oxygen delivery to the myocardium. These observations at high altitude suggest that right ventricular overload, per se, does not interfere with left ventricular function unless pulmonary hypertension is severe and accompanied by severe hypoxemia.

At sea level, cor pulmonale is not associated with left ventricular enlargement as long as arterial hypoxemia is modest in degree, but in pulmonary disorders associated with severe hypoxemia, left ventricular enlargement and malfunction may occur. In the latter group, a complicated interplay seems to be involved in the pathogenesis of abnormal left ventricular performance: independent disease of the left ventricle, particularly arteriosclerotic heart disease, aggravated by the direct effects of inadequate oxygen delivery to the myocardium plus the noxious effect of severe hypoxemia and acidosis on the myocardium. In turn, the respiratory insufficiency, which initiated the impaired myocardial performance by causing abnormal levels of arterial blood gases, is intensified if left ventricular failure causes interstitial and alveolar pulmonary edema.

CLINICAL MANIFESTATIONS OF COR PULMONALE

The likelihood that a physician will recognize that a patient has cor pulmonale depends on his or her awareness that the underlying respiratory disorder can culminate in pulmonary hypertension. The diagnosis is generally straightforward in obliterative diseases of the pulmonary circulation, e.g., multiple pulmonary emboli. It is much more elusive in obstructive disease of the airways because chronic bronchitis and bronchiolitis are not always self-evident, and clinical indexes of pulmonary hypertension are not always reliable. Therefore, the cor pulmonale that follows chronic bronchitis may be appreciated only retrospectively, i.e., after an episode of overt right ventricular failure. Detection may be particularly difficult if the systemic venous congestion and peripheral edema develop insidiously, over days to weeks, rather than suddenly in the course of an acute bronchopulmonary infection. This situation has been dramatically demonstrated by the increased clinical detection of cor pulmonale and right ventricular failure that has accompanied the increased awareness of the sleep apnea syndromes and of the high incidence of cor pulmonale as a complication.

DIFFERENTIAL DIAGNOSIS Cor pulmonale is particularly important to recognize in the elderly patient who is old enough to have arteriosclerotic heart disease, has had cough and sputum for many years ("chronic bronchitis"), and clearly manifests right ventricular failure. Analyses of arterial blood gases are then most helpful in deciding whether the primary cardiac disorder is in the right or left ventricle, since appreciable arterial hypoxemia, hypercapnia, and acidosis are unusual in left-sided heart failure unless frank pulmonary edema is also present.

Support for the diagnosis of cor pulmonale may be adduced from roentgenographic and electrocardiographic evidence of right ventricular enlargement. Rarely is catheterization of the right side of the heart needed to settle the question, once suspicion of cor pulmonale is aroused. But, if necessary, cardiac catheterization will typically show pulmonary arterial hypertension, normal left atrial ("pulmonary wedge") pressures, and the classic hemodynamics of right ventricular failure.

The conventional signs of right ventricular enlargement include a cardiac thrust along the left sternal border, or immediately below the sternum, and a fourth heart sound arising in the hypertrophied ventricle. Concomitant pulmonary hypertension is suggested by a thrust in the second left interspace adjacent to the sternum, an unusually loud second component of the second heart sound in the same area, and occasionally the murmur of pulmonary valvular insufficiency. If the right ventricle fails, tricuspid insufficiency and a right ventricular gallop sound are often added. Hydrothorax is uncommon, even after the advent of overt right ventricular failure. Permanent arrhythmias, such as atrial flutter or fibrillation, are unusual, but transitory arrhythmias are common during severe hypoxia or when respiratory alkalosis has been induced by mechanical hyperventilation.

The diagnostic value of the *electrocardiogram* in cor pulmonale depends on the underlying pulmonary or ventilatory disorder (Table 262-3). It is most valuable in pulmonary vascular or interstitial disease, particularly if unassociated with obstructive disease of the airways, or in alveolar hypoventilation with normal lungs. Conversely, because of the hyperinflated lungs and the episodic nature of the pulmonary hypertension and right ventricular overload, patterns diagnostic of right ventricular hypertrophy are uncommon in cor pulmonale secondary to chronic bronchitis and emphysema. Consequently, even if right ventricular enlargement in the course of chronic bronchitis and emphysema is marked, as during a bout of acute upper respiratory infection, electrocardiographic evidence may be inconclusive because of rotation and displacement of the heart, widened distances between electrodes and the cardiac surface, and the predominance of dilatation over hypertrophy in the cardiac enlargement. Thus a reliable diagnosis of right ventricular enlargement can be expected in one-third of patients with chronic bronchitis and emphysema whose hearts show right ventricular hypertrophy at autopsy, whereas the diagnosis is easily and reliably made in the great majority of patients with cor pulmonale originating in pulmonary disorders other than chronic bronchitis and emphysema. With these qualifications in mind, the more reliable criteria for right ventricular hypertrophy in a patient who has chronic bronchitis and emphysema have proved to be an S_1Q_3 pattern; right axis deviation $\geq 110°$; an $S_1S_2S_3$ pattern; and an R/S ratio in $V_6 \leq 1.0$. Combinations of these criteria enhance their diagnostic sensitivities.

Roentgenography has more diagnostic value in arousing suspicion of or confirming than in detecting enlargement of the right ventricle. Suspicion is aroused by evidences of an ante-

TABLE 262-3
ECG patterns in chronic cor pulmonale

1 Chronic obstructive lung disease (suggestive, but not diagnostic, of right ventricular enlargement)*
  - *a* "P pulmonale" (in leads II, III, aVF)
  - *b* Right axis deviation $\geq 110°$
  - *c* R/S ratio in $V_6 \leq 1$
  - *d* rRS′ in right chest leads
  - *e* Right bundle branch block (partial or complete)

2 Pulmonary vascular or interstitial disease; general alveolar hypoventilation (diagnostic of right ventricular enlargement)
  - *a* Classic pattern in V_1 or V_3R (dominant R or R′ with inverted T waves in right chest leads)
  - *b* Often associated with "suggestive" criteria above

* *Among the "suggestive" criteria, it is difficult to distinguish right ventricular enlargement (hypertrophy and dilatation) from changes in the anatomic and electrical positions of the heart produced by the hyperinflated lungs. Consequently, the "suggestive" criteria are more useful as confirmatory, than as diagnostic, evidence.*

cedent predisposing pulmonary disorder coupled with large central pulmonary arteries and a pruned peripheral arterial tree, i.e., evidence of pulmonary hypertension. Serial x-rays are generally more useful than a single examination for heart size, particularly in obstructive disease of the airways, where dramatic changes in heart size may occur between a bout of acute respiratory insufficiency and recovery.

Echocardiography has recently come into play as a tool for detecting pulmonary hypertension on the basis of movements of the pulmonary valve. The technique is not easy but is gaining in popularity.

CLINICAL FORMS OF COR PULMONALE AND THEIR TREATMENT

Regardless of the mechanism of initiation—anatomic, vasomotor, or both—chronic pulmonary hypertension tends to be self-perpetuating because of continuing narrowing and obliteration of the pulmonary vascular bed by muscular hypertrophy of small arteries and arterioles, arteriosclerosis, thrombosis, and, less commonly, tortuous malformations in the course of small arteries and arterioles ("plexiform lesions").

ANATOMIC INCREASE IN PULMONARY VASCULAR RESISTANCE These abnormalities may be sorted into two general categories (Table 262-2): vascular disease and extravascular disease, as described below.

Vascular disease; occlusive disease of the small pulmonary arteries In these disorders, widespread occlusion of the small pulmonary vessels takes place over months to years. Most often, the cause is multiple pulmonary emboli (Chap. 282); less common are multiple thromboses such as those which complicate sickle cell anemia. A rare cause is primary (unexplained) pulmonary hypertension (Chap. 281).

Tachypnea, persisting during sleep, is an outstanding feature of multiple pulmonary emboli. This increase in respiratory frequency is associated with alveolar hyperventilation as indicated by characteristically low values for alveolar and arterial P_{CO_2} and for serum bicarbonate. Incapacitating breathlessness occurs on mild exertion. Precordial or thoracic pain is not uncommon: occasionally the pain mimics angina; at other times it is clearly pleuritic, intensifying during inspiration. The clinical roentgenographic and electrocardiographic signs of right ventricular enlargement are present. Cyanosis, which is rarely impressive before heart failure, usually becomes striking after the right ventricle fails. Objective evidence for pulmonary emboli is conventionally sought by photoscanning and pulmonary angiography (Chaps. 272 and 282).

Of all patients who develop cor pulmonale, those with multiple pulmonary emboli or primary pulmonary hypertension have the highest pulmonary arterial pressures; these may equal or even exceed systemic arterial pressures. The cardiac output tends to be low. Mild arterial hypoxemia is the rule and seems to arise from shunting within the lungs. Whether the shunts represent blood flow through recanalized vessels (e.g., glomus formations) that are no longer in contact with alveoli, or too-rapid passage of the entire cardiac output through unoccluded and dilated portions of the pulmonary vascular tree, or blood flow through anatomic pulmonary arteriovenous channels that are ordinarily inoperative, is conjectural. During right-sided heart failure, these shunts cause profound arterial hypoxemia because the shunted (mixed venous) blood has an extremely low O_2 content.

Once pulmonary hypertension is fixed, treatment directed at the process in the lungs is rarely effective, since organization of emboli has led to irreversible occlusions of innumerable small arteries. Continuous administration of O_2-enriched mixtures is standard. Caution must be exercised to avoid oxygen toxicity by administering as little additional oxygen as possible. Unfortunately, compromises are often required, since arterial blood is not easily restored toward normal levels of oxygenation because of the magnitude of the venous shunts.

The grim outlook for treating the cor pulmonale of multiple pulmonary emboli, as well as the ever-present prospect of catastrophic pulmonary embolization, has emphasized the need for prophylactic measures in patients judged to be candidates for pulmonary emboli (Chap. 282). Heart failure is treated by the usual cardiotonic measures in conjunction with measures directed at improving arterial oxygenation. Rarely does it respond dramatically as long as the hemodynamic overload persists.

Diffuse interstitial fibrosis and granuloma Among the diverse entities included in this category are (1) sarcoidosis, berylliosis, and the "nonspecific" granulomatoses (Chap. 280); (2) scleroderma of the lung (Chap. 280), (3) the various interstitial or alveolar-septal fibroses such as "fibrosing alveolitis," radiation fibrosis, or pulmonary asbestosis, and the special progressive form of interstitial disease known as the Hamman-Rich syndrome (Chap. 280); (4) immunopathologic disease of the lungs, exemplified by "farmer's lung" (Chap. 274); and (5) diffuse carcinomatous infiltration of the lung, such as "alveolar-cell" or lymphangitic carcinoma (Chap. 284).

Clinically, the respiratory difficulty often begins with an acute respiratory illness that fails to resolve. Tachypnea persists. The roentgenogram shows fine nodular or fibrotic lesions widely disseminated throughout both lung fields. In the resting subject, the arterial P_{O_2} is sustained at near-normal levels by chronic hyperventilation; during exercise, it drops precipitously. The arterial P_{CO_2} is normal or slightly low, reflecting the balance between the augmented ventilation, the oxygen consumption, which is often increased, and the partition of the augmented ventilation between the alveoli and the dead space.

As long as hypoxemia is mild, pulmonary hypertension is modest. But as the disease progresses and as hypoxemia increases—in part because of ventilation-perfusion abnormalities—the level of pulmonary hypertension also increases, and cor pulmonale begins to evolve. Right ventricular failure generally occurs late in the course of the disease. At first, it responds well to oxygen mixtures and a cardiotonic program (Chap. 253). Oxygen therapy is quite useful since it affords relief of dyspnea and improves oxygenation without threat of carbon dioxide retention. However, oxygen dependence may become marked, and the hazards of oxygen toxicity increase pari passu with the increasing concentrations of inspired oxygen and the duration of exposure.

Relief of heart failure is usually transient unless the initiating mechanism is controlled. Rarely is the underlying lesion in the lung reversible, even though steroids occasionally have been associated with dramatic benefit, especially in some of the granulomatoses and "fibrosing alveolitis." More apt to be rewarding is the successful treatment of superimposed respiratory infection which has toppled a stable patient into heart failure.

VASOMOTOR INCREASE IN PULMONARY VASCULAR RESISTANCE For convenience, alveolar hypoventilation, a prime cause of elevated pulmonary vascular resistance, can be identified by a value for arterial P_{CO_2} greater than 45 mmHg; the disorder may be regarded as either "general" or "net."

Alveolar hypoventilation: general The critical importance of abnormal values for blood gases in the pathogenesis of cor pulmonale is illustrated by the syndrome of alveolar hypoventilation coexistent with normal lungs ("general alveolar hypoventilation"). In these patients, some abnormality, either in the regulation of ventilation or in the neuromuscular apparatus, rather than intrinsic pulmonary disease, is responsible for the hypoxia and hypercapnia. The syndrome may have diverse etiologies. The particular category of sleep apnea syndromes is currently receiving considerable attention. These disorders and the pathways by which they lead to alveolar hypoventilation and cor pulmonale are considered in Chap. 286.

Alveolar hypoventilation: net The common denominator in this group of disorders is the imbalance between alveolar ventilation, blood flow, and diffusion, resulting in hypercapnia and hypoxemia. In contrast to *general* alveolar hypoventilation, in which the same abnormalities of arterial blood gas levels occur despite normal lungs, intrinsic lung disease is the basis for the abnormal values for blood gases in *net* alveolar hypoventilation.

The assortment of obstructive airways diseases predisposing to cor pulmonale has been pictured as a spectrum of bronchopulmonary disorders, ranging from pure obstruction of the airways at one end to pure emphysema at the other; between the two ends are the mixtures which are most prevalent (Chap. 279). Most likely to develop cor pulmonale is the patient with bronchitis and bronchiolitis, usually with some emphysema, in whom obstructive disease of the airways has so deranged the balance between alveolar ventilation, blood flow, and diffusion as to cause the characteristic syndrome of cyanosis (hypoxemia), somnolence (hypercapnia), and right ventricular failure; these are the "blue bloaters." In contrast, the "pink puffers," with comparable degrees of airways obstruction by conventional tests, do not develop hypoxia in the course of their breathless existence; only during an intercurrent respiratory infection, as hypoxia is superimposed, do they become candidates for cor pulmonale. Emphysema without bronchitis is rarely associated with cor pulmonale since alveolar ventilation and capillary blood flow seem to be commensurately curtailed, as after pulmonary resection, so that neither hypoxia nor pulmonary hypertension becomes appreciable.

Successful treatment of the "blue bloater" with cor pulmonale depends on relieving the bronchitis and bronchiolitis (Chap. 287). Cardiotonic agents are useless unless oxygenation is improved. If the patient succeeds in maintaining good oxygenation, digitalis and diuretics can usually be discontinued. Relief of airways obstruction is more readily accomplished in some disorders than in others. For example, it is generally easier in chronic bronchitis than in cystic fibrosis, in which most of the airways remain plugged with abnormal thick, tenacious sputum despite heroic therapeutic efforts.

Cor pulmonale is uncommon in uncomplicated silicosis or tuberculosis. On the other hand, it is not uncommon when silicosis, anthrosilicosis, or long-standing fibrotic tuberculosis is complicated by extensive, conglomerate, massive fibrosis, distorted adjacent parenchyma, shrunken lobes, and bronchitis. The likelihood of cor pulmonale is increased further by chronic pleurisy, fibrothorax, or excisional surgery. In such cases, a combination of anatomic restriction of the vascular bed and disturbances in gas exchange is involved in the pathogenesis of the pulmonary hypertension. Indeed, the disturbances in gas exchange, often brought to clinical levels by an acute respiratory infection, are the most reversible element of this disorder.

Although it is convenient to separate "net" from "general" alveolar hypoventilation on pathogenetic grounds, the therapeutic principles are basically the same for both and are described in Chap. 287. The present section will deal only with the circulatory abnormalities.

Since the pulmonary hypertension in the most prevalent pulmonary disorders is rarely anatomically fixed but arises mainly from hypoxia and acidosis, relief of alveolar hypoventilation is usually remarkably successful in restoring the circulation to normal. Measures to improve alveolar ventilation vary considerably. In mild cases, simple measures, such as hydration, antibiotics, and bronchodilators, often suffice; in more severe degrees of hypoxemia and hypercapnia, in which heart failure is associated with respiratory insufficiency, mechanical aids to respiration are usually needed.

It has been noted above that treatment of right-sided heart failure is less important than restoring the blood gas values to tolerable levels. The usual therapeutic measures for heart failure (Chap. 253) apply: low-salt regimen, digitalis, diuretics. However, measures to decrease the circulating blood volume (and hematocrit) are of greater importance. Several phlebotomies, each draining 300 to 400 ml, may be needed within a period of 2 to 3 weeks to bring hematocrit and blood volume back to normal; repeated phlebotomies at monthly or bimonthly intervals may have to be instituted to prevent return of the hypervolemia. Diuretics have to be given with more care than usual because the metabolic alkalosis, which may complicate the use of potent diuretics such as ethacrynic acid, aggravates ventilatory insufficiency by depressing the effectiveness of the CO_2 stimulus on the respiratory centers.

The effects of vigorous therapy, directed mainly to the pulmonary disorder, are often dramatic in improving the blood gas abnormalities and heart failure. Other manifestations usually clear more slowly. Indeed, several weeks to a month may elapse before the arterial blood gases, the hematocrit, cardiac output, and pulmonary arterial pressures return to optimal levels. But therapy throughout is guided by the fact that the final outcome in cor pulmonale usually depends on the ability to cope with the underlying respiratory disorder rather than with the changes in the heart and circulation.

Vasodilators in pulmonary hypertension and cor pulmonale In recent years, vasodilator agents, such as hydralazine, have been given to patients with pulmonary hypertension of diverse etiologies, including diffuse interstitial fibrosis, on the assumption that a vasoconstrictor component may be contributing to the pulmonary hypertension. These trials have not been undertaken without some trepidation, particularly in patients with intrinsic lung disease, in whom relaxation of vascular tone in diseased areas might exaggerate ventilation–blood flow abnormalities and, thereby, increase arterial hypoxemia. To date, this fear has not been realized. Instead, arterial oxygenation is not adversely affected, whereas cardiac output and oxygen delivery to the tissues do increase at the same time that pulmonary hypertension decreases. Symptomatic improvement, at rest and during exercise, accompanies the increase in cardiac output and oxygen delivery. It is important to note that this improved performance is not always accompanied by a drop in pulmonary arterial pressure, raising questions about the extent to which the evolution of cor pulmonale is influenced by the use of pulmonary vasodilators.

REFERENCES

Battesti JP et al: Chronic cor pulmonale in pulmonary sarcoidosis. Thorax 33:76, 1978

Fishman AP: Dynamics of the pulmonary circulation, in *Handbook of Physiology*, vol 2: *Circulation*, WF Hamilton, P Dow (eds). Washington, DC, American Physiological Society, 1963

———: Chronic cor pulmonale. State of the art. Am Rev Respir Dis 114:775, 1976

——— (ed): *Pulmonary Diseases and Disorders.* New York, McGraw-Hill, 1980

———: Primary pulmonary hypertension: More light or more tunnel? Ann Intern Med 94(6):815–817, 1981

FOWLER NO: Cor pulmonale caused by lung disease, in *Cardiac Diagnosis and Treatment,* 3d ed, NO Fowler (ed). New York, Harper & Row, 1980, chap 55, p 915

HEATH D, WILLIAMS DR: *Man at High Altitude.* Edinburgh, Churchill Livingstone, 1977

KOERNER SK, MALOVANY RJ: Acute respiratory insufficiency and cor pulmonale: Pathophysiology, clinical features and management. Am Heart J 88:115, 251, 1974

MCFADDEN ER, BRAUNWALD E: Cor pulmonale and pulmonary thromboembolism, in *Heart Disease,* 2d ed, E Braunwald (ed). Philadelphia, Saunders, 1983, chap 46

RUBIN LJ, PETER RH: Hemodynamics at rest and during exercise after oral hydralazine in patients with cor pulmonale. Am J Cardiol 47:116, 1981

STERN RC et al: Heart failure in cystic fibrosis. Am J Dis Child 134:267, 1980

WAGENVOORT CA, WAGENVOORT N: *Pathology of Pulmonary Hypertension.* New York, Wiley, 1977

WEBER KT, JANICKI JS: Interdependence of cardiac function, coronary flow, and oxygen extraction. Am J Physiol 235:H784, 1978

263 THE CARDIOMYOPATHIES AND MYOCARDITIDES

JOSHUA WYNNE
EUGENE BRAUNWALD

CARDIOMYOPATHY

The cardiomyopathies are diseases involving the myocardium primarily, not as the result of hypertension or of congenital, valvular, coronary arterial, or pericardial abnormalities.[1] When the cardiomyopathies are classified on an etiologic basis, two fundamental forms are recognized: (1) a primary type, consisting of heart muscle disease of unknown cause; (2) a secondary type, consisting of myocardial disease of known cause, or associated with a disease involving other organ systems (Table 263-1). From a clinical point of view, however, it is more desirable to classify the cardiomyopathies on the basis of differences in their pathophysiology and clinical presentation (Tables 263-2 and 263-3). The distinction between the functional categories is not absolute, however, and there is often some overlap.

DILATED (CONGESTIVE) CARDIOMYOPATHY Systolic pump function is impaired, leading to cardiac enlargement and often producing symptoms of congestive heart failure. Mural thrombi are often present, particularly in the left ventricular apex. Histologic examination reveals extensive areas of interstitial and perivascular fibrosis, with minimal necrosis and cellular infiltration. Although no etiology is apparent in many cases, dilated cardiomyopathy (formerly called congestive cardiomyopathy) is probably the end result of myocardial damage produced by a variety of toxic, metabolic, or infectious agents. A reversible form of dilated cardiomyopathy may be found with selenium deficiency and hypophosphatemia.

TABLE 263-1
Etiologic classification of cardiomyopathies

I Primary myocardial involvement
- *A* Idiopathic (D,R,H)
- *B* Familial (D,H)
- *C* Eosinophilic endomyocardial disease (R)
- *D* Endomyocardial fibrosis (R)

II Secondary myocardial involvement
- *A* Infective (D)
  - *1* Viral myocarditis
  - *2* Bacterial myocarditis
  - *3* Fungal myocarditis
  - *4* Protozoal myocarditis
  - *5* Metazoal myocarditis
- *B* Metabolic (D)
- *C* Familial storage disease (D,R)
  - *1* Glycogen storage disease
  - *2* Mucopolysaccharidoses
- *D* Deficiency (D)
  - *1* Electrolytes
  - *2* Nutritional
- *E* Connective tissue disorders (D)
  - *1* Systemic lupus erythematosus
  - *2* Polyarteritis nodosa
  - *3* Rheumatoid arthritis
  - *4* Scleroderma
  - *5* Dermatomyositis
- *F* Infiltrations and granulomas (R,D)
  - *1* Amyloidosis
  - *2* Sarcoidosis
  - *3* Malignancy
  - *4* Hemochromatosis
- *G* Neuromuscular (D)
  - *1* Muscular dystrophy
  - *2* Myotonic dystrophy
  - *3* Friedreich's ataxia (H,D)
  - *4* Refsum's disease
- *H* Sensitivity and toxic reactions (D)
  - *1* Alcohol
  - *2* Radiation
  - *3* Drugs
- *I* Peripartum heart disease (D)
- *J* Endocardial fibroelastosis (R)

NOTE: *The principal clinical manifestation(s) of each etiologic grouping is denoted by D (dilated), R (restrictive), or H (hypertrophic cardiomyopathy).*
SOURCE: *Adapted from the WHO/ISFC task force report on the definition and classification of cardiomyopathies, 1980.*

Clinical manifestations Symptoms of left- and right-sided congestive failure, manifested by dyspnea on exertion, fatigue, orthopnea, paroxysmal nocturnal dyspnea, peripheral edema, and palpitations, develop gradually in most patients. Some patients have left ventricular dilatation for months and even years before becoming symptomatic.

PHYSICAL EXAMINATION Variable degrees of cardiac enlargement and findings of congestive heart failure are noted. The pulse pressure is small, and the jugular venous pressure is elevated in the presence of failure of the right side of the heart. Third and fourth heart sounds are common, and mitral or tricuspid regurgitation may occur. Diastolic murmurs, valvular calcification, hypertension, and changes of vascular disease in the optic fundi mitigate strongly *against* the diagnosis of cardiomyopathy.

LABORATORY EXAMINATIONS The chest roentgenogram demonstrates left ventricular enlargement, although generalized

TABLE 263-2
Clinical classification of cardiomyopathies

1 Dilated (congestive): Left and/or right ventricular enlargement, impaired systolic function, congestive heart failure, arrhythmias, emboli
2 Restrictive: Endomyocardial scarring or myocardial infiltration resulting in restriction to left and/or right ventricular filling
3 Hypertrophic: Disproportionate left ventricular hypertrophy, typically involving septum more than free wall, with or without obstruction to ventricular outflow; usually of a nondilated left ventricular cavity

[1] *Diffuse myocardial fibrosis secondary to multiple myocardial scars produced by extensive coronary arterial narrowing and occlusion can impair left ventricular function and is frequently referred to as ischemic cardiomyopathy. According to the definition given above, however, the term* cardiomyopathy *should be restricted to a condition* primarily *involving heart muscle.*

TABLE 263-3
Laboratory evaluation of the cardiomyopathies

	Dilated (congestive)	*Restrictive*	*Hypertrophic*
Chest roentgenogram	Moderate to marked cardiac enlargement Pulmonary venous hypertension	Mild cardiac enlargement	Mild to moderate cardiac enlargement
Electrocardiogram	ST-segment and T-wave abnormalities	Low-voltage Conduction defects	ST-segment and T-wave abnormalities Left ventricular hypertrophy Abnormal Q waves
Echocardiogram	Left ventricular dilatation and dysfunction	Increased left ventricular wall thickness Normal systolic function	Asymmetric septal hypertrophy (ASH) Systolic anterior motion (SAM) of the mitral valve
Radionuclide studies	Left ventricular dilatation and dysfunction (RVG)	Normal systolic function (RVG)	Vigorous systolic function (RVG) Asymmetric septal hypertrophy (RVG or ^{201}Tl)
Cardiac catheterization	Left ventricular dilatation and dysfunction Elevated left- and often right-sided filling pressures Diminished cardiac output	Normal systolic function Elevated left- and right-sided filling pressures	Vigorous systolic function Dynamic left ventricular outflow obstruction Elevated left- and right-sided filling pressures

NOTE: *RVG = radionuclide ventriculogram; ^{201}Tl = thallium 201.*

cardiomegaly is often seen, sometimes due to a concomitant pericardial effusion. The lung fields may demonstrate evidence of pulmonary venous hypertension and interstitial or alveolar edema. The electrocardiogram often shows sinus tachycardia or atrial fibrillation, ventricular arrhythmias, left atrial enlargement, diffuse nonspecific ST-T-wave changes, and sometimes intraventricular conduction defects. Echocardiography and radionuclide ventriculography show left ventricular enlargement, with normal or minimally thickened walls, and systolic dysfunction (reduced ejection fraction); a pericardial effusion is often noted.

Hemodynamic studies reveal a cardiac output which is moderately or severely reduced at rest, and which does not increase normally with exercise. The left ventricular end-diastolic, left atrial, and pulmonary capillary wedge pressures usually are elevated; when failure of the right side of the heart supervenes, the right ventricular end-diastolic, right atrial, and central venous pressures are also elevated. Angiography reveals a dilated, diffusely hypokinetic left ventricle, often with some degree of mitral regurgitation; the coronary arteries are normal, thereby excluding so-called ischemic cardiomyopathy.

TREATMENT Most patients pursue an inexorably downhill course, and the majority, particularly those over 55 years of age, die within 2 years of the onset of symptoms. Systemic embolization is common, and all patients without contraindications should receive anticoagulants. Since the cause of primary dilated cardiomyopathy is, by definition, unknown, specific therapy is not possible. Prolonged strict bed rest for up to 1 year or more has been advocated for the optimal management of these patients, but the effectiveness of this form of therapy remains controversial and such therapy is not feasible in most patients; strenuous exertion should, however, be interdicted. Standard therapy of heart failure with salt restriction, diuretics, digitalis, and vasodilators may produce symptomatic improvement, at least in the initial phases of the illness; however, these patients appear to be at increased risk of digitalis toxicity. Newer experimental cardiotonic agents, such as amrinone, may provide additional clinical improvement (Chap. 253). Antiarrhythmic agents may be used to treat symptomatic or serious arrhythmias, although they may be extremely resistant to the usual agents. Occasionally, in appropriate patients, cardiac transplantation may be an alternative.

The preceding discussion emphasized clinical features of the dilated cardiomyopathies, regardless of whether they are primary or secondary in etiology. Many cases of dilated cardiomyopathy are primary (without a definable cause), but a number of specific conditions may also cause dilated cardiomyopathy secondarily. Since some of these conditions are reversible, features peculiar to these disorders will be considered in turn.

Alcoholic cardiomyopathy Individuals who consume large quantities of alcohol over many years may develop a clinical picture identical to idiopathic dilated cardiomyopathy; indeed, alcoholic cardiomyopathy is the major form of secondary dilated cardiomyopathy in the western world. Ceasing alcohol consumption before severe heart failure has developed may halt the progression, or even reverse the course of this disease, unlike the idiopathic variety which is marked by progressive deterioration. Thus, the key to the treatment of alcoholic cardiomyopathy is total and permanent abstinence. Although thiamine deficiency may be present in many of these patients, alcoholic cardiomyopathy is associated with a low cardiac output and systemic vasoconstriction. In contrast, beriberi heart disease (Chaps. 83 and 264) is characterized by elevated cardiac output and diminished peripheral vascular resistance, so that thiamine deficiency per se does not appear to cause alcoholic cardiomyopathy.

Peripartum cardiomyopathy Cardiac dilatation and congestive heart failure of unexplained cause may develop during the last month of pregnancy or within the first few months after delivery. The etiology of this disorder is unknown but may relate to a preexisting cardiomyopathy which was not apparent prior to pregnancy. Necropsy shows cardiac enlargement, often with mural thrombi, along with histologic evidence of myocardial degeneration and fibrosis. The patient who develops peripartum cardiomyopathy is typically multiparous, black, and over the age of 30. While some patients are malnourished, there is no conclusive evidence that dietary deficiencies are etiologically involved. The symptoms, signs, and treatment are similar to those in patients with idiopathic dilated cardiomyopathy. The prognosis in these patients appears to be closely related to whether the heart size returns to normal after the first episode of congestive heart failure. If the peripartum heart returns to normal size, subsequent pregnancies may sometimes be well tolerated; if the heart remains enlarged, however, further pregnancies frequently produce increasing myocardial damage, ultimately leading to refractory congestive heart failure and death. Those who recover should be encouraged to avoid further pregnancies, particularly if cardiomegaly persists.

Neuromuscular disease Cardiac involvement is common in many of the muscular dystrophies. In *Duchenne's progressive muscular dystrophy,* myocardial involvement is most frequently indicated by a distinctive and unique electrocardiographic pattern. The characteristic electrocardiographic abnormality consists of tall R waves in right precordial leads with an R/S ratio greater than 1.0, often associated with deep Q waves in the limb and lateral precordial leads, and is not found in other forms of muscular dystrophy. Rapidly progressive congestive heart failure may supervene after years of apparent circulatory stability during which the only detectable abnormalities are in the electrocardiogram. *Myotonic dystrophy* is characterized by a variety of electrocardiographic abnormalities, especially disorders of impulse formation and conduction, but other overt clinical evidence of heart disease is uncommon. Because of the abnormalities of impulse generation and conduction, syncope and sudden death are major hazards; in appropriate patients, insertion of a permanent pacemaker may be efficacious. In *limb-girdle* and *fascioscapulohumeral dystrophy,* cardiac involvement is uncommon and seldom severe.

Drugs A variety of pharmacologic agents may damage the myocardium acutely, producing a pattern of inflammation (myocarditis), or they may lead to chronic damage of the type seen with idiopathic dilated cardiomyopathy. Certain drugs produce only electrocardiographic abnormalities, while others may precipitate fulminant congestive heart failure and death. The anthracycline derivatives, particularly *doxorubicin* (Adriamycin), are powerful antineoplastic agents, which, when given in high doses (more than 550 mg/m^2 for doxorubicin), may produce fatal heart failure. Factors that potentiate the cardiotoxicity of these agents include radiation to the heart and prior, concurrent, or subsequent treatment with other antineoplastic agents, particularly *cyclophosphamide.* Radionuclide ventriculography (Chap. 250) may document preclinical deterioration of left ventricular function and allow appropriate dose adjustments; half of asymptomatic patients treated with standard doses may demonstrate left ventricular dysfunction for years after treatment. Electrocardiographic changes and arrhythmias may result from treatment with tricyclic antidepressants, the phenothiazines, emetine, lithium, and various aerosol propellants.

RESTRICTIVE CARDIOMYOPATHY The hallmark of the restrictive cardiomyopathies is abnormal diastolic function; the ventricular walls are excessively rigid and impede ventricular filling. Myocardial fibrosis, hypertrophy, or infiltration secondary to a variety of etiologies is usually responsible. The infiltrative diseases, which represent important etiologies for secondary restrictive cardiomyopathy, may also show some impairment of systolic function. Myocardial involvement with *amyloid* is a common cause of restrictive cardiomyopathy, although restriction is also seen in hemochromatosis, glycogen deposition, endomyocardial fibrosis, fibroelastosis, the eosinophilias, neoplastic infiltration, and myocardial fibrosis of diverse causes. In many of these conditions, particularly those with substantial concomitant endocardial involvement, partial obliteration of the ventricular cavity by fibrous tissue and thrombus contributes to the abnormally elevated resistance to ventricular filling. As a result of persistently elevated venous pressure these patients commonly have dependent edema, ascites, and an enlarged, tender liver. The jugular venous pressure is elevated and does not fall normally, or it may rise with inspiration (Kussmaul's sign). The heart sounds may be distant, and third and fourth heart sounds are common. In contrast to constrictive pericarditis, which these diseases resemble, the apex impulse is usually easily palpable. The electrocardiogram shows low-voltage, nonspecific ST-T-wave changes and various arrhythmias. Pericardial calcification on x-ray, which would suggest constrictive pericarditis, is absent. Echocardiography typically reveals symmetrically thickened left ventricular walls and normal or slightly reduced systolic function. Cardiac catheterization shows a decreased cardiac output, elevation of the right and left ventricular end-diastolic pressures, and a dip and plateau configuration of the diastolic portion of the ventricular pressure pulse resembling that seen in constrictive pericarditis.

Differentiation from constrictive pericarditis, at the bedside and even after cardiac catheterization, may be difficult or impossible (Chaps. 251 and 265). This distinction is of importance because the latter condition is potentially curable by operation. Right ventricular transvenous endomyocardial biopsy may be helpful in the differentiation of these two diseases by revealing interstitial infiltration or fibrosis in restrictive cardiomyopathy, but exploratory thoracotomy is occasionally necessary to distinguish restrictive cardiomyopathy from chronic constrictive pericarditis.

Endomyocardial fibrosis This is a progressive disease of unknown etiology, which occurs most commonly in children and young adults residing in tropical and subtropical Africa, particularly Uganda and Nigeria. The disease is characterized by fibrous endocardial lesions of the inflow portion of the right or left ventricle (or both) and often involves the atrioventricular valves, producing valvular regurgitation. The apex of the ventricles may be obliterated by a mass of thrombus and fibrous tissue. In many ways this disease resembles eosinophilic endomyocardial disease, although they occur in quite different geographic areas and age groups. Endomyocardial fibrosis is a frequent cause of heart failure in Africa, accounting for up to a quarter of deaths due to heart disease.

The clinical picture depends upon which ventricle and atrioventricular valve show predominant involvement; left-sided involvement results in symptoms of pulmonary congestion, while predominant right-sided disease presents features of a restrictive cardiomyopathy. Medical treatment is often disappointing, and surgical excision of the fibrotic endocardium and replacement of the involved atrioventricular valve has led to substantial symptomatic improvement in a small number of patients.

Eosinophilic endomyocardial disease Also called *Loeffler's endocarditis* and *fibroplastic endocarditis,* this disease appears to be a subcategory of the hypereosinophilic syndrome in which the heart is predominantly involved (Chap. 57). Typically, the endocardium of either or both ventricles thickens markedly, with involvement of the underlying myocardium. Large mural thrombi may develop in either ventricle, thereby compromising the size of the ventricular cavity and serving as a source of pulmonary and systemic emboli. Hepatosplenomegaly and localized eosinophilic infiltration of other organs are usually present. Once the disease becomes clinically evident, survival is usually brief, although recent reports have suggested a more benign course, with average survival exceeding 5 years. The reason for this improvement in prognosis is unclear but may be related to therapy with corticosteroids and immunosuppressive drugs.

Differential diagnosis Involvement of the heart is the most frequent cause of death in *primary amyloidosis* (Chap. 66), while clinically significant cardiac involvement is uncommon in the secondary form. Biopsy of the rectal mucosa, gingiva, liver, kidney, and myocardium permits the diagnosis to be made antemortem in over three-quarters of cases. The heart is firm, rubbery, and noncompliant, and four clinical presentations (alone or in combination) are seen: (1) diastolic dysfunction (restrictive cardiomyopathy); (2) systolic dysfunction; (3) arrhythmias; and (4) orthostatic hypotension. The two-dimensional echocardiogram may be helpful in making the diagnosis of amyloidosis and may show a thickened myocardial wall with a distinctive "speckled" appearance. *Hemochromatosis* (Chap. 97) should be suspected if cardiomyopathy occurs in the setting of diabetes mellitus, hepatic cirrhosis, and increased skin pigmentation. Phlebotomy may be of some benefit if employed early in the course of the disease. Continuous subcutaneous administration of desferrioxamine may reduce body iron stores in advanced cases, but whether this produces clinical improvement is unclear. Myocardial *sarcoidosis* (Chap. 235) is generally associated with other manifestations of systemic disease and may have restrictive as well as congestive features, since cardiac infiltration by sarcoid granulomata results not only in increased stiffness of the myocardium but also in diminished systolic contractile function. *Endocardial fibroelastosis* is a disease seen in infants, characterized by a thickened endocardium that shows proliferation of elastic tissue. It is most unusual in adult patients, although small patches of it may be found in patients with endomyocardial fibrosis.

Transvenous biopsy of the endocardium (Chap. 251), usually right ventricular, has been used increasingly to obtain specimens for histologic and electron microscopic study. This relatively simple and safe technique is becoming important in the diagnosis of myocardial disease, particularly in the recognition of infiltrative diseases such as amyloidosis, hemochromatosis, and sarcoidosis.

HYPERTROPHIC CARDIOMYOPATHY This disease is characterized by left ventricular hypertrophy, typically of a nondilated chamber, without obvious antecedent cause. The hypertrophy is thus not secondary to a cardiovascular or systemic disease, such as hypertension or aortic stenosis, that places a hemodynamic burden on the left ventricle. Two features of the disease have attracted the greatest attention: (1) asymmetric septal hypertrophy (ASH), wherein the upper portion of the interventricular septum is preferentially hypertrophied in comparison to the thickness of the posterobasal left ventricular free wall; and (2) dynamic left ventricular outflow tract obstruction, due to narrowing of the subaortic area usually resulting from the midsystolic apposition of the anterior mitral valve leaflet against the hypertrophied septum. Initial studies of this disease emphasized the dynamic obstructive features, and it has been termed idiopathic hypertrophic subaortic stenosis (IHSS), hypertrophic obstructive cardiomyopathy (HOCM), and muscular subaortic stenosis. It has become clear, however, that many and perhaps most patients with hypertrophic cardiomyopathy do not, in fact, demonstrate outflow tract obstruction. The ubiquitous pathophysiologic abnormality is not systolic but rather *diastolic* dysfunction, characterized by increased stiffness of the hypertrophied muscle. This results in elevated diastolic filling pressures and is present despite a hypercontractile left ventricle.

The pattern of hypertrophy is distinctive in hypertrophic cardiomyopathy and differs from that seen in secondary hypertrophy (as in hypertension). Most patients demonstrate a ventricular septum whose thickness is disproportionately increased when compared with the free wall. All, however, show a bizarre and disorganized arrangement of cardiac muscle cells in the septum, whether or not obstruction is present. Patients without obstruction may demonstrate similar derangements of the left ventricular free wall, while these findings are often lacking in patients with obstruction.

Most cases of hypertrophic cardiomyopathy appear to be transmitted as autosomal dominants with a high degree of penetrance, although sporadic cases are seen. Echocardiographic studies have confirmed that up to one-half the first-degree relatives (i.e., parents, siblings, and children) of hypertrophic cardiomyopathic patients have evidence of septal involvement, although many are without evidence of obstruction and are asymptomatic.

In contrast to the obstruction produced by a fixed narrowed orifice, such as valvular aortic stenosis, the obstruction in hypertrophic cardiomyopathy, when present, is dynamic and may change between examinations and even from beat to beat. Obstruction appears to result from further narrowing of an already small left ventricular outflow tract by systolic anterior motion (SAM) of the mitral valve against the hypertrophied septum. While SAM may be found in a variety of other conditions besides hypertrophic cardiomyopathy, it is *always* found when obstruction is present in hypertrophic cardiomyopathy. Three basic mechanisms are involved in the production of dynamic obstruction: (1) increased left ventricular contractility, which reduces ventricular systolic volume and increases the ejection velocity of the blood moving through the outflow tract, thus drawing the anterior mitral valve leaflet against the septum as a result of reduced distending pressure; (2) decreased ventricular volume (preload) which reduces the size of the outflow tract; and (3) decreased aortic impedance and pressure (afterload), which increases the velocity of flow through the subaortic area and also reduces ventricular systolic volume. Interventions which increase myocardial contractility, such as exercise, isoproterenol, and digitalis glycosides, and those that reduce ventricular volume, such as the Valsalva maneuver, sudden standing, nitroglycerin, amyl nitrite, or tachycardia, all may result in an increase in obstruction. Conversely, elevation of arterial pressure by phenylephrine, squatting, augmentation of venous return by raising the legs, and expansion of the blood volume all increase ventricular volume and ameliorate the obstruction. Sometimes the hypertrophied septum bulges into the outflow tract of the right ventricle, thereby impeding the ejection of blood from this chamber as well. Hypertrophic cardiomyopathy has been found in association with *lentiginosis* and other disorders of neural crest tissue. A similar hemodynamic pattern may be found in the infants of diabetic mothers and in patients with *Friedreich's ataxia*.

Clinical features Many patients with hypertrophic cardiomyopathy are asymptomatic and may be relatives of patients with known disease. Unfortunately, the first clinical manifestation of the disease may be sudden death, frequently occurring in children and young adults, often during or after physical exertion. In symptomatic patients the most common complaint is dyspnea, largely due to increased stiffness of the left ventricular walls, which impairs ventricular filling and leads to elevated diastolic pressures. Other symptoms include angina pectoris, fatigue, and syncope. Symptoms are not related to the presence or severity of outflow obstruction. Most patients with obstruction demonstrate a double or triple apical impulse, a rapidly rising carotid arterial pulse, and a fourth heart sound. The hallmark of obstructive hypertrophic cardiomyopathy is a systolic murmur, which is typically harsh, diamond-shaped, and begins well after the first heart sound, since ejection is unimpeded early in systole. The murmur is best heard at the lower left sternal border as well as at the apex, where the murmur is often more holosystolic and blowing in quality, no doubt due to the mitral regurgitation which usually accompanies obstructive hypertrophic cardiomyopathy.

LABORATORY EVALUATION The *electrocardiogram* commonly shows left ventricular hypertrophy and widespread, deep, broad Q waves that suggest an old myocardial infarction but apparently result from the abnormal electrophysiologic properties of the septal myocardium. Many patients demonstrate arrhythmias, both atrial (supraventricular tachycardia or atrial fibrillation) as well as ventricular (ventricular tachycardia) during ambulatory (Holter) monitoring. *Chest roentgenography* may be normal, although mild to moderate left ventricular enlargement is common. Aortic root enlargement and valvular calcification are not seen, helping to differentiate this condition from valvular aortic stenosis. The mainstay of the diagnosis of hypertrophic cardiomyopathy is the *echocardiogram,* which demonstrates left ventricular hypertrophy, typically with the septum 1.3 or more times the thickness of the high posterior left ventricular free wall. The septum may demonstrate an unusual ground-glass appearance, probably related to its abnormal cellular architecture and myocardial fibrosis. A rare form of hypertrophic cardiomyopathy is characterized by massive apical hypertrophy, often associated with giant negative T waves on the electrocardiogram. The left ventricular cavity is typically small in hypertrophic cardiomyopathy, with vigorous posterior wall motion, but reduced septal excursion. Systolic anterior motion of the mitral valve is found in patients with obstruction. The indirectly recorded *carotid arterial pulse* tracing rises unusually rapidly and often displays a "spike-and-dome" configuration.

The two typical hemodynamic features are elevated left ventricular diastolic pressures due to diminished left ventricular compliance and, when obstruction is present, a pressure gradient between the body of the left ventricle and the subaortic region. When a gradient is not present, it often can be induced by provocative maneuvers such as infusion of isoproterenol, inhalation of amyl nitrite, or the Valsalva maneuver. Radionuclide scintigraphy with thallium 201 and blood pool scans permits visualization of the size and orientation of the interventricular septum.

Treatment Beta-adrenergic blockers are often used and may ameliorate the symptoms of angina pectoris and syncope. Resting intraventricular pressure gradients are usually unchanged, although these drugs may limit the increase in the gradient which occurs during exercise. However, there is no evidence that beta blockers protect against sudden death, which is presumably arrhythmic in origin; whether antiarrhythmic agents are efficacious in this setting remains unestablished. The calcium channel blocking drugs, particularly verapamil and nifedipine, are promising new agents which may reduce the stiffness of the ventricle and reduce the elevated diastolic pressures. Surgical myotomy/myectomy of the hypertrophied septum may result in lasting symptomatic improvement, but the mortality of about 10 percent limits the operation to severely symptomatic patients with high-grade obstruction unresponsive to medical management. Digitalis, diuretics, nitrates, and beta-adrenergic agonists are best avoided if possible, particularly in patients with known left ventricular outflow tract pressure gradients.

PROGNOSIS The natural history of hypertrophic cardiomyopathy is variable, although most patients demonstrate an improvement or stabilization of symptoms with time. Atrial fibrillation is common; its onset usually leads to a striking increase in symptoms, presumably due to loss of the atrial contribution to filling of the thickened ventricle. Infective endocarditis occurs in less than 10 percent of patients, and endocarditis prophylaxis is indicated, particularly in patients with resting obstruction and mitral regurgitation. Progression of obstructive hypertrophic cardiomyopathy to left ventricular dilatation and dysfunction without an outflow gradient has been reported but is unusual. The major cause of mortality in hypertrophic cardiomyopathy is sudden death, which may occur in asymptomatic patients or interrupt an otherwise stable course in symptomatic ones. Paradoxically, younger patients and those with mild or no obstruction appear to be at particular risk of sudden death. Since sudden death typically occurs during or just after physical exertion, strenuous exercise should be avoided in all patients, regardless of symptoms. Although hemodynamic factors may play a role, it is likely that most deaths, particularly those that are sudden, are due to a ventricular arrhythmia. Beta-adrenergic blockade appears to be ineffective in preventing sudden death. The protective effect of calcium channel blockers or antiarrhythmic agents has not been established.

MYOCARDITIS

Myocarditis is said to be present when the heart is involved in an inflammatory process. Most commonly the result of an infectious process, myocarditis may also be present in hypersensitivity states such as acute rheumatic fever (Chap. 257) or may be caused by radiation, chemicals, physical agents, and drugs. Myocarditis may be acute or chronic. In an unknown number of cases, acute myocarditis progresses to chronic dilated cardiomyopathy. While almost every infectious agent is capable of producing myocarditis, clinically significant acute myocarditis in the United States is caused most commonly by viruses. Coxsackie B is the most frequent etiologic agent of viral myocarditis, but Coxsackie A, poliomyelitis, influenza, adeno, echo, rubeola, and rubella viruses also cause the disease. In most cases, the presence of myocarditis is inferred only by the finding of transient electrocardiographic ST-T-wave abnormalities, but arrhythmias, heart failure, and death may occur in fulminant cases, particularly in infants and pregnant women. Myocarditis is frequently associated with acute pericarditis, particularly when it is caused by Coxsackie B strains or echoviruses (Chap. 205).

Physical examination may be normal in patients who have only electrocardiographic abnormalities, although more severe cases may show a muffled first heart sound, along with a third heart sound and a murmur of mitral regurgitation. A pericardial friction rub may be audible in patients with associated pericarditis.

Experimental studies suggest that exercise may be deleterious in patients with myocarditis, and strenuous activity should be proscribed until the electrocardiogram has returned to normal. Prolonged bed rest has been advocated for more severe cases, although its efficacy remains to be established. Patients who develop congestive heart failure respond to the usual measures (digitalis, diuretics, salt restriction), but they appear to be unusually sensitive to digitalis. Arrhythmias are common and are occasionally difficult to manage. Deaths attributed to heart failure, tachyarrhythmias, and heart block have been reported, and it seems prudent to monitor patients with arrhythmias, especially during the acute illness.

Though viral myocarditis is most often self-limited and without sequelae, active disease may recur, and it is likely that acute viral myocarditis occasionally progresses to a chronic form. Patients with viral myocarditis often give a history of a preceding upper respiratory febrile illness, and viral nasopharyngitis or tonsillitis may be evident clinically. The isolation of virus from the stool, pharyngeal washings, or other body fluids, and changes in specific antibody titers are helpful clinically. It is possible that many instances of apparent *idiopathic* dilated cardiomyopathy (page 1449) in fact arise from mild or subclinical episodes of myocarditis. While corticosteroids may exacerbate heart damage in animals with acute viral myocarditis, a small number of humans with congestive heart failure and inflammatory myocarditis appear to respond to an experimental protocol utilizing immunosuppression with prednisone and azathioprine. Serial right ventricular endomyocardial biopsies have shown regression of inflammatory infiltrates in patients so treated.

Chagas' disease Chagas' disease, caused by the protozoan *Trypanosoma cruzi* (Chap. 220), produces an extensive myocarditis which typically becomes evident years after the initial infection. It is one of the most common causes of heart disease encountered in Central and South America; in rural areas up to 20 percent of the population may be affected. Although only a minority of infected individuals have an acute illness, upwards of one-third develop chronic myocardial damage, typically appearing 20 years after the initial infection. The chronic form is characterized by dilatation of several cardiac chambers, fibrosis and thinning of the ventricular wall, aneurysm formation in the areas of thinning (especially at the apex), and mural thrombi. Chronic progressive heart failure, often predominantly right-sided, is the rule. The electrocardiogram typically shows right bundle branch block and left anterior hemiblock, which may progress to complete atrioventricular block. The echocardiogram may reveal a unique pattern of hypokinesis of the posterior left ventricular wall and relatively preserved septal motion. Ventricular arrhythmias are common and are seen particularly during and after exertion. The cause of death is either intractable congestive heart failure or an arrhythmia. Therapy is directed toward amelioration of the congestive heart failure and arrhythmias.

GIANT-CELL MYOCARDITIS This rare myocarditis of unknown etiology is characterized by the presence of multinucleated giant cells in the myocardium. It usually causes rapidly fatal congestive heart failure and arrhythmia in young to middle-aged adults. At necropsy, the distinctive features include grossly visible serpiginous areas of myocardial necrosis in both ventricles and microscopic evidence of giant cells within an extensive inflammatory infiltrate. The cause of giant-cell myocarditis remains obscure, although it occurs in association with thymoma, systemic lupus erythematosus, and thyrotoxicosis.

LYME CARDITIS Lyme disease is a newly described condition, apparently caused by the elaboration of circulating immune complexes in response to a tick-borne agent. Conduction abnormalities are the most common manifestations of cardiac involvement and may progress to complete atrioventricular block with syncope. Concomitant myopericarditis is not uncommon, and mild left ventricular dysfunction may occur. Prednisone may be efficacious in ameliorating the heart block; penicillin or tetracycline is used to treat the accompanying skin rash.

RADIATION MYOCARDITIS A variety of acute and chronic cardiac complications may result from the use of ionizing radiation in the treatment of carcinoma of the lung or breast, lymphoma, or Hodgkin's disease. Only an occasional patient manifests acute cardiac abnormalities; typically such an abnormality consists of acute pericarditis. The most common presentation is that of chronic pericardial effusion or constriction occurring months or years after exposure (in rare cases up to 10 years) (Chap. 265). Myocardial fibrosis, resulting from damage to the microvasculature, often with formation of atherosclerotic plaques of the epicardial coronary arteries, is also common.

REFERENCES

BROSIUS FC III et al: Radiation heart disease. Am J Med 70:519, 1981

FUSTER V et al: The natural history of idiopathic dilated cardiomyopathy. Am J Cardiol 47:525, 1981

GOTTDIENER JS et al: Doxorubicin cardiotoxicity: Assessment of late left ventricular dysfunction by radionuclide cineangiography. Ann Intern Med 94:430, 1981

JOHNSON RA et al: An occidental case of cardiomyopathy and selenium deficiency. N Engl J Med 304:1210, 1981

LORELL BH et al: Improved diastolic function and systolic performance in hypertrophic cardiomyopathy after nifedipine. N Engl J Med 303:801, 1980

MARON BJ, EPSTEIN SE: Hypertrophic cardiomyopathy. Recent observations regarding the specificity of three hallmarks of the disease: Asymmetric septal hypertrophy, septal disorganization and systolic anterior motion of the anterior mitral leaflet. Am J Cardiol 45:141, 1980

MCKENNA WJ et al: Arrhythmias in hypertrophic cardiomyopathy: Exercise and 48 hour ambulatory electrocardiographic assessment with and without beta adrenergic blocking therapy. Am J Cardiol 45:1, 1980

OLSEN EGJ: The pathology of cardiomyopathies. A critical analysis. Am Heart J 98:385, 1979

STEERE AC et al: Lyme carditis: Cardiac abnormalities of Lyme disease. Ann Intern Med 93:8, 1980

WYNNE J: Hypertrophic cardiomyopathy: A broadened concept of the disease and its management, in *Update III: Harrison's Principles of Internal Medicine,* KJ Isselbacher, et al (eds). New York, McGraw-Hill, 1982, pp 129–146

———, BRAUNWALD E: The cardiomyopathies and myocarditides, in *Heart Disease: A Textbook of Cardiovascular Medicine,* 2d ed, E Braunwald (ed). Philadelphia, Saunders, 1983, chap 41

264
CARDIAC TUMORS, CARDIAC MANIFESTATIONS OF SYSTEMIC DISEASES, AND TRAUMATIC CARDIAC INJURY

WILSON S. COLUCCI
EUGENE BRAUNWALD

TUMORS OF THE HEART

PRIMARY TUMORS Primary tumors of the heart are rare and are often classified as "benign" histologically (Table 264-1). However, since all cardiac tumors have the potential for causing life-threatening complications, and many are now curable by surgery, it is important that this diagnosis be made whenever possible. Primary cardiac tumors are similar to those that may occur in other mesenchymal structures. Approximately three-quarters are *histologically* benign, and the remainder are malignant, in almost all cases sarcomas.

Clinical presentation Cardiac tumors may present with a wide array of cardiac and noncardiac manifestations. There may be signs and symptoms of all the more common forms of heart disease, including chest pain, syncope, heart failure, murmurs, arrhythmias, conduction disturbances, and pericardial effusion or tamponade. The specific signs and symptoms produced are most closely related to the location of the tumor.

Myxoma Myxomas are the most common type of primary cardiac tumor, accounting for one-third to one-half of all cases. They occur at all ages, show no sex preference, and may be familial. Most authorities consider the myxoma a true neoplasm, while others have suggested that it is formed by organization of an intracardiac thrombus attached to the endocardium. The large majority of myxomas are located in the atria, particularly the left, and arise from the interatrial septum in the vicinity of the fossa ovalis, but they may also occur in the ventricles or be multiple in location. Most myxomas are pedunculated on a fibrovascular stalk and average 4 to 8 cm in diameter. The most common clinical presentation resembles that of mitral valve disease, either stenosis as a result of tumor prolapse into the mitral orifice during diastole or regurgitation as a consequence of injury to the valve by tumor-induced trauma. Ventricular myxomas may cause outflow obstruction and may therefore mimic subaortic or subpulmonic stenosis. Characteristically, the symptoms and signs are highly dependent on position, intermittent, and sudden in onset as a result of changes in tumor position with gravity. On auscultation, a characteristic low-pitched sound, termed a "tumor plop," is audible during early or middiastole and is thought to result from the tumor abruptly stopping as it strikes the ventricular wall. Myxomas may also present with peripheral or pulmonary emboli, or any of several noncardiac signs and symptoms including fever, weight loss, cachexia, malaise, arthraliga, rash, clubbing, Raynaud's phenomenon, hypergammaglobulinemia, anemia, polycythemia, leukocytosis, elevated erythrocyte sedimentation rate, thrombocytopenia, or thrombocytosis. Not surprisingly, myxomas are frequently misdiagnosed as endocarditis, collagen vascular disease, or noncardiac tumor.

Both M-mode and two-dimensional echocardiography are useful in the diagnosis of cardiac myxoma, the latter having the advantage of allowing determination of the site of tumor attachment and tumor size, important considerations in the planning of surgical excision. While cardiac catheterization and angiography are generally performed prior to surgery, catheterization of the chamber from which the tumor originates is attended by the risk of dislodgment of tumor emboli, and in many centers is no longer considered mandatory when adequate noninvasive information is available.

Surgical excision utilizing cardiopulmonary bypass is indicated in all patients and is generally curative. Occasional reports of tumor recurrence are most likely due to inadequate excision of multiple tumor sites.

TABLE 264-1
Relative incidence of primary tumors of the heart

Type	*Percent*
BENIGN	
Myxoma	30.5
Lipoma	10.5
Papillary fibroelastoma	9.9
Rhabdomyoma	8.5
Fibroma	4.0
Hemangioma	3.5
Teratoma	3.3
Mesothelioma of the AV node	2.8
Other benign tumors	2.1
Total	75.1
MALIGNANT	
Sarcomas	18.6
Lymphoma	1.6
Other malignant tumors	4.7
Total	24.9

SOURCE: *Modified from HA McAllister, JJ Fenoglio, in Atlas of Tumor Pathology, Washington, Armed Forces Institute of Pathology, 1978, fasc 15, 2d series.*

Other benign tumors Cardiac *lipomas,* although relatively common, are usually incidental findings at postmortem examination and seldom result in symptoms. However, they may grow as large as 15 cm and present with symptoms due to mechanical interference with cardiac function, arrhythmias, or conduction disturbances, or as an abnormality of the cardiac silhouette on chest x-ray. *Papillary fibroelastomas,* similarly, are relatively common findings on cardiac valves or the adjacent endothelium but seldom result in clinical symptoms. Occasionally, these growths may cause mechanical interference with valvular function. *Rhabdomyomas* and *fibromas,* the most frequent tumors in infants and children, most commonly occur in the ventricles, and therefore produce signs and symptoms by mechanical obstruction which may mimic valvular stenosis, congestive heart failure, restrictive or hypertrophic cardiomyopathy, and pericardial constriction. Rhabdomyomas are probably hamartomatous growths, are multiple in about 90 percent of cases, and may be associated with tuberous sclerosis, adenoma sebaceum, and benign kidney tumors. *Hemangiomas* and *mesotheliomas* are generally small tumors, most often intramyocardial in location, and not infrequently cause atrioventricular conduction disturbances and even sudden death as a result of their propensity for location in the region of the AV node.

Sarcomas Cardiac sarcomas may be of several histologic types but in general are characterized by a rapidly downhill course leading to the patient's death in weeks to months from the time of presentation as a result of hemodynamic compromise, local invasion, or distant metastases. Sarcomas commonly involve the right side of the heart, and because of their rapid growth, invasion of the pericardial space and obstruction of the cardiac chambers or venae cavae are common. At the time of presentation these tumors have often spread too extensively for surgical excision. While there are scattered reports of palliation with surgery, radiotherapy, and chemotherapy, the overall experience with cardiac sarcomas is poor. The one exception to this appears to be cardiac lymphosarcomas which may respond well to a combination of chemo- and radiotherapy.

TUMORS METASTATIC TO THE HEART Tumors metastatic to the heart are several times more common than primary tumors, and as the life expectancy of patients with various forms of malignant neoplasms is extended by more effective therapy, it is likely that the frequency of cardiac metastases will also increase. Although cardiac metastases occur in all tumor types with an incidence ranging from 1 to 20 percent, the incidence is especially high in malignant melanoma, and to a somewhat lesser extent in leukemia and lymphoma. In absolute numbers, cardiac metastases are most common in carcinoma of the breast and lung, reflecting the high incidence of these cancers. Cardiac metastases almost always occur in the setting of widespread primary disease, and most often there is either primary or metastatic disease elsewhere in the thoracic cavity. Nevertheless, occasionally a cardiac metastasis may be the initial presentation of a tumor elsewhere in the body.

Cardiac metastases reach the heart via the bloodstream, lymphatics, or direct invasion and are small, firm nodules; although diffuse infiltrations may also occur, especially with sarcomas or hematologic neoplasms. The pericardium is most often involved, followed by myocardial involvement of any chamber, and, rarely, by involvement of the endocardium or cardiac valves.

Cardiac metastases result in clinical manifestations only about 10 percent of the time, and rarely are they the cause of death. In most patients they are *not* the cause of the presenting clinical features but occur in the setting of a previously recognized malignant neoplasm. While cardiac metastases may present a large number of nonspecific signs and symptoms, the most common are dyspnea, a new systolic murmur, signs of acute pericarditis, cardiac tamponade, a rapid increase in the cardiac silhouette on chest x-ray, the new onset of an ectopic tachyarrhythmia, AV block, and congestive heart failure. As with primary cardiac tumors, the clinical presentation is more closely related to the location and size of the tumor than to its histological type. Many of these signs and symptoms may also occur with myocarditis, pericarditis, or cardiomyopathy resulting from radiotherapy or chemotherapy.

The electrocardiographic findings are entirely nonspecific and may include ST-T-wave changes, decreased QRS voltage, arrhythmias, and conduction disturbances. On chest roentgenography the cardiac silhouette is most often normal but may reveal a pericardial effusion or bizarre contour. Echocardiography is useful for the diagnosis of pericardial effusion and the visualization of larger metastases. Angiography may delineate discrete lesions, and pericardiocentesis can allow a specific cytologic diagnosis. Since most patients with cardiac metastases have widespread disease, therapy generally consists of pericardiocentesis, when there is hemodynamic compromise, and treatment directed at the primary tumor. The removal of a malignant effusion by pericardiocentesis with or without concomitant instillation of a sclerosing agent (e.g., tetracycline) often prevents reaccumulation of the effusion.

CARDIAC EFFECTS OF CANCER THERAPY See Chap. 263.

CARDIOVASCULAR MANIFESTATIONS OF SYSTEMIC DISEASES

DIABETES MELLITUS (See Chap. 114) In patients with insulin-dependent diabetes mellitus there is an increased incidence of large-vessel atherosclerosis and myocardial infarction, and diabetics are more likely to have an abnormal or absent pain response to myocardial ischemia, probably as a result of generalized autonomic nervous system dysfunction. Diabetic patients may also have myocardial dysfunction characteristic of a restrictive cardiomyopathy in the absence of large-vessel coronary artery disease, as evidenced by elevated left ventricular filling pressures and an abnormally large fall in stroke volume in response to an increase in cardiac afterload. Histologically, these patients have increased amounts of collagen, glycoprotein, triglycerides, and cholesterol in the myocardial interstitium, and in some cases intimal thickening, hyaline deposition, and inflammatory changes have been observed in small intramural arteries. While these changes alone seldom result in clinical heart failure, it is likely that they contribute to the excessive cardiovascular morbidity and mortality of diabetics.

MALNUTRITION AND THIAMINE DEFICIENCY (BERIBERI)
Malnutrition (see Chap. 78) In patients whose intake of protein, calories, or both is severely deficient, the heart may become thin, pale, and flabby with myofibrillar atrophy and interstitial edema. The systolic pressure and cardiac output are low, and the pulse pressure narrow. Generalized edema is common and is due to a combination of factors, including reduced serum oncotic pressure and myocardial dysfunction. Such profound states of malnutrition, termed *marasmus* in the case of caloric deficiency, or *kwashiorkor* in the case of relative protein deficiency, are most common in underdeveloped countries. However, significant nutritional heart disease may also occur in developed nations, particularly in patients with severe cardiac failure in whom gastrointestinal hypoperfusion and venous congestion may cause anorexia and malabsorption. Open-heart surgery poses an increased risk in such patients, who may benefit from preoperative intensive hyperalimentation. Deficient nutrients and minerals should be replaced gradually since rapid expansion of the intravascular space may stress the weakened heart and result in overt congestive heart failure.

Thiamine deficiency (see Chap. 83) In many cases, malnutrition is accompanied by thiamine deficiency, although this hypovitaminosis may also occur in the presence of an adequate protein and caloric intake, particularly in the far east where polished rice deficient in thiamine is a major dietary component. The widespread use of thiamine-enriched flour in western nations confines this disease primarily to alcoholics and food faddists. Clinically, there is usually evidence of generalized malnutrition, peripheral neuropathy, glossitis, and anemia. The characteristic cardiovascular syndrome is that of high-output heart failure with tachycardia, increased cardiac output, and often elevated filling pressures in the left and right side of the heart. It appears that the major cause of the high-output state is vasomotor depression, the precise mechanism of which is not understood, but which leads to a reduced systemic vascular resistance. The cardiac examination reveals a wide pulse pressure, tachycardia, a third heart sound, and, frequently, a systolic murmur at the apex. The electrocardiogram may show decreased voltage, a prolonged QT interval, and T-wave abnormalities; the chest x-ray generally shows a large heart with signs of congestive heart failure. The response to thiamine is often dramatic, with diuresis and a reduction in heart size. Although the response to digitalis and diuretics may be poor prior to thiamine therapy, these agents may be important *after* thiamine is given since the left ventricle may not be capable of dealing with the increased work load presented by the return of vascular tone.

OBESITY (See Chap. 79) Although not defined as a disease per se, severe obesity is associated with an increase in cardiovascular morbidity and mortality, due in part to hypertension and atherosclerotic coronary artery disease, both of which are more prevalent in obese patients. In addition, these patients have a distinct abnormality of the cardiovascular system characterized by increases in total and central blood volumes, cardiac output, and left ventricular filling pressure. It appears that cardiac output is elevated in order to help supply the metabolic needs of the excessive adipose tissue. Left ventricular filling pressure is often at the upper limits of normal and rises excessively with exercise. As a result of chronic volume and pressure overload, abnormal ventricular function may develop. Pathologically, there is left and, in some cases, right ventricular hypertrophy and generalized cardiac enlargement, which is not due simply to fatty infiltration of the myocardium. Clinically, these patients may develop pulmonary congestion, peripheral edema, and exercise intolerance, findings which may be difficult to recognize in massively obese patients. Weight reduction is the most effective therapy and results in reduction in blood volume and in return of cardiac output toward normal. Digitalis, sodium restriction, and diuretics may also be useful. This form of heart disease should be distinguished from the Pickwickian syndrome (Chap. 286), which may share several of the cardiovascular features but, in addition, frequently has components of central apnea, hypoxemia, pulmonary hypertension, and cor pulmonale.

THYROID DISEASE (See Chap. 111) Thyroid hormone exerts a major influence on the cardiovascular system by a number of direct and indirect mechanisms, and not surprisingly, cardiovascular effects are prominent in both hypo- and hyperthyroidism. Thyroid hormone causes increases in total body metabolism and oxygen consumption which indirectly place an increased work load on the heart. In addition, although the exact mechanism has not been defined, thyroid hormone exerts direct inotropic and chronotropic effects which are similar to those seen with adrenergic stimulation (e.g., tachycardia, increased cardiac output). It has been shown that thyroid hormone increases the synthesis of myosin and of sodium/potassium ATPase, as well as the density of myocardial beta-adrenergic receptors.

Hyperthyroidism Excess thyroid hormone results in increases in heart rate, cardiac output, and pulse pressure. Patients may present with palpitations, systolic hypertension, fatigue, or, in patients with underlying heart disease, angina or heart failure. Sinus tachycardia is found in about 40 percent of patients, and atrial fibrillation in about 15 percent. Other findings include a hyperactive precordium, an increase in the intensity of the first heart sound and the pulmonic component of the second heart sound, a third heart sound, and, in some cases, a midsystolic murmur heard best at the left sternal border with or without a systolic ejection click. A systolic scratchy sound, the *Means-Lerman* scratch, may occasionally be heard at the left second intercostal space during expiration and is thought to result from the rubbing of the hyperdynamic pericardium against the pleura. Elderly patients with hyperthyroidism may present with only the cardiovascular manifestations of thyrotoxicosis, which may be resistant to therapy until the hyperthyroidism is controlled. Both angina pectoris and congestive heart failure are unusual, unless there is coexistent underlying heart disease, and in many cases will resolve with therapy of the hyperthyroidism.

Hypothyroidism There is a reduction in cardiac output, stroke volume, heart rate, blood pressure, and pulse pressure. In about one-third of patients there is a pericardial effusion which only rarely results in tamponade. Clinically, there is cardiomegaly, bradycardia, weak arterial pulses, and distant heart sounds. Biochemical abnormalities, including elevations of CK, GOT, and LDH, may lead to a mistaken diagnosis of myocardial infarction. The electrocardiogram generally shows sinus bradycardia and low voltage and may show prolongation of the QT interval, decreased P-wave voltage, prolonged AV conduction time, intraventricular conduction disturbances, and nonspecific ST-T-wave abnormalities. Chest x-ray shows cardiomegaly, often with a "water bottle" configuration, pleural effusions, and, in some cases, evidence of congestive heart failure. Pathologically, the heart is pale, dilated, and flabby, often with myofibrillar swelling, loss of striations, and interstitial fibrosis.

Patients with hypothyroidism frequently have elevations of cholesterol and triglycerides and severe atherosclerotic coronary artery disease. Prior to treatment with thyroid hormone, patients with hypothyroidism usually do not have angina pectoris and appear to have relatively few myocardial infarctions, presumably because of the low metabolic demands made by their condition. However, such patients, especially when elderly, are prone to angina and myocardial infarction during replacement of thyroid hormone, and this should always be done with extreme care, starting with very low doses which are increased gradually.

MALIGNANT CARCINOID (See Chap. 131) These tumors elaborate a variety of vasoactive amines, kinins, indoles, and other substances which are believed to be responsible for the diarrhea, flushing, and labile blood pressure seem in these patients. The cardiac lesions due to gastrointestinal carcinoids are almost exclusively in the right side of the heart and occur only when there are hepatic metastases, suggesting that the substance responsible for the cardiac lesions is inactivated by passage through the liver and lungs. Similar lesions occur in the left side of the heart when there is a right-to-left shunt or the tumor is located in the lungs. Fibrous plaques are found on the endothelium of the cardiac chambers, valves, and great vessels. These plaques, which result in distortion of the cardiac valves, consist of smooth-muscle cells imbedded in a stroma of acid mucopolysaccharide and collagen, and presumably result from healing of endothelial injury. The clinical syndrome is most often that of tricuspid regurgitation, pulmonic stenosis, or both. In some cases a high-output state may occur, presumably as a result of a decrease in systemic vascular resistance due to a vasoactive substance released by the tumor. Progression of the cardiac lesions does not appear to be affected by treatment with serotonin antagonists, and in some cases valve replacement is indicated.

PHEOCHROMOCYTOMA (See Chap. 113) In addition to causing hypertension, which may be labile or sustained, the high circulating levels of catecholamines may also cause direct myocardial injury. Focal myocardial necrosis and inflammatory cell infiltration are seen in about 50 percent of patients who die with pheochromocytoma and may contribute to clinically significant left ventricular failure and pulmonary edema. In addition, hypertension results in left ventricular hypertrophy.

RHEUMATOID ARTHRITIS AND THE COLLAGEN VASCULAR DISEASES **Rheumatoid arthritis** (see Chap. 346) There may be inflammation of any or all parts of the heart in patients with rheumatoid arthritis. *Pericarditis* is the most common cause of clinically apparent disease and may be found in 30 to 50 percent of all patients with rheumatoid arthritis, particularly those with subcutaneous nodules, if carefully searched for by echocardiography or at postmortem examination. However, only a small fraction of these patients will have clinical evidence of pericarditis, which usually follows a benign course, but occasionally may progress to cardiac tamponade or constrictive pericarditis. The pericardial fluid is generally an exudate, with decreased concentrations of complement and glucose and elevated cholesterol. Treatment is directed at the underlying rheumatoid arthritis and may include corticosteroids. Pericardiectomy is usually required in cases of tamponade or persistent effusion. *Coronary arteritis* with intimal inflammation and edema is present in about 20 percent of cases but only rarely results in angina pectoris or myocardial infarction. The cardiac valves, most often the mitral and aortic, may be involved by inflammation and granuloma formation which in some cases may cause clinically significant regurgitation due to valve deformity. Myocarditis rarely results in cardiac dysfunction.

Seronegative arthropathies The seronegative arthropathies (Chaps. 347 and 348), ankylosing spondylitis, Reiter's syndrome, psoriatic arthritis, and the arthritides associated with ulcerative colitis and regional enteritis may be accompanied by a pancarditis with tachycardia, cardiomegaly, and prolongation of the AV conduction time. These patients are particularly likely to develop aortic regurgitation due to an aortitis and consequent dilatation of the aortic root and AV block, both of which are more common in patients with peripheral joint involvement and long-standing disease. Up to one-fifth of patients with peripheral joint involvement and disease for more than 30 years have significant aortic regurgitation. Occasionally, aortic regurgitation precedes the onset of arthritis, and, therefore, the diagnosis of a seronegative arthritis should be considered in young males with isolated aortic regurgitation.

Systemic lupus erythematosus (SLE) (see Chap. 70) Pericarditis is common, occurring in about two-thirds of patients, and generally pursues a benign course, although rarely tamponade or constriction may result. The characteristic *endocardial lesions* of SLE, described by Libman and Sacks, consist of wart-like lesions most often located at the angles of the AV valves or on the ventricular surface of the mitral valve. Although arteritis of large coronary arteries may rarely result in myocardial ischemia, there is also an increased frequency of coronary atherosclerosis which may be related to hypertension or corticosteroid therapy.

TRAUMATIC HEART DISEASE

Cardiac damage may be due to both penetrating and nonpenetrating injuries. The most frequent cause of a *nonpenetrating injury* is impact of the chest against the steering wheel of an automobile. Serious injury of the heart may ensue even though no external sign of thoracic trauma is evident. Although the commonest injury is myocardial contusion, any structure of the heart may be affected by the trauma. If the valvular apparatus is ruptured, a loud heart murmur produced by valvular regurgitation may appear, followed by the development of rapidly progressive heart failure. The most serious consequence of nonpenetrating injury is rupture, either of the atria or of the ventricles, which is generally fatal. Hemopericardium may also follow tearing of a pericardial vessel or coronary artery.

Myocardial contusion may cause arrhythmias, bundle branch block, or electrocardiographic abnormalities resembling those of infarction, and so it is important to bear trauma in mind as a cause of otherwise unexplained electrocardiographic changes. Similarly, myocardial contusion may produce positive radionuclide scans and regional impairment of ventricular function, as occurs in patients with acute myocardial infarction (Chap. 250). Pericardial effusion may occur weeks or even months after the accident. In these cases, the pericardial effusion is a manifestation of the postcardiac injury syndrome, which resembles the postpericardiotomy syndrome (Chap. 265).

Acute myocardial failure resulting from rupture of a valve usually requires operative correction. Myocardial infarction due to trauma is treated similarly to that due to ischemic heart disease (Chap. 261). Pericardial hemorrhage often leads to constriction which must be treated by decortication.

Penetrating injuries of the heart, produced by bullets or stab wounds, usually result in immediate or very rapid death because of hemopericardium or massive hemorrhage. However, sometimes the patient survives the acute incident and presents with a cardiac murmur and congestive heart failure. A left-to-right shunt due to traumatic ventricular septal defect, aortopulmonary artery fistula, or coronary arteriovenous fistula may be suspected and confirmed by cardiac catheterization and angiocardiography. Operation is indicated if hemodynamically significant abnormalities are present or if a foreign body, e.g., a bullet, is lodged in the heart. Immediate thoracotomy should be carried out if there is cardiac tamponade and/or shock, whether the trauma was penetrating or nonpenetrating. Pericardiocentesis may be helpful in patients with tamponade, but usually only as a holding maneuver.

Rupture of the aorta is a common consequence of chest trauma. Indeed, rupture of the aorta at the isthmus or just above the aortic valve is the most common vascular deceleration injury. The clinical presentation is similar to that in aortic dissection (Chap. 268). The arterial pressure and pulse amplitude may be increased in the upper extremities and decreased in the lower extremities, and on chest roentgenogram there may be widening of the mediastinum. Occasionally, the rupture is limited by the aortic adventitia and results in a silent false aneurysm which may be discovered months or years after the injury. When great vessel rupture is due to a penetrating injury, there is usually a hemothorax and, less often, a hemopericardium. Hematoma formation may compress major vessels, and arteriovenous fistulae may be formed, sometimes resulting in high-output congestive heart failure.

REFERENCES

BULKLEY BH, ROBERTS WC: The heart in systemic lupus erythematosus and the changes induced in it by corticosteroid therapy. A study of 36 necropsy patients. Am J Med 58:243, 1975

COHN PF, BRAUNWALD E: Traumatic heart disease, in *Heart Disease,* 2d ed, E Braunwald (ed). Philadelphia, Saunders, 1983, chap 44

COLUCCI WS, BRAUNWALD E: Primary tumors of the heart, in *Heart Disease,* 2d ed, E Braunwald (ed). Philadelphia, Saunders, 1983, chap 42

KALTMAN AJ, GOLDRING RM: Role of circulatory congestion in the cardiorespiratory failure of obesity. Am J Med 60:645, 1976

KAWAI C et al: Reappearance of beriberi heart disease in Japan. A study of 23 cases. Am J Med 69:383, 1980

LEVEY GS: The heart and hyperthyroidism. Med Clinics North Am 59:1193, 1976

LEVINE HD: Compromise therapy in the patient with angina pectoris and hypothyroidism. Am J Med 69:411, 1980

LOCKWOOD WB, BROGHAMER WL JR: The changing prevalence of secondary cardiac neoplasms as related to cancer therapy. Cancer 15:2659, 1980

PAINO TD et al: Coronary arterial surgery in patients with incapacitating angina pectoris and myxedema. Am J Cardiol 40:226, 1977

REGAN TL et al: Evidence for cardiomyopathy in familial diabetes mellitus. J Clin Invest 60:885, 1977

ROBERTS WC, SJOERDSMA A: The cardiac disease associated with the carcinoid syndrome. Am J Med 36:5, 1969

STOLLERMAN E: Rheumatic fever, connective tissue disorders and heart disease, in *Heart Disease,* 2d ed, E Braunwald (ed). Philadelphia, Saunders, 1983, chap 48

WILLIAMS LT et al: Thyroid hormone regulation of beta-adrenergic receptor number. J Biol Chem 252:2787, 1977

265 PERICARDIAL DISEASE

EUGENE BRAUNWALD

NORMAL FUNCTIONS OF THE PERICARDIUM

The visceral pericardium is a serous membrane, separated by a small amount of fluid, an ultrafiltrate of plasma, from a fibrous sac, the parietal pericardium. The pericardium prevents sudden dilatation of the cardiac chambers during exercise and hypervolemia, and as the result of the development of a negative intrapericardial pressure during ejection it facilitates atrial filling during ventricular systole. The pericardium also restricts the anatomic position of the heart, minimizes friction between the heart and surrounding structures, prevents displacement of the heart and kinking of the great vessels, and probably retards the spread of infections from the lungs and pleural cavities to the heart. Notwithstanding the foregoing, total absence of the pericardium does not produce obvious clinical disease. In partial left pericardial defects the main pulmonary artery and left atrium may bulge through the defect; rarely herniation and subsequent strangulation of the left atrium may cause sudden death.

It is useful to classify the types of pericarditis both clinically and etiologically (Table 265-1), as this disorder is by far the most common pathological process involving the pericardium.

ACUTE PERICARDITIS

Pain, a pericardial friction rub, electrocardiographic changes, and pericardial effusion with cardiac tamponade and paradoxic pulse are cardinal manifestations of many forms of acute pericarditis and will be considered prior to a discussion of the most common varieties.

Pain is an important but not invariable symptom in various forms of acute pericarditis; it is usually present in the acute infectious types and in many of the forms presumed to be related to hypersensitivity or autoimmunity. Pain is often absent in a slowly developing tuberculous, postirradiation, neoplastic or uremic pericarditis. The pain of pericarditis is often severe; its character and location have been described in Chap. 4. It is characteristically in the center of the chest, referred to the back and the trapezius ridge. Often the pain is pleuritic, i.e., sharp and aggravated by inspiration, coughing, and changes in body position, but occasionally it is a steady, constrictive pain, which radiates into either arm or both arms and resembles that of myocardial ischemia; confusion with myocardial infarction is common. Characteristically, however, the pain is relieved by sitting up and leaning forward. This problem becomes even more perplexing when, with acute pericarditis, the serum transaminase level rises to about 80 units. However, the MB isoenzyme of creatine kinase does not rise in acute pericarditis.

The *pericardial friction rub* is the most important physical sign; it may have up to three components per cardiac cycle, as described in Chap. 248, and can sometimes be elicited only when firm pressure with the diaphragm of the stethoscope is applied to the chest wall. It is heard most frequently during expiration, but an independent pleural friction rub may be audible during inspiration, with the patient leaning forward or in the left lateral decubitus position. The rub is likely to be inconstant and transitory, and a loud to-and-fro leathery sound may disappear within a few hours, possibly to reappear the following day.

The *electrocardiogram* in acute pericarditis without massive effusion usually displays widespread elevation of the ST segments, involving two or three standard limb leads and V_2 to V_6, with reciprocal depressions only in aVR and V_1 and without significant changes in QRS complexes, except occasionally for some diminution in voltage. Several days later, the ST segments return to normal and the T waves then become inverted. In contrast, in acute myocardial infarction, reciprocal depression of ST segments is usually more prominent; QRS changes occur, particularly the development of Q waves; and T-wave inversions usually occur before the ST segments have become isoelectric. Sequential electrocardiograms are useful in distinguishing acute pericarditis from acute myocardial infarction and from early repolarization (see also Chap. 249). Depression of the PR segment (below the T-P segment) also is common in acute pericarditis. With large pericardial effusion, the QRS voltage is reduced. Atrial premature beats and atrial fibrillation are sometimes noted.

PERICARDIAL EFFUSION Usually associated with one or more of the above-mentioned manifestations of pericarditis and an enlargement of the cardiac silhouette, pericardial effusion is especially important when it develops within a relatively short time. Differentiation from cardiac enlargement may be difficult, but heart sounds tend to become faint; the friction rub may disappear or remain clearly audible, and the apex impulse may vanish, but sometimes it is felt well within the left border of cardiac dullness. The chest roentgenogram may show a "water bottle" configuration of the cardiac silhouette. Lucent pericardial fat lines may be seen deep within the cardiopericardial silhouette. Fluoroscopic examination may show the ventricular pulsations to be diminished. When the effusion is large, an area of dullness and tubular breath sounds is often encountered at the angle of the left scapula, probably caused by compression of the lung (Ewart's sign).

Diagnosis of pericardial effusion Echocardiography (Chap. 250) is the most effective laboratory technique available, since it is sensitive, specific, simple, innocuous, and noninvasive, and may be performed at the bedside. The presence of pericardial fluid is recorded as a relatively echo-free space between the posterior pericardium and the posterior left ventricular epicardium in patients with small effusions and such a space between the anterior right ventricle and the parietal pericardium just

TABLE 265-1
Classification of pericarditis

I Clinical classification
- *A* Acute pericarditis (<6 weeks)
  - *1* Fibrinous
  - *2* Effusive (or bloody)
- *B* Subacute pericarditis (6 weeks to 6 months)
  - *1* Constrictive
  - *2* Effusive-constrictive
- *C* Chronic pericarditis (>6 months)
  - *1* Constrictive
  - *2* Effusive
  - *3* Adhesive (nonconstrictive)

II Etiologic classification
- *A* Infectious pericarditis
  - *1* Viral
  - *2* Pyogenic
  - *3* Tuberculous
  - *4* Mycotic
  - *5* Other infections (syphilitic, parasitic)
- *B* Noninfectious pericarditis
  - *1* Acute myocardial infarction
  - *2* Uremia
  - *3* Neoplasia
    - *a* Primary tumors (benign or malignant)
    - *b* Tumors metastatic to pericardium
  - *4* Myxedema
  - *5* Cholesterol
  - *6* Chylopericardium
  - *7* Trauma
    - *a* Penetrating chest wall
    - *b* Nonpenetrating
  - *8* Aortic aneurysm (with leakage into pericardial sac)
  - *9* Postradiation
  - *10* Associated with atrial septal defect
  - *11* Associated with severe chronic anemia
  - *12* Infectious mononucleosis
  - *13* Familial Mediterranean fever
  - *14* Familial pericarditis
    - *a* Mulibrey nanism*
  - *15* Sarcoidosis
  - *16* Acute idiopathic
- *C* Pericarditis presumably related to hypersensitivity or autoimmunity
  - *1* Rheumatic fever
  - *2* Collagen vascular disease
    - *a* Systemic lupus erythematosus
    - *b* Rheumatoid arthritis
    - *c* Scleroderma
  - *3* Drug-induced
    - *a* Procainamide
    - *b* Hydralazine
    - *c* Other
  - *4* Postcardiac injury
    - *a* Postmyocardial infarction (Dressler's syndrome)
    - *b* Postpericardiotomy

* *An autosomal recessive syndrome, characterized by growth failure, muscle hypotonia, hepatomegaly, ocular changes, enlarged cerebral ventricles, mental retardation, and chronic constrictive pericarditis.*

beneath the anterior chest wall with larger effusions (Fig. 265-1). In patients with large effusions the heart may swing freely within the pericardial sac; when severe, this motion may be associated with electrical alternans. While M-mode echocardiography is usually adequate for the diagnosis of pericardial effusion, two-dimensional echocardiography is often superior since it allows more precise localization and estimation of the quality of pericardial fluid. The diagnosis of pericardial fluid or thickening may be confirmed by one of the following:

1 *Cardiac catheterization.* A catheter is introduced into the right atrium and rotated so that its tip makes contact with the lateral right atrial wall. In the presence of an effusion, or pericardial thickening, the tip of the catheter is seen to be separated from the radiolucent lungs by an opaque band.
2 *Angiocardiography.* Contrast medium is injected rapidly into the right atrium; again the lateral wall is separated from the edge of the cardiac silhouette.

When examination of pericardial fluid is deemed essential, exploration of the pericardium may be required. To accomplish this, a needle should be attached to a properly grounded electrocardiographic lead, and intrapericardial pressure should be measured, utilizing the same apparatus employed for measuring cerebrospinal fluid pressure during lumbar puncture. When an effusion develops, the fluid nearly always has the physical characteristics of an exudate. Bloody fluid is commonly due to tuberculosis or tumor, but it may also be found in the effusion of rheumatic fever or in the post-cardiac injury syndrome (see below). Occasionally, bloody fluid may be found in the effusion of uremic pericarditis and in the hemopericardium following myocardial infarction, especially following the administration of anticoagulants.

CARDIAC TAMPONADE The accumulation of fluid in the pericardium in an amount sufficient to cause serious obstruction to the inflow of blood to the ventricles results in cardiac tamponade. The amount of fluid necessary to produce this critical state may be as small as 250 ml, when the fluid develops rapidly; or it may be over 1000 ml in slowly developing effusions when the pericardium has had the opportunity to stretch and adapt to the increasing volume of fluid. The volume of fluid required to produce tamponade varies directly with the thickness of the ventricular myocardium and inversely with the thickness of the parietal pericardium. Tamponade results most often from bleeding into the pericardial space following cardiac operations, trauma (including cardiac perforation during diagnostic procedures), tuberculosis, and tumor (most commonly carcinoma of the lung and breast and lymphoma), but it may occur in acute viral or idiopathic pericarditis, postradiation pericarditis, renal failure during dialysis, and hemopericardium which may result when a patient with any form of acute pericarditis is treated with anticoagulants.

The clinical manifestations are due to the fall in cardiac output and to systemic venous congestion. However, the classic findings of falling arterial pressure, rising venous pressure, and a small quiet heart with faint heart sounds usually are seen only with severe tamponade occurring within minutes, as happens with cardiac trauma. More frequently, tamponade develops more slowly and the clinical manifestations, resembling those of heart failure, include dyspnea, orthopnea, hepatic engorgement, and jugular venous hypertension. A high index of suspicion is required, since, in many instances, no obvious cause for pericardial disease is apparent, and tamponade should be considered in any patient with hypotension and elevation of jugular venous pressure with a prominent x descent; often the y descent is absent. A widening of the area of flatness to percussion across the anterior aspect of the chest wall, a paradoxical pulse (see below), relatively clear lung fields, diminished pulsations of the cardiac silhouette on fluoroscopy, reduction in amplitude of the QRS complexes, and *electrical alternans* should raise the suspicion of cardiac tamponade. Since immediate treatment may be lifesaving, prompt measures to establish the diagnosis, i.e., echocardiography, followed by cardiac catheterization, should be undertaken. The latter reveals elevation of the right atrial pressure with a prominent x but no y descent. When measured, the pericardial pressure is also elevated and equal to the right atrial pressure. The pulmonary artery wedge is equal, or close, to right atrial, right ventricular, and pulmonary artery diastolic pressures. The "square root" sign in the ventricular pressure pulses characteristic of constrictive pericarditis (see below) is usually absent.

Paradoxical pulse This important clue to the presence of cardiac tamponade consists of *a greater than normal (10 mmHg) inspiratory decrease in systolic arterial pressure.* When severe, it may be detected by palpating weakness or disappearance of the arterial pulse during inspiration, but usually sphygmomanometric measurement of systolic pressure during slow respiration is required (Fig. 265-2).

The mechanism of paradoxical pulse in cardiac tamponade is complex. Normally, the inspiratory decline in intrathoracic pressure enhances right ventricular filling by virtue of the increased pressure gradient between the extrathoracic veins and

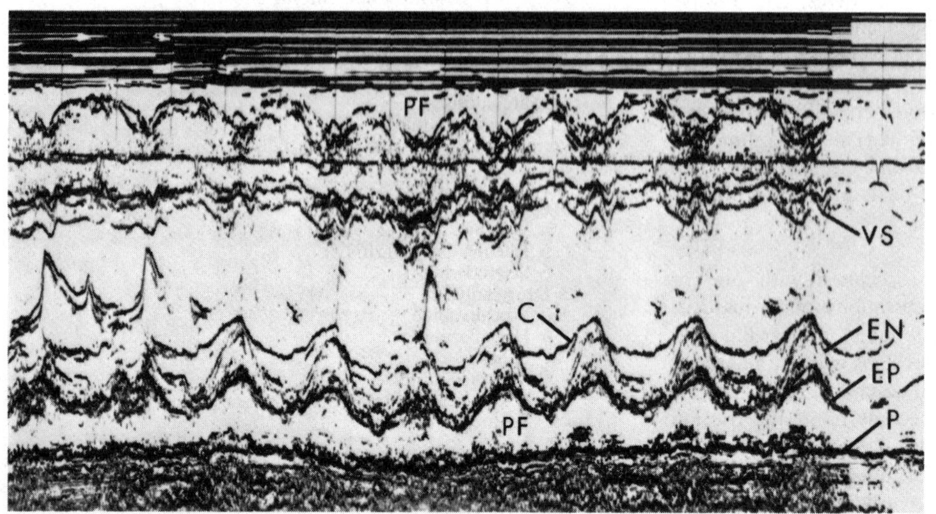

FIGURE 265-1
Patient with moderate pericardial effusion (idiopathic). Echogram demonstrates anterior (smaller) and posterior (larger) echo-free spaces. The motion of the anterior wall of the right ventricle, ventricular septum, and left ventricular posterior wall is normal; i.e., during ventricular systole the right ventricular anterior wall and ventricular septum move posteriorly as the left ventricular posterior wall moves anteriorly. PF, pericardial fluid; C, chordae tendineae; VS, ventricular septum; EN, endocardium; EP, epicardium; P, pericardium. (Reproduced with permission from AJ Tajir, Am J Med 63:34, 1977.)

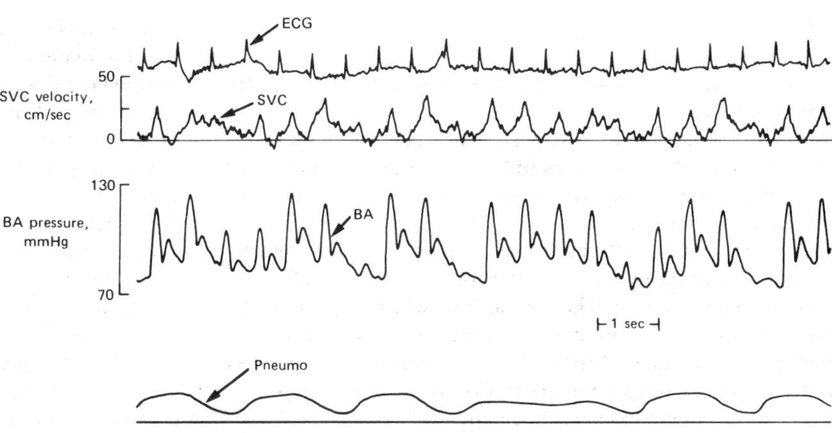

FIGURE 265-2
Simultaneous recording of electrocardiogram (ECG), blood flow velocity in the superior vena cava (SVC), brachial arterial pressure (BA), and the pneumogram (Pneumo) in a patient with cardiac compression and paradoxical pulse. A downward deflection of the pneumogram denotes significant inspiration, when SVC blood velocity rises and arterial pressure falls (paradoxical pulse). Arterial pressure is maintained during prolonged expiratory pause.

the chambers of the right side of the heart. Right ventricular volume and stroke output increase, but since both ventricles are enclosed in a common chamber, the pericardial sac, an increase in right ventricular volume results in a reduction in left ventricular volume. Also, left ventricular afterload rises during inspiration (as intrapericardial pressure declines), and left ventricular stroke volume and therefore arterial pressure decline slightly during inspiration. In cardiac tamponade, since both ventricles share a tight incompressible covering, the inspiratory augmentation of right ventricle volume results in a reciprocal reduction in left ventricle volume. Also, respiratory distress increases the fluctuations in intrathoracic pressure, which, in addition to exaggerating the mechanism just described, are also transmitted directly to the intrathoracic aorta and hence to the peripheral arterial bed.

Low-pressure tamponade refers to mild tamponade in which the intrapericardial pressure is increased from its slightly subatmospheric levels to +5 to +10 mmHg and the central venous pressure is slightly elevated; arterial pressure is unaffected. The patients are asymptomatic or complain of mild weakness and dyspnea. The diagnosis is aided by echocardiography, and both hemodynamic and clinical manifestations improve following mild pericardiocentesis.

Paradoxical pulse occurs in only approximately one-third of patients with constrictive pericarditis. It is important to bear in mind that paradoxical pulse is not pathognomonic of pericardial disease because it may be observed in various forms of restrictive cardiomyopathies (Chap. 263) and, in some cases of hypovolemic shock, chronic obstructive airways disease, and severe bronchial asthma.

TREATMENT All patients with acute pericarditis should be observed frequently and carefully for the possibility of a developing effusion or, if effusion is already present, for signs of tamponade. In the presence of an effusion, arterial and venous pressures and heart rate should be monitored continuously or carefully followed and serial echocardiograms and chest roentgenograms obtained. If manifestations of tamponade appear, pericardiocentesis must be carried out at once, since relief of the intrapericardial pressure may be lifesaving.

VIRAL OR IDIOPATHIC FORM OF ACUTE PERICARDITIS This disorder is an important clinical entity because of its frequency and because it may be confused with other more serious illnesses. In some cases an A or B coxsackievirus or the virus of influenza, echovirus type 8, mumps, herpes simplex, chickenpox, or adenovirus has been isolated from pericardial fluid and/or appropriate elevations in viral antibody titers have been noted; in other instances, acute pericarditis has occurred in association with illnesses of known viral origin and, presumably, was caused by the same agent. More commonly there is an antecedent infection of the respiratory tract, but in many patients such an association is not evident and viral isolation and serologic studies are negative. Most frequently, a viral causation cannot be established nor can it be excluded; the term *acute idiopathic pericarditis* is then appropriate. However, regardless of the specific causative factor, the clinical manifestations are similar. This form of acute pericarditis occurs at all ages but is more frequent in young adults; it is often associated with pleural effusions and pneumonitis. The appearance of fever and precordial pain at about the same time, often 10 to 12 days after a presumed viral illness, constitutes an important feature in the differentiation of acute pericarditis from myocardial infarction, in which pain precedes fever. The constitutional symptoms are usually mild to moderate, but occasionally the initial symptoms are stormy, the temperature rising to 40°C. The disease ordinarily runs its course in a few days to 2 weeks, but occasionally after the patient has apparently recovered he or she may have one or several recurrences, weeks or even months later. Tamponade is unusual, although accumulation of some pericardial fluid is common, and constrictive pericarditis develops rarely. A pericardial friction rub is often audible. The ST-T wave alterations in the electrocardiogram are usually transitory, but the abnormal T waves may persist for several years or indefinitely, constituting a subsequent source of confusion in persons without a clear history of pericarditis. Pleuritis and pneumonitis frequently accompany pericarditis. The erythrocyte sedimentation rate is elevated. Granulocytosis followed by lymphocytosis is common.

There is no specific therapy, but anti-inflammatory treatment with aspirin, if necessary up to 900 mg qid, may be given. If this is ineffective, indomethacin (25 to 75 mg qid) or corticosteroids (prednisone, 20 to 80 mg daily) effectively suppress the clinical manifestations of the acute illness and may be useful in patients who do not respond to supportive nonspecific therapy after the purulent and tuberculous forms of pericarditis have been excluded. After the patient has been asymptomatic for 1 week, the dose of the anti-inflammatory agent is gradually tapered. Recurrences occur in about one-fourth the patients, but the tendency to relapse decreases within 2 years after the initial episode. When recurrences persist beyond this period, pericardiectomy may be effective in terminating the illness.

POST-CARDIAC INJURY SYNDROME During the past few years, it has been recognized that a number of disorders, identical in their clinical manifestations, may appear under a variety of circumstances. They have one common feature: previous injury to the myocardium, with blood in the pericardial cavity. The syndrome has been observed when the injury has been induced in the course of a cardiac operation (postpericardiotomy syndrome or, as it was originally designated, postcommissurotomy syndrome). It may also follow myocardial infarction (Dressler's syndrome) or develop after trauma of the heart (e.g., stab wound, contusions following a nonpenetrating blow to the chest, and following perforation of the heart with a pacemaker catheter).

The principal symptom is pain, which usually develops after an interval of 1 to 4 weeks following the cardiac injury but sometimes appears only after a lapse of months. Recurrences are common and may occur up to 2 years or more after the injury. Fever up to 40°C, pericarditis, pleuritis, and pneumonitis are the outstanding features, the bout of illness usually subsiding in 1 or 2 weeks. The pericarditis, which appears to be the most constant lesion, may be of the fibrinous variety, or it may be a pericardial effusion, which is often serosanguineous and sometimes causes tamponade. Concomitantly, arthralgias, leukocytosis, an increased sedimentation rate, and typical electrocardiographic changes may occur.

The mechanism whereby the clinical manifestations are induced is not certain, but there is a likelihood that they are the result of a hypersensitivity reaction in which the antigen originates from injured myocardial tissue and/or pericardium; the suggested designation of post-cardiac injury syndrome for this group of disorders implies that they may have a common pathogenetic mechanism. Circulating autoantibodies to myocardium occur frequently, but their precise role in this syndrome has not been defined. Viral infection may also play an etiologic role, since antiviral antibodies are often elevated in patients who develop this syndrome following cardiac surgery.

The clinical picture mimics acute viral or acute idiopathic pericarditis. Moreover, it is possible that the recurrences that occur so frequently in the latter condition are not always caused by an exacerbation of the original (presumably viral) infection, but that the original injury may have initiated the sequence of events that culminates in the post-cardiac injury syndrome.

Often no treatment is necessary aside from aspirin or analgesics. The management of pericardial effusion and tamponade has already been discussed. When the illness is severe and is followed by a series of disabling recurrences, therapy with indomethacin or corticosteroids is usually effective.

Differential diagnosis Differential diagnosis of *acute idiopathic pericarditis* is primarily one of exclusion, as there is no specific test for this disorder. Consequently all other disorders that may be associated with acute fibrinous pericarditis must be considered. When associated with *acute myocardial infarction,* acute fibrinous pericarditis may be confused with acute viral or idiopathic pericarditis; this complication of infarction, described on page 1442, must be differentiated by the occurrence of fever, pain, and a friction rub in the first 4 days following the development of the infarct. Electrocardiographic abnormalities (such as the appearance of Q waves and earlier T-wave changes in myocardial infarction), the extent of the elevations of myocardial enzymes, and the total clinical picture are helpful in the identification of the pericarditis of acute myocardial infarction. A common error is assuming that acute viral or idiopathic pericarditis represents acute myocardial infarction.

Acute pericarditis occurring as a component of the *post-cardiac injury* syndrome is most likely to be confused with acute idiopathic pericarditis when it follows myocardial infarction or a nonpenetrating bruise to the chest. Such pericarditis is differentiated from acute idiopathic pericarditis chiefly by timing. If it occurs within a few weeks of an infarction or a chest blow, concluding that the two are probably related is justified. If the infarct has been silent or the chest blow forgotten, the relationship to the pericarditis may not be recognized.

It is important to distinguish *pericarditis due to collagen disease* from acute idiopathic pericarditis. Most important in the differential diagnosis is the pericarditis due to systemic lupus erythematosus (Chap. 70). Sometimes the latter appears as an asymptomatic effusion; more often pain is present, and rarely tamponade develops. Very rarely, when pericarditis occurs in the absence of other evidence of any underlying disorder, differentiation from acute viral and idiopathic pericarditis or tuberculous pericarditis may be made on discovery of lupus erythematosus (LE) cells, a rise in antinuclear antibodies, or by the specific methods for diagnosing tuberculosis. Acute pericarditis is also an occasional complication of *rheumatoid arthritis, scleroderma,* and *periarteritis nodosa,* but again, other evidence of these diseases is usually obvious. Asymptomatic pericardial effusion is also frequent in these disorders. It is important to question every patient with acute pericarditis about the ingestion of procainamide, hydralazine, isoniazid, cromolyn, and minoxidil, since these drugs can cause this syndrome.

The pericarditis of *acute rheumatic fever* is generally associated with evidence of severe pancarditis and with cardiac murmurs (Chap. 257). *Pyogenic (purulent) pericarditis* is usually secondary to cardiothoracic operations, immunosuppressive therapy, rupture of the esophagus into the pericardial sac, and rupture of a ring abscess in a patient with infective endocarditis and with septicemia occurring in a patient with an aseptic pericarditis. It is now uncommonly due to pneumococcal pneumonia and pleuritis, previously the most common cause. *Uremic pericarditis* (Chap. 291) occurs in up to one-third of patients with chronic uremia; it is seen most frequently in patients undergoing chronic hemodialysis. It may be fibrinous or associated with a bloody effusion. A friction rub is common; pain may be absent. Treatment with an anti-inflammatory agent and intensification of hemodialysis is usually adequate therapy. Occasionally, when tamponade occurs, pericardiocentesis is required. When pericarditis is recurrent or persistent, pericardiectomy is necessary. Pericarditis due to *neoplastic diseases* results from mediastinal irradiation or extension of primary or metastatic tumors (most commonly carcinoma of the lung and breast, malignant melanoma, and lymphoma) to the pericardium or from invasion by a lymphomatous or leukemic process; pain, atrial arrhythmias, and tamponade are complications which occur occasionally. Unusual causes of acute pericarditis include syphilis, fungous infection (histoplasmosis, blastomycosis, aspergillosis, and candidiasis), and parasitic infestation (amebiasis, toxoplasmosis, echinococcosis, trichinosis).

TUBERCULOUS PERICARDIAL EFFUSION Tuberculous involvement of the pericardium may present as an acute fibrinous pericarditis, but more frequently it presents as a chronic pericardial effusion. With the acute form, the history of precordial pain is inconstant and there may be no other evidence of tuberculosis (Chap. 174). The symptoms are often those of a chronic, systemic illness in an individual with effusion. It is important to bear this condition in mind when a middle-aged or elderly person with fever has an apparent enlargement of the heart of undetermined origin, with or without elevation of venous pressure. Weight loss, fever, and fatigability are sometimes observed. Inasmuch as effective specific methods of therapy have now reduced strikingly the mortality rate from the previous figures of about 70 percent, overlooking a tuberculous pericardial effusion is a serious error. Consequently, no method of examination should be omitted to establish this diagnosis. Included are chest roentgenograms for pulmonary tuberculosis and a search for tuberculosis in other organs; tuberculin skin tests, repeated after several weeks; cultures and smears of gastric washings and of pleural and pericardial fluid. Finally, if the diagnosis is still obscure, a pericardial biopsy, preferably by a limited thoracotomy, should be performed after 1 or 2 weeks of preliminary antituberculous chemotherapy. If definitive evidence is then still lacking, but the specimen shows caseation necrosis, antituberculous chemotherapy for at least 24 months is justified (Chap. 174). Pericardiectomy should be carried out in order to prevent the development of constriction if the biopsy specimen shows a thickened pericardium.

Differential diagnosis of chronic pericardial effusion *Tuberculosis* is the most common cause of chronic pericardial effusion.

Myxedema may be responsible for a pericardial effusion that is sometimes massive but rarely, if ever, causes cardiac tamponade. The other manifestations of myxedema should clarify the diagnosis, but unfortunately, even when they are present the diagnosis is frequently overlooked. It is important, therefore, to carry out appropriate tests for thyroid function (Chap. 111) in patients with an enlarged cardiac outline of undetermined origin. The cardiac silhouette is markedly enlarged and an echocardiogram is necessary to distinguish cardiomegaly from pericardial effusion. *Cholesterol pericardial disease* produces large pericardial effusions with a high cholesterol content, which may induce an inflammatory response and constrictive pericarditis.

Neoplasms, systemic lupus erythematosus, rheumatoid arthritis, mycotic infection, radiation therapy, pyogenic infections, severe chronic anemia, and chylopericardium may also cause chronic pericardial effusion.

Aspiration and analysis of the pericardial fluid may often be helpful in diagnosis. In infections the organism can be identified by smear or on culture. Grossly sanguineous pericardial fluid results most commonly from a neoplasm, tuberculosis, uremia, or slow leakage from an aortic aneurysm.

CHRONIC CONSTRICTIVE PERICARDITIS

This disorder results when the healing of an acute fibrinous or serofibrinous pericarditis is followed by obliteration of the pericardial cavity, with the formation of granulation tissue which gradually contracts and forms a firm scar, encasing the heart and interfering with filling of the ventricles. In some reports, a high percentage of all cases has been of tuberculous origin. In other series, particularly those reported in the last decade, tuberculosis has been an infrequent cause. The condition also may follow purulent infection, trauma, radiation, histoplasmosis, neoplastic disease, and acute viral or idiopathic pericarditis, rheumatoid arthritis, lupus erythematosus, and chronic renal failure with uremia treated by chronic dialysis. In many patients the cause of the pericardial disease is undetermined, and in them it is presumed that an asymptomatic or forgotten bout of acute pericarditis, acute or idiopathic, was the inciting event. Rarely, routine fluoroscopic or radiographic examination may reveal calcification of the pericardium in a person who is free of all symptoms referable to the heart.

The basic physiological abnormality in symptomatic patients with chronic constrictive pericarditis, as in those with cardiac tamponade, is the inability of the ventricles to fill adequately during diastole because of the limitations imposed by the rigid, thickened pericardium or the tense pericardial fluid. Stroke volume is diminished, and the end-diastolic pressures in both ventricles, as well as the mean pressures in the atria, pulmonic veins, and systemic veins, are elevated to about the same levels. Despite these hemodynamic changes myocardial function may be normal; instead, the ventricles may be considered to be underloaded. In constrictive pericarditis the central venous and right and left atrial pressure pulses display an M-shaped contour, with prominent x and y descents; the y descent is the most prominent deflection and is interrupted by a rapid rise in pressure during early diastole, when ventricular filling is impeded by the constricting pericardium. In cardiac tamponade the pressure contour differs in that the most prominent deflection is the x trough, while the y descent is usually absent. These characteristic changes are transmitted to the jugular veins, where they may be recorded or recognized by inspection. In constrictive pericarditis, but not in cardiac tamponade, both ventricular pressure pulses exhibit characteristic "square root" signs during diastole. These hemodynamic changes, although characteristic, are not pathognomonic of constrictive pericarditis but are also observed in cardiomyopathies characterized by restriction of ventricular filling, as discussed on page 1451.

CLINICAL FINDINGS Weakness, fatigue, weight loss, and anorexia are common. The patients often appear to be chronically ill with decreased muscle mass, a protuberant abdomen, and peripheral edema. Contrary to a widely held impression, dyspnea, though absent or slight at rest, is often present on exertion, and orthopnea is common in chronic constrictive pericarditis, although it is not severe. Attacks of acute left ventricular failure (acute pulmonary edema) practically never occur. The cervical veins are distended and may remain so even after intensive diuretic treatment, and in about one-third of the cases a paradoxical pulse may be observed; this may be associated with failure of venous pressure to decline during inspiration (Kussmaul's sign). Congestive hepatomegaly is pronounced and may impair hepatic function; ascites is common and is usually more prominent than dependent edema. In about half the patients, the heart is normal in size; if it is enlarged, the enlargement is rarely extreme. The apical pulse is reduced in intensity. The heart sounds may be distant, an early third heart sound, i.e., a pericardial knock, occurring 0.06 to 0.12 s after aortic valve closure, is often conspicuous, and murmurs are usually absent. The apex beat is poorly defined, and cardiac pulsations under fluoroscopic examination are diminished. Because of the high sustained venous pressure, congestive splenomegaly may be sufficiently pronounced to make the spleen palpable. In the absence of infective endocarditis or tricuspid valve disease, splenomegaly in a patient with congestive heart failure should arouse suspicion of constrictive pericarditis. Protein-losing gastroenteropathy due to impaired lymphatic drainage from the small intestine, and the nephrotic syndrome or sometimes only marked proteinuria or hypoalbuminemia, may complicate chronic constrictive pericarditis. The electrocardiogram frequently displays low voltage of the QRS complex and flattening or inversion of the T waves in most leads; P mitrale is frequently found in patients with sinus rhythm; atrial fibrillation is present in about one-third of these patients.

Systemic and/or pulmonary venous congestion is initially the result of impaired filling of the ventricles caused by the restrictive action of the inelastic pericardium. However, the fibrotic process may extend into the myocardium, and venous congestion may then be due to the combined effects of the myocardial and pericardial lesions. The interference with filling reduces the work of the heart and perhaps this leads to myocardial atrophy. The latter probably accounts for the delayed beneficial effects of operative treatment observed in some patients with advanced disease.

Inasmuch as the usual physical signs of cardiac disease (murmurs, cardiac enlargement) may be inconspicuous or entirely lacking, hepatic enlargement and dysfunction associated with intractable ascites may lead to a mistaken diagnosis of cirrhosis of the liver. This error should be avoided if the neck veins are inspected carefully in all patients with ascites and hepatomegaly. *Given a clinical picture resembling that of cirrhosis, but with the added feature of distended neck veins, careful search for calcification of the pericardium by chest roentgeno-*

grams and fluoroscopy should be carried out and may disclose a curable or remediable form of heart disease. Calcification occurs in only about one-half of these patients and usually not in those that are not of long-standing. Therefore, surgical exploration of the pericardium is justifiable if the clinical picture and cardiac catheterization findings are suggestive even in the absence of pericardial calcification.

DIFFERENTIAL DIAGNOSIS Like cor pulmonale (Chap. 262), chronic constrictive pericarditis may be associated with severe systemic venous hypertension but with little or no pulmonary congestion; the heart may not appear to be enlarged, and a striking inspiratory fall in arterial pressure may be present. However, in cor pulmonale advanced parenchymal pulmonary disease is evident and venous pressure falls during inspiration. *Tricuspid stenosis* may also simulate the picture of chronic constrictive pericarditis; congestive hepatomegaly and ascites may be equally prominent, and the manifestations of left-sided heart failure may be inconspicuous. However, in tricuspid stenosis, the characteristic murmur, the frequent coexistence of mitral stenosis, the absence of a paradoxic pulse, as well as the absence, in the jugular venous pulse, of the steep, deep *y* descent followed by a rapid ascent (manifested by the diastolic shock on palpation and its audible equivalent, the pericardial knock), should make the clinical differentiation possible.

It is of the greatest importance, though often difficult, to distinguish chronic constrictive pericarditis from various forms of heart disease which are characterized by a similar physiologic abnormality, i.e., restriction of ventricular filling, leading to a similar clinical picture. Described in Chap. 263, these include endomyocardial fibrosis, infiltrative cardiomyopathies such as amyloidosis, hemochromatosis, sarcoidosis, scleroderma and idiopathic myocardial hypertrophy, in which the marked thickening of the ventricular wall is responsible for the diminished compliance.

The features favoring the diagnosis of one of the above forms of cardiomyopathy are a well-defined apex beat, conspicuous enlargement of the heart, and pronounced orthopnea with attacks of acute left ventricular failure, left ventricular hypertrophy, bundle branch block, or significant Q waves in the electrocardiogram. At catheterization, patients with chronic constrictive pericarditis usually have left atrial or pulmonary arterial wedge pressure equaling right atrial pressure, the latter often exceeding 15 mmHg following intensive medical treatment for heart failure; the pulmonary artery systolic pressure is often less than 50 mmHg, and the right ventricular end-diastolic pressure often reaches one-third of the systolic pressure; the cardiac output is slightly depressed. In contrast, in patients with cardiomyopathy, the left atrial usually exceeds the right atrial pressures by more than 5 mmHg, the mean right atrial pressure usually falls to below 15 mmHg following treatment, the pulmonary artery systolic pressure often exceeds 50 mmHg, and the right ventricular end-diastolic pressure is usually less than one-third the systolic pressure, while the cardiac output is markedly depressed. The volumes of both ventricles, as determined by angiography or echocardiography (Chap. 251), are characteristically reduced or normal in constrictive pericarditis, and the ejection fractions are normal; the left ventricular end-diastolic volume may be normal in some cardiomyopathies but is frequently elevated in others, in whom the ejection fraction is reduced; the latter finding militates strongly against the diagnosis of constrictive pericarditis. The echocardiogram in chronic constrictive pericarditis characteristically shows pericardial thickening, i.e., a distinct echo posterior to the left ventricular wall, and paradoxical septal motion. The left ventricular wall moves sharply outward in early diastole and then remains flat. The diagnosis of restrictive cardiomyopathy, when it is due to an infiltrative disease, such as amyloidosis, can often be made by endomyocardial biopsy.

The lesson to be learned is that when a patient has progressive, disabling, and unresponsive congestive failure, and if he or she displays any of the phenomena of constrictive heart disease, the most careful and detailed clinical and laboratory studies must be carried out in order to detect or exclude constrictive pericarditis. In many instances cardiac catheterization, selective angiocardiography, coronary arteriography, and even endomyocardial biopsy may be required. However, when even these examinations do not yield a definitive diagnosis, surgical exploration of the pericardium is the only decisive method of determining whether constrictive pericarditis is responsible for the clinical manifestations of heart failure.

Occult constrictive disease Patients with this condition may have unexplained fatigue, dyspnea, and chest pain. No overt manifestations of pericardial disease are present, but following the rapid intravenous infusion of 1 liter of saline solution, atrial and ventricular pressure pulses and diastolic equilibration of intracardiac pressures, as in overt constrictive pericarditis, occur. Although symptomatic improvement may follow pericardiectomy, this procedure should not be carried out in asymptomatic persons.

TREATMENT Surgery is the only definitive treatment of constrictive pericarditis, but diuretics and sodium restriction are useful during preoperative preparation for pericardial resection. Digitalis may be beneficial in the prevention of heart failure when resection of the thickened pericardium permits an increased inflow into the ventricles and hence places an enhanced burden on an atrophic myocardium. The benefits derived from a complete cardiac decortication are often striking, and frequently the improvement, though slight at first, is progressive over a period of many months.

Many instances of constrictive pericarditis are of tuberculous origin. Antituberculous therapy during the phase of effusion may prevent the development of constriction, and such therapy should be carried out before and after operation, if a tuberculous origin is suspected or cannot be excluded in a patient with chronic constrictive pericarditis (Chap. 174).

SUBACUTE EFFUSIVE-CONSTRICTIVE PERICARDITIS This form of pericardial disease is characterized by tense effusion into a free pericardial space, as well as by constriction of the heart by thickened pericardium, and thus it shares a number of features both with pericardial effusion producing cardiac compression and with pericardial constriction. It may be caused by tuberculosis, multiple attacks of acute idiopathic pericarditis, radiation, traumatic pericarditis, uremia, and scleroderma. The heart is generally enlarged, and there are a paradoxical pulse and a prominent *x* descent in the atrial pressure pulse. Following pericardiocentesis, the physiologic findings may change from those of cardiac tamponade to those of pericardial constriction. In many patients the condition progresses to the chronic constrictive form of the disease. Wide excision of both the visceral and parietal pericardium is usually effective.

OTHER DISORDERS OF THE PERICARDIUM

Pericardial cysts appear as rounded or lobulated deformities of the cardiac silhouette, most commonly at the right cardiophrenic angle. They do not cause symptoms, and their major clinical significance lies in the possibility of confusion with a tumor, ventricular aneurysm, or massive cardiomegaly. *Tumors* involving the pericardium are most commonly secondary to malignant neoplasms originating in or invading the mediastinum, including carcinoma of the bronchus and breast, lymphoma, and melanoma. The most common *primary* malignant tumor is the mesothelioma. The usual clinical picture of malignant pericardial tumor is an insidiously developing, often bloody, pericardial effusion. Surgical exploration is required to establish a definitive diagnosis and to carry out definitive or, more commonly, palliative treatment.

REFERENCES

BOVE AA, SANTAMORE WP: Ventricular interdependence. Prog Cardiovasc Dis 23:365, 1981

BUSH CA et al: Occult pericardial disease. Circulation 56:924, 1977

HANCOCK EW: Subacute effusive-constrictive pericarditis. Circulation 43:183, 1971

HURST JW et al (eds): Pericardial disease, in *The Heart: Arteries and Veins,* 5th ed. New York, McGraw-Hill, 1982, p 1363

LOVELL B, BRAUNWALD, E: Pericardial disease, in *Heart Disease,* 2d ed. Philadelphia, Saunders, 1983, chap 43

REDDY et al (eds): *Pericardial Disease.* New York, Raven, 1982

ROBERTS WC, SPRAY TL: Pericardial heart disease. Curr Probl Cardiol 2:3, 1977

SHABETAI R: *The Pericardium.* New York, Grune & Stratton, 1981

section 2 | Disorders of the vascular system

266
ATHEROSCLEROSIS AND OTHER FORMS OF ARTERIOSCLEROSIS

EDWIN L. BIERMAN

Arteriosclerosis, a generic term for thickening and hardening of the arterial wall, is responsible for the majority of deaths in the United States and most westernized societies. One type of arteriosclerosis is *atherosclerosis,* the disorder of the larger arteries that underlies most *coronary artery disease, aortic aneurysm,* and *arterial disease of the lower extremities* and also plays a major role in *cerebrovascular disease.* Atherosclerosis is by far the leading cause of death in the United States, both above and below age 65 (Table 266-1).

Other types of arteriosclerosis include focal calcific arteriosclerosis (*Mönckeberg's arteriosclerosis*) and *arteriolosclerosis.* The major arterial diseases other than arteriosclerosis include *congenital structural defects, inflammatory* or granulomatous diseases (e.g., syphilitic aortitis), and disorders affecting mainly the smaller vessels, such as *hypersensitivity* or autoimmune diseases.

THE NORMAL ARTERY

STRUCTURE The normal artery wall consists of three reasonably well-defined layers: the intima, the media, and the adventitia.

Intima A single continuous layer of *endothelial cells* lines the lumen of all arteries. The intima is delimited on its outer aspect by a perforated tube of elastic tissue, the *internal elastic lamina.* This tube of elastic tissue is particularly prominent in the large elastic arteries and the medium-caliber muscular arteries, and it disappears in capillaries. The endothelial cells are attached to one another by a series of junctional complexes and are also attached, apparently somewhat tenuously, to an underlying meshwork of loose connective tissue, the *basal lamina.* These lining endothelial cells normally form a barrier that controls the entry of substances from the blood into the artery wall. Such substances usually enter the cells by specific transport systems. Normally, no other cell type is present in the intima of most arteries.

Media The media consists of only one cell type, the *smooth-muscle cell,* arranged in either a single layer (as in small muscular arteries) or multiple lamellae (as in elastic arteries). These cells are surrounded by small amounts of collagen and elastic fibers, which they elaborate, and usually take the pattern of diagonal concentric spirals through the vessel wall. They are closely apposed to one another and may be attached by junctional complexes. The smooth-muscle cell appears to be the major connective tissue–forming cell of the artery wall, producing collagen, elastic fibers, and proteoglycans. In that sense it is analogous to the fibroblast in skin, the osteoblast in bone, and the chondroblast in cartilage. The media is bounded on the luminal side by the internal elastic lamina and on the abluminal side by a less continuous sheet of elastic tissue, the *external elastic lamina.* In *elastic arteries,* like the aorta and the major pulmonary arteries, elastic lamellae are prominent. Such arteries expand and increase their elastic tension with the pulse of systole. In diastole, the elastic fibers recoil, helping to propel the blood distally and progressively dampening the pulsatile character of flow toward more terminal vessels. In *muscular arteries,* in which smooth-muscle cells predominate, peripheral flow is regulated, particularly in arterioles, by contraction (vasoconstriction) and relaxation (vasodilatation). Located about midway through the media of most arteries is a "nutritional watershed." The outer portion is nourished from the small blood vessels (vasa vasorum) in the adventitia; the inner layers receive their nutrients from the lumen.

TABLE 266-1
Deaths, by cause, in the United States, 1978

	No. of deaths, thousands			
	Below age 65		*Age 65 and above*	
Causes of death	*Male*	*Female*	*Male*	*Female*
All causes	390	217	640	634
All cardiovascular diseases	142	60	363	401
Ischemic heart disease	107	34	250	251
Cerebrovascular disease	14	12	61	89
Hypertensive disease*	2	2	5	7
All infectious disease	5	5	5	5
All cancer	83	72	133	109
Accidents	62	20	13	11

* *A substantial proportion of deaths of hypertensive persons occurs with ischemic heart disease or cerebrovascular disease; such deaths are classified in those categories.*

SOURCE: *National Center for Health Statistics, Vital Statistics Report, Final Mortality Statistics, 1978.*

Adventitia The outermost layer of the artery is the adventitia, which is delimited on the luminal aspect by the external elastic lamina. This external coat consists of a loose interwoven admixture of collagen bundles, elastic fibers, smooth-muscle cells, and fibroblasts. This layer also contains the vasa vasorum and nerves.

METABOLISM AND FUNCTION The artery wall is a metabolically active organ that must meet a steady demand for energy to maintain smooth-muscle tension and endothelial cell function, and to repair and replenish tissue constituents. The mechanical forces on the arterial wall are complex, and considerable tensile stresses are imposed on it, mainly by hydraulic force. Shear or frictional stresses are especially prominent near the entrance regions of branches. The form and manner in which these forces are dissipated depend upon flow, the amount of elastic tension developed, and the tethering or external support provided by surrounding structures. Arteries are also permeable pipes, which constantly exchange fluid and solutes with the blood they carry.

Maintenance of the endothelial cell lining is critical. Endothelial cell turnover occurs at a slow rate but may be accelerated in focal areas by changing patterns of flow along the vessel wall. When intact, these cells selectively control the passage of circulating substances by active transport (endocytosis and exocytosis) through their cytoplasm and elaborate connecting tissue components to form their own substratum. In addition, intact endothelial cells function to prevent clotting partly by elaboration of a particular prostaglandin (prostacyclin or PGI_2) that inhibits platelet function, thereby enhancing unimpeded flow of blood. When the lining is damaged, platelets adhere to it, in part as the result of production of a different class of prostaglandins, the thromboxanes, and form a clot; endothelial cells function in the clotting process by elaboration of key substances, including factor VIII.

The metabolism of arteries reflects the biochemistry of smooth-muscle cells. Arterial smooth-muscle cells form abundant collagen, elastic fibers, soluble and insoluble elastin, and glucosaminoglycans (mainly dermatan sulfate). Multiple anabolic and catabolic pathways are present. These cells metabolize glucose by both anaerobic and aerobic glycolysis. A variety of catabolic enzymes are present including fibrinolysins, mixed-function oxidases, and lysosomal hydrolases. Because of the prominence of lipids in atherosclerotic lesions, much attention has been directed to lipid metabolism in arteries. Arterial wall cells can synthesize fatty acids, cholesterol, phospholipids, and triglycerides from endogenous substrates to satisfy their structural needs (membrane replenishment), but smooth-muscle cells appear preferentially to utilize lipids from plasma lipoproteins transported into the wall. Circulating lipoproteins traverse endothelial cells in pinocytotic vesicles. Smooth-muscle cells possess specific high-affinity surface receptors for certain apoproteins on the surface of lipid-rich lipoproteins, thus facilitating the entry of lipoproteins into the cell by adsorptive endocytosis. As has been shown for cultured skin fibroblasts, in arterial smooth-muscle cells these vesicles fuse with lysosomes, resulting in catabolism of lipoprotein components (Chap. 103). Free cholesterol entering the cell in this manner inhibits endogenous cholesterol synthesis, facilitates its own esterification, and partially limits further entry of cholesterol by regulating the number of lipoprotein receptors.

Thus, many complex and interrelated metabolic processes are present in arterial wall cells. Although some of these may play a role in the production of arteriosclerosis, no one biochemical reaction can be singled out as culpable. Physiological factors, such as transfer processes across the endothelial lining, the flux of oxygen and substrates from both the luminal and adventitial sides of the wall, and the reverse flow of catabolic products, need to be considered as well. The ability of the arterial wall to maintain the integrity of its endothelium, prevent platelet aggregation, and ensure the nutrition of its middle portion may be the critical determinants of the arteriosclerotic process.

CHANGES WITH AGING The major change that occurs with normal aging in the arterial wall in humans is a slow, apparently continuous, symmetrical increase in the thickness of the intima. This intimal thickening results from a gradual accumulation of smooth-muscle cells (presumably resulting from migration of these cells from the media and their subsequent proliferation), surrounded by additional connective tissue. In the nondiseased artery wall, lipid content, mainly cholesterol ester and phospholipid (particularly sphingomyelin), also progressively increases with age. Phospholipid synthesis rises with aging (perhaps in response to the need for more membrane formation for plasma membranes, vesicles, lysosomes, and other intracellular organelles) followed by a compensatory increase in activity of all phospholipases except sphingomyelinase. While most of the phospholipid in the normal artery wall appears to be derived from in situ synthesis, the cholesterol ester that accumulates with aging appears to be derived from plasma, since it contains principally linoleic acid, the major plasma cholesterol ester fatty acid. Furthermore, low-density lipoproteins (LDL) are immunologically detectable in the intima of normal arteries in direct relation to their concentration in plasma. It has been estimated that between the second and sixth decade, the normal intima accumulates approximately 10 mg cholesterol per gram of tissue. Thus, as the normal artery ages, smooth-muscle cells and connective tissue accumulate diffusely in the intima, leading to progressive thickening of this layer, coupled with progressive accumulation of sphingomyelin and cholesterol linoleate. This diffuse age-related intimal thickening is to be distinguished from focal discrete raised fibromuscular plaques, a characteristic feature of atherosclerosis.

Functionally, these changes with aging result in gradual increasing rigidity of vessels. The larger arteries may become dilated, elongated, and tortuous, and aneurysms may form in areas of an encroaching degenerating arteriosclerotic plaque. Such "wear-and-tear" changes are frequently proportional to the vessel diameter and correlated with branching, curvature, and anatomic points of attachment. The amount of external support also determines the ability of vessels, weakened by loss of elasticity, to withstand hydrostatic pressure. The unsupported cerebral arteries may be particularly vulnerable in this regard. Although senescence is accompanied by the intimal thickening that is a feature of localized atheromatosis, the changes of aging and arteriosclerosis appear to be separate and distinct processes.

NONATHEROMATOUS FORMS OF ARTERIOSCLEROSIS

Atherosclerosis involves primarily the intimal layer and occurs most commonly in the abdominal aorta and its large renal and lower extremity branches, the coronary arteries and the cerebral vasculature. It may accompany or accelerate the other major forms of arteriosclerosis, *focal calcification* and *arteriolosclerosis* (Table 266-2).

FOCAL CALCIFICATION Not to be confused with atherosclerosis is focal calcification of the media, particularly in the medium-sized muscular arteries. This type of arteriosclerosis is called *Mönckeberg's sclerosis* and is common in the lower extremities, upper extremities, and the arterial supply of the genital tract in both sexes. This disorder is rare in individuals below age 50 and affects both sexes indiscriminately. The process involves degeneration of smooth-muscle cells, followed by calcium deposition. The vessels become hard and tortuous, so that palpable vessels such as the radial artery can be felt as rigid tubes. Its characteristic radiological appearance consists of regular concentric calcifications, commonly seen in pelvic and femoral vessels. The medial changes alone do not narrow the lumen, have little effect on the circulation, and have relatively little clinical significance. However, in the lower extremities, medial sclerosis is often associated with atherosclerosis, leading to arterial occlusion. These changes are common in the elderly, and in patients on long-term corticosteroid therapy, but in individuals with diabetes mellitus, focal calcification may be accelerated and severe.

Focal calcification also can produce the arteriosclerotic aortic valve in the elderly. Progressive calcium deposition occurs on the aortic surface of normal trileaflet aortic valves with age, resulting in a spectrum of clinical findings ranging from an innocent systolic murmur to severe calcific aortic stenosis (Chap. 258).

ARTERIOLOSCLEROSIS This disorder involves hyaline and degenerative changes affecting both the intima and media of small arteries and arterioles, particularly in the spleen, pancreas, adrenal, and kidney. In the kidney, but not necessarily elsewhere, arteriolosclerosis is almost invariably associated with hypertension. Lesser degrees of sustained hypertension characteristically cause *hyalinization* of renal arterioles; more severe or malignant hypertension produces a typical *fibrous and elastic hyperplasia,* and even necrosis, of the media and intima.

ATHEROSCLEROSIS

LESIONS Morbid anatomy Atherosclerosis is a patchy nodular type of arteriosclerosis. The lesions are commonly classified as *fatty streaks, fibrous plaques,* and *complicated lesions.* Fatty streaks may be the earliest lesions of atherosclerosis but the evidence is very uncertain. They are characterized by an accumulation of lipid-filled smooth-muscle cells and macrophages (foam cells) and fibrous tissue in focal areas of the intima. They are stained distinctly by fat-soluble dyes, but may be visible without staining as yellowish or whitish patches on the intimal surface. The lipid is mainly cholesterol oleate, partly derived from synthesis in situ. The fatty streak is usually sessile and causes little obstruction and no symptoms. The lesion is universal, appearing in various segments of the arterial tree at different ages beginning in the aorta in infancy. In all children, regardless of race, sex, or environment, fatty streaks are present in the aorta by age 10 and increase to occupy as much as 30 to 50 percent of the aortic surface by age 25, but they do not appear to extend further with aging. Despite a presumed relation between fatty streaks and fibrous atherosclerotic plaques, aortic fatty streaks are not correlated with the location and extent of fibrous lesions. In the coronary arteries, the extent of fatty streaks may be a better indicator of the development of clinically significant raised lesions later in life. They are usually observed by age 15 and continue to involve more surface area with increasing age. Fatty streaks in the cerebral arteries are also present in all populations, develop during the third and fourth decade, and are more extensive in those populations having a higher incidence of cerebrovascular disease. It is generally believed that fatty streaks may be reversible, but the evidence is inconclusive.

Fibrous plaques, also called raised lesions or pearly plaques, are palpably elevated areas of intimal thickening and represent the most characteristic lesion of advancing atherosclerosis. They do not share with fatty streaks the ubiquitous distribution among populations. These plaques first appear in the abdominal aorta, coronary arteries, and carotid arteries in the third decade and increase progressively with age. They appear in men before women, in the aorta before the coronary arteries, and much later in the vertebral and intracranial cerebral arteries. Reasons for the difference in susceptibility of various segments of the arterial tree and the nonuniform distribution of lesions are not known. Typically, the fibrous plaque is firm, elevated, and dome-shaped, with an opaque glistening surface that bulges into the lumen. It consists of a central core of extracellular lipid and necrotic cell debris ("gruel") covered by a fibromuscular layer or cap containing large numbers of smooth-muscle cells, macrophages, and collagen. Thus the plaque is much thicker than normal intima. Although the lipid, like that of fatty streaks, is mainly cholesterol ester, linoleic rather than oleic is the principal esterified fatty acid. Thus plaque cholesterol ester composition differs from fatty streaks but resembles plasma lipoproteins.

The *complicated lesion* is a calcified fibrous plaque containing various degrees of necrosis, thrombosis, and ulceration. These are the lesions frequently associated with symptoms. With increasing necrosis and accumulation of gruel, the arterial wall progressively weakens, and rupture of the intima can occur, causing aneurysm and hemorrhage. Arterial emboli can form when fragments of plaque dislodge into the lumen. Stenosis and impaired organ function result from gradual occlusion as plaques thicken and thrombi form.

Localization Although the term *generalized atherosclerosis* is commonly used clinically, lesions are actually irregularly distributed; different vessels are involved at different ages and to varying degrees. The aorta, especially its abdominal portion, is involved earliest and most severely by atherosclerotic lesions, and it is the bellweather of lesions elsewhere. The *aorta* is usually most heavily involved in its abdominal portion, about the orifices of its branches, particularly at the level of the coronary and intercostal arteries, in the aortic arch, and frequently at its bifurcation into the iliac arteries. There is more atherosclerosis in the lower than in the upper limbs. In the legs, the incidence decreases peripherally, as the musculoelastic vessels give way to large muscular arteries and these become smaller vessels, such as the plantar or digital arteries. Plaques and thrombosis are particularly common in the *femoral* artery, in Hunter's canal, and in the *popliteal* artery just above the knee joint. The *anterior* and *posterior tibial* arteries are often occluded together, but in different sites—the posterior where it rounds the

TABLE 266-2
Disorders associated with early arteriosclerosis

ATHEROSCLEROSIS
Diabetes mellitus
Hypertension
Familial hypercholesterolemia
Familial combined hyperlipidemia
Familial dysbetalipoproteinemia
Hypothyroidism
Werner's syndrome
Cholesterol ester storage disease
Systemic lupus erythematosus

NONATHEROMATOUS ARTERIOSCLEROSIS
Diabetes mellitus
Chronic renal insufficiency
Chronic vitamin D intoxication
Pseudoxanthoma elasticum
Idiopathic arterial calcification in infancy
Aortic valvular calcification in the elderly
Werner's syndrome
Homocystinuria

internal malleolus and the anterior where it is superficial and becomes the dorsalis pedis artery. The peroneal artery, which is well embedded in muscle, often escapes when other major vessels are occluded, and it may be the main blood supply to the extremity (*peroneal leg*). Atherosclerosis in abdominal branches, except for the renal and mesenteric arteries, causes less difficulty than in coronary and cerebral vessels.

In the *coronary arteries,* raised lesions are most prominent in the main stems, the highest incidence being a short distance beyond the ostia. Atherosclerosis is nearly always found in the epicardial (extramural) portions of the vessels, while the intramural coronary arteries are spared. Coronary atherosclerosis is often diffuse. The degree to which the lumen is narrowed varies, but once the process is present, all the intima of the extramural portions of the vessel is usually involved. A single tiny plaque occluding an otherwise normal coronary artery is rare. Selective involvement of the coronary arteries may relate to the unique hemodynamic forces unlike those of other major arteries, resulting from greater flow in diastole than systole. The implications of these flow patterns for atherogenesis are as yet unknown. Typical atheromatous fibrous plaques also develop in saphenous vein aortocoronary bypass grafts.

In the cervical and cerebral arteries the distribution of atherosclerosis is patchy, as it may be in other arteries. It first appears in the base of the brain in the carotid, basilar, and vertebral arteries. The proximal portion of the internal carotids in the neck is a site of special predilection. There is a concentration of lesions near bifurcations. Atherosclerosis in the *pulmonary artery* bears no relation to the severity of the disease in the aorta or other systemic arteries. There is some involvement in about half of adults over 50 years of age who have no reason to have pulmonary hypertension. Pulmonary hypertension per se, however, is associated with medial hypertrophy, intimal thickening, and great acceleration of atheroma formation.

THEORIES OF ATHEROGENESIS One generally accepted theory for the pathogenesis of atherosclerosis consistent with a variety of experimental evidence is the *reaction to injury* hypothesis. According to this idea the endothelial cells lining the intima are exposed to repeated or continuing insults to their integrity. The injury to the endothelium may be subtle or gross, resulting in a loss of the ability of the cells to attach to one another and to the underlying connective tissue. The cells then become susceptible to the shearing stress of the blood flow and they may desquamate. Examples of types of "injury" to the endothelium include chemical injury, as in chronic hypercholesterolemia or homocystinemia, mechanical stress associated with hypertension, and immunologic injury, as may be seen after cardiac or renal transplantation. Loss of endothelial cells at susceptible sites in the arterial tree would lead to exposure of the subendothelial tissue to increased concentrations of plasma constituents, and a sequence of events including platelet adherence, platelet aggregation and formation of microthrombi, and release of platelet granular components, including a potent mitogenic factor. This platelet factor, in conjunction with other plasma constituents, including lipoproteins and hormones such as insulin, could stimulate both the migration of medial smooth-muscle cells into the intima and their proliferation at these sites of injury. These proliferating smooth-muscle cells would deposit a connective tissue matrix and accumulate lipid, a process that would be particularly enhanced with hyperlipidemia. Macrophages derived from circulating blood monocytes might enter the arterial wall and also accumulate lipid. Thus repeated or chronic injury could lead to a slowly progressing lesion involving a gradual increase in smooth-muscle cells, macrophages, connective tissue, and lipid. Areas where the shearing stress on endothelial cells is increased, such as branch points or bifurcation of vessels, would be at greater risk. As the lesions progress and the intima becomes thicker, blood flow over the sites will be altered and potentially place the lining endothelial cells at even greater risk for further injury, leading to an inexorable cycle of events culminating in the complicated lesion. However, a single or a few injurious episodes may lead to a proliferative response that could regress, in contrast to continued or chronic injury. This reaction to injury hypothesis thus is consistent with the known intimal thickening observed during normal aging, would explain how many of the etiologic factors implicated in atherogenesis might enhance lesion formation, might explain how inhibitors of platelet aggregation could interfere with lesion formation, and fosters some optimism regarding the possibility of interrupting progression, or even producing regression of these lesions.

Other theories of atherogenesis are not mutually exclusive. The *monoclonal hypothesis* suggests, on the basis of single isoenzyme types found in lesions, that the intimal proliferative lesions result from the multiplication of single individual smooth-muscle cells, as do benign tumors. In this manner, mitogenic, and possibly mutagenic, factors that might stimulate smooth-muscle cell proliferation would act on single cells. Focal *clonal senescence* may explain how intrinsic aging processes contribute to atherosclerosis. According to this theory, the intimal smooth-muscle cells that proliferate to form an atheroma are normally under feedback control by diffusible agents (mitosis inhibitors) formed by the smooth-muscle cells in the contiguous media, and this feedback control system tends to fail with age as these controlling cells die and are not adequately replaced. This is consistent with the recent observation that cultured human arterial smooth-muscle cells, like fibroblasts, show a decline in their ability to replicate as a function of donor age. If this loss of replicative potential applies to a controlling population of smooth-muscle cells, then cells that are usually suppressed would be able to proliferate.

The *lysosomal theory* suggests that altered lysosomal function might contribute to atherogenesis. Since lysosomal enzymes can accomplish the generalized degradation of cellular components required for continuing renewal, this system has been implicated in cellular aging and the accumulation of lipofuscin or "age pigment." It has been suggested that increased deposition of lipids in arterial smooth-muscle cells may be related in part to a relative deficiency in the activity of lysosomal cholesterol ester hydrolase. This would result in increased accumulation of cholesterol esters within the cells, perhaps accentuated by lipid overloading of lysosomes, eventually leading to cell death and extracellular lipid deposition. Consonant with this idea, patients with the rare cholesterol ester storage disease, caused by a defect in lysosomal cholesterol ester hydrolase, may have accelerated atherosclerosis. However, lipid droplets in foam cells are often cytoplasmic rather than lysosomal.

RECOGNITION OF ATHEROSCLEROSIS Angiographic visualization of deformity in the lumen of a vessel remains the best presumptive test of silent atherosclerosis. Coronary angiography now permits visualization and assessment of arteries as small as 0.5 mm in diameter. Several sophisticated noninvasive techniques have been developed for demonstrating its presence. Doppler probes for measuring velocity and amount of blood flow have been used noninvasively and adapted to determine vessel outlines. Ultrasonic techniques are not yet clinically useful for detection of plaques in the coronary arteries.

Functional tests based on pathophysiological or metabolic effects of a narrowed arterial lumen often give indirect clues. Assessment of electrocardiographic changes induced after standardized exercise is a relatively simple noninvasive aid to the diagnosis of coronary atherosclerosis with significant narrowing. Similarly, myocardial perfusion defects demonstrable with imaging techniques using radionuclides are usually attributable to atherosclerosis (Chap. 250). Digit plethysmography with exercise often unmasks significant atherosclerotic involvement of lower extremity arteries.

Radiographic demonstration of calcification in the location of arteries does not always indicate the presence of atherosclerosis. Although calcified coronary vessels usually indicate atherosclerosis, complete luminal obstruction may occur in the absence of any calcification. Calcification or beading of peripheral arteries is not correlated directly with atherosclerosis. Abnormalities in retinal arterioles evident upon funduscopic examination are not well correlated with atherosclerosis in arteries. Thus despite the availability of a variety of tests, detection of atherosclerosis usually awaits one of the clinical complications attending a critical decrease of blood flow in an involved vessel. As yet there is no blood test for atherosclerosis. Knowledge of the prevalence and incidence of arteriosclerosis and most of the inferences concerning its causes are derived from tabulations of the appearance of its complications.

Ischemic heart disease (IHD), synonymous with *coronary heart disease* or *arteriosclerotic heart disease* (Chap. 260), is the most useful indicator of atherosclerosis available today. Practically all patients with myocardial infarction, as defined by electrocardiographic and enzyme changes, have coronary atherosclerosis. Rare exceptions are due to congenital anomalies of the coronary vessels, emboli, or ostial occlusion due to other types of cardiac or vascular disease. Nontraumatic *sudden death* (Chap. 30) makes up a sizable portion of all deaths eventually certified as due to IHD. At autopsy, evidence of fresh myocardial infarction or of *coronary thrombosis* is usually absent. While ventricular fibrillation may have been due to sudden closure of a partially compromised vessel by a small thrombus or embolus, or to *spasm*, none of these need have preceded a fatal arrhythmia. The majority of victims of sudden death have had a previous diagnosis of IHD; the number who had diabetes or hypertension is also significant. In epidemiologic studies of IHD, *angina pectoris* and electrocardiographic changes attributable to ischemia without infarction are considered "softer end points" and treated separately.

Cerebrovascular disease (stroke) is a less reliable criterion for the presence of atherosclerosis. It includes *cerebral hemorrhage* and *cerebral thrombosis* (Chap. 356). Cerebral thrombosis, including infarction or softening without evidence of embolus, is usually due to atherosclerosis. On the other hand, cerebral hemorrhage is most often the result of congenital aneurysms or of vascular defects peculiar to hypertension and diabetes. Dissections of the aorta (Chap. 268), *peripheral vascular disease* (Chap. 269), thrombosis of other major vessels, and ischemic renal disease (Chap. 298) likewise are not used to determine the prevalence of atherosclerosis in a population or as an index of atherosclerosis elsewhere. Therefore, from an epidemiologic standpoint, consideration of atherosclerosis focuses on IHD.

INCIDENCE AND PREVALENCE According to the National Health Examination Survey, about 5 million Americans have IHD. It is the leading cause of death in males after age 35 and in all persons after age 45. Premature deaths from IHD, arbitrarily defined as appearing before age 65, occur preponderantly in men, and a third of all deaths from IHD in males occur before age 65. In fact nearly all the excess premature mortality in American males is due to IHD. Between the ages of 35 and 55 the death rate is five times higher in white men than in white women in the United States. The exceptions are women with hypertension, diabetes, hyperlipidemia, or premature (usually iatrogenic) menopause, who are at increased risk and often share the risk of the male. For both sexes, there is more than a fivefold increase in the average annual incidence of myocardial infarction between ages 40 and 60. A distressing higher mortality rate in younger nonwhite women is probably due mainly to a greater incidence of hypertension in blacks. There is less difference between men and women in the prevalence of angina pectoris than in that of myocardial infarction; after age 65 more women than men have angina without a history of infarction.

Changing death rates Death rates in the United States from IHD rose appreciably between 1940 and 1960. Mortality peaked in 1963 and started to decline with the rate of decline accelerating in recent years for all ages, for both sexes, and for whites and nonwhites. This recent decline in mortality from coronary atherosclerosis (Table 266-3) is the first recorded in American history and is almost unique among industrialized countries. In other parts of the world, including the Soviet Union, Japan, and many countries in Europe, IHD death rates are still climbing. In 1976 the reduction in IHD death rate averaged more than 20 percent for persons age 35 to 74. The trend remains unexplained, but there has been a concurrent change in living habits including reduced smoking among middle-aged males, decreased consumption of animal fats and cholesterol, better control of hypertension, and improved treatment of IHD.

International comparisons In most industrialized countries, IHD is the major single cause of premature cardiovascular deaths. There are, however, marked differences in premature death rates among them. The seven having the highest rates in males between 45 and 54 years of age are Finland, the United States, Scotland, Northern Ireland, Australia, New Zealand, and Canada. Much lower age-adjusted death rates from IHD are found in Latin America and Japan. The rates in Japan are about one-fifth of those in the United States. Subsamples obtained in many countries convey the strong impression that upper socioeconomic classes that have adopted the culture of western industrialized countries have far more IHD than lower socioeconomic classes. Among the most obvious cultural differences between these groups are total calories, fat content of the diet, and amount of physical work. Extensive epidemiologic studies have not revealed the reasons for differences between cultures that are superficially similar. Migrants to the United States tend to have a higher risk of death from premature IHD than age-matched relatives who remain at home. Although there are many instances in which different ethnic groups in the same locality have widely differing prevalences of IHD, the available data suggest that cultural factors are more important than genetic determination of IHD. Nevertheless,

TABLE 266-3
Age-adjusted death rates by cause in the United States, 1968 and 1978

	Rate per 100,000 population		
Cause of death	*1968*	*1978*	*Percent change*
All deaths	743.8	606.1	−18.5
All cardiovascular diseases	361.8	267.9	−26.0
Ischemic heart disease	241.6	180.9	−25.1
Cerebrovascular disease	71.3	45.3	−36.5
Rheumatic heart disease	7.2	4.5	−37.5
Cancer	129.2	133.8	+3.6
Accidents and violence	76.5	67.8	−9.4

SOURCE: *The National Center for Health Statistics, Vital Statistics Report, Final Mortality Statistics, 1978.*

genetic heterogeneity undoubtedly underlies many of the striking differences in susceptibility seen among individuals sharing the same ethnic and cultural setting.

ETIOLOGIC FACTORS A number of conditions and habits present more frequently in individuals who develop atherosclerosis than in the general population; these factors have been termed *risk factors.* The majority of people below age 65 afflicted with atherosclerosis have one or more identifiable risk factors other than aging per se (Table 266-4). The risk factor concept implies that a person with at least one risk factor is more likely to develop a clinical atherosclerotic event and to do so earlier than a person with no risk factors. The presence of multiple risk factors further accelerates atherosclerosis. They vary in terms of importance in the population of the United States. There is general agreement from an epidemiologic perspective that hypercholesterolemia, hypertension, and cigarette smoking may be the most potent factors involved in causation of atherosclerosis. Risk factors also vary in terms of their potential reversibility with current techniques of preventive management.

Thus age, sex, and genetic factors are currently considered to be irreversible risk factors, whereas continually emerging evidence suggests that elimination of cigarette smoking and treatment of hypertension reverses the high risk for atherosclerosis attributable to those factors. Life insurance policyholder data suggest that reduction of marked obesity reduces total mortality, presumably by diminishing the sequelae of atherosclerosis. Potentially reversible factors currently under study include hyperglycemia and the various forms of hyperlipidemia.

These factors are not mutually exclusive since they clearly interact. For example, obesity appears to be causally associated with hypertension, hyperglycemia, hypercholesterolemia, and hypertriglyceridemia. Genetic factors may play a role by exerting direct effects on arterial wall cell structure and metabolism, or they may act indirectly via such factors as hypertension, hyperlipidemia, diabetes, and obesity. Aging appears to be one of the more complex factors associated with the development of atherosclerosis, since many of the risk factors in themselves are related to aging, e.g., elevated blood pressure, hyperglycemia, and hyperlipidemia. Thus in addition to the possible involvement of intrinsic aging in atherogenesis (perhaps through effects on arterial wall metabolism), a variety of associated metabolic factors are also age-dependent.

Hyperlipidemia Both *hypercholesterolemia* and *hypertriglyceridemia* appear to be important risk factors for atherosclerosis. While there is no absolute quantitative definition of hyperlipidemia, statistical definitions, based on the upper 5 or 10 percent of the distribution of plasma lipid levels within a population, are often used. Such definitions are likely to detect affected individuals from families with one of the familial hyperlipidemias or hyperlipidemia associated with other diseases or drugs, and also are useful for prediction of emergence of premature atherosclerosis and institution of preventive measures. However, these upper limits of "normality" are too high for defining those cholesterol and triglyceride levels that are correlated with increasing risk of IHD in whole populations. Thus, correlations between the cholesterol concentrations in young men in North America and the incidence of premature IHD indicate that an increasing risk can be detected when the cholesterol level is higher than 220 mg/dl, a value close to the mean for men from 40 to 49 years of age in this population. Extrapolation of similar data from other populations suggests that a cholesterol level at birth averages 60 mg/dl. Within a month the average has risen to about 120 and by the first year to 175. A second rise begins in the third decade and continues to about age 50 in men and somewhat later in women.

A similar age-related increase in plasma triglyceride levels is also observed. The increases in cholesterol are associated mainly with a rise in *low-density lipoprotein* (LDL) concentrations, the increases in triglyceride with a rise in *very low density lipoproteins* (VLDL). Adiposity may play a key role in this age-associated rise in triglyceride and cholesterol levels since the increases in triglyceride, cholesterol, and body weight with age in whole populations occur concurrently. In primitive people who remain thin throughout adulthood, plasma lipids do not increase with age. Metabolic mechanisms have been postulated whereby obesity, which is associated with insulin resistance of peripheral tissues and compensatory hyperinsulinemia, promotes enhanced production of triglyceride- and cholesterol-rich lipoproteins by the liver. Current concepts of plasma lipoprotein transport suggest that accumulation of cholesterol in the circulation may in part be secondary to excessive production of triglyceride-rich lipoproteins.

Hypercholesterolemia is associated unequivocally with increased incidence of premature IHD; however, its importance varies in relation to age. In the Framingham study, cholesterol levels in males below age 40 were closely related to the future development of IHD; this relation was much less pronounced in older individuals. For both sexes combined, the relative incidence of myocardial infarction in individuals between the ages of 30 and 49 with cholesterol levels greater than 260 mg/dl was three to five times that for individuals with cholesterol levels less than 220. There appears to be a continuous gradient of risk as the cholesterol level ascends. These data are supported by comparisons of the prevalence of IHD and cholesterol (or LDL) in many other populations. The relationship of triglycerides and VLDL to IHD is confounded by a rise in cholesterol as VLDL increases. Nevertheless, in several, but not all, population studies, increased triglycerides (or VLDL) are independently correlated with premature IHD.

Hypertriglyceridemia may be associated with premature atherosclerosis in some specific disorders; this association may not be apparent in studies of whole populations. Patients with high VLDL who come from families with familial combined hyperlipidemia appear to be at the same increased risk as those affected members of these families with elevated LDL levels. In contrast, patients with comparably elevated VLDL levels who come from families with pure monogenic familial hypertriglyceridemia do not appear to have an increased risk. In addition, high VLDL may increase the risk for premature atherosclerosis when associated with other risk factors for coronary artery disease such as in diabetes, and in patients on chronic hemodialysis who smoke and are hypertensive. Individuals in whom remnant lipoproteins accumulate, with resulting elevations in both cholesterol and triglycerides (Chap. 103), also seem to be at risk for early development of atherosclerosis.

TABLE 266-4
Risk factors for atherosclerosis

1 Not reversible
- *a* Aging
- *b* Male sex
- *c* Genetic traits—positive family history of premature atherosclerosis

2 Reversible
- *a* Cigarette smoking
- *b* Hypertension
- *c* Obesity

3 Potentially or partially reversible
- *a* Hyperlipidemia—hypercholesterolemia and/or hypertriglyceridemia
- *b* Hyperglycemia and diabetes mellitus
- *c* Low levels of high-density lipoproteins (HDL)

4 Other possible factors
- *a* Physical inactivity
- *b* Emotional stress and/or personality type

Some of these relationships were clarified in a comprehensive study in Seattle of the role of the genetics of hyperlipidemia in clinical atherosclerosis in which 500 consecutive survivors of myocardial infarction were tested. Hyperlipidemia was present in about one-third of the group. Approximately one-half of the males and two-thirds of the females below age 50 had either hypertriglyceridemia, hypercholesterolemia, or both. On the other hand, in individuals over age 70 the prevalence of atherosclerotic coronary disease was very high, yet virtually no males (and only about one-fourth of the females) had hyperlipidemia. Thus, in both sexes there appeared to be a progressive decline with age in the association of hyperlipidemia with myocardial infarction. More than half of the hyperlipidemic atherosclerotic survivors appeared to have simple monogenic familial disorders inherited as an autosomal dominant trait (*familial combined hyperlipidemia, familial hypertriglyceridemia,* and *familial hypercholesterolemia,* in descending order of frequency, Table 266-5). These simply inherited hyperlipidemias (particularly hypercholesterolemia) were more frequent in myocardial infarction survivors below age 60 than in those who were older. In contrast, nonmonogenic forms of hyperlipidemia occurred with equal frequency above and below age 60. Thus it appears that genes associated with the simply inherited hyperlipidemias accelerate changes seen with age, leading to atherosclerosis at an earlier age than usual. All studies indicate that hyperlipidemia is a more meaningful risk factor below age 50 and that it operates independently of, and in addition to, hypertension, diabetes, obesity, and other factors. For men and women over age 65, there is no evidence of a correlation between hyperlipidemia and atherosclerosis or its complications.

When the screening of individuals for hyperlipidemia occurs after a myocardial infarction, it is several decades too late. Screening at birth or in childhood for genetic hyperlipidemia is not practical or useful except in the instance of familial hypercholesterolemia, which may affect about 1 in 1000 children. This is detectable by LDL elevations in cord blood when one already knows that a parent is affected. Other genetic or nongenetic primary hyperlipidemia is often not apparent until the third decade. *Today, good health maintenance practice includes a test for detection of hyperlipidemia in all persons between 20 and 30 years of age. It is especially important in all young persons who have a family history of premature IHD.*

Hyperlipidemia is best detected by measurement of the concentration of cholesterol and triglycerides in serum or plasma in a sample obtained after an overnight fast. The measurements should be made by a reliable laboratory that follows a program of standardization. Routine use of lipoprotein electrophoresis provides little additional information, is nonspecific, and is not recommended for screening or for management. In adults less than 55 years of age, a cholesterol concentration (C) greater than 250 mg/dl or a triglyceride concentration (TG) greater than 200 mg/dl clearly indicates hyperlipidemia sufficient to require some attention by the physician to the items listed in Table 266-6. If hyperlipidemia is absent, the tests need not be repeated for several years in an adult who maintains body weight and does not otherwise change in health or life-style. Vigor in pursuing the "causative factors" in Table 266-6 should increase in proportion to the degree of hyperlipidemia. If causes of *secondary hyperlipidemia* or offending drugs are absent, attention to the origin of *primary hyperlipidemia* turns mainly to diet and genetic causes. Severe hyperlipidemia (C $>$ 350 mg/dl or TG $>$ 400 mg/dl) usually reflects a genetic disorder; when xanthomas are present, it practically always does. Diagnosis always includes examination of first-degree relatives and proceeds according to information contained in Chap. 103.

Direct proof is still lacking that reduction of hyperlipidemia results in a decrease in progression of atherosclerosis in humans. It has been demonstrated directly in other primates, however, and several controlled trials of different diets which have been accompanied by fall in mean cholesterol levels in small test populations have shown a favorable effect on incidence of the overall complications of IHD. In a recent trial, the drug clofibrate given to a normal population reduced the incidence of nonfatal myocardial infarctions associated with a reduction of cholesterol levels; however, total mortality was not lowered. The weight of evidence strongly favors conservative measures to control hyperlipidemia in patients through middle age.

The first step in treatment of primary hyperlipidemia is attention to diet. All patients with mild to moderate hyperlipidemia should first be brought to normal weight if they exceed it, and then be maintained on a diet emphasizing decreases in intake of saturated fat and cholesterol. If hypertriglyceridemia is present, alcohol intake should be limited or eliminated. A single dietary approach to all forms of hyperlipidemia, including reduced intake of calories, cholesterol, and saturated fat, is appropriate for most patients. The degree of dietary restriction would be proportional to the degree and nature of the hyperlipidemia. The maximum effect of such a regimen will be observed within 2 months after body weight has stabilized. If at that time C is greater than 300 mg/dl, a 2-month trial of a bile acid binding resin (cholestyramine or colestipol) should be considered. If TG remains greater than 300 mg/dl, clofibrate may be tried. These two drugs may be used simultaneously if both C and TG are high; their use remains empirical. In patients with familial hypercholesterolemia (Chap. 103) com-

TABLE 266-5
Frequency of hyperlipidemia in survivors of myocardial infarction

	% of total myocardial infarction survivors		
Disorder	*Under age 60*	*Over age 60*	*Ratio*
1 Monogenic hyperlipidemias	20.6	7.5	—
a Familial hypercholesterolemia	4.1	0.7	6:1
b Familial hypertriglyceridemia	5.2	2.7	2:1
c Familial combined hyperlipidemia	11.3	4.1	3:1
2 Polygenic hypercholesterolemia	5.5	5.5	1:1
3 Sporadic hypertriglyceridemia	5.8	6.9	1:1

SOURCE: *Goldstein et al.*

TABLE 266-6
Factors to consider in patients with hyperlipidemia

1 Disorders to which hyperlipidemia is secondary
- *a* Uncontrolled diabetes mellitus (insulin deficiency)
- *b* Hypothyroidism
- *c* Uremia
- *d* Nephrotic syndrome (hypoproteinemia)
- *e* Obstructive liver disease
- *f* Dysproteinemia (multiple myeloma, lupus erythematosus)

2 Drugs producing or aggravating hyperlipidemia
- *a* Oral contraceptives
- *b* Estrogens
- *c* Glucocorticoids
- *d* Antihypertensives

3 Dietary factors
- *a* Caloric intake (recent weight gain)
- *b* Content of saturated fats and cholesterol
- *c* Alcohol intake

4 Genetic disorders (primary hyperlipidemias)
- *a* Family history of hyperlipidemia or xanthomas
- *b* History of pancreatitis or recurrent abdominal pain

bined therapy with a resin and nicotinic acid has achieved dramatic normalization of LDL cholesterol levels. Continued therapy with any hypolipidemic drug is dependent upon the demonstration that, when added to diet at stable weight, it is associated with at least a 15 percent further decrease in hyperlipidemia. However, further studies are needed to define the long-term efficiency of hypolipidemic agents in the prevention of atherosclerosis and its sequelae. The long-term effects of these drugs used before puberty are unknown, and their use during pregnancy is not advocated.

High-density lipoproteins (HDL) HDL, a complex family of particles that carry about 20 percent of the total plasma cholesterol, is inversely associated with the development of premature atherosclerosis, and therefore can be considered an "antirisk factor." HDL levels can be assessed simply by measurement of cholesterol in the supernatant fluid after the other lipoproteins in plasma have been precipitated. Thus individuals whose HDL cholesterol is elevated may be less likely to develop IHD; conversely low HDL cholesterol is associated with increased risk of IHD. In the Framingham study, low HDL cholesterol was a more potent lipid risk factor than was high cholesterol or LDL. At least five diverse population studies have confirmed a close correlation between IHD and low HDL, independent of other factors.

Consistent with differences in risk between the sexes, HDL cholesterol averages about 25 percent higher in women than in men. Estrogens tend to raise and androgens tend to lower HDL levels. In women, low HDL, particularly when associated with diabetes and obesity, markedly raises the risk of IHD. Octogenarians tend to have high HDL which may be partly familial. Of interest for preventive measures, cigarette smoking decreases and regular strenuous exercise increases HDL cholesterol. Regular exercise increases HDL even in individuals after myocardial infarction. A small daily intake of alcohol has been associated with both reduced risk of IHD and high HDL levels. Mechanisms for these effects remain unknown.

HDL cholesterol measurements are usually not very helpful since the analytical error in most laboratories exceeds the differences in HDL levels associated with risk. HDL measurements are most helpful in individuals, especially women, with only a mild increase in plasma cholesterol and normal triglyceride levels to determine whether the increase is in HDL rather than in LDL. Because of the close inverse relationship between plasma triglycerides (or VLDL) and HDL, HDL in hypertriglyceridemic persons, with or without hypercholesterolemia, will be predictably low and gives little additional useful information.

Hypertension (see Chap. 267) High blood pressure is an important risk factor for atherosclerosis, mainly IHD and cerebrovascular disease. The risk increases progressively with increasing blood pressure; in the Framingham Study, IHD incidence in middle-aged men with blood pressures exceeding 160/95 was more than five times that in normotensive men (blood pressure 140/90 or less). Hypertensive men and women are both affected, with the diastolic pressure perhaps being more important. In industrialized populations, blood pressure appears to increase inexorably with age; however, the nature of this age relation varies among populations, since there are remote primitive populations that age without any changes in blood pressure levels. The age-associated blood pressure increase might be related to physical activity or dietary factors, particularly sodium and total caloric content. In contrast to the other age-related risk factors, hypertension appears to increase atherosclerosis throughout the age span. Thus, after the age of about 50, hypertension may be more potent than hypercholesterolemia as a risk factor.

Conversely, the risk for atherosclerosis appears diminished by therapeutic reduction of blood pressure. Recent intervention studies have shown convincingly that reduction of diastolic levels greater than 105 mmHg significantly reduces the incidence of strokes, IHD, and congestive heart failure in men. Even when patients with diastolic elevations between 90 and 105 mmHg are similarly maintained on adequate treatment, the incidence of some of these complications may be reduced. Special urgency for relief of hypertension obtains when hyperlipidemia or other risk factors are present.

Cigarette smoking Not only is cigarette smoking one of the more potent risk factors for atherosclerosis, it is also one of the factors that when reduced or eliminated clearly decreases the risk of developing atherosclerosis. Ample statistical evidence supports a mean increase of about 70 percent in the death rate, and a three- to fivefold increase in risk of IHD, in men who smoke one pack of cigarettes per day compared with nonsmokers. In general, the increase in death rate is proportional to the amount smoked and decreases with age. Excess morbidity from myocardial infarction is also present in women smokers, but the relationship is somewhat less firm than in men. However, there is an impressive accentuation of IHD mortality in women over age 35 taking oral contraceptives who in addition smoke cigarettes. In some atherosclerosis-prone populations, such as patients maintained on long-term hemodialysis, cigarette smoking interacts with other risk factors, resulting in a marked enhancement of atherosclerosis mortality. Such interaction is also likely for diabetic and hypertensive populations.

The association of smoking and increased IHD remains unexplained. Pipe and cigar smokers have a lesser increase in risk of IHD, presumably because less smoke is inhaled. Smokers dying of causes other than IHD have been found at autopsy to have more coronary atherosclerosis than nonsmokers. The major influence of smoking is upon the incidence of sudden death, however. Those who stop smoking show a prompt decline in risk and may reach the risk level of nonsmokers as early as after 1 year of abstention.

Hyperglycemia and diabetes mellitus (see Chap. 114) Studies in a variety of populations have shown an association of hyperglycemia with clinically evident atherosclerotic disease suggesting a role of hyperglycemia in atherogenesis. In known diabetics, both insulin-dependent and non-insulin-dependent types, there is at least a twofold increase in incidence of myocardial infarction compared with nondiabetics. This risk is markedly increased in younger diabetics, and diabetic women are even more prone to IHD than are diabetic men. There is an increased tendency toward cerebral thrombosis and infarction but not toward cerebral hemorrhage in diabetes. Gangrene of the lower extremities has been variously estimated to be from 8 to 150 times as frequent in diabetics as in nondiabetics. Diabetes is associated with an increase in atherosclerosis observed at autopsy in a variety of populations worldwide, whether the prevalence of atherosclerosis in a particular population is high or low. The approximately twofold increase in the frequency of hypertension among diabetics, particularly adult females, may accentuate the risk. This relationship is presumably associated with obesity.

The risk for atherosclerotic disease, however, does not appear to be grossly related to the degree of hyperglycemia among diabetics. Results in the University Group Diabetes Program Study have suggested that reduction of blood glucose by insulin does not appear to influence mortality from established atherosclerosis during a 5-year period. Thus, hyperglycemia and atherosclerosis are associated, since there is an increased prevalence of large vessel disease in known diabetics and, conversely, an increased prevalence of hyperglycemia in association with atherosclerotic disease. These associations remain unexplained and reversibility undocumented. Clinical and experimental studies also support a role for high circulating insulin levels in IHD. The capillary microangiopathy, pathognomonic of diabetes and causing important dysfunction of the kidneys and retina, has unknown clinical significance in relation to atherosclerotic disease in larger arteries.

Obesity In general, morbidity and mortality from IHD are higher in direct relation to the degree of overweight beyond about 30 percent. Furthermore, from data obtained in the Framingham study, it appears that obesity may accelerate atherosclerosis since its effect is more apparent before age 50. Nevertheless, some of the major epidemiologic studies of coronary heart disease have not demonstrated an independent relationship between this condition and anything less than very severe obesity. However, obesity is a disorder closely associated with four other potent risk factors, i.e., hypertriglyceridemia, hypercholesterolemia, hyperglycemia, and hypertension. The relationship between obesity and atherosclerosis is thus multifaceted; and since in practice obesity does not occur "independently," it is of considerable importance as a risk factor.

Physical inactivity Study of the relationship of the prevalence of IHD to daily (occupational) physical activity is made difficult because so many variables are involved. Among prospective studies the Framingham data do indicate that the less sedentary an individual is, the less susceptible that individual is to sudden death. Physical work may be the major determinant of greatly differing incidences of IHD in Southern black and white males and in populations that move from rural areas to urbanized environments. How physical activity may operate to decrease death from IHD, or possibly atherogenesis, is not known. Beyond ameliorating hyperlipidemia by increasing caloric expenditure, no mechanism has been demonstrated. The meaning of the physical activity–induced increase in HDL, the antirisk factor for IHD, remains mysterious. Physical training has been shown to improve exercise performance in patients with IHD and angina pectoris. Regular physical activity is supported as a desirable element in a program of preventive health maintenance.

Stress and personality There is a valid clinical impression that psychic or emotional stress and anxiety are associated with precipitation of overt IHD and sudden death. Debate continues as to whether there may be distinct personality types prone to and relatively immune from premature IHD (the so-called personality types A and B), and whether the presumably more deleterious type is amenable to correction beyond elimination of cigarette smoking, adverse dietary patterns, and avoidance of stressful life situations. Many social and demographic analyses have so far failed to reach any agreement about the etiologic relationships of occupation and similar situational factors and the incidence of IHD.

Genetic factors Premature atherosclerosis often appears to be familial. In many instances this can be attributed to the inheritance of risk factors such as hypertension, diabetes mellitus, and hyperlipidemia. Occasionally, families with excessive premature vascular disease can be found in which none of the known risk factors appears to be operating. Genetic determinants of protective factors, such as HDL, need to be understood; undoubtedly other important determinants remain to be discovered. Nevertheless, family history is one of the more important factors to be weighed in assessment of risk in helping the physician to avoid missing treatable risk factors, and in institution of appropriate preventive measures.

ROLE OF DIET IN RISK FOR ATHEROSCLEROSIS The relationship of diet to IHD remains an area of intense interest and persistent controversy. In epidemiologic studies, no population habitually subsisting on a diet low in saturated fat and cholesterol has an appreciable amount of IHD. These populations also tend to have lower plasma lipid concentrations. There is a general upward shift of average cholesterol and triglyceride levels in highly developed countries, which is an effect of change in total culture and life-style as well as in diet. Dietary changes in migrant populations who move from more primitive to more industrialized societies commonly include increased intake of total calories, animal fats, cholesterol, and salt, leading to a diet-accentuated emergence of risk factors such as obesity, hyperlipidemia, and hypertension. There is no question that the plasma cholesterol (and LDL) level is sensitive to the amount of saturated fat and cholesterol in the diet. The "average" adult in the United States eats about 140 g fat per day and about 500 mg cholesterol. The mixture of fats ingested usually contains about three times as much saturated fatty acids (mainly palmitic and stearic) as polyunsaturated fatty acids (mainly linoleic and linolenic). If a healthy young adult switches from this diet to one containing the same amount of total fat in which the ratio of polyunsaturates to saturates is closer to unity and the cholesterol content is less than 300 mg per day, the cholesterol concentration will usually drop by 10 to 15 percent within 2 weeks, and remain depressed on continuation of the diet.

The average cholesterol level in most populations is most closely related to the amount of animal fats (meat, eggs, and milk products, major sources of long-chain saturated fatty acids and cholesterol) in the diet. Increased animal fat consumption also tends to be correlated with a greater proportion of dietary fats being saturated and with lesser intake of complex carbohydrates and vegetable fibers; these are dietary changes that may lead to a rise in plasma cholesterol levels. The average triglyceride level is more sensitive to total caloric balance and to alcohol intake. It is important to note that physical activity, emotional stress, smoking, and intake of coffee or tea have only weak or indirect influences on total cholesterol and triglyceride concentrations.

In experimental animals added dietary cholesterol and fat are essential for the production of atherosclerosis. Typical American diets fed to nonhuman primates produce aortic and coronary atherosclerosis which is reversible when a cholesterol-free diet is fed. Controlled metabolic studies in humans show a direct relation between dietary and plasma cholesterol below intakes of about 600 mg per day; no relation is observed at higher intakes when plasma cholesterol is already high. There appear to be marked genetic variations in the ability of dietary cholesterol to influence plasma cholesterol among individuals and among populations. The relation between dietary polyunsaturated/saturated fat ratio (P/S) and both cholesterol and triglyceride levels also has been amply established.

A definitive prospective study of the effect of diet on IHD in the general population has never been undertaken. Nevertheless, preliminary reports of newer studies of alterations of diet in high-risk populations, coupled with published findings of studies in selected populations, provide strong evidence of a reversible relation among diet, plasma lipids, and IHD. On this basis, although without definite proof of effectiveness, numerous authoritative nutrition councils have recommended prudent dietary modifications for the general population of western countries to be instituted early in life and to include a caloric intake adjusted to achieve and maintain ideal body weight, a reduction in total fat calories to 30 to 35 percent of total calories achieved by a substantial reduction in dietary saturated fat to less than 10 percent of total calories, and a reduction in cholesterol intake to less than 300 mg per day. Although a causal relationship in humans between sodium intake and hypertension has not been firmly established, avoidance of excessive dietary sodium has also been recommended.

RISK FACTORS AND MECHANISMS OF ATHEROGENESIS *Adiposity* produces insulin resistance in peripheral tissues (mainly muscle and adipose), which leads to compensatory hyperinsulinemia. The liver is not resistant to some effects of insulin, and enhanced production of triglyceride-rich lipoproteins results, leading to elevated plasma triglyceride and cholesterol levels. Thus it has been demonstrated that body weight is related not only to triglyceride levels but also to cholesterol levels. Concomitantly, obesity is associated with increased total body cholesterol synthesis. Obesity produces higher circulating levels of insulin, both in the basal state and after stimulation with glucose or other secretagogues. Since obesity is related to atherosclerosis—both directly and via hypertension, hypertriglyceridemia, hypercholesterolemia, and hyperglycemia—it is not surprising that many studies show a relationship between serum insulin levels, particularly after oral glucose intake, and atherosclerotic disease of the coronary and peripheral arteries. A few studies, however, suggest that this association between insulin and atherosclerosis occurs independently of obesity. It has been postulated that insulin may directly affect arterial wall metabolism, leading to increased endogenous lipid synthesis and thus predisposing to atherosclerosis. Insulin has been shown in physiological concentrations to stimulate proliferation of arterial smooth-muscle cells and enhance binding of LDL and VLDL to fibroblasts; it therefore may be one of the plasma factors gaining increased access to the intima and media after endothelial injury and thus may be an additional factor in atheroma formation.

Hypertension may enhance atherogenesis by directly producing injury via mechanical stress on endothelial cells at specific high-pressure sites in the arterial tree. This would allow the sequence of events in the chronic injury hypothesis of atherogenesis to take place. In addition, hypertension might allow more lipoproteins to be transported through intact endothelial lining cells by altering permeability. Hypertension markedly increases lysosomal enzyme activity, presumably owing to stimulation of the cellular disposal system by the internalization of increased amounts of plasma substances. This might lead to increased cell degeneration and release of the highly destructive enzymes (within the lysosomes) into the arterial wall. Experimental hypertension also increases the thickness of the intimal smooth-muscle layer in the arterial wall and increases connective tissue elements. It is still not known if continued high pressure within the artery produces changes in the ability of smooth-muscle cells or stem cells to proliferate.

Diabetes could provide a unique contribution to atherogenesis. Although the fundamental genetic abnormality in human diabetes mellitus remains unknown, it has been suggested that genetic diabetes in humans represents a primary cellular abnormality intrinsic to all cells, resulting in a decreased life span of individual cells, which in turn results in increased cell turnover in tissues. If arterial endothelial and smooth-muscle cells are intrinsically defective in diabetes, accelerated atherogenesis can be readily postulated on the basis of any one of the current theories of pathogenesis. Platelet dysfunction in diabetes might also play a role.

The role of glucose in atheroma formation, if any, is poorly understood. Hyperglycemia is known to affect aortic wall metabolism. Sorbitol, a product of the insulin-independent aldose reductase pathway of glucose metabolism (the polyol pathway) accumulates in the arterial wall in the presence of high glucose concentrations, resulting in osmotic effects including increased cell water content and decreased oxygenation. Increased glucose also appears to stimulate proliferation of cultured arterial smooth-muscle cells.

The development of atherosclerosis accelerates in approximate quantitative relation to the degree of *hyperlipidemia*. A long-established theory suggests that the higher the circulating levels of lipoprotein the more likely they are to gain entrance to the arterial wall. By an acceleration of the usual transendothelial transport, large concentrations of lipoproteins within the arterial wall could overwhelm the ability of smooth-muscle cells to metabolize them. Lipoproteins have been immunologically identified in atheroma, and in humans there is a close relationship between plasma cholesterol and arterial lipoprotein cholesterol concentration. Chemically modified lipoproteins, possibly produced in hyperlipidemic disorders, could gain access to the scavenger arterial wall macrophages leading to formation of foam cells as in xanthomas. It is possible that the lipid that accumulates in the arterial wall with increasing age results from infiltration of plasma lipoproteins. However, atheromatous lesions are associated with a more marked increase in arterial wall lipids, which may result in part from injury to the endothelium possibly produced by chronic hyperlipidemia, as demonstrated in cholesterol-fed monkeys. A further mechanism for accelerated atherogenesis in hyperlipidemia is related to the ability of LDL to stimulate proliferation of arterial smooth-muscle cells.

The effect of *chronic smoke inhalation* from cigarettes could result in repetitive injury to endothelial cells, thereby accelerating atherogenesis. Hypoxia stimulates proliferation of cultured human arterial smooth-muscle cells; thus, since cigarette smoking is associated with high levels of carboxyhemoglobin and low oxygen delivery to tissues, another mechanism for atherogenesis is suggested. Hypoxia could produce diminished lysosomal enzyme degradative ability, as evidenced by impaired degradation of LDL by smooth-muscle cells, causing LDL to accumulate in the cells. Consistent with this suggestion is the fact that aortic lesions that resemble atheroma have been produced in experimental animals by systemic hypoxia, and lipid accumulation in the arterial wall of cholesterol-fed rabbits and monkeys appears to be increased by hypoxia.

RISK FACTOR REVERSAL AND REGRESSION OF ATHEROSCLEROSIS Although the emergence of clinical consequences of atherosclerosis can be lessened, no convincing instance of regression or interruption of progression of atherosclerosis, determined by direct or indirect examination of lesions, by removal or reversal of any single or group of risk factors has yet been proved in humans. Nevertheless, feasibility of such demonstrations is becoming established, and preliminary results are encouraging. Through mass-media educational efforts, whole communities can be influenced to reduce smoking, change diet, and lower blood pressure levels. Adult males in the United States have lowered cigarette consumption, although increases among teenage girls have kept total usage high. There has been a trend toward lower cholesterol and saturated fat consumption in the United States, coupled with increasing attention to reducing overweight and the use of exercise programs. Concomitantly, and perhaps causally, there has been the noted decline in IHD mortality. Treatment of hyperlipidemia in some instances has been shown to reduce atherosclerotic involvement of peripheral vessels by both invasive and noninvasive measurement. There is also some encouraging evidence in animals, most notably in primates, that relatively complicated plaques induced by hyperlipidemia will regress, and that further progression of atherosclerosis will cease when hyperlipidemia is removed. Therefore efforts to prevent atherogenesis, to interrupt progression, and perhaps to promote regression of existing lesions by risk factor reduction seem warranted.

PREVENTION Although premature IHD is overall the most costly and common of the untimely complications of atherosclerosis, preoccupation with IHD should not obscure the fact that angina pectoris and myocardial infarction are expressions of late-stage atherosclerotic lesions. Factors precipitating these clinical events may be independent of those leading to initiation of plaque formation or its progression to a complicated lesion. Steps taken to prevent recurrence of myocardial infarction or fatal arrhythmia, termed *secondary prevention,* will not necessarily be the same as those taken to delay or prevent formation of atherosclerosis (*primary prevention*). Since atherosclerotic plaques have been detected in the coronary arteries of American males as early as the second decade in autopsy studies of Korean and Vietnam war deaths, primary prevention of atherosclerosis must begin early in life, long before there is any suspicion of IHD.

Thus, *prevention of atherosclerosis, rather than treatment, is the goal.* Although an effective program has not been established with certainty, enough is known to guide both in identification of those with a higher risk and in development of conservative measures that probably will reduce that risk. Thus prevention currently is equated with risk factor reduction.

The decline of American death rates from premature IHD today coincides with two trends in health practices. One is the increasing acceptance of the importance of detecting and attempting to correct some of the risk factors correlated with atherosclerosis. The other is a greater awareness of the dietary sources of cholesterol and saturated fats and a tendency of the public to restrict their intake somewhat. Whether these trends are causally related to the decline in death rate is not known. While a rigorous approach to changes in life-style for the general population may be debatable, it is desirable to continue finding and helping those most susceptible to early atherosclerosis. The physician's role in risk factor reduction involves treatment of hypertension and advice regarding diet, body weight, smoking, and exercise. Drug treatment of hyperlipidemia should be limited to those individuals at risk who do not respond adequately to dietary management. Although preliminary trials are encouraging, the long-term value of antiplatelet drugs in reducing either the mortality rate or incidence of myocardial infarction in individuals with IHD remains unproved, and trials are continuing.

TREATMENT There is no agent proven to have any value in "treatment" of atherosclerosis unless it clearly reduces severe hyperlipidemia or obvious hypertension. In fact, there is no treatment of atherosclerosis, only of its complications. While end-stage treatment technology has reduced morbidity (Chap. 260), prevention remains the long-term goal of both research and health care practice.

REFERENCES

BIERMAN EL, ROSS R: Aging and atherosclerosis, in *Atherosclerosis Reviews,* R Paoletti, AM Gotto Jr (eds). New York, Raven, 1977, pp 79–111

BROWN MS et al: Regulation of plasma cholesterol by lipoprotein receptors. Science 217:628, 1981

BRUNZELL JD et al: Pathophysiology of lipoprotein transport. Metabolism 27:1109, 1978

GLUECK CJ, CONNOR WE: Diet–coronary heart disease relationships reconnoitered. Am J Clin Nutr 31:727, 1978

GOLDSTEIN JL et al: Hyperlipidemia in coronary heart disease. J Clin Invest 52:1533, 1544, 1973

GORDON T et al: Diabetes, blood lipids, and the role of obesity in coronary heart disease risk for women. The Framingham Study. Ann Intern Med 87:393, 1977

——— et al: High density lipoprotein as a protective factor against coronary heart disease. The Framingham Study. Am J Med 62:707, 1977

GOTTLIEB AI: Smooth muscle and endothelial cell function in the pathogenesis of atherosclerosis. Can Med Assoc J 126:903, 1982

MCGILL HC JR (ed): The geographic pathology of atherosclerosis. Invest 18:463, 1968

REAVEN GM et al (eds): Proceedings of a conference on diabetes and atherosclerosis. Diabetes, vol 30 (Suppl 2), 1981

ROSS R: The arterial wall and atherosclerosis. Annu Rev Med 30:1, 1979

267 HYPERTENSIVE VASCULAR DISEASE

GORDON H. WILLIAMS
EUGENE BRAUNWALD

An elevated arterial pressure is probably the more important public health problem in developed countries—being common, asymptomatic, readily detectable, usually easily treatable, and often leading to lethal complications if left untreated. As a result of extensive educational programs in the late 1960s and 1970s by both private and governmental agencies, the number of undiagnosed and/or untreated patients has been significantly reduced. This factor may be the most important one responsible for the decline in cardiovascular mortality which has taken place during the latter half of the 1970s (Chap. 266). Although our understanding of the pathophysiology of an elevated arterial pressure has increased, in 90 to 95 percent of cases the etiology (and thus potentially the prevention or cure) is still unknown.

DEFINITION

Since there is no dividing line between normal and high blood pressure, arbitrary levels have been established to define those who have an increased risk of developing a morbid cardiovascular event and/or will clearly benefit from medical therapy. These definitions should consider not only the level of diastolic pressure but also systolic pressure, age, sex, and race. For example, patients with a diastolic pressure greater than 90 mmHg will have a significant reduction in morbidity and mortality with adequate therapy. These, then, are patients who have hypertension and who should be considered for treatment.

The level of *systolic* pressure is also important in assessing arterial pressure's influence on cardiovascular morbidity. Males with normal diastolic pressures ($<$ 82 mmHg) but elevated systolic pressures ($>$ 158 mmHg) have a $2\frac{1}{2}$-fold increase in their cardiovascular mortality rates when compared with individuals with similar diastolic pressures but whose systolic pressures are normal ($<$ 130 mmHg).

Other significant factors which modify blood pressure's influence on the frequency of morbid cardiovascular events are age, race, and sex with young black males being most adversely affected by hypertension.

Thus, even though in an adult hypertension is usually defined as a pressure greater than or equal to 150/90, in men under 45 years of age a pressure greater than or equal to 130/90 mmHg may be elevated.

Individuals can be classified as being *normotensive* if arterial pressure is less than the levels noted above and as having *sustained* hypertension if the diastolic pressure always exceeds these levels. Arterial pressure fluctuates in most persons, whether they are normotensive or hypertensive. Those who are classified as having *labile* hypertension are patients who sometimes but not always have arterial pressures within the hypertensive range. These patients are often considered to have borderline hypertension.

Sustained hypertension can become accelerated or enter a malignant phase. Though a patient with *malignant hypertension* often has a blood pressure above 200/140, it is papilledema, usually accompanied by retinal hemorrhages and exudates, and not the absolute pressure level, that defines this condition. *Accelerated hypertension* signifies a significant recent increase over previous hypertensive levels associated with evidence of vascular damage on funduscopic examination but without papilledema.

FREQUENCY The prevalence of hypertension depends on both the racial composition of the studied population and the criteria used to define the condition. In a Caucasian suburban population as used in the Framingham Study, nearly 20 percent would have blood pressures greater than 160/95 while 45 percent would have pressures greater than 140/90. An even higher prevalance has been documented in the nonwhite population.

ETIOLOGY

The cause of elevated arterial pressure is unknown in most cases. The prevalence of various forms of secondary hypertension depends on the nature of the population studied and how extensive the evaluation is. There are no available data to define the frequency of secondary hypertension in the general population, although in middle-aged males it has been reported to be 6 percent. On the other hand, in referral centers where patients undergo an extensive evaluation, it has been reported to be as high as 35 percent. The various forms of hypertension are outlined in Table 267-1, and their relative frequencies are given in Table 267-2.

ESSENTIAL HYPERTENSION Patients with arterial hypertension and no definable cause are said to have *primary, essential,* or *idiopathic hypertension.* By definition, the underlying mechanism(s) is unknown; however, the kidney probably plays a central role (see Chap. 29). Undoubtedly, this group represents a spectrum of diseases and includes as yet undefined forms of secondary hypertension. There are characteristics common to many patients in this group, however, including a positive family history for hypertension and evidence for increased vascular reactivity.

Heredity Genetic factors have long been assumed to be important in the genesis of hypertension. Data supporting this view can be found in animal studies as well as population studies in humans. One approach has been to assess the correlation of blood pressures within families (familial aggregation). From these studies the minimum size of the genetic factor can be expressed by a correlation coefficient of approximately 0.2. Most studies would also support the concept that the inheritance is probably multifactoral.

Environment A number of environmental factors have been specifically implicated in the development of hypertension including salt intake, obesity, occupation, family size, and crowding. These factors have all been assumed to be important in the increase in blood pressure with age in more affluent societies, in contrast to the decline in blood pressure with age in more primitive cultures. Indeed, even the familial aggregation of blood pressure has been suggested as being related, at least in part, to environmental rather than genetic factors. However, since adopted children do not demonstrate familial aggregation of blood pressure, this phenomenon is probably almost entirely the result of genetic factors.

Factors modifying the course of essential hypertension Age, race, sex, smoking, serum cholesterol, glucose intolerance, weight, and perhaps renin activity may all alter the prognosis of this disease. The younger the patient when hypertension is first noted, the greater the reduction in life expectancy if left untreated. In the United States, urban blacks have about twice the prevalence rate for hypertension as whites and more than four times the hypertension-induced morbidity rate. At all ages and in both white and nonwhite populations, females with hypertension fare better than males. Yet, females with hypertension run the same relative risk of a morbid cardiovascular event compared with their normotensive counterparts as males do. Accelerated atherosclerosis is an invariable companion of hypertension. Thus, it is not surprising that independent risk factors associated with the development of atherosclerosis, e.g., an elevated serum cholesterol, glucose intolerance, and/or cigarette smoking, significantly enhance the effect of hypertension on mortality rates regardless of age, sex, or race. There is no question that there is a positive correlation between obesity and arterial pressure. A gain in weight is associated with an

TABLE 267-1
Classification of arterial hypertension

I Systolic hypertension with wide pulse pressure
- *A* Decreased compliance of aorta (arteriosclerosis)
- *B* Increased stroke volume
  - *1* Arteriovenous fistula
  - *2* Thyrotoxicosis
  - *3* Hyperkinetic heart disease
  - *4* Fever
  - *5* Psychogenic factors
  - *6* Aortic regurgitation
  - *7* Patent ductus arteriosus

II Systolic and diastolic hypertension (increased peripheral vascular resistance)
- *A* Renal
  - *1* Chronic pyelonephritis
  - *2* Acute and chronic glomerulonephritis
  - *3* Polycystic renal disease
  - *4* Renovascular stenosis or renal infarction
  - *5* Most other severe renal disease (arteriolar nephrosclerosis, diabetic nephropathy, etc.)
  - *6* Renin-producing tumors
- *B* Endocrine
  - *1* Oral contraceptives
  - *2* Adrenocortical hyperfunction
    - *a* Cushing's disease and syndrome
    - *b* Primary hyperaldosteronism
    - *c* Congenital or hereditary adrenogenital syndromes (17α-hydroxylase and 11β-hydroxylase defects)
  - *3* Pheochromocytoma
  - *4* Myxedema
  - *5* Acromegaly
- *C* Neurogenic
  - *1* Psychogenic
  - *2* "Diencephalic syndrome"
  - *3* Familial dysautonomia (Riley-Day)
  - *4* Poliomyelitis (bulbar)
  - *5* Polyneuritis (acute porphyria, lead poisoning)
  - *6* Increased intracranial pressure (acute)
  - *7* Spinal cord section
- *D* Miscellaneous
  - *1* Coarctation of aorta
  - *2* Increased intravascular volume (excessive transfusion, polycythemia vera)
  - *3* Polyarteritis nodosa
  - *4* Hypercalcemia
- *E* Unknown etiology
  - *1* Essential hypertension (>90% of all cases of hypertension)
  - *2* Toxemia of pregnancy
  - *3* Acute intermittent porphyria

TABLE 267-2
Prevalence of various forms of hypertension in the general population and in specialized referral clinics*

Diagnosis	*General population, %*	*Specialty clinic, %*
Essential hypertension	92–94	65–85
Renal hypertension:		
Parenchymal	2–3	4–5
Renovascular	1–2	4–16
Endocrine hypertension:		
Primary aldosteronism	0.3	0.5–12
Cushing's syndrome	<0.1	0.2
Pheochromocytoma	<0.1	0.2
Oral contraceptive-induced	2–4	1–2
Miscellaneous	0.2	1

* *Estimates based on a number of reports in the literature.*

increased frequency of hypertension in subjects with normal pressures, and weight loss in obese subjects with hypertension lowers their arterial pressure and, if they are being treated, the intensity of therapy required to maintain them normotensive. However, there are no convincing data that obesity adversely affects the hypertension-associated mortality rate. Plasma renin activity has also been reported by some to influence and correlate with the development of morbid cardiovascular events in patients with hypertension.

Natural history Because essential hypertension is a heterogenous disorder, variables in addition to the level of arterial pressure modify its course. Thus, the probability of developing a morbid cardiovascular event with a given arterial pressure may vary by as much as twentyfold depending on whether associated risk factors are present (Table 267-3). Although exceptions have been reported, most untreated adults with hypertension will have an increase in their arterial pressure with time. Furthermore, both from actuarial data and from experience in the era prior to effective therapy, it has been documented that untreated hypertension is associated with a shortening of life by 10 to 20 years, usually related to an acceleration of the atherosclerotic process, with the rate of acceleration in part related to the severity of the disease. Even individuals with relatively mild disease, i.e., without evidence of end organ damage, left untreated for 7 to 10 years have a high risk of developing significant complications. Nearly 30 percent will exhibit atherosclerotic complications, and more than 50 percent will have end organ damage related to the hypertension itself, e.g., cardiomegaly, congestive heart failure, retinopathy, a cerebrovascular accident, and/or renal insufficiency. Thus, even in its mild forms, hypertension is a progressively lethal disease, if left untreated.

TABLE 267-3
Factors indicating an adverse prognosis in hypertension

I Black race
II Youth
III Male
IV Persistent diastolic pressure >115 mmHg
V Smoking
VI Diabetes mellitus
VII Hypercholesterolemia
VIII Obesity
IX Evidence of end organ damage
- *A* Cardiac
  - *1* Cardiac enlargement
  - *2* ECG changes of ischemic or left ventricular strain
  - *3* Myocardial infarction
  - *4* Congestive heart failure
- *B* Eyes
  - *1* Retinal exudates and hemorrhages
  - *2* Papilledema
- *C* Renal: impaired renal function
- *D* Nervous system: cerebrovascular accident

SECONDARY HYPERTENSION As noted earlier, in only a small minority of patients with an elevated arterial pressure can a specific cause be identified. Yet, they should not be ignored for at least two reasons: (1) with correction of the cause their hypertension may be cured, and (2) the secondary forms may provide insight into the etiology of essential hypertension. Nearly all the secondary forms are related to an alteration in hormone secretion and/or renal function and are discussed in detail in other chapters.

Renal hypertension (see also Chap. 298) Hypertension produced by renal disease is the result of either (1) a derangement in the renal handling of sodium and fluids leading to volume expansion or (2) an alteration in renal secretion of vasoactive materials resulting in a systemic or local change in arteriolar tone. The main subdivisions of renal hypertension are renovascular hypertension, including preeclampsia and eclampsia, and renal parenchymal hypertension. A simple explanation for *renal vascular hypertension* is that decreased perfusion of renal tissue due to stenosis of a main or branch renal artery activates the renin-angiotensin system described in Chap. 112. The angiotensin elevates arterial pressure by direct vasoconstriction, by stimulation of aldosterone secretion with resultant sodium retention (Chap. 29), and/or by stimulating the adrenergic nervous system. In actual practice only about one-half of patients with renovascular hypertension have elevated absolute levels of renin activity in peripheral plasma, although when renin measurements are referenced against an index of sodium balance, a much higher fraction have inappropriately high values.

In recent years the use of the competitive angiotensin antagonist, saralasin (1-sar, 8-ala angiotensin II), has further clarified the role of angiotensin in the genesis of the hypertension in this disease. Nearly all patients with surgically correctable disease have exhibited a reduction of arterial pressure when given these agents in the sodium- or volume-depleted state.

Activation of the renin-angiotensin system also has been offered as an explanation for the hypertension in both acute and chronic *renal parenchymal disease.* In this formulation the only difference between renovascular and renal parenchymal hypertension is that the decreased perfusion of renal tissue in the latter case results from inflammatory and fibrotic changes involving multiple small intrarenal vessels. There are enough differences between the two conditions, however, to suggest that there are other mechanisms active in renal parenchymal disease: (1) peripheral plasma renin activity is elevated far less frequently in renal parenchymal than in renovascular hypertension; (2) cardiac output is said to be normal in the renal parenchymal type (unless uremia and anemia are present), but slightly elevated in renovascular hypertension; (3) circulatory responses to tilting and to the Valsalva maneuver are exaggerated in the latter condition; and (4) blood volume tends to be high in patients with severe renal parenchymal disease and low in patients with severe renovascular hypertension. Alternate explanations for the hypertension in renal parenchymal disease include the possibilities that the damaged kidneys (1) produce an unidentified vasopressor substance other than renin, (2) fail to produce a necessary humoral vasodilator substance (perhaps prostaglandin or bradykinin), (3) fail to inactivate circulating vasopressor substances, and/or (4) are ineffective in disposing of sodium, and the retained sodium is responsible for the hypertension as outlined earlier. Though all these explanations, including participation of the renin-angiotensin system, probably have some validity in individual patients, the hypothesis involving sodium retention is particularly attractive. It is supported by the observation that those patients with chronic pyelonephritis or polycystic renal disease who are salt wasters do not develop hypertension, and by the observation that removal of salt and water by dialysis or diuretics is effective in controlling arterial pressure in the majority of patients with renal parenchymal disease.

A recently described form of renal hypertension results from the excess secretion of renin by juxtaglomerular cell tumors or nephroblastomas. The initial presentation has been similar to that of hyperaldosteronism with hypertension, hypokalemia, and overproduction of aldosterone. However, in contrast to primary aldosteronism, peripheral renin activity is *elevated instead of subnormal.* This disease can be distinguished from other forms of secondary aldosteronism by the presence of normal renal function and with unilateral increases in renal vein renin concentration without a renal artery lesion.

Endocrine hypertension ADRENAL HYPERTENSION Hypertension is a feature of a variety of adrenal cortical abnormalities. In *primary aldosteronism* (Chap. 112) there is a clear relationship between the aldosterone-induced sodium retention and the hypertension. Normal individuals given aldosterone develop hypertension only if they also ingest sodium. Since aldosterone causes sodium retention by stimulating renal tubular exchange of sodium for potassium, hypokalemia is a prominent feature in most patients with primary aldosteronism, and the measurement of serum potassium provides a simple screening test. The effect of sodium retention and volume expansion in chronically suppressing plasma renin activity is critically important for the definitive diagnosis. In most clinical situations plasma renin activity and plasma or urinary aldosterone levels parallel each other, but in patients with primary aldosteronism, aldosterone levels are high and relatively fixed because of autonomous aldosterone secretion, while plasma renin activity levels are suppressed and respond sluggishly to sodium depletion. Primary aldosteronism may be secondary either to a tumor or bilateral adrenal hyperplasia. It is important to distinguish between these two conditions preoperatively, as usually the hypertension in the latter is not modified by operation (Chap. 112).

The sodium-retaining effect of large amounts of glucocorticoids also offers an explanation for the hypertension in severe cases of *Cushing's syndrome* (Chap. 112). Moreover, increased production of mineralocorticoids also has been documented in some patients with Cushing's syndrome. However, the hypertension in many cases of Cushing's syndrome does not seem volume dependent, leading investigators to speculate that it may be secondary to glucocorticoid-induced production of renin substrate (angiotensin-mediated hypertension) or a steroid-induced change in vascular reactivity. In the forms of the adrenogenital syndrome due to C-11 or C-17 hydroxylase deficiency (Chap. 112) deoxycorticosterone accounts for the sodium retention and the resultant hypertension, which is accompanied by suppression of plasma renin activity.

In patients with *pheochromocytoma* increased secretion of epinephrine and norepinephrine by a tumor most often located in the adrenal medulla causes excessive stimulation of adrenergic receptors, which results in peripheral vasoconstriction and cardiac stimulation. This diagnosis is confirmed by demonstrating increased urinary excretion of epinephrine and norepinephrine or their metabolites (Chap. 113).

ACROMEGALY (see also Chap. 109) Hypertension, coronary atherosclerosis, and cardiac hypertrophy are frequent complications of this condition.

HYPERCALCEMIA (see also Chap. 338) The hypertension which occurs in up to one-third of patients with hyperparathyroidism ordinarily can be attributed to renal parenchymal damage due to nephrolithiasis and nephrocalcinosis. However, increased calcium levels can also have a direct vasoconstrictive effect. In some cases, the hypertension disappears when the hypercalcemia is corrected.

ORAL CONTRACEPTIVES The most common cause of endocrine hypertension is that resulting from the use of estrogen-containing oral contraceptives. Indeed, this may be the most common form of secondary hypertension. The mechanism producing the hypertension is likely to be secondary to activation of the renin-angiotensin-aldosterone system. Thus, both volume (aldosterone) and vasoconstrictor (angiotensin II) factors are important. The estrogen component of oral contraceptive agents stimulates the hepatic synthesis of the renin substrate angiotensinogen, which in turn favors the increased production of angiotensin II and secondary aldosteronism. Women taking oral contraceptives have increased plasma concentrations of angiotensin II and aldosterone with some increase in arterial pressure. However, only about 5 percent actually have an increase in arterial pressure to greater than 140/90, and in about half of these the hypertension will remit within 6 months of stopping the drug.

Why some women taking oral contraceptives develop hypertension and others do not is unclear but may be related to (1) increased vascular sensitivity to angiotensin II, (2) the presence of mild renal disease, (3) familial factors (over one-half have a positive family history for hypertension), (4) age (hypertension is significantly more prevalent in women over age 35), and/or (5) obesity. Indeed some investigators have suggested that the oral contraceptives are simply unmasking patients with essential hypertension.

Coarctation of the aorta (see also Chap. 256) The hypertension associated with coarctation may be caused by the constriction itself, or perhaps by the changes in the renal circulation which result in an unusual form of renal arterial hypertension. The diagnosis of coarctation is usually evident from physical examination and routine x-ray findings.

Low-renin essential hypertension Approximately 20 percent of patients who by all other criteria have essential hypertension have suppressed plasma renin activity. This occurs more frequently in black than in white patients. Though these patients are not hypokalemic, they have been reported to have expanded extracellular fluid volumes, and it is tempting to implicate sodium retention and renin suppression due to excessive production of an unidentified mineralocorticoid. Involvement of the adrenal cortex is suggested by the observation that large doses of spironolactone, the mineralocorticoid antagonist, and the inhibition of steroidogenesis by aminoglutethimide can result in sodium loss and lowering of blood pressure in these patients. A search for other mineralocorticoids occasionally reveals increased secretion of 18-hydroxy-11-deoxycorticosterone or 16-hydroxydehydroepiandrosterone in some patients. However, the frequency of these abnormalities is no greater than in patients with normal renin hypertension. Recent studies have suggested that many of these patients have an increased sensitivity to angiotensin II which may be the underlying mechanism. Since this altered sensitivity has been reported even in patients with normal renin hypertension, it is likely that patients with low-renin hypertension are not a distinct subset but rather form part of a continuum of patients with essential hypertension.

High-renin essential hypertension Approximately 15 percent of patients with essential hypertension have plasma renin levels elevated above the normal range. It has been suggested that plasma renin plays an important role in the pathogenesis of the elevated blood pressure in these patients. However, most studies have documented that saralasin significantly reduces blood pressure in less than half of these patients. This has led some investigators to postulate that the elevated renin levels and blood pressure may both be secondary to an increased activity of the adrenergic system. It has been proposed that, in those patients with angiotensin-dependent high-renin hypertension whose arterial pressures are lowered by saralasin, the mechanism responsible for the increased renin and, therefore, the hypertension is a compensatory hyperreninemia secondary to a decreased adrenal responsiveness to angiotensin II.

EFFECTS OF HYPERTENSION

For nearly 70 years it has been known that patients with hypertension die prematurely. The most common cause of death is heart disease, with strokes and renal failure also frequently occurring, particularly in those with significant retinopathy.

EFFECTS ON HEART Cardiac compensation for the excessive work load imposed by increased systemic pressure is at first sustained by left ventricular hypertrophy. Ultimately, the function of this chamber deteriorates, it dilates, and the symptoms and signs of heart failure appear (Chap. 253). Angina pectoris may also occur because of accelerated coronary arterial disease and/or increased myocardial oxygen requirements as a consequence of the increased myocardial mass, which exceeds the capacity of the coronary circulation. On physical examination the heart is enlarged and has a prominent left ventricular impulse. The sound of aortic closure is accentuated, and there may be a faint murmur of aortic regurgitation. Presystolic (atrial, fourth) heart sounds appear frequently in hypertensive heart disease, and a protodiastolic (ventricular, third heart) sound or summation gallop rhythm may be present. Electrocardiographic changes of left ventricular hypertrophy (Chap. 249) are common; evidence of ischemia or infarction may be observed late in the disease. The majority of deaths due to hypertension result from myocardial infarction or congestive heart failure.

NEUROLOGIC EFFECTS The neurologic effects of long-standing hypertension may be divided into retinal and central nervous system changes. Because the retina is the only tissue in which the arteries and arterioles can be examined directly, repeated ophthalmoscopic examination provides the opportunity to observe the progress of the vascular effects of hypertension. The Keith-Wagener-Barker classification of the *retinal changes* in hypertension has provided a simple and excellent means for serial evaluation of the hypertensive patient. Increasing severity of hypertension is associated with focal spasm and progressive general narrowing of the arterioles, as well as the appearance of hemorrhages, exudates, and papilledema. These retinal lesions often produce scotomata, blurred vision, and even blindness, especially in the presence of papilledema or hemorrhages of the macular area. Hypertensive lesions may develop acutely and, if therapy results in significant reduction of blood pressure, may show rapid resolution. Rarely, these lesions resolve without therapy. In contrast, retinal arteriolosclerosis results from endothelial and muscular proliferation, and it accurately reflects similar changes in other organs. Sclerotic changes do not develop as rapidly as hypertensive lesions, nor do they regress appreciably with therapy. As a consequence of increased wall thickness and rigidity, sclerotic arterioles distort and compress the veins as they cross within their common fibrous sheath, and the reflected light streak from the arterioles is changed by the increased opacity of the vessel wall.

Central nervous system dysfunction also occurs frequently in patients with hypertension. Occipital headaches, most often in the morning, are among the most prominent early symptoms of hypertension. Dizziness, lightheadedness, vertigo, tinnitus, and dimmed vision or syncope may also be observed, but the more serious manifestations are due to vascular occlusion or hemorrhage (Chap. 356).

The pathogeneses of these two disorders are quite different. *Cerebral infarction* is secondary to the increased atherosclerosis observed in hypertensive patients, while *cerebral hemorrhage* is the result of both the elevated arterial pressure and the development of cerebral vascular microaneurysms (Charcot-Bouchard aneurysms). Only age and arterial pressure are known to influence the development of the microaneurysms. Thus, it is not surprising that the association of arterial pressure with cerebral hemorrhage is so much better than with either cerebral or myocardial infarction.

RENAL EFFECTS (See also Chap. 298) Arteriolosclerotic lesions of the afferent and efferent arterioles and the glomerular capillary tufts are the most common renal vascular lesions in hypertension and result in decreased glomerular filtration rate and tubular dysfunction. Proteinuria and microscopic hematuria occur because of glomerular lesions, and approximately 10 percent of the deaths secondary to hypertension result from renal failure. Blood loss in hypertension occurs not only from renal lesions; epistaxis, hemoptysis, and metrorrhagia also occur most requently in these patients.

APPROACH TO THE PATIENT WITH HYPERTENSION

In evaluating patients with hypertension, the initial history, physical examination, and laboratory tests should be directed at (1) uncovering correctable secondary forms of hypertension (Table 267-1), (2) establishing a pretreatment base line, (3) assessing factors which may influence the type of therapy or which may be adversely modified by therapy, and (4) determining whether other risk factors for the development of arteriosclerotic cardiovascular disease are present (Chap. 266).

SYMPTOMS AND SIGNS The majority of patients with hypertension have no symptoms referable to their blood pressure elevation and will be identified only in the course of a physical examination. When symptoms do bring the patient to the physician, they fall into three categories. They are related to (1) the elevated pressure itself, (2) the hypertensive vascular disease, and (3) the underlying disease in the case of secondary hypertension. Though popularly considered a symptom of elevated arterial pressure, headache is characteristic only of severe hypertension; most commonly it is localized to the occipital region, is present when the patient awakens in the morning, and subsides spontaneously after several hours. Other possibly related complaints include dizziness, palpitations, and easy fatigability. Complaints referable to vascular disease include epistaxis, hematuria, blurring of vision owing to retinal changes, episodes of weakness or dizziness due to transient cerebral ischemia, angina pectoris, and dyspnea due to cardiac failure. Pain due to dissection of the aorta or to a leaking aneurysm is an occasional presenting symptom.

Examples of symptoms related to the underlying disease in secondary hypertension are polyuria, polydipsia, and muscle weakness secondary to hypokalemia in patients with primary aldosteronism, or weight gain and emotional lability in patients with Cushing's syndrome. The patient with a pheochromocytoma may present with episodic headaches, palpitations, diaphoresis, and postural dizziness.

CLINICAL EVALUATION History A strong family history of hypertension, along with the reported finding of intermittent pressure elevation in the past, favors the diagnosis of essential hypertension. Secondary hypertension often develops before the age of 35 or after the age of 55 years. The history of use of adrenal steroids or estrogens is of obvious significance. A history of repeated urinary tract infections suggests chronic pyelonephritis, although this condition may occur in the absence of symptoms; nocturia and polydipsia suggest renal or endocrine disease, while trauma to either flank or an episode of acute flank pain may be a clue to the presence of renal injury. A history of weight gain is compatible with Cushing's syndrome, while weight loss suggests pheochromocytoma. A number of aspects of the history aid in determining whether vascular disease has progressed to dangerous stages. These include chest pain due to myocardial ischemia and symptoms of cerebrovascular insufficiency, of congestive heart failure, and/or of peripheral vascular insufficiency. Other risk factors that could be elicited include cigarette smoking, diabetes mellitus, lipid disorders, and a family history of early deaths due to cardiovascular disease.

Physical examination The physical examination starts with the patient's general appearance. For instance, are the round face and trunkal obesity of Cushing's syndrome present? Is muscular development in the upper extremities out of proportion to that in the lower extremities, suggesting coarctation of the aorta? The next step is to compare the blood pressures and pulses in both upper extremities. Also, measurements in the supine position should be compared with measurements taken during standing. A rise in diastolic pressure when the patient goes from the supine to the standing position is most compatible with essential hypertension; a fall, in the absence of antihypertensive medications, suggests other forms of secondary hypertension. Detailed examination of the ocular fundi is mandatory, since funduscopic findings provide one of the best indications of the duration of hypertension and of prognosis. The Keith-Wagener-Barker classification of funduscopic changes (Table 267-4) is useful; the specific changes should be recorded and a grade assigned. Palpation and auscultation of the carotid arteries for evidence of stenosis or occlusion are important; narrowing of a carotid artery may be a manifestation of hypertensive vascular disease, and it may also be a clue to the presence of a renal arterial lesion, since these two lesions may occur together. In examination of the heart and lungs, one should search for evidence of left ventricular hypertrophy and cardiac decompensation. Is there a left ventricular lift? Are third and fourth heart sounds present? Are there pulmonary rales? Chest examination also includes a search for extracardiac murmurs and palpable collateral vessels that may result from coarctation of the aorta. The most important part of the abdominal examination is auscultation for bruits originating in stenotic renal arteries. Bruits due to renal arterial narrowing nearly always have a diastolic component or may be continuous and are best heard just to the right or left of the midline above the umbilicus, or in the flanks; they are present in many patients with renal artery stenosis due to fibrous dysplasia and in 40 to 50 percent of those with functionally significant stenosis due to arteriosclerosis. The abdomen also should be palpated for abdominal aneurysm and for the enlarged kidneys of polycystic renal disease. The femoral pulses must be carefully felt, and, if they are decreased and/or delayed, blood pressure in the lower extremities must be measured. Even if the femoral pulse is normal to palpation, arterial pressure in the lower extremities should be recorded at least once in patients in whom hypertension is discovered before the age of 30 years. Finally examination of the extremities for edema and a search for evidence of a previous cerebrovascular accident and/or other intracranial pathology should be performed.

Laboratory investigation Controversy exists as to what laboratory studies should be performed in patients presenting with hypertension. In general, the disagreement resides in how extensively to evaluate the patient for secondary forms of hypertension. In the following discussion laboratory studies are divided into those which should be performed in all patients with sustained hypertension (basic group) and those which should be added if (1) from the initial evaluation a secondary form of hypertension is suggested and/or (2) arterial pressure is not controlled after first-step therapy.

TABLE 267-4
Classification of hypertensive and arteriolosclerotic retinopathy

	Hypertension					*Arteriolosclerosis*	
	Arterioles						
Degree	*General narrowing AV ratio**	*Focal spasm†*	*Hemorrhages*	*Exudates*	*Papilledema*	*Arteriolar light reflex*	*AV crossing‡ defects*
Normal	3:4	1:1	0	0	0	Fine yellow line, red blood column	0
Grade I	1:2	1:1	0	0	0	Broadened yellow line, red blood column	Mild depression of vein
Grade II	1:3	2:3	0	0	0	Broad yellow line, "copper wire," blood column not visible	Depression or humping of vein
Grade III	1:4	1:3	+	+	0	Broad white line, "silver wire," blood column not visible	Right-angle deviation, tapering, and disappearance of vein under arteriole Distal dilatation of vein
Grade IV	Fine, fibrous cords	Obliteration of distal flow	+	+	+	Fibrous cords, blood column not visible	Same as grade III

* *This is the ratio of arteriolar to venous diameters.*
† *This is the ratio of diameters of region of spasm to proximal arteriole.*
‡ *Arteriolar length and tortuosity increase with severity.*

BASIC STUDIES Renal status is evaluated by assessing the presence of protein, blood, and glucose in the urine and measuring serum creatinine and/or blood urea nitrogen (BUN). Microscopic examination of the urine is also helpful. A serum potassium level is needed both as a screen for mineralocorticoid-induced hypertension and as a base line prior to initiating diuretic therapy.

Other blood chemistries may also be useful particularly since they can often be ordered as a battery of automated tests at minimal cost to the patient. For example, a blood glucose is helpful both because diabetes mellitus may be associated with accelerated arteriosclerosis, resultant renal vascular disease, and diabetic nephropathy, and because primary aldosteronism, Cushing's syndrome, and pheochromocytoma all can be associated with hyperglycemia. Furthermore, since subsequent antihypertensive therapy with diuretics can raise the blood glucose level, it is important to establish a base line. The possibility of hypercalcemia may also be investigated. Serum uric acid is useful because of the increased incidence of hyperuricemia in patients with renal and essential hypertension and because, as with blood glucose, the level subsequently may be raised by treatment with diuretics. Serum cholesterol and triglycerides may be measured to identify other factors which predispose to the development of arteriosclerosis. An electrocardiogram should be obtained in all cases as an assessment of cardiac status, particularly if left ventricular hypertrophy is present, and as a base line. The chest roentgenogram may also be helpful by providing the opportunity to identify aortic dilatation or elongation and the rib notching that occurs in coarctation of the aorta.

SECONDARY STUDIES (Table 267-5) Certain clues from the history, physical examination, and basic laboratory studies suggest an unusual cause for the hypertension and dictate the need for special studies. For example, the abrupt onset of severe hypertension and/or the onset of hypertension of any severity under the age of 25 or after the age of 50 years should lead to laboratory tests to exclude renovascular hypertension and pheochromocytoma (Table 267-5). A history of headaches, palpitations, anxiety attacks, unusual sweating, and weight loss should lead to tests to exclude pheochromocytoma (as well as hyperglycemia). The presence of an abdominal bruit should lead to workup for renovascular hypertension, and the finding of bilateral upper abdominal masses on physical examination, consistent with polycystic renal disease, should lead to the performance of an intravenous pyelogram (Chap. 299). An elevated creatinine or blood urea nitrogen, associated with proteinuria and hematuria, should initiate a detailed workup for renal insufficiency (Chap. 289). Special studies are also indicated if there is therapeutic failure on the first-step drug program. The specific diagnostic measures depend on the most likely causes of secondary hypertension.

Pheochromocytoma. The easiest and best screening procedure for pheochromocytoma is the measurement of catecholamines or their metabolites in a 24-h urine collected during the time the patient is hypertensive. Measurement of plasma catecholamine levels may also be useful. This test may be indicated even in patients who do not have spells, as over half the patients with pheochromocytoma have fixed hypertension. Provocative tests are seldom if ever indicated (Chap. 113).

Cushing's syndrome. A 24-h urine test for 17-hydroxysteroids and/or 17-ketosteroids or a plasma cortisol level can be used to screen for the presence of this condition; however, the more definitive test involves the administration of 1 mg dexamethasone at bedtime, followed by measurement of plasma cortisol at 7 to 10 A.M. Suppression of the plasma cortisol level to below 5 μg/dl effectively rules out Cushing's syndrome (Chap. 112).

Renovascular hypertension. The standard screening test for renal vascular hypertension has been the rapid-sequence intravenous pyleogram (IVP). Features suggestive of renal ischemia include (1) unilateral delayed appearance and excretion of contrast material, (2) a difference in kidney size greater than 1.5 cm, (3) irregular contour of the renal silhouette, suggesting partial infarction or atrophy, (4) indentations on the ureter or renal pelvis, possibly due to dilated ureteral arteries (collateral notching), and (5) hyperconcentration of contrast medium in the collecting system of the smaller kidney. When these criteria are used, the false-positive rate is 11 percent and the false-negative rate 12 percent. The isotope renogram, which measures differential uptake and excretion by the two kidneys of one of several isotope-labeled substances, can be used as a further screening procedure. Its sensitivity may be somewhat greater but its reliability is probably somewhat less than the IVP. The most recently developed screening test is the blood pressure response to the angiotensin II antagonist saralasin. The false-positive rate, i.e., a fall in systolic arterial pressure exceeding 10 mmHg, appears to be the same or lower than with an IVP with a comparable false-negative rate. Since it is considerably easier to administer and less expensive than an IVP, it may be a better screening test for renovascular hypertension. Split renal function tests and measurements of random peripheral plasma renin activity are less useful and have been almost entirely replaced by one or more of the other three screening tests.

The definitive test of surgically correctable renal disease is the combination of a renal angiogram and renal vein renin determinations. The renal arteriogram both establishes the presence of a renal arterial lesion and aids in determining whether the lesion is due to atherosclerosis or to one of the fibrous or fibromuscular dysplasias. It does not, however, prove that the lesion is responsible for the hypertension, nor does it permit prediction of the chances of surgical cure; it must be noted that (1) renal artery stenosis is a frequent finding by angiography and at postmortem in normotensive individuals, and (2) essential hypertension is a common condition and may occur in combination with renal arterial stenosis which actually may not be responsible for the hypertension. Bilateral renal vein catheterization for measurement of plasma renin activity is, therefore, used to assess the functional significance of any lesion noted on arteriography. When one kidney is ischemic and the other is normal, all the renin released comes from the involved kidney. In the most straightforward situation, the ischemic kidney has a significantly higher venous

TABLE 267-5
Laboratory tests and special studies for evaluation of hypertension

I Basic studies
- *A* Always included
  - *1* Urine for protein, blood, and glucose
  - *2* Hematocrit
  - *3* Serum potassium
  - *4* Serum creatinine and/or blood urea nitrogen
  - *5* Electrocardiogram
- *B* Usually included, depending on cost and other factors
  - *1* Microscopic urinalysis
  - *2* White blood cell count
  - *3* Serum glucose, cholesterol, and triglycerides
  - *4* Serum calcium, phosphate, and uric acid
  - *5* Chest x-ray

II Special studies to screen for secondary hypertension
- *A* Renovascular: rapid sequence IVP, radioisotope renogram, and/or saralasin test
- *B* Pheochromocytoma: 24-h urine for creatinine, metanephrines, and catecholamines or plasma catecholamines
- *C* Cushing's syndrome: overnight dexamethasone suppression test

plasma renin activity than the normal kidney by a factor of 1.5 or more. Moreover, the renal venous blood draining the uninvolved kidney exhibits levels similar to those in the inferior vena cava below the entrance of the renal veins. Significant benefit from operative correction may be anticipated in at least 80 percent of patients with the findings described above. When obstructing lesions in the *branches* of the renal arteries are demonstrated by arteriography, an attempt to obtain blood samples from the main *branches* of the renal vein should be made in an effort to identify a localized intrarenal arterial lesion responsible for the hypertension.

Primary aldosteronism. The diagnosis of this cause of secondary hypertension is discussed in Chap. 112. These patients almost always exhibit hypokalemia. Diuretic therapy often complicates the picture when the hypokalemia is first observed and needs to be assessed. Given hypokalemia, the relation between plasma renin activity and the aldosterone level becomes the key to the diagnosis of primary aldosteronism. The aldosterone concentration or excretion is high and plasma renin activity is low in primary aldosteronism, and these levels are relatively unaffected by changes in sodium balance. A critical part of the evaluation after primary aldosteronism has been established is to determine whether unilateral or bilateral disease is present since surgical removal of the lesion usually reduces arterial pressure only in those with unilateral disease.

Plasma renin activity measurements. Some studies have suggested that most hypertensive patients should have a plasma renin level measured and indexed against a 24-h urine sodium excretion rate to assess whether high, low, or normal levels are present. This information, it is argued, may be important for both therapeutic and prognostic reasons. However, it is unclear, on the basis of presently available data and treatment programs, that these measurements are really useful except in patients with findings suggestive of renal vascular disease or mineralocorticoid excess in whom lateralizing renal vein renin levels or suppressed peripheral renin levels may be of diagnostic and/or therapeutic significance.

TREATMENT Virtually every patient with a diastolic arterial pressure exceeding 90 mmHg is a candidate for diagnostic studies and for subsequent treatment. Furthermore, at any given level of blood pressure elevation, the risk of developing hypertensive vascular complications is greater in men than in women, and in younger persons than in older ones. It may be argued, then, that it is hard to justify producing the uncomfortable side effects of therapy in, for example, an asymptomatic woman over 70 years of age with a diastolic pressure of 90 mmHg. On the other hand, it is easy to justify side effects in a man of 30 with a diastolic pressure of 104 mmHg, because such a person may be expected to receive the greatest benefit from therapy. Fortunately, the choice of treatment is such that a satisfactory program to control arterial pressure with minimal side effects can be developed for most patients. A reasonable guideline would be that all patients with diastolic pressure repeatedly above 90 mmHg should be treated unless specific contraindications exist. There is controversy regarding the advisability of treating isolated *systolic* hypertension. Until the results of a well-controlled prospective study provide evidence to the contrary, treatment of isolated systolic hypertension is not recommended. Patients with labile hypertension or isolated systolic hypertension who are not treated should have regular follow-up examinations at 6-month intervals, because of the frequent development of progressive and/or sustained hypertension.

The identification of an operable form of secondary hypertension does not automatically mean that surgical treatment is indicated. The decision depends upon the age and general health of the patient, the natural history of the lesion, and the response of the pressure to drug therapy. In patients with renovascular hypertension the feasibility of vascular repair versus nephrectomy and the degree of overall renal function impairment must be considered. Age and general health are important in patients with renovascular hypertension due to arteriosclerosis, because there is no evidence that repair of the stenosis increases life expectancy in the elderly patient with other evidence of vascular disease. Knowledge of the natural history of the disease is especially important when approaching the decision in the young patient with renal-artery stenosis due to fibrous dysplasia. If the arteriographic appearance suggests that the stenosis is due to intimal or subadventitial fibroplasia, the lesion may be expected to progress and operation is required. Medial fibroplasia, on the other hand, often remains stable, and operation may not be necessary if pressure can be controlled by drug therapy. The decision regarding operation should also be considered carefully in patients with primary aldosteronism when bilateral adrenal venography does not demonstrate a tumor, because such patients may prove to have multinodular hyperplasia. This means that bilateral adrenalectomy would be required to eliminate the aldosterone excess, and, even then, hypertension usually persists. If hypokalemia can be controlled by spironolactone or other drug therapy, and arterial pressure lowered with antihypertensive agents, then it is reasonable to withhold operative treatment.

General measures (Table 267-6) Nondrug therapeutic intervention is probably indicated in all patients with sustained hypertension and probably most with labile hypertension. The general measures employed include (1) relief of stress, (2) diet, (3) regular exercise, and (4) control of other risk factors contributing to the development of arteriosclerosis. Relief of emotional and environmental stress is one of the reasons for the improvement in hypertension that occurs when the patient is hospitalized. Though it is usually impossible to extricate the hypertensive patient from all internal and external stresses, he or she should be advised to avoid any unnecessary tensions. In rare instances, it may be appropriate to recommend a change of job or of life-style. Recently it has been suggested that relaxation techniques may also lower arterial pressure. However, it is uncertain that these techniques alone have much long-term effect.

Dietary management has three aspects:

1 Because of the documented efficacy of sodium restriction and volume contraction in lowering blood pressure, patients previously were instructed to curtail sodium intake drastically. The advent of effective oral diuretics provided an additional method of decreasing body sodium stores and led some to suggest that sodium restriction was no longer neces-

TABLE 267-6
Treatment of patients with hypertension

GENERAL MEASURES

1 Relief of stress (relaxation techniques)
2 Dietary control
  a Restrict sodium chloride to 4 to 6 g per day
  b Restrict calories
  c Restrict cholesterol and saturated fats
3 Regular isotonic exercise
4 Stop cigarette smoking

DRUG THERAPY

Step 1: Thiazide diuretic
Step 2: Add an antiadrenergic agent: β blocker, methyldopa, or reserpine
Step 3: Add a vasodilator: hydralazine or captopril
Step 4: Add guanethidine or substitute clonidine or prazosin for a step 2 drug

sary. However, a number of reports have documented that while mild sodium restriction has little, if any, direct action on blood pressure, it significantly potentiates the effectiveness of nearly all antihypertensive agents. Thus, the most practical approach now is to advise mild dietary sodium restriction (up to 5 g NaCl per day).

2 Caloric restriction should be urged for the patient who is overweight. Some obese patients will show a significant reduction in pressure simply as a consequence of weight loss.

3 A moderate restriction in intake of cholesterol and saturated fats is recommended on the suggestive evidence that such a diet may diminish the incidence of arteriosclerotic complications. Regular exercise is indicated within the limits of the patient's cardiovascular status. Not only is exercise helpful in controlling weight, but in addition there is evidence that physical conditioning itself may lower arterial pressure. Isotonic exercises (jogging, swimming) are better than isometric exercises (weight lifting) since, if anything, the latter raises arterial pressure. The dietary management outlined above is aimed at the control of other risk factors. Probably the most significant additional step that could be taken in this area would be to convince the smoker to give up cigarettes.

Drug therapy (Table 267-7) To make rational use of antihypertensive drugs, the sites and mechanisms of their action must be understood. In general, there are four classes of drugs: diuretics, antiadrenergic agents, vasodilators, and angiotensin blockers.

DIURETICS (see also Chap. 253) Drugs active on the renal tubules affect arterial pressure primarily by causing sodium diuresis and volume depletion. The thiazides are the most frequently used and most extensively investigated members of this group, and their early effect certainly is related to the diuresis. A reduction in peripheral vascular resistance also has been reported by some workers to be important in the long term. Thiazide diuretics form the cornerstone of most therapeutic programs designed to lower arterial pressure and are usually effective within 3 to 4 days. Their most frequent side effects are hypokalemia due to renal potassium loss, hyperuricemia due to uric acid retention, and carbohydrate intolerance. The more potent diuretics, furosemide and ethacrynic acid, also have been shown to be antihypertensive but have been less extensively used for this purpose primarily because of their shorter duration of action. Spironolactone causes renal sodium loss by blocking the effect of endogenous mineralocorticoids, and therefore it may be more effective in patients whose mineralocorticoids are present in excess, e.g., primary or secondary aldosteronism. Although they do not compete directly with aldosterone, triamterene and amiloride act at the same site as spironolactone to impede sodium reabsorption and are effective in the same situations as spironolactone. Any of these three potassium-sparing diuretics can also be given along with thiazide diuretics to minimize renal potassium loss.

ANTIADRENERGIC AGENTS (see also Chap. 73) These drugs act at one or more sites either centrally on the vasomotor center, in peripheral neurons modifying catecholamine release, or by blocking adrenergic receptor sites on target tissue. Drugs that appear to have predominant *central actions* are *clonidine* and *methyldopa.* These drugs and their metabolites are predominantly alpha-receptor agonists. Stimulation of alpha receptors in the vasomotor centers of the brain *reduces* sympathetic outflow, thereby reducing arterial pressure. Usually a fall in cardiac output and heart rate also occurs, more commonly with clonidine, but the baroreceptor reflex is intact. Thus, postural symptoms are absent. However, rebound hypertension may rarely occur when these drugs, particularly clonidine, are stopped. This is probably secondary to the increase in norepinephrine release which had been inhibited by these agents secondary to their agonist effect on presynaptic alpha receptors.

Another class of antiadrenergic agents is the *ganglionic blocking* drugs. These compounds block ganglionic transmission in the autonomic nervous system. They have little effect when the patient is supine, but they prevent reflex vasoconstriction in the upright position. Ganglionic blocking agents interfere with parasympathetic as well as sympathetic function, and this results in such side effects as impairment of visual accommodation, paralytic ileus, retention of urine, and failure of erection and ejaculation. Because of these problems, ganglionic blocking agents are now usually reserved for the rapid lowering of arterial pressure by parenteral administration of the short-acting agent *trimethaphan* in patients with severe hypertension.

Various drugs act at *postganglionic nerve endings.* The *rauwolfia alkaloids* are the oldest members of the group; their long-term effect results from their ability to inhibit the storage of norepinephrine within the vesicles in adrenergic nerve endings, thus leading to depletion of catecholamine stores. When given parenterally, they also have a direct effect on vascular smooth muscle. The rauwolfia alkaloids, like the other drugs of this class, exhibit the side effects that result from the unopposed activity of the parasympathetic nervous system, including nasal congestion, diarrhea, impairment of sexual function, and increased gastric secretion. Depression is the most serious side effect of the rauwolfia alkaloids; this is most likely to occur in elderly patients. The rauwolfia alkaloids are most helpful in treatment by the oral route of mild to moderate hypertension. *Guanethidine* blocks the release of norepinephrine from the sympathetic nerve endings. It has a greater postural effect than the other drugs that work at the nerve endings, and orthostatic hypotension is a frequent side effect. However, centrally mediated side effects (sedation, depression) are infrequently observed since guanethidine has a low lipid solubility and, therefore, only poorly enters the central nervous system.

The last group of drugs affecting the adrenergic system are those which block the *peripheral adrenergic receptors,* either alpha or beta. *Phentolamine* and *phenoxybenzamine* block the action of norepinephrine at *alpha*-adrenergic receptor sites. While the above two compounds block both pre- and postsynaptic alpha receptors, the former action accounts for the tolerance which develops, while *prazosin* is more effective because it selectively blocks only the *postsynaptic alpha* receptor. Thus, presynaptic alpha action remains, suppressing norepinephrine release.

A variety of effective *beta-adrenergic receptor blocking agents* are available which block sympathetic effects on the heart and should be most effective in reducing cardiac output and in lowering arterial pressure when there is increased cardiac sympathetic nerve activity. In addition, they block the adrenergic nerve-mediated release of renin from the renal juxtaglomerular cells, and this action may be an important component of their blood pressure–lowering action. Beta-adrenergic blockers are particularly useful when employed in conjunction with vascular smooth-muscle relaxants, which tend to evoke a reflex increase in myocardial contractility, and with diuretics, the administration of which often results in an elevation of circulating renin activity. In practice, beta blockers appear to be effective even when there is no evidence of increased sympathetic tone with about one-half or more of all patients showing a fall in pressure. However, these agents can precipitate congestive heart failure and asthma in susceptible

TABLE 267-7

Drugs used in treatment of hypertension—listed according to site of action

Site of action	*Drug*	*Dosage*	*Indications*	*Contraindications*	*Frequent or peculiar side effects*
DIURETICS					
Renal tubule	Thiazides	Depends on specific drug	Mild hypertension, as adjunct in treatment of moderate to severe hypertension	Diabetes mellitus, hyperuricemia, primary aldosteronism	Potassium depletion, hyperglycemia, hyperuricemia, dermatitis, purpura
	Hydrochlorothiazide	Oral: 25–50 mg daily or twice daily			
	Furosemide	Oral: 20–40 mg daily or twice daily	Mild hypertension, as adjunct in severe or malignant hypertension	Hyperuricemia, primary aldosteronism	Potassium depletion, hyperuricemia, nausea, vomiting, diarrhea
	Ethacrynic acid	Oral: 25–50 mg daily or twice daily	Mild hypertension, as adjunct in severe or malignant hypertension	Hyperuricemia, primary aldosteronism	Potassium depletion, hyperuricemia, diarrhea
	Spironolactone	Oral: 25–100 mg three or four times daily	Hypertension due to hypermineralocorticoidism, adjunct to thiazide therapy	Renal failure	Hyperkalemia, diarrhea, gynecomastia, menstrual irregularities
	Triamterene	Oral: 100 mg one to three times daily	Hypertension due to hypermineralocorticoidism, adjunct to thiazide therapy	Renal failure	Hyperkalemia, nausea, vomiting, leg cramps
	Amiloride	Oral: 5–20 mg daily			
ANTIADRENERGIC AGENTS					
Central	Clonidine	Oral: 0.1–0.6 mg two to four times daily	Mild to moderate hypertension, renal disease with hypertension		Postural hypotension, drowsiness, dry mouth, rebound hypertension after abrupt withdrawal
	Methyldopa (also acts by blocking sympathetic nerves)	Oral: 250–750 mg three or four times daily IV: 250–1000 mg every 4–6 h (tolerance may develop)	Mild to moderate hypertension (oral), malignant hypertension (IV)	Pheochromocytoma, active hepatic disease (IV), during MAO inhibitor administration	Postural hypotension, sedation, fatigue, diarrhea, impaired ejaculation, fever, gynecomastia, lactation, positive Coombs tests (occasionally associated with hemolysis)
	Sedatives and tranquilizers		Tense or anxious patient with hypertension		Drowsiness, fatigue
	Phenobarbital	Oral: 15–30 mg three or four times daily			
	Diazepam	Oral: 2–10 mg four times daily			
Autonomic ganglia	Trimethaphan	IV: 1–10 mg/min	Severe or malignant hypertension	Severe coronary artery disease, cerebrovascular insufficiency, diabetes mellitus (on hypoglycemic therapy), glaucoma, prostatism	Postural hypotension, visual symptoms, dry mouth, constipation, urinary retention, impotence
Nerve endings	Rauwolfia alkaloids		Mild to moderate hypertension in young patient	Pheochromocytoma, peptic ulcer, depression, during MAO inhibitor administration	Depression, nightmares, nasal congestion, dyspepsia, diarrhea, impotence
	Reserpine	Oral: 0.1–0.5 mg daily			
	Guanethidine	Oral: 10–300 mg daily	Moderate to severe hypertension	Pheochromocytoma, severe coronary artery disease, cerebrovascular insufficiency, during MAO inhibitor administration	Postural hypotension, bradycardia, dry mouth, diarrhea, impaired ejaculation, fluid retention
Alpha receptors	Phentolamine	IV: 1–5 mg	Suspected or proved pheochromocytoma	Severe coronary artery disease	Tachycardia, weakness, dizziness, flushing
	Phenoxybenzamine	Oral: 10–50 mg once or twice daily (tolerance may develop)	Proved pheochromocytoma		Postural hypotension, tachycardia, miosis, nasal congestion, dry mouth
	Prazosin	Oral: 1–5 mg two or three times daily	Mild to moderate hypertension		Sudden syncope, headache, sedation dizziness, tachycardia
Beta receptors	Propranolol	Oral: 10–120 mg two to four times daily	Mild to moderate hypertension (especially with evidence for hyperdynamic circulation), adjunct to hydralazine therapy	Congestive heart failure, asthma, diabetes mellitus (on hypoglycemic therapy), during MAO inhibitor administration	Dizziness, depression, bronchospasm, nausea, vomiting, diarrhea, constipation, heart failure
	Metoprolol	Oral: 50–225 mg twice daily			
	Nadolol	Oral: 40–320 mg daily			
	Atenolol	Oral: 50–100 mg daily			

TABLE 267-7 *(continued)*
Drugs used in treatment of hypertension—listed according to site of action

Site of action	*Drug*	*Dosage*	*Indications*	*Contraindications*	*Frequent or peculiar side effects*
VASODILATORS					
Vascular smooth muscle	Hydralazine	Oral: 10–75 mg four times daily IV or IM: 10–50 mg every 6 h (tolerance may develop)	As adjunct in treatment of moderate to severe hypertension (oral), malignant hypertension (IV or IM), renal disease with hypertension	Lupus erythematosus, severe coronary artery disease	Headache, tachycardia, angina pectoris, anorexia, nausea, vomiting, diarrhea, lupus-like syndrome
	Minoxidil	Oral: 5–50 mg daily	Severe hypertension	Severe coronary artery disease	Tachycardia, aggravates angina, marked fluid retention, hair growth on face and body, coarsening of facial features, possible pericardial effusions
	Diazoxide	IV: 300 mg rapidly	Severe or malignant hypertension	Diabetes mellitus, hyperuricemia, congestive heart failure	Hyperglycemia, hyperuricemia, sodium retention
	Nitroprusside	IV: 0.5–8 (μg/kg)/min	Malignant hypertension		Apprehension, weakness, diaphoresis, nausea, vomiting, muscle twitching
ANGIOTENSIN-CONVERTING ENZYME INHIBITOR					
	Captopril	Oral: 10–150 mg three times daily	Treatment-resistant hypertension; renal artery stenosis	Renal failure (reduction of dose)	Leukopenia, pancytopenia, proteinuria, nephrotic syndrome, membranous glomerulopathy, urticarial rash, fever, loss of taste

individuals and must be used with caution in diabetics receiving hypoglycemic therapy because they inhibit the usual sympathetic responses to hypoglycemia. Cardioselective beta-blocking agents (so-called $beta_1$ blockers) have been developed (metoprolol, atenolol) which may be superior to nonselective beta blockers such as propranolol in patients with bronchospasm. Nadolol, a nonselective beta blocker, unlike other drugs of this class is excreted unchanged in the urine and has a half-life of 14 to 20 h. Therefore, only one dose a day is required. Atenolol may also need to be given only once a day.

VASODILATORS *Hydralazine* is the most versatile of the drugs that cause direct relaxation of vascular smooth muscle; it is effective both orally and parenterally, acting mainly on arterial resistance, rather than on venous capacitance vessels, as evidenced by lack of postural changes. Unfortunately, the effect of hydralazine on peripheral resistance is partly negated by reflex increases in sympathetic discharges that raise heart rate and cardiac output. These limit the usefulness of hydralazine, especially in patients with severe coronary artery disease. However, the efficacy of hydralazine can be increased if it is given in conjunction with beta blockers or drugs such as methyldopa, clonidine, or reserpine, all of which block reflex sympathetic stimulation of the heart. A serious side effect of doses of hydralazine exceeding 300 mg per day has been the production of a lupus erythematosus-like syndrome.

Minoxidil is even more potent but unfortunately produces significant hirsutism and, therefore, is mainly limited to patients with severe hypertension and renal insufficiency.

An interesting drug in the same category as hydralazine but restricted in its application to acute situations is the thiazide derivative *diazoxide.* It is not a diuretic; in fact, it causes sodium retention. However, like the other thiazides, it reduces carbohydrate tolerance. It must be given rapidly intravenously to guarantee effect. It begins to act immediately to lower blood pressure, and its effects may last for several hours. *Nitroprusside* given intravenously also acts as a direct vasodilator, with onset and offset of actions that are almost immediate. These latter two drugs are useful only for the treatment of hypertensive emergencies (Table 267-9).

ANGIOTENSIN BLOCKERS Drugs from several of the categories discussed above have been shown to possess an additional action resulting in inhibition of renin secretion. These include clonidine, reserpine, methyldopa, and propranolol, with clonidine and propranolol being the most effective. There is also a group of analogues of angiotensin II, e.g., saralasin, that act by antagonizing the effects of angiotensin II; these polypeptides require parenteral administration and are not useful for chronic management. A third group of drugs in this class are those which inhibit the enzyme converting angiotensin I into angiotensin II, e.g., captopril. Data on these converting-enzyme inhibitors are still limited. However, these agents are extremely promising because they not only inhibit the generation of a potent vasoconstrictor (angiotensin II) but also retard the degradation of a potent vasodilator (bradykinin) and may alter prostaglandin production. They are especially useful in renal or renovascular hypertension, as well as in accelerated and malignant hypertension. Their value in milder, uncomplicated hypertension will depend on the incidence and severity of adverse effects with prolonged use.

Approach to drug therapy (Table 267-6) The aim of drug therapy is to use the agents just described, alone or in combination, to return arterial pressure to normal levels with minimal side effects. When used in combination, drugs should be chosen for their different sites of action. Since many effective antihypertensive agents are available, a number of useful therapeutic regimens have been developed. The approach recommended is a modification of the step-care program suggested by the Joint National Committee on Detection, Evaluation and Treatment of High Blood Pressure. In general this approach can be used in most patients with hypertension. Those who have significant hypertension, however (average diastolic pressure of 130 mmHg or more), will require more intensive therapy with several drugs simultaneously. The following plan is suggested for patients without contraindications to specific agents, such as those listed in Table 267-7. The first drug employed is a thiazide diuretic. Even if not effective by itself, it potentiates the action of other hypotensive agents. It should be started at less than maximal doses and gradually increased at 2- to 4-week intervals until either arterial pressure is reduced to normal, maximum levels are reached, or side effects become significant. Reduction of serum potassium levels below 3.3 meq per liter or the simultaneous administration of cardiac glycosides will require potassium supplementation or the addition of a potassium-sparing diuretic. Asymptomatic hyperuricemia (less than 10 mg/dl) usually does not require treatment.

If arterial pressure is not controlled and other reasons for poor therapeutic response are not present (Table 267-8), then the addition of a second drug is appropriate. Prior to this step a search for possible secondary forms of hypertension should be made by performing the following studies (if not previously obtained): rapid-sequence IVP, isotope renogram and/or saralasin test; microscopic urinalysis and urine culture; serum calcium and phosphate; serum potassium; 24-h urine for creatinine, metanephrines, and catecholamines; and, if appropriate, overnight dexamethasone suppression test. If these studies are normal, then one of the antiadrenergic drugs, usually a beta blocker, should be added. Again therapy should begin with small doses, gradually increased until either the hypertension is controlled or a maximum dose is reached (Table 267-7).

If arterial pressure is still not controlled, then the addition of a vasodilator (hydralazine) or, with caution, captopril is indicated. Adequate diuretic therapy and sodium restriction are again important, as is the simultaneous use of a sympathetic blocking drug when vasodilators are used. Hydralazine and minoxidil should be used cautiously in patients with coronary artery disease (angina) since they may increase cardiac rate. There are only a few patients in whom blood pressure cannot be adequately controlled with the above approach. In these, use of other drugs discussed in the previous section should be considered. Failure to obtain adequate pressure control may be due to insufficient volume depletion, and more vigorous dietary sodium restriction and diuretic administration may be helpful in resistant cases. In those few patients who are still resistant, a fourth step is necessary. This consists of giving a different antiadrenergic agent such as clonidine or prazosin, in place of the initial one, or substituting or adding guanethidine or captopril in increasing doses.

TABLE 267-8
Reasons for poor therapeutic response in patients with hypertension

1 Inadequate patient compliance
2 Volume expansion
  a Excessive sodium intake
  b Secondary to nondiuretic antihypertensive agent
3 Inadequate doses
4 Drug antagonism
  a Cold remedies
  b Sympathomimetics
  c Oral contraceptives (estrogens)
  d Adrenal steroids
5 Secondary forms of hypertension
  a Pheochromocytoma
  b Renal disease
6 Inappropriate combination therapy

While the recommendations outlined above are satisfactory for the majority of patients, it is important to use a flexible approach since individual patients may respond differently to each combination of drugs. For those patients requiring multiple drugs, once the appropriate combination has been found, the use of a single pill with the appropriate combination of drugs may simplify the regimen and thereby increase compliance. Every effort should be made to reduce the number of times each day the patient must interrupt his or her schedule for the medication.

As noted earlier, in those patients who present with markedly elevated diastolic pressure—greater than 125 mmHg—an accelerated treatment program is needed including the initial use of maximum therapeutic doses of two or more drugs.

Reduction of arterial pressure in hypertensive patients with impaired renal function is often accompanied by an initial increase in serum creatinine. This change does not represent further structural renal damage and should not deter continuation of therapy, since achievement of blood pressure control may eventually reduce the value toward normal. Therapy in the azotemic patient should emphasize the use of those drugs that have the least propensity to lower renal blood flow, namely, captopril and to a lesser extent hydralazine, clonidine, and methyldopa. However, captopril and methyldopa may accumulate in the presence of renal failure, and the dosage might have to be reduced.

Probably fewer than one-third of hypertensive patients in the United States are being treated effectively. Only a small number of these failures is related to drug unresponsiveness. The majority is related to (1) failure to detect hypertension, (2) failure to institute effective treatment of the asymptomatic hypertensive subject, and (3) failure of the asymptomatic hypertensive subject to adhere to therapy. In order to improve this deficiency, patients must be educated to continue treatment once an effective regimen has been identified. Side effects and inconveniences of treatment must be minimized or counteracted in order to obtain the patient's continued cooperation.

MALIGNANT HYPERTENSION

In addition to marked blood pressure elevation in association with papilledema and retinal hemorrhages and exudates, the full-blown picture of malignant hypertension may include manifestations of hypertensive encephalopathy, such as severe headache, vomiting, visual disturbances (including transient blindness), transient paralyses, convulsions, stupor, and coma. These have been attributed to spasms of cerebral vessels and to cerebral edema. In some patients who have died, multiple small thrombi have been found in the cerebral vessels. Cardiac decompensation and rapidly declining renal function are other critical features of malignant hypertension. Oliguria may, in fact, be the presenting feature. The vascular lesion characteristic of malignant hypertension is fibrinoid necrosis of the walls of small arteries and arterioles, and this can be reversed by effective antihypertensive therapy.

The pathogenesis of malignant hypertension is unknown. However, at least two independent processes, dilatation of cerebral arteries and generalized arteriolar fibrinoid necrosis, contribute to the associated signs and symptoms. The cerebral arteries dilate because the normal autoregulation of cerebral blood flow decompensates secondary to the markedly elevated arterial pressure. As a result, cerebral blood flow is excessive, producing the encephalopathy associated with malignant hypertension. Many patients also show evidence of a microangiopathic hemolytic anemia, but this appears to be a secondary phenomenon, which could, however, contribute to the deterioration of renal function. Most patients also have elevated levels of peripheral plasma renin activity and increased aldosterone production, and these may be involved in causing vascular damage.

About 1 percent of hypertensive patients develop the malignant phase, which occurs in the course of both essential and secondary hypertension. Rarely it is the first recognized manifestation of the blood pressure problem. The average age at diagnosis is 40, and men are more often affected than women. Prior to the availability of effective therapy, life expectancy after diagnosis of malignant hypertension was less than 2 years, with most deaths being due to renal failure, cerebral hemorrhage, or congestive heart failure. With the advent of effective antihypertensive therapy, at least half of patients survive for more than 5 years.

Malignant hypertension is a medical emergency and requires immediate therapy. The initial aim of therapy should be to reduce diastolic pressure toward, but not below, 90 mmHg. The drugs available for treatment of malignant hypertension can be divided into two groups on the basis of time of onset of action (Table 267-9). Those in the first group act within a few minutes but are not satisfactory for long-term management. If the patient is having convulsions, if arterial pressure must be reduced rapidly, then one from the immediate-acting group should be used. *Diazoxide* is the easiest to administer, for no individual titration of dosage is required. A dose of 300 mg is given rapidly intravenously, and the antihypertensive effect is noted in 1 to 2 min. The same dose can be repeated when the pressure begins to rise, usually after several hours. In an occasional patient, pressure may drop below normal levels after diazoxide administration. Because of this, some physicians use a modified program, giving 150 mg rather than 300 mg initially, followed by a second 150-mg dose in 5 min if the blood pressure response has been minimal. It should not be used in patients who may have a dissecting aneurysm. The other two agents in this group require continuous infusion and close monitoring. *Nitroprusside* is given by continuous intravenous infusion at a dose of 0.5 to 8.0 (μg/kg)/min. It has the advantage over the ganglionic blockers of not being associated with the development of tachyphylaxis and can be utilized for days with few side effects. The dosage must be controlled with an infusion pump. *Trimethaphan,* a ganglionic blocker, is given at a rate of 1 to 15 mg/min. The patient should be in the sitting position, and the pressure should be monitored closely, preferably in an intensive care unit.

Patients given any of these agents should also receive other medications effective for long-term control. Those in the second group require 30 min or more to obtain full effect, but have the advantage of being satisfactory for subsequent oral administration and for long-term management of the patient's hypertension (Table 267-9). If such a delay in attainment of full effect is acceptable, intravenous *methyldopa* is an effective drug with which to begin therapy if symptoms of encephalopathy are absent. A dose of 500 mg in 100 to 200 ml 5% dextrose in water is given intravenously over 30 min; if the effect is inadequate in 2 to 4 h, a second dose of 500 to 1000 mg is given. Additional intravenous doses may then be given every 6 h until the pressure is stabilized. Intravenous *hydralazine* is effective in many patients within 10 min; an effective protocol involves giving 10-mg doses intravenously every 10 to 15 min until the desired effect has been obtained or until a total of 50 mg has been administered. The total required for response may then be repeated intramuscularly or intravenously every 6 h. Hydralazine should be used with caution in patients with significant coronary artery disease and should be avoided in patients evidencing myocardial ischemia or dissecting aneurysm. The converting-enzyme inhibitor, *captopril,* while promising in preliminary studies, is still under investigation.

The potent diuretics furosemide and ethacrynic acid are important adjuncts to the therapy just discussed. Given either orally or intravenously, they serve to maintain sodium diuresis in the face of a falling arterial pressure, and thus will speed recovery from encephalopathy and congestive heart failure as well as maintain sensitivity to the primary antihypertensive drug. Digitalis (Chap. 253) also is indicated if there is evidence of cardiac decompensation.

In patients with malignant hypertension in whom the existence of pheochromocytoma is suspected, urine should be collected for measurement of the products of catecholamine metabolism, and drugs which might release additional catecholamines, such as methyldopa, reserpine, and guanethidine, must be avoided. The parenteral drug of choice in these patients is phentolamine administered with care to avoid a precipitous reduction in arterial pressure.

There is hope even for patients who fail to respond sufficiently to any of the forms of therapy and who show progressive deterioration in renal function. In some, a period of peritoneal dialysis or hemodialysis to deplete extracellular fluid has resulted in better blood pressure control and eventual improvement in renal function. In other patients with refractory hypertension and renal failure who do not respond to volume depletion or hypotensive therapy, including minoxidil, particularly those with marked elevation of plasma renin activity, bilateral nephrectomy has resulted in amelioration of hypertension; subsequently these patients have been maintained on chronic dialysis or have received renal homografts. However,

TABLE 267-9
Therapeutic agents used to treat malignant hypertension

Drug	*Route*	*Time course of action*			*Oral preparation available*
		Onset	*Peak*	*Duration*	
IMMEDIATE ONSET					
Diazoxide	IV bolus	1–3 min	2–4 min	4–12 h	No
Nitroprusside	Continuous IV	<1 min	1–2 min	2–5 min	No
Trimethaphan	Continuous IV	<1 min	1–2 min	2–5 min	No
DELAYED ONSET					
Hydralazine	IV, IM	10–20 min	20–40 min	2–6 h	Yes
Methyldopa	IV	1–3 h	3–5 h	2–12 h	Yes
Reserpine	IM	2–3 h	3–4 h	6–24 h	Yes

bilateral nephrectomy should be avoided where possible since (1) the loss of renal erythropoietin will contribute to the associated anemia, (2) vitamin D metabolism may be adversely affected, and (3) all residual renal function will be lost.

REFERENCES

Atkinson AB et al: Captopril in clinical hypertension. Changes in components of renin angiotensin system and in body composition in relation to fall in blood pressure with a note on measurement of angiotensin II during converting enzyme inhibition. Br Heart J 44:290, 1980

Bennett PN et al: Thirty years of drugs for hypertension. Brit J Clin Pharmacol 13:1, 1982

Berglund G et al: Prevalence of primary and secondary hypertension: Studies in a random population sample. Br Med J 2:554, 1976

Campese VM et al: Role of sympathetic nerve inhibition and body sodium-volume state in the antihypertensive action of clonidine in essential hypertension. Kidney Int 18:351, 1980

Dluhy RG et al: Abnormal adrenal responsiveness and angiotensin II dependency in high renin essential hypertension. J Clin Invest 64:270, 1979

Fujita T et al: Factors influencing blood pressure in salt-sensitive patients with hypertension. Am J Med 69:334, 1980

Genest J et al: Role of the adrenal cortex and sodium in the pathogenesis of human hypertension. Can Med J 118:538, 1978

Hegeland A: Treatment of mild hypertension: A five year controlled drug trial. The Oslo study. Am J Med 5:725, 1980

Hollenberg NK et al: Renin, angiotensin and an angiotensin antagonist: Response to saralasin in essential and secondary hypertension. Medicine 58:115, 1979

Huang CM et al: Comparison of antihypertensive effects of captopril and propranolol in essential hypertension. JAMA 245:478, 1981

Hypertension Detection and Follow-up Program Cooperative Group: Five year findings, JAMA 242:2562, 1979

Kaplan NM: *Clinical Hypertension,* 3d ed. Baltimore, Williams & Wilkins, 1983

Klahr S, Massry SG: *Contemporary Nephrology.* New York, Plenum, 1981

Linas SL et al: Minoxidil. Ann Intern Med 94:61, 1981

Ram CVS et al: Moderate sodium restriction and various diuretics in the treatment of hypertension. Arch Intern Med 141:1015, 1981

Strandgaard S: Autoregulation of cerebral blood flow in hypertensive patients. Circulation 53:720, 1976

268 DISEASES OF THE AORTA

JAMES E. DALEN

The walls of the aorta must withstand the shearing effect of each systolic thrust of blood. With its large diameter, the aorta is under greater tension than the rest of the arterial system because wall tension is a direct function of both diameter and pressure. For this reason, the effects of hypertension are particularly deleterious. In addition, the aorta is subject to infection, trauma, necrosis of the media, and, most notably, arteriosclerosis, which has replaced syphilis as the most frequent disease affecting the aorta. Arising from these stresses are four major diseases of the aorta: aneurysm, dissection, arteriosclerotic occlusive disease, and aortitis. The number of deaths due to disease of the aorta is uncertain because other cardiovascular disease, ischemic heart disease, hypertensive disease, and cerebrovascular disease often coexist and take priority in the coding of death certificates.

ANEURYSMS A "true" aortic aneurysm is an abnormal widening that involves all three layers of its wall. The basic defect is destruction of elastic fibers in the media, which permits the remaining fibrous tissue to stretch and leads to an increase in diameter, which in turn raises wall tension. As this process leads to further enlargement, rupture becomes increasingly possible. "False" aneurysms, which are usually caused by trauma, are those disruptions of the inner and medial segments of the wall which permit expansion of the aorta so that the wall of the aneurysm consists of only adventitia and/or perivascular clot.

The commonest aneurysms are *fusiform,* in which a segment of the aorta becomes diffusely dilated, its total circumference being affected. In contrast, *saccular* aneurysms involve a portion of the circumference and consist of an outpouching with a mouth.

The commonest underlying cause of aneurysm is arteriosclerosis, but cystic medial necrosis, trauma, and syphilis and other infections must also be noted as causes.

Aneurysms of the abdominal aorta Three-fourths of all aortic aneurysms occur in the abdominal aorta, just below the renal arteries. Nearly all aneurysms in the abdominal aorta are caused by arteriosclerosis. The majority of victims are men older than age 60; more than half have associated hypertension. The incidence is increased in cigarette smokers.

The *diagnosis* is often made by physical examination, which reveals a pulsating mass in the midepigastrium. The diagnosis may first be suspected by x-ray of the abdomen, which demonstrates curvilinear calcification in the wall of the aneurysm. The diagnosis is confirmed by *ultrasound.* Continuous ultrasonic B scanning can visualize the abdominal aorta in longitudinal and transverse sections. This permits delineation of the size of the abdominal aorta and the thickness of its walls. It also allows detection of intraluminal clot. Its noninvasive nature permits serial estimation of the size of the aneurysm. Computed tomography can also accurately delineate abdominal aneurysms and may identify those that are at risk of rupture. Most patients are asymptomatic when the diagnosis is first made. When symptoms do occur, they consist of abdominal or low back pain.

The *prognosis* depends upon the size of the aneurysm and, very importantly, the presence of other arteriosclerotic cardiovascular diseases. The diameter of the normal abdominal aorta is 2.5 cm. When the diameter of the aneurysm is greater than 6 cm, the probability of rupture in a 10-year period is 45 to 50 percent, whereas it is only 15 to 20 percent when the diameter is less than 6 cm.

Ischemic arteriosclerotic heart disease, which is present in about one-half of patients with abdominal aneurysm, has a profound impact on the prognosis. In one series of patients who had not had surgery, 5-year survival without clinically evident associated coronary disease was 50 percent. With ischemic heart disease, 5-year survival was only 20 percent. Follow-up of patients without surgery for abdominal aneurysms has shown that about one-third die of rupture of the aneurysm and one-third die of associated cardiovascular disease.

In properly selected patients operation prolongs life by preventing rupture. Symptomatic or expanding aneurysms and aneurysms more than 6 cm in diameter should have prompt surgical correction. The therapeutic decision for patients with asymptomatic aneurysms of moderate size (4 to 6 cm) is more difficult. Operative mortality with elective surgery, that is, before rupture, is about 5 to 10 percent. It is influenced by the size of the aneurysm but far more by the presence of associated cardiovascular disease. If there is no significant associated cardiovascular disease, small (4 to 6 cm) asymptomatic aneurysms should usually have surgical correction. With significant associated disease, it may be appropriate to follow the patient with serial ultrasound examinations. Surgery should be performed if symptoms occur, or if there is a significant increase in the size of the aneurysm.

Some patients with ruptured aneurysms survive long enough to become candidates for emergency surgical repair. They usually present, in shock, with severe pain in the abdomen, the lower back, or both. A tender pulsatile mass may be palpated. The salvage rate with emergency surgery in these circumstances is about 50 percent.

Aneurysms of the descending aorta The second most frequent site of aortic aneurysms is in the descending aorta just distal to the origin of the left subclavian artery. These aneurysms are usually fusiform and due to arteriosclerosis. Many patients with an aneurysm of the descending aorta also have an aneurysm of the abdominal aorta. Most patients are asymptomatic when the diagnosis is first suspected by chest x-ray and then confirmed by fluoroscopy or aortography. Resection of thoracic aneurysms is more difficult than is resection of abdominal aneurysms. The risk of operation is in large part determined by associated cardiovascular or pulmonary disease. Operative therapy to prevent rupture is indicated if the aneurysm is symptomatic, larger than 10 cm in transverse diameter, or enlarging rapidly, unless associated cardiovascular disease presents a prohibitive risk.

Traumatic, false aneurysms of the descending aorta may occur in patients who survive rupture of the aorta. The most frequent cause is deceleration injuries suffered in automobile accidents. Rupture usually occurs at the site of the ligamentum arteriosum. These patients usually note chest and back pain, similar to that associated with dissection. Blood pressure may be increased in the upper extremities, but absent or decreased in the lower extremities. Chest x-ray usually shows mediastinal widening. The diagnosis is confirmed by computed tomography and angiography. These patients are likely to be young and without associated cardiovascular disease. Surgical resection is indicated.

Less frequently, aneurysms of the descending aorta are saccular owing to *lues* or other *infection* (mycotic aneurysms). Saccular aneurysms are particularly likely to rupture and should be treated surgically.

Aneurysms of the ascending aorta In a prior era, nearly all aneurysms of the ascending aorta were due to *syphilis*. They were readily recognized by x-ray by the presence of calcification in the wall of the ascending aorta. Luetic aneurysms can become huge, causing signs and symptoms by compression of adjacent structures. At the present time, the commonest cause of aneurysms of the ascending aorta is *cystic medial necrosis*, which may occur in association with Marfan's syndrome or as a response to hypertension and/or aging of the aorta, or it may be of unknown etiology.

Aneurysms of the ascending aorta, particularly when they are due to cystic medial necrosis, may cause aortic regurgitation and lead to left ventricular failure. In this circumstance, resection of the aneurysm and replacement of the ascending aorta and aortic valve and coronary reimplantation are indicated.

The most common symptom of large aneurysms of the ascending aorta is chest pain, usually described as a deep, diffuse, aching sensation. The decision to resect an asymptomatic aneurysm to prevent rupture depends upon its size, the presence and severity of aortic regurgitation, and the presence of associated cardiovascular disease.

Aneurysms of the aortic arch These aneurysms—the least frequent of all—are the most likely to cause symptoms because they compress adjacent structures, thus causing dysphagia, dry cough, hoarseness, dyspnea, or pain. Arch aneurysms may be fusiform due to arteriosclerosis, or saccular due to syphilis or other infection. Surgical correction of aneurysms of the aortic arch carries an operative risk as high as 40 to 50 percent.

Management of concurrent hypertension Hypertension, which is present in more than half of patients with aortic aneurysms, needs optimal management. Persistent systolic hypertension abets further enlargement of aneurysms and may predispose to their rupture. In addition to standard antihypertension medications, propranolol is appropriate to help control hypertension and, in addition, decrease stress to the aortic wall by blunting myocardial contractility.

DISSECTION OF THE AORTA This occurs when the intima is interrupted so that blood enters the wall of the aorta and separates its layers. Dissection is the most frequent and the most important acute disease involving the aorta and, without treatment, is almost always fatal. With prompt diagnosis and appropriate therapy, the majority of patients survive.

As with aneurysm of the aorta, the basic defect that permits dissection is disease of the media. The commonest disorder of the media that predisposes to dissection is *cystic medial necrosis*, which, in some instances, may be associated with Marfan's syndrome or, more commonly, with disorders that increase the hemodynamic stress on the aorta such as hypertension, pregnancy, coarctation, or bicuspid aortic valve. A far less common cause of disease of the media predisposing to dissection is arteriosclerosis.

Nearly all aortic dissections begin as a tear in the intima at one of two sites: the ascending aorta (2 to 5 cm above the aortic valve) or the descending aorta, just distal to the origin of the left subclavian artery. The aorta is relatively fixed in each of these two positions, but is mobile on each side. Thus, at these two points, the hemodynamic stress of each systolic pressure wave is maximal, and the intima overlying diseased media may tear there, permitting blood to enter and separate the layers of the aorta.

The signs and symptoms and, importantly, the therapeutic implications are quite different when dissection involves the ascending aorta as opposed to dissection limited to the descending aorta.

Dissection of the ascending aorta Dissection usually begins as an intimal tear in the proximal ascending aorta and extends antegrade around the arch into the descending and abdominal aorta. This type of aortic dissection is the most common and the most lethal. In other cases, the intimal tear may occur in the aortic arch or descending aorta, and the dissection may progress retrograde to involve the ascending aorta. The majority of these patients are men under age 60. About one-half have hypertension.

Dissection of the ascending aorta is heralded by the abrupt onset of very severe chest pain (Chap. 4). Unlike the pain of myocardial infarction, the pain is maximal at the onset. The pain is most frequent in the anterior chest, but may radiate to, or even be limited to, the midscapular area of the back. The pain is nearly always initially attributed to acute myocardial infarction. There are several ways that the appropriate diagnosis may be made. Since dissection of the ascending aorta involves the great vessels in the majority of cases, a discrepancy between the carotid pulses, or a difference in the blood pressure in the two arms, should lead to a search for other evidence of aortic dissection. Dissection involving the carotids can cause a sudden neurologic deficit that may be intermittent. If the dissection compromises the right coronary artery, arrhythmias may occur, and occasionally there may be electrocardiographic signs of acute myocardial infarction. In approximately one-half of patients, the dissection causes acute aortic regurgitation. The presence of a new murmur of aortic regurgitation in the setting of apparent myocardial infarction should suggest the possibility of dissection of the ascending aorta. In the most severe cases, dissection causes hemopericardium. The appearance of a pericardial friction rub may be rapidly followed by pericardial tamponade.

Chest x-ray provides the most important clue to the presence of dissection of the ascending aorta. The most consistent finding is widening of the superior mediastinum. The ascending aorta may be enlarged out of proportion to the descending aorta. Once dissection is suspected by physical examination or chest x-ray, preparations for aortography to confirm the diagnosis should be made at once. Dissection of the ascending aorta can also be recognized by computed tomography. Unless hypotension is present, medical treatment, aimed at lowering blood pressure and depressing myocardial contractility, should be begun. This is most appropriately effected by beginning an infusion of trimethaphan (Arfonad), 1 to 2 mg/min, or nitroprusside, 20 to 400 ng/min, with intraarterial pressure monitoring in place.

Aortography or cineangiography, performed by the retrograde arterial technique will usually demonstrate a false lumen, and possibly an intimal flap separating the true and false lumina in the ascending aorta. If the blood in the false lumen has clotted, the principal finding will be an abnormal narrowing of the true lumen.

Once the diagnosis of dissection involving the ascending aorta has been established by aortography, the majority of patients should have surgical correction, which consists of resection of the portion of the aorta containing the intimal tear and replacement with a prosthetic graft. Concomitant aortic valve replacement is frequently required if severe aortic regurgitation is present. Surgical correction can be performed at a risk of about 20 percent. Although medical treatment is vital to stabilize the patient prior to operation, it rarely is definitive in patients with dissection involving the ascending aorta because the majority develop life-threatening complications, such as hemopericardium, hypotension, compromise of the carotid or coronary arteries, or aortic regurgitation. Without treatment, death is usually due to rupture into the pericardium.

Dissection of the descending aorta Dissection limited to the descending aorta is most likely to occur in elderly hypertensive patients. Dissection ordinarily begins with an intimal tear just beyond the origin of the left subclavian artery and the hematoma proceeds distally to the diaphragm or into the abdominal aorta. Dissection of the descending aorta usually does not proceed in retrograde fashion. Therefore, aortic regurgitation and hemopericardium do not occur. The carotid pulses and blood pressure in the arms are usually not altered. The primary symptom is the sudden onset of chest pain, often interscapular, often radiating to the anterior chest. The prime supporting evidence of dissection is to be found in the chest roentgenogram, which usually shows a widening of the superior mediastinum and may show the descending to be larger than the ascending aorta. If there is intimal calcification in the aortic knob, its distance from the outer border of the aortic shadow may be increased.

The diagnosis of dissection of the descending aorta should be confirmed by aortography. As with dissection involving the ascending aorta, hypotensive treatment should begin when the diagnosis is first suspected. Trimethaphan or nitroprusside, in a continuous intravenous drip at an infusion rate sufficient to keep systolic pressure at 100 to 120 mmHg, are the ideal first drugs. Propranolol or reserpine should also be begun.

Patients with dissection of the descending aorta usually do not have urgent indications for surgical correction. Medical treatment to lower systolic pressure, and to depress myocardial contractility so as to blunt the force of systole, may control the dissection. If medical treatment does not relieve the pain, or if there is evidence of progression of the dissection by x-ray or the appearance of a left pleural effusion (due to hemothorax), surgical resection should be performed. Surgical correction of dissection of the descending aorta poses a higher risk than dissection of the ascending aorta because the patients are older and are more likely to have associated cardiovascular disease. Elective surgical correction may be indicated after the dissection is controlled with medical therapy.

Prolonged, optimal control of hypertension is essential in patients with dissection of the ascending or descending aorta. In the absence of overt or latent congestive heart failure, it is advisable to include propranolol in the regimen to help prevent recurrent dissection.

ARTERIOSCLEROTIC OCCLUSIVE DISEASE The majority of adults in the United States have some degree of arteriosclerosis of the aorta. However, the disease remains silent unless it causes aneurysm, or unless it is sufficiently advanced to cause occlusive disease. The mildest form of arteriosclerosis of the aorta, longitudinal fatty streaks of the intima, may be seen in children (Chap. 266). Elevated intimal plaques begin to appear in adult life. Occlusive disease of the aorta may occur if these plaques are complicated by hemorrhage, ulceration, calcification, or overlying thrombus formation.

Arteriosclerotic occlusive disease is most frequent in the abdominal aorta, where it involves the terminal part of the aorta and extends for a variable distance into the iliac and femoral arteries. Arteriosclerosis of the aorta may be complicated by superimposed thrombosis. Depending upon the adequacy of collateral circulation, arteriosclerotic occlusive disease may cause ischemia of the lower extremities.

The classic symptom is claudication, which is present in the buttocks and thighs or in the calves. If the occlusive disease is severe, or the collateral circulation is poor, severe ischemia may lead to pain at rest or tissue necrosis and gangrene. Impotence may also occur. The femoral pulses are absent or diminished in the majority of cases. Arteriography is needed to delineate the extent of the disease.

Surgical treatment consists of aortic-femoral bypass grafting. Endarterectomy may be indicated when the disease is limited to the terminal aorta and proximal iliac arteries. The results of operation are usually excellent; symptoms are relieved or decreased in more than 90 percent of the patients in some series. Patency rates of 80 to 90 percent at 5 years have been reported. As with aneurysms, operative and late mortality is usually due to associated ischemic heart disease, which is present in up to one-half of the patients. The status of coronary and cerebrovascular circulations should be assessed prior to operation.

Symptomatic arteriosclerotic occlusive disease is rare in the ascending or descending thoracic aorta but may occur in the arch, where it becomes symptomatic by compromising the origin of one or more of the arch vessels. The carotid pulses, and/or pulses of the upper extremities, may be obliterated; thus, arteriosclerotic occlusive disease is one of the causes of the aortic arch syndrome. Other causes of this syndrome (also called "pulseless disease") include Takayasu's arteritis, syphilis, trauma, and neoplasm. Symptoms may include ischemia of the upper extremities or, more commonly, cerebrovascular ischemia, dependent upon the location of the disease. Surgical correction is usually feasible; utilizing an extraanatomic bypass graft; however, its appropriateness depends upon the extent of the disease, and the status of the coronary and cerebral circulations.

AORTITIS Several different diseases may cause aortitis, i.e., an inflammatory process involving the wall of the aorta. The pathophysiology of aortitis depends on the severity of the process and upon its location. Aortitis becomes most evident when it involves the origins of the vessels of the aortic arch. Under these circumstances, it can, as noted above, cause the aortic arch syndrome.

The best understood cause of aortitis is *syphilis.* Only 10 percent of patients with luetic aortitis develop complications that permit its detection during life: saccular thoracic aneurysms, aortic valvulitis causing aortic regurgitation, and stenosis of the coronary ostia. Uncomplicated luetic aortitis is recognized at postmortem as a chronic panarteritis that causes patchy destruction of smooth muscle and elastic tissue of the media, endarteritis obliterans of the vasa vasorum, and intimal atherosclerosis. The process is most marked in the ascending aorta because of the predilection of treponemas for its rich lymphatic supply. The only clinical correlates of uncomplicated luetic aortitis are dilatation of the ascending aorta with or without calcification and a tambour-like aortic second sound.

TAKAYASU'S DISEASE Takayasu's disease is a nonspecific obstructive arteritis that has a particular predilection for the aortic arch of young females. It is more common in the orient than in the west. Although it is suspected to be an autoimmune disease, its exact etiology is unknown. In the majority of cases, the disease begins in the second or third decade of life. In its initial stage, constitutional symptoms may occur. These may include fever, malaise, anorexia, weight loss, night sweats, and at times arthralgias.

These constitutional symptoms are then replaced by signs and symptoms secondary to involvement of the large arteries, particularly the aortic arch and its main branches. The pathologic lesion is a panarteritis that seems to begin with inflammation of the adventitia, with subsequent disruption and fibrotic changes in the media, and marked proliferation of the intima. Involvement of the arch vessels may be heralded by local pain and the presence of bruits. Progression of the aortitis causes stenosis at, or obliteration of, the origins of the arch vessels, thereby causing the aortic arch syndrome. Obstruction of the carotid arteries causes blurred vision, syncope, and dizziness secondary to cerebral ischemia. Involvement of the subclavian arteries causes paresthesias, intermittent claudication, and loss of pulses of the upper extremities. The pulmonary arteries may be involved in some cases. Hypertension occurs in the majority of cases owing to involvement of the renal arteries or to suprarenal obstruction of the aorta. The presence of hypertension, with absent pulses in the upper extremities, has caused this syndrome to be called *reversed coarctation.* The diagnosis is confirmed by angiographic study of the aorta.

Reconstructive vascular surgery may relieve symptoms; however, the disease follows a relentless course so that death from congestive failure or stroke usually occurs within 5 years of diagnosis. Although some studies have shown that corticosteroid therapy may alleviate some of the constitutional symptoms of this disease, there is no evidence that treatment improves life expectancy.

REFERENCES

BAHNSON HT et al: The aorta, in *Gibbon's Surgery of the Chest,* 3d ed, DC Sabiston, FC Spencer (eds). Philadelphia, Saunders, 1976, p 878

BERNSTEIN EF et al: Growth rates of small abdominal aortic aneurysms. Surgery 80:765, 1976

DALEN JE et al: Dissection of the aorta: Pathogenesis, diagnosis, and treatment. Prog Cardiovasc Dis 23:237, 1980

DEBAKEY ME et al: Aneurysms of the thoracic aorta. Mod Concepts Cardiovasc Dis 10:53, 1975

ISHIKAWA K: Natural history and classification of occlusive thromboaortopathy (Takayasu's disease). Circulation 57:27, 1978

LUPI-HERRERA E et al: Takayasu's arteritis: Clinical study of 107 cases. Am Heart J 93:94, 1977

MALONE JM et al: The natural history of bilateral aortofemoral bypass grafts for ischemia of the lower extremities. Arch Surg 110:1300, 1975

MILLER DC et al: Operative treatment of aortic dissections: Experience with 125 patients over a sixteen-year period. J Thorac Cardiovasc Surg 78:365, 1979

SLATER EE, DESANCTIS RW: Disease of the aorta, in *Heart Disease,* 2d ed, E Braunwald (ed). Philadelphia, Saunders, 1980, chap 45

SMUCKLER AL et al: Echocardiographic diagnosis of aortic root dissection by M-mode and two-dimensional techniques. Am Heart J 103:897, 1982

SZILAGYI DE et al: Contribution of abdominal aortic aneurysmectomy to prolongation of life. Ann Surg 164:678, 1966

THOMPSON JE et al: Surgical management of abdominal aortic aneurysms. Ann Surg 181:654, 1975

WHEAT MW: Acute dissecting aneurysms of the aorta: Diagnosis and treatment—1979. Am Heart J 99:373, 1980

269 VASCULAR DISEASES OF THE EXTREMITIES

D. EUGENE STRANDNESS, JR.

The correct approach to patients with suspected peripheral vascular disease is to identify the system involved (arterial, venous, or lymphatic), estimate the degree of disability, and determine if special tests are required to clarify further the extent of the involvement. The therapy employed depends upon a knowledge of the natural history of the disorder as related to known risk factors, the potential for further complications, and the likelihood that available therapy will be successful.

ARTERIAL DISORDERS

ACUTE ARTERIAL OCCLUSION Sudden interruption of the blood supply results in a spectrum of symptoms and signs which are dependent upon the location and extent of the occlusion and existing collateral circulation. The major causes are embolism, thrombosis, and injury. In the arm, the heart is the source of emboli in 95 percent of the patients. Less common causes include emboli from ulcerated plaques in the subclavian artery, aneurysms of the arch vessels, and paradoxical emboli via a patent foramen ovale.

In the leg, the heart is again the most common source of emboli, but they may also arise from ulcerated plaques and aneurysms of the thoracic, abdominal, femoral, and popliteal arteries. Over half of the large emboli from the heart lodge in the femoral or popliteal arteries. The iliac arteries are involved in approximately one-fifth, the abdominal aorta in one-sixth. The remainder will occlude the tibial or peroneal vessels.

When the heart is the source, the causes include mural thrombi from the left atrium or ventricle and the aortic or mitral valve. Mural thrombi arise secondary to atrial fibrillation or on the endocardial surface of the ventricle secondary to myocardial infarction. A prosthetic valve in either the aortic or mitral position may also be the source. While uncommon, the possibility of an atrial myxoma must always be kept in mind. When emboli arise from ulcerated plaques or aneurysms, they are often small and lodge in the small arteries of the distal limb. When they arise from the abdominal or thoracic aorta, bilateral involvement is the rule.

Arterial thrombosis occurs secondary to injury, arteriosclerosis obliterans, femoral or popliteal aneurysms, collagen vascular diseases, myeloproliferative disorders, disseminated intravascular coagulation, and the dysproteinemias.

Symptoms and signs Acute arterial occlusion results in symptoms and signs related to the site of involvement and the immediately available collateral circulation. If the pressure distal to the obstruction falls to below 40 mmHg, the clinical picture will be dramatic. The initial complaint is pain in the most distal part of the limb, followed by pallor, coldness, and a sensation of numbness. Cutaneous sensation is lost within the first hour. Within 6 h, ischemic muscular contracture develops associated with subcutaneous hemorrhage and focal areas of gangrene. Fixed staining of the skin is the most certain sign of irreversible tissue death.

If limb viability is not in question, pallor, a decrease in temperature, and numbness may be the only complaints. The appearance of rest pain in the digits and forefoot indicates that arterial inflow is marginal. Pulses are absent distal to the site of occlusion.

Though the diagnosis is rarely difficult when the extent of the ischemia is as outlined above, there are important variations in the clinical picture. If the immediately available collateral circulation is sufficient to maintain viability, the patient may complain only of a sensation of numbness, usually accompanied by a decrease in the temperature of the part. Under these circumstances, the circulation will nearly always improve, with these minor symptoms disappearing over the course of several hours.

Diagnosis The most important elements include the history of the sudden onset of pain, coldness, and numbness. If a combination of pain, pallor, and paralysis is noted, limb viability will be lost unless the responsible lesion can be corrected within a time frame of 6 h or less. If the limb remains viable, the only complaints may be coldness and numbness. Detection of a bruit is common when an arterial plaque or aneurysm is the source of the embolus.

When the leg is affected, it is important to determine if there is a history of intermittent claudication since under these circumstances, the acute ischemia may be due to thrombosis on an ulcerated plaque. When cholesterol emboli occur, the symptoms may be confusing depending upon the source. The most common situation is the "blue-toe" syndrome, which may be bilateral if the origin is the abdominal or thoracic aorta. Ischemic rest pain is often present and accompanied by prominent livedo reticularis of the feet. Peripheral pulses are nearly always present, since emboli rarely pass through collateral arteries in sufficient quantity to produce serious foot ischemia. When these tiny emboli originate from the thoracic aorta, abdominal pain and hematuria may also occur. Aneurysms of the femoral and popliteal arteries must always be kept in mind. The initial manifestation is often thrombosis or embolization. The diagnosis may be suspected by physical examination and verified by B-mode ultrasound.

Arteriography is rarely necessary to make the diagnosis of major artery occlusion and results in needless, dangerous delay when severe ischemia is present.

Treatment When limb viability is threatened, immediate operation is required for occlusion of the major arteries. Embolectomy is nearly always feasible and can be performed under local anesthesia. Heparin is always given immediately and continued until oral anticoagulation can be accomplished. Operative arteriography is often required not only to verify the diagnosis but also to evaluate the success of the procedure. In the case of thrombosis on a plaque, thrombectomy alone is often not successful, and some form of bypass grafting may be required.

In the arm, occlusions of the radial, ulnar, or brachial artery may often be treated nonoperatively with good results. However, patients with brachial artery occlusions may later have arm claudication if their occupation requires heavy physical labor. In the leg, isolated occlusions distal to the popliteal artery rarely require operative intervention. If the obstruction is in or proximal to the popliteal artery, embolectomy should be carried out (with few exceptions) not only because of a higher incidence of limb loss but also because of subsequent development of intermittent claudication.

Long-term anticoagulation must be used to prevent recurrence of the embolism. If a cardiac lesion is found, serious consideration should be given to operative correction of the underlying problem. Patients with microemboli should be treated expectantly with aspirin and dipyridamole (Persantine). While controversial, surgery should be reserved for those patients in whom aneurysms (particularly femoral and popliteal) are the source of emboli. Vasodilator drugs are not helpful during either the acute or chronic phases of therapy.

ARTERIOSCLEROSIS OBLITERANS The primary lesion of arteriosclerosis is the intimal plaque, which progressively narrows and, in many instances, leads to complete occlusion of large and medium-sized arteries (Chap. 266). In the abdomen the disease has its highest incidence in the aorta and common iliac arteries. The external iliac arteries are often spared. Distal to the inguinal ligament, occlusions are most common in the adductor canal, with the popliteal artery itself down to the level of its three major branches having a much lower incidence of involvement. In the lower leg, the posterior tibial artery at the ankle and the anterior tibial at its origin are most commonly diseased. Arteriosclerosis obliterans is usually a segmental disease, with marked variation from patient to patient in its extent.

Clinical features Unless complicated by thrombosis, the symptoms and signs that develop secondary to arteriosclerosis obliterans rarely have an abrupt onset, since the process is a gradual, progressive one. The most common symptom occurs with exercise and is termed *intermittent claudication*, i.e., the pain that occurs in a muscle(s) with an inadequate blood supply that is stressed by exercise. The patient often describes the discomfort as a cramp which disappears within 1 or 2 min after stopping the exercise. Occasionally, profound weakness will be noted as exercise progresses. The walking distance required to produce the claudication is usually quite constant from day to day. The pain is more severe and the walking distance is always shortened when the patient walks upstairs and up a hill.

A point not often appreciated is that with arteriosclerosis obliterans claudication does not occur with occlusions in the anterior tibial, posterior tibial, or peroneal arteries. The location of the involved muscle group(s) is useful in predicting the most proximal level of occlusion. For example, calf and thigh claudication suggests that the primary involvement is proximal to the origin of the thigh muscles, i.e., the profunda femoris artery. The combination of hip, thigh, and buttock claudication with impotence in the male indicates terminal aortic occlusion, the *Leriche syndrome.*

The second important group of symptoms consists of those which occur at rest and are the result of either multiple levels of occlusion or involvement of a critical arterial segment where the major collaterals are also obstructed. Paresthesias and indeed numbness may occur but are less common than continuous pain in the toes or foot, which may be partially or completely relieved by dependency. Ulceration and gangrene of the toes and distal foot are a common occurrence when the disease reaches this advanced stage.

The patient with diabetes mellitus often presents variations in the clinical picture. Approximately 30 percent of patients with diabetes have a peripheral neuropathy which results in loss of deep pain sensation and sympathetic tone. When diabetics with a neuropathy develop ulcers with or without arterial occlusion, the lesions are typically painless. The combination of chronic arterial occlusion, peripheral neuropathy, and a nonhealing ulcer is a difficult therapeutic problem.

The physical examination is useful in substantiating the diagnosis and localizing the levels of disease. Patients with single occlusions in the aortoiliac or superficial femoral artery often have limbs which are normal in appearance. Patients with far-advanced disease secondary to multiple levels of disease often have ulcers, gangrene, loss of hair, trophic nail changes, and dependent rubor. Chronic arterial narrowing and occlusion lead to loss of pulses distal to the most proximal level of disease. The pulses should be examined in the groin in the popliteal fossa, and at the level of the ankle. If the involvement results in narrowing only, bruits are commonly heard which are transmitted for varying distances downstream from the stenosis. Auscultation should be performed from the level of the midabdomen to the popliteal artery; one should listen for the characteristic sound which is diagnostic of arterial narrowing.

Special diagnostic tests The magnitude of the physiologic derangement can be assessed simply by measuring the ankle systolic blood pressure at rest and following exercise to the point of claudication. Since arterial occlusion forces the blood to follow alternate pathways (collaterals) whose resistance to flow exceeds that of the normal vessel, an abnormal pressure gradient develops which lowers the pressure recorded at the ankle. The pressure may be measured by a variety of plethysmographs or the ultrasonic velocity detector. In general, if the systolic pressure at the ankle is greater than one-half that recorded from the arm, occlusion of one segment is most likely. Ankle pressures less than one-half of the arm systolic pressure are most often observed with multiple levels of disease.

When the patient with intermittent claudication exercises to the point of pain, the postexercise ankle blood pressure falls, often to unrecordable levels, requiring several minutes to return to the prewalking level. With exercise there is a marked fall in arterial resistance in the muscle. The amount of inflow available through the collateral arteries is inadequate, because of their high resistance to flow. As a consequence, distal arterial pressure falls and blood is shunted away from the foot. These changes explain the pallor in the foot which is so commonly observed during and immediately following exercise to the point of claudication. This test is most useful in following the progress of disease with and without therapy and is the most sensitive index of change available. Its great utility lies in the fact that each patient can serve as his or her own control.

Arteriography is essential prior to operation to localize precisely the disease and the extent of the involvement. However, it is rarely required to establish the diagnosis of arterial narrowing or occlusion secondary to arteriosclerosis obliterans.

Differential diagnosis It is rarely difficult to make the diagnosis of chronic arterial narrowing or occlusion if the clinical picture is combined with measurements of ankle blood pressure. There is a recently recognized entity, referred to as "pseudoclaudication," which may be secondary to neurospinal disease. The features of the symptom complex which are useful in distinguishing it from true intermittent claudication include the following: (1) the exercise-pain-rest cycle is not constant; (2) the symptoms may include numbness, tingling, weakness, incoordination, and clumsiness; (3) patients with pseudoclaudication may have to sit down or even lie down for relief; and (4) the time required for the pain to disappear often exceeds the few minutes observed in claudication due to arterial occlusion.

Therapy Patients with mild or moderate intermittent claudication may benefit from a rigorous, daily exercise training program. The essential features of this program include (1) repetitive daily walks to 75 percent of the claudication distance with interspersed periods of rest (1 to 2 min); (2) weekly retesting of maximum walking time with readjustment of walking distance; and (3) continuation of the exercise program—this is essential, since evidence suggests that cessation of the daily walking periods will result in loss of improvement. Vasodilator drugs have been advocated and used for the treatment of intermittent claudication, but evidence supporting their efficacy is lacking.

Weight reduction can be useful in patients with intermittent claudication by simply reducing the workload involved. It is also important that *smoking be stopped* entirely. All patients with arteriosclerosis should have their serum lipid levels determined, since they may be found to have a treatable disorder (Chap. 266). Direct arterial surgery may be effective in bypassing or removing areas of occlusion but should be reserved for those patients with disabling claudication.

Most patients with ischemic rest pain, ulcers, or gangrene present serious problems which can be helped only by direct arterial surgery. Lumbar sympathectomy may be useful but should be used *only* in patients with mild rest pain. If the rest pain is controlled by nonnarcotic analgesics and transient dependency, about 50 percent of these patients can obtain permanent pain relief by lumbar sympathectomy.

The majority of patients with arteriosclerosis obliterans will never require surgical therapy even though they do suffer some disability. The nondiabetic will have a limb loss rate of about 2 percent per year; this rate increases to 7 percent per year if the patient has diabetes mellitus. Meticulous foot care, which includes properly fitting shoes, and immediate attention to cuts and blisters are critical in proper management. This is particularly true in patients with diabetes and a peripheral neuropathy who are unable to appreciate deep pain.

Selected patients with isolated stenoses of the iliac arteries or superficial femoral artery may be candidates for transluminal dilation with a balloon catheter. The early results are promising, but its performance must be a joint decision between the radiologist and vascular surgeon.

THROMBOANGIITIS OBLITERANS (BUERGER'S DISEASE) In 1908 Buerger described a nonatheromatous lesion involving arteries, veins, and nerves occurring in young males and frequently leading to nonhealing ulcers and gangrene. Though there has been some controversy concerning the existence of this disease as a specific entity, sufficient evidence is available to recommend its continued recognition. The exact pathogenesis is obscure, but there appears to be a definite relationship with tobacco smoking or chewing.

The disease typically occurs in young males and has a characteristic location and set of clinical manifestations. Whereas arteriosclerosis obliterans is a segmental disease of large and medium-sized arteries, Buerger's disease starts in the smaller arteries of the hands and feet. There is usually an intense inflammatory component, which in later stages results in arterial and venous occlusion as well as fibrous encasement of the entire neurovascular bundle.

Clinical features The diagnosis of Buerger's disease should be suspected when male patients in the 20- to 40-year age range give the following history. A superficial, migratory nodular phlebitis may occur early in the disease. These nodules are well localized, associated with cutaneous erythema, and tender to touch. Cold sensitivity of the Raynaud's type occurs in about one-half the patients and is frequently confined to the hands. The fingers turn white when exposed to cold, then blue, and finally red—the so-called triphasic color response.

One of the most characteristic and typical symptoms of Buerger's disease is *instep claudication*. Exercise results in pain in the instep, promptly relieved by rest. Calf claudication may occur but is unusual, since the disease does not commonly progress proximally to involve and occlude either the popliteal or superficial femoral artery. When there is hand involvement, the occlusions may be bilateral, are often symmetric, and may lead to the development of hand claudication and fingertip ulcers which are exquisitely painful and difficult to heal.

The following findings during *physical examination* should lead one to suspect Buerger's disease: (1) intense rubor of the feet; (2) absent foot pulses in the presence of a normal femoral and popliteal pulse; and (3) reduction or absence of the radial and/or ulnar pulses.

Therapy There is only one effective treatment, and that is permanent, complete abstinence from tobacco. However, for some unknown reason, patients with Buerger's disease rarely discontinue smoking even though amputation is usually the inevitable consequence and the only method available of controlling the severe rest pain and ulceration which ultimately develop.

ARTERIOVENOUS FISTULAS Acquired Most acquired arteriovenous fistulas occur secondary to penetrating injuries; however, they may in certain circumstances occur secondary to blunt trauma. Malignancy, infection, and arterial aneurysms have also been responsible for the development of arteriovenous communications.

CLINICAL PICTURE Patients with penetrating injuries of an extremity should all be suspected of having an arteriovenous fistula. Initially there are no distinguishing symptoms which alert the physician to the presence of the fistula. The diagnosis is made by noting a continuous murmur and palpable thrill over the abnormal communication. Compression of the feeding artery will obliterate the murmur and thrill. With large fistulas compression of the feeding artery results in an abrupt slowing of the heart rate (Branham's sign). In rare instances distal arterial perfusion may be so severely impaired that gangrene develops.

With chronic fistulas the clinical manifestations may mimic those of venous disease, with varicose veins, stasis pigmentation, and cutaneous ulcers. Cardiac enlargement with or without failure may be seen in long-standing fistulas. Infection (bacterial endarteritis) may complicate large fistulas.

THERAPY The proper treatment of arteriovenous fistulas is division of the communication with maintenance of arterial continuity. Immediate operation may be indicated with large fistulas between such vessels as the abdominal aorta and inferior vena cava where cardiac failure may develop very quickly.

Congenital The development of anomalous communications between arteries and veins can pose both diagnostic and therapeutic difficulties. When there is an arrest in the development of the circulation during the stage of an undifferentiated capillary network, a *cavernous hemangioma* results. There is at this period an interlacing system of blood spaces which contain mixed blood, and it is impossible to distinguish the arterial and venous components.

When the development is arrested at the stage of differentiation, intercommunicating arteriovenous channels may persist. If the fistulas are large enough to be visualized arteriographically, the term used is congenital *macrofistulous arteriovenous* aneurysm. When the fistulas are too small to be visualized by arteriography, the term *microfistulous communication* should be used. This classification, based upon the size of the communications, is useful from a therapeutic standpoint.

CLINICAL MANIFESTATIONS The clinical manifestations are extremely variable and largely depend upon the location and extent of the abnormal communications. The most common symptoms are (1) cosmetic changes due to the presence of the fistulas in the subcutaneous tissue and skin, (2) limb swelling and hypertrophy, (3) visible pulsations in some cases with macrofistulous communications, and (4) varicose veins in atypical locations. In long-standing cases stasis pigmentation and cutaneous ulcers may develop in response to the continued venous hypertension.

DIAGNOSIS The presence of arteriovenous fistulas should be suspected when the following findings are presented: (1) unilateral leg or arm swelling, (2) cutaneous hemangioma of the "port-wine" variety, (3) varicose veins in atypical locations, and (4) an increase in temperature of the part. An important syndrome which may be confused with congenital arteriovenous fistulas is the *Klippel-Trénaunay* syndrome. The triad of this syndrome consists of varicose veins, "port-wine" hemangioma of the skin, and bone and soft-tissue hypertrophy. The arteriovenous communications are rarely demonstrable by arteriography.

THERAPY The management of congenital arteriovenous fistulas depends entirely upon location, extent, and clinical manifestations. Treatment is largely conservative, with support stockings used to control the venous hypertension and valvular incompetence which often produce symptoms identical with those of the postphlebitic syndrome. If the fistulas are limited in extent, it may be possible to excise the lesions in their entirety, but this is usually not feasible.

THORACIC OUTLET SYNDROMES The neurovascular bundle, by virtue of its course from the neck and thorax, is subject to compression by both muscular and skeletal structures. Traditionally, the bases for the symptoms and signs have been subdivided into the underlying anatomic defect(s), which include the scalenus anticus, cervical rib, costoclavicular, and the hyperabduction syndromes. From a diagnostic standpoint, obliteration of the radial pulse in a variety of arm positions has been considered the distinguishing feature of the underlying problem. This should no longer be considered the key diagnostic test since it frequently occurs in normal subjects. Further, the symptoms are generally due to compression of the brachial plexus and not the subclavian artery.

Those patients with the most prominent symptoms and signs will have cervical ribs with an associated fibrous band which attaches to the first rib producing compression of the neurovascular bundle. The key diagnostic features in these patients are (1) prompt appearance of paresthesias and numbness with the arm abducted to 90° and externally rotated, (2) appearance of a prominent bruit in the supraclavicular fossa, and (3) immediate disappearance of the symptoms when the arm is returned to the neutral position. There is little doubt that chronic arterial compression can lead to aneurysmal dilatation of the subclavian artery with occlusion and/or emboli, but this is rare.

In the absence of a *clear-cut* relationship between arm position and the symptoms, it is essential to rule out other causes for the clinical picture, which includes a cervical disk, degenerative joint disease, and the carpal tunnel syndrome. If cold sensitivity is also present, the vasospastic syndromes discussed in the next section must be ruled out. Removal of the first rib is performed too frequently and must be reserved for only those patients in whom the diagnosis is clear and other causes have been ruled out. The best results will be obtained in patients with cervical ribs in whom the relationship between arm position and neurovascular compression is easily demonstrated.

VASOSPASTIC DISORDERS The diseases in this category include primary and secondary cold sensitivity of the Raynaud's type, livedo reticularis, and acrocyanosis. The challenge in dealing with these entities is not in making the correct diagnosis but rather in determining if there is an associated disease responsible for the symptoms and signs. Those that are primary, e.g., without underlying disease, are generally benign, rarely lead to digit ulcers, and never terminate fatally.

Cold sensitivity of the Raynaud's type To establish this diagnosis, it is necessary to determine if a "triphasic" color response occurs, i.e., pallor, cyanosis, and rubor in that sequence. The most important element is the pallor, during which the digits turn absolutely white.

Livedo reticularis Livedo reticularis presents with a persistent cyanotic mottling of the skin which has a typical "fishnet" appearance. In contrast to Raynaud's disease, a phenomenon which is confined to the digits, livedo reticularis may involve all parts of the extremities and trunk. This cutaneous pattern is often accentuated by exposure to cold.

Acrocyanosis The most uncommon of the vasospastic disorders is acrocyanosis, which is characterized by a persistent diffuse cyanosis of the fingers, hands, toes, and feet. This disease is benign and not associated with an underlying disorder. The involved parts are nearly always cold, with excessive perspiration being a common accompanying feature.

Diagnosis Primary cold sensitivity of the Raynaud's type is more common in women, often starting in the late teens, is bilateral and symmetric, and rarely leads to fingertip ulcers or gangrene. The hands are more commonly affected than the feet. Those factors which should lead the clinician to suspect an underlying disorder include (1) abrupt onset with rapid progression to tissue necrosis; (2) late onset in life (age greater than 50 years), particularly in men; (3) unilateral or asymmetric involvement; and (4) associated symptoms compatible with a systemic disease.

Sorting out the underlying causes is often difficult because of the wide variety of diseases which may have cold sensitivity as a part of their clinical picture. The following diseases must be kept in mind: (1) chronic arterial disease, most particularly thromboangiitis obliterans; (2) the collagen vascular disorders, with scleroderma being the most common; (3) occupational and industrial exposure to vibrating instruments; (4) poisoning with lead and arsenic; (5) ingestion of drugs, namely, the ergotamine preparations, methysergide, and propranolol; (6) hematologic disorders, namely, cryoglobulins, cold agglutinins, and dysproteinemias; (7) bilateral thoracic outlet syndromes; (8) late sequelae of bilateral cold injury; (9) primary pulmonary hypertension; and (10) occult carcinoma.

The secondary causes of livedo reticularis include (1) collagen diseases, in particular periarteritis nodosa and disseminated lupus erythematosus; (2) hematologic disorders, i.e., hyperviscosity syndrome, macroglobulinemia, and cryoglobulinemia; (3) cholesterol emboli arising from ulcerated plaques in the thoracic and abdominal aorta; (4) Cushing's syndrome; (5) drug ingestion, i.e., adrenal corticosteroids; (6) prolonged dependency or immobilization; (7) late result of cold injury; and (8) prolonged exposure to or the local application of heat.

Therapy The primary forms of cold sensitivity, i.e., livedo reticularis and acrocyanosis, rarely require treatment other than assurance and instruction relative to the dangers of prolonged exposure to cold. Sympathectomy has been widely applied, with inconsistent results, in the treatment of Raynaud's disease. Lumbar sympathectomy, probably because of the higher incidence of permanent denervation, is more likely to give good results than cervicodorsal sympathectomy. Sympathectomy, particularly in the upper extremity, should be performed only when conservative measures fail to control the symptoms. Vasodilator drugs have been used but with limited success. Biofeedback techniques may be used to lessen the severity of the attacks. When an underlying disease has been found, treatment is directed at the cause of the problem.

ERYTHROMELALGIA This rare disorder of unknown etiology expresses itself as burning, tingling, and often itching of the foot and lower leg which appears as the ambient temperature increases. There is usually a critical temperature for each patient above which the symptoms appear [usually in the range of 31.7 to 36.1°C (89 to 97°F)]. During the attack the patient's feet and lower legs become bright red. The patient quickly finds that the symptoms are related to temperature and will assiduously avoid those circumstances which bring out the symptoms. Characteristically, patients wear sandals, avoid stockings, sleep with their feet outside the bedcovers, and use fans to reduce the skin temperature.

The *diagnosis* is established by the history and the examination of the extremities during an attack. The pedal pulses are intact, and the skin is warm and bright red. The disease is usually primary but has, in rare instances, been associated with myeloproliferative disorders.

Therapy is usually unsuccessful, but some patients have reported relief with aspirin or methysergide maleate.

VENOUS DISORDERS

VARICOSE VEINS Varicose veins are dilated, tortuous superficial veins with incompetent valves. The greater and lesser saphenous systems are most commonly involved, but it is not unusual for secondary branches of the superficial system of veins also to become dilated. They most often appear after the age of 20, but in women often develop in relation to puberty, during pregnancy, and with commencement of the menopause. In men there is a fairly even distribution in the onset of symptoms by decades up to age 70.

The etiology remains largely obscure, but varicose veins are known to be aggravated by hormonal factors in the female, increased intraabdominal pressure, and in rare instances, arteriovenous fistulas. Hereditary factors are important but have been poorly studied.

Classification It is important to classify varicose veins as either primary or secondary. Primary varicose veins occur in the absence of deep venous disease and generally have a benign course. Varicosities which occur secondary to obstruction and valvular incompetence of the deep venous system are much more serious.

Clinical features Primary varicose veins are brought to the attention of the patient first by the cosmetic deformity and second by the symptoms which develop with prolonged standing. The patient complains of a feeling of heaviness in the leg, combined with fatigue, that gets progressively worse toward the end of the day. Elevation of the legs will result in rapid and impressive relief from the symptoms. When the varicose veins are secondary to deep venous obstruction, loss of valves, and incompetent perforating veins, the symptoms are more severe and accompanied by swelling (see "Postthrombotic Syndrome" below).

Diagnosis The diagnosis of primary varicose veins is made largely by inspection of the legs in the upright position. The varicosities appear as dilated, often tortuous channels which are most commonly observed in the greater and lesser saphenous systems. When isolated clusters are observed in atypical locations, the possibility of an underlying incompetent perforating vein or arteriovenous fistula should be considered. To assess whether or not incompetent perforating veins are contributing factors, the Trendelenburg test may be employed. With the legs elevated and the superficial veins empty, a tourniquet is applied about the thigh close to the groin. The patient then quickly stands, and the pattern of filling is noted. If the superficial veins do not fill in 30 s, it is unlikely that incompetent perforating veins are contributing to the etiology of the varicose veins.

Therapy The majority of patients with symptomatic primary varicose veins should be treated initially with compression stockings. If the deep veins and perforating channels are patent and competent, it is very unusual for primary varicose veins to lead to stasis pigmentation and ulceration. In those rare instances in which treatment with compression stockings is inadequate, high ligation and stripping of the long and/or short saphenous veins may be required.

ACUTE VENOUS OCCLUSION Obstruction of superficial or deep veins occurs in two settings. The first is associated with an intense inflammatory component as usually observed with involvement of superficial veins. More common and potentially lethal is thrombosis of the deep veins where inflammation as either the inciting event or a clinical manifestation is uncommon. Thus, it is appropriate to separate these two entities since the clinical course and treatment are different.

Superficial thrombophlebitis Except for so-called chemical phlebitis secondary to direct intimal injury, the etiology remains obscure, but the clinical presentation is dramatic. The involved vein is exquisitely tender with surrounding erythema and edema. A fever is often present. While concern has been expressed regarding propagation of the thrombus into the deep venous system with subsequent pulmonary embolization, this rarely occurs. Treatment is directed at local measures to reduce the inflammation—application of heat, elevation of legs, and administration of anti-inflammatory agents such as indomethacin. It is important to be certain that the presenting symptoms are not signs due to a bacterial cellulitis or lymphangitis. The Doppler velocity detector is useful in distinguishing the above, since thrombophlebitis is always associated with thrombosis of the involved segment.

Acute venous thrombosis The most common in-hospital vascular disorder is thrombosis of the minor and major deep veins of the leg. In the initial stages, the soleus plexus of veins and sinus of the venous valve are the sites most commonly involved. When the thrombi remain confined to these areas, they are not detectable unless prospective screening with ^{125}I-labeled fibrinogen has been carried out (Chap. 282).

Upper extremity thrombosis is uncommon but may be associated with strenuous effort. The site of involvement is most commonly at the level of the axillary-subclavian vein as it enters the thorax.

ETIOLOGY There are definite known precipitating factors, which include trauma and bacterial infection, but these are not the most common causes. The much larger group of patients who develop this problem fall into one or more of the following categories: (1) prolonged bed rest associated with a medical or surgical illness; (2) malignancy, particularly of the pancreas, lung, or gastrointestinal system; (3) administration of estrogens including oral contraceptives; (4) disseminated intravascular coagulation; (5) the postpartum period; and (6) paralysis.

CLINICAL FEATURES The most important factor concerning the symptoms and signs that develop is that they are not specific and may result from a variety of other diseases. Although edema and local tenderness with associated pain have been considered the most important findings, they are not sufficient to warrant either making the diagnosis of venous thrombosis or instituting therapy. Pulmonary embolization (Chap. 282) may, in fact, be the first clue that deep venous thrombosis is present.

DIAGNOSIS The bedside diagnosis of deep venous thrombosis is so inaccurate that it *must* be established by some independent means. The ^{125}I-labeled fibrinogen test is used for prospective studies but has limited application since it must be given prior to the initiation of the thrombosis. The most useful available noninvasive tests include Doppler ultrasound and plethysmography. Properly used, these tests have a rate of false-positive and false-negative results in the range of 5 to 10 percent. These methods are insensitive to thrombi confined to the muscular veins but can be used for sequential study to detect propagation into the major deep veins. If a vascular laboratory is present which has experience with these noninvasive tests, therapy can be based upon the results. However, if the tests are unavailable or the findings equivocal, contrast venography should be performed. A promising new approach is to carry out radionuclide venography with simultaneous lung scanning. This diagnostic test provides two critically important bits of information: the status of the major deep veins and a base-line perfusion lung scan.

THERAPY The treatment is directed at control of the thrombotic process already initiated. There is agreement that intravenous heparin is the most effective therapy. The preferred method is continuous administration, starting with a loading dose of 5000 to 10,000 units and varying the dosage depending upon the partial thromboplastin time, which should be kept between two and three times the control time. The two major advantages of this approach are a more uniform level of anticoagulation and a lower incidence of hemorrhagic complications.

The duration of heparin therapy depends upon the degree of involvement and whether pulmonary embolization has occurred. With the latter, treatment must be continued for 10 to 14 days and even longer if the patient remains at risk. Oral therapy with one of the coumarin preparations should be started while the patient is still on heparin, which is discontinued only when a satisfactory level of anticoagulation has been achieved. The maintenance level varies considerably between 2 to 15 mg daily but must be carefully controlled to keep the one-stage prothrombin time approximately two times the control time.

Fibrinolytic therapy may be of value in that small group of patients with spontaneous venous thrombosis not associated with surgery or trauma. Streptokinase has been shown to be effective in lysing thrombi which have been present fewer than 14 days.

The duration of oral anticoagulation is dependent upon the severity of the problem. For isolated calf vein thrombosis, therapy of 4 to 6 weeks is sufficient. However, for femoropopliteal or iliofemoral thrombosis, with or without pulmonary embolism, anticoagulation should be continued for 3 to 6 months.

PROPHYLACTIC MEASURES There is conflicting evidence that low-dose heparin (5000 units subcutaneously 2 h prior to operation, then three times daily) is effective in reducing the incidence of deep venous thrombosis as well as the occurrence of fatal and nonfatal pulmonary embolism.

Operative therapy is usually applied to patients who either have sustained pulmonary embolism that is not controlled by adequate doses of heparin or have sustained hemorrhagic complications. The more commonly used procedures include ligation or partial occlusion of the inferior vena cava by a plastic clip. Patients who are not candidates for the direct operative approach may benefit from the transvenous placement of an "umbrella" in the vena cava just below the renal veins.

POSTTHROMBOTIC SYNDROME Patients who have single or multiple episodes of deep venous thrombosis will frequently have irreversible changes in the veins which lead to further morbidity. The acute venous thrombosis often leads to residual chronic occlusion and destruction of the venous valves.

The loss of the valvular mechanism in the deep venous system forces the blood to follow abnormal pathways, particularly during exercise. In the standing position or during walking the muscle pump pushes the blood proximally, distally, and out through the perforating veins into the superficial system. By increasing venous and capillary pressures, this sequence of events, over a period of many years, leads to edema, and to rupture of small superficial veins in the vicinity of the perforating veins. The subcutaneous hemorrhage leads to deposition of hemosiderin pigment (stasis pigmentation), subcutaneous fibrosis, cutaneous atrophy, and lymphatic obstruction. These chronic changes lead to the development of stasis ulcers, which are difficult to manage.

Clinical features and diagnosis The important features of this disorder consist of swelling which is always worse at the end of the day, pain, cutaneous pigmentation (usually in the region of the medial malleolus), and nonhealing ulcers which develop secondary to minor trauma. Repeated trauma, subcutaneous hemorrhage, and cellulitis can produce changes in the skin and subcutaneous tissues that are indistinguishable from those of the postphlebitic state. In questionable cases venography is useful in establishing the cause of the problem.

Therapy The most important factor in the treatment of the postphlebitic syndrome is to reduce the hydrostatic pressure and to prevent "high-pressure leaks" through the perforating veins when the patient is erect. This can best be accomplished by a tailored pressure-gradient stocking, which must be worn at all times that the patient is ambulatory, and by elevating legs when possible.

When an ulcer is present, healing may be accomplished by applying an impregnated gauze dressing from the base of the toes to below the knee. This is changed weekly and permits healing in 90 percent of patients. The remaining patients require excision of the ulcer with skin grafting. Support stockings must be worn regardless of the therapy directed at the ulcer, because the deep venous system remains incompetent and edema will continue to develop without adequate external support.

LYMPHATIC DISORDERS

LYMPHEDEMA Lymphedema, an abnormal accumulation of lymph in the extremities, occurs from multiple causes which include (1) lymphedema from organisms such as *Wuchereria bancrofti*; (2) infectious lymphedema resulting in thrombosis of lymphatics; (3) congenital lymphedema with arrest in lymph growth, which is apparent at birth or shortly thereafter; (4) traumatic lymphedema secondary to direct injury, burns, operations, and radiation; (5) essential lymphedema—so-called Milroy's disease, which appears at puberty and is most commonly observed in women; (6) allergic lymphedema occurring secondary to exposure to drugs and pollens; (7) postthrombotic lymphedema, which represents combined venous and lymphatic obstruction; and (8) malignant lymphedema, which occurs secondary to either direct invasion or obstruction of the lymphatics by tumor cells.

Clinical features Painless swelling of the involved extremity is the earliest and most common symptom and sign with most types of lymphedema. The swelling usually starts in the foot and ankle and then progresses proximally. Initially the swelling tends to subside somewhat at night, but as the process progresses, the swelling becomes permanent secondary to fibrosis of both the skin and subcutaneous tissues. Skin color and texture are normal until the late stages, when the skin becomes thickened and brown and has multiple papillary projections—so-called lymphostatic verrucosis.

Diagnosis The location and nature of the edema readily separate lymphedema from edema due to other causes. In the legs, the dorsa of the toes and foot are nearly always involved; this is uncommon in other causes of swelling. The edema is often brawny in character and pits only with difficulty. Though the other forms of edema often improve with bed rest, elevation, and diuretics, lymphedema, even in early stages, responds poorly to these measures. In later stages when fibrosis develops in the skin and subcutaneous tissues, these conservative measures are of little, if any, value. Lymphangiography in selected cases may be of value in localizing and elucidating the cause of the lymphedema.

Therapy Therapy is directed at minimizing the amount of edema and preventing recurrent attacks of cellulitis when this is a problem. Pressure-gradient stockings and the use of intermittent-pressure devices at night are helpful in controlling the edema. Since recurrent attacks of cellulitis due to the beta-hemolytic streptococcus are not uncommon and always result in further lymphatic destruction, prophylactic penicillin should be used indefinitely. Excision of the edematous tissue is reserved for only the most advanced stage of the disease when there is marked, irreversible swelling and disfigurement.

ANTERIOR TIBIAL COMPARTMENT SYNDROMES

Acute swelling of the anterior tibial compartment may occur secondary to intensive exercise, increased capillary permeability (with ischemia), or hematoma in the enclosed space. When arterial revascularization has been successful for prolonged ischemia, muscular swelling resulting in an increase in compartment pressure may lead to nerve damage, and muscle necrosis. This is recognized by the severe pain in the compartment, swelling, and local tenderness. If the anterior compartment is involved, there is anesthesia of a triangular area on the dorsum of the foot at the base of the first and second toes. *Immediate* fasciotomy is indicated, since a delay of even a few hours may result in irreversible changes.

REFERENCES

BERNSTEIN EF (ed): *Noninvasive Diagnostic Techniques in Vascular Disease.* St Louis, Mosby, 1981

FREEMAN LM, BLAUFOX MD: Thrombosis detection. Semin Nucl Med 7:3, July 1977

PERCUTANEOUS TRANSLUMINAL ANGIOPLASTY: Special section. Am J Roetgen, November, 1980

RUTHERFORD RF (ed): *Vascular Surgery.* Philadelphia, Saunders, 1977

STRANDNESS DE JR: The case against low-dose heparin, in *Current Controversies in Cardiovascular Disease,* E Rapaport (ed). Philadelphia, Saunders, 1980

———, Thiele BL: *Selected Topics in Venous Disorders.* New York, Futura, 1981

——— et al: Present status of acute venous thrombosis. Surg Gynecol Obstet 145:433, 1977

TAYLOR LM et al: Finger gangrene caused by small artery occlusive disease. Ann Surg 193:453, 1981

WESSLER SW: The case for low-dose heparin, in *Current Controversies in Cardiovascular Disease,* E Rapaport (ed). Philadelphia, Saunders, 1980

section 3 | Disorders of the respiratory system

Diagnostic methods

270 APPROACH TO THE PATIENT WITH DISEASE OF THE RESPIRATORY SYSTEM

EUGENE BRAUNWALD

As in other branches of medicine, a careful and detailed history and physical examination are the cornerstones of an accurate diagnosis in patients with disorders of the respiratory system. In addition, the roentgenographic examination occupies a particularly important role in the evaluation of patients with lung disease. Since abnormalities of the respiratory system are frequently a manifestation of a systemic process, attention must be focused not only on the chest; a comprehensive evaluation of the patient's entire health status is essential. For example, the presence of a pulmonary lesion on x-ray may be due to metastatic disease, and hemoptysis may be due to a disorder of hemostasis. Diffuse scleroderma may result in diffuse pulmonary infiltrative disease (Chaps. 280 and 352), and multiple pulmonary cavities may be a manifestation of Wegener's granulomatosis (Chap. 69). All of the so-called collagen vascular diseases may have prominent pulmonary manifestations. Carcinoma of the lung (Chap. 284) may be accompanied by prominent extrathoracic manifestations, which may overshadow the pulmonary lesion. These include myopathy, peripheral neuropathy, hypertrophic pulmonary osteoarthropathy, and a variety of endocrine and metabolic manifestations, including Cushing's syndrome, the carcinoid syndrome, a hyperparathyroid-like picture, inappropriate secretion of antidiuretic hormone, gonadotropin (Chap. 122), and increased frequency of pulmonary infections.

HISTORY In eliciting the history of patients with pulmonary disease, it must be appreciated that an increasing fraction of the population is exposed to materials which are potentially toxic to the lung (Chap. 275). The history must therefore contain a detailed *occupational and personal history* with a description of exposure to hazards such as asbestos, coal, silica, beryllium, bagasse, iron oxide, tin oxide, cotton dust, titanium oxide, silver, nitrogen dioxide, animals, moldy hay, air conditioners, and furnace humidifiers. It is useful to construct a work history, which includes the patient's duties, duration of exposure, use of protective devices, and illness in fellow workers. The occupational history should include information on a job-by-job basis as well as the military service. Contact with both wild and domestic animals may result in pulmonary symptoms, such as bronchospasm in the subject allergic to a pet, or, less commonly, acute pneumonitis in patients with ornithosis (Chap. 194), tularemia (Chap. 159), or Q fever. Because it is such an important risk factor for many forms of lung disease, history of tobacco consumption must be sought and should be quantified. Aspiration pneumonia and pneumococcal and *Klebsiella* pneumonia occur in alcoholics, and lung abscess occurs in intravenous drug abusers. A record of the patient's *previous residence* is of considerable importance in the diagnosis of histoplasmosis (the south and midwestern United States), coccidioidomycosis (the southwestern United States), tropical eosinophilia, and South American blastomycosis. For example, pulmonary mass lesions in patients in the Mediterranean Basin may be due to hydatid cysts, hemoptysis in patients from central China may be caused by paragonimiasis (Chap. 231), and cor pulmonale in Egypt frequently results from schistosomiasis (Chap. 228).

The *family history* should consider pulmonary diseases which may be genetic, such as cystic disease of the lung, pulmonary emphysema due to $alpha_1$ antitrypsin deficiency, cystic fibrosis, asthma, hereditary telangiectasia, Kartagener's syndrome, and alveolar microlithiasis, as well as infections due to the tubercle bacilli, fungi, and schistosoma where exposure to involved family members is important.

Dyspnea is a cardinal manifestation of diseases involving the respiratory and cardiovascular systems (Chap. 26). A detailed physical examination of both organ systems is therefore mandatory in every patient with this symptom. Dyspnea secondary to cardiac disease is often recognized by the presence of other evidence of heart failure, such as cardiac enlargement, gallop rhythms, and cardiac murmurs. It may be difficult to differentiate paroxysmal nocturnal dyspnea due to pulmonary edema of cardiac origin from nocturnal attacks of bronchial asthma, but a detailed description of the circumstances in which this symptom occurs is most useful. Dyspnea also is a common functional complaint, and an important clue in the identification of this form is the observation that shortness of breath often occurs at rest and is relieved during exertion; the opposite is the case in patients in whom this symptom is secondary to disease of the lungs or heart. Equally important in the differential diagnosis is a careful elucidation of the relationship of dyspnea to other symptoms such as cough or angina pectoris.

Patients with diseases involving the respiratory system may also present with *chest pain* which is frequently caused by inflammation of the pleura, occurring in pneumonia, pulmonary thromboembolism, tuberculosis, and malignancy (Chap. 4). Pleuritic pain is usually localized to one side of the chest and is related to movements of the thorax and to respiration. Lesions confined to the pulmonary parenchyma do not produce pain, while diseases involving the organs in the mediastinum (Chap. 285) may cause local discomfort with radiation characteristic of the specific organ. Pain may also originate in or be referred to the chest wall; it may be due to intercostal neuritis, as in herpes zoster, or to compression of the intercostal nerves as they leave the spinal cord. Such pain is often superficial in character and may be related to coughing and straining. Thoracic pain may also be due to myositis, costochondral disturbances, myocardial ischemia, pericarditis, esophageal disease, and aortic dissection and aneurysm (Chap. 4).

Cough and *expectoration* are also cardinal features of pulmonary disease (Chap. 25). Few patients can describe the severity of cough or quantity of expectoration reliably, and it is therefore desirable for the physician to inspect a 24-h collection of sputum. Cough is often precipitated by foreign materials irritating nerve endings in airways and is frequently caused by inflammation of the bronchi; the latter may be persistent (as in patients with a cigarette cough and chronic bronchitis) or acute (as in a variety of viral and bacterial infections). The time of occurrence of the cough and the character and quantity of expectorated material may point to the diagnosis. For example, bronchiectasis and lung abscess produce purulent sputum which may have an offensive odor or be streaked with blood (Chaps. 276 and 277). In pulmonary edema, the sputum is pink, frothy, and watery (Chap. 26). Mucoid (translucent, viscid, shiny, white or gray) or mucopurulent (mucoid with flecks of yellow or green pus) sputum is characteristic of acute and chronic bronchitis. Sputum is bloody or rusty in pneumonia; it is thick, gelatinous, and brick red, laced with pus, in *Klebsiella* pneumonia. Paroxysmal cough may also be the presenting feature in patients with bronchial asthma, in whom physical examination reveals wheezing respirations and squeaking musical sounds (Chap. 273), as well as in patients with left ventricular failure, in whom it generally occurs at night and in the recumbent position (Chap. 253). Pulmonary tuberculosis (Chap. 174), though less common than previously, remains a common cause of chronic cough, as does neoplasm of the lung (Chap. 284). A change in the character of a chronic cough, unaccompanied by an acute infection, should alert the physician to the need of carrying out a detailed examination.

Hemoptysis is often a frightening symptom (Chap. 25). Faint streaking of the sputum with blood may be observed in acute infections of the respiratory tract. However, many patients with bloody sputum have serious disease, such as pulmonary thromboembolism, tuberculosis, critical mitral stenosis, neoplasm of the lung, or bronchiectasis. In all instances it is necessary to exclude sources of blood in the nasopharynx and bleeding of gastric or esophageal origin. The character of the bloody expectorate should be defined, since it may be helpful in identifying the underlying disease process. Sputum which is frankly bloody without mucus or pus may be due to pulmonary thromboembolism (Chap. 282). When pus is present, pneumonia, bronchiectasis, or lung abscess should be considered. Dilute, pink, frothy sputum should suggest acute pulmonary edema (Chap. 26).

PHYSICAL EXAMINATION In addition to a careful examination of the thorax, a meticulous *general physical examination* is mandatory in patients with disorders of the respiratory system. Disturbances of mentation or even coma occur in patients with acute carbon dioxide retention and hypoxemia. Telltale stains on the fingers point to heavy cigarette smoking; infected teeth and gums may occur in patients with aspiration pneumonitis and lung abscess; characteristic cutaneous lesions may point to the presence of sarcoidosis (Chap. 235), collagen vascular disease, Wegener's granulomatosis, and berylliosis, all of which may have prominent pulmonary manifestations. Clubbing of the fingers, or when advanced, osteoarthropathy (Chap. 353) may point to carcinoma (Chap. 284) or suppurative disease (Chap. 276) of the lung; chronic hypoxemia, as occurs in patients with chronic bronchitis (Chap. 279); pulmonary arteriovenous fistula; or congenital heart disease with right-to-left shunt (Chap. 256). However, clubbing is also seen in some patients with biliary cirrhosis, regional enteritis, and ulcerative colitis. A careful search for infection in the teeth, gums, tonsils, or sinuses is recommended in patients known to have or to be suspected of having bronchiectasis or lung abscess. Neurologic findings including headache, drowsiness, papilledema, and other evidence of increased intracranial pressure may occur in patients with pulmonary disease who have hypoxemia and hypercapnia. Vascular collapse is a late complication of carbon dioxide intoxication and is characterized by hypotension, flushed skin, sweating, and tachycardia.

DIAGNOSTIC TESTS The *roentgenographic examination* of the chest represents the cornerstone of the diagnostic workup of the patient with suspected pulmonary disease, and it is the integration of the information obtained from the clinical examination and the roentgenogram which often provides the key to diagnosis. Unfortunately, physical examination of the chest has been deemphasized, largely because of the recognition of the enormous value of radiographic techniques. However, abnormalities such as small or moderate amounts of fluid in the alveoli or in the mediastinum, bronchospasm, and pleural effusions can often be detected more accurately by physical examination than by chest roentgenography. Tracheal deviation can be readily recognized on physical examination and may be observed in obstruction of a major bronchus and in atelectasis.

Chest roentgenograms obtained in the lateral decubitus position frequently reveal small pleural effusions not evident in the upright position. A number of other abnormalities may be associated with normal roentgenograms. These include solitary lesions less than 6 mm in diameter, acute pulmonary thromboembolism without infarction, early interstitial pneumonia, diffuse granulomatous disease such as miliary tuberculosis, interstitial disease such as scleroderma and systemic lupus erythematosus, bronchiectasis, acute chronic bronchitis, mild to moderate emphysema, endobronchial masses only partially obstructing the airways, and the majority of instances of hypoventilation due to disorders of the central nervous system or neuromuscular disease. On the other hand, gross abnormalities of thoracic structure; pulmonary, mediastinal, and pleural masses; parenchymal consolidation, cysts, cavities, and abnormalities of the pulmonary vascular bed are all detected more reliably by roentgenographic than by physical examination.

An abnormal chest roentgenogram may be the presenting feature in an asymptomatic patient. In such circumstances the physician must make every effort to obtain earlier films in order to determine whether the lesion is new or old. Laminography, computerized tomography, angiocardiography, and pulmonary scintigraphy are additional procedures which may be helpful in establishing a diagnosis in a patient with an abnormality on the plain chest roentgenogram.

A variety of other diagnostic procedures are helpful in the workup of the patient with known or suspected pulmonary disease. These are presented in Chap. 272 and include skin tests for tuberculosis; scratch or intradermal tests to detect atopic reactions; appropriate serum complement fixation tests; and examination and culture of the sputum, pleural fluid, and bronchial washings. Bronchoscopy, bronchial brushings, and bronchoscopic biopsy have been greatly facilitated by the development of the fiberoptic bronchoscope. Mediastinoscopy, scalene node and mediastinal node biopsy, and pleural and lung biopsy may also be instrumental in establishing a diagnosis in an otherwise asymptomatic patient. Particularly important points which must be investigated in the history of the asymptomatic patient with a lesion discovered on a routine chest roentgenogram include exposure to individuals with tuberculosis; previous tuberculin and fungous skin tests; residence in or visits to areas where fungal disease is endemic; a history of smoking and of exposure to dusts; and symptoms of systemic disease such as fever, sweat, fatigue, and weight loss. Physiologic (lung function) studies (Chap. 271) are of limited value in establishing an etiologic diagnosis in the patient with pulmonary diseases. They are, however, very helpful in assessing the physiologic consequences of disorders of the respiratory system and chest wall, as well as in following the effects of their progression or remission. Simple functional tests, such as observing the patient climbing one or two flights of stairs, are often valuable in determining whether or not the patient is grossly disabled.

In the approach to a patient with pulmonary disease, consideration must be given to the observation that substantial changes in the relative incidence of disease affecting the respiratory system have taken place in the United States during the past three decades. Chronic infectious disorders such as tuberculosis, lung abscess, and bronchiectasis have decreased. On the other hand, patients with chronic bronchitis and with emphysema now survive longer and form an increasing fraction of patients with chronic respiratory disease, as do patients with environmental lung disease and with drug-induced disease. Modern intercontinental travel has increased the appearance in the lung of parasitic infestations in the western world. Also, the reduction of immunologic competence which occurs in diabetics as well as in the treatment of patients with a variety of malignancies and following organ transplantation (Chap. 292) has led to an increasing incidence of opportunistic infections of the lungs with a variety of microorganisms rarely pathogenic in the past.

REFERENCE

Fishman AP (ed): *Pulmonary Diseases and Disorders.* New York, McGraw-Hill, 1980

Snider GL (ed): *Clinical Pulmonary Medicine.* Boston, Little, Brown, 1981

271
DISTURBANCES OF RESPIRATORY FUNCTION

JOHN B. WEST

The prime function of the lung is to exchange gas between the inspired air and the venous blood. A convenient starting point, therefore, for a discussion of disturbances of respiratory function is the alveolar membrane across which gas exchange occurs (Fig. 271-1). This blood-gas barrier is less than 1 μm thick and has a surface area of some 100 m^2. It is therefore ideally suited to its gas exchange function.

FIGURE 271-1
The functional lung unit. The alveolar membrane across which gas exchange takes place has alveolar gas on one side and pulmonary capillary blood on the other.

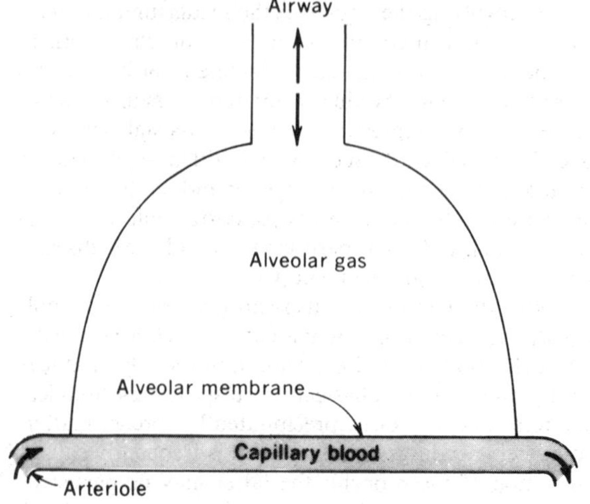

Air is pumped to one side of this membrane and blood to the other. The air flows through conducting tubes, the bronchi; these are not lined with blood capillaries, with the result that no gas exchange can occur within them. These conducting airways, therefore, comprise a *dead space*. Beyond these airways is the *alveolar gas*, which makes up most of the volume of the lung. This gas is in a constant state of agitation because of molecular diffusion, and thus all the alveolar gas has access to the capillary blood via the alveolar membrane.

On the other side of the membrane, blood is pumped from the right side of the heart to the pulmonary capillaries. These delicate vessels have diameters of only about 10 μm, so that the blood is spread out in a thin film, one or two red blood cells thick, around the air sacs.

It is worth emphasizing two features of the basic lung unit shown in Fig. 271-1: (1) its symmetry, i.e., air and blood are equally important in the central process of gas exchange (this simple fact is sometimes forgotten in clinical medicine, where the patient's difficulties in moving air in and out of the lung often dominate the picture); (2) the simplicity of the lung unit compared with, say, the nephron. The structure of the lung is simple because its main role is simple, i.e., bringing together air and blood so that gas exchange can occur by passive diffusion. By contrast, the kidney carries out many functions involving active transport, and its structure is correspondingly complicated.

VENTILATION

This is the process of moving inspired air into the alveolar gas compartment, where the gas exchange with the blood occurs. It is worth attaching some typical values for ventilation to the lung shown in Fig. 271-1. A normal breath is about 500 ml, so that with a breathing frequency of 15 per minute some 7 to 8 liters of air enters the lung each minute. However, because the volume of the conducting airways (dead space) is about 150 ml, only 350 of the 500 ml of air inhaled with each breath reaches the alveolar gas compartment. The rest remains behind in the airways and is subsequently exhaled. Thus, the volume of fresh gas entering the alveoli each minute is about 350 ml $\times$ 15, or some 5 liters. This is known as the *alveolar ventilation* and is of key importance to gas exchange. Of the 5 liters of air entering the alveoli, some 300 ml of oxygen moves across into the blood each minute to be replaced by about 250 ml of carbon dioxide. Thus less than 5 percent of the gas volume inhaled is exchanged with the gas in the blood.

The above figures apply to resting conditions. On exercise, the oxygen uptake may rise as high as 4 to 6 liters per minute and the minute volume of air inspired may increase twentyfold. This is accomplished by an increase in both tidal volume and the frequency of breathing.

It should be noted that inspired air passes only a limited distance down the airways by ordinary bulk flow. Before it gets to the alveoli, its forward velocity is reduced to something like a millimeter per second, because of the enormous combined cross-sectional area of the small airways. In addition, the volume of gas in the bronchioles is so large that the alveoli and their ducts have completed their expansion before the fresh inspired air reaches them. The last few millimeters of its travel are therefore accomplished by molecular diffusion within the small airways. This process is very rapid for gas molecules but exceedingly slow for dust particles if they are over 0.5 μm in diameter. For this reason most inhaled dusts and aerosols never reach the alveoli, and many are deposited in the region of the terminal bronchioles.

MEASUREMENT OF VENTILATION The total volume of air passing the lips is easily measured by connecting a large bag or spirometer to the patient via a mouthpiece and one-way valve. The resting and exercise ventilations are increased when disease impairs the efficiency of pulmonary gas exchange, but the measurement of ventilation by itself is not often useful because it is partly under voluntary control and is often changed by the stress of the measurement.

CONTROL OF VENTILATION The rhythmic act of breathing is initiated in the respiratory centers of the pons and medulla. The level of ventilation is controlled by the arterial P_{CO_2}, P_{O_2}, and pH, and by reflexes originating in the lung and elsewhere. The chief regulation is carried out by the medullary chemoreceptors which respond to changes in the partial pressure of carbon dioxide P_{CO_2} in arterial blood. There is evidence that these chemoreceptors are exquisitely sensitive to a fall in pH of the cerebrospinal fluid near them, which occurs when carbon dioxide diffuses across the blood-brain barrier. This dissolved gas moves easily across the blood-brain barrier, whereas H^+ and HCO_3^- do not.

Arterial hypoxemia also increases the ventilation through its action on the peripheral chemoreceptors in the carotid bodies. This hypoxic stimulus is normally relatively weak and variable but may dominate during chronic hypoxemia, for example, following ascent to high altitude. This is also often the situation in patients with chronic respiratory failure, with the result that the administration of oxygen may cause hypoventilation and severe carbon dioxide retention.

The pH of the arterial blood has an effect on ventilation which is independent of the P_{CO_2}. This is why ventilation may be increased during metabolic acidosis, thus reducing the arterial P_{CO_2}.

Reflexes from the lung from stretch receptors, irritant receptors and receptors situated in the alveolar walls (juxtacapillary or J) also influence ventilation under some conditions.

HYPOVENTILATION When inspired air reaches the alveoli, oxygen is removed from it and carbon dioxide is added. The concentrations, or partial pressures, of these two gases in the alveoli depend on a balance between two processes. On the one hand, the removal of oxygen from (or addition of carbon dioxide to) the alveolar gas is determined by the metabolic demands of the body. On the other hand, the addition of oxygen to (or removal of carbon dioxide from) the alveolar gas depends on the amount of alveolar ventilation. Thus, if the alveolar ventilation is low in relation to oxygen uptake and carbon dioxide output, the partial pressure of oxygen in alveolar gas and arterial blood falls, and the level of carbon dioxide rises. This is hypoventilation.

Hypoventilation is commonly caused by disease outside the respiratory system and often exists in the presence of normal lungs. Causes include depression of the respiratory center by drugs or anesthesia, damage to the medulla by disease, diseases affecting the nerve supply to the muscles of the thorax or the muscles themselves, injury to the chest wall, and obstruction to the airways. Because the lungs themselves are often normal, the prognosis may be excellent if the precipitating cause is removed. However, hypoventilation can also be caused by primary disease of the lungs. Note that hypoventilation always causes both hypoxemia and hypercapnia, although the first can be abolished by adding oxygen to the inspired air. The carbon dioxide retention can be relieved only by increasing the ventilation, e.g., by using a ventilator. Disorders leading to hypoventilation are discussed in more detail in Chap. 286.

HYPERVENTILATION If the alveolar ventilation is abnormally high for the carbon dioxide production of the body, the arterial P_{CO_2} falls. This may occur in metabolic acidosis, e.g., uremia, in which the chemoreceptors respond to the low blood pH. Hysterical hyperventilation is also not uncommon. For more information on hyperventilation see Chap. 286. The sensation of respiratory distress, or *dyspnea,* which should be clearly distinguished from *hyperpnea,* is considered in detail in Chap. 26.

DIFFUSION ACROSS THE BLOOD-GAS BARRIER

Oxygen and carbon dioxide move across the blood-gas barrier by a process of simple physical diffusion from a region of high partial pressure to one of low, just as water runs downhill. Consider a red blood cell as it enters a pulmonary capillary. The P_{O_2} in mixed venous blood (in the pulmonary artery) is typically about 40 mmHg, and as the cell enters the capillary, the P_{O_2} in alveolar gas less than 1 μm away is approximately 100 mmHg. Oxygen therefore moves rapidly across the barrier into the cell to combine with hemoglobin, and the P_{O_2} rises. As a consequence, the oxygen pressure difference between the cell and the alveolar gas falls, and the rate of inflow of oxygen is reduced. However, under normal conditions, the diffusion properties of the alveolar membrane are so good and the rate of combination of oxygen with hemoglobin so rapid that before the cell has spent more than about a third of its time in the capillary, its P_{O_2} has virtually reached that of the alveolar gas. This transfer of oxygen is helped by the shape of the oxygen dissociation curve; the nearly flat upper part of the curve (see Fig. 54-1) ensures that the driving pressure difference is maintained until almost all the oxygen is moved across. Thus, under ordinary circumstances, there is no measurable difference between the P_{O_2} of alveolar gas and that of the blood at the end of the pulmonary capillary. Indeed, the normal lung has plenty of reserve diffusion in hand.

Two factors which stress the diffusion ability of the lung are exercise and alveolar hypoxemia. During strenuous exercise, the time spent by the red blood cells in the capillaries is greatly reduced, perhaps to a third of that at rest, so that the time available for the diffusion process is curtailed. Even so, the P_{O_2} in the capillary blood almost reaches that of the alveolar gas, except possibly during the most exhausting work. Additional stress occurs if the lung inspires a low oxygen mixture, thus reducing the alveolar P_{O_2}. Because the pressure difference between the oxygen in the gas and that in the red blood cells as they enter the capillary is lowered, the rate of movement of oxygen across the membrane is slowed. There is evidence that heavy work when the inspired P_{O_2} is very low (e.g., at high altitude) causes lowering of the arterial P_{O_2} because of inadequate diffusion into the pulmonary capillary. It is generally argued that carbon dioxide transfer is never limited by diffusion across the alveolar membrane because of the much higher diffusion rate of this gas, but recent work suggests that this may not always be the case.

MEASUREMENT OF DIFFUSING CAPACITY This can be done using carbon monoxide. The subject inspires a low concentration (approximately 0.1 percent), and the rate of uptake of the gas by the blood is calculated from the difference between the inspired and expired concentrations. The measurement can be made during the course of a single 10-s breath-holding period, or over a minute or so of steady breathing. In both cases, the diffusing capacity is expressed as the milliliters per minute of carbon monoxide taken up by the lung per millimeter of mercury of partial pressure of carbon monoxide in the alveolar gas. Normal values are in the region of 20 (ml/min)/mmHg at rest, rising to 60 (ml/min)/mmHg or more on exercise.

The reason the uptake of carbon monoxide measures the diffusing capacity is the remarkable avidity of blood for this gas. This means that appreciable amounts of carbon monoxide can be combined with hemoglobin in the blood at an exceedingly low partial pressure. As a result, the rise in partial pressure of carbon monoxide in the red blood cells as they pass along the pulmonary capillaries is negligible, and the amount of the gas which is transferred into the blood is determined only by the diffusion properties of the alveolar membrane and the rate of combination of carbon monoxide with hemoglobin. The latter depends on the P_{O_2} in the alveoli; by measuring the carbon monoxide uptake at various inspired oxygen partial pressures, it is possible to determine separately the diffusing capacity of the alveolar membrane itself and the volume of blood in pulmonary capillaries. In patients who smoke, the level of carboxyhemoglobin in the blood may not be negligible and should be allowed for.

The measurement of carbon monoxide uptake is a relatively simple procedure, and there is no problem in following changes of diffusing capacity in the normal lung under a variety of conditions. Unfortunately, however, it is very difficult to say how far the carbon monoxide uptake reflects the true diffusion characteristics of the alveolar membrane and the capillary blood in the presence of appreciable lung disease. The reason for this is that inequality of ventilation, diffusion characteristics, and blood volume reduce the carbon monoxide in an unpredictable way. For this reason, the test when used in the clinic is sometimes said to measure the *transfer factor* of the lung for carbon monoxide and should be looked upon as a general index of the efficiency of gas exchange in the lung rather than as a specific test of diffusion.

IMPAIRMENT OF DIFFUSION The diffusion properties of the alveolar membrane depend on its thickness and area. Thus, the diffusing capacity is reduced by diseases in which the thickness is increased, including diffuse interstitial fibrosis (Chap. 280), sarcoidosis (Chap. 235), asbestosis (Chap. 275), and alveolar cell carcinomatosis (Chap. 284). The diffusing capacity also falls when the area of the membrane is reduced. This occurs following pneumonectomy and in emphysema. In addition, as we saw above, the diffusing capacity falls when the capillary blood volume or the number of red blood cells in the capillaries is reduced. This is the case in anemia and in diseases such as pulmonary embolism.

The importance of diffusion impairment as a cause of hypoxemia has long been disputed. In those lung diseases such as diffuse interstitial fibrosis in which microscopically the alveolar wall is thickened, it is tempting to attribute any hypoxemia to defective diffusion. The term *alveolar-capillary block* was coined for this situation, and it is certainly an easy one to remember. However, recent work indicates that impaired diffusion is not the principal cause of the hypoxemia in these patients. It is probably impossible for normal ventilation and blood flow to occur in an alveolus which has a thickened wall, and several investigators have shown marked inequality of ventilation and blood flow in the lung in these conditions. Studies in which it is possible to assess the extent of ventilation-perfusion inequality in patients with interstitial lung disease using a multiple inert gas technique indicate that, at rest, all the hypoxemia can be attributed to uneven ventilation and blood flow. However, on exercise, a small component of the hypoxemia is apparently caused by diffusion impairment. Thus, most of the hypoxemia in patients with so-called alveolar-capillary block must be attributed to ventilation-perfusion inequality.

BLOOD FLOW

Mixed venous blood is pumped to the pulmonary capillaries directly from the right side of the heart so that the total *pulmonary blood flow* is equal to the cardiac output, say 5 or 6 liters per minute in a normal adult. We saw earlier that the volume of fresh inspired air entering the alveoli each minute, the *alveolar ventilation,* is some 5 liters. Thus, the overall ratio of ventilation to blood flow, or *ventilation/perfusion ratio,* is about 1.

Even though the volumes of fresh gas and blood reaching the alveoli each minute are about the same, the volumes involved in exchanging gas at any instant are very different. Thus, while the alveolar gas volume is 2 to 3 liters at the end of a normal expiration, the capillary blood volume is only some 70 ml. This is why the lung microscopist sees chiefly air.

The pressures in the pulmonary circulation have long been considered the domain of the cardiologist, but they have an important bearing on gas exchange in the lung. The normal pulmonary arterial pressure is only just sufficient to raise blood to the top of the upright lung; if the pressure is reduced, as in hemorrhagic shock, the upper part of the lung is unperfused and gas exchange is impaired. Alterations in the pulmonary venous pressure, too, affect the distribution of blood flow in the lung.

VENTILATION-PERFUSION RELATIONSHIPS

Up to this point, we have been assuming that all lung units behave identically. Thus, Fig. 271-1 has been taken to refer to an alveolus, a group of alveoli with their duct, a lobe, or even the whole lung. In fact, however, the lung is not homogeneous, and the differences in behavior between the millions of units are responsible for the great bulk of the hypoxemia and hypercarbia seen in clinical practice. We shall see that even in the normal lung, there are marked regional differences in blood flow and ventilation which affect gas exchange, while in diseased states, the inhomogeneity becomes so severe that respiratory failure may ultimately develop.

NORMAL DISTRIBUTION OF BLOOD FLOW It is possible to measure the regional distribution of blood flow and ventilation in the lung by using radioactive gases. In one technique, the inert gas xenon 133 is employed. To measure blood flow, the xenon is dissolved in saline and injected into a peripheral vein. On reaching the lung, it is evolved into alveolar gas because of its poor solubility; there it remains during breath holding, and its radiation can be detected by external counters. To measure ventilation, the patient inhales a single breath of the radioactive gas and again its regional distribution is measured. In both instances, a further measurement after a period of rebreathing of xenon allows a correction for lung volume to be made.

In the normal upright lung, blood flow per unit volume decreases rapidly from bottom to top, reaching very low values at the apex. This pattern is affected by change of posture and exercise. When the subject lies supine, the apical and basal blood flows become the same, but the posterior (dependent) part of the lung has a higher blood flow than the anterior region. In the lateral position, the dependent regions are best perfused. On exercise in the upright position, both apical and basal blood flows increase, so that the proportion of the total flow going to the apex rises.

The cause of this uneven distribution of blood flow lies in the hydrostatic pressure differences within the lung. The pulmonary circulation is unique in that air and blood are separated by a very delicate membrane over a vertical distance of some 30 cm in the upright position, and consequently, the hydrostatic effect of this large column of blood determines the caliber of the small vessels. The distribution of blood flow depends on the relative magnitudes of the pulmonary arterial, venous, and alveolar pressures. In particular, if pulmonary arterial pressure falls (as in hemorrhage, shock, and anesthesia) or alveolar pressure is raised (as in positive-pressure ventilation), the distribution of blood flow becomes more uneven. The normal pattern is also commonly affected by both heart and lung disease.

NORMAL DISTRIBUTION OF VENTILATION Ventilation also increases down the upright lung, though the changes are less marked than for blood flow. This distribution of ventilation which is seen under normal resting conditions is altered at low lung volumes. It has been shown that when a normal subject exhales as far as possible (to residual volume) and then gradually inhales in small steps, initially very little air goes into the lower zones, but the upper zones are well ventilated. However, before this subject reaches a normal resting lung volume (functional residual capacity), this distribution is reversed and the lower zones are better ventilated than the upper. This pattern is then maintained right up to maximal volumes. The poor ventilation of the dependent regions of the lung at low lung volumes is seen in the erect, supine, and lateral situations, and it has important implications in clinical situations in which the lung volume is low, e.g., in obesity or following abdominal surgery. Since the dependent regions are the best perfused, the impairment of gas exchange may then be severe.

The cause of the normal uneven distribution of ventilation has to do with the way the lung is supported inside the chest. It is known that the expanding pressure on the lung is less in the dependent zones, presumably because these regions help to support the lung above them. Thus, the intrapleural pressure is less negative at the bottom of the lung than at the top. The reason for the greater ventilation of the dependent regions at normal volumes is twofold: (1) these alveoli have a smaller resting volume, and (2) their increase in volume is relatively large because, having a smaller volume, they are more distensible. By contrast, these dependent regions are poorly ventilated at low lung volumes because the expanding forces on them are then too weak to inflate them. Indeed, under these conditions, the airways to these alveoli may close and the alveoli become unventilated.

The volume at which the lower zone airways close (the *closing volume*) is considerably less than the functional residual capacity in normal young subjects. However, as the lung ages, and especially in the presence of chronic obstructive lung disease, the closing volume increases until it encroaches on the normal breathing range. Thus elderly normal subjects and patients with chronic bronchitis and emphysema frequently close their lower zone airways during resting breathing; this results in a poorly ventilated region which impairs gas exchange.

The closing volume can be measured from the single-breath nitrogen test (see "Measurement of Ventilation Inequality" below). There is some evidence that the measurement of closing volume is a sensitive test of early disease affecting the small airways. For example, cigarette smokers may have an increased closing volume when other tests of lung function are still normal.

VENTILATION/PERFUSION RATIO We have seen that while blood flow increases greatly down the upright lung, the change in ventilation is less. As a result, the ventilation/perfusion ratio varies from a high value at the top of the lung to a low value at the bottom. The ventilation/perfusion ratio is of key importance because it determines the gas exchange which occurs in any part of the lung.

Consider a lung unit as shown in Fig. 271-1. It can readily be seen that the partial pressure of oxygen in the alveolar gas (and therefore in the end-capillary blood) will be set by a balance between the rate of its removal by the blood flow, on the one hand, and the rate of its replenishment by the ventilation on the other. Thus, if the ventilation is gradually reduced but the blood flow is maintained, the oxygen partial pressure will gradually fall. The limit is reached when the unit is not ventilated and the P_{O_2} becomes that of venous blood. This is a ventilation/perfusion ratio of zero. By contrast, if perfusion is gradually reduced, the P_{O_2} will rise. The limit now occurs when the unit is unperfused and the P_{O_2} in the alveolus is the same as that of inspired air. This is a ventilation/perfusion ratio of infinity.

Thus, the crucial factor determining the oxygen partial pressure is the ventilation/perfusion ratio; this is also true for the partial pressure of carbon dioxide, and indeed of any other gas that might be present. It can be shown that regional differences of gas exchange occur in the normal upright lung as a consequence of the uneven ventilation/perfusion ratios.

OVERALL GAS EXCHANGE Though such regional differences in gas exchange are of interest, more important is the effect of uneven ventilation/perfusion ratios on overall gas exchange, i.e., the ability of the lung to take up oxygen and put out carbon dioxide. The reason gas transfer is impaired by uneven ventilation and blood flow is that those lung units which are overperfused in relation to their ventilation, and which therefore have a low P_{O_2}, contribute a disproportionate amount of the blood flow to the systemic arterial system. The net result is that the arterial P_{O_2} is depressed because it is loaded with less well oxygenated blood. In the same way, because these lung units have a relatively high P_{CO_2}, they tend to elevate the arterial P_{CO_2}. It is as if uneven ventilation/perfusion ratios set up a barrier between the gas and the blood, with the result that the arterial P_{O_2} is depressed and the P_{CO_2} is raised.

There is an additional reason why the arterial P_{O_2} is reduced by ventilation/perfusion ratio inequality. Though the oxygen content of blood draining from alveoli with a low ventilation/perfusion ratio is always abnormally low, alveoli with a high ventilation/perfusion ratio are not able to oxygenate their blood much more than normal alveoli. This is because the blood is normally almost fully saturated with oxygen owing to the shape of the oxygen dissociation curve. This additional reason does not apply to carbon dioxide.

In the normal lung, the effects of uneven ventilation/perfusion ratios on overall gas exchange are trivial; the arterial P_{O_2} is reduced by only a few millimeters of mercury and the P_{CO_2} is raised by less than 1 mmHg, if all else remains the same. Both these liabilities can be met if the total ventilation of the lung and thus its overall ventilation/perfusion ratio are increased. Indeed, the level of overall ventilation is normally set by the medullary respiratory center via the arterial P_{CO_2}. Thus, if uneven ventilation/perfusion ratios elevate the arterial P_{CO_2}, this is brought back by the increased respiratory drive and the consequently higher overall ventilation.

In the diseased lung, the effects of ventilation/perfusion ratio inequality on gas transfer may be very severe because the degree of uneven ventilation and blood flow is far greater than in the normal lung. The arterial P_{O_2} may be depressed by 50 mmHg or more, and in practice no amount of increased ventilation can return it to its normal level. The P_{CO_2}, however, is often maintained at the normal level by an increase in total ventilation. The reason an increase in ventilation to diseased lungs can reduce the arterial P_{CO_2} but not increase the P_{O_2} to normal levels lies in the different shapes of the two dissociation curves. If the ventilation is not increased, the P_{CO_2} remains elevated. Ventilation/perfusion ratio inequality is much the commonest cause of hypoxemia and hypercapnia in generalized lung disease.

MEASUREMENT OF VENTILATION/PERFUSION INEQUALITY Unfortunately, it is difficult to derive much information about the pattern of uneven ventilation and blood flow in the diseased lung. Because much of the inequality is at the microscopic level, radioactive gas detectors which "see" relatively large regions of lung give little indication of the extent of the unevenness. The best method as yet which is suitable for clinical practice is the analysis of expired gas and arterial blood.

We have seen that the P_{O_2} of arterial blood is depressed in the presence of ventilation/perfusion ratio inequality because it is loaded with less well oxygenated blood from those alveoli which are overperfused in relation to their ventilation. By contrast, the expired alveolar gas receives a disproportionately high contribution from lung units which are overventilated in relation to their blood flow, where the P_{O_2} is high. An alveolar-arterial oxygen difference therefore develops, and the magnitude of this difference is a measure of the amount of ventilation/perfusion ratio inequality.

Though arterial blood can be collected by puncture, a representative sample of mixed alveolar gas is often impossible to obtain in the diseased lung because of its disturbed pattern of emptying. An alternative is to collect all the expired gas (including that from the dead space of the bronchi), using a valve box and a large bag or spirometer, and to calculate what is called the *ideal alveolar* P_{O_2}. This is the value which the alveolar gas would have in the absence of ventilation/perfusion ratio inequality. This calculation is made using the arterial P_{CO_2} and the alveolar gas equation.

The P_{O_2} difference between ideal alveolar gas and arterial blood chiefly reflects those alveoli with an abnormally *low* ventilation/perfusion ratio, i.e., the alveoli which are overperfused in relation to their ventilation. These alveoli cause the hypoxemia, and their presence has the same effect as the admixture of some venous blood with arterial blood. Indeed, it is possible to express their contribution *as if* a certain proportion of the venous blood bypassed the lung altogether and was then added to the arterial blood. This is called *venous admixture,* physiologic shunt, or wasted blood flow, and is calculated from the P_{O_2} difference between ideal alveolar gas and arterial blood. Normally, calculated venous admixture is only about 2 percent of the pulmonary blood flow, but it may rise to 30 percent or higher in the presence of severe ventilation/perfusion ratio inequality.

The alveoli with an abnormally *high* ventilation/perfusion ratio, i.e., those which are overventilated in relation to their perfusion, mainly affect carbon dioxide elimination. They behave as if a certain proportion of the inspired gas bypassed the alveoli altogether, i.e., as if the dead space were increased in size, thus resulting in wasted ventilation. Their contribution can be calculated from the P_{CO_2} of arterial blood and mixed expired gas, using Bohr's equation. This gives a value for the *physiologic dead space,* which includes not only the volume of the bronchi but also the so-called alveolar dead space attributable to the overventilated alveoli. Normally the physiologic dead space is less than 30 percent of the tidal volume at rest, but it may rise to 50 percent or more in the presence of severe disease. Both venous admixture and physiologic dead space are typically increased in chronic obstructive pulmonary disease (Chap. 279) and interstitial diseases of the lung (Chap. 280); in pulmonary thromboembolism (Chap. 282), an increase in dead space predominates.

Another method of measuring ventilation/perfusion inequality has recently been described. Rather than measuring the partial pressures of oxygen and carbon dioxide in arterial blood and expired gas, this method uses a continuous infusion of six foreign inert gases into the venous blood. After a steady state of gas exchange has been established, the consequent partial pressures in arterial blood and expired gas are then measured. From this information, it is possible to derive an almost continuous distribution of ventilation/perfusion ratios. Young normal subjects have very narrow distributions centered on the normal value of about 1. Patients with chronic obstructive lung disease and asthma, for example, often have bimodal distributions with substantial amounts of blood flow going to lung units with very low ventilation/perfusion ratios. As yet, this method is confined to the clinical research setting.

MEASUREMENT OF VENTILATION INEQUALITY Because the measurement of ventilation/perfusion ratio inequality is a relatively difficult procedure, the simpler measurement of uneven ventilation is often made. Although it would be theoretically possible for a patient to have ventilatory inequality but no mismatch of ventilation and blood flow, this is not seen in practice.

The simplest method of measuring uneven ventilation is the single-breath nitrogen wash-out test. For this, the patient takes a single inspiration of pure oxygen and then exhales fully. A rapid nitrogen meter at the lips measures expired nitrogen concentration, and expired volume is recorded simultaneously. After 750 ml has been expired (sufficient to clear the dead space), the rise in nitrogen concentration over the next 500 ml is measured. This is less than 1.5 percent in normal subjects. However, in patients with uneven ventilation, the nitrogen concentration rises more rapidly because the degree of dilution of the nitrogen by the inhaled oxygen varies throughout the lung, and also because the poorly ventilated regions (which receive little oxygen and therefore have the most nitrogen) always empty last. This is a simple, quick, and useful test, and it may also be used to give the closing volume (see earlier under "Normal Distribution of Ventilation").

Uneven ventilation can also be detected by a multibreath nitrogen wash-out test, but this is now seldom used.

VENTILATION/PERFUSION RATIO INEQUALITY IN DISEASE Virtually all generalized diseases of the lung, such as emphysema, chronic bronchitis, diffuse interstitial fibrosis, and the pneumoconioses, result in mismatch of ventilation and blood flow. As yet little is known about the pattern of unevenness in these conditions, though it is not difficult to imagine that an area of fibrosis or a bulla, for example, must interfere with both ventilation and blood flow.

There is evidence that, in general, areas of the lung which are poorly ventilated are also poorly perfused. One reason for this is that local pathologic change tends to disturb both processes by its mechanical effects. However, there are other physiologic mechanisms which reduce the mismatch of ventilation and perfusion. One is the reduction in blood flow to a poorly ventilated, hypoxic region of the lung, which has now been demonstrated on many occasions. The precise mechanism is unknown, but it appears to be a local response to alveolar hypoxemia, since it occurs in the isolated denervated lung. Another mechanism is the reduction of ventilation which has been shown to follow obstruction to a branch of the pulmonary artery. This is apparently due to an increase in resistance of the small airways caused by a fall in P_{CO_2} in the region. This mechanism is weak in human beings.

How far these two mechanisms operate in practice is unknown, but it has been shown that the administration of various bronchodilator and vasodilator drugs to patients with generalized lung disease can exaggerate their hypoxemia. For example, isoproterenol (by aerosol) and epinephrine and aminophylline (by injection) have been shown to reduce the arterial P_{O_2} of some patients with chronic obstructive lung disease and bronchial asthma. It is possible that one of the actions of these drugs is to interfere with these active mechanisms which reduce ventilation/perfusion ratio inequality.

MECHANICS OF BREATHING

The bellows function of the lung is one of the easiest to measure and also one of the most informative measurements in practice. Serious malfunction of the lung is almost always accompanied by a reduced ventilatory capacity.

LUNG AND CHEST WALL The lung is elastic and collapses if it is not held expanded. The pressure *inside* the lung (alveolar pressure) is the same as atmospheric pressure at the end of inspiration or expiration if the glottis is open. The pressure *outside* the lung (intrapleural pressure) is less than atmospheric pressure, or "negative." This pressure keeps the lung inflated and is developed by the chest wall, which is also elastic and tends to bow outward. If air is introduced into this space and a pneumothorax is produced, the lung collapses inward and the chest wall moves outward.

During quiet breathing, inspiration is produced chiefly by the action of the diaphragm assisted by the intercostal muscles, and expiration results from the passive elastic recoil of the lungs. During deep breathing, the accessory muscles such as the sternomastoids and scaleni are called upon, and patients with diseased lungs may use these even at rest. Under these conditions, expiration is often assisted by the abdominal muscles.

COMPLIANCE This is a term used to describe the elastic properties of the lung and chest wall. The normal lungs expand by about 200 ml when the expanding pressure (intrapleural pressure) changes by 1 cmH_2O. Thus the compliance (or distensibility) of the lungs is said to be 200 ml/cmH_2O. In fact, this figure only applies at normal resting lung volumes; at high lung volumes, the lungs are less easy to expand and their compliance falls. A more complete description of the elastic properties of the lungs, therefore, is the pressure-volume curve over the whole range of lung volumes; for this reason, this measurement is preferred in many pulmonary function laboratories. The compliance of the normal chest wall is about the same as that of the lungs, and the compliance of both lung and chest wall together is therefore about half this value, i.e., 100 ml/cmH_2O.

The compliance of lung depends very much on how much tissue is present. A single lobe, for example, will clearly not change its volume by as much as a whole lung for the same change in expanding pressure. Compliance is therefore sometimes corrected for lung volume and called *specific compliance.*

The normal elastic behavior of the lungs is only partly caused by the elastic tissue within it. An important component is the surface tension of the fluid lining the alveoli. The lungs may be regarded as composed of 300 million tiny bubbles which tend to collapse for the same reason that a soap bubble on the end of a bubble pipe does. The surface forces which tend to reduce the area of the surface thus tend to reduce the volume of the bubble. These surface forces therefore contribute to the elastic force of the lung. Fortunately some of the cells lining the alveoli produce a phospholipid which lowers the surface tension of the lining fluid to extremely low values. The substance is known as a *surfactant.* This lowering of the surface tension is of great physiologic importance, because it helps to maintain the stability of the alveoli and discourage atelectasis.

About half the normal elastic recoil force of the lung is due to these surface forces.

The normal elastic behavior of the lung is disturbed by many diseases. Diffuse pulmonary fibrosis, pleural thickening, healed tuberculosis with scarring, and atelectasis all reduce the compliance of the lung. Heart disease, such as mitral stenosis and left ventricular failure, also commonly lowers compliance, although it is often difficult to be certain whether the volume of ventilating lung is reduced by edema in the airways, for example, or whether the elastic behavior of the lung tissue itself is altered. An absence of surfactant is thought to be responsible for the alveolar collapse and the stiff lungs seen in hyaline membrane disease of the newborn. In emphysema and old age, the lungs become more compliant and have an abnormally large volume at normal expanding pressures.

AIRWAY RESISTANCE So far we have been looking at the static forces involved in maintaining the expansion of the lung. However, during ventilation, additional forces are required to move air along the airways, because of the resistance offered to flow. This is expressed as the pressure difference between the alveoli and the mouth per unit of airflow rate. The normal value is in the vicinity of 1 to 2 cmH_2O per liter per second of flow at normal flow rates. The resistance rises at higher flow rates.

Until recently it was thought that the chief site of resistance was the small airways. However, it is now known that most of the resistance lies in the medium-sized bronchi and that the bronchioles less than 2 mm in diameter contribute less than 20 percent of the total airway resistance. The reason for this is the prodigious number of small airways. As a consequence, substantial increases in resistance of these bronchioles will not be detected by the usual pulmonary function tests, and they are said to constitute a "silent zone." There is currently a good deal of interest in tests designed to detect changes in the small airways. These include the single-breath nitrogen test, the measurement of closing volume referred to above, and the measurement of "frequency-dependent compliance," i.e., the apparent fall in lung compliance which occurs at high breathing rates. Whether these tests are better at detecting early airway disease than the time-honored forced expiratory volume (see below under "Measurements of Mechanics") has not yet been established.

Various factors alter airway resistance. For example, the resistance is higher during expiration than inspiration, and it is greater at small lung volumes because the airways are then not held open so much. A single deep inspiration often reduces the resistance, but the inhalation of cigarette smoke or other irritants increases it, through reflex contraction of airway smooth muscle following stimulation of irritant receptors located in the airway wall.

A dramatic increase in airway resistance occurs during forced expiration. The cause of this is collapse of the airways, so-called dynamic compression. The explanation is that the high intrapleural pressure is applied not only to the alveoli in an effort to empty them but also to the outside walls of the airways which lie within the chest. Consequently the airways are compressed, and as a result, the expiratory flow rate is independent of respiratory effort over a large range, since the greater the effort, the more the collapse. In normal subjects, this phenomenon takes place only during forced expirations, but it occurs much more readily in patients with chronic bronchitis and emphysema. This is because the airway walls are diseased and weakened, or because the airways lose their support by radial traction from the surrounding lung.

Diseases which increase airway resistance during normal breathing include bronchial asthma and chronic bronchitis. The resistance may rise to many times its normal value and even during clinical remissions of the disease can be shown to be abnormally high. Lung volume increases in these conditions, and this has two helpful consequences: the airways are pulled open more, thus limiting the increase in resistance, and the higher passive recoil pressure of the lung assists expiration.

WORK OF BREATHING To move the lungs and chest wall and force air along the airways, work is required and the respiratory muscles must consume oxygen. In normal subjects, the work of breathing is very small except during the large ventilation of heavy exercise. In patients with obstructive lung disease, however, the frictional resistance to airflow is high even at rest and the work of breathing is much increased, perhaps to 5 or 10 times its normal value. Under these conditions, the oxygen cost of breathing may become an appreciable fraction of the total oxygen consumption.

Patients with a reduced compliance of the lungs or chest wall have a higher work of breathing, because the stiffer structures are more difficult to move. These patients tend to use rapid shallow breaths, which reduces their oxygen cost of ventilation. However, if breathing becomes too shallow, the volume of air merely moved in and out of the bronchial dead space becomes disproportionately high, and gas exchange is consequently impaired. A compromise is therefore reached.

MEASUREMENTS OF MECHANICS One of the most useful tests in the armamentarium of the pulmonary function laboratory is the analysis of a single forced expiration. The patient makes a full inspiration and then exhales as hard and as fast as possible into a lightweight spirometer. Typical records are shown in Fig. 271-2. It can be seen that for a normal subject the total volume exhaled is large. This is called the vital capacity or, preferably, the *forced vital capacity* (FVC). (The word "forced" is added because the volume may be less than the vital capacity measured with a slow expiration.) Also, about 80 percent of this volume is exhaled in 1 s. This is called the *forced expiratory volume,* or FEV_1. In *obstructive lung disease,* e.g., chronic bronchitis and emphysema, the forced vital capacity is reduced because the airways close and limit expiration before the patient has breathed out fully. In addition, the FEV_1 is grossly reduced as is the FEV/FVC percentage. This is because of the high airway resistance, which slows down the rate of expiration. In *restrictive lung disease,* e.g., ankylosing spondylitis, the FVC is low because of the limited expansion of the lung or chest wall. However, the FEV_1 is often not reduced proportionately, because airway resistance is normal. Thus the FEV/FVC percentage is normal or high. Normal values for lung volumes and spirometric tests are found in the appendix.

Other indexes of ventilatory function can be derived from a forced expiration. One is the maximal midexpiratory flow ($FEF_{25-75\%}$), which is obtained by dividing the volume between 75 percent and 25 percent of the vital capacity by the corresponding elapsed time (Fig. 271-2). This correlates well with the FEV_1 but may be a more sensitive measure of airway obstruction in early chronic obstructive lung disease.

Impaired lung function is almost always associated with a reduced FEV_1, and the test is therefore a valuable screening procedure. It is also useful in assessing the efficacy of bronchodilator therapy and in following the progress of patients with asthma or chronic obstructive lung disease.

Other lung volumes can also be measured at the same time. The *total lung capacity* is the total volume of gas in the lung at full inspiration. The *inspiratory capacity* is the maximum volume which can be inspired from the resting volume of the lungs, which is called the *functional residual capacity.* The maximum volume which can be expired from the resting level

FIGURE 271-2
Measurement of the forced expiratory volume, FEV_1; forced vital capacity, FVC; and maximum midexpiratory flow, $FEF_{25-75\%}$. The patient makes a full inspiration and then exhales as hard and as fast as possible. As the patient exhales the pen moves down. The FEF_1 is the volume exhaled in 1 s; the FVC is the total volume exhaled. The $FEF_{25-75\%}$ is the mean flow rate measured over the middle half of the FVC. Note the differences between the normal, obstructive, and restrictive patterns.

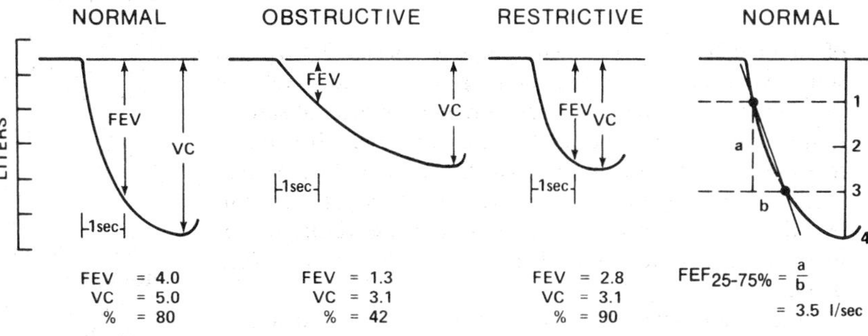

is the *expiratory reserve volume.* This leaves the *residual volume* still in the lungs, and this and the functional residual capacity can be measured only indirectly. One technique is to connect the patient to a spirometer circuit containing helium and measure the degree of dilution of this gas which occurs after several minutes of rebreathing. Another is to use a body plethysmograph (see below).

These volumes are often altered by disease. The functional residual capacity and residual volume are typically increased in diseases in which there is an increased airway resistance, for example, in emphysema, chronic bronchitis, and asthma. Indeed, at one time an elevated residual volume was regarded as an essential feature of emphysema, but less emphasis is placed on this test now. A reduced functional residual capacity and residual volume are often seen in patients with a reduced lung compliance, for example, in diffuse interstitial fibrosis. Here the lung is stiff and tends to recoil to a much smaller resting volume.

The measurement of compliance and airway resistance is more difficult. In order to determine lung compliance, i.e., volume change per unit of pressure change, the pressure expanding the lungs must be known. In practice this can be found by passing a small latex balloon connected to a manometer down into the esophagus. Esophageal pressure is then taken as a measure of intrapleural pressure. To measure airway resistance, i.e., the pressure drop along the airways per unit of airflow, alveolar pressure must be known. This can be found by seating the patient in a large airtight box, or plethysmograph. First, the patient is asked to try to breathe against a complete obstruction, and from the change in box pressure, lung volume can be calculated. Next, the patient is asked to pant, and again box pressure is recorded. Alveolar pressure can then be derived and airway resistance calculated. This equipment is available only in specialized centers.

Aging has an important influence on lung function. With increasing age there is a fall in vital capacity and forced expiratory volume and an increase in functional residual capacity, residual volume, and closing volume. Some inequality of ventilation and ventilation/perfusion ratios develops and the arterial P_{O_2} falls almost linearly with age. It is therefore important to take account of the age of the patient when interpreting many pulmonary function tests.

ACID-BASE DISTURBANCES If pulmonary gas exchange is impaired, the P_{CO_2} in the arterial blood may rise, thus tending to depress the pH and causing *respiratory acidosis.* The compensatory mechanisms which are then brought into play are discussed in Chap. 44.

MEASUREMENT OF BLOOD GASES Blood gas measurements play a vital role in the management of respiratory failure. Arterial blood can be obtained by direct puncture, and the oxygen and carbon dioxide partial pressures and the pH can be measured by electrodes. Oxygen saturation can be derived by spectrophotometry.

HYPOXEMIA

The four main causes of a low arterial P_{O_2} are (1) ventilation/perfusion ratio inequality, (2) right-to-left shunt, (3) hypoventilation, and (4) impaired diffusion. In addition, living at high altitude or deliberately inspiring a low oxygen mixture causes hypoxemia.

1 *Ventilation/perfusion ratio inequality* is the commonest cause and is responsible for almost all the hypoxemia seen in chronic lung disease. Specific tests of ventilation/perfusion inequality are not generally available, although the multiple inert gas infusion technique referred to earlier can be used in specialized centers. The demonstration of ventilatory inequality (see above) is a useful pointer. Mild degrees of ventilation/perfusion ratio inequality may be present without hypoxemia, and considerable inequality may exist without hypercapnia if overall ventilation is increased. However, carbon dioxide retention almost always develops eventually. The hypoxemia is eventually abolished by the administration of 100% oxygen. However, with severe inequality, the arterial P_{O_2} may take so many minutes to rise to normal values because of very poorly ventilated areas that, in practice, the levels seen in normal subjects may not be attained. Exercise may or may not aggravate the hypoxemia and hypercapnia (see Table 271-1). The response of the arterial P_{O_2} to exercise depends to a large extent on the changes in total ventilation and blood flow.
2 *Shunted blood,* i.e., blood which has bypassed ventilated areas of the lung, causes hypoxemia. Patients with right-to-left shunts through congenital heart defects or a pulmonary arteriovenous fistula belong to this group. Patients with ventilation/perfusion ratio inequality often have some parts of the lung completely unventilated, and the contribution of these regions is indistinguishable from that of a shunt. The hypoxemia due to shunt is not abolished (although it is reduced) by administering 100% oxygen, and this test will distinguish it from the other causes of hypoxemia. The level of the arterial P_{O_2} under these conditions allows the percentage

TABLE 271-1
Features helpful in distinguishing the various causes of hypoxemia and hypercapnia

	Hypoxemia	*Hypercapnia*	*Hypoxemia on exercise*	*Hypercapnia on exercise*	*Hypoxemia on 100% O_2*
Ventilation/perfusion ratio inequality	Yes	Yes or no	Yes	Yes or no	No
Shunt	Yes	No	Yes	Possible	Yes
Hypoventilation	Yes	Yes	Often severe	Often severe	No
Impaired diffusion	Yes (rarely)	No	Often severe	No	No

of shunted blood to be measured. The arterial P_{O_2} rises to some extent because of the addition of dissolved oxygen to the pulmonary blood, and a measurement of arterial saturation may not permit detection of the hypoxemia. It is therefore important to measure P_{O_2}. The hypoxemia of shunt may be exaggerated by exercise. Hypercapnia does not occur unless the shunt is very gross, because the respiratory center increases the ventilation, thus holding the arterial P_{CO_2} down.

3 *Hypoventilation* always causes both hypoxemia and hypercapnia. Because of the shape of the oxygen dissociation curve, which means that a substantial fall in arterial P_{O_2} can occur with little reduction in oxygen saturation (see Fig. 54-4), considerable carbon dioxide retention may be present without recognizable cyanosis. If the patient is inhaling an enriched oxygen mixture, e.g., in the anesthetic recovery room, hypoxemia is not present but the hypercapnia may be severe.

4 *Impaired diffusion* rarely causes hypoxemia but not hypercapnia. The hypoxemia is accentuated by exercise but abolished if an enriched oxygen mixture is administered. As we have seen, diffusion impairment may occur in normal subjects during work at very high altitude, but its importance as a cause of hypoxemia in disease is minimal.

HYPERCAPNIA

The two chief causes of carbon dioxide retention are ventilation/perfusion ratio inequality and hypoventilation. Ventilation/perfusion ratio inequality is the commonest cause, although many patients have some degree of uneven ventilation and blood flow without hypercapnia. A combination of the two causes can occur.

Why does a patient with chronic lung disease develop hypercapnia? Progressive lung disease (perhaps aggravated by an acute infection) causes increasing mismatch of blood flow and ventilation and greater impairment of carbon dioxide transfer. For a time, the respiratory center is able to hold the arterial P_{CO_2} down to the normal level by increasing the ventilation, but the work of breathing is usually high because of airway obstruction, so that eventually a compromise is reached and the arterial and alveolar partial pressures rise. This has the advantage that more carbon dioxide is put out for the same ventilation, so it may be looked upon as a compensatory mechanism, albeit a hazardous one. As the ventilation/perfusion ratio inequality becomes worse, the tendency is for the arterial P_{CO_2} to rise further.

A particularly dangerous situation may arise if such a patient is given oxygen to breathe. The chief stimulus to ventilation in these patients is often hypoxemia, and when this is suddenly relieved, the ventilation may drop precipitously and the arterial P_{CO_2} climb rapidly. The carbon dioxide retention and acidosis may then cause clouding of consciousness, muscular twitching, and a raised intracranial pressure. Drugs which depress the respiratory center may produce a similar effect. Thus while oxygen administration is indicated in these patients because of their severe hypoxemia, it should be given with caution.

Another hazardous situation often arises when these patients are taken off oxygen because they are retaining too much carbon dioxide. Since the body stores of carbon dioxide are so large, many minutes elapse before the alveolar P_{CO_2} returns to reasonable levels. During this recovery period, this high alveolar carbon dioxide dilutes the alveolar oxygen and may cause profound hypoxemia.

METABOLIC FUNCTIONS OF THE LUNG

In addition to its primary function of gas exchange, the lung has significant metabolic functions. One of the most important of these is the synthesis of phospholipids such as dipalmitoyl lecithin, a constituent of surfactant (see earlier under "Compliance"). In addition the lung modifies various substances circulating within the blood. For example, it converts the relatively inactive polypeptide angiotensin I into the potent vasoconstrictor angiotensin II. Also the lung inactivates circulating serotonin, bradykinin, and some prostaglandins, while it takes up norepinephrine and histamine to some degree.

In disease, the lung has a remarkable potential for hormone production and secretion. For example, neoplasms such as bronchial carcinomas can produce a variety of polypeptide hormones.

REFERENCES

COTES JF: *Lung Function*, 4th ed. St Louis, Mosby, 1979

FISHMAN AP: Assessment of pulmonary performance, in *Pulmonary Diseases and Disorders*, AP Fishman (ed). New York, McGraw-Hill, 1980, pp 359–416

WEST JB: *Pulmonary Pathophysiology—the Essentials*, 2d ed. Baltimore, Williams & Wilkins, 1982

272
FIBEROPTIC BRONCHOSCOPY AND OTHER DIAGNOSTIC PROCEDURES

KENNETH M. MOSER

In seeking a definitive diagnosis in the patient with respiratory disease, a wide choice of diagnostic procedures is available. These procedures vary considerably, not only in diagnostic reliability and specificity, but also in terms of the discomfort and hazard to the patient. Hence, an orderly sequence of test selection is mandatory. This sequence should begin with procedures involving little risk and move on to those which entail higher morbidity and mortality rates only if necessary.

NONINVASIVE PROCEDURES

RADIOGRAPHIC PROCEDURES The *chest roentgenogram* serves two major roles in the search for a diagnosis in the patient with respiratory disease: *detector* and *guide.* Often, in its role as a detector, the routine chest roentgenogram initiates the diagnostic search by disclosing an abnormality in an asymptomatic individual. More commonly, it permits detection of pulmonary involvement in someone already ill. Rarely, detection may coincide with diagnosis; e.g., in spontaneous pneumothorax or when a radiopaque foreign body has been aspirated.

Far more frequently, however, the roentgenogram, having detected potential disease, provides a guide to the selection of subsequent diagnostic procedures. Many radiographic findings are quite characteristic of certain diseases. A number of radiographic patterns are sufficiently repetitive to warrant descriptive names, such as bilateral hilar adenopathy, solitary pulmonary nodule, diffuse interstitial infiltrate, alveolar filling pattern, multinodular lesion, and honeycomb lung. Thus, a particular radiographic finding, combined with other pertinent data, often permits establishment of a reasonable list of possible diagnoses. For example, the roentgenographic detection of bilateral hilar adenopathy in an asymptomatic, 26-year-old black male immediately places sarcoidosis at the top of the list. A chest roentgenogram disclosing upper lobe cavities in a febrile male whose brother recently was admitted to a tuberculosis sanitarium would make tuberculosis the most likely entity. Or a "diffuse interstitial" infiltrate—for which more than 100 causes exist—may yield a prompt diagnosis of varicella pneumonia when combined with the classical skin lesions.

In some instances, special radiographic techniques may provide valuable diagnostic insights.

Fluoroscopy allows visualization of the thoracic contents in a dynamic rather than static manner and also permits a wide range of special views. It also indicates whether a lesion is pulsatile, what its precise location in the thorax is, whether the hemidiaphragms move normally, i.e., whether they are fixed or move paradoxically, and how various zones of the lung behave during inspiration and expiration. Image intensification, permanent recording of fluoroscopy on videotape, and quantification of lung density from such recordings (videodensitometry) are extending the diagnostic capabilities of this simple procedure.

Tomography (laminagraphy, planigraphy) is a radiographic technique by which a sequence of roentgenograms, each representing a "slice of the lung" at a different depth, is obtained. Ordinarily, "cuts" are made at 0.5- to 1-cm distances through the area of interest. Tomograms can identify a number of features which were not appreciated on the "routine" roentgenogram, including the presence of calcium or cavity in a lesion; the presence of hilar or mediastinal adenopathy; abnormalities in configuration of the trachea and major bronchi; and the contours of masses in the mediastinal area.

Thoracic *computerized tomography (CT) scanning,* using the whole-body device, may provide useful information not available by other techniques for the definition of pleural lesions (e.g., differentiating fluid from tumor), lesions in the mediastinum (nodes, tumors, vascular structures), multiple lung nodules, and perhaps lesions in the major pulmonary arteries. As the technique becomes more widely used, its value and limitations in each of these contexts will become established. For example, the sensitivity of the CT scan in detecting pulmonary nodules not evident on the chest roentgenogram will be a mixed diagnostic blessing until it is known how many "normal" individuals may have such nodules and how these small, benign, hitherto "unseen" lesions can be distinguished (by size, density, or location) from neoplastic lesions.

SKIN TESTS Having arrived at a tentative list of diagnostic possibilities based on the history, physical examination, and radiographic appearance, the physician should move to other procedures. One of the simplest and most commonly overlooked is the application of *skin tests* with specific antigens. Antigens are now available to assist in the diagnosis of tuberculosis, histoplasmosis, coccidioidomycosis, blastomycosis, trichinosis, toxoplasmosis, and certain forms of aspergillosis. These tests vary with respect to sensitivity and cross-reactivity, and attention to scrupulous technique in performance and interpretation is vital. Also, some antigens (e.g., histoplasmosis) may confound serologic tests performed subsequently. A negative battery of skin tests, particularly if it incorporates antigens such as mumps, streptokinase-streptodornase, *Trichophyton,* and *Monilia,* may provide a diagnostic clue by suggesting disorders associated with depressed cell-mediated immunity, such as Hodgkin's disease, sarcoidosis, disseminated tuberculosis, or coccidioidomycosis.

SEROLOGIC TESTS These tests also may be useful in the diagnosis of histoplasmosis, blastomycosis, coccidioidomycosis, toxoplasmosis, *Mycoplasma* pneumonia, Legionnaires' disease, a variety of other infectious diseases involving the lungs, and certain immunologically mediated lung diseases. Often, more extensive diagnostic procedures can be avoided if appropriate serologic tests are obtained. However, there is substantial interinstitutional variability with respect to the sensitivity, specificity, and types of serologic tests.

SPUTUM EXAMINATION Another rapid, innocuous diagnostic procedure is *sputum examination.* It is important that the specimen contain sputum, not saliva. The gross nature of the sputum—color, odor, and the presence of blood—may provide valuable clues. Carefully stained smears of the sputum should be examined next, for these may disclose the causative organism in many bacterial pneumonias, in tuberculosis, and in some fungous infections. Sputum eosinophilia can suggest the presence of reversible airway disease responsive to corticosteroids; hemosiderin-laden macrophages suggest the possibility of Goodpasture's syndrome. Often valuable time is lost because the sputum smear is not examined and results of culture are awaited instead.

Culture of expectorated sputum (spontaneous or induced) has fallen into disrepute because of uncertain yield and, particularly, because of frequent and unavoidable contamination by the oropharyngeal bacterial flora. Although such cultures are invaluable for identification of organisms responsible for tuberculous and fungous infections, their utility in detection of other bacterial agents responsible for pulmonary infection is often uncertain and can be misleading, particularly in patients who are immunocompromised, intubated, or receiving antimicrobial therapy. Four procedures, described below, are now gaining wide acceptance because they limit oropharyngeal contamination and/or obtain representative samples of lung secretions from the area of lung involvement: (1) catheter-brush sampling, (2) transtracheal aspiration, (3) transbronchial lung biopsy, and (4) percutaneous needle aspiration of the lung.

Exfoliative cytology of the sputum is helpful in the diagnosis of carcinoma of the lung (Chap. 284). Proper handling of such specimens is essential. Sputum samples often can be obtained in patients who are not coughing by having them inhale a heated mixture of a mildly irritative solution which induces cough.

PULMONARY FUNCTION TESTS (see also Chap. 271) Certain "patterns" of derangement in spirometric tests, arterial blood gases, diffusing capacity, and other functional parameters are particularly suggestive of certain pulmonary diseases. For example, diffuse interstitial fibrotic diseases of the lungs (Chap. 280) produce a "restrictive" spirometric defect, reduced pulmonary compliance, a reduced diffusing capacity, and an alveolar-arterial oxygen tension difference which is widened at rest and widens further with exercise. Emphysema (Chap. 279) characteristically causes expiratory obstruction, lung hyperinflation, decreased static elastic recoil (increased compliance), and a reduced diffusing capacity.

PULMONARY SCINTIPHOTOGRAPHY Scintiphotographs ("scans") of intrathoracic structures are obtained by a variety of "scanning" devices which record the pattern of intrathoracic radioactivity after intravenous injection or inhalation of gamma-emitting radionuclides. Direct photographic or computer-derived images, or digital data, reflecting radionuclide distribution are used for diagnostic purposes. The most commonly used images are those which reflect the distribution of pulmonary blood flow (perfusion) and ventilation. Such scans have multiple diagnostic applications. For example, a normal perfusion scan casts great doubt on the diagnosis of acute pulmonary embolism (Chap. 282). When perfusion scans showing defects are combined with ventilation scans, ventilation-perfusion patterns are provided which assist in the diagnosis of parenchymal lung diseases and vascular occlusive disorders, including pulmonary embolism.

Another type of scan involves intravenous injection of radionuclides which have an affinity for intrathoracic inflammatory and neoplastic tissues. Concentration of gamma-emitting nuclides, defined by scanning, may permit detection of neoplastic or inflammatory disease in the lungs or mediastinal lymph nodes. Uptake by the lungs may reflect the extent of inflammatory activity associated with diffuse interstitial pneumonitis, sarcoidosis, and granulomatous infections. Concentrations in bones or soft tissues may assist in the detection of disseminated (extrapulmonary) foci in patients with pulmonary granulomatous and neoplastic diseases.

New radionuclides continue to emerge which, when complexed with such materials as platelets, white blood cells (e.g. indium 111), fibrinogen, and albumin, may allow imaging of intrathoracic vessels, thrombi, inflammation, and neoplasms. Tomographic and other image-processing methods are emerging which may further extend the value of these techniques. Gallium 67 is the most useful of these radionuclides now available.

All the above procedures involve minimal risks and discomfort to the patient. Where applicable, these approaches should be considered before the more invasive techniques discussed below are considered, unless the condition of the patient demands immediate diagnosis.

INVASIVE PROCEDURES

BRONCHOSCOPY The primary objectives of bronchoscopy include direct visualization of the tracheobronchial tree, including abnormalities such as tumors or granulomatous lesions; biopsy of suggestive or obvious endobronchial lesions; and brushing, washing, or biopsy of lung regions for cultural and cytologic examinations. Both the *diagnostic reach of* and *accessibility to* bronchoscopy have been expanded by the flexible fiberoptic bronchoscope (FOB). This can be understood best by comparing the FOB with the "standard" rigid bronchoscope.

The rigid bronchoscope is a wide-bore metal tube which incorporates a lighted mirror-lens system. The FOB is composed of fiberoptic bundles which provide both illumination and visualization pathways. A small channel with a diameter of 1 to 3 mm traverses the FOB, through which instruments can be passed, fluids delivered, and suction applied. The rigid bronchoscope comes in various external diameters limited only by the feasibility of introducing the rigid device orally and through the larynx. Biopsy and other procedures are carried out through the rather capacious interior of the rigid tube. The FOB also is available in various external diameters, but all are substantially smaller than rigid bronchoscopes (since no "wall" exists in the FOB). The distal tip of the FOB can be *flexed* easily to 90° and usually to 130° or more from the vertical.

Thus, the rigid bronchoscope permits visualization only of lobar bronchi and the orifices of some segmental bronchi. The flexible, smaller FOB extends the range of *view* to all segmental and subsegmental bronchi and the range for *biopsy and sampling* to the pulmonary parenchyma itself. A biopsy forceps, catheter, or brush passed through the FOB can be directed well beyond the tip of the bronchoscope itself, permitting *transbronchial lung biopsy, brushings,* or *aspiration of secretions* for culture and cytologic examination from the most distal regions of the lung. Indeed, both forceps and brush can reach and perforate the pleura, leading to pneumothorax. Therefore, when the lesion being approached is distal, fluoroscopic guidance is essential. Not only does this permit placement of the FOB, forceps, catheter, or brush directly into the area of interest, but also it assures that the pleura will not be inadvertently reached and punctured. The FOB also allows *regional* lung lavage to obtain materials for cytologic examination and culture. The use of specially designed catheters (see below) placed through the FOB is quite useful in obtaining representative, noncontaminated secretions for culture, thus avoiding the problems mentioned previously with expectorated sputum.

Thus, the FOB has sharply increased the limited diagnostic reach previously available with rigid bronchoscopy. Equally important, the FOB has made bronchoscopy more available to the physician and more acceptable to the patient. The performance of rigid bronchoscopy requires the supine position for peroral insertion of the device; can be performed safely by a relatively few trained surgeons; and is often carried out under general anesthesia in an operating room. Therefore, it has been a procedure requiring significant preparation and hence delay. Fiberoptic bronchoscopy can be performed in the sitting or supine position, since the FOB is easily inserted transnasally; can be performed by a large number of trained pulmonary specialists as well as surgeons; usually requires only local anesthesia; and can be performed safely on the wards, in diagnostic rooms equipped with a "dentist-type" chair, and in intensive care units. The FOB can be used easily in intubated patients on ventilators with simple "side-arm" adapters attached to the endotracheal tube. Therefore, when bronchoscopy is indicated, it is not surprising that fiberoptic bronchoscopy is now commonly the first choice. The roomier rigid bronchoscope is now usually reserved for situations in which the small biopsy-suction channel in the FOB may be inadequate (e.g., for removal of large foreign bodies). The FOB also has a widening range of therapeutic applications including aspiration or lavage of secretions in patients with airway obstruction or atelectasis due to retained secretions; obstruction of bleeding areas of the lung, with a wedged FOB itself or with a balloon catheter passed via the FOB, in patients who are poor surgical risks; removal of small foreign bodies; and placement of radionuclides in tumors.

The hazards of bronchoscopy are modest but should be recognized. In addition to the risk of general anesthesia which rigid bronchoscopy usually requires, they can include hypoxemia, laryngospasm, bronchospasm, pneumothorax, and, of course, bleeding following biopsy. Proper management before, during, and after bronchoscopy should prevent most of these complications. There is no absolute contraindication to FOB. Even in the presence of massive hemoptysis, FOB with appropriate precautions can yield useful information. Patients with bronchospasm (or a history of bronchospasm) are at particular risk of acute enhancement of spasm and should be approached after good preparation and with resources for intubation-ventilation at hand. The primary contraindication to both rigid and fiberoptic bronchoscopy is the same: performance by inexperienced personnel. Lack of experience sharply reduces diagnostic and therapeutic yield while increasing risks.

BRONCHOGRAPHY In this method, radiopaque material is instilled into the tracheobronchial tree via a catheter or bronchoscope. Positioning of the patient and catheter permits the material to coat all portions of the tracheobronchial tree for a sufficient period so that their outline can be recorded on chest roentgenograms. Bronchography is indicated for the diagnosis of bronchiectasis, for the identification of obstruction in distal bronchi, and for the detection of other types of congenital and acquired forms of tracheobronchial distortion or malformation. Like FOB, bronchography may induce bronchospasm; also, the irritative effects of the contrast medium may persist for some days.

TRANSTRACHEAL, CATHETER-BRUSH, AND PERCUTANEOUS NEEDLE ASPIRATION OF THE LUNG All three of these procedures are used to obtain material for culture and microscopic examination. In the case of culture, all three techniques bypass the oropharyngeal flora, though transtracheal aspiration is the least certain in this regard.

Transtracheal aspiration involves needle puncture of the cricothyroid membrane, insertion of a plastic cannula, and installation of a saline solution, followed by suctioning of a sample. The procedure cannot be performed in intubated patients; contamination rates are high in previously intubated patients or those who have aspirated oropharyngeal contents. Because the procedure entails risks, although these are minimized by meticulous technique and experience, clear indications for its use should exist. These include patients with apparent pulmonary infection who are unable to cough, in whom cough is nonproductive, or in whom there has been a lack of response to therapy based on smears or cultures from expectorated sputum.

In these same contexts, *catheter-brush devices* specially designed with a distal plug to avoid oropharyngeal contamination can be used. These are manipulated (through an FOB or without it) under fluoroscopic guidance into the involved lung area. The distal absorbable plug is then ejected and the inner brush or catheter advanced for sampling. Finally, an alternative procedure is direct percutaneous aspiration, which can be performed using a small (23- or 25-gauge), thin-walled, *noncutting* needle. The needle, connected to a syringe, is introduced percutaneously into the area of the lung of interest; 2 to 3 ml saline is injected and then aspirated into the syringe and the needle withdrawn. Both the catheter-brush and needle approaches are high-yield, low-contamination procedures. In experienced hands, the risks are low, consisting chiefly of pneumothorax and bleeding. Patients should be carefully monitored for both.

The presence of an hemorrhagic diathesis is a relative contraindication to all three of the above procedures.

THORACENTESIS AND PLEURAL BIOPSY Thoracentesis should be performed to obtain pleural fluid in all pleural effusions of uncertain etiology and may be indicated for relief of symptoms in some patients with effusion of known cause. In effusions of uncertain cause, closed (needle) pleural biopsy should be performed as part of the same procedure.

When pleural fluid is small in amount or when its presence or location is uncertain from routine or lateral decubitus roentgenograms, performance of the thoracentesis and biopsy under fluoroscopic, ultrasound, or CT scan guidance enhances both yield and safety. Pleural fluid obtained should be examined for specific gravity, white blood cell count and differential, protein and glucose concentrations, lactic acid dehydrogenase (LDH), pH, P_{CO_2} (sample collected anaerobically), and amylase. Gram stain, cultures, and exfoliative cytologic specimens should be obtained; and in some instances, rheumatoid factor and complement levels are measured. The gross appearance of the fluid, the quantity obtained, and the precise location of the thoracentesis should be recorded. A combination of a pleural fluid LDH above 200 IU, a pleural fluid/serum protein ratio greater than 0.5, and a pleural fluid/serum LDH ratio greater than 0.6 all indicate that an "exudative" rather than "transudative" process is present. A low pH ($<$ 7.20) indicates that an empyema, probably requiring tube drainage, is present (Chap. 285). Specific diagnostic findings in pleural fluid may include the opalescent, pearly fluid characteristic of chylothorax; positive smears or cultures for tuberculosis or other infections; a marked elevation of amylase indicative of effusion secondary to pancreatitis or a ruptured esophagus; and the very low glucose values often seen in effusions associated with rheumatoid arthritis.

As already noted, closed (needle) pleural biopsy should follow thoracentesis whenever the diagnosis is uncertain. It is important to leave some fluid in the pleural space as this makes biopsy easier and safer. Bleeding, pneumothorax, and bronchopleural fistula induced by cutting through the visceral pleura are all more likely in the absence of fluid, and a satisfactory biopsy specimen is less likely to be obtained. Several special needles are available for biopsy of the parietal pleura. All have a cutting edge and some device for retaining the biopsy. The needle is inserted into the pleural effusion, then withdrawn until it is seated on the parietal pleura, from which a biopsy is obtained with the cutting edge. Usually, three biopsies are taken from different sites at the same session. Care should be exercised to place the needle in a position least likely to impinge on the intercostal vessels. All fluid to be used for diagnosis should be removed before biopsy since postbiopsy bleeding may obscure the true character of the fluid.

Pleuroscopy, using a modified FOB inserted through an intercostal trocar, also can be used for both direct inspection and biopsy of the pleura. In the absence of a pleural effusion, two other options exist for obtaining tissue from pleural-based lesions: aspiration needle biopsy and open biopsy. The technique for aspiration biopsy is the same as that described above, although some physicians use "cutting" needles (see "Lung Biopsy" below). Open pleural biopsy involves a limited thoracotomy, requiring anesthesia. A small intercostal incision is made, and the parietal pleura is biopsied under direct visualization. The incision is then closed, often without an intercostal tube. Open biopsy has several advantages because a larger specimen is obtained and the pleura and underlying lung can be seen and palpated. When pleural involvement is "spotty," open biopsy increases the possibility of establishing a diagnosis.

PULMONARY AND BRONCHIAL ANGIOGRAPHY Radiopaque materials are injected rapidly by vein or via a catheter into the systemic veins, right heart chambers, or the pulmonary artery. Magnification techniques allow visualization of smaller pulmonary vessels. Digital subtraction methods for recording and processing images may permit satisfactory angiography after injection of small quantities of contrast medium via peripheral veins. Angiography is frequently used to detect pulmonary emboli and a variety of congenital and acquired lesions of the pulmonary vessels. The procedure is not without risk, particularly in patients with pulmonary hypertension, and clear indication for it must exist as well as personnel experienced in its performance and interpretation.

Angioscopy, an experimental technique for direct visualization of the right cardiac chambers and pulmonary arterial system, can be accomplished by insertion of a fiberoptic device via a peripheral vein. The diagnostic role of this procedure in embolic and other disorders remains to be defined.

Bronchial arteriography is now used in some centers to identify otherwise unidentified bleeding sites in the lungs. Transarterial placement of a catheter into the orifices or parent vessels of bronchial arteries can be accomplished by experienced operators. Radiopaque material is then injected so that these arteries can be visualized. If a bleeding site is identified, emboli can be injected via the catheter as a means for halting hemoptysis.

MEDIASTINOSCOPY AND MEDIASTINOTOMY Another favored site for biopsy is the lymph nodes in the mediastinum. Because they receive lymphatic drainage from the lungs, these nodes often disclose intrathoracic diseases such as carcinoma, granulomatous infections, and sarcoidosis. Biopsy of these nodes is accomplished during mediastinoscopy. This involves insertion of a lighted mirror-lens system, much like a bronchoscope, through an incision at the base of the neck anteriorly. The instrument is advanced under visual control into the mediastinum, where inspection and biopsy can be carried out. Because of its higher yield of diagnostic lymph nodes, mediastinoscopy has virtually replaced biopsy of the *scalene fat pad* for nodes of interest on the right side of the mediastinum. However, for anatomic reasons, mediastinoscopy on the left is less satisfactory and more hazardous. Nodes in this location are usually approached through a limited left anterior thoracotomy (mediastinotomy) or, occasionally, by scalene fat pad biopsy. Mediastinoscopy and mediastinotomy are low-risk, high-yield procedures. They are invaluable in the "staging" of patients with known or suspected pulmonary malignancy.

LUNG BIOPSY Finally, if the diagnosis still remains unclear, biopsy of the lung may be required. Again, "closed" and "open" approaches are available. Closed biopsies are of three types: transbronchial, aspiration, and "cutting needle." Transbronchial biopsy, carried out through the fiberoptic bronchoscope, is a highly useful procedure, particularly since larger forceps have been introduced and the taking of multiple biopsies during one procedure has become routine.

However, when lesions are small and/or anatomically located beyond the reach of the FOB, direct aspiration needle biopsy is often more rewarding. *Aspiration* biopsy, mentioned previously, provides cytologic material but does not actually obtain a specimen of lung whose architecture can be examined, a feature which may be necessary to establish a diagnosis. Various "cutting" needles are available which do provide a "core" of the involved lung. However, this approach has waned in popularity because of the high incidence of pneumothorax and bleeding, occasional deaths due to air embolism, and the small size of the biopsy specimen, which may limit diagnostic interpretation. Fluoroscopic guidance is essential in all these closed approaches, and they are contraindicated if pulmonary hypertension or a hemorrhagic diathesis is present.

Open lung biopsy, requiring thoracotomy, is the final diagnostic resort. It is, however, a relatively safe procedure even in patients with respiratory failure, hemorrhagic diathesis, or pulmonary hypertension if meticulous surgical and anesthetic techniques are observed. Direct visualization allows selection of an optimum biopsy site, and of course, a specimen of adequate size is obtained. In selecting among these closed and open options, consideration of local expertise in their performance is a key factor.

All specimens obtained by biopsy should be both cultured and processed for pathologic examination.

REFERENCES

ANDERSON HA, FABER LP: Diagnostic and therapeutic applications of the bronchoscope. Chest 73(Suppl):685, 1978

BARTLETT JG, FINEGOLD SM: Bacteriology of expectorated sputum with quantitative culture and wash technic compared to transtracheal aspirates. Am Rev Resp Dis 117:1019, 1979

BORDOW RA et al: *Manual of Clinical Problems in Pulmonary Medicine.* Boston, Little, Brown, 1980

HANSON R et al: Transbronchial biopsy via flexible fiberoptic bronchoscope: Results in 164 patients. Am Rev Resp Dis 114:67, 1976

HAYES DA et al: Evaluation of two bronchofiberoscopic methods of culturing the lower respiratory tract. Am Rev Resp Dis 122:319, 1980

JOST RG et al: Computed tomography of the thorax. Radiology 126:125, 1978

PALMER DL et al: Needle aspiration of the lung in complex pneumonias. Chest 78:16, 1980

POE RH: Sensitivity and specificity of the non-specific transbronchial lung biopsy. Am Rev Resp Dis 119:25, 1979

PRATTER MR, IRWIN RS: Transtracheal aspiration. Chest 76:518, 1979

SACKNER MA (ed): *Diagnostic Technics in Pulmonary Disease.* New York, Marcel Dekker, 1981

SEGELMAN SS et al: *Pulmonary System: Practical Approaches to Pulmonary Diagnosis.* New York, Grune & Stratton, 1980

SNIDER GL (ed): *Clinical Pulmonary Medicine.* Boston, Little, Brown, 1981

Lung disease caused by immunologic and environmental injury

273 ASTHMA

E. R. McFADDEN, JR.
K. FRANK AUSTEN

DEFINITION Asthma is a disease of airways that is characterized by increased responsiveness of the tracheobronchial tree to a multiplicity of stimuli. Asthma is manifested physiologically by a widespread narrowing of the air passages which may be relieved spontaneously or as a result of therapy. Asthma is manifested clinically by paroxysms of dyspnea, cough, and wheezing. It is an episodic disease, acute exacerbations being interspersed with symptom-free periods. Typically, most attacks are short-lived, lasting minutes to hours, and after them the patient seems to recover completely clinically. However, there can be a phase in which the patient experiences some degree of airway obstruction daily. This phase can be mild, with or without superimposed severe episodes, or much more serious, with severe obstruction persisting for days or weeks, a condition known as *status asthmaticus.*

PREVALENCE AND ETIOLOGY The prevalence and incidence of asthma in various parts of the world is difficult to assess with certainty because of the lack of reliable population-based figures which have used uniform diagnostic criteria. However, data from a national health survey indicate that 3 percent of the population of the United States suffers from this disease. Similar figures have been reported from other countries. Bronchial asthma occurs at all ages but predominantly in early life. About one-half of the cases develop before age 10 and another third occur before age 40. In childhood, there is a 2:1 male/female preponderance which equalizes by age 30.

From an etiologic standpoint, asthma is a heterogeneous disease, and attempts to define it in etiologic or pathologic terms have proved difficult. It is useful for epidemiologic and clinical purposes to classify the forms of this disease by the principal stimuli that incite or are associated with acute episodes. However, it is important to emphasize that the common denominator underlying the asthmatic diathesis is a nonspecific hyperirritability of the tracheobronchial tree. Thus, the distinction between various types of asthma may often be artificial, and the response of a given subclassification may be initiated by more than one type of stimulus. With this reservation in mind, one can describe two broad groups: allergic and idiosyncratic.

Allergic asthma is often associated with a personal and/or family history of allergic diseases such as rhinitis, urticaria, and eczema; positive wheal-and-flare skin reactions to intradermal injection of extracts of airborne antigens; increased levels of IgE in the serum; and/or positive response to provocation tests involving the inhalation of specific antigen. Immunologic mechanisms appear to be causally related to the development of asthma in 25 to 35 percent of all cases, and contributory in perhaps another third. Allergic asthma is frequently seasonal, and it is most often observed in children and young adults. A nonseasonal form may result from allergy to feathers, animal danders, molds, and other antigens present continuously in the environment.

A significant segment of the asthmatic population will present with negative family or personal histories of allergy, negative skin tests, and normal serum levels of IgE, and therefore cannot be classified on the basis of defined immunologic mechanisms. These we term *idiosyncratic*. Many of these will develop a typical symptom complex upon contracting an upper respiratory illness. The initial insult may be little more than a common cold, but after several days the patient begins to develop paroxysms of wheezing and dyspnea that can last for days to months. These individuals should not be confused with the so-called infective asthmatics or with persons in whom the symptoms of bronchospasm are superimposed upon chronic bronchitis (see Chap. 279).

Unfortunately, many patients will not clearly fit into either of the above categories but will fall into a mixed group with features of each. In general, those patients whose onset of disease is in early life will tend to have a strong allergic component to their illness while those who develop their asthma late tend to be nonallergic or to have mixed etiologies.

STIMULI THAT PROVOKE ACUTE EPISODES OF ASTHMA

Allergens Allergic asthma is dependent upon an IgE response controlled by T and B lymphocytes and activated by the interaction of antigen with mast cell–bound IgE molecules. Most of the allergens that provoke asthma are airborne, and in order to induce a state of sensitivity, they must be reasonably abundant for considerable periods of time. Once sensitization has occurred, however, the patient can then exhibit exquisite responsivity, so that minute amounts of the offending agent can produce significant exacerbations of the disease. The mechanism by which an inhaled antigen can provoke an acute episode of asthma in a susceptible individual is unknown, and several paradoxes remain to be solved. The first is that most aeroallergens are too large to stay suspended in the airstream when respired and are effectively removed by the filtering action of the nose and mouth. Second, even when directly applied to the nose or inhaled through the mouth, whole pollen grains fail to induce measurable airway obstruction in asthmatic subjects who respond vigorously to an aerosol of a solution of the same antigen. Third, because tight intercellular bridges in the lining epithelium of the airways prevent movement of large molecules from the lumen into the submucosa, a dilemma exists about how the antigen can rapidly reach a submucosal mast cell to initiate an acute reaction. Along these same lines, it has also been difficult to explain the findings that substances such as charcoal dust, which are chemically and immunologically inert, can induce changes in airflow resistance in asthma.

Sufficient data that provide at least a partial insight into these problems have accumulated. It now seems likely that plant debris other than pollen may provide sufficiently small antigenic particles to allow penetration of the lung's defenses. Once this occurs, recent evidence demonstrates that there may be two converging pathways in the initial reaction sequence, and that a stimulus may have a direct effect upon the smooth muscle of an airway while simultaneously activating subepithelial vagal receptors, thereby provoking reflex bronchoconstriction as well. Precise details on how these effects are elicited are lacking, but it is now known that mast cells and sensory nerve endings are also located intramucosally in the airway lumen and not only submucosally as formerly thought. Thus, mast cell–antigen interaction can occur initially at the mucosal surface of the airway, and the chemical products of that interaction can facilitate penetration of additional antigen to the more numerous submucosal mast cells by opening the tight junctions. As this occurs, neural receptors can be activated so as to amplify the response. When this occurs, the released neurotransmitter can then enter into a positive feedback by its action on both mast cells and tight junctions. In addition, it is possible that the inflammatory changes resulting from chronic antigen-induced release of chemical mediators lowers the response threshold of the airway irritant or rapidly adapting stretch receptors and so changes airway responsivity to a variety of stimuli.

Aspirin and related substances In a group of patients ingestion of aspirin or other nonsteroidal anti-inflammatory agents such as indomethacin, mefenamic acid, ibuprofen, fenoprofen, flufenamic acid, naproxen, and propoxyphene makes the asthma worse. These patients are usually adults with the triad of severe unremitting asthma, nasal polyposis, and sinusitis. However, aspirin sensitivity can be found in the absence of this triad and has also been reported in children. Other drug allergies are common in such patients, and, while they are sensitive to acetylsalicylic acid, they generally tolerate sodium salicylate. The reaction, which is sometimes alarming, usually occurs within 2 h of ingestion of as little as 300 mg aspirin. (In the laboratory 15 to 30 mg can induce the response.) In its most severe form, it is characterized by acute rhinitis, wheezing, skin flushing, pruritus, urticaria, hypotension, and syncope. An immunologic basis has not been demonstrated. Consequently, this reaction may be idiosyncratic; however, data are beginning to accumulate that suggest that the products of arachidonic acid metabolism are involved. Further, the possibility of asthmatics coming into contact with substances related to aspirin in food additives (e.g., tartrazine yellow) and elsewhere in the environment is so great because of the widespread use of these compounds that this sensitivity may be the cause of the reaction rather than merely an exacerbating factor.

Environmental factors An additional group of persons will become symptomatic when confronted with environmental conditions which promote the concentration of airborne pollutants and antigens. This type of asthma, the so-called Tokyo-Yokohama or New Orleans asthma, tends to occur in individuals living in heavy industrial or dense urban areas during thermal inversions, or in other situations associated with stagnant air masses. Such atmospheric conditions generally make all types of asthma worse, but they also cause the de novo development of symptoms in some individuals who are not otherwise troubled. The reaction may be idiosyncratic, but it may also be toxic, resulting from exposure to chemicals like SO_2 that depress lung function in anyone if inhaled in sufficient concentration. Alternatively, inhalation of polluted air could open tight junctions and so alter the threshold of the irritant receptors in the airways of a latent asthmatic so as to create a response to other less noxious stimuli.

Occupational factors A variety of compounds used in industry can cause asthma in susceptible individuals. Various names have been applied to this condition, such as meat wrappers' asthma, bakers' asthma, woodworkers' asthma, and they give some indication of the heterogeneity of the jobs in which reversible airway disease can be found. The agents causing occupational asthma can be grouped into six categories: metal salts; wood and vegetable dusts; industrial chemicals and plastics; pharmaceutical agents; biological enzymes; and animal and insect dusts, serums, and secretions. The underlying mechanisms appear to be three in number: (1) in some cases the offending agent results in the formation of a specific IgE, and the cause seems immunologic; (2) materials being employed, in other cases, cause a direct liberation of bronchoconstrictor substances; and (3) work-related irritant substances, in still other cases, directly or reflexly stimulate the airways of either latent or frank asthmatics. In this form of asthma, the patients give a characteristic cyclic history. They are well when they arrive at work; symptoms develop toward the end of the shift, progress after leaving the work site, and then regress. Absence from work during weekends or vacation periods brings about a remission. Frequently, there are similar symptoms in fellow employees.

Infections Respiratory infections are the most common of the stimuli that evoke acute exacerbations of asthma. For many years, it was believed that bacterial infection was of prime importance, but well-controlled investigations have rather conclusively demonstrated that respiratory viruses are the major factors. In young children, the most important infectious agents are respiratory syncytial virus and parainfluenza virus. In older children and adults, rhinovirus and influenza virus predominate as pathogens. Most studies indicate that simple colonization of the tracheobronchial tree is insufficient to evoke acute episodes of bronchospasm and that attacks of asthma occur only when symptoms of an ongoing respiratory tract infection are, or have been, present. The mechanism by which viruses induce asthma is unknown, but the weight of current evidence suggests that the resulting inflammatory changes in the airway mucosa produce a disruption of tight junctions and a reduction in the firing thresholds of the subepithelial receptors. Supporting evidence for this concept is derived from the fact that the airway responsiveness of normal nonasthmatic subjects to aerosols of histamine and methacholine are dramatically, but transiently, increased after a viral respiratory infection.

Exercise Asthma can also be induced or made worse by physical exertion. Provocation of bronchospasm by exercise is probably operative to some extent in every asthmatic patient, and in some it may be the only trigger mechanism that will produce symptoms. In the latter circumstance, when such patients are followed for sufficient periods of time, one can often observe the development of recurring episodes of airway obstruction independent of exercise: thus, the onset of this problem can frequently serve as the first manifestation of the full-blown asthmatic syndrome. Exercise-induced asthma is particularly troublesome in children and young adults because of their usual high level of physical activity. The mechanism by which exercise produces acute exacerbations of asthma is related to the degree of cooling of intrathoracic airways that develops as heat and water are transferred from the mucosa to the inspired air to bring the latter to body conditions before it reaches the alveoli. The higher the ventilation and the colder, hence drier, the inspired air, the more the airway temperature falls, and so there is a significant interaction between the stress of the exercise task and the climatic environment in which it is performed with the magnitude of the postexertional obstruction. Thus, for the same inspired air conditions, running will produce a more severe attack of asthma than will walking. Conversely, for a given task, the inhalation of cold air during its performance will markedly enhance the response, while warm, humid air will blunt or abolish it. Consequently, activities such as ice hockey, cross-country skiing, or ice skating are more provocative than is swimming in an indoor heated pool.

Emotional stress Abundant objective data now exist that demonstrate that psychological factors can interact with the asthmatic diathesis to worsen or ameliorate the disease process. The pathways and nature of the interactions are complex but probably operational to some extent in almost half of the patients studied. Changes in airway caliber seem to be mediated through modification of vagal efferent activity. The most frequently studied variable has been that of suggestion, and the weight of current evidence is that it can be quite an important influence in selected asthmatics. Recent investigations have shown that when responsive individuals are given the appropriate suggestion, they can actually decrease or increase the pharmacologic effects of adrenergic and cholinergic stimuli on their airways. The extent to which psychological factors participate in the induction and/or continuation of any given acute exacerbation is unknown but probably varies from patient to patient and in the same patient from episode to episode.

PATHOLOGY In a patient who has died of acute asthma, the most striking feature of the lungs at necropsy is their gross overdistention and failure to collapse when the pleural cavities are opened. When the lungs are cut, numerous gelatinous plugs of exudate are found in the majority of the bronchial branches down to the terminal bronchiole. Histologic examination shows hypertrophy of the bronchial smooth muscle, mucosal edema, denudation of the surface epithelium, pronounced thickening of the basement membrane, and eosinophilic infiltrates in the bronchial wall. In asthmatic patients who die from trauma and causes other than asthma itself, mucous casts, basement membrane thickening, and eosinophilic infiltrates are frequently observed. In both situations there is an absence of any of the well-recognized forms of destructive emphysema.

IMMUNOPATHOLOGY The concurrence of allergic rhinitis and asthma in many patients with a familial background of such disorders, and the presence in the serum of passive transfer activity to the clinical allergen led Coca and Cooke in 1923 to introduce the term *atopy* for the propensity to develop an altered state of reactivity after "natural" exposure to specific allergens. As presently used, atopy implies a familial tendency to manifest alone or in combination such conditions as asthma, rhinitis, urticaria, and eczematous (atopic) dermatitis; and the passive transfer factor is now known to be immunoglobulin E (IgE). The importance of specific IgE in atopic diseases is that this immunoglobulin fixes to tissue mast cells. When this occurs, these cells become the target of further antigen exposure and mast cell–derived mediators appear to be the effector principles of the subsequent symptom complex. Mast cells are located in respiratory tissues in both mucosal and deeper perivenular sites and can be triggered by immune and, perhaps also, by nonimmune mechanisms. In skin the end result of the allergen-induced release of preformed and newly generated chemical mediators is an acute response followed in some individuals by a delayed subacute reaction. The early phase is edematous and acellular with an influx of plasma proteins, and the later response is characterized by the influx of specific phagocytic cells. The pulmonary response to aerosol allergen challenge can also be biphasic in some subjects, but the pathologic correlates are, of course, not determined. The natural regulation of this process is multifactorial and includes the intensity and persistence of the event activating the mast cell, the intracellular controls regulating the generation and release of the mediators, feedback mechanisms by which released mediators modulate subsequent mast cell response, the reaction to mediator activity, and the rate at which the released mediators undergo biodegradation. Thus, because of their contents and strategic locations, tissue mast cells may well be immunologically specific gatekeepers at sites of potential host penetration. Such a postulate also implies a potential for serving the host in either a beneficial or an adverse manner, depending upon the appropriateness of activation and capability for containment of the response.

The elicitation of asthma by nonsteroidal anti-inflammatory agents in patients who are not allergic to defined airborne allergens and who manifest no IgE-mediated sensitivity to the agents suggests that the mast cell may not be the only source of chemical mediators of reversible bronchoconstriction. It seems likely that the inhibition of the oxidative metabolism of arachidonic acid (see below) via the cyclooxygenase pathway without attenuation of utilization by the 5-lipoxygenase pathway creates an imbalance in the product profile to which some patients are exquisitely bronchoreactive.

Chemical mediators of immediate hypersensitivity The chemical mediators of immediate hypersensitivity presumably relevant to human disease have been identified (Tables 273-1 and 273-2) by in vitro and in vivo approaches. Granule-associated substances are considered the primary mediators of immediate hypersensitivity and consist of histamine; heparin proteoglycan; a tryptic neutral protease termed *tryptase;* acid hydrolases such as β-hexosaminidase, β-glucuronidase, and arylsulfatase A; a pair of eosinophilotactic tetrapeptides; and high-molecular-weight neutrophil chemotactic factor.

Those mediators which are not stored preformed in the mast cell and appear as a result of coupled activation-secretion of the granule are considered to be secondary. Thus, they can be by-products of that reaction, or of the perturbation of a second cell by the primary mediators, or both. Prostaglandin D_2 (PGD_2) is the major mast cell product of the oxidative metabolism of arachidonic acid after stereospecific perturbation of the IgE receptor of human or rat mast cells. Further, in patients with systemic mastocytosis, metabolites of PGD_2 appear in urine along with histamine at concentrations manyfold the normal values. An activator, previously termed *slow-reacting substance of anaphylaxis* (SRS-A), has been resolved into three structurally defined leukotriene (LT) products of the oxidative metabolism of arachidonic acid via the 5-lipoxygenase pathway (Fig. 273-1). Although the vasoactive and spasmogenic SRS-A leukotrienes C, D, and E are generated by IgE-dependent activation of pulmonary fragments, nasal polyp fragments, and dispersed pulmonary lung cells, it seems likely that their source includes both mast cells and secondarily recruited nonmast cells.

Role of the chemical mediators It has been known for about 20 years that the airways of individuals with asthma have an exquisite hyperreactivity to a wide variety of inhaled stimuli, including such chemical mediators as histamine, acetylcholine, prostaglandin $F_{2\alpha}$ ($PGF_{2\alpha}$), and crude SRS-A. Furthermore, the response is augmented in the presence of beta-adrenergic blockers such as propranolol. Increased airway hyperreactivity has recently been demonstrated in a portion of clinically unaffected family members in large kindreds with asthmatic members, suggesting that overt clinical disease may require the presence of both airway hyperreactivity and a trigger such as

TABLE 273-1
Primary mediators of immediate-type hypersensitivity reactions in human tissues

Mediators	*Structural characteristics*	*Other functions*
Histamine	β-Imidazolethylamine	Constriction of airways (H_1); increased venular permeability (H_1 and H_2); down regulation of inflammatory cellular function (H_2)
Heparin	Proteoglycan	Anticoagulant; anticomplementary
Tryptase	Neutral protease	
β-Hexosaminidase	Acid hydrolase	Exoglycosidase
β-Glucuronidase	Acid hydrolase	Exoglycosidase
Arylsulfatase	Acid hydrolase	Exosulfatase
Eosinophilotactic factors (ECF)	Ala(Val)-Gly-Ser-Glu; acidic peptides; acidic polypeptides	Deactivation of eosinophils; augmentation of C3b receptor function of eosinophils
High-molecular-weight neutrophil chemotactic factor	Neutral macromolecule	Deactivation of neutrophils

TABLE 273-2
Secondary mediators of immediate-type hypersensitivity reactions in human tissues

Mediators	*Chemical Structure*	*Other functions*
Prostaglandin D_2 (PGD_2)	9α,15(*S*)-Dihydroxy-11-ketoprosta-5-*cis*-13-*trans*-dienoic acid	Constriction of airways; vasodilation; chemokinetic for neutrophils
Leukotriene B (LTB_4)*	5*S*,12*R*-Dihydroxy-6,14-*cis*-8,10-*trans*-eicosatetraenoic acid	
Leukotriene C (LTC_4)	5(*S*)-Hydroxy-6(*R*)-*S*-glutathionyl-7,9-*trans*-11,14-*cis*-eicosatetraenoic acid	Constriction of airways; increased venular permeability
Leukotriene D (LTD_4)	5(*S*)-Hydroxy-6(*R*)-*S*-cysteinylglycyl-7,9-*trans*-11,14-*cis*-eicosatetraenoic acid	As for LTC_4
Leukotriene E (LTE_4)†	5(*S*)-Hydroxy-6(*R*)-*S*-cysteinyl-7,9-*trans*-11,14-*cis*-eicosatetraenoic acid	As for LTC_4

* *The listing of LTB_4 is presumptive and based on the presence of low-molecular-weight, nonpeptide eosinophilotactic activity in the diffusate of IgE-activated human lung fragments.*

† *The listing of LTE_4 is presumptive and based upon the progressive conversion of $LTC_4 \rightarrow LTD_4 \rightarrow LTE_4$ in human plasma or peripheral blood leukocyte preparations.*

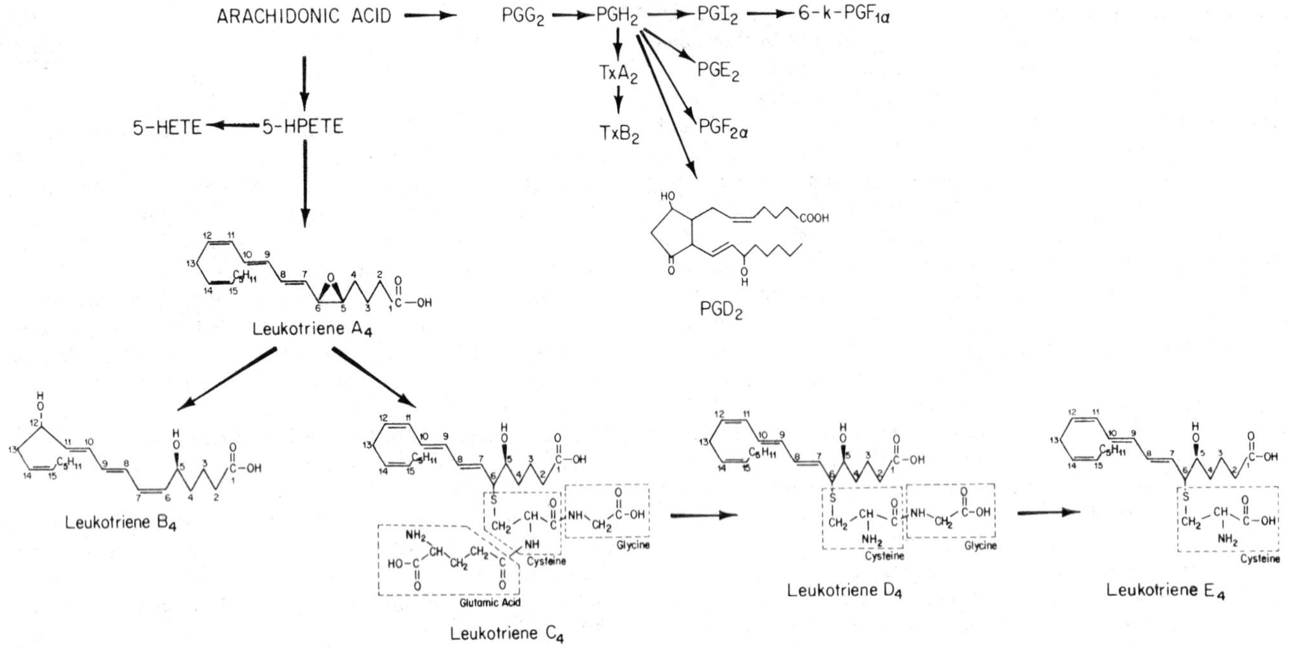

FIGURE 273-1

Structural depiction of the leukotriene products of the oxidative metabolism of arachidonic acid and of PGD_2. The arrow to the right of arachidonic acid depicts the formation of the prostaglandins (PG) and thromboxanes (TX) via the cyclooxygenase pathway. The arrow pointing downward represents the generation of the leukotrienes through the lipoxygenase pathway. 5-Hydroperoxyeicosatetraenoic acid (5-HPETE) is an intermediate step that can be metabolized to 5-hydroxyeicosatetraenoic acid (5-HETE) or to leukotriene A_4.

episodic allergic mediator release. Whether persistent mediator release alone is sufficient to establish an acquired hyperreactivity is unknown. However, the capacity of mast cells to serve as a trigger is supported by their intraepithelial location and the arguments developed earlier in this chapter in the section on allergens.

Histamine has both direct effects and indirect cholinergic reflex effects on bronchomotor tone. It also increases the permeability of veins to proteins. Histamine-induced changes in bronchomotor tone and mucosal edema could contribute to lowering the threshold of the irritant receptors to nonspecific stimuli, but it seems unlikely that histamine alone is sufficient. In fact, histamine may decrease mediator release from primary and perhaps secondary target cells through a feedback mechanism involving the stimulation of membrane-associated histamine-2 receptor sites linked to adenylate cyclases.

The leukotriene constituents of SRS-A (LTC_4, LTD_4, and LTE_4) exert profound effects on the tracheobronchial tree as assessed in vitro or in vivo. Taken together, the available data from several species indicate that SRS-A leukotrienes are substantially more potent in humans and animals than histamine or prostaglandins in inducing bronchoconstriction, have a greater duration of action, and exhibit a preference for peripheral airways.

PGD_2 constricts central and peripheral airways in the dog, but marked overproduction in humans with mastocytosis is characterized by episodic hypotension without wheezing. Although there is no information on PGD_2 aerosol administration to normal humans, it may be relevant that a cyclooxygenase product such as $PGF_{2\alpha}$ (Fig. 273-1) is less potent by several orders of magnitude than is LTC_4 in eliciting alterations in pulmonary mechanics.

The likely possibility that histamine and the SRS-A leukotrienes are the mediators of reversible airways changes in bronchial asthma still leaves unanswered the mechanism(s) of persistent, underlying airway hyperirritability. Although there is controversy as to whether or not seasonal allergic asthma is associated with increased nonspecific airway reactivity, the release of neutral protease and acid hydrolases from mast cell activation in response to antigen exposure could damage structural proteoglycans, and the influx of inflammatory cells in response to chemotactic and chemokinetic factors could also contribute to inflammation and injury of the airways. Hence, an acute reaction has the potential of damaging epithelial defenses and thus setting the stage on which other stimuli can act. In addition, the prolonged acquisition of airway hyperreactivity after certain viral infections of the respiratory tract also suggests that injurious processes might account for the acquired, as opposed to the inborn, airway hyperirritability essential for an asthmatic response. The characteristic association of mast cell–dependent allergic reactions with local eosinophilia is now attributed to the presumptive generation of LTB_4 along with the eosinophilotactic peptides. Indeed, the Charcot-Leyden crystal, characteristically present in asthmatic sputum, along with eosinophils in allergic patients, is composed solely of an eosinophil membrane protein, lysophospholipase. While the eosinophil may inhibit the effects of mast cell activation by its capacity to inactivate histamine, SRS-A leukotrienes and lysolecithin, the release of its highly cationic major basic protein (MBP) may have a direct cytotoxic action on mucosal and other cells.

The immunopharmacologic data thus suggest that chronic allergic bronchial asthma may be regarded as the superimposition of acute and subacute inflammatory events upon a base line of airway hyperirritability. Circumvention of the endogenous regulatory mechanisms of mast cell activation would supply an obvious trigger in allergic asthma, but this cell may also be involved in the pathobiologic response to nonimmunologic stimuli.

PATHOPHYSIOLOGY AND CLINICAL CORRELATES The pathophysiologic hallmark of asthma is a reduction in airway diameter brought about by contraction of smooth muscle, edema of the bronchial wall, and thick tenacious secretions. Although the relative contributions of each component to the patient's ventilatory impairment are unknown, the net result is an increase in airway resistance, decreased forced expiratory volumes and flow rates, hyperinflation of the lungs and thorax, increased work of breathing, changes in elastic recoil, abnormal distribution of both ventilation and pulmonary blood flow, mismatched ratios, and altered arterial blood gases. Thus, although asthma is considered to be primarily a disease of airways, virtually all aspects of pulmonary function are compromised during an acute attack. In addition, in very symptomatic patients there frequently is electrocardiographic evidence of right ventricular hypertrophy. Pulmonary hypertension can be found, and the patient may develop a paradoxical pulse. This sign and that of the use of the accessory muscles of respiration have been found to be extremely valuable in indicating the severity of the obstruction. In the presence of either, pulmonary function tends to be significantly more impaired than in its absence. It is important to note that the development of these signs depends upon the generation of large negative intrathoracic pressures. Thus, if the patient is breathing shallowly, they could be absent even though obstruction is quite severe.

The other signs and symptoms of asthma imperfectly reflect the physiologic alterations that are present, so much so that if one relies upon the loss of subjective complaints, or even the sign of wheezing, as being the end point at which therapy for an acute attack should be terminated, an enormous reservoir of residual disease is missed.

Hypoxia is a universal finding during acute exacerbations, but frank ventilatory failure is relatively uncommon. Most asthmatics who present for treatment have hypocapnia and a respiratory alkalosis. Statistically, the finding of normal arterial carbon dioxide tension tends to be associated with quite severe levels of obstruction, and consequently when found in a symptomatic individual, should be viewed as impending respiratory failure and treated as such. Usually, there are no clinical counterparts to the derangements in blood gases. Cyanosis is a very late sign. Thus, a dangerous level of hypoxia can go undetected. Likewise the signs which are attributable to carbon dioxide retention such as sweating, tachycardia, and wide pulse pressure do not tend to be of great value in predicting the presence of hypercapnia in individual patients, for they are too frequently seen in anxious patients with more moderate disease to be of much use. Consequently, trying to judge the state of an acutely ill patient's ventilatory status on clinical grounds alone can be extremely hazardous, and should not be relied upon with any confidence. Arterial blood gas tensions, therefore, must be measured.

The symptoms of asthma consist of a triad of dyspnea, cough, and wheezing, the latter often being regarded as the sine qua non. In its most typical form asthma is an episodic disease, and all three symptoms coexist. Attacks often occur at night, for reasons which are not clear but may relate to fluctuations in airway receptor thresholds that may result from circadian variations in the circulating levels of endogenous catecholamines and histamine. Attacks may also abruptly follow exposure to a specific allergen, physical exertion, a viral respiratory infection, or emotional excitement. At the onset the patient experiences a sense of constriction in the chest, often with a nonproductive cough. Respiration becomes audibly harsh, and wheezing in both phases of respiration becomes prominent. Patients frequently have tachypnea, and expiration becomes prolonged. The lungs rapidly become overinflated, and the anterior-posterior diameter of the thorax increases. If the attack is severe or prolonged, the accessory muscles become visibly active. Termination of the episode is frequently marked by a cough producing thick stringy mucus which often takes the form of casts of the distal airways (Curschmann's spirals), and when examined microscopically often shows eosinophils and Charcot-Leyden crystals. In extreme situations, wheezing may markedly lessen or even disappear completely, cough may become extremely ineffective, and the patient may begin a gasping type of respiratory pattern. These findings imply extensive mucous plugging and impending suffocation. Ventilatory assistance by mechanical means may be required. Atelectasis due to inspissated secretions may occasionally occur with asthmatic attacks, but spontaneous pneumothorax and/or mediastinal emphysema are rare.

Less typically, a patient with asthma may complain of intermittent episodes of nonproductive cough or dyspnea only on exertion. Unlike other asthmatics when examined during their symptomatic periods, these patients tend to have normal breath sounds but will wheeze after repeated forced exhalations and will show dynamic ventilatory impairments when tested in the laboratory.

The differentiation of asthma from other diseases associated with dyspnea and wheezing is usually not difficult, particularly if the patient is seen during an acute episode. The physical findings and symptoms listed above, and the history of periodic attacks, are quite characteristic. A personal or family history of allergic diseases such as eczema, rhinitis, or urticaria is valuable contributory evidence. *Upper airway obstruction by tumor* or *laryngeal edema* can occasionally be confused with asthma. Typically, such a patient will present with stridor, and the harsh respiratory sounds can be localized to the area of the trachea. Diffuse wheezing throughout both lung fields is usually absent. However, differentiation can sometimes be difficult, and indirect laryngoscopy or bronchoscopy may be required.

Persistent wheezing localized to one area of the chest in association with paroxysms of cough indicates *endobronchial disease* such as foreign-body aspiration, neoplasms, or bronchial stenosis.

The signs and symptoms of *acute left ventricular failure* can occasionally mimic asthma, but the findings of moist basilar rales, gallop rhythms, blood-tinged sputum, and other signs of heart failure (Chap. 253) allow the appropriate diagnosis to be reached.

Recurrent episodes of bronchospasm can occur with *carcinoid tumors* (Chap. 131), *recurrent pulmonary emboli* (Chap. 282), and *chronic bronchitis* (Chap. 279). In the latter there are no true symptom-free periods in that one can usually obtain a history of chronic cough and sputum production as a background upon which acute attacks of wheezing are superimposed. Recurrent emboli, particularly in young women on oral contraceptives, are occasionally very difficult to separate from asthma. Frequently, these patients will present with episodes of breathlessness, particularly on exertion, and they can sometimes wheeze. Pulmonary function studies may show evidence of peripheral airway obstruction (Chap. 271), and when these changes are present, lung scans may also be abnormal. The therapeutic response to bronchodilators, discontinuation of the contraceptives, and institution of anticoagulant therapy may be helpful, but pulmonary angiography may be necessary in order to establish the correct diagnosis.

Eosinophilic pneumonias (Chap. 274) are often associated with asthmatic symptoms as are various chemical pneumonias and exposures to insecticides and cholinergic drugs. Bronchospasm can occasionally be a manifestation of *polyarteritis* with pulmonary involvement.

LABORATORY FINDINGS It is difficult to establish the diagnosis of asthma in the laboratory, for no single test is conclusive. Positive wheal-and-flare reactions to skin tests can be demonstrated to various allergens, but that finding does not necessarily correlate with the intrapulmonary events. Sputum and blood eosinophilia are also helpful but are not specific for asthma. Chest roentgenograms showing hyperinflation are nondiagnostic, as are tests of pulmonary function. The latter, however, are quite useful in that one can measure the degree of obstruction present, document its reversible nature, and, when combined with provocational challenges, demonstrate the airway hyperirritability so characteristic of this disease. Furthermore, the performance of forced vital capacity maneuvers is very helpful in the evaluation of acute asthmatic attacks. A reduction in the 1-s forced expiratory volume (FEV_1) to less than 25 percent of that predicted or to less than 750 ml with little or no response following the administration of a bronchodilator indicates that the patient should receive very careful surveillance in conjunction with intensive treatment.

THERAPY Elimination of the causative agent(s) from the environment of an allergic asthmatic is the most successful means available of treating this condition (for details on avoidance see Chap. 67). Desensitization or immunotherapy with extracts of the suspected allergens has enjoyed widespread favor, but controlled studies are limited and have not proved it to be highly effective.

Drug treatment The drugs used in the treatment of asthma may be conveniently broken down into five major categories: methylxanthines, beta-adrenergic agonists, glucocorticoids, chromones, and anticholinergics. This array attests to the fact that the perfect agent has yet to be developed, and because there are few controlled trials that have conclusively demonstrated the superiority of one regimen over the other, specific recommendations for therapy are difficult to make. Thus, the treatment for a given patient is often determined empirically and is based on the overall severity and chronicity of the illness, and the response to the chosen intervention. Since the degree of relief of airway obstruction is frequently incomplete with the use of a single agent, multiple drug regimens are commonplace.

METHYLXANTHINES Theophylline is the only agent of this class used for its bronchodilating activity, and it is a competitive inhibitor of phosphodiesterase, an enzyme that inactivates cyclic adenosine monophosphate (AMP). The action of this drug is thought to be mediated by an increase in intracellular cyclic AMP levels, although this is still debated. The therapeutic plasma concentrations of theophylline lie between 10 and 20 μg/ml, but the dosage required to achieve this plasma level varies widely from patient to patient due to differences in the disposition of the drug. Therefore, therapy must be individualized. Theophylline half-lives are prolonged in liver disease, in the elderly, and in the presence of a high carbohydrate diet. They can be appreciably shortened in cigarette smokers.

In contrast to the large number of oral compounds, aminophylline is the only preparation available for intravenous use. The current recommendations are 5.6 mg per kilogram of body weight as a loading dose followed by one of three maintenance schedules: 0.9 (mg/kg)/h in young patients; 0.68 (mg/kg)/h in those over 50 years of age; and 0.45 (mg/kg)/h in patients with liver disease or congestive heart failure. In patients who have taken the drug sporadically, half the loading dose is used, and it is best to eliminate it completely if the patient was on a seemingly adequate oral regimen. Methylxanthines are medium-potency bronchodilators and in acute situations tend to improve FEV_1 by only 20 to 25 percent.

ADRENERGIC STIMULANTS This class of compounds consists of catecholamines, resorcinols, saligenins, and ephedrine, which have their effects through stimulation of alpha-, $beta_1$-, and $beta_2$-adrenergic receptors (Chap. 73). Only the beta agonists are useful in the treatment of asthma. They produce their physiologic effects by activating adenyl cyclase and through that elevate cellular levels of cyclic AMP. The perfect bronchodilator of this class would be one with pure $beta_2$ activity. It would dilate airways, but would not have the undesirable effects of cardiac stimulation.

The catecholamines are norepinephrine, epinephrine, isoproterenol, and isoetharine. Since norepinephrine is predominantly an alpha agonist, it is not employed to treat asthma. The other drugs are useful bronchodilators, but they are short acting and not effective by oral administration. Epinephrine is about equal in its alpha and beta effects. The usual dose is 0.3 to 0.5 ml of a 1:1000 solution administered subcutaneously. Isoproterenol is devoid of alpha activity and is the most potent agent of this group. It is usually administered in a 1:200 solution by inhalation. Controlled studies have shown that repetitive doses of epinephrine or isoproterenol are considerably more efficacious than the use of methylxanthines in the therapy of acute exacerbations of asthma. Isoproterenol has been used by the intravenous route in the management of status asthmaticus. In these circumstances, extremely careful monitoring of heart rate, rhythm, and blood pressure is an absolute requirement; and this therapy is not recommended save for very dire emergencies. Isoetharine is the most $beta_2$-selective compound of this class, but is a relatively weak bronchodilator. It is employed as an aerosol and supplied as a 1% solution. Ephedrine is not a catecholamine but its action in large part is mediated by enhancing the release of endogenous sympathomimetics. It therefore has both alpha and beta activity, and its usefulness is further limited by the possibility of self-blockade of its catecholamine-releasing effects.

Manipulation of the catecholamine molecule gives rise to the resorcinols and saligenins. These alterations confer more $beta_2$ selectivity and give these compounds longer duration of action and make them suitable for oral administration. Resorcinols in widespread clinical use include metaproterenol and terbutaline, while salbutamol, a saligenin, is a highly selective $beta_2$ agonist available only in aerosol form in the United States. Oral terbutaline and salbutamol appear equipotent and more effective than metaproterenol. Both have durations of action in excess of 6 h. A frequent side effect of these drugs is tremor. Aerosols of these three agents provide almost as much bronchodilation as does isoproterenol but with much less cardiac stimulation.

GLUCOCORTICOIDS Glucocorticoids have been used for over 25 years in the treatment of asthma, but controversy still surrounds such basic issues as their specific indication and dose. Although it is difficult to provide precise recommendations because objective data are lacking, there are several situations in the management of acute and chronic asthma in which all would agree that steroids should be employed. In acute illness, that is when severe airway obstruction is not resolving, or is even worsening despite intense optimal bronchodilator therapy, and in chronic disease, steroids are most helpful when there has been failure of a previously optimum regimen with frequent recurrences of symptoms of progressive severity.

Although many dosage schedules have been proposed, few objective data on pulmonary function are available to support them. Those that are indicate that plasma cortisol levels above 100 μg/dl may be required to produce an effect. In acute situations, this can be achieved by the intravenous administration of 4 mg per kilogram of body weight of hydrocortisone as a loading dose, followed several hours later by an infusion regulated to deliver 3 mg/kg every 6 h. It should be emphasized that the effects of steroids in acute asthma are not immediate and may not be seen for 6 h or more after their initial administration. Consequently, it is mandatory to continue vigorous bronchodilator therapy during this interval. After 24 to 72 h, depending upon response, the patient can be switched to oral agents. A usual starting point is 60 mg prednisone as a single daily morning dose. The amount can then be reduced by 5 mg every third or fourth day. In situations in which it appears that continued steroid therapy will be needed, an alternate-day schedule should be instituted to minimize side effects. This is particularly important in children, since continuous corticosteroid administration interrupts growth. Long-acting preparations such as dexamethasone should not be used in this approach for they defeat the purpose of alternate-day schedules by causing prolonged suppression of the pituitary-adrenal axis.

Inhaled steroids of high topical potency are available. Of the compounds studied, beclomethasone appears to combine maximum antiasthmatic effect with a minimum of systemic absorption. The usual dose is two puffs (100 μg) four times daily, but double this amount has been used without hyperadrenal corticism or adrenal suppression. The major side effect is symptomatic oropharyngeal candidiasis.

CHROMONES Cromolyn sodium is not a bronchodilator, but has its effect by inhibiting degranulation of mast cells, thereby preventing the release of the chemical mediators of anaphylaxis. The drug does not inhibit the combination of antigen with antibody, nor does it affect the fixation of IgE to mast cells. Cromolyn has been shown to be of use in atopic and nonatopic asthmatics, and it blunts exercise-induced asthma in both children and adults. Numerous trials have shown that about 75 percent of patients derive worthwhile benefits from the drug in terms of reduction of medications and improvement in symptoms. Therapy is best initiated between attacks or in periods of relative remission. If no response is noted by 4 to 6 weeks, the drug can be discontinued.

ANTICHOLINERGICS Anticholinergic drugs, such as atropine, are known to produce bronchodilatation in patients with asthma, but their use has been limited by systemic side effects. Recently, newer nonabsorbable aerosol agents have undergone extensive trials and have been found to be both effective and remarkably free of untoward effects. These agents, when available, may be of particular benefit in patients with asthma and coexistent heart disease, in whom use of methylxanthines and beta stimulants may be dangerous.

MISCELLANEOUS Opiates, sedatives, and tranquilizers should be absolutely avoided in the acutely ill asthmatic because the risk of depressing alveolar ventilation is great and respiratory arrest has been reported to occur shortly after their use. Admittedly most individuals are anxious and frightened, but experience has shown that they can be calmed equally well by the physician's presence and reassurances. Beta-adrenergic blockers and parasympathetic agonists should be avoided, or used with great caution, for they can cause marked deterioration in lung function.

Expectorants and mucolytic agents have enjoyed great vogue in the past, but there is little evidence available to indicate that they add significantly to the treatment of the acute or chronic phases of this disease. Mucolytic agents such as acetylcysteine may actually produce bronchospasm when administered to susceptible asthmatics. This can be overcome by aerosolizing them in solution with a beta-adrenergic agent. The use of intravenous fluids in the treatment of acute asthma has also been advocated. There is little evidence to indicate that this adjunct hastens recovery, but it may prevent dehydration and through that forestall the inspissation of secretions, by replacing the larger insensible water losses that could occur with prolonged hyperventilation.

PROGNOSIS AND CLINICAL COURSE Death from asthma is uncommon. Mortality statistics for the United States for the year 1973 reveal 1912 deaths from asthma at all ages. In the age group 5 to 34 years, the ages in which few other diseases are likely to be confused with asthma, there were 250 deaths, yielding a death rate of approximately 0.3 per 100,000 persons.

The available information on the clinical course of asthma suggests that somewhere between 50 to 80 percent of all patients can expect to have a reasonably good prognosis, particularly those whose disease is mild and develops in childhood. The number of children still having asthma 7 to 10 years after the initial diagnosis varies from 26 to 78 percent with an average of 46 percent; however, the percentage who continue to have severe disease is relatively low (6 to 19 percent). The natural course of asthma in adult life has been little investigated. Some studies suggest that spontaneous remissions occur in approximately 20 percent of those who develop the disease as adults and 40 percent or so can be expected to improve with less frequent and severe attacks as they grow older.

REFERENCES

ATKINS PC, ZWEIMAN B: Pharmacologic therapy of asthma, in *Update: Pulmonary Diseases and Disorders*, AP Fishman (ed). New York, McGraw-Hill, 1982, pp 336–348

AUSTEN KF: Biologic implications of the structural and functional characteristics of the chemical mediators of immediate hypersensitivity, in *The Harvey Lectures, Series 73*, New York, Academic, 1977–78, p 93

FELDMAN NT, MCFADDEN ER: Asthma: Therapy old and new. Med Clin North Am 61:1239, 1977

MCFADDEN ER et al: Acute bronchial asthma: Relations between clinical and physiological manifestations. N Engl J Med 288:221, 1973

MIDDLETON E et al (eds): *Allergy: Principles and Practice*. St. Louis, Mosby, 1978

SAUNDERS NA, MCFADDEN ER: Asthma. An Update. Disease-a-Month 24:1, 1978

SEGAL MS, WEISS EB (eds): *Asthma: Mechanisms and Therapeutics*. Boston, Little, Brown, 1976

WINSLOW CM, AUSTEN KF: Enzymatic regulation of mast cell activation and secretion by adenylate cyclase and cyclic AMP-dependent protein kinases. Fed Proc 41:22, 1982

274
HYPERSENSITIVITY PNEUMONITIS

JORDAN N. FINK

Sensitization by the inhalation route most commonly results in the IgE-mediated allergic respiratory disease immunologic asthma (Chap. 273). However, it has been recognized that immunologic respiratory diseases involving other immune mechanisms may result from the inhalation of and subsequent sensitization to environmental antigens. A wide variety of biologic dusts may induce an immunologically mediated interstitial pneumonitis involving the medium-size and terminal airways as well as the alveoli and interstitium. This disease, hypersensitivity pneumonitis, or extrinsic allergic alveolitis, may occur in several forms and may be reversible or may lead to irreversible pulmonary damage depending on the amount and duration of exposure to the offending agent, the nature of the inhaled dust, and the immune response of the patient.

Any of a wide variety of inhalable organic dusts may result in hypersensitivity pneumonitis in approximately 2 to 10 percent of exposed individuals (Table 274-1). The antigens are usually small enough to enter the alveoli (less than 5 μm), although the absorption of soluble antigens from large particles deposited in the airways may also be important in the induction of disease.

ANTIGENS

Pulmonary disease suggestive of hypersensitivity pneumonitis was first recognized in grain workers by Ramazzini in 1713. Modern studies began in 1932 when Campbell described farmer's lung and in 1965 when thermophilic actinomycetes were identified as the offending antigen in this disease. Thermophilic actinomycetes are bacteria of less than 1 μm in size found in the soil, grain, compost, and forced-air heating and cooling systems. The most common organisms involved in hypersensitivity pneumonitis include *Micropolyspora faeni, Thermoactinomyces vulgaris, T. viridis, T. sacchari,* and *T. candidus.* They thrive best at 56 to 60°C, temperatures which are commonly reached during composting or in heating systems. Individuals working with compost (farmers, sugarcane workers, mushroom workers) or living in environments with contaminated forced-air systems are thus at risk for the development of hypersensitivity pneumonitis. (See also Table 275-1.)

Other organisms associated with hypersensitivity pneumonitis are saprophytes common to the natural environment or to a particular environment and ranging in size from 1 to 10 μm. Fungi present in particular environments include *Alternaria* sp. in wood chips, *Penicillium* sp. in cork or cheese factories, and *Aspergillus* sp. in the malting industry.

Serum proteins which may be inhaled by susceptible individuals are also important antigens. Avian proteins from dried excreta of caged pigeons, chickens, parakeets, love birds, or turkeys may be inhaled, and some individuals in close contact with these birds become ill following repeated exposure. Protein antigens from bovine and porcine serum and pituitary powder may be inhaled by patients with diabetes insipidus and result in pulmonary disease.

TABLE 274-1
Etiology of hypersensitivity pneumonitis

Disease	*Source of antigen*	*Antigen*
	THERMOPHILIC ACTINOMYCETES	
Farmer's lung	Moldy vegetable compost	*Micropolyspora faeni, Thermoactinomyces vulgaris, T. sacchari, T. candidus, T. viridis*
Bagassosis		
Mushroom worker's lung		
Ventilation pneumonitis	Contaminated forced-air systems	
	FUNGI	
Malt worker's lung	Moldy malt	*Aspergillus* sp.
Wood worker's lung	Moldy wood dust	*Alternaria* sp.
Suberosis	Moldy cork dust	*Penicillium frequentans*
Cheese worker's lung	Moldy cheese	*Penicillium caseii*
Sequoiosis	Moldy wood	*Pullularia* sp.
	ANIMAL PROTEINS	
Bird breeder's lung	Avian dust	Avian proteins
Pituitary snuff lung	Pituitary snuff	Bovine and porcine proteins
Animal handler lung	Rat and mouse urine	Rat and mouse urinary proteins
	AMOEBAE	
Ventilation pneumonitis	Contaminated system	*Naegleria gruberi, Acanthamoeba castellani*
	CHEMICALS	
Paint refinisher's disease	Paint catalyst	Toluene diisocyanate
Plastic worker's lung	Plastic ingredients	Phthalic anhydride

Recently recognized sources of inhaled antigens which may induce sensitization are forced-air heating and cooling systems. The design of devices such as humidifiers, spray wash (as contrasted to refrigeration coil) air conditioning systems and vaporizers favors stagnation of water and subsequent growth of a variety of contaminants. In heated systems, thermophilic actinomycetes may proliferate, while in unheated systems fungi, bacteria, and amoebas may be the predominant antigens. Inhalation of aerosols from contaminated systems may thus result in an immune response and pulmonary disease, such as has been described in miniepidemics occurring in office buildings. More recently, chemicals widely used in the plastics industry have been recognized as causing hypersensitivity pneumonitis. These antigens are less soluble than fungal or bacterial antigens and include phthalic anhydride, toluene diisocyanate, and trimellitic anhydride.

It is likely that with the recognition of more sources of antigen exposure, as well as heightened physician awareness, the number of cases of hypersensitivity pneumonitis which are diagnosed will increase.

IMMUNOLOGIC FEATURES

The characteristic immunologic finding in hypersensitivity pneumonitis is the occurrence of serum precipitating antibodies against the offending antigen. Agar gel immunodiffusion techniques may be utilized to demonstrate the serum antibodies which are present in nearly all ill individuals but also in the serum of up to 50 percent of similarly exposed and asymptomatic persons. The precipitating antibodies are of the IgG class of immunoglobulins, but IgA and IgM antibodies have also been detected.

Skin tests may be carried out with certain of the offending antigens, though some antigens are irritating and produce nonspecific reactions. Immediate wheal-and-flare skin reactions can be demonstrated, followed by an area of erythema, edema, and induration in 6 to 8 h. The former reaction suggests an anaphylactic or IgE-mediated reaction, while the late-onset reaction is typical of a localized immune-complex vasculitis. No skin reactions suggestive of tuberculin or cellular-type sensitivity have been demonstrated. While such skin reactions are found in most ill individuals, they may also be present in well but exposed persons. Therefore, the serum precipitin and skin reactions indicate an immune response to an environmental antigen and require clinical correlation to be meaningful.

Pigeon breeders are regularly exposed to avian antigens and may develop hypersensitivity pneumonitis. Studies of the peripheral cells of these individuals have demonstrated lymphokine generation and thymidine uptake stimulated by antigen in most symptomatic and a few asymptomatic breeders. Recent studies have also demonstrated normal suppressor T-cell activity in asymptomatic pigeon breeders, while symptomatic breeders have depressed suppressor T-cell activity.

ALVEOLAR LAVAGE The technique of bronchoalveolar lavage has provided a useful method for the study of the antigen–antibody cell interaction within the lung which may be separate and distinct from the peripheral responses. Fluid obtained by lung lavage from pigeon breeders contains relatively high titers of specific antibody of the IgG and IgA class of immunoglobulins and elevated IgM levels.

Studies of the cellular components of the lung fluids from pigeon breeders have demonstrated increased numbers of T lymphocytes. Increased blastogenesis in response to a specific antigen has been detected to a greater degree with the lung lymphocytes of symptomatic breeders. The pulmonary lymphocyte responses correlate better with disease than the cellular or humoral studies of the serum or peripheral cells.

PATHOGENESIS

It is generally acknowledged that hypersensitivity pneumonitis is an immunologic disorder, but the immunologic mechanisms involved in the pathogenesis of the disease have not been clarified. Recent studies suggest that multiple mechanisms may be associated with the disease.

Thermophilic actinomycete antigens activate complement components by the alternate pathway, and chemotactic and alveolar macrophage activating factors such as C3b or other complement split products may be elaborated from complement proteins by the inhaled material. The relative insolubility and continued presence of the antigens such as *M. faeni* spores may also promote amplification of the complement sequence. Activation of macrophages by the antigens may release lysosomal enzymes, chemotactic factors, and other inflammatory components inducing pulmonary lesions. Such activation may be enhanced by the presence of immune complexes resulting from the local immune response following repeated antigen challenge. Sensitized T cells activated by antigens secrete lymphokines, which then participate in the inflammatory process via macrophage activation and chemotaxis. Thus, alveolar and interstitial inflammation of hypersensitivity pneumonitis may occur by several routes and mechanisms. While an immediate wheal-and-flare skin reaction to injected antigen is detectable and bronchial challenge may result in an immediate response in some ill individuals, a role for IgE in hypersensitivity pneumonitis has not been demonstrated. IgE levels are usually not elevated, and the immediate skin reactivity can be demonstrated in asymptomatic individuals.

The role of immune complexes in the pathogenesis of hypersensitivity pneumonitis also warrants consideration. Complement-fixing precipitating antibodies are the hallmark of the disease, and skin reactivity and pulmonary responses to antigen present as an immediate and late-onset reaction. Immunofluorescent studies of a lung biopsy specimen have revealed the presence of immunoglobulin and complement in a neutrophilic eosinophilic and plasma cell vasculitis. Further, insoluble complexes of antigen and antibody may lead to granuloma formation of the nature seen in hypersensitivity pneumonitis, and recently immune complexes have been detected in the circulation of asymptomatic and symptomatic breeders after exposure.

Cellular immune reactions are also probably important in the pathogenesis of hypersensitivity pneumonitis. In vitro production of lymphokines such as migration inhibition factor has been more consistently detected in antigen-stimulated peripheral lymphocytes from symptomatic than from asymptomatic pigeon breeders. Studies of bronchoalveolar cells have detected an increase in total numbers of T cells and antigen-reactive T cells in symptomatic breeders. Such local cellular immunity may be essential for induction of lesions irrespective of the presence of peripheral cellular or humoral immune responses.

CLINICAL FEATURES OF HYPERSENSITIVITY PNEUMONITIS

The presentation of the patient with hypersensitivity pneumonitis depends on several factors, including (1) the intrinsic nature of the inhaled dust, such as particle size, solubility, and immunogenicity; (2) the frequency and intensity of inhalation exposure; and (3) the local pulmonary and probably systemic immune response of the exposed individual. Other factors, such as the occurrence of pulmonary inflammation simultaneous with antigen exposure, have also been suspected as important influences on the development of hypersensitivity pneumonitis.

The presentation of the clinical illness is usually similar irrespective of the type or nature of the inhaled dust or chemical. The time required for sensitization by inhalation is variable and may take many months or years of exposure.

ACUTE FORM The clinical features of the acute and most common form of hypersensitivity pneumonitis occur suddenly, a number of hours after exposure to antigen.

Symptoms of this form of hypersensitivity pneumonitis are both respiratory and systemic, occurring 4 to 8 h after inhalation exposure to the organic dust or chemical. Prominent features include cough, dyspnea, chills, high fever, myalgia, and malaise. The symptoms may persist up to 8 h, and the subsequent recovery is usually rapid and spontaneous, though in some cases, mild symptoms may persist for days. The episodes recur each time the patient is exposed to the offending antigen. The severity of the attack is variable, depending on the degree of exposure and sensitivity of the individual. The episodes are frequently confused with an acute viral disease such as influenza, and broad-spectrum antibiotics have been administered for suspected bronchitis or bronchopneumonia. If the episodes are frequent and severe, anorexia, weight loss, chronic cough, and progressive dyspnea may occur.

Physical examination during the acute episode reveals an acutely ill, dyspneic patient. Suffusion of the conjunctivae, irritability, and an unwillingness to be examined are often found. Characteristically, bibasilar end-inspiratory rales are heard and may persist for days or even weeks after the attack subsides.

Laboratory features include a leukocytosis up to 25,000 white cells per cubic millimeter with a left shift and up to 10 percent eosinophils. Immunoglobulin levels are elevated, except for IgE, and rheumatoid factor may be detected in 65 percent of patients. The acute laboratory features return to normal with subsidence of the attack, and all clinical abnormalities disappear with avoidance of exposure.

Pulmonary function The pulmonary function abnormalities seen during the period after exposure, while the acute episode is evolving, may be of several types. The most common response occurs within 6 h after exposure and consists of a restrictive pattern manifested by a reduction in forced vital capacity and 1-s forced expiratory volume with little alteration in the ratio of these two parameters. Expiratory flow rates change little, but diffusing capacity and arterial oxygen tensions often decrease, reductions that are accentuated by exercise. These abnormalities suggest interstitial inflammation, and they resolve as the clinical features subside. However, if sufficient parenchymal damage has occurred, the abnormalities in volume and flow as well as hypoxia and hypercapnia may be detected during asymptomatic phases.

A second type of response observed in patients with hypersensitivity pneumonitis occurs in two phases. There is an immediate obstructive response with reductions in forced vital capacity and forced expiratory flow rates. The response is short-lived, followed by a several-hour period of normalcy, and then the late-phase reaction described above occurs.

Controlled challenge studies using pertinent antigens have demonstrated that the immediate reaction is responsive, while the late phase is resistant to the action of beta agonists. Further, pretreatment of the challenged subjects with corticosteroids blocks both responses. These findings indicate that different physiologic or immunologic mechanisms may be involved in the different types of pulmonary function responses to challenge.

Chest x-ray Roentgenographic findings in patients with hypersensitivity pneumonitis are variable, depending on the frequency of acute attacks and the temporal relationship between the attack and the taking of the x-ray (Fig. 274-1). If the acute episodes are widely spaced, the x-ray may be normal. Often, a finely defined reticular pattern and general coarsening of the bronchovascular markings are demonstrable between episodes. During an acute episode, soft, patchy, ill-defined densities which tend to coalesce may be seen in the parenchyma. As the disease progresses, diffuse fibrosis, parenchymal contraction, and honeycombing may be present.

Pathologic features Lung biopsy of patients with recurrent acute episodes of hypersensitivity pneumonitis has demonstrated the infiltration of alveolar walls with plasma cells, macrophages, and occasional eosinophils occluding alveolar spaces. With progression of disease, fibrosis and obliteration of the alveolar spaces along with obliteration of the bronchiolar lumina occurs.

Sarcoid-like granulomas with Langhans' giant cells may be seen with lymphocytic infiltrations. The presence of inter- and intraalveolar foam-laden macrophages, or histiocytes, may be characteristic of this group of diseases. Fluorescent studies of lung biopsies have demonstrated the presence of antigen in alveolar septa and on bronchial epithelium, but immunoglobulin or complement component deposition has not been consistently demonstrated.

CHRONIC FORM Prolonged antigen exposure has resulted in a chronic form of the disease with irreversible pulmonary damage in some patients without recurrent explosive acute episodes. These patients are often exposed to low levels of antigen for prolonged periods and develop symptoms of progressive dyspnea, cough, malaise, weakness, and weight loss. This form of hypersensitivity pneumonitis has been described in bird breeders who have kept one or two birds in the house or in some cases of ventilation pneumonitis where there is almost continuous exposure to contaminated forced-air systems. Chronic disease has not yet been recognized in chemically induced hypersensitivity pneumonitis, nor have the reasons for its development been elucidated.

FIGURE 274-1
Diffuse bibasilar infiltrates in patient with ventilation pneumonitis from contaminated humidifier.

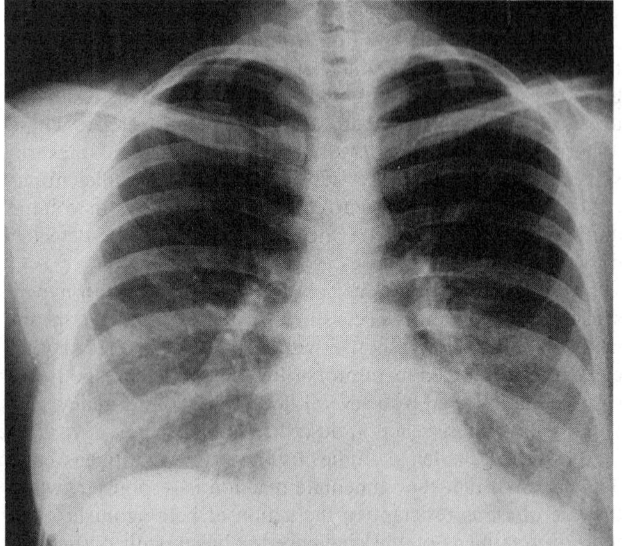

On the other hand, some farmers with years of recurrent acute episodes of pneumonitis related to exposure to molding hay develop chronic pulmonary symptoms of dyspnea which may be a manifestation of irreversible parenchymal fibrotic disease occurring even after cessation of exposure.

Patients with the chronic form develop a predominant restrictive pulmonary defect with marked diminution of diffusion capacity. The chest x-ray usually demonstrates diffuse fibrosis. The lung biopsy demonstrates fibrotic changes without the prominent cellular reaction of lymphocytic and plasma cell infiltration. Granulomas may be dispersed throughout the parenchyma. The bronchiolar walls are thickened by collagen and lymphocytic infiltrates and their lumina are obstructed by granulation tissue. This obstruction may lead to destruction of peripheral alveolar walls with subsequent honeycombing.

While patients with the acute form of hypersensitivity pneumonitis respond well to avoidance of the offending antigen or to short courses of corticosteroids, patients with the chronic form respond less, if at all, presumably because of the irreversible pulmonary parenchymal changes that have occurred.

DIAGNOSIS

Physician awareness is most important in determining the presence of hypersensitivity pneumonitis. A history of environmental exposure to a possible source of antigen, along with symptoms of "recurrent flu" or chronic cough and dyspnea temporally related to that environment, should make the physician aware of the possibility of hypersensitivity pneumonitis. The characteristic physical, laboratory, and pulmonary function abnormalities described above are also helpful in distinguishing hypersensitivity pneumonitis from other interstitial diseases.

Environmental cultures isolating thermophilic actinomycetes or antigenic fungi may also be useful, as would be the demonstration of serum precipitating antibody to these organisms. Careful inhalation challenge with the suspect environmental antigen may identify the source of the disease by inducing an acute episode. An alternative method of challenge would be the measurement of pulmonary function before, during, and after exposure to the suspect environment. Significant changes in function related to exposure would be diagnostic. Lung biopsy may be necessary in difficult cases; however, with increased diagnostic ability, that procedure is less needed than was previously the case.

TREATMENT

Avoidance of the offending antigen is essential in the treatment of hypersensitivity pneumonitis, as it is in other allergic respiratory diseases. Environmental manipulations such as the use of masks, air filters, alterations in forced-air ventilation systems, or even changes in the patients' habits or occupations may be necessary to achieve control. Improving ventilation of pigeon coops, avoidance of contact with birds, or alterations in farming practices are some of the environmental manipulations which may be useful in returning the patient to normal function.

Pharmacologic measures may be needed if the offending antigen cannot be avoided or if the disease is progressing even with avoidance. The use of bronchodilators such as theophylline and beta agonists or antihistamines is generally not of value. Cromolyn sodium is of questionable value in preventing acute episodes of hypersensitivity pneumonitis. Corticosteroids remain the main therapeutic approach. They should be utilized in doses up to 80 mg of prednisone per day in recurrent acute episodes with significant interepisode pulmonary function and chest x-ray abnormalities. They can be tapered rapidly once clinical improvement has begun and avoidance of the offending antigen has been instituted. The clinical and laboratory responses to corticosteroids are usually dramatic, and the duration and dose should be determined by the patient's clinical and laboratory evaluation. Long-term use of corticosteroids should be reserved for chronic disease where irreversible changes can be demonstrated. However, despite their effectiveness these drugs should not be used in place of avoidance of antigen. Early detection of hypersensitivity pneumonitis and identification of the antigen and its source with subsequent avoidance are still most important.

ALLERGIC BRONCHOPULMONARY ASPERGILLOSIS

Allergic bronchopulmonary aspergillosis was described in 1952 and, until recently, was thought to be limited to Great Britain. Through the work of Patterson, the disease has been recognized with increasing frequency in the United States. Allergic bronchopulmonary aspergillosis usually occurs as a complication of allergic asthma in individuals whose airways become a culture medium for *Aspergillus fumigatus* for unexplained reasons. The disease has also been shown to occur in asymptomatic individuals or in patients with minimal symptoms, and fatal cases due to progressive pulmonary destruction have been reported.

CLINICAL FEATURES Asthma which may be associated with intermittent chills, fever, and malaise is characteristic. The episodes are associated with transient or fixed soft pulmonary infiltrates on chest x-ray and a central bronchiectasis. Sputum cultures demonstrate *A. fumigatus* in approximately 75 percent of the cases, and precipitating antibodies against the organism can be demonstrated in the serum of most patients. Sputum and blood eosinophilia are characteristic, as are markedly elevated serum IgE levels. Immediate wheal and flare and late-onset erythema and edema can usually be detected on skin testing with *A. fumigatus* extract. Most of these clinical abnormalities wane in between acute episodes.

The diagnosis of the disease is made by careful history, physical, x-ray, and laboratory examination of asthmatics with recurrent severe episodes of respiratory distress or transient "pneumonia." Chest tomograms may be useful in detecting the characteristic central bronchiectasis. Serum IgE levels appear to fluctuate with disease activity and may thus be useful in diagnosis and continuous evaluation of patients with the disease.

TREATMENT The treatment of allergic bronchopulmonary aspergillosis is directed toward the underlying asthma (see Chap. 273) and its complication, colonization of the respiratory tree with *A. fumigatus*. Corticosteroids remain the drug of choice. Prednisone may be used in dosages of up to 60 mg per day, depending on the severity of the aspergillosis. The drug may be tapered slowly until, with continued relief of symptoms, it can be discontinued. If a flare of aspergillosis recurs, it may be necessary to reinstitute corticosteroid therapy. There is some evidence that such flares of the disease are preceded by elevations of total IgE levels. Thus, corticosteroids may be used when IgE levels increase in order to prevent an acute flare of aspergillosis. Only through continuous monitoring and appropriate therapy of the patient with allergic bronchopulmonary aspergillosis can the severe sequelae of the disease be prevented.

DRUG-INDUCED HYPERSENSITIVITY LUNG DISEASE

Drugs can induce a variety of pulmonary diseases by immunologic mechanisms mediated by antibodies, sensitized cells, or both. The symptoms of drug-induced pulmonary disease are usually nonspecific and consist of acute or insidious cough and dyspnea, with or without fever. Chest x-ray abnormalities include diffuse or fleeting soft infiltrations, and pulmonary function abnormalities range from a restrictive pattern with decreased diffusion to obstruction. A wide variety of drugs may cause pulmonary disease, and the disorder should be suspected in a patient who develops unexplained respiratory and/or systemic symptoms while on drug therapy.

Nitrofurantoin has been most commonly reported to induce pulmonary disease. The immunologic mechanism involved has been demonstrated to include sensitized cells, since lymphokine generation could be detected from patients' lymphocytes stimulated with the drug. The drug may induce a reaction consisting of an acute pleural effusion associated with chills, fever, cough, and dyspnea occurring several days after onset of therapy. Eosinophilia is characteristic. A diffuse alveolar or alveolar-interstitial infiltrate is evident but clears shortly after the drug is withdrawn.

In the chronic form of the disease, fever, pleural effusion, and eosinophilia are absent. There is insidious cough and dyspnea with a diffuse interstitial pattern on x-ray which may reverse with cessation of drug and use of corticosteroids.

Diffuse interstitial pulmonary disease of suspected immunologic origin is associated with the use of *busulfan,* an alkylating agent; *methotrexate,* an antimetabolite used in therapy of leukemia; or *bleomycin,* used in the therapy of certain carcinomas. Symptoms include dyspnea, cough, and fever, occurring months to years after onset of therapy, which may progress to irreversible fibrosis or resolve.

Pulmonary infiltration with eosinophils may be associated with drugs, though usually the cause of the disorder is not discovered. The patient may present with chills, fever, cough, dyspnea, and asthma. Eosinophilia is present in the sputum and in as high as 50 percent of cases in the peripheral blood. The chest x-ray demonstrates diffuse, often peripheral, infiltrates which clear, as do the symptoms, with cessation of the drug or with use of corticosteroids. The drugs most commonly associated with this disorder include *sulfonamides, chlorpropamide,* and *penicillin.*

Methysergide is used as prophylaxis for migraine. It may be associated with chronic pleural effusion, as well as pulmonary or pleural fibrosis and localized pleuropulmonary fibrosis. Retroperitoneal fibrosis, however, is the most common adverse effect of the chronic use of the drug. The mechanism of the fibrotic reaction is unknown and is usually only partially reversible, if at all, with cessation of use.

Pulmonary manifestations of drug-induced systemic lupus, such as pleurisy, pleural effusion, and diffuse interstitial pneumonitis, occur as a part of the systemic disorder. A wide variety of drugs may induce the disorder, and the disease usually remits when the drug is discontinued.

Asthma of immunologic origin may be a manifestation of a drug reaction. Allergy to *penicillin* and its derivatives may be manifested by bronchospasm. *Propranolol* can induce bronchospasm in the asthmatic by further enhancing the beta-adrenergic blockade present.

Aspirin and the other *nonsteroidal anti-inflammatory agents* can cause an acute asthmatic episode in susceptible individuals. The mechanism of the reaction may be related to enhancement of production of prostaglandins with bronchoconstrictor activity by interference with arachidonic acid metabolic pathways.

The therapy of choice in drug-induced asthma is avoidance.

DIAGNOSIS AND THERAPY The diagnosis of drug-induced hypersensitivity lung disease rests largely on the history revealing a temporal relationship between the pulmonary signs and symptoms and the onset of drug therapy. In some patients it may be necessary to discontinue all drugs and then observe for resolution of the disease in order to clarify the diagnosis. In patients on multiple drugs, sequential discontinuance of drugs for periods up to 2 weeks each may be useful.

The therapy for drug-induced hypersensitivity lung disease is primarily avoidance of the inciting agent. If resolution does not occur, corticosteroids (prednisone in doses up to 40 to 60 mg daily) may be of value. The corticosteroid should be tapered off as soon as the signs and symptoms abate.

REFERENCES

Atkinson GW, Israel HL: Pulmonary aspergillosis, in *Update: Pulmonary Diseases and Disorders,* AP Fishman (ed). New York, McGraw-Hill, 1982, pp 66–86

Banaszak EF et al: Hypersensitivity pneumonitis due to contamination of an air conditioner. N Engl J Med 283:271, 1970

Fink JN et al: Pigeon breeder's disease—A clinical study of a hypersensitivity pneumonitis. Ann Intern Med 68:1205, 1968

———: Immune reactions of the lung. Hosp Prac 16:51, 1981

McCombs RP: Diseases due to immunologic reaction in the lungs. N Engl J Med 286:1186, 1973

Schatz M et al: Immunologic lung disease. N Engl J Med 300:1310, 1979

Schlueter DP: Response of the lung to inhaled antigens. Am J Med, 57:476, 1974

Schoenberger CI, Crystal RG: Drug induced lung disease, in *Update IV: Harrison's Principles of Internal Medicine,* KJ Isselbacher et al (eds). New York, McGraw-Hill, 1983, pp 49–74

Winterbauer RH, Hammar SP: Diffuse hypersensitivity disorders of the lung, in *Update: Pulmonary Diseases and Disorders,* AP Fishman (ed). New York, McGraw-Hill, 1982, pp 205–229

275 ENVIRONMENTAL LUNG DISEASES

FRANK E. SPEIZER

This chapter is designed to provide a perspective on the approaches used to assess pulmonary diseases for which environmental causes are suspected. This assessment is important because removal of the patient from a harmful environment is often the only intervention that might prevent further significant deterioration or lead to improvement in a patient's condition. Furthermore, the identification of an environmentally associated disease in a single patient may lead to primary preventive strategies in other similarly exposed people who have not yet developed disease. Unless the physician specifically considers environmental exposures, these diseases will go undetected.

The exact magnitude of the problem is unknown, but there is no question that large numbers of people are at risk of developing serious respiratory disease as a result of occupational or environmental exposures. For example, even if only 5 percent (a conservative estimate) of workers currently exposed to asbestos, cotton dust, or silica are to suffer from respiratory disease as a result of their exposure, this represents more than 100,000 individuals in the United States. Although industries are required to spend substantial amounts of capital in efforts to protect their workers, occupationally related respiratory diseases continue to occur. These diseases are often attributed to exposures in the distant past at a time when we were not aware of or at least did not consider worker protection to the degree that we do today. We have, as a society, elected to pay compensation to affected individuals, and the physician is often called upon to judge not only the physical condition of such a patient but also the degree to which the illness can be related to, or aggravated by, a particular occupational exposure.

HISTORY AND PHYSICAL EXAMINATION The patient history is of paramount importance in assessing any potential occupational or environmental exposure. Often one is dealing with potential exposures in industries or environmental settings in which the physician has little personal experience. The physician must, therefore, ask the patient to describe a suspected environmental exposure in detail.

Inquiry into specific work practices should include questions about specific contaminants involved, the availability and use of personal respiratory protection devices, the size and ventilation of work spaces, the numbers of other workers potentially at risk of exposure, and whether other coworkers have similar complaints. In addition, the patient must be questioned about alternative sources for potentially toxic exposures, including hobbies or other environmental exposures at home. Short-term exposures to potential toxic agents in the distant past also must be considered. This information can be best elicited by a detailed occupational history which inquires about every job (beginning even with part-time jobs during schooling), about the nature of the work, the materials handled, and the duration and chronological years of employment.

Fortunately, very active worker education campaigns in the 1960s and 1970s have made many people aware of the potential hazards in their work places. In some industries management makes a specific effort to inform employees about potentially hazardous exposures. These efforts include the provision of specific educational materials, the availability and instruction in the use of personal protective equipment, and information on environmental control procedures. Reminders posted in the work place may warn workers about hazardous substances. Protective clothing, lockers, and shower facilities may be considered necessary parts of the job. However, even in these ideal settings, the introduction of new processes, particularly when related to the use of new chemical compounds, may change exposure significantly, and often only the employee on the production line is aware of the change. For the physician who regularly sees patients from a particular industry, a visit to the work site can be very instructive.

The physical examination of patients with environmentally related lung diseases may help to determine the nature and severity of the pulmonary condition. Unfortunately, the pulmonary response to most injurious agents is the development of a limited number of nonspecific physical signs. These findings do not point to the specific causative agent, and other types of information must be used to arrive at an etiologic diagnosis.

PULMONARY FUNCTION TESTS AND CHEST RADIOGRAPH The use of pulmonary function tests and radiographic examinations of the chest can provide insight into the nature of the exposures which have led to the current condition of the patient and the level of impairment. Many mineral dusts produce characteristic alterations in the mechanics of breathing and lung volumes, which clearly indicate a restrictive pattern (Chaps. 271 and 280). On the other hand, exposures to a number of organic dusts or chemical agents capable of producing occupational asthma result in pronounced obstructive patterns of pulmonary dysfunction that may be reversible (Chap. 273). Standardized approaches for measuring the mechanics of breathing and diffusion across the alveolar membrane (Chap. 271) have been proposed for screening large industrial groups to look for these abnormalities. Measurement of change in FEV_1 before and after a working shift can be used to detect an acute bronchoconstrictive response. An acute decrement of FEV_1 over the Monday work shift is a characteristic feature of cotton textile workers with byssinosis.

For many years the chest radiograph has been used to detect and monitor the pulmonary response to mineral dusts. To provide a standardized way of recording judgments about the kind and severity of radiographic abnormalities, the International Labor Organization (ILO)/International Classification of Radiographs of Pneumoconioses was developed. The ILO scheme involves classifying chest roentgenograms according to the nature and size of opacities seen and the extent of involvement of the parenchyma. Extensive description of the ILO system is beyond the scope of this chapter; however, it is important to note that small, rounded opacities can result from inhalation of inert (inorganic) dusts, such as iron oxide and barium, or potentially fiber-producing dusts, such as coal, or highly reactive dusts, such as silica. When shadows become large (radiographic lesions greater than 1 cm in diameter), the condition is termed *complicated pneumoconiosis,* sometimes called *progressive massive fibrosis* (PMF). Recent reviews of data collected over the last 30 years suggest that generally only progressive massive fibrosis is associated with a significant excess decline in pulmonary function in coal worker's pneumoconiosis.

Judgments based only on chest radiographs may over- or underestimate the functional impact of pneumoconiosis. With dusts causing rounded, regular opacities, such as in coal worker's pneumoconiosis, the degree of involvement on the chest radiograph may be quite extensive, while pulmonary function may be only minimally impaired. In contrast, in pneumoconiosis causing linear, irregular opacities, as seen in asbestosis, the radiograph may lead to underestimation of the severity of the impairment. It is possible to have a history of exposure, moderately reduced FVC, and a reduced diffusion in asbestosis, with a relatively normal chest radiograph. The radiographic findings of irregular or linear opacities are simply more difficult to separate from normal markings until relatively late in the disease.

Other diagnostic procedures of use in identifying environmentally induced lung disease include evaluating heavy metal exposures (arsenic, cadmium in battery plant workers); bacteriological studies (tuberculosis in medical care personnel, anthrax in wool sorters); fungal studies (coccidioidomycosis in southwestern farm workers, histoplasmosis in poultry or pigeon handlers); or serologic studies (psittacosis in pet shop workers or owners of sick birds, Q fever in tanners or slaughterhouse workers). Ultimately, a lung biopsy may be required both to make a specific morphological diagnosis of the underlying pulmonary disease and to attempt to identify the etiologic agent by use, for example, of x-ray diffraction for metal content.

MEASUREMENT OF EXPOSURE If reliable environmental sampling data are available, these sources of information should be used in assessing a patient's exposure. Since many of the chronic diseases result from exposure over many years, current environmental measurements should be combined with work histories to arrive at estimates of past exposure. However, the dose of any environmental agent is a complex interaction of chemical reaction, both at the emission source and in the ambient atmosphere, and phsyiological factors, including ventilation rate and depth, which may affect transport and deposition of aerosols and gases in the lung. Even in acute conditions, when monitoring of exposure may be possible, little may be known about the actual dose received by the lung. Most of the research on health effects of air pollutants (discussed later in this chapter) has relied upon fixed-station monitoring of outdoor air, often at locations somewhat distant from the residences of the people being studied. In addition, most people spend less than 20 percent of their time outdoors. Efforts to determine the penetration rate of outdoor contaminants into the indoors suggest that these penetration rates are highly pollutant specific. Therefore, outdoor measurements can be used only in a relative sense, and they cannot be relied upon to estimate actual dose.

In situations where individual exposure to specific agents has been determined, either in a work setting or for ambient air pollutants, transport of these agents through the airways may be an important factor affecting dose. The upper airways are remarkably effective filters of both particles and gases. For example, virtually 100 percent of sulfur dioxide, a highly soluble gas, is absorbed in the upper airways in concentrations as high as 35 parts per million (ppm) during quiet breathing, and even during exercise sulfur dioxide is unlikely to penetrate beyond the large bronchi. On the other hand, nitrogen dioxide, which is less soluble, may reach the bronchioles and alveoli in sufficient quantities to result in an acute life-threatening disease in farmers exposed even briefly to the gas evolved from moldy hay in silos (silo filler's disease).

Particle size and chemistry of air contaminants also must be considered. Particles above 10 to 15 μm, because of their settling velocities in air, do not penetrate beyond the upper airways. These larger particles are often referred to as "fugitive dusts" and include pollens, other windblown dusts, and dusts resulting from mechanical industrial processes. They have little or no role in chronic respiratory disease except as possibly related to cancer (see below).

Particles below 10 μm in size are created by the burning of fossil fuel or high-temperature industrial processes resulting in condensation products from gases, fumes, or vapors. These particles are divided into two size fractions on the basis of their chemical characteristics. Particles approximately 2.5 to 10 μm (coarse-mode fraction) contain crustal elements, such as silica, alumium, and iron. These particles mostly deposit relatively high in the tracheobronchial tree. Particles less than approximately 2.5 μm (fine-mode fraction or accumulation mode) contain sulfates, nitrates, and organic compounds. The deposition of the fine-mode particles is more often in the terminal bronchioles and alveoli. The smallest particles, those less than 0.1 μm in size, remain in the airstream and deposit in the lung only on a random basis as they come into contact with the alveolar walls through thermal forces and/or Brownian movement.

Besides the size characteristics of particles and the solubility of gases, the actual chemical composition, mechanical properties, and immunogenicity or infectivity of inhaled material determine in large part the nature of the diseases found among exposed persons.

OCCUPATIONAL EXPOSURES AND PULMONARY DISEASE

INORGANIC DUSTS Asbestos exposure Except in localized regions with single industrial exposures, such as coal-mining or granite-quarrying regions, the most frequent inorganic dust–related chronic pulmonary diseases are associated with industries using *asbestos fibers.* Asbestos is a generic term for several different mineral silicates, including chrysotile, amosite, anthophyllite, and crocidolite. Approximately 1.4 million workers in the United States have had exposure to the various forms of asbestos fibers. Besides mining, milling, and manufacturing of asbestos products, exposures occur in the construction trades (pipe fitters, boiler makers) because of the exceptional properties of asbestos fibers for use in thermal and electric insulation. In addition, asbestos is used in the manufacture of fire-smothering blankets and safety garments, as filler for plastic materials, in cement and floor tiles, and in friction materials, such as brake and clutch linings.

Exposure to asbestos is not limited to persons who directly handle the material. Cases of asbestos-related diseases have been encountered in individuals with only moderate exposure, such as the painter or electrician who works alongside the insulation worker in a shipyard, or the housewife who does no more than shake out and wash her husband's work clothes. Community exposure has probably resulted from the use of asbestos-containing material sprayed on steel girders in many large buildings as a safety feature to prevent buckling in case of fire. Clusters of cases of mesothelioma have been noted in the neighborhood of an asbestos plant in London and in the communities near asbestos mines in South Africa.

Asbestos was first used extensively in the 1940s. Starting in 1975 it has been replaced with alternatives, such as fiberglass or slag wool. The major health effects from exposure to asbestos are pulmonary fibrosis (asbestosis) and cancers of the respiratory tract and pleura.

Asbestosis is a diffuse interstitial fibrosing disease of the lung which is directly related to the intensity and duration of exposure. Except for a history of exposure to asbestos (generally in a work setting), asbestosis resembles the other forms of diffuse interstitial fibrosis (Chap. 280). Usually at least 10 years of moderate to severe exposure have occurred before the disease becomes manifest.

The patient presents with a dry cough, chest tightness, and breathlessness on exertion. The characteristic physical signs include dry, crackling inspiratory rales, particularly at the lung bases. Late manifestations, generally with more than 20 years of exposure, include cyanosis and clubbing of the nail beds. Physiologic studies reveal a restrictive pattern with a decrease in lung volumes. Flow rates are commonly reduced less than would be predicted on the basis of the volume reduction. An early sign of severe disease may be a reduction in diffusing capacity.

The chest radiograph can be used to determine a number of manifestations of asbestos exposure, as well as to identify specific lesions. Past exposure is specifically indicated by pleural plaques, which are characterized by either thickening or calcification along the parietal pleura, particularly along the lower lung fields, the diaphragm, and the cardiac border. Without additional manifestations, pleural plaques imply only exposure, not pulmonary impairment. The radiographic diagnosis of asbestosis depends upon the presence of irregular or linear opacities, usually first noted in the lower lung fields and spreading into the middle and upper lung fields as the disease becomes progressively worse. An indistinct heart border or a "ground glass" appearance in the lung fields is seen in some cases. As the fibrotic changes in the parenchyma begin to coalesce, the patient develops obliteration of entire acinar units with eventual formation of the classical honeycombed lung which appears on chest radiographs as coarse infiltrates with small (about 7 to 10 μm) air spaces.

Pulmonary fibrosis occurs following exposure to any of the four common types of asbestos fiber. The fibrotic lesions do not appear to relate to either shape or chemical composition of any of the four, although the prevalence of disease may be influenced by fiber type. Recent studies indicate that during phagocytosis of the asbestos fiber, the membrane of the macrophage is damaged, which results in the release of lysosomes containing enzymes which may act on the lung parenchyma.

Lung cancer (Chap. 284), either squamous-cell or adenocarcinoma, is the most frequent cancer associated with asbestos exposure. The excess frequency of lung cancer in asbestos workers is associated with a minimum lapse of 15 to 19 years between first exposure and development of the disease. Persons with more exposure are at greater risk of disease. In addition, there appears to be a significant multiplicative effect which leads to a far greater risk of lung cancer in persons who are cigarette smokers and have asbestos exposure than would be expected by taking the sum of both risks.

Mesotheliomas (Chap. 285), both pleural and peritoneal, are also associated with asbestos exposure. In contrast to lung cancer there does not appear to be any association with smoking. Relatively short-term exposures of 1 to 2 years or less occurring some 20 to 25 years in the past have been associated with the development of mesotheliomas (which stresses the point of obtaining a complete environmental exposure history). The risk for this type of tumor peaks 30 to 35 years after initial exposure. Although approximately 50 percent of mesotheliomas metastasize, the tumor generally is locally invasive, and death usually results from local extension. Most patients present with effusions that may obscure the underlying pleural tumor. The major diagnostic problem is differentiation from peripherally spreading pulmonary adenocarcinoma or adenocarcinoma metastatic to pleura from an extrathoracic primary site. A needle or even open biopsy is helpful in diagnosis.

One concern in making a definitive diagnosis of a mesothelioma relates to potential compensation to the survivors of a patient with this usually fatal disease. Since epidemiologic studies have shown that up to 80 percent of mesothelioma may be associated with asbestos exposure, documented mesothelioma in a worker with occupational exposure to asbestos may be compensable in many parts of the United States.

Silicosis In spite of the technical adequacy of existing protective equipment, *free silica* (SiO_2), or crystalline quartz, is still a major occupational hazard. In the United States estimates of potential numbers of exposed workers range between 1.2 to 3 million people. The major occupational exposures include mining, stone cutting, abrasive industries, blasting, road and building construction, farming, and quarrying, particularly of granite. Most often the progressive pulmonary fibrosis (silicosis) occurs in a dose-response fashion after many years of exposure.

Workers exposed to sandblasting in confined spaces, tunneling through rock with high quartz content (15 to 25 percent), and in the manufacture of abrasive soaps may develop acute silicosis with as little as 10 months exposure. The disease may be rapidly fatal in less than 2 years in spite of the worker being removed from exposure. A radiographic picture of profuse miliary infiltration or consolidation is characteristic of acute silicosis.

In long-term, relatively less intense exposure, radiographic changes of rounded, small opacities in the upper lobes with retraction and hilar adenopathy classically appear after 15 to 20 years of exposure. Calcification of hilar nodes may occur in as many as 20 percent of cases. These changes may be preceded by or be associated with a reticular pattern of irregular densities which are uniformly present throughout the upper lung zones.

The nodular fibrosis may be progressive in the absence of further exposure, with coalescence and formation of nonsegmental conglomerates of irregular masses in excess of 1 cm in diameter. These masses become quite large and are characteristic of progressive massive fibrosis (PMF). Significant functional impairment with both restrictive and obstructive components may be associated with this form of silicosis. In the late stages of the disease ventilatory failure may develop. Patients with silicosis are at greater risk of acquiring *Mycobacterium tuberculosis* infections (silicotuberculosis), although tuberculosis is not always involved in the progression of the disease to PMF. Because the frequency with which tuberculosis has been found at autopsy in patients with PMF exceeds considerably the frequency of premorbid diagnosis, treatment for tuberculosis is indicated in any patient with silicosis and a positive tuberculin test.

Other less hazardous silicates include fuller's earth, kaolin, mica, diatomaceous earths, silica gel, soapstone, carbonate dusts, and cement dusts. The production of fibrosis in workers exposed to these agents is believed to be related to either the free silica content of these dusts or, for substances which contain no free silica, to the potentially large dust loads to which these workers may be exposed.

Other silicates, including *talc dusts,* may be contaminated with asbestos and/or free silica. Accidental exposure to significant quantities of talc may result in an acute syndrome with cough, cyanosis, and labored breathing (acute talcosis). Severe progressive fibrosis with respiratory failure may ensue within a few years. Far more common is the fibrosis and/or pleural or lung cancer associated with chronic exposure in rubber workers who use commercial talc as a lubricant in tire molds. Pure talc does not produce fibrosis; thus, it is difficult to sort out whether the effects are due to the contamination of commercial talc by asbestos or by free silica.

Coal worker's pneumoconiosis (CWP) *Coal dust* is associated with CWP, which has enormous social, economic, and medical significance in every nation in which coal mining is an important industry. Simple radiographically identified CWP is seen in 12 percent of all miners and in as many as 50 percent of anthracite miners with more than 20 years work on the coal face. The prevalence of disease is lower in workers in bituminous coal mines. Since much of the western United States coal is bituminous, CWP is less prevalent in that region.

Much of the symptomatology associated with simple CWP appears to be similar and additive to the effects of cigarette smoking on the development of chronic bronchitis and obstructive ventilatory disease (Chap. 279). In the early stages of simple CWP, radiographic abnormalities consist of small, irregular opacities (reticular pattern). With prolonged exposure, one sees small, rounded, regular opacities, 1 to 5 mm in diameter (nodular pattern). Calcification is generally not seen, although approximately 10 percent of older anthracite miners have calcified nodules.

Complicated CWP is manifested by the appearance on the chest radiograph of nodules ranging from 1 cm in diameter to an entire lobe, generally confined to the upper half of the lungs. This condition, considered a form of PMF, is associated with premature mortality and is accompanied by significant reduction in diffusing capacity. In contrast to patients with silicosis, only a relatively small percentage of underground miners with simple CWP (5 to 15 percent, depending on the type of coal) develop PMF.

The mechanism whereby PMF occurs in CWP is not fully understood. Several hypotheses have been proposed, including (1) sufficient free silica is present in the dust to be responsible; (2) normal clearance mechanisms are unable to clear the excessive dust loads; (3) an interplay occurs between an intrinsic immunologic mechanism and the dust and/or damaged lung tissue; and (4) atypical reactions to *Mycobacterium tuberculosis* occur. As previously described, PMF in silicosis is associated with prolonged duration and high intensity of exposure to free silica. Heavy exposure to carbon particles free of silica occurs in carbon black, graphite, and charcoal workers. The prolonged exposure of these workers may result in sufficient accumulation of carbon in the lung to produce PMF. The mechanism appears to relate to a breakdown of the clearance capacity of the airways.

Caplan's syndrome, which includes seropositive rheumatoid arthritis with characteristic PMF, is consistent with an immunopathologic mechanism. The syndrome was first described in coal miners but subsequently has been found in a number of pneumoconioses. Similarly, the high prevalence of antinuclear antibodies in sandblasting workers with silicosis and the elevation of gamma globulin levels in silicotic individuals suggest an immunologic mechanism. Although mycobacterial infections are found more often in coal miners than PMF is found in silicotic patients, tuberculosis does not appear to be associated with most of the cases of PMF in coal miners.

Berylliosis Beryllium may produce an acute pneumonitis or, far more commonly, a chronic interstitial pneumonitis. Histologically, it may be difficult to differentiate the chronic form of the disease from sarcoidosis (Chap. 235). Nonspecific pulmonary function tests may be normal or indicate evidence of restrictive disease, between 2 and 15 years of exposure depending on its intensity. Unless one inquires specifically about occupational exposures to beryllium in the manufacture of alloys, ceramics, and, before the 1950s, in the production of fluorescent lights, one may miss entirely the etiologic relationship to an occupational exposure.

Rarely, other hard metals, including aluminum powders, chromium, cobalt, titanium dioxide, and tungsten, may produce pulmonary fibrosis.

Other inorganic dusts Other dusts are considered *nuisance dusts* because their major impact seems to be reduction in visibility and irritation of eyes, ears, nasal passages, and other mucous membranes. If they penetrate to the lower airways, they do not affect the architecture of the terminal bronchioles or acinar spaces or destroy collagen. Generally, any effects are reversible. Pulmonary function tests are usually normal unless another disease process coexists. If radiodense, macular collections of these dusts may produce striking radiographic pictures which are so characteristic that patients with a history of significant exposure are easily diagnosed as having the condition which bears the name reflecting the nature of the dust. Examples are iron and iron oxides from welding or silver finishing (*siderosis*); tin oxide used in metallurgy, color stabilization, printing, and the manufacture of porcelain, glass, and fabric (*stannosis*); and barium sulfate used as a catalyst for organic reactions, drilling mud components, and electroplating (*baritosis*). Metal dusts producing similar radiodense pictures include *cerium dioxide* and *antimony salts.*

Most of the inorganic dusts discussed thus far are associated with the production of either dust macules or interstitial fibrotic changes in the lung. Another set of dusts (see Table 275-1), along with some of the dusts previously discussed, is associated with chronic mucus hypersecretion (chronic bronchitis), with or without reduction of expiratory flow rates. These conditions may be caused by cigarette smoking, and any effort to attribute some component of the disease to occupational and environmental exposures must take cigarette smoking into account. In some studies the evidence suggests an additive effect of dust exposure and smoking. Those exposures associated with obstructive syndromes are generally represented by one or two studies of specific occupational groups with a small number of affected nonsmokers. Cigarette smoke

TABLE 275-1
Selected occupational dusts believed to be associated with mucus hypersecretion and/or obstructive airway disease and other respiratory diseases*

Agent	*Exposure*	*Mucus hypersecretion*	*Obstruction*	*Other conditions†*
INORGANIC DUST				
Arsenic	Manufacture of pesticides, pigments, glass, alloys	X		C
Barium and compounds including BaO, $BaSO_4$, $BaCO_3$	Catalyst, drilling mud, electroplating	X		P
Cadmium dust	Electroplating, battery manufacture, welding, smelting, aluminum soldering	X	X	P
Cement dust	Construction trades, manufacture of cement blocks	X	X	
Chromium and CrO_3, CrF_2	Corrosion inhibitor pigment, metallurgy, electroplating	X		C
Coal dust	Mining	X		P
Coke oven emissions	Retort house, coke ovens	X	X	P, C
Graphite	Steelmaking, lubricants, pencils, paints, stove polish	X	X	P
Iron dust	Steel and nonferrous foundry workers, welding	X		P
Mica	Insulation, roofing shingles, oil refining, rubber manufacturing	X		P
Rock dusts	Miners, tunnelers, quarry workers	X		P
Vanadium pentoxide	Welding electrodes, additive to steel, by-product in ash from oil burning	X	X	
ORGANIC DUST (see Chap. 274)				
Cotton dust, flax, hemp	Manufacture of yarns for linen, rope, cotton; ginning, cottonseed crushing; waste fiber processing	X	X	
Grain dusts	Farmers, workers in grain elevators, barge and grain ship crewmembers	X	X	
Moldy hay	Farmers, other animal attendants	X		HP

* *The table excludes agents associated with asthma as the primary disease (see Chap. 273).*
† *Other conditions include hypersensitivity pneumonitis (HP), pneumoconiosis (P), and cancers (C).*

is usually the more noxious agent, and dust effects may be discernible only in nonsmokers.

ORGANIC DUSTS Some of the specific diseases associated with organic dusts are discussed in detail in the chapters on asthma (Chap. 273) and on hypersensitivity pneumonitis (Chap. 274). Many of these diseases are named for the specific setting in which the disease is found, e.g., farmer's lung, malt worker's disease, or mushroom worker's disease. Occupational and other environmental exposures must be sought when these conditions are suspected. Often the temporal relation of symptoms to exposure furnishes the best evidence for the diagnosis, and removal or minimizing of exposure may be an effective component of intervention. Three occupational groups are singled out for discussion because they represent the largest proportion of people affected by the diseases resulting from organic dusts.

Cotton dust (byssinosis) Estimates of the number of exposed persons in the United States vary, but probably over 800,000 are exposed occupationally to cotton, flax, or hemp in the production of yarns for cotton, linen, and rope making. Although this discussion focuses on cotton, the same syndrome to a somewhat lesser degree has been reported in exposure to flax, hemp, and jute.

Although cotton dust–related disease was first described in the seventeenth century, it is only in the last 30 to 40 years that the disease has been recognized as a worldwide problem in the textile industry. Exposure occurs throughout the manufacturing process but is most pronounced in those portions of the factory involved with the treatment of the cotton prior to spinning—i.e., blowing, mixing, and carding (straightening of fibers). Cases reported from spinning rooms are believed to be due to secondary contamination from carding rooms. Recent attempts to control dust levels by use of exhaust hoods, general increase in ventilation, and wetting procedures in some settings have been highly successful. However, respiratory protective equipment appears to be required during certain operations to prevent workers from being exposed to levels of dust that exceed the current United States cotton dust standard.

Byssinosis is characterized clinically as occasional (early stage) and then regular (late stage) chest tightness toward the end of the first day of the workweek (Monday chest tightness). In epidemiologic studies, up to 80 percent of carding room employees may show a significant drop in their FEV_1 over the course of a Monday shift, depending on the level of exposure in the carding room air.

Initially the symptoms do not recur on subsequent days of the week. However, in 10 to 25 percent of workers, the disease may be progressive with chest tightness recurring or persisting throughout the workweek. After more than 10 years of exposure, workers with recurrent symptoms are more likely to have an obstructive ventilatory pattern on pulmonary function testing. These higher grades of impairment are seen in workers exposed both to high levels of dust and for the greatest duration. There is an additive effect of cotton dust exposure plus cigarette smoking. The highest grades of impairment are generally seen in smokers.

Treatment in the early stages of the disease is directed toward reversing the bronchospasm with bronchodilators; however, the chest tightness appears at least in part to relate to histamine release, and antihistamines have been shown to lessen anticipated fall in FEV_1 the first day of the week. Clearly, reduction of dust exposure is of primary importance. All workers with persistent symptoms or significantly reduced levels of pulmonary function should be moved to areas of lower risk of exposure. Regular surveillance of pulmonary function in the industry has made it easier to identify affected persons. Persons with reduced pulmonary function, a personal history of respiratory allergy, and positive history of continued cigarette smoking should be considered at increased risk of developing byssinosis in association with working in the cotton industry.

Grain dust Although the exact number of workers at risk in the United States is not known, at least 500,000 people work in grain elevators, and over 2 million farmers are potentially at risk. The presentation of disease in grain elevator employees or workers in flour or feed mills is virtually identical to the characteristic finding in cigarette smokers, i.e., persistent cough, mucus hypersecretion, wheeze and dyspnea on exertion, and reduced FEV_1 and FEV_1/FVC ratio (Chap. 271).

Dust concentrations in grain elevators vary greatly but appear to be in excess of 10,000 $\mu g/m^3$ with approximately one-third of the particles by weight being in the respirable range. The effect of grain dust exposure is additive to that of cigarette smoking with approximately 50 percent of workers who smoke having symptoms. Among nonsmoking grain elevator operators, approximately a quarter have mucus hypersecretion, about five times the number that would be expected in unexposed nonsmokers. However, evidence of obstruction is observed only in workers who smoke. It is not clear if this results from an enhancement of cigarette smoking effect in exposed workers, or if smokers are more susceptible to the effects of grain dust.

Farmer's lung This results from exposure to moldy hay containing spores of thermophilic actinomycetes that produce a hypersensitivity pneumonitis (Chap. 274). There are few good population-based estimates of the frequency of occurrence of this condition in the United States. However, among farmers in Great Britain the rate of disease ranges from approximately 10 to 50 per 1000. The prevalence of disease varies in association with rainfall, which determines the amount of fungal growth, and with differences in agricultural practices related to turning and stacking hay.

The patient with acute farmer's lung presents 4 to 8 h after exposure with fever, chills, malaise, cough, and dyspnea without wheezing. The history of exposure is obviously essential to separate this disease from similar symptoms that might occur in influenza or pneumonia. In the chronic form of the disease, the history of repeated attacks after similar exposure is important to separate this syndrome from other causes of patchy fibrosis, e.g., scarcoidosis.

Other diseases associated with organic dusts are summarized in Table 275-1. For patients who present with hypersensitivity pneumonitis, specific and careful inquiry about occupations, hobbies, or other home environmental exposures will, in most cases, reveal the source of the etiologic agent.

ASSESSMENT OF DISABILITY Significant reduction of dust levels in coal mines has resulted from federal legislation, enacted in the United States in 1969, which requires that respirable dust levels in underground mines be reduced to less than 2000 $\mu g/m^3$. This same legislation authorized payment to coal miners (or their survivors) who are totally disabled by CWP. The criteria for disability from CWP remain unclear and arbitrary. Much of the difficulty relates to the inability to determine in an individual with simple CWP what proportion of an observed respiratory impairment is related to coal dust and what proportion is due to cigarette smoking. The law as currently interpreted suggests that to be eligible for payment of a claim, one need only show that an underlying condition (i.e., chronic bronchitis with obstruction, presumably due to cigarette smoking) is aggravated by CWP. The variability of the interpretation results in substantial variability in the disposition of claims, with the physician often asked by advocates on one side or the other to try to make definitive statements in the face of uncertainty. Similar separate bills have been introduced into Congress to deal with other single occupational diseases, such as asbestosis and byssinosis. Thus, it becomes critical that physicians involved in occupational lung disease claim cases be aware of detailed exposure histories of their patients, both in terms of occupational exposures and other environmental exposures (cigarette smoking). In addition, these physicians must understand that the extent to which the level of physiologic impairment incapacitates an individual may not be the sole criterion for determining disability. To assess disability properly may require input not only from physicians but also from experts in ergonomics and vocational rehabilitation, lawyers, and employer and employee representatives.

TOXIC CHEMICALS Exposure to toxic chemicals affecting the lung generally occurs in the form of gases and vapors. A common accident is one in which the victim is trapped in a confined space where the chemicals have accumulated to toxic levels. In addition to the specific toxic effects of the chemical, the victim will often sustain considerable anoxia, which can play a dominant role in determining whether the individual recovers.

Table 275-2 lists a variety of toxic agents which can produce acute and sometimes life-threatening reactions in the lung. All of these agents in sufficient concentrations have been demonstrated, at least in animal studies, to affect the lower airways and disrupt alveolar architecture, either acutely or as a result of chronic exposure. Some of these agents may be generated acutely in the environment. For example, when plastics burn, a number of compounds, including hydrogen cyanide and hydrochloric acid, may be formed and released. The effects and treatment of exposure to these toxic gases are discussed elsewhere (Chap. 238).

Fire fighters and fire victims are at risk of *smoke inhalation,* a numerically important cause of acute cardiorespiratory failure. Smoke inhalation kills more fire victims than does thermal injury. Smoke inhalation victims may suffer some degree of lower respiratory tract inflammation, similar to that seen with exposure to irritant gases, e.g., chlorine. Severe cases may develop pulmonary edema. Carbon monoxide poisoning with resulting significant hypoxemia can be life-threatening (Chap. 238). Fire fighters may inappropriately use the "blackness" of the smoke to indicate the degree to which incomplete combustion and, thus, elevation of carbon monoxide levels are present. Because of the increased use of synthetic materials (plastics, polyurethanes), the color of smoke may be significantly altered and fire fighters may not use appropriate available protective equipment. In addition, they may be exposed to other toxic agents with which they are unfamiliar.

Fire fighters and victims also may be exposed to large quantities of particulate smoke. Significant long-term effects are not clearly associated with this particulate exposure except as related to the production of irritating effects on the upper airways. Studies attempting to demonstrate either an increased risk of cardiovascular events, presumably from recurrent exposure to carbon monoxide, or excess of chronic respiratory disease from repeated smoke inhalation, are inconclusive, partly because of the difficulties in measuring exposure.

Some agents used in the manufacture of synthetic materials such as plastics, polyurethanes, and other polymers have resulted in some workers being sensitized to extremely low levels of *isocyanates, aromatic amines,* or *aldehydes.* Repeated exposure to these agents causes some workers to develop chronic cough and sputum production, asthma, or episodes of low-grade fever and malaise. Occasionally, as in byssinosis, these symptoms occur early in the workweek, but usually recur with-

TABLE 275-2
Selected common toxic chemical agents

Agents	*Selected exposures*	*Acute effects from high or accidental exposure*	*Chronic effects from relatively low exposure*
Acid fumes; H_2SO_4, HNO_3	Manufacture of fertilizers, chlorinated organic compounds, dyes, explosives, rubber products, metal etching, plastics	Mucous membrane irritation, followed by chemical pneumonitis 2–3 days	No data
Ammonia	Refrigeration, petroleum refining, manufacture of fertilizers, explosives, plastics, and other chemicals	Same as acid fumes	Chronic bronchitis
Cyanides	Electroplating, extraction of gold or silver, manufacture of mirrors, fumigants, photo supplies	Increase respiratory rate followed by respiratory arrest, lactic acidosis, pulmonary edema, death	No data
Diazomethane	Methylating agent for acid compounds; laboratory workers	Violent coughing, dyspnea, wheezing, pulmonary edema	No data
Formaldehyde	Manufacture of resins, leathers, rubber, metals, & woods; laboratory workers, embalmers; emission from urethane foam insulation	Same as acid fumes	Cancers in one species of animals; no data on humans
Halides (Cl, Br, F)	Bleaching in pulp, paper, textile industry; manufacture of chemical compounds; synthetic rubber, plastics, disinfectant, rocket fuel, gasoline	Mucous membrane irritation, pulmonary edema; possible reduced FVC 1–2 yrs after exposure	Dryness of mucous membrane, epistaxis, dental fluorosis, tracheobronchitis
Hydrogen sulfide	By-product of many industrial processes, oil, other petroleum processes and storage	Low: conjunctival irritation; higher: respiratory paralysis similar to cyanides	Chronic bronchitis, recurrent pneumonitis
Ozone	Arc welding, flour bleaching, deodorizing, emissions from copying equipment, photochemical air pollutant	Mucous membrane irritant, pulmonary hemorrhage and edema	Chronic eye irritation
Phosgene	Organic compound, metallurgy, volatization of chlorine-containing compounds	Delayed onset of bronchiolitis and pulmonary edema	Chronic bronchitis
Phthalic anhydride	Manufacture of resin esters, polyester resins, thermoactivated adhesives	Nasal irritation, cough	Asthma, chronic bronchitis
Nitrogen dioxide	Silage, metal etching, explosives, rocket fuels, welding, by-product of burning fossil fuels	Cough, dyspnea, pulmonary edema may be delayed 4–12 h; possible result from acute exposure: bronchiolitis obliterans in 2–6 wks	Emphysema in animals, ? chronic bronchitis
Sulfur dioxide	Manufacture of sulfuric acid, bleaches, coating of nonferrous metals, food processing, refrigerant, burning of fossil fuels, wood pulp industry	Mucous membrane irritant, epistaxis	? Chronic bronchitis

out workweek periodicity. In the case of exposure to diisocyanate in the production of polyurethane, chronic and persistent asthma in selected individuals appears to result from exposure to concentrations well below the recognized industrial standard. Methods to identify susceptible individuals are needed. At present, challenge testing is being used to determine if a given patient is sensitive. These challenges can be carried out in special environmental chambers where the physician can simulate the work exposure. Alternatively, nonspecific challenges with either pharmacologic agents, such as methacholine and histamine, or isocapneic cold air breathing are being used to identify patients with hyperreactive airways. The usefulness of this nonspecific approach as a method to screen potential workers has yet to be established.

An unusual route of exposure occurs in *polymer fume fever.* Polymers, notably fluorocarbons, which at normal temperatures produce no reaction, may be transmitted from a worker's hands to his or her cigarettes. Upon burning the cigarette, the polymer is volatilized, and the inhaled agent causes a characteristic syndrome of fever, chills, malaise, and occasionally mild wheezing. The same condition occurs in workers exposed to heated polymers without cigarette use. The syndrome is obviously controlled by proper attention to hygiene in the work place. A similar self-limited, influenza-like syndrome—*metal fume fever*—results from acute exposure to fumes or smoke of zinc, copper, magnesium, and other volatilized metals. The fever may begin several hours after work and resolves within 24 h, only to return on repeated exposure. A proper occupational history should make the diagnosis evident.

ENVIRONMENTAL RESPIRATORY CARCINOGENS Historically, it has been the astute clinician who has recognized a higher incidence of malignant tumors associated with certain environmental exposures. When these observations are linked to an occupational setting, they must be pursued by epidemiologic studies of relatively large groups of both current and former workers. Often the concentration and/or exact nature of the substances contained in the putative exposures cannot be determined. Rarely, the possibility that a substance can play an etiologic role in cancer is supported by observing that a few cases of a very rare tumor in a particular group represent "an epidemic." The best examples of this are nasal sinus cancer in nickel workers and angiosarcomas in vinyl chloride workers.

Only in those few cases in which animal studies have been carried out can one confirm that a given suspected agent is really a carcinogen. For example, bis(chloromethyl) ether (BCME) has been shown to produce tumors in animals and oat-cell cancer of the lung in humans. In this particular case,

BCME, used as a chemical intermediary in the manufacture of a number of organic compounds, was known to produce tumors in animals almost before the substance was introduced into industry. (This case is one of the prime examples of why federal legislation was enacted in the United States in the 1970s to control the release of toxic substances, particularly new chemicals.)

In addition to the asbestos trades, other occupational exposures associated with either proven or suspected respiratory carcinogens include work with arsenic compounds, beryllium (animal studies only), chromium, coke ovens (exposure to polycyclic hydrocarbons), iron oxide, mustard gas, production of pure nickel from various ores, talc (possible asbestos contamination in both mining and milling), welding, woodworking (nasal cancer only), and uranium. The occurrence of excess cancers in uranium miners raises the possibility that there exist a large number of workers at risk by virtue of exposure to similar radiation hazards. This includes not only workers involved in processing uranium, up to and including its use in nuclear power plants and in military nuclear hardware, but also workers exposed in underground mining operations where radon daughters may be emitted from rock formations. In the latter case, the levels of exposure are generally considered to be relatively low. However, specific consideration must be given to the possibility of excess exposure for any hard rock miner.

GENERAL ENVIRONMENTAL EXPOSURES

AIR POLLUTION Dramatic and disastrous episodes of air pollution inversions have been documented in many industrialized centers in the world. Each of these episodes has been associated with excess acute mortality in the very old, the very young, and in those with chronic cardiopulmonary diseases. The most dramatic event was the London fog of 1952, in which approximately 4000 excess deaths occurred over a 2-week period following 5 days of severe cold and dense fog. Similar episodes in the United States, although less dramatic in terms of total deaths, occurred in Donora, Pennsylvania, in 1948, and in New York City in the 1960s. In these episodes, generally associated with cold temperature and air stagnation, patients with underlying cardiopulmonary disease were most severely affected.

In addition to significant excess mortality during these episodes, a large number of people required medical care for cardiorespiratory complaints. Subsequent follow-up studies failed to implicate these episodic disasters in the etiology of chronic respiratory disease in adults. On the other hand, many epidemiologic studies of both international and regional differences in the prevalences of chronic respiratory disease suggest that long-term exposures in polluted areas in the early to middle part of the twentieth century were associated with excess chronic respiratory disease.

In 1970, the federal government established air quality standards for several pollutants believed to be responsible for excess cardiorespiratory diseases. Primary standards designed to protect the public health with an adequate margin of safety exist for sulfur dioxide, total suspended particulates, nitrogen dioxide, ozone, lead, and carbon monoxide. These standards vary in their averaging times and levels, in part related to the differences in the known physiologic responses to each pollutant.

Pollutants are generated from both stationary sources (power plants and industrial complexes) and mobile sources (automobiles), and none of the pollutants occur in isolation. Thus, except for the change in carboxyhemoglobin from carbon monoxide exposure, it becomes extremely difficult to relate any specific health effect to any single pollutant. Furthermore, pollutants may be changed by chemical reactions after being emitted. For example, reducing agents, such as sulfur

dioxide and particulate matter from a power plant stack, may react in air to produce acid sulfates and aerosol (acid rain), which can be transported long distances in the atmosphere. Oxidizing substances, such as oxides of nitrogen and oxidants from automobile exhaust, may react with sunlight to produce ozone. This reaction is a particular problem in those portions of the southwest where air stagnation is in part related to local geographic conditions combined with increased sources of emissions.

The symptoms and diseases most commonly associated with air pollution are the same as those commonly associated with cigarette smoking. In addition, respiratory illness in early childhood has been associated with chronic exposure to levels of SO_2 and total suspended particulates in excess of about two to three times the current standard for the annual average of the 24-h levels. It is not known if persistent chronic exposure to a relatively constant level of pollutant(s) and recurrent short-term peak exposures which average to the same mean level have different effects. For a patient with significant cardiopulmonary impairment, one can only advise the individual to stay indoors during periods when pollution exceeds current standards.

INDOOR EXPOSURES Because of increased concern about energy costs, efforts are underway to reduce air exchange rates in all indoor environments. The effects of these efforts will be to increase exposures to a variety of air contaminants heretofore not considered important. Three examples of potential health effects from exposure to indoor pollutants are discussed to indicate the magnitude of possible problems.

For many years little attention, beyond its nuisance effect, has been given to the effects of *passive cigarette smoking*. The implication has been that passive smoking exposures were too low to be of any consequence. Recent studies have shown that the respirable particulate load in any household is directly proportional to the number of cigarette smokers living in the home. The potential health effects are discussed in Chap. 244.

Other indoor pollutants of increasing concern are the oxides of nitrogen (NO_2 and N_2O_4) generated by the oxidation of nitrogen in air above the flame of gas cook stoves. One-hour averages of NO_2 in the range of 300 to 700 $\mu g/m^3$ can be measured in kitchens of households using gas stoves. Studies of children living in such households (compared to children from households with electric stoves) suggest an excess rate of respiratory illness before age 2. A few studies of both children and adults failed to find any association between respiratory illness and gas stoves. A slight but significant reduction in pulmonary function has been found in children living in households with gas stoves compared to children from households with electric stoves. Whether these effects in children are important in the later development of chronic respiratory disease requires further study.

A novel source of indoor exposure to *formaldehyde* results from the curing process involved in the placement of urea-formaldehyde insulating foam or in several wood products used in modern furniture and the construction of mobile homes. Natural "degassing" of formaldehyde occurs during the first few months after the foam has been blown into the walls, with concentrations of formaldehyde as high as 5 ppm rapidly dropping off to less than 0.1 ppm. Chronic exposure to low levels of urea-formaldehyde (generally less than 1 ppm) may result if the foam is improperly installed. Patients apparently sensitive to concentrations of formaldehyde generally well below 1 ppm will complain of upper airway irritation with occasional epistaxis, sore throats, chest pain, and wheeze. Lower respiratory complaints, however, are uncommon, and often the most disturbing complaints are mild memory and mood disorders.

PORTAL OF ENTRY The lung is a primary source of entry into the body for a number of toxic agents that affect other organ systems. For example, the lung is the route of entry for benzene (bone marrow), carbon disulfide (cardiovascular and nervous systems), cadmium (kidney), and mercury (kidney, central nervous system). Thus, in any disease state of obscure origin, it is important to consider possible inhaled environmental agents. Such consideration can sometimes furnish the clue needed to identify a specific external cause for a disorder that might otherwise be labeled "idiopathic."

REFERENCES

American Thoracic Society: *Health Effects of Air Pollution.* New York, American Lung Association, 1978

Becklake MR: Asbestos-related fibrosis of the lungs (asbestosis) and pleura, in *Update: Pulmonary Diseases and Disorders,* AP Fishman (ed). New York, McGraw-Hill, 1982, pp 167–192

Cochrane AL, Moore FA: A 20-year follow-up of men aged 55-64 including coal-miners and foundry workers in Stavley, Derbyshire. Br J Ind Med 37:226, 1980

Craighead JE, Mossman BT: The pathogenesis of asbestos-associated diseases. N Engl J Med 306:1446, 1982

Dauber JH: Silicosis, in *Update: Pulmonary Diseases and Disorders,* AP Fishman (ed). New York, McGraw-Hill, 1982, pp 149–166

Ferris BG Jr: Epidemiology Standardization Project. Am Rev Respir Dis 118(6)(2):1, 1978

Division of Lung Diseases, National Heart, Lung and Blood Institute: *Report of Task Force on Epidemiology of Respiratory Diseases.* USPHS, Washington, NIH Publication 81-2019, 1980

Guidelines for the Use of INTERNATIONAL LABOUR OFFICE Classification of Radiographs of Pneumoconiosis. Occupational Safety and Health Sciences 22 (Revised 1980), Geneva, ILO, 1980

National Institute for Occupational Safety and Health: *Occupational Diseases, a Guide to Their Recognition.* USPHS, Washington, DHEW Publication 77-81, 1977

Parkes WR: *Occupational Lung Disorders,* 2d ed. London, Butterworth, 1981

Pulmonary infections

276 PNEUMONIA AND LUNG ABSCESS

JAN V. HIRSCHMANN
JOHN F. MURRAY

PNEUMONIA

DEFINITION Pneumonia is defined as inflammation in the lung parenchyma, the portion distal to the terminal bronchioles and comprising the respiratory bronchioles, alveolar ducts, alveolar sacs, and alveoli. While the inflammation may have many different causes and varying durations, the term *pneumonia* most commonly refers to acute infections.

PATHOGENESIS Organisms reach the lung to cause pneumonia by one of four routes: (1) inhalation of microbes present in the air, (2) aspiration of organisms from the naso- or oropharynx, the most common cause of bacterial pneumonia, (3) hematogenous spread from a distant focus of infection, or rarely, (4) direct spread from a contiguous site of infection.

Lung defense mechanisms Although inhalation of organisms and aspiration of oropharyngeal contents are probably common, even in healthy people, the airway distal to the larynx is normally sterile or possesses a sparse flora because of several protective mechanisms. The glottis reflexly closes when material is aspirated; whatever reaches the trachea and large bronchi usually evokes coughing, which expels the material from the tracheobronchial tree. The airway from the larynx to the terminal bronchioles is further protected by its lining of mucus-covered ciliated epithelium, which propels trapped inhaled matter from the smaller to the larger airways, where it can be eliminated by expectoration or swallowing.

The immunoglobulins constitute another defense mechanism. IgA, present in high concentrations in the upper respiratory tract, protects against viral infection. It is less abundant in the lower respiratory secretions, where it may help agglutinate bacteria, neutralize microbial toxins, and reduce bacterial attachment to mucosal surfaces. IgG in the serum and lower respiratory tract agglutinates and opsonizes bacteria; activates complement, promoting chemotaxis of granulocytes and macrophages; neutralizes bacterial toxins and viruses; and lyses gram-negative bacteria. Also present in the alveoli are alveolar macrophages, which ingest and kill organisms, and alveolar lining material, which may enhance phagocytic function. In addition, neutrophils, which ingest and kill organisms, and lymphocytes, providing humoral and cell-mediated immunity, are available from the bloodstream to help combat infection.

Predisposing conditions Pneumonia may occur in healthy people but is usually associated with conditions that impair one or more of the defense mechanisms listed above. Altered consciousness from alcoholism, cranial trauma, seizures, general anesthesia, drug overdose, cerebrovascular disease, or other causes, and old age depress the cough and glottic reflexes, allowing the aspiration of oropharyngeal contents. Pain from trauma or thoracic or upper abdominal surgery; weakness from malnutrition or neuromuscular disease; thoracic cage deformities such as serious kyphoscoliosis; or severe obstructive lung disease may prevent the full inspiration and brisk expiration necessary to generate an effective cough. An endotracheal tube or tracheostomy eliminates glottic closure and impedes effective coughing.

Mucociliary transport is impaired by alcohol, cigarette smoke, old age, and preceding viral respiratory infections, which may cause necrosis and desquamation of the tracheobronchial epithelium. Endobronchial obstruction from tumor, foreign body, or other causes compromises effective clearance mechanisms. Thick mucus from cystic fibrosis or chronic bronchitis makes the transport system less effective. Indeed, in chronic bronchitis, the tracheobronchial tree is typically colonized with an abundant flora, especially pneumococci and *Hemophilus influenzae.*

Lymphocyte disorders, including congenital and acquired immunodeficiencies, and granulocyte abnormalities may predispose to pneumonia (see Chaps. 57, 64, and 137). Pulmonary infection may also occur when alveolar macrophage function is impaired by cigarette smoke, hypoxia, starvation, anemia, pulmonary edema, and viral respiratory infections.

Oropharyngeal flora Most pneumonias arise from the aspiration of oropharyngeal flora, normally a complex assortment of aerobic and anaerobic bacteria. Which of these organisms causes the pneumonia seems to depend upon the identity of the microbes present and the quantity of material aspirated. *Streptococcus pneumoniae, H. influenzae, Staphylococcus aureus,* and even *Neisseria meningitidis,* all potential pathogens, are often found in the oropharynx of healthy adults. Each of these organisms, as single agents, may cause pneumonia when aspirated into alveoli. Anaerobes, however, which outnumber aerobes severalfold in the oral cavity, are weak pathogens individually and usually cause infection by an interaction among several species. These organisms, therefore, are likely to cause pneumonia, usually as a polymicrobial infection, only when aspirated in relatively large quantities.

Coliforms, such as *Escherichia coli, Klebsiella,* and *Proteus,* are uncommon in the oropharynx of healthy adults. Several conditions, especially hospitalization, however, favor their growth. Serious underlying illness, confinement in an intensive care unit, the use of an endotracheal tube or tracheostomy, contaminated respiratory equipment, and antimicrobial therapy, which frequently selects out organisms resistant to the agents used, especially encourage colonization with coliforms present in the hospital environment. Certain illnesses, such as acute granulocytic leukemia, alcoholism, and diabetes mellitus, are associated with an increased frequency of oropharyngeal colonization with aerobic gram-negative bacilli whether or not the patient is hospitalized.

CLINICAL MANIFESTATIONS The major symptoms of pneumonia, occurring in varying combinations, are cough, fever, chest pain, dyspnea, and the production of sputum, which may be mucoid, purulent, or even bloody. In some patients, extrapulmonary features such as confusion or disorientation may predominate, and occasionally, especially in elderly, alcoholic, or neutropenic patients, respiratory symptoms and signs are absent altogether. Important in the history are inquiries about prodromal symptoms, the type of onset (abrupt or gradual), the presence of rigors and pleuritic chest pain, similar illness in family members or acquaintances, animal exposure, and recent travel.

Common physical findings are fever, tachycardia, and tachypnea. Severely hypoxemic patients may be cyanotic. On chest examination there may be decreased respiratory excursion on the affected side because of pleuritic pain and dullness to percussion from pneumonic consolidation or an accompanying pleural effusion. Among the earliest auscultatory findings is the presence of high-pitched, end-inspiratory crackles, originating from fluid-filled alveoli, that are often increased by, or heard only after, coughing. Secretions in the airways may cause lower-pitched, early or mid-inspiratory crackles. Consolidated lung surrounding a patent bronchus often gives rise to bronchial breath sounds, an accentuation of both the inspiratory and expiratory phases of breathing. In some patients, despite impressive roentgenographic abnormalities, physical examination of the chest is entirely normal. In patients whose pneumonia is secondary to hematogenous spread, the primary site of infection may be apparent. Alternatively, bacteremia arising from pneumonia may cause infection in distant sites, such as meningitis, septic arthritis, or pustular skin lesions.

The arterial blood gases commonly reveal hypoxemia and, in the absence of other pulmonary disease, hypocarbia and respiratory alkalosis. These abnormalities result from ventilation-perfusion inequality, particularly the continued perfusion of the poorly ventilated areas affected by the pneumonia.

ROENTGENOGRAPHIC FINDINGS The microbial etiology of a pneumonia cannot be accurately predicted by its roentgenographic characteristics. Nevertheless, certain appearances are more typical of some organisms than others. Pneumonias tend to conform to one of three pathological and roentgenographic patterns (see Fig. 276-1): (1) alveolar or air space pneumonia, (2) bronchopneumonia, or (3) interstitial pneumonia. In air space pneumonia the organism causes an inflammatory exudate that spreads from one alveolus to the next via the communicating channels, known as the pores of Kohn, and the canals of Lambert. Segmental boundaries are not preserved, and the bronchi, relatively uninvolved, remain patent. The roentgenographic result is nonsegmental consolidation with air bronchograms, the classic example being pneumococcal pneumonia. Some organisms produce bronchopneumonia, which consists of inflammation in the conducting airways, especially terminal and respiratory bronchioles, and the surrounding alveoli. Because interalveolar spread in the peripheral air spaces is minimal, the pneumonia tends to maintain a distribution corresponding to the involved pulmonary segment. Inflammation affects the bronchi themselves, sometimes causing atelectasis, and air bronchograms are absent. An example is staphylococcal pneumonia. *Mycoplasma pneumoniae* and viruses often cause an interstitial pneumonia, where inflammation is predominantly in the alveolar septa, producing a reticular radiographic appearance.

DIAGNOSTIC TECHNIQUES Among the most useful procedures to define a pneumonia's etiology is the microscopic examination of a Gram-stained sputum specimen. Although precise speciation of bacteria is impossible by Gram's stain alone, the appearance of organisms allows reasonable inferences about their identity. An acceptable sputum sample, one genuinely arising from the lower respiratory tract rather than the oropharynx, has more than 25 leukocytes per low-power field (100×). Squamous epithelial cells from the oropharynx are sparse, and alveolar macrophages are often present. Specimens that fail to meet these standards represent mostly saliva and are useless for further examination or culture. Acceptable specimens should be cultured on appropriate media.

Adequate staining of acceptable specimens is crucial for accurate interpretation. If cells, including the nuclei of leukocytes, are not gram-negative (red), the sample is underdecolorized. If gram-positive (blue) organisms are present near the gram-negative leukocytes, the stain is suitable. If the cells and all the organisms are gram-negative, the slide may be overdecolorized and may require restaining. The slide should be examined carefully for the predominant organism; bacteria overlying squamous epithelial cells should be disregarded.

Usually, sputum expectorated after a deep cough is acceptable for stain and culture by the criteria outlined above. When the patient cannot produce a satisfactory specimen, inhalation of ultrasonically nebulized saline or suctioning with a catheter introduced through the nose into the posterior pharynx will often induce coughing and provide an adequate sample. Since sputum that is expectorated or obtained by nasotracheal suction is unavoidably contaminated by oropharyngeal flora,

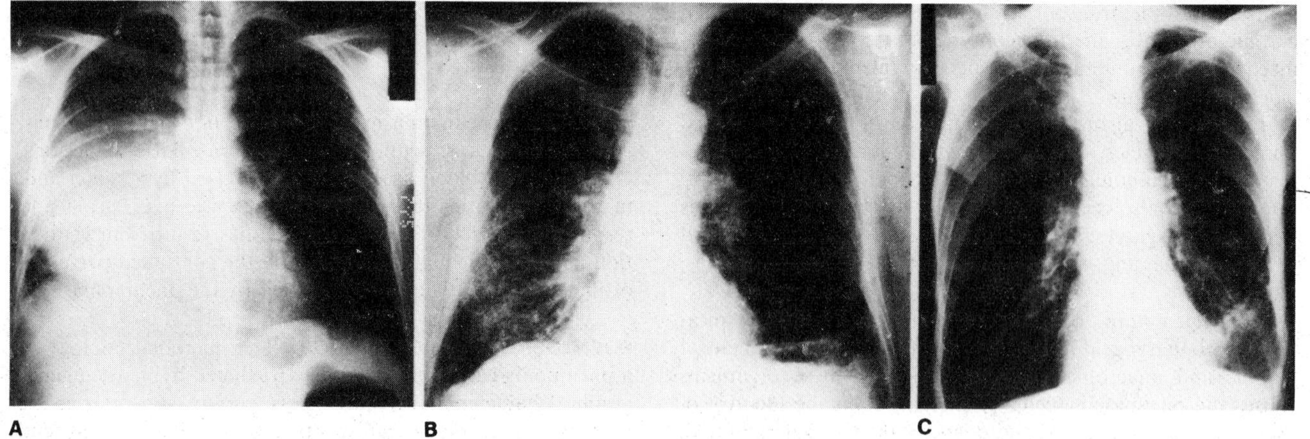

FIGURE 276-1
Roentgenographic appearances of pneumonia. A. Air space pneumonia. There is a dense, homogeneous, nonsegmental consolidation in the right lower lobe with a visible air bronchogram. B. Interstitial pneumonia. A linear or reticular pattern involves the lower lung fields bilaterally, more on the right. C. Bronchopneumonia. A segmental infiltrate without a visible air bronchogram appears in the left lower lung field.

which normally contains anaerobic organisms, it is not appropriate for anaerobic cultures.

Another method of obtaining sputum is transtracheal aspiration with a polyethylene catheter inserted into the trachea through the cricothyroid membrane. This procedure is generally safe but should be accompanied by oxygen administration in those with hypoxemia and avoided in those with serious clotting disorders or platelet defects. This method avoids contamination with the abundant, complex mouth flora and yields a specimen suitable for anaerobic culture. An alternate way of obtaining lower respiratory secretions is transthoracic aspiration of the lung with a spinal needle attached to a syringe. The major complications are pneumothorax or pulmonary hemorrhage. Lower respiratory secretions may also be obtained by bronchoscopy. Because contamination with oropharyngeal flora is generally unavoidable, even with preceding endotracheal intubation, these specimens are approximately equivalent to good expectorated sputum samples, unless specially designed catheters, which may provide uncontaminated specimens, are used.

Occasionally, lung biopsy may be necessary for accurate diagnosis and treatment, especially in immunocompromised patients. This procedure is discussed later in the chapter under "Treatment, Pneumonia in the Compromised Host."

Since bacteremia sometimes accompanies pneumonia, blood cultures taken from two separate venipuncture sites may grow the responsible organism. Similarly, the presence of a pleural effusion requires a thoracentesis, which may yield infected fluid. Skin lesions, joint effusions, and cerebrospinal fluid should be cultured if these areas appear infected.

Although viruses, *M. pneumoniae, Coxiella burnetti, Legionella pneumophila,* and *Francisella tularensis,* may grow from sputum specimens cultured on appropriate media, pneumonias due to these agents are usually diagnosed by serology. Acute and convalescent serum samples should be obtained when these agents are suspected; seroconversion to *L. pneumophila* may take 6 weeks. Legionnaires' disease may also be diagnosed by direct immunofluorescence of respiratory tract secretions (see Chap. 162).

DIFFERENTIAL DIAGNOSIS Community-acquired pneumonias Pneumococcal pneumonia (see Chap. 146), the most common bacterial pneumonia, in its classic form frequently follows an upper respiratory infection and begins abruptly with a single shaking chill, fever, pleuritic chest pain, and a cough productive of purulent, often bloody sputum. In some patients, especially the elderly and those with serious underlying disorders such as alcoholism or chronic obstructive lung disease, the illness is often considerably less dramatic, with the insidious onset of fever, cough, and dyspnea or extrapulmonary features such as confusion or weakness. The white blood cell count is usually elevated, with increased immature forms, but may be normal or low. The typical sputum Gram's stain shows numerous neutrophils and abundant, gram-positive lancet-shaped diplococci as the predominant organism. The chest roentgenogram characteristically demonstrates a unilateral, homogeneous, nonsegmental air space consolidation, usually abutting against a visceral pleural surface. Unilateral or bilateral multilobar involvement may occur, and in patients with emphysema the consolidation may have an inhomogeneous appearance of multiple "holes" from the radiolucent, uninvolved bullae. Cavitation rarely occurs, but pleural effusions, usually small but occasionally voluminous, are frequent.

Pneumonia from *S. pyogenes* (see Chap. 148) is very uncommon. It may follow pharyngitis or a viral illness, especially influenza, or occasionally occurs as outbreaks in closed populations, such as military recruits. The onset is typically abrupt, with multiple rigors, fever, a productive cough, and pleuritic chest pain. Pharyngitis is often present. The white blood cell count is commonly elevated, and immature forms increased. The sputum Gram's stain shows multiple neutrophils and gram-positive cocci in chains. The chest roentgenogram usually reveals unilateral bronchopneumonia and large pleural effusions, which develop rapidly after the onset of illness.

Pneumonia from *S. aureus* (see Chap. 147), also quite uncommon, tends to follow an influenza attack. The onset is generally abrupt and the course rapid, with fever, multiple rigors, purulent sputum production, and pleuritic chest pain. The white blood cell count is elevated, and immature forms are increased. The sputum smear shows numerous neutrophils and gram-positive cocci in clumps. The chest roentgenogram reveals bronchopneumonia, often bilateral, frequently with cavitation and pleural effusions. Pneumatoceles, thin-walled cystic spaces, may develop, primarily in children.

Pneumonia due to *N. meningitidis* (see Chap. 149) may occur in sporadic cases, following viral respiratory infections, or especially in military recruits. The onset may be abrupt, resembling pneumococcal pneumonia, or more gradual, with cough, fever, sore throat, and chest pain. Meningitis or cutaneous evidence of meningococcemia is uncommon, and blood cultures are typically sterile. Neutrophilic leukocytosis is usual. The sputum smear shows gram-negative diplococci that are often present within the cytoplasm of neutrophils. The chest film most commonly demonstrates patchy alveolar consolidation, predominantly in the lower lobes. Pleural effusions and pulmonary cavitation are rare.

Although *H. influenzae* (see Chap. 156) pneumonia may occur in healthy young adults, the typical patient is over 50 years old and has chronic obstructive lung disease or alcoholism. The onset may be abrupt but is more frequently gradual. The major complaints are fever, productive cough, chills, dyspnea, and pleuritic chest pain. Neutrophilic leukocytosis is usual. The sputum smear shows abundant neutrophils and many pleomorphic gram-negative organisms that range from cocci to bacilli of various sizes and are often especially predominant in the cytoplasm of the white blood cells. The bacilli are slender, unlike the typical plump appearance of enteric organisms. The chest film usually discloses diffuse bronchopneumonia, often bilateral, although air space consolidation sometimes occurs. Pleural effusions developing rapidly in the course of disease are common, but lung abscess formation is rare.

Klebsiella pneumoniae (see Chap. 151) pneumonia is very uncommon. It typically occurs in middle-aged or elderly patients with underlying chronic disease, especially alcoholism and diabetes mellitus. The illness begins abruptly with fever, rigors, productive cough, and dyspnea. Neutrophilic leukocytosis is usual, although neutropenia occasionally occurs. The sputum may be tenacious and bloody. Plump gram-negative bacilli of uniform size are visible on the sputum smear. The chest roentgenogram shows an air space pneumonia usually in one of the upper lobes and frequently complicated by abscess formation and a pleural effusion. The inflammatory exudate in the lung may be so voluminous that the interlobar fissure bulges, a characteristic, but not pathognomonic, finding.

Pneumonia from *anaerobic organisms* (see Chap. 173) usually occurs in patients with periodontal disease, which increases their number in the mouth, and in patients with a propensity to aspirate because of swallowing disorders, altered consciousness, or other causes. The onset may be abrupt but is usually gradual, with several days to weeks of fever, weight loss, and a productive cough. The sputum may be foul smelling, a feature diagnostic of anaerobic infection. The sputum smear typically shows many neutrophils, and several different organisms, usually both gram-positive and gram-negative, are profuse. Many anaerobic bacteria have a characteristic appearance. *Actinomyces,* eubacterium, and Bifidobacterium are filamentous, branching, thin gram-positive rods. Peptostreptococci are tiny gram-positive cocci in chains. *Fusobacterium* appears as a long, fusiform gram-negative rod with pointed ends, while *Bacteroides* are pleomorphic gram-negative bacilli that range from coccoid to long, filamentous structures. Understandably, aerobic cultures typically fail to grow a likely pathogen. Chest films demonstrate consolidation in the segments where gravitation favors the flow of aspirated material. These are the posterior segments of the upper lobes and the superior segments of the lower lobes, when aspiration has occurred in the supine position, and the basilar segments of the lower lobes for the upright position. Single or multiple areas of cavitation and pleural effusions are very common.

Pneumonia due to *L. pneumophila* (Legionnaires' disease, see Chap. 162) may occur in outbreaks or sporadically. The first symptoms of myalgia and headache are followed by fever, chills, and a cough that is nonproductive or yields small amounts of mucoid sputum. Diarrhea, chest pain that is often pleuritic, and confusion or delirium are common. Sputum smears show few leukocytes and rare bacteria. The organism itself is not visible on Gram's stain. The chest film reveals air space consolidation that may develop into unilateral or bilateral, poorly marginated, rounded opacities. Pleural effusions, if present, are usually small, and cavitation rarely occurs.

Pneumonia due to *Francisella tularensis* (see Chap. 159) follows tick bites or exposure to infected animals. A cutaneous ulcer and regional lymphadenopathy may be present but are absent in the typhoidal form. The illness typically begins abruptly with fever, chills, headache, and cough, which is usually nonproductive. The leukocyte count is usually normal but may be elevated. The sputum smear may show neutrophils, but the organism is rarely seen. The chest roentgenogram typically shows a bronchopneumonia, often with hilar adenopathy, a finding seldom seen in other bacterial pneumonias. Sometimes the pneumonia appears as a distinctive, oval, homogeneous consolidation. Pleural effusions are common, but cavitation is rare.

The most frequent cause of community-acquired, nonpyogenic pneumonia is *M. pneumoniae* (see Chap. 190). It occurs most commonly in children or young adults, but may develop in older persons, especially during outbreaks in a family group. It differs from the bacterial pneumonias described above in many respects. It has an insidious, rather than abrupt, onset and a cough that is nonproductive or yields only small amounts of mucoid sputum. Pleuritic chest pain, rigors, and hemoptysis are distinctly uncommon. The temperature is generally less than 38.9°C (102°F), and headache is a prominent symptom. As in other nonpyogenic pneumonias, the sputum smear typically demonstrates mononuclear leukocytes or neutrophils but few organisms, since the agent is not visible on Gram's staining. The white blood cell count is usually normal or only mildly elevated, with a normal differential. The chest roentgenogram demonstrates segmental bronchopneumonia, or sometimes a predominant interstitial pattern, mostly affecting the lower lung fields. Bilateral involvement is common, but, unlike many bacterial pneumonias, substantial pleural effusions or cavitation are rare. The extent of radiographic involvement is often more impressive than the clinical examination would suggest.

Other community-acquired nonpyogenic pneumonias are Q fever, psittacosis, and viral pneumonia. Q fever (see Chap. 189) occurs from the inhalation of aerosolized particles containing *Coxiella burnetti,* the usual sources being placental tissues, amniotic fluid, milk, and feces of infected cattle, sheep, and goats. It is largely an occupational disease of those exposed to livestock. It begins abruptly with headache, fever, chills, and myalgias. Chest pain, often pleuritic, and a nonproductive cough follow. The white blood cell count is usually normal, and the chest film typically shows segmental consolidation that is predominantly in the lower lobes.

Psittacosis (see Chap. 194), also an occupational disease, occurs in those exposed to infected birds. Fever, an excruciating headache, myalgias, and an unproductive cough are the predominant symptoms. Splenomegaly, rare in most pneumonias, is frequent. The white blood cell count is usually normal. The roentgenographic appearance varies from homogeneous to patchy consolidation, which may be segmental or lobar in distribution. Sometimes the chest film shows nodular or miliary opacities.

Viral pneumonias are quite uncommon in civilian adults who are not immunosuppressed, and this diagnosis should be made only with strong clinical or epidemiologic evidence, supported by viral cultures and serologic studies. The overwhelming majority of pneumonias in adults are due to the agents discussed above, not viruses. The most frequent viral pneumonia is *influenza* (see Chap. 198), which tends to occur in patients with underlying cardiac or pulmonary disease. It begins as typical influenza, with fever, myalgias, and headache. Twelve to thirty-six hours later dyspnea and cyanosis may develop rapidly and often proceed to a fatal outcome. The chest roentgenogram shows diffuse, patchy, unilateral or bilateral air space pneumonia. Even with these typical clinical features, a bacterial superinfection, especially with pneumococci or *S. aureus,* may be responsible for the pneumonia, instead of the virus itself.

Varicella (see Chap. 204) can cause pneumonia in adults and typically begins 2 to 3 days after the vesicular eruption appears. Fever, cough, dyspnea, hemoptysis, and pleuritic chest pain are the major symptoms. The chest film demonstrates patchy, diffuse, generally discrete air space consolidations that are coarsely nodular.

Measles (see Chap. 200) pneumonia in adults generally occurs in military recruits and may begin just before, with, or after the skin rash. The chest film shows a diffuse bilateral reticular pattern.

Adenovirus (see Chap. 197) pneumonia also occurs predominantly in military recruits. Fever, cough, rhinitis, and pharyngitis are the major features. The chest film shows patchy consolidation, generally in the lower lung fields.

In endemic areas the fungi *Coccidioides immitis* and *Histoplasma capsulatum* (see Chap. 183) must be considered in the differential diagnosis of community-acquired pneumonia. The diagnosis is usually established by serology.

Hospital-acquired pneumonia Because of changes in oropharyngeal flora with hospitalization, hospital-acquired pneumonias, unlike community-acquired ones, are likely to be due to a wide variety of aerobic gram-negative bacilli with varying antimicrobial susceptibilities and, less frequently, *S. aureus,* pneumococci, or *H. influenzae.* Only rarely is it possible to distinguish among pneumonias caused by different species of gram-negative rods on the basis of the clinical or roentgenographic features. Adequate sputum Gram's stains and cultures, therefore, are especially important in defining the etiologic agent and suggesting the appropriate antibiotic therapy.

Hospitalized patients with endotracheal tubes or tracheostomies receiving mechanical ventilation are an important group in whom the diagnosis of pneumonia is particularly difficult to make. Shortly after intubation, the tracheobronchial tree becomes colonized with organisms, and a purulent tracheobronchitis commonly ensues. Even though there is purulent sputum with plentiful organisms, this tracheobronchitis requires no antimicrobial therapy, which only encourages the growth of drug-resistant organisms, unless pneumonia is present. The diagnosis of pneumonia requires evidence of parenchymal lung involvement and in this setting depends upon the presence of purulent tracheobronchial secretions *plus* fever, leukocytosis, and a new or progressive pulmonary infiltrate on chest films. Inspection of a gram-stained sputum specimen is useful in differentiating between colonization of the lower respiratory tract, in which case bacteria are absent or scanty, and true infection, in which case bacteria are numerous.

TREATMENT Community-acquired pneumonia Patients whose history or physical examination suggests the likelihood of pneumonia should have a chest roentgenogram to confirm the diagnosis and delineate the pattern and extent of pulmonary involvement. Most patients with mild to moderate disease on clinical and radiologic assessment can be treated as outpatients. In them, a white blood cell count may be useful in the differential diagnosis, but routine blood cultures and arterial blood gases are unnecessary, The clinical and radiographic features and the sputum Gram stain should dictate the choice of antimicrobial therapy. If sputum is unobtainable or unhelpful and the other information inconclusive, oral erythromycin, 500 mg qid, is a good choice. It is effective against pneumococci and *M. pneumoniae,* the two most frequent causes of community-acquired pneumonia, but also should be satisfactory to treat Legionnaires' disease, and many cases of *H. influenzae* pneumonia and anaerobic pneumonias. Auxiliary measures should include adequate hydration, analgesics to relieve chest pain, if present, and cough suppressants for those with the harassing, unproductive cough characteristic of *M. pneumoniae.* In patients with good clinical improvement, a repeat chest film after 6 weeks is appropriate to document radiographic resolution. Failure to resolve by then indicates possible endobronchial obstruction and the necessity for bronchoscopy.

Reasons for hospitalization include severe dyspnea or hypoxemia; evidence of empyema or extrapulmonary foci of infections, such as meningitis; shock; serious underlying disease, especially cardiac or pulmonary; severe systemic manifestations such as delirium, whose presence warrants a lumbar puncture to exclude concomitant meningitis; or social circumstances making treatment at home unfeasible. These patients should have two blood cultures obtained from separate venipuncture sites; a complete blood count, including white blood cell differential; and arterial blood gas measurements if there is marked tachypnea, severe dyspnea, altered mental status potentially attributable to hypoxemia, cyanosis, or serious underlying cardiopulmonary disease. The clinical and radiographic features and, especially, the sputum Gram's stain should indicate the proper antibiotic choice. Since the most common community-acquired pneumonia requiring hospitalization is pneumococcal, the appropriate agent usually is penicillin, 2.4 million units daily, intramuscularly or intravenously. If the sputum smear is unsatisfactory or unobtainable by expectoration or nasotracheal suctioning, transtracheal aspiration may be indicated, particularly if the patient has an underlying illness like alcoholism that makes gram-negative pneumonia more likely.

In patients with unobtainable or uninformative sputum, the following recommendations provide guidelines for initial therapy in patients requiring hospitalization. Penicillin remains the drug of choice in most circumstances, including suspected anaerobic infections following the aspiration of large quantities of oropharyngeal contents. Reasonable alternatives include clindamycin, 300 mg intravenously every 6 h, or parenteral cefazolin, 500 mg every 8 h. In drug addicts and in patients developing pneumonia after an influenza attack, pneumococcus and *S. aureus* are the likely pathogens, and a semisynthetic penicillinase-resistant penicillin like oxacillin or nafcillin, 8 to 12 g daily intravenously, is indicated. Alternatives include vancomycin, 2 g intravenously daily, or cephalothin, 8 to 12 g intravenously daily. In patients with chronic bronchitis complicated by acute pneumonia, penumococcus and *H. influenzae* are the most common causes, and ampicillin, 2 to 6 g daily intravenously, is a good choice for therapy in the unusual patient whose sputum sample is inadequate for diagnosis. Alternatives include tetracycline, 2 g daily; chloramphenicol, 2 g daily; or cefamandole, 2 g daily, all given intravenously. In patients with suspected Legionnaire's disease, erythromycin, 1 g intravenously every 6 h, is the drug of choice.

Auxiliary measures include adequate hydration, the administration of humidified oxygen, relief of chest pain by adequate analgesics, and the encouragement of coughing to expectorate sputum. Intermittent positive pressure breathing (IPPB), however, is not helpful, and postural drainage should generally be reserved for those with bronchiectasis or lung abscess. Mechanical ventilation is required when the diffuseness of the pneumonia or the severity of underlying cardiopulmonary disease prevents adequate oxygenation with spontaneous respiration and supplemental oxygen by mask or nasal prongs.

Hospital-acquired pneumonia Since the range of organisms causing hospital-acquired pneumonias is so wide and their antimicrobial susceptibilities so variable, precise bacteriologic diagnosis is crucial. Patients with hospital-acquired pneumonias should have blood cultures, and vigorous attempts must be made to obtain sputum by expectoration, nasotracheal suctioning, or, if these are unsuccessful, transtracheal aspiration. When gram-negative rods are the predominant organism on Gram's stain, an aminoglycoside effective against *Pseudomonas aeruginosa*, like gentamicin, should be given. If gram-positive cocci resembling *S. aureus* are present, a penicillinase-resistant penicillin is appropriate. If a mixture of these organisms is present or no sputum is obtainable, a combination of an aminoglycoside plus a penicillinase-resistant penicillin or a cephalosporin is a good choice. Determination of the precise agents used should be guided by knowledge of the local hospital flora and its antimicrobial sensitivities. The regimen should be altered later according to the identity and susceptibility of the organisms isolated. If the sputum smear reveals organisms characteristic of pneumococci, anaerobes, or *H. influenzae*, which sometimes cause nosocomial pneumonias, the appropriate therapy for these organisms recommended in Chap. 141 should be given.

Pneumonia in compromised hosts (see also Chap. 137) Compromised hosts with pneumonia require special consideration. Patients who are severely neutropenic from acute leukemia or from cytotoxic agents generally develop pneumonia from aerobic gram-negative bacilli. Unless the Gram's stains strongly indicate otherwise, these patients should receive an aminoglycoside effective against *P. aeruginosa* and either carbenicillin or ticarcillin until the culture results return.

In severely immunosuppressed patients without neutropenia, the possible causes of fever and a new pulmonary infiltrate are legion. They fall into four categories: (1) the disease itself, such as Hodgkin's disease of the lung; (2) the effects of treatment, such as radiation pneumonitis or pulmonary toxicity from agents like methotrexate; (3) infections; and (4) miscellaneous disorders such as pulmonary emboli and intrapulmonary hemorrhage. Possible infectious causes include not only bacteria but also fungi, like *Candida* or *Aspergillus*; viruses, especially cytomegalovirus; and protozoa, particularly *Pneumocystis carinii* (see Chap. 222). In these patients unless the initial evaluation, including sputum smears, strongly indicates a specific diagnosis, further information obtained by bronchoscopic biopsy, transthoracic needle aspiration, or, preferably, open-lung biopsy is necessary for definitive diagnosis.

For safe performance, all these procedures require correction of severe thrombocytopenia and clotting disorders. *Transthoracic needle aspiration* may be useful in peripheral, localized disease, but because it fails to provide tissue specimens, it is not recommended for diffuse infiltrates, where histologic examination rather than stains and cultures of aspirated material is so frequently necessary for specific diagnosis. Pneumothorax occurs in about 20 percent, requiring chest tube placement in about 10 percent; significant pulmonary hemorrhage develops in about 5 percent. Contraindications include uncorrectable hypoxemia, lack of patient cooperation, bullous lung disease, and mechanical ventilation. *Fiberoptic bronchoscopy* with washings, sterile brushings, and transbronchial biopsy is appropriate for both localized and diffuse processes, but the quantity of tissue obtained is small and may be unrepresentative, especially in diffuse disease. The procedure yields a specific diagnosis in about 50 percent of cases. Pneumothorax or significant hemorrhage each occurs in about 5 to 10 percent, with about one-half of pneumothoraxes requiring chest tube drainage. Contraindications include uncorrectable hypoxemia or an uncooperative patient. Bleeding complications are considerably greater in uremia, although it is not an absolute contraindication. *Open-lung biopsy* yields accurately representative tissue in nearly all patients. A specific diagnosis is established in about 70 percent of patients; in the remaining 30 percent nonspecific inflammation and fibrosis are found whose cause is unknown and for which there is no effective therapy. Such a finding allows antimicrobial agents to be withheld or discontinued. Open-lung biopsy is remarkably safe, with a mortality rate of less than 1 percent in these very ill patients. It can be performed even in patients requiring mechanical ventilation.

While many clinicians initiate these invasive diagnostic procedures as soon as the initial, rapid clinical evaluation and examination of sputum smears prove inconclusive, others reserve them for patients who fail to respond to "empiric" therapy within 48 to 72 h. Empiric treatment is initiated with an aminoglycoside combined with a cephalosporin, carbenicillin, or ticarcillin. With diffuse infiltrates sulfamethoxazole-trimethoprim is added to treat *P. carinii*. For those patients who fail to respond and are unable to undergo invasive diagnostic procedures, amphotericin B is added for focal infiltrates, especially if the patient has recently received prolonged broad-spectrum antibiotic therapy and is leukopenic. This empiric approach is usually less advisable than obtaining a specific diagnosis with invasive techniques.

LUNG ABSCESS

DEFINITION A lung abscess is a necrotic area of lung parenchyma containing purulent material. An etiologic classification appears in Table 276-1.

PATHOGENESIS The pathogenesis of infectious lung abscesses is nearly identical to that of pneumonia as discussed earlier in this chapter. Most arise from the aspiration of naso- or oropharyngeal contents. The development of a lung abscess, instead of just pneumonia, depends upon the infecting organism's ability to cause necrosis of lung tissue. Pneumococci, *H. influenzae*, *M. pneumoniae*, and viruses rarely cause necrosis, but it is common in pulmonary infections due to *K. pneumoniae* and other enteric gram-negative bacilli and *S. aureus*. Anaerobic organisms are the most frequent cause of pyogenic lung abscesses and tend to occur when large quantities of oropharyngeal material are aspirated because of disordered consciousness or impaired swallowing.

Less frequently, abscesses arise from hematogenous spread of organisms to the lung. This may occur during bacteremia originating from a distant site of infection or as a result of septic emboli either from right-sided endocarditis or from septic thrombophlebitis associated with infections in the extremities or the abdominal cavity.

Patients with tuberculosis (see Chap. 174), pulmonary fungal infections (see Chaps. 183 and 184), and pleuropulmonary

TABLE 276-1
Classification of lung abscesses according to cause

1 Necrotizing infections
- *a* Pyogenic bacteria (*S. aureus, Klebsiella*, group A streptococcus, *Bacteroides, Fusobacterium*, anaerobic and microaerophilic cocci and streptococci, other anaerobes, *Nocardia*)
- *b* Mycobacteria (*Mycobacterium tuberculosis, M. kansasii, M. intracellularis*)
- *c* Fungi (*Histoplasma, Coccidioides, Aspergillus*)
- *d* Parasites (amoebas, lung flukes)

2 Cavitary infarction
- *a* Bland embolism
- *b* Septic embolism (various anaerobes, *Staphylococcus, Candida*)
- *c* Vasculitis (Wegener's granulomatosis, periarteritis)

3 Cavitary malignancy
- *a* Primary bronchogenic carcinoma
- *b* Metastatic malignancies (very uncommon)

4 Other
- *a* Infected cysts
- *b* Necrotic conglomerate lesions (silicosis, coal miner's pneumoconiosis)

amebiasis (see Chap. 217) may develop one or more areas of lung necrosis. Although usually labeled "cavities," these lesions are really abscesses. While the clinical course typically distinguishes these conditions from pyogenic lung abscess, there may be many similarities that cause confusion in the differential diagnosis.

CLINICAL MANIFESTATIONS Anaerobic lung abscess The clinical features of pulmonary infections due to staphylococci, streptococci, and aerobic gram-negative bacilli are discussed earlier in this chapter and in the chapters dealing with the specific organisms. These are usually acute, rapidly progressive infections.

Although the spectrum of illness in anaerobic lung abscess may vary from a mild productive cough to acute disease with severe systemic manifestations, the onset is usually insidious, with the symptoms gradually worsening over several weeks. The most common feature is a cough productive of moderate to large amounts of purulent sputum that is often fetid and bloody. Fever, pleuritic or dull chest pain, dyspnea, weakness, anorexia, and weight loss, which can be considerable, are common. A condition predisposing to aspiration, such as alcoholism or epilepsy, is usually present.

Most patients are febrile. Oral examination usually discloses poor dentition, with caries, gingivitis, and periodontal infection, conditions which increase the number of anaerobes in the oral cavity. The chest examination may be normal or may include signs of consolidation, rales, and, occasionally, amphoric or cavernous breath sounds over the involved area. Patients with an associated empyema may have dullness to percussion and decreased breath sounds. Clubbing, although uncommon, may occur. Neutrophilic leukocytosis with an increase in immature forms is usual, and, if the infection has persisted for several weeks, anemia and hypoalbuminemia may be present. The medical history, physical findings, and routine laboratory results are often nonspecific; foul-smelling sputum present in about half the patients, however, clearly indicates an anaerobic pulmonary infection. Definitive diagnosis rests on the demonstration of an abscess cavity on chest films and the identification of the causative organisms on culture.

The chest roentgenogram reveals an area of consolidation containing a radiolucency. Not all radiolucent areas are abscess, however, and either a wall or a border completely surrounding the lucent area or a fluid level within it should be present to diagnose an abscess cavity. Even these criteria are not definitive, since infected bullae or cysts or an empyema with a bronchopleural fistula may have an identical appearance. The abscess cavities are located in those segments that are most dependent at the time of aspiration: the posterior segment of the upper or superior segment of the lower lobes, especially on the right, when the patient is supine or the basilar segments of the lower lobes when upright.

Examination of the sputum by both microscopy and culture is essential to establish the correct diagnosis. In staphylococcal and aerobic gram-negative bacillary infections, the single causative organism clearly predominates on smear and culture. Gram's stain of sputum from an anaerobic abscess reveals abundant neutrophils and numerous organisms, including gram-positive cocci and rods and gram-negative rods of varying size and configuration. Since expectorated sputum is unavoidably contaminated by the normal anaerobic oral flora, anaerobic sputum cultures are appropriate only for specimens obtained by transtracheal or transthoracic aspiration. Secretions aspirated through the fiberoptic bronchoscope are unsuitable because the instrument is contaminated as it passes through the naso- or oropharynx, even with preceding endotracheal intubation. Appropriately collected and cultured sputum specimens usually grow two or more anaerobic organisms, most commonly *Peptococcus, Peptostreptococcus, Fusobacterium nucleatumi*, and *Bacteroides melaninogenicus.* In about 60 percent of cases the infecting flora is exclusively anaerobic; in 40 percent both aerobes and anaerobes are present. The most common aerobic isolates are *S. aureus* and enteric gram-negative bacilli.

Associated pleural effusions should be aspirated and cultured aerobically and anaerobically. Blood cultures are usually sterile.

Septic pulmonary emboli In patients with septic pulmonary emboli, the site of origin is usually tricuspid valve endocarditis, particularly in intravenous drug abusers, or septic thrombophlebitis, which may occur in the arm veins of patients with infected intravenous catheter sites, infected injection sites from intravenous drug abuse, or infected arteriovenous shunts used in hemodialysis. Other areas of septic thrombophlebitis include pelvic veins with postpartum or postoperative pelvic infections, peritonsillar and internal jugular veins with pharyngeal infections, and veins adjacent to undrained suppuration, such as soft tissue infections or osteomyelitis. Rigors, high fever, dyspnea, cough, tachycardia, and tachypnea are the major clinical manifestations in these acutely ill patients. Neutrophilic leukocytosis is usual. The chest film typically discloses multiple, bilateral, round, or wedge-shaped opacities. These frequently and rapidly excavate to form thin-walled cavities, often without fluid levels. Small pleural effusions on one or both sides are common. Blood cultures are usually positive. Patients may not produce sputum, but if they do, it usually reveals the responsible organism, most commonly *S. aureus,* on Gram's stain and culture.

TREATMENT The history, physical examination, chest roentgenograms, and most importantly, Gram's and acid-fast sputum stains usually indicate whether an abscess is caused by aerobic organisms, anaerobes, or tubercle bacilli. Abscesses caused by aerobic organisms or tubercle bacilli should be treated according to the recommendations outlined in the chapters dealing with them.

Where septic pulmonary emboli from septic thrombophlebitis are suspected, it is important not only to institute appropriate antimicrobial therapy but also to identify the source. Removal of catheters, incision and drainage of systemic abscesses or infected veins, or ligation of the inferior vena cava may be necessary to prevent further embolization.

When the clinical findings and the sputum Gram's stain suggest an anaerobic abscess, penicillin is the drug of choice. It is usually given intravenously in doses of 5 to 10 million units daily until clinical improvement (return of appetite, defervescence) occurs. Oral penicillin V in doses of about 500 mg four times daily is then given for the duration of therapy. Some clinicians use oral medication from the start. Penicillin is effective in virtually all cases, even when *B. fragilis,* which is resistant in vitro to penicillin, is isolated as part of the anaerobic flora. It is also effective when there is a mixture of aerobic and anaerobic organisms. Alternative agents for penicillin-allergic patients or the rare case that fails to respond to penicillin are clindamycin and chloramphenicol. Because of relapses with shorter courses, antibiotics are usually given for at least 6 weeks. The optimal duration of therapy is unknown, but some clinicians continue treatment until the chest roentgenogram is clear or shows a stable residual lesion.

Ancillary measures include postural drainage and chest physiotherapy to help drain the abscess cavity. The role of bronchoscopy is unsettled. Some physicians believe that every patient with a lung abscess deserves bronchoscopy; others reserve its use for patients who fail to respond as anticipated to antibiotic therapy, who have evidence of an obstructing tumor or foreign body, or who have poorly communicating cavities that fail to drain adequately.

Except for the tube thoracostomy drainage of an associated empyema, surgery for lung abscess is rarely necessary. Incomplete roentgenographic resolution is not a sufficient reason for resectional surgery since delayed closure is common. Resection is indicated for massive hemoptysis, malignancy, or associated symptomatic bronchiectasis. Rarely, tube thoracostomy or some other form of surgical drainage may be necessary to manage uncontrolled sepsis arising from a poorly draining abscess.

REFERENCES

Pneumonia

BARTLETT JG: Anaerobic bacterial pneumonitis. Am Rev Respir Dis 119:19, 1979

FRASER RG, PARE JAP: *Diagnosis of Diseases of the Chest.* Philadelphia, Saunders, 1978, vol II, chap 6

GREEN GM et al: Defense mechanisms of the respiratory membrane. Ann Rev Respir Dis 115:479, 1977

KNIGHT V: *Viral and Mycoplasmal Infections of the Respiratory Tract.* Philadelphia, Lea & Febiger, 1973, chaps 5, 6, 14

MUFSON MA: Pneumococcal vaccine, in *Update: Pulmonary Diseases and Disorders,* AP Fishman (ed). New York, McGraw-Hill, 1982, pp 34–44

PIERCE AK, SANFORD JP: Aerobic gram-negative bacillary pneumonias. Am Rev Respir Dis 110:647, 1974

———: The gram-negative bacillary pneumonias, in *Update IV: Harrison's Principles of Internal Medicine,* KJ Isselbacher et al (eds). New York, McGraw-Hill, 1983, pp 75–86

REYNOLDS HY (ed): Respiratory infections. Clin Chest Med 2:1, 1981

Lung abscess

BARTLETT JG et al: Bacteriology and treatment of primary lung abscess. Am Rev Respir Dis 109:510, 1974

ESTRERA AS et al: Primary lung abscess. J Thorac Cardiovasc Surg 79:275, 1980

JOHANSON WG et al: Aspiration pneumonia, anaerobic infections, and lung abscess. Med Clin N Am 64:385, 1980

277 BRONCHIECTASIS AND BRONCHOLITHIASIS

JOHN F. MURRAY

These disorders both involve branches of the tracheobronchial system, have numerous, rather than single, underlying causes, and occasionally coexist. However, the pathogenesis, clinical manifestations, treatment, and prognosis of the two conditions are remarkably different.

BRONCHIECTASIS

DEFINITION Bronchiectasis can be defined as a permanent abnormal dilatation of one or more large (greater than 2 mm in diameter) bronchi due to destruction of the elastic and muscular components of the bronchial wall. This definition is not completely satisfactory because bronchi are also abnormally dilated in chronic bronchitis. Thus chronic bronchitis merges into bronchiectasis, and the distinction between them depends upon the *degree* of dilatation. The semantic problem is complicated further by the fact that the two conditions frequently coexist.

Classification is therefore difficult and is not useful in indicating the clinical severity of the disease; however, certain descriptive terms are commonly used to describe the appearance of bronchi displayed by bronchography. *Saccular (cystic) bronchiectasis* occurs mainly in the proximal large bronchi; affected airways show marked dilatation ending in large sacs at about the fourth bronchial division. *Cylindrical (fusiform) bronchiectasis* involves airways from the sixth to the tenth generation; the bronchographic appearance shows mild to moderate uneven widening, without a great increase in diameter, of bronchi that often look beaded and end squarely and abruptly. *Varicose bronchiectasis* is intermediate between saccular and cylindrical changes and is used to describe bronchi that resemble varicose veins. Saccular, varicose, and cylindrical bronchiectasis represent stages in a continuum of involvement, and all three may be present in the same patient.

Although "true" bronchiectasis is not reversible, the concept of reversibility is an important one, because abnormalities displayed by bronchography in some patients with reversible lung diseases (atelectasis, tracheobronchitis) may simulate bronchiectasis. Atelectasis causes shortening and tortuosity of airways in the involved region, producing an accordion-like appearance on bronchography. Similarly, ulcerations of the bronchial mucosa, which are common in viral infections of the lower respiratory tract, appear as an irregular pattern on bronchography. Both conditions resemble cylindrical bronchiectasis. Reexpansion of the collapsed lung and/or regeneration of the epithelium results in reversibility of the "pseudobronchiectasis." Thus bronchography, if indicated, should be delayed for several months after an episode of tracheobronchitis, pneumonia, or atelectasis.

PATHOGENESIS Since bronchiectasis is defined by the presence of morphologic changes in the caliber of large bronchi, its pathogenesis depends on antecedent factors that either cause or lead to necrosis of the bronchial wall and supporting tissues. The origin of the destructive process is nearly always a bacterial infection, but other factors—hereditary, congenital, or mechanical—that predispose to the development of the infection are often also present. Thus, the infection may be a primary event, such as suppurative necrotizing pneumonia, or it may be secondary to local or systemic abnormalities that impair defense mechanisms (i.e., cellular, humoral, and tracheobronchial clearance) and promote bacterial growth. Now, because the use of vaccines and antibiotic drugs has resulted in a marked decline in the incidence of severe necrotizing pneumonias and their bronchiectatic complications, this sequence is infrequently encountered; however, bronchiectasis as a complication of underlying systemic disorders appears to be increasing.

Hereditary and congenital factors Several hereditary and congenital disorders have been identified in which there is a high incidence of secondary bronchiectasis. *Congenital bronchiectasis* occurs at the site of a pre- or postnatal development defect of the bronchial system. The formation of cysts, cul-de-sacs, or bronchomalacia leads to pooling of secretions and bacterial infection. The generalized disorder of exocrine gland secretions in patients with *cystic fibrosis,* discussed in Chap. 278, affects the physical properties of tracheobronchial mucus and/or the adequacy of mucociliary clearance; this causes retention of secretions, with partial or complete plugging of airways, that provides a nidus for implantation and growth of bacteria. Most deaths (95 percent) of patients with cystic fibrosis who survive beyond 1 year of age are now caused by the consequences of bronchiectasis and accompanying chronic bronchopulmonary suppuration. The diffuse bronchiectasis rarely encountered with patients with *atopic bronchial asthma*, in whom there is often a strong familial association (Chap. 273), presumably is related to diffuse obstruction, as described below.

A variety of hereditary *immune-deficiency diseases*, secondary to either cellular or humoral defects, is associated with a high incidence of bacterial infections. Involvement of the sinuses and airways is particularly common, and the tendency for infections to recur in the lower airways often leads to bronchiectasis in patients with impaired immunologic mechanisms.

A newly designated group of genetically determined disorders called the *immotile cilia syndrome*, which includes *Kartagener's syndrome* (bronchiectasis, dextrocardia, and sinusitis) is characterized by ultrastructural changes causing immotility of cilia in the respiratory tract epithelium, sperm, and other cells. These abnormalities lead to recurrent sinopulmonary infections, infertility, and presumably disturbances during embryogenesis.This syndrome has recently been broadened to include patients with chronic sinobronchial disease from impaired mucociliary clearance who had "ciliary dyskinesia," not immotile cilia. The high incidence of unexplained bronchiectasis in Eskimo families and in the Maoris of New Zealand may also be hereditary in origin.

Obstruction Postobstructive bronchiectasis was much commoner in preantibiotic years than it is today. The availability of antimicrobial therapy and corrective surgical procedures accounts for the decreased incidence in this form of the disease. It is now recognized that obstruction per se does *not cause* bronchiectasis but *favors its development* by impairing clearance mechanisms, which enhances bacterial infection. Any process that leads to bronchial obstruction, therefore, may be associated with bronchiectasis distal to the site of involvement. Since the disorders causing obstruction are usually confined to one part of the bronchial system, postobstructive bronchiectasis is of the localized rather than the diffuse variety found in most forms of congenital-hereditary bronchiectasis. An exception is the bronchiectasis associated with diffuse obstruction of airways in patients with chronic bronchitis, atopic asthma, and cystic fibrosis. Patients with atopic asthma are liable to have secondary infections with *Aspergillus*, which produces the syndrome of bronchopulmonary aspergillosis characterized by proximal airway bronchiectasis, eosinophilia, and recurrent bouts of mucous plugging (Chap. 273).

Endobronchial tumors or foreign bodies, compression of airways from enlarged hilar lymph nodes or tumor masses, and bronchostenosis from endobronchial inflammatory disease (especially tuberculosis) all cause bronchial obstruction and may favor the development of postobstructive bronchiectasis.

Necrotizing inflammation Virtually all forms of bronchiectasis are associated with bacterial infections. If it were not for the presence of infection, the complications of bronchiectasis would be negligible. Although the development of the causative infection(s) is often favored by the presence of a hereditary disorder and/or bronchial obstruction that predisposes the patient to secondary bacterial involvement, bronchiectasis can occur as the result of necrotizing infections in a previously healthy individual. This presumably is the mechanism underlying the bronchiectasis that follows tuberculosis and the staphylococcal or other suppurative pneumonias; furthermore, the tendency for necrotizing pneumonias occasionally to complicate measles, pertusis, adenovirus infections, and influenza accounts for the frequency of bronchiectasis as a sequela of these disorders.

In rare instances, bronchiectasis may follow the introduction of corrosive chemical substances, commonly hydrocarbons, into the tracheobronchial tree. Similarly, the repeated aspiration of gastric fluid into the lungs may cause bronchiectasis. Since ulceration from chemical causes is invariably associated with secondary bacterial infection, it is difficult to dissociate the contributions of these two factors.

CLINICAL MANIFESTATIONS The signs and symptoms of bronchiectasis depend on the extent, severity, location, and presence of complications of the disease, but the hallmarks of the disease are chronic cough with sputum production, hemoptysis, and recurrent pneumonia. Even these vary greatly in frequency and severity and may be absent if the disease is mild or involves only the upper lobes of the lung.

The most frequent symptom is a *chronic cough* that produces sputum. The amount of sputum varies considerably but may be voluminous and is apt to be purulent during bouts of intercurrent infections. Streaks of blood in the sputum are common, and frank hemoptysis of large amounts of blood may develop if necrosis of the mucosa is severe. Exacerbation of chronic bronchial infection is frequent and may progress to pneumonia, occasionally with lung abscess or empyema formation. Associated systemic features of bronchiectasis are fever, weight loss, anemia, and weakness; these usually indicate the presence of active sepsis from severe disease or untreated intercurrent bacterial infection.

In what was once the typical patient with bronchiectasis, symptoms developed during infancy or early childhood; the onset was usually acute and followed suppurative pneumonia or pulmonary infection complicating measles or pertussis. However, because of the success of antimicrobials and vaccines in treating or preventing these disorders, acute onset of bronchiectasis at an early age is becoming infrequent, except in those areas of the United States and other countries where, owing to isolation or poverty, good medical care is not available.

Although chronic childhood bronchiectasis is decreasing, another group of patients with a different form of the disease appears to be increasing: these patients have recurrent lower respiratory tract infections that initially respond to treatment, with symptom-free intervals between episodes. The infections usually begin during childhood or young adulthood. As the number of recurrent bouts increases, the time between them tends to shorten and the response to treatment becomes less complete. Finally, chronic symptoms of cough and sputum develop. Patients in this category are likely to have cystic fibrosis, immune-deficiency diseases, immotile cilia, or atopic asthma.

Sinusitis is a common accompaniment of diffuse bronchiectasis and may be an expression of the vulnerability of the entire respiratory tract in these patients. Development of digital clubbing, metastatic abscesses (often brain), and amyloidosis were common complications in the past but are less frequent now. If the disease is widespread, it may resemble other forms of chronic obstructive lung disease, with generalized wheezing and ultimate progression to cor pulmonale; this constellation is particularly apt to occur in patients with underlying systemic abnormalities that lead to diffuse pulmonary involvement.

DIAGNOSIS Bronchiectasis is defined as a morphologic disorder; hence its diagnosis depends on demonstrating the abnormal anatomy of the bronchial system. Ordinarily this is accomplished by roentgenographic techniques, usually *bronchography*. The diagnosis should be *suspected* in any patient with chronic productive cough, especially if the sputum intermittently becomes more purulent and streaked with blood. Physical examination seldom reveals the severity and extent of distribution of the disease. Inspiratory rales are often the only evidence of pulmonary involvement. Occasionally, advanced cases of saccular bronchiectasis can be diagnosed by routine (plain) chest roentgenography; in such cases multiple 1- to 2-cm cystic lesions or fluid levels in poorly delineated sacs can be seen. More often, however, plain chest roentgenograms show only streaky infiltrations and loss of volume in involved areas; at times the chest roentgenograms may appear completely normal.

Bronchography (Chap. 272) should not be performed routinely in all patients with suggestive symptoms but is indicated primarily in the evaluation of patients for possible operation, those with recurrent, localized pneumonias or severe hemoptysis. Since the information from bronchography contributes little to the management of patients in whom surgery is contraindicated, such as those with minimal disability, with generalized involvement, or with obstructive airways disease, the procedure should be avoided in these patients because of its hazards. When bronchography is indicated, it should not be performed in patients during exacerbations of their cough and sputum production, but only after the manifestations have been thoroughly treated (see next section) and the volume of secretions is minimal. It is safer and advisable to study one lung at a time, owing to alterations in pulmonary function and to occasional inflammatory reactions induced by the procedure. Filling must be adequate and all segments must be visualized if the study is to be considered satisfactory for diagnostic purposes.

Bronchoscopy does not establish the diagnosis of bronchiectasis but may be useful in identifying the source of secretions in patients with cough and sputum and in determining the site of bleeding in patients with hemoptysis.

All patients with multiple episodes of sinopulmonary infections should have an immunologic survey to detect immune-deficiency diseases. Similarly, patients with suspected cystic fibrosis should have measurements of the concentrations of sodium and chloride in two or more samples of sweat (Chap. 278). Electron photomicrographic studies of sperm or mucosal biopsies from the respiratory tract reveal characteristic abnormalities in patients with the immotile cilia syndrome in whom tracheobronchial clearance is delayed or absent. Patients with asthma and suspected bronchiectasis from bronchopulmonary aspergillosis should have sputum cultures for *Aspergillus* and serologic studies for aspergillin precipitins.

The sputum volume, color, cellular content, and bacterial inhabitants are useful guides to the presence of active infection. The concentration of albumin in the sol phase of bronchopulmonary secretions correlates roughly with clinical estimates of the severity of bronchiectasis; in patients with severe disease an exudative sputum presumably indicates persistent underlying inflammation. Sputum eosinophilia provides a clue to the presence of asthma and/or bronchopulmonary aspergillosis. During exacerbations of the disease, the sputum increases in volume, becomes more purulent, and contains large numbers of polymorphonuclear leukocytes and bacteria that can be identified by Gram's stain. Culture of the sputum often reveals normal nasopharyngeal flora and, less commonly, *Diplococcus pneumoniae* or *Hemophilus influenzae.* Fetid sputum signifies the presence of anaerobic microorganisms. Sputum from patients receiving prolonged or frequent treatment with broad-spectrum antibiotic drugs may grow *Staphylococcus* species or a mucoid strain of *Pseudomonas aeruginosa;* this finding is especially common in patients with cystic fibrosis.

The blood count is usually within the normal range but may reveal anemia, reflecting chronic infection, or leukocytosis, signifying active suppuration. The urinalysis is normal except in the rare instances of *amyloidosis,* when proteinuria occurs. The electrocardiogram is normal until the late stages, when *cor pulmonale* may supervene and right ventricular hypertrophy develops. Owing to the wide variations in the extent and severity of the disease, only broad generalizations about pulmonary function abnormalities are possible, although a correlation exists between the overall impairment of lung function and the number of involved segments. Vital capacity and expiratory flow rates tend to be reduced but may be within normal limits if the disease is mild. In the late stages of diffuse bronchiectasis severe airflow obstruction can occur. A mild to moderate reduction in arterial oxygen tension (P_{O_2}) reflects regional abnormalities in the distribution of ventilation with respect to perfusion. Mismatching of ventilation and perfusion is the physiologic hallmark of bronchiectasis and can now be examined in regions of the lung by the use of radioactive gases, e.g., ^{133}Xe (Chap. 271). Pulmonary function studies are helpful in defining the extent and severity of abnormalities, in assessing the effects of therapy, and in evaluating patients for surgery.

TREATMENT Since bacterial infections are associated with most forms of bronchiectasis initially and are responsible for its exacerbation, antibiotics are the major weapons for its prevention and treatment. The choice of antimicrobial agents should be guided by the results of sputum culture; however, as indicated, these may reveal "normal flora" and no conspicuous pathogen. The drug of choice for patients with this finding is ampicillin or one of its derivatives; patients allergic to the penicillins usually respond to trimethoprim-sulfamethoxazole or one of the tetracyclines. When pneumococci are present, it is best to avoid the tetracycline drugs, as some pneumococcal strains are resistant to these agents. Antibiotics should be given until sputum production becomes minimal and purulence disappears; this desirable therapeutic result is usually achieved swiftly (5 to 7 days) if antibiotics are started early in the course of an exacerbation—as soon as the patient's cough increases and becomes productive of sputum in greater quantity and purulence than customary—but much longer periods are required if the infection is well established. Continuous treatment with antimicrobials on "prophylactic" schedules such as 1 week per month has not been shown to be beneficial and promotes the development of resistant organisms. Antibiotics should be administered either orally or by injection, *not* by nebulization (owing to failure of delivery, inactivation of the antibiotic, and risk of sensitization).

Adjuvant medical measures are useful in diminishing the consequences of bronchiectasis. Postural drainage and physical therapy are recommended for those with thick or tenacious sputum, especially if present in large amounts. Bronchodilators are indicated in patients with documentable bronchospasm. Expectorants and humidifiers are of questionable value. Adequate hydration is probably just as effective as the administration of expectorants. Fiberoptic bronchoscopy is useful in identifying sites of endobronchial disease (Chap. 272) and sources of secretions and hemoptysis and permits removal of secretions by aspiration under direct vision. Repeated bronchoscopies are helpful in the management of the unusual patient with problems of sputum retention. Similarly, bronchial lavage has been tried as a "last resort" in patients with large volumes of inspissated secretions. Oxygen should be given to patients with hypoxia during acute exacerbations; it can be administered outside the hospital to patients who are severely and chronically hypoxic. Inflammation from any cause will aggravate the effects of chronic bronchiectasis; therefore, smoking should be prohibited, exposure to air which is excessively polluted should be avoided, and influenza and pneumococcal vaccines should be administered yearly.

Resectional surgery, once the mainstay of treatment, is used far less often now than previously for two reasons: (1) medical management is very effective in controlling bronchiectasis and preventing disability from it; (2) many patients with bronchiectasis have a generalized disorder that makes their entire tracheobronchial system vulnerable; although their bronchiectasis may appear well localized when evaluated initially, new sites of involvement may appear later. Operation should be considered in patients with localized (i.e., resectable) lesions who do not respond to medical management or who are so disabled by complications that either their livelihood or their emotional life is impaired. Bouts of hemoptysis, especially if massive, and recurrent localized pneumonias are the usual complications that require hospitalization, cause repeated disability, and indicate the need for surgery.

PREVENTION The best approach to bronchiectasis is prevention. Patients with heritable diseases that predispose to bronchiectasis and their families should obtain genetic counseling to minimize the incidence of these disorders. Prompt diagnosis and effective antimicrobial treatment of bacterial infections of the lower respiratory tract constitute the best way of avoiding their potential chronic sequelae. The eradication of measles and pertussis by vaccines should eliminate these diseases as harbingers of bronchiectasis.

Prompt removal of foreign bodies, tumors, and other causes of bronchial obstruction should diminish postobstructive bronchiectasis.

BRONCHOLITHIASIS

The term *broncholith* has two meanings: in a general sense it indicates any calcification that impinges on and distorts the wall of a bronchus; in a restricted sense it refers to a calcified tissue fragment that is loose within the lumen of a bronchus. Intraluminal broncholiths can form in three ways: (1) calcification of aspirated food or tissue that was retained in the airway for a long time, (2) protrusion into the lumen and fragmentation of a calcified bronchial cartilage because of necrosis of the bronchial wall in bronchietasis, and (3) erosion of a contiguous calcified granuloma through the wall. Numerous disorders leave calcified deposits that can be detected by chest roentgenography, but clinically significant broncholithiasis is rare. It is usually a late complication of one of the three common granulomatous infections: tuberculosis, histoplasmosis, and coccidioidomycosis. Of these, histoplasmosis has the greatest tendency to heal with multiple residual calcifications, and coccidioidomycosis has the least; hence broncholithiasis in the United States, especially in the central and eastern regions, is most likely to be related to previous infection with *Histoplasma capsulatum;* in Europe half the cases are caused by tuberculosis.

The clinical consequences of broncholithiasis are related to the movement of stones through the airway wall and their release into the lumen. The process of erosion is often accompanied by paroxysms of cough, intermittent hemoptysis, and bronchopulmonary infection. The overlying inflammatory reaction impairs bronchial clearance and narrows the lumen; these conditions may lead to distal bronchiectasis or, if the obstruction is complete, atelectasis. The hallmark of broncholithiasis is the coughing and expectoration of chalky sediment, sandy (gritty) particles, or stones. Such episodes are usually single but may be multiple.

Broncholithiasis should be suspected in any patient with recurrent cough and hemoptysis whose chest roentgenograms show multiple calcifications in the lung and/or mediastinal lymph nodes. The diagnosis can be established by recovering stones in the sputum, by visualizing broncholiths penetrating the bronchial wall at the time of bronchoscopy, or by establishing that calcified particles have disappeared on serial chest x-ray films. Tomography may be helpful in determining with greater precision than routine roentgenograms the presence and location of calcifications in and around bronchi.

Treatment depends on the magnitude of the symptoms. The disorder is self-limiting once the stone has eroded into the lumen and is coughed up; however, ulceration of the particle may be slow and attended by significant symptoms. Antimicrobial agents are useful in the treatment of associated bacterial infection. Bronchoscopy should be performed and the stone removed if possible. At times, thoracotomy and lung resection are necessary, usually for obstructive complications or massive hemoptysis.

REFERENCES

Bronchiectasis

BASS H et al: Regional structure and function in bronchiectasis: A correlative study using bronchography and ^{133}Xe. Am Rev Resp Dis 97:598, 1968

BROGAN TD et al: Composition of bronchopulmonary secretions from patients with bronchietasis. Thorax 35:624, 1980

CROFTON J: Diagnosis and treatment of bronchiectasis: I. Diagnosis. II. Treatment and prevention. Br Med J 1:721 & 783, 1966

DAVIS AL: Bronchiectasis, in *Pulmonary Diseases and Disorders,* AP Fishman (ed). New York, McGraw-Hill, 1980, chap 111, pp 1209–1219

FIELD CE: Bronchiectasis: Third report on a follow-up study of medical and surgical cases from childhood. Arch Dis Child 44: 551, 1969

STURGESS JM et al: Transposition of ciliary microtubules. Another cause of impaired ciliary motility. N Engl J Med 303:318, 1980

Broncholithiasis

ARRIGONI MG et al: Broncholithiasis. J Thorac Cardiovasc Surg 62:231, 1971

Case Records of the Massachusetts General Hospital (Case 23–1978). N Engl J Med 298:1353, 1978

278
CYSTIC FIBROSIS

HARRY SHWACHMAN

DEFINITION Cystic fibrosis (CF), a condition known in Europe as *mucoviscidosis,* is an autosomal recessive disease characterized by abnormally thick secretions from mucous glands, pancreatic insufficiency in approximately 80 percent of patients, and a three- to fivefold increase in the concentration of sodium and chloride in eccrine sweat in 97 percent of all cases. The main clinical features are related to the dysfunction of the pancreas and to a chronic, diffuse, obstructive, infectious pulmonary process. Although the disease is commonly diagnosed and treated by pediatricians, an increasing number of patients with mild disease survive into adulthood or are initially diagnosed at that time.

ETIOLOGY AND EPIDEMIOLOGY The disease occurs predominantly in Caucasians, with a frequency of 1 in 1600 births in this race. The gene frequency in the Caucasian population is 1 in 20. It is less than one-tenth as common in Negroes. Although both sexes are equally affected, males survive longer than females. In the past, cystic fibrosis was considered a fatal disease of infancy and childhood. As a result of early diagnosis and the detection of mild cases combined with improved medical management, the life expectancy has increased from approximately 2 years in 1948 to 20 years at present.

There is no reliable test to detect the heterozygote, although many studies offer the promise that this might be accomplished in the near future. The pathogenesis of this disease remains obscure, and there is a considerable body of conflicting reports in the literature. Many investigators believe that there is a "CF factor" in the form of an abnormal alpha$_2$ macroglobulin complex in serum which characterizes the disease. The absence of an isoenzyme of arginine esterase has been detected. Some investigators believe that the transport of electrolytes is abnormal and that the defect in the sweat glands is due to a substance that inhibits sodium transport within the lumen of the duct. The chemical composition of the mucus secreted by the various glands may reveal minor differences from the normal in that the ratio of fucose to sialic acid differs. One group of investigators suspects this to be a disorder of lysosomes, in spite of the fact that there is no appreciable accumulation of a metabolite within the cell. Studies utilizing cultured skin fibroblasts have yielded a great deal of information about differences in the biological behavior when compared with control cultures. There is considerable controversy concerning many of the metabolic aspects of this disease.

AGE OF DIAGNOSIS In our clinic approximately 85 percent of cases are diagnosed under 15 years of age. In a series of 75 patients who exceeded 25 years of age, 12 were observed in whom the diagnosis was established beyond 20 years of age. The author has recently seen two healthy, well-nourished 39-year-old men, married 14 and 15 years. They were referred because of sterility and both were found to have cystic fibrosis. They showed minimal alterations in pulmonary function tests and work full time. They have a negative family history. One patient had a history of pneumonia on two occasions with a cholecystectomy and gravel in the gallbladder and the other a history of duodenal ulcer with no other gastrointestinal complaints. These are most unusual patients because they enjoyed a normal childhood and adolescence and were detected late in life because of sterility. These cases illustrate the marked variation in the clinical manifestations of the disease.

CLINICAL MANIFESTATIONS Cystic fibrosis has diverse clinical manifestations (Table 278-1). The initial manifestation occurs in the newborn in the form of intestinal obstruction or meconium ileus, which occurs in approximately 10 percent of all cases of cystic fibrosis. When the intestinal obstruction is uncomplicated, the sticky meconium can be displaced by carefully administered meglumine diatrizoate (Gastrografin) enemas. In the presence of complications such as volvulus, secondary atresia, or perforation, surgical correction is necessary. With rare exceptions survivors develop the typical clinical manifestations of the disease. However, the mortality rate for infants with meconium ileus is high and varies from 20 to 60 percent. In the CF clinic at the Boston Children's Hospital eight patients who had surgery for meconium ileus at birth survived beyond 30 years of age. The meconium in cystic fibrosis has a high content of albumin and an increase in activity of lactase. These characteristics are used as signals in screening for cystic fibrosis in the neonate. The meconium from babies with CF is highly viscous. These characteristics of meconium are being used in screening babies for CF. There is no universally accepted screening test at present.

The early clinical findings include a rapid respiratory rate and a faint, hacking cough. The cough often becomes persistent and may induce vomiting. At times the cough is paroxysmal and resembles pertussis. Failure to gain weight and the passage of large, frequent bowel movements accompanied by an excessive appetite are characteristic features in early life. Many gastrointestinal complications, including rectal prolapse, steatorrhea and creatorrhea, pot belly, hypoproteinemia, anemia and hypoprothrombinemia, growth retardation, and other features secondary to malabsorption can be avoided by early recognition of the disease and administration of appropriate therapy (see below).

Although the lungs are normal at birth, the pulmonary lesions may be progressive. The earliest defects include infection and the elaboration of a thick mucus which results in either complete or partial obstruction of the bronchioles. Although infection supervenes, fever is rarely present. Patchy atelectasis, irregular aeration, and air trapping are seen as the earliest changes in the chest x-ray. The infection persists and the initial bacterial flora, which usualy includes *Staphylococcus aureus*, is later replaced by gram-negative bacteria. *Pseudomonas aeruginosa* becomes the predominant inhabitant, and the rough strain may soon be accompanied or replaced by a mucoid strain. Thus *P. aeruginosa* and staphylococci, usually coagulase-positive, are the predominant microorganisms isolated

TABLE 278-1
Principal clinical manifestations of cystic fibrosis

- *I* Viscid secretions—small duct obstruction
  - *A* Respiratory
    - *1* Atelectasis
    - *2* Emphysema
    - *3* Bronchitis, bronchopneumonia, bronchiectasis, lung abscesses, aspergillosis
    - *4* Sinusitis, nasal polyposis
    - *5* Hemoptysis, mild to massive
    - *6* Pneumothorax
    - *7* Pulmonary hyptertension
    - *8* Cor pulmonale
    - *9* Respiratory failure
- *II* Intestinal
  - *A* Delayed passage of meconium at birth
    - *1* Meconium ileus
    - *2* Volvulus
    - *3* Peritonitis
    - *4* Ileal atresia
    - *5* Rectal prolapse
    - *6* Secondary intussusception
    - *7* Obstruction due to fecal impaction
    - *8* Pneumatosis intestinales
  - *B* Pancreas
    - *1* Nutritional and growth failure due to pancreatic insufficiency
    - *2* Steatorrhea and creatorrhea
    - *3* Diabetes mellitus
    - *4* Vitamin deficiencies; vitamins A, D, E, and K
    - *5* Pancreatic calcification (rare)
- *III* Hepatobiliary
  - *A* Mucous hypersecretion
  - *B* Atrophic gallbladder, cholelithiasis
  - *C* Loss of bile salts
  - *D* Focal biliary cirrhosis
  - *E* Laennec's cirrhosis
  - *F* Bile plugging of ductules
  - *G* Hepar lobatum
  - *H* Portal hypertension
  - *I* Esophageal varices
  - *J* Hypersplenism
- *IV* Reproductive system
  - *A* Males: sterility; absent or defective vas deferens, epididymis, and seminal vesicles in about 99 percent of males
  - *B* Females: decreased fertility; increased viscosity of vaginal secretions
- *V* Skeletal
  - *A* Retardation of bone age
  - *B* Demineralization
  - *C* Hypertrophic osteoarthropathy
- *VI* Other
  - *A* Nasal polyposis, recurrent
  - *B* Sinusitis, generalized
  - *C* Salt depletion
  - *D* Heat stroke
  - *E* Salivary gland hypertrophy
  - *F* Retinal hemorrhage
  - *G* Hypertrophy of apocrine glands
  - *H* Iatrogenic complications

SOURCE: *After H Shwachman, RJ Grand, Gastrointestinal Disease, M Sleisenger, J Fordtran (eds). Philadelphia, Saunders, 1978.*

from the lungs at postmortem. Other pathogens such as *Escherichia coli, Proteus,* and *Aspergillus* may also occur. The mucoid strain of *P. aeruginosa* is rarely encountered in other disease states and has been considered pathognomonic of cystic fibrosis pulmonary infection.

The pulmonary complications include pneumonia, bronchiectasis, atelectasis, abscesses of varying sizes, empyema, pneumothorax, and hemoptysis. The immune response appears intact and septicemia is rare, even in the presence of extensive pulmonary infection.

With longer survival of patients with cystic fibrosis new complications have been observed. The clinical challenges of dealing with these patients consist in recognizing and treating these complications. Either a viral or a bacterial infection or some environmental condition may set off the process which leads to an exacerbation of the pulmonary manifestations. There may be no increase in susceptibility to infection, but once the infection becomes established, it is apt to become more severe and prolonged. Death in cystic fibrosis is primarily due to the extensive pulmonary infection which leads to respiratory failure. Cor pulmonale is a common late complication. Pulmonary function tests combined with a clinical evaluation and chest roentgenogram provide an indication of the severity of the disease.

Although the liver reveals changes in approximately 10 percent of cases, it seldom accounts for jaundice in the neonatal period. The earliest change is a focal biliary cirrhosis; bile plugging and proliferation of the bile ductules are pathognomonic. Fatty infiltration may occur. The lesion may progress to a multilobular cirrhosis. Portal hypertension occurs in approximately 5 percent of patients, and this may be followed by hypersplenism. Most of these patients have pancreatic insufficiency. Portal hypertension has not been seen in the 20 percent of the CF population with persistent pancreatic function. Rarely, patients may present with portal hypertension as the initial complaint.

The male genital tract is of special importance in CF since the great majority of adult males with CF (approximately 99 percent) are sterile, owing to structural defects in the Wolffian duct derivatives, the vas deferens, the seminal vesicles, and the epididymis. However, sexual function and secondary sex characteristics are normal. The female may be unable to become pregnant because of the increased viscosity of cervical mucus or the presence of a mucus cervical plug. The fertility rate is approximately one-fifth that of healthy women of the same age group. However, births to well over 120 women with CF have been recorded in the United States. The chances of having a baby with CF in mothers with CF are 1 in 40, and three such cases have been observed. The vast majority of the babies born to mothers who have cystic fibrosis have had normal sweat tests and are healthy, they are obligate heterozygotes.

A small group of patients have an incomplete expression of the disease. The major features are the typical pulmonary lesion, normal or borderline sweat electrolytes, sterility in the adult male, and minimal or no pancreatic disease.

DIAGNOSIS Clinical suspicion must be high to suggest this disease. A positive family history is helpful, but the most accurate diagnostic test for CF is the sweat test, which should be performed in a laboratory known for its accuracy. The level of sweat electrolytes does not reflect the severity of the disease, although a number of cases with borderline sweat electrolytes have mild disease. A variety of sweat tests is available, but unfortunately many results are not reliable because of inaccuracy, lack of experience, or unstandardized procedures and equipment. The recommended procedure is the quantitative pilocarpine iontophoresis method, in which sweat from the forearm (stimulated by pilocarpine iontophoresis) is absorbed into a weighed gauze pad and eluted, and the Na and Cl concentrations are determined. This procedure requires approximately 40 min. The least amount of sweat for analysis should be 50 mg. Patients with CF should yield values of at least 65 meq per liter for both Na and Cl. A positive sweat test does not establish a diagnosis but will confirm the diagnosis in a patient with the clinical features of the disease. Thus, the diagnosis of CF cannot be made in the presence of elevated sweat electrolytes in a patient who is asymptomatic and has a clear chest x-ray.

The sweat test must be standardized, since one can achieve high electrolyte values by a variety of stimuli including exercise or exposure to heat or any method that produces a rapid sweat rate. Although the values for healthy adults are greater than those for healthy children, the quantitative pilocarpine procedure will identify the adult with CF. A number of procedures have been used, including the chloride ion electrode and conductivity methods. In expert hands these methods are valid and reproducible, but in the hands of the average technician, erratic results are very common. In view of the profound medical and personal implications of the diagnosis of CF, it should be made only with a great deal of circumspection, and a second sweat test is recommended for confirmation.

THERAPY Since the disease varies greatly from mild to severe, treatment must be individualized. The management of pancreatic insufficiency includes the use of a potent pancreatic preparation with each meal, such as pancreatin (Viokase) or pancrelipase (Cotazym) or pancrease, the reduction of fat in the diet, the liberal use of multivitamins, and a high caloric intake (Chap. 325). The use of added salt should be considered in hot weather or with fever, or whenever sweating is excessive. This will prevent heat exhaustion and salt depletion. In those patients with adequate pancreatic function no dietary restriction is necessary. Chronic recurrent pancreatitis has been noted in patients with some pancreatic function.

The management of the pulmonary disease includes postural drainage, an exercise program, and the use of antibiotics either singly or in combination to combat the pulmonary infection. Aerosols are also advocated in patients with early bronchiectasis; these include *N*-acetylcysteine (Mucomyst), neomycin or colistin, and isoproterenol (Isuprel). Bronchodilators may be used if there is evidence of bronchospasm.

Attention must be paid to the social, emotional, and financial aspects; assistance through various agencies may be necessary. The cooperation of social workers, nutritionists, physical therapists, and nurses is important in the continuing care of these patients. Constant encouragement and education are essential. Hb A_1C should be followed routinely in patients with CF since diabetes mellitus occurs in nearly 10 percent of patients.

REFERENCES

INGRAM RH JR, MCFADDEN ER: Pulmonary performance in cystic fibrosis, in *Pulmonary Diseases and Disorders,* AP Fishman (ed). New York, McGraw-Hill, 1980, pp 614–620

MANGOS JA: Cystic fibrosis, in *Physiology of Membrane Disorders,* TE Andreoli et al (eds). New York, Plenum, 1978, chap 46, pp 941–953

MARK EJ, SHWACHMAN H: Progressive repsiratory failure in a 46-year-old man with a positive sweat test. N Engl J Med 296:1519, 1977

MATHEWS LW ET AL: Cystic fibrosis, in *Pulmonary Diseases and Disorders,* AP Fishman (ed). New York, McGraw-Hill, 1980, pp 600–613

NADLER HL ET AL: Cystic fibrosis, in *The Metabolic Basis of Inherited Disease,* 4th ed, JB Stanbury et al (eds). New York, McGraw-Hill, 1978, p 1683

SHWACHMAN H et al: Cystic fibrosis: A new outlook. 70 patients above 25 years of age. Medicine 56:129, 1977

———: Cystic fibrosis, in *Current Problems in Pediatrics,* L Gluck (ed). Chicago, Year Book, August, 1978, vol 8, pp 1–72

Diffuse lung disease

279
CHRONIC BRONCHITIS, EMPHYSEMA, AND AIRWAYS OBSTRUCTION

ROLAND H. INGRAM, JR.

Chronic bronchitis and emphysema are two distinct processes, often present in combination in patients with chronic airways obstruction. The diagnosis of chronic bronchitis is made by history, chronic airways obstruction is assessed physiologically, and emphysema can be diagnosed with certainty only by histologic examination of sections of whole lung fixed at inflation. Although the relationships between clinical characteristics, physiologic derangements, and morphologic changes have been diligently studied for many years, reasonably certain and uniform clinical criteria are still not available. Definitions and classifications have evolved, but these are not universally accepted. Nonetheless, the following definitions along with brief qualifications and descriptions are currently used by most persons involved in the diagnosis, treatment, and epidemiology of the chronic obstructive airways syndromes.

DEFINITIONS *Chronic bronchitis* is a condition associated with excessive tracheobronchial mucus production sufficient to cause cough with expectoration for at least 3 months of the year for more than 2 consecutive years. Several subclassifications have been proposed. *Simple chronic bronchitis* describes a condition characterized by mucoid sputum production. *Chronic mucopurulent bronchitis* is characterized by persistent or recurrent purulence of sputum in the absence of localized suppurative diseases such as bronchiectasis. Since there may or may not be obstruction as assessed by the use of the forced expiratory vital capacity maneuver, *chronic bronchitis with obstruction* deserves a separate classification. There is a further subset of patients with chronic bronchitis and obstruction who experience severe dyspnea and wheezing in association with inhaled irritants or during acute respiratory infections. Such patients are said to have *chronic infective asthma* or *chronic asthmatic bronchitis.* Confusion is possible between patients with this condition and those with asthma (Chap. 273) who may also have *chronic airways obstruction.* The patient with chronic asthmatic bronchitis has a long history of cough and sputum production with a later onset of wheezing, whereas the asthmatic with chronic obstruction gives a long history of wheezing with later onset of chronic productive cough.

Emphysema is defined as distention of the air spaces distal to the terminal bronchiole with destruction of alveolar septa. *Chronic obstructive lung disease* is defined as a condition in which there is chronic obstruction to airflow due to chronic bronchitis and/or emphysema (see below). Although the degree of obstruction may be less when the patient is free from respiratory infection and may improve somewhat with bronchodilator drugs, some obstruction is always present.

PREVALENCE Approximately 20 percent of adult males have chronic bronchitis, yet only a minority are clinically disabled. According to all surveys males are more often affected than females. Although cigarette smoking is the single most important etiologic factor, occupational and environmental exposures are now receiving more attention.

Since no criteria have been agreed upon for making the diagnosis of emphysema during life, the incidence data are derived solely from postmortem surveys. It is rare to find adult lungs completely free of emphysema. There is a distinct increase in the extent of emphysema in the fifth decade with further increases through the seventh decade and little increase after that. Approximately two-thirds of adult males and one-fourth of females (most without recognized dysfunction) will have well-defined emphysema, which is often limited in extent. Therefore, the majority of those with emphysema will not have had disability or even symptoms associated with it. The situation is analogous to atherosclerosis in that the morphologic changes are far more frequent than the clinical manifestations attributable to the changes.

PATHOLOGY *Chronic bronchitis* is associated with hyperplasia and hypertrophy of the mucus-producing glands found in the submucosa of large cartilaginous airways. Quantitation of this anatomic change, known as the *Reid index,* is based upon the ratio of the thickness of the submucosal glands to that of the bronchial wall. In persons without a history of chronic bronchitis the mean ratio is 0.44 with a standard deviation ± 0.09, whereas those with such a history have a mean ratio of 0.52 ± 0.08. Although a low index is *rarely* associated with symptoms and a high index is commonly associated with symptoms during life, there is a great deal of overlap. Therefore many persons will have morphologic changes in large airways without having had chronic bronchitis.

Perhaps more important than the abnormalities in large airways are the changes often found in the small noncartilaginous airways. Goblet-cell hyperplasia, mucosal and submucosal inflammatory cells, and edema, peribronchial fibrosis, intraluminal mucus plugs, and increased smooth muscle are characteristic findings in small airways. The frequency of these latter findings in relation to premortem clinical and functional status has not been determined. However, in lungs from patients with chronic obstructive lung disease which have been studied at postmortem, the major site of airflow obstruction has been shown to be in the small airways.

Emphysema is classified according to the pattern of involvement of the gas-exchanging units (acini) of the lung distal to the terminal bronchiole. Although several morphologic patterns have been described, the two most important in the context of this discussion are those involving the respiratory bronchioles and alveolar ducts in the center of the acinus (centriacinar emphysema) and those involving the entire acinus (panacinar emphysema). Quite often both morphologic patterns are present in a single lung of a patient dying from chronic obstructive lung disease, although one type may predominate over the other.

With centriacinar emphysema the distention and destruction are mainly limited to the respiratory bronchiole and alveolar ducts, with relatively less change peripherally in the acinus. Because of the large functional reserve in the lung, many units must be involved in order for overall dysfunction to be detectable. The centrally destroyed regions of the acinus have a high ventilation/perfusion ratio because the capillaries are missing yet ventilation continues. This results in increased wasted ventilation (Vd/Vt), while the peripheral portions of the acinus have crowded and small alveoli with intact, perfused capillaries giving a low ventilation/perfusion ratio. This results in wasted blood flow to give a high alveolar-arterial P_{O_2} difference ($P_{A_{O_2}} - Pa_{O_2}$) (Chap. 271). Mild degrees of centriacinar emphysema, often limited to the lung apices, are extremely common in lungs from persons above age 50 and are practically considered a normal finding.

Panacinar emphysema involves both the central and peripheral portions of the acinus which results, if the process is extensive, in a reduction of the alveolar-capillary gas exchange surface and loss of elastic recoil properties. When emphysema is severe, it may be difficult to distinguish between the two types which most often coexist in the same lung.

CONTRIBUTORY FACTORS **Smoking** Cigarette smoking is the most commonly identified correlate with both chronic bronchitis during life and extent of emphysema at postmortem. Experimental studies have shown that prolonged cigarette smoking impairs ciliary movement, inhibits function of alveolar macrophages, and leads to hypertrophy and hyperplasia of mucus-secreting glands; massive exposure in dogs can produce emphysematous changes. In addition to these chronic effects it is probable that smoke causes polymorphonuclear leukocytes to release proteolytic enzymes acutely. Inhaled cigarette smoke can produce an acute increase in airways resistance due to vagally mediated smooth-muscle constriction, presumably by way of stimulating submucosal irritant receptors. The relationship of such recurrent episodes of acute bronchial constriction to the development and progression of chronic airways obstruction is uncertain. Recent studies, however, indicate that increased airways reactivity is associated with more rapid progression in those with chronic airways obstruction.

It is now well established that some young asymptomatic smokers have considerable obstruction in small airways without there being either an increase of airway resistance or a diminution in the forced expiratory volume in 1 s. Since small airways, because of their large total cross-sectional areas, contribute very little to overall airflow resistance, more sensitive tests must be used to detect mild degrees of small-airways obstruction. Some tests, such as a decrease in compliance and resistance at rapid breathing rates, are based upon nonuniform behavior of the lung which is apparent only at increased frequencies. Obstruction of small airways also results in airways closure at higher lung volumes than in persons of the same age with unobstructed airways (Chap. 271). The measurements of closing volume and frequency dependence of resistance and compliance require special equipment not often available to clinicians. However, the simple spirogram is useful since flow rates at or below the midvital capacity range are often diminished in persons with mild small-airways obstruction. It has been shown that obstruction of small airways is the earliest demonstrable mechanical defect in young cigarette smokers and that the obstruction may disappear after cessation of smoking. It is possible, but has not been established with certainty, that those with small-airways obstruction are at greater risk of developing disabling chronic airways obstruction at some future time.

Not only is cigarette smoking the most common single factor leading to chronic airways obstruction, it also interacts with virtually every other contributory factor to be discussed below.

Air pollution The incidence and mortality rates of both chronic bronchitis and emphysema may be higher in heavily industrialized urban areas. Exacerbations of bronchitis are clearly related to periods of heavy pollution with sulfur dioxide (SO_2) and particulate matter. While nitrogen dioxide (NO_2) can produce small-airways obstruction (bronchiolitis) in experimental animals exposed to high concentrations, there are no data convincingly implicating NO_2, at even the highest pollutant levels, in the pathogenesis or worsening of airways obstruction in humans (Chap. 275).

Occupation Chronic bronchitis is more prevalent in workers who engage in occupations exposing them to either inorganic or organic dusts or to noxious gases. Epidemiologic surveys have succeeded in demonstrating an accelerated decline in lung function in many such workers—e.g., workers in plastics plants exposed to toluene diisocyanate and carding room workers in cotton mills (Chap. 275)—suggesting that their occupational exposure contributes to their future disability.

Infection Morbidity, mortality, and frequency of acute respiratory illnesses are higher in patients with chronic bronchitis. Many attempts have been made to relate these illnesses to infection with viruses, mycoplasmas, and bacteria. However, only the rhinovirus is found more often during exacerbations; that is to say, pathogenic bacteria, mycoplasmas, and viruses other than rhinovirus are found just as often between as during exacerbations. It is intuitively appealing to assign some role to respiratory infections in the pathogenesis and progression of chronic obstructive lung disease, and although this question is under study, there has been no conclusion to date. Recent epidemiologic studies, however, implicate acute respiratory illness as one of the major factors associated with the etiology as well as the progression of chronic airways obstruction. It has been shown that cigarette smokers may either transitorily develop or worsen small-airways obstruction in association with even mild viral respiratory infections. There is also some evidence that severe viral pneumonia early in life may lead to chronic obstruction, predominantly in small airways.

Familial and genetic factors Familial aggregation of chronic bronchitis has been well demonstrated in the past. Recent surveys have shown that children of smoking parents may experience more frequent and severe respiratory illnesses and have a higher prevalence of chronic respiratory symptoms. In addition, nonsmokers who remain in the presence of cigarette smokers have increased blood levels of carbon monoxide which indicates that they are significantly exposed to smoke. Thus a part of the familial aggregation may be related to home air pollution generated by smoking family members. However, some studies of monozygotic twins have suggested some genetic predisposition to the development of chronic bronchitis independent of personal or familial smoking habits. The exact genetic mode of transmission, if it exists at all, is uncertain.

The protease inhibitor alpha$_1$ antitrypsin is an acute-phase reactant, and normally the serum levels rise in association with many inflammatory reactions and with estrogen administration. Either deficient or absent serum levels of alpha$_1$ antitrypsin are found in some patients with the early onset of emphysema. By use of the techniques of acid starch gel and immunoelectrophoresis, genetic typing of the protease inhibitor (Pi) types has been possible. Most of the normal population have two M genes, designated as Pi type MM, and have alpha$_1$ antitrypsin levels in excess of 250 mg/dl serum. Several genes are associated with alterations in levels of serum alpha$_1$ antitrypsin, but the commonest ones associated with emphysema are the Z and S genes. Individuals who are homozygous ZZ or SS have serum levels often near 0 but always less than 50 mg/dl and develop severe panacinar emphysema in the third and fourth decades of life. The panacinar process predominates at the lung bases. Progressive dyspnea with minimal cough characterizes the clinical presentation, although chronic bronchitis is prominent in smokers. The MZ and MS heterozygotes have intermediate levels of serum alpha$_1$ antitrypsin (i.e., between

50 and 250 mg/dl); hence the genetic expression is that of an autosomal codominant allele. It is a matter of some controversy whether the heterozygous state is associated with lung function abnormalities. Published studies are in direct conflict on this point, and further data are needed to be certain. The matter is of some importance, since the heterozygous state is common, with incidence estimates varying between 5 and 14 percent of the general population.

The precise way in which antitrypsin deficiency produces emphysema is unclear. In addition to inhibition of trypsin, $alpha_1$ antitrypsin is an effective inhibitor of elastase and collagenase, as well as several other enzymes. There is experimental evidence that the structural integrity of lung elastin and collagen depends upon this antienzyme which protects the lung from proteases released from leukocytes. It is tempting to speculate that recurrent inflammatory reactions related to infection and pollutants play some role in pathogenesis by calling forth leukocytes whose released proteases are uninhibited and are free to cause the damage.

PATHOPHYSIOLOGY On the basis of the use of flow rates from forced expiratory vital capacity maneuvers and more sophisticated measures of airways resistance and elastic recoil properties of the lung, it has become clear that both chronic bronchitis and emphysema can exist without evidence of obstruction. However, by the time a patient begins to experience dyspnea as a result of these processes, obstruction is always demonstrable. Since chronic bronchitis and emphysema are usually combined, it might appear fruitless to determine the role of each in producing an individual patient's disability. However, one process may dominate over the other, and to the extent that inflammatory airways disease, secretions, and bronchospasm are present, there are therapeutic possibilities with some hope for improvement. Therefore it is of value to understand the mechanisms of airways obstruction in order to guide therapy and anticipate results.

Both chronic bronchitis and emphysema result in airways narrowing. In addition to the primary airways processes of chronic bronchitis, loss of elastic recoil of the lung in emphysema accounts for a decrease in airways caliber through loss of radial traction on airways. Narrowing of airways is often associated with both an increase in airways resistance and a diminution in maximal expiratory flow rates.

There are occasions in which a normal or only slightly elevated airways resistance is accompanied by low maximal expiratory flow rates. Under such circumstances an increase in the dynamic collapsibility of intrathoracic airways during forced exhalation is a possible explanation. Also in this context, the elastic recoil pressure of the lung must be considered in a slightly different way. In addition to providing radial support to airways during quiet breathing, the elastic recoil properties of the lung serve as a major determinant of maximal expiratory flow rates. The static recoil pressure of the lung is the difference between alveolar and intrapleural pressure. During forced exhalations, when alveolar and intrapleural pressures are high, there are points in the airway at which bronchial pressure equals pleural pressure. Flow does not increase with higher pleural pressure after these points become fixed so that the effective driving pressure between alveoli and such points is the elastic recoil pressure of the lung (Fig. 279-1). Hence maximal expiratory flow rates represent a complex and dynamic interplay between airways caliber, elastic recoil pressures, and collapsibility of airways. As a direct consequence of the altered pressure-airflow relationships, the work of breathing is increased in bronchitis and emphysema. Since flow-resistive work is flow rate–dependent, there is a disproportionate increase in the work of breathing with increased ventilation.

The designated subdivisions of the lung volume outlined in Chap. 271 are abnormal to varying degrees in both bronchitis and emphysema. The residual volume (RV) and functional residual capacity (FRC) are almost always higher than normal. Since the normal FRC is the volume at which the inward recoil of the lung is balanced by the outward recoil of the chest wall, loss of elastic recoil of the lung would clearly result in a higher static FRC. In addition, prolongation of expiration in association with obstruction would lead to a dynamic increase in FRC if inspiration is initiated before the respiratory system reaches its static balance point. Elevations of total lung capacity (TLC) are frequent. The exact cause is uncertain, but increases in TLC are often found in association with decreases in the elastic recoil of the lung. The vital capacity is frequently decreased, yet significant airways obstruction can be present with a normal to near-normal vital capacity.

The consequences of the airways and parenchymal processes are far more extensive than just the mechanical alterations discussed above. Maldistribution of inspired gas and blood flow is always present to some extent. When the mismatching is severe, impairment of gas exchange is reflected in abnormalities of arterial blood gases. There are regions of the lung with ventilation in excess of perfusion which increase the wasted ventilation ratio (that is, *Vd/Vt;* Chap. 271). At a nor-

FIGURE 279-1

A. A schematic diagram of the lung and intrathoracic airways with no airflow. The alveolar pressure (Palv) is greater than pleural pressure (Ppl) by an amount equal to the elastic recoil pressure of the lung (Pel)—i.e., Palv is the algebraic sum of Ppl + Pel. With no airflow Palv = P atmospheric, and for all of the intrathoracic airways, pressure outside is less than the pressure inside due to the Pel. B. The same schematic lung during *forced exhalation when pleural pressure becomes quite positive. Palv is still greater than Ppl by an amount equal to Pel. However, there is a pressure drop along the airway associated with flow, and at some point Ppl equals local bronchial pressure (so-called equal pressure point, EPP). Mouthward from this point, Ppl* exceeds *local bronchial pressure and hence acts to compress the airways. C. Pressure within the airways from alveoli to the intrathoracic trachea as a dashed line (---) and Ppl is shown as a constant (———). Therefore, the driving pressure from alveoli to EPP is equal to Pel, and a decrease in Pel (i.e., loss of elastic recoil) would mean a smaller driving pressure and smaller flow rates.*

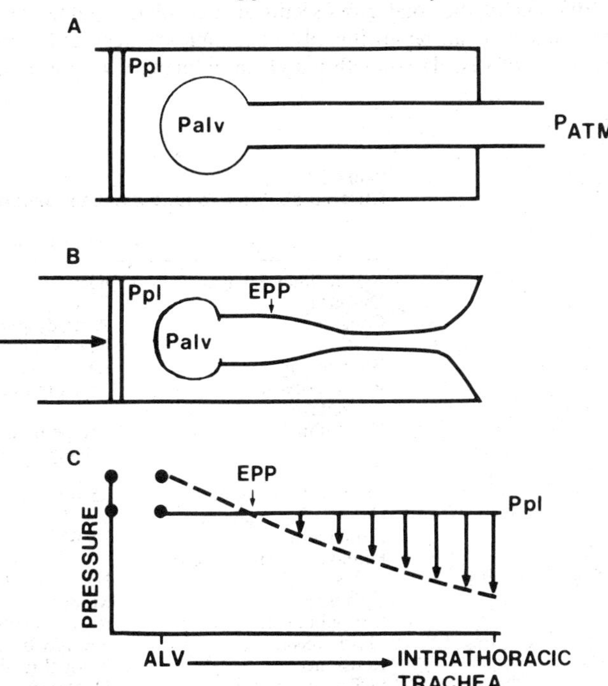

mal resting CO_2 production, the net effective alveolar ventilation, as reflected by the arterial P_{CO_2}, may be excessive, normal, or insufficient depending upon the relationship of the overall minute volume to the wasted ventilation ratio. The net contribution of regions with perfusion in excess of ventilation can be assessed by either estimating or measuring the alveolar-arterial P_{O_2} difference (that is, $P_{A_{O_2}} - Pa_{O_2}$; Chap. 271). Whatever the clinical syndrome associated with chronic bronchitis and emphysema, there are to some degree increases in both wasted ventilation and wasted blood flow.

The clinical manifestations depend, in large part, upon the ventilatory response to the disordered lung function. Some patients, at the cost of extremely high effort of breathing and chronic dyspnea, will maintain a strikingly increased minute volume, which results both in a normal to low arterial P_{CO_2}, despite the high Vd/Vt, and a relatively high arterial P_{O_2}, despite the high difference, $P_{A_{O_2}} - Pa_{O_2}$. Other patients with only modest increases in effort of breathing and less dyspnea will maintain a normal to only moderately elevated minute volume at the cost of accepting a high arterial P_{CO_2} and a severely depressed arterial P_{O_2}.

Factors which account for clear differences in ventilatory responses between patients have been studied and debated for years. The bulk of available evidence suggests that those patients who maintain relatively normal or low arterial P_{CO_2} levels are those with an increased ventilatory drive relative to their blood gas values and those who chronically maintain high arterial P_{CO_2} and lower P_{O_2} levels have a diminished ventilatory drive in relation to their more severely deranged blood gas values. It is not at all certain whether individual differences are accounted for by variations in peripheral or central chemoreceptor sensitivity or through other afferent pathways. Perhaps of more immediate value is the fact that patients with predominant emphysema are either normally or excessively responsive both to hypercapnia and to exercise, whereas those with predominant bronchitis are less responsive to both, despite similar degrees of airways obstruction by spirometry.

The pulmonary circulation malfunctions not only in terms of regional distribution of blood flow but in terms of abnormal overall pressure-flow relationships. There is often mild to severe pulmonary hypertension at rest with further increases disproportionate to cardiac output elevations during exercise. A reduction in the total cross-sectional area of the pulmonary vascular bed can be attributed to anatomic changes and constriction of vascular smooth muscle in pulmonary arteries and arterioles as well as destruction of alveolar septa with loss of capillaries. Rarely does loss of capillaries alone lead to severe pulmonary hypertension with cor pulmonale, except as a terminal event. Of more importance is the constriction of pulmonary vessels in response to alveolar hypoxia. The constriction is reversible upon increase in alveolar P_{O_2} with therapy. There is a synergism between hypoxia and acidosis which assumes importance during episodes of acute or chronic respiratory insufficiency. Chronic hypoxia leads not only to pulmonary vascular constriction but also to secondary erythrocytosis. The latter, although not proved to be a significant contributor to pulmonary hypertension, could add an unfavorable rheologic load. As discussed in Chap. 262, the chronic afterload on the right ventricle leads to hypertrophy and, in association with disordered blood gases, ultimately to failure.

CLINICAL-FUNCTIONAL CORRELATIONS Dyspnea and impairment of physical work capacity are characteristic only of severe to moderately severe airways obstruction. There is considerable variation among patients, and those with predominant emphysema have greater dyspnea and restriction of physical activity with lesser degrees of obstruction than those in whom chronic bronchitis predominates. The majority of patients have functionally mixed disease, will usually experience exertional dyspnea when the forced expiratory volume in 1 s (FEV_1) falls below 50 percent of that predicted, and will have dyspnea at rest when the FEV_1 is less than 25 percent of that predicted. In addition to dyspnea at rest, carbon dioxide retention and cor pulmonale frequently occur when the FEV_1 falls to 25 percent of that predicted. However, those with predominant bronchitis often have carbon dioxide retention and cor pulmonale with FEV_1 values above 25 percent of normal, in contrast to patients with predominant emphysema whose FEV_1 usually falls well below that level before the onset of carbon dioxide retention and cor pulmonale. With a respiratory infection, small changes in the degree of obstruction can make a large difference in symptoms and gas exchange. Thus small therapeutic gains have rewarding results.

In general, the more severe the obstruction, the poorer the prognosis. Despite the general relationship, 20 to 30 percent of patients with severe obstruction and carbon dioxide retention will survive beyond 5 years.

CLINICAL SYNDROMES It is clear that the clinical presentation can vary in severity from simple chronic bronchitis without disability to the severely disabled state with chronic respiratory failure. From a practical standpoint, it is well to

TABLE 279-1
Chronic obstructive lung disease: Salient features of the two types

	Predominant emphysema	*Predominant bronchitis*
Age at time of diagnosis	60±	50±
Dyspnea	Severe	Mild
Cough	After dyspnea starts	Before dyspnea starts
Sputum	Scanty, mucoid	Copious, purulent
Bronchial infections	Less frequent	More frequent
Respiratory insufficiency episodes	Often terminal	Repeated
Chest film	"Hyperinflation" ± bullous changes, small heart	Increased bronchovascular markings at bases, large heart
Chronic Pa_{CO_2}, mmHg	35–40	50–60
Chronic Pa_{O_2}, mmHg	65–75	45–60
Hematocrit, %	35–45	50–55
Pulmonary hypertension:		
Rest	None to mild	Moderate to severe
Exercise	Moderate	Worsens
Cor pulmonale	Rare, except terminally	Common
Elastic recoil	Severely decreased	Normal
Resistance	Normal to slight increase	High
Diffusing capacity	Decreased	Normal to slight decrease

consider that any symptom or any measurable abnormality may foreshadow the development of severe disabling disease; hence cessation of smoking and avoidance of environmental irritants and toxins are to be advised. However, the advice to modify behavior and life patterns is rarely taken, and most physicians are called upon to categorize and treat patients with fully developed, chronic airways obstruction. Thus the approach taken here is to describe two polar opposite types of fully developed, chronic obstructive pulmonary disease with the realization that the majority of patients will have some features of both types. The salient features of each type are outlined in Table 279-1.

Predominant emphysema These patients often give a long history of exertional dyspnea with minimal cough which is productive of only small amounts of mucoid sputum. Mucopurulent exacerbations in association with infections are not frequent. The body build is asthenic with evidence of weight loss. The patient appears distressed with obvious use of accessory muscles of respiration which serve to lift the sternum in an anterosuperior direction with each inspiration. There is tachypnea with a relatively prolonged expiration through pursed lips, or expiration is begun with a grunting sound. While sitting, these patients often lean forward, extending the arms to brace themselves. The neck veins may be distended during expiration, yet they collapse briskly with inspiration. The lower intercostal spaces retract with each inspiration, and by palpation the lower lateral chest wall can be felt to move inward. The percussion note is hyperresonant, and by auscultation the breath sounds are diminished, with faint, high-pitched rhonchi heard toward the end of expiration. The cardiac impulse, if at all visible, is seen only in the xiphoid and subxiphoid regions, and cardiac dullness is either absent or severely reduced. By palpation there is frequently a sustained forward and downward right ventricular impulse in the subxiphoid region, and a presystolic gallop accentuated during inspiration is commonly heard.

The arterial P_{O_2} is often in the mid-70s (mmHg), and the P_{CO_2} is low to normal. Because of the maintained increase in minute volume and the maintenance of arterial P_{O_2} sufficient to nearly saturate hemoglobin, these patients have been referred to as "pink puffers."

The TLC and RV are invariably increased, the vital capacity is low, and the maximal expiratory flow rates are diminished. The elastic recoil properties of the lung are severely impaired, and in direct proportion to this impairment, the capacity of the lung to transfer carbon monoxide is lowered.

On radiographic examination the diaphragms are low and flattened, the bronchovascular shadows do not extend to the periphery of the lung, and the cardiac silhouette is lengthened and narrowed. These findings in association with a large retrosternal translucency on lateral chest radiographs are interpreted as hyperinflation which correlates well with increases in TLC and loss of elastic recoil. Peripheral attenuation of bronchovascular markings and increased retrosternal lucency correlate best with subsequent postmortem demonstration of extensive and severe emphysema which is predominantly of the panacinar type.

It is fortunate that the patient with predominant emphysema is less prone to mucopurulent relapses than is the patient with predominant bronchitis, since such relapses frequently lead to severe respiratory failure and death. That is to say, right-sided heart failure and hypercapnic respiratory failure are often terminal events in those patients with predominant emphysema. In the absence of such relapses, the clinical course is characterized by severe and progressive dyspnea for which little can be done. The physician's role is to seek out and treat any factor that is possibly reversible and strive to avoid pollutants and infections.

Predominant bronchitis The patient with predominant bronchitis usually has an impressive history of cough and sputum production for many years with an immodest history of cigarette smoking. Initially the cough is present only in the winter months, and the patient is apt to seek medical attention, if at all, only during the more severe of the frequent mucopurulent relapses. Over the years the cough progresses from hibernal to perennial, and mucopurulent relapses increase in frequency, duration, and severity. After beginning to experience exertional dyspnea, the patient often seeks medical help and will be found to have a severe degree of obstruction. Occasionally such a patient will seek out a physician only after the onset of peripheral edema secondary to overt right ventricular failure. More rarely the initial medical contact is made by family members who present the physician with a deeply cyanotic, edematous, and stuporous patient with acute respiratory insufficiency.

The patient with predominant bronchitis is often overweight and cyanotic. There is usually no apparent distress at rest, the respiratory rate is normal or only slightly increased, and there is no apparent usage of accessory muscles. The chest percussion note is normally resonant, and by auscultation, one can usually hear coarse rhonchi and wheezes which change in location and intensity after a deep and productive cough. There may be a sustained heave along the lower left sternal border which indicates right ventricular hypertrophy. In the presence of right ventricular failure there are often an early diastolic gallop and occasionally a holosystolic murmur, both of which are accentuated by inspiration. The latter finding is indicative of functional tricuspid regurgitation which is frequently accompanied by neck vein distention characterized by large *v* waves and brisk *y* descents. With right ventricular failure the cyanosis deepens and peripheral edema becomes prominent. Clubbing of the digits is unusual.

With or without right ventricular failure, the minute volume is only slightly increased. Failure to increase minute volume greatly in the face of significant proportions of wasted ventilation and blood flow results in severely deranged arterial blood gases, with arterial P_{CO_2} values which are chronically increased to the range of the high 40s to low 50s (mmHg). The lowered P_{O_2} produces desaturation of hemoglobin, serves to stimulate erythropoiesis, and results in hypoxic pulmonary vasoconstriction. Desaturation and erythrocytosis combine to produce the cyanosis, and hypoxic pulmonary vasoconstriction accentuates the right-sided heart failure. Because of cyanosis and edema secondary to heart failure, such patients have been referred to as "blue bloaters." It has been proposed, with some supporting data, that one of the pathophysiologic events in the blue bloaters is the occurrence of repeated episodes of severe nocturnal oxygen desaturation in association with sleep apnea.

The TLC is often normal, and there is a moderate elevation of RV. The vital capacity is mildly diminished, and maximal expiratory flow rates are invariably low. The elastic recoil properties of the lung are normal or only slightly impaired, and the capacity of the lung to transfer carbon monoxide is either normal or minimally decreased.

On radiographic examination the diaphragms are well rounded, the bronchovascular markings are increased in the lower lung fields, and the cardiac silhouette is somewhat enlarged. In association with right ventricular failure the cardiac silhouette enlarges further, pulmonary arteries become more prominent, and an antigravity distribution of perfusion is apparent.

Despite well-planned management (see below) the patient with predominant bronchitis may experience many episodes of respiratory failure from which recovery is frequent with proper therapy (see Chap. 287). The ability to recover from such repeated episodes in those patients is in striking contrast to the frequently fatal outcome of such events in those with predominant emphysema. Ultimately, the lungs at postmortem will be found to have severe bronchitic changes in both large and small airways and only moderate emphysema, predominantly of the centriacinar variety.

PRINCIPLES OF MANAGEMENT Intelligent management must be based upon as complete knowledge as possible of the degree of obstruction, the extent of disability, and the relative reversibility of the patient's illness. To the extent that obstructive processes in the airways are contributory, there is a chance for treatment to be effective. Since emphysema is an irreversible process, prevention of progression and avoidance of acute insults constitute the only approach. History, physical examination, and chest radiographs should be supplemented by tests of lung function performed during a symptomatically stable period. Ideally, complete spirometry, plethysmographic lung volumes, airways resistance, transfer of carbon monoxide, arterial blood gases, and lung elastic recoil properties should be measured. Spirometry, lung volumes, and resistance should be remeasured after the administration of bronchodilators in order to assess the degree of acutely reversible airways obstruction. Failure to see an acute change with bronchodilator drugs does not rule out the possibility of improvement with more prolonged administration of these agents. In instances in which the degree of exertional dyspnea appears to be disproportionately greater than the degree of obstruction, measurements of blood gases, minute volume, CO_2 production, and O_2 consumption during exercise are indicated in order to determine whether impaired lung function is sufficient to account for the symptoms. After the initial assessment the physician has some idea of the relative emphasis to be placed upon patient education, preventive measures, and direct therapeutic interventions in management of the patient and the illness.

Cessation of smoking is the only certain means of influencing the progression of the chronic obstructive airways syndromes, and such behavior modification is most effective at early stages of the disease processes. In the instances in which occupational or environmental exposures are thought to play a significant role, change of occupation or relocation of dwelling is advisable. The validity of such advice should be carefully considered since the impact on both the patient and the family is likely to be great. A simpler environmental change is that of eliminating aerosol sprays such as deodorants, hair sprays, and insecticides from the household. Hair sprays have been shown to produce acute airways responses even in normal subjects. Other preventive measures include yearly vaccination against the common or expected influenza virus strains, and every third to fourth year, the patient should be given pneumococcal polysaccharide vaccine.

Infections cannot be totally avoided, and the patient should be made aware that increasing purulence, viscosity, or volume of secretions signals the onset of an infection which should be treated early. The commonest pathogenic bacteria found are *Hemophilus influenzae* and *Streptococcus pneumoniae.* As mentioned above, however, the role of such bacteria is in question since they are just as often isolated during periods of relative clinical quiescence. Nonetheless, tetracycline or ampicillin should be given for a 7- to 10-day course. It is practical to have the patient keep a 7- to 10-day supply of antibiotics at home and to begin treatment at the onset of symptoms. In Great Britain it is common practice to give continuous antibiotic therapy during winter months in order to prevent mucopurulent relapses. Although there is evidence that viruses are frequent causes of mucopurulent relapses, clinical studies have shown that the standard antibiotic regimens decrease the duration and severity of infective episodes unrelated to culturable bacterial pathogens. Microscopic examination and culture of sputum are indicated if there are chills, fever, or chest pain or if purulence fails to respond to usually administered antibiotics.

It has been shown repeatedly that exercise programs, although not accompanied by measurable improvement in lung function, result in increased exercise tolerance and an improved sense of well-being. The improvement is usually task-specific, so that most physicians advise walking in preference to the use of special apparatus, such as stationary bicycles or wall gyms.

Bronchodilator drugs are often quite helpful in alleviating symptoms, especially in those patients who respond to them acutely in the laboratory. These drugs form three categories: the methylxanthines, sympathomimetics with strong beta-adrenergic-stimulating properties, and anticholinergics. Theophylline, the most commonly used methylxanthine, can be given orally, rectally, or parenterally; in addition to bronchodilatation, it stimulates respiration and has cardiotonic and diuretic properties. The most commonly used beta-adrenergic agent, isoproterenol, is given mainly as an aerosol. More selective $beta_2$-stimulating drugs have recently been developed, and these can be given both orally and by aerosol with fewer cardiac side effects. Anticholinergic agents such as atropine have been avoided in the past because of their tendency to desiccate secretions, but such drugs are effective bronchodilators; new analogues that are given by inhalation with less effect on secretions are now being developed and tested and may be found useful in the future.

The use of glucocorticosteroids is, at our present state of knowledge, based upon very little scientific data from properly controlled clinical trials. Since these agents have time- and dose-related side effects that vary from deleterious to catastrophic, the almost invariable subjective benefit must be supported by objective measurements. There is little room for doubt in the minds of physicians that some patients respond well, even dramatically, to these agents in both objective and subjective terms. The real problem is how to select those most likely to benefit. Eosinophilia in the sputum, rather than in the blood, appears to help identify that subgroup in advance. However, the best guidelines are, first, to try these agents only after maximal bronchodilator and bronchopulmonary drainage measures have been tried without success; second, to begin prednisone 30 mg once per day; third, to confirm the objective change in terms of spirometry and gas exchange, stopping these agents if no objective benefit is seen; and fourth, to decrease to the smallest dose that will maintain the improved level of function.

Bronchopulmonary drainage should be maintained in patients with hypersecretion. If the coughing mechanism is either ineffective or if paroxysms of coughing are exhausting, postural drainage is often a useful adjunct. Although liquefaction of secretions by means of orally administered expectorants or aerosol delivery of mucolytic agents is an appealing idea, it has never been shown by properly designed trials to be more effective than simple maintenance of total-body hydration.

Intermittent positive pressure breathing (IPPB) devices have long been advocated for home management. The various rationales include diminution in the work of breathing, promotion of bronchopulmonary drainage, and more efficient delivery of bronchodilator drugs. The first of the rationales has been shown to have no basis in fact, and the goals of the last two have been shown to be as well accomplished by postural drainage and use of less elaborate aerosol generators. Hence the use of IPPB for home management cannot be justified.

When arterial hypoxia is persistent and severe (Pa_{O_2} <55 mmHg) in association with cor pulmonale (see Chap. 262) and signs of right heart failure, portable oxygen therapy is indicated. The available data indicate that supplemental oxygen improves both exercise tolerance and neuropsychological function and alleviates pulmonary hypertension and right heart failure. Although there are not sufficient data, those to date suggest that the need for hospitalization occurs less frequently and life span is lengthened by the use of supplemental oxygen. In view of the expense of such therapy and the dangers of uncontrolled oxygen delivery (see below), it should be given only when it can be carefully monitored and its beneficial effects objectively verified.

Since most patients with chronic airways obstruction, especially those with features of predominant bronchitis, can be shown to decrease their Pa_{O_2} values significantly during sleep, most prominently during the REM phase, nocturnal oxygen administration has been suggested. While the rationale is clear and the results quite good, a recent cooperative clinical trial that compared nocturnal with continuous O_2 supplementation in severly hypoxic patients found that continuous O_2 administration was associated with a significantly lower mortality rate. Patients in both treatment groups experienced neuropsychological and hemodynamic benefits. Thus, supplemental nocturnal oxygen is better than none, but continuous oxygen is better than nocturnal in such severely ill patients.

Secondary erythrocytosis with the hematocrit in excess of 50 percent is most easily viewed as a mechanism allowing greater oxygen delivery to compensate for the chronically lowered arterial P_{O_2}; hence improvement in oxygenation through improved lung function or by oxygen administration is the most physiologic means to reverse erythrocytosis. Since erthrocytosis results in elevation of blood viscosity at all shear rates, the proposal has been made that pulmonary vascular hypertension is aggravated by its presence. However, no study has demonstrated an objective improvement in hemodynamics, lung mechanics, or gas exchange following phlebotomy. Nonetheless, some patients who complain of headaches and a sense of head fullness show a favorable subjective response to periodic phlebotomy when the hematocrit is in excess of 55 percent. In support of this subjective improvement is the demonstration that, following phlebotomy, cerebral blood flow, previously diminished, returns toward normal.

ACUTE RESPIRATORY FAILURE

DIAGNOSIS Although it may be strongly suspected on clinical grounds, the firm diagnosis of acute respiratory failure in chronic airways obstruction is based upon measurements of arterial blood gas (Pa_{O_2}, Pa_{CO_2}) and pH values that must be interpreted in relation to the patient's chronic status. Since many patients will have chronically lowered Pa_{O_2} levels and increased Pa_{CO_2} values, the diagnosis is based upon the degree of change from the usual state of the individual patient. With regard to oxygenation, an acute decrease in Pa_{O_2} from a usual mid-70 mmHg range to the low 60s (mmHg) is just as indicative of acute respiratory failure as is an acute drop from a chronic mid-50 mmHg range to the mid-40s (mmHg). Thus a drop in Pa_{O_2} equal to or greater than 10 to 15 mmHg indicates acute failure.

Since renal compensation for chronic hypercapnia results in adjustment of arterial pH to near-normal values, the acuteness of the increase in Pa_{CO_2} can often be judged by the pH, unless there is a concomitant metabolic acidemia. As a practical guide, any level of hypercapnia associated with an arterial pH value less than 7.30 should be considered as acute respiratory failure.

PRECIPITATING FACTORS Increases in volume, viscosity, and/or purulence of secretions, presumably due to infection of the tracheobronchial tree, are the most common antecedents of acute respiratory failure in chronic obstructive lung disease. Increasing airways obstruction with airways inflammation and secretion, especially in association with a relatively blunted ventilatory drive, leads to worsening hypoxia and increasing CO_2 retention. Agitation, insomnia, and increasing dyspnea with impending respiratory failure are occasionally treated, mistakenly, with either sedatives or narcotics, and these, too, may precipitate frank respiratory failure. In fact such depressant drugs which impair ventilatory drive should be avoided at all times in patients with severe chronic obstructive lung disease. Major episodes of air pollution can also lead to respiratory failure, and the physicians responsible for patients with severe bronchitis and emphysema should be alert to these environmental events.

Pneumonia, thromboembolism, left ventricular failure, and pneumothorax occasionally precipitate acute respiratory failure and are extremely difficult to detect unless considered and specifically sought. As a minimum, chest radiographs, electrocardiograms, and sputum examinations should be obtained in addition to arterial blood gas measurements in all patients with respiratory failure.

TREATMENT OF RESPIRATORY FAILURE The treatment of respiratory failure consists of two simultaneous processes: (1) maintaining acceptable levels of oxygenation and ventilation; and (2) treatment of infection, removal of secretions, and reversing any airway constriction present.

With regard to the first, these patients *need* oxygen when they are severely hypoxic, and while fears of respiratory depression due to the removal of the hypoxic respiratory stimulus are realistic, O_2 must be used, yet in the smallest concentration possible to give a Pa_{O_2} in the mid-50 mmHg range while the patient's Pa_{CO_2}, pH, and clinical status are carefully monitored. It is best to begin with only modest increases in FI_{O_2} to approximately 0.24 (cf. air at 0.21), which can be accomplished using nasal prongs with O_2 flows at 1 to 2 liters per minute or, more precisely, with the use of a 0.24 Venturi mask. These latter masks, based upon Bernoulli's principle, deliver a fixed concentration of O_2 irrespective of the O_2 flow rate by entraining air in direct proportion to O_2 flow rate. They are high-flow masks (oxygen plus air entrained from the room), each designed for a specific FI_{O_2} (0.24, 0.28, 0.35, 0.40). Even small increases in Pa_{O_2} when starting from low levels result in significant increases in arterial oxygen content due to the shape of the oxygen-hemoglobin saturation curve over this range (Chap. 54). With improved oxygenation some patients will concomitantly increase their Pa_{CO_2} values. The standard explanation has been that this increase is due to the removal of the hypoxic drive to ventilation leading to further hypoventilation. While this is the most important mechanism, recent data indicate that worsening ventilation-perfusion relationships (Chap. 271) occur with O_2 treatment. This is attributed to reversal of hypoxic pulmonary arterial constriction in the more initially hypoxic, less well ventilated regions, which in turn leads to decreased perfusion of initially less hypoxic, better ventilated regions. The result is an increase in the wasted ventilation ratio (Vd/Vt,

Chap. 271) leading to a smaller effective alveolar ventilation. In either case, the $F_{I_{O_2}}$ should be increased as little as possible to achieve a Pa_{O_2} in the mid-50 mmHg range. Some increase in Pa_{CO_2} can be expected and should not cause alarm if the patient is alert. The majority of patients can be managed in this conservative way with excellent results. However, occasionally large increases in Pa_{CO_2} occur and lead to stupor and coma. This can be explained by CO_2-induced cerebral vascular dilatation with increased intracranial pressure, including the development of papilledema, combined with the effect of hypercapnia and hypoxia on cerebral function. It must be emphasized that if stupor and coma supervene, stopping the administration of oxygen is the *worst possible* course of action. When CO_2 narcosis is present, respirations are sufficiently depressed from the CO_2 itself so that the patient will no longer respond to the rapidly worsening hypoxia, and fatal arrhythmias, generalized seizures, and death may ensue. The only alternative is to intubate the trachea and provide mechanical ventilatory support. Mechanical ventilators are described in Chap. 287.

Once mechanical ventilation has been instituted, the tidal volume and frequency should be set gradually to decrease the Pa_{CO_2} only down to the chronically elevated level rather than attempt to decrease it to or below a normal value. Since such patients have renal compensation for their chronic hypercapnia, Pa_{CO_2} values at or below the normal level result in significant alkalemia which in turn can lead to severe tachyarrhythmias and generalized seizures.

As mentioned above, maintaining oxygenation and ventilation serves to buy time while secretion removal, bronchial dilatation, and treatment of infection are instituted. Removal of secretions is accomplished by urging the patient to cough or by passing suction catheters into the trachea which, in addition to removing secretions that are present, stimulate cough that brings more secretions up to the region of the catheter tip. The advantage, if any, from the use of mucolytic agents in this process has yet to be demonstrated. However, beta-adrenergic bronchodilating agents have been shown to increase the rate of transport of particles by the mucociliary blanket, and, thus, in addition to bronchodilatation, such agents should improve the clearance of airway secretions. Postural drainage and chest percussion are other often used adjuncts that have been shown, especially when secretions are voluminous, to improve tracheobronchial clearance, to increase sputum volume beyond that produced by cough, and to reduce airways obstruction.

Bronchodilatation with aminophyllin given orally or by infusion and beta-adrenergic agonists by inhalation or subcutaneous injection has assumed a prominent role in treatment of acute respiratory failure in chronic airways obstruction. In addition to bronchodilatation these agents improve bronchopulmonary clearance and may help induce diuresis and hemodynamic improvement when there is cor pulmonale with failure (Chap. 262). Unless there is clearly an acute pneumonia, the use of antibiotics is more controversial in the setting of acute respiratory failure than in mucopurulent relapses without failure. Nonetheless, broad-spectrum antibiotics, if no single agent is suspected or isolated, or erythromycin, if legionellae or mycoplasma are suspected, should be added to the regimen.

Complications arising in the course of treatment for acute respiratory failure are cardiac arrhythmias, most often multifocal supraventricular tachycardias, left ventricular failure, pulmonary emboli, and gastrointestinal hemorrhage from stress ulceration. Cardiac arrhythmias resulting from rapid decreases in oxygenation or increases in pH due to overventilation can be readily avoided. However, when giving multiple drugs having cardiotonic properties, the question always arises as to whether the arrhythmias are related to these. Keeping serum theophylline levels in the 10 to 20 mg/per liter range and using relatively selective beta agonists, such as isoetharine by inhalation, can minimize these effects.

Left ventricular failure, usually attributable to coronary atherosclerosis with acute myocardial infarction, systemic hypertension, or aortic valvular disease, is difficult to detect in the presence of cor pulmonale. Fortunately, improving lung function and oxygenation most often reverse the pulmonary hypertension and right ventricular failure (Chap. 262) and induce a brisk diuresis. If signs of congestive failure persist or worsen after providing adequate oxygenation, consideration must be given to left ventricular failure; an assessment in such patients is best made through echocardiography or radioventriculography since the usual physical and radiographic findings are obscured in such patients. Only in the presence of adequate gas exchange and only with either the firm demonstration of, or strong clinical suspicion of, left ventricular failure should digitalis be used. Diuretic agents should also be reserved for left ventricular failure. They almost invariably produce hypokalemic, hypochloremic metabolic alkalemia that results in depression of ventilatory drive and interference with removal from mechanical ventilatory support.

Pulmonary emboli are suspected to be common in the setting of acute respiratory failure and are extremely difficult to detect since the lung scan is totally nonspecific and signs of cor pulmonale fluctuate in concert with the degree of lung dysfunction. Hence low-dose heparin prophylaxis should be used to prevent this complication. Gastrointestinal hemorrhage commonly complicates acute respiratory failure and is thought to be due to stress ulceration of the gastric mucosa. Awareness of this complication enhances the ability to detect it and act quickly. Antacids, nasogastric suction, and/or cimetidine have been used to diminish the frequency.

For those patients who have required mechanical ventilatory support, the process of removal from that support is largely empirical. In general, improving gas exchange and lung mechanics along with alertness and responsiveness of the patient signal that the support can be removed. Data such as maximal voluntary inspiratory mouth pressures greater than 20 cmH_2O, vital capacity greater than 10 ml per kilogram of body weight, and spontaneous tidal volume greater than 5 ml per kilogram of body weight are reassuring. However, many patients can be removed from such support with lesser values than these.

Failure to maintain gas exchange after removal of mechanical ventilatory support can usually be explained. *First* on the list is the continued administration or persistence of sedative and tranquilizing drugs that may have been prescribed earlier for agitation. These should be discontinued and time allowed for their metabolism. *Second* is the possibility that the endotracheal tube is of small bore and imposes a resistive load. If so, it should be replaced by a larger one. *Third* is worsening airways obstruction and accumulation of secretions; continued bronchial dilatation and airway suctioning avoid these. *Fourth* is a metabolic alkalemia, with or without diuretic therapy, that should be treated with potassium chloride. *Fifth* is having maintained a Pa_{O_2} and Pa_{CO_2} while being on mechanical ventilation that are too high and too low, respectively. This can be avoided by using an $F_{I_{O_2}}$ just sufficient to keep the Pa_{O_2} around 60 mmHg and using the assist mode with small enough tidal volumes to keep the Pa_{CO_2} at the expected chronic level (i.e., that associated with a normal or slightly low arterial pH) before discontinuing mechanical support. *Sixth* is poor nutrition, hypokalemia, or neuromuscular disease, making the patient too weak to maintain breathing or resulting in fatigue of the respiratory muscles. Nutrition, of course, is a longer range problem that should be anticipated, while hypokalemia is often handled along with the metabolic alkalemia. Muscle fatigue, especially diaphragmatic, has received a great deal of attention recently. From a practical standpoint, paradoxical (inward) movement of the upper abdomen with inspiration is the key clinical finding. Recent experimental evidence suggests that therapeutic levels of aminophylline reverse the manifestations of fatigue. Hypothyroidism is a metabolic condition with neuromuscular consequences and is difficult to detect in this clinical setting. Thus any prolonged and difficult weaning process should lead to the assessment of thyroid function.

PROGNOSIS On the average, data collected on large populations demonstrate a slow and relentless diminution in ventilatory function in patients with chronic airways obstruction. Although slow, the decrement in function with time far exceeds the rate of change seen with normal aging. In general, the likelihood of episodes of acute respiratory failure increases when the FEV_1 falls below 25 percent of predicted normal values. Although the in-hospital mortality rate averages 30 percent for a single episode and the 5-year survival rate after the initial episode of respiratory failure averages only 15 to 20 percent, the clinical syndrome is extremely important in determining both the short- and long-range prognosis. As noted above, those patients with predominant emphysema have a poorer prognosis after the onset of respiratory failure than do those with predominant bronchitis.

BULLOUS EMPHYSEMA Confluent air spaces with diameters in excess of 1 cm are occasionally congenital but most often are found in association with generalized emphysema or progressive fibrotic processes. Gradual increases in size of such air spaces (or bullae) result from traction applied by regions with better elastic recoil properties, and such regions lose volume as the bullae become enlarged. If disability is severe, if the bulla is extremely large, and if either lobar gas sampling or ventilation and perfusion scans demonstrate that sufficient function remains in the nonbullous regions, surgical excision of the bulla may lead to functional improvement. Usually, however, improvement is relatively transitory because other emphysematous regions gradually enlarge into bullae after surgery.

VARIANTS OF EMPHYSEMA In addition to the centriacinar and panacinar forms of emphysema described above, other structural patterns have been described but are functionally less important. Often there is overdistention and alveolar septal destruction in lung regions surrounding scar tissue (paracicatricial or scar emphysema) or along the borders of the acinus (paraseptal emphysema). The latter form, when it occurs at the visceral pleural surface, may predispose to episodes of spontaneous pneumothorax (Chap. 285). Infants rarely develop a check valve mechanism in a lobar bronchus which leads to rapid and life-threatening overdistention (congenital lobar emphysema). Unilateral emphysema may be an incidental radiographic finding (Macleod's or Swyer-James's syndromes). Since, in this condition, the airways are normal in number and structure but the alveoli are reduced in number, this form of unilateral emphysema has been attributed to disease occurring before the age of 8 years when alveoli are normally increasing in number. Overdistention and alveolar septal destruction are not present, and so this condition does not fit the definition of true emphysema. Most often the pulmonary artery on the affected side is hypoplastic. Although usually an incidental finding, the affected lung may become repeatedly infected so that surgical excision may be indicated.

REFERENCES

AUBIER M et al: Effects of the administration of O_2 on ventilation and blood gases in patients with chronic obstructive pulmonary disease during acute respiratory failure. Am Rev Resp Dis 122:747, 1980

BLOCK ER: Oxygen therapy, in *Update: Pulmonary Diseases and Disorders,* AP Fishman (ed). New York, McGraw-Hill, 1982, pp 349–365

COSIO M et al: The relations between structural changes in small airways and pulmonary function tests. N Engl J Med 298:1277, 1978

DIENER CF, BURROWS B: Further observation on the course and prognosis of chronic obstructive lung disease. Am Rev Resp Dis 111:719, 1975

HUGH-JONES P, WAIMSTER W: The etiology and management of disabling emphysema: State of the art. Am Rev Resp Dis 117:343, 1978

MATTHAY RA (ed): *The Medical Clinics of North America: Symposium on Chronic Obstructive Lung Diseases.* Philadelphia, Saunders, 1981

SCIENTIFIC BASIS OF IN-HOSPITAL RESPIRATORY THERAPY. Conference proceedings. Am Rev Resp Dis 122 5(2):1, 1980

THURLBECK WM: A pathologist's approach to clinical bronchitis and emphysema, in *Update: Pulmonary Diseases and Disorders,* AP Fishman (ed). New York, McGraw-Hill, 1982, pp 137–148

———, SIMON G: Radiographic appearance of the chest in emphysema. Am J Roentgenol 130:429, 1978

280 DIFFUSE INFILTRATIVE DISEASES OF THE LUNG

JOHN F. MURRAY

Infiltration means the diffusion into, or accumulation in, a tissue of substances not normal to it. Infiltrates of the lung are usually either cellular (e.g., inflammatory or neoplastic infiltration) or noncellular (e.g., infiltration by edema fluid, collagen, or other substances). Numerous clinicopathologic entities, therefore, are associated with diffuse infiltration of the lung (Table 280-1), and the differential diagnosis includes more than 100 entities. Although these disorders differ considerably in their pathogenesis—which is obscure in many instances—they share the common features of widespread structural involvement and characteristic alterations in pulmonary function. Because of these similarities, they are often accompanied by identical signs, symptoms, and roentgenographic changes.

In most large series of patients who presented with clinical, radiographic, and physiologic evidence of chronic diffuse infiltrative diseases of the lung, no underlying cause or associated condition could be identified in about half the cases, despite thorough evaluation. Thus, in this discussion brief descriptions of the major categories of disorders included in the differential diagnosis of diffuse infiltrative diseases of the lung are provided, but emphasis is placed on the important entity known as *diffuse idiopathic pulmonary fibrosis.*

It follows from these considerations that the number of diffuse infiltrative diseases of the lung is large. Table 280-1 lists the most important causes but is by no means inclusive.

PATHOGENESIS **Infections** Several members of each of the major classes of infectious agents are known to cause diffuse infiltration of the lung parenchyma. Viruses that affect the lower respiratory tract cause an acute interstitial inflammatory infiltration of lymphocytes, histiocytes, and plasma cells that may be accompanied by occasional hyaline membranes. Although most viral interstitial pneumonias resolve without significant residual lesions, experimental and clinical evidence has linked viruses with chronic, progressive diffuse interstitial disease, perhaps because, in some instances, they are capable of initiating an immunologic response that perpetuates the injury.

TABLE 280-1
Causes of diffuse infiltrative diseases of the lungs

1 Infections*
  a Viruses: influenza, cytomegalovirus, measles, varicella-zoster
  b Bacteria: miliary tuberculosis, staphylococcal infection, streptococcal infection, *Klebsiella* infection, mycoplasma infection, brucellosis, salmonellosis, shigellosis, tularemia, glanders, pneumonic plague, pertussis, psittacosis (ornithosis), lymphopathia venereum, Q fever, Rocky Mountain spotted fever, nocardiosis
  c Fungi: histoplasmosis, coccidioidomycosis, blastomycosis, cryptococcosis, candidiasis, aspergillosis, geotrichosis, sporotrichosis
  d Parasites: schistosomiasis, *Pneumocystis carinii* infection, filariasis, toxoplasmosis, paragonimiasis, ascariasis, trichinosis, hookworm infestation, strongyloides, visceral larva migrans, amebiasis, echinococcosis

2 Occupational causes
  a Mineral dusts: silicosis; asbestosis; berylliosis; coal miner's pneumoconiosis; Shaver's disease (bauxite); diatomaceous earth disease; talc pneumoconiosis; siderosis (arc welder's disease); pneumoconiosis from barium, silver, tin, vanadium, manganese
  b Chemical fumes: nitrogen dioxide (silo-filler's disease), chlorine, ammonia, sulfur dioxide, phosgenes, acetylene, kerosene, carbon tetrachloride, bromine, hydrogen fluoride, hydrochloric acid, nitric acid, picric acid

3 Neoplastic causes: bronchioloalveolar carcinoma, hematogenous metastases, lymphangitic carcinomatosis, leukemia, lymphoma, polycythemia vera

4 Congenital or familial causes: cystic fibrosis, Niemann-Pick disease, Gaucher's disease, neurofibromatosis, tuberous sclerosis, familial dysautonomia (Riley-Day syndrome), pulmonary alveolar microlithiasis, familial idiopathic pulmonary fibrosis (congenital cystic disease with pulmonary fibrosis and familial fibrocystic pulmonary dysplasia)

5 Metabolic causes: uremic pneumonitis, hypercalcemia, paraquat poisoning

6 Physical agents: postirradiation fibrosis, thermal injury, oxygen toxicity, blast injury

7 Circulatory causes
  a Thromboembolic: multiple pulmonary emboli, fat embolism, lymphangiography, sickle-cell anemia, foreign-body vasculitis (drug addicts, schistosomiasis)
  b Hemodynamic: pulmonary edema, chronic passive congestion with fibrosis (possibly with hemosiderosis and/or bone deposition)

8 Immunologic causes
  a Goodpasture's syndrome
  b Collagen diseases: scleroderma, rheumatoid arthritis, lupus erythematosus, periarteritis nodosa, Wegener's granulomatosis, dermatomyositis, Sjögren's syndrome
  c Hypersensitivity pneumonia: inhaled antigens, farmer's lung, bagassosis, bird fancier's disease, maple bark disease, sequoiosis, mushroom grower's disease, malt worker's lung, pneumonitis from pituitary snuff, exposure to *Bacillus subtilis* enzymes (detergent manufacturing), or smallpox vaccine
  d Sarcoidosis

9 Drug reactions: sensitivity to hydralazine, busulfan, nitrofurantoin, hexamethonium, mecamylamine, methysergide, bleomycin, cyclophosphamide, and procainamide

10 Unknown origin
  a Histiocytosis X: Letterer-Siwe disease, Hand-Schüller-Christian disease, eosinophilic granuloma
  b Idiopathic hemosiderosis
  c Pulmonary alveolar proteinosis
  d Diffuse idiopathic pulmonary fibrosis (synonyms: organizing interstitial pneumonia, usual interstitial pneumonia, chronic interstitial pneumonitis, idiopathic interstitial pulmonary fibrosis, acute diffuse interstitial fibrosis of the lungs, diffuse fibrosing alveolitis, cryptogenic fibrosing alveolitis, chronic diffuse sclerosing alveolitis, chronic Hamman-Rich syndrome, bronchiolar emphysema, and muscular cirrhosis of the lung)

* *Infections are not a common cause of diffuse infiltrative disease of the lungs. More commonly they cause focal processes.*

Diffuse parenchymal calcifications are known to follow varicella pneumonia. Necrotizing pyogenic bacterial infections that may heal with permanent scarring are usually focal rather than diffuse because they are acquired by aspiration through the tracheobronchial tree. In contrast, hematogenous infections, such as miliary tuberculosis, disseminated mycoses, and the migration of certain parasites, typically cause widespread pulmonary involvement. *Pneumocystis carinii* and/or cytomegalovirus are being recognized with increasing frequency; these infections are a particular problem in the immune compromised host. However, infections are not a common cause of *diffuse* infiltration of the lung, but they are important to recognize because most of them are treatable.

Occupational causes A wide variety of mineral dusts and chemical fumes may be inhaled (Chap. 275). Whether or not disease is produced depends on a number of factors, including the duration of exposure and concentration of the agent, its chemical properties (e.g., whether or not it is inert, fibrogenic, granuloma-inducing), and the susceptibility (including immunologic responsiveness) of the host. The long-standing notion that a "host factor" exists has received support from the presence of rheumatoid factor and antinuclear factor in the serum of many patients with various pneumoconioses, particularly of a severe or accelerated variety.

Diffuse parenchymal infiltration results from the tissue injury produced by the toxic substances and the cellular response they provoke and from the subsequent organization and evolution of the reaction. Once exposure ceases, the process may remain stable, as in early ("simple") silicosis, or it may progress slowly and become clinically apparent only many years later, as in asbestosis. The growth and conglomeration of the early small infiltrates in patients with coal miner's pneumoconiosis or silicosis into progressive massive fibrosis may occur spontaneously but often signifies the presence of either rheumatoid disease (Caplan's syndrome or rheumatoid pneumoconiosis) or coexisting infection with *Mycobacterium tuberculosis* or other mycobacteria.

Neoplastic disease Widespread pulmonary neoplasms (Chap. 284) are an important cause of diffuse pulmonary infiltrations that may occur in three different locations: (1) the surface epithelium, (2) the blood vessels and lymph channels and their surrounding spaces, and (3) the interstitial tissues. Bronchioloalveolar carcinoma is a primary lung cancer that may cause either focal tumor deposits or extensive epithelial infiltration (pulmonary adenomatosis). Some varieties grow slowly and are not invasive; others spread rapidly and are highly malignant. The lung parenchyma may become diffusely infiltrated by hematogenous or lymphatic metastases from a primary tumor anywhere in the body. Similarly, widespread interstitial pulmonary involvement may occur during the course of Hodgkin's or non-Hodgkin's lymphomas, in mycosis fungoides, and in Kaposi's sarcoma.

Infiltration of the lung with leukemic cells can be identified microscopically in a high proportion of patients with leukemia, but the involvement, in most cases, is not associated either with radiographically recognizable lesions or with clinically significant symptoms. Acute and chronic lymphatic leukemias are much more likely than myelogenous leukemias to cause pulmonary infiltrations. Fever and detectable pulmonary infiltrations in a patient with leukemia usually indicate the presence of an infection, often by an "opportunistic" organism; these conditions should not be regarded as leukemic, and a thorough search should be made for potential pathogens. Untreated polycythemia vera is often associated with congestion of the pulmonary circulation and occasionally has been reported to cause interstitial pulmonary fibrosis.

Congenital or familial diseases Several unrelated congenital or familial diseases are associated with diffuse pulmonary infiltration; most are systemic disorders, and the pulmonary component may be overshadowed by involvement of other organs that are more important and frequent sources of morbidity and mortality. *Familial dysautonomia* may be associated with pulmonary scarring secondary to pneumonitis resulting from frequent aspiration caused by autonomic nervous system dysfunction. Diffuse pulmonary fibrosis has been found in 10 to

20 percent of patients with *tuberous sclerosis* or *neurofibromatosis* (von Recklinghausen's disease). In *Niemann-Pick disease* and *Gaucher's disease* (usually in infantile form), chest roentgenograms may reveal fine reticulonodular shadows that reflect the presence of diffuse infiltration by histiocytes containing the abnormal lipids that characterize the diseases. Diffuse parenchymal scarring occurs in *cystic fibrosis* secondary to widespread bronchiectasis and recurrent pyogenic infections.

Pulmonary microlithiasis is a sporadic or familial disease in which there are innumerable intraalveolar calcified particles. The disorder presumably begins at an early age and is often recognized accidentally by chest roentgenography in an asymptomatic patient. There are no identifiable alterations in calcium and phosphorus metabolism, but local physicochemical abnormalities in lung tissue may account for the deposition of calcium salts. *Familial idiopathic pulmonary fibrosis* is identical to the more commonly observed sporadic variety (described in more detail later) but has, in addition, a definite familial incidence and a tendency to afflict younger persons.

Metabolic disorders Two relatively common clinical disorders, uremia and hypercalcemia, are associated with diffuse pulmonary infiltration. The pathologic findings in *uremic pneumonitis* consist of a fibrinous exudate in the alveoli (most marked in the hilar regions of the lung), often organized into dense hyaline membranes, and an interstitial pneumonia with varying degrees of organization. It is possible that chronic left ventricular failure contributes to or causes these changes and that uremic pneumonitis is not a discrete entity.

Hypercalcemia from virtually any cause, e.g., hyperparathyroidism, extensive bone malignancy, and hypervitaminosis D, may be associated with multiple deposits of calcium salts in the lungs. The lung, like the gastric mucosa and renal tubules, is a preferred site of involvement, presumably owing to local changes in pH which favor calcification. Although metastatic calcification of the lung parenchyma may be extensive when examined microscopically, it is often undetectable by chest roentgenography and seldom produces symptoms. A peculiar type of diffuse nodular calcification has been observed in patients undergoing chronic dialysis.

Accidental or deliberate ingestion of the herbicide *paraquat* produces injury in several organs, including the lung. If the patient survives the acute episode, chronic lung disease may result, consisting of diffuse inflammatory thickening of the interalveolar septa and interstitial fibrosis. The mechanism of tissue injury is not clear but may involve induction of metabolic abnormalities in type II alveolar epithelial cells.

Physical agents *Radiation pneumonitis* results from the cytotoxic effects of irradiation of the lung. The areas of involvement are usually sharply confined to the target sites, but if either the area irradiated or the secondary scatter is extensive, much of the lung parenchyma may be involved. The pathologic process consists of varying degrees of capillary congestion, interstitial edema, cellular infiltration, lymphangiectasis, and hyaline membrane formation. In the chronic phase, dense interstitial fibrosis develops, and blood vessels become narrowed or obliterated. Virtually every patient who acquires radiation pneumonitis also develops radiation fibrosis; however, fibrosis may occur in the absence of a clinically significant acute phase, presumably through the organization of a subacute and more indolent reaction. Use of certain drugs may potentiate the effects of irradiation, but this does not completely account for the wide variation in the response of patients to a given dose, suggesting that "host factors" may also be important. *Thermal and blast injuries* initiate a similar series of pathogenetic events: diffuse parenchymal injury, followed by organization and repair. There is also abundant experimental and clinical

evidence that *oxygen*, given in high concentrations for several days, also injures the lung. The concentration of oxygen and the duration of exposure are clearly important, but it is likely that toxicity is modified by other factors such as age, drugs, and the underlying disease. Exposure to high concentrations of oxygen damages pulmonary capillary endothelium and initiates an acute infiltrative-edematous phase, often with hyaline membrane formation, followed by a proliferative phase leading to fibrosis and collagen deposition. An analogous chronic condition called *bronchopulmonary dysplasia* that develops in newborn infants with respiratory distress is also believed to be related to oxygen toxicity.

Circulatory disorders Numerous thromboembolic conditions and a variety of hemodynamic complications of disorders of the left side of the heart and the pulmonary venous system may cause obliteration of, or leakage from, small pulmonary blood vessels. Diffuse pulmonary infiltrations ensue if *thromboemboli* elicit a perivascular inflammatory response or if abnormal hydrostatic forces cause chronic accumulation of fluid in the interstitium; when excessive fluid is retained in the lung parenchyma for prolonged periods, as in *mitral stenosis* and *chronic left ventricular failure*, hemosiderin is deposited, and possibly it or other factors cause slowly progressive interstitial fibrosis. At times, focal organization may progress to bone deposition.

Immunologic disorders The disorders in this category are believed to be caused by aberrant immunologic mechanisms. Although definitive proof is lacking in some instances, four major subgroups can be differentiated on the basis of their clinical manifestations and immunologic characteristics.

GOODPASTURE'S SYNDROME (see also Chap. 295) There is convincing evidence that this syndrome, which afflicts chiefly men 16 to 25 years of age, is related to a type II immunologic reaction. Antibody that cross-reacts with both glomerular and alveolar-capillary basement membranes can be found in the bloodstream and eluted from the lungs of affected persons; these observations are reinforced by the demonstration of a linear pattern of immunofluorescence in lungs and kidneys, which is consistent with the binding of antibody to basement membrane antigen. Clinical manifestations are related to hemoptysis and anemia from extensive intrapulmonary hemorrhage and to rapidly progressive renal failure.

"COLLAGEN DISEASES" Diseases in this group share such common features as multisystem involvement, considerable overlap in organ dysfunction (e.g., arthritis, nephritis), and the presence of excessive quantities of immunoglobulins and circulating non-organ-specific "autoantibodies." There is good evidence that the nephritis and probably the diffuse interstitial pneumonitis of lupus erythematosus are caused by a type III immunologic reaction. Deposition of immune complexes in alveolar walls is supported by an irregular staining pattern on immunofluorescence and electron-dense deposits on ultrastructural examination. Whether or not this mechanism accounts for the diffuse interstitial fibrosis found in patients with lupus erythematosus, scleroderma, rheumatoid arthritis, dermatomyositis, and Sjögren's syndrome is uncertain. Furthermore, vascular lesions have also been observed at times in all of these disorders, and vasculitis is the principal lesion in periarteritis nodosa (and related disorders like Churg-Strauss allergic granulomatosis) and Wegener's granulomatosis. Signs and symptoms of diffuse pulmonary infiltration may be overshadowed by those of involvement of other organ systems; at times, however, dyspnea and respiratory disability are profound.

HYPERSENSITIVITY PNEUMONIA (see also Chap. 274) A good example of how numerous apparently varied disorders express themselves through a common pathogenetic mechanism can be found in hypersensitivity pneumonia (also called extrinsic allergic alveolitis and allergic interstitial pneumonitis). The factors that determine the pathogenesis of pulmonary infiltration following inhalation of an organic dust include the immunologic reactivity of the host, the nature and size of the particles, and the degree and duration of exposure. The onset may be acute if exposure is great or if the patient is exquisitely sensitive to the antigen; conversely, the onset may be insidious in weakly sensitized subjects or when exposure is mild.

Hypersensitivity to a suspected (specific) antigen and components of a type III immunologic reaction can be established by demonstrating precipitating or complement fixing antibodies in the patient's serum and by the presence of a positive intermediate skin reaction (Arthus type) 4 to 8 h after intradermal testing. Finding precipitating antibodies alone is not diagnostic because they are often found in exposed persons without lung disease. Evidence for an etiologic role for the antigen is obtained by reproducing an acute attack, with attendant pulmonary function abnormalities, following inhalation of an aerosol containing the antigen. Evidence such as the presence of granulomas and sensitized T lymphocytes implicates type IV cell-mediated immune responses, in addition to type III immune-complex phenomena, in the pathogenesis of hypersensitivity pneumonitis. These findings can be reconciled by postulating that deposition of immune complexes causes the acute responses associated with the disorder, whereas chronic granuloma formation underlies the subacute and chronic manifestation. Specific examples of immunologic disorders involving the lung are detailed in Chap. 274.

SARCOIDOSIS Sarcoidosis (Chap. 235) is a multisystem disease with characteristic, but *not* pathognomonic, noncaseating granulomas commonly involving the lungs, lymph nodes, and liver. Interalveolar and interstitial granulomas may be undetectable roentgenographically but can be recognized by sensitive tests of pulmonary function. There is increasing evidence that sarcoidosis is caused by a type IV (cellular immune) reaction. Studies of lymphocytes recovered from the bloodstream and from bronchial lavage have reconciled the apparent paradox between the cellular immune responses that are exaggerated in the lung and other involved organs and those that are depressed elsewhere.

Drug reactions Many different drugs have been linked to the development of diffuse infiltrative diseases of the lung. The most common agents are listed in Table 280-1. The mechanism of action is uncertain, but because several drugs (e.g., the antineoplastic agents) have a radiomimetic effect, direct damage of lung tissue is possible; others (e.g., hydralazine and procainamide) may cause injury by an immunologic reaction. The onset may be acute with fever and, at times, eosinophilia or chronic with or without associated clinical and serologic features of the lupus erythematosus syndrome. Recognition of the role of drugs in the pathogenesis of diffuse infiltrative lung disorders is essential because continued administration of the offending drug will worsen the process, whereas removal is sometimes associated with significant improvement.

Unknown origin Although the basic pathogenesis of many of the diseases just discussed (e.g., drug reactions, congenital disorders, immunologic diseases) is not known, they can be classified according to major subject headings that allow inferences to be made concerning their etiology. There remain several important diffuse infiltrative diseases of the lung that cannot be conveniently grouped and so are listed separately under disorders of unknown origin.

HISTIOCYTOSIS X Histiocytosis X is a generic term that includes *Letterer-Siwe disease, Hand-Schüller-Christian disease, eosinophilic granuloma,* and their variants. The disorder is characterized by proliferation of, and infiltration by, histiocytes into various tissues. The stimulus for the histiocytic proliferation is unknown, and inflammatory, immunologic, and neoplastic causes have been considered. Tissue eosinophilia may occur, and the presence of foam cells, collagenization, and fibrosis indicates older organizing lesions. The major variations of histiocytosis X depend on the age of the patient, the extent of involvement, and the duration of the disease. The pulmonary complications vary, therefore, in a manner analogous to the progression in sarcoidosis, from acute cellular infiltration to chronic extensive scarring of the lung parenchyma.

IDIOPATHIC PULMONARY HEMOSIDEROSIS This uncommon disease affects infants and children and is extremely rare in persons more than 20 years of age; its chief manifestations are diffuse pulmonary infiltration, anemia, and hemoptysis. Bleeding into the lung interstitium accounts for the anemia and, when brisk, for the hemoptysis. Hemosiderin-filled macrophages, the clinical hallmark of the disease, can be found in the sputum during exacerbations and are abundant in the lung at all times. The presence of blood or blood products appears to initiate a fibrogenic response that leads to an increase in reticulum, collagen, and, ultimately, fibrous tissue. The prognosis is poor, and death usually occurs during an acute episode of bleeding; however, if the patient survives for several years, extensive interstitial fibrosis may result. Theories about etiology have included immunologic mechanisms, vascular defects, and abnormal iron storage, but none is proved.

PULMONARY ALVEOLAR PROTEINOSIS This rare entity is characterized by diffuse pulmonary infiltrations, which, in contrast to the disorders described earlier, are confined to alveolar spaces; alveoli in involved areas are filled with a dense granular material that stains vividly with the periodic acid Schiff technique. The material has been identified as a lipoprotein with many chemical similarities to pulmonary surfactant, but with different physical properties. Although hyperplasia of alveolar epithelium is usually present, inflammation and fibrous thickening of the interalveolar septa are conspicuously absent, and, in the absence of infection, fibrous tissue organization to the stage of honeycombing has been reported only once. In contrast to the relatively uniform roentgenographic and pathologic appearance of the lungs in pulmonary alveolar proteinosis, the clinical manifestations are extremely varied; they range from asymptomatic involvement to total disability or death from hypoxia, cor pulmonale, or secondary infection (often with "opportunistic" microorganisms, notably *Nocardia*). The etiology is unknown, and the natural history is poorly defined and appears to be variable: both spontaneous resolution and worsening have been reported.

DIFFUSE IDIOPATHIC PULMONARY FIBROSIS The lack of specificity of the pulmonary pathologic reaction in the large number of diffuse pulmonary infiltrative disorders is best illustrated by the many known causes of or associations with diffuse interstitial fibrosis. *Identical* pathologic findings have been documented in cases caused by infections, occupational exposure, hypersensitivity reactions, a variety of familial disorders, irradiation or oxygen inhalation, prolonged circulatory failure, and "collagen disease." The term "*usual* organizing interstitial pneumonia" (UIP) has been recommended for all these disorders, because it correctly describes the predominance of the fibrotic reaction with a minimal cellular infiltrate that occurs in all of them. But this designation is not completely satisfactory because it ignores what is known about etiology and pathogenesis. In most large series of cases of UIP, the etiology or pathogenesis can be identified in about half. The remaining patients in whom a specific diagnosis cannot be made have been described by a variety of terms, but the most common one used in the United States is diffuse idiopathic pulmonary fibrosis. The confusion about nomenclature is reflected in the number of synonyms listed in Table 280-1 that are mainly descriptive, each having some advantages and some disadvantages over the others. The term *Hamman-Rich disease* should be reserved for patients with acute rapidly progressive diffuse interstitial pneumonitis with fibrosis; this variant is much less common than chronic idiopathic pulmonary fibrosis.

Until recently, *desquamative interstitial pneumonia* (DIP) was considered sufficiently distinct to warrant classification as a separate entity. In patients with DIP, there is striking hyperplasia of the type II alveolar epithelial cells and filling of alveolar spaces with macrophages; in addition, there is an impressive interstitial cellular infiltration and an interstitial fibrotic reaction of varying severity. Evidence of progression from DIP to UIP on serial biopsies has led to the belief that the DIP is probably an early stage in the development of the more commonly observed UIP.

CLINICAL MANIFESTATIONS The symptoms, signs, and results of laboratory tests obviously vary, depending on the extent of the pulmonary process and its rate of progress. In addition, pulmonary involvement is substantially augmented by the presence of secondary complications—infection, cor pulmonale, and pneumothorax.

The predominant complaint caused by pulmonary infiltration is *dyspnea,* which is usually insidious in development, related primarily to exercise at its onset, and progressive. Weakness and fatigue often occur and are difficult to dissociate from breathlessness. Cough is present much less commonly than in other pulmonary diseases, and, if productive, especially if associated with fever, signifies the coexistence of bronchopulmonary infection. A variety of uncharacteristic and variable pleuritic and substernal chest pains may develop during the evolution of the disorder. Findings on physical examination may be unremarkable, especially in the early stages. The most characteristic findings are increased transmission of breath sounds and showers of superficial crackling rales at the lung bases. Clubbing of the digits and cyanosis indicate more severe involvement; signs of cor pulmonale (loud pulmonary second sound, parasternal heave, venous distention, hepatomegaly, and peripheral edema) imply advanced lung dysfunction with hypoxia and obliteration of the pulmonary vascular bed.

Chest roentgenographic findings depend on the stage of involvement. In early disease the roentgenogram may not show any abnormalities or the lungs may have a homogeneous "ground glass" haziness. Later, the pattern is one of diffuse reticular or reticulonodular densities. With progression of the process, the linear densities become coarser; small cystic lesions appear (honeycombing); marked loss of lung volume occurs (shown primarily by elevation of the diaphragm); and central pulmonary arterial dilatation and right ventricular enlargement may become apparent. Pleural effusions and hilar adenopathy do not occur in uncomplicated cases.

Routine laboratory studies are not very helpful. The most consistent abnormality is an elevated sedimentation rate. Antinuclear antibodies, circulating immune complexes, latex-agglutinating antibodies, or cryoglobulins can be found in as many as 40 percent of patients with diffuse idiopathic pulmonary fibrosis. Polycythemia may be present if hypoxia has been severe and prolonged. Pulmonary function studies, however, provide valuable documentation of the severity of impairment that is useful in deciding whether lung disease is present in symptomatic patients with normal chest roentgenograms, whether treatment is indicated, and in defining prognosis; they are also useful in following the course of the disease and objectively determining its response to treatment. However, pulmonary function studies do *not* delineate etiology or pathogenesis, because, as might be anticipated from the similar pathologic involvement of the lungs in the various disorders, the functional impairment is also similar.

Patients with diffuse idiopathic pulmonary fibrosis characteristically have a decrease in lung volumes, especially vital capacity and total lung capacity, and in diffusing capacity. Occasionally, however, these tests may be within normal limits in patients with biopsy-proven disease. The most consistently abnormal finding is a widened alveolar-arterial oxygen tension difference: increased values are usually found in patients at rest, but they are invariably found during exercise.

Unwarranted emphasis has been placed on the contribution of impaired diffusion of oxygen (the so-called alveolar-capillary block syndrome) to the alveolar-arterial oxygen tension difference, which is now recognized as being caused by mismatching of the distribution of inspired air and blood flow (ventilation-perfusion imbalance) (Chap. 271). However, in about 20 percent of patients the barrier to diffusion contributes to the characteristic finding of a worsening of arterial oxygen tension observed in these patients during exercise. In advanced disease, the presence of substantial right-to-left shunts of blood augment the hypoxia and make it relatively refractory to the administration of oxygen.

A corollary finding is alveolar hyperventilation (presumably owing to stimuli from hypoxia and intrapulmonary reflexes) that occurs despite an increased physiologic dead space. Arterial carbon dioxide tension is thereby reduced while the disease process progresses through most of its course; carbon dioxide tension becomes normal and finally elevated only in the terminal stages of the illness.

Another basic functional disturbance of the lungs of patients with diffuse interstitial infiltrative disorders is a decrease in pulmonary compliance (i.e., the lungs become stiffer). The increased stiffness of the lungs is also reflected in an increase in maximum static transpulmonary (recoil) pressure, especially when the patient's total lung capacity is taken into account (i.e., the coefficient of retraction).

DIAGNOSIS Careful historical examination is essential to the diagnosis of occupational lung diseases and hypersensitivity pneumonias. Chills, fever, weight loss, fatigue, and other nonspecific symptoms suggest that either an infectious process or a systemic disorder underlies the diffuse pulmonary infiltration. Physical examination seldom contributes to the differential diagnosis of those disorders confined to the lungs but may reveal important evidence of multisystem involvement in infectious, neoplastic, familial, metabolic, immunologic, and circulatory diseases as well as in sarcoidosis and histiocytosis X.

The results of routine blood counts, urinalysis, and blood chemistries are not likely to reveal important abnormalities or provide clues to the etiology of the underlying pulmonary disorder. Infections may be identified by appropriate cultural or serologic studies; hypersensitivity and immunologic diseases may be established by finding circulating antibodies or immune complexes; and neoplasms may be diagnosed by cytologic examination of the sputum. However, specific diagnosis of most diffuse infiltrative diseases, if it can be made at all, requires examination of tissue.

Biopsy is often the only method of documenting the type and cause of pulmonary disorder. The source of biopsy material is determined by the likelihood of obtaining diagnostic tissue and by the risks inherent in the procedure. Skin, lymph nodes, marrow, and liver are useful biopsy sites in disseminated infections, neoplasms, and at times sarcoidosis. However, the best way to diagnose pulmonary sarcoidosis when other sites of involvement are not readily available is by mediastinal node or lung biopsy. If cervical or supraclavicular lymph nodes are palpable, they should be examined histologically and culturally. If nodes are not palpable, but paratracheal or mediastinal nodes are evident roentgenographically, mediastinoscopy is indicated. At times, anterior mediastinotomy provides a useful approach to hilar nodes.

The majority of diffuse pulmonary infiltrative diseases are not associated with significant lymphadenopathy; if a diagnosis cannot be documented by other means, lung biopsy is indicated. Three types of lung biopsy are available: percutaneous, transbronchial, and open. Transbronchial biopsy has gradually replaced percutaneous biopsy and has proved useful in patients with diffuse infiltrative disease of the lung. However, the amount of tissue sampled is small, which limits diagnostic investigation. For this reason, open lung biopsy is recommended because it allows removal of a suitable piece of selected lung tissue that can be cultured and examined histologically by light and electron microscopy; in addition, a portion can be frozen for special studies at a later date (virus cultures, chemical or spectroscopic analysis). Open biopsy is the procedure of choice in the seriously ill patient with severe hypoxia and/or mechanical ventilation because it can be carried out under controlled conditions and will ensure maximum diagnostic reliability.

Histologic findings in patients with idiopathic pulmonary fibrosis span a continuum from those with a rich interstitial and alveolar cellular infiltration and minimal interstitial fibrosis (the DIP type) to those with mainly a fibrotic reaction and little inflammatory response (the UIP type). But there are variations to these basic patterns, and the findings may differ from one region to another in the same specimen. These patients do not have vasculitis, granulomas, or evidence of minerals or foreign matter in their lungs.

Recently, it has been shown that the uptake of radioactive gallium by the lungs, assessed by external counters, correlates with the cellularity found on lung biopsy. Similarly, the cellular and immunoglobulin composition of fluid lavaged from the lung during fiberoptic bronchoscopy has been correlated with the cellularity of the infiltrative process. At present, the results of these procedures do not appear to have diagnostic specificity but may indicate responsiveness to anti-inflammatory drugs and provide a means of assessing the influence of therapy.

TREATMENT The majority of diffuse pulmonary infiltrations do not respond well to therapy, but some are eminently treatable, and the value of making an etiologic diagnosis lies in determining which of the many available therapeutic agents should be used. Specific chemotherapy is available for most infectious agents. Removal from exposure diminishes the risk of occupational pulmonary diseases and may allow clearing of hypersensitivity pneumonias. Lung lavage is indicated in severely disabled patients with pulmonary alveolar proteinosis. Plasmapheresis to remove circulating anti-basement membrane antibodies has proved effective in controlling Goodpasture's syndrome.

Corticosteroids are useful in the treatment of many of the causes of organizing interstitial pneumonia, especially when administered early. They are helpful in patients with hypersensitivity pneumonias, chemical injuries of the lungs, sarcoidosis, and histiocytosis X; their role in idiopathic hemosiderosis is questionable. They are seldom of benefit in the treatment of collagen diseases, diseases due to occupational dusts, and chronic diffuse interstitial fibrosis of known or idiopathic origin and they are contraindicated in alveolar proteinosis.

The response of patients with diffuse idiopathic pulmonary fibrosis is highly variable and difficult to predict. In general, compared with patients who do not respond, those who do are younger, have a predominant cellular infiltration in biopsied tissues, and have circulating immune complexes, polymorphonuclear leukocytes recoverable by lung lavage, and, as a corollary observation, appreciable uptake of gallium in the lung. All of these findings point to an early stage of development that precedes the inherently irreversible later phase of widespread fibrosis.

When corticosteroids are used, they should be given in sufficient doses to ensure that a response will occur if one can be elicited. Patients with idiopathic pulmonary fibrosis should be given a trial of prednisone: 1 mg/kg per day up to 80 mg in a single daily oral dose for 6 weeks and thereafter decreasing by 0.05 mg/kg per week until 0.25 mg/kg per day is reached. The patient's response must be followed objectively by serial chest roentgenograms and, more importantly, by appropriate tests of pulmonary function (arterial blood gases, lung volumes, diffusing capacity), since subjective responses to corticosteroids are notoriously unreliable. Measurements of gas exchange during exercise, such as the change in arterial P_{O_2} or alveolar-arterial P_{O_2} difference divided by the change in O_2 consumption, are reported to be the most sensitive tests of responsiveness to treatment.

Immunosuppressive drugs have been suggested as useful adjuncts to corticosteroid therapy of patients with idiopathic pulmonary fibrosis; however, preliminary results of a controlled trial with azathioprine are unimpressive.

In contrast, immunosuppressive therapy has produced striking long-term remissions of severe forms of Wegener's granulomatosis, usually a progressive and fatal disease. Rheumatoid arthritis and lupus erythematosus nephritis have responded to cytotoxic drugs in short-term controlled trials, but whether the fibrotic pulmonary infiltrations associated with these diseases will resolve remains to be determined. Thus far, the results from uncontrolled trials are not encouraging. Drugs that inhibit fibrogenesis are being tried in controlled studies, but none is available for routine use.

PROGNOSIS It follows from the information presented in previous sections that the course and prognosis of diffuse infiltrative diseases of the lung are extremely variable. The outlook is determined by the natural history of the underlying cause of the disorder, how far advanced it is when diagnosed, its response to therapy, and the presence of complications. The prognosis is favorable in those diseases with a reversible component, either spontaneous or induced by easily tolerated therapy (infections, chemical injuries, hypersensitivity pneumonias, and sarcoidosis). The prognosis is poor in most collagen diseases, progressive occupational dust diseases, chronic diffuse idiopathic interstitial fibrosis, and in any condition that has advanced to severe lung fibrosis and honeycombing; these disorders are associated with slow but relentless lung destruction, with progressive hypoxia, and finally with death from cor pulmonale or secondary bronchopulmonary infection.

REFERENCES

Basset F et al: Pulmonary histiocytosis X. Am Rev Resp Dis 118:811, 1978

CARRINGTON CB et al: Natural history and treated course of usual and desquamative interstitial pneumonia. N Engl J Med 298:801, 1978
CRYSTAL RG et al: Idiopathic pulmonary fibrosis: Clinical, histologic, radiographic, physiologic, scintigraphic, cytologic, and biochemical aspects. Ann Intern Med 85:769, 1976
DREISIN RB et al: Circulating immune complexes in the idiopathic interstitial pneumonias. N Engl J Med 298:353, 1978
EPLER GR et al: Normal chest roentgenograms in chronic diffuse infiltrative lung disease. N Engl J Med 298:934, 1978
FULMER JD et al: Morphologic-physiologic correlates of the severity of fibrosis and degree of cellularity in idiopathic pulmonary fibrosis. J Clin Invest 63:665, 1979
HUNNINGHAKE GW, FAUCI AS: Pulmonary involvement in the collagen vascular diseases, in *Update IV: Harrison's Principles of Internal Medicine,* KJ Isselbacher et al (eds). New York, McGraw-Hill, 1983, p 147

KAO D et al: Advances in the treatment of pulmonary alveolar proteinosis. Am Rev Resp Dis 111:361, 1975
LINE BR et al: Gallium-67 citrate scanning in the staging of idiopathic pulmonary fibrosis: Correlation with physiologic and morphologic features and bronchoalveolar lavage. Am Rev Resp Dis 118:355, 1978
MATTHAY RA et al: Pulmonary manifestations of systemic lupus erythematosus: Review of twelve cases of acute lupus pneumonitis. Medicine 54:397, 1975
TURNER-WARWICK M et al: Cryptogenic fibrosing alveolitis: Response to corticosteroid treatment and its effect on survival. Thorax 35:593, 1980

Vascular diseases of the lung

281 PRIMARY PULMONARY HYPERTENSION

JOHN ROSS, JR.

Primary (or idiopathic) pulmonary hypertension is an uncommon disease, the diagnosis of which can be established only after a thorough search for the usual causes of pulmonary hypertension. The patient with primary pulmonary hypertension typically is a young female between the ages of 20 and 40, although older and younger patients of either sex have been described. The clinical and laboratory features of severe pulmonary hypertension are present, but there is no evidence of parenchymal pulmonary disease or of primary heart disease, nor is there evidence for the occurrence of pulmonary emboli. Anatomic verification often has been necessary to distinguish clearly the primary form of pulmonary hypertension from that due to multiple pulmonary emboli, although angiography and radioisotope scanning methods have facilitated this differentiation considerably.

PATHOLOGY The findings on pathologic examination of patients with primary pulmonary hypertension usually are confined to the right side of the heart and lungs. The right atrium often is enlarged and the right ventricle is hypertrophied. Frequently, the large pulmonary arteries exhibit atherosclerotic plaques. The disease process involves the small pulmonary arteries (between 40 and 300 μm in diameter), which exhibit muscular hypertrophy and intimal hyperplasia, sometimes with fibrosis. On occasion, a necrotizing arteritis may be encountered. Other histologic studies have shown a reduced number of small arteries, as well as fewer capillaries in the alveolar wall. Electron-microscopic studies have documented an increase in thickness of the endothelial cells and basement membranes of alveolar capillaries, and some capillaries are blocked by the abnormal epithelial cells. Medial hypertrophy of muscular pulmonary arteries may be the first response to prolonged pulmonary vasoconstriction, but in later stages of the disease concentric laminar intimal fibrosis and plexiform lesions appearing as cellular, intraluminal tufts (so-called plexogenic pulmonary arteriopathy) may develop. Patients with recurrent pulmonary thromboembolism may clinically resemble patients with primary pulmonary hypertension, but histologic sections of the lung exhibit various degrees of organization of pulmonary thromboemboli; some may be recanalized, there may be fibrous septa and eccentric fibrosis in the vessels; secondary medial hypertrophy of muscular arteries may be marked, but plexiform lesions are not present. In infants and young children with pulmonary venoocclusive disease the clinical picture may suggest primary pulmonary hypertension, and the pulmonary wedge pressure may be normal. Organized thrombotic disease is found in the venules and small veins, together with proximal hypertrophy of the muscular venous wall and secondary medial hypertrophy in the pulmonary arterioles.

Rarely, disease of the systemic arterial vascular bed resembling that found in the pulmonary blood vessels has been described. The syncope and sudden death which may occur in this disease have been attributed in some patients to involvement of the coronary arterial branch supplying the sinoatrial node.

ETIOLOGY The cause of primary pulmonary hypertension is unknown, but a number of possible etiologic factors have been suggested. A few patients with primary pulmonary hypertension have been reported in whom minimal changes were found in the pulmonary vessels on pathologic examination, and this observation has raised the possibility that a neurohumoral vasoconstrictor mechanism is involved. Support for this view has been provided by the observation that the pulmonary vascular resistance can be acutely reduced in some patients with this disease by the intrapulmonary injection of vasodilators, or by breathing oxygen. A febrile illness may precede the onset of the disease by a variable period and has been implicated in the etiology. The occurrence of the disease in young females has prompted the suggestion that unrecognized thromboemboli or amniotic fluid emboli during pregnancy may play a role. In other patients, it seems quite possible that the disease may represent an end stage of earlier, unrecognized emboli originating from the legs or pelvic veins. An apparent association between an increased occurrence of primary pulmonary hypertension and use of the anoretic agent aminorex fumarate (Menocil), an agent having structural similarity to ephedrine, was observed in Europe between 1967 and 1970. The alkaloids in many species of crotalaria plants used in herbal brews may cause pulmonary hypertension in humans, as demonstrated experimentally in rats. The use of oral contraceptives may bear a relation to the occurrence of pulmonary hypertension, particularly in patients with predisposing factors such as systemic lupus erythematosus or a family history of primary pulmonary hypertension.

Raynaud's phenomenon precedes the onset of primary pulmonary hypertensive disease by a number of years in an appreciable number of patients. This association and the occurrence of Raynaud's disease in scleroderma, disseminated lupus erythematosus, rheumatoid arthritis, and dermatomyositis have led to the speculation that primary pulmonary hypertension may represent a form of collagen vascular disease. Moreover, primary pulmonary hypertension and collagen vascular disease, including lupus erythematosus, have been reported to occur simultaneously in a number of patients. It also has been suggested that the disease may be congenital and present from birth; however, the closely packed, parallel elastic fibers in the main pulmonary arteries in patients having Eisenmenger's syndrome from birth, described by some investigators, usually have not been observed in patients with primary pulmonary hypertension. Finally, primary pulmonary hypertension has been reported in a number of families; sometimes more than two members and up to three generations have been affected. A fibrinolytic defect was reported in one family study.

PATHOPHYSIOLOGY Some studies have suggested that the response of the pulmonary vascular bed is labile early in the course of this disease, as evidenced by a response to vasodilating agents and oxygen. It also has been proposed that the disease tends to progress. Thus, serial cardiac catheterizations have shown a tendency for the pulmonary vascular resistance to increase and to become fixed. With the development of severe pulmonary vascular disease, abnormal elevation of the pulmonary arterial pressure occurs, often to a striking degree, and the pulmonary arterial pressure may be equal to that in the systemic arterial bed. The pulmonary arterial wedge pressure is normal in patients with primary pulmonary hypertension, the cardiac output is normal or reduced, and no intracardiac shunts are detected. In many patients the mean right atrial pressure is elevated, and the *a* wave in the right atrium may be markedly elevated, an indication of the forceful atrial contraction necessary to fill the hypertrophied right ventricle. With the long-standing overload on the right side of the heart, right ventricular failure finally develops. In some patients, peripheral cyanosis occurs secondary to reduced cardiac output, and occasionally central cyanosis becomes evident at the end stage of the disease because of right-to-left shunting through a patent foramen ovale. Mild systemic arterial desaturation is quite common, even in the absence of heart failure, and may be due to shunting within the lungs. Pulmonary function in patients with primary pulmonary hypertension generally is normal, although hyperventilation often is present, resulting in hypocapnia and a decreased serum bicarbonate concentration. A low carbon monoxide–diffusing capacity has been described in some patients.

CLINICAL PICTURE The patient, usually a young female, gives a history of relatively recent onset of symptoms. Ordinarily, the natural course of the disease encompasses less than 5 years, but occasionally survival for 25 years or more has been reported. Not uncommonly, patients with primary pulmonary hypertension are classified as neurotic early in the course of their disease because of the hyperventilation, chest discomfort, and the relative paucity of objective findings. Precordial pain on exertion occurs in from 25 to 50 percent of patients, and occasionally severe chest pain has been associated with a dissection of the main pulmonary artery. Other common symptoms are weakness, fatigue, exertional dyspnea, and effort syncope. Hoarseness may be noted because of compression of the left recurrent laryngeal nerve by the enlarged pulmonary artery. Unexplained sudden death occurs relatively often. Sudden death also has occurred during cardiac catheterization or surgical procedures and after the administration of barbiturates or anesthetic agents. The terminal course usually is characterized by right-sided heart failure. Very rarely, spontaneous regression of the disease has been reported.

On physical examination, the jugular venous pulse usually shows a prominent *a* wave, there is a right ventricular heave, and an impulse may be felt over the region of the main pulmonary artery. An ejection click may be audible at the pulmonic area, the second heart sound is narrowly split, and the pulmonic closure sound is markedly accentuated and may be palpable. Often, an atrial gallop sound is heard at the lower left sternal border, and in some patients there is an ejection murmur at the pulmonic area, or the early diastolic murmur of pulmonic regurgitation. The chest roentgenogram may show cardiac enlargement with right ventricular and right atrial prominence, and there is marked dilatation of the pulmonary artery segment. Peripherally, the pulmonary arteries taper sharply, and the lung fields may appear oligemic. The electrocardiogram almost always shows some evidence of right ventricular enlargement, with right axis deviation, right ventricular hypertrophy in the precordial leads, and sometimes inverted T waves over the right precordium. Right atrial enlargement also may be evident on the electrocardiogram.

DIFFERENTIAL DIAGNOSIS It is imperative that the diagnosis of primary pulmonary hypertension not be made until potentially treatable causes of elevated pulmonary arterial pressure have been excluded. The presence of pulmonary hypertension and cor pulmonale caused by chronic pulmonary disease can be established readily by finding abnormalities in pulmonary function. In particular, interstitial lung diseases with fibrosis, such as sarcoidosis, and pneumoconioses, such as silicosis, as well as hypoxic pulmonary hypertension associated with impaired ventilation should be excluded. Cardiac catheterization studies are necessary to search for a primary cardiac defect, and angiography or radioactive lung-scanning studies also may be indicated to detect pulmonary emboli (Chap. 282). In performing pulmonary arteriography, the use of small amounts of contrast medium, preferentially injected selectively into the branches of the main pulmonary artery, is advisable since sudden death has occasionally occurred. Patients having chronic emboli to the lungs are difficult to distinguish from those with primary pulmonary hypertension, but the distinction is important because anticoagulants, inferior vena caval interruption, and pulmonary embolectomy sometimes have been effective in patients with embolic disease. The lung scan and pulmonary arteriogram are typically normal in primary pulmonary hypertension, but with thromboembolic pulmonary hypertension, perfusion defects on lung scan or pulmonary arterial occlusions and filling defects on angiography often are visible. With pulmonary embolism, serial chest x-rays may show evidence of pulmonary infarction. Open lung biopsy has been used occasionally to differentiate primary pulmonary hypertension from the thromboembolic variety. Sometimes a site of origin for emboli cannot be identified in the leg veins, and other possible sources should be considered, such as right atrial thrombus, or ovarian and pelvic vein thromboses. Occasionally, pulmonary hypertension is due to parasitic disease, such as schistosomiasis or filariasis, or to multiple pulmonary artery thromboses consequent to sickle cell disease.

Several congenital cardiac conditions must be considered and excluded by appropriate cardiac catheterization studies. Valvular pulmonic stenosis usually can be distinguished from pulmonary hypertension by identification of the delayed, soft pulmonic closure sound, but peripheral stenoses of the pulmonary arteries may be associated with an increased second heart sound. A left-to-right shunt at the pulmonary arterial, ventricular, or atrial levels should be sought. The wide, fixed splitting of the second heart sound should be helpful in identifying patients with atrial septal defect. Eisenmenger's syndrome in a patient with ventricular septal defect or patent ductus arteriosus (Chap. 256) may be confused with primary pulmonary hypertension, but usually in Eisenmenger's syndrome cyanosis, polycythemia, and clubbing are present, and at cardiac catheterization a large right-to-left shunt at the ventricular or pulmonary arterial level can be demonstrated.

The murmurs of tricuspid or pulmonic regurgitation and the atrial gallop sounds heard in patients with primary pulmonary hypertension may be mistaken for the murmurs of rheumatic mitral and aortic valve disease, or vice versa. Before making the diagnosis of primary pulmonary hypertension, the presence of left atrial hypertension due to undetected mitral stenosis, or to a more unusual lesion such as left atrial myxoma or cor triatriatum, should be specifically sought and excluded. This can be done by echocardiography, by obtaining pulmonary arterial wedge pressure tracings, or by catheterization of the left side of the heart, with angiography if necessary.

THERAPY In many patients with primary pulmonary hypertension the downhill course is progressive despite treatment, and therapy must be palliative. The use of anticoagulants is of doubtful value, provided chronic pulmonary embolic phenomena can be excluded. Right-sided heart failure should be treated with a cardiotonic and diuretic regimen (Chap. 253). Since there is no hypocapnia in these patients, the hypoxia which may accompany heart failure can be treated safely with oxygen therapy.

Recent reports have indicated that in some patients pharmacologic therapy can produce clinical and hemodynamic improvement. Although long-term observations concerning prolongation of life are not available, four categories of drugs have been found useful in small groups of patients: (1) direct vascular smooth-muscle relaxants (nitroprusside, diazoxide, and hydralazine); (2) beta agonists (sublingual isoproterenol, oral terbutaline); (3) alpha-adrenergic blocking agents (phentolamine and phenoxybenzamine); (4) calcium antagonists (nifedipine and verapamil). Immunosuppressive agents, prostaglandin antagonists (indomethacin), or PGI_2 have rarely been used.

In some patients, favorable hemodynamic effects from orally administered drugs such as diazoxide or hydralazine have been sustained for many months, with clinical improvement manifested by relief of severe dyspnea and reduction in the number of syncopal episodes. Prior to instituting long-term therapy with such drugs, measurement of the acute responses of the pulmonary artery pressure, pulmonary vascular resistance, cardiac output, and arterial pressure is usually indicated in order to assess efficacy and to detect unfavorable effects. In some patients hemodynamic deterioration has been reported following the use of vasodilators.

Transplantation of the heart and lungs has now been successfully accomplished and in the future may offer hope for some patients with primary pulmonary hypertension. Long-term follow-up of patients subjected to this procedure is not yet available.

REFERENCES

Alpert JS, Braunwald E: Primary pulmonary hypertension, in *Heart Disease*, E Braunwald (ed). Philadelphia, Saunders, 1980, pp 1633–1642

Camerini F et al: Primary pulmonary hypertension: Effects of nifedipine. Br Heart J 44:352, 1980

Edwards WD, Edwards JE: Clinical primary pulmonary hypertension. Three pathologic types. Circulation 56:884, 1977

Fishman AP: Primary pulmonary hypertension: More light or more tunnel? Ann Intern Med 94:815, 1981

Follath F et al: Drug-induced pulmonary hypertension? Br Med J 1:265, 1971

Lupi-Herrera E et al: The role of hydralazine therapy for pulmonary arterial hypertension of unknown cause. Circulation 65:645, 1982

Rubin LJ, Peter RH: Primary pulmonary hypertension: New approaches to therapy. Am Heart J 100:757, 1980

Voelkel N, Reeves JT: Primary pulmonary hypertension, in *Pulmonary Vascular Diseases*, KM Moser (ed). New York, Marcel Dekker, 1979

Wagenvoort CA, Wagenvoort N: *Pathology of Pulmonary Hypertension*. New York, Wiley, 1977, p 345

Wang SWS et al: Diazoxide in treatment of primary pulmonary hypertension. Br Heart J 40:572, 1978

282
PULMONARY THROMBOEMBOLISM

KENNETH M. MOSER

Pulmonary thromboembolism (PTE) is a leading cause of morbidity and mortality, and can appear in many clinical contexts. Epidemiologic surveys indicate that PTE is responsible for more than 50,000 deaths in the United States annually. However, available data suggest that less than 10 percent of all pulmonary emboli result in death. Thus, the incidence of fatal plus nonfatal emboli in this nation probably exceeds 500,000 annually. This overall incidence seems verified by autopsy statistics. Evidence of recent or old embolism is detected in 25 to 30 percent of routine autopsies; with special techniques, this figure exceeds 60 percent. Even these data underestimate incidence, since many emboli resolve without trace and are not found at postmortem examination. The high incidence of PTE at autopsy contrasts sharply with the incidence of antemortem diagnosis. Available information suggests that an antemortem diagnosis has been made in only 10 to 30 percent of all cases in which old or recent embolism is demonstrated at autopsy.

VENOUS THROMBOSIS

PATHOGENESIS Available data indicate that more than 95 percent of pulmonary emboli arise from thrombi in the deep venous system of the lower extremities. Thrombi occurring in the right cardiac chambers or in other veins account for the remainder. In situ pulmonary arterial thrombosis is rare. Thus, embolism should be viewed as a *complication* of deep venous thrombosis (DVT). Furthermore, it appears that the larger leg veins (those above the knee) are the most common source of those pulmonary emboli which reach clinical attention. These facts have several important implications with respect to PTE: (1) prevention of DVT is the most effective approach to prevention of embolism; (2) prompt treatment of DVT may limit the frequency of embolism; (3) techniques which allow the diagnosis of DVT in the leg veins will allow identification of the vast majority of patients at high risk of embolism.

The three factors which promote DVT (and, therefore, embolic risk) are stasis, abnormalities of the vessel wall, and alterations in the blood coagulation system. Coagulation alterations have been studied extensively, but as yet there is no reliable test for a state of "hypercoagulability," i.e., a test which will predict the risk of DVT (except for the rare patients with antithrombin III deficiency or cystinuria). In the absence of such a test, the risk of DVT is best assessed by recognizing the presence of known "clinical" risk factors. Conditions associated with a high risk of venous thromboembolism include the postpartum period, left and right ventricular failure, fractures or other injuries of the lower extremities, chronic deep venous insufficiency of the legs, prolonged bed rest, carcinoma, and obesity.

NATURAL HISTORY In the contexts noted above, deep venous thrombi usually develop in the region of a venous valve. Platelets aggregate, forming a nidus (white thrombus), followed by development of a large fibrin (red) thrombus. The process is apparently a rapid one; large, extensive thrombi can develop within minutes. Growth occurs by continued fibrin and platelet accretion. Beyond formation, two processes may contribute to resolution: fibrinolysis and organization. Fibrinolysis may result in complete resolution within hours to several days. Any remaining thrombus undergoes organization, leaving behind a fibrotic zone that becomes reendothelialized. Valves are often rendered incompetent by this process, and modest or extensive luminal narrowing may occur. Once thrombus growth has halted, fibrinolysis/organization reaches a stable state in 7 to 10 days. It is during the first few days after formation, therefore, that embolic risk is highest.

DETECTION The clinical diagnosis of DVT is difficult. DVT is frequently present in the absence of clinical signs (e.g., pain, heat, swelling), and it is absent in 50 percent of patients in whom clinical signs or symptoms suggest its presence. Therefore a number of diagnostic tests have been developed. There are three noninvasive procedures available for the early detection and follow-up of DVT: (1) impedance plethysmography, which detects venous outflow obstruction, is highly sensitive to above-knee thrombosis, but fails to detect many below-knee thrombi; (2) the Doppler technique, which is highly operator dependent; (3) the radiofibrinogen method, which is very sensitive to thrombus formation in calf veins and lower thigh veins, but not sensitive to thrombi which form in the upper thigh or above (also, 24 h is required for a definitive answer). The impedance and radiofibrinogen tests correlate well with the definitive (but invasive) standard for the diagnosis of DVT, i.e., *ascending contrast phlebography*. The combination of impedance plethysmography and radiofibrinogen leg scanning is equal in accuracy to contrast venography.

PROPHYLAXIS Application of these noninvasive approaches to the early diagnosis and follow-up of patients at high risk of DVT has led to significant changes in the approach to the prevention of DVT (and therefore of PTE). One validated prophylactic method is the use of small doses of subcutaneous heparin. Multiple studies, utilizing chiefly radiolabeled fibrinogen, have shown the high incidence of DVT in certain groups: patients over the age of 40 years with fractures of the pelvis and/or lower extremities; patients with myocardial infarction and/or severe congestive heart failure; patients undergoing major abdominal, thoracic, or gynecologic surgery. Furthermore, in the last group of patients, investigations have demonstrated a significant reduction in the incidence of DVT, PTE, and lethal PTE when heparin is given subcutaneously, in a dose of 5000 units every 12 h, beginning *before* operation (or on admission to the hospital) and continued until the patient is ambulatory. There is general agreement that this prophylactic approach, which has limited effect on coagulation tests and is associated with little risk of hemorrhage, should also be applied to *medical* patients at high risk of DVT and PTE. In the case of acute myocardial infarction, high risk would be imposed by the development of congestive failure, the presence of severe obesity, chronic venous insufficiency, or a prior history of DVT or PTE. Mechanical leg compressive devices appear to be promising for prophylaxis in patients at risk of hemorrhage with low-dose heparin (neurosurgery, spinal cord trauma) or in whom low-dose heparin has proved ineffective (hip surgery, prostate surgery).

NATURAL HISTORY OF EMBOLISM

THE ACUTE EVENTS The immediate result of thromboembolism is complete or partial obstruction of the pulmonary arterial blood flow to the distal lung. This obstruction leads to a series of pathophysiologic events which can be categorized as the "respiratory" and "hemodynamic" consequences of PTE.

Respiratory consequences Embolic obstruction produces a zone of the lung which is ventilated but not perfused—an intrapulmonary "dead space" (Chap. 271). Because it cannot participate in the process of gas exchange, ventilation of this nonperfused area is "wasted," in the functional sense. A potential consequence of embolic obstruction is constriction of the air spaces and airways in the affected lung zone. In animal experiments in which each lung is ventilated separately, this "pneumoconstriction" appears to be due to the marked bronchoalveolar hypocapnia that results from cessation of pulmonary capillary blood flow because it is abolished by inhalation of carbon dioxide–enriched air. This probably occurs very rarely in patients who inhale dead space air (rich in carbon dioxide) into embolized lung zones.

Another disturbance caused by embolic obstruction—loss of alveolar surfactant—does not occur immediately. This surface-active lipoprotein is required to maintain alveolar stability. In its absence, alveolar collapse occurs. Cessation of pulmonary capillary blood flow leads to reduction in surfactant within 2 or 3 h, which becomes severe at 12 to 15 h. Frank atelectasis—the morphologic expression of alveolar instability—can be detected at 24 to 48 h after interruption of blood flow.

Arterial hypoxemia is a common, though by no means universal, consequence of embolism. Several mechanisms can contribute to hypoxemia: ventilation-perfusion disturbances; cardiac failure with a lowered mixed venous P_{O_2} (widened arteriovenous difference); and obligatory perfusion through hypoventilated (and normally vasoconstricted) lung zones.

Hemodynamic consequences The primary hemodynamic consequence of thromboembolic obstruction is a reduction in the cross-sectional area of the pulmonary arterial bed. This loss of vascular capacity increases the resistance to pulmonary blood flow, which, if marked, leads to pulmonary hypertension and acute failure of the right ventricle. Tachycardia and often a decline in cardiac output also occur.

The factors which determine the severity of these hemodynamic changes have been the subject of continued debate. There is agreement that the *extent of embolic obstruction* is a key factor. However, the reserve capacity of the pulmonary arteriocapillary bed is so extensive that more than 50 percent of the vascular area must be obstructed before significant elevation in pulmonary arterial pressure results. Because pulmonary hypertension occurs in some patients with occlusion of lesser extent, investigators have searched for reflex or humoral vasoconstrictor mechanisms associated with embolism. Despite long and careful search for such mechanisms, their extent and frequency in human PTE remains unknown. Hence, some workers maintain that the degree of embolic obstruction itself is the only determinant of hemodynamic impairment. They suggest that instances of apparent disparity between the extent of embolism and clinical response reflect only clinical underestimation of the magnitude of the embolism. Other investigators, however, have presented compelling evidence to support the occurrence of pulmonary vasoconstriction with embolism. Some have demonstrated that constriction is associated with obstruction of the smaller, but not the larger, pulmonary arterial vessels. Another thesis holds that serotonin, a known pulmonary vasoconstrictive-bronchoconstrictive substance, is released from platelets, coating fresh emboli as they lodge in the pulmonary tree. This thesis introduces the attractive concept that an embolus might be regarded, in part, as a packet with pharmacologic, as well as obstructive, potential. A consensus view is that, while the extent of embolism is a key factor, humoral and/or reflex influences probably operate in certain patients and compromise the pulmonary circulation to a greater extent than might be expected on an anatomic basis alone.

The cardiopulmonary status of the patient prior to embolism is also critical in determining the clinical severity of embolism. A small embolus may have limited impact upon an otherwise healthy individual but may have serious consequences in someone with advanced cardiac or pulmonary disease.

Both experimental and clinical studies have established that infarction—death of lung tissue—rarely accompanies embolic occlusion. It is likely that less than 10 percent of emboli in humans lead to infarction. That infarction rarely follows embolism should occasion little surprise. The lung has three avenues for obtaining oxygen: the pulmonary arterial circulation, the bronchial arterial circulation, and the airways. Thus, infarction occurs infrequently, and its appearance usually is associated with compromise of bronchial arterial flow and/or airways to the involved area. Such compromise is promoted by the existence of other cardiac or pulmonary diseases, such as left ventricular failure, mitral stenosis, and chronic obstructive lung disease. Thus, infarction may occur in 30 percent or more of such patients, while it is quite rare in individuals who are free of cardiopulmonary disease.

BEYOND THE ACUTE STATE The vast majority of pulmonary emboli resolve, and resolve rather quickly. Resolution of fresh emboli begins within the first few days and is well advanced in 10 to 14 days. As in DVT, two mechanisms promote restoration of vascular patency: the fibrinolytic system and the process of organization. However, the fibrinolytic system appears capable of more rapid dissolution of emboli than of venous thrombi.

The availability of these two efficient mechanisms raises the question as to why not all emboli resolve. There may be some impairment of the intrinsic fibrinolytic system. The emboli may have been well organized prior to their lodgment in the lung so that they are subject to neither fibrinolytic attack nor further organization. Alternatively, some emboli may be recurrent, so that their failure to resolve is more apparent than real.

Another important element of the natural history of thromboembolism is the development of bronchial arterial collateral circulation. If pulmonary arterial obstruction persists, bronchial arterial flow increases substantially over a period of several weeks, restoring flow to the capillary bed. With the return of flow, surfactant production is restored, so that alveolar stability is regained and atelectasis resolves.

DIAGNOSTIC FEATURES

Sudden onset of unexplained dyspnea should suggest the diagnosis of embolism. This symptom, related to the sudden addition of alveolar "dead space," is usually the only one which occurs. *Pleuritic chest pain and hemoptysis are present only when infarction has occurred* and, because bland embolism rarely leads to infarction, are usually absent. With extensive embolism, severe substernal oppressive discomfort may be present, probably due to right ventricular ischemia. Patients also may present with syncope, suggesting a neurologic disorder. The most reliable symptom, however, is breathlessness. Severe, persistent dyspnea is an ominous sign, for it usually indicates extensive embolic occlusion.

PHYSICAL EXAMINATION Findings on physical examination, like the history, may be deceptively normal. Examination of the lungs may disclose a few atelectatic rales; localized wheezes rarely are heard. A pleural friction rub or evidence of pleural effusion will not be present unless infarction has occurred.

On cardiac examination, the single consistent finding is tachycardia. Only in the rare cases of massive embolism will signs such as a right ventricular gallop, a palpable "lift" over the right ventricle, a loud pulmonary closure sound, or prominent *a* waves in the jugular venous pulse be found. A scratchy systolic ejection-type murmur may be heard in the pulmonic area. Also, a systolic or continuous murmur accentuated by inspiration may be audible over the lung fields. These murmurs appear to be generated by turbulence of flow in vessels partially obstructed by emboli since they disappear after resection or resolution of emboli. They should be carefully sought in any patient suspected of having PTE. Wide splitting of the second heart sound may be present. This indicates extensive embolic obstruction and implies both severe pulmonary hypertension and right ventricular failure. As embolic resolution occurs, this finding disappears. Absence of an accentuated pulmonic closure sound is not a reliable guide to the severity of PTE, since, when embolism is sufficiently massive to reduce cardiac output, pulmonary closure may be normal or diminished.

The detection of *deep venous thrombosis* qualifies as an excellent clue to the diagnosis of embolism, but its absence does not exclude embolism. Even when sought with diligence, *clinical* evidence of thrombophlebitis is found in less than half of patients with PTE. *Fever* in patients with pulmonary embolism is uncommon without complicating infection or infarction. With infarction, fever of 37.8 to 38.3°C (oral) is the rule; but temperature elevations to 39°C or above may occur, making the differentiation between pulmonary infarction and infection difficult.

On clinical grounds alone, then, a firm diagnosis of embolism cannot be made; the clinical *suspicion* of embolism requires confirmation by laboratory studies.

LABORATORY STUDIES Routine laboratory studies contribute little toward the diagnosis. Leukocytosis and elevation of the sedimentation rate are rarely present in the absence of infarction. A variety of other blood tests, such as assay for specific fibrinopeptides, fibrin degradation products, or enzymes, have been proposed; none has been shown to be diagnostically sensitive or specific.

Aside from tachycardia, the *electrocardiogram* is normal in most patients. With extensive embolization, there may be evidence of acute pulmonary hypertension, rightward shift of the QRS axis, a tall, peaked P wave, and ST-T changes indicative of right ventricular strain (Chap. 249). These changes are often transient, lasting minutes to hours, but when persistent, suggest severe pulmonary vascular obstruction.

The *chest roentgenogram* may show a parenchymal infiltrate and evidence of a pleural effusion if *infarction* has occurred. Characteristically, the infiltrates caused by infarction abut against the pleura. However, their shape varies, and they do not usually appear until 12 to 36 h after the embolism has occurred. The effusion, which often precedes the infiltrate, is characteristically small. Thoracentesis usually, but by no means invariably, yields hemorrhagic fluid, with the characteristics of an exudate.

The radiographic findings with embolism alone are more subtle. *Differences in diameter between vessels which should be of equivalent size* should raise the suspicion of embolism. For example, embolic obstruction of the right main pulmonary artery can lead to dilation of the left main pulmonary artery because that vessel must accept the entire pulmonary flow. There may be *abrupt "cutoff"* of a vessel; i.e., as the vessel is traced distally, it suddenly disappears. Clot has the same radiodensity as blood, accounting for the proximal shadow; the absence of flow beyond the clot explains the sudden radiographic "disappearance" of the vessel.

Organization of a clot within a pulmonary artery may lead to retraction of the vessel's walls and a so-called rattail configuration, in which the vessel is relatively normal proximally and suddenly tapers to a sharp point. Finally, there may be *abnormal radiolucency* in some lung zones due to absent or decreased flow. Such abnormally lucent areas, indicative of proximal arterial obstruction, are best appreciated by examining comparable areas in the two lung fields.

Even in embolization without infarction, the roentgenogram may show small infiltrates, which appear in about 24 h and reflect atelectasis secondary to surfactant depletion. They are not associated with effusion, may fail to touch a pleural surface, and disappear without the linear scarring characteristic of infarction. It should be emphasized that a *normal chest roentgenogram does not exclude the diagnosis of PTE.* Indeed, a *normal* chest roentgenogram is the *most common* finding in embolic disease.

Analysis of arterial blood gases Massive embolism is commonly associated with arterial hypoxemia, hypocapnia, and respiratory alkalosis. In addition, the difference between alveolar P_{CO_2} and arterial P_{CO_2} ($P_{A_{CO_2}} - P_{a_{CO_2}}$) may be widened owing to the increase in alveolar dead space (Chap. 271). However, a normal P_{O_2} does not exclude the diagnosis.

The laboratory tests discussed thus far are often negative in PTE and are relatively nonspecific. Therefore, it is usually necessary to proceed to two more definitive techniques: pulmonary perfusion and ventilation radiophotoscans and the pulmonary angiogram.

Pulmonary perfusion and ventilation scintiphotography Perfusion scintiphotographs (photoscans) are obtained by gamma camera imaging of the distribution of intravenously injected, gamma-emitting radionuclides. The most commonly used radionuclides are microspheres or macroaggregates of albumin (MAA), labeled with a gamma-emitting isotope such as technetium 99m. The radioactive particles, 50 to 100 μm in diameter, are trapped in the pulmonary capillary bed because the pulmonary capillaries approximate 10 μm in diameter. Alternatively, xenon 133 gas, dissolved in saline solution, may be used, but patients must hold their breath. The distribution of labeled particles entrapped in capillaries, or of xenon 133 evolved from them, accurately depicts the distribution of pulmonary blood flow.

The camera-generated perfusion image can be recorded on radiographic film, on special photographic film, on a television screen, or on videotape. Normal scans exhibit homogeneous distribution of radioactivity, smooth margins, and a configuration which corresponds to the normal anatomy of the lungs. Any deviation from these characteristics requires explanation because it represents an abnormality in blood flow distribution.

The perfusion lung photoscan is quite valuable in the diagnosis of embolism. A properly performed perfusion scan which is *normal* excludes the diagnosis of clinically significant pulmonary embolism. On the other hand, a scan demonstrating zones of absent or sharply decreased radioactivity in the patient whose other findings are compatible with PTE keeps the diagnosis of embolism among the possibilities. Scanning is simple, safe, and rapid. It can be repeated to define the resolution, or recurrence, of obstructive vascular phenomena. Like any laboratory test, however, the photoscan must be applied and interpreted with care. It is important, for example, to obtain multiple scan views because lesions not apparent in one view may be easily detected in another. Furthermore, the lung photoscan demonstrates only abnormalities of the *distribution of blood flow*. It does not provide anatomic information. Many disorders other than PTE are associated with abnormalities in the distribution of pulmonary blood flow. Any disease process, such as pneumonia, atelectasis, or pneumothorax, which reduces the ventilation of a lung zone will decrease its perfusion. Parenchymal diseases, such as emphysema, sarcoidosis, bronchogenic carcinoma, and tuberculosis, can all produce scan defects. Therefore a perfusion defect lacks specificity. The chest x-ray may aid in assessing the perfusion scan since a perfusion defect which occurs in the same area as an x-ray infiltrate does not point to a pulmonary embolus but may represent pneumonia, atelectasis, or infarction. However, despite the presence of an x-ray infiltrate, a perfusion scan may be useful in disclosing defects in other, clear lung zones. It must also be appreciated that a perfusion defect in a zone "clear" by chest x-ray may occur not only with embolism but also with such diverse disorders as emphysema and sarcoidosis.

When a perfusion defect does occur in a lung zone that is normal by chest x-ray, its specificity can be enhanced by also assessing the distribution of *ventilation* in the region(s) of abnormal blood flow. This is accomplished by performing a ventilation scan. This is achieved by having the patients breathe a radioactive gas such as xenon 133 or xenon 127. If vascular obstruction (e.g., embolism) is present, scans will demonstrate normal wash-in and, more important, normal wash-out of radioactivity from the embolized lung zones. However, if parenchymal disease is responsible for the perfusion abnormality, washin and/or washout will be abnormal. Thus, "mismatch" of perfusion and ventilation is characteristic of vascular obstruction; "match" is indicative of parenchymal disease. When perfusion defects are limited to areas of roentgenographic infiltration, however, ventilation scanning is of no value since the ventilation defect will always match the perfusion defect.

Pulmonary angiography This is the only means for providing anatomic information about the pulmonary vasculature. Injection of radiopaque material, preferably through a cardiac catheter advanced into the pulmonary artery, allows recording of a visual image of the pulmonary vessels. Cardiac catheterization and angiography require specialized personnel, a reasonable period for preparation and performance, and they entail more risk than the procedures discussed above. However, the procedure has the advantage of providing valuable hemodynamic data which may be necessary for therapeutic decisions. Interpretive limitations of angiography are of three types: (1) *Injection artifacts* may occur which suggest absence of flow to a vessel. Injection should be repeated whenever the question of such artifacts exists. (2) The inability to evaluate the patency of small vessels is another limitation. Emboli in vessels below the resolving capability of the method cannot be detected with certainty, although magnification techniques can extend resolving capability. (3) Interpretive errors may also be a consequence of *not looking for the proper type of defect.* There are only two diagnostic findings. One is the *abrupt "cutoff"* of a vessel at the point of embolic impaction. However, complete embolic obstruction is uncommon. Therefore, *filling defects* are the most frequent finding; i.e., the embolus creates a "negative" shadow as the radiopaque material flows around it. The major contraindication to angiography is the absence of personnel who are experienced in both performing the procedure and interpreting the results. Serious diagnostic errors are commonplace if optimal techniques are not used or the complexities of interpretation are not appreciated. However, the risks of angiography are low in experienced hands. Injection of large boluses of contrast medium into the main pulmonary artery should be avoided in favor of small injections into vessels supplying lung regions identified as abnormal on the perfusion scan.

How far one should proceed down the diagnostic pathway outlined above depends on many factors, the major ones being the severity of the patient's symptoms and the hazards of contemplated therapy. Both condition the need for precise diagnosis. If misdiagnosis in either direction carries high risk, precision is mandatory. If this is not provided by photoscanning, then there should be no hesitancy in proceeding to angiography. However, if local expertise is lacking in either scanning or angiography, that procedure which is most reliable should be performed—or the patient should be transferred to a facility where such procedures are known to be reliable.

TREATMENT

Initial intravenous administration of heparin is the therapy of choice for PTE. With a strong *suspicion* of embolism based on clinical and routine laboratory tests, such therapy should be instituted immediately, without awaiting diagnostic confirmation, unless the initial dose of heparin places the patient at clear risk (i.e., in patients with recent or active bleeding or a known hemostatic defect). Except in such patients, heparin therapy should not await diagnostic confirmation; one can always stop therapy if such confirmation is not forthcoming.

There is consensus regarding the goals of therapy in both DVT and PTE: (1) immediate inhibition of the growth of thromboemboli, (2) promotion of thromboembolic resolution, and (3) prevention of recurrence. Heparin achieves the first goal; it encourages the second by allowing fibrinolytic dissolution to be achieved unopposed by thrombus growth; and it assists in, although it does not assure, prevention of recurrence. In addition, heparin inhibits platelet aggregation (and therefore serotonin release) at the embolic site, and its anticoagulant action is promptly reversible.

There is *not* consensus, however, regarding (1) heparin regimens which best combine safety and efficacy; (2) the need for, and type of, tests for monitoring coagulation behavior during heparin therapy; (3) how long, and with what agents, antithrombotic therapy should be maintained; or (4) in which patients thrombolytic therapy should antedate antithrombotic therapy.

REGIMENS In DVT, three methods of heparin administration have been advocated by various investigators: continuous intravenous, intermittent intravenous, intermittent subcutaneous. Continuous intravenous heparin is usually given in a dose of approximately 1000 units per hour. Intermittent intravenous heparin is commonly given in a dose of approximately 5000 units every 4 h or 7500 every 6 h. Subcutaneous heparin has been recommended as a dose of 5000 units every 4 h, 10,000 every 8 h, or 20,000 every 12 h. Studies exist which indicate that each of these regimens is more efficacious, safer, or both. Therefore, at this time, one can conclude only that *each* of these regimens (which approximate 30,000 units per 24 h) represents an acceptable treatment regimen. At present, the continuous intravenous regimen, delivered by an infusion pump, is the most popular. *Intramuscular* injection of heparin is to be avoided because hematomas will develop.

In PTE, the same options for heparin therapy exist. The only additional question is whether an initial large intravenous bolus (10,000 to 20,000 units) should be given to inhibit the aggregation (and release reaction) of platelets adherent to the embolus. Most workers advocate such a dose, with one of the "standard" regimens being started 2 to 4 h later.

MONITORING The value of clotting times (CT), partial thromboplastin times (PTT), or other coagulation tests to monitor heparin effect and guide alterations in dose is not clearly established. The risk of hemorrhage (the principal complication of heparin therapy) is not clearly related to coagulation test alterations; rather, it appears related to factors such as the coexistence of other diseases associated with bleeding risk (gastric or duodenal ulcer, coagulopathies, uremia) and advanced age. Likewise, achievement of the desired effect of heparin (cessation of thrombus growth in vivo) has not been related to coagulation tests. Therefore, it is questionable whether monitoring with such tests is superior to empiric use of one of the regimens described above. If done improperly or poorly timed, these tests are worthless and may be misleading. If used appropriately, the usual objective is to keep the CT or PTT, measured *just prior to the next* intermittent dose, at 1.5 to 2.0 times the base-line CT or PTT and at 1.5 to 2.5 times control with continuous infusion.

DURATION OF THERAPY In DVT, one of the "full-dose" regimens is usually maintained for 7 to 10 days, the rationale being that this is the period required for dissolution and/or organization of the thrombus. In PTE, for the same reasons, a similar duration of therapy is advised. Bed rest is indicated until cardiopulmonary or leg symptoms subside. Carefully applied elastic support hose should be used (to encourage venous flow) as soon as leg pain, if present, subsides.

Beyond the acute phase, there are three therapeutic options available: cessation of heparin, maintenance of low-dose heparin, or initiation of therapy with *prothrombinopenic drugs.* In deciding among these options, it should be recognized that the question being addressed is: does the patient need continued protection against the risk of *recurrent* DVT (and, therefore, PTE)? If the risk factor(s) that precipitated the acute episode of DVT-PTE is no longer present, the patient is asymptomatic, and impedance plethysmography is normal, it is acceptable to reduce heparin to a lower dose starting on day 7, ambulate the patient, and, if no symptoms develop, discontinue heparin on day 9 or 10. If these criteria are not met, prolonged prophylactic therapy seems warranted. There is no consensus regarding the optimal duration of such therapy because firm data on this point are lacking. If *reversible* risk factors are present (e.g., immobilization after a leg fracture), therapy should be continued until the risk factors present have resolved. If the risk factors present are nonreversible (e.g., severe left and/or right ventricular failure) or if the IPG remains positive, empiric decisions are made. At a minimum, 3 months of therapy seems wise because recurrence is relatively common during this period. Beyond 3 months, however, continuation depends upon the balance between specific risk factors exhibited by the patient and the risks of continued therapy. In some instances, this balance may warrant lifetime maintenance on anticoagulant drugs.

Prothrombinopenic drugs are not suitable for initial therapy in thromboembolism. Their only role is in maintaining anticoagulant protection for prolonged periods. If prothrombinopenic drugs are to be used, the patient should be "in range" as defined by a prothrombin time 1.5 to 2.5 times the control time for 3 to 5 days before heparin is discontinued. An alternative to the prothrombinopenic agents is the use of self-injected subcutaneous heparin. Current data suggest that a dose of 5000 to 10,000 units every 12 h is adequate for this type of prophylaxis, is well tolerated, and need not be monitored with coagulation tests.

These post-PTE prophylactic regimens should be maintained until the risk factor(s) favoring recurrence has subsided.

Thrombolytic (fibrinolytic) agents such as streptokinase and urokinase can hasten the resolution of venous thrombi and pulmonary emboli. They do not replace antithrombotic therapy. When used, thrombolytic agents must be followed by a standard course of antithrombotic therapy. Despite extensive study and a clear demonstration that these agents can enhance the speed of resolution, it has not been established that their use alters the short- or long-term morbidity or mortality rates among patients with either DVT or PTE. Both drugs are associated with hemorrhagic risk, particularly in patients who recently have had, or require, any invasive procedure (e.g., venipuncture, arterial puncture, angiography, Swan-Ganz catheterization). If they do offer a therapeutic advantage, it would appear to be (1) in patients with extensive, large-vein DVT (e.g., iliofemoral); and (2) in patients with massive embolism and persistent systemic hypotension in whom embolectomy would otherwise be contemplated.

Surgical therapy for DVT (thrombectomy) is now rarely considered because the results have not been encouraging. In PTE, surgical therapy should be reserved for those patients in whom heparin therapy is deemed inadequate or impractical. Anticoagulant therapy may be contraindicated by the presence of a bleeding diathesis, or the patient may be in such critical condition that it is felt unwise to await a response to medical therapy. In such instances *venous interruption* and *pulmonary embolectomy* must be considered.

The objective of venous interruption is to prevent immediate recurrence of embolism. Ligation of the superficial femoral vein offers no protection against embolization from the deep femoral venous system, and ligation of the common femoral vein is unacceptable because of severe obstruction to venous drainage. Furthermore, these procedures must be bilateral to grant protection from a suspected embolic focus in the legs. For these reasons, interruption of the inferior vena cava has replaced more distal ligation procedures. A number of surgical procedures have been applied to the inferior vena cava: simple ligation; plication, in which fine channels are preserved; and the application of totally or partially occlusive clips or filters. Nonsurgical interruption also can be accomplished by introducing "umbrella" or balloon devices, attached to catheters, into the inferior vena cava via neck or upper-extremity veins. Each procedure has advantages and disadvantages. For example, total interruption leads to a transient fall in cardiac output and variable degrees of edema of the legs; successful plication does not prevent small emboli from reaching the lungs; devices introduced into the inferior vena cava may migrate upward or be badly placed. Unfortunately, no form of inferior vena caval interruption precludes embolic recurrence. There are several reasons for this; sizable collateral channels develop weeks to months after interruption of the cava, through which embolization may recur; thromboembolism may originate at the site of caval manipulation; caval blockade does not prevent embolization from foci within the right cardiac chambers. Therefore, because most pulmonary emboli do resolve, caval interruption should be regarded as a *lifesaving procedure* to be restricted to patients who could not tolerate an *immediate* embolic recurrence. To elect this procedure, definite evidence of cardiopulmonary compromise by embolism is required, and there should be reasonable assurance that the embolic source is in the caval drainage area.

Caval interruption is not a formidable surgical procedure but may be associated with substantial morbidity. It should be used therefore only when required, and with recognition that it does not necessarily provide long-term protection. There is one instance, however, in which prompt caval ligation is the therapy of choice: septic thrombophlebitis of pelvic origin with multiple septic pulmonary emboli. If these patients do not respond promptly to a heparin-antibiotic regimen, they may die unless caval (and left ovarian vein) ligation is carried out promptly.

Two criteria should be met before emergency pulmonary embolectomy is performed: (1) there must be evidence of severe hemodynamic compromise due to embolism which is not responsive to supportive measures, particularly sustained systemic hypotension; and (2) the personnel and equipment required for embolectomy carried out with the aid of cardiopulmonary bypass must be available.

SPECIAL CONSIDERATIONS Total resolution of emboli does not always occur. If residual vascular obstruction is substantial, the patient may present, months or years after the actual embolic events, with dyspnea and pulmonary hypertension of uncertain cause. Multiple undetected recurrent small emboli may produce the same picture. The latter condition may be misdiagnosed as "chronic lung disease" or "primary" pulmonary hypertension (Chap. 281) or cor pulmonale of unclear etiology (Chap. 262).

Such patients should be studied by appropriate techniques, since larger emboli are potentially resectable (thromboendarterectomy), even after having been present for months to years. These conditions are potentially curable forms of otherwise fatal pulmonary hypertensive disease.

Embolism should also be suspected in other clinical contexts: as a precipitating cause for cardiac arrhythmia; as a reason for sudden or progressive worsening of congestive heart failure (Chap. 253); as an explanation for sudden deterioration in the patient with chronic obstructive pulmonary disease; and as a possible alternative to the diagnosis of "psychic" hyperventilation.

PROGNOSIS IN PULMONARY EMBOLISM The prognosis of the patient with pulmonary embolism *in whom therapy is promptly instituted* is excellent. As stated at the outset of this chapter, less than 1 embolic event in 10 is lethal. The majority of these deaths occur suddenly and can be avoided only by prophylaxis (see above). The remainder appear to be due to embolic extension or recurrence, which therapy can moderate. Thus, for patients who survive long enough to reach medical attention and receive heparin, the outlook is quite good. Morbidity following embolism is uncommon since embolic resolution is the rule and few patients develop the pulmonary hypertensive problem noted above.

Limited reliable data are available regarding recurrence rates in the months and years after a single embolic event (with or without prolonged postembolic anticoagulant therapy). In the absence of risk factors, recurrence appears to be uncommon, but more precise data are needed.

NONTHROMBOTIC EMBOLISM

Because the lung vasculature serves as a filter of the venous circulation, it is the recipient of diverse materials which can gain entry into venous blood, including bone marrow, foreign bodies, parasites, and tumor cells. The most frequently encountered form of nonthrombotic embolism is *fat embolism*. This dramatic and controversial entity follows the introduction of neutral fat into the venous circulation, most commonly after bone trauma or fracture (marrow fat), but occasionally after trauma to adipose tissue or liver infiltrated by fat. The clinical sequence is characteristic. After a latent period of 12 to 36 h or more, during which the patient is asymptomatic, sudden cardiopulmonary and neurologic deterioration appears. Mental aberrations, delirium, and coma develop. Dyspnea, tachypnea, and tachycardia occur, and the chest roentgenographic and physiologic components of the "adult respiratory distress syndrome" appear (see Chap. 287). Anemia and thrombocytopenia are common, as are petechiae on the upper thorax and arms. The pathogenesis of the syndrome is not clear, but it seems likely that two events occur: release of free fatty acids (by action of lipases on the neutral fat) which induces a toxic vasculitis, followed by platelet-fibrin thrombosis; and actual obstruction of small pulmonary arteries by macroaggregates of fat. Several forms of therapy have been proposed (corticosteroids, heparin, ethanol), but none has proved effective; treatment remains supportive and mortality rate high.

Another dramatic form of nonthrombotic embolism is *amniotic fluid embolism*. This occurs during both spontaneous delivery and cesarean section. Sudden and massive obstruction of the pulmonary microvasculature occurs, leading to shock and, often, death. With survival of the initial phase of the disease, the picture of disseminated intravascular coagulation appears. The syndrome is due to the entrance of a significant quantity of amniotic fluid into the venous circulation. This fluid is a potent thromboplastic agent which induces thrombosis in the pulmonary vasculature and elsewhere. The fluid also contains particulates which lodge in the lung. Treatment consists of supportive measures.

Nonembolic pulmonary arterial obstruction due to *vasculitis* has become a common problem among intravenous drug users. This vasculitis, caused by the drugs per se or materials (e.g., talc) mixed with the drugs, can induce thrombosis. This entity may be difficult to distinguish from PTE. Repetitive episodes may lead to irreversible and severe pulmonary hypertension.

REFERENCES

BELL WR, MEEK AG: Guidelines for the use of thrombolytic agents. N Engl J Med 301:1266, 1979

CHEELY R et al: The role of noninvasive tests versus pulmonary angiography in the diagnosis of pulmonary embolism. Am J Med 70:17, 1981

CONTI S, DASCHBACH M: Venous thromboembolism prophylaxis. Arch Surg 117:1036, 1982

DAILY PO et al: Surgical management of chronic pulmonary embolism: Surgical technic and late results. J Thorac Cardiovasc Surg 79:523, 1980

HAVIG GO: Source of pulmonary emboli. Acta Hir Scand 478(Suppl):42, 1977

HULL R et al: Adjusted subcutaneous heparin versus warfarin sodium in the long-term treatment of venous thrombosis. N Engl J Med 305:189, 1982

KAKKAR VV et al: Prevention of post-operative embolism by low-dose heparin: An international multicenter trial. Lancet 2:45, 1975

MCFADDEN ER, BRAUNWALD E: Cor pulmonale and pulmonary thromboembolism, in *Heart Disease*, 2d ed, E Braunwald (ed). Philadelphia, Saunders, 1983

MOSER KM, LEMOINE JR: Is embolic risk conditioned by location of deep venous thrombosis? Ann Intern Med 94:439, 1981

———: Pulmonary vascular obstruction due to embolism and thrombosis, in *Pulmonary Vascular Disease*, KM Moser (ed). New York, Dekker, 1979, pp 341–386

———: Diagnostic approaches to pulmonary embolism. J Resp Dis 2:78, 1981

SASAHARA AA, DALEN JE: Controversy: Should fibrinolytic drugs be used to treat acute pulmonary embolism? J Cardiovasc Med 5:793, 1980

Urokinase-Streptokinase Embolism Trial. Phase 2 results. JAMA 229:1606, 1974

WILSON JE et al: Heparin therapy in venous thromboembolism. Am J Med 70:808, 1981

Other abnormalities of the respiratory tract

283

DISEASES OF THE UPPER RESPIRATORY TRACT

LOUIS WEINSTEIN

Disorders of the upper respiratory tract (nose, nasopharynx, paranasal sinuses, and larynx) are among the commonest forms of human illness. In most instances, they result in discomfort which is more annoying and distracting than disabling, and while they may interfere with the individual's function sufficiently to prevent participation in normal activities, usually they are not life-threatening and do not lead to serious chronic disability. Less commonly, more serious disorders may present with symptoms referable to the upper respiratory tract.

NOSE

ANOSMIA Total loss of olfactory sense is most common as a transient manifestation of acute infections of the upper respiratory tract. It may be present with chronic nasal obstruction due to edema of the mucosa or marked swelling of the turbinates and with congenital defects, ozena, tumors (see below), trauma involving the olfactory nerves, and nasal polyps.

RHINITIS AND NASAL OBSTRUCTION Intermittent or persistent nasal discharge may be caused by a variety of disorders, including hay fever, vasomotor rhinitis and complicating nasal polyposis, acute coryza, and other forms of viral rhinitis, the upper respiratory manifestations of measles, syphilis (the "snuffles" of the congenital disease), tuberculosis, and nasal diphtheria, intranasal foreign bodies, and chronic use of vasoconstrictor drugs.

Acute and self-limited nasal obstruction is usually associated with acute upper respiratory tract infections, most commonly viral. Hypertrophy and inflammation of the turbinates leading to nasal obstruction, with or without persistent nasal discharge, may be caused by allergic reactions. A common reason for difficulty in breathing through the nose is a *deviated septum.* Menstruation is associated, in some instances, with bogginess of the turbinates to a degree sufficient to produce retardation of airflow through the nose; pregnancy may produce the same phenomenon.

RHINORRHEA Although unilateral nasal discharge may be caused by intranasal foreign bodies, when it is intermittent or persistent, the possibility that it is due to *cerebrospinal fluid (CSF) rhinorrhea* must be considered. This condition may be diagnosed by injecting a marker such as a dye (fluorescein) or a radioactive tracer into the CSF and following its appearance in nasal secretions. A positive reaction for glucose indicates that the nasal discharge is cerebrospinal fluid.

OZENA This is a severe chronic rhinitis of unknown cause, characterized by thick, greenish discharge, mucosal crusts, atrophy of the turbinates, and an offensive odor. Patients eventually become anosmic. Even when the nasal passages are widened and resistance to airflow is decreased, obstruction is a constant complaint. Cultures grow gram-negative bacilli (*Klebsiella, Pseudomonas,* etc.). Treatment, aimed at reducing the odor, includes use of local or systemic antibiotics and large doses of vasodilators [tolazoline (Priscoline), nicotinic acid]. Local cleansing by means of repeated saline irrigation is extremely important to eliminate foul-smelling crusts.

EPISTAXIS Probably the commonest cause is nose picking, leading to tearing of the rich network of veins in the anterior nares (Kiesselbach's plexus). Among the infections in which acute nosebleed may develop are typhoid fever, unilateral nasal diphtheria, pertussis, and malaria. Minor epistaxis may also appear in the course of viral infections of the upper respiratory tract. Other causes of intermittent or repeated episodes of epistaxis are atheromas of the nasal vessels, hypertension, vicarious menstruation, bleeding diatheses including thrombocytopenia of different etiologies and deficiencies of clotting factors, polycythemia vera, rhinoliths, acute sinusitis especially involving the ethmoid sinus with thrombosis of the ethmoidal vein, tumors of the nose and paranasal sinuses, and nasal angiomas. Episodes of bleeding or the severity of attacks are frequently increased in patients receiving aspirin. Vitamin C and prothrombin deficiency are *not* associated with isolated epistaxis, although this may occur with bleeding from other sites. In hereditary hemorrhagic telangiectasia (Osler-Rendu-Weber syndrome) the only site of bleeding may be the nose; a family history of repeated hemorrhages from this and other sites should suggest this diagnosis.

NASAL FURUNCULOSIS Furuncles involving the internal or external surfaces of the nose pose potential threats to life because of the possibility of spread to the cavernous sinus via the draining veins. When seen in their early stage, they respond rapidly to antimicrobial therapy which should be directed primarily against *Staphylococcus aureus* and given in large doses (Chap. 147). Oral treatment may be adequate in the early stages of the disease, but parenteral therapy is necessary when the constitutional reaction is severe and there is marked edema of the intra- or extranasal tissues. *Under no circumstances should these lesions be squeezed* because of the danger of spread of organisms to intracranial venous sinuses. Also, incision for drainage should not be carried out unless pain becomes severe or the lesion has become large.

NASAL TUMORS Basal-cell carcinoma of the skin covering the nose is the commonest malignant tumor of this organ. Rodent ulcer resulting from local spread of a basal-cell lesion may involve not only the skin over the external nasal surface and adjacent areas of the face, but may also invade intranasally and produce marked destruction of the internal structures.

PHARYNX

ACUTE PHARYNGITIS The outstanding symptom of acute pharyngitis, regardless of cause, is a sore throat. About two-thirds of all acute illnesses in families are viral infections of the upper respiratory tract, with varying degrees of pharyngeal discomfort present. The acute pharyngitides can be classified into three groups: (1) treatable infections, (2) untreatable infections, and (3) noninfectious disorders (Table 283-1).

Physical examination of the pharyngeal mucosa may reveal changes varying in intensity from mild redness and congestion of blood vessels (many viral infections) to intense red-purple color, patchy yellow exudate, hypertrophy of all the lymphoid tissue, and marked vascular injection (e.g., severe disease due to group A *Streptococcus pyogenes*). Symptoms may be variable and may range from a complaint of "scratchy throat" to pain so severe that swallowing of saliva is difficult. The presence of exudate does not establish a specific etiology and may be noted in infections due to *S. pyogenes, Hemophilus influenzae, H. parainfluenzae* (children), *Corynebacterium diphtheriae, Streptococcus pneumoniae* (rare) as well as in some viral diseases, such as those caused by adenovirus and Epstein-Barr (EB) virus. Ulcerations involving the posterior pharyngeal wall and/or tonsils are characteristically present in fusobacterial infections (Plaut-Vincent's angina), pharyngeal tularemia, syphilis (primary chancre), tuberculosis, following local trauma to the pharynx, and in immunosuppressed and agranulocytic patients in whom invasion by fusobacteria or other members of the indigenous pharyngeal microflora takes place. The presence of limited or extensive pseudomembrane does not always indicate a specific microbial cause. While most characteristic of faucial diphtheria, such lesions may be present in infectious mononucleosis (EB virus), agranulocytosis, staphylococcal pharyngitis, and diffuse injury to the pharyngeal mucosa following direct trauma or chemical or thermal burns.

The tonsils are often involved in the course of viral and bacterial pharyngitis; they may be markedly reddened and swollen and contain exudate in the crypts.

The etiologic diagnosis of acute pharyngitis is difficult to establish on the basis of visual examination of the throat. However, in some instances in which characteristic findings are present, such as the typical pseudomembrane and suggestive odor of diphtheria, severe group A streptococcal infection, the ulceration and anaerobic odor of fusobacterial disease, or the white irregular patches overlying shallow ulcers produced by *Candida,* a specific cause may be suspected.

Cultures of the pharyngeal mucosa, tonsils, or exudate will usually reveal the bacteria responsible for the disease and determine the choice of antimicrobial agent. It should be stressed, however, that these are not always rewarding. For example, only 70 percent of single throat cultures yield group A *S. pyogenes,* even when pharyngitis due to this organism is severe. Patients suspected of having streptococcal pharyngitis but whose throat cultures fail to yield the organism should be treated if this kind of disease is known to be present in the community in which they live at the time they present. The sore throat of subacute thyroiditis may be relieved occasionally by the administration of thyroid hormone or prednisone. None of the viral pharyngitides is treatable.

Gonococcal pharyngitis is almost always the result of orogenital contact. The incidence of the disease in heterosexual men varies from 0.2 to 1.4 percent. It ranges from 5 to 25 percent in homosexual males; 20 percent of those with genital infection have simultaneous involvement of the throat. From 5 to 18 percent of women with other manifestations of gonorrhea have pharyngitis; in 1 to 3 percent this is the only disease. While mild to severe sore throat is present in about 30 percent of patients, the majority are asymptomatic. Because the clinical features of gonococcal pharyngitis may mimic disease produced by other organisms, the diagnosis is based on isolation and identification of *Neisseria gonorrhoeae.* This is accomplished by culturing pharyngeal secretions on Thayer-Martin medium immediately after they are obtained; incubation in an atmosphere of 5% CO_2 is required. The isolated organism must be confirmed as the gonococcus by its biological properties because of the presence of other *Neisseria* in the pharynges of most normal individuals.

PERITONSILLAR CELLULITIS AND ABSCESS (QUINSY) This condition is most often a complication of acute pharyngitis. The organisms commonly involved are group A *S. pyogenes* and *S. aureus.* The first sign of this disease is marked enlargement of the tonsils, which are surrounded by red, edematous pillars. The tonsillar and peritonsillar hypertrophy may progress to a degree threatening occlusion of the upper airway. High-grade fever and leukocytosis are present, and severe rigors may occur. In its early stages, the process is a cellulitis, but, in the absence of therapy, abscess develops as infection progresses and involves one or both tonsils; at this time, soft grayish-white exudate may cover the tonsillar surfaces. The diagnosis is made on the basis of the physical findings. If detected early when only peritonsillar cellulitis is present, administration of a properly selected antimicrobial agent may clear the infection and abort the development of abscess. Antimicrobial therapy alone is inadequate after abscess has developed. The optimal treatment at this stage is incision and drainage of the involved tonsil(s).

PARAPHARYNGEAL SPACE ABSCESS This syndrome is always a complication of acute pharyngitis. Primary or secondary bacterial invasion of one of the tonsils results in the development of an intratonsillar abscess accompanied by considerable edema and inflammatory reaction in the parapharyngeal space. The lesion is usually unilateral and the involved tonsil protrudes toward the midline; there is frequently very little pharyngeal discomfort, but there is marked tenderness at the angle of the jaw on the same side as the tonsillar abscess. The remainder of the throat frequently has a benign appearance. There is usually considerable fever and leukocytosis. If unrecognized and not treated early in its course, the infection spreads through the tonsillar veins to the jugular vein, where it produces thrombophlebitis. Septic emboli from this source may be widely disseminated and cause widespread metastatic thrombosis and infection with single or multiple abscesses of the lungs, a highly fatal syndrome termed *postanginal sepsis.* Early recognition and institution of therapy before spread to the jugular vein results in rapid clearing of the infection.

RETROPHARYNGEAL ABSCESS Infection of the retropharyngeal lymph nodes occurs most often as a complication of acute bacterial pharyngitis in children 3 years of age or younger; these nodes disappear rapidly after this age. Adults usually acquire the disease as a result of injury to the posterior pharyngeal wall by a sharp object, as a complication of neglected acute infections of the middle ear, during the course of tuberculosis, or secondary to suppurative parotitis. A universal symptom is the sensation of a "lump in the throat that cannot be swallowed." Dyspnea that is present in the sitting position and absent when patients lie on their back and pain on swallowing are common. The voice has a characteristic quality that has been likened to the cry of a duck (*cri du canard*). Coughing, snoring, choking, and stertorous breathing are often present. As the abscess enlarges, progressive airway obstruction develops, marked edema and redness of the entire posterior pharynx and cervical lymphadenopathy are common, and there is usually high fever. When recognized early, most retropharyngeal abscesses respond promptly to antimicrobial therapy. Because most of the organisms involved are gram-positive cocci, parenteral administration of a penicillinase-resistant penicillin or a cephalosporin compound is usually effective; in young children, therapy must include agents effective against *H. influenzae.* If the abscess comes to attention late in its course or if obstruction of the airway is progressing rapidly, the lesion must be drained surgically and chemotherapy must be given before, during, and after the procedure. Tracheostomy may be necessary in far-advanced cases.

TUMORS OF THE TONSILS Carcinoma of the tonsil is the second commonest tumor of the upper airway (osteoma being the commonest; see below). Other neoplastic tonsillar lesions include lymphoma and Hodgkin's disease. Persistence of pain in one enlarged firm tonsil, in the absence of an infectious

TABLE 283-1
Etiology of pharyngitis

- *I* Infections
  - *A* Treatable
    - *1* Group A *Streptococcus pyogenes*
    - *2* *Hemophilus influenzae*
    - *3* *H. parainfluenzae*
    - *4* *Neisseria gonorrhoeae*
    - *5* *N. meningitidis*
    - *6* *Corynebacterium diphtheriae*
    - *7* *Spirochaeta pallida*
    - *8* *Fusobacterium*
    - *9* *F. tularensis*
    - *10* *Candida*
    - *11* *Cryptococcus*
    - *12* *Histoplasma*
    - *13* *Mycoplasma pneumoniae*
    - *14* *Streptococcus pneumoniae* (?)
    - *15* *Staphylococcus aureus* or gram-negative bacilli are rare and are usually found in neutropenic patients or those treated with antibiotics
  - *B* Untreatable
    - *1* Primary
      - *a* Influenza virus
      - *b* Rhinovirus
      - *c* Coxsackievirus A
      - *d* Epstein-Barr virus
      - *e* Echovirus
      - *f* Herpes simplex
      - *g* Reovirus
    - *2* Manifestation of systemic disease
      - *a* Poliomyelitis
      - *b* Measles
      - *c* Chickenpox
      - *d* Smallpox
      - *e* Viral hepatitis
      - *f* Rubella
      - *g* Pertussis
- *II* Noninfectious
  - *A* Trauma by heat, sharp objects, etc.
  - *B* Inhalation of irritants
  - *C* Dehydration—mouth breathing
  - *D* Glossopharyngeal neuralgia
  - *E* Subacute thyroiditis (tends to be prolonged or frequently recurrent, often associated with low-grade fever)
  - *F* Psychogenic
  - *G* Monomyelocytic leukemia
  - *H* Immunosuppressed state

process, is an indication for biopsy. The presence of fever does not rule out a neoplastic lesion, because considerable elevation of the temperature may be present when lymphoma is the cause.

LINGUAL TONSILS These are situated on the posterior borders of the tongue and extend from the circumvallate papillae to the epiglottis. Infection produces lingual pain that may be severe and markedly increased by movement of the tongue. Sore throat is often absent or mild; when the responsible organism is *S. pyogenes,* fever is present. Examination of the posterior tongue reveals swelling and redness of the lymphoid masses; yellow exudate is present in the crypts when group A streptococci are the cause of the disease. The pharynx may appear normal or only slightly reddened.

SINUSES

ACUTE SINUSITIS The organisms most often responsible for acute sinusitis are *S. pneumoniae,* group A *S. pyogenes, S. aureus,* and *H. influenzae.* Other bacteria may be involved in patients receiving immunosuppressive therapy, in those who have received antibiotics, or in whom penetrating trauma, local tumors, or vasculitis is a predisposing factor. The etiology of chronic sinusitis may be the same as that of the acute form, but more than one pathogen may be present. In many instances, however, cultures yield only members of the indigenous microflora of the upper respiratory tract.

The commonest predisposing factor of acute purulent sinusitis is viral infection of the upper respiratory tract, which may lead to obstruction of drainage of the paranasal sinuses and the development of localized pain, tenderness, and low-grade fever. These manifestations usually clear as the viral disease subsides. In a number of instances, however, invasion by pyogenic bacteria supervenes and is responsible for the development of purulent sinusitis. Obstruction of meatal drainage of any type or direct introduction of bacteria into the sinuses may lead to the development of acute infection of the paranasal sinuses. Abscesses of the roots of the upper bicuspid or molar teeth that rupture into the maxillary sinuses, swimming and diving, and direct local injury may be inciting mechanisms. Fractures of the bones encompassing the sinuses, especially the frontals and ethmoids, may be followed by infection. Wegener's granulomatosis and tumors of the meatuses of the turbinates may produce the clinical picture of acute or chronic sinusitis. In some of these patients, bacterial infection is superimposed, and these patients are studied only after infection develops, the underlying lesion often being overlooked. This underscores the fact that recurrent or prolonged episodes of sinusitis that are refractory to antimicrobial therapy, or that relapse soon after treatment is discontinued, must be investigated thoroughly for the presence of a noninfectious obstructing lesion.

The diagnosis of acute purulent sinusitis is usually made when constitutional manifestations are present, such as fever, chills, pain and tenderness of the involved sinuses, nasal obstruction, and recurrent headaches that change in intensity with position and disappear shortly after getting out of bed. Isolation of a pathogenic organism from the nasal secretions or from material draining into the meatuses of the nasal turbinates may help to solidify the diagnosis. When there is marked swelling of the turbinates, they can be shrunk by the local application of cocaine or other potent vasoconstrictors. This exposes the meatuses and permits the collection of exudate draining directly from the involved sinus. Transillumination of the sinuses is also helpful, while radiologic study is of value in identifying the specific sinus involved.

Frontal sinusitis is characterized by pain over the forehead approximately in the area of the underlying sinus. Although the overlying site is usually normal, it may be swollen and reddened over an area outlining the sinuses. Pressure applied over the sinuses and on the lateral edge of the orbital ridges produces pain. Examination of the nasal turbinates shows purulent exudate in the middle or superior meatus if drainage is not prevented by swelling of these structures. Pain, swelling, and tenderness in the anterior portions of the maxillae are the outstanding features of *maxillary sinusitis.* When the infection is severe, pain may be referred to the upper teeth which may become loosened, and hemorrhage may be present in the surrounding tissues. Pus is visible in the middle meatus of the turbinates. The symptoms and signs of *ethmoid sinusitis* are pain in the upper lateral areas of the nose, frontal headache, and redness of the skin and tenderness to pressure over the upper lateral areas of the nasal bones adjacent to the inner canthi of the eyes. Pus is visible in the middle meatus when the anterior cells of the sinus are involved, and in the superior meatus if the posterior cells are infected; in most instances, both areas of the sinus are involved and exudate is present in both meatuses. The manifestations of infection of the *sphenoid sinus* are tenderness and pain over the vertex of the skull, the mastoid bones (in the presence of normal tympanic membranes), and the occipital portion of the head. Rarely, streaks of redness may be detectable over both zygomas as a result of irritation of the maxillary branch of the trigeminal nerve that lies in close proximity to the sinus.

Osteomyelitis of the frontal bone is a rare complication of frontal sinusitis. This is characterized by fever, chills, leukocytosis, frontal headache, and the presence of cool, pale edema over the forehead (Pott's puffy tumor). Involvement of the bone in which the ethmoid sinus lies may be manifested by unilateral or bilateral exophthalmos when one or both sinuses are involved. This is usually due to a sterile or pyogenic orbital cellulitis secondary to a "sympathetic" inflammation or perforation of the lamina papyracea, the lateral wall of the sinus, and the medial wall of the orbit. Impairment of venous return from the orbits may lead to the development of retinal hemorrhages. Intracranial spread of infection from the sinuses through the diploic veins may lead to meningitis, infection, and thrombosis of the superficial cerebral veins or cavernous and sagittal venous sinuses, cranial nerve palsies, and extradural abscess.

Bacterial meningitis is also a rare complication of purulent sinusitis, usually involving the frontal sinuses, and associated with cranial osteomyelitis and subdural and brain abscess. Sudden onset of convulsions, hemiplegia, and aphasia in a patient with acute frontal sinusitis should suggest the possibility of subdural abscess with thrombophlebitis of the sagittal sinus or superficial cerebral veins. Infections of the ethmoid sinus may be complicated by paralysis of the third cranial nerve due to invasion of the dural sinuses, or profuse epistaxis as a result of thrombosis of the ethmoidal veins that drain into the cavernous sinus, which may become thrombosed. Chronic or recurrent purulent sinusitis may eventually be responsible for the development of bronchiectasis. An unusual form of chronic sinusitis in association with bronchiectasis and situs inversus is *Kartagener's syndrome.* Patients with these disorders have been noted to have delayed mucociliary transport in the lower airways—the immotile ciliary syndrome; this is accompanied in men by lack of motility of sperm, the numbers of which are normal.

CHRONIC SINUSITIS It is difficult to establish the diagnosis of chronic sinusitis in the absence of documented recurrences of acute purulent infection. Many patients complaining of headaches, often frontal in nature, and troubled by obstruction of the nasal airway, may have some degree of tenderness over any of the paranasal sinuses. X-ray examinations of the sinuses often reveal thickening of the mucous membranes. Cultures of the nose or nasal discharge frequently yield no pathogenic organisms. In many instances, an allergic background is present in individuals with this syndrome; in these cases, relief of symptoms is often produced by the judicious use of nasal vasoconstrictors, and treatment is directed to the specific allergy. Occasionally, chronic sinusitis is due to persistent infection, as demonstrated by repeated isolation of a pathogenic organism. However, there is considerable experience to suggest that the manifestations presented by many patients are not related to chronic infection, but are due to other factors such as irritating dusts or gases or excessive exposure to tobacco smoke.

Effective management of acute sinusitis rests on demonstration of a specific pathogenic organism in the secretion present in the nose or drained from the sinuses, testing of the organism for sensitivity to a variety of antimicrobial agents, and administration of the most active agent in adequate dose. The antibiotics most effective for the bacteria most frequently involved in this disease are discussed in Chap. 141. Vasoconstrictors are of help in producing transient relief of symptoms, but must not be used excessively. Surgical drainage may be indicated when infection becomes prolonged or local or intracranial complications develop.

TUMORS OF THE SINUSES The commonest benign tumor of the paranasal sinuses is osteoma. Fifty percent of cases involve the frontal, 40 percent the ethmoid, and 10 percent the maxillary and sphenoid sinuses. The malignant tumors include carcinoma of the maxilla, sarcoma, Burkitt's lymphoma, myeloma, and adenocarcinoma. Melanoma of the nasal cavity may extend into the paranasal sinuses. Other malignant diseases originating in the sinuses may invade the nasal cavity and, because they produce obstruction, lead to consideration of the nose as the primary site of the lesion. A neoplastic lesion should be ruled out in patients who experience repeated episodes of acute sinusitis or who have chronic symptoms, particularly repeated epistaxis in the absence of an identifiable pathogenic organism.

LARYNX

SYMPTOMS AND SIGNS OF LARYNGEAL DISEASE There are three main causes of laryngeal disease: (1) intralaryngeal lesions, (2) extralaryngeal processes that produce other manifestations by direct pressure on either the larynx or the nerves that supply the vocal cords, and (3) disorders in which either local or diffuse disease of the nervous system leads to dysfunction of the vocal cords. A differential diagnosis of the various disorders of the larynx is presented in Table 283-2.

Hoarseness is the commonest symptom of disorders of the larynx, regardless of etiology. The common denominator of the numerous causes of this symptom is interference with normal phonatory function of the larynx. Both inflammatory and noninflammatory diseases of this organ as well as functional disturbances (hysterical aphonia) may be causative factors. Although hoarseness is usually of short duration with acute self-limited processes such as infections, it may persist for long periods.

Cough is common with any type of laryngeal disease. *Pain* occurs occasionally, while *stridor* and *dyspnea* are uncommon manifestations of laryngeal involvement. However, when present, the latter are ominous because they indicate the development of airway obstruction which may rapidly become complete. Obstruction to breathing is not only associated with intralaryngeal lesions or those which exert pressure directly on this organ but may also occur as a result of neurologic disorders in which paralysis of both vocal cords develops.

The exact cause of laryngeal obstruction can be detected only by direct or indirect examination of the larynx. *This is usually necessary when manifestations have persisted for longer than 2 or 3 weeks.* However, if serious obstruction of the airway develops rapidly in acute disorders of the larynx, laryngoscopic examination should be carried out promptly and tracheostomy performed if necessary.

TABLE 283-2
Differential diagnosis of hoarseness and other manifestations of laryngeal dysfunction

I Intralaryngeal disease
- *A* Infectious
  - *1* Common cold
  - *2* Viral laryngitis
  - *3* *Hemophilus influenzae*
  - *4* Membranous laryngitis *(Streptococcus pyogenes, Pseudomonas, Fusobacterium)*
  - *5* Diphtheria (laryngeal membrane)
  - *6* Herpes simplex
  - *7* Actinomycosis
  - *8* Candidiasis
  - *9* Blastomycosis
  - *10* Tuberculosis (ulcers)
  - *11* Syphilis (secondary stage, chondritis, gumma)
  - *12* *Mycoplasma pneumoniae*
  - *13* *Syngamus laryngeus*
- *B* Noninfectious
  - *1* Trauma (edema or hematoma)
  - *2* Vocal cord nodules (singer's nodes)
  - *3* Papillomas of vocal cords
  - *4* Pachyderma of vocal cords
  - *5* Inhalation of smoke, fire, irritating gases, tobacco smoke
  - *6* Leukoplakia of vocal cords
  - *7* Rheumatoid arthritis (involvement of cricoarytenoid joint)
  - *8* Chronic alcoholism
  - *9* Benign tumors
  - *10* Cancer
  - *11* Foreign bodies

II Extralaryngeal disease
- *A* Lesions in neck [produce hoarseness because of (1) pressure on larynx that interferes with movement of vocal cords, (2) edema secondary to decreased venous and lymphatic drainage, and (3) impingement on laryngeal nerves with paresis or paralysis of cords]
  - *1* Hemorrhages and/or edema due to trauma, severe traction of neck, thyroidectomy, tracheostomy, and biopsy of scalene node
  - *2* Tumors of hypopharynx
  - *3* Tumors of carotid body
  - *4* Thrombophlebitis of jugular bulb
- *B* Local and systemic disorders outside neck (produce hoarseness by pressure on laryngeal nerves anywhere along the course outside the neck, or paresis or paralysis of the vocal cords as a manifestation of generalized neurologic dysfunction)
  - *1* Local lesions
    - *a* Bacterial meningitis
    - *b* Meningovascular syphilis
    - *c* Infectious mononucleosis (enlarged mediastinal nodes)
    - *d* Angioneurotic edema
    - *e* Mitral stenosis (enlarged pulmonary artery)
    - *f* Aneurysms of arch of aorta, carotid or innominate arteries
    - *g* Ligation of patent ductus arteriosus
    - *h* Tumors of mediastinal structures
    - *i* Tumors of parotid gland
    - *j* Relapsing polychondritis
    - *k* Neoplastic disease of meninges
    - *l* Fracture of base of skull
    - *m* Cancer or nodules of thyroid
    - *n* Goiter
  - *2* Systemic disorders
    - *a* Diphtheria (peripheral neuritis)
    - *b* Poliomyelitis (bulbar)
    - *c* Infectious mononucleosis (nervous system involvement)
    - *d* Herpes zoster
    - *e* Mucoviscidosis
    - *f* Myxedema
    - *g* Acromegaly
    - *h* Wegener's granulomatosis
    - *i* Lupus erythematosus
    - *j* Diabetic neuropathy
    - *k* Poisoning by lead, mercury, arsenic, botulinus toxin

The disorders of the larynx described below require specific and early diagnosis because of their life-threatening potential.

ACUTE EPIGLOTTITIS Acute infections of the epiglottis are most commonly caused by *H. influenzae* in children; this organism, as well as the pneumococcus and group A streptococci, may be responsible for the disease in all age groups. Although a rare cause of acute epiglottitis in normal adults, *S. pneumoniae* is involved in this disease more commonly in patients with Hodgkin's disease, leukemia, and multiple myeloma. The onset of symptoms is often very rapid and is characterized by varying degrees of fever, severe sore throat, pooling of pharyngeal secretions, drooling, and dysphagia. Stridor is rapidly followed by increasing difficulty in breathing as airway obstruction develops. If untreated, there is increasing use of the accessory muscles of respiration followed by cyanosis, prostration, and finally shock.

Examination of the hypopharynx reveals a markedly swollen, cherry red epiglottis, which may be necrotic when *S. pyogenes* is involved. Treatment must be undertaken early, preferably before there is evidence of severe respiratory distress. In such instances, the administration of ampicillin or any other antimicrobial agent effective against the organisms most often involved, together with inhalation of moist air and oxygen, will often prevent progression of the disease. When it is clear that the airway is seriously threatened, tracheostomy, in addition to chemotherapy, is urgently indicated.

CANDIDAL LARYNGITIS This disease is uncommon but occurs occasionally in patients with mucocutaneous candidiasis and those who have been receiving antibiotics or are immunosuppressed. Because it is almost always associated with candidal esophagitis, it has been suggested that all persons with involvement of the esophagus by *Candida* undergo laryngoscopy. Hoarseness is not common. Scarring of the larynx may develop if antifungal therapy is not administered.

TUBERCULOUS LARYNGITIS Although decreasing in incidence over many years, infection of the larynx by *Mycobacterium tuberculosis* is still a problem. Many of the clinical features of this disease have changed over the last 40 years. It is now most common in older patients (50 to 59 years), more frequent in men than in women (3:1), and may be present in the absence of radiographic evidence of pulmonary disease. Hoarseness is present in almost all cases. While multiple ulcers, present primarily on the posterior aspect of the vocal cords, were common in the past, they are now relatively infrequent. The vocal cords are involved in 50 percent of cases; disease of the false cords and ventricles is next most common. In some cases, only hyperemia and edema are present; this may lead to a misdiagnosis of nonspecific laryngitis.

SYNGAMOSIS OF THE LARYNX This disease, caused by the worm, *Syngamus laryngeus,* is a problem in the Caribbean islands, Brazil, and the Philippines. The vectors of the parasite are domestic and wild birds and cattle. Infestation is initiated by inhalation of the male and female forms of the worm, which then attach to the mucosa of the larynx, pharynx, or trachea. Symptoms include severe, paroxysmal, nonproductive cough, fever and nausea of short duration, occasional hemoptysis, and a "crawling" sensation in the larynx; these symptoms persist for 4 or more months. The white blood count is normal, without eosinophilia. There are no pulmonary lesions. Diagnosis is established by washing out the trachea and demonstrating the characteristic eggs. The male and female worms, which are attached to each other in constant copulation, may be coughed up; they may also be removed by direct laryngoscopy. There is no specific treatment. The disease usually clears when the eggs and worms are coughed out. Although it has been suggested that thiabendazole or mebendazole may be effective, this has not been documented.

FOREIGN BODY Inhalation of a foreign body rapidly produces symptoms. *Pain* is "sticking" in quality and localized to the larynx. *Laryngeal spasm* is usually present. *Dyspnea* may develop as a result of edema and lead to a degree of obstruction sufficient to compromise the airway. There is often a *change in the quality of the voice;* complete *aphonia* may occur. If the inhaled object is sharp, as a chicken bone, there is rapid development of local swelling and progressive obstruction to breathing. Perforation of the larynx may occur and lead to infection that extends from the local site to other areas in the neck and mediastinum. Suspicion of a foreign body makes mirror or laryngoscopic examination an emergency procedure.

CANCER OF THE LARYNX This lesion develops at an average age of 60 years and is 10 times more common in men than in women. Cancers of the larynx are of two types: *intrinsic,* arising on the anterior segment of the vocal cords (70 percent of the cases), and *extrinsic,* extending beyond the vocal cords. Although hoarseness develops early in the course of intrinsic lesions, it is frequently late in onset with extrinsic ones. The treatment of choice for this disease is surgery.

Small lesions of the middle third of the cord often respond to radiation alone. Total or partial laryngectomy is required in the majority of cases. When the cancer involves the epiglottis and/or the false cords, partial supraglottic laryngectomy is the preferred operative procedure because it does not result in loss of normal speech and has a high chance of cure. In some instances, preoperative irradiation of the larynx and surrounding lymph nodes may help in the eradication of the tumor. About 90 percent of cancers of the larynx are cured if detected and treated early.

REFERENCES

Bailey CM, Windle-Taylor PC: Tuberculous laryngitis: A series of 37 patients. Laryngology 91:93, 1981

Dudley JP et al: *Candida* laryngitis in chronic mucocutaneous candidiasis. Its association with *Candida* esophagitis. Ann Otol Rhin Laryngol 89:574, 1981

Eliasson R et al: The immotile-cilia syndrome. A congenital ciliary abnormality as an etiologic factor in chronic airway infections and male sterility. N Engl J Med 297:1, 1977

Kessler HA et al: Acute pneumococcal epiglottitis in immunocompromised adults. Scand J Infect Dis 12:209, 1980

Ossoff RM, Wolff AP: Acute epiglottitis in adults. JAMA 244:2639, 1980

Paparella MM, Shumrick DA: *Otolaryngology.* Philadelphia, Saunders, 1980

Weinstein L, Molavi A: *Syngamus laryngeus* infection. Ann Intern Med 74:577, 1971

284
NEOPLASMS OF THE LUNG

JOHN D. MINNA

In 1982, primary carcinoma of the lung affected more than 85,000 males and 32,000 females in the United States, most of whom died within 1 year. The peak incidence occurs between ages 55 and 65 years, and lung cancer is the leading cause of cancer death in men and the second leading cause of death in women. The incidence is increasing, causing the age-adjusted lung cancer death rate for both sexes to double every 15 years. At the time of diagnosis, only 20 percent of all lung cancer patients will have local disease, while 25 percent will have disease spread to regional lymph nodes, and 55 percent will have distant metastatic sites. Even in those patients with supposedly localized disease, overall 5-year survival is only 30 percent for males and 50 percent for females, and this survival rate has not changed significantly over the past 20 years. Thus, primary carcinoma of the lung is a major health problem with a generally grim prognosis. However, an orderly approach to diagnosis, staging, and treatment based on knowledge of the clinical behavior of lung cancer, combined with a critical review of clinical treatment trials, allows selection of the best therapy for individual patients for either potential cure or optimal palliation. This approach should be multidisciplinary, involving the interaction of medical internists or chest physicians, medical, radiation, and surgical oncologists, pathologists, as well as diagnostic and supportive care personnel.

PATHOLOGY

The histologic classification of primary lung neoplasms recommended by the World Health Organization in 1977 should be used (see Table 284-1). Four major cell types make up 95 percent of all primary lung neoplasms. These are squamous or epidermoid carcinoma, small-cell (also called "oat-cell") carcinoma, adenocarcinoma (including bronchioloalveolar), and large-cell (also called large-cell anaplastic) carcinoma. The various cell types have different natural histories and responses to therapy and thus a correct histologic diagnosis by an experienced pathologist is the first step to correct treatment.

Major treatment decisions are made on the basis of whether the tumor is histologically classified as a small-cell carcinoma or one of the "non-small-cell" varieties (which include epidermoid, adenocarcinoma, large-cell carcinoma, bronchioloalveolar carcinoma, and mixed versions of these). Some of these distinctions are summarized in Tables 284-2 and 284-3.

In general, small-cell carcinoma has spread beyond the bounds of resectional surgery at the time of presentation and is primarily managed with chemotherapy with or without radiotherapy, while if they are found to be localized at the time of presentation, the non-small-cell varieties should be considered for a curative attempt with either surgery or radiotherapy.

Epidermoid cancer is the most common histologic type found in males, while adenocarcinoma is the most common type found in females. Ninety percent of patients with lung cancer of all histologic types are cigarette smokers, while the rare nonsmoking patient who develops lung cancer usually has adenocarcinoma. However, in nonsmokers with adenocarcinoma involving the lung, the possibility of other primary sites, particularly breast cancer, should be considered. Epidermoid and small-cell cancers usually present as central masses with endobronchial growth, while adenocarcinomas and large-cell cancers tend to present as peripheral nodules or masses with pleural involvement. Epidermoid and large-cell cancers cavitate in 20 to 30 percent of cases. Bronchioloalveolar carcinoma can present as a single mass, a diffuse, multinodular lesion, or as a fluffy infiltrate.

TABLE 284-1
World Health Organization (WHO) classification of malignant pleuropulmonary neoplasms

I Epidermoid carcinoma
II Small-cell carcinoma (including fusiform, polygonal, lymphocyte-like, and others)
III Adenocarcinoma (including acinar, papillary, and bronchioloalveolar)
IV Large-cell carcinoma (including solid tumors with and without mucin and giant-cell and clear-cell tumors)
V Combined epidermoid and adenocarcinomas
VI Carcinoid tumors
VII Bronchial gland tumors (including cylindromas and mucoepidermoid tumors)
VIII Papillary tumors of the surface epithelium
IX "Mixed" tumors and carcinosarcomas
X Sarcomas
XI Unclassified
XII Mesotheliomas (including localized and diffuse)
XIII Melanomas

ETIOLOGY

The large majority of lung cancers is associated with and probably caused by cigarette smoking; benzo[*a*]pyrene is a major carcinogen in tobacco smoke. There is a dose-response relationship between the lung cancer death rate and the total amount (often expressed in "cigarette pack years") of cigarettes smoked, such that the risk is increased sixty- to seventyfold for the man smoking two packs a day for 20 years compared to the nonsmoker. Conversely, the chance of developing lung cancer decreases with cessation of smoking but may never return to the nonsmoker level. The increase in lung cancer in women is also associated with a rise in female cigarette smoking. In contrast, pipe smoking does not appear to be related to lung cancer. As a preventive measure, efforts to get persons to stop smoking should continue. Other suggested lung cancer carcinogens include ionizing radiation or uranium ore exposure, asbestos, the halo ethers [bis(chloromethyl) ether and chloromethyl methyl ether], chromates, metallic iron and iron oxides, nickel, beryllium, and arsenic. Radiation and halo ether exposures are particularly associated with small-cell and epidermoid lung cancer. Probably there is a cocarcinogenic effect of smoking and these industrial or environmental pollutants, particularly in uranium miners and asbestos workers. Also, peripheral adenocarcinomas occur more frequently in areas of chronic scarring caused by chronic inflammatory changes, chronic interstitial fibrosis, or scleroderma.

CLINICAL MANIFESTATIONS AND MODE OF PRESENTATION

The natural history of lung cancer begins with cytologic changes of atypia in bronchial epithelial cells progressing through carcinoma in situ to frank invasion. These changes usually occur before signs or symptoms have developed and

TABLE 284-2
Incidence, frequency of metastases, and surgical resectability of the major lung cancer histologic types

Cell type	*Incidence in autopsy series, %*	*Necropsy frequency of distant metastases when clinically localized, %**	*Resectability rate (AJC Study), %†*	*5-year survival after curative resection, %*
Non-small-cell carcinoma:				
Epidermoid	33	17	60	37
Adenocarcinoma	25	40	38	27
Large-cell carcinoma	16	14	38	27
Small-cell carcinoma	25	63	11	<1

* *Determined from autopsy studies of patients dying of causes other than cancer within 30 days following an apparent curative surgical resection.*
† *AJC = American Joint Committee Study for Cancer Staging and End Results Reporting, indicating percentage of cases thought to undergo a curative resection.*
SOURCE: *Adapted from Minna et al, 1981.*

are only seen in cytology (e.g., sputum and bronchial washings) or biopsies. Lung cancer gives rise to chest radiograph findings and other signs and symptoms from local tumor growth, invasion or obstruction of adjacent structures, growth in regional nodes via lymphatic spread, growth in distant metastatic sites after hematogenous dissemination, or as a remote effect of the tumor (paraneoplastic syndrome) usually resulting from peptide hormone secretion by the tumor. Appropriate identification of these signs and symptoms as tumor-related will guide further evaluation and therapy and be of prognostic importance.

If mass screening programs are excluded, 5 to 15 percent of patients are detected while asymptomatic, usually on a routine chest radiograph, while the vast majority of patients present with some sign or symptom. Signs and symptoms secondary to central or endobronchial growth of the primary tumor include cough, hemoptysis, wheeze and stridor, dyspnea, and pneumonitis (fever and productive cough) from obstruction. Signs and symptoms secondary to the peripheral growth of the primary tumor include pain from pleural or chest wall involvement, cough, dyspnea on a restrictive basis, and symptoms of lung abscess resulting from tumor cavitation. Signs and symptoms related to the regional spread of tumor in the thorax by contiguity or by metastasis to regional lymph nodes include tracheal obstruction, esophageal compression with dysphagia, recurrent laryngeal nerve paralysis with hoarseness, phrenic nerve paralysis with elevation of the hemidiaphragm and dyspnea, and sympathetic nerve invasion and paralysis with Horner's syndrome. *Pancoast's,* or *superior sulcus tumor, syndrome* results from local extension of a tumor (usually epidermoid) growing in the apex of the lung with involvement of the eighth cervical and first and second thoracic nerves, with shoulder pain which characteristically radiates in the ulnar distribution of the arm, and often with radiologic destruction of the first and second ribs. Often Horner's syndrome and Pancoast's syndrome will coexist. Other problems of regional spread include *superior vena cava syndrome* from vascular obstruction; pericardial and cardiac extension with resultant tamponade, arrhythmia, or cardiac failure; lymphatic obstruction with resultant pleural effusion; and lymphangitic spread through the lungs with hypoxemia and dyspnea. In addition, bronchioloalveolar carcinoma can spread transbronchially, producing tumor growing along multiple alveolar surfaces with resultant impairment of oxygen transfer, respiratory insufficiency, dyspnea, hypoxemia, and production of large amounts of sputum.

Extrathoracic metastatic disease is found at autopsy in over 50 percent of patients with epidermoid carcinoma, 80 percent of patients with adeno- and large-cell carcinoma, and over 95 percent of patients with small-cell cancer. These autopsy studies have found lung cancer metastases in virtually every organ system. Thus, the majority of lung cancer patients eventually need therapy to palliate symptoms. Common clinical problems related to metastatic disease of lung cancer include brain metastases with neurologic deficits; bone metastases with pain and pathologic fractures; bone marrow invasion with cytopenias or leukoerythroblastosis; liver metastases causing biochemical liver dysfunction, anorexia, biliary obstruction, and pain; lymph node metastases in the supraclavicular region and occasionally in the axilla and groin that can be painful and ulcerate; and spinal cord compression syndromes from epidural or bone metastases.

Remote effects of cancer or *paraneoplastic syndromes* are common in lung cancer patients and may be the presenting finding or first sign of recurrence. In addition, paraneoplastic syndromes may mimic metastatic disease and, unless detected, lead to inappropriate palliative rather than curative treatment. Often the paraneoplastic syndrome may be relieved with successful treatment of the tumor, and tumor treatment is the basis for correcting such syndromes. In some cases the pathophysiology of the paraneoplastic syndrome is known, particularly when a hormone with biologic activity is secreted by a tumor (Chap. 122). However, in many cases the pathophysiology is unknown. *Systemic symptoms* of anorexia, cachexia, and weight loss (seen in 30 percent of patients), fever (20 percent), and suppressed immunity are paraneoplastic syndromes of unknown etiology. *Endocrine syndromes* are seen in 12 percent of patients and have the best understood pathophysiology, including hypercalcemia and hypophosphatemia resulting from ectopic parathyroid hormone production by epidermoid cancer; hyponatremia with the syndrome of inappropriate secretion of antidiuretic hormone by small-cell cancer; and Cushing's syndrome resulting from ectopic secretion of ACTH by small-cell cancer. *Skeletal connective tissues syndromes* include clubbing in 30 percent (usually non-small-cell), and hypertrophic pulmonary osteoarthropathy (in 1 to 10 percent, usually adenocarcinomas) with periostitis and clubbing giving pain, tenderness, and swelling over the affected bones, and a positive bone scan. *Neurologic-myopathic syndromes* are seen in only 1 percent of patients but are dramatic and include the myasthenic *Eaton-Lambert syndrome* with small-cell cancer, peripheral neuropathies, subacute cerebellar degeneration, cortical degeneration, and polymyositis. *Coagulation, thrombotic, and hematologic manifestations* occur in 1 to 8 percent of patients and include migratory venous thrombophlebitis (*Trousseau's syndrome*); nonbacterial thrombotic (marantic) endocarditis with arterial emboli; disseminated intravascular coagulation with hemorrhage; and anemia, granulocytosis, and leukoerythroblastosis. *Cutaneous manifestations* such as dermatomyositis and acanthosis nigricans are uncommon (1 percent or less) as are the *renal manifestations* of nephrotic syndrome or glomerulonephritis (1 percent or less).

TABLE 284-3
Comparison between small-cell and "non-small-cell" lung cancers

	Small-cell	*Non-small cell*
HISTOLOGY		
	Scant cytoplasm, indistinct nucleoli, small hyperchromatic nuclei	Abundant cytoplasm, prominent nucleoli, enlarged, pleomorphic nuclei
BIOCHEMICAL		
	L-Dopa decarboxylase, neuron-specific enolase, creatinine kinase BB isoenzyme	Keratin (epidermoid) Mucin (adenocarcinoma)
CYTOGENETICS		
	Deletion 3p(14–23)	No known specific defect
HORMONE PRODUCTION		
	ACTH, AVP, calcitonin, bombesin	PTH (epidermoid)
RESPONSE TO RADIOTHERAPY		
	+ + + (often complete)	+ (uncommonly complete)
RESPONSE TO COMBINATION CHEMOTHERAPY		
Overall regression rate	90%	30%
Complete regression rate	50%	5%

DIAGNOSIS AND STAGING

EARLY DIAGNOSIS Screening persons at high risk (males over 45 years of age smoking 40 or more cigarettes per day) for lung cancer with sputum cytologies and chest radiographs every 4 months has shown a prevalence rate of lung cancer in asymptomatic patients of 4 to 8 cases per 1000 persons. With follow-up screening, 4 new cases of lung cancer are found per 1000 persons followed per year. These lung cancers are detected 72 percent of the time by radiographs alone, 20 percent by cytology alone, while 6 percent are detected by both methods. In contrast to nonscreened patients, 90 percent of these screened patients who develop lung cancer are asymptomatic, 62 percent have resectable lung cancer, and 53 percent of all the new cases are American Joint Commission (AJC) postsurgical stage I (see below) with a 5-year survival probability of 45 percent. These results are being prospectively compared to a randomized control group not receiving this intensive screening. If the lung cancer death rate is reduced significantly in the screened group, screening should be generally practiced in high-risk patients.

ESTABLISHING A TISSUE DIAGNOSIS OF LUNG CANCER Once signs, symptoms, or screening studies suggest lung cancer, it is necessary to establish a tissue diagnosis of malignancy, determine the histologic cell type, and stage the patient for appropriate treatment. In the case of the solitary pulmonary nodule or other local lesion, the tissue diagnosis will be made with definitive surgical resection, while in larger lesions tumor tissue or tumor cells in washings may be obtained at fiberoptic bronchoscopy with bronchial biopsy. Other routes of obtaining tissue include a mediastinal node biopsy at mediastinoscopy; percutaneous biopsy of an enlarged supraclavicular lymph node, soft tissue mass, or lytic bone lesion; bone marrow biopsy; or cytologic examination of pleural fluid or needle biopsy of the involved pleura. In poor-risk or unresectable patients, a transthoracic fine-needle aspiration biopsy or transbronchial forceps biopsy can be used, particularly with peripheral lesions.

STAGING PATIENTS WITH LUNG CANCER Lung cancer staging consists of two parts, first, a determination of the location of tumor (anatomic staging) and second, an assessment of a patient's ability to withstand various antitumor treatments (physiologic staging). For example, in a patient with non-small-cell lung cancer it is crucial to determine if the tumor can be resected by a standard surgical procedure such as a lobectomy or pneumonectomy (determination of "resectability") based on the anatomic stage of the tumor and whether the patient could tolerate such a surgical procedure (determination of "operability") based on the cardiopulmonary condition of the patient.

Staging system for non-small-cell lung cancer The TNM (tumor size, or T factor; regional nodal involvement, or N factor; and presence or absence of distant metastases, M factor) staging system developed by the AJC on End Results Reporting should be used in non-small-cell lung cancer, particularly in preparing patients for curative attempts with surgery or radiotherapy (Table 284-4). The various T, N, and M factors are combined to form three different groups (stages I, II, and III) and a fourth group consisting of occult carcinoma detected on screening cytology exams but with no other evidence of tumor (Table 284-4). This stage grouping can be performed at different times.

Staging for small-cell lung cancer A simple two-stage system adapted from the Veterans Administration Lung Cancer Study Group is used. In this two-stage system, *limited stage disease* (about 40 percent of all small-cell cancer patients) is defined as disease confined to one hemithorax and regional lymph nodes (including mediastinal, contralateral hilar, and usually ipsilateral supraclavicular nodes), while *extensive stage disease* (about 60 percent of all patients) is defined as disease beyond this. In part, the definition of *limited stage* relates to whether the known tumor can be encompassed within a tolerable radiation therapy port. Thus, ipsilateral pleural effusion, recurrent laryngeal nerve involvement, and superior vena caval obstruction can all be limited stage disease. However, cardiac tamponade and bilateral pulmonary parenchymal involvement are generally scored as extensive stage disease because of the size of the radiation therapy port required to cover all known disease.

GENERAL STAGING PROCEDURES All lung cancer patients should have a complete history and physical examination, with evaluation of all other medical problems and a determination of performance status and weight loss.

An ear, nose, and throat examination is necessary because of the frequent occurrence of second cancers in this area. Chest roentgenograms are needed to evaluate tumor size and nodal involvement, and it is very useful, if not mandatory, to obtain any old x-ray films for comparison. Tomograms are only used for specific diagnostic problems, and while chest CT scans are in wide use, they should not be used alone for staging or primary treatment decisions until more published data on their accuracy are available.

A complete blood count with platelet determination, routine blood chemistries, skin test for tuberculosis, electrocardiogram, and pulmonary function studies are obtained. Arterial blood gas measurements are obtained if any signs or symptoms of respiratory insufficiency are present. If signs or symptoms suggest organ involvement by tumor, appropriate radionuclide

TABLE 284-4
TNM classification of lung cancer

PRIMARY TUMOR (T)	
TX	Occult cancer; only evidence in bronchial washings cytologically
T1	Less than 3 cm, surrounded by lung or visceral pleura, and without bronchoscopic invasion proximal to a lobar bronchus
T2	Tumor more than 3 cm; or tumor with atelectasis or pneumonitis extending to hilum but less than entire lung, within a lobar bronchus, and more than 2 cm distal to carina; no pleural effusion
T3	Tumor of any size with extension into parietal pleura, chest wall, diaphragm, mediastinum; less than 2 cm from carina; or atelectasis, pneumonitis of entire lung; pleural effusion with or without malignant cells
REGIONAL LYMPH NODES (N)	
N0	Negative hilar and mediastinal nodes
N1	Positive ipsilateral hilar nodes
N2	Positive mediastinal nodes (also scored when vocal cord paralysis, SVC obstruction, and trachea or esophageal compression are present, all of which strongly indicate mediastinal node invasion)
DISTANT METASTASIS (M)	
M0	No known distant metastasis
M1	Distant metastasis present with site specified (e.g., brain)
STAGE GROUPING	
Occult carcinoma	TX, N0, M0
Stage I	T1, N0, M0; T1, N1, M0; T2, N0, M0
Stage II	T2, N1, M0
Stage III	T3 with any N or M; N2 with any T or M; M1 with any T or N

ans (e.g., brain, liver, or bone) are performed, as well as ra-
diographs of any suspicious bony lesions. Routine radionuclide scans are not obtained in the asymptomatic patient because of the high frequency of false-positive and false-negative studies. Any accessible lesions suspicious for cancer should be biopsied if a histologic diagnosis has not already been made, or if treatment or staging decisions would be based on whether or not the lesion contained cancer. In candidates for curative surgery or radiotherapy, a barium swallow is performed, if esophageal symptoms are present, followed by esophagoscopy if abnormalities are found.

In patients over 30 years of age presenting with a *solitary pulmonary nodule* (defined as an x-ray density completely surrounded by normal aerated lung, with circumscribed margins, smooth contour, and minimal if any associated atelectasis, pneumonitis, or regional adenopathy) the general procedures, fiberoptic bronchoscopy, and prethoracotomy medical evaluation should be done. In nearly all instances (irrespective of nodule calcifications or duration on x-ray follow-up) these nodules should be removed surgically if the patient can tolerate thoracotomy since 35 percent will be malignant. This is particularly true if the patient smokes. If the patient is not an operative candidate, transthoracic fine-needle biopsy and radiation therapy are used.

In patients presenting with a mass lesion on chest x-ray and no obvious contraindications to a curative approach with surgery or radiotherapy after the initial evaluation and fiberoptic bronchoscopy (see below), the mediastinum must be investigated. This varies between different centers and includes (1) gallium 67 citrate scanning first (which will localize in over 70 percent of lung cancers and thus strongly suggest mediastinal metastases), followed by mediastinoscopy in patients with positive scans or computed tomography plus tomograms, and if these are positive, mediastinoscopy; (2) proceeding directly to mediastinoscopy (right-sided tumors) or lateral mediastinotomy (left-sided lesions) on all patients; (3) proceeding directly to thoracotomy. In patients presenting with disease confined to the chest but not resectable, thus making them candidates for curative radiotherapy, other tests such as fiberoptic bronchoscopy are only done as indicated to evaluate specific symptoms such as hemoptysis.

Pretreatment staging for patients with histologically documented small-cell lung cancer include the initial general lung cancer evaluation as well as fiberoptic bronchoscopy with washings and biopsies to determine the tumor extent before therapy; bone marrow biopsy and aspiration since 20 to 30 percent of patients have tumor in the bone marrow; and radionuclide scans of liver, brain, and bone if symptoms or other findings are suggestive of disease involvement in these areas. Percutaneous or peritoneoscopy-directed liver biopsy may be performed if other findings are suggestive but not diagnostic of the presence of tumor in the liver, particularly if this would alter the planned therapy.

If signs or symptoms of spinal cord compression or leptomeningitis develop at any time in lung cancer patients of any histologic type, a myelogram and examination of the cerebrospinal fluid cytology are performed to determine the need for local therapy to the site of compression (usually with radiotherapy), and intrathecal chemotherapy (usually with methotrexate) if malignant cells are detected. In addition, a radionuclide brain scan or brain CT scan are performed to search for brain metastases that are often associated with compression or leptomeningitis.

STAGING OF NON-SMALL-CELL LUNG CANCER WITH METASTATIC DISEASE In patients presenting with disease that is not curable by either surgery, radiotherapy, or their combination, all of the general procedures are done plus fiberoptic bronchoscopy as indicated to evaluate hemoptysis, obstruction, or pneumonitis; and pleurocentesis and cytologic examination if fluid is present.

A variety of other staging procedures including gallium 67 citrate scanning, computed tomography, tomograms, angiograms, venograms, scintiscans, sonography, and blind nodal biopsies at present should not be part of the routine staging evaluation of the lung cancer patient.

DETERMINATION OF RESECTABILITY AND OPERABILITY In patients with non-small-cell lung cancer, the following are major contraindications to curative attempts by surgery or radiotherapy alone using standard treatment methods: extrathoracic distant metastases; superior vena cava syndrome; vocal cord and, in most cases, phrenic nerve paralysis; malignant pleural effusion; cardiac tamponade; tumor within 2 cm of the carina (not curable by surgery but potentially curable by radiotherapy); metastasis to the contralateral lung; bilateral endobronchial tumor (potentially curable by radiotherapy); metastasis to the supraclavicular lymph nodes; lymph node metastasis in the contralateral mediastinum (potentially curable by radiotherapy); involvement of the main stem pulmonary artery; and a histologic diagnosis of small-cell lung cancer. While some chest surgeons would argue that patients with ipsilateral mediastinal lymph node involvement can be cured with surgery (and adjuvant radiotherapy), nearly all would agree that any extracapsular nodal involvement or fixation of the nodes in the mediastinum precludes surgical cure.

PHYSIOLOGIC STAGING Patients with lung cancer often have cardiopulmonary and other medical problems related to chronic obstructive pulmonary disease as well as other medical problems. Since it is not always possible to predict whether a lobectomy or pneumonectomy will be required until the time of operation, a conservative approach is to restrict resectional surgery to patients who could potentially tolerate a pneumonectomy. In addition to nonambulatory performance status, a myocardial infarction within the past 3 months is a contraindication to thoracic surgery because 20 percent of patients will die of reinfarction alone, while an infarction in the past 6 months is a relative contraindication. Other major contraindications include uncontrolled major arrhythmias; maximum breathing capacities of less than 40 percent predicted; an FEV_1 less than 1 liter, while a FEV_1 over 2.5 liters allows pneumonectomy (recommending surgery when the FEV_1 is 1.1. to 2.4 liters requires careful judgment); CO_2 retention (which is more serious than hypoxemia); and severe pulmonary hypertension. In patients with borderline pulmonary status or a question of pulmonary hypertension, split pulmonary function testing by ventilation-perfusion lung scans or bronchospirometry and right heart catheterization study with temporary unilateral pulmonary artery occlusion can define physiologic operability.

TREATMENT

NON-SMALL-CELL LUNG CANCER: LOCALIZED DISEASE In patients with non-small-cell lung cancer of AJC clinical stages I and II (Table 284-4), who can tolerate operation, the treatment of choice is pulmonary resection. In rare stage III cases with favorable age, cardiopulmonary function, and anatomy (such as a small tumor or ipsilateral mediastinal node involvement without capsular extension) resection should also be considered. The extent of resection is a matter of surgical judgment based on findings at exploration. In general, conservative resection that encompasses all known tumor gives survival equal to that obtained with more extensive procedures. Thus, lobectomy is preferred to pneumonectomy, while wedge resections and segmentectomies are reserved for patients with poor pulmonary reserve and small peripheral lesions. Approximately 43 percent of all lung cancer patients will undergo thoracotomy. Of these, 77 percent will have a definitive resection, 12 percent will only be explored for disease extent, and 12 percent will have a palliative procedure with known disease left behind. The fraction of long-term survivors following definitive surgical therapy is remarkably consistent throughout major centers performing lung cancer surgery in the United States. Approximately 30 percent of all patients resected for cure survive 5 years, and 15 percent survive 10 years. The 30-day hospital mortality following pulmonary resection at major centers is also very constant, ranging from 4 to 9 percent for lobectomy and 9 to 11 percent for pneumonectomy. The 5-year survivals following resection for the different histologic types are epidermoid, 33 percent; adenocarcinoma, 26 percent; large-cell carcinoma, 28 percent; bronchioloalveolar carcinoma, 51 percent; and small-cell carcinoma, less than 1 percent. As a function of postsurgical treatment stage the AJC 5-year survival data for stages I, II, III (N0–N1, M0), and III (N2, M0), respectively, are epidermoid, 54 percent, 35 percent, 19 percent, 13 percent; adenocarcinoma and large-cell carcinoma, 51 percent, 18 percent, 10 percent, 2 percent. Thus, the majority of patients who were initially thought to have a "curative" resection ultimately died of metastatic disease (usually within 2 years of surgery), indicating the need for some form of adjuvant treatment.

Management of occult carcinoma When sputum cytology screening indicates malignant cells but a normal chest radiograph is found (TX tumor stage), the lesion must be localized. Over 90 percent can be localized by meticulous examination of the bronchial tree with a fiberoptic bronchoscope under general anesthesia and collection of a series of differential brushings and biopsies.

Often carcinoma in situ or multicentric lesions are found. Thus, current recommendations are for the most conservative surgical resection, allowing removal of the cancer and conservation of lung parenchyma even if the bronchial margins are positive for carcinoma in situ. The 5-year survival estimate for these occult cancers is approximately 60 percent.

Radiotherapy Those patients who are AJC stage III M0, as well as those with AJC stages I and II disease who refuse surgery or appear not to be candidates for pulmonary resection for medical reasons, should be considered for radiation therapy with curative intent. The decision to administer high-dose and potentially curative radiotherapy is based upon the extent of disease and the volume of the chest that requires irradiation. Patients with distant metastases, positive supraclavicular nodes, pleural effusion, or cardiac involvement are generally not considered for such curative radiation treatment. The median survival for unresectable patients with non-small-cell lung cancer localized to the chest undergoing primary radiotherapy with curative intent is less than 1 year. However, 5-year survival data show up to 6 percent of patients alive when treated with radiotherapy alone. In addition to potential cure, radiotherapy, by controlling the primary tumor, may increase the quality and length of life of noncured patients, although there are few data to support this latter consideration directly. Treatment usually involves midplane doses of 55,000 to 60,000 mGy (5500 to 6000 rad), and the major concern is the amount of lung parenchyma and other organs in the thorax included within the treatment plan, including the spinal cord, heart, and esophagus. Patients with a major degree of underlying pulmonary disease may have to have the treatment plan compromised because of the deleterious effect of radiation on pulmonary function. Either split course or continuous fraction radiotherapy can be given with similar survival results. The development of radiation pneumonitis is proportional to the dose of radiation and volume of lung incorporated within the radiation field. Acute radiation esophagitis occurs during treatment but usually is self-limited, while spinal cord injury should be avoided by careful treatment planning.

Combined modality therapy At present there appears to be no consensus for the use of pre- or postoperative radiation therapy (despite cure rates with radiotherapy alone at 6 percent) or adjuvant chemotherapy. Currently, these forms of combined modality therapy should only be administered as part of approved clinical trials. One exception to this is the management of carcinomas of the superior pulmonary sulcus producing *Pancoast's syndrome.* These patients should have the usual preoperative staging procedures, including mediastinoscopy as well as CT scans to determine tumor extent and neurologic examination with electromyography to document neurologic findings. Often a histologic diagnosis is not made, and with the constellation of tumor location and pain distribution the diagnostic accuracy for cancer is better than 90 percent. If mediastinoscopy is negative, two curative approaches may be used in treating a Pancoast's syndrome tumor. The first preoperative irradiation [30,000 mGy (3000 rad) in 10 treatments] is given to the area followed by an en bloc resection of the tumor and involved chest wall 3 to 6 weeks later. At 3 years, survival figures of 42 percent for epidermoid and 21 percent for adeno- and large-cell carcinomas have been reported. The second approach involves radiotherapy alone in curative doses and standard fractionation with similar survival to combined modality therapy reported.

MANAGEMENT OF PATIENTS WITH DISSEMINATED NON-SMALL-CELL LUNG CANCER The 70 percent of patients who turn out to have unresectable non-small-cell cancer have a poor prognosis. For example, median survivals of 34, 25, 17, 8, and 4 weeks are seen for patients with performance status scores of 0 (asymptomatic), 1 (symptomatic, fully ambulatory), 2 (in bed $<$ 50 percent of the time), 3 (in bed $>$ 50 percent of the time), and 4 (bedridden), respectively. Standard medical management, the judicious use of pain medications, and the appropriate use of radiotherapy form the cornerstone of management. Patients whose primary tumors are causing symptoms such as bronchial obstruction with pneumonitis, hemoptysis, or upper airway or superior vena caval obstruction should, in general, have radiotherapy to the primary tumor. The case for prophylactic treatment of the asymptomatic patient is to prevent major symptoms from occurring within the thorax, if follow-up is uncertain. However, if the patient can be followed closely, deferring treatment until the development of symptoms is appropriate. Usually a course of 30,000 to 40,000 mGy (3000 to 4000 rad) over 2 to 4 weeks is given to the tumor. The frequencies of relief by radiation therapy of intrathoracic symptoms are hemoptysis, 84 percent; SVC syndrome, 80 percent; dyspnea, 60 percent; cough, 60 percent; atelectasis, 23 percent; and vocal cord paralysis, 6 percent. Other symptoms of metastatic disease treated with radiotherapy include cardiac tamponade (treated with pericardiocentesis and radiation therapy to the entire cardiac silhouette); painful bony metastases (with relief in 66 percent of cases); and brain, spinal cord compression, or brachial plexus involvement. Usually, with brain and cord compression, dexamethasone (25 to 100 mg total per day in 4 divided doses) is also given and then rapidly tapered to the lowest dosage which relieves neurologic symptoms. In all cases, the key to effective palliation is to detect the complication and begin radiotherapy at the earliest possible time. Pleural effusions are common and are usually treated with thoracentesis as needed, but without radiotherapy. If they recur and are symptomatic, chest tube drainage with a sclerosing agent such as intrapleural tetracycline is used. The chest is first completely drained. Then 1000 mg of tetracycline is dissolved in 100 ml of normal saline, and 50 ml of 1% xylocaine added, and this is injected via the chest tube. The chest tube is clamped and the patient rotated onto different sides to distribute the sclerosing agent. Twenty-four to forty-eight hours later the chest tube is pulled when there is little drainage (usually less than 100 ml/12 h).

Anticancer chemotherapy is not yet standard therapy for non-small-cell lung cancer and, in general, should only be given as part of clinical trials approved by the local institutions. Approximately 10 to 20 percent of patients will have objective tumor shrinkage with the most active single agents, and 30 to 40 percent of patients will respond to combination chemotherapy. However, a complete clinical regression of tumor occurs (a "complete response") in less than 5 percent of cases. Those patients whose tumors respond to chemotherapy have significantly longer survivals (around 30 to 40 weeks median survival) compared to those patients who do not respond to therapy (10 to 20 weeks median). The problem is that the responding patients also have better prognostic features (such as good performance status) and it is difficult to separate the effect of these on survival from that of chemotherapy. In those patients with non-small-cell lung cancer who desire nonprotocol chemotherapy, it is reasonable to give chemotherapy if the patient is fully ambulatory, has an evaluable tumor mass (to follow response to therapy), has not received prior chemotherapy or radiotherapy, and is able to understand and accept the potential benefits and toxicities from such therapy. The chemotherapy should be delivered by a physician or medical oncologist, and one of the standard regimens such as "CAP" [cyclophosphamide, doxorubicin (Adriamycin), *cis*-platin] or vindesine (an experimental drug) or vinblastin plus *cis*-platin should be used. However, there is little to distinguish these from many other reported regimens except their differing toxicities.

MANAGEMENT OF SMALL-CELL LUNG CANCER The goal of initial treatment is to obtain a complete clinical regression of tumor documented by repeating the initial positive staging procedures, particularly fiberoptic bronchoscopy with washings and biopsy. This initial response, determined 6 to 12 weeks after the start of therapy, predicts both median and long-term survival and potential cure. Patients obtaining a complete clinical regression of tumor survive longer than patients with an objective but only partial regression (tumor shrinkage of more than 50 percent of visible disease with no sign of tumor progression elsewhere), who in turn survive longer than patients with no response. In addition, all long-term (over 3 years) survivors come from the complete response group. Untreated patients with small-cell lung cancer have median survivals of only 6 to 17 weeks, and randomized trials have shown that radiotherapy alone is superior to surgery alone, that chemotherapy is superior to radiotherapy, and that chemotherapy plus radiotherapy is superior to radiotherapy alone. Randomized trials comparing chemotherapy plus radiotherapy to chemotherapy alone are currently underway. Thus, the correct integration of chemotherapy with or without radiotherapy or surgery is the cornerstone of the treatment of small-cell cancer.

Following initial staging, patients are grouped into the limited or extensive disease stages and classified as being physiologically able or not able to tolerate intensive combination chemotherapy or combined modality chemoradiotherapy. Such intensive therapy should be reserved for ambulatory patients (PS 2 or better), with no prior chemotherapy or radiotherapy, no other major medical problems, and adequate heart, liver, renal, and bone marrow function. The arterial P_{O_2} on room air should be above 50 mmHg, and there should be no CO_2 retention. All patients with some or more of these limitations must have their initial chemoradio- or chemotherapy modified to prevent undue toxicity. The overall mortality rate from initial high-dose combination chemotherapy even in these selected patients is about 5 percent at major centers. This figure is comparable to the operative mortality rate for pulmonary resection and indicates the need for physiologic staging of patients before chemotherapy.

In appropriate patients, high-dose combination chemotherapy with or without radiotherapy should be given ("induction therapy"). This must be coupled with supportive care for infectious, hemorrhagic, and other medical complications. Meticulous attention to the details of therapy and the day to day management of the patient through the initial 6 to 12 weeks of treatment is essential if therapy-related mortality is to be kept low. Because of this the induction period should be supervised by a medical oncologist. The current principles of primary chemotherapy may be summarized as follows: first, combination chemotherapy using three or four of the known active agents concurrently should be used. A variety of combination chemotherapies have been reported, including CMC (cyclophosphamide + methotrexate + CCNU), alternating with VAP (vincristine + doxorubicin + procarbazine); CAV (cyclophosphamide + doxorubicin + vincristine); CCMV (cyclophosphamide + CCNU + methotrexate + vincristine); CAVP-16 (cyclophosphamide + doxorubicin + VP-16). At present there is no evidence that any one regimen is better than another if adequate drug dose and schedules are given. Second, the initial combination chemotherapy is given in high doses during the first 6 to 8 weeks such that severe granulocytopenia (e.g., granulocyte counts less than 500 per microliter) and moderate to severe thrombocytopenia (platelets less than 50,000 per microliter) are to be expected. Following the initial intense (or "induction") therapy, patients should be restaged to determine if they have entered a "complete clinical remission," including complete disappearance of all clinically evident lesions and paraneoplastic syndromes, or a "partial remission"; or have "no response" or tumor progression (seen in 10 percent of patients or less). Following this, "maintenance" chemotherapy is given to responding patients for periods of 6 to 12 months in 3-, 4-, or 6-week cycles, depending on the combination of chemotherapy used. Appropriate drug dose modifications are made to keep the white blood count above 2000 per microliter and the platelet count above 50,000 per microliter. The patients are restaged between 6 and 12 months, depending on the individual regimens; if they are still in a complete remission, chemotherapy is stopped. The value of more prolonged chemotherapy is not documented. Patients with a partial tumor regression are generally kept on chemotherapy until the time of objective tumor progression and then switched to new chemotherapy (either with known activity or on an experimental protocol). Patients not responding or with objective tumor progression should be switched to new chemotherapy, preferably with a non-cross-resistant combination in an attempt to get an objective tumor response. High-dose [40,000 mGy (4000 rad)] radiotherapy to the whole brain should be given to patients with documented brain metastases. Prophylactic cranial radiotherapy may be given to patients with objective tumor responses, particularly those with complete responses, as this will significantly decrease the development of brain metastases (occurring in 60 to 80 percent of patients living 2 or more years who do not receive such prophylactic radiotherapy), but such prophylactic therapy has not been shown to prolong survival. In the case of symptomatic progressive lesions in the chest or at other critical sites, if radiotherapy has not yet been given to these areas, it may be administered in full doses (e.g., 40,000 mGy to the chest tumor mass). The management of other metastatic disease is similar to that for non-small-cell lung cancer.

There are definite toxicities of both an acute and chronic nature that should be expected with combined modality chemoradiotherapy, particularly if chemo- and radiotherapy are given concurrently. Thus, the role of radiotherapy in the primary treatment of small-cell lung cancer is still undergoing clinical investigation. However, retrospective analysis of long-term survivors, and analysis of local failures in the chest following chemotherapy alone, are suggestive that chest radiotherapy is of benefit. If radiotherapy is to be given to the primary lesion, patients should be selected (limited stage disease with PS 0–1 and initial good pulmonary function) such that radiotherapy can be given in full doses, by conventional fractionation, and in a manner that will not compromise the needed combination chemotherapy or sacrifice too much lung. The radiation oncologist must be prepared to deliver tailored radiotherapy with shaping of fields during treatment, much the same as is done for Hodgkin's disease. In extensive stage disease, the routine use of chest radiotherapy is to be avoided. However, if chemotherapy is inadequate to relieve local tumor symptoms, a course of radiotherapy can be added.

Applying these principles, several centers around the world have reported potential cure rates of 15 to 25 percent for limited stage disease and 1 to 5 percent for extensive stage disease. Overall, approximately 50 percent of patients with limited stage and 30 percent with extensive stage disease will enter a complete remission, and 90 to 95 percent of all patients will have some objective tumor shrinkage (complete or partial response). These responses increase the median survival from 2 to 4 months for untreated patients to 10 to 12 months for extensive stage and 14 to 18 months for limited stage patients. In addition, most patients have relief of their tumor-related symptoms and improvement of performance status. However, the maintenance of good performance status by the patient while receiving outpatient chemotherapy requires judgment and skill on the part of the medical oncologist delivering the chemotherapy so as to avoid undue therapeutic toxicity. A variety of new drug treatments are being tried (such as new drug combinations, alternating combinations of drugs, very intensive initial or "reinduction" therapy with autologous bone marrow infusion), as well as novel forms of combining chemo- and radiotherapy and surgery, but these should all be reserved for approved clinical protocols.

A special case arises when a resected pulmonary cancer is determined on pathology review to be small-cell carcinoma. A small number of such patients have been randomized on surgical adjuvant trials to chemotherapy, and such patients had improved survival compared to placebo controls. Thus, it would be prudent either to enter such patients on clinical trials or to treat them with adjuvant chemotherapy, particularly if the mediastinal nodes are positive.

IMMUNOTHERAPY

Lung cancer patients frequently have severe immunosuppression, and conversion from an anergic to a reactive state can occur. This change in immune status may be associated with improvement in survival. All of this suggests that immunosuppression may represent a paraneoplastic syndrome associated with lung cancer. However, a large number of randomized and unrandomized trials have not confirmed the value of "immunotherapies" such as intrapleural BCG, levamisole, *Cornyebacterium parvum,* allogenic irradiated tumor cells, "tumor associated antigens," other adjuvants, or thymosin. Thus, immunotherapy should only be given as part of approved clinical trials.

CLINICAL TRIALS AND BIOLOGIC STUDIES

The current poor prognosis for most lung cancer patients requires the continued performance of well-designed clinical trials to test new forms of therapy. In addition, the development of methods to culture tumor cells directly from patients will allow (1) the prospective testing of tumor sensitivity in vitro to drugs, radiation therapy, and biologic response modifiers such as monoclonal antibodies; (2) the analysis of tumor cell growth factors, hormone and other nutritional requirements; and (3) the biochemical and genetic study of lung cancer cells, including the characterization of paraneoplastic syndromes. All of these should provide a more rational basis for treatment.

BRONCHIAL ADENOMAS

Bronchial adenomas are slowly growing intrabronchial lesions which represent 1 percent of all pulmonary neoplasms. Eighty to ninety percent are carcinoids, 10 to 15 percent are adenocystic tumors (or cylindromas), and 2 to 3 percent are mucoepidermoid tumors. Adenomas present in patients 15 to 60 years old (average age 45) as intrabronchial lesions and are often symptomatic for several years. Patients may have chronic cough, recurrent hemoptysis, or obstruction with atelectasis, lobar collapse, or pneumonitis and abscess formation. Bronchial carcinoids, which usually follow a benign course, and small-cell lung cancers, which are highly malignant, are both derived from the same normal bronchial epithelial component, the Kulchitsky cell. This cell is part of the amine precursor uptake and decarboxylation (APUD) system. Carcinoids, like small-cell lung cancers, may secrete other hormones such as ACTH or arginine vasopressin and thus cause paraneoplastic syndromes. In addition, bronchial carcinoids may produce the carcinoid syndrome, with cutaneous flush, bronchoconstriction, diarrhea, and cardiac valvular lesions (see Chap. 131), which small-cell lung cancer does not. Occasionally pathologists may have difficulty in distinguishing carcinoids from small-cell lung cancers, and carcinoid tumors appearing more aggressive histologically (referred to as "atypical carcinoids") metastasize in 70 percent of cases to regional nodes, liver, or bone, compared to only a 5 percent metastasis rate of carcinoids with typical histology.

Bronchial adenomas of all types, because of their endobronchial and often central location, are usually visible via fiberoptic bronchoscopy, and tissue for histologic diagnosis is obtained in this manner. Surgical excision is the primary treatment for all types of bronchial adenomas. The extent of surgery is determined at operation and should be as conservative as possible. Often bronchotomy with local excision, sleeve rejection, segmental resection, or lobectomy is sufficient. Five-year survival rates following surgical resection are 95 percent, decreasing to 70 percent if regional nodes are involved.

METASTATIC PULMONARY TUMORS

The lung is frequently the site of metastatic disease from primary cancers outside the lung. Usually such metastatic disease is considered incurable. However, two special situations may arise. First is the development of a solitary pulmonary shadow on chest x-ray in a patient known to have an extrathoracic neoplasm. This may represent a metastasis or a new primary lung cancer. Because the natural history of lung cancer is worse than for most other primary tumors, it is wise to approach the single pulmonary nodule in a patient with a known extrathoracic tumor as though the nodule were a primary lung cancer, particularly if the patient is over 35 years of age and a smoker. This means a vigorous evaluation looking for other sites of active cancer and, if none are found, surgical resection of the nodule. Second, multiple pulmonary nodules may be resected for cure as well. This is usually recommended if, after careful staging, (1) the patient can tolerate the contemplated pulmonary resection; (2) the primary tumor has been definitively and successfully treated; and (3) all known metastatic disease can be encompassed by the projected pulmonary resection. The key is selection and screening of patients to exclude patients with uncontrolled primary tumors and extrapulmonary metastases. Primary tumors whose pulmonary metastases have been successfully resected for cure include osteogenic sarcoma; colon, rectal, uterine, cervix, and corpus tumors; and bladder and kidney tumors. Five-year survival rates of 20 to 30 percent have been found in carefully selected patients, and the most dramatic results have been seen in osteogenic sarcomas where resection of pulmonary metastases (sometimes requiring several thoracotomies) is becoming a standard curative treatment approach.

REFERENCES

BUNN PA JR, IHDE DC: Small cell bronchogenic carcinoma: A review of therapeutic results, in *Lung Cancer,* RB Livingston (ed). The Hague/Boston/London, Martinus Nijhoff, 1981

LICHTER AS, BUNN PA: The management of small-cell cancer of the lung, in *Update: Pulmonary Diseases and Disorders,* AP Fishman (ed). New York, McGraw-Hill, 1982, pp 300–317

MATTHEWS MJ, GORDON PR: Morphology of pulmonary and pleural malignancies, in *Lung Cancer Clinical Diagnosis and Treatment,* MJ Straus (ed). New York, Grune & Stratton, 1977

MINNA JD et al: Lung cancer, in *The Principles and Practice of Oncology,* VT DeVita et al (eds). Philadelphia, Lippincott, 1981

———, BUNN PA JR: Paraneoplastic syndromes, in *The Principles and Practice of Oncology,* VT DeVita et al (eds). Philadelphia, Lippincott, 1981

MUGGIA FM, ROZENCWEIG M (eds): *Progress in Cancer Research and Therapy,* vol 11: *Lung Cancer.* New York, Raven, 1979

MOUNTAIN CF: Assessment of the role of surgery for control of lung cancer. Ann Thorac Surg 24:365, 1977

STANLEY KE: Prognostic factors for survival in patients with inoperable lung cancer. J Nat Cancer Inst 65:25, 1980

285
DISEASES OF THE PLEURA, MEDIASTINUM, AND DIAPHRAGM

ROLAND H. INGRAM, JR.

THE PLEURA

The visceral and parietal pleurae form a continuous membrane that encloses a potential space which normally contains only a small amount of liquid. This liquid is dynamic, and, as with all movements of liquid between the vascular and extravascular compartments, the principles of the Starling equation (Chap. 26) apply. Under normal circumstances, the liquid is filtered out of the parietal pleura which is supplied by systemic capillaries at a mean pressure of 30 cmH_2O and most is taken up at the visceral pleura supplied by the pulmonary circulation that has a mean capillary pressure of 11 cmH_2O. For the removal of macromolecules plus some liquid there are, in addition, lymphatic stomata in the diaphragmatic and basilar portions of the parietal pleura. Abnormal accumulations of liquid, designated as pleural effusions, occur with changes in hydrostatic and oncotic forces (transudation) or with alterations in membrane permeability (exudation) such as occurs with inflammation or neoplastic involvement.

The parietal pleura is supplied by segmental nerves and when inflamed gives rise to pain which is referred to superficial regions supplied by the intercostal nerves and the thoracic segments. This pain is sharp and superficial, and is aggravated during inspiration (Chap. 4). Since the location of the pain is determined by the distribution of the somatic afferents, pain may be referred to the shoulder if the diaphragmatic pleura (C3 to C5) is involved or to the upper abdomen if the lower thoracic intercostals are affected. The visceral pleura is supplied by visceral afferents that do not produce sharp and localizable pain.

The patient with pleuritic chest pain frequently has shallow, rapid breathing, and there may be lesser excursion of the affected hemithorax than the unaffected side (splinting). Inflammation of the pleural surfaces may also cause a pleural friction rub which may be localized or may be best heard at the lower thorax posteriorly, the region where there is greatest respiratory excursion. A pleural friction rub has a harsh, scratchy quality and is heard throughout the respiratory cycle; it is maximal toward the end of inspiration and early in expiration.

PLEURITIS Inflammation of the pleura can occur with or without apparent underlying pulmonary disease and has many causes, including pneumonia, tuberculosis, pulmonary infarction, and neoplasm. Pleural pain in the *absence of physical and roentgenographic findings* suggests the diagnosis of epidemic pleurodynia (Bornholm's disease, Chap. 205), other viral infections of the pleura, or connective tissue disorders such as systemic lupus erythematosus. The *presence of parenchymal disease on the chest roentgenogram* in a patient with pleuritic chest pain and fever suggests an infectious process such as acute bacterial pneumonia (Chap. 276). Pulmonary infarction secondary to pulmonary embolism (Chap. 282) may also cause inflammation of the pleural surface. Under these circumstances, hemoptysis is a common presenting feature. The finding of a *pleural effusion in the absence of parenchymal disease* suggests postprimary tuberculosis, subdiaphragmatic abscess, mesothelioma, or primary bacterial infection of the pleural space.

Treatment of pleuritis is directed toward the underlying disease and relief of pain. Analgesics frequently suppress pain, but generally they do not completely eradicate the pain associated with deep breaths and coughing. If pain prevents the patient from coughing up secretions, regional anesthesia by blockade of the appropriate intercostal nerves with a medium-duration local anesthetic is helpful. Occasionally, acute pleuritis leads to chronic adhesive pleuritis as a sequela of tuberculosis, empyema, or hemothorax. Adhesive pleuritis is characterized by marked thickening of the pleura, which may interfere with pulmonary function. Under these circumstances, the thickened pleura encases the lung and "traps" it, so that the lung behaves as if it were small and stiff, despite having intrinsically normal mechanical properties. If symptoms such as dyspnea are severe, surgical removal of the thickened pleura (decortication) may be indicated.

PLEURAL EFFUSION Pleural effusions may or may not be associated with disease of the pleura. In general, effusions due to pleural disease more nearly resemble plasma (exudates), while those occurring with a normal pleura are ultrafiltrates of the plasma (transudates). Effusions in association with pleuritis are due to increased permeability of the parietal pleura secondary to inflammatory or neoplastic involvement. A good example of pleural effusion with a normal pleura is that associated with congestive heart failure. Both increased liquid formation from the parietal pleura due to systemic capillary hypertension and decreased reabsorption from the visceral pleura secondary to elevations in pulmonary capillary pressure account for the abnormal collection of pleural liquid in this condition. Hypoalbuminemia, as occurs in nephrosis or cirrhosis, also leads to increased formation and decreased resorption of pleural liquid on the basis of decreased intravascular oncotic pressures. An additional mechanism, lymphatic obstruction, also leads to effusions in the absence of pleural disease. In this case the sharp distinction between exudates and transudates may become fuzzy. Since the lymphatic channels provide the only route for reabsorption of protein from the pleural space, protein concentrations in the effusion are often high, even though the pleura is not abnormally permeable.

The extent to which a pleural effusion compromises lung volume will depend in part on the relative stiffness of the lung and chest wall. At lung volumes in the normal breathing range, the chest wall tends to recoil outward while the lung tends to recoil inward. Many pleural effusions are asymptomatic, but patients may complain of shortness of breath, pleuritic chest pain, or a dull sensation in the chest. The physical signs include deviation of the trachea away from the affected side, dullness to percussion, and diminished breath sounds over the affected side. Egophony may be heard at the upper border of the effusion.

The most common appearance of a pleural effusion on chest roentgenogram is obliteration of the sharp angle between the diaphragm and rib cage (costophrenic angle) with an upward concavity of the liquid level. Occasionally, effusions lie underneath the lung (*subpulmonic effusion*) and give the appearance of an elevated hemidiaphragm. A chest roentgenogram in the lateral decubitus position (affected side down) will show the pleural liquid layering out along the lateral chest wall, provided the liquid is not loculated. A clue to the presence of a subpulmonic effusion in the left hemithorax from the chest roentgenograph taken in the upright posture is a wide density between the gastric air bubble and the apparent upper border of the diaphragm. Pleural effusions may be missed on anteroposterior roentgenograms taken in the supine posture since the liquid layers out posteriorly. In this case it produces a generally hazy shadow that is difficult to detect when unilateral and impossible to detect when bilateral. Occasionally, effusions may form between lobes of the lungs and produce a rounded opacity on the chest roentgenogram that resembles a solitary nodule. Since these often disappear with resolution of the effusion, they are referred to as *phantom tumors.*

FIGURE 285-1
Approach to the diagnosis of pleural effusions.

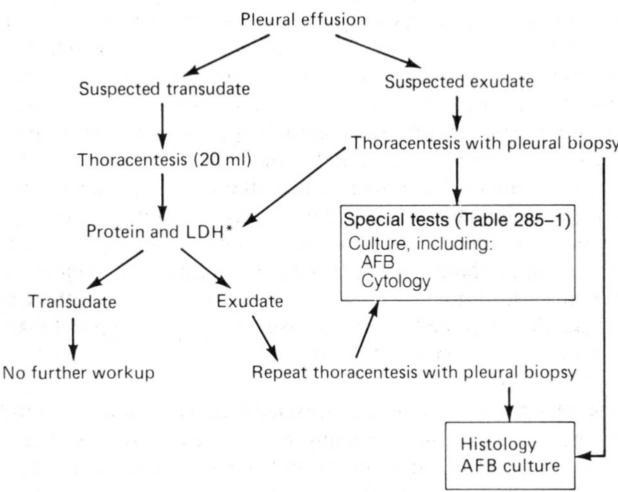

Aspiration of the pleural effusion under local anesthesia should always be performed if the etiology of the effusion is in doubt, or if the effusion is causing dyspnea. If the diagnosis of neoplasm or tuberculosis is seriously considered, closed pleural biopsy with an Abrams or Cope needle should be performed at the time of the initial thoracentesis.

Pleural liquid that is bloodstained is suggestive of neoplasm or pulmonary infarction; however, blood may also be present in effusions due to infection, congestive heart failure, and trauma. The differentiation of pleural effusions into *transudates* and *exudates* is of considerable diagnostic importance. Many different tests on the pleural liquid have been advocated (Table 285-1); however, no single test is diagnostic. Effusions which have a high protein content, high pleural liquid-to-serum LDH activity ratios, and many white blood cells are indicative of exudates. However, transudates secondary to congestive heart failure may have high protein contents after the volume of the effusion decreases with diuresis; any effusion that contains cellular debris may have a high pleural liquid-to-serum LDH ratio; and there is no absolute leukocyte count that clearly differentiates transudates from exudates. Clearly the diagnosis depends on interpretation of the test results in the context of the patient's illness. In addition to chemical tests, exudative pleural liquid should receive complete cytologic and microbiologic examinations. Figure 285-1 presents an approach to the evaluation of pleural effusions. Despite an orderly and complete approach, no cause will be found for the pleural effusion in up to 25 percent of patients.

Postprimary tuberculous effusions present as isolated pleural effusions in the absence of radiologically demonstrable paren-

TABLE 285-1
Constituents of pleural effusions

	Transudate	*Exudate*
ROUTINE TESTS		
Protein	$<$3.0 g/100 ml	$>$3.0 g/100 ml
Lactic dehydrogenase	Low	High
Pleural fluid/serum LDH ratio	$<$0.6	$>$0.6
SPECIAL TESTS		
RBC	$<$10,000/mm^3	$>$100,000/mm^3 suggests neoplasm, infarction, trauma $>$10,000, $<$100,000/mm^3 indeterminant
WBC	$<$1000/mm^3	Usually $>$1000/mm^3
Differential WBC	Usually $>$50% lymphocytes or mononuclear cells	$>$50% lymphocytes (tuberculosis, neoplasm) $>$50% polymorphonuclear (acute inflammation)
pH	$>$7.3	$<$7.3 (inflammatory)
Glucose	Same as blood ($\pm$)	Low (infection) Extremely low (rheumatoid arthritis, occasionally neoplasm)
Amylase		$>$500 units/ml (pancreatitis; occasionally neoplasm, infection)
Specific proteins		Low C3, C4 components of complement (SLE, rheumatoid arthritis) Rheumatoid factor Antinuclear factor

chymal disease and occur within months of primary subclinical infection. The patient may be asymptomatic or, more commonly, presents with fever, malaise, and weight loss. Occasionally, high fever and pleuritic chest pain are present. More than 90 percent of patients have a positive tuberculin skin test. Thoracentesis reveals an *exudative* effusion, with predominant lymphocytosis. Acid-fast bacilli are rarely seen on direct smear, and cultures are positive in fewer than 20 percent of pleural effusions due to tuberculosis. The diagnostic yield is higher with closed pleural biopsy, which will reveal noncaseating granulomas and/or positive culture material in more than 50 percent of the cases.

Neoplastic pleural effusions are common; they are usually exudative. *Bronchogenic carcinoma* is the commonest malignancy causing pleural effusions and may do so by direct extension to the pleural surface, obstruction to lymphatic drainage (secondary to mediastinal spread), or by pleural inflammation secondary to pneumonia behind an obstructed bronchus. Patients usually present with symptoms referable to the primary lesion (Chap. 284) but may present with dyspnea or pleuritic chest pain. The effusion is invariably an exudate with or without blood. Pleural liquid cytology and pleural biopsy will confirm the diagnosis in up to 60 percent of cases. *Metastatic carcinoma,* most commonly from the breast, may also cause pleural effusions and is a more frequent cause of bilateral pleural effusions than bronchogenic carcinoma. *Lymphoma* may directly involve the pleura or may obstruct lymphatic drainage leading to a pleural effusion. Malignant effusions reaccumulate rapidly after aspiration, and repeated aspirations are not warranted. Instillation of sclerosing compounds such as tetracycline or cytotoxic agents may succeed in producing adhesions between parietal and visceral pleural surfaces and decrease the rate of liquid accumulation.

Rheumatoid arthritis (Chap. 346) may cause exudative pleural effusions with or without nodular changes in the pulmonary parenchyma or on the pleural surface. Patients are most often males, and subcutaneous nodules are usually associated with the arthritis. The pleural liquid is characteristically turbid and greenish yellow and has a very low glucose concentration (less than 20 mg/dl) due to impaired glucose transport into the pleural liquid. These effusions are usually asymptomatic and do not require specific therapy. However, on occasion pleuritic chest pain and fever herald the onset of rheumatoid effusions, and, because of the acute presentation along with low glucose levels in the liquid, infectious empyema must be ruled out. Mononuclear pleocytosis and negative Gram stains and cultures aid in eliminating empyema.

Symptoms and signs referable to the chest very frequently accompany *subphrenic* (*subdiaphragmatic*) *abscess.* Fever, pleuritic chest pain, and an exudative pleural effusion are common. The chest roentgenogram usually reveals elevation of the hemidiaphragm, a small pleural effusion, and basal atelectasis, but is rarely diagnostic. Thoracentesis usually reveals sterile liquid, but an empyema due to direct extension of the infection may be present. It should be emphasized that pleural effusions following abdominal surgery are very common and should not be taken as a sign of a subdiaphragmatic abscess in the absence of other clinical features.

In *pancreatitis,* a left-sided pleural effusion may be present in up to 15 percent of patients with acute pancreatitis or pancreatic pseudocysts. Effusions are typically exudative and have a high amylase concentration. A high pleural fluid amylase concentration has occasionally been reported in neoplasm and infection, and may also be found in cases of esophageal rupture where the amylase is of salivary origin. No specific therapy of pleural effusion secondary to pancreatitis is indicated. An exception is the occurrence of a chronic effusion due to a fistula connecting a pancreatic pseudocyst to the pleural space. Surgical management of the primary pancreatic problem is indicated.

Pleural effusion and ascites in association with nonmetastatic pelvic tumors in women has been designated as *Meigs's syndrome.* The pleural effusion is most commonly right sided, may be an exudate or transudate, and is thought to develop from movement of ascitic liquid across the diaphragm. Both the ascites and pleural liquid dramatically resolve following removal of the pelvic tumor.

Eosinophilic pleural effusion is defined as the finding of eosinophils in excess of 10 percent in the pleural liquid; this attention-getting yet nonspecific finding may be present in effusions due to acute bacterial pneumonia, viral pleuritis, pancreatitis, neoplasm, and trauma.

Patients have been described with the triad of *yellow nails, lymphedema of the extremities, and pleural effusions.* The effusions have a high protein concentration and are thought to be due to impaired lymphatic drainage of the pleural space rather than to pleural disease.

CHYLOTHORAX Leakage of thoracic duct lymph into the pleural space may be due to trauma to the thoracic duct or obstruction of the duct by a malignant process (lymphoma, mediastinal spread of bronchogenic carcinoma) or mediastinal fibrosis. A rare disorder, *lymphangiomyomatosis,* is frequently accompanied by chylothorax. Thoracentesis reveals a milky white liquid which is characteristically an exudate. Fat globules may be seen microscopically on staining with Sudan III dye. Total fat content ranges from 1 to 4 g/dl. In cases of traumatic rupture of the thoracic duct, conservative management by repeated aspiration or thoracostomy-tube drainage and by cessation of oral feedings is tried initially. If this fails, lymphangiography followed by surgical ligation of the thoracic duct may be indicated. A chylothorax secondary to malignancy should not be repeatedly aspirated, since it reaccumulates rapidly.

Pseudochylous effusions do not contain fat globules but have a cloudy, milky appearance due to high concentrations of cholesterol in the pleural liquid. Cholesterol crystals may give a metallic sheen to the pleural liquid. This condition most frequently occurs in long-standing pleural effusions, and the most frequent underlying diagnoses are tuberculosis and rheumatoid lung disease.

HEMOTHORAX Hemothorax due to frank bleeding into the pleural space most commonly follows blunt or penetrating trauma to the chest. A small amount of bleeding may complicate a spontaneous pneumothorax, producing a hemopneumothorax when preexisting adhesions are disrupted as air separates the parietal and visceral pleurae. Patients with hematologic disorders or who are taking anticoagulants may bleed into the pleural space following procedures such as closed pleural biopsy; therefore, a pleural biopsy should never be performed without first assuring that the patient's coagulation status is adequate. Treatment of hemothorax is directed toward adequate drainage of the pleural space. Continued bleeding, inadequate drainage, or shock unresponsive to blood replacement require thoracotomy. Inadequate drainage of a hemothorax may lead to an intense, fibrous reaction (fibrothorax) where the thickened pleura encases the lung (trapped lung); early decortication is indicated.

EMPYEMA The presence of infected liquid or frank pus in the pleural space is termed an empyema. In the majority of cases it is the result of spread of infection from a contiguous structure and may complicate the course of bacterial pneumonia, subdiaphragmatic abscess, lung abscess, or esophageal perforation. Up to 20 percent of empyemas follow thoracic surgery or instrumentation of the pleural space (thoracentesis, inadvertent entry of the pleural space during puncture of the subclavian vein). Direct infection of the pleural space without involvement of the underlying lung by hematogenous spread of organisms from a distant site accounts for the remaining cases and is more common in children than adults. Bacteria implicated in the etiology of empyema include *Staphylococcus aureus* (most common in all ages), *Pseudomonas aeruginosa, Klebsiella pneumoniae, Escherichia coli, Pneumococcus* spp., and anaerobic bacteria.

Chest pain, fever and night sweats, cough, and weight loss are common complaints. These symptoms may be mild if an empyema develops during the course of antibiotic treatment for bacterial pneumonia; hence the empyema may go unrecognized. Signs of a pleural effusion will be present, and the chest roentgenogram will reveal pleural liquid and usually underlying parenchymal disease. Thoracentesis may reveal thick, purulent liquid, but in the early stages of the disease, thin, serous liquid with a high leukocyte count (>5000 per cubic millimeter; polymorphonuclear cells predominate), high protein content (>3 g/dl), and low glucose concentration (<20 mg/dl) may be obtained. Gram's stain usually reveals the causative organism.

Treatment is directed at providing adequate drainage of the pleural space in addition to appropriate antimicrobial therapy. If the pleural liquid is thin, drainage may occasionally be achieved by repeated thoracenteses. Most commonly, closed thoracostomy-tube drainage will be required. Prospective studies have suggested that if the initial pleural liquid pH is <7.0, tube thoracostomy will be needed irrespective of the other characteristics of the liquid. If closed drainage of the pleural space does not result in the disappearance of fever and general improvement of the patient within 4 to 5 days, a limited thoracotomy is indicated, at which time resection of a small portion of the overlying rib and manual breakdown of pleural adhesions is performed. If this approach fails, or if treatment has been delayed, decortication with removal of the thick, fibrous tissue covering the lung (pleural peel) may be necessary to obtain lung expansion and obliteration of the empyema cavity. Rarely, an unrecognized empyema may rupture through the chest wall and spontaneously drain onto the body surface (*empyema necessitans*).

The mortality rate of empyema is high among patients who are elderly, who have serious underlying disease, or in whom treatment is delayed.

PNEUMOTHORAX A pneumothorax is a collection of gas in the pleural space that results in complete or partial collapse of the lung. Normally, the pressure in the pleural space at the end of a quiet breath is subatmospheric due to a balance between the tendency of the lung to recoil inward and the tendency of the chest wall to recoil outward (Chap. 271). The lung may therefore be thought to be held in an expanded position by the surrounding negative pleural pressure much as a balloon would be held inflated when surrounded by a vacuum. When air enters the pleural space, pleural pressure in the affected hemithorax tends toward atmospheric pressure; the less negative the pleural pressure, the greater the degree of lung collapse. The mediastinum shifts toward the unaffected side as a result of the normal elastic recoil of the unaffected lung. If pressure inside the pneumothorax becomes above atmospheric, as may occur with a one-way leak into the pleural space ("ball-valve" leak) or when a pneumothorax occurs as a complication of positive pressure ventilation, a *tension pneumothorax* is present. Under these circumstances the affected lung is compressed, the mediastinum is further shifted toward the unaffected side, and cardiac output may be severely compromised due to the positive intrathoracic pressure decreasing venous return to the heart. Tension pneumothorax is a medical emergency.

A pneumothorax may occur spontaneously or may be secondary to underlying lung disease, chest trauma, mechanical ventilation, or perforated esophagus.

Spontaneous pneumothorax Spontaneous pneumothorax most commonly occurs in previously healthy adults between 20 and 40 years of age. In such patients there is a strong tendency toward recurrence of the pneumothorax. Air leaks into the pleural space due to rupture of small blebs on the surface of the visceral pleura; the etiology of these blebs is unclear. They tend to be at the apex of the lung, perhaps due to the more negative pleural pressure around the lung apex. Some patients have been found to have small pleural nodules consisting of histiocytes, giant cells, and other inflammatory cells (*reactive eosinophilic pleuritis*). These lesions should be differentiated from pulmonary eosinophilic granuloma.

Pleuritic chest pain and dyspnea are the commonest complaints in patients with pneumothorax. Physical examination reveals tachypnea, asymmetrical expansion of the chest on the affected side (due to outward recoil of the chest wall as the lung collapses), mediastinal shift with deviation of the trachea and apex beat away from the pneumothorax, and hyperresonance to percussion and diminished breath sounds over the affected side. The chest roentgenogram reveals a visible visceral pleural edge with no lung markings between this edge and the chest wall. Chest roentgenograms should be taken in the upright position before a pneumothorax can be excluded, since in the supine posture upward movement of air with approximation of visceral and parietal pleurae laterally may obscure its presence. Small pneumothoraxes may be more easily seen if the chest roentgenogram is taken at the end of a maximal expiration. If pneumothorax is associated with tearing of adhesions in the pleural space, *hemopneumothorax* may develop, with a gas-liquid level visible in the pleural space.

Treatment depends on the size of the pneumothorax. A small pneumothorax needs only close observation, since the air leak has usually sealed by the time the patient presents. The air in the pleural space will be reabsorbed spontaneously, since the sum of the partial pressures of the gases in the pleural space (i.e., air = 760 mmHg at sea level) is greater than the sum of the partial pressures of gases in the end-capillary blood due to the low end-capillary P_{O_2}. Larger pneumothoraxes should be aspirated or treated with closed thoracostomy-tube drainage. Failure of the lung to reexpand, despite application of suction to the chest tube, indicates that the lung is "trapped," that a major bronchus is occluded, or that there is a large continuing air leak through a major communication between the pleural space and lung (*bronchopleural fistula*). A bronchopleural fistula rarely occurs spontaneously unless there is underlying lung disease such as rupture of a lung abscess into the pleural space or necrotizing pneumonia, but may occur following lung resection or chest trauma or during mechanical ventilation (barotrauma). Spontaneous *tension* pneumothorax is unusual, but if present, it should be treated by immediate aspiration through a wide-bore needle placed in the pleural space at the level of the second intercostal space anteriorly at the midclavicular line. If there is circulatory collapse and severe dyspnea, tension pneumothorax should be suspected and treated without waiting for roentgenographic confirmation.

Approximately 50 percent of patients with spontaneous pneumothorax have a recurrence, and the incidence of further recurrence is even higher following the second episode. Repeated spontaneous pneumothorax should be treated surgically by application of irritants to the pleural surfaces so that they adhere to each other (*pleurodesis*) or by performing a *parietal pleurectomy*. Because of the tendency of pneumothorax to recur, if both sides are ever involved, even at different times, surgical intervention is indicated.

Patients with pneumothorax should not be moved in unpressurized aircraft because the decrease in atmospheric pressure may result in enlargement of the pneumothorax to an extent that it may seriously compromise ventilatory and cardiac function. Similarly, patients with a history of spontaneous pneumothorax should not pilot aircraft or undertake scuba diving. Should a pneumothorax occur underwater, enlargement of the pneumothorax on ascent may be catastrophic.

Pneumothorax may occur spontaneously in patients with a wide variety of lung diseases, such as asthma, emphysema, lung abscess, neoplasm, eosinophilic granuloma, and the adult respiratory distress syndrome. In the presence of underlying lung disease closed thoracotomy-tube drainage will almost always be needed. *Catamenial pneumothorax* is a rare disorder characterized by spontaneous pneumothorax at the time of the menstrual period. The right side is more frequently, but not invariably, affected. The pathogenesis of this disorder is not understood but may be related to intrathoracic endometriosis. Hormonal therapy with suppression of ovulation is usually successful.

PLEURAL TUMORS Two types of *mesothelioma,* a rare tumor of the visceral and parietal pleurae, are recognized. The *localized form* is a solitary growth on the pleural surface that only occasionally causes a pleural effusion and may be cured by surgical resection. Patients are often asymptomatic or may complain of chest pain and cough. The *diffuse mesothelioma* is a highly malignant tumor that is usually associated with a serous or blood-stained pleural effusion. There is no effective therapy for this tumor. Clubbing of the digits and hypertrophic pulmonary osteoarthropathy are associated with pleural-based tumors. The diagnosis of mesothelioma may be obtained from cytologic examination of the pleural liquid or closed pleural biopsy, but difficulty may be encountered distinguishing this tumor histologically from adenocarcinoma. There is an increased incidence of pleural and peritoneal mesotheliomas among persons exposed to asbestos; a higher incidence is found among those engaged in the processing and use of asbestos products than those in the mining industry. The interval between exposure and tumor development often exceeds 20 years; continuous exposure to asbestos is not necessary. In addition to primary tumors, the pleura is a common site for *metastases* from neoplasms of the bronchus, breast, ovary, and gastrointestinal tract.

MEDIASTINUM

The mediastinum occupies the central portion of the chest and is anatomically defined by the thoracic inlet above, the diaphragm below, the mediastinal pleura laterally, the paravertebral gutter and ribs posteriorly, and the sternum anteriorly. The mediastinum is divided into four compartments for descriptive purposes (Fig. 285-2). The *superior mediastinum* is bounded above by the plane of the first rib and below by an imaginary line drawn anteroposteriorly from the sternal angle to the lower edge of the fourth thoracic vertebra. It contains the trachea, upper esophagus, thymus gland, thoracic duct, great veins, arch of the aorta and its branches, and the phrenic, vagus, and left recurrent laryngeal nerves. Below the superior mediastinum lie three further compartments. The *anterior mediastinum* contains fibroareolar tissue and lymph nodes, but no major structures. The *middle mediastinum* contains the heart, ascending aorta, great veins, pulmonary artery, and phrenic nerves. The *posterior mediastinum* contains the esophagus, thoracic duct, descending aorta, sympathetic chain, and intercostal and vagal nerves.

TUMORS AND CYSTS The commonest mediastinal masses in adults are metastatic carcinomas (most commonly bronchogenic carcinoma) and lymphomas. Neurogenic tumors, teratodermoids, thymomas, and bronchogenic cysts account for approximately two-thirds of the remaining mediastinal masses.

One-third of patients are asymptomatic, with the mediastinal mass detected on a routine chest roentgenogram. In the remainder, chest pain, cough, dyspnea, and symptoms due to compression or invasion of structures in the mediastinum may be present (e.g., dysphagia, hoarseness due to recurrent laryngeal nerve involvement, superior vena caval obstruction). Symptoms are more common with malignant tumors.

Investigation of a mediastinal mass begins with posteroanterior and lateral chest roentgenograms to which are added oblique views, a contrast study of the esophagus, and tomography, if needed, to define more clearly the anatomic location and borders of the mass. The anatomic site of the lesion is of diagnostic importance, and may determine the next step in the diagnostic workup (Fig. 285-2). Computerized tomography of the chest with injection of contrast material into a peripheral vein, or angiography of the pulmonary circulation or aorta may be needed to distinguish vascular from nonvascular lesions, a differentiation of particular importance if biopsy of the mass is considered. A further value of computerized tomography is the detection of the cystic nature of a lesion, a finding that strongly indicates that it is benign. Mediastinoscopy and biopsy are useful in the diagnosis of mediastinal masses if metastatic carcinoma, lymphoma, or sarcoidosis are considered likely. Lymph nodes behind the trachea and below the aortic arch on the left side are not accessible for biopsy using this approach. Scalene lymph node biopsy in the absence of palpable nodes may provide the diagnosis if lymphoma or metastatic carcinoma is suspected. Bronchoscopy is unlikely to be helpful in the diagnostic workup unless there are symptoms suggestive of an endobronchial lesion (e.g., hemoptysis) or unless there is evidence of lobar collapse, consolidation, or a mass lesion in the lung parenchyma on chest roentgenograph. Special tests such as radionuclide scanning with ^{131}I to detect an active retrosternal goiter may also be helpful.

FIGURE 285-2
Common sites for mediastinal masses.

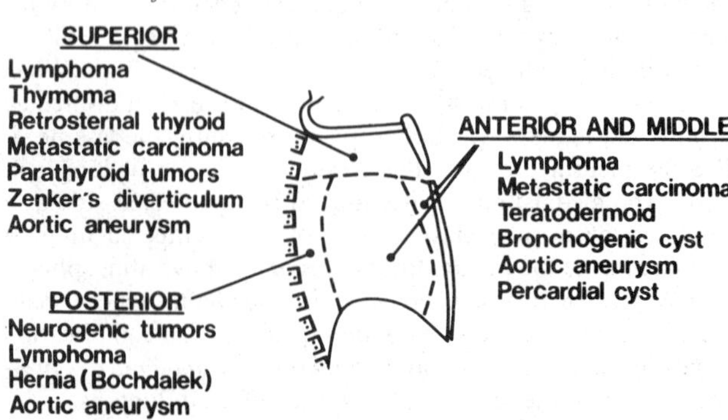

Neurogenic tumors are the most common primary mediastinal neoplasms and are found almost exclusively in the posterior mediastinum near the paravertebral gutter. The majority of these neoplasms are benign; neurofibromas, schwannomas, and ganglioneuromas are the commonest tumors seen. Vague chest pain and cough may be present, but "root" pain is an infrequent complaint. *Paravertebral abscesses* also appear in the posterior mediastinum, and the clinical picture of infection often gives the major clue. Neurofibromas may occur singly or in association with von Recklinghausen's disease (Chap. 365). Occasionally these are accompanied by hypertrophic pulmonary osteoarthropathy. *Ganglioneuromas* arise from the sympathetic chain and, together with *neuroblastomas,* may secrete hormones which lead to diarrhea, flushing, and hypertension. Vanillylmandelic acid (VMA) may be found in the urine. Mediastinal *neuroblastoma* usually occurs in children, is particularly responsive to irradiation, and has a better prognosis than neuroblastomas of the abdomen or retroperitoneal space. *Pheochromocytoma* is a rare mediastinal tumor which may secrete catecholamines and present the same clinical picture as the more common (but still rare) abdominal form (Chap. 113). The treatment of all neurogenic tumors of the mediastinum is surgical, with postoperative irradiation for patients with neuroblastomas.

Teratodermoids most commonly arise in the anterior mediastinum. Most of these tumors are detected in early adult life and approximately 10 to 20 percent undergo malignant changes. Teratodermoids frequently contain linear calcification of the lining of a cyst, and bone and teeth may be evident on chest roentgenogram. They are treated by surgical excision.

Thymomas account for 10 percent of primary mediastinal neoplasms and are found in the superior and anterior mediastinum. Approximately one-fourth are malignant, but they rarely metastasize. Myasthenia gravis (Chap. 372) occurs in about 50 percent of patients with thymoma; however, the majority of patients with myasthenia gravis do not have a thymic tumor. Agammaglobulinemia, pure red blood cell aplasia, and Cushing's syndrome have been reported to be associated with thymoma. Because of compression of the trachea by the tumor, patients may complain of dyspnea in the supine posture. Symptoms may also arise from local invasion or compression of other surrounding structures. Treatment is by surgical excision; malignant thymomas are usually radiation-sensitive.

Lipomas can develop almost anywhere but most often are seen in the superior or anterior mediastinum. Computerized tomography almost always allows a noninvasive diagnosis.

Benign cysts most commonly arise in the anterior and middle mediastinum. Most do not produce symptoms and are detected only on routine chest roentgenography. *Bronchogenic cysts* most commonly develop in the paratracheal area or near the carina. The cysts are lined with ciliated respiratory epithelium and contain smooth muscle and cartilage in their walls. They are liquid-filled and therefore have a uniform density on chest roentgenogram, where they appear as rounded or tear-shaped opacities. Usually the cysts have no demonstrable communication with the tracheobronchial tree; however, they may become infected. *Enteric cysts* occur along the esophagus and are lined by gastric or intestinal epithelium. As with bronchogenic cysts, infection and abscess formation may occur. If the cyst contains acid-secreting cells, ulcer formation, perforation, and hemorrhage may occur. The *pericardial cyst* is a developmental anomaly and is attached to the pericardium but only rarely communicates with the pericardial cavity.

Hernias through the diaphragm produce mediastinal masses that may or may not contain intestinal gas. The commonest is through the esophageal hiatus as discussed below. More rarely a defect in the posterolateral portion (so-called foramen of Bochdalek) of the diaphragm allows herniation of intestine into the left side of the chest. More often presenting as a mediastinal mass is a retrosternal herniation through the foramen of Morgagni.

SUPERIOR VENA CAVAL SYNDROME Obstruction of the superior vena cava (SVC) secondary to compression or infiltration by superior mediastinal tumors results in a characteristic constellation of physical findings with dilatation of collateral veins of the upper thorax and neck, plethora and edema of the face and neck, conjunctival edema, and headache. Visual disturbances and alterations in the state of consciousness may occur. Compression of the adjacent esophagus and trachea may cause dysphagia, wheeze, and shortness of breath.

Obstruction of the SVC is almost invariably due to malignant disease, approximately 75 percent of the cases being due to *bronchogenic carcinoma. Lymphoma* accounts for almost all the remaining cases. Right-sided tumors much more frequently produce the syndrome as would be expected on an anatomic basis. Rarely, this syndrome occurs with *fibrosing mediastinitis* that is either idiopathic or secondary to histoplasmosis or occurs in association with methylsergide ingestion. *Retrosternal thyroid* and *aortic aneurysms* are among the other benign causes of SVC obstruction. Using invasive diagnostic procedures such as bronchoscopy, esophagoscopy, and mediastinoscopy in an attempt to obtain a tissue diagnosis is contraindicated due to the risk of bleeding during the procedure. Unless clinical examination and noninvasive investigations suggest a benign cause for the obstruction, or unless there is tissue elsewhere to biopsy (e.g., lymphadenopathy, skin lesions), the patient should receive irradiation or chemotherapy before attempts are made to obtain a tissue diagnosis. Corticosteroids are sometimes given during the initial stages of management in an effort to decrease edema at the site of obstruction.

PNEUMOMEDIASTINUM (MEDIASTINAL EMPHYSEMA) Air within the planes of the mediastinum may appear spontaneously or may be secondary to chest trauma, perforation of the trachea, bronchus, or esophagus, spread of air from the fascial planes of the neck or pharynx, or from dissection of air from the retroperitoneal space. When pneumomediastinum occurs with no apparent cause, it is referred to as a *spontaneous pneumomediastinum.* In contrast to spontaneous pneumothorax, as discussed above, there is no tendency for recurrence. Air is thought to dissect from alveoli to the interstitial space and into the vascular adventitia to the hilum. From there it moves into the mediastinum, neck, or retroperitoneal space. Occasionally mediastinal air ruptures into the pleural space, giving a small pneumothorax, most often on the left side. Predisposing factors include raised intrathoracic pressure, as with coughing, vomiting, and Valsalva maneuvers. Rapid decompression such as occurs with sudden ascent during diving has also been implicated. Pneumomediastinum may also occur spontaneously during an attack of asthma. The patient with pneumomediastinum may be asymptomatic but usually complains of retrosternal pain and dyspnea; less commonly there is sore throat due to dissection of air into the retropharyngeal space. Examination may reveal subcutaneous crepitus in the upper body, and a crunching sound synchronous with the heart beat may be heard over the precordium (Hamman's sign). Fever and mild leukocytosis are common with uncomplicated pneumomediastinum. Occasionally, cardiac function is compromised with physical signs of cardiac tamponade (Chap. 265). A lateral chest roentgenogram should always be obtained if pneumomediastinum is suspected since abnormalities may be seen only on this view. Air is seen outlining the pulmonary artery trunk and root of aorta and may be seen tracking into the neck.

Pneumomediastinum secondary to *esophageal perforation* may follow endoscopy or may occur with vomiting (Boerhaave's syndrome). Esophageal perforation is a surgical emergency and should be suspected if there is increasing pain aggravated by swallowing or fever and when signs of increasing mediastinal width and left pleural effusion occur on chest roentgenogram. Acute and fulminant mediastinitis is a frequent sequela and should be treated with immediate surgical drainage, closure of the perforation site, and broad-spectrum antibiotic therapy.

THE DIAPHRAGM

The diaphragm is the major muscle of inspiration and is derived embryonically from the septum transversum and the pleuroperitoneal membranes. Its motor nerve supply is from the phrenic nerves (C3 to C5); the afferent supply is derived both from the phrenic and lower intercostal nerves. When the diaphragm contracts, intrathoracic pressure is lowered and intraabdominal pressure is increased. Thus, the diaphragm acts as if it were "pulling" on the lung (by lowering intrathoracic pressure) and "pushing" on the rib cage (by raising abdominal pressure), resulting in an increase in lung volume and outward movement of both rib cage and abdomen as it descends on inspiration.

DIAPHRAGMATIC PARALYSIS *Unilateral diaphragmatic paralysis* is usually the result of injury to a phrenic nerve secondary to trauma or tumor in the mediastinum. The lesion is usually asymptomatic, but the patient may complain of dyspnea in the supine posture when the diaphragm, weakened by unilateral paralysis, must work against the added load of the abdominal contents. Unilateral paralysis results in only a small decrease in vital capacity. The diagnosis is suggested by the finding of an elevated hemidiaphragm on chest roentgenogram and can be confirmed by fluoroscopy. Paradoxical (i.e., upward) motion of the affected hemidiaphragm occurs when the patient is asked to sniff, a maneuver that suddenly lowers intrathoracic and raises intraabdominal pressure.

Bilateral diaphragmatic paralysis is less common than unilateral paralysis, but it has far greater consequences on respiration. Bilateral paralysis may be due to high cervical cord injury, motor neuron disease, poliomyelitis, polyneuropathies, or bilateral involvement of the phrenic nerve by mediastinal lesions. Recently the use of ice slush in the pericardium for cardioplegia during cardiac surgery has been associated with bilateral paralysis due to cold injury of the phrenic nerves. The patient with bilateral diaphragmatic paralysis usually has severe shortness of breath, particularly in the supine position, and often hypercapnic respiratory failure is present. In most of these patients there is paradoxical (i.e., inward) motion of the abdomen on inspiration, a finding easily observed at the bedside, particularly with the patient supine. This is due to passive ascent of the diaphragm as intrathoracic pressure is lowered by the intercostal and accessory muscles. In a few patients paradoxical abdominal motion may not be obvious with the patient erect due to use of the abdominal muscles during expiration. Here, abdominal motion will appear normal as contraction of the abdominal muscles causes inward abdominal motion on expiration and relaxation results in outward abdominal motion on inspiration. Under these circumstances the diaphragm may appear to move normally at fluoroscopy, and the diagnosis of diaphragmatic paralysis will be missed.

The vital capacity which is reduced in the upright posture is even more severely reduced when the patient is supine because the paralyzed diaphragm is sucked upward during a maximal inspiration with displacement of abdominal contents into the thorax. The diagnosis of bilateral diaphragmatic paralysis is established by assessment of transdiaphragmatic pressure obtained by comparison of simultaneous measurements of esophageal and gastric pressures. Treatment of this disorder may be conservative, using a rocking bed at night; in patients with intact phrenic nerves, electrical pacing of those nerves has been successful.

ELEVATION OF THE HEMIDIAPHRAGM ON CHEST ROENTGENOGRAPH Normally, the right side of the diaphragm is approximately 4 cm higher than the left due to displacement by the liver. *Apparent elevation* of one hemidiaphragm is due to a subpulmonic pleural effusion, and a lateral decubitus chest roentgenogram will establish this diagnosis. *True elevation* of one hemidiaphragm is most commonly due to upward displacement secondary to intraabdominal masses or ascites, or it may be due to loss of lung volume on the affected side secondary to pulmonary collapse or fibrosis. *Eventration of the diaphragm* is a rare congenital disorder more common on the left side. The anterior two-thirds of the diaphragm is replaced by a thin membrane, resulting in upward movement of abdominal contents into the thoracic cage. Patients are usually asymptomatic, and the diagnosis is made following a routine chest roentgenogram. No treatment is necessary. Rarely, eventration of the diaphragm may seriously compromise ventilatory function in the newborn. Plication of the hemidiaphragm is then performed. Eventration must be distinguished from *diaphragmatic hernias* through which abdominal contents are displaced into the chest. The most common location is at the esophageal hiatus with displacement of part of the stomach into the posterior mediastinum (Chap. 305).

MISCELLANEOUS DISEASES OF THE DIAPHRAGM Neoplasms of the diaphragm are rare; they include lipomas, fibromas, neurofibromas, and cysts. These benign tumors are approximately 1 to $1\frac{1}{2}$ times more frequent than the malignant fibrosarcoma. The diaphragm may be involved by direct extension of primary lung or abdominal tumors and may be the site of metastases from distant tumors.

REFERENCES

BLACK LF: Pleural disease. Basics of RD. Am Thorac Soc News 6:26, 1978

LIGHT RW et al: Parapneumonic effusions. Am J Med 69:507, 1980

MARVASTA MA et al: Misleading density of mediastinal cysts on computed tomography. Ann Thorac Surg 31:167, 1981

NEWSOM DJ et al: Diaphragm function and alveolar hypoventilation. Q J Med 177:87, 1976

SILVERMAN NA, SABISTON, DC: Mediastinal masses. Surg Clin N Am 60:757, 1980

286
DISORDERS OF VENTILATION

JOHN B. WEST

The principles governing pulmonary ventilation and its regulation are discussed in Chap. 271. The fine control of ventilation is normally carried out by the central chemoreceptors near the ventral surface of the medulla which respond to changes in pH

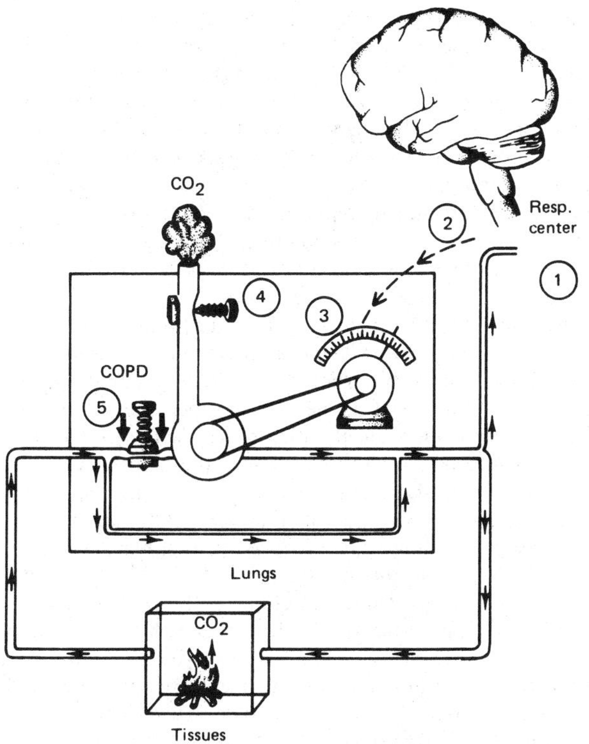

FIGURE 286-1
Scheme to illustrate the various causes of carbon dioxide retention. These include (1) disorders of the respiratory center or (2) of the supplying nerves or (3) of muscles of ventilation or (4) some mechanical problem in lung or chest wall, including obstruction to the upper airways. All these conditions result in hypoventilation. However, chronic obstructive pulmonary disease (5) in effect diverts blood from the ventilated regions, so that carbon dioxide retention occurs in spite of a normal (or high) ventilation. In addition, the ventilatory response is inappropriate for the level of carbon dioxide in these patients because of the increased work of breathing and sometimes also because of a reduced sensitivity of the respiratory center.

of the extracellular fluid around them. The composition of this fluid is mainly determined by the cerebrospinal fluid. For example, a fall in pH caused by diffusion of carbon dioxide across the blood-brain barrier increases respiratory drive, thus holding the arterial P_{CO_2}[1] within close limits (Fig. 286-1). The extreme sensitivity of this feedback control is seen when a normal subject inhales air containing carbon dioxide. Typically the ventilation may double for a rise in P_{CO_2} of only 2 to 3 mmHg.

Arterial hypoxemia constitutes a coarse control through its action on the peripheral chemoreceptors in the carotid bodies. Although this control is minor under normal conditions, it becomes very important during chronic hypoxemia, as in people living at high altitude, or in patients with chronic lung disease. Under these conditions the increased ventilation lowers the P_{CO_2} of the arterial blood and cerebrospinal fluid, but the pH of the cerebrospinal fluid is reset to its normal level of about 7.32 by outward movement of bicarbonate.

Additional control is afforded by changes in pH of the arterial blood irrespective of its P_{CO_2}. This relatively weak regulation apparently occurs through stimulation of the peripheral chemoreceptors, and although it is seldom seen under normal conditions, it may dominate in the control of ventilation in metabolic acidosis. Reflexes originating in the lung and elsewhere also affect ventilation under some circumstances.

Disorders of the regulation of respiration include hypoventilation, hyperventilation, and abnormal patterns of breathing. A cardinal feature of hypoventilation is carbon dioxide retention (Table 286-1), and indeed these terms are often used virtually interchangeably. This can be misleading, but following common usage, the various types of carbon dioxide retention are grouped here under the heading of hypoventilation.

[1] *Unless otherwise stated, the partial pressures refer to arterial blood.*

HYPOVENTILATION

CARBON DIOXIDE RETENTION CAUSED BY PURE HYPOVENTILATION (NORMAL LUNGS) In this group of diseases, the amount of air going into the lungs each minute is reduced. Strictly it is the volume of air entering the alveoli, or *alveolar ventilation*, which is crucial (Chap. 271). However, in practice, the volume of the conducting airways remains fairly constant so that, if the amount of air passing the lips is abnormally low, hypoventilation is said to be present.

The alveolar ventilation and alveolar P_{CO_2} are related by the following equation:

$$\text{Alveolar } P_{CO_2} = \frac{CO_2 \text{ output}}{\text{alveolar ventilation}}$$

In normal lungs, the P_{CO_2} of arterial blood is virtually the same as that in alveolar gas, and the carbon dioxide output at rest remains fairly constant. Thus the expression implies that if the alveolar ventilation is halved, the arterial P_{CO_2} is doubled.

The level of alveolar ventilation also influences the P_{O_2}. As the ventilation falls and the P_{CO_2} rises, the P_{O_2} falls. An important practical point is that, if the P_{CO_2} is considerably increased by pure hypoventilation, say to 70 mmHg, the P_{O_2} may still be well above the level at which cyanosis can be detected clinically. Thus a patient may have serious carbon dioxide retention and yet appear a "healthy" pink color. Note also that if a patient is given an oxygen-enriched mixture to breathe, the hypoxemia will be abolished, but the hypercapnia remains (Chap. 287).

Conditions affecting the respiratory center During normal *sleep*, the P_{CO_2} rises by 3 or 4 mmHg. Patients with idiopathic hypoventilation or with the "Pickwickian syndrome" (see below) are particularly likely to develop depressed breathing when they are asleep. One of the commonest causes of hypoventilation is depression of the respiratory center by *drugs*.

TABLE 286-1
Causes of carbon dioxide retention

1 Pure hypoventilation (normal lungs)
- *a* Respiratory center depression—morphine derivatives, barbiturates, some general anesthetics
- *b* Diseases of the brainstem—encephalitis, hemorrhage, trauma, neoplasm (rare)
- *c* Abnormalities of spinal cord conducting pathways—high cervical dislocation
- *d* Anterior horn cell disease—poliomyelitis
- *e* Diseases of nerves to respiratory muscles—Guillain-Barré syndrome, diphtheria
- *f* Diseases of the myoneural junction—myasthenia gravis, anticholinesterase poisoning
- *g* Diseases of the respiratory muscles—progressive muscular dystrophy
- *h* Thoracic cage abnormalities—crushed chest, kyphoscoliosis (lungs may be abnormal)
- *i* Upper airway obstruction—thymoma, aortic aneurysm
- *j* Hypoventilation associated with extreme obesity (Pickwickian syndrome)
- *k* Idiopathic hypoventilation
- *l* Other causes—metabolic alkalosis

2 CO_2 retention associated with chronic lung disease

These include many anesthetics, the barbiturates, and morphine and its derivatives. Respiratory center depression is often seen in the recovery room, before the effects of anesthetic and preoperative sedatives have worn off, and also in the emergency room in patients who have taken an overdose of barbiturate. In these circumstances, the arterial P_{CO_2} should be measured, and assisted ventilation following endotracheal intubation or tracheostomy may be lifesaving. Depression of the respiratory center is often accompanied by impairment of the cough reflex and difficulties with swallowing, so that aspiration of fluid into the lungs may occur and lead to pneumonia. An additional advantage of intubation is that it allows the airways to be sucked free of secretions and inhaled material (Chap. 287).

Brainstem abnormalities Conditions which may cause hypoventilation include inflammation, hemorrhage, trauma, and rarely neoplasms. Encephalitis and acute bulbar poliomyelitis (in the absence of involvement of the respiratory muscles) may cause slowing and shallowness of respiration. Irregularities of rhythm and periods of apnea may develop. The first signs of these abnormalities often appear during sleep. The ventilatory response to inhaled CO_2 mixtures is depressed. These patients can return their blood gases to normal by voluntarily increasing their ventilation, and indeed they can sometimes be managed by being reminded to breathe when periods of apnea develop. However, they may die because of apnea during sleep. Respiratory depression may be associated with loss of the cough and swallowing reflexes and consequent accumulation of secretions.

Neuromuscular disorders Neuromuscular disorders affecting the spinal conducting pathways, the anterior horn cells, the nerves to the respiratory muscles, and the respiratory muscles themselves are important causes of hypoventilation (Table 286-1). Examples include compression of the cervical cord, poliomyelitis, the Guillain-Barré syndrome, and myasthenia gravis. The most important muscle of respiration is the diaphragm, and patients with progressive disease often do not complain of dyspnea until the diaphragm is involved. By then their ventilatory reserve is severely compromised, and they must be carefully observed. The converse also occurs. Patients with neurologic disease such as amyotrophic lateral sclerosis may complain of dyspnea as their initial symptom at a time when their neurologic findings may be extremely subtle. The progress of the disease can be monitored by measuring the vital capacity and the arterial blood gases. Again, the treatment of hypoventilation in these conditions is assisted ventilation either by oropharyngeal intubation in acute states, or with a tracheostomy for long-term management (Chap. 287). Patients with chronic paresis of their respiratory muscles are likely to develop chest infections because of their difficulty in getting rid of secretions.

Thoracic cage abnormalities CRUSHED CHEST An increasingly common cause of hypoventilation is trauma to the thoracic cage resulting from automobile accidents. Frequently this is caused by impact of the steering wheel with the sternum, or the chest is crushed when a wheel of a car runs over it. Usually there are multiple injuries. There may be dissociation of movement of the chest wall, so that one region is sucked in while the remainder of the chest wall moves out during inspiration ("flail chest"). Prompt intubation and assisted ventilation is often required, and careful monitoring of the arterial blood gases is mandatory.

SCOLIOSIS Bony deformity of the chest can lead to respiratory failure with a raised arterial P_{CO_2}. *Scoliosis* refers to lateral curvature of the spine, and kyphosis to posterior curvature. The effects of scoliosis on cardiopulmonary function are the more serious, especially if the angulation is situated high in the vertebral column. Scoliosis is frequently associated with rotation of the spine and backward protuberance of the ribs, giving the appearance of an added kyphosis. In fact, the term *kyphoscoliosis* is often used for this condition, although true kyphoscoliosis is rare. Some 80 percent of cases of scoliosis are idiopathic in origin. The rest are caused by neuromuscular disorders such as poliomyelitis or are congenital in origin.

The initial complaint is dyspnea on exertion. Later hypoxemia develops; eventually carbon dioxide retention and signs of failure of the right side of the heart may supervene. Sometimes bronchitis may complicate the picture, especially in smokers. The chief cause of the CO_2 retention is the deformity of the chest wall which leads to an inefficient action of the respiratory muscles and a great increase in the work of breathing. The compliance of the chest wall is reduced (it is stiffer), especially in older patients, and this results in rapid, shallow breathing, so that an increasingly large fraction of the tidal volume is wasted in the dead space of the bronchi. The hypoventilation causes not only hypercapnia but also hypoxemia. Pulmonary vasoconstriction results, pulmonary artery pressure rises, and the work of the right side of the heart increases. This is exaggerated by the polycythemia which develops (Chap. 262).

It should be noted, however, that these patients also have abnormal lungs. These tend to be remarkably small, and the restricted pulmonary vascular bed probably also plays a role in the development of pulmonary hypertension. Areas of atelectasis are common, presumably because the volume of the thoracic cage is greatly reduced. Uneven ventilation of the lungs has been demonstrated in many cases, so that ventilation-perfusion inequality contributes to the hypoxemia.

Pulmonary function tests show a reduction in all lung volumes; indeed the total lung capacity may be reduced to half the predicted normal value. Some of the inequality of ventilation can be explained by airway closure in dependent regions of the lung as a result of the gross reduction of lung volume. Airway resistance in relation to lung volume is approximately normal, but the maximum breathing capacity is reduced because of the restricted vital capacity. The diffusing capacity of the lung for carbon monoxide is not markedly abnormal when related to lung volume. In advanced disease, a reduced ventilatory response to inhaled carbon dioxide can be demonstrated. This is probably related to the large increase in the work of breathing caused by the deformity of the chest wall. Not only is the chest wall stiff, but the respiratory muscles operate inefficiently.

Little specific therapy is available. Just as the cause of most cases of the disease is unknown, so are the factors determining its progression poorly understood. Some help can be obtained from orthopedic braces such as the Milwaukee brace, in the early stages of the disease. Corrective surgery such as the Harrington procedure during adolescence improves the appearance and may relieve back pain. However, the long-term effects on cardiopulmonary function are unknown. Any pulmonary infection should be promptly and vigorously treated with appropriate antibiotics. If hypoxemia is severe and O_2 therapy is required (Chap. 287), the patient should be carefully watched for evidence of increasing hypoventilation. Cor pulmonale and right-sided heart failure should be treated with diuretics, digitalis, and perhaps phlebotomy if the polycythemia is severe.

OTHER CONDITIONS Also associated with an abnormal chest wall are ankylosing spondylitis and pectus excavatum. In *ankylosing spondylitis* (Chap. 347) there is immobility of the vertebral joints and fixation of the ribs, so that movement of the chest wall may be grossly reduced. There is a reduction of vital capacity and total lung capacity, but good movement of the diaphragm is preserved so that the ventilatory capacity is unimpaired. Some fall in the compliance of the chest wall has been reported and also some uneven ventilation, the latter possibly caused by the reduced lung volume. In general, however, the lungs are virtually normal and do not show the pathologic changes seen in kyphoscoliosis. Hypoventilation is not a feature, and secondary heart failure does not occur.

Pectus excavatum is a congenital abnormality in which the lower part of the sternum is depressed toward the spine. In spite of the bizarre appearance of the chest, little interference with pulmonary function is the rule. There may be a slight reduction in vital capacity, total lung capacity, and maximum breathing capacity, but gas exchange is virtually normal, and hypoventilation does not occur. Surgical correction for cosmetic reasons may be considered.

Obstruction to the upper airways Tracheal stenosis can be caused by neoplasms such as thymoma in structures adjacent to the trachea, by scarring following injury, by aortic aneurysm, or by a congenital abnormality. Tumors originating in the upper airways and foreign bodies may also be responsible for airways obstruction. Hypoventilation with CO_2 retention may occur, and this may be of long standing. It is possible to distinguish tracheal obstruction from the airway obstruction of chronic obstructive lung disease by the stridor and by the flow patterns of maximal inspiration and expiration. In addition, pulmonary function tests show no inequality of ventilation. Intermittent upper airway obstruction may occur in obese and other people during sleep (see "Sleep Apnea" below).

Hypoventilation associated with extreme obesity ("Pickwickian syndrome") Some extremely obese patients hypoventilate, and the association of obesity, somnolence, polycythemia, and excessive appetite has been dubbed the *Pickwickian syndrome,* after the fat boy, Joe, in Charles Dickens's *Pickwick Papers.* Apart from the obesity, the clinical features are similar to those in patients with idiopathic hypoventilation (see below). In the fully developed form they include marked obesity (body weight typically over 130 kg), somnolence, twitching, cyanosis, periodic respiration, secondary polycythemia, right ventricular hypertrophy, and right-sided heart failure.

The obesity may have been present for years, but in some cases a recent rapid gain in weight has been described. The somnolence may be a striking feature, the patient sometimes dozing off halfway through a sentence. The cyanosis and periodic breathing are particularly marked during sleep. Sleep apnea may occur (see below), and in some patients this is caused by upper airway obstruction as a result of collapse of the pharyngeal walls. Ankle edema is a common symptom, and an enlarged liver and engorged neck veins are seen.

Blood gas measurements show an elevated P_{CO_2} and depressed P_{O_2}; the former may be as high as 70 mmHg. Lung function tests show a reduction in lung volumes, particularly in the expiratory reserve volume (the volume which can be forcibly exhaled from normal end-expiration). The vital capacity is also reduced, as is the compliance of the chest cage. The abdominal pressure is raised, especially when the patient is supine, thus forcing the diaphragm into the chest. There are no indications of airway obstruction and little inequality of ventilation, but the energy cost of moving the chest wall is abnormally high. The ventilatory response to inhaled CO_2 is therefore generally greatly decreased. In these respects the syndrome is similar to kyphoscoliosis. However, in addition, some patients have a diminished sensitivity of the respiratory center to CO_2. The reduction of lung volume causes airway closure in the dependent regions of the lung, and this contributes to the hypoxemia. There is an increase in the resting oxygen consumption of these patients which aggravates the effects of their impaired ventilation.

A striking feature of this syndrome is the dramatic improvement that takes place in all symptoms when the patient loses weight. Objective indices of improvement include a fall in arterial P_{CO_2}, rise in P_{O_2}, increases in vital capacity, total lung capacity, and total ventilation, and an enhanced ventilatory response to inhaled CO_2. In addition, signs of heart failure often disappear. Even a loss of 15 to 20 kg is often sufficient to bring about a remarkable improvement in well-being. Treatment by caloric restriction is indicated. In addition, recent work shows that some patients respond well to progesterone. If upper airway obstruction causes sleep apnea, tracheostomy is often very beneficial.

It is important to note that not all extremely obese patients develop hypoventilation. Some investigators have suggested that the Pickwickian individual is simply a patient with idiopathic hypoventilation who happens to be obese. The term *Pickwickian syndrome* is often used rather loosely. It should be reserved for very obese patients who have an increased P_{CO_2} without evidence of lung disease. The cause of the hypoventilation is not clear but presumably is related to the high energy cost of moving the chest wall. In addition the reduction in lung volumes caused by elevation of the diaphragm causes shallow, inefficient breathing. However the association of marked somnolence and voracious appetite suggests that, in some patients at least, there is an abnormality in the central nervous system.

Idiopathic hypoventilation Idiopathic, or primary, hypoventilation is a rare disease of unknown cause occurring in patients whose lungs and chest wall are normal. A colorful name sometimes given to this condition is Ondine's curse after the fairy whose human lover lost the ability to breathe automatically and had to will himself to do so. Most of the reported patients have been between 20 and 60 years of age, and there has been a preponderance of males. Typical symptoms include lack of energy, somnolence, headache, and some breathlessness on exertion. Cyanosis, especially when the patient is asleep, is a common observation, this being caused by a combination of the hypoxemia and polycythemia. Periodic breathing is often noted at night. Occasionally unusual sensitivity to sedatives or hypnotic drugs given preoperatively has been a feature. In some cases, an acute respiratory infection has prompted awareness of the condition. Several patients have had a past history of encephalitis, neurosyphilis, or schizophrenia. Signs of heart failure including engorged neck veins, enlarged heart, palpable liver, and peripheral edema have been described in severe cases.

The P_{CO_2} is elevated, generally in the range of 55 to 80 mmHg, and the P_{O_2} is depressed; these can rapidly be restored to near normal by asking the patient to increase ventilation voluntarily. Indeed some observers have found considerable variability in the P_{CO_2}, because, when the patients are tested and become aware of their breathing, they tend to breathe more. For this reason the finding of a raised plasma bicarbonate may be a useful diagnostic pointer. The hematocrit is typically between 50 and 70 percent. The ventilatory response to inhaled CO_2 is greatly impaired, though the work of breathing is not increased. Tests of pulmonary function are generally normal with no indication of airway obstruction. The pulmonary arterial pressure is typically increased because of the alveolar hypoxemia.

No specific pathologic changes have been found in the central nervous system of these patients. Congestive heart failure and respiratory infections should be treated vigorously.

Metabolic alkalosis A few patients with metabolic alkalosis hypoventilate, although this causes no symptoms and is difficult to detect clinically. The commonest causes include severe vomiting, and potassium and chloride loss such as that caused by diuretics or steroid therapy. The arterial pH is always raised, indicating only partial respiratory compensation. Many patients with metabolic alkalosis do not hypoventilate at all.

Sleep apnea Over the last 10 years a number of patients have been described in whom breathing periodically stops during sleep. Sleep apnea is defined as cessation of airflow at the nostrils and mouth for at least 10 s. This can occur in normal subjects up to 10 times a night and then only during rapid eye movement (REM) sleep. But in the patients with sleep apnea syndrome there are usually over 10 apneic periods per hour of sleep.

Sleep apnea is of two types: obstructive and central. In *obstructive sleep apnea,* airflow (as measured by thermistors at the nose and mouth) ceases despite persistent respiratory efforts as shown by abdominal and thoracic inspiratory movements. These movements can be recorded by transducers around the abdomen and chest. Sometimes the patient seeks medical advice because of loud snoring and daytime somnolence. The airway obstruction can be caused by backward movement of the tongue, narrowing of upper airway by obesity, collapse of the pharyngeal walls due to failure of the genioglossus muscle, or greatly enlarged tonsils or adenoids. Arterial oxygen saturation (measured by ear oximeter) falls during the apneic periods, cardiac arrhythmias may develop, and acute elevations in systemic and pulmonary artery pressures can occur. There is often chronic sleep deprivation, and the patient may exhibit daytime somnolence, chronic fatigue, and morning headaches. Personality disturbances such as paranoia, hostility, and agitated depression may develop. Long-term tracheostomy has been shown to be beneficial in some of these patients. Weight loss is valuable if the patient is obese. Methoxyprogesterone has been used as a respiratory stimulant, but its value is uncertain.

Central sleep apnea is caused by a transient cessation of inspiratory muscle activity. It is recognized by the absence of both airflow and respiratory movements. Patients who tend to hypoventilate (see Table 286-1) may develop apneic episodes during sleep when respiratory drive is depressed. It is now known that during REM sleep breathing is often irregular and unresponsive to chemical and vagal drives. The exception is hypoxemia, which remains a powerful stimulus to breathe. Even during hypoxemia, irregular breathing and periods of apnea may develop if normal respiratory drive is altered by sleep. This is seen to a striking degree in the Cheyne-Stokes breathing of normal subjects at high altitude.

Sudden infant death syndrome This is sometimes known as "crib death." Typically the infant is found dead in the crib with no apparent cause. The etiology of this is still obscure, but some investigators believe that this is a special case of the sleep apnea syndrome described above. In addition it is known that the rib cage collapses easily in some young infants and there may be paradoxical movement of the chest wall, that is, the rib cage moves in rather than out during inspiration. This may be accentuated by poor coordination of the respiratory muscles as a result of immaturity of the nervous system. It has also been shown that infants do not respond to transient airway obstruction by increasing their respiratory efforts, as occurs in the normal adult. This would make them abnormally vulnerable to upper respiratory tract infections. Finally, it is possible that some deaths are caused by cardiac arrhythmias during an apneic period.

CARBON DIOXIDE RETENTION ASSOCIATED WITH CHRONIC LUNG DISEASE The commonest clinical situation in which CO_2 retention is seen is chronic lung disease. Patients with this condition are often said to be "hypoventilating," but the cause of their hypercapnia is clearly very different from that in patients with normal lungs whom we have considered so far. Historically it is easy to see how the term hypoventilation came to be applied so indiscriminately. When in the late 1950s it became possible to measure the P_{CO_2} of arterial blood in the clinical setting, CO_2 retention was found to be a common and serious complication of chronic lung disease which could always be abolished by artificially increasing the ventilation. Thus it was natural to say that these patients had a reduced ventilation, and this term had the advantage of keeping an important therapeutic option in the forefront.

It is important to understand the factors leading to CO_2 retention in these patients if their disease is to be managed most effectively. Figure 286-1 shows a scheme of the factors determining CO_2 elimination in patients with lung disease. CO_2 is produced in the tissues at a rate which depends on the level of metabolic activity; at rest there is little variation. It is transported to the lungs in the venous blood and pumped out by the ventilation. The speed of the pump is normally set by the level of the P_{CO_2} via the medullary chemoreceptors. In the presence of lung disease, the efficiency of the pump is impaired. Thus, for the same level of ventilation, less CO_2 is eliminated. This is principally because ventilation and blood flow are unevenly matched within the lung (see Chap. 271). In any event the result is that for a normal level of ventilation, inadequate amounts of CO_2 are excreted, and CO_2 retention occurs.

When the increased arterial P_{CO_2} causes a fall in the cerebrospinal fluid pH which is sensed by the medullary chemoreceptors, the ventilation is increased. This usually returns the P_{CO_2} to normal, because fortunately even lungs with grossly mismatched ventilation and blood flow can greatly increase their elimination of CO_2 when their ventilation is raised. (Contrast this with the behavior of O_2, where uneven ventilation and blood flow invariably result in low P_{O_2}; this follows from the shape of the O_2 dissociation curve as discussed in Chap. 271.) Thus a common end result is a normal P_{CO_2}, but at the expense of increased ventilation. However, in the presence of severe disease, the ventilation may not be increased enough to restore the P_{CO_2} to normal, and CO_2 retention therefore occurs.

The ventilatory response to CO_2 in these patients can be reduced for two reasons. One is an increased work of breathing. It has been shown that if normal subjects breathe through a resistance, their ventilatory response to inhaled CO_2 is depressed. Indeed, the relationship between increase in ventilation and inspired CO_2 concentration may become indistinguishable from that observed in patients with chronic airway obstruction. In most cases of chronic obstructive lung disease, the resistance to airflow is high so that the increase in ventilation for a given rise in arterial P_{CO_2} is depressed. Such patients may have a normal neural output of the respiratory center in response to an increased P_{CO_2}, but nevertheless the ventilatory response is impaired.

However, some patients also have a reduced neural output of the respiratory center in response to an increased arterial P_{CO_2}. This can be established by specialized tests such as measurement of the mechanical work performed during inspiration or the inspiratory pressure developed during a brief period of airway occlusion. The reason for the diminished sensitivity of the respiratory center in these patients is not understood, though in some cases it may be congenital. There is evidence that the sensitivity of the respiratory center to CO_2 (and hypoxemia) varies considerably among normal subjects. It may be that those patients who have good respiratory center sensitivity are more distressed by dyspnea, while those who respond weakly may succumb to CO_2 retention and respiratory failure.

When CO_2 retention becomes established, the respiratory center becomes reset at a higher arterial P_{CO_2}. This can be explained by an increase in bicarbonate concentration in the cerebrospinal fluid because of transport of bicarbonate across the blood-gas barrier. As a result the pH of the cerebrospinal fluid is returned to near its normal value of 7.32 in spite of its increased P_{CO_2}. Since this pH apparently chiefly determines the response of the medullary chemoreceptors, respiratory drive may then not be much increased despite the raised P_{CO_2}.

Further CO_2 retention occurs in some patients with chronic lung disease, especially following the administration of oxygen. These patients have chronic hypercapnia and hypoxemia but a near normal pH in their arterial blood (compensated respiratory acidosis) and in their cerebrospinal fluid. Their main stimulus to ventilation may be the arterial hypoxemia via the peripheral chemoreceptors, so that, when this is relieved, ventilation almost ceases. The ensuing rise in P_{CO_2} may further depress ventilation because of the narcotic effect of high levels of carbon dioxide. This extremely dangerous situation should be avoided by giving carefully controlled O_2 concentrations, for example, 24 to 28 percent, assiduously watching the patient, and measuring the arterial P_{CO_2} from time to time. CO_2 retention in chronic obstructive lung disease is considered in Chap. 279, and the treatment of acute and chronic respiratory failure in Chap. 287.

HYPERVENTILATION

Hyperventilation is most commonly caused by lesions of the central nervous system, metabolic acidosis, and anxiety states. In addition, hyperventilation may be seen in salicylate poisoning, acute or chronic hypoxemia (as at high altitude), severe hypoglycemia, and hepatic coma. A patient with severe cerebral hemorrhage causing coma may exhibit deep, regular respirations of a mechanical nature. This causes a reduced P_{CO_2} in the arterial blood, which initially shows a high pH and a normal base excess. Irregularities of breathing such as Cheyne-Stokes respiration may also occur. In metabolic acidosis caused, for example, by uncontrolled diabetes mellitus or by chronic renal insufficiency, deep regular respiration known as *Kussmaul breathing* is frequently seen. Active rather than passive expiratory movements are a feature of this pattern. Here the low P_{CO_2} is accompanied by reduction in base excess and a low pH (see Chap. 44).

In the hyperventilation of anxiety states, the patient may be very apprehensive and complain of shortness of breath, difficulty in taking a deep breath, a feeling of chest tightness, or a sense of suffocation. The patient is often a nervous, anxious woman who has other functional disturbances due to tension. There are often accompanying symptoms such as numbness in the limbs, palpitations, and epigastric discomfort. The fall in P_{CO_2} and the consequent alkalosis may be severe and cause tetany with carpopedal spasm. The reduced plasma bicarbonate level and relatively normal arterial pH (compensated respiratory alkalosis) distinguish chronic hyperventilation from the acute hyperventilation with fall in P_{CO_2} which frequently accompanies an arterial puncture. The patient may complain of fainting spells and blurring of vision; these are probably related to the reduction in cerebral blood flow caused by low P_{CO_2}. The finding of slow waves of high voltage in the EEG suggests that these changes may be the result of hypoxemia. The changes can be reversed by hyperbaric oxygenation. The serum calcium level remains normal. It is likely that some of the cardiovascular symptoms are related to the release of epinephrine.

These patients are usually not aware of the overbreathing, although they may admit to periods of sighing. It is often possible to reproduce many of the symptoms of an attack by encouraging them to overbreathe spontaneously. It is also useful to demonstrate to these patients that they can hold a breath for a considerable period even during an attack. An attack can sometimes be terminated by having the patient breathe in and out of a plastic bag, or inhale a 5% CO_2 mixture. However, attention to the underlying anxiety state is indicated.

Hyperventilation also occurs in some types of lung disease, including interstitial lung disease and pulmonary edema. The hyperventilation of interstitial disease is particularly marked on exercise where the breathing is typically rapid and shallow, and the arterial P_{CO_2} may fall to the 20s. The cause of the hyperventilation is uncertain, but stimulation of the juxtacapillary (J) receptors in the alveolar wall by the process involving the lung has been implicated. Part of the hyperventilation may also be explained by the stimulation of the peripheral chemoreceptors by the severe arterial hypoxemia which may occur in these conditions.

ABNORMAL PATTERNS OF VENTILATION

CHEYNE-STOKES BREATHING This is a form of periodic breathing characterized by alternating periods of apnea and hyperpnea. The patient often lies motionless for 15 to 20 s and then begins to breathe shallowly at first, then with increasing amplitude, and finally shallowly again. The respirations during this period of breathing are regular in time.

The cause of this disturbance presumably lies in some delay in the control process which results in "hunting" for the equilibrium condition. Periodic breathing can be produced in experimental animals by lengthening the distance over which blood travels from the thorax to the brain. As a result, the response of the medullary chemoreceptors lags behind the blood gas changes produced by the lungs, and a cyclical chain of events is created. Conditions in which Cheyne-Stokes breathing is seen include congestive heart failure when the circulation time is prolonged (Chap. 253), brain damage caused by trauma or cerebral hemorrhage, and chronic hypoxemia. It occurs in normal subjects living at high altitude, especially during sleep.

BIOT'S BREATHING This is another form of periodic breathing in which periods of apnea are punctuated by a few deep breaths which may be irregular and which do not have the waxing and waning pattern of Cheyne-Stokes respiration. It is most frequently associated with brain damage.

OTHER TYPES Brain injury can result in bizarre patterns of ventilation. These include apneustic breathing, which is characterized by a postinspiratory pause (rather than the usual postexpiratory), and ataxic breathing, which is irregular in timing and depth.

REFERENCES

Burwell CS et al: Extreme obesity associated with alveolar hypoventilation—A Pickwickian syndrome. Am J Med 21:811, 1956

FISHMAN AP: The syndrome of chronic alveolar hypoventilation. Bull Physio-Pathol Resp 8:971, 1972 (contains some 25 papers from a symposium on hypoventilation)

GUILLEMINAULT C, DEMENT WC: *Sleep Apnea Syndromes.* New York, Alan R Liss, 1978

ROUSSOS C, MAKLEM PT: Disorders of the respiratory muscle function, in *Update III: Harrison's Principles of Internal Medicine,* KJ Isselbacher et al (eds). New York, McGraw-Hill, 1982, pp 83–100

WEST JB: *Pulmonary Pathophysiology—The Essentials,* 2d ed. Baltimore, Williams & Wilkins, 1982

287 ADULT RESPIRATORY DISTRESS SYNDROME

ROLAND H. INGRAM, JR.

Adult respiratory distress syndrome is a descriptive term that has been applied to many acute, diffuse infiltrative lung lesions of diverse etiologies when they are accompanied by severe arterial hypoxemia. The term was chosen because of several clinical and pathologic similarities between such acute illnesses in adults and the neonatal respiratory distress syndrome. However, in the neonatal form, immaturity of alveolar surfactant production and a highly compliant chest wall are primarily involved in the pathophysiology, whereas in the adult, alveolar surfactant changes are secondary to the primary process, and the chest wall is not compliant. Despite the large number of causes (Table 287-1), the clinical characteristics, respiratory pathophysiologic derangement, and current techniques for management of these acute abnormalities are remarkably similar. It has been argued that the "lumping" of such processes of different etiologies obscures the unique features of each in terms of pathogenesis, prevention, and specificity of treatment. It is clear that the conditions listed do not always lead to respiratory failure and that specific treatment of the underlying processes will often be different. Therefore, the reader is urged to refer to the appropriate sections of this text for the unique characteristics of each condition and to recognize that only the common features at the onset of respiratory failure will be focused upon in this chapter. It should be further emphasized that many of the listed conditions are often present in combination and may come into play at different times in the clinical course of the adult respiratory distress syndrome.

TABLE 287-1
Conditions which may lead to the adult respiratory distress syndrome

1 Diffuse pulmonary infections (e.g., viral, bacterial, fungal, *Pneumocystis*)
2 Aspiration (e.g., gastric contents with Mendelson's syndrome, water with near drowning)
3 Inhalation of toxins and irritants (e.g., chlorine gas, NO_2, smoke, ozone, high concentrations of oxygen)
4 Narcotic overdose pulmonary edema (e.g., heroin, methadone, morphine, dextropropoxyphene)
5 Nonnarcotic drug effects (e.g., nitrofurantoin)
6 Immunologic response to host antigens (e.g., Goodpasture's syndrome, systemic lupus erythematosus)
7 Effects of nonthoracic trauma with hypotension ("shock lung")
8 In association with systemic reactions to processes initiated outside the lung (e.g., gram-negative septicemia, hemorrhagic pancreatitis, amniotic fluid embolism, fat embolism)
9 Postcardiopulmonary bypass ("pump lung," "postperfusion lung")

PATHOPHYSIOLOGY Regardless of the initiating process, the adult respiratory distress syndrome is invariably associated with increased liquid in the lungs. Thus it is a form of pulmonary edema, yet it is distinct from cardiogenic pulmonary edema because pulmonary capillary hydrostatic pressures are not elevated (Chap. 26). Initially there is injury to the alveolar-capillary membrane that results in leakage of liquid, macromolecules, and cellular components from the blood vessels into the interstitial space and, with increasing severity, into the alveoli. The increasing vascular permeability to proteins (decreased reflection coefficient, σ, discussed in Chap. 26) leaves the hydrostatic gradient unopposed so that even mild elevations in capillary pressures greatly increase interstitial and alveolar edema. Alveolar collapse occurs secondary to the effect of the alveolar liquid, especially its fibrinogen, that interferes with normal surfactant activity and because of possible impairment of further surfactant production by injury to the granular pneumocytes. Though radiographically diffuse, the regional dysfunction is nonhomogeneous; it leads to severe ventilation-perfusion imbalance and the shunting of blood through regions in which alveoli are collapsed or filled with liquid. The lungs become less compliant—i.e., stiffen because of interstitial edema, alveolar collapse, and increase in surface forces. Because of the decreased compliance, large inspiratory pressures must be generated by the respiratory muscles so that the work of breathing is elevated. The large mechanical loads lead to fatigue of the muscles of breathing with resulting diminution in tidal volumes and worsening gas exchange. Both hypoxemia and the stimulation of receptors in the stiff lung parenchyma cause an increase in respiratory frequency, decrease in tidal volume, and deterioration in gas exchange.

PATHOLOGY In the absence of specific demonstrable pathogens, the pathology is remarkably similar among the various conditions leading to the adult respiratory distress syndrome, since the lung has a limited number of ways in which it reacts to an almost limitless number of injuries. Grossly, the lungs are heavy, edematous, and almost airless with regions of hemorrhage, atelectasis, and consolidation. By light microscopy there is edema and cellular infiltration of interalveolar septa and interstitial spaces surrounding airways and blood vessels, atelectasis and hyaline membranes in many regions, engorgement of vessels with red blood cells, and aggregates of platelets along with interstitial and alveolar hemorrhage. In addition, both hyperplasia and dysplasia of the granular pneumocytes are often present.

If the illness has been prolonged beyond 10 days, there is often a surprising amount of fibrosis in addition to the acute changes. In instances of recovery and subsequent death from another cause, significant interstitial fibrosis and emphysematous changes may be found in the lung. A significant number of patients, however, will recover completely and have normal pulmonary function with no respiratory symptoms. Hence aggressive clinical management is both indicated and often rewarding.

CLINICAL CHARACTERISTICS At the time of initial injury and for several hours thereafter the patient may be free of respiratory symptoms or signs. The earliest sign often is an increase in respiratory frequency followed shortly by dyspnea. Arterial blood gas measurement in the earlier period will disclose a depressed P_{O_2} despite a decreased P_{CO_2} so that the alveolar-arterial difference for oxygen (Chap. 271) is increased. At this early stage, administration of oxygen by mask or nasal prongs results in a significant increase in the arterial P_{O_2}. The brisk rise in P_{O_2} indicates that ventilation-perfusion mismatching and, possibly, diffusion impairment account for the widened alveolar-arterial P_{O_2} difference ($PA_{O_2}-Pa_{O_2}$) initially. Physical examination may be unremarkable, although a few fine inspiratory rales may be audible. Radiographically the lung fields may be clear or demonstrate only minimal and scattered interstitial infiltrates. With progression, the patient becomes cyanotic and increasingly dyspneic and tachypneic. Rales are more prominent and are easily heard throughout both lung fields along with regions of tubular breath sounds; the chest radiograph demonstrates diffuse, extensive bilateral interstitial and alveolar infiltrates (Fig. 287-1). At this point hypoxemia cannot be corrected by the simple expedient of increasing the oxygen concentration of the inspired gas, and mechanical ventilatory support must be started. Right-to-left shunting of blood through collapsed or filled alveoli becomes the major mechanism for arterial hypoxemia at this more advanced stage. In contrast to ventilation-perfusion mismatching and diffusion impairment, with right-to-left shunts, $P\text{A}_{O_2} - Pa_{O_2}$ remains high with breathing of pure oxygen. Positive end-expiratory pressure (PEEP) serves to increase lung volume, which in turn opens collapsed alveoli and decreases shunting. With further progression, and if mechanical ventilator and PEEP therapy are delayed, the combination of increasing tachypnea and decreasing tidal volumes results in alveolar hypoventilation, a rising P_{CO_2}, and worsening hypoxemia; these represent a near-terminal constellation of findings.

MANAGEMENT OF HYPOXEMIC RESPIRATORY FAILURE The brief description given above contains the salient principles of management, integrated with the clinical events that lead to escalation of therapeutic interventions. Implicit in that description is that the simplest method and the lowest inspired fraction of oxygen ($F\text{I}_{O_2}$) should be used to give the desired result. The oxyhemoglobin dissociation curve (Fig. 54-4) gives some guide as to the Pa_{O_2} for which to aim. At a P_{O_2} of 60 mmHg, hemoglobin is approximately 90 percent saturated. Therefore, a reasonable objective is to achieve a Pa_{O_2} of 60, since higher levels add little to oxygenation and introduce the risk of oxygen toxicity to the lung. In contrast to respiratory failure complicating chronic airways obstruction (Chap. 279), depression of ventilation is not an issue in hypoxemic respiratory failure.

There are multiple means to deliver O_2, in order of increasing effectiveness: soft nasal prongs, simple face masks, and face masks with inspiratory reservoir bags. The effective $F\text{I}_{O_2}$ (that is actually entering the trachea) will be determined by the concentration of O_2 delivered from the tank or wall device, its flow rate, and the minute ventilation of the patient. In the hypoxemic form of respiratory failure, it is reasonable to start with moderate flow rates (5 to 10 liters per minute of 100% O_2) and monitor arterial blood gases, adjusting flow rates and O_2 concentrations depending upon results.

If adequate oxygenation cannot be maintained with these less invasive measures, endotracheal intubation should be carried out and mechanical ventilatory support should be instituted. The rationale behind mechanical ventilatory support in a patient who is hyperventilating is *not* to increase ventilation but to increase mean lung volume, thereby opening previously closed airways and improving oxygenation. This is done by using large tidal volumes (approximately 15 ml per kilogram of lean body weight) at a slower breathing rate (12 to 15 breaths per minute) than the spontaneous one of the patient. Most often, at this juncture, the respiratory system is sufficiently stiff that high inflation pressures are required and a volume-cycled ventilator (in contrast to the pressure-cycled ones) is needed. If the patient makes expiratory efforts during the inflation cycle, peak inspiratory pressures will increase, possibly enough to activate the high-pressure pop-off valve, which results in delivery to the patient of a smaller tidal volume than selected. Under these circumstances consideration is often given to sedation and/or neuromuscular paralysis. However, a much more logical way to proceed is to institute synchronized intermittent mandatory ventilation (SIMV). In the SIMV mode, the patient is allowed to breathe spontaneously with periodic delivery of mandatory breaths that are synchronized with spontaneous inspiratory efforts. If the spontaneous breathing rate is so rapid that expiratory efforts occur before the mandatory breath is fully delivered, only then should sedation and/or paralysis be used.

Should the Pa_{O_2} be greater than 60 mmHg, the next step is to lower the $F\text{I}_{O_2}$. If the $F\text{I}_{O_2}$ can be lowered to 0.6 or less with a Pa_{O_2} equal to or greater than 60 mmHg, the mechanical ventilation should proceed at that $F\text{I}_{O_2}$ as long as necessary. There are two basic indications for the addition of positive end-expiratory pressure (PEEP), the basic rationale for which is to increase lung volume further, thereby opening previously closed alveoli. First, if the $F\text{I}_{O_2}$ cannot be lowered to or below 0.6, then PEEP should be added to allow a decrease of the $F\text{I}_{O_2}$ below the toxic range. Second, if the Pa_{O_2} cannot be increased to or above 60 mmHg with an $F\text{I}_{O_2}$ of 1.0, PEEP should be added. The optimal magnitude of the PEEP is determined by the response of the Pa_{O_2} and the extent of the cardiovascular alterations resulting from the higher pressure. The major alteration is a decrease in cardiac output due to two mechanisms. First, increased intrapleural pressures serve to impede venous return directly, an effect which is, to a variable extent, offset by peripheral venoconstriction. Second, increases in lung volume may increase pulmonary vascular resistance, leading to increased pressure and dilatation of the right ventricle, which in turn displaces the interventricular septum toward the left. This displacement, in effect, decreases left ventricular diastolic com-

FIGURE 287-1
A standard posteroanterior chest radiograph from a patient with the adult respiratory distress syndrome secondary to a severe viral pneumonitis. Such a diffuse radiographic change is typical of all conditions listed in Table 287-1 when they are severe enough to cause acute hypoxemic respiratory failure. A similar radiographic picture is also seen in pulmonary edema due to left ventricular failure (Chap. 26). Often in such acutely ill patients, the radiograph must be taken with a portable unit and the film exposed from the anterior direction. Both the anteroposterior exposure and the failure to take a deep inspiration result in an apparent enlargement of the cardiac silhouette which further obscures the reliable detection of left ventricular failure.

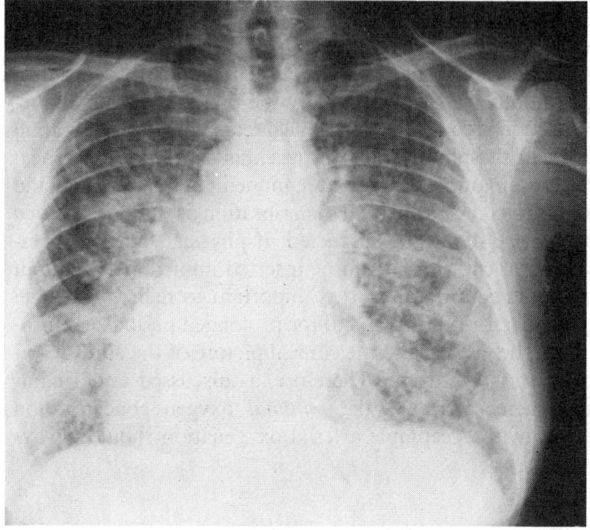

pliance; hence less filling leads to smaller stroke volumes. In a physiological sense optimal levels of PEEP are those associated with the greatest delivery of O_2 to the body; the latter is the product of cardiac output and arterial oxygen content.

In patients who are critically ill and/or unstable, insertion of a catheter into a radial artery and a balloon-tipped (Swan-Ganz) catheter into the pulmonary artery can provide valuable information in guiding supportive therapy such as requirements for intravenous fluids, the need for diuresis, and assessment of the effects of mechanical ventilation. From the Swan-Ganz catheter it is possible to measure pulmonary arterial and pulmonary capillary wedge pressures, cardiac output by the thermodilution technique, and to sample mixed venous blood as a means to assess the adequacy of O_2 delivery in relation to demand. Recognition of over-damping and accelerative artifacts in the pulmonary arterial pressure signal and learning the criteria for true wedging are essential if serious misinterpretations are to be avoided. Even with accurate pressure measurements, there is an additional precaution that must be taken with regard to interpretation of intrathoracic vascular pressures referenced to atmosphere when PEEP is being used. If pleural pressure is greater than atmospheric, as is most often the case with PEEP, the true effective (i.e., intravascular minus pleural) pressure will be overestimated and could lead to errors in both assessment and management. A reasonable estimate of the true value is gained by examining vascular pressures just before inflation and subtracting from these pressures an amount equal to one-half the value of PEEP. In view of the leaky alveolocapillary membrane it is best to keep the pulmonary capillary wedge pressure as low as is compatible with a reasonable cardiac output, arterial pressure, and urinary output.

Mixed venous blood P_{O_2} values have long been considered to indicate the adequacy of oxygen delivery relative to demand. A low value (e.g., < 20 mmHg) surely indicates that there is tissue hypoxemia irrespective of measured cardiac output and Pa_{O_2}. However, a high value does not exclude serious hypoxemia of the tissues, especially in gram-negative bacillary septicemia, in which systemic low-resistance shunts can develop and leave several capillary beds underperfused.

Recent attention has been focused on the effect of body position on the degree of arterial oxygenation. Although patients with the adult respiratory distress syndrome have diffuse lung disease, there may be some regional variation in the extent of disease such that one side is more severely involved than the other. In this instance the less involved lung should be the more dependent one when the patient is in a lateral position. Since the distribution of pulmonary blood flow is so heavily determined by gravity (Chap. 271), having the more involved lung, with its minimal ventilation, in the more dependent position results in a measurable increase in intrapulmonary shunt, manifested as a striking fall in Pa_{O_2}. The possible contribution of a positional effect on arterial oxygenation should always be considered before escalating therapeutic interventions.

Occasionally PEEP must be gradually increased to levels in excess of 20 cmH_2O in an attempt to maintain arterial oxygenation. At these high levels of PEEP there may be a paradoxical decrease in Pa_{O_2}. The explanation for this paradox is as follows: high levels of PEEP may not open some of the closed airways but will overdistend those units already open. Overdistention of units increases the vascular resistance in these regions and results in more blood perfusing regions with closed airways, thereby increasing the degree of shunt. The only alternative is to decrease PEEP back to that level associated with the greatest delivery of oxygen to the body (product of cardiac output and arterial oxygen content).

In the situations where maximal PEEP with $F_{I_{O_2}}$ of 1.0 does not supply sufficient oxygen, the possibility of utilizing extracorporeal membrane oxygenators (ECMO) has been both considered and tried. Despite the logical appeal of this form of supportive therapy, a randomized, large prospective study of ECMO therapy has demonstrated that, while it can support gas exchange, there is no effect on survival in acute hypoxemic respiratory failure.

Complications Increasing severity of the clinical illness and continued radiographic progressions in association with the primary process often obscure complications that arise during the course of acute hypoxemic respiratory failure. The development of *left ventricular failure* is a good example of a common, easily missed complication. This is because all patients are likely to have diffuse rales and rhonchi, even without left ventricular failure, and these sounds also serve to make it difficult to detect gallop rhythms. An additional difficulty is that portable chest films are taken in the anteroposterior direction, often at less than full lung inflation, so that the cardiac silhouette appears enlarged. Thus the ordinary physical and radiographic assessments are difficult to rely on. With deterioration, therefore, left ventricular failure should be suspected; it is helpful to insert a Swan-Ganz (see above) catheter which can be used to monitor pulmonary arterial pressure continuously and intermittently to assess pulmonary capillary wedge pressure and oxygen content of mixed venous blood.

With a diffuse radiographic pattern, a secondary bacterial infection is easily overlooked; therefore, frequent sputum smears and cultures should be obtained, especially when there is fever. With many conditions—e.g., gram-negative septicemia, acute hemorrhagic pancreatitis, and "shock lung"—there may be associated *disseminated intravascular coagulation,* which leads to gastrointestinal and intrapulmonary hemorrhage (Chap. 318). Frequent monitoring of platelet count, fibrinogen level, and partial thromboplastin and prothrombin times is helpful in the early detection of this complication and in guiding treatment.

Bronchial obstruction by endotracheal or tracheostomy tubes often occurs. These tubes, when too long or poorly anchored, slide into one main bronchus, usually the right one because of its less angulated origin from the trachea. The tube then blocks ventilation of the other main bronchus, and atelectasis may ensue. Such an event usually causes abrupt deterioration in the patient with respiratory failure. It is detected readily by physical examination, which reveals the absence of breath sounds over the occluded lung. The tube should immediately be pulled back slowly if this complication is suspected. Finally, in the course of treating the illness with mechanical ventilators and high inflation pressures, *pneumothorax* or *pneumomediastinum* may develop and may be impossible to detect except radiologically. Occasionally the presence of subcutaneous emphysema provides a clinical clue. Any deterioration should lead the physician to suspect this complication, repeat the chest radiograph, and institute immediate treatment should pneumothorax be present. If deterioration is sudden, *tension pneumothorax* should be suspected; if physical signs are present, a pleural catheter should be inserted immediately without radiographic confirmation. It is important to realize that high oxygen concentrations (>0.60) for prolonged periods can produce both the lesions and the clinical picture of the adult respiratory distress syndrome. Therefore, as discussed under clinical management above, the *minimal* oxygen concentration associated with acceptable arterial oxygenation should always be used.

Discontinuation of mechanical ventilatory support The ability of the patient to maintain adequate gas exchange without the support of a mechanical ventilator is most often heralded by a decreasing $F_{I_{O_2}}$ requirement, smaller inflation pressures for mandatory or assisted breaths, and a spontaneous respiratory rate below 30 per minute. Other useful guidelines are a spontaneous tidal volume $\geq$ 5 ml per kilogram of lean body weight, a vital capacity $\geq$ 15 ml/kg, and the ability to generate a static inspiratory pressure $\geq$ 20 cmH_2O. Despite these indicators and guidelines, some patients are unable to support themselves for long periods of time so that multiple weaning "trials" guided by mechanical and gas exchange data are carried out in a semiempirical way. Synchronized intermittent mandatory ventilation (SIMV) as described above has been advocated as a logical transitional mode whereby the frequency of the mandatory breaths is gradually decreased. There is a great deal of intuitive appeal to this approach, but it has not been appropriately tested and compared with more abrupt, intermittent withdrawal trials. As in patients with hypercapnic respiratory failure, the six mechanisms for failure to wean should be considered in these patients as well.

Prognosis Given the diversity of the etiologies and the frequency of associated diseases, it is difficult, if not impossible, to give meaningful prognostic figures for the adult respiratory distress syndrome. If all recently published series are taken together, the mortality rate runs between 50 and 60 percent. This represents an improved survival rate over the virtual 100 percent mortality rate of a few years ago and is a result of the application of modern treatment techniques described above. If the syndrome is due to drug overdose, the mortality rate is low; if associated with shock, the chances of a fatal outcome are much greater. Other etiologies and associated diseases are between these two extremes. The following factors appear to be associated with a poor outcome: an increase in $P_{A_{O_2}} - Pa_{O_2}$, requiring increasing inspired O_2 concentrations and

PEEP; decreasing compliance, requiring greater inflation pressures; either low or falling colloid osmotic pressures; and the onset of systemic arterial hypotension not responding to intravascular volume replacement.

In survivors with previously normal lung function, the long-term prognosis for recovery appears to be remarkably good. Lung volumes and arterial blood gases have been shown to return to normal levels within 4 to 6 months after respiratory failure. There are instances, however, when the fibrotic residua are sufficiently great that complete recovery is unlikely.

REFERENCES

ELLIOT GC et al: Pulmonary function and exercise gas exchange in survivors of adult respiratory distress syndrome. Am Rev Resp Dis 123:492, 1981

FERNANDEZ E, CHERNIACK RM: The use and abuse of drugs, in *Update II: Harrison's Principles of Internal Medicine,* KJ Isselbacher et al (eds). New York, McGraw-Hill, 1982

FISHMAN AP: Down with the good lung. N Engl J Med 304:537, 1981

GERHARDT RE: Ultrafiltration in the management of the adult respiratory distress syndrome, in *Update: Pulmonary Diseases and Disorders,* AP Fishman (ed). New York, McGraw-Hill, 1982, pp 387–395

HUREWITZ A, BERGOFSKY EH: Adult respiratory distress syndrome: Physiologic basis of treatment. Med Clin N Am 65:33, 1981

JARDIN F et al: Influence of positive end-expiratory pressure on left ventricular performance. N Engl J Med 304:387, 1981

STAUB NC: Pulmonary edema due to increased microvascular permeability. Ann Rev Med 32:291, 1981

WOOD LDH, PREWITT RM: Cardiovascular management in acute hypoxemic respiratory failure. Am J Cardiol 47:963, 1981

ZAPOL WM et al: Extracorporeal membrane oxygenation in severe acute respiratory failure: A randomized prospective study. JAMA 242:2193, 1979

section 4 | Diseases of the kidney and urinary tract

288

APPROACH TO THE PATIENT WITH DISEASES OF THE KIDNEYS AND URINARY TRACT

FREDRIC L. COE
BARRY M. BRENNER

Diseases affecting the kidneys or the lower urinary tract can often be detected, even in asymptomatic patients, from clues derived from routine clinical and laboratory examination. Physicians have long appreciated that specific lesions of the urinary tract frequently give rise to a consistent array of clinical signs, symptoms, and laboratory findings which, when taken together, constitute syndromes that effectively narrow the range of causal entities to be considered in the search for an exact diagnosis. Ten such nephrological syndromes have been recognized and are listed in Table 288-1. Although the findings derived from routine evaluation are often sufficient to suggest the presence of one of these syndromes, they are rarely adequate for precise diagnosis. Instead, additional biochemical, serologic, radiological, and/or urologic evaluation is usually required, as is sequential clinical observation. Occasionally, even these approaches prove inadequate, and precise diagnosis must await the results of renal biopsy or exploratory laparotomy. Nevertheless, these syndromes serve as useful frameworks upon which an orderly system of diagnostic nephrology can be based. The purpose of this chapter is to present the general features of these syndromes and the clinical and laboratory data base required for their recognition. Succeeding chapters in this section will then be concerned with detailed descriptions of the various disease entities known to cause the syndromes.

THE MAJOR SYNDROMES IN NEPHROLOGY **Acute or rapidly progressive renal failure** This syndrome exists in patients in whom glomerular filtration rate (GFR) falls drastically over a period of days (acute) to several weeks (rapidly progressive). Severe oligoanuria and progressive azotemia often accompany the decline in GFR, adding further to the notion of acuteness, since life could not have been sustained for very long with such inadequate renal function. Acute tubular necrosis, considered in detail in Chap. 290, whether due to sepsis, exposure to a known nephrotoxin, or to any of a number of other causes, is usually responsible for acute renal failure. Extracapillary proliferative (crescentic) glomerulonephritis,[1] due to glomerular immunological injury or to vasculitis, leads to deterioration of renal function in a period of weeks to a few months and is, therefore, also an important cause of this syndrome (Chap. 294).

A number of clinical and laboratory abnormalities can be recognized in patients with the syndrome of acute or rapidly progressive renal failure (Table 288-1). Proof for the existence of the syndrome, however, requires documentation of severe oliguria or anuria and a rapid decline in GFR. If these findings are not present, the other clinical and laboratory abnormalities listed in Table 288-1 can be regarded only as clues consistent with, but not proof of, the existence of this syndrome. Ultimately the syndrome of acute or rapidly progressive renal failure can be established only by serial observations, and especially serial determinations of urine flow rate and blood urea nitrogen (BUN) or serum creatinine levels. The causes of this important syndrome and the steps required to invoke or exclude them in a given patient are considered principally in Chap. 290, while other potentially important causes of acute or rapidly progressive renal failure including rapidly progressive glomerulonephritis (Chap. 294), acute interstitial edema (Chap. 297), major renal vascular accidents (Chap. 298), and urinary tract obstruction (Chap. 301) are discussed elsewhere in this section.

[1] *The term* rapidly progressive glomerulonephritis *is often used to denote renal failure associated with extensive extracapillary proliferation in glomeruli, which leads to crescent formation.*

Chronic renal failure Chronic renal failure is a syndrome which results from progressive and irreversible destruction of nephrons, regardless of cause (Chap. 291). This syndrome may be considered to exist when GFR is found to be reduced and is known to have been reduced for at least 3 to 6 months (Table 288-1). Often, in fact, a gradual decline in GFR can be documented over a period of years. Proof of chronicity is also provided by the demonstration by abdominal scout film, ultrasonography, intravenous pyelography, or tomography of

TABLE 288-1
Initial clinical and laboratory data base for defining major syndromes in nephrology

Syndromes	*Important clues to diagnosis*	*Findings which are common but not of diagnostic value*	*Location of discussion of diseases causing syndrome*
Acute or rapidly progressive renal failure	Anuria Oliguria Documented recent decline in GFR	Hypertension, hematuria Proteinuria, pyuria Casts, edema	Chaps. 290, 294, 297, 298, 301
Chronic renal failure	Azotemia for > 3 months Prolonged symptoms or signs of uremia Symptoms or signs of renal osteodystrophy Kidneys reduced in size bilaterally Broad casts in urinary sediment	Hematuria, proteinuria Casts, oliguria Polyuria, nocturia Edema, hypertension Electrolyte disorders	Chaps. 289, 291
Acute nephritis	Hematuria, RBC casts Azotemia, oliguria Edema, hypertension	Proteinuria Pyuria Circulatory congestion	Chaps. 293 to 295
Nephrotic syndrome	Proteinuria > 3.5 g per 1.73 m^2 per 24 h Hypoalbuminemia Hyperlipidemia Lipiduria	Casts Edema	Chaps. 294, 295
Asymptomatic urinary abnormalities	Hematuria Proteinuria (below nephrotic range) Sterile pyuria, casts		Chap. 294
Urinary tract infection	Bacteriuria > 10^5 colonies per milliliter Other infectious agent documented in urine Pyuria, leukocyte casts Frequency, urgency Bladder tenderness, flank tenderness	Hematuria Mild azotemia Mild proteinuria Fever	Chap. 296
Renal tubule defects	Electrolyte disorders Polyuria, nocturia Symptoms or signs of renal osteodystrophy Large kidneys Renal transport defects	Hematuria "Tubular" proteinuria Enuresis	Chaps. 297, 299
Hypertension	Systolic/diastolic hypertension	Proteinuria Casts Azotemia	Chaps. 29, 267, 298
Nephrolithiasis	Previous history of stone passage or removal Previous history of stone seen by x-ray Renal colic	Hematuria Pyuria Frequency, urgency	Chap. 300
Urinary tract obstruction	Azotemia, oliguria, anuria Polyuria, nocturia, urinary retention Slowing of urinary stream Large prostate, large kidneys Flank tenderness	Hematuria Pyuria Enuresis, dysuria	Chap. 301

bilateral reduction of kidney size. Other findings consistent with long-standing renal failure, such as renal osteodystrophy or signs and symptoms of uremia, also help to establish this syndrome (Table 288-1). Several laboratory abnormalities are often regarded as reliable indicators of chronicity of renal disease, such as anemia, hyperphosphatemia, or hypocalcemia, but these are not specific and may be misleading (Chap. 289). In contrast, the finding of broad casts in the urinary sediment (Chap. 40) is quite specific for chronic renal failure, the wide diameters of these casts reflecting the compensatory dilatation and hypertrophy of surviving nephrons. Proteinuria is a frequent but nonspecific finding, as is hematuria. Chronic obstructive uropathy, polycystic and medullary cystic diseases, analgesic nephropathy, and the inactive end stage of any chronic tubulointerstitial nephropathy are excellent examples of conditions in which the urine often contains little or no protein, cells, or casts even though nephron destruction has progressed to the stage of chronic renal failure.

When acute renal failure occurs and there is also clear evidence of chronic renal failure, the acute component must be evaluated as if chronic renal failure were not present, largely because the acute component is potentially reversible. In most instances, depletion of extracellular fluid volume accounts for the acute deterioration of renal function, but other factors such as urinary tract obstruction, drug-induced nephrotoxicity, or exacerbation of the underlying renal disease may also be responsible (Chap. 291).

Acute nephritis A number of diseases involve the glomeruli and, to a generally lesser extent, the tubules in an acute but *transient* inflammatory process, manifested clinically by acute reduction in GFR, rapidly progressive azotemia, oliguria, and salt and water retention. The resulting expansion of the extracellular volume, if marked, leads to hypertension, pulmonary vascular congestion, and facial and peripheral edema (Chap. 294). Damage of the glomerular wall is usually severe enough in almost all causes of this syndrome to permit red blood cells and plasma proteins to gain access to the urinary space (Chap. 40). Gross or microscopic hematuria, red blood cell casts, and proteinuria, therefore, occur with great regularity; their absence should alert the physician to other diagnostic possibilities. In the acute nephritic syndrome these various clinical and laboratory abnormalities (Table 288-1) exhibit a remarkable tendency to wax and wane in synchrony over a period of from several days to a few weeks.

Acute poststreptococcal glomerulonephritis due to infection with group A streptococci is the prototype of the syndrome of acute nephritis (Chap. 294). Immune complexes become deposited in the subepithelial region of the glomerular capillary wall, between the basement membrane and the visceral epithelial cells that separate the membrane from the urinary space. The process is usually self-limited, with renal function returning to normal within weeks to months in the vast majority of affected patients. Acute nephritis can occur during the course of a wide variety of other bacterial and viral infections (Chap. 294), with deposition of immune complexes again believed to be responsible for the usually transient renal damage that occurs. Immune complexes are also believed to be critical to the pathogenesis of lupus nephritis, membranoproliferative glomerulonephritis, and Henoch-Schönlein purpura (Chaps. 293 to 295).

It is important to recognize that all the forms of acute glomerulonephritis and vasculitis that cause acute or rapidly progressive renal failure may mimic the syndrome of acute nephritis at their onset, largely because hematuria, proteinuria, and fluid retention occur commonly during all forms of acute renal failure. But in many of these disorders, the features of renal failure do not wane. This distinction highlights the transient character of the acute nephritic syndrome, because progression to chronic renal failure is uncommon. Acute tubulointerstitial nephritis (Chap. 297), mixed IgG/IgM cryoglobulinemia (Chap. 295), and membranoproliferative glomerulonephritis (Chap. 294) are exceptions to this general principle, however, and often cause chronic renal failure.

Patients with the acute nephritic syndrome usually have a proliferative form of glomerulonephritis, and the prognosis and treatment are influenced strongly by the precise histological and ultrastructural pattern, as well as the types of immune complexes and immunoglobulins deposited in the renal tissues. Renal biopsy is, therefore, a cornerstone in the evaluation of most patients with this syndrome.

Nephrotic syndrome This syndrome is generally held to be present when a patient demonstrates massive proteinuria (usually defined as more than 3.5 g protein per 1.73 m^2 per 24 h and consisting mainly of albumin), reduced serum albumin concentration, edema, and hyperlipidemia (Table 288-1). Massive proteinuria alone has come to define the syndrome since this finding connotes serious renal disease whether or not the protein losses lead to hypoalbuminemia, lipid disturbances, or edema (Chap. 40). Provided the proteins appearing in the urine are not abnormal paraproteins readily excreted by the normal kidney (e.g., light chains in multiple myeloma), massive proteinuria must be evaluated carefully and completely, irrespective of the physiologic consequences of protein loss.

Common causes of the nephrotic syndrome include lipoid nephrosis, idiopathic membranous nephropathy, focal glomerulosclerosis, and diabetic glomerulosclerosis (Chaps. 294 and 295). These diseases typically cause less inflammation than is seen in diseases associated with the acute nephritic syndrome; therefore, the urine contains fewer cellular elements. Acute changes in GFR and urine volume are also uncommon. Hematuria may be a frequent manifestation of some forms of nephrotic syndrome, however, especially chronic membranoproliferative glomerulonephritis (Chap. 294). The presence of many cellular or granular casts should suggest lupus nephritis (Chap. 295) or one of the several known causes of acute nephritis associated with massive proteinuria (Chap. 294).

Asymptomatic urinary abnormalities As indicated in Table 288-1, mild degrees of microscopic hematuria, pyuria, casts, or less than 3.5 g protein per 1.73 m^2 per 24 h may be present in the urine of a patient lacking concurrent evidence of other nephrological syndromes. By exclusion, these patients are best considered to belong to the syndrome of asymptomatic urinary abnormalities. Isolated hematuria or proteinuria, or unexplained pyuria, are the most frequent abnormalities that occur in this syndrome.

Isolated hematuria, without proteinuria or casts, may be the sole clue to the presence of neoplasm, stone, or infection (e.g., tuberculosis) in any part of the urinary tract (Chaps. 40, 296, 300, and 302). Isolated hematuria may also arise from renal papillae in analgesic and sickle cell nephropathies (Chaps. 297 and 298). Persistent isolated hematuria often requires intravenous pyelography, cystoscopy, and, occasionally, renal arteriography, to identify the source of bleeding. *Nephronal hematuria,* in which red blood cells or hemoglobin pigment is present in casts, indicates damage to the nephron (Chap. 40). It occurs without proteinuria, mainly in benign recurrent hematuria and Berger's disease (Chap. 294). *Nephronal hematuria and proteinuria* occur together in many specific renal diseases that may eventually lead to chronic renal failure (Chap. 291). In general, the combination of nephronal hematuria and proteinuria suggests a worse prognosis than either one alone.

Isolated proteinuria, without red blood cells or other formed elements in the urinary sediment, is characteristic of many renal diseases which manifest little or no inflammatory reaction within the glomeruli (e.g., diabetes mellitus, amyloidosis). Less than nephrotic-range proteinuria is common in mild forms of all the diseases that can cause overt nephrotic syndrome (Chaps. 294 and 295). "Tubular" proteinuria (Chap. 40) is the rule in cystinosis; in heavy metal intoxication from cadmium, lead, or mercury, and in the peculiar Balkan nephropathy localized to only a small region along the Danube River (Chap. 297).

Pyuria may also be a sole urinary abnormality and frequently reflects infection or inflammation of the lower urinary tract, rather than intrinsic parenchymal renal disease. Nevertheless, prominent pyuria can occur in any inflammatory disease of the kidneys, especially tubulointerstitial nephritis, lupus nephritis, pyelonephritis, and renal transplant rejection, but usually in association with mild proteinuria or hematuria. The finding of leukocyte casts (Chap. 40) establishes the kidney as the site of the inflammatory reaction.

Pyuria associated with urine that is sterile on routine bacteriological culture presents a special problem. Certain causes of "sterile pyuria" that are clinically obvious include (1) recent bacterial urinary infection being treated with antibiotics, (2) adrenocortical steroid therapy, (3) acute febrile episodes, (4) cyclophosphamide administration, (5) hemodialysis treatment, (6) pregnancy, (7) renal transplant rejection, (8) recent genitourinary trauma, and (9) prostatitis and cystourethritis. Leukocytes from vaginal secretions may contaminate the urine, so a midstream, clean-catch urine sample should be collected to substantiate a urinary origin. Pyuria associated with proteinuria, nephronal hematuria (Chap. 40), or casts probably signifies inflammatory disease of the renal glomeruli, tubules, interstitium, or microcirculation, and evaluation should focus not upon the pyuria but upon identifying the nature of the renal disease.

Persistent sterile pyuria that cannot be ascribed to any of the foregoing causes has a narrow differential diagnosis. Unusual infections, such as tuberculosis, fungi, atypical mycobacteria, *Hemophilus influenzae,* anaerobic bacteria, fastidious bacteria that grow only on enriched media, and L forms, all must be sought. Intravenous pyelography is needed to detect causes such as urinary tract calculi, papillary necrosis, and renal infiltration by lymphoma or myeloma cells. The latter is usually suspected because of other evidence of myeloma or lymphoma, for both rarely involve only the kidneys. If all tests are negative, cystoscopy may reveal cystitis or trigone inflammation.

Urinary tract infection This syndrome is defined by the demonstration in urine of pathogenic organisms, either bacteria, tubercle bacilli, or fungi (Chap. 296). When urine specimens are obtained for culture, the condition under which the urine is collected must minimize contamination from external genitourinary surfaces. Women should void into a wide-mouthed sterile container after preliminary cleansing of the vulva with a moist, sterile gauze pledget. In men, midstream collection is usually adequate. Bacterial colony counts of 10^5 organisms per milliliter or greater in urine generally indicate urinary tract colonization and infection. Levels between 10^4 and 10^5 colonies per milliliter are usually viewed as suspicious and require reculture. When the urinary tract is anatomically normal, *Escherichia coli* is the usual bacterial pathogen. After prolonged antibiotic treatment of persistent infections, particularly when urinary drainage is impaired or stones are present, *Klebsiella, Enterobacter,* and *Proteus* species predominate.

As discussed in Chap. 296, the presence of a positive urine culture need not imply that an organism is producing tissue inflammation or injury. In some patients, tissue effects may be trivial; in others, injury may be occurring even though symptoms or urinary abnormalities are not present at the time of evaluation. When bacteriuria is associated with tissue inflammation or injury, clinical manifestations usually depend upon the site(s) involved. Dysuria, frequency, urgency, and suprapubic tenderness are common symptoms of bladder and urethral inflammation (Chap. 42 and Table 288-1). Prostatitis also leads to frequency, dysuria, and urgency, and the prostate may be boggy and tender on rectal examination. Flank pain, chills, fever, nausea and vomiting, hypotension from sepsis, and leukocyte casts all suggest true renal parenchymal infection, i.e., pyelonephritis (Chap. 296).

Whether or not remediable causes are found, predisposing factors and visible sequelae of urinary tract infection must be sought because they alter prognosis and, therefore, the approach to treatment. The approaches involved and the basis for decision making in this common clinical syndrome are discussed in Chap. 296.

Renal tubule defects This syndrome encompasses a large number of acquired and hereditary disorders, all of which tend to affect tubules more than glomeruli. Hereditary anatomic defects, including such entities as polycystic renal disease, medullary cystic disease, and medullary sponge kidney, are readily detected by intravenous pyelography, which is usually performed because of hematuria, bacteriuria, flank pain, or unexplained azotemia (Chap. 299).

Defects in tubule transport functions, on the other hand, tend not to be associated with prominent renal anatomic defects and arise either as inherited traits (Chap. 299) or during the course of acquired renal disease (Chap. 297). In general, these functional defects impair secretion and/or reabsorption of electrolytes and organic solutes, or limit urinary concentrating and diluting ability (Table 288-1). Typical manifestations of such functional disturbances include polyuria and nocturia (Chap. 41), metabolic acidosis (Chap. 44), and various disorders of fluid and electrolyte balance (Chap. 43). Such defects are defined by direct physiological measurements; their elucidation requires a sound understanding of normal renal physiology.

Hypertension The syndrome of hypertension is considered to exist when the average of a series of reliable blood pressure measurements exceeds 145 mmHg systolic or 95 mmHg diastolic (Table 288-1). The pathogenetic mechanisms, clinical and laboratory manifestations, and therapeutic approaches are discussed in detail elsewhere (Chaps. 29 and 267). In addition, a number of renal complications of hypertension are reviewed in Chap. 298, as is the entity of renal artery stenosis, an infrequent but potentially curable cause of hypertension.

Nephrolithiasis This syndrome is established with certainty when a stone is passed, visualized by x-ray, or removed at surgery or cystoscopy (Table 288-1 and Chap. 300). Less certain, but highly suggestive, evidence of nephrolithiasis exists in the patient with renal colic, painful hematuria, or unexplained pyuria, dysuria, and urinary frequency (Chap. 42). Colic varies in its symptomatology but usually begins suddenly in one flank, radiates downward toward the groin, and is excruciatingly painful.

Most renal stones are composed of calcium, uric acid, cystine, or struvite (magnesium ammonium phosphate). All are radiopaque except for those composed solely of uric acid and are, therefore, visible by routine abdominal radiography. Uric acid stones appear as radiolucent filling defects and can be mistaken for tumor or blood clot. The causes of stones are diverse; the approach to their detection, treatment, and prevention is discussed in Chap. 300.

Urinary tract obstruction Documentation of the various structural or functional causes of urinary tract obstruction usually requires radiological or surgical visualization. The manifestations of obstruction, which initiate the search for its causes, are numerous (Table 288-1) and are reviewed in Chap. 301. Anuria in an adult is almost always due to obstruction of bladder outflow. Less commonly, blockage of upper urinary drainage from both kidneys, or from a solitary functioning kidney, accounts for total or near-total cessation of urine flow. A large bladder after voiding is a sign of outflow obstruction, usually due to urethral stricture, tumor, stone, neurogenic causes, or prostatic hypertrophy. Nocturia, frequency and overflow incontinence, and slowing or hesitancy of micturition are also suggestive of outflow obstruction (Chaps. 41 and 42). Upper tract obstruction often produces few clinical manifestations. When it is incomplete or unilateral urine volume may be normal, or even elevated because of a loss of renal concentrating ability (Chap. 41). Urinary stasis secondary to obstruction commonly predisposes to recurrent urinary tract infection.

MISCELLANEOUS DISORDERS In addition to the 10 major syndromes of nephrology that serve as the basis for organization of subsequent chapters in this section, tumors of the urinary tract (Chap. 302) and a variety of vascular disorders that affect the kidneys (Chap. 298) are also considered in this section. The entities considered in these two chapters are heterogeneous, in both their pathogenesis and clinical expression and, therefore, do not lend themselves readily to the syndromic approach.

REFERENCES

Black DAK: Diagnosis and renal disease, in *Renal Disease*, 4th ed, DAK Black (ed). St. Louis, Blackwell, 1980

Cameron JS: The natural history of glomerulonephritis, in *Renal Disease*, 4th ed, DAK Black (ed). St. Louis, Blackwell, 1980, p. 329

Coe FL: The clinical and laboratory assessment of the patient with renal disease, in *The Kidney*, 2d ed, BM Brenner, FC Rector Jr (eds). Philadelphia, Saunders, 1981, p 1135

289

DISTURBANCES OF RENAL FUNCTION

BARRY M. BRENNER
THOMAS H. HOSTETTER

Near constancy of the composition of the internal environment, including the volume and compartmental distribution of the body fluids, is a condition essential to human survival. With unrelenting acquisition of food and fluids, which vary from day to day in amount as well as composition, preservation of the internal environment requires the continuous excretion of the by-products of these substances, and in amounts that balance precisely the quantities acquired by ingestion and metabolic transformation. Although losses from skin, lungs, and intestine normally contribute to this excretory capacity, by far the greatest responsibility for solute and water excretion is borne by the kidneys.

The kidneys operate primarily to maintain the integrity of the *extracellular* environment. The continuous exchange of water and solutes that takes place across all cell membranes during life, however, permits the kidneys to contribute signifi-

cantly to the regulation of the volume, composition, and tonicity of the *intracellular* fluids as well. To accomplish these tasks, the human kidney has evolved a number of physiological mechanisms that enable the individual to excrete any excesses of water and nonmetabolized solute contained in the diet, as well as the nonvolatile end products of nitrogen metabolism, such as urea and creatinine. By contrast, when faced with deficits of water and/or any of the other major constituents of the body fluids, renal excretion of these substances can be curtailed, reducing the likelihood of severe volume or solute depletion. The purpose of this chapter is to review the major functions of the normal kidney and to examine the way these functions are affected by disorders that impair the operations of this organ in humans.

MECHANISMS OF RENAL EXCRETORY FUNCTION WITH NORMAL AND REDUCED NEPHRON MASS

The volume of urine excreted per day (about 1.5 liters, or roughly 1 ml/min) is the small residuum of two very large, and in many ways opposing, processes—namely, *ultrafiltration* of 180 liters or more fluid per day (approximately 125 ml/min) across glomerular capillaries on the one hand and, on the other, *reclamation* (or *reabsorption*) of more than 99 percent of this ultrafiltrate by transport processes operating in the renal tubules. The enormity of the initial step in this process in humans is underscored by the fact that, in humans under resting conditions, about 20 percent of the cardiac output passes through the kidneys, which together comprise less than 1 percent of body weight. Hence, per unit weight of tissue, the rate of blood flow to the kidneys is much greater than that to other solid organs generally considered to be well perfused, including the heart, brain, and liver.

GLOMERULAR ULTRAFILTRATION Urine formation begins with the elaboration of a protein-free ultrafiltrate of plasma across the walls of the glomerular capillaries. The rate of ultrafiltration (glomerular filtration rate, GFR) is determined by three factors: (1) the balance of pressures acting across the capillary wall (the glomerular capillary hydrostatic and Bowman's space oncotic pressures tend to favor filtration, while glomerular capillary oncotic and Bowman's space hydrostatic pressures tend to retard it), (2) the rate at which plasma flows through the glomeruli, and (3) the permeability and the total surface area of the filtering capillaries. A decrease in GFR can be expected when (1) glomerular hydrostatic pressure is reduced (as in hypotensive shock), (2) tubule (hence, Bowman's space) hydrostatic pressure is increased (ureteral or bladder neck obstruction), (3) plasma oncotic pressure rises to unusually high levels (hemoconcentration due to dehydration; multiple myeloma or other dysproteinemias), (4) renal (hence, glomerular) blood and plasma flow are decreased (circulatory collapse, profound heart failure), and (5) permeability and/or total filtering surface area is reduced (acute or chronic glomerulonephritis).

Despite the extraordinarily high rate of water movement across the glomerular capillary wall, all but the smallest of the circulating plasma proteins are normally excluded from passage through this barrier. Molecules the size of inulin (approximately 5200 mol wt), or smaller, normally appear in glomerular urine in the same concentrations as in plasma water, whereas the transport of substances of increasingly greater size diminishes progressively, normally approaching very low values as the size of serum albumin is approached. The *glomerular capillary basement membrane* and the *slit-like diaphragms* that connect adjacent epithelial cell foot processes on the urinary aspect of the glomerular capillary wall (Fig. 40-1, page 214) are believed to serve as major barriers to protein filtration. In addition to these mechanical gates, *electrostatic factors* also serve to retard the filtration of plasma proteins, especially albumin. The albumin molecule behaves as a polyanion in physiological solution, and is therefore retarded by the highly anionic glycoproteins contained in the various component layers of the glomerular wall. With disruption of these mechanical and electrostatic barriers, as seen in many forms of glomerular injury (see Chaps. 293 to 295), abnormally large quantities of plasma proteins gain access to the urine.

BIOLOGICAL CONSEQUENCES OF SUSTAINED REDUCTIONS IN GFR Measurement of total GFR of both kidneys provides a sensitive and commonly employed index of overall renal excretory function. When renal excretory function is impaired, either acutely or chronically, one or more of the determinants of GFR in affected nephrons is altered unfavorably so that total GFR declines. The magnitude of the decline is determined by the sum of the impairments of function of individual glomeruli. Initially, the effect of such impairments in single-nephron GFR (SNGFR), no matter how small, is to reduce the total rate of excretion of water and those solutes normally contained in the glomerular ultrafiltrate. In the steady state, these reduced rates of filtration, when accompanied by comparably reduced rates of excretion, lead to *retention* and *accumulation* of the unexcreted substances in the body fluids. Further reduction in GFR augments the degree to which these substances are retained.

Figure 289-1 depicts the major patterns of response to these impairments in filtration. The degree of reduction in total GFR is plotted on the abscissa, expressed as a percentage of normal (100 percent). For the various solutes normally contained in glomerular filtrate, three general types of response are common, depicted by curves A, B, and C. Curve A describes the pattern seen with substances, such as creatinine and urea, which normally depend largely on glomerular filtration for their excretion into the urine; i.e., secretion fails to influence urinary excretion appreciably. Therefore, as GFR falls, plasma levels of creatinine, urea, and other substances normally excreted largely by filtration rise progressively, albeit in the nonlinear manner illustrated.

FIGURE 289-1

Representative patterns of adaptation for different types of solutes in body fluids in chronic renal failure. (After NS Bricker et al, in Brenner and Rector.)

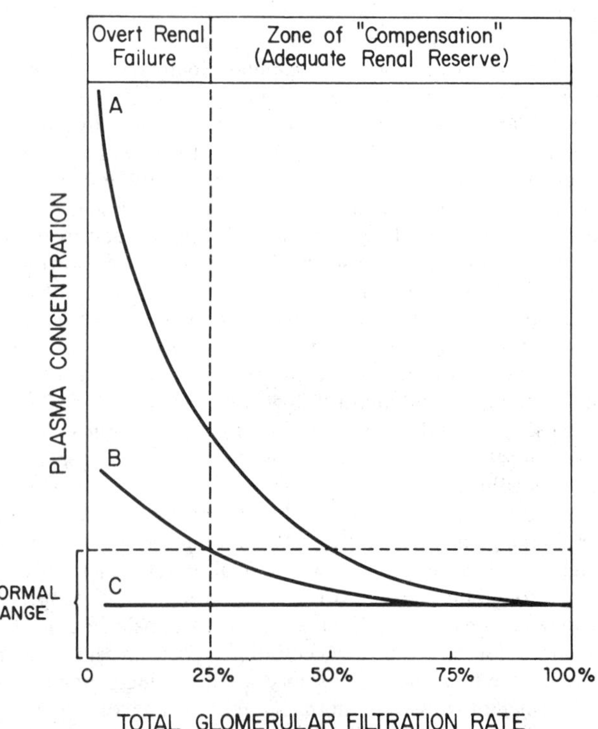

The clinical course of chronic renal failure (CRF) usually also conforms to the pattern described by *curve A.* Patients with CRF usually pass from a long asymptomatic period of "compensation" to a more accelerated and clinically symptomatic terminal phase. In other words, chronic forms of renal injury which lead to slow but inexorable destruction of nephron mass usually lead to progressive but modest elevations in creatinine and urea levels in plasma, but not to levels beyond the range of normal, despite loss of as much as 50 percent of total GFR. With further loss of nephron mass, and further reduction in GFR, however (even though the rate of nephron destruction may not be accelerated), the limits of renal reserve are exceeded, and continued accumulation of *curve A type solutes* leads to plasma concentrations clearly beyond the range of normal (Fig. 289-1). Because these retained solutes are believed to exert "toxic" effects on virtually all organ systems, manifestations of CRF now become overt. As a result, for patients with reduced renal mass, even small additional decrements in total GFR may spell the difference between "compensation" and overt uremia.

Despite this tendency for *curve A type solutes* to accumulate with progressive renal failure, external balance for these solutes can still be achieved. In the case of creatinine, for example, assuming a constant rate of creatinine production, a 50 percent reduction in GFR results in an approximate doubling of the plasma creatinine concentration. The latter restores the filtered load of creatinine (that is, GFR × plasma creatinine concentration) to the preillness level, and urinary excretion rate again becomes equivalent to the rate of creatinine production. Unfortunately, since no mechanism exists for augmenting creatinine excretion beyond this level, elimination of retained creatinine is not possible, and plasma concentration remains twice normal. With progressive reduction in GFR, plasma creatinine levels rise further, due both to the most recent loss of function and to the retention associated with earlier nephron destruction (Fig. 289-1). *In practice, so long as the net rates of acquisition and production remain reasonably constant, the inverse relationship between plasma concentrations of solutes such as creatinine and urea and GFR is sufficiently reliable and predictable to allow plasma levels of such solutes to serve as useful clinical indexes of GFR.*

In contrast to solutes of the *curve A type,* plasma levels of substances such as phosphate, urate, and potassium (K^+) and hydrogen (H^+) ions usually fail to rise above the normal range until GFR falls to a small percentage of normal. With progressive renal failure this pattern of response, depicted by *curve B* in Fig. 289-1, reflects the participation of tubule transport mechanisms that contribute to the excretion of these substances. In other words, *as GFR declines, the tubules facilitate the excretion of progressively greater fractions of the filtered load of these solutes, either by enhancing their net secretion or by diminishing their net reabsorption.* Plasma levels of *curve B type solutes,* therefore, rise much less than do those of *curve A* because, with progressive reduction in GFR, *excretion rate per nephron* and, therefore, *fractional excretion* both increase. Eventually, however, enhanced fractional excretion can no longer offset the inevitable retention of these solutes caused by a markedly diminished GFR, and plasma levels rise above the normal range (Fig. 289-1). For urate, phosphate, and K^+ at least, increased fractional excretion usually serves to maintain normal plasma levels until GFR falls to less than one-fourth of normal.

Finally, for certain solutes, such as sodium chloride (NaCl), concentrations in plasma remain virtually constant, and at normal levels, throughout the entire course of CRF, despite continued ingestion of these substances in normal amounts. Such solutes conform to the pattern described by *curve C* in Fig. 289-1. The extent of compensation is nearly complete and represents a fundamental adaptation to renal injury. To illustrate the magnitude of the adaptation involved, it is useful to compare the pattern of Na^+ excretion in an individual with normal renal excretory function (GFR of 125 ml/min) with that in an individual with advanced renal insufficiency (GFR of 2 ml/min). Both subjects are allowed to ingest a diet containing 7 g salt per day (120 meq Na^+). With a normal serum Na^+ concentration of 140 meq per liter, external Na^+ balance is achieved in the normal individual by excreting approximately 0.5 percent of the filtered load of Na^+. By contrast, for external balance to be maintained in the patient with CRF, fractional excretion of Na^+ must rise to 30 percent. *In other words, external balance for* Na^+ *demands that the same quantity of* Na^+ *(120 meq) be excreted into the urine each day in the subject with CRF as in the normal subject.* Given the drastic reduction in GFR faced by the patient with CRF, external balance can be achieved only by a progressive transformation of the Na^+ reabsorptive processes in surviving tubules, so that a progressively larger fraction of the filtered load of Na^+ escapes reabsorption and appears in final urine. In short, *the rate of excretion of* Na^+ *per surviving nephron increases in inverse proportion to the composite GFR of surviving nephrons.*

MECHANISMS OF TUBULE TRANSPORT WITH NORMAL AND REDUCED NEPHRON MASS Loss of renal function with nearly all forms of progressive renal disease is usually attended by a progressive distortion of renal morphology and architecture. Despite this structural disarray, glomerular and tubular functions often remain as closely integrated (i.e., *glomerulotubular balance*) in the diseased kidney as they do in the normal organ, at least until the final stages of CRF. A fundamental feature of this *intact nephron hypothesis* is that following loss of nephron mass, residual renal function derives primarily from the operation of surviving healthy nephrons, while the diseased nephrons are believed to cease functioning. Despite progressive nephron destruction, there is considerable evidence to suggest that many of the mechanisms that contribute to the maintenance of solute and water balance differ only quantitatively, and not qualitatively, from those believed to govern fluid and solute homeostasis under normal physiological conditions. The most important of these are considered below.

Tubule transport of sodium chloride and water in health Most of the filtered water and Na^+ salts are reabsorbed by the tubules, leaving small and variable amounts, equivalent on a day-to-day basis to the quantities ingested, to reach the final urine. About two-thirds of the glomerular ultrafiltrate is reabsorbed in the *proximal tubule* without changing the osmolality or Na^+ concentration of the unreabsorbed fraction (Fig. 289-2). In other words, fluid reabsorption in the proximal tubule is *isosmotic.* Reabsorption of Na^+ across the proximal tubule cell involves a two-step process. Since the Na^+ concentration in the cell is lower, and the voltage more negative, than in either the tubule lumen or peritubular fluid, the movement of Na^+ from lumen to cell proceeds down electrochemical gradients and is therefore a passive process. Efflux of Na^+ from tubule cell to peritubular interstitial fluid is believed to be due to an active, energy-dependent process, although the mechanism involved is not well understood. According to current concepts, salts of Na^+ enter proximal tubule cells through the luminal brush border membrane and then are transported from the cells into *lateral intercellular channels.* As a result, salt concentration (and osmolality) within the channels exceeds that in adjacent tubule cells or surrounding interstitium, causing movement of water from tubule lumen and cell interior into the channels by osmosis. As a consequence, the hydrostatic pressure within the channels rises, driving fluid into the surrounding peritubular interstitium.

The rate of reabsorption of fluid from proximal convoluted tubules and peritubular interstitium is sensitive to the effects of *physical factors,* i.e., the hydrostatic and colloid osmotic (or oncotic) pressures acting across the walls of the peritubular capillaries. Because the plasma proteins in glomerular capillaries are concentrated by ultrafiltration, there is a marked rise in the oncotic pressure as plasma flows along the glomerular capillary network. This step-up in plasma oncotic pressure is transmitted largely unchanged to the peritubular capillaries, via the efferent arterioles. These resistance vessels cause a substantial drop in hydrostatic pressure, however, so that when the plasma reaches the peritubular capillaries, oncotic pressure greatly exceeds hydrostatic pressure. These *Starling forces* are therefore oriented in an *uptake mode,* in contrast to the *filtration mode* at the glomerulus, where hydrostatic pressure exceeds oncotic. The extent to which oncotic pressure exceeds hydrostatic pressure in the peritubular capillary network is thought to modulate the overall rate of reabsorption of fluid by the proximal tubules. Therefore, when peritubular oncotic pressure falls, or hydrostatic pressure rises, uptake of fluid by these capillaries is reduced. As a result, fluid is retained in the interstitial space, altering the hydrostatic pressure in the space, and ultimately retarding the egress of fluid from the lateral intercellular channels. Without an adequate route of drainage, fluid in the channels leaks back into the tubule lumen and diminishes *net fluid reabsorption* by this tubule segment. The opposite occurs in states in which peritubular oncotic pressure increases (increased filtration fraction), or hydrostatic pressure decreases (enhanced efferent arteriolar tone). Under these circumstances, peritubular capillary uptake of reabsorbate is augmented, leading ultimately to *enhanced net fluid reabsorption* by the proximal tubule.

In contrast to the proximal tubule, active outward transport of NaCl from tubule lumen to peritubular blood has not been established for the *thin limbs of Henle's loop.* However, passive outward salt transport does occur, as indicated in Fig. 289-2. In the next segment of the nephron, the *medullary thick ascending limb of Henle,* the concentration of NaCl is reduced below the level that prevails at the beginning of this segment. Here the means for lowering the salt concentration involves the *active transport of* Cl^-, with Na^+ following passively to preserve electroneutrality. Since the ascending limb of Henle is always impermeable to water, net NaCl reabsorption not only generates hypotonic tubule fluid, but also gives rise to the high NaCl concentration of the outer medullary interstitium (Fig. 289-2).

The fluid leaving the thick ascending limb of Henle is normally low in NaCl concentration, a condition largely independent of the organism's diet or state of hydration. In the *distal convoluted tubule,* water reabsorption is variable, depending on the state of hydration or, more specifically, on the presence or absence of the *antidiuretic hormone (ADH)* in plasma. In the absence of ADH, this and more distal nephron segments are impermeable to water, so that the hypotonic fluid entering this segment is excreted as *dilute urine.* Indeed, continued salt reabsorption along the distal convoluted tubule results in further dilution of the urine. In the presence of ADH, the permeability of the late portion of this segment to water increases, and as a result, the osmolality of the late distal tubule fluid rises to a value close to that of plasma. NaCl continues to be reabsorbed from the tubule lumen, against moderately steep chemical and electrical gradients. The reabsorptive process for NaCl at this site is enhanced by *aldosterone.*

The *cortical collecting tubule* possesses an extremely low permeability to water in the absence of ADH, whereas this permeability increases greatly in the presence of the hormone. The sensitivity of this segment to ADH appears to be more pronounced than is that of the distal convoluted tubule. As with the distal convoluted tubule, the cortical collecting tubule is capable of further net reabsorption of NaCl.

The terminal segment of the distal nephron is the highly branched *papillary collecting duct.* Continued electrolyte transport in this segment results in the large ion concentration dif-

FIGURE 289-2

Transport functions of the various anatomic segments of the mammalian nephron. Fluid reabsorption across the proximal tubule is isosmotic and accounts for reabsorption of approximately two-thirds of the filtered Na^+ and H_2O. The major portions of the filtered HCO_3^-, amino acids, and glucose are reabsorbed in the early proximal convoluted tubule. Reabsorption of glucose and amino acids is coupled to Na^+ transport and thereby generates a negative potential difference within the tubule lumen. At the same time, HCO_3^- is reabsorbed by a nonelectrogenic mechanism, most likely via H^+ secretion. The active transport of these solutes results in transepithelial concentration and effective osmotic pressure gradients promoting H_2O flow across the proximal tubule, into the peritubular capillaries. The rise in tubule fluid Cl^- concentration is a necessary reciprocal consequence of the decreased luminal HCO_3^- concentration. The resultant high concentration of Cl^- becomes an important force for the outward passive transport of Cl^- down its concentration gradient, resulting in a lumen positive potential difference in the late proximal convoluted tubule. The pars recta of the proximal tubule is capable of active electrogenic transport of Na^+ independent of organic solute transport. Under normal conditions, approximately one-third of the glomerular filtrate enters the descending limb of Henle's loop. Because the thin descending limb is incapable of active outward NaCl transport and is characterized by low permeability to Na^+ but high H_2O permeability, H_2O is abstracted passively as the fluid approaches the bend of Henle's loop. Hypertonic fluid with a greater NaCl concentration but lower urea concentration than the surrounding medullary interstitium thus enters the thin ascending limb of Henle. This segment differs from the descending limb in that it is largely impermeable to H_2O and urea but highly permeable to NaCl. These characteristics allow for passive diffusion of NaCl out of the ascending limb. Active electrogenic Cl^- transport across the water-impermeable thick ascending limb of Henle, with Na^+ following passively, allows for separation of solute and water. In consequence tubule fluid becomes dilute, and the medullary interstitium hypertonic. Irrespective of the final osmolality of the urine, the fluid that enters the distal convoluted tubule is always hypoosmotic. This segment exhibits active Na^+ reabsorption. All but the terminal portion of the distal convoluted tubule is water impermeable, even in the presence of ADH. Aldosterone exerts its effect in this segment by enhancing Na^+ reabsorption, which is variably coupled to K^+ and H^+ secretion. The cortical and papillary portions of the collecting duct are sites where ADH exerts its principal effect. The permeability of these segments to H_2O in the absence of ADH is very low but can be greatly enhanced in the presence of ADH. These segments are also characterized by active Na^+ reabsorption, which appears to depend on the presence of mineralocorticoid. In the absence of ADH, the collecting tubule is water impermeable so that hypotonic tubule fluid courses through it. However, in the presence of ADH, water is avidly reabsorbed here, resulting in hypertonic final urine.

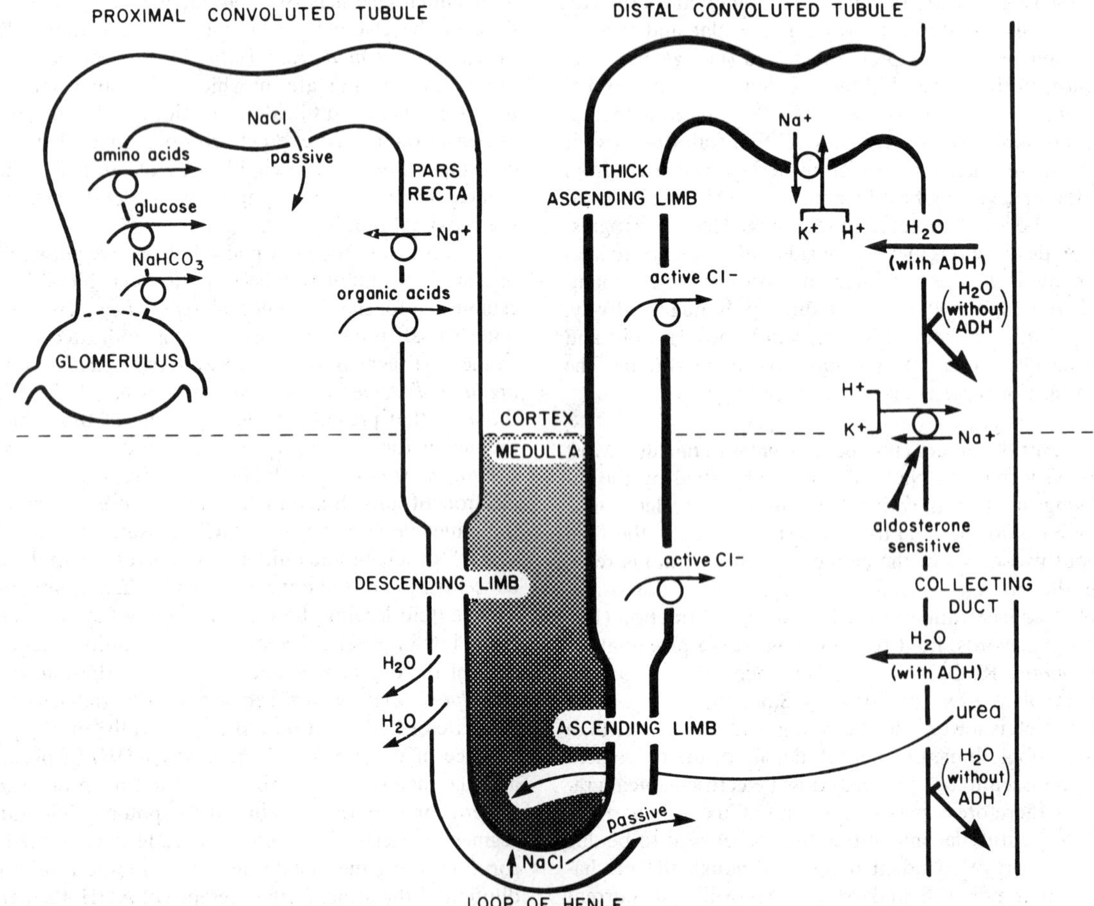

ferences that normally exist between urine and plasma. As in the cortical collecting tubule, Na^+ transport appears to be active since reabsorption proceeds against sizable electrochemical gradients. The rate of Na^+ transport in this segment depends on the diet and on the load of Na^+ delivered from more proximal segments, and is affected by aldosterone. The permeability of this segment to water also increases markedly in the presence of ADH.

Effects of reduced nephron mass on sodium chloride transport in surviving nephrons With progressive destruction of nephrons, *maintenance of external balance for NaCl requires that fractional salt excretion increases as GFR decreases.* Very likely several mechanisms contribute to this adaptive increase in fractional salt excretion. With losses of functioning nephron units, peritubular capillary hydrostatic and oncotic pressures are probably altered in directions that serve to suppress proximal tubule reabsorption of NaCl and water. For example, a rise in peritubular capillary hydrostatic pressure, which tends to inhibit net proximal fluid reabsorption, might be anticipated with arterial hypertension, a common feature of renal insufficiency. Similarly, peritubular oncotic pressure might be expected to decline with renal injury, owing both to reductions in filtration fraction and to hypoalbuminemia. While such alterations in peritubular factors clearly account for diminution in proximal fluid reabsorption in response to falling levels of GFR in animals, such alterations have not been established with certainty in humans. Aldosterone, normally an important determinant of Na^+ reabsorption in distal portions of the nephron, is probably not a major factor responsible for reducing fractional Na^+ reabsorption, since aldosterone levels in plasma are rarely reduced in CRF. Furthermore, external Na^+ balance has been shown to be preserved in bilaterally adrenalectomized uremic dogs maintained on fixed doses of mineralocorticoid hormones. Yet another factor that has received attention in contributing to the suppression of fractional NaCl reabsorption in CRF relates to the retention of solutes as GFR declines. In addition to urea and creatinine, a host of *organic acids* (including *hippurates*) also accumulate. These substances are normally excreted by both filtration and tubule secretion; the latter process involves a carrier-mediated organic acid transport system in proximal tubule epithelia. When GFR is reduced and plasma levels of these organic acids increase, sufficient fluid may accompany the secretion of these organic anions into the proximal tubule lumen (by osmosis) to diminish net fluid reabsorption, and even favor net fluid secretion. Evidence in support of this intriguing mechanism derives from studies in which uremic serums were capable of inducing net fluid secretion in isolated proximal tubules of rabbits studied in vitro.

It has also been suggested that NaCl transport across the mammalian renal tubule may be governed, at least in part, by a *natriuretic hormone.* In support of this possibility, serums and urine from patients and dogs with uremia have been reported to contain factors capable of inhibiting NaCl transport across frog skin, toad bladder, and rat renal tubule. However, accumulation of natriuretic factors in uremia may not be without cost; the "trade-off" for maintenance of external Na^+ balance is the possibility of abnormalities occurring in Na^+ transport across cell membranes, which often occurs in advanced renal insufficiency. This possibility is discussed in greater detail in Chap. 291.

The obligatorily high rate of solute excretion per surviving nephron (so-called osmotic diuresis due to urea and other retained solutes) may also contribute to enhancing fractional NaCl excretion, much as occurs in normal subjects following administration of nonreabsorbable solutes such as mannitol. Finally, certain forms of CRF tend to be associated with unusually pronounced salt losses in urine. These *salt-wasting nephropathies* include chronic pyelonephritis and other tubulointerstitial diseases (see Chap. 297) as well as polycystic and medullary cystic diseases. These disorders have in common greater destruction of medullary and interstitial, than cortical and glomerular, portions of the renal parenchyma. Preferential impairment of tubule reabsorptive function, rather than a primary reduction in GFR, may, therefore, underlie the salt-losing tendency in these disorders. A number of clinical derangements associated with the altered renal handling of NaCl in CRF (including hypo- and hypervolemia, hypertension, etc.) are considered in Chap. 291.

Effects of reduced nephron mass on water reabsorption in surviving nephrons As with NaCl, there is a progressive increase in the fractional excretion of water with advancing renal insufficiency, so that even the patient with a total GFR of 5 ml/min or less can usually maintain external water balance. The adaptations in the handling of water by the tubules of the diseased kidney are of importance in the pathogenesis of the urinary concentrating defect and, hence, of the polyuria and nocturia seen commonly in CRF (see Chap. 41). To appreciate the mechanisms involved, the responses of a normal and a uremic subject in maintaining external water balance need to be compared. Assuming that both subjects ingest the same diet and also the same amount of fluid, total solute and volume excretion in each subject should be identical as well. If the *obligatory solute load* to be excreted in each is assumed to be 600 mosmol per day, and urine osmolality is 300 mosmol/kg, a urine volume of 2 liters per day will be required to excrete the total solute load in each subject. If GFR in normal and uremic subjects is 180 and 4 liters per day, respectively, urinary volume excretion of 2 liters per day represents excretion of slightly more than 1 percent of the filtered water in the normal individual, compared with a much larger value, 50 percent, in the uremic subject. Since the range of urine osmolalities that the diseased kidney can achieve (250 to 350 mosmol/kg) is much narrower than in the normal (40 to 1200 mosmol/kg), the individual with normal function is able to excrete the obligatory daily solute load of 600 mosmol in as little as 500 ml urine per day or as much as 15 liters per day, compared with the much narrower range in the patient with renal insufficiency, from about 1.7 to 2.4 liters per day.

In CRF, the limited ability to concentrate the urine usually correlates closely with other measures of impaired renal function. Isosthenuria is, therefore, a nearly universal finding when GFR falls below 25 ml/min. At this level of GFR and below, urine osmolality becomes insensitive even to supramaximal doses of ADH, suggesting that the concentrating defect is related not only to loss of diseased nephrons but also to impaired concentrating ability in surviving nephrons. As has been discussed, with diminution in functioning nephron mass, there is a concurrent increase in fractional excretion of a number of solutes. As a consequence, solute diuresis per nephron obligates a nearly isosmotic amount of water and prevents the elaboration of hypertonic urine, even in the presence of adequate amounts of ADH. Disease-induced abnormalities of the architecture of the renal medulla (loops of Henle, vasa rectae), aberrations in renal medullary blood flow, and defective transport of NaCl in the ascending limb of Henle undoubtedly also contribute to this defect in urine concentration. Finally, there is suggestive evidence that uremia per se may impair the responsiveness of terminal nephron segments to ADH.

Since patients with renal insufficiency are usually unable to excrete concentrated urine, they must have access to adequate amounts of water in order to ensure the excretion of total daily solute loads. For this reason, restriction of fluid intake may prove extremely hazardous in patients with CRF. Likewise, impairment of diluting capacity may prevent many patients from excreting large amounts of ingested fluids. The consequences of the abnormal water excretion patterns in CRF, including the tendencies to development of hypo- and hypernatremia, are considered in Chaps. 43 and 291.

Tubule transport of phosphate with normal and reduced nephron mass Under normal physiological conditions, about 80 to 90 percent of the filtered load of phosphate is reabsorbed, mainly in the proximal tubule. *Parathyroid hormone (PTH)* augments phosphate excretion by inhibiting this proximal reabsorptive process (Chap. 338). Hence, with enhanced PTH secretion, reabsorption of phosphate can fall markedly, to as little as 15 percent of the amount filtered. By modifying phosphate reabsorption, PTH plays a key role in phosphate homeostasis. In normal humans, when dietary phosphate intake increases, a *transient* rise in plasma phosphate concentration is usually observed. This results in a similarly transient reduction in the plasma ionized calcium concentration (due largely to calcium-phosphate deposition in bone), which, in turn, stimulates PTH secretion. By enhancing fractional phosphate excretion, PTH restores external phosphate balance and normophosphatemia. This then enables plasma ionized calcium levels to return to normal, thereby removing the stimulus to PTH release, and restoring all elements of the phosphate control system to the original steady state.

With advancing renal disease, and constant dietary intake of phosphate, external phosphate balance is achieved by progressive reduction in fractional phosphate reabsorption. Enhanced PTH secretion is an important determinant of this phosphaturic response to reduced nephron mass. Figure 289-3 provides a schematic summary of the mechanisms believed to be involved. As shown, with each succeeding decrement in GFR, the total amount of phosphate filtered by surviving glomeruli is reduced, leading to transient retention of phosphate and, therefore, a rise (albeit small) in the phosphate concentration in extracellular fluid, including plasma. This rise in plasma phosphate concentration leads to a reciprocal small decline in plasma ionized calcium concentration and a corresponding increase in PTH secretion. Although the phosphaturic response of surviving tubules to this elevation in circulating PTH is thought to restore plasma phosphate and, therefore, calcium levels to normal (at least in the "compensated" stage of CRF described by the relatively flat portion of curve B in Fig. 289-1), the biological cost of this return to normophosphatemia and normocalcemia is a *persistent elevation in the plasma PTH level.* As shown in Fig. 289-3, with successive decrements in GFR, each stage in this overall process is repeated, but at an ever-increasing cost, namely, *progressive elevation in the circulating level of PTH.* At least two additional processes are thought to contribute to elevated PTH levels in renal failure. One relates to the skeletal resistance to the calcemic effect of PTH seen in uremia. This resistance necessitates a greater than normal level of circulating PTH to effect an increment in serum calcium concentration. The other derives from the finding that reductions in renal mass impair the ability of the kidneys to degrade circulating PTH. The fact that phosphate conforms more to a curve B than curve C type solute in Fig. 289-1 indicates that these forms of adaptation are limited; ultimately phosphate retention occurs when GFR falls below about 25 ml/min.

FIGURE 289-3
The "Bricker" model for return to external phosphate balance in chronic renal failure. (From NS Bricker et al, in Brenner and Rector.)

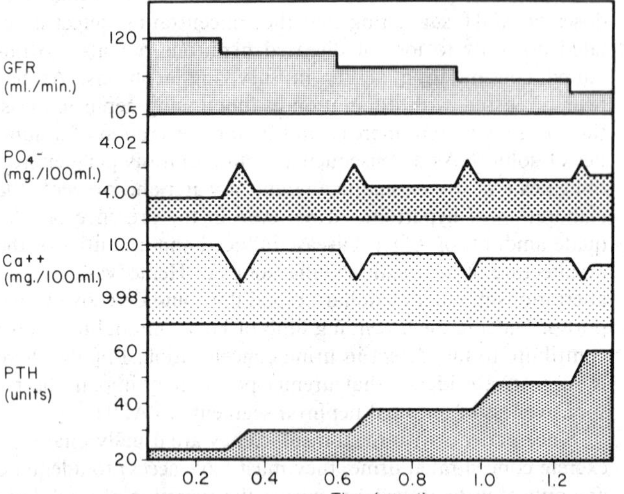

Since PTH exerts major biological effects on bone, as well as renal tubules, the external balance of phosphate in CRF is achieved at the expense of elevated PTH levels, which, in turn, account for many of the bone changes of renal osteodystrophy (i.e., *secondary hyperparathyroidism,* Fig. 291-1). In support of this ingenious *trade-off hypothesis,* studies in animals with CRF suggest that when dietary phosphate intake is reduced in proportion to the reduction in GFR, external balance of phosphate no longer requires augmentation of fractional phosphate excretion in surviving nephrons. Accordingly, circulating PTH levels no longer rise, and the typical bone changes of secondary hyperparathyroidism are diminished, if not prevented.

Destruction of renal mass also impairs phosphate, calcium, and skeletal metabolism by mechanisms largely independent of impaired excretory function. The kidneys are normally the major site of *metabolic conversion of vitamin D to its active metabolites.* Whereas the tendency to secondary hyperparathyroidism begins, at least theoretically, when a single nephron unit is destroyed, impaired vitamin D biotransformation is not usually apparent until GFR falls to below 25 percent of normal. As discussed in detail in Chap. 340, precursors of the active form of vitamin D, synthesized in skin or acquired from foods, undergo initial hydroxylation in the liver to form 25-hydroxyvitamin D_3 [25-(OH)D_3]. The kidney is the site of a second important hydroxylation step, to form 1,25-dihydroxyvitamin D_3 [1,25-$(OH)_2D_3$]. This activated form of vitamin D operates to enhance intestinal calcium and phosphate absorption, as well as to promote resorption of these ions from bone. In addition, 1,25-$(OH)_2D_3$ probably opposes the phosphaturic action of PTH at the level of the renal tubule, by augmenting, rather than diminishing, phosphate reabsorption. With advancing renal disease, reduction in renal mass causes vitamin D hydroxylation to be impaired; phosphate retention has also been shown to suppress this important hydroxylation reaction. Reduction in circulating 1,25-$(OH)_2D_3$ levels, by suppressing calcium absorption from gut, contributes further to the development of the hypocalcemia and PTH excess of CRF, the consequences of which are considered in Chap. 291.

Hydrogen and bicarbonate transport with normal and reduced nephron mass As discussed in Chap. 44, the pH of extracellular fluid in humans is normally maintained within a narrow range, 7.36 to 7.44, despite day-to-day variations in the quantity of acids entering the body fluids from dietary and metabolic sources (approximately 1 meq H^+/kg per day). These acids consume buffer, of which bicarbonate (HCO_3^-) is the most important. Such buffering minimizes the changes in pH that would otherwise occur. The HCO_3^- buffer system would be of little long-term benefit were it not for homeostatic mechanisms, however, since with unrelenting acquisition of nonvolatile acids from dietary and metabolic sources, buffering capacity would ultimately be exhausted, eventually culminating in fatal acidosis. The kidneys normally function to prevent this possibility by *regenerating* HCO_3^- and, thereby, maintaining the concentration of HCO_3^- in the plasma. In addition to generating HCO_3^-, the kidneys also *reclaim* essentially all the HCO_3^- present in the glomerular ultrafiltrate. This reabsorptive process takes place in the proximal tubule and is virtually complete below a critical serum HCO_3^- concentration—the threshold concentration—which in humans is normally about 26 meq per liter, identical to the concentration of HCO_3^- in plasma. As a consequence, urinary wastage of HCO_3^- is prevented. Alternatively, when plasma HCO_3^- concentration rises above this threshold level, reabsorption of HCO_3^- becomes less complete, and the excess HCO_3^- escapes into the final urine, returning the plasma HCO_3^- concentration to the threshold level. Despite reabsorption of all the filtered HCO_3^-, metabolic acidosis would still ensue if HCO_3^- consumed in buffering nonvolatile strong acids were not constantly regenerated.

The *reabsorption* of filtered HCO_3^- and the *regeneration* of new HCO_3^- occur by a single mechanism. In proximal tubule cells, H^+, formed by the splitting of water into H^+ and OH^-, is secreted into the tubule lumen, very likely in exchange for Na^+. The OH^- ion, under the influence of *carbonic anhydrase*, combines with CO_2 to form HCO_3^-, which diffuses across the peritubular cell membrane to enter the extracellular HCO_3^- pool. The H^+ secreted into the tubule lumen combines with a filtered HCO_3^-, forming H_2CO_3. Dehydration of the latter in the proximal tubule lumen leads to the formation of CO_2 which also diffuses from lumen to peritubular blood. As a result, *a filtered HCO_3^- ion is reclaimed.* Secreted H^+ ions are also free to combine with non-HCO_3^- buffers (e.g., phosphate or ammonia) in the tubule fluid and to be excreted in these forms in the final urine. HCO_3^-, the other original product of the breakdown of H_2CO_3, formed within the tubule cell, enters the peritubular blood, and *a HCO_3^- ion is regenerated.*

Hydrogen ions in the urine are bound primarily to filtered buffers (e.g., phosphate) in an amount (the so-called titratable acid) equivalent to the amount of alkali required to titrate the pH of the urine to the pH of blood. It is usually not possible, however, to excrete all the daily acid load as titratable acid alone. To serve as additional buffer, the cells of the renal tubules generate ammonia (NH_3), largely from the hydrolysis of glutamine. NH_3 diffuses from these cells into the tubule lumen where it combines with H^+ to form NH_4^+. As noted above, each mole of NH_4^+ excreted into the urine is associated with the regeneration of 1 mol of HCO_3^-. *Ammoniagenesis,* a process which occurs within proximal tubule cells, is responsive to the acid-base needs of the individual. When faced with an acute acid burden and an increased need for HCO_3^- regeneration, the rate of renal ammonia synthesis increases sharply.

The quantity of hydrogen ions excreted as titratable acid and NH_4^+ is equal to the quantity of HCO_3^- regenerated in tubule cells and added to the plasma. Under steady-state conditions, the quantity of net acid excreted into the urine (the sum of titratable acid and NH_4^+ minus HCO_3^-) must equal the quantity of acid gained by the extracellular fluid from all sources. Metabolic acidosis and alkalosis result when this delicate balance is perturbed, the former the result of *insufficient* net acid excretion, the latter due to *excessive* acid excretion.

Progressive loss of renal function usually causes little or no change in arterial pH, plasma bicarbonate concentration, or arterial carbon dioxide tension (P_{CO_2}) until GFR falls below 50 percent of normal. Thereafter, all three quantities tend to decline as *metabolic acidosis* ensues. In general, the metabolic acidosis of CRF is not due to overproduction of endogenous acids, but is largely a reflection of the reduction in renal mass, which limits the amount of NH_3 (and therefore HCO_3^-) that can be generated. Although surviving nephrons are probably capable of generating supernormal quantities of NH_3 *per nephron,* the diminished nephron population causes overall NH_3 production to be reduced to an extent inadequate to permit sufficient buffering of H^+ in urine. Though patients with CRF may acidify the urine normally (i.e., urine pH as low as 4.5), the defect in NH_3 production limits total daily acid excretion to 30 to 40 meq, or half to two-thirds the quantity of nonvolatile acid formed in the same time period. Metabolic acidosis is the inevitable consequence of this positive balance for H^+, which in most patients with stable CRF is relatively mild and nonprogressive (arterial pH of approximately 7.33 to 7.37).

Given this substantial daily accumulation of H^+, and the typically stable and nonprogressive nature of the resulting acidosis, including the observed relative constancy of the plasma HCO_3^- concentration (albeit at reduced levels of 14 to 20 meq per liter), it follows that some large tissue source of buffering must account for the stability of the acidosis in CRF. Bone is the most likely candidate, particularly in view of its large reservoir of alkaline salts (calcium phosphate and calcium carbonate). Dissolution of this buffer source probably contributes to the osteodystrophy of CRF (see Fig. 291-1).

Although the acidosis of CRF is a consequence of the reduction in total renal mass and is therefore tubular in origin, it nevertheless depends to a large extent on the level of GFR. When GFR is reduced to only a moderate extent (i.e., to about 50 percent of normal), retention of anions, principally sulfates and phosphate, is not pronounced, so that as the plasma HCO_3^- level falls owing to tubular dysfunction, retention of Cl^- by the kidneys leads to the development of *hyperchloremic acidosis.* At this stage, therefore, *the anion gap is normal.* With further reduction in GFR and more pronounced azotemia, however, retention of phosphates, sulfates, and other *unmeasured* anions is the rule, and plasma Cl^- concentration falls to normal levels despite the reduction in plasma HCO_3^- concentration. *A moderate to large anion gap therefore develops.*

Tubule potassium transport with normal and reduced nephron mass As with H^+, the concentration of K^+ in extracellular fluid is normally maintained within a relatively narrow range, 4 to 5 meq per liter. Ninety-five percent or more of total body K^+ is in the intracellular fluid compartment, where the intracellular concentration is approximately 160 meq per liter. Normal individuals maintain external K^+ balance by excreting into the urine an amount of K^+ per day equivalent to the amount ingested, minus the relatively small amounts lost in stool and sweat. K^+ is freely filtered at the glomerulus, although the amount excreted usually represents no more than about 20 percent of the quantity filtered. The great bulk of the filtered K^+ is *reabsorbed* in the early portions of the nephron, about two-thirds in the proximal tubule, and an additional 20 to 25 percent in the loop of Henle. A K^+ *secretory process* operates in the distal tubule and terminal nephron segments. This process is largely dependent on exchange of K^+ for Na^+, the reabsorbed Na^+ creating an electrical gradient across the tubule wall, lumen negative. K^+ therefore diffuses from the cell interior into the lumens of distal tubules and collecting ducts, down this electrochemical gradient.

The ability to maintain external K^+ balance and normal plasma K^+ concentration as well, until relatively late in the course of CRF, is a consequence primarily of a progressive increase in fractional excretion of K^+. Greatly enhanced rates of K^+ secretion in distal portions of surviving tubules appear to underlie this adaptation. The augmented secretion rate of aldosterone is believed to contribute to enhanced tubule secretion of K^+, as do the increased distal tubule flow rates in residual functioning nephrons and the enhanced luminal electronegativity created by the increased concentration of highly impermeable anions such as phosphate and sulfate. Aldosterone also stimulates net entry of K^+ into the lumen of the colon, a mechanism known to be enhanced in CRF. More detailed discussions of the abnormalities in K^+ homeostasis in acute and chronic forms of renal failure are given in Chaps. 290 and 291.

REFERENCES

BRENNER BM, RECTOR FC JR (eds): *The Kidney,* 2d ed. Philadelphia, Saunders, 1981

BRICKER NS: On the pathogenesis of the uremic state: An exposition of the "trade-off" hypothesis. N Engl J Med 286:1093, 1972

HAYSLETT JP: Functional adaptation to reduction in renal mass. Physiol Rev 59:137, 1979

HOSTETTER TH, BRENNER BM: Glomerular adaptations to renal injury, in *Contemporary Issues in Nephrology,* vol 8: *Chronic Renal Failure.* New York, Churchill Livingstone, 1981

MAXWELL MH, KLEEMAN CR: *Clinical Disorders of Fluid and Electrolyte Metabolism,* 3d ed. New York, McGraw-Hill, 1980

ROSE BD: *Clinical Physiology of Acid-Base and Electrolyte Disorders.* New York, McGraw-Hill, 1977

290
ACUTE RENAL FAILURE

ROBERT J. ANDERSON
ROBERT W. SCHRIER

Acute renal failure is broadly defined as a rapid deterioration in renal function sufficient to result in accumulation of nitrogenous wastes in the body. The causes of such deterioration include renal hypoperfusion, obstructive uropathy, and intrinsic renal disease such as acute glomerulonephritis. After exclusion of these entities, there remains a group of patients in whom acute renal failure is potentially reversible with time. Although the histologic findings of tubular necrosis are not consistently present in these patients, the term *acute tubular necrosis* has been used to describe this form of renal failure. Many clinicians use the terms acute renal failure and acute tubular necrosis interchangeably to denote the clinical syndrome of potentially reversible intrinsic acute renal failure.

ETIOLOGY Sixty percent of all cases of acute renal failure are related to surgery or trauma. Forty percent occur in a medical setting, and 1 to 2 percent are related to pregnancy. The most common general cause of acute renal failure is *renal ischemia.* Clinical conditions associated with renal ischemia include severe hemorrhage, profound volume depletion, intraoperative hypotension, cardiogenic shock, and operative procedures associated with interruption of renal circulation. The duration of the renal ischemia is very important in the occurrence of acute renal failure. If ischemia is brief, then correction of the course of ischemia can restore renal function (i.e., prerenal azotemia). With longer duration of renal hypoperfusion, acute tubular necrosis may supervene. Recent studies suggest that removal of the vasodilating influence of renal prostaglandins with nonsteroidal anti-inflammatory agents can enhance renal ischemia. Thus, use of these agents in patients with diminished basal renal blood flow (cardiac failure, hepatic cirrhosis, nephrotic syndrome, glomerulonephritis) may precipitate acute renal failure.

Nephrotoxic agents are a frequent cause of acute renal failure. In the past, heavy metals, organic solvents, and glycols were common inducers of acute renal failure. Although these toxins are less frequently encountered currently, their occasional occurrence serves to illustrate the importance of seeking a history of occupational and environmental toxin exposure in each patient with acute renal failure. More recent studies suggest that *aminoglycoside antibiotics* are now the leading nephrotoxic cause of acute renal failure. The acute renal failure associated with these drugs is enhanced by depletion of intravascular volume, advancing age, the presence of underlying renal disease, potassium depletion, and the concomitant use of other nephrotoxic agents or potent diuretics. Some anesthetic agents (methoxyflurane and enflurane) and radiographic contrast agents also may induce acute renal failure. Contrast agent–induced nephrotoxicity is especially common in dehydrated patients with underlying diabetic nephropathy.

Release of large amounts of *myoglobin* into the circulation is now recognized with increasing frequency as a cause of acute renal failure. Rhabdomyolysis and myoglobinuria are often due to extensive trauma with crush injuries. However, nontraumatic rhabdomyolysis associated with increased muscle oxygen consumption (heat stroke, severe exercise, and seizures), decreased muscle energy production (hypokalemia, hypophosphatemia, and genetic enzymatic deficiencies), muscle ischemia (arterial insufficiency, drug overdosage with resultant coma and muscle compression), infections (influenza), and direct toxins (alcohol) also can produce rhabdomyolysis resulting in acute renal failure. Careful questioning of patients with acute renal failure for muscular symptoms as well as examination for tender, swollen muscles is therefore important, although many of these patients may have muscle necrosis without muscle symptoms. The exact mechanism whereby myoglobinuria results in acute renal failure is uncertain. There is substantial evidence that myoglobin is not directly nephrotoxic. However, direct nephrotoxicity of other muscle breakdown products, as well as tubular obstruction due to myoglobin precipitation and cast formation, has been proposed. Most patients with rhabdomyolysis-associated acute renal failure also have concomitant depletion of intravascular volume and renal hypoperfusion.

Intravascular hemolysis may also cause acute renal failure. Although pure hemoglobin per se is not a potent nephrotoxin, toxic substances from red blood cell stroma and concomitant renal hypoperfusion may act synergistically to induce acute renal failure. Lastly, in spite of intensive investigation, experienced clinicians are often unable to establish a definite etiology for some cases of acute renal failure. In other cases, multiple etiologies are likely, as in patients with shock who are volume-depleted, have received blood transfusions, are septic, and have received nephrotoxic antibiotics.

PATHOPHYSIOLOGY Current pathogenic theories of acute renal failure have been developed largely in animal models. These theories can be divided into those suggesting either a tubular or a vascular basis for acute renal failure. One tubular theory suggests that casts and cellular debris obstruct tubular lumina with resultant increases in intratubular pressure sufficient to decrease net filtration pressure. Alternatively, some investigators feel that "back-leak" of glomerular filtrate across damaged renal tubular epithelium is responsible for azotemia in acute renal failure. Proponents of a vascular basis for acute renal failure suggest that either marked decreases in renal perfusion pressure or severe afferent arteriolar constriction reduces glomerular plasma flow and hydrostatic pressure sufficient to diminish glomerular filtration. This vascular theory has led some proponents to suggest that *vasomotor nephropathy* might be the preferred term for many cases of acute renal failure. Another theory of acute renal failure suggests that alterations in the permeability properties of the glomerular capillary wall are responsible for acute renal failure. While a precise pathogenic schema of acute renal failure is not available at present, it seems likely that both tubular and vascular events interact to cause acute renal failure. For example, ischemia may cause a lower glomerular capillary pressure, which then predisposes to slow tubular flow, sludging debris, and ultimately secondary tubular obstruction. Additional studies are required to define the relative importance of each factor and to differentiate between mechanisms that are involved in the initiation (early) and maintenance (late) phases of acute renal failure.

PATHOLOGY The histopathologic alterations observed in kidneys of patients with acute renal failure are variable. Frequently, no overt abnormalities are observed on light microscopy. However, varying degrees of tubular necrosis with disrupted, necrotic, or regenerating tubular epithelium, intratubular casts, interstitial edema, and interstitial cellular infiltration can be seen. Tubular collapse and dilated tubules both can be observed. Unless either disseminated intravascular coagulation or severe, prolonged ischemic insults are present, intrarenal blood vessels and glomeruli are normal by light and electron microscopy. Microdissection studies demonstrate two general types of renal lesions. Following direct nephrotoxic injury, a uniform, diffuse necrosis of proximal tubular cells, especially of proximal convoluted tubules, is observed. The tubular basement membrane is unaltered. In contrast, following renal ischemia, mild, patchy necrosis occurs throughout the nephron, which tends to be most marked in distal tubular segments at the corticomedullary junction. Disruption of tubular basement membrane is also observed. Despite these histologic differences, the clinical courses of nephrotoxic and ischemic acute renal failure are similar. A striking lack of correlation between renal histopathologic changes and renal functional parameters is often noted in acute renal failure. Renal biopsies performed after recovery from acute renal failure either demonstrate minor abnormalities or are normal.

DIFFERENTIAL DIAGNOSIS (See Table 290-1) The diagnosis of acute renal failure is one of exclusion since prerenal (renal hypoperfusion), postrenal (obstruction of urine flow), and other intrarenal disorders (glomerulonephritis, renal interstitial and vascular diseases) may all lead to an identical clinical syndrome of deteriorating renal function. In contrast to acute renal failure, however, prerenal, postrenal, and other intrarenal glomerular or vascular disorders may be specifically treatable.

Impaired renal perfusion from extrarenal causes may result in sufficient reduction in glomerular filtration so that the daily endogenous load of nitrogenous wastes cannot be excreted. The azotemia can be reversed if the cause of the renal ischemia is corrected. This may require expansion of extracellular fluid volume, improvement in cardiac output, or restoration of normal renal perfusion pressure. A careful history with regard to volume loss or sequestration and symptoms of impaired cardiac output then is necessary in patients with declining renal function. In addition, physical examination with specific attention to orthostatic hypotension and tachycardia, jugular venous pressure, cardiac function, skin turgor, and mucous membranes should be an initial undertaking in any patient with renal deterioration.

Obstruction to urine flow at any level of the urinary tract must be considered in every patient with renal failure. This form of acute deterioration in renal function is often reversible and will be encountered in 1 to 10 percent of patients with decreasing renal function. Urinary retention secondary to anatomic (prostatic disease) or functional (organic or drug-induced neuropathy) bladder neck obstruction is a relatively common cause of renal failure and can be evaluated by suprapubic palpation and percussion as well as by a single bladder catheterization to measure postvoiding residual volume. Obstruction of the upper urinary tract is a less common cause of renal failure since it requires simultaneous obstruction of both ureters or unilateral ureteric obstruction with absence of, or severe disease in, the contralateral kidney. Causes of bilateral urinary tract obstruction include retroperitoneal fibrosis and space-occupying processes such as tumor or abscess, surgical accident, and bilateral intraureteric occlusion (stones, papillary tissue, blood clots, or pus). A careful rectal and pelvic examination is essential in evaluation for postobstruction renal failure. A plain film of the abdomen may help detect retroperitoneal disease or radiopaque calculi. If obstruction of the upper urinary tract cannot be excluded by infusion pyelography, then ultrasound, computerized tomography (CT scanning), or investigation of the patency of the ureter(s) by retrograde pyelography may be required. Obstruction to urine flow can also occur within the kidney. Such intrarenal obstruction is usually due to intratubular precipitation of poorly soluble material such as uric acid (tumor chemotherapy), oxalic acid (ethylene glycol overdose, methoxyflurane anesthesia, small bowel bypass), methotrexate (insoluble metabolites), sulfonamides (out-

TABLE 290-1
Major causes of acute renal failure

Disorder	*Example*
PRERENAL FAILURE	
Hypovolemia	Skin, gastrointestinal, or renal volume loss; hemorrhage; sequestration of extracellular fluid (burns, pancreatitis, peritonitis)
Cardiovascular failure	Impaired cardiac output (infarction, tamponade); vascular pooling (anaphylaxis, sepsis, drugs)
POSTRENAL FAILURE	
Extrarenal obstruction	Urethral occlusion; bladder, pelvic, prostatic, or retroperitoneal neoplasms; prostatism; surgical accident; medications; calculi; pus; blood clots
Intrarenal obstruction	Crystals (uric acid, oxalic acid, sulfonamides, methotrexate)
Bladder rupture	Trauma
SPECIFIC RENAL DISEASES	
Vascular diseases	Vasculitis; malignant hypertension; thrombotic thrombocytopenic purpura; scleroderma; arterial and/or venous occlusion
Glomerulonephritis	Immune-complex disease; antiglomerular basement membrane disease
Interstitial nephritis	Drugs; hypercalcemia; diffuse infection
ACUTE TUBULAR NECROSIS	
Postischemic	All conditions listed above for prerenal failure
Pigment-induced	Hemolysis (transfusion reaction, malaria); rhabdomyolysis (trauma, muscle disease, coma, heat stroke, severe exercise, potassium or phosphate depletion)
Toxin-induced	Antibiotics; contrast material; anesthetic agents; heavy metals; organic solvents
Pregnancy-related	Septic abortion; uterine hemorrhage; eclampsia

dated, long-acting insoluble compounds), and perhaps myeloma proteins.

Once pre- and postrenal disorders have been excluded, it is appropriate to consider specific renal disorders such as renal vascular disorders, glomerulonephritis, and interstitial nephritis (Table 290-1). The frequency with which these specific renal disorders will be encountered as a cause of deteriorating renal function depends on the patient's age. In adults, only 5 to 10 percent of all cases of decreasing renal function can be attributed to these specific disorders, while this figure may be as high as 40 to 60 percent in the pediatric population. Although these disorders are less frequent than acute tubular necrosis, they are often amenable to specific therapy and should be considered in each case of deterioration in renal function.

The initial presentation of the patient with end-stage renal failure may be confused with acute renal failure when there is no information about renal function prior to presentation. Under these circumstances, the presence of uremic osteodystrophy, uremic neuropathy, small kidney size on abdominal films, and unexplained anemia suggests chronic renal failure. However, some end-stage renal diseases such as amyloidosis, polycystic disease, diabetic glomerulosclerosis, scleroderma, and rapidly progressive glomerulonephritis may have normal-sized or enlarged kidneys, necessitating time for continued observation and rarely renal biopsy to distinguish between potentially reversible forms of acute renal failure and end-stage chronic renal failure.

Observation of the pattern of urine flow may provide a diagnostic clue as to the cause of declining renal function. Complete anuria (no urine by catheterization) is rare in acute tubular necrosis. Potential causes of total anuria include complete bilateral ureteric obstruction, diffuse cortical necrosis, rapidly progressive glomerulonephritis, and bilateral renal artery occlusion. Wide fluctuations in daily urine output suggest intermittent obstructive uropathy. Polyuria (> 3 liters per day) can be a hallmark of partial urinary tract obstruction. This occurs secondary to the accompanying defect in renal concentrating ability. Although oliguria (< 400 ml per day) has been considered to be a cardinal feature of acute renal failure, a substantial portion of patients have urine volumes of greater than 1 liter per day. This situation has been termed nonoliguric acute renal failure.

Examination of the urinary sediment is of great value in the differential diagnosis of acute impairment of renal function. Sediment containing few formed elements or only hyaline casts strongly suggests prerenal azotemia or obstructive uropathy. With acute tubular necrosis, brownish pigmented cellular casts and many renal tubular epithelial cells are observed in over 75 percent of patients. Red blood cell casts suggest the presence of glomerular or vascular inflammatory diseases of the kidney and rarely, if ever, occur with acute tubular necrosis. The presence of large numbers of polymorphonuclear leukocytes, singly or in clumps, suggests acute diffuse pyelonephritis or papillary necrosis. Eosinophilic casts on Wright's stain of urine sediment supports a diagnosis of acute allergic interstitial nephritis. The combination of brownish pigmented granular casts and positive occult blood tests on urine in the absence of hematuria indicates either hemoglobinuria or myoglobinuria. In acute renal failure, the finding in fresh, warm urine of large numbers of uric acid crystals may suggest a diagnosis of acute uric acid nephropathy, while the finding of large numbers of oxalic acid or hippuric acid crystals suggests ethylene glycol toxicity. The presence of large numbers of broad casts (greater than two to three white blood cells in diameter) suggests chronic renal disease. Chemical analysis of urine composition is also helpful in differentiating acute tubular necrosis from prerenal azotemia and is depicted in Table 290-2. It is important to recall that other disorders associated with abrupt deterioration in renal function and intact renal tubular integrity, such as glomerulonephritis and early (few hours) obstructive uropathy, have urine chemical values similar to those encountered in prerenal azotemia. Prior administration of diuretic agents, osmotic diuresis due to glycosuria, bicarbonaturia, and ketonuria may interfere with avid renal tubular reabsorption of sodium and water and thus alter urinary chemical indexes. A urinary uric acid/creatinine concentration ratio of greater than 1 suggests that acute uric acid nephropathy may be the cause of the acute renal failure.

Rarely, the cause of declining renal function will not be readily apparent. In other cases, features considered atypical for acute tubular necrosis (gradual onset of renal failure; anuria in the absence of obstructive uropathy; the presence of marked hypertension, heavy proteinuria, significant hematuria, underlying systemic disease, and prolonged oliguria) will be present. Since such atypical features may indicate the presence of a potentially treatable form of renal parenchymal disease, e.g., secondary Wegener's disease, systemic lupus erythematosus, Goodpasture's syndrome, or rapidly progressive glomerulonephritis, a diagnostic renal biopsy may be indicated when the cause of renal failure is not apparent or such atypical features are present.

TABLE 290-2
Urine findings in prerenal azotemia and acute renal failure

Laboratory test	*Prerenal azotemia*	*Acute renal failure*
Urine osmolality (mosmol/kg)	>500	<400
Urine sodium (meq/liter)	<20	>40
Urine/plasma creatinine	>40	<20
Renal failure index†	<1	>2
Fractional excretion‡ of filtered sodium	<1	2
Urine sediment	Normal or occasional granular casts	Brown granular casts, cellular debris

† $\dfrac{\textit{Urine Na (meq/liter)}}{\textit{Urine/plasma creatinine}}$

‡ $\dfrac{\textit{Urine Na/serum Na}}{\textit{Urine creatinine/serum creatinine}}$

CLINICAL COURSE The clinical course in acute tubular necrosis can be divided into an initiating phase, a maintenance phase, and a recovery phase. The initiating phase is the period of time between the precipitating event and the appearance of acute renal failure which is no longer reversible by alteration in extrarenal factors. Recognition of the initiating phase of acute renal failure is extremely important since early correction of the underlying cause of renal failure may theoretically prevent the development of the maintenance phase. However, the initiating phase of acute renal failure may be evident to the clinician only in retrospect because it lacks characteristic signs and symptoms.

Oliguria has been considered the cardinal feature of the initiating and maintenance phases of acute renal failure. However, recent studies suggest that 25 to 50 percent of all patients with acute renal failure are nonoliguric (urine volume > 400 ml per day). Although progressive acute renal failure without oliguria can result from any type of renal insult, including both ischemic and toxic insults, this form of renal failure appears to be particularly frequent following nephrotoxic (e.g., aminoglycoside) drug administration. Progressive azotemia occurs in nonoliguric patients owing to the marked impairment in glomerular filtration rate and renal concentrating capacity. For example, maximal urine osmolality of the nonoliguric patient averages only 350 mosmol per kilogram of water. Therefore, with a urine output of 1000 ml per day, a maximum of 350 mosmol solute can be excreted daily. In acute renal failure, daily solute loads may be increased from normal values of 600 mosmol to values as high as 1000 mosmol. Thus, a positive solute (predominately urea and creatinine) balance and azotemia would occur despite a daily urine output of 1 liter.

Oliguria characterizes the maintenance phase of acute renal failure in more than 50 percent of cases. When oliguria occurs, it starts shortly following the inciting event and lasts an average of 10 to 14 days. However, the oliguric phase may be as short as a few hours or as long as 6 to 8 weeks. Prolonged oliguria is common in the elderly patient with underlying vascular disease. If oliguria persists for longer than 4 weeks, the diagnosis of acute tubular necrosis should be reconsidered, and entities such as diffuse cortical necrosis, rapidly progressive glomerulonephritis, renal artery occlusion, and renal vasculitis are possible. Anuria is not characteristic of acute tubular necrosis. However, several days of severe oliguria with urine volume less than 100 ml per day may be encountered with acute tubular necrosis.

Urinary elimination of nitrogenous wastes, water, electrolytes, and acid is impaired in the initiating and maintenance phases of acute renal failure. The magnitude of resultant abnormalities in blood chemistry depends on whether the patient is oliguric or nonoliguric and on the catabolic state of the patient. Nonoliguric patients have higher levels of glomerular filtration than do oliguric patients and thus excrete more nitrogenous waste, water, and electrolytes in their urine. Hence, abnormalities in blood chemistry are generally milder in nonoliguric than oliguric patients with acute renal failure.

In the afebrile, noncatabolic, oliguric patient with acute renal failure, the daily increments in blood urea nitrogen (BUN) and serum creatinine average 10 to 20 and 0.5 to 1.0 mg/dl, respectively. In catabolic patients with fever, sepsis, or extensive trauma, daily increments in BUN and serum creatinine may be as high as 40 to 100 and 2 to 5 mg/dl, respectively. In patients with acute renal failure due to rhabdomyolysis, the daily increment in serum creatinine may be disproportionately higher compared with the BUN. This is due to the release from muscle of creatine which is converted by nonenzymatic hydrolysis to creatinine.

Salt and water overload with resultant hyponatremia, edema, and pulmonary congestion are ever-present dangers in patients with acute renal failure, particularly in oliguric patients. Hyponatremia results from excessive water intake, and edema from excessive sodium and water intake. If urinary losses are not replaced, the nonoliguric patient with a relatively high rate of urine flow and high concentration of urine sodium will develop intravascular volume depletion which may retard recovery of renal function.

Hyperkalemia due to decreased renal elimination of potassium occurring with continued tissue potassium release is a frequent accompaniment of acute renal failure. The usual rate of increase in serum potassium in the noncatabolic, oliguric patient is 0.3 to 0.5 meq per day. Higher rates of rise in serum potassium concentration should suggest the possibility of an endogenous (tissue destruction, hemolysis) or exogenous (medication, diet, blood transfusion) potassium load or of cellular shift of potassium due to acidemia. Generally, hyperkalemia is asymptomatic until serum potassium increases to values greater than 6.0 to 6.5 meq per liter. Above that level, electrocardiographic abnormalities (bradycardia, recent appearance of left axis deviation, peaked T waves, prolonged QRS complexes, prolonged PR interval, and decreased amplitude of the P waves) and ultimately cardiac arrest can occur. Hyperkalemia can also result in muscle weakness and flaccid quadriparesis.

Hyperphosphatemia, hypocalcemia, and mild *hypermagnesemia* are usually present in acute renal failure. Hyperphosphatemia results from decreased renal phosphorus elimination in the presence of continued release of phosphorus from tissues. The serum phosphorus is usually in the range of 6 to 8 mg/dl, but much higher values may be encountered in the traumatized, catabolic patient as well as the patient with rhabdomyolysis. Hypocalcemia in the range of 6 to 9 mg/dl often develops during acute renal failure. The reason for this decrease in serum calcium concentration is not clear. Asymptomatic increases in serum magnesium to levels of 2 to 3 mg/dl are often observed in acute renal failure. The serum magnesium elevation is mild unless magnesium-containing compounds such as antacids are ingested.

Metabolic acidosis is a regular accompaniment of acute renal failure. The daily production of approximately 1 meq per kilogram of body weight of nonvolatile acid from endogenous metabolic sources can no longer be eliminated by the damaged kidney. A retention of organic acids results which is sufficient to produce a daily decrease of 1 to 2 meq in plasma bicarbonate and metabolic acidosis with an anion gap.

Hyperuricemia in the range of 9 to 12 mg/dl due to decreased renal uric acid excretion is usually present in acute renal failure. In catabolic patients with extensive tissue damage, much higher values of serum uric acid may be observed. Elevation of serum amylase due to impaired renal amylase excretion may be observed in the absence of clinical evidence of pancreatitis. The elevations of amylase are mild and are usually less than twice the upper limit of normal.

Abnormalities in the hematologic examination are usually present in acute renal failure. A normocytic normochromic anemia occurs shortly following the onset of significant azotemia, and the hematocrit usually stabilizes between values of 20 to 30 volume percent. This anemia is due to impaired erythropoiesis as well as to a mild and variable degree of shortened red blood cell survival. Additional factors that often contribute to anemia include hemodilution, gastrointestinal blood loss, and suppressed erythropoiesis due to infections or drug administration. White blood cell production is not severely disturbed in acute renal failure. However, since acute renal failure usually occurs in the setting of stress and tissue damage, mild leukocytosis is usually present. Leukocytosis persisting after the initial week of acute renal failure should suggest the possibility of infection. Mild degress of thrombocytopenia due to reduction of bone marrow platelet production may be observed early in the course of acute renal failure. Qualitative defects in platelet function occur and, in association with additional poorly defined coagulation disturbances, contribute to the bleeding tendency of acute renal failure. Acute renal failure may follow intravascular hemolysis and may also be a complication of several primary hematologic or vascular disorders that have major hematologic manifestations such as disseminated intravascular coagulation, thrombotic thrombocytopenic purpura, hemolytic uremic syndrome, and systemic lupus erythematosus.

Cardiovascular complications of acute renal failure involve circulatory congestion, hypertension, arrhythmias, and pericarditis. Circulatory congestion is usually due to excessive sodium and water administration. Mild hypertension is seen in 15 to 25 percent of cases and usually appears in the second week of oliguria. This hypertension is usually a manifestation of extracellular fluid volume overload; however, the increased activity of the renin-angiotensin system may also be involved in some instances. Supraventricular arrhythmias may complicate 20 to 30 percent of cases of acute renal failure. Known causes for these arrhythmias include congestive heart failure, electrolyte abnormalities, digitalis intoxication, pericarditis, and anemia. Pericarditis currently occurs infrequently, probably because of the early institution of dialytic therapy.

Neurological abnormalities are common in acute renal failure. In undialyzed patients, lethargy, somnolence, confusion, disorientation, asterixis, agitation, myoclonic muscle twitching, and generalized seizures may be observed. These neurological abnormalities are most often encountered in the elderly patient and generally respond well to dialytic therapy. In addition to uremia per se, drug administration, metabolic and electrolyte abnormalities, and primary neurological disease should be considered as potential causes of neurological disturbances in the patient with acute renal failure.

Gastrointestinal complications of acute renal failure are common and include anorexia, nausea, vomiting, ileus, and poorly defined abdominal complaints. The combination of stress of acute illness and hemostatic abnormalities can lead to gastrointestinal hemorrhage in 10 to 30 percent of patients. Fortunately, the gastrointestinal hemorrhage is usually mild in nature and easily controlled with conservative therapy. Recently, administration of cryoprecipitates has also been suggested to be of value in treating bleeding associated with uremia.

Infections complicate 30 to 70 percent of all cases of acute renal failure and are a leading cause of morbidity and mortality. The sites of infection include the respiratory tract, operative sites, and urinary tract. Resultant septicemia is frequent, and both gram-positive and gram-negative organisms are encountered. Although the exact factors responsible for the high rate of infection remain to be determined, disruption of normal anatomic barriers with intravenous infusions and indwelling catheters may play a role. There is also evidence of impaired host defenses including leukocyte dysfunction in the setting of uremia.

The recovery phase of acute renal failure commences when the glomerular filtration rate increases so that the BUN and serum creatinine concentrations no longer continue to increase. In oliguric acute renal failure, the recovery phase is heralded by a progressive increase in urine volume. Generally, in the first days the urine volume may double daily, and in some cases a daily urine volume of greater than 2 liters may be observed for a few days. In nonoliguric patients, a marked diuretic phase is usually not observed. The duration of the recovery phase in patients with BUN and serum creatinine concentrations greater than 50 and 5 mg/dl, respectively, averages 15 to 25 days in oliguric patients and 5 to 10 days in nonoliguric patients. The major complications of acute renal failure, such as infections, gastrointestinal hemorrhage, fluid and electrolyte disturbances, and cardiovascular dysfunction, may persist or first appear during the recovery phase of acute renal failure. In addition, during the recovery phase, persistent abnormalities in glomerular and tubular function can lead to over- or underhydration or electrolyte disturbances unless careful daily weight, intake and output, biochemical, and clinical monitoring are continued during the recovery phase of acute renal failure, especially in patients with rhabdomyolysis. The cause of this complication remains obscure.

Although the major improvement in renal function occurs within the first 1 to 2 weeks of the recovery phase, renal function continues to improve for up to a year following acute renal failure. Sensitive tests of glomerular and tubular function also suggest that some mild defects in renal function may persist indefinitely following acute tubular necrosis. However, the vast majority of patients achieve clinically normal renal function, and there is no evidence of later progression of renal dysfunction or of complications such as hypertension.

The mortality rates in large series of patients with acute renal failure vary from 30 to 60 percent. The mortality rates are highest in postoperative or traumatized patients (50 to 70 percent), intermediate in patients with acute renal failure encountered in a medical setting (30 to 50 percent), and lowest in acute renal failure observed in an obstetrical setting (10 to 20 percent). Advanced age, the presence of serious underlying illness, and the development of multiple medical complications during the course of acute renal failure are associated with higher mortality rates. Nonoliguric acute renal failure is associated with a lower morbidity and mortality rate than oliguric acute renal failure. Infections, complications resulting from fluid and electrolyte disturbances, gastrointestinal hemorrhage, and progression of the primary underlying disease are the major causes of mortality in acute renal failure.

MANAGEMENT The first principle of therapy in acute renal failure is to exclude causes of deterioration in renal function which are potentially remedial. A search for prerenal factors, obstructive uropathy, glomerulonephritis, renal vascular and interstitial disease, and intrarenal crystal precipitation should be performed. Once the diagnosis of acute tubular necrosis is made by exclusion, little specific therapy is available. Dialysis for the removal of nephrotoxins, such as carbon tetrachloride, ethylene glycol, and heavy metals following chelation therapy, may be indicated. Even in the presence of acute tubular necrosis, any prerenal factors should be corrected both to improve the circulation and to avoid delay in the onset of the recovery phase. In the oliguric patient in whom prerenal factors have been corrected, it has become common clinical practice to administer either a potent loop diuretic or mannitol in an attempt to enhance urine flow. The rationale for such therapy is based on the thought that there is an early phase of renal failure during which the correction of prerenal factors and establishment of urine flow can lead to a nonoliguric state. Prospective studies have demonstrated lower morbidity and mortality rates in nonoliguric as compared with oliguric acute renal failure. However, a prospective controlled study of the utility of potent diuretics in early acute renal failure to convert oliguric to nonoliguric renal failure with attendant decrease in morbidity and mortality rates is needed.

Conservative therapy is capable of controlling many of the manifestations of acute renal failure. After any defects in intravascular volume have been corrected, fluid intake should equal measured output plus estimated insensible losses. Sodium and potassium administration should not exceed measured losses. Daily monitoring of fluid balance and body weight allow assessment of the patient's volume status. A daily weight loss of 0.2 to 0.3 kg occurs in the well-managed patient with acute renal failure. Greater weight loss suggests hypercatabolism or volume depletion, and lesser weight loss suggests excessive salt and water administration. The serum sodium concentration provides a guideline for water administration. A decrease in serum sodium concentration indicates that an excess of total body water is present, while an abnormally high serum sodium concentration indicates a deficiency of body water.

In an effort to minimize catabolism, daily intake should include at least 100 g of carbohydrate. Recently some studies suggest that central intravenous administration of a mixture of amino acids and hypertonic glucose improves morbidity and mortality in patients with acute renal failure following surgical procedures or trauma. Since parenteral hyperalimentation may be associated with significant complications, this form of nutrition should be reserved for catabolic patients in whom the enteral routine of alimentation does not prove to be satisfactory. In the past, anabolic androgens have been utilized in an effort to decrease protein catabolism and diminish the rate of rise of BUN. Such therapy is not generally utilized at present. Additional means of minimizing catabolism include early removal or debridement of necrotic tissue, control of pyrexia, and early, specific antimicrobial therapy.

The mild metabolic acidosis associated with acute renal failure is generally not treated unless serum bicarbonate falls to below 10 meq per liter. Rapid correction of acidemia by acute alkali administration may decrease ionized calcium concentrations and precipitate tetany. Hypocalcemia is usually asymptomatic and rarely requires specific therapy. Hyperphosphatemia should be controlled with 30 to 60 ml aluminum hydroxide administered orally 4 to 6 times per day, since a high calcium-phosphorus product (>70) may cause soft-tissue calcification. For the occasional patient with profound hyperphosphatemia, early dialysis therapy and intravenous alimentation may help control elevated serum phosphate concentration. Unless acute uric acid nephropathy is a diagnostic consideration, the secondary hyperuricemia of acute renal failure is usually not treated with allopurinol. Because of the decreased glomerular filtration rate, the filtered load of uric acid, and thus intratubular deposition, is low. Also, for unknown reasons, clinical gout rarely complicates acute renal failure, despite hyperuricemia. Careful observation of the hematocrit and stool for occult blood is important in the early detection of gastrointestinal blood loss. If a rapid decrease in hematocrit occurs which appears to be out of proportion to the degree of renal failure, alternative causes of anemia should be sought.

Congestive heart failure and hypertension indicate the presence of volume overload and should be treated accordingly, recognizing, of course, that many drugs such as digoxin are largely excreted by the kidneys. As suggested earlier, hypertension occasionally may persist in the absence of volume overload, thus factors such as hyperreninemia may contribute to the hypertension. Selective histamine-2 receptor blockade (cimetidine) therapy has been of benefit in preventing gastrointestinal bleeding in some seriously ill patients but has not yet been studied in acute renal failure. Avoidance and early detection of infection require minimization of interruption of normal anatomic barriers, including avoidance of long-term catheterization of the urinary bladder, provision of mouth and skin care, promotion of early mobilization, utilization of aseptic techniques for intravenous and tracheostomy sites, and close clinical monitoring. Fever and suspected infection should be promptly evaluated with careful inspection of lung, wounds, urinary tract, and intravenous sites. Since the metabolism and elimination of many drugs are impaired in acute renal failure, careful monitoring of medication records and adjustment of drug doses are required.

Hyperkalemia is an ever-present threat in acute renal failure. Mild elevations of serum potassium (< 6.0 meq per liter) can best be treated by withdrawal of all sources of potassium and by continued close laboratory observation. If serum potassium increases to values greater than 6.5 meq per liter and particularly if any electrocardiographic changes appear, active therapy should be instituted. Therapy of such hyperkalemia can be divided into emergent and nonemergent forms. Emergent therapy includes intravenous administration of calcium (5 to 10 ml of 10% calcium chloride solution intravenously over 2 min with electrocardiographic monitoring) and of bicarbonate (44 meq intravenously over 5 min), insulin and glucose (200 to 300 ml of 20% glucose with 20 to 30 units regular insulin given intravenously over 30 min). Nonemergent therapy includes administration of potassium-binding ion exchange resins such as sodium polystyrene sulfonate (Kayexalate). This can be administered orally every 3 to 4 h in 25- to 50-g doses with 100 ml 20% sorbitol to avoid constipation. Alternatively, in the patient who cannot take oral medications, 50 g sodium polystyrene sulfonate and 50 g sorbitol in 200 ml water can be given as a retention enema at 1- to 2-h intervals. With refractory hyperkalemia, hemodialysis may be necessary.

Some patients with acute renal failure, particularly those who are nonoliguric and noncatabolic, can be successfully managed with minimal or no dialytic therapy. There has been an increasing tendency to use dialysis therapy early in acute renal failure in an attempt to minimize the development of complications. Early (prophylactic) use of dialysis frequently simplifies management, allowing more liberal fluid and potassium intake and improvement of the general well-being of the patient. Absolute indications for dialysis include symptomatic uremia (usually manifested by central nervous system and/or gastrointestinal symptomatology), development of resistant hyperkalemia, severe acidemia or fluid overload not responsive to medical therapy, and pericarditis. In addition, many centers attempt to keep predialysis levels of BUN and serum creatinine less than 100 and 8 mg/dl, respectively. Adequate prevention of uremic symptoms may require infrequent dialysis in the noncatabolic, nonoliguric patient or daily dialysis in the catabolic, traumatized patient. In some circumstances peritoneal dialysis is an acceptable alternative to predialysis. However, because of the relative lack of efficiency of peritoneal dialysis, its use is contraindicated in the catabolic patient, and it is most useful in the noncatabolic patient when the need for infrequent dialysis is anticipated.

PREVENTION Because of the high mortality and morbidity of acute renal failure, prophylactic therapy deserves special mention. A fivefold reduction in deaths secondary to acute renal failure occurred from the Korean war to the Vietnamese conflict. This reduction in the acute renal failure mortality rate paralleled earlier evacuation from the field and early expansion of intravascular volume. Thus, identification of patients at high risk for the development of acute renal failure is important. Such high-risk patients include those with multiple trauma, burns, rhabdomyolysis, and intravascular hemolysis; those receiving potential nephrotoxins; and those undergoing operative procedures necessitating interruption of renal blood flow. In these patients, particular attention should be given to maintaining optimal intravascular volume, cardiac output, and urine flow rates. Care in the use of potential nephrotoxic drugs, early therapy of cardiogenic shock, sepsis, and eclampsia of pregnancy may also reduce the occurrence of acute renal failure.

ACUTE RENAL FAILURE IN PREGNANCY When acute renal failure occurs during pregnancy, it is usually in either the earlier or later stages of gestation. During the first trimester of pregnancy, acute renal failure usually occurs in the setting of nontherapeutic, nonsterile abortion. In these cases, volume depletion, sepsis, and nephrotoxins contribute to the acute renal failure. This form of acute renal failure has markedly declined with the current widespread availability of sterile abortion.

Acute renal failure can also occur because of either excessive postpartum hemorrhage or preeclampsia in the latter stages of pregnancy. The majority of patients with this type of acute renal failure generally recover total renal function. A small number of pregnant patients with acute renal failure, however, have not recovered renal function, and in these cases histological evidence of diffuse cortical necrosis is found. This entity usually complicates the severe hemorrhage of abruptio placentae and is associated with clinical and laboratory evidence of intravascular coagulation.

A rare form of acute renal failure occurring 1 to 12 weeks following uncomplicated pregnancy has been described and termed postpartum glomerulosclerosis. This form of renal failure is usually characterized by irreversible, rapidly progressive renal failure, although milder cases have been described. All of these patients have an associated microangiopathic hemolytic anemia. The renal histopathologic changes are indistinguishable from malignant hypertension or scleroderma. The pathophysiology of this disorder has not been defined. No therapeutic modality is consistently successful, although heparin therapy has been advocated.

HEPATORENAL SYNDROME The hepatorenal syndrome is a serious complication of advanced liver disease in which renal failure occurs in the absence of clinical, laboratory, or anatomic evidence of other causes of renal dysfunction. The renal failure is usually associated with oliguria, an unremarkable urinary sediment, and low urinary sodium concentrations (< 10 meq per liter). Generally, the renal failure occurs in the setting of advanced hepatic cirrhosis complicated by jaudice, ascites, and hepatic encephalopathy. Occasionally, this syndrome may complicate fulminant hepatitis. The mechanism of the renal failure is not known. The lack of consistent histopathologic alterations in kidneys of patients with this syndrome and the restoration of normal renal function when kidneys from donors with hepatorenal syndrome are transplanted into recipients without liver disease suggest a functional defect.

Treatment of the hepatorenal syndrome is usually unsuccessful. Care should be taken in the cirrhotic patient not to induce major changes in intravascular volume by large paracentesis or aggressive diuresis, maneuvers which may precipitate hepatorenal syndrome. Since this syndrome mimics prerenal azotemia, a cautious trial of expansion of intravascular volume is warranted. In a few cases, recovery has followed either portacaval shunting or insertion of an abdominal-venous (Leveen) shunt. These treatment modalities have not been subjected to controlled trials. The abdominal-venous shunt may be associated with peritonitis, intravascular coagulation, and pulmonary congestion. Improvement in hepatic function often results in parallel improvement in renal function. Every effort should be made to ensure that more specifically treatable causes of concomitant liver and renal dysfunction, such as infections (leptospirosis, hepatitis with immune-complex disease), toxins (aminoglycosides, carbon tetrachloride), and circulatory disorders (severe heart failure, shock), are not present. It should also be recalled that jaundiced patients with liver disease may be particularly susceptible to acute tubular necrosis.

REFERENCES

LEVINSKY NG et al: Acute renal failure, in *The Kidney,* BM Brenner, FC Rector Jr. (eds). Philadelphia, Saunders, 1981, p 1181

BRENNER BM, STEIN JH (eds): Acute renal failure, in *Contemporary Issues in Nephrology.* New York, Churchill-Livingstone, 1980, vol 6

SCHRIER RW, CONGER JD: Acute renal failure: Pathogenesis, diagnosis and management, in *Renal and Electrolyte Disorders,* RW Schrier (ed). Boston, Little, Brown, 1980, p 375

FINN WF: Acute renal failure, in *Diseases of the Kidney,* LE Earley, CW Gottschalk (eds). Boston, Little, Brown, 1979, p 167

CRONIN RE: The patients with acute azotemia, in *Manual of Nephrology. Diagnosis and Therapy,* RW Schrier (ed). Boston, Little, Brown, 1981, p 135

291
CHRONIC RENAL FAILURE: PATHOPHYSIOLOGIC AND CLINICAL CONSIDERATIONS

BARRY M. BRENNER
J. MICHAEL LAZARUS

In contrast to the remarkable capacity of the kidney to regain function following the various forms of acute renal injury discussed in the preceding chapter, renal injury of a more sustained nature is often not reversible but leads instead to progressive destruction of nephron mass. Glomerulonephritis, tubulointerstitial diseases, diabetic nephropathy, and nephrosclerosis are among the most common causes of chronic renal failure. These and other progressive forms of renal disease are considered in detail in the remaining chapters of this section. Irrespective of cause, the eventual impact of severe reduction in nephron mass is an alteration in function of virtually every organ system in the body. *Uremia* is the term generally applied to the clinical syndrome observed in patients suffering from profound loss of renal function. Although the cause(s) of the syndrome remain unknown, the term uremia was adopted originally because of the presumption that the abnormalities seen in patients with chronic renal failure (CRF) resulted from *retention* in the blood of urea and the other end products of metabolism normally excreted into the urine. It is clear that the uremic state represents more than failure of renal excretory function alone, because a host of metabolic and endocrine functions normally subserved by the intact kidney are also impaired in CRF. Furthermore, the inexorably progressive course to renal failure is often accompanied by severe malnutrition, impaired metabolism of carbohydrates, fats, and proteins, and defective utilization of energy. Because CRF involves more than just retention of normal urinary constituents in blood, the term *uremia* in current usage is devoid of any pathophysiologic connotation, but is employed instead to refer, in a general sense, to the constellation of signs and symptoms associated with CRF, regardless of etiology.

The presentation and severity of signs and symptoms of uremia often vary greatly from patient to patient, depending, at least in part, on the magnitude of the reduction in functioning renal mass as well as the rapidity with which renal function is lost. As discussed in Chap. 289, in the relatively early stage of CRF [i.e., when total glomerular filtration rate (GFR) is reduced but not to levels below about 35 to 50 percent of normal], overall renal function is sufficient to maintain the patient symptom-free, although renal reserve may be diminished. At this stage of renal impairment base-line excretory, biosynthetic, and other regulatory functions of the kidney are generally well maintained. At a somewhat later stage in the course of CRF (GFR about 20 to 35 percent of normal), *azotemia* occurs, and initial manifestations of renal insufficiency usually appear, with *hypertension* and *anemia* being the most common early abnormalities. Other derangements include *carbohydrate intolerance, hyperuricemia, hypertriglyceridemia,* and impaired ability to elaborate concentrated urine, the latter leading to *polyuria* and *nocturia* (see Chap. 41). Although patients are relatively asymptomatic at this stage, renal reserve is diminished sufficiently that any sudden stress, such as intercurrent infection, urinary tract obstruction, dehydration, or administration of a nephrotoxic drug, may compromise renal function still further, often leading to signs and symptoms of overt uremia. Return to a more stable base line can frequently be achieved in such patients by prompt correction of the underlying acute disturbance. With further loss of nephron mass (GFR below 20 to 25 percent of normal), the patient develops *overt renal failure,* which, in addition to increased severity of the anemia and hypertension, is characterized by *metabolic acidosis, fluid overload,* and various disturbances of the *gastrointestinal, cardiovascular,* and *nervous systems.* At this stage there is still sufficient capacity to excrete potassium so that clinically significant hyperkalemia is not a problem. Uremia may be viewed as the final stage in this inexorable process, when many of or all the untoward manifestations of CRF become evident clinically. In this chapter the causes and clinical characteristics of the disturbances of the various organ systems seen in patients with CRF will be considered.

PATHOPHYSIOLOGY AND BIOCHEMISTRY OF UREMIA

ROLE OF RETAINED TOXIC METABOLITES The finding that serums from patients with uremia exert toxic effects in a variety of biological test systems has motivated a diligent search to identify the responsible toxin(s). The most likely candidates thought to qualify as toxins in uremia are the *by-products of protein and amino acid metabolism.* Unlike fats and carbohydrates, which are eventually metabolized to carbon dioxide and water, substances which are easily excreted even in uremic subjects via lungs and skin, the products of protein and amino acid metabolism depend largely on the kidneys for excretion. A vast number of such products have been identified, with urea being quantitatively the most important. *Urea* represents some 80 percent or more of the total nitrogen excreted into the urine in patients with CRF maintained on diets containing 40 or more grams of protein per day. The *guanidino compounds* are the next most abundant of the nitrogenous end products of protein metabolism and include substances such as guanidine, methyl- and dimethylguanidine, creatinine, creatine, and guanidinosuccinic acid. As with urea, guanidines are derived, at least in part, from urea cycle amino acids. Other metabolic products of amino acid and protein catabolism that have been implicated as possible uremic toxins include *urates and other end products of nucleic acid metabolism, aliphatic amines,* a variety of *peptides,* and, finally, several *derivatives of the aromatic amino acids tryptophan, tyrosine, and phenylalanine.* The role of these substances in the pathogenesis of the clinical and biochemical abnormalities seen in CRF is unclear. It is generally believed that uremic symptoms correlate only in a rough and inconsistent way with concentrations of urea in blood. Nevertheless, although urea is probably not a major cause of overt uremic toxicity, it may account for some of the less serious clinical abnormalities, including anorexia, malaise, vomiting, and headache. On the other hand, elevated levels of plasma *guanidinosuccinic acid,* by interfering with activation of platelet factor III by adenosine diphosphate (ADP), have been shown to contribute to the impaired platelet function seen in CRF. *Creatinine,* generally regarded as a nontoxic substance, may cause adverse effects in uremic subjects following conversion to more toxic metabolites such as sarcosine and methylguanidine. Whether these substances, as well as *creatine,* a metabolic precursor of creatinine, and the other compounds cited above, are of clinical importance in the pathogenesis of uremic toxicity remains to be established.

Nitrogenous compounds of larger molecular weight are also retained in CRF. A toxic role for these substances has been suggested, on the impression that patients treated with intermittent peritoneal dialysis are less troubled with neuropathy than patients maintained on chronic hemodialysis, despite higher levels of urea and creatinine in blood. Since the clearance of small molecules depends mainly upon blood and dialysate flow rates, which are higher with hemodialysis, whereas clearance of larger molecules depends more on membrane surface area and time, which are greater with peritoneal dialysis, this form of therapy may be a more effective means of removing these substances of larger molecular weight. Using a variety of chemical separation procedures, several groups of workers have obtained evidence in support of this "middle-molecule hypothesis" by observing differences in composition between normal and uremic plasmas, with prominent abnormal "uremic peaks" in the molecular weight range of about 300 to 3500. Evidence from amino acid analysis suggests that these substances of larger molecular weight are polypeptides. Despite the foregoing, proof that efficient removal of middle molecules is associated with objective evidence of clinical well-being, and improvement in neuropathy in particular, remains to be provided. On the other hand, when there is insufficient removal of substances of smaller molecular weight (e.g., urea), symptoms of uremia are frequently aggravated.

Not all these middle-sized molecules accumulate in uremic plasma because of decreased renal excretion alone. The kidney normally *catabolizes* a number of circulating plasma proteins and polypeptides; with reduced renal mass, this capacity may be impaired greatly. Furthermore, plasma levels of many polypeptide hormones [including parathyroid hormone (PTH), insulin, glucagon, growth hormone, luteinizing hormone, and prolactin] rise with advancing renal failure, often markedly so, not only because of impaired renal catabolism but also because of enhanced endocrine secretion. The consequences of high circulating levels of many of these hormones in CRF are considered below and in Chap. 289.

EFFECTS OF UREMIA ON CELLULAR FUNCTIONS

Alterations in the composition of intracellular and extracellular fluids in CRF have long been recognized. Such abnormalities are believed to be a consequence, at least in part, of *defective ion transport* across cell membranes generally, with retained uremic toxins possibly mediating these alterations in transmembrane ion transport. Integrity of cellular volume and composition depends to a large extent on the active outward transport of Na^+ from cell interior to exterior, the resulting intracellular fluid being relatively low in Na^+ and high in K^+, whereas the reverse is true for extracellular fluid. Active Na^+ transport is a metabolically costly process, accounting for a major fraction of basal energy utilization and oxygen consumption. The consequences of this efflux of Na^+ from cells are many and include, most notably, (1) the generation of a resting electrical potential difference across the cell membrane (with this transcellular voltage oriented so that cell interior is electronegative to cell exterior), and (2) a mechanism for enhancing the influx of K^+ into cells.

In experimental animals, partial inhibition of this active efflux mechanism for Na^+ across cell membranes leads to alterations in body composition and cell functions similar to those demonstrable in erythrocytes, leukocytes, skeletal muscle, and other tissues obtained from uremic subjects. These include increased and decreased intracellular concentrations of Na^+ and K^+, respectively, and reduction in magnitude of the transcellular voltage. These alterations have been shown to be largely reversed by efficient hemodialysis and, for erythrocytes at least, to be recreated when cells from normal subjects are incubated in uremic serums. Other derangements in cellular function have also been implicated as causes for altered body composition in uremia. For example, *Na^+- and K^+-stimulated ATPase activity* has been shown to be decreased in erythrocytes and brain tissue derived from uremic patients and animals, respectively. Whether the "uremic toxins" which account for these derangements in cellular function represent abnormally retained products of metabolism which fail to be excreted, or normal substances present in increased quantities in response to reduced renal mass, remains unknown. *Parathyroid and natriuretic hormones,* examples of this category of substances, are discussed in this context in Chap. 289.

EFFECTS OF UREMIA ON WHOLE-BODY COMPOSITION

What is the impact of these disturbances in active transcellular Na^+ transport on the uremic organism as a whole? From the pathophysiologic considerations already discussed, CRF is likely to lead to abnormally high intracellular Na^+ concentrations, and hence to osmotically induced overhydration of cells generally, whereas these same cells are thought to be relatively deficient in K^+. With the inevitable onset of malaise, anorexia, nausea, vomiting, and diarrhea, patients with CRF may eventually develop classic protein-calorie malnutrition and negative nitrogen balance, often with profound losses of lean body mass and fat deposits. Owing to the concomitant tendency for salt and water retention, these losses often go unnoticed until the late stages of CRF. Whereas a large fraction of the increase in total body water in uremia is the result of expansion of intracellular volume, extracellular volume expansion also is observed commonly. With initiation of intermittent hemodialysis or renal transplantation, there is often an immediate and substantial loss of body weight, due primarily to correction of this overhydration. With successful transplantation, the initial diuresis is followed by a period of impressive weight gain, due to restoration of lean body mass and fat deposits to preillness levels. For patients on chronic dialysis, the anabolic response is less dramatic, even when therapy is regarded as optimal, involving mainly reaccumulation of fat deposits. The failure to restore lean body mass to normal with chronic dialysis may reflect insufficient intake of protein, which, in adequately dialyzed patients, should be maintained at levels of 0.8 to 1.4 g/kg per day.

The occurrence of deficits in intracellular K^+ concentration in CRF has already been mentioned and may result from inadequate intake (poor diet or overzealous K^+ restriction by the physician), excessive losses (vomiting, diarrhea, diuretics), reduction of Na^+- and K^+-stimulated ATPase, or a combination of these. In addition to promoting losses of K^+ into urine (which may be substantial if urine volume remains relatively normal in uremic subjects), the high levels of plasma aldosterone often seen in CRF may also augment net secretion of K^+ into the colon, thereby contributing to marked K^+ losses in stool or diarrheal fluids. Despite deficits in intracellular K^+ concentration, serum K^+ is usually normal or high in CRF, owing most often to metabolic acidosis, which induces an efflux of K^+ from cells. Additionally, uremic patients are relatively resistant to the action of insulin (see below), a hormone which normally enhances K^+ uptake by skeletal muscle.

EFFECTS OF UREMIA ON METABOLISM

HYPOTHERMIA In experimental animals injections of urine, urea, or other retained toxic metabolites can induce hypothermia, and basal heat production diminishes soon after nephrectomy. Since active Na^+ transport across cell membranes accounts for a major proportion of basal energy production, it is generally believed that the inverse relationship between body temperature and degree of azotemia is due, in part, to inhibition of the sodium pump by some retained toxin(s). Dialysis usually returns body temperature to normal.

CARBOHYDRATE METABOLISM The ability to metabolize an exogenous glucose load is impaired in most patients with CRF. The defect largely involves a slowing of the rate at which blood glucose concentration declines to the normal range after administration of a glucose load. Fasting blood sugar levels are usually normal or only slightly elevated; severe hyperglycemia and/or ketosis is uncommon. Consequently, the *glucose intolerance of CRF* usually does not require specific therapy (hence the term *azotemic pseudodiabetes*). Because insulin depends to a large extent on the kidney for its removal from plasma and eventual degradation, circulating insulin levels tend to be increased in uremia. Whereas insulin levels in plasma are only slightly to moderately increased in most fasting uremic subjects, levels considerably in excess of normal are usually found in response to a glucose load. The response to intravenous insulin in patients with CRF is also abnormal, and the rate of utilization of glucose by peripheral tissues often is diminished substantially. The glucose intolerance of uremia is thought to result largely from this peripheral resistance to the action of insulin.

In normal subjects, deficits of K^+ induced by administration of cation exchange resins or thiazide diuretics may result in glucose intolerance. The possibility exists, therefore, that in uremia the intracellular deficits of K^+ (described above) may also contribute to carbohydrate intolerance. It is likely that metabolic acidosis also contributes to impaired carbohydrate metabolism in uremia since this acid-base disturbance has been shown to depress glycolysis, impair glucose utilization, and interfere with the peripheral action of insulin. A role for *glucagon* in the abnormal carbohydrate metabolism of uremia has also been suggested, on the observation that plasma glucagon levels are usually increased in CRF and the fact that glucagon plays a major role in hepatic glycogenolysis. In part, hyperglucagonemia may be a consequence of reduced renal mass since this hormone, as does insulin, depends on the kidneys for its clearance and catabolism. Finally, the possible contributions of other hormones in the pathogenesis of this glucose intolerance, including catecholamines, growth hormone, and prolactin, as well as the myriad of potentially toxic metabolites retained in CRF, remain to be determined.

NITROGEN AND LIPID METABOLISM Given that the capacity to eliminate the nitrogenous end products of protein catabolism is reduced drastically, CRF may be regarded as a state of *protein intolerance.* As discussed above, retention of these end products of nitrogen metabolism is thought to represent a dominant cause of the signs and symptoms of uremic toxicity.

Hypertriglyceridemia and decreased high-density lipoprotein cholesterol are common in uremia, whereas cholesterol levels in plasma are usually normal. Whether uremia accelerates triglyceride production by the liver and intestine is unknown. The well-known lipogenic effect of hyperinsulinism may contribute to increased triglyceride synthesis. The rate of removal of triglycerides from the circulation, which depends in large part on the enzyme *lipoprotein lipase,* has been shown to be depressed in uremia, an effect not corrected appreciably by hemodialysis. The high incidence of premature atherosclerosis seen in patients on chronic dialysis (see "Cardiovascular and Pulmonary Abnormalities" below) may be related, at least in part, to these abnormalities in lipid metabolism.

CLINICAL SPECTRUM OF ABNORMALITIES IN UREMIA

As noted earlier, CRF leads ultimately to disturbances in function of every organ system in the body. With the advent and increasingly greater application of chronic dialysis in the past two decades, the incidence and severity of these disturbances have been modified enormously, so that virtually everywhere that modern medicine is practiced, the overt and florid manifestations of uremia have largely disappeared. Unfortunately, however, even optimal dialysis therapy is not a panacea for the patient with CRF, because, as indicated in Table 291-1, some disturbances resulting from impaired renal function fail to respond fully, while others may even progress despite dialysis treatment. Furthermore, as with many modern and complex therapeutic modalities, intermittent dialysis may be responsible for the appearance of unique abnormalities not seen prior to initiation of therapy; these abnormalities should be viewed as complications of dialysis.

FLUID, ELECTROLYTE, AND ACID-BASE DISORDERS (See also Chaps. 43 and 44) **Sodium and volume homeostasis** In most patients with stable CRF, modest increases in total body Na^+ and water content can be documented, although objective signs of extracellular fluid (ECF) volume expansion may not be apparent clinically. With ingestion of excessive amounts of salt and water, however, control of excess volume becomes an important clinical and therapeutic consideration. In general, excessive *salt* ingestion contributes to, or aggravates, congestive heart failure, hypertension, ascites, and edema formation. On the other hand, hyponatremia and weight gain are the typical consequences of excessive ingestion of *water*, abnormalities which in most patients are relatively mild and asymptomatic. In the majority of patients, daily intake of fluid equal in volume to urine volume per day plus about 500 ml usually will maintain the serum Na^+ concentration at normal levels. Hypernatremia is encountered relatively infrequently in CRF, although its occurrence has been noted during peritoneal dialysis when high glucose concentrations are added to the dialysate. In dialysis patients with evidence of extracellular volume expansion, management should include ultrafiltration and restriction of salt and water intake between dialyses. In the patient with CRF not maintained on dialysis, diuretics and modest restriction of salt and water intake are the mainstays of therapy.

Patients with CRF have grossly impaired renal mechanisms for conserving Na^+ and water (discussed in detail in Chap. 289). When confronted with an *extrarenal* cause for increased fluid loss (e.g., vomiting, diarrhea, fever), these patients are prone to develop ECF volume depletion, with signs and symptoms of dry mouth and other mucous membranes, dizziness, syncope, tachycardia, decreased filling of jugular veins, orthostatic hypotension, and even vascular collapse. Depletion of extracellular fluid volume typically results in deterioration of residual renal function and, in the previously stable and asymptomatic patient with mild CRF, signs and symptoms of overt uremia. Cautious fluid repletion usually restores extracellular and intravascular volumes to normal and often, but not always, returns renal function to previously stable levels.

Potassium homeostasis Derangements in K^+ balance (see also Chaps. 43 and 289) are occasionally documented by laboratory analysis in patients with CRF, but are rarely responsible for clinical symptoms unless GFR is below 5 ml/min or an endogenous (hemolysis, trauma, infection) or exogenous (stored blood, K^+-containing medications) K^+ load is administered. Despite progression of renal failure, most patients maintain normal serum K^+ concentrations until the final stages of uremia. As discussed in Chap. 289, this ability to sustain K^+ balance with advancing renal failure is due to adaptations in the renal distal tubules and colon, sites where aldosterone and other factors serve to enhance K^+ secretion. Not surprisingly, oliguria, or disruption of key adaptive mechanisms, can lead to *hyperkalemia* and its potentially ominous effects on cardiac function. Antikaliuretic drugs, such as spironolactone or triamterene, should be used with extreme

TABLE 291-1
Clinical spectrum of abnormalities in uremia*

FLUID AND ELECTROLYTE DISTURBANCES
Volume expansion and contraction (I)
Hypernatremia and hyponatremia (I)
Hyperkalemia and hypokalemia (I)
Metabolic acidosis (I)
Hyperphosphatemia and hypophosphatemia (I)
Hypocalcemia (I)
ENDOCRINE-METABOLIC DISTURBANCES
Renal osteodystrophy (I or P)
Secondary hyperparathyroidism (I or P)
Carbohydrate intolerance (I)
Hyperuricemia (I or P)
Hypothermia (I)
Hypertriglyceridemia (P)
Protein-calorie malnutrition (I or P)
Impaired growth and development (P)
Infertility and sexual dysfunction (P)
Amenorrhea (P)
NEUROMUSCULAR DISTURBANCES
Fatigue (I)
Sleep disorders (P)
Headache (I or P)
Impaired mentation (I)
Lethargy (I)
Asterixis (I)
Muscular irritability (I)
Peripheral neuropathy (I or P)
Restless legs syndrome (I or P)
Paralysis (I or P)
Myoclonus (I)
Seizures (I or P)
Coma (I)
Muscle cramps (D)
Dialysis disequilibrium syndrome (D)
Dialysis dementia (D)
CARDIOVASCULAR AND PULMONARY DISTURBANCES
Arterial hypertension (I or P)
Congestive heart failure (I)
Pericarditis (I)
Cardiomyopathy (I or P)
Uremic lung (I)
Accelerated atherosclerosis (P or D)
DERMATOLOGIC DISTURBANCES
Pallor (I or P)
Hyperpigmentation (I or P)
Pruritus (P)
Ecchymoses (I or P)
Uremic frost (I)
GASTROINTESTINAL DISTURBANCES
Anorexia (I)
Nausea and vomiting (I)
Uremic fetor (I)
Gastroenteritis (I)
Peptic ulcer (I or P)
GI bleeding (I, P, or D)
Hepatitis (D)
Refractory ascites (D)
HEMATOLOGIC AND IMMUNOLOGIC DISTURBANCES
Normocytic, normochromic anemia (P)
Lymphocytopenia (P)
Bleeding diathesis (I or D)
Increased susceptibility to infection (I or P)
Splenomegaly and hypersplenism (P)
Leukopenia (D)
Hypocomplementemia (D)

* *Virtually all the abnormalities contained in this table are completely reversed by successful renal transplantation. The response of these abnormalities to intermittent hemo- or peritoneal dialysis therapy is more variable. I denotes an abnormality which usually improves with an* optimal *program of intermittent dialysis and related therapy. P denotes an abnormality which tends to persist, or even progress, despite an* optimal *dialysis program. D denotes an abnormality which develops only after initiation of dialysis therapy.*

caution in CRF. Hyperkalemia in CRF may also be induced by abrupt lowering of arterial blood pH, since acidosis is associated with efflux of K^+ from intracellular to extracellular fluids. A clinically useful index of the magnitude of this hydrogen-potassium exchange is that for every 0.1 unit change in blood pH, there will be a reciprocal change in serum K^+ concentration of approximately 0.6 meq per liter. Correction of acidosis-induced hyperkalemia with sodium bicarbonate is the treatment of choice. Intravenous insulin and dextrose are useful in lowering serum potassium acutely, while the ion exchange resin sodium polystyrene sulfonate (Kayexalate) is useful in longer-term control of hyperkalemia. Patients in whom hyperkalemia persists in the absence of excessive K^+ intake, oliguria, or acute acidosis should be evaluated for the possibility of *hyporeninemic hypoaldosteronism.* Patients with this syndrome have reduced circulating levels of renin and aldosterone in the plasma and often also have diabetes mellitus.

Hypokalemia due to diminished ability of the kidneys to conserve K^+ is uncommon in most forms of CRF. When hypokalemia occurs in these patients, poor dietary K^+ intake, usually in association with excessive diuretic therapy or gastrointestinal losses, is likely to be the underlying cause. When hypokalemia occurs as a result of primary K^+ wasting in urine, it may represent a solitary renal reabsorptive defect or, more commonly, be associated with other solute transport abnormalities, as in Fanconi's syndrome, renal tubular acidosis, or other forms of hereditary or acquired tubulointerstitial diseases (see Chaps. 297 and 299). A detailed discussion of the clinical consequences and management of hypokalemia and hyperkalemia is given in Chap. 43.

Metabolic acidosis With advancing renal failure, total daily acid excretion falls below the level needed to maintain external balance of hydrogen ions. Metabolic acidosis is the inevitable result, and the mechanisms involved are considered in Chap. 289. In most patients with stable renal insufficiency, administration of 20 to 30 meq sodium bicarbonate or sodium citrate per day will usually correct the acidosis. In response to a sudden acid challenge (whether from an endogenous or exogenous source), however, patients with CRF are particularly susceptible to profound acidosis, which requires more substantial quantities of alkali for correction. Administration of sodium must be carried out with careful attention to the patient's volume status.

Phosphate, calcium, and bone As discussed in detail in Chap. 289, serum phosphate concentration begins to rise when GFR falls below about 25 percent of normal. Calcium deposition in bone is critically dependent upon the availability of phosphate; retention of phosphate in plasma, therefore, facilitates calcium entry into bone and thereby contributes to the *hypocalcemia* and *elevations in plasma PTH* levels seen in CRF. Hypocalcemia in CRF also results from the impaired ability of the diseased kidney to synthesize *1,25-dihydroxyvitamin* D_3 [1,25-$(OH)_2D_3$], the active metabolite of vitamin D (Fig. 291-1). Reabsorption of calcium in the gut is impaired when circulating levels of this active metabolite are low. Finally, in patients with advanced CRF, the ability of PTH to mobilize calcium salts from bone may be altered. Despite these various causes of hypocalcemia, symptoms such as tetany are rare unless patients are treated with large amounts of alkali.

Overproduction of parathyroid hormone, disordered vitamin D metabolism, chronic metabolic acidosis, and excessive fecal losses of calcium all contribute to the occurrence of bone diseases in uremia (Fig. 291-1). *Renal* and *uremic osteodystrophy* are broad and imprecise terms that encompass a number of distinct skeletal abnormalities, including osteomalacia, osteitis fibrosa cystica, osteosclerosis, and, in children especially, impaired bone growth. Although clinical symptoms of bone disease are uncommon, occurring in less than 10 percent of patients with advanced renal failure, radiological and histological abnormalities are observed in about 35 and 90 percent, respectively. Renal osteodystrophy is seen more often in growing children than in adults, and especially in patients with congenital renal anomalies associated with very slowly progressive renal insufficiency. On radiological examination, three types of lesions can be identified: (1) changes analogous to those described in children with nutritional rickets, namely, widened osteoid seams at the growth margin of bones (so-called renal rickets); (2) the bone changes of *secondary hyperparathyroidism* (*osteitis fibrosa cystica*), characterized by osteoclastic bone resorption and manifested by subperiosteal erosions, especially of the phalanges, long bones, and distal ends of the clavicles; and (3) *osteosclerosis,* often best noted by enhanced bone density in the upper and lower margins of vertebrae, producing the so-called rugger jersey spine. Since patients with osteosclerosis are usually in negative calcium balance, sclerosis is due mainly

FIGURE 291-1
Pathogenesis of bone diseases in chronic renal failure.

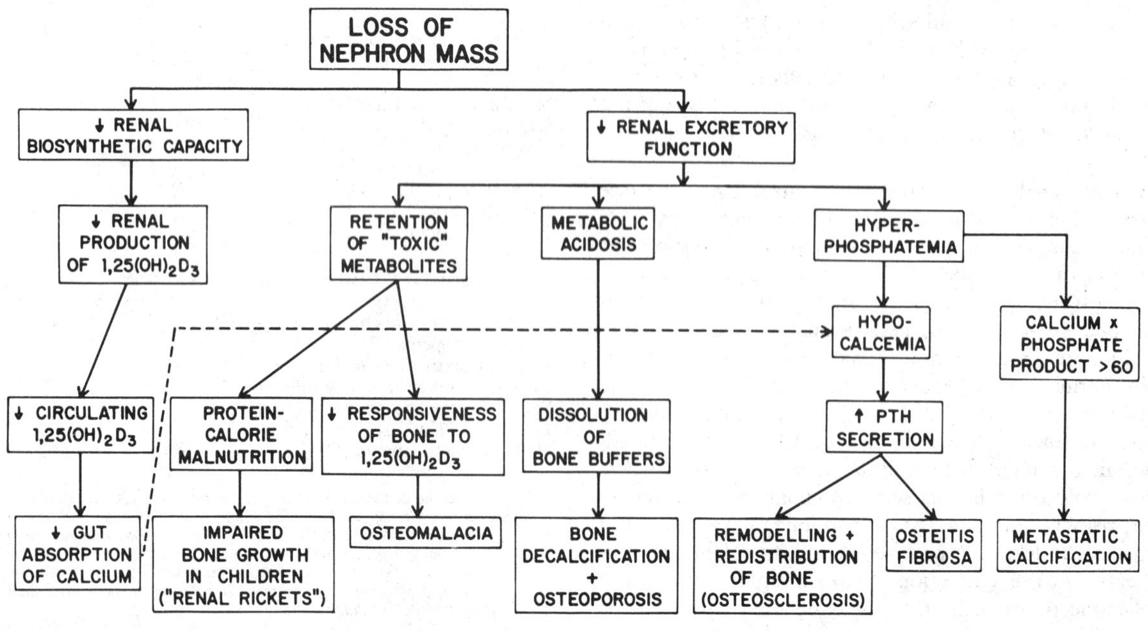

to bone remodeling and redistribution. With very rapid mobilization of skeletal calcium, as occurs in dialysis when the bath is low in calcium, or following prolonged bed rest, osteosclerosis is usually replaced by loss of bone density and osteoporosis.

With renal osteodystrophy there is a tendency to *spontaneous fractures,* which are often slow to heal. The ribs are most commonly involved. Painful joints may occur in association with renal osteodystrophy due to calcium deposition in bursas and other periarticular structures. When bone pain is severe, a proximal *myopathy* may coexist, giving rise to gait abnormalities and even leading to cessation of ambulation. The incidence of *aseptic necrosis of the hip* is increased in renal transplant recipients, probably related to such factors as chronic corticosteroid therapy, secondary hyperparathyroidism, and altered vitamin D metabolism. In CRF there is often a tendency to *extraosseous,* or *metastatic, calcification,* especially when the calcium-phosphate product exceeds 60. Medium-sized blood vessels; subcutaneous, articular, and periarticular tissues; myocardium; eyes; and lungs are common sites of metastatic calcification.

Management of patients with renal osteodystrophy includes reduction in dietary phosphate available for absorption through the use of aluminum hydroxide binding agents. When such treatment is instituted early in CRF, signs and symptoms of renal osteodystrophy and parathyroid gland hypertrophy may largely be prevented. Daily vitamin D supplementation, in the form of 1,25-dihydroxycholecalciferol or dihydrotachysterol, is also of value, particularly to improve osteomalacia, osteitis fibrosa cystica, and myopathy. Supplementation of dietary calcium intake (to 1 to 1.5 g per day) as well as judicious increases in calcium ion concentration in the dialysate is also useful for treating or preventing hypocalcemia, but should not be instituted until hyperphosphatemia is corrected. Close monitoring of serum calcium and phosphate concentrations is required to avoid serious hypercalcemia and metastatic calcification.

Other solutes Other inorganic solute derangements in CRF include *hyperuricemia* and *hypermagnesemia.* Uric acid retention is a common feature of CRF but rarely leads to symptomatic gout. Hypophosphatemia is usually a consequence of overzealous oral administration of phosphate-binding gels. Because serum magnesium levels tend to rise in CRF, magnesium-containing antacids and cathartics should be avoided.

CARDIOVASCULAR AND PULMONARY ABNORMALITIES Fluid retention in uremic patients often results in congestive heart failure and/or pulmonary edema. A unique form of pulmonary congestion and edema may be seen in uremia even in the absence of volume overload and is typically associated with normal or mildly elevated intracardiac and pulmonary wedge pressures. This entity, referred to as *uremic lung,* is characterized radiologically by perihilar vascular congestion (the peripheral lung regions appear uninvolved), giving rise to the impression of a "butterfly wing" distribution. Uremic lung, as well as cardiopulmonary abnormalities associated with circulatory overload, usually respond promptly and dramatically to vigorous dialysis.

Arterial hypertension is the most commonly observed complication of end-stage renal disease. When it is not present, the patient is either receiving antihypertensive therapy or is volume-depleted, the latter condition usually due to excessive gastrointestinal fluid losses, overzealous or surreptitious diuretic therapy, or salt-wasting forms of renal disease (e.g., polycystic or medullary cystic disease or chronic pyelonephritis). Since fluid overload is the major cause of hypertension in uremic subjects, the normotensive state can usually be restored by dialysis. Nevertheless, some patients remain hypertensive, despite rigorous salt and water restriction and ultrafiltration, because of hyperreninemia. In the majority of these cases, antihypertensive drug therapy is effective. A small minority of these patients develop *accelerated or malignant hypertension,* manifested by markedly elevated systolic and diastolic pressures, severe hyperreninemia, encephalopathy, seizures, retinal changes, and papilledema. Use of more potent drugs such as minoxidil and nitroprusside may prove useful; however, in the exceptional patient in whom malignant hypertension fails to respond to maximum antihypertensive therapy and rigorous dialysis, bilateral nephrectomy should be considered.

As is likely with uremic lung, retained metabolic toxins contribute to the occurrence of *pericarditis* in patients with CRF. The clinical presentation of pericarditis in uremic subjects is generally similar to that of other etiologies (Chap. 265), except that pericardiocentesis for effusions usually yields hemorrhagic fluid. Treatment with intensive dialysis is recommended, and systemic anticoagulation should be avoided to minimize the possible occurrence of hemorrhagic tamponade. Oral indomethacin may be useful for pericarditis. In some patients, pericardiocentesis with intrapericardial instillation of air or steroids is effective for pericardial tamponade. Pericardiectomy should be considered only after more conservative treatment has failed.

Clinical experience with chronically dialyzed patients followed for the past decade or more has revealed the disturbing occurrence of *accelerated atherosclerosis,* leading to development of significant coronary, cerebral, and peripheral vascular disease. There are seemingly ample causes for these complications, including long-term hypertension, hyperlipidemia, glucose intolerance, and metastatic vascular and myocardial calcification, which, by interfering with the atrioventricular conduction system of the heart, have been known to cause cardiac arrhythmias and sudden death.

HEMATOLOGIC ABNORMALITIES *Normochromic, normocytic anemia* occurs regularly in CRF and contributes to fatigability and listlessness in these patients. Erythropoiesis is depressed in CRF, due both to the effects of retained toxins on bone marrow and to diminished biosynthesis of erythropoietin by the diseased kidney. *Hemolysis* also occurs and involves an extracorpuscular defect since survival of erythrocytes from normal subjects is reduced when these cells are transfused into uremic patients, and erythrocytes from patients with CRF have relatively normal survival times when transfused into normal individuals. Gastrointestinal and chronic dialyzer *blood loss* contributes to anemia, as does *hypersplenism* in the occasional patient. Blood loss is exaggerated in hemodialysis patients because of the need for heparin (during dialysis) and oral anticoagulants (between dialyses) to minimize clotting of vascular access devices. Transfusions may contribute to suppression of erythropoiesis in CRF and, due to increased risk of hepatitis and hemosiderosis, should be avoided unless anemia aggravates other underlying disorders (for example, coronary or cerebrovascular disease). Androgen therapy has been shown to improve erythropoiesis in some dialysis patients not previously subjected to nephrectomy. Parenteral or oral iron therapy and vitamin supplementation are also indicated in most patients, the former to correct deficits due to chronic blood loss (especially when blood transfusions are withheld) and the latter, especially folic and ascorbic acids and the soluble B vitamins, to offset chronic losses of these substances through dialyzer membranes.

Abnormal hemostasis is another common hematologic derangement in CRF, characterized by a tendency to abnormal bleeding and bruising. Bleeding into gastrointestinal tract, pericardial sac, and intracranial vault, in the form of subdural hematoma or intracerebral hemorrhage, is of greatest concern. Prolongation of bleeding time, decreased platelet factor III activity, abnormal platelet aggregation and adhesiveness, and impaired prothrombin consumption contribute to the clotting defects in uremia. The abnormality in factor III correlates with increased plasma levels of guanidinosuccinic acid and can largely be corrected by dialysis.

A wide variety of changes in leukocyte formation and function also occur in uremia leading to *enhanced susceptibility to infection.* Lymphocytopenia and atrophy of lymphoid structures occur in CRF, whereas neutrophil production is relatively unimpaired. Nevertheless, there is evidence to suggest that all leukocyte cell types are affected adversely by uremic serum. Decreased chemotaxis is among the best documented of the defects occurring in uremic leukocytes, with resulting impairment of acute inflammatory response and decreased delayed hypersensitivity. There is a tendency for uremic patients to have less fever in response to infection. For these reasons, infections may be more difficult to recognize in uremia. Leukocyte function may also be impaired in patients with CRF because of such coexisting factors as acidosis, hyperglycemia, protein-calorie malnutrition, and serum and tissue hyperosmolarity (due to azotemia). Mucosal barriers to infection may also be defective, and, in dialysis patients, vascular access devices also serve as common portals of entry for pathogens, particularly staphylococci. Anti-inflammatory steroids and immunosuppressive drugs add further to the risk of serious infection in many of these patients.

NEUROMUSCULAR ABNORMALITIES Subtle disturbances of central nervous system function, including inability to concentrate, drowsiness, and insomnia, are among the earliest symptoms of uremia. Mild behavioral changes, loss of memory, and errors in judgment soon follow, and often are associated with signs of neuromuscular irritability, including hiccups, cramps, and fasciculations and twitching of large muscle groups. Asterixis, myoclonus, and chorea are common in terminal uremia, as are stupor, seizures, and coma. Many of these neuromuscular complications of severe uremia resolve with dialysis, although nonspecific EEG abnormalities may persist.

Peripheral neuropathy is a relatively common complication of advanced CRF. Initially, sensory nerve involvement exceeds motor, lower extremities are involved more than the upper, and the distal portions of the extremities more than proximal. The "restless legs syndrome," characterized by ill-defined sensations of discomfort in the feet and lower legs and frequent leg movement, is a disturbing complication in some uremic patients. If dialysis is not instituted soon after onset of sensory abnormalities, motor involvement follows, often leading to loss of deep tendon reflexes, weakness, peroneal nerve palsy (foot drop), and, eventually, flaccid quadriplegia. Accordingly, early evidence of peripheral neuropathy is generally taken as a firm indication to initiate dialysis or transplantation.

Two types of neurological disturbances appear to be unique to patients on chronic dialysis. One is the syndrome of *dialysis dementia,* seen in patients who have been on dialysis for a number of years. This syndrome is characterized by speech dyspraxia, myoclonus, dementia, and eventually seizures and death. The possibility of aluminum intoxication has been suggested, with aluminum contamination of dialysate as the likely source. The other disturbance occurs during the first few dialyses, in association with rapid reduction of blood urea levels. Nausea, vomiting, drowsiness, headache, and even grand mal seizures have been attributed to the more rapid (dialysis-induced) reduction in osmolality of extracellular than intracellular fluids within the cranium, leading to cerebral edema and raised intracranial pressure—hence the term *dialysis disequilibrium syndrome.*

GASTROINTESTINAL ABNORMALITIES Anorexia, hiccups, nausea, and vomiting are common and early manifestations of uremia and contribute to the protein-calorie malnutrition of this disorder. *Uremic fetor,* a uriniferous odor to the breath, derives from the breakdown of urea in saliva to ammonia and is often associated with unpleasant taste sensation. Mucosal ulcerations leading to blood loss can occur at any level of the gastrointestinal tract in very late stages of CRF—so-called uremic gastroenteritis. Peptic ulcer disease is particularly common, occurring in as many as one-fourth of uremic subjects. Whether this high incidence is related to increased gastric acidity, hypersecretion of gastrin, or secondary hyperparathyroidism is unknown. Most of the gastrointestinal symptoms, except those related to peptic ulcer disease, usually improve with dialysis.

Viral hepatitis (see also Chaps. 138 and 318), though not a complication of uremia per se, is a common problem encountered in chronic dialysis patients because of frequent blood transfusions. Recent studies in the United States have reported detecting hepatitis B type antigen in 5 to 10 percent of chronic dialysis patients and in 2 percent of dialysis support personnel. This prevalence is higher than in the general population and indicates transmission between patients and support staff. Viral hepatitis in dialysis patients tends to be milder, indeed, often subclinical, in comparison with nonuremic victims. Jaundice and hyperbilirubinemia are uncommon; the abnormalities consist of mild hepatomegaly, modest elevations in SGOT, SGPT, and alkaline phosphatase, and moderate sodium sulfobromophthalein (Bromsulphalein) retention. Type B antigen is usually present and may persist long after other features of the illness have resolved. In addition to serum hepatitis, hemodialysis patients are also susceptible to other infectious forms of hepatitis, particularly that caused by cytomegalovirus (Chap. 211). Hepatitis associated with hypersensitivity or toxic reactions to commonly employed drugs and solvents may also occur.

ENDOCRINE-METABOLIC DISTURBANCES The common disturbances in parathyroid function, glucose, and insulin metabolism, as well as the lipid, protein-calorie, and other nutritional abnormalities of uremia have already been considered. In general, pituitary, thyroid, and adrenal gland functions are relatively normal, often despite measurable abnormalities in circulating thyroxine, growth hormone, aldosterone, and cortisol levels. In women, amenorrhea and inability to carry pregnancies to term are early manifestations of uremia. While menses frequently reappear after chronic dialysis is initiated, successful pregnancies remain rare. In men with CRF, including those on chronic dialysis, impotence, oligospermia, and germinal cell dysplasia are common, as are reduced plasma testosterone levels. As with growth, sexual maturation is often impaired in adolescent children, even among those on chronic dialysis.

DERMATOLOGIC ABNORMALITIES The skin shows many abnormalities. This is not surprising in view of anemia (pallor), defective hemostasis (ecchymoses and hematomas), calcium deposition and secondary hyperparathyroidism (pruritus, excoriations), dehydration (poor skin turgor, dry mucous membranes), and the general cutaneous consequences of protein-calorie malnutrition. A sallow, yellow cast may reflect the combined influences of anemia and retention of a variety of pigmented metabolites, or *urochromes.* In advanced uremia urea concentrations in sweat may reach sufficiently high levels that, after evaporation, a fine white powder can be found on the skin surface—so-called uremic (urea) frost. Although many of these cutaneous abnormalities improve with dialysis, *uremic pruritus* may persist and is usually resistant to most systemic and topical therapies. Regular bathing and lubrication of the skin with bland ointments are helpful in preventing superficial infection and excessive dryness.

REFERENCES

BRICKER NS: On the pathogenesis of the uremic state: An exposition of the "trade off" hypothesis. N Engl J Med 286:1093, 1972

DEFRONZO RA et al: Carbohydrate metabolism in uremia: A review. Medicine 52:469, 1973

DELUCA HF: The kidney as an endocrine organ involved in the function of vitamin D. Am J Med 58:39, 1975

ERSLEV AJ: Management of the anemia of chronic renal failure. Clin Nephrol 2:174, 1974

FELDMAN HS, SINGER I: Endocrinology and metabolism in uremia and dialysis: A clinical review. Medicine 54:345, 1975

GOLDBLUM SE, REED WP: Host defenses and immunologic alterations associated with chronic hemodialysis. Ann Intern Med 93:597, 1980

KARLINSKY ML et al: Preservation of renal function in experimental glomerulonephritis. Kidney Intern 17:293, 1980

KOPPLE JD, COBURN JW: Metabolic studies of low protein diets in uremia: Nitrogen and potassium. Medicine 52:583, 1973

MONTGOMERIE JZ et al: Renal failure and infection. Medicine 47:1, 1968

NOLPH KD: Short dialysis, middle molecules and uremia. Ann Intern Med 86:93, 1977

TYLER HR: Neurologic disorders in renal failure. Am J Med 44:734, 1968

WEIDMANN P et al: Plasma renin activity and blood pressure in terminal renal failure. N Engl J Med 285:757, 1971

ZELNICK EB, GOYAL RK: Gastrointestinal manifestations of chronic renal failure. In Seminars in Nephrol 1:124, NA Kurtzman (ed). Grune & Stratton, 1981

292
DIALYSIS AND TRANSPLANTATION IN THE TREATMENT OF RENAL FAILURE

CHARLES B. CARPENTER
J. MICHAEL LAZARUS

Over the past three decades, dialysis and transplantation have become effective treatment modalities in prolonging the life of patients with renal insufficiency. Such treatment, however, alters the disease process and has created new disease entities (see Chap. 291). The approach to treatment in acute renal failure is different from chronic renal failure because of the irreversible nature of the latter. Conservative medical management, hemodialysis, or peritoneal dialysis are the mainstays of therapy for acute renal failure; transplantation can be added to this treatment regimen for patients with chronic renal failure. Options for treatment of patients with chronic or irreversible renal failure are outlined as follows:

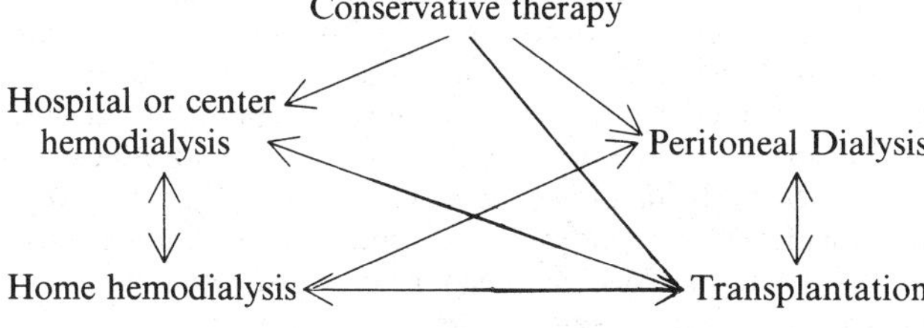

Initially patients are managed with conservative therapy, but eventually they require hemodialysis, peritoneal dialysis, or

cadaver or related donor transplantation. Because of limited success with each of these treatment modalities this chronic disease should be approached with the concept of moving from one form of therapy to another as indicated by the degree of success and incidence of complications with each form of treatment.

Therapy for renal failure should be initiated at a time in the disease process when complications will be moderate, but not when the patient is completely asymptomatic. The advanced complications of uremia, as noted in Chap. 291, should be avoided by early treatment. Early dialysis is especially applicable to patients with acute renal failure in whom resumption of renal function can be expected and to patients with chronic renal failure who have a good immunologic match with a related donor in whom transplantation can lead to resumption of normal renal function. In the remainder of patients, the clinical judgment to move from conservative treatment to dialysis or transplantation is determined by the patient's quality of life and whether or not the benefits of treatment outweigh the risks.

Selection of patients to receive dialysis and/or transplantation is a matter of much debate. Because of the reversible nature of acute renal failure, *all* patients with this diagnosis should be supported with dialysis, at least for some period of time, to allow return of renal function. In patients with irreversible or chronic renal failure, criteria for selection for transplantation are generally more stringent than those for dialysis and are guided by the possibility of complications related to immunosuppressive therapy. Most transplant programs limit the upper age to approximately 55 to 60 years because of increased complications and mortality in the elderly, particularly when cadavers are utilized for transplantation. Any disease process which may be aggravated by prednisone, azathioprine, cyclophosphamide, or other immunosuppressive agents or any patient with medical complications so severe that they likely might not survive surgery and drug therapy should obviously not be offered transplantation. Clearly, the quality of life and long-term results are superior in the totally *successful* renal transplant recipient. Criteria for treatment with hemodialysis or peritoneal dialysis are more liberal since dialysis has less morbidity than transplantation in older patients and those with major medical complications. Because of the cost of these programs, some have suggested restricted entry. These decisions, based on moral and social issues, continue to generate debate. In most areas of the world today, the cost of medical care for chronic renal failure is borne by government. In the United States, chronic renal failure is the only major illness in patients under the age of 65 which is covered by Medicare. With economic support from the government for dialysis and transplantation programs, both in this country and abroad, rules and regulations have been and will continue to be generated which will affect the practice of medicine in this group of patients with regard to their selection and the type of treatment employed.

CONSERVATIVE TREATMENT Conservative (nondialytic, nontransplant) therapy should be instituted early to control symptoms, minimize complications, prevent long-term sequelae of uremia, and slow the progression of renal insufficiency, if possible. Every effort should be made to correct any of the numerous reversible components which agggravate renal impairment. In patients with acute renal failure, prerenal factors, such as volume depletion, decreased cardiac output, or renal artery stenosis, or postrenal components, such as urethral or ureteral obstruction, must be sought and corrected. Such pre-

and postrenal components may exacerbate underlying parenchymal disease in patients with chronic renal insufficiency and must be treated in this group as well. Most important is treatment of the underlying disease or complications of renal insufficiency which further hasten the loss of nephrons. Hypertension, urinary tract infections, nephrolithiasis, structural abnormalities of the urinary tract, or those forms of glomerulonephritis which may respond to therapy should be treated aggressively. Preventive aspects include avoidance of nephrotoxic drugs and large doses of radiopaque agents in the patient with already compromised renal insufficiency.

Modification of diet is an important aspect of conservative therapy. Early restriction of sodium and fluid may be important in the treatment of hypertension. As renal insufficiency progresses, restriction of foods high in phosphate and potassium is necessary. Reduction of protein content reduces anorexia, nausea, and vomiting and has been suggested by some to retard progression of the disease. Adult patients should receive no less than 0.6 g of protein per kilogram per day to avoid negative nitrogen balance. Supplementation of low protein diets with essential ketoamino acid therapy may be useful in prolonging the period of conservative therapy by allowing utilization of urea as a source of nonessential nitrogen. Correction of electrolyte imbalance, e.g., use of sodium bicarbonate or calcium carbonate to correct mild acidosis, or bicarbonate, dextrose and insulin, and potassium exchange resins for treatment of hyperkalemia, will be necessary in more advanced states of uremia. Some chemical abnormalities occurring with renal failure do not require or are not amenable to treatment; hypermagnesemia, hyperamylasemia, hypertriglyceridemia, or mild carbohydrate intolerance generally do not require therapy. Treatment of hyperuricemia may be in order if the patient suffers from gout. However, hyperuricemia alone has not been shown to be detrimental. It has been suggested that secondary hyperparathyroidism may accentuate progression of renal failure. Whether this is due to hyperphosphatemia, an elevated calcium-phosphorus product, or parathormone itself is not clear. Nonetheless, vigorous efforts using aluminum-containing antacids to lower phosphorus and calcium supplements and vitamin D products (dihydrotachysterol or 1,25-dihydroxycholecalciferol) to maintain the serum calcium are effective in suppressing parathyroid stimulation, perhaps in slowing renal insufficiency, and likely avoiding severe bone disease later (see Chap. 339). To avoid visceral and vascular calcification it is important to maintain the calcium-phosphorus product below 60. Fluid, sodium, potassium, phosphate, and protein restriction offer the patient a very restricted and often unacceptable diet. This, coupled with the administration of multiple medications, often occurs at a time when the complications of uremia appear and consideration for dialysis and/or transplantation is in order.

While conservative measures are being carried out, it is necessary to prepare the patient with an intensive educational program to explain the possibilities of eventual renal failure and the various forms of therapy available. The more knowledgeable patients are concerning hemodialysis, peritoneal dialysis, and transplantation, the easier and more appropriate will be their decisions at a later time. With hemodialysis, the major method of obtaining blood for treatment is through an arteriovenous fistula. Since these devices often take several months to develop, prophylactic placement of a fistula in a patient planning for hemodialysis is important in minimizing future complications of circulatory access. For those patients who select peritoneal dialysis, placement of the peritoneal catheter does not require preparation, and therapy can be instituted as soon as uremic signs and symptoms develop. In those patients who may perform home dialysis or undergo transplantation, early education of family members for selection and preparation as a home dialysis helper or a related donor for transplantation should occur well before the onset of symptomatic renal failure. In those patients who may have a good antigenic match with a willing donor, transplantation without intervening hemodialysis or peritoneal dialysis should be considered.

HEMODIALYSIS Hemodialysis employs the process of diffusion across a semipermeable membrane to remove unwanted substances from the blood while adding desirable components. A constant flow of blood on one side of the membrane and a cleansing solution–dialysate on the other allows removal of waste products in a fashion grossly similar to that of glomerular filtration. By altering the composition of the dialysate, the method of exposure of blood and dialysate (geometry of the dialyzer), the type and surface area of dialysis membrane, and the frequency and duration of exposure, patients without renal function can be maintained in a relatively healthy state. Hemodialysis equipment is composed of three components—the blood delivery system, the composition and delivery system of the dialysate, and the dialyzer itself. Blood is pumped to the dialyzer by a roller pump through lines with appropriate equipment to measure flow and pressures within the system; blood flow should be approximately 200 to 300 ml/min. Hydrostatic pressure within the system can be manipulated to achieve desirable fluid removal, so-called ultrafiltration. The dialysate is delivered to the dialyzer from a storage tank or proportioning system which manufactures dialysate on line. In most systems dialysate passes once across the membrane, countercurrent to blood flow at a rate of 500 ml/min, or it may be recirculated multiple times at higher flow rates. The composition of the dialysate may be altered depending upon the patient's needs, but in a particular dialysis unit it is usually a fixed formula. There are three principal types of dialyzers—the flat plate dialyzer, in which flat sheets of cellophane are layered one on another with intervening plastic templates; the coil dialyzer, in which cylindrical tubes of cellophane are coiled around a plastic mesh support; and the hollow fiber or capillary dialyzer, in which membrane material is spun into fine capillaries, thousands of which are packed into bundles with blood flowing through the capillaries while dialysate is circulated on the outside of the fiber bundle.

Most patients require between 10 and 15 h of dialysis per week, equally divided into several sessions. The time depends upon body size, residual renal function, dietary intake, complicating illnesses, and the degree of anabolism or catabolism. The time, frequency of treatments, type and size of dialyzer, and dialysate composition, blood, or dialysate flow may all be altered to accomplish specific needs.

The Achilles' heel of hemodialysis is access to the circulation. In the early 1960s, development of the arteriovenous shunt made chronic dialysis possible. This device has had a high failure rate because of infection and thrombosis and led in 1966 to the development of the arteriovenous (AV) fistula. The fistula is preferably created from a native vein, but if not available, a prosthetic conduit (Dacron, extended polytetrafluoroethylene, bovine carotid arteries) between an artery and a nearby vein may be utilized. Cannulation of arteriovenous fistulas with large-bore needles allows blood flow sufficient to carry out hemodialysis. Unfortunately, infection, thrombosis, and aneurysm formation also occur in the arteriovenous fistula, particularly in prosthetic devices. There is a relatively high incidence of septicemia and septic embolization associated with shunt and fistula infection; the most common infecting agent is *Staphylococcus aureus*.

Advantages of hemodialysis are the relatively short treatment time and minimal interruption of life-style between treatments. It is more efficient than peritoneal dialysis, allowing rapid changes in abnormal serum values. Hemodialysis can be performed in the home, but the patient requires an assistant during treatment. It is the most widely available form of dialysis and is used in approximately 90 percent of patients with end-stage renal disease.

Many complications in the chronic dialysis patient are related to underlying disease or those uremic conditions not reversed by dialytic therapy. These and other related problems of hemodialysis are discussed in Chap. 291. Septicemia and septic embolization are the major complications of AV fistula failure. However, a significant psychological impact is related to the failure of the AV fistula. Depression and altered self-image are other common psychiatric problems. The rapid flux in osmolality may cause a disequilibrium syndrome, while rapid changes in electrolytes (particularly potassium) may lead to arrhythmia during dialysis. Hypotension is a common phenomenon during hemodialysis and is due to many factors—the extracorporeal circulation, degree of ultrafiltration, change in serum osmolality, presence of autonomic neuropathy, concomitant use of antihypertensive agents, removal of catecholamines, or infusion of acetate (used as the dialysate buffer) which is a cardiac depressant and vasodilator. Mechanical and/or iatrogenic complications such as hemolysis, air embolus, blood leaks, and contaminated dialysate have become less common with improved equipment. Device-induced adverse reactions may occur, as exemplified by complement-mediated leukopenia and hypoxemia due to exposure of blood to cellophane. Heparin, necessary during the hemodialysis procedure, may lead to complications such as subdural hematoma and retroperitoneal, gastrointestinal, pericardial, and pleural hemorrhage. One of the major concerns in long-term dialysis patients is the high incidence of mortality related to myocardial infarction and cerebral vascular accidents. These are likely due to the preexistence and continuation of common risk factors in the uremic patient such as hypertension, hyperlipidemia, vascular calcification due to hyperparathyroidism, and high cardiac output due to anemia, among others. The potential for complications should cause the physician to evaluate the risk/benefit ratio with dialysis treatment before proceeding in the individual patient.

PERITONEAL DIALYSIS Peritoneal dialysis, like hemodialysis, may be performed in various settings and with a number of different techniques. In patients with acute renal failure, peritoneal dialysis is usually performed by placement of a stylet-type catheter, and peritoneal lavage is constantly performed for 24 to 72 h. One- to two-liter exchanges every 20 to 60 min can be carried out until the desired clinical and/or chemical improvements are achieved. The catheter is then removed and the patient observed until symptoms or laboratory results dictate the need for a further 1 to 3 days of peritoneal dialysis. Chronic peritoneal dialysis has been attempted since the late 1940s but was relatively unsuccessful until development of a permanent peritoneal catheter in 1968—the Tenckhoff catheter. Use of this indwelling catheter and closed continuous-cycle dialysate delivery equipment led to treatment protocols with which patients were treated 2 to 3 times per week for a total of 30 to 40 h to achieve clearances and fluid removal similar to those of hemodialysis. In 1978, the concept of constant peritoneal lavage with prolonged dwell times led to the development of continuous ambulatory peritoneal dialysis (CAPD), which differs from intermittent peritoneal dialysis in that patients instill fluid into the peritoneal cavity, seal the catheter, continue in an ambulatory mode, and every 4 to 6 h empty the peritoneal cavity and replace the dialysate. This technique utilizes 2-liter containers of dialysate and obviates the need for dialysis equipment. Modification of the technique using a cyclic dialysate delivery device to exchange dialysate during the night with chronic dwelling of fluid during the waking hours may be more acceptable to some patients.

Twenty-four- to seventy-two-hour peritoneal dialysis using a stylet-catheter is usually performed in a hospital setting. Intermittent peritoneal dialysis may be performed in a center or at home (usually overnight), while continuous ambulatory dialysis is performed anywhere. As with hemodialysis, the composition of the dialysate can be modified to accommodate ultrafiltration and clearance needs. The major difference in peritoneal dialysate formulas is the larger quantity of dextrose used as an osmotic agent to achieve fluid removal. Advantages of peritoneal dialysis are avoidance of heparinization and vascular surgery and a slower clearance rate which may be advantageous in some patients with cardiovascular instability. It is more amenable to total self-treatment. Disadvantages include the longer treatment time—either longer periods intermittently or continuous involvement. It should not be used in patients with recent abdominal surgery or pulmonary compromise. Inadequate clearance may occur in some patients, e.g., those with scleroderma, vasculitis, or malignant hypertension. Complications include catheter tunnel infection, peritonitis, and moderate protein loss. CAPD requires a higher degree of patient compliance and has a higher rate of peritonitis than intermittent peritoneal dialysis because of multiple entries into the system.

RESULTS At the end of 1980, approximately 48,000 patients were on chronic dialysis, while over the past 10 years, nearly 30,000 patients have undergone renal transplantation in the United States. Approximately 85 to 90 percent of patients are on hemodialysis, while 10 to 15 percent perform some type of peritoneal dialysis. Of all new patients with end-stage renal disease, approximately 35 to 50 percent are physically and psychologically suitable for renal transplantation. Many of these patients are sensitized with high antibody titers and are on hemodialysis and peritoneal dialysis awaiting availability of a cadaver kidney. An acutely ill or medically complicated patient will likely undergo dialysis in a hospital dialysis unit or intensive care unit, while stable patients may be dialyzed as outpatients in the hospital dialysis unit, in an out-of-hospital dialysis center, or at home. Most centers attempt to have patients participate in their own care, so-called self-dialysis. The percentage of patients performing home dialysis varies from 12 to 40 percent, depending upon the area of the country and factors such as population density, economics, and social issues. Home dialysis is preferable for many because of self-reliance and freedom from hospital or center dialysis schedules. Patient motivation is the primary factor in selection of home or in-center self-dialysis. Dialysis performed in the hospital setting is most expensive, while home dialysis with a nonpaid family assistant or alone (peritoneal dialysis only) is somewhat less expensive than in-center dialysis.

The mean age for patients on dialysis is the late fifties, partly because nephrosclerosis and eventual renal failure from other parenchymal diseases occur in older patients, but more likely because the selection process favors transplantation in younger patients.

Approximately 10 to 20 percent of patients with chronic renal failure are totally rehabilitated by dialysis, and another

30 to 40 percent of nondiabetic patients may be expected to be rehabilitated to a functional status even if not employed. Twenty percent of patients will be returned to a level of function not considered rehabilitated but able to care for themselves. The remainder (approximately 20 percent) are fully dependent on support from others. Diabetics, who have a rehabilitation rate and survival rate significantly lower than that of nondiabetic patients, make up much of the latter two groups. Determination of mortality rates is variable because of age and the disease process; however, most chronic dialysis programs have annual mortality rates of approximately 10 percent per year.

TRANSPLANTATION

Transplantation of the human kidney is now a justified procedure for the treatment of advanced chronic renal failure. Worldwide, tens of thousands of such procedures have been performed and occur at the rate of 50 or more per year in some medical centers. The results with properly matched familial donors are superior to those obtained with organs from cadaveric donors, with 75 to 90 percent compared to 50 to 60 percent graft survival rates at 1 year, respectively. Grafts functioning at 1 year are rejected at a much slower rate over the subsequent years, although occasionally a graft may suffer an acute irreversible rejection episode after many months of good function. The most striking improvement in clinical renal transplant results in recent years is in patient morbidity and mortality rates, the latter declining to less than 5 percent in a number of centers. These findings represent an increasing tendency on the part of transplant teams to decrease immunosuppressive therapy so that in the case of severe rejection the kidney rather than the patient is lost. The figures for graft survival, however, show little overall improvement since 1970, suggesting that methods of immunosuppressive therapy, which have been uniformly utilized from 1970 to the present, remain relatively inadequate. Most striking are the accumulated data showing clear beneficial effects of blood transfusions in the preconditioning of potential recipients. Nontransfused recipients are at highest risk for rejecting their grafts, while multiple random transfusions or transfusions from specific donors can greatly improve chances for graft survival. An increasing number of second and even third transplants are being performed, and the overall results are comparable to those with first transplants; in other words, rejection of a graft does not necessarily prejudice the results of another transplant attempt.

SELECTION OF RECIPIENTS FOR KIDNEY TRANSPLANTATION Table 292-1 lists practical considerations in the selection of a recipient for a human renal allograft. Such a procedure should be undertaken only when conservative treatment has failed, when there are no reversible elements in the patient's renal failure, and when the patient is too ill to be maintained comfortably with the usual methods of treatment. However, morbidity is lessened if transplantation is performed before the patient is critically ill. Provision of adequate amounts of transfused blood prior to transplantation is of major importance. Transplantation should not be utilized in an attempt to salvage patients from failure to thrive on dialysis. On the other hand, when no well-matched related donor is available, the patient and physician should consider carefully the relative risks against those of continued dialysis and this will depend upon the specifics of each case. Overall, approximately 4 to 7 percent of dialysis or transplant patients of comparable age and general condition die each year. The recipient should be free of life-threatening extrarenal complications such as cancer, severe coronary artery disease, and cerebrovascular disease. Provided that diffuse vascular involvement is not present, diabetes itself is not a contraindication. Oxalosis can be expected to recur in relatively short order in a transplanted kidney. Although age may be a limiting factor, it is advanced "physiologic" rather than the chronologic age which contraindicates transplantation. Although abnormalities of the bladder and urethra present additional hazards, successful renal allografts have been placed in individuals with these abnormalities by prior construction of an artificial bladder (i.e., ileal conduit) into which the donor ureter is placed.

DONOR SELECTION Donor sources are cadavers or volunteer blood-related living donors. Living volunteer donors should be normal on physical examination and of the same major ABO blood group, because there is good evidence that crossing major blood group barriers prejudices survival of the allograft. It is, however, possible to transplant a kidney of a type O donor into an A, B, or AB recipient. Selective renal arteriography should be performed on volunteer donors to rule out the presence of multiple or abnormal renal arteries, because the surgical procedure is inordinately difficult and the ischemic time of the transplanted kidney prohibitively long when vascular abnormalities exist. Cadaveric donors should be free of malignant neoplastic disease because of the possible transmission of cancer to the recipient.

A coordinated regional or national system of computerized information sharing and logistical support for the transportation of cadaver kidneys to suitable recipients is under development. It is now possible to remove cadaver kidneys and to maintain them for up to 48 h on cold pulsatile perfusion or simple flushing and cooling. This should permit adequate time for various typing, cross matching, transportation, and selection problems to be solved.

TISSUE TYPING AND CLINICAL IMMUNOGENETICS Matching for antigens of the HLA major histocompatibility gene complex (Chap. 60) has long been accepted as an ideal criterion for selection of donors for renal allografts. Each mammalian species studied has shown evidence for a single chromosomal region which encodes the strong, or major, transplantation antigens, and the analogous sixth chromosomal region is called *HLA* in human beings. Other antigens, called "minor," may nevertheless play crucial roles, especially the ABH blood groups and a newly defined endothelial antigen which is shared with blood monocytes, but not lymphocytes. Evidence for designation of HLA as the genetic region encoding strong transplantation antigens comes from the success rate in living related donor renal and bone marrow transplantation, with superior results in HLA-identical sibling pairs. Nevertheless,

TABLE 292-1
Contraindications to kidney transplantation

1 Absolute contraindications
- *a* Reversible renal involvement
- *b* Ability of conservative measures to maintain useful life
- *c* Advanced forms of major extrarenal complications (cerebrovascular or coronary disease, neoplasia)
- *d* Active infection
- *e* Oxalosis
- *f* Active glomerulonephritis
- *g* Previous sensitization to donor tissue

2 Relative contraindications (see text)
- *a* Age
- *b* Presence of vesical or urethral abnormalities
- *c* Iliofemoral occlusive disease
- *d* Diabetes mellitus
- *e* Psychiatric problems

10 to 15 percent of HLA-identical renal allografts are rejected, often within the first weeks after transplantation. It is likely, though not proved, that these failures represent states of prior sensitization to non-HLA antigens. Non-HLA antigens are relatively weak and therefore suppressible by conventional immunosuppressive therapy. Once priming has occurred, however, secondary responses are much more refractory to treatment. In fact, ABH incompatibilities are hazardous because of the presence of natural anti-A and anti-B antibodies.

Living related donors Among first-degree relatives, the general level of expected graft success is in direct proportion to matching for 2,1, or no HLA haplotypes, as defined by HLA serologic typing and the presence or absence of a proliferative response in the mixed lymphocyte culture (MLC) (Chap. 60). HLA-incompatible siblings do barely better than the overall average with cadaveric donors (50 to 60 percent at 1 year), while HLA semi-identicals (haploidentical) are in the 70 to 75 percent range. Since a number of poorly matched grafts in fact do quite well, it is apparent that matching does not necessarily provide a measure of the degree of incompatibility. Intrafamilial MLCs among haploidenticals can be a measure of responsiveness. Low responder donor-recipient pairs have a 1-year graft survival rate of 90 percent, while vigorous responders are at the level of 55 percent. The MLC is a relatively imprecise technique, but when carefully performed, it may be useful for selection of those living related HLA-haploidentical donors whose organs will be better tolerated.

Cadaveric donors The overall success rate for unrelated donors is 50 to 60 percent of grafts functioning at 1 year. It has been extremely difficult to assess the role of HLA matching in cadaveric donor grafting because of considerable variation in overall results from center to center, including, until recently, relatively high mortality rates. The so-called full-house match of two HLA-A and two HLA-B antigens between unrelated individuals does not ensure matching for other loci adjacent to HLA-A and -B, in contrast to first-degree relatives where the HLA-A and -B antigens are excellent markers for the other linked loci. The degree to which two-A and two-B antigen matching improves cadaveric renal graft survival is in the range of 10 percent and is most likely attributable to the fact that some of these matches will also include compatibility for HLA-D because of the nonrandomness of the association of linked alleles (linkage disequilibrium) in the population (Chap. 60). The more racially homogeneous the population, the greater the chances that any given marker will be in linkage disequilibrium with another.

HLA-D and -DR are not strictly identical (Chap. 60). The availability of reagents to type for HLA-DR antigens, as expressed on peripheral blood B lymphocytes and monocytes, makes rapid approximation of HLA-D compatibility feasible. The results seem to confirm the importance of matching for both DR alleles, with 10 percent or more improvement over one or no matches. Although some additional benefit may be gained by HLA-A and -B matching, the major effect so far seems to be with consideration of DR alone. Rapid assessment (e.g., 24 h) of the MLC response for HLA-D is currently not possible.

Presensitization A positive cross match of recipient serum with donor T lymphocytes is usually predictive of an acute vasculitic event termed *hyperacute* rejection. A few years ago it was thought that patients making such antibodies against a surrogate panel of normal lymphocytes were at high risk for accelerated, if not hyperacute, rejection, even when the donor-specific cross match was negative. That this is no longer so can be attributed to the greater efforts being made in monitoring patients on dialysis, defining not only the presence or absence of antibodies but also the HLA antigens to which they are directed. Patients sustained by hemodialysis often show fluctuating antibody titers and specificity patterns, sometimes, but not always, temporally related to receipt of blood transfusions. At the time of assignment of a cadaveric kidney, cross matches are performed with more than one highly reactive serum, and the previously analyzed antibody specificities are also taken into account. Another advance has been the finding that presensitization to antigens expressed on B lymphocytes, but not T lymphocytes, is not a contraindication to transplantation. Many of these antibodies are anti-DR, while others are non-HLA IgM antibodies active in the cold and at room temperature, which may also be autoreactive.

Endothelial-monocyte system In some cases of unexpected accelerated rejection, antibodies with reactivity to renal endothelium and blood monocytes have been found, both in the circulation and in eluates from rejected grafts. Practical techniques of typing and cross matching for this non-HLA system are under development. Second transplants following rapid loss of the first graft seem to be particularly at risk.

Overview of transplantation immunogenetics In addition to the ABO blood groups, the important histocompatibility antigens presently known are HLA-A, -B, -C, -DR, and the endothelial-monocyte system (Table 292-2 and Chap. 60). The best current data suggest that major immunogenicity lies in the DR antigens, while A, B, C, and endothelial-monocyte antigens provide the major targets for effector IgG, and in the case of A, B, and C, at least, for killer T lymphocytes. Hence the current emphasis is on A, B, and C cross matching and DR matching.

Blood transfusions At a time when it appeared that transfusion-induced sensitization against a random lymphocyte panel was predictive of a high graft failure rate, a number of transplantation units undertook a policy of withholding blood from as many dialysis patients as possible. The clinical need for blood was found to be less than originally thought, especially in nonnephrectomized patients, and avoidance of possible exposure to hepatitis was also a consideration. The overall experience with the nontransfused patients has been a dramatic one, confirmed many times over: such patients are at the *highest risk* for graft failure. Still at issue is the number of transfused units needed for optimal graft survival, with the bulk of the evidence showing that more than 10 units is optimal (Fig. 292-1), although some studies claim an effect with 1 or 2 units, given in advance or at the time of transplantation. Data are presently lacking on the question of using fresh vs. frozen vs. washed cells, as well as the precise methods of storage em-

TABLE 292-2
Histocompatibility in renal transplantation
RELATIVE IMPORTANCE OF TYPING AND CROSS MATCHING FOR SEROLOGICALLY DEFINED ANTIGENS

Antigens	*Typing (antigen matching)*	*Cross matching*
Class I (HLA-A, -B, -C)	+	+++
Class II (HLA-DR)	+++	−
Endothelial-monocyte (non-HLA)	?−	+++

ployed. As in many areas of clinical transplantation, there are not a sufficient number of cases and/or carefully randomized trials. Nevertheless, the large number of cases included in prospective studies has already provided impressive overall evidence that the greater the number of pretransplant transfusions the better the graft survival.

The mechanisms of the transfusion effect are unknown but may involve a selection process of screening out responders to certain HLA antigens, or, alternatively, transfusions may induce states of specific suppression. Assessment of the combined effects of transfusions and DR matching shows that they are not additive. If there is a good match for HLA-DR antigens, prior priming to induce low responsiveness appears to be unnecessary. Alternatively, if the recipient is exposed to multiple units of blood, HLA-DR matching adds no further benefit. Living donor haploidentical grafts also benefit from blood transfusions. In particular, the use of blood from the intended donor on three occasions prior to transplantation results in superior graft survival in those 70 percent of recipients who do not become sensitized to HLA. Part of the effect is one of selection of antibody nonresponders; in addition, it is likely that specific suppression is induced. The preliminary data with donor-specific transfusions show a success rate of greater than 90 percent at 1 year, in the range attained by HLA identical grafts.

IMMUNOLOGY OF REJECTION Knowledge of the immunology of tissue transplantation stems largely from animal experimentation. However, enough evidence has accumulated in humans, particularly in kidney transplantation, to indicate that the evidence is similar though not identical for the different species. The immunological mechanisms are not qualitatively different from those found in other areas of immunology (Chap. 61). The evidence is that early rejection is associated with T lymphocytes (Tc) having direct antigen-specific cytotoxicity against donor antigens. However, significant numbers of B lymphocytes, null cells, and macrophages appear in the early infiltrate, and cells capable of mediating antibody-dependent cell-mediated cytotoxicity (ADCC) are also present (Fig. 292-2). Later in the process of rejection, antigen-specific cytotoxic cells appear, which do not bear the usual T-cell markers. B lymphocytes are not only present, but many of them also produce immunoglobulins. The spectrum of cellular and humoral response and graft injury is quite varied, depending upon specific genetic differences between donor and recipient and states of presensitization. All of the processes shown in Fig. 292-2 are possible, but their relative contribution varies from case to case. Further dissection of the heterogeneity of the human allograft response, utilizing newer techniques for identification of lymphocyte subsets, may add to the value of graft biopsy as a guide to therapy and prognosis.

The failure of transplanted kidneys after 2 or even 3 years of adequate function is due to a form of "chronic rejection." In such kidneys the development of nephrosclerosis, with proliferation of the vascular intima of renal vessels, and intimal fibrosis, with marked decrease in the lumen of the vessels, takes place (Fig. 292-3). The result is renal ischemia, hypertension,

FIGURE 292-1
Beneficial effect of blood transfusions from random donors prior to grafting from a cadaveric renal donor. There is a significant increase in graft survival rates with increasing numbers of units transfused, shown on the right in steps from 0 to >20 units. The numbers in parentheses are the total numbers of cases at risk in each transfusion category. The numbers of cases observed at 3 months are indicated next to the curves. These data, confirmed in several other studies, are from the 8th International Histocompatibility Workshop, 1980. (From Opelz and Terasaki.)

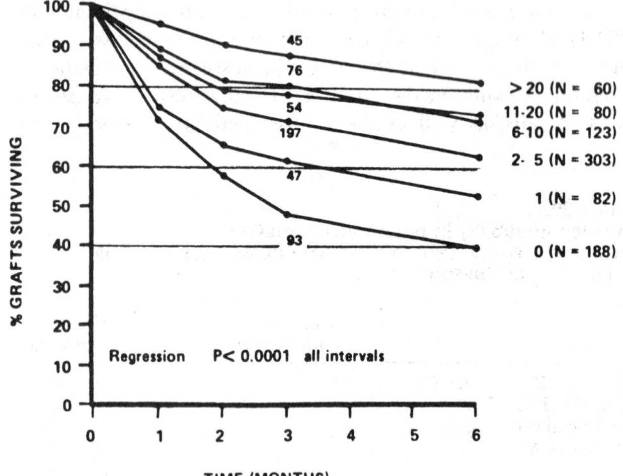

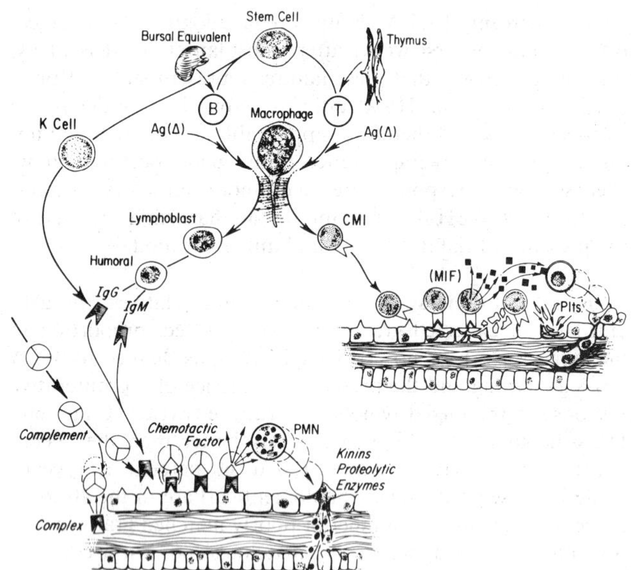

FIGURE 292-2
Overall scheme of the development of effector mechanisms in graft rejection. Bone marrow stem cells differentiate under the influence of the thymus gland into mature thymus-derived (T) lymphocytes, or under the influence of an equivalent to the avian bursa of Fabricius into mature bone-marrow-derived (B) lymphocytes. Exposure to antigen (Δ) results in an interaction between T cells and B cells, and often involves macrophages. The sensitized B cells, after mitoses, develop into immunoglobulin-secreting cells (e.g., plasma cells), illustrated here by IgG and IgM. Such immunoglobulins may form immune complexes with antigen in the circulation which activate the complement sequence, or they may react directly with antigens on the blood vessel surface. Elaboration of secondary mediators, including the products of complement activation, results in vascular damage as illustrated. Sensitized T lymphocytes are the primary effector cells in cell-mediated immunity (CMI) and may react directly with antigens in the graft to exert a cytotoxic effect. In addition, T cells release factors, such as macrophage migration inhibition factor (MIF), which may accelerate the rate of mononuclear cell infiltration. It has also been shown that unsensitized non-T cells (K cells) can be activated to exert cytotoxic effects by the fixation of IgG to target cells, followed by interaction of the IgG (Fc portion) with a receptor on the K cell. Finally, platelet aggregation and thrombosis can occur following the endothelial damage induced by any of these mechanisms.

widespread tubular atrophy, interstitial fibrosis, and glomerular atrophy with eventual renal failure.

IMMUNOSUPPRESSIVE TREATMENT When histocompatibility differences exist between donor and recipient, it is necessary to modify or suppress the immune response in order to enable the recipient to accept a graft. Immunosuppressive therapy, in general, suppresses all immune responses, including those to bacteria, fungi, and even malignant tumors. In the 1950s when clinical renal transplantation began, sublethal total-body irradiation was employed. Currently, immunosuppression is more safely induced pharmacologically. Agents used in humans to suppress the immune response are the following:

Drugs *Azathioprine* (Imuran), an analogue of mercaptopurine, is the keystone to immunosuppressive therapy in humans. This agent can inhibit synthesis of deoxyribonucleic acid (DNA), ribonucleic acid (RNA), or both. Because cell division and proliferation are a necessary part of the immune response to antigenic stimulation, suppression by this agent may be mediated by the inhibition of mitosis of immunologically competent lymphoid cells, interfering with synthesis of DNA. Alternatively, immunosuppression may be brought about by blocking the synthesis of RNA (possibly messenger RNA), to inhibit processing of antigens prior to lymphocyte stimulation. This drug has little effect in suppressing a secondary immune response, however. Therapy with azathioprine is generally instituted 2 days prior to transplantation in the recipient of a living donor kidney and on the day of transplantation in the case of a cadaveric donor kidney recipient at a level of 4 mg/kg per day. The drug is later tapered to levels of 1.5 to 3 mg/kg per day, as long as the allograft functions. Because the drug is rapidly metabolized by the liver, its dosage need not be varied directly in relation to renal function, even though renal failure results in retention of the metabolites of azathioprine. Some patients are unusually sensitive to this drug, particularly when renal function is compromised, and reduction in dosage is required because of leukopenia and occasionally thrombocytopenia. Excessive amounts of azathioprine may also cause jaundice, anemia, and alopecia. If it is essential to administer allopurinol concurrently, the azathioprine dose must be drastically reduced, since inhibition of xanthine oxidase delays degradation. This combination is best avoided.

FIGURE 292-3
Biopsy of the renal cadaveric allograft illustrating obliterative endarteritis. Loss of the media is associated with intimal thickening. The elastic tissue shows dissolution of the elastica. The evidence for arteritis with subsequent thrombosis is typically the gaps in the elastica and media. The intimal thickening probably represents organization of a thrombus formed in response to the arteritis. [From GJ Dammin, JP Merrill, in Structural Basis for Renal Disease, EL Becker (ed), New York, Hoeber-Harper, 1968.]

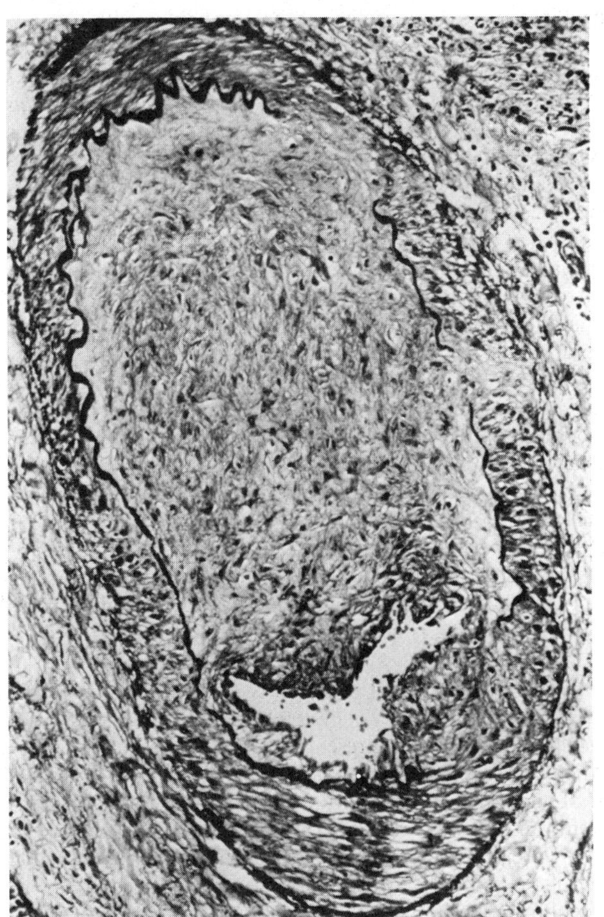

The *glucocorticosteroids* are important adjuncts to immunosuppressive therapy. Of all the agents employed, prednisone has effects that are easiest to assess, and in large doses it is unquestionably the most effective agent for the reversal of rejection. In general, 30 to 40 mg prednisone is given immediately prior to or at the time of transplantation, and the dosage is gradually reduced. The well-known side effects of the glucocorticosteroids, particularly impairment of wound healing and predisposition to infection, make it desirable to taper the dose as rapidly as possible in the immediate postoperative period. Customarily methylprednisolone, 1 to 2 g intravenously, is administered immediately upon diagnosis of beginning rejection and continued once daily for 3 days. When the drug is effective, the results are usually apparent within 48 to 96 h. Such "pulse" doses are less effective in the slow rejection process, which may not become apparent until 2 to 3 years after transplantation. Most patients whose renal function is stable after 6 months or a year do not require large doses of prednisone; maintenance doses of 15 or 20 mg per day are the rule. Many patients tolerate an alternate-day course of steroids better than daily doses without an increased risk of rejection.

The mechanisms of steroid effects are uncertain. Although lymphopenia results from large doses of corticosteroids, this is primarily due to sequestration of recirculating blood lymphocytes to lymphoid tissue. There is recent evidence that steroids block clonal expansion of effector T cells by preventing production of T-cell growth factor (Interleukin 2).

When jaundice or nephritis appears in patients maintained on azathioprine, *cyclophosphamide* may be substituted. It appears to be as effective in the maintenance of renal allografts as azathioprine and somewhat more effective in hepatic allografts. Leukopenia, alopecia, cystitis, ovarian fibrosis, and aspermia may result if the dosage is not carefully regulated. Prospective cadaveric *donors* have been treated with massive doses of cyclophosphamide and methylprednisolone in an attempt to decrease the antigenicity of the graft by eliminating "passenger leukocytes." The results of this technique are somewhat uncertain.

Cyclosporin A is a fungal peptide having potent antilymphocytic activity in animals and in in vitro systems. It appears to have a preferential effect upon early activation of helper-inducer T lymphocytes, thereby augmenting suppressor T-cell responses. Assessment of this agent in human renal transplantation is currently under way in a number of trials. Early results are encouraging, although it seems to work well only in conjunction with corticosteroids. Some incidence of nephrotoxicity, hepatotoxicity, and lymphomas has been reported.

Antilymphocyte globulin (ALG) When serum from animals made immune to host lymphocytes is injected into the recipient, a marked suppression of cellular immunity to the tissue graft results. The action upon cell-mediated immunity is considerably greater than upon humoral immunity. A globulin fraction of the serum is the agent generally employed. For use in humans, peripheral human lymphocytes, thymocytes, or lymphocytes from spleens or thoracic duct fistulas have been injected into horses, rabbits, or goats to produce antilymphocyte serum, from which the globulin fraction is then separated. Although ALG, or ATG (antithymocyte globulin), is unquestionably effective in prolonging grafts in experimental animals, its efficacy in the transplantation of human tissue is somewhat less clear. Heterologous antibody against defined T-lymphocyte subsets, in the form of mouse antihuman monoclonal IgG, may offer a more precise approach to this form of therapy.

Other techniques Among other techniques of immunosuppression, thymectomy and splenectomy have not been widely accepted. Local irradiation of the transplanted kidney in two or three doses of 3500 mGy (350 rads) each has also been utilized. This technique may result in fewer early rejection episodes in cadaveric transplants than in nonirradiated controls. Fractional total lymph node irradiation, as employed in the therapy of Hodgkin's disease, is an interesting new modality currently under investigation.

CLINICAL COURSE AND MANAGEMENT OF THE RECIPIENT

Bilateral nephrectomy at some point prior to transplantation is performed for a specific cause but not as a routine. Hypertension which is difficult to control or infection involving the end-stage kidneys are the two most common indications. Nephrectomized patients maintain a much lower hematocrit level, but this is no longer considered a disadvantage per se, because blood transfusions need not be avoided in preparation for transplantation. Difficulties do arise when these multiply transfused patients become sensitized and must remain on dialysis. Nephrectomy per se does not appear to affect the survival of subsequent renal allografts.

Adequate hemodialysis should be performed within 48 h of surgery, and care should be taken that the serum potassium level is not markedly elevated so that intraoperative cardiac arrhythmias can be averted. The diuresis that commonly occurs postoperatively must be carefully monitored; in many instances it may be massive, reflecting the inability of ischemic tubules to regulate sodium and water excretion. Massive potassium losses may occur and occasionally result in cardiac arrhythmias. Most chronically uremic patients have some excess of extracellular fluid, and some degree of negative balance should be accomplished, provided circulatory hemodynamics remain stable. Acute tubular necrosis (ATN) may cause immediate oliguria or may follow an initial short period of graft function. ATN is most likely to occur when cadaveric donors have been hypotensive, or if the interval between cessation of blood flow and organ harvest (warm ischemic time) has been more than a few minutes. Recovery usually occurs within 3 weeks, although periods as long as 6 weeks have been reported. Superimposition of rejection upon ATN is common, and the differential diagnosis may be difficult.

The rejection episode Early diagnosis of rejection allows prompt institution of therapy to preserve renal function and prevent irreversible damage due to fibrosis. Clinical evidence of rejection may be characterized by fever, swelling, and tenderness over the allograft, and by significant reduction in urine volume. In patients whose renal function is good initially, oliguria may be accompanied by decreased urinary sodium concentration and increased osmolarity. These changes may not be present in the more chronic stages of rejection or when renal function is impaired at the onset of rejection.

Arteriography and radioactive iodohippurate sodium (Hippuran) renograms of the transplanted kidney may be useful in ascertaining changes in the renal vasculature and in renal blood flow, even in the absence of urinary flow. Diagnostic ultrasound has become the procedure of choice to rule out urinary obstruction or to confirm the presence of perirenal collections of urine, blood, or lymph. When renal function has been good initially, a rise in the serum creatinine level and a decrease in the creatinine clearance is the most sensitive and reliable indicator of rejection.

Management problems Modification of the usual clinical manifestations of infection by immunosuppressive therapy is a major problem in the posttransplant period. The signs and symptoms of infection may be masked and distorted, and fever without obvious cause is common. Only after days or weeks will it become apparent that it has a viral or fungal origin. The importance of blood cultures in such patients cannot be overemphasized, because systemic infection without obvious foci is frequent, although wound infections with or without urinary fistulas are most common. Particularly important are rapidly occurring pulmonary lesions, which may result in death within 5 days of onset. When these become apparent, immunosuppressive agents should be discontinued except for maintenance doses of prednisone. In the case of *Pneumocystis carinii* (Chap. 222) trimethoprim-sulfamethoxazole is the treatment of choice; amphotericin B has been used effectively in systemic fungal infections. Involvement of the oropharynx with *Candida* (Chap. 184) may be treated with local nystatin. Small doses (a total of 300 mg) of amphotericin given over a period of 2 weeks may be effective in refractory oral candidiasis. *Aspergillus* (Chap. 184), *Nocardia* (Chap. 182), and cytomegalovirus (CMV) (Chap. 211) infections also occur. The latter are particularly common in transplant recipients, and active CMV infection is frequently associated with rejection episodes. The complications of corticosteroid therapy are well known and include gastrointestinal bleeding, hemorrhagic pancreatitis, impairment of wound healing, osteoporosis, diabetes, and cataract formation. The treatment of jaundice in transplant patients should include cessation of azathioprine therapy. It is surprising that total cessation of azathioprine therapy often does not result in rejection of a graft. In some instances of jaundice, cyclophosphamide may be substituted for azathioprine. Antiplatelet agents and anticoagulants, although effective in theory, have not been successful in the prevention of the chronic vascular lesion.

In spite of the potential teratogenic effects of immunosuppressive agents, both women and men have become parents after transplantation. The incidence of congenital abnormalities in the offspring is not unusual.

Glomerular lesions Even identical twins who do not require immunosuppression may develop glomerular lesions after transplantation. These represent recurrence of a glomerulonephritic process. Glomerular lesions may occur in 10 to 15 percent of allografts, even when the original disease was accidental removal of a solitary kidney. The pathogenesis is related to a chronic rejection process. In other cases the lesions resemble those of the patient's own original disease. The recurrence of the nephrotic syndrome with "nil disease" in transplanted kidneys whose recipient's original nil disease had progressed to renal failure with focal sclerosis, and the recurrence in renal allografts of the classic lesions of IgA nephropathy and of membranoproliferative glomerulonephritis with electron-dense deposit disease are classic examples. In the last of these, the incidence of recurrence has been reported to be as high as 30 to 40 percent. In most instances, however, the recurrence of the original renal lesions represents no threat to the patient's immediate prognosis, and a primary diagnosis of glomerulonephritis is rarely taken as a contraindication to transplantation.

Malignancy The incidence of tumors arising in patients on immunosuppressive therapy is 5 to 6 percent, or approximately 100 times greater than that observed in the general population in the same age range. The most common lesions are cancer of the skin and lips and carcinoma in situ of the cervix, as well as lymphomas, particularly reticulum cell sarcoma in the central nervous system and gastrointestinal tract.

Other complications *Hypercalcemia* after transplantation may indicate failure of hyperplastic parathyroid glands to regress. Aseptic necrosis of the head of the femur is probably due to preexisting hyperparathyroidism. With improved management of calcium and phosphorus metabolism during chronic dialysis the incidence of parathyroid-related complications has fallen dramatically.

Both chronic dialysis and renal transplant patients have a higher incidence of death from myocardial infarction and stroke than in the population at large, and this is particularly true in diabetics. Contributing factors are hypertension and hypertriglyceridemia. Depressed high-density lipoprotein cholesterol (HDL) concentrations in dialysis patients may persist after transplantation.

REFERENCES

CARPENTER CB et al: Renal transplantation: Immunobiology, in *The Kidney,* B Brenner, F Rector (eds). Philadelphia, Saunders, 1981, pp 2544–2598

GOTCH FA: Progress in hemodialysis. Clin Nephrol 9:144, 1978

HOLLENBERG NK, TILNEY NL: Renal transplantation: Donor selection and surgical aspects, in *The Kidney,* B Brenner, F Rector (eds). Philadelphia, Saunders, 1981, pp 2599–2617

LAZARUS JM: Complications in hemodialysis: An overview. Kidney Intern 18:783, 1980

———, KJELLSTRAND CM: Dialysis: Medical aspects, in *The Kidney,* B Brenner, F Rector (eds). Philadelphia, Saunders, 1981, pp 2491–2543

MANIS T, FREIDMAN EA: Dialytic therapy for irreversible uremia. N Engl J Med 301:1321, 1979

MERRILL JP: Dialysis versus transplantation in the treatment of end stage renal disease. Ann Rev Med 29:343, 1978

MORRIS PJ (ed): *Kidney Transplantation. Principles and Practice.* New York, Grune & Stratton, 1979

NOLPH KD et al: Continuous ambulatory peritoneal dialysis: Three-year experience at one center. Ann Intern Med 92:609, 1980

OPELZ G, TERASAKI PI: International Histocompatibility Workshop on Renal Transplantation, in *Histocompatibility Testing 1980,* PI Terasaki (ed). UCLA Tissue Typing Laboratory, 1980, pp 592–624

STROM TB et al: Renal transplantation: Clinical management of the transplant recipient, in *The Kidney,* B Brenner, FC Rector (eds). Philadelphia, Saunders, 1981, pp 2618–2658

293 IMMUNOPATHOGENETIC MECHANISMS OF RENAL INJURY

RICHARD J. GLASSOCK
BARRY M. BRENNER

Recognition of the important role played by aberrant immunologic processes in many forms of renal injury, especially those involving the glomerular circulation, constitutes one of the most significant conceptual advances made in the understanding of renal diseases during the last quarter century. Although the fine details of these abnormal processes have been elucidated for many disease entities, large gaps in knowledge still exist concerning both the initiating events and the etiological factors involved in renal disease.

In its broadest conceptual framework the immunopathogenesis of renal injury can be simplified to a few fundamental mechanisms, which are presented in Chap. 63. One involves the reaction of a circulating antibody with its respective renal antigen in situ. The antigen may be either an intrinsic constituent of the kidney or one which has been bound to the tissue by some special biochemical or immunological reaction. Antigens in basement membranes of glomerular capillaries or renal tubules and antibodies to these basement membranes are prime components of this mechanism. A variety of antigenic components of the glomerular capillary walls and renal tubules are now recognized. Binding of circulating antibody to these tissue antigens gives rise to several distinctive structural alterations and immunohistochemical appearances, as will be discussed below. This category of immune processes is often referred to as the *antitissue antibody–mediated diseases.*

Another pathogenetic category, by far the most prevalent in human renal disease, involves the localization of circulating macromolecular aggregates composed of antigens and antibodies (i.e., circulating immune complexes) within renal structures, principally glomeruli. This mechanism is referred to as *immune-complex–mediated disease.* The immune complexes need not bear any special immunochemical relationships to renal structures; thus the kidney can be viewed as a passive participant or an innocent party, damaged by processes originating elsewhere. The source of the antigen may be either *endogenous* (*autologous*) or *exogenous* (*environmental*). Further, exogenous antigens may be biologically inert or derived from an organism capable of self-replication (e.g., bacteria, viruses, etc.). Under special circumstances environmental agents may also combine with autologous substances to result in new antigenic compounds (hapten-protein conjugates), which may act in concert with antibodies to form immune complexes. In contrast to the above mechanisms, *cell-mediated* immune processes are far less well established as possible mechanisms in glomerular and vascular diseases of the kidney. Finally, certain human glomerular diseases are prominently associated with abnormal activation of the *alternative pathway of the complement cascade.*

IMMUNOPATHOGENETIC MECHANISMS Once initiated, immune injury is mediated by the interaction of a number of humoral and cellular factors. Activation of the complement (C) cascade may lead to the direct cytolysis of the cellular constituents of the glomerulus or may lead to the production of biologically active fragments capable of enhancing vascular permeability or attracting polymorphonuclear leukocytes and other cellular constituents. Coagulation may be directly initiated by alterations in the endothelial surface and exposure of collagen matrix, followed by localized platelet aggregation. Interactions between the complement cascade and coagulation are numerous and complex. Complement activation may trigger coagulation and vice versa. Activation of the Hageman factor may initiate the kallikrein-kinin system. Potent vasoactive peptides may thus be released and play a role in alterations in local and systemic hemodynamics observed in conjunction with immunologically induced renal diseases. Polymorphonuclear leukocytes, eosinophils, and monocytes (macrophages), and platelets all may be called forth to participate in immune-mediated injury to varying degrees. Polymorphonuclear leukocytes and monocytes appear to participate in glomerular injury by virtue of their ability to release factors locally which are capable of degrading basement membrane glycoproteins enzymatically. Platelet deposition may be involved in the proliferation of glomerular cells via the release of a platelet-derived growth factor. Under certain circumstances structural and/or functional alterations of the glomerulus may occur solely as a result of the interaction of antibody with tissue antigens or the deposition of immune complexes without the necessary participation or activation of other hormonal or cellular factors.

ANTITISSUE ANTIBODY-MEDIATED RENAL INJURY Anti-basement membrane antibody disease This form of renal injury is relatively rare in humans, accounting for less than 5 percent of all immunologically mediated glomerulonephritides. The experimental prototype of this mechanism is nephrotoxic serum nephritis. Here an antibody to glomerular basement membrane (GBM) of one species (e.g., rat) is raised in another species (e.g., rabbit). The anti-GBM antibody is then administered intravenously to the species originally providing the immunogen (e.g., rat). The *heterologous* antibody binds rapidly to its respective antigen in the GBM. In this instance the antigen is a noncollagen glycoprotein which is uniformly distributed along the glomerular capillary wall as repeating subunits. Therefore, the deposited immunoglobulin (Ig) will assume a linear pattern by immunofluorescence microscopy (Fig. 293-1*A*). If sufficient heterologous antibody has been administered and bound, various mediator factors are induced. These include the complement and coagulation cascades, vasoactive peptides and amines, and polymorphonuclear leukocytes and macrophages (monocytes). These mediators act to disturb the functional and anatomical integrity of the glomerular capillary wall, leading to proteinuria. Proliferation of cellular elements within the glomerulus, by causing capillary luminal obstruction and hemodynamic alterations, results in a reduction in the glomerular filtration rate. Local enzyme release from storage sites in infiltrating cells may lead to fragmentation of the GBM and leakage of macromolecules, such as fibrinogen, as well as migration of cellular elements, such as macrophages and erythrocytes, into Bowman's space. In the presence of severe glomerular capillary wall damage there may be associated extracapillary proliferation (crescents). Under many circumstances such extracapillary proliferation is dependent upon the polymerization of fibrin within Bowman's space. Although the activation of the complement cascade facilitates injury by virtue of chemotactic and cytolytic effects, glomerular injury may occur independent of complement activation. For example, by virtue of surface receptors for an altered Fc portion of Ig, cells such as polymorphonuclear leukocytes and macrophages are attracted to sites of antibody deposition. This *heterologous phase* of nephrotoxic serum nephritis would be self-limited were it not for the fact that the deposited Ig is foreign to the host and therefore quite distinct from the original GBM antigen reacting with the heterologous antibody. As a consequence, a host-directed response to the deposited foreign Ig perpetuates the glomerular injury and leads to chronic disease. This is referred to as the *autologous phase* of nephrotoxic serum nephritis. Remarkably little "foreign" antigen is required to initiate this phase, so little in fact that amounts, classes, or subunits of

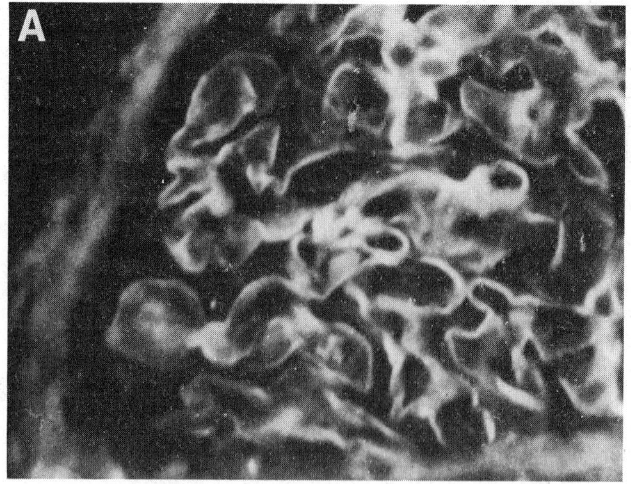

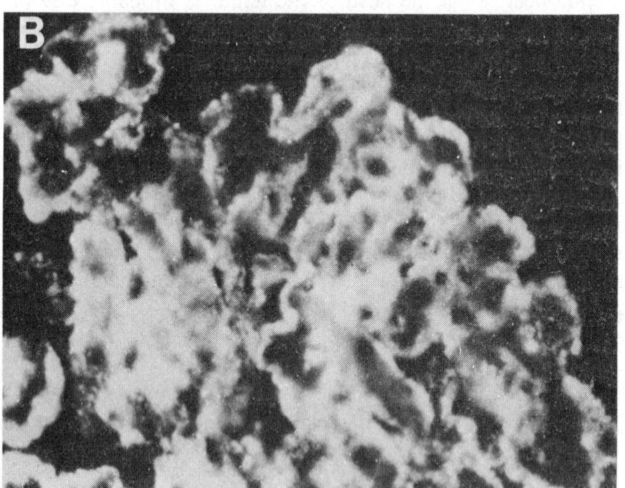

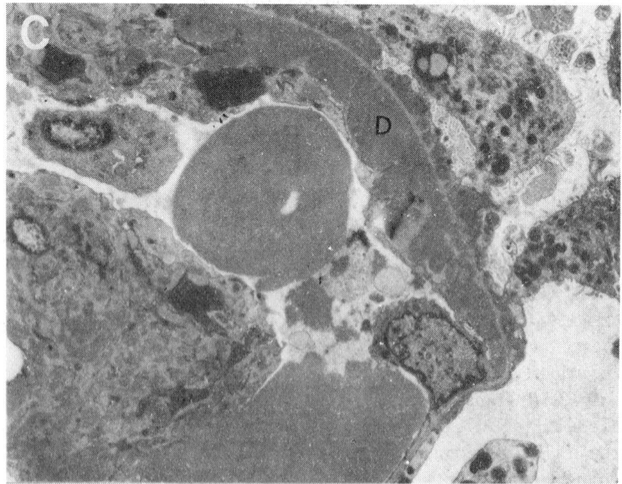

FIGURE 293-1

A. Immunofluorescence photomicrograph of a portion of a glomerulus from a patient with antiglomerular basement membrane antibody–mediated glomerular injury. Note the linear deposits (fluorescein-labeled anti-human IgG). B. Immunofluorescence photomicrograph of a portion of a glomerulus from a patient with immune-complex–mediated glomerular injury. Note the irregular, granular deposits (fluorescein-labeled anti-human IgG). C. Electron micrograph of a portion of a glomerular capillary from a patient with immune-complex–mediated glomerular injury. Note the electron-dense deposits (D).

heterologous antibody to GBM incapable of initiating injury in their own right can induce an autologous phase if the host response is magnified by preimmunization to foreign Ig. Both humoral and cellular immune mechanisms participate in the perpetuation of glomerular injury in the autologous phase.

Glomerular injury of the type seen in the laboratory model of nephrotoxic serum nephritis rarely occurs in humans. However, in the early days of renal transplantation some preparations of heterologous antilymphocyte serum used to suppress allograft rejection were contaminated with antibodies to human GBM antigens, and nephrotoxic serum nephritis was inadvertently produced in transplant recipients in the treatment of rejection with these preparations.

The formation of antibodies to autologous renal structures may also be induced by intentional immunization of animals with renal antigens (e.g., GBM or tubule basement membranes, TBM), usually in conjunction with adjuvants. Under most circumstances the antigen consists of semipurified extracts of homologous or heterologous GBM or TBM. These antigens possess some degree of cross reactivity with autologous antigens. It is also theoretically possible that altered autologous antigens, released into the circulation consequent to tissue injury, might induce antibody production to normal autologous antigens. The active induction of antitissue autoantibody disease by immunization with organ extracts and adjuvants is a well-studied phenomenon. Such immunization results in the termination of natural tolerance to autologous tissue antigens. The precise mechanism by which this is brought about is unknown, but may involve the calling forth of T-helper cells to interact with dormant B cells already genetically programmed to synthesize antibody to self-constituents. The expansion of autoreactive clones of B cells leads to production of circulating antibody. Other mechanisms may also be involved, including modulation of the activity of T-suppressor cells. In any case, the primary distinction between *active* and *passive* models of antitissue antibody diseases involves the source of antibody. Since in the former the antibody is endogenous and not immunogenetic in the ordinary sense, an autologous phase does not occur, unless, of course, anti-idiotype or antiantibody production develops. By and large, progressive injury in the active models is dependent upon a continuing source of antibody or induction of cell-mediated immunity to constituents of the glomerulus. Mediation of injury presumably occurs by pathways similar to those operating in the passively induced models of nephritis. Recent studies have strongly implicated bone marrow–derived monocytes as playing an important role.

Certain diseases occurring in humans virtually duplicate the events which transpire in the model of actively induced anti-basement membrane antibody–mediated renal disease. The best studied is the clinicopathologic entity known as *Goodpasture's syndrome,* or pulmonary hemorrhage and glomerulonephritis (see also Chap. 295). This syndrome is generally believed to be mediated by antibody to GBM; however, the etiologic factors are largely unknown. It has been suggested that exposure to viral infection may release altered autologous antigens capable of abrogating natural tolerance. Goodpasture's syndrome fulfills the criteria of an anti-basement membrane antibody–induced disease, namely,

1 Circulating antibody to normal human GBM is present. This antibody also reacts to a limited extent with primate GBM and to basement membrane antigens of alveoli and renal tubules.
2 "Linear" deposits of IgG, and rarely IgA, are found deposited in diseased tissue.
3 Eluates of diseased tissue contain antibody to normal GBM.
4 Circulating or eluted antibody is capable of inducing glomerular disease in subhuman primates.
5 Renal transplant recipients may acquire the disease if transplantation is performed when the disease is active.

The pulmonary manifestations set Goodpasture's syndrome apart from the experimental models of anti-basement membrane antibody disease in which such manifestations usually do not occur, despite the fact that there is extensive cross reaction between GBM and alveolar capillary basement membrane. Linear Ig deposits are found along the alveolar basement membrane, serum and eluates of lung tissue will react in vivo with normal lung and kidney basement membranes, and serum and eluates of kidney react in vitro with normal lung alveolar basement membrane. The precise mechanisms responsible for pulmonary hemorrhage in anti-basement membrane antibody–induced disease are not well understood. The level of circulating anti-basement membrane antibody does not relate well to the severity of pulmonary hemorrhage. Although GBM antigens are the principal targets of the immune response in this disease, TBM antigens may also be the site of deposition of antibody. "Linear" deposits of Ig along TBM, circulating anti-TBM antibody, and eluates containing anti-TBM antibody are characteristically present. The development of an anti-TBM antibody response without concomitant anti-GBM antibody production has been recorded occasionally in human diseases: most notably in occasional cases of acute methicillin-induced hypersensitivity interstitial nephritis, in rare cases of poststreptococcal glomerulonephritis, in chronic idiopathic interstitial nephritis, and in renal allograft rejection.

Other nonglomerular basement membrane–related antitissue antibody diseases It now seems clear that the glomerular capillary wall and mesangium are composed of a number of potentially immunogenic glycoproteins other than the classic GBM glycopeptide mentioned above in the context of nephrotoxic serum nephritis and Goodpasture's syndrome. These antigens are distributed in various patterns along the glomerular capillary wall and/or within the mesangium and are probably biochemically distinct structural components of the glomerulus. Binding in situ of passively administered heterologous antibody or the actively induced autoantibody to these antigens will therefore produce differing patterns of immunoglobulin localization. Certain of these antigens, some seemingly closely related to renal tubule epithelial antigens, are localized to the external (subepithelial) aspect of the glomerular capillary wall and are distributed in a discontinuous fashion. Thus, passively administered heterologous antibody will localize in a granular or discontinuous pattern as the antigen-antibody interaction occurs in situ along the glomerular capillary wall. This sequence of events is observed in a model of experimental glomerulonephritis known as *passive Heymann nephritis* or *heterologous immune-complex glomerulonephritis.* This model is induced by the *passive* administration of a heterologous IgG containing antibodies directed against antigenic determinants of renal tubule epithelial antigens which cross react with glomerular capillary wall antigen. In a fashion quite similar to that observed in the autologous phase of nephrotoxic serum nephritis, an antibody response to the heterologous IgG deposited along the glomerular capillary wall may sustain and augment glomerular injury. Whether a similar sequence of events can be induced by *active* immunization with a renal tubule epithelial antigen is a matter of some current controversy; however, much experimental evidence is available to suggest that an autoantibody reacting with the same or similar antigens in the subepithelial aspect of the glomerular capillary wall may be involved in an experimental disease induced by active immunization with renal tubule epithelial antigens in a complete Freund's adjuvant. This model is referred to as *active Heymann nephritis* or *autologous immune-complex glomerulonephritis.* Because the antigen-antibody interaction takes place at the site of injury, these models are often referred to as *in situ immune-complex diseases.* Other intrinsic renal antigens distributed in other patterns or at other sites along the glomerular capillary wall or mesangium may be involved in evoking renal disease in experimental animals and in humans.

Furthermore, it is also now well recognized that circulating endogenous or environmental substances having special biological or biochemical affinity for glomerular structures, including the glomerular capillary wall or mesangium, may deposit in these structures in a nonimmunological fashion and thus act as a "planted" antigen. Examples of such planted antigens thus far described include certain drugs, lectins, and deoxyribonucleic acid. Reaction of such substances with glomerular structures could evoke disease in which antibody is not directed to a native tissue constituent but rather to a constituent artificially planted within the glomerular structures. Several experimental models of this pathogenetic sequence have been described, but there is little definitive information concerning the prevalence of this mechanism in human renal disease.

IMMUNE-COMPLEX–MEDIATED RENAL INJURY Circulating immune-complex disease The deposition in the kidney of immune complexes formed in the circulation accounts for over 75 percent of all diseases of the kidney for which there is clear evidence of participation of some immunologic process. At the experimental level a multitude of models have been studied, each illustrating important points regarding the details of the pathogenetic processes involved. The best studied of these models, illustrative of the exogenous, nonreplicating category, has been that of *acute and chronic serum sickness.* These models are developed by single or multiple injections, respectively, of soluble immunogenic foreign serum protein. Figure 293-2 depicts the sequence of events which occurs following the intravenous injection of a single dose of such foreign serum proteins. Initially the protein equilibrates with the intra- and extravascular fluids and undergoes slow metabolic degradation. Subsequently, as a clone of specifically activated B cells begins to secrete antibody into the extracellular fluid, the rate of elimination of the antigen from the circulation will accelerate (i.e., immune elimination) and circulating immune complexes will be formed. At first these immune complexes will be generated in a large excess of antigen and therefore will be relatively small and highly soluble. Few of these complexes possess properties which favor tissue localization and little disease results. With clonal expansion, antibody secretion accelerates still further, so that the ratio of antibody to antigen will approach equivalence and favor the formation of soluble aggregates of increasing size and complexity. A small portion of these will then localize within the glomerular mesangium; in the walls of peripheral capillaries; and in joints, heart valves, choroid plexus, splenic sinusoids, and larger blood vessels, particularly at sites of turbulent flow. The localization of these complexes depends in part on changes in capillary permeability brought about by the release of vasoactive amines, such as histamine, from cellular storage sites. In experimental animals, platelets, basophils, and IgE antibody interact to bring about this release of permeability factors. Once deposited, these complexes possess unique properties which evoke an inflammatory response at the site of deposition. This appears to be especially true of complexes localized within the microvasculature outside the kidney. If the antibody is capable of fixing C1q, the classical complement cascade will be activated; complement components will then be consumed in the process. The antigen itself may also be involved in complement activation. Polysaccharide antigens may be independently capable of initiating complement activation via the alternative pathway.

FIGURE 293-2

Circulating antigen, antibody, antigen-antibody complexes, and hemolytic complement activity following intravenous injection of soluble serum protein (e.g., bovine serum albumin). Ordinate (log scale) refers to percent of injected antigen remaining in circulation; amount of free antibody as micrograms of antigen bound per milliliter of serum; antigen-antibody complexes as percent injected antigen in immune complexes; complement as percent of normal serum. [After FJ Dixon, in Immunological Diseases, 2d ed, M Samter (ed), Boston, Little, Brown, 1971.]

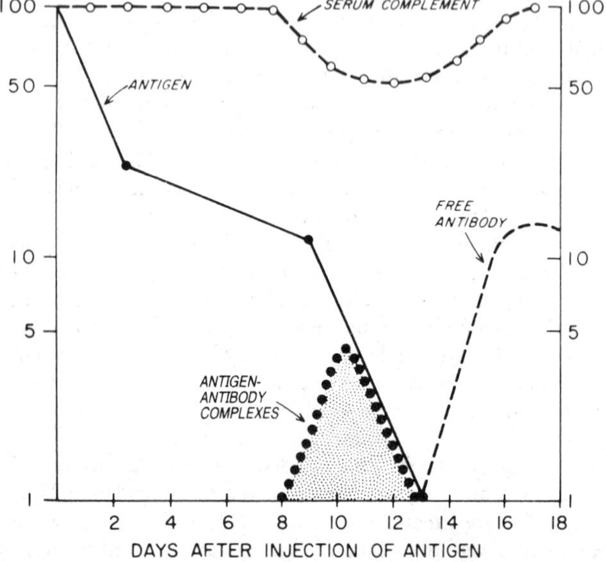

Ultimately the supply of antigen is exhausted. However, antibody synthesis proceeds unabated, leading eventually to a state of antibody excess, which, in the case of multivalent antigens such as soluble serum proteins, favors extensive polymerization of the immune complex, the formation of a lattice network, and a great increase in the size of the immune complex. These immune complexes formed in antibody excess are then treated as particulate material by the mononuclear-phagocyte system and removed rapidly. Once all the antigen is eliminated, only free antibody can be detected in the circulation. The immune complexes deposited in the kidney during the immune elimination phase will be metabolized and degraded by infiltrating monocytes and polymorphonuclear cells, and the inflammatory process will eventually subside spontaneously.

On the other hand, if the antigen is administered repeatedly (thus resembling the situation which prevails when antigens are released from endogenous sites or from replicating organisms), then the opportunity exists for the development of a continuing or fluctuating level of soluble circulating immune complexes of varying molecular composition and phlogistic activity. In this circumstance, modifying the function of the mononuclear phagocyte system, the release of factors which alter glomerular capillary permeability, the rate of antigen egress into the vascular fluids, or the rate of antibody formation all would be expected to have far-reaching consequences on the amount of immune complexes localizing and/or persisting within renal structures.

Although this formulation presupposes that immune complexes form within the circulation and then are deposited in vascular structures, it is also possible for immune complexes to be formed in the extravascular (interstitial) compartment by virtue of diffusion into this fluid compartment of cell-derived antigens and circulating antibody. Such a phenomenon may explain the deposition of immune complexes in the interstitial areas of the kidney, with relative sparing of the glomerular circulation. Regardless of the nature of the antibody or antigen or the particular circumstances surrounding the immunologic events, a valuable clue to the presence of immune-complex deposition is the morphologic pattern found when tissues are examined by immunofluorescence or electron microscopic techniques. Granular, discontinuous, and irregular deposits of Ig, often in conjunction with complement components, are found by immunofluorescence (Fig. 293-1*B*), whereas electron-dense deposits are seen by electron microscopy (Fig. 293-1*C*). Sometimes these deposits acquire a definite substructure, but for the most part they are rather homogeneous. The deposits may develop in several locations within the glomerulus: beneath the epithelial cells (subepithelial), within the basement membrane (intramembranous), beneath the endothelium (subendothelial), and within the mesangial matrix. Immune complexes may also localize in the peritubular capillary network. The precise reason for localization at these differing sites is not well understood but may involve factors such as size or charge of the complexes, receptors for the Fc or complement components within glomerular structures, or local hemodynamic events. The deposits appear to increase in size by aggregation, and there is some evidence that glomerular cells may participate in their removal. The persistence of deposits is related to the rate of formation balanced by the activity of removal systems. Once deposited in glomeruli, circulating immune complexes evoke local inflammatory and functional changes, which at least for the glomerular circulation may be relatively independent of complement or polymorphonuclear leukocytes. Infiltrating monocytes may play a critical role in mediating glomerular injury. The morphologic lesions which result from immune-complex deposition may vary considerably, from diffuse proliferative to nonproliferative membranous or sclerosing lesions. Coagulation, platelet aggregation, activation of the complement cascade, and release of vasoactive amines may participate in determining the pattern of morphologic response.

The *exogenous* antigens involved in circulating immune-complex–mediated disease are derived chiefly from infectious agents such as bacteria, viruses, or parasites. Replication of the organism provides a continuing source of antigen. The best-studied examples of these in humans are *infective endocarditis, leprosy, syphilis, hepatitis B,* and *malaria.* The *endogenous* antigens involved in human disease vary considerably and include *DNA, thyroglobulin, autologous immunoglobulins, erythrocyte stroma, renal tubule antigens,* and *tumor-specific* or *tumor-associated* antigens.

COMPLEMENT-ASSOCIATED GLOMERULAR INJURY Although there is little evidence that complement activation, independent of antitissue antibody or circulating immune complexes, can bring about glomerular injury, there are certain associations between complement and renal disease in humans. The clinicopathologic entity known as *idiopathic membranoproliferative glomerulonephritis* (see also Chap. 294) may be associated with patterns of serum complement component deposition within glomeruli suggestive of involvement of the alternative pathway of complement activation, perhaps independent of immune-complex deposition. These patterns are not, however, necessarily unique to this group of disorders since they may also be observed in a wide variety of postinfectious glomerulonephritides and in certain collagen-vascular diseases.

As discussed in greater detail in Chap. 63, the alternative pathway mechanism of complement activation depends upon the interaction of aggregated or immune-complex IgA, polysaccharides, or lipopolysaccharides with factors B, D of the alternative pathway system, and C3 of the classical complement cascade. Subsequently, an enzyme capable of cleaving native C3 is assembled, composed of a fragment of C3 (C3b) and an altered form of factor B (Bb). This alternative pathway C3 convertase is analogous to the C3 convertase generated in the classical pathway of complement activation. The alternative pathway C3 convertase is stabilized by binding to properdin and degraded by several inactivators (C3b inactivator, β1H). Alternative pathway C3 convertase cleaves C3 into C3a (anaphylatoxin I) and C3b, which is further cleaved by C3 inactivator into C3c and C3d, biologically inactive fragments. The C3b formed in this manner can also autocatalytically form additional alternative pathway C3 convertase in the presence of factors B, D, and Mg^{2+}. The hallmarks of activation of the alternative pathway are depressed serum levels of native C3, circulating fragments of C3 (C3c, C3d), low levels of factor B, and circulating fragments of B (Bb), all occurring in the absence of perturbations in the early classical components C1q, C4, and C2. The terminal complement components C5 through C9 may also be activated and even result in lysis of cells in the absence of antibody. Depression of the synthesis of C3 may also contribute to diminished serum levels, since circulating fragments of C3 may reduce cellular production.

In *idiopathic membranoproliferative glomerulonephritis,* particularly the subset known as "dense deposit disease," serum C3 levels are depressed; C4, C1, and C2 levels tend to be normal; and C3 may be deposited in glomeruli without Ig (see also Chap. 294). In addition, an oligoclonal autoantibody (an immunoconglutinin) to alternative pathway C3 convertase is frequently found in the circulation. This autoantibody reacts with a conformational neoantigen of the alternative pathway C3 convertase and acts to stabilize this enzyme from the influence of C3b inactivator and β1H in a fashion similar to properdin. As a result serums containing this autoantibody are capable of inducing C3 cleavage in vitro by permitting the assembly of a stable fluid phase C3 convertase. This antibody is also known as C3 nephritic factor (C3NeF), and was first described in the serums of patients with glomerulonephritis and persistent depression of C3 levels.

The relationship between these aberrations in the complement pathway and glomerular injury is uncertain. No experimental models of persistent activation of the alternative pathway have been associated with glomerulonephritis; thus, glomerular injury may be a closely associated but pathogenetically unrelated phenomenon, perhaps genetically determined. On the other hand, some have suggested that persistent hypocomplementemia may interfere with the normal removal processes for environmental antigens such as viruses. Such a defect might favor the persistence of these antigens in the circulation and enhance the likelihood of formation of circulating immune complexes.

CELL-MEDIATED IMMUNITY IN GLOMERULAR AND TUBULOINTERSTITIAL DISEASES The roles of specifically sensitized cells acting independently of antibody (i.e., T-killer cells) and antibody-dependent lymphoid cell–mediated (ADCC) or "armed" macrophages in the pathogenesis of glomerular and tubulointerstitial diseases have been difficult to establish firmly except in one clear-cut example. The rejection of renal allografts in nonsensitized recipients is clearly a cell-mediated process. This subject is dealt with in greater detail in Chap. 292.

It is true that by utilizing a variety of in vitro techniques cell-mediated hypersensitivity to both environmental and endogenous antigens may be demonstrable in several diseases of the kidney, including glomerulonephritis. The precise role such "sensitized" cells play in the actual tissue injury is unclear, especially in human glomerular disease. No doubt the burgeoning knowledge in the field of cell-cell interactions will eventually clarify these uncertainties. It is very likely that some diseases which do not fit into an antibody or immune-complex–mediated category will find an explanation in reactions of the cell-mediated variety. One likely candidate for this category is so-called minimal change disease, one of the morphological subsets of idiopathic nephrotic syndrome. Furthermore, because of the prominence of lymphoid cell infiltration, various forms of chronic tubulointerstitial nephritis have also been suggested as examples of cell-mediated reactions (see Chap. 297).

REFERENCES

ANDRES GA et al: Tubular and interstitial disease due to immunologic mechanisms. Kidney Intern 7:271, 1975

COUSER WG et al: In-situ immune complex formation and glomerular injury. Kidney Intern 17:1, 1980

GLASSOCK RJ: Immunologically mediated renal disease, in *Contemporary Nephrology,* S Klahr (ed). New York, Plenum, 1981

MCCLUSKY RT, ANDRES GA (eds): *Immunologically Mediated Renal Diseases. Criteria for Diagnosis and Treatment.* New York, Dekker, 1978

WILSON CB et al: Antiglomerular basement membrane induced glomerulonephritis. Kidney Intern 3:74, 1973

———: Immunologic mechanisms of renal disease, in *Contemporary Issues in Nephrology,* CB Wilson, BM Brenner, JH Stein (eds). New York, Churchill Livingstone, 1979, vol 3

———, DIXON FJ: The renal response to immunological injury, in *The Kidney,* 2d ed, BM Brenner, FC Rector Jr (eds). Philadelphia, Saunders, 1981

294
THE MAJOR GLOMERULOPATHIES

RICHARD J. GLASSOCK
BARRY M. BRENNER

Disease-induced alterations of the structural and functional integrity of the glomerular capillary circulation are often associated with the findings, either singly or in combination, of hematuria, proteinuria, reduced glomerular filtration rate (GFR), and hypertension. Five major glomerulopathic syndromes are recognized: *acute glomerulonephritis, rapidly progressive glomerulonephritis, chronic glomerulonephritis,* the *nephrotic syndrome,* and *asymptomatic urinary abnormalities.* This chapter deals with each of these syndromes in some detail, describing diseases in which the kidney is either the sole or predominant organ involved (i.e., the primary glomerulopathies) or is involved as a complication of infection or drug exposure. Glomerular injury associated with multisystem disorders or heredofamilial conditions is discussed in Chap. 295.

ACUTE GLOMERULONEPHRITIS (AGN)

The causes of AGN are given in Table 294-1. The "acute nephritic syndrome" consists of the abrupt onset of *hematuria* and *proteinuria,* accompanied by evidence of *azotemia* (i.e., reduced GFR) and renal *salt and water retention.* If GFR is reduced markedly, oligoanuria may be present (see also Chap. 290). Salt and water retention leads to circulatory congestion, hypertension, and edema. Fluid retention appears to be due both to diminished GFR and to exaggerated salt and water reabsorption, particularly in distal nephron segments.

The edema of acute glomerulonephritis tends to appear initially in areas of low tissue pressure, such as the *periorbital* areas, but may subsequently progress to involve dependent portions of the body and lead to *ascites* and/or *pleural effusions. Circulatory congestion* is manifested by an increase in systemic and pulmonary vascular pressures, normal or increased cardiac output, and a shortened circulation time. In the absence of underlying valvular, myocardial, or coronary artery disease or severe diastolic hypertension there is little likelihood that true left ventricular congestive heart failure will develop. If pulmonary capillary pressure rises above the opposing plasma oncotic pressure, however, pulmonary edema may ensue. *Arterial diastolic hypertension* is the consequence of several factors, including extracellular fluid volume expansion, enhanced cardiac output, and modest increases in peripheral vascular resistance. Plasma renin activity, aldosterone, and the sympathetic nervous system are relatively suppressed. Hypertension may at times be accompanied by encephalopathy, particularly in young children.

The extent and severity of urinary abnormalities in AGN vary considerably. Gross (macroscopic) *hematuria* is the most common, and is often described by the patient as smoky, coffee, or cola-colored urine. Lesser degrees of hematuria may go unrecognized by the patient or parent; for this reason, the features of fluid retention and hypertension may be ascribed erroneously to other illnesses if a careful examination of the urine sediment is omitted from the initial laboratory evaluation. Hematuria is often, but not invariably, accompanied by the excretion of *red cell casts.* Leukocyturia and leukocyte casts may also occur, indicating the presence of inflammation in the glomerulus and interstitium. The degree of *proteinuria* varies according to the nature and severity of the underlying glomerular lesions. Rarely, protein excretion rates may fall within the normal range, but generally are between 0.2 and 3 g per day. If proteinuria is marked and sustained, features of the nephrotic syndrome may appear (see below).

The short-term evolution of acute nephritis generally depends upon the nature of the underlying glomerular lesion; however, within a week or so of onset most patients with postinfectious AGN will begin to experience spontaneous resolution of fluid retention and hypertension. Urinary abnormalities often take longer to resolve. A few patients with the acute nephritic syndrome will go on in the ensuing weeks or months to develop a rapidly progressive form of renal failure (i.e., rapidly progressive glomerulonephritis, discussed below). The long-term outlook for patients with AGN is considered below in the context of treatment of specific lesions.

ACUTE POSTSTREPTOCOCCAL GLOMERULONEPHRITIS (PSGN) Clinical features and diagnosis This disorder can be viewed as the archetype of AGN. PSGN follows in the wake of *pharyngeal or cutaneous infection* with one of a limited number of strains of *group A beta-hemolytic streptococci.* These potentially "nephritogenic" streptococci may be identified by serotyping of a cell wall antigen (M protein). Among outbreaks of infection with proved "nephritogenic" strains of streptococci the PSGN attack rate is relatively uniform, but because of variation in the nephritogenicity among group A streptococci, attack rates among outbreaks of infection may vary considerably. Among families, asymptomatic episodes of PSGN exceed symptomatic episodes by a factor of 3 or 4 to 1. Immunity to M protein is type-specific, long-lasting, and protective. Repeated episodes of PSGN are therefore unusual. Outbreaks of pharyngeal infection–associated PSGN are commonest in children aged 6 to 10. AGN following cutaneous streptococcal infection is more commonly associated with factors such as poor personal hygiene, overcrowding, and concomitant cutaneous disease, such as scabies infestation. Seasonal and geographic variations in prevalence of PSGN are more marked for pharyngeal than for cutaneous associated disease.

An important feature of PSGN is the existence of a *latent period* between the earliest manifestations of infection and the onset of recognizable signs and symptoms of nephritis. The latent period is more apparent following pharyngeal infections, where it usually is 6 to 10 days in duration. Cutaneous infections are associated with longer latent periods, averaging about 2 weeks. Definitive signs of glomerular inflammation occurring at the same time as, or shortly after, infection usually indicate an *exacerbation* of a preexisting chronic glomerular disease such as Berger's disease (IgA nephropathy) (see below).

The diagnosis of PSGN rests upon the demonstration of at least two of the following features: (1) The presence of a group A beta-hemolytic streptococcus of a potentially nephritogenic M-protein type in a throat or skin lesion. (2) The demonstration of an immune response to one or more of the streptococcal *exoenzymes,* including anti-streptolysin O (ASO), antistreptokinase (ASK), anti-deoxyribonuclease B (ADNAase B), anti-nicotinyl adenine dinucleotidase (ANADase), or antihyaluronidase (AH). ASO responses are typically brisk in pharyngeal infections, but often absent in cutaneous infection; whereas AH, ADNAase, and ANADase responses occur after the latter. Testing for multiple antibody responses and serial determinations is necessary to achieve a diagnostic accuracy of 90 percent. Early antimicrobial therapy may prevent the antibody response to exoenzymes and render throat cultures negative, but may not interfere with the development of PSGN; this makes accurate serologic diagnosis difficult or impossible. (3) The demonstration of a transient decline in the serum concentration of C3 component of complement, with a return to normal within 8 weeks after the first signs of renal disease. Other complement components (i.e., C1q and C4) are frequently less depressed. In addition to these laboratory features it is desirable to document a latent period appropriate to the nature of the infection. Furthermore, the patient should not have any known preexisting renal disease.

Other laboratory features commonly observed in PSGN include transient cryoimmunoglobulinemia, positive tests for circulating immune complexes, and circulating high-molecular-weight fibrinogen complexes. The erythrocyte sedimentation rate is usually elevated, while C-reactive protein and rheumatoid factor are generally normal or absent. Mild anemia and hypoalbuminemia, both largely dilutional in origin, may be present. Severe hypoalbuminemia may be encountered if heavy proteinuria is present and prolonged. Excretion rates of urinary protein in excess of 3.5 g per day occur in less than 20 percent of hospitalized patients. Proteinuria is usually of a nonselective character and frequently contains high concentrations of fibrin-degradation products (FDP) and C3 protein, particularly during the diuretic phase. Hyponatremia, hyperkalemia, and metabolic acidosis may be seen in azotemic or oliguric patients, especially those having free access to water or potassium. Urinary sodium concentration is usually low, reflecting avid salt reabsorption in the distal nephron. Abdominal films reveal normal or enlarged kidneys. The chest x-ray may be normal or reveal a slightly enlarged heart, often accompanied by signs of pulmonary congestion. The electrocardiogram may reveal nonspecific T-wave abnormalities. Rheumatic fever rarely coexists with acute PSGN.

The differential diagnosis of PSGN includes other infectious or primary renal diseases which may produce an identical acute nephritic syndrome (Table 294-1). Multisystem diseases such as SLE, Schönlein-Henoch purpura, and vasculitis may present initially as acute nephritis (Chap. 295). Predominantly nonglomerular diseases, including thrombotic thrombocytopenic purpura, hemolytic-uremic syndrome, and acute hypersensitivity interstitial nephritis may also present the features of the acute nephritic syndrome (Chaps. 297 and 298).

Pathology and pathogenesis Renal biopsies performed early in the course of PSGN reveal *diffuse, endocapillary proliferative glomerulonephritis.* Infiltration of glomeruli with polymorphonuclear leukocytes and monocytes is also common. The glomerular capillary walls are usually thin and delicate and free of necrosis. Occasional discrete proteinaceous deposits projecting from the outer aspects of the capillary wall toward the urinary space (humps) may be recognized by light microscopy and coincide with the electron-dense deposits seen by electron microscopy. Segmental extracapillary proliferation (crescents) may involve a few glomeruli, but diffuse crescent formation is uncommon except among a subset of patients presenting with severe and rapidly progressive acute renal failure (see section below on rapidly progressive glomerulonephritis). Extraglomerular vessels and tubulointerstitial areas are usually normal. Red blood cells are frequently seen in the lumens of distal tubules, where they form red blood cell casts.

By immunofluorescence microscopy, granular deposits of IgG are seen in peripheral capillary loops and mesangium, nearly always accompanied by C3 and properdin, but less commonly by C1q and C4 (Chap. 293). These deposits may also be recognized by electron microscopy and probably represent immune complexes, although the precise nature of the antigen-antibody systems involved remains unknown. Most likely the antigen is derived from the streptococcal organism itself, but this has been difficult to verify. The profile of altered serum complement components described above, and the prominent C3 and properdin deposition in glomeruli, are suggestive of involvement of the alternative pathway of complement activation (Chap. 293).

Course and treatment The ultimate *prognosis* for PSGN appears to differ between sporadic and epidemic forms and between adults and children. *Epidemic* forms of the disease in *children* have a uniformly favorable short- and long-term prognosis. Few patients die of complications of renal failure (fewer than 1 percent), and nearly all experience a spontaneous resolution of abnormal clinical signs within a week after the onset of illness. Abnormalities in the urinary sediment and protein excretion subside slowly in the ensuing months; in a few cases, several years elapse before the urinary sediment becomes consistently normal. Among children with PSGN during epidemics of streptococcal infection, and in whom some form of preexisting chronic glomerular disease was absent, long-term follow-up has revealed little or no evidence of progression to chronic renal disease. A very small percentage may develop extensive crescentic glomerulonephritis with its relentlessly progressive course. The site of the streptococcal infection, the

TABLE 294-1
Causes of acute glomerulonephritis

I Infectious diseases
  A Poststreptococcal glomerulonephritis
  B Nonpoststreptococcal glomerulonephritis
    1 Bacterial: Infective endocarditis, "shunt nephritis," sepsis, pneumococcal pneumonia, typhoid fever, secondary syphilis, meningococcemia
    2 Viral: Hepatitis B, infectious mononucleosis, mumps, measles, varicella, vaccinia, echovirus, and coxsackievirus
    3 Parasitic: Malaria, toxoplasmosis

II Multisystem diseases: Systemic lupus erythematosus, vasculitis, Schönlein-Henoch purpura, Goodpasture's syndrome

III Primary glomerular diseases: Membranoproliferative glomerulonephritis, Berger's disease, "pure" mesangial proliferative glomerulonephritis

IV Miscellaneous: Guillain-Barré syndrome, irradiation of Wilms's tumor, self-administered diphtheria-pertussis-tetanus vaccine, serum sickness

type of M protein, the severity in abnormalities of complement components or urinary sediment, or the extent of the rise in antibody response to exoenzymes have little or no bearing on the ultimate prognosis of PSGN. Prolonged and persistent heavy proteinuria and/or abnormal GFR imply a more unfavorable outcome. *Sporadic* cases of PSGN among *children* may have more serious long-term consequences, although this remains controversial. After the subsidence of the acute disease, some children subsequently develop slowly progressive glomerular capillary obliteration (glomerulosclerosis), reduced GFR, and hypertension; after several decades, end-stage renal failure from chronic glomerulonephritis may result. The persistence of abnormal proteinuria is the rule in such cases.

The prognosis for *adults* with PSGN seems to be less favorable than for children. The reason for this apparent age difference is poorly understood. Although the overall prognosis for PSGN in *epidemics* seems good, *sporadic* PSGN in adults appears to be associated with lasting and/or progressive deterioration in renal function in as many as one-third to one-half of all cases. This may take the form of persistent proteinuria and/or hematuria, or of slowly progressive glomerulosclerosis and renal failure, often accompanied by hypertension. This evolution seems more likely to occur when the initial disease has been unusually severe. Whether milder forms of sporadic PSGN can lead to chronic disease is an important but unresolved issue (see "Chronic Glomerulonephritis" below).

The *treatment* of acute PSGN is supportive. It seems reasonable to recommend bed rest until the signs of glomerular inflammation and circulatory congestion (primarily hypertension) subside, but prolonged forced periods of inactivity are of no demonstrable benefit in the healing process. Fluid retention, circulatory congestion, and edema may be treated with sodium and fluid restriction, or loop diuretics. Diuresis alone will often ameliorate mild to moderate hypertension. If severe hypertension is present, vasodilator drugs such as nitroprusside, hydralazine, or diazoxide may be useful. Encephalopathy and pulmonary congestion will generally improve with lowering of blood pressure and the relief of circulatory overload. Digitalis preparations should be avoided except in instances of well-documented organic heart disease with congestive failure. Treatment with ion exchange resins and/or dialysis may be required for cases of severe oliguria, fluid overload, and hyperkalemia. Mild protein restriction is desirable for azotemic patients. A 7- to 10-day course of antimicrobials (e.g., penicillin or erythromycin) should be given if streptococcal infection is documented. Long-term chemoprophylaxis is not indicated. Steroids and cytotoxic drugs have not been shown to be of value.

NONSTREPTOCOCCAL ACUTE GLOMERULONEPHRITIS

Clinical features and diagnosis A variety of infectious illnesses other than those caused by group A beta-hemolytic streptococci may also be associated with AGN (Table 294-1). These include *bacteremic states* and various *viral* and *parasitic* diseases. Ordinarily these diseases can be diagnosed by the presence of typical extrarenal clinical features or by bacteriologic or serologic findings. Infective endocarditis, visceral sepsis, typhoid fever, infectious mononucleosis, acute viral hepatitis (hepatitis B), falciparum malaria, and toxoplasmosis represent examples of infectious diseases capable of evoking AGN. A substantial body of evidence indicates that circulating immune complexes play an important role in the pathogenesis of AGN in these diseases. Bacteremic states are frequently associated with persistent depression of serum concentrations of complement components C1q, C4, and C3, elevated levels of rheumatoid factor, circulating cryoimmunoglobulins, and strongly positive tests for circulating immune complexes. Control of infection usually results in the resolution of the signs of glomerular inflammation, although, in occasional instances, rapidly progressive or chronic glomerulonephritis may ensue.

RAPIDLY PROGRESSIVE GLOMERULONEPHRITIS (RPGN)

A minority of patients with AGN develop azotemia, which is *transient,* usually in association with a short period of oliguria. A diuresis usually follows within days or a few weeks and GFR returns to normal. On the other hand, some cases of AGN are characterized by a *rapidly progressive* form of renal failure, which often develops abruptly and displays little tendency for spontaneous or complete recovery. The clinical term *rapidly progressive glomerulonephritis* (*RPGN*) is often applied to this group to connote the development of renal failure in a period of weeks to months, rather than years or decades, as is typical of chronic glomerulonephritis (see below). Usually, but not invariably, extensive *extracapillary* (*crescentic*) *glomerulonephritis* is found as the pathologic lesion underlying the syndrome of RPGN, and the two terms are often used interchangeably.

RPGN can arise in three clinical settings (Table 294-2): (1) as a renal complication of an acute or subacute infectious disease, (2) as a renal complication in many multisystem diseases, and (3) as a primary or idiopathic glomerular disease. The first category is discussed in Chap. 293, the second in Chap. 295, and the third will be considered here.

IDIOPATHIC RAPIDLY PROGRESSIVE GLOMERULONEPHRITIS

Clinical features and diagnosis This disorder affects individuals in a broad age distribution and has a predilection for males. Wide geographic differences in the prevalence of the disease have been noted, and outbreaks ("miniepidemics") may occur. Some patients have had recent heavy exposure to volatile hydrocarbons, but there is little evidence to support a cause-and-effect relationship. While a flu-like or viral prodrome may occur, frank arthritis, sinusitis, otitis, skin rash, neuritis, or encephalopathy are uncommon and are more in keeping with a multisystem disease. Symptoms of weakness, nausea, and vomiting (indicative of azotemia) usually dominate the clinical picture. Oliguria, abdominal or flank pain, and hemoptysis may also be present (see "Goodpasture's Syndrome," Chap. 295). The blood pressure is usually normal or only modestly elevated. Urinalysis typically reveals hematuria and red cell casts, but exceptional cases with relatively benign urine sediments have been observed. Proteinuria is always present and may occasionally be massive. Other biochemical features of the nephrotic syndrome are uncommon, probably because of the concomitant reduction in GFR. Proteinuria is typically nonselective, and high concentrations of FDP are found in urine. Azotemia develops early and tends to progress at a rapid rate. Other clinical and laboratory features relate to the underlying pathology and pathogenesis.

Pathology and pathogenesis It is clear that idiopathic RPGN is far from a homogeneous disease. By light microscopy the characteristic abnormality found in the kidneys is *extensive extracapillary proliferation,* i.e., *crescents.* The extent and degree of glomerular involvement varies considerably; however, among patients with rapid deterioration of renal function it is usual for more than 70 percent of glomeruli to be involved with circumferential crescents. Endocapillary proliferation may also be seen, but if very prominent, suggests the presence of antigen-antibody complexes. Fibrin-related antigens are nearly always demonstrable within the crescents by special stains or by immunofluorescence. Gaps or focal discontinuities in the glomerular basement membrane (GBM) are observed in association with crescents.

Variations in the underlying pathogenetic mechanisms responsible for RPGN are revealed by immunofluorescence studies of renal biopsies (Chap. 293). In approximately one-third of cases, *linear deposits* of IgG, often accompanied by C3, indicate involvement of *anti-GBM antibodies.* Circulating anti-GBM antibodies are found in this group by indirect immunofluorescence, hemagglutination, or radioimmunoassay techniques. Patients falling into this pathogenetic subgroup tend to have normal serum complement levels and a marked tendency to develop hemoptysis (see also "Goodpasture's Syndrome," Chap. 295). About one-third of cases will have findings indicative of *immune-complex–mediated disease,* namely, *granular deposits* of immunoglobulin by immunofluorescence microscopy and electron-dense deposits by electron microscopy. This mechanism of RPGN tends to occur in older individuals, to produce more constitutional symptoms, and to result in more disturbances of the complement pathways than does anti-GBM antibody–mediated disease. Hemoptysis may also occur, but circulating anti-GBM antibodies are absent. The remainder of cases of RPGN reveal scanty or no immunoglobulins or complement by immunofluorescence; their pathogenesis is unknown. This group also tends to include older individuals, in whom serum complement concentrations are normal and anti-GBM antibodies are absent. Occasionally, mild hemoptysis may occur.

It is obvious from the foregoing discussion that lung hemorrhage may be observed in a variety of circumstances associated with RPGN. This subject is covered in greater detail in the section on Goodpasture's syndrome in Chap. 295. As noted in Table 294-2, other idiopathic (primary) renal diseases may, from time to time, be accompanied by a prominent tendency for crescent formation and a rapidly progressive course.

Course and treatment In general, the prognosis for preservation of renal function in RPGN is poor. Patients with crescent formation in 70 percent or more of glomeruli, oliguria or severe reduction in GFR (less than 5 ml/min) at the time of presentation, or an anti-GBM antibody–mediated process have the worst prognosis. Although advances in treatment are changing the outlook for patients with RPGN, at least one-half to two-thirds of patients currently require maintenance hemodialysis within 6 months of discovery of the illness. Exceptional patients with crescentic glomerulonephritis will have a more protracted illness. Spontaneous resolution is very uncommon, except among patients with infection as the basis for formation of antigen-antibody complexes, where removal of antigen can take place.

The treatment of RPGN is currently undergoing reevaluation. *Corticosteroids,* in the form of "pulses" of parenteral methylprednisolone in high doses, or continuous oral prednisone daily, often combined with *cytotoxic agents* (azathioprine or cyclophosphamide), have yielded varying degrees of success, particularly in the patients revealing granular or minimal Ig deposits in glomeruli. Since no controlled studies have yet been conducted, however, it is difficult to verify the exact value of these approaches. The addition of *anticoagulants* (heparin or Coumadin) and antithrombotic agents (cyproheptadine, dipyridamole, sulfinpyrazone) seems rational on the basis of evidence suggesting involvement of the coagulation process in the genesis of crescent formation. However, objective evidence of benefit from such therapies in animals afflicted with experimentally induced crescentic glomerulonephritis has been inconsistent, in part because of variations in the severity of the disease models, the timing of treatment, and the nature of the anticoagulant or antithrombotic agent used. Anticoagulants may be hazardous in patients with advanced renal failure. *Ancrod,* a fibrinogenolytic agent not yet released in the United States, may prove to be the most effective agent. Very recently, *intensive plasma exchange* (plasmapheresis—2 to 4 liters of plasma daily or three times weekly), combined with steroids and cytotoxic agents, has been employed in patients with RPGN with very encouraging preliminary results, especially in patients revealing linear Ig deposits in glomeruli (anti-GBM antibody–mediated disease). Beneficial effects appear to be greatest when such combined therapy is instituted early in the course of disease, before glomerular abnormalities are advanced. Despite aggressive therapy, patients with oliguria continue to do poorly. Clearly, treatment must be individualized, and because regular dialysis therapy and/or transplantation are available to virtually all patients with RPGN, one should probably err on the side of a conservative approach, unless compelling evidence in support of potential reversibility is present.

RPGN may recur in the renal transplant. It is difficult to be certain of the precise risk in individual cases. At present it seems prudent to recommend that, after initiating dialysis, a period of 3 to 6 months be allowed to elapse before undertaking renal transplantation in patients who have circulating anti-GBM antibodies. There is no convincing evidence that bilateral nephrectomy in advance of transplantation reduces the risk of recurrent disease in the transplant.

THE NEPHROTIC SYNDROME (NS)

In its overt form, NS is characterized by *albuminuria, hypoalbuminemia, hyperlipidemia,* and *edema.* These abnormalities are direct or indirect consequences of excessive glomerular leakage of plasma proteins into the urine (see also Chaps. 28 and 40). The abnormality of the glomerular capillary wall underlying the excessive filtration of plasma protein can arise as a consequence of a wide variety of disease processes, including immunological disorders, toxic injuries, metabolic abnormalities, biochemical defects, and vascular disorders. Thus, nephrotic syndrome should be viewed as a common endpoint of a variety of disease processes damaging the permeability properties of the glomerular capillary wall. *Heavy proteinuria* is the hallmark of the nephrotic state. Arbitrarily, protein excretion rates in excess of 3.5 g per 1.73 m^2 per day are considered to be in the nephrotic range, primarily because proteinuria of this magnitude is seldom observed in tubulointerstitial and vascular diseases of the kidney. Sustained heavy proteinuria is often, but not invariably, accompanied by *hypoalbuminemia.* Excessive urinary losses, increased renal catabolism, and inadequate hepatic synthesis of albumin all contribute to this depression of plasma albumin. The resulting decrease in plasma oncotic pressure leads to a disturbance in the Starling forces acting across peripheral capillaries. Intravascular fluid migrates into

TABLE 294-2
Causes of rapidly progressive glomerulonephritis

I Infectious diseases
  A Poststreptococcal glomerulonephritis
  B Infective endocarditis
  C Occult visceral sepsis
II Multisystem diseases
  A Systemic lupus erythematosus
  B Schönlein-Henoch purpura
  C Vasculitis (including Wegener's granulomatosis)
  D Goodpasture's syndrome
  E Essential cryoimmunoglobulinemia
  F Malignancy (rare)
III Primary glomerular diseases
  A Idiopathic crescentic glomerulonephritis
  B Membranoproliferative glomerulonephritis
  C Berger's disease (rare)
  D Membranous glomerulopathy complicated by anti-glomerular basement membrane antibody formation (rare)

the interstitial tissue (i.e., *edema*), particularly in areas of low tissue pressure. These disturbances initiate a series of homeostatic adjustments designed to correct the resulting deficit in effective plasma volume. These include activation of the renin-angiotensin-aldosterone system, enhanced antidiuretic hormone secretion, stimulation of the sympathetic nervous system, and perhaps a reduction in the secretion of a postulated "natriuretic hormone." These and other poorly understood adjustments lead to renal sodium and water retention, primarily because of avid reabsorption in distal nephron segments, resulting in unrelenting edema. The severity of edema correlates with the level of serum albumin and with the extent of urinary protein losses. The extent and severity of edema is significantly conditioned by the presence of other factors such as heart disease or peripheral vascular disease. Profound hypoalbuminemia may occasionally be associated with severe plasma volume reduction, postural hypotension, syncope, and shock. Very occasionally acute renal failure may occur.

The diminished plasma oncotic pressure also appears to stimulate hepatic lipoprotein synthesis, and *hyperlipidemia* is a frequent accompaniment of the nephrotic state. Low-density lipoproteins and cholesterol are elevated most frequently, but as the plasma oncotic pressure falls to very low levels, very low density lipoproteins and tryglycerides also increase. Excessive urinary losses of plasma protein factors regulating lipoprotein synthesis or disposal may also contribute to the hyperlipidemic state. Whether these lipid abnormalities contribute to accelerated atherosclerosis remains controversial. Lipid bodies (fatty casts, oval fat bodies) commonly appear in the urine.

Urine losses of plasma proteins other than albumin are also of importance in NS. Loss of thyroxine-binding globulin may produce abnormalities in thyroid function tests, including a low T4 and an enhanced resin T3 uptake. Loss of cholecalciferol-binding protein may lead to a vitamin D deficiency state, secondary hyperparathyroidism, and bone disease, and also may contribute to the hypocalcemia and hypocalciuria seen commonly in NS. Enhanced urinary excretion of transferrin may produce an iron-resistant microcytic, hypochromic anemia. Zinc and copper deficiency may result from urinary losses of metal binding proteins. Loss of antithrombin III (heparin cofactor) in the urine may be associated with increased coagulability, which may or may not be balanced by losses of procoagulant factors in the urine. If it is not, it may produce a hypercoagulable state, and the increased tendency to thrombosis may lead to renal vein thrombosis.

Some patients with NS develop severe IgG deficiency, in part due to urinary losses and hypercatabolism. Low-molecular-weight complement components may also be lost in the urine and contribute to defects in the opsonization of bacteria. Various drug-binding proteins (chiefly albumin) may be decreased, altering the pharmacokinetic and toxicity properties of many drugs. Cellulose acetate electrophoresis of serum reveals, in addition to diminished albumin levels, increases of alpha and beta globulins.

COMPLICATIONS AND MANAGEMENT OF THE NEPHROTIC SYNDROME *Edema* should be managed cautiously and conservatively. Overly vigorous diuresis with potent loop diuretics (furosemide or ethacrynic acid) may result in a further lowering of effective plasma volume, and GFR, and lead to postural hypotension. Severe extracellular volume depletion may predispose to the development of acute renal failure. The temptation to administer concentrated salt-poor albumin should be resisted, as nearly all the administered protein will be excreted in 24 to 48 h, so that any beneficial effect on plasma oncotic pressure will be transient. However, such treatment may be necessary in severely hypoalbuminemic patients suffering from profound postural symptoms or very refractory anasarca.

The treatment of *hyperlipidemia* is difficult at best and its influence on morbidity and mortality uncertain. Most agents effective in reducing cholesterol and/or triglyceride levels are either too toxic (e.g., clofibrate) or poorly tolerated (e.g., cholestyramine) for chronic use. The value of newer agents in the management of hyperlipidemia in NS is not well established.

The *thromboembolic complications* of NS are reasonably common and have a broad range of clinical manifestations, including spontaneous peripheral venous and/or arterial thromboses, as well as pulmonary arterial and renal venous occlusions. *Renal vein thrombosis,* either unilateral or bilateral, is a particularly distressing complication of NS. In the past, this was regarded as a cause rather than a consequence of NS, a conclusion no longer held to be true. Certain glomerular lesions are more likely than others to be associated with renal vein thrombosis. These include membranous nephropathy, membranoproliferative glomerulonephritis, and amyloidosis. Features which are suggestive of acute renal vein thrombosis include unilateral or bilateral flank or loin pain, gross hematuria, left-sided varicocele, widely fluctuating GFR and urinary protein excretion rates, and asymmetry of renal size and/or function. Scalloping of the ureters (due to collateral circulation) and evidence of pulmonary emboli and/or infarction (Chap. 298) may occur in chronic renal vein thrombosis. However, chronic forms of renal vein thrombosis are commonly asymptomatic. Renal vein thrombosis is best documented by selective renal venous angiography. The presence of a documented thromboembolic complication of NS is usually regarded as a clear indication for long-term oral anticoagulation. The effectiveness of heparin may be impaired by concomitant antithrombin III deficiency, a plasma factor required for the full expression of the heparin-induced antithrombin effect.

To offset protein malnutrition, a diet rich in protein of high biological value should be provided unless marked azotemia is present. Correction of transport protein deficiencies is not fea-

TABLE 294-3
Causes of the nephrotic syndrome

I Primary glomerular diseases
- *A* Minimal change disease
- *B* Mesangial proliferative glomerulonephritis*
- *C* Focal and segmental glomerulosclerosis
- *D* Membranous glomerulopathy
- *E* Membranoproliferative glomerulonephritis
  - *1* Type I
  - *2* Type II
  - *3* Other variants
- *F* Other uncommon lesions
  - *1* Crescentic glomerulonephritis
  - *2* Focal and segmental* unclassifiable lesions
  - *3* Unclassifiable lesions

II Secondary to other diseases
- *A* Infections: Poststreptococcal glomerulonephritis, endocarditis, "shunt nephritis," secondary syphilis, leprosy, hepatitis B, infectious mononucleosis, malaria, schistosomiasis, filariasis
- *B* Drugs: Organic gold; inorganic, organic, and elemental mercury; penicillamine; "street" heroin; probenecid; captopril; Tridione; mesantoin; perchlorate; antivenom; antitoxins; contrast media
- *C* Neoplasia: Hodgkin's disease, lymphomas, leukemia, carcinomas, melanoma, Wilms's tumor
- *D* Multisystem: Systemic lupus erythematosus, Schönlein-Henoch purpura, vasculitis, Goodpasture's syndrome, dermatomyositis, dermatitis herpetiformis, amyloidosis, sarcoidosis, Sjögren's syndrome, rheumatoid arthritis
- *E* Heredofamilial: Diabetes mellitus, Alport's syndrome, sickle cell disease, Fabry's disease, nail-patella syndrome, lipodystrophy, congenital nephrotic syndrome
- *F* Miscellaneous: Preeclamptic toxemia, thyroiditis, myxedema, malignant obesity, renovascular hypertension, chronic interstitial nephritis with vesicoureteric reflux, chronic allograft rejection, beestings

* *Includes Berger's disease (IgA nephropathy).*

sible. Supplemental vitamin D might be desirable if overt deficiency is present, but this has not been evaluated clinically. In rare circumstances, profound protein malnutrition or other complications of massive proteinuria may justify ablation of renal function by medical or surgical means.

A classification of the causes of NS is provided in Table 294-3. The multisystemic, heredofamilial, neoplastic, and metabolic causes are discussed in Chap. 295. The primary (idiopathic) glomerular diseases associated with NS, as well as the diseases secondary to infectious or drug etiologies, are considered below.

IDIOPATHIC NEPHROTIC SYNDROME This diagnosis is arrived at by exclusion of known causes of NS, such as infections, drug exposure, multisystem disease, or hereditary disorders. The idiopathic forms of NS are further classified according to the morphologic features found on renal biopsy (Table 294-4). Performance of a renal biopsy, at least among adults, is required for the accurate diagnosis of idiopathic NS and for the formulation of a rational plan of treatment. Children need not always be subjected to renal biopsy since careful clinical study can often lead to accurate diagnosis.

Minimal change disease This is often referred to as *lipoid nephrosis, nil lesion,* or *foot process disease.* In this form of idiopathic NS, although little or no alterations of the glomerular capillaries are demonstrable by light microscopy (hence the designation "minimal change"), *diffuse epithelial foot process effacement*[1] is evident by electron microscopy. Immunofluorescence microscopy reveals absent or irregular and nonspecific deposits of immunoglobulin and complement components. Minimal change disease is the most frequently encountered form of idiopathic NS in children, accounting for more than 70 to 80 percent of cases diagnosed before the age of 8. This lesion is not rare in adults, representing 15 to 20 percent of cases of idiopathic NS in patients over the age of 16. There is a slight predilection for males. Typically patients present with overt NS, normal blood pressure, normal or slightly reduced GFR, and a "benign" urinary sediment. Varying degrees of microscopic hematuria are found in up to 20 percent of cases. Urinary protein is typically highly selective in children (e.g., it contains principally albumin and minimal amounts of high-molecular-weight plasma proteins such as IgG, $alpha_2$ macroglobulin, or C3) but is variable in adults. Fibrin split products and C3 are absent in the urine. Serum levels of complement components are normal, except for a slight reduction in C1q. IgG concentrations are often quite depressed during relapse, whereas IgM levels are modestly increased, both during remission and relapse. Some cases may have associated allergic diathesis (e.g., to milk, pollens, etc.), a history of recent immunization, or upper respiratory infection. Circulating immune complexes may be found in some patients using certain assays. The histocompatibility antigen HLA-B12 is more prevalent when minimal change disease is associated with atopy, indicating a possible genetically based predisposition to this disease. Thromboembolic manifestations occur, but renal vein thrombosis is uncommon.

[1] *The term "fusion" is often used to describe these changes in foot processes, although true fusion of cell membranes does not occur.*

TABLE 294-4
Idiopathic nephrotic syndrome
SELECTED FEATURES OF UNDERLYING PRIMARY GLOMERULAR LESIONS

	*Morphology**			*Approximate prevalence in children/ adults, %*			
Lesion	*LM*	*IFM*	*EM*		*Common clinical/ lab features*	*Response to therapy†*	*Likelihood of maintaining renal function‡*
Minimal change	Normal or very mild proliferation	Negative-trace IgM	Foot process fusion, no deposits	70+/15–20	Highly selective proteinuria,§ *normal* C3, decreased IgG, increased IgM	Steroids++ Cytotoxic drugs+ (cyclophosphamide, chlorambucil) Frequent relapses	95+
Mesangial proliferative	Diffuse proliferation	Negative or variable mesangial IgM, IgG, C3	Mesangial deposits	15–20/5–10	Hematuria, *normal* C3	Steroids± Cytotoxic drugs (?)	80 (?)
Focal sclerosis	Focal and segmental sclerosis	Focal and segmental IgM, C3	Foot process fusion, sclerosis, hyaline	10/10	Hematuria, leukocyturia, poorly selective proteinuria, *normal* C3	Steroids− Cytotoxic drugs− Anticoagulants (?)	45–50
Membranous glomerulopathy	Thick capillary wall, spikes of BM material	Diffuse granular capillary wall IgG	Subepithelial deposits	<5/30–40	Variable protein selectivity, *normal* C3, renal vein thrombosis	Steroids+ Cytotoxic drugs (?)	50–70
Membranoproliferative							
Type I	Mesangial interposition, lobular change	Diffuse C3; variable IgG, IgM	Subendothelial deposits	8/<5	Hematuria, *reduced* C3 (intermittent)	Steroids (?) Anticoagulants (?) Cytotoxic drugs (?)	60
Type II	Mesangial interposition	C3 capillary wall and mesangial nodules	Intramembranous deposits	3/<5	Hematuria, *reduced* C3 (persistent), +C3NF	Steroids− Cytotoxic drugs−	45

* *LM = light microscopy, IFM = immunofluorescence microscopy, EM = electron microscopy, BM = basement membrane.*
† *Response to therapy: ++ = highly responsive, + = variably responsive, ± = occasionally responsive, − = unresponsive.*
‡ *Percent of patients maintaining sufficient renal function to obviate need for chronic dialysis or transplantation.*
§ *Protein selectivity = differential protein clearance, e.g., IgG/transferrin clearance ratio. Highly selective = <0.1, moderately selective = 0.11 to 0.20, poorly selective = >0.20.*

Spontaneous remissions and relapses of heavy proteinuria may occur, usually for reasons which are unexplained. Interestingly, an identical lesion is encountered in patients with Hodgkin's disease, in whom NS develops, suggesting a role for lymphocytes in its pathogenesis. Except for patients who develop focal and segmental sclerosing lesions (see below), a progressive decline in GFR does not occur. Acute renal failure is rare. In the preantibiotic era infection with encapsulated organisms (e.g., pneumococci) was a leading cause of death, but now the mortality rate is exceedingly low and most deaths are associated with complications of treatment rather than the disease itself. Rarely, acute renal failure may occur even in the absence of profound hypovolemia. The mechanism of this phenomenon is obscure but could relate to tubular obstruction from heavy proteinuria or severe glomerular epithelial cell effacement. The renal failure is responsive to steroids and diuretics.

Since the etiology and pathogenesis are unknown, treatment is empirical and symptomatic. A large body of evidence indicates that corticosteroids markedly enhance the natural tendency for this disease to undergo spontaneous remission. Daily and alternate-day oral steroid therapy seem to be equally effective, the latter associated with fewer steroid-related complications. Daily prednisone (60 mg/m^2 in children, 1 to 1.5 mg/kg in adults) for 4 weeks, followed by alternate-day prednisone (35 to 40 mg/m^2 in children, 1 mg/kg in adults) for 4 additional weeks is a regimen often recommended for initial treatment of this disorder. The vast majority of patients who respond do so within the first 4 weeks of treatment, but occasionally a favorable response requires more prolonged therapy. The absence of a response within 8 weeks is usually indicative of an error in diagnosis and should provoke a review of the renal biopsy. In many patients who respond, withdrawal of steroid treatment is often accompanied by relapse; this usually occurs within the first year after cessation of treatment. Such relapses may be re-treated with the initial regimen as described above, but with gradual withdrawal of prednisone and low-maintenance doses of 5 to 10 mg daily or on alternate days for 3 to 6 months. A steroid-dependent patient or one with multiple relapses may be benefited by a brief course of cyclophosphamide (1 to 2 mg/kg per day) or chlorambucil (0.1 to 0.2 mg/kg per day) for 8 to 12 weeks. When given with steroids to patients to induce remissions, either of these agents reduces the likelihood of a subsequent relapse. However, these agents have serious adverse effects on bone marrow, and in the case of cyclophosphamide, the gonads and urinary bladder. They may also be oncogenic. Azathioprine has been demonstrated to be ineffective in inducing prolonged remissions. The use of cytotoxic agents should be reserved for patients who develop serious or life-threatening complications of multiple courses of steroid therapy. The long-term prognosis of patients with the minimal change lesion is excellent; a 10-year survival in excess of 90 percent can be expected, but a few develop renal failure usually as a consequence of the lesion described in the next section.

MESANGIAL PROLIFERATIVE GLOMERULONEPHRITIS The lesion is characterized by a mild to moderate diffuse, but distinct, increase in the cellularity of the glomerular capillary bed. The peripheral glomerular capillary walls are thin and delicate, and extracapillary proliferation is not seen. The precise nature of the proliferating cells is not clearly understood but may represent combinations of proliferating mesangial cells, endothelial cells, and infiltrating mononuclear cells. Glomerular involvement is usually reasonably uniform, although there may be some segmental accentuation of hypercellularity. Necrosis of glomerular tufts is absent. Deposits of proteinaceous material, if seen, are confined to the mesangial areas. Interposition of mesangial cells and cytoplasm into the periphery of the glomerular capillary wall is not seen. By immunofluorescence, a variety of patterns are observed. If granular IgA deposits in the mesangium predominate, accompanied by C3 and fibrin-reactive antigens but not the early acting components of the complement cascade, then the lesion is categorized as IgA nephropathy, or Berger's disease (see below). Other patterns of immunofluorescence may be observed, including a predominance of IgM deposits in a granular pattern diffusely throughout the mesangium, isolated mesangial C3 deposits, scattered mesangial IgG deposits, and no immunoglobulin or complement deposits. Thus, the light-microscopic appearance of mesangial proliferative glomerulonephritis represents an extremely heterogeneous category of glomerular diseases with respect to underlying pathogenesis and undoubtedly to etiology. Some patients presenting with this morphologic lesion may in fact represent instances of resolving postinfectious glomerulonephritis, hereditary nephritis, or other multisystem diseases such as Henoch-Schönlein purpura, vasculitis, or systemic lupus erythematosus. Electron-microscopic findings are nonspecific. Occasionally small electron-dense paramesangial deposits may be observed. The findings of large electron-dense deposits in the mesangium in association with the morphologic appearance of mesangial proliferative glomerulonephritis should heighten the suspicion of a multisystem disease or Berger's IgA nephropathy.

This lesion accounts for approximately 10 percent of instances of idiopathic nephrotic syndrome in adults and 15 percent in children. It tends to be more common in older children and young adults. Males tend to be affected slightly more often than females. Hematuria, either gross or microscopic, is commonly observed. Loin pain, bilateral or unilateral, may be seen in the idiopathic disorder but is more frequently observed in patients who have underlying IgA nephropathy. Laboratory features are not distinctive. Renal function may be modestly decreased at the time of diagnosis but is most often normal. Complement component levels are most often normal. IgG levels may be modestly reduced. IgA levels may be increased in IgA nephropathy. Circulating immune complexes may be found in some patients. Anti-streptolysin O titers are usually normal. Proteinuria is most often nonselective. No association with HLA antigens has yet been described for that category of patients who do not display predominant IgA mesangial deposits. The pathogenesis of this lesion is unknown and almost certainly the result of diverse pathogenetic processes. The presence of mesangial immunoglobulin deposits and circulating immune complexes in some, but not all, patients suggests an immune-complex pathogenesis, although the antigen(s) is unknown.

Among patients with well-developed nephrotic syndrome and moderate to severe diffuse mesangial proliferation, there is a tendency for persistence of proteinuria and progression to renal insufficiency. This is particularly true if areas of focal and segmental glomerular sclerosis are noted to be superimposed on the mesangial proliferative lesion at the time of the initial renal biopsy. Patients with milder forms of mesangial proliferative glomerulonephritis, particularly when unassociated with mesangial immunoglobulin deposition, may follow a more benign course. Some patients behave in a fashion quite similar to those with the minimal change lesion. Since renal biopsies from patients with the minimal change lesion may display mild degrees of glomerular hypercellularity, the apparently benign course followed by this subset of patients may indicate that they should be categorized as examples of minimal change lesion with more prominent mesangial proliferation rather than separately categorized under the heading of mesangial proliferative glomerulonephritis. Patients with well-developed mesangial proliferative lesions, particularly in association with mesangial IgM deposits, tend to be unresponsive to corticosteroid therapy and to evolve with time into those of focal and segmental glomerular sclerosis. Indeed, the lesion of mesangial proliferative glomerulonephritis may be a predecessor of the lesion of focal and segmental glomerulosclerosis. Patients with mesangial proliferative glomerulonephritis who have complete remissions of proteinuria following treatment with corticosteroids in a fashion similar to that described for the minimal change lesion tend to do well with little inclination toward progressive renal insufficiency. Exacerbations and remissions of proteinuria may occur. Steroid-unresponsive patients with persistent nephrotic syndrome have a tendency to progress to renal insufficiency at variable rates. The role of adjunctive cytotoxic therapy (cyclophosphamide, chlorambucil, or azathioprine) has not yet been established in this category of lesions. Some studies have indicated that long-term therapy with indomethacin may be of benefit in this category of lesions, but no suitably controlled long-term studies have yet been performed.

Because of the highly variable pathogenesis in mesangial proliferative glomerulonephritis and its relative rarity, long-term prospective studies of natural history and therapy have not yet been conducted. Many patients, particularly those with mild degrees of proliferation and a remitting course following corticosteroid therapy, will have a very benign prognosis. Other patients, particularly those with steroid unresponsiveness and focal and segmental glomerulosclerosing lesions on the initial biopsy, will have a poor prognosis, often developing end-stage renal failure in 5 to 10 years following the initial diagnosis.

Focal and segmental glomerulosclerosis (focal sclerosis) This lesion is characterized by sclerosis and hyalinization of some, but not all, glomeruli (hence the term *focal*). Among affected glomeruli, only a portion of the glomerular tuft is abnormal (hence, *segmental*). There is a predilection for these lesions initially to affect the *juxtamedullary glomeruli* and to be associated with progressive tubulointerstitial damage. By immunofluorescence, granular and nodular deposits of IgM and C3 are found in the segmental sclerosing lesion. By electron microscopy, focal basement membrane collapse and denudation of epithelial surfaces are noted. All glomeruli reveal diffuse epithelial foot process effacement. This lesion accounts for 10 to 15 percent of cases of idiopathic NS seen among children and adults. Males tend to be affected slightly more often than females. Many investigators believe that focal sclerosis represents a stage in the evolution of a subgroup of patients with minimal change disease or "pure" mesangial proliferative glomerulonephritis (see above). In more than two-thirds of cases of focal sclerosis overt NS will be present at the time of diagnosis; in the remainder only isolated proteinuria in the nonnephrotic range is present. Hypertension, reduced GFR, abnormal tubule function, and abnormal urinary sediment occur commonly. It is important to emphasize that focal sclerosis may have clinical features indistinguishable from either minimal change disease, mesangial proliferative glomerulonephritis, or membranous glomerulopathy (see below). Proteinuria is nearly always nonselective or becomes so on follow-up. FDP and C3 may be present in the urine. Serum levels of C3 are normal and IgG levels are reduced, but not as severely as in minimal change disease. Similar lesions may be seen in association with "street" heroin abuse, vesicoureteral reflux, and renal allograft rejection and may complicate a variety of other primary glomerular diseases in the late stages. The occurrence of focal and segmental glomerulosclerosis in remnant glomeruli after extensive renal ablation has led to the suggestion that hyperfiltration (or some hemodynamic determinants thereof) may play a causative role in pathogenesis. Abnormalities in the prevalence of HLA antigens have not been consistently described. Renal vein thrombosis is uncommon.

There is little tendency for spontaneous remission, except among children. A progressive decline in GFR is the rule, albeit at variable rates. A subset of patients with focal sclerosis, who have extremely heavy proteinuria (i.e., greater than 15 to 20 g per day) and profound hypoalbuminemia, progress quite rapidly to end-stage renal failure, occasionally in a period of only a few months. Rarely, acute renal failure without recovery occurs.

The etiology and pathogenesis of focal sclerosis are unknown. Immune-complex–mediated disease has been postulated, primarily on the basis of immunofluorescence findings, and circulating immune complexes have been found in a small minority of cases.

There is no convincing evidence that any form of treatment is effective in forestalling the ultimate development of end-stage renal failure among patients with documented focal sclerosis. Some patients may experience a reduction in daily protein excretion with steroid therapy. The effect of cytotoxic drugs and anticoagulants requires further study. Partial remissions of proteinuria, i.e., reductions to less than 2 g per day, seem to be associated with an improved long-term prognosis. At least 50 percent of patients with persistent heavy proteinuria develop end-stage renal failure or die of intercurrent illnesses within 10 years of diagnosis. The prognosis is much poorer for those patients with persistent NS in whom azotemia or hypertension is evident at time of diagnosis. This lesion has been found to recur in renal allografts, occasionally within a few hours of transplantation, suggesting the possibility of a circulating glomerular permeability "toxin" in its pathogenesis.

Membranous glomerulopathy This lesion is characterized by the presence of irregular, discontinuous proteinaceous deposits along the outer (or subepithelial) aspect of the glomerular capillary wall. These deposits contain IgG and appear dense by electron microscopy. Unlike focal sclerosis, *all glomeruli are involved uniformly*. At an early stage all glomeruli may appear normal by light microscopy, but as the disease progresses, immune deposits coalesce, causing the capillary wall to thicken. Eventually, increased amounts of basement membrane material project outward between deposits toward the urinary space, giving the appearance of "spikes." There is little proliferation of capillary endothelial or mesangial cells, although mesangial sclerosis may occur in advanced cases. Tubulointerstitial atrophy and vascular lesions are other late manifestations.

This disorder accounts for 30 to 40 percent of cases of idiopathic NS in adults but is quite rare in children. In over 80 percent of cases overt NS is present. In the remainder only isolated proteinuria is found. Males tend to be affected more often than females. Blood pressure, GFR, and urinary sediment tend to be normal early in the course, making it extremely difficult to distinguish membranous glomerulopathy from minimal change disease on clinical grounds alone. Urinary protein selectivity is quite variable. Serum complement components are normal, but IgG levels are usually modestly depressed. Membranous glomerulopathy may develop in association with systemic lupus erythematosus (Chap. 295), certain chronic infections (e.g., malaria, hepatitis B), solid tumors (e.g., melanoma and cancer of the lung and colon), or after exposure to heavy metals (gold, mercury) or drugs (penicillamine). A careful search for these causes is warranted in every case of idiopathic NS due to membranous glomerulopathy. There appears to be a high frequency of renal vein thrombosis in affected patients (see above).

Spontaneous complete remissions of NS are quite common

in children with membranous nephropathy but take place in only 20 to 25 percent of adults. Steroid treatment does not greatly influence the development of lasting complete remissions, but may induce a reduction of proteinuria to nonnephrotic levels. A beneficial effect of steroids is still a source of controversy, since spontaneous partial remissions also occur, although somewhat less frequently than in steroid-treated patients. There is presently no agreement about optimal dosage and duration of therapy; however, alternate-day steroid therapy seems to be the safest approach. Cytotoxic agents appear to be of no benefit but are deserving of further study.

Slowly progressive renal functional impairment occurs almost exclusively among those patients with persistent proteinuria in the nephrotic range. Recently, controlled trials of short-term alternate-day prednisone therapy have demonstrated a reduction in the tendency for progressive renal failure. Partial or complete spontaneous or treatment-associated remissions provide nearly complete protection from renal failure. Complete or partial remissions occur at variable times after the discovery of the disease, but renal failure is unlikely to develop in the first few years. Within 10 years of the time of the diagnosis, however, 35 to 50 percent of patients will die of intercurrent illness or develop end-stage renal failure. The vast majority of survivors will have had complete or partial remission of proteinuria. Rare cases have recurred in renal transplants. A few patients are known to have developed superimposed anti-GBM antibody–mediated disease and RPGN.

Membranoproliferative glomerulonephritis This group of disorders is characterized by proliferation of mesangial cells, often with segmental or diffuse interposition of these cells or their cytoplasm into peripheral capillary loops. There is evidence of increased synthesis of mesangial matrix as well. The glomerular capillary wall is irregularly thickened, by virtue of the mesangial extensions and the attendant synthesis of basement membrane–like material. This group of disorders is also known as *mesangiocapillary* or *lobular glomerulonephritis.* Several immunofluorescence and electron-microscopic patterns are present and are believed to reflect heterogeneous mechanisms of pathogenesis. In the ultrastructural *type I* lesion, subendothelial electron-dense deposits are present. C3 is deposited in a granular pattern indicative of immune-complex pathogenesis, but IgG and the early components of complement are present inconsistently. In the ultrastructural *type II* lesion the lamina densa of the GBM is transformed into an extremely electron-dense character, giving rise to the term *dense deposit disease.* Basement membranes in Bowman's capsules and in tubules are similarly affected. C3 is found irregularly in the GBM and in granules or rings in the mesangium. Small amounts of Ig (typically IgM) are present, but the early acting complement components are absent from the deposits. Properdin deposition is variable. Additional ultrastructural variants, based upon location of deposit and basement membrane changes, have also been described.

Membranoproliferative glomerulonephritis, types I and II, is found in 5 to 10 percent of cases of idiopathic NS in children, particularly between the ages of 8 to 16 years, and somewhat less commonly in adults. Type I accounts for at least two-thirds of cases. Sexes are affected equally. In 50 to 75 percent of patients, a full-blown NS is present, often with features of AGN. In the remainder, proteinuria is in the nonnephrotic range and is nearly always accompanied by microscopic hematuria. Blood pressure and GFR are frequently abnormal, and the urinary sediment is typically active. Functional abnormalities of the renal tubules are common. Urinary protein selectivity is usually poor; FDP and C3 are found in the urine. Serum C3 levels are reduced in 70 to 80 percent of cases of type I and in over 90 percent of type II disease. The early acting complement components C1q, C4, and C2 are often normal, however, especially in type II disease. This pattern may be indicative of activation of the alternate complement pathway (see Chap. 293). C3 nephritic factor (C3NF) is often found in the serum of patients with type II, especially if the C3 level is quite low. Circulating immune complexes are found in type I. Lesions similar to type I membranoproliferative glomerulonephritis may also be found in SLE, hemolytic-uremic syndrome, transplant rejection, chronic hepatitis B antigenemia, and "shunt" nephritis. Renal vein thrombosis may occur. Type II nephritis may be associated with partial lipodystrophy.

Spontaneous remissions are uncommon. There is little evidence favoring a beneficial effect of any form of therapy, but long-term, alternate-day steroid therapy (0.3 to 0.5 mg/kg every other day) may delay the progression of the disease. Treatment regimens which combine steroids and cytotoxic agents are not of proven value. Recently, preliminary evidence suggesting a beneficial effect of anticoagulants and inhibitors of platelet aggregation has appeared. Larger scale trials involving longer follow-up periods will be required before this approach can be widely recommended. The course is usually relentlessly progressive, and approximately one-half of patients die or develop end-stage renal failure within 10 years of the diagnosis. The prognosis for type II lesions seems somewhat worse than for type I. Type II disease almost invariably recurs in the transplanted kidney but does not always result in the premature loss of the allograft.

Other forms of idiopathic nephrotic syndrome In a small percentage of adults and children with idiopathic NS (i.e., 5 to 10 percent) other lesions are encountered on renal biopsy. These include *crescentic glomerulonephritis* and *focal* and *segmental proliferative glomerulonephritis.* The pathogenetic mechanisms responsible for these lesions vary. For example, some of the cases of focal and segmental glomerulonephritis may have extensive mesangial IgA deposits and fit into the category of Berger's disease (see below). Serum C3 levels are usually normal. The clinical characteristics, natural history, and response to treatment of these lesions are not well defined. Hematuria is common and may be recurrent. Proteinuria tends to be nonselective. Spontaneous remissions of NS are uncommon. Since no controlled studies have been conducted, it is not possible to evaluate the effectiveness of treatment. Crescentic glomerulonephritis is likely to have a poor prognosis, whereas mesangial and focal and segmental proliferative glomerulonephritis have a more favorable long-term outlook.

NEPHROTIC SYNDROME CAUSED BY INFECTIOUS AGENTS, DRUGS, OR CHEMICALS Table 294-3 lists the common infectious and drug-related etiologies of NS. In many instances, NS will abate following cure of the infection or withdrawal of the offending medication. In patients receiving organic gold therapy for rheumatoid arthritis, or in those exposed to inorganic, organic, or elemental mercury or to penicillamine therapy, membranous glomerulopathy is usually the lesion responsible for NS. NS is known to follow immunization and antiserum treatment of tetanus or snakebite and to occur in situations associated with atopy.

ASYMPTOMATIC URINARY ABNORMALITIES

This group of patients is identified principally by the findings of *proteinuria in the nonnephrotic range and/or hematuria,* unaccompanied by edema, reduced GFR, or hypertension. Abnormalities are often discovered incidentally and may be persistent or recurrent. This syndrome may, of course, be but a phase in the natural history of other glomerulopathic syndromes, especially nephrotic syndrome or chronic glomerulonephritis. Common glomerular disorders which present as asymptomatic proteinuria and/or hematuria at some point in their natural history are listed in Table 294-5. The heredofamilial and multisystem diseases are discussed in Chap. 295.

IDIOPATHIC RENAL HEMATURIA (See also Chap. 40) **Berger's disease (IgA nephropathy)** This disorder was first described by Berger and Hinglais in 1968 and is characterized by recurrent episodes of gross or microscopic hematuria. The diagnosis depends on the finding of prominent IgA deposits in the mesangium by immunofluorescence microscopy. Berger's disease is the most common cause of recurrent hematuria of glomerular origin. It most commonly affects young adults, mostly males. Typically, episodes of macroscopic hematuria are associated with minor flu-like illnesses or vigorous exercise. Patients frequently complain of vague constitutional symptoms, but skin rash, arthritis, and abdominal pain are absent. Urine protein excretion rates are usually less than 3.5 g per day; not uncommonly protein excretion is normal or only mildly increased. The nephrotic syndrome develops occasionally. Blood pressure, GFR, and serum albumin are normal, at least early in the disease. Serum IgA levels are increased in about 50 percent of cases, while serum complement component levels remain normal. Biopsy of the skin of the volar surface of the forearm will often reveal dermal capillary deposits of IgA, C3, and fibrin, but not early acting complement components or IgA secretory fragments. Similar skin biopsy findings may be encountered in Schönlein-Henoch purpura (Chap. 295). Indeed, Berger's disease may be a monosymptomatic form of Schönlein-Henoch purpura.

Renal biopsy reveals a spectrum of changes by light microscopy, but diffuse mesangial proliferative or focal and segmental proliferative glomerulonephritis is found most often. In some cases glomerular morphology may be normal by light microscopy; rarely, crescents may be found. The distinguishing feature is the finding by immunofluorescence microscopy of *diffuse mesangial deposition of IgA,* often accompanied by lesser amounts of IgG and nearly always by C3 and properdin, but not by C1q or C4. Fibrin reactive antigens are also commonly demonstrable in the mesangium or in association with crescents if the latter are present. The pathogenesis of IgA nephropathy is unknown, but the systemic character of the IgA deposits (skin and glomerular capillaries), the presence of circulating IgG and IgA complexes in the majority of cases, and its similarity to Schönlein-Henoch purpura suggest that it is an immune-complex–mediated disease. The nature and source of the antigen are unknown.

The prognosis is variable, but, in general, the disease tends to progress slowly. It has been estimated that approximately 50 percent of patients can be expected to develop end-stage renal failure within 25 years of the time of diagnosis. Azotemia, hypertension, or proteinuria in the nephrotic range at the time of diagnosis are associated with a poor prognosis. At present, there is no evidence to suggest that any form of therapy greatly influences the natural history. Some have suggested that intermittent steroid therapy may reduce the frequency of episodes of gross hematuria.

Other primary renal hematurias Some cases of recurrent hematuria do not reveal the typical immunofluorescence findings seen in Berger's disease. This group of patients is poorly defined, and in them the etiology and pathogenesis is varied. Some may represent resolving episodes of acute glomerulonephritis or early examples of membranoproliferative or hereditary glomerulonephritis (Alport's syndrome, see Chap. 295). The morphologic lesions most commonly encountered are focal and segmental or diffuse mesangial proliferative glomerulonephritis, although mild and nonspecific glomerular changes may also be observed. Immunofluorescence studies reveal varying degrees of immunoglobulin and/or complement component deposition (principally IgM and/or C3) in the mesangium. Some cases show linear deposits of IgG, suggesting a possible anti-GBM antibody pathogenesis. Electron microscopy may reveal dense deposits in the mesangium. Overall, this group of patients is believed to have an excellent prognosis, with spontaneous permanent remissions of recurrent hematuria. Progressive renal insufficiency is unusual. Because of the benign prognosis no treatment is indicated.

ISOLATED NONNEPHROTIC PROTEINURIA OF GLOMERULAR ORIGIN (See also Chap. 40) The discovery of mild to moderate degrees of proteinuria (i.e., greater than 150 mg but less than 2.0 g per day), unaccompanied by abnormalities in the urinary sediment or evidence of hypertension or reduced renal function, is a common problem in internal medicine. Such patients may display other features of heredofamilial or multisystem diseases, including diabetes mellitus, amyloidosis, rheumatoid arthritis, or cancer. Among cases of isolated proteinuria consequent to primary glomerular disease the abnormality may either be persistent or evanescent. Proteinuria may occur primarily in the upright posture (*orthostatic proteinuria*) or be present both in recumbent and erect positions. Persistent nonnephrotic proteinuria, demonstrable in both orthostatic and recumbent positions, generally indicates the presence of some significant and readily demonstrable glomerular pathology. Some of the lesions which might be encountered have been discussed in the context of idiopathic nephrotic syndrome. Other patients may prove to have a clinically unsuspected disease such as amyloidosis or diabetes mellitus. In the remainder, the lesions are usually trivial and nonspecific and their long-term significance is quite uncertain. In the case of primary glomerular diseases, so long as urinary protein excretion remains modest, the prognosis is excellent and deterioration of renal function is uncommon. On the other hand, orthostatic proteinuria is more often than not associated with mild and entirely nonspecific glomerular alterations which have little tendency for progression. Furthermore, orthostatic proteinuria commonly disappears during prolonged follow-up. Renal biopsy is commonly undertaken in patients with persistent and isolated proteinuria, largely as a means of accurately estimating long-term prognosis.

TABLE 294-5
Glomerular causes of asymptomatic urinary abnormalities

I Hematuria with or without proteinuria
- *A* Primary glomerular diseases
  - *1* Berger's disease (IgA nephropathy)
  - *2* Membranoproliferative glomerulonephritis
  - *3* Other primary glomerular hematurias accompanied by "pure" mesangial proliferation, focal and segmental proliferative glomerulonephritis, or other lesions
- *B* Associated with multisystem or heredofamilial diseases
  - *1* Alport's syndrome and other "benign" familial hematurias
  - *2* Fabry's disease
  - *3* Sickle cell disease
- *C* Associated with infections
  - *1* Resolving poststreptococcal glomerulonephritis
  - *2* Other postinfectious glomerulonephritides

II Isolated nonnephrotic proteinuria
- *A* Primary glomerular diseases
  - *1* "Orthostatic" proteinuria
  - *2* Focal and segmental glomerulosclerosis
  - *3* Membranous glomerulopathy
- *B* Associated with multisystem or heredofamilial diseases
  - *1* Diabetes mellitus
  - *2* Amyloidosis
  - *3* Nail-patella syndrome

CHRONIC GLOMERULONEPHRITIS (CGN)

The syndrome of CGN is characterized chiefly by *persistent urinary abnormalities* (e.g., proteinuria and/or hematuria) and by *slowly progressive impairment of renal function,* eventuating in hypertension, contracted granular kidneys, and end-stage renal failure. With the possible exception of the minimal change lesion associated with idiopathic nephrotic syndrome (see above) all the disorders described in this chapter and in Chap. 295 can lead eventually to CGN. The pathophysiology of the syndrome of CGN as it appears in the context of renal failure is described in Chaps. 289 and 291.

The glomerular structural alterations that underlie this syndrome may be categorized as *proliferative* (including mesangial, endo- and/or extracapillary proliferative glomerulonephritis, and focal and segmental proliferative glomerulonephritis), *sclerosing* (including focal and diffuse glomerular sclerosis), and *membranous.* Such lesions are found in the vast majority of patients with CGN. In the small remainder, the underlying lesions are not readily categorized morphologically. These are often referred to as *chronic "nonspecific" glomerulonephritis.*

The clinical characteristics of the specific lesions are described in other sections of this chapter. The etiologic and pathogenetic origins of chronic nonspecific glomerulonephritis are unknown but are undoubtedly heterogeneous. Complicating vascular disease contributes to the glomerular obliteration seen in this group of disorders. It is quite reasonable to suspect that some of the patients categorized as having chronic nonspecific glomerulonephritis may have had an earlier unrecognized or undiagnosed episode of acute PSGN. However, such patients usually fail to recall a specific episode of acute nephritis.

The detection of CGN usually occurs in one of several ways: (1) by the incidental finding of abnormal urine, impaired renal function, or hypertension during multiphasic screening of asymptomatic individuals or during evaluation of such individuals for an unrelated illness; (2) as the result of the insidious onset of progressive symptoms or signs of advanced renal disease, especially anemia and hypertension; or (3) after an exacerbation of glomerulonephritis, usually during the course of a nonspecific viral or bacterial illness. In advanced stages of the syndrome, the clinical separation of CGN from other causes of renal failure may be difficult; however, the presence of symmetrically contracted kidneys, moderate to heavy proteinuria, abnormal urinary sediment (especially red blood cell casts), and x-ray evidence of normal pyelocalyceal systems are all suggestive of CGN.

The evolution of CGN varies considerably, depending upon the nature of the underlying disease and the presence or absence of complications, especially hypertension. Ten, fifteen, twenty, or more years may elapse from the first discovery of an abnormal urine sediment until the development of end-stage renal failure. Renal biopsy is necessary to define the precise nature of the underlying glomerular lesion. The principal advantage of a morphologic evaluation among patients presenting with the syndrome of CGN is to determine prognosis rather than therapy.

Treatment of patients with CGN is supportive and symptomatic. Despite many years of controlled and uncontrolled trials, unequivocal evidence of a favorable effect of treatment with steroids, cytotoxic agents, nonsteroidal anti-inflammatory agents, and anticoagulants has yet to be provided. The management of specific lesions is discussed in greater detail in the relevant sections of this chapter. Hypertension and symptomatic urinary tract infections should be treated vigorously, taking care to avoid nephrotoxic agents. Diuretics should generally be employed only as adjuncts to antihypertensive management or to deal with debilitating degrees of edema. Fluid and sodium should be provided according to the dictates of blood pressure control. Rigorous salt restriction is usually unnecessary and may be hazardous. In the absence of congestive heart failure or marked hypoalbuminemia, severe edema rarely occurs in CGN until the terminal phases of the illness. Potassium restriction is usually unnecessary.

REFERENCES

CAMERON JS: Pathogenesis and treatment of membranous glomerulonephritis. Kidney Intern 15:88, 1979

———: The natural history of glomerulonephritis, in *Renal Disease,* 4th ed, D Black, NF Jones (eds). Oxford, Blackwell Scientific, 1980

DROZ D: Natural history of primary glomerulonephritis with mesangial deposits of IgA. Contrib Nephrol 2:150, 1976

GLASSOCK RJ: A clinical and immunopathologic dissection of rapidly progressive glomerulonephritis. Nephron 22:253, 1978

——— et al: Primary glomerular diseases, in *The Kidney,* 2d ed, BM Brenner, FC Rector Jr (eds). Philadelphia, Saunders, 1981

———, COHEN AH: Secondary glomerular diseases, in *The Kidney,* 2d ed, BM Brenner, FC Rector Jr (eds). Philadelphia, Saunders, 1981

HOSTETTER TH, RENNKE HG, BRENNER BM: Compensatory renal hemodynamic injury: A final common pathway of residual nephron destruction. Am J Kidney Dis 1:310, 1982

KINCAID-SMITH P et al (eds): *Progress in Glomerulonephritis.* New York, Wiley, 1979

LIEN JWK, MATHEW TH, MEADOWS R: Acute post-streptococcal glomerulonephritis in adults—a long-term study. Q J Med 40:99, 1979

295
GLOMERULOPATHIES ASSOCIATED WITH MULTISYSTEM DISEASES

RICHARD J. GLASSOCK
BARRY M. BRENNER

Glomerular injury may be a prominent feature of diseases which affect multiple organs and systems. By and large the etiologies of these diseases are unknown, but aberrant immunologic processes, neoplasia, metabolic disturbances, and genetically based biochemical abnormalities are believed to be dominant factors in their pathogenesis.

IMMUNOLOGICALLY MEDIATED MULTISYSTEM DISEASES

SYSTEMIC LUPUS ERYTHEMATOSUS (See also Chap. 70) Systemic lupus erythematosus (SLE) is the archetype of an immunologically mediated multisystem disease (see Chap. 293) and is representative of the group of multisystem diseases in which renal involvement is extremely common. The etiology of SLE is unknown; however, a growing body of evidence suggests that viral infection, genetic factors, and abnormal immune responsiveness interact to produce the disease. The principal pathogenetic mechanism responsible for tissue injury in SLE appears to be the deposition of circulating immune complexes, although other mechanisms in all likelihood also play a role, including antitissue antibody, "planted" antigens, and in situ immune-complex formation (see Chap. 293). The circulating immune complexes may be composed of a wide variety of endogenous antigens combined with autoantibodies. Viral-antiviral immune complexes (retroviral antigens) may also be present. DNA (single-stranded and double-stranded) is a major antigenic component of immune complexes. The prevalence of clinically evident renal involvement in SLE has been variously reported, ranging from as low as 35 percent to more than 90 percent. Clinical manifestations of renal disease range from mild abnormalities of the urinary sediment (predominantly hematuria) to massive proteinuria, and from chronic indolent glomerulonephritis to a fulminant inflammatory process leading to rapidly progressive renal failure.

Morphological evidence of renal involvement may exist with or without clinical manifestations. If immunofluorescence and electron-microscopic studies of renal tissue are performed, abnormalities are present in virtually every patient with SLE. The diagnosis and extrarenal manifestations of SLE are more fully described in Chap. 70. This section will deal with the clinical features of the various forms of renal involvement of SLE. Although extrarenal features often dominate the clinical picture, SLE may present initially solely with renal manifestations. The abnormal glomerular morphological lesions observed in SLE form a spectrum which may be divided, somewhat arbitrarily, into several categories based upon correlative light- and electron-microscopic and immunofluorescence studies of renal biopsies.

Minimal lupus glomerular lesion This pattern is characterized by few or no changes by light microscopy. Immunofluorescence studies reveal moderate immunoglobulin (Ig) and complement deposits exclusively in mesangium. Scattered electron-dense deposits are found in mesangium by electron microscopy. Clinical renal manifestations may include mild proteinuria and microscopic hematuria. Glomerular filtration rate (GFR) is almost always normal. Serologic manifestations vary according to activity of extrarenal disease. Antibodies to DNA are usually found in low titer, and levels of C3 and C4 may be decreased, especially if dermatitis is severe. Circulating immune complexes may be detected in patients with this lesion.

Mesangial lupus glomerulonephritis This pattern is characterized by mild to moderate diffuse mesangial cell proliferation and/or mesangial sclerosis. Immunofluorescence studies reveal immunoglobulins (IgG, IgM, and IgA) and complement components (C1q, C4, C3) deposited in a granular pattern exclusively in the mesangium. Electron-dense deposits are also confined to the mesangium by electron microscopy. This morphological appearance may be found in the absence of clinical evidence of renal disease or may be associated with only minor abnormalities in the urinary sediment and modest proteinuria. GFR is almost always normal. Hypertension may or may not be present. It is thought that mesangial lupus glomerulonephritis may be the initial stage of renal involvement in SLE, from which all other patterns evolve. Associated serologic abnormalities depend upon the degree of extrarenal activity. These include positive antinuclear antibodies (ANA); increased levels of antibody to denatured, single-stranded (ssDNA) or native, double-stranded (dsDNA); depressed serum levels of C3, C4, and C1q; and detectable levels of circulating immune complexes (CIC) (Table 295-1).

Focal and segmental lupus glomerulonephritis This pattern is characterized by focal and segmental cellular proliferation, often associated with necrosis, superimposed on diffuse mesangial hypercellularity. Granular deposits of immunoglobulins and complement components are more extensive than in the mesangial form and involve both the mesangium and occasional glomerular capillary loops. By electron microscopy subendothelial dense deposits are found in the mesangium and in a few peripheral capillary loops. Clinical and laboratory evidence of renal injury is observed more commonly than in mesangial lupus glomerulonephritis. Nephrotic syndrome may occur in 10 to 20 percent of patients, but in general GFR is well preserved. This lesion may persist, resolve, or progress to diffuse proliferative lupus glomerulonephritis. Serologic features of active disease are often present in untreated patients. A recent study suggests that patients in this category who have necrosis of glomerular capillary loops have the same prognosis as those with diffuse glomerulonephritis.

Diffuse proliferative lupus glomerulonephritis This pattern is characterized by diffuse mesangial and endothelial cell proliferation which may include extensive peripheral capillary wall interposition of mesangial cells (i.e., membranoproliferative glomerulonephritis; see Chap. 294). In addition focal cellular necrosis, hematoxylinophilic bodies, fibrinoid necrosis, and "wire loops" (capillaries whose basement membranes are thickened markedly owing to subendothelial deposits) may be present. Extensive extracapillary proliferative (crescentic) glomerulonephritis, vasculitis, and interstitial nephritis may also be found. Granular deposits of immunoglobulins and complement components are extensive and involve the mesangium and nearly every capillary loop. Electron microscopy reveals extensive subendothelial and mesangial electron-dense deposits as well as occasional intramembranous or subepithelial deposits. Most patients will have an active urinary sediment,

TABLE 295-1
Serologic findings in selected multisystem diseases

Disease	*C3*	*Ig*	*FANA*	*Anti-dsDNA*	*Anti-GBM*	*Cryo-Ig*	*CIC*
Systemic lupus erythematosus	+ to +++	↑ IgG	+++	++	−	++	+++
Goodpasture's syndrome	−	−	−	−	+++	−	±
Henoch-Schönlein purpura	−	↑ IgA	−	−	−	±	++
Polyarteritis	+	↑ IgG	+	±	−	++	+++
Wegener's granulomatosis	±	↑ IgA, IgE	−	−	−	±	++
Cryoimmunoglobulinemia	++	±	−	−	−	+++	++
Multiple myeloma	−	↓↑IgG, IgA, IgD, IgE	−	−	−	+	±
Waldenström's macroglobulinemia	−	↑ IgM	−	−	−	−	−
Amyloidosis	−	± Ig	−	−	−	−	−

NOTE: *C3 = C3 component of complement; Ig = immunoglobulin levels; FANA = fluorescent antinuclear antibody assay; anti-dsDNA = antibody to double-stranded (native) DNA; anti-GBM = antibody to glomerular basement membrane antigens; cryo-Ig = cryoimmunoglobulin; CIC = circulating immune complexes; − = normal; + = occasionally slightly abnormal; ++ = often abnormal; +++ = severely abnormal.*

heavy proteinuria, and progressive impairment of renal function; occasionally, however, clinical evidence of renal involvement is lacking. In the untreated patient evidence of serologic activity is usually present, including positive ANA, markedly depressed serum C3 and C4 concentrations, high levels of precipitating and nonprecipitating complement-fixing antibody to dsDNA, cryoimmunoglobulinemia, and circulating immune complexes (CIC). This lesion usually is associated with an ominous prognosis, although vigorous treatment may greatly modify the course (see below).

Membranous lupus glomerulopathy This pattern is nearly identical to that described for idiopathic membranous glomerulopathy (Chap. 294), except that mesangial deposits and mesangial proliferation are seen more frequently. There is thickening of the glomerular capillary wall due to the presence of immunoglobulin and complement-containing electron-dense deposits in the subepithelial space, often associated with a spike-like basement membrane reaction. Nearly all patients manifest heavy proteinuria and the nephrotic syndrome. Although GFR may be normal initially, most patients ultimately develop progressive renal failure. A proliferative lesion may occasionally evolve in these patients, and the prognosis then assumes that of the diffuse proliferative form of glomerulonephritis. Serologic features of SLE may or may not be present at the time of diagnosis of this nephropathy. Antibody to dsDNA tends to be nonprecipitating. Some patients with membranous lupus glomerulopathy may be erroneously categorized as having idiopathic membranous glomerulopathy (see Chap. 294). Careful serial serologic investigations, measurement of the level of antibody to dsDNA or ssDNA, circulating immune complexes, and biopsies of skin for dermal-epidermal deposits of Ig ("lupus band test") may prove helpful for diagnosis in such cases.

Sclerosing or end-stage lupus glomerulonephritis This pattern is characterized by obliterative and sclerosing lesions of portions of the glomeruli, and probably represents a late stage of proliferative lesions. Immunofluorescence studies may be only weakly positive for immunoglobulins; subendothelial deposits are seen infrequently. Hypertension and impaired renal function are common. Serologic parameters of activity of SLE may or may not be present.

Prognosis and treatment The prognosis and treatment of SLE with renal involvement depends to a large extent upon the nature of the underlying renal lesion. Patients with milder forms of renal disease (e.g., minimal, mesangial, or focal lupus glomerulonephritis) tend to do well if treatment is primarily directed to control of the extrarenal manifestations of the disease. Corticosteroids in modest doses, salicylates, or antimalarials are usually sufficient. Potent nonsteroidal, anti-inflammatory agents may cause functional depression of GFR and should be used with caution in patients with known renal involvement. Serologic parameters, including anti-dsDNA and complement components (C3, C4), should be followed serially. Fluorescent antinuclear antibody tests have little value in prognosis or in following the effectiveness of treatment in patients with SLE. A return to normal values for antibody to dsDNA and/or complement components is a favorable sign; however, persistently abnormal serologic features do not necessarily indicate worsening or progressive renal involvement, especially in patients with active extrarenal manifestations. For patients with mild lesions which have not evolved into diffuse proliferative lupus glomerulonephritis, overall survival is excellent, and 85 percent or more of patients can be expected to survive at least 10 years. Patients with membranous lupus glomerulopathy who receive treatment directed primarily at the extrarenal features also have favorable long-term prognosis. On the other hand, patients with diffuse proliferative lupus glomerulonephritis do less well and, therefore, warrant a more aggressive approach toward ameliorating the renal disease. Unfortunately, it has been difficult to prove unequivocally that aggressive forms of treatment, such as high doses of oral or parenteral steroids or combinations of steroids and cytotoxic drugs (immunosuppressive therapy), are truly beneficial in the management of these patients. It has been suggested that high doses of steroids, either given as "pulses" of parenteral methylprednisolone (10 to 20 mg/kg for 3 to 5 doses) or oral prednisone (1 to 2 mg/kg per day) for weeks or months, are required to suppress clinical manifestations of glomerular disease (restore GFR, improve urine sediment, and reduce proteinuria). Unfortunately, some patients will continue to manifest active and progressive renal disease despite such aggressive steroid therapy. A large body of experience, mostly uncontrolled, has suggested that the addition of a cytotoxic agent (i.e., azathioprine, cyclophosphamide, or chlorambucil) will exert a "steroid-sparing" effect and act to bring the disease under better control. This suggestion has been difficult to confirm in controlled studies. Cytotoxic agents have serious side effects (e.g., enhanced susceptibility to infections, bladder irritation, damaging effects on the gonads, and possible oncogenic potential). These very real hazards notwithstanding, selected patients with diffuse proliferative glomerulonephritis treated with a combination of steroids and cytotoxic drugs seem to have done better than would be expected. A trial of such therapy seems indicated providing no contraindications exist, fully informed consent is obtained, and there is sufficient histopathologic evidence to support the notion that the renal lesions are, in fact, potentially reversible. Little is to be gained by using a combined steroid-cytotoxic approach in patients with advanced renal failure due to progressive glomerular capillary obliteration and sclerosis. These patients are best referred for dialysis and/or transplantation. The role of intensive plasma exchange accompanied by immunosuppressive therapy for fulminating disease has not yet been established, but early experience appears extremely promising. In some centers an aggressive steroid-cytotoxic drug approach has been associated with an approximate 85 percent 5-year survival in diffuse proliferative lupus glomerulonephritis. Serologic studies, especially serial measurements of antibody to dsDNA, complement components, and circulating immune complexes, are useful parameters to follow in patients under therapy. Normalization of these parameters usually indicates satisfactory control of disease and provides reassurance that drug dosage can be safely diminished. These measurements also need to be monitored in order to guide resumption of more aggressive therapy.

Overall, long-term prognosis for patients with SLE and renal involvement has improved steadily over the past decade. Whether improvements in methods of diagnosis, serologic monitoring, or treatment are responsible is unknown. Progression to end-stage renal disease is now relatively uncommon even for patients with diffuse proliferative glomerulonephritis. Cerebral involvement and infectious complications of therapy now loom as major causes of morbidity and mortality in SLE. Patients with SLE seem to do well on regular chronic dialysis; moreover, as uremia develops, some patients have noted remissions of extrarenal activity. In transplanted patients, recurrence of SLE in the renal allograft has been quite uncommon. These observations indicate that patients with SLE and nephritis are satisfactory candidates for both dialysis and transplantation.

GOODPASTURE'S SYNDROME This disorder consists of a triad of findings: *pulmonary hemorrhage, glomerulonephritis,* and *antibody to basement membrane antigens.* Its etiology is unknown. Goodpasture's syndrome typically affects young males but may appear at any age. Pulmonary hemorrhage may be extremely mild and easily overlooked, or severe and life-threatening. The initial manifestations of pulmonary involvement are cough, mild shortness of breath, and hemoptysis. Hilar pulmonary infiltrates may be seen by chest x-ray, and hypoxia is frequent. With marked intraalveolar hemorrhage pulmonary carbon monoxide uptake is increased, and the pulmonary clearance of radioactive carbon monoxide is depressed. Pulmonary iron sequestration may be documented by scanning of the lungs with ^{59}Fe. Hemosiderin-laden macrophages may be seen in the sputum, but this is a nonspecific finding. Iron-deficiency anemia may result if pulmonary bleeding is prolonged and severe. A history of recent inhalation of volatile hydrocarbons or viral influenza may be obtained. Fever, arthralgias, and other systemic symptoms are generally mild or absent at the time of presentation. Pulmonary hemorrhage may also be associated with renal failure in SLE, polyarteritis, Wegener's granulomatosis, cryoimmunoglobulinemia, Henoch-Schönlein purpura, pulmonary embolism consequent to renal vein thrombosis, Legionnaires' disease, and as a feature of congestive heart failure occurring in patients with end-stage renal disease. These disorders can ordinarily be differentiated from Goodpasture's syndrome by their extrarenal clinical features and by typical serologic findings (Table 295-1).

The appearance of glomeruli in Goodpasture's syndrome ranges from normal or nearly normal to focal proliferative and necrotizing glomerulonephritis; most often there is extensive extracapillary proliferation (crescents). Rapidly progressive renal failure is the most common clinical feature of the syndrome, although patients may initially present only with microscopic abnormalities in the urinary sediment and normal renal function. Immunofluorescence studies of renal biopsy material reveal the typical *linear deposits* of anti-basement membrane antibody, often but not necessarily always accompanied by C3 deposition. Anti-basement membrane antibodies can be eluted from such tissue by appropriate in vitro techniques. Electron-microscopic studies do not reveal electron-dense deposits.

Circulating antibody to basement membrane (glomerular, alveolar, and tubular) antigens are found in over 90 percent of cases if serums are examined early in the course of the disease by such sensitive assays as immunofluorescence or radioimmunoassay (Table 295-1). The level of circulating antibody does not correlate well with the severity of the renal or pulmonary manifestations. Measurements of circulating antibody are principally of diagnostic value and have no established prognostic significance. Serum complement components are nearly always normal; CIC and cryoimmunoglobulins are absent.

The course of the disorder is quite variable. Patients surviving an initial bout of severe hemoptysis may undergo long-term remissions of pulmonary disease or may have repeated bouts of pulmonary hemorrhage. Mild forms of glomerular injury may not progress, and the principal clinical problems may be related to recurrent hemoptysis. The diagnosis in such patients may be confused clinically with idiopathic pulmonary hemosiderosis. More commonly the renal disease is progressive, sometimes fulminant, leading to oliguric renal failure in a matter of a few weeks or months (i.e., rapidly progressive glomerulonephritis).

The treatment of Goodpasture's syndrome is undergoing a rapid and dramatic change. Life-threatening degrees of pulmonary hemorrhage may respond temporarily to high doses of parenteral methylprednisolone (10 to 15 mg/kg) given over short periods. The effectiveness of such steroid therapy in reversing extensive crescentic glomerular lesions is not well established. Anticoagulants are contraindicated in the face of active pulmonary hemorrhage. Intensive plasma exchange (2 to 4 liters of plasma per day), employed in combination with cytotoxic drugs and modest doses of steroids, has been associated with dramatic remissions of pulmonary hemorrhage and improvement of the glomerular lesions. This is particularly true if treatment is initiated early in patients with relatively acute disease in whom oliguria has not yet developed. The duration and frequency of plasma exchanges need to be individualized, depending upon the clinical response of the patient and results of monitoring levels of circulating antibody to glomerular basement membrane antigens. Renal biopsy is helpful in guiding the management, but even in the presence of very extensive crescent formation satisfactory responses have been obtained. If irreversible glomerular obliteration, extensive interstitial fibrosis, and tubular atrophy are found, especially in the oliguric patient with long-standing disease, intensive plasma exchange offers little hope for improving the renal lesion. Such patients are best referred for regular hemodialysis and/or transplantation. Although recurrences may occasionally develop after renal transplantation, Goodpasture's syndrome is not a contraindication to transplantation so long as transplantation is delayed until circulating anti-basement membrane antibody has fallen to undetectable levels.

HENOCH-SCHÖNLEIN PURPURA (See also Chap. 333) This disorder is characterized by the development of nonthrombocytopenic purpura, arthralgias, abdominal pain, and glomerulonephritis. Renal involvement is very common and is manifested chiefly by hematuria and proteinuria. In some instances renal involvement is severe, leading to rapidly progressive glomerulonephritis or nephrotic syndrome. The onset of the disease may resemble acute postinfectious glomerulonephritis. Serum complement component levels are usually normal. Serum IgA levels are increased in about half the patients (Table 295-1). Renal biopsy reveals a spectrum of abnormalities depending upon the severity of clinical renal disease. Mild diffuse mesangial cell proliferation and/or focal and segmental proliferative glomerulonephritis is noted most commonly when bouts of macroscopic hematuria accompanied by modest proteinuria are found clinically. More severe and diffuse proliferative glomerulonephritis, sometimes accompanied by extracapillary proliferation (crescents), is seen among patients with heavy proteinuria and/or rapidly diminishing GFR. Characteristically, immunofluorescence studies reveal mesangial and peripheral capillary granular deposits of IgA, IgG, C3, properdin, and fibrinogen but not C1q, C4, IgA secretory piece, or IgM. Similar immunofluorescence findings are noted in the dermal capillaries of biopsies of involved and uninvolved skin. Electron microscopy reveals electron-dense deposits principally confined to the mesangium. These findings suggest that Henoch-Schönlein purpura is due to circulating IgA-containing immune complexes. Circulating cryoimmunoglobulins and immune complexes have been noted in some instances; however, the nature of the antigen and the antibody reactivity of the IgA are unknown. Although food allergies and upper respiratory infections may be present, there is no clear-cut etiologic relationship. *Berger's disease* (IgA nephropathy, Chap. 294) may represent a form of Henoch-Schönlein purpura.

The diagnosis of Henoch-Schönlein purpura is ordinarily not difficult when the typical clinical features mentioned above are present. The differential diagnosis includes SLE, polyarteritis, infective endocarditis, postinfectious glomerulonephritis, and essential cryoimmunoglobulinemia.

The course is benign in the majority of cases; however, in some patients progressive renal failure may occur. Renal biopsy is a useful prognostic tool. Patients with persistent urinary abnormalities may experience deterioration of renal function several years after diagnosis. Treatment is symptomatic and there is no convincing evidence that steroid or immunosuppressive therapy is beneficial for the renal lesion, although these treatments may ameliorate some of the extrarenal features. Patients with rapidly progressive (crescentic) glomerulonephritis may be benefited by intensive plasma exchange or immunosuppressive drugs combined with anticoagulant and antithrombotic agents (see Chap. 294).

SYSTEMIC NECROTIZING VASCULITIS (See also Chap. 69) Glomerular involvement is common in the heterogeneous group of disorders which result from widespread inflammatory and necrotizing lesions of blood vessels. Several clinical and pathological variations are recognized, including microscopic polyarteritis (hypersensitivity angiitis), macroscopic polyarteritis (periarteritis nodosa), Wegener's granulomatosis, allergic granulomatous arteritis, rheumatoid vasculitis, temporal arteritis, and Takayasu's syndrome. Henoch-Schönlein purpura and SLE can also be considered as examples of vasculitis.

Renal involvement in *macroscopic polyarteritis* consists principally of inflammatory lesions of the relatively large blood vessels. Lesions of various ages are found. Fibrotic vascular occlusion, intrarenal aneurysms, and segmental renal infarctions may be noted. Hypertension tends to be severe and may be associated with a microangiopathic hemolytic anemia. Glomerular lesions of ischemia or necrosis may be seen. The disorder tends to affect older males, and there may be a history of drug abuse (amphetamines) or concomitant chronic hepatitis B infection. Fever, neuritis, cutaneous ulcers, purpura, abdominal pain, central nervous system disturbances, and coronary artery disease may also be found. Complement component levels are variable, but tests for CIC are often positive (Table 295-1). Renal failure is usually slowly progressive in nature and late in onset. The pathogenesis is presumed to be related to vascular deposits of circulating immune complexes; in some instances these complexes are composed of hepatitis B surface antigens, antibody, and complement.

Microscopic polyarteritis (hypersensitivity angiitis) tends to involve smaller vessels of the kidney and other organs. Pulmonary involvement is particularly common so that this disease superficially resembles the anti-basement membrane antibody-mediated diseases (Goodpasture's syndrome). Eosinophilia is found commonly in patients with pulmonary involvement. Renal disease is often rapidly progressive and is associated with segmental or diffuse glomerular capillary necrosis and extensive crescent formation. Deposits of IgG or IgM may be seen in affected glomeruli, but, in general, such deposits are scanty and evanescent.

Some patients with macroscopic or microscopic forms of polyarteritis may have long-standing underlying rheumatoid arthritis. For reasons that are only poorly understood, the disseminated vasculitis accompanying rheumatoid arthritis seldom affects the kidney. Renal involvement in Takayasu's syndrome and in temporal arteritis is likewise unusual.

The overall prognosis for microscopic and macroscopic forms of polyarteritis is poor with or without renal involvement. Therapy with corticosteroids, combined with cytotoxic agents, is likely to exert a beneficial effect, especially if applied early in the course of disease, before irreversible vascular damage with occlusion and fibrosis has occurred. Patients with rapidly progressive renal failure may benefit from aggressive therapy including high-dose parenteral methylprednisolone and/or plasma exchange if such treatment is instituted early.

Wegener's granulomatosis (see also Chap. 69) is a special variety of systemic necrotizing vasculitis characterized by its predilection to affect the upper and lower respiratory tract and the kidneys. Hemoptysis may be present; thus, these cases may be confused with Goodpasture's syndrome. Serum levels of IgA and IgE may be increased, and complement component levels are usually normal (Table 295-1). Pathologically, a granulomatous necrotizing vasculitis is seen in kidneys, lungs, and other organs. Immunofluorescence studies reveal scattered granular deposits of immunoglobulin and complement, suggesting an immune-complex–mediated pathogenesis. The antigen and antibody systems are unknown. The prognosis of untreated patients with Wegener's granulomatosis is very poor. The use of steroids and cytotoxic drugs, particularly cyclophosphamide, has radically altered the course of this disease. Long-term survival and prolonged disease-free intervals have been produced by aggressive treatment with cyclophosphamide. Response of the pulmonary lesion is especially dramatic.

Allergic granulomatous arteritis (Churg and Strauss syndrome) is a rare form of vasculitis in which severe asthma, fever, and eosinophilia are associated with necrotizing granulomas and extensive tissue infiltration with eosinophils. Necrotizing glomerulonephritis may be found. Steroids seem to be effective in the treatment of this disorder.

MISCELLANEOUS IMMUNOLOGICALLY MEDIATED MULTISYSTEM DISEASES **Mixed connective tissue disease (MCTD)** In this disorder, which is described in Chap. 352, renal disease is uncommon and, if present, is usually mild. Clinical manifestations include hematuria and proteinuria and occasionally nephrotic syndrome. Pathologically, membranous glomerulopathy or membranoproliferative glomerulonephritis is seen. The prognosis is generally favorable, and treatment is directed at extrarenal manifestations.

Rheumatoid arthritis Several forms of glomerular injury may occur in rheumatoid arthritis (Chap. 346). Secondary amyloidosis occurs in 5 to 10 percent of patients with long-standing arthritis. Nephrotic syndrome may arise as a complication of both gold therapy and penicillamine (see Chap. 294). In addition, the kidney may share in the vasculitis seen occasionally in patients with severe rheumatoid arthritis. Finally, patients with rheumatoid arthritis (untreated with gold or penicillamine) may develop a mild proliferative glomerulitis or diffuse membranous glomerulopathy which resembles lesions seen in SLE. Proteinuria, sometimes with nephrotic syndrome, is the principal clinical feature of these lesions.

Other disorders *Sjögren's syndrome* (Chap. 346) may be associated with nephrotic syndrome due to membranous or membranoproliferative glomerulonephritis (type I). More frequently, interstitial nephritis is seen. *Sarcoidosis* is rarely complicated by membranous nephropathy. *Partial or total lipodystrophy* may be associated with membranoproliferative glomerulonephritis (type II, dense deposit disease) (see Chap. 294). Complement abnormalities are found, consisting of depressed C3 levels, normal C1q and C4 levels, and circulating C3 lytic factors (i.e., C3 nephritic factor).

Chronic liver disease may be complicated by glomerular disease. The nephrotic syndrome may appear in the course of *chronic active hepatitis* associated with persistent hepatitis B surface antigenemia. Glomerular lesions include membranous glomerulopathy or membranoproliferative (type I) glomerulonephritis. Immunofluorescence studies in such patients reveal granular deposits of immunoglobulins, complement components, and hepatitis B surface antigen, indicating an immune-complex disease. Serum C3 levels are often reduced, and tests for CIC and cryoimmunoglobulins are frequently positive. Occasionally patients will have little clinical evidence of liver disease, yet develop distinct glomerular lesions secondary to chronic hepatitis B infection. *Acute viral hepatitis* may be associated with transient hematuria or proteinuria and resemble other postinfectious glomerulonephritides (see Chap. 294). Severe *chronic liver disease* (cirrhosis) may be associated with diffuse glomerulosclerosis. Few clinical manifestations of glomerular disease are found. Prominent mesangial IgA deposits, of unknown pathogenetic significance, have been noted in patients with cirrhosis.

MULTISYSTEM DISEASES ASSOCIATED WITH PARAPROTEINEMIA AND NEOPLASIA **Essential (mixed) cryoimmunoglobulinemia** This disorder is associated with high serum levels of circulating cold precipitable immunoglobulins (cryoimmunoglobulins), usually consisting of IgG and IgM; the latter possess rheumatoid factor activity. Purpura, necrotizing skin lesions in cold-exposed areas, arthralgias, fever, and hepatosplenomegaly are found frequently. Hepatitis B infection and other occult fungal, bacterial, or viral infections may be the cause of this syndrome. Cryoimmunoglobulins are also found in the circulation in many diseases, particularly chronic infections, and probably represent circulating immune complexes with unusual physical properties. Glomerular disease is common, resulting from the precipitation of the cryoimmunoglobulin in the glomerular capillaries. Acute renal failure, rapidly progressive (crescentic) glomerulonephritis, or the nephrotic syndrome may result. Serum complement components are depressed, and CIC are present (Table 295-1). Pathologically, a diffuse proliferative glomerulonephritis may be seen, with immunofluorescence findings consistent with the deposition of the circulating cryoimmunoglobulin. Eradication of the underlying infection, if possible, is of great value in treatment. Intensive plasma exchange, accompanied by steroids and cytotoxic agents, has been used with some success in severe cases.

Monoclonal gammopathies *Multiple myeloma* (Chap. 65) may be associated with at least three types of glomerular injury. Amyloidosis (Chap. 66) (see below) occurs in 10 to 15 percent of patients with proved multiple myeloma. Lesions resembling nodular diabetic glomerular sclerosis are seen occasionally. Monoclonal cryoimmunoglobulins occasionally may be deposited in glomeruli. Proteinuria and the nephrotic syndrome are common clinical features of glomerular injury in multiple myeloma. *Waldenström's macroglobulinemia* may be associated with acute renal failure when the homogeneous IgM paraprotein precipitates in glomerular capillaries as "thrombi." Intensive plasma exchange, accompanied by therapy with alkylating agents, may be beneficial. Hyperviscosity may occasionally result in functional alterations in GFR. Renal amyloidosis occurs uncommonly. *Benign monoclonal gammopathies* are seldom associated with glomerular complications, except for mild asymptomatic proteinuria and, rarely, nephrotic syndrome. Excessive production of *light chains of Ig* (especially kappa type) may evoke glomerular alterations (nodular glomerulosclerosis, focal sclerosis) due to deposition of the abnormal protein in mesangium or along the subendothelial aspect of the glomerular capillary wall.

Amyloidosis (see also Chap. 66) This disorder may occur in the absence of systemic disease (primary amyloidosis), may be secondary to chronic inflammatory processes (e.g., rheumatoid arthritis, osteomyelitis, paraplegia), multiple myeloma, other neoplastic diseases, or may occur in a heredofamilial form (e.g., familial Mediterranean fever). All forms may affect the glomeruli.

Primary amyloidosis commonly affects the kidneys. It usually occurs in older age groups. Proteinuria, often of nephrotic proportions, is the most common clinical manifestation of renal involvement. The urine sediment tends to be benign. The degree of proteinuria is not necessarily related to the extent of glomerular deposition of amyloid. Enlarged kidneys may be noted in patients with well-preserved renal function, but this is a nonspecific finding. The blood pressure is normal unless advanced uremia is present. Pathologically, the classic features include hypocellular glomeruli infiltrated with amorphous deposits which are positive with Congo red stains and reveal apple green birefringence under polarized light. The typical fibrillar nature of the amyloid deposits can be demonstrated by electron microscopy. The fibrils in primary amyloidosis are related immunologically to the immunoglobulin light chain. A similar immunochemical relationship is noted in multiple myeloma. Immunofluorescence studies reveal amorphous deposits of immunoglobulin and complement in glomeruli. Renal vein thrombosis may complicate the course of amyloidosis.

Renal amyloidosis is a progressive disease for which there is no established form of treatment. Remissions may occur in secondary amyloidosis if the cause can be found and eliminated. Remissions in primary amyloidosis have been exceedingly rare; however, a few reports describe remissions following the use of cytotoxic agents. Overall the 5-year survival for patients with primary amyloidosis is less than 20 percent. Azotemia, persistent nephrotic syndrome, and clinically evident myocardial involvement confer an even more ominous prognosis.

Neoplastic disease Glomerular alterations may develop in close association with a variety of neoplastic diseases. *Carcinomas,* especially adenocarcinoma of lung, colon, stomach, and breast, may be accompanied by glomerular lesions resembling idiopathic membranous glomerulopathy, although, on occasion, crescentic or focal and segmental proliferative glomerulonephritis or amyloidosis may be seen. Nephrotic syndrome is the most common clinical renal manifestation. Approximately 6 to 10 percent of patients with idiopathic nephrotic syndrome associated with membranous glomerulopathy harbor an underlying malignancy. Successful treatment of the tumor, especially by surgical means, may lead to a remission of the clinical findings. Presumably the glomerular lesions arise because of the deposition of circulating immune complexes, which are composed of tumor antigen and antitumor antibody. Amyloidosis may occasionally occur.

Lymphomas and leukemias may also give rise to glomerular abnormalities. Hodgkin's disease is most commonly associated with the findings of idiopathic nephrotic syndrome (minimal change disease). Other glomerular lesions including membranous glomerulopathy, focal proliferative and sclerosing glomerulonephritis, and amyloidosis may also be seen. The mechanism of the association of Hodgkin's disease with minimal change disease is unknown, but an underlying T-cell abnormality has been suggested. The nephrotic syndrome is the chief clinical manifestation of glomerular involvement in Hodgkin's disease. Proteinuria may wax and wane with fluctuations in the clinical activity of the Hodgkin's disease. Remissions may be produced by local x-ray irradiation of involved lymph nodes or by systemic chemotherapy.

METABOLIC, BIOCHEMICAL, AND HEREDITARY DISORDERS

DIABETIC NEPHROPATHY (See also Chap. 114) Diabetes mellitus affects the structure and function of the kidney in many ways. *Diabetic nephropathy* is a generic term which encompasses all the lesions occurring in the kidneys of patients with diabetes mellitus. These lesions include *glomerulosclerosis* (diffuse or nodular), *arterionephrosclerosis, chronic interstitial nephritis, papillary necrosis,* and various tubular lesions. Diabetic nephropathy is associated with a variety of clinical syndromes, including mild asymptomatic proteinuria, nephrotic syndrome, progressive renal failure (acute, rapidly progressive, or chronic), and hypertension. Glomerular lesions are particularly common and account for the majority of abnormal clinical findings referable to the kidney. *Diffuse diabetic glomerulosclerosis* (diffuse intercapillary glomerulosclerosis) is the most common lesion and can be identified in the vast majority of diabetic patients regardless of the presence or absence of abnormal clinical findings referable to the kidney. This lesion consists of a mild diffuse increase in mesangial matrix accompanied by an increased width of the glomerular basement membrane. Various exudative lesions, such as capsular drops and fibrin caps, may also be present. Hyaline arteriosclerosis, particularly of the efferent arteriole, is also found commonly. Taken together, these lesions strongly suggest the diagnosis of diabetes mellitus, but individually they are not specific. *Nodular glomerulosclerosis* (Kimmelstiel-Wilson lesion), on the other hand, is reasonably specific for juvenile onset or islet-cell antibody-positive diabetes mellitus. This lesion consists of PAS-positive, laminated, intercapillary nodules developing on a background of a diffuse increase in mesangial matrix. At the periphery of the nodules open glomerular capillary loops are found. The nodules are relatively acellular, in contrast to the cellular lesions sometimes seen in membranoproliferative glomerulonephritis (often referred to as *lobular glomerulonephritis*). A variable percentage of glomeruli may be affected.

The pathogenesis of diffuse or nodular diabetic glomerulosclerosis is poorly understood. Evidence supporting a role for both the abnormal diabetic milieu (e.g., insulinopenia, hyperglycemia, glycosuria) and genetic factors is reviewed in Chap. 114.

The principal clinical manifestation of diabetic glomerular disease is proteinuria. Initially proteinuria is mild and asymptomatic. Overt carbohydrate intolerance nearly always precedes the development of proteinuria by one or more decades; however, in exceptional cases proteinuria either develops in concert with overt hyperglycemia or even may precede the clinical appearance of diabetes mellitus. GFR is often increased in early diabetic glomerulopathy. The diastolic blood pressure is normal initially. The urine sediment is typically benign, although pyuria may be present if urinary tract infection coexists. An active urinary sediment suggests the chance occurrence of another form of glomerulopathy. Diabetic retinopathy strongly indicates the presence of underlying glomerulopathy, but exceptions have been recorded. With the passage of time, the quantity of protein excreted increases, often with the development of overt nephrotic syndrome. Hypertension appears and progressively worsens but seldom is of malignant proportions. Typically, plasma renin activity is normal or decreased. Acquired hyporeninemic hypoaldosteronism, with persistent hyperkalemia and mild hyperchloremic metabolic acidosis, is common. From the time of appearance of proteinuria, progressive loss of GFR and end-stage renal failure can be expected to occur within 5 to 7 years. For reasons that are unknown, the rate of loss of GFR in diabetic nephropathy exceeds that of many of the common primary glomerulopathies, including membranoproliferative glomerulonephritis, membranous glomerulopathy, and focal glomerular sclerosis.

Until the cause (or causes) of diabetes mellitus is (are) found, prevention of the glomerulopathy will not be feasible. If the abnormal diabetic milieu is responsible for the vascular complications (including glomerular disease), as some have suggested, then very precise regulation of blood sugar (e.g., meticulous attention to diet, exercise, insulin dosage, servo-feedback devices for insulin administration) may be effective in reducing the development of diabetic nephropathy. Once developed to a clinically recognizable stage, no form of treatment has unequivocally altered the natural history of diabetic nephropathy. Patients with end-stage renal failure due to diabetic nephropathy may be poor candidates for long-term dialysis, primarily because of concomitant multiple organ dysfunction secondary to widespread arteriovascular disease. Mortality rates among diabetics on chronic dialysis are three to five times higher than among similarly treated nondiabetics of comparable age. Renal transplantation has been successfully undertaken in the younger diabetic, especially if a living related donor is available. The success rate is somewhat less than in the nondiabetic population, but transplantation is a viable alternative to dialysis in selected patients. Recurrence of typical diabetic glomerular lesions has been documented in renal allografts, but thus far, with short-term follow up, progressive loss of GFR secondary to recurrent disease has not been noted.

ALPORT'S SYNDROME This disorder consists of sensorineural deafness associated with hereditary nephritis. Renal disease manifests itself at an early age, principally as recurrent hematuria. Males are more frequently and severely affected than females. Slowly progressive renal insufficiency, terminating in end-stage renal disease in the second to third decade, is common among males. There is no clear-cut relationship between the onset or severity of the hearing abnormality and the clinical extent of renal disease. Other associated abnormalities include two related ophthalmological complications, spherophakia and lenticonus, as well as thrombocytopathia, hyperprolinemia, and cerebral dysfunction. Complement component levels are normal. Family studies have indicated an X-linked mode of inheritance, with variable penetrance and expressivity, perhaps due to the influence of the Lyon hypothesis effect on the X chromosome. The pathogenesis of this disorder is unknown but may be due to defective synthesis of glycopeptide (noncollagenous) components of glomerular and tubular basement membranes.

The pathological features by light microscopy are nonspecific, and a diagnosis cannot be established by optical microscopy alone. Both glomerular and interstitial lesions are present. Focal and diffuse glomerular proliferation, with segmental sclerosis, is common. Interstitial foam cells are nonspecific findings. Electron microscopy reveals thinning, splitting, and delamination of both glomerular and tubular basement membranes, thought by some to be specific for Alport's syndrome. Immunofluorescence studies fail to reveal deposits of immunoglobulins or complement components. The autoantibody to basement membrane antigens found in patients with Goodpasture's syndrome does not react with the glomeruli of some patients with Alport's syndrome. Treatment is supportive; steroids and cytotoxic agents are ineffective. The disease is not known to recur following transplantation.

FABRY'S DISEASE (See also Chap. 104) This disorder, angiokeratoma corporus diffusum, is an X-linked inborn error of glycosphingolipid metabolism which leads to the accumulation of neutral glycosphingolipids in many tissues including the kidney. A specific deficiency of alpha galactosidase, ceramide trihexosidase A has been described. Renal manifestations include hematuria and modest proteinuria, often associated with slowly progressive renal failure. Light-microscopic findings include foamy alterations of the epithelial cells of the glomerulus. Staining of these cells with Sudan black reveals them to contain lipid. Electron microscopy reveals these same cells to contain intracellular rounded laminated bodies ("myelin figures"). The disorder is untreatable unless replacement of the deficient enzyme can be ensured. Some investigators have claimed that successful renal transplantation corrects the enzyme deficiency. Perhaps transplantation of other tissues (e.g., bone marrow) may ultimately become the treatment of choice.

NAIL-PATELLA SYNDROME This disorder is an autosomal dominant disease, linked to the ABO blood groups and characterized by dystrophic nails, absence of one or both patellae, iliac horns, and renal disease. The renal manifestations include isolated proteinuria and hematuria, and occasionally the nephrotic syndrome. Progressive renal failure is relatively uncommon. Glomerular lesions by light microscopy are nonspecific, but electron microscopy reveals a characteristic moth-eaten appearance of the glomerular basement membrane associated with intramembranous collagen fibrils. The prognosis is generally favorable. No treatment is known to be effective.

CONGENITAL NEPHROTIC SYNDROME This disorder is an autosomal recessive trait characterized by the development of nephrotic syndrome at the time of or shortly after birth. It occurs with highest frequency in families of Finnish extraction. Affected individuals have very large placentas, low birth weight, anasarca, polycythemia, and an initially normal GFR. α-Fetoprotein levels are increased in amniotic fluid and maternal serum. Proteinuria is usually heavy and very nonselective. Nephrotic syndrome appearing several months after birth is usually due to other causes, especially minimal change disease or focal glomerular sclerosis (Chap. 294). Congenital syphilis or congenital toxoplasmosis may produce a similar syndrome and must be excluded. Pathologically, microcystic transformation of the cortical nephrons, due to proximal tubular dilatation, is found. Glomerular changes are nonspecific. Extensive effacement of the foot processes and sclerosis of the glomerular tufts are seen by electron microscopy. Immunofluorescence findings are either negative or nonspecific. The course is progressive, and few patients survive the first year of life. Death is usually due to inanition, infection, or renal failure. All forms of treatment have been ineffective. A few patients may survive long enough to be considered for renal transplantation.

SICKLE CELL DISEASE (See also Chaps. 298 and 330) This disorder is an autosomal dominant trait characterized by the development of an abnormal hemoglobin (hemoglobin S). Glomerular lesions occur infrequently in homozygous sickle-cell disease. The medulla seems to be preferentially affected, leading to impaired concentrating ability and acid excretion and, occasionally, papillary necrosis. Some patients develop mainly glomerular lesions, often accompanied by proteinuria and a nephrotic syndrome. These glomerular lesions are either membranous or membranoproliferative glomerulonephritis. Immunofluorescence findings are usually positive, with both immunoglobulin and complement components deposited in a granular pattern suggesting immune-complex–mediated disease. In a few instances, renal tubuloepithelial antigens have been localized in these deposits, suggesting that ischemic damage of the kidney may release autologous renal antigens to provoke the immune-complex disease. The course in patients with sickle cell disease complicated by glomerulopathy is often relentlessly progressive, leading ultimately to the development of end-stage renal disease. No form of treatment is known to be effective. Transplantation has been successful occasionally.

REFERENCES

BALDWIN DS et al: Lupus nephritis. Clinical course as related to morphologic forms and their transitions. Am J Med 62:12, 1977

CRAWFURD MD, TOGHILL PJ: Alport's syndrome of hereditary nephritis with deafness. Q J Med 37:563, 1968

GLASSOCK RJ, COHEN AJ: Secondary glomerular diseases, in *The Kidney*, 2d ed, BM Brenner, FC Rector Jr (eds). Philadelphia, Saunders, 1981

O'NEILL WM et al: Hereditary nephritis: A re-examination of its clinical and genetic features. Ann Int Med 88:176, 1978

SUKI WN, EKNOYAN G (eds): *The Kidney in Systemic Disease*, 2d ed. New York, Wiley, 1981

296 URINARY TRACT INFECTION, PYELONEPHRITIS, AND RELATED CONDITIONS

WALTER E. STAMM
MARVIN TURCK

DEFINITIONS Acute infections of the urinary tract can be subdivided into two general anatomic categories: lower tract infection (urethritis, cystitis, and prostatitis) and upper tract infection (acute pyelonephritis). The latter term should be reserved for acute bacterial infections that involve the renal interstitium; it should not be used to refer to lower urinary tract infections. Cystitis and acute pyelonephritis may occur together or independently. Either infection may be asymptomatic or present as the clinical syndromes outlined below.

Recurrent infections can be classified as relapses (a recurrence with the same strain, as judged by species identification, serotype, and antibiogram, that occurs within 1 to 2 weeks of stopping antibiotic therapy) or reinfections (a recurrence with a new strain). Most relapses are thought to result from unresolved renal infection.

Symptoms of dysuria, urgency, and frequency unaccompanied by significant bacteriuria have been termed the acute urethral syndrome. Although widely used, this term lacks anatomic precision because many cases of urethral syndrome are in actuality bladder infections.

Chronic pyelonephritis refers to chronic interstitial nephritis believed to result from bacterial infection of the kidney (see Chap. 297). Many noninfectious diseases also cause an interstitial nephritis indistinguishable pathologically from chronic pyelonephritis.

Microbiologically, urinary tract infection exists when pathogenic microorganisms are detected in the urine, urethra, kidney, or prostate. In most instances, more than 10^5 organisms per milliliter grown from a properly collected midstream "clean catch" urine sample indicate infection. However, significant bacteriuria may be absent in some circumstances when true urinary infection exists. Especially in symptomatic patients, a smaller number of bacteria (10^2 to 10^4 per milliliter of midstream urine) may accompany infection. In urine specimens obtained by suprapubic aspiration or "in and out" catheterization, or from a patient with an indwelling catheter, colony counts of 10^2 to 10^4 per milliliter generally indicate infection.

ACUTE INFECTIONS OF THE URINARY TRACT: CYSTITIS, ACUTE PYELONEPHRITIS, URETHRAL SYNDROME

EPIDEMIOLOGY Acute urinary tract infections are very common, involving at least 15 percent of all females at some time during their lives. Some studies show that 20 percent of adult women, regardless of age, experience dysuria each year. However, only 50 percent, mostly younger women, seek medical attention. Males rarely develop symptomatic urinary tract infections until after age 45 unless urologic abnormalities are present.

Many urinary tract infections remain asymptomatic. Approximately 1 percent of male infants and fewer female infants acquire asymptomatic bacteriuria. After infancy, asymptomatic bacteriuria occurs in fewer than 1 percent of males until age 45 to 50; in older males, up to 5 percent have bacteriuria. During childhood, 1 to 2 percent of females have asymptomatic bacteriuria. This increases to 2 to 5 percent during the childbearing years, 2 to 10 percent during pregnancy, and 5 to 15 percent in older women.

ETIOLOGY Many different microorganisms can infect the urinary tract, but by far the most common agents are the gram-negative bacilli. *Escherichia coli* causes approximately 90 percent of acute infections in patients without urologic abnormalities or calculi. Other gram-negative rods, including *Proteus, Klebsiella, Enterobacter, Serratia,* and *Pseudomonas* account for a smaller proportion of uncomplicated infections. These organisms assume increasing importance in recurrent infections and infections associated with urologic manipulation, calculi, or obstruction. They play a major role in nosocomial, catheter-associated infections (see below). *Proteus* species, by virtue of urease production, and *Klebsiella* species, through production of extracellular slime and polysaccharides, predispose to stone formation and are isolated more frequently from patients with calculi.

Gram-positive cocci play a lesser role in urinary tract infections. Enterococci and *Staphylococcus aureus* often cause infections in patients with renal stones or previous instrumentation. Isolation of *S. aureus* should arouse suspicion of bacteremic infection of the kidney. *Staphylococcus saprophyticus,* a novobiocin-resistant, urease-positive, coagulase-negative staphylococcus, has been recognized as an important cause of acute symptomatic urinary tract infections in young females.

About one-third of women with dysuria and frequency have either a nonsignificant number of bacteria in midstream urine cultures or completely sterile cultures, and have been defined as having the urethral syndrome. About three-quarters of these women have significant pyuria, while one-quarter have no pyuria and little objective evidence of infection. In the women with pyuria, two groups of pathogens account for the majority of infections. Low quantities (10^2 to 10^4 bacteria per milliliter) of coliforms or staphylococci in midstream urine specimens are found in some women, and these bacteria are probably the causative agents because they can usually be isolated from a suprapubic aspirate, as well as from urethral and vaginal cultures. Further, such low-count bacteriuria is usually associated with pyuria and responds to appropriate antimicrobial therapy. In other women who have the acute urethral syndrome, pyuria, and sterile urine (even on suprapubic aspiration), *Chlamydia trachomatis* appears to be an important etiologic agent.

Viruses can produce pyelonephritis in animals and may increase the kidney's susceptibility to infection with coliform bacteria. In humans, viruses are most commonly recovered from the urine without evidence of acute urinary disease, although some adenoviruses have been implicated as a cause of hemorrhagic cystitis. Similarly, *Candida* and other fungi may colonize the urine of catheterized patients or diabetics, but they rarely cause acute symptomatic infection.

PATHOGENESIS AND SOURCES OF INFECTION The urinary tract should be viewed as a single anatomic unit connected by a continuous column of urine that extends from the urethra to the kidney. In the vast majority of infections, bacteria gain access to the bladder via the urethra. Ascent of bacteria from the bladder may then follow and is probably the usual pathway for most renal parenchymal infections. However, at least 50 percent of patients with bacteriuria do not have evidence of pyelonephritis.

The distal urethra is normally colonized with diphtheroids, streptococcal species, and staphylococcal species but not with the enteric gram-negative bacilli that commonly cause urinary tract infections. In females prone to development of cystitis, however, enteric gram-negative organisms residing in the bowel colonize the introitus, the periurethral skin, and the distal urethra prior to and during episodes of bacteriuria. Factors predisposing to periurethral colonization with coliforms remain poorly understood but may involve alteration of normal perineal flora, absence of local antibody, and/or enhanced attachment of organisms to the epithelial cells of infection-prone women. A small number of periurethral bacteria probably gain entry to the bladder frequently, perhaps facilitated in some women by trauma during intercourse. Whether infection ensues then depends upon a number of factors, including the pathogenicity of the strain, the inoculum size, and local and systemic host defense mechanisms.

Under normal circumstances, bacteria placed in the bladder are rapidly cleared in humans or experimental animals. This results partly from the flushing and dilutional effects of voiding, but also from direct antibacterial properties of urine and the bladder mucosa. Due mostly to high urea concentration and high osmolarity, the bladder urine of many normal persons inhibits or kills bacteria. Prostatic secretions possess antibacterial properties as well. Polymorphonuclear leukocytes in the bladder wall also appear to play a role in clearing bacteriuria. The role of locally produced antibody remains unclear. Hematogenous pyelonephritis occurs most often in debilitated patients who either have chronic illnesses or who are receiving immunosuppressive therapy. Staphylococcal pyelonephritis may follow bacteremia from distant foci of infection in the bone, skin, endothelium, or elsewhere.

CONDITIONS AFFECTING PATHOGENESIS **Sex** The female urethra appears particularly prone to colonization with colonic gram-negative bacilli, owing to its proximity to the anus, its short length (about 4 cm), and its termination beneath the labia. Urethral trauma, as occurs during sexual intercourse, may cause introduction of bacteria into the bladder. The precise role of intercourse in the pathogenesis of urinary infections remains unclear, however. In males, prostatitis or urethral obstruction due to prostatic hypertrophy are important factors predisposing to bacteriuria.

Pregnancy Depending on socioeconomic status, urinary infections are detected in 2 to 8 percent of pregnant women. In particular, symptomatic infections occur more commonly during pregnancy; fully 20 to 40 percent of pregnant women with asymptomatic bacteriuria subsequently develop pyelonephritis. Bladder catheterization during or after delivery causes additional infections. Cystitis and pyelonephritis are no more common in women with toxemia of pregnancy than in other pregnant women. Increased prematurity and newborn mortality may result from urinary infections during pregnancy.

Obstructive uropathy Any impediment to the free flow of urine—tumor, stricture, stone, or prostatic hypertrophy—results in hydronephrosis and greatly increased frequency of urinary tract infection. Infection superimposed on urinary tract obstruction may lead to rapid destruction of renal tissue. It is of utmost importance, therefore, when infection is present to repair obstructive lesions. On the other hand, with minor degrees of obstruction that are not progressive or associated with infection, great caution must be exercised in attempting surgical correction. The introduction of infection in such patients may be more damaging than uncorrected minor obstructions which do not significantly impair renal function.

Neurogenic bladder dysfunction Interference with the nerve supply to the bladder, as in spinal cord injury, tabes dorsalis, multiple sclerosis, diabetes, or other diseases, may be associated with urinary tract infection. The infection may be initiated by the use of catheters for bladder drainage and is favored by the prolonged standing of urine in the bladder. An additional factor often present in these patients is bone demineralization due to immobilization, which causes hypercalciuria, calculus formation, and obstructive uropathy.

Vesicoureteral reflux This condition is defined as reflux of urine from the bladder cavity up into the ureters and sometimes into the renal pelvis. It occurs during voiding or with elevation of pressure in the bladder. In practice, vesicoureteral reflux exists when retrograde movement of radiopaque or radioactive material can be demonstrated. However, since a fluid connection between the bladder and kidney always exists in the patent urinary system, during infections some retrograde movement of bacteria probably occurs normally but is not detected by radiologic techniques. An anatomically impaired ureterovesical junction facilitates reflux of bacteria.

Vesicoureteral reflux is common in children with anatomic abnormalities of the urinary tract and in children with anatomically normal but infected urinary tracts. In the latter group, reflux disappears with advancing age and probably results from rather than causes urinary infection. Follow-up of children with urinary tract infection who were found to have reflux establishes that renal damage correlates with massive reflux, not with infection.

The routine search for reflux would be aided by development of noninvasive tests applicable to young children, where the need is greatest. In the meantime, it appears reasonable to search for massive reflux in anyone with unexplained failure of renal growth or renal scarring, because urinary tract infection per se is an insufficient explanation for these abnormalities. On the other hand, it is doubtful that all children with recurrent urinary tract infections but normal tracts on pyelography should be subjected to voiding cystoureterography merely to detect the rare patient with massive reflux that did not reveal itself on the intravenous pyelogram.

Renal disease and hypertension Experimental and clinical evidence indicate that various renal diseases may increase the kidney's susceptibility to infection. These include diabetic nephropathy, gout, nephrocalcinosis, sickle cell disease, hypercalcemia, and hypokalemia. In surveys of nonhospital populations, mean blood pressure levels are likely to be slightly higher in women with urinary infections than in those without infections. However, whether hypertension or urinary infection is primary remains unclear. Because persons with abnormal urinalyses or hypertension often undergo urinary tract instrumentation, thereby providing access of bacteria to the urinary tract, it is possible that repeated catheterizations rather than underlying renal disease predispose these patients to infection.

Diabetes mellitus Despite reports that chronic pyelonephritis at autopsy is very common in diabetics, clinical surveys of hospital and nonhospital populations have failed to document any convincing difference in the prevalence of urinary tract infections in diabetic and nondiabetic persons of the same age. This suggests either that diabetics with urinary infections are more likely to develop pyelonephritis or that in the presence of severe vascular and glomerular lesions in diabetic kidneys, morphologic changes result which are similar to those of bacterial infection. The problem requires further study. Irritation of the vulva in women with heavy uncontrolled glucosuria probably increases the rate of false-positive voided cultures and may predispose to bladder infection. When diabetic neuropathy has interfered with normal bladder function, persistent infections of the urine are frequent.

Urinary tract infections in diabetics may produce difficulties in the regulation of carbohydrate metabolism and may precipitate diabetic acidosis. The risk of additional renal disease caused by infection in persons already subject to severe vascular and glomerular disease must, of course, be avoided whenever possible. Diabetics are also likely to develop necrotizing papillitis, a fulminating form of renal disease usually associated with infection (see below).

EXPERIMENTAL EVIDENCE Urinary tract infections can be produced in experimental animals by inoculation of bacteria into the renal pelvis or into the bladder urine. Certain organisms such as *Pseudomonas*, enterococci, staphylococci, and *Candida* are capable of causing infection in the normal kidney when they are injected by the intravenous route. Coliform organisms will generally not do this unless intrarenal hydronephrosis or acute obstruction of the ureter is present. Renal damage resulting from a viral or staphylococcal infection can also render the kidney susceptible to infection by coliforms injected intravenously.

Clinical and experimental evidence has shown that the papillae and medulla of the kidney are particularly susceptible to bacterial infection. Bacterial multiplication in animals with pyelonephritis begins in the medulla, and in this normally hypertonic environment at least some host defense mechanisms such as leukocyte migration, phagocytosis, and complement activity are likely to be impaired. In addition, cell wall defective bacteria can survive in the hypertonic environment of the renal medulla, whereas they are lysed in tissues isotonic to plasma. In patients without urinary obstruction, decreasing the osmolarity of the papillae by drinking large quantities of water would be expected to increase resistance to infection. However, experiments testing the effect of water diuresis on urinary infections vary in outcome, depending on animal species, test organism, means by which bacteria gain access to the urinary tract, and presence of underlying renal disease. In humans, water diuresis may temporarily lower the concentration of bacteria in the urine, but the long-term consequences of water diuresis on the natural history of urinary infections or on the outcome of antibiotic treatment are unknown.

Infections involving the upper urinary tract usually cause a significant rise in serum antibodies directed against the O antigen of the infecting strain. They also produce a temporary defect in renal concentrating ability in many patients, and may be associated with formation of leukocyte casts. Lower tract infections rarely result in increased antibody titers, concentrating defects, or white cell casts. Unfortunately, these methods of distinguishing renal parenchymal infection from cystitis are neither reliable nor convenient enough for routine clinical use. More sensitive tests for distinguishing pyelonephritis from cystitis (bilateral ureteral catheterization and the bladder washout technique originated by Fairley) are inherently invasive and too complex for clinical practice. The development of a simpler and clinically applicable test to separate upper and lower tract infections based upon antibody coating of bacteria in the urine appears to be an important advance. In this test, bacteria from patients with pyelonephritis demonstrate antibody coating on their surface when they have been exposed to a fluorescein-labeled antihuman globulin and are viewed under a fluorescence microscope. No surface antibodies can be visualized on bacteria from patients with cystitis. This antibody response consists mainly of IgG and can be reproduced in an experimental pyelonephritis model in animals. However, false-negative results occur in 15 to 20 percent of patients who have upper tract infection as judged by direct localization procedures. These false-negatives probably occur because antibody production, particularly in first infections, requires 10 to 15 days, and many patients require treatment before this length of time elapses. False-positive results occur in males with prostatitis and women with hemorrhagic cystitis, heavy proteinuria, and vaginal or fecal contamination of midstream urine. Infections with yeast or *Pseudomonas* cause false-positives due to autofluorescence and because staphylococci with protein A nonspecifically bind human immunoglobulin.

CLINICAL PRESENTATION Clinical signs and symptoms cannot be relied upon to diagnose urinary tract infection correctly or to localize the site of infection. Approximately one-half of patients with significant bacteriuria (including some with upper tract infection) have no symptoms at all. Of those with significant bacteriuria and symptoms, about one-half have cystitis and one-half have pyelonephritis. Clinical symptoms and signs, though often suggestive, cannot reliably distinguish between upper and lower tract infection. Furthermore, among women presenting with dysuria and frequency, only 60 to 70 percent have significant bacteriuria.

Enumeration of the number of bacteria in the urine is therefore an extremely important diagnostic procedure. In symptomatic infections of the urinary tract, bacteria are usually demonstrable in the urine in large numbers. Quantitative estimation of the number of bacteria in voided urine specimens, as a rule, makes it possible to distinguish contaminants from true bacteriuria, and 10^5 or more bacteria per milliliter has been the criterion traditionally used for this purpose. However, in symptomatic women with pyuria, counts of 10^2 to 10^4 coliforms per milliliter of midstream urine usually indicate infection, not contamination, and should not be disregarded. In asymptomatic or minimally symptomatic patients, two or three urine specimens should be examined bacteriologically before instituting therapy, and 10^5 or more per milliliter of a single species should be demonstrable in the repeated specimens. A quantitative estimate can be made by means of Gram's stain or microscopic examination of uncentrifuged, freshly voided urine. If bacteria can be found by this method, it may be assumed that the number present approximates 100,000 per milliliter. Since the large number of bacteria in the bladder urine is due in part to bacterial multiplication during residence in the bladder cavity, samples of urine from the ureters or renal pelvis might contain fewer than 10^5 bacteria per milliliter and yet indicate infection. Similarly, the presence of bacteriuria of any degree in suprapubic aspirates or of 10^2 or more per milliliter of urine obtained by catheterization usually indicates infection. In some circumstances (antibiotics, high urea concentration, high osmolarity, low pH), urine will inhibit bacterial multiplication, resulting in a lower number of bacteria in the presence of infection. For this reason, antiseptic solutions should not be used in washing the periurethral area prior to collection of the urine specimen. Water diuresis or recent voiding also reduces the bacterial counts in urine.

Cystitis Many physicians refer to significant bacteriuria associated with dysuria, frequency, urgency, and suprapubic pain as cystitis. In actuality, both urethritis and cystitis are usually present. The urine often becomes grossly cloudy, malodorous, and, in about 50 percent of cases, bloody. Pyuria without leukocyte casts and bacteria should be present on examination of the unspun urine. Physical examination generally reveals only a reddened, tender urethra or suprapubic tenderness. If a purulent urethral discharge or a vaginal discharge is present, especially with fewer than 10^5 bacteria per milliliter on culture, other causes of urethritis, vaginitis, or cervicitis such as *C. trachomatis*, gonorrhea, *Trichomonas, Candida,* and *Herpesvirus hominis* should be ruled out. Prominent systemic manifestations like fever over 101°F, nausea, vomiting, and costovertebral angle tenderness usually indicate concomitant renal infection. However, the absence of these findings does not ensure that infection is limited to the bladder and urethra.

Acute pyelonephritis Symptoms generally develop rapidly over a few hours or a day and include fever which is often 103°F or greater, shaking chills, nausea, vomiting, and diarrhea. Symptoms of cystitis may or may not be present. Besides fever, tachycardia, and generalized muscle tenderness, physical examination reveals marked tenderness on deep pressure in one or both costovertebral areas or on deep abdominal palpation. In some patients, signs and symptoms of gram-negative sepsis predominate. Most patients have significant leukocytosis, pyuria with leukocyte casts in the urine, and bacteria on a Gram's stain of unspun urine. Hematuria may be present during the acute phase of the disease, but if it persists after acute manifestations of infection have subsided, a stone, tumor, or tuberculosis should be considered.

Except in individuals with papillary necrosis or urinary obstruction, the manifestations of acute pyelonephritis usually subside within a few days, even without specific antibacterial therapy. However, despite the absence of symptoms, bacteriuria or pyuria may persist. With severe pyelonephritis, fever subsides more slowly and may not disappear for several days, even after appropriate antibiotic treatment has been instituted.

Urethral syndrome Approximately 30 to 40 percent of women with dysuria and frequency have midstream urine cultures that show either no growth or nonsignificant growth. Clinically, these women with the acute urethral syndrome cannot be readily distinguished from those with cystitis. In women with the acute urethral syndrome in whom pyuria is initially demonstrated, distinction should be made between those having sexually transmitted pathogens such as *C. trachomatis* or *Neisseria gonorrhoeae* and those having low-count coliform or staphylococcal infection. Women with a gradual onset of illness, no hematuria, no suprapubic pain, and a history of more than 7 days of symptoms should be suspected of having chlamydial infection. The additional history of a recent sex partner change, especially if the patient's partner has recently had chlamydial or gonococcal urethritis, should heighten the suspicion of a sexually transmitted infection, as would the finding of mucopurulent cervicitis. Gross hematuria, suprapubic pain, abrupt onset of illness, a duration of illness of 3 to 4 days, and a history of previous urinary tract infections favor coliform infection.

Catheter-associated urinary tract infections Bacteriuria frequently occurs in hospitalized patients with indwelling urethral catheters. *Proteus, Pseudomonas, Klebsiella,* and *Serratia,* in addition to *E. coli,* usually cause these infections. Many infecting strains show marked antimicrobial resistance compared with organisms that cause community-acquired urinary infections.

Infection occurs when bacteria reach the bladder by migrating through the column of urine in the catheter lumen or up the mucous sheath outside the catheter. Hospital-acquired pathogens reach the patient's catheter or urine-collecting system on the hands of hospital personnel, in contaminated solutions or irrigants, and via contaminated instruments or disinfectants. In addition, the patient's own bowel flora often migrate to the perineal skin and periurethral area and reach the bladder via the conduit provided by the catheter.

Most catheter-associated infections appear to be benign. They cause minimal symptoms, no fever or pyuria, and often resolve after withdrawal of the catheter. The frequency of upper tract infection associated with catheter-induced bacteriuria remains unknown. Gram-negative bacteremia, which follows 1 to 2 percent of cases of catheter-associated bacteriuria, is the most significantly recognized complication of catheter-induced urinary infections.

These infections can be partially prevented in patients catheterized less than 2 weeks by use of a sterile closed collecting system, attention to aseptic technique during insertion and care of the catheter, and by measures to minimize cross infection. Despite these precautions, the majority of patients catheterized longer than 2 weeks develop bacteriuria. The optimal treatment for such patients has not been established. Removal of the catheter and a short course of antibiotics to which the organism is susceptible is probably the best course of action and nearly always eradicates the bacteriuria. If the catheter cannot be removed, antibiotic therapy usually proves to be unsuccessful and may result in infection with a more resistant strain. In this situation, the bacteriuria should be ignored unless the patient develops symptoms or is at high risk of developing bacteremia. In these cases, systemic antibiotics or urinary bladder antiseptics may reduce the degree of bacteriuria and the likelihood of bacteremia.

TREATMENT Several therapeutic principles should underlie treatment of urinary tract infections:

1 Quantitative urine cultures should be obtained to diagnose infections before starting treatment.
2 Antimicrobial sensitivity testing should be used to direct therapy in patients with recurrent infections.
3 Factors predisposing to infection, such as obstruction, neurogenic bladder, calculi, etc., should be identified and corrected if possible.
4 Relief of clinical symptoms does not indicate bacteriologic cure, and follow-up cultures after therapy should be obtained.
5 After completion of therapy and follow-up cultures, each treatment episode should be classified as failure (bacteriuria not eradicated during therapy or upon the immediate posttreatment culture) or a cure (elimination of bacteriuria). Recurrent infections should be classified as relapses or reinfections.
6 In general, uncomplicated infections confined to the lower urinary tract respond to low doses and short courses of therapy, while upper tract infections require longer periods of treatment. Relapses usually indicate an upper tract focus of infection while reinfection more often indicates lower tract infection.
7 Community-acquired infections, especially initial infections, are nearly always due to antibiotic-sensitive strains.
8 Patients with repeated infections, instrumentation, or recent hospitalization should be suspected of harboring resistant strains.

Until recently, most antibiotic trials did not distinguish lower urinary tract infections from upper tract infections in assessing therapeutic outcome. In such trials, many antibiotics (ampicillin, sulfonamides, tetracyclines, penicillin, cephalosporins, nitrofurantoin, aminoglycosides, and others) achieved cure rates of approximately 80 percent. However, data utilizing the antibody-coated bacteria method suggest that the location of a urinary tract infection greatly influences success or failure of a therapeutic agent. Bladder bacteriuria can usually be eliminated with nearly any regimen to which the infecting strain is sensitive, and as little as a single dose of 500 mg intramuscular kanamycin will eliminate bladder bacteriuria in most patients. A 7-day course of therapy with oral drugs appears more than adequate. With upper tract infections, however, single-dose therapy fails in the majority of cases and even a 7-day course will be unsuccessful in many patients. Longer periods of treatment (2 to 6 weeks) aimed at eradicating a persistent focus of infection may be necessary in cases of relapse.

For patients with *acute uncomplicated cystitis,* a 7-day course of a sulfonamide, ampicillin, nitrofurantoin, nalidixic acid, or tetracycline has proved highly effective. More than 90 percent of these infections are due to *E. coli,* and although resistance patterns vary geographically, most strains are sensitive to many antibiotics. Development of the antibody-coated bacteria test has provided new impetus for assessing single-dose treatment of acute uncomplicated cystitis since it allows localization studies to be done in large numbers of acutely symptomatic patients. It has been shown that a single 3-g oral dose of amoxicillin was comparable to conventional 10-day therapy in eradication of lower tract infection. Subsequently, single-dose ampicillin (3.5 g), trimethoprim-sulfamethoxazole (four single-strength tablets), and sulfa alone have been successfully used to treat acute uncomplicated episodes of cystitis due to coliforms. The advantages of single-dose therapy include lesser expense, assured compliance, fewer side effects, and perhaps less intense selective pressure for emergence of resistant organisms in the gut, vaginal, or perineal flora. Although further study aimed at defining the limitations of single-dose therapy is needed, it does appear safe and efficacious for women presenting with acute uncomplicated cystitis. Since the antibody-coated bacteria test is not generally available for routine clinical purposes, single-dose therapy should be used without localization studies, the response to therapy itself serving as a means of localization. Single-dose therapy should be used only in reliable patients where posttreatment follow-up can be ensured, and in patients in whom symptoms have been present for less than 10 days. It should not be used in women with symptoms or signs of pyelonephritis or in women with urologic abnormalities or stones. In women with previous infections due to antibiotic-resistant organisms, single-dose therapy may be less appropriate. Further evaluation of single-dose therapy in children and pregnant women with bacteriuria is needed before it can be recommended in these populations. Males with urinary tract infection often have urologic abnormalities or prostatic involvement and positive antibody-coated-bacterial bacteriuria, and hence are not candidates for single-dose therapy.

Treatment of the acute urethral syndrome depends upon the etiologic agent involved. Women with urethral syndrome due to low-count coliforms should be managed as are women with acute cystitis. Although further study is needed, these women appear to respond well to single-dose therapy. In women with chlamydial infection, tetracycline (500 mg orally qid for 7 days) should be used. Women with the acute urethral syndrome and no pyuria have not responded to antimicrobial agents.

Acute pyelonephritis without accompanying clinical evidence of calculi or urologic disease is due to *E. coli* in most cases. Although the optimal route and duration of therapy have not been established, a 10- to 14-day course of trimethoprim-sulfamethoxazole, cephalosporin, or ampicillin usually provides adequate therapy. Intravenous antibiotics, at least for the first several days of treatment, should probably be given to all but minimally symptomatic patients. Some patients relapse following therapy and should be investigated to determine whether unrecognized calculi or urologic disease is present. If not, treatment should be extended to 2 to 6 weeks to eliminate a presumed upper tract focus causing recurrent bacteriuria.

When suspected *gram-negative sepsis* complicates acute pyelonephritis, hospitalization, prompt parenteral therapy with an aminoglycoside, and ancillary measures to treat sepsis should be provided (see Chap. 139). When the antibiotic sensitivities of the infecting strain are available, therapy can be changed to a less toxic agent. Similar therapy should be used for infected patients with calculi or urologic abnormalities who have suspected sepsis.

Optimal treatment regimens for patients with *catheter-associated urinary tract infections* have not been well established. These infections often remit spontaneously or with short-term antibiotic therapy if the catheter can be removed. If the catheter cannot be removed, systemic antibiotics or urinary antiseptics may reduce bacteriuria, but do not usually eliminate it. Asymptomatic bacteriuria in catheterized patients can probably be left untreated in most patients who are not immunosuppressed or who are not at high risk for sepsis because of old age, severe underlying disease, diabetes, or pregnancy.

PROGNOSIS In patients with uncomplicated cystitis or pyelonephritis, treatment ordinarily results in complete resolution of symptoms. In fact, symptoms usually remit even without specific therapy. Lower tract infections in adult women are of concern mainly because they cause discomfort, minor morbidity, and time lost from work. Cystitis may also result in upper tract infection or in bacteremia (especially during instrumentation), but there is little evidence to suggest that renal impairment follows. When repeated episodes of cystitis occur, they are nearly always reinfections, not relapses. Why a subpopulation of adult women develops a predisposition to multiple recurrent infections remains poorly understood. In some cases, residual urine, urethral stenosis, or other anatomic explanations exist, but most women with recurrent infections have no such demonstrable abnormality.

Uncomplicated acute pyelonephritis in adults rarely progresses to functional impairment and chronic renal disease. Repeated upper tract infections often indicate relapse rather than reinfection, and a vigorous search for renal calculi or an underlying urologic abnormality should be undertaken. If neither is found, 6 weeks of chemotherapy may be useful in eradicating an unresolved focus of infection.

Repeated symptomatic urinary tract infections in children, and in adults with obstructive uropathy, neurogenic bladder, structural renal disease, or diabetes more often progress to chronic renal disease. Asymptomatic bacteriuria in these groups, as well as in adults without urologic disease or obstruction, predisposes to increased episodes of symptomatic infection but does not result in renal impairment in most instances.

PREVENTION Patients with frequent symptomatic infections may benefit from long-term low-dose antibiotics directed at preventing recurrences. A single dose of trimethoprim-sulfamethoxazole (80 mg trimethoprim and 400 mg sulfamethoxazole daily), trimethoprim alone (100 mg daily), or nitrofurantoin (50 mg daily) have been particularly effective. Suppressive therapy should be initiated only after bacteriuria has been eradicated with a full-dose treatment regimen. Women having more than two infections every 6 months should be considered for preventive antibiotics. Low-dose antibiotics (nitrofurantoin 50 to 100 mg) after sexual intercourse may also be of benefit in preventing episodes of symptomatic infections. Other situations in which prophylaxis appears to have some merit include men with chronic prostatitis; patients undergoing prostatectomy, both during the operation and postoperative periods; and pregnant women with asymptomatic bacteriuria.

CHRONIC PYELONEPHRITIS

Chronic interstitial nephritis thought to result from bacterial infection of the kidney has been termed *chronic pyelonephritis.* It may occur in patients with predisposing urologic abnormalities (obstruction, vesicoureteral reflux, or neurogenic bladder) or in patients with apparently normal urinary tracts. Unlike acute urinary tract infections, for which simple diagnostic criteria and characteristic clinical syndromes exist, no pathognomonic clinical, laboratory, or pathologic criteria can be used to identify cases of chronic pyelonephritis, and few reliable data on the incidence or prevalence of this condition have been collected. Many patients with renal lesions that fulfill the pathologic criteria for chronic pyelonephritis at autopsy have sterile urine cultures and were not known to have had clinical episodes of bacterial urinary tract infection or urinary obstruction during life. Such cases suggest that other forms of renal injury result in morphologic changes indistinguishable from those produced by bacterial infection. Conversely, relatively few individuals with acute urinary infection develop chronic infection or progressive renal impairment. Most often, this occurs in patients with anatomic obstruction, neurogenic bladder, or vesicoureteral reflux.

Patients with many episodes of urinary tract infection; impaired renal function; pyuria with white cell casts; bacteriuria; an intravenous pyelogram showing an irregularly outlined renal pelvis with caliectasis and cortical scars; and typical pathologic changes can be diagnosed as having chronic pyelonephritis. In less typical patients, the relationship of infection to renal damage is uncertain and the diagnosis often remains unclear.

PATHOLOGY Characteristically, the kidneys are asymmetric in size, scarred, and irregularly pitted on the surface. Pathologic changes usually begin in the interstitial tissue of the medulla and papillae, with connective tissue, lymphocytes, and plasma cells completely replacing interstitium and tubules. Foci of active interstitial inflammation may be seen throughout the medulla, and leukocyte casts are found in some tubules. Other tubules contain large amounts of eosinophilic material and colloid casts, and may be dilated. Early in the disease, most glomeruli appear relatively normal. A proliferative endarteritis may be present. With progression, involvement of glomeruli and vessels becomes more pronounced and uniform, eventually resulting in an "end-stage" kidney.

None of the foregoing changes is pathognomonic for chronic pyelonephritis. Similar morphologic features may result from the nephropathy of chronic hypokalemia, nephrocalcinosis, chronic analgesic abuse, primary vascular disease of the kidneys, obstruction, diabetes mellitus, and Balkan nephropathy (see Chap. 297).

CLINICAL FEATURES Early signs and symptoms are minimal and nonspecific and often include hypertension. Later, as glomerular filtration and renal blood flow decline, the characteristic clinical and laboratory features of uremia appear (see Chap. 291).

The appearance of white blood cell casts in the urine suggests the diagnosis of chronic pyelonephritis. However, bacteria, leukocytes, and leukocyte casts may appear only intermittently and often are not present during the chronic stage of the disease. Intravenous pyelography is often normal early in the course of the disease but subsequently shows bilateral small kidneys with irregular outlines, calyceal blunting or dilatation, and cortical scarring. Renal biopsy may be normal owing to the focal nature of the disease early in its course.

PROGNOSIS The course of chronic pyelonephritis may be prolonged and compatible with a comfortable life even after considerable impairment of renal function. Associated hypertension generally worsens the prognosis. In perhaps no other renal disease can fluctuations in renal function be so marked or frequent. During acute infections or episodes of dehydration, renal decompensation may progress to the stage of advanced uremia; yet the patient may recover and regain adequate renal function for years. Correction of obstructing lesions may prevent progression of the disease.

TREATMENT Surgically approachable obstructive lesions should be promptly corrected. Antibiotic therapy for proved infections should be given and should be based on antimicrobial sensitivity tests. Hypertension should be controlled to reduce renal vascular complications. The treatment of chronic renal failure is discussed in Chap. 291.

PAPILLARY NECROSIS

The renal papilla is of major importance in the pathogenesis of chronic interstitial nephritis and, when complicated by bacterial infection, pyelonephritis. The peculiar susceptibility of the renal papilla to bacterial infection has been discussed earlier in this chapter (see "Experimental Evidence"). It has become evident that a variety of underlying conditions cause primary renal papillary damage, resulting eventually in the renal lesions of chronic interstitial nephritis. When urinary infection does not supervene, the resulting renal disease may progress slowly and silently to the point of renal insufficiency. The pathology of this renal injury may be indistinguishable from that of pyelonephritis. In addition to common diseases such as gout and diabetes mellitus, which cause renal papillary damage, many medications, which achieve enormous concentrations in the urine traversing the renal papilla, may be toxic for that zone of the kidney. The best known of these are phenacetin-containing analgesic mixtures. This problem is much more common than generally recognized, and diagnosis requires careful attention to historical information obtained from the patient.

It is not known how many other substances may be important in the pathogenesis of primary renal papillary disease. However, in view of the benignity of urinary infection in persons without underlying renal papillary damage, it is reasonable to assume the presence of primary underlying renal papillary damage in any patient with urinary infection who shows the development or progression of renal damage.

When severe infection of the renal pyramids is present in association with vascular diseases of the kidney or with urinary tract obstruction, renal papillary necrosis is likely to result. Patients with diabetes, sickle cell disease, chronic alcoholism, and vascular disease seem peculiarly susceptible to this complication. Hematuria, pain in the flank or abdomen, and chills and fever are the most common presenting symptoms. Acute renal failure with oliguria or anuria sometimes occurs. Rarely, sloughing of a pyramid may take place without symptoms in a patient with chronic urinary infection, and the diagnosis is made when the necrotic tissue is passed in the urine or identified as a "ring shadow" on pyelography. If renal function deteriorates suddenly in a diabetic or a patient with chronic obstruction, the diagnosis of renal papillary necrosis should be entertained, even in the absence of fever or pain. Although renal papillary necrosis is often bilateral, when it is unilateral, nephrectomy may be lifesaving in the management of overwhelming infection.

RENAL AND PERINEPHRIC ABSCESS

See Chap. 140.

PROSTATITIS

The term *prostatitis* designates various inflammatory conditions affecting the prostate, including acute and chronic infections with specific bacteria and, more commonly, instances in which signs and symptoms of prostatic inflammation are present but no specific organisms can be detected (prostatosis). Patients in this category usually have low back pain and perineal or testicular discomfort; less often, mild dysuria may be present. Microscopic pyuria or hematuria without any other evidence of genitourinary disease may be the only manifestation of prostatic disease. Such patients may respond to prostatic massage and warm sitz baths. Antibiotic therapy produces variable results.

ACUTE BACTERIAL PROSTATITIS This disease generally affects young male adults when it occurs spontaneously, but it may be associated with an indwelling urethral catheter. It is characterized by fever, chills, dysuria, and a tense or boggy, extremely tender, prostate. Palpation of the prostate is the key to diagnosis. Although prostatic massage usually produces purulent secretions with a large number of bacteria on culture, bacteremia may result from manipulation of the inflamed gland. For this reason, and because the etiologic agent can usually be identified on urine culture, massage should be avoided unless antibiotic treatment has been instituted. The infection is generally due to one of the common gram-negative urinary tract pathogens or *Staphylococcus aureus*, and response to therapy should be guided by the antimicrobial sensitivity pattern of the infecting strain. Initially, intravenous ampicillin, cephalosporins, or aminoglycosides can be utilized if gram-negative rods are seen in the urine Gram stain, and a cephalosporin or nafcillin if gram-positive cocci are seen. Although these drugs do not readily diffuse into the noninflamed prostate gland, the response to antibiotics is usually prompt, perhaps because the drugs penetrate more readily into the acutely inflamed prostate. The long-term prognosis is good, although in some instances acute infection may result in abscess formation, epididymoorchitis, seminal vesiculitis, septicemia, and residual chronic bacterial prostatitis. Since the advent of antibiotics, the frequency of acute bacterial prostatitis has diminished markedly. Many so-called cases of acute prostatitis are probably posterior urethritis.

CHRONIC BACTERIAL PROSTATITIS This entity is less well defined and is difficult to diagnose. It is a major cause of recurrent bacteriuria in males. Symptoms are usually absent, the prostate feels normal on palpation, and although many white blood cells may be seen in the urinary sediment, results of conventional bacteriologic studies are negative. A small number of bacteria may be cultured from the expressed prostatic secretion or postmassage urine. The presence of these bacteria can be determined only by careful quantitative bacteriologic techniques when the bladder urine is sterile. The method used by Stamey and colleagues should be employed. The usual symptoms of frequency and dysuria occur when infection spreads to the bladder urine. Antibiotics are of limited value in eradicating the focus of chronic infection in the prostate, but they usually do relieve the symptoms of the acute exacerbations promptly. The relative ineffectiveness of antimicrobials in part results from the poor penetration of most antibiotics into the prostate because the low pH which prevails in this organ precludes solubility of most drugs. The macrolide group of drugs (erythromycin) do enter the prostatic secretions, but these agents are generally ineffective against gram-negative organisms. Sulfonamide-trimethroprim has been employed successfully in some of these infections. Patients with frequent episodes of acute cystitis should be treated with prolonged courses of antimicrobials with a view toward suppressing symptoms and keeping the bladder urine sterile. Total prostatectomy produces cure of chronic prostatitis but is associated with considerable morbidity. Transurethral prostatectomy is safer but cures only one-third of patients.

Urinary infections are much less common in men than in women, perhaps because of the antibacterial properties of prostatic fluid. The pattern of recurrent bladder infection in the male with chronic bacterial prostatitis is clinically not very different from that seen in the recurrent cystourethritis of the female. It has been suggested that this pattern of infection in women is due to chronic bacterial infection of the paraurethral glands and ducts, which are, in fact, vestigial remnants of the prostate.

REFERENCES

BRUMFITT W, ASSCHER AW: *Urinary Tract Infection.* New York, Oxford University Press, 1973

FANG LST et al: Efficacy of single-dose and conventional therapy in urinary tract infection localized by the antibody-coated bacteria technique. N Engl J Med 298:413, 1978

JONES SR et al: Localization of urinary tract infection by detection of antibody-coated bacteria in urine sediment. N Engl J Med 290:591, 1975

KRAFT JK, STAMEY TA: The natural history of symptomatic recurrent bacteriuria in women. Medicine 56:55, 1977

KUNIN CM: *Detection, Prevention and Management of Urinary Tract Infections,* 3d ed. Philadelphia, Lea & Febiger, 1979

RONALD AR, HARDING GKM: Urinary prophylaxis in women. Ann Intern Med 94:268, 1981

SANFORD JP: Urinary tract symptoms and infection. Ann Rev Med 26:485, 1975

STAMEY TA: *Urinary Infections.* Baltimore, Williams & Wilkins, 1972

STAMM WE et al: Causes of the acute urethral syndrome in women. N Engl J Med 303:409, 1980

Symposium on Urinary Infections. Kidney Int, vol 4 (suppl), 1975

297 TUBULOINTERSTITIAL DISEASES OF THE KIDNEY

BARRY M. BRENNER
THOMAS H. HOSTETTER

A large and etiologically diverse group of bilateral renal diseases can be distinguished from those considered in Chaps. 294 and 295 because the histological and functional abnormalities involve the tubules and interstitium to a greater degree than the glomeruli and renal vasculature (see Table 297-1). Morphologically, acute forms of these tubulointerstitial disorders are characterized predominantly by interstitial edema, often associated with cortical and medullary infiltration by polymorphonuclear leukocytes and patchy areas of tubule cell necrosis. In more chronic forms, interstitial fibrosis predominates, inflammatory cells are typically mononuclear, and abnormalities of the tubules tend to be more widespread, as evidenced by atrophy, luminal dilatation, and thickening of tubule basement membranes. In the past, the diagnosis of chronic pyelonephritis was almost universally applied when these chronic tubulointerstitial abnormalities were found. It is now apparent that only a small proportion of these lesions results from infection. Nonbacterial factors, including exogenous toxins and metabolic and immunologic derangements, constitute the major pathogenetic mechanisms thought to be involved. Because of the nonspecific nature of the histology, particularly in chronic tubulointerstitial diseases, biopsy specimens rarely provide a specific diagnosis. The urine sediment is also unlikely to be diagnostic, except in allergic forms of acute tubulointerstitial disease in which eosinophils may predominate in the urinary sediment (see below).

Defects in tubule function often accompany these alterations of tubule and interstitial structure. Proximal tubule dysfunction may be manifested as selective reabsorptive defects leading to hypokalemia, aminoaciduria, glycosuria, phosphaturia, uricosuria, or bicarbonaturia (proximal or type II renal tubular acidosis, see Chap. 299). In combination these defects constitute the *Fanconi syndrome.* Protein excretion is usually modest, rarely exceeding 2 g per 24 h. The excreted proteins are typically of low molecular weight and include beta$_2$ microglobulin, lysozyme, and immunoglobulin light chains. Defective proximal tubule reabsorption of these readily filtered small-molecular-weight proteins accounts for their augmented excretion in these disorders. Tubule sodium reabsorption may also be deranged in patients with advanced tubulointerstitial diseases, predisposing them to the tendency to salt wasting and the threat of overt hypovolemia. One or more of these reabsorptive defects are commonly encountered with heavy metal poisoning, multiple myeloma, and other tubulointerstitial processes affecting the renal cortex diffusely.

Defects in urinary acidification and concentrating ability often represent the most troublesome of the tubule dysfunctions encountered in patients with tubulointerstitial disease. Metabolic acidosis of the hyperchloremic type often develops at a relatively early stage in the course of the renal insufficiency. Patients with this finding generally elaborate urine of maximal acidity (pH of 5.3 or less). In such patients the defect in acid excretion usually proves to be caused by a reduced capacity to generate and excrete ammonia due to the reduction in renal mass. Preferential damage to the collecting ducts, as in amyloidosis or chronic obstructive uropathy, may also predispose to distal or type I renal tubular acidosis, characterized by abnormally high urine pH ($>$5.5) during spontaneous or NH_4Cl-induced metabolic acidosis. Patients with tubulointerstitial diseases affecting medullary and papillary structures predominantly may also evidence substantial concentrating defects, with resultant nocturia and polyuria. The impairment in maximal concentration is typically unresponsive to the administration of antidiuretic hormone, hence a form of nephrogenic diabetes insipidus. Analgesic nephropathy and sickle cell disease are prototypes of this form of injury.

Although the major structural defects originate in the tubules and interstitium, progressive reduction in glomerular filtration rate (GFR) is a common functional accompaniment of most, if not all, forms of tubulointerstitial damage, reflecting secondary injury to glomeruli and other elements of the renal microcirculation.

TOXINS

A number of factors make the renal tubules and interstitium particularly prone to toxic injury. Although the kidneys constitute less than 1 percent of total body mass, they receive approximately 20 percent of the cardiac output, and 90 percent or more of this very large renal blood flow is distributed to the renal cortex. Exposure of tubules and interstitium of the renal cortex to circulating toxins is, therefore, quantitatively greater than is that of most other tissues. Transport processes operating in renal tubules contribute further to the intrarenal accumulation of toxins, thereby enhancing local concentrations of noxious agents. Furthermore, the urinary concentrating mechanism can establish high levels of toxins within medullary and papillary portions of the kidney, predisposing these regions to chemical injury. Finally, the relatively acid pH of the fluid within most nephron segments may affect the ionization characteristics of potentially toxic compounds and thereby influence local concentration and solubility. Although these normal physiological processes render the kidney particularly vulnerable to toxic injury, the role of nephrotoxins in the causation of renal damage often goes unrecognized, largely because the manifestations of such injury are usually nonspecific in nature and insidious in onset. Diagnosis largely depends upon obtaining a history of exposure to a certain toxin, a difficult matter since exposure may be occult. Particular attention should, therefore, be paid to the patient's occupational history, as well as to an assessment of exposure, current as well as remote, to pharmaceutical agents, especially antibiotics and analgesics. The clinical recognition of a potential association between a patient's renal disease and exposure to a nephrotoxin is of crucial importance because, unlike many other forms of renal disease, progression of the functional and morphological abnormalities associated with toxin-induced nephropathies may be prevented, and even reversed, simply by eliminating additional exposure.

EXOGENOUS TOXINS **Analgesic nephropathy** Over the past three decades, numerous studies have established that individuals who ingest large quantities of analgesic drugs are particularly prone to develop tubulointerstitial damage and papillary necrosis. Indeed, in Australia, Switzerland, and Sweden, analgesic abuse ranks as one of the most common causes of chronic renal failure, and it is now recognized as an important cause of renal insufficiency in the United States as well. Studies in animals have demonstrated that *phenacetin* and *aspirin* can induce papillary necrosis when either of these drugs is given in quantities far in excess of usual therapeutic doses. However, these chemicals are far more likely to cause renal damage, and clinically apparent renal disease, when ingested in combination. Epidemiologic studies leave no doubt that the chronic ingestion of mixtures of these analgesics produces permanent and irreversible renal injury in humans.

Morphologically, analgesic nephropathy is characterized by papillary necrosis and tubulointerstitial inflammation. At an early stage prior to overt papillary necrosis, damage to the vascular supply of the inner medulla (vasa recta) leads to a local interstitial inflammatory reaction and, eventually, to papillary ischemia, necrosis, fibrosis, and calcification. Destruction of papillae usually precedes extension of the tubulointerstitial abnormalities to the renal cortex and, therefore, occurs before renal size and GFR are reduced significantly. It is important to recognize that although papillary necrosis is a common finding in patients with the nephropathy of analgesic abuse, necrosis of papillae may also be seen in patients with chronic pyelonephritis, diabetes mellitus, sickle cell disease, and obstructive uropathy. The susceptibility of the renal papillae to damage by analgesic compounds which contain phenacetin is believed to be related to the establishment of a renal corticomedullary gradient for the phenacetin metabolite *acetaminophen,* resulting in papillary tip concentrations which are more than tenfold higher than those present in renal cortex. Hydration serves to dissipate this gradient and may explain the protective effect of this maneuver in preventing phenacetin-induced papillary necrosis in animals. The aspirin in these analgesic compounds is also believed to contribute to renal injury, by uncoupling oxidative phosphorylation in renal mitochondria and by inhibiting the synthesis of renal prostaglandins, which are potent endogenous renal vasodilator hormones. Both effects of aspirin favor hypoxia in renal tissues and, therefore, enhance the susceptibility of the inner medulla to nephrotoxic injury.

Clinically, analgesic nephropathy occurs some three to five times more commonly in women than men. A direct relationship exists between the total amount of analgesic compounds ingested and the degree of renal impairment. An intake of 1.0 g phenacetin per day for 1 to 3 years, or total ingestion of 2 kg phenacetin in combination with other analgesics, appears to represent minimum requirements for the development of analgesic nephropathy. In such patients, renal function usually declines gradually, in association with chronic necrosis of papillae and diffuse tubulointerstitial damage to the renal cortex. Occasionally, papillary necrosis may be associated with gross hematuria, and even renal colic, due to obstruction of a ureter by a fragment of necrotic tissue. More than half of patients with analgesic nephropathy have pyuria, which, if persistently associated with sterile urine, provides an important clue to the diagnosis. Nonetheless, active pyelonephritis may coexist in patients with analgesic nephropathy. Proteinuria, if present, is typically mild (less than 1 g per 24 h). Patients with analgesic nephropathy are usually unable to generate maximally concentrated urine, reflecting the underlying medullary and papillary damage. An acquired form of distal renal tubular acidosis has been described and may contribute to the development of *nephrocalcinosis.* The occurrence of anemia out of proportion to the degree of azotemia may also provide a useful clue to the diagnosis of analgesic nephropathy. Occult gastrointestinal bleeding (usually secondary to analgesic-induced gastritis) and, in an occasional patient, hemolysis (particularly in those with glucose 6-phosphate dehydrogenase deficiency) are believed to contribute to the severity of the anemia. Vague abdominal complaints, as well as nonspecific headaches and arthralgias, are common in these patients. Moderate hypertension is also a common finding. It progresses to a malignant phase in only a small minority of patients. When analgesic nephropathy has progressed to the stage of moderate to severe renal insufficiency, the kidneys usually appear bilaterally shrunken on intravenous pyelography, and the calyces are deformed. A "ring sign" on the pyelogram is pathognomonic of papillary necrosis and represents the radiolucent sloughed papilla surrounded by the radiodense contrast material which fills the calyx. Also, transitional cell carcinoma may develop in the urinary pelvis or ureters as a late complication of analgesic abuse.

Every effort must be made to convince the patient who ingests excessive quantities of analgesics to discontinue this hazardous practice. When renal damage is at an early stage, cessation of drug abuse will usually arrest the progression of the nephrotoxic process; not infrequently, overall renal function will improve with time. With continued abuse of these drugs, however, progressive renal damage leads invariably to chronic renal failure.

TABLE 297-1
Principal causes of tubulointerstitial disease of the kidney

- *I* Toxins
  - *A* Exogenous toxins
    - *1* Analgesic nephropathy
    - *2* Lead nephropathy
    - *3* Miscellaneous nephrotoxins (e.g., antibiotics, radiographic contrast media, heavy metals)
  - *B* Metabolic toxins
    - *1* Acute uric acid nephropathy
    - *2* Gouty nephropathy
    - *3* Hypercalcemic nephropathy
    - *4* Hypokalemic nephropathy
    - *5* Miscellaneous metabolic toxins (e.g., hyperoxaluria, cystinosis, Fabry's disease)
- *II* Neoplasia
  - *A* Lymphoma
  - *B* Leukemia
  - *C* Multiple myeloma
- *III* Immune disorders
  - *A* Hypersensitivity nephropathy
  - *B* Sjögren's syndrome
  - *C* Amyloidosis (see also Chap. 66)
  - *D* Transplant rejection (see Chap. 292)
  - *E* Tubulointerstitial abnormalities associated with glomerulonephritis (see also Chaps. 294 and 295)
- *IV* Vascular disorders (see Chaps. 290 and 298)
  - *A* Arteriolar nephrosclerosis
  - *B* Atheroembolic disease
  - *C* Sickle cell nephropathy
  - *D* Acute tubular necrosis
- *V* Hereditary renal diseases
  - *A* Hereditary nephritis (Alport's syndrome) (see Chap. 295)
  - *B* Medullary cystic disease (see Chap. 299)
  - *C* Medullary sponge kidney (see Chap. 299)
- *VI* Infectious injury (see Chap. 296)
  - *A* Acute pyelonephritis
  - *B* Chronic pyelonephritis
- *VII* Miscellaneous disorders
  - *A* Chronic urinary tract obstruction (see Chap. 301)
  - *B* Vesicoureteral reflux
  - *C* Radiation nephritis
  - *D* Balkan nephropathy

Lead nephropathy (see also Chap. 239) Children and adults suffering from lead intoxication often develop a chronic form of tubulointerstitial renal disease. In children, lead poisoning usually results from ingestion of lead-based paints (pica). The oxide of lead liberated from paint, or present in the vapor arising from the welding of metals covered with lead-based paint, may be inhaled in substantial quantities, thereby constituting an industrial form of exposure in adults. Alcohol, illegally distilled in an apparatus constructed from automobile radiators (so-called moonshine), is yet another source of lead poisoning. Tubule transport processes enhance the accumulation of lead within renal cells, particularly of the proximal convoluted tubule, leading to cell degeneration, mitochondrial swelling, and eosinophilic intranuclear inclusion bodies rich in lead. In addition to tubule degeneration and atrophy, lead nephropathy is associated with ischemic changes in the glomeruli, fibrosis of the adventitia of small renal arterioles, and focal areas of cortical scarring. Eventually, the kidneys become grossly atrophic. In addition to progressive azotemia, abnormalities of tubule function may occur, particularly *renal glycosuria* and *aminoaciduria.* Urinary excretion of lead, bile pigments, and porphyrin precursors, particularly δ-aminolevulinic acid, coproporphyrin, and urobilinogen, may be increased. Patients with chronic lead nephropathy are characteristically *hyperuricemic,* a consequence of enhanced reabsorption of filtered urate. Acute gouty arthritis (so-called saturnine gout) occurs in about 50 percent of patients with lead nephropathy, in striking contrast to other forms of chronic renal failure in which gout is rare. Hypertension is also a frequent complication of this disorder. Therefore, in any patient with slowly progressive renal failure, atrophic kidneys, gout, and hypertension, the diagnosis of lead intoxication should be seriously considered. In addition to these manifestations, patients with chronic lead poisoning often complain of frequent episodes of abdominal colic and have evidence of anemia, peripheral neuropathy, and encephalopathy. The diagnosis may be suspected by finding elevated serum levels of lead. However, because blood levels may not be elevated even in the presence of a toxic total-body burden of lead, the quantitation of lead excretion following a standardized infusion of the chelating agent calcium disodium ethylenediaminetetraacetic acid (EDTA) is a more reliable indicator of serious lead exposure. Urinary excretion of more than 0.6 mg of lead per day is indicative of overt or potential toxicity. Treatment includes removing the patient from the source of exposure and augmenting lead excretion with a chelating agent such as calcium disodium EDTA.

Miscellaneous nephrotoxins Many agents which commonly lead to acute renal failure are also capable of producing tubulointerstitial injury (see Chap. 290). These include antibiotics (e.g., aminoglycosides, amphotericin B), radiographic contrast agents, various hydrocarbons (e.g., carbon tetrachloride), and heavy metals (e.g., mercury, cadmium, and bismuth). Nonsteroidal anti-inflammatory drugs including fenoprofen and ibuprofen have also been implicated. Of note, the tubulointerstitial nephropathy which develops in some patients taking these and other nonsteroidal anti-inflammatory drugs may be associated with nephrotic-range proteinuria and histological evidence of minimal change glomerulopathy.

METABOLIC TOXINS Acute uric acid nephropathy Disorders characterized by acute overproduction of uric acid and extreme hyperuricemia often lead to a rapidly progressive form of renal insufficiency, so-called acute uric acid nephropathy. This tubulointerstitial disease is usually seen in patients given cytotoxic drugs for the treatment of lymphoproliferative or myeloproliferative disorders, but may also occur in these patients even before such treatment is begun. The pathological changes associated with acute uric acid nephropathy are largely the result of deposition of uric acid crystals in the kidneys and their collecting systems leading to partial or complete obstruction of collecting ducts, renal pelvis, or ureter. Since obstruction is often bilateral, patients typically show the clinical course of acute renal failure, characterized by oliguria and rapidly rising serum creatinine concentration. In the early phase of this disorder, uric acid crystals can often be found in urine, usually in association with microscopic or gross hematuria. Peak serum uric acid levels vary but are almost always above 20 mg/dl and may even exceed 60 mg/dl.

Prevention of hyperuricemia in patients at risk, by treatment with allopurinol in doses of 200 to 800 mg per day prior to cytotoxic therapy, greatly reduces the danger of acute uric acid nephropathy. Once hyperuricemia develops, however, efforts should be directed to preventing deposition of uric acid within the urinary tract. Increasing urine volume with potent diuretics (furosemide or mannitol) effectively lowers intratubular uric acid concentrations, and alkalinization of the urine to pH 7 or greater with sodium bicarbonate and/or a carbonic anhydrase inhibitor (acetazolamide) enhances uric acid solubility. If these efforts, together with allopurinol therapy, are ineffective in preventing acute renal failure, dialysis should be instituted to lower the serum uric acid concentration as well as to treat the acute manifestations of uremia. The combination of conservative therapy and hemodialysis allows most patients with acute uric acid nephropathy to survive this form of acute renal failure and ultimately recover renal function essentially completely.

Gouty nephropathy Patients with less severe but more prolonged forms of hyperuricemia are predisposed to a more chronic tubulointerstitial disorder, often referred to as *gouty nephropathy.* Since other conditions associated with hyperuricemia, such as hypertension, nephrolithiasis, pyelonephritis, and even lead poisoning, may contribute to renal damage, the effect of chronic hyperuricemia per se on renal function is unsettled. Nevertheless, the severity of renal involvement in this disorder correlates well with the duration and magnitude of the elevation of the serum uric acid concentration. Histologically, the distinctive feature of gouty nephropathy is the presence of crystalline deposits of uric acid and monosodium urate salts in kidney parenchyma. These deposits are believed to represent the primary pathogenetic process in gouty nephropathy, with intraluminal crystallization of uric acid taking place in distal tubules and collecting ducts where urine pH is generally quite low and where uric acid concentrations are considerably in excess of levels in plasma. These deposits not only cause intrarenal obstruction, but also incite an inflammatory response, leading to lymphocytic infiltration, foreign-body giant-cell reaction, and eventual fibrosis, especially of medullary and papillary regions of the kidney. Bacteriuria and pyelonephritis occur in about one-fourth of cases, presumably as complications of intrarenal urinary stasis. Since patients with gout frequently suffer from hypertension and hyperlipidemia, degenerative changes of the renal arterioles may constitute a striking feature of the histological abnormality, often out of proportion to other morphological defects. Clinically, gouty nephropathy is an insidious cause of renal insufficiency. Early in its course, GFR may be near normal, often despite focal morphological changes in medullary and cortical interstitium, proteinuria, and diminished urinary concentrating ability. Whether reducing serum uric acid levels with allopurinol exerts a beneficial effect on the kidney remains to be demonstrated. Although such undesirable consequences of hyperuricemia as gout and uric acid stones respond well to allopurinol, use of this drug in asymptomatic hyperuricemia has not been shown to improve renal function consistently. On the other hand, uricosuric agents such as probenecid, which may increase uric acid stone production, clearly have no role in the treatment of renal disease associated with hyperuricemia.

Hypercalcemic nephropathy Chronic hypercalcemia, as occurs in primary hyperparathyroidism, sarcoidosis, multiple myeloma, vitamin D intoxication, or metastatic bone disease, is a well known cause of tubulointerstitial damage and progressive renal insufficiency. Pathologically, the earliest renal lesion induced by hypercalcemia is a focal degenerative change in renal epithelia, primarily in collecting ducts, distal convoluted tubules, and loops of Henle. Tubule cell necrosis leads to nephron obstruction and stasis of intrarenal urine, favoring local precipitation of calcium salts and infection. Dilatation and atrophy of tubules eventually occur, as do interstitial fibrosis, mononuclear leukocyte infiltration, and interstitial calcium deposition (nephrocalcinosis). Calcium deposition may also occur in glomeruli and the walls of renal arterioles. Clinically, the most striking defect is an inability to concentrate the urine maximally, resulting in polyuria and nocturia. Defective transport of chloride in the ascending limb of Henle's loop is believed to be responsible, at least in part, for this concentrating defect. Additionally, reduced collecting duct responsiveness to ADH may contribute to this abnormality. Reductions in GFR and renal blood flow also occur, both in states of acute severe hypercalcemia as well as with prolonged hypercalcemia of lesser severity. Distal renal tubular acidosis and sodium and potassium wasting have also been described in these chronic states. Eventually, uncontrolled hypercalcemia leads to severe tubulointerstitial damage and overt renal failure. Urinalysis is rarely a clue to the presence of hypercalcemic renal failure, but abdominal x-rays may demonstrate nephrocalcinosis as well as nephrolithiasis, the latter due to the hypercalciuria which often accompanies hypercalcemia. Treatment for hypercalcemic nephropathy consists of reducing the serum calcium concentration toward normal and correcting the primary abnormality of calcium metabolism. The management of hypercalcemia is discussed in Chap. 339. Prognosis for recovery of renal function depends upon the severity of the renal lesion at the time hypercalcemia is corrected. Renal dysfunction of recent onset secondary to acute hypercalcemia may be completely reversible. Gradual, progressive renal insufficiency related to chronic hypercalcemia, however, may not improve with correction of the calcium disorder. Nonetheless, every effort should be made to return serum calcium concentration to normal in order to minimize further loss of renal function.

Hypokalemic nephropathy Disturbances of renal structure and function are observed commonly in patients with moderate to severe potassium depletion of at least several weeks' duration. Histologically, renal epithelial cells are often seen to contain numerous vacuoles, most marked in proximal, and to a lesser extent, distal convoluted tubules. These findings usually disappear with potassium repletion. Glomeruli and blood vessels are usually uninvolved. Whether prolonged or recurrent potassium deficiency results in irreversible tubulointerstitial fibrosis, scarring, and atrophy is still a controversial issue. Loss of urinary concentrating ability is the most commonly encountered functional defect. Experimental studies in animals have shown that this urinary concentrating abnormality is preceded by a period of primary polydipsia. The reduced concentrating capacity which eventually develops is due, at least in part, to defective operation of the countercurrent multiplier system. Elevated rates of intrarenal prostaglandin synthesis may also contribute to this concentrating defect, since prostaglandins are known to antagonize the hydroosmotic action of antidiuretic hormone on collecting-duct epithelium. Symptoms of nocturia, polyuria, and polydipsia are frequently encountered in patients with chronic potassium depletion, although, occasionally, patients with severe hypokalemia have no complaints referable to the urinary tract. It has been suggested that patients with hypokalemic nephropathy have an enhanced susceptibility to pyelonephritis, but this issue remains unresolved. The polydipsia is probably due to both the impaired renal concentrating ability and a primary disorder of the thirst mechanism, which is believed to be a common feature of most chronic potassium depletion states. Urinalysis often reveals no abnormalities except for mild proteinuria. Serum creatinine and urea nitrogen concentrations usually remain within normal limits. Treatment should be directed at repleting body potassium stores and correcting the primary process responsible for potassium loss. With correction of body potassium stores, functional and histological abnormalities of the kidneys usually disappear, although maximum urinary concentrating ability may not return to normal for several months.

Miscellaneous metabolic toxins Urinary oxalate, derived from the metabolism of glycine and, to a variable extent, from ingested oxalate, may deposit as insoluble intratubular calcium oxalate crystals and result in chronic tubulointerstitial damage in patients with hereditary or acquired forms of *hyperoxaluria. Cystinosis* and *Fabry's disease* are other hereditary depositional disorders affecting the renal tubules and interstitium. The reader is referred to Chaps. 295, 299, and 300 for more detailed discussions of these and other uncommon metabolic causes of tubulointerstitial injury.

NEOPLASIA

In addition to being the site of origin of several benign and malignant neoplasms (see Chap. 302), the kidneys are frequently affected by neoplasms arising outside the urinary tract. Except for the glomerulopathies associated with lymphomas and several solid tumors (see Chap. 294), the renal manifestations of primary extrarenal neoplastic processes are confined mainly to the interstitium and tubules. Although metastatic renal involvement by solid tumors is unusual, the kidneys are often invaded by neoplastic cells in various lymphomas and leukemias and in multiple myeloma. In postmortem studies of patients with *lymphoma,* renal involvement is found in approximately one-half of cases. The involvement may be focal, in the form of multiple discrete nodules, or diffuse, with lymphomatous infiltration throughout the renal parenchyma. Diffuse infiltration is seen most commonly in lymphomas other than Hodgkin's disease. There may be flank pain related to massive renal infiltration, and x-rays may show enlargement of one or both kidneys. Renal insufficiency occurs in a distinct minority of cases, and overt uremia is rare. Treatment of the primary disease may improve renal function in these cases.

The kidneys are also commonly involved in various forms of *leukemia.* At postmortem examination, bilateral renal involvement can be demonstrated in approximately 50 percent of cases. As with lymphoma, uremia is rarely, if ever, a consequence of leukemic infiltration of the kidneys. The kidneys can also be involved in leukemias because of the associated high incidence of hyperuricemia, hypercalcemia, and lysozymuria. The myelogenous leukemias, particularly of the monocytic type, may be complicated by tubule defects involving potassium and magnesium wasting.

In contrast, infiltration of the kidneys with *myeloma* cells is infrequent. When it occurs, the process is usually focal, so that renal insufficiency from this cause is also uncommon. The more usual lesion is *"myeloma kidney,"* which is characterized histologically by atrophic tubules, many with eosinophilic intraluminal casts, and numerous multinucleated giant cells within tubule walls as well as in the interstitium. The frequent occurrence of myeloma kidney in patients with Bence-Jones proteinuria has suggested a causal relation. Bence-Jones proteins are thought to cause myeloma kidney through direct toxicity to renal tubule cells. In addition, Bence-Jones proteins may precipitate within the distal nephron where the high concentrations of these proteins and the acid composition of the tubule fluid favor intraluminal cast formation and intrarenal obstruction. Indeed, positive immunofluorescence staining for light chains can often be demonstrated in casts found in myeloma kidneys. Occasionally, acute renal failure occurs after intravenous pyelography in patients with multiple myeloma and is believed to result from the further precipitation of Bence-Jones proteins induced by dehydration prior to radiographic study. Routine dehydration of the patient with myeloma in preparation for intravenous pyelography should, therefore, be avoided. Multiple myeloma may also affect the kidneys indirectly. Hypercalcemia or hyperuricemia may occur and lead to the nephropathies described above. Proximal tubule disorders are also seen occasionally in patients with myeloma, including type 2 proximal renal tubular acidosis and the Fanconi syndrome. Additionally, intrarenal deposits of *amyloid* (see below) may contribute to impaired excretory function in patients with multiple myeloma.

IMMUNE DISORDERS

HYPERSENSITIVITY NEPHROPATHY An acute diffuse tubulointerstitial reaction may result from hypersensitivity to a number of drugs. First reported after the use of sulfonamides, acute tubulointerstitial damage is now seen most often with the antibiotic *methicillin,* although other drugs, including *ampicillin, penicillin, cephalothin, phenindione, thiazides,* and *furosemide,* have also been implicated. Grossly, the kidneys are usually enlarged. Histologically, the glomeruli appear normal. The principal pathological abnormalities are in the interstitium of the kidney, which reveals pronounced edema and infiltration with polymorphonuclear leukocytes, lymphocytes, plasma cells, and, in some cases, large numbers of eosinophils. If the process is severe, tubule cell necrosis and regeneration may also be apparent. Immunofluorescence studies in a number of cases either have been unrevealing or have demonstrated a linear pattern of immunoglobin and complement deposition along tubule basement membranes. In a few cases of methicillin-induced acute tubulointerstitial disease, circulating antitubule basement membrane antibodies have also been found, suggesting that autoantibody formation may have been induced by the penicilloyl hapten of methicillin (by conjugation of hapten with tubule basement membrane proteins, thereby altering the native antigenicity of the basement membrane). Evidence for an immunologic basis for these various drug-related nephropathies also derives from the facts that the onset of nephropathy does not appear to be dose-related, often follows a second exposure to the drug presumed to be responsible for the renal injury, and often is associated with increased levels of serum IgE. In the case of methicillin, the patients usually develop evidence of renal injury after about 2 weeks of drug administration. Hematuria, fever, skin rash, and eosinophilia are prominent. Many patients develop azotemia which typically resolves after withdrawal of the offending drug. Proteinuria and pyuria often accompany the hematuria, and occasionally eosinophils are found in the urine sediment. The clinical picture may be confused with acute glomerulonephritis, but when acute azotemia and hematuria are accompanied by eosinophilia, skin rash, and a history of drug exposure, a hypersensitivity reaction leading to acute tubulointerstitial nephritis should be regarded as the leading diagnostic possibility. Discontinuation of the drug usually results in complete reversal of the renal injury; rarely, renal damage may be irreversible. Corticosteroids have been used, but their value in this disorder has not been established with certainty.

SJÖGREN'S SYNDROME (See also Chap. 346) Keratoconjunctivitis sicca, or Sjögren's syndrome, is an immunologic disorder characterized by dryness of mucous membranes and mononuclear cell infiltration of salivary and lacrimal glands; it is often seen in patients with rheumatoid arthritis. When the kidneys are involved in Sjögren's syndrome, the predominant histological findings are those of chronic tubulointerstitial disease. Interstitial infiltrates are composed primarily of lymphocytes, causing the histology of the renal parenchyma in these patients to resemble that of the salivary and lacrimal glands. Renal functional defects associated with this disorder include diminished urinary concentrating ability and distal renal tubular acidosis. Urinalysis may show pyuria (predominantly lymphocyturia) and mild proteinuria.

AMYLOIDOSIS (See also Chaps. 66 and 295) Glomerular pathology usually predominates and leads to heavy proteinuria and azotemia. However, tubule function may also be deranged, giving rise to a nephrogenic form of diabetes insipidus and to distal renal tubular acidosis. In several cases these functional abnormalities have been correlated with peritubular deposition of amyloid, particularly in areas surrounding vasa rectae, loops of Henle, and collecting ducts. Bilateral enlargement of the kidneys, especially in a patient with massive proteinuria and evidence for tubule dysfunction, should raise the possibility of amyloid renal disease.

TUBULOINTERSTITIAL ABNORMALITIES ASSOCIATED WITH GLOMERULONEPHRITIS A number of primary glomerulopathies may also be associated with damage to tubules and interstitium. Pathogenetically, the extraglomerular component in these renal disorders often involves the same mechanisms that are responsible for the more pronounced glomerular injury. For example, in more than half of patients with the nephropathy associated with systemic lupus erythematosus, deposits of immune complexes can be identified in tubule basement membranes, usually accompanied by an interstitial mononuclear inflammatory reaction. Similarly, in many patients with glomerulonephritis associated with antiglomerular basement membrane antibody, the same antibody can be shown to be reactive against tubule basement membranes as well.

MISCELLANEOUS DISORDERS

VESICOURETERAL REFLUX (See also Chaps. 296 and 301) Normally, the junction of the terminal ureter with the urinary bladder provides a competent sphincter so that during micturition urine leaves the bladder only via the urethra. However, when the function of the ureterovesical junction is impaired, urine may reflux into the ureters due to the high intravesical pressure that develops during voiding. Clinically, reflux is often detected on the voiding and postvoiding films obtained during intravenous pyelography, although voiding cystourethrography may be required for definitive diagnosis. Bladder infection may ascend the urinary tract to the kidneys through incompetent ureterovesical sphincters. Not surprisingly, therefore, reflux is often discovered in patients with acute and/or chronic urinary tract infections. In children particularly, reflux of minor degree may disappear with time and standard therapy of intercurrent urinary infection. With more severe degrees of reflux, characterized by marked dilatation of ureters and renal pelves, progressive renal damage often appears, and although active infection may also be present, uncertainty exists as to the necessity of infection in producing the scarred kidney of reflux nephropathy. In contrast to those with other forms of chronic tubulointerstitial disease, patients with renal insufficiency and scarring due to reflux often demonstrate substantial proteinuria. Indeed, in such cases glomerular lesions similar to those of idiopathic focal glomerulosclerosis (Chap. 294) are often present in addition to the more usual changes of chronic tubulointerstitial disease. Surgical correction of reflux is usually necessary only with the more severe degrees of reflux since renal damage appears to best correlate with the extent of reflux. Obviously, if extensive glomerulosclerosis already exists, urological repair may no longer be warranted.

RADIATION NEPHRITIS Clinical renal dysfunction can be expected to occur if 2300 R or more of x-ray irradiation is administered to both kidneys during a period of 5 weeks or less. Histological examination of the affected kidneys reveals hyalinized glomeruli, atrophic tubules, extensive interstitial fibrosis, and hyalinization of the media of renal arterioles. Radiation-induced renal ischemia is believed to be the main pathogenetic factor responsible for the widespread tubulointerstitial damage, which may not become evident clinically for weeks to months after completion of irradiation. The clinical presentation of acute radiation nephritis includes rapidly progressive azotemia, moderate to malignant hypertension, anemia, and proteinuria, which may reach the nephrotic range. More than 50 percent of these cases progress to chronic renal failure. A more insidious form of radiation nephritis may also occur; it is characterized by slower development of azotemia, anemia, and nephrotic syndrome. Malignant hypertension has also been known to follow unilateral renal irradiation and to resolve with ipsilateral nephrectomy. Radiation nephritis in recent years has all but vanished because of heightened awareness of its pathogenesis by radiotherapists.

BALKAN NEPHROPATHY Balkan nephropathy is an acquired, endemic disorder restricted to the small geographic region where Yugoslavia, Romania, and Bulgaria meet to form the Danubian basin. The renal lesions seen in affected patients from this region progress from focal tubular atrophy, interstitial edema, and mononuclear cell infiltration to diffuse interstitial fibrosis, leading eventually to bilaterally shrunken, atrophic kidneys. Epidemiologic studies point to an environmental toxin as the cause, but the offending agent has not yet been identified. Defects in urinary concentrating ability, low-molecular-weight ("tubular") proteinuria, and renal tubular acidosis are common. In most cases, the disease is progressive, leading eventually to chronic renal failure. A high incidence of papillary transitional carcinoma of the renal pelvis and upper ureter appears to be a late complication in patients with this endemic nephropathy.

REFERENCES

Batumen V et al: The role of lead in gout nephropathy. New Engl J Med 304:520, 1981

Cotran RS: Tubulo-interstitial diseases, in *The Kidney,* 2d ed, BM Brenner, FC Rector Jr (eds). Philadelphia, Saunders, 1981, chap 29

———, Pennington JE: Urinary tract infection, pyelonephritis, and reflux nephropathy, in *The Kidney,* 2d ed, BM Brenner, FC Rector Jr (eds). Philadelphia, Saunders, 1981, chap 28

———: Glomerulosclerosis in reflux nephropathy. Kidney Int 21:528, 1982

Ditlove J et al: Methicillin nephritis. Medicine 56:483, 1977

Hall PW, Dammin GJ: Balkan nephropathy. Nephron 22:281, 1978

Kincaid-Smith P (ed): Symposium on analgesic nephropathy. Kidney Int 13:1, 1978

Murray T, Goldberg M: Chronic interstitial nephritis: Etiologic factors. Ann Intern Med 82:453, 1975

Porter GA, Bennett WM: Toxic nephropathies, in *The Kidney,* 2d ed, BM Brenner, FC Rector Jr (eds). Philadelphia, Saunders, 1981, chap 39

Torres VE et al: The progression of vesicoureteral reflux nephropathy. Ann Intern Med 92:776, 1980

Wilson CB, Dixon FJ: The renal response to immunologic injury, in *The Kidney,* 2d ed, BM Brenner, FC Rector Jr (eds). Philadelphia, Saunders, 1981, chap 25

298 VASCULAR INJURY TO THE KIDNEY

NORMAN K. HOLLENBERG

Processes ranging from renal artery stenosis and occlusion to arteriolar nephrosclerosis, polyarteritis nodosa, the hemolytic uremic syndromes, scleroderma, and preeclampsia share a sufficient number of clinical features, morphological characteristics, and pathogenetic consequences to justify their consideration together. The clinical, functional, and morphological expressions of interrupting the renal blood supply depend on the degree of obstruction to flow, the rate at which the occlusion occurs, the level of vessel or vessels involved, and the total mass of ischemic parenchyma. Because the intrarenal arterial tree is made up of end arteries, sudden occlusion results in infarction with clinical manifestations that vary with the level at which the occlusion occurs. More gradual partial occlusion, on the other hand, results in ischemic atrophy and a different functional and clinical picture.

Renal blood flow, averaging 4.0 (ml/g)/min, exceeds by three- to fivefold the flow in such metabolically active organs as the heart, liver, and brain. Renal blood flow is not adjusted to satisfy metabolic need, but rather to provide the plasma flow and pressure to the glomerular capillary bed required to sustain glomerular filtration. Renal perfusion is also an important determinant of sodium handling by the kidney. For these reasons, a reduction in renal blood flow too small to result in cell death has important consequences including a reduction in filtration rate, increased sodium reabsorption, increased renin release, and hypertension. To a varying extent all are features common to the syndromes resulting from abnormalities in the renal circulation.

ACUTE ARTERIAL OCCLUSION Acute, complete occlusion of the main renal artery or a major intrarenal arterial branch may follow blunt trauma to the abdomen or back or embolism in patients with mitral stenosis and atrial fibrillation, infective endocarditis, mural thrombi overlying myocardial infarcts, or ulcerating atherosclerotic disease of the aorta. The kidneys receive about one-fifth of the cardiac output, making embolic occlusion of the small intrarenal arteries relatively common. Acute occlusion results in coagulation necrosis in the region supplied by the obstructed artery, the size of the wedge-shaped infarct varying with the level of the occlusion.

The clinical features also depend on the size of the infarct. Small infarcts, involving a portion of the renal cortex, are often clinically silent. Larger infarcts may induce a sudden, sharp unremitting pain in the flank or upper abdomen associated with fever, leukocytosis, and gross or microscopic hematuria. The impact on renal function also varies. Even total occlusion of one main renal artery may leave the blood urea nitrogen (BUN) and serum creatinine in the normal range in the presence of a healthy contralateral kidney which can undergo hypertrophy. When the patient has only a solitary functioning kidney, arterial occlusion enters the differential diagnosis of acute oliguric renal failure. Although total destruction of the kidney will generally occur within hours of occlusion, at least a dozen case reports of restoration of renal function after days to weeks of total occlusion have appeared, generally in a setting in which prior partial occlusion has led to a rich collateral arterial blood supply sufficient for nutrition although inadequate to maintain renal function. Angiography is necessary to establish the diagnosis. Evidence of collateral filling of the intrarenal arterial tree suggests that operation may restore renal function.

RENAL ARTERY STENOSIS (See also Chap. 267) Partial occlusion of the renal artery or its major branches by atherosclerotic narrowing or by fibromuscular dysplasia is responsible for about 1 to 2 percent of cases of hypertension; its importance lies in the fact that it represents the most common curable form of hypertension. *Renal arterial atherosclerosis,* as with atherosclerosis elsewhere, is more frequent in males, and its incidence increases with advancing age, previous hypertension, or diabetes mellitus. The *fibromuscular dysplasias* of the renal artery are a heterogeneous group of lesions in which fibrous or fibromuscular thickening may involve the intima, the media, or the subadventitial region. The process is frequently bilateral and may extend into the intrarenal tree. The fibrous dysplasias are 10 times more common in females, appear most often in the third and fourth decades, and, presumably because the individuals are younger, are associated with a lower surgical morbidity and a higher cure rate than are atherosclerotic renal arterial lesions.

The clinical features which may be helpful in detecting renal artery stenosis include a history of the onset of hypertension at an age which is unusual for essential hypertension, i.e., under 30 or over 50 years of age, or of a poor response to medical therapy. Physical examination may reveal a bruit in the flank or upper abdominal region. Routine laboratory evaluation often reveals evidence of secondary hyperaldosteronism including hypokalemia and metabolic alkalosis. As in primary aldosteronism, hypokalemia may be masked by a restricted sodium intake.

The intravenous pyelogram (IVP) and the radionuclide Hippuran renogram are the most widely used screening tests for renovascular hypertension. Characteristics in the pyelogram suggesting renal artery stenosis include a reduction in renal size of at least 1.5 cm compared with the opposite kidney, a delay in the appearance of contrast in the involved kidney when films are obtained at 1, 2, and 3 min after injection of the contrast agent, hyperconcentration of contrast on the involved side in the late films, and filling defects in the renal pelvis and ureter reflecting the local effects of dilated collateral arteries. In the Cooperative Study on Renovascular Hypertension, the characteristic triad of the late appearance of contrast medium in a small kidney, which showed late hyperconcentration of contrast in the renal pelvis, was never seen in patients with essential hypertension. Unfortunately, only 22 percent of patients with renovascular hypertension had this triad, and so it was relatively insensitive. The presence of any single abnormality was found in 78 percent of patients with renovascular hypertension, but with a sharp reduction in specificity since 11 percent of patients with essential hypertension had at least one of these manifestations, most commonly a significant difference in renal size. The characteristics of a radiohippuran renogram which suggest renal artery stenosis include a delay in the rate of rise of the tracer in the kidney, a delay in the time to reach the peak, and a reduced rate of disappearance from the kidney. The renogram identified 75 percent of patients with renovascular hypertension, with a false-positive rate of 24 percent. Because both the IVP and the renogram compare the two kidneys, they are less often positive when stenosis is bilateral.

Because of the high incidence of hypertension and the low yield of renovascular hypertension when a detailed evaluation is undertaken, the clinical indications for laboratory investigations in search of renovascular hypertension are gradually undergoing modification. No more than 1 to 2 percent of patients with hypertension have a curable renal arterial lesion. The evaluation is costly. Finally, operation, especially in patients with atherosclerosis, carries considerable risk. For these reasons a detailed evaluation for renal artery stenosis is currently recommended only when the yield is likely to be high, including patients in whom the onset of hypertension has occurred before the age of 30 years, in the presence of a bruit, or when hypertension is severe and responds poorly to medical therapy.

Identification of renal artery stenosis can be accomplished only by arteriography. Because all arterial lesions are not hemodynamically significant, ancillary tests are used to assess the hemodynamic significance of the stenosis. The most widely used test involves the measurement of renin activity in blood samples obtained from both renal veins and either the lower inferior vena cava or the aorta. A positive test, strongly suggestive of curable renovascular hypertension, reveals a plasma renin activity from the involved renal veins which exceeds the contralateral renal vein concentration by at least 50 percent, and evidence of suppression of renin-release from the intact contralateral kidney, i.e., identical renin activity in the arterial and contralateral renal venous plasma. With these criteria the false-positive rate is only 7 percent, but there is a quantitatively important false-negative rate. There is considerable interest in the potential utility of angiotensin antagonists in identifying curable, renin-mediated renovascular hypertension. Preliminary data obtained suggest that a 10-mmHg fall in diastolic pressure following the injection of saralasin (Sarenin) will identify 86 percent of curable patients, with a false-positive rate of 8.5 percent, which compares favorably with the available alternatives. At present we employ renal arteriography and renal vein renin determinations as the standard approach in patients in whom the history, physical examination, and preliminary laboratory evaluation make renovascular hypertension likely.

The Cooperative Study on Renovascular Disease has provided a clear picture of the current results of operation. When renal artery stenosis was due to fibromuscular disease, the cure rate exceeded 90 percent with a mortality of no more than 3 percent—probably reflecting the youth of the population which was largely free of additional systemic disease. In patients with atherosclerotic disease, on the other hand, the mortality was 9 percent and the failure rate exceeded 25 percent. For these reasons evaluation for renal artery surgery in older patients who are likely to have atherosclerotic disease is restricted in many centers to patients in whom medical management fails.

The converting enzyme inhibitor captopril (Capoten) is particularly effective in renovascular hypertension and is recommended for the patient with hypertension which is resistant to a standard regimen. Medical therapy, while it may control the hypertension, will not prevent the progress of the renal arterial lesion. Percutaneous transluminal angioplasty, in which a balloon-tipped catheter is employed to dilate the stenotic area during renal arteriography, has provided encouraging preliminary results but must be considered experimental as the duration of follow-up in the patients treated has been short.

ARTERIOLAR NEPHROSCLEROSIS Small-vessel changes in the kidney are so intimately associated with both long-standing hypertension and the normal aging process that it is difficult to define the boundary between normal and disease and to discuss the vascular lesion without discussing hypertension. At least some degree of small-vessel lesion is found in about 70 percent of normotensive individuals who die after the age of 60 years. The frequency and severity of the arteriolar and small-artery lesions are increased in younger age groups with predisposing factors, which include hypertension and diabetes. Large and medium-sized arteries at the interlobar and arcuate levels show intimal thickening of variable degree. Typically, more widespread and more severe abnormalities are seen in the small arteries and arterioles where, in addition, there is an eosinophilic hyalin thickening which results in a variable degree of vascular narrowing. As a consequence there is patchy ischemic atrophy. The severity of the ischemic atrophy and glomerular sclerosis, in general, parallels that of the vascular change.

The vascular changes presumably account for most of the loss of renal function which accompanies normal aging and which is accentuated in the patient with hypertension. The reductions in renal plasma flow and glomerular filtration rate account for the loss of an element of functional reserve, making older individuals more prone to develop azotemia when faced with volume depletion or surgical stress. The increased incidence of drug-induced complications in the elderly presumably reflects the important role played by glomerular filtration in the excretion of drugs and metabolites. Some examples are the propensity of the elderly to develop eighth nerve toxicity with streptomycin and to be particularly sensitive to digoxin. Other features of arteriolar nephrosclerosis include a moderate loss of concentrating power and often mild proteinuria. Occasionally more profound renal functional abnormalities occur, but marked renal insufficiency is uncommon.

On the other hand, "accelerated nephrosclerosis" associated with malignant hypertension is a dramatic complication of all forms of hypertension in which an abrupt change in course, renal insufficiency, and a uremic death were common before effective therapy became available (Chap. 267). The onset of the malignant phase is characterized by a sharp increase in blood pressure, with diastolic pressures typically exceeding 130 mmHg. In essential hypertension, the malignant phase is usually preceded by a benign period of variable duration, but occasionally occurs de novo. This process also occurs as a complication of all forms of secondary hypertension including glomerulonephritis, pyelonephritis, vasculitis, renal artery stenosis, scleroderma, polycystic kidney disease, Cushing's syndrome, pheochromocytoma, and hypertension associated with use of oral contraceptives. Until recently it was suggested that accelerated nephrosclerosis does not complicate the course of primary aldosteronism, but several well-documented cases now exist. In pheochromocytoma accelerated hypertension is typically associated with preserved renal function.

The morphological hallmarks of the renal lesion of malignant hypertension include petechial hemorrhages of the cortical surface, responsible for the characteristic "flea-bitten" appearance; fibrinoid necrosis of afferent arterioles; a hyperplastic endarteritis of the interlobular and arcuate arteries; and severe ischemic atrophy or infarction distal to the abnormal vessels. Immunofluorescent and electron-microscopic studies have shown that the amorphous material in the arteriolar wall consists of fibrin. Several lines of investigation suggest that the severe hypertension, per se, is responsible for the vascular necrosis, probably due to endothelial injury and leakage of fibrin and other plasma constituents into the arteriolar wall.

The clinical features include severe hypertension, neuroretinopathy with blurring of vision, retinal hemorrhages, exudates, and papilledema. Hypertensive encephalopathy is evidenced by severe headache, changes in the sensorium, and seizures. Congestive heart failure and rapidly progressive uremia are common. The renal manifestations include gross or microscopic hematuria, marked proteinuria, and a rapid rise in BUN and creatinine. As in renal artery stenosis, evidence of secondary aldosteronism is common with hypokalemia and a metabolic alkalosis, until the metabolic acidosis of renal failure supervenes.

Prior to the availability of effective therapy for the hypertension, the mortality in patients with this syndrome approximated 50 percent in 3 months and 90 percent within 1 year. In the past two decades, the availability of effective antihypertensive therapy (Chap. 267) has greatly improved the prognosis of accelerated nephrosclerosis. In the early 1950s a BUN which exceeded 30 mg/dl at the time the diagnosis was made guaranteed a rapid demise. Today a patient with a BUN which exceeds this level by three- or fourfold may have a stable course with effective therapy.

SCLERODERMA (PROGRESSIVE SYSTEMIC SCLEROSIS) (See also Chap. 352) The renal aspects of scleroderma are considered in some detail here because renal involvement is second only to that of heart and lungs as a cause of death, and the characteristic morphological lesions and clinical course closely resemble those associated with accelerated nephrosclerosis.

As in accelerated nephrosclerosis, the morphological features include kidneys which are generally normal or only slightly reduced in size even in patients who have died with renal failure. Petechial hemorrhages and wedge-shaped cortical infarcts are common. The most striking and distinctive abnormality is seen at the level of the intralobular arteries which are markedly narrowed or occluded as a result of fibrinoid change and deposition of fibrin and acid mucopolysaccarides. The afferent arterioles in some patients also show fibrinoid necrosis and occasional occlusion by fibrin thrombi. Distal to the occlusion ischemic atrophy and infarction are evident. It has been suggested, in part because of the similarity to the changes in accelerated nephrosclerosis, that the renal vascular lesions are secondary to the hypertension, but such vascular changes have been well documented at necropsy in patients with scleroderma who have never been hypertensive.

Renal involvement is rarely the presenting feature. In one study renal involvement was found at presentation in only 3 percent of patients with scleroderma. However, in a 20-year longitudinal survey, 47 percent of patients ultimately developed a clinically important renal lesion. There is uniform agreement that renal failure contributes to or is primarily responsible for 40 to 50 percent of all deaths. Renal involvement is associated with a poor prognosis in patients with this condition; most patients with clinically evident renal disease die in less than 1 year and often within 3 months. Indeed, in the aforementioned longitudinal study only 10 percent of patients without renal involvement died, whereas 60 percent of patients with proteinuria, azotemia, or hypertension succumbed.

Renal involvement in scleroderma is usually characterized clinically by an abrupt onset and an explosive course; accelerated hypertension is followed by oliguria and a uremic death within months. Clinical evidence of major renal involvement is typically noted 3 to 5 years after the onset of manifestations in the skin and other systems. Occasionally, however, renal disease antedates obvious skin involvement.

A second, less distinct clinical expression of renal involvement is also being recognized. Isolated proteinuria unaccompanied by either hypertension or azotemia adversely affects prognosis but less strikingly than does the syndrome of malignant hypertension. Mild hypertension, without proteinuria or azotemia, occurs with greater frequency in scleroderma than would be anticipated from known prevalence of essential hypertension. Mild hypertension without proteinuria or azotemia occurs later than the malignant form and has a much less grave prognosis.

No specific therapy exists for scleroderma. In the past 3 years a series of reports have indicated that very aggressive antihypertensive therapy makes renal failure avoidable. Presumably because the hypertension is renin-mediated, the converting enzyme inhibitor, captopril, has been especially effective. Renal transplantation has been successful in a limited number of patients with scleroderma.

SICKLE CELL NEPHROPATHY (See also Chaps. 295 and 330) Sickle cell disease, sickle cell trait, sickle thalassemia, and other combinations of hemoglobin S with abnormal hemoglobins often have clinically important disorders of renal structure and function. The most dramatic of the renal manifestations is gross painless hematuria. A history of mild trauma to the renal area may be obtained. The bleeding arises from miliary gross and microscopic infarcts in the papillae, renal pelvis, and renal cortex. For unknown reasons the bleeding occurs from the left side in 80 percent of cases and, despite the systemic nature of the primary process, is bilateral in only 11 percent. Abnormalities in the IVP, most commonly a pelvic filling defect, are frequent and have led to unnecessary surgical intervention. Most cases remit spontaneously. Because causes other than sickle cell anemia may be responsible for hematuria in these patients, a complete urologic assessment is generally performed (Chap. 40). When filling defects are found, serial studies are recommended; surgical exploration should be considered only if they persist. Operation may also be required in rare instances of life-threatening hemorrhage.

Failure of urinary concentration is the most consistent feature of sickle cell nephropathy. In very young children with sickle cell anemia the concentrating defect can be reversed by multiple transfusions, but the capacity for improvement is lost with age, becoming negligible in patients after 15 years of age. In older adults the maximum concentration of the urine rarely exceeds 400 mosmol per liter. The failure of urinary concentration is typically attributed to a disorder of perfusion of the renal medulla. This, in turn, may be due to the sickling process per se or to an abnormality of the microvasculature. Because both hypoxia and an increased osmolality precipitate the sickling phenomenon and because sickle cells increase blood viscosity significantly, this condition may impede the normal circulation through the vasa recta which normally have a very high resistance to flow. In addition, microangiographic studies have revealed obliteration and distortion of the remaining vasa recta.

Appreciable proteinuria is common in sickle cell disease and occurred in 31 percent of patients in one series. On occasion proteinuria is sufficiently severe that the nephrotic syndrome develops. Distal renal tubular acidosis has also been reported as an uncommon complication.

With increasing age, the growing number and size of cortical infarcts result in a progressive reduction in glomerular filtration rate and renal plasma flow, which are typically higher than normal in the young patients with sickle cell disease. Deterioration of renal function caused by sickle cell anemia to the point at which dialysis becomes necessary has not been described. However, it has been shown that patients with sickle cell disease can be maintained on chronic hemodialysis without encountering undue complications.

HEMOLYTIC-UREMIC SYNDROME (See also Chap. 329) The coincidence of acute renal failure, hemolytic anemia, and thrombocytopenia has emerged as a clearly defined, relatively common entity in which infants or children develop acute anemia, signs of renal and central nervous system injury, and gastrointestinal bleeding after a prodrome of digestive, respiratory, and systemic symptoms. The hallmarks of the syndrome are hemolysis due to red blood cell fragmentation, a reduction in platelet count, and biochemical and pathological evidence of intravascular coagulation. The differential diagnosis includes thrombotic thrombocytopenic purpura, renal cortical necrosis as part of the Shwartzman reaction in gram-negative sepsis, severe vasculitis, and "necrotizing glomerulonephritis." Differentiation among these entities may be extremely difficult, even at necropsy.

Initially only severe, generally fatal cases were recognized, but with increasing familiarity patients with mild or moderate lesions have been identified. The immediate prognosis is related to the degree of renal failure and the severity of involvement of the central nervous system. If the patient survives, the hematologic abnormality is short-lived and does not recur. In some patients the extent of renal destruction precludes prolonged survival without dialysis. In a few others severe neurological sequelae have been permanently disabling. In many patients the renal lesions heal completely, but on occasion slowly progressive renal failure occurs after the initial insult.

Although primarily a disease of children, there has been increasing recognition of this syndrome in adults. In adults the prodrome, which resembles a nondescript viral illness, is less striking, but associations have been found with pregnancy and the postpartum period, use of oral contraceptive agents, and infection, including typhoid fever, gram-negative bacteremia, mumps, and infectious mononucleosis. The clinical manifestations are similar to those in children, and the prognosis appears to be poorer.

Because chemical evidence of coagulation disturbances and fibrin deposition in small arteries and arterioles is common and because the syndrome is accompanied by a microangiopathic hemolytic anemia, there is widespread belief that disseminated intravascular coagulation plays a major role. The commonly observed coagulation disturbances include thrombocytopenia, a prolonged prothrombin time, and accumulation of fibrin degradation products in the serum. For unknown reasons the kidney is the most extensively involved organ in the hemolytic-uremic syndrome. Because in adults pregnancy and oral contraceptive agents appear to predispose to cortical necrosis and pregnancy also predisposes to the Shwartzman reaction induced by endotoxin in animals, it has been suggested that the Shwartzman reaction and the hemolytic-uremic syndrome share a common mechanism. The morphological lesions are also strikingly similar; immunofluorescent studies have revealed intense staining with antibody to fibrin in both conditions.

The treatment is largely supportive. There is major controversy as to whether heparin therapy modifies the natural history. Controlled studies have been disappointing, but in individual patients heparin therapy has been temporally associated with improvement in renal function. Other forms of therapy including steroids, immunosuppressive agents, antimetabolites, exchange transfusions, and dextran have met with equivocal results.

RENAL VEIN THROMBOSIS Thrombosis of one or both of the renal veins is an uncommon cause of the nephrotic syndrome. Occlusion of both renal veins usually, but not necessarily, implies thrombosis of the inferior vena cava as well. Renal vein thrombosis is most commonly associated with membranous glomerulonephritis. It is not clear whether the glomerulonephritis predisposes to renal vein thrombosis or vice versa, but the weight of evidence favors the former (Chap. 294). Other causes of renal vein thrombosis include local trauma, invasion of the renal vein by hypernephroma, and severe dehydration, especially in children.

Clinical features and morphological change depend on the availability of an adequate collateral venous drainage. Sudden complete thrombosis of a renal vein, without adequate collateral drainage, causes severe lumbar pain, hematuria, and loss of function of the involved kidney. The kidney is enlarged and suffers hemorrhagic infarction. When the process is bilateral or involves a solitary kidney, this sequence leads to oliguria and renal failure. If the occlusion is more gradual, especially if adequate collateral venous channels develop, renal function is preserved, and massive proteinuria results in the nephrotic syndrome. Hypertension is uncommon, and the urinary sediment may be entirely normal or contain only a few red blood cells.

The diagnosis is suggested by a history of trauma, pain, or a predisposing factor such as prolonged travel in a cramped position. A history of pulmonary embolism should also lead to suspicion of this diagnosis. Physical examination may reveal a venous collateral map on the anterior abdominal wall if the inferior vena cava is involved. The intravenous pyelogram may show filling defects in the renal pelvis and ureter reflecting collateral draining veins. The diagnosis is established by inferior vena caval and selective renal venography. Diagnostic ultrasound is playing an increasing role in diagnosis.

Surgical removal of a clot from the renal venous system has been successful in a small number of patients, especially in children in whom the onset is often in association with dehydration and occurs acutely. In most circumstances, however, medical management with anticoagulants has been used. Recanalization of the renal veins has led to amelioration of the nephrotic syndrome in occasional patients. Typically, however, anticoagulants are employed to prevent pulmonary embolism and extension of the thrombus into the open collateral veins.

PREECLAMPSIA AND ECLAMPSIA: TOXEMIAS OF PREGNANCY Toxemia of pregnancy is characterized by the appearance, during gestation or within 7 days of delivery, of a constellation of abnormalities which includes hypertension, edema, and proteinuria (preeclampsia). When hypertension is more severe, convulsions and coma may occur (eclampsia). Preeclampsia usually begins after the thirty-second week of pregnancy but may begin earlier, particularly in women with preexisting renal disease or hypertension. Preeclampsia in the first trimester occurs in hydatidiform mole. Toxemia has a bimodal frequency with peak incidence in the young primipara and in multiparous women over 35 years of age. In the United States toxemia occurs in approximately 7 percent of pregnancies. Perhaps as a reflection of an increased prevalence in the economically underprivileged, the incidence reaches 30 percent in Puerto Rico. Most series include many patients in whom preexisting renal disease or hypertension either begins during or is exacerbated by pregnancy, but there is clearly, in addition, a specific process affecting the kidney and the vascular system which in most patients improves dramatically when, or soon after, pregnancy is terminated.

The morphological features in the kidney include reversible generalized swelling of the glomerular tufts and apparent thickening of the glomerular basement membrane due to an increase of the cytoplasm of the endothelial cells with narrowing of the capillary lumina, a finding termed *glomerular endotheliosis,* and sub- or interendothelial fibrinoid deposition. In patients who die of acute toxemia of pregnancy, necrosis of renal tubules and of liver cells is frequent, along with evidence of disseminated intravascular coagulation and petechial hemorrhage in the brain.

The pathogenesis is not clearly understood. Sodium retention and an increase in blood volume are normal concomitants of pregnancy. Considerable evidence suggests that plasma volume is *lower* in the toxemic than in the normal pregnancy, and from this observation debate about the role of too little or too much sodium intake has emerged. Whether the reduced plasma volume is a cause or consequence of the process is unclear. The evidence suggests that uteroplacental ischemia occurs with toxemia. The uterus, like the kidney, synthesizes both vasoconstrictors (renin) and vasodilators (prostaglandins of the E series). One current hypothesis is that the release of small amounts of renin from the uterus in a setting of increased sensitivity to angiotensin is responsible for the severe hypertension.

The onset is typically insidious but may be abrupt. Because arterial blood pressure normally falls during pregnancy, pressures which exceed 125/75 mmHg should be considered abnormal, especially if they are rising. In association, headache, visual disturbances, epigastric distress, and apprehension are frequent. Edema usually appears coincident with hypertension; it is typically generalized, being particularly evident in the face and hands. Proteinuria generally follows the onset of the syndrome within several days but occasionally precedes the hypertension and edema. Examination of the optic fundi reveals segmental arteriolar narrowing and a glistening retinal sheen indicative of edema. Hemorrhages and exudates occur late and only in severe cases.

Examination of the urine reveals from a trace to 10 g protein per 24 h, as well as granular and hyalin casts, but red blood cells and cellular casts are infrequent. Because of the physiological increase of glomerular filtration rate and reduction in serum urea and creatinine concentration which occurs in a normal pregnancy, a blood urea nitrogen of 20 mg/dl is usually indicative of a sharp diminution in filtration rate. A more striking increase in blood uric acid is common, reflecting a reduction in urate clearance.

Treatment varies with the severity of the process. In patients with mild hypertension and minimal proteinuria, antihypertensive agents are routinely used: whether restriction of sodium intake, which is required to control edema, may be a precipitating factor in preeclampsia is the subject of debate. If the process is more severe, patients are admitted to the hospital for bed rest and closer control of sodium intake and blood pressure. Involvement of the central nervous system with convulsions and marked hypertension are unequivocal indications for termination of pregnancy, which is usually followed by prompt improvement of the mother. Emptying of the uterus is the most effective treatment. Proteinuria and hypertension usually disappear within 1 or 2 weeks but on occasion may persist for as long as 6 months. A substantial fraction of patients with preeclampsia are left with a process which is indistinguishable from essential hypertension. Whether such patients were candidates for development of essential hypertension which became apparent during, or was precipitated by, pregnancy is not yet clear.

POLYARTERITIS NODOSA (See also Chaps. 69 and 295) The genre *necrotizing vasculitis* includes polyarteritis nodosa, hypersensitivity angiitis (also known as the microscopic form of polyarteritis), and allergic granulomatous angiitis. Because renal involvement occurs in at least 80 percent of patients with polyarteritis nodosa and contributes to death in a substantial number, they are considered here. Other vasculitides such as rheumatic arteritis and temporal arteritis rarely involve the kidney. Various attempts at classification reflect a sorting of clinical syndromes, primarily by site and size of vessel involved, major presenting symptoms, and clinical course. They are not based on an understanding of the etiology or pathogenesis, and no classification is totally satisfactory. Moreover, attempts at classification have been made primarily by information based on necropsy, and distinctions among polyarteritis nodosa, hypersensitivity angiitis, and granulomatous angiitis are indistinct in many patients because of overlap of these syndromes.

Polyarteritis nodosa is a recurrent or progressive, necrotizing inflammatory disease of the medium and small-sized muscular arteries. The kidney is the most common organ involved, with estimates ranging upward of 70 percent, and renal failure is one of the major causes of death. Hypertension occurs in about 50 percent of patients and is usually a late manifestation, probably reflecting renal ischemia which develops during the healing phase. The hypertension often terminates in a malignant phase with hypertensive encephalopathy or heart failure. Renal involvement may be manifested by proteinuria, microscopic or gross hematuria, urinary casts, azotemia, and edema.

In polyarteritis nodosa, the lesions involve only the medium and small muscular arteries, especially at sites of branching. There is disagreement concerning the involvement of capillaries and veins. Classically there are subendothelial and medial edema and fibrinoid necrosis; infiltration of all vessel coats with an inflammatory exudate including polymorphonuclear leukocytes, eosinophils, lymphocytes, and plasma cells; destruction of the media and internal elastica; proliferation of fibroblasts, which generally starts in the adventitia and progresses during a stage of granulation through the vessel wall with healing, and a reduction in the acute inflammatory process; and healed lesions in which the vessel wall is replaced by fibrous tissue and the lumen is generally narrowed or occluded. Glomerular lesions consisting of focal or diffuse proliferative changes or ischemic necrosis are common. Any or all of these stages may be present at any time in the kidney. Renal insufficiency and hypertension characteristically develop during the healing stages. Because larger vessels are involved, a renal biopsy of the cortex may miss the characteristic lesion.

The pathogenetic factors responsible for polyarteritis are becoming clearer. Multiple lines of evidence have implicated an immunologic mechanism, and since 1970 a number of studies have implicated hepatitis B as the responsible antigen in as many as 30 percent of patients with necrotizing vasculitis and the polyarteritis nodosa syndrome. A vasculitis indistinguishable from polyarteritis nodosa is also being recognized in an increasing number of young drug abusers. Because of the multiplicity of the chemical agents injected, and the high probability of contamination, the exact etiologic agent has not been unequivocally defined, but methamphetamine appears to be a common denominator.

Hypersensitivity angiitis differs from classic polyarteritis nodosa. It is often a fulminating illness characterized by an acute necrotizing inflammatory process involving small arteries, arterioles, capillaries, and venules; the involvement in all vessels appears to be at the same stage. Proteinuria and hematuria are present in virtually every patient, but hypertension is generally absent.

Allergic granulomatous angiitis is also a diffuse systemic vascular disease, but, in addition, there are widespread extravascular granulomatous, necrotizing lesions. Azotemia occurs in some cases but with less frequency than in hypersensitivity angiitis or classic polyarteritis. In addition there may be focal glomerular lesions and fibrosis.

Therapy of the vasculitides is discussed in Chap. 69. General supportive measures include control of hypertension, which is required in most patients with renal involvement. Corticosteroids are widely employed and with immunosuppressive agents are the only presently available therapy of any potential value. In patients with renal involvement, steroids may have an initial adverse effect on the clinical course because vascular healing is frequently associated with obliteration of arteries, resulting in focal renal infarction, increasing hypertension, and azotemia. A recent report suggests that the addition of cyclophosphamide may be useful in the patient in whom steroids are ineffective, especially when there is renal involvement.

REFERENCES

ALFREY AC: The renal response to vascular injury, in *The Kidney*, 2d ed, BM Brenner, FC Rector Jr (eds). Philadelphia, Saunders, 1981, chap 30

ALLEYNE GAQ et al: The kidney in sickle cell anemia. Kidney Int 7:371, 1975

FAUCI AS et al: Cyclophosphamide therapy of severe systemic necrotizing vasculitis. N Engl J Med 301:235, 1979

FERRIS TF: Toxemia and hypertension, in *Medical Complications during Pregnancy*, GN Burrow, TF Ferris (eds). Philadelphia, Saunders, 1975

GIANANTONIO CA et al: The hemolytic-uremic syndrome. Nephron 11:174, 1973

LLACH F et al: The clinical spectrum of renal vein thrombosis: Acute and chronic. Am J Med 69:819, 1980

LOPEZ-OVEJERO JA et al: Reversal of vascular and renal crises of scleroderma by oral angiotensin-converting-enzyme blockade. N Engl J Med 300:1417, 1979

MAXWELL MH: Cooperative study of renovascular hypertension: Current status. Kidney Int 8:S153, 1975

OLIVER JA, CANNON PJ: The kidney in scleroderma. Nephron 18:141, 1977

SERGENT JS et al: Vasculitis with hepatitis B antigenemia: Long-term observations in nine patients. Medicine 55:1, 1976

299
HEREDITARY TUBULAR DISORDERS

SATISH KATHPALIA
FREDRIC L. COE

POLYCYSTIC RENAL DISEASE IN ADULTS

ETIOLOGY AND PATHOLOGY This disease is found in 1 in 500 autopsies and 1 in 3000 hospital admissions and accounts for approximately 5 percent of all instances of end-stage renal failure. Inheritance is autosomal dominant, and penetrance is nearly 100 percent in carriers who survive until the eighth decade. The cortex and medulla of both kidneys are usually filled with thin-walled, spherical cysts, ranging from millimeters to several centimeters in diameter, that enlarge the organs and interfere with their functioning, presumably by compressing the nephrons and causing localized intrarenal obstruction. The cysts, which are lined by a low cuboidal epithelium, contain straw-colored fluid that becomes hemorrhagic with trauma or infection. The intervening renal parenchyma may be normal or show changes of nephrosclerosis or interstitial nephritis.

CLINICAL FEATURES Symptoms usually begin in the third or fourth decades. Flank pain is the most frequent symptom. Other common symptoms include gross and microscopic hematuria, especially after trauma, and nocturia due to impaired osmotic concentrating ability. Ten percent of patients pass renal calculi whose composition and pathogenesis have not been well studied. Stones and blood clots both cause renal colic. Usually the kidneys are palpable and asymmetrical and have a knobby surface. Hypertension develops in 75 percent of patients, and progression to chronic renal failure usually occurs.

Proteinuria is the most common laboratory abnormality, but it rarely exceeds 2 g per day. Urinary infection ultimately occurs in most patients, especially as a consequence of instrumentation and renal calculi, while erythrocytosis may occur because of high circulating erythropoietin levels; in other patients anemia may result from the hematuria.

Acute renal failure can result from infection, ureteral obstruction due to clots or stone, or sudden angulation of a ureter by a nearby cyst. Azotemia progresses slowly in the absence of these complications. Patients with end-stage chronic renal failure tend to have higher hematocrits than their counterparts with other renal diseases. Fluid overload is infrequent because of a tendency for renal salt wasting.

Hepatic cysts are present in about 30 percent of patients with polycystic kidneys. Hepatic function is usually normal, and the liver cysts usually are asymptomatic but can cause epigastric discomfort or biliary colic, or can become infected. Cysts also may occur in the spleen, pancreas, lungs, ovaries, testes, epididymis, thyroid, uterus, broad ligament, and bladder. Subarachnoid hemorrhage from an intracranial aneurysm is the cause of death in about 9 percent of patients.

DIAGNOSIS Palpable kidneys, hypertension, or asymptomatic urinary abnormalities are often the only manifestations. Excretory or retrograde urography typically shows large kidneys with elongated pelvises and flat calyces that are indented by cysts. Ultrasonography and radioisotopic renal scanning can both demonstrate the cysts quite well. Gray scale sonography may be an alternative to intravenous pyelography for screening individuals with an affected parent, especially when genetic counseling is desired. Computerized tomography may be complementary.

TREATMENT Superimposed renal damage such as that produced by analgesics, obstruction, urinary infection, nephrotoxic antibiotics, and hypertension must be guarded against. Dehydration and inadequate intake of sodium chloride (less than 100 m*M* per day) should be avoided. The management of chronic renal failure is simplified because fluid overload is not a usual problem and the hypertension is usually amenable to treatment, but the cysts can cause special problems, such as pain, bleeding, infection, or ureteral obstruction. Puncture of cysts, and in some instances even nephrectomy, may be necessary for treatment.

POLYCYSTIC RENAL DISEASE IN INFANTS AND CHILDREN The *infantile form* manifests itself at birth by diffusely enlarged kidneys, renal failure, and maldevelopment of intrahepatic bile ducts. The *childhood form* consists of medullary ductal ectasia which is usually asymptomatic, in association with congenital hepatic fibrosis and portal hypertension. Inheritance of both the infantile and childhood forms is autosomal recessive. Renal failure develops frequently in both forms, but death usually results as a consequence of hepatic disease in the childhood form.

Morphology In the infantile form, the distal tubules and collecting ducts are dilated into elongated cysts that are arranged in a radial fashion, particularly in the cortex, and make the kidneys very large and spongy. In the childhood form, cysts are fewer in number, cortical collecting ducts are less involved, and the kidneys are not as large. Small intrahepatic bile ducts are irregularly dilated, and large interconnecting spaces, lined by hyperplastic epithelium, fill the portal areas. There is portal fibrosis rather than dilatation and proliferation of small bile ducts, and portal hypertension is the rule by late childhood.

DIAGNOSIS AND TREATMENT Infantile polycystic kidneys may be large enough to cause dystocia. At birth they do not function, and oliguric renal failure, respiratory distress, hypertension, and congestive heart failure appear. Intravenous pyelography may reveal a mottled nephrogram with variable retention of contrast material in cysts that correspond to dilated cortical and medullary collecting ducts. On retrograde urography the calyces are blunted, and abnormal pyelotubular reflux may be seen. In the childhood type the intravenous pyelogram may suggest medullary sponge kidney, because medullary tubular ectasia is prominent. Renal failure is an inconstant feature, though chronic infection is common.

MEDULLARY SPONGE KIDNEY

PATHOLOGY In this condition the ducts of Bellini, i.e., the terminal collecting ducts that reach to the ends of the papillae and drain the final urine into the renal pelvis, are dilated to cystic proportions and frequently contain small calcium oxalate calculi. The kidneys are involved asymmetrically, and the more abnormal kidney is usually the larger of the two. One or more medullary cysts are found near the tip of each involved papilla, and calculi form in the terminal collecting ducts in, or proximal to, the cysts (Fig. 299-1). Parenchymal alterations are secondary to intrarenal obstruction. The cysts are lined by cuboidal and, sometimes, by pseudostratified and stratified squamous epithelium.

CLINICAL DIAGNOSIS AND TREATMENT Medullary sponge kidney has been found in 1 of 200 unselected intravenous pyelograms. Although most cases are sporadic, familial instances with autosomal dominant inheritance have been described. The disease has a bimodal pattern of appearance, the first in adolescence and the second during the third and fourth decades. Calculi, infection, and hematuria occur in 60, 35, and 30 percent of patients, respectively. Papillary nephrocalcinosis due to clusters of stones in cysts is a common feature. Hypercalciuria occurs in nearly half of stone-forming patients but is equally frequent in other forms of calcium stone disease (Chap. 300). Hypertension is no more common than in the general population. Renal failure is rare, unless nephrolithiasis and/or renal infections are unusually severe.

The diagnosis of medullary sponge kidney is made by intravenous urography. The magnitude of pyelotubular backflow may vary from a simple papillary blush to frank tubular ectasia at the tips of the papillae. Small pyramidal cysts and nephrocalcinosis are frequent, and papillary concretions are obscured by the urographic contrast medium. Ectatic collecting ducts are usually difficult to fill during retrograde pyelography, and so the contrast material remains separate from papillary concretions in the cysts.

Asymptomatic patients require no treatment except advice to avoid dehydration and thereby reduce the risk of stone formation. The metabolic etiology of stones should be sought and treated conventionally, while infection and urological consequences of stones should be treated as described in Chap. 300. Medullary sponge kidneys are abnormally vulnerable to infection, and urological instrumentation should, therefore, be minimized.

MEDULLARY CYSTIC DISEASE (NEPHRONOPHTHISIS COMPLEX)

ETIOLOGY This is a mixture of hereditary medullary cystic diseases that have similar morphology but differing patterns of inheritance. The recessive form is associated with renal failure before 20 years of age (early-onset type), whereas the dominant form causes renal failure only after the second decade (adult-onset type). Both sexes are affected. When renal disease is associated with retinal degenerative changes (renal retinal dysplasia), inheritance is always recessive, but renal failure occurs during adult life.

PATHOLOGY In either form, most of the cysts are in the medulla and the corticomedullary region and have been localized by microdissection to collecting ducts and distal convoluted tubules. Cysts have a low, frequently atrophic, epithelium and range from microscopic dimensions to several millimeters in size. The kidneys usually are asymmetrically scarred and shrunken. Both tubular atrophy and periglomerular fibrosis are present, but the former is more severe than the latter. In advanced cases, glomeruli become sclerotic and hyalinized, cortical fibrosis and cellular interstitial infiltration appear, and the histology becomes difficult to differentiate from that of chronic interstitial nephritis.

DIAGNOSIS AND TREATMENT Concentrating ability, acid excretion, and sodium conservation are defective as might be expected from a lesion that damages late segments of the nephron. The disease is marked by polyuria, progressive renal failure, stunted growth, severe anemia, hyperchloremic metabolic acidosis, and poor sodium conservation. In adults, the inability to conserve sodium may cause a salt-wasting syndrome that resembles Addison's disease but that is unresponsive to mineralocorticoids. Hypertension usually is a terminal event. The urinalysis is normal at first, but mild proteinuria may develop. On intravenous pyelography, the kidneys are small, scarred, and without calcification. The calyces are distorted by numerous cysts in the corticomedullary area.

In the presence of acidosis, high sodium and water intake and alkali replacement are needed. Treatment of infections, anemia, hypertension, and other aspects of end-stage renal failure are as discussed in Chap. 291. Genetic counseling may be helpful in family planning and in selection of a related donor for renal transplantation.

FUNCTIONAL TUBULAR DISORDERS

BARTTER'S SYNDROME In 1962, Bartter described a syndrome consisting of hypokalemia due to renal potassium wasting, elevated plasma renin activity and aldosterone secretion, normotension, hyporesponsiveness of blood pressure to infused angiotensin II, and hyperplasia of the granular cells of the juxtaglomerular apparatus. Weakness, or periodic paralysis, and polyuria occur because of chronic potassium depletion. Hyperplasia of renal medullary interstitial cells, which produce prostaglandins (PG) E and F, has been described in some patients, along with very elevated PGE_2 production. Inheritance is autosomal recessive, and manifestations commonly begin in childhood.

Pathogenesis While the pathogenetic sequence has not been proved with certainty, there is some evidence for a defect of tubular chloride or potassium transport. Either may produce hypokalemia, which stimulates release of prostaglandins E_2 and I_2, which in turn results in increased secretion of renin, leading to enhanced concentration of circulating angiotensin II and thus aldosterone. Both angiotensin II and aldosterone increase renal kallikrein, which increases plasma bradykinin, while aldosterone enhances potassium loss further. The normalcy of blood pressure results from the vasodepressor actions of PGE_2 and bradykinin, despite increased production of renin, angiotensin, and aldosterone.

Excessive production of PGE_2 resulting from hypokalemia, a known stimulator of PGE_2 synthesis, may therefore be a secondary consequence of the syndrome. In some cases blockade of PGE_2 production with indomethacin lowered renin levels and restored vascular response to angiotensin II infusion, but did not reduce potassium wasting. This observation supports the notion that overproduction of PGE_2 may be a secondary phenomenon.

Treatment The dietary intake of sodium chloride and potassium should be liberal; often potassium supplements are required despite a high dietary intake. Pharmacological blockade of aldosterone effects on distal tubules with spironolactone can prevent potassium wasting, though sodium intake must be increased. Inhibition of prostaglandin synthesis with indomethacin, ibuprofen, or aspirin has met with varying success, as indicated above. Beta-adrenergic blockade has also been used, with some success, to lower renin production.

LIDDLE'S SYNDROME (PSEUDOHYPERALDOSTERONISM) This rare inherited disorder is characterized by hypertension, hypokalemic alkalosis, and negligible aldosterone secretion. It appears to be due to an unusual tendency of distal tubules or collecting ducts to conserve sodium and excrete potassium despite the virtual absence of aldosterone. No other biochemical abnormalities have been described. However, transport rates

FIGURE 299-1

A. Radiographic appearance of medullary sponge kidney. Abdominal flat plate reveals multiple bilateral calcifications. B. Radiographic contrast material accumulates in the dilated and cystic terminal collecting ducts and obscures the calcifications.

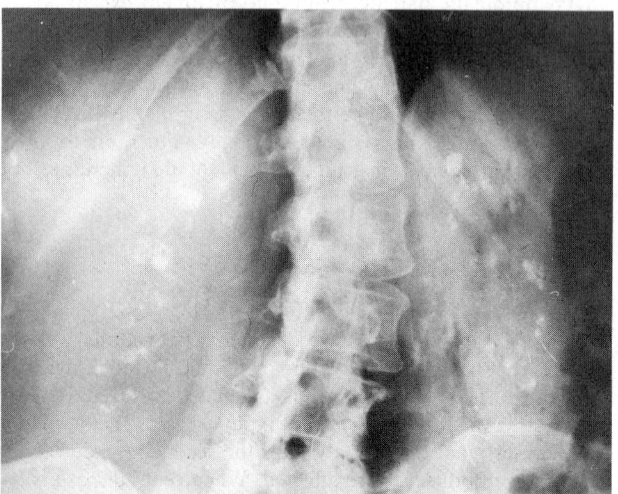

A

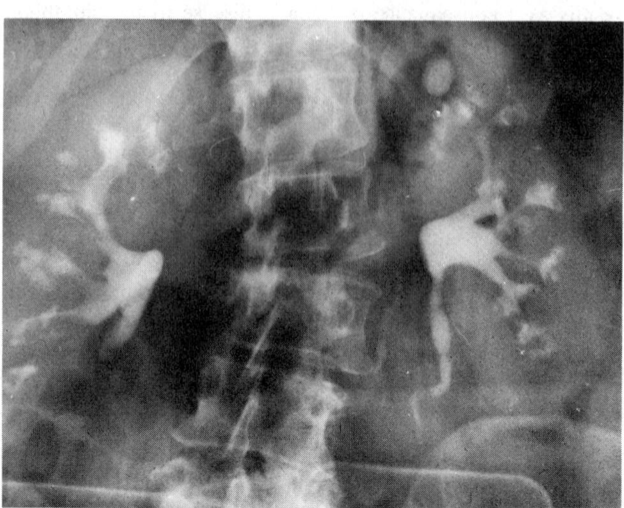

B

of sodium in red blood cells are altered. These patients respond to 100 mg per day of triamterene (Chap. 253), a diuretic agent that blocks sodium and potassium exchange in the distal tubule.

FAMILIAL NEPHROGENIC DIABETES (DI)

In this disease the distal tubules and collecting ducts are unresponsive to vasopressin because of a sex-linked recessive disease, with variable penetrance in heterozygous females. Affected individuals excrete large volumes of very hypotonic urine even when plasma osmolality and vasopressin concentration are both high. Polyuria, polydipsia, and hypertonic dehydration following restriction of fluid intake all result from renal tubular insensitivity to antidiuretic hormone (ADH). Unresponsiveness to vasopressin may be due to reduced production of cyclic adenosine 5′-monophosphate (cyclic AMP) in the epithelium of the collecting ducts, to the inability of cyclic AMP to increase the permeability of collecting duct luminal cell membranes to water, or to a combination of the two. Other hereditary tubular defects such as juvenile nephronophthisis, medullary cystic and polycystic diseases, as well as cystinosis and congenital or acquired chronic urinary tract obstruction can cause vasopressin-resistant (nephrogenic) DI, but in these syndromes the characteristic findings of the underlying disorder are obvious.

Affected infants easily become dehydrated, hypernatremic, and hyperthermic, and damage of the central nervous system and resultant mental retardation may result. In the absence of dehydration, overall renal function is normal. On intravenous pyelography the renal pelvis, ureters, and bladder are dilated, as in any form of DI, because of massive diuresis.

Oral hydration usually is adequate treatment except during early infancy, when hypotonic parenteral fluids may be required. Vasopressin and its synthetic analogues are ineffective, but diuretic agents such as chlorothiazide reduce polyuria. This drug inhibits NaCl reabsorption in the cortical portions of the thick ascending limb of the loop of Henle, thereby reducing production of free water. In addition, chlorothiazide produces a diuresis that causes contraction of extracellular fluid volume which, in turn, stimulates reabsorption of NaCl and water in the proximal tubule and limits their delivery to the thick ascending limb. Sodium restriction enhances its effect.

RENAL TUBULAR ACIDOSIS (RTA)

In this group of disorders renal excretion of acid is reduced out of proportion to any reduction of glomerular filtration rate that may be present. Metabolic acidosis results, but in contrast to renal failure the anions that accompany surplus hydrogen ions in the blood, such as sulfate and phosphate, are excreted normally and are unavailable to balance any fall in serum bicarbonate that occurs. Therefore, the kidneys reabsorb chloride in unusually large amounts, and serum chloride rises to preserve electroneutrality in the extracellular fluid. The result is *hyperchloremic acidosis,* and the unmeasured anion gap is normal. There is general agreement that four types of RTA exist. Types 1 and 2 are often hereditary. Type 3 is a rare mixture of types 1 and 2. Type 4 is acquired and is associated with either hyporeninemic hypoaldosteronism or tubular hyporesponsiveness to circulating mineralocorticoid hormones.

TYPE 1 (DISTAL) RTA Sporadic cases occur, but autosomal dominant inheritance is usually present. The kidney does not lower urine pH normally, either because the collecting ducts permit excessive back-diffusion of hydrogen ions from lumen to blood or fail to transport hydrogen ions against a steep pH gradient. Since titration of urine buffers and diffusion trapping of NH_4^+ in the tubules both depend upon a low intraluminal pH, excretion of acid is deficient. Urinary osmotic concentration and potassium conservation also tend to be impaired.

Chronic acidosis lowers tubule reabsorption of calcium, causing renal hypercalciuria and mild secondary hyperparathyroidism. The hypercalciuria, alkaline urine, and low levels of urine citrate—which normally complexes about 40 percent of urine calcium and is deficient during systemic acidosis—cause calcium phosphate stones and papillary nephrocalcinosis. Growth is stunted in children because of rickets; this growth defect responds dramatically to amelioration of the acidosis with sodium bicarbonate or other alkali. In the adult bone disease takes the form of osteomalacia. In both children and adults, bone disease may result, at least in part, from acidosis-induced loss of bone mineral as well as from inadequate production of 1,25-dihydroxyvitamin D_3 [1,25-$(OH)_2D_3$]. Since the kidney does not conserve potassium or concentrate the urine normally, polyuria and hypokalemia occur. Given the stress of an intercurrent illness, acidosis and hypokalemia can become life-threatening.

The diagnosis is suggested by osteomalacia or rickets, hyperchloremic acidosis associated with alkaline urine, and calcium phosphate stones or nephrocalcinosis. To prove that the urine pH cannot be lowered normally, the oral ammonium chloride (NH_4Cl) loading test should be carried out: 0.1 g (1.9 mmol) NH_4Cl per kilogram is administered, and the course of blood and urine pH are followed. Although systemic acidosis worsens, urine pH does not fall below 5.5. Urinary infection must not be present during this test because bacteria may possess urease which hydrolyzes urea to ammonia and produces a very alkaline urine. When hyperchloremic acidosis is severe and the urine is grossly alkaline, the test is unnecessary.

A clinically confusing situation may occur when type 1 RTA results from nephrocalcinosis due to hereditary idiopathic hypercalciuria. In this circumstance, stones usually are composed of calcium oxalate, and hypokalemia is absent. Other hereditary diseases that cause RTA, medullary sponge kidney, galactosemia, Ehler-Danlos syndrome, Fabry's disease, and hereditary elliptocytosis, can be excluded by clinical findings. The relatives of patients with type 1 RTA should be screened because they may have this treatable cause of renal damage.

Treatment Sodium bicarbonate tablets (10 grains = 7.2 meq base) and Shohl's solution (1 meq base per milliliter, as Na and K citrate) are both convenient for treatment; the dose should be 0.5 to 2.0 meq/kg in four or five divided doses daily. The total dose of alkali should be raised until acidosis and hypercalciuria are both eliminated, and the patients should then be followed by measurements of serum chloride and CO_2 content and of urine calcium excretion approximately twice yearly. Potassium supplementation usually is not required. Requirements for alkali usually increase during intercurrent illnesses.

TYPE 2 (PROXIMAL) RTA Proximal RTA usually occurs as part of a generalized disorder of proximal tubule function. It can be a transient disorder of infancy, which usually disappears in childhood. An isolated form, i.e., without accompanying phosphaturia, aminoaciduria, and uricosuria, has been described in a single family. The pathophysiology of proximal RTA is the same whether isolated or part of a generalized disorder. Bicarbonate reabsorption in the proximal tubule is defective, and renal bicarbonate wasting occurs at a normal concentration of plasma bicarbonate. As plasma bicarbonate falls, the filtered load drops to a level that the defective tubule can reabsorb. Then the urine is free of bicarbonate and has a low pH. Potassium wasting and hypokalemia occur, especially when supplementary alkali is given, because bicarbonate is excreted in the urine partly as the potassium salt. There is moderate hypercalciuria, and stone formation is rare. During the NH_4Cl loading test, urine pH falls below 5.5.

Treatment is often not required. When it is, because of severe acidosis, bicarbonate must be given in large amounts daily, often above 4 meq/kg, and even up to 10 meq/kg per day, because bicarbonate is rapidly excreted in the urine. Another approach is to use thiazides and a low-salt diet, which induce mild volume depletion and enhance proximal bicarbonate reabsorption, thereby reducing the required dose. Potassium supplements are needed during treatment because excessive sodium bicarbonate reaches the distal nephron where much of the sodium is exchanged for potassium, which is then lost in the urine.

VITAMIN D DISORDERS

FAMILIAL X-LINKED HYPOPHOSPHATEMIC VITAMIN D-REFRACTORY RICKETS (See also Chap. 341) Reduced tubular reabsorption of phosphate by the proximal tubule and hypophosphatemia occur in this sex-linked dominant disease, which can also be termed *renal phosphate leak.* Although they may be asymptomatic, patients usually are short and their bones rachitic; their legs are particularly short and deformed, and they develop osteomalacia in adult life. Bone age and dentition are retarded, and the teeth are poorly developed. The skull becomes deformed, and the maxillofacial region may develop abnormally. Overgrowth of bone at sites of muscular attachment can limit movement or compress nerves. Bony abnormalities are less common in females. Serum alkaline phosphatase levels are elevated, serum parathyroid levels are normal or high, while serum calcium concentration is usually normal, and urinary calcium excretion rate is normal or low.

The hypophosphatemia arises in part from decreased tubular reabsorption of phosphate and increased fractional excretion of phosphate. Intestinal absorption of calcium and phosphate may be decreased in untreated patients but increased during treatment with vitamin D. Although glycinuria and mild glucosuria have been reported, most patients exhibit only a defect in excretion of phosphate. Absence of hyperchloremic acidosis and a normal serum calcium concentration help to exclude RTA, malabsorption syndrome, and nutritional rickets.

Treatment requires oral neutral phosphate, 1 to 4 g daily, in divided doses, and 10,000 to 50,000 units of vitamin D; one must watch for hypercalcemia. Combination of oral phosphate with 1α-$(OH)D_3$ or $1,25(OH)_2D_3$ may be more beneficial. Bony deformities require orthopedic management, but corrective surgery, except for genu valgum, should be postponed until active growth is completed.

VITAMIN D-DEPENDENT RICKETS (See also Chap. 340) Also known as hereditary pseudovitamin D-deficiency rickets, this disease is inherited as an autosomal recessive trait, and there is a high incidence of parental consanguinity. Defective production of $1,25$-$(OH)_2D_3$ by the kidneys, perhaps because of a genetic defect in 25-hydroxycholecalciferol 1α-hydroxylase, has been proposed as the basis for the disease. But the dose of $1,25$-$(OH)_2D_3$ or 1α-hydroxyvitamin D_3 [1α-$(OH)D_3$] required to heal rickets is higher than that for vitamin D-deficiency rickets, suggesting an attenuated response to, or excessive degradation of, $1,25$-$(OH)_2D_3$.

Rickets usually appears before 2 years of age. Serum calcium is low, parathyroid hormone concentration and alkaline phosphatase are high, and plasma phosphorus is variable. Urinary calcium is decreased, fecal calcium is increased, and tubular phosphate reabsorption is reduced. Serum levels of $1,25$-$(OH)_2D_3$ are undetectable. Aminoaciduria and hyperchloremic acidosis can occur, but urinary cyclic AMP increases normally in response to PTH infusion.

The 1α-hydroxylated metabolites of vitamin D bypass the enzyme defect and produce a dramatic healing of rickets. Vitamin D_2, 10,000 to 40,000 units per day, is also effective, but oral calcium, 0.5 to 2.0 g per day, is needed as well. The need for vitamin D persists throughout life. $1,25$-$(OH)_2D_3$, an ideal replacement therapy, may prove to be the drug of choice, but one must watch for hypercalcemia.

RENAL GLUCOSURIA

See Chap. 93.

ISOLATED HYPOURICEMIA (See also Chap. 93)

This disorder, in which there is a defect in proximal tubular reabsorption of sodium urate, is familial and appears to be inherited in an autosomal recessive pattern. Hypouricemia can occur in the Fanconi syndrome, Hartnup's disease, and Wilson's disease, but may also appear as an isolated trait. Uric acid clearance is high, and urine oxypurine levels are normal, excluding hereditary xanthinuria. Patients are asymptomatic except for occasional uric acid nephrolithiasis. No specific treatment is needed except the avoidance of dehydration. Coexistent hypercalciuria and decreased bone density have been described in a few patients, who may have a related disease with recessive inheritance.

SELECTIVE DISORDERS OF AMINO ACID TRANSPORT

CYSTINURIA (See also Chap. 93) Proximal tubular and jejunal transport of cystine and the other dibasic amino acids, lysine, arginine, and ornithine, are defective, and excessive amounts are lost in the urine. Clinical disease is due solely to the insolubility of cystine, which forms stones. Patients are short, probably because of a linked inherited tendency rather than amino acid losses. Cystinuria is transmitted as an autosomal recessive trait whose prevalence in newborns is 1 in 7000.

Pathogenesis The weight of available evidence indicates that cystinuria occurs because of defective transport of amino acids by the brush borders of renal tubule and intestinal epithelial cells. Cystine, lysine, arginine, and ornithine appear to share a common renal transport pathway, because infusion of lysine decreases tubular reabsorption of the other three. But cystine also seems to be transported by a separate transport mechanism, because cystinuria and dibasic aminoaciduria can each occur independently. The inheritance of the brush border transport defects is complex. The intestinal defects are not similar in all patients who are homozygous for cystinuria, and the extent of aminoaciduria in those relatives of cystinuric patients who are heterozygous carriers of the defect, for example, their siblings, varies from family to family. Thus far three types of inheritance have been described (Table 299-1).

Diagnosis and treatment Cystine stones are formed only by patients with cystinuria, but 10 percent of stones formed by cystinuric patients do not contain cystine; therefore, every stone former should be screened for the disease. The sediment from a first morning urine specimen in many patients with homozygous cystinuria reveals typical flat hexagonal platelike cystine crystals. Cystinuria can also be detected using the sodium nitroprusside test on a urine sample. The test gives a positive response to 75 to 125 mg cystine per gram of creati-

TABLE 299-1
Classification of cystinuria into three types

	Type I	*Type II*	*Type III*
Intestinal transport:			
Cystine	0	↓↓	N−↓
Lysine	0	0	↓
Arginine	0	—	—
Urine excretion in heterozygotes:			
Cystine	N	↑	↑
Lysine	N	↑	↑

NOTE: ↑ = *increased;* ↓ = *reduced;* ↓↓ = *very reduced; 0 = absent transport; N = normal urinary excretion rates;* — = *not known.*

nine, a concentration lower than that found in the urine of patients with homozygous cystinuria but well above the levels encountered in normal urine. Because the test is sensitive, it will be positive in many individuals who are heterozygous for cystinuria, most of whom do not form cystine stones (Table 299-1). A positive nitroprusside test or the finding of cystine crystals in the urine sediment should be evaluated by measurement of daily cystine excretion. Normal adults excrete 40 to 60 mg per gram of creatinine; heterozygotes usually excrete less than 300 mg/g; and patients with homozygous cystinuria almost always excrete above 250 mg/g.

Treatment consists of a high fluid intake, even at night. Daily urine volume should exceed 3 liters (Chap. 300). Raising urine pH with alkali is helpful, provided the resulting daily urine pH exceeds 7.5. Because drug side effects are frequent, D-penicillamine, which forms the soluble mixed disulfide cysteine-penicillamine, should be used only when fluid loading and alkali therapy have been ineffective. *N*-Acetyl-D-penicillamine has a similar mode of action and may have fewer side effects, but is not available for routine use. Mercaptopropinylglycine has been used to dissolve renal calculi by perfusion of the renal pelvis and has been given by mouth to prevent stones, but also is experimental. Low methionine diets have not proved to be practical for clinical use.

HARTNUP'S DISEASE (See also Chap. 93) In this rare autosomal recessive disorder, renal and intestinal transport of monoamino-monocarboxylic amino acids are defective. An erythematous, scaly, pellagra-like rash appears after exposure to sunlight, and episodic cerebellar ataxia, emotional instability, delirium, and aminoaciduria all occur. The prevalence is 1 in 15,000 newborns and is higher in the offspring of consanguineous marriages.

Dietary monoamino-monocarboxylic amino acids remain in the intestinal lumen where they undergo bacterial degradation. At the same time, they are lost in the urine. Inadequate tryptophan availability limits nicotinamide synthesis and leads to pellagra. The products of tryptophan degradation appear to cause central nervous system symptoms. Decreased absorption and urine loss of the other monoamino-monocarboxylic amino acids can cause generalized malnutrition.

The diagnosis is based upon demonstration of massive urine losses of alanine, serine, threonine, asparagine, glutamine, valine, leucine, isoleucine, phenylalanine, tyrosine, tryptophan, histidine, glycine, and citrulline. Hypouricemia may also occur. Renal function is otherwise normal. Most patients respond to treatment with oral nicotinamide, 40 to 200 mg per day, and a high-protein diet to compensate for amino acid malabsorption and loss. The ultimate prognosis is good, and the disease often improves with adulthood.

FAMILIAL IMINOGLYCINURIA (See also Chap. 93) This autosomal recessive trait is characterized by excessive urinary excretion of proline, hydroxyproline, and glycine despite normal plasma levels of these amino acids, probably because of deletion or alteration of a membrane transport protein of the renal tubule cells. The patients are well. Iminoglycinuria can occur in normal newborn infants for up to 3 months.

FANCONI SYNDROME

Fanconi syndrome is a constellation of transport defects in the proximal tubule involving amino acids, monosaccharides, sodium, potassium, calcium, phosphate, bicarbonate, uric acid, and proteins. Generalized aminoaciduria, glucosuria, salt wasting, hypercalciuria, hypophosphatemia, proximal renal tubular acidosis, hypouricemia, and tubular proteinuria (Chap. 40) all may result. Fanconi syndrome can be acquired or arise from systemic inherited diseases such as cystinosis, tyrosinemia, galactosemia, fructose intolerance, glycogen storage disease (type 1), Wilson's disease, familial nephrosis, and hereditary amyloidosis. Lowe's (or oculocerebrorenal) syndrome is an X-linked recessive form of the Fanconi syndrome associated with ocular and cerebral abnormalities.

An autosomal recessive disease, *adult Fanconi syndrome,* occurs in the absence of any systemic disorder. The term *adult* is misleading since cases are recognized in childhood, but no abnormalities are apparent at birth. Dwarfism and hypophosphatemic rickets occur along with the laboratory abnormalities of Fanconi syndrome. Renal failure is rare, and the prognosis is usually good when the systemic effects of Fanconi syndrome are treated. Typically, there is a "swan neck" deformity of the initial portion of the proximal tubule which, in all probability, is the anatomic basis of this tubular disorder. There is cellular atrophy in the deformed tubular segment. The consequences of each of the transport defects that involve water, sodium, potassium, acid, and phosphate excretion often require treatment. Water, sodium, and potassium intake must be liberal, and phosphate supplements may be needed. Metabolic acidosis may be corrected by the administration of alkali. Vitamin D may be needed to help promote bone healing. Glucosuria, uricosuria, and tubular proteinuria do not require treatment.

REFERENCES

AVIOLI LV: Vitamin D–resistant rickets, in *Diseases of the Kidney,* 3d ed, LE Earley, CW Gottschalk (eds). Boston, Little, Brown, 1979, p 1055

BARDGETTE JJ et al: Bartter's syndrome: Mechanisms, diagnosis, and treatment, in *Update II: Harrison's Principles of Internal Medicine,* KJ Isselbacher et al (eds). New York, McGraw-Hill, 1981

BATLLE DC, ARRUDA JAL: Renal tubular acidosis syndromes. Mineral Electrolyte Metab 5:83, 1981

BERNSTEIN J, KISSANE JM: Hereditary disorders of the kidney, part 1: Parenchymal defects and malformations. Perspect Ped Pathol 1:117, 1973

BRENES LG et al: Familial proximal renal tubular acidosis. Am J Med 52:244, 1977

CHAN JCM: Bartter's syndrome. Nephron 26:155, 1980

CULPEPPER RM, HEBERT SC, ANDREOLI TE: Nephrogenic diabetes insipidus, in *The Metabolic Basis of Inherited Disease,* 5th ed, JB Stanbury et al (eds). New York, McGraw-Hill, 1982, p 1867

DANOVITCH GM: Clinical features and pathophysiology of polycystic disease in man, in *Cystic Diseases of the Kidney,* KD Gardner (ed). New York, Wiley, 1976, p 123

DEFRONZO FA, THIER SO: Inherited disorders of renal tubule function, in *The Kidney,* 2d ed, BM Brenner, FC Rector Jr (eds). Philadelphia, Saunders, 1981, p 1816

HALPERIN EC, THIER SO: Cystinuria, in *Contemporary Issues in Nephrology,* BM Brenner, JH Stein (eds), FL Coe (guest ed). New York, Churchill Livingstone, 1980, vol 5, p 208

Jepson JB: Hartnup disease, in *The Metabolic Basis of Inherited Disease,* 5th ed, JB Stanbury et al (eds). New York, McGraw-Hill, 1982, p 1804

Kupier JJ: Medullary sponge kidney, in *Cystic Diseases of the Kidney,* KD Gardner Jr (ed). New York, Wiley, 1976, p 151

Liddle GW et al: A familial renal disorder simulating primary aldosteronism but with negligible aldosterone secretion. Trans Ann Am Phys 76:199, 1963

McSherry E: Renal tubular acidosis in childhood. Kid Int 20:799, 1981

Rasmussen H, Anast C: Familial hypophosphatemic rickets and vitamin D-dependent rickets, in *The Metabolic Basis of Inherited Disease,* 5th ed, JB Stanbury et al (eds). New York, McGraw-Hill, 1982, p 1743

Scriver CR: Familial iminoglycinuria, in *The Metabolic Basis of Inherited Disease,* 5th ed, JB Stanbury et al (eds). New York, McGraw-Hill, 1982, p 1792

——— et al: Genetic aspects of renal tubular transport: Diversity and topology of carriers. Kid Int 9:149, 1976

Segal S: Disorders of renal amino acid transport. N Engl J Med 294:1044, 1976

Steele BT, Lirenman DS, Beattie CW: Nephronophthisis. Am J Med 68:531, 1980

Tofuku Y, Kuroda M, Takeda R: Hypouricemia due to renal urate wasting: Two types of tubular transport defects. Nephron 30:39, 1982

300 NEPHROLITHIASIS

FREDRIC L. COE
MURRAY J. FAVUS

TYPES OF STONES

Calcium salts, uric acid, cystine, and struvite ($MgNH_4PO_4$) are the basis of virtually all kidney stones formed by patients residing in the western hemisphere. Calcium oxalate and calcium phosphate stones comprise 75 to 85 percent of the total (Table 300-1) and may be admixed in the same stone. Calcium phosphates in stones are usually hydroxyapatite [$Ca_5(PO_4)_3OH$] or, less commonly, brushite ($CaHPO_4$).

Calcium stones are formed mainly by men; the average age of onset is the third decade. Most persons who form a single calcium stone will eventually form another, and the intervals between successive stones shorten or remain constant, suggesting that stone-forming activity usually does not wane with time. The average rate of new stone formation in patients who have previously formed a stone is about one stone every 2 or 3 years. Calcium stone disease is strongly familial.

In the urine, calcium oxalate monohydrate crystals (whewellite) usually grow as biconcave ovals that resemble red blood cells in shape and size, but also occur in a larger, "dumbbell" form. In polarized light the crystals appear bright against a dark background with an intensity dependent upon orientation, a property known as *birefringence.* Calcium oxalate dihydrate crystals (weddellite) are bipyramidal and only weakly birefringent. Apatite crystals do not exhibit birefringence and appear amorphous, because the actual crystals are too small to be resolved by light microscopy. Brushite produces elongated lathlike (narrow, long, rectangular) crystals.

Uric acid stones are radiolucent, account for 5 to 8 percent of all stones (Table 300-1), and are also formed mainly by men. Half of the patients who form uric acid stones have gout; whether or not gout is present, uric acid lithiasis is familial. In urine, uric acid crystals become red-orange colored because they adsorb the pigment uricine. Anhydrous uric acid produces very small crystals that appear amorphous by light microscopy. They are indistinguishable from apatite crystals, except for their birefringence. Uric acid dihydrate tends to form teardrop-shaped crystals as well as flat, square plates; both are strongly birefringent. Uric acid gravel appears like red dust, and the stones are also orange or red on some occasions. *Cystine stones* are very uncommon (less than 1 percent of all stones), are lemon yellow, and sparkle; they are radiopaque because they contain sulfur. Cystine crystals appear in the urine as flat, hexagonal plates.

Struvite ($MgNH_4PO_4$) *stones* are common (Table 300-1) and potentially dangerous. These stones, formed mainly by women, result from urinary tract infection with bacteria that possess urease, usually *Proteus* species. The stones can grow to a large size and fill the renal pelvis and calyces to produce a "staghorn" appearance. They are radiopaque and have a variable internal density. In urine, struvite crystals are rectangular prisms that have been likened to coffin lids.

MANIFESTATIONS OF STONES

As stones grow upon the surfaces of the renal papillae or within the urinary collecting system, they need not produce symptoms. Accordingly, asymptomatic stones are often discovered during the course of abdominal radiographic studies undertaken for unrelated reasons. Sometimes stones cause only gross or microscopic hematuria. In fact, stones rank, along with benign and malignant neoplasms, renal cysts, and genitourinary tuberculosis, as among the most common causes of isolated hematuria. Much of the time, however, stones break loose and enter the ureter, or occlude the ureteropelvic junction, causing pain and obstruction.

STONE PASSAGE A stone can traverse the ureter without symptoms, but most of the time passage produces pain and bleeding. The pain begins gradually, usually in the flank, but increases over the next 20 to 60 min to become very severe, and narcotic drugs are often needed for its control. The pain may remain in the flank or spread downward and anteriorly toward the loins, testicles, or vulva. Pain that migrates downward always indicates that the stone has passed to the lower third of the ureter, but if the pain does not migrate, the position of the stone cannot be predicted. A stone in the portion of the ureter within the bladder wall causes frequency, urgency, and dysuria that may be confused with urinary tract infection. Hematuria is the rule with passage of a stone.

OTHER SYNDROMES **Staghorn calculi** Struvite, cystine, and uric acid stones often grow too large to enter the ureter. They gradually fill the renal pelvis and may extend outward through the infundibula to the calyces themselves.

Nephrocalcinosis Calcium stones grow on the renal papillae. Most break loose and cause colic, but sometimes they remain in place so that multiple papillary calcifications are found by x-ray, a condition termed *nephrocalcinosis.* Papillary nephrocalcinosis is very common in hereditary distal renal tubular acidosis and in other states characterized by severe hypercalciuria. In medullary sponge kidney disease (Chap. 299) calcification may occur in dilated distal collecting ducts.

Sludge There can be enough uric acid or cystine in the urine to plug both ureters with precipitate. Calcium oxalate crystals do not do this because usually less than 100 mg oxalate is excreted daily in the urine in even severe hyperoxaluric states, compared with 1000 mg uric acid in patients with ordinary hyperuricosuria and 200 to 400 mg cystine in patients with homozygous cystinuria. Calcium phosphate crystals can render the urine milky but do not plug the urinary tract.

INFECTION Although urinary tract infection is not a direct consequence of stone disease, it is a frequent complication that arises from instrumentation and surgery of the urinary tract, which are frequently required in the treatment of stone disease. Stone disease and urinary infection can enhance the seriousness of one another and interfere with treatment. Obstruction of an infected kidney by a stone may lead to sepsis and extensive damage of renal tissue, since it converts the urinary tract proximal to the obstruction into a closed, or partially closed, space that can become an abscess. On the other hand, some forms of infection, those due to bacteria that possess the enzyme urease, can produce stones composed of struvite.

ACTIVITY OF STONE DISEASE *Active disease* means that new stones are forming or that preformed stones are growing. Sequential radiographs of the renal areas are needed to document the growth or appearance of new stones and to assure that stones which pass are actually newly formed, not preexistent ones.

PATHOGENESIS OF STONES

Urinary stones usually arise because of the breakdown of a delicate balance. On the one hand the kidneys must conserve water, but they must also excrete materials that have a low solubility. These two opposing requirements must be balanced against one another during adaptation to a particular combination of diet, climate, and activity. The problem is mitigated to some extent by the fact that urine contains some substances that inhibit crystallization of calcium salts and others that bind calcium in soluble complexes. But these protective mechanisms are less than perfect. When the urine becomes saturated with insoluble materials, because their excretion rates are excessive, and/or because water conservation is extreme, crystals form and may grow and aggregate with one another to form a stone.

SUPERSATURATION Consider a solution that is in equilibrium with crystals of calcium oxalate. The product of the chemical activities of the calcium and oxalate ions in the solution is termed the *equilibrium solubility product,* because it is the activity product that is unique to the equilibrium condition. If the crystals are removed, and if either calcium or oxalate is added to the solution, the activity product will rise, but the solution will remain clear; no new crystals form. Such a solution is considered to be *metastably supersaturated.* If new calcium oxalate seed crystals are now added, they will grow in size. Ultimately, the activity product will reach a critical value at which a solid phase begins to develop spontaneously. This value is called the *upper limit of metastability,* or the *formation product.* Stone growth in the urinary tract requires a urine that, on the average, is above the equilibrium solubility product.

TABLE 300-1
Major cause of renal stones

Stone type and causes	*Percent of all stones**	*Percent occurrence of specific causes**	*Ratio of men to women*	*Etiology*	*Diagnosis*	*Treatment*
Calcium stones	75–85		2:1 to 3:1			
Idiopathic hypercalciuria		50–55	2:1	Hereditary (?)	Normocalcemia, unexplained hypercalciuria†	Thiazide diuretic agents
Hyperuricosuria		20	4:1	Diet	Urine uric acid > 750 mg per 24 h (women), > 800 mg per 24 h (men)	Allopurinol or diet
Primary hyperparathyroidism		5	3:10	Neoplasia	Unexplained hypercalcemia	Surgery
Distal renal tubular acidosis		Rare	1:1	Hereditary	Hyperchloremic acidosis, minimum urine pH > 5.5	Alkali replacement
Intestinal hyperoxaluria		~1–2	1:1	Bowel surgery	Urine oxalate > 50 mg per 24 h	Cholestyramine or oral calcium loading
Hereditary hyperoxaluria		Rare	1:1	Hereditary	Urine oxalate and glycolic or L-glyceric acid increased	Fluids and pyridoxine
Idiopathic stone disease		20	2:1	Unknown	None of the above present	Oral phosphate, fluids
Uric acid stones	5–8					
Gout		~50	3:1 to 4:1	Hereditary	Clinical diagnosis	Alkali to raise urine pH
Idiopathic		~50	1:1	Hereditary (?)	Uric acid stones, no gout	Allopurinol if daily urine uric acid above 1000 mg
Dehydration		?	1:1	Intestinal, habit	History, intestinal fluid loss	Alkali, fluids, reversal of cause
Lesch-Nyhan syndrome		Rare	Men	Hereditary	Reduced hypoxanthine guanine phosphoribosyltransferase level	Allopurinol
Malignant tumors		Rare	1:1	Neoplasia	Clinical diagnosis	Allopurinol
Cystine stones	1		1:1	Hereditary	Stone type; elevated cystine excretion	Massive fluids, alkali, D-penicillamine if needed
Struvite stones	10–15		2:10	Infection	Stone type	Antimicrobial agents and judicious surgery

* *Values are percent of patients who form a particular type of stone and who display each specific cause of stones.*
† *Urine calcium above 300 mg per 24 h (men), 250 mg per 24 h (women), or 4 mg/kg per 24 h either sex. Hyperthyroidism, Cushing syndrome, sarcoidosis, malignant tumors, immobilization, vitamin D intoxication, rapidly progressive bone disease, and Paget's disease all cause hypercalciuria and must be excluded in diagnosis of idiopathic hypercalciuria.*

Persistence of a stone requires an average activity product at least equal to the solubility product. In general there is agreement that excessive supersaturation is a factor common to the formation of most stones.

Calcium, oxalate, and phosphate form many stable soluble complexes among themselves and with other substances in urine, such as calcium citrate. As a result, their free ion activities are considerably below their chemical concentrations and can be measured only by indirect techniques. Urine supersaturation can be increased by dehydration or by overexcretion of calcium, oxalate, or phosphate. Supersaturation of the urine with cystine or uric acid also rises when overexcretion or low urine volume is present. Urine pH can also be an important factor; phosphate and uric acid are weak acids that dissociate readily over the physiological range of urine pH. Alkaline urine contains more urate and dissociated phosphate, favoring deposits of sodium hydrogen urate, octocalcium phosphate, and apatite. Below a urine pH of 5.5, uric acid crystals (p*K* 5.47) predominate, whereas phosphate crystals are rare. The solubility of calcium oxalate, on the other hand, is not influenced by changes in urine pH. Measurements of supersaturation in a 24-h urine sample are averages that probably underestimate the risk of precipitation. Transient dehydration or postprandial bursts of overexcretion may cause values that are considerably above the average.

NUCLEATION **Homogeneous nucleation** When urine is supersaturated with respect to calcium oxalate, clusters of ions form at random as supersaturation rises. Most of them disperse when their mass is small because the internal forces between ions that tend to hold the clusters together are too weak to overcome the random tendency of ions to move away. Clusters of over 100 ions can remain stable because attractive forces balance surface losses. Once they are stable, nuclei can grow at a supersaturation far below that needed for their creation. The formation product marks the point at which stable nuclei become frequent enough to create a permanent solid phase.

Heterogeneous nucleation If a supersaturated urine is seeded with preformed nuclei of a crystal that is similar in structure to calcium oxalate, calcium and oxalate ions in solution will precipitate on the crystal's surface as they would upon a seed crystal of calcium oxalate itself. The organized growth of one crystal on the surface of another is called *epitaxial growth*, and the seeding of a supersaturated solution by foreign nuclei is called *heterogeneous nucleation*. Sodium hydrogen urate, uric acid, and hydroxyapatite crystals can serve as heterogeneous nuclei for calcium oxalate. Brushite ($CaHPO_4 \cdot 2H_2O$) can be transformed to hydroxyapatite and cause heterogeneous nucleation of sodium hydrogen urate; as a consequence, calcium oxalate stones can form even if urine calcium oxalate supersaturation never exceeds the metastable limit.

INHIBITORS OF CRYSTAL GROWTH AND AGGREGATION Stable nuclei must grow and aggregate to produce a stone of clinical significance. Urine contains potent inhibitors of both of these processes for calcium oxalate and calcium phosphate, but not for uric acid, cystine, or struvite crystals. Inorganic pyrophosphate is a potent inhibitor which appears to affect calcium phosphate more than calcium oxalate crystals. Other urine inhibitors that appear to be glycoproteins strongly inhibit the growth of calcium oxalate crystals. Slowing of crystal growth must raise the apparent upper limit of metastability, because the critical growth of ion clusters into stable nuclei is hindered. As a consequence of the presence of these inhibitors, crystal growth in urine is very slow compared with simple salt solutions, and the upper limit of metastability is higher.

EVALUATION AND TREATMENT OF PATIENTS WITH NEPHROLITHIASIS

A majority of patients with nephrolithiasis harbor remediable metabolic disorders that cause stones and can be detected by chemical analysis of the serum and urine. A practical outpatient evaluation consists of three 24-h urine collections, each with a corresponding blood sample. Serum and urine calcium, uric acid and creatinine, urine oxalate and serum electrolyte measurements should be made. Whenever possible, the composition of kidney stones should be determined because treatment depends on stone type (Table 300-1). No matter what disorders are found, every patient should be counseled to avoid dehydration and to drink six to eight glasses of water daily. Since treatment is prolonged, the use of medications must be justified by the activity and severity of stone disease and the desire the patient may have for protection against new stones.

The management of stones that are already present in the kidneys or urinary tract requires a combined medical and surgical approach. The specific treatment for any individual patient depends upon the details of the location of the stone, the extent of obstruction, the function of the affected and unaffected kidneys, the presence or absence of urinary tract infection, the progress of stone passage, and the risk of operation or anesthesia, given the overall clinical state of the patient. In general, when severe obstruction, infection, intractable pain, or serious bleeding occur, removal of a stone by operation upon the kidney, renal pelvis, or ureter or by passing a flexible basket retrograde up the ureter from the bladder during the course of cystoscopy is usually attempted. This dictum applies whether the stone is small and in the ureter or is a large staghorn calculus that fills the renal pelvis.

CALCIUM STONES **Idiopathic hypercalciuria** (see also Chap. 339) This condition appears to be hereditary, and its diagnosis is straightforward (Table 300-1). In some patients, primary intestinal hyperabsorption of calcium causes transient postprandial hypercalcemia that suppresses secretion of parathyroid hormone. The renal tubules are deprived of their most potent normal stimulus to reabsorb calcium at the same time that the filtered load of calcium is increased. In other patients, reabsorption of calcium by the renal tubules appears to be defective, and secondary hyperparathyroidism is evoked by urinary losses of calcium. Renal activation of 1,25-dihydroxyvitamin D is increased, producing intestinal hyperabsorption of calcium. Hypercalciuria contributes to stone formation by raising urine saturation with respect to calcium oxalate and calcium phosphate.

Thiazide diuretics lower urine calcium in both types of hypercalciuria and are very effective in preventing the formation of stones. The drug effect requires slight contraction of the extracellular fluid volume, and massive use of NaCl will reduce its therapeutic effect.

Hyperuricosuria About 20 percent of calcium oxalate stone formers are hyperuricosuric, primarily because of an excessive intake of purine from meat, fish, and poultry. The mechanism of stone formation probably is heterogeneous nucleation of calcium oxalate by crystals of sodium hydrogen urate or uric acid that lodge in the terminal ends of the collecting ducts and produce an anchored site on which calcium oxalate can deposit. A change in diet is ideal treatment but difficult for many patients to achieve. The alternative is allopurinol, usually 100 mg bid. Some patients eventually alter their diets so that allopurinol can be withdrawn.

Primary hyperparathyroidism (see also Chap. 339) The diagnosis of this condition, which is more common in women than men, is aided by the finding of unexplained phosphate stones and is established by documenting hypercalcemia that cannot be otherwise explained accompanied by inappropriately elevated serum concentrations of parathyroid hormone. Hypercalciuria, which is usually present, raises the urine supersaturation of calcium phosphate and/or calcium oxalate (Table 300-1). It is important to establish the diagnosis since parathyroidectomy is effective treatment and should be carried out before renal damage has occurred.

Distal renal tubular acidosis (see also Chap. 299) The defect in this condition seems to reside in the distal nephron, which cannot establish a normal pH gradient between urine and blood, leading to hyperchloremic acidosis. The minimum urine pH in response to an oral challenge with NH_4Cl, 1.9 mmol/kg, is above 5.5. Hypercalciuria, an alkaline urine, and a low urine citrate concentration cause supersaturation with respect to calcium phosphate. Calcium phosphate stones are formed, nephrocalcinosis is common, and osteomalacia or rickets may occur. Renal damage is frequent, and a gradual fall in glomerular filtration rate usually occurs. Treatment with supplemental alkali reverses hypercalciuria and limits the production of new stones. The usual dose of sodium bicarbonate is 0.5 to 2.0 meq/kg, in four to six divided doses. An alternative is Shohl's solution, which contains citrate and citric acid.

Hyperoxaluria Overabsorption of dietary oxalate and consequent oxaluria, i.e., so-called intestinal oxaluria, has been ascribed to fat malabsorption (Chap. 308). The latter can be caused by a variety of conditions, including bacterial overgrowth syndromes, chronic disease of the pancreas and biliary tract, jejunoileal bypass in treatment of obesity, or ileal resection greater than 22 cm for inflammatory bowel disease. With fat malabsorption, calcium in the bowel lumen is bound by fatty acids instead of precipitating with oxalate, which is left free for excessive absorption in the colon. Delivery of unabsorbed fatty acids and bile salts to the colon may injure the colonic mucosa and permit excessive oxalate absorption. Dietary excess of oxalate, ascorbic acid loading, and hereditary hyperoxaluric states due to overproduction of oxalate are much less common causes of hyperoxaluria. Ethylene glycol intoxication and methoxyflurane, an anesthetic agent, can also cause oxalate overproduction and hyperoxaluria. Hyperoxaluria from any cause can produce tubulointerstitial nephropathy (Chap. 297) and lead to stone formation.

Cholestyramine, a resin that can bind oxalate, at a dose of 8 to 16 g per day, correction of fat malabsorption, and a low-fat diet are effective treatments for oxaluria secondary to intestinal absorption. Calcium lactate, 8 to 14 g per day, which acts by precipitating oxalate in the gut lumen is an alternative form of therapy. There is no effective treatment for hereditary hyperoxaluria, a disorder characterized by an enzymatic defect involving the metabolism of the precursor of oxalate and transmitted as an autosomal recessive. A high fluid intake, phosphate, and pyridoxine (200 mg per day) are recommended, but irreversible renal failure secondary to recurrent stone formation usually occurs before the age of 20 years.

Idiopathic calcium lithiasis At least 20 percent of patients have no obvious cause for stones (Table 300-1). The best treatment for them appears to be a high fluid intake, so that the urine specific gravity remains below approximately 1.005 throughout the day and night. Oral phosphate at a dose of 2 g phosphorus daily may lower urine calcium and increases urine pyrophosphate excretion, and thereby may bring about a reduction in the rate of recurrence of stones. Orthophosphate causes mild nausea and diarrhea initially, but tolerance may improve with continued intake. Thiazide treatment to reduce calcium excretion and allopurinol to diminish uric acid output may also be helpful. There are no adequate studies to support the use of supplemental magnesium, pyridoxine, or methylene blue, commonly mentioned remedies.

URIC ACID STONES These stones form because the urine becomes supersaturated with undissociated uric acid. In gout, idiopathic uric acid lithiasis, and dehydration, the average pH is abnormally low, usually below 5.4, and often below 5.0. Undissociated uric acid (pK 5.35, in urine), which is very insoluble and cannot be dissolved in urine in concentrations exceeding 200 to 300 mg per liter, predominates. Hyperuricosuria, when present, increases supersaturation; but urine of low pH can be excessively supersaturated with undissociated uric acid even though the daily excretion rate is normal. Myeloproliferative syndromes, chemotherapeutic treatment of malignant tumors, and the Lesch-Nyhan syndrome cause such massive production of uric acid and consequent hyperuricosuria that stones and uric acid sludge occur even at a normal urine pH. The renal collecting tubules can be plugged by uric acid crystals with consequent acute renal failure.

The two goals of treatment are to raise urine pH and to lower urine uric acid excretion, when it is very high, i.e., above 1000 mg per day. Supplemental alkali, 1 to 3 meq/kg per day, should be given in three or four evenly spaced divided doses, one of which should be reserved for bedtime. If the overnight urine pH is below 5.5, the evening dose of bicarbonate may be raised, or 250 mg acetazolamide added at bedtime. With massive overexcretion of uric acid, high doses of allopurinol, exceeding 300 mg daily, may be needed. Treatment with allopurinol should be instituted before chemotherapy of highly cellular tumors, since massive hyperuricosuria can be expected. Alkali treatment must be avoided if hypercalciuria is also present.

CYSTINE STONES (See also Chap. 299) Like uric acid, cystine is more soluble in alkaline than in acid urine. However, improvement in solubility begins only above pH 7; therefore, alkali confers only limited benefits. The major treatment is sufficient water to create 3 to 4 liters urine per day, and deliberate nocturia is an unavoidable part of treatment. If fluids and alkali are insufficient, D-penicillamine may be added. The side effects of this drug, i.e., anosmia and loss of taste, usually respond to replacement of zinc. Development of the nephrotic syndrome is a common serious side effect of D-penicillamine that contraindicates further use of the drug.

STRUVITE STONES These stones are always a result of urinary infection with bacteria, usually *Proteus* species, which possess urease, an enzyme that degrades urea to NH_3 and CO_2. The NH_3 hydrolyzes to NH_4^+ and raises pH, usually to 8 or 9. The CO_2 hydrates to H_2CO_3 and then dissociates to CO_3^{2-} which precipitates with calcium as $CaCO_3$. The NH_4^+ precipitates PO_4^{3-} and Mg^{2+} to form the triple salt $MgNH_4PO_4$. The result is a stone of calcium carbonate admixed with struvite. It is impossible to form struvite in urine without infection, because NH_4^+ concentration is very low in urine that is alkaline in response to physiological stimuli. Chronic *Proteus* infection can occur because of impaired urinary drainage, infection of retained stones of any type, urologic instrumentation or surgery, and especially chronic antibiotic treatment, which can favor the emergence of *Proteus* as the predominant urinary tract flora.

Treatment Mandelamine, which lowers urine pH and liberates formaldehyde, is used for chronic suppression of infection when a stone is present. More extreme lowering of urine pH with chronic administration of NH_4Cl may retard stone growth but may also raise urine calcium level and promote the formation of calcium oxalate stones. Antimicrobial treatment is best reserved for dealing with acute exacerbation of infection and for maintenance of a sterile urine after surgery, in the hope of preventing recurrence or minimizing stone growth. Surgery should be reserved for severe obstruction, intractable pain, bleeding, or serious manifestations of urinary infection. Since stones can regrow from any infected fragment which is left behind, recurrences following operation are quite common.

REFERENCES

COE FL: Nephrolithiasis: Pathogenesis and treatment. Chicago, Year Book, 1978

——— et al: Effect of low calcium diet on urine calcium excretion, parathyroid function, and serum $1,25(OH)_2D_3$ levels in patients with idiopathic hypercalciuria and in normal subjects. Am J Med 72:25, 1982

FLEISCH H et al (eds): *Urolithiasis Research.* New York, Plenum, 1976

———, FAVUS MJ: Disorders of stone formation, in *The Kidney,* 2d ed, BM Brenner, FC Rector Jr (eds). Philadelphia, Saunders, 1981

PAK CYC (ed): Urolithiasis. Kidney Int 13:341, 1978

STRAUSS AL et al: Factors that predict relapse of calcium nephrolithiasis during treatment. Am J Med 72:25, 1982

301
URINARY TRACT OBSTRUCTION

BARRY M. BRENNER
H. DAVID HUMES
EDGAR L. MILFORD

Obstruction to the flow of urine, with attendant stasis and elevation in urinary tract pressure, impairs renal and urinary conduit functions and represents a common cause of acute and chronic renal failure. With early relief of obstruction, these defects in function usually disappear completely. However, chronic obstruction may produce profound and permanent loss of renal mass (renal atrophy) and excretory capability, as well as enhanced susceptibility to local infection and stone formation. Early and accurate diagnosis and prompt and appropriate therapy are, therefore, essential to minimize the otherwise devastating effects of obstruction on urinary tract structure and function.

ETIOLOGY Obstruction to urine flow can result from *intrinsic* or *extrinsic mechanical blockade* as well as from *functional defects* not associated with fixed occlusion of the urinary drainage system. Lesions causing mechanical obstruction can occur at any level of the urinary tract, from the renal calyces to the external urethral meatus. Normal points of narrowing, such as the ureteropelvic and ureterovesical junctions, bladder neck, and urethral meatus, are common sites of obstruction. When blockage is above the level of the bladder, unilateral dilatation of the ureter (*hydroureter*) and renal pyelocalyceal system (*hydronephrosis*) occur; when the lesion is at or below the level of the bladder, bilateral involvement is the rule.

Common forms of mechanical obstruction are listed in Table 301-1. In childhood, *congenital malformations,* including marked narrowing of the ureteropelvic junction, anomalous (retrocaval) location of the ureter, and posterior urethral valves predominate. The latter defect is the most common cause of bilateral hydronephrosis in the male child. Children may also have bladder dysfunction secondary to congenital urethral stricture, urethral meatal stenosis, or bladder neck obstruction. In adults, urinary tract obstruction is due mainly to *acquired defects.* Pelvic tumors, calculi, and urethral stricture predominate. Ligation of, or injury to, the ureter during pelvic or colonic surgery can lead to hydronephrosis which, if unilateral, may remain relatively silent and undetected. Obstructive uropathy may also result from extrinsic neoplastic (carcinoma of cervix or colon, retroperitoneal lymphoma) or inflammatory disorders. One such inflammatory disorder is retroperitoneal fibrosis, a process of unknown cause seen most commonly in middle-aged males, which occasionally leads to bilateral ureteral obstruction. Occurring in some patients taking methysergide for relief of migraine, retroperitoneal fibrosis must be distinguished from other retroperitoneal causes of ureteral obstruction, particularly lymphomas and pelvic neoplasms.

Functional impairment of urine flow usually results from disorders which involve both the ureter and bladder. Common functional lesions include neurogenic bladder, often with adynamic ureter, and vesicoureteral reflux. Reflux of urine from bladder to ureter(s) is more common in children than adults and may result in severe unilateral or bilateral hydroureter and hydronephrosis. Abnormal insertion of the ureter into the bladder is the most common cause of vesicoureteral reflux in children. Reflux occurring in the absence of urinary tract infection or bladder neck obstruction usually does not lead to renal parenchymal damage and often resolves spontaneously as the child matures. Surgical reinsertion of the ureter into the bladder is indicated if reflux is severe and unlikely to improve spontaneously, if renal function deteriorates, or if urinary tract infections recur despite chronic antimicrobial therapy.

TABLE 301-1
Common mechanical causes of urinary tract obstruction

*Ureter**	*Bladder outlet†*	*Urethra†*
CONGENITAL		
Ureteropelvic junction narrowing or obstruction	Bladder neck obstruction	Posterior urethral valves
Ureterovesical junction narrowing or obstruction	Ureterocele	Anterior urethral valves
Ureterocele		Stricture
Retrocaval ureter		Meatal stenosis
		Phimosis
ACQUIRED INTRINSIC DEFECTS		
Calculi	Benign prostatic hypertrophy	Stricture
Inflammation	Cancer of prostate	Tumor
Trauma	Cancer of bladder	Calculi
Sloughed papillae	Calculi	Trauma
Tumor	Diabetic neuropathy	Phimosis
Blood clots	Spinal cord disease	
Uric acid crystals		
ACQUIRED EXTRINSIC DEFECTS		
Pregnant uterus	Carcinoma of cervix, colon	Trauma
Retroperitoneal fibrosis	Trauma	
Aortic aneurysm		
Uterine leiomyomata		
Carcinoma of uterus, prostate, bladder, colon, rectum		
Retroperitoneal lymphoma		
Accidental surgical ligation		

* *Lesions are typically associated with unilateral obstruction.*

CLINICAL FEATURES Pain is the symptom which most commonly provokes the need for medical attention. The pain of urinary tract obstruction is due to distention of the collecting system or renal capsule. The severity of the pain is influenced more by the rate at which distention develops than the degree of distention. Acute supravesical obstruction, as from a stone lodged in a ureter (Chap. 300), is associated with excruciatingly severe pain, usually called *renal colic.* This pain is relatively steady and continuous, with little fluctuation in intensity, and often radiates to the lower abdomen, testes, or labia. The patient with renal colic is usually restless and unable to remain still. By contrast, more insidious causes of obstruction, such as chronic narrowing of the ureteropelvic junction, may produce little or no pain, yet result in total destruction of the affected kidney. Flank pain which comes on only with micturition is pathognomonic of vesicoureteral reflux.

Symptoms of *polyuria* and *nocturia* commonly accompany chronic partial urinary tract obstruction and result from impaired renal concentrating ability. This defect usually does not improve with administration of exogenous vasopressin and is therefore a form of acquired nephrogenic diabetes insipidus. Disturbances in chloride transport in the ascending limb of Henle and, in azotemic patients, the osmotic (urea) diuresis per nephron lead to decreased medullary hypertonicity and, hence, a concentrating defect. Partial obstruction, therefore, may be associated with increased rather than decreased urine output. Indeed, wide fluctuations in urinary output in a patient with azotemia should always raise the possibility of intermittent or partial urinary tract obstruction. If fluid intake becomes inadequate in these patients, severe dehydration and hypernatremia may develop. On the other hand, complete and bilateral obstruction, or complete unilateral obstruction in a patient with only one previously functioning kidney, results in *total anuria.* Hesitancy and straining to initiate the urinary stream, postvoid dribbling, urinary frequency, and (overflow) incontinence are complaints common to patients with obstruction at or below the level of the bladder (see Chap. 42).

In addition to loss of urinary concentrating ability and azotemia, partial bilateral urinary tract obstruction often results in other derangements of renal function, including *acquired distal renal tubular acidosis* and *renal salt wasting.* These defects in tubule function are often accompanied by histological evidence of widespread renal tubulointerstitial damage. Morphological abnormalities appear early in the course of obstruction; initially the interstitium becomes edematous and infiltrated with mononuclear inflammatory cells. With continued obstruction, the interstitium becomes fibrotic; scarring and atrophy of the papillae and medulla occur and precede these processes in the cortex.

The possibility of urinary tract obstruction must always be considered in patients with urinary tract infections or urolithiasis. Urinary stasis encourages the growth of organisms as well as the formation of crystals, especially magnesium ammonium phosphate (struvite). Systemic manifestations of urinary tract obstruction include *hypertension* and *polycythemia.* Hypertension is seen frequently in acute and subacute forms of unilateral obstruction and is usually a consequence of increased release of renin by the involved kidney. Chronic unilateral or bilateral hydronephrosis, in the absence of extracellular volume expansion or other forms of renal disease, rarely results in significant hypertension. Polycythemia, an infrequent complication of obstructive uropathy, is probably secondary to increased erythropoietin production by the obstructed kidney.

DIAGNOSIS A history of difficulty in voiding, pain, infection, or changes in urinary volume is common. Evidence for distention of the kidney or urinary bladder often can be obtained by palpation and percussion of the abdomen. A careful rectal examination may reveal enlargement or nodularity of the prostate, abnormal rectal sphincter tone, or a rectal or pelvic mass. The penis should be inspected for evidence of meatal stenosis or phimosis. In the female, vaginal, uterine, and rectal lesions responsible for urinary tract obstruction are usually revealed by inspection and palpation.

Urinalysis and examination of the urine sediment may reveal hematuria, pyuria, and bacteriuria. Often, however, the urine sediment is devoid of abnormal elements, even when obstruction leads to marked azotemia and extensive structural damage. An abdominal scout film should be obtained to evaluate the possibility of nephrocalcinosis or a radiopaque stone at any level of the urinary collecting system. If urinary tract obstruction is suspected, abdominal ultrasonography should be performed to evaluate renal and bladder size, as well as pyelocalyceal and ureteral contours. If distention of these structures is absent, functionally significant urinary tract obstruction can safely be excluded in differential diagnosis.

Intravenous pyelography is the recommended procedure to employ if an obstructive abnormality is revealed by ultrasound. If the patient is not azotemic, a standard dose of contrast medium usually provides adequate information. With renal insufficiency, however, high-dose (drip-infusion) pyelography with nephrotomography is usually required for adequate visualization. In the presence of obstruction, the appearance time of the nephrogram is often delayed but eventually becomes more dense than normal because of slow tubular fluid flow rate which results in enhanced water reabsorption by the nephrons and greater concentration of contrast medium within tubules. The kidney involved by an acute obstructive process is usually slightly enlarged, and there is dilatation of the calyces, renal pelvis, and ureter above the obstruction. The ureter, however, is not tortuous, as is the case when the obstruction is chronic. In comparison with the nephrogram, the pyelogram may be extremely faint, especially if the dilated renal pelvis is voluminous, causing dilution of the contrast medium. The radiographic study should be continued until the site of obstruction is determined or the contrast medium is excreted. Delayed films taken as long as 48 h after contrast administration may be necessary to determine the exact site of obstruction.

Patients suspected of having intermittent ureteropelvic obstruction (whether functional or mechanical) should have radiological evaluation while they are in pain, since a normal pyelogram is commonly seen during asymptomatic periods. Hydration or mannitol infusion often helps to provoke a symptomatic attack. Patients with obstruction at or below the level of the bladder exhibit thickening, trabeculation, and diverticula of the bladder wall. Postvoiding films reveal residual urine. Voiding cystourethrography is of great value in the diagnosis of vesicoureteral reflux and bladder neck and urethral obstructions. If these radiographic studies fail to provide adequate information for diagnosis, endoscopic visualization by the urologist often permits precise identification of lesions involving the urethra, prostate, bladder, and ureteral orifices. To facilitate visualization of a suspected lesion in a ureter or renal pelvis, *retrograde* or *antegrade pyelography* should be attempted. The former approach involves catheterization of the involved ureter under cystoscopic control, while the antegrade technique necessitates placement of a catheter into the renal pelvis via a needle inserted percutaneously under ultrasonic or fluoroscopic guidance. While the antegrade approach carries the added advantage of providing immediate and certain decompression of a unilateral obstructing lesion, many urologists initially attempt the retrograde approach and resort to the antegrade method only when attempts at retrograde catheterization have been unsuccessful.

TREATMENT AND PROGNOSIS An individual with any form of urinary tract obstruction complicated by infection requires relief of obstruction as soon as possible to prevent development of generalized sepsis and progressive renal damage. On a temporary basis, depending on the site of obstruction, drainage is often satisfactorily achieved by nephrostomy, ureterostomy, or ureteral, urethral, or suprapubic catheterization. When infection is not present, immediate surgery often is not required, even in the presence of complete obstruction and anuria (because of the availability of dialysis), at least until acid-base, fluid and electrolyte, and cardiovascular status have been restored to normal. Nevertheless, the site of obstruction should be ascertained as soon as feasible, in part because of the possibility that sepsis may occur and necessitate prompt urologic intervention. Elective relief of obstruction is usually recommended in patients with urinary retention, recurrent urinary tract infections, persistent pain, or progressive loss of renal function. Infrequently, mechanical obstruction can be alleviated by nonsurgical means, as with radiation therapy for retroperitoneal lymphoma. Likewise, functional obstruction secondary to neurogenic bladder may be decreased with the combination of frequent voiding and cholinergic drugs. The approach to obstruction secondary to renal stones is discussed in Chap. 300.

With relief of obstruction, the *prognosis* regarding return of renal function depends largely upon whether irreversible renal damage has occurred. When obstruction is not relieved, the patient's course will depend mainly on whether the obstruction is complete or incomplete, bilateral or unilateral, and whether urinary tract infection is also present. Complete obstruction with infection can lead to total destruction of the kidney within days. Experimental studies in dogs suggest that relief of complete obstruction of 1 and 2 weeks' duration restores glomerular filtration rate to 60 and 30 percent of normal, respectively; after 8 weeks, recovery does not occur. Nevertheless, in the absence of definitive evidence of irreversibility, every effort should be made to facilitate decompression in the hope of restoring renal function at least partially.

POSTOBSTRUCTIVE DIURESIS Relief of bilateral, but not unilateral, complete urinary tract obstruction commonly leads to a postobstructive diuresis, characterized by polyuria, which may be massive. The urine is usually hypotonic and may contain a large amount of sodium chloride. The natriuresis is due, at least in part, to the excretion of retained urea, which acts as a poorly reabsorbable solute and diminishes salt and water reabsorption in the tubules (osmotic diuresis). The increase in intratubular pressure very likely also contributes to the impairment in net sodium chloride reabsorption, especially in the terminal nephron segments. It has been suggested that natriuretic factors (other than urea) also accumulate during uremia induced by obstruction and serve to depress tubule salt and water reabsorption when urine flow is reestablished. In the vast majority of patients this diuresis is physiological, resulting in the *appropriate* excretion of the excesses of salt and water retained during the period of obstruction. When extracellular volume and composition return to normal, the diuresis usually abates spontaneously. Therefore, replacement of urinary losses should serve only to prevent hypovolemia, hypotension, or disturbances in serum electrolyte concentrations. Occasionally, iatrogenic expansion of extracellular volume, secondary to administration of excessive quantities of intravenous fluids, is responsible for, or sustains, the diuresis observed in the postobstructive period. Replacement of no more than two-thirds of urinary volume losses per day is usually effective in avoiding this complication. In a rare patient, however, relief of obstruction may be followed by urinary salt and water losses severe enough to provoke profound dehydration and vascular collapse. In these patients, an intrinsic defect in tubule reabsorptive function is probably responsible for the marked diuresis. Appropriate therapy in such patients includes intravenous administration of large quantities of salt-containing solutions to replace sodium and volume deficits.

REFERENCES

GUGGENHEIM SJ, SCHRIER RW: Obstructive nephropathy: Pathophysiology and management, in *Renal and Electrolyte Disorders*, 2d ed, RW Schrier (ed). Boston, Little, Brown, 1980

HARRIS RH, YARGER WE: The pathogenesis of post-obstructive diuresis. J Clin Invest 56:880, 1975

KAYE AD, POLLACK HM: Diagnostic imaging approach to the patient with obstructive uropathy. Semin Nephrol 2:55, 1982

WILSON DR: Renal function during and following obstruction. Annu Rev Med 28:329, 1977

WRIGHT FS, HOWARDS SS: Obstructive injury, in *The Kidney*, 2d ed, BM Brenner, FC Rector Jr (eds). Philadelphia, Saunders, 1981, chap 38

302
TUMORS OF THE URINARY TRACT

BARRY M. BRENNER
H. DAVID HUMES
EDGAR L. MILFORD

TUMORS OF THE KIDNEY

BENIGN RENAL TUMORS Several benign tumors are known to arise in renal parenchyma. They usually remain small in size and are recognized as incidental findings at autopsy or nephrectomy, the latter performed for other reasons. *Adenomas* are the most common benign renal tumors, occurring as small (5- to 10-mm) nodules in from 10 to 20 percent of all kidneys examined grossly. With other less frequently encountered benign lesions, including hamartomas (angiomyolipomas) and hemangiopericytomas, adenomas may be responsible for recurrent painless hematuria. Since adenomas are believed to undergo malignant transformation and are histologically indistinguishable from some renal-cell carcinomas, nephrectomy is appropriate when they are detected clinically. *Hamartomas* are observed commonly in patients with tuberous sclerosis but also occur in individuals without this ectodermal defect. Hamartomas may be unilateral or bilateral, contain vascular, fat, and smooth-muscle components, and rarely, if ever, undergo malignant change. By angiography, these highly vascular lesions often reveal multiple small arterial aneurysms. *Hemangiopericytomas* are uncommon benign renal tumors arising from capillary pericytes in the region of the juxtaglomerular apparatus. They have been associated with increased renin production and hypertension, both of which usually disappear with resection of the tumor.

MALIGNANT RENAL TUMORS **Renal-cell carcinoma (hypernephroma, adenocarcinoma of kidney)** This is the most common renal neoplasm, occurring almost exclusively in adults over age 20. The yellow color of this fleshy tumor initially led to the erroneous impression that it arises from "adrenal rests"—hence the term *hypernephroma.* Instead, renal-cell carcinoma is of tubular epithelial origin, with tumor cells often arranged in a tubular or cord-like distribution.

CLINICAL FEATURES Renal-cell carcinoma has been called the "internist's tumor" because the lesion is often diagnosed, even in the absence of metastases, from *systemic* rather than urologic manifestations. The triad of *gross hematuria, flank pain,* and a *palpable abdominal mass,* although considered as classic evidence for the clinical diagnosis of renal-cell carcinoma, is encountered relatively infrequently, appearing in less than 10 percent of cases. Clinically, the most common presenting abnormality is *hematuria,* which occurs in about 60 percent of cases. Unfortunately, although microscopic hematuria is a consistent abnormality of the urinary sediment examination, bleeding is not usually evident grossly, so that the tumor often grows to large size before symptoms appear. These include pain and a sensation of fullness in the flank. By this time, the tumor has often invaded the renal capsule and local renal veins which provide the main route to distant metastases, especially to lungs, brain, and bone. Local spread to liver and perirenal lymph nodes is also common.

Systemic symptoms of *fatigability, weight loss,* and *cachexia* are found in about half the patients with renal-cell carcinoma. *Intermittent fever,* unassociated with evidence of infection, occurs occasionally and may be the only sign of this renal neoplasm. *Anemia* is common and is a presenting sign in approximately 50 percent of cases. *Erythrocytosis,* on the other hand, seen in about 5 percent of patients, is almost certainly due to erythropoietin production by tumor cells. *Eosinophilia, leukemoid reactions, thrombocytosis,* and *increased erythrocyte sedimentation rate* are other hematologic abnormalities associated with this tumor. Renal-cell carcinomas are capable of producing a number of hormones or hormone-like substances, including *parathyroid hormone* and *prostaglandins* (which, in turn, may lead to hypercalcemia), *prolactin* (galactorrhea), *renin* (hypertension), *gonadotropins* (feminization or masculinization), and *glucocorticoids* (Cushing's syndrome). In very vascular tumors, *intrarenal arteriovenous fistulas* may predispose to high-output congestive heart failure. Tumor invasion of the renal vein and inferior vena cava may result in symptomatic left *varicocele* and *dependent edema,* respectively. Alternatively, hepatic vein occlusion by tumor, with or without vena caval obstruction, may lead to *hepatosplenomegaly* and *ascites* formation. Reversible disturbances in liver function are sometimes found in affected patients, even in the absence of liver metastases. These include Bromsulphalein retention, elevated alkaline phosphatase, hypoalbuminemia, and prolongation of the prothrombin time. Finally, nearly two-thirds of patients with von Hippel-Lindau disease, characterized by hereditary vascular malformations of the retina and cerebellum, develop renal-cell carcinomas, which are often multiple and bilateral.

DIAGNOSIS Although intrarenal calcifications and/or alterations in renal contours seen on the abdominal scout film may suggest the presence of a renal-cell carcinoma, excretion urography (with nephrotomography) is the primary examination by which most renal masses are detected and initially evaluated. In this evaluation, it is essential to differentiate between benign cystic lesions and renal neoplasms. Cysts are usually radiolucent and exhibit a thin, well-defined margin, whereas carcinomas tend to have thick, irregular walls and are usually radiopaque. Ultrasound studies of the kidney provide additional means for distinguishing between cyst and tumor since the latter are far more echogenic than the former. Since cystic necrosis can occur within an otherwise solid tumor and a tumor can arise from the wall of a cyst, all sonolucent masses should be evaluated by percutaneous needle aspiration, under ultrasonic guidance, and the collected fluid submitted to cytologic examination and lipid analysis. Renal neoplasms tend to have a high content of neutral fats, phospholipids, and cholesterol. Contrast material should also be injected into the cyst cavity to evaluate the wall contour, which is usually irregular in carcinomas.

Masses which are found to be radiopaque by pyelography are best evaluated by selective renal angiography, which reveals abnormal tumor vessels (neovascularization) in approximately 95 percent of patients with renal-cell carcinoma. Other renal arteriographic abnormalities associated with this neoplasm include arteriovenous communications (pooling of contrast media in venous sinusoids within the tumor mass) and evidence of tumor invasion of the major renal veins and inferior vena cava. Whereas nontumor vasculature undergoes brisk vasoconstriction in response to local renal arterial infusion of epinephrine, the abnormal tumor vessels fail to constrict and, therefore, persist as a "tumor blush" when epinephrine is infused. Computer-assisted tomography also gives detailed information about the three-dimensional relationship of the mass to perirenal structures and is therefore a very useful adjunct to arteriography. Indeed, urological surgeons have recently begun to substitute the CT scan for the arteriogram in the preoperative evaluation of the patient with an echogenic renal mass.

Examination of urinary cytology, although useful in the diagnosis of neoplasms of the renal pelvis, ureter, and bladder, has not been helpful in renal-cell carcinoma. Once the diagnosis of renal-cell carcinoma is established, chest x-ray and scans of bone, liver, and brain should be obtained to evaluate the possibility of metastatic involvement.

PROGNOSIS AND TREATMENT The prognosis in patients with renal-cell carcinoma is largely dependent upon the extent of tumor involvement at the time of diagnosis. The current overall 5-year survival rate is about 45 percent. If distant metastases are not evident, this survival rate increases to nearly 65 percent. The conventional approach to treatment in patients without evidence of metastases is *radical nephrectomy.* An aggressive approach has also been endorsed by some surgeons for patients having evidence of a solitary metastasis. Although scattered reports in the literature suggest the possibility of spontaneous regression of various metastatic foci following surgical removal of the primary lesion, it is generally believed that nephrectomy in patients with disseminated disease should be employed mainly to relieve symptoms resulting from the primary tumor, such as severe pain or bleeding. The response of metastatic renal-cell carcinoma to treatment with chemotherapy, hormonal agents, or radiotherapy has generally been unsatisfactory.

Nephroblastoma (Wilms's tumor) Nephroblastoma is the second most common malignant tumor of the kidney and is the most common malignancy of the urinary tract in children. Fewer than 150 cases have been reported in adults. The tumor often reaches very large size, may be bilateral, and presents as a palpable mass in 50 percent or more of cases. Hematuria, pain, fever, and hypertension are other common abnormalities noted at time of diagnosis. All these manifestations of nephroblastoma respond favorably to nephrectomy. Although once considered an incurable tumor, aggressive programs of pre- and postoperative irradiation and postoperative chemotherapy with actinomycin D (often in combination with vincristine) have improved the prognosis markedly, and the 5-year survival now exceeds 75 percent.

TUMORS OF THE URINARY COLLECTING SYSTEM

Tumors of the renal pelvis, ureter, and urinary bladder, derived from transitional epithelia, account for 10 to 15 percent of all primary malignancies in adults. These *urothelial* carcinomas are multicentric in nature and often occur (and recur) at multiple sites in the lower urinary tract in an affected patient. The wall of the urinary bladder is the most common site of involvement. Epidemiologic studies have confirmed a markedly increased incidence of bladder cancer in workers exposed to various aromatic amines employed in the dyeing, chemical, and rubber industries. It has been suggested that exposure to synthetic sweeteners, food colors, tobacco, and coffee may account for a large proportion of other cases.

Hematuria is the sole presenting complaint in nearly all cases, irrespective of the exact level of urinary tract involvement. When the tumor arises in the renal pelvis or upper ureter, gross hematuria may be associated with signs and symptoms of *ureteral colic,* due to obstruction by blood clots. Intravenous and/or retrograde pyelography, cystoscopy with biopsy, and urine cytology are the main approaches to establishing the site, nature, and extent of involvement of tumors of the collecting system. Endoscopic brush biopsy is used for upper tract lesions. Urothelial tumors tend to spread by local invasion. Prognosis is, therefore, dependent upon extent of invasion and degree of anaplasia at time of diagnosis, with patients with bladder carcinoma having less than a 30 percent chance for 5-year survival when tumor extends beyond the bladder wall. The prognosis is considerably better when the tumor is confined to the bladder and is treated with cystectomy, usually in combination with local radiotherapy. Nephroureterectomy is the treatment of choice for urothelial tumors of the renal pelvis or ureter.

Squamous-cell carcinoma is a less frequent neoplasm of the renal pelvis than is the papillary, transitional-cell variety and has an extremely poor prognosis. Squamous-cell tumors have been shown to occur more commonly in patients with recurrent nephrolithiasis and upper urinary tract infections. A high incidence of bladder cancer of the squamous type has been found in patients with chronic parasitic infestation due to *Schistosoma haematobium.*

Benign hypertrophy and adenocarcinoma of the prostate, extremely common disorders in men beyond age 50, are considered in Chap. 117.

REFERENCES

CAMPBELL MF, HARRISON JH (eds): *Urology,* 4th ed. Philadelphia, Saunders, 1978

CRONIN RE et al: Renal cell carcinoma: Unusual systemic manifestations. Medicine 55:291, 1976

RICHIE JP, SKINNER DG: Renal neoplasia, in *The Kidney,* 2d ed, BM Brenner, FC Rector Jr (eds). Philadelphia, Saunders, 1981, chap 40

RIESELBACH RE, GARNICK MG (eds): *Cancer and the Kidney.* Philadelphia, Lea & Febiger, 1982

STANLEY RJ et al: Computed tomography of the genitourinary tract. J Urol 119:780, 1978

section 5 | Disorders of the alimentary tract

303 APPROACH TO THE PATIENT WITH GASTROINTESTINAL DISEASE

KURT J. ISSELBACHER
ROGER J. MAY

GENERAL CONSIDERATIONS Gastrointestinal symptoms occur not only with primary gastrointestinal tract disease but frequently as manifestations of other systemic diseases. Thus anorexia, nausea, and vomiting may be seen in congestive failure and uremia, and diarrhea or constipation may be seen as a consequence of metabolic derangements such as electrolyte changes or alterations in thyroid function. With today's technical advances one finds too often that the physician is willing to diagnose (or misdiagnose) gastrointestinal disease simply by relying on routine x-ray studies of the upper and lower parts of the gastrointestinal tract. Such an overwhelming dependence on technical procedures often leads to great pitfalls. In order to define the most probable and profitable area to study, the proper approach requires careful attention to the history and physical examination before ordering the appropriate diagnostic tests.

IMPORTANCE OF THE HISTORY To evaluate gastrointestinal symptoms, a careful history is crucial. Pain or indigestion is the most common intestinal complaint. Correlation between pain and gastrointestinal function must of necessity be chronologic. There should be a meticulous inquiry as to the frequency and specificity of the complaint. The questioning should include the location of the pain and whether it is circumscribed or diffuse. It is important to determine what factors aggravate or relieve the discomfort. *Does eating produce the symptom?* If so, determine whether the discomfort occurs *while eating* (as in esophageal disorders and abdominal angina), shortly *after the meal* (as often occurs in biliary tract disease), or *30 to 90 min later* (as typically seen with peptic ulcer). *Does eating relieve the symptom,* and if so, for how long? Temporary relief of epigastric pain is characteristic of gastritis and peptic ulceration. Many patients have tried or taken antacids by the time they come to the physician, and a history indicating relief of epigastric pain by antacids is suggestive of peptic disease of the upper part of the intestine. *What is the relation of pain to bowel movements?* The patient with ulcerative colitis often obtains temporary relief from lower abdominal cramps by defecation.

Attention should be paid to *anorexia* and weight *loss;* their combined occurrence should make one suspicious of an underlying malignancy. If weight loss is accompanied by an increased appetite, one must consider the diagnosis of malabsorption or maldigestion as well as a hypermetabolic state, such as thyrotoxicosis. If *diarrhea* is present, one should determine the average number of the stools, their consistency, and their timing. To some patients, diarrhea means an increased number of stools, even though they are relatively normal in consistency; to others, diarrhea means watery stools. The occurrence of nocturnal diarrhea is suggestive of organic rather than functional bowel disease. In a patient with diarrhea one should ask about stool *odor* (malodorous stools being typical of pancreatic insufficiency and sprue), change in stool *color* (light-colored stools are seen with steatorrhea or cholestasis), and whether blood or mucus has been noted (blood is characteristic of ulcerative colitis but is hardly ever noted in functional bowel disease).

Finally, careful attention must be given to a "drug history." We are living in a "medicated society." Unless asked, patients may forget to mention that they take aspirin almost daily for headache, and this may indeed account for occult blood in the stool. Many patients take daily laxatives, which may explain chronic diarrhea and colonic changes on x-ray.

PHYSICAL EXAMINATION AND ENDOSCOPY A vague history of abdominal distress may be brought into focus by a thorough physical examination. Upper abdominal distress together with tenderness in the right upper quadrant suggests that cholecystitis or hepatitis may be present. The history of intermittent abdominal pain together with a palpable mass or tender loop of bowel in the right lower quadrant should make one suspicious of regional enteritis. All too often, however, in gastrointestinal diseases the routine physical examination is negative, and other techniques for examining the intestine are needed. Among the techniques which should almost be routine as an extension of the physical examination is *sigmoidoscopy*. This technique is important in the diagnosis of colonic cancer because (1) approximately 50 percent of large-intestine malignancies are within the reach of the sigmoidoscope; and (2) small rectosigmoid tumors may be missed on examination after a barium enema because of the tortuosity and redundancy of the intestine in this area. Sigmoidoscopy also permits inspection of the mucosa for edema, erythema, friability, or ulceration. In a patient with diarrhea due to nonspecific causes, the mucosa may be normal; with dysentery due to agents such as *Shigella*, the mucosa may become friable, edematous, and hyperemic; if the latter findings are combined with extensive ulcerations, ulcerative or amebic colitis may be present.

With the advent of *fiberoptic instruments*, it has become much easier and less hazardous to perform endoscopic procedures. Gastroscopy is valuable in helping to determine whether a gastric ulcer is benign or malignant. Endoscopy has become an increasingly routine technique in the approach to selected patients with upper gastrointestinal bleeding. Colonoscopy with fiberoptic equipment permits direct examination of mucosa beyond the customary 25 cm of the rigid sigmoidoscope. (For details see Chap. 304.)

RADIOLOGIC EXAMINATION Perhaps in no other organ system is the use of x-ray examination as important to diagnosis as in disorders of the intestinal tract. In fact, with few exceptions, investigation of the patient with gastrointestinal symptoms is not complete without appropriate x-ray examination. However, all too often x-ray examination is ordered by the physician without attention to a number of important factors.

Initial considerations by the internist To obtain the best and most effective use of gastrointestinal x-rays, the physician must decide (1) which *organ system* is most likely to be involved, (2) in what *sequence* to perform the x-rays, and (3) whether there are any *contraindications* to the proposed radiologic study.

After ordering an upper gastrointestinal series and finding the results negative, the physician may decide to order a barium enema only to learn that it must be delayed because of the presence of barium from the prior study. Therefore, if a thorough study of the intestinal tract is contemplated, the sequence should be (1) oral cholecystogram, (2) barium enema, and (3) upper gastrointestinal series. Preparation or prior cleansing of the intestinal tract is important for a proper barium enema examination, but the physician must keep in mind that with obstructing lesions of the colon or small intestine or in the presence of active ulcerative colitis, the use of strong cathartics may be hazardous and even life-threatening. *No x-ray preparation should be considered routine.* In fact, the barium examination itself may aggravate an acute ulcerative colitis or precipitate colonic perforation or the onset of toxic megacolon. Similarly, if partial obstruction of the intestine is detected by plain x-ray of the abdomen, the physician must be wary of introducing barium from above for fear of producing further or complete intestinal obstruction.

Consultation with the radiologist One cannot overemphasize the importance of providing the radiologist with as much information as possible about the nature of the disease process under investigation. Though this can be done in writing (on the x-ray requisition), it is often preferable to do it verbally. In fact, in difficult cases it is advantageous for the physician to join the radiologist during the study. In addition, the radiologist may suggest, for example, that instead of barium an iodinated radiopaque dye may be preferable; that the study should be supplemented with angiography, especially in the patient with gastrointestinal bleeding or portal hypertension; or that the examination be repeated with more adequate preparation of the patient.

Interpretation All too often the busy physician allows a negative x-ray report to be the decisive factor in the diagnosis. If the patient has had weight loss and a change in bowel habits and the physician suspects a colonic neoplasm, inspection of the x-rays (personally or preferably with the radiologist) may in fact reveal that the patient had too much retained fecal material in his colon or that the area of concern was never well visualized. Similarly, if the patient has typical ulcer symptoms or a classic history of biliary colic, the physician should not discard the diagnosis merely because of a negative x-ray report.

On the other hand the physician must be able to determine whether the abnormal finding is causally related to the symptoms. This is especially true in older patients where the presence of a hiatus hernia, gallstones, or diverticulosis is not unusual and hence may be coincidental.

DIAGNOSTIC APPROACHES Problems of swallowing The approach should be as follows:

1 Careful visual and *neurologic examination* of the pharynx, with tests for myasthenia gravis if indicated.
2 *Routine esophageal x-rays* in the upright and lateral or Trendelenburg position. The horizontal views are essential for demonstration of the swallowing mechanism, unaided by gravity, and of the esophagogastric junction. For details of the pharyngoesophageal area cineradiography is necessary because of the rapidity with which the contrast media passes through. Hiatus hernia is extremely common (in 15 to 35 percent of persons over 50) and often asymptomatic unless spontaneous reflux of gastric contents can be demonstrated to occur repeatedly.
3 *Esophagoscopy* is desirable to describe lesions suggested by x-ray, or if the lesion is unsuspected, to obtain biopsies from masses or abnormal mucosa, and to obtain washings for exfoliative cytologic study. The diagnosis of peptic esophagitis is best made endoscopically. Esophageal varices can be identified by this approach when they are too small to be seen radiologically, although the latter technique will pick up 70 percent of large varices.
4 *Manometric studies* of the upper esophagus, particularly in conjunction with cineradiography, at present offer the best differential between disorders primary in the central nervous

system, primary pharyngeal muscular disease, and cricopharyngeal dystonia. Manometry of the lower esophagus is useful in the diagnosis of diffuse esophageal spasm, achalasia, and infiltrative diseases which can alter esophageal motility.

Peptic or digestive disorders The approaches to these disorders include:

1 *Insertion of a nasogastric tube.* This is used to establish whether significant gastric retention (more than 75 ml of gastric contents in the fasting state) exists, and whether there is acid, bile, blood, or other material in these contents. If pyloric obstruction or gastric atony is present, the tube is used to maintain suction while the patient's electrolyte and fluid balance is restored to normal; the stomach is kept as clean as possible so that reliable radiologic investigation may be carried out.
2 *Radiologic examination* of stomach, duodenum, and the upper part of the jejunum is the most important single procedure in this area. The single examination of the stomach carries an overall accuracy of about 80 percent if the lumen is carefully cleaned out beforehand; duodenal lesions are most precisely identified (90 percent). However, gastritis and superficial ulcers of the duodenum may be missed with routine barium studies.
3 When lesions are noted radiographically in the stomach, *upper intestinal endoscopy* may be very helpful in identifying the diffuseness of the mucosal response in gastritis or, together with biopsy and brushings for cytology, in differentiating between peptic and neoplastic ulcerating lesions. Gastroscopy may permit the diagnosis of superficial erosive gastritis and the Mallory-Weiss syndrome as a cause of bleeding when the x-ray examination is negative. It may identify a specific bleeding site in clinical situations where several potential bleeding sites could exist, such as in the patient with portal hypertension. Gastroscopy is also particularly helpful in inspecting the postoperative stomach, especially in detecting stomal ulceration or alkaline reflux gastritis. The first and second portions of the duodenum can also be examined with the fiberoptic gastroscope, and important information about ulcers and other lesions can be obtained by this procedure.
4 *Gastric acid secretory studies* are useful in the diagnosis of the Zollinger-Ellison syndrome or atrophic gastritis, and for determination of completeness of vagotomy. Suspected gastric carcinoma is better diagnosed directly through gastroscopy and biopsy than indirectly through acid secretory studies (achlorhydria). They should not be obtained for the routine diagnosis of uncomplicated duodenal ulcer. There is no convincing evidence that acid studies are useful in determining the type of surgery for duodenal ulcer.

The only reliable technique for measuring rates of gastric acid production employs an indwelling tube and requires careful attention to details of tube placement, handling of samples, and analysis. Presently this method is used in one of two ways: (1) *Basal secretion* is that obtained in the morning after an overnight fast in an unstimulated stomach; it measures vagal plus hormonal factors acting on the gastric mucosa. After discarding the first aspirate, four samples are taken over a period of an hour, while the patient expectorates any saliva. (2) *Maximum acid output* is assessed by collecting samples every 15 min for an hour in a patient who has previously received the histamine analogue betazole parenterally (2 mg/kg). Alternatively, one may give pentagastrin (6 μg/kg) intramuscularly. With these drugs one attempts to obtain maximal stimulation of parietal cells. The maximum output is proportional to the total "parietal cell mass." Achlorhydria is defined as the failure of the stomach so stimulated to produce a juice with a pH less than 6. The normal basal fasting secretion is 30 to 70 ml/h, with acid production being 1 to 5 meq/h. Average maximal acid output is 20 meq/h with the upper limit of normal approximately 40 meq/h. The finding of undetectable basal acid secretion or a maximal acid secretion less than 12.5 meq/h is considered incompatible with active duodenal ulcer disease. In the Zollinger-Ellison syndrome basal acid secretion is usually greater than 10 meq/h and exceeds 60 percent of the maximal acid output. Increased serum gastrin level may confirm the diagnosis.

Obstructive and vascular disorders of the small intestine When intestinal problems present as obstructive syndromes, the plain x-ray of the abdomen is the most important diagnostic adjunct to careful physical examination. Patterns of dilatation of individual loops of intestine may be characteristic, as in volvulus or acute pancreatitis; erect and decubitus views will often show fluid levels in the affected segments. Air under the diaphragm is diagnostic of a perforated viscus; air in the portal vein usually results from intestinal necrosis secondary to mesenteric vascular occlusion. The diagnostic accuracy of the plain x-ray in all types of intestinal obstruction is about 75 percent. Celiac artery angiography is of particular value in the diagnosis of mesenteric vascular disease.

Inflammatory and neoplastic diseases of small and large intestine Patients with these conditions are usually identified by history, physical examination, and careful examination of the stools for exudate and blood. Sigmoidoscopy is valuable in identifying mucosal and neoplastic lesions of the lower 25 cm of the colon. The mucosal surface of the entire colon and terminal ileum can be examined directly and biopsied through the fiberoptic colonoscope. This technique is valuable in differentiating between inflammatory and neoplastic stricture, or in evaluating polypoid lesions beyond the reach of the sigmoidoscope. The radiologic examination of the small intestine is highly reliable in identifying the prestenotic and stenotic lesions of Crohn's disease. In the colon a single examination in a well-prepared patient has a diagnostic accuracy of 80 to 85 percent; the addition of air-contrast technique brings the accuracy up over 90 percent, but none of these figures is meaningful if the patient is poorly prepared for the examination. In the demonstration of small polyps the degree of accuracy is understandably not so high, but for polyps larger than 1 cm, which are of greater clinical importance, it is satisfactory. The cecal area is the hardest to examine adequately because of its anatomy; flat plaquelike lesions on the posterior wall are particularly hard to demonstrate. The rectal area is usually better visualized proctoscopically than it is radiologically. The immunologic assay for the carcinoembryonic antigen has not proved to be specific for colonic cancer; nevertheless, it does contribute to the evaluation of the extent of tumor and to the detection of residual or recurrent disease in postoperative patients.

Peroral biopsy of the small intestine and forceps biopsy of the rectosigmoid are of considerable importance in revealing mucosal disease. Rectal biopsy is an excellent means of demonstrating amyloidosis, schistosomiasis, and amebiasis. Submucosal disease is not seen in these superficial biopsies. Hirschsprung's disease is histologically diagnosed by a deep surgical biopsy of the lower part of the rectum.

Malabsorption syndromes Malabsorption may be suspected on the basis of history and physical examination and is confirmed by examination of the stools. Radiologic examination is of general help in ruling out local lesions and suggesting motor and secretory dysfunction, but it is rarely diagnostic unless an abnormal small-bowel mucosa or fistulas between intestine and stomach are demonstrated.

The tests useful in the diagnosis of malabsorption are discussed in Chap. 307. A simple screening test for excessive fat in the stools can be accomplished by the microscopic examination of a stool specimen stained with Sudan. Chemical analysis of 3-day stool collection for fat, with the patient on a standard diet, is used to establish the diagnosis of malabsorption. The D-xylose absorption test is about 90 percent accurate in separating mucosal disease from pancreatic insufficiency. Peroral biopsy of the small intestine is of value in the diagnosis of celiac disease, and may show the less common infiltrations of the mucosa by amyloid or bacterial mucoproteins (Whipple's disease). Leakage of protein into the intestinal lumen may cause hypoproteinemia and can be demonstrated by the recovery in stools of intravenously administered markers such as albumin labeled with iodine or chromium isotopes.

Pancreas The pancreas is difficult to study directly because of its anatomic location and relative inaccessibility. Calcification of the pancreas on a plain abdominal film is highly suggestive of chronic pancreatitis and may be associated with fat malabsorption. Pancreatic exocrine insufficiency can be documented by intubation of the duodenum and collection of pancreatic juice after stimulation with secretin or a test meal. The pancreatic duct can be cannulated via the fiberoptic duodenoscope; pancreatic juice can then be collected for cytology, or the duct visualized by the injection of a radiopaque dye. This latter is helpful in the diagnosis of pancreatic tumors and cysts. Angiography, abdominal ultrasound, and computerized tomography may also be useful in the diagnosis of pancreatic disease. See Chaps. 324 and 325.

304 GASTROINTESTINAL ENDOSCOPY

FRED E. SILVERSTEIN
CYRUS E. RUBIN

Fiberendoscopes have revolutionized the examination of the gastrointestinal tract. Because of the flexibility of the fiberoptic bundles and because of controllability of the instrument tip, the operator can steer the instrument around multiple bends under visual control. A side channel permits passage of a variety of endoscopic tools such as biopsy forceps, foreign-body forceps, cytology brushes, wash tubes, and electrocautery snares. The viewing window and the light at the instrument's distal end can be washed free of obscuring material. Fluid can be aspirated from hollow organs, and air can be insufflated as needed to improve visualization.

The usefulness of fiberendoscopy in diagnosing gastrointestinal disease is well established. Shallow lesions such as erosions or healing ulcers are missed by single-contrast x-ray but not by endoscopy. The brilliant success of polypectomy via the colonoscope has led to the development of other endoscopic methods of treatment which may replace some invasive surgical techniques; the most significant advances in the future will probably be in this area.

Although esophagogastroduodenoscopy (EGD) is not a procedure for the occasional operator, it should be available in every general hospital. It is a relatively easy procedure to perform technically, but training and continued experience are necessary for optimal diagnostic accuracy. Complications are most frequent when the operator is inexperienced. Before the procedure the competent endoscopist always takes a history and examines the patient. Prior evaluation of cardiac status and clotting mechanisms is also essential.

The more complex procedures such as colonoscopy and endoscopic retrograde cholangiopancreatography (ERCP) require special dexterity, a substantial investment of time for learning, and constant practice to maintain adequate skill; they are probably best accomplished by subspecialists. Colonoscopy, one hopes, will be simplified so that it can be as widely available as esophagogastroduodenoscopy.

UPPER GASTROINTESTINAL ENDOSCOPY Forward-viewing, oblique, and side-viewing instruments may be used for EGD. After a careful explanation of the procedure to the patient, pharyngeal topical anesthesia with viscous lidocaine is followed by intravenous diazepam to the point of mild sedation. With the newer, small-caliber instruments less or no diazepam is needed. The tip of the endoscope is placed at the upper cricopharyngeal sphincter of the esophagus and the patient is encouraged to swallow while gentle pressure is exerted. Small amounts of air are passed through the endoscope to visualize the esophageal lumen. The endoscope is then passed under direct vision into the stomach. The gastric body and antrum are carefully examined. The instrument tip is retroflexed to view the gastric cardia and the whole lesser curvature. The pylorus is traversed, and the first and second portions of the duodenum are visualized. The whole examination is repeated as the instrument is withdrawn. Visualized lesions can be recorded on still photographs, movies, or videotape. Biopsies and brush cytological examinations can be obtained from suspicious areas.

EGD is a relatively safe procedure in experienced hands. Several large surveys suggest a risk of serious complications during diagnostic EGD of approximately 1 in 500 and a risk of death of approximately 1 in 5000. The risks are higher in emergency procedures and in the elderly or seriously ill. In a survey of patients examined by endoscopy during bleeding, 1 in 200 had serious complications and 1 in 700 died from the procedure. A nationwide survey revealed a morbidity of 0.13 percent and a mortality of 0.004 percent. The main causes of mortality were cardiopulmonary complications and perforations by the instrument. Upper endoscopy is usually substituted for x-ray in the urgent diagnosis of gastrointestinal illness in women who might be pregnant.

Peptic regurgitant esophagitis Esophagitis is one of the commonest benign diseases of the upper gastrointestinal tract. Esophageal pain may be confused with cardiac disease, or esophagitis may present as painless blood loss. Because esophagitis usually involves only the superficial mucosa, it cannot be diagnosed by routine single-contrast x-ray. At endoscopy, the diffuse bleeding, linear erosions, friability, and ulcerations of erosive esophagitis are clearly visible. Not every patient with heartburn requires esophagoscopy, but the procedure is indicated if x-ray shows a stricture, a mass, or an ulcer, if the patient's symptoms persist despite therapy, or if antireflux surgery is contemplated.

The squamous mucosa of the esophagus is far more vulnerable to peptic digestion than the columnar epithelium of the stomach. Thus, bleeding esophagitis is located on the squamous side of the esophagogastric junction and is most severe in the distal esophagus where the squamous mucosa is most exposed to regurgitated acid and pepsin from the stomach. Discrete peptic ulceration of the esophagus is uncommon.

A short area of esophagitis or a stricture can be seen at levels as high as the arch of the aorta. This is explained by progressive replacement of distal eroded squamous mucosa with metaplastic gastric epithelium, which is more resistant to peptic digestion (Barrett's epithelium). This finding can be documented by biopsy. Such epithelium is more prone to malignant transformation and, therefore, may merit regular surveillance with esophagoscopy and/or exfoliative cytology every 12 to 24 months.

Esophagitis may progress to scarring and stricture formation. The endoscopic appearance of a benign stricture is characteristic but not diagnostic because a malignancy can be missed and should be ruled out before medical treatment is undertaken with dilation and antacids; therefore, the whole length of the stricture should be sampled by biopsy and cytological brushing to rule out cancer, if necessary, at repeat endoscopy after dilatation. Endoscopy is often indicated in an esophageal ulcer, with biopsy of the rim of the ulcer to rule out cancer.

Dilations of difficult strictures are best initiated by passing a flexible-tipped guide wire via the side channel of the endoscope through the stricture under direct vision. The endoscope can then be withdrawn over the wire, which serves as a guide for passage of progressively larger metal olives through the stricture under fluoroscopic control.

Peptic ulcer It is now generally agreed that esophagogastroduodenoscopy is more accurate than upper gastrointestinal x-ray in detecting ulcers. It has been suggested that x-ray be abandoned entirely in favor of endoscopy for detecting ulcers. This makes sense when seeking the source of acute upper gastrointestinal bleeding if urgent surgical intervention is being considered; in such situations, obscuring barium would make endoscopy impossible. However, in the workup of the patient with less pressing ulcer complaints, an upper gastrointestinal x-ray is still often used as the initial diagnostic test. As more radiologists routinely use air contrast to obtain better mucosal detail, diagnostic sensitivity for superficial lesions will increase. The greater expense and discomfort of endoscopy are justified if the x-ray is equivocal, if the ulcer is possibly malignant, if the x-ray is negative but the clinical picture is suggestive of peptic ulceration, or if the patient is about to be operated for ulcer and there is a need to be sure that an ulcer is present and that other lesions have not been missed. Patients with duodenal ulcers by x-ray or with classic ulcer deformities of the duodenal bulb do not require endoscopy for diagnosis if the presenting symptoms are characteristic and if the symptomatic response to strict antacid or cimetidine treatment is good. Some feel that screening endoscopy using the new small-diameter endoscopes may be the preferable initial approach to the symptomatic patient. These instruments can be passed easily, often without sedation, for rapid and complete upper gastrointestinal examinations. When used in this manner the cost of the endoscopy should be reduced.

There are some situations in which x-ray reveals ulcers missed by endoscopy, e.g., ulcers in hourglass constrictions of the stomach or in small duodenal bulbs incompletely visualized by currently available instruments. Fiberendoscopy is especially useful in visualizing postbulbar ulcers, giant duodenal ulcers, and stomal ulceration after partial gastrectomy, all of which can be missed by x-ray. Endoscopy may be of use in determining the cause of gastric outlet obstruction. In most circumstances, patients with duodenal ulcers do not need another endoscopy to see if the ulcer has healed.

In the enthusiasm for fiberendoscopy one must not forget that visual interpretation of gross pathology is subjective—one observer's ulcer is another's erosion. An erosion is confined to the mucosa and heals without a trace, whereas an ulcer is deeper and usually implies a chronic recurrent disease. Endoscopically, erosions are superficial, small, and multiple; ulcers are deeper and larger and tend to be solitary. In the future it is likely that lesions seen endoscopically will be easily recorded for review on videotape or disk, just as currently all lesions seen fluoroscopically are demonstrated in spot films.

Cancer The endoscopic appearance of upper gastrointestinal cancer may seem obvious, especially if there is a mass growing into the lumen. On the other hand, malignant ulcers, infiltrative carcinomas, or small early carcinomas are frequently impossible to diagnose by their gross appearance. The biopsies obtained with currently available forceps are very small, and deeper lesions can be missed. Only one of multiple biopsies may reveal the cancer. Therefore, it is recommended that six to eight biopsies be taken from the rim of a gastric ulcer. A larger particle of tissue may be removed from a suspicious elevated mucosal lesion with an electrocautery snare or with a "jumbo" biopsy forceps passed via the large channel of a special endoscope, and this may facilitate diagnosis. Experience and skill in choosing the biopsy site improve the accuracy. An exfoliative or cytological examination of the lavage or brush specimen adds to the diagnostic accuracy in all areas of the upper gastrointestinal tract (see Chap. 307).

It may be impossible to differentiate severe esophagitis from infiltrative cancer by the gross appearance at esophagoscopy. Biopsies from patients with cancer may show only the associated inflammation. Thus, all such lesions should have careful cytological examination, either by lavage or by brushing. Because chronic inflammation may predispose to esophageal cancer, patients with lye stricture, peptic regurgitant esophagitis, or the stasis esophagitis of achalasia merit esophagoscopy and cytological examination when they are first seen and whenever their symptom patterns change.

Radiological demonstration of healing of a benign-appearing gastric ulcer is very reassuring but not infallible in excluding cancer. A history of ingesting ulcerogenic drugs increases the likelihood of benignancy. Often ulcers in such patients are followed to complete healing radiologically after discontinuing the ulcerogenic drug. Diagnostic accuracy in differentiating benign from malignant gastric ulcer by exfoliative cytological lavage, endoscopic biopsy, or brush cytology depends very much upon the combined skills of endoscopists, cytologists, and pathologists. Among North American communities accuracy in diagnosing cancer may vary from 70 to 90 percent. Physicians must individually decide which patients should be examined by methods that have proved accurate in their own community, and which patients should be referred to centers with greater resources. The effort expended in diagnosing gastric cancer tends to be proportional to the frequency of the disease in a community. What is done in Japan may not be justified in the United States (see Chap. 307).

Primary gastric lymphoma is a diagnosis well worth making because the 5-year survival rate is far higher than for adenocarcinoma. It can mimic benign gastric ulcer or adenocarcinoma by gastroscopy or x-ray. It can be diagnosed by biopsy or cytology, although the accuracy is not as high as in adenocarcinoma.

If a polypoid lesion of the stomach is covered by mucosa that appears normal by gastroscopy, the likelihood of malignancy is very small. Such lesions are often intramural, extramucosal benign tumors such as leiomyomas or pancreatic rests. Polyps covered by abnormal-appearing mucosa can be benign or malignant. Random biopsy can miss carcinoma within a polyp. If technically feasible, polyps should, therefore, be removed in their entirety by snare cautery for histological examination. If over 2 cm in diameter, they are more likely to contain cancer (see Chap. 307).

Ampullary carcinoma may be diagnosed by biopsy and brush cytology during duodenoscopy. Other primary duodenal malignancies are very rare. Extensions from pancreatic or biliary tract cancer are difficult to diagnose because the tumor may not have extended into the mucosa and may therefore not be accessible for biopsy or cytological examination. In these secondary tumors, diagnosis must depend upon some combination of echography, hypotonic duodenography, selective pancreatic angiography, and endoscopic retrograde cholangiopancreatography, with cytological examination of ductal contents.

Upper gastrointestinal bleeding (see also Chap. 37) Endoscopy within the first 12 to 24 h of an upper gastrointestinal hemorrhage can be very helpful in planning rational therapy by visualizing the bleeding source. Shallow lesions not visible by x-ray may be seen (esophagitis, Mallory-Weiss tear, erosive gastritis, shallow stress ulcer, and telangiectasia). Lesions which are visible by x-ray may not be the source of bleeding. Only endoscopy can determine the actual bleeding site, which may affect treatment. For example, visualization of a spurting artery which is flooding the stomach indicates massive ongoing bleeding requiring prompt operative intervention. Several studies have shown that the demonstration at endoscopy of any bleeding whatsoever or a nonbleeding vessel in the ulcer base makes a poor outcome more likely.

A conservative estimate of the diagnostic accuracy of emergency endoscopy in upper gastrointestinal bleeding is 80 to 85 percent, which is far superior to emergency x-ray examination. Endoscopic diagnoses of bleeding erosive gastritis may be made too frequently when blood from another unsuspected source spreads over the gastric mucosa or when trauma from overly vigorous antecedent lavage creates ecchymoses. To avoid overdiagnosis of erosive gastritis, portions of the gastric wall should be washed free of blood to determine the true appearance of the underlying gastric mucosa.

Every patient having endoscopy for upper gastrointestinal bleeding merits a complete endoscopic examination of the esophagus, stomach, and duodenum. Finding a potential bleeding lesion is not proof that this is the source of hemorrhage unless active bleeding is seen. Approximately one-half of patients with esophageal varices can be shown endoscopically to be bleeding from another source such as erosive gastritis, duodenal ulcer, or gastric ulcer. Occasionally it is not possible to diagnose the exact lesion which is bleeding, but localizing the area of bleeding can be very helpful; for example, bright red arterial blood may be seen pouring from the duodenum when the esophagus and stomach are relatively free of blood.

There are three controversial areas. First, *do all bleeders need endoscopy?* The authors feel that endoscopy is indicated in all patients who may require surgery because of continual bleeding or rebleeding. Although 85 percent of upper gastrointestinal bleeders stop spontaneously, it is impossible to predict which ones will; therefore, endoscopy is recommended for most bleeders. Second, *how early should endoscopy be performed in the acutely bleeding patient?* Most studies suggest that the diagnostic accuracy of esophagogastroduodenoscopy remains high for the first 12 to 24 h after the bleeding episode. All would agree that it is desirable to delay endoscopy until vital signs have been stabilized after adequate blood replacement. Upper endoscopy is usually performed during waking hours at a time during the first day of bleeding when the patient's vital signs are stable and when the full endoscopic team is available. Emergency endoscopy at night should be reserved for those patients with continued massive bleeding or rebleeding requiring an immediate decision regarding surgery or other treatment. If the patient is exsanguinating, endoscopy can follow induction of anesthesia just preceding surgery. Thus, the patient's airway is protected by an endotracheal tube. Finally, *does endoscopy affect the clinical outcome?* Current studies suggest that it does not. This may be more a reflection on the inadequacies of medical therapy and the dangers of nonelective surgical treatment of bleeding patients who are severely ill than on the usefulness of more accurate endoscopic detection of the bleeding source. If endoscopic or pharmacologic methods of stopping bleeding prove to be safe and effective in controlled trials, more accurate endoscopic diagnosis may indeed affect the outcome favorably.

Emergency endoscopy is not for the inexperienced. It requires considerable technical skill and interpretative experience and the best available instruments.

Other indications Upper endoscopy is usually substituted for x-ray in the urgent diagnosis of gastrointestinal illness in *pregnancy.* Most patients with *dysphagia* merit esophagoscopy because the cause is frequently organic and may be missed by x-ray. On the other hand, dysphagia caused by esophageal spasm or dysrhythmia is best diagnosed by manometry or cineradiography. *Painful swallowing* (odynophagia), especially in immunosuppressed or diabetic patients, may merit esophagoscopy because biopsy and scrapings of the involved esophageal wall may reveal monilial, herpetic, or cytomegalic virus infections. Soon after ingestion of a corrosive agent, limited and gentle esophagoscopy is useful in evaluating the severity of injury. Many impacted foreign bodies can be removed from the esophagus or stomach with a snare or forceps; sharp foreign bodies are usually best removed by pulling them into the lumen of a rigid tubular esophagoscope or by pulling them into a protective overtube around a fiberoptic endoscope. Careful esophagoscopy after removal of a foreign body is important to determine whether there is an underlying lesion which caused the impaction (e.g., cancer, benign stricture, peptic esophagitis).

In the postoperative stomach, gastroscopy is especially useful in detecting carcinoma, recurrent ulceration, retrograde intussusception, and stomal stricture. Several European studies indicate a definite threat of carcinoma developing in the gastric stump 10 to 20 years after a Billroth II gastrectomy. The diagnosis of such postoperative carcinomas may require many biopsies of seemingly normal mucosa near the anastomosis. Prospective data on the natural history of this condition in the United States are badly needed because, if the European studies are confirmed, such patients should be examined by endoscopy and biopsied on a regular basis.

When the duodenal bulb shows reddening or nodularity, many endoscopists diagnose "duodenitis." There is little evidence to suggest that this picture is of significance. On the other hand, diffuse and bleeding erosions of the duodenal bulb merit a diagnosis of "erosive duodenitis," especially after ingestion of gastric irritants such as aspirin; such erosions may also be a precursor of frank ulcerations. A nodular or narrow duodenum will occasionally yield granulomas on biopsy, indicative of Crohn's disease.

ENDOSCOPIC RETROGRADE CHOLANGIOPANCREATOGRAPHY (ERCP) This endoscopic technique involves placing a side-viewing instrument in the descending duodenum. The papilla of Vater is cannulated, contrast medium is injected, and the pancreatic ducts and hepatobiliary tree are visualized radiologically. Skilled operators can visualize 90 to 95 percent of pancreatic ducts and 80 to 85 percent of biliary ducts.

ERCP is performed on an x-ray table. The oropharynx is usually anesthetized with topical lidocaine, and most endoscopists sedate the patient with intravenous diazepam. Atropine and glucagon are given intravenously to induce duodenal hypotonia. The pancreatic duct is usually visualized first and gently filled throughout its entire length with 2 to 5 ml contrast material (Fig. 304-1*A*). Injection is continued until the first side branches are seen or until the patient complains of pain. Overfilling is avoided. By insertion of the cannula at a more acute cephalad angle, the common bile duct and the whole biliary tract including the gallbladder are visualized (Fig. 304-1*B*).

At present not all indications for ERCP are clearly established. Those for the hepatobiliary tree are clearer than those for the pancreatic duct. Because ERCP is not without risk, it is justified only to seek an operable lesion or to prevent an unnecessary operation. Asymptomatic amylase elevations occur in 30 to 40 percent of patients after the procedure and are rarely of clinical significance. Pancreatitis occurs in only 1 percent of patients but is usually benign and self-limited. By monitoring the pancreas during injection using a high-resolution TV screen, the force of injection can be limited to avoid filling of pancreatic acini. This probably minimizes the complication of pancreatitis. In a nationwide survey of complications, the morbidity rate was 3 percent and mortality rate 0.2 percent. It is significant that the complication rate was highest for the inexperienced operator (7 percent). The morbidity and mortality rates are substantially lower from large centers with great experience. The main serious complication is retained, nonsterile contrast material proximal to an obstructed duct causing cholangitis or pancreatic sepsis. Patients suspected of having bile duct obstruction are started on systemic antibiotics prior to the ERCP. Furthermore, if bile duct or pancreatic duct obstruction is first revealed by ERCP, antibiotic coverage is indicated to reduce the incidence of bacteremia; such patients should be drained surgically within 36 h. No patient should have ERCP unless advance arrangements for possible operation have been made with the patient and a surgical consultant.

Retrograde cholangiography This procedure is especially useful in patients with persistent jaundice whose cause cannot be established by conventional diagnostic methods. The important differential diagnosis is between "surgical" and "medical" jaundice. When the cause of jaundice is unclear, approximately 15 percent of patients thought to have "medical" jaundice prove to have extrahepatic biliary obstruction requiring surgery, and, conversely, the same percentage of patients thought to have "surgical" jaundice prove to have an open ductal system by ERCP and can be spared unnecessary surgery.

Remediable causes of obstructive jaundice which can be diagnosed by retrograde cholangiography include common duct stones (Fig. 304-1*C*), gallbladder stones, benign strictures, and, occasionally, resectable ductal carcinomas. In jaundiced patients with suspected primary liver disease, such as sclerosing cholangitis or primary biliary cirrhosis, ERCP can relieve the worry that an operable obstruction is being missed.

In addition to ERCP, there are four other methods of visualizing the biliary tree in the jaundiced patient. Which test to use first depends on the clinical situation, the availability of equipment, and the experience of the specialists using the tech-

FIGURE 304-1
A. A tapering pancreatic duct (arrow) of normal diameter is seen and may be compared with the endoscope (E) 1 cm in diameter. B. Normal cholangiogram. The diameter of the common duct (CD) is normal. The intrahepatic ducts branch normally, and the gallbladder (GB) can be seen. The endoscope (E) is seen in the duodenum. C. Three stones (arrows) are visible in an obstructed, dilated common duct (CD). The intrahepatic ducts (IHD) are also grossly dilated. Regurgitated contrast material is seen in the duodenum (DUO). D. The sharp cutoff (arrow) of the pancreatic duct (P) is caused by a carcinoma of the body of the pancreas.

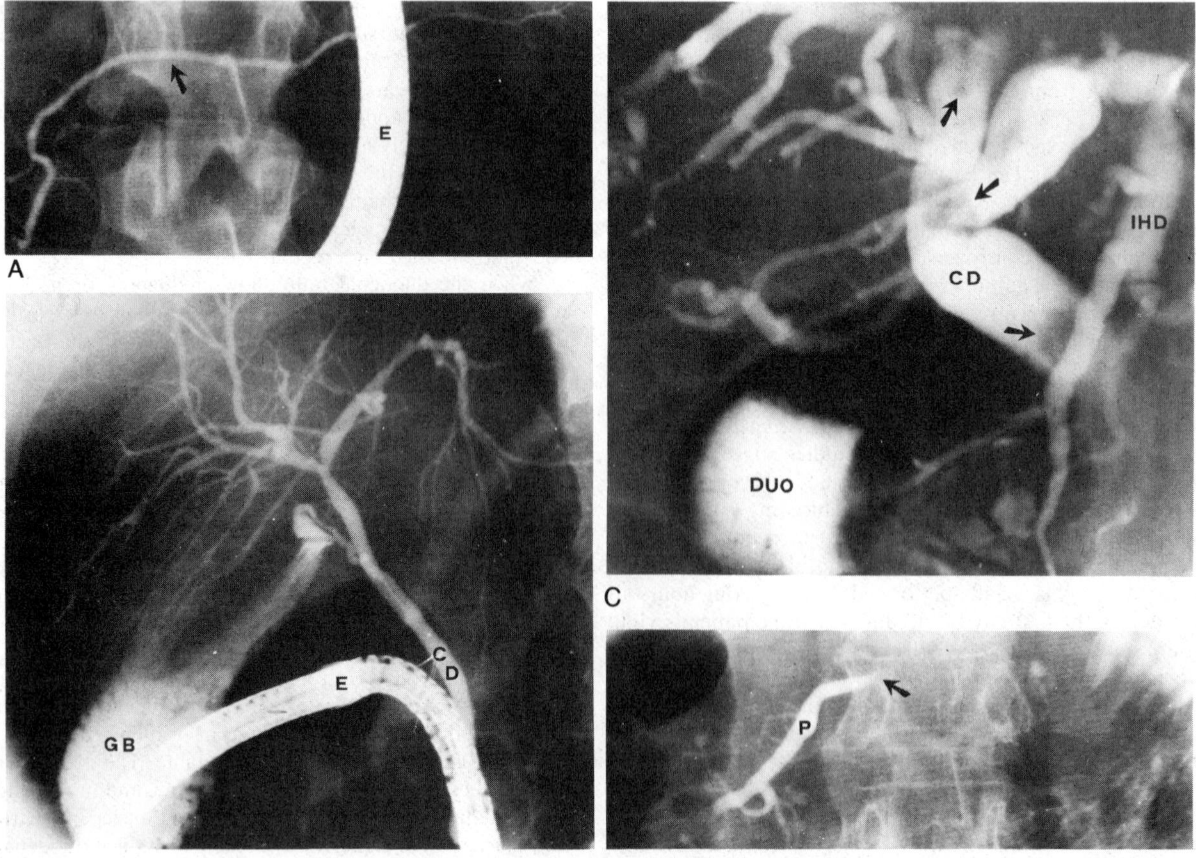

niques. The first method is *percutaneous transhepatic cholangiography* (*PTC*), in which contrast material is injected from the exterior via a "skinny" needle into the intrahepatic bile ducts under fluoroscopic control; success in visualizing the ducts is 90 to 100 percent if the ducts are dilated, but only approximately 66 percent if they are not dilated. PTC is generally safe, but complications do occur (sepsis, bleeding, bile leak, etc.); precise morbidity and mortality figures are not yet established. The three other methods, which are noninvasive, use *ultrasound* (echo), *computerized tomography* (CT scan), and *PIPIDA scans* (^{99m}Tc-labeled paraisopropyliminodiacetic acid). The first two techniques employ sound waves or x-rays to visualize organs and any stones, cysts, or solid masses within them. They can also be used to determine whether the biliary ducts or gallbladder are enlarged. The PIPIDA scans are used to determine patency of the cystic and common ducts and to study gallbladder emptying after administration of cholecystokinin (CCK).

The relative usefulness of these five tests is not established. Many physicians first try the noninvasive echo or CT scan to see whether the biliary ducts are dilated and to seek a clear cause of the patient's jaundice (stones, pancreatic mass, etc.). The PIPIDA scan will determine if the cystic duct and bile ducts are patent. Direct visualization is undertaken if the diagnosis is not established, PTC first if the hepatic ducts are dilated, and ERCP if not. In the event of a technical failure or incomplete information resulting from either ERCP or PTC, one of the other techniques is tried. This approach detects most lesions requiring surgical intervention.

ERCP or PTC can also be useful in patients with biliary pain, cholangitis, or impaired liver function after previous biliary surgery. Remediable postoperative lesions such as strictures can be discovered, and their precise anatomy outlined so that reoperation is less difficult.

Retrograde pancreatography Patients with recurrent or chronic pancreatitis may merit retrograde pancreatography to seek a lesion which can be approached surgically, such as cyst, localized pancreatitis in the tail, or ductal pathology amenable to drainage, which may be found in nearly 50 percent of these patients. Finding concomitant unsuspected stones in the gallbladder or common duct may direct surgical intervention to this underlying problem.

Patients with symptoms, signs, or laboratory findings suggesting pancreatic carcinoma may have pancreatograms suggesting malignancy with a narrowed, encased, or sharply "cutoff" pancreatic duct (Fig. 304-1*D*). Differentiation of such pancreatic ductal findings from benign inflammatory disease can be difficult. Cytological examination of pancreatic duct contents obtained during ERCP may prove helpful. Unfortunately, most patients with symptomatic pancreatic cancer diagnosed by ERCP are inoperable.

Patients presenting with painless steatorrhea of pancreatic origin may be shown to have a ductal pattern suggesting chronic pancreatitis or pancreatic carcinoma. Some of these carcinomas may be resectable, although it is as yet unknown whether this represents palliation or the more remote possibility of cure.

Pancreatography has not been useful in the study of obscure upper abdominal pain. Pancreatic cysts can be better diagnosed by noninvasive techniques such as echography, and pancreatography should be reserved for those cases where the diagnosis is unclear or when the surgeon desires precise outlining of the anatomy immediately prior to surgery. Pancreatography alone does not seem promising as a method of screening for early pancreatic carcinoma, although cytological examination of ductal fluid may prove useful.

Therapeutic ERCP Successful endoscopic papillotomy of the sphincter of Vater with extraction of retained stones has now been reported by several groups. An electrosurgical wire attached to the ERCP catheter can be used to cut the sphincter of Vater. Certainly this approach will be used increasingly in patients who are poor operative risks. The overall success rate is approximately 90 percent, with a mortality rate of about 0.8 percent and a complication rate of about 7 percent. Complications include bleeding, perforation, pancreatitis, cholangitis, and stone impaction. These results compare favorably with surgery, especially in the high-risk patient with previous biliary surgery. Endoscopic papillotomy may also permit nonoperative biliary drainage via transnasal tubes or stints placed into the common bile duct. Manometry of the sphincter presents certain technical difficulties, but it may yet prove invaluable in the diagnosis of periampullary stenosis.

Other diagnostic techniques Critical comparative studies are needed of the various approaches to biliary tree disorders and to pancreatic diseases (ERCP, PTC, angiography, CT scanning, and ultrasound).

COLONOSCOPY The interior of the entire length of the colon from anus to cecum can be visualized by the experienced colonoscopist. This method may prove to be the most significant diagnostic and therapeutic application of fiberoptic endoscopy because it can diagnose potentially curable colonic cancers missed by other techniques.

Approximately one-half of colonoscopies are performed because of an abnormal barium enema showing a polyp or a narrowing or filling defect suggesting carcinoma. Approximately one-quarter of colonoscopies are done because of chronic occult gastrointestinal bleeding. The ability to examine the whole colon is proving valuable in the management of some patients with inflammatory bowel disease.

Patients are prepared for colonoscopy with a liquid diet for 2 days, magnesium citrate laxation the evening before examination, and tap water enemas the morning of the procedure. Another method of preparing the colon is a total-gut lavage with physiologic saline. This method prepares the patient without laxatives or enemas and only requires a few hours. Immediately before the procedure the patients are lightly sedated with intravenous diazepam and meperidine. Intravenous anticholinergics and glucagon are used when needed to relax local spasm. Vasovagal bradycardial reactions can be reversed quickly by intravenous anticholinergics.

The main complications of colonoscopy are hemorrhage and perforation (morbidity rate is 0.5 to 1.3 percent; mortality rate is 0.02 percent). The complication rate for polypectomy is 1 to 2 percent. The complication rate is higher during the first 40 procedures by a new colonoscopist. Diverticular or ischemic disease and prior irradiation make the procedure more difficult and hazardous. The risk of perforation is also increased in the patient with very active colitis, and colonoscopy should be avoided during the acute phase.

Polyps A polyp seen on barium enema merits colonoscopy for several reasons: it may be an artifact or a cancer, and a second polyp or cancer may have been missed. The polyp can usually be excised, with lower morbidity and mortality rates than with surgery. The best way to rule out cancer within a polyp is to remove it completely for histological examination. The most common colonic polyps are hyperplastic histologically, and they do not develop cancer; colonic polyps which show benign neoplasia histologically may become malignant (adenomatous and villous polyps). The risk of neoplastic polyps being cancerous increases with their size. The risk is also higher in villous adenomas. Pedunculated polyps with cancer confined to the mucosa and with an uninvolved stalk can be cured by removal with an electrocautery snare during colonoscopy. Thus, most colonoscopists will remove all polyps more than 0.5 cm in diameter. It is more difficult to know what to do with polyps smaller than 0.5 cm in diameter because some are adenomatous, although most are hyperplastic. A coagulating biopsy technique can be used to both biopsy and destroy even the smallest adenomatous polyp in the hope that the subsequent risk of developing colonic cancer will be reduced. The wisdom of this course of action is suggested by a sigmoidoscopic study in which the removal of all polyps reduced the expected incidence and invasiveness of subsequently developing cancers. Most agree that the patient with adenomatous polyps is more likely to develop another polyp or cancer and therefore merits some regular screening program. The optimal frequency of follow-up examinations after polypectomy is not yet established, although studies in progress will hopefully soon provide valid guidelines.

Cancer screening by x-ray All filling defects on barium enema merit evaluation by colonoscopy. If the lesion is a pedunculated polyp, it can be removed for histological examination; if its appearance suggests a cancer, it can be biopsied and brushed for histological and cytological confirmation. When a polyp or a carcinoma is found, the remainder of the colon should be screened for additional polyps and synchronous carcinoma. This avoids multiple colotomies to search for a second lesion and reduces surgical morbidity. Approximately 10 percent of lesions diagnosed as carcinoma by x-ray are not present on colonoscopy or are found to be caused by other diseases.

Narrowing by x-ray An etiologic diagnosis of segmental narrowing may be difficult by x-ray. Colonoscopy often determines the cause of segmental narrowing and differentiates adenocarcinoma from inflammation secondary to ischemia, irradiation, diverticular disease, or Crohn's colitis. Even the most classic "apple-core" lesion by x-ray may be covered by normal mucosa at colonoscopy, suggesting an extrinsic inflammatory lesion. Narrowed segments present on x-ray are not visualized (in 10 to 30 percent of patients) during colonoscopy, probably because they are areas of temporary spasm. Such findings avoid unnecessary operations.

Chronic bleeding (x-ray and sigmoidoscopy negative) This condition leads to approximately 25 percent of colonoscopies. The cause of bleeding is found in approximately 40 percent of such patients. The common bleeding sources are adenomatous polyp (15 percent), adenocarcinoma (15 percent), and Crohn's disease (7 percent). Many of these carcinomas are resectable, and this group may benefit most from colonoscopy. If no bleeding source is found, a search may be appropriate for an upper gastrointestinal source with an upper gastrointestinal x-ray and/or upper endoscopy. Narrowing or masses on x-ray can be studied colonoscopically to see if they are due to inflammation, malignancy, or an artifact.

Inflammatory bowel disease Colonoscopy is not routinely indicated in patients with inflammatory bowel disease. Colonoscopy may help in the initial diagnosis, especially in differentiating Crohn's colitis from ulcerative colitis. It can aid the surgeon in assessing the activity and extent of the disease before surgery. Colonoscopy can evaluate radiographic abnormalities suggesting cancer, such as strictures, polyps, or masses. Colonoscopy may be indicated in patients with ulcerative colitis of more than 10 years' duration because of the increased risk of carcinoma; it is hoped that repeated colonoscopies will serve to detect these malignancies earlier than x-ray and while the lesions are still curable. The frequency of colonoscopy and/or double-contrast barium enema examination in such patients is not yet established. The prognostic value of "precancer" or "dysplastic" changes revealed by multiple colonic biopsies in patients with long-standing ulcerative colitis remains to be established. Preparation for colonoscopy must often be modified for patients with inflammatory bowel disease. Colonoscopy is contraindicated in patients with toxic megacolon, very active disease, or a possible intestinal perforation.

Other indications The short fiberoptic colonoscope may replace the rigid 25-cm sigmoidoscope for routine screening because it can be passed to 40 to 60 cm with minimal preparation. There is less discomfort and a higher diagnostic yield. However, the question remains whether flexible sigmoidoscopy will pick up significant lesions missed by screening stools for occult blood. At this time, rigid sigmoidoscopy remains an important method of evaluating colorectal symptoms. After segmental colonic resection for carcinoma, colonoscopy may detect early mucosal recurrence and differentiate it from benign anastomotic strictures or bleeding suture granulomas. Colonoscopy is occasionally used during laparotomy to assist the surgeon in ruling out other lesions. The colonoscope can be advanced to the cecum rapidly with the surgeon's assistance, and additional polyps removed without colotomy. The authors believe that the best diagnostic approach to acute bleeding is selective angiography; this may be useful not only for finding lesions such as angiodysplasia and bleeding diverticulas but also for permitting treatment with vasoconstrictors. Visualizing a bleeding site by colonoscopy may be difficult when there is massive bleeding.

Colonoscopy detects some carriers of the dominant familial polyposis gene before diagnosis by barium enema and sigmoidoscopy. Such information is useful for genetic counseling of patients regarding their decision to have children. Carcinoma is a great threat only in those familial syndromes which produce many adenomatous polyps (familial polyposis and Gardner's syndrome); in these conditions, polypectomy is useful for diagnosis, but colectomy is the only treatment which prevents development of carcinoma. Peutz-Jeghers syndrome and generalized juvenile polyposis produce mostly hamartomatous polyps and, therefore, have a very much lower incidence of gastrointestinal carcinoma; the cancers that develop in these patients may be related to occasional polyps undergoing adenomatous change.

Malignant tumors develop in 2 to 3 percent of patients with Peutz-Jeghers syndrome, and they are mostly located in the stomach and duodenum. Thus these patients may merit regular upper endoscopy and prophylactic polypectomy.

CONTRAINDICATIONS All types of fiberoptic endoscopy are contraindicated in certain clinical situations, including the uncooperative or combative patient, a patient with an acute myocardial infarction, or a patient with an acute perforation of the intestine.

CONSCIOUS LAPAROSCOPY The potentialities for laparoscopy in conscious patients have not been as fully appreciated in North America as they have been in other countries where it has been used widely for over 20 years. This procedure has extremely low mortality and morbidity rates in experienced hands. The instrument used for laparoscopy is a stiff tube with a lens system that provides a superb view. Under local anesthesia pneumoperitoneum is gradually induced with air or nitrous oxide. To avoid intraabdominal trauma, the extent of the gas cavity must be determined by probing with a spinal needle before the sharp trocar is carefully pushed through the abdominal wall into this cavity. The sharp obturator is removed and the laparoscope introduced through the airtight trocar to visualize the peritoneal cavity.

Much of the exterior of the liver, gallbladder, spleen, peritoneum, diaphragm, and pelvic organs can be clearly visualized. Portions of the colon and small bowel can also be seen, depending upon the location and size of the greater omentum. Lesions can be biopsied under direct vision, and any resultant bleeding controlled by electrocoagulation. Furthermore, in centers with extensive experience contrast material can be injected into the liver to visualize vascular, lymphatic, and biliary systems.

Laparoscopy should be considered an indispensable diagnostic tool. It permits one to make a difficult diagnosis without resorting to laparotomy by biopsying localized hepatic disease under direct vision, and can often help differentiate "medical" from "surgical" jaundice. It may also enable staging of malignant disease without laparotomy.

REFERENCES

BECK K et al (eds): *Color Atlas of Laparoscopy.* New York, Schattauer Verlag, 1970

COTTON PB, BEALES JSM: Endoscopic pancreatography in management of relapsing acute pancreatitis. Br Med J 1:608, 1974

COTTON PE, WILLIAMS CB: *Practical Gastrointestinal Endoscopy.* Oxford, Blackwell, 1980

KOCH H: Operative endoscopy. Gastrointest Endosc 24:65, 1977

PETERSON WL et al: Routine early endoscopy in upper gastrointestinal tract bleeding: A randomized, controlled trial. N Engl J Med 304:925, 1981

Proceedings of the NIH Consensus Workshop. Dig Dis Sci 26:1s, 1981

SAFRANY L: Duodenoscopic sphincterotomy and gallstone removal. Gastroenterology 72:330, 1977

TEAGUE RH et al: Colonoscopy for investigation of unexplained rectal bleeding. Lancet 1:1350, 1978

305
DISEASES OF THE ESOPHAGUS

RAJ K. GOYAL

The two major functions of the esophagus are the transport of the food bolus from the mouth to the stomach and the prevention of retrograde flow of gastrointestinal contents. Retrograde flow is prevented by the two esophageal sphincters, which remain closed between swallows and which are functional rather than distinct anatomical entities. The upper esophageal sphincter remains closed by the elastic properties of its wall and by contraction of the cricopharyngeus and inferior pharyngeal constrictor muscles due to continuous neural excitation. Many neuromuscular disorders involving these muscles result in reduction in resting sphincter pressure and consequent esophagopharyngeal reflux. In contrast, the lower esophageal sphincter remains closed because of its intrinsic myogenic tone, and vagal (parasympathetic) innervation causes its relaxation. A reflex increase in the lower sphincter pressure occurs with an increase in intraabdominal pressure and ingestion of a protein meal. Fatty meals, smoking, and beverages with a high xanthine content (tea, coffee, cola) cause a reduction in sphincter pressure. Many hormones and neurotransmitters can modify lower sphincter pressure. Cholinergic muscarinic agonists, alpha-adrenergic agonists, gastrin, pancreatic polypeptide, substance P, and prostaglandin $F_{2\alpha}$ cause contraction; in contrast ganglionic stimulants, beta-adrenergic agonists, dopamine, cholecystokinin, secretin, vasoactive intestinal polypeptide, ATP, and adenosine cause relaxation of the sphincter. Effects of many of these agents are pharmacological rather than physiological. Reduced lower sphincter pressure may lead to gastroesophageal reflux and reflux esophagitis.

SYMPTOMS

DYSPHAGIA See Chap. 32.

ESOPHAGEAL PAIN *Heartburn,* or pyrosis, is characterized by burning retrosternal discomfort that may move up and down the chest like a wave. When severe, it may radiate to the sides of the chest, neck, and angles of the jaw. Heartburn is a characteristic symptom of reflux esophagitis and may be associated with regurgitation or a feeling of warm fluid climbing up the throat. It is aggravated by bending forward, straining, or lying recumbent and is worse after meals. It is relieved by upright posture, by swallowing of saliva or water, or, more reliably, by antacids. Heartburn appears to be produced by heightened mucosal sensitivity and can be reproduced by infusion of dilute (0.1 *N*) hydrochloric acid (Bernstein test) or neutral hyperosmolar solutions into the esophagus.

Odynophagia, or painful swallowing, is characteristic of nonreflux esophagitis, particularly monilial and herpes esophagitis. Odynophagia may also occur with peptic ulcer of the esophagus (Barrett's ulcer), carcinoma with periesophageal involvement, caustic damage of the esophagus, and esophageal perforation. Odynophagia is unusual in uncomplicated reflux esophagitis.

Chest pain other than heartburn and odynophagia occurs when the esophageal muscle contracts with excessive force, for a long duration, and repetitively, as in diffuse esophageal spasm. Chest pain due to periesophageal involvement caused by carcinoma or peptic ulcer may be constant and agonizing. Sometimes different types of esophageal pains exist together in the same patient, and frequently patients are not able to describe the pain accurately enough to allow its classification.

REGURGITATION Regurgitation is the effortless appearance of gastric or esophageal contents in the mouth. In distal esophageal obstruction and stasis, as in achalasia or a large diverticulum, the regurgitated material consists of tasteless mucoid fluid or undigested food. Regurgitation of sour or bitter-tasting material occurs in severe gastroesophageal reflux and is associated with incompetence of both the upper and lower esophageal sphincters. Regurgitation may result in laryngeal aspiration, with spells of coughing and choking that awaken the patient from sleep, and aspiration pneumonia. Water brash is reflex salivary hypersecretion which occurs in response to peptic esophagitis; it should not be confused with regurgitation.

DIAGNOSTIC TESTS

RADIOLOGICAL STUDIES Barium swallow with fluoroscopy and esophogram is the most widely used test for diagnosis of esophageal disease and can be used to evaluate both structural and motor disorders. The pharynx is examined to detect stasis of barium in the valleculae and pyriform sinuses and regurgitation of barium into the nose and tracheobronchial tree. Since the pharyngeal phase of swallowing lasts no more than a second, cineradiography may be necessary to permit detection and analysis of abnormalities of pharyngeal function. Spontaneous reflux of barium from the stomach into the esophagus should be sought in patients with suspected reflux esophagitis. Esophageal peristalsis is best studied in the recumbent position since in the upright position the passage of most of the barium occurs by gravity alone. A double-contrast esophagram, obtained by coating the esophageal mucosa with barium and distending the esophageal lumen with air using effervescent granules, is particularly useful in demonstrating mucosal ulcers and early cancers. Figures 305-1 and 305-2 illustrate the radiographic appearance of some esophageal lesions.

ESOPHAGOSCOPY Fiberoptic esophagogastroduodenoscopy is described in Chap. 304. Esophagoscopy is the direct method of establishing the cause of mechanical dysphagia and of identifying mucosal lesions, such as superficial ulcers and esophagitis, which may not be identified by the usual barium swallow. In the presence of marked luminal narrowing, examination can be achieved by using a smaller caliber endoscope, although on occasion a stricture must be dilated prior to a complete endoscopic examination. Transendoscopic biopsies are useful in diagnosing carcinoma, reflux esophagitis, or other mucosal diseases. Obtaining cells by scraping the mucosa with a Teflon brush during endoscopy may enable the cytologist to detect carcinoma missed by mucosal biopsies.

ESOPHAGEAL MOTILITY Esophageal motility entails simultaneous recording of pressures from different sites in the esophageal lumen. This is usually done with a train of 3 to 4 water-filled catheters connected to pressure transducers. The assembly is passed by mouth or nose through the esophagus into the stomach and then gradually withdrawn 1 cm at a time until pressures from each centimeter of the esophagus and pharynx are recorded at rest and during swallowing. The upper and lower esophageal sphincters appear as zones of high pressure which relax on swallowing. The esophageal body shows peristaltic waves with each swallow.

Esophageal motility studies are very helpful in the diagnosis of achalasia, diffuse esophageal spasm and its variants, scleroderma, and other motor disorders of the esophagus, as well as neuromuscular disorders of the upper esophagus and pharynx (Fig. 305-3) but are of no value in the diagnosis of mechanical dysphagia. In patients with reflux esophagitis, esophageal manometry is useful in quantitating lower esophageal competence and providing information on the status of the esophageal body motor activity. The information obtained by manometry is quantitative and cannot be obtained by barium swallow or endoscopy.

Special tests for the evaluation of reflux esophagitis are described later.

MOTOR DISORDERS

STRIATED MUSCLE Pharyngeal paralysis Pharyngeal paralysis is characterized by dysphagia, nasal regurgitation, and tracheobronchial aspiration during swallowing. It occurs in a variety of neuromuscular disorders (see Table 32-2). Some of these disorders may also involve laryngeal and orofacial muscles. When the suprahyoid muscles are also paralyzed, the opening of the upper sphincter with swallowing is also impaired, causing severe dysphagia.

Barium swallow and cineradiography reveal stasis of barium in the valleculae and pyriform sinuses as well as nasal and tracheobronchial aspiration (Fig. 305-1). Pharyngeal motility studies demonstrate reduced amplitude of pharyngeal and upper esophageal contractions and reduced basal upper esophageal sphincter pressure without further relaxation on swallowing (Fig. 305-3). Patients with myasthenia gravis and polymyositis respond to treatment for these diseases (see Chap. 372). Dysphagia in patients with cerebrovascular accident improves with time, although not completely. Treatment in most instances is mainly supportive, consisting of nasogastric tube feeding and physiotherapy. Cricopharyngeal myotomy is sometimes performed but its usefulness is unproved.

FIGURE 305-1
Radiographic appearance of some motor disorders of the pharynx and esophagus. (1) Pharyngeal paralysis with tracheal aspiration (arrow). (2) Cricopharyngeal achalasia. Note the prominent cricopharyngeus which is recognized by its smoothness and location in the posterior wall. (3) Diffuse esophageal spasm. Note typical corkscrew appearance of the lower part of the esophagus. (4) Achalasia showing dilatation of esophageal body with air fluid level and closed lower esophageal sphincter. (5) Muscular (contractile) lower esophageal ring. Note a nice symmetrical contraction in 5A that has disappeared in 5B obtained during the same examination. (6) Scleroderma esophagus showing dilated esophagus with a stricture in 6A and reflux of barium from the stomach into the esophagus in 6B. (Courtesy of Dr Harvey Goldstein.)

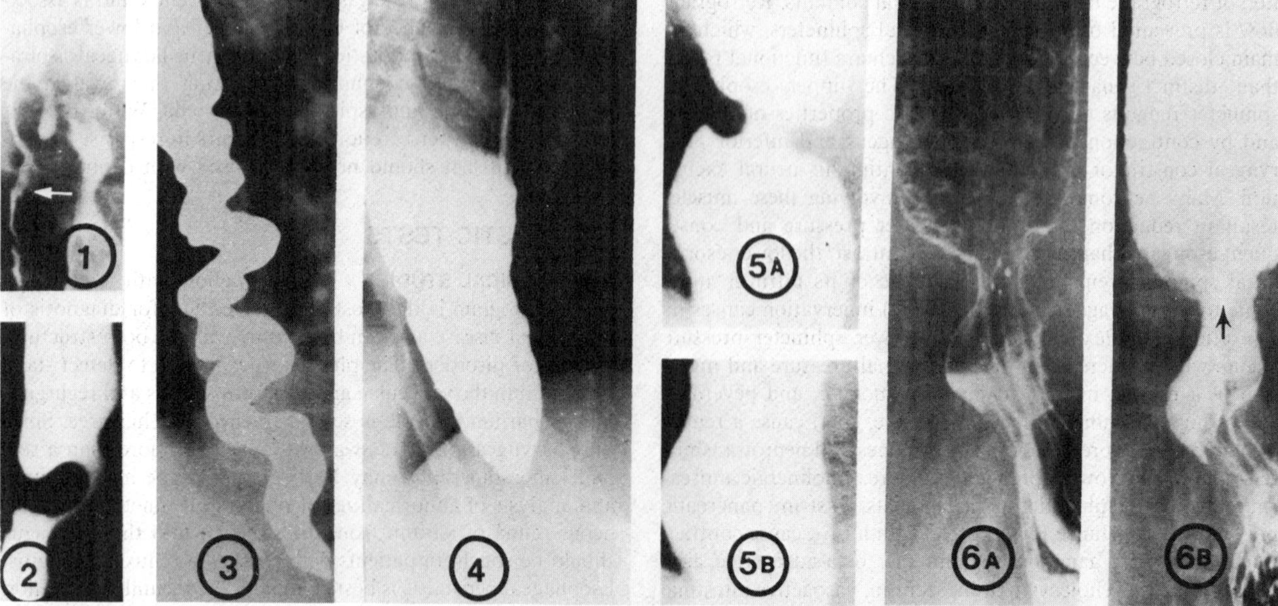

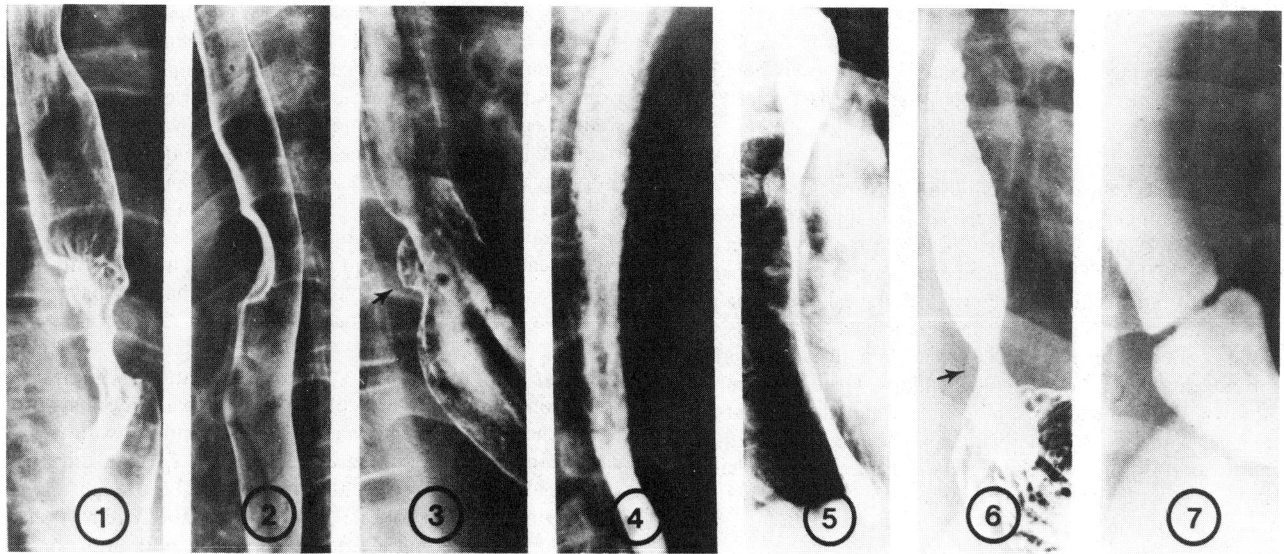

FIGURE 305-2
Radiographic appearance of selected structural lesions of the esophagus. (1) Carcinoma of the esophagus. Note the typical annular narrowing with overhanging margins and destruction of the mucosa. (2) Leiomyoma of the esophagus. Note the smooth filling defect and right angles of origin from the esophageal wall. (3) Esophageal ulcer in columnar-cell-lined esophagus (Barrett's esophagus). (4) Monilial esophagitis. Note irregular plaque-like filling defects. (5) Long stricture secondary to lye ingestion. (6) Peptic stricture which is short and tubular. Note the associated hiatus hernia. (7) Mucosal lower esophageal mucosal (Schatzki) ring. Note a thin weblike annular constriction at the esophagogastric junction. It is associated with a small hiatal hernia. (Courtesy of Dr Harvey Goldstein.)

Extensive operative procedures to prevent aspiration are rarely needed. Death is often due to pulmonary complications.

Cricopharyngeal achalasia Failure of the cricopharyngeus to relax on swallowing leads to a contracted cricopharyngeus, which appears as a prominent bar on the posterior wall of the pharynx on barium swallow (Fig. 301-1*A*). A transient cricopharyngeal bar is seen in up to 5 percent of subjects without dysphagia undergoing upper gastrointestinal studies; it can be produced in normal subjects during a Valsalva maneuver. When contraction is persistent, patients may complain of food sticking in their throats. Cricopharyngeal myotomy may be helpful, but it is contraindicated in the presence of gastroesophageal reflux because in such patients this procedure may lead to pharyngeal and pulmonary aspiration.

Globus hystericus A sensation of a constant lump in the throat but with no difficulty during swallowing occurs especially in subjects with emotional disorders, particularly in women. Barium studies are normal, but manometry shows a hypertensive upper sphincter. Treatment is primarily one of reassurance.

SMOOTH MUSCLE Achalasia Achalasia is a motor disorder of the esophageal smooth muscle in which the lower esophageal sphincter does not relax properly with swallowing and the normal peristalsis of the esophageal body is replaced by abnormal contractions. Based upon the changes in the esophageal body, achalasia can be of two types: in *classic achalasia* simultaneous contractions of small amplitude occur, while in *vigorous achalasia* contractions are simultaneous in onset, large in amplitude, and repetitive, resembling those seen in diffuse esophageal spasm.

PATHOPHYSIOLOGY The underlying abnormality is defective innervation of the esophagus. Histopathological studies in achalasia show a marked reduction in myenteric neurons, particularly the argyrophilic neurons. Primary idiopathic achalasia accounts for most of the patients seen in the United States. Secondary achalasia may be caused by gastric carcinoma infiltrating the esophagus; lymphoma; Chagas' disease; neuropathic, chronic intestinal pseudoobstruction syndrome; irradiation; and certain toxins and drugs.

CLINICAL FEATURES Achalasia affects patients of all ages and both sexes. Dysphagia, chest pain, and regurgitation are the main symptoms. Dysphagia occurs early with both liquids and solids and is worsened by emotional stress and hurried eating. Various maneuvers, including the Valsalva, designed to increase intraesophageal pressure, may help passage of the bolus into the stomach. Chest pain is more pronounced in vigorous achalasia than in classic achalasia. Regurgitation and pulmonary aspiration occur because of retention of large volumes of saliva and ingested food in the esophagus. The presence of heartburn and gastroesophageal reflux argues against achalasia. The overall course is usually chronic with progressive dysphagia and weight loss over months to years.

DIAGNOSIS Chest x-ray shows absence of the gastric air bubble and sometimes a tubular mediastinal mass beside the aorta. The presence of an air-fluid level in the mediastinum in the upright position represents unpassed food in the esophagus and is characteristic. Barium swallow shows esophageal dilatation, and in advanced cases the esophagus may become so dilated as to warrant the term *sigmoid dilatation.* On fluoroscopy normal peristalsis is lost in the lower two-thirds of the esophagus. The terminal part of the esophagus shows a persistent beak-like narrowing representing the nonrelaxing lower esophageal sphincter (Fig. 305-1*B*). In patients with vigorous achalasia, there may be pronounced nonperistaltic contractions without a dilated esophagus.

Manometry shows normal or elevated basal lower esophageal sphincter pressure and swallow-induced relaxation which is absent or reduced in degree, duration, and consistency (Fig. 305-3). The esophageal body shows elevated resting pressure. In response to swallows, primary peristaltic waves are replaced by simultaneous-onset contractions. These contractions may be of poor amplitude (classic achalasia) or of large amplitude and long duration (vigorous achalasia). Administration of the cholinergic muscarinic agonist mecholyl causes a marked increase in esophageal resting pressure. Endoscopy is helpful in excluding the secondary causes of achalasia, particularly gastric carcinoma.

TREATMENT Medical treatment using soft foods, sedatives, nitrates, and anticholinergic drugs is usually unsatisfactory. Calcium channel antagonists such as nifedipine have been used with some success. The best available therapy involves balloon dilation to reduce the basal lower esophageal sphincter pressure by tearing muscle fibers. In experienced hands this technique is effective in about 85 percent of patients. Perforation and bleeding are potential complications. Heller's extramucosal myotomy of the lower sphincter, in which the circular muscle layer is incised, is equally effective. Reflux esophagitis and peptic stricture may follow successful treatment of achalasia. However, this complication is more frequent with myotomy than with balloon dilation.

Diffuse esophageal spasm and related motor disorders Diffuse esophageal spasm is a motor disorder of the esophageal smooth muscle characterized by multiple spontaneous contractions and by swallow-induced contractions that are of simultaneous onset, large amplitude, long duration, and repetitive occurrence. Variants of diffuse esophageal spasm show only some but not all of these motor abnormalities.

PATHOPHYSIOLOGY The pathogenesis of the various abnormalities in peristalsis in diffuse esophageal spasm is not known. Histopathological studies show patchy neural degeneration localized to nerve processes rather than the prominent degeneration of nerve cell bodies seen in achalasia.

FIGURE 305-3

Motility patterns in selected esophageal and pharyngeal disorders. In normal subjects, the upper and lower esophageal sphincters appear as zones of high pressure. With a swallow (indicated by ↑), pressure in the sphincters falls and a contraction wave starts in the pharynx and progresses down the esophagus. In scleroderma, the lower part of the esophagus (smooth muscle) shows reduced amplitude of contractions, which may be peristaltic or simultaneous in onset, and hypotension of the lower sphincter. In achalasia, the lower part of the esophagus shows reduced amplitude of contractions that are simultaneous in onset. In contrast to scleroderma, the lower esophageal sphincter in achalasia is hypertensive and fails to relax in response to a swallow. In diffuse esophageal spasm the lower part of the esophagus shows simultaneous onset, large amplitude, long duration, and repetitive contractions. In polymyositis, the smooth-muscle part of the esophagus is normal. The skeletal muscle part shows reduced amplitude of contractions. The upper esophageal sphincter is hypotensive and may not relax normally on swallowing due to associated weakness of the suprahyoid muscles.

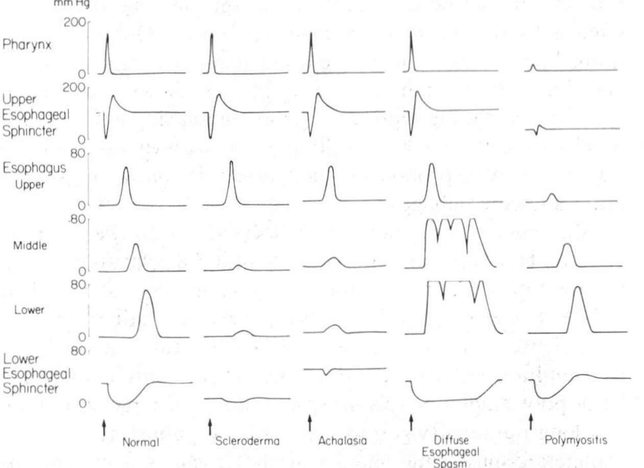

Variants of diffuse esophageal spasm frequently occur as a primary disease or in association with a variety of diseases as well as emotional stress and aging. These variants are more frequent in clinical practice than the fully developed diffuse esophageal spasm. Reflux esophagitis, irradiation esophagitis, collagen vascular diseases, and esophageal obstruction can cause esophageal motor abnormalities. The relationship between reflux esophagitis and motor abnormalities is controversial. Overlapping features of diffuse esophageal spasm and achalasia occur in vigorous achalasia.

CLINICAL FEATURES The symptomatic patient with diffuse spasm or its variants presents with chest pain, dysphagia, or both. Chest pain is particularly marked in patients with esophageal contractions of large amplitude and of long duration. Chest pain usually occurs at rest but may be brought on by swallowing or by emotional stress. The pain is retrosternal; may radiate to the back, sides of the chest, both arms, or the sides of the jaw; and lasts for a few seconds to several minutes. It may be acute and severe, mimicking the pain of myocardial ischemia. Dysphagia for solids and liquids may occur with or without chest pain.

Diffuse esophageal spasm must be differentiated from other causes of chest pain, particularly ischemic heart disease with atypical angina. Often a complete cardiac workup is done before the esophageal etiology is seriously considered. The presence of dysphagia in association with pain should point to the esophagus as the site of disease. Symptoms of esophageal spasm should be carefully distinguished from those of reflux esophagitis; sometimes the two may coexist.

DIAGNOSIS Barium swallow shows that normal sequential peristalsis below the aortic arch is replaced by uncoordinated simultaneous contractions that produce the appearance of curling or multiple ripples in the wall, sacculations, and pseudodiverticula—the "corkscrew" esophagus (Fig. 305-1*C*). Sometimes an esophageal contraction obliterates the lumen, and barium is pushed away in both directions. The lower esophageal sphincter opens normally.

Manometry reveals the characteristic prolonged large amplitude and repetitive contractions of simultaneous onset in the lower part of the esophagus (Fig. 305-3). Only one or two of these abnormalities may be present in variants of diffuse spasm. The lower sphincter relaxes normally. Manometry may be normal at the time of study; therefore, several techniques (including a cold water swallow and pharmacologic agents such as mecholyl, bethanechol, and pentagastrin) are used to provoke changes in esophageal spasm, although the usefulness of these tests is limited. Many patients who have chest pain and/or dysphagia have minor esophageal motor abnormalities in their basal study. These patients reproduce their chest pain with administration of a cholinergic drug or ergonovine and develop obvious motor abnormalities on motility studies. Ergonovine should be used with caution because it may produce spasm of the coronary arteries and may be dangerous in patients with coronary artery disease.

TREATMENT Anticholinergics are usually of limited value because the nerves that mediate esophageal contractions are noncholinergic. Agents which relax smooth muscle provide symptomatic relief. Sublingual nitroglycerin, long-acting nitrates, and isoproterenol may be helpful in some cases, but hydralazine and nifedipine may be more effective. Esophageal dilation with mercury-filled rubber dilators may produce symptomatic relief as a result of distention of the lower esophagus, but this is largely a placebo effect. Reassurance and tranquilizers are helpful in allaying patients' apprehension. Balloon dilation is sometimes attempted but can be hazardous; its usefulness is uncertain. In severe cases resistant to all therapy, a longitudinal myotomy of esophageal circular muscle is performed; it relieves pain in two-thirds of patients.

Scleroderma involving the esophagus The esophageal lesions in systemic sclerosis consist of muscular atrophy of the smooth muscle portion, with weakness of contraction in the lower two-thirds of the esophageal body and incompetence of the lower esophageal sphincter. The esophageal wall is thin and atrophic with or without areas of patchy fibrosis. Patients present with dysphagia to solids and to liquids in the recumbent position. They may also present with heartburn and regurgitation due to gastroesophageal reflux and esophagitis, which in turn may lead to stricture formation and more pronounced dysphagia. Barium swallow shows dilatation and loss of peristaltic contractions in the middle and distal portions of the esophagus. The lower esophageal sphincter is patulous, and gastroesophageal reflux may occur freely (Fig. 305-1*E*). Mucosal changes from esophageal ulceration may be detected, and esophageal stricture may be present. Motility studies show marked reduction in the amplitude of smooth-muscle contractions, which may be peristaltic or nonperistaltic. Lower esophageal sphincter resting pressure is subnormal, but with normal relaxation (Fig. 305-3). Currently, there is no effective treatment for the motor difficulty. Reflux esophagitis and its complications should be treated aggressively as described under reflux esophagitis.

INFLAMMATORY DISORDERS

GASTROESOPHAGEAL REFLUX AND ESOPHAGITIS Reflux esophagitis consists of esophageal mucosal damage resulting from reflux of gastric or intestinal contents into the esophagus. Depending on the causative agent, it is referred to as peptic, bile, or alkaline esophagitis.

Pathophysiology Three considerations involved in the pathophysiology of reflux esophagitis are (1) the pathogenesis of the esophageal reflux episode, (2) the cumulative, or net, esophageal reflux, and (3) the pathogenesis of esophagitis.

Two conditions must be met for a *reflux episode* to occur: the gastrointestinal contents must be "ready" to reflux, and the antireflux mechanism at the lower end of the esophagus must be compromised. Gastrointestinal contents are most likely to reflux (1) when gastric volume is increased (after meals, with pyloric obstruction or gastric stasis syndrome, and in acid hypersecretory states), (2) when the gastric contents are located near the gastroesophageal junction (due to recumbency or bending), and (3) when gastric pressure is increased (with obesity, pregnancy, ascites, or tight binders or girdles).

The normal antireflux mechanisms consist of the lower esophageal sphincter (LES) and the anatomic configuration of the gastroesophageal junction. Reflux occurs only when the LES–gastric pressure gradient is lost. It can be caused by increased intragastric pressure or a transient or sustained decrease in the sphincter tone itself. Most patients with reflux have lower than normal LES pressures. The incompetence of the LES may be primary or secondary. The secondary causes include scleroderma-like diseases; a myopathic type of chronic intestinal pseudoobstruction syndrome; pregnancy; female sex hormones; smoking; smooth-muscle medications such as atropine, beta-adrenergics, aminophylline, nitrates, calcium channel antagonists, and other smooth-muscle relaxants; destruction of the sphincter by surgical resection, myotomy, or balloon dilation; and esophagitis. The importance of the anatomic configuration of the esophagogastric junction is not fully known at present. However, the role of a sliding hiatal hernia in the impairment of the reflux barrier is not felt to be so important as was once thought.

The net or *cumulative esophageal reflux*, i.e., the amount and duration of refluxed material remaining in the esophagus, is dependent on (1) the amount of refluxed material per episode and frequency of episodes; (2) the clearing of the esophagus by gravity and peristaltic contraction; and (3) neutralization by salivary secretion.

Esophagitis is a complication of reflux, and it develops when the mucosal defenses that normally counteract the effect of injurious agents on the esophageal mucosa succumb to the onslaught of the refluxed acid pepsin or bile. *Histologic esophagitis* shows microscopic changes of mucosal infiltration with granulocytes or eosinophils, hyperplasia of basal cells, and elongation of dermal pegs. It can occur with or without endoscopic abnormalities. *Erosive esophagitis* shows endoscopically visible damage to the mucosa in the form of marked redness, friability, bleeding, superficial linear ulcers, and exudates. *Peptic stricture* results from fibrosis that causes constriction of the esophageal lumen. The fibrosis is predominantly submucosal, but it may involve the whole wall. Peptic strictures occur in about 10 percent of patients with reflux esophagitis. Short peptic strictures caused by spontaneous reflux are usually 1 to 3 cm long and are present in the distal esophagus near the squamocolumnar junction (Fig. 305-2*B*). Long and tubular peptic strictures are the result of persistent vomiting or prolonged nasogastric intubation. Replacement of the squamous epithelium of the esophagus by columnar epithelium *(Barrett's esophagus)* may also result from reflux esophagitis. Columnar-cell lined-esophagus may be further complicated by peptic ulcer or peptic stricture high up in the lower or midesophagus, and adenocarcinoma may develop in 2 to 5 percent.

Clinical features Heartburn is the characteristic symptom and is produced by the contact of refluxed material with the inflamed esophageal mucosa. However, this symptom may be absent in some patients. Dysphagia suggests development of peptic stricture. In peptic strictures, the usual history is of several years of heartburn preceding dysphagia. However, in one-third of patients dysphagia may be the presenting symptoms. Progressive dysphagia and weight loss may indicate development of adenocarcinoma in Barrett's esophagus. Bleeding occurs due to mucosal erosions or Barrett's ulcer. Reflux in the absence of esophagitis is usually asymptomatic. Severe reflux may reach the pharynx and mouth and result in pulmonary aspiration. Recurrent pulmonary aspiration can cause aspiration pneumonia and pulmonary fibrosis.

Diagnosis Evaluation of reflux esophagitis is designed to assess the presence and severity of reflux, nature of refluxant, presence and severity of esophagitis, and pathophysiology of reflux. History, barium swallow, esophagoscopy, mucosal biopsy, esophageal motility, and a variety of special tests are utilized.

Presence of reflux is suggested by history. Spontaneous reflux from the stomach into the esophagus on barium examination suggests advanced reflux. Reflux of barium induced by stressful maneuvers is not very helpful, however, because of a high incidence of false-positive and false-negative results. Recently, scintiscan using radiolabeled 99^{m} technetium sulfur colloid has been used to quantitate gastroesophageal reflux. Several tests that utilize the recording of esophageal luminal pH with a small pH electrode have been proposed to detect and quantitate reflux of gastric acid. In these tests the pH electrode is swallowed, positioned in the stomach, gradually withdrawn across the LES, and then fixed at 5 cm above the sphincter. In the standard acid reflux test, a diagnosis of reflux can be made by failure of the pH to rise as the electrode enters the esophagus and by a decrease in esophageal pH with straining maneuvers. Quantitative information on the acid reflux is obtained by long-term (24-h) esophageal pH recording. The pH recordings are helpful only in the evaluation of acid reflux. The presence of bile or alkaline reflux is suggested by the occurrence of reflux symptoms in the absence of gastric acid and by the demonstration of bile in the aspirate of esophageal reflux.

The *presence and complications of reflux esophagitis* are assessed by barium swallow, esophagoscopy, mucosal biopsy, and the Bernstein test. Barium swallow is usually normal in uncomplicated esophagitis but may reveal the complication of stricture or ulcer formation. A high esophageal peptic stricture, deep ulcer, and adenocarcinoma suggest complications of Barrett's esophagus. Uncomplicated Barrett's esophagus is not diagnosed by barium studies. Esophagoscopy reveals the presence of erosive esophagitis, ordinary distal peptic stricture, or columnar cell–lined lower esophagus with or without a proximally located peptic stricture, ulcer, or adenocarcinoma. Esophagoscopy may be normal in many patients with esophagitis; in such patients mucosal biopsies and Bernstein tests are helpful. The mucosal biopsies should be obtained 5 cm above the LES because in the distal esophagus mucosal changes are quite frequent in normal subjects. False-positive and false-negative results occur in approximately 10 percent of biopsies. Patients with Barrett's esophagus will show columnar mucosa lining the esophagus which may be of gastric fundic, cardiac, or specialized type. The Bernstein test consists of an infusion of solutions of 0.1 *N* HCl and normal saline into the esophagus. It is useful in diagnosing reflux esophagitis which is not endoscopically obvious. In patients with reflux esophagitis, infusion of acid, but not of saline, reproduces the symptoms of heartburn. Infusion of acid in normal subjects produces no symptoms. Reflux esophagitis should be included in the differential diagnosis of chest pain, esophagitis, upper gastrointestinal bleeding, and dysphagia.

The *causative and predisposing factors* are assessed by history, esophageal motility, and esophageal clearance studies. Esophageal motility studies may provide useful quantitative information on the competence of the LES and of esophageal motor function. Barium swallow and scintiscans can be used to study esophageal clearance. An esophageal acid clearance test using a pH electrode quantifies the number of swallows necessary to clear the esophagus of 10 ml of instilled dilute 0.1 *N* HCl.

Full diagnostic evaluation is not necessary in every patient with reflux esophagitis. In transient and mild cases who give a clear-cut history of reflux esophagitis, a therapeutic trial may be sufficient. In persistent cases, and in those in whom the diagnosis is not clear, barium swallow, esophagoscopy, and esophageal motility with pH monitoring are indicated.

Treatment The main principle of treatment is neutralization of the offending material (antacids and H_2-receptor antagonists in peptic esophagitis; cholestyramine and aluminum hydroxide in bile esophagitis). In general, management of uncomplicated cases includes weight reduction, sleeping on a bed with elevation of the head of the bed, antacids (80 meq) 1 and 3 h after meals, cimetidine 300 mg at bedtime, elimination of factors that increase abdominal pressure, and avoidance of smoking and harmful medications. Patients should avoid fatty foods, coffee, chocolate, alcohol, mint, orange juice, and any other foods they find that exacerbate their symptoms. Anticholinergic drugs should not be used since they may reduce LES pressure and impair esophageal clearance.

In moderate to severe cases, the above measures are more strictly enforced, particularly elevation of the head end of the bed usually by 6 to 8 or sometimes as much as 12 in. Cimetidine, 300 mg qid, may be added. Long-acting H_2-receptor antagonists, such as ranitidine, may be more convenient to use. In the case of bile esophagitis, cholestyramine or aluminum hydroxide antacid is used. If the patient does not fully respond, metoclopramide (10 mg qid) or bethanecol (25 mg qid) can be prescribed to raise sphincter pressure, hasten gastric emptying, and improve esophageal clearance. Their usefulness, however, is limited. The role of coating agents such as sucralfate remains to be determined. Patients with reflux esophagitis with complications such as Barrett's esophagus with or without deep ulcer should be vigorously treated. Patients who have an associated peptic stricture are treated with dilators to relieve dysphagia in addition to vigorous treatment for reflux.

Antireflux surgery (Belsey repair, Nisson's fundoplication, and Hill repair), in which the gastric fundus is wrapped around the esophagus, increases the lower sphincter pressure and should be considered in resistant and complicated cases of reflux esophagitis that do not fully respond to medical therapy and in which there is persistently inadequate lower sphincter pressure but normal peristaltic contractions in the esophageal body.

Close follow-up is indicated in patients with complications of Barrett's esophagus because some of them may develop adenocarcinoma.

HERPES ESOPHAGITIS (See also Chap. 210) Herpes simplex virus may be normally present in saliva and may cause esophagitis in patients who are debilitated and immunosuppressed. Many patients are asymptomatic, while others complain of the acute onset of odynophagia and dysphagia. Bleeding may occur in severe cases, and systemic manifestations such as fever, chills, and mild leukocytosis may be present. Herpes blisters on the lips provide a clue to the diagnosis. Endoscopy shows vesicles and small, discrete, punched-out superficial ulcerations with or without fibrinous exudate. In later stages of the disease there is diffuse erosive esophagitis caused by enlargement and coalescence of the ulcers. Mucosal cells from biopsy of the edge of an ulcer show ballooning degeneration, ground-glass change in the nuclei with eosinophilic intranuclear inclusions (Cowdry type A), and giant-cell formation. These changes may also be detected in cytological specimens. Culture of the tissue for herpes simplex virus is required for definitive diagnosis. Examination of serial serum specimens for rising titers of complement-fixing antibodies to herpes simplex type I is helpful in diagnosis. Treatment is supportive because herpes esophagitis is a self-limited disease lasting 5 to 7 days. Viscous lidocaine is helpful in providing relief of odynophagia. Adequate fluid, electrolyte, and calorie intake should be ensured. The usefulness of antiviral agents such as vidarabine and acyclovir is not known.

***CANDIDA* (MONILIAL) ESOPHAGITIS** Many *Candida* species are normal inhabitants of the throat but become pathogenic and produce esophagitis in the setting of malignant neoplasms (particularly lymphoma and leukemia); treatment with immunosuppressive agents, steroids, and broad-spectrum antibiotics; diabetes mellitus; hypoparathyroidism; systemic lupus erythematosus; hemoglobinopathy; and corrosive esophageal injury. Occasionally monilial esophagitis occurs in the absence of any of the above predisposing factors. Patients may be asymptomatic or complain of odynophagia and dysphagia. Oral thrush or other evidence of mucocutaneous moniliasis may be absent. Systemic invasion with *Monilia* may occur.

Barium swallow may be normal or may show multiple nodular filling defects of various sizes (Fig. 305-2). Large nodular defects may resemble clusters of grapes. Endoscopy shows small yellow-white raised plaques with surrounding erythema in mild disease. In extensive disease, confluent linear and nodular plaques are seen. Diagnosis is made by demonstration of yeast or hyphal forms in the plaques using 10% KOH. Biopsies are not always positive. Culture is helpful in confirming the species and, if needed, the drug sensitivities of the yeast (see Chap. 184).

Nystatin oral suspension (100,000 units per milliliter) given in the dose of 4 to 6 ml every 4 h is the treatment of choice. In poorly responsive patients it can be administered every 2 h. The suspension can be made viscous in methylcellulose. Parenteral amphotericin B (total dose, 500 mg) is indicated in patients whose organisms are resistant to mycostatin, or who are toxic and in whom the presence of invasion is suspected. Flucytosine should not be used alone because of the potential development of tolerance. Microconazole and ketoconazole have been used successfully in some cases. Oral (viscous) lidocaine is used for temporary relief of pain.

OTHER TYPES OF ESOPHAGITIS *Irradiation esophagitis* is a common occurrence during radiation treatment for lung, mediastinal, or esophageal carcinoma. The frequency of esophagitis increases with the amount of radiation to the area. Dysphagia and odynophagia are the main symptoms and may last several weeks to several months after the conclusion of therapy. The esophageal mucosa becomes erythematous, edematous, and friable. Superficial erosions coalesce to form larger superficial ulcers. Submucosal fibrosis and degenerative changes in the blood vessels, muscles, and myenteric neurons may be present. The treatment is relief of pain with viscous lidocaine. Esophageal stricture may develop, causing severe dysphagia. Strictures are treated by dilation with rubber dilators. *Corrosive esophagitis* occurs following ingestion of caustic agents, such as strong alkalis, acids, or initiating medications accidentally or in suicide attempts. When severe, corrosive injury may lead to esophageal perforation, bleeding, and death. Healing is usually associated with stricture formation. Caustic strictures are usually long and rigid (Fig. 305-2). They can be dilated by passing a metal dilator of increasing diameter over a guide wire through the stricture. *Esophagitis associated with mucocutaneous disease* occurs in epidermolysis bullosa, pemphigoid, Behçet's syndrome, and Stevens-Johnson syndrome. Esophageal involvement in these disorders is indicated by development of odynophagia and dysphagia. Esophageal involvement responds to treatment of primary conditions.

TUMORS OF THE ESOPHAGUS

BENIGN TUMORS Benign tumors of the esophagus account for less than 10 percent of all esophageal tumors. The most common benign tumor is leiomyoma; less common ones are lipoma, fibrovascular polyp, squamous papilloma, and lymphangioma. These tumors are usually polypoid and frequently asymptomatic, although dysphagia occurs in a few patients when the esophageal lumen is severely compromised. Benign tumors must be distinguished from malignant tumors, although often this distinction cannot be made with certainty prior to surgical removal. Endoscopic mucosal biopsies are not helpful in the diagnosis of leiomyoma, lipoma, or fibrovascular polyps because of their submucosal location.

MALIGNANT TUMORS The primary malignant tumors of the esophagus are squamous-cell carcinoma (90 percent) and adenocarcinoma (less than 10 percent). Adenocarcinomas usually arise from metaplastic columnar epithelium (Barrett's esophagus) but may rarely arise from esophageal glands. Other uncommon tumors include carcinosarcoma, pseudosarcoma, melanoma, and verrucous squamous-cell carcinoma. In addition, adenocarcinoma of the stomach may spread to the esophagus by direct extension. Local spread from carcinoma of the lung or thyroid is unusual. Metastatic lesions from malignancies of remote organs are rare. Esophageal involvement may occur in up to 25 percent of patients with lymphoma, although symptomatic esophageal involvement occurs in less than 5 percent of these patients.

Squamous-cell carcinoma Squamous-cell carcinoma of the esophagus is the fifth most common cancer in adult males. There is considerable geographical variation with a very high incidence in certain regions of China, Iran, and Russia. In the United States it is more common in males than in females and three to four times more common in blacks than in whites.

Alcohol and smoking are important predisposing factors in the United States. Esophageal tumors may occur with higher frequency in association with carcinoma of the head and neck, lye strictures, ionizing radiation exposure, achalasia, Plummer-Vinson syndrome, and tylosis, a rare genetic disease in which the skin of the hands and feet is thickened.

CLINICAL FEATURES Progressive dysphagia and weight loss of short duration are characteristic. Dysphagia begins with solid foods and gradually progresses to include semisolids and liquids. In eccentric tumors and those arising from the stomach, dysphagia may be mild and may not occur until late in the disease. Dysphagia is rarely present for more than 1 year. Chest pain occurs as the tumor spreads to periesophageal tissues. Weight loss is usually profound because of anorexia and dysphagia. Bleeding from the tumor is usually slow, but brisk bleeding may occur. Rarely, invasion of the tumor into the aorta causes rapid exsanguination. Pulmonary aspiration, pneumonia, and, rarely, lung abscess can result from esophageal obstruction and aspiration or from tracheoesophageal fistula. Hoarseness may result from recurrent laryngeal nerve involvement. Physical examination is usually not striking except for evidence of recent weight loss. Supraclavicular nodes and an enlarged liver may be found when the tumor has spread to these sites. Signs of pulmonary aspiration may be present. Hypercalcemia may result from tumor production of a parathyroid hormone-like substance.

DIAGNOSIS The disease is usually advanced when the diagnosis is first made, and early detection is unusual. Carcinoma must be excluded by careful workup in all patients with persistent dysphagia and/or weight loss of short duration. Patients with gastric carcinoma involving the terminal esophagus may present themselves with symptoms suggestive of reflux esophagitis, while others may have what appears as achalasia or diffuse esophageal spasm. Recent development of any such symptoms in subjects over 40 years old should be carefully investigated.

The esophogram is the mainstay of diagnosis. Adequate esophageal distention and multiple views may be needed to diagnose early lesions. Double-contrast studies may also be helpful. An ulcerating lesion should be distinguished from a peptic ulcer in the columnar-cell-lined esophagus. Any esophageal ulcer that occurs without associated columnar-cell-lined esophagus should be considered carcinoma until proved otherwise. An infiltrating lesion may resemble a peptic stricture or may produce a picture resembling achalasia. Polypoid lesions should be distinguished from various benign neoplasms and from other types of carcinoma.

Endoscopy should be performed in all patients to detect suspected cases that may be missed on barium studies and to obtain tissue confirmation of cases that have been diagnosed on x-ray. Multiple biopsies and brush cytologies should be obtained. A thorough examination of the fundus of the stomach by turning the endoscope back on itself is imperative in all cases.

Computerized tomography has been helpful in determining extraesophageal spread to mediastinal structures and paraaortic abdominal lymph nodes.

TREATMENT Surgical therapy is indicated in resectable carcinoma of the lower third of the esophagus in relatively young subjects with otherwise good general health. Adenocarcinoma is also preferentially treated with surgery. Postoperatively, patients should be given radiation therapy. In other patients, radiation alone is given. Advanced cases are treated with radiotherapy and other conservative methods to keep the esophageal lumen patent so the patient can swallow saliva and other liquids. These maneuvers include esophageal dilation and insertion of a prosthesis, such as a Celestin tube. The prognosis is poor, and the overall 5-year survival rate is less than 5 percent.

OTHER ESOPHAGEAL DISORDERS

PHARYNGEAL AND ESOPHAGEAL DIVERTICULA Diverticula are outpouchings of the wall of the esophagus. *Zenker's diverticula* appear in the natural weakness in the posterior hypopharyngeal wall and cause halitosis and regurgitation of saliva and food particles consumed several days previously. When they become large and filled with food, they may compress the esophagus and cause dysphagia or complete obstruction. *Midesophageal diverticula* may be caused by traction from old adhesions or by propulsion associated with esophageal motor abnormalities. *Epiphrenic diverticula* may be associated with achalasia. Small- or medium-sized diverticula and midesophageal and epiphrenic diverticula are usually asymptomatic. *Diffuse intramural diverticulosis* of the esophagus is due to dilatation of the esophageal glands. This may be associated with a stricture high up in the esophagus. These patients may present with dysphagia.

Symptomatic Zenker's diverticula are treated by cricopharyngeal myotomy with or without diverticulectomy. Very large symptomatic esophageal diverticula are removed surgically. When they are associated with motor abnormalities, distal myotomy is performed. Stricture associated with diffuse intramural diverticulosis is treated with rubber dilators.

ESOPHAGEAL WEBS Weblike constrictions of the esophagus are usually congenital but may be acquired. Asymptomatic hypopharyngeal webs are demonstrated in up to 10 percent of normal individuals. When concentric, they cause intermittent dsyphagia to solids. Symptomatic hypopharyngeal webs with iron-deficiency anemia in middle-aged women constitute Plummer-Vinson syndrome. The clinical importance of this syndrome is uncertain. Midesophageal webs are rare. Symptomatic webs are treated by rupture of the web with a rubber dilator.

LOWER ESOPHAGEAL RINGS Lower esophageal *mucosal ring* (Schatski ring) is a thin weblike constriction located at the squamocolumnar mucosal junction at or near the border of the lower esophageal sphincter (Fig. 305-2). It invariably produces dysphagia when the diameter is less than 1.3 cm. The dysphagia to solids is the only symptom and it is usually episodic. Asymptomatic rings may be present in about 10 percent of normal individuals. Lower esophageal ring is one of the common causes of dysphagia. Treatment is simple rupture of the ring with a large-diameter rubber dilator.

Lower esophageal *muscular ring* (contractile ring) is located proximal to the site of mucosal rings and may represent the abnormal uppermost segment of the lower esophageal sphincter. These rings are characterized by a change in size and shape from one time to another (Fig. 305-1). They may also cause dysphagia and should be differentiated from peptic strictures, achalasia, and lower esophageal mucosal rings. They are treated with rubber dilators.

HIATAL HERNIA Hiatal hernia is a herniation of a part of the stomach into the thoracic cavity through the esophageal hiatus in the diaphragm. A *sliding hiatal hernia* is one in which the gastroesophageal junction and fundus of the stomach slide upward. A sliding hernia may result from weakening of the anchors of the gastroesophageal junction to the diaphragm, longitudinal contraction of the esophagus, or increased intraabdominal pressure. Small sliding hernias can be demonstrated commonly during barium studies if intraabdominal pressure is increased. Their incidence increases with age; in the sixth decade of life the prevalence of such hernias is around 60 percent. It is unlikely that a small sliding hiatal hernia by itself produces any clinical symptoms, and its role in the pathogenesis of reflux esophagitis is uncertain.

A *paraesophageal* hernia is one in which the esophagogastric junction remains fixed in its normal location and a pouch of stomach herniates beside the gastroesophageal junction through the esophageal hiatus. A paraesophageal or mixed paraesophageal and sliding hernia may become incarcerated and strangulate. This situation is manifested by acute chest pain, dysphagia, and a mediastinal mass, and requires prompt operative treatment. A herniated gastric pouch may cause dysphagia and may be the site of gastritis and ulceration causing chronic blood loss. A large paraesophageal hernia should be repaired because of a high rate of complications.

ESOPHAGEAL RUPTURE Perforation of the esophagus may be caused by (1) iatrogenic damage from instrumentation of the esophagus or external trauma; (2) increased intraesophageal pressure associated with forceful vomiting or retching (this is also called spontaneous rupture or Boerhaave's syndrome); or (3) diseases of the esophagus such as corrosive ingestion, peptic ulcer, neoplasm, and, rarely, esophagomalacia. The site of perforation is variable and depends on the cause. Instrumental perforation occurs in the pharynx and the lower esophagus. Iatrogenic perforation is usually a tear, 1 to 8 cm in length, which is present just above the diaphragm in the posterolateral wall.

Esophageal perforation causes severe retrosternal chest pain which may be worsened by swallowing. Free air enters the mediastinum and spreads to neighboring structures and causes palpable subcutaneous emphysema in the neck, mediastinal cracking sounds on auscultation, and pneumothorax. Pleural effusion and hydropneumothorax may ensue, and severe cases are associated with shock. With time secondary infection supervenes, and mediastinal abscess and pleuropulmonary suppurative complications may develop. Esophageal perforation associated with vomiting usually deposits gastric contents in the mediastinum and causes severe mediastinal complications. On the other hand, instrumental perforation may be mild and free of severe complications.

Spontaneous rupture of the esophagus may mimic myocardial infarction, pancreatitis, or ruptured abdominal viscus. Symptoms of chest pain may be mild, particularly in the elderly, and mediastinal emphysema may develop late. X-ray of the chest shows abnormalities in the majority of patients, and diagnosis is confirmed by barium swallow.

Treatment includes esophageal and gastric suction and parenteral broad-spectrum antibiotics. Surgical drainage and repair of the laceration should be performed as soon as possible. In patients with terminal carcinoma, surgical repair may not be feasible, and those with minor instrumental perforations can be treated conservatively. Extensive corrosive damage may require esophageal diversion and subsequent excision.

MALLORY-WEISS SYNDROME Vomiting and retching may cause a tear that involves only the mucosa and is not transmural. The tear usually involves the gastric mucosa near the squamocolumnar mucosal junction, but it may also involve the esophageal mucosa. Patients present with upper gastrointestinal bleeding which may be severe. Most patients recover with only conservative management, but those with severe arterial bleeding require surgery.

FOREIGN BODIES Foreign bodies may lodge in the cervical esophagus just beyond the upper esophageal sphincter, around the aortic arch, or above the lower esophageal sphincter. Impaction of a bolus of food, particularly a piece of meat or bread, may occur when the esophageal lumen is narrowed due to stricture, carcinoma, or a lower esophageal ring. Acute impaction causes complete inability to swallow and severe chest pain. Both foreign bodies and food boluses may be removed endoscopically. Use of meat tenderizer to facilitate passage of an obstructed meat bolus is to be discouraged because of potential digestion of the esophagus itself.

REFERENCES

BEHAR J et al: Cimetidine in the treatment of symptomatic gastroesophageal reflux. A double blind controlled trial. Gastroenterology 74:441, 1978

BOZYMSKI EM et al: Barrett's esophagus. Ann Intern Med 97:103, 1982

CEDERQVIST C et al: Cancer of the oesophagus: I. 1002 cases. Survey and survival; II. Therapy and outcome. Acta Chir Scand 144:227, 1978

COHEN S: Motor disorders of the esophagus. N Engl J Med 301:184, 1979

DODDS WJ et al: Pathogenesis of reflux esophagitis. Gastroenterology 81:376, 1981

GOYAL RK, RATTAN S: Neurohumoral, hormonal and drug receptors for the lower esophageal sphincter. Gastroenterology 74:598, 1973

KILMAN WJ, GOYAL RK: Disorders of pharyngeal and upper esophageal sphincter motor function. Arch Intern Med 136:592, 1976

OWENSBY LC, STAMMER JL: Esophagitis associated with herpes simplex infection in an immunocompetent host. Gastroenterology 74:1305, 1978

PARKER EF, MOERTEL CC: Carcinoma of the esophagus: Is there a role for surgery? Am J Dig Dis 23:730, 1978

RICHTER JE, CASTELL DO: Gastroesophageal reflux: Pathogenesis, diagnosis and therapy. Ann Intern Med 97:93, 1982

VANTRAPPEN G, HELLEMANS J: Treatment of achalasia and related motor disorders. Gastroenterology 79:144, 1980

306
PEPTIC ULCER

JAMES E. McGUIGAN

The term *peptic ulcer* is used to refer to a group of ulcerative disorders of the upper gastrointestinal tract which appear to have in common the participation of acid-pepsin in their pathogenesis. The major forms of peptic ulcer are chronic duodenal and gastric ulcer. The Zollinger-Ellison syndrome, which is caused by gastrin-releasing tumors (gastrinomas), may also be considered a form of peptic ulcer.

Although our present knowledge of the etiology of peptic ulcer is incomplete, information from studies in humans and in experimental animals indicates that acid-pepsin is crucial for development of peptic ulcer. The presence or absence of peptic ulcer is determined by the delicate interplay between gastric acid secretion and mucosal resistance. Peptic ulcer is produced when the aggressive effects of acid-pepsin dominate the protective effects of gastric or duodenal mucosal resistance. Why do not all humans develop peptic ulcer? The normal capacity of gastric and proximal duodenal mucosa to resist the corrosive effects of acid-pepsin is extraordinary and unique. This resistance to acid-pepsin is not shared by other tissues—hence the susceptibility of the esophageal mucosa to injury when exposed to refluxed gastric juice and the almost inevitable ulceration of the small intestine at the site of surgical attachment to actively secreting gastric mucosa.

Much has been learned concerning the mechanisms regulating gastric secretion and about a variety of factors which appear important in the development of peptic ulcer. Consideration of gastric physiology provides an understanding of some elements responsible for producing peptic ulcer as well as a rational basis for its treatment.

GASTRIC PHYSIOLOGY RELATED TO PEPTIC ULCER

The gastric mucosa possesses an extraordinary capacity to secrete acid. Parietal (oxyntic) cells secrete hydrochloric acid by a process involving oxidative phosphorylation. Parietal cells, located in mucosal glands in the body and fundus of the stomach, can secrete hydrogen ions at a concentration 3 million times that found in blood. The estimated concentration of HCl secreted directly by parietal cells is approximately 160 m*M*. Each secreted hydrogen ion (H^+) is accompanied by a chloride ion (Cl^-). With increased gastric hydrogen ion secretion, there is a reciprocal decrease in sodium ion secretion. For each hydrogen ion secreted into the gastric lumen, one bicarbonate ion (HCO_3^-) is returned via the gastric venous circulation, accounting for the *alkaline tide,* which directly reflects the magnitude of gastric H^+ secretion. Bicarbonate is released from carbonic acid; the latter is generated from carbon dioxide by parietal cell carbonic anhydrase. The two-component hypothesis for secretion of gastric juice proposes that parietal cells secrete pure HCl, which is mixed (in various proportions) with nonparietal cell alkaline secretions, similar in ionic composition to extracellular fluid.

Multiple *chemical, neural,* and *hormonal* factors participate in regulation of gastric acid secretion. Acid secretion is stimulated by gastrin and by cholinergic postganglionic vagal fibers via muscarinic receptors on parietal cells. Gastrin, the most potent known stimulant of gastric acid secretion, is present in cytoplasmic secretory granules in gastrin cells (or G cells) which are interspersed among other epithelial cells in the mid and deeper portions of the antral pyloric glands. Gastrin, as many other peptides, is present in multiple molecular forms (Fig. 306-1). The major form of tissue gastrin is heptadecapeptide gastrin (G-17) which contains 17 amino acid residues. Gastrin II is the form of gastrin in which the tyrosyl residue at position 12 is sulfated, and gastrin I is the nonsulfated form. Approximately two-thirds of circulating gastrin consists of a larger molecular species of gastrin, namely, "big gastrin," or G-34. This species of gastrin contains 34 amino acids, the final 17 of which are identical to heptadecapeptide gastrin and may also be present in sulfated (G-34 II) or nonsulfated (G-34 I) forms. G-17 has a shorter half-life than G-34. Although most circulating gastrin is G-34, the major hormonal stimulus to gastric acid secretion after feeding is due to G-17. On a molar basis circulating G-17 is approximately six times as potent as G-34 in stimulating gastric acid secretion.

More than 90 percent of antral mucosal gastrin is in the form of G-17. Gastrin is also present in duodenal mucosa, the highest concentration being in the most proximal duodenum (approximately 10 percent of the antral concentration). The mucosal concentration of gastrin and the proportion as G-17 decrease with progression down the duodenum. The effects of gastrin and the vagus on gastric acid secretion are intimately related. Vagal stimulation increases gastric acid secretion by (1) directly stimulating parietal cells, (2) stimulating release of gastrin into the circulation, and (3) lowering the parietal cell threshold to circulating gastrin concentrations. There is also evidence that some possibly noncholinergic vagal branches or fibers may inhibit gastrin release.

Histamine is present in large concentrations in mast cells in the lamina propria of the parietal cell–containing regions of the gastric mucosa. Histamine-containing mast cells are in close proximity to parietal cells, with a ratio of one mast cell to every two or three parietal cells. Views on the importance of histamine in stimulating gastric acid secretion have differed enormously, with some suggesting that histamine is the "final common pathway" for cholinergic and gastrin stimulation of parietal cell acid secretion, while others were skeptical about any role of histamine in this process.

Interest in the role of histamine on acid secretion was renewed by the discovery of H_2-receptor antagonists which inhibit the action of histamine on H_2-receptors (located on gastric parietal, cardiac atrial, and uterine smooth-muscle cells). These drugs exert negligible effect on H_1-receptors, which are readily inhibited by conventional antihistamines. H_2-receptor antagonists (e.g., cimetidine) inhibit basal acid secretion and secretory responses to feeding, gastrin, histamine, hypoglycemia, and vagal stimulation. Most of the presently available information supports the conclusions that (1) histamine does play an important role in stimulating acid secretion, (2) it acts in concert with gastrin and cholinergic activity on parietal cells, which bear receptors for histamine, gastrin, and acetylcholine, but (3) it is probably *not* the final common effector molecule in the stimulation of parietal cell secretion.

Food ingestion is the major physiological stimulus of gastric acid secretion. Traditionally, gastric acid secretion has been classified into three phases—cephalic, gastric, and intestinal. This classification is of some value in examining the multiple factors which regulate gastric acid secretion. The *cephalic phase* represents the gastric acid secretory response to the sight, smell, taste, and anticipation of food. The *gastric phase* is induced by the presence of food in the stomach. The *intestinal phase* is due to the entry or presence of food within the lumen of the small intestine. Although these three phases are convenient for considering the diverse contributions to gastric acid secretion, each phase is complex and not necessarily due to a single stimulatory control mechanism.

The cephalic phase appears to be mediated primarily by the vagus, which increases gastric acid secretion by stimulation of parietal cells directly and by stimulating the release of gastrin into the circulation. The gastric phase involves stimulation of chemical and mechanical receptors in the gastric wall by luminal contents. Mechanical distention of the stomach stimulates gastric acid secretion but not gastrin release; this mechanical effect is inhibited by atropine and appears to be mediated by vagal reflexes. Food in the stomach promotes acid secretion by increasing gastrin release, principally due to the *protein* content and the *products* of *protein digestion* contained in the meal; oral glucose and fat cause slight increases in serum gastrin but do no stimulate gastric acid secretion. Food in the proximal small intestine stimulates the intestinal phase of gastric acid secretion. A peptone meal introduced into the small intestine stimulates gastric acid secretion but not gastrin release. It has been proposed that food in the small intestine induces release of an intestinal hormone, presumably a polypeptide, which stimulates gastric acid secretion. This substance is believed to be distinct from gastrin and, unlike gastrin, appears to be degraded substantially during its portal transit through the liver.

Ingestion of both caffeine-containing and caffeine-free *coffee* stimulates gastric acid secretion: both forms of coffee stimulate gastrin release. In humans *ethanol* ingestion does not stimulate gastrin release or acid secretion; in fact, at concentrations sufficient to interrupt the gastric mucosal barrier (i.e., greater than 14 percent), ethanol reduces gastric acid output. Intravenous *calcium* stimulates acid secretion and produces minimal increases in serum gastrin levels. Oral calcium has been reported to stimulate gastric acid secretion directly, i.e., without an increase in serum calcium or gastrin concentrations. Except in patients with gastrinoma, hypercalcemia is usually not associated with acid hypersecretion or increases in serum gastrin.

Inhibition of gastric acid secretion can be produced by several mechanisms. Acid secretion may be inhibited by acid in the stomach or duodenum, by hyperglycemia, or by hypertonic fluids or fat in the duodenum. Reduction of the intragastric pH to 3.0 produces partial inhibition of gastrin release; further reduction to pH 1.5 or below blocks the release of gastrin to almost all stimuli. There is evidence that inhibition of gastrin release by intraluminal acid is due to the action of *somatostatin,* which is present in high concentrations in antral mucosal D cells. Somatostatin reduces gastric acid secretion by inhibition of gastrin release and by direct inhibition of parietal cell secretion. Acid in the duodenum also inhibits gastric acid secretion; this may be secondary to stimulation of release of secretin and/or other peptides capable of inhibiting gastric acid secretion. *Secretin* is a linear polypeptide which contains 27 amino acids and bears structural similarities to glucagon. Secretin is released from S cells in the mucosa of the small intestine in response to mucosal acidification. Fat in the duodenum also inhibits gastric acid secretion; gastric inhibitory peptide (GIP) has been proposed as a candidate for this enterogastrone action; however, this role for GIP is yet to be proved. The mechanisms by which hyperglycemia or intraduodenal hyperosmolality inhibits gastric acid secretion are not known. Additional peptides identified in the mucosa of the

Big Gastrin (G 34)	Glu-Leu-Gly-Pro-Gln-Gly-Pro-Pro-His-Leu-Val-Ala-Asp-Pro-Ser-Lys-Lys- -Gln-Gly-Pro-Trp-Leu-Glu-Glu-Glu-Glu-Glu-Ala-Tyr*-Gly-Trp-Met-Asp-Phe-NH_2
Heptadecapeptide Gastrin (G 17)	Glu-Gly-Pro-Trp-Leu-Glu-Glu-Glu-Glu-Glu-Ala-Tyr*-Gly-Trp-Met-Asp-Phe-NH_2
Minigastrin (G 14)	Trp-Leu-Glu-Glu-Glu-Glu-Glu-Ala-Tyr*-Gly-Trp-Met-Asp-Phe-NH_2
C-Terminal pentapeptide	Gly-Trp-Met-Asp-Phe-NH_2

FIGURE 306-1
*Amino acid sequences of gastrin peptides, all of which contain the common C-terminal pentapeptide amide. (*Tyrosyl is sulfated in gastrin II and nonsulfated in gastrin I molecules.)*

gastrointestinal tract which have the capacity to inhibit gastric acid secretion include glucagon-like peptides, vasoactive intestinal peptide (VIP), and urogastrone; the latter appears to be structurally and functionally identical to epidermal growth factor. The extent to which these peptides contribute to the overall regulation of gastric acid secretion is not clear.

The proteolytic effect of *pepsin* and the corrosive effects of acid appear to be integral components in the tissue injury which leads to peptic ulceration. Acid autocatalytically cleaves inactive pepsinogen molecules to active pepsins and also provides the pH required for pepsin activity. Pepsin activity is substantially reduced above pH 4.0, and these enzymes are inactivated irreversibly at neutral or alkaline pH. There are a variety of pepsinogens and pepsins in gastric juice. Pepsinogens (and their corresponding active pepsins) have been classified by immunochemical techniques as either PG I (pepsinogens 1 through 5) or PG II (pepsinogens 6 and 7). Pepsinogen I is present in chief and mucous cells in the body and fundus of the stomach. Pepsinogen II is located in cells of the pyloric glands, Brunner's glands of the duodenum, mucous cells of the gastric cardiac glands, and the same cells in which PG I is found. Both PG I and PG II are found in plasma, while only PG I can be detected in urine. A high degree of correlation exists between serum concentrations of PG I and maximal gastric acid secretion. In general, agents which stimulate gastric acid secretion also stimulate pepsinogen secretion. Cholinergic action is particularly potent in promoting pepsinogen secretion. Secretin, although it inhibits gastric acid secretion, stimulates pepsinogen secretion.

Parietal cells also secrete *intrinsic factor.* Agents which stimulate gastric acid secretion also lead to secretion of intrinsic factor.

The precise mechanism or mechanisms which comprise *mucosal resistance,* by which the normal stomach and duodenum resist the corrosive effects of acid-pepsin, have not been defined. The importance of gastric mucus to mucosal resistance is uncertain. Gastric mucus, secreted by gastric mucous cells, is a gelatinous material which coats the mucosal surface of the stomach. Mucus secretion is enhanced by mechanical or chemical irritation and by cholinergic stimulation. Gastric mucus is a polymer which contains four protein subunits. Depolymerization of the glycoprotein subunits of mucus, which may be produced by peptic digestion or disruption of disulfide bonds, renders the glycoprotein incapable of forming a viscous gel. This mucus coating serves as an unstirred layer through which the diffusion of acid and pepsin is reduced. Bicarbonate ions are secreted by gastric surface epithelial cells and enter the unstirred layer of mucus gel; this mechanism facilitates the development of a substantial hydrogen ion gradient between major gastric luminal contents and the apical surfaces of gastric mucosal cells.

Gastric mucus contains glycoprotein blood group substances. Approximately three-fourths of the population secrete gastric juice containing AB(H) substances and are referred to as *secretors.* Normally the gastric luminal epithelial cell surfaces and intercellular tight junctions provide an almost completely impermeable barrier to back-diffusion of hydrogen ions from the lumen. This *gastric mucosal barrier* may participate in mucosal resistance to acid-peptic ulceration. This barrier may be interrupted by various agents including bile acids, salicylates, alcohol, and weak organic acids, thus permitting *back-diffusion of hydrogen ions* from the lumen to intra- and intercellular sites. Such back-diffusion may result in cellular injury, release of histamine from mast cells, further stimulation of acid secretion, damage to small blood vessels, mucosal hemorrhage, and superficial ulceration. Interruption of the gastric mucosal barrier may be responsible (at least in part) for the hemorrhagic erosive gastritis associated with salicylate and ethanol ingestion and may also contribute to other forms of gastric mucosal injury. *Decreased mucosal blood flow,* accompanied by back-diffusion of available hydrogen ions, also appears to contribute to gastric mucosal damage. *Prostaglandins* are present in abundant quantities in the gastric mucosa. Various prostaglandins have been shown to inhibit gastric mucosal injury due to a wide variety of agents. It is possible that endogenous prostaglandins contribute to mucosal resistance and have a cytoprotective function.

The relationship between the gastric mucosal barrier and mucosal resistance to chronic peptic ulcer has not been completely elucidated. Other mucosal factors, some of which are genetic, apparently contribute to the ability of the gastric mucosa to resist or permit the development of peptic ulceration.

MEASUREMENT OF GASTRIC ACID SECRETION

Since HCl secretion by the stomach appears to be an important factor in the production of peptic ulcer disease, measurement of basal and stimulated acid secretion by the stomach may be of value in the assessment of peptic ulcer patients. In general, basal and stimulated acid outputs in females are approximately two-thirds to three-fourths those found in males. The range of values for normal subjects is extremely broad and overlaps substantially with that found in patients with duodenal ulcer, gastric ulcer, and even the Zollinger-Ellison syndrome. Mean basal acid output (BAO) in normal males without known ulcer disease is about 1.5 to 2.0 meq/h. In duodenal ulcer patients mean basal acid output averages from 4 to 6 meq/h, again with a wide degree of variation. Patients with gastric ulcer tend to have gastric acid secretory rates which are normal or even slightly below those of normal subjects.

Measurement of gastric acid output is not helpful in either diagnosing peptic ulcer or excluding it. Thus measuring gastric acid secretion is clearly not necessary in all patients with duodenal ulcer disease. However, detection of gastric acid hypersecretion is of value when the Zollinger-Ellison syndrome is suspected. Measurement of gastric acid output is useful to detect achlorhydria, as found in patients with pernicious anemia. Since patients with benign gastric ulcer virtually always secrete some acid, pentagastrin-fast achlorhydria in a patient with a gastric ulcer almost always indicates malignancy. Measurement of gastric acid secretion is indicated in the search for the cause of ulcer recurrence after surgery for peptic ulcer.

In order to measure gastric acid output, a radiopaque gastric tube is passed so that its tip is located in the most dependent portion of the stomach. With the patient in a reclining or semirecumbent position on the left side, the position of the tube is verified by fluoroscopy. Gastric contents are aspirated and discarded. Basal gastric acid secretions are then collected in four consecutive 15-min intervals to determine the 1-h basal acid output. Secretion volume and acid concentration (titrated with 0.1 *N* sodium hydroxide to pH 7.0) are measured, and acid output is expressed as milliequivalents per hour.

A variety of substances have been used to produce maximal acid output (MAO) by the stomach. These have included *histamine, betazole* (Histalog)—a structural analogue of histamine—and *pentagastrin* (Peptavlon). Histamine, the first standard stimulant to be used for gastric acid secretory testing, requires the simultaneous administration of an antihistaminic agent to inhibit untoward systemic side effects. Betazole possesses fewer of the undesired side effects of histamine and does not require the concomitant administration of an antihistamine. Pentagastrin (*N-tert*-butyloxycarbonyl-β-Ala-Try-Met-Asp-Phe-NH_2) contains the biologically active carboxyl-terminal tetrapeptide amide portion of the gastrin molecule and is currently the preferred agent to induce maximal acid secretion. Gastric juice is collected for four additional consecutive 15-min periods after the subcutaneous injection of pentagastrin (6 μg/kg). The MAO is the expression of the milliequivalents of acid aspirated during the 1 h after pentagastrin administration. Peak acid output (PAO) is calculated by combining the two highest consecutive 15-min acid outputs following pentagastrin injection and multiplying by 2.

DUODENAL ULCER

GENERAL CONSIDERATIONS Duodenal ulcer is a chronic and recurrent disease. The ulcer is usually deep and sharply demarcated. It tends to penetrate through the submucosa and often into the muscularis propria. The ulcer floor contains no intact epithelium and usually consists of a zone of eosinophilic necrosis resting on a base of granulation tissue surrounded by variable amounts of fibrosis. The ulcer bed may be clear or contain either blood or a proteinaceous exudate with entrapped erythrocytes and acute and chronic inflammatory cells. More than 95 percent of duodenal ulcers occur in the first portion of the duodenum, and approximately 90 percent of these are located within 3 cm of the junction of the pyloric and duodenal mucosa. Duodenal ulcers are usually round or oval, but they may be irregular or elliptic. They are usually less than 1 cm in diameter. Rarely, duodenal ulcers may be extremely large (3 to 6 cm in diameter) and may be mistaken radiographically for the entire duodenal bulb. These giant ulcers are usually identified directly by endoscopy or at surgery or postmortem examination.

The absolute prevalence of duodenal ulcer in the population is not known. Estimates have ranged from 6 to 15 percent. This variation may be related to the populations examined, differences in study design and diagnostic methods (e.g., endoscopy vs. radiological examination), and perhaps to actual changes in frequency of duodenal ulcer disease. The best current estimates suggest that approximately 10 percent of the population has clinical evidence of duodenal ulcer at some time in their lifetimes. Duodenal ulcer is approximately two to three times as common in males as in females and is four times as frequent as clinically recognized gastric ulcer. The frequency of duodenal ulcer and its recognized complications has been decreasing in the United States and England during the past 30 years. The reason or reasons for this reduction are not known.

Duodenal ulcer is both chronic and recurrent. It has been estimated that approximately 50 percent of duodenal ulcers recur within 1 year and from 80 to 90 percent within 2 years. Although much is now known concerning factors which contribute to the development of duodenal ulcer, we do not completely understand its pathogenesis. Acid secretion by the stomach is required for production of a duodenal ulcer, but the factors which render the acid-secreting subject susceptible to duodenal ulceration are not completely understood. As a group, duodenal ulcer patients secrete more acid than normal; however, from one-half to two-thirds of duodenal ulcer patients have gastric acid secretory rates, both BAO and MAO, within the normal range. Duodenal ulcer patients have been shown to have, on the average, approximately 1.9 billion parietal cells, with a maximum capacity to secrete approximately 42 meq of gastric acid per hour, which contrasts with 1.0 billion parietal cells and 22 meq/h for nonduodenal ulcer subjects. However, the variations between both groups are so large that most duodenal ulcer patients are within the normal range. As a group, duodenal ulcer patients also have comparable increases in gastric secretion of pepsin and in serum pepsinogen I levels. Peptic ulcer appears to develop when there is an unfavorable balance between gastric acid-pepsin secretion and gastric or duodenal mucosal resistance. In duodenal ulcer disease, the evidence favors the etiologic importance of absolute or, in most instances, relative gastric acid hypersecretion. However, in patients with gastric ulcer, defective mucosal resistance appears to be the major permissive etiologic factor.

Fasting *serum gastrin* concentrations are normal in duodenal ulcer patients. However, in response to a protein-containing meal, more gastrin is released into the circulation in duodenal ulcer patients than in normal subjects. Duodenal ulcer patients also have a greater gastric acid secretory response to gastrin than normal persons. Thus given doses of pentagastrin or gastrin produce more acid secretion, and smaller doses of pentagastrin or gastrin are required to achieve the same fraction (50 percent) of the maximal acid secretory response in duodenal ulcer patients compared with normal subjects. In addition, in duodenal ulcer patients intragastric acid is less effective in inhibiting both gastrin release and gastric acid secretion. Therefore, although fasting serum gastrin levels are normal in duodenal ulcer patients, gastrin may still play an important role in their often observed acid hypersecretion. Duodenal ulcer patients tend to empty their stomachs more rapidly than do nonduodenal ulcer patients. This phenomenon, together with acid hypersecretion, may contribute to greater hydrogen ion concentrations in the first part of the duodenum in patients with duodenal ulcer.

Genetic factors appear to be important. Duodenal ulcers are approximately three times as common in first-degree relatives of duodenal ulcer patients when compared with the population at large. Patients with duodenal ulcers have an increased frequency of blood group O and of the nonsecretory status [those who do not secrete AB(H) antigens in their gastric juice], but these associations are weak. An increased incidence of HLA-B5 antigen in white male subjects with duodenal ulcer has also been shown. Elevated serum pepsinogen I (PG I) levels have been found in approximately 50 percent of patients with duodenal ulcer. Increases in serum pepsinogen appear to be inherited as an autosomal dominant trait. Individuals with this trait have a frequency of duodenal ulcer eight times greater than the general population. Thus an elevated PG I level may prove to be a valuable subclinical marker of the duodenal ulcer diathesis in families with this autosomal dominant form of peptic ulcer disease.

Cigarette smoking has been associated with increased duodenal ulcer frequency, decreased responses to therapy, and an increased mortality (from duodenal ulcer). Cigarette smoking does not increase gastric acid secretion. It has been suggested that the increased incidence of duodenal ulcer among cigarette smokers may be secondary to the demonstrated effects of cigarette smoking in inhibiting pancreatic bicarbonate secretion (a neutralizer of secreted gastric acid) and/or by acceleration of gastric emptying of acid into the duodenum. The incidence of duodenal ulcer is also increased in patients with chronic renal failure, alcoholic cirrhosis, renal transplantation, hyperparathyroidism, systemic mastocytosis, and chronic obstructive pulmonary disease. Antibodies to herpes simplex have been reported to be higher in titer and more frequent in serums of patients with duodenal ulcer than in normals.

The importance of *psychological factors* in the pathogenesis of duodenal ulcer remains controversial. Contrary to earlier views, there is no single characteristic duodenal ulcer personality. There is no identifiable differences in frequency of duodenal ulcer among different socioeconomic classes or occupation groups. Chronic anxiety and psychological stress may, however, be factors in exacerbation of ulcer activity.

CLINICAL FEATURES Epigastric pain is by far the most frequent symptom of duodenal ulcer. The pain is often described as burning or gnawing. Just as frequently, however, the pain may be ill-defined, boring, or aching, or is perceived as abdominal pressure or fullness, or as a sensation of hunger. In approximately 10 percent of patients the pain is located to the right of the midepigastrium. The pain characteristically occurs from 90 min to 3 h after eating. It frequently awakens the patient at night. Pain on awakening before breakfast is sufficiently rare in patients with duodenal ulcer as to challenge the diagnosis. The pain is usually relieved within a few minutes by food or antacids. The severity of pain varies substantially from patient to patient, and symptoms tend to be recurrent and episodic. Duodenal ulcer may recur in the absence of pain. Episodes of pain may persist for periods of several days to weeks or months. Periods of remission may last from weeks to years and are almost always longer than the episodes of pain. In some patients the disease is more aggressive, with frequent persistent symptoms and development of complications. Pain relief (whether with antacids or food) is believed to result from acid neutralization. Ingestion of food leads to a transient partial neutralization of gastric acid, which is followed by gastrin release and resultant stimulation of acid secretion. With subsequent gastric emptying and increasing gastric acid secretion, a sufficiently low pH is achieved that pain results. Acid-induced pain in patients with duodenal ulcer is believed due to (1) acid stimulation of chemical receptors and/or (2) alterations in gastric motility.

Changes in the character of the pain may signal the development of complications. For example, ulcer pain which becomes constant, is no longer relieved by food or antacids, or radiates to the back or either upper quadrant may herald *penetration* of the ulcer (often into the pancreas). Ulcer pain which is accentuated rather than relieved by food, and/or is accompanied by vomiting, often indicates *gastric outlet obstruction.* Abrupt, severe, or generalized abdominal pain is characteristic of free *perforation* into the peritoneal cavity. Weight loss, in the absence of some degree of gastric outlet obstruction, is unusual. Duodenal ulcer may cause acute gastrointestinal *hemorrhage,* with vomiting of blood or coffee-grounds material, or with melena, and the passage of black tarry stools or even frank red blood, if the bleeding is massive.

It is important to emphasize that *many patients with active disease have no ulcer symptoms.* This leads to a significant, although not quantifiable, underestimation of duodenal ulcer frequency and recurrence in the population. Recent studies, especially those using duodenoscopy, indicate that there is poor correlation between ulcer activity, resolution of symptoms, and ulcer healing. Since many duodenal ulcer patients are asymptomatic, the absence of ulcer-type pain does not exclude duodenal ulcer as a potential cause for gastrointestinal hemorrhage or symptoms due to gastric outlet obstruction or abrupt ulcer perforation.

On *physical examination* epigastric tenderness is by far the most frequent abnormal finding. The area of tenderness is usually in the midline, often midway between the umbilicus and the xiphoid process. In 20 to 30 percent of patients the tender area is to the right of the midline. Acute free perforation of the ulcer into the peritoneal cavity often produces a rigid, boardlike abdomen, usually with generalized rebound tenderness. In patients with gastric outlet obstruction caused by a duodenal or pyloric channel ulcer one may find a "succussion splash" due to fluid and air in the distended stomach. Tachycardia or hypotension, in some instances demonstrable only by orthostatic maneuvers, may reflect acute hemorrhage from duodenal ulcer. Cutaneous and mucosal pallor may result from anemia from acute or chronic blood loss.

Only about 5 percent of duodenal ulcers are located distal to the duodenal bulb, and most of these are in the immediate postbulbar portion of the first part of the duodenum. Most immediate postbulbar ulcers are of the common duodenal ulcer variety. However, postbulbar ulceration, when located in or beyond the second portion of the duodenum, suggests the Zollinger-Ellison syndrome. Postbulbar ulcer pain may be located in the right upper quadrant or radiate through to the back. Obstruction and hemorrhage are more frequent with postbulbar ulcers than with those in the duodenal bulb.

The pyloric channel, which is 1 to 2 cm in length, is the narrowest portion of the gastric outlet. Ulcers in this location may produce symptoms similar to those of a duodenal ulcer; however, symptoms due to channel ulcer tend to be less responsive to food and antacids. With pyloric channel ulcers food may accentuate rather than relieve ulcer pain and may result in vomiting secondary to partial gastric outlet obstruction. In general, surgery is required more frequently with channel ulcers than with those in the duodenal bulb.

DIAGNOSIS Epigastric pain readily relieved by food or antacids strongly suggests duodenal ulcer. However, many patients with ulcer-like symptoms may have no evidence of an ulcer even after careful radiographic and endoscopic examination. Barium examination of the upper gastrotintestinal tract is of value in identifying duodenal ulcer and is the usual method used to establish the diagnosis. The proportion of ulcers identified radiographically depends on the skill, persistence, enthusiasm, and diagnostic criteria of the radiologist. Using conventional barium contrast techniques, 70 to 80 percent of duodenal ulcers visualized by endoscopy can be identified by x-ray examination. With newer double-contrast barium examinations, it is possible to detect approximately 90 percent of duodenal ulcers. On x-ray the typical duodenal ulcer appears as a discrete crater in the proximal portion of the duodenal bulb. Marked deformity of the duodenal bulb, common in patients with chronic recurrent duodenal ulcer, may make radiographic identification of the ulcer difficult or impossible (Figs. 306-2 and 306-3).

FIGURE 306-2
Deformed duodenal bulb with ulcer crater.

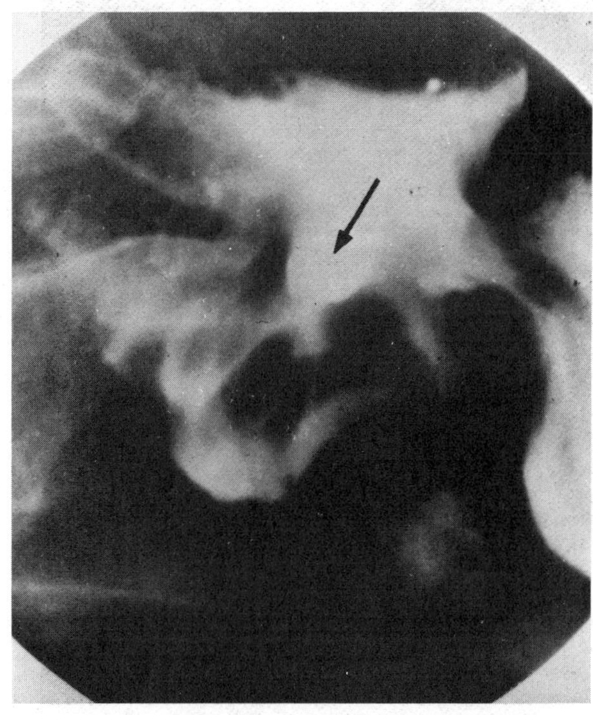

Use of fiberoptic endoscopic examination of the upper gastrointestinal tract has facilitated accurate diagnosis of duodenal ulcer disease. Duodenoscopy is not required for diagnosis of duodenal ulcer when it has been established by barium radiographic examination. Endoscopy may be of great value, however, (1) in detecting suspected duodenal ulcer in the absence of radiographically demonstrable ulcer and in patients with radiographic deformity and uncertainty regarding ulcer activity, (2) in identifying ulcers too small or too superficial to be recognized by x-ray, and (3) in identifying an ulcer as the source of active gastrointestinal hemorrhage. Duodenoscopy also permits direct visualization and photographic documentation of the character of the ulcer, its size, shape, and location, and it may provide a reference basis for the assessment of healing. Endoscopic studies have shown that 85 percent of duodenal ulcers are less than 1 cm in diameter, with approximately 70 percent having a diameter between 0.5 and 1 cm.

Measurement of gastric acid secretion is not necessary in most patients with clinical features of a typical duodenal ulcer. Determination of serum gastrin is recommended in those patients in whom surgery is planned or gastrinoma is suspected.

MEDICAL TREATMENT Major objectives of therapy are relief of pain and ulcer healing. Prevention of ulcer recurrence and complications are additional objectives. In the past enthusiasm has been expressed for virtually every mode of treatment which has ever been tried for this disease. In many instances conclusions regarding the effectiveness of therapy have been obscured by spontaneous healing, an intrinsic component of the natural history of the disease, and imprecise methods to assess ulcer activity. Specific agents currently available and recommended for use in treatment of duodenal ulcer are considered below.

FIGURE 306-3
Distortion of the duodenal bulb with "cloverleaf" deformity.

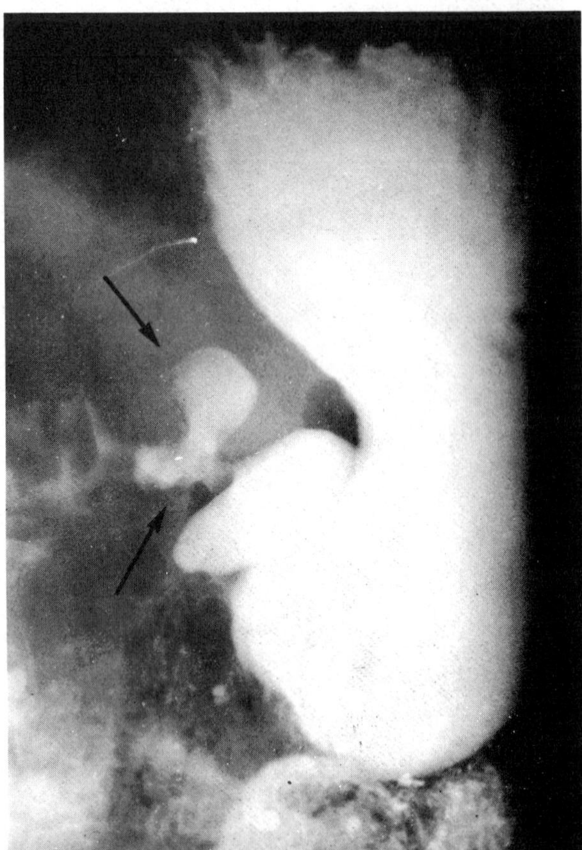

Antacids Traditionally, administration of antacids has been the major accepted form of treatment for duodenal ulcer. Studies with endoscopic verification of ulcer activity have established the effectiveness of antacids in duodenal ulcer healing. Many types of antacids are available and have been used in the treatment of duodenal ulcer. The ideal antacid should be potent in neutralizing acid, inexpensive, not adsorbed from the gastrointestinal tract, and contain negligible amounts of sodium. The ideal antacid should be sufficiently palatable to be readily tolerated with repeated dosage and should be free from side effects. Although the ideal antacid is yet to be developed, a number of preparations are available which can be used in treatment of patients with duodenal ulcer. Individual antacids differ substantially in their capacities to neutralize acid, their sodium contents, their absorption properties, and their potential adverse effects (see Table 306-1).

Calcium carbonate is a potent and inexpensive antacid. In neutralizing acid, it is converted to calcium chloride in the stomach. Approximately 10 percent of calcium ingested as calcium carbonate is absorbed from the proximal small intestine. Unfortunately, chronic calcium carbonate administration may be associated with the milk-alkali syndrome, producing elevations of serum calcium, phosphate, blood urea nitrogen, creatinine, and bicarbonate. These patients may develop renal calcinosis and progressive renal insufficiency. Calcium carbonate is unique among antacids in that its ingestion is followed by stimulation of gastric acid secretion (a genuine "acid rebound" phenomenon). This is due to the direct action of calcium in stimulating parietal cell acid secretion and, perhaps to a lesser extent, to calcium-mediated stimulation of gastrin release. Because of its potential adverse effects, calcium carbonate is not recommended for use as an antacid for treatment of patients with peptic ulcer.

Sodium bicarbonate is a potent, rapidly acting, inexpensive antacid. However, because of its tendency to induce systemic alkalosis and its high sodium content, it should not be used as an antacid in treatment of peptic ulcer.

The most widely used antacid preparations are mixtures of aluminum hydroxide and magnesium hydroxide, in some in-

TABLE 306-1
Relative potency of liquid antacid preparations

Antacid	*Contents*	*meq/30 ml**
Delcid	Al and Mg hydroxides	256
Mylanta II	Mg and Al hydroxides, simethicone	124
Titralac	Glycine, Ca carbonate	118
Camalox	Al and Mg hydroxides, Ca carbonate	108
Basaljel	Al carbonate	100
Aludrox	Al hydroxide gel, Mg hydroxide	84
Maalox	Mg and Al hydroxide	78
Cremalin	Hexitol-stabilized Al hydroxide gel, magnesium hydroxide	78
Di-Gel	Al and Mg hydroxides, simethicone	76
Mylanta	Mg and Al hydroxides, simethicone	72
Silain-Gel	Mg and Al hydroxides, simethicone	70
Marblen	Mg and Ca carbonates, Al hydroxide, Mg phosphate, Mg trisilicate	70
WinGel	Al and Mg hydroxides, hexitol stabilized	70
Gelusil M	Mg trisilicate, Al hydroxide, Mg hydroxide	66
Riopan	Mg and Al hydroxides	66
Amphojel	Al hydroxide gel	58
A-M-T	Mg trisilicate, Al hydroxide gel	54
Kolantyl Gel	Bentyl, Al hydroxide, Mg hydroxide, methylcellulose	52
Trisogel	Mg trisilicate, Al hydroxide gel	52
Malcogel	Mg trisilicate, Al hydroxide gel	48
Gelusil	Mg trisilicate, Al hydroxide gel	40
Robalate	Dihydroxyaluminum aminoacetate	34
Phosphaljel	Al phosphate gel	12

* *Indicates the capacity, expressed in milliequivalents, to raise the pH of 0.1 N HCl and maintain it at pH 3.0 for 2 h.*
SOURCE: *After Fordtran et al.*

stances with additional agents. *Aluminum hydroxide* neutralizes hydrochloric acid with the production of aluminum chloride and water. Use of aluminum hydroxide tends to produce constipation. Aluminum binds phosphate within the gut lumen, thereby facilitating its excretion. As a consequence, prolonged and regular use of aluminum hydroxide may induce systemic phosphate depletion with resultant weakness, malaise, and anorexia. This complication is probably restricted to, and must be considered in, patients with a phosphate-deficient diet, e.g. dietary deficiency associated with chronic alcoholism or other states of reduced dietary protein intake.

Magnesium hydroxide is a potent antacid which neutralizes hydrochloric acid to produce magnesium chloride and water. Magnesium hydroxide may produce loosening of the stools. This laxative effect and the constipating effects of aluminum hydroxide can be overcome by using these agents in combination, or by alternating their use. Antacid combinations vary enormously in their capacities to neutralize hydrochloric acid. Table 306-1 provides examples of some available liquid antacid preparations and their neutralizing capacities, as defined by their ability to increase and maintain the pH of 0.1 *N* hydrochloric acid at 3.0 for 2 h. *Magnesium trisilicate,* which is frequently included in various antacid mixtures, is a slow-acting weak antacid. In general, tablet preparations of magnesium hydroxide–aluminum hydroxide are less potent than their liquid forms.

Acceptance of the crucial role of acid in the pathogenesis of duodenal ulcer provides a rational basis for the use of antacids in treatment of patients with duodenal ulcer. There have been controlled studies on the effects of antacids on duodenal ulcer healing, in which vigorous antacid therapy has been compared with placebo, and ulcer response has been verified by endoscopy. Four weeks of treatment with a potent magnesium and aluminum hydroxide antacid mixture has been shown to increase duodenal ulcer healing. Ulcer healing occurred in 45 percent of patients receiving placebo and in 78 percent of those treated with 30 ml antacid (144 meq) given 1 and 3 h after meals and at bedtime.

H_2-receptor antagonists It has been known for decades that conventional antihistamines, which readily block the actions of histamine on smooth muscle of the gut or bronchi, do not inhibit histamine-stimulated gastric acid secretion. The parietal cell receptor for histamine has been classified as the H_2-receptor and that blocked by classic antihistamines as the H_1-receptor. The H_2-receptor antagonist *cimetidine* is used widely in the treatment of duodenal ulcer. Cimetidine is related structurally to histamine (Fig. 306-4), sharing the same imidazole ring, but bearing an extended side chain which contains a cyanoguanidine group. Cimetidine, at a dose of 300 mg, inhibits basal acid secretion by more than 80 percent and meal-stimulated acid secretion by approximately 70 percent. It strikingly reduces acid secretory responses to histamine, caffeine, insulin, hypoglycemia, and gastrin. Cimetidine has been shown to be more effective than placebo in promoting endoscopically verified duodenal ulcer healing. Its effectiveness in promoting duodenal ulcer healing appears to be comparable with that of vigorous antacid therapy. The recommended oral dose of cimetidine for treatment of patients with duodenal ulcer is 300 mg four times daily, with meals and at bedtime. Treatment of active duodenal ulcer with cimetidine is continued for periods from 4 to 8 weeks. Chronic administration of cimetidine, in doses of 400 mg at bedtime or 400 mg twice each day, has been shown to reduce duodenal ulcer recurrence during the 12-month period of treatment. Considering the enormous numbers of patients who have been treated with cimetidine, few serious adverse effects have been experienced. Cimetidine administration has been associated with slight and reversible increases in serum transaminase and creatinine levels. Instances of diarrhea, fatigue, and skin rash have also been described. Central nervous system abnormalities (confusion, agitation, coma, disorientation, and seizures) may occur, especially in elderly patients, in those receiving large doses or when there is substantial hepatic or renal functional impairment. Tender gynecomastia may occur in patients treated with large doses for prolonged periods of time; this is believed to be caused by the weak antiandrogenic effects of cimetidine. Brief increases in serum prolactin (2 to 3 h) have been shown to follow intravenous and oral cimetidine. Cimetidine inhibits the activity of certain hepatic microsomal enzymes and may, therefore, reduce the elimination rate and increase the actions of drugs such as diazepam and warfarin.

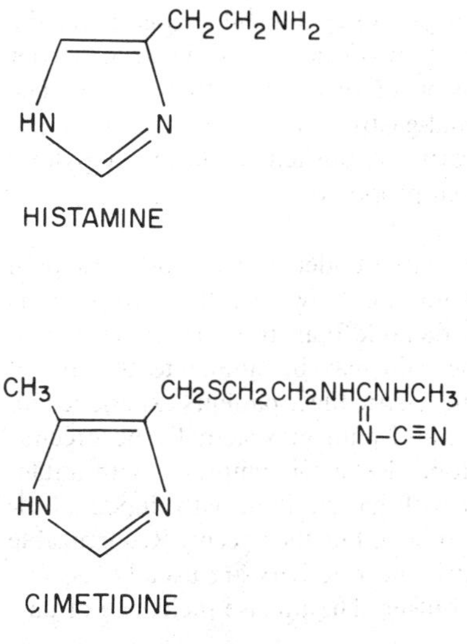

A variety of other H_2-receptor antagonists are under development and evaluation but are not yet available for general use. Some of these may be more potent and have longer biological half-lives than cimetidine and may prove to be associated with even fewer adverse effects.

FIGURE 306-4
Chemical structures of histamine and the H_2-receptor antagonist cimetidine. Note the common imidazole ring and the cyanoguanidine group in the cimetidine side chain.

$CH_2CH_2NH_2$
HN N
HISTAMINE

CH_3 $CH_2SCH_2CH_2NHCNHCH_3$
N–C≡N
HN N
CIMETIDINE

Anticholinergic agents Anticholinergic drugs act by inhibiting the effects of acetylcholine on muscarinic receptors. These agents decrease gastric acid secretion, but not as effectively as H_2-receptor antagonists. Anticholinergics reduce basal gastric acid secretion by approximately 50 percent, histamine- or gastrin-stimulated acid secretion by 40 percent, and postprandial acid secretion by 30 percent. They also delay gastric emptying. Most studies have *not* shown that anticholinergic agents hasten healing or improve symptoms of duodenal ulcer; therefore, they are not recommended as primary therapy for duodenal ulcer. However, anticholinergic agents may prove to be useful when combined in a program of treatment with antacids or cimetidine. Side effects of anticholinergic agents include dryness of mouth, blurring of vision, cardiac arrhythmias, and urinary retention. They should not be used in patients with glaucoma, impaired gastric emptying, or history or symptoms of urinary retention.

Diet Many different dietary programs have been recommended and used for treatment of patients with duodenal ulcer. There is no evidence that bland diets reduce gastric acid secretion, promote healing, or relieve symptoms in patients with duodenal ulcer. Similarly soft diets or diets free of spices or fruit juices have not been proved to be of benefit. Traditionally, milk and cream have been prescribed in the treatment of ulcer patients. There is no evidence that ulcer healing is benefited by milk and cream diets. These diets may contribute to the development of the milk-alkali syndrome and may be associated with increased atherogenesis. Furthermore, they may stimulate gastric acid secretion by milk protein and calcium.

What dietary measures, if any, should be recommended in the treatment of duodenal ulcer? Clearly, strict diet control is not necessary. Milk should not be used as a component of treatment for patients with duodenal ulcer. It is reasonable to suggest that if patients experience symptoms after ingestion of certain foods, these should be avoided. A regular diet can be combined with antacids as described below. Because of their effects on gastric secretion it is probably wise for duodenal ulcer patients to avoid coffee, with or without caffeine, as well as other caffeine-containing beverages. It is probably also wise to restrict alcohol intake in patients with duodenal ulcer.

Possible drugs for the future An assortment of drugs have been shown in some studies to promote healing of duodenal or gastric ulcer. These agents may become available for general use and will be described briefly. *Colloidal bismuth* compounds have been thought to aid ulcer healing by forming (in an acid medium) a bismuth-protein coagulum which protects the ulcer from acid-peptic digestion. *Sucralfate,* a basic aluminum salt of a sulfated disaccharide, forms an adherent chemical complex with proteins at the ulcer base, presumably creating a protective barrier for the ulcer against potentially harmful effects of acid and pepsin. *Sulpiride* is an orthopramide, which is structurally related to metoclopramide, possesses antiemetic and antidepressant properties, and has been used in the treatment of duodenal ulcer patients. *Pruglumide,* a derivative of isoglutamic acid, is believed to block gastrin receptors, reduce acid secretion, and increase mucosal resistance. Studies are underway to evaluate the efficacy of several *prostaglandins* in ulcer healing; their use is based on their cytoprotective effects and their capacity to reduce gastric acid secretion.

General therapeutic considerations How does one integrate available information concerning treatment of duodenal ulcer to construct a reasonable therapeutic formulation? Clinical studies have verified the effectiveness of *antacids* and of H_2-receptor antagonists, such as *cimetidine,* in the promotion of duodenal ulcer healing. On the basis of present knowledge, there appear to be two primary approaches to the medical treatment for duodenal ulcer—namely, either the neutralization of gastric acid by the frequent use of potent antacids or the inhibition of secreted gastrin acid by H_2-receptor antagonists.

Antacid treatment of duodenal ulcer should consist of frequent doses of a potent liquid antacid. However, the minimal or optimal doses of antacids required for duodenal ulcer healing are not precisely known. On the basis of an antacid program which has been shown to be effective, it is recommended that the antacid (100 to 140 meq of neutralizing activity; for most antacids this equals 30 to 60 ml) be given 1 and 3 h after each meal and at bedtime. Such a regimen should be continued for approximately 6 weeks. Symptom recurrence may be treated by shorter periods of therapy, at similar dose levels. When *cimetidine* is used, a 300-mg tablet is recommended with each meal and at bedtime for 6 to 8 weeks. When anticholinergics are used in conjunction with antacids or cimetidine, they are administered either once a day at bedtime or four times a day (i.e., before meals and at bedtime).

GASTRIC ULCER

INCIDENCE AND ANATOMIC LOCATION The peak incidence for gastric ulcer is in the sixth decade, approximately 10 years later than for duodenal ulcer. Gastric ulcers, just as duodenal ulcers, are more common in males. They are also similar histologically to duodenal ulcers. Characteristically, gastric ulcers are deep and extend beyond the mucosa of the stomach. Almost all benign gastric ulcers are located in the *antrum,* in a zone immediately distal to the junction of the antral mucosa with the acid-secreting mucosa of the body of the stomach. The location of this junction is variable, especially on the lesser gastric curvature. In general, the antrum extends approximately two-thirds of the way up the lesser curvature and one-third of the way up the greater curvature of the stomach. Benign gastric ulcers are rare in the fundus of the stomach. Benign gastric ulcers are almost always accompanied by gastritis and variable amounts of mucosal atrophy involving the antrum. Gastritis may be present or absent with aspirin-associated gastric ulcers; ulcers associated with salicylate ingestion are usually located in the antrum, but they are not confined to the junction of the antral and parietal cell mucosa, as are common gastric ulcers.

ETIOLOGY AND PATHOGENESIS Acid-pepsin appears to be important in the pathogenesis of gastric ulcer. In contrast to duodenal ulcer, however, gastric ulcer patients generally have acid secretory rates which are normal, or even reduced, when compared with nonulcer subjects. Although many patients with gastric ulcer have reduced rates of acid secretion, *true achlorhydria* in response to stimulation *almost never occurs* in patients with *benign* gastric ulcer. Ten to twenty percent of patients with gastric ulcer also have duodenal ulcer disease. Patients with both duodenal and gastric ulcers tend to have acid secretory patterns which parallel those of duodenal ulcer. Patients with pyloric channel ulcers have acid secretory rates and clinical patterns similar to those found with common duodenal ulcer.

Various factors have been considered to be involved in the pathogenesis of gastric ulcer. Most evidence supports the importance of primary defects in gastric mucosal resistance and/or direct gastric mucosal injury as the most important elements. Serum gastrin levels are increased in some gastric ulcer patients, but these increases are limited to those with gastric acid hyposecretion. Gastric emptying has also been shown to be delayed. It has been suggested that regurgitation of duodenal contents, especially those containing bile, may induce gastric mucosal injury and subsequent gastric ulceration. Gastric ulcer patients have been shown to have increased duodenal-gastric reflux of bile and greater concentrations of bile in their stomachs when compared with nonulcer subjects or duodenal ulcer patients. It has been proposed that bile acids injure the gastric mucosa by interruption of the gastric mucosal barrier with resultant back-diffusion of secreted hydrogen ions. The factors producing duodenal-gastric reflux in gastric ulcer patients have not been clearly established; a defect in pyloric sphincter function has been proposed.

CLINICAL FEATURES As with duodenal ulcer, epigastric pain is the most common symptom. However, this symptom is much less typical and predictable than those in patients with duodenal ulcer. While the pain may be similar to that noted with duodenal ulcers, some gastric ulcer patients experience no relief of pain with eating, and pain may actually be precipitated or accentuated by food. Relief of symptoms with antacids is also less consistent with gastric than with duodenal ulcers. Gastric ulcers tend to heal, but then recur. Recognizable episodes of recurrent gastric ulcer activity are usually less frequent than with duodenal ulcer. The precise incidence of gastric ulcer is not known, since many gastric ulcer patients are asymptomatic. Although duodenal ulcer is identified clinically as more frequent than gastric ulcer, most autopsy studies show an equal or greater proportion of gastric ulcers when compared with duodenal ulcers. This may be due in part to more acute preterminal events but also may reflect the often asymptomatic clinical course of gastric ulcer. While nausea and vomiting almost always indicate gastric outlet obstruction in duodenal ulcer patients, these symptoms may occur in patients with gastric ulcer in the absence of mechanical obstruction. Weight loss occurs in about 40 percent of patients due to anorexia or to food aversion from discomfort produced by eating.

Gastric outlet obstruction may develop with ulcers in the pyloric channel or most distal antrum. Hemorrhage is a common complication, occurring in approximately 25 percent. Gastric ulcer perforation is less frequent than hemorrhage. Mortality with perforation of gastric ulcers is approximately three times that which occurs with duodenal ulcers. This increased mortality is due only in part to the increased age of gastric ulcer patients. The greater mortality may also be due to uncertainty and delay in diagnosis, as well as to greater soilage of the peritoneum with gastric ulcer perforation. Mortality is also greater in patients with hemorrhage due to gastric ulcer than when associated with duodenal ulcer.

DIAGNOSIS The history may be of value in suspecting gastric ulcer, but it is not as characteristic as in duodenal ulcer. The two major methods for diagnosis are barium examination of the upper gastrointestinal tract and endoscopy. Gastric ulcer can usually be identified by the standard barium examination with an accuracy that approaches 90 percent. Superficial ulcerations and erosions, however, may escape radiographic identification. Approximately 4 percent of gastric ulcers which appear benign radiographically prove to be malignant (by endoscopic biopsy or at surgery). Both benign and malignant gastric ulcers occur more commonly on the lesser than on the greater curvature (Fig. 306-5). Radiation of gastric mucosal folds from the margin of the ulcer crater suggests a benign lesion. Large gastric ulcers, i.e., those greater than 3 cm in diameter, are more often malignant than smaller ones. An ulcer within a mass, as defined radiographically, also suggests malignancy. Because of false-positive and false-negative errors, radiographic appearance cannot be used as the sole criterion for the benign or malignant nature of a gastric ulcer.

Endoscopic visualization of the ulcer allows one to define its size, location, and, by biopsy, its histological characteristics. At gastroscopy at least six biopsies should be obtained from the inner margin of the ulcer and from the ulcer bed. If accurate cytology is available, brushings of the ulcer should be performed prior to biopsy. By application of combined radiographic, endoscopic, and histological techniques, distinguishing a malignant from a benign gastric ulcer should be possible with greater than 95 percent confidence.

Gastric ulcer in association with histamine- or pentagastrin-fast achlorhydria, is rare. As a result, it almost always indicates that one is dealing with a gastric carcinoma. However, it should be empahsized most patients with gastric carcinoma (about two-thirds to three-fourths) are capable of secreting some gastric acid, although it is usually less than normal.

MEDICAL TREATMENT At present, antacid administration is the most widely accepted primary treatment for gastric ulcer. The ideal dosage and frequency for antacid therapy for gastric ulcer healing are not known. However, since acid hypersecretion is not characteristic of the disease, smaller doses of antacid may possibly be required than for treatment of duodenal ulcer. It is suggested that 15 to 30 ml of a potent liquid antacid be taken 1 and 3 h after meals and at bedtime. Anticholinergic agents have been recommended by some physicians. However,

because of substantial side effects of anticholinergic drugs, their tendency to reduce gastric emptying, which is already impaired in these patients, the fact that gastric ulcer patients are often older and, therefore, more susceptible to the complications of these agents, and the lack of evidence for their benefit, the use of anticholinergic drugs in gastric ulcer treatment does not appear justified. Some studies suggest that hospitalization and/or cessation of smoking are of benefit in gastric ulcer healing.

Experience with the use of H_2-receptor antagonists in the treatment of patients with gastric ulcer is limited but suggests that drugs such as cimetidine may be of value when administered in a dose of 300 mg four times per day, with meals and at bedtime. It remains to be determined whether cimetidine treatment is comparable to antacid administration as primary therapy for benign gastric ulcer.

Since salicylate ingestion has been associated with the development of gastric ulcers, patients with gastric ulcer should not ingest salicylates. Alcohol, because of its injurious effects on the gastric mucosa, should also be avoided. Milk and cream, as well as bland or homogenized diets, have not been shown to be of value in treatment. In general, it is probably sufficient to recommend that patients take a diet of their own choice. Since coffee (caffeine-containing or caffeine-free) and other caffeine-containing liquids stimulate gastric acid secretion, it may be of benefit to omit these beverages.

Carbenoxolone has been used in many countries (but not in the United States) in the treatment of patients with gastric

FIGURE 306-5
Benign lesser curvature gastric ulcer. Note ulceration beyond the projected margins of the stomach and the collar of edema.

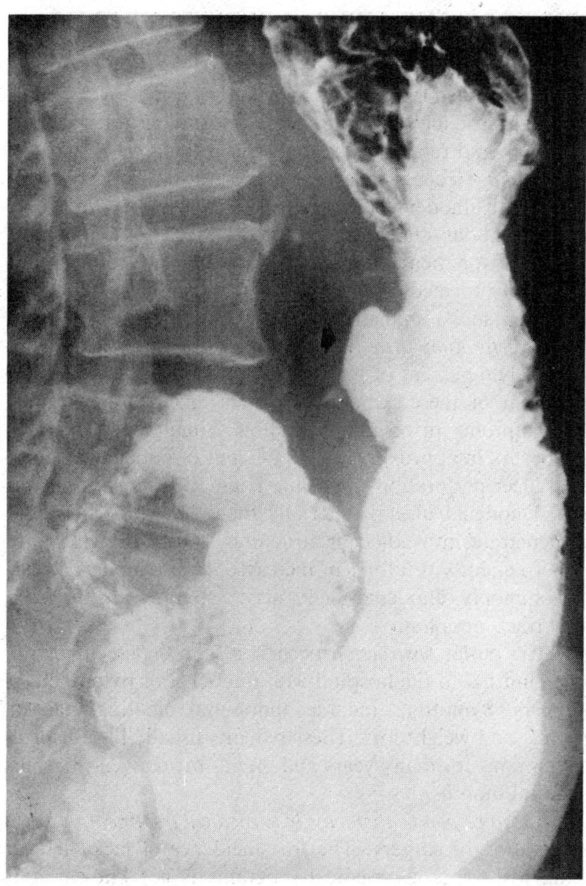

ulcer. This drug is a hydrolytic product of glycyrrhizic acid (derived from licorice) and has been shown to improve symptoms and increase the rate of gastric ulcer healing. Carbenoxolone is not an antacid and does not decrease gastric acid secretion. It increases the life span of gastric mucosal epithelial cells and increases the secretion and viscosity of gastric mucus. Carbenoxolone possesses aldosterone-like effects, and thus sodium and water retention tend to occur. It is possible to inhibit the aldosterone-like effects of carbenoxolone by use of aldosterone antagonists; however, the latter also abolish the beneficial effects of carbenoxolone in gastric ulcer healing. Problems with sodium and water retention and the availability of alternative drugs have led to its decreased use worldwide.

The failure of gastric ulcer to decrease satisfactorily in size and to heal with antacid treatment has been used to suggest gastric malignancy. Benign gastric ulcers should heal completely after 3 months of vigorous antacid therapy. Upper gastrointestinal barium examination or gastroscopy should be performed after 4 weeks of antacid therapy, at which time definite healing should be demonstrable in benign gastric ulcers—the diameter of most ulcers should be reduced by more than 50 percent. If at 4 weeks the ulcer is not reduced in size, malignancy must be suspected and sought for by appropriate biopsies of the ulcer and exfoliative cytology. If the ulcer has not healed completely at 8 weeks, x-ray and endoscopic examination should be repeated in another month, at which time most benign gastric ulcers should have healed. In general, large gastric ulcers heal more slowly than smaller ones. One must be alert, however, to the occasional "healing" of an ulcerating gastric carcinoma with treatment with antacids or cimetidine. Apparent complete healing does not assure the benign nature of a gastric ulcer since approximately 70 percent of gastric ulcers eventually found to be malignant will undergo significant healing with medical treatment.

COMPLICATIONS AND SURGERY FOR PEPTIC ULCER

Surgery is reserved for patients with complications of duodenal ulcer and gastric ulcer. These include hemorrhage, obstruction, perforation, and refractoriness to medical therapy.

Hemorrhage occurs in approximately 15 to 20 percent of patients with duodenal ulcers; there may be a recurrence of bleeding in about 40 percent of patients with an initial hemorrhage. In most patients hemorrhage from peptic ulcer responds satisfactorily to medical management—including gastric suction and antacid administration.

Free *perforation* into the peritoneal cavity occurs in approximately 6 percent of patients with duodenal ulcer. Five to ten percent of these patients will have had no recognizable ulcer symptoms prior to perforation. Simultaneous hemorrhage occurs in approximately 10 percent of patients with duodenal ulcer perforation; mortality is greatly increased in this group. Duodenal ulcers, especially those located posteriorly, may penetrate into adjacent structures, most often the pancreas—frequently resulting in increased serum amylase levels. Less commonly, duodenal ulcers may penetrate into the liver, biliary tract, or colon.

Gastric outlet *obstruction* occurs in 2 to 4 percent of patients admitted to the hospital with duodenal or pyloric channel ulcers. Symptoms include abdominal bloating, nausea, vomiting, and weight loss. These patients usually have had ulcer symptoms for many years and often obstructive symptoms for several months.

Failure to respond satisfactorily to medical treatment requires consideration of surgery. The true incidence of lack of ulcer healing with vigorous medical programs is not known; it is clear, however, that most patients with peptic ulcer can be treated successfully without surgery.

Decisions regarding surgery for patients with complications of peptic ulcer must be individualized. Risks of surgery must be balanced with risks of the disease. The patient's discomfort, costs of medical care and hospitalization, and time lost from work must be weighed in relation to the morbidity and possible mortality associated with surgery and anesthesia, risks of recurrent ulcer, and long-term postoperative sequelae. The skill and experience of the surgeon must be weighed as major factors in considering operation.

SURGERY FOR DUODENAL ULCER No single surgical procedure has been accepted universally as the most satisfactory duodenal ulcer operation. At present the most commonly performed surgical procedures are *vagotomy with antrectomy, vagotomy with pyloroplasty, and parietal cell vagotomy* (also referred to as *proximal gastric or superselective vagotomy*) without a gastric drainage procedure. With conventional (truncal) vagotomy and antrectomy, the vagal trunks are transected, the antrum is removed, and gastrointestinal continuity is reestablished by anastomosis of the remaining stomach with the proximal duodenum (Billroth I anastomosis) or with a loop of the jejunum (Billroth II anastomosis). Vagotomy and antrectomy is an effective procedure with a low recurrence rate (approximately 1 percent). Morbidity and mortality with vagotomy and antrectomy are variable, depend upon patient selection and the skill of the surgeon, but are probably slightly greater than with vagotomy and pyloroplasty.

When the procedure of vagotomy and pyloroplasty is selected, pyloroplasty is performed to facilitate gastric drainage after truncal or selective vagotomy. Vagotomy is performed to inhibit vagal stimulation of gastric acid secretion. Vagotomy does not inhibit gastrin release; in fact, release of gastrin is enhanced after vagal interruption. As indicated above, three types of vagotomy are now used in the surgical treatment of duodenal ulcer and pyloric channel ulcer, namely, *truncal vagotomy, selective vagotomy,* and *parietal cell vagotomy.* Pyloroplasty with truncal vagotomy, which is still the most commonly performed method of vagal transection in the United States, is associated with approximately 1 percent mortality. Ulcer recurrence during the 5 years after surgery is about 5 to 8 percent. With selective vagotomy only the branches of the vagus which supply the stomach are transected, preserving the vagal innervation of the other abdominal viscera. Selective vagotomy has been found by some surgeons to result in a more complete vagotomy, less ulcer recurrence, and fewer postvagotomy complications than truncal vagotomy. Parietal cell vagotomy spares the branches of the vagus which innervate the antrum, and a gastric drainage procedure is unnecessary. Both immediate and late postoperative complications are less common with parietal cell vagotomy than with truncal vagotomy, and reductions in acid secretion with parietal cell vagotomy are generally comparable with those produced with truncal or selective vagotomy. Mortality with parietal cell vagotomy is less than 1 percent. Most studies indicate that with experience in the performance of parietal cell vagotomy, recurrence is comparable to that with other forms of vagotomy with pyloroplasty. This procedure, which is being used with increasing frequency, appears to be an effective and safe surgical therapy for duodenal ulcer.

SURGERY FOR GASTRIC ULCER Surgical treatment is required for gastric ulcer patients who do not respond satisfactorily to medical therapy or who develop complications similar to those described for duodenal ulcer. With the available diagnostic accuracy of careful radiographic examination, endoscopy, biopsy of the ulcer margins, and exfoliative cytology, it should rarely be necessary to operate because of a remaining uncertainty regarding the malignant or benign nature of the ulcer. The recommended surgical procedure for the treatment of gastric ulcer is antrectomy with gastroduodenal (Billroth I) anastomosis. It is not necessary to perform a vagotomy when antrectomy is performed for gastric ulcer (not located in the pyloric channel).

CONSEQUENCES AND SYNDROMES AFTER PEPTIC ULCER SURGERY

Modern surgery for peptic ulcer is effective in both the treatment of ulcer complications and in the prevention of ulcer recurrence. However, numerous postoperative sequelae and syndromes may occur.

RECURRENT ULCERATION Recurrent ulceration has been reported in approximately 5 percent of all patients after surgery for peptic ulcer. Approximately 95 percent of these recurrences follow surgery for duodenal ulcer disease. The risk of development of recurrent ulcer is 3 to 10 percent after surgery for duodenal ulcer and approximately 2 percent after gastric ulcer surgery. Recurrence is more common after vagotomy and pyloroplasty and after parietal cell vagotomy than after vagotomy and antrectomy. When ulcers occur after partial gastric resection, the site is usually at the anastomosis or immediately distal to it in the small intestine. Abdominal pain is the most common symptom in patients with a stomal (or marginal) ulcer. The pain is usually epigastric but is often not characteristic of common duodenal ulcer. It is usually, but not always, relieved by meals or antacids and, in general, tends to be more persistent and progressive than that observed with unoperated duodenal ulcer. Hemorrhage or anemia due to blood loss, nausea and vomiting from obstruction, weight loss, or symptoms from perforation may occur. The development of a stomal ulcer after duodenal ulcer surgery usually indicates that an incomplete vagotomy was performed. Inadequate gastric resection, when performed without vagotomy, may also result in stomal ulceration. Additional causes for the development of recurrent ulcer include an excessively long jejunal afferent loop, an inadvertently performed gastroileal or gastrocolic anastomosis, poor gastric drainage, and ingestion of ulcerogenic drugs. Less commonly, a marginal ulcer may be caused by gastrinoma or by acid hypersecretion secondary to retained antrum. If patients with gastrinomas are treated by gastroenterostomy, stomal ulceration is almost inevitable.

Radiographic examination with barium is of limited diagnostic value and identifies only from 50 to 65 percent of stomal ulcerations. Surgical deformity at the anastomotic site may often mimic stomal ulcer in its absence, or conceal it when present. When suspected, endoscopic examination is required to identify stomal ulceration. Medical treatment with antacids is almost always unsatisfactory in patients with stomal ulcer. Cimetidine has been used successfully in inducing healing of recurrent ulcer. The long-term effects of cimetidine on recurrent ulcers and the prevention of their further recurrence remain to be established. Surgery is usually necessary for treatment of ulcer recurrence and it is usually, but not invariably, successful. In patients with recurrent ulcer provocative tests should be performed with infusions of calcium or secretin and measurements of serum gastrin to identify or exclude gastrinoma (see below).

RECURRENT ULCER DUE TO RETAINED ANTRUM Recurrent ulcers have been described in a small number of patients after antrectomy with gastrojejunostomy (Billroth II anastomosis) in which the antral resection was not complete. In these patients the distal antrum, inadvertently not resected, remains in continuity with the duodenum after surgery. These patients usually develop or continue to have gastric acid hypersecretion due to gastrin release by the residual antral mucosa which is no longer in contact with gastric acid, the normal inhibitor of gastrin release. In these patients fasting serum gastrin levels may be normal to moderately increased. Patients with retained antrum can be distinguished from those with gastrinoma by intravenous injection of secretin with measurements of serum gastrin. Gastrinoma patients exhibit paradoxical increases in serum gastrin, whereas in those with retained antrum, serum gastrin levels decrease after secretin administration (see Table 306-2). These patients can be treated successfully by surgical removal of the remaining antrum.

AFFERENT LOOP SYNDROMES Patients with partial gastric resection with gastrojejunostomy (Billroth II anastomosis) may experience abdominal bloating and pain 20 min to 1 h after eating, frequently followed by nausea and vomiting. The vomitus often contains large amounts of bile. Characteristically, the bloating and abdominal discomfort are relieved by vomiting. This type of afferent loop syndrome, which is very uncommon, is believed to be caused by distention of an incompletely draining afferent intestinal loop by pancreatic and biliary secretions which are stimulated by eating. Serum amylase levels may be mildly or moderately increased. Because of partial obstruction it is often difficult to demonstrate the afferent loop by barium meal examination. Treatment is surgical correction of the incomplete afferent loop obstruction, and, in some instances, revision to a gastroduodenal anastomosis.

A second form of afferent loop dysfunction is that due to stasis with bacterial overgrowth within the afferent loop. These patients may exhibit the same characteristics as are found with other forms of small intestinal bacterial overgrowth or blind loop syndromes (see Chap. 308). These include malabsorption, especially of fat and vitamin B_{12}. Correction of the afferent loop bacterial overgrowth syndrome can be accomplished by surgical revision of the afferent loop.

BILE REFLUX GASTRITIS After peptic ulcer surgery a small proportion of patients experience early satiety, abdominal discomfort, and vomiting, which is believed due to reflux of duodenal contents into the stomach. Endoscopic examination usually reveals regurgitated bile in the stomach and diffuse gas-

TABLE 306-2
Provocative gastrin tests*

Disorder	*Gastrin response (change from basal level)* *After secretin injection*	*After calcium infusion*	*After test meal*
Zollinger-Ellison (gastrinoma)	Increase (usually greater than 200 pg/ml)	Increase (usually more than 50% or more than 400 pg/ml)	Little or no increase (increase less than 50%)
Common duodenal ulcer	Decrease or no change	Small increase (usually less than 50%; always less than 400 pg/ml)	Moderate increase (often slightly more than normal, but less than in gastrin cell hyperplasia)
Antral gastrin cell hyperplasia	Decrease	May or may not increase greater than 50%	Striking increase (greater than 300%)

* *Responses and results are based on currently available data and are subject to change as further information becomes available.*

tritis, often involving the entire gastric remnant. Various terms assigned to this entity include *alkaline reflux gastritis, bile reflux gastritis, duodenogastric reflux,* and *bilious vomiting.* The mechanisms or materials contained in the refluxed intestinal contents accounting for these symptoms have not been defined. Although the term bile reflux gastritis has been used, there is no certainty that regurgitated bile is responsible for the syndrome. Administration of cholestyramine, intended to bind bile acids and facilitate their excretion, has not been of benefit in this disorder. Some surgeons have reported successful treatment of bile reflux gastritis by diversion of duodenal contents from proximity to the stomach with a Roux en Y anastomosis.

DUMPING SYNDROME Following peptic ulcer surgery some patients experience an assortment of vasomotor symptoms after eating. These include palpitation, tachycardia, lightheadedness, diaphoresis, and, less frequently, postural hypotension. Abdominal discomfort and vomiting may also occur. The vasomotor symptoms, referred to as the *early dumping syndrome,* are usually experienced within 30 min after eating and are believed to result from rapid emptying of hyperosmolar gastric contents into the proximal small intestine. This leads to a shift of fluid into the gut lumen and produces intestinal distention and contraction of plasma volume. Additional proposed mechanisms for these symptoms include stimulation of autonomic reflexes secondary to small intestinal distention and/or release of hormones from the gut in response to rapid entry of gastric contents into the duodenum or jejunum.

The *late dumping syndrome* refers to a symptom complex comprising dizziness, lightheadedness, palpitation, diaphoresis, confusion, and, in rare instances, syncope, occurring 90 min to 3 h after eating. The symptoms can often be precipitated by meals rich in simple carbohydrates, especially sucrose. The syndrome appears to be caused by hypoglycemia due to insulin release stimulated by abrupt increases in blood glucose secondary to rapid emptying of sugar-containing meals into the proximal small intestine.

Both forms of the dumping syndrome are treated by dietary measures. These include limitation of simple sugar-containing liquids and solids (sweets), elimination of liquids at mealtime, and frequent small meals. Most patients have not been benefited by surgical procedures such as insertion of reversed jejunal loops and isoperistaltic jejunal interposition.

POSTVAGOTOMY DIARRHEA A significant number of patients experience diarrhea after peptic ulcer surgery, especially with a procedure including truncal vagotomy. Diarrhea usually occurs within 2 h of eating. Although the mechanism is not clear, interruption of vagal fibers to the abdominal viscera appears to play an important role in the production of the diarrhea. Diarrhea has been estimated to occur in 20 to 30 percent of patients after truncal vagotomy with drainage, in 4 to 20 percent with selective vagotomy and drainage, and in only 1 to 8 percent of those with parietal cell vagotomy (without drainage). Rapid emptying of gastric contents into the small intestine, resulting in increased fluid volume within the intestinal lumen, due to the osmotic action of the meal, may also contribute to the diarrhea.

HEMATOLOGIC COMPLICATIONS Intrinsic factor secreted by gastric parietal cells is necessary for active absorption of vitamin B_{12} by the distal ileum. Patients who have had total gastrectomy invariably will develop malabsorption of vitamin B_{12} and should receive monthly intramuscular injections of vitamin B_{12} (50 to 100 μg indefinitely). Megaloblastic anemia due to vitamin B_{12} deficiency is rare after partial gastric resection; however, reduced serum vitamin B_{12} levels have been observed in about 14 percent of these patients. Even more rarely vitamin B_{12} deficiency may be produced by bacterial overgrowth in a stagnant afferent loop following Billroth II anastomosis. Gastritis in the remaining stomach develops in more than 60 percent of duodenal ulcer patients after vagotomy and antrectomy or vagotomy and pyloroplasty. This may result in decreased vitamin B_{12} absorption. Inasmuch as the stomach secretes intrinsic factor in excess of need by approximately 100 times, peptic ulcer patients treated with partial gastric resection do not develop vitamin B_{12} deficiency secondary to the amount of stomach resected. (In addition, the resected portion of the stomach is almost always principally antrum, which contains few parietal cells.) However, after peptic ulcer surgery patients may develop decreased serum vitamin B_{12} levels due to reduced absorption of food-bound vitamin B_{12}; these patients will often have normal absorption of free vitamin B_{12}, as used in the Schilling test. The precise mechanism for the malabsorption of food-bound vitamin B_{12} is not known. It may be due in part to rapid emptying of gastric contents, with reduced efficiency of intrinsic factor binding of vitamin B_{12}. Anemia after peptic ulcer surgery may also result from deficiency produced by malabsorption of iron or folate. A combined deficiency of vitamin B_{12}, iron, and folate is common in patients with anemia following partial or subtotal gastric resection. Iron deficiency is the most common single hematologic defect after peptic ulcer surgery and may result from either blood loss (e.g., with persistent or recurrent ulcer) or from iron malabsorption. Patients with gastric resection malabsorb dietary iron but have normal absorption of iron salts, therefore they will respond favorably to treatment with therapeutic oral iron preparations. Folate deficiency may result from either reduced dietary intake or impaired folate absorption. Except for the anemia associated with early recurrent ulcer disease, the development of anemia after peptic ulcer surgery is gradual, usually occurring several years postoperatively.

The nature of the anemia after ulcer surgery should be clarified by determination of the red blood cell morphology and by measurements of serum iron, folate, and vitamin B_{12}. Iron or folate deficiency may be treated by oral replacement. Vitamin B_{12} deficiency should be treated with monthly intramuscular injections of the vitamin.

OSTEOMALACIA AND OSTEOPOROSIS Osteoporosis and osteomalacia may develop after partial or complete gastrectomy but occur rarely after vagotomy and pyloroplasty. Osteomalacia is extremely frequent following gastrojejunostomy or Billroth II anastomosis. These bone changes are believed to result from malabsorption of calcium and vitamin D. Patients may develop bone pain and have pathological fractures. The incidence of bone fractures in men following gastric resection has been estimated to be almost twice that of control subjects of similar age. Reduced bone density requires years to develop and can be identified by x-ray. Patients with osteomalacia usually have increased levels of serum alkaline phosphatase and may have reduced serum calcium concentrations. These patients should be treated by supplemental oral vitamin D and calcium.

GENERAL MALABSORPTION (See Chap. 308) Mild, chemically demonstrable steatorrhea is common in patients after ulcer surgery. Weight loss is more common after partial gastric resection than with vagotomy without resection and occurs in approximately 60 percent of patients in whom a portion of the stomach has been removed. The major cause of weight loss after peptic ulcer surgery is reduced food intake. On a 100-g fat diet, loss of stool fat seldom exceeds 15 g per day (normal individuals, less than 7 g per day). The causes of maldigestion and malabsorption after peptic ulcer surgery include rapid gastric emptying, reduced dispersion of food in the stomach, reduced bile concentrations in the gut lumen, increased rate of transit of the meal through the small intestine, and reduced or delayed pancreatic secretory responses to feeding. Steatorrhea and weight loss, sometimes accompanied by vitamin B_{12} malabsorption, may develop as a result of bacterial overgrowth, especially in patients with afferent loop bacterial stasis. Overt symptoms and other manifestations of malabsorption appearing after surgery for peptic ulcer may also be due to other preexisting conditions, including latent celiac sprue and chronic pancreatitis.

CARCINOMA AFTER PARTIAL GASTRECTOMY Several studies have documented an increased incidence of adenocarcinoma of the stomach in duodenal ulcer patients following partial gastric resection and after vagotomy and drainage without resection. This usually develops 10 or more years after ulcer surgery. The possibility of carcinoma of the stomach should be considered when abdominal symptoms, which may be similar to or distinct from those due to the original ulcer, appear many years after apparently successful surgery.

ZOLLINGER-ELLISON SYNDROME (GASTRINOMA)

In 1955 Zollinger and Ellison described the syndrome which bears their name, i.e., ulcer disease of the upper gastrointestinal tract, marked increase of gastric acid secretion, and nonbeta islet-cell tumors of the pancreas.

ETIOLOGY AND PATHOGENESIS Zollinger and Ellison, in their original description of the syndrome, suggested that the ulcer disease in these patients resulted from liberation of a secretagogue from the islet-cell tumors which accounted for the often enormously increased rates of gastric acid secretion. Their proposal was proved correct when in 1960 extracts of Zollinger-Ellison tumors were shown to stimulate gastric acid secretion. Subsequently, it was found that the pancreatic tumors contained gastrin and that large amounts of this hormone were released into the circulation, producing the pathophysiologic characteristics of the syndrome. These gastrin-containing tumors are, therefore, now referred to as *gastrinomas.* Gastrin has been demonstrated in these tumors by chemical isolation of polypeptides with amino acid compositions and peptide mapping patterns identical to those of human gastrin molecules. In addition, large amounts of gastrin have been demonstrated by radioimmunoassay in gastrinomas and in serums of patients with the Zollinger-Ellison syndrome.

Most gastrinomas are found within the pancreas. Multiple, apparently primary, tumors are common. Pancreatic gastrinomas may be single or multiple and may vary in size from 2 mm to more than 20 cm in diameter. In from one-half to two-thirds of patients multiple gastrinomas are present within the pancreas; however, more than half of these are not identified at surgery. Pancreatic gastrinomas are most common in the body or tail of the pancreas. Approximately 13 percent of patients with this syndrome have tumors in the wall of the proximal duodenum. Gastrinomas have also been located less commonly in other sites, including the hilum of the spleen and the stomach. In rare instances, the Zollinger-Ellison syndrome has resulted from ectopic gastrin-containing tumors, e.g., parathyroid and ovarian adenomas. A small number of gastrin-containing islet-cell tumors have been described which contained multiple hormones, for example, adrenocorticotropic hormone, glucagon, insulin, pancreatic polypeptide, and vasoactive intestinal peptide. The absolute frequency of multiple hormones contained in or released by these tumors is not known. Approximately one-third of patients with gastrinomas have increases in serum concentrations of *pancreatic polypeptide.* About two-thirds are histologically or biologically malignant, and about half have spread to the liver when the tumor is identified. Malignant gastrinomas usually grow slowly. From one-half to two-thirds of patients with gastrinomas have metastases, most commonly to regional lymph nodes and liver; spread may also be to peritoneal surfaces, spleen, bone, skin, or mediastinum. Gastrinomas have light-microscopic similarities to carcinoid tumors and may be mistaken for carcinoid tumors, especially when arising from the mucosa of the small intestine or stomach. Pancreatic islet-cell hyperplasia occurs in approximately 10 percent of patients with the Zollinger-Ellison syndrome. Hyperplasia of the islets, accompanying recognizable or unidentified gastrinoma, appears to be a consequence rather than a cause of excess gastrin release, since gastrin is not present in the hyperplastic tissue.

In most gastrinomas approximately 90 to 95 percent of gastrin is in the form of heptadecapeptide gastrin (G-17 or little gastrin), with most of the remainder being big gastrin (G-34). In contrast, approximately two-thirds of circulating gastrin in gastrinoma patients is G-34; most of the remainder of circulating gastrin is G-17. However, smaller amounts of even larger forms of gastrin and smaller gastrin fragments can be detected in the serum. The parietal cell mass is substantially expanded to from three to six times normal, secondary to the trophic effects of gastrin on parietal cells.

In from 20 to 25 percent of patients with the Zollinger-Ellison syndrome, the gastrinoma is a component of the multiple endocrine adenomatosis type I (MEA-I) syndrome, an autosomal dominant disorder with a high degree of penetrance and great variability in expressivity. Patients with MEA-I may have hyperplasia, adenomas, or carcinoma involving the parathyroid glands, pancreatic islets, and pituitary: the organs involved are in that order of frequency. Hyperparathyroidism is present in 87 percent of patients with the MEA-I syndrome, and gastrinoma is present in approximately half of these patients (see Chap. 123).

While the true incidence of the Zollinger-Ellison syndrome is not known, estimates are that it accounts for 0.1 to 1 percent of peptic ulcers. The Zollinger-Ellison syndrome may occur at any age, but initial manifestations are most common between ages 30 and 60.

CLINICAL FEATURES From 90 to 95 percent of patients with gastrinomas develop ulceration of the gastrointestinal tract at some point during the course of their disease. Profound gastric hypersecretion is found in most, but not all, patients. Symptoms are often similar to those seen in patients with typical peptic ulcer disease. However, the ulcer symptoms may be more fulminant, progressive, and persistent, and usually respond poorly to usual medical and surgical peptic ulcer treatment programs. The anatomic site of the ulcers in patients with gastrinoma is similar, but not identical, to that of patients with common types of peptic ulcer. About 75 percent of gastrinoma patients have ulcers in the first portion of the duodenum or in the stomach; these are usually single, but may be multiple. When multiple ulcers occur, they are frequently located not only in the first portion of the duodenum, but also in the remainder of the duodenum or even the jejunum. In one large series, 14 percent of the ulcers were found in the duodenum beyond its first portion, and 11 percent in the jejunum. Prompt recurrence of ulcer, often with hemorrhage or perforation, after peptic ulcer surgery without total gastrectomy (in which the Zollinger-Ellison syndrome had not been recognized) is characteristic of gastrinoma.

Diarrhea occurs in about 40 percent of patients, and about 7 percent of patients with gastrinoma may have diarrhea in the absence of ulcer disease. The diarrhea is due to the outpouring of large amounts of hydrochloric acid into the proximal duodenum and can be reduced or eliminated by aspiration of gastric juice. The excessive acid has been shown to reduce the pH within the lumen of the proximal and distal jejunum to as low as 1 and 3.6, respectively. Inflammatory changes may develop in the mucosa of the small intestine, presumably secondary to the injurious effect of the increased amounts of acid and pepsin. Steatorrhea, which is less common than diarrhea, appears to result from inactivation of pancreatic lipase by the large concentration of acid in the proximal small intestine and from decreases in luminal bile salts. The decrease in bile salt concentration of the intraluminal contents is caused by precipitation of the major bile acids at low pH. This leads to impaired micelle formation which, in turn, reduces the intestinal absorption of fatty acids and monoglycerides (see Chap. 308). Vitamin B_{12} malabsorption, not correctable by addition of intrinsic factor, has been detected in some patients with the Zollinger-Ellison syndrome. Although the secretion of intrinsic factor appears normal, the reduced pH within the gut interferes with intrinsic factor mediation of vitamin B_{12} absorption. This can be corrected by neutralization of the intestinal contents. The mechanism by which low pH in the gut interferes with intrinsic factor action is not known.

Diarrhea in patients with gastrinoma is invariably accompanied by gastric acid *hypersecretion.* (This does not occur in patients with common duodenal ulcer with similar rates of hypersecretion of gastric acid; the reason for this difference is not known.) Severe diarrhea is also seen with nonbeta islet-cell tumors of the pancreas, but these tumors are usually associated with *hyposecretion* of gastric acid or even achlorhydria [pancreatic cholera or WDHA (watery diarrhea, hypokalemia, and achlorhydria) syndrome]. In most cases, the pancreatic cholera syndrome appears to be due to tumor release of VIP (see Chaps. 123 and 325).

DIAGNOSIS The presence of a gastrinoma should be suspected in patients with a compatible clinical history, especially in those with evidence of marked acid hypersecretion. Two-thirds of gastrinoma patients have basal gastric acid outputs (BAO) which exceed 10 meq/h. However, as stated earlier, there is substantial overlap in the rates of gastric acid secretion among patients with gastrinoma, duodenal ulcer, and normal subjects. Gastrinoma patients often have basal acid output rates which are greater than 60 percent of those induced by maximal stimulation (MAO). In most normal subjects and duodenal ulcer patients basal acid secretory rates are less than 60 percent of maximal secretion. However, because of frequent patient variations, with exceptions to these guidelines by patients with gastrinomas and common duodenal ulcers, the use of the BAO/MAO ratio is of no value in the certain identification of gastrinoma patients.

Some radiographic features may suggest and support the diagnosis of the Zollinger-Ellison syndrome. Large mucosal folds may be demonstrated in the stomach, duodenum, and, in some instances, the jejunum. The lumen of the stomach and small intestine often contains large amounts of fluid. Radiographic features of most ulcers in these patients, except when they are multiple or distal in location, are similar to the common peptic ulcer. Arteriography is of limited value in identifying patients with gastrinoma; primary tumors or hepatic metastases demonstrated at surgery have been identified in only from 20 to 30 percent of gastrinoma patients. Some reports suggest that computerized axial tomography may be of greater value in identifying primary or metastatic gastrinoma. Endoscopic retrograde pancreaticoduodenography (ERCP) has not proved to be of assistance in the diagnosis or exclusion of pancreatic gastrinomas.

The diagnosis in a patient with clinical features consistent with the Zollinger-Ellison syndrome depends upon the demonstration of *increased serum gastrin levels* by radioimmunoassay. Fasting serum gastrin levels in normal subjects and patients with typical duodenal ulcer average approximately 60 pg/ml and usually do not exceed 160 pg/ml. Patients with gastrinoma almost always have fasting serum gastrin levels which are greater than 200 pg/ml and have been reported as high as 450,000 pg/ml.

Several provocative tests are of value, especially in patients who do not exhibit pronounced hypergastrinemia (i.e., serum gastrin greater than 1000 pg/ml). These tests involve the measurement of serum gastrin levels in response to intravenous calcium infusion, secretin injection, or ingestion of a standard test meal (see Table 306-2).

The *calcium infusion test* involves constant 3-h intravenous infusion of calcium gluconate (5 mg calcium per kilogram per hour). Serum samples for gastrin measurements are obtained before and at 30-min intervals for 4 h after initiation of infusion. In gastrinoma patients serum gastrin concentrations usually increase above the basal serum gastrin by at least 50 percent or by more than 400 pg/ml. In the *secretin injection test,* secretin (GIH secretin, 2 units per kilogram) is given intravenously over 30 to 60 s. (Boots secretin is approximately one-sixth as potent as GIH secretin supplied by the Karolinska Institute, Stockholm. Boots secretin should not be used, since it contains large amounts of gastrin-like material which is immunoreactive with antibodies to gastrin and, therefore, can spuriously increase serum gastrin concentrations.) Gastrin is measured in serum samples obtained before injection of secretin and at 5-min intervals thereafter for 30 min. In normal individuals and duodenal ulcer patients secretin produces either no change or small reductions in serum gastrin levels. In contrast, in gastrinoma patients intravenous secretin induces paradoxical increases in serum gastrin. The gastrin levels increase promptly, usually at 5 min, by at least 200 pg/ml. The third provocative test involves the *feeding of a standard meal;* gastrin is measured in serum samples obtained before the meal and at 15-min intervals for 90 min. In gastrinoma patients peak serum gastrin levels do not increase (or increase minimally) and never reach values 50 percent greater than fasting levels (see Table 306-2).

The precise frequency with which gastrinoma patients conform to the criteria suggested for these provocative tests remains to be established. However, with what information is now available, the following conclusions appear warranted. *The secretin infusion test appears to be the provocative test of greatest value in identifying gastrinoma patients.* Positive serum gastrin responses to intravenous secretin are detected in more than 90 percent of patients with gastrinoma. Using the criteria suggested, paradoxical increases in serum gastrin following secretin injection have not been detected in nongastrinoma patients. Exaggerated release of gastrin in response to calcium infusion has been found in more than 80 percent of gastrinoma patients; however, this exaggerated response to calcium infusion has been observed in some nongastrinoma patients with hypergastrinemia (e.g., achlorhydria with or without pernicious anemia). In gastrinoma patients enhanced gastrin release with calcium infusion is rarely, if ever, observed in the absence of paradoxical gastrin release in response to secretin.

In a very small proportion of duodenal ulcer patients (less than 1 percent), gastric acid hypersecretion may be accompanied by increased serum gastrin levels due to hyperfunction and/or hyperplasia of antral gastrin cells (G cells). These can be distinguished from gastrinoma patients by the secretin and meal stimulation tests. In patients with this antral gastrin cell abnormality, intravenous secretin reduces serum gastrin and ingestion of the test meal leads to striking increases in serum gastrin levels, exceeding the fasting serum gastrin concentration by more than 200 percent.

TREATMENT Except for cimetidine, these patients have been resistant to conventional forms of medical and surgical ulcer treatment. Antacids produce transient symptomatic relief but seldom induce ulcer healing or sustained relief of symptoms. Incomplete gastric resection (with or without vagotomy or pyloroplasty with vagotomy) is almost invariably followed by prompt and often fulminant ulcer recurrence. Many patients with gastrinoma have had multiple surgical procedures, particularly when the diagnosis was not established initially. Mortality has been lowest when gastrectomy has been performed as the initial surgical procedure. For this reason, total gastrectomy has been considered the surgical procedure of choice; subtotal gastric resections should not be performed.

The H_2-receptor antagonist cimetidine has been used successfully in the medical treatment of patients with gastrinoma. Improvement in clinical symptoms, ulcer healing, and decreases in gastric acid output occur in 80 to 85 percent of patients so treated. Many, but not all, of these patients have responded sufficiently well to cimetidine so as to not require surgery. Cimetidine must be administered at approximately 6-h intervals. The dose required is often 1.5 to 3 times that used in the treatment of common duodenal ulcer. Cimetidine therapy must be continued indefinitely, since even temporary discontinuance of it is usually followed by ulcer recurrence. H_2-receptor antagonists, like cimetidine, are indicated in patients who are not satisfactory candidates either for total gastrectomy or for surgical attempts at tumor resection, as well as preoperatively prior to total gastrectomy. A small number of Zollinger-Ellison patients have been treated effectively with parietal cell vagotomy and cimetidine; however, more data are needed to assess the merits of this treatment program. The use of longer acting and potentially more potent H_2-receptor antagonists, prostaglandins, and other agents reducing acid secretion may prove to be of value in these patients in the future.

In selecting the best therapy, the biological behavior of these tumors and the clinical manifestations of the syndrome in the given patient must be taken into consideration. Therapeutic doses of cimetidine are indicated in the period during which the diagnosis is being established and the location and extent of tumor are being determined, and also as treatment in preparation for surgery. Cimetidine is certainly indicated for patients who are not satisfactory operative candidates, for those who refuse surgery, and for those in whom surgery is not possible. When metastatic gastrinoma is present, several factors must be considered. Control of the ulcer disease may be achieved in most instances with cimetidine and/or total gastric resection. However, there is no convincing evidence that tumor progression is influenced by gastrectomy. Patients with progressive invasive gastrinoma may be benefited somewhat by streptozotocin and with 5-fluorouracil which may reduce tumor bulk and partially reduce serum gastrin levels.

The most difficult treatment decisions are in those patients in whom the location and extent of the tumor have not been defined. With more general use of gastrin radioimmunoassay, patients with gastrinomas are being detected earlier in the course of their disease. Prior studies indicated that the morbidity and mortality in patients with the Zollinger-Ellison syndrome were largely due to the complications of the severe ulcer disease. However, with earlier diagnosis, effective antiulcer treatment and longer follow-up, more frequent consequences of the invasive properties of malignant gastrinoma are being recognized. Although complete surgical removal of gastrinoma, with cure, has been achieved in less than 10 percent of patients with gastrinoma, earlier detection may make it possible to improve upon these results.

STRESS ULCERS AND EROSIONS

A variety of acute ulcerative lesions of the gastrointestinal tract are distinct clinically from chronic peptic ulcer. Among these are the acute upper gastrointestinal erosions and ulcerations which are often observed in patients with shock, burns, sepsis, and severe trauma. These are often referred to as *stress erosions* and *ulcers*. These lesions, which are frequently multiple, are most common in the acid-secreting portion of the stomach, but they may also occur in the antrum and duodenum. Acute stress erosions and ulcerations are usually superficial, with necrosis limited to the mucosa.

These erosions and superficial ulcers are extremely frequent and occur in about 90 percent of patients with massive injuries and burns. The most common clinical finding in patients with acute erosions or ulcerations is painless gastrointestinal hemorrhage. Blood loss is usually minimal but may be substantial. Erosions develop most frequently approximately 24 h after trauma. Small amounts of blood loss may be detected in the first 24 to 48 h after trauma. However, when massive hemorrhage occurs, it is usually more than 2 or 3 days after the acute insult. The diagnosis is best established by upper gastrointestinal endoscopy. The erosive lesions are frequently too superficial to be recognized by barium examination of the upper gastrointestinal tract. Acute ulcerations and erosions should be suspected when there is evidence of upper gastrointestinal bleeding in patients with severe injuries, burns, infections, and shock.

Many theories have been proposed to explain stress-associated acute mucosal ulceration, but the mechanism for the mucosal injury is still not clear. Gastric acid appears to be involved in the production of these acute stress erosions and ulcers, although there is usually no evidence of acid hypersecretion. The lesions cannot be produced in experimental animals in the absence of acid. The two major mechanisms which have been proposed are mucosal ischemia and enhanced back-diffusion of hydrogen ions. Investigation of the gastric mucosal barrier indicates that it is intact after severe burns and injuries. A number of studies support the conclusion that mucosal ischemia may be the most important element in the production of stress ulceration.

The treatment of acute stress ulcerations and erosions is principally preventive. In high-risk patients the frequency of stress ulcerations can be diminished by the vigorous use of antacids to neutralize gastric contents. While anticholinergics are of no value, there is preliminary evidence that inhibition of acid secretion by cimetidine may be effective in prevention of stress ulceration: however, cimetidine does not appear as effective as vigorous (every 30 to 60 min) therapy with antacids. Intravenous vasopressin infusion or its selective intraarterial infusion into the left gastric artery has been found to decrease hemorrhage in patients with stress erosions. When medical therapy fails to arrest bleeding, surgical approaches have varied from pyloroplasty and vagotomy to total gastrectomy.

The term *Cushing's ulcer* has been applied to acute ulceration of the upper gastrointestinal tract associated with intracranial injury or increases in intracranial pressure, e.g., with brain tumors. These ulcers may involve the stomach, proximal duodenum, or esophagus, and frequently lead to hemorrhage or perforation. They do not differ histologically from acute stress ulceration. Treatment includes correction of increased intracranial pressure, when possible, and the usual measures for treatment of acute erosions and ulcerations.

DRUG-ASSOCIATED ULCERS AND EROSIONS

Gastric and duodenal ulcers have been described following administration of many drugs. Salicylate ingestion has been shown to be associated with an increased incidence of gastric ulcer and is a frequent cause of hemorrhagic gastric erosions. There is no evidence of an increased frequency of duodenal ulcer among patients treated with salicylates. The mechanism by which salicylates induce, or are associated with, gastric ulcer has not been established. It has been suggested that salicylates contribute to the development of gastric ulcer by mucosal injury induced by interruption of the gastric mucosal barrier, the principal mechanism by which salicylates appear to produce erosive gastritis. An additional mechanism by which salicylates may injure the gastric mucosa is by their capacity to inhibit prostaglandin synthesis, since various prostaglandins have been shown to have cytoprotective properties, by which they prevent damage to the gastric mucosa in response to a variety of agents. Patients with gastric ulcer should avoid salicylates, and many physicians also withhold recommending salicylates in patients with duodenal ulcer.

Administration of corticosteroids has been reported to be associated with development of ulcer disease of the upper gastrointestinal tract. Although for the most part this proposal has been widely accepted, there are no firm data conclusively establishing the association between corticosteroids and gastric or duodenal ulcers. Most controlled studies have failed to demonstrate an increased incidence of ulcers in patients treated with corticosteroids for a variety of disorders. Some studies have suggested an increased incidence of ulcer disease in patients with rheumatoid arthritis: these patients may often be receiving other potentially ulcerogenic drugs, which may account for the apparent increase in ulcer frequency when these patients are treated with corticosteroids. At present a direct association between treatment with corticosteroids and an increased incidence of duodenal or gastric ulcer has not been established.

Other drugs which have been reported to be associated with ulceration of the upper gastrointestinal tract include indomethacin, phenylbutazone, and reserpine. It is uncertain whether these drugs are responsible for the associated ulcer disease and, if so, by what mechanism the ulceration is produced. Because of the potential suspected ulcerogenicity of corticosteroids, indomethacin, phenylbutazone, and reserpine, most physicians limit their use, when possible, in patients with known peptic ulcer disease. In addition to these agents, gastric ulcer and acute gastric erosions have been reported after ingestion of other anti-inflammatory agents used in the treatment of arthritis, including ibuprofen and naproxen. When possible, their use should also be limited in patients with ulcer disease.

REFERENCES

Bardhan KD et al: Double blind comparison of cimetidine and placebo in the maintenance and healing of chronic duodenal ulceration. Gut 20:158, 1979

Elashoff JD, Grossman MI: Trends in hospital admissions and death rates for peptic ulcer in the United States from 1970 to 1978. Gastroenterology 78:280, 1980

Fordtran JS et al: In vivo and in vitro evaluation of liquid antacids. N Engl J Med 288:923, 1973

Isenberg JI et al: Increased sensitivity to stimulation of acid secretion by pentagastrin in duodenal ulcer. J Clin Invest 55:330, 1975

Johnston D: Treatment of peptic ulcer and its complications, in *Recent Advances in Surgery*, S Taylor (ed). Edinburgh, Churchill Livingstone, 1980, p 355

Lamers CBH, Van Tongeren JHM: Comparative study of the value of calcium, secretin, and meal stimulated increase in serum gastrin to the diagnosis of the Zollinger-Ellison syndrome. Gut 18:128, 1977

McCarthy DM: The place of surgery in the Zollinger-Ellison syndrome. N Engl J Med 302:1344, 1980

McGuigan JE, Trudeau WL: Differences in rates of gastrin release in normal persons and patients with duodenal ulcer. N Engl J Med 288:64, 1973

Martin F et al: Comparison of the healing capacities of sucralfate and cimetidine in the short-term treatment of duodenal ulcer: A double blind randomized study. Gastroenterology 82:401, 1982

Peterson WL et al: Healing of duodenal ulcer with an antacid regime. N Engl J Med 297:341, 1977

Priebe HJ et al: Antacid versus cimetidine in preventing acute gastrointestinal bleeding. N Engl J Med 302:426, 1980

Richardson CT: Sucralfate. Ann Int Med 97:269, 1982

Robert A: Cytoprotection by prostaglandins. Gastroenterology 77:761, 1979

Rotter JI et al: Duodenal ulcer disease associated with elevated serum pepsinogen I. An inherited autosomal disorder. N Engl J Med 300:63, 1979

Walsh JH, Grossman MI: Gastrin. N Engl J Med 292:1324, 1975

Winship DH: Cimetidine in the treatment of duodenal ulcer. Review and commentary. Gastroenterology 74:402, 1978

307 CANCER, BENIGN TUMORS, GASTRITIS, AND OTHER GASTRIC DISEASES

WALTER C. MacDONALD
CYRUS E. RUBIN

CANCER

CARCINOMA Throughout the world gastric cancer is one of the most common lethal malignancies. Although its frequency is decreasing in the United States, it still causes about 15,000 deaths each year. Because symptoms in the early, potentially curable phase are often minimal or nonexistent, patients usually seek medical advice too late. Thus, less than 15 percent of patients survive 5 years, despite improved diagnostic and surgical techniques.

Epidemiology Whereas gastric cancer is very common in Japan, the Central and South American Andes, and parts of eastern Europe, it is uncommon in the United States, Mexico, and Malaysia. Over the past 40 years in the United States there has been a remarkable but unexplained fall in the annual mortality from 30 to 8 per 100,000. A lesser decline is apparent in western Europe. Some pathologists separate gastric cancer into two histologic types for epidemiological purposes: intestinal and diffuse. These pathologists believe that the reduction in the incidence of the intestinal type accounts for the overall fall in the incidence of gastric cancer in the United States and certain other countries. Japanese migrating to the United States continue to have a high incidence, but their children have a much lower incidence, suggesting the importance of environmental factors in pathogenesis. Throughout the world, men are affected about twice as often as women. The mean age usually quoted is 55 years, but the patients are even older in some North American series. Only 5 percent of patients are less than 40 years of age.

Etiology The cause of gastric cancer is unknown, but diet has been implicated. Gastric cancer can be readily induced in some animals by the oral administration of *N*-methyl-N^1-nitrosoguanidine. It has been suggested that gastric cancer may be related to the formation of *N*-nitroso compounds by the conversion of food nitrates to nitrites, which then interact in the stomach with secondary or tertiary amines. Interestingly, this reaction is inhibited by ascorbic acid.

Predisposing factors Gastric cancer is two to four times more common in first-degree relatives of patients with the disease than in a control population. The concordance rate is greater for identical than dizygotic twins. The disease is marginally more common in persons with blood group A. These data suggest a small genetic element in pathogenesis.

Atrophic gastric mucosa, especially when associated with intestinal metaplasia, probably increases the risk of gastric cancer. Such mucosal changes are invariably seen in Addisonian pernicious anemia, and 6 percent of these patients develop stomach cancer. Comparison of Japanese and American autopsy results shows that the high-risk Japanese have more extensive atrophic gastritis and intestinal metaplasia than the low-risk Americans. Serial biopsy studies also suggest that persons with atrophic gastritis are more likely to develop gastric cancer than those with normal mucosa. It must, however, be recognized that atrophic gastritis is common in normal older people without cancer, and that some patients with gastric cancer have no gastritis in the uninvolved portions of the stomach.

Adenomatous gastric polyps either contain adenocarcinoma or are associated with carcinoma elsewhere in the stomach in as often as 30 percent of cases. It is not known whether these uncommon adenomatous polyps contain cancer from the onset or whether they were originally benign. Certainly most gastric cancers do not begin as polyps. Patients with gastric polyps are also predisposed to cancer elsewhere in the stomach, but to a lesser degree. This predisposition is possibly related to the atrophic gastritis which is regularly seen surrounding both kinds of polyps.

Benign gastric ulcer without operation has not been shown to be a precursor of gastric cancer. European studies have shown that there is an increased risk of gastric cancer 10 to 20 years after surgical treatment for peptic ulcer, especially if a Billroth II partial gastrectomy was done.

Pathology Gastric cancers are almost always adenocarcinomas. Gross and microscopic classification of these carcinomas is frequently impossible because many are of mixed pattern. In general, there are five macroscopic types: polypoid, ulcerative, combined ulcerative and infiltrative, diffuse infiltrative (linitis plastica), and superficial spreading. Microscopic classification is particularly difficult, but three cell types are discernible: intestinal, gastric (pylorocardiac), and diffuse (mucous cell). In the Laurén classification, only two cell types are recognized: intestinal and diffuse. When classifiable, the gross and microscopic categorizations have limited prognostic value. Polypoid, ulcerative, and superficial spreading cancers are often less malignant than the infiltrative types. Microscopically, the intestinal cell type has a slightly better prognosis than the diffuse mucous cell variety. However, the most important morphologic factors in prognosis are the depth of invasion and the presence or absence of metastases. Stromal reaction with lymphocytes, plasma cells, and young fibroblasts is indicative of host resistance and improves the prognosis.

Cancer originates with equal frequency in the antrum and body of the stomach and involves the lesser curvature more often than the greater. Ten to twenty percent occur at the cardia. The cancer spreads by direct extension along the gastric wall and through it to the perigastric tissues. Sometimes direct extension involves the pancreas, colon, or liver. Proximal gastric tumors often invade the esophagus, but distal ones less commonly cross the pylorus into the duodenum. Lymph node metastases to the perigastric nodes are usually present; nodes in the preaortic area, porta hepatis, and hilum of the spleen are often involved as well. Spread via the thoracic duct can involve the left supraclavicular (Virchow's) lymph nodes. Peritoneal metastases are evident in about 20 percent of patients at laparoscopy or operation. Intraabdominal metastases may be confined to the ovary or prerectal pouch. Blood-borne metastases to the liver are apparent in about 30 percent of patients at operation; less often, the lungs, brain, or other organs are involved.

Clinical features The history is of little help in distinguishing benign from malignant gastric ulcer because many of the varied symptoms may be seen in both diseases. Approximately 25 percent of patients with cancer have classic ulcer symptoms. The most common presenting complaint, however, is upper abdominal discomfort of insidious onset. This is often mild but varies greatly in severity from a vague, postprandial fullness to a severe, steady pain. Anorexia, often with slight nausea, is very common but is not the usual presenting complaint. Weight loss is observed in about 50 percent of patients. Nausea and vomiting are particularly prominent with tumors of the pylorus, but can occur with advanced disease elsewhere in the stomach. Dysphagia is the major symptom of cardia tumors. Weakness, hematemesis, melena, and alteration in bowel habits are other presenting complaints. Some patients suffer from the symptoms of anemia, or their anemia may be discovered on routine examination. Occasionally, an ulcerating carcinoma perforates, and rarely a gastrocolic fistula develops.

The initial symptoms may be related to metastases. These include abdominal distention by malignant ascites; jaundice from biliary tract obstruction by nodes at the porta hepatis or by intrahepatic metastases; pain from bone involvement; neurologic symptoms secondary to brain metastases; and shortness of breath from lung spread. Mechanical bowel obstruction can be secondary to peritoneal metastases, and pelvic symptoms can result from ovarian spread.

The duration of symptoms before patients see a physician is remarkably variable but averages 6 months. Symptoms of several years' duration are not uncommon. Some patients with long-standing functional gastrointestinal complaints may notice a change in their pain pattern. In North America, less than 10 percent of patients with symptoms have disease confined to the mucosa or submucosa. Screening studies in Japan confirm that most patients with early curable gastric cancer are asymptomatic, although some have mild epigastric distress.

An epigastric mass is palpable in only a minority of patients; it is a poor prognostic sign but does not exclude the possibility of cure. Abdominal tenderness is found in about one-third of patients. Pallor or cachexia may be observed, and occasionally a gastric succussion splash is demonstrable. Physical signs suggesting metastases should be carefully sought because distant metastases that are proved by biopsy exclude curative surgery. These include hepatomegaly, jaundice, enlargement of left supraclavicular (Virchow's) or scalene nodes, a shelf-like mass in the prerectal pouch above the prostate or cervix (Blumer's shelf), an ovarian mass on vaginal or abdominal examination (Krukenberg's tumor), ascites, an umbilical mass, and skin nodules. A low-grade fever may occur with advanced disease, particularly with liver metastases. Rarely gastric cancer is associated with dermatomyositis, acanthosis nigricans, neuromyopathy, hypoglycemia, or multiple seborrheic keratoses.

Laboratory findings Iron-deficiency anemia because of occult bleeding is found in about two-thirds of patients. Occasionally the cancer is associated with pernicious anemia. Rarely a pancytopenia is caused by bone marrow replacement. A "leukemoid" reaction and disseminated intravascular coagulation are other rare findings. Occult blood is demonstrable in the stools in about 80 percent of patients if repeated tests are done. Elevation of 5′-nucleotidase suggests the presence of liver metastases, which can be confirmed by liver scan. The serum albumin may be low because of protein leakage from the involved gastric mucosa. Measurement of gastric secretion is considered less helpful than in the past. Achlorhydria after stimulation with pentagastrin usually excludes a benign peptic ulcer, but the test is of limited value because most patients with a malignant ulcer secrete some acid. A rise in the carcinoembryonic antigen (CEA) after treatment suggests recurrence of carcinoma, but the test is of little initial diagnostic value.

Diagnosis In North America x-ray of the stomach is the initial method used for detecting gastric carcinoma. In more than 90 percent of symptomatic patients, x-ray detects a gastric abnormality. However, experienced radiologists fail to differentiate benign from malignant gastric lesions in approximately 25 percent of cases. Thus, gastroscopy with biopsy and brush or exfoliative cytology must be used to confirm or exclude a diagnosis of cancer (see Chap. 304). It may be more important to the patient to exclude gastric cancer than it is to diagnose it because unnecessary emotional trauma and surgical morbidity or mortality can be avoided by definitive diagnosis of benign disease.

The diagnostic accuracy of x-ray is greatest when it is used wisely. Equivocal examinations should always be repeated. The use of double contrast techniques helps to detect small lesions by improving mucosal detail. The stomach should be distended at some time during every x-ray examination because decreased distensibility may be the only indication of a diffuse infiltrative carcinoma. Although gastric ulcers can be detected fairly easily, it may be impossible to distinguish benign from malignant ulcers radiologically. Differential x-ray diagnosis is also difficult when the antrum is narrowed or when mucosal folds are enlarged. Cancer of the proximal stomach invading the neural plexuses of the esophagus may mimic achalasia by x-ray. In cancer of the cardia the x-ray appearance may be considered normal or may be confused with benign mucosal distortion secondary to a hiatus hernia. It is impossible to differentiate adenocarcinoma from lymphoma radiologically. Cancer of the pancreas or colon invading the stomach may be confused with primary gastric neoplasm.

Fiberoptic gastroscopy with biopsy and brush cytology is especially useful for confirming the diagnosis of cancer suspected by x-ray, differentiating cancer from lymphoma, clarifying equivocal radiologic findings, and checking suspicious clinical findings despite negative x-rays. At least six biopsies should be taken from suitable areas of a suspected neoplasm; if the tissue is serially sectioned and thoroughly examined by an expert, accuracy in the diagnosis of cancer approaching 90 percent can be achieved. The addition of brush cytology raises the accuracy in detecting cancer even higher but slightly raises the risk of a false diagnosis of cancer. Diffuse infiltrative tumors and recurrent cancers can be impossible to diagnose even by these methods because malignant cells may not be present in the biopsied mucosal layer. Expertly performed exfoliative cytology by "blind" gastric lavage yields cancer cells in over 85 percent of patients with a false-positive rate of less than 1 percent. The procedure is particularly useful in elderly or poor-risk patients and in those in whom endoscopy is unsuccessful or equivocal. If all techniques are used, gastric cancer is seldom missed, but occasionally laparoscopy or laparotomy is required for diagnosis.

The x-ray demonstration of a benign-appearing gastric ulcer presents special problems. Some physicians feel that gastroscopy is not mandatory if the x-ray features are typically benign, if healing at 6 weeks is complete by x-ray, and if a follow-up x-ray examination several months later is negative. Other physicians, however, feel that gastroscopic biopsy and brush cytology are required for all patients with a gastric ulcer in order to exclude carcinoma or lymphoma. The marked drop in the incidence of malignant gastric ulcers in North America has raised the question whether it is cost-effective to endoscope all patients with gastric ulcer rather than to perform endoscopy only in those with a suspicious x-ray or clinical course.

Using x-ray and intragastric photography for mass screening, the Japanese have detected many early curable cancers of the stomach. In North America, such screening methods are probably not cost-effective because the disease is relatively uncommon. However, special attention must be paid to patients over 40 years of age who are predisposed to gastric cancer because of pernicious anemia, the presence or history of an adenomatous gastric polyp, a family history of gastric cancer, Billroth II gastrectomy 10 to 20 years previously, or birth in countries where gastric cancer is common. In addition, one must be certain that all gastric ulcers treated medically are indeed benign.

Treatment Surgical removal of the tumor offers the only chance for cure. A careful evaluation for evidence of distant metastases will avoid unnecessary surgery. Physical examination is supplemented by chest x-ray, liver function tests, liver scan, and, in selected cases, abdominal ultrasound (echo). The use of computerized tomography (CT scan) has increased the accuracy of preoperative staging. Suspected areas of metastasis should be sampled, for example, lymph nodes or liver and pleural or peritoneal effusions. If metastases are suspected but unproved, laparoscopy under local anesthesia with direct biopsy of suspected areas of metastasis is particularly helpful in assessing operability. Cancer of the distal and midstomach is usually treated by subtotal gastrectomy; removal of the regional lymph nodes requires resection of the greater and lesser omentum and sometimes the spleen. Tumors of the proximal stomach are usually treated by distal esophagectomy and proximal gastrectomy. Total gastrectomy is indicated only occasionally. If obstruction is present or if bleeding is a problem, palliative resection may be worthwhile even though the disease is found to be incurable at operation. The operative mortality rate for gastric cancer is still as high as 10 percent in many hospitals.

It is often difficult to assess the reported results of surgical treatment. Careful and standardized descriptions by surgeon and pathologist would facilitate comparison of different series. These should include depth of tumor penetration, extent of lymph node involvement, and presence of distant metastases. More than 80 percent of cancers confined to the mucosa or submucosa are curable, compared with 10 to 20 percent when the tumor extends through the serosa. Up to 50 percent survive 5 years after curative resection if the lymph nodes are not involved. Tumor diameter of less than 2 cm and a long history of symptoms are good prognostic signs. However, in North America only 10 to 15 percent survive 5 years after diagnosis. Rarely, patients live for 5 years without treatment or for many years after a palliative resection.

Chemotherapy with 5-fluorouracil (5-FU) causes some tumor regression in about 10 percent of patients. Combination chemotherapy [e.g., 5-FU, doxorubicin (Adriamycin), and mitomycin C] induces a response in a higher percentage of patients, but the median survival is still less than 1 year. There are, however, occasional very worthwhile responses to chemotherapy. The effectiveness of adjuvant radiotherapy, or chemotherapy, remains to be proved of long-term value. Palliative radiotherapy may be useful to control bleeding and to alleviate pain from bone metastases. Other palliative measures include replacement of iron and vitamin B_{12}, dilatation of obstructing cardia tumors with or without placement of plastic tubular stents, treatment of postgastrectomy problems, and the judicious use of analgesics and antiemetics.

LYMPHOMA Primary gastric lymphomas account for about 5 percent of gastric malignancies and about 60 percent of gastric sarcomas. Most are histiocytic lymphomas (reticulum-cell sarcomas) or lymphocytic lymphomas; Hodgkin's disease is relatively uncommon, and plasmacytoma is rare. Some gastric lymphomas present a varied histologic picture that defies classification. Gastric involvement secondary to disseminated lymphoma is more common than the primary form. In one large series, one-third of histiocytic lymphomas and one-sixth of lymphosarcomas eventually spread to the stomach. The sexes are affected equally, and the mean age is about 55 years.

The symptoms are indistinguishable from those of gastric ulcer or cancer. Hematemesis (20 percent) and perforation (10 percent) occur more often than with carcinoma. An abdominal mass is palpable in approximately one-third of patients. Approximately half of patients have iron-deficiency anemia, usually with occult blood demonstrable in the stools.

X-ray studies usually show an abnormality which can seldom be distinguished from adenocarcinoma. Large rigid folds, multiple ulcers, or duodenal involvement suggest the possibility of lymphoma. The x-ray appearance may also be confused with that of Ménétrier's disease or benign peptic ulcer. The tumor is usually obvious at gastroscopy, but its gross appearance is seldom diagnostic. A preoperative diagnosis can often be made by the combination of endoscopic biopsy and cytologic examination, but even these methods may fail. Pseudolymphoma cannot be distinguished from true lymphoma prior to surgical excision.

Primary gastric lymphoma is most often treated by a combination of surgical excision and radiation therapy. Usually surgery precedes radiotherapy, but it may be advantageous to shrink large tumors with radiation before attempting to excise them. Thirty to fifty percent of patients so treated survive 5 years. Survival is particularly good if the tumor does not penetrate the serosa or involve the perigastric nodes. A careful search for evidence of disseminated disease should be made before operation. Laparoscopy is especially useful for such staging. Lymphangiography, CT scan, and bone marrow biopsy are also useful for staging in selected cases. Some patients with nonresectable tumors have survived 5 years after treatment with radiotherapy alone. There is some evidence that radiotherapy without operation may be suitable treatment, at least in selected cases. The role of chemotherapy for primary gastric lymphoma is not well defined. Disseminated lymphoma with gastric involvement is treated by chemotherapy and radiotherapy as discussed in Chap. 125.

LEIOMYOSARCOMA These tumors account for 1 to 3 percent of gastric malignancies. The mean age of the persons affected is about 60 years, and the sexes are affected equally. The tumors are usually large, spherical, and in the upper half of the stomach; they tend to ulcerate and become necrotic in their center. The tumor may spread to the peritoneum or liver but rarely to lymph nodes. Most patients complain of pain. The majority are anemic, and massive bleeding occurs in about one-third. A mass is palpable in more than 50 percent. X-ray studies show a large, smooth tumor, often with central ulceration and sometimes with a sinus tract to the center of the neoplasm. It is impossible to differentiate leiomyosarcoma by x-ray from benign leiomyoma except that leiomyosarcomas tend to be larger. Endoscopic biopsy rarely provides a correct preoperative diagnosis, but brush cytology of the ulceration may. Treatment is by wide surgical excision if feasible; about 25 to 40 percent of patients are cured. Expert chemotherapists have used Adriamycin in combination with various other agents to achieve modest palliation in a minority of patients with advanced disease. Radiotherapy is ineffective.

Carcinoid tumors and other malignancies Gastric carcinoids are uncommon. Like carcinoids elsewhere, they may be multiple. They are often symptomless but can cause bleeding or epigastric pain. The roentgenographic appearance is that of a smooth, rounded, sessile filling defect sometimes with ulceration. About 25 percent are malignant, but only a small minority cause the malignant carcinoid syndrome. Small carcinoids can be excised locally; those larger than 2 cm and those that are malignant require partial gastrectomy. The chemotherapy of malignant carcinoids and the treatment of the carcinoid syndrome are described in Chap. 131.

Rare primary gastric malignancies include carcinosarcoma, hemangiopericytoma, neurogenic sarcoma, fibrosarcoma, and liposarcoma. Approximately 10 percent of leiomyoblastomas are malignant. Metastases to the stomach most often originate from generalized lymphoma, lung cancer, breast cancer, or malignant melanoma.

BENIGN TUMORS

EPITHELIAL POLYPS After cancer, benign epithelial polyps are the most common tumors of the stomach (5 to 10 percent). There is considerable confusion regarding the nomenclature of these epithelial polyps. What is important to remember is that 80 to 90 percent of them are not neoplastic, and probably never become malignant. The most common nonneoplastic polyp is called *hyperplastic;* it is composed almost completely of normal surface mucous cells, and at times of mucus-secreting pyloric glands. The glands are intermingled with smooth-muscle fibers and may be cystic. Greater than 90 percent of such polyps are less than 1.5 cm in diameter and do not enlarge with the passage of time. They may be single or multiple or pedunculated or sessile and can occur in any part of the stomach. They are covered with normal-appearing mucosa and frequently have a superficial ulceration on their tip. The mucosa surrounding them often shows nonerosive gastritis or atrophy. Although hyperplastic polyps almost never become malignant, carcinoma in other parts of the same stomach may occur, but less frequently than with adenoma.

Ten to twenty percent of benign epithelial polyps are composed of neoplastic epithelium and are called *adenomas.* In general they resemble adenomatous polyps of the colon. They are usually larger than 2 cm in diameter and do enlarge with the passage of time. As many as 40 percent of all adenomatous gastric polyps are already malignant when first diagnosed and the rest may become malignant. They can be pedunculated but are more often sessile and are solitary in two-thirds of cases. They are covered with abnormal reddened velvety mucosa which may be lobulated or mammillated. Most are located in the antrum. The mucosa surrounding them is usually atrophic, and carcinoma elsewhere in the stomach is common (30 percent or more in various series).

Both hyperplastic and adenomatous polyps occur more frequently in patients over 50 years of age, and 80 percent or more of these patients are achlorhydric. From 6 to 20 percent of patients with pernicious anemia have epithelial polyps. Occult bleeding is the most important clinical manifestation and at times is associated with vague epigastric distress. Rarely, vomiting results from prolapse of a large, pedunculated antral polyp into the duodenum. Radiologically, the polyps appear as smooth, rounded, or lobulated filling defects, with or without a stalk. Although those greater than 2 cm in diameter are more likely to be adenomas or polypoid carcinomas, exceptions are not uncommon.

Hyperplastic polyps may have a different gross appearance from adenomas at endoscopy, but one cannot differentiate between the two with certainty even after sampling them by forceps biopsy. To determine the histologic nature of a polyp and to exclude malignancy, the whole lesion is best examined. Most pedunculated or small sessile polyps can be removed with an electrocautery snare during gastroscopy by an experienced endoscopist. It may be dangerous to attempt endoscopic removal of larger sessile polyps or those with a broad pedicle. Such lesions can be biopsied endoscopically by removing a sizable superficial portion of the polyp with a coagulating cautery snare, or the diagnosis can be established by surgical excision. Once the histological diagnosis of adenoma has been made, excision is the appropriate treatment. Because of the high risk of cancer in the surrounding mucosa, such patients must be followed regularly with endoscopic and cytologic examinations. Partial or even total gastrectomy may eventually be needed.

Rare hamartomatous gastric polyps are made up of the various benign epithelial cells normally present in the gastric mucosa. They are usually part of two familial polyposis syndromes: Peutz-Jeghers and juvenile polyposis. Twenty-five percent of Peutz-Jeghers cases involve the stomach or duodenum and 2 to 3 percent develop gastric or duodenal carcinoma. Malignant change in gastric juvenile polyposis is either very rare or absent. Cronkhite-Canada syndrome is a rare cause of benign gastric retention polyps composed of dilated cystic glands with markedly edematous stroma.

Diffuse gastric polyposis is a rare and poorly defined condition in which the gastric mucosa is covered with numerous sessile or pedunculated epithelial polyps. Multiple gastric polyps are usually proved to be hyperplastic by snare excision. Such patients should be followed by regular endoscopic and cytologic examinations because of the higher frequency of cancer in the surrounding mucosa. Multiple gastric adenomas are very rare. They may be seen in familial polyposis or Gardner's syndrome. Because of the high risk of cancer they may require partial or even total gastrectomy.

LEIOMYOMAS AND RARE BENIGN TUMORS Most leiomyomas are tiny and of no clinical significance. Larger ones, usually 3 cm or more in diameter, may cause massive or occult bleeding or epigastric pain. The x-ray appearance is that of a smooth, rounded, sessile filling defect, often with a central ulcer. The gastroscopic appearance is highly suggestive but not diagnostic. Mucosal biopsies are usually too superficial for diagnosis, but brush cytology of the ulcerated area may help rule out leiomyosarcoma. Small symptomatic lesions may be treated by local surgical excision, and larger ones by partial gastrectomy. Other rare benign gastric tumors include lipomas, schwannomas, leiomyoblastomas, hemangiomas, lymphangiomas, adenomyomas, and fibromas.

PSEUDOTUMORS A number of gastric conditions other than peptic ulcer simulate neoplasms by x-ray. These include hypertrophic pyloric stenosis; antral gastritis; inflammatory polyps; Ménétrier's disease and other gastric hyperplasias; pseudolymphoma; heterotopic pancreas; gastric eosinophilic granuloma; Crohn's disease; gastric varices; hematoma; deformity after fundoplication (Nissen repair); extrinsic pressure by the liver, pancreas, or spleen; and bezoars or retained food. Often endoscopic evaluation and consideration of the total clinical picture solve these problems, but in rare cases surgical exploration is necessary to exclude malignancy.

GASTRITIS

EROSIVE GASTRITIS Erosive gastritis (also known as hemorrhagic gastritis or multiple gastric erosions) is a frequent cause of upper gastrointestinal bleeding, but it is rarely severe. Erosions may be completely asymptomatic. By endoscopy, multiple bleeding erosions are distributed diffusely throughout the gastric mucosa or are localized to the fundus, body, or antrum. The intervening mucosa may appear reddened and friable, or it may appear normal.

Histologically, the mucosal destruction by erosions does not extend below the muscularis mucosae; characteristically, the mucosal lesions heal completely. At any one time, different erosions can be observed in various stages of evolution and regression. Erosions may occur in flat mucosa or on the crests of small mucosal mounds. Between erosions there may be areas of surface epithelium depleted of mucus and focal or diffuse extravasation of blood into the lamina propria. Erosions may develop in mucosa that is histologically normal or that shows changes of any type of gastritis. If the process persists, erosions may deepen and extend below the muscularis mucosae into the submucosa to form acute ulcers (Chap. 306); then bleeding may become severe.

Erosive gastritis can occur for no apparent reason. Many cases, however, are associated with aspirin ingestion. The low pK_a of aspirin facilitates its gastric absorption in the acid milieu of the gastric lumen because it is un-ionized and liposoluble at a low pH and is therefore absorbed readily by passive nonionic diffusion. At the neutral intracellular pH of the gastric surface epithelium aspirin becomes an ionized acid which can destroy the cells and provide an entry point for acid-peptic digestion. When aspirin is given with sodium bicarbonate or an enteric coating, it may not be injurious because it cannot be absorbed by the gastric mucosa in its ionized form. Acute alcoholism and ingestion of certain anti-inflammatory prostaglandin inhibitors such as phenylbutazone or indomethacin may also be associated with erosive gastritis. Chronic blood loss from erosions or gastric ulcers may occur in patients who regularly take large doses of aspirin or other nonsteroid anti-inflammatory drugs. Portal hypertension also may predispose to erosive gastritis.

Severe stress secondary to burns, sepsis, trauma, surgery, shock, or respiratory, renal, or liver failure often causes gastric erosions or acute ulcers. Their pathogenesis is poorly understood and probably varies with different predisposing conditions. There are data suggesting that alterations in mucosal blood flow lead to areas of microinfarction with further evolution of the lesion dependent upon acid-peptic digestion. Now that hyperalimentation and a strict antacid regimen are regularly used in severely stressed patients, erosions infrequently progress to ulcers with resultant severe hemorrhage or even perforation.

Patients present with hematemesis and/or melena. Many have no other symptoms, but some notice mild epigastric discomfort or nausea. The diagnosis is best made by gastroscopy on the same day as the bleeding episode, because otherwise the lesions may have healed and disappeared. Standard x-ray examination is of no help because the lesions are too superficial to change the barium silhouette. They may, however, be demonstrated by double-contrast studies. Many clinical diagnoses of erosive gastritis are made in patients with upper gastrointestinal bleeding and negative x-rays. Unfortunately, such presumptive diagnoses can be wrong. Erosive gastritis is best diagnosed by early gastroscopy.

The usual measures for restoring circulating blood volume should be undertaken promptly (Chap. 40). Not uncommonly, the bleeding has stopped by the time a tube is passed. If not, lavage of the stomach with iced isotonic saline through a large-diameter Ewald tube is traditional, but its efficacy is unproved in this spontaneously remitting illness. In any event, such lavage may facilitate diagnostic gastroscopy by washing out the stomach. Gravity drainage, *not suction*, should be used for emptying the iced saline from the stomach, lest suction artifacts be produced which are indistinguishable from acute erosions endoscopically.

If bleeding stops, a regimen of hourly antacids and cimetidine is instituted. If bleeding continues, or if rebleeding fails to respond to iced saline lavage, an attempt at control by selective infusion of Pitressin into the left gastric artery may stop the bleeding. In the rare case in which bleeding continues and is life-threatening, the erosions have usually progressed to deeper acute ulcers and emergency operation is necessary. Antrectomy with vagotomy appears to be the most effective surgical treatment but is not always successful. Very rarely persistent severe bleeding requires total gastrectomy.

NONEROSIVE GASTRITIS This is a histologic diagnosis and not a clinically recognizable entity because it probably does not cause symptoms. In fact, histologic evidence of gastritis is frequent in asymptomatic individuals, especially as they get older. Thus, the assumption that most nonulcer dyspepsia is caused by gastritis is unjustified. The diagnosis of gastritis can be made with certainty only by biopsy. There are two main types: fundal gland gastritis and pyloric gland gastritis (antral gastritis). In many persons, however, both gastric areas are involved, often in a patchy manner.

Nonerosive fundal gland gastritis This condition diffusely affects the mucosa of the body and fundus but may spare the antrum. There are three pathologic patterns: superficial gastritis, atrophic gastritis, and gastric atrophy. In addition, there may be metaplasia to the mucous cells of the pyloric glands, or to the goblet and absorptive cells of the intestine. In superficial gastritis, acute and chronic inflammation and epithelial abnormalities are confined to the superficial nonglandular mucosa. In atrophic gastritis there is partial loss of fundal glands and more chronic inflammation manifested by an increased number of lymphocytes and plasma cells within the lamina propria. To varying degrees the chief and parietal cells of the fundal glands may be replaced by intestinal or mucous cells. In gastric atrophy, the fundal glands have mostly disappeared and are almost completely replaced by mucous or intestinal cells, the mucosa is often thinned, and there is usually no histologic evidence of inflammation. Severe fundal gland atrophy is invariably present in Addisonian pernicious anemia. The relationship, if any, between the three types of nonerosive fundal gastritis is uncertain, although some biopsy studies suggest that the superficial type sometimes progresses to atrophic gastritis and atrophy.

Nonerosive fundal gland gastritis is a very common histologic finding in the general population, particularly in older age groups. The atrophic type is especially common in patients with thyroid disease or idiopathic iron-deficiency anemia and in relatives of patients with pernicious anemia. Nonerosive fundal gland gastritis does not have a characteristic gross appearance by barium x-ray or gastroscopy unless there is severe mucosal atrophy; then, the fold pattern may be flattened in the fundus and body by x-ray, and pallor, absent folds, and submucosal vessels may be seen by gastroscopy.

Patients with superficial fundal gland gastritis usually have normal or slightly reduced acid secretion. Those with atrophic fundal gastritis are hypochlorhydric, and those with fundal atrophy are achlorhydric. In pernicious anemia the parietal cells which secrete intrinsic factor are virtually absent, and as a result food vitamin B_{12} is not absorbed. Serum gastrin levels are high in patients with pernicious anemia and in some patients with severe atrophic fundal gastritis because the uninvolved antrum secretes gastrin continuously in the absence of acid to inhibit it. Antibodies to parietal cells are present in the serum of about 60 percent of persons with atrophic gastritis and 80 to 90 percent of those with pernicious anemia. Antibodies to intrinsic factor are present in the serum or gastric juice of most patients with pernicious anemia but are not found in patients with superficial or atrophic gastritis. The relationship between these immunologic phenomena and the gastric mucosal atrophy of pernicious anemia is uncertain.

Ordinarily, superficial or atrophic fundal gastritis requires no treatment. After adequate investigation has excluded other disease, those patients who have abdominal distress should be reassured. It is essential to rule out vitamin B_{12} malabsorption in persons who are found to be achlorhydric. If pernicious anemia is proved, it is treated as discussed in Chap. 327. The iron-deficiency anemia which may be associated with atrophic gastritis responds to medicinal iron.

Although severe atrophic gastritis and especially gastric fundal atrophy predispose to gastric cancer, diagnostic screening of patients so affected has not been productive. It is prudent nonetheless to investigate thoroughly unexplained abdominal symptoms in such patients.

Nonerosive pyloric gland gastritis So-called antral or pyloric gland gastritis is common in asymptomatic persons. It too has superficial and atrophic patterns. With age, this type of gastritis probably tends to extend proximally and replaces some fundal glands. It appears to be more common in alcoholics. Patients with benign gastric ulcer almost invariably have pyloric gland gastritis surrounding much of the ulcer. In aspirin-related gastric ulcers, the rim may be free of gastritis. If the peptic ulcer is located in the upper stomach, pyloric gland gastritis may extend far proximally. Gastric cancer is often associated with pyloric and fundal gland gastritis, as well as metaplasia to the intestinal type of glands. Acid secretion may be normal or low, depending upon the extent of fundal gland involvement. In pyloric gland gastritis, unlike fundal gastritis, serum gastrin levels tend to be low, and antibodies to gastrin-producing cells are present, rather than antibodies to parietal cells. It has been postulated that regurgitation of duodenal contents, particularly bile salts, into the stomach causes pyloric gland gastritis.

In most cases, pyloric gland gastritis does not cause symptoms and does not require treatment. Occasionally, it is associated with narrowing of the antrum suggestive of malignancy on x-ray examination; often such patients complain of ulcer-like pain and may indeed prove to have ulcers subsequently. At gastroscopy, normal antral motility suggests pliability, and malignancy can usually be excluded. The symptoms often respond to antacids.

GASTRIC HYPERPLASIA ("HYPERTROPHIC" GASTRITIS) Hypertrophic gastritis is a histologic misnomer. The individual mucosal epithelial cells are not enlarged (hypertrophic), but there are more of them (hyperplasia), and thus the mucosa is thickened. There are three causes for gastric mucosal hyperplasia: Ménétrier's disease, hypersecretory gastropathy, and Zollinger-Ellison syndrome (gastrinoma; see Chap. 306). Most hyperplastic mucosal conditions produce enlarged gastric folds which are often indistinguishable by x-ray or endoscopy from infiltrative cancer, lymphoma, or a functional abnormality.

Ménétrier's disease This is an uncommon type of gastric mucosal hyperplasia of unknown cause. It is characterized grossly by tortuous enlargement of the gastric mucosal folds resembling cerebral convolutions, and histologically by a thickened mucosa with hyperplasia of mucous cells and loss of most parietal and chief cells. The gastric pits are markedly elongated and tortuous and often exhibit cystic dilatation; these cysts may penetrate through the muscularis mucosae into the submucosa. The lamina propria often contains increased numbers of lymphocytes. Intestinal metaplasia may be present. The mucosal involvement may be localized or diffuse, and tends to be most prominent on the greater curvature.

Epigastric pain is the most common complaint. Anorexia, nausea, vomiting, weight loss, or diarrhea are other symptoms. Bleeding is not uncommon because of superficial erosions. Some patients develop a gastric ulcer. Carcinoma may develop rarely. Loss of protein through the mucosa often causes hypoalbuminemia, and sometimes edema. The gastric juice contains little or no hydrochloric acid and often excessive mucus. X-ray studies show very large folds and sometimes hypomotility. Ménétrier's disease is difficult to differentiate radiologically from the heavy folds of cancer, lymphoma, Zollinger-Ellison syndrome, or from a functional variation seen in normal persons. The diagnosis can usually be made from clinical, radiologic, and laboratory data supplemented by gastroscopy, preferably using one of the newer, larger biopsy forceps to get the deeper biopsy needed for diagnosis, and brush cytology to rule out cancer. Occasionally, laparotomy with full-thickness biopsy of the stomach is necessary to establish the diagnosis and to exclude malignancy.

There is no specific treatment, but frequent small meals may give some symptomatic relief. Those with gastric ulcers should receive antacids or cimetidine. A high-protein diet should be given to patients with hypoalbuminemia, but intravenous human albumin may be necessary for those with severe edema. Treatment with anticholinergic drugs or cimetidine may reduce protein loss. Partial gastrectomy may be helpful for intractable symptoms if the disease is sufficiently well localized. Rarely, total gastrectomy may be necessary. This gesture of desperation should be deferred as long as possible because spontaneous improvement or complete reversal of chronic disease is well documented in some individuals.

Hypersecretory gastropathy This is a far more common cause of gastric mucosal hyperplasia than Ménétrier's disease or gastrinoma. There is some question whether it is really a separate entity. The majority of these patients probably represent the upper end of the spectrum of increased fundal gland mass seen in patients with duodenal ulcer. Patients with this syndrome differ from those with classic Ménétrier's disease because they secrete gastric acid normally or excessively, but not at the high rate seen in gastrinoma; furthermore, their blood gastrin levels are normal. Grossly, the gastric mucosa is indistinguishable from that found in Ménétrier's disease, but histologically it shows lengthened fundal glands composed of increased numbers of parietal and chief cells. Ulcer symptoms may improve after antacids or cimetidine, but some patients may require surgery. Substantial loss of protein through the mucosa occurs only rarely; when present, it may be difficult to control unless the disease remits spontaneously.

Gastrinoma (Zollinger-Ellison syndrome) This is a fundal gland hyperplasia caused by excessive gastrin secretion by a gastrinoma, usually located in the pancreas. The pathogenesis, clinical features, and treatment are described in the previous chapter on peptic ulcer.

POSTGASTRECTOMY GASTRITIS After partial gastrectomy, gastritis often develops in the gastric remnant, especially if the stomach has been connected to the jejunum as in a Billroth II operation. Inflammation is usually accompanied by loss of parietal and chief cells, resulting in hypochlorhydria or achlorhydria, which protects against recurrent ulceration. Occasionally, secretion of intrinsic factor is insufficient for adequate vitamin B_{12} absorption. The pathogenesis of the gastritis is not well understood, but it is probably caused by reflux of bile and pancreatic juice through the large stoma and by loss of the trophic effect of gastrin secondary to antrectomy.

Usually, the histologic evidence of gastritis is not associated with symptoms. Occasionally, severe inflammation, especially near the stoma, is associated with epigastric pain, which may be aggravated by eating. Bilious vomiting and symptoms of regurgitant esophagitis may also be present. Similar symptoms occasionally occur after vagotomy and pyloroplasty, even though gastritis is usually less severe. Gastroscopy often shows a red, edematous mucosa, a finding which appears to correlate better with symptoms than does histologic evidence of gastritis. Precise data regarding the diagnosis of symptomatic postgastrectomy gastritis remain scarce.

Asymptomatic patients require no treatment but should be observed for evidence of iron deficiency, which is common, and for vitamin B_{12} deficiency, which is uncommon. Some symptomatic patients respond to six small meals daily and, strangely enough, to the frequent use of antacids. The head of the bed should be raised if there is any suggestion of esophageal reflux. Attempts to bind the presumably irritating bile salts with cholestyramine have been disappointing. Surgical diversion of bile from the stoma by a Roux en Y loop may relieve severe symptoms unresponsive to medical management, but it is impossible to predict which patients will respond favorably to surgical treatment.

Alarming reports from Europe of frequent precancerous dysplasia and carcinoma within the residual gastric mucosa 10 to 20 years after Billroth II gastrectomy raise the question of the desirability of endoscopy with biopsy and cytology at regular intervals in all such patients. Postoperative carcinoma is probably less frequent in North America, but this impression remains to be confirmed by careful study.

CORROSIVE GASTRITIS The accidental or suicidal ingestion of strong alkali, such as lye, or of acids, such as hydrochloric or carbolic, can cause necrosis of the gastric wall, particularly in the prepyloric region. Alkali usually injures the esophagus more severely than the stomach, whereas the reverse tends to occur with acid. The degree of gastric injury varies with the quantity and concentration of irritant ingested and the amount of food present in the stomach. Patients complain of burning of the mouth, throat, and retrosternal area. With gastric injury, there is severe epigastric pain, often with vomiting. Perforation, peritonitis, or massive hemorrhage may occur shortly after corrosive ingestion, or may be delayed. Later, scarring may cause esophageal or pyloric stenosis.

If the patient is seen shortly after ingesting a corrosive, the stomach should be gently emptied via a small, soft rubber tube. Orange juice or dilute vinegar can be given for alkali and antacids for acid. Intravenous therapy, sedation, analgesia, supportive measures, and careful observation are instituted. Corticosteroids may be helpful if edema threatens the airway, and antibiotics may help treat aspiration pneumonia. If perforation or peritonitis is suspected, laparotomy should be performed, and a partial gastrectomy done if full-thickness injury to the wall is found. Surgical treatment may be necessary also for acute massive bleeding or for late obstruction caused by scarring.

PHLEGMONOUS GASTRITIS This rare condition should be considered when a patient presents with acute upper abdominal pain, signs of peritonitis, fever, purulent ascitic fluid, nausea or vomiting, and a normal serum amylase. It is a bacterial infection of the gastric wall, most often caused by streptococci, although staphylococci, pneumococci, *Escherichia coli,* or gas-forming bacteria can be responsible. Alcoholism, upper-respiratory or other infection, peptic ulcer, and gastric surgery are predisposing conditions. Vigorous antibiotic therapy including penicillin should be followed immediately by laparotomy which is both diagnostic and therapeutic. Depending upon the operative findings, drainage or partial gastrectomy should be performed. Without surgery the mortality is nearly 100 percent; with surgery it is approximately 20 percent.

OTHER GASTRIC DISEASES

ACUTE GASTRIC DILATATION This is an uncommon but serious condition. The use of nasogastric suction has greatly reduced its frequency in the postoperative period. Gastric dilatation may also occur after trauma, the use of body casts, pneumonia, diabetic acidosis, or large doses of anticholinergic drugs. It is a rare complication of many diseases and also may occur for no apparent reason. The patient complains of anorexia and epigastric fullness and often vomits small amounts of fluid. Increasing abdominal distention with tympany, especially in the left hypochondrium, and a succussion splash are demonstrable. Untreated, large volumes of fluid are sequestered in a gastric "third space" with resultant saline and potassium depletion. The patient becomes restless and listless; hypovolemia, tachycardia, reduced urine output, and, finally, shock develop. Aspiration pneumonia may occur. A plain x-ray film of the abdomen shows massive gastric distention with an air-fluid level. Continuous nasogastric suction and restoration of fluid and electrolyte balance result in rapid improvement.

ADULT HYPERTROPHIC PYLORIC STENOSIS In this uncommon condition, the pyloric muscle is enlarged because of hypertrophy and possibly hyperplasia of the fibers of the circular layer. Many cases are associated with a peptic ulcer near the pylorus. In others, the pyloric muscle hypertrophy has been attributed to associated antral gastritis or neoplasm. A minority of cases without other gastric disease may be due to unrecognized infantile hypertrophic pyloric stenosis. Most often symptoms of pyloric obstruction such as nausea, vomiting, and gastric retention develop in mid-adult life, although occasionally mild symptoms are lifelong. An epigastric mass is not palpable in adults as it is in infants. Barium x-ray studies show a long, narrowed pyloric canal, often with triangular outpouchings within the canal. Gastroscopy shows a narrowed pylorus that is fixed in the open position. Although the diagnosis often appears highly likely from the above studies, an infiltrating cancer often cannot be excluded without operation. A limited gastric resection is said to give better symptomatic relief than a pyloromyotomy, and in addition provides an exact histologic diagnosis. The frequently associated juxtapyloric ulcers merit vagotomy.

MALLORY-WEISS SYNDROME A longitudinal laceration in the cardioesophageal region is the cause of about 5 to 10 percent of massive episodes of upper gastrointestinal bleeding. About 60 percent of tears are located just below the gastroesophageal junction; the remainder involve the cardioesophageal junction and least frequently the esophagus alone. The tear is often related to retching, although other causes of increased abdominal pressure have been implicated. These include severe coughing, straining, convulsions, trauma, and childbirth. Often the patients are alcoholic. Many have a hiatus hernia. A history of vomiting normal gastric contents followed by hematemesis or melena suggests the diagnosis. Not uncommonly, however, the history is not helpful. The diagnosis is best made by endoscopy. If endoscopic visualization is inadequate, then the site of bleeding can often be determined by arteriography. Barium x-ray examination is almost always negative. The initial treatment is supportive and expectant. Most often the bleeding stops spontaneously. If it stops, it rarely recurs. If bleeding continues, selective arteriography with infusion of pitressin can be tried. In a minority of cases, persistent bleeding requires that the laceration be sutured through a gastrotomy. Treatment of perforation complicating an esophageal tear is discussed in Chap. 305.

BEZOARS AND FOREIGN BODIES Conglomerates of food and mucus or phytobezoars composed of vegetable matter sometimes form in the gastric remnant after partial gastrectomy, especially if a vagotomy was also performed. They occur less often after vagotomy and pyloroplasty. Autonomic neuropathy associated with diabetes mellitus is another predisposing condition. Rarely yeast bezoars have been found. Patients complain of anorexia, epigastric fullness, nausea, or vomiting. The diagnosis is often apparent from the barium x-ray examination, but endoscopy may be needed to distinguish the food mass from a neoplasm. The food conglomerate or bezoar can often be removed by vigorous and repeated gastric lavage. Fragmenting the lesion at gastroscopy may facilitate removal by lavage. Some phytobezoars can be partially digested with cellulase and then broken up successfully by lavage. Occasionally surgical removal is necessary. If the mass passes into the small bowel, it can cause obstruction requiring surgery. Treatment with metoclopramide and a low-fiber diet may be tried to prevent recurrence.

Bezoars in the intact stomach are rare. Phytobezoars are most common, a well-known type being the persimmon ball. Trichobezoars are composed of hair. Concretions of inorganic substances such as shellac, asphalt, or calcium carbonate are occasionally seen. Bezoars of the intact stomach often require surgical removal, although nonoperative methods may be successful for phytobezoars. Persimmon balls have responded to treatment with papain and sodium bicarbonate.

Small foreign bodies such as coins, marbles, or even closed safety pins usually pass through the stomach and bowel without difficulty. Elongated, sharp objects such as needles, toothpicks, or open safety pins may hold up at some point and cause obstruction, ulceration, bleeding, abscess, or peritonitis. Occasionally, large objects such as forks or knives are swallowed by emotionally disturbed persons. Patients who have swallowed dangerous objects should be promptly referred to an experienced endoscopist who may elect endoscopic removal, observation, or surgical treatment, depending on the circumstances.

GASTRIC DIVERTICULA These uncommon lesions usually occur just below the cardia on the posterior wall near the lesser curvature. Almost all are asymptomatic and require no treatment. Pain, bleeding, or perforation is a very rare complication. Surgery should not be undertaken except for severe intractable symptoms that cannot be attributed to another cause. The x-ray appearance is usually diagnostic, but occasionally gastroscopy is needed to distinguish the lesion from a peptic ulcer.

GASTRIC VOLVULUS OR TORSION Rarely the stomach can twist about its longitudinal axis, thus turning itself upside down and obstructing the lower esophagus. The volvulus may be acute or more often chronic. It tends to be associated with a paraesophageal hernia or eventration of the diaphragm. The stomach can also twist about the vertical axis of the gastrohepatic omentum to produce a torsion rather than a true volvulus. Acute volvulus is associated with severe upper abdominal pain and retching which produces saliva rather than gastric or duodenal contents. Passage of a nasogastric tube beyond the cardia is usually impossible. Plain x-ray films of the abdomen show distention of the stomach; the finding of two separate fluid levels is diagnostic. Acute volvulus may be of short duration and subside spontaneously or may be associated with strangulation and require emergency surgical treatment. Those with chronic volvulus may be asymptomatic or have intermittent pain, often associated with eating. Severe symptoms may require surgical correction of the volvulus, including repair of an associated paraesophageal hernia, if present.

RARE GASTRIC DISEASES Pseudolymphoma This benign lymphoid hyperplasia may involve the stomach. Grossly the lesion is usually single and ulcerated. Some lesions are nodular; others may present as enlarged folds. Multiple tumor nodules seen with true lymphoma are not found. There is a marked lymphocytic infiltration of the gastric wall. The lesion is distinguished from true lymphoma by the maturity of the germinal centers and by the presence of inflammatory cells other than lymphocytes. The x-ray and endoscopic findings usually suggest malignancy or peptic ulcer. Partial gastrectomy is usually required for diagnosis and treatment.

Eosinophilic gastroenteritis The antrum may be involved in this condition which is usually associated with marked peripheral eosinophilic leukocytosis. The diagnosis can be made by mucosal biopsy, and chronic treatment with small doses of corticosteroids is usually effective.

Eosinophilic granuloma This is usually a circumscribed lesion of the antrum and is not associated with peripheral eosinophilic leukocytosis. It does not respond to corticosteroid treatment and may require excision because of pyloric obstruction or other symptoms.

Other specific gastritides Tuberculosis and tertiary syphilis rarely affect the stomach. The diagnosis can sometimes be made from the clinical picture and endoscopic biopsy, but more often operation is needed to exclude malignancy. Appropriate antibiotic therapy is effective. Other rare gastric infections include CMV, herpes simplex, candidiasis, and histoplasmosis. Crohn's disease may involve the stomach and produce epithelioid granulomas indistinguishable from sarcoid. Unlike Crohn's, with its predilection for the small and large bowel, gastrointestinal sarcoid involves mostly the stomach.

REFERENCES

DUPONT JB et al: Adenocarcinoma of the stomach: Review of 1497 cases. Cancer 41:941, 1978

GREEN PHR et al: Early gastric cancer. Gastroenterology 81:247, 1981

HERMAN R et al: Gastrointestinal involvement in nonHodgkin's lymphoma. Cancer 46:215, 1980

IMAI T et al: Chronic gastritis in Japanese with reference to high incidence of gastric carcinoma. J Natl Cancer Inst 47:179, 1971

KREUNING J et al: Gastric and duodenal mucosa in "healthy" individuals, an endoscopic and histopathological study of 50 volunteers. J Clin Pathol 31:69, 1978

LAURÉN P: The two histologic main types of gastric carcinoma: Diffuse and so-called intestinal carcinoma. Acta Pathol Microbiol Scand 64:31, 1965

MACDONALD JS et al: 5-Fluorouracil, doxorubicin and mitomycin (FAM) combination chemotherapy for advanced gastric cancer. Ann Intern Med 92:533, 1980

MING S: Tumors of the esophagus and stomach, in *Atlas of Tumor Pathology*, 2d ser. Washington, DC, Armed Forces Institute of Pathology, 1971, fasc 7

SCHRUMPF E et al: Mucosal changes in the gastric stump 20–25 years after partial gastrectomy. Lancet 2:467, 1977

308 DISORDERS OF ABSORPTION

NORTON J. GREENBERGER
KURT J. ISSELBACHER

MECHANISMS OF ABSORPTION

Diseases of the small intestine are frequently accompanied by alterations in intestinal function, and clinically this impaired function is seen as the malabsorption syndrome. In order to obtain a better appreciation of the derangements which occur in the many disorders of intestinal function, the processes of normal absorption will first be reviewed.

It is important to distinguish between digestion and absorption, since an increased loss of nutrients in the stool may be a reflection of a derangement of either process. Digestion involves the breakdown or hydrolysis of nutrients to smaller molecules in order to prepare the ingested substances for absorption, or transport across the intestinal cell. It will be recalled that most of the digestive process is initiated in the stomach by acid and pepsin and is continued in the upper small intestine primarily by the action of pancreatic enzymes such as lipase, amylase, and trypsin. As a result of these digestive actions carbohydrates are broken down to monosaccharides and disaccharides, proteins to peptides and amino acids, and fats to monoglycerides and fatty acids. In the adult it is in this form that nutrients are, to a large extent, transported across the epithelial surface of the intestinal cell.

ANATOMIC AND PHYSIOLOGIC FACTORS The intestine has an enormous surface area. This can be attributed in large part to its length, which in the adult is more than 12 ft, and to the foldings of the surface plicae. At the light microscopic level, the villi of the small intestine provide additional surface area, which is further augmented by the presence of microvilli (approximately 2×10^8 per square centimeter) on the outer, or brush border, region of epithelial cells. Thus the total absorptive area of the small intestine is enormous.

Motility (contractility) of the bowel is an important process which permits nutrients to remain in intimate contact with the intestinal cells and possibly influences the continued movement of the nutrients *into* and along the absorbing channels, such as the lymphatics. Two types of motility aid in this process: the gross motility of the intestine itself and the motility of individual villi. Entrance of the nutrients into the general circulation is achieved via the capillaries into the portal system or via the lacteals into the intestinal lymphatics.

TYPES OF ABSORPTION Four mechanisms have been considered to be important in the transport of substances across the intestinal cell membrane, namely, active transport, passive diffusion, facilitated diffusion, and endocytosis.

Active transport involves the transport of a substance across the cell against an electric or chemical gradient; this process requires energy, is carrier-mediated, and is subject to competitive inhibition. *Passive diffusion* is the opposite of this process; energy is not required, transport is with (rather than against) the electric or chemical gradient, the process is not carrier-mediated, and it does not show properties of competitive inhibition. Thus active transport may be viewed as "uphill" transport, whereas passive diffusion is equivalent to "downhill" transport. *Facilitated diffusion* is similar to passive diffusion except that such a process shows evidence of being carrier-mediated and frequently subject to competitive inhibition.

Endocytosis is a process akin to phagocytosis. By this mechanism nutrients (soluble or particulate) upon entering the cell are surrounded by the components of the outer plasma cell membrane. In the intestinal tract endocytosis occurs in the neonatal period and, contrary to earlier belief, also occurs to a limited extent in the adult organism. While quantitatively limited, it appears to account, for example, for uptake of antigens.

SITES OF ABSORPTION While many substances are absorbed throughout the length of the small intestine, certain nutrients tend to be absorbed more in one region than in other regions. The proximal intestine is a major area for the absorption of iron, calcium, water-soluble vitamins, and fat (monoglycerides and fatty acids). Sugars are absorbed in the proximal and also midintestine. While the amino acids appear to be absorbed primarily in the middle of the small intestine or jejunum, some absorption also occurs in the upper and lower areas. The distal small intestine appears to be the *major* absorptive area for bile salts and vitamin B_{12}. As is emphasized below, this factor is of clinical significance in circumstances where there has been removal or disease of the ileum.

The colon is important for the absorption of water and electrolytes, a process which occurs predominantly in the cecum. Although the rectum is not a usual site for absorption of ingested foodstuffs, drugs introduced by rectum may be absorbed there. Thus drugs introduced by this route, such as salicylates or steroids, may be absorbed systemically.

ABSORPTION OF SPECIFIC NUTRIENTS Carbohydrate absorption Much of the carbohydrate we ingest is in the form of starch, a complex polysaccharide consisting of many hexose units (attached either in a 1,4 or 1,6 linkage). By the action of salivary and pancreatic amylase, starch is hydrolyzed to oligosaccharides and then to dissacharides (mostly maltose). While monosaccharides such as glucose are readily absorbed, disaccharides are not. Disaccharides are split enzymatically into their component sugars by disaccharidases (or oligosaccharidases) located on or within the microvilli of intestinal epithelial cells. The two types of disaccharidases are β-galactosidases (lactase) and α-glucosidases (sucrase, maltase). By the action of these enzymes, lactose is split into glucose and galactose, sucrose into glucose and fructose, and maltose into two molecules of glucose. The resultant monosaccharides are then transported through the cell into the portal circulation. Most disaccharides are hydrolyzed so rapidly by brush border enzymes that the capacity of the transport mechanism is exceeded and some monosaccharides diffuse back into the intestinal lumen. Lactose, however, is hydrolyzed at a slower rate, and thus lactose hydrolysis is the rate-limiting step in lactose absorption.

Sugars such as glucose and galactose are absorbed by an active transport mechanism. The transport rate of sugars can be related to the substrate concentration by the expression K_t, where K_t stands for the monosaccharide substrate concentration that produces half the maximal transport rate. Published K_t values for glucose transport have varied widely, partly because of failure to consider the unstirred water layer, which constitutes a diffusion barrier for solutes.

Glucose (and galactose) entry into the cell is largely coupled to sodium ions (so-called symport); both sodium and glucose appear to bind to the hexose carrier in the microvillus membrane. Energy is required for the movement of glucose into the cell, which seems largely to come from the sodium pump and the Na^+-K^+-ATPase of the basolateral membrane (see below).

Protein and amino acid absorption Dietary proteins are initially subject to degradation in the stomach by pepsin. However, complete hydrolysis is largely achieved by the action of the pancreatic enzymes trypsin, chymotrypsin, and carboxypeptidase. By these enzymatic processes oligopeptides, dipeptides, and amino acids are formed. Just as there are disaccharidases in mucosal cells to digest disaccharides, there are also oligopeptidases to split small peptides. Dipeptidases are located in the cytoplasm as well as on the microvilli. Dipeptides are absorbed more rapidly than amino acids, and presumably their uptake involves a separate mechanism. As indicated above, contrary to earlier beliefs proteins can also be absorbed by the adult intestine. Although quantitatively limited, protein absorption probably is immunologically significant.

Most naturally occurring amino acids are L-amino acids, and these are subject to a number of different transport processes. *Neutral* amino acids seem to share a common carrier mechanism; thus amino acids such as tryptophan and alanine show competitive inhibition. Among the *dibasic* amino acids which appear to have a distinct transport mechanism are arginine, ornithine, and lysine. The neutral amino acid cystine shares this mechanism. There is also a separate transport system for *glycine* and the *imino acids* proline and hydroxyproline. There is also a transport system for *dicarboxylic* acids such as glutamic and aspartic acids. Therefore, in genetic disorders, such as cystinuria, one will find impaired absorption not only of cystine but also of arginine, ornithine, and lysine. Similarly in Hartnup disease, a defect in the transport of neutral amino acids (especially of tryptophan, phenylalanine, histidine) is found. In these genetic disorders uptake and absorption of dipeptides is normal.

The actual mechanism of the absorption of amino acids by the intestine has not been elucidated. As in the case of carbohydrates, sodium ions appear to be required for the entry of these acids and the energy needed for their concentration within the cell. Some amino acids have affinity for more than one mechanism. For example, glycine may be transported by both the neutral and imino acid transport systems.

Fat absorption (Fig. 308-1) Most of the ingested dietary fats are in the form of long-chain triglycerides. These triglycerides contain both saturated fatty acids (such as palmitic and stearic) and unsaturated fatty acids (such as oleic and linoleic). The particle size of the fat is decreased largely by the churning action of the stomach. The entry of fat into the duodenum plus the presence of acid causes release of secretin and pancreozymin-cholecystokinin, which in turn leads to a stimulation of the flow of bile and pancreatic juice.

ROLE OF PANCREATIC LIPASE The hydrolysis of triglycerides by pancreatic lipase is a complex process involving lipase, colipase, and bile salts. Pancreatic lipase is an enzyme that binds to the oil-water interface of an emulsified triglyceride substrate. The detergent properties of bile salts permit pancreatic lipase to gain access to water-insoluble lipids. One of the important functions of bile salts is to clear the oil-water interface of dietary fat from proteins of exogenous and endogenous origin, thus making it available for pancreatic lipolysis. Colipase, a protein present in pancreatic juice, is also essential for the action of lipase; its function is to anchor the lipase close to the surface of the triglyceride droplet. All three components, i.e., pancreatic lipase, colipase, and bile salts, form a *ternary complex*, which generates lipolytic products that diffuse away from the complex and are absorbed. With colipase present, lipase remains at the interface and forms 2-monoglycerides and fatty acids, which are the major end products of triglyceride hydrolysis. Less than 5 percent of ingested fat remains in the form of diglycerides and triglycerides. Without colipase, bile acids would actually wash pancreatic lipase away from the interface and its hydrolytic rate would be reduced.

ROLE OF BILE SALTS (Fig. 308-2) Bile salts play an important role in the digestion and absorption of fat. They are synthesized in the liver (approximately 200 to 600 mg daily) from cholesterol and excreted in the bile in the form of their glycine or taurine conjugates. In humans the principal bile acids excreted are conjugates of cholic and chenodeoxycholic acid. Bile salts are good detergents, because they have both polar (hydrophilic) and nonpolar (hydrophobic) groups. During digestion the concentration of conjugated bile salts in the lumen is in the range of 5 to 15 μmol/ml, and at these concentrations the bile salts aggregate to form *micelles.* Fatty acids and monoglycerides enter these micelles, forming mixed micelles. An emulsion of triglyceride is turbid; mixed micelles containing bile salts, fatty acids, and monoglycerides are clear solutions. The formation of *mixed micelles* and hence the solubilization of fatty acids and monoglycerides are much more effectively achieved with *conjugated bile salts* at the pH which normally exists in the intestinal lumen (Fig. 308-2).

Most conjugated bile salts are absorbed in the ileum and after entering the portal vein are subject to an enterohepatic circulation. By this process about 90 percent of the conjugated bile salts reaching the ileum are reabsorbed. As a consequence only about 200 to 600 mg bile salts is excreted in the feces per day, while, as part of the enterohepatic circulation, as much as 20 to 30 g bile salts recirculates daily between the liver and intestine. When the enterohepatic circulation is intact, the size of the bile salt pool is largely determined by the frequency of the enterohepatic circulation, i.e., the number of cycles per day (see also Chap. 323). If the ileum is diseased or removed, absorption of bile salts is impaired, and a significant fecal loss of bile salts will occur. As a consequence of this bile salt depletion, the concentration of bile salts in the intestinal lumen will also decrease, leading to further impairment of fat absorption. A similar result will occur if bile salt reabsorption is prevented by chelating agents, such as cholestyramine (see "Regional Enteritis" below).

INTRAMUCOSAL ASPECTS OF FAT ABSORPTION (Fig. 308-1) After the hydrolysis of fatty acids to monoglycerides and their interaction with bile salts to form mixed micelles, the lipids pass through an "unstirred" water layer covering the cell surface. The mixed micelles apparently do not enter the cell, but instead the component fatty acids and monoglycerides are released from the micellar phase and then enter the cell by diffusion. In aqueous duodenal contents, large bile salt mixed micelles saturated with products of lipolysis coexist with larger liquid crystal liposomes of the same lipids saturated with free fatty acids and mixed bile salts. These phases are interconvertible and both may be important in fat digestion and absorption. Upon entry into the mucosal cell, fatty acids may interact with specific binding proteins. The subsequent fate of the intracellular lipid is strongly influenced by the fatty acid chain length. Fatty acids and monoglycerides derived from long-chain triglycerides (i.e., containing C-16 to C-18 fatty acids) are promptly *reesterified to triglycerides* by enzymes of the endoplasmic reticulum. These triglycerides then interact with specific apolipoproteins plus cholesterol and phospholipid to form chylomicrons and very low density lipoproteins. These initially accumulate in the Golgi region of the cell and then are secreted into the lacteals and the intestinal lymph. There are thus four major steps in the absorption of long-chain fatty acids and monoglycerides: (1) mucosal uptake and interaction with binding proteins, (2) reesterification to triglycerides, (3) lipoprotein formation, and (4) secretion into lymph.

By contrast, fatty acids derived from medium-chain triglycerides (i.e., containing C-8 and C-12 fatty acids) are *not reesterified* to any significant extent within the cell and are not incorporated into lipoproteins. Instead, they rapidly enter the portal venous system, where they are transported as fatty acids bound to albumin. The major aspects of fat absorption are summarized in Fig. 308-1.

Absorption of cholesterol and fat-soluble vitamins (A, D, E, K) In addition to contributing significantly to the total-body synthesis of cholesterol, the intestine also plays an active role in the absorption of cholesterol and its esters. Within the lumen, cholesterol esters from the bile and diet are hydrolyzed by a pancreatic esterase. There is also a separate cholesterol esterase in the intestinal microvilli, which completes this hydrolysis. As a result only free cholesterol appears to enter the intestinal cell. However, just as in the case of long-chain fatty acids, much of the cholesterol is reesterified and is then secreted primarily into lymph.

The absorption mechanisms of the fat-soluble vitamins A, D, E, and K are not well understood. The intestine is able to convert β-carotene into vitamin A. The vitamin A thus formed or absorbed from the lumen is esterified in the mucosa primarily with palmitic acid, transported in the chylomicrons of the lymph, and stored as retinol palmitate in the liver. The other lipid-soluble vitamins also appear in lymph chylomicrons, but esterification with fatty acids does not appear to be necessary for their transport.

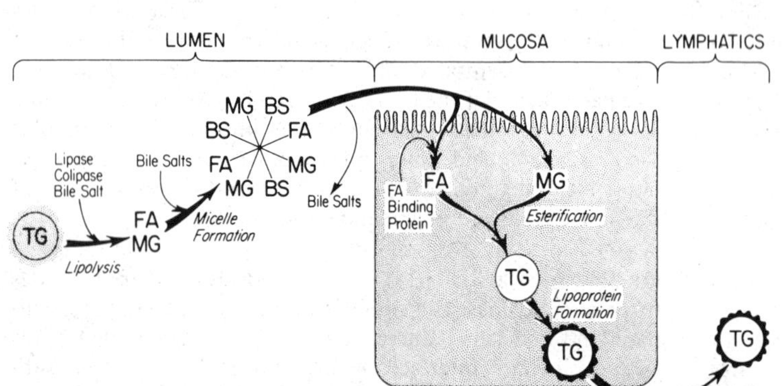

FIGURE 308-1
Scheme of intestinal digestion, absorption, esterification, and transport of dietary triglycerides. TG = triglycerides; FA = fatty acids; MG = monoglyceride; BS = bile salts.

Water and sodium absorption In spite of extensive investigations the main mechanisms of water and electrolyte transport are not well understood. There are two pathways by which water and ions cross the intestinal mucosa: the paracellular and transcellular pathways. Individual intestinal mucosa cells are joined near their apex by a "tight junction," and ions and water traverse this *paracellular* pathway during absorption and secretion. It is believed that the tight junction pathway contains aqueous-filled channels or pores. Such intercellular spaces are closed in the resting state and dilated during absorption. Considerable evidence has accumulated indicating that pumps and carriers are involved in intestinal water and solute transport. For example, the basolateral membrane contains a Na^+ pump which actively transports Na^+ out of the mucosal cell and into the intercellular space. *Transcellular* transport requires passage of ions through two membrane barriers, i.e., the apical plasma membrane and the basolateral membrane. After Na^+ and Cl^- are transported across the brush border membrane into the cell, Na^+ is pumped across the basolateral membrane and Cl^- either follows passively or is also pumped into the intercellular space. Since Na^+-K^+-ATPase is present in the basolateral but not in the brush border membrane, it could be the biochemical mediator of this pump. Bulk water movement obviously influences the movement of Na^+, K^+, and Cl^-. This "solvent drag" effect is explained by two mechanisms: (1) solutes may be caught in a moving stream of water and transported across a membrane, and (2) water movement results in increased concentration of solute on the side of the membrane from which water was transported, which causes solute to diffuse through the direction of flow. Diarrhea can be simply defined as impaired net absorption of water and electrolytes by the small intestine or colon. Some mechanisms producing diarrhea are listed in Table 308-1.

TABLE 308-1
Some mechanisms in the production of diarrhea

- *I* Secretory diarrhea
  - *A* Secretory agents associated with adenylate cyclase system
    - *1* Enterotoxin-producing bacteria *(Vibrio cholerae, Escherichia coli)*
    - *2* Methylxanthines (caffeine, theophylline)
    - *3* Prostaglandins
    - *4* Vasoactive intestinal peptide (VIP)
    - *5* Dihydroxy bile acids (affect colon primarily; effects seen after ileal resection)
  - *B* Secretory agents *not associated* with adenylate cyclase system
    - *1* Glucagon, secretin, cholecystokinin-pancreozymin, serotonin, calcitonin, gastrin inhibitory polypeptide (GIP)
    - *2* Some laxatives* (ricinoleic acid, bisacodyl, phenolphthalein, dioctyl sodium sulfosuccinate)
    - *3* Bacterial enterotoxins *(Shigella, Staphylococcus aureus, Clostridium perfringens)*
  - *C* Mucosal injury, altered cell permeability
    - *1* *Salmonella, Shigella,* invasive *E. coli,* gastroenteritis viruses
    - *2* Celiac sprue
    - *3* Inflammatory bowel disease (ulcerative colitis, regional enteritis)
  - *D* Neoplasms with or without hormone production
    - *1* Gastrinoma (gastrin)
    - *2* Carcinoid syndrome (serotonin, prostaglandins)
    - *3* Medullary carcinoma thyroid (calcitonin, prostaglandins)
    - *4* Pancreatic cholera syndrome (? VIP)
    - *5* Villous adenoma
- *II* Osmotic diarrhea
  - *A* Impaired carbohydrate absorption
    - *1* Disaccharidase deficiency (lactose or sucrose-isomaltose intolerance)
    - *2* Glucose-galactose malabsorption
  - *B* Laxative ingestion or abuse
    - *1* Nonabsorbable osmotically active agents (lactulose, sorbitol, mannitol)
    - *2* Saline purgatives (magnesium phosphate, magnesium hydroxide-containing antacids)
  - *C* Postsurgical
    - *1* Vagotomy and pyloroplasty*
    - *2* Gastrojejunostomy* (Billroth I and II)
- *III* Motility disorders
  - *A* Laxative abuse*
  - *B* Irritable bowel syndrome
  - *C* Diverticular disease of the colon
  - *D* Diabetic diarrhea with visceral neuropathy

* *Multiple mechanisms involved in production of diarrhea.*

Calcium absorption Calcium is actively transported by the small intestine, and this process is intimately linked to the active form of vitamin D_3, namely, 1,25-dihydroxycholecalciferol. The role of two other intestinal cell proteins, calcium-binding protein and calmodulin, in the absorption of calcium remains unclear.

Iron absorption The formation of soluble iron complexes is important for maintaining intraluminal iron in an absorbable form. Gastric acid facilitates the chelation of inorganic iron with substances such as ascorbic acid, sugars, amino acids, and bile; these macromolecular complexes then remain soluble in the more alkaline duodenum and jejunum. Iron intake with the average western diet averages 15 to 25 mg per day; iron absorption averages 0.5 to 1.0 mg per day in men and 1.0 to 2.0 mg per day in women during their reproductive years. A regulatory mechanism for the absorption of inorganic iron appears to exist within the small-intestinal mucosal cells. Iron is actively transported by the small intestine, and the duodenum is the principal site of iron absorption. The absorption of elemental iron in humans and animals involves at least two distinct

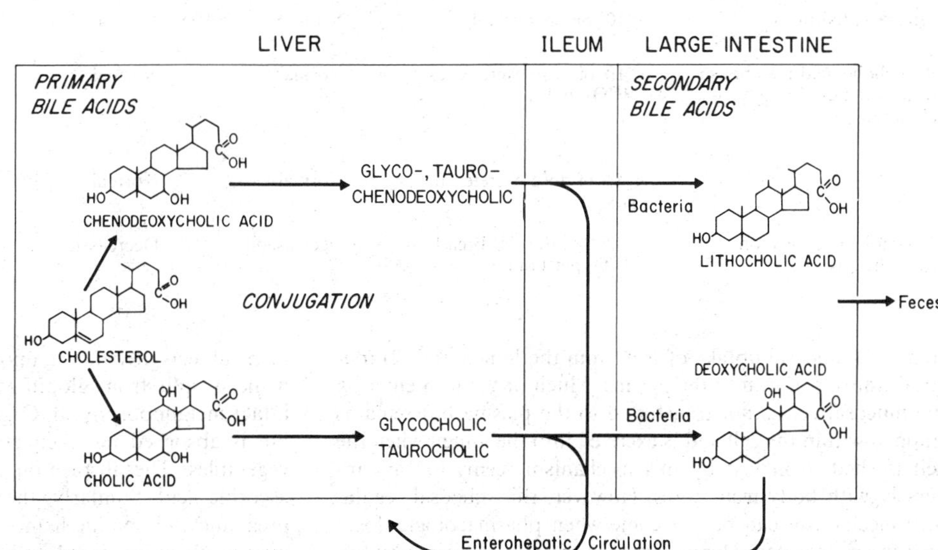

FIGURE 308-2
Scheme of hepatic and intestinal metabolism of bile salts and the enterohepatic circulation (from ileum to liver). Note that bacteria lead to the formation of secondary bile acids; of the latter, only deoxycholic acid is absorbed to any appreciable extent.

TABLE 308-2
Tests useful in the diagnosis of malabsorptive disorders

Test	*Normal values*	*Typical findings in:* *Malabsorption (nontropical sprue)*	*Maldigestion (pancreatic insufficiency)*	*Comment*
Quantitative determination of stool fat	<6 g/24 h; >95% coefficient of fat absorption	>6 g/24 h	>6 g/24 h	Best test for establishing presence of steatorrhea
D-Xylose absorption (25-g oral dose)	5-h urinary excretion >4.5 g; peak blood level >30 mg/dl	↓	Normal	A good screening test for carbohydrate absorption
Small-intestinal x-rays		Malabsorption pattern	Normal or minimal malabsorption pattern; occasionally pancreatic calcification	Moulage sign and other abnormalities may be present in several disorders (see text)
Small-intestinal mucosal biopsy		Abnormal	Normal	A specific diagnosis can be established in a small number of disorders (see text)
Schilling test for vitamin B_{12} absorption	>8% urinary excretion in 48 h	Frequently ↓	Frequently ↓	Useful in determining whether vitamin B_{12} malabsorption is due to gastric or small-intestinal disorders
Secretin test	Volume >1.8 (ml/kg)/h Bicarbonate concentration >80 meq/liter	Normal	Abnormal	See discussion of pancreatic insufficiency in Chaps. 324 and 325
Serum calcium	9–11 mg/dl	Frequently ↓	Usually normal	
Serum albumin	3.5–5.5 g/dl	Frequently ↓	Usually normal	Decreased levels of both serum albumin and globulins should raise the question of protein-losing enteropathy
Serum cholesterol	150–250 mg/dl	↓	Frequently ↓	Usually decreased in disorders associated with significant steatorrhea
Serum iron	80–150 μg/dl	Frequently ↓	Normal	Low values may reflect decreased body iron stores
Serum carotenes Serum vitamin A	>100 IU/dl >100 IU/dl	↓ ↓	Usually ↓	Fairly satisfactory screening tests for malabsorption
Prothrombin time	70–100%; 12–15 s	Frequently ↓	Frequently ↓	
Urine 5-hydroxyindoleacetic acid (5-HIAA)	2–9 mg/24 h	↑	Normal	Slightly increased level (12–16 mg/24 h) characteristically found in nontropical sprue
Breath H_2 (after 50 g lactose)	Minimal breath H_2	May be ↑	Normal	Secondary to lactase deficiency (see text)
Duodenal fluid analysis:				
Conjugated bile salts	> 2 mmol/ml	Normal	Normal	May be decreased with bacterial overgrowth, ileal resection, or ileal inflammatory disease
Unconjugated bile salts	Not present	Normal	Normal	Increased with bacterial overgrowth
Micellar lipid	>50% ingested lipid in micellar phase	Normal or decreased	Decreased	Decreased with a deficiency of conjugated bile salts or pancreatic lipase
Bacteria (culture)	$<10^3$ organisms/ml	Normal	Normal	$>10^5$ organisms/ml indicates bacterial overgrowth
Glycocholic acid metabolism (oral glycine-1-[^{14}C]glycocholate)	<1% of dose excreted as $^{14}CO_2$ in 4 h	Normal	Normal	Increased $^{14}CO_2$ excretion with bacterial overgrowth or bile acid malabsorption (due to ileal resection or inflammatory disease)
	<4% of dose excreted in stools	Normal	Normal	Increased fecal excretion of ^{14}C in bile acid malabsorption
[^{14}C]Triolein absorption (breath test)	>3.5% of dose as breath $^{14}CO_2$ per hour	Decreased	Decreased	Correlates well with chemical stool fat; recently introduced test

steps: (1) mucosal uptake of iron from the lumen and (2) mucosal transfer of iron to the plasma. Much of the iron entering the mucosal cell is not transferred to the plasma but remains trapped within the cell and is excreted into the lumen when the cell is shed. Iron lost by this mechanism seems to vary inversely with body iron stores. However, this mucosal regulatory mechanism can be overcome when pharmacologic doses of iron are ingested. Hemoglobin iron is also absorbed by human subjects, depending upon body requirements for iron; the heme is split from globin in the lumen and absorbed as an intact metalloporphyrin. Organic iron in the form of hemoglobin is absorbed more effectively than iron from cereals and vegetables. The absorption of inorganic iron is increased by ascorbic acid. Similarly, the presence of anemia, liver injury, pregnancy, idiopathic hemochromatosis, or a portacaval shunt may result in increased iron absorption. Conversely, the prior ingestion of large doses of iron and the presence in the lumen of phosphates, carbonates, and phytates may lead to decreased absorption of inorganic iron. Impaired absorption of iron is frequent in disorders (such as nontropical sprue) which involve the duodenal mucosa.

Water-soluble vitamins *Vitamin B_{12} absorption* is discussed in Chap. 327. In the case of *folic acid absorption,* it should be emphasized that folates exist in food conjugated with glutamyl peptides. These *polyglutamates* must be deconjugated (by folic deconjugase) to monoglutamates for absorption to occur. Certain drugs (such as oral contraceptives, sulfasalazine, diphenylhydantoin, trimethoprim, and pyrimethamine) inhibit the absorption of dietary folate and hence can cause folate deficiency. Sulfasalazine, for example, competitively inhibits three enzymes important in the intestinal metabolism of folate, i.e., dehydrofolate reductase, methylene tetrahydrofolate reductase, and serine transhydroxymethylase. Thiamine and riboflavin appear to be absorbed by passive diffusion.

TESTS USEFUL IN THE DIAGNOSIS OF MALABSORPTION

Most of the tests useful in the diagnosis of malabsorption indicate the presence of abnormal absorptive or digestive function, and only a few tests may suggest a specific diagnosis. Accordingly, it is frequently necessary to employ a combination of tests to establish a diagnosis. To illustrate the use of various tests, the characteristic findings in nontropical sprue, an example of a primary malabsorptive disorder, and pancreatic insufficiency, an example of impaired digestion, are compared in Table 308-2.

Stool fat The qualitative examination of the stool for undigested muscle fibers, neutral fat, and split fat is a simple and reliable screening test for steatorrhea. The finding of an increased number of muscle fibers indicates impaired intraluminal digestion. Properly performed, the qualitative microscopic examination of a stool specimen with the Sudan III stain is of value and correlates well with the quantitative determination of fecal fat by the Van de Kamer method. The latter remains the most reliable measurement of steatorrhea. A normal fecal fat excretion is less than 6 g for 24 h, or less than 6 percent of ingested fat.

Oral [^{14}C]triolein can also be used as an effective test for fat absorption. During the digestive process the triolein is hydrolyzed, and the labeled glycerol is absorbed and metabolized by the liver. The $^{14}CO_2$ produced is exhaled and can then be measured hourly (for 6 h) in the expired air. Normally more than 3.5 percent of the administered label [0.185 MBq (5 μCi)] appears in the breath per hour.

Xylose absorption In the most commonly employed form of the xylose absorption test, the patient ingests 25 g D-xylose. A 5-h urine xylose excretion of 4.5 g or greater is considered normal. There is some decreased renal excretion with age, and over age sixty-five 3.5 g is the normal value. Low values may be obtained in patients with ascites, intestinal bacterial overgrowth, or renal insufficiency, after administration of certain drugs (e.g., aspirin, indomethacin), and most commonly if the urine collection is incomplete. To obviate difficulties in interpreting the test, it is advisable to determine the blood xylose level 2 h after ingestion of xylose. A blood xylose level of 30 mg/dl or greater indicates normal absorption of D-xylose. An abnormal D-xylose absorption test is found most frequently in disorders affecting the mucosa of the proximal small intestine, such as nontropical and tropical sprue.

Gastrointestinal x-ray studies All patients with malabsorption should have radiographic examinations of the small intestine and, in many cases, of the esophagus, stomach, and colon as well. Occasionally, the latter two examinations may provide important clues to the presence of such disorders as gastroileostomy, scleroderma, Zollinger-Ellison syndrome, ulcerative colitis, and intestinal fistulas. The typical small-bowel radiographic abnormalities in patients with a malabsorption syndrome are a breaking up of the barium column with segmentation, clumping, and coarsening of the mucosal folds. Segmentation or clumping of the barium in a small-bowel loop is often termed a *moulage sign.* Less frequently there is dilatation of the proximal small bowel and loss of a normal mucosal pattern. Collectively, these changes have been referred to as a *malabsorption pattern.* These findings are nonspecific and may be found in several of the disorders listed in Table 308-3. Some representative examples of abnormal small-bowel radiographs are shown in Fig. 308-3.

Small-intestinal biopsy The most commonly used instruments for obtaining peroral biopsy specimens from the small intestine include the Rubin and Shiner tubes and the Crosby, Carey, and Ross-Moore capsules. Examination of small-bowel biopsy specimens has proved to be of considerable value in the differential diagnosis of malabsorptive disorders. Table 308-3 lists disorders associated with abnormalities in intestinal biopsies, and Fig. 308-4 depicts some illustrative lesions.

Schilling test for vitamin B_{12} absorption The Schilling test is valuable in the differential diagnosis of malabsorption and is frequently carried out in three stages: (1) without intrinsic factor, (2) with intrinsic factor, and (3) after a course of treatment with antibiotics. Since vitamin B_{12} is absorbed primarily in the distal ileum, an abnormal Schilling test may indicate a pathologic condition of the distal small bowel. In disorders affecting the terminal ileum such as regional enteritis and lymphomas, the first-stage Schilling test is frequently abnormal. The ileal

TABLE 308-3
Disorders associated with abnormalities in small-bowel biopsy specimens

I Disorders in which biopsy is of diagnostic value (diffuse lesions)
- *A* Whipple's disease: Lamina propria infiltrated with macrophages containing PAS-positive glycoproteins
- *B* Abetalipoproteinemia: Villus structure normal; epithelial cells vacuolated due to excess fat
- *C* Agammaglobulinemia: Flattened or absent villi; increased lymphocyte infiltration; absence of plasma cells

II Disorders in which biopsy may be of diagnostic value (patchy lesions)
- *A* Intestinal lymphoma: Infiltration of lamina propria and submucosa with malignant cells
- *B* Intestinal lymphangiectasia: Dilated lacteals and lymphatics in lamina propria; clubbed villi
- *C* Eosinophilic enteritis: Diffuse or patchy eosinophilic infiltration in lamina propria and mucosa
- *D* Amyloidosis: Presence of amyloid confirmed by special stains
- *E* Regional enteritis: Noncaseating granulomas
- *F* Parasitic infestations: Parasitic invasion of mucosa; adherence of trophozoites to mucosal surface, as in giardiasis
- *G* Systemic mastocytosis: Mast cell infiltration of lamina propria

III Disorders in which biopsy is abnormal but not diagnostic
- *A* Celiac sprue: Shortened or absent villi; hypertrophied crypts; damaged surface epithelium; mononuclear infiltrate
- *B* "Collagenous" sprue: Indistinguishable from celiac sprue; extensive subepithelial collagen deposition
- *C* Tropical sprue: Lesion similar to celiac sprue with shortened or absent villi; lymphocyte infiltration
- *D* Folate deficiency: Shortened villi; megalocytosis; decreased mitoses in crypts
- *E* Vitamin B_{12} deficiency: Similar to folate deficiency
- *F* Acute radiation enteritis: Similar to folate deficiency
- *G* Systemic scleroderma: Fibrosis around Brunner's glands
- *H* Bacterial overgrowth syndromes: Patchy damage to villi and increased lymphocyte infiltration

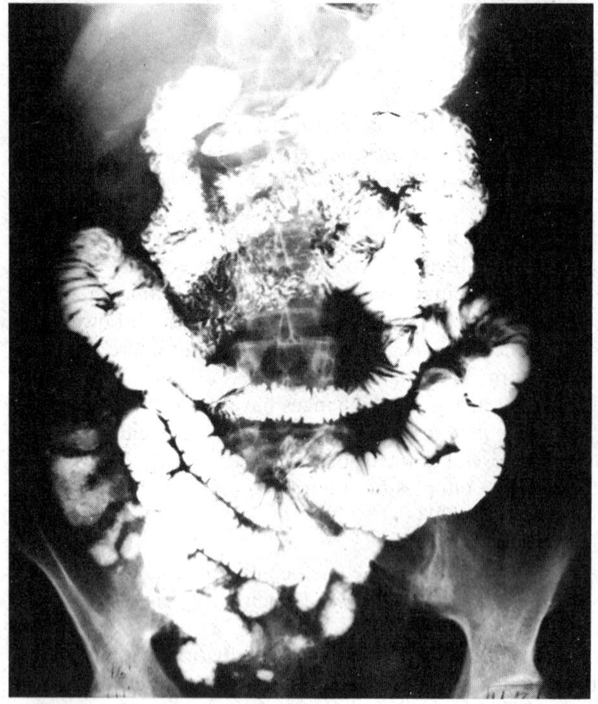

A

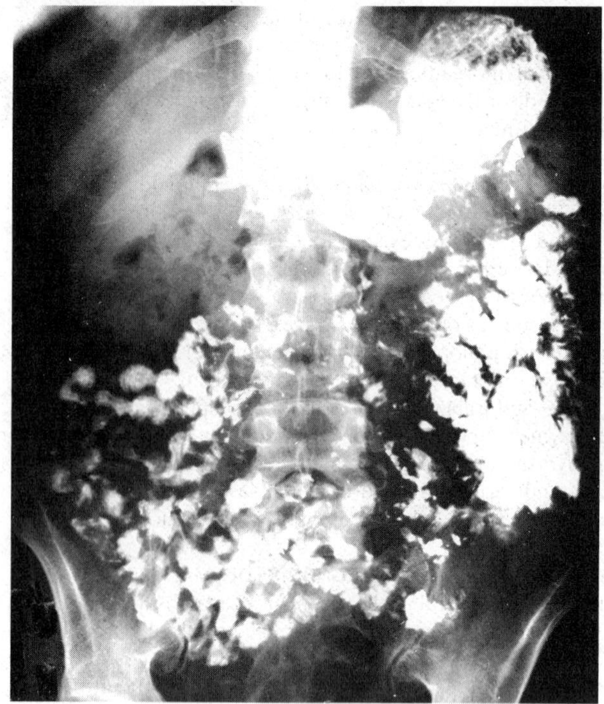

B

FIGURE 308-3

A. X-ray of a normal small intestine showing good mucosal pattern. B. Intestinal x-ray of a patient with nontropical sprue. Note dilatation of small bowel, lack of mucosal markings, and segmentation and clumping of barium. C. Intestinal x-ray of patient with obstructed lymphatics due to Köhlmeier-Degos disease. Note "accordion-pleated" pattern at lower edge of film.

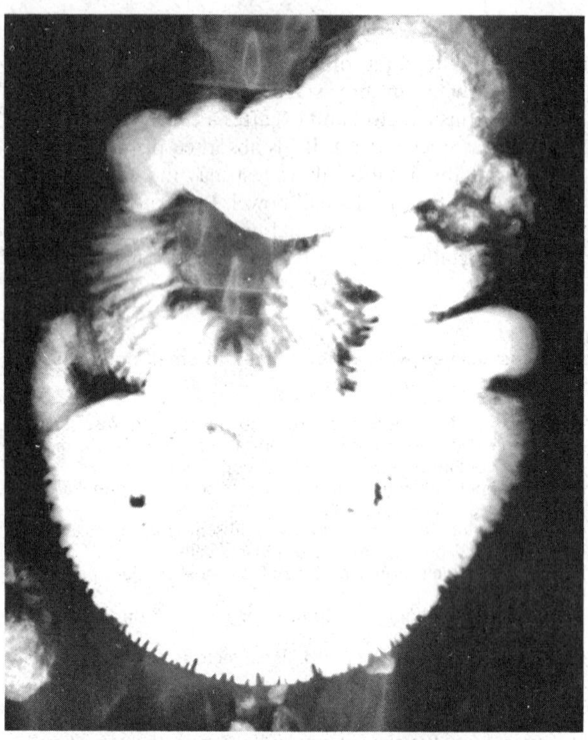

C

receptor site appears to be damaged in these disorders, and the impaired absorption of B_{12} is not corrected by the addition of intrinsic factor or the use of antibiotics. The Schilling test may also be useful in establishing a diagnosis of abnormal bacterial overgrowth of the small bowel, which may be present in disorders such as blind loop syndrome, scleroderma, and multiple small-bowel diverticula (see below). In the blind loop syndrome, for example, the bacteria can actually take up vitamin B_{12} with resultant impaired absorption of B_{12}. Under these conditions the first-stage Schilling test is frequently abnormal, as is the second stage. After appropriate antibiotic treatment the Schilling test usually returns to normal. Vitamin B_{12} absorption is frequently abnormal in patients with exocrine pancreatic insufficiency (see Chap. 325).

Secretin test The secretin test, secretin pancreozymin test, and intraduodenal perfusion with essential amino acids, which may be useful in establishing a diagnosis of pancreatic insufficiency, are discussed in detail in Chap. 324.

Serum calcium, albumin, cholesterol, magnesium, and iron Abnormal serum calcium, albumin, cholesterol, magnesium, and iron values may be found in several malabsorptive disorders. The primary value of such tests is to suggest that abnormal intestinal absorptive function may be present. These tests are usually of limited value in the *differential diagnosis* of malabsorption, but if abnormal, may be helpful in supporting this diagnosis.

FIGURE 308-4

Typical peroral intestinal biopsies.

A. Jejunal mucosa of patient with nontropical sprue. Note virtual absence of villi, elongated crypts (some are cut in cross section), mononuclear infiltrate, cuboidal instead of columnar epithelium on top of villi (300×).

B. Biopsy from the same patient as in A, after 9 months on a gluten-free diet. Note the reappearance of villi with normal-appearing columnar cells, and reduction in infiltrate and crypt height (300×).

C. Biopsy from patient with agammaglobulinemia. The features bear a striking resemblance to those of nontropical sprue. There is a marked mononuclear infiltration, some of it in aggregates (200×).

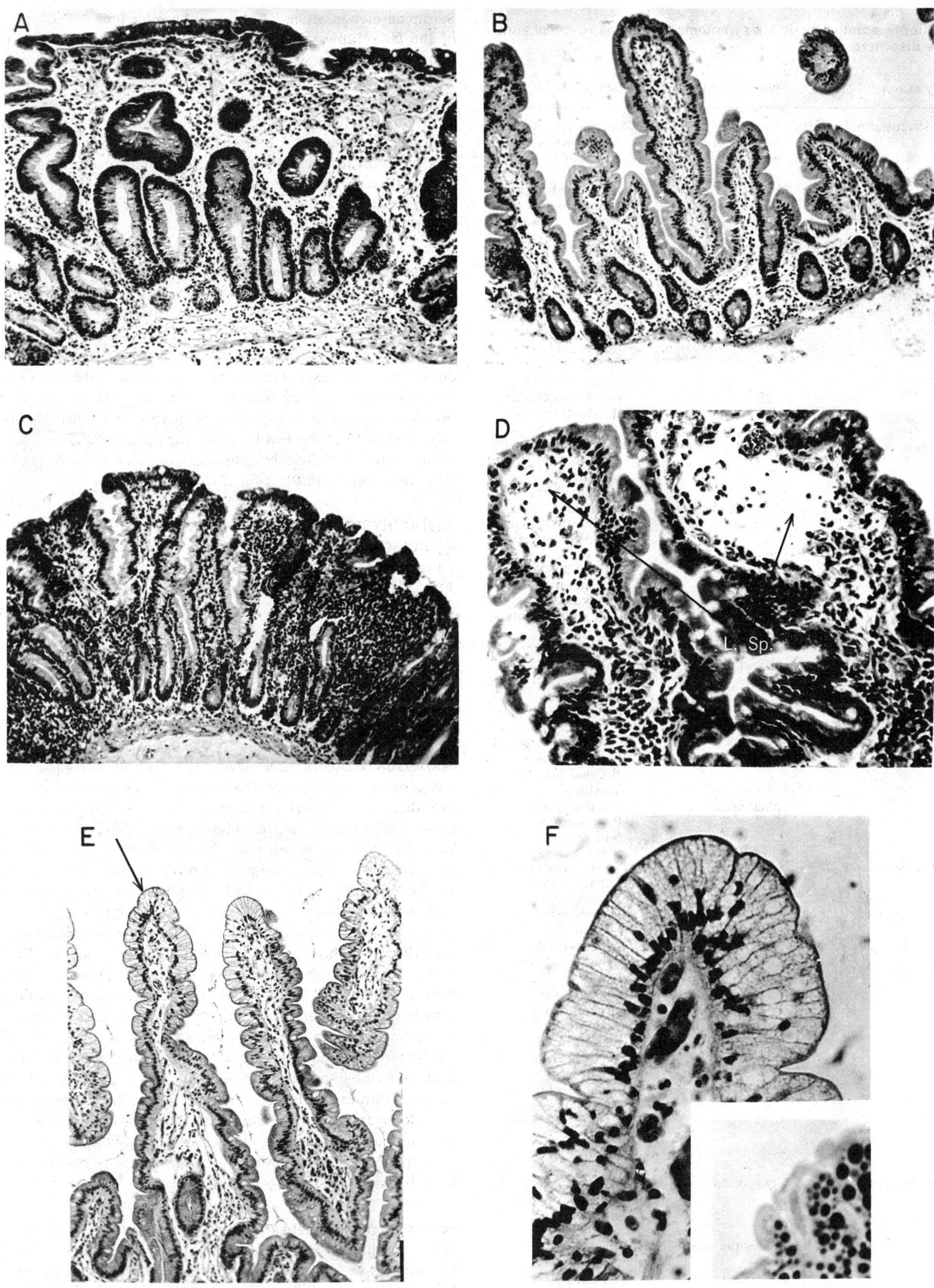

D. Close-up of villi of patient with protein-losing enteropathy. Tips of villi are broadened and dilated. Lymphatic spaces are present (arrows) (450×).

E. Intestinal biopsy from patient with abetalipoproteinemia. The villus tips have a "lacy" appearance (arrow) due to retained fat (300×). (This is more apparent at the higher magnification shown in F.)

F. High-power micrograph of villus from patient with abetalipoproteinemia. The vacuoles are filled with lipid (750×). Insert shows dark-staining (osmium) lipid droplets in mucosal cells (osmium counterstained with Giemsa; 800×).

TABLE 308-4
Pathophysiologic basis for symptoms and signs in malabsorptive disorders

Organ system	*Symptom or sign*	*Pathophysiology*
Gastrointestinal	Generalized malnutrition and weight loss	Malabsorption of fat, carbohydrate and protein → loss of calories
	Diarrhea	Impaired absorption or increased secretion of water and electrolytes; unabsorbed dihydroxy bile acids and fatty acids → decreased absorption of water and electrolytes; excess load of fluid and electrolytes presented to the colon may exceed its absorptive capacity
	Flatus	Bacterial fermentation of unabsorbed carbohydrate
	Glossitis, cheilosis, stomatitis	Deficiency of iron, vitamin B_{12}, folate, and other vitamins
Genitourinary	Nocturia	Delayed absorption of water, hypokalemia
	Azotemia, hypotension	Fluid and electrolyte depletion
	Amenorrhea, ↓ libido	Protein depletion and "caloric starvation" → secondary hypopituitarism
Hematopoietic	Anemia	Impaired absorption of iron, vitamin B_{12}, and folic acid
	Hemorrhagic phenomena	Vitamin K malabsorption → hypoprothrombinemia
Musculoskeletal	Bone pain	Protein depletion → impaired bone formation → osteoporosis
		Calcium malabsorption → demineralization of bone → osteomalacia
	Osteoarthropathy	Cause uncertain
	Tetany, paresthesias	Calcium malabsorption → hypocalcemia; magnesium malabsorption → hypomagnesemia
	Weakness	Anemia; electrolyte depletion (hypokalemia)
Nervous system	Night blindness	Impaired absorption vitamin A → vitamin A deficiency
	Xerophthalmia	Vitamin A deficiency
	Peripheral neuropathy	Vitamin B_{12}, thiamine deficiency
Skin	Eczema	Cause uncertain
	Purpura	Vitamin K deficiency
	Follicular hyperkeratosis and dermatitis	Deficiency of vitamin A, zinc, essential fatty acids, and other vitamins

Serum carotenes, vitamin A, and prothrombin time Absorption of the fat-soluble vitamins A, D, K, and E is frequently impaired in patients with steatorrhea. Measurements of serum carotene and vitamin A levels are useful as screening tests for malabsorption. However, other tests not only are more sensitive but often give more specific information than the serum carotene and vitamin A levels. The blood prothrombin time is an important test, since patients with malabsorption may present with abnormal bleeding due to vitamin K deficiency. If the decreased prothrombin activity is due to malabsorption, it should be readily correctable with parenteral vitamin K.

Breath tests The bile acid breath test utilizing [^{14}C]cholylglycine is a reasonably reliable screening test for bacterial overgrowth syndromes. Approximately two-thirds of patients with a positive small-bowel culture will have an abnormal bile acid breath test. However, in patients with suspected malabsorption of bile acids the test is rather insensitive without the additional determination of fecal bile acid excretion. The excretion of breath hydrogen after ingestion of lactose is a sensitive, specific, and noninvasive test for detecting lactase deficiency. Lactulose and [^{14}C]xylose breath tests for bacterial overgrowth have also been found helpful.

PATHOPHYSIOLOGIC BASIS FOR SYMPTOMS AND SIGNS IN MALABSORPTIVE DISORDERS The common symptoms and signs found in malabsorptive disorders are listed in Table 308-4. The most frequent symptoms are those of malnutrition, weight loss, and diarrhea. However, in each of the clinical settings listed in Table 308-4, it is important to consider the cause of the malabsorption.

DISORDERS ASSOCIATED WITH MALABSORPTION (See Table 308-5)

INADEQUATE DIGESTION **Liver and biliary tract disease** It is not generally appreciated that patients with acute or chronic liver disease may develop malabsorption due to impaired intraluminal digestion. Steatorrhea has been described in acute viral hepatitis, chronic extrahepatic biliary tract obstruction, primary biliary cirrhosis, and postnecrotic and nutritional cirrhosis. Absorption of D-xylose and vitamin B_{12} are usually normal, and small-intestinal mucosal biopsy specimens are generally unremarkable. The steatorrhea associated with liver and biliary tract disease is thought to be due to impaired hepatic synthesis or excretion of conjugated bile salts, resulting in impaired formation of micellar lipid. In addition to steatorrhea, patients with liver disease may have impaired absorption of vitamin D and calcium, resulting in severe metabolic bone disease. This is particularly common in patients with primary biliary cirrhosis. Skeletal roentgenograms may show increased porosity of bone, cortical thinning, vertebral compression, and spontaneous pathologic fractures. Patients with alcohol-induced liver disease may also have exocrine pancreatic insufficiency. Accordingly, pancreatic function should be evaluated in patients with liver disease and malabsorption.

Postgastrectomy malabsorption The presence of a malabsorption syndrome has been documented frequently in patients after subtotal gastrectomy. Steatorrhea is more common with a Billroth II than a Billroth I type of anastomosis. Usually the fat loss is minimal, ranging from 7 to 10 g per 24 h. Patients with gross steatorrhea usually have impaired intraluminal fat digestion due to several factors: (1) With a Billroth II anastomosis the duodenum is bypassed, and there is a decreased entry of stomach contents into the proximal duodenum (i.e., afferent loop). This leads to a decreased stimulus for the release of *secretin* and *pancreozymin* from the duodenum and may result in a depressed pancreatic enzyme response. (2) There may be *inadequate mixing* of the pancreatic enzymes and bile salts secreted into the proximal duodenum with the gastric contents entering the jejunum. (3) There may be *stasis* of intestinal contents in the afferent loop, resulting in abnormal bacterial proliferation in the proximal small bowel. This in turn may lead to abnormalities in bile salt metabolism (see "Pathophysiology" below). (4) The presence of maldigestion may lead to *protein depletion*, which in turn may produce further impairment in pancreatic function. (5) The *loss of the reservoir function of the stomach* may result in decreased intestinal transit time. Perhaps the most important factor is rapid gastric emptying, which results in low luminal concentrations of digestive secretions for the first 60 to 80 min after a meal. Such a disorder has been described in patients with subtotal gastrectomy and duodenostomy (Billroth I), gastrojejunostomy (Billroth II), and truncal vagotomy and pyloroplasty (V&P). That gastric emptying rates are somewhat slower in patients with V&P may account for the overall less severe nutritional deficiencies in such patients. In some patients treatment with pancreatic enzymes may lead to significant improvement. Specimens of duodenal or jejunal fluid should be obtained for culture of both aerobic and anaerobic organisms and appropriate antibiotic therapy instituted if there is evidence of abnormal bacterial overgrowth (colony count of greater than 10^7 per milliliter of jejunal fluid). Because the duodenum is the principal site of absorption of iron and calcium, in patients with a Billroth II anastomosis impaired absorption of calcium and iron may also develop. Occult metabolic bone disease occurs frequently in this setting.

TABLE 308-5
Classification of the malabsorption syndromes

- *I* Inadequate digestion
  - *A* Postgastrectomy steatorrhea*
  - *B* Deficiency or inactivation of pancreatic lipase
    - *1* Exocrine pancreatic insufficiency
      - *a* Chronic pancreatitis
      - *b* Pancreatic carcinoma
      - *c* Cystic fibrosis
      - *d* Pancreatic resection
    - *2* Ulcerogenic tumor of the pancreas (Zollinger-Ellison syndrome, gastrinoma)*
- *II* Reduced intestinal bile salt concentration (with impaired micelle formation)
  - *A* Liver disease
    - *1* Parenchymal liver disease
    - *2* Cholestasis (intrahepatic or extrahepatic)
  - *B* Abnormal bacterial proliferation in the small bowel
    - *1* Afferent loop stasis
    - *2* Strictures
    - *3* Fistulas
    - *4* Blind loops
    - *5* Multiple diverticula of the small bowel
    - *6* Hypomotility states (diabetes, scleroderma, intestinal pseudoobstruction)
  - *C* Interrupted enterohepatic circulation of bile salts
    - *1* Ileal resection
    - *2* Ileal inflammatory disease (regional ileitis)
  - *D* Drugs (by sequestration or precipitation of bile salts)
    - *1* Neomycin
    - *2* Calcium carbonate
    - *3* Cholestyramine
- *III* Inadequate absorptive surface
  - *A* Intestinal resection or bypass
    - *1* Mesenteric vascular disease with massive intestinal resection
    - *2* Regional enteritis with multiple bowel resections
    - *3* Jejunoileal bypass
  - *B* Gastroileostomy (inadvertent)
- *IV* Lymphatic obstruction
  - *A* Intestinal lymphangiectasia
  - *B* Whipple's disease*
  - *C* Lymphoma
- *V* Cardiovascular disorders
  - *A* Constrictive pericarditis
  - *B* Congestive heart failure
  - *C* Mesenteric vascular insufficiency
  - *D* Vasculitis
- *VI* Primary mucosal absorptive defects
  - *A* Inflammatory or infiltrative disorders
    - *1* Regional enteritis*
    - *2* Amyloidosis
    - *3* Scleroderma*
    - *4* Lymphoma*
    - *5* Radiation enteritis
    - *6* Eosinophilic enteritis
    - *7* Tropical sprue
    - *8* Infectious enteritis (e.g., salmonellosis)
    - *9* Collagenous sprue
    - *10* Nonspecific ulcerative jejunitis
    - *11* Mastocytosis
    - *12* Dermatologic disorders (e.g., dermatitis herpetiformis)
  - *B* Biochemical or genetic abnormalities
    - *1* Nontropical sprue (gluten-induced enteropathy); celiac sprue
    - *2* Disaccharidase deficiency
    - *3* Hypogammaglobulinemia
    - *4* Abetalipoproteinemia
    - *5* Hartnup disease
    - *6* Cystinuria
    - *7* Monosaccharide malabsorption
- *VII* Endocrine and metabolic disorders
  - *A* Diabetes mellitus*
  - *B* Hypoparathyroidism
  - *C* Adrenal insufficiency
  - *D* Hyperthyroidism
  - *E* Ulcerogenic tumor of the pancreas (Zollinger-Ellison syndrome, gastrinoma)*
  - *F* Carcinoid syndrome

* *Malabsorption caused by multiple defects.*

INADEQUATE ABSORPTIVE SURFACE (SHORT BOWEL SYNDROME) Extensive intestinal resection often results in the short bowel syndrome. The most common disorders resulting in short bowel syndrome are (1) massive intestinal resection following a vascular insult to the small intestine, (2) regional enteritis with multiple bowel resections, and (3) jejunoileal bypass for morbid obesity. In general, the absorption of nutrients will be influenced by the extent and site of small bowel resected, the presence of the ileocecal valve, and adaptation of the remaining small bowel. Resection of 40 to 50 percent of the small bowel is usually well tolerated, provided the proximal duodenum, the distal half of the ileum, and the ileocecal valve are spared. By contrast, resection of the ileum and the ileocecal valve alone may induce severe diarrhea and malabsorption, even though less than 30 percent of the small intestine is resected.

Several measures are important in the management of short bowel syndrome: (1) The diet should contain at least 2500 cal and consist primarily of carbohydrate and protein with fat restricted to less than 40 g per day. A fat-restricted diet is effective in reducing diarrhea, presumably because there is decreased production of hydroxy fatty acids from long-chain fats. Such hydroxy fatty acids, in essence, are cathartics and increase net secretion of water and electrolytes by the colon as well as the small bowel. (2) It is often necessary to provide vitamin and mineral supplements, which usually include K^+, Cl^-, Mg^{2+}, Ca^{2+}, trace metals (Zn, Cd, Mn), iron, folate, vitamin B_{12}, other vitamins (A, D, E, K, B_1, B_2, B_6, biotin), and essential fatty acids. (3) Specific drugs (for example, belladonna alkaloids, diphenoxylate, loperamide, and codeine), which decrease intestinal motility and prolong mucosal contact time, are helpful in controlling diarrhea. These agents also decrease ileostomy outputs. (4) A bile salt–sequestering agent such as cholestyramine blunts the effects of bile salts, which stimulate net secretion of water and electrolytes by the colon. (5) Patients with short bowel syndrome may have gastric acid hypersecretion, which results in dilution of pancreatic secretions as well as inactivation of pancreatic enzymes. Under these conditions, the histamine H_2-receptor antagonist, cimetidine, is useful because it will suppress gastric acid secretion and decrease the volume of fluid entering the proximal small bowel, thus leading to an increased concentration of pancreatic enzymes. In addition, supplemental pancreatic enzyme therapy may be required. (6) A bypassed colon can be used to receive infusions of fluid and electrolytes since a portion of the colon can still absorb 1000 to 1500 ml fluid per day. Finally, (7) total parenteral nutrition is frequently required during the first 6 months after massive intestinal resection until some degree of adaptation has occurred. Such patients may also require long-term parenteral hyperalimentation with a silicone rubber catheter in the superior vena cava, and this can be done at home.

For a discussion of regional enteritis see Chap. 309.

MALABSORPTION DUE TO BACTERIAL OVERGROWTH OF THE SMALL BOWEL The proximal small intestine is usually bacteriologically sterile because of three factors: (1) the acid milieu of the stomach; (2) intestinal peristalsis, which sweeps bacteria to the distal small bowel; and (3) secretion into the lumen of the intestine of immunoglobulins, which may serve as coproantibodies. When bacteria are isolated from the upper small bowel, they are frequently contaminants transported from the mouth and upper respiratory tract, and the colony count rarely exceeds 10^4 per milliliter of jejunal fluid. The major mechanism limiting the growth of bacteria in the small intestine is normal peristalsis. Any disorder leading to impaired intestinal motility may result in abnormal stasis of intestinal contents with ineffective mechanical cleansing of bacteria. This in turn may lead to abnormal bacterial proliferation and malabsorption. Several malabsorptive disorders have been associated with bacterial overgrowth of the small bowel, and these are listed in Table 308-6.

Pathophysiology Bacterial overgrowth may result in changes in bile salt metabolism, and these are believed directly and indirectly to account for the steatorrhea. First, bacteria (especially anaerobic gram-positive bacteria) may lead to the intraluminal deconjugation of bile salts with a consequent production of free bile acids. In contrast to conjugated bile salts, unconjugated bile salts may be absorbed in the proximal small bowel by nonionic diffusion, resulting in decreased intraluminal concentrations of bile salts in the jejunum. Second, the decreased bile salt concentrations, the increase of unconjugated bile salts, and the decrease of the conjugated salts all serve to contribute to impaired intraluminal micelle formation and hence fat malabsorption. In addition to abnormalities in bile salt metabolism, intestinal mucosal lesions have been demonstrated in patients with intestinal stasis. Such lesions are often patchy in distribution, and the histologic appearance ranges in severity from minimal changes in villous architecture to severe lesions with virtual absence of villi. The etiology of these lesions is unclear; possible causes include damage caused by bacterial invasion, bacterial toxins, or metabolic products such as unconjugated bile salts. In this regard, certain bacteria such as *Bacteroides* elaborate proteases which solubilize brush border proteins and destroy disaccharidases such as sucrase and maltase. The impaired absorption of vitamin B_{12} is not related to the disturbed bile salt metabolism but appears to be due to uptake of vitamin B_{12} by microorganisms.

Many of the above abnormalities in bile salt metabolism may be reversed by appropriate antibiotic therapy. When such treatment is instituted, unconjugated bile salts in the jejunal fluid decrease, an increase in the micellar lipid phase will occur, and steatorrhea diminishes or disappears. In addition, significant improvement in the absorption of vitamin B_{12} will occur with broad-spectrum antibiotics such as tetracycline.

TABLE 308-6
Causes of intestinal bacterial overgrowth (intestinal colonization)

I Structural abnormalities producing stasis of intestinal contents
- *A* Multiple small-bowel diverticula
- *B* Strictures
  - *1* Regional enteritis*
  - *2* Radiation enteritis*
  - *3* Occlusive vascular disease; vasculitis
- *C* Billroth II subtotal gastrectomy with afferent loop stasis*
- *D* Multiple laparotomies resulting in adhesions and partial small-bowel obstruction

II Fistulas
- *A* Gastrocolic, gastroileal, jejunoileal, jejunocolic

III Motor abnormalities resulting in intestinal hypomotility
- *A* Scleroderma*
- *B* Amyloidosis*
- *C* Diabetes mellitus*
- *D* Hypothyroidism
- *E* Vagotomy
- *F* Intestinal pseudoobstruction (see Table 308-7)

IV Miscellaneous
- *A* Hypogammaglobulinemia*
- *B* Nodular lymphoid hyperplasia
- *C* Pernicious anemia
- *D* Pancreatic insufficiency

V No underlying disorder detected

* *Multiple mechanisms may contribute to malabsorption in these disorders*

Clinical manifestations Breath tests, i.e., ^{14}C-labeled bile acid, [^{14}C]xylose, and lactulose, are useful screening tests for malabsorption syndrome due to abnormal bacterial overgrowth of the small intestine. A definitive diagnosis is established by demonstrating larger numbers of microorganisms (greater than 10^7 per milliliter) and a polymicrobial flora in cultures of duodenal or jejunal fluid. Other clinical features include the following: (1) steatorrhea of a moderate degree, usually in the range of 15 to 30 g fecal fat per 24 h; (2) macrocytic anemia with a megaloblastic bone marrow; (3) impaired absorption of vitamin B_{12} which is not corrected by intrinsic factor; and (4) correction of steatorrhea and impaired vitamin B_{12} absorption by antibiotic therapy. Absorption of D-xylose, peroral small-intestinal biopsy specimens, and other tests of absorptive function (Table 308-2) may be normal in these patients. A single course or intermittent courses (2 to 3 a week per month) of therapy with antibiotics such as tetracycline, ampicillin, or trimethoprim-sulfamethoxazole (Bactrim) are usually given.

Chronic intestinal pseudoobstruction (see also Chap. 310) Chronic intestinal pseudoobstruction is a heterogeneous syndrome with a variety of causes (Table 308-7). Primary or idiopathic intestinal pseudoobstruction is a chronic illness characterized by recurrent episodes of intestinal obstruction in which all known causes of mechanical obstruction and other illnesses known to produce intestinal pseudoobstruction have been excluded. In addition to abnormalities in small-bowel motility, derangements in esophageal, gastric, and colonic motility have also been described. Malabsorption, secondary to stasis of intestinal contents with resultant abnormal bacterial proliferation in the small bowel, is frequently present.

Tropical sprue Tropical sprue is a malabsorptive disorder of unknown cause affecting residents or visitors to tropical regions. Both epidemic and endemic forms of the disease have been recognized. The etiology of the disorder has not been elucidated, but it might well result from one or more of the following: (1) a nutritional deficiency, (2) a transmissible infectious microorganism, and (3) a toxin elaborated by a microorganism or contained in the diet. It is of interest that coliform organisms, shown to produce an enterotoxin causing fluid secretion, have been isolated from the jejunum of tropical sprue patients but not from other patients with bacterial overgrowth of the proximal small bowel. Anorexia, diarrhea, weight loss, symptoms of anemia, sequelae of nutritional deficiency (Table 308-4), and abdominal distention are common findings. Patients are frequently deficient in iron as well as vitamin B_{12} and folate. Laboratory studies usually reveal anemia (megaloblastic in 60 percent of cases) and impaired absorption of fat, xylose, and vitamin B_{12}. Malabsorption of at least two nutrients is considered essential for the diagnosis. Jejunal biopsy classically reveals shortened and thickened villi, increased crypt depth, and increased infiltration of mononuclear cells in the lamina propria and epithelium (Table 308-3). However, these biopsy findings are not specific, and the lesion may be patchy; in addition, interpretation is difficult because "control" biopsies from asymptomatic residents in the same tropical region are often considered abnormal when compared with normal biopsies from patients in temperate zones. Such histological findings have been termed *tropical jejunitis.* Treatment with vitamin B_{12}, folate, and antibiotics have all been effective in inducing a remission. A short course, i.e., 2 to 4 weeks, of therapy with a sulfonamide or tetracycline is usually given. Occasional patients require more prolonged antibiotic therapy.

Scleroderma Although there are numerous reports of small-intestinal involvement in scleroderma, frank malabsorption has been reported infrequently. It has been suggested that malabsorption may be due to several factors: (1) lymphatic obstruction; (2) reduced arterial blood supply to the gut; (3) impaired intestinal motility leading to relative stasis of intestinal contents and hence bacterial overgrowth; and (4) involvement of the intestinal wall by the disease. At present there is little evidence to support the first two postulated mechanisms. In some cases abnormal bacterial proliferation in the upper small bowel has been documented, and in these patients antibiotic therapy has resulted in decrease in steatorrhea, gain in weight, and increased absorption of vitamin B_{12}. In the intestinal wall there may also be extensive deposition of collagen, especially in the muscular mucosa, submucosa, and muscularis externa, with significant muscle atrophy. Studies of duodenal myoelectric activity in scleroderma revealed normal slow-wave frequency and propagation velocity but decreased excitability of the bowel to mechanical stimuli such as distention and humoral stimuli such as pentagastrin and secretin. This motor dysfunction may be an important factor in the dilatation, atony, and stasis of intestinal contents in scleroderma.

DISORDERS ASSOCIATED WITH LYMPHATIC OBSTRUCTION

Whipple's disease This is a rare disorder characterized clinically by arthralgia, abdominal pain, diarrhea, progressive weight loss, and impaired intestinal absorption. Wasting, low-grade fever, increased skin pigmentation, and peripheral lymphadenopathy are frequently present. In addition, central nervous system manifestations including confusion, memory loss, focal cranial nerve signs, nystagmus, and ophthalmoplegia may be present. Laboratory examination usually reveals the presence of steatorrhea, impaired xylose absorption, abnormal small-bowel x-rays, hypoalbuminemia, and anemia. Hypoalbuminemia is due to excessive loss of serum albumin into the gastrointestinal tract as well as impaired synthesis of albumin.

The diagnosis is established by demonstrating the presence in the mucosa of macrophages containing large cytoplasmic granules which give a brilliant magenta stain with periodic acid Schiff reagent (PAS). Such macrophages may also be seen in other tissues such as lymph nodes, spleen, or liver. The finding of PAS-positive macrophages in the lamina propria is not specific for Whipple's disease, but virtual replacement of most cellular elements in the lamina propria by these macrophages has been seen only in this disorder. In addition to the PAS-positive macrophages, jejunal biopsies frequently show dilated lymphatics and some degree of blunting of the intestinal mucosal villi.

Electron microscopic studies have revealed the presence of rod-shaped structures (or bacilliform bodies) 0.3 by 1.5 to 2.5 μm within and adjacent to the macrophages in the lamina propria as well as within epithelial cells, and polymorphonuclear leukocytes. The ultrastructural features of these bacilliform bodies suggest that they are microorganisms. It is of particular interest that after treatment with antibiotics the bacilliform bodies decrease or disappear together with a decrease in the number of PAS-positive macrophages. In addition, the reappearance of the bacteria often heralds the onset of a clinical relapse after antibiotics have been withdrawn.

Whipple's disease at one time was thought to be invariably fatal. However, it is now clear that therapy with antibiotics, with or without corticosteroids, will usually induce a clinical remission. In a few cases there has been complete reversal of the histologic abnormalities in the jejunal mucosa, and some of these cases have been followed for 10 years. It is recommended that patients with Whipple's disease be treated with antibiotics such as tetracycline for at least 1 year and then followed closely with serial small-bowel biopsies. The most important parameter for following the disease and predicting its course is the presence or absence of bacilli in sections of small-bowel biopsies.

Intestinal lymphoma Steatorrhea is a manifestation of *primary* intestinal lymphoma. The disease occurs predominantly in men, and the mean age of onset of symptoms is about 50 years. The diagnosis should be suspected in patients with malabsorption with the following findings: (1) a malabsorption syndrome in which clinical and biopsy features resemble those of nontropical sprue but in which there is an incomplete response to a gluten-free diet, (2) the presence of *abdominal pain* and *fever,* and (3) signs and symptoms of intestinal obstruction. The usual stigmata of generalized lymphoma are frequently absent. Hepatomegaly, splenomegaly, palpable abdominal masses, and peripheral adenopathy are usually not found. Lymphangiography may reveal abnormal intraabdominal nodes. The diagnosis can be established by laparotomy and often may be made by thorough examination of multiple mucosal biopsy specimens obtained perorally. There may be a total absence of villi or lesser degrees of blunting and shortening of the villi. In contrast to nontropical sprue, the lamina propria is usually massively infiltrated with lymphoid cells. Malignancy may be diagnosed by demonstrating lymphoid cells with the cytologic features of malignancy, the presence of reticulum cells outside germinal centers, and infiltration and destruction of crypts by pleomorphic lymphoid cells. Some patients elaborate or secrete a fragment of the heavy chain of IgA immunoglobulins (*α-chain disease*). The latter is probably a variant of intestinal lymphoma.

TABLE 308-7
Causes of chronic intestinal pseudoobstruction

I Primary: Idiopathic
II Secondary
- *A* Collagen vascular disease
  - *1* Scleroderma
  - *2* Dermatomyositis/polymyositis
  - *3* Systemic lupus erythematosus
- *B* Amyloidosis
- *C* Endocrine disorders
  - *1* Myxedema
  - *2* Diabetes mellitus
- *D* Neurological diseases
  - *1* Chagas' disease
- *E* Others
  - *1* Jejunoileal bypass
  - *2* Jejunal diverticulosis
  - *3* Drugs (tricyclic antidepressants, clonidine, etc.)

The mechanism of malabsorption in intestinal lymphoma may be related to several factors: (1) diffuse involvement of the small-intestinal mucosa; (2) involvement of the bowel wall with lymphatic obstruction; and (3) localized stenosis with stasis of intestinal contents and bacterial overgrowth. It should be emphasized that it is often difficult, by clinical and morphologic features alone, to distinguish nontropical sprue from intestinal lymphoma. Indeed, there is evidence to suggest that lymphoma may develop as a late complication of nontropical sprue.

The course of intestinal lymphoma has ranged from 4 months to 4 years from the onset of symptoms. Perforation, bleeding, and intestinal obstruction are common terminal complications. There is insufficient evidence to determine whether radiation therapy, chemotherapy, or localized surgical resection modify the natural course of the disease.

CARDIOVASCULAR DISORDERS Steatorrhea has been described in patients with chronic congestive heart failure, superior mesenteric artery insufficiency, and constrictive pericarditis. Abnormal dilated mucosal lymphatics and excessive enteric loss of protein have been demonstrated in patients with constrictive pericarditis. The mechanism of steatorrhea in patients with chronic heart failure remains uncertain. It might be due to congestion and edema of the mucosa, mucosal hypoxia, or abnormalities in pancreatic function. Although pronounced steatorrhea is uncommon in congestive heart failure, these patients are frequently anorectic, and a low fat intake could mask a latent steatorrhea. Steatorrhea is quite infrequent in patients with vasculitis and is thought to be due to segmental infarction of the small bowel in addition to intestinal ischemia.

DEFECTS IN MUCOSAL FUNCTION

INFLAMMATORY OR INFILTRATIVE DISORDERS **Regional enteritis** The clinical features of regional enteritis are described in Chap. 309. Malabsorption in regional enteritis may result from several factors: (1) interruption of the enterohepatic circulation of bile salts by ileal disease or resection; (2) deconjugation of bile salts due to bacterial overgrowth, in turn related to strictures and/or fistulas; (3) active inflammatory bowel disease causing impaired mucosal cell function; (4) inadequate absorptive surface resulting from intestinal resection or fistulas; and (5) severe protein depletion producing impaired exocrine pancreatic function. Active ileal disease and/or ileal resection resulting in an interrupted enterohepatic circulation of and deficiency of conjugated bile salts appears to be the major factor responsible for steatorrhea as well as impaired absorption of vitamin B_{12}. Small-bowel absorptive function has been correlated with the extent of ileal disease or resection. When the length of ileal dysfunction exceeds 90 to 100 cm, virtually all patients will have steatorrhea and vitamin B_{12} malabsorption. After intestinal resection, the functional capacity of the remaining small bowel will depend on the site and extent of resection as well as the presence of residual inflammatory disease. Massive intestinal resection usually results in impaired absorption of all food constituents. When the malabsorption is due to strictures and blind loops as a result of previous surgical therapy, antibiotic therapy may be helpful, but surgical removal of these areas is usually necessary for long-term improvement. With diffuse inflammatory disease a florid malabsorption syndrome may occur with steatorrhea, hypocalcemia, impaired vitamin B_{12} absorption, and hypoalbuminemia due to increased enteric protein loss. Treatment with sulfasalazine and corticosteroid drugs may be beneficial (see Chap. 309).

After *ileal resection,* patients frequently have bothersome diarrhea. This appears to be due to *interruption of the enterohepatic circulation* whereby increased amounts of bile salts reach the colon, where they interfere with water and electrolyte absorption and thus have a cathartic effect. The *bile salt–induced diarrhea* after ileal resection may respond to treatment with cholestyramine, an exchange resin which binds bile salts and causes them to lose their biochemical effect on the bowel. Patients with ileal resection of less than 100 cm and fecal fat excretion less than 20 g per day show the best symptomatic response to cholestyramine.

Chronic nongranulomatous ulcerative jejunoileitis This disorder is characterized by abdominal pain, weight loss, fever, diarrhea, steatorrhea, hypoalbuminemia, and protein-losing enteropathy. Clinical features mimic those found in both regional enteritis and celiac sprue. Indeed, the intestinal lesion may be indistinguishable from celiac sprue. However, exclusion of gluten from the diet does not result in any benefit. Corticosteroid treatment has resulted in transient improvement, but long-term effects are unpredictable.

Amyloidosis This disorder is discussed in detail in Chap. 66.

Radiation injury to the small bowel Extensive morphologic damage of the small-intestinal mucosa often follows normal or excessive abdominal irradiation. These changes include a decrease in crypt mitoses, marked shortening of the villi, megalocytosis of epithelial cells, and inflammatory cell infiltration of the lamina propria. This may be associated with transient diarrhea and impaired intestinal absorption. However, restoration of normal intestinal architecture is usually complete within 2 weeks after cessation of therapy. Persistent diarrhea and malabsorption may develop shortly after x-ray therapy, or there may be a latent period of several years before the onset of diarrhea. Steatorrhea, ranging from 10 to 40 g per day, has been frequently observed, but impaired absorption of calcium, iron, D-xylose, or vitamin B_{12} is less common. In some patients intestinal strictures may develop following irradiation, and thus stasis of intestinal contents and abnormal bacterial proliferation may occur. In others, intestinal lymphangiectasia, presumably due to lymphatic obstruction, has been documented. Diarrhea and malabsorption may be refractory to all methods of management. Treatment with antibiotics, pancreatic enzymes, gluten-free diet, adrenal corticosteroids, anticholinergic drugs, and opiates has met with but limited success.

Eosinophilic enteritis Eosinophilic gastroenteritis is a disorder of the stomach, small bowel, and colon of unknown etiology characterized by peripheral blood eosinophilia and eosinophilic infiltration of the gut wall but without evidence of vasculitis. The clinical manifestations, usually recurrent, are protean and relate to the site of gastrointestinal tract involvement. Three main patterns have been identified: (1) Predominant mucosal disease manifested by iron-deficiency anemia, hypoalbuminemia due to protein-losing enteropathy, and mild steatorrhea. Patients in this group often present with a malabsorption syndrome and a history of intolerance to specific foods. (2) Predominant muscle layer disease characterized by marked thickening and rigidity of the stomach and proximal small bowel with obstructive symptoms and radiologic features of pyloric narrowing and obstruction. The obstructive form of eosinophilic gastroenteritis accounts for half of the reported cases since 1970. Accordingly, eosinophilic enteritis should be considered in the differential diagnosis of gastric outlet obstruction, diffuse small-bowel disease, and ileocolitis. Indeed, eosinophilic enteritis often mimics regional enteritis. (3) Predominant subserosal disease in which the cardinal manifestation is ascites with marked eosinophilia in the ascitic fluid. Although the above classification based on tissue layer of major involvement is useful in understanding the principal manifestations, it should be emphasized that multiple clinical forms, e.g., ascites (serosal involvement) and obstruction (muscular involvement), also occur.

Previous reports have emphasized food allergy and mucosal features of this disease. However, food sensitivity is related to symptoms in less than 20 percent of patients. In such patients fasting serum IgE levels are often elevated, and challenge with offending foods frequently evokes symptoms of abdominal pain and diarrhea in addition to a marked increase in serum IgE levels. In most patients with eosinophilic enteritis, however, immunological studies including serum immunoglobulins, serum complement, lymphocyte quantitation, and lymphocyte response to nonspecific nitrogens reveal no abnormalities. Thus, both IgE-mediated and IgE-dependent mechanisms may be operative in different patients with eosinophilic gastroenteritis. Several nonreaginic factors influence peripheral blood and tissue eosinophilia. It seems clear that evidence of allergy or food sensitivity is often absent and is not required for the diagnosis of eosinophilic enteritis. In addition, even in patients with food allergies, elimination diets are frequently ineffective and such patients may require prolonged corticosteroid therapy to remain well. Surgical treatment for relief of obstructive symptoms and corticosteroids are the mainstays of therapy.

Dermatitis and malabsorption A malabsorption syndrome, usually mild, has been reported in patients with a variety of dermatological disorders, including psoriasis, eczematoid dermatitis, and dermatitis herpetiformis. Proximal intestinal mucosal abnormalities are almost invariably found in patients with dermatitis herpetiformis. In one study 21 of 22 patients had lesions ranging in severity from a completely "flat" to an almost normal intestinal mucosa. The mucosal lesions were often patchy in distribution. Clinical and laboratory evidence of significant malabsorption was infrequent, possibly due to the limited length of small intestine involved in this skin disorder. In some patients with dermatitis herpetiformis, blunted and flattened intestinal mucosal lesions, and steatorrhea, there may be a striking improvement in villous architecture and regression of steatorrhea after withdrawal of gluten from the diet. Further, in patients with dermatitis herpetiformis and a morphologically normal small-intestinal mucosa, administration of a high-gluten diet may result in blunted and flattened mucosal lesions indistinguishable from those of nontropical sprue. As in the latter disease, an increased frequency of HLA-B8 is also seen. These observations raise the interesting question as to whether certain patients with dermatitis herpetiformis and a malabsorption syndrome have latent nontropical sprue.

BIOCHEMICAL OR GENETIC ABNORMALITIES Nontropical sprue DEFINITION Nontropical sprue is a disorder characterized by malabsorption, abnormal small-bowel structure, and intolerance to gluten, a protein found in wheat and wheat products. It has been appropriately referred to as *gluten-induced enteropathy.* Celiac disease in children and nontropical sprue of the adult are probably one and the same disorder with the same pathogenesis.

There are insufficient data to provide an accurate estimation of the incidence of nontropical sprue in any population. This is largely because the severity of the disease varies greatly and individuals may have typical mucosal change and yet have no overt symptoms. Seventy percent of the cases in most reported series are women. The incidence in siblings appears to be many times higher than that in the general population, and it has been suggested that sprue may be inherited through a dominant gene of incomplete penetrance. Celiac sprue patients have an increased frequency of serum histocompatibility antigens, particularly of the HLA-B8 and HLA-Dw3 types. The HLA-B8 phenotype has been found in 85 to 90 percent of sprue patients as compared with 20 to 25 percent in normal subjects. The HLA-B8 antigen may be linked to immune response genes which may determine the immunologic recognition of certain substances. It has been suggested that such genetic factors may predispose to immunologic tolerance of dietary proteins such as the peptides in gluten or to the production of pathogenic antigluten antibodies which could result in binding of gluten to epithelial cells with subsequent tissue damage.

PATHOPHYSIOLOGY Gluten and the related substance gliadin are high-molecular-weight proteins found especially in wheat. These proteins, as well as the larger peptide hydrolysis products (containing glutamine), are toxic when administered to patients with sprue in remission. The exact mechanism for this effect is not clear, but two theories have been proposed, namely, a "toxic" and an immunologic theory. One possible mechanism is that patients with sprue lack a specific mucosal peptidase, so that gluten or its larger glutamine-containing peptides are not effectively hydrolyzed to smaller peptides (i.e., dipeptides or amino acids). As a consequence "toxic" peptides might accumulate in the mucosa. It has been demonstrated that patients with sprue in remission will develop steatorrhea and typical mucosal changes when they are given gluten. Similar results will occur with the administration of peptide hydrolysates containing at least eight amino acids with a terminal glutamine residue. It has been shown that when gluten is instilled into the *ileum* of sprue patients, histologic changes begin to occur within hours, but not in the upper jejunum, suggesting that the effect is immediate and local rather than systemic. After noxious gluten fractions damage surface absorptive cells, the damaged cells are sloughed rapidly from the mucosal surface into the gut lumen. To compensate for this, cell proliferation increases, crypts hypertrophy, and cell migration is accelerated to replace the damaged and sloughed epithelial cells. This more rapid than normal epithelial cell renewal can be reversed by a gluten-free diet. The intestinal mucosa of patients with sprue shows many enzyme alterations, including decreased levels of disaccharidases, alkaline phosphatase, and peptide hydrolases, as well as impaired ability to digest gluten peptides. However, these abnormalities usually revert toward normal after successful treatment with a gluten-free diet. There is additional evidence supporting the concept of toxicity of gluten and gluten breakdown products in sprue. First, gliadin is toxic to sprue mucosa maintained in organ culture, causing ultrastructural changes and depression of disaccharidase activity. Second, sprue mucosa hydrolyzes a specific fraction of a gliadin digest (i.e., fraction 9) in a defective manner, and fraction 9 is selectively toxic to sprue mucosa. Third, specific fractions of gluten fed to sprue patients cause transient alterations in mucosal histology and depression of disaccharidase activity, but full recovery is observed in 72 h. The rapid onset of these changes and prompt recovery are consistent with a direct toxic effect. Despite intensive study, however, no persistent, specific, or selective peptidase deficiency has been demonstrated.

It has also been suggested that gluten or gluten metabolites may initiate an *immunologic reaction* in the intestinal mucosa. The presence of a mononuclear inflammatory cell infiltrate in the lamina propria of the mucosa, the beneficial response to corticosteroid drugs, the finding of abnormal antibodies to gliadin in the serum of sprue patients, the synthesis of increased amounts of antigliadin antibody by sprue mucosa maintained in organ culture, and the elaboration of lymphokines such as migration inhibitory factor (MIF) by sprue mucosa incubated with gliadin have all been cited as evidence in support of this hypothesis. However, the evidence indicating that an abnormal (immune) mechanism is important in initiating or perpetuating this disease process remains to be determined.

Jejunal biopsy specimens from patients with nontropical sprue usually show a characteristic lesion. There is blunting and flattening of the mucosal surface, with villi either absent or broad and short. The crypts are elongated, and there is generally a dense infiltration of inflammatory cells in the lamina propria. The surface epithelium is altered with a sparse brush border, cuboidal rather than the normal columnar cells, and infiltration of inflammatory cells in the epithelial layer. These changes are usually most severe in the proximal small bowel, presumably because this area of the bowel is exposed to the highest gluten concentration. The typical morphologic changes illustrated in Fig. 308-4 are characteristic of nontropical sprue but are not specific. Similar changes have been described in other conditions, including lymphoma, tropical sprue, and hypogammaglobulinemia associated with malabsorption. Many biochemical abnormalities have been demonstrated in mucosal biopsy specimens from nontropical sprue patients. Impaired esterification of fatty acids to triglycerides, decreased uptake of amino acids, and decreased activity of intestinal disaccharidases (especially lactase) have been well documented. The latter observation may account for the high incidence of milk intolerance in untreated sprue patients or those in relapse. However, the greater abundance of undifferentiated crypt cells may be important, since crypt cells normally have a decreased capacity for nutrient uptake than villus cells.

Since the mucosa is damaged and altered in patients with nontropical sprue, there may be *decreased release of pancreatic tropic hormones* (secretin and cholecystokinin-pancreozymin). This results in decreased stimulation of the pancreas with lower than normal intraluminal levels of pancreatic enzymes in response to a meal. In addition, the gallbladder appears to be resistant to the action of cholecystokinin, resulting in absent or minimal contractions of the gallbladder, in turn leading to sequestration of bile salts in an inert gallbladder. These two defects may result in impaired intraluminal digestion of fat and protein, which will be superimposed on the defect in intestinal transport caused by a damaged mucosa.

Diarrhea is common in sprue patients and is due to a number of factors, including *impaired absorption* of salt and water by duodenum and jejunum, net *secretion* of water and electrolytes by an abnormally permeable jejunal mucosa, and net colonic secretion of water and electrolytes induced by unabsorbed fatty acids and hydroxy fatty acids. However, the distal small intestine in sprue has the ability to adapt to the damage and loss of absorptive capacity in the proximal small intestine. Indeed, increased ileal absorption of sodium, chloride, and water has been demonstrated in sprue patients.

CLINICAL FEATURES Most patients with nontropical sprue will have a typical malabsorption syndrome characterized by weight loss, abdominal distention and bloating, diarrhea, steatorrhea, and abnormal tests of absorptive function. The characteristic alterations in tests of intestinal absorption are outlined in Table 308-2. It should be emphasized, however, that some sprue patients may present with isolated abnormalities which initially do not suggest the diagnosis of nontropical sprue. Thus, a patient may be admitted for investigation of iron-deficiency anemia without apparent blood loss or of abnormal bleeding due to hypoprothrombinemia, but not have diarrhea or overt steatorrhea. Likewise, sprue patients may present with puzzling metabolic bone disease without diarrhea or steatorrhea. Such patients usually complain of bone pain and tenderness and frequently are found to have extensive demineralization of bone, compression deformities, kyphoscoliosis, and Milkman's fractures. Emotional disturbances are common in these patients, and many individuals with a diagnosis of weight loss initially considered related to severe anxiety and depression are subsequently found to have nontropical sprue. In each of the above clinical settings, the diagnosis of sprue should be considered in the differential diagnosis.

Since there is no specific diagnostic test, three criteria should be met in order to establish a definite diagnosis of nontropical sprue: (1) evidence of malabsorption; (2) an abnormal small-bowel (jejunal) biopsy showing blunting and flattening of the villi along with changes in the surface epithelium; and (3) clinical, biochemical, and histologic improvement after institution of a gluten-free diet. In equivocal cases, the patient can be challenged with 30 to 50 g gluten orally, and if this promptly results in increased diarrhea and steatorrhea, the diagnosis of gluten-induced enteropathy is established. It should be emphasized that tests of intestinal absorption may reveal abnormalities which range from very minimal alterations to severe changes. Abnormalities in absorption tests have been shown to correlate reasonably well with the length of small-bowel involvement and to a lesser extent with the severity of the proximal lesion. A possible variant of celiac sprue is *collagenous* sprue. In this disorder small-bowel biopsy specimens characteristically reveal a blunted and flattened mucosa and large masses of eosinophilic hyalin material in the lamina propria. In one study of 349 jejunal biopsy specimens from 145 patients with celiac sprue, 45 (31 percent) showed basement membrane thickening often associated with collagen deposition, but dense collagen deposition was found in only 11 patients. Interestingly, fatal, unremitting malabsorption developed in four of the latter patients. These observations suggest that collagenous membrane thickening is a fairly frequent finding in jejunal biopsies from patients with sprue but that dense collagen deposits are an unusual feature and may indicate a poor prognosis.

TREATMENT Despite the uncertainties concerned with the diagnosis of nontropical sprue, approximately 80 percent of the patients improve after institution of a *gluten-free diet.* Symptomatic improvement usually occurs within a few weeks, but improvement in tests of absorptive function and small-bowel histologic characteristics may not occur for months. It has been repeatedly demonstrated that strict adherence to a gluten-free diet more consistently results in improvement than does suboptimal gluten restriction. Nevertheless, even with strict diet adherence some cases show little improvement in intestinal histologic features. Patients with nontropical sprue treated with corticosteroids but continuing a normal gluten-containing diet have shown symptomatic improvement as well as improvement in intestinal histology and tests of intestinal absorptive function. The mechanism by which corticosteroids protect the mucosa from the effects of gluten is not clear.

If a patient with nontropical sprue does not respond to a gluten-free diet, other possibilities or complicative factors must be considered: (1) the diagnosis is incorrect; (2) the patient is not adhering strictly to the diet; (3) there may be another concurrent disease, such as pancreatic insufficiency; (4) the patient may have ulceration of the jejunum or ileum; (5) lactase deficiency may be present with resultant milk intolerance; (6) the patient may have collagenous sprue; or (7) he or she may have developed intestinal lymphoma, a disease which appears to occur more frequently in sprue than in the general population. Finally, it should be emphasized that a small number of patients show a markedly delayed response to a gluten-free diet, with significant improvement occurring only after 24 to 36 months of therapy. Approximately 50 percent of patients with refractory sprue respond to corticosteroids; such patients may also require parenteral hyperalimentation.

Disaccharidase deficiency syndromes As indicated above, the hydrolysis of disaccharides occurs on or within the brush border (microvilli) of intestinal epithelial cells by specific disaccharidases located there. As would be anticipated, both primary (genetic or familial) and secondary (acquired) deficiencies of these disaccharidases have been observed.

LACTASE DEFICIENCY IN THE ADULT Instances of isolated deficiency of mucosal lactase occur which are associated with symptoms of lactose intolerance. Since lactose is the principal carbohydrate of milk, such individuals show milk intolerance with symptoms of abdominal cramps, bloating or distention, and diarrhea. Similar symptoms will occur following the ingestion of lactose. The symptoms are due to the fact that lactose when not hydrolyzed is not absorbed, and its osmotic effect in the lumen leads to shifts of fluid into the intestinal tract. The pH of the stool will also decrease because of the production of lactic acid and short-chain fatty acids from the fermentation of lactose by colonic bacteria. Although primary intestinal lactase deficiency seems to be hereditary, lactose or milk intolerance may not become clinically evident until puberty or late adolescence. There are significant racial differences in the incidence of this entity. It would appear that about 5 to 15 percent of the adult white population shows intestinal lactase deficiency, but in American Negroes, Bantus, and Orientals, the incidence has been reported as high as 80 to 90 percent.

The diagnosis may be suspected when one obtains a history of gastrointestinal symptoms following milk ingestion. It should be emphasized that the ingestion of only moderate amounts of lactose, e.g., 5 to 12 g or the amount contained in 100 to 240 ml milk, often results in symptoms. Bloating, cramps, and flatulence, but not diarrhea, are usually produced with ingestion of small to moderate amounts of lactose. The vast majority of lactose-intolerant patients are aware that they are milk-intolerant and avoid milk. That these symptoms are not due to allergic reactions to the proteins in milk (i.e., milk allergy or hypersensitivity) can be demonstrated by performing a lactose tolerance test. This test consists of administering an oral dose of lactose (usually from 0.75 to 1.5 g per kilogram of body weight) and obtaining serial blood samples for measurements of blood glucose. In a positive test, intestinal symptoms occur, and the blood glucose increases less than 20 mg/dl above the fasting level. However, false-positive and -negative tests occur in 20 percent of normal subjects because the test is influenced by gastric emptying and glucose metabolism. Measurement of breath hydrogen after ingestion of 50 g lactose is a more sensitive and specific test. The rationale for this test is that unabsorbed lactose is converted to hydrogen by colonic bacteria and breath hydrogen excretion subsequently rises. The test is noninvasive and is not influenced by gastric emptying or metabolic factors.

Acquired lactase deficiency is often seen in association with a variety of gastrointestinal diseases, in many of which there is histologic evidence of mucosal damage. The disorders in which lactose intolerance and lactase deficiency may occur include nontropical and tropical sprue, regional enteritis, bacterial infections of the intestinal tract, giardiasis, abetalipoproteinemia, cystic fibrosis, and ulcerative colitis.

DEFICIENCY OF OTHER DISACCHARIDASES Damage to the intestinal mucosa may produce decreased levels of other disaccharidases such as sucrase-isomaltase, but usually these are not as depressed as lactase, and symptoms of specific intolerance, such as sucrose intolerance, are uncommon. There are instances of primary and apparently hereditary sucrose intolerance, but these always occur in association with sucrase-isomaltase deficiency.

Hypogammaglobulinemia Malabsorption may be associated with hypogammaglobulinemia or agammaglobulinemia. The hypogammaglobulinemia may be of the congenital or the acquired type, with the onset either in childhood or adulthood. When malabsorption has been noted, it has included impaired absorption of fat, D-xylose, and vitamin B_{12}. Peroral intestinal biopsy may reveal changes comparable to those seen in nontropical sprue, but often one finds a more striking mononuclear infiltrate giving a nodular appearance to the mucosa both microscopically and macroscopically. Diarrhea and steatorrhea may precede or follow the development of hypogammaglobulinemia, and these may worsen during infections and subside after the infection is controlled with antibiotics. Intestinal infestation with *Giardia lamblia* is common in hypogammaglobulinemic patients. Meticulous collection and culture of intestinal fluids has revealed excessive numbers of anaerobic bacteria in the small bowel of some patients with hypogammaglobulinemia. However, the relationship between such overgrowth with anaerobes and diarrhea and steatorrhea remains to be clarified. Arthritis, resembling rheumatoid arthritis, and thymoma have also been described in patients with this syndrome. In some patients improvement in diarrhea and malabsorption may occur spontaneously, whereas in others improvement may follow treatment with a gluten-free diet, corticosteroids, antibiotics, injections of gammaglobulin, and cholestyramine. These forms of therapy have not been uniformly successful. Although transient improvement is common, complete cessation of symptoms is distinctly unusual.

The relationship between hypogammaglobulinemia and malabsorption remains obscure. There is no evidence to date indicating that excessive enteric loss of gammaglobulin or alteration of the intestinal microflora occurs, but abnormalities in IgA metabolism may be important in this syndrome. This immunoglobulin is the predominant one in the intestinal mucosa and is found in many exocrine secretions, including tears, saliva, gastric juice, and intestinal juice. A few patients have been described with malabsorption and selective deficiency of IgA.

Abetalipoproteinemia See Chap. 103.

Hartnup disease, cystinuria See Chap. 93.

ENDOCRINE AND METABOLIC DISORDERS Diabetes mellitus The occurrence of diarrhea and steatorrhea in patients with diabetes mellitus has been well documented. When steatorrhea accompanies diabetes, it may be due to the presence of (1) exocrine pancreatic insufficiency, (2) coexistent nontropical sprue, (3) abnormal bacterial proliferation in the proximal small bowel, or (4) severe and uncontrolled diabetes per se (e.g., so-called diabetic diarrhea). Patients falling into the first three categories will usually respond in a satisfactory manner to treatment with pancreatic extracts, a gluten-free diet, and antibiotics, respectively. The pathogenesis of diarrhea and steatorrhea in patients in the fourth category remains poorly understood, and the response to various forms of therapy has been quite variable. It has been demonstrated that patients with diabetic diarrhea and steatorrhea may have involvement of the autonomic nervous system with degenerative changes in the sympathetic and parasympathetic nerves and ganglia. In some patients bacterial overgrowth in the stomach and proximal small bowel may occur and contribute to the diarrhea and steatorrhea.

The clinical features in patients with diarrhea and steatorrhea due to diabetes per se seem to be fairly uniform. Diabetes usually develops at a young age and is often severe and difficult to control. There is a distinct predominance of males. Several signs of autonomic neuropathy are usually present, including postural hypotension, anhydrosis, impotence, and bladder irregularities. Peripheral vascular disease and peripheral neuropathy are also common. Gastrointestinal x-rays may show delayed gastric emptying and disordered transit through the small bowel. Peroral small-bowel biopsy specimens are normal. Tests of intestinal absorptive function are normal except for steatorrhea and azotorrhea. There has been no consistent response to therapy with pancreatic extracts, gluten-free diet, or corticosteroids. When bacterial overgrowth is present, broad-spectrum antibiotics may be helpful.

Hypoparathyroidism Steatorrhea has been documented in several patients with idiopathic hypoparathyroidism. In addition to hypocalcemia, impaired absorption of D-xylose and vitamin B_{12}, decreased serum iron values, and abnormal small-intestinal roentgenograms have been demonstrated in some cases. In such patients the serum phosphorus level is elevated (due to the hypoparathyroidism) rather than low (as in primary malabsorption). The cause of malabsorption in this disorder is unclear.

Adrenal insufficiency Although there are few studies on fat excretion in adrenal insufficiency in man, malabsorption, especially of fat, appears to occur more frequently than has been generally appreciated. Patients with adrenal insufficiency have been found to have steatorrhea which was corrected by therapy with adrenal corticosteroids.

Hyperthyroidism There are few detailed studies on intestinal absorptive function in patients with hyperthyroidism. Mild to moderate steatorrhea and hypoalbuminemia have been reported, but absorption of D-xylose and vitamin B_{12} is frequently normal. Steatorrhea usually remits after successful treatment of hyperthyroidism. Clinical studies suggest that steatorrhea in hyperthyroidism is not due to any defect of pancreatic, biliary, or small-intestinal mucosal function, but is a result of hyperphagia with ingestion of unusually large amounts of fat occurring in association with rapid gastric emptying and intestinal transit.

Ulcerogenic tumor of the pancreas (Zollinger-Ellison syndrome) The clinical features of ulcerogenic tumor of the pancreas are described in Chap. 306. Malabsorption is frequently found in this disease. The acidification and dilution of intestinal contents caused by gastric acid hypersecretion leads to major disturbances in fat digestion and absorption. Impaired formation of micellar lipid due to inactivation of pancreatic lipase is probably the major factor in the production of steatorrhea. Other factors contributing to fat malabsorption in this disorder include (1) precipitation of glycine conjugated bile salts due to low intraluminal pH, (2) alteration of the intestinal mucosa with ulceration and metaplasia, and (3) impaired fatty acid esterification and chylomicron formation.

Carcinoid syndrome (see Chap. 131) Although diarrhea is common in the carcinoid syndrome, malabsorption with significant steatorrhea is unusual. In many of the cases of carcinoid syndrome with steatorrhea there has been a prior intestinal resection (usually ileal), and in these cases the resection is the important factor in the causation of steatorrhea. However, direct involvement of the bowel wall and mesentery by the carcinoid tumor have been well documented. That abnormalities in serotonin metabolism may also be important is suggested from the decrease in the steatorrhea observed in some of these patients when treated with the antiserotonin drug methysergide. Although side effects may occur, for control of diarrhea and steatorrhea, patients may be given a trial of 8 to 12 mg methysergide per day.

DRUG-INDUCED ABSORPTIVE DEFECTS See Table 308-8.

PROTEIN-LOSING ENTEROPATHY The gastrointestinal tract has been shown to play a significant role in the metabolism and physiologic degradation of plasma proteins. The exact magnitude of the normal gastrointestinal protein loss in man has remained unclear, but studies with ^{125}I-labeled and ^{51}Cr-labeled albumin have suggested that between 10 and 20 percent of the normal turnover of albumin may be accounted for by enteric protein loss. However, under certain pathologic conditions, excessive gastrointestinal protein loss may develop. An extensive number of disorders have been found to be associated with intestinal protein loss. Some of these are listed in Table 308-9.

Pathophysiology Several mechanisms have been proposed for the passage of plasma proteins across the gastrointestinal mucosa, both normally and in certain disease states. First, plasma proteins may pass into the gastrointestinal tract through an inflamed or ulcerated mucosa and account for the protein loss occasionally seen in regional enteritis and ulcerative colitis. Second, plasma protein loss may occur as a result of disordered mucosal cell structure. For example, patients with nontropical sprue have abnormal villous structure and surface epithelium, and these changes could facilitate the diffusion of plasma protein between the cells. Third, in the presence of increased lymphatic pressure, there may be increased passage of plasma proteins into the lumen via the intercellular spaces of the mucosal epithelium. This might be expected to occur in disorders in which there is granulomatous or neoplastic involvement of lymphatics. Fourth, dilated lymph vessels in the mucosa may rupture through the surface epithelium, discharging their contents into the intestinal lumen. This is thought to be important in the pathogenesis of steatorrhea and hypoproteinemia in patients with idiopathic intestinal lymphangiectasia (see "Intestinal Lymphangiectasia" below).

Several techniques have been developed for the detection and quantitation of gastrointestinal protein loss. Most of these involve the use of intravenously administered radioactive-labeled macromolecules such as ^{125}I-labeled serum albumin, $^{51}CrCl_3$, ^{51}Cr-labeled albumin, and indium 111. ^{111}In-labeled transferrin and $^{51}CrCl_3$ (which rapidly become attached to cir-

TABLE 308-8
Some drug-induced absorptive defects

Drug	*Absorptive defect*
Antacids	Phosphorus
Anticonvulsants	Folates
Biguanides (DBI)	Glucose, amino acids, vitamin B_{12}
Cholestyramine	Warfarin, thyroid hormone, cardiac glycosides, phenylbutazone
Colchicine	Xylose, vitamin B_{12}, cholesterol
Ethanol	Xylose, vitamin B_{12}, folate, glucose, amino acids
Methotrexate	Xylose, folic acid
Neomycin	Fatty acids, xylose, vitamin B_{12}
p-Aminosalicylic acid (PAS)	Cholesterol, vitamin B_{12}
Sulfasalazine	Folate
Tetracycline	Ferrous ions

SOURCE: *Longstreth and Newcomer.*

TABLE 308-9
Disorders associated with protein-losing enteropathy

I Stomach
- *A* Gastric carcinoma
- *B* Giant hypertrophy of the gastric mucosa
- *C* Atrophic gastritis
- *D* Postgastrectomy syndrome

II Small intestine
- *A* Intestinal lymphangiectasia
- *B* Nontropical sprue
- *C* Tropical sprue
- *D* Regional enteritis
- *E* Whipple's disease
- *F* Lymphoma
- *G* Intestinal tuberculosis
- *H* Acute infectious enteritis
- *I* Scleroderma
- *J* Jejunal diverticulosis
- *K* Allergic gastroenteropathy

III Colon
- *A* Colonic neoplasm
- *B* Ulcerative colitis
- *C* Granulomatous colitis
- *D* Megacolon

IV Cardiac
- *A* Congestive heart failure
- *B* Constrictive pericarditis
- *C* Interatrial septal defect
- *D* Primary cardiomyopathy

V Miscellaneous
- *A* Esophageal carcinoma
- *B* Gastrocolic fistula
- *C* Agammaglobulinemia
- *D* Nephrosis

culating transferrin) are the compounds available commercially for clinical use. After the intravenous administration of 0.93 to 1.11 MBq (25 to 30 μCi) of the labeled compound to normal subjects, between 0.1 and 0.7 percent of the administered radioactivity is recovered in the stool over a 4-day period. Patients with excessive enteric protein loss may excrete from 2 to 40 percent of the injected radioactive label. False-positive results may be obtained if the stool specimen is contaminated with urine.

Using intravenously administered radioiodinated albumin, the decline in radioactivity in the serum and whole body can be followed, and the rate of albumin synthesis and degradation determined. Such studies carried out in patients with protein-losing enteropathies have demonstrated a reduced circulating (intravascular) and total-body pool of albumin, a normal or increased rate of albumin synthesis, markedly shortened albumin survival, and increased fecal protein loss. Whereas normal subjects catabolize 5 to 10 percent of their intravascular albumin pool each day (the fractional catabolic rate), patients with excessive enteric protein loss may have fractional catabolic rates of 50 to 60 percent.

Studies utilizing radioiodinated immunoglobulins have demonstrated a decreased intravascular globulin pool and increased fractional catabolic rate. However, the synthesis of IgG is usually normal, suggesting that a decreased level of IgG and increased enteric protein loss is not a potent stimulus for IgG synthesis. The increase in fractional catabolic rate is comparable for albumin, IgG, and IgM immunoglobulins, further suggesting that there is bulk loss of plasma proteins into the intestinal tract and not a selective loss of certain proteins. The finding of decreased globulins often is an ancillary aid in excluding renal, cardiac, and hepatic cases of hypoalbuminemia.

Abnormalities in albumin and globulin metabolism in patients with a protein-losing enteropathy may be reversed or diminished within a few months after the institution of appropriate therapy. It is obviously important that a specific etiologic diagnosis should be established in all patients with treatable disorders, who may be expected to have a remission induced by the appropriate therapy for the underlying disease. The intestinal protein loss in patients with nontropical sprue, Whipple's disease, constrictive pericarditis, regional enteritis, ulcerative colitis, and Ménétrier's disease has been ameliorated by therapy appropriate for the underlying disorder.

Intestinal lymphangiectasia PATHOPHYSIOLOGY The disorder intestinal lymphangiectasia is characterized by increased enteric loss of protein, hypoproteinemia, edema, lymphocytopenia, malabsorption, and abnormal dilated lymphatic channels in the small intestine. The high incidence of chylous effusions and abnormal peripheral, retroperitoneal, and thoracic lymphatics indicates that intestinal lymphangiectasia is part of a generalized congenital disorder of the lymphatic system. It has been suggested that the hypoplastic visceral lymphatic channels result in obstruction to lymph flow, with the subsequent development of increased intestinal lymphatic pressure. This in turn may lead to dilated lymphatic vessels throughout the small-bowel wall and mesentery. Hypoproteinemia and steatorrhea are thought to be due to rupture of the dilated lymphatic vessels with discharge of lymph into the bowel lumen. In adults approximately 1500 ml lymph, containing 70 g fat and 50 g albumin, passes through the thoracic duct each day. The leakage of a small amount of this lymph might be expected to result in considerable loss of protein and fat into the intestinal lumen. In addition, absorption of dietary long-chain triglycerides stimulates lymph flow, and this may increase further the retrograde leakage of intestinal lymph into the lumen. Three lines of evidence support the concept of intestinal leakage of lymph in intestinal lymphangiectasia: (1) chylous fluid has been recovered from the duodenum in these patients; (2) retrograde passage of contrast material from retroperitoneal lymphatics into the duodenum and jejunum has been documented; and (3) significant steatorrhea may persist in patients after institution of a completely fat-free diet, suggesting an increased enteric loss of endogenous fat present in lymph.

CLINICAL FEATURES The disease affects primarily children and young adults. All patients have edema, which may be asymmetrical because of hypoplastic peripheral lymphatics. Chylous effusions and diarrhea are common symptoms. The primary laboratory finding is hypoproteinemia with decreased serum levels of albumin, immunoglobulins IgG, IgA, and IgM, transferrin, and ceruloplasmin. Despite moderate to severe hypogammaglobulinemia there does not appear to be an increased incidence of pyogenic bacterial infections. In addition, circulating antibody response to challenge with *Brucella* and typhoid antigens is normal. Steatorrhea is usually mild, although in some instances fat loss may be as much as 40 g per day. Some patients have hypocalcemia and impaired absorption of vitamin B_{12}. Lymphocytopenia (due to the loss of lymphocytes in lymph) is common, with lymphocyte counts ranging from 400 to 1000 per milliliter (normal: 1500 to 4000 per milliliter). This is associated with abnormal delayed hypersensitivity, as evidenced by prolonged homograft survival and impaired cutaneous responsiveness to antigens such as mumps and monilia.

Small-bowel roentgenograms are frequently abnormal, showing changes of mucosal edema and a malabsorption pattern. Lymphangiograms may demonstrate hypoplastic peripheral and visceral lymphatics with the absence of groups of retroperitoneal lymph nodes. Specimens of jejunal mucosa characteristically reveal dilated and telangiectatic lymphatic vessels in the lamina propria and submucosa. The villi may be club-shaped because of distortion from grossly dilated lymphatics (Fig. 308-4). Such changes in the intestinal mucosa may be reversed after appropriate therapy. The diagnosis of intestinal lymphangiectasia is therefore established by

(1) small-intestinal biopsy and (2) demonstration of increased enteric protein loss using radioactive macromolecules.

TREATMENT A low-fat diet, by decreasing lymph flow, usually results in significant improvement with decreased fecal fat excretion, decreased enteric protein loss, increased serum calcium and albumin levels, and an increased half-life of injected ^{125}I-labeled albumin. Similar results may be obtained by the substitution of medium-chain triglycerides (MCT) for dietary long-chain triglycerides, since MCT are transported as medium-chain fatty acids by the portal vein rather than via the lymph.

REFERENCES

AMENT ME et al: Structure and function of the gastrointestinal tract in primary immunodeficiency syndromes. Medicine 52:227, 1973

BAYLESS TM et al: Lactose and milk intolerance: Clinical implications. N Engl J Med 292:1156, 1975

BOND JH, LEVITT MD: Use of breath hydrogen (H_2) in the study of carbohydrate absorption. Am J Dig Dis 22:379, 1977

CALDWELL JH et al: Eosinophilic gastroenteritis with obstruction. Immunological studies of seven patients. Gastroenterology 74:825, 1978

CHUNG YC et al: Protein digestion and absorption in human small intestine. Gastroenterology 76:1415, 1979

COOPER BT et al: Celiac disease and malignancy. Medicine 59:249, 1980

GASKIN KJ et al: Colipase and maximally activated pancreatic lipase in normal subjects and patients with steatorrhea. J Clin Invest 69:368, 1982

GRAY GM: Carbohydrate digestion and malabsorption, in *Physiology of the Gastrointestinal Tract,* LR Johnson et al (eds). New York, Raven, 1981

HOWDLE PD et al: Cell-mediated immunity to gluten within the small intestinal mucosa in coeliac disease. Gut 23:115, 1982

KLIPSTEIN FA: Tropical sprue in travelers and expatriates living abroad. Gastroenterology 80:590, 1981

LONGSTRETH GF, NEWCOMER AD: Drug-induced malabsorption. Mayo Clin Proc 50:284, 1975

MACGREGOR I et al: Gastric emptying of liquid meals and pancreatic and biliary secretion after subtotal gastrectomy or truncal vagotomy and pyloroplasty in man. Gastroenterology 72:195, 1977

NEWCOMER AD et al: Triolein breath test. A sensitive and specific test for fat malabsorption. Gastroenterology 76:6, 1979

RIEPE SP et al: Effect of secreted *Bacteroides* proteases on human intestinal brush border hydrolases. J Clin Invest 66:314, 1980

TRIER JS et al: Celiac sprue and refractory sprue. Gastroenterology 75:307, 1978

WESER E et al: Short bowel syndrome. Gastroenterology 77:572, 1979

309 INFLAMMATORY BOWEL DISEASE

Ulcerative colitis and Crohn's disease

ROBERT M. GLICKMAN

DEFINITION

Inflammatory bowel disease (IBD) is a general term for a group of chronic inflammatory disorders of unknown etiology involving the gastrointestinal tract. Since there are no pathognomonic features or specific diagnostic tests, in a strict sense, these disorders remain diagnoses of exclusion. Their features are sufficiently characteristic, however, to permit accurate diagnosis in the majority of cases. Chronic IBD may be divided into two major groups, chronic nonspecific *ulcerative colitis* and *Crohn's disease.* The original description of the disease by Crohn, Ginzberg, and Oppenheimer in 1932 localized the disease to segments of ileum. However, the same process may involve the buccal mucosa, esophagus, stomach, and duodenum as well as the jejunum and ileum. Crohn's disease of the small bowel is also known as *regional enteritis.* In addition, a similar inflammatory picture may occur in the colon, either alone or with accompanying small-intestinal involvement. In most instances, this form of colitis can be distinguished clinically and pathologically from ulcerative colitis and is also referred to as *Crohn's disease of the colon.* Granulomatous colitis is a less accurate term since only a portion of cases exhibit granulomas. Clinically these disorders are characterized by recurrent inflammatory involvement of intestinal segments with diverse clinical manifestations and often resulting in a chronic, unpredictable course.

EPIDEMIOLOGY

The epidemiologic and etiologic considerations in ulcerative colitis and Crohn's disease share many features in common and will be discussed together. These diseases are more common in Caucasians than in blacks and orientals with an increased incidence (three- to sixfold) in Jews compared to non-Jews. Both sexes are equally affected.

The incidence and prevalence of the two diseases differ slightly with most studies showing ulcerative colitis to be more common. When analyzed in western Europe and the United States, ulcerative colitis (including ulcerative proctitis) has an incidence of approximately 6 to 8 cases per 100,000 population and an estimated prevalence of approximately 70 to 150 cases per 100,000 population. Estimates of the incidence of Crohn's disease (colonic plus small bowel) are approximately 2 cases per 100,000 population; the prevalence is estimated at 20 to 40 per 100,000 population. Although there is no firm documentation, many believe the incidence of Crohn's disease (especially colonic) to be increasing.

While peak occurrence of both diseases is between ages 15 and 35, it has been reported in every decade of life. A familial incidence of IBD has been recorded with estimates that 2 to 5 percent of persons with Crohn's disease or ulcerative colitis will have one or more relatives affected. There is no specificity however, for a given form of IBD within a given family. Such epidemiologic clustering of cases could argue for either genetic or common environmental influences on the development of these diseases (see below). It has been suggested that there is a probable hereditary basis for these disorders plus a strong environmental component.

ETIOLOGY AND PATHOGENESIS

While the cause of ulcerative colitis and Crohn's disease remains unknown, certain features of these diseases have suggested several areas of possible etiologic importance. These include familial or genetic, infectious, immunologic, and psychological factors.

Inflammatory bowel disease is more common in whites, occurs with an increased frequency in Jews, and exhibits some familial clustering. This suggests that there may be a *genetic* predisposition to the development of the disease. In addition, the disease has been described in monozygotic twins. A search for genetic markers which might be of value in identifying susceptible individuals has not identified any single marker (i.e., histocompatibility antigen) in patients with inflammatory bowel disease.

The chronic inflammatory nature of these diseases has prompted a continuing search for a possible *infectious etiology.*

In spite of numerous attempts to find known bacterial, fungal, or viral agents, no etiologic agent has thus far been isolated. Preliminary reports of isolates of cell wall variants of *Pseudomonas* or of transmissible agents producing cytopathic effects in tissue culture have yet to be confirmed. Efforts to produce specific granulomatous tissue reactions with filtrates from Crohn's disease tissue have yielded conflicting and nonreproducible results. As discussed below, many infectious agents can produce *acute* colitis or ileitis; however, there is no evidence that these agents are involved in *chronic* inflammatory bowel disease.

The theory that an *immune* mechanism may be involved is based on the concept that the extraintestinal manifestations which may accompany these disorders (e.g., arthritis, pericholangitis) may represent autoimmune phenomena and that therapeutic agents, such as corticosteroids and azathioprine, may exert their effects via immunosuppressive mechanisms. Patients with inflammatory bowel disease may have *humoral antibodies* to colon cells, bacterial antigens such as *Escherichia coli*, lipopolysaccharide, and foreign proteins such as cow milk protein. In general, the presence and titer of these antibodies does not correlate with disease activity. It is likely that these antigens gain access to immunocompetent cells secondary to epithelial damage. In addition, IBD has been described in association with agammaglobulinemia as well as IgA deficiency, casting further doubt on the pathogenetic role of humoral antibodies. *Immune complexes* have also been invoked to explain extraintestinal manifestations of IBD. While there are well-defined examples of tissue injury resulting from immune complexes, studies utilizing specific detection techniques have failed to demonstrate an increased frequency of immune complexes in patients with IBD.

Associated abnormalities of *cell-mediated immunity* include cutaneous anergy, diminished responsiveness to various mitogenic stimuli, and decreases in the number of peripheral T cells. Since many of these changes may revert to normal when the disease is quiescent, it is likely that they are secondary phenomena. Experimental colitis has been produced in laboratory animals by prior sensitization with dinitrochlorobenzene, suggesting a T-cell–dependent mechanism of tissue injury. It remains to be determined whether the regulation of immune function (e.g., suppressor T cells) is of pathogenic importance in the etiology of IBD. Thus far, none of the altered immunologic findings have been specific for either ulcerative colitis or Crohn's disease.

FIGURE 309-1
Ulcerative colitis. Resected colon with portion of terminal ileum. The specimen showed uniform inflammation, erythema, and hemorrhage and a normal terminal ileum.

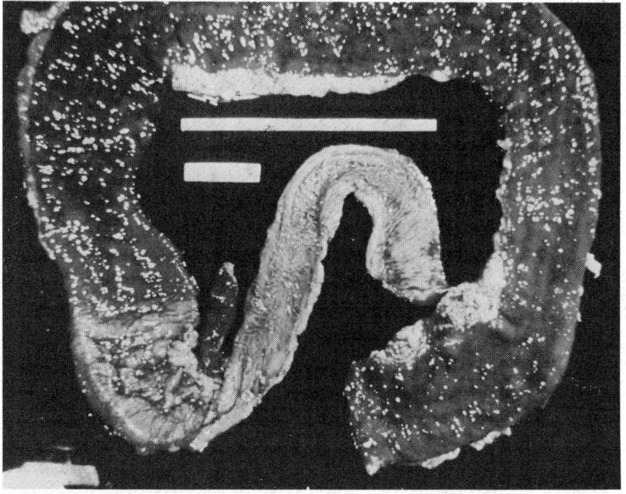

The *psychological* features of patients with inflammatory bowel disease have also been stressed. It is not uncommon for these diseases to present initially or to flare in association with major psychological stresses such as the loss of a family member. It has been suggested that patients with IBD have a characteristic personality which renders them susceptible to emotional stresses which in turn may precipitate or exacerbate their symptoms. While there is little evidence directly relating possible emotional factors to the etiology of inflammatory bowel disease, there is little doubt that a chronic disease of unknown etiology affecting individuals in the prime of their life often results in feelings of anger, anxiety, and some degree of depression. These reactions are undoubtedly important factors in modifying the course of these diseases and in the response to therapy.

PATHOLOGY

In ulcerative colitis there is an inflammatory reaction primarily involving the colonic mucosa. Grossly, the colon appears ulcerated, hyperemic, and usually hemorrhagic (Fig. 309-1). A striking feature of the inflammation is that it is *uniform* and *continuous* with no intervening areas of normal mucosa. The rectum is usually involved (95 percent of cases) and the inflammation extends proximally in a continuous fashion but for a variable distance. When there is involvement of the entire colon, there may be minimal involvement of a few centimeters of the terminal ileum, referred to as "backwash ileitis." This involvement never leads to the thickening and narrowing characteristic of Crohn's disease. The surface mucosal cells as well as the crypt epithelium and submucosa are involved in an inflammatory reaction with neutrophilic infiltration (Fig. 309-2*A*). This progresses to epithelial damage with loss of surface epithelial cells resulting in multiple ulcerations. Infiltration of the crypts with neutrophils results in characteristic (but not specific) small crypt abscesses and their eventual destruction. There may also be loss of crypt epithelium with a loss of goblet (mucus-producing) cells and submucosal edema. With repetitive cycles of inflammation, mild submucosal fibrosis develops. Regenerative activity is evidenced by irregular crypt epithelium often showing bifurcation at the base of the crypts. It is important to stress that unlike Crohn's disease, deeper layers of the bowel beneath the submucosa usually are not involved. In severe ulcerative colitis, as seen with toxic megacolon, the bowel wall may become extremely thin, the mucosa denuded with inflammation extending to the serosa leading to dilatation and subsequent perforation.

Recurrent inflammation may lead to characteristic features of chronicity. Fibrosis and longitudinal retraction result in shortening of the colon. Loss of the normal haustral pattern leads radiologically to a smooth, "lead-pipe" appearance of the colon. Regenerating islands of mucosa surrounded by areas of ulceration and denuded mucosa appear as "polyps" protruding into the lumen of the colon. However, these protrusions are inflammatory in nature and not neoplastic and are therefore called pseudopolyps (Fig. 309-2*B*).

With long-standing ulcerative colitis, the surface epithelium may show features of *dysplasia.* Changes of nuclear and cellular atypia are thought to represent a premalignant change occurring in the setting of long-standing ulcerative colitis. Marked dysplasia in colonic biopsies in the setting of long-standing colitis is associated with a significant risk of a coexistent carcinoma elsewhere in the colon and may influence the decision to advise colectomy.

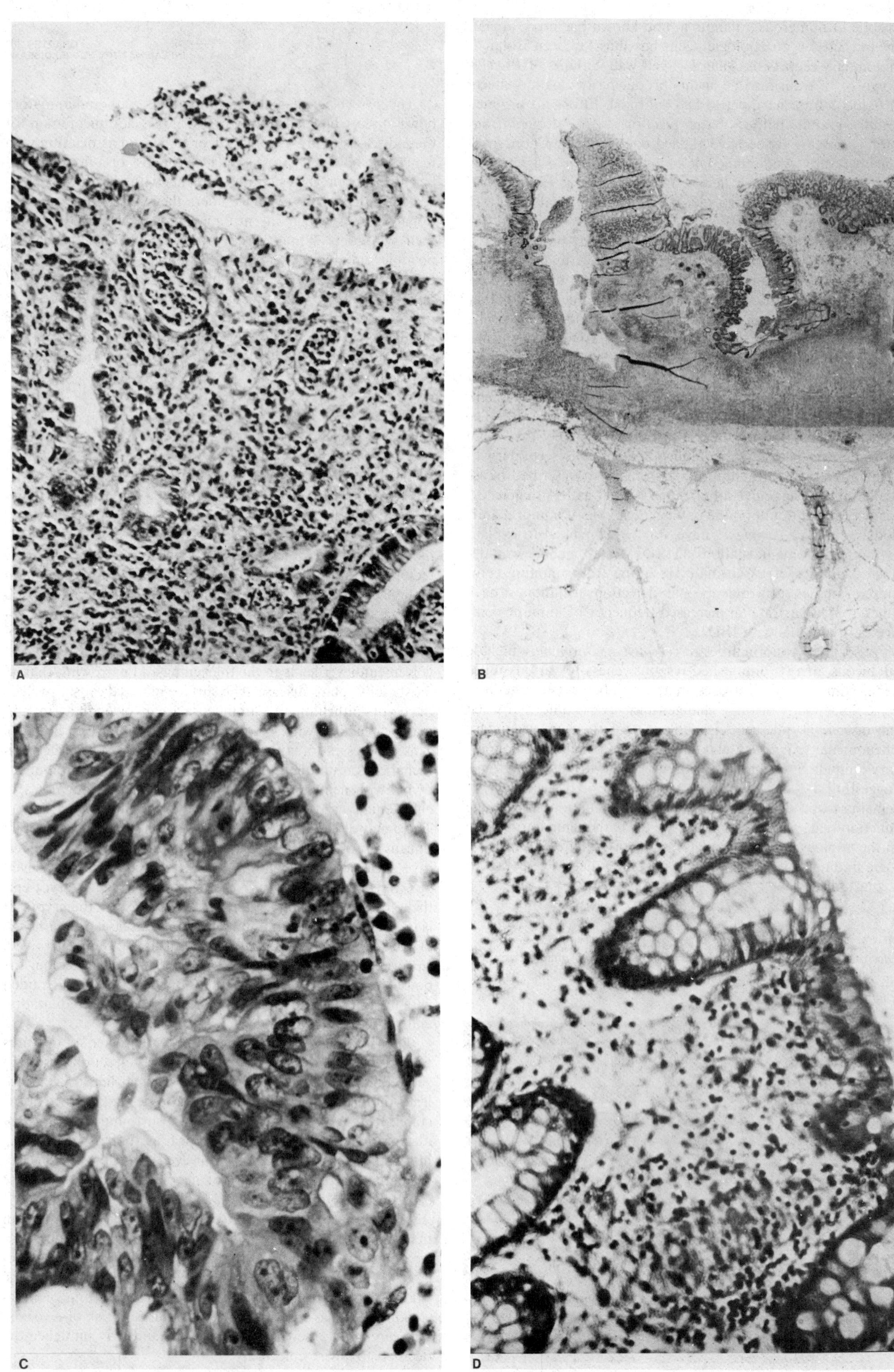
A
B
C
D

Crohn's disease, in contrast to ulcerative colitis, is characterized by chronic inflammation extending through *all layers of the intestinal wall* and involving the mesentery as well as regional lymph nodes. Whether or not the small bowel or colon is involved, the basic pathologic process is the same.

The earliest pathologic changes in Crohn's disease are poorly defined since surgery is usually not electively undertaken early in the course of the disease. At laparotomy, the terminal ileum appears hyperemic and boggy, with mesentery and mesenteric lymph nodes swollen and reddened. At this early stage, the bowel wall, although edematous, is usually pliable. While some patients with this initial presentation will subsequently develop typical regional enteritis, a significant number will recover completely. This acute form of ileitis will undoubtedly be shown to have diverse etiologies. Indeed, approximately 80 percent of patients with this presentation have been shown to be infected with *Yersinia enterocolitica,* an organism capable of producing a self-limited, acute inflammatory ileitis.

As the disease progresses, the gross appearance assumes a characteristic picture. The bowel appears greatly thickened and leathery with the lumen narrowed (Fig. 309-3). This characteristic stenosis can occur in any portion of the intestine and may be associated with varying degrees of intestinal obstruction. The mesentery appears greatly thickened, fatty, and often extends over the serosal surface of the bowel in characteristic finger-like projections. The appearance of the mucosa is variable, depending on the severity and stage of the disease, but may appear relatively normal in sharp contrast to ulcerative colitis. In more advanced cases, the mucosa has a nodular, "cobblestoned" look. This is the result of submucosal thickening and mucosal ulceration, often linear in the long axis of the bowel at the base of mucosal folds. These ulcerations may penetrate into the submucosa and muscularis and coalesce to form intramural channels which become manifested as fistulas and fissures.

There are other morphological features distinguishing Crohn's disease from ulcerative colitis. In Crohn's disease, the disease is often *discontinuous;* severely involved segments of bowel are separated from each other with intervening segments of apparently normal bowel, producing "skip areas." In approximately 50 percent of Crohn's disease of the colon, the rectum may be spared. In sharp contrast, in ulcerative colitis the involvement is contiguous and the rectum is almost always involved. In addition, in Crohn's disease the transmural inflammatory process, involving serosa and mesentery, also accounts for the characteristic fistula and abscess formation. As a result of serosal inflammation, adjacent loops of small intestine may become adherent and matted together by a fibrinous peritoneal reaction, leading to palpable mass, most often in the right lower quadrant. Fistula formation may occur between adherent loops of intestine, colon, or other adjacent organs such as the bladder or vagina. Fistulous tracts may also lead to the skin or end blindly within the peritoneum or retroperitoneum, surrounded by adherent loops of bowel and inflammatory tissue. Fistula formation is not seen in ulcerative colitis.

Microscopically, granulomas are most helpful in distinguishing Crohn's disease from other forms of inflammatory bowel disease; they do not occur in ulcerative colitis. They may be seen in rectal or colonoscopic biopsies (Fig. 309-2*D*). While granulomas are a helpful finding when present, it is the chronic inflammation involving all layers of the intestinal wall which is most characteristic.

In most series reporting the distribution of Crohn's disease, approximately 30 percent will involve the small intestine (usually the terminal ileum) without colonic disease, 30 percent with only colonic involvement, and 40 percent with ileocolic involvement usually of the ileum and right colon. In a small number of patients (mostly children and adolescents) there may be diffuse and extensive ulceration of the jejunum and ileum.

While there often are sufficient features to enable the distinction between ulcerative colitis and Crohn's disease of the colon (Table 309-1), in 10 to 20 percent of cases this distinction may not be possible.

FIGURE 309-2
Colonic biopsies in inflammatory bowel disease. A. Ulcerative colitis. The surface mucosa is destroyed and the submucosa is diffusely infiltrated with polymorphonuclear leukocytes. Crypt abscesses are also present. B. Pseudopolyp. Regenerating island of mucosa with adjacent area of ulceration. C. Ulcerative colitis. Severe dysplasia occurring in long-standing chronic ulcerative colitis. Note atypical changes in the nuclei and marked palisading of nuclei of the crypt epithelium. D. Crohn's disease of the colon. Note the relatively intact mucosa with a solitary granuloma in the submucosa.

CLINICAL FEATURES

ULCERATIVE COLITIS The major symptoms of ulcerative colitis are bloody diarrhea and abdominal pain, often with fever and weight loss in more severe cases. With mild disease, there may be one or two semiformed stools containing little blood and with no systemic manifestations. In contrast, the patient with severe disease may have frequent liquid stools containing blood and pus, complain of severe cramps, and demonstrate symptoms and signs of dehydration, anemia, fever, and weight loss. With predominantly rectal involvement, constipation rather than diarrhea may be present, and tenesmus may be a major complaint. On occasion, intestinal symptoms may be overshadowed by fever, weight loss, or one of the extracolonic manifestations of the disease (see below).

The physical findings in ulcerative colitis are usually nonspecific; there may be some abdominal distention or tenderness along the course of the colon. In mild cases, the general

TABLE 309-1
Pathologic and clinical features of IBD

	Ulcerative colitis	*Crohn's disease*
PATHOLOGIC		
Segmental	0	++
Transmural involvement	+/−	++
Granulomas	0	+/++ (50%)
Fibrosis	+	++
Fissuring, fistulas	+/−	++
Mesenteric fat, lymph node involvement	0	++
CLINICAL		
Diarrhea	++	++
Rectal bleeding	++	+
Abdominal pain	+	++
Palpable mass	0	++
Fistulas	+/−	++
Strictures	+	++
Small-bowel involvement	+/− ("backwash ileitis")	++
Rectal involvement	++ (95%)	+/++ (50%)
Extracolonic disease	+	+
Toxic megacolon	+	+/−
Recurrence after colectomy	0	+
Malignancy (with long-standing disease)	+	+/−

NOTE: *0 = never; +/− = rare; + = occasional; ++ = Frequent, common.*

physical examination will be normal. Extracolonic manifestations include arthritis, skin changes, or evidence of liver disease. Fever, tachycardia, and postural hypotension are usually associated with more severe disease. The laboratory findings are often nonspecific and usually reflect the degree and severity of bleeding and inflammation. There may be anemia which reflects chronic disease as well as iron deficiency from chronic blood loss. Leukocytosis with a left shift and an elevated sedimentation rate are often seen in the severely ill, febrile patient. Electrolyte abnormalities, especially hypokalemia, reflect the degree of diarrhea. Hypoalbuminemia is common with extensive disease and usually represents luminal protein loss through an ulcerated mucosa. An elevated alkaline phosphatase may indicate associated hepatobiliary disease (see below).

The clinical course of ulcerative colitis is variable. The majority of patients will suffer a relapse within 1 year of the first attack, reflecting the recurrent nature of the disease. There may, however, be prolonged periods of remission with only minimal symptoms. In general, the severity of symptoms reflects the extent of colonic involvement and the intensity of the inflammation. At one end of the spectrum are patients who present with limited involvement of the rectum (ulcerative proctitis) or rectum and sigmoid (ulcerative proctosigmoiditis). Consistent with this limited colonic involvement, the disease is usually mild, with minimal systemic or extracolonic manifestations. The major symptoms are rectal bleeding and tenesmus. Most of these patients, especially those with only rectal involvement, will not develop more extensive disease. In the remainder, the disease may extend proximally with variable involvement. Most patients with ulcerative colitis (perhaps 85 percent) will have mild to moderate disease of an intermittent nature and can be managed without hospitalization. In approximately 15 percent of patients, the disease assumes a more fulminant course, involves the entire colon, and presents with severe bloody diarrhea and systemic signs and symptoms. The patients are at risk to develop toxic dilatation and perforation of the colon (described below) and represent a medical emergency.

CROHN'S DISEASE As discussed above, the basic pathologic features of Crohn's disease are the same whether the disease involves the small bowel or colon. The clinical presentation, however, will largely reflect the anatomic location of the disease and to some degree will predict which complications of the disease may develop. The clinical features of ulcerative colitis and Crohn's disease are compared in Table 309-1.

The major clinical features of Crohn's disease are fever, abdominal pain, diarrhea often without blood, and generalized fatigability. There may be associated weight loss. With *colonic involvement* diarrhea and pain are the most frequent symptoms. Rectal bleeding is distinctly less common than with ulcerative colitis and reflects (1) sparing of the rectum in many patients, and (2) the transmural nature of the disease with only irregular mucosal involvement. There may be associated severe anorectal complications such as fistulas, fissures, and perirectal abscess. Such features may antedate the clinical onset of colitis and should always raise the suspicion of associated Crohn's disease. With recurrent perirectal inflammation the anal canal may be thickened and perianal fistulas or scarring may be present. With extensive colonic involvement, dilatation of the colon may occur, since Crohn's disease often results in a thickened colonic wall. However, this is less common with Crohn's disease than with ulcerative colitis. Extracolonic manifestations (discussed below), particularly arthritis, are seen more commonly with colonic than with small-bowel Crohn's disease (regional enteritis).

With involvement of the *small bowel* there may be additional presenting signs and symptoms. Typically, the disease has its onset in a young adult with a history of fatigue, variable weight loss, right lower quadrant discomfort or pain, and diarrhea. Low-grade fever, anorexia, nausea, and vomiting may also be present. The abdominal pain may be steady and localized to the right lower quadrant or may assume a colicky or crampy pattern, reflecting variable degrees of intestinal stenosis. The diarrhea is often moderate, usually without gross blood; if there is no rectal involvement, tenesmus is absent. Physical examination at this time often reveals right lower quadrant tenderness with an associated fullness or mass reflecting adherent loops of bowel. At this time the patient may have mild anemia, mild to moderate leukocytosis, and an elevated sedimentation rate.

Since acute ileitis may have an abrupt onset with fever, leukocytosis, and right lower quadrant pain, the clinical picture may be indistinguishable from acute appendicitis. The diagnosis can be made only at laparotomy, when the characteristic beefy red terminal ileum, boggy mesenteric fat, and succulent mesenteric lymph nodes indicate that appendicitis alone could not produce this picture.

While the symptoms of diarrhea and abdominal pain will usually alert the clinician to the possibility of regional enteritis, other symptoms may dominate the clinical presentation. In children, and the aged, fever of undetermined origin and unexplained weight loss may be prominent and initially may cause one to suspect underlying malignancy. In some patients, the

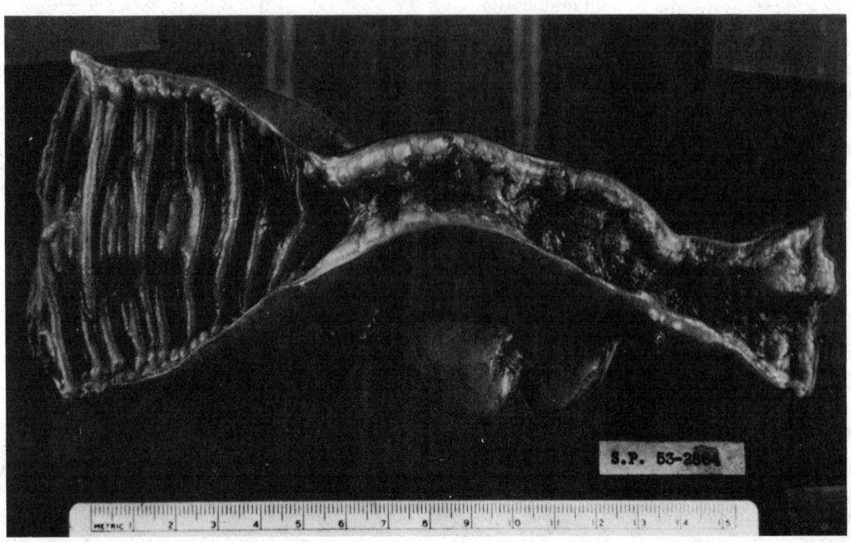

FIGURE 309-3
Regional enteritis. Resected specimen of terminal ileum demonstrates thickened bowel wall and chronically inflamed mucosa. Note the relatively sharp demarcation of the diseased segment with grossly normal mucosa on the left.

first manifestation of the disease may be intestinal obstruction; in others the disease may present with fistula formation in the form of perianal sepsis or urinary tract infection resulting from an enterovesical fistula. Similarly, right ureteral obstruction and hydronephrosis may occur due to external compression of the ureter by a right lower quadrant inflammatory mass. On occasion, often in the setting of extensive small-bowel involvement, features of malabsorption may be prominent. These features, along with anorexia and the catabolic effects of the chronic inflammatory process, may combine to produce striking degrees of weight loss.

The complications of the disease are often local, resulting from intestinal inflammation and involvement of adjacent structures.

Intestinal obstruction is a frequent complication, occurring in 20 to 30 percent of patients during the course of the disease. In the initial stages, the obstruction usually is due to the acute inflammation and edema of the involved intestinal segment, usually the terminal ileum. However, as the disease progresses and fibrosis develops, obstruction may be due to a fixed narrowing of the bowel.

Fistula formation is a frequent complication of chronic regional enteritis as well as Crohn's disease of the colon. Fistulas may occur between contiguous segments of intestine; they may also burrow into the retroperitoneal spaces and present as cutaneous fistulas or indolent abscesses. In a significant number of patients, the first indication of the disease may be the presence of persistent rectal fissures, a perirectal abscess, or a rectal fistula. Although uncommon, pneumaturia should raise the suspicion of enterovesical fistula and is often associated with a persistent urinary tract infection.

Since Crohn's disease is a transmural disease with the bowel wall greatly thickened, free *intestinal perforation* is uncommon. In a small number of cases, however, it may be the presenting feature, and the disease is first discovered at the time of laparotomy for a perforated viscus. The passage per rectum of bright red blood should alert one to the possible coexistence of rectal involvement (i.e., ileocolitis). Crohn's disease may also involve the *stomach* and *duodenum.* The involvement is usually of the antrum and/or the first and second portions of the duodenum. Symptoms may include pain mimicking peptic ulcer disease. Later in the course of the disease, chronic scarring may produce gastric outlet or duodenal obstruction.

There are increasing reports of *small-bowel* and *colonic malignancy* developing in the setting of long-standing Crohn's disease. Although the risk of developing malignancy is statistically increased, the complication is uncommon when compared with the frequency of malignancy in ulcerative colitis (see below). As in other chronic inflammatory diseases, patients with long-standing Crohn's disease may rarely develop secondary *amyloidosis,* which may manifest itself with hepatosplenomegaly or significant proteinuria. The presence of extensive ileal disease, resulting in *bile salt malabsorption,* is associated with a decreased bile salt pool and an increased lithogenicity of bile (see Chap. 308). Up to 30 percent of patients with extensive ileal disease will develop gallstones. Also, in the setting of ileal disease, there is increased intestinal absorption of dietary oxalate with resultant hyperoxaluria and the development of *urinary oxalate stones.*

DIAGNOSIS

The diagnosis of IBD should be entertained in all patients presenting with diarrhea or bloody diarrhea, persistent perianal sepsis, and abdominal pain. There may be atypical presentations such as fever of unexplained origin in the absence of bowel symptoms or with extracolonic manifestations such as arthritis or liver disease antedating or overshadowing the bowel involvement. Since Crohn's disease may also involve the small intestine, it should be considered in the differential diagnosis of all types of malabsorption syndromes, intermittent intestinal obstruction, and abdominal fistulas.

The laboratory examination is usually nonspecific and reflects the extent and severity of the inflammatory reaction. In addition, when Crohn's disease involves the small bowel, laboratory features of malabsorption may be present. There may be a variable degree of anemia, from occult blood loss or the effect of chronic inflammation on the bone marrow. Folate or vitamin B_{12} malabsorption may also contribute to the anemia. While the Schilling test may be abnormal in patients with extensive ileal disease, frank macrocytic anemia due to vitamin B_{12} malabsorption alone is unusual, attesting to the marked efficiency of ileal absorption of the vitamin. When there is significant diarrhea, electrolyte abnormalities (hypokalemia, hypomagnesemia) may be prominent. Hypocalcemia may reflect extensive mucosal involvement and malabsorption of vitamin D. Hypoalbuminemia may result from amino acid malabsorption as well as from protein-losing enteropathy. Variable degrees of steatorrhea may result from bile salt depletion and mucosal damage. Mild abnormalities of liver function (especially an increased serum alkaline phosphatase) may reflect the development of a fatty liver in the malnourished patient or a coexisting pericholangitis. Significant jaundice is unusual. Proteinuria may reflect secondary amyloidosis, a rare complication.

Sigmoidoscopy and *radiologic* studies of the bowel are most important in establishing the diagnosis of inflammatory bowel disease. Sigmoidoscopy must be performed in all patients presenting with chronic diarrhea and in all instances of rectal bleeding. While meticulous air-contrast barium enema examination of the perfectly prepared colon may disclose the earliest mucosal changes in either ulcerative colitis or Crohn's disease (see below), a conventional barium enema examination is often "normal" in early disease. Direct visualization of the colonic mucosa combined with biopsy is the most sensitive way of determining whether rectal inflammation is present. It can often be performed without prior enema preparation in the patient actively having diarrhea. The goal of sigmoidoscopy is to establish *whether* mucosal inflammation is present and not necessarily to determine its full *extent* at the initial examination. Thus, if sigmoidoscopic changes are encountered within the first 8 to 10 cm, it is not necessary to pass the instrument to its full length which may cause discomfort when the bowel is acutely inflamed. In ulcerative colitis, findings include a loss of mucosal vascularity, diffuse erythema, friability of the mucosa, and often an exudate consisting of mucus, blood, and pus. The most characteristic feature is mucosal friability, best demonstrated by lightly wiping the surface of the mucosa with a cotton swab and observing the mucosa for the appearance of diffuse, small bleeding points. Equally characteristic is the uniformity of involvement. Once diseased mucosa is encountered (usually in the rectum), there are no areas of intervening normal mucosa before the proximal extent of the disease is reached. Ulceration is shallow, may be small or confluent, but invariably occurs in segments of active colitis. Rectal biopsy may corroborate mucosal inflammation. With more chronic disease, the mucosa may show a granular appearance and pseudopolyps may be present.

Sigmoidoscopy is also of value in the diagnosis of colonic Crohn's disease. The findings are of ulcerations which may be tiny, aphthous erosions or deep, longitudinal fissures. They usually occur in segments of otherwise normal mucosa. Since the mucosa is not uniformly involved, friability and diffuse granularity, which are hallmarks of ulcerative colitis, are not characteristic of Crohn's colitis. Rather a cobblestone appearance, which is a coarse irregularity of the mucosal surface, reflects submucosal inflammation and is characteristic of Crohn's disease. Pseudopolyps, edema, and strictures may be seen in Crohn's colitis as well as in ulcerative colitis. Colonic mucosal biopsy reveals granulomas in 30 to 50 percent of specimens taken from involved areas. Features such as crypt abscesses, infiltration with inflammatory cells, or ulcerations are nonspecific but compatible features. Sigmoidoscopic or colonoscopic examination is also indicated when Crohn's disease appears to involve the small bowel, since ileal biopsy is usually not feasible and coexisting colonic involvement occurs in a significant number of cases. Perianal inflammatory lesions as well as areas of rectal disease seen at sigmoidoscopy will often show granulomatous inflammation. Rectal biopsy of seemingly "uninvolved" areas may also show microscopic evidence of granulomatous inflammation in only 15 percent of patients.

The *radiologic evaluation* of the bowel provides essential information in the diagnosis of IBD. Barium enema, in ulcerative colitis, may reveal the extent of the disease and help define associated features such as stricture, pseudopolyposis, or carcinoma. The earliest features seen in ulcerative colitis are irritability and incomplete filling due to associated inflammation. Fine ulcerations may be seen at this time as serrations along the contour of the bowel producing a hazy margin (Fig. 309-4). The ulcerations may become deeper and with more fulminant disease produce a grossly ragged and irregular contour. Polypoid defects appear as a result of edematous mucosa between ulcerations. The diffuse pattern of ulceration is best seen on the evacuation film or on air-contrast barium enema. In the chronic stage of the disease (Fig. 309-5), the characteristic features are shortening of the bowel, depression of the flexures, narrowing of the bowel lumen, and rigidity. The bowel has a symmetrical, ahaustral, tubular appearance with a decreased mucosal pattern. Although strictures are uncommon, when they occur they have a concentric lumen with fusiform tapering margins. Eccentricity should raise the suspicion of an associated carcinoma.

Barium enema examination in Crohn's disease of the colon has features which usually distinguish it from ulcerative colitis. Features characteristic of Crohn's disease include rectal sparing, the presence of skip lesions, and the finding of small ulcerations occurring on small irregular nodules. The small ulcerations often extend to produce longitudinal ulcers (Fig. 309-6) and transverse fissures which in reality are limited sinus tracts. These may extend into adjacent tissues to produce fistulas. Irregular thickening and fibrosis may lead to stricture formation which may be multiple. In 10 to 15 percent of cases the disease may uniformly involve the entire colon, making differentiation from ulcerative colitis more difficult. Reflux of barium into the terminal ileum during barium enema may reveal characteristic ileal changes of regional enteritis.

When Crohn's disease involves the small intestine, the terminal ileum is most characteristically involved with features similar to colonic involvement. Careful x-ray examination of the small bowel may demonstrate loss of mucosal detail and rigidity of involved segments resulting from submucosal edema or stenosis. The submucosal inflammation may lead to the characteristic radiologic cobblestoned appearance of the mucosa (Fig. 309-7), and fistulous tracts may be seen, especially in the ileocecal area (Fig. 309-8). Involvement of the stomach and duodenum usually appears radiologically as stiffening and infiltration of the mucosa and can mimic an infiltrative tumor. If such an appearance is due to regional enteritis, there is almost always coexistent involvement of either the jejunum or ileum.

FIGURE 309-4

Acute ulcerative colitis, air-contrast study. Note the diffuse fine ulceration involving the entire colon producing a fine serration along the contour of the bowel. (Courtesy of Dr R Gold, Columbia Presbyterian Medical Center.)

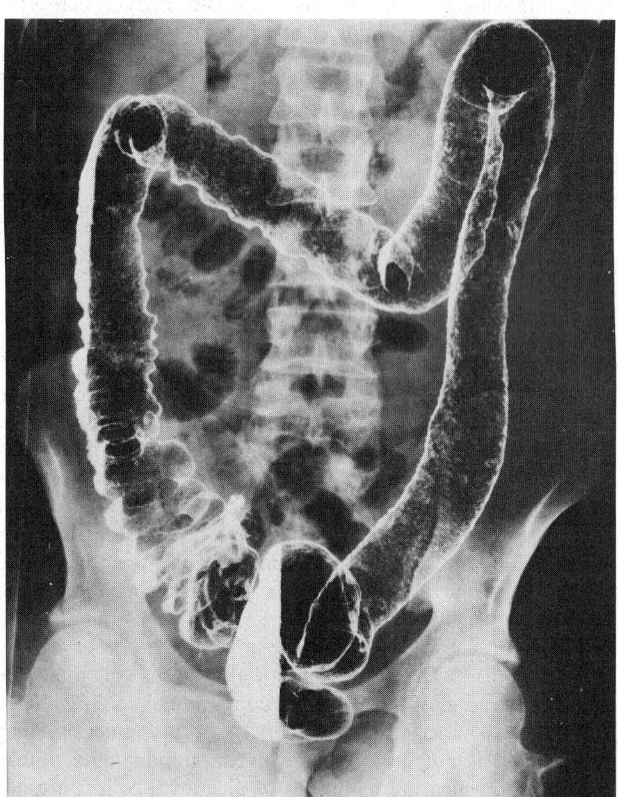

FIGURE 309-5

Chronic ulcerative colitis. Note the loss of haustrations and the fusiform stricture in the transverse colon. (Courtesy of Dr R Gold, Columbia Presbyterian Medical Center.)

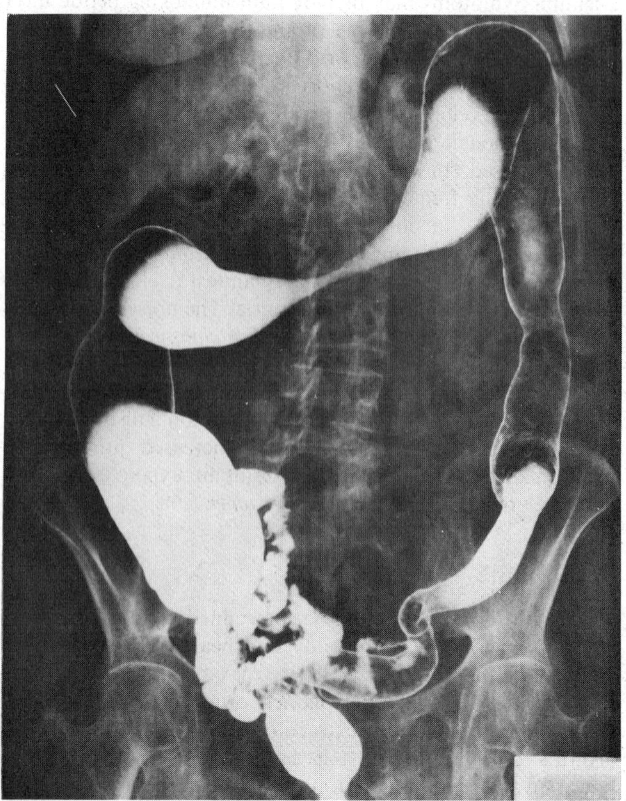

While barium studies often provide information on the pattern and extent of inflammatory bowel disease, caution must be exercised in obtaining these studies in the acutely ill patient with severe colitis in whom barium study and the bowel cleansing which precedes it may result in a worsening of the disease and can precipitate toxic dilatation of the colon.

Fiberoptic colonoscopy has added greatly to the diagnosis of colonic inflammatory bowel disease. Areas formerly beyond the reach of the sigmoidoscope can now be directly visualized and biopsy material obtained. Early in the course of colonic inflammation, endoscopic examination and biopsy are the most sensitive techniques to demonstrate mucosal involvement. Polypoid lesions, strictures, and unclear x-ray features can usually be fully defined. Periodic colonoscopic examination and biopsy are being increasingly used in cancer surveillance in patients with long-standing inflammatory bowel disease (see below).

FIGURE 309-6
Crohn's colitis. Air-contrast study.

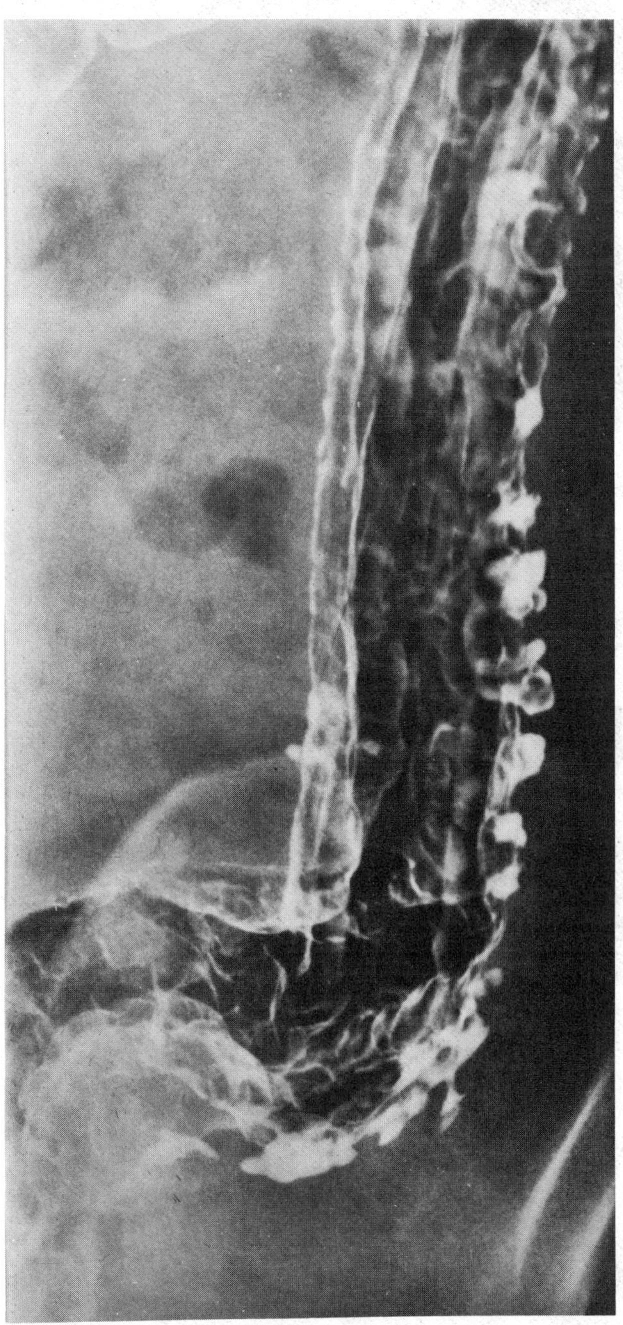

DIFFERENTIAL DIAGNOSIS

Many entities must be considered in the differential diagnosis in IBD. The focus of the differential diagnosis will in large measure be determined by the presenting features of the disease. When *rectal bleeding* is the presenting complaint, a colonic source should be considered. While *hemorrhoids* are commonly found, they must be considered a tentative source of bleeding until sigmoidoscopy and barium enema have eliminated other colonic lesions. Colonic *neoplasms* (carcinoma, adenomatous polyps) may also present with rectal bleeding and can usually be diagnosed by barium enema with subsequent sigmoidoscopic or colonoscopic biopsy. It should be remembered that carcinoma may complicate long-standing colitis. Rectal bleeding from *colonic diverticula* or *arteriovenous malformations* usually present no problem in differential diagnosis since radiologic and endoscopic features of inflammatory bowel disease are absent. *Radiation proctitis,* which may present as a localized area of colitis, is usually found in the setting of pelvic irradiation. The onset may, however, occur at variable (months to years) periods of time after irradiation. Characteristic features on sigmoidoscopy include mucosal atrophy and telangiectasia along with friability and small ulcerations. A colitis sometimes indistinguishable from ulcerative colitis may occur in Behçet's syndrome and is associated with aphthous oral ulceration, uveitis, and urethritis.

Acute colitis may be caused by a variety of *infectious* agents (Chap. 142). Often presenting with bloody diarrhea, infectious colitis may be difficult to distinguish from IBD at initial presentation. A listing of these agents is given in Table 309-2.

Amebiasis may present with bloody diarrhea and at sigmoidoscopy be indistinguishable from idiopathic ulcerative colitis. A history of recent foreign travel or homosexual exposure should always be sought. Since specific amebicidal therapy is necessary to eradicate this infection and corticosteroids may be detrimental, every effort should be made to exclude this diagnosis in appropriate individuals. Acute *bacillary dysentery* may be caused by *Shigella* and *Salmonella* or *Campylobacter,* all easily diagnosed by stool culture. *Yersinia enterocolitis,* which often presents as acute ileitis, can also produce a self-limited colitis, sometimes with granulomatous reaction. Infectious agents may cause acute proctitis indistinguishable from idiopathic ulcerative proctitis. Such infections, often seen in homosexuals, may be due to *gonorrhea* or *lymphogranuloma venereum* (LGV) as well as *amebiasis.* Recently, in homosexual men, non-LGV strains of *Chlamydia* have been shown to produce a granulomatous proctitis closely resembling Crohn's disease of the rectum.

Pseudomembranous colitis (antibiotic-associated colitis) is caused by a necrolytic toxin elaborated by *C. difficile* which under certain circumstances proliferates within the bowel. Most often the disease is a result of antibiotic therapy which presumably upsets the normal ecologic balance of the bowel

TABLE 309-2
Microbiological causes of colitis

Shigella
Salmonella
Amebiasis
Yersinia
Campylobacter
Lymphogranuloma venereum (LGV)
"Non-LGV" *Chlamydia*
Gonorrhea
Pseudomembranous colitis (*Clostridium difficile* toxin)
Tuberculosis

flora permitting *C. difficile* to proliferate. Almost every antibiotic has been implicated, although cases related to the use of vancomycin or aminoglycosides are rare. Most often diarrhea is profuse and watery, although bloody diarrhea occurs in 5 percent of cases. Characteristic lesions are seen on sigmoidoscopy and appear as multiple, discrete yellowish plaques which on biopsy show features of acute inflammation and ulceration with a pseudomembrane of fibrin and necrotic material. On occasion lesions may be beyond reach of the sigmoidoscope and require colonoscopy. Diagnosis is best made by either culturing the organisms directly from stool or by detecting *C. difficile* toxin in the stool. Treatment is either directed at binding the toxin or at eradicating the *C. difficile* organisms. Anion exchange resins such as cholestyramine (4 g PO qid for 5 days) will bind the toxin and may be used in mild cases. Vancomycin (250 mg PO qid for 7 to 14 days) is the treatment of choice for more severely ill patients and should produce clinical improvement within 5 days. Since vancomycin therapy is expensive, alternative therapies have been proposed. Metronidazole (500 mg PO tid) or bacitracin (25,000 units PO qid) have been suggested as alternative therapies. With all forms of therapy, relapse rates (15 to 30 percent) have been observed and may require a subsequent course of therapy to eradicate the organism. On occasion, infectious causes of colitis will be superim-

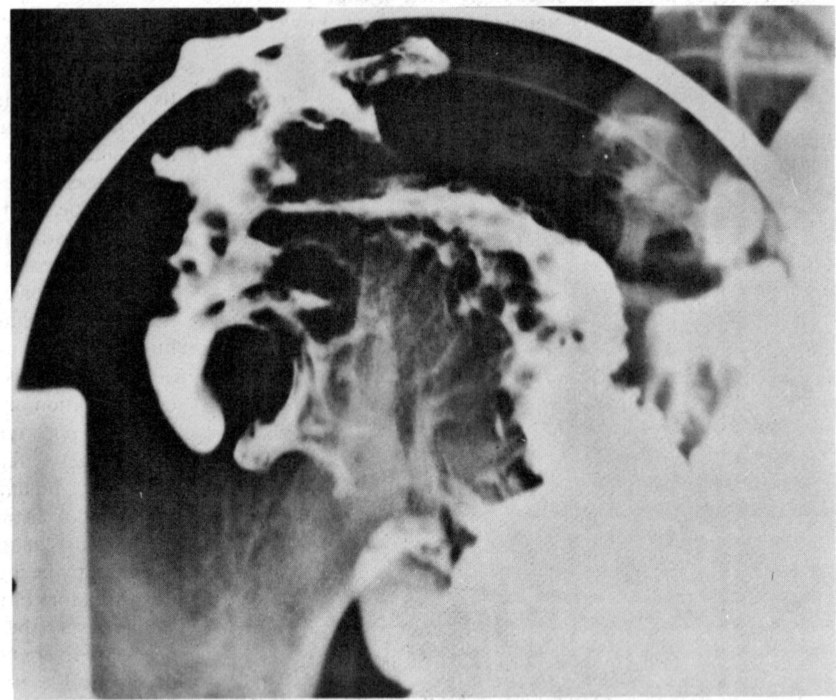

FIGURE 309-7
Crohn's ileocolitis. Note the nodularity and ulceration of the terminal ileum and the deformity of the cecum.

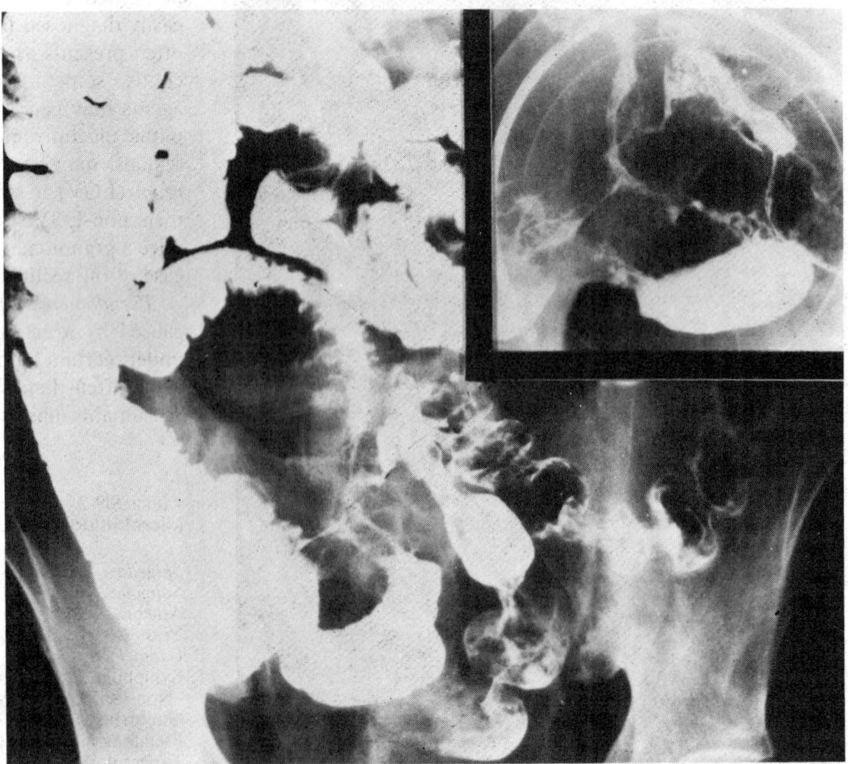

FIGURE 309-8
Regional enteritis. X-ray showing fistulas between loops of bowel. Insert is a compression film of this area; note fistulas between adjacent loops of bowel.

posed on ulcerative colitis or Crohn's disease. In this case, once the acute infection has subsided, symptoms and inflammatory mucosal changes may persist, raising the possibility of associated idiopathic IBD. Similar considerations apply to the patient with IBD who uncommonly may develop associated *pseudomembranous* colitis. The finding of *C. difficile* toxin in the stool and subsequent treatment will serve to clarify this presentation.

Abdominal pain in association with rectal bleeding, especially in the older age group, may be due to *ischemic colitis.* Because of an excellent collateral circulation, the rectum is usually spared. Radiologic features are often characteristic.

Inflammatory bowel disease may be difficult to distinguish from functional diarrhea early in the course of disease. The presence of constitutional symptoms such as fatigue, fever, and weight loss, coupled with laboratory features of anemia, elevated erythrocyte sedimentation rate, or occult blood in the stool should alert the clinician to the possibility of IBD. Similarly, finding leukocytes in a stained stool specimen points to an inflammatory basis for the diarrhea. In all cases, stool cultures and parasitologic examination of the stool are required to rule out enteric bacterial pathogens or amebiasis. In the *irritable bowel syndrome* sigmoidoscopy, rectal biopsy, and barium enema examination are all normal.

Once the diagnosis of idiopathic IBD has been established, the distinction between ulcerative colitis and Crohn's disease of the colon is usually possible. Differential diagnostic features are shown in Table 309-1.

With small-intestinal involvement (regional enteritis) the differential diagnosis should include disorders presenting with intraabdominal abscesses, fistulas, intestinal obstruction, and malabsorption. The finding of associated colonic involvement in patients with ileal disease will often serve to distinguish Crohn's disease from other ileal disorders. With diffuse involvement of the jejunum and ileum, regional enteritis must be distinguished from *nongranulomatous ulcerative jejunoileitis.* Abdominal pain and diarrhea are prominent features of this disorder, and weight loss, malabsorption, and hypoproteinemia tend to be more prominent than in regional enteritis. Small-bowel biopsy shows a more diffuse lesion with flattened villi (similar to celiac sprue), infiltration of the lamina propria, and mucosal ulceration. *Abdominal lymphoma* may likewise present with clinical and radiologic features difficult to distinguish from regional enteritis. Hepatosplenomegaly and peripheral adenopathy, when present, are helpful clues, but often disease is confined to the intestine. In such cases, laparotomy is usually required to make the definitive histologic diagnosis.

The advanced presentation of regional enteritis with areas of stenosis and draining fistulas may also be confused with *chronic fungal infection of the bowel,* including actinomycosis, aspergillosis, and blastomycosis. These infections often are seen in debilitated patients with impaired host defenses. Fungal skin tests and examination of fistula drainage and biopsy material for characteristic granules and fungi are helpful in making the diagnosis.

Intestinal tuberculosis characteristically produces stenotic lesions, usually in the terminal ileum, also often involving the contiguous cecum and ascending colon. Unlike regional enteritis, "skip areas" are unusual. Histologically, the granulomatous inflammation seen with *Mycobacterium* tuberculosis may be indistinguishable from regional enteritis; acid-fast stains and cultures are required. Fortunately in western countries primary intestinal tuberculosis is now rare; when intestinal involvement does occur, it invariably is associated with pulmonary tuberculosis.

TABLE 309-3
Some systemic complications of inflammatory bowel disease

1 Nutritional and metabolic
- *a* Weight loss, ↓ muscle mass, growth retardation (children)
- *b* Electrolyte deficiency (K^+, Ca^{2+}, Mg^{2+})
- *c* Hypoalbuminemia (↓ nutrition, protein-losing enteropathy)
- *d* Anemia (chronic disease, iron deficiency; rarely folate or vitamin B_{12} deficiency in Crohn's disease)
- *e* Bile salt deficiency with ileal disease (steatorrhea and fat-soluble vitamin deficiency; ↑ colonic oxalate absorption → renal stones; ↑ lithogenicity of bile → gallstones)

2 Musculoskeletal
- *a* Peripheral arthralgia, arthritis
- *b* Ankylosing spondylitis, sacroileitis
- *c* Granulomatous myositis (rare)

3 Hepatobiliary disease
- *a* Fatty liver
- *b* Cholelithiasis
- *c* Pericholangitis, biliary cirrhosis (rare)
- *d* Sclerosing cholangitis
- *e* Bile duct carcinoma
- *f* Chronic active hepatitis and cirrhosis

4 Skin and mucous membrane
- *a* Erythema nodosum
- *b* Pyoderma gangrenosum
- *c* Aphthous stomatitis
- *d* Crohn's disease of buccal mucosa, gingiva, vagina

5 Eye
- Iritis, uveitis, episcleritis

6 Venous thrombosis and thromboembolism (hypercoagulability, dehydration, stasis)

COMPLICATIONS OF INFLAMMATORY BOWEL DISEASE

The complications of IBD may be classified as local, which are a direct reflection of mucosal inflammation and its extension or systemic complications (Table 309-3). Local complications of IBD such as fistulas, abscesses, and strictures have been described above. In addition, perforation, toxic dilatation, and the development of carcinoma may complicate both ulcerative colitis and Crohn's disease.

PERFORATION Intestinal perforation can occur in severe ulcerative colitis since with extensive ulceration the bowel wall may become extremely thin. The clinical features are those of acute peritonitis with signs of peritoneal inflammation and the demonstration of free air under the diaphragm on upright film of the abdomen. These are an indication for immediate colectomy.

Toxic dilatation of the colon may occur in Crohn's colitis but is more common in ulcerative colitis. This complication can best be considered as a severe form of ulcerative colitis with the additional feature of colonic dilatation. It is thought that the neuromuscular tone of the bowel is affected by the severe inflammation resulting in dilatation. Injudicious use of hypomotility agents (codeine, diphenoxylate, loperamide, paregoric, anticholinergic agents) to treat diarrhea in the setting of acute colitis can precipitate this complication. Similarly, cathartic preparation and barium enema examination as well as superimposed hypokalemia may be contributing factors. Clinically, features of severe colitis are present with high fever, tachycardia, volume depletion, electrolyte imbalance, and abdominal pain. On examination, the patient appears toxic, and colonic dilatation may be evident. There is abdominal tenderness and if perforation has already occurred, peritoneal signs are present. Diarrhea may actually decrease markedly due to colonic atony, creating the false impression that the colitis is clinically improved. Plain film of the abdomen will show colonic dilatation with the colonic diameter more than 6 cm. There may be air in the wall of the colon and irregular, ulcerated islands of mucosa may be silhouetted against the air shadow. While the transverse colon is the most common site of dilatation, this is probably largely positional, since with the patient supine, this is the highest portion of the colon. This presentation of colitis represents a true medical emergency and is associated with a mortality of greater than 30 percent if perforation has occurred. Appropriate therapy is discussed below.

CARCINOMA AND INFLAMMATORY BOWEL DISEASE There is an increased incidence of carcinoma in patients with chronic IBD when compared to the general population, especially in patients who have more extensive mucosal involvement (i.e., pancolitis) and those who have had their disease for extended periods of time. Cumulative risk of cancer rises steadily with the duration of disease. It has been estimated that with pancolitis there is a risk of cancer of 12 percent at 15 years, 23 percent at 20 years, and 42 percent at 24 years. In children, the risk of cancer appears to rise more sharply after the first 10 years of disease, perhaps reflecting the higher incidence of pancolitis in children. Limited involvement of the colon (i.e., proctitis) has a low risk of malignant degeneration. Malignancy developing in Crohn's disease of the colon or small bowel is less well documented, but the incidences of both small- and large-bowel malignancies are increased compared to the general population. The incidence, however, is less than in ulcerative colitis.

The development of colon carcinoma arising in the setting of IBD demonstrates important differences when compared to carcinoma arising in a noncolitic population. Clinically, many of the earlier warning signs of a colonic neoplasm (i.e., rectal bleeding, change in bowel habits) will be difficult to interpret in the setting of colitis. In colitic patients the distribution of carcinomas is more uniform throughout the colon than in noncolitic patients; in the latter the majority of carcinomas are in the rectosigmoid within reach of the sigmoidoscope. In colitis patients the tumors are more often multiple, flat, and infiltrating and appear to have a higher grade of malignancy. There is some evidence to suggest that these features may reflect the younger age at which they occur rather than the associated colitis. Further adding to the difficulty in diagnosis is the frequent occurrence of mucosal irregularities, ulcerations, and pseudopolyps, making a small carcinoma difficult to diagnose radiologically or endoscopically.

Efforts have been directed to devise effective screening procedures to detect carcinoma developing in the setting of IBD. Carcinoembryonic antigen (CEA) may be elevated nonspecifically in ulcerative colitis and therefore is of limited value. Periodic barium enemas and/or sigmoidoscopy or colonoscopy have been suggested, but interpretation is sometimes hampered by abnormalities related to the colitis itself. The addition of colonic mucosal biopsy may add a significant dimension. It was originally suggested that a generalized precancerous lesion may be present in high-risk patients with colitis who either harbor an occult malignancy or who will develop cancer. Subsequent studies of rectal biopsies in patients with long-standing colitis showed that if dysplasia was present, there was approximately a 50 percent chance that an associated malignancy was present in those patients who subsequently came to colectomy. Complicating these findings was the fact that dysplastic changes were only found in rectal biopsies 60 percent of the time, making colonoscopy with multiple biopsies desirable. In addition, in some patients not undergoing colectomy, dysplasia was not a consistent finding on subsequent biopsies. While more information is needed on the prognostic significance and reproducibility of finding dysplastic changes on mucosal biopsy, it seems prudent to examine patients with colonic IBD of greater than 8 to 10 years' duration with colonoscopy and multiple mucosal biopsies at regular intervals. The frequency of such examinations has not been established, with recommendations varying from 6 months to 2 years. If severe dysplasia is found, then confirmation at less than 6-month intervals seems prudent. While most authorities would not advise "prophylactic" colectomy in the patient with long-standing colitis, the finding of severe dysplasia may well identify a subgroup who already harbor an occult carcinoma or who are at high risk of its development. There can be no uniform recommendation for this small group of patients, but many physicians will advise colectomy in this setting.

EXTRAINTESTINAL MANIFESTATIONS OF INFLAMMATORY BOWEL DISEASE

There are a variety of nonintestinal symptoms and signs which may be associated with IBD and occur in both ulcerative colitis and Crohn's disease (Table 309-3). Since some of these manifestations may not coincide with, or may overshadow, the underlying bowel disease, they may on occasion pose difficult diagnostic problems. Their etiology is currently unknown.

Joint manifestations are common in patients with IBD (~25 percent incidence). These may range from arthralgia only to an acute arthritis with painful, swollen joints.

The nondeforming arthritis is mono- or polyarticular and often migratory. Knees, ankles, and wrists are most commonly involved, but any joint may be affected. Joint fluid, if aspirated, reveals findings of an acute arthritis without crystals or evidence of infection. Tests for specific forms of arthritis (rheumatoid factor, antinuclear antibody, and LE factor) are negative. Typically, the arthritis correlates with activity of the underlying bowel disease. Rarely, peripheral arthritis may truly antecede clinical bowel symptoms. Arthritis is more commonly found in patients with colonic than with small-bowel involvement alone (regional enteritis).

In contrast, the central arthritis or ankylosing spondylitis associated with IBD is unrelated to the activity of the underlying bowel disease. It may antedate the bowel disease by years and persist after surgical or medical remission of the disease has been achieved. Symptoms are of low backache and stiffness with eventual limitation of motion. This may be associated with sacroileitis as well. X-rays usually reveal characteristic changes. In contrast to the peripheral arthritis, there is a strong association of HLA-B27 with ankylosing spondylitis, whether or not IBD is present.

Like the peripheral arthritis *skin manifestations* are more common with colonic disease. They occur in about 15 percent of patients, and when present the severity correlates with activity of the bowel disease. *Erythema nodosum* may be seen and heals without scarring. *Pyoderma gangrenosum,* an ulcerating lesion often occurring on the trunk, is relatively painless and may heal with scarring. In the rare patient, the lesion may persist even after colectomy for ulcerative colitis. *Aphthous ulcers* resemble "canker sores" of the mouth, and in approximately 5 to 10 percent of patients they are present during periods of active disease and then resolve. Their etiology is unknown and they are treated symptomatically. *Ocular manifestations* such as episcleritis, recurrent iritis, and uveitis occur in approximately 5 percent of patients and may represent a severe manifestation of the disease. In general, their activity parallels the course of the bowel disease, and the lesions may respond dramatically when colectomy is done for other indications.

Abnormalities of *liver function* are common in IBD. In the severely ill, malnourished patient, mild abnormalities of serum aminotransferases and alkaline phosphatase are often seen and represent nonspecific focal hepatitis or fatty infiltration. Factors favoring fatty infiltration of the liver in the severely ill patient are poor nutrition and often concomitant steroid therapy. The lesion is not progressive and resolves with disease remission. *Pericholangitis* is characterized histologically by portal tract inflammation, some bile ductular proliferation, and concentric fibrosis around bile ductules. Most often, the lesion is clinically insignificant, and its sole manifestation is an elevated serum alkaline phosphatase. It is usually nonprogressive and requires no therapy. Rarely, there may be an apparent progression to cirrhosis of either the postnecrotic or biliary type. Uncommonly, patients with IBD may develop *sclerosing cholangitis* (Chap. 323), a chronic inflammation of unknown etiology involving the extrahepatic and intrahepatic bile ducts which may produce varying degrees of extrahepatic biliary obstruction. Corticosteroids and immunosuppressive therapy are not beneficial. Reversal of the disease after colectomy is an inconsistent result and should not form the sole indication for colectomy. Cholangiocarcinoma, arising in the extrahepatic biliary tree, has an increased incidence in patients with chronic ulcerative colitis. Such patients will present with extrahepatic biliary obstruction which must be distinguished from sclerosing cholangitis. Finally, *chronic active hepatitis* which may progress to *cirrhosis* may be seen in IBD, although the exact relationship between these disorders is unknown. The evaluation and therapy are similar to the disease occurring in noncolitic patients. There is no clear evidence that colectomy influences the course of this form of liver disease.

TREATMENT

In general, the treatment of ulcerative colitis and Crohn's disease shares certain common principles. Initial treatment of all forms of uncomplicated IBD is primarily medical, and the principles of medical therapy are similar. Surgery is reserved for (1) specific complications and (2) intractability of disease. There are certain important differences, however, between ulcerative colitis and Crohn's disease; namely, the response to drug therapy may differ, complications often differ, and the prognosis after surgical therapy is not the same.

ULCERATIVE COLITIS **Medical therapy** Once the diagnosis is established, the severity of the disease must be assessed. Mild ulcerative colitis, including ulcerative proctitis, can usually be treated on an ambulatory basis. More severe disease, especially at initial presentation, is best treated in a hospital setting. The disease can rapidly worsen, and the course of a given attack cannot be predicted at the outset. The aims of therapy are to control the inflammatory process and replace nutritional losses. A certain degree of improvement usually follows intravenous correction of fluid and electrolyte disturbances. Blood transfusions may be required in severe anemia, especially when there is continued active bleeding. Agents to control diarrhea (diphenoxylate, loperamide, codeine, anticholinergics) should be used with extreme caution for fear of precipitating colonic dilatation and toxic megacolon. The decision to institute specific nutritional replacement therapy will be determined by the nutritional status of the patient and whether a protracted clinical course can be anticipated. In the severely ill patient, even clear liquids orally may stimulate colonic activity, and it is often wise to give the patients nothing by mouth. In this setting, intravenous alimentation, either peripheral or central, has been used as interim nutritional replacement therapy (see Chap. 82). While there is no evidence that intravenous alimentation is effective as primary therapy, it is an important component of a treatment program. In the less severely ill patients able to tolerate fluids by mouth, the use of elemental oral diets may be beneficial providing supplemental nutrition with low fecal volume. While milk is not contraindicated in ulcerative colitis, diarrhea will be exacerbated if there is an associated lactase deficiency.

The principal drugs used in the therapy of ulcerative colitis are the *anti-inflammatory agents, sulfasalazine* (Azulfidine) and *adrenal corticosteroids* or ACTH. Sulfasalazine consists of a sulfonamide (sulfapyridine) moiety chemically bound to a salicylate (5-aminosalicylate); it undergoes bacterial cleavage in the colon. The liberated sulfapyridine is efficiently absorbed and largely excreted in the urine; the liberated 5-aminosalicylate believed to be the active component remains largely in the colon and is excreted in the stool. The salicylate moiety is thought to exert its action through inhibition of prostaglandin synthesis. While most physicians are familiar with the use of sulfasalazine to prevent recurrences of ulcerative colitis, it is less well appreciated that this agent is effective in the therapy of acute ulcerative colitis of mild to moderate severity. Therapeutic doses of 4 to 6 g daily are required. The drug is usually started at a dose of 500 mg bid and then increased daily or every other day by 1 g until the therapeutic dose is achieved.

In the severely ill patient who may not tolerate oral medication and where a more rapid time frame of therapy is often desired, initial therapy is begun with corticosteroids or ACTH. While some physicians still prefer ACTH to corticosteroids, these agents appear equally effective when given in equivalent dosages and by comparable routes of administration. The choice is one of individual preference; however, oral prednisone (45 to 60 mg daily) is often employed initially. Alternatively, intravenous ACTH may be given (40 to 60 units) over an 8-h drip infusion. In the severely ill patient, parenteral administration of corticosteroids is preferable to avoid the uncertainty of adequate oral absorption. Improvement is usually noted after 7 to 10 days of such therapy by a reduction in fever, decreased bloody diarrhea, and an improvement in appetite.

After initial improvement low-roughage oral feedings can be resumed. At this point the dose of steroids can be tapered, or if ACTH was used initially, oral prednisone at reduced dosage can be started. There is no specific schedule for tapering corticosteroids. The guiding principle, however, is that once clinical remission is achieved, there is no evidence that chronic steroid administration favorably influences the long-term outlook of the disease or that recurrences can be prevented by chronic steroid therapy. In practice, steroid therapy can be tapered and discontinued over a 2- to 3-month period after discharge. In some patients (10 to 15 percent) efforts to completely eliminate steroids may be associated with a flare of the disease, and low to moderate steroids (10 to 15 mg of prednisone daily) may be required to suppress disease activity. This should not be confused with the prophylactic administration of steroids to patients in remission, but rather represents incompletely responsive disease. Once the acutely ill patient is taking oral feedings, sulfasalazine should be added as described above in a daily dose of 2 g. Controlled trials have shown that this dose of sulfasalazine, when administered chronically to patients with ulcerative colitis, is effective in decreasing the frequency of relapses and should be continued chronically after corticosteroids have been discontinued. Patients with glucose phosphate dehydrogenase deficiency or those exhibiting allergic reactions to the drug unfortunately cannot be maintained on it.

The use of immunosuppressive therapy with drugs such as azathioprine is less well established in ulcerative colitis. As a single agent in the therapy of acute ulcerative colitis, the drug is ineffective. However, the drug may be added to the regimen at a dose of 1.5 to 2.0 mg/kg when corticosteroids fail or when the steroid dose needed to reduce inflammation is too high. It is desirable to monitor the blood count and observe the patient carefully for infection. Azathioprine may also have a limited role as a "steroid-sparing agent" in the patient with chronic ulcerative colitis who must be maintained on corticosteroids to control disease activity.

Toxic megacolon is a major complication of severe ulcerative colitis which requires rapid, intensive management best carried out jointly by the internist or gastroenterologist and surgeon. Once the diagnosis is established, prompt and vigorous use of intravenous fluids, electrolyte replacement therapy, and blood transfusions is indicated. Because of the fear of perforation and high likelihood that bacteremia and occult perforation have occurred, many physicians will institute broad-spectrum antibiotic coverage after appropriate cultures have been obtained. The patient is given nothing by mouth, and nasogastric suction is often instituted. Full intravenous corticosteroid therapy is also begun. Majority opinion favors an initial period of medical stabilization for the first 24 to 48 h. If significant objective improvement has not occurred and if perforation seems imminent, emergency colectomy should be carried out. While it is certainly true that some patients, under maximal medical therapy, may slowly improve and thus avoid colectomy, the risk of this course of action must be carefully considered. If perforation occurs, mortality rates rise sharply, approaching 50 percent in those who subsequently go on to colectomy.

At the other end of the spectrum is the patient with mild ulcerative colitis, limited to the rectum or rectosigmoid, who is managed on an ambulatory basis. Therapy is initiated with sulfasalazine, 0.5 to 1.0 g four times a day with meals. If rectal symptoms such as tenesmus are prominent, topical steroids in the form of small enemas may produce marked improvement. The equivalent of 100 mg hydrocortisone (20 mg prednisone) in 60 to 100 ml saline is used as a bedtime enema. On occasion the use of steroid foam preparations may be better tolerated in the patient with severe tenesmus. Retention enemas have been shown to deliver medication as far as the descending colon, and absorption of steroid is small (~ 10 to 20 percent). If large doses of rectal steroids are required for control, it is preferable to use oral prednisone at a moderate dosage (20 mg daily).

Psychotherapy The elements of trust and mutual understanding combined with the compassion and expertise of the physician are essential in the therapy of any chronic disease and are particularly important in the long-term management of patients with inflammatory bowel disease. Often these patients are intelligent young adults who are frequently resentful of a disease affecting them during the most productive years. Through the vigorous participation of the physician many patients are able to lead reasonably stable and productive lives. More formal psychiatric assistance may be required in the chronically ill patient, in particular children or adolescents, or in the elderly where severe depressive reactions are common. This is particularly true when colectomy is being advised and in the emotional adjustment which must be made after colectomy.

Pregnancy and ulcerative colitis While many physicians are apprehensive about the management and prognosis of ulcerative colitis in the pregnant patient, the outcome for the patient and the fetus is excellent. In general, the pregnancy is not threatened by coexistent colitis, with no increase in stillbirths or premature deliveries when compared to the general population. When patients with inactive colitis become pregnant, approximately 50 percent may have an exacerbation of their disease with some clustering of these flares during the first trimester and in the postpartum period. The therapy of ulcerative colitis during pregnancy is largely the same as in the nonpregnant patient. Sulfasalazine is used to treat mild to moderate disease since there is no evidence that the drug is harmful to the fetus or leads to increased incidence of fetal malformations. Women with inactive colitis who enter a pregnancy on maintenance sulfasalazine should be continued on the drug. Since sulfapyridine appears in breast milk, in the newborn with unconjugated hyperbilirubinemia from other causes, breast feeding should be discontinued or the drug stopped if the colitis is inactive. In most situations, however, the drug should be continued to protect the mother during the postpartum period from a relapse of disease. Corticosteroids should be used in the same dosage and for the same indications as in the nonpregnant patient.

Thus, it is clear that the patient with colitis can realistically plan to have a family. It is prudent, however, to bring active disease under control before pregnancy is undertaken to ensure the most optimal physical and emotional setting for the pregnancy. Similar conclusions apply to the management of Crohn's disease during pregnancy.

Surgical therapy Approximately 20 to 25 percent of patients with ulcerative colitis will require colectomy during the course of their disease. A major indication for colectomy is failure to respond to intensive medical management. Such patients, although not showing colonic dilatation, may fail to improve after 7 to 10 days of optimal medical therapy. Fever, persistent bloody diarrhea, and severe fatigue may persist, and consideration should be given to semielective colectomy. Elective colectomy may be performed in patients whose disease remains chronically active and who require continuous corticosteroid administration. Such patients are at risk of developing the complications of chronic steroid therapy. After colectomy these patients often feel more energetic and usually gain back weight to their preillness level. As discussed above the patient with long-standing colitis is at high risk for colonic cancer. While most authorities do not advise "prophylactic" colectomy in the patient with quiescent disease, the finding of marked dysplasia on colonoscopic biopsies done as a part of a surveillance program should make the physician think seriously about advising colectomy.

The decision to advise colectomy in other than emergency circumstances is difficult for both patient and physician. Many patients have an understandable reluctance to undergo colectomy and have difficulty in conceptualizing life with an ileostomy. In most metropolitan centers there are ileostomy groups who visit patients preoperatively and can provide answers to many practical questions. It is also desirable for the patient to be visited by a nurse familiar with stoma care to instruct the patient on the practical aspects of handling the ileostomy.

While total proctocolectomy with permanent ileostomy is the procedure of choice for almost all patients undergoing colectomy, several alternative approaches have been suggested. The *continent ileostomy* is an ileal loop reservoir fashioned under the skin with a nipple valve to prevent spilling of ileal contents. Ileal effluent collects in this reservoir which must be emptied with a soft rubber catheter. Only a small stoma is externally visible, thus eliminating an external ileostomy appliance. Problems with this procedure include a failure of continence, irritation of the mucosa of the ileal reservoir from stasis ("pouchitis"), and bacterial overgrowth which may lead to mild malabsorption. Repeat operations are common, and this procedure should only be done by skilled surgeons familiar with the technique. *Ileorectal anastomosis* with *mucosal stripping* of the rectal segment is sometimes done in children who require colectomy for ulcerative colitis but is rarely carried out in adults.

CROHN'S DISEASE The medical management of colonic Crohn's disease is similar in most respects to that of ulcerative colitis. In a multicenter study (National Cooperative Crohn's Disease Study) sulfasalazine was shown to be effective in the therapy of active colonic disease. Corticosteroids also were efficacious but less so than with small-bowel involvement. The indications and dosages of these medications are similar to ulcerative colitis. Since in Crohn's disease, intraabdominal sepsis can result from fistula or abscess formation, corticosteroids must be used with caution and constant attention is required to detect evidence of sepsis, which can be masked by these agents. In general, the disease is less explosive in onset, and although toxic dilatation and perforation can occur, they are less common that in ulcerative colitis. The principles of management are the same. Because of the indolent nature of the disease, the response to therapy is often less complete than in ulcerative colitis, and the disease tends to progress despite apparent clinical inactivity. It may be more difficult to achieve a clinical remission and to withdraw steroids completely. As in ulcerative colitis, controlled studies have shown no benefit to continuing steroids after remission since the frequency of recurrence is not altered by prophylactic steroid therapy. Disappointingly, sulfasalazine did not decrease recurrence rates in Crohn's disease.

While response to therapy of the initial attack of Crohn's colitis may be satisfactory, many patients continue to have persistently active disease. This may express itself as progressive weight loss, diarrhea, and deterioration of general health. Perianal disease with predominantly left-sided colonic involvement (fistula formation and perirectal abscesses) may constitute a recurrent problem. In one controlled study, *metronidazole* (20 mg/kg per day in divided dosage) resulted in marked improvement in 10 of 18 patients with chronic perineal fistulas associated with Crohn's disease. It is not clear whether the drug is active because of its antibacterial properties or through another mechanism. It is possible that this drug may prove to be of value in the therapy of the perineal complications of Crohn's disease before surgical therapy is attempted. The role of immunosuppressive therapy such as azathioprine has been controversial in Crohn's disease. The multicenter United States study (National Cooperative Study) found azathioprine to be ineffective as a single agent in the therapy of active Crohn's disease. Yet there have been reports of dramatic improvement in a small percentage of patients when azathioprine (1.5 to 2 mg/kg) is added to a maximal program in the nonresponding patient. Some investigators have found 6-mercaptopurine (the active metabolite of azathioprine) effective in controlling disease activity when added to corticosteroids and sulfasalazine. However, a beneficial response may take 6 to 8 months in some patients.

The management of Crohn's disease of the small intestine (regional enteritis) is similar to that for colonic Crohn's disease, and as noted many patients have concomitant small and large bowel disease. Several additional considerations are pertinent however. *Intestinal obstruction* is not uncommonly a presenting feature with ileal involvement. Initially, this may be secondary to acute inflammation and will respond to corticosteroids. With recurrent involvement and the development of fibrosis, steroid therapy is less effective and surgical decompression is required. *Nutritional problems* often are more severe with involvement of the small intestine than with colonic involvement alone. Added to the general catabolic nature of the disease may be loss of absorptive surface which may result from progressive involvement or because of surgical resection. Refinements in the technique of parenteral alimentation have made it possible to provide a patient's total daily caloric intake intravenously for a period of weeks or even months (see Chap. 82). Parenteral alimentation has been employed with increasing frequency in the severely ill patient as a means of placing the gastrointestinal tract "at rest" and in preparing the malnourished patient for surgery. With this approach the disease may become quiescent, and the drainage from fistulas may decrease. However, disease activity frequently recurs when oral feedings are resumed. On occasion, prolonged intravenous alimentation, administered at home, may be required when oral

feedings are not effective or in children exhibiting severe growth failure associated with Crohn's disease. Most often it is possible to design a dietary program of oral supplementation to nourish the patient adequately.

In patients with extensive small-bowel involvement or in those with a short bowel resulting from extensive intestinal resection, supplementation of electrolytes, minerals, and vitamins will be required. Extensive ileal disease or resection often results in diarrhea induced by bile salts and in malabsorption; cholestyramine may be needed to control the diarrhea and medium-chain triglycerides added to reduce fat malabsorption (see Chap. 308). In patients with stenotic segments of intestine, a low-residue (low-fiber) diet should be recommended. A lactose-free diet should be instituted if there is an associated lactase deficiency. Other dietary modifications have not been shown to have any beneficial effect on the primary disease process. Patients should be encouraged to eat a nutritious, appealing diet of their own choosing. *Surgical therapy* is generally reserved for the complications of Crohn's disease rather than as a primary form of therapy. In contrast to ulcerative colitis, more patients with Crohn's disease will require surgery in the chronic management of the disease. Approximately 70 percent of patients will require at least one operation during the course of their disease. Although each case and situation must be individualized, in general, surgery may be required (1) for persistent or fixed bowel narrowing or obstruction; (2) for symptomatic fistula formation to the bladder, vagina, or skin; (3) for persistent anal fistulas or abscesses; and (4) for intraabdominal abscesses, toxic dilatation of the colon, or perforation. In contrast to ulcerative colitis, where colectomy is curative, in Crohn's disease surgical resection of the small or large intestine is followed by a high rate of recurrence. With resection of segments of small bowel or ileum and reanastomosis a recurrence rate of 50 to 75 percent over a 5-year period is not unusual. Recurrence of disease is invariably proximal to the created anastomosis. When total colectomy and ileostomy are performed for Crohn's disease of the colon without significant small-intestinal involvement, recurrence rates are lower, varying from 10 to 30 percent. Despite these recurrences, most patients do not develop a short bowel syndrome and usually can expect significant improvement. Faced with the possibility of recurrent disease many physicians are reluctant to advise surgery in Crohn's disease, except for the type of clear-cut complications described above. Alternatively, patients with persistently active disease may require chronic maintenance on unacceptably high levels of corticosteroids and with the appreciable risk of steroid side effects. Just as a failure of medical therapy should lead to colectomy in ulcerative colitis, such should be the conclusion in the patient with Crohn's colitis without major small-bowel involvement. While in this setting there is also a definite rate of recurrence, such recurrences are often not disabling. When extensive small-bowel disease is present, surgical therapy is often not feasible and should only be reserved for specific disease complications.

The therapy of Crohn's disease in children presents special problems since normal growth and development may be retarded in the presence of active disease. In addition to conventional drug therapy, intensive nutritional therapy or the judicious use of surgery may be required.

PROGNOSIS

The overall prognosis of IBD has been favorably affected by the use of corticosteroids and sulfasalazine, as well as by supportive techniques such as intravenous alimentation. In *acute* ulcerative colitis these therapeutic modalities can result in a remission in almost 90 percent of patients. The mortality of an initial acute attack is approximately 5 percent. Poor prognostic factors and an increased mortality rate are likely when there is total colonic involvement, when the onset occurs over age 60, and when toxic megacolon develops.

The long-term prognosis of *chronic* ulcerative colitis is more difficult to assess due to the variable and intermittent nature of the disease and improvements in therapy. Left-sided colitis and ulcerative proctitis have a very favorable prognosis and probably no increase in mortality; similarly the long-term prognosis for extensive colitis has improved greatly. Older studies suggested a poor prognosis for extensive colitis, with less than 50 percent of patients surviving 15 years after onset. More recent observations (longest follow-up 11 years) show a 10-year mortality rate of between 5 and 10 percent for severe first attacks (excluding toxic megacolon). Approximately 75 percent of patients will experience relapses, and 20 to 25 percent will require colectomy. The problem of carcinoma developing in the setting of long-standing chronic ulcerative colitis is an important factor in determining the long-term prognosis of ulcerative colitis. As discussed above, periodic surveillance with colonoscopy and multiple biopsies to detect dysplastic changes is indicated to detect a high-risk group for which to advise colectomy.

The prognosis for Crohn's disease is not as favorable as for ulcerative colitis. An exception is *acute regional enteritis,* often discovered during laparotomy for suspected appendicitis; this has an excellent prognosis. More than two-thirds of such patients may show no subsequent evidence of regional enteritis, and this form of acute ileitis may well be due to different mechanisms than those responsible for Crohn's disease. Prevailing surgical opinion favors a conservative approach in this situation, and in most instances operative resection is not advised.

In the majority of patients with Crohn's disease the course is chronic and intermittent regardless of the site of involvement. The disease responds less well to medical therapy with time, and over two-thirds of patients develop complications requiring surgery at some point in their disease. In contrast to ulcerative colitis, where mortality appears greatest early in the disease, in Crohn's disease the mortality rate increases with the duration of the disease, and probably ranges from 5 to 10 percent. Most deaths occur from peritonitis and sepsis. As indicated above, following surgery patients with Crohn's disease often have recurrence and relapses. Nevertheless, the therapy of Crohn's disease will result in reasonably stable and productive lives for most Crohn's disease patients.

REFERENCES

General

KIRSNER JB, SHORTER RG (eds): *Inflammatory Bowel Disease,* 2d ed. Philadelphia, Lea & Febiger, 1980

———, ———: Recent developments in "nonspecific" inflammatory bowel disease. N Engl J Med 306:775, 837, 1982

SLEISENGER MH, FORDTRAN JS (eds): *Gastrointestinal Diseases,* 2d ed. Philadelphia, Saunders, 1978

Etiology and diagnostic aspects

BEEKEN WL: Transmissible agents in inflammatory bowel disease. Med Clin N Am 64:1031, 1980

BLASER MJ, RELLER LB: *Campylobacter* enteritis. N Engl J Med 305:1444, 1981

GOODMAN MJ et al: The usefulness of rectal biopsy in inflammatory bowel disease. Gastroenterology 72:952, 1977

GREENSTEIN AJ et al: The extraintestinal complications of ulcerative colitis and Crohn's disease. A study of 700 patients. Medicine 55:401, 1976

JESS P: Acute terminal ileitis. A review of recent literature on the relationship to Crohn's disease. Scand J Gastroenterol 16:321, 1981

QUINN TC et al: *Chlamydia trachomatis* proctitis. N Engl J Med 305:195, 1981

TRNKA YM, LAMONT JT: Association of *Clostridium difficile* toxin with symptomatic relapse of chronic inflammatory bowel disease. Gastroenterology 80:693, 1981

VAN TRAPPEN G et al: *Yersinia enteritis* and enterocolitis: Gastroenterological aspects. Gastroenterology 72:220, 1977

Therapy of inflammatory bowel disease

AZAD KHAN AK et al: Optimum dose of sulphasalazine for maintenance treatment in ulcerative colitis. Gut 12:232, 1980

BERNSTEIN LH et al: Healing of perineal Crohn's disease with metronidazole. Gastroenterology 79:357, 1980

GREENSTEEN AJ et al: Reoperation and recurrence in Crohn's colitis and ileocolitis. N Engl J Med 293:658, 1975

GYDE SN et al: Malignancy in Crohn's disease. Gut 21:1024, 1980

KELTS DG et al: Nutritional basis of growth failure in children and adolescents with Crohn's disease. Gastroenterology 76:720, 1979

LENNARD JONES JE et al: Cancer in colitis: Assessment of the individual risk by clinical and histological criteria. Gastroenterology 73:1280, 1977

LOCK MR et al: Recurrence and reoperation for Crohn's disease. N Engl J Med 304:1586, 1981

PRESENT DH et al: Treatment of Crohn's disease with 6-mercaptopurine. N Engl J Med 302:981, 1980

SUMMERS RW et al: National cooperative Crohn's disease study: Results of drug treatment. Gastroenterology 77:849, 1979

URSING B et al: A comparative study of metronidazole and sulfasalazine for active Crohn's disease. The Cooperative Crohn's Disease Study in Sweden. Gastroenterology 83:550, 1982

310 DISEASES OF THE SMALL AND LARGE INTESTINE

J. THOMAS LaMONT
KURT J. ISSELBACHER

SYMPTOMS OF INTESTINAL DISEASE

SYMPTOMS OF DISEASES OF THE SMALL INTESTINE The major clinical manifestations of small-bowel disease are *motility disturbances,* abdominal *pain* and *distention,* gastrointestinal *bleeding,* and *malabsorption.*

An alteration in the normal propulsive activity of the small intestine is a common manifestation of a variety of diseases. The presentation may be one of decreased motility, such as paralytic ileus resulting from metabolic disturbance or peritonitis, or intestinal obstruction caused by tumors, adhesions, volvulus, or intussusception (Chap. 311). Diarrhea frequently accompanies small-bowel disease (Chap. 36) resulting from direct involvement of the mucosa by inflammatory or infiltrative lesions (sprue, regional enteritis). The associated malabsorption of fat and bile salts is an important factor in the pathogenesis of diarrhea in these conditions (Chaps. 36 and 308).

Abdominal pain due to small-intestinal disease is usually periumbilical or supraumbilical and often poorly localized. With obstruction, pain is classically described as intermittent or colicky. As the intestine becomes progressively dilated with loss of muscular tone, the colicky nature of the pain may become less apparent. Acute inflammation of the small intestine which involves the visceral or parietal peritoneum is associated with steady, aching pain, usually located directly over the inflamed area and often accompanied by guarding and rebound tenderness. *Gastrointestinal bleeding* due to small-bowel disease may be detected as occult bleeding or, less commonly, brisk hemorrhage. In general, blood from a source distal to the ligament of Treitz is not acted on by gastric acid and appears as a dark maroon color in contrast to the black, tarry melena which often results from gastric or duodenal bleeding. Obviously, the appearance of blood in the stool depends not only on site of bleeding but also on the briskness of the hemorrhage and the rapidity of transit; thus localization of the bleeding site by stool appearance alone may be misleading.

An important clue to the presence of small-bowel disease is the demonstration of malabsorption of fat. With extensive mucosal damage or lymphatic obstruction, the presenting symptoms may relate to any of the features of a malabsorption syndrome or protein-losing enteropathy (Chap. 308) and should direct attention to the small intestine.

SYMPTOMS OF COLONIC DISEASE The major symptoms of colonic disease are *alteration in bowel habit, rectal bleeding,* and *pain.* Alteration in bowel habit implies a change from previous patterns of defecation; hence a detailed history is important. Most normal individuals have one to three movements of well-formed stools each day. *Diarrhea* means the passage of watery or loose stools usually with increased frequency, while *constipation* implies infrequent passage of hard, dry stools; *obstipation* is the absence of spontaneous bowel movements. A persistent change in bowel habit, particularly in older individuals with no previous irregularity, is usually an important early symptom of organic disease of the colon and should never be labeled *functional* unless a thorough diagnostic evaluation is negative. The appearance of the stool may also provide important diagnostic clues. Blood coating the exterior of a formed stool implies a lesion in the anal canal or rectum, while blood admixed with the feces indicates a bleeding source higher in the colon. Brisk hemorrhage from the colon or distal small intestine results in passage of fresh blood, called *hematochezia.* This may appear as fresh blood and clots if the lesion is in the left colon, or darker maroon-colored blood if the bleeding source is in the right colon.

Pain resulting from colonic disease is usually localized to either of the lower abdominal quadrants, as opposed to pain of small-intestinal origin, which is localized to the periumbilical area or higher. Rectal pain is often felt deep in the pelvis, while pain in the anal canal is accurately localized to the perineum. The mechanisms of colonic pain are similar to those in other intestinal viscera (see Chap. 5). Distention from gas or fluid causes crampy or colicky pain from stretching of the muscle layers and resulting contraction or spasm. Pain of this type is often relieved by passage of flatus or stool. Pain may also result if the colonic wall is inflamed or infiltrated by tumor. Acute colonic inflammation which involves the visceral or parietal peritoneum produces sharply localized pain, which may be accompanied by abdominal guarding and rebound tenderness. An important symptom of rectal disease is *tenesmus,* or painful straining at stool, with a sensation of incomplete emptying after defecation. This symptom can be caused by retention of stool in the rectum, by tumors of the rectum which simulate retained stools, or by colonic inflammation.

DIAGNOSTIC PROCEDURES

PHYSICAL EXAMINATION Careful *examination* of the abdomen may disclose a mass or fistula associated with inflammatory or neoplastic disease, localized tenderness, or abdominal distention resulting from ileus or intestinal obstruction. The physical examination and findings in the patient with acute abdominal pain are discussed in Chap. 5.

Thorough examination may also reveal extraintestinal findings associated with small-intestinal diseases. Thus buccal pigmentation or telangiectasia may indicate coexistent small-bowel polyposis or telangiectasia and may clarify episodes of abdominal pain or chronic bleeding. Similarly, evidence of iritis, arthritis, or erythema nodosum may suggest the presence of inflammatory bowel disease.

Perhaps the most important part of the physical examination in the diagnosis of colonic diseases is the *digital rectal examination.* This procedure should never be omitted for reasons of modesty or fear of embarrassment because it is essential in the diagnosis of perianal, sphincteric, and ampullary lesions; prostatic and uterine abnormalities; and even small rectal masses. A metastatic tumor may be felt in the perirectal tissues as a shelf-like deformity (Blumer's shelf), especially anteriorly above the prostate. The fecal material on the glove should be immediately tested chemically for occult blood. Approximately one-half of all rectal carcinomas lie within reach of the index finger, and omission of the rectal examination may delay diagnosis and worsen the prognosis.

STOOL EXAMINATION Abnormal stools constitute important objective evidence of colonic disease. Stools should be examined by the physician as soon as possible after defecation for the presence of visible blood on the surface or within the specimen. A small sample should be tested for occult blood. Microscopic examination of fresh stool is important in the diagnosis of parasitic diseases, particularly in amoebic colitis when motile trophozoites can be seen in fresh, warm stool suspensions. Stool suspensions can also be stained with a drop of methylene blue for polymorphonuclear leukocytes, which indicate the presence of an acute inflammatory exudate characteristic of ulcerative colitis, amoebic colitis, and bacillary dysentery. Fixed and stained slides of stool may also reveal amoebas and other parasites, while stool culture is essential for the diagnosis of bacillary dysentery. Sudan III stain of stool is a useful screening test for steatorrhea.

BARIUM STUDIES The considerable length of the small intestine (some 12 to 22 ft in the adult) makes *radiologic studies* of the small bowel of prime importance and usually forms the basis for the diagnosis of small-bowel diseases. *Small-bowel x-rays* are not usually part of a routine upper gastrointestinal series and must be specifically requested. In view of the length of the small bowel and wide variations in transit time, it is essential to provide the radiologist with as much information as possible, since the precise nature of the problem may determine various technical aspects of the examination. It is only through sequential examination of the barium column as it progresses through the small bowel that localized abnormalities such as tumors, fistulas, areas of ischemia, or inflammatory bowel disease may be apparent.

Barium enema is an extremely accurate diagnostic tool for the identification of structural abnormalities of the colon. A careful study in a well-prepared patient can demonstrate mucosal lesions as small as 0.5 cm. For high-quality resolution of subtle lesions, such as small polyps or early changes of ulcerative colitis, an air-contrast barium enema is useful. In this study the mucosa is outlined by a thin coat of barium, after which air is injected to enhance contrast and outline small lesions. The combined use of the digital examination, stool guaiac test, proctosigmoidoscopy, and barium enema will identify 95 percent of significant colonic lesions. Negative results of these procedures constitute strong evidence that a functional disorder may be present.

SIGMOIDOSCOPY Contrary to the general impression, the technique of sigmoidoscopy is not difficult to master, and with practice the discomfort to the patient is minimal. The physician should learn to evaluate mucosal friability (one of the earliest signs of proctitis and colitis) and to recognize abnormal vascular patterns, edema, ulcerations, and polyps. Ninety percent of tumors of the rectum and rectosigmoid can be directly visualized with this instrument. Approximately half of all tumors of the large intestine lie within the terminal 25 cm of the colon and within the reach of the sigmoidoscope. It is important to remember that the distal 20 to 25 cm of the colon is difficult to examine by barium enema. A rectal carcinoma can be missed on routine barium enema yet easily visualized and biopsied through the sigmoidoscope. Furthermore, the earliest changes of ulcerative colitis may not be demonstrated radiographically but may be obvious through the sigmoidoscope. Rectal biopsy is easily and painlessly accomplished through the instrument and is associated with minimal morbidity except in the presence of bleeding disorders.

INTESTINAL ENDOSCOPY See Chap. 288.

MESENTERIC ANGIOGRAPHY Angiography is helpful in the diagnosis of two conditions: intestinal ischemia and gastrointestinal hemorrhage. Patients suspected of having acute intestinal ischemia from arterial embolus as well as chronic ischemia (intestinal angina) should undergo angiography to locate the site of blockage. Angiography is also very helpful in some patients with acute gastrointestinal blood loss. The success of this technique is related to the rate of blood loss, being most successful when bleeding exceeds 0.5 ml/min.

DISORDERS OF INTESTINAL MOTILITY

A major function of the intestinal tract is to propel the intestinal contents (food, secretions, chyme, feces) from stomach toward anus. Abnormalities of motility comprise the most common intestinal diseases: diverticulosis, megacolon, constipation, and irritable bowel syndrome. Although these conditions share a common abnormality, i.e., dysmotility, their clinical features are quite diverse.

DIVERTICULOSIS Diverticula may be either congenital or acquired and may affect either the small or large intestine. Congenital diverticula are herniations of the entire thickness of intestinal wall, while the more common acquired diverticula consist of herniations of the mucosa through the muscularis, generally at the site of a nutrient artery.

Small-intestinal diverticula Diverticula may occur in any portion of the small intestine; however, with the exception of Meckel's diverticulum, the most common locations are in the duodenum and jejunum. Most often diverticula are asymptomatic and discovered incidentally on upper gastrointestinal x-rays. On occasion, however, they may cause symptoms either because of their anatomic proximity to other structures or rarely from inflammation or bleeding.

Duodenal diverticula arise singly from the medial surface of the second portion of the duodenum. In most patients, they cause no symptoms. Rarely, they may present as acute diverticulitis with abdominal pain, fever, gastrointestinal bleeding or, most rarely, perforation. Adjacent structures, such as the bile or pancreatic ducts, may become involved; cases of common-duct obstruction and pancreatitis have been reported. Jejunal diverticula, while less common, may also be the site of acute inflammation, bleeding, or perforation with resulting abscess or peritonitis.

Multiple jejunal diverticula may be associated with a malabsorption syndrome related to bacterial overgrowth within the diverticula, similar to other situations where intestinal stasis (i.e., blind loops) permits bacterial proliferation. The consequences of bacterial proliferation with resultant mucosal damage, deconjugation of bile salts, and vitamin B_{12} malabsorption are discussed in Chap. 308.

Meckel's diverticulum, a persistent omphalomesenteric duct, is the most frequent congenital anomaly of the digestive tract, occurring in approximately 2 percent of autopsied adults. The diverticulum is wide-mouthed, about 5 cm long, and arises from the antimesenteric border of the ileum, usually within 100 cm of the ileocecal valve. The sac may be lined with normal ileal mucosa (approximately 50 percent) or contain gastric, duodenal, pancreatic, or colonic mucosa. While rarely symptomatic in adults, Meckel's diverticulum may produce hemorrhage, inflammation, and obstruction in children and young adults.

Hemorrhage occurs almost exclusively before age 10 and invariably results from septic ulceration of ileal mucosa adjacent to a Meckel's diverticulum lined with gastric mucosa. The diagnosis may be established by isotope scanning of the abdomen after injection of technetium, which is taken up by the ectopic gastric mucosa in the diverticulum (Fig. 310-1). In older children and young adults inflammation of the diverticulum may mimic acute appendicitis. Mechanical obstruction may also occur if the diverticulum intussuscepts into the lumen of the bowel or twists on a fibrous remnant of the omphalo-

FIGURE 310-1
Meckel's diverticulum (technetium abdominal scan). After the intravenous administration of ^{99m}Tc, the abdominal scan shows the isotope concentrated in the gastric mucosa (s), the urinary bladder (b), and in an ectopic area (m) surgically proved to be Meckel's diverticulum. (Courtesy of S Treves.)

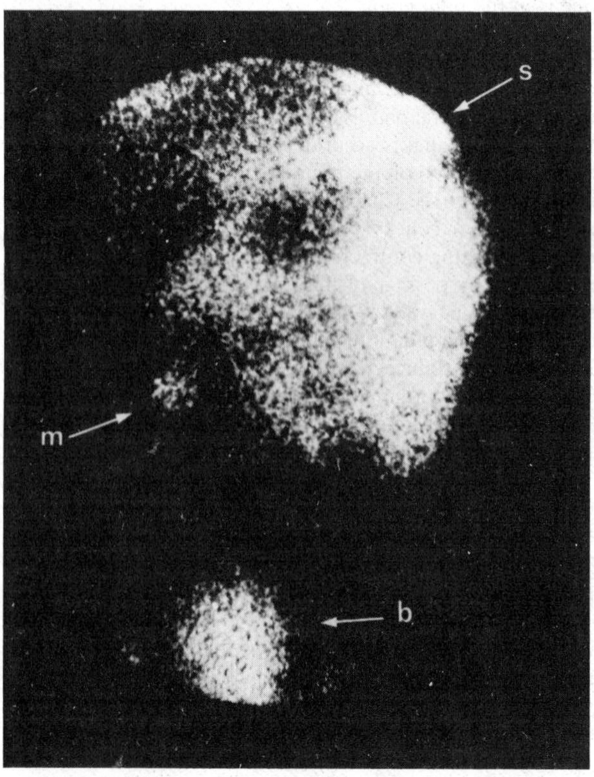

mesenteric duct which extends from the diverticulum to the abdominal wall. The treatment of any of these complications of Meckel's diverticulum is surgical excision.

Colonic diverticula Diverticula of the colon are herniations or saclike protrusions of the mucosa through the muscularis, at the point where a nutrient artery penetrates the muscularis. Diverticula occur most commonly in the sigmoid colon and decrease in frequency in the proximal colon. They increase with age, and the incidence ranges between 20 and 50 percent in western populations over age 50. The exact mechanism for their formation is unknown but may be related to an increase in intraluminal pressure. Thickening of the muscle coat of the colon in most patients with diverticula suggests that herniations of mucosa are caused by increased pressure produced by colonic muscle contractions. The rarity of colonic diverticula in underdeveloped nations in contrast to their frequent occurrence in western countries has led to the speculation that diverticula result from the highly refined western diet, which is deficient in dietary fiber or roughage. It is proposed that such diets result in decreased fecal bulk, narrowing of the colon, and an increase in intraluminal pressure in order to move the smaller fecal mass. The role of dietary fiber in the etiology and treatment of diverticular disease remains to be determined.

Colonic diverticula are usually asymptomatic and are an incidental finding on barium enema performed for other reasons. The major complications are inflammation, both acute and chronic, and hemorrhage. Since diverticulosis is quite common in older patients, one must avoid the temptation of attributing symptoms to the diverticula unless other conditions, especially colonic neoplasm, have been excluded.

Diverticulitis Inflammation can occur in or around the diverticular sac. The cause of diverticulitis is probably mechanical, related to retention in the diverticula of undigested food residues and bacteria, which may form a hard mass called a *fecalith.* This compromises the blood supply to the thin-walled sac (made up solely of mucosa and serosa) and renders it susceptible to invasion by colonic bacteria. The inflammatory process may vary from a small intramural or pericolic abscess to generalized peritonitis. Some attacks are accompanied by minimal symptoms and seem to heal spontaneously. Studies of resected specimens indicate that most perforations of the diverticular sac are small and result in inflammation of the sac itself and the corresponding serosal surface. Diverticulitis occurs more often in men than women, and three times as often in the left than in the right colon. This suggests that diverticulitis may be related to the higher intraluminal pressures and the more solid fecal material in the sigmoid and descending colon.

Acute diverticulitis is a disease of variable severity characterized by lower abdominal pain and tenderness. The clinical features are lower abdominal pain, made worse by defecation, and signs of peritoneal irritation—muscle spasm, guarding, rebound tenderness, fever, and leukocytosis. Rectal examination may reveal a tender mass if the area of inflammation is close to the rectum. Although constipation may not have been noted prior to the onset of the illness, the inflammation around the colon often results in some degree of constipation. Rectal bleeding, usually microscopic, is noted in 25 percent of cases; it is rarely massive. Complications include free perforation, which results in acute peritonitis, sepsis, and shock, particularly in the elderly. The perforation may be walled off by adherent omentum or neighboring structures such as the bladder or small bowel. Abscess formation or fistulas then occur as the inflammatory mass burrows into other organs (Fig. 310-2). Severe pericolitis may cause a dense, fibrous reaction or stricture around the bowel which can be associated with colonic obstruction. Repeated attacks of diverticulitis in the same area generally require surgical resection.

DIFFERENTIAL DIAGNOSIS In the less acute situation differential diagnosis is principally that of a neoplasm in the area of the diverticulosis. Sigmoidoscopy may show an acutely inflamed mucosa over an apparent extrinsic mass; passing the instrument through the contracted lumen is usually impossible. During the acute phase of diverticulitis, barium enema may be hazardous, since contrast material under pressure may lead to rupture of an inflamed diverticulum and convert a walled-off

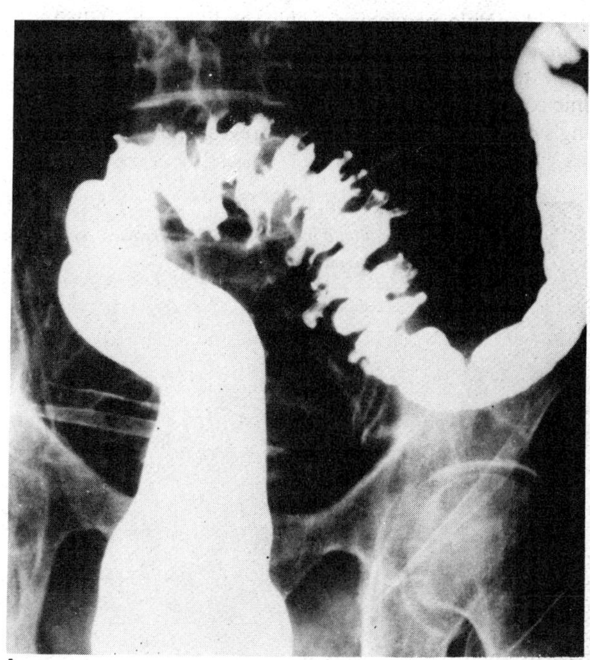

A

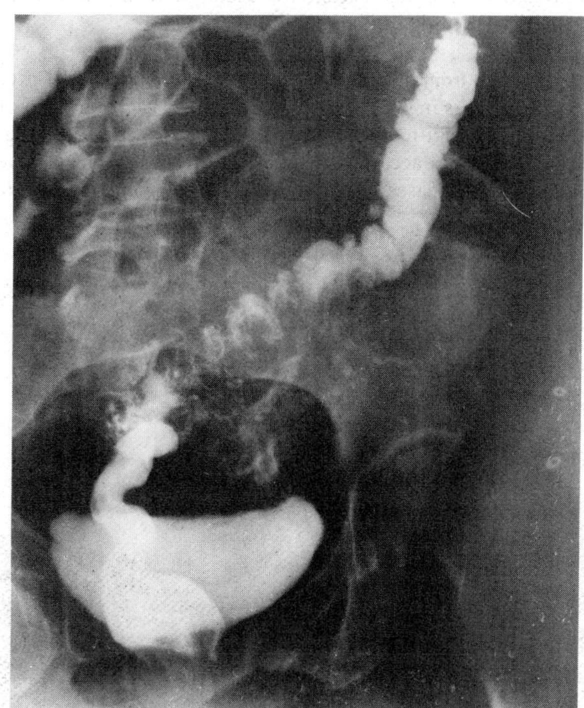

B

inflammatory lesion to a free perforation. The examination is usually safe after adequate treatment and healing of the diverticulitis. The radiologic findings on barium enema suggestive of diverticulitis are leakage of barium from a diverticular sac, stricture formation, and the presence of a pericolic inflammatory mass. In many patients, the distortion caused by inflammation prevents a clear distinction between cancer and diverticulitis; surgical excision may be required for accurate diagnosis.

TREATMENT For the mild case without signs of perforation, treatment consists of bed rest, stool softeners, liquid diet, and a wide-spectrum antibiotic such as tetracycline or ampicillin. Repeated attacks of diverticulitis in the same area generally require surgical resection. Severe attacks with acute peritoneal signs, suspected abscess, or perforation require intravenous antibiotics directed against gram-negative anaerobic bacteria, followed by surgical drainage or resection. The usual procedure is a diverting colostomy with resection of the involved colon; reanastomosis is then performed at a second operation.

Painful diverticular disease without diverticulitis Some patients with diverticulosis develop recurrent left lower quadrant colicky pain without clinical or pathologic evidence of acute diverticulitis. They often have bouts of alternating constipation and diarrhea, and the pain may be relieved by defecation or passage of flatus. These features suggest the coexistence of the irritable bowel syndrome (see below). Examination during a bout of pain reveals tenderness of the sigmoid colon, but signs of peritoneal inflammation such as rebound tenderness, muscle guarding, fever, and leukocytosis are absent. Barium enema shows typical diverticula without evidence of inflammation and stricture, plus a "sawtooth" irregularity of the lumen reflecting associated muscle spasm. In some patients the pain is severe enough to warrant observation in hospital and restriction of food since feeding aggravates the pain by causing colonic contraction. Anticholinergics, which reduce sigmoid contractions, and mild sedation are usually all that is required. The patient should be started on a high-residue diet or given a bulk laxative such as hemicellulose, unprocessed bran, or psyllium extract. Surgical excision is usually not indicated unless acute diverticulitis or its complications occur.

Hemorrhage from diverticula This rare complication of diverticulosis occurs in elderly patients and is caused by erosion of a vessel by a fecalith within the diverticular sac. The bleeding is painless and not accompanied by signs or symptoms of diverticulitis. Most cases of mild or moderate hemorrhage stop spontaneously with bed rest and blood transfusion. In patients with severe hemorrhage mesenteric angiography can be both diagnostic in localizing the bleeding site and therapeutic since vasoconstrictive drugs infused intraarterially can effectively control hemorrhage. The angiographer can direct the surgeon to the area of bleeding if surgery is required for continued or recurrent bleeding. The location of bleeding diverticula demonstrated at angiograph in several series has been more commonly in the right colon, particularly the ascending colon, in contrast to the sigmoid colon, where diverticula are more numerous.

MEGACOLON Megacolon, or giant colon, is characterized by massive distention of the colon usually accompanied by severe constipation or obstipation. This condition can be either congenital or acquired and is seen in all age groups. Acute toxic megacolon is a severe complication of chronic ulcerative colitis (see Chap. 309).

Aganglionic megacolon (Hirschsprung's disease) This is a congenital disorder which becomes manifest in early infancy, occurring more frequently in males, and is often familial. These infants have massive abdominal distention, absent bowel movements, and impaired nutrition due to chronic obstruction of the colon. In some individuals with less severe symptoms the disease may not be diagnosed until adolescence or early adulthood. The inability to defecate is caused by the absence of ganglion cells (Meissner's and Auerbach's plexuses) in a small segment of the distal colon. This aganglionic segment is unable to relax to permit passage of stool, causing the normal colon proximal to it to become greatly dilated. On rectal examination the ampulla is empty of feces and the anal sphincter is normal. Barium enema reveals a narrowed segment in the rectosigmoid area, with massive dilatation above (Fig. 310-3). Diagnosis is made by deep surgical biopsy under anesthesia and demonstration of absent ganglion cells in the diseased segment. In most patients the aganglionic segment is in the rectosigmoid colon; in rare instances the lesion may involve more proximal bowel or even the entire colon. The treatment is usually surgical, although milder cases may be treated by enemas to empty the colon. The most effective operation is a pull-through procedure in which normally innervated colon is anastomosed to the distal rectum just above the internal sphincter, thus bypassing the contracted aganglionic segment.

Chronic idiopathic megacolon This condition, also called *psychogenic megacolon,* has its onset later in childhood, usually at the time toilet training begins. It is characterized by severe chronic constipation and distention, and in contrast to Hirschsprung's disease, digital examination reveals the rectal ampulla

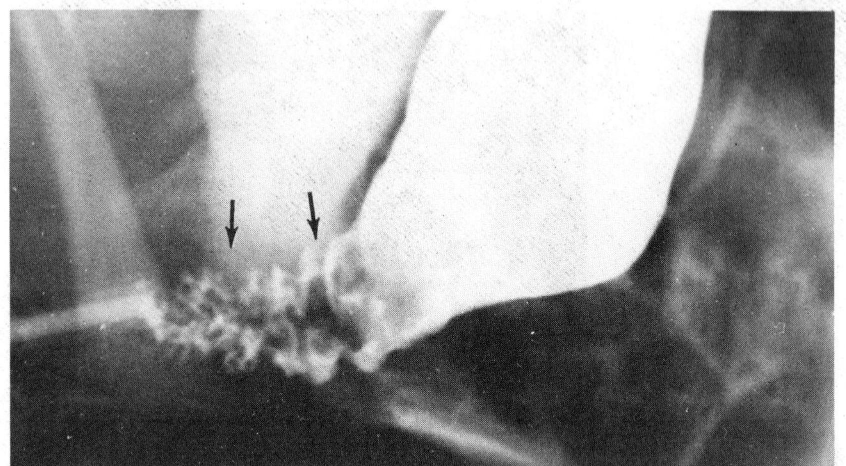

FIGURE 310-3
Aganglionic megacolon with narrowed rectal segment (arrows).

to be invariably distended with feces. Barium enema shows the entire colon to be distended with stools, no narrowed segment is seen, and rectal biopsy discloses the normal complement of ganglion cells in Auerbach's plexus. Treatment is based on education in normal bowel habits, but a long course of enemas or large doses of mineral oil may be required until the patient acquires more normal bowel movements.

Acquired megacolon In Central and South America infection with *Trypanosoma cruzi* (Chagas' disease) can result in destruction of the ganglion cells of the colon, producing a clinical picture similar to congenital megacolon, except that the onset is in adult life rather than childhood. A number of other diseases are associated with megacolon in adults. Patients with schizophrenia or depression, particularly institutionalized patients, may have obstipation and massive colonic dilatation. Severe neurologic disorders including cerebral atrophy, spinal cord injury, and parkinsonism may also cause megacolon. Myxedema, infiltrative diseases such as amyloidosis, and scleroderma can also reduce colonic motility and produce marked colonic distention. Narcotic drugs, particularly morphine and codeine, can cause severe constipation, especially when administered to bedridden patients. Digital rectal examination of adults with acquired megacolon reveals a rectum distended with feces, as opposed to the empty rectum in aganglionic megacolon. Treatment is aimed at the underlying disease as well as the careful use of enemas and cathartics.

INTESTINAL PSEUDOOBSTRUCTION Intestinal pseudoobstruction is a chronic motility disorder of the intestinal tract characterized by recurrent attacks of nausea, vomiting, abdominal pain, and distention of the small and large intestine mimicking mechanical obstruction. Pseudoobstruction can be either primary or secondary. In primary (idiopathic) pseudoobstruction no other disease entity is present, and the cause of the motility disorder is obscure. Secondary pseudoobstruction has been described in patients with scleroderma, amyloidosis, diabetes, sprue, muscular dystrophy, Parkinson's disease, and following intestinal bypass. The pathogenesis of the idiopathic variety involves poor peristalsis as demonstrated by esophageal and small-intestinal motility tracings. An abnormality of physiologic neural responses to distention has been postulated; however, no morphologic abnormality of enteric nerves or smooth-muscle fibers is demonstrable.

The diagnosis of idiopathic pseudoobstruction is based on a history of recurrent attacks of obstructive symptoms with no evidence of mechanical obstruction, abnormal (aperistaltic) esophageal motility, and exclusion of other entities which can alter intestinal motility. Barium studies reveal dilatation of the small bowel and delayed transit. During an acute attack air fluid levels are seen in the small and occasionally in the large bowel. Steatorrhea due to bacterial overgrowth of the small bowel is not uncommon.

The medical management of idiopathic intestinal pseudoobstruction is unsatisfactory because of our lack of basic understanding of its causes. The acute attacks generally respond to intestinal intubation, preferably with a Miller-Abbott tube, to decompress the small intestine; parenteral alimentation is used to maintain nutritional status. Stimulation of intestinal peristalsis with metoclopramide, neostigmine (Prostigmin), or bethanechol may be helpful in some patients. Chronic antibiotic therapy should be tried in those patients with bacterial overgrowth and steatorrhea. Long-term home parenteral hyperalimentation may be necessary for patients with chronic pain and distention who are resistant to all other therapy. Once the diagnosis is established, surgical exploration should be carefully avoided, as most patients are made worse by laparotomy except when a mechanical obstruction is relieved. On the other hand, surgical exploration may be required in patients with signs or symptoms of peritonitis. In addition, some patients with idiopathic pseudoobstruction may develop true mechanical obstruction from adhesions arising from previous explorations or from volvulus of dilated, atonic bowel loops. The prognosis of idiopathic intestinal pseudoobstruction is unfavorable due to the lack of satisfactory treatment. Death from malnutrition, steatorrhea, and electrolyte disturbances is not uncommon.

IRRITABLE BOWEL SYNDROME The irritable bowel syndrome (IBS) is the most common gastrointestinal disease in clinical practice, and although not a life-threatening illness, it causes great distress to those afflicted and a feeling of helplessness and frustration for the physician attempting to treat it. The patient with irritable bowel syndrome may present with one of *three clinical variants.* Patients with so-called spastic colitis complain primarily of chronic abdominal pain and constipation. A second group has chronic intermittent watery diarrhea, often without pain. Some patients have both features and complain of alternating constipation and diarrhea.

The basic pathophysiologic abnormality in the irritable bowel syndrome is an alteration of intestinal motility. Patients with the spastic colon variant (pain and constipation) have *increased* resting colonic motility; in contrast those presenting primarily with diarrhea have *decreased* resting colonic motility. Both groups have an increase in colonic motility after injection of cholinergic drugs or cholecystokinin; motility may also be increased in association with psychological stress. It has been suggested that cholecystokinin may be a normal stimulus of intestinal motility and that the spastic colon may result from an exaggerated response to the normal release of cholecystokinin after eating.

Patients with the irritable bowel syndrome also exhibit an abnormal basic electrical rhythm in the colon, characterized by an increase in 3-cycle-per-minute (cpm) slow-wave activity. It is not certain, however, whether these abnormalities of smooth-muscle contraction are primary or secondary to another underlying abnormality of intestinal neuromuscular function.

Many investigators have described evidence of significant psychological disturbances in the majority of patients with irritable bowel syndrome. Depression, hysteria, and obsessive-compulsive traits are common, and psychological stress frequently triggers an exacerbation of symptoms. It should be noted, however, that in normal individuals colonic motility is altered by stress. For example, increased intracolonic pressure has been observed in normal volunteers during a stressful interview. These observations suggest that psychological stress may be a nonspecific trigger of symptoms in the irritable bowel syndrome, as is the case in many other illnesses of diverse etiology.

Clinical features The irritable bowel syndrome is a disease of young or middle-aged adults; female/male ratio is 2:1. The predominant feature is a history of chronic constipation, diarrhea, or both. The typical patient describes watery diarrhea occurring *intermittently* for months or years. The diarrhea is usually worse in the morning upon arising or after breakfast. After the passage of three or four loose stools with excessive mucus the patient may feel well for the remainder of the day. Diarrhea throughout the day or especially nocturnal diarrhea is most unusual. The diarrhea may last for weeks or months and then disappear spontaneously for variable periods of time. Some patients describe "pencil-like" pasty stools rather than diarrhea.

Another typical presentation is that of chronic abdominal pain with constipation, or with alternating constipation and diarrhea. These patients describe intermittent crampy lower abdominal pain, often over the sigmoid colon, which is usually relieved by passage of flatus or stool. A variety of other complaints, such as heartburn, excessive bloating, back pain, weakness, faintness, and palpitations, are frequent in patients with irritable bowel syndrome.

Physical examination reveals these patients to be anxious but otherwise normal. During intense pain, the abdomen may be distended, but no visible peristalsis is noted; the abdominal musculature is relaxed, and a tender sigmoid full of feces may be palpated in the left lower quadrant. Characteristically, the rectal ampulla is empty of feces. Sigmoidoscopic examination is usually normal or at most shows a prominent vascular pattern. There may be difficulty in negotiating the rectosigmoid curve at 13 to 15 cm from the anus because of spasm. Large amounts of clear mucus are frequently encountered during the examination.

The *diagnosis* of the irritable colon syndrome is suggested by the chronic intermittent nature of symptoms without obvious signs of physical deterioration, the relation of symptoms to environment or emotional stress, and the exclusion of other conditions. The evaluation should include a careful history, complete physical examination including sigmoidoscopy, stool examination (for occult blood, parasites, and pathogenic bacteria), and a barium enema. The latter study serves to rule out other lesions since there are no diagnostic x-ray findings for this syndrome, although spasticity of the sigmoid, accentuated haustra, and a tubular appearance to the descending colon may be observed when the patient is symptomatic. Lactase deficiency may masquerade as irritable colon syndrome and should be excluded by a trial of milk restriction, a lactose tolerance test, or a lactose breath hydrogen test (see Chap. 308). Thyrotoxicosis is easily confused with irritable bowel syndrome and should be excluded by appropriate laboratory studies.

Treatment of the irritable colon syndrome requires both skill and patience. It is important that the patient be reassured that this condition normally does not lead to the development of inflammatory bowel disease (i.e., ulcerative colitis) or colonic malignancy. It is also important for both the patient and the physician to realize that the condition is chronic, and while it may be alleviated, it cannot be cured. The patient should be encouraged to adapt to the symptoms so as to minimize their impact on life-style. The physician should not imply that the symptoms are largely emotional or psychological in origin, since this is usually rejected by the patient. It is appropriate, however, to emphasize the relationship between psychological stress and the onset of severity of symptoms, as this may allow the patient to better deal with the disease. After the diagnosis is established, frequent x-rays and endoscopies are not necessary; general physical examinations, hemograms, and stool examinations, however, should be carried out at regular intervals.

Drug treatment is aimed at altering the abnormal colonic motility in this disease. Patients with constipation may respond to an increase in dietary bulk in the form of unprocessed bran or other nonabsorbed bulk laxatives. Mild sedation with phenobarbital or tranquilizers may be indicated, and anticholinergic drugs are useful in some patients. Troublesome diarrhea may respond to diphenoxylate (Lomotil) or paregoric. Unfortunately, no specific drug or dietary regimen affords good relief in all patients, and thus a number of therapeutic maneuvers need to be tried.

CHRONIC CONSTIPATION In Chap. 36 the mechanism of defecation is discussed. Disorders involving the sensory or motor components of this mechanism may arise from destruction of the nerves subserving these functions, from invasion or inflammation of the rectosigmoid itself, or from central nervous system lesions. Most cases of chronic constipation arise from habitual neglect of afferent impulses, failure to initiate defecation, and accumulation of large, dry fecal masses in the rectum. This voluntary suppression of the call to stool may arise during the period of toilet training in childhood, or later in life because of a sense of social impropriety, unaccustomed surroundings, uncomfortable toilet facilities, or illnesses which require confinement to bed. As constant distention of the rectum with feces becomes chronic, the patient grows less aware of rectal fullness. Bowel movements become progressively more difficult, and painful hemorrhoids or anal fissures reinforce suppression of the urge to defecate. To avoid these problems, the patient begins the chronic use of laxatives or enemas, without which defecation becomes impossible.

Treatment The physician should make every attempt to educate the patient about the chain of events which has led to chronic constipation. Attempts should be made to alter patterns of many years' duration, and the patient must recognize the importance of responding to, rather than suppressing, the urge to defecate. It is helpful to initiate a routine whereby defecation is attempted at a given time each day. In most individuals the call to stool occurs in the morning after breakfast. Physical exercise such as a brisk walk just before attempts at defecation may be helpful. Patients are instructed to increase dietary bulk with foods rich in fiber, such as green vegetables and unprocessed cereal grains, or by the regular use of bulk laxatives, such as hemicellulose, psyllium extract, and powdered unprocessed bran. The success of such a regimen depends to some extent on the duration of symptoms. Elderly patients with long-standing constipation and reliance on enemas or laxatives are more resistant to these measures than younger patients whose bowel patterns are less established. Moreover, poor muscle tone, reduced physical activity, and increased incidence of other medical conditions make the problem more difficult in the older age group. Bedridden elderly patients often develop severe constipation and even fecal impaction unless preventive measures are taken. This applies not only to patients with previous constipation but also to those with regular bowel movements prior to their confining illness. Regular administration of stool softeners, bulk laxatives, or mild cathartics is necessary until full ambulation and a normal diet are resumed. The onset of fecal impaction in bedridden patients is heralded by a feeling of rectal distention, urgency of defecation, or tenesmus. Occasionally the fecal impaction will result in low-grade chronic obstruction with dilatation and increased fluid content proximal to the impaction; "paradoxical diarrhea" may thus occur as fluid moves past the obstructing fecal mass. This situation will be aggravated if antidiarrheal drugs are given because the underlying constipation will be worsened. The appropriate maneuver is to disimpact the rectum manually or to administer gentle enemas if the impaction is beyond the reach of the finger.

VASCULAR DISORDERS OF THE INTESTINE

Ischemia is the end result of interruption or reduction of the blood supply of the intestine. However the clinical manifestations of intestinal ischemia range from mild chronic symptoms to catastrophic episodes, depending on the segment involved, the degree of involvement, and the rapidity of the process. Thus, the clinician should be aware of a spectrum of intestinal ischemia ranging from mild chronic symptoms to catastrophic episodes. The gut derives its arterial blood supply from the celiac axis and the superior and inferior mesenteric arteries. The small intestine is supplied by the celiac and superior mesenteric arteries; the colon is supplied by branches of the superior and inferior mesenteric arteries. A rich network of anastomotic vessels and the possible development of collateral circulation determine the clinical picture of acute or chronic intestinal arterial insufficiency.

MESENTERIC ISCHEMIA AND INFARCTION Acute small-intestinal ischemia may be classified as *occlusive* or *nonocclusive.* Occlusion may result from arterial thrombus or embolus of the celiac or superior mesenteric arteries, or from venous occlusion in the same distribution. Arterial embolus occurs most commonly in patients with chronic or recurrent atrial fibrillation, artificial heart valves, or valvular heart disease, while arterial thrombosis is associated with extensive atherosclerosis or low cardiac output. Venous occlusion is quite rare and is occasionally seen in women taking oral contraceptives. Approximately two-thirds of patients with mesenteric ischemia do not have a definite occlusion of a major vessel, a condition referred to as *nonocclusive* ischemia. The exact cause of nonocclusive disease is obscure; systemic arterial hypotension, cardiac arrhythmias, prolonged heart failure, dehydration, and endotoxemia have been suggested as contributing factors.

The outstanding clinical feature of acute mesenteric ischemia is severe abdominal pain, often colicky and periumbilical at the onset, later becoming diffuse and constant. Vomiting, anorexia, diarrhea, and constipation are also frequent but of little diagnostic help. Examination of the abdomen may reveal tenderness and distention. Bowel sounds are often normal even in the face of severe infarction. Some patients have a surprisingly normal abdominal examination in spite of severe pain. Mild gastrointestinal bleeding is often detected by guaiac examination of stool, but gross hemorrhage is unusual except in ischemic colitis (see below). Late in the course of the disease (24 to 72 h) gangrene of the bowel occurs with diffuse peritonitis, sepsis, and shock. Abdominal plain films in patients with mesenteric ischemia may reveal air fluid levels, distention, and evidence of thick mucosal folds ("thumbprinting"). Barium study of the small intestine again reveals only nonspecific dilatation, poor motility, and mucosal thickening.

Acute mesenteric ischemia is a grave condition with a high morbidity and mortality. Patients suspected of having acute arterial embolus should undergo immediate celiac and mesenteric angiography to localize the embolus, followed by embolectomy. Restoration of normal circulation may allow complete recovery if performed before irreversible necrosis or gangrene has occurred. Unfortunately infarction and transmural necrosis are frequently found at surgery, necessitating resection. Arterial or venous thrombosis is not generally amenable to surgical removal of the thrombus, and resection of the affected bowel is required. Similarly, patients with nonocclusive ischemia are not candidates for corrective vascular surgery (as major vessels are patent). These individuals often have extensive necrosis of the small or large intestine because of the widespread nature of the ischemic event. The decision to operate on patients with suspected mesenteric ischemia is a difficult one as the typical patient is a poor surgical risk owing to advanced age, dehydration, sepsis, and other serious medical conditions.

Chronic arterial insufficiency may precede acute vascular insufficiency, producing so-called abdominal angina. As in angina pectoris, there are symptoms of chronic mesenteric insufficiency under conditions where there is a need for increased splanchnic blood flow. The patient complains of intermittent dull or cramping midabdominal pain 15 to 30 min after a meal, lasting for several hours postprandially. Significant weight loss is primarily due to a decreased food intake; however, chronic intestinal ischemia may also produce mucosal damage and malabsorption, which in turn aggravates the weight loss. Since abdominal angina may progress to bowel infarction, serious consideration should be given to performing arteriographic studies to confirm the diagnosis in those patients who are candidates for abdominal vascular surgery. The only definitive treatment is surgical removal of the obstruction or the construction of bypass arterial grafts to the ischemic bowel.

A variety of systemic conditions are associated with *vasculitis* of the large and small arteries supplying the intestine. Most often, these disorders can be recognized by the associated extraintestinal manifestations as in polyarteritis nodosa, lupus erythematosus, dermatomyositis, Henoch-Schönlein purpura (allergic vasculitis), and rheumatoid vasculitis. When larger arteries are involved, as in polyarteritis nodosa, the picture of acute intestinal infarction is similar to embolic or atherosclerotic vascular occlusion. Often the involvement of smaller vessels leads to areas of intramural hemorrhage and edema leading to abdominal pain, variable degrees of intestinal obstruction, and bleeding. Plain abdominal x-rays may show "thumbprinting" and "spiculation" due to localized edema, hemorrhage, and ulceration. In many instances, treatment of the underlying disorder may lead to regression of symptoms. If signs of an acute abdomen develop, surgical exploration is usually indicated.

Intramural small-intestinal hemorrhage may occur with vasculitis, trauma, or impaired coagulation, especially in patients receiving anticoagulants. The clinical and radiologic features resemble those seen with vasculitis and local mucosal hemorrhage.

ISCHEMIC COLITIS Ischemia of the colon most often affects the elderly population because of the greater frequency of vascular disease in that group. Nearly all patients with ischemic colitis have nonocclusive disease, that is, obstruction of major vessels is not seen. Shunting of blood away from the mucosa may contribute to this condition, but the mechanism of ischemia is not known.

The clinical picture depends upon the degree of ischemia and the rate of its development. In *acute fulminant ischemic* colitis the major manifestations are severe lower abdominal pain, rectal bleeding, and hypotension. Dilatation of the colon and physical signs of peritonitis are seen in severe cases. Plain abdominal films may reveal thumbprinting from submucosal hemorrhage and edema. Barium enema is hazardous in the acute situation because of the risk of perforation. Sigmoidoscopy or colonoscopy may detect ulcerations, friability, and bulging folds from submucosal hemorrhage. Angiography is not helpful in the management of patients with presumed ischemic colitis since a remedial occlusive lesion is very rarely found. Surgical resection may be required in some patients with fulminant ischemic colitis to remove gangrenous bowel; others with lesser degrees of ischemia may respond to conservative medical management.

Subacute ischemic colitis, the most common clinical variant of ischemic colonic disease, produces lesser degrees of pain and bleeding, often occurring over several days or weeks. The left colon may be involved, but the rectum is usually spared because of collateral blood flow, a distinguishing feature from acute ulcerative colitis. Barium enema reveals edema, cobblestoning, thumbprinting, and occasionally superficial ulceration. Angiography is not indicated as almost all cases are nonocclusive. Occasionally *stricture formation* may follow a bout of ischemic colitis or may present de novo without a history of antecedent pain or bloody diarrhea. Most cases of nonocclusive ischemic colitis resolve in 2 to 4 weeks and do not recur. Surgery is not required except for obstruction secondary to postischemic stricture.

PRIMARY NONSPECIFIC ULCERATION OF THE SMALL INTESTINE

Although the existence of rare solitary and unexplained ulcers of the small intestine has been recognized for many years, a recent increased incidence has suggested vascular factors producing ischemic necrosis of the mucosa in one or more areas of the small bowel. Most of these ulcers occur in patients receiving enteric-coated drugs known to be irritating to the mucosa; the most commonly implicated agent is potassium chloride, given to patients on chronic diuretic therapy. The symptoms are those of abdominal pain and obstruction, rarely with peritonitis and perforation. Surgical excision of the ulcerated or stenotic intestinal segment is generally required.

TUMORS OF THE SMALL INTESTINE

Small-bowel tumors comprise only 3 to 6 percent of gastrointestinal neoplasms. Because of their rarity, the diagnosis is often delayed. Abdominal symptoms are usually vague and poorly defined, and conventional x-ray studies of the upper and lower intestinal tract are usually normal. Small-bowel tumors should be considered in the following situations: (1) recurrent, unexplained episodes of crampy abdominal pain; (2) intermittent bouts of intestinal obstruction, especially in the absence of inflammatory bowel disease or prior abdominal surgery; (3) intussusception in the adult; and (4) evidence of chronic intestinal bleeding in the face of negative conventional x-rays. A careful small-bowel barium study is the diagnostic procedure of choice. The diagnostic accuracy is improved by infusing barium through a nasogastric tube placed in the duodenum (enteroclysis).

BENIGN TUMORS In general, the histology of benign small-bowel tumors is difficult to predict on clinical and radiologic grounds alone. The symptomatology of benign tumors is not distinctive, with pain, obstruction, and hemorrhage being the most frequent symptoms. These tumors are usually discovered in the fifth and sixth decades of life, more often in the distal rather than the proximal small intestine. The most common benign tumors are adenomas, leiomyomas, lipomas, and angiomas.

Adenomas These tumors include those of the islet cells and Brunner's glands as well as polypoid adenomas. *Islet-cell adenomas* are occasionally located outside the pancreas, and the associated syndromes are discussed in Chap. 116. *Brunner's gland adenomas* are not truly neoplastic but represent a hypertrophy or hyperplasia of submucosal duodenal glands. These appear as small nodules in the duodenal mucosa. Most often this is an incidental finding on x-ray not associated with any clinical disorder.

Polypoid adenomas Approximately 25 percent of benign small-bowel tumors are polypoid adenomas. They may present as single polypoid lesions or less commonly as papillary villous adenomas. As in the colon, the sessile or papillary form of the tumor is sometimes associated with coexistent carcinoma. Multiple polypoid tumors may occur throughout the small bowel in the Peutz-Jeghers syndrome (Chap. 52) and are usually hamartomas. The malignant potential of these lesions is low.

Leiomyomas These arise from smooth-muscle components of the intestine and are usually intramural lesions affecting the overlying mucosa. Ulceration of the mucosa may cause gastrointestinal hemorrhage of varying severity.

Lipomas These tumors occur with greatest frequency in the distal ileum and at the ileocecal valve. Their radiolucent appearance on x-ray is characteristic. They are usually intramural and asymptomatic but may on occasion be associated with bleeding.

Angiomas While uncommon these are important small-bowel tumors since a high percentage of patients with these lesions will have evidence of intestinal bleeding. They may take the form of telangiectasia or hemangiomas. Multiple intestinal telangiectasia occurs in a nonhereditary form confined to the gastrointestinal tract or as a part of the hereditary Osler-Rendu-Weber syndrome. The latter syndrome is described in Chap. 333. Vascular tumors may also take the form of isolated hemangiomas, most commonly in the jejunum. Angiography, especially during a bout of bleeding, is the procedure of choice in evaluating these lesions.

MALIGNANT TUMORS While not too common, small-bowel malignancies occur in patients with long-standing regional enteritis and celiac sprue with greater frequency than in the general population. In contrast to benign tumors, malignant tumors of the small bowel are frequently associated with fever, weight loss, anorexia, bleeding, and an abdominal mass on physical examination. After ampullary carcinomas [many of which arise from the bile or pancreatic duct (see Chap. 325)], the most frequent small-bowel malignancies are adenocarcinomas, lymphomas, leiomyosarcomas, and carcinoid tumors.

Adenocarcinomas These occur with highest frequency in the distal duodenum and proximal jejunum, where they tend to ulcerate and cause hemorrhage or obstruction. Radiologically, they may be confused with chronic duodenal ulcer disease or Crohn's disease if the patient has long-standing regional enteritis. The diagnosis is best made by endoscopy and biopsy under direct vision.

Leiomyosarcomas Large, bulky tumors, leiomyosarcomas often are greater than 5 cm in diameter and may be palpable on abdominal examination. Bleeding, obstruction, or perforation are the most common manifestations.

Lymphomas All histologic types of lymphomas may involve the small bowel, either primarily or secondarily. In both instances, lymphosarcomas and reticulum-cell sarcomas are more common than Hodgkin's disease. Involvement is more common in the jejunum and ileum than in the duodenum. Grossly, lymphomas may infiltrate the bowel wall or present as a large polypoid mass, often with central ulceration. Involvement of the adjacent mesentery and lymph nodes is common. Occasionally the small intestine may be diffusely involved, leading to malabsorption. This type of involvement, which for unknown reasons is more common in the Middle East, may be difficult to differentiate from celiac disease, since in the latter there is an increased incidence of lymphomas. An uncommon variant of Mediterranean lymphoma is *α-chain disease,* found primarily in young people of Mediterranean origin. It leads to severe diarrhea, malabsorption, and often hypoproteinemia. The intestine is infiltrated with plasma cells, and fragments of the IgA heavy chains are found in blood and urine.

In most instances laparotomy is required for the diagnosis of primary intestinal lymphomas. Infiltrating lymphomas of the distal bowel must be distinguished from benign infiltrating lesions such as regional enteritis. Stenosis of bowel segments, involvement of both large and small bowel, and the extracolonic manifestations of inflammatory bowel disease suggest regional enteritis. Peroral intestinal biopsy and lymphangiography are useful in the diagnosis of diffuse intestinal lymphoma. Treatment of localized lymphoma is surgical resection, with good survival if the disease has not spread. Chemotherapy and radiotherapy are employed in the management of more extensive disease, but with discouraging results.

Carcinoid tumors Among the most common epithelial tumors of the small intestine are carcinoid tumors. They arise from argentaffin cells of the crypts of Lieberkühn and are most commonly found from the midduodenum to the transverse colon, areas embryologically derived from the midgut. The appendix is the most common location for gastrointestinal carcinoid, where the tumor is found incidentally at the time of appendectomy. Most intestinal carcinoids are asymptomatic and of low malignant potential, but invasion and metastases may occur and lead to the carcinoid syndrome (see Chap. 131).

TUMORS OF THE LARGE INTESTINE

Neoplasms of the colon, either benign or malignant, are very commonly encountered in clinical practice. The clinician must be alert to the possibility that a variety of colonic symptoms, particularly blood in the stools, can indicate the presence of a polyp or carcinoma. It is also of importance to recognize the settings in which colonic malignancy is more prevalent and to strive for earlier diagnosis in order to increase the 5-year survival rate.

POLYPS OF THE COLON A polyp is a structure arising from a mucosal surface and projecting into the lumen. This definition includes benign lesions, while the designation *polypoid carcinoma* refers to a malignant lesion which resembles a polyp. The most common polyp is the *adenomatous polyp*, which may be solitary or multiple, sessile (flat, not on a stalk), or pedunculated (on a stalk as in Fig. 310-4). Single adenomatous polyps are believed to occur in 2 to 15 percent of the adult population and should not be confused with small hyperplastic mucosal tags which are very common and of no clinical or pathologic significance. Adenomatous polyps occur more commonly in the rectum and sigmoid colon (80 percent) compared with the rest of the colon (20 percent). Adenomatous polyps are usually silent; when they produce symptoms, these usually consist of recurrent episodes of bleeding or intermittent obstruction if the polyp is large. The clinical significance of adenomatous polyps relates primarily to their relationship to colon cancer. Most pathologists now believe that a small percentage of adenomatous polyps undergo malignant degeneration based on the facts (1) that foci of atypia or carcinoma in situ are occasionally found in polyps, (2) that the incidence follows a similar age and anatomic distribution, and (3) that patients with multiple congenital polyposis of the colon have a marked increase in incidence of colon cancer.

FIGURE 310-4
Adenomatous polyp of sigmoid colon on a long stalk.

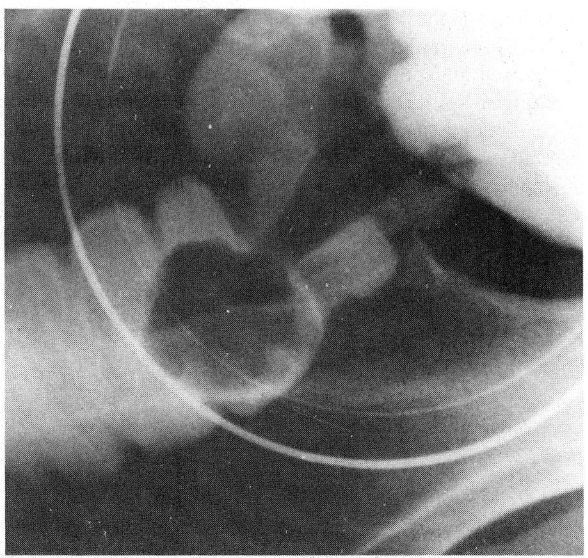

Treatment of polyps in adults is influenced by their possible malignant transformation. Polyps in the sigmoid colon or rectum should be removed via the sigmoidoscope whenever possible. Polyps higher in the colon which are less than 1 cm in diameter are rarely malignant. However, recent experience with colonoscopic polypectomy has shown that even small polyps or polyps on stalks may be malignant. For this reason removal of polyps via the colonoscope is recommended unless there is some contraindication to the procedure. This spares the patient a laparotomy and may occasionally detect a tumor in what otherwise would have been considered a benign polyp. In 40 to 50 percent of patients who have had polyps removed, new polyps will develop in the subsequent decade. Therefore, follow-up barium enemas or colonoscopies should be performed periodically (every 2 to 3 years) to detect new polyps.

Villous adenoma is a polypoid lesion with a much higher rate of malignancy than adenomatous polyps. The majority of these occur in the rectum or sigmoid and usually are larger than adenomatous polyps. They are soft, frond-like masses which are quite friable and bleed easily. The histologic pattern is one of atypical cells which resemble surface epithelial cells; evidence of malignant degeneration is present in 40 to 60 percent. Rarely these tumors will cause protracted watery diarrhea with excessive potassium loss leading to profound hypokalemia and dehydration. Most villous adenomas call attention to their presence by bleeding or passage of mucus per rectum. Proper treatment involves surgical resection with follow-up sigmoidoscopies and barium enema examinations to detect recurrence.

HEREDITARY POLYP SYNDROMES *Familial colonic polyposis* is a rare autosomal dominant disorder characterized by the appearance of numerous (often 1000 or more) adenomatous polyps involving the entire colon. Occasional cases appear to have no family history and presumably result from a spontaneous mutation. The polyps are not present at birth but appear in childhood and adolescence, giving rise to diarrhea or rectal bleeding. Once this disease is diagnosed, it is imperative that the entire family be examined by sigmoidoscopy and barium enema. The probability of cancer of the colon occurring in affected individuals is nearly 100 percent by age 40. Hence prophylactic colectomy is indicated, usually after the patient has attained full adult growth. Most surgeons prefer total colectomy and ileostomy, while others leave the rectum, which allows the patient to have normal bowel movements. These patients require careful follow-up sigmoidoscopy and removal of all polyps in the rectal stump. However, the rate of carcinoma in the rectal stump is so high that total colectomy should probably be considered the treatment of choice.

Gardner's syndrome refers to the coexistence of multiple colonic adenomatous polyps and various benign tumors elsewhere, such as lipomas, fibromas, sebaceous cysts, and osteomas, particularly of the jaw and skull bones. The colonic polyps develop at a later age than in multiple colonic polyposis, but the malignant potential is the same and thus colectomy is also recommended. Some patients with Gardner's syndrome have gastric and duodenal polyps, and malignancies of the duodenum have been reported in some of these individuals.

An entity easily confused with multiple colonic polyposis is *juvenile polyposis*, in which inflammatory polyps occur in the colon or in both large and small bowel. Histologically these polyps are composed of columnar epithelium and mucus cysts; inflammatory cells are often present and account for the designation "inflammatory polyp." Juvenile polyposis coli also occurs in kindreds and causes rectal bleeding or features of growth retardation, making differentiation from multiple adenomatous polyps difficult. However, the risk of malignancy is not increased, and hence colectomy is not recommended. The *Peutz-Jeghers* syndrome is characterized by multiple hamartomatous polyps of the entire gastrointestinal tract, associated with melanotic spots on the skin, lips, and buccal mucosa. Although the polyps in this syndrome are most prevalent in the small intestine, colonic polyps also occur. Several cases of malignant degeneration of duodenal polyps have been reported. Clinical features alone do not allow accurate differentiation of the various hereditary polyp syndromes (see Table 310-1). For this reason, careful histologic examination of polyps from several areas should always be obtained prior to colectomy in patients with suspected polyposis coli.

CANCER OF THE COLON Cancer of the large bowel, the second most common site for carcinoma in both males and females, accounts for about 20 percent of all deaths due to malignant disease in the United States. Unfortunately, the death rate for this disease has not changed for the past 40 years and will undoubtedly remain the same until methods for earlier detection and improved treatment are available.

Etiology The cause of colon cancer is unknown. The greater incidence in western society suggests that dietary factors may be involved, but the association may be circumstantial rather than causal. The risk of colon cancer is definitely increased in patients with familial adenomatous polyps, ulcerative colitis, and Crohn's disease of the colon. However, in most patients with colon cancer no predisposing condition or factor can be identified. As with other malignant diseases, familial aggregates of the disease are well documented.

Pathology Colon carcinomas affect men and women approximately equally. The peak incidence is in the fifth, sixth, and seventh decades, except in patients with polyposis or inflammatory bowel disease. The cecum and ascending colon are involved in 15 percent of all carcinomas of the large bowel; the transverse colon in 10 percent; and the descending colon, rectosigmoid, and rectum in 75 percent. Approximately half of all cancers of the large intestine are within reach of the sigmoidoscope. About 3 percent of patients will have two primary colon cancers.

Adenocarcinoma is the most common type of colon cancer. The degree of differentiation varies widely but is not well correlated with degree of invasiveness or rapidity of growth. Classifications of the tumors according to their microscopic appearance—papillary, medullary, scirrhous, or colloid—are not of great assistance to the physician. The most important pathologic finding is the extent of spread of the tumor at the time of surgery, as this is closely correlated with prognosis. Those patients whose tumor is confined to the bowel wall have an excellent chance for cure following surgical resection, as indicated by a 5-year survival rate of greater than 95 percent. In patients with extension of the tumor to the serosa and mesenteric fat, the 5-year survival rate following resection is 80 percent. With lymph node metastases 5-year survival rate is reduced further to 40 percent, while the presence of distant metastases to liver, lung, bone, or brain reduces the 5-year survival rate to zero.

Clinical features Symptoms of colon carcinoma are usually vague and nonspecific at the outset. Weight loss and malaise are common and often disregarded by the patient. It is convenient to divide cancers of the colon into those affecting the right and left sides. Cancers of the cecum and ascending colon are usually flat or polypoid and often "silent" clinically because they do not obstruct the lumen or cause visible melena. Cancer of the rectosigmoid may obstruct the lumen or bleed and hence cause the patient to seek medical advice. The following symptoms are important clues to the presence of colonic carcinoma.

1 *Changes in bowel habits* are most frequent when carcinoma affects the left colon. These changes are often minimal but progressive and include diarrhea, constipation, and a sensation of incomplete rectal emptying (tenesmus).
2 *Rectal bleeding* occurs in left-sided lesions in about 70 percent of cases and is usually noticed by the patient. When the lesion is in the ascending colon or cecum, fewer than 25 percent of patients notice any blood in the stools, no doubt because the blood is thoroughly admixed with the fecal slurry in the right colon. Rectal bleeding should never be attributed to hemorrhoids or rectal fissures, especially in older individuals, unless a malignancy has been ruled out by barium enema and proctosigmoidoscopy.
3 *Pain* in the lower part of the abdomen is occasionally a symptom of lesions of the cecum or ascending colon. Pain in left colonic lesions may be related to varying degrees of bowel obstruction above a constricting carcinoma. Occasionally a sigmoid carcinoma may present as an acute bowel obstruction or acute perforation with peritonitis.
4 Symptoms of *anemia* are frequent in right-sided colonic cancer. Cardiac failure or angina pectoris may be the presenting symptoms.
5 *Anorexia, weight loss,* and *malaise* may occur at any time.

Diagnosis Carcinoma of the colon is one of the most common malignancies, and the physician must be alert to symptoms such as weight loss, blood in the stool, or change in bowel habit. The potentially serious nature of these symptoms must be recognized and not attributed to hemorrhoids or other minor conditions until carcinoma has been definitely excluded. It must be stressed that cancer of the large bowel is curable if discovered early in the course and that delay in diagnosis is the most significant factor in poor prognosis.

The most efficient and economical screening procedure for

TABLE 310-1
Hereditable gastrointestinal polyp syndromes

Syndrome	*Distribution of polyps*	*Histologic type*	*Malignant degeneration*	*Associated lesions*
Familial colonic polyposis	Large intestine	Adenoma	100%	None
Gardner's syndrome	Large intestine	Adenoma	100%	Osteomas, fibromas, lipomas, epidermoid cysts
Peutz-Jeghers syndrome	Small and large intestine	Hamartoma	Rare	Mucocutaneous pigmentation
Juvenile polyposis	Small and large intestine	Inflammatory polyp	Absent	None

colon cancer involves testing the stool for occult blood (guaiac test). Most colonic malignancies bleed slowly into the lumen even before they reach sufficient size to cause symptoms. Thus the presence of occult blood in the stool should alert the physician to the possibility of colon cancer, particularly in individuals above the age of 40. As usually performed, the guaiac test suffers from variable sensitivity due to instability of the dye. Commercially prepared cards impregnated with the dye (Hemoccult test) are available in which the dye appears to be stable and the number of false-positive tests are reduced. False-positive tests can also be diminished if patients do not eat meat for several days prior to the test. A screening protocol for colon cancer has been devised which involves Hemoccult testing of six stool samples while the patient is on a meat-free diet. This simple screening technique appears to increase the detection of presymptomatic colon cancers amenable to surgical cure.

The *digital rectal examination* is the most important aspect of the physical examination, since approximately half of rectal cancers are within reach of the finger. Physical findings such as ascites, jaundice, or palpable abdominal masses indicate metastatic disease. Iron-deficiency anemia is present in over half of patients with right-sided lesions. Patients with left-sided lesions may also be anemic but less frequently and to a much less severe degree, since their blood loss is more easily appreciated by the appearance of the stools. In the presence of liver metastases the serum alkaline phosphatase and 5′-nucleotidase retention are elevated. The carcinoembryonic antigen (CEA) is not specific for colon cancer, and a normal level does not exclude the diagnosis. It is useful, however, in following patients after surgery, since return to normal of previously elevated CEA levels indicates successful removal of tumor, while persistently elevated or increasing CEA levels postoperatively suggest residual tumor or metastatic spread.

Any patient suspected of having a colonic carcinoma should undergo sigmoidoscopy. This procedure is particularly useful in the diagnosis of low-lying rectal cancers which can be missed on barium enema. Sigmoidoscopy also allows for the diagnosis of other bleeding lesions in the rectum or sigmoid colon, particularly hemorrhoids, polyps, and proctitis.

A careful barium enema in a well-prepared colon is the next diagnostic maneuver. Important aspects of this examination are the following: (1) Tumors may project into the bowel, giving rise to a filling defect in the barium column (Fig. 310-5). (2) They may partially or completely encircle the bowel, producing a narrowing of the barium column proximal to which the bowel is often dilated (Fig. 310-6). (3) They may, by contiguous infiltration, distort the position of the colon, so that the barium is not free to follow gravity during the radiologist's examination of the patient. (4) After the barium has been expelled, films of the mucosal relief may show defects due to tumor which has not penetrated the muscular coat. (5) Some tumors give rise to no specific defects but interfere with peristalsis, so that irritability, fluid retention, and spasticity may be noted. It is worth emphasizing that the accuracy of barium enema in the diagnosis of low-lying rectal cancer is not high. It is imperative, therefore, that a careful sigmoidoscopic examination precede the barium enema. Colonoscopy and biopsy are recommended for all suspicious lesions seen on barium enema which are above the reach of the sigmoidoscope.

FIGURE 310-5
Filling defect in the cecum produced by a carcinoma.

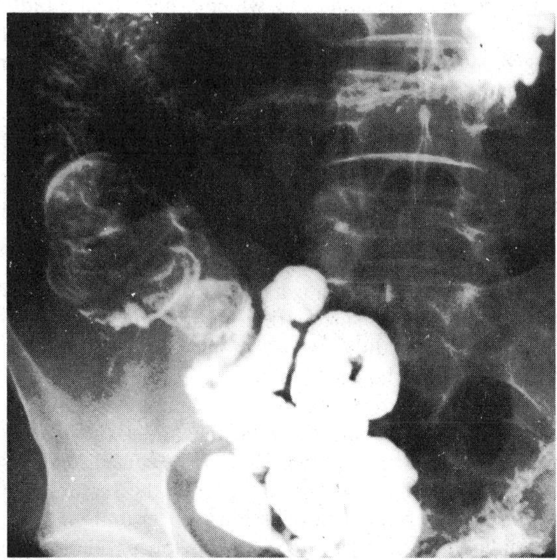

Differential diagnosis of colon cancer includes almost all the entities which affect that organ because changes in bowel habit and bleeding are common symptoms. Thus colitis, diverticular disease, polyps, and ischemic disease can be easily confused with colon carcinoma. Even more important is the fact that these diseases can coexist with or lead to malignancy. Filling defects of the cecum can occur in amoebic colitis, owing to the presence of a large inflammatory mass (amoeboma). This is rare except in patients with long-standing chronic amebiasis. Tuberculosis, endometriosis, lymphogranuloma venereum, carcinoid tumors, and lymphoma may all masquerade as colon carcinoma. Metastatic cancer from other organs can occasionally involve the colon extrinsically and produce symptoms. Thus metastases to the perirectal area can produce diarrhea or obstructive symptoms. Such tumors produce extrinsic compression of the lumen and may be palpated through the rectum as a shelf (Blumer's shelf) or mass.

Complications Since it is characteristic for tumors to invade, many tumors of the colon are first diagnosed because of a com-

FIGURE 310-6
Obstructing carcinoma of the sigmoid.

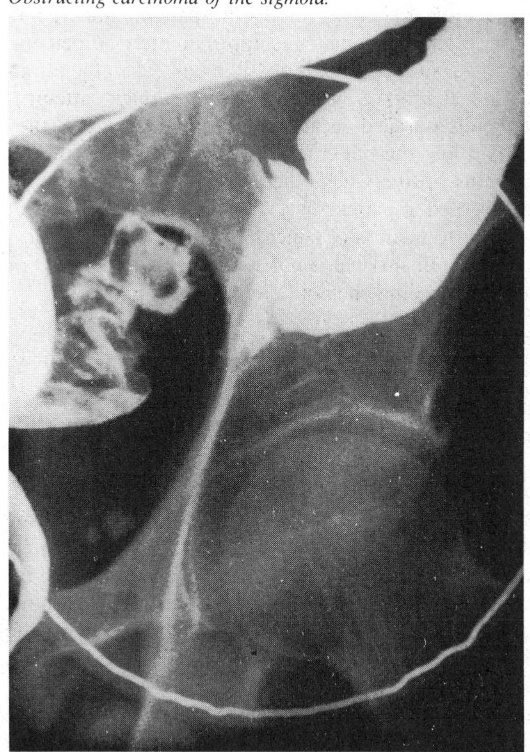

plication of the original lesion. The tumor may perforate the bowel wall, giving rise to acute peritonitis; may perforate slowly and wall itself off, giving rise to a local inflammatory mass and localized peritonitis; or may invade blood vessels to produce an episode of brisk rectal bleeding. More often, the tumor partially obstructs the bowel lumen for a long period of time, during which the colon proximal to the tumor dilates slowly without dramatic change in symptoms until frank obstruction occurs. This happens most often when the tumor is in the sigmoid, where the stool is driest. Tumors also weaken the colonic wall in such a way that an intussusception may occur, the tumor leading the intussusception. Similarly, fixation of the bowel wall by a tumor may produce a volvulus, which is most frequently seen in the sigmoid colon. Very large and slowly growing tumors may produce symptoms by pressure on neighboring organs such as uterus, bladder, or ureters. Inguinal hernias may become apparent as the first sign of such increased pressure. Fistulas between the colon and pelvic organs should lead to a thorough search for an underlying neoplastic infiltration. Abscesses inside the peritoneal cavity and cellulitis of the abdominal wall secondary to tumor infiltration are occasionally seen.

Treatment The current approach to treatment of colon cancer is primarily surgical. Some surgeons prefer preoperative radiation therapy to prevent metastases, but it has not been convincingly demonstrated that this improves survival. Surgeons generally prefer abdominoperineal resection and colostomy for tumors located below the peritoneal reflection; above this area there is considerably more freedom of choice, depending primarily on the size and extent of the lesion. Even patients with obvious metastases usually benefit from a limited palliative resection, since this will relieve or prevent painful obstruction and hemorrhage. The overall operative mortality for colectomy is about 5 percent, except for emergency resections for perforation or obstruction. The operative mortality is somewhat higher for lesions in the left colon and for tumors which have perforated. Discussion of the complications of surgical therapy and the management of colostomies can be found in surgical texts.

The overall 5-year survival rate for all patients undergoing resection for colonic malignancy is approximately 50 percent. As already noted, surgical cure is possible only when the tumor is confined to the bowel wall. Palliative surgical attempts should not be discouraged because the symptomatic relief they produce may allow the patient to live in comfort for the remaining months of life. Chemotherapy with 5-fluorouracil or other agents is used in patients with metastases to the liver, but temporary improvement is obtained only in 25 percent or less of cases, and overall survival is not significantly affected. (For further details regarding chemotherapy, see Chap. 125.)

ANORECTAL PROBLEMS

HEMORRHOIDS The internal hemorrhoidal plexus of veins is located in the submucosal space above the valves of Morgagni. The anal canal separates it from the external hemorrhoidal venous plexus, but the two spaces communicate under the anal canal, the submucosa of which is attached to underlying tissue to form the interhemorrhoidal depression. Whenever the internal hemorrhoidal plexus is enlarged, there is associated increase in supporting tissue mass, and the resultant venous swelling is called an *internal hemorrhoid.* When veins in the external hemorrhoidal plexus become enlarged or thrombosed, the resultant bluish mass is called an *external hemorrhoid.*

Both types of hemorrhoids are very common and are associated with increased hydrostatic pressure in the portal venous system, such as during pregnancy, straining at stool, or with cirrhosis. When internal hemorrhoids enlarge, pain is not a usual feature until the situation is complicated by thrombosis, infection, or erosion of the overlying mucosal surface. Most persons complain of bright red blood on the toilet tissue or coating the stool, with a feeling of vague anal discomfort. The discomfort is increased when the hemorrhoid enlarges or prolapses through the anus; prolapse is often accompanied by edema and sphincteric spasm. Prolapse, if not treated, usually becomes chronic as the muscularis stays stretched, and the patient complains of constant soiling of underclothing with very little pain. Prolapsed hemorrhoids may become infected or thrombosed; the overlying mucous membrane may bleed profusely as the result of the trauma of defecation.

External hemorrhoids, because they lie under the skin, are quite often painful, particularly if there is a sudden increase in their mass. These episodes result in a tender blue swelling at the anal verge due to thrombosis of a vein in the external plexus and need not be associated with enlargement of the internal veins. Since the thrombus usually lies at the level of the sphincteric muscles, anal spasm often occurs.

The diagnosis of internal and external hemorrhoids is made by inspection, digital examination, and direct vision through the anoscope and proctoscope. Since such lesions are very common, they must not be regarded as the cause of rectal bleeding or chronic hypochromic anemia until a thorough investigation has been made of the more proximal gastrointestinal tract. Acute blood loss can occasionally be attributed to internal hemorrhoids. Chronic anemia in the presence of large but not definitely bleeding hemorrhoids should provoke a search for a polyp, cancer, or ulcer.

Most hemorrhoids respond to conservative therapy such as sitz baths or other forms of moist heat, suppositories, stool softeners, and bed rest. Internal hemorrhoids which remain permanently prolapsed are best treated surgically; milder degrees of prolapse or enlargement with pruritus ani or intermittent bleeding can be successfully handled by the injection of sclerosing solutions. External hemorrhoids which become acutely thrombosed are treated by incision, extraction of the clot, and compression of the incised area following clot removal. No surgical procedure should be carried out in the presence of acute inflammation of the anus, ulcerative proctitis, or ulcerative colitis. Both proctoscopy and barium enema should always be performed before a patient is subjected to hemorrhoidectomy.

ANAL INFLAMMATION Perianal inflammatory lesions may be primary or may be associated with inflammatory bowel disease or diverticular disease as mentioned above. Anal *fissures* are superficial erosions of the anal canal which usually heal rapidly with conservative therapy. Anal *ulcers* are more chronic and deep and give symptoms largely as the result of painful spasm of the external anal sphincter during and after defecation. Bleeding may occur with either fissure or ulcer; healing of the ulcer often is associated with a hypertrophied anal papilla and some degrees of anal contracture. *Fistula in ano,* a tract leading from the rectal lumen to the perianal skin, usually results from local crypt abscesses; fewer than 5 percent of such lesions found in medical practice in the United States are due to tuberculosis or cancer. The fistula is a chronically inflamed canal made up of fibrous tissue surrounding granulation tissue, the lumen of which may be difficult to demonstrate. Perirectal *abscesses* often represent the tracking down into the anal area of purulent material escaping from the rectosigmoid; diverticulitis, Crohn's disease, or colitis may be the underlying cause. Previous anal or rectal surgical therapy may be causal. Fistulas between the rectum and vagina and between the rectum and bladder represent serious complications of granulomatous, septic, or malignant disorders and require the patient to be hospitalized for definitive diagnostic and therapeutic procedures.

REFERENCES

Disorders of motility

ALMY TP, HOWELL DA: Diverticular disease of the colon. N Engl J Med 302:324, 1980

DROSSMAN DA et al: The irritable bowel syndrome. Gastroenterology 73:811, 1977

SCHUFFLER MD et al: Chronic intestinal pseudo-obstruction. Medicine 60:173, 1981

SWARBRICK ET et al: Site of pain from the irritable bowel. Lancet 2:443, 1980

Intestinal ischemia

MARSHAK RH et al: Ischemia of the colon. Mount Sinai J Med 48:180, 1981

OTTINGER LW: The surgical management of acute occlusion of the superior mesenteric artery. Ann Surg 188:721, 1978

RENTON CJ: Nonocclusive intestinal infarction. Gastroenterology 1:655, 1972

Intestinal neoplasia

BUNTAIN WL et al: Collective review: Premalignancy of polyps of the colon. Surg Gynecol Obstet 134:499, 1972

BURKITT DP: Epidemiology of cancer of the colon and rectum. Cancer 28:2, 1971

BUSSEY HJ et al: Genetics of gastrointestinal polyposis. Gastroenterology 74:1325, 1978

FREUND H et al: Primary neoplasms of the small bowel. Am J Surg 135:757, 1978

LIPKIN M et al: Nondegradation of fecal cholesterol in subjects at high risk for cancer of the large intestine. J Clin Invest 67:304, 1981

NAGVI MS et al: Lymphomas of the gastrointestinal tract: Prognostic guides based on 162 cases. Ann Surg 170:221, 1969

WINAWER SJ et al: Screening for colon cancer. An overview. Cancer 45:1093, 1980

311
ACUTE INTESTINAL OBSTRUCTION

WILLIAM SILEN

ETIOLOGY AND CLASSIFICATION Intestinal obstruction may be *mechanical* or *nonmechanical* (resulting from neuromuscular disturbances which produce either *adynamic* or *dynamic ileus*). The causes of mechanical obstruction of the lumen are conveniently divided into (1) lesions *extrinsic* to the intestine, e.g., adhesive bands, internal and external hernias; (2) lesions *intrinsic* to the wall of the intestine, e.g., diverticulitis, carcinoma, regional enteritis; and (3) obturation of the lumen, e.g., gallstone obstruction, intussusception. From the clinical standpoint, however, it is most useful to consider whether the obstructive mechanism involves the small or large intestine, because the causes, symptoms, and treatment are different (see below). Adhesions and external hernias are the most common causes of obstruction of the small intestine, constituting 70 to 75 percent of cases of this type. Adhesions, however, almost never produce obstruction of the colon, while carcinoma, sigmoid diverticulitis, and volvulus, in that order, are the most common etiologies and together account for about 90 percent of the cases.

Adynamic ileus is probably the most common overall cause of obstruction. Recent studies indicate that the development of this condition is mediated via the hormonal component of the sympathoadrenal system. Adynamic ileus will occur after any peritoneal insult, and its severity and duration will be dependent to some degree on the type of peritoneal injury. Hydrochloric acid, colonic contents, and pancreatic enzymes are among the most irritating substances, whereas blood and urine are less so. Adynamic ileus occurs to some degree after any abdominal operation, and its severity varies directly with the amount of intestinal handling and the length of the operation; it usually lasts 2 to 3 days after most operative procedures. Retroperitoneal hematomas, particularly associated with vertebral fracture, commonly cause severe adynamic ileus and the latter may occur with other retroperitoneal conditions such as ureteral calculus or severe pyelonephritis. Thoracic diseases including lower-lobe pneumonia, fractured ribs, and myocardial infarction frequently produce adynamic ileus, as do electrolyte disturbances, particularly potassium depletion. Finally intestinal ischemia, whether the result of vascular occlusion or intestinal distention itself, may perpetuate an adynamic ileus. Spastic or dynamic ileus is very uncommon and results from extreme and prolonged contraction of the intestine. It has been observed in heavy metal poisoning, uremia, porphyria, and extensive intestinal ulcerations.

PATHOPHYSIOLOGY Distention of the intestine is caused by the accumulation of gas and fluid proximal to and within the obstructed segment. Seventy to eighty percent of intestinal gas consists of swallowed air, and because this is composed mainly of nitrogen, which is poorly absorbed from the intestinal lumen, removal of air by continuous gastric suction is an important adjunct in the treatment of intestinal distention. The accumulation of fluid proximal to the obstructing mechanism results not only from ingested fluid, swallowed saliva, gastric juice, and biliary and pancreatic secretions but also from interference with normal sodium and water transport. During the first 12 to 24 h of obstruction there is a marked depression of flux from lumen to blood of sodium and consequently water in the distended proximal intestine. After 24 h, there is also movement of sodium and water into the lumen, contributing further to the distention and fluid losses. Intraluminal pressure rises from a normal of 2 to 4 cmH_2O to 8 to 10 cmH_2O. During peristalsis, when simple obstruction or a "closed loop" is present, pressures reach 30 to 60 cmH_2O. Closed-loop obstruction of the small intestine results when the lumen is occluded at two points by a single mechanism such as a hernial ring or adhesive band, thus producing a closed loop whose blood supply is often obstructed at the same time. Strangulation of the loop itself is thus common in association with marked distention proximal to the involved loop. A form of closed-loop obstruction is encountered when complete obstruction of the colon exists in the presence of a competent ileocecal valve (85 percent of individuals). Although the blood supply of the colon is not entrapped within the obstructing mechanism, distention of the cecum is extreme because of its greater diameter (LaPlace's law), and impairment of the intramural blood supply is considerable with consequent gangrene of the cecal wall, usually anteriorly. Necrosis of the small intestine may occur by the same mechanism of interference with intramural blood flow when distention is extreme, but this sequence is uncommon in the small intestine. Once impairment of blood supply occurs, bacterial invasion supervenes and subsequent peritonitis develops. The systemic effects of extreme distention include elevation of the diaphragms with restricted ventilation and subsequent atelectasis. Venous return via the inferior vena cava may also be impaired.

The loss of fluids and electrolytes may be extreme, and unless replacement is prompt, leads to hemoconcentration, hypovolemia, renal insufficiency, shock, and death. Vomiting, accumulation of fluids within the lumen by the mechanisms described above, and the sequestration of fluid into the edematous intestinal wall and peritoneal cavity as a result of impairment of venous return from the intestine all contribute to massive loss of fluid and electrolytes. As soon as significant impedance to venous return is present, the intestine becomes severely congested, and blood begins to seep into the intestinal lumen. Blood loss may reach significant levels when long segments of intestine are involved.

SYMPTOMS *Mechanical small-intestinal obstruction* is characterized by cramping midabdominal pain which tends to be more severe the higher the obstruction. The pain occurs in paroxysms, and the patient is relatively comfortable in the intervals between the pains. Audible borborygmi are often noted by the patient simultaneously with the paroxysms of pain. The pain may become less severe as distention progresses, probably because motility is impaired in the edematous intestine. When strangulation is present, the pain is usually more localized and may be steady and severe without a colicky component, a fact which often causes delay in diagnosis of obstruction. Vomiting is almost invariable, and it is earlier and more profuse the higher the obstruction. The vomitus initially contains bile and mucus and remains as such if the obstruction is high in the intestine. With low ileal obstruction, the vomitus becomes feculent, i.e., orange-brown in color with a foul odor, which results from the overgrowth of bacteria proximal to the obstruction. Singultus is common. Obstipation and failure to pass gas by rectum are invariably present when the obstruction is complete, although some stool and gas may be passed spontaneously or after an enema shortly after onset of the complete obstruction. Diarrhea is occasionally observed in partial obstruction. Blood in the stool is rare, even in the completely obstructed patient, but does occur in cases of intussusception. Other than some minor but inconsistent differences in pain patterns noted above, the symptoms of strangulating obstructions cannot be distinguished from those of nonstrangulating obstructions.

Mechanical colonic obstruction produces colicky abdominal pain similar in quality to that of small-intestinal obstruction but of much lower intensity. Complaints of pain are occasionally absent in stoic elderly patients. Vomiting occurs late, if at all, particularly if the ileocecal valve is competent. Paradoxically, feculent vomitus is very rare. A history of recent alterations in bowel habits and blood in the stool is common because carcinoma and diverticulitis are the most frequent causes. Constipation becomes progressive, and obstipation with failure to pass gas ensues. Acute symptoms may develop over a period of a week.

In *adynamic ileus,* colicky pain is absent, and only discomfort from distention is evident. Vomiting may be frequent but is rarely profuse. It usually consists of gastric contents and bile and is almost never feculent. Complete obstipation may or may not occur. Singultus is very common.

PHYSICAL FINDINGS *Abdominal distention* is the hallmark of all forms of intestinal obstruction. It is least marked in cases of obstruction high in the small intestine and most marked in colonic obstruction. Early in the course of the disease, especially in closed-loop strangulating small-bowel obstruction, distention may be barely perceptible or absent. Tenderness and rigidity are usually minimal; the temperature is rarely above 100°F in nonstrangulating obstruction of the small and large intestine. Contrary to popular belief the same is true of strangulating obstruction until very late in the course of the disease, a fact which has often resulted in unfortunate delay in treatment. Signs and symptoms of shock also occur *very late* in strangulating obstruction. The appearance of shock, tenderness, rigidity, and fever often means that there has been contamination of the peritoneum with infected intestinal content. The presence of a palpable abdominal mass usually signifies a closed-loop strangulating small-bowel obstruction because the tense fluid-filled loop is the palpable lesion. Auscultation may reveal loud high-pitched borborygmi coincident with the colicky pain, but this classic finding is often not present late in strangulating or nonstrangulating obstruction. A quiet abdomen does not eliminate the possibility of obstruction, nor does it necessarily establish the diagnosis of adynamic ileus.

LABORATORY AND X-RAY FINDINGS Leukocytosis, with shift to the left, usually occurs when strangulation is present, but a normal white blood cell count does not exclude strangulation. Elevation of the serum amylase is encountered occasionally in all forms of intestinal obstruction, especially the strangulating variety.

The x-ray is extremely valuable but under certain circumstances may also be misleading. In nonstrangulating complete small-bowel obstruction, x-rays are almost completely reliable. Distention of fluid- and gas-filled loops of small intestine usually arranged in a "stepladder" pattern with air-fluid levels and an absence or paucity of colonic gas are pathognomonic (Fig. 311-1). These findings, however, are absent in slightly over half the cases of strangulating small-bowel obstruction, especially early in the disease. A general haze due to peritoneal fluid and sometimes a "coffee-bean" shaped mass are seen in strangulating obstruction. Occasionally the films are normal, but when symptoms are consistent with obstruction of the small intestine, a normal film should suggest strangulation. Roentgenographic differentiation of partial mechanical small-bowel obstruction from adynamic ileus may be impossible since gas is present in both small and large intestine; however, colonic distention is usually more prominent in adynamic ileus. A radiopaque dye given by mouth is useful in making this distinction.

FIGURE 311-1

Acute mechanical obstruction of small intestine (upright film). Note air-fluid levels, marked distention of bowel loops, and absence of colonic gas.

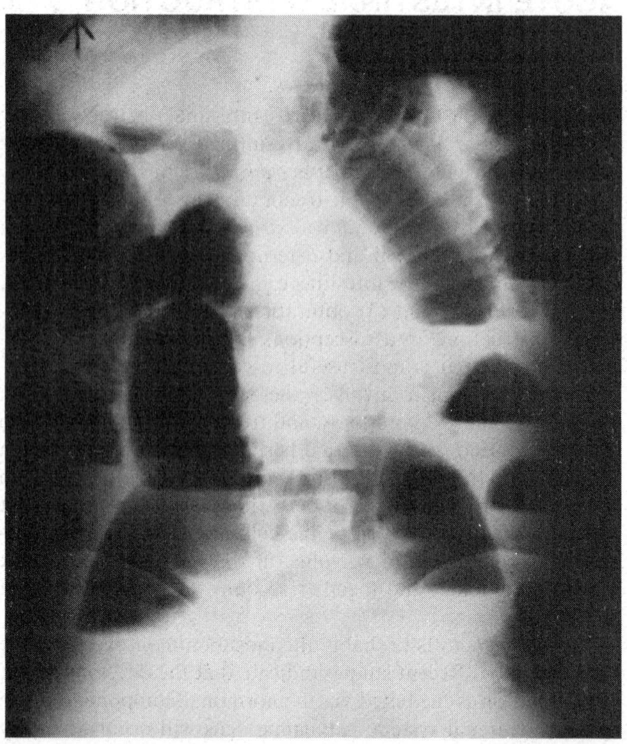

Colonic obstruction with a competent ileocecal valve is easily recognized because distention with gas is mainly confined to the colon. Barium enema is usually advisable to determine the nature of the lesion except when concomitant perforation is suspected, a rare occurrence. When the ileocecal valve is incompetent, the films resemble those of partial small-bowel obstruction or adynamic ileus, and barium enema is necessary to establish the correct diagnosis. Barium given by mouth is perfectly safe when obstruction is in the small intestine since the barium sulfate does not become inspissated in this location. *Barium should never be given by mouth to a patient with possible colonic obstruction* until that possibility has been excluded by barium enema.

MESENTERIC VASCULAR OCCLUSION This term refers to a form of intestinal obstruction in which there is no mechanical occlusion of the intestine but ischemia is the basic feature. About 50 percent of cases result from occlusion of the superior mesenteric artery due to emboli or atherosclerotic narrowing. An additional 40 percent of cases are due to nonocclusive ischemia, a condition which usually occurs in elderly patients with congestive heart failure taking digitalis glycosides. The latter drugs have been shown to decrease splanchnic blood flow. The remainder are cases of pure venous mesenteric occlusion due to thrombi. Any patient with severe heart disease, particularly in the presence of auricular fibrillation, who complains of abdominal pain should be considered to have intestinal ischemia until proved otherwise. Over 70 percent of cases have a 2- to 3-day history of low-grade colicky abdominal pain, often with diarrhea containing microscopic blood; this is followed by catastrophic shock, severe abdominal tenderness, rigidity, leukocytosis, and fever. Only in venous infarction, the rarest form of mesenteric vascular occlusion, are these findings encountered early. X-ray examination shows a nonspecific adynamic ileus, but selective angiography is usually diagnostic. Occasionally, barium enema is useful if the lesion is confined to the colon and shows characteristic "thumbprinting," representing edematous and hemorrhagic mucosal folds most often in the region of the splenic flexure (see also Chap. 310).

PROGNOSIS AND TREATMENT **Small-intestinal obstruction** The overall mortality rate for obstruction of the small intestine is about 10 percent, even under the most optimal conditions. While the mortality rate for nonstrangulating obstruction is as low as 5 to 8 percent, that for strangulating obstruction has been reported to be between 20 and 75 percent. Well over half of the deaths from small-bowel obstruction occur in those with strangulation; however, the latter constitute only one-fourth to one-third of the cases. Careful studies indicate that the clinical, laboratory, and x-ray findings are not reliable in distinguishing strangulating from nonstrangulating obstruction when obstruction is complete. Complete obstruction is suggested when there has been a total cessation in the passage of gas or stool per rectum and when gas is absent in the distal intestine by x-ray. Since strangulating small-bowel obstruction is always complete, operation should always be undertaken in such patients after suitable preparation. Prior to operation, fluid and electrolyte balance should be restored, and decompression instituted by means of a nasogastric tube. Six to eight hours of preparation may be necessary. During this period broad-spectrum antibiotics are indicated if strangulation is felt to be likely, but operation should not be delayed unless there is unequivocal clinical and roentgenographic evidence of resolution of the obstruction during the period of preparation. Attempts to pass a long tube into the small intestine usually fail while putting the patient through uncomfortable unproductive manipulations which delay appropriate fluid replacement and decompression. *There are probably few if any indications for the use of a long intestinal tube.* Procrastination of operation because of improvement in well-being of the patient during resuscitation and gastric decompression usually leads to unnecessary and hazardous delay in proper treatment. Purely nonoperative therapy is safe only in the presence of incomplete obstruction and is best utilized in patients with (1) repeated episodes of partial obstruction, (2) recent postoperative partial obstruction, and (3) partial obstruction following a recent episode of diffuse peritonitis.

Colonic obstruction The mortality rate for colonic obstruction is about 20 percent. As in small-bowel obstruction, nonoperative treatment is contraindicated unless the obstruction is incomplete. Occasionally, but not always, when the obstruction is incomplete, nonoperative therapy may result in sufficient decompression that a definitive operative procedure can be undertaken at a later date. This can usually be accomplished by discontinuation of all oral intake and perhaps by nasogastric suction, although attempts to decompress a *completely* obstructed colon by intubation are almost invariably futile. A long intestinal tube will not decompress an obstructed colon with a competent ileocecal valve. When obstruction is complete, early operation is mandatory, especially when the ileocecal valve is competent; cecal gangrene is likely if the cecal diameter exceeds 10 cm on plain abdominal film. For obstruction on the left side of the colon, the most common site, preliminary operative decompression by cecostomy or transverse colostomy followed by definitive resection of the primary lesion is the treatment of choice. For a lesion of the right or transverse colon, primary resection and anastomosis can safely be performed because distension of the ileum with consequent discrepancy in size and hazard in suture are not present.

Adynamic ileus This type of ileus usually responds to nonoperative continuous decompression and adequate treatment of the primary disease. The prognosis is usually good. Rarely, adynamic colonic distention may become so great that cecostomy is required if cecal gangrene is feared. Spastic ileus usually responds to treatment of the primary disease.

Mesenteric vascular occlusion The mortality for mesenteric vascular occlusion usually is greater than 80 percent. For occlusive mesenteric ischemia, early operation is mandatory. Vascular reconstruction with resection of nonviable intestine is the procedure of choice unless intestinal gangrene is irreversible, in which case resection alone is indicated. If diffuse nonocclusive ischemia can be diagnosed by selective angiography, treatment involves adequate volume replacement and 24-h perfusion of the superior mesenteric artery with vasodilating agents, followed by operation to resect intestine of questionable viability. Although some instances of survival have been reported in this condition, these are rare.

REFERENCES

BECKER WF: Acute adhesive ileus: A study of 412 cases with particular reference to the abuse of tube decompression in treatment. Surg Gynecol Obstet 95:472, 1952

BOLEY S et al: Initial results from an aggressive roentgenologic and surgical approach to acute mesenteric ischemia. Surgery 82:848, 1977

COHN I, ATIK M: Strangulation obstruction: Closed loop studies. Ann Surg 153:94, 1961

DUBOIS A et al: Postoperative ileus: Physiopathology, etiology and treatment. Ann Surg 178:781, 1973

FAULK DL et al: Chronic intestinal pseudoobstruction. Gastroenterology 74:922, 1978

Gough IR: Strangulating adhesive small bowel radiographs. Br J Surg 65:431, 1978

Marston A et al: Ischaemic colitis. Gut 7:1, 1966

Shields R: The absorption and secretion of fluid and electrolytes by the obstructed bowel. Br J Surg 52:774, 1965

Silen W: *Cope's Early Diagnosis of the Acute Abdomen,* 15th ed. London, Oxford, 1979

312
ACUTE APPENDICITIS

WILLIAM SILEN

INCIDENCE AND EPIDEMIOLOGY The maximum incidence of acute appendicitis occurs in the second and third decades of life. While the disease may be encountered at any time of life, it is relatively rare at the extremes of age. Males and females are equally affected except between puberty and age 25, when males predominate in a 3:2 ratio. Perforation is relatively much more common in infancy and in the aged, during which periods mortality rates are highest. The mortality rate has decreased steadily in Europe and the United States from 8.1 per 100,000 of the population in 1941 to less than 1 per 100,000 in 1970. The absolute incidence of the disease also decreased by about 40 percent between 1940 and 1960 but since then has remained unchanged. Although various factors such as changing dietary habits, altered intestinal flora, and better nutrition and intake of vitamins have been suggested to explain the reduced incidence, the exact reasons have not been elucidated. Of interest is that the overall incidence of appendicitis is much lower in underdeveloped countries, especially parts of Africa, and in lower socioeconomic groups.

PATHOGENESIS The primary pathogenetic hallmark has always been thought to be luminal obstruction. While obstruction can be identified by careful examination in 30 to 40 percent of cases, recent studies have shown that ulceration of the mucosa is the initial event in the majority. The causation of the ulceration is unknown, although a viral etiology has been postulated. Whether the inflammatory reaction attendant with ulceration is sufficient to obstruct the tiny appendiceal lumen even transiently is also not clear. Obstruction, when present, is most commonly caused by a fecalith which results from accumulation and inspissation of fecal matter around vegetable fibers. Enlarged lymphoid follicles associated with viral infections (e.g., measles), inspissated barium, worms (e.g., pinworms, *Ascaris,* and *Taenia*), and tumors (e.g., carcinoid or carcinoma) may also obstruct the lumen. Secretion of mucus distends the organ, which has a capacity of only 0.1 to 0.2 ml, and luminal pressures rise as high as 60 cmH_2O. Luminal bacteria multiply and invade the appendiceal wall as venous engorgement and subsequent arterial compromise result from the high intraluminal pressures. Finally, gangrene and perforation occur. If the process evolves slowly, adjacent organs such as the terminal ileum, cecum, and omentum may wall off the appendiceal area so that a localized abscess will develop, whereas rapid progression of vascular impairment may cause perforation with free access to the peritoneal cavity. Subsequent rupture of primary appendiceal abscesses may produce fistulas between the appendix and bladder, small intestine, sigmoid, or cecum. Occasionally, acute appendicitis may be the first manifestation of Crohn's disease. While chronic infection of the appendix with tuberculosis, amebiasis, and actinomycosis may occur, a useful clinical aphorism states that *chronic appendiceal inflammation is not usually the cause of prolonged abdominal pain of weeks or months duration.* In contrast, it is clear that recurrent acute appendicitis does occur, often with complete resolution of inflammation and symptoms between attacks. Recurrent acute appendicitis may become more frequent as antibiotics are dispensed more freely.

CLINICAL MANIFESTATIONS The history and sequence of symptoms are among the most important diagnostic features of appendicitis. The initial symptom is almost invariably *abdominal pain* of the visceral type, resulting from appendiceal contractions or distention of the lumen. It is usually poorly localized in the periumbilical or epigastric regions. There is often an accompanying urge to defecate or pass flatus, neither of which relieves the distress. This visceral pain is mild, often cramping, and rarely catastrophic in nature, usually lasting 4 to 6 h, but may not be noted by stoic individuals or by some patients during sleep. As inflammation spreads to the parietal peritoneal surfaces, the pain becomes somatic, steady, and more severe, aggravated by motion or cough and usually located in the *right lower quadrant. Anorexia* is so frequent that the presence of hunger should arouse serious suspicion of the diagnosis of acute appendicitis. *Nausea* and *vomiting* occur in 50 to 60 percent of cases, but vomiting is rarely profuse and protracted. The development of nausea and vomiting before the onset of pain is extremely rare. Change in bowel habit is of little diagnostic value since any or no alteration may be observed, although the presence of diarrhea caused by an inflamed appendix in juxtaposition to the sigmoid may cause serious diagnostic difficulties. Urinary frequency and dysuria occur if the appendix lies adjacent to the bladder. The typical sequence of symptoms (poorly localized periumbilical pain followed by nausea and vomiting with subsequent shift of pain to the right lower quadrant) occurs in only 50 to 60 percent of patients, and some variations are considered below.

Physical findings vary with time after onset of the illness and according to the location of the appendix, which may be situated deep in the pelvic cul-de-sac, in the right lower quadrant in any relation to the peritoneum, cecum, and small intestine, in the right upper quadrant, or even in the left lower quadrant. *The diagnosis cannot be established unless tenderness can be elicited.* While tenderness is sometimes absent in the early visceral stage of the disease, it ultimately always develops and is found in any location corresponding to the position of the appendix. Abdominal tenderness may be completely absent if a retrocecal or pelvic appendix is present, in which case the sole physical finding may be tenderness in the flank or on rectal or pelvic examination. Percussion, rebound tenderness, and referred rebound tenderness are often, but not invariably, present; they are most likely to be absent early in the illness. Flexion of the right hip and guarded movement by the patient are due to parietal peritoneal involvement. Hyperesthesia of the skin of the right lower quadrant and a positive psoas or obturator sign are often late findings and are rarely of diagnostic value. When the inflamed appendix is in close proximity to the anterior parietal peritoneum, muscular rigidity is present, yet is often minimal early. The temperature is usually normal or slightly elevated (99 to 100.5°F), but a temperature above 101°F should always suggest the presence of perforation. Tachycardia is commensurate with the elevation of the temperature. Rigidity and tenderness become more marked as the disease progresses to perforation and localized or diffuse peritonitis. Distention is rare unless severe diffuse peritonitis has developed. The alleged disappearance of pain and tenderness just prior to perforation is extremely unusual. A mass may develop if localized perforation has occurred but usually will not be detectable before 3 days after onset of the disease. Earlier presence of a mass suggests carcinoma of the cecum or

Crohn's disease. Perforation is rare before 24 h after onset of symptoms but may be as high as 80 percent after 48 h.

Laboratory examination does not establish the diagnosis since the latter is based primarily on clinical grounds. Although moderate leukocytosis of 10,000 to 18,000 cells per cubic millimeter is frequent (with a concomitant shift to immature cells), the absence of leukocytosis does not eliminate the possibility of acute appendicitis. Leukocytosis of greater than 20,000 cells per cubic millimeter should alert the clinician to the probability of perforation. Anemia and blood in the stool suggest a primary diagnosis of carcinoma of the cecum, especially in elderly individuals. The urine may contain a few white or red blood cells without bacteria if the appendix lies close to the right ureter or bladder.

Urinalysis is most useful, however, in excluding genitourinary conditions which may mimic acute appendicitis. X-rays are rarely of value except when an opaque fecalith (5 percent of patients) is observed in the right lower quadrant (especially in children) together with other clinical findings consistent with appendicitis. Consequently there is no routine need to obtain films of the abdomen unless there is a possibility of other conditions such as intestinal obstruction or ureteral calculus.

While the typical historical sequence and physical findings are present in 50 to 60 percent of cases, it is obvious that a wide variety of atypical patterns of disease are encountered, especially at the age extremes and during pregnancy. The 70 to 80 percent incidence of perforation and generalized peritonitis in infants under 2 years of age is dramatic testimony to the importance of the history in the early detection of the disease. Any infant or child with diarrhea, vomiting, and abdominal pain is highly suspect. Fever is much more common in this age group, and abdominal distention is often the only physical finding. In the elderly, pain and tenderness are often obtunded, and thus the diagnosis is frequently delayed. A 30 percent incidence of perforation in patients over 70 attests to the importance of this delay. Elderly patients often present themselves initially with a slightly painful mass (a primary appendiceal abscess), or sometimes appear with adhesive intestinal obstruction 5 or 6 days after a previously undetected perforated appendix. Appendicitis occurs about once in every 1000 pregnancies and is the most common extrauterine condition requiring abdominal operation. The diagnosis may be missed or delayed because of the frequent occurrence of mild abdominal discomfort and nausea and vomiting during pregnancy. During the last trimester when the mortality rate from appendicitis is highest, uterine displacement of the appendix to the right upper quadrant and laterally leads to confusion in diagnosis.

DIFFERENTIAL DIAGNOSIS A listing of the differential diagnoses of acute appendicitis would produce an encyclopedic compendium of all conditions which cause abdominal pain since appendicitis may simulate any of these diseases. Diagnostic accuracy is about 75 to 80 percent for experienced clinicians and must be based solely on the clinical criteria outlined above. It is probably better to err slightly in the direction of overdiagnosis since delay is associated with perforation and increased morbidity and mortality. In unperforated appendicitis the mortality rate is 0.1 percent, little more than that associated with general anesthesia; for perforated appendicitis there is an overall mortality of 3 percent, a figure which increases to 15 percent in the elderly. Four to six hours of observation in doubtful cases is always more beneficial than harmful, however. The most common conditions discovered at operation when acute appendicitis is erroneously diagnosed are, in rough order of frequency, mesenteric lymphadenitis, no organic disease, acute pelvic inflammatory disease, ruptured graafian follicle or corpus luteum cyst, and acute gastroenteritis. In addition, acute cholecystitis, perforated ulcer, acute pancreatitis, acute diverticulitis, strangulating intestinal obstruction, ureteral calculus, and pyelonephritis frequently present diagnostic difficulties.

It is useful to consider separately some of the more common and difficult diagnostic possibilities, especially in the female. Differentiation of *pelvic inflammatory disease* from acute appendicitis may be virtually impossible. Gram-negative intracellular diplococci on cervical smear are not pathognomonic unless *Neisseria gonorrhea* can be cultured. Pain on movement of the cervix is not specific and may occur in appendicitis if perforation has occurred or if the appendix lies adjacent to the uterus or adnexa. *Rupture of a graafian follicle* (mittelschmerz) occurs at midcycle with spill of blood and fluid to produce pain and tenderness more diffuse and usually of a less severe degree than in appendicitis. Fever and leukocytosis are usually absent. *Rupture of a corpus luteum cyst* is identical clinically to rupture of a graafian follicle but develops about the time of menstruation. The presence of an adnexal mass and evidence of blood loss help differentiate *ruptured tubal pregnancy. Twisted ovarian cyst* and *endometriosis* occasionally are difficult to distinguish from appendicitis.

Acute mesenteric lymphadenitis is the appellation usually given when enlarged, slightly reddened lymph nodes at the root of the mesentery and a normal appendix are encountered at operation. Whether this is a single, discrete entity is unclear since the causative factor is not known. The diagnosis is essentially impossible clinically, although retrospectively there often appears to have been more diffuse pain and tenderness, perhaps associated with lymphocytosis. Children seem to be affected more frequently than adults. Operation should be undertaken unless there is rapid resolution of all symptoms and findings. *Acute gastroenteritis* usually causes profuse watery diarrhea, often with nausea and vomiting but without localized findings. Between cramps, the abdomen is completely relaxed. In salmonella gastroenteritis the abdominal findings are similar, although the pain may be more severe and more localized, and fever and chills are common. The occurrence of similar symptoms among other members of the family may be helpful. When the diagnosis of acute pelvic appendicitis with perforation has been missed, gastroenteritis is the most common previous working diagnosis. Persistent abdominal or rectal tenderness should eliminate the diagnosis of gastroenteritis. *Regional enteritis* (Crohn's disease) is usually associated with a more prolonged history, often with previous exacerbations regarded by the patient or physician as episodes of gastroenteritis unless the diagnosis has been established previously. *Meckel's diverticulitis* usually cannot be distinguished from acute appendicitis but is very rare.

TREATMENT Cathartics and frequent enemas should be avoided if appendicitis is under consideration, and antibiotics should not be administered when the diagnosis is in question, as they will only mask the presence or development of perforation. The treatment is early operation and appendectomy as soon as the patient can be prepared. Preparation rarely takes more than 1 to 2 h in early appendicitis but may require 6 to 8 h in cases of severe sepsis and dehydration associated with late perforation. The *only* circumstance in which operation is *not* indicated is the presence of a palpable mass 3 to 5 days after the onset of symptoms. Should operation be undertaken at that time, a phlegmon rather than a definitive abscess will be found, and complications from dissection of such a phlegmon are frequent. Such patients treated with broad-spectrum antibiotics, parenteral fluids, and rest usually show resolution of the mass and symptoms within 1 week. *Interval appendectomy* can and should be done safely 3 months later. Should the mass enlarge or the patient become more toxic, drainage of the abscess is necessary. The complications of subphrenic, pelvic, or other intraabdominal abscesses usually follow perforation with generalized peritonitis, and can be avoided by early diagnosis of the disease.

REFERENCES

BOLTON JP: Assessment of the value of the white cell count in management of suspected acute appendicitis. Br J Surg 62:906, 1975

CANTRELL JR, STAFFORD ES: The diminishing mortality from appendicitis. Ann Surg 141:749, 1955

FITZ RH: Perforating inflammation of the vermiform appendix: With special reference to its early diagnosis and treatment. Trans Assoc Am Physicians 1:107, 1886

HYMAN P, WESTRING DW: Leukocytosis in acute appendicitis: Observed racial differences. JAMA 229:1630, 1974

SAKOVER RP, DEL FAVA RL: Frequency of visualization of normal appendix with barium enema examination. Am J Roentgenol Radium Ther Nucl Med 121:312, 1974

SISSON RG et al: Superficial mucosal ulceration and pathogenesis of acute appendicitis. Am J Surg 122:378, 1971

THOMAS DR: Conservative management of appendix mass. Surgery 73:677, 1973

THORBJARNARSON B: Acute appendicitis in patients over the age of 60. Surg Gynecol Obstet 125:1277, 1967

313
DISEASES OF THE PERITONEUM AND MESENTERY

KURT J. ISSELBACHER
J. THOMAS LaMONT

ACUTE PERITONITIS Peritonitis is a localized or generalized inflammatory process of the peritoneum that may appear in both acute and chronic forms. In the acute form the motor activity of the intestine is decreased, and the intestinal lumen becomes distended with gas and fluid. Fluid accumulates as a result of failure to reabsorb the 7 or 8 liters normally secreted daily into the lumen and absorbed from the distal small bowel and colon. There is also accumulation of fluid in the peritoneal cavity as well as decreased oral intake. These combined losses can lead to rapid depletion of the plasma volume with impaired cardiac and renal function.

Etiology Peritonitis may be due to entry of bacteria into the peritoneal cavity from a perforation in the gastrointestinal tract or from an external penetrating wound. It may be secondary to severe chemical reactions from the release of pancreatic enzymes, the digestive juices of the upper gastrointestinal tract, or bile as a result of injury or perforation of the intestine or biliary tract. Patients with systemic lupus erythematosus may have bouts of peritonitis during attacks of their disease.

The most common causes of bacterial peritonitis are appendicitis, perforations associated with diverticulitis, peptic ulcer, gangrenous gallbladder, and gangrenous obstruction of the small bowel from adhesive bands, incarcerated hernia, or volvulus. Any lesion leading to the escape of intestinal bacteria may be a source, including a perforating carcinoma, foreign body, and ulcerative colitis. The peritoneal cavity is remarkably resistant to contamination, and unless continuing contamination occurs, the disease process becomes localized. Patients with alcoholic cirrhosis and ascites have an increased susceptibility to spontaneous bacterial peritonitis, usually from enteric pathogens. This complication occurs in the absence of recognizable perforation of a viscus, and may be due to leakage of bacteria through the intestinal wall.

Clinical features These usually consist of increasing abdominal pain, distention, nausea and vomiting, inability to pass feces or flatus, fever, hypotension, tachycardia, thirst, and oliguria. On physical examination the patient appears acutely ill, febrile, and has a variable degree of abdominal distention. The abdomen is usually acutely tender and tympanitic, often with rebound tenderness. The location of the pain and tenderness depends on the underlying cause and whether the inflammation is localized or generalized. In *localized* peritonitis, as seen in uncomplicated appendicitis or diverticulitis, the physical findings are limited to the area of inflammation. With widespread peritoneal inflammation there is *generalized* peritonitis with diffuse abdominal tenderness and rebound.

Peristalsis may be present initially but usually disappears as the illness progresses. Hypotension is common, as is leukocytosis, which often is greater than 20,000 cells per cubic millimeter. X-ray examination of the abdomen shows dilatation of the large and small bowel with edema of the small-bowel wall as evidenced by the distance between adjacent loops of gas-filled small intestine. Diagnostic paracentesis is valuable in determining the nature of the exudate as well as whether bacteria can be demonstrated or cultured. Lead colic, gastric crises of syphilis, and acute porphyria may cause severe abdominal symptoms that resemble the picture of acute peritonitis.

GONOCOCCAL PERITONITIS This usually involves an extension of gonococcal infection from a primary focus in the female reproductive tract. The signs of inflammation usually are limited to the pelvis, but there may be findings of a mild generalized peritonitis. Occasionally the patient has right upper quadrant pain and tenderness caused by gonococcal perihepatitis involving the liver capsule and adjacent peritoneum (Fitz-Hugh–Curtis syndrome; see also Chap. 150).

STARCH PERITONITIS An acute granulomatous peritonitis can develop in some patients as a foreign-body reaction to cornstarch used to powder surgical gloves. The clinical picture is that of acute abdominal pain and fever 10 to 30 days after an abdominal operation. The diagnosis can be made by paracentesis and demonstration of starch granules in monocytes. However, most patients are reexplored because of the fear of abscess or bacterial peritonitis, with the finding of foreign-body granuloma studding the peritoneum.

PSEUDOMYXOMA PERITONEI This is a rare condition resulting from rupture of a mucocele of the appendix or of a mucinous ovarian cyst. The abdomen becomes filled with masses of jelly-like material. Occasionally, with removal of the mucocele or the ovarian cyst and most of the myxomatous material, a cure may ensue. In other cases, however, the mucoid material recurs, leading to progressive wasting and eventual death. Colloid carcinoma arising from the stomach or colon with peritoneal implants may resemble pseudomyxoma at laparotomy. The course of this type of highly malignant tumor is one of rapid cachexia and early death. The diagnosis can usually be made by the appearance of many highly malignant cells in the peritoneal implants.

CANCER OF THE PERITONEUM Aside from mesothelioma, which in most patients is caused by previous exposure to asbestos, cancer of the peritoneum is usually secondary to a neoplasm within the abdomen, most commonly of the stomach and ovary. Invariably this type of metastatic malignancy is associated with progressive ascites with a high specific gravity and high protein content, often with large numbers of red blood cells or even gross blood. The diagnosis is established by demonstrating malignant cells in the fluid. The clinical progress of this malignant spread can sometimes be arrested by installations of radioactive gold, nitrogen mustard, or chloroquine.

FAMILIAL MEDITERRANEAN FEVER See Chap. 236.

PNEUMATOSIS CYSTOIDES INTESTINALIS This is a condition in which multiple gas-filled blebs or cysts accumulate in the intestinal wall beneath the serosal surface of the bowel. The exact source of the gas has not been explained satisfactorily. In some instances, this disease is associated with specific ulceration of the intestinal mucosa, in particular peptic ulcer with outlet obstruction. Cysts in the wall of the small bowel are seen as an occasional complication of mesenteric vascular occlusion. In the large bowel, these cysts are usually benign, may be seen with a variety of other disorders, and usually disappear in time.

There are no specific physical findings secondary to the pneumatosis, and the diagnosis is made either by x-ray or at laparotomy. Occasionally the subserosal cysts may rupture, resulting in pneumoperitoneum.

CHYLOUS ASCITES This term refers to the accumulation of chyle (intestinal lymph) in the peritoneal cavity. The condition is sometimes associated with chylothorax. The fluid in the peritoneal cavity appears milky or creamy because of the presence of chylomicrons. This fat may be demonstrated microscopically by staining with Sudan III and may be removed by acidification of the fluid followed by extraction with ether. The chyle (lipid) will then go into the ether phase. Many conditions may be associated with the cloudy or milky-appearing peritoneal fluid, so-called pseudochylous ascites. The milky or turbid appearance is usually due to the presence of protein and desquamated cells. The turbidity of this fluid will not be removed with the ether but will clear with addition of alkali.

The causes of chylous ascites include (1) penetrating or nonpenetrating trauma that damages the main duct in the lymphatic system within the abdomen, (2) intestinal obstruction if it is associated with rupture of a major lymphatic channel, (3) congenital lymphangiectasia, (4) malignant disease or tuberculous infection that obstructs the intestinal lymphatics, (5) filariasis, or (6) cirrhosis.

The sudden accumulation of chyle in the peritoneal cavity often results in abdominal pain, signs of peritoneal irritation, and leukocytosis. These symptoms gradually subside, leaving the patient with a distended but nontender, fluid-filled abdomen. Lymphangiography is of value in determining the location of the leak or site of obstruction to the lymphatic channels. The course depends upon the underlying etiologic factors.

MESENTERIC LIPODYSTROPHY This is a rare disorder usually affecting middle-aged women and characterized pathologically by infiltration of the mesentery with lipid-laden macrophages and fibrous tissue. These patients present with ill-defined abdominal pain and occasionally an abdominal mass. The diagnosis is made at laparotomy by demonstration of thick fibrofatty masses at the root of the mesentery with retraction and distortion of the bowel loops.

REFERENCES

CONN HO: Spontaneous bacterial peritonitis. Multiple revisitations. Gastroenterology 70:455, 1976

KIPFER RE et al: Mesenteric lipodystrophy. Ann Intern Med 80:582, 1974

LIMBER GK et al: Pseudomyxoma peritonei. Ann Surg 1978:587, 1973

SCHWARTZ SI et al: *Principles of Surgery,* 3d ed. New York, McGraw-Hill, 1979

WARSHAW AL: Diagnosis of starch peritonitis by paracentesis. Lancet 2:1054, 1972

section 6 | Disorders of the hepatobiliary system

314
APPROACH TO THE PATIENT WITH LIVER DISEASE

KURT J. ISSELBACHER

GENERAL CONSIDERATIONS While disease of the liver or biliary tract may be directly responsible for the symptoms that bring the patient to the physician, examination for nonhepatic complaints may occasionally provide the clues to otherwise asymptomatic or occult hepatobiliary disease. Liver function studies and other diagnostic procedures such as biopsy (as discussed in Chap. 316) are crucial, but much valuable information as to the possible nature and extent of liver disease can be obtained by a carefully elicited history and thorough physical examination.

Importance of clinical history Since laboratory tests often do not establish the specific cause of liver disease, the history is of the greatest significance. *Family history* is important with respect to jaundice, anemia, splenectomy, or cholecystectomy; a positive history may be helpful in diagnosing hemolytic anemia, congenital or familial hyperbilirubinemia, or gallstones. In Wilson's disease (hepatolenticular degeneration), there may be a family history of tremor or neurologic abnormalities. *Occupation* should be reviewed in detail, and *environmental factors* need to be examined. Note should be made of any contact with rats or other animals possibly carrying Weil's disease and of exposure to toxins such as carbon tetrachloride, beryllium, or vinyl chloride. The patient should be asked about travel to other countries, especially to areas where hepatitis may be endemic. Careful questioning regarding alcohol intake is important in most cases. Since the alcoholic often denies or understates the amounts consumed, it is desirable to check the validity of the history with close friends or relatives of the patient.

Contact with jaundiced patients (including intimate or sexual relations) should be noted. If the patient has had any *injections* in the previous 6 months, hepatitis B or non-A, non-B infection may be the underlying disease. Injections include blood tests, blood or plasma transfusions, tattooing, and dental treatment. The patient should be asked about narcotics, hallucinogens, or stimulant *drugs* taken parenterally, as well as about agents taken orally, such as chlorpromazine or estrogen-containing drugs known to affect liver function.

A previous history of indigestion and right upper quadrant pain suggests cholelithiasis or choledocholithiasis. Jaundice following shortly after operation on the biliary tract suggests residual stone, that which occurs within 6 months suggests hepatitis B or posttransfusion hepatitis, and that occurring after 1 or more years may be due to stricture of the common bile duct. Postoperative jaundice may be due to the anesthetic, especially after multiple uses of halothane, or to the impaired hepatic excretory function resulting from relative hypoxemia of liver cells during the operative or postoperative period.

The *onset of the illness* should be noted. The relatively abrupt onset of nausea, anorexia, and aversion to smoking followed by progressive jaundice suggests viral hepatitis. A gradual development of jaundice associated with pruritus suggests cholestasis. Intermittent right upper quadrant abdominal pain followed by cholestatic jaundice points to gallstone disease, while the gradual onset of painless jaundice with weight loss is suggestive of tumor, such as carcinoma of the head of the pancreas. Jaundice associated with fever and chills makes cholangitis and extrahepatic biliary obstruction likely possibilities.

The patient with hepatitis generally feels ill, and dark urine and light stools occur before the appearance of scleral or skin icterus. In cholestatic hepatitis, the patient may feel relatively well and complain only of symptoms due to the obstruction, such as pruritus.

Physical examination Jaundice is looked for in the sclera as well as the skin. Pallor indicative of anemia may be a reflection of hemolysis, cirrhosis, or neoplasm. Significant cachexia, especially of the extremities, may be associated with cancer or active cirrhosis. In the alcoholic, one should look for stigmas of cirrhosis such as parotid gland enlargement, Dupuytren's contracture, gynecomastia, testicular atrophy, and diminished axillary or pubic hair.

The *skin examination* may reveal ecchymoses due to prothrombin deficiency, or purpura due to thrombocytopenia. *Palmar erythema* or *spider angiomas* may reflect acute or chronic liver disease. Spider angiomas are usually found above the umbilicus and especially on the face, neck, shoulders, forearms, and dorsum of the hands. The presence of a few spider angiomas is not abnormal in women, especially during pregnancy. However, their appearance in men is always abnormal and should be carefully searched for. In chronic cholestasis, *scratch marks, finger clubbing,* and *xanthoma* of the eyelids and extensor surfaces of the tendons of the wrists and ankles may be found. A *slate color* to the skin due to increased melanin should suggest the presence of hemochromatosis.

Evaluation of the *mental state* and *neurologic function* is important. Slight deterioration of the intellect and minimal personality changes may suggest hepatocellular disease or the presence of portal-systemic venous shunts, but care must be taken to exclude other causes such as neurologic disease. The presence of flapping tremor of the hands (asterixis) may be found in association with portal-systemic encephalopathy or impending hepatic coma.

Abdominal examination may reveal ascites, which, together with dilated periumbilical veins, suggests cirrhosis and extensive portal collateral circulation. A very large nodular and rock-hard liver suggests the presence of hepatoma or hepatic metastases. Careful percussion is necessary to evaluate the size of a nonpalpable liver. A small liver may indicate cirrhosis (especially postnecrotic); a small liver which diminishes in size suggests severe hepatitis or massive hepatic necrosis. In the alcoholic, fatty infiltration and cirrhosis often produce a uniform enlargement of the liver. The liver edge is tender in hepatitis, in congestive heart failure, and occasionally in malignant disease and with alcoholism (especially "alcoholic hepatitis").

A palpable and sometimes visibly enlarged gallbladder (Courvoisier's sign) suggests extrahepatic biliary obstruction often due to pancreatic cancer. A tender gallbladder and positive Murphy's sign suggests cholelithiasis or choledocholithiasis. A palpable spleen may indicate hepatitis or cirrhosis; significant splenomegaly may be a reflection of portal hypertension.

Abdominal auscultation may reveal the presence of a venous hum over dilated collateral veins radiating from the umbilicus, the so-called caput medusae. In advanced cirrhosis this venous hum is virtually diagnostic of significant portal hypertension. A bruit may sometimes be heard over large regenerating nodules in cirrhosis, and occasionally over hepatomas and metastatic nodules in the liver. The presence of a friction rub strongly suggests neoplastic disease or a hepatic abscess. A friction rub may occasionally be heard over hepatomas and metastatic liver nodules.

Liver function tests Serum assays for biochemical markers of liver disease are an integral part of the proper evaluation of liver and biliary tract disease. In general, the serum bilirubin is measured to confirm the presence and severity of the jaundice and determine the degree of bilirubin conjugation. Transaminase (aminotransferase) elevations reflect the severity of active hepatocellular damage, and the alkaline phosphatase elevations are found with cholestasis and hepatic infiltrates. Serum albumin and the prothrombin time are determined as indexes of hepatic synthetic function. These and other tests are reviewed in Chaps. 38 and 316.

Diagnostic procedures (see Chap. 316) The further evaluation of patients with hepatobiliary disease should be individualized depending on the history, physical findings, and initial screening laboratory tests. Hepatocellular disease such as hepatitis is often sufficiently clear so that no additional tests are needed. However in severe, chronic, or ambiguous cases scintiscans or liver biopsy may be needed to determine the nature of the liver disease. When hepatic tumors are suspected, an ultrasound and scintiscan study is usually performed followed by liver biopsy, angiography, or laparoscopy for a more specific diagnosis. When biliary obstruction is suspected, the first examination is usually an ultrasound study to determine the size of the bile ducts, whether gallstones are present, or whether there is the suggestion of a mass in the head of the pancreas. Frequently more information is needed and thus a percutaneous endoscopic cholangiogram or exploratory laparotomy may be performed.

CLASSIFICATION OF LIVER DISEASE The classification of the various types of liver disease has been difficult because in many instances the etiology and pathogenetic mechanism are obscure. As a consequence, one finds an abundance of labels and names applied to hepatic disorders. Some individuals use the term *hepatitis* to imply viral infection, others simply to connote evidence of hepatic inflammation. One finds ambiguity in the use of the words *acute, subacute,* and *chronic. Chronicity* should refer to continuing or recurrent disease (i.e., duration).

TABLE 314-1
Classification of liver disease

I Parenchymal
  A Hepatitis (viral, drug-induced, toxic)
    1 Acute
    2 Chronic (persistent or active)
  B Cirrhosis
    1 Alcoholic (portal, nutritional, Laennec's cirrhosis)
    2 Postnecrotic
    3 Biliary
    4 Hemochromatosis
    5 Rare types (e.g., Wilson's disease, galactosemia, cystic fibrosis of pancreas, $alpha_1$-antitrypsin deficiency)
  C Infiltrations
    1 Glycogen
    2 Fat (neutral fat, cholesterol, gangliosides, cerebrosides)
    3 Amyloid
    4 Lymphoma, leukemia
    5 Granuloma (e.g., sarcoidosis, tuberculosis, idiopathic)
  D Space-occupying lesions
    1 Hepatoma, metastatic tumor
    2 Abscess (pyogenic, amoebic)
    3 Cysts (polycystic disease, *Echinococcus*)
    4 Gummas
  E Functional disorders associated with jaundice
    1 Gilbert's syndrome
    2 Crigler-Najjar syndrome
    3 Dubin-Johnson and Rotor syndromes
    4 Cholestasis of pregnancy and benign recurrent cholestasis
II Hepatobiliary
  A Extrahepatic biliary obstruction (by stone, stricture, or tumor)
  B Cholangitis
III Vascular
  A Chronic passive congestion and cardiac cirrhosis
  B Hepatic vein thrombosis (Budd-Chiari syndrome)
  C Portal vein thrombosis
  D Pylephlebitis
  E Arteriovenous malformations

Activity should refer to evidence of the presence of perpetuation of liver cell injury; this is most readily identified on biopsy by the degree of hepatocellular necrosis and by serum transaminase elevations.

Because of the difficulties involved in defining the etiology of many types of liver disease, in most instances the process is best defined and described by an examination of the morphologic character of the lesion. Therefore, a *morphologic classification* of liver disease, as outlined in Table 314-1, appears at present more practical than one based on etiology.

REFERENCES

SCHIFF L: *Diseases of the Liver,* 4th ed. Philadelphia, Lippincott, 1975

SHERLOCK S: *Diseases of the Liver and Biliary System,* 6th ed. Philadelphia, Davis, 1981

WRIGHT R et al: *Liver and Biliary Disease.* London, Saunders, 1979

315 DERANGEMENTS OF HEPATIC METABOLISM

DANIEL K. PODOLSKY
KURT J. ISSELBACHER

The liver plays a central role in the maintenance of metabolic homeostasis. It is therefore not surprising that the development of clinically important liver disease is accompanied by diverse systemic manifestations of disordered metabolism. The liver has considerable reserve capacity, so minimal or even moderate cell injury may not be reflected by measurable changes in its metabolic function. However, some functions of the liver are more sensitive than others, and a variety of defects may be seen, depending on the nature and extent of the initial insult.

The biochemical functions in which the liver plays a major role include (1) the intermediate metabolism of amino acids and carbohydrates, (2) synthesis and degradation of proteins and glycoproteins, (3) metabolism and degradation of drugs and hormones, and (4) regulation of lipid and cholesterol metabolism. The derangements of these functions are discussed in connection with their occurrence in various forms of parenchymal liver disease. Alterations of bilirubin, porphyrin, and bile salt metabolism are discussed elsewhere (Chaps. 37, 99, 308).

Metabolic derangements are most evident in the patient with advanced liver disease, and the manifestations are similar regardless of the initial etiologic insult. To a varying degree similar abnormalities are observed in patients with severe chronic hepatitis, micronodular cirrhosis, and postnecrotic cirrhosis. Since the many functions of the liver may be affected to varying degrees in individual patients, no single test effectively measures the overall state of liver function. The proper interpretation of liver function tests is discussed in Chap. 316.

CARBOHYDRATE METABOLISM Although the pathways of normal carbohydrate intermediate metabolism are presented in Chap. 89, several salient features pertinent to hepatic function should be emphasized. The liver functions to maintain normal levels of blood sugar by a combination of glycogenesis, glycogenolysis, glycolysis, and gluconeogenesis. These pathways are regulated by a number of hormones including insulin, glucagon, growth hormone, and certain catecholamines. The exquisite sensitivity of the hepatocytes to insulin is responsible for the uptake of an oral glucose load by the liver and its subsequent utilization for glycogen synthesis, triglyceride formation, and, to a small extent, glycolysis. In the fasting state, the liver contributes to glucose homeostasis by glycogenolysis and gluconeogenesis in response to hypoinsulinemia and hyperglucagonemia. Maintenance of normal blood glucose levels through gluconeogenesis is ultimately related to catabolism of muscle protein which provides the necessary amino acid precursors, especially alanine (see Chap. 89). In a complementary fashion, in the postprandial state, the liver directs alanine and branched-chain amino acids to the peripheral tissues, where they are then incorporated into muscle protein. These reciprocal pathways form a glucose-alanine shuttle which is modulated by ambient changes in the hormones mentioned above (Fig. 315-1).

Abnormalities of glucose homeostasis are common in cirrhosis (Table 315-1). Most frequently hyperglycemia and glucose intolerance are observed. Glucose intolerance is associated with normal or increased levels of plasma insulin (except

TABLE 315-1
Alteration of glucose metabolism in cirrhosis

Factors leading to hyperglycemia:
  Decreased hepatic glucose uptake
  Decreased hepatic glycogen synthesis
  Hepatic resistance to insulin
  Portal-systemic glucose shunting
  Peripheral insulin resistance
  Hormonal abnormalities (serum)
    ↑ Glucagon
    ↓ Cortisol
    ↓ Insulin (hemochromatosis)
Factors leading to hypoglycemia:
  Decreased gluconeogenesis
  Decreased hepatic glycogen content
  Hepatic resistance to glucagon
  Poor oral intake
  Hyperinsulinemia secondary to portal-systemic shunting

in patients with hemochromatosis), suggesting that insulin resistance rather than insulin deficiency may be responsible. One of the factors that may play a role in the apparent insulin resistance is an absolute decrease in the liver's ability to metabolize a glucose load because of a decrease in functioning hepatocellular mass. In addition, hyperglucagonemia may be present due to decreased hepatic clearance of this hormone resulting from portal-systemic shunting. In patients with hemochromatosis, insulin levels, however, may indeed be low due to pancreatic involvement, and as a result carbohydrate intolerance is often more severe than in alcoholic cirrhosis. Patients with cirrhosis may also have elevated serum lactate levels reflecting the decreased capacity of the liver to utilize this substrate for gluconeogenesis.

Hypoglycemia, although more common in acute fulminant hepatitis, may also be seen in the patient with end-stage cirrhosis. Glycogen in the liver accounts for 5 to 7 percent of the normal tissue weight. Because the capacity of the liver to store glycogen is limited (approximately 70 g) and glucose consumption continues at a constant rate (approximately 150 g per day), hepatic glycogen stores are depleted after 1 day of fasting. Hypoglycemia in end-stage cirrhosis may be due to decreased hepatic glycogen stores, diminished glucagon responsiveness, or decreased capacity to synthesize glycogen due to extensive parenchymal destruction.

AMINO ACID AND AMMONIA METABOLISM Through a variety of anabolic and catabolic processes, the liver is the major site of amino acid interconversion. Amino acids utilized for hepatic protein synthesis are derived from dietary protein, metabolic turnover of endogenous protein (primarily from muscle), and direct synthesis in the liver. Most of the amino acids entering the liver via the portal vein are catabolized to urea (except for the branched-chain amino acids leucine, isoleucine, and valine). A lesser amount is released into the general circulation as free amino acids, and these may play an important role in the glucose-alanine cycle mentioned above. In addition, amino acids are utilized for the synthesis of liver intracellular proteins, plasma proteins, and special compounds such as glutathione, glutamine, taurine, carnosine, and creatine. Disruption of normal amino acid metabolism may be reflected in altered plasma amino acid concentrations. In general, levels of aromatic amino acids normally metabolized by the liver are elevated, while those of the branched-chain amino acids, largely utilized by skeletal muscle, tend to be normal or depressed. It has been suggested by some investigators that an alteration in the ratio of these two types of amino acids plays a role in the development of hepatic encephalopathy (see below), but there is not agreement on this concept.

Hepatic catabolism or degradation of amino acids involves two major reactions: transamination and oxidative deamination. Transamination, the process by which the amino group of an amino acid is transferred to a keto acid, is catalyzed by aminotransferases. These enzymes are found in very high amounts in liver but are also present in other tissues, such as kidney, muscle, heart, lung, and brain. Glutamic-oxaloacetic acid transaminase (alanine aminotransferase, ALT) has been studied most extensively, and increased levels are found in the serum secondary to various types of liver injury (e.g., acute viral and drug-induced hepatitis). As a result of transamination, amino acids can enter the citric acid cycle and then function in the intermediary metabolism of carbohydrates and lipids (see Chap. 89). Most of the nonessential amino acids are also synthesized in the liver by transamination. Oxidative deamination, which results in conversion of amino acids to keto acids (and ammonia), is catalyzed by L-amino-acid oxidase with two exceptions: glycine oxidation is catalyzed by glycine oxidase, and glutamic oxidation is catalyzed by glutamic dehydrogenase. With severe liver damage (e.g., massive hepatic necrosis), utilization of amino acids is impaired, free amino acids in the bloodstream increase, and an "overflow" type of amino aciduria may occur.

Urea production is intimately related to the metabolic pathways outlined above, providing a means for disposal of ammonia, the toxic product of nitrogen metabolism. Disruption of this process is of particular clinical importance in the patient with severe acute and chronic liver disease. The fixation of amino acid–derived NH_3 in the form of urea is carried out via the Krebs-Henseleit cycle. The final step of this cycle, the formation of urea by arginase, is irreversible. In advanced liver disease urea synthesis is often depressed, leading to an accumulation of NH_3, usually with a significant reduction in blood urea nitrogen (BUN), an ominous sign of liver failure. This finding may be obscured by superimposed renal impairment, which often develops in patients with severe hepatic failure. Urea is mostly excreted by the kidney, but approximately 25 percent is diffused into the intestine where it is converted to NH_3 by bacterial urease. The intestinal production of ammonia also occurs from the bacterial deamination of unabsorbed amino acids and of protein derived from the diet, exfoliated cells, or blood in the gastrointestinal tract.

Gut NH_3 is absorbed and transported to the liver via the

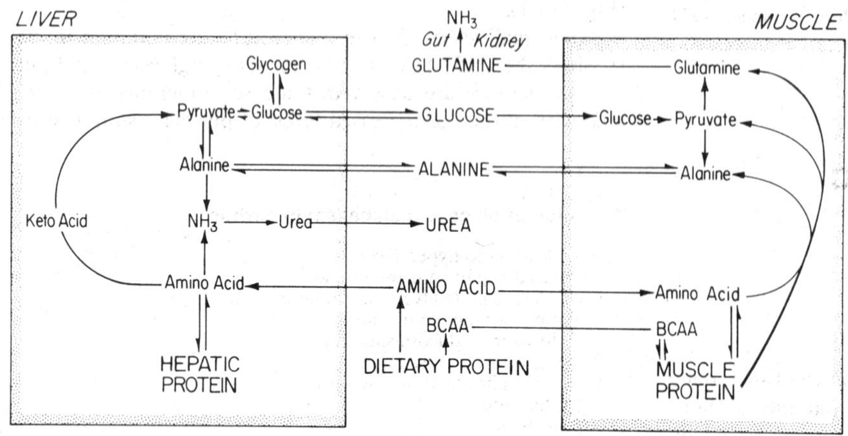

FIGURE 315-1
Carbohydrate-protein exchange between muscle and liver. After an overnight fast there is net release of amino acids by muscle (predominantly alanine and glutamine). These are derived from transamination of pyruvate, degraded amino acids, and glucose. Branched-chain amino acids (BCAA) are particularly important as a source of nitrogen for alanine synthesis. Alanine is utilized for gluconeogenesis by the liver, and urea is formed as a by-product. The kidney and the gut are the main sites of glutamine uptake, where it is used both for ammonia production and as a possible source of energy, respectively. Following ingestion of dietary protein, skeletal muscle goes into an anabolic phase; there is selective hepatic escape and muscle uptake of dietary BCAA, reduced muscle output of alanine and glutamine, and a reduced rate of hepatic gluconeogenesis. Hepatic tissue protein also goes into an anabolic phase following protein ingestion.

portal vein, where it is again converted to urea. The kidney also produces varying amounts of NH_3, largely by the deamination of glutamine. The contributions of the gut and kidney to ammonia synthesis have important implications for the management of the hyperammonemic state frequently seen in patients with advanced liver disease or with portal-systemic shunting of blood.

While the exact chemical mediators of hepatic encephalopathy remain unknown, elevated levels of blood NH_3 generally correlate with the degree of encephalopathy, although approximately 10 percent of such patients have normal levels of blood ammonia. In addition, therapeutic measures that reduce serum NH_3 levels also usually lead to clinical improvement. The several mechanisms known to lead to increased blood NH_3 levels in patients with cirrhosis are illustrated in Fig. 315-2 and include the following: (1) If there is excessive nitrogenous material in the intestine (from bleeding or dietary protein), excessive amounts of NH_3 will be formed by bacterial deamination of amino acids. (2) If renal function declines (as in the hepatorenal syndrome), blood urea nitrogen rises, leading to increased diffusion of urea into the intestinal lumen, where bacterial urease converts it to NH_3. (3) If hepatic function is significantly depressed, diminished urea synthesis may occur with a resultant decrease in the removal of NH_3. (4) If alkalosis (often due to central hyperventilation) and hypokalemia accompany hepatic decompensation, there may be a decrease in the renal availability of H^+ ions; as a result, the NH_3 produced from glutamine by the action of renal glutaminase is permitted to enter the renal vein (rather than being excreted as NH_4^+) leading to increased peripheral blood NH_3 levels. In addition hypokalemia itself leads to increased NH_3 production. (5) If portal hypertension is present and anastomoses exist between the portal vein and systemic venous channels, these portal-systemic shunts will allow NH_3 from the gut to bypass hepatic detoxification, leading to elevated blood NH_3 levels. Thus, with portal-systemic shunting of blood, elevated NH_3 levels may develop even with relatively little hepatocellular dysfunction.

An additional factor important in determining whether a given NH_3 level in the blood will be detrimental to the central nervous system is the blood pH. The more alkaline the pH, the more toxic a given level of NH_3 is likely to be. At 37°C the pK of NH_3 is 8.9; this is close enough to the pH of blood so that minor changes in pH can affect the NH_4^+/NH_3 ratio. Because un-ionized NH_3 crosses membranes more readily than NH_4^+ ions, alkalosis favors the entry of ammonia into the brain (with subsequent changes in cell metabolism) by shifting the equilibrium of the following reaction to the right

$$NH_4^+ + OH \rightleftharpoons NH_3 + HOH$$

As a result, alkalosis not only increases peripheral blood NH_3 levels by renal mechanisms but also increases tissue levels by influencing the diffusion of NH_3 across membranes.

FIGURE 315-2

Major factors (steps 1 to 4) influencing the level of blood ammonia. In cirrhosis with portal hypertension, venous collaterals allow ammonia to bypass the liver (step 5), permitting the entry of ammonia into the systemic circulation (portal-systemic shunting).

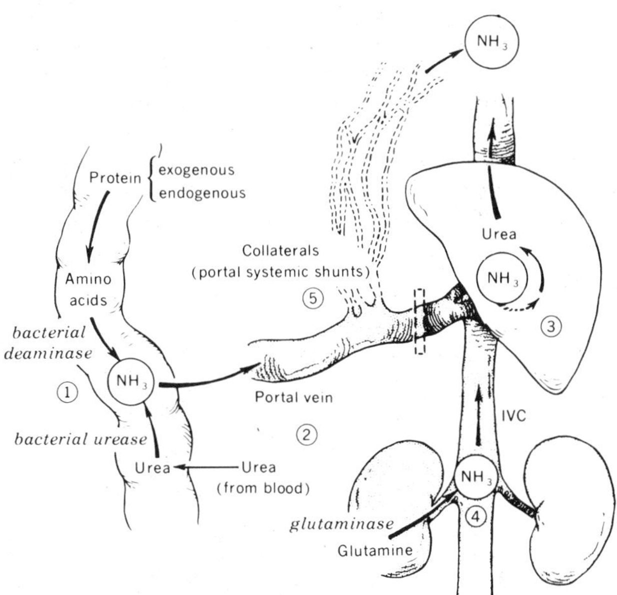

PROTEIN SYNTHESIS AND DEGRADATION The liver is an important site of protein synthesis and degradation. Although the body muscle mass produces the greatest total amount of protein, the liver has the highest rate of synthesis per gram of tissue. The liver synthesizes not only the proteins it needs, but also and perhaps more importantly it produces numerous export proteins. Among the latter, albumin is the most important; *it is produced at a rate of approximately 12 g per day,* representing 25 percent of total hepatic protein synthesis and half of all exported protein. The average normal half-life of serum albumin is 17 to 20 days. The proportion of hepatocytes carrying out active albumin synthesis varies from 10 to 60 percent depending on the body's requirements. Approximately 60 percent of albumin is found in the extravascular spaces, but plasma albumin is still the most abundant circulating protein. Although albumin secreted by the hepatocytes lacks significant carbohydrate, it may undergo nonenzymatic glucosylation in the circulation as a reflection of ambient serum glucose concentrations.

Albumin contributes significantly to the plasma oncotic pressure. In addition, it is the principal binding and transport protein for numerous substances including some hormones, fatty acids, trace metals, tryptophan, bilirubin, and other organic anions of both endogenous and exogenous origin. Despite the many important functions of albumin, rare individuals with congenital analbuminemia appear to have no major physiological derangements other than the excessive accumulation of extravascular fluid. While many of the less hydrophobic ligands may be transported in the unbound form, this suggests that other serum proteins may also have the potential for functioning in binding and transport.

Much has been learned about the mechanisms involved in the synthesis of secretory proteins, especially of albumin (see Fig. 315-3). Polyribosomes bound to the rough endoplasmic reticulum (RER) of the hepatocyte are the principal site of translation of messenger ribonucleic acid (mRNA) coding for export proteins; in contrast proteins destined for intracellular use, such as ferritin, are synthesized on free rather than bound polyribosomes in the cytoplasm. After a short-term fast, there is a decrease in the amount of albumin mRNA associated with the RER; instead more mRNA is found in the cytosol and in a state dissociated from polyribosomes. Albumin, like secretory proteins produced by other organs, appears to be synthesized initially as a larger precursor, preproalbumin. This precursor molecule contains an additional 24 extra amino acid residues on the N-terminus, referred to as a "signal peptide," which undergoes two sequential cleavages (or "processing"); the molecule is then transported to the Golgi apparatus prior to secretion. The "pre" portion of preproalbumin is cleaved within the RER even before protein synthesis is completed; the "pro" segment is removed within the lumen of the ER. Once synthesis and processing are completed, albumin is transported from the Golgi vesicles to the hepatocyte surface by mechanisms which are unclear but almost certainly involve the microfilaments and microtubule apparatus of the cell. Although the hepatic lymph space of Disse provides a potential avenue for the newly released albumin, most secreted proteins enter the plasma.

Albumin synthesis is subject to a number of regulatory influences. These include the rate of transcription of specific mRNAs and the availability of the substrate tRNA (transfer RNA). At the translational level, the integrity of polyribosomes and their synthetic abilities is modified by factors affecting initiation, elongation, and release of peptides and proteins as well as by the availability of ATP, GTP, and magnesium ions. The rate of albumin synthesis is also influenced by the availability of amino acid precursors, especially tryptophan, the scarcest of the essential amino acids. Indeed in patients with large carcinoid tumors albumin synthesis may decrease precipitously when tryptophan is shunted from albumin production into the pathway leading to 5-hydroxytryptophan (serotonin) synthesis (see Chap. 91). The rate of albumin synthesis is also affected by colloid oncotic pressure with increased production occurring in response to falling oncotic pressure. Finally, hormonal influences on hepatic protein metabolism such as insulin and glucagon are closely integrated with the nutritional factors discussed above.

The liver also produces a wide variety of other secretory proteins, most of which have a synthetic pathway and processing procedure similar to albumin (Fig. 315-3). The presence of a *signal peptide,* such as the "prepro" segment of albumin, which is subsequently removed during protein maturation appears to be a general mechanism for orienting proteins in the membranes of the ER and directing them for export rather than for intracellular use or degradation. Most proteins undergo even further modification in the form of sequential *glycosylation* in the RER and Golgi apparatus. The carbohydrate moieties of these glycoproteins appear to be important in determining their site of action and their rate of tissue uptake after secretion. Some of the clinically important secretory glycoproteins include ceruloplasmin, $alpha_1$ antitrypsin, and most other alpha and beta globulins. While the site of albumin catabolism is uncertain, the removal of terminal sialic acid residues after secretion and the resultant exposure of penultimate galactose or *N*-acetylglucosamine residues appear to result in receptor-mediated uptake of "aged" proteins by hepatocytes and Kupffer cells, followed by their subsequent degradation.

One of the clinically most important derangements in protein metabolism is the development of hypoalbuminemia, which results largely from reduced synthetic activity. Decreased synthesis may be caused by a decrease in the number as well as the function of hepatocytes. A decrease in the dietary supply of amino acids can also contribute to deficient synthesis. To some extent the body attempts to compensate for decreased albumin synthesis by reducing the rate of degradation. Attempts to raise the serum albumin level by intravenous infusions are often futile because this compensatory mechanism can be blunted and the decrease in albumin degradation may not occur. The reduced degradation of albumin is not a general phenomenon in chronic liver disease because other proteins such as fibrinogen are degraded more rapidly than normal. The degree of hypoalbuminemia is also augmented in the patient with ascites, where large amounts of the body's albumin are present in the ascitic fluid. When there is increased hepatic venous pressure (as in postsinusoidal or hepatic vein outflow block) there may be increased hepatic lymph production with extravasation into the peritoneal cavity.

Other proteins produced by the liver include many of the blood-clotting factors: fibrinogen (factor I), prothrombin (factor II), and factors V, VII, IX, and X as well as inhibitors of both coagulation and fibrinolysis. Factors II, VII, IX, and X are vitamin K–responsive and are dependent upon normal intestinal fat absorption. Vitamin K activates an enzyme system in liver endoplasmic reticulum which catalyzes the γ-carboxylation of selected glutamyl residues in clotting factor precursors. The γ-carboxylation enhances the Ca^{2+} and phospholipid binding capacity of prothrombin and permits its rapid conversion to thrombin in the presence of factors V and X (Chap. 334).

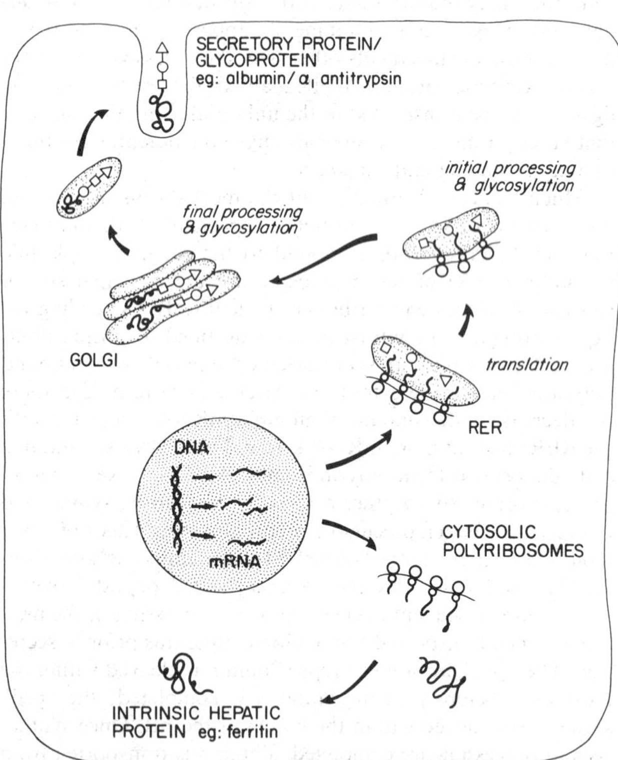

FIGURE 315-3
Schematic diagram illustrating major steps in synthesis, processing, and secretion of proteins and glycoproteins by the liver. Ribosomal subunits and mRNA form polysome complexes to initiate protein synthesis. Polyribosomes synthesizing proteins destined for export (e.g., albumin) associate with membranes to form membrane-bound polysomes [i.e., the rough endoplasmic reticulum (RER)]. Synthesis of precursor molecule (e.g., "preproalbumin") occurs and is followed by stepwise proteolytic cleavage and secretion from the cell. Other export proteins (e.g., $alpha_1$ antitrypsin) are first glycosylated in the RER and Golgi prior to secretion. Proteins produced for intracellular use (e.g., ferritin) are synthesized on nonmembrane-bound cytosolic polyribosomes and processed by stepwise proteolytic cleavage and secretion from the cell.

The liver is involved in the process of hemostasis by virtue of both anabolic and catabolic functions. As expected, severe liver disease leads to reduced synthesis of prothrombin, a vitamin K–dependent clotting factor. The presence of malnutrition, the use of broad-spectrum antibiotics, or concomitant impairment of fat absorption due to reduction in intestinal bile salt concentration (e.g., cholestasis) may accentuate hypoprothrombinemia by decreasing the amount of vitamin K that can be absorbed from the intestine. In these situations, the prothrombin levels may be at least partially corrected by parenteral vitamin K administration. However, when the coagulopathy results from impaired hepatocellular function and not cholestasis or intestinal factors, exogenous vitamin K is unlikely to correct or improve prothrombin synthesis. The vitamin K–dependent clotting proteins have a substantially shorter serum half-life than albumin; therefore, hypoprothrombinemia usually precedes the development of hypoalbuminemia, especially in the patient with acute hepatocellular disease. In cirrhosis, coagulopathy may be further aggravated by the thrombocytopenia resulting from hypersplenism.

Since the liver is also the site of production of non-vitamin K–dependent clotting factors, severe liver disease injury may lead to decreased plasma concentrations of factor V in addition to factors II, VII, IX, and X. It is unusual for fibrinogen to be reduced significantly, unless there is an associated disseminated intravascular coagulation (DIC). For unclear reasons, the liver may actually produce increased amounts of fibrinogen as well as other proteins such as acute-phase reactants (C-reactive proteins, haptoglobin, ceruloplasmin, and transferrin). The latter are produced both in response to liver injury (e.g., severe chronic active hepatitis) and in association with systemic illnesses such as cancer, rheumatoid arthritis, bacterial infections, burns, and myocardial infarctions. However, while the diseased liver may produce normal or increased amounts of fibrinogen, the molecules themselves may be qualitatively abnormal (i.e., structurally and functionally), reflecting more subtle derangements in protein synthesis. These functionally abnormal fibrinogen molecules may contribute to the altered hemostasis frequently found in patients with chronic liver disease.

DETOXIFICATION MECHANISMS Water-soluble drugs and endogenous substances usually are excreted unchanged in the urine or bile. However, lipid-soluble compounds tend to accumulate in the body and affect cellular processes, unless they are converted to less active compounds or to more soluble metabolites which are more easily excreted. The liver has an important role in the metabolism of many exogenous drugs and endogenous hormones by virtue of several enzyme systems involved in biochemical transformation. There are two major types of reactions. The first, *phase I reactions,* result in chemical modification of reactive groups by oxidation, reduction, hydroxylation, sulfoxidation, deamination, dealkylation, or methylation. Such modifications usually involve one of several enzymatic systems, including the mixed function oxidases, cytochromes b_5 and P_{450} (microsomal), and the glutathione *S*-acyltransferases (cytoplasmic). These biochemical reactions usually lead to *inactivation* of drugs such as barbiturates and benzodiazepines. However, *activation* may also occur. For example, cortisone is activated to cortisol and prednisone to prednisolone (both products being more potent than the parent compounds); imipramine, a depressant, is converted to desmethylimipramine, an antidepressant. On the other hand, phase I reactions may convert a nontoxic compound to a toxic one as in the metabolism of isoniazid and acetaminophen. Similarly, some carcinogens may be activated by formation of highly reactive epoxide intermediates in the liver, while other carcinogens may be detoxified.

The enzymes responsible for phase I reactions, especially those involving the cytochrome P_{450} system, can be induced by drugs such as ethanol, barbiturates, haloperidol, and glutethimide. Conversely, hepatic microsomal enzymes may be inhibited by agents such as chloramphenicol, cimetidine, disulfiram, dextropropoxyphene, allopurinol, and, paradoxically, by ethanol. The concomitant administration of two drugs metabolized by the same microsomal enzyme may result in modification, potentiation, or diminution of the pharmacologic efficacy of either or both drugs.

Phase II reactions may follow phase I reactions or proceed independently; these involve the conversion of substances to their glucuronide, sulfate, acetyl, taurine, or glycine derivatives, thereby converting lipophilic substances to water-soluble derivatives and permitting their excretion in bile or urine. Conjugation catalyzed by microsomal UDPglucuronyltransferases to form glucuronide derivatives is one of the most common phase II reactions. In general, the conjugates are more soluble than the parent compound and are pharmacologically inactive.

Important in the clinical management of patients with chronic liver disease is an awareness that there may be varying degrees of impairment in the hepatic uptake, detoxification, and excretion of certain drugs. Portal-systemic shunting of blood may decrease the "first-pass effect" of drugs absorbed from the gut. In cirrhosis, altered intrahepatic hemodynamics due to a disordered liver architecture may also reduce the rates of hepatic drug clearance. Hypoalbuminemia will permit drugs, usually bound to albumin, to be present in increased concentrations of their unbound form in the circulation and extracellular spaces; this may result in an increased activity of such drugs. Most importantly, a decrease in the amount of function of microsomal enzymes responsible for phase I and phase II reactions will result in slower rates of drug inactivation and elimination. Drugs for which there may be a decreased clearance in patients with liver disease include anticonvulsants (e.g., phenytoin, phenobarbital), anti-inflammatory agents (e.g., acetaminophen, phenylbutazone, corticosteroids), minor tranquilizers, cardioactive drugs (e.g., lidocaine, quinidine, propranolol), and antibiotics (e.g., nafcillin, chloramphenicol, tetracyclines, clindamycin, trimethoprim, rifampin, pyrazinamide). This will lead to decreased dosage requirements and a narrowing of the range between therapeutic and toxic drug levels. In the future, the aminopyrine clearance test may permit an assessment of the degree of impairment of detoxification mechanisms in individual patients. In this test, orally administered [^{14}C]aminopyrine is absorbed from the gut and metabolized by the hepatic cytochrome P_{450} system releasing [^{14}C]O_2, which is excreted and easily measured in the breath. In hepatocellular disease, the rate of [^{14}C]O_2 production will be reduced. Finally, in addition to an alteration in drug metabolism, the patient with chronic liver disease may also possess an increased central nervous system sensitivity to opiates and other sedatives.

The difficulties in safely administering pharmacologic agents to patients with both acute and chronic liver disease are underscored by the frequency with which administration of benzodiazepines is cited as precipitating hepatic coma. It may be very difficult clinically to determine whether agitation, confusion, and irrational behavior are due to early hepatic encephalopathy or related to the concurrent use of benzodiazepines, opiates, barbiturates, and other depressants.

The mechanism by which some agents may exert a hepatotoxic effect can involve the same metabolic pathways responsible for normal drug detoxification. The mechanism of acetaminophen (Tylenol) toxicity is particularly illustrative. Acetaminophen is metabolized and detoxified by the hepatic mixed-function oxygenase system, but one of the intermediate products is a potent free radical (postulated metabolite *N*-acetylimidoquinone) which can inactivate many enzymes and proteins by binding irreversibly to their sulfhydryl groups. Normally this interaction can be prevented by reduced glutathione. In the presence of excessive amounts of the acetaminophen free radical (e.g., from overdosage or underlying liver disease), the glutathione levels of the hepatocytes are readily exhausted and the excess free radicals can lead to inactivation of cellular proteins and produce widespread hepatocellular necrosis. In the case of acetaminophen overdosage, the very early administration of sulfhydryl groups in the form of *N*-acetylcysteine can often prevent this drug-induced liver injury.

HORMONE METABOLISM In addition to its role in the metabolism of diverse pharmacologic agents, the liver is also responsible for inactivation or modification of several endogenous hormones; therefore, chronic liver disease may be accompanied by signs of apparent hormonal imbalance. Some hormones (e.g., insulin and glucagon) are inactivated in the liver by proteolysis or deamination. Thyroxine and triiodothyronine are metabolized in the liver by reactions involving deiodination. Steroid hormones, such as corticosteroids and aldosterone, are first inactivated to their tetrahydro derivative (by reduction of the Δ^4 double bond and the 3-keto group), followed by conjugation, mostly with glucuronic acid. Testosterone is metabolized to the isomeric 17-ketosteroids, androsterone and etiocholanolone, and excreted in the urine mostly as sulfate conjugates. Estrogens, such as estradiol, may be converted to estriol and estrone and then conjugated with glucuronic acid or sulfate. Abnormalities in estrogen (and testosterone) metabolism are believed to be involved in the development of spider angiomas, loss of axillary or pubic hair, and testicular atrophy frequently seen in patients with chronic liver disease. In addition, increased portal-systemic shunting of testosterone and androstenedione secondary to portal hypertension may lead to the development of gynecomastia in cirrhotic males due to increased peripheral conversion to estradiol and estrone. In patients with alcoholic liver disease, feminization may also be related to the direct toxic effects of alcohol on the gonadal-pituitary-hypothalamic axis. Similar effects are also seen in patients with hemochromatosis due to deposition of iron in these sites.

Estrogens also act directly on the liver to impair hepatic secretory activity. Estradiol and related estrogens, such as those present in contraceptive pills, interfere with sodium sulfobromophthalein (Bromsulphalein, BSP) and bile salt excretion and worsen the preexisting defect in secretion of conjugated bilirubin in patients with Dubin-Johnson syndrome; they may also elevate plasma alkaline phosphatase levels (see Chap. 316). Related steroids such as etiocholanolone and pregnanediol have been shown to stimulate δ-aminolevulinic acid (ALA) synthetase activity leading to increased porphobilinogen excretion. Since these steroids exert these effects only in their unconjugated form, the increased hepatic levels of δ-aminolevulinic acid synthetase in patients with alcoholic cirrhosis may be secondary to the action of gonadal steroids.

LIPID METABOLISM: FATTY ACIDS AND TRIGLYCERIDES Under normal conditions, most of the fatty acids taken up by the liver and esterified to triglyceride are derived from adipose tissue or the diet. Some fatty acids (especially saturated ones) are synthesized in the liver from acetate. The fatty acids may then be converted enzymatically to triglyceride, esterified with cholesterol, incorporated into phospholipids, or oxidized to CO_2 or ketone bodies. Most of the triglyceride is produced for export, but in order to be secreted it must be converted to lipoproteins by combining with relatively specific apoprotein moieties. This emphasizes the importance of protein synthesis for the release and secretion of triglyceride from the liver. With the exception of cholestatic disease (see below), clinically significant alterations in lipoprotein and cholesterol metabolism are usually not found in patients with chronic liver disease.

Studies on the production of fatty liver have shown that singly or in combination, one or more of the steps depicted in Fig. 315-4 may be involved. An increased influx of fatty acids mobilized from adipose tissue due to drugs (e.g., ethanol or corticosteroids) or secondary to diabetic ketosis may lead to a fatty liver. Similarly, increased levels of fatty acids in the liver, either from enhanced fatty acid synthesis or from decreased fatty acid oxidation may lead to increased triglyceride formation. In some instances (e.g., ethanol excess) there may also be increases in the carbohydrate backbone, α-glycerophosphate, involved in fatty acid esterification to triglyceride. Since release of triglyceride involves the formation of lipoproteins, lipid accumulation may occur because of decreased apoprotein synthesis. This appears to be the case in fatty livers seen in patients with protein-calorie malnutrition (kwashiorkor) and due to toxins such as carbon tetrachloride, phosphorus, or ethionine, as well as following excessive doses of antibiotics like tetracycline that can inhibit protein synthesis. Finally, there may be impaired lipoprotein secretion from the liver. Alcohol is perhaps the most common agent leading to a fatty liver, but the mechanism(s) whereby alcohol leads to increased liver triglyceride is not clear. Depending on factors such as dose or duration, alcohol ingestion may affect any of the seven steps shown in Fig. 315-4; however, the primary factor for the production of the alcohol-induced fatty liver remains to be determined. The alterations in the redox state due to excessive accumulation of NADH resulting from oxidation of alcohol may also contribute.

In addition to the changes leading to fatty liver, there are many metabolic alterations which may be found in the blood of patients following the ingestion of large amounts of alcohol. These include, among others, *increased* plasma levels of lactate, proline, urate, and triglycerides and *decreased* plasma levels of glucose, magnesium, phosphate, and triiodothyronine (T_3).

CHOLESTEROL Cholesterol and bile acid synthesis is carried out primarily by the liver. Cholesterol exists either free or com-

FIGURE 315-4

Factors in the uptake and esterification of fatty acids to triglyceride by the liver, including the formation and release of triglyceride as lipoprotein. The numbers refer to steps, which, if altered, may result in increased liver triglyceride (i.e., fatty liver).

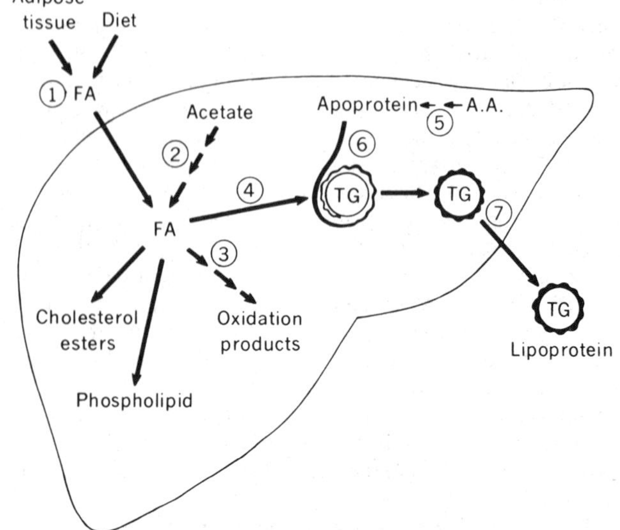

bined with fatty acids in the form of cholesterol esters; in the plasma both are found primarily in association with β-lipoproteins. The plasma and liver also contain lecithin–cholesterol acyltransferase (LCAT), an enzyme involved in the conversion of free cholesterol to its esterified form. Since there is exchange of free cholesterol between tissues, changes in plasma cholesterol levels reflect changes in total body cholesterol. However, decreases in plasma cholesterol esters may reflect hepatic damage and impaired hepatic cholesterol esterification.

Severe liver injury often leads to a decrease in *total* serum cholesterol levels, including both free and esterified fractions. This may be due to decreased synthesis of cholesterol and cholesterol esters, decreased apoprotein synthesis, or both. In cholestasis (either intra- or extrahepatic) total serum cholesterol often increases strikingly. Disorders of cholestasis are associated with marked abnormalities of lipoprotein metabolism. In primary biliary cirrhosis there are pronounced elevations in serum free cholesterol and low density lipoproteins (LDL); conversely, serum HDL is reduced and may disappear from the serum in patients with long-standing disease. Similar but less marked changes are seen in other cholestatic conditions.

The increase in serum free cholesterol (and phospholipid) and the concomitant decrease in esterified cholesterol in cholestasis may be related to a decrease in the hepatic production of LCAT. Reduced levels of LCAT are also correlated with the appearance of an abnormal LDL, referred to as lipoprotein X (LP-X). Although LP-X, which has a high content of free cholesterol and triglyceride, was originally thought to be a specific indicator of biliary tract obstruction, it is evident that it appears in any cholestatic condition. While the depressed hepatic production of LCAT may be responsible for altered lipid content and composition of lipoproteins, the factors leading to the overall increase in total serum cholesterol are not clear. In experimental animals, bile duct ligation results in a net increase in hepatic cholesterol synthesis, and in "regurgitation" of bile salts, cholesterol, and LP-X into venous radicals. However, it is difficult to translate these experimental findings to the patient with primary biliary cirrhosis unless any insult to cells lining the biliary canaliculi and ductules can impair the delicate balance of lipid synthesis and removal.

Most of the derangements of hepatic metabolism discussed above are evident only in patients with severe or long-standing liver disease. Indeed, in all but the most severe cases of acute viral hepatitis, hepatic metabolic functions are remarkably well preserved, and in most cases of mild to moderate acute viral hepatitis, it is uncommon to observe clinically important alterations in carbohydrate, protein, and lipid metabolism. However, in the patients with severe or fulminant hepatitis, whether from a viral or toxic agent, the metabolic derangements may be similar to those seen in more chronic disease. For example, in fulminant hepatitis there may be pronounced hypoprothrombinemia and impaired coagulation, hypoalbuminemia, and the relatively acute development of ascites, as well as hyperammonemia and encephalopathy. However, in contrast to patients with cirrhosis, abnormalities in carbohydrate metabolism are more likely to lead to profound hypoglycemia rather than to hyperglycemia. This hypoglycemia appears to reflect both a marked decrease in hepatic glycogen stores as well as diminished glucagon responsiveness. There may also be poor oral intake due to nausea and anorexia together with increased glucose utilization secondary to hyperinsulinemia (due to portal-systemic shunting and decreased insulin degradation).

REFERENCES

ALBERTI KGMM: Some metabolic aspects of liver disease, in *Topics in Gastroenterology,* SC Truelove, J Trowell (eds). London, Blackwell, 1975, vol 2, p 341

FLANNERY DB et al: Current status of hyperammonemic syndromes. Hepatology 2:495, 1982

HOYUMPA AM et al: Hepatic encephalopathy. Gastroenterology 77:803, 1979

ONSTAD GR, ZIEVE L: What determines blood ammonia? Gastroenterology 77:803, 1979

OWEN OE et al: Hepatic, gut and renal substrate flux rates in patients with hepatic cirrhosis. J Clin Invest 68:240, 1981

POPPER H, SCHAFFNER F: *Progress in Liver Diseases,* New York, Grune & Stratton, 1979, vol 6

SHAFRITZ DA, ISSELBACHER KJ: Current concepts of hepatic protein synthesis, in *The Liver and Its Diseases,* F Schaffner et al (eds). New York, Intercontinental Medical Book, 1974, pp 45–53

SHERLOCK S: *Diseases of the Liver and Biliary System,* 6th ed. London, Blackwell, 1981

SMITH AR et al: Alteration in plasma and CSF amino acids, amines and metabolites in hepatic coma. Ann Surg 187:343, 1978

TRIGER DR: Hyperglobulinemia in liver disease, in *Topics in Gastroenterology,* SC Truelove, J Trowell (eds). London, Blackwell, 1975, vol 2, p 320

WRIGHT R et al: *Liver and Biliary Disease.* Philadelphia, Saunders, 1979

316 DIAGNOSTIC PROCEDURES IN LIVER DISEASE

KURT J. ISSELBACHER
J. THOMAS LaMONT

Prompt recognition of liver disease and determination of its nature and extent require an understanding of the physiologic bases of a wide variety of techniques that assess liver function. Since no "battery" of tests is universally applicable, those most appropriate to a given clinical problem must be selected, their potential value and risk considered, and the results interpreted in relation to the clinical findings.

LIVER FUNCTION TESTS

Many liver function tests are based on a wide variety of biochemical reactions, such that the clinician can select combinations of tests that often measure different aspects of hepatic function. Many tests, however, are still empiric and semiquantitative, and no single test is universally helpful in diagnosis. Some methods are too sensitive and lack diagnostic specificity, others are affected by nonhepatic factors, and many simply do not measure any true physiologic function of the liver.

The physician concerned with clinical liver disease should be guided by several practical principles: (1) the tests selected should assess different parameters of liver function; (2) liver function tests should be used *serially* in order to evaluate the evolution or course of the disease; and (3) all such tests should be interpreted within the total clinical context with the recognition that any laboratory test may be fallible. The discussion that follows deals with representative and commonly used tests and should be read in conjunction with Chaps. 38 and 315.

SERUM BILIRUBIN (See also Chaps. 38 and 317) Spectrophotometric determinations of serum bilirubin in the clinical laboratory measure two pigment fractions: (1) the water-soluble conjugated fraction that gives a *direct reaction* with the diazo reagent and consists largely of conjugated bilirubin (as the mono- and diglucuronide), and (2) the lipid-soluble *indirect-reaction* fraction (total minus direct) that represents primarily unconjugated bilirubin. The serum of normal adults (when measured by the van den Bergh reaction) contains less than 0.25 mg direct-reacting bilirubin per deciliter and 1 mg or less of total bilirubin per deciliter. As noted in Chap. 38, in classifying the type of jaundice it is initially helpful to measure both the direct and total serum bilirubin in order to determine whether the patient has predominantly unconjugated or conjugated hyperbilirubinemia.

URINE BILIRUBIN Bilirubinuria causes the urine to become smoky or tea-colored; this appearance is also caused by hemoglobin or myoglobin in the urine, which can be differentiated by appropriate tests. Clinically significant concentrations of urine bilirubin are measured by the foam test, Harrison spot test, or the Ictotest tablet method. One can also use a dye-impregnated strip which changes color when dipped into a bilirubin-containing urine. Bilirubinuria occurs only when there is an increase in the serum direct or conjugated bilirubin. This is an important point in the diagnosis of conditions characterized by unconjugated hyperbilirubinemia in which bilirubinuria is not noted. Bilirubinuria occurs with even minimal degrees of jaundice, and in fact may be detected before the patient becomes jaundiced.

URINE UROBILINOGEN Although of limited usefulness as a test of liver function and now rarely performed, semiquantitative measurements of urobilinogen can be made on a freshly collected 2-h urine specimen by the Watson method (normal values 0.2 to 1.2 units). In complete bile duct obstruction there is no excretion of bilirubin into the gut; hence, there is no conversion of bilirubin to urobilinogen by intestinal bacteria. This results in disappearance of urobilinogen from the urine.

BROMSULPHALEIN (BSP) EXCRETION BSP is a dye which is taken up by the hepatocytes and secreted into the bile. The BSP test is now rarely utilized because enzymes such as the aminotransferases are easier to perform and better indicators of hepatocellular dysfunction. Furthermore, the agent has not been available in the United States in recent years. Perhaps its only value would be in the diagnosis of the Dubin-Johnson syndrome (see Chap. 317). The test is performed by injecting intravenously 5 mg BSP per kilogram of body weight and obtaining a sample of venous blood from another venous site after 45 min. The result is expressed as the percentage of injected dye remaining, which in normal persons is less than 5 percent.

SERUM ENZYME ASSAYS Measurements of many serum enzymes have been used to quantify liver damage or to distinguish between hepatocellular (i.e., functional) and mechanical cholestasis. No specific or truly diagnostic test has been devised to solve either problem, but the enzymatic liver function tests described below have proved helpful in the clinical study of many hepatobiliary diseases.

Alkaline phosphatase Serum contains alkaline phosphatase, an enzyme which hydrolyzes synthetic phosphate esters at pH 9. As indicated in Chap. 315, this enzyme is produced by many tissues, especially bone, intestine, liver, and placenta, and is excreted in bile. Most of the enzyme present in normal serum is derived from bone. In hepatobiliary disease, there is an increased release of the hepatic enzyme into the bloodstream, apparently owing to increased enzyme synthesis. In the absence of bone disease and pregnancy, an elevated serum alkaline phosphatase level generally reflects impaired hepatic excretory function.

Several methods of comparable accuracy and sensitivity are available to measure alkaline phosphatase activity. The most widely used are international units (normal: 25 to 85 units), Bodansky units (normal: 1.5 to 4.5 units), and the King-Armstrong method (normal: 4 to 13 units). Growing children and women in late pregnancy have serum levels that may be twice normal.

Slight to moderate increases in alkaline phosphatase (1 to 2 times normal) occur in many patients with parenchymal liver disorders such as hepatitis and cirrhosis, and transient increases may occur in all types of liver disease. The most striking increases (3 to 10 times normal) occur with extrahepatic biliary obstruction or in intrahepatic cholestasis, such as drug cholestasis or primary biliary cirrhosis. The alkaline phosphatase is almost always mildly elevated in metastatic liver disease, and in many cases is the only abnormality on routine liver function tests. As already noted, the enzyme may be elevated in incomplete biliary obstruction or obstruction of one hepatic duct, namely, under conditions when the serum bilirubin is normal or only slightly elevated. Since bone is a source of the enzyme, extensive Paget's disease, bony metastases, and other diseases associated with increased osteoblastic activity may produce high levels of alkaline phosphatase in the absence of liver disease. However, one can distinguish the two enzymes by their heat stability; liver alkaline phosphatase is heat-stable, while the bone enzyme is heat-labile.

5′-Nucleotidase This enzyme is another phosphatase which originates largely in the liver and is used clinically to determine whether an elevation of the alkaline phosphatase is caused by liver or bone disease. In hepatic disease both 5′-nucleotidase and alkaline phosphatase are elevated, while in primary bone disease the alkaline phosphatase is elevated but the 5′-nucleotidase is usually normal. However, there are exceptions to this observation, and other liver function tests are usually required to establish the presence or absence of liver disease.

Transaminases (aminotransferases) Assays of many serum enzymes have been proposed as measures of hepatocellular damage. Of these, the serum aspartate aminotransferase (AST, SGOT) and alanine aminotransferase (ALT, SGPT) have proved to be the most practical. GOT is found in all body tissues, especially in heart, liver, and skeletal muscle. GPT is present primarily in the liver and to a lesser extent in kidney and skeletal muscle. Although many studies have shown that the height and duration of serum enzyme elevations parallel the extent of liver cell damage (i.e., necrosis or altered cell permeability), precise quantitative correlations cannot be made in most clinical conditions (Chap. 315). Normal serum contains less than 40 Karmen units of AST and less than 40 Karmen units of ALT.

In the absence of acute necrosis or ischemia of other organs such as the myocardium, high AST and ALT levels suggest liver cell damage. With extensive acute hepatic necrosis, as in severe viral hepatitis, serum enzyme levels of 1000 to 3000 units may be found. Less severe necrosis produces transient levels of 500 to 1000 units. Mild chronic or focal liver diseases (e.g., subclinical or anicteric viral hepatitis, Laennec's cirrhosis, granulomatous infiltrations, and tumor invasion) may be associated with transaminase levels of 50 to 200 units. With intrahepatic or extrahepatic cholestasis (in the absence of hepatic cell necrosis) AST and ALT levels usually are not significantly elevated and rarely exceed 300 units. In acute viral hepatitis the ALT level is generally higher than AST, while in alcoholic hepatitis AST tends to be higher than ALT.

Serial determinations of SGOT and SGPT are helpful in following the course of a patient with liver disease, especially with acute or chronic hepatitis. Caution is needed in the interpretation of abnormal levels. Serum transaminases may actually *decrease* in some patients with fulminant hepatitis, because of the previous excessive release of enzymes from the liver. Laennec's cirrhosis and postnecrotic cirrhosis may be associated with only slightly elevated or even normal transaminase levels.

Lactic dehydrogenase (LDH) Measurement of total serum LDH is usually not helpful in diagnosing liver disease because it is present in all organs and released into the serum from a variety of tissue injuries. Fractionation of LDH into its five tissue-specific isoenzymes may give useful information about the site of origin of the LDH elevation. Moderate elevations of LDH levels are common in acute viral hepatitis and in cirrhosis; biliary tract disease may produce slight elevations. High serum levels may be found in metastatic carcinoma of the liver.

Other enzymes A very sensitive enzyme for the detection of minimal hepatocellular damage is γ-glutamyl transpeptidase (GGT). This enzyme is found in high concentration in kidney and liver, and is elevated in the serum of almost all patients with hepatobiliary disorders. An elevated level is often observed in the serum of heavy drinkers before other liver function tests are abnormal. Ornithine carbamyl transferase (OCT) is a urea cycle enzyme present only in liver and intestinal tissue. Elevation of this enzyme occurs primarily in liver disease; however, it is not specific for any particular type of liver disease, and its diagnostic usefulness is therefore limited.

SERUM PROTEINS Albumin, prothrombin, fibrinogen, and several other serum proteins are synthesized exclusively by liver cells, and extensive liver damage may lead to decreased blood levels of these proteins. The level of serum immunoglobulins, produced by lymphocytes and plasma cells, varies widely in hepatobiliary disease and reflects inflammatory or immune responses rather than liver cell dysfunction. Thus, analyses of the various serum proteins may provide helpful insights into the nature and extent of liver disease. However, as noted in Chap. 315, many nonhepatic factors also affect the metabolism of these proteins.

Albumin and globulins Total concentrations of serum albumin (normally 3.5 to 5 g/dl) and globulin (normally 2 to 3.5 g/dl) may be determined chemically. The level of each should be evaluated separately, because the *albumin/globulin (A/G) ratio* has no physiologic significance. Concentrations of $alpha_1$, $alpha_2$, beta, and gamma globulins are usually measured by electrophoretic methods.

Hypoalbuminemia may occur in subacute and massive hepatic necrosis, chronic active hepatitis, cirrhosis, and other disorders with significant destruction or replacement of liver cells. The serum albumin level also serves as a useful guide to prognosis and therapy in these diseases. *Hyperglobulinemia* suggests the presence of chronic inflammatory disorders such as cirrhosis and chronic active hepatitis. Neoplastic and inflammatory diseases of the liver may produce increased levels of $alpha_2$ globulins, and some patients with bile duct obstruction have high beta globulin levels.

Immunoglobulins Nonspecific immunoglobulin abnormalities occur in a variety of acute and chronic liver diseases. The major immunoglobulin fractions may be increased slightly in the course of acute viral hepatitis. Increased concentrations of IgA and IgG are common in Laennec's cirrhosis, striking elevations of IgG levels are characteristic of chronic active hepatitis, and high levels of IgM may be seen in primary biliary cirrhosis. None of these changes, however, is specific or diagnostic.

Clotting factors The serum activities of several clotting factors are useful indicators of hepatic synthetic function and are important in patients with liver disease who are bleeding or about to undergo surgery. The *one-stage prothrombin time,* which reflects the activities of prothrombin, fibrinogen, and factors V, VII, and X, is dependent upon both hepatic synthesis of these factors and intestinal uptake of vitamin K. Prolongation of the prothrombin time may occur in severe hepatocellular necrosis as in hepatitis or cirrhosis and usually reflects a decrease in factor VII, the rate-limiting step in the prothrombin time. Obstruction of the bile duct or prolonged intrahepatic cholestasis may cause vitamin K deficiency because of impaired lipid absorption. Parenteral injection of vitamin K (10 mg per day) will cause normalization of the prothrombin time in 48 h if the liver's synthetic function is normal. Thus, vitamin K will not improve the prothrombin time if there is extensive hepatocellular disease or dysfunction. The *partial thromboplastin time,* which reflects the activities of fibrinogen, prothrombin, and factors V, X, VIII, IX, XI, and XII, may also be prolonged in patients with liver disease. It is necessary to assess the clotting mechanism in all patients with liver disease before any surgical procedure including liver biopsy. This can be accomplished by measuring the prothrombin time, partial thromboplastin time, platelet count, and bleeding time (see Chaps. 55 and 334).

SERUM AMMONIA Ammonia is elevated in the blood of some patients with liver disease, either acute or chronic. In acute fulminant hepatitis a markedly elevated serum ammonia reflects severe hepatocellular necrosis and the consequent inability of the liver to convert ammonia to urea. Cirrhotic patients, in particular those who have undergone a portacaval shunt, may also have varying degrees of hyperammonemia and hepatic encephalopathy. In these patients the ammonia produced by colonic bacteria and carried in portal venous blood is shunted around the liver and enters the systemic circulation. There is only a rough correlation between the serum ammonia levels and the degree of hepatic encephalopathy. Some patients will function normally with a twofold elevation, while others will be stuporous at the same level. Serum ammonia levels may also increase before the onset of coma and return to normal some 48 to 72 h before improvement of the neurologic status. This lag between the elevation of ammonia levels and onset of encephalopathy may indicate the relatively slow transport of ammonia into the central nervous system. However, metabolites other than ammonia also appear to be important in the pathogenesis of hepatic encephalopathy, and this may help to explain the observed lack of correlation between ammonia levels and hepatic coma.

BLOOD LIPIDS Measurements of serum total cholesterol (normal: 130 to 230 mg/dl) and cholesterol esters (normal: 50 to 70 percent of total cholesterol) are frequently made in patients with liver disease. Acute or chronic diffuse liver disease often results in decreased total values and a decrease in the ester fraction; cholestasis, whether functional or mechanical, characteristically produces moderate to extreme elevations of the total cholesterol level but with a decrease in the percent esterified. In cholestasis one also finds variable elevations of serum triglycerides and of an abnormal lipoprotein (lipoprotein X).

IMMUNOLOGIC TESTS Immunologic derangements occur in a variety of liver diseases. Antimitochondrial antibodies are frequently found in primary biliary cirrhosis (85 percent of cases), although they may also be positive in some patients with chronic active hepatitis and drug hepatitis. In chronic active hepatitis the LE cell test may be positive, and antinuclear as well as anti-smooth-muscle antibodies may be present in the blood. Immunologic methods are the key to the detection of the hepatitis B surface antigen (HBsAg) in long-incubation or serum hepatitis and are discussed in detail in Chap. 318. Alpha fetoprotein is of value in the diagnosis of hepatoma. Measurements of alpha$_1$ antitrypsin should be performed in infants with cirrhosis or hepatitis since they may have a hereditary deficiency of this enzyme.

RADIOLOGIC PROCEDURES

ABDOMINAL ROENTGENOGRAM Films of the upper abdomen and lower thorax rarely provide accurate estimates of liver size and shape, but gross hepatomegaly and hepatic masses that elevate or distort the diaphragm may be detected. However, the abdominal film is more accurate in determining the presence of splenomegaly and is often helpful in detecting minimal degrees of splenic enlargement. Plain films of the abdomen may reveal calcific densities in the gallbladder, biliary tree, pancreas, or liver (as echinococcal cysts, hemangioma, or, rarely, a metastatic tumor mass).

BARIUM STUDIES OF THE GASTROINTESTINAL TRACT An upper gastrointestinal series should be performed in suspected cases of portal hypertension, because esophagogastric varices can be demonstrated with about 70 to 90 percent accuracy when they are present. Enlargement of the left lobe of the liver (as with tumor, abscess, or cirrhosis) may displace the barium-filled stomach laterally and anteriorly. Tumors of the head of the pancreas often produce displacement or irregularity of the second portion of the duodenum. The radiologist can increase the diagnostic accuracy of a search for lesions involving the head of the pancreas or papilla of Vater by performing a hypotonic duodenogram. This involves injection of an anticholinergic drug or glucagon to inhibit motility; it often permits a better view of the mucosa and provides data concerning the distensibility of the duodenum.

CHOLECYSTOGRAPHY AND CHOLANGIOGRAPHY *Oral cholecystography* is useful primarily in the diagnosis of diseases of the gallbladder, especially gallstones. The dye tablets [iopanoic acid (Telepaque)] are given the night before the study, absorbed from the intestine, and excreted by hepatocytes into the bile. Thus the test cannot be performed in the presence of hepatic excretory dysfunction or diarrhea (with decreased absorption of the dye). Nonvisualization of the gallbladder after a single dose of dye usually indicates gallbladder disease, but in some patients a second dose of the dye will show normal gallbladder opacification. A second dose study is required in at least 10 or 15 percent of patients who initially have inadequate visualization. This requirement limits the usefulness of oral cholecystography, especially in comparison to ultrasound which does not depend upon hepatic excretory function.

Intravenous cholangiography requires the administration of dye as an intravenous bolus and, like oral cholecystography, requires hepatic excretion to visualize the bile ducts and gallbladder. Unfortunately even mild impairment of liver function may prevent adequate visualization of this technique, thus limiting its application in the evaluation of patients with serum bilirubin levels greater than 2.5 to 3 mg/dl.

Percutaneous transhepatic cholangiography with a very thin needle is sometimes used to distinguish between mechanical biliary obstruction and intrahepatic cholestasis. This approach is used when decreased liver function precludes the use of intravenous cholangiography. With experience and proper precautions, dilated major ducts proximal to an obstructing lesion can be cannulated and visualized in up to 90 percent of cases; the normal or small ducts associated with intrahepatic cholestasis are more difficult to demonstrate, but with modern techniques, they can be demonstrated in up to 75 percent of cases.

Endoscopic retrograde cholangiopancreatography (ERCP) with the fiberoptic duodenoscope is another method of demonstrating the bile ducts radiographically in jaundiced patients. The papilla of Vater is cannulated under direct vision, and contrast material is injected into the biliary and pancreatic ducts. ERCP is particularly useful in jaundiced patients with suspected lesions of the head of the pancreas or ampulla of Vater, since in addition to contrast studies one may also obtain washings or brushings for cytology, or biopsies of intraduodenal mass lesions. ERCP does not rely upon dilatation of the bile ducts for success, and since the liver itself is not punctured, there is no risk of bile peritonitis in patients with high-grade biliary obstruction. However, acute pancreatitis may result from injection of contrast material into the pancreatic duct.

ANGIOGRAPHY An increasingly useful and effective approach for visualizing the hepatic and portal circulation involves *selective angiography* of the celiac, superior mesenteric, and hepatic arteries. In most centers it has replaced splenoportography since by injection of these arteries one can visualize both the arterial (hepatic) and venous (hepatic and portal) systems. Selective arteriography is quite safe. It is useful (1) in demonstrating the hepatic arterial circulation which will be deranged in cirrhosis and in the diagnosis of primary and secondary liver tumor masses, and (2) in visualizing the portal circulation for evidence of a collateral circulation, venous obstruction, anomalous vessels, etc. In major medical centers, this angiographic method is increasingly used as a diagnostic tool for the study of chronic liver disease and portal hypertension.

RADIOISOTOPE LIVER SCANS (SCINTISCANS) Hepatic scintiscans are performed with gamma-emitting isotopes that are extracted selectively by the liver, followed by external radiation scanning of the upper abdomen. There are basically three types of liver scans: the colloidal scan which depends on uptake of labeled colloid by Kupffer cells, the HIDA or PIPIDA scans in which the dye is taken up and excreted by hepatocytes, and the gallium scan in which the radionuclide ^{67}Ga is concentrated in neoplastic and inflammatory cells to a greater degree than in hepatocytes. Hence, a hepatoma or liver abscess will produce an area of reduced uptake or "hole" using a colloid or HIDA or PIPIDA scans, but there will be an area of increased uptake or "hot spot" with a gallium scan. The colloidal scan with ^{198}Au colloidal gold or ^{99m}Tc sulfur colloid is most commonly used. This technique can demonstrate filling defects greater than 2 to 3 cm in diameter; hence, in metastatic liver disease with smaller diffuse deposits, the scan will be falsely negative. False-positive scans are frequently observed in cirrhosis, because the distorted lobular architecture will result in irregular uptake and sometimes produce filling defects. The gallium scan may be helpful in diagnosing neoplastic infiltration in the patient with cirrhosis since the tumor will show increased uptake, while fibrous bands will show decreased uptake. The HIDA or PIPIDA scans (^{99m}Tc-labeled-*N*-substituted iminoacetic acids) have been used as a method of differentiating intrahepatic cholestasis from extrahepatic obstruction. With complete biliary obstruction there is failure of the isotope to enter the duodenum, while in intrahepatic cholestasis some isotope will be seen in the lumen of the small bowel. However, a clear-cut distinction of these entities with the HIDA or PIPIDA scans is unusual, and in this situation they have limited clinical usefulness in differentiating intra- from extrahepatic cholestasis. The major application of HIDA or PIPIDA liver scans is in the diagnosis of acute cholecystitis, where failure of the nuclide to enter the gallbladder is considered evidence of cystic duct or common bile duct obstruction.

ULTRASONOGRAPHY (See also Chaps. 323 to 325) Modern diagnostic ultrasound of the gallbladder is probably more accurate than oral cholecystography in detecting gallstones and has the added advantage of being independent of liver function. It can therefore be used to detect gallstones in the gallbladder or biliary tree in patients with jaundice. Ultrasound is also very useful in detecting mass lesions such as tumors, cysts, or liver abscess. Lesions as small as 1 to 2 cm can be visualized with this technique. Ultrasound of the upper abdomen is also quite useful in evaluating the possible causes of extrahepatic biliary obstruction. Abdominal computerized tomography (CT) scanning and ultrasound are approximately equal in their diagnostic sensitivity in evaluating patients with suspected mass lesions, gallstones, or obstructive jaundice. In general, ultrasound is the procedure of choice since it is less expensive than CT scanning and does not expose the patient to radiation.

COMPUTERIZED TOMOGRAPHY (CT SCAN) The CT scan of the abdomen provides a visual image of the abdominal viscera without injection of contrast material. This technique is particularly useful in the diagnosis of mass lesions in the liver or pancreas, where it has an accuracy and sensitivity comparable to that obtained with ultrasound. The test is particularly useful in differentiating intrahepatic fluid collections such as cysts, abscesses, and hematomas, since the density of the fluid can be determined with relative accuracy. Dilatation of the gallbladder, extrahepatic bile ducts or portal vein can be diagnosed on the CT scan. The major advantage of CT scanning is the ability to obtain an excellent image of solid intraäbdominal organs such as pancreas, liver, and spleen with modest doses of radiation, thus avoiding more invasive techniques such as angiography, cholangiography, or ERCP.

OTHER DIAGNOSTIC PROCEDURES

PORTAL AND HEPATIC VEIN MANOMETRY Estimation of the wedged hepatic venous pressure (WHVP, an approximation of the postsinusoidal intrahepatic venous pressure) by *hepatic vein catheterization* is useful in the study of patients with known or presumed portal hypertension. While determination of the WHVP is not a routine procedure, the demonstration of a normal or slightly elevated WHVP in a patient with clinical evidence of portal hypertension serves to localize the obstruction to the extrahepatic portion of the portal vein, the portal inflow system (as in schistosomiasis), or the presinusoidal vessels (as in some cases of fatty liver or portal fibrosis) rather than to the sinusoids or hepatic veins. Measurement of the splenic pulp pressure (a reliable reflection of the actual portal venous pressure) by *percutaneous portal manometry* is rarely performed. A WHVP greater than 10 mmHg above inferior vena cava pressure is indicative of portal hypertension.

PERCUTANEOUS NEEDLE BIOPSY OF THE LIVER Percutaneous needle biopsy is a safe, simple, and valuable method of diagnosing liver disease. Although the needle biopsy sample is small, *diffuse parenchymal disorders* such as cirrhosis, hepatitis, and drug reactions may be diagnosed with remarkable accuracy. In *disseminated focal diseases* (such as granulomas or tumor infiltrates) serial sections may demonstrate the lesion.

The biopsy is performed under local anesthesia, usually with the Menghini (aspiration), Klatskin, or Vim-Silverman (cutting) needle, by means of either the transpleural or subcos-

tal approach. If the operator is skillful and the patient is carefully selected, morbidity should be low and limited to occasional postbiopsy pain or vasovagal reactions. The mortality of liver biopsy as reported in several large series is approximately 1 death in 5000 biopsies when the Menghini technique is used.

Some of the major indications for needle biopsy are (1) unexplained hepatomegaly or hepatosplenomegaly, (2) cholestasis of uncertain cause, (3) persistently abnormal liver function tests, (4) suspected systemic or infiltrative diseases such as sarcoidosis, miliary tuberculosis, or fever of unknown origin, and (5) suspected primary or metastatic liver tumor.

Needle biopsy should not be performed if (1) the patient is not able to cooperate; (2) clinical or laboratory evidence indicates impaired hemostasis (for example, the one-stage prothrombin time is prolonged by 3 s or more over control), thrombocytopenia (less than 80,000 to 100,000 platelets per cubic millimeter) or purpura is present, or the partial thromboplastin time or bleeding time is prolonged; (3) there is infection of the right pleural space or septic cholangitis; (4) profound anemia or tense ascites is present; or (5) compatible blood is not available for transfusion in case of hemorrhage. Amyloidosis and carcinoma of the liver may increase the hazard of postbiopsy hemorrhage. Although biopsy in mechanical biliary obstruction may lead occasionally to the escape of bile and localized bile peritonitis, this complication is uncommon. With the increasing use of CT and ultrasonography, it is possible to perform aspiration biopsies with very thin needles which can be "directed" to the site of the lesion with the aid of one of these imaging procedures. The aspirated material can then be used for cytology (tumors) and culture (abscesses).

PERITONEOSCOPY (LAPAROSCOPY) With this technique the serosal lining, liver, gallbladder, spleen, and other abdominal organs can be visualized with minimum discomfort and hazard. Diagnosis may be made by inspection or directed needle biopsy. Peritoneoscopy is useful in the study of patients with suspected intraabdominal malignancy since it may obviate the need for exploratory laparotomy to establish a diagnosis.

LAPAROTOMY When the most thorough clinical, laboratory, and biopsy studies fail to define the precise nature of hepatobiliary disease, exploratory laparotomy may be necessary. However, it must be reemphasized that when there is evidence of significant hepatocellular necrosis (e.g., markedly elevated SGOT levels), laparotomy will often be accompanied by an increased morbidity and mortality owing to postoperative liver decompensation. When laparotomy is performed, the medicosurgical team should be prepared to obtain full benefit from this direct approach, using biopsy, culture, cholangiography, and angiography as required.

REFERENCES

BRENSILVER HL, KAPLAN MM: Significance of elevated liver alkaline phosphatase in serum. Gastroenterology 68:1556, 1975

LOMAS F et al: Increased specificity of liver scanning with the use of ^{67}gallium citrate. N Engl J Med 286:1323, 1972

MAURO MA et al: Hepatobiliary scanning with ^{99m}Tc-PIPIDA in acute cholecystitis. Radiology 142:193, 1982

OKUDA K: Advances in hepatobiliary ultrasonography. Hepatology 1:662, 1981

PEREIRAS R et al: Percutaneous transhepatic cholangiography with the "skinny" needle. Ann Intern Med 86:562, 1977

Rosali SB: Enzyme tests in diseases of the liver and hepatobiliary tract, in *The Principles and Practice of Diagnostic Enzymology*, JH Wilkinson (ed). Chicago, Year Book, 1976, pp 303–360

Sabesin SM: Cholestatic lipoproteins—Their pathogenesis and significance. Gastroenterology 83:704, 1982

Wittenberg J, Ferrucci J: Computed body tomography. Gastroenterology 74:287, 1978

317
DISTURBANCES OF BILIRUBIN METABOLISM

KURT J. ISSELBACHER

The normal metabolism of bilirubin and the approach to the patient with jaundice have been presented in Chap. 38. With a consideration of these pathways, the disorders of bilirubin metabolism can be divided into four major categories, namely, those due to (1) increased pigment production, (2) reduced hepatic uptake of bilirubin, (3) impaired hepatic conjugation, and (4) decreased excretion of the conjugated pigment from the liver into bile. The first three of these disorders are associated with predominantly unconjugated hyperbilirubinemia (i.e., more than 80 percent of serum bilirubin is unconjugated, or indirect-reacting). The fourth group, defective excretion, is associated with predominantly conjugated hyperbilirubinemia (i.e., more than 50 percent of serum bilirubin is conjugated, or direct-reacting) and with bilirubinuria.

DISORDERS CAUSING PREDOMINANTLY UNCONJUGATED HYPERBILIRUBINEMIA

The plasma concentration of unconjugated bilirubin is determined by (1) the rate at which newly synthesized bilirubin enters the plasma (bilirubin turnover) and (2) the rate of irreversible removal of bilirubin by the liver (hepatic bilirubin clearance). The latter can result from derangements of hepatic bilirubin uptake, conjugation, or both. Measurements of these variables, although not routinely available, permit a classification of patients into those with *increased bilirubin turnover* (e.g., hemolysis), those with *decreased bilirubin clearance* (e.g., Gilbert's syndrome), and those in whom both mechanisms operate.

OVERPRODUCTION OF BILIRUBIN (INCREASED TURNOVER)

Increased destruction of circulating erythrocytes (intravascular and extravascular hemolysis) In disorders associated with hemolysis, most commonly the hemolytic anemias, the rate of bilirubin production is increased and may even exceed the amount that can be removed by a normal liver. The resulting jaundice is primarily an unconjugated hyperbilirubinemia. There is often also a small but definite increase in the serum conjugated bilirubin, when the amount of bilirubin glucuronide formed exceeds the amount that the liver can excrete (see Chap. 38). If there is significant anemia or if other adverse factors are present (e.g., fever, sepsis, hypoxemia, or vascular collapse), the ability of the liver to handle the pigment load will be compromised, and the degree of jaundice will be greater.

The clinical and diagnostic features of the various hemolytic anemias are described in Chap. 329. The presence of reticulocytosis, shortened red blood cell survival, and increased fecal urobilinogen, in the absence of clinical and laboratory evidence of liver disease, strongly suggest hemolysis and overproduction of bilirubin as the cause of the jaundice. It is obvious, however, that in some cases (e.g., cirrhosis, tumors, and sepsis), hemolysis *plus* deranged liver function may be present. In most cases of uncomplicated hemolytic states, the mean serum bilirubin level will be in the range of 3 to 5 mg/dl; rarely, levels up to 10 mg/dl may be seen.

Jaundice due to increased pigment production may also be seen as a consequence of *tissue infarction* (e.g., pulmonary infarcts) and large *collections of blood in tissues* (e.g., leakage from blood vessels after catheterization studies, rupture of an aortic aneurysm). If hypotension and hypoxemia also supervene, jaundice is usually more pronounced, and the resulting impairment of liver function may also lead to a significant increase in the serum conjugated bilirubin level (see "Postoperative Jaundice" below).

Except in early infancy, elevations of serum unconjugated bilirubin levels are not generally harmful per se, and the prognosis is that of the hemolytic process itself. However, in the neonatal state and infancy, unconjugated bilirubin levels above 20 mg/dl may lead to *kernicterus* due to bilirubin deposition in the lipid-rich basal ganglia (see Chap. 362). Chronic overproduction of bilirubin may result in the formation of gallstones composed predominantly of bilirubin ("pigment stones"). In this situation, all the potential complications of calculus disease of the biliary tract (Chap. 323) may be superimposed on the chronic hemolytic state which produced it.

Increased production of bilirubin from sources other than circulating erythrocytes As indicated in Chap. 38, about 15 to 20 percent of the circulating bilirubin is normally derived from sources other than the destruction of circulating red blood cells. This represents the so-called early-labeled fraction; it includes the synthesis of bilirubin from nonhemoglobin heme in the liver and from hemoglobin heme in the marrow.

In some conditions, jaundice results from an increased destruction of red blood cells or their precursors in the marrow—a process referred to as *ineffective erythropoiesis* (see Chaps. 38 and 54). In patients with thalassemia, pernicious anemia, and congenital erythropoietic porphyria, such an increased rate of formation of the early-labeled bilirubin fraction has been demonstrated. It is possible that some cases of unexplained unconjugated hyperbilirubinemia may be caused by an increased hepatic production of bilirubin from nonhemoglobin heme, but this phenomenon has not yet been demonstrated clinically.

IMPAIRED HEPATIC UPTAKE OF BILIRUBIN Drugs While numerous drugs may theoretically interfere with uptake of bilirubin by the liver, only a few agents have been definitely shown to influence this process. Flavaspidic acid, used in the treatment of tapeworm infestation, may cause unconjugated hyperbilirubinemia, as well as impairment of sodium sulfobromophthalein (Bromsulphalein, BSP) clearance, during its administration. The jaundice readily subsides following treatment. Flavaspidic acid competes with bilirubin for intrahepatic binding proteins (ligandins), leading thereby to unconjugated hyperbilirubinemia. The jaundice which may occur with novobiocin and some cholecystographic dyes is also apparently due to an interference in bilirubin uptake.

Gilbert's syndrome Some cases of this syndrome of chronic unconjugated hyperbilirubinemia may be due to a defect in hepatic uptake (as reflected by alteration in BSP kinetics). In most cases, however, a deficiency of bilirubin glucuronyl transferase can be demonstrated. Hence this syndrome is best considered as a defect in bilirubin conjugation. (For discussion, see below.)

IMPAIRED BILIRUBIN CONJUGATION (DECREASED ACTIVITY OF BILIRUBIN GLUCURONYL TRANSFERASE) Neonatal jaundice (physiological jaundice of the newborn) Almost every infant exhibits some transient unconjugated hyperbilirubinemia between the second and fifth days of life. While during gestation the placenta serves to clear bilirubin from the fetus, after birth infants must detoxify the pigments themselves. However, at this stage the hepatic enzyme system is still "immature" and inadequate for the task. As a result, unconjugated bilirubinemia develops, usually not exceeding 5 mg per deciliter of serum. The activity of glucuronyl transferase increases within several days to 2 weeks after birth, and concomitantly the serum bilirubin returns to normal. In the premature infant the glucuronyl transferase activity is less, and the neonatal jaundice may be more pronounced. The "maturation" of the fetal and neonatal liver may be enhanced by treatment of the pregnant mother or the newborn infant with phenobarbital or related drugs. This results in a clear-cut reduction of the degree and duration of unconjugated hyperbilirubinemia in the newborn. In infants with a superimposed hemolytic process (e.g., erythroblastosis), the excessive pigment load leads to more pronounced jaundice, and bilirubin levels may exceed 20 mg per deciliter of serum. It should be emphasized that neonatal jaundice is not present at the time of delivery; if jaundice is present at birth, other causes must be considered.

Two soluble, low-molecular-weight cytoplasmic liver cell proteins (ligandins Y and Z) have been described. These appear to be involved in the normal binding of bilirubin and drugs by the liver (Chap. 38). In experimental animals the Y protein which appears to bind bilirubin is low in the neonatal state and increases with age. It has been proposed that deficiency of this protein may contribute to neonatal jaundice.

An additional facet of the "immature" liver is a concomitant defect in the excretion of *conjugated* bilirubin. Rarely this defect persists beyond the time needed for the development of adequate glucuronide conjugation and may explain the occasional presence of conjugated hyperbilirubinemia in infants with erythroblastosis (*inspissated-bile syndrome*).

When in the neonatal state unconjugated bilirubin levels approach 20 mg/dl, the infants may develop and die of *kernicterus.* This condition results from unconjugated bilirubin deposition in the lipid-rich basal ganglia. In the past treatment consisted of exchange transfusions, and albumin infusions were used to increase binding of bilirubin in the circulation and diminish its entry into the brain. The current approach is *phototherapy;* intense illumination of these patients with strong white or blue light leads to the photoisomerization of bilirubin to water-soluble isomers that are rapidly excreted in the bile without the prior need of conjugation.

TABLE 317-1
Hereditary unconjugated hyperbilirubinemias with deficiency of glucuronyl transferase

Features	*Mild (Gilbert's syndrome)*	*Moderate (Crigler-Najjar syndrome type II)*	*Severe (Crigler-Najjar syndrome type I)*
Inheritance	Unclear*	Dominant†	Recessive
Serum bilirubin, mg/dl	1–6	6–20	20–45
Kernicterus	No	Rare	Yes
Conjugated bilirubin in bile	Yes (↑ monoconjugates)	Yes (↑↑ monoconjugates)	No
Response to phenobarbital	Yes	Yes	No
Bilirubin conjugation	↓‡	↓↓	Absent

* *Many cases are without familial incidence.*
† *Variable expressivity.*
‡ *Other defects such as occult hemolysis and ↓ bilirubin uptake may coexist.*

Hereditary glucuronyl transferase deficiency There are currently three syndromes that fall into this category. As indicated in Table 317-1, they reflect progressive decreases in the activity of glucuronyl transferase and thus may be part of a spectrum, i.e., from minimal deficiency to complete absence of bilirubin glucuronyl transferase.

GILBERT'S SYNDROME Since the original report by Gilbert in 1907, there has been an increased recognition of this benign but chronic disorder characterized by mild, persistent, unconjugated hyperbilirubinemia. The patient usually does not manifest this disorder until after the second decade and is often unaware of the jaundice until it is detected by physical examination or routine laboratory testing. The total serum bilirubin level usually ranges and fluctuates from 1.2 to 3 mg/dl and rarely exceeds 5 mg/dl. With the van den Bergh diazo reaction, less than 20 percent of the bilirubin gives a direct reaction; however, studies using more accurate methods (such as high-pressure liquid chromatography) show that the serum bilirubin in patients with Gilbert's syndrome is all unconjugated. Typically the jaundice fluctuates and is exacerbated following prolonged fasting (see below), surgery, fever or infection, and excessive exertion or alcohol ingestion. Liver function tests are normal, and the liver cells usually appear normal by light microscopy.

With the exception of hemolytic anemias, this disorder is probably the most common cause of mild unconjugated hyperbilirubinemia. Detailed studies show these patients to have a partial deficiency of bilirubin glucuronyl transferase. Some patients also manifest decreased bilirubin uptake and increased hemolysis. Decreased glucuronyl transferase alone or together with a decrease in bilirubin uptake appears to account for the observed *decrease in hepatic bilirubin clearance.* A decreased clearance and hepatic uptake of bile salts has also been shown.

Previously Gilbert's syndrome was traditionally defined as mild, chronic, unconjugated hyperbilirubinemia occurring in the absence of hemolysis. However, with the use of radiobilirubin kinetics and erythrocyte half-life studies, at least two forms of Gilbert's syndrome have been described. One group includes patients with decreased bilirubin clearance and *no hemolysis.* A second group includes those who also have *evidence of hemolysis* (often occult) and hence increased bilirubin turnover. It would appear that the simultaneous presence of both derangements is a chance occurrence of two not uncommon disorders occurring in the same patient and does not imply a causal relationship. There is increasing evidence of the heterogeneity of patients with Gilbert's syndrome. Some patients have an increase in hepatocyte lipofuscin and an increase in the smooth endoplasmic reticulum (SER); others show an increase in hepatic lysosomal enzymes.

A feature of Gilbert's syndrome which can be useful diagnostically is the increase in serum bilirubin following prolonged fasting or calorie deprivation. Thus, patients with this disorder, when placed on 300 cal per day for 2 days, will increase their serum bilirubin by 1.5 mg/dl or more, with the major increase being in the unconjugated fraction. It appears that a decrease in glucuronyl transferase activity is needed in order to obtain this effect. Patients with hemolysis do not show an increase in serum bilirubin with fasting. As a reflection of the mild decrease in glucuronyl transferase (1) their bilirubin levels will decrease when the enzyme activity is enhanced following phenobarbital administration, and (2) their bile shows a modest increase in monoconjugates of bilirubin (see Table 317-1).

In general, the diagnosis of this benign but not uncommon disorder is made by exclusion. The diagnosis is suspected in a patient with low-grade unconjugated hyperbilirubinemia when there are (1) no systemic symptoms, (2) *no overt* or clinically recognizable hemolysis, (3) normal tests of routine liver function, and (4) a liver biopsy (although usually not necessary) that is normal by light microscopy.

CRIGLER-NAJJAR SYNDROME (TYPES I AND II) This disorder is known to exist in two forms. Type I is the clinically *severe* form (originally described by Crigler and Najjar) and is due to *absence of glucuronyl transferase.* Type II has more *moderate* clinical findings due to *partial deficiency of glucuronyl transferase.* The major differences between the two variants are summarized in Table 317-1.

Type I (Crigler-Najjar) is a rare disorder. Infants develop high unconjugated bilirubin levels in the serum (20 to 45 mg/dl). Absence of the enzyme can be demonstrated in the liver. Routine liver function tests are normal, as is the liver histology. Because of the absence of glucuronyl transferase no conjugated bilirubin is formed by the liver; hence no bilirubin is secreted by the liver, and the bile is colorless.

Phototherapy may temporarily and transiently reduce the unconjugated bilirubin level. Phenobarbital has no effect since the enzyme defect is complete and no drug "induction" is therefore possible. Affected infants usually die within the first year of life, although some patients have survived to the second or third decade of life. Death is usually from kernicterus.

A strain of rats (Gunn rat) with the type I defect exists and is widely used as an animal model of the Crigler-Najjar syndrome.

Type II patients have a partial deficiency of glucuronyl transferase, and their disorder is less severe. Serum unconjugated bilirubin levels are lower (6 to 20 mg/dl), jaundice may not appear until adolescence, and neurological complications are uncommon. The bile contains variable amounts of conjugated bilirubin with a significant increase in monoconjugates. Phenobarbital is effective in lowering the serum bilirubin level in type II patients. However, the disorder is relatively benign in those patients whose bilirubin is less than 18 to 20 mg/dl.

Acquired deficiency of glucuronyl transferase As with any enzyme, glucuronyl transferase is susceptible to inhibition by a variety of agents, and because of the decreased activity of the enzyme in the neonatal state, such inhibition may be more evident at that time. Neonatal jaundice may be aggravated or prolonged in infants treated with *drugs* such as chloramphenicol or novobiocin, or with *vitamin K.* In some breast-fed infants jaundice has been ascribed to the presence in *breast milk* of pregnane-3β,20α-diol, a good inhibitor of glucuronyl transferase. When the infant is removed from the breast, the "breast-milk jaundice" subsides.

Hypothyroidism delays the normal "maturation" of glucuronyl transferase. In cretins, neonatal jaundice may be prolonged for weeks or months. In fact, the presence of prolonged unconjugated hyperbilirubinemia after birth may be a clue to an underlying hypothyroidism.

In the infant, as well as in the adult, *liver cell damage* leads to impairment in glucuronide conjugation as a result of decreased transferase activity. However, since excretion is probably the rate-limiting step in bilirubin metabolism and since this step is always interfered with to a greater extent than conjugation in parenchymal liver disease, the pigment which accumulates in the blood is predominantly conjugated bilirubin.

DISORDERS CAUSING PREDOMINANTLY CONJUGATED HYPERBILIRUBINEMIA

In jaundice due to primary liver disease, the plasma usually exhibits elevated levels of both conjugated and unconjugated bilirubin, and *urine contains bilirubin.* The relative proportions of the two pigments are highly variable. In many familial hepatic abnormalities (described below) and in some forms of drug-induced liver injury, the jaundice is almost entirely due to conjugated hyperbilirubinemia, 60 to 80 percent of the serum bilirubin giving a direct van den Bergh reaction. Such a pigment pattern is also seen with extrahepatic biliary obstruction.

In jaundice associated with diffuse liver cell damage, as in hepatitis and cirrhosis, the conjugated bilirubin levels may be somewhat less than in the above cholestatic syndromes, with the direct-reacting values ranging from 50 to 70 percent of the total serum bilirubin. However, the pattern is quite variable, and in all the above hepatic disorders, once the serum bilirubin components have been measured, repeated fractionation during the course of the disease is of little diagnostic or prognostic value. One cannot differentiate intrahepatic and extrahepatic causes of jaundice from either the levels or proportions of the two pigment types (i.e., unconjugated and conjugated bilirubin) in plasma. Thus the main purpose of the initial fractionation of the plasma bilirubin is to distinguish hepatic parenchymal and biliary obstructive disease from the disorders associated with predominantly unconjugated hyperbilirubinemia.

FAMILIAL DEFECTS IN HEPATIC EXCRETORY FUNCTION Dubin-Johnson syndrome This disorder, also called *chronic idiopathic jaundice,* is a benign, autosomally inherited hyperbilirubinemia characterized by the presence of a dark pigment in the centrilobular region of the liver cells. Functionally there exists a *defect in biliary excretion* of bilirubin, cholephilic dyes, and porphyrins. Using the diazo method for measuring bilirubin, the serum pigment in these patients typically has been observed to be in the range of 3 to 10 mg/dl and predominantly of the conjugated type. However, with the newer and more accurate method (alkaline methanolysis and high-pressure liquid chromatography), homozygous patients with the Dubin-Johnson syndrome have been shown to have *unconjugated bilirubin* as the major serum pigment. This finding may in part reflect pigment which, after conjugation by the liver, is deconjugated in the hepatobiliary system and refluxed into the plasma. Moreover, the serum contains more diconjugated than monoconjugated bilirubin, just the reverse of what is seen in acquired hepatobiliary disease. This reverse ratio is believed to be characteristic and diagnostic for homozygous patients.

Patients with Dubin-Johnson syndrome may be asymptomatic or have vague constitutional or gastrointestinal symptoms. Not infrequently the liver is slightly enlarged; in about one-fourth of the cases there is mild hepatic tenderness. Oral and intravenous cholangiography fails to visualize the biliary tract. There is typically and characteristically a late rise in the plasma BSP elimination curve at *90 min.* This is caused by the reflux from the liver of the conjugated dye and reflects the defect in the hepatic excretory transport maximum (T_m). It is noteworthy that there is no secondary rise in plasma when dyes which are not conjugated by the liver are given, such as indocyanine green. When bile salts such as ursodeoxycholic acid are given, these patients show a decreased hepatic uptake and clearance. In the liver the striking feature is the presence of a brown or black pigment in the hepatocytes. Earlier findings suggested that this unique pigment was melanin; however, electron spin resonance studies have not confirmed this. In fact, in some patients who also developed hepatitis, the pigment disappears from the liver and is excreted in the urine.

These patients also show an abnormality in coproporphyrin excretion. Normal urine contains mostly coproporphyrin III and small amounts of coproporphyrin I; Dubin-Johnson patients show a reversal of this pattern, i.e., a predominant excretion of coproporphyrin I. Heterozygotes show an intermediate excretory pattern.

There is impaired excretion of many metabolites, including conjugated bilirubin, BSP, and iodinated dyes. Excretion of bile acids, however, is normal. Oral contraceptive agents may accentuate hyperbilirubinemia or may produce jaundice for the first time. Features of cholestasis such as pruritus or steatorrhea are usually lacking, but serum alkaline phosphatase levels are *not* elevated. Impairment in the excretion of epinephrine metabolites may account for the accumulation of the melanin pigments. The overall prognosis of the disorder is excellent.

Rotor syndrome is similar in many respects to the Dubin-Johnson syndrome. However, *there is no pigment in the liver cells,* the gallbladder is usually visualized on cholecystography, and there is an increase in the total urinary coproporphyrins, but not an increased percentage excretion of coproporphyrin I. The BSP excretion pattern does *not* show a secondary rise at 90 min. The impairment in excretion which is typical of Dubin-Johnson syndrome is not present; instead in most cases of the Rotor syndrome there is impairment of *hepatic storage capacity* (*S*). This rare syndrome is inherited as an autosomal recessive trait and is genetically distinct from Dubin-Johnson syndrome.

Benign familial recurrent cholestasis This is a relatively rare syndrome characterized by recurrent attacks of pruritus and jaundice. During an attack the serum alkaline phosphatase and bile acid levels are markedly elevated, and liver biopsy shows the morphological features of cholestasis. However, at laparotomy, biliary obstruction is not found, and operative cholangiography reveals a patent and apparently normal biliary tree. Remissions are the rule, and at such times hepatic function tests and liver morphological features are usually normal. The cause of the disorder is unknown; cirrhosis does not develop, and the disorder is benign. A congenital origin has been postulated on the basis of the early age of onset and familial incidence.

Recurrent jaundice of pregnancy This form of jaundice is also known as *intrahepatic cholestasis of pregnancy.* During a normal pregnancy some changes in liver function occur, especially during the last trimester. Usually these consist of slight increases in BSP retention and of serum alkaline phosphatase. This mild increase in alkaline phosphatase during pregnancy is normally of placental rather than hepatic origin. Bilirubin increases never exceed 2 mg per deciliter of serum and usually are hardly detectable.

In a small number of pregnant women an intrahepatic cholestasis may appear. This usually occurs in the third trimester but may develop any time after the seventh week of gestation. The clinical features consist primarily of pruritus and jaundice. Serum bilirubin levels are usually less than 6 mg/dl and rarely higher than 8 mg/dl. The serum alkaline phosphatase and cholesterol levels are elevated significantly, while other liver function tests are only mildly deranged. Histologically the liver shows varying degrees of cholestasis but only a few parenchymal cell changes. The clinical and laboratory abnormalities subside promptly after delivery and are usually completely normal within 7 to 14 days.

This condition has been seen more frequently in Scandinavia and Europe than in the United States. Since steroid hormones and specifically estrogens can induce changes in hepatic excretory function in normal individuals (see Chap. 315), these patients probably have an increased susceptibility or sensitivity to the hepatic effects of estrogenic and progestational hormones. The intrahepatic cholestasis is usually termed *recurrent,* since the syndrome often (but not always) reappears in subsequent pregnancies. The process is benign and self-limited, and treatment is usually not needed, but cholestyramine administration will diminish the pruritus. This disorder must be distinguished from the many other causes of jaundice not unique to pregnancy, such as viral hepatitis. It must also be distinguished from the idiopathic *acute fatty liver of pregnancy* and the *tetracycline-induced* fatty liver. The latter two conditions are rare, occur in the last trimester, and have a high fatality rate: however, in these disorders there is evidence of diffuse parenchymal damage and not just cholestasis.

ACQUIRED DEFECTS OF HEPATIC EXCRETORY FUNCTION

Drug-induced cholestasis A condition entirely analogous to the intrahepatic cholestasis of pregnancy may occur in some women following the use of oral contraceptive agents. A significant number of individuals using these drugs show mild increases in BSP retention, and even more have decreased BSP excretory capacity as measured by infusion tests. In some, mild cholestatic jaundice may occur, liver function returns to normal when the drugs are withdrawn, and chronic liver disease does not appear to result. It is relevant that one-third of the reported patients with jaundice due to oral contraceptives also have a history of recurrent intrahepatic cholestasis of pregnancy.

The nature of these changes produced by the natural and synthetic female sex hormones is very similar to those resulting from the administration of certain testosterone analogues, especially those with α substitutions at the 17 position of the steroid nucleus. These agents (such as methyltestosterone and norethandrolone) commonly cause BSP retention and less commonly cause jaundice or significant changes in other liver functions. However, unlike the female hormones, these agents have been implicated as a cause of chronic liver disease, especially biliary cirrhosis.

Because of these phenomena, synthetic steroid sex hormones should not be used in patients with liver disease. Conversely, in individuals using these agents the appearance of jaundice or elevations in serum aminotransferase (transaminase) levels or alkaline phosphatase contraindicates their further use. However, mild to moderate increases in BSP retention alone are probably not of clinical significance, although liver function tests should be carried out periodically.

As is discussed in detail in Chap. 318, there are many drugs which may produce not simply cholestasis but liver injury resembling acute hepatitis or cholestatic hepatitis. In contrast to the jaundice produced by the steroid hormones, the clinical features are those of fever, rash, arthralgia, and eosinophilia, with the liver showing a pronounced inflammatory reaction. These features suggest that such reactions are *allergic* or *toxic* in nature and therefore differ from the effects caused by the steroid hormones, which probably represent an exaggerated response by the liver to the normal action of these hormones.

Postoperative jaundice The occurrence of postoperative jaundice is a problem of increasing importance. It is perhaps seen more frequently now than in earlier years, because patients are able to undergo major surgical procedures (i.e., cardiac surgery, repair of ruptured aneurysms) and survive. In approaching this problem the possible pathogenic mechanisms listed in Table 317-2 need to be considered. The patient may have *pigment overload,* especially from blood transfusions (due to he-

TABLE 317-2
Conditions causing or contributing to postoperative jaundice

I Increased pigment load
- *A* Hemolytic anemia
- *B* Transfusions (especially of stored blood)
- *C* Resorption of hematomas, blood in extravascular spaces

II Impaired hepatocellular function
- *A* Hepatitis-like picture
  - *1* Halothane anesthesia
  - *2* Drugs
  - *3* Shock
  - *4* Infection with hepatitis viruses
- *B* Cholestatic picture
  - *1* Hypotension, hypoxemia
  - *2* Drugs
  - *3* Sepsis

III Extrahepatic obstruction
- *A* Bile duct injury
- *B* Choledocholithiasis

molysis of stored blood), from resorption of blood in extravascular spaces, and less commonly from hemolytic anemia. *Hepatocellular damage* and decreased liver cell function may occur due to concurrent use of hepatotoxic drugs (Chap. 318) or anesthetics such as halothane. Hepatocellular necrosis may follow profound shock; with lesser degrees of hypotension or hypoxemia, morphological damage may be slight, but significant impairment of function may occur. Hence, prior shock or hypotension plus pigment overload may produce significant jaundice. Extensive sepsis can also produce jaundice, often of a cholestatic type. Concurrent renal impairment due to hypotension and hypoxemia may enhance the degree of jaundice because the renal excretion of conjugated bilirubin is decreased. *Extrahepatic obstruction* due to surgical damage or stones needs to be considered, but may be difficult to exclude.

A form of jaundice referred to as *benign postoperative intrahepatic cholestasis* may be seen. In the typical case the patient has had major and prolonged surgery for a catastrophic event such as a ruptured aortic aneurysm complicated by hypotension and hypoxemia, extensive blood loss into tissues, and massive blood replacement. Jaundice may be noted on the second or third postoperative day, and the serum bilirubin, predominantly conjugated, may reach 20 to 40 mg/dl by the eighth to tenth day. Serum alkaline phosphatase levels may be elevated three- to tenfold. Typically the SGOT is only mildly elevated. The liver morphology is striking in that necrosis is not seen but only cholestasis and erythrophagocytosis.

The cause of this type of postoperative cholestatic jaundice is uncertain. However, in all likelihood it reflects (1) increased pigment load, (2) decreased liver function due to hypoxemia and hypotension, and (3) decreased renal bilirubin excretion due to varying degrees of tubular necrosis as a result of shock. This diagnostic possibility must be considered in the postoper-

TABLE 317-3
Laboratory features in icteric states

	Serum bilirubin			
Bilirubin disorder	*Unconjugated*	*Conjugated*	*Urine bilirubin*	*Comments*
I Overproduction				
A Hemolysis (intra- and extravascular	↑	N	0	↑ Bilirubin turnover
B Ineffective erythropoiesis	↑	N	0	Splenomegaly; normal RBC survival; normoblasts in marrow
II Defective hepatic uptake	↑	N	0	Normal liver biopsy; direct/total serum bilirubin <20%
A Some drugs (e.g., flavaspidic acid, novobiocin)				
B Gilbert's syndrome (some cases)				
III Defective conjugation	↑	Low	0	
A Neonatal jaundice				↓ Glucuronyl transferase; ? ↓ ligandins
B Gilbert's syndrome				↓ Glucuronyl transferase and ↓ bilirubin uptake; some may have ↑ hemolysis; bile contains ↑ monoconjugates
C Conjugated nonhemolytic jaundice (types I and II)				Type I = absence of transferase Type II = deficiency of transferase; bile contains ↑↑ monoconjugates
IV Defective excretion				
A Intrahepatic obstruction				
1 Familial syndromes				
a Dubin-Johnson	↑	↑↑	+	Abnormal BSP curve, hepatic lipochrome pigment; ↑ urinary coproporphyrin type I
b Rotor				No liver pigment; ↑ total urinary coproporphyrin
2 Drugs (e.g., chloramphenicol, methyltestosterone)	↑	↑↑	+	↑ Alkaline phosphatase but other function tests usually normal
3 Benign recurrent cholestasis	↑	↑↑	+	↑ Alkaline phosphatase
4 Recurrent jaundice of pregnancy (third trimester)	↑	↑↑	+	↑ Alkaline phosphatase; may be reproduced in afflicted subjects by estrogens or progesterone
B Extrahepatic obstruction (tumors, stone, stricture of bile duct)				↑↑ Alkaline phosphatase (often > fourfold
1 Partial	↑	↑↑	+	
2 Complete	↑	↑↑	+	
V Hepatocellular disease*				
A Hepatitis	↑	↑↑	+	Direct/total serum bilirubin >50–70%; liver biopsy important for diagnosis
B Cirrhosis: Same as hepatitis	↑	↑↑		

* *Note that in hepatocellular disease there is generally an interference in all pathways of bilirubin metabolism (i.e., impaired uptake, conjugation, and excretion).*

ative patient with marked cholestatic jaundice. The course of the jaundice is self-limited and will subside if the other systemic complications do not predominate and lead to death.

Hepatitis and cirrhosis These disorders, discussed in detail in Chaps. 318 to 320, constitute the *most common disorders associated with jaundice.* As has been stated previously, when the liver cell is damaged, as in viral hepatitis, there is often impairment in all three major hepatic phases of bilirubin metabolism, namely, uptake, conjugation, and excretion. Since the excretory step is the one which is rate-limiting and most readily affected by injury, significant amounts of conjugated bilirubin reenter the systemic circulation. There are also usually lesser increases in the serum unconjugated bilirubin. The latter is probably a reflection of the impaired uptake and conjugation, and is due in part to the shortened life span of red blood cells often found in liver disease. In most patients with hepatitis and cirrhosis, the total serum bilirubin levels tend not to exceed 50 mg/dl, but on rare occasions levels of up to 90 or 95 mg/dl have been described. (For a summary of laboratory features in icteric states, see Table 317-3.)

EXTRAHEPATIC BILIARY OBSTRUCTION Anatomic or mechanical obstruction of the bile ducts is most commonly due to stones, tumors, or strictures. The clinical picture is quite similar to that of intrahepatic cholestasis with pronounced elevation of the alkaline phosphatase level. Usually, but not always, fever, pain, and chills may be present. While the amount of direct-reacting (conjugated) bilirubin predominates in the serum, the amount of the total serum bilirubin which is direct-reacting is variable (60 to 80 percent) and of no real diagnostic or prognostic significance. In contrast to hepatitis and cirrhosis, the serum bilirubin level often tends to plateau and rarely exceeds levels of 35 mg/dl. The reason for this plateau is not clear but may be related to renal excretion of conjugated bilirubin or alternative pathways of bilirubin catabolism in obstructive jaundice.

REFERENCES

Benign familial recurrent cholestasis

DePagter AGF et al: Familial benign intrahepatic cholestasis. Gastroenterology 71:202, 1976

Endo T et al: Bile acid metabolism in benign recurrent intrahepatic cholestasis. Gastroenterology 76:1002, 1979

Dubin-Johnson and Rotor syndromes

Berk PD et al: Inborn errors of bilirubin metabolism. Med Clin North Am 59:803, 1975

Rosenthal P et al: Homozygous Dubin-Johnson syndrome exhibits a characteristic serum bilirubin pattern. Hepatology 1:540, 1981

Swartz HM et al: On the nature and excretion of the hepatic pigment in the Dubin-Johnson syndrome. Gastroenterology 76:958, 1979

Wolkoff AW et al: Rotor's syndrome: A distinct inheritable pathophysiologic entity. Am J Med 60:173, 1976

Wolpert E et al: Abnormal sulfobromophthalein metabolism in Rotor's syndrome and obligate heterozygotes. N Engl J Med 206:1099, 1977

Glucuronyl transferase deficiency states

Berthelot P, Dhumeaus D: New insights into the classification and mechanisms of hereditary, chronic, non-hemolytic hyperbilirubinemia. Gut 19:474, 1978

Dawson J et al: Gilbert's syndrome: Evidence of morphologic heterogeneity. Gut 20:848, 1979

Felsher BF, Carpio NM: Caloric intake and unconjugated hyperbilirubinemia. Gastroenterology 69:42, 1975

Fevery J et al: Unconjugated bilirubin and an increased proportion of bilirubin monoconjugates in the bile of patients with Gilbert's syndrome and Crigler-Najjar disease. J Clin Invest 60:970, 1977

Ohkubo H et al: Ursodeoxycholic acid oral tolerance test in patients with constitutional hyperbilirubinemias and effect of phenobarbital. Gastroenterology 81:126, 1981

——— et al: Effects of corticosteroids on bilirubin metabolism in patients with Gilbert's syndrome. Hepatology 1:168, 1981

Postoperative jaundice

Koff RS: Postoperative jaundice. Med Clin North Am 59:823, 1975

LaMont JT, Isselbacher KJ: Postoperative jaundice, in *Liver and Biliary Disease,* R Wright et al (eds). Philadelphia, Saunders, 1979

318 ACUTE HEPATITIS

JULES L. DIENSTAG
JACK R. WANDS
RAYMOND S. KOFF

ACUTE VIRAL HEPATITIS

Acute viral hepatitis is a systemic infection affecting the liver predominantly. Classically two types of viruses (A and B) had been implicated as the etiologic agents in this systemic infection; however, recently others (non-A, non-B) have been described. Viruses A and B can now be distinguished by their antigenic properties but are known to produce clinically similar diseases in humans. Synonyms used to describe hepatitis A include infectious hepatitis, short-incubation hepatitis, and MS-1 hepatitis. Hepatitis B has also been referred to as serum hepatitis, long-incubation hepatitis, MS-2 hepatitis, or hepatitis B surface antigen (HBsAg)-positive hepatitis.

ANTIGENIC PROPERTIES OF HEPATITIS VIRUSES Hepatitis A Hepatitis A virus (HAV) is a nonenveloped 27-nm (Fig. 318-1), heat-, acid-, and ether-resistant RNA virus with biophysical characteristics of the enterovirus subgroup of picornaviruses. Inactivation of viral activity can be achieved by boiling for 1 min, by contact with formaldehyde and chlorine, or by ultraviolet irradiation. All strains of this virus identified to date are immunologically indistinguishable and belong to one serotype. The virus is present in the liver, bile, stools, and blood during the late incubation period and acute preicteric phase of illness, but viral shedding in feces and viremia diminish rapidly once jaundice becomes apparent. Hepatitis A virus has been grown in tissue culture and remains the only human hepatitis virus to be cultivated in vitro.

Hepatitis B This viral infection is unique in that concentrations of viral antigen in the blood may reach 500 μg/ml. Electron microscopic studies of serum have demonstrated the morphologic appearance of the various particles related to hepatitis B infection (see Fig. 318-1). Three types of particles have been observed (Table 318-1). The most numerous are the 22-nm particles which appear as spherical or long filamentous forms; these are antigenically identical with the outer surface or coat of the hepatitis B virus and are thought to represent excess viral coat protein. Less frequently seen in serum are large 42-nm spherical Dane particles, which are believed to represent the intact hepatitis B virus (HBV). These large particles characteristically have an outer coat and an inner icosahedral core measuring 27 nm in diameter. Previous studies have shown that antiserum obtained from hemophiliacs, who were presumably repeatedly exposed to hepatitis viruses through multiple blood transfusions, would form a precipitin line by diffusion in agar gel with an antigen present in hepatitis serum. This antigen was originally called the Australia antigen or hepatitis-associated antigen and subsequently referred to as hepatitis B surface antigen (HBsAg). These observations provided the first serologic test to distinguish hepatitis B from non-B hepatitis. Isolation from serum of the various virus-associated particles related to hepatitis B infection and detection of antibodies to the antigens associated with these particles have permitted a more complete understanding of the antigenic composition of the hepatitis B virus (see Table 318-1). The long, tubular and small, spherical particles (22 nm) possess HBsAg, which is also present on the surface of the 42-nm Dane particle. HBsAg can be measured in clinical laboratories and is specific for hepatitis B infection. "Spurs" of immunoprecipitate are produced by certain combinations of HBsAg and antibody reactants in double immunodiffusion studies. Analysis of these reactions has led to the recognition of a number of different antigenic determinants. There is a common group-reactive antigen, *a*, shared by all HBsAg-positive serums. In addition, HBsAg may contain several subtype-specific antigens—namely, *d* or *y*, *w* or *r*, as well as others. These HBsAg *subtypes* provide additional epidemiologic markers in evaluating the transmission of hepatitis B infection in that subtypes "breed true." For example, studies of hepatitis outbreaks among patients and staff in hemodialysis units have shown that index cases and their contacts have identical HBsAg subtypes. Clinical course and outcome, however, are independent of subtype.

The intact 42-nm virion can be disrupted by mild detergents and the 27-nm core particle isolated. Naked core particles do not circulate in serum. The antigen is referred to as hepatitis B core antigen (HBcAg), and the corresponding antibody is anti-HBc. HBcAg does not cross-react with HBsAg. Within the core particle is a predominantly double stranded DNA which is associated with a DNA polymerase; the latter presumably directs replication or repair of viral DNA. Thus, *hepatitis B virus can be classified as a DNA virus.* Genetic material from HBV cores has been cloned in bacterial, yeast, and mammalian cell vectors, genetic and amino acid maps have been plotted, and synthetic HBsAg polypeptides have been produced in the laboratory.

A number of laboratory techniques are employed for the measurement of HBsAg in serum. The least sensitive is Ouchterlony gel diffusion. Counterimmunoelectrophoresis (CIEP) is approximately 10 times more sensitive. *Radioimmunoassay* is the most sensitive and preferred technique for the measurement of HBsAg in serum. It is approximately 1000 times more sensitive than gel diffusion. Recently, enzyme immunoassays for the detection of HBsAg comparable in sensitivity to radioimmunoassays have been released.

A third antigen associated with hepatitis B is *hepatitis B e antigen* (*HBeAg*). HBeAg is a soluble, nonparticulate antigen, which is found only in HBsAg-positive serum, which is immunologically and biochemically distinct from HBsAg, DNA polymerase, and intact HBcAg, but appears to be an internal component of the core of HBV. This antigen has not been completely characterized. Originally HBeAg and its antibody (anti-HBe) were detected by a relatively insensitive gel immunodiffusion technique, but very sensitive radioimmunoassays and enzyme immunoassays are used currently. HBsAg-positive serum containing HBeAg is more likely to be highly infectious and to be associated with the presence of HBV virions and DNA polymerase than HBeAg-negative or anti-HBe-positive serum. For example, asymptomatic HBsAg carrier mothers who are HBeAg-positive almost invariably transmit hepatitis B infection to their offspring. Every individual with acute hepatitis B infection develops HBeAg transiently, early in the course of illness, but persistent HBeAg positivity correlates with ongoing viral replication, may be associated with chronic hepatitis, and its disappearance may be a harbinger of

FIGURE 318-1

Electron micrograph of (left) 27-nm hepatitis A virus particles purified from stool of a patient with acute hepatitis A virus infection and aggregated by hepatitis A antibody, and (right) concentrated serum from a patient with acute hepatitis B infection demonstrating the 42-nm virion, tubular forms, and spherical 22-nm particles of hepatitis B surface antigen (132,000×).

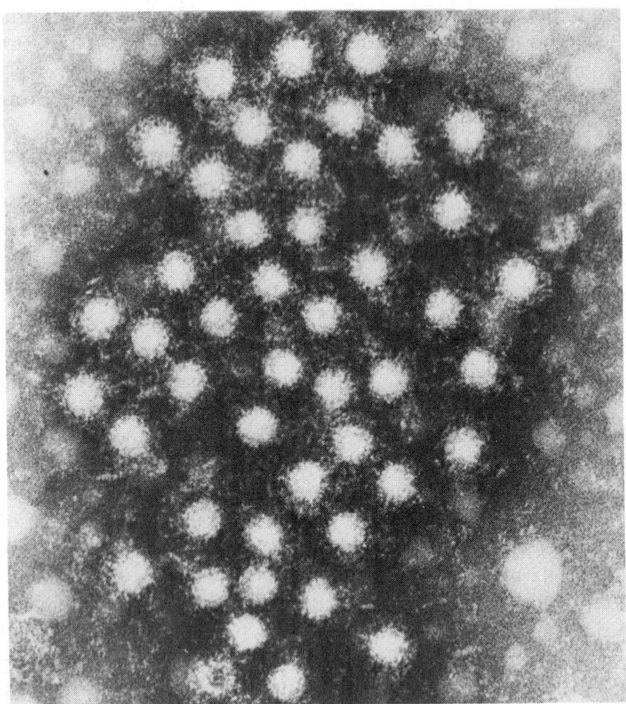

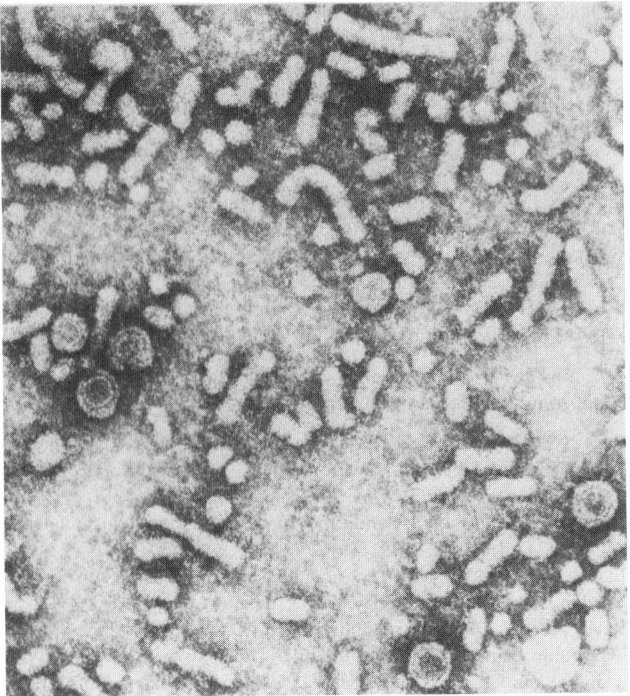

biochemical improvement and resolution of infection. Unfortunately HBeAg is not a sufficiently discriminating marker to support prognostic predictions or to substitute for morphologic evaluation of severity in patients with chronic hepatitis.

Non-A, non-B hepatitis Sensitive serologic tests for identifying both types A and B hepatitis have led to the identification of hepatitis cases with incubation periods and modes of transmission consistent with an infectious disease but without serologic evidence of hepatitis A or B infection. Identified initially among recipients of transfused blood, these cases of so-called non-A, non-B hepatitis have not been associated serologically with Epstein-Barr virus or cytomegalovirus (except in rare instances) or with other viruses known to involve the liver. One or more of these non-A, non-B viruses exist and have been implicated in a variety of epidemiologic forms of hepatitis transmission (see below). Although the virus(es) or virus antigens have not been identified definitively, chimpanzees are a susceptible host and may prove useful in the isolation, characterization, and serologic identification of these agents.

HUMORAL RESPONSE TO HEPATITIS VIRUS INFECTION

There is a nonspecific increase in serum immunoglobulins during acute viral hepatitis. Serum IgG and IgM are elevated in about one-third of patients during the acute phase of infection, but serum IgM elevation is seen more characteristically during acute type A hepatitis. During the acute phase of viral hepatitis, antibodies to smooth muscle and other cell constituents may be present, and low titers of rheumatoid factor, antinuclear antibody, and heterophile antibody can also be found occasionally. These antibodies are nonspecific and can also be associated with other viral and systemic diseases. In contrast, virus-specific antibodies, which appear during and after hepatitis virus infection, are serologic markers of diagnostic importance.

Antibodies of hepatitis A Anti-HAV can be detected during acute illness when serum transaminase activity is elevated and fecal HAV shedding is still occurring. This early antibody response is predominantly of the IgM class and persists for several months. During convalescence, however, anti-HAV of the IgG class becomes the predominant antibody (Fig. 318-2). Therefore, the diagnosis of hepatitis A is made during acute illness by demonstrating high-titer anti-HAV of the IgM class. Alternatively, diagnosis can be based on an increase in anti-HAV titers between acute and convalescent serum samples. Following acute illness, anti-HAV remains detectable indefinitely, and patients with serum anti-HAV are immune to reinfection. Indeed, the anti-HAV present in immune globulin preparations accounts for the protection it affords against hepatitis A infection.

In the general population, anti-HAV increases in prevalence as a function of increasing age and of decreasing socioeconomic status. Serologic evidence of prior hepatitis A infec-

TABLE 318-1
Nomenclature and features of hepatitis antigens and antibodies

*Hepatitis type**	*Particle diameter, nm*	*Description*	*Antigen (abbreviation)*	*Corresponding antibody (abbreviation)*	*Remarks*
A	27	Icosahedral virus particle	Hepatitis A virus (HAV)	Hepatitis A antibody (anti-HAV)	RNA-type virus; present in stool and serum early in course of hepatitis A
B	42	Intact virion (surface and core); spherical (Dane particle)	Hepatitis B surface antigen (HBsAg) Hepatitis B core antigen (HBcAg)	Hepatitis B surface antibody (anti-HBs) Hepatitis B core antibody (anti-HBc)	DNA-type virus; found in serum
	27	Core of virion, icosahedral	HBcAg	Anti-HBc	Core contains DNA and DNA polymerase; present in hepatocyte nuclei but not in serum Anti-HBc detected in serum during and after acute infection with virus
	22	Appear as spherical and filamentous forms; both have same antigenic properties as surface of virion; represent excess viral coat material	HBsAg	Anti-HBs	HBsAg detectable in > 90% of patients with acute hepatitis B; found in serum, body fluids, and hepatocyte cytoplasm Anti-HBs appears following B infection; protective antibody
		Antigen subtypes:			
		Group reactive	/a	Anti-/a	Antigen common to all HBsAg particles
		Type specific	/*d* or *y; w* or *r*	Anti-; *d* or *y; w* or *r*	Useful in epidemiologic investigation
	Nonparticulate	Soluble protein	HBeAg	Anti-HBe	HBeAg found in HBsAg-positive serum only, correlates with infectivity and presence of intact virus particles; HBeAg is an internal component of the HBV core

* *Non-A, non-B hepatitis viruses are transmissible hepatitis agents, but no immunologic marker or virus particle has yet been satisfactorily demonstrated.*

tion occurs in about 40 percent of urban populations, fewer than 5 percent of whom recall having had a symptomatic case of hepatitis. In older age groups (>50 years) evidence of previous hepatitis A infection approaches 80 percent, regardless of socioeconomic class. In developing countries, exposure, infection, and subsequent immunity is almost universal in childhood.

Antibodies to hepatitis B Specific antibody to HBsAg in serum (anti-HBs) has been demonstrated by radioimmunoassay in both the general population and patients convalescing from acute hepatitis B. Both IgM and IgG anti-HBs responses have been demonstrated in prospectively studied adult patients. The appearance of IgM anti-HBs after primary exposure is *transient,* whereas IgG anti-HBs persists for years after infection. In volunteer blood donors, the prevalence of anti-HBs ranges from 5 to 10 percent, but the prevalence is higher in lower socioeconomic strata, older age groups, and persons frequently exposed to blood products.

A *primary immune response* with the production of anti-HBs occurs after acute infection or immunization. A subsequent and more pronounced rise in anti-HBs titers suggests an *anamnestic response.* Such a presumed anamnestic anti-HBs response has been observed in patients and medical personnel with preexisting anti-HBs following their reexposure to HBsAg, either through blood transfusions or hospital contacts. These individuals do not develop biochemical or clinical evidence of acute hepatitis B following this exposure, suggesting that *anti-HBs protects against reinfection with hepatitis B virus.*

There is significant variability in the time of appearance of anti-HBs following exposure to HBsAg or acute hepatitis B infection. In some patients, anti-HBs is detectable 2 weeks to 2 months after HBsAg disappears from the serum; however in many instances anti-HBs is not detectable until 4 to 6 months or more after the disappearance of HBsAg. Measurement of serum anti-HBs is clinically and epidemiologically useful in documenting previous clinical or subclinical hepatitis B infection and may aid in documenting reexposure to HBsAg. Anti-HBs is rarely detectable in chronic carriers of HBsAg.

Antibody to the core antigen (anti-HBc) appears in the serum in high titer approximately 2 weeks after the appearance of HBsAg; it precedes detectable levels of anti-HBs by weeks to months (Fig. 318-3). During the "gap" between disappearance of HBsAg and the emergence of anti-HBs, anti-HBc may be the only serologic marker of recent HBV infection. This interval may be brief, as with acute infection, or may last many months or even years following resolution of chronic infection. In the absence of HBsAg and anti-HBs, anti-HBc in high titer reflects ongoing viral replication; such anti-HBc–positive blood has been implicated in the development of transfusion-associated type B hepatitis in a small number of recipients. Following recovery, however, the anti-HBc titer is generally low, and anti-HBs is present as well. In some persons, however, years after infection anti-HBc may persist in the circulation longer than anti-HBs. Therefore anti-HBc alone does not necessarily indicate active virus replication. Immune individuals who are reexposed to hepatitis B develop a secondary anamnestic anti-HBs response, but the anti-HBc titer does not change.

Antibody to HBeAg appears after the disappearance of HBeAg, usually later than anti-HBc but earlier than anti-HBs (Fig. 318-3). Its appearance in HBsAg-positive serum correlates with relatively low infectivity.

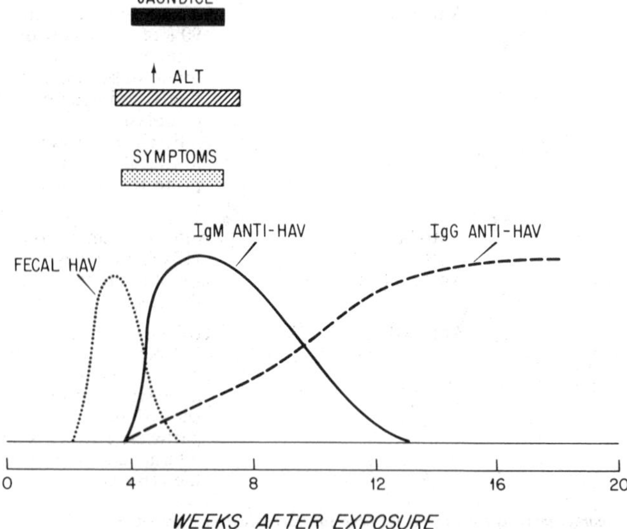

FIGURE 318-2
Scheme of typical clinical and laboratory features of viral hepatitis type A.

Antibodies to non-A, non-B agents Acceptable serologic tests to identify antigens and antibodies associated with non-A, non-B virus have not been developed. Details of the humoral immune response remain to be described.

IMMUNOPATHOGENIC MECHANISM IN ACUTE VIRAL HEPATITIS While data on the immunopathogenesis of hepatitis A are very limited, there is increasing evidence that the clinical manifestations of acute hepatitis B are determined by the immunologic responses of the host. Immune-complex–mediated tissue damage appears to play a major pathogenetic role in the extrahepatic manifestations of acute hepatitis B. The occasional prodomal "serum sickness-like" syndrome observed in acute hepatitis B appears to be related to the deposition in tissue blood vessel walls of circulating immune complexes leading to activation of the complement system. The clinical consequences are rash, angioedema, and arthritis. In these patients during the early prodrome of hepatitis B, HBsAg in high titer in association with small amounts of anti-HBs leads to the formation of soluble, circulating immune complexes (in antigen excess). Complement components in the serum are depressed during the arthritic phase of the illness and are also detectable in the circulating immune complexes. In addition to complement components, these complexes contain the intact virus, tubules, and 22-nm spheres (HBsAg), anti-HBs, IgG, IgM, and IgA. These immune complexes disappear after recovery from the serum sickness-like syndrome.

In patients who become chronic carriers of HBsAg following acute hepatitis, other types of immune-complex diseases may be seen. *Glomerulonephritis* with the nephrotic syndrome is occasionally observed: HBsAg, immunoglobulins, and C3 deposition has been found on the glomerular basement membrane. Twenty to thirty percent of patients with *polyarteritis nodosa* have HBsAg in serum, and in these patients the affected small and medium-sized arterioles have been shown to contain HBsAg, immunoglobulins, and complement components.

Cellular immunity (delayed hypersensitivity) may be important in the host's response to hepatitis B infection. Patients with depressed T-lymphocyte function have a high frequency of chronic infection with hepatitis B virus. In addition, lymphocytes from patients with hepatitis B have been shown to be cytotoxic for isolated liver cells or liver-derived cell lines in vitro. Other evidence suggests that alterations in the host's cellular immune response may be important in the development of the HBsAg carrier state and progression from acute hepatitis B to chronic active hepatitis.

PATHOLOGY The typical morphologic lesions of hepatitis A and B and non-A and non-B are often similar and consist of panlobular infiltration with mononuclear cells, hepatic cell necrosis, hyperplasia of Kupffer cells, and variable degrees of cholestasis. Hepatic cell regeneration is present, as evidenced by numerous mitotic figures, multinucleated cells, and "rosette" or "pseudoacinar" formation. The mononuclear infiltration consists primarily of small lymphocytes, although plasma cells and eosinophils are occasionally seen. Liver cell damage consists of hepatic cell degeneration and necrosis, cell dropout, ballooning of cells, and acidophilic degeneration of hepatocytes (so-called Councilman bodies). Large hepatocytes with a ground-glass appearance of the cytoplasm may be seen in chronic but not acute hepatitis B; these cells have been shown to contain HBsAg and can be identified histochemically with orcein or aldehyde fuchsin. In uncomplicated viral hepatitis the reticulin framework is preserved.

A more severe histologic lesion, *bridging hepatic necrosis*, also termed *subacute* or *confluent necrosis*, is occasionally observed in some patients with acute hepatitis. "Bridging" between lobules results from large areas of hepatic cell dropout, with collapse of the reticulin framework. Characteristically, the "bridge" consists of condensed reticulum, inflammatory debris, and degenerating liver cells that span adjacent portal areas, portal to central veins, or central vein to central vein. This lesion had been thought to have prognostic significance; many of the originally described patients with this lesion had a subacute course terminating in death within several weeks to months or developed chronic active hepatitis and postnecrotic cirrhosis. More recent investigations have failed to uphold the association between bridging necrosis and such a poor prognosis in patients with acute hepatitis. Although the frequency of bridging may be higher among hospitalized patients with severe acute hepatitis, and although cirrhosis, chronic hepatitis, and even death have been observed in this group, the frequency of bridging necrosis in uncomplicated acute viral hepatitis is probably on the order of 1 to 5 percent. Prospective studies have failed to demonstrate a difference in prognosis between patients with acute hepatitis who have bridging necrosis and those who do not. Therefore, although demonstration of this lesion in patients with chronic hepatitis has prognostic significance (see Chap. 319), its demonstration during acute hepatitis is less meaningful, and liver biopsies to identify this lesion are no longer undertaken routinely in patients with acute hepatitis. When confluent necrosis is more severe and spans several lobules, the lesion is called *multilobular hepatic necrosis*. This lesion appears to be associated with a poor prognosis. In *massive hepatic necrosis* (fulminant hepatitis, acute yellow atrophy), the striking feature at postmortem examination is the finding of a small, shrunken, and soft liver. Histologic examination reveals massive necrosis and dropout of liver cells of most lobules with extensive collapse and condensation of the reticulin framework.

Immunofluorescence antibody studies have been instrumental in localizing HBsAg to the cytoplasm of infected liver cells. In contrast, HBcAg predominates in the nucleus but occasionally scant amounts are also seen in the cytoplasm. Electron-microscopic studies of liver biopsy material have demonstrated the presence of HBsAg particles in the cytoplasm and HBcAg particles in the nucleus of liver cells during hepatitis B infection. These morphologic observations suggest that DNA is synthesized and packaged within core particles in the nucleus, while the surface coat is assembled in the cytoplasm, resulting in the formation of the intact hepatitis B virus.

EPIDEMIOLOGY Traditionally, viral hepatitis had been classified into two epidemiologically distinct types: infectious hepatitis (hepatitis A) and serum hepatitis (hepatitis B). These distinctions were based on earlier observations that hepatitis A had a shorter incubation period (15 to 45 days), high contagion rate, and usually a fecal-oral route of transmission; while hepatitis B had a longer incubation period (30 to 180 days), was less contagious, and was thought to be transmitted only by the parenteral route. It is now recognized that *a clear distinction between hepatitis A and B cannot be made solely by clinical or epidemiologic features* (Table 318-2), that modes of transmission overlap, and, moreover, that other hepatitis viruses exist besides hepatitis A and B. The most accurate means to distinguish the various types of viral hepatitis involves specific serologic testing.

Hepatitis A is transmitted almost exclusively by the fecal-oral route. Spread of this virus is enhanced by poor personal hygiene and overcrowding, and large outbreaks as well as sporadic cases have been traced to contaminated food, water, milk, and shellfish. Intrafamily and intrainstitutional spread are also common. Early epidemiologic observations suggested that there is a predilection for hepatitis A to occur in late fall and early winter. In temperate zones, epidemic waves had been recorded every 5 to 20 years as new segments of nonimmune population appeared; however, in developed countries, the incidence of type A hepatitis has been declining, presumably as a function of improved sanitation, and these cyclic patterns are no longer being observed. No HAV carrier state has been identified after acute type A hepatitis; perpetuation of the virus in nature depends presumably on nonepidemic, inapparent subclinical infection.

It has long been recognized that a major route of hepatitis B transmission is percutaneous, but the designation "serum hepatitis" is an inaccurate label for the epidemiologic spectrum of HBV infection recognized today. As detailed below, most of the hepatitis transmitted by blood transfusion is not caused by HBV, and, moreover, in approximately 50 percent of patients with acute type B hepatitis, there is no history of an identifiable percutaneous exposure. This group of hepatitis cases had been labeled "infectious hepatitis" and had been attributed to HAV, until serologic tests became available with which to establish HBV as the causative agent. Therefore, we now recognize that many cases of type B hepatitis result from less obvious modes of nonpercutaneous or covert percutaneous transmission. HBsAg has been identified in almost every body fluid from infected persons—saliva, tears, seminal fluid, cerebrospinal fluid, ascites, breast milk, synovial fluid, gastric juice, pleural fluid, urine, and even rarely in feces. Although there is

FIGURE 318-3
Scheme of typical clinical and laboratory features of acute viral hepatitis type B.

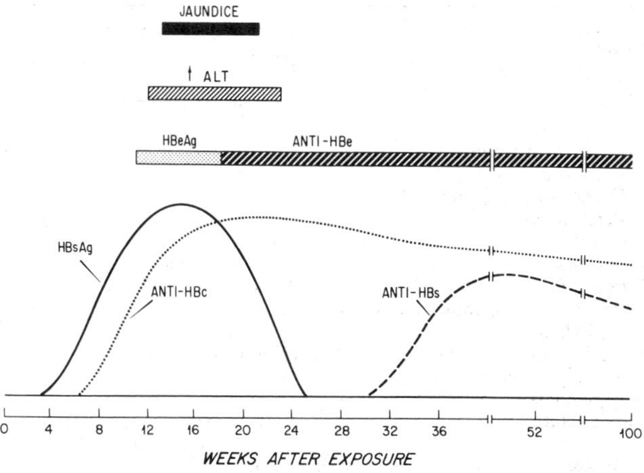

abundant evidence to suggest that feces are not infectious, at least some of these body fluids—most notably semen and saliva—have been shown to be infectious when administered percutaneously or nonpercutaneously to experimental animals. Among the nonpercutaneous modes of HBV transmission, oral ingestion has been documented as a potential route of exposure, but one whose efficiency is quite low; when successful, oral inoculation is followed by a prolonged incubation period. On the other hand, the two nonpercutaneous routes considered to have the greatest impact are intimate (especially sexual) contact and perinatal transmission. High attack rates of HBV infection occur in spouses of acutely infected persons, in residents and staff of institutions for the mentally retarded, and, to a lesser extent, in family members of chronically infected patients. In sub-Saharan Africa, intimate contact among toddlers is considered instrumental in maintaining the high frequency of HBs antigenemia in the population. Perinatal transmission occurs primarily in infants born to HBsAg carrier mothers or mothers with acute hepatitis B during the third trimester of pregnancy or during the early postpartum period. Perinatal transmission is rare in North America and western Europe but occurs with great frequency and is the most important mode of HBV perpetuation in the far east and developing countries. Although the precise mode of perinatal transmission is unknown, epidemiologic evidence suggests that infection occurs approximately at the time of delivery and is not a function of breast-feeding. Likelihood of perinatal transmission of HBV correlates with HBe antigenemia; HBeAg-positive mothers almost always and anti-HBe-positive mothers almost never transmit HBV infection to their offspring. In most cases, acute infection in the neonate is clinically asymptomatic, but the child is very likely to become an HBsAg carrier.

The over 200 million HBsAg carriers in the world constitute the main reservoir of hepatitis B in human beings. Serum HBsAg is infrequent (0.1 to 0.5 percent) in normal populations in the United States and western Europe; however, a prevalence of up to 5 to 15 percent has been found in the far east and in some tropical countries, and as high as 30 percent in patients with Down's syndrome, lepromatous leprosy, leukemia, Hodgkin's disease, polyarteritis nodosa, in patients with chronic renal disease on hemodialysis, and in needle-using drug addicts.

Routine screening of blood donors for HBsAg and the elimination of commercial blood sources has markedly decreased the incidence of hepatitis B after transfusion, but *posttransfusion hepatitis* still remains a significant medical problem. The incidence of posttransfusion hepatitis has been reported to be from 0.3 to 9 cases per 1000 transfused units, or between 0.5 and 13 cases per 100 patients transfused. The risk of anicteric hepatitis following transfusion is much greater than that of clinical hepatitis with jaundice. The risk of viral hepatitis after transfusion of blood derivatives is dependent on the methods by which these products are processed. The *greatest risk* follows the use of multiple pooled donor products such as concentrates of factors II, VII, VIII, IX, and X. Hepatitis has developed in 20 to 30 percent of individuals receiving these pooled products for the first time. Blood products associated with an *average risk* include whole blood, packed red blood cells, single donor platelets, and plasma. Products involving *no risk* include human albumin and immune and hyperimmune globulin because of prior treatment of these substances by heating to 60°C and cold ethanol extraction. It had been suggested that frozen glycerol-treated red blood cells may carry a reduced risk of hepatitis, but this has not been confirmed. Elimination of HBsAg-negative blood that is positive for anti-HBc may prevent the few residual cases of transfusion-associated type B hepatitis, but this would lead to the loss of many noninfectious units and compromise the available blood supply. More of a problem than the relatively rare posttransfusion type B hepatitis is the occurrence of non-A, non-B posttransfusion hepatitis, which accounts for approximately 90 percent of cases following transfusion of voluntarily donated blood prescreened for HBsAg. The fact that it is transmitted by transfused blood from asymptomatic donors (Table 318-2) and that it can be transmitted to chimpanzees by blood from patients with chronic hepatitis suggests that there is a carrier state for non-A, non-B hepatitis. Currently, the frequency of posttransfusion non-A, non-B hepatitis approaches 10 percent of blood recipients, especially among recipients of multiple units of blood products. Unfortunately, there is no acceptable serologic screening test to identify non-A, non-B hepatitis agents in blood, and elimination of transfusion-associated non-A, non-B hepatitis will remain an elusive goal until a sensitive, specific test is developed. As an interim measure, however, blood banks may begin to screen for serum alanine aminotransferase (ALT), elevations of which in donor blood have been associated with an increased frequency of hepatitis in recipients. Discarding donor blood with elevated ALT activity, it has been estimated, would eliminate approximately 30 percent of transfusion-associated non-A, non-B hepatitis, but at a cost

TABLE 318-2
Comparisons of type A, type B, and non-A, non-B hepatitis

Feature	*Hepatitis A (infectious hepatitis, MS-1, short-incubation hepatitis)*	*Hepatitis B (serum hepatitis, MS-2, long-incubation hepatitis)*	*Non-A, non-B hepatitis*
Incubation	15–45 days (mean 30)	30 to 180 days (mean 60–90)	15–160 (mean 50)
Onset	Acute	Often insidious	Insidious
Seasonal incidence	Fall, winter	Year round	Year round
Age preference	Children, young adults	Any age	Any age but more common in adults
Transmission route:			
Fecal-oral	+++	−	Unknown
Other nonpercutaneous*	+/−	++	++
Percutaneous	+/−	+++	+++
Severity	Mild	Often severe	Moderate
Prognosis	Generally good	Worse with age, debility	Moderate
Progression to chronicity	None	Occasional (5–10%)	Occasional (10–50%)
Immune serum globulin (ISG) prophylaxis	Good	Partial	?
Hepatitis B immune globulin (very high titer anti-HBs) prophylaxis	(Not applicable)	Good after needle stick, sexual contact, maternal-neonatal contact	(Not applicable)
Carrier state	Rare, if ever	0.1–1.0%	Exists but prevalence unknown

* *For example, sexual or maternal-neonatal contact.*

of 1 to 2 percent of the national blood supply and a loss of many noninfectious units of blood.

In addition to being transmitted by transfusion, non-A, non-B hepatitis cases have been observed in other settings of percutaneous and nonpercutaneous exposure (e.g., intrafamily contact, intravenous drug abuse, occupational contact, nosocomial infection, hemodialysis units, renal transplantation, and intrainstitutional contact). Non-A, non-B hepatitis accounts for approximately 20 percent of sporadic cases presenting for medical evaluation. Occurrence of multiple bouts of non-A, non-B hepatitis among drug abusers and hemophiliacs and of cases with either short or long incubation periods and cross-challenge studies in chimpanzees suggest that there may be more than one non-A, non-B hepatitis agent.

CLINICAL AND LABORATORY FEATURES **Symptoms and signs** The *prodromal symptoms* of acute viral hepatitis are variable and systemic. Constitutional symptoms of anorexia, nausea and vomiting, fatigue, malaise, arthralgias, myalgias, headache, photophobia, pharyngitis, cough, and coryza may precede the onset of jaundice by 1 to 2 weeks. The nausea, vomiting, and anorexia are frequently associated with alterations in olfaction and taste. A low-grade fever between 100 and 102°F is more often present in hepatitis A than in B, except when hepatitis B is heralded by a serum sickness-like syndrome; rarely a fever of 103 to 104°F may accompany the constitutional symptoms. Dark urine and clay-colored stools may be noticed by the patient from 1 to 5 days prior to the onset of clinical jaundice.

With the onset of *clinical jaundice* the constitutional prodromal symptoms usually diminish, but in some patients mild weight loss (2.5 to 5 kg) is common and may continue during the entire icteric phase. The liver becomes enlarged and tender and may be associated with right upper quadrant pain and discomfort. Infrequently, patients present with a cholestatic picture, suggesting extrahepatic biliary obstruction. Splenomegaly and cervical adenopathy are present in 10 to 20 percent of patients with acute hepatitis. Rarely, a few spider angiomas appear during the icteric phase and disappear during convalescence. During the *recovery phase,* constitutional symptoms disappear, but usually some liver enlargement and abnormalities in hepatic function are still evident. The duration of the posticteric phase is variable, ranging from 2 to 12 weeks, and usually is more prolonged in acute hepatitis B and in non-A, non-B hepatitis. Complete clinical and biochemical recovery is to be expected 3 to 4 months after the onset of jaundice in three-quarters of uncomplicated cases. In the remainder biochemical recovery may be delayed.

Laboratory features The serum transaminases SGOT and SGPT (also designated aminotransferases, AST and ALT) show a variable increase during the prodromal phase of acute viral hepatitis and precede the rise in bilirubin level (see Figs. 318-2 and 318-3). The actual level of these enzymes, however, does not correlate well with the degree of liver cell damage. Peak levels vary from 400 to 4000 IU or more; these levels are usually reached at the time the patient is clinically icteric and progressively diminish during the recovery phase of acute hepatitis. The diagnosis of *anicteric* hepatitis is difficult and requires a high index of suspicion; it is often based solely on transaminase elevations, although mild increases in conjugated bilirubin may also be found.

Jaundice is usually visible in the sclera or skin when the serum bilirubin value exceeds 2.5 mg/dl. When jaundice appears, the serum bilirubin typically rises to levels ranging from 5 to 20 mg/dl. The serum bilirubin may continue to rise despite falling serum transaminase levels. In most instances the total bilirubin is equally divided between the conjugated and unconjugated fractions. The absolute level of the serum bilirubin appears to have some prognostic significance; levels above 20 mg/dl extending and persisting late into the course of viral hepatitis may indicate more severe disease. In certain patients with underlying hemolytic anemia, however, such as glucose 6-phosphate dehydrogenase deficiency and sickle cell anemia, high serum bilirubin is common, resulting from superimposed hemolysis. In such patients bilirubin levels greater than 30 mg/dl have been observed and do not necessarily indicate a worse prognosis.

Neutropenia and lymphopenia are transient and are followed by a relative lymphocytosis. Atypical lymphocytes (varying between 2 and 20 percent) are common during the acute phase. These atypical lymphocytes are indistinguishable from those seen in infectious mononucleosis. It is important to measure the *prothrombin time* (PT) in patients with acute viral hepatitis, for a prolonged value may signify extensive hepatocellular necrosis and indicate a worse prognosis. Occasionally a prolonged PT may occur with only mild increases in the serum bilirubin and transaminase levels. A blood sugar determination is often helpful in patients with symptoms of *hypoglycemia.* Prolonged nausea and vomiting, inadequate carbohydrate intake, and poor hepatic glycogen reserves may contribute to very rare episodes of hypoglycemia in the patient with uncomplicated viral hepatitis. Serum alkaline phosphatase may be normal or only mildly elevated to levels of 80 to 240 IU. A diffuse but mild elevation of the gamma globulin fraction is common. In some patients mild and transient steatorrhea has been noted as well as slight microscopic hematuria and minimal proteinuria.

A number of serologic tests are available to establish a diagnosis of type B or type A hepatitis. After infection with HBV, the first serologic marker detectable in serum is HBsAg. Circulating HBsAg precedes elevations in serum aminotransferase activity and clinical symptoms (Fig. 318-3) and remains detectable during the entire icteric phase of acute hepatitis B and beyond. In typical cases, HBsAg becomes undetectable 1 to 2 months following the onset of jaundice; HBs antigenemia rarely lasts longer than 6 months. Infrequently, levels of HBsAg are too low to be detected during acute HBV infection; in these approximately 10 percent of cases, tests for anti-HBc and anti-HBs during acute illness and convalescence may help establish the diagnosis of hepatitis B.

The titer of HBsAg bears little relationship to the severity of clinical disease. Indeed, there is an inverse correlation between the serum concentration of HBsAg and the degree of liver cell damage. Titers are *highest* in immunosuppressed patients and in normal carriers, lower in chronic liver disease (but higher in chronic persistent than in chronic active hepatitis), and *very low* in acute fulminant hepatitis. These observations suggest that in hepatitis B the degree of liver cell damage and the clinical course are probably related to variations in the patient's immune response to hepatitis B virus rather than to the amount of circulating HBsAg.

Another serologic indicator which may be of value in patients with hepatitis B is HBeAg. Its principal clinical usefulness is as an indicator of relative infectivity of the patient with hepatitis B.

Tests for fecal or serum hepatitis A virus are not routinely available. Therefore, a diagnosis of type A hepatitis is based on detection of anti-HAV of the IgM class (or rising titers of anti-HAV) (Fig. 318-2).

Because there are no serologic tests for non-A, non-B hepatitis, a diagnosis of non-A, non-B hepatitis is made by serologic exclusion of HAV and HBV infection in the setting of a compatible history.

PROGNOSIS Virtually all previously healthy patients with hepatitis A recover completely from their illness with no clinical sequelae. Similarly in acute hepatitis B, 90 percent of patients have a favorable course and recover completely. There are, however, certain clinical and laboratory features which suggest a more complicated and protracted course. Patients with advanced age and serious underlying medical disorders, such as congestive heart failure, severe anemia, diabetes mellitus, and malignancy, may have a prolonged course and are more likely to develop severe hepatitis. Initial presenting features such as ascites, peripheral edema, and symptoms of hepatic encephalopathy suggest a poorer prognosis. In addition, a prolonged prothrombin time, low serum albumin, hypoglycemia, and serum bilirubin values greater than 20 mg/dl suggest severe hepatocellular disease. Patients with these clinical and laboratory features deserve prompt hospital admission. The case fatality rate in hepatitis A and B is very low (<0.1 percent), but the case fatality rate in hepatitis A and B is significantly increased by age and underlying debilitating disorders. Non-A, non-B hepatitis is less severe in the acute phase than type B hepatitis and is more commonly anicteric, but the case fatality rate is not known.

COMPLICATIONS AND SEQUELAE During the prodromal phase of acute hepatitis B some patients may develop a serum sickness-like syndrome characterized by arthralgia or arthritis, rash, angioedema, and rarely hematuria and proteinuria. This syndrome occurs prior to the onset of clinical jaundice, and these patients are often erroneously diagnosed as having rheumatoid arthritis or other rheumatologic diseases such as systemic lupus erythematosus. This syndrome occurs in about 5 to 10 percent of hepatitis B patients. The diagnosis can be established by measuring the serum transaminase values, which are almost invariably elevated, and serum HBsAg.

The most feared complication of viral hepatitis is *fulminant hepatitis* (massive hepatic necrosis); fortunately this is a rare event. This is primarily seen in hepatitis B, less frequently in non-A, non-B hepatitis, and only occasionally in hepatitis A. Patients usually present with signs and symptoms of encephalopathy and, in fact, many progress to deep coma. The liver is usually small, and the prothrombin time excessively prolonged. The combination of a rapidly shrinking liver size, rapidly rising bilirubin levels, and significant prolongation of the prothrombin time, together with clinical signs of confusion, disorientation, somnolence, ascites, and edema indicates that the patient has hepatic failure with encephalopathy. Cerebral edema is common; evidence of brainstem compression as well as gastrointestinal bleeding, sepsis, respiratory failure, cardiovascular collapse, and renal failure are terminal events. The mortality is exceedingly high (greater than 80 percent in patients with deep coma), but patients who survive may have a complete biochemical and histologic recovery.

After acute type B hepatitis, approximately 10 percent of patients remain HBsAg-positive for more than 6 months. Most of these individuals clear the antigen from their circulation during the next several years, but a small percentage remain chronically HBsAg-positive. In their serum, anti-HBc is present in high titer, but anti-HBs is rarely detected. These patients may (1) be asymptomatic carriers, (2) have low-grade chronic persistent hepatitis, or (3) have chronic active hepatitis. The likelihood of becoming an HBsAg carrier after acute HBV infection is especially high among neonates, persons with Down's syndrome, chronically hemodialyzed patients, and other immunosuppressed patients. After non-A, non-B hepatitis, as many as 40 to 50 percent of patients with transfusion-associated disease, much less frequently in patients with sporadic hepatitis, will have biochemical indicators of abnormal liver function for more than a year. In contrast, hepatitis A virus infection does not cause chronic liver disease.

Chronic active hepatitis is a major late complication of acute hepatitis B occurring in approximately 3 percent of cases (see Chap. 319). This complication rarely, if ever, occurs after hepatitis A but may occur in patients with transfusion-associated, non-A, non-B hepatitis. Certain clinical and laboratory features suggest progression of acute hepatitis to chronic active hepatitis: (1) lack of complete resolution of clinical symptoms of anorexia, weight loss, and fatigue and the persistence of hepatomegaly; (2) the presence of "bridging" or multilobular hepatic necrosis on liver biopsy during protracted, severe acute viral hepatitis; (3) failure of the serum transaminase, bilirubin, and alkaline phosphatase levels to return to normal within 6 to 12 months following the acute illness; and (4) the *continued presence of HBsAg* 6 months or more after acute hepatitis, suggesting chronic viral infection of the liver.

Rare complications of viral hepatitis include pancreatitis, myocarditis, atypical pneumonia, aplastic anemia, transverse myelitis, and peripheral neuropathy. *Lifelong carriers* of HBsAg appear to have an enhanced risk of developing hepatocellular carcinoma (see Chap. 321). In children, hepatitis B may rarely present with anicteric hepatitis, a nonpruritic papular rash of the face, buttocks, and limbs, and lymphadenopathy (papular acrodermatitis of childhood or Gianotti-Crosti syndrome).

DIFFERENTIAL DIAGNOSIS Viral diseases such as infectious mononucleosis; those due to cytomegalovirus, herpes simplex, and coxsackievirus; and toxoplasmosis may share certain clinical features with viral hepatitis and cause elevation in the serum transaminase and less commonly the serum bilirubin levels. Tests such as the differential heterophile and serologic tests for these agents may be helpful in the differential diagnosis, if the HBsAg, anti-HBc, and IgM anti-HAV determinations are negative. A complete drug history is particularly important, for many drugs can produce either a picture of acute hepatitis or cholestasis (see below). Equally important is a past history of unexplained "repeated episodes" of acute hepatitis. This should alert the physician to the possibility that the underlying disorder is chronic active hepatitis. Alcoholic hepatitis must also be considered, but usually the serum transaminases are not as markedly elevated, other stigmata of alcoholism may be present, and the finding on liver biopsy of fatty infiltration, a neutrophilic inflammatory reaction, and "alcoholic hyalin" would be consistent with alcohol-induced rather than viral liver injury. Because acute hepatitis may present with right upper quadrant abdominal pain, nausea and vomiting, fever and icterus, it is often confused with acute cholecystitis, common duct stone, or ascending cholangitis. Patients with acute viral hepatitis tolerate surgery poorly; therefore it is important to exclude this diagnosis, and a percutaneous liver biopsy may be necessary prior to laparotomy. Viral hepatitis in the elderly is often misdiagnosed as obstructive jaundice due to common duct stone or carcinoma of the pancreas. Because acute hepatitis in the elderly may be quite severe and the operative mortality high, a thorough evaluation including laboratory tests, radiographic studies of the biliary tree, and even liver biopsy may be necessary to exclude primary parenchymal liver disease. Another clinical constellation that may mimic acute hepatitis is right ventricular failure with passive hepatic congestion. Physical examination is usually sufficient to distinguish between the two entities.

MANAGEMENT AND PREVENTION **Treatment of acute attack** There is no specific treatment for *typical acute viral hepatitis.* Hospitalization may be required to establish the correct diagnosis, for clinically severe illness, and for the elderly patient because of the high mortality. Most patients, however, do not require hospitalization. Forced and prolonged bed rest is not essential for full recovery, but many patients will feel better with restricted physical activity. A high-calorie diet is desirable, and because many patients may experience nausea late in the day, the major caloric intake is best tolerated in the morning. Intravenous feeding is necessary in the acute stage if the patient has persistent vomiting and cannot maintain oral intake. Drugs capable of producing adverse reactions such as cholestasis or those metabolized by the liver should be avoided. If significant pruritus is present, the use of a bile-salt-sequestering resin, such as cholestyramine, will usually alleviate this symptom. Corticosteroid therapy has no value in uncomplicated typical acute viral hepatitis.

Physical isolation of patients with hepatitis to a single room and bathroom is rarely necessary except in the case of fecal incontinence for hepatitis A, or uncontrolled, voluminous bleeding for hepatitis types B and non-A, non-B. Because most patients hospitalized with hepatitis A excrete little if any HAV, the likelihood of HAV transmission from these patients during their hospitalization is low. Therefore, burdensome enteric precautions are no longer recommended. Although gloves should be worn when handling the bedpans or fecal material of patients with hepatitis A, these precautions do not represent a departure from sensible procedure for all hospitalized patients. For patients with types B and non-A, non-B hepatitis, emphasis should be placed on blood precautions, i.e., avoiding direct, ungloved hand contact with blood and other body fluids. Enteric precautions for these agents are unnecessary. The importance of simple hygienic precautions, such as hand washing, cannot be overemphasized.

Patients may be discharged from the hospital when there is substantial symptomatic improvement, a significant downward trend in the serum transaminase and bilirubin values, and normal prothrombin time. Mild transaminase elevations should not be considered contraindications to the gradual resumption of normal activity.

For patients with acute *severe clinical hepatitis,* or "bridging necrosis," corticosteroid therapy has often been used; however, controlled studies have failed to demonstrate the effectiveness of steroids in treating this form of severe hepatitis and have suggested that steroid therapy may, in fact, be hazardous to some patients.

In *fulminant hepatitis,* the goal of therapy is to support the patient by maintenance of fluid balance and an open airway, support of circulation, control of bleeding, correction of hypoglycemia, and treatment of other complications of the comatose state in anticipation of liver regeneration and repair. Protein intake should be restricted and oral neomycin or lactulose administered, but such therapy has been shown in controlled trials to be ineffective. Massive doses of corticosteroids have been administered. Likewise, exchange transfusion, plasmapheresis, human cross-circulation, porcine liver cross-perfusion, and hemoperfusion have not been proved to enhance survival.

Hazards to medical and paramedical personnel Sporadic outbreaks of acute viral hepatitis, primarily type B, have been reported in blood bank employees, laboratory technicians, nurses, physicians, and dentists. Exposure to hepatitis viruses may result from contact with blood or other body fluids by pipeting, starting and maintaining intravenous cannulas, drawing blood, changing surgical dressings, emptying bedpans, caring for catheters, handling surgical instruments and pathologic specimens, and other patient care procedures. Defective gloves are common after long surgical procedures, and point source epidemics of acute hepatitis B have been reported among surgeons. Similarly, outbreaks of acute hepatitis have occurred in physicians and nurses working in hemodialysis and oncology units and in clinical laboratory employees; prevalence of exposure to hepatitis B in such health care settings is related directly to the extent of contact with blood or body fluids rather than with patients per se.

Approximately 15 to 20 percent of health care workers have one or more serologic markers of HBV infection, and 1 percent are HBsAg-positive. Transmission of HBV infection in health care settings, however, appears to be unidirectional from patients to staff. Most evidence collected to date suggests that, with rare exceptions, HBsAg-positive health care workers do not increase the risk of HBV infection for their patient contacts.

Asymptomatic HBsAg-positive carriers represent the greatest risk to health personnel because there are no readily identifiable clinical features, such as jaundice, that allow recognition and subsequent precautionary measures. Approximately 1 percent of all admissions to large metropolitan hospitals are HBsAg-positive, but 90 percent of these are not identified routinely. Patients with a past history of hepatitis or multiple transfusions; patients from areas of the world where hepatitis B is endemic; and those with parenteral drug abuse, chronic liver disease, chronic renal failure, leukemia, Hodgkin's disease, polyarteritis nodosa, Down's syndrome, and leprosy should have routine HBsAg determinations performed because of the high frequency of the HBsAg carrier state in these groups. If positive, they should be treated as potentially infectious, and appropriate precautions should be employed during operative or other acute care procedures. In dialysis units introduction of patient and staff education, routine periodic screening for HBsAg and transaminase elevations, and segregation of HBsAg-positive from susceptible patients have greatly reduced the incidence of hepatitis in both patients and medical personnel.

Prophylaxis All preparations of immune globulin (IG) contain anti-HAV, although the titers may vary. When administered before exposure or during the early incubation period, IG is effective in preventing clinically apparent type A hepatitis. In some cases, IG does not abort infection but, by ameliorating it, renders it inapparent. As a result long-lasting "passive-active" immunity occurs; however, this is now considered to be the exception rather than the rule. For intimate contacts (household, institutional) of hepatitis A patients, administration of 0.02 ml/kg is recommended. It is not necessary for casual contacts (office, factory, school, hospital) nor for elderly individuals who are almost invariably immune. By the time common-source outbreaks of type A hepatitis are recognized, it is usually too late in the incubation period for IG to be effective; however, prophylaxis may prevent illness in secondary cases. For travelers to tropical and developing countries, IG prophylaxis is recommended. When such travel lasts less than 3 months, 0.02 ml/kg is given; for longer travel, a dose of 0.05 ml/kg every 4 to 6 months is recommended.

For passive immunoprophylaxis against hepatitis B, both standard IG (with very modest levels of anti-HBs) and a high anti-HBs titer hepatitis B immune globulin (HBIG) have been evaluated. Currently HBIG is recommended for postexposure prophylaxis of persons who have sustained an accidental needle stick with or who have ingested HBsAg-positive material. A dose of 0.06 ml/kg is given as soon after exposure as possible. This dose should be repeated 1 month later. Although official recommendations are lacking, most authorities advise postexposure prophylaxis with HBIG for the spouse or other sexual contact of a patient with acute type B hepatitis. In the only study reported, one dose of HBIG was superior to one dose of IG. Postexposure prophylaxis with HBIG is also recommended for infants born to HBsAg-positive mothers. *Immediately after birth,* these infants should receive 0.5 ml of HBIG intramuscularly, and the same dose should be repeated at 3 and 6 months of age. For preexposure prophylaxis against hepatitis B in endemic settings (e.g., travel to endemic areas, staff and patients of custodial institutions for the developmentally handicapped, hemodialysis patients and staff), IG is as effective as HBIG in preventing acute infection. In these settings, however, environmental and hygienic measures may be sufficient to abort hepatitis B virus transmission. When this is not the case, however, IG should be given at a dose of 0.05 to 0.07 ml/kg at 4-month intervals. Anti-HBs-positive persons require no immunoprophylaxis. All these indications for globulins are being reevaluated since active immunization with an HBV vaccine has become available. Immunogenicity, safety, and efficacy trials have been conducted with a vaccine prepared from purified, noninfectious 22-nm spherical forms of HBsAg derived from the plasma of chronic carriers. The vaccine has been shown to be safe and highly effective in preventing the transmission of HBV infection in high-risk populations.

For non-A, non-B hepatitis the effectiveness of IG prophylaxis has not been demonstrated consistently. The only effective measures thus far which have reduced posttransfusion hepatitis are elimination of commercially obtained blood and screening for HBsAg. Screening donor blood for ALT, as noted above, may also be useful in reducing the frequency of transfusion-associated non-A, non-B hepatitis.

COMMON PROBLEMS IN CLINICAL PRACTICE Expert opinion is divided regarding the *indications for liver biopsy* in the hospitalized patient with acute viral hepatitis. Most agree, however, that a liver biopsy is indicated when there is (1) a question about the diagnosis or (2) clinical evidence suggesting chronic active hepatitis. Liver biopsy should be performed only by physicians thoroughly familiar with this procedure in order to ensure adequate tissue for pathologic examination and to minimize the risk to the patient.

Serum HBsAg may persist for variable periods of time or indefinitely following hepatitis B infection. For example, immunosuppressed transplant recipients and patients with myeloproliferative and lymphoproliferative disorders are particularly susceptible to the acquisition of HBsAg from repeated blood transfusions; 10 to 30 percent of these patients become carriers of HBsAg but may have little, if any, clinical evidence of liver disease. In contrast, the occasional persistence of HBsAg following acute icteric or anicteric hepatitis in normal individuals may be associated with the development of chronic liver disease. Therefore, it is particularly important to document the disappearance of serum HBsAg following apparent clinical recovery from acute hepatitis B. If HBsAg is detectable 6 to 12 months after acute hepatitis B, and serum transaminases remain elevated, a liver biopsy may be indicated to exclude the development of chronic active hepatitis and differentiate this disorder from chronic persistent hepatitis (see Chap. 319) or asymptomatic HBsAg carriage with normal liver morphology.

Routine screening of blood donors by blood banks has identified numerous carriers of HBsAg who are often then referred to a physician for evaluation. Typically, such individuals are asymptomatic and have no signs of liver disease on physical examination. Liver function studies are either normal or show only mild abnormalities. Follow-up examinations will establish whether the patient is in the early prodrome of anicteric or icteric acute hepatitis B. If, however, there is evidence on clinical examination of chronic liver disease and abnormal liver function tests, a diagnostic liver biopsy should be performed. If the patient is entirely asymptomatic with a normal examination and liver function tests are normal on several separate determinations, then the patient is probably a chronic carrier of HBsAg, and liver biopsy is not necessarily indicated, since progression to chronic liver disease is very unusual. In asymptomatic patients with mild elevations in the serum transaminase or alkaline phosphatase, bilirubin, and gamma globulin determinations, a liver biopsy may be indicated to exclude chronic active hepatitis.

TOXIC AND DRUG-INDUCED HEPATITIS

Liver injury may follow the inhalation, ingestion, or parenteral administration of a number of chemical agents. These include industrial toxins (e.g., carbon tetrachloride, trichloroethylene, yellow phosphorus), the toxic cyclic peptides of certain species of *Amanita* and *Galerina* (mushroom poisoning), and, more commonly, pharmacologic agents used in medical therapy. It is essential that any patient presenting with jaundice or impaired liver function be questioned carefully about exposure to chemicals used in work or at home and drugs taken by prescription or bought "over the counter." In general, two major types of chemical hepatotoxicity have been recognized: (1) direct toxic and (2) idiosyncratic.

As shown in Table 318-3, toxic hepatitis is one which occurs with predictable regularity in individuals exposed to the offending agent and is dose-dependent. The latent period between exposure and liver injury is usually short (often several hours), although clinical manifestations may be delayed for 24 to 48 h. Agents producing toxic hepatitis are generally systemic poisons or are converted in the liver to toxic metabolites. The direct hepatotoxins result in morphologic abnormalities which are reasonably characteristic and reproducible for each toxin. For example, carbon tetrachloride and trichloroethylene characteristically produce a centrilobular zonal necrosis, whereas yellow phosphorus poisoning typically results in periportal injury. *Amanita phalloides* toxin usually produces massive hepatic necrosis. Tetracycline, when administered in intravenous doses greater than 1.5 g daily, leads to microvesicular fat deposits in the liver. Liver injury is often only one facet of the toxicity produced by the direct hepatotoxins, and it may go unrecognized until jaundice appears.

In idiosyncratic drug reactions the occurrence of hepatitis is usually infrequent and unpredictable, the response is not dose-dependent and may occur at any time during or shortly after exposure to the drug. Idiosyncratic reactions may be due to unique host susceptibility (metabolic reactivity) to specific agents or may be immunologically mediated. Immunologic evidence of classic hypersensitivity mechanisms (i.e., the demonstration of specific circulating or tissue-fixing antibodies) is not available. Similarly, a role for lymphocyte-mediated immune mechanisms in drug-induced hepatitis has been postulated but not proved. However, extrahepatic manifestations of hypersensitivity are common in some drug reactions and include arthralgias, rashes, fever, leukocytosis, and eosinophilia. Idiosyncratic reactions lead to a morphologic pattern that is more variable than those produced by direct toxins; a single agent is often capable of causing a variety of lesions, although certain patterns tend to predominate. Depending on the agent involved, idiosyncratic hepatitis may result in a clinical and morphologic picture indistinguishable from viral hepatitis (e.g., halothane) or may clinically simulate extrahepatic bile duct obstruction with morphologic evidence of cholestasis and minimal hepatocellular damage (e.g., chlorpromazine). Morphologic alterations may also include bridging hepatic necrosis (e.g., methyldopa), or, infrequently, hepatic granulomas (e.g., sulfonamides).

Not all adverse hepatic drug reactions can be described as either toxic or idiosyncratic in type. For example, oral contraceptives, which combine estrogenic and progestational com-

TABLE 318-3
Some features of toxic and drug-induced hepatic injury

	Direct toxic effect		*Idiosyncratic*			*Other*
Features	*(Carbon tetrachloride, e.g.)*	*(Acetaminophen, e.g.)*	*(Halothane, e.g.)*	*(Isoniazid, e.g.)*	*(Chlorpromazine, e.g.)*	*(Oral contraceptive agents, e.g.)*
Predictable and dose-related toxicity	+	+	0	0	0	+
Latent period	Short	Short	Variable	Variable	Variable	Variable
Arthralgia, fever, rash, eosinophilia	0	0	+	0	+	0
Liver morphology	Necrosis, fatty infiltration	Centrilobular necrosis	Similar to viral hepatitis	Similar to viral hepatitis	Cholestasis *with* portal inflammation	Cholestasis *without* portal inflammation

pounds, may result in impairment of hepatic function and occasionally in jaundice. However they do not produce necrosis or fatty change (in lower species), manifestations of hypersensitivity are generally absent, but genetic susceptibility to the development of oral contraceptive–induced cholestasis is well documented.

Because viral hepatitis is often a presumptive diagnosis and many adverse drug reactions produce a clinicopathologic picture resembling it, evidence of a causal relationship between the use of a drug and subsequent liver injury may be most difficult. The relation is most convincing for the direct hepatotoxins for which the frequency of hepatic impairment is usually high and the latent period between the start of therapy and impaired function is short. Idiosyncratic reactions may be reproduced, in some instances, when rechallenge, after an asymptomatic period, results in a recurrence of signs, symptoms, and morphologic and biochemical abnormalities. Rechallenge is often ethically unfeasible, and documentation of adverse hepatic reactions must often await the collection of other clinical cases.

Treatment of toxic and drug-induced hepatic disease is largely supportive as in acute viral hepatitis. Withdrawal of the suspected agent is indicated at the first sign of an adverse reaction. In the case of the direct toxins, liver involvement should not divert attention from renal or other organ involvement which may also threaten survival.

In Table 318-4, several classes of chemical agents are listed together with examples of the pattern of liver injury produced by them. It should be noted that certain drugs appear to be responsible for the development of chronic as well as acute hepatic injury. For example, oxyphenisatin, α-methyldopa, and isoniazid have been associated with chronic active hepatitis, and halothane and methotrexate have been implicated in the development of cirrhosis. A syndrome resembling primary biliary cirrhosis has been described following treatment with chlorpromazine, methyl testosterone, tolbutamide, and other drugs. Portal hypertension in the absence of cirrhosis may result from alterations in hepatic architecture produced by vitamin A or arsenic intoxication, industrial exposure to vinyl chloride, or administration of thorium dioxide (Thorotrast). The latter three agents have also been associated with angiosarcoma of the liver. Oral contraceptives have been implicated in the development of hepatic adenoma and, rarely, hepatic cell carcinoma and occlusion of the hepatic vein. Another unusual lesion, peliosis hepatis (blood cysts of the liver), has been observed in some patients treated with oral contraceptives or anabolic steroids. The existence of these hepatic disorders expands the spectrum of liver injury induced by chemical agents and emphasizes the need for a thorough drug history in all patients with liver dysfunction.

The following are the patterns of adverse hepatic reactions for some prototypic agents.

ACETAMINOPHEN HEPATOTOXICITY (DIRECT TOXIN) Acetaminophen (Tylenol), an analgesic and antipyretic that is available without a prescription, has caused severe centrilobular hepatic necrosis when ingested in large amounts in suicide attempts or accidently by children. A single dose of 10 to 15 g, occasionally less, may produce clinical evidence of liver injury. Fatal fulminant disease is usually associated with ingestion of 25 g or more, although not invariably. Blood levels of acetaminophen correlate with the severity of hepatic injury (levels above 300 μg/ml at 4 h after ingestion are predictive of the development of severe damage). Nausea, vomiting, diarrhea, abdominal pain, and shock are early manifestations occurring 4 to 12 h after ingestion. Twenty-four to forty-eight hours later, when these features are abating, hepatic injury becomes apparent. Maximal abnormalities and hepatic failure may not be evident until 4 to 6 days after ingestion. Renal failure and myocardial injury may be present.

Acetaminophen hepatotoxicity is mediated by a toxic reactive metabolite formed from the parent compound by the cytochrome P_{450} mixed-function oxidase system of the hepatocyte. This metabolite is detoxified by binding to glutathione. When excessive amounts of the metabolite are formed, glutathione levels in liver fall, and the metabolite is covalently bound to nucleophilic hepatocyte macromolecules. The latter process is believed to lead to hepatocyte necrosis; the precise sequence and mechanism are unknown. Hepatic injury may be potentiated by prior administration of alcohol or other drugs which stimulate the mixed-function oxidase system, or alternately by conditions, such as starvation, which reduce hepatic glutathione levels.

Treatment of acetaminophen overdosage includes gastric lavage, supportive measures, and oral administration of acti-

TABLE 318-4
Principal alterations of hepatic morphology produced by some commonly used drugs and chemicals

Principal morphologic change	*Class of agent*	*Example*
Cholestasis	Anabolic steroid	Methyl testosterone*
	Antithyroid	Methimazole
	Chemotherapeutic	Erythromycin estolate
	Oral contraceptive	Norethynodrel with mestranol
	Oral hypoglycemic	Chlorpropamide
	Tranquilizer	Chlorpromazine*
Fatty liver	Chemotherapeutic	Tetracycline
Hepatitis	Anesthetic	Halothane†
	Anticonvulsant	Phenytoin
	Antihypertensive	Methyldopa†
	Chemotherapeutic	Isoniazid†
	Diuretic	Chlorothiazide
	Laxative	Oxyphenisatin†
Toxic (necrosis)	Hydrocarbon	Carbon tetrachloride
	Metal	Yellow phosphorus
	Mushroom	*Amanita phalloides*
	Analgesic	Acetaminophen

* *Rarely associated with primary biliary cirrhosis-like lesion.*
† *Occasionally associated with chronic active hepatitis or bridging hepatic necrosis and cirrhosis.*

vated charcoal or cholestyramine to prevent absorption of residual drug. Neither of the latter agents appears to be effective if given more than 30 min after acetaminophen ingestion; if they are used, the stomach should be lavaged before other agents are administered orally. In patients with high acetaminophen blood levels, measured 4 to 10 h after ingestion, the administration of sulfhydryl compounds (e.g., cysteamine, cysteine, or *N*-acetylcysteine) within 12 h of ingestion appears to reduce the severity of hepatic necrosis. These agents act either by repleting hepatic glutathione, binding the reactive metabolite, or inhibiting its production. Late administration of sulfhydryl compounds is of uncertain value.

Although survivors of acute acetaminophen overdose usually have no evidence of hepatic sequelae, in a few patients prolonged or repeated administration of acetaminophen in therapeutic doses has led to the development of chronic active hepatitis and cirrhosis.

HALOTHANE HEPATOTOXICITY (IDIOSYNCRATIC REACTION) Halothane, a nonexplosive fluorinated hydrocarbon anesthetic agent, structurally similar to chloroform, has been reported to result in severe hepatic necrosis in a small number of individuals, many of whom have previously been exposed to this agent. The failure to produce similar hepatic lesions in animals, the rarity of the hepatic impairment in humans, and the delayed appearance of hepatic injury suggest that halothane is not a direct hepatotoxin but may be a sensitizing agent. However, manifestations of hypersensitivity are seen in fewer than 25 percent of cases. A genetic predisposition leading to an idiosyncratic metabolic reactivity has been postulated. Adults, obese people, and women appear to be particularly susceptible to halothane-induced injury. Fever, moderate leukocytosis, and eosinophilia may occur in the first week following halothane administration. Jaundice usually is noted 7 to 10 days after exposure but may occur earlier in previously exposed patients. Nausea and vomiting may precede the onset of jaundice. Hepatomegaly is often mild, but liver tenderness is common. The serum transaminases are elevated. The pathologic changes at autopsy are indistinguishable from massive hepatic necrosis due to viral hepatitis. The case fatality rate of halothane hepatitis is not known but may vary from 20 to 40 percent in cases with severe liver involvement. In rare instances cirrhosis has been observed following repeated bouts of halothane hepatitis. It is strongly suggested that patients in whom unexplained spiking fever, especially delayed fever, or jaundice develops after halothane anesthesia not receive this agent again. Because cross-reactions between halothane and methoxyfluorane have been reported, the latter agent should probably not be used after halothane reactions.

METHYLDOPA HEPATOTOXICITY (TOXIC AND IDIOSYNCRATIC REACTION) Minor alterations in liver tests are reported in about 5 percent of patients treated with this antihypertensive agent. These trivial abnormalities typically resolve despite continued drug administration. In less than 1 percent of patients acute liver injury, resembling viral hepatitis or chronic active hepatitis, or rarely a cholestatic reaction is seen 1 to 20 weeks after methyldopa is started. In 50 percent of cases the interval is less than 4 weeks. A prodrome of fever, anorexia, and malaise may be noted for a few days before the onset of jaundice. Rash, lymphadenopathy, arthralgia, and eosinophilia are rare. Serologic markers of autoimmunity are infrequently detected, and less than 5 percent of patients have a Coombs-positive hemolytic anemia. In about 15 percent of patients with methyldopa hepatotoxicity the clinical, biochemical, and histological features are those of chronic active hepatitis with or without bridging necrosis and macronodular cirrhosis. With discontinuation of the drug the disorder usually resolves, although progression has been seen in a few patients.

ISONIAZID HEPATOTOXICITY (TOXIC AND IDIOSYNCRATIC REACTION) Approximately 10 percent of patients treated with the antituberculosis agent isoniazid will develop elevated serum transaminase levels during the first few weeks of therapy; this appears to represent a toxic reaction to a metabolite of the drug. Whether or not isoniazid is continued, these values (usually < 200 units) return to normal in a few weeks. About 1 percent of treated patients develop an illness indistinguishable from viral hepatitis; approximately half of these occur within the first 2 months of treatment, while in the remainder clinical disease may be delayed for many months. Liver biopsy reveals morphologic changes similar to viral hepatitis or bridging hepatic necrosis. The disease may be severe, with a case fatality rate of 10 percent. Important liver injury appears to be age-related; the highest frequency is in patients over age 50, the lowest under the age of 20. Fever, rash, eosinophilia, and other manifestations of drug allergy are distinctly unusual. A correlation of liver injury with rapid acetylation of isoniazid has been suggested. A picture resembling chronic active hepatitis has been observed in a few patients.

CHLORPROMAZINE HEPATOTOXICITY (CHOLESTATIC IDIOSYNCRATIC REACTION) In about 1 percent of patients receiving chlorpromazine, intrahepatic cholestasis with jaundice develops after 1 to 4 weeks of treatment. In rare instances, jaundice has been reported after a single exposure. Anicteric reactions are frequent. The onset may be abrupt with fever, rash, arthralgias, lymphadenopathy, nausea, vomiting, and epigastric or right upper quadrant pain. Pruritus may precede the appearance of jaundice, dark urine, and light stools. Eosinophilia with or without mild leukocytosis may be present, and conjugated hyperbilirubinemia, moderately elevated serum alkaline phosphatase, and mildly elevated serum transaminase levels (100 to 200 units) are noted. Liver biopsy reveals cholestasis, bile plugs in dilated bile canaliculi, and a dense portal infiltrate of polymorphonuclear, eosinophilic, and mononuclear leukocytes. Occasionally, scattered foci of hepatic parenchymal necrosis may be evident. Jaundice and pruritus usually subside within 4 to 8 weeks following cessation of therapy, without sequelae, and fatalities are rare. Cholestyramine may be of value in relieving severe pruritus. In a small number of patients, jaundice is prolonged for several months to years; rarely, a disorder resembling primary biliary cirrhosis may develop.

ORAL CONTRACEPTIVE HEPATOTOXICITY (CHOLESTATIC REACTION) The administration of oral contraceptive combinations of estrogenic and progestational steroids results in significant BSP retention in a high proportion of patients, and, to a far lesser extent, elevation of serum alkaline phosphatase. Weeks to months after taking these agents, intrahepatic cholestasis with pruritus and jaundice is noted in a small number of patients. Especially susceptible seem to be patients with recurrent idiopathic jaundice of pregnancy, severe pruritus of pregnancy, or a family history of these disorders. Laboratory studies, with the exception of liver function tests, are normal, and extrahepatic manifestations of hypersensitivity are absent. Liver biopsy reveals cholestasis with bile plugs in dilated canaliculi and striking bilirubin staining of liver cells. In contrast to chlorpromazine-induced cholestasis, portal inflammation is absent. The lesion is reversible on withdrawal of the agent, and sequelae have not been reported. The two steroid components appear to act synergistically on hepatic function, although the estrogen may be primarily responsible. Oral contraceptives are contraindicated in patients with a history of recurrent jaundice of pregnancy. As indicated above, neoplasms of the liver and hepatic vein occlusion have also been associated with oral contraceptive therapy.

17,α-ALKYL-SUBSTITUTED ANABOLIC STEROIDS (CHOLESTATIC REACTION) The majority of patients receiving these agents, used mainly in the treatment of bone marrow failure, develop mild hepatic dysfunction. Impaired excretory function is the predominant defect, but the precise mechanism is uncertain. Only a minority of patients develop jaundice, which appears to be dose-related. Jaundice may be the sole clinical manifestation of hepatotoxicity, although anorexia, nausea, and malaise are described in some patients. Pruritus is not a prominent feature. Serum transaminases are usually less than 100 units, and serum alkaline phosphatase levels are normal, mildly elevated, or, in less than 5 percent of patients, three or more times the upper value of normal. Examination of liver tissue reveals cholestasis without inflammation or necrosis. Hepatic sinusoidal dilatation and peliosis hepatitis have been found in a few patients. The cholestatic disorder is usually reversible on cessation of treatment, although fatalities have been linked to peliosis. An association with hepatic adenoma and hepatocellular carcinoma has been reported.

REFERENCES

Viral hepatitis

ALTER HJ (ed): Hepatitis B. Semin Liver Dis 1:1, 1981

DIENSTAG JL et al: Hepatitis A virus infection: New insights from seroepidemiologic studies. J Infect Dis 137:328, 1978

———: Non-A, non-B hepatitis. Adv Intern Med 26:187, 1980

———, ISSELBACHER KJ: Therapy of acute and chronic hepatitis. Arch Intern Med 141:1419, 1981

FAVERO MS et al: Guidelines for the care of patients hospitalized with viral hepatitis. Ann Intern Med 91:872, 1979

GREGORY PB et al: Steroid therapy in severe viral hepatitis: A double blind, randomized trial of methyl-prednisolone versus placebo. N Engl J Med 294:681, 1976

IMMUNIZATION PRACTICES ADVISORY COMMITTEE: Immune globulins for protection against viral hepatitis. Ann Intern Med 96:193, 1982

KOFF RS: *Viral Hepatitis.* New York, Wiley, 1978

ROBINSON WS: The enigma of non-A, non-B hepatitis. J Infect Dis 145:387, 1982

SEEFF LB, HOOFNAGLE JH: Immunoprophylaxis of viral hepatitis. Gastroenterol 77:161, 1979

SZMUNESS W et al: Hepatitis B vaccine: Demonstration of efficacy in a controlled clinical trial in a high-risk population in the United States. N Engl J Med 303:833, 1980

——— et al (eds): *Viral Hepatitis: 1981 International Symposium.* Philadelphia, Franklin Institute Press, 1982

WANDS JR et al: Immunodiagnosis of hepatitis B with high-affinity IgM monoclonal antibodies. Proc Natl Acad Sci USA 78:1214, 1981

Drug-induced hepatitis

BLACK M et al: Isoniazid-associated hepatitis in 114 patients. Gastroenterology 69:389, 1975

ISHAK KG, IREY NS: Hepatic injury associated with the phenothiazines: Clinicopathologic and follow-up study of 36 patients. Arch Pathol 93:283, 1972

MITCHELL JR, JOLLOW DJ: Metabolic activation of drugs to toxic substances. Gastroenterology 68:392, 1975

ZIMMERMAN HJ: *Hepatotoxicity.* New York, Appleton-Century-Crofts, 1978

——— (ed): Drug-induced liver disease. Semin Liver Dis 1:91, 1981

319 CHRONIC ACTIVE HEPATITIS

JACK R. WANDS
RAYMOND S. KOFF
KURT J. ISSELBACHER

DEFINITION Chronic active hepatitis is a disorder of diverse etiologies characterized by continuing hepatic necrosis, active inflammation, and fibrosis which may lead to or be accompanied by cirrhosis. While signs and symptoms of chronic liver disease are typical, manifestations of systemic involvement are common, and extrahepatic features and seroimmunologic abnormalities may dominate the clinical presentation. The prominence of these manifestations has led to the use of a variety of terms to describe this disorder. These terms include autoimmune hepatitis, lupoid hepatitis, acute juvenile cirrhosis, plasma cell hepatitis, subacute hepatitis, and chronic active liver disease. Chronic active hepatitis seems to be the most appropriate designation for this clinicopathologic entity, regardless of the etiology and the clinical variations.

PATHOLOGY Although chronic active hepatitis may be suspected from the clinical history and the physical findings, *liver biopsy is necessary to establish the diagnosis.* The cardinal histopathologic features observed in the liver include (1) a dense mononuclear and plasma cell infiltration of the portal zones which greatly expands these areas with extension of the inflammatory infiltrate into the liver lobule; (2) destruction of the hepatocytes at the periphery of the lobule (so-called piecemeal necrosis) with erosion of the limiting plate surrounding the portal triads; (3) connective tissue septa extending from the portal zones into the lobule, isolating parenchymal cells into clusters and enveloping bile ducts; and (4) evidence of hepatic regeneration with "rosette" formation, thickened liver-cell plates, and regenerative "pseudolobules." This process may be patchy, and individual liver lobules may remain uninvolved. Councilman-like bodies, which represent necrosis of single liver cells, may be seen in the periportal areas. The lesion of bridging hepatic necrosis may be seen in some patients with chronic active hepatitis. This lesion or its more extensive variant, multilobular bridging hepatic necrosis, suggests the presence of severe disease.

There is substantial morphologic evidence that in some instances chronic active hepatitis will progress to or is accompanied by the development of cirrhosis. On liver biopsy, cirrhosis can be demonstrated in 20 to 50 percent of patients, even early in the course of the disease, and at autopsy postnecrotic cirrhosis may be found. It is also possible that many cases of so-called cryptogenic cirrhosis are the result of chronic active hepatitis after inflammation and necrosis have subsided. In other patients fibrosis is not progressive and morphologic evidence of cirrhosis cannot be found.

Chronic persistent hepatitis is often confused with chronic active hepatitis. While the clinical features of chronic persistent and chronic active hepatitis may be somewhat similar, the important distinction between these two entities is that chronic persistent hepatitis rarely if ever progresses to cirrhosis or produces portal hypertension or parenchymal liver failure. The diagnosis can be established with certainty only by liver biopsy. In typical chronic persistent hepatitis there is infiltration of the portal areas with mononuclear cells, but there is no erosion of the limiting plate (piecemeal necrosis) or extension of the inflammation into the liver lobule. A "cobblestone" arrangement of liver cells, indicative of hepatic regenerative activity, is a common feature. Minimal fibrosis may be observed, but cirrhosis is characteristically absent. The morphologic features of chronic active hepatitis and chronic persistent hepatitis are compared in Table 319-1.

ETIOLOGY Multiple etiologic agents may initiate chronic active hepatitis. Probably the most important and common triggering factors are infection with hepatitis B virus or the non-A, non-B hepatitis viruses. In about one-third of patients the disease begins abruptly following an illness typical of acute viral hepatitis. Persistence of the hepatitis B surface antigen (HBsAg) in the serum is found in 20 to 30 percent of patients with chronic active hepatitis, suggesting that persistent hepatitis B virus infection may be related to the development of chronic active hepatitis. Many of these HBsAg-positive patients also have positive tests for the hepatitis B e antigen (HBeAg) (see Chap. 318). Similarly persistent non-A, non-B hepatitis virus infections may be responsible for cases of chronic active hepatitis following transfusion-associated and sporadic non-A, non-B hepatitis. Furthermore, the transition of hepatitis B–induced bridging hepatic necrosis (see Chap. 318) to chronic active hepatitis has been observed, and infection by non-A, non-B agents may be involved in the pathogenesis of some cases of chronic active hepatitis observed in immunosuppressed renal transplant recipients. Drugs are involved in the pathogenesis of some cases. Features typical of chronic active hepatitis have been found in some patients in association with the ingestion of laxative preparations containing oxyphenisatin. In these patients challenge with oxyphenisatin has led to increased activity of the disease, while discontinuance has resulted in clinical, biochemical, and histologic improvement. Methyldopa, isoniazid, nitrofurantoin, and other drugs have also been incriminated as etiologic agents in a few patients with chronic active hepatitis. Thus, chemical as well as viral agents may play a role in the production of chronic active hepatitis. The existence of other triggering factors seems likely, but their nature and mechanisms of action remain to be determined.

IMMUNOPATHOGENESIS There is increasing evidence that the progressive parenchymal-cell destruction in patients with chronic active hepatitis involves an interaction with the immune system conditioned or controlled by genetic factors. Evidence to support this concept includes the following facts: (1) In the liver the histopathologic lesions are composed predominantly of *small lymphocytes* and plasma cells in association with progressive liver-cell destruction and replacement by fibrous tissue. (2) A variety of circulating "autoantibodies" are frequently detected, such as anti-smooth-muscle, antimitochondrial, and antithyroid antibodies (see Table 319-2). (3) The persistence of HBsAg in the serum and the hepatitis B core antigen (HBcAg) in the liver cell following an attack of acute hepatitis B is frequently associated with the development of chronic active or chronic persistent hepatitis. (4) Other "autoimmune" diseases such as thyroiditis, ulcerative colitis, Coombs-positive hemolytic anemia, proliferative glomerulonephritis, and Sjögren's syndrome may be associated with chronic active hepatitis or are observed in relatives of affected patients. (5) Histocompatibility antigen HLA-B1 or -B8 and DRw3 and DRw4 are more prevalent than expected in patients with chronic active hepatitis without HBsAg. (6) Finally, the use of corticosteroids, believed to be effective in a variety of immunologic and autoimmune disorders, is often beneficial in the treatment of severe chronic active hepatitis.

There is increasing evidence that cellular immune reactions may be important in the pathogenesis of chronic active hepatitis. It has been suggested that lymphocytes become sensitized to altered or new antigens present on the surface membranes of hepatocytes. This hypothesis is supported in part by studies demonstrating that circulating lymphocytes may have the capability of causing liver cell damage in vitro.

Humoral immune mechanisms may be responsible for some of the clinical manifestations of chronic active hepatitis. In particular, extrahepatic features such as arthralgias, arthritis, rash, and glomerulonephritis appear to be mediated by the deposition of circulating immune complexes. Furthermore, complement activation, as demonstrated by low serum complement levels, and the presence of complement components in immune complexes suggest that circulating immune complexes may be involved in mediating extrahepatic inflammation and tissue damage.

TABLE 319-1
Distinguishing features of chronic active and chronic persistent hepatitis

Features	*Chronic active hepatitis*	*Chronic persistent hepatitis*
Clinical:		
Onset like acute viral hepatitis	30%	70%
Recurrent acute episodes	Common	Infrequent
Extrahepatic involvement (e.g., arthralgias, pleuritis, colitis)	Common	Rare
Prognosis	Variable	Good
Liver histology:		
Piecemeal necrosis	Characteristic	Inconstant
Site of inflammation	Portal extending into lobule	Portal
Lobular architecture	Distorted	Preserved
Fibrosis	Common	Slight
Progression to cirrhosis	Common	Rare

CLINICAL FEATURES The clinical spectrum of chronic active hepatitis extends from asymptomatic illness at one end to fatal hepatic failure at the other. It affects all age groups, but chronic active hepatitis of undetermined etiology is more common in young women and adolescents. In approximately two-thirds of patients the disease has an *insidious onset* over a period of several weeks to months. In a number of individuals the disease is discovered incidentally, and the duration of the illness is uncertain. In the remainder an abrupt onset similar to acute viral hepatitis is seen, but features of chronic active hepatitis usually develop during the ensuing 12 to 24 months. The clinical and laboratory features suggesting progression from acute hepatitis to chronic active hepatitis are discussed in Chap. 318. *Fatigue* is a common symptom. Persistent or recurrent *jaundice* is noted in about 80 percent of typical cases. Intermittent deepening of jaundice and recurrent symptoms of *malaise, anorexia,* and *low-grade fever,* suggestive of a superimposed acute hepatitis, are common throughout the course of the illness. In some patients complications of cirrhosis, such as ascites, variceal bleeding, encephalopathy, coagulopathy, or hypersplenism, may first bring the patient to medical attention. In others the extrahepatic features dominate the clinical picture, and liver disease is entirely unsuspected. Extrahepatic presenting features may include amenorrhea, bloody diarrhea (due to associated ulcerative colitis), abdominal pain, arthralgia or arthritis, macular or papular eruptions, acne, erythema nodosum, pleurisy, pericarditis, anemia, azotemia, and sicca syndrome (of keratoconjunctivitis and xerostomia). These extrahepatic features and abnormal serologic reactions tend to be more frequent in women than men and in patients without serologic evidence of preceding hepatitis B.

The *course* of chronic active hepatitis is variable, and the disease may persist for long periods without clinically overt liver disease. This appears to be particularly true of chronic active hepatitis associated with hepatitis B or non-A, non-B hepatitis. The condition may occasionally remit into a clinically inactive phase, although continuing hepatocellular necrosis or progression to cirrhosis may also occur. The histologic lesion may reverse itself completely before the development of cirrhosis in some HBsAg-positive patients after their antigen-

TABLE 319-2
Serologic abnormalities in chronic active hepatitis

Serologic tests or reactions	*Frequency, %*
Increased serum IgG, IgM, IgA	50–70
Smooth-muscle antibodies	40–80
Antinuclear antibodies	20–50
Antimitochondrial antibodies	10–20
Lupus erythematosus (LE) cells	10–20
Rheumatoid factor	10–20
Heterophile reaction	5–10
Antigastric, antithyroid, antiadrenal antibodies	<5
False-positive syphilis test	<5

emia has spontaneously cleared or following the loss of HBeAg and the development of anti-HBe. If untreated, the case fatality rate may be high (50 to 75 percent) during the first few years of illness, especially in patients with clinically severe disease and histologically confirmed chronic active hepatitis with cirrhosis and in those with bridging or multilobular hepatic necrosis, when death occurs as a result of liver failure and hepatic coma. Later death is often due to a complication of cirrhosis—variceal hemorrhage or intercurrent infection. Primary hepatocellular carcinoma is an uncommon complication of HBsAg-negative chronic active hepatitis even when the disease has progressed to postnecrotic cirrhosis. This finding is in contrast to long-term HBsAg carriers with chronic active hepatitis and/or cirrhosis in whom the incidence of liver carcinoma is increased (see Chap. 317). In a small number of patients clinical and histologic features of primary biliary cirrhosis may be noted during the course of typical chronic active hepatitis. Thus there is a clinical similarity between these two liver disorders, particularly in the early phase of illness. In most instances, however, a clinical and histologic distinction between these conditions can eventually be made.

LABORATORY FINDINGS Liver function tests are invariably abnormal but may not correlate with the clinical severity or histopathologic findings in the individual case. In fact, some patients have normal serum bilirubin, alkaline phosphatase, and globulin determinations with only minimal transaminase (aminotransferase) elevations or HBsAg positivity and yet have a liver biopsy consistent with severe chronic active hepatitis. In typical cases the serum bilirubin is moderately elevated (3 to 10 mg/dl). Serum aspartate aminotransferase (SGOT) and alanine aminotransferase (SGPT) levels are increased and fluctuate in the range of 100 to 1000 units in most cases, although values as high as 4000 units have been reported.

The hepatitis B surface antigen may be found in 20 to 30 percent of patients with chronic active hepatitis and more commonly in men than women. Hypergammaglobulinemia (> 2.5 g/dl) is common, particularly in patients with extensive plasma-cell infiltration of the liver. Mild hypoalbuminemia occurs in patients with active disease or in those with advanced cirrhosis. Serum alkaline phosphatase levels may be moderately elevated or near normal. The prothrombin time is often prolonged, particularly late in the disease or during active phases.

A variety of abnormal serologic reactions and circulating "autoantibodies" are found in chronic active hepatitis. Some of these serologic reactions are nonspecific and may be seen in other viral diseases. Circulating autoantibodies against DNA, IgG, smooth muscle, and mitochondria support the concept that chronic active hepatitis is indeed a systemic disease. Table 319-2 depicts some of the abnormal serologic reactions observed in chronic active hepatitis.

DIFFERENTIAL DIAGNOSIS Early in the course of chronic active hepatitis the disease may resemble typical *acute viral hepatitis*. However, the persistence of symptoms, including biochemical abnormalities such as elevated serum transaminase and bilirubin levels or circulating HBsAg over the ensuing months indicates that a chronic liver disorder is present. The major entity which is often confused with chronic active hepatitis is *chronic persistent hepatitis*. As indicated in Table 319-1, in chronic persistent hepatitis the onset of the illness frequently resembles acute hepatitis. The transaminase enzymes are usually elevated to a mild degree in chronic persistent hepatitis, and HBsAg may be present in serum. Fatigue, anorexia, malaise, right upper quadrant discomfort, and hepatomegaly may be associated with either chronic persistent or chronic active hepatitis. Thus, a definitive diagnosis can only be established by liver biopsy since a *differentiation between chronic active and chronic persistent hepatitis cannot be made by clinical and biochemical criteria*. This distinction is important because chronic persistent hepatitis is not a progressive disorder, rarely if ever results in cirrhosis, and requires no therapy.

The presence of extrahepatic manifestations in chronic active hepatitis such as pleuritis, arthritis, and arthralgias may cause confusion with *connective tissue disorders* such as rheumatoid arthritis and systemic lupus erythematosus. The existence of clinical and biochemical features suggestive of progressive liver disease clearly distinguishes chronic active hepatitis from these disorders. In adolescence, *Wilson's disease* may present with features of chronic active hepatitis before the neurologic manifestations become apparent; serum ceruloplasmin, serum and urinary copper determination, and measurement of the liver copper levels will establish the diagnosis. Late in the course of chronic active hepatitis some patients may present with *postnecrotic cirrhosis* without evidence of active hepatitis. This lesion, termed cryptogenic cirrhosis, may also represent an end stage of other destructive liver diseases (e.g., primary biliary cirrhosis). *Primary biliary cirrhosis*, as previously mentioned, may share histologic similarities with chronic active hepatitis particularly early in the disease. However, in primary biliary cirrhosis the prominence of pruritus plus markedly elevated serum alkaline phosphatase and cholesterol levels, the presence of high titers of antimitochondrial antibodies (in contrast to the low levels seen in chronic active hepatitis), and the pattern of histologic progression will usually permit differentiation from chronic active hepatitis.

MANAGEMENT During episodes of active disease the patient should be managed as in acute viral hepatitis with general supportive care. Hospitalization may be required to define the severity and extent of disease, to verify the presence of extrahepatic involvement, and to confirm the diagnosis by percutaneous liver biopsy. Restriction of activity is indicated during active phases, but prolonged bed rest following remission is unnecessary. Corticosteroid therapy is the treatment of choice in symptomatic HBsAg-negative chronic active hepatitis and bridging or multilobular hepatic necrosis. Corticosteroids have been shown to be effective in prolonging survival of these patients during the first few years of illness when the mortality rate is high. A therapeutic response characterized by a complete clinical, biochemical, and histologic remission is to be expected in 60 to 80 percent of patients. Either prednisone or prednisolone therapy should be initiated at a dose of 40 to 60 mg daily. This dose can usually be gradually tapered within 2 to 3 months to 15 to 20 mg daily. The beneficial effects of corticosteroid treatment on the course and prognosis of patients with mild or asymptomatic chronic active hepatitis (in the absence of cirrhosis or multilobular necrosis) remain to be determined.

The effect of corticosteroids on the natural course of

HBsAg-positive chronic active hepatitis is less clear. It is difficult to justify treatment of *asymptomatic* HBsAg carriers who have evidence only of chronic active hepatitis on liver biopsy. In such patients, the disease may be mild and corticosteroid therapy is often associated with little improvement in aminotransferase values and liver histology. Similarly, in *symptomatic* HBsAg-positive patients with chronic active hepatitis the value of corticosteroids has not been shown with certainty, and a deleterious effect has in fact been reported in some patients. Close follow-up examinations and a repeat liver biopsy 6 months to 1 year following the initial evaluation are often helpful to establish the natural course of the disease and to determine whether fibrosis or cirrhosis has developed. If the disease has progressed, a trial of corticosteroids may be warranted. However, if objective improvement in the clinical and biochemical features of the disease is not apparent after several months of therapy, corticosteroids should be discontinued. In some patients cessation of corticosteroids has been followed by clinical, biochemical, and histologic improvement.

When corticosteroids are used, improvement of fatigue and anorexia is usually noted within days to several weeks. Biochemical improvement is to be expected over several weeks to months, with a fall in serum bilirubin and globulin levels and a rise in serum albumin. The serum transaminase level usually drops promptly, but the absolute value of the transaminase *alone* does not appear to be a useful marker of recovery in the individual patient. Histologic improvement, characterized by a decrease in mononuclear infiltration and subsequent improvement in the extent of hepatocellular necrosis, may be delayed for 6 to 24 months. After a favorable clinical and biochemical response, repeat liver biopsy may show features consistent with chronic persistent hepatitis. Despite this histologic improvement, relapses are common when corticosteroids are discontinued.

Reduction of the suppressive corticosteroid doses should be performed cautiously, particularly at lower prednisone levels, since even small decrements in therapy may be associated with clinical worsening, and increasing dosage may be needed for control of spontaneous exacerbation. Unless major complications require discontinuation of corticosteroids, they should be prescribed for at least 12 months or longer in order to reduce the risk of relapse.

Other therapeutic approaches have been used in the treatment of chronic active hepatitis, particularly in the elderly and in patients with major side effects from corticosteroids. An initial prednisone dosage of 30 mg, tapered down to 10 to 20 mg in combination with 50 to 75 mg azathioprine has been demonstrated to be effective; this treatment avoids the adverse effects of high dosage of corticosteroids. However, *azathioprine alone is not effective* in the treatment of chronic active hepatitis. Alternate-day prednisone therapy diminishes steroid side effects but usually does not provide adequate therapy. Antiviral chemotherapy with interferon or vidarabine may be useful in the management of HBsAg-positive chronic active hepatitis. Controlled clinical trials of this experimental therapy are in progress.

REFERENCES

Berman M et al: The chronic sequelae of non-A, non-B hepatitis. Ann Intern Med 91:1, 1979

Czaja AJ et al: Laboratory assessment of severe chronic active liver disease during and after corticosteroid therapy. Correlation of serum transaminase and gamma globulin levels with histologic features. Gastroenterology 80:667, 1981

Hodges JR et al: Chronic active hepatitis: The spectrum of disease. Lancet 1:550, 1982

Koretz RL et al: Hepatitis B surface antigen carriers—To biopsy or not to biopsy. Gastroenterology 75:860, 1978

Lam KC et al: Deleterious effect of prednisolone in HBsAg-positive chronic active hepatitis. N Engl J Med 304:380, 1981

Mackay IR, Tait BD: HLA associations with autoimmune-type chronic active hepatitis: Identification of B8-DRw3 haplotypes by family studies. Gastroenterology 79:95, 1980

Maddrey WC et al: Drug induced liver disease. Gastroenterology 72:1348, 1977

Summerskill WH et al: Prednisone for chronic active liver disease: Dose titration, standard dose, and combination with azathioprine compared. Gut 16:876, 1976

Wands JR et al: Arthritis associated with chronic active hepatitis: Complement activation and characterization of circulating immune complex. Gastroenterology 69:1286, 1975

Weller IVD et al: Effects of prednisone/azathioprine in chronic hepatitis B viral infection. Gut 23:650, 1982

320 CIRRHOSIS

J. THOMAS LaMONT
RAYMOND S. KOFF
KURT J. ISSELBACHER

DEFINITION Morphologic The essential morphologic features of cirrhosis are (1) an increase in fibrous tissue and (2) nodular regeneration. These processes cause progressive distortion of the vascular bed of the liver and disorganization of the normal lobular architecture. The basic precursor of cirrhosis is believed to be diffuse liver cell death; however, evidence of necrosis may no longer be apparent when liver tissue is examined. The network of scars, the regenerating cell masses, and the changes in hepatic circulation develop secondarily. Less constant pathologic features of most types of cirrhosis include intralobular or portal inflammation, focal or widespread cholestasis, and proliferation of bile ductules.

Clinical and functional The morphologic elements of cirrhosis often have dramatic clinical counterparts. Progressive reduction of liver cell mass may produce jaundice, ascites and edema, central nervous system dysfunction, and cachexia—the syndrome of hepatic insufficiency. The advancing fibrosis leads to distortion of the intrahepatic vasculature, which in turn contributes to the development of portal venous hypertension with resultant esophageal and gastric varices and splenomegaly. Nodular regeneration often leads to distortion of liver shape and compression of intrahepatic venous and lymphatic radicles, which also contribute to portal hypertension and ascites. No clinical, etiologic, or morphologic classification of cirrhosis is satisfactory at present. Clinical signs and symptoms may not reflect accurately the extent and precise nature of the cirrhotic process or its stage of evolution or activity. In addition, pathologic patterns may represent nonspecific hepatic responses to many different forms of liver cell injury, while a variety of morphologic patterns may be produced by a specific etiology in a single patient. However, in spite of these limitations, it is possible to categorize most cases of cirrhosis clinically, adding qualifying morphologic or etiologic terms when possible. Most types of cirrhosis can be classified as follows: (1) alcoholic, (2) postnecrotic, (3) biliary (either primary or secondary), (4) hemochromatosis, (5) cardiac or congestive, or (6) rare forms and cirrhosis of uncertain etiology.

ALCOHOLIC LIVER DISEASE AND CIRRHOSIS

DEFINITION Alcoholic liver disease is the term used to describe the spectrum of liver injury associated with acute and chronic alcoholism. Three components are recognized: (1) alcoholic fatty liver, (2) alcoholic hepatitis, and (3) alcoholic cirrhosis. These entities may exist independently, or coexist in the same liver. Furthermore, while fatty liver is a regular feature of both acute and chronic alcoholism, available evidence suggests that by itself fatty liver does not lead to the development of cirrhosis. On the other hand alcoholic hepatitis in some cases appears to be the precursor of alcoholic cirrhosis, although progression to cirrhosis is not invariable. Since alcohol may stimulate fibrogenesis and collagen synthesis in the liver, it is possible that cirrhosis may occur, at least in some instances, without preceding alcoholic hepatitis.

Alcoholic cirrhosis, the most common variety encountered in North America and many parts of western Europe and South America, is characterized by diffuse fine scarring, a fairly uniform loss of liver cells, and small (often less than lobule-sized) islands of preserved or regenerating parenchyma. The terms *Laennec's, micronodular, portal,* and *fatty cirrhosis* have also been used to describe this type of chronic liver disease. While the eponym has some historical value, each of the other terms has misleading implications: etiologic factors other than alcohol may lead to micronodular cirrhosis and in late stages of alcoholic disease macronodular lesions may predominate; the fibrosis and scarring may not be centered about the portal triads; and cirrhosis may develop in the absence of important fatty infiltration of liver cells.

ETIOLOGY Experimental studies of both normal and alcoholic subjects have shown that ethanol (in moderate to large doses) produces liver dysfunction and fatty infiltration (Chap. 315) despite the ingestion of a well-balanced diet. This pattern of liver injury (*alcoholic fatty liver*) is completely reversible on cessation of alcoholism. If alcoholism continues, fatty liver persists. Most alcoholics with fatty liver do not develop alcoholic hepatitis or cirrhosis. However, some individuals develop an inflammatory reaction with polymorphonuclear infiltration and liver cell necrosis in addition to fatty changes. This lesion of *alcoholic hepatitis* may be the forerunner of cirrhosis, because healing with fibrosis distorts the normal lobular architecture. Many epidemiologic studies have implicated chronic alcoholism as the major cause of alcoholic cirrhosis: between 10 and 20 percent of chronic alcoholic patients in the United States have clinical or morphologic evidence of cirrhosis. The quantity and duration of drinking necessary to cause cirrhosis is unknown, but average social usage is not sufficient to cause permanent liver damage. The typical alcoholic with cirrhosis has consumed a pint or more of whisky, several quarts of wine, or an equivalent amount of beer per day for at least 10 years. The amount of ethanol, rather than the type of alcoholic beverage, is the determinant factor.

Most chronic alcoholics consume protein- and vitamin-poor diets and may develop other clinical syndromes clearly related to faulty nutrition (exemplified by folate deficiency or Korsakoff-Wernicke's disease); moreover, treatment of cirrhotic patients with protein-rich diets often produces clinical and morphologic improvement. For these and other reasons, including the observation of a hepatic lesion closely resembling alcoholic injury in patients undergoing intestinal bypass operations for the control of obesity, absolute or relative *malnutrition* is regarded as a contributing factor to the evolution of cirrhosis. Although malnutrition per se does not lead to cirrhosis, a reasonable concept, based on much circumstantial evidence, is that a combination of *chronic alcohol ingestion plus impaired nutrition* leads to alcoholic hepatitis and cirrhosis.

Intercurrent bacterial *infections* are common in cirrhotic patients and seem, on occasion, to accelerate the course of the disease. There are, however, no firm data to implicate overt or latent infection in the pathogenesis of alcoholic cirrhosis. Icteric or anicteric bridging hepatic necrosis, presumably of viral origin, may occasionally lead to the development of a finely nodular cirrhosis resembling alcoholic cirrhosis in its general morphologic character, perhaps explaining the frequent reports of portal cirrhosis in nonalcoholic patients in England. Serial biopsies in these cases do not show many of the characteristic histologic features of progressive alcoholic cirrhosis (see below), and such cases may represent variants of postnecrotic cirrhosis.

Although rates of ethanol metabolism are under genetic control, no *metabolic defect* has been identified in cirrhotic patients or their families to suggest a unique "susceptibility" to ethanol or its toxic effects. Nonetheless, it is clear that individual tolerance to ethanol and its capacity to induce cirrhosis varies widely and that a true biologic predisposition to ethanol-induced liver diseases may exist.

PATHOLOGY AND PATHOGENESIS **Alcoholic fatty liver** The liver is enlarged, yellow, greasy, and firm. The parenchymal cells are usually diffusely abnormal, and many are distended by cytoplasmic fat vacuoles. When large, these triglyceride-containing vacuoles may push the hepatocyte nucleus to the periphery of the cell and flatten it against the cell membrane. The accumulation of fat in the liver of the alcoholic results from a number of alterations in fat metabolism; however, decreased mitochondrial fatty acid oxidation may play a key role. Triglyceride disappears with therapy and abstinence and recurs promptly after resumption of alcohol ingestion.

Alcoholic hepatitis Morphologic features include hepatic cell degeneration and necrosis, often with ballooned cells, accompanied by an infiltrate consisting of polymorphonuclear leukocytes and lymphocytes. The polymorphonuclear cells may encircle damaged hepatocytes which contain intracytoplasmic *Mallory bodies* or *alcoholic hyaline.* These irregular, dendritic, or beadlike clumps of perinuclear, deeply eosinophilic material have a fibrillar or tubular appearance on electron microscopy. They may represent aggregates of cystoskeletal intermediate filaments. In some patients Mallory bodies and hepatic cell necrosis are prominent in the centrilobular region, producing the lesion of *sclerosing hyaline necrosis.* In patients with cirrhosis and recurrent or continuing alcoholic hepatitis the Mallory bodies tend to be found in liver cells at the periphery of nodules. Mallory bodies are highly suggestive of, but *not specific* for, alcoholic hepatitis since morphologically similar material has been seen in occasional patients with Wilson's disease, primary biliary cirrhosis, hepatocellular carcinoma, and following intestinal bypass surgery. They are commonly found in Indian juvenile cirrhosis.

Immunological mechanisms may have a role in the pathogenesis of alcoholic hepatitis. Thymus-derived (T) lymphocytes are sequestered in the liver and may be reduced in the peripheral blood. Sensitization of T lymphocytes and a humoral response to alcoholic hyaline antigens have been described. The precise responsible mechanism remains to be determined.

Alcoholic cirrhosis As alcoholism continues and the liver disease advances, hepatocytes are destroyed, fibroblasts (including myofibroblasts with contractile properties) are found at the sites of injury, and collagen formation is stimulated. *Web-like septa of connective tissue appear in periportal and pericentral zones.* These fibrous septa become denser and more confluent, connecting portal triads and central veins. The fine connective tissue network contains small vessels, lymphatics, and other remnants of portal triads and surrounds small masses of liver cells. These lobular remnants undergo regeneration and form nodules. Inflammation is usually minimal and transient, but may be a prominent morphologic feature during acute exacerbations of alcoholic hepatitis. As the liver cell mass diminishes, the liver shrinks in size, acquires a finely nodular (hobnail) appearance, and becomes hard.

Alcoholic cirrhosis is basically a progressive disease, but appropriate therapy and strict avoidance of alcohol may arrest the disease at most stages and permit repair and functional improvement. Continued loss of liver cells by focal necrosis due to alcoholic hepatitis or continued stimulation of collagen formation results in progressive stromal collapse, fibrosis, and vascular distortion. Although regeneration occurs within the small remnants of parenchyma, cell loss eventually exceeds replacement, the liver cell mass dwindles, and a phase of irreversible, or end-stage, cirrhosis is reached.

CLINICAL FEATURES **Signs and symptoms** Clinical manifestations of alcoholic *fatty liver* are usually minimal or entirely absent, and the disorder may not be recognized unless another illness (e.g., alcoholic pancreatitis) brings the patient to medical attention. Hepatomegaly may be the only finding which signals the presence of alcoholic fatty liver. Jaundice, ascites, and edema are usually absent unless more serious liver injury is present.

The extremely broad spectrum of alcoholic hepatitis varies from a mild asymptomatic illness to severe, sometimes fatal hepatic insufficiency. Initial episodes are more likely to be clinically silent than recurrent or continuing bouts of alcoholic hepatitis in which clinical manifestations may be striking. Clinical features resemble those of viral or toxic liver injury. Anorexia, nausea and vomiting, malaise, weight loss, abdominal distress, and jaundice are common presenting complaints. Fever may be seen in about 50 percent of patients. Tender hepatomegaly is the most common physical finding. Arterial "spider" angiomata, jaundice, ascites, and edema are common, and the spleen is enlarged in about a third of cases.

In many patients alcoholic hepatitis is superimposed upon or presents concurrently with alcoholic cirrhosis, but it is the former which is responsible for clinical manifestations. Jaundice and other signs of hepatic dysfunction may subside with therapy, but continued alcoholic excess and poor dietary habits lead to further episodes of hepatic decompensation. Acute acceleration of alcoholic liver damage may follow protracted drinking bouts. Fever, nausea and vomiting, deepening jaundice, hepatic encephalopathy, and ascites may occur rapidly in association with widespread liver cell loss and inflammation. Although some patients die during the acute exacerbations, most recover after several weeks or months. A few patients experience one or more transient episodes of cholestatic jaundice during the course of alcoholic liver disease. Clinical and laboratory studies may suggest the presence of mechanical biliary obstruction, but liver biopsy and the response to conservative therapy usually support the diagnosis of intrahepatic cholestasis.

Alcoholic cirrhosis also may be clinically silent, and about 10 percent of cases are discovered incidentally at laparotomy or autopsy. Men are affected more frequently than women, but this sex difference has decreased steadily in recent years as drinking habits have changed in many western countries. Although the average age of onset of symptoms is about 50 years, cirrhosis may be found in alcoholic patients in the third or fourth decade of life.

Typically, after 10 or more years of alcohol excess, progressive liver dysfunction, fluid retention, and portal hypertension may become evident. After a period of weeks or months, the patient notes gradually increasing weakness and fatigability, anorexia, slight weight loss, jaundice, intermittent ankle edema, and increasing abdominal girth due to ascites. A firm and enlarged liver may be the only sign of disease, but additional typical findings include muscle wasting, jaundice, spider angiomas, gynecomastia and testicular atrophy (in men), menstrual irregularity or amenorrhea (in women), palmar erythema, splenomegaly, and ascites. Loss of body hair, parotid gland enlargement, purpura, clubbing of the fingers, and diffuse hyperpigmentation of the skin are common but less specific clinical signs. Dupuytren's contractures are not infrequent in alcoholics but are not specifically related to cirrhosis. Low-grade fever without shaking chills is frequent.

Over a period of 3 to 5 years, the cirrhotic patient becomes emaciated, weak, and chronically jaundiced; and ascites and signs of portal hypertension become increasingly prominent. Most patients with advanced cirrhosis die in hepatic coma, often precipitated by hemorrhage from esophageal varices or intercurrent infection. Acute and chronic pancreatitis and peptic ulceration occur with greater frequency in cirrhotic patients than in normal subjects. Gram-negative bacteremia, acute bacterial peritonitis, and hepatocellular carcinoma are late complications.

Laboratory findings Laboratory studies are often unremarkable in alcoholic fatty liver except for minimal SGOT (aspartate aminotransferase, AST) elevations. In more severe alcoholic liver disease laboratory abnormalities are characteristic. Anemia is often present. The etiology is almost always complex, and acute and chronic gastrointestinal blood loss, folic acid deficiency, hypersplenism, and a direct toxic effect of alcohol on the bone marrow are contributing causes. Hemolytic anemia accompanied by hypercholesterolemia and unusual spur-like projections of the erythrocyte membrane (acanthocytosis) have been described in some alcoholics with cirrhosis. Leukopenia and thrombocytopenia may result from hypersplenism or be a direct effect of alcohol on the bone marrow. Many patients have marked leukocytosis and a leukemoid reaction may be seen in a few. Liver function tests reveal hyperbilirubinemia and variable elevations of serum alkaline phosphatase. The SGOT is usually less than 250 units, although the SGPT (alanine aminotransferase, ALT) is usually lower and may be nearly normal. (A ratio of SGOT/SGPT greater than 2 is found more frequently in patients with alcoholic hepatitis than with viral hepatitis.) In patients with the lesion of sclerosing hyaline necrosis, SGOT levels may be considerably higher and may exceed 500 units. The serum albumin is usually depressed, while globulins are increased. Quantitative immunoglobulin determinations reveal elevations of all classes, especially IgG. In severe cases clotting factor deficiencies are common, as manifested by prolongation of the prothrombin and partial thromboplastin times. Elevated blood ammonia levels reflect a combination of impaired liver function and shunting of portal blood around the liver into the systemic circulation.

A diabetic type of glucose intolerance may occur in cirrhosis and appears to be a reflection of endogenous insulin resistance; however, clinical diabetes is uncommon. Respiratory alkalosis is frequently present, and reflects a tendency to hyperpnea seen in these patients. Hypomagnesemia is also common, and results from dietary deficiency and increased urinary losses. Dilutional hyponatremia and hypokalemia from excessive urinary loss are frequent in patients with ascites and edema, and reflect secondary hyperaldosteronism.

DIAGNOSIS Alcoholic fatty liver should be suspected in alcoholic patients with hepatomegaly. Alcoholic hepatitis should be considered in an alcoholic with recent heavy drinking who presents with an enlarged tender liver, jaundice, fever, and ascites. This variant of alcoholic liver disease can be fatal; and variceal bleeding, infection, and hepatic encephalopathy are common.

Alcoholic cirrhosis should be strongly suspected in patients with a history of prolonged or excessive alcohol intake, hepatomegaly and other signs of chronic liver disease, plus laboratory evidence of hepatic dysfunction. If there are no contraindications, most patients should have a percutaneous needle biopsy of the liver to confirm the diagnosis as well as to determine the stage and activity of the disease process. When the course of an otherwise stable cirrhotic patient changes without obvious explanation, complicating conditions such as occult bleeding, infection, hepatocellular carcinoma, and portal vein thrombosis should be sought.

PROGNOSIS Both retrospective and prospective studies of the natural history of severe alcoholic liver disease show that early, vigorous, and meticulous medical care will prolong life, decrease morbidity, and delay or prevent the appearance of certain complications. Patients with cirrhosis who abstain from alcohol and consume nutritious diets have a 5-year survival rate of about 60 percent, whereas those who continue to drink have a 40 percent 5-year survival rate. Mortality rates are higher in patients with complications, such as variceal bleeding or ascites, in whom abstinence may not improve survival rates. Massive variceal hemorrhage is a major direct or contributing cause of death in many patients. Although surgical shunts are effective in reducing portal hypertension, the overall prognosis remains poor in patients with advanced, irreversible liver disease.

TREATMENT Alcoholic hepatitis and cirrhosis are serious illnesses that require prolonged medical supervision and management. In most instances it is desirable to hospitalize the patient for initial study and assessment of the response to therapy as well as for dietary and medical instruction.

In the absence of signs of impending hepatic coma, a *diet* containing at least 1 g protein per kilogram of body weight and 2000 to 3000 cal per day should be prescribed. Because the patient with alcoholic hepatitis is often anorectic or nauseated, these dietary aims may be achieved by offering the patient three or four small meals with supplemental feedings of eggnog or ice cream. Vitamin supplements, in the form of multivitamin capsules, may be given, but there is no rationale for the clinical use of lipotropic agents. In the presence of Wernicke-Korsakoff disease (see Chap. 362) the patient should receive large parenteral doses of thiamine. The patient should understand clearly that neither nutritious diet nor added vitamins will protect the liver against the effects of further alcohol ingestion. *Therefore, alcohol should be absolutely forbidden.*

Ascites and edema may disappear with bed rest alone. More persistent fluid retention should be treated with *salt restriction,* utilizing diets that contain 1 to 2 g sodium chloride per day. Water restriction, limiting fluid intake to volumes that equal the measured fluid loss of the prior day, may be necessary if hyponatremia is present. In patients with active disease (i.e., jaundice, or signs of hepatic insufficiency) diuretics should be used with great caution in order to prevent electrolyte depletion, hypovolemia, and hepatic encephalopathy (see "Ascites" later in this chapter).

Confusion, drowsiness, or other signs of impending *hepatic coma* should be treated by prompt decrease in protein intake to levels of 20 to 30 g daily of less. A careful search for intercurrent bacterial infection and for gastrointestinal hemorrhage should be made, including the aspiration of gastric contents, and appropriate therapy to control infection or bleeding should be instituted. Possible offending drugs, especially diuretics and sedatives, should be omitted and any electrolyte imbalance corrected promptly (see "Hepatic Encephalopathy" below). Despite randomized studies from several studies the role of corticosteroids in acute alcoholic hepatitis remains controversial. In several studies a beneficial response was observed with prednisone or prednisolone 40 mg per day, while other investigators have been unable to confirm this. Preliminary studies suggest that intravenous infusion of insulin and glucagon may be helpful, but this experimental therapy remains to be proved effective or safe.

Anemia should be characterized and corrected by appropriate means. Folic acid deficiency is particularly common in alcoholics and requires replacement therapy. *Fever,* especially when low-grade and unaccompanied by chills or other signs of infection, may be a manifestation of alcoholic hepatitis. However, the presence of hectic or persistent fever or shaking chills requires a vigorous search for septic processes, especially urinary tract infection, pneumonia, gram-negative bacteremia, or peritonitis.

POSTNECROTIC CIRRHOSIS

DEFINITION This form of chronic liver disease, the most common type of cirrhosis on a worldwide basis, is characterized morphologically by (1) confluent, often extensive loss of liver cells, (2) stromal collapse and fibrosis that produce broad bands of connective tissue containing the remains of many triads, and (3) irregular, large nodules, varying in size from microscopic to grossly visible, of intact or regenerating parenchyma. This pattern, which may vary considerably in extent and severity, results from an overall but unequal injury to the liver. As with other forms of cirrhosis, the appearance of advanced postnecrotic disease offers little insight into the original or potentiating causes of the liver cell damage.

The terms *toxic cirrhosis, coarsely nodular cirrhosis, posthepatic cirrhosis, cryptogenic cirrhosis,* and *multilobular cirrhosis,* are synonymous with postnecrotic cirrhosis.

ETIOLOGY The cause of postnecrotic cirrhosis is still unknown, but epidemiologic and serologic evidence suggests that viral hepatitis is an antecedent factor in many instances. In the United States, about 25 percent of patients with postnecrotic cirrhosis have a history compatible with recent or remote attacks of acute viral hepatitis. Furthermore, the progression of bridging hepatic necrosis through chronic active hepatitis (see Chap. 319) to postnecrotic cirrhosis is well documented. Approximately 5 to 20 percent of patients with established postnecrotic disease have positive serologic tests for HBsAg. A few patients with postnecrotic cirrhosis associated with hepatitis B have negative blood tests but have hepatitis B antigens present in liver tissue. Non-A, non-B viral hepatitis may be responsible for some cases, but hepatitis A is not an established cause.

A small percentage of cases stem from documented *intoxications* with industrial *chemicals* (e.g., phosphorus), poisons (e.g., *Amanita phalloides* toxins), or drugs (oxyphenisatin, α-methyldopa). Finally, certain *infections* (e.g., brucellosis), *parasitic infections* (clonorchiasis), *metabolic disorders* (hepatolenticular degeneration), and *advanced alcoholic liver disease* may produce confluent cell loss and result in postnecrotic cirrhosis.

PATHOLOGY AND PATHOGENESIS Typically, the postnecrotic liver is small, grossly distorted in shape, and composed of nodules of liver cells separated by dense, wide, sunken scars. Microscopically, the established lesion includes (1) large islands of parenchymal cells with rounded (inactive) or ragged (active) margins; (2) interdigitating broad to thin fibrous septa containing distorted vessels, lymphatics, and bile ducts derived from many portal areas; and (3) prominent mononuclear inflammatory infiltrates, often in the form of follicles or clusters. In some sections of liver, lobular architecture appears nearly normal, but central veins are absent or markedly displaced.

Current evidence suggests that infectious, toxic, metabolic, or nutritional factors initiate the postnecrotic process. The destruction appears to progress as the result of similar repeated or persistent insults or possibly on the basis of "autoimmune" liver cell injury.

CLINICAL FEATURES Postnecrotic cirrhosis affects women at least as often as men and should be suspected in nonalcoholic patients with evidence of chronic liver disease, especially in those in the younger age group. Like those with alcoholic cirrhosis, a few patients with postnecrotic disease may have little clinical evidence of advanced cirrhosis, the diagnosis being made at operation or postmortem examination or by a needle biopsy performed to investigate asymptomatic hepatosplenomegaly. About 25 percent of patients present with signs and symptoms suggesting active hepatitis, but often with atypical features such as prolonged illness, intense and protracted jaundice, ascites, or manifestations of portal hypertension. Splenomegaly may be the only sign of postnecrotic cirrhosis, and hypersplenism may be prominent. Some patients have bouts of upper abdominal pain, the sudden onset of unexplained ascites, episodes of hepatic encephalopathy, or massive variceal hemorrhage as the major or initial clinical feature. The signs and symptoms of postnecrotic cirrhosis resemble those of alcoholic cirrhosis and reflect the loss of liver cell reserve, advancing portal hypertension, and disorders of salt and water metabolism. In general, however, patients with postnecrotic cirrhosis show less wasting and more persistent jaundice early in their clinical illness than do patients with alcoholic cirrhosis.

The results of hematologic and liver function tests resemble those of alcoholic cirrhosis, but protracted and pronounced hyperbilirubinemia, persistent moderate elevations of serum transaminases (aminotransferases), and hypergammaglobulinemia (3 to 4 g per deciliter of serum) are often present.

DIAGNOSIS AND PROGNOSIS Postnecrotic cirrhosis should be suspected in young persons and nonalcoholic adults with signs and symptoms of cirrhosis or portal hypertension. Most laboratory and radiologic studies are nondiagnostic, and needle or operative liver biopsies are the definitive diagnostic procedures, but nonuniformity of the pathologic process may result in confusing sampling errors. About 75 percent of cases tend to progress despite supportive therapy and after 1 to 5 years terminate in death from exsanguinating variceal hemorrhage, hepatic coma, or superimposed hepatocellular carcinoma.

TREATMENT Because the primary cause of this disease is rarely detectable or treatable, long-term care must include appropriate rest, control of ascites (see below), avoidance of drugs or excessive protein intake that may induce hepatic coma (see below), prompt treatment of infections, and surgical treatment of portal hypertension (see below) if life-threatening variceal hemorrhage occurs. Patients with coexistent or antecedent chronic active hepatitis and cirrhosis may respond to therapy as described in Chap. 319.

BILIARY CIRRHOSIS

DEFINITION *Biliary cirrhosis* refers to a disorder characterized by clinical and chemical signs of chronic impairment of bile excretion and morphologic evidence of progressive liver destruction centered about the intrahepatic bile ducts. Major clinical concomitants of impaired bile excretion (cholestasis) include protracted itching, progressive and prolonged jaundice, steatorrhea, the development of cutaneous xanthelasmas and xanthomas, hepatomegaly, and marked elevations of serum alkaline phosphatase, cholesterol, and other lipid fractions. Morphologically, most forms of biliary cirrhosis evolve from chronic inflammatory lesions of the interlobular ducts, bile ductules, and periportal liver cells. True cirrhosis represents a *late* and often nonspecific phase.

Biliary cirrhosis can be *primary*, in which case the process is related to chronic inflammation and fibrosis of the intrahepatic bile ductules, or *secondary* to obstruction of the common bile duct or its large branches.

ETIOLOGY The cause of *primary biliary cirrhosis* is still unknown. The observation that 90 percent of cases occur in middle-aged women strongly suggests an endocrine contribution. The occasional onset of primary biliary cirrhosis following a bout of atypical (so-called cholestatic) hepatitis has led to speculation that viral destruction of liver and duct cells initiates the disease process. Supporting serologic data are lacking, however. Although no drug has produced a picture typical of progressive biliary cirrhosis, the occasional appearance of many elements of the syndrome in patients treated with phenothiazine suggests that drug hypersensitivity may be one etiologic factor. Hepatic copper levels are elevated, but this appears to be a nonspecific, secondary phenomenon resulting from impaired hepatic excretion of copper into bile due to chronic cholestasis. The occasional association of this form of cirrhosis with calcinosis, Raynaud's phenomenon, sclerodactyly, and telangiectasia (so-called CRST syndrome) suggests that in some cases abnormalities of connective tissue may be related to primary biliary cirrhosis.

The "Sicca complex" of dry eyes and dry mouth, autoimmune thyroiditis, and renal tubular acidosis also may be present and indicate that primary biliary cirrhosis may be a systemic disorder.

Primary biliary cirrhosis is associated with a number of specific and nonspecific immunologic abnormalities:

1 A circulating mitochondrial antibody (IgG) is present in the serum of more than 95 percent of patients with primary biliary cirrhosis and only rarely in other forms of liver disease.
2 Elevated serum levels of IgM are seen in about 80 percent of patients with primary biliary cirrhosis, and cryoproteins, composed of IgM or IgM and IgG, are present in 90 to 95 percent. These cryoproteins consist of complement-fixing immune complexes which appear to activate the alternate complement pathway.
3 Circulating antibodies that react with bile canaliculi and the cytoplasm of bile ductular cells have been demonstrated in primary biliary cirrhosis. However, similar antibodies occur in many patients with acute hepatitis.
4 Impaired lymphocyte transformation has been documented in some patients, suggesting derangement of cell-mediated immune responses.

These observations suggest strongly that disordered immune responses play a major role in the initiation or progression of the chronic hepatic lesion of biliary cirrhosis, but the exact mechanisms involved are unclear.

Most instances of *secondary biliary cirrhosis* result from partial or total obstruction of the common bile duct or its major branches for more than a year. In adults, chronic bile duct obstruction by postoperative strictures or by gallstones, usually with superimposed infectious cholangitis, is the most common cause of this type of biliary cirrhosis. Tumors of the pancreas, biliary tree, or gallbladder that produce obstruction of the common bile duct occasionally induce cirrhosis but only rarely permit survival to this stage. A few patients with the peculiar pericholangitis of ulcerative colitis or with idiopathic sclerosing cholangitis develop secondary biliary cirrhosis. Congenital atresia of the intra- or extrahepatic bile duct system, a relatively common anomaly, induces rapidly advancing periportal fibrosis in infants; most cases are inoperable and eventually fatal. In neither acquired nor congenital biliary obstruction is the exact pathogenesis of the cirrhotic process understood. Simple effects of pressure, local toxicity of bile constituents, or secondary infection do not alone appear to explain the morphologic events satisfactorily.

PATHOLOGY AND PATHOGENESIS The earliest recognizable lesion of *primary biliary cirrhosis* might be termed "chronic nonsuppurative destructive cholangitis," a diffuse necrotizing and inflammatory process centered about the portal triads. This is characterized by destruction of medium and small bile duct cells, infiltration with acute and chronic inflammatory cells, local fibroblastic reaction, and variable bile stasis. At times, periductal granuloma and lymph follicles may be seen. Mallory (hyaline) bodies may be present in periportal hepatocytes. Progression of this process over a period of months to years (usually 3 to 5 years) leads to loss of liver cells, the formation of pseudolobules, expansion of periportal fibrosis into a network of connective tissue scars, with apparent loss of interlobular ducts and the development of cirrhosis with a micronodular configuration. However, end-stage primary biliary cirrhosis may be indistinguishable from postnecrotic cirrhosis in its gross and microscopic appearance.

Unrelieved obstruction of the extrahepatic bile ducts leads to (1) centrilobular bile stasis, cell degeneration, and focal areas of necrosis; (2) proliferation and dilatation of the portal ducts and ductules; (3) sterile or infected cholangitis with accumulation of polymorphonuclear infiltrates around bile ducts; and (4) progressive expansion of portal tracts by edema and fibrosis. Extravasation of bile from ruptured canaliculi, ductules, or ducts leads to the formation of "bile lakes" surrounded by cholesterol-rich pseudoxanthomatous cells. These changes are followed by a finely nodular cirrhosis with isolated islands of hepatocytes surrounded by dense fibrous septa. The duration of biliary obstruction necessary to cause cirrhosis is at least 1 year, and relief of the blockage is frequently accompanied by biochemical and morphological improvement. In both primary and secondary biliary cirrhosis, the liver is initially enlarged and greenish-yellow in appearance, but evolves to a smaller, firmer, more coarsely nodular organ as the disease progresses.

CLINICAL FEATURES Signs and symptoms Many patients with *primary biliary cirrhosis* are asymptomatic, and the disease is initially detected by the finding of a raised serum alkaline phosphatase on screening examination. The disease may remain clinically silent for many years. Although not diagnostic, the early clinical course of primary biliary cirrhosis is quite characteristic. The patient typically is a middle-aged woman who develops persistent generalized itching (the earliest symptom in about 50 percent of cases), followed by dark urine, pale stools, and jaundice, with some darkening (melanosis) of the exposed areas of the skin. In contrast to many other forms of cirrhosis, there are few early signs of liver cell failure and hepatic fibrosis, and most of the features reflect impaired bile excretion. Steatorrhea with associated malabsorption of lipid-soluble vitamins often produces purpura, diarrhea, and osteomalacia; the last may be manifested by backache and bone pain. Protracted elevation of serum lipids, especially cholesterol, leads to the deposit of yellowish plaques or nodules in the subcutaneous tissues in the form of periorbital xanthelasmas and xanthomas over joints, in skin folds, and at sites of trauma. Over a period of months to years, the itching, jaundice, and hyperpigmentation slowly increase. At that time the pruritus and skin lipid deposits may decrease, ascites and edema usually appear, and signs of liver cell failure and portal hypertension supervene. Most symptomatic patients die within 5 to 10 years from the first signs of the illness. However, asymptomatic patients discovered primarily on the basis of finding an elevated serum alkaline phosphatase have a much better prognosis, and may remain asymptomatic for 10 years or more. Death usually results from hepatic insufficiency and is often precipitated by variceal bleeding, intercurrent infection, or surgical procedures.

Physical examination may be entirely normal in the early phase of the disease, when pruritus is the sole complaint. Later there may be jaundice of varying intensity, hyperpigmentation of the exposed skin areas, xanthelasmas and xanthomas, moderate to striking hepatomegaly, splenomegaly, and clubbing of the fingers. Fever and chills are rare and usually indicate mechanical biliary obstruction or other associated diseases. Muscle wasting, spider angiomas, palmar erythema, ascites and edema, the bony tenderness of osteomalacia, and the vertebral compression fractures of osteoporosis appear in advanced stages of the disease.

Secondary biliary cirrhosis, which may be difficult to differentiate from primary biliary cirrhosis on the basis of clinical features alone, should be strongly considered in patients with a history of previous biliary tract surgery or gallstones, bouts of ascending cholangitis, and right upper quadrant pain.

Laboratory findings Biliary cirrhosis is frequently diagnosed at a presymptomatic stage because of the widespread use of blood chemistry screening tests. The earliest laboratory abnormality is a two- to fivefold elevation of the serum alkaline phosphatase, accompanied by normal or slightly increased bilirubin and transaminases. As the disease evolves, the bilirubin becomes progressively elevated and in the final stages may reach 30 mg/dl or more. Transaminase (aminotransferase) values rarely exceed 150 to 200 units. Marked elevation of IgM is frequent in primary biliary cirrhosis; elevation of IgG also occurs. Hyperlipidemia is common, the most striking elevation being in unesterified cholesterol. An abnormal, unique lipoprotein (lipoprotein X) found in the plasma of patients with cholestasis is also present in this disorder. Serum bile salts (especially trihydroxy) are increased, but neither serum nor skin levels can be correlated with the intensity of itching. Hypoprothrombinemia and mild to moderate steatorrhea result from a deficiency of bile salts in the gut and impaired absorption of the fat-soluble vitamins and dietary lipids. The mitochondrial antibody test is positive in most cases of primary but usually not in secondary biliary cirrhosis. Patients with primary biliary cirrhosis have elevated liver copper levels; however, the relation of these derangements in copper metabolism to the pathogenesis of this disease is not clear.

DIAGNOSIS Biliary cirrhosis should be considered in any patient with signs, symptoms, and laboratory evidence of protracted obstruction to bile flow. Liver biopsy may be diagnostic of primary biliary cirrhosis. A positive mitochondrial antibody test suggests the presence of primary biliary cirrhosis. However, since false-positive results occur, this test should not be used by itself to make the diagnosis but rather be combined with liver biopsy, cholangiography, or laparotomy. The major diagnostic challenge, regardless of the duration of symptoms, is to exclude remediable causes of mechanical bile duct obstruction before permanent liver damage has occurred. This can usually be accomplished by either a transhepatic cholangiogram or by ERCP. If these attempts are unsuccessful or if the situation is confusing, an exploratory laparotomy with an operative cholangiogram may be required.

TREATMENT Complete correction of any mechanical obstruction to bile flow is the most important step in the prevention and therapy of *secondary biliary cirrhosis.* There is no known medical therapy which alters the slowly progressive course of primary biliary cirrhosis. Therapeutic efforts are therefore directed at the many bothersome symptoms or complications of the disease as they develop. Itching may be helped by antihistamines or topical lotions containing menthol. Systemic corticosteroids and various synthetic androgen compounds may decrease itching but are accompanied by serious side effects (especially exacerbation of osteopenia) and do not alter the course of the disease. Azathioprine is ineffective. The bile salt–sequestering resin *cholestyramine,* in doses of 8 to 12 g per day, usually relieves itching. Penicillamine, the copper-chelating agent, appears to enhance copper excretion in patients with primary biliary cirrhosis and has been prescribed by some, but its effect on the overall course of the disease is still unclear. Steatorrhea can be treated by reduction in dietary long-chain triglycerides and substitution of medium-chain triglycerides which do not require bile salts for absorption. The *fat-soluble vitamins* D, A, and K should be given by parenteral injection at regular intervals to help prevent or correct osteomalacia and hypoprothrombinemia. Salt restriction and judicious use of oral diuretic agents usually prevent disabling ascites and edema (see "Ascites" later in this chapter). The occurrence of esophagogastric variceal hemorrhage may require surgery or endoscopic sclerosis.

HEMOCHROMATOSIS

See Chap. 97.

CARDIAC CIRRHOSIS

DEFINITION *Cardiac cirrhosis* is a relatively rare complication of severe right-sided congestive heart failure of long-standing duration in patients with cor pulmonale, tricuspid insufficiency, or constrictive pericarditis. Cardiac cirrhosis must be distinguished from *acute passive congestion* of the liver which occurs in the setting of acute heart failure, and is reversible upon correction or improvement of the heart disease.

PATHOLOGY Acute heart failure of any cause may produce acute passive congestion of the liver. This results from elevation of right ventricular pressure which is transmitted to the liver via the inferior vena cava and hepatic veins. The acutely congested liver is tensely swollen and the hepatic sinusoids are dilated and engorged with blood. In the presence of superimposed hypotension or hypoxemia there may be centrilobular necrosis of hepatocytes. These morphologic changes are transient, and full recovery occurs if the heart disease can be corrected. Severe and prolonged heart failure causes fibrosis around the central veins, which extends outward as stellate scars, ultimately producing nodular regeneration and cirrhosis.

CLINICAL FEATURES In acute passive congestion the liver is enlarged and tender, and the patient may complain of severe right upper quadrant pain due to stretching of Glisson's capsule. Abnormalities of liver function are quite variable, ranging from mild elevations of bilirubin and transaminases to a syndrome resembling acute viral hepatitis with a bilirubin of 10 mg or greater and transaminases greater than 1000 units per deciliter of serum. Serum albumin and prothrombin are usually normal, except in severe centrilobular necrosis. In long-standing right-sided heart failure the liver is enlarged, firm, and usually nontender. Splenomegaly may result from simple passive congestion and does not necessarily indicate cirrhosis. In cases of tricuspid insufficiency the liver may be pulsatile, but this finding disappears as cirrhosis develops. Cardiac cirrhosis is infrequently diagnosed antemortem because the signs and symptoms of heart failure greatly overshadow the liver disease. Bleeding from esophageal varices is rarely observed.

DIAGNOSIS The findings of a firm, enlarged liver with mild abnormalities of liver function tests, ascites, and peripheral edema in a patient with valvular heart disease, constrictive pericarditis, or cor pulmonale of long duration (greater than 10 years) should suggest the diagnosis of cardiac cirrhosis. Heart failure and hepatomegaly are quite common in hemochromatosis and amyloidosis, but these entities can be easily differentiated by appropriate blood tests and liver biopsy.

Budd-Chiari syndrome or occlusion of the hepatic veins is easily confused with congestive hepatomegaly, particularly the acute variety. In this condition the liver is grossly enlarged and tender, and severe intractable ascites is present. However, signs and symptoms of heart failure are notably absent. The clinical course may be indolent if the obstruction is gradual, or may be rapidly downhill in acute obstruction. The usual cause is thrombosis of the hepatic veins, often in the setting of polycythemia rubra vera or hypernephroma invading the inferior vena cava; occasionally congenital fibrous webs occlude the main hepatic veins. Hepatic venography or liver biopsy showing centrilobular congestion and necrosis and sinusoidal dilatation in the absence of right-sided heart failure establishes the diagnosis.

TREATMENT Prevention or treatment of cardiac cirrhosis depends on proper diagnosis and therapy of the underlying cardiovascular disorder. If constrictive pericarditis is present and pericardectomy is possible, liver function may improve within 6 to 12 months and fibrous bands will become narrower and avascular.

FORMS OF CIRRHOSIS OF UNKNOWN ETIOLOGY

Clinical, etiologic, and morphologic classifications of cirrhosis do not encompass all cases. Classification criteria for the study of patients with cirrhosis vary widely throughout the world, but *unexpected and unexplained cirrhosis accounts for about 10 percent of chronic liver disease* seen at autopsy. Equally important, many patients with cirrhosis are "classified" improperly during life, and small and unrepresentative biopsy specimens from patients with a poor history often account for the errors in diagnosis.

Cirrhosis may be found in association with the following diseases:

1 *Metabolic disorders:* galactosemia, hereditary fructose intolerance, glycogen storage diseases, hereditary tyrosinemia, alpha$_1$-antitrypsin deficiency, and the Fanconi syndrome
2 *Infectious diseases:* brucellosis, schistosomiasis, neonatal cytomegalovirus, and toxoplasma infections
3 *Infiltrative diseases:* sarcoidosis

4 *Gastrointestinal disorders:* chronic inflammatory bowel disease and cystic fibrosis of the pancreas
5 *Chemical intoxications:* pyrrolidizine alkaloids (venoocclusive disease) and arsenic

NONCIRRHOTIC FIBROSIS OF THE LIVER

Several diseases, either congenital or acquired, may be associated with localized or generalized hepatic fibrosis. The clinical manifestations in such cases may suggest on occasion the diagnosis of true cirrhosis, but the absence of clinical and functional evidence of hepatocellular damage, the lack of nodular regenerative activity, and the localized nature of the scarring usually serve to distinguish these conditions from true cirrhosis.

IDIOPATHIC PORTAL HYPERTENSION (NONCIRRHOTIC PORTAL FIBROSIS) Not infrequently patients with portal hypertension and splenomegaly have no clinical or morphologic evidence of cirrhosis. Instead of cirrhosis, careful inspection of the liver often shows some fibrosis in the portal areas and variable thickening of the walls of the portal vein branches in the liver. There appear to be three variants of the process. Some patients have only *intrahepatic phlebosclerosis* and *fibrosis,* others have in addition segmental thickening or *sclerosis of the portal and splenic veins,* and a third group may show actual *thrombosis* of these vessels. Such cases have been reported from many parts of the world, some of them under the term "Banti's syndrome." In the United States cases of noncirrhotic portal fibrosis have been associated with chronic ingestion of arsenicals.

SCHISTOSOMIASIS (See also Chap. 228) The ova of *Schistosoma mansoni* elicit granulomatous and fibrotic reactions along the portal tracts, the result of a delayed hypersensitivity reaction modulated by an antigen-antibody immune-complex reaction. The characteristic hepatic lesion of schistosomiasis is, therefore, noncirrhotic portal ("pipestem") fibrosis, which produces progressive occlusion of the portal venules with resultant presinusoidal portal hypertension. In advanced cases sinusoidal portal hypertension may be seen. True cirrhosis may be present in some cases, but nutritional deficiencies and other factors, e.g., hepatitis B infection, contribute to this process. Clinically, the signs of portal hypertension predominate and variceal hemorrhage is the usual presentation. The liver and spleen are moderately enlarged. Hepatocellular function is usually normal, but jaundice and serum alkaline phosphatase elevations may be noted.

CONGENITAL HEPATIC FIBROSIS This rare variant of polycystic disease of the liver is probably transmitted as an autosomal recessive trait and may be associated with cystic renal disease. Typically, the patient is young, has no history or signs of hepatocellular disease, and presents with unexplained hepatosplenomegaly, hemorrhage from esophagogastric varices due to presinusoidal portal hypertension, or renal failure. Surgical correction of the portal hypertension may permit long-term survival in patients without renal involvement because progressive liver failure is rare. The biopsy findings are distinctive; normal masses of liver parenchyma are separated by mature fibrous bands containing networks of bile ducts; large cysts (typical of polycystic disease) are not found. The cellular damage, inflammation, and nodular regeneration of cirrhosis are notably absent.

MAJOR SEQUELAE OF CIRRHOSIS

Patients with any form of cirrhosis, with its progressive loss of liver cell function and advancing distortion of intrahepatic vasculature, are threatened by three major complications: *portal hypertension* and its associated complications of variceal hemorrhage and splenomegaly, disabling *fluid retention* in the form of ascites and edema, and *hepatic encephalopathy (hepatic coma).* One-third of deaths in patients with alcoholic cirrhosis are related to variceal hemorrhage; ascites occurs in 60 to 85 percent of cases of advanced cirrhosis; and about 50 percent of patients with cirrhosis die in hepatic coma. Other complications include portal vein thrombosis and hepatocellular carcinoma (especially in postnecrotic cirrhosis and hemochromatosis).

PORTAL HYPERTENSION **Definition** The normal adult liver is perfused by about 1500 ml blood per minute. Approximately two-thirds of hepatic blood flow and one-half of the oxygen supply is provided by the portal vein; the remainder is derived from the hepatic artery. Normally the pressure in the portal vein is quite low (10 and 15 cm saline), since the vascular resistance in the hepatic sinusoids is also low. The nodular regeneration and distortion of the lobular architecture of the cirrhotic liver produce an increase in vascular resistance in the portal venous bed, and a rise in portal venous pressure (portal hypertension) owing to the impairment of blood flow. Portal hypertension is defined as a portal pressure of over 30 cm saline when measured at surgery, a direct percutaneous transhepatic portal vein pressure greater than 8 mmHg above inferior vena cava pressure, or a wedged hepatic vein pressure greater than 4 mmHg above the inferior vena cava pressure.

Pathogenesis Portal hypertension usually results from obstruction to portal blood flow. Anatomically this obstruction can occur at three levels: (1) hepatic veins (Budd-Chiari syndrome), (2) intrahepatic (cirrhosis, metastatic tumors), (3) portal vein (thrombosis, tumor involvement). Portal hypertension can also result from increased portal blood flow in the absence of obstruction, as in myeloid metaplasia with massive splenomegaly.

The commonest cause of portal hypertension in the United States is *cirrhosis,* which produces impedance of blood flow through the liver by fibrosis, thrombosis, and nodular regeneration. About 30 to 60 percent of patients with cirrhosis have an important degree of portal hypertension. The second most common cause of portal hypertension is *mechanical obstruction* of the extrahepatic portal vein, usually the result of thrombosis or tumor invasion. *Occlusion of the major hepatic veins* (Budd-Chiari syndrome) or their small intrahepatic branches (as in venoocclusive disease) may lead to portal hypertension. About 5 percent of patients with cirrhosis and portal hypertension have associated *portal vein thrombosis.* As mentioned above, a small number of patients with sustained portal hypertension have no evidence of cirrhosis but show variable degrees of fibrosis and sclerosis of the intrahepatic portal veins (noncirrhotic portal fibrosis).

Clinical features Many patients with portal hypertension of intra- or extrahepatic origin have symptoms or signs related only to the primary disease, and portal hypertension is tolerated without incident for years. Four major clinical consequences of portal hypertension may, however, lead to its recognition: (1) the development of extensive *portal-systemic venous collaterals,* with gastrointestinal hemorrhage; (2) the appearance of *congestive splenomegaly* with hypersplenism; (3) the onset of episodic stupor or *hepatic (portal-systemic) encephalopathy;* and (4) the development of *ascites.*

The development of collateral channels between the portal

and systemic venous beds is the most characteristic consequence of portal hypertension. Major sites of collateral flow involve dilated veins around the rectum (hemorrhoids), cardioesophageal junction (esophagogastric varices), and retroperitoneal space and the falciform ligament of the liver (periumbilical or abdominal wall collaterals). Although hemorrhoids bleed frequently and varices of the bowel rupture occasionally, massive hemorrhage from thin-walled varices in the upper stomach and lower esophagus is the major complication of portal hypertension. Variceal bleeding occurs without obvious precipitating cause and presents usually as painless massive hematemesis or melena. Abdominal wall collaterals are helpful clinical signs of portal hypertension and appear as slightly tortuous epigastic vessels (caput medusae) that radiate from the umbilicus toward the xiphoid and rib margins. Vascular bruits may be heard over the upper abdomen. *Splenomegaly*, the result of passive congestion, fibrosis, and siderosis, is present in most patients with significant and long-standing portal hypertension. The absence of splenomegaly does not rule out portal hypertension, because splenic size correlates poorly with the level of portal pressure. As noted in Chap. 336, splenic enlargement may be accompanied by abnormal sequestration and destruction of the circulating blood cells (hypersplenism). Patients with portal hypertension and with extensive portal-systemic venous shunting may experience bouts of *hepatic (portal-systemic) encephalopathy or hepatic coma.* These episodes are often precipitated by gastrointestinal hemorrhage and a moderate to high protein diet. Ascites is not a feature of portal vein obstruction or other forms of presinusoidal portal hypertension but is a common occurrence in portal hypertension associated with cirrhosis or hepatic venous blockade.

Diagnosis The diagnosis of portal hypertension is usually based on indirect evidence such as the presence of esophageal varices, abdominal collateral veins, or hypersplenism or ascites in a patient with cirrhosis. Esophageal varices are visualized in the majority of cases by a careful *barium swallow* or *fiberoptic endoscopy.* The finding on a liver scan of significant uptake of radioactivity in the spleen and bone marrow suggest shunting of blood away from the liver and is suggestive of cirrhosis. Direct measurement of portal venous pressure by percutaneous transhepatic "skinny needle" catheterization is available in some medical centers. In patients with variceal bleeding and in certain patients with suspected portal vein thrombosis or previous portacaval shunt surgery it is useful to obtain measurement of portal pressure and visualization of the portal system prior to operation. Splenoportography, which requires percutaneous needle puncture of the spleen, is not widely used because it is technically difficult and hazardous. When percutaneous transhepatic catheterization of the portal vein is not feasible, mesenteric and hepatic angiography are frequently obtained prior to shunt surgery to visualize the hepatic arterial bed as well as the portal system during the venous runoff phase. This allows the surgeon to plan the operative approach, and also provides valuable information regarding the presence of unsuspected lesions such as hepatocellular carcinoma or Budd-Chiari lesions. In addition, measurement of wedged hepatic vein pressure (WHVP) can be obtained by wedging the catheter into the hepatic parenchyma. Elevation of WHVP occurs in portal hypertension due to cirrhosis, while WHVP is normal in portal vein thrombosis.

Treatment GENERAL Vigorous treatment of patients with alcoholic hepatitis superimposed on alcoholic cirrhosis, chronic active hepatitis, and other liver diseases may lead to a fall in portal pressure and to the disappearance of varices. As a rule, however, portal hypertension caused by established cirrhosis or portal vein occlusion is not reversible, and variceal hemorrhage remains a grave threat, particularly in patients with large varices. No precise prognosis can be made in individual cases, but more than 30 percent of patients with cirrhosis and varices experience a major hemorrhage within 5 years and have an overall mortality of 60 to 80 percent. In contrast, patients with normal liver function and variceal hemorrhage secondary to portal vein block tolerate episodes of hemorrhage relatively well. Despite technical improvements in surgical methods of portal vein or variceal decompression, shunts should be reserved for patients who bleed from varices.

ACUTE VARICEAL HEMORRHAGE Prompt and effective care of the patient with massive hematemesis or melena from a ruptured varix requires coordinated medical-surgical efforts. The basic elements of management include the following:

Quantitative replacement of blood loss is essential to prevent further deterioration of liver function. It is often advisable to use fresh blood if massive replacement therapy is required. *Demonstration of esophageal varices, location of the actual bleeding site,* and *exclusion of other causes of gastrointestinal hemorrhage* by endoscopy or radiography are critical. It should not be assumed that cirrhotics with proved or probable varices are bleeding from the varices, because at least one-third have other potential bleeding sites in the upper gastrointestinal tract.

Temporary control of variceal bleeding may be achieved by vasopressin infusions, balloon tamponade, left gastric vein occlusion, or endoscopic sclerosis of varices. Continuous infusion of 0.4 unit of vasopressin per minute through a peripheral vein may lead to a temporary decrease or cessation in variceal hemorrhage by lowering splanchnic blood flow and portal pressure. Vasopressin dosage is then tapered and discontinued 48 h after bleeding has stopped. Transient decreases in cardiac output, cardiac arrhythmias, and water retention may make the use of vasopressin hazardous to patients with ischemic heart disease. Mesenteric angiography is useful in both diagnosis and treatment of variceal bleeding. The injection of contrast material into the mesenteric, celiac, or gastric arteries is used to localize the site of hemorrhage. Temporary control of bleeding can be achieved in a high percentage of patients by infusion of vasopressin directly into the splanchnic bed via the superior mesenteric artery. This method has no clear advantage over peripheral vein infusion. The Sengstaken-Blakemore tube or a modified single-balloon tube may be inserted into the stomach, inflated, and attached to traction to provide local compression of the submucosal veins. Although often effective in producing temporary control of massive hemorrhage, this device is difficult to place accurately and is uncomfortable for the patient; and its use is often complicated by rebleeding, esophageal erosions, airway obstruction, or aspiration. The use of balloon tamponade or vasopressin infusion should be regarded as temporary therapy with a significant incidence of relapse. If both methods fail to control bleeding, transhepatic catheterization and occlusion of the left gastric vein may result in the cessation of variceal hemorrhage. Another method to control acute bleeding is direct injection of sclerosing solutions (such as ethanolamine oleate) into the varices via the endoscope. The efficacy and safety of this approach are still being evaluated.

Evaluation of liver function and *assessment of operative risk* are important but difficult. No single clinical test of liver function can predict accurately the immediate postoperative morbidity and mortality. In general, however, patients with compensated or stable cirrhosis have a much more favorable outlook than those with deepening jaundice, ascites, or signs of encephalopathy. Careful medical management for 2 or 3 weeks or longer may permit considerable recovery of liver function in patients with active alcoholic cirrhosis.

Emergency surgical shunting procedures to arrest bleeding may be performed within a few days. The mortality is 25 to 50 percent in the typical patient, but the operation does prevent exsanguination, usually prevents future variceal bleeding, and may permit considerable recovery of liver function.

In many patients, *elective shunt surgery* may be advisable. The results of large clinical series indicate that effective portacaval shunt surgery does not improve longevity but does prevent recurrent variceal hemorrhage. The type of surgical shunt procedure (e.g., portacaval, splenorenal) often depends on the experience and judgment of the surgeon. Portal decompression does not usually correct the pancytopenia of hypersplenism. In infants and in other patients with extensive portal vein disease, effective portal-systemic shunts may be constructed, using other branches of the portal vein and the trunk of the inferior vena cava. Late complications in patients with functioning portacaval shunts include hepatic coma (15 to 20 percent), peptic ulceration (10 to 15 percent), slight unconjugated hyperbilirubinemia, and, rarely, accumulation of iron within the cirrhotic liver. A *selective*, distal splenorenal shunt with portal-azygous ligation appears to decompress varices without dramatically altering portal pressure and may be relatively free of the complication of disabling encephalopathy.

ASCITES See also Chap. 39.

Definition Ascites, the accumulation of excessive volumes of fluid within the peritoneal cavity, frequently accompanies cirrhosis and other types of diffuse parenchymal liver disease. The development of ascites is often accompanied by hemodilution, edema, and decreased urine volume. These and other clinical findings reflect the complex abnormalities of electrolyte, water, and protein metabolism that may complicate severe liver disease and other disturbances of the hepatic circulation.

Pathogenesis The physician detects ascites when 500 ml or more of fluid has accumulated in the peritoneal cavity. Ultrasonographic examination of the abdomen is useful in verifying the presence of smaller amounts of fluid. Ascites results from disturbances of both local and systemic mechanisms that regulate the passage of fluid and solutes across vascular and serosal membranes. The *local or intraabdominal factors* favoring ascites formation in cirrhosis include the following:

1 *Portal hypertension.* The contribution of portal hypertension to the formation of ascites is not clearly understood, as patients with portal hypertension due to extrahepatic portal vein block do not generally have ascites. On the other hand reduction in portal vein pressure by a side-to-side portacaval anastomosis often results in improvement in ascites. Undoubtedly portal hypertension combined with other factors contributes to the formation and persistence of ascites in the cirrhotic patient.
2 *Increased flow of hepatic lymph.* Weeping of lymph from the surface of the cirrhotic liver can be observed at surgery. This presumably results from distortion and blockage of the hepatic sinusoids and lymphatics resulting in extravasation of protein-rich lymph into the peritoneal cavity. This mechanism may be quite important in the formation of ascites in the Budd-Chiari syndrome, in which the ascitic fluid has a high protein level.

The most important systemic factors include the following:

1 *Decreased plasma colloid oncotic pressure.* Low serum albumin in cirrhosis results from a combination of expansion of the plasma volume, causing dilution of serum proteins, impaired hepatic synthesis, and loss of albumin from the vascular space into the peritoneal cavity. Up to one-fourth of total body albumin may be present in the ascitic fluid. Hypoalbuminemia in turn reduces the plasma oncotic pressure and leads to loss of water into the extravascular space.
2 *Hyperaldosteronism.* Secondary hyperaldosteronism is common in the cirrhotic patient with ascites and leads to excessive reabsorption of sodium in the distal tubule. Hyperaldosteronism results from increased aldosterone secretion by the adrenal gland, presumably due to a reduction in renal blood flow and impaired hepatic metabolism and excretion of aldosterone.
3 *Impaired water excretion.* Patients with ascites have impaired renal excretion of a water load, secondary to reduced renal vascular flow and in some patients due to excessive serum levels of antidiuretic hormone.

Treatment In some patients with reversible liver disease, particularly acute alcoholic hepatitis or chronic active hepatitis, improvement in liver function may be accompanied by spontaneous diuresis. However, in patients with stable cirrhosis liver function may not improve significantly after a period of observation, and therapy directed against the ascites is indicated. It should be remembered that ascites develops quite slowly, and *must be removed slowly* in order to avoid acute changes in plasma volume, which can be disastrous. The goal of therapy should be the loss of not more than 1.0 kg per day if both ascites and peripheral edema are present, or no more than 0.5 kg per day in patients with ascites only. Fluid loss during treatment can be monitored by accurate daily weights.

Bed rest and strict fluid and sodium restriction are the first measures to be tried in the cirrhotic patient with ascites. Sodium intake should be restricted to 30 meq per day and fluid intake may be limited to 1500 ml per day if hyponatremia is marked. Not surprisingly, patients do not tolerate this degree of sodium restriction, and caloric intake may decline. It is therefore important to supply adequate low-sodium snacks or supplements to ensure an adequate intake of calories and protein essential for healing of the damaged liver. If after 1 week there has been no change in weight, spironolactone 25 mg four times daily is added. If this dose is inadequate, spironolactone is increased in stepwise increments every 4 days until a maximum dose 100 mg four times daily is reached. If the ascites is still refractory, one may cautiously try furosemide 40 to 80 mg per day. Aggressive diuretic therapy may be complicated by depletion of plasma volume and reduction of renal function. Brisk diuresis may also cause hypokalemic alkalosis, which in turn enhances hepatic encephalopathy. Therefore frequent assessment of fluid and electrolyte status is mandatory, and restoration of plasma volume with infusions of albumin may be required if significant intravascular volume depletion occurs.

The conservative management of ascites is successful in the majority of cirrhotics, especially in the hospital setting, if sodium and water intake are strictly limited. In general, diuresis is more likely to occur in those patients in whom improvement in liver function occurs. A minority of patients with advanced cirrhosis fail to respond, despite intensive medical therapy. In some of these patients with intractable ascites a side-to-side portacaval shunt may result in improvement in ascites, presumably due to reduction of portal pressure. However, these patients are extremely poor surgical risks, and operative mortality and morbidity are high. Surgical implantation of a plastic shunt between the peritoneal cavity and the superior vena cava has also been used successfully to reduce intractable ascites. This type of peritoneovenous shunt (LeVeen) has a pressure-sensitive, one-way valve which allows ascites fluid to flow from the abdominal cavity to the superior vena cava. Although this technique may be useful in obtaining short-term control of ascites, it is accompanied by significant complications, including infection and disseminated intravascular coagulation; its overall efficacy remains to be determined.

Therapeutic *paracentesis* may be required in patients with respiratory embarrassment or impending rupture of an umbilical hernia due to massive ascites. Up to 3 liters of fluid may be removed over a 4-h period using a plastic indwelling catheter or small-bore needle. Since the ascites usually reaccumulates within several days, it may be necessary to repeat the procedure until a diuresis can be initiated. Repeated therapeutic paracenteses should not be performed in patients with cirrhosis, since this may be complicated by infection of the ascites, chronic ascites leak, hemorrhage, and volume and protein depletion.

Hepatorenal syndrome is a serious complication of cirrhosis, characterized by advancing azotemia, oliguria, and intractable ascites. This may follow a bout of severe gastrointestinal bleeding, sepsis, and too rapid attempts at diuresis or paracentesis; or it may occur without a recognized precipitant. The urine output falls to 200 to 400 ml per day, with gradual elevation of the serum creatinine and marked sodium retention. Death may occur from uremia, gastrointestinal bleeding, or hepatic coma. The exact cause of renal failure in cirrhosis is unknown, but altered renal hemodynamics appears to be responsible for this functional disorder. Contributing factors include decrease in renal cortical perfusion, marked hyperaldosteronism, decreased effective circulating plasma volume, and increased intraabdominal pressure from tense ascites. The kidneys are structurally intact; urinalysis, pyelography, and renal biopsy are usually normal. Treatment is usually unsuccessful, although some patients with hypotension and decreased plasma volume may respond to infusions of salt-poor albumin with increasing urine output and gradual loss of ascites. Salt and water restriction are also usually employed, but recovery seems to be most closely correlated with improvement in liver function. In a few patients, recovery has followed a portacaval shunt or liver transplantation; however, most patients are extremely poor candidates for major surgery because of their severe liver disease and precarious general condition. It has been suggested but not proved that peritoneovenous shunt may reverse renal failure in some patients.

SPONTANEOUS BACTERIAL PERITONITIS Patients with ascites and cirrhosis, particularly alcoholic cirrhosis, may develop acute bacterial peritonitis without an obvious precipitating event. The classic presentation is the abrupt onset of fever, chills, generalized abdominal pain, and rebound tenderness accompanied by cloudy ascitic fluid with a high white cell count and bacteria. However, a more common presentation is that of fever of unknown origin with mild abdominal pain which may be attributed to other causes. The diagnosis of spontaneous bacterial peritonitis is based upon careful examination of the ascites fluid. The presence of a white cell count greater than 300 cells per cubic millimeter, with more than 75 percent polymorphonuclear leukocytes, should suggest the diagnosis; this should be confirmed by demonstrating bacteria by Gram's stain and by culture. Enteric gram-negative bacilli are found in the majority of cases; pneumococci and other gram-positive organisms are occasionally found. The mechanism by which bacteria infect the ascites fluid is not known. Hematogenous spread during spontaneous bacteremia or leakage of bacteria from the intestinal tract are possible sources of infection. In the majority of cases a focus of infection is not present elsewhere in the body and the route of contamination remains unknown.

Bacterial peritonitis is a serious complication of cirrhosis, with a significant morbidity and mortality; not uncommonly the infection results in hepatic encephalopathy and worsening of liver function. The patient with suspected bacterial peritonitis should be treated initially with broad-spectrum antibiotics effective against gram-negative and gram-positive organisms. More specific antibiotics may be selected after the results of culture and sensitivity tests are available.

HEPATIC ENCEPHALOPATHY Definition Hepatic (portal-systemic) encephalopathy is a complex organic brain syndrome characterized by disturbances in consciousness, fluctuating neurologic signs, asterixis or "flapping tremor," and distinctive electroencephalographic changes. This metabolic disorder of the nervous system may appear in the course of acute or chronic hepatocellular disease or as a complication of portal-systemic venous shunting. It may be *acute* and self-limiting or *chronic* and progressive.

Pathogenesis No single biochemical or physiologic defect has been shown to be the actual cause of hepatic encephalopathy or coma. Most studies have shown that hepatic coma and its associated disorders of cerebral function result from (1) the shunting of portal blood directly into the systemic circulation, so that the blood largely bypasses the liver, and (2) severe hepatocellular damage and dysfunction. Both circumstances have a common result: various toxic substances absorbed from the intestine are not metabolized by the liver, thus allowing them to accumulate within the brain. Ammonia is one such compound, and many, but not all, patients with hepatic encephalopathy have elevated systemic arterial and venous blood levels of ammonia. Hyperammonemia is most often found in patients with portal-systemic venous shunting and in hepatic cell failure.

Undoubtedly, "toxic" substances other than ammonia are involved in the genesis of hepatic encephalopathy. The administration of methionine to patients with portal-systemic shunts has been shown to precipitate stupor or encephalopathy in the absence of hyperammonemia. Other putative factors include mercaptans, short-chain fatty acids, false neurotransmitter substances, and alterations in plasma levels of aromatic and branched-chain amino acids. The liver also is believed to produce substances that are essential for normal brain metabolism, and in liver failure these may be reduced. Decreased cerebral oxygen uptake and impaired intermediary metabolism of glucose in the brain are common but nonspecific features of hepatic encephalopathy.

Most patients with chronic forms of hepatic encephalopathy have distinctive enlargement and proliferation of protoplasmic astrocytes in many areas of the brain, and a few develop band-like cerebral cortical necrosis. These findings suggest that the syndrome may progress from a functional to a structural or irreversible phase.

PRECIPITATING FACTORS In the patient with stable inactive cirrhosis, hepatic encephalopathy often follows a precipitating event. Perhaps the most common predisposing factor is *gastrointestinal bleeding,* which causes an increase in the production of ammonia and other nitrogenous substances in the colon. *Increased dietary protein* may also result in a similar increase in nitrogenous substances by colonic bacteria. *Electrolyte disturbances,* particularly hypokalemic alkalosis secondary to excessive diuresis or vomiting, may precipitate hepatic encephalopathy. Systemic alkalosis causes an increase in the relative concentration of uncharged ammonia (NH_3) and a decrease in ammonium ions (NH_4^+) (see Chap. 315). The uncharged ammonia can more readily cross the blood-brain barrier and accumulate in the central nervous system. Hypokalemia also increases renal ammonia production, some of which enters the systemic circulation by the renal vein. Acute *infections* often trigger hepatic encephalopathy, although the mechanisms involved are not clear. The features of encephalopathy may overshadow the signs of infection and delay diagnosis and treatment. Therefore all patients in hepatic coma should be carefully evaluated for precipitating conditions, such as pneumonia, peritonitis, urinary tract infections, or pancreatitis. *Deterioration of liver function* from any cause will usually precipitate hepatic encephalopathy in the stable cirrhotic. Acute viral hepatitis, alcoholic hepatitis, or extrahepatic obstruction all cause worsening liver function and impairment of the liver's metabolic capacity. Liver function may also worsen after surgery, or in the presence of other diseases such as heart failure or infection.

Diagnosis The recognition of hepatic encephalopathy or coma depends on four major elements: (1) The patient should have evidence of advanced hepatocellular disease, extensive portal-systemic collateral shunts, or both. The liver disease may be acute and massive, as in toxic or fulminant viral hepatitis; or chronic and advanced, as in cirrhosis. The portal-systemic venous shunts, which must permit a significant portion of the portal blood to bypass the liver, may be either *spontaneous* (e.g., naturally developing collaterals) or *surgical* (e.g., large portacaval anastomoses). Most of the patients who develop hepatic encephalopathy have, in fact, elements of both liver disease and portal-systemic shunting. (2) Disturbances of awareness and mentation are characteristic, and forgetfulness and confusion progress to stupor and finally to deep coma. (3) Mental changes are accompanied by shifting combinations of neurologic signs, which include rigidity, hyperreflexia, extensor plantar signs, and, rarely, seizures. Asterixis, or "liver flap," which is a nonrhythmic asymmetric lapse in voluntary sustained posture of extremities, head, and trunk, is often seen in precoma and in advancing hepatic encephalopathy but cannot be elicited in the presence of coma. This neurologic picture is nonspecific and is encountered also in patients with uremia, ventilatory failure, drug intoxication, and other forms of metabolic brain disease. (4) Most patients with the clinical features of hepatic coma have characteristic symmetrical, high-voltage, slow-wave (2 to 5 per second) patterns on the electroencephalogram. *Fetor hepaticus,* a unique musty odor of the breath and urine, may be noted in patients with hepatic coma and also in those with extensive collateral circulation. Several clinical variants of the "classic" syndrome of hepatic encephalopathy have been recognized. *Chronic progressive hepatocerebral degeneration,* which may develop in patients with stable liver disease or with portacaval anastomoses, is characterized by a slow decline in intellectual function, psychiatric symptoms, cerebellar ataxia, tremor, and choreoathetosis. Isolated signs of *myelopathy,* including spasticity and hyperreflexia of the legs, may antedate the other elements of hepatic coma by several months. Both of these conditions must be distinguished from other nonhepatic causes of deranged nervous system function, as well as from Wilson's disease.

A number of conditions can mimic the clinical features of hepatic encephalopathy, particularly in the alcoholic patient with cirrhosis. Acute alcoholic intoxication, delirium tremens, Wernicke's encephalopathy, and Korsakoff's psychosis are accompanied by confusion and tremor and thus are easily confused with hepatic encephalopathy. *Subdural hematoma* is common in the alcoholic and may present with stupor or coma unaccompanied by localizing neurologic signs. *Meningitis* may produce alteration of consciousness without the usual clinical features. For example, lack of a febrile response to acute infection is quite common in the cirrhotic and may lead to delayed diagnosis. *Drug overdose,* particularly with sedatives, tranquilizers, or narcotics, may result from altered hepatic excretion of these agents, and can produce confusion or stupor. *Hypoglycemia* caused by poor nutrition, inadequate glycogen stores in the liver, and alcohol-induced impairment of gluconeogenesis occasionally occurs in the cirrhotic and may be accompanied by alteration of mental function. The diagnosis of hepatic encephalopathy is usually one of exclusion. A careful neurologic examination and judicious use of lumbar puncture, brain scan, skull films, and computerized tomography (CT scan) are generally required to eliminate intracranial hemorrhage or infection, while hypoglycemia, drug overdose, or alcohol intoxication are diagnosed by appropriate blood measurements.

Treatment Early recognition and prompt treatment of hepatic encephalopathy are essential as the condition may progress rapidly to death. Alterations in personality, mood disturbances, slight confusion, deterioration in self-care and handwriting, unusual somnolence, and asterixis are early diagnostic clues. Number-connection tests are simple, sensitive, and reliable bedside methods for assessing the degree of encephalopathy and response to treatment. It also may be desirable to grade or classify the stages of hepatic encephalopathy, since this is often helpful in charting the course of the illness and gauging the effects of therapy. One useful classification is based on the severity of mental signs, the presence of asterixis, and EEG abnormalities (see Table 320-1).

The patient with severe hepatic encephalopathy requires careful attention to the usual supportive measures for the comatose patient, including a nasogastric tube and urinary catheter. Careful monitoring of fluid intake and output is essential. The deeply comatose patient with an absent gag reflex should undergo endotracheal intubation to avoid aspiration pneumonia and ensure adequate delivery of oxygen.

Specific treatment of hepatic encephalopathy is aimed at (1) decreasing ammonia production in the colon and (2) elimination or treatment of precipitating factors. In the presence of acute gastrointestinal bleeding the blood in the bowel lumen should be promptly evacuated with enemas and laxatives in order to reduce the nitrogen load. Ammonia production can also be decreased by oral administration of neomycin, a poorly absorbed antibiotic, at a dosage of 0.5 g every 6 h. Ammonia absorption can be decreased with oral administration or enemas of lactulose, a nonabsorbable disaccharide. The sugar enters the colon where it is metabolized by colonic bacteria to organic acids, which lower the pH in the colon. The excess hydrogen ions convert ammonia (NH_3) to ammonium (NH_4^+), which, because of its positive charge, is not readily absorbed, and bacterial assimilation of NH_3 appears to be increased. Lactulose usually produces a reduction in serum ammonia and improvement in encephalopathy within 24 to 48 h. Lactulose is administered in a loading dose of 50 ml syrup (65 g/dl) every 2 h until diarrhea occurs; thereafter the dose is adjusted so that the patient has two to four loose stools per day.

Elimination or treatment of precipitating factors is of prime importance in the treatment of hepatic encephalopathy. Bleeding from the upper gastrointestinal tract must be promptly controlled to prevent worsening encephalopathy. This is usually difficult in the typical cirrhotic with bleeding varices or

TABLE 320-1
Clinical stages of hepatic encephalopathy

Stage	*Mental status*	*Asterixis*	*EEG*
I	Euphoria/depression, mild confusion, slurred speech, disordered sleep	±	Usually normal
II	Lethargy, moderate confusion	+	Abnormal
III	Marked confusion, incoherent speech, sleeping but rousable	+	Abnormal
IV	Coma; may or may not respond to noxious stimuli	−	Abnormal

hemorrhagic gastritis who represents a poor surgical risk. Temporary elimination of all dietary protein is required until the patient improves to the point at which protein can be tolerated. Fluid and electrolyte abnormalities, particularly hypokalemic alkalosis, should be corrected promptly. Sedatives, analgesics, and tranquilizers should be discontinued, and antibiotics administered as indicated to patients with evidence of infection. Heroic measures such as extracorporeal charcoal column perfusion or exchange transfusion have not been convincingly shown to benefit the acutely encephalopathic patient.

Chronic hepatic encephalopathy is best treated with modest protein restriction (30 or 40 g per day) accompanied by small doses of either neomycin or lactulose. Treatment is adjusted to obtain a reasonable functional level of the patient with the least amount of protein restriction and neomycin or lactulose.

REFERENCES

Alcoholic and postnecrotic cirrhosis

BOROWSKY SA et al: Continued heavy drinking and survival in alcoholic cirrhotics. Gastroenterology 80:1405, 1981

THEODOSSI A et al: Controlled trial of methylprednisolone therapy in severe acute alcoholic hepatitis. Gut 23:75, 1982

VAN THIEL DH et al: Gastrointestinal and hepatic manifestations of chronic alcoholism. Gastroenterology 81:594, 1981

ZETTERMAN RK, SORRELL MF: Immunologic aspects of alcoholic liver disease. Gastroenterology 81:616, 1981

Biliary and other types of cirrhosis

CHRISTENSEN E et al: Clinical pattern and course of disease in primary biliary cirrhosis based on an analysis of 236 patients. Gastroenterology 78:236, 1980

GALBRAITH RM: High prevalence of seroimmunologic abnormalities in relatives of patients with active chronic hepatitis or primary biliary cirrhosis. N Engl J Med 290:64, 1974

MATLOFF DS et al: A prospective trial of D-penicillamine in primary biliary cirrhosis. N Engl J Med 306:319, 1982

WANDS JR et al: Circulating immune complexes and complement activation in primary biliary cirrhosis. N Engl J Med 298:233, 1978

Hepatic encephalopathy

ATTERBURY CE et al: Neomycin-sorbitol and lactulose in the treatment of acute portal-systemic encephalopathy. Am J Digest Dis 23:398, 1978

CONN HO et al: Comparison of lactulose and neomycin in the treatment of chronic portal-systemic encephalopathy: A double-blind controlled trial. Gastroenterology 72:573, 1977

FISHER J: Amino acids in hepatic coma. Dig Dis Sci 27:97, 1982

HOYUMPA AM, SCHENKER S: Perspectives in hepatic encephalopathy. Lab Clin Med 100:477, 1982

ZIEVE L: The mechanism of hepatic coma. Hepatology 1:360, 1981

Portal hypertension and ascites

CLARK AW et al: Prospective controlled trial of injection sclerotherapy in patients with cirrhosis and recent variceal hemorrhage. Lancet 2:552, 1980

CONN HO et al: Distal splenorenal shunt vs portal systemic shunt. Hepatology 1:151, 1981

EPSTEIN M: Deranged sodium homeostasis in cirrhosis. Gastroenterology 76:607, 1979

LEBREC D et al: The effect of propranolol on portal hypertension in patients with cirrhosis. Hepatology 2:523, 1982

MACDOUGALL BRD et al: Increased long-term survival in variceal haemorrhage using injection sclerotherapy. Results of a controlled trial. Lancet 1:124, 1982

SHERLOCK S: Portal circulation and portal hypertension. Gut 19:70, 1978

321
TUMORS OF THE LIVER

ELLIOT ALPERT
KURT J. ISSELBACHER

PRIMARY CARCINOMA Carcinomas arising within the liver may be of liver cell (*hepatocellular*), bile duct cell (*cholangiocellular*), or mixed origin. Hepatocellular carcinoma (primary liver cell carcinoma) accounts for 80 to 90 percent of liver carcinomas. There is, however, little practical purpose in distinguishing between the two types, since both may be found in different parts of the same tumor and the clinical courses are similar.

Epidemiology and etiology Primary liver cancers account for only 1 to 2 percent of malignant tumors found at autopsy in North and South America and Europe. However, in parts of Africa and Asia they may account for up to 20 to 30 percent of all types of malignancy. Liver cell carcinoma occurs two to four times more frequently in men than in women. The peak incidence occurs in the fifth and sixth decades of life in the United States, but one to two decades earlier in areas with a high prevalence of liver carcinoma. Cirrhosis, usually macronodular or postnecrotic, is found in 60 to 75 percent of autopsied patients with primary liver cell carcinoma in all parts of the world.

There is wide variation in the incidence of hepatocellular carcinoma in different parts of the world, and a number of etiologic factors may be important.

1 *Chronic liver disease* of any etiology also appears to predispose to the development of carcinoma. A variety of metabolic, alcoholic, viral, or idiopathic chronic liver diseases can lead to liver cell carcinoma. Alpha$_1$-antitrypsin deficiency and hereditary tyrosinosis, with active liver disease since birth, have a high incidence of developing into carcinoma. In the adult age group, *hemochromatosis* has the highest risk of malignant degeneration, presumably owing to the long duration of the chronic liver inflammation. However, alcoholic and postnecrotic cirrhosis are the most common forms of underlying liver disease in patients with liver carcinoma in the United States.

2 *Viral hepatitis* is endemic in many areas of Africa and Asia. The prevalence of hepatitis B antigenemia in the normal population is 1 to 10 percent in some parts of Africa. In these areas, most patients with hepatocellular carcinoma superimposed on chronic liver disease will have serologic evidence of hepatitis B infection. There is also evidence of the integration of the hepatitis B virus DNA (HBV-DNA) into the genome of liver cells in some patients with prior HB infection, some patients with long-standing HBV infection including those who have developed a superimposed carcinoma. Therefore, hepatitis B virus infection is probably an important cause of chronic liver disease and subsequent liver carcinoma in many parts of the world.

3 *Mycotoxins*, metabolites of saprophytic fungi, including certain known hepatic carcinogens (e.g., aflatoxins), are continuously ingested in foodstuffs in small amounts and are found in high concentrations in foods in parts of Africa and Asia, where liver cell carcinoma is found more frequently. Ingested mycotoxins and viral inflammation can act synergistically to increase the risk of malignant hepatocellular transformation.

4 The male predominance in liver cancer and the effect of sex hormones on experimental carcinogenesis suggest that *hormonal factors* may be important. Significantly, hepatocellular carcinoma has been reported in some patients on long-term androgenic therapy.

5 *Iatrogenic factors* include thorium dioxide (Thorotrast), an agent widely used for radiological images for about 20 years until the mid-1950s. Since there is lifelong hepatic storage and virtually no decay of this radioisotope, the liver is exposed to continuous low-level radiation. After a 15- to 20-year latent period, angiosarcoma or chronic liver disease with carcinoma can develop. Long-term use of the contraceptive pill rarely may lead to development of hepatic cell adenoma, a benign but highly vascular tumor with a tendency to bleed internally or intraperitoneally. Malignant transformation into carcinoma has been reported in a few instances.

Clinical features Hepatic cancers may escape clinical recognition during life because they often occur in patients with underlying cirrhosis, and the symptoms and signs may initially suggest a progression of the underlying liver disease. *Hepatomegaly,* with *pain* or *tenderness,* usually moderate in degree and localized to the upper abdomen or the right upper quadrant, is a major complaint in more than half the cases. Other clinical features which should alert the clinician to the diagnosis include a *mass* in the liver, particularly if tender; the presence of a *friction rub* or *bruit* over the liver; and *blood-tinged ascites* (hemoperitoneum) which occurs in about 20 percent of cases. On rare occasions one may find metabolic disturbances such as polycythemia, hypoglycemia, acquired porphyria, hypercalcemia, and dysglobulinemia. Jaundice is characteristic of cholangiocarcinoma but is relatively uncommon in hepatocellular carcinoma in the absence of active liver disease.

Anemia and elevated alkaline phosphatase levels are common laboratory findings. In a patient with cirrhosis, a disproportionately high serum alkaline phosphatase in relation to other abnormal liver function tests is often a clue to an infiltrating or partially obstructing liver carcinoma.

Diagnosis The clinical features outlined above should suggest the possibility of primary liver carcinoma. Liver scintiscans may indicate the presence of one or more hepatic masses but frequently cannot distinguish between regenerating nodules in a cirrhotic liver and primary or metastatic liver tumors. Gallium 67 scans showing hepatocellular uptake in the abnormal area may be more helpful than ^{99m}Tc scans. Ultrasound or CT scan can demonstrate lesions with a density different from normal liver tissue. These noninvasive techniques also help in directing percutaneous biopsy for definitive diagnosis. Hepatic artery *angiography* may reveal distortion or obstructions of vessels or "tumor blushes" characteristic of neovascularization and usually can define the extent of the tumor and its resectability. Angiography cannot, however, distinguish between types of tumor and may not be able to differentiate benign from malignant solitary tumors.

A unique fetal alpha$_1$ globulin, *alpha-fetoprotein* (AFP), is found in the serum of almost all patients with hepatocellular carcinoma. Very high levels, between 500 ng/ml and 5 mg/ml, occur in 70 to 90 percent of patients. The serum AFP may be slightly elevated in about 5 to 10 percent of patients with large hepatic metastases from gastrointestinal tumors, and in about one-third of patients with acute or chronic viral hepatitis, but only rarely to levels over 500 ng/ml in these conditions. Minimally elevated levels of AFP may persist in some patients with chronic hepatitis. AFP is also elevated up to 500 ng/ml in maternal serums during normal pregnancy. Higher levels can occur in maternal serums with fetal distress or death. The detection and persistence of *high levels* of serum AFP (over 500 or 1000 ng/ml) in an adult with liver disease and without an obvious gastrointestinal tract tumor strongly suggest the presence of primary liver carcinoma. Ectopic hormones, such as chorionic gonadotropin are rarely found. Several variant isoenzymes (including aldolase, alkaline phosphatase, and 5′-nucleotide phosphodiesterase) have been reported in some liver cancer patients and also may be helpful diagnostically when present.

Percutaneous *liver biopsy* can be diagnostic, especially if the biopsy is taken in the area of a palpable nodule or mass localized by ultrasound or CT scans. False-negatives may occur in as many as one-fourth of patients if the biopsy is performed in a routine, blind manner with the intercostal approach. Cytologic examination of ascitic fluid is invariably negative for tumor cells. *Laparoscopy* or *laparotomy* with open liver biopsy is often required for diagnosis. This direct approach has the additional advantage of identifying the occasional patient with localized resectable tumor who may be suitable for partial hepatectomy.

Course and management The course of the disease is fatal and usually rapid. Most patients die within 3 to 6 months from gastrointestinal hemorrhage, progressive cachexia, or hepatic failure.

If the patient is young, in good general health, and has no obvious extrahepatic involvement, solitary hepatic lesions may be excised, or *partial hepatectomy* carried out, but the 5-year survival rate is low. Persistently high or rising levels of AFP after excision of the tumor are indicative of residual or recurrent tumor. Hepatocellular carcinoma may respond for brief periods to systemic or intraarterial chemotherapy, particularly doxorubicin hydrochloride (Adriamycin) or a combination of chemotherapeutic agents. However, the results are still poor, and further trials of combined drug therapy are in progress. Liver transplantation has been attempted in the treatment of hepatic cancer, but recurrence of tumor and frequent appearance of metastases after transplantation have limited the usefulness of this procedure. It is possible that, in the future, aggressive surgery or transplantation may prove to be of value in the treatment of small, localized tumors if diagnosed early.

OTHER BENIGN AND MALIGNANT TUMORS These tumors are very rare. Hepatoblastomas are histologically distinct primary malignant tumors of the liver occurring only in infancy and early childhood and characteristically have very high levels of serum AFP. Since they are usually solitary masses, they are more usually resectable and have a higher 5-year survival rate than hepatocellular carcinoma. *Hemangiomas,* the most common of the benign tumors, are usually single and small, but may present as a large hepatic nodule. Percutaneous needle liver biopsy is contraindicated if the diagnosis is suspected because of the danger of hemorrhage. The diagnosis can be made by angiography. Surgical excision is usually not indicated unless the tumors are large and symptomatic or a malignant lesion cannot be excluded. *Hemangioendotheliomas* or *angiosarcomas* are rare malignant vascular tumors. They have occurred in some patients in association with chronic *vinyl chloride* exposure. These rare tumors have also begun to occur 15 to 20 years after the administration of Thorotrast.

Benign hepatic adenomas and focal nodular hyperplasia, although quite rare, have been reported with increasing frequency, particularly in women taking oral contraceptives for long periods. These lesions may regress when the pill is discontinued. Other rare tumors include benign cholangiomas, rhabdomyomas, and rhabdomyosarcomas. These tumors usually present as a palpable mass in the liver or with intraabdominal hemorrhage. They can be visualized and their extent defined by angiography. Surgical exploration and open biopsy or resection are usually required for definitive diagnosis.

METASTATIC TUMORS Metastatic malignant tumors of the liver are common in clinical practice, ranking second only to cirrhosis as a cause of fatal liver disease. In the United States the incidence of clinically significant metastatic carcinoma is at least 20 times greater than that of primary carcinoma. Hepatic metastases have been reported at autopsies in 30 to 50 percent of patients dying from malignant disease.

Pathogenesis The liver is uniquely vulnerable to invasion by tumor cells: its size, high rate of blood flow, and double perfusion by hepatic artery and portal vein combine to make it the most common site of metastases except for the lymph nodes. In addition, local tissue factors appear to support the growth of metastatic implants. Virtually all types of neoplasms except those primary in the brain may metastasize to the liver. The most common primary tumors are those of the gastrointestinal tract, lung, and breast, and melanomas. Less common are metastases from tumors of the thyroid, prostate, and skin.

Clinical features Most patients with metastatic malignancy of the liver present with (1) symptoms referable only to the primary tumor, with asymptomatic hepatic involvement discovered in the course of clinical evaluation; (2) nonspecific symptoms of weakness, weight loss, fever, sweating, and loss of appetite; or rarely, with (3) features indicating active hepatic disease, especially abdominal pain, hepatomegaly, ascites, or jaundice.

Patients with widespread metastatic liver involvement usually have suggestive clinical signs of cancer and hepatic enlargement; some have localized induration or tenderness of the liver; signs of portal hypertension may be present; or a friction rub may be found, usually over tender areas of the liver.

Abnormal liver function tests are frequent but often mild and nonspecific. They reflect the effects of fever and wasting, as well as the infiltrating neoplastic process itself. An increase in serum alkaline phosphatase is the most common and frequently the only abnormality noted. Hypoalbuminemia, anemia, and occasional mild elevation of transaminase levels may also be found with more widespread disease. Greatly elevated serum levels of CEA are usually found when the metastases are from primary malignancies in the gastrointestinal tract, breast, or lung.

Diagnosis Evidence of metastatic invasion of the liver should be sought actively in any patient with a primary malignancy, especially of the lung, gastrointestinal tract, or breast, before resection of the primary lesion is undertaken. Abnormal liver function tests, particularly an elevated alkaline phosphatase, or demonstration of a mass by liver scintiscan, ultrasound, or CT may provide a presumptive diagnosis. Blind percutaneous needle biopsy of the liver will result in a positive diagnosis in only 60 to 80 percent of cases with established metastases. Serial sectioning of specimens, two or three repeat biopsies, or cytologic examination of biopsy smears may increase the diagnostic yield by 10 to 15 percent. The yield is greatly increased when biopsies are directed by ultrasound or CT or obtained by laparoscopy.

Treatment Most metastatic carcinomas respond poorly to all forms of treatment, which is usually only palliative. Surgical removal of a single large metastasis is rarely feasible. Systemic chemotherapy with combinations of different chemotherapeutic agents briefly may slow tumor growth and reduce symptoms in some patients but does not significantly alter the prognosis. It remains to be determined whether newer drugs or combination chemotherapy eventually will prove to be more effective.

REFERENCES

ALPERT E: Alpha-fetoprotein: Developmental biology and clinical significance, in *Progress in Liver Disease*, vol 5, H Popper, F Schaffner (eds). New York, Grune & Stratton, 1975

———: Primary hepatic tumor. Gastroenterology 74:759, 1978

BEASLEY RP et al: Hepatocellular carcinoma and hepatitis B virus. Lancet 2:1129, 1981

BRECHOT C et al: Evidence that hepatitis B virus has a role in liver cell carcinoma in alcoholic liver disease. N Engl J Med 306:1384, 1982

JOHNSON PJ et al: Hepatocellular carcinoma in Great Britain: Influence of age, sex, HBsAg status, and etiology of underlying cirrhosis. Gut 19:1022, 1978

KLATSKIN G: Hepatic tumors: Possible relationship to use of oral contraceptives. Gastroenterology 73:386, 1977

MARGOLIS S, HOWEY C: Systemic manifestations of hepatoma. Medicine 51:381, 1972

OMATA M et al: Hepatocellular carcinoma in the USA: Etiologic considerations. Localization of hepatitis B antigens. Gastroenterology 76:279, 1979

SELIKOFF IJ, HAMMOND EC (eds): Toxicity of vinyl chloride–polyvinyl chloride. Ann NY Acad Sci 246:1975

SHAFRITZ DA et al: Integration of hepatitis B virus DNA into the genome of liver cells in chronic liver disease and hepatocellular carcinoma. N Engl J Med 305:1067, 1981

SZMUNESS W: Hepatocellular carcinoma and hepatitis B virus: Evidence for a causal association. Prog Med Virol 24:49, 1978

WOGAN G: Aflatoxin in carcinogenesis and its implications in man, in *Hepatocellular Carcinoma*, K Okuda, RL Peters (eds). New York, Wiley, 1976

322 INFILTRATIVE AND METABOLIC DISEASES AFFECTING THE LIVER

KURT J. ISSELBACHER
J. THOMAS LaMONT

Many disseminated, systemic, or metabolic diseases involve the liver in a diffuse manner by the infiltration of abnormal cells or the accumulation of chemical substances or metabolites. Although infiltrative diseases may vary widely in their etiology and extrahepatic manifestations, the findings in the liver may be quite similar. Generalized enlargement and firmness of the liver, gradual and nonspecific deterioration of liver function, and, less often, signs of portal hypertension or ascites are typical features of this group of diseases. Differential diagnosis by clinical means may be difficult on occasion, but the diffusely infiltrated liver provides an excellent source of tissue for diagnostic purposes.

The infiltrative process may involve one or more of the structural components of the liver: the hepatocytes, the Kupffer cells and other elements of the reticuloendothelial system, the interstitial tissue, or the blood vessels.

LIPID INFILTRATIONS

FATTY LIVER Slight to moderate enlargement of the liver due to diffuse infiltration of liver cells by neutral fat (triglyceride) is a common clinical and pathologic finding. Although minimal fatty changes are often transient and have no clinical significance, persistent or extensive fatty infiltration may produce dysfunction and symptoms that require careful evaluation.

Etiology The major causes of fatty liver encountered in clinical practice depend on the age, geographic location, and metabolic-nutritional status of the patient population. *Chronic alco-*

holism is the most common cause of fatty liver in this country and in other countries with a high alcohol intake. The severity of fatty involvement is roughly proportional to the duration and degree of alcoholic excess. *Protein malnutrition,* especially in infancy and early childhood, accounts for most cases of severe fatty liver in the tropical zones of Africa, South America, and Asia. The hepatic changes may be associated with other clinical and pathologic features of kwashiorkor. Patients with adult-onset *diabetes mellitus,* especially those who are overweight and are poorly controlled, often have fatty livers. *Obesity* is commonly associated with fatty infiltration of the liver, which recedes as weight reduction occurs. However, *jejunoileal bypass* for surgical treatment of morbid obesity is sometimes associated with severe fatty liver and hepatic failure which may be fatal. In patients with Cushing's syndrome and in those receiving large doses of corticosteroids, fatty infiltration of the liver may occur. In many *chronic illnesses,* especially those complicated by impaired nutrition or malabsorption, increased fat is found in liver cells. For example, patients with ulcerative colitis, chronic pancreatitis, or protracted heart failure frequently have moderately fatty livers at the time of death. Patients maintained on prolonged *intravenous hyperalimentation* may also develop a fatty liver.

Acute fatty liver is caused by a number of hepatotoxins and is frequently accompanied by signs and symptoms of liver failure. Carbon tetrachloride intoxication, DDT poisoning, and ingestion of substances containing yellow phosphorus result in severe fatty liver. Acute and prolonged alcohol ingestion may also be considered in this category and may be associated with a rapidly enlarging and fat-laden liver. Minor degrees of fatty infiltration are seen following acute alcoholic intoxication, but this is rarely of clinical significance. Two types of acute fatty liver deserve special comment: *Acute fatty liver of pregnancy,* a rare but often fatal condition seen during the third trimester of pregnancy, is characterized by nausea, vomiting, abdominal pain, renal failure, and coma. *Massive tetracycline therapy,* in amounts of 3 to 12 g administered intravenously, is a rare cause of acute fatty liver and fatal hepatic coma, especially during pregnancy.

Pathogenesis The hepatic lipid deposits, which consist largely of triglycerides and lesser amounts of phospholipid and cholesterol, appear as vacuoles of varying size within the cytoplasm of liver cells. In extreme cases, every liver cell is involved, and lipids comprise up to 30 to 40 percent of the total liver weight.

The biochemical mechanisms leading to hepatic triglyceride accumulation are described in Chap. 315. Fatty infiltration has been produced in experimental animals by a variety of toxic agents and drugs, such as alcohol, carbon tetrachloride, and orotic acid. Dietary deficiencies, such as choline deficiency, readily lead to increased fat in the liver in the rat. However, with few exceptions these experimental studies cannot be used directly to explain the pathogenesis of fatty liver in clinical disease. Moderate doses of ethanol may produce both acute and chronic fatty changes in human subjects, probably by its direct effects on hepatic triglyceride and fatty acid metabolism (Chap. 315). Protein deficiency seems to account for the fatty liver of kwashiorkor, and impaired protein synthesis for the fat accumulation following tetracycline and carbon tetrachloride administration. In diabetes mellitus and in starvation, increased mobilization of fatty acids from adipose tissue may be involved.

Clinical features The signs and symptoms of fatty liver are related to the degree of fat infiltration, the time course of its accumulation, and the underlying cause. The obese or diabetic patient with chronic fatty liver is usually asymptomatic and has only mild tenderness over the enlarged liver. The liver function tests are normal or show mild elevations of alkaline phosphatase, transaminases, or aminotransferases. In contrast, alcoholic patients with acute fatty liver following a bout of heavy drinking may have right upper quadrant pain and tenderness with laboratory evidence of cholestasis. The clinical presentation of acute fatty liver of pregnancy or fatty liver from hepatotoxins is that of fulminant hepatic failure of any cause, with evidence of hepatic encephalopathy, marked elevations of prothrombin time and transaminases, and variable degrees of jaundice.

Diagnosis The findings of a firm, nontender, and generally enlarged liver with minimal hepatic dysfunction in a patient with chronic alcoholism, malnutrition, poorly controlled diabetes mellitus, or obesity should suggest a fatty liver. Needle biopsy of the liver will demonstrate the increased fatty content and possibly the underlying primary disorder. In acute fatty liver of pregnancy and in most cases of Reye's syndrome (see below), fat accumulates in small vacuoles (microvesicular fat), rather than in large cytoplasmic droplets. The reason for the morphologic appearance of the fat in these two disorders is unclear.

Treatment Attention to nutritional factors, removal of alcohol or offending toxins, and correction of any associated metabolic disorders usually result in recovery. There is no clinical rationale for the use of lipotropic agents such as choline. When indicated, attention should be directed to abstinence from alcohol, careful control of diabetes, weight loss, or correction of intestinal absorptive defects. In the alcoholic fatty liver there is gradual disappearance of fat from the liver after 4 to 8 weeks of adequate diet and abstinence from alcohol.

REYE'S SYNDROME (FATTY LIVER WITH ENCEPHALOPATHY)

This acute illness has been described in children up to 15 years of age. It is characterized by vomiting, progressive central nervous system damage, signs of hepatic injury, hypoglycemia, and morphologically by extensive fatty vacuolization of the liver and renal tubules. The cause is unknown, although viral and toxic agents, especially salicylates, have been implicated. Cases have been reported from several countries; infants and children of either sex are affected and familial occurrences have been described. An association between salicylate ingestion and Reye's syndrome was suggested soon after the disease was first described. Epidemiologic evidence reveals increased aspirin use and much higher serum salicylate levels in children with this illness than in the general population during outbreaks of Reye's syndrome. However, it seems clear that this illness may also occur in the absence of exposure to salicylates. In fatal cases, the liver is enlarged and yellow, with striking diffuse fatty microvacuolization of cells. Peripheral zonal hepatic necrosis has also been present in some cases. Fatty changes of the renal tubular cells, cerebral edema, and neuronal degeneration of the brain are the major extrahepatic changes.

The onset often follows an upper respiratory tract infection in a previously healthy child. Within 1 to 3 days persistent vomiting occurs together with stupor, which usually progresses rapidly to generalized convulsions and coma. The liver is enlarged, but *jaundice is characteristically absent or minimal.* Marked increases in serum transaminases and prothrombin time, hypoglycemia, metabolic acidosis, and elevated serum ammonia levels are the major laboratory findings. The mortality rate in Reye's syndrome is approximately 50 percent. Therapy consists of infusions of glucose and fresh frozen plasma, as well as intravenous mannitol, to reduce the cerebral edema. Chronic liver disease has not been reported in survivors.

Since the disease appears typically to follow apparent upper respiratory tract infections, chickenpox, or influenza, virologic studies have been carried out. Isolations from stool and tissues have included coxsackievirus, influenza viruses, echovirus 11, and adenovirus type 3. The role of these viral agents in the pathogenesis of the disease is still unclear. Electron-microscopic studies show structural alterations of the mitochondria of liver, brain, and muscle. Hyperammonemia in Reye's syndrome results in part from a transient dysfunction of several hepatic mitochondrial enzymes which convert ammonia to urea. As indicated, it is very suggestive that in many cases aspirin plays a role in the pathogenesis of this disorder. Salicylates in high doses are known to uncouple mitochondrial oxidative phosphorylation and in animals to reduce brain glucose before the appearance of hypoglycemia. Thus, it is possible that in a postviral state some children when given salicylates (with the development of high blood levels) may get structural and functional damage to mitochondria in organs such as liver, kidney, and brain. Therefore, the clinical manifestations of Reye's syndrome may result from the combination of a viral agent and salicylates producing damage to mitochondria. Conceivably this occurs only in metabolically susceptible individuals. In any event, *salicylates should be avoided* during outbreaks of Reye's syndrome and not prescribed if the diagnosis is suspected.

NIEMANN-PICK DISEASE (See Chap. 56) This rare heritable disorder, found mainly in Jewish infants, is characterized by the accumulation of sphingomyelin and cholesterol in reticuloendothelial cells of the liver, spleen, bone marrow, and brain. Hepatomegaly and splenomegaly are present, but jaundice and other evidence of hepatic dysfunction are rare. The liver shows clusters of lipid-filled, foamy Kupffer cells. Diagnosis is made by lipid analysis of the tissue.

GAUCHER'S DISEASE (See Chap. 56) Accumulations of large reticuloendothelial cells containing glucocerebrosides (Gaucher's cells) in the liver and spleen account for the characteristic moderate to massive hepatosplenomegaly. Rarely, ascites or portal hypertension is produced by compression of the intrahepatic vasculature. The diagnosis may be made readily by liver biopsy and demonstration of the Gaucher's cells.

WOLMAN'S AND CHOLESTEROL ESTER STORAGE DISEASES Wolman's disease is a rare and fatal familial lipidosis of infancy producing hepatosplenomegaly and stippled calcification of the adrenal glands. Liver biopsy shows clusters of foam cells (reticuloendothelial cells filled with cholesterol ester and triglycerides), hepatocytes containing fat, and patchy fibrosis. A related but less severe genetic disorder is cholesterol ester storage disease. In this condition there is hypercholesterolemia and accumulation of both cholesterol esters and triglycerides in hepatic lysosomes. Both these storage disorders are associated with hepatic deficiencies of cholesterol ester hydrolase and triglyceride lipase.

Other rare lipid disorders associated with hepatomegaly and increased fat in the liver include abetalipoproteinemia (Chap. 103), Tangier disease (Chap. 103), Fabry's disease (Chap. 103), and types I and V hyperlipoproteinemia (Chap. 103).

HEPATIC GLYCOGEN ACCUMULATION

DIABETIC GLYCOGENOSIS Hepatic enlargement caused by distention of liver cells with glycogen is present in some poorly controlled and often juvenile diabetic patients. Ketoacidosis and vigorous insulin therapy may further enhance hepatic enlargement and glycogen deposition. In the absence of cirrhosis, the hepatomegaly usually decreases with careful control of the diabetes.

GLYCOGEN STORAGE DISEASE (See Chap. 100) The normal liver contains 1 to 5 percent glycogen (by weight). In types I, II, and VI hereditary glycogen storage disease, increased amounts of glycogen (and fat) are found. Types III and IV are associated with derangements of glycogen structure, and cirrhosis may be present. Enzymatic and chemical analysis of liver tissue is usually needed for diagnosis.

WILSON'S DISEASE (See also Chap. 98) This rare disease, predominantly of young people, is characterized by cirrhosis, softening and degeneration of the basal ganglia, and pigmentation of the cornea (Kayser-Fleischer rings). Increased copper deposition in the tissues seems to be responsible for the liver and basal ganglia changes. Liver cells are ballooned and show increased glycogen with glycogen vacuolization in the nuclei. The liver shows all grades of changes from minimal to severe periportal or macronodular cirrhosis. The details of the clinical features are discussed in Chap. 98.

GALACTOSEMIA (See also Chap. 101)

Hepatic changes are common in patients with unrecognized or untreated galactosemia. In early weeks of life fatty infiltration and cholestasis may be noted in acutely ill infants. If the disease goes unrecognized for months or years, cirrhosis may develop.

OTHER INFILTRATIVE DISEASES

HURLER'S SYNDROME (See Chap. 106) This is an uncommon hereditary disease that is characterized by the widespread tissue deposition of mucopolysaccharide (chondroitin sulfate B and heparin sulfate) in many tissues. The liver is frequently enlarged and firm. Microscopically, Kupffer cells and other macrophages are enlarged and filled with metachromatic granular material. Cirrhosis may be a late complication.

ALPHA$_1$ ANTITRYPSIN DEFICIENCY (See also Chap. 279) Patients with homozygous deficiency of serum alpha$_1$ antitrypsin (α_1-AT) are prone to develop emphysema in adult life. The disease is suggested by the absence of alpha$_1$ globulin on serum electrophoresis and confirmed by direct measurement of α_1-AT. The exact phenotype can then be determined by starch electrophoresis. Hepatocytes of some patients with this deficiency contain periodic acid Schiff (PAS)–positive globules which have been shown to be alpha$_1$ trypsin. Approximately 10 percent of children with homozygous deficiency (PiZZ phenotype) of α_1-AT will develop significant liver disease including neonatal hepatitis and progressive cirrhosis. It has been suggested that 15 to 20 percent of all chronic liver disease in infancy may be attributed to α_1-AT deficiency. Some adults have PAS-positive globules and portal fibrosis or cirrhosis. The occurrence of liver disease in these patients is not dependent upon the development of lung disease.

RETICULOENDOTHELIAL DISORDERS (See also Chaps. 56 and 130)

Moderate to massive hepatomegaly and splenomegaly occur frequently in the various types of leukemia and lymphoma. Jaundice, when present, is usually slight and results from hemolysis. Deep and protracted jaundice is distinctly rare and is caused by obstruction of the intrahepatic or extrahepatic bile ducts by tumor. Liver biopsy specimens reveal portal and sinusoidal infiltrates in most cases of leukemia, but the cellular pattern may be mixed and nonspecific. Liver biopsy is diagnostic in only 5 percent of patients with Hodgkin's disease. This percentage is increased in those with advanced disease or splenomegaly. Directed biopsy at laparoscopy or laparotomy is more likely to be positive than "blind" needle biopsy. Nonspecific histologic changes in the liver have been described in patients with lymphoma and may contribute to the abnormal liver function tests.

Myeloid metaplasia and other myeloproliferative disorders associated with extramedullary hematopoiesis produce hepatomegaly which may reach huge proportions, especially following splenectomy. Bromosulphalein (BSP) retention and alkaline phosphatase elevations are often found. Ascites and portal hypertension, apparently caused by diffuse involvement of portal venules and lymphatics, are rare complications.

GRANULOMATOUS INFILTRATIONS

Systemic granulomatous diseases, including sarcoidosis, miliary tuberculosis, histoplasmosis, brucellosis, schistosomiasis, berylliosis, and drug reactions, produce focal infiltrative hepatic lesions with great regularity. In addition, isolated granulomas of no diagnostic importance may be found occasionally in patients with various forms of cirrhosis and hepatitis. The liver infiltrated by granulomas may be slightly enlarged and firm, but hepatic dysfunction is usually limited to BSP retention and increased serum alkaline phosphatase levels. In a few patients with sarcoidosis or brucellosis portal hypertension may develop, and extensive postnecrotic scarring or postnecrotic cirrhosis may follow healing of the granulomatous lesions.

Needle biopsy of the liver reveals granulomas and often provides the first definite evidence of a systemic or disseminated granulomatous disease. In patients with sarcoidosis who have neither clinical nor laboratory evidence of hepatic involvement, needle biopsy is positive in about 80 percent of cases. In cases of suspected miliary tuberculosis a portion of the biopsy should be cultured and stained for mycobacteria. The organism can be detected in the majority of cases, particularly when caseating granulomas are present. Serial sections of the biopsy specimen should be examined if granulomas are not apparent. Individual granulomas are rarely specific in their microscopic appearance, and final diagnosis usually requires other clinical, laboratory, or histologic data.

AMYLOIDOSIS (See also Chap. 66)

Systemic amyloidosis, whether primary and idiopathic, familial, or secondary to chronic inflammatory or neoplastic diseases, often involves the liver. Grossly, the liver infiltrated with amyloid is enlarged and pale and rubbery in consistency. Microscopically, the birefringent amyloid deposits appear as homogeneous waxy material within the space of Disse, often being concentrated in the periportal areas with atrophy of adjacent liver cell plates. Selective involvement of the walls of blood vessels, especially of the hepatic arterioles, may be a striking feature of primary amyloidosis. With this possible exception, however, the hepatic lesions are the same in all forms of amyloidosis and are present in 60 to 90 percent of cases.

An enlarged and firm liver is found in about 60 percent of patients, and ascites occurs in advanced stages of the disease in about 20 percent. Jaundice, portal hypertension, and other signs of chronic liver disease are usually absent. Liver function changes, although frequent, correlate poorly with the extent of liver infiltration. Hypoalbuminemia, BSP retention, and elevated serum alkaline phosphatase levels are common. On hepatic scan, multiple filling defects simulate metastases. The diagnosis is established by biopsy of rectum, skin, liver, or other involved organs.

REFERENCES

Bagley CM et al: Liver biopsy in Hodgkin's disease. Ann Intern Med 76:219, 1972

Glenner GG: Amyloid deposits and amyloidosis. The β-fibrilloses. N Engl J Med 302:1283, 1980

Irani SK, Dobbins WO III: Hepatic granulomas: A review of 73 patients from one hospital and survey of the literature. J Clin Gastroent 1:131, 1979

Maddrey WC et al: Sarcoidosis and chronic hepatic disease: A clinical and pathologic study of 20 patients. Medicine 49:375, 1970

Partin J et al: Serum salicylate concentrations in Reye's disease: A study of 130 biopsy-proven cases. Lancet 1:191, 1982

Partin JC: Reye's syndrome (encephalopathy and fatty liver). Gastroenterology 69:511, 1975

Spechler SJ, Koff RS: Wilson's disease: Diagnostic difficulties in the patient with chronic hepatitis and hyperceruloplasminemia. Gastroenterology 78:103, 1980

Sveger T: Liver disease in α_1-antitrypsin deficiency. N Engl J Med 294:1316, 1976

323 DISEASES OF THE GALLBLADDER AND BILE DUCTS

MARK S. McPHEE
NORTON J. GREENBERGER

PHYSIOLOGY OF BILE PRODUCTION AND FLOW

BILE SECRETION AND COMPOSITION Bile formed in the hepatic lobules is secreted into a complex network of canaliculi, small bile ductules, and larger bile ducts which run with lymphatics and branches of the portal vein and hepatic artery in portal tracts situated between hepatic lobules. These interlobular bile ducts coalesce to form larger septal bile ducts that join to form the right and left hepatic ducts, which in turn unite to form the common hepatic duct. The common hepatic duct is joined by the cystic duct of the gallbladder to form the common bile duct which enters the duodenum (often after joining the main pancreatic duct) through the ampulla of Vater.

Hepatic bile is a pigmented isotonic fluid with an electrolyte composition resembling blood plasma. The electrolyte composition of gallbladder bile differs from that of hepatic bile since most of the inorganic anions, chloride and bicarbonate, have been removed by reabsorption across the basement membrane.

Major components of bile by weight include water (82 percent), bile acids (12 percent), lecithin and other phospholipids (4 percent), and unesterified cholesterol (0.7 percent). Other constituents include conjugated bilirubin, proteins (IgA, by-products of hormones, and other proteins metabolized in the liver), electrolytes, mucus, and, often, drugs and their metabolic by-products.

The total daily basal secretion of hepatic bile is approximately 500 to 600 ml. The metabolic products of hepatocyte uptake and synthesis are secreted into the bile canaliculi which are lined by microvillus membrane components associated with microfilaments of actin, microtubules, and other contractile elements. Within the hepatocyte, conjugation of many of the bile constituents may occur, while other components of bile such as primary bile acids, lecithin, and some cholesterol are synthesized de novo. Three mechanisms are important in regulating bile flow: (1) active transport of bile acids from hepatocytes into the canaliculi, (2) bile acid–independent ATPase-mediated transport of sodium, and (3) ductular secretion. The last is a secretin-mediated and cyclic AMP–dependent phenomenon which appears to result from the active transport of sodium and bicarbonate into the ductule with resulting passive movement of water across the cell membrane.

THE BILE ACIDS The primary bile acids, cholic and chenodeoxycholic acids, are synthesized from cholesterol in the liver, conjugated with glycine or taurine and excreted into the bile. Secondary bile acids, including deoxycholate and lithocholate, are formed in the colon as bacterial metabolites of the primary bile acids. However, lithocholic acid is much less efficiently absorbed from the colon than deoxycholic acid. Other secondary bile acids, found in trace amounts, which include ursodeoxycholic acid (a stereoisomer of chenodeoxycholate) and a variety of other unusual or "aberrant" bile acids, may be produced in increased amounts in patients with chronic cholestatic syndromes. In normal bile, the ratio of glycine to taurine conjugates is about 3:1, while in patients with cholestasis, increased concentrations of sulfate and glucuronide conjugates of bile acids are often found.

Bile acids are detergents which in aqueous solutions and above a critical concentration of about 2 m*M* form molecular aggregates called micelles. Cholesterol alone is poorly soluble in aqueous environments, and its solubility in bile depends upon both the lipid concentration and the relative molar percentages of bile acids and lecithin. Normal ratios of these constituents favor the formation of solubilizing "mixed micelles," while abnormal ratios promote the precipitation of cholesterol crystals in bile.

In addition to facilitating the biliary excretion of cholesterol, bile acids are necessary for the normal intestinal absorption of dietary fats via a micellar transport mechanism (see Chap. 308). Bile acids also serve as a major physiologic driving force for hepatic bile flow and aid in water and electrolyte transport in the small bowel and colon.

ENTEROHEPATIC CIRCULATION Bile acids are efficiently conserved under normal conditions. Conjugated and unconjugated bile acids are absorbed by *passive diffusion* along the entire gut. Quantitatively much more important for bile salt recirculation, however, is the *active transport* mechanism for conjugated bile acids in the distal ileum (see Chap. 308). The reabsorbed bile acids enter the portal bloodstream and are taken up rapidly by hepatocytes, reconjugated and resecreted into bile (enterohepatic circulation).

The normal bile acid pool size is approximately 2 to 4 g. During digestion of a meal, the bile acid pool undergoes at least one or more enterohepatic cycles depending upon the size and composition of the diet. Normally the bile acid pool circulates approximately 5 to 10 times daily. Intestinal absorption of the pool is about 95 percent efficient, so that fecal loss of bile acids is in the range of 0.3 to 0.6 g per day. This fecal loss is compensated by an equal daily synthesis of bile acids by the liver, and thus the size of the bile salt pool is maintained. Bile acids returning to the liver suppress de novo hepatic synthesis of primary bile acids from cholesterol by inhibiting the rate limiting enzymes, 7α-hydroxylase. While the loss of bile salts in stool is usually matched by increased hepatic synthesis, the maximum rate of synthesis is approximately 5 g per day, which may be insufficient to replete the bile acid pool size when there is pronounced impairment of intestinal bile salt reabsorption.

GALLBLADDER AND SPHINCTERIC FUNCTIONS In the fasting state, the sphincter of Oddi offers a high pressure zone of resistance to bile flow from the common bile duct into the duodenum. This tonic contraction serves to (1) prevent reflux of duodenal contents into the pancreatic and bile ducts, and (2) promote bile filling of the gallbladder. The major factor controlling the evacuation of the gallbladder is the peptide hormone cholecystokinin which is released from the duodenal mucosa in response to the ingestion of fats and amino acids. Cholecystokinin produces (1) powerful contraction of the gallbladder, (2) decreased resistance of the sphincter of Oddi, (3) increased hepatic secretion of bile, and thus (4) enhanced flow of biliary contents into the duodenum.

Hepatic bile is "concentrated" within the gallbladder by energy-dependent transmucosal absorption of water and electrolytes. Almost the entire bile acid pool may be sequestered in the gallbladder following an overnight fast for delivery into the duodenum with the first meal of the day. The normal capacity of the gallbladder is 30 to 75 ml of bile.

DISEASES OF THE GALLBLADDER

CONGENITAL ANOMALIES Anomalies of the biliary tract may be found in 10 to 20 percent of the population, including abnormalities in number, size, and shape (e.g., agenesis of the gallbladder, duplications, rudimentary or oversized "giant" gallbladders, and diverticula). Phrygian cap is a clinically innocuous entity in which a partial or complete septum (or fold) separates the fundus from the body. Anomalies of position or suspension are not uncommon and include left-sided gallbladder, intrahepatic gallbladder, retrodisplacement of the gallbladder, and "floating" gallbladder. The latter condition predisposes to acute torsion, volvulus, or herniation of the gallbladder.

GALLSTONES Pathogenesis of gallstones Gallstones are quite prevalent in most western countries. In the United States, autopsy series have shown gallstones in at least 20 percent of women and in 8 percent of men over the age of 40. It is estimated that 16 to 20 million persons in the United States have gallstones and that approximately 1 million new cases of cholelithiasis develop each year.

Gallstones are crystalline structures formed by concretion or accretion of normal or abnormal bile constituents. These stones are divided into three major types: cholesterol and mixed stones account for 80 percent of the total, with pigment stones comprising the remaining 20 percent. Mixed and cholesterol gallstones usually contain more than 70 percent cholesterol monohydrate plus an admixture of calcium salts, bile acids and bile pigments, proteins, fatty acids, and phospholipids. Pigment stones are primarily composed of calcium bilirubinate; they contain less than 10 percent cholesterol.

CHOLESTEROL AND MIXED STONES The solubility of cholesterol in bile depends upon the relative molar concentrations of cholesterol, bile acids, and lecithin. These concentrations may be expressed on triangular coordinates as a "phase diagram" of bile composition (Fig. 323-1). As noted above, cholesterol is relatively water insoluble and normally is kept in solution (in the form of mixed micelles) by bile salts and phospholipids.

The most important mechanism in the formation of lithogenic (stone-forming) bile is increased biliary secretion of cholesterol. This may occur in association with obesity, high caloric diets, or drugs (e.g., clofibrate) and may result from increased activity of hydroxymethylglutaryl-coenzyme A (HMG-CoA) reductase, the rate-limiting enzyme of hepatic cholesterol synthesis. In some patients, impaired hepatic conversion of cholesterol to bile acids may also occur, resulting in a decrease of the lithogenic cholesterol/bile acid ratio. Lithogenic bile also results from decreased hepatic secretion of bile salts and phospholipids which may follow impaired hepatic synthesis (e.g., rare inborn errors of metabolism such as cerebrotendinous xanthomatosis) or defects affecting the enterohepatic circulation of these constituents (e.g., ileal disease or resection). In addition, most patients with gallstones appear to have reduced activity of hepatic cholesterol 7α-hydroxylase, the rate-limiting enzyme for primary bile acid synthesis.

Stone formation in bile supersaturated with cholesterol requires both nucleation and the production of cholesterol monohydrate crystals, which may grow by accretion or concretion to form macroscopic aggregates. The major known predisposing factors to cholesterol stone formation are summarized in Table 323-1.

PIGMENT STONES Gallstones composed largely of calcium bilirubinate are much more common in the orient than in western countries. The presence of increased amounts of unconjugated, insoluble bilirubin in bile results in the precipitation of bilirubin which may aggregate to form pigment stones or may fuse to form the nidus for growth of mixed cholesterol gallstones. In western countries, chronic hemolytic states (with increased conjugated bilirubin in bile) or alcoholic liver disease are associated with an increased incidence of pigment stones. Deconjugation of soluble bilirubin mono- and diglucuronide may be mediated by the enzyme β-glucuronidase, which is sometimes produced when bile is chronically infected by bacteria. Pigment stone formation is especially prominent in orientals and is often associated with infections in the biliary tree (see Table 323-1).

Diagnosis of gallstones Procedures of potential use in the diagnosis of cholelithiasis and other diseases of the gallbladder are detailed in Table 323-2. The plain abdominal film may detect gallstones containing sufficient calcium to be radiopaque (10 to 15 percent of cholesterol and mixed stones and approximately 50 percent of pigment stones). Plain radiography may also be of use in the diagnosis of emphysematous cholecystitis, porcelain gallbladder, limey bile, and gallstone ileus.

Oral cholecystography (OCG) is a useful procedure for the diagnosis of gallstones but is rapidly being replaced by ultrasound (see below). False-positive results are rare, but the oral cholecystogram may be falsely negative (when good opacification is achieved) in approximately 5 to 10 percent of patients with gallstones. Factors which may produce nonvisualization of the OCG are summarized in Table 323-2. When these can be excluded, nonvisualization of the gallbladder following a second dose of oral contrast agent is highly correlated with underlying cystic duct obstruction or chronic inflammation of the gallbladder.

Ultrasonography of the gallbladder is very accurate in the identification of cholelithiasis and has some advantages over oral cholecystography (see Fig. 323-2*A*). The gallbladder is easily visualized with the technique, and, in fact, failure to image the gallbladder successfully in a fasting patient correlates well with the presence of underlying gallbladder disease. Stones as small as 2 mm in diameter may be confidently identified provided that firm criteria are used [e.g., acoustic "shadowing" of opacities that are within the gallbladder lumen and that change with position (gravity)]. In major medical centers the false-negative and false-positive rates for ultrasound in gallstone patients are about 2 to 4 percent.

Radiopharmaceuticals, such as ^{99m}Tc-labeled *N*-substituted iminodiacetic acids (HIDA, DIDA, PIPIDA, etc.), are rapidly extracted from the blood and are excreted into the biliary tree in high concentration even in the presence of mild to moderate serum bilirubin elevations. Failure to image the gallbladder may indicate cystic duct obstruction, acute or chronic cholecystitis, or surgical absence of the organ. Such scans have their greatest application in the diagnosis of acute cholecystitis.

FIGURE 323-1
Phase diagram of bile composition. The relative concentrations of cholesterol, bile acids, and lecithin are expressed on triangular coordinates as mole percentages totaling 100 percent. The equilibrium limit of solubility for cholesterol is denoted by the solid line. Hatchmarks indicate the metastable zone, where slow precipitation of cholesterol from supersaturated bile may occur. Point A represents a micellar solution in which cholesterol is solubilized in mixed micelles. Point B, on the equilibrium limit of solubility line, indicates bile saturated with cholesterol. Point C depicts cholesterol supersaturated bile, a composition leading to the precipitation of cholesterol crystals.

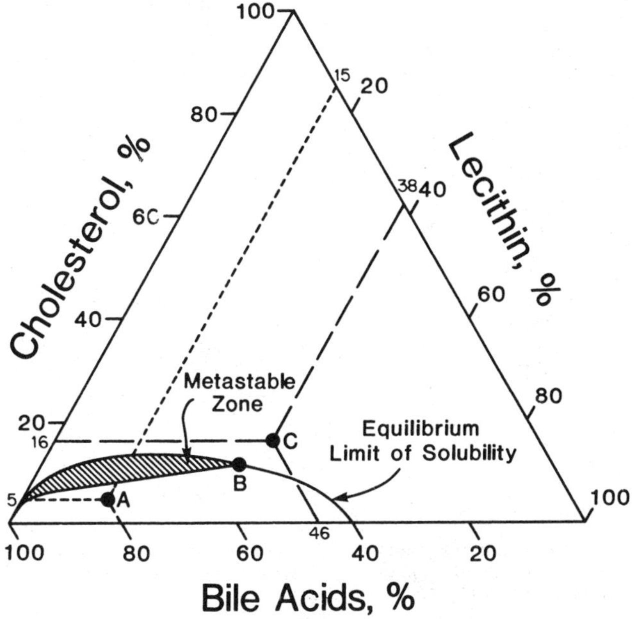

Symptoms of gallstone disease Gallstones usually produce symptoms by causing inflammation or obstruction following their migration into the cystic duct or common bile duct. The most specific and characteristic symptom of gallstone disease is biliary colic. Obstruction of the cystic duct or common bile duct by a stone produces increased intraluminal pressure and distention of the viscus which cannot be relieved by repetitive biliary contractions. The resultant visceral pain is characteristically a severe, steady aching or pressure in the epigastrium or

TABLE 323-1
Predisposing factors for cholesterol and pigment gallstone formation

1 Cholesterol and mixed stones
- *a* Demography: northern Europe and North and South America greater than orient; probable familial, hereditary aspects
- *b* Obesity, high calorie diet (↑ cholesterol output)
- *c* Clofibrate therapy (↑ cholesterol output)
- *d* Malabsorption of bile acids (e.g., ileal disease or resection) (↓ bile salt secretion)
- *e* Female sex hormones: women > men after puberty; oral contraceptives and other estrogens (↓ bile salt secretion)
- *f* Age, especially among males
- *g* Other factors: pregnancy, diabetes mellitus, dietary polyunsaturated fats (↑ cholesterol output)

2 Pigment stones
- *a* Demographic/genetic factors: orient, rural setting
- *b* Chronic hemolysis
- *c* Alcoholic cirrhosis
- *d* Chronic biliary tract infection, parasite infestation
- *e* Increasing age

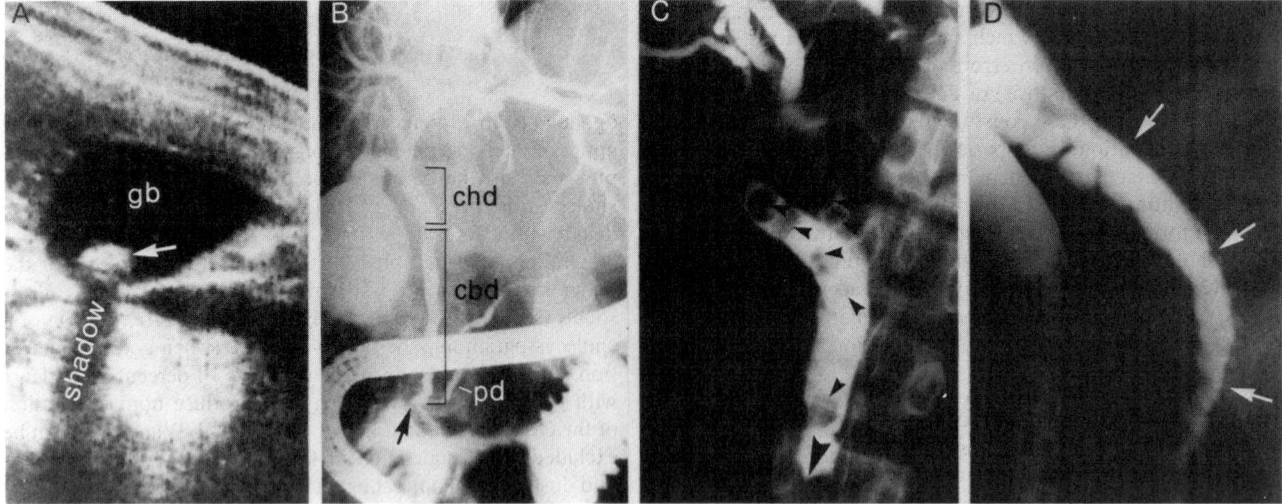

FIGURE 323-2
Examples of ultrasound and radiologic studies of the biliary tract. A. An ultrasound study showing a distended gallbladder containing a single large stone (arrow) which casts an acoustical shadow. B. Endoscopic retrograde cholangiopancreatogram (ERCP) showing normal biliary tract anatomy. In addition to the endoscope and large vertical gallbladder filled with contrast dye, the common hepatic duct (chd), common bile duct (cbd), and pancreatic duct are shown. The arrow points to the ampulla of Vater. C. Percutaneous transhepatic cholangiogram (PTHC) showing choledocholithiasis. The biliary tract is dilated and contains multiple radiolucent calculi (small arrows). The dilatation is due to obstruction by a large stone in the distal portion of the duct (large arrow). D. ERCP showing sclerosing cholangitis. The common bile duct is to the right of the endoscope. Following retrograde cholangiography, the common bile duct shows thickening of the wall with a narrow, beaded lumen typical of sclerosing cholangitis.

right upper quadrant of the abdomen with frequent radiation to the interscapular area, right scapula, or shoulder.

Biliary colic begins quite suddenly and may persist with severe intensity for 1 to 4 h, subsiding gradually or rapidly. An episode of biliary pain is sometimes followed by a residual mild ache or soreness in the right upper quadrant which may persist for 24 h or so. Nausea and vomiting frequently accompany episodes of biliary colic, and mild elevations of serum bilirubin (not exceeding 5 mg/dl) occur in 25 percent of patients. Persistent jaundice or a high serum bilirubin level suggests common duct stones. Fever or chills (rigors) with biliary colic usually implies an underlying complication, i.e., cholecystitis, pancreatitis, or cholangitis. Complaints of vague epigastric fullness, dyspepsia, eructation, or flatulence, especially following a fatty meal, should not be confused with biliary colic. Such symptoms are frequently elicited from patients with gallstone disease but are not specific for biliary calculi. Biliary colic may be precipitated by eating a fatty meal or by consumption of a large meal following a period of prolonged fasting.

TABLE 323-2
Diagnostic evaluation of the gallbladder

Procedure	*Diagnostic advantages*	*Diagnostic limitations*	*Comment*
Plain abdominal x-ray	Low cost Readily available	Relatively low yield ?Contraindicated in pregnancy	Pathognomonic findings in: Calcified gallstones Limey bile, porcelain GB Emphysematous cholecystitis Gallstone ileus
Oral cholecystogram (OCG)	Low cost Readily available Accurate identification of gallstones (90–95%) Identification of GB anomalies, hyperplastic cholecystoses Identification of chronic GB disease after nonvisualization on double dose	?Contraindicated in pregnancy ?Contraindicated with history of reaction to iodinated contrast Nonvisualization with: Serum bilirubin >2–4 mg/dl Failure to ingest or absorb tablets Impaired hepatic excretion Very small stones may be undetected More time consuming than GBUS	Often initial procedure of choice in identification of gallstones
Gallbaldder ultrasound (GBUS)	Rapid Accurate identification of gallstones (>95%) Simultaneous scanning of GB, liver, bile ducts, pancreas "Real-time" scanning allows assessment of GB volume, contractility Not limited by jaundice, pregnancy May detect very small stones	Bowel gas Massive obesity Ascites Recent barium study	Procedure of choice for detection of stones if diagnostic limitations prevent OCG
Radioisotope scans (HIDA, PIPIDA, etc.)	Accurate identification of cystic duct obstruction Simultaneous assessment of bile ducts	?Contraindicated in pregnancy Serum bilirubin >6–12 mg/dl Cholecystogram of low resolution	Indicated for confirmation of suspected cholecystitis

Natural history of gallstones Gallstone disease discovered in an asymptomatic patient or in a patient whose symptoms are not referable to cholelithiasis is a common clinical problem. The natural history of "silent" or asymptomatic gallstones has occasioned much debate. In contrast to previous reports, a recent study of silent gallstone patients suggests that the cumulative risk for the development of symptoms or complications requiring surgery is relatively low—10 percent at 5 years, 15 percent at 10 years, and 18 percent at 15 years. Patients remaining asymptomatic for 15 years were unlikely to develop symptoms during further follow-up, and most patients who did develop complications from their gallstones experienced *prior* warning symptoms.

Complications requiring cholecystectomy appear to be much more common in gallstone patients who have developed symptoms. Patients found to have gallstones at a young age are more likely to develop symptoms from cholelithiasis than patients older than 60 years at the time of initial diagnosis. Patients with diabetes mellitus and gallstones appear to be particularly susceptible to septic complications. In addition, asymptomatic gallstone patients with nonvisualization of the gallbladder on OCG appear to have an increased tendency to develop symptoms and complications.

Treatment of gallstones SURGICAL THERAPY Although the management of "silent" gallstones remains controversial, the risk of developing symptoms or complications requiring surgery is quite small (in the range of 1 to 2 percent per year) in most asymptomatic gallstone patients. Thus, a recommendation for prophylactic cholecystectomy in a patient with gallstones should probably be based on assessment of three factors: (1) the presence of symptoms which are frequent enough or severe enough to interfere with the patient's general routine; (2) the presence of a prior complication of gallstone disease, i.e., history of acute cholecystitis, pancreatitis, gallstone fistula, etc.; or (3) the presence of an underlying condition predisposing the patient to increased risk of gallstone complications (e.g., diabetes mellitus, calcified or porcelain gallbladder, cholesterolosis, adenomyomatosis, nonvisualizing gallbladder on oral cholecystography, and/or a previous attack of acute cholecystitis regardless of current symptomatic status). Patients with very large gallstones (over 2 cm in diameter) and patients having gallstones in a congenitally anomalous gallbladder might also be considered for prophylactic cholecystectomy. Although age under 50 years is a worrisome factor in asymptomatic gallstone patients, few authorities would now recommend routine cholecystectomy in all young patients with silent stones.

MEDICAL THERAPY—GALLSTONE DISSOLUTION Treatment with oral chenodeoxycholic acid (CDCA, chenic acid) or its 7β-epimer, ursodeoxycholic acid (UDCA),[1] to dissolve cholesterol or mixed gallstones has resulted in complete or partial dissolution of such stones in approximately 50 to 60 percent of patients with radiolucent gallstones. Biliary secretion of these agents following oral bile acid administration alters the bile acid/cholesterol/lecithin ratio in bile (the lithogenic index). The major therapeutic effect of CDCA, however, is thought to be secondary to a decrease in HMG-CoA reductase activity, which in turn results in decreased hepatic cholesterol synthesis.

Oral bile acid therapy is much less effective in dissolving (1) pigment gallstones, which represent approximately 20 percent of radiolucent stones; (2) radiopaque or calcified gallstones; (3) gallstones greater than approximately 1.5 cm in diameter; and (4) gallstones in gallbladders poorly opacified following oral cholecystography. In patients with multiple, small, radiolucent gallstones in a functioning gallbladder, success rates for CDCA therapy up to 80 percent have been reported if daily doses of 10 to 15 mg/kg of CDCA are used over a 1- to 3-year treatment period. However, lower daily doses of CDCA, i.e., 5 to 10 mg/kg, have resulted in much lower complete dissolution (5 to 15 percent) as well as partial dissolution rates (40 percent). Further, some massively obese patients may require doses as high as 20 to 25 mg/kg per day of CDCA to achieve cholesterol desaturation of bile. After successful dissolution of stones and withdrawal of CDCA treatment, *recurrence* of cholelithiasis is likely unless factors initially producing lithogenesis have been altered in the interim. The results of the U.S. National Cooperative Gallstone Study are summarized in Table 323-3.

Chenodeoxycholic acid therapy is usually associated with self-limited diarrhea in most patients given an optimal therapeutic dose. In addition, approximately 25 percent of patients treated with CDCA acid develop mild (two- to three-fold) and transient (less than 6 months) elevations of serum transaminase levels. Although hepatic injury has been described, biopsy and liver function studies in humans have shown serious CDCA-induced hepatotoxicity in only a small percentage of patients.

Ursodeoxycholic acid is therapeutically effective at lower doses (5 to 10 mg/kg per day) than chenodeoxycholic acid and has not been associated with the relatively high incidence of diarrhea and serum transaminase elevations seen in CDCA-treated patients.

[1] *Neither CDCA nor UDCA has as yet been approved for clinical use by the U.S. Food and Drug Administration.*

ACUTE AND CHRONIC CHOLECYSTITIS Acute cholecystitis Acute inflammation of the gallbladder wall usually follows obstruction of the cystic duct by a stone. Inflammatory response can be evoked by three factors: (1) *mechanical inflammation* produced by increased intraluminal pressure and distention with resulting ischemia of the gallbladder mucosa and wall; (2) *chemical inflammation* caused by the release of lysolecithin (due to the action of phospholipase on lecithin in bile) and other local tissue factors; and (3) *bacterial inflammation* which may play a role in 50 to 85 percent of patients with acute cholecystitis. The organisms most frequently isolated by culture of gallbladder bile in these patients include *Escherichia coli, Klebsiella* species, group D *Streptococcus, Staphylococcus* species, and *Clostridium* species.

Acute cholecystitis often begins as an attack of biliary colic which progressively worsens. Approximately 60 to 70 percent of patients report having experienced prior attacks which resolved spontaneously. As the episode progresses, however, the pain of acute cholecystitis becomes more generalized in the right upper abdomen. As with biliary colic, the pain of chole-

TABLE 323-3
Chenodeoxycholic acid (CDCA) and gallstone dissolution
RESULTS OF U.S. NATIONAL GALLSTONE STUDY

1 Patients—916 with radiolucent stones, treated 24 months
  a Placebo
  b Low-dose CDCA; 375 mg per day
  c High-dose CDCA; 750 mg per day
2 Results—best with high dose
  a Complete dissolution, 13.5%
  b Partial dissolution, 27.3%; complete plus partial 40.8%
  c Best results—women, thin patients, small stones
3 Side effects
  a Mild diarrhea
  b Changes in hepatic structure, function; 3% clinically significant liver damage
  c Elevation (10%) of serum LDL cholesterol
4 Recurrence—likely when CDCA stopped

SOURCE: *Schoenfield et al.*

cystitis may radiate to the interscapular area, right scapula, or shoulder. Peritoneal signs of inflammation such as increased pain with jarring or on deep respiration may be apparent. The patient is anorectic and often nauseated. Vomiting is relatively common and may produce symptoms and signs of volume depletion. Jaundice is unusual early in the course of acute cholecystitis but may occur when edematous inflammatory changes involve the bile ducts and surrounding lymph nodes.

A low-grade fever is characteristically present, but shaking chills or rigors are not uncommon. The right upper quadrant of the abdomen is almost invariably tender to palpation. An enlarged, tense gallbladder is palpable in one-quarter to one-half of patients. Deep inspiration or cough during subcostal palpation of the right upper quadrant usually produces increased pain and inspiratory arrest (Murphy's sign). A light blow delivered to the right subcostal area may elicit a marked increase in pain. Localized rebound tenderness in the right upper quadrant is common, as are abdominal distention and hypoactive bowel sounds from paralytic ileus, but generalized peritoneal signs and abdominal rigidity are usually absent unless perforation has occurred.

The diagnosis of acute cholecystitis is usually made on the basis of a characteristic history and physical examination. The triad of sudden onset of right upper quadrant tenderness, fever, and leukocytosis is highly suggestive. Typically, leukocytosis in the range of 10,000 to 15,000 cells per cubic millimeter with a left shift on differential count is found. The serum bilirubin is mildly elevated (less than 5 mg/dl) in 45 percent of patients, while 25 percent have modest elevations in serum transaminases (usually less than a fivefold elevation). The radionuclide (e.g., HIDA) biliary scan may be confirmatory, but not diagnostic, if bile duct imaging is seen without visualization of the gallbladder. Cholecystography by oral or intravenous technique is almost always nonvisualizing.

Approximately 75 percent of patients treated medically have remission of acute symptoms within 2 to 7 days following hospitalization. In 25 percent, however, a complication of acute cholecystitis will occur despite conservative treatment (see below). In this setting, prompt surgical intervention is required. Of the 75 percent of patients with acute cholecystitis who undergo remission of symptoms, approximately one-quarter will experience a recurrence of cholecystitis within 1 year, and 60 percent will have at least one recurrent bout within 6 years. In view of the natural history of the disease, acute cholecystitis is best treated by early surgery whenever possible.

ACALCULOUS CHOLECYSTITIS In 5 to 10 percent of patients with acute cholecystitis, calculi obstructing the cystic duct are not found at surgery. In over 50 percent of such cases an underlying explanation for acalculous inflammation is not found. An increased risk for the development of acalculous cholecystitis is especially associated with serious trauma or burns, with the postpartum period following prolonged labor, and with orthopedic and other nonbiliary major surgical operations in the postoperative period. Other precipitating factors include vasculitis, obstructing adenocarcinoma of the gallbladder, diabetes mellitus, torsion of the gallbladder, "unusual" bacterial infections of the gallbladder (e.g., *Leptospira, Streptococcus, Salmonella,* or *Vibrio cholerae*), and parasitic infestation of the gallbladder. Acalculous cholecystitis may also be seen with a variety of other systemic disease processes (sarcoidosis, cardiovascular disease, tuberculosis, syphilis, actinomycosis, etc.) and may possibly complicate periods of prolonged parenteral hyperalimentation.

Although the clinical manifestations of acalculous cholecystitis are indistinguishable from those of calculous cholecystitis, the setting of acute gallbladder inflammation complicating severe underlying illness is characteristic of acalculous disease. Ultrasound, CT scanning, or radionuclide examinations demonstrating a large, tense, static gallbladder without stones and with evidence of poor emptying over a prolonged period may be diagnostically useful in some cases. The complication rate for acalculous cholecystitis exceeds that for calculous cholecystitis. Successful management of acute acalculous cholecystitis appears to depend primarily upon early diagnosis and surgical intervention with meticulous attention to postoperative care.

EMPHYSEMATOUS CHOLECYSTITIS So-called emphysematous cholecystitis is thought to begin with acute cholecystitis (calculous or acalculous) followed by ischemia or gangrene of the gallbladder wall and infection by gas-producing organisms. Bacteria most frequently cultured in this setting include anaerobes such as *Clostridium welchii,* or *perfringens,* and aerobes such as *E. coli.* This condition occurs most frequently in elderly men and in patients with diabetes mellitus. The clinical manifestations are essentially indistinguishable from those of nongaseous cholecystitis. The diagnosis is usually made on plain abdominal film by the finding of gas within the gallbladder lumen, dissecting within the gallbladder wall to form a gaseous ring, or in the pericholecystic tissues. The morbidity and mortality rates with emphysematous cholecystitis are considerable. Prompt surgical intervention coupled with appropriate antibiotics is mandatory.

Chronic cholecystitis Chronic inflammation of the gallbladder wall is almost always associated with the presence of gallstones and is thought to result from repeated bouts of subacute or acute cholecystitis or from persistent mechanical irritation of the gallbladder wall. The presence of bacteria in the bile occurs in approximately one-quarter of patients with chronic cholecystitis. Although the presence of bactibilia in a patient with *chronic* cholecystitis undergoing elective cholecystectomy probably adds little to the operative risk, intraoperative Gram's staining and routine culturing of bile has been advocated to identify those patients whose gallbladder is colonized with *Clostridium* species. Appropriate antibiotics intra- and postoperatively are recommended in such patients because colonization with these organisms may be associated with devastating septic complications following surgery. Chronic cholecystitis may remain asymptomatic for years, may progress to symptomatic gallbladder disease or to acute cholecystitis, or may present with one of the complications detailed below.

Complications of cholecystitis EMPYEMA AND HYDROPS Empyema of the gallbladder usually results from progression of acute cholecystitis with persistent cystic duct obstruction to superinfection of the stagnant bile with a pus-forming bacterial organism. The clinical picture resembles that of cholangitis with high fever, severe right upper quadrant pain, marked leukocytosis, and, often, prostration. Empyema of the gallbladder carries a high risk of gram-negative sepsis and/or perforation. Emergency surgical intervention with proper antibiotic coverage is required as soon as the diagnosis is suspected.

Hydrops or mucocoele of the gallbladder may also result from prolonged obstruction of the cystic duct, usually by a large solitary calculus. In this instance, the obstructed gallbladder lumen is progressively distended, over a period of time, by mucus (mucocoele) or by a clear transudate (hydrops) produced by mucosal epithelial cells. A visible, easily palpable, nontender mass often extending from the right upper quadrant into the right iliac fossa may be found on physical examination. The patient with hydrops of the gallbladder frequently remains asymptomatic, although chronic right upper quadrant pain also may occur. Cholecystectomy is indicated since empyema, perforation, or gangrene may complicate the condition.

GANGRENE AND PERFORATION Gangrene of the gallbladder results from ischemia of the wall and patchy or complete tissue necrosis. Underlying conditions often include marked distention of the gallbladder, vasculitis, diabetes mellitus, empyema, or torsion resulting in arterial occlusion. Gangrene usually predisposes to perforation of the gallbladder, but perforation may also occur in chronic cholecystitis without premonitory warning symptoms. *Localized perforations* are usually contained by the omentum or by adhesions produced by recurrent inflammation of the gallbladder. Bacterial superinfection of the walled-off gallbladder contents results in abscess formation. Most patients are best treated with cholecystectomy, but some seriously ill patients may be managed with cholecystostomy and drainage of the abscess. *Free perforation* is less common but is associated with a mortality rate of approximately 30 percent. Such patients may experience a sudden transient relief of right upper quadrant pain as the distended gallbladder decompresses; this is followed by signs of generalized peritonitis.

FISTULA FORMATION AND GALLSTONE ILEUS *Fistulization* into an adjacent organ adherent to the gallbladder wall may result from inflammation and adhesion formation. Fistulas into the duodenum are most common, followed in frequency by those involving the hepatic flexure of the colon, stomach or jejunum, abdominal wall, and renal pelvis. Clinically "silent" biliary-enteric fistulas occurring as a complication of chronic cholecystitis have been found in up to 5 percent of patients undergoing cholecystectomy. Asymptomatic cholecystoenteric fistulas may sometimes be diagnosed by finding gas in the biliary tree on plain abdominal films. Barium contrast studies or endoscopy of the upper gastrointestinal tract or colon may demonstrate the fistula, but oral cholecystography will almost never result in opacification of either the gallbladder or the fistulous tract. Treatment in the symptomatic patient usually consists of cholecystectomy, common bile duct exploration, and closure of the fistulous tract.

Gallstone ileus refers to mechanical intestinal obstruction resulting from the passage of a large gallstone into the bowel lumen. The stone customarily enters the duodenum through a cholecystoenteric fistula at that level. The site of obstruction by the impacted gallstone is usually at the ileocecal valve, provided that the more proximal small bowel is of normal caliber. The majority of patients do not give a history of either prior biliary tract symptoms or complaints suggestive of acute cholecystitis or fistulization. Large stones over 2.5 cm in diameter are thought to predispose to fistula formation by gradual erosion through the gallbladder fundus. Diagnostic confirmation may occasionally be found on the plain abdominal film (e.g., small intestinal obstruction with gas in the biliary tree and a calcified, ectopic gallstone) or following an upper gastrointestinal series (cholecystoduodenal fistula with small bowel obstruction at the ileocecal valve). Emergency laparotomy is indicated with enterolithotomy and careful palpation of the more proximal small bowel and gallbladder to exclude other stones.

LIMEY (MILK OF CALCIUM) BILE AND PORCELAIN GALLBLADDER Calcium salts may be secreted into the lumen of the gallbladder in sufficient concentration to produce calcium precipitation and diffuse, hazy opacification of bile or a layering effect on plain abdominal roentgenography. This so-called limey bile or milk of calcium bile is usually clinically innocuous, but cholecystectomy is recommended since limey bile most often occurs in an hydropic gallbladder. In the entity called porcelain gallbladder, there is calcium salt deposition within the wall of a chronically inflamed gallbladder which may be detected on the plain abdominal film. Cholecystectomy is advised in all patients with porcelain gallbladder since in a high percentage of cases this finding appears to be associated with the development of carcinoma of the gallbladder.

Treatment of cholecystitis MEDICAL THERAPY Although surgical intervention remains the mainstay of therapy for acute cholecystitis and its complications, a period of in-hospital stabilization may be required before cholecystectomy. Oral intake is eliminated, nasogastric suction is initiated, and extracellular volume depletion and electrolyte abnormalities are repaired. Meperidine or pentazocine are usually employed for analgesia since they may produce less spasm of the sphincter of Oddi than drugs such as morphine. Intravenous antibiotic therapy is usually indicated in patients with severe acute cholecystitis even though bacterial superinfection of bile may not have occured in the early stages of the inflammatory process. Postoperative complications of wound infection, abscess formation, or sepsis are reduced in antibiotic-treated patients. Effective single-agent antibiotics include ampicillin, cephalosporins, chloramphenicol, or aminoglycosides, but in diabetic or debilitated patients and in those with signs of gram-negative sepsis, combination antibiotic treatment may be preferable (see also Chap. 145).

SURGICAL THERAPY The optimal timing of surgical intervention in patients with acute cholecystitis remains controversial. Urgent (emergency) cholecystectomy or cholecystostomy is probably appropriate in most patients in whom a complication of acute cholecystitis such as empyema, emphysematous cholecystitis, or perforation is suspected or confirmed. In uncomplicated cases of acute cholecystitis up to 30 percent of patients fail to resolve their symptoms on appropriate medical therapy, and progression of the attack or a supervening complication leads to the performance of early operation (within 24 to 72 h). The technical complications of surgery are not increased in patients undergoing early as opposed to delayed cholecystectomy. Delayed surgical intervention is probably best reserved for (1) patients in whom the overall medical condition imposes an unacceptable risk for early surgery, and (2) cases in which the diagnosis of acute cholecystitis is in doubt. Early cholecystectomy is the treatment of choice for most patients with acute cholecystitis. Mortality figures for emergency cholecystectomy in most centers approach 3 percent, while the mortality risk for elective or early cholecystectomy approximates 0.5 percent in patients under age 60. Of course, the operative risks increase with age-related diseases of other organ systems and with the presence of long-term or short-term complications of gallbladder disease. Seriously ill or debilitated patients with cholecystitis may be managed with cholecystostomy and tube drainage of the gallbladder. Elective cholecystectomy may then be done at a later date.

Postcholecystectomy complications Early complications following cholecystectomy include atelectasis and other pulmonary disorders, abscess formation (often subphrenic), external or internal hemorrhage, biliary-enteric fistula, and bile leaks. Jaundice may indicate absorption of bile from an intraabdominal collection following a biliary leak, or mechanical obstruction of the common bile duct by retained calculi, intraductal blood clots, or extrinsic compression. Routine performance of intraoperative cholangiography during cholecystectomy has helped to reduce the incidence of these early complications.

Overall, cholecystectomy is a very successful operation which provides total or near-total relief of presurgical symptoms in 75 to 90 percent of patients. The most common cause of persistent postcholecystectomy symptoms is an overlooked extrabiliary disorder (e.g., reflux esophagitis, peptic ulceration, postgastrectomy syndrome, pancreatitis or irritable bowel syndrome). In a small percentage of patients, however, a disorder of the extrahepatic bile ducts may result in persistent symptomatology. These so-called postcholecystectomy syndromes may be due to (1) biliary strictures, (2) retained biliary calculi, (3) cystic duct stump syndrome, (4) stenosis or dyskinesia of the sphincter of Oddi, or (5) bile salt–induced diarrhea or gastritis.

CYSTIC DUCT STUMP SYNDROME In the absence of cholangiographically demonstrable retained stones, symptoms resembling biliary colic or cholecystitis in the postcholecystectomy patient have frequently been attributed to disease in a long (> 1 cm) cystic duct remnant (cystic duct stump syndrome). Careful analysis, however, reveals that postcholecystectomy complaints are attributable to other causes in almost all patients in whom the symptom complex was originally thought to result from the existence of a long cystic duct stump. Accordingly, considerable care should be taken to investigate the possible role of other factors in the production of postcholecystectomy symptoms before attributing them to cystic duct stump syndrome.

BILE SALT–INDUCED CATHARSIS AND GASTRITIS Postcholecystectomy patients may develop symptoms and signs of gastritis which has been attributed to duodenogastric reflux of bile. However, firm data linking an increased incidence of bile gastritis with surgical removal of the gallbladder are lacking. Similarly, the occurrence of cholestyramine-responsive diarrhea in a small number of patients following cholecystectomy has been attributed to an alteration of the enterohepatic circulation of bile acids induced or unmasked by removal of the gallbladder.

THE HYPERPLASTIC CHOLECYSTOSES The term *hyperplastic cholecystoses* is used to denote a group of disorders of the gallbladder characterized by excessive proliferation of normal tissue components.

Adenomyomatosis is characterized by a benign proliferation of gallbladder surface epithelium with gland-like formations, extramural sinuses, transverse strictures, and/or fundal nodule ("adenoma" or "adenomyoma") formation. Outpouchings of mucosa termed Rokitansky-Aschoff sinuses may be seen on oral cholecystography in conjunction with hyperconcentration of contrast medium. Characteristic dimpled filling defects may also be seen.

Cholesterolosis is characterized by abnormal deposition of lipid, especially cholesterol esters, in the lamina propria of the gallbladder wall. In its diffuse form ("strawberry gallbladder"), the gallbladder mucosa is brick red and speckled with bright yellow flecks of lipid. The localized form shows solitary or multiple "cholesterol polyps" studding the gallbladder wall. Cholesterol stones of the gallbladder are found in nearly half the cases. Cholecystectomy is indicated in both adenomyomatosis and cholesterolosis when cholelithiasis is present.

CANCER OF THE GALLBLADDER Most cancers of the gallbladder develop in conjunction with stones rather than polyps. Necropsy series show a prevalence of gallbladder cancer of 0.43 percent, rising to approximately 1 percent in patients with gallstones. In the United States, adenocarcinomas comprise the vast majority of the estimated 6500 new cases of gallbladder cancer diagnosed each year. The female/male ratio is 4:1 and the mean age at diagnosis is approximately 70 years. The clinical presentation is most often one of unremitting right upper quadrant pain associated with weight loss, jaundice, and a palpable right upper quadrant mass. Cholangitis may supervene. The gallbladder rarely visualizes on OCG, and preoperative diagnosis of the condition is rare. Once symptoms have appeared, spread of the tumor outside the gallbladder by direct extension or by lymphatic or hematogenous routes is almost invariable. Over 75 percent of gallbladder carcinomas are unresectable at the time of surgery, the exceptions being tumors discovered incidentally at laparotomy. The 1-year mortality rate for this disease is 90 percent, and only 5 percent of patients survive 5 years or more from the time of diagnosis. Radical operative resection does not appear to improve survival. Results of trials with radiation and chemotherapy of primary gallbladder cancer have also been disappointing (see Chap. 141).

DISEASES OF THE BILE DUCTS

CONGENITAL ANOMALIES Biliary atresia and hypoplasia Atretic and hypoplastic lesions of the extrahepatic and major intrahepatic bile ducts are the most common biliary anomalies of clinical relevance encountered in infancy. The clinical picture is one of severe obstructive jaundice during the first month of life, with pale stools. The diagnosis is confirmed by surgical exploration with operative cholangiography. Approximately 10 percent of cases of biliary atresia are treatable with Roux en Y choledochojejunostomy, with the Kasai procedure (hepatic portoenterostomy) being attempted in the remainder in an effort to restore some bile flow. Most patients, even those having successful biliary-enteric anastomoses, eventually develop chronic cholangitis, extensive hepatic fibrosis, and portal hypertension.

Choledochal cysts Cystic dilatation may involve the free portion of the common bile duct, i.e., choledochal cyst, or may present as diverticulum formation in the intraduodenal segment. In the latter situation chronic reflux of pancreatic juice into the biliary tree can produce inflammation and stenosis of the extrahepatic bile ducts leading to cholangitis or biliary obstruction. Because the process may be gradual, approximately 50 percent of patients present with onset of symptoms after age 10. The diagnosis may be made by ultrasound, abdominal CT, or cholangiography. Surgical treatment involves excision of the "cyst" and biliary-enteric anastomosis. Patients with choledochal cysts are at increased risk for the subsequent development of cholangiocarcinoma.

Congenital biliary ectasia Cystic dilatation of the intrahepatic bile ducts may involve either the major intrahepatic radicles (Caroli's disease) or the inter- and intralobular ducts (congenital hepatic fibrosis) or both. In Caroli's disease, clinical manifestations include recurrent cholangitis, abscess formation in and around the affected ducts, and, sometimes, gallstone formation within portions of ectatic intrahepatic biliary radicles. The CT scan and cholangiographic pattern is diagnostic, and treatment with ongoing antibiotic therapy is usually undertaken in an effort to limit the frequency and severity of recurrent bouts of cholangitis. Progression to secondary biliary cirrhosis with portal hypertension, amyloidosis, extrahepatic biliary obstruction, cholangiocarcinoma, or recurrent episodes of sepsis with hepatic abscess formation is common.

CHOLEDOCHOLITHIASIS Pathophysiology and clinical manifestations Passage of gallstones into the common bile duct occurs in approximately 10 to 15 percent of patients with cholelithiasis. The incidence of common duct stones increases with increasing age of the patient, so that up to 25 percent of elderly patients may have calculi in the common duct at the time of cholecystectomy. Undetected duct stones are left behind in approximately 1 to 5 percent of cholecystectomy patients. The overwhelming majority of bile duct stones are cholesterol or mixed stones formed in the gallbladder which then migrate into the extrahepatic biliary tree through the cystic duct. Primary calculi arising de novo in the ducts are usually pigment stones developing in patients with (1) chronic hemolytic diseases; (2) hepatobiliary parasitism or chronic, recurrent cholangitis; (3) congenital anomalies of the bile ducts (especially Caroli's disease); or (4) dilated, sclerosed, or strictured ducts. Common duct stones may remain asymptomatic for years, may pass spontaneously into the duodenum, or (most often) may present with biliary colic or a complication.

Complications CHOLANGITIS Cholangitis may be acute or chronic, and symptoms result from inflammation which usually requires at least partial obstruction to the flow of bile. Bacteria are present on bile culture in approximately 75 percent of patients with acute cholangitis early in the symptomatic course. The characteristic presentation of acute cholangitis involves biliary colic, jaundice, and spiking fevers with chills (Charcot's triad). Blood cultures are frequently positive and leukocytosis is typical. *Nonsuppurative* acute cholangitis is most common and may respond relatively rapidly to supportive measures and to treatment with antibiotics (see Chap. 145). In *suppurative* acute cholangitis, however, the presence of pus under pressure in a completely obstructed ductal system leads to symptoms of severe toxicity—mental confusion, bacteremia, and septic shock. Response to antibiotics alone in this setting is relatively poor, multiple hepatic abscesses are often present, and the mortality rate approaches 100 percent unless prompt surgical correction of the obstructing lesion and drainage of infected bile is carried out.

OBSTRUCTIVE JAUNDICE Gradual obstruction of the common bile duct over a period of weeks or months usually leads to initial manifestations of jaundice or pruritus without associated symptoms of biliary colic or cholangitis. Painless jaundice may occur in patients with choledocholithiasis, but this manifestation is much more characteristic of biliary obstruction secondary to malignancy of the head of pancreas, bile ducts, or ampulla of Vater.

In patients whose obstruction is secondary to choledocholithiasis, associated chronic calculous cholecystitis is very common and the gallbladder in this setting may be relatively indistensible. The absence of a palpable gallbladder in most patients with biliary obstruction from duct stones is the basis for *Courvoisier's law,* i.e., that the presence of a palpably enlarged gallbladder suggests that the biliary obstruction is secondary to an underlying malignancy rather than to calculous disease. Biliary obstruction causes progressive dilatation of the intrahepatic bile ducts as intrabiliary pressures rise. Hepatic bile flow is suppressed, and regurgitation of conjugated bilirubin into the bloodstream leads to jaundice accompanied by dark urine (bilirubinuria) and light-colored (acholic) stools.

Common bile duct stones should be suspected in any patient with cholecystitis whose serum bilirubin level exceeds 5 mg/dl. The maximum bilirubin level is seldom over 15.0 mg/dl in patients with choledocholithiasis unless concomitant hepatic disease or another factor leading to marked hyperbilirubinemia exists. Serum bilirubin levels of 20mg/dl or more should suggest the possibility of neoplastic obstruction. The serum alkaline phosphatase level is almost always elevated in biliary obstruction. A rise in alkaline phosphatase often precedes clinical jaundice and may be the only abnormality in routine liver function tests. There may be a two- to tenfold elevation of serum transaminases, especially in association with acute obstruction. Following relief of the obstructing process, serum transaminase elevations usually return rapidly to normal, while the serum bilirubin level may take 1 to 2 weeks to return to normal. The alkaline phosphatase usually falls slowly, lagging behind the decrease in serum bilirubin.

PANCREATITIS The most common associated entity discovered in patients with nonalcoholic acute pancreatitis is biliary tract disease. Biochemical evidence of pancreatic inflammation complicates acute cholecystitis in 15 percent of cases and choledocholithiasis in over 30 percent, and the common factor appears to be the passage of gallstones through the common duct. Coexisting pancreatitis should be suspected in patients with symptoms of cholecystitis who develop (1) back pain or pain to the left of the abdominal midline, (2) prolonged vomiting with paralytic ileus, or (3) a pleural effusion, especially on the left side. Surgical treatment of gallstone disease is usually associated with resolution of the pancreatitis.

SECONDARY BILIARY CIRRHOSIS Secondary biliary cirrhosis may complicate prolonged or intermittent duct obstruction with or without recurrent cholangitis. Although this complication may be seen in patients with choledocholithiasis, it is more common in cases of prolonged obstruction from stricture or neoplasm. Once established, secondary biliary cirrhosis may be progressive even after correction of the obstructing process, and increasingly severe hepatic cirrhosis may lead to portal hypertension or to hepatic failure and death. Prolonged biliary obstruction may also be associated with clinically relevant deficiencies of the fat-soluble vitamins A, D, and K.

Diagnosis and treatment The diagnosis of choledocholithiasis is usually made by cholangiography (see Table 323-4), either preoperatively or intraoperatively at the time of cholecystectomy (see Fig. 325-2*C*). The incidence of coexisting common duct stones in patients with cholelithiasis is relatively high. Operative cholangiography should be performed routinely during surgical procedures on the biliary tract. Preoperative indications for common duct exploration include (1) cholangiographic demonstration of ductal stones, (2) jaundice or cholangitis preceding operation, (3) a history of gallstone-related pancreatitis, and (4) cholangiographic evidence of a markedly enlarged common bile duct. Operative indications for exploration of the duct include (1) manual palpation of stones in the common bile duct, (2) positive intraoperative cholangiogram, (3) enlargement of the common bile duct or cystic duct at operation, (4) multiple small stones or "sand" in the gallbladder, and (5) a gallbladder empty of stones at surgery in a patient with previously documented gallstones.

In most cases of choledocholithiasis, the treatment of choice is cholecystectomy with choledocholithotomy and T-tube drainage of the bile ducts. A T-tube cholangiogram is usually performed prior to T-tube removal on or before the tenth postoperative day. Retained calculi seen on T-tube cholangiography may be removed percutaneously by placement of a steerable basket catheter under radiographic guidance through the matured T-tube sinus tract. Endoscopic sphincterotomy followed by spontaneous or basket stone extraction is an additional nonsurgical alternative in the management of patients with common duct stones, especially in elderly or poor-risk patients.

TRAUMA, STRICTURES, AND HEMOBILIA Benign strictures of the extrahepatic bile ducts result from surgical trauma in approximately 95 percent of cases and occur in about 1 in 500 cholecystectomies. Strictures may present with bile leak or abscess formation in the immediate postoperative period or with biliary obstruction or cholangitis as long as 2 years or more following the inciting trauma. The diagnosis is established by percutaneous or endoscopic cholangiography. Successful operative correction by a skillful surgeon with duct to bowel anastomosis is usually possible, although mortality rates from surgical complications, recurrent cholangitis, or secondary biliary cirrhosis are high.

Hemobilia may follow traumatic or operative injury to the liver or bile ducts, intraductal rupture of an hepatic abscess or aneurysm of the hepatic artery, biliary or hepatic tumor hemorrhage, or mechanical complications of choledocholithiasis or hepatobiliary parasitism. Diagnostic procedures such as liver biopsy, percutaneous transhepatic cholangiography (PTHC), and transhepatic biliary drainage catheter placement may also be complicated by hemobilia. Patients often present with a classical triad of biliary colic, obstructive jaundice, and melena or occult blood in the stools. The diagnosis is sometimes made by cholangiographic evidence of blood clot in the biliary tree, but selective angiographic verification may be required. Although minor episodes of hemobilia may resolve without operative intervention, surgical ligation of the bleeding vessel is frequently required.

EXTRINSIC COMPRESSION OF THE BILE DUCTS Partial or complete biliary obstruction may sometimes be produced by extrinsic compression of the ducts. The most common cause of this form of obstructive jaundice is carcinoma of the head of the pancreas. Biliary obstruction may also occur as a complication of either acute or chronic pancreatitis or involvement of lymph nodes in the porta hepatis by lymphoma or metastatic carcinoma. The latter should be distinguished from cholestasis resulting from massive replacement of the liver by tumor.

HEPATOBILIARY PARASITISM Infestation of the biliary tract by adult helminths or their ova may produce a chronic, recurrent pyogenic cholangitis with or without multiple hepatic abscesses, ductal stones, or biliary obstruction. This condition is relatively rare but does occur in inhabitants of southern China and elsewhere in southeast Asia. The organisms most commonly involved are trematodes or flukes, including *Clonorchis sinensis, Opisthorchis viverrini* or *felineus,* and *Fasciola hepatica.* The biliary tract may also be involved by intraductal migration of adult *Ascaris lumbricoides* from the duodenum or by intrabiliary rupture of hydatid cysts of the liver produced by *Ech-*

TABLE 323-4
Diagnostic evaluation of the bile ducts

Procedure	*Diagnostic advantages*	*Diagnostic limitations*	*Contraindications*	*Complications*	*Comment*
Hepatobiliary ultrasound (HBUS)	Rapid Simultaneous scanning of GB, liver, bile ducts, pancreas Accurate identification of dilated bile ducts Not limited by jaundice, pregnancy Guidance for fine-needle biopsy	Bowel gas Massive obesity Ascites Barium Partial bile duct obstruction Poor visualization of distal CBD	None	None	Initial procedure of choice in investigating possible biliary obstruction
Computerized body tomography (CT)	Simultaneous scanning of GB, liver, bile ducts, pancreas Accurate identification of dilated bile ducts, masses Not limited by jaundice, gas, obesity, ascites High-resolution image Guidance for fine-needle biopsy	Extreme cachexia Movement artifact Ileus Partial bile duct obstruction High cost May not be readily available	Pregnancy	Reaction to iodinated contrast, if used	Indicated for evaluation of hepatic or pancreatic masses Procedure of choice in investigating possible biliary obstruction if diagnostic limitations prevent HBUS
Intravenous cholangiogram (IVC)	Noninvasive Readily available	Serum bilirubin >3 mg/dl Misses 40% of common duct stones Poor resolution even with tomography	Pregnancy History of reaction to iodinated contrast	Reaction to iodinated contrast	Few indications unless other cholangiography techniques not available or have failed
Percutaneous transhepatic cholangiogram (PTHC)	Extremely successful when bile ducts dilated Best visualization of proximal biliary tract Possible separate visualization of obstructed left ductal system Bile cytology/culture Percutaneous transhepatic drainage	Nondilated or sclerosed ducts	Pregnancy Uncorrectable coagulopathy Massive ascites ? Hepatic abscess	Bleeding Hemobilia Bile peritonitis Bacteremia, sepsis	Usually, initial cholangiogram of choice when bile ducts are dilated
Endoscopic retrograde cholangio-pancreatogram (ERCP)	Simultaneous pancreatography Visualization/biopsy of ampulla and duodenum Best visualization of distal biliary tract Bile or pancreatic cytology Endoscopic sphincterotomy and stone removal ? Biliary manometry Not limited by ascites, coagulopathy, abscess	Gastroduodenal obstruction ? Roux en Y biliary-enteric anastomosis	Pregnancy ? Acute pancreatitis ? Severe cardiopulmonary disease	Pancreatitis Cholangitis, sepsis Infected pancreatic pseudocyst Perforation (rare) Hypoxemia, aspiration	Cholangiogram of choice in: Absence of dilated ducts ? Pancreatic, ampullary or gastroduodenal disease Prior biliary surgery PTHC contraindicated or failed Endoscopic sphincterotomy a treatment possibility

inococcus species. The diagnosis is made by cholangiography and the presence of characteristic ova on stool examination. When obstruction is present, the treatment of choice is laparotomy under antibiotic coverage, with common duct exploration and a biliary drainage procedure. It should be emphasized that in the orient, one also sees cholangiohepatitis associated with pigment lithiasis, which may, in fact, be more common than cholangitis due to parasites.

SCLEROSING CHOLANGITIS Primary or idiopathic sclerosing cholangitis is a disorder characterized by a progressive, inflammatory, sclerosing and obliterative process affecting the extrahepatic and, often, the intrahepatic bile ducts. The lesion may appear as an isolated entity or may occur in association with inflammatory bowel disease, especially ulcerative colitis, or with multifocal fibrosclerosis syndromes such as retroperitoneal, mediastinal, and/or periureteral fibrosis, Riedel's struma or pseudotumor of the orbit. Secondary sclerosing cholangitis may occur as a long-term complication of choledocholithiasis, cholangiocarcinoma, operative or traumatic biliary injury, or contiguous inflammatory processes.

Patients with sclerosing cholangitis often present with signs and symptoms of chronic or intermittent biliary obstruction: jaundice, pruritus, right upper quadrant abdominal pain, or acute cholangitis. Late in the course, complete biliary obstruction, secondary biliary cirrhosis, hepatic failure, or portal hypertension with bleeding varices may occur. The diagnosis is usually established by finding thickened ducts with narrow, beaded lumina on cholangiography (see Fig. 323-2*D*). Endoscopic retrograde cholangiopancreatogram (ERCP) is probably the cholangiographic technique of choice in suspected cases since intrahepatic ductal involvement may make PTHC difficult or impossible. When a diagnosis of sclerosing cholangitis has been established, a search for associated diseases, especially for chronic inflammatory bowel disease, should be carried out.

Therapy with cholestyramine may help control symptoms of pruritus, and antibiotics are useful when cholangitis complicates the clinical picture. Corticosteroids have not been shown to be efficacious. In cases where complete or high-grade biliary obstruction has occurred, surgical intervention may be appropriate. Efforts at biliary-enteric anastomosis or stent placement may, however, be complicated by recurrent cholangitis and further progression of the stenosing process. The role of colectomy in patients with sclerosing cholangitis complicating chronic ulcerative colitis is uncertain. The prognosis is unfavorable, with a mean survival of 4 to 10 years following the diagnosis, regardless of therapy.

CHOLANGIOCARCINOMA Benign tumors of the extrahepatic bile ducts are extremely rare causes of mechanical biliary obstruction. The majority of these are papillomas, adenomas, or cystadenomas which present with obstructive jaundice or hemobilia. Adenocarcinoma of the extrahepatic ducts is relatively more common. There is a slight male preponderance (60 percent), and the peak age incidence is in the fifth to seventh decades. Apparent predisposing factors include (1) some chronic hepatobiliary parasitic infestations, (2) congential anomalies, ectactic ducts, (3) sclerosing cholangitis and chronic ulcerative colitis, and (4) occupational exposure to possible biliary tract carcinogens (workers in rubber or automotive plants). Cholelithiasis is not clearly associated with cholangiocarcinoma as a predisposing factor. The lesions may be diffuse or nodular; the latter often arise at the confluence of the hepatic ducts (Klatskin tumors).

Patients with cholangiocarcinoma usually present with biliary obstruction, painless jaundice, pruritus, weight loss, and acholic stools. A deep-seated, vaguely localized right upper quadrant pain may be an associated complaint. Hepatomegaly and a palpable, distended gallbladder are frequent accompanying signs. Fever is unusual unless associated with ascending cholangitis. Because the obstructing process is gradual, the cholangiocarcinoma is often far advanced by the time it presents clinically. The diagnosis is most frequently made by cholangiography following ultrasound demonstration of dilated intrahepatic bile ducts. Any focal strictures of the bile ducts should probably be considered malignant until proved otherwise. Long-term palliation of the tumor is possible in some cases when radiation and/or chemotherapy are combined with palliative drainage of the biliary tree.

PAPILLARY STENOSIS AND BILIARY DYSKINESIA Symptoms of biliary colic accompanied by signs of recurrent, intermittent biliary obstruction may occasionally be produced by dysfunction of the sphincter of Oddi. Papillary stenosis is thought to result from acute or chronic inflammation of the papilla of Vater or from glandular hyperplasia of the papillary segment. Criteria for the diagnosis of papillary stenosis are highly debatable, and preoperative identification of the lesion may be extremely difficult. Endoscopic, cholangiographic, and manometric findings during ERCP may suggest the diagnosis. Intraoperative palpation of the ampulla with operative cholangiography, probing of the sphincter, and/or operative manometry may be required for attempted confirmation in strongly suspected cases. Treatment consists of surgical sphincteroplasty to ensure wide patency of the distal portions of both the bile and pancreatic ducts.

Criteria for diagnosing dyskinesia of the sphincter of Oddi are even more controversial than those of papillary stenosis. Proposed mechanisms include spasm of the sphincter, denervation sensitivity resulting in hypertonicity, and abnormalities of the sequencing or frequency rates of sphincteric contraction waves. When thorough evaluation has failed to demonstrate another cause for the pain, and when cholangiographic and manometric criteria suggest a diagnosis of biliary dyskinesia, medical treatment with nitrites or anticholinergics to attempt pharmacologic relaxation of the sphincter has been proposed. Surgical sphincteroplasty may occasionally be indicated in patients who fail to respond to a 2- to 3-week trial of medical therapy.

CARCINOMA OF THE PAPILLA OF VATER The ampulla of Vater may be involved by extension of tumor arising elsewhere in the duodenum or may itself be the primary site of origin of sarcomas, carcinoid tumors, or adenocarcinomas. Papillary adenocarcinomas are associated with slow growth and a more favorable clinical prognosis than diffuse, infiltrative cancers of the ampulla, which are more frequently widely invasive. The presenting clinical manifestation is usually obstructive jaundice. ERCP is probably the preferred diagnostic technique when ampullary carcinoma is suspected, because it allows for direct endoscopic inspection and biopsy of the ampulla as well as for performance of pancreatography to exclude a diagnosis of pancreatic malignancy. Cancer of the papilla is usually treated by wide, often radical, surgical excision. Lymph node or other metastases are present at the time of surgery in approximately 20 percent of cases, and the 5-year survival rate following surgical therapy in this group is only 5 to 10 percent. In the absence of metastases, however, radical pancreaticoduodenectomy (Whipple procedure) is associated with 5-year survival rates as high as 40 percent, and several long-term survivors have been reported.

REFERENCES

BACHRACH WH, HOFMANN AF: Ursodeoxycholic acid in the treatment of cholesterol cholelithiasis. Dig Dis Sci 27:737, 833, 1982

BENNION LJ, GRUNDY SM: Risk factors for the development of cholelithiasis in man. N Engl J Med 299:1161, 1221, 1978

BISMUTH H, MALT RA: Carcinoma of the biliary tract. N Engl J Med 301:704, 1979

CHAPMAN RWG et al: Primary sclerosing cholangitis: A review of its clinical features, cholangiography and hepatic histology. Gut 2:870, 1980

COTTON PB: ERCP. Gut 18:316, 1977

FERRUCCI JT JR, MUELLER PR: Interventional radiology of the biliary tract. Gastroenterology 82:974, 1982

GRACIE WA, RANSOHOFF DF: The natural history of silent gallstones. The innocent gallstone is not a myth. N Engl J Med 307:798, 1982

HOWARD RJ: Acute acalculous cholecystitis. Am J Surg 141:194, 1981

MCPHEE MS, SCHAPIRO RH: Biliary obstruction: Current approaches to diagnosis and treatment, in *Update I: Harrison's Principles of Internal Medicine,* KJ Isselbacher et al (eds). New York, McGraw-Hill, 1981, pp 1–22

SCHOENFIELD LS et al: Chenodiol (chenodeoxycholic acid) for dissolution of gallstones: The National Cooperative Gallstone Study. A controlled trial of efficacy and safety. Ann Intern Med 95:257, 1981

SOLOWAY RD et al: Pigment gallstones. Gastroenterology 72:167, 1977

WELCH CE, MALT RA: Abdominal surgery. N Engl J Med 300:705, 1979

section 7 | Disorders of the pancreas

324
APPROACH TO THE PATIENT WITH PANCREATIC DISEASE

NORTON J. GREENBERGER
PHILLIP P. TOSKES

GENERAL CONSIDERATIONS

Inflammatory disease of the pancreas may be acute, relapsing, or chronic. Although good data exist concerning the frequency of acute pancreatitis (about 5000 new cases per year in the United States with a mortality rate of about 10 percent), the number of patients who suffer with relapsing pancreatitis or chronic pancreatitis is largely undefined. The relative inaccessibility of the pancreas to direct examination and the nonspecificity of the abdominal pain associated with pancreatitis make the diagnosis of pancreatitis difficult and usually dependent on elevation of blood amylase levels. Many patients with relapsing pancreatitis and the majority of patients with chronic pancreatitis do not have elevated blood amylase levels. Some patients with chronic pancreatitis develop signs and symptoms of pancreatic exocrine insufficiency, and thus objective evidence for pancreatic disease can be demonstrated. However, greater than 90 percent of the pancreas must be damaged before maldigestion of fat and protein is manifested. Obviously there is a very large reservoir of pancreatic exocrine function, and the signs and symptoms usually associated with exocrine insufficiency are late manifestations, depending on virtually complete destruction of the gland. Even the secretin stimulation test, which is the most sensitive method of assessing pancreatic exocrine function, is probably abnormal only when greater than 75 percent of exocrine function has been lost. Thus, the number of patients who have subclinical exocrine dysfunction (i.e., less than 90 percent loss of function) is unknown.

The clinical manifestations of acute and chronic pancreatitis and pancreatic insufficiency are protean. Thus, patients may present with hyperlipidemia, vitamin B_{12} malabsorption, hypercalcemia, hypocalcemia, hyperglycemia, ascites, pleural effusions, and chronic abdominal pain with normal amylase levels. Indeed, if the clinician considers pancreatitis as a possible diagnosis only when presented with a patient having classic symptoms (i.e., severe, constant epigastric pain that radiates through to the back, along with an elevated blood amylase level), only a minority of the patients with pancreatitis will be correctly diagnosed.

As emphasized in Chap. 325, the etiologies as well as the clinical manifestations are quite varied. Although it is well appreciated that *pancreatitis* is frequently secondary to alcohol abuse and biliary tract disease, pancreatitis is also caused by drugs, trauma, and viral infections, and is associated with metabolic and connective tissue disorders. In addition, in 10 to 20 percent of patients with chronic pancreatitis, the etiology is obscure.

The incidence of *pancreatic cancer* in the United States has increased threefold since 1930. Associations have been made with cigarette smoking, exposure to some industrial carcinogens, and diabetes. The outlook for early diagnosis and effective treatment remains dismal.

Cystic fibrosis is usually considered a disease of childhood. However, an appreciable number of children with this disease reach adulthood because of more effective therapy for pulmonary complications. Eighty-five percent of patients with cystic fibrosis have pancreatic exocrine insufficiency; in some, pancreatic impairment may represent the primary clinical defect. This disease, in which the metabolic defect has not yet been clearly defined, affects many organ systems in addition to the gastrointestinal tract.

TESTS USEFUL IN THE DIAGNOSIS OF PANCREATIC DISEASE

Several tests have proved of value in the evaluation of pancreatic exocrine function. Examples of specific tests and usefulness in the diagnosis of acute and chronic pancreatitis are summarized in Table 324-1.

PANCREATIC ENZYMES IN BODY FLUIDS The serum amylase is widely used as a screening test for acute pancreatitis in the patient with acute abdominal or back pain. A value greater than 150 Somogyi units per deciliter should raise the question of acute pancreatitis; levels greater than 300 units make the diagnosis more likely. In acute pancreatitis the serum amylase is usually elevated within 24 h and remains so for 1 to 3 days.

TABLE 324-1

Tests useful in the diagnosis of acute and chronic pancreatitis

Test	Principle	Comment
I Pancreatic enzymes in body fluids		
A Amylase		
1 Serum	Pancreatic inflammation leads to increased enzyme levels	Simple; reliable; false-negatives and -positives
2 Urine	Renal clearance of amylase is increased in acute pancreatitis	May be abnormal when serum levels normal; false-negatives and -positives
3 Amylase/creatinine clearance ratio (C_{am}/C_{cr})	Renal clearance of amylase greater than clearance of creatinine	No more sensitive than the serum amylase
4 Ascitic fluid	Disruption of gland or main pancreatic duct leads to increased amylase	Can establish diagnosis of pancreatitis; false-positives with intestinal obstruction and perforated ulcer
5 Pleural fluid	Exudative pleural effusion with pancreatitis	False-positives with carcinoma of the lung and esophageal perforation
6 Isoenzymes	P isoamylases arise from the pancreas; S isoamylases are from other sources	Useful in identifying nonpancreatic causes of hyperamylasemia
B Serum lipase	Pancreatic inflammation leads to increased enzyme levels	New methods of determination greatly simplified; positive in 60–70% of cases
II Studies pertaining to pancreatic structure		
A Radiological and radionuclide tests		
1 Plain film of the abdomen	Abnormal in acute and chronic pancreatitis	Simple; normal in more than 50% of both acute and chronic pancreatitis
2 Upper gastrointestinal x-rays	Displacement of stomach or widening of duodenal loop suggests a pancreatic mass (inflammatory, neoplastic, cystic)	Simple; frequently normal; largely superseded by ultrasonography and CT scanning
3 Ultrasonography	Echographic appearances can provide information on edema, inflammation, calcification, pseudocysts, and mass lesions	Simple, noninvasive; sequential studies quite feasible; procedure of choice for diagnosis of pseudocyst
4 Computerized tomography (CT scan)	Permits detailed visualization of pancreas and surrounding structures	Useful in the diagnosis of pancreatic calcification, dilated pancreatic ducts, and pancreatic tumors; may not be able to distinguish between inflammatory and neoplastic mass lesions; high cost
5 Selective angiography	Can identify pancreatic neoplasms (1) by sheathing of celiac or superior mesenteric branches by tumor or (2) by tumor straining; displacement of vessels by tumor	Angiography indicated with (1) suspected islet-cell tumors and (2) proposed pancreatic or duodenal resection; most reliable angiographic features reflect nonresectable pancreatic cancer
B Endoscopic retrograde cholangiopancreatography (ERCP)	Cannulation of pancreatic and common bile duct permits visualization of pancreatic-biliary ductal system	Provides diagnostic data in 60–85% of cases; differentiation of chronic pancreatitis from pancreatic carcinoma may be difficult
C Pancreatic biopsy with ultrasound guidance	Percutaneous biopsy with skinny needle and localization of lesion by sonography	High diagnostic yield; laparotomy avoided; requires special technical skills
III Tests of exocrine pancreatic function		
A Direct stimulation of the pancreas with analysis of duodenal contents		
1 Secretin-pancreozymin (CCK-PZ) test	Secretin leads to increased output of pancreatic juice and HCO_3^-; CCK-PZ leads to increased output of pancreatic enzymes; pancreatic secretory response related to functional mass of pancreatic tissue	Sensitive enough to detect occult disease; duodenal intubation; fluoroscopy; poorly defined normal enzyme response; overlap in chronic pancreatitis; large secretory reserve capacity of the pancreas
B Indirect stimulation of pancreas with measurement of pancreatic enzymes		
1 Lundh test meal	Test meal (fat, carbohydrate, and protein) causes increased release of CCK-PZ, which causes increased enzyme output; trypsin concentration measured	Useful in patients with pancreatic exocrine insufficiency; false-negatives with delayed gastric emptying; false-positives in patients with primary mucosal disease of the gut and choledocholithiasis; does not measure secretory capacity
2 Benzoyl-tyrosyl-*p*-aminobenzoic (Bz-Ty-PABA, tripeptide hydrolysis) test	Synthetic peptide (Bz-Ty-PABA) specifically cleaved by chymotrypsin, liberating PABA which is absorbed and excreted in the urine	Simple and reliable test of pancreatic exocrine function; sensitivity and specificity not yet fully defined
C Measurement of intraluminal digestion products		
1 Microscopic examination of stool for undigested meat fibers and fat	Lack of proteolytic enzymes causes decreased digestion of meat fibers	Simple, reliable; not sensitive enough to detect milder cases of pancreatic insufficiency
2 Quantitative stool fat determination	Lack of lipolytic enzymes brings about impaired fat digestion	Reliable, reference standard for defining severity of malabsorption; does not distinguish between maldigestion and malabsorption
3 Fecal nitrogen	Lack of proteolytic enzymes leads to impaired protein digestion, causing increase in stool nitrogen	Does not distinguish between maldigestion and malabsorption
D Measurement of pancreatic enzymes in feces		
1 Chymotrypsin	Pancreatic output of proteolytic enzymes	May be useful in evaluating cystic fibrosis patients; tedious; 10% false-positives and false-negatives

Levels return to normal within 3 to 5 days unless there is extensive pancreatic necrosis, incomplete ductal obstruction, or pseudocyst formation. Approximately 75 percent of patients with acute pancreatitis will have an elevated serum amylase. Normal values, however, may occur if (1) there is a delay (2 to 5 days) in obtaining blood samples, (2) the underlying disorder is relapsing chronic pancreatitis rather than acute pancreatitis, and (3) hypertriglyceridemia is present. Patients with hypertriglyceridemia and proven pancreatitis have been found to have spuriously low levels of amylase activity presumably because of a circulating amylase inhibitor; serial dilutions of plasma will correct this abnormality and permit identification of hyperamylasemia.

The serum amylase is often elevated in other conditions (Table 324-2), in part because the enzyme is found in many organs in addition to the pancreas (salivary glands, liver, small intestine, kidney, fallopian tube) and can be produced by various tumors (carcinoma of the lung, esophagus, and ovary). Isoenzymes of amylase fall into two general categories, those arising from the pancreas (P isoamylases) and those from nonpancreatic sources (S isoamylases). The measurement of serum isoamylases appears to be of clinical importance. For example, in certain conditions, such as the postoperative state, acute alcohol intoxication, and diabetic ketoacidosis, it had been assumed that elevations in serum amylase indicated acute pancreatitis. However, the elevation of serum amylase in such conditions has been shown to actually be of the S type. The relative complexity of procedures for determining isoamylases has prevented extensive clinical use of this test, but with the development of more simplified assays widespread use of this determination is now possible.

Urine amylase is increased in acute pancreatitis and may be elevated for 7 to 10 days after serum values have returned to normal. The finding that the renal clearance of amylase is increased in acute pancreatitis has led to the suggestion that the amylase/creatinine clearance ratio (C_{am}/C_{cr}) may be a more specific test for the diagnosis of acute pancreatitis. It also may serve to identify patients with pancreatitis who do not have hyperamylasemia. The ratio is calculated by the following formula:

$$\frac{C_{am}}{C_{cr}} = \frac{\text{urine amylase}}{\text{serum amylase}} \times \frac{\text{serum creatinine}}{\text{urine creatinine}} \times 100$$

The normal range of C_{am}/C_{cr} is 1 to 5 percent. In acute pancreatitis, the ratio usually exceeds 5 percent and may range up to 14 percent. However, experience with the C_{am}/C_{cr} has demonstrated that it is no more sensitive than the serum amylase. In addition, the specificity of the C_{am}/C_{cr} has been seriously questioned because the ratio is also increased in a number of other disorders, e.g., diabetic ketoacidosis, burns, pancreatic neoplasms, renal failure, and the postoperative state. The mechanism of increased renal amylase clearance in acute pancreatitis is secondary to a reversible renal tubular defect which results in decreased amylase reabsorption.

Elevation of ascitic fluid amylase occurs in acute pancreatitis as well as (1) in pancreatogenous ascites due to disruption of the main pancreatic duct of a leaking pseudocyst and (2) in other abdominal disorders which simulate pancreatitis (e.g., intestinal obstruction, intestinal infarction, and perforated peptic ulcer). Elevation of pleural fluid amylase occurs in acute pancreatitis, chronic pancreatitis, carcinoma of the lung, and esophageal perforation.

In the past, serum lipase levels were not frequently performed because of methodological problems. However, newer methods are now available. In a representative study, lipase levels were elevated in 63 percent of patients with acute pancreatitis, amylase levels in 70 percent, and both enzymes in 83 percent. Increased lipase levels have also been found in ascitic fluid in patients with acute pancreatitis.

TABLE 324-2
Causes of hyperamylasemia and hyperamylasuria

I Pancreatic disease
- *A* Pancreatitis
  - *1* Acute
  - *2* Chronic: ductal obstruction
  - *3* Complications of pancreatitis
    - *a* Pancreatic pseudocyst
    - *b* Pancreatogenous ascites
    - *c* Pancreatic abscess
- *B* Pancreatic trauma
- *C* Pancreatic carcinoma

II Nonpancreatic disorders
- *A* Renal insufficiency
- *B* Salivary gland lesions
  - *1* Mumps
  - *2* Calculus
  - *3* Irradiation sialadenitis
  - *4* Maxillofacial surgery
- *C* "Tumor" hyperamylasemia
  - *1* Carcinoma of the lung
  - *2* Carcinoma of the esophagus
  - *3* Ovarian carcinoma
- *D* Macroamylasemia
- *E* Burns
- *F* Diabetic ketoacidosis
- *G* Pregnancy
- *H* Renal transplantation
- *I* Cerebral trauma
- *J* Drugs: morphine

III Other abdominal disorders
- *A* Biliary tract disease: cholecystitis, choledocholithiasis
- *B* Intraabdominal disease
  - *1* Perforated or penetrating peptic ulcer
  - *2* Intestinal obstruction or infarction
  - *3* Ruptured ectopic pregnancy
  - *4* Peritonitis
  - *5* Aortic aneurysm
  - *6* Chronic liver disease
  - *7* Postoperative hyperamylasemia

SOURCE: *After WB Salt II, S Schenker, Medicine 55:269, 1976.*

STUDIES PERTAINING TO PANCREATIC STRUCTURE **Radiologic tests** Plain films of the abdomen provide useful information in 30 to 50 percent of patients with acute pancreatitis. The most frequent abnormalities include (1) a localized ileus usually involving the jejunum ("sentinel loop"); (2) a generalized ileus with air-fluid levels; (3) the "colon cutoff sign," which results from isolated distention of the transverse colon; (4) duodenal distention with air-fluid levels; and (5) a mass, which is frequently a pseudocyst. In chronic pancreatitis, an important radiographic finding is pancreatic calcification, which characteristically is localized adjacent to and superimposed on the second lumbar vertebra (see Fig. 325-1).

Upper gastrointestinal x-rays may reveal displacement of the stomach by the retroperitoneal mass (see Fig. 325-2*A*) or widening and effacement of the duodenal C loop, which also suggests the presence of a pancreatic mass that could be an inflammatory, cystic, or neoplastic process. The use of hypotonic duodenography or good-quality air-contrast studies increases the diagnostic yield of upper gastrointestinal x-rays in patients with carcinoma of the head of the pancreas.

Ultrasonography (echography) can provide important information in patients with acute pancreatitis, chronic pancreatitis, pancreatic calcification, pseudocyst, and pancreatic carcinoma. Echographic appearances can indicate the presence of edema, inflammation, and calcification (not obvious on plain films of the abdomen), as well as pseudocysts and mass lesions (see Figs. 325-1 to 325-3). In acute pancreatitis the pancreas is characteristically enlarged. In pancreatic pseudocyst the usual appearance is that of an echo-free, smooth, round fluid collection. Pancreatic carcinoma distorts the usual landmarks, and mass lesions greater than 3.0 cm are usually detected as localized, echo-free solid lesions. *Ultrasound should be the initial investigation for most patients with suspected pancreatic disease.* However, obesity, excess small- and large-bowel gas, and recently performed barium-contrast examinations can interfere with ultrasound studies.

Computerized tomography (CT scan) is useful in the detection of pancreatic tumors, fluid-containing lesions such as pseudocysts and abscesses, and calcium deposits. Most lesions are characterized by (1) enlargement of the pancreatic outline, (2) distortion of the pancreatic contour, or (3) fluid-containing lesions that have different attenuation coefficients than normal pancreas. However, it is occasionally difficult to distinguish between inflammatory and neoplastic lesions. Oral water-soluble contrast agents may be used to opacify the stomach and duodenum during CT scans; this permits more precise delineation of various organs as well as mass lesions.

Selective catheterization of the celiac and superior mesenteric arteries combined with superselective catheterization of others such as the hepatic, splenic, and gastroduodenal arteries permits visualization of the pancreas and detection of pancreatic neoplasms and pseudocysts. Pancreatic neoplasms can be identified by the sheathing of blood vessels by a mass lesion (see Fig. 325-3). Hormone-producing pancreatic tumors are especially likely to exhibit increased vascularity and tumor staining. Angiographic abnormalities are noted in many patients with pancreatic carcinoma but are uncommon in patients without pancreatic disease. Angiography complements ultrasonography and endoscopic retrograde cholangiopancreatography (ERCP) in the study of a patient with a suspected pancreatic lesion and is often carried out if ERCP is either unsuccessful or nondiagnostic.

The radiologic approach to the patient with suspected pancreatic disease is summarized in Table 324–3.

Endoscopic retrograde cholangiopancreatography ERCP may provide useful information on the status of the pancreatic ductal system and thus aid in the differential diagnosis of pancreatic disease (see Figs. 325-2 and 325-3). Pancreatic carcinoma is characterized by stenosis or obstruction of either the pancreatic duct or common bile duct; both ductal systems are often abnormal. In chronic pancreatitis ERCP abnormalities include (1) luminal narrowing, (2) irregularities in the ductal system with stenosis, dilatation, sacculation, and ectasia, and (3) blockage of the pancreatic duct by calcium deposits. Differentiation from carcinoma may be difficult because of similar overlapping features, i.e., ductal stenosis and irregularity. Elevated serum amylase levels following ERCP have been reported in 25 to 75 percent of patients, but clinical pancreatitis is uncommon. In a series of 300 patients pancreatitis occurred in only five patients following ERCP.

TABLE 324-3
Radiologic approach to the patient with suspected pancreatic disease

	Suspected disease	*Initial diagnostic study*	*Supplemental study*
I	Acute pancreatitis		
	A Acute pancreatitis, uncomplicated	US	CT
	B Pseudocyst	US	CT
	C Suspected pancreatic abscess	CT	
II	Chronic pancreatitis	CT	ERCP
III	Mass lesions, tumors		
	A Epigastric mass	US	CT
	B Carcinoma, head	US	CT or ERCP or PTC
	C Carcinoma, body or tail	CT	ERCP
	D Functioning islet cell tumor	Angiography	CT
	E Obstructive jaundice	US	ERCP or PTC

SOURCE: *After JT Ferrucci Jr, J Wittenberg, in Update II: Harrison's Principles of Internal Medicine, KJ Isselbacher et al (eds), New York, McGraw Hill, 1981.*
NOTE: *US = ultrasonography; CT = computerized tomography; ERCP = endoscopic retrograde cholangiopancreatography; PTC = percutaneous transhepatic cholangiography.*

Pancreatic biopsy with radiologic guidance Percutaneous aspiration biopsy of the pancreas under ultrasound or CT guidance can provide a definitive diagnosis of pancreatic neoplasms.

TESTS OF EXOCRINE PANCREATIC FUNCTION

(See Table 324-1)

Pancreatic function tests can be divided into the following categories:

1 *Direct stimulation of the pancreas* by intravenous infusion of secretin or secretin plus cholecystokinin (CCK) followed by collection and measurement of duodenal contents
2 *Indirect stimulation of the pancreas* utilizing nutrients or amino acids, fatty acids, and synthetic peptides followed by assay of proteolytic, lipolytic, and amylolytic enzymes
3 Study of *intraluminal digestion products* such as undigested meat fibers, stool fat, and fecal nitrogen
4 *Measurement of fecal pancreatic enzymes* such as chymotrypsin

The secretin test, used to detect diffuse pancreatic disease, is based on the physiological principle that the pancreatic secretory response is directly related to the functional mass of pancreatic tissue. In the standard assay, secretin is given intravenously in a dose of 1 clinical unit (CU) per kilogram, either as a bolus or continuous infusion. Obviously, results will vary with the secretin preparation used, dose, mode of administration, and completeness of collection of duodenal contents. Normal values for the standard secretin test are (1) volume output > 2.0 ml/kg in 80 min, (2) bicarbonate (HCO_3^-) concentration > 80 meq per liter, and (3) HCO_3^- output > 10 meq in 30 min. The most reproducible measurement having the highest level of discrimination between normal subjects and patients with chronic pancreatitis appears to be the maximal bicarbonate concentration.

The *combined secretin-CCK test* permits measurement of pancreatic amylase, lipase, trypsin, and chymotrypsin. Although there is overlap in the distribution of enzyme output in normal subjects and patients with pancreatitis, markedly decreased enzyme outputs suggest advanced damage and destruction of acinar cells. With frank exocrine pancreatic insufficiency there is usually an overall reduction in both HCO_3^- concentration and output of several enzymes. However, with lesser degrees of pancreatic damage there may be a dissociation between HCO_3^- concentration and enzyme output. There may also be a dissociation between the results of the secretin test and other tests of absorptive function. For example, patients with chronic pancreatitis often have abnormally low outputs of HCO_3^- after secretin but normal fecal fat excretion. Thus, the secretin test measures the secretory capacity of ductular epithelium, while fecal fat excretion indirectly reflects intraluminal lipolytic activity. Steatorrhea does not occur until intraluminal levels of lipase are markedly reduced, underscoring the fact that only small amounts of enzymes are necessary for intraluminal digestive activities. An abnormal secretin test should suggest only that chronic pancreatic damage is present; it will not consistently distinguish between chronic pancreatitis and pancreatic carcinoma.

Another test of exocrine pancreatic function, which indirectly reflects intraluminal chymotrypsin activity, has been evaluated in patients with pancreatic disease. This test (the *tripeptide hydrolysis test*) utilizes a synthetic peptide, *N*-benzoyl-L-tyrosyl-*p*-aminobenzoic acid (Bz-Ty-PABA), that is specifically cleaved by chymotrypsin to Bz-Ty and PABA. Normally, after oral administration, the peptide reaches the small intestine, where it is hydrolyzed by chymotrypsin with the liberation of PABA, which is rapidly absorbed and excreted in the urine. Results in several hundred patients with chronic pancreatitis and other disorders indicate that PABA excretion is significantly lower in chronic pancreatitis compared with controls. The overall sensitivity and specificity of the test remains to be determined.

Measurement of *intraluminal digestion products,* i.e., undigested muscle fibers, stool fat, and fecal nitrogen, is discussed in Chap. 308. Measurement of chymotrypsin in stool reflects pancreatic output of this proteolytic enzyme. Decreased chymotrypsin activity in stool has been reported in patients with chronic pancreatitis and cystic fibrosis. However, normal values may occur in patients with pancreatic insufficiency, and false-positive results have been reported in up to 10 percent of normal individuals.

Tests useful in the diagnosis of exocrine pancreatic insufficiency and the differential diagnosis of malabsorption are also discussed in Chaps. 308 and 325.

325
DISEASES OF THE PANCREAS

NORTON J. GREENBERGER
PHILLIP P. TOSKES
KURT J. ISSELBACHER

BIOCHEMISTRY AND PHYSIOLOGY OF PANCREATIC EXOCRINE SECRETION

GENERAL CONSIDERATIONS The pancreas secretes 1500 to 3000 ml isosmotic alkaline (pH > 8.0) fluid per day containing about 20 enzymes and zymogens. The pancreatic secretions provide the enzymes needed to effect the major digestive activity of the gastrointestinal tract and provide an optimum pH for the function of these enzymes.

REGULATION OF PANCREATIC SECRETION Hormonal and neural mechanisms The exocrine pancreas is under both hormonal and neural control, with hormonal control being of primary importance. Gastric *acid* is the stimulus for the release of secretin, a peptide with 27 amino acids. Sensitive radioimmunoassay studies for secretin suggest that the pH threshold for the release of secretin from the duodenum and jejunum is 4.5. Secretin stimulates the secretion of pancreatic juice rich in *water and electrolytes.* Release of cholecystokinin-pancreozymin (CCK-PZ) from duodenum and jejunum is largely produced by long-chain fatty acids, certain essential amino acids (tryptophan, phenylalanine, valine, methionine), and acid itself. CCK-PZ (a peptide with 33 amino acids) evokes an *enzyme-rich secretion from the pancreas.* Gastrin, although it shares an identical terminal tetrapeptide with CCK-PZ, is a weak stimulus for pancreatic enzyme output. The *parasympathetic nervous system* (via the vagus) exerts some control over pancreatic secretion. Part of this is mediated by the release of gastrin, and part is secondary to a direct effect of acetylcholine on the pancreatic acinar cell. In addition, vagal stimulation effects release of vasoactive intestinal peptide (VIP), a secretin agonist. Vagal control of pancreatic secretion seems to be most important following a truncal vagotomy, but even in such patients severe maldigestion does not ensue. Bile salts also stimulate pancreatic secretion, thereby integrating the functions of the biliary tract, pancreas, and small intestine.

Pancreatic secretion at the cellular level There appear to be two functionally distinct pathways by which secretagogues can stimulate pancreatic secretion. Studies with isolated pancreatic acinar cells indicate that secretin, VIP, and cholera toxin interact with receptors on the acinar cell, leading to an increase in cellular cyclic adenosine monophosphate (cyclic AMP). CCK-PZ, acetylcholine, gastrin, and various other peptides (e.g., bombesin, caerulein, litorin, physalaemin, and eledoisin) react with other receptors on the acinar cell to cause the release of membrane calcium and induce changes in the electrical properties of the pancreatic acinar cell surface and junctional membranes. When a secretagogue that increases cyclic AMP is added to a secretagogue that increases calcium outflux, potentiation of enzyme secretion occurs.

WATER AND ELECTROLYTE SECRETION Although sodium, potassium, chloride, calcium, zinc, phosphate, and sulfate are found within pancreatic secretion, *bicarbonate is the ion of primary physiological importance.* In the acini and in the ducts, secretin causes the cells to add water and bicarbonate to the fluid. In the ducts an exchange occurs between bicarbonate and chloride. There is a good correlation between the maximal bicarbonate output after stimulation with secretin and the pancreatic mass. The bicarbonate output of 120 to 300 meq per day neutralizes gastric acid production and creates the appropriate pH for the activity of the pancreatic enzymes.

ENZYME SECRETION The pancreas secretes amylolytic, lipolytic, and proteolytic enzymes. Amylolytic enzymes such as amylase hydrolyze starch to oligosaccharides and to the disaccharide maltose. The *lipolytic enzymes* include lipase, phospholipase A, and cholesterol esterase. Bile salts *inhibit* lipase, but colipase, another constituent of pancreatic secretion, binds to lipase and prevents this inhibition. Bile salts *activate* phospholipase A and cholesterol esterase. *Proteolytic enzymes* include *endopeptidases* (trypsin, chymotrypsin), which act on the internal peptide bonds of proteins and polypeptides; exopeptidases (carboxypeptidases, aminopeptidases), which act on the free carboxyl terminal end and free amino terminal end of peptides, respectively; and elastase. The proteolytic enzymes are secreted as inactive precursors (zymogens). Ribonucleases (deoxyribonucleases, ribonuclease) are also secreted. *Enterokinase,* an enzyme found within the duodenal mucosa, cleaves the lysine-isoleucine bond of trypsinogen to form trypsin. Trypsin then activates the other proteolytic zymogens in a cascade phenomenon. All pancreatic enzymes have pH optima in the alkaline range.

AUTOPROTECTION OF THE PANCREAS Autodigestion of the pancreas is prevented by the packaging of proteases in precursor form and by the synthesis of protease inhibitors. These protease inhibitors are found within the acinar cell, the pancreatic secretions, and the alpha$_1$- and alpha$_2$-globulin fractions of plasma.

EXOCRINE-ENDOCRINE RELATIONSHIPS Pancreatic glucagon (29 amino acid residues) has a high degree of structural similarity to secretin. It decreases volume and enzyme secretion by the pancreas but not bicarbonate secretion. Glucose, in large concentrations, may also inhibit pancreatic exocrine secretion. The choleretic and insulinotropic effects of secretin are shared by glucagon.

ACUTE PANCREATITIS

GENERAL CONSIDERATIONS Pancreatic inflammatory disease may be classified as follows: (1) acute pancreatitis, (2) relapsing acute pancreatitis, (3) relapsing chronic pancreatitis,

TABLE 325-1
Causes of acute pancreatitis

I Alcohol ingestion (acute and chronic alcoholism)
II Biliary tract disease (gallstones)
III Postoperative (abdominal, nonabdominal)
IV Post-endoscopic retrograde cholangiopancreatography (ERCP)
V Trauma (especially blunt abdominal type)
VI Metabolic
- *A* Hyperlipidemia
- *B* Hypercalcemia, e.g., hyperparathyroidism
- *C* Renal failure
- *D* After renal transplantation*
- *E* Acute fatty liver of pregnancy†

VII Hereditary pancreatitis
VIII Infections
- *A* Mumps
- *B* Viral hepatitis
- *C* Other viral infections (coxsackievirus, echovirus)
- *D* Ascariasis
- *E* Mycoplasma

IX Drug-associated
- *A* Definite association
  - *1* Azathioprine
  - *2* Sulfonamides
  - *3* Thiazide diuretics
  - *4* Furosemide
  - *5* Estrogens (oral contraceptives)
  - *6* Tetracycline
- *B* Probable association
  - *1* Chlorthalidone
  - *2* Corticosteroids
  - *3* Ethacrynic acid
  - *4* Procainamide
  - *5* Iatrogenic hypercalcemia
  - *6* L-Asparaginase
  - *7* Valproic acid

X Connective tissue disorders with vasculitis
- *A* Systemic lupus erythematosus
- *B* Necrotizing angiitis
- *C* Thrombotic thrombocytopenic purpura

XI Penetrating duodenal ulcer
XII Obstruction of the ampulla of Vater
- *A* Regional enteritis
- *B* Duodenal diverticulum

XIII Pancreas divisum
XIV Recurrent bouts of acute pancreatitis without obvious cause
- *A* Consider
  - *1* Occult disease of the biliary tree or pancreatic ducts
  - *2* Drugs
  - *3* Hyperlipidemia
  - *4* Pancreas divisum

XV Other

* *Pancreatitis occurs in 3 percent of renal transplant patients and is due to many factors including surgery, hypercalcemia, drugs (corticosteroids, azathioprine, L-asparaginase, diuretics), and viral infections.*
† *Pancreatitis also occurs in otherwise uncomplicated pregnancy and is most often associated with cholelithiasis.*

and (4) chronic pancreatitis. This classification is based primarily on clinical criteria with the obvious difference between the acute and chronic varieties; restoration of normal function occurs in the former and permanent residual damage occurs in the latter. The pathologic spectrum of acute pancreatitis varies from *edematous pancreatitis,* which is usually a mild and self-limited disorder, to *necrotizing pancreatitis,* in which the degree of pancreatic necrosis correlates with the severity of the attack and its systemic manifestations. *Hemorrhagic pancreatitis* is less meaningful because variable amounts of interstitial hemorrhage can be found in pancreatitis as well as in other disorders such as pancreatic trauma, pancreatic carcinoma, and severe congestive heart failure.

The incidence of pancreatitis varies in different countries and depends upon etiological factors, e.g., alcohol, gallstones, metabolic factors, and drugs (Table 325-1). In the United States, for example, acute pancreatitis is related to alcohol ingestion more commonly than to gallstones; in England the opposite obtains. Epidemiologic data based on autopsy data indicate that in the United States the overall prevalence of acute pancreatitis is approximately 0.5 percent. An upward trend has been noted in the crude death rate in recent years from 1.0 per 100,000 in 1955 to 1.3 in 1965.

ETIOLOGY AND PATHOGENESIS There are many causative factors in the pathogenesis of acute pancreatitis (Table 325-1), but the mechanisms by which these conditions trigger pancreatic inflammation have not been identified. Alcoholic patients with pancreatitis may represent a special subset, since most alcoholics do not develop pancreatitis. The list of identifiable causes is growing, and it is likely that pancreatitis related to viral infections and drugs is more common than heretofore recognized.

Autodigestion is one pathogenetic theory which proposes that proteolytic enzymes (e.g., trypsinogen, chymotrypsinogen, proelastase, and phospholipase A) are activated within the pancreas rather than in the intestinal lumen. A variety of factors (such as endotoxins, exotoxins, viral infections, ischemia, anoxia, and direct trauma) are believed to activate these proenzymes. Activated proteolytic enzymes, especially trypsin, not only digest pancreatic and peripancreatic tissues but also can activate other enzymes such as elastase and phospholipase. The active enzymes then digest cellular membranes and cause proteolysis, edema, interstitial hemorrhage, vascular damage, coagulation necrosis, fat necrosis, and parenchymal cell necrosis. Cellular injury and death result in the liberation of activated enzymes. In addition, activation and release of bradykinin peptides and vasoactive substances (e.g., histamine) are believed to produce vasodilatation, increased vascular permeability, and edema. There is thus a cascade of events culminating in the development of acute necrotizing pancreatitis.

The autodigestion theory has largely eclipsed two older theories. The "common channel" theory holds that such an anatomic arrangement facilitates reflux of bile into the pancreatic duct, and this results in activation of pancreatic enzymes. (Actually, a common channel with free communication between the common bile duct and main pancreatic duct is infrequently encountered.) The second theory is that obstruction and hypersecretion are pivotal in the development of pancreatitis. Obstruction of the main pancreatic duct, however, produces pancreatic edema but not pancreatitis.

CLINICAL FEATURES *Abdominal pain* is the major symptom of acute pancreatitis. Pain may vary from a mild and tolerable discomfort to severe, constant, and incapacitating distress. Characteristically, the pain which is steady and boring in character, is located in the epigastrium and periumbilical region and often radiates to the back as well as to the chest, flanks, and lower abdomen. The pain is frequently more intense when the patient is supine, and patients often obtain relief by sitting with the trunk flexed and knees drawn up. Nausea, vomiting, and abdominal distention due to gastric and intestinal hypomotility and chemical peritonitis are also frequent complaints.

Physical examination frequently reveals a distressed and anxious patient. Low-grade fever, tachycardia, and hypotension are fairly common. Shock is not unusual and may result from (1) hypovolemia secondary to exudation of blood and plasma proteins into the retroperitoneal space, i.e., a "retroperitoneal burn"; (2) increased formation and release of kinin peptides which cause vasodilatation and increased vascular permeability; (3) systemic effects of proteolytic and lipolytic enzymes released into the circulation; and (4) impairment of myocardial contractility by kinins and other poorly characterized peptides. Jaundice occurs infrequently; when present it usually is due to edema of the head of the pancreas with compression of the intrapancreatic portion of the common bile duct. Erythematous skin nodules due to subcutaneous fat necrosis may occur. In 10 to 20 percent of patients there are pulmonary findings, including basilar rales, atelectasis, and pleural effusion, the latter most frequently left-sided. Abdominal tenderness and muscle rigidity are present to a variable degree, but compared with the intense pain, these signs may be unimpressive. Bowel sounds are usually diminished or absent. A pancreatic pseudocyst may be palpable in the upper abdomen. A faint blue discoloration around the umbilicus (Cullen's sign) may occur as the result of hemoperitoneum and a blue-red-purple or green-brown discoloration of the flanks (Turner's sign) reflects tissue catabolism of hemoglobin. The latter two findings, which are uncommon, indicate the presence of a severe necrotizing pancreatitis.

LABORATORY DATA The diagnosis of acute pancreatitis is usually established by the presence of an increased serum amylase exceeding 200 Somogyi units. However, there appears to be no definite correlation between the severity of pancreatitis and the degree of serum amylase elevation. After 48 to 72 h, even with continuing evidence of pancreatitis, amylase values tend to return to normal. It will be recalled that amylase elevations in serum and urine occur in many conditions other than pancreatitis (Table 324-2). The C_{am}/C_{cr} ratio is usually elevated in patients with severe obvious pancreatitis. Serum lipase activity increases in parallel with amylase activity, and measurement of both enzymes increases the diagnostic yield. Markedly increased levels of peritoneal or pleural fluid amylase ($>$5000 units per deciliter) are also helpful, if present, in establishing the diagnosis.

Leukocytosis (15,000 to 20,000 leukocytes per cubic millimeter) occurs frequently. More severe cases may show hemoconcentration with hematocrit values exceeding 50 percent because of loss of plasma into the retroperitoneal space and peritoneal cavity. *Hyperglycemia* is common and is due to multiple factors that include decreased insulin release, increased glucagon release, and increased output of adrenal glucocorticoids and catecholamines. *Hypocalcemia* occurs in approximately 25 percent of cases and its pathogenesis is incompletely understood. While earlier studies suggested that the parathyroid gland response to a decrease in serum calcium is impaired, subsequent observations have failed to confirm this. Intraperitoneal saponification of calcium by fatty acids in areas of fat necrosis occurs as well as increased plasma levels of glucagon and calcitonin, but it is felt that these abnormalities do not adequately explain the hypocalcemia. *Hyperbilirubinemia* (serum bilirubin $>$ 4.0 mg/dl) occurs in approximately 10 percent of patients. However, jaundice is transient and serum bilirubin levels return to normal in 4 to 7 days. Serum alkaline phosphatase and aspartate aminotransferase (SGOT) levels are also transiently elevated and parallel serum bilirubin values. Serum albumin is decreased to $\leq$ 3.0 g/dl in about 10 percent of cases and is associated with more severe pancreatitis and an increased mortality rate (Table 325-2). Methemalbumin, a circulating heme metabolite attached to albumin, has been considered as a useful index of severe necrotizing pancreatitis. Its usefulness, however, has been limited by its nonspecificity for pancreatitis (it occurs, for example, in abdominal trauma, bone fractures, soft-tissue trauma, and retroperitoneal hematoma) and its absence in the majority of cases of severe necrotizing pancreatitis. *Hypertriglyceridemia* occurs in 15 to 20 percent of cases, and serum amylase levels in such patients are often spuriously normal (see Chap. 324). Most patients with hypertriglyceridemia and pancreatitis, when subsequently examined, show evidence of an underlying derangement in lipid metabolism which probably antedated the pancreatitis. Approximately 25 percent of patients have *hypoxemia* (arterial $P_{O_2} \leq$ 60 mmHg), which may herald the onset of adult respiratory distress syndrome. Finally, the electrocardiogram is occasionally abnormal in acute pancreatitis with ST-segment and T-wave abnormalities simulating myocardial ischemia.

Radiologic studies useful in the diagnosis of acute pancreatitis are listed in Table 324-1 and discussed in Chap. 324. Although one or more of the abnormalities are found in over 50 percent of patients, the findings are inconstant and nonspecific. Conventional x-rays have been superseded, to a large extent, by *ultrasonography* and CT scanning; their chief value in acute pancreatitis is to help exclude other diagnoses, especially a perforated viscus. While earlier studies suggested that oral cholecystography performed shortly after an attack of pancreatitis failed to opacify the gallbladder in more than half of patients, more recent studies indicate that in nonjaundiced, alcoholic patients with acute pancreatitis not caused by gallstones, oral cholecystography *after resumption of a solid diet* and *before hospital discharge* is successful in opacifying the gallbladder in 90 percent of patients.

DIAGNOSIS Any severe acute pain in the abdomen or back should suggest acute pancreatitis. The diagnosis is usually entertained when a patient with a possible predisposition to pancreatitis presents with severe and constant abdominal pain, nausea, emesis, fever, tachycardia, and abnormal findings on abdominal examination. Laboratory studies frequently reveal leukocytosis, abnormal x-rays of the abdomen and chest, hypocalcemia, and hyperglycemia. The diagnosis is usually confirmed by finding an elevated serum amylase. Obviously, not all the above features have to be present for the diagnosis to be established.

The *differential diagnosis* should include consideration of the following disorders: (1) perforated viscus, especially peptic ulcer; (2) acute cholecystitis and biliary colic; (3) acute intestinal obstruction; (4) mesenteric vascular occlusion; (5) renal colic; (6) myocardial infarction; (7) dissecting aortic aneurysm; (8) connective tissue disorders with vasculitis; (9) pneumonia; and (10) diabetic ketoacidosis. A penetrating duodenal ulcer can usually be identified by upper gastrointestinal x-rays and/or endoscopy. A perforated duodenal ulcer is readily diagnosed by the presence of free intraperitoneal air. It may be difficult to differentiate acute cholecystitis from acute pancreatitis since an elevated serum amylase may be found in both disorders. Pain of biliary tract origin is more right-sided and gradual in onset, and ileus is usually absent. Intestinal obstruction due to mechanical factors can be differentiated from pancreatitis by the history of colicky pain, findings on abdominal examination, and x-rays of the abdomen showing characteristic changes of mechanical obstruction. Acute mesenteric vascular occlusion is usually evident in elderly debilitated patients with brisk leukocytosis, abdominal distention, and bloody diarrhea, in whom paracentesis shows sanguinous fluid and arteriography shows vascular occlusion. Serum as well as peritoneal fluid amylase levels are increased, however, in patients with intestinal infarction. Systemic lupus erythematosus and polyarteritis nodosa may be confused with pancreatitis, espe-

TABLE 325-2
Factors adversely influencing survival in acute pancreatitis*

I Risk factors identifiable upon admission to hospital
- *A* Increasing age
- *B* Hypotension
- *C* Tachycardia
- *D* Abnormal pulmonary findings
- *E* Abdominal mass
- *F* Fever
- *G* Leukocytosis
- *H* Hyperglycemia
- *I* First attack of pancreatitis

II Risk factors identifiable during initial 48 h of hospitalization
- *A* Fall in hematocrit $>$ 10 percent with hydration and/or hematocrit $<$ 30 percent
- *B* Necessity for massive fluid and colloid replacement
- *C* Hypocalcemia
- *D* Hypoxemia with or without adult respiratory distress syndrome
- *E* Hypoalbuminemia
- *F* Azotemia

* *Increased mortality with three or more risk factors.*

cially since pancreatitis may develop as a complication of those diseases. Diabetic ketoacidosis is often accompanied by abdominal pain and elevated serum amylase levels, thus closely mimicking acute pancreatitis. The serum lipase is not elevated in diabetic ketoacidosis.

COURSE OF THE DISEASE AND COMPLICATIONS There is an increased mortality rate with three or more risk factors identifiable either at the time of admission to hospital or during the initial 48 h of hospitalization (see Table 325-2). It is important to identify the patient with acute pancreatitis with an increased risk of dying. In one large series such a subgroup was characterized by at least three of the following features: (1) respiratory failure requiring intubation, (2) shock, (3) massive colloid replacement, and (4) serum calcium < 8.0 mg/dl. The survival rate was only 29 percent in the patients treated with medical measures but increased to 64 percent with operative treatment. The high mortality of such severely ill patients, despite maximal medical treatment, suggests that alternative therapeutic approaches such as peritoneal lavage or early surgical intervention merit broader consideration.

The local and systemic complications of acute pancreatitis are listed in Table 325-3. Patients frequently develop an inflammatory mass in the first 2 to 3 weeks after pancreatitis. These may be phlegmons, abscesses, or pseudocysts (see below). Systemic complications include pulmonary, cardiovascular, hematologic, renal, metabolic, and central nervous system abnormalities. Pancreatitis, hypertriglyceridemia, and alcoholism constitute a triad in which cause and effect remain incompletely understood. However, several reasonable conclusions can be drawn. First, hypertriglyceridemia can precede and apparently cause the development of pancreatitis. Second, the vast majority ($>$ 80 percent) of patients with acute pancreatitis do not have hypertriglyceridemia. Third, almost all patients with pancreatitis and hypertriglyceridemia are *either* alcoholics who have been drinking shortly before the onset of pancreatitis *or* patients with preexistent hypertriglyceridemia. Finally, many of the patients with this triad have persistent hypertriglyceridemia after recovery from pancreatitis and abstention from alcohol.

Purtscher's retinopathy, a relatively unusual complication, refers to the sudden and severe loss of vision in patients with acute pancreatitis. It is characterized by a peculiar funduscopic appearance with cotton-wool spots and hemorrhages confined to an area limited by the optic disk and macula; it is believed to be due to posterior retinal artery occlusion with aggregated granulocytes.

TREATMENT In most patients (approximately 85 to 90 percent) with acute pancreatitis, the disease is self-limited and subsides spontaneously, usually within 2 to 5 days after treatment is instituted. Medical therapy is aimed at reducing pancreatic secretion and, in essence, "putting the pancreas at rest." Conventional measures include (1) analgesics for pain, (2) intraveneous fluids and colloids to maintain normal intravascular volume, (3) no oral alimentation, and (4) nasogastric suction to decrease gastrin release from the stomach and prevent gastric contents from entering the duodenum. Recent controlled trials, however, have shown that nasogastric suction offers no clear-cut advantages in the treatment of mild to moderately severe acute pancreatitis. Its use, therefore, must be considered elective rather than mandatory.

Anticholinergic drugs have previously been considered standard therapy in patients with acute pancreatitis, the rationale being to blunt stimulation of the pancreas. However, there are no controlled trials, demonstrating that anticholinergic drugs are superior to placebo. Moreover, anticholinergics may make it difficult to determine whether tachycardia, decreased urine output, bowel hypomotility, need for additional fluid replacement, and signs of toxicity are due to the drugs or to a worsening of the pancreatitis. Accordingly, their use is not recommended. Although antibiotics have been used in the treatment of acute pancreatitis, two recent randomized prospective trials have shown no benefit from the use of antibiotics in acute pancreatitis of mild to moderate severity. However, because secondary infection of necrotic pancreatic tissue (phlegmon, abscess, pseudocyst) or obstructed biliary passages (ascending cholangitis, complicating choledocholithiasis) contributes to much of the late mortality, appropriate *antibiotic therapy of established infection* is obviously quite important. Previous reports suggested that glucagon was useful in acute pancreatitis, but controlled trials have not provided convincing evidence of effectiveness. Similarly, aprotinin (Trasylol) and cimetidine have not proved effective.

The patient with mild to moderate pancreatitis usually requires treatment with intravenous fluids, fasting, and possibly nasogastric suction for 2 to 4 days. A clear liquid diet is fre-

TABLE 325-3
Complications of acute pancreatitis

I Local
- *A* Pancreatic phlegmon
- *B* Pancreatic abscess
- *C* Pancreatic pseudocyst
  - *1* Pain
  - *2* Rupture
  - *3* Hemorrhage
  - *4* Infection
- *D* Pancreatic ascites
  - *1* Disruption of main pancreatic duct
  - *2* Leaking pseudocyst
- *E* Involvement of contiguous organs by necrotizing pancreatitis
  - *1* Massive intraperitoneal hemorrhage
  - *2* Thrombosis of blood vessels
  - *3* Bowel infarction
- *F* Obstructive jaundice

II Systemic
- *A* Pulmonary
  - *1* Pleural effusion
  - *2* Atelectasis
  - *3* Mediastinal abscess
  - *4* Pneumonitis
  - *5* Adult respiratory distress syndrome
- *B* Cardiovascular
  - *1* Hypotension
    - *a* Hypovolemia
    - *b* Hypoalbuminemia
  - *2* Sudden death
  - *3* Nonspecific ST-T changes in electrocardiogram simulating myocardial infarction
  - *4* Pericardial effusion
- *C* Hematologic
  - *1* Disseminated intravascular coagulation (DIC)
- *D* Gastrointestinal hemorrhage *
  - *1* Peptic ulcer disease
  - *2* Erosive gastritis
  - *3* Hemorrhagic pancreatic necrosis with erosion into major blood vessels
  - *4* Portal vein thrombosis, variceal hemorrhage
- *E* Renal
  - *1* Oliguria
  - *2* Azotemia
  - *3* Renal artery and/or renal vein thrombosis
- *F* Metabolic
  - *1* Hyperglycemia
  - *2* Hypertriglyceridemia
  - *3* Hypocalcemia
  - *4* Encephalopathy
  - *5* Sudden blindness (Purtscher's retinopathy)
- *G* Central nervous system
  - *1* Psychosis
  - *2* Fat emboli
- *H* Fat necrosis
  - *1* Subcutaneous tissues (erythematous nodules)
  - *2* Bone
  - *3* Miscellaneous (mediastinum, pleura, nervous system)

* Aggravated by coagulation abnormalities (DIC).

quently started on the third to fifth day and a regular diet by the fifth to seventh day. The patient with unremitting *fulminant pancreatitis* usually requires inordinate amounts of fluid and close attention to complications such as cardiovascular collapse and respiratory insufficiency. Removal of toxic pancreatic exudate from the peritoneal cavity appears to alter the course of this lethal situation. This can be accomplished by either *peritoneal lavage* via a percutaneous dialysis catheter or *laparotomy* with wide sump drainage. If peritoneal lavage does not halt the patient's deterioration, laparotomy should be considered. The use of parenteral nutrition makes it possible to give nutritional support to patients with severe, acute, or protracted pancreatitis who are unable to eat normally.

PANCREATIC PHLEGMON, ABSCESS, AND PSEUDOCYST The *phlegmon* is a solid mass of swollen, inflamed pancreas often containing patchy areas of necrosis; it may be present for 1 to 2 weeks. This prolonged inflammatory process should not be confused with a pseudocyst, a differentiation which is usually accomplished by sonography. Occasionally, extensive areas of pancreatic necrosis develop in phlegmons and require incision and drainage. Phlegmons may also be secondarily infected, resulting in abscess formation. The latter occurs in 5 to 10 percent of patients with acute pancreatitis. Severe pancreatitis with the presence of three or more risk factors, postoperative pancreatitis, early oral feeding, early laparotomy, and perhaps injudicious use of antibiotics predispose to the development of pancreatic abscess. Pancreatic abscess may also develop because of communication of a pseudocyst with the colon, after inadequate surgical drainage of a pseudocyst, or after needling of a pseudocyst. The characteristic signs of abscess are fever, leukocytosis, ileus, and rapid deterioration in a patient initially recovering from pancreatitis. However, the only manifestations may be persistent fever and signs of continuing pancreatic inflammation. Laparotomy with radical sump drainage is mandatory because the mortality for undrained pancreatic abscess approaches 100 percent. Multiple abscesses are common and reoperation is frequently required.

Pseudocysts of the pancreas are collections of tissue, fluid, debris, pancreatic enzymes, and blood, which develop over a period of 1 to 4 weeks after the onset of acute pancreatitis. In contrast to true cysts, pseudocysts do not have epithelial lining and the walls consist of necrotic tissue, granulation tissue, and fibrous tissue. Disruption of the pancreatic ductal system is common. However, the subsequent course of this disruption varies widely, namely, from spontaneous healing to continuous leakage of pancreatic juice causing tense ascites. Pseudocysts are preceded by pancreatitis in 90 percent of cases and by trauma in 10 percent. Approximately 85 percent are located in the body or tail of the pancreas and 15 percent in the head. Some patients have two or more pseudocysts. Abdominal pain, with or without radiation to the back, is the usual presenting complaint. A palpable, tender mass may be found in the middle or left upper abdomen. The serum amylase is elevated in 75 percent of cases some time in their course and may fluctuate markedly.

Pseudocysts displace some portion of the gastrointestinal tract on x-ray examination in 75 percent of cases (Fig. 325-1). Sonography, however, has proved to be reliable in detecting pseudocysts and should be the initial diagnostic procedure in a patient suspected of having a pseudocyst (Fig. 325-1). Sonography also permits differentiation between an edematous and an inflamed pancreas (pancreatic phlegmon), which can give rise to a palpable mass and an actual pseudocyst. Furthermore, serial ultrasound studies will indicate whether a pseudocyst has resolved. Computerized tomography (CT scanning) complements the use of ultrasound in the diagnosis of pancreatic pseudocyst (Fig. 325-2), especially when it is infected.

The management of pseudocysts is compromised by incomplete knowledge of the natural history of this disorder. Thus, in some patients there may be spontaneous resolution of pseudocysts, however, the frequency of this is not clear. In others, serious complications may occur such as (1) pain caused by expansion of the lesion and pressure on other viscera, (2) rupture, (3) hemorrhage, and (4) abscess. Rupture of a pancreatic pseudocyst is a particularly serious complication. Shock almost always supervenes and mortality rates range from 14 percent if the rupture is not associated with hemorrhage to over 60 percent if hemorrhage has occurred. Rupture and hemorrhage are the prime causes of mortality in pancreatic pseudocyst. A triad of findings, e.g., increase in size of the mass, localized bruit over the mass, and a sudden decrease in hemoglobin and hematocrit levels without obvious signs of external blood loss should alert one to the diagnosis of hemorrhage from a pseudocyst. Thus, in pseudocyst patients who are stable and uncomplicated, and in whom serial ultrasound studies show a decreasing pseudocyst, conservative therapy is indicated. Conversely, patients with a pseudocyst which is expanding and which is complicated by rupture, hemorrhage, and abscess should be operated on. Surgical therapy consists of internal or external drainage of the cyst. Prolonged observation of a nonresolving pancreatic pseudocyst exposes the patient to increased risks which exceed those of elective surgery.

PANCREATIC ASCITES AND PANCREATIC PLEURAL EFFUSIONS Pancreatic ascites is usually due to disruption of the main pancreatic duct, often associated with an internal fistula between the duct and the peritoneal cavity (see also Chap. 39). The diagnosis of pancreatic ascites is suggested in a patient with an elevated serum amylase who also has increased levels of albumin ($>$ 3.0 g/dl) and amylase in the ascitic fluid. In addition, endoscopic retrograde cholangiopancreatography (ERCP) will often demonstrate passage of contrast material from a major pancreatic duct or a pseudocyst into the peritoneal cavity. As many as 15 percent of patients with pseudocysts have concurrent pancreatic ascites. The differential diagnosis should include intraperitoneal carcinomatosis, tuberculous peritonitis, constrictive pericarditis, and Budd-Chiari syndrome.

If the pancreatic duct disruption is posterior, an internal fistula may develop between the pancreatic duct and pleural space producing a pleural effusion, which is usually left-sided and often massive.

Treatment usually involves placing the patient on nasogastric solution and parenteral alimentation to decrease pancreatic secretion. In addition, paracentesis is performed to keep the peritoneal cavity free of fluid and hopefully effect sealing of the leak. If ascites continues to recur after 2 to 3 weeks of medical management, the patient should be operated on following pancreatography to define the anatomy of the abnormal duct.

CHRONIC PANCREATITIS AND PANCREATIC EXOCRINE INSUFFICIENCY

GENERAL AND ETIOLOGICAL CONSIDERATIONS Chronic inflammatory disease of the pancreas may take the form of relapsing chronic pancreatitis or chronic pancreatitis. In relapsing chronic pancreatitis there are episodes of acute inflammation superimposed upon a previously injured pancreas. The causes of relapsing chronic pancreatitis are similar to those of acute pancreatitis (Table 325-2), except that there is an appreciable incidence of cases of undetermined origin. In addition, the pancreatitis associated with gallstones is predominantly acute or relapsing acute in nature. A cholecystectomy is almost always performed in patients after the first or second attack of gallstone-associated pancreatitis. Patients with chronic pancreatitis may present with persistent abdominal pain, with or

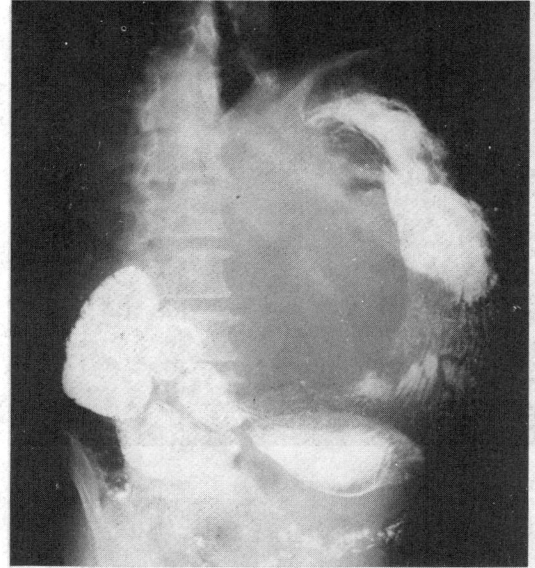

A

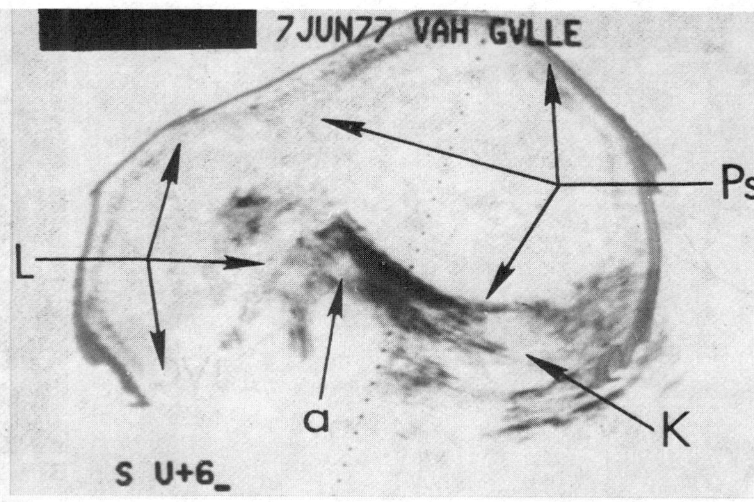

B

C

FIGURE 325-1
Pseudocyst of the pancreas. A. Upper gastrointestinal x-ray showing displacement of stomach by pseudocyst. B. Sonogram showing pseudocyst (Ps), K = kidney, a = aorta, L = liver. C. CT scan showing pseudocyst compressing left kidney.

without steatorrhea, and some may present with steatorrhea and no pain.

Patients with chronic pancreatitis who develop extensive destruction of the pancreas (i.e., less than 10 percent of exocrine function remaining) will demonstrate steatorrhea and azotorrhea. In the adult in the United States, alcoholism is the most common cause of clinically apparent pancreatic exocrine insufficiency, while cystic fibrosis is the most frequent cause in children. In other parts of the world, severe protein calorie malnutrition is a common etiology. Table 325-4 lists other causes of pancreatic exocrine insufficiency, but they are relatively uncommon.

PATHOPHYSIOLOGY Unfortunately, the events that initiate an inflammatory process within the pancreas are still not well understood, and the many hypotheses will not be reviewed. In the case of alcohol-induced pancreatitis, however, it has been suggested that the primary defect may be the precipitation of protein (inspissated enzymes) within the ducts. The resulting ductal obstruction can lead to duct dilatation, diffuse atrophy of the acinar cells, fibrosis, and eventual calcification of some of the protein plugs. While patients with alcohol-induced pancreatitis generally consume large amounts of alcohol, some consume very little (i.e., 50 g or less per day). Thus, prolonged consumption of "socially acceptable" amounts of alcohol is compatible with the development of pancreatitis. In addition, the finding of extensive pancreatic fibrosis in patients who have expired during their first attack of clinical acute alcohol-induced pancreatitis supports the concept that such patients already have chronic pancreatitis.

CLINICAL FEATURES Patients with relapsing chronic pancreatitis may present with symptoms identical with those found in acute pancreatitis, but their pain may be continuous or intermittent, or pain may be absent. The pathogenesis of this pain is poorly understood. Although the classic description is that of epigastric pain radiating through the back, the pain pattern is often atypical. The pain may be maximal in the right or left upper quadrants in the back or diffuse throughout the upper abdomen; it may even be referred to the anterior chest or flank. Characteristically, the pain is persistent, deep-seated, and unresponsive to antacids. It often is increased by alcohol and ingestion of heavy meals (especially foods rich in fat). Often the pain is so severe as to require the frequent use of narcotics.

Weight loss, abnormal stools, and other signs of symptoms suggestive of malabsorption (Table 308-5) are common in chronic pancreatitis. However, clinically apparent deficiencies of fat-soluble vitamins are surprisingly rare. The physical findings in these patients are usually not impressive such that there is a disparity between the severity of the abdominal pain and the paucity of physical signs (save some abdominal tenderness and mild temperature elevation).

DIAGNOSTIC EVALUATION (See Chap. 324) In contrast to patients with relapsing acute pancreatitis, the serum amylase and lipase levels are usually not elevated. Elevations of the serum bilirubin and alkaline phosphatase may indicate cholestasis secondary to chronic inflammation around the common bile duct (Fig. 325-3). Many patients demonstrate impaired glucose tolerance, and some may have an elevated fasting blood glucose level.

The classic triad of pancreatic calcification, steatorrhea, and diabetes mellitus usually establishes the diagnosis of chronic pancreatitis and exocrine pancreatic insufficiency but is found in less than one-third of chronic pancreatitis patients. Accordingly, it is often necessary to perform the *secretin stimulation test,* which usually becomes abnormal when 75 percent or more of pancreatic exocrine function has been lost. Approximately

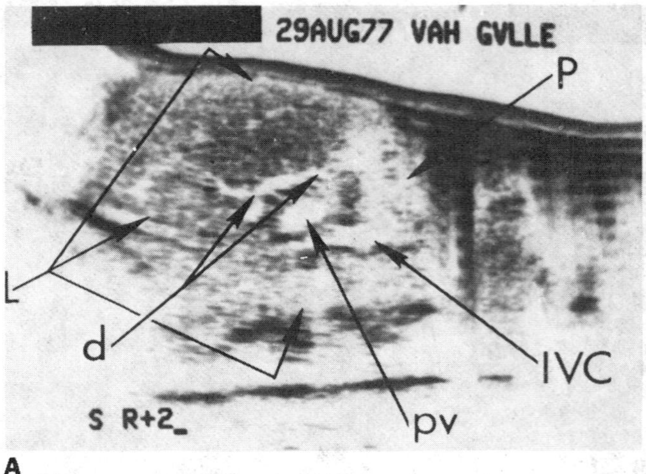

A

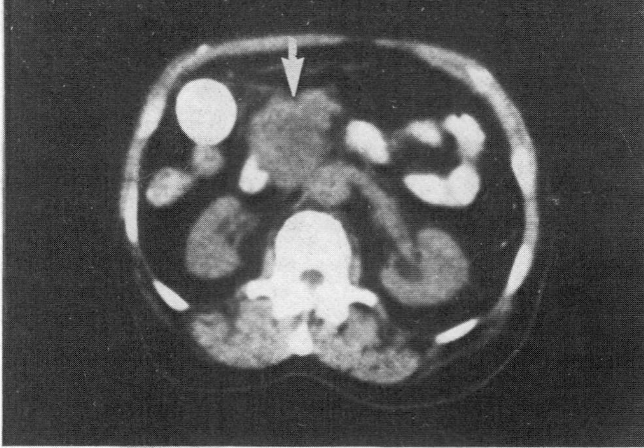
B

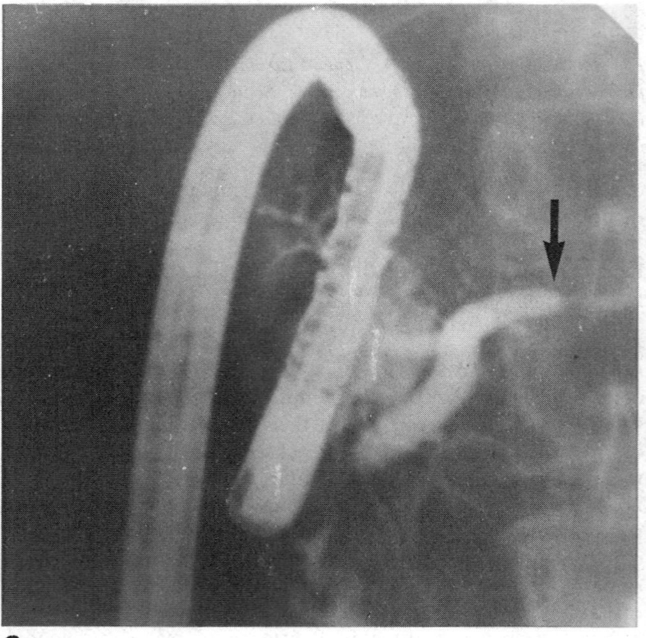
C

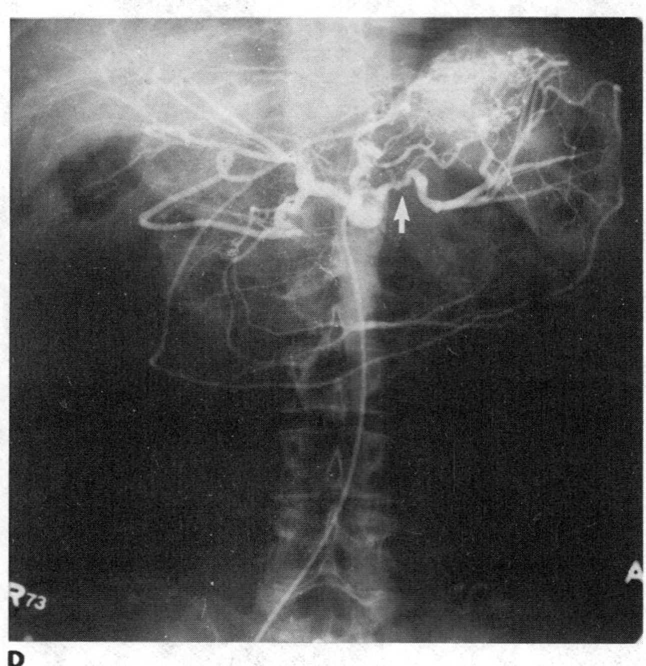

D

FIGURE 325-2

Carcinoma of the pancreas. A. Sonogram showing pancreatic carcinoma (P), dilated intrahepatic bile ducts (d), dilated portal vein (pv), and inferior vena cava (IVC). B. CT scan showing pancreatic carcinoma (arrow). C. ERCP showing abrupt cut off of the duct of Wirsung (arrow). D. Arteriogram showing sheathing of splenic artery by tumor encasement (arrow).

TABLE 325-4
Causes of pancreatic exocrine insufficiency

I Alcohol, chronic alcoholism
II Cystic fibrosis
III Severe protein calorie malnutrition with hypoalbuminemia
IV Pancreatic and duodenal neoplasms
V Pancreatic resection
VI Gastric surgery
  A Subtotal gastrectomy with Billroth II anastomosis
  B Subtotal gastrectomy with Billroth I anastomosis
  C Truncal vagotomy and pyloroplasty
VII Gastrinoma (Zollinger-Ellison syndrome)
VIII Hereditary pancreatitis
IX Traumatic pancreatitis
X Hemochromatosis
XI Shwachman's syndrome (pancreatic insufficiency and bone marrow dysfunction)
XII Trypsinogen deficiency
XIII Enterokinase deficiency
XIV Isolated deficiencies of amylase, lipase, or proteases
XV Alpha$_1$-antitrypsin deficiency
XVI Idiopathic pancreatitis

40 percent of patients with chronic pancreatitis have *cobalamin* (*vitamin B_{12}*) *malabsorption* which is corrected by the administration of oral pancreatic enzymes. There is usually a marked excretion of fecal fat (see Chap. 308), which can be reduced with the administration of oral pancreatic extract. The *tripeptide* function test (Chap. 324) and D-xylose urinary excretion test are useful in patients with "pancreatic steatorrhea," since the tripeptide test will be abnormal and the D-xylose excretion usually normal.

The radiographic hallmark of chronic pancreatitis is the presence of scattered calcification throughout the pancreas (Fig. 325-3). Pancreatic calcification indicates that significant damage has occurred and obviates the need for the secretin test. Alcohol by far is the most common cause of pancreatic calcification, but it may also be seen in severe protein calorie malnutrition, hyperparathyroidism, hereditary pancreatitis, posttraumatic pancreatitis, and islet-cell tumors.

Special techniques such as sonography, CT scanning, and

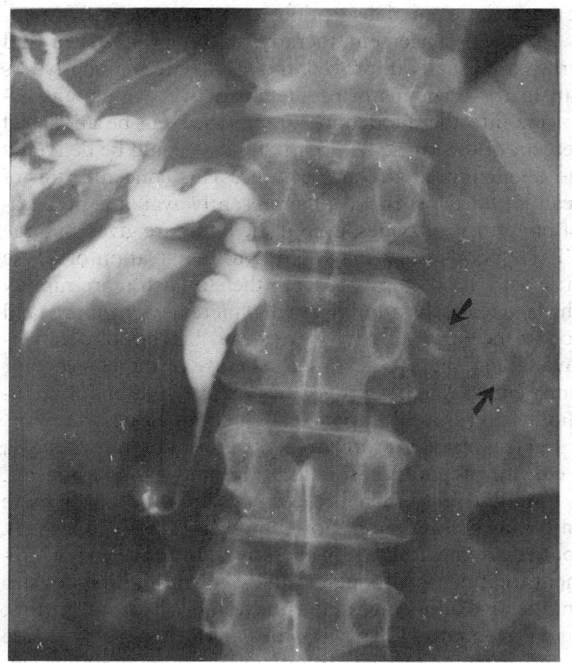
A

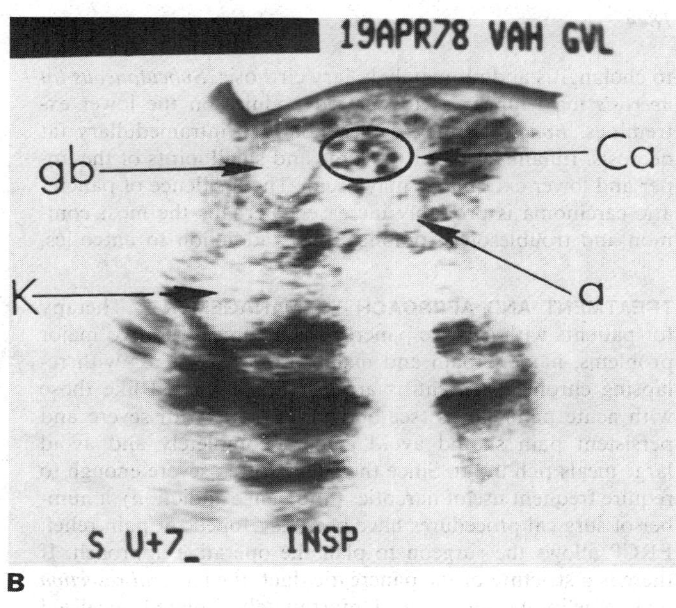

B

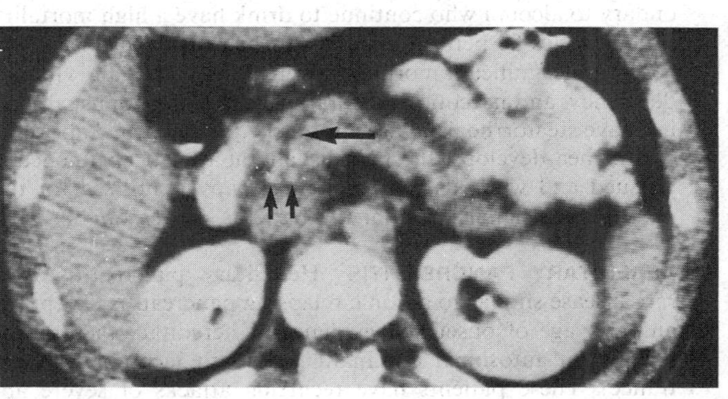
C

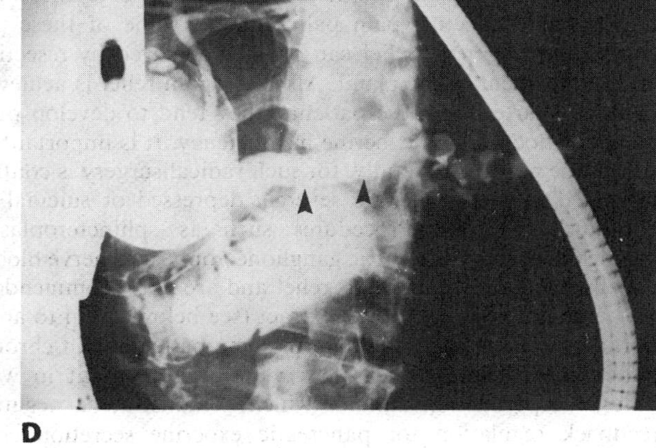
D

FIGURE 325-3
Radiological abnormalities in chronic pancreatitis. A. Pancreatic calcification (arrows) and stenosis (tapering) of the intrapancreatic portion of the common bile duct demonstrated by percutaneous transhepatic cholangiography. B. Pancreatic calcification (Ca) demonstrated by sonography. gb = gallbladder; K = kidney; a = aorta. C. Pancreatic calcification (vertical arrows) and dilated pancreatic duct (horizontal arrow) demonstrated by CT scan. D. Endoscopic retrograde cholangiopancreatogram shows grossly dilated pancreatic ducts (arrows) in a patient with long-standing pancreatitis.

ERCP have added new dimensions to the diagnosis of pancreatic disease. In addition to excluding pseudocysts and pancreatic cancer, sonography may show calcification or dilated ducts associated with chronic pancreatitis (Fig. 325-3). Similar benefits can be derived from CT scans, but the availability and lower cost make sonography preferable at present. ERCP is the only nonoperative technique which provides a direct view of the pancreatic duct. In patients with alcohol-induced pancreatitis, ERCP may reveal a pseudocyst missed by sonography or CT scan.

COMPLICATIONS OF CHRONIC PANCREATITIS The complications of chronic pancreatitis are protean. *Cobalamin malabsorption* occurs in 40 percent of patients with alcohol-induced chronic pancreatitis and virtually all with cystic fibrosis. The vitamin B_{12} malabsorption is consistently corrected by the administration of pancreatic enzymes (containing proteases). The cobalamin malabsorption may be due to excessive binding of cobalamin by nonintrinsic factor B_{12}–binding proteins. The latter are ordinarily destroyed by pancreatic proteases, but with pancreatic insufficiency the nonspecific binding proteins escape degradation and compete with intrinsic factor for vitamin B_{12} binding. Although the majority of patients show *impaired glucose tolerance*, the development of diabetic ketoacidosis and coma is uncommon. Similarly, end organ damage (retinopathy, neuropathy, nephropathy) is also uncommon, and the appearance of these complications should raise the question of concomitant genetic diabetes mellitus. A nondiabetic retinopathy, peripheral in location and secondary to vitamin A and/or zinc deficiency, is common in these patients. High amylase containing *effusions* occur within the pleura, pericardium, or peritoneum. *Gastrointestinal bleeding* may occur from ruptured varices secondary to splenic vein thrombosis due to inflammation of the tail of the pancreas. *Icterus* may occur, owing to either edema of the head of the pancreas compressing the common bile duct or chronic cholestasis secondary to chronic inflammatory reaction around the intrapancreatic portion of the common bile duct (Fig. 325-3). This chronic obstruction may lead to cholangitis and ultimately biliary cirrhosis. *Subcutaneous fat necrosis* may appear as tender red nodules on the lower extremities. *Bone pain* may be secondary to intramedullary fat necrosis. Inflammation of the large and small joints of the upper and lower extremities may occur. The incidence of pancreatic carcinoma is probably increased. Perhaps the most common and troublesome complication is addiction to narcotics.

TREATMENT AND APPROACH TO MANAGEMENT Therapy for patients with chronic pancreatitis is directed to two major problems, namely, pain and malabsorption. Patients with relapsing chronic pancreatitis are essentially treated like those with acute pancreatitis (see above). Patients with severe and persistent pain should avoid alcohol completely and avoid large meals rich in fat. Since the pain is often severe enough to require frequent use of narcotics (and hence addiction), a number of surgical procedures have been developed for pain relief. ERCP allows the surgeon to plan the operative approach. If there is a stricture of the pancreatic duct, then a *local resection* may ameliorate the pain. Unfortunately isolated localized strictures are not common. In most patients with alcohol-induced disease, the pancreas is diffusely involved and surgically correctible localized ductal disease is rare. When there is primary ductal obstruction, side-to-side pancreaticojejunostomy may provide effective pain palliation. In some of these patients, however, pain relief can only be achieved by resecting 50 to 95 percent of the gland. Although pain relief is achieved in three-quarters of these patients, they tend to develop pancreatic endocrine and exocrine insufficiency. It is important to screen the patients carefully, for such radical surgery is contraindicated in those who are severely depressed or suicidal or continue to drink. Procedures such as sphincteroplasty, splanchnicectomy and celiac ganglionectomy, and nerve blocks usually bring only temporary relief and are not recommended.

Large doses of pancreatic extract (see below) seem to ameliorate and even abort the pain in some patients with chronic pancreatitis. These clinical observations seem to fit in with data in experimental animals which demonstrate a negative feedback regulation for pancreatic exocrine secretion controlled by the amount of proteases within the lumen of the proximal small intestine. It seems reasonable to approach the patient with severe persistent or continuous abdominal pain thought to be secondary to chronic pancreatitis in the following manner. After other causes of abdominal pain (peptic ulcer, gallstones, etc.) have been appropriately excluded, a pancreatic *sonogram* should be done. If no mass is found, a *secretin test* may be performed, since with chronic pancreatitis and pain this test will be abnormal. If the secretin test is abnormal (i.e., decreased bicarbonate concentration or volume output) a 3- to 4-week *trial of pancreatic extract* is appropriate. If no relief is obtained, and especially if the volume secreted during the secretin test is very low, *ERCP* should be performed. If a pseudocyst or a localized ductal obstruction is found, appropriate surgery should be considered. A provocative study from South Africa questions the significance of the relationship of dilated ducts and/or strictures to pain. The finding of an appreciable obstruction or stricture in 65 percent of the patients who were pain-free more than 1 year, compared with 79 percent of the group with pain, suggests that factors other than duct obstruction or narrowing may be important in the pathogenesis of pain. It may be that the most important factors in the relief of pain are abstinence from alcohol and progressive pancreatic dysfunction rather than the surgical procedure per se. If no surgically remedial lesion is found and severe pain continues despite abstinence from alcohol, subtotal pancreatic resection may be necessary.

The treatment of malabsorption rests upon the use of pancreatic enzyme replacement therapy. Although diarrhea and steatorrhea are usually improved, the results are frequently less than satisfactory. The major problem is delivery of enough active enzyme into the duodenum. Steatorrhea can be abolished if 10 percent of the normal amount of lipase could be delivered into the duodenum at the proper time. This concentration of lipase cannot be achieved with the presently available preparations of pancreatic enzymes, even if the latter are given in large doses. These poor results may be due to inactivation of lipase by gastric acid, food emptying from the stomach more rapidly than the exogenously administered pancreatic enzymes, and variation in the enzyme activity of various batches of commercially available pancreatic extracts. The use of the H_2-receptor antagonist cimetidine has proved to be a useful adjunct in patients failing to respond to pancreatic extract alone.

For the usual patient three to eight tablets or capsules of a potent enzyme preparation should be administered with meals. If this program fails, then the enzymes may be given more frequently (in the same total dose but every 2 h while awake). Some patients require adjuvant therapy to improve enzyme replacement treatment. Although initially cimetidine was considered an effective adjuvant, studies have failed to confirm this. Sodium bicarbonate (1.3 g with meals) is effective, but side effects and expense restrict its use. Antacids containing calcium carbonate or magnesium hydroxide are not effective.

Patients with severe exocrine pancreatic insufficiency secondary to alcohol who continue to drink have a high mortality (in one series 50 percent were dead when followed for 5 to 12 years) and significant morbidity (weight loss, lassitude, vitamin deficiency, and narcotic addiction). Those with pain usually do not have steatorrhea and are approached as described above. If steatorrhea develops, the pain usually abates. If abstinence is pursued and vigorous replacement therapy is utilized for the maldigestion-malabsorption, the patients do reasonably well.

HEREDITARY PANCREATITIS Hereditary pancreatitis is a rare disease similar to chronic relapsing pancreatitis except for an early age of onset and evidence of hereditary factors (involving an autosomal dominant gene with incomplete penetrance). These patients have recurring attacks of severe abdominal pain which may last from a few days to a few weeks. The serum amylase and lipase levels may be elevated during acute attacks. Patients frequently develop pancreatic calcification, diabetes mellitus, and steatorrhea, and in addition, they have an increased incidence of pancreatic carcinoma. Abdominal complaints in relatives of patients with hereditary pancreatitis should raise the question of pancreatic disease.

CYSTIC FIBROSIS

GENERAL CONSIDERATIONS Cystic fibrosis is the most common hereditary lethal disease in Caucasian children. It is transmitted as an autosomal recessive trait, with a prevalence of 1 per 1500 to 2500 births and with approximately 1 in 20 Caucasians being heterozygous for the condition. Patients with cystic fibrosis have a dysfunction of the mucus-producing exocrine glands in the bronchi, pancreas, liver, and intestine. However, the basic metabolic defect is unknown. This disease is no longer one of childhood and adolescence. With improvement in the therapy of patients with cystic fibrosis, an increasing number of patients are reaching adulthood. Twenty years ago the mean survival was only 1 year; presently, the mean survival is 16 years.

CLINICAL FEATURES Although the triad of recurrent pulmonary infections, maldigestion-malabsorption, and an abnormal sweat test are characteristic, patients are frequently seen without these classical manifestations. Approximately 85 percent of patients with cystic fibrosis have impairment of pancreatic exocrine function. Steatorrhea is often marked and accompanied by deficiencies of fat-soluble vitamins (e.g., low prothrombin levels). A small number of patients may have recurrent pancreatitis with abdominal pain and elevated amylase levels. Biliary cirrhosis develops in 5 to 10 percent. Approximately 15 percent of patients may develop intestinal obstruction at birth because of the thick, tenacious intestinal secretions. Similarly, children or adults may develop small- or large-bowel obstruction, ileocolic intussusception, cecal or sigmoid volvulus, rectal impaction, and rectal prolapse. Cobalamin and bile acid malabsorption are common but correctable by oral pancreatic extract. Cobalamin deficiency is rare, perhaps due to the almost universal administration of pancreatic extract to these patients beginning at an early age. The incidence of gallstones is increased. Although frank diabetes is uncommon, glucose intolerance may be present in 40 percent of patients. Nearly all males have aspermia because of a failure in development of the vas deferens, epididymis, and seminal vesicles.

DIAGNOSIS A properly performed and interpreted sweat test (quantitative pilocarpine iontophoresis) is essential for the diagnosis of cystic fibrosis. In almost all patients the sweat chloride is greater than 60 meq per liter. Secretin or CCK-PZ tests will usually demonstrate severe impairment of bicarbonate output and pancreatic enzymes, respectively. The tripeptide hydrolysis test (Chap. 324) is usually abnormal. Suction biopsy of the rectum will often show dilated crypts containing excessive amounts of mucus, but the specificity of these findings has been questioned.

THERAPY Treatment includes antibiotics for recurrent pulmonary infections, inhalation and physical therapy, pancreatic extracts, and vitamin supplementation, as well as psychological and emotional support. Although complete correction of fat malabsorption is usually not achieved, satisfactory weight gain is often attained. Elevated blood and urine uric acid levels may occur in children taking excessive doses of pancreatic extract, but this is reversible with reduction in dosage.

CANCER OF THE PANCREAS

GENERAL CONSIDERATIONS Carcinoma of the pancreas is now the fourth commonest cancer causing death in the United States; only cancer of the lung, colon, and breast occur more frequently. It accounts for 10 percent of all tumors of digestive organs and over 20,000 deaths per year. The incidence has increased 300 percent since 1930 to approximately 11 per 100,000 population. The disease is more common in males than females (1.5:1), and the peak incidence is between the ages of 60 to 70. Although the etiologic factors in most cases are not known, incidence of carcinoma of the pancreas is 2.0 to 2.5 times greater in *smokers* than in nonsmokers, and about 2 times greater in patients with *diabetes mellitus.* Patients with *calcific pancreatitis* also have an increased incidence of pancreatic carcinoma. Some reports have suggested an association between heavy coffee intake and increased risk of pancreatic cancer, but whether a true causal relationship exists is uncertain. The tumors are usually adenocarcinomas arising from ductal epithelium. The head of the pancreas is involved in about 65 percent, the body and tail in 30 percent, and the tail alone in 5 percent. At the time of diagnosis the tumor is confined to the pancreas in only 15 percent of patients; 25 percent demonstrate local invasion or regional lymph node spread, and the remaining 60 percent exhibit distinct metastases.

CLINICAL FEATURES Weight loss, abdominal pain, anorexia, and jaundice are the classic symptoms. Nausea, weakness and fatigue, vomiting, diarrhea, dyspepsia, and back pain are also fairly common. The weight loss in carcinoma is extensive (average total loss about 25 lb) and is not fully explained by anorexia and maldigestion. The weight loss in patients with lesions in the body and tail, in whom malabsorption should be minimal, is often as pronounced as when the carcinoma is in the head of the pancreas.

Pain occurs at some time in the course of the disease in 75 to 90 percent of patients. With tumors of the head of the pancreas, the pain is likely to be in the epigastrium and right upper quadrant; with lesions in the body of the pancreas, pain often localizes in the midline, whereas with lesions in the tail, pain may be referred to the left upper quadrant. Abdominal pain may be vague or be a steady dull, aching, or boring pain often radiating through to the back. Severe and unrelenting pain suggests extension into the retroperitoneal area with invasion of the neural plexus around the celiac axis ganglion.

Jaundice occurs some time in the course of the disease in 80 to 90 percent of patients with carcinoma of the head, and in 10 to 40 percent in patients with tumors of the body and tail. When it occurs it is progressive and accompanied by pruritus. Both constipation and diarrhea have been cited as the predominant alteration of bowel habits. Emotional disturbances frequently occur in cancer of the pancreas and may take the form of insomnia, restlessness, rage, anxiety, depression, suicidal tendencies, and a sense of impending doom.

Physical examination frequently reveals evidence of weight loss, jaundice, and enlarged liver and abdominal tenderness. Although the gallbladder is usually enlarged, it is palpable in only 15 to 40 percent of cases (Courvoisier's sign). The finding of an enlarged gallbladder in a jaundiced patient without biliary colic should suggest malignant obstruction of the extrahepatic biliary tree. Splenomegaly may result from compression, invasion, and thrombosis of the portal venous system, especially the splenic vein. Erosion of the duodenal mucosa may cause occult or frank gastrointestinal bleeding. In carcinoma of the body and tail, an abdominal mass can be felt in 40 to 50 percent of patients; hepatomegaly is less common than in tumors of the head of the pancreas, and obvious hepatic enlargement should suggest hepatic metastasis. An important physical finding is an abdominal bruit which is usually heard in the periumbilical area and left upper quadrant, and this is due to invasion and/or compression of the splenic artery by tumor. Thrombophlebitis occurs in approximately 10 percent of patients and is more common with the tumors of the body or tail of the pancreas. In acinar-cell carcinomas, which are uncommon, tender subcutaneous nodules due to subcutaneous fat necrosis and polyarthralgia occur.

The diagnosis of pancreatic carcinoma should be suspected in patients past the age of 50 who present with any of the following findings: (1) unexplained weight loss greater than 10 percent of normal body weight; (2) unexplained upper abdominal pain, especially with a negative upper gastrointestinal tract workup; (3) unexplained back pain; (4) an attack of pancreatitis without an obvious cause; (5) sudden onset of diabetes mellitus without a predisposing cause such as obesity or family history; and (6) jaundice with obstructive features. Carcinoma of the hepatic duct bifurcation, of the ampulla of Vater, and of the duodenum also need to be considered in the differential diagnosis, but these all occur quite infrequently.

LABORATORY FINDINGS Laboratory data are only occasionally helpful in suggesting the diagnosis of pancreatic carcinoma. The serum amylase and lipase values are abnormal in only 10 percent of cases. About 20 percent of patients have fasting hyperglycemia or glycosuria, although the glucose tolerance test is abnormal in 50 percent. Anemia, which occurs in one-third of patients, and occult blood in the stool, which occurs in one-half of patients, are usually due to erosion of the duodenal mucosa by tumor. Although the stools may have a greasy or pultaceous consistency, frank steatorrhea occurs in only about 10 percent of patients. Carcinoma of the head of the pancreas with bile duct obstruction is accompanied by hyperbilirubinemia and clay-colored stools. By contrast, the blood, urine, and feces in patients with carcinoma of the body and tail of the pancreas are often normal. The serum alkaline phosphatase is usually elevated in patients with jaundice (and may antedate the hyperbilirubinemia). It is elevated in about 35 percent of cases without jaundice.

DIAGNOSTIC PROCEDURES (See Table 325-5) Although standard gastrointestinal x-rays may suggest the presence of carcinoma of the head of the pancreas, the tumor is usually of considerable size before it distorts the duodenal mucosa and the configuration of the duodenal loop. Thus, only 50 percent of patients with carcinoma of the head of the pancreas have an abnormal examination. The frequency of abnormal exams is even lower with lesions in the body and tail of the pancreas.

Ultrasound is valuable in the diagnosis of pancreatic carcinoma, especially as an initial screening procedure; abnormalities are found in 70 to 90 percent of patients with pancreatic carcinoma. Sonography is most likely to be positive if the tumor is over 2 cm in diameter and lies in the head or body of the pancreas; lesions in the body and tail of the pancreas are more difficult to recognize.

If available, tests of exocrine pancreatic function with duodenal intubation and aspiration of duodenal contents after intravenous injection of secretin or secretin plus cholecystokinin are useful. Such tests are abnormal in approximately 80 percent of cases. However, pancreatic function tests do not permit discrimination between chronic pancreatic carcinoma and chronic pancreatitis. Cytologic examination of pancreatic fluid and pancreatic secretory studies obtained after secretin-cholecystokinin stimulation should theoretically be useful but practically has been found not to be reliable enough to diagnose pancreatic cancer.

CT scanning is frequently abnormal in pancreatic carcinoma; in most series of proved cases, CT scans detected the lesion in over 80 percent. False-positive results have been reported in about 5 to 10 percent of cases where no tumor was found at laparotomy. Such false-positive results will perhaps be less in the future. CT scanning has slight advantages over ultrasound, such as better definition of the body and tail of the pancreas as well as contiguous organs, but the cost is considerably greater. Selective and superselective angiography is of definite value in some patients. Advantages of angiography include (1) detection of carcinoma in the body and tail of the pancreas by observing vessel sheathing (Fig. 325-2), vessel displacement, and vascular occlusion; (2) detection of metastatic spread to the liver; and (3) assessment of the degree of involvement of huge pancreatic vessels which may be an important consideration preoperatively. When the arteriogram is positive, about 85 percent of patients can be expected to have pancreatic cancer; however, false negatives occur in about 15 percent of patients.

ERCP may be diagnostic in 75 to 85 percent of cases. The characteristic findings are stenosis or obstruction of either the pancreatic or the common bile duct; both duct systems are abnormal in over half the cases. The differentiation, however, between carcinoma and chronic pancreatitis by ERCP can be quite difficult if both diseases are present. False-negative results with ERCP are quite low (less than 5 percent). Finally, *percutaneous aspiration biopsy of the pancreas* under ultrasonic guidance is a new procedure which can provide a definitive diagnosis and may obviate surgical exploration.

Of the many serologic markers available, only two, the LAI assay and galactosyltransferase isoenyzme II (GT-II), appear promising. Serum GT-II may be useful by itself and in combination with imaging techniques in distinguishing benign from malignant pancreatic disease. The combination of GT-II with ultrasound, CT scanning, or ERCP increases the sensitivity of detecting pancreatic cancer to greater than 90 percent. However, GT-II does not distinguish between pancreatic carcinoma and other gastrointestinal neoplasms. Finally, the value of these tests in detecting asymptomatic patients with pancreatic cancer remains to be determined.

Patients with carcinoma of the pancreas are frequently investigated for several months before a diagnosis is established. Even laparotomy may not provide a definitive diagnosis because chronic pancreatitis may produce a hard mass in the head of the pancreas indistinguishable from carcinoma by palpation. Furthermore, biopsy of such a mass may not show neoplastic tissue and reveal only evidence of pancreatitis because the carcinoma is often surrounded by edematous, inflamed, and fibrotic tissue, e.g., changes of chronic pancreatitis.

TREATMENT AND COURSE When the diagnosis is confirmed at laparotomy, the tumor is usually inoperable. The resectability rate in most series is only about 15 to 20 percent. If the tumor is localized and has not spread to portal lymph nodes, and is not fixed to other structures (e.g., portal vein, superior mesenteric vein, and common bile duct), the lesion should be considered resectable. Resection under these circumstances offers an opportunity for palliation, although survival does not appear to be prolonged. In many patients, just palliative bypass of biliary tract obstruction should be performed. Importantly, the mortality rate with a Whipple procedure (pancreatoduodenal resection) is about 20 percent in most series. The

TABLE 325-5
Diagnostic procedures for pancreatic carcinoma*

Location of carcinoma	*Sonography*	*Exocrine pancreatic function tests*	*Cytologic examination duodenal fluid*	*Computerized tomography (CT scan)*	*Endoscopic retrograde cholangiopancreatography (ERCP)*	*Percutaneous transhepatic cholangiogram (PTC)*	*Selective arteriography*	*Percutaneous pancreatic biopsy with radiologic guidance*	*Upper gastrointestinal x-rays*
Head	++	++	+	+++	+++	+++	+++	++++	+
Body	++	++	+	+++	+++	+	+++	++++	+
Tail	++	++	+	+++	+++	0	+++	++++	+

* *If the ultrasound examination shows a pancreatic mass with dilated intrahepatic ducts, a PTC is the logical next step. If the patient has a mass on ultrasound examination but without dilated ducts, ERCP should be done. If clinical suspicion is high or exocrine pancreatic function tests are abnormal, ERCP should be considered. If ERCP is unsuccessful, selective arteriography is recommended. If arteriography shows encasement of vessels or hepatic metastases, percutaneous pancreatic biopsy should be considered as an alternative to laparotomy. See also Table 324-1A.*

NOTE: + = *helpful occasionally* (<50 *percent cases*); ++ = *useful, especially as initial screening procedure;* +++ = *frequently* (> 50 *percent cases*) *abnormal;* ++++ = *often diagnostic.*

median survival is 6 months from the time of diagnosis. Approximately 10 percent of patients survive 1 year, and in most reported series, the 5-year survival rate is a dismal 1 to 2 percent. Multicenter studies on patients with inoperable pancreatic cancer suggest that either high-dose small-volume radiation therapy or multidrug chemotherapy (fluorouracil, cyclophosphamide, methotrexate, and vincristine followed by fluorouracil and mitomycin for maintenance) significantly prolongs survival in 15 to 30 percent of patients.

PANCREATIC ENDOCRINE TUMORS

Pancreatic endocrine tumors are summarized in Table 325-6 and discussed in Chap. 116.

OTHER CONDITIONS

ANNULAR PANCREAS When there is a failure in communication of the ventral and dorsal anlage of the pancreas, a ring of pancreatic tissue encircles the duodenum. Such an annular pancreas may cause intestinal obstruction in the neonate or the adult. Symptoms of postprandial fullness, epigastric pain, nausea, and vomiting may be present for years before the diagnosis is entertained. The radiographic findings are symmetric dilatation of the proximal duodenum with bulging of the recesses on either side of the annular band, effacement of the duodenal mucosa without destruction of the mucosa, accentuation of the findings in the right anterior oblique position, and the lack of change on repeated examinations. The differential diagnosis should include duodenal webs, tumors of the pancreas or duodenum, postbulbar peptic ulcer, regional enteritis, and adhesions. Patients with annular pancreas have an increased incidence of pancreatitis and peptic ulcer. Because of these and other potential complications, the treatment is surgical even though the condition has been present for years. Retrocolic duodenojejunostomy is the procedure of choice, although some surgeons advocate Billroth II gastrectomy, gastroenterostomy, and vagotomy.

PANCREAS DIVISUM Pancreas divisum occurs when the embryologic ventral and dorsal parts of the pancreas fail to fuse so that pancreatic drainage is accomplished mainly through the accessory papilla. This condition should be thought of in patients with recurrent pancreatitis without obvious cause, in patients who develop pancreatitis after ingesting small amounts of alcohol, and in patients having ERCP who complain of abdominal pain immediately following the injection of small amounts of contrast material (due to overdistention of the small duct of Wirsung). Since the accessory papilla in the duct of Santorini is too small to accept total pancreatic secretion, obstructive pain and pancreatitis may result. An awareness of this condition is also important because the radiographic appearances of ventral pancreas may be mistaken for ductal obstruction secondary to carcinoma, and failure to recognize it may result in inappropriate surgery.

MACROAMYLASEMIA Macroamylasemia is a condition whereby amylase is circulating in the blood in a polymer form too large to be easily excreted by the kidney. The patient with this condition will demonstrate an elevated serum amylase value, a low urinary amylase, and a C_{am}/C_{cr} of less than 1 percent. The presence of macroamylase can be documented by chromatography of the serum. The prevalence of macroamylasemia is 1.5 percent of the nonalcoholic general adult hospital population. Usually macroamylasemia is an incidental finding and is not related to disease of the pancreas or other organs. It is important to be aware of this condition so that patients with macroamylasemia will not be needlessly evaluated and treated for pancreatic disease.

TABLE 325-6
Pancreatic endocrine tumors

Syndrome	*Hormone(s) produced*	*Primary hormone effects*	*Pathologic features*	*Clinical features*
Zollinger-Ellison	Gastrin	Gastric acid hypersecretion with basal acid outputs usually >15 meq/h	Non-beta-cell islet tumors; 10% aberrant (duodenal); 60% malignant	Severe peptic ulcer disease often refractory to therapy; ectopic ulcers; diarrhea; multiple endocrine adenomas (parathyroid, pituitary, adrenal, thyroid)
Insulinoma	Insulin	Hypoglycemia with inappropriately increased serum insulin levels	Beta-cell islet tumors; 80–90% benign	Hypoglycemic symptoms
Glucagonoma	Glucagon	Hyperglucagonemia →glucose intolerance	Alpha-cell islet tumors; 60% malignant	Slow growing pancreatic tumor; hyperglycemia; bullous and eczematoid dermatitis; weight loss; anemia
Somatostatinoma	Somatostatin	Somatostatin inhibition of insulin, gastrin and pancreatic enzyme secretion	Delta-cell islet tumor	Pancreatic tumor; diarrhea; anemia
Pancreatic cholera	Vasoactive intestinal peptide (VIP) ? Gastrin ? Glucagon ? Gastric inhibitory polypeptide	Hormones cause altered salt and water transport by gut	? Delta-cell tumor; > 50% malignant	Pancreatic tumor with severe watery diarrhea, flushing; weight loss, hypercalcemia; hypochlorhydria; inordinate fecal water and electrolyte losses
Carcinoid	Serotonin Prostaglandins	Altered gut motility; diarrhea	Non-beta-cell islet tumors	Carcinoid syndrome with flushing; wheezing; diarrhea; alcohol intolerance; hepatomegaly

REFERENCES

ARVANITAKIS C et al: Diagnostic tests of exocrine pancreatic function and disease. Gastroenterology 74:932, 1978

BRADLEY EL et al: The natural history of pancreatic pseudocysts: A unifying concept of management. Am J Surg 137:135, 1979

DIMAGNO EP et al: Relations between pancreatic enzyme outputs and malabsorption in severe pancreatic insufficiency. N Engl J Med 288:813, 1973

——— et al: A prospective comparison of current diagnostic tests for pancreatic cancer. N Engl J Med 297:737, 1977

FERRUCCI JT JR, WITTENBERG J: Radiologic imaging of the pancreas: 1982, in *Update II: Harrison's Principles of Internal Medicine,* KJ Isselbacher et al (eds). New York, McGraw-Hill, 1982

FOULIS AK et al: Endotoxemia and complement activation in acute pancreatitis. Gut 23:656, 1982

FRIESEN SR: Tumors of the endocrine pancreas. N Engl J Med 306:580, 1982

LANKISCH PG: Exocrine pancreatic function tests. Gut 23:777, 1982

MALLORY A, KERN F: Drug-induced pancreatitis: A critical review. Gastroenterology 78:813, 1980

MORGAN RGH, WORMSLEY KG: Progress report. Cancer of the pancreas. Gut 18:550, 1977

RANSON JHG et al: Diagnostic signs in the role of operative management in acute pancreatitis. Surg Gynecol Obstet 139:67, 1974

RUSSELL JGB et al: Ultrasonic scanning in pancreatic disease. Gut 19:1027, 1978

SARLES H: Chronic calcifying pancreatitis—chronic alcoholic pancreatitis. Gastroenterology 66:604, 1974

SCHWACHMAN H et al: Cystic fibrosis: A new outlook: 70 patients above 25 years of age. Medicine 56:129, 1977

SINGH M, WEBSTER PD: Neurohormonal control of pancreatic secretion. A review. Gastroenterology 74:193, 1978

WARSHAW A: Acute pancreatitis. Viewpoints Dig Dis, vol 9, no 5, November 1977

section 8 | Disorders of the hematopoietic system

Red blood cell disorders

326 IRON-DEFICIENCY AND IRON-LOADING ANEMIAS

ANDREW I. SCHAFER
H. FRANKLIN BUNN

Among the transition metals that are essential to life, iron is the most abundant and important, being used in a broad repertoire of biochemical reactions. When complexed with porphyrin and inserted into an appropriate protein, iron not only binds oxygen reversibly but also participates in a number of vital oxidation-reduction reactions. Since inorganic iron is highly toxic, specific processes have evolved for its assimilation, transport, and storage. Under normal circumstances iron homeostasis is precisely maintained but can go awry in a variety of clinical settings, leading either to iron deficiency or iron overload.

IRON METABOLISM The amount of iron obtained from the diet must replace the obligatory losses from the skin and gastrointestinal and genitourinary tracts; these losses generally do not exceed 1 mg daily in the adult male or nonmenstruating female. Additional iron requirements due to menstrual blood loss vary greatly but average about 0.5 mg daily. The amount of iron present in the diet, about 10 to 20 mg daily in the United States, greatly exceeds that required to meet physiologic demands, and the widespread prevalence of iron deficiency is due in part to the inefficient absorption of dietary iron. Heme iron is better absorbed than nonheme iron. Unfortunately, the diet of most of the population of the world is virtually devoid of meats and hence of heme iron. Even in the more developed countries, only 5 to 10 percent of the iron in the diet is absorbed.

Absorption Because there is no major physiologic route for the excretion of iron, body iron content normally is largely determined by its absorption. Iron is absorbed mainly in the duodenum and proximal jejunum. The absorption of nonheme iron is modified by several factors in the diet and in gastrointestinal secretions. Iron-binding anions in food, such as ethylenediaminetetraacetic acid (EDTA), which is used as a preservative in a number of foodstuffs, tannates (contained in tea), carbonates, oxalates, and phosphates all inhibit iron absorption. Medicinal antacids, such as magnesium trisilicate, and clay may also impair iron absorption. In contrast, other substances in the diet, including ascorbic acid, citric acid, amino acids, and sugars, enhance iron absorption. Gastric secretions and hydrochloric acid facilitate nonheme iron absorption by poorly understood mechanisms which probably involve the stabilization of ionic iron, thereby preventing its precipitation as insoluble ferric hydroxide. Most of these dietary and secretory factors do not affect the absorption of heme iron, which is taken up by the mucosal cells as the intact metalloporphyrin.

Intestinal iron absorption depends on both the amount and bioavailability of dietary iron and is controlled by the gut mucosal "setting" which is responsive to the state of body iron stores. The amount of iron entering the mucosal cell and passing into the portal circulation is regulated to maintain a normal body iron content. The signals which determine this "mucosal intelligence" are largely unknown. However, when the demand for iron is increased by depletion of body reserves due to growth spurts, pregnancy, or menstrual and pathologic hemorrhage, the efficiency of iron absorption can increase to about 10 to 20 percent. Conversely, when excessive body stores of iron are present, intestinal iron absorption is markedly reduced.

Distribution The distribution of iron in normal adults is shown in Fig. 326-1. Most of the body iron is found in red cells as the iron porphyrin complex of hemoglobin. Smaller quantities of iron are utilized in various tissues in the form of myoglobin as well as heme and nonheme enzymes. Excess iron is stored in the body as ferritin and hemosiderin, primarily in mononuclear-phagocyte cells of the spleen, liver, and bone marrow and in hepatic parenchymal cells. Exchange of iron between these communicating tissue compartments is effected by the carrier plasma protein transferrin, a beta globulin synthesized in the liver.

Transport The major destination of plasma transferrin-bound iron is the erythron, where immature red cell precursors assimilate the iron for hemoglobin synthesis. A much smaller amount of transferrin iron is delivered to other sites, particularly the parenchymal cells of the liver. When transferrin iron saturation is increased, parenchymal iron uptake is increased. Virtually no iron is deposited in mononuclear-phagocyte cells from the plasma transferrin pool. These cells derive most of their iron from the phagocytosis of senescent red cells. Following phagocytosis, the iron is liberated from the porphyrin ring by heme oxygenase and is either released to the plasma to be bound by transferrin or is stored in the form of ferritin and hemosiderin. Therefore, the passage of iron through the mononuclear-phagocyte system is unidirectional (see Fig. 326-1). Iron metabolism is characterized by conservation of body iron, so that the iron of hemoglobin degradation is continually reutilized for erythropoiesis. Storage iron is readily mobilized in response to increased demand by the erythron, but chronic infection, inflammation, or malignancy can interfere with the release of iron from mononuclear-phagocyte stores.

LABORATORY EVALUATION In the laboratory assessment of body iron status, the most direct and sensitive tests involve *examination of tissues for iron content.* Depletion of bone marrow iron stores is the earliest stage in the development of iron deficiency and can be detected by the absence of Prussian blue–stainable iron in an aspirate of bone marrow. Histochemical assessment of increased bone marrow iron does not correlate as well with body iron stores in disorders of transfusional iron overload, and it is an unreliable index of iron overload in idiopathic hemochromatosis. The most sensitive test of iron loading in hemochromatosis (Chap. 97) is quantitative measurement of liver iron content in a liver biopsy specimen. Computerized tomography can show increased density of the liver.

FIGURE 326-1

The distribution of iron in normal adults and internal iron kinetics. Bold arrows indicate major pathways of iron movement.

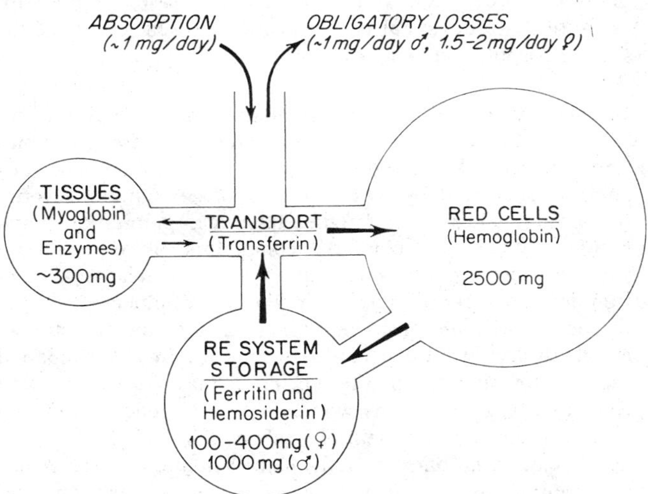

Measurement of *serum iron and total iron-binding capacity* (or transferrin) is useful in the diagnosis of both iron deficiency and overload states (Fig. 326-2, Table 326-1). The degree to which transferrin is saturated with iron represents a reliable indicator of iron supply to the developing red cell. Transferrin is normally about 20 to 45 percent saturated. The serum iron is characteristically decreased both in iron deficiency and in association with chronic disorders; however, in the latter the iron-binding capacity is generally also decreased to maintain a transferrin saturation of over 15 percent, while in the former it is usually increased so that transferrin saturation falls below 10 percent. In hypoproliferative and iron-overload states, serum iron is elevated and transferrin saturation may approach 100 percent.

Assay of *serum ferritin* correlates closely with total-body iron stores. The finding of a low ferritin level is diagnostic of iron deficiency and obviates the need to perform bone marrow aspiration for the purpose of assessing stainable iron. Measurement of serum ferritin is also useful in detecting and determining the degree of iron overload, although it may underestimate iron stores in some patients with early hemochromatosis. The serum ferritin level depends not only on tissue iron stores but also on the rate of release of ferritin from the tissues. Therefore, in cases of extensive tissue damage, as may occur in patients with inflammation, liver disease, and certain malignancies, the ferritin level is usually elevated in the absence of iron overload and may be normal in the presence of coexisting iron deficiency.

Ferrokinetics *Ferrokinetic studies,* using tracer amounts of a radioactive isotope of iron, provide a more dynamic laboratory assessment of iron supply to the marrow and erythropoiesis in general than do the static methods described above. Radioactive iron (^{59}Fe) bound to plasma transferrin in vitro is injected intravenously. From serial samples of the peripheral blood following injection the plasma iron turnover can be determined as well as the subsequent incorporation of iron into the hemoglobin of circulating red cells. In normal subjects, injected radioiron disappears rapidly and exponentially from plasma, with a half-time of 60 to 90 min. Figure 326-3*A* shows the linear clearance of plasma radioiron when it is plotted semilogarithmically. Plasma iron turnover (PIT) is the measure of the absolute amount of iron released from plasma transferrin per unit of time and is calculated from the rate of disappearance of iron label from the plasma, the plasma iron content, and the plasma volume. In normal individuals 30 to 40 mg of iron leaves the plasma daily. The PIT reflects the rate of *total* erythropoiesis. The *effectiveness* of erythropoiesis is indicated by the extent that the iron label is incorporated into hemoglobin in circulating red cells (Fig. 326-3*B*). In about a week, red cells normally accumulate 80 to 90 percent of the injected dose of radioiron.

TABLE 326-1
Stages in the development of iron deficiency

	Normal	*Mild*	*Moderate*	*Severe*
Hemoglobin:	15 g/dl	13 g/dl	10 g/dl	5 g/dl
MCV	N	↓	↓	↓↓
MCHC	N	N	↓	↓↓
Marrow Fe stores	Present	Absent	Absent	Absent
Serum Fe/TIBC, μg/dl	100/300	~75/300	~50/450	~25/600
Fe enzymes	N	N	N	↓

NOTE: *MCV = mean corpuscular volume; MCHC = mean corpuscular hemoglobin concentration; TIBC = total iron-binding capacity; N = normal.*

In conditions of bone marrow failure (hypoplastic anemias) plasma iron clearance is slow, PIT is decreased, and there is very little incorporation of ^{59}Fe into hemoglobin. In iron deficiency, ^{59}Fe is removed from plasma more rapidly than normal and is almost entirely utilized by the hemoglobin of newly formed red cells. A similar pattern of ferrokinetics is seen in polycythemia vera, which is characterized by increased effective erythropoiesis. In hemolytic states, radioiron is rapidly cleared from the plasma and rapidly appears in circulating red cells, but because of the premature removal of red cells from the circulation, the apparent maximal recovery is less than normal. In disorders of hemoglobin synthesis, such as thalassemia and the sideroblastic anemias, plasma iron clearance is likewise rapid and PIT is increased; however, because of ineffective erythropoiesis, red cell radioiron utilization is low. A similar ferrokinetic profile is seen in megaloblastic anemias and myeloid metaplasia, which are likewise characterized by ineffective erythropoiesis.

IRON-DEFICIENCY ANEMIA When the supply of iron to the bone marrow falls short of that required for the production of red blood cells, anemia will ensue. Iron deficiency is the most common cause of anemia throughout the world. This condition is particularly prevalent in tropical areas where the dietary intake of meat is low and where infestation with hookworm is endemic. In the United States, about 20 percent of women in the childbearing age group are iron-deficient, while the overall prevalence in adult males is about 2 percent.

Etiology The development of iron deficiency depends upon one or more of the following factors: (1) increased requirements, (2) inadequate dietary intake, (3) decreased intestinal absorption, and (4) blood loss. Accordingly, certain groups of individuals can be readily identified to be at increased risk for developing iron deficiency.

Increased requirements for iron occur during the growth spurts of infancy and adolescence and during pregnancy. Up to 10 percent of pre-school-age children in the United States are iron-deficient, with a peak incidence at 1 to 2 years of age. The increased demand for iron during infancy is not adequately met by a diet rich in milk and cereals and poor in meat and vegetables. The iron content of such a diet is low, and assimilation may be further impaired by the presence of iron-binding anions, particularly phosphates. Accordingly, an infant's diet should be supplemented with iron. During adolescence, iron intake also may be compromised owing to irregular dietary habits and the current predilection for "junk food." During pregnancy the growing fetus usurps about 500 mg of iron from the mother, even if she is already iron-deficient. The daily iron requirement increases about threefold during pregnancy. Currently, the vast majority of pregnant women who seek medical attention are routinely given prophylactic treatment with iron salts. Among pregnant women who do not receive adequate antenatal care, the incidence of iron deficiency exceeds 50 percent.

Inadequate intake of iron is prevalent in certain parts of the world where diets are low in animal proteins. The decreased iron content of the diets of infants and adolescents is mentioned above. Among indigent and elderly individuals, iron intake is often suboptimal, owing to a combination of economic constraints, poor dentition, and apathy.

Decreased absorption of iron can occur in many clinical settings. After partial or total gastrectomy, the assimilation of dietary iron is impaired, owing primarily to increased motility and bypass of the proximal intestine, which is the primary site of iron absorption. Achlorhydria also contributes to decreased iron absorption. Patients with chronic diarrhea or intestinal malabsorption may also develop iron deficiency, particularly if the duodenum and proximal jejunum are involved. Sometimes iron-deficiency anemia is a harbinger of nontropical (celiac) sprue.

Blood loss is by far the most important cause of iron deficiency in adults. Among women in the childbearing age group, menstrual blood loss is responsible for most cases of iron deficiency. Women who take estrogen-progesterone birth control pills tend to have reduced menstrual blood loss, whereas those with intrauterine devices have increased menstrual blood flow.

Gastrointestinal blood loss is the primary cause of iron deficiency among adult males but must be carefully considered in any iron-deficient patient. The testing of stool for occult blood is an indispensable part of the evaluation of all patients with iron deficiency or unexplained anemia. Since gastrointestinal bleeding can be intermittent, it may be necessary to test multiple specimens over an extended time span. The most common causes of gastrointestinal blood loss are peptic ulcer, hiatus hernia, diverticulosis, and cancer. Hemorrhoids and salicylate ingestion are often responsible for the presence of occult blood in the stool but rarely cause significant blood loss. In about 15 percent of patients with documented gastrointestinal bleeding, no source can be determined, even after extensive radiologic and endoscopic investigation. In tropical areas parasitic infestations, particularly hookworm, are a major cause of blood loss.

Occasionally, as in patients with hereditary telangiectasia or in those with a bleeding diathesis, gastrointestinal bleeding arises from multiple sites. Thrombocytopenia, qualitative platelet disorders, and von Willebrand's disease are more apt to cause gastrointestinal bleeding than are deficiencies of the soluble coagulation factors.

FIGURE 326-2

Serum iron and iron-binding capacity in various disorders.

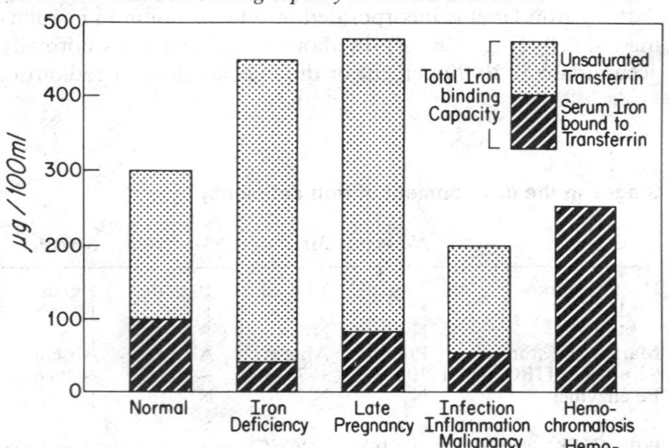

Clinical findings Because iron deficiency usually develops insidiously, anemic patients are often relatively free of symptoms. In general, the signs and symptoms of iron-deficiency anemia are shared by other anemias of comparable severity (Chap. 54). Weakness, fatigue, lassitude, palpitations, and lightheadedness are common complaints. It is uncertain whether these symptoms are due solely to anemia or whether iron deficiency per se exerts an independent influence, perhaps through depletion of iron-containing enzymes and cofactors in certain tissues. Iron-deficient rats continue to have impaired exercise tolerance even after their anemia is corrected with transfused red cells. Many women with iron deficiency but no significant anemia complain of weakness and fatigue, but such nonspecific symptoms are difficult to evaluate. Iron deficiency is sometimes associated with pica, a desire to gnaw on solid substances. Patients develop a craving for clay (geophagia), cornstarch (amylophagia), or ice (pagophagia). This peculiar symptom subsides when iron deficiency is corrected. Iron deficiency may also be associated with a variety of gastrointestinal symptoms. Following severe and prolonged deficiency, patients sometimes develop dysphagia owing to thin membranous webs at the postcricoid area (Plummer-Vinson syndrome). More commonly, iron-deficient patients develop a variety of less specific gastrointestinal symptoms, such as anorexia, nausea, eructation, and constipation, but it is uncertain whether these complaints are caused by iron deficiency per se. Those with prolonged iron deficiency often have achlorhydria and gastric atrophy. Menorrhagia is a common symptom in iron-deficient women. Gastric atrophy and menorrhagia may contribute toward the development of iron deficiency rather than being sequelae.

Physical findings may include pallor, tachycardia, and a "hemic" flow murmur, signs shared by patients with other types of anemia. Those with prolonged iron deficiency often have dry, brittle, and ridged nails which occasionally assume a concave surface (koilonychia). The epithelium at the edges of the lips may be cracked (angular stomatitis), and the tongue may become atrophic and even tender (glossitis). The spleen is seldom enlarged. The nonhematologic manifestations of iron deficiency such as koilonychia, angular stomatitis, glossitis, and esophageal webs are rarely encountered nowadays, probably because iron deficiency is more readily diagnosed and more promptly treated than in earlier times.

Laboratory findings A variety of laboratory tests can be used to assess varying degrees of iron deficiency (Table 326-2). Prior to the development of anemia, iron stores become depleted. A bone marrow aspirate, stained with Prussian blue, will show markedly reduced or absent deposits of iron in macrophages. This finding is accompanied by a decrease in the level of serum ferritin. As iron deficiency progresses, the serum iron falls while the iron-binding capacity of the serum increases. As a result, the fractional saturation of transferrin falls markedly. With the development of anemia, red cells become microcytic and hypochromic. The mean corpuscular hemoglobin concentration is usually higher when determined by an electronic counter than the more accurate measurement obtained from a packed cell volume. The development of hypochromic red cells is accompanied by an increase in free erythrocyte protoporphyrin. Protoporphyrin IX accumulates in the red cell because there is insufficient iron to convert it to heme (see Fig. 54-2). This fluorometric assay is a reliable and cost-effective way of screening large groups of individuals such as schoolchildren for iron deficiency.

In well-developed iron deficiency anemia, the red cells become more severely hypochromic and microcytic (Plate 9–4). Often, only a thin rim of cytoplasm appears on the periphery of the red cell. Small fragments and bizarre poikilocytes are also seen. Such misshapen red cells have shortened survival in the circulation. The percentage of reticulocytes is usually normal but may increase temporarily following an acute episode of blood loss. The white count is usually normal, while the platelet count is normal or increased. The bone marrow displays moderate erythroid hyperplasia. Many of the late normoblasts appear to have scanty cytoplasm.

Differential diagnosis In a patient with hypochromic microcytic anemia, the major diagnostic possibilities are iron deficiency, thalassemia, anemia of chronic inflammation, and sideroblastic anemia. Several laboratory tests (shown in Table 326-2) are useful in the differential diagnosis. Mild iron deficiency may be readily confused with β-thalassemia trait or with the two-deletion forms of α thalessemia ($\alpha\alpha^0/\alpha\alpha^0$ or $\alpha^0\alpha^0/\alpha\alpha$) (Chap. 330). In these mild forms of thalassemia, microcytosis is much more marked than hypochromia; accordingly the mean corpuscular hemoglobin concentration (MCHC) is usually normal. The red cell size distribution is more uniform than that in iron deficiency. Target cells and basophilic stippling are usually more prominent in thalassemia than in iron deficiency. Hemoglobin A_2 is elevated in β-thalassemia trait and decreased in iron deficiency and α thalassemia. β-Thalassemia trait may be masked by the finding of a normal level of hemoglobin A_2 if the patient has coexisting iron deficiency. The serum iron is normal or elevated in the thalassemias and decreased in both iron deficiency and in the anemia of chronic disease. However, as Fig. 326-2 shows, the transferrin level is also decreased in the latter. The laboratory tests shown in Table 326-2 are not very helpful in determining whether a patient with a chronic inflammatory disease, such as rheumatoid arthritis, has become iron-deficient. The finding of a low serum ferritin level or absent iron stores in a bone marrow aspirate would be diagnostic of iron deficiency. A trial of iron therapy may be necessary to settle the issue. The diagnosis of sideroblastic anemia rests on the demonstration of ringed sideroblasts in the bone marrow. These patients often have a population of hypochromic microcytic red cells, even though the red cell indexes are usually normal.

FIGURE 326-3
Ferrokinetics in normal subjects and patients with disorders of erythropoiesis. A. Plasma radioiron clearance. B. Red cell radioiron utilization.

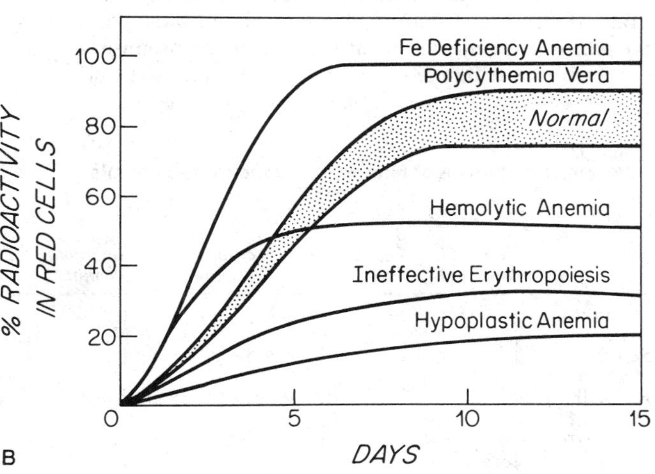

Treatment Iron-deficiency anemia responds very effectively to iron therapy. However, an equally important part of management is to elicit and, if possible, correct the cause of the iron deficiency. Unless the patient has a clear-cut history of menorrhagia or bleeding from an obvious local site such as prolonged epistaxis or hemorrhoids, the gastrointestinal tract must be evaluated with appropriate radiologic and endoscopic studies.

Among the many iron preparations available, ferrous sulfate taken by mouth is the simplest and preferred treatment for most patients. The addition of extraneous minerals (copper, molybdenum) or vitamins adds to the cost of the preparation but little to its efficacy. In some prenatal multivitamin preparations, calcium carbonate and magnesium oxide may actually interfere with the absorption of the iron. Most patients respond well to ferrous sulfate, 300 mg (60 mg elemental iron) three times daily. Absorption is somewhat enhanced if the iron is administered between meals. Conversely, patients experience less gastric distress if the iron is taken with meals. Some patients tolerate therapy better if it is begun with only one tablet per day and gradually increased over several days. About 15 percent of orally administered iron is absorbed during the first 3 weeks of therapy. Thereafter, absorption decreases, averaging about 5 percent. Treatment for at least 6 months is needed in most cases if body stores are to be replenished.

The response to treatment is generally very satisfactory. A peak reticulocytosis is generally seen at about day 10 with a gradual increase in hemoglobin and correction of red cell indexes.

Failure to respond to therapy usually means that (1) the diagnosis was incorrect; (2) the patient has failed to take the prescribed iron; (3) blood loss has exceeded the buildup of hemoglobin; (4) erythropoiesis has been suppressed by infection, inflammation, or tumor; (5) the iron has not been properly absorbed.

Parenteral therapy is rarely required. When iron is absorbed poorly, as in some patients who have undergone gastrectomy or those with proximal intestinal disease, particularly celiac sprue, iron-dextran may be given intramuscularly. The first dose should be limited to 50 mg because severe reactions sometimes occur. By repeated injections, a total of 1.5 to 2.0 g may be given in this way. Although more likely to produce an adverse reaction, intravenous administration is also possible in patients who cannot tolerate intramuscular injections. The iron-dextran solution can be given by direct infusion, or it can be diluted in about 20 ml sterile saline and administered by intravenous drip. One or two drops should be given intravenously, and then, if no untoward symptoms develop in the next 5 min, 500 mg is infused slowly. The total amount of parenteral iron that should be given is based on the calculated deficit in red blood cell mass, plus an additional 1000 mg to replenish iron stores. Transfusion of blood is seldom indicated, unless the patient has evidence of cardiovascular compromise, such as congestive heart failure or coronary or cerebral ischemia.

TABLE 326-2
Differential diagnosis of microcytic hypochromic anemia

	Iron deficiency	*β-Thalassemia trait*	*Anemia of chronic disease*	*Sideroblastic anemia*
Serum iron	↓	N	↓	↑
TIBC	↑	N	↓	N
Serum ferritin	↓	N	↑	↑
Red cell protoporphyrin	↑	N	↑	↑ or N
HbA_2	↓	↑	N	↓

IRON-LOADING ANEMIAS Dependence on multiple blood transfusions by some patients with acquired or congenital anemias can lead to a state of generalized iron overload. One unit of blood contains about 200 to 250 mg iron. Therefore, in a patient with failure of bone marrow erythroid activity who requires about 4 units of blood every month, at least 20 g of elemental iron can be expected to accumulate within 2 years; this is enough iron to produce clinical symptoms in some patients with idiopathic hemochromatosis. Hyperabsorption of dietary iron in idiopathic hemochromatosis (Chap. 97), in which excess iron is distributed predominantly in parenchymal cells, leads to earlier signs of clinical organ damage than transfusional iron loading, in which excess iron initially is deposited in the mononuclear-phagocyte system. However, most patients who have received more than 100 units of blood exhibit evidence of organ damage in a pattern which resembles that observed in idiopathic hemochromatosis.

In anemias associated with ineffective erythropoiesis, transfusional iron overload is compounded by excessive intestinal iron absorption. The importance of this factor is exemplified by patients with sideroblastic anemia or thalassemia intermedia who can develop advanced hemochromatosis even in the absence of transfusions. The mechanisms responsible for the inappropriate hyperabsorption of dietary iron in patients with ineffective erythropoiesis are unknown, but iron absorption can be reduced if the anemia is corrected and erythropoiesis is suppressed by transfusion. Thalassemia is discussed in Chap. 330.

Sideroblastic anemia Sideroblastic anemia consists of a group of disorders of diverse etiologies (Table 326-3) characterized by ringed sideroblasts in the bone marrow comprising at least 10 percent of the nucleated red cell population. Ringed sideroblasts are normoblasts which contain iron deposits within mitochondria. The partial or complete rings of Prussian blue–staining granules are produced by the perinuclear distribution of these iron-laden mitochondria. A number of metabolic abnormalities have been noted in the sideroblastic anemias, including defects in one or more of the enzymatic steps in heme synthesis. Since the initial and terminal steps in heme porphyrin synthesis are localized in the mitochondria, it is difficult to determine whether such abnormalities are the cause or the result of mitochondrial iron loading. In addition to the presence of ringed sideroblasts in the bone marrow, these disorders share certain other characteristics: a population of microcytic and hypochromic red cells in the peripheral smear due to defective heme synthesis; bone marrow erythroid hyperplasia as a result of ineffective erythropoiesis; increased levels of red cell porphyrins; and marked increase in the serum iron and transferrin saturation often accompanied by evidence of generalized iron overload.

Hereditary sideroblastic anemia may be either X-linked or autosomal recessive and is often pyridoxine-responsive. Severe anemia is usually first noted in young adulthood, although the age of onset may vary greatly even within a single kindred. Large doses of vitamin B_6 result in at least a partial correction of the anemia in patients with hereditary pyridoxine-responsive sideroblastic anemia. The genetic lesion may affect the

TABLE 326-3
The sideroblastic anemias

1 Hereditary or congenital sideroblastic anemias
2 Acquired sideroblastic anemias
  a Associated with drugs and toxins (e.g., alcohol, lead, isoniazid, chloramphenicol)
  b Associated with neoplastic and inflammatory disease (e.g., carcinoma, leukemia, myeloproliferative disorders, Hodgkin's disease, other lymphomas, myeloma, rheumatoid arthritis)
  c Idiopathic refractory sideroblastic anemia

first and rate-limiting enzyme of porphyrin synthesis, δ-aminolevulinic acid synthetase (ALA-S), either directly or through metabolism of its essential cofactor, pyridoxal 5′-phosphate.

A variety of drugs and toxins can cause a reversible sideroblastic anemia which usually resolves following removal of the offending agent. These include isoniazid (INH) and alcohol, which cause abnormalities in pyridoxine metabolism, and lead, which interferes with several reactions in the pathway of heme synthesis. Sideroblastic anemia occurs in about 30 percent of hospitalized alcoholics; ringed sideroblasts in the bone marrow disappear within several days after cessation of alcohol ingestion. Secondary sideroblastic anemia has also been observed occasionally in association with a variety of inflammatory, neoplastic, and preleukemic states; in these disorders the clinical picture is dominated by the underlying illness.

Sideroblastic anemia is a common form of refractory anemia in older patients, in whom other associated diseases, drugs, or toxins cannot be identified. Many of these patients have an indolent course and die of nonhematologic causes. However, some patients become transfusion-dependent and develop complications of iron overload. Unlike the other types of sideroblastic anemia, this can be a preleukemic disorder, which is frequently associated with chromosomal abnormalities and transforms into acute nonlymphocytic leukemia in approximately 10 percent of cases.

Treatment In cases of secondary sideroblastic anemia, withdrawal of the offending drug or toxin or treatment of the underlying disease is usually beneficial. Patients with acquired idiopathic sideroblastic anemia rarely respond to pyridoxine, although a 2- to 3-month trial of this vitamin in a dose of 200 mg daily should be attempted. A trial of androgens, in a regimen similar to that used in aplastic anemia, may ameliorate the anemia in some cases. In idiopathic refractory sideroblastic anemia, therapy is usually supportive. Many patients require frequent blood transfusions, and measures to reduce transfusional iron loading are required.

While phlebotomy is the most effective treatment for hemochromatosis, in anemic patients with transfusional iron overload, in whom phlebotomy is precluded, elimination of excess iron can be achieved only with iron-chelating agents. Deferoxamine is presently the only clinically effective iron chelator available. Deferoxamine-chelated iron is excreted primarily in the urine. Because the drug is not well absorbed when given orally and has a short half-life, it should be administered by continuous parenteral infusion. Deferoxamine can be administered to ambulatory patients by means of a subcutaneous infusion delivered by a portable pump. Doses are generally 1.5 to 2.5 g daily, infused over 16 to 24 h; however, there is considerable individual variation, and the optimal regimen should be established for individual patients. Adverse effects from deferoxamine are unusual. Patients may develop cataracts after long-term use, and periodic slit-lamp eye examinations are indicated in patients on chronic therapy. Local erythema and discomfort at the subcutaneous injection site can usually be prevented by the addition of hydrocortisone to the deferoxamine solution. Hypersensitivity reactions occur rarely.

Oral ascorbic acid supplementation may markedly enhance the iron-chelating efficiency of deferoxamine, presumably by liberating more free intracellular iron to become available for chelation. However, increased amounts of free iron may also damage cells by generating free oxygen radicals. This may be manifested clinically by cardiac irritability or congestive heart failure. Therefore, the administration of ascorbic acid to patients with iron overload may be hazardous.

Manipulation of blood transfusions to infuse selectively young red cells (neocytes), and thereby prolong the interval between transfusions, is a promising measure for the avoidance of iron overload in transfusion-dependent patients, but its application to adult patients has not been established.

REFERENCES

BOTHWELL TH et al: *Iron Metabolism in Man.* Oxford, Blackwell Scientific, 1979

CROSBY WH: Current concepts in nutrition: Who needs iron? N Engl J Med 297:543, 1977

DALLMAN PR et al: Effects of iron deficiency exclusive of anaemia. Br J Haematol 40:179, 1978

FINCH CA, HUEBERS H: Perspectives in iron metabolism. N Engl J Med 360:1520, 1982

KUSHNER JP, CARTWRIGHT GE: Sideroblastic anemia. Adv Intern Med 22:229, 1977

——— et al: Idiopathic refractory sideroblastic anemia. Medicine 59:139, 1971

PROPPER RD et al: New approaches to the transfusion management of thalassemia. Blood 55:55, 1980

SCHAFER AI: Iron overload, in *Current Hematology.* New York, Wiley, 1981 vol 1, chap 5

——— et al: Clinical consequences of acquired transfusional iron overload in adults. N Engl J Med 304:319, 1981

327 MEGALOBLASTIC ANEMIAS

BERNARD M. BABIOR
H. FRANKLIN BUNN

The megaloblastic anemias are disorders caused by impaired deoxyribonucleic acid (DNA) synthesis. Cells primarily affected are those having a relatively rapid turnover, especially hematopoietic precursors and the gastrointestinal epithelial cells. Cell division is sluggish, but cytoplasmic development progresses normally, so megaloblastic cells tend to be large, with an increased ratio of ribonucleic acid (RNA) to DNA. Megaloblastic cells tend to be destroyed in the marrow in excessive numbers, an abnormality termed *ineffective erythropoiesis* (Chaps. 54 and 326).

Most megaloblastic anemias are due to a deficiency of vitamin B_{12} and/or folic acid. The various clinical entities associated with megaloblastic anemia are listed in Table 327-1. This classification is easier to comprehend if the physiological and biochemical principles discussed below are kept in mind.

PHYSIOLOGICAL CONSIDERATIONS

FOLIC ACID Folic acid is the common name for pteroylmonoglutamic acid. It is synthesized by many different plants and bacteria. Fruits and vegetables constitute the primary dietary source of the vitamin. Some forms of dietary folic acid are labile and may be destroyed by cooking. The minimum daily requirement is normally about 50 μg but may be increased severalfold during periods of enhanced metabolic demand such as pregnancy.

The assimilation of adequate amounts of folic acid is dependent on the nature of the diet and its means of preparation. Folates in various foodstuffs are largely conjugated to polyglutamic acid. This highly polar side chain impairs the intestinal absorption of the vitamin. However, conjugases (γ-glutamyl carboxypeptidases) in the lumen of the gut convert polyglutamates to mono- and diglutamates, which are readily absorbed in the proximal jejunum.

There are binding proteins in plasma for folates, but their physiological significance is unclear. Plasma folate is primarily in the form of N^5-methyltetrahydrofolate, a monoglutamate. N^5-Methyltetrahydrofolate is transported into cells by a carrier which is specific for the tetrahydro forms of the vitamin. Once in the cell, the folate is reconverted to the polyglutamate form, after removal of the N^5-methyl group in a vitamin B_{12}–requiring reaction (see below). The polyglutamate form may be useful for retention of folate by the cell.

Normal individuals have about 5 to 20 mg folic acid in various body stores, half in the liver. In light of the minimum daily requirement, it is not surprising that a deficiency will occur within months if dietary intake or intestinal absorption is curtailed.

VITAMIN B_{12} This vitamin is a complex organometallic compound in which a cobalt atom is situated within a corrin ring, a

TABLE 327-1
Classification of the megaloblastic anemias

I Vitamin B_{12} deficiency
- *A* Inadequate intake: vegetarians (rare)
- *B* Malabsorption
  - *1* Inadequate production of intrinsic factor (IF)
    - *a* Pernicious anemia
    - *b* Gastrectomy
    - *c* Congenital absence or functional abnormality of IF (rare)
  - *2* Disorders of terminal ileum
    - *a* Tropical sprue
    - *b* Nontropical sprue
    - *c* Regional enteritis
    - *d* Intestinal resection
    - *e* Neoplasms and granulomatous disorders (rare)
    - *f* Selective vitamin B_{12} malabsorption (Imerslund's syndrome) (rare)
  - *3* Competition for vitamin B_{12}
    - *a* Fish tapeworm
    - *b* Bacteria: blind loop syndrome
  - *4* Drugs: *p*-Aminosalicylic acid, colchicine, neomycin
- *C* Other
  - *1* Nitrous oxide
  - *2* Transcobalamin II deficiency (rare)

II Folic acid deficiency
- *A* Inadequate intake: Unbalanced diet (common in alcoholics, teenagers, some infants)
- *B* Malabsorption
  - *1* Tropical sprue
  - *2* Nontropical sprue
  - *3* Drugs: Phenytoin, barbiturates, (?) ethanol
- *C* Increased requirements
  - *1* Pregnancy
  - *2* Infancy
  - *3* Malignancy
  - *4* Increased hematopoiesis (chronic hemolytic anemias)
  - *5* Chronic exfoliative skin disorders
  - *6* Hemodialysis
- *D* Impaired metabolism
  - *1* Inhibitors of dihydrofolate reductase: Methotrexate, pyrimethamine, triamterene, pentamidine, etc.
  - *2* Alcohol
  - *3* Rare enzyme deficiencies: Formiminotransferase, dihydrofolate reductase, etc.

III Other causes
- *A* Drugs which impair DNA metabolism
  - *1* Purine antagonists: 6-mercaptopurine, azathioprine, etc.
  - *2* Pyrimidine antagonists: 5-fluorouracil, cytosine arabinoside, etc.
  - *3* Others: Procarbazine, hydroxyurea
- *B* Metabolic disorders (rare)
  - *1* Hereditary orotic aciduria
  - *2* Others
- *C* Megalobastic anemia of unknown etiology
  - *1* Refractory megalobastic anemia
  - *2* Di Guglielmo's syndrome*

* *A form of acute nonlymphocytic leukemia with atypical, dysplastic changes in erythroid series.*

structure similar to the porphyrin from which heme is formed (Fig. 54-1). As with heme, both δ-aminolevulinic acid and porphobilinogen are precursors in the biosynthesis of vitamin B_{12}. However, unlike heme, vitamin B_{12} cannot be synthesized in the human body and must be supplied in the diet. The only dietary source of vitamin B_{12} is animal products: meat and dairy foods. The minimum daily requirement for vitamin B_{12} is about 2.5 μg.

During gastric digestion, vitamin B_{12} in food is released and forms a stable complex with gastric R binder, one of a group of closely related glycoproteins of unknown function which are found in secretions (e.g., saliva, milk, gastric juice, bile), granulocytes, and plasma. On entering the duodenum, the vitamin B_{12}–R binder complex is digested, releasing the vitamin B_{12}, which then binds to intrinsic factor (IF). This glycoprotein of molecular weight 50,000 is produced by the parietal cells of the stomach. The secretion of intrinsic factor generally parallels that of hydrochloric acid. The vitamin B_{12}–intrinsic factor complex is resistant to proteolytic digestion and travels to the distal ileum, where specific receptors on the mucosal brush border bind the vitamin B_{12}–intrinsic factor complex, thereby enabling the vitamin to be absorbed. Thus, intrinsic factor serves as a cell-directed carrier protein. Vitamin B_{12} is transferred from the ileal receptor across the mucosa to the capillary circulation where it binds initially to another transport protein, transcobalamin II (TC II). The vitamin B_{12}–TC II complex is rapidly taken up by the liver, the bone marrow, and other proliferating cells. Normally, about 2 mg vitamin B_{12} is stored in the liver, and another 2 mg is stored elsewhere in the body. In view of the minimum daily requirement, about 3 to 6 years would be required for a normal individual to become deficient in vitamin B_{12} if absorption were to cease abruptly.

Although TC II is the acceptor for newly absorbed vitamin B_{12}, most circulating vitamin B_{12} is bound to transcobalamin I (TC I), a glycoprotein closely related to gastric R binder. TC I appears to be derived in part from leukocytes. The paradox that most circulating vitamin B_{12} is bound to TC I rather than TC II, even though TC II receives all the vitamin B_{12} which is absorbed by the intestine, is explained by the fact that vitamin B_{12} bound to TC II is rapidly cleared from the blood ($t_{\frac{1}{2}}$ about 1 h), while clearance of vitamin B_{12} bound to TC I requires many days. The function of TC I is unknown.

BIOCHEMICAL CONSIDERATIONS

FOLATE The *prime function* of this vitamin is to transfer one-carbon moieties such as methyl and formyl groups to various organic compounds (see Fig. 327-1). The source of these one-carbon moieties is usually serine, which reacts with tetrahydrofolate to produce glycine and $N^{5,10}$-methylenetetrahydrofolate. An alternative source is formiminoglutamic acid, an intermediate in histidine catabolism, which gives up its formimino group to tetrahydrofolate to yield N^5-formiminotetrahydrofolate and glutamic acid. These derivatives provide entry into an interconvertible donor pool consisting of tetrahydrofolate derivatives carrying one-carbon various moieties (see Fig. 327-1). The constituents of this pool can donate their one-carbon moieties to appropriate acceptor compounds to form metabolic intermediates which are ultimately converted to building blocks used in the synthesis of biological macromolecules. The most important such building blocks are (1) purines, in which the C-2 and C-8 atoms are introduced in folate-dependent reactions; (2) deoxythymidylate monophosphate (dTMP), synthesized from $N^{5,10}$-methylenetetrahydrofolate and deoxyuridylate monophosphate (dUMP); and (3) methionine, formed by the transfer of a methyl group from N^5-methyltetrahydrofolate to homocysteine. Vitamin B_{12} is also required for the formation of methionine from homocysteine (see below).

In all but one of the one-carbon transfer reactions, tetrahydrofolate is produced. It can immediately accept a one-carbon moiety and reenter the donor pool. The single exception is the thymidylate synthetase reaction (dUMP → dTMP), in which dihydrofolate is the product (Fig. 327-1). This must be reduced to tetrahydrofolate by the enzyme dihydrofolate reductase before it can reenter the donor pool. A number of drugs are able to inhibit dihydrofolate reductase, thereby diverting folate from the donor pool and producing what amounts to a state of folate deficiency in the face of normal tissue folate concentrations.

VITAMIN B_{12} In humans there are two metabolically active forms of vitamin B_{12}, identified by the alkyl group attached to the sixth coordination position of the cobalt atom: adenosylcobalamin and methylcobalamin. The vitamin preparation which is used therapeutically is cyanocobalamin. Cyanocobalamin has no known physiological role and must be converted to a biologically active form before it can be used by tissues.[1]

Adenosylcobalamin is required for the conversion of methylmalonyl coenzyme A (CoA) to succinyl CoA. Lack of this cofactor leads to large increases in the tissue levels of methylmalonyl CoA and its precursor, propionyl CoA. As a consequence, nonphysiological fatty acids containing an odd number of carbon atoms are synthesized and incorporated into neuronal lipids. This biochemical abnormality may underlie the neurological complications of vitamin B_{12} deficiency (see below).

Methylcobalamin is an essential cofactor in the conversion of homocysteine to methionine (Fig. 327-2). When this reaction is deficient, folate metabolism is deranged, and it is this derangement which is thought to underlie the defect in DNA synthesis and the megaloblastic maturation pattern in patients who are deficient in vitamin B_{12} (see Fig. 327-2). What appears to happen in vitamin B_{12} deficiency is that the unconjugated N^5-methyltetrahydrofolate newly taken from the bloodstream cannot be converted to other forms of tetrahydrofolate by methyl transfer. This is the so-called folate trap hypothesis. Since N^5-methyltetrahydrofolate is a poor substrate for the conjugating enzyme (this has been shown in rats but has not yet been demonstrated in humans), it largely remains in the unconjugated form and slowly leaks from the cell. Tissue folate deficiency therefore develops, and this results in megaloblastic hematopoiesis. This hypothesis explains the fact that tissue folate stores in vitamin B_{12} deficiency are substantially reduced, with a disproportionate reduction in conjugated as compared with unconjugated folates, despite normal or supranormal serum folate levels. It also explains why large doses of folate can produce a partial hematologic remission in patients with vitamin B_{12} deficiency.

[1] *Strictly speaking, vitamin B_{12} refers only to cyanocobalamin. However, in this chapter, the term* vitamin B_{12} *will refer to both cyanocobalamin and biologically active cobalamins.*

FIGURE 327-1
Scheme of folate metabolism.

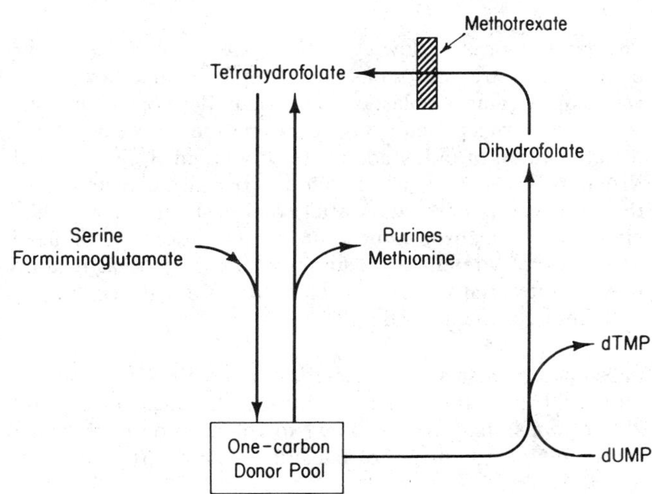

CLINICAL DISORDERS

CLASSIFICATION OF MEGALOBLASTIC ANEMIAS The etiology of megaloblastic anemia varies in different parts of the world. In temperate zones, folate deficiency in alcoholics and pernicious anemia are the common types of megaloblastic anemias. In certain areas close to the equator, tropical sprue is endemic and an important cause. In Finland, megaloblastic anemia is sometimes secondary to infestation by the fish tapeworm *Diphyllobothrium latum.*

The dietary intake of vitamin B_{12} is more than adequate for the body's requirements, except in true vegetarians (individuals who live on a purely vegetable diet) and their breast-fed infants. Thus, deficiency of vitamin B_{12} is almost always due to malabsorption. As explained in the section above, the absorption of vitamin B_{12} depends upon a specific binding protein produced in the stomach and uptake by a specific receptor in the mucosa of the distal ileum. Accordingly, several steps in this process can go awry and lead to malabsorption. These are listed in Table 327-1. In contrast, the dietary intake of folic acid is marginal in many parts of the world. Furthermore, since the body's stores of folate are relatively low, folic acid deficiency can arise rather suddenly during periods of decreased dietary intake or increased metabolic demand. Finally, folic acid deficiency may be due to malabsorption. Often two or more of these factors coexist in a given patient.

Combined deficiencies of vitamin B_{12} and folic acid are not uncommon. Patients with tropical sprue are often deficient in both vitamins. The biochemical lesion that results in megaloblastic maturation of bone marrow cells also causes structural and functional abnormalities of the rapidly proliferating epithelial cells of the intestinal mucosa. Thus, severe deficiency of one vitamin can lead to malabsorption of the other. Furthermore, as discussed above, a deficiency of vitamin B_{12} causes a secondary reduction in cellular folic acid.

Finally, megaloblastic anemias may occasionally be induced by factors unrelated to a vitamin deficiency. Most such cases are caused by one or more of the many drugs which produce megaloblastic anemia as a side effect. Less common causes include certain acquired defects of hematopoietic stem cells. Rarest of all are certain congenital enzyme deficiencies in which megaloblastic anemia is characteristically encountered.

FIGURE 327-2
Diagram showing the interrelationship between vitamin B_{12} (methylcobalamin) and folate metabolism within the cell.

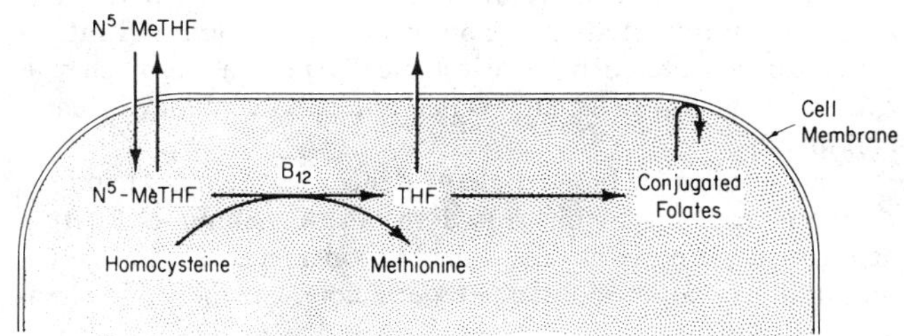

VITAMIN B_{12} DEFICIENCY There are many conditions in which vitamin B_{12} deficiency may develop. Although each has its own characteristic manifestations, certain clinical features are common to all. These clinical features involve the blood, the gastrointestinal tract, and the nervous system.

The hematologic manifestations are almost entirely the result of the anemia which characterizes vitamin B_{12} deficiency, although very rarely purpura may appear, due to thrombocytopenia. Symptoms may include weakness, lightheadedness, vertigo, and tinnitus, as well as palpitations, angina, and the symptoms of congestive failure. On physical examination, the patient with florid vitamin B_{12} deficiency is pale, with slightly icteric skin and eyes. The pulse is rapid, and the heart may be enlarged; auscultation will reveal a systolic flow murmur. The spleen and liver may be somewhat enlarged. There may be a slight fever.

The gastrointestinal manifestations reflect the effect of vitamin B_{12} deficiency on the rapidly turning over gastrointestinal epithelium. The patient sometimes complains of a sore tongue, which on inspection will be smooth and beefy red. Anorexia with moderate weight loss may also be evident, possibly accompanied by diarrhea and other gastrointestinal symptoms. These latter manifestations may be in part caused by megaloblastosis of the small intestinal epithelium, which results in malabsorption.

The neurological manifestations are the most worrisome of all, because they often fail to remit completely on treatment. They begin pathologically with demyelination, followed by axonal degeneration and eventual neuronal death; the final stage, of course, is irreversible. Sites of involvement include peripheral nerves, the spinal cord, where the posterior and lateral columns undergo demyelination, and the cerebrum itself. Signs and symptoms include numbness and paresthesias in the extremities (the earliest neurological manifestations), weakness, ataxia, and poor finger coordination. There may be sphincter disturbances. Reflexes may be diminished or increased. The Romberg and Babinski signs may be positive, and position sense will be diminished. Disturbances of mentation will vary from mild irritability and forgetfulness to severe dementia or frank psychosis. It should be emphasized that occasionally *neurological disease may occur in a patient with a normal hematocrit.*

In the usual patient, in whom hematologic problems predominate, the blood and bone marrow show characteristic megaloblastic changes which are described under "Diagnosis" below. The anemia may be very severe—hematocrits of 15 to 20 are not infrequent—but is surprisingly well tolerated by the patient because it develops so slowly.

Pernicious anemia The most common cause of vitamin B_{12} deficiency in temperate climates is pernicious anemia, in which intrinsic factor secretion ceases owing to atrophy of the gastric mucosa. It is most frequently seen in individuals of northern European descent and is much less common in southern Europeans, blacks, and Orientals. Men and women are equally affected. It is a disease of the elderly, the average patient presenting near age 60; it is rare under 30, although typical pernicious anemia can be seen in children under 10 (juvenile pernicious anemia). An inherited condition in which an abnormal intrinsic factor is secreted by a histologically normal stomach will cause vitamin B_{12} deficiency which appears in infancy or early childhood.

On the basis of incomplete evidence, pernicious anemia is currently thought to be caused by an autoimmune reaction against gastric parietal cells. There is considerable evidence for immunologic abnormalities in pernicious anemia. The incidence of pernicious anemia is substantially increased in patients with other diseases thought to be of immunologic origin, including Graves' disease, myxedema, thyroiditis, idiopathic adrenocortical insufficiency, vitiligo, and hypoparathyroidism. Patients with pernicious anemia also have abnormal circulating antibodies related to their disease: 90 percent have antiparietal cell antibody while 60 percent have anti-intrinsic factor antibody. Antiparietal cell antibody is also found in 50 percent of patients with gastric atrophy without pernicious anemia as well as in 10 to 15 percent of an unselected patient population, but anti-intrinsic factor antibody is usually absent from these patients. Relatives of patients with pernicious anemia show an increased incidence of the disease, and even clinically unaffected relatives may have anti-intrinsic factor antibody in their serum. A final point supporting an immunologic basis for pernicious anemia is the fact that corticosteroids have been reported to reverse the disease both pathologically and clinically.

The destruction of parietal cells in pernicious anemia is thought to be mediated by the cellular immune system. Humoral factors such as anti-intrinsic factor antibody probably have little role in the pathogenesis of the disease, a view supported by the observation that pernicious anemia is unusually common in patients with agammaglobulinemia.

Pathologically, the most characteristic finding in pernicious anemia is gastric atrophy which involves only the acid- and pepsin-secreting portion of the stomach; the antrum is spared. Other pathological changes, which are secondary to the deficiency of vitamin B_{12}, include megaloblastoid alterations in the gastric and intestinal epithelium and the neurological changes described above. The abnormalities in the gastric epithelium are evident as cellular atypia in gastric cytology specimens, a finding which must be carefully distinguished from the cytological abnormalities seen in gastric malignancy.

The *clinical manifestations* are primarily those of vitamin B_{12} deficiency, as described above. The disease is of insidious onset and progresses slowly. An additional physical finding is the tendency of patients with pernicious anemia to be fair-haired or prematurely gray. Laboratory examination will reveal pentagastrin-fast achlorhydria as well as the hematologic and other laboratory abnormalities discussed below in "Diagnosis."

Through appropriate replacement therapy, patients with pernicious anemia should experience complete and lifelong correction of all abnormalities which are due to vitamin B_{12} deficiency, except to the extent that irreversible changes in the nervous system may have occurred prior to treatment. These patients, however, are unusually subject to certain gastric problems, including gastric polyps and cancer of the stomach. In view of the latter complication, patients should be followed with frequent stool guaiac examinations together with further diagnostic studies when indicated.

Postgastrectomy Following total gastrectomy or extensive damage to gastric mucosa as, for example, by ingestion of corrosive agents, megaloblastic anemia may develop because the source of intrinsic factor has been removed. In such patients the absorption of orally administered vitamin B_{12} is impaired. Megaloblastic anemia may also follow partial gastrectomy, but the incidence is lower than after total gastrectomy, in which vitamin B_{12} malabsorption occurs in 100 percent of patients. The cause of vitamin B_{12} deficiency after partial gastrectomy may be intestinal overgrowth of bacteria, but it does not always respond to antibiotics.

Intestinal organisms The macrocytic anemia seen in association with intestinal strictures, diverticula, anastomoses, and "blind loops" may be attributed to colonization of the small intestine by large masses of bacteria which divert vitamin B_{12}

from the host. Steatorrhea may also be seen under these circumstances, because bile salt metabolism is disturbed when the intestine is heavily colonized with bacteria. Hematologic responses have been observed after administration of oral antibiotics such as tetracycline and ampicillin.

Megaloblastic anemia is seen, in Finland especially, in persons harboring the tapeworm *D. latum.* The anemia has been attributed to competition by the worm for vitamin B_{12}. Destruction of the worm eliminates the problem.

Ileal abnormalities Vitamin B_{12} deficiency is commonly found in tropical sprue, while it is an unusual complication of nontropical sprue (gluten-sensitive enteropathy; see Chap. 308). Virtually any disorder which compromises the absorptive capacity of the distal ileum can result in vitamin B_{12} deficiency. Specific entities include regional enteritis, Whipple's disease, and tuberculosis. Segmental involvement of the distal ileum by disease can cause megaloblastic anemia without any other manifestations of intestinal malabsorption such as steatorrhea. Vitamin B_{12} malabsorption is also seen after ileal resection. The Zollinger-Ellison syndrome (intense gastric hyperacidity due to a gastrin-secreting tumor) may cause vitamin B_{12} malabsorption by acidifying the small intestine. This will retard the transfer of the vitamin from R binder to intrinsic factor and will impair the binding of the vitamin B_{12}–intrinsic factor complex to the ileal receptors. Chronic pancreatitis may also cause vitamin B_{12} malabsorption by impairing the transfer of the vitamin from R binder to intrinsic factor. This abnormality can be detected by tests of vitamin B_{12} absorption (see below, Schilling test), but it is invariably mild and never causes clinical vitamin B_{12} deficiency. Finally, there is a rare congenital disorder, described by Imerslund, in which a selective defect in vitamin B_{12} absorption is accompanied by proteinuria.

FOLIC ACID DEFICIENCY Patients with folic acid deficiency are more apt to be malnourished than those with vitamin B_{12} deficiency. Accordingly, they are likely to appear wasted. The gastrointestinal manifestations are similar to but may be more widespread and more severe than those of pernicious anemia. Diarrhea is often present, and cheilosis and glossitis are also encountered. However, in contrast to vitamin B_{12} deficiency, neurological abnormalities do not occur.

The hematologic manifestations of folic acid deficiency are the same as those of vitamin B_{12} deficiency. Folic acid deficiency can generally be attributed to one or more of the following factors: increased demand for folate, inadequate intake, and malabsorption.

Increased demand Tissues with a relatively high rate of cell division such as the bone marrow or gut mucosa have a large requirement for folate. Therefore, patients with chronic hemolytic anemias or other causes of very active erythropoiesis may become deficient if their high folate requirement is not met by dietary intake. Likewise, a pregnant woman may become deficient in folic acid because of the high demand of the developing fetus. Folate deficiency may also occur during the growth spurts of infancy and adolescence.

Inadequate intake of folic acid is commonly encountered among a number of groups. Alcoholics frequently become folate-deficient because their main source of caloric intake is in the form of alcoholic beverages. Distilled spirits are virtually devoid of folic acid, while beer and wine do not contain enough of the vitamin to satisfy the daily requirement. In addition, alcohol may interfere with folate metabolism. Narcotic addicts are also prone to become folate-deficient because of malnutrition. In general, indigent and elderly individuals who subsist primarily on canned foods or "tea and toast" and teenagers whose diet consists of soft drinks and potato chips are likely to develop folate deficiency.

Malabsorption syndromes Folic acid deficiency is a common accompaniment of tropical sprue. Both the gastrointestinal symptoms and malabsorption are improved by the administration of either folic acid or antibiotics by mouth. Patients with nontropical sprue (gluten-sensitive enteropathy) may also develop significant folic acid deficiency which parallels other parameters of malabsorption. Similarly, alcohol-related folate deficiency may be due in part to malabsorption. In addition, other primary small-bowel disorders are sometimes associated with vitamin deficiency. These entities are all discussed in Chap. 308.

DRUGS Next to deficiency of folate or vitamin B_{12}, the most common cause of megaloblastic anemia is drug ingestion. Drugs which cause megaloblastic anemia do so by interfering with DNA synthesis, either directly or by antagonizing the action of folate. They can be classified as follows:

1 *Direct inhibitors of DNA synthesis.* The drugs in this category are used in the treatment of malignancy. Their efficacy depends on their ability to disrupt DNA synthesis. They include alkylating agents (nitrogen mustard, cyclophosphamide, etc.), purine and pyrimidine analogues (5-fluorouracil, cytosine arabinoside, 6-thioguanine, 6-mercaptopurine, etc.), and other drugs which interfere with DNA synthesis by a variety of mechanisms (Adriamycin, bleomycin, hydroxyurea).

2 *Folate antagonists.* The most toxic of these is methotrexate, an exceedingly powerful inhibitor of dihydrofolate reductase which is used in the treatment of certain malignancies. Much less toxic, but still capable of inducing a megaloblastic anemia, are several weak dihydrofolate reductase inhibitors which are used to treat a variety of nonmalignant conditions. These include pentamidine, trimethoptrine, triamterene, and pyrimethamine.

The megaloblastic changes in methotrexate poisoning appear to result from the following sequence of events. In methotrexate-poisoned cells, the methylation of dUMP to dTMP is grossly impaired. As a consequence, the phosphorylation of dUMP to dUTP, normally a very minor reaction, becomes a major route of dUMP metabolism. The capacity of a highly specific dUTP pyrophosphatase to degrade dUTP back to dUMP is exceeded under these conditions, and dUTP accumulates in the cell. This dUTP is incorporated into newly synthesized DNA, because DNA polymerase cannot distinguish between dUTP and the closely related normal substrate, dTTP. As a result, defective strands of DNA are produced in which T is partly replaced by U. The U-containing regions of these defective strands are recognized by a specific repair system, which excises them and attempts to replace them with normal DNA. In methotrexate-poisoned cells, however, there is so much dUTP and so little dTTP that the new DNA is also likely to be defective. It is this futile cycle of faulty replication, error excision, faulty repair, etc., which explains the megaloblastic pattern of DNA synthesis in methotrexate-poisoned cells. The megaloblastic changes in folate and vitamin B_{12} deficiency might have a similar biochemical origin.

3 *Nitrous oxide.* Nitrous oxide inhalation causes the destruction of endogenous vitamin B_{12}. As ordinarily used, this anesthetic does not destroy enough of the vitamin to cause clinical manifestations. Repeated or protracted exposure, however, may lead to a megaloblastic anemia. Fatal megaloblastic anemia has been reported in patients with tetanus who were given nitrous oxide continuously for weeks.

4 *Others.* A number of drugs antagonize folate by mechanisms which are poorly understood but are thought to involve an effect on absorption of the vitamin by the intestine. In this category are certain anticonvulsants [phenytoin (Dilantin), primidone (Mysoline)], and phenobarbital (Luminal). Megaloblastic anemia induced by these agents is mild.

OTHER Hereditary Megaloblastic anemia may be seen in several hereditary disorders. It is a regular feature of orotic aciduria, a defect in pyrimidine metabolism which is also characterized by retarded growth and development as well as the excretion of large amounts of orotic acid, and which is due to a deficiency of orotidylic decarboxylase and phosphorylase. Megaloblastic anemia has been reported in a single case of the Lesch-Nyhan syndrome, a condition resulting from a deficiency of hypoxanthine-guanine phosphoribosyltransferase whose clinical manifestations include gout, mental retardation, and self-mutilation. Congenital folate malabsorption also causes megaloblastic anemia, accompanied by ataxia and mental retardation. Megaloblastic anemia has been reported to accompany the congenital deficiency of other folate-metabolizing enzymes including formiminotransferase, dihydrofolate reductase, and N^5-methyltetrahydrofolate reductase. These deficiencies are less well documented than is congenital folate malabsorption. Megaloblastic changes as well as multinuclearity of red blood cell precursors are seen in the marrow of certain patients with congenital dyserythropoietic anemia, a group of inherited disorders characterized by mild to moderate anemia presenting at any age and pursuing a benign course.

Transcobalamin II deficiency, as well as the congenital abnormalities in vitamin B_{12} absorption described previously, causes pronounced deficiencies in vitamin B_{12} in infancy or early childhood, with all the accompanying manifestations. Megaloblastic anemia is not seen in hereditary transcobalamin I deficiency, nor is it a prominent feature of the methylmalonic acidurias, a group of conditions in which vitamin B_{12} metabolism is severely deranged.

Acquired idiopathic anemia Some patients with acquired sideroblastic anemia and other forms of refractory anemia show megaloblastic erythropoiesis. Megaloblastic changes are restricted to the red blood cell series; large granulocyte precursors and giant metamyelocytes are not seen (see below). Both are associated with an increased incidence of acute leukemia.

Megaloblastic changes are seen in erythremic myelosis and acute erythroleukemia (di Guglielmo) where red blood cell precursors are prominently involved. Here, the marrow is characterized by bizarre erythroid maturation, with multinuclearity and multipolar mitotic figures in the red blood cell precursors. Erythremic myelosis is discussed further in Chap. 128.

DIAGNOSIS The finding of significant macrocytosis [mean corpuscular volume (MCV) $>$ 96 fl] suggests the presence of a megaloblastic anemia. Other causes of macrocytosis include hemolysis, liver disease, alcoholism, hypothyroidism, and aplastic anemia. If the macrocytosis is marked (MCV $>$ 110 fl), the patient is much more likely to have a megaloblastic anemia. The reticulocyte count is low, and the leukocyte and platelet count may also be decreased, particularly in severely anemic patients. The blood smear (Plate 9-2) demonstrates marked anisocytosis and poikilocytosis, together with macroroovalocytes, large, oval, fully hemoglobinized erythrocytes, typical of megaloblastic anemias. There is some basophilic stippling, and an occasional nucleated red blood cell may be seen. In the white blood cell series, the neutrophils show hypersegmentation of the nucleus. This is such a typical finding that a single cell with a nucleus of six lobes or more should raise the immediate suspicion of a megaloblastic anemia. A rare myelocyte may also be seen. Bizarre, misshapen platelets are also observed. The bone marrow examination is very helpful in the diagnosis of megaloblastic anemia. The marrow is hypercellular with a decreased myeloid/erythroid ratio and abundant stainable iron. Red blood cell precursors are abnormally large and have nuclei that appear much less mature than would be expected from the development of the cytoplasm (nuclear-cytoplasmic asynchrony). The nuclear chromatin is more dispersed than it should be and consequently stains less intensely than normal. To the extent that it is aggregated, it condenses in a peculiar fenestrated pattern which is very characteristic of megaloblastic erythropoiesis. Abnormal mitoses may be seen. Granulocyte precursors are also affected, many being larger than normal, including giant bands and metamyelocytes. Megakaryocytes are decreased and show abnormal morphology.

Megaloblastic anemias are characterized by ineffective erythropoiesis (Chaps. 54 and 326). In a severely megaloblastic patient as many as 90 percent of the red blood cell precursors may be destroyed before they are released into the bloodstream, compared with 10 to 15 percent in the normal subject. Enhanced intramedullary destruction of erythroblasts results in an increase in unconjugated bilirubin and lactic acid dehydrogenase (isoenzyme 1) in plasma. Abnormalities in iron kinetics also attest to the presence of ineffective erythropoiesis, with increased iron turnover but low incorporation of labeled iron into circulating red blood cells.

In evaluating a patient with megaloblastic anemia, it is important to determine whether there is a deficiency of vitamin B_{12} or of folate. In many hospitals, specific assays for serum vitamin B_{12} and folate are available. Radioisotopic dilution techniques are easier to perform than microbiologic assays. However, the radioisotopic measurement of serum vitamin B_{12} may give falsely high values when an impure vitamin B_{12} binding protein is used. This problem is not encountered with the microbiologic assay. The normal range of vitamin B_{12} in serum is 200 to 900 pg/ml; values less than 100 pg/ml indicate clinically significant deficiency.

The normal serum concentration of folic acid ranges from 6 to 20 ng/ml; values of 4 ng/ml or less are generally considered to be diagnostic of folate deficiency. However, it must be remembered that the organisms used for the microbiological assay of folic acid are affected by many antibiotics. Thus, a serum sample from a patient who is on antibiotics may occasionally give a falsely low reading. Unlike serum vitamin B_{12}, serum folate levels may reflect recent alterations in dietary intake. Measurement of red blood cell folate occasionally provides useful information since it is not subject to short-term fluctuations in folate intake and is, therefore, a better index of tissue folate stores than serum folate.

A test which is occasionally used in the diagnosis of megaloblastic anemia is the deoxyuridine (dU) suppression test. This test is based on the observation that the uptake of tritiated thymidine by bone marrow cells, suppressed sharply (10 times or more) by deoxyuridine under normal circumstances, is affected to a much smaller extent in megaloblastic anemia. The abnormality in deoxyuridine suppression is probably related in some way to alterations in nucleotide pool sizes in megaloblastic cells.

Once vitamin B_{12} deficiency has been established, its pathogenesis can be delineated by means of a Schilling test. A patient is given radioactive vitamin B_{12} by mouth followed shortly thereafter by an intramuscular injection of unlabeled vitamin B_{12}. The proportion of the administered radioactivity excreted in the urine during the next 24 h provides an accurate measure of absorption of vitamin B_{12}, assuming that a complete urine sample has been collected. Since vitamin B_{12} deficiency is almost always due to malabsorption (Table 327-1), this first stage of the Schilling test should be abnormal. The patient is then given labeled vitamin B_{12} bound to intrinsic factor. Absorption of the vitamin will now approach normal if the patient has pernicious anemia or some other type of intrinsic factor deficiency. If vitamin B_{12} absorption is still decreased, the patient may have bacterial overgrowth (blind loop syndrome) or ileal disease including an ileal absorptive defect secondary to vitamin B_{12} deficiency. The former type of vitamin B_{12} malabsorption can usually be corrected by the administration of antibiotics. The Schilling test can provide equally reliable information after the patient has had adequate therapy with parenteral vitamin B_{12}.

Patients with pernicious anemia have atrophic gastritis with pentagastrin-fast achlorhydria and hypergastrinemia. As discussed in "Pernicious Anemia" above, these individuals have a very high incidence of antiparietal cell antibody and a somewhat lesser incidence of anti-intrinsic factor antibody.

TREATMENT

VITAMIN B_{12} DEFICIENCY Apart from specific therapy related to the underlying disorder (e.g., antibiotics for intestinal overgrowth with bacteria), the mainstay of treatment for B_{12} deficiency is replacement therapy. Since the defect is one of absorption, replacement should be administered parenterally, specifically in the form of intramuscular cyanocobalamin. (If intramuscular administration is contraindicated or refused, vitamin B_{12} deficiency can be managed by oral replacement therapy, but at doses of 300 to 1000 μg daily, it is an exceedingly expensive mode of treatment which requires very close medical supervision to avoid relapse.) Treatment should be started with 100 μg vitamin B_{12} per day for a week. The frequency of administration of the vitamin may then be decreased, the goal being to give a total of 2000 μg during the first 6 weeks. The patient may then be placed on 100 μg cyanocobalamin intramuscularly every month, a regimen that must be maintained for the rest of the patient's life. If necessary, larger doses may be given at less frequent intervals (e.g., 1 mg every 2 to 4 months), but the risk of relapse is substantially greater than if the vitamin is given monthly.

The response to treatment is gratifying. Shortly after treatment is begun, and several days before a hematologic response is evident in the peripheral blood, the patient will experience an increase in strength and an improved sense of well-being. Marrow morphology begins to revert toward normal within a few hours after treatment is initiated. Reticulocytosis begins 4 to 5 days after therapy is started and peaks at about day 7 (Fig. 327-3), with subsequent remission of the anemia over the next several weeks. If a reticulocytosis does not occur, or if it is less brisk than expected from the level of the hematocrit, a search should be made for other factors contributing to the anemia (e.g., infection, coexisting folate deficiency, or hypothyroidism). The sudden development of hypokalemia and salt retention may occur early in the course of therapy; usually these are of no consequence, but occasionally they may represent clinical problems.

FIGURE 327-3
Hematologic response of a patient with pernicious anemia to an intramuscular injection of 100 μg vitamin B_{12} on day 0. (From A Erslev, TG Gabuzda, Pathophysiology of Blood, Philadelphia, Saunders, 1975.)

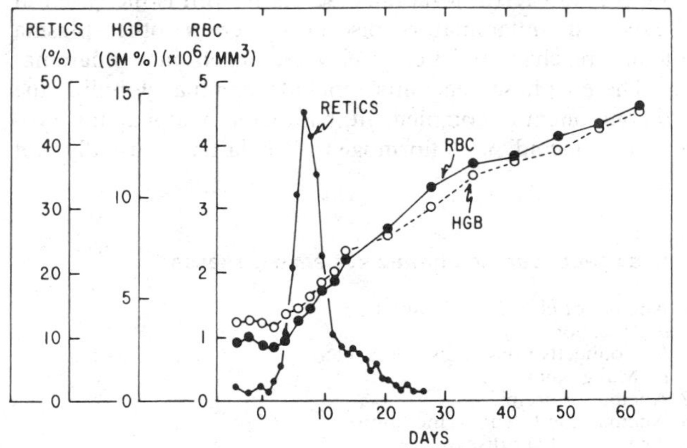

In most cases, replacement therapy is all that is needed for the treatment of vitamin B_{12} deficiency. Occasionally, however, a patient with a severe anemia will have such a precarious cardiovascular status that emergency transfusion is necessary. This must be done with great care, since it is very easy to precipitate florid congestive failure in such patients by fluid overload. Blood must be administered slowly in the form of packed cells, with very close observation, giving as an initial dose no more than 100 ml. This small volume will frequently be enough to ameliorate the cardiovascular problems sufficiently that further therapy can be restricted to vitamin B_{12} replacement. If necessary, blood may be administered by exchanging patient blood (mostly plasma) for packed cells.

With lifelong treatment, patients should experience no further manifestations of B_{12} deficiency. As previously stated, neurological symptoms may not be fully corrected even by optimal therapy. The potential for late development of gastric carcinoma in pernicious anemia necessitates careful follow-up of the patient.

FOLATE DEFICIENCY Like vitamin B_{12} deficiency, folate deficiency is treated by replacement therapy. The usual dose of folate is 1 mg per day, by mouth, but higher doses (up to 5 mg per day) may be required for folate deficiency due to malabsorption. Parenteral folate is rarely necessary. The hematologic response is similar to that seen after replacement therapy for vitamin B_{12} deficiency—that is, a brisk reticulocytosis after about 4 days, followed by correction of the anemia over the next 1 to 2 months. The duration of therapy depends on the basis of the deficiency state. Patients with a continuously increased requirement (such as patients with hemolytic anemia) or those with malabsorption or chronic malnutrition should continue to receive oral folic acid indefinitely. In addition, the patient should be encouraged to maintain an optimal diet containing adequate amounts of folate.

Folate, particularly in large doses, can correct the megaloblastic anemia of vitamin B_{12} deficiency without altering the neurological abnormalities. The neurological manifestations may even be aggravated by folate therapy. Vitamin B_{12} deficiency can thus be masked in patients who for one reason or another are taking large doses of folate. For this reason, a hematologic response to folate must never be used to rule out vitamin B_{12} deficiency in a given patient; vitamin B_{12} deficiency can be excluded only by appropriate laboratory evaluation.

OTHER CAUSES OF MEGALOBLASTIC ANEMIA Megaloblastic anemia due to drugs can be treated, if necessary, by reducing the dose of the drug or eliminating it altogether. The effects of folate antagonists which inhibit dihydrofolate reductase can be counteracted by folinic acid (citrovorum factor) in a dose of 100 to 200 mg per day. Since folinic acid is a derivative of tetrahydrofolate, it circumvents the block in folate metabolism imposed by dihydrofolate reductase inhibitors, replenishing the tissues with a form of folate which can directly enter the one-carbon donor pool.

Certain of the congenital megaloblastic anemia–producing

enzyme deficiencies can be treated by appropriate specific therapeutic regimens. The anemia of orotic aciduria is corrected by uridine, and the anemia in one case of Lesch-Nyhan syndrome responded to adenine. Both congenital folate malabsorption and homocystinuria have been treated successfully with oral folate, the former with very large doses (40 mg per day). Transcobalamin II deficiency can be treated with cyanocobalamin, but the vitamin has to be administered parenterally in very large large doses so that it can enter cells by mass action without the aid of TC II.

For the megaloblastic forms of sideroblastic anemia, pyridoxine in pharmacologic doses (as high as 300 mg per day) should be tried. A few patients will respond to this therapy. Simple supportive measures are all that appear to be in order for treatment of refractory megaloblastic anemia. Acute erythroleukemia (di Guglielmo's disease) is usually treated like other types of acute nonlymphocytic leukemia (see Chap. 128).

REFERENCES

ALLEN RH: The plasma transport of vitamin B_{12}. Brit J Haematol 36:153, 1976

BECK WS: The megaloblastic anemias, in *Hematology*, WJ Williams et al (eds). New York, McGraw-Hill, 1983

CHANARIN I: *The Megaloblastic Anemias*, 2d ed. Oxford, Blackwell, 1979

——— et al: How vitamin B_{12} acts. Brit J Haematol 47:487, 1981

ERBE R: Inborn errors of folate metabolism. N Engl J Med 293:753, 807, 1975

KOLHOUSE JF et al: Cobalamin analogues are present in human plasma and can mask cobalamin deficiency because current radioisotope dilution assays are not specific for true cobalamin. N Engl J Med 299:785, 1978

LAWSON DH et al: Early mortality in the megaloblastic anemias. Q J Med 41:1, 1972

LINDENBAUM J: Aspects of vitamin B_{12} and folate metabolism in malabsorption syndromes. Am J Med 67:1037, 1979

———: Folate and vitamin B_{12} deficiencies in alcoholism. Semin Hematol 17:119, 1980

SCOTT JM, WEIR DG: Drug induced megaloblastic change. Clin Haematol 9:587, 1980

328
ANEMIA ASSOCIATED WITH CHRONIC DISORDERS

H. FRANKLIN BUNN

Among the most commonly encountered anemias are those that accompany a variety of chronic underlying diseases. They can be corrected only if the primary condition is reversible. As shown in Table 328-1, these anemias can be subdivided into several groups. Those associated with chronic inflammation are characterized by an abnormality in iron metabolism.

ANEMIA OF CHRONIC INFLAMMATION

CLINICAL DESCRIPTION Patients who have a chronic systemic inflammatory disorder persisting more than a month usually develop an anemia which is of mild or moderate severity. The extent of the anemia is roughly proportional to the duration and severity of the inflammatory process. These disorders include chronic infections such as subacute infective endocarditis, osteomyelitis, lung abscess, tuberculosis, and pyelonephritis. Among noninfectious causes of anemia of chronic inflammation, the most common is rheumatoid arthritis. Other noninfectious inflammatory disorders often associated with chronic anemia include systemic lupus erythematosus, vasculitides (such as temporal arteritis), sarcoidosis, regional enteritis, and tissue injury such as fractures.

This kind of anemia is also commonly encountered in neoplastic disorders, including Hodgkin's disease and a variety of solid tumors such as carcinoma of the lung and breast. Other factors may contribute to the development of more severe anemia in cancer patients. In those with gastrointestinal cancer, blood loss can be the predominant factor. Chronic gastrointestinal bleeding will lead to iron deficiency. Furthermore, cancer patients may develop progressive anemia if the bone marrow is invaded with tumor cells. Myelophthisic anemia is discussed in detail in Chap. 331. Cancer patients are often malnourished and may develop folate deficiency. Rarely, patients with disseminated malignancy develop severe microangiopathic hemolytic anemia (Chap. 329). Finally, suppression of hematopoiesis by chemotherapeutic agents or radiation therapy may aggravate anemia.

HEMATOLOGIC DESCRIPTION Hemoglobin values generally range between 9 and 11 g/dl. A hemoglobin level less than 8 g/dl indicates the presence of one or more of the aggravating factors mentioned above. Although this group of anemias is generally classified as normocytic-normochromic, red blood cells often contain a subnormal amount of hemoglobin and may be microcytic. It is not uncommon for the mean corpuscular volume to be as low as 70 fl. Examination of the bone marrow reveals normal erythroid maturation. However, the red blood cell precursors have less stainable iron than normal (i.e., fewer sideroblasts), while the macrophages in the marrow usually contain increased amounts of iron. Myeloid hyperplasia and an increase in plasma cells may be seen in certain chronic infections.

The reticulocyte count is usually normal ($<$ 3 percent). Careful measurement of red blood cell survival generally reveals moderately shortened erythrocyte life span. Cross-transfusion studies point to an extracorpuscular mechanism, perhaps hyperplasia of the mononuclear-phagocyte system. There is seldom any other evidence of significant hemolysis. However, in certain chronic infections such as subacute infective endocarditis and miliary tuberculosis, splenomegaly can contribute to further shortening of the red blood cell life span, thereby increasing the severity of the anemia. In this setting spherocytes are often seen on the blood smear.

Serum iron is characteristically subnormal in this group of anemias, and, in contrast to iron deficiency, the total transferrin level is also reduced but to a lesser extent (see Fig. 326-1). Hence the fractional saturation of transferrin is slightly lower than normal. The serum iron falls within hours or days following the onset of the inflammation, whereas several weeks elapse before the transferrin level falls. Serum ferritin is increased in patients with inflammatory disorders. Certain other plasma proteins are characteristically elevated in chronic inflammation. These "phase reactants" include gamma globulin, the third component of complement, haptoglobin, $alpha_1$ antitrypsin, orosomucoid, and fibrinogen. The latter is usually not

TABLE 328-1
Anemias secondary to chronic systemic diseases

1 Anemia of chronic inflammation
  a Infection
  b Connective tissue disorders, etc.
  c Malignancy
2 Anemia of uremia
3 Anemia due to endocrine failure
4 Anemia of liver disease

measured since protein electrophoresis is routinely done on serum rather than plasma. Elevation of these proteins is responsible for the increased rate of red blood cell sedimentation which is so commonly observed.

It is often difficult to detect iron deficiency in a patient with chronic inflammation. The serum iron is low, and red blood cell protoporphyrin is increased in both conditions. When iron deficiency is superimposed on a chronic inflammatory state, the serum ferritin falls and transferrin level rises, usually to within normal limits. Under such circumstances, the amount of storage iron in the bone marrow is unpredictable. This problem is commonly encountered in patients with rheumatoid arthritis who may have developed iron deficiency owing to gastrointestinal blood loss. Because of this diagnostic uncertainty, it is often prudent to give such a patient a trial of iron and ascertain whether the hemoglobin level increases. However, it is important to avoid prolonged administration of iron unless a true deficiency state persists.

PATHOGENESIS The anemia of chronic inflammation is primarily due to defective red blood cell production and failure to compensate for the slightly decreased red blood cell life span. The subnormal amounts of iron in erythroblasts, in spite of an abundance of storage iron, suggests a defect in the transfer of iron to the developing erythroid cells. The cells that are formed are somewhat "iron deficient," and therefore tend to be small and pale. As in true iron deficiency, increased red blood cell protoporphyrin reflects the reduced availability of iron for heme synthesis. This defect can be quantitated by iron kinetic studies. If radioactive iron bound to transferrin is administered, there is normal uptake into erythroblasts and incorporation into circulating red cells. In contrast, if hemoglobin labeled with radioactive iron is injected, the incorporation of label into circulating red cells is only half normal. The hyperplastic mononuclear phagocyte system which is responsible for decreased survival of circulating red cells probably traps the hemoglobin iron and prevents its transfer to the bone marrow. For unexplained reasons, erythropoietin levels tend to be lower than expected for the degree of anemia. However, erythropoietin levels are not as low as in the anemia of renal failure (see below) and may not play a significant role in the pathogenesis of the anemia.

MANAGEMENT The anemia of chronic inflammation is not responsive to hematinic agents such as iron, folic acid, or vitamin B_{12}. Since the anemia is seldom severe, blood transfusion is rarely indicated. Efforts should be directed toward correcting the underlying disorder. In addition, if the anemia is more severe than expected, it is essential to search for other factors such as blood loss or drug-induced myelosuppression that could contribute to the reduction of red blood cell mass.

ANEMIA OF UREMIA

Anemia almost always accompanies the uremic syndrome. Although the hemoglobin level is highly variable among uremic patients, the severity of the anemia is roughly proportional to the degree of azotemia. The etiology of the renal failure usually has little bearing on the extent of anemia. However, for any level of serum creatinine patients with polycystic disease tend to be less anemic than those with other types of renal disease. In contrast to anemias associated with other chronic disorders discussed in this chapter, the anemia of uremia can be very severe, with hemoglobin levels as low as 4 g/dl. However, patients often tolerate such marked anemia remarkably well. This is largely due to compensatory adjustments such as redistribution of blood flow and a decrease in the oxygen affinity of the blood (see Chap. 54).

The anemia of uremia is normochromic and normocytic. Examination of the bone marrow seldom reveals any abnormalities. Red blood cell morphology is usually normal. In about one-third of patients, so-called burr cells are seen in the peripheral blood smear. These red blood cells have a characteristic evenly scalloped border (see Plate 9-9). Neither the degree of anemia nor the red blood cell life span is influenced by the presence of burr cells. In most patients the reticulocyte count is normal and the red blood cell survival is only modestly decreased. Thus the low red blood cell mass is due to decreased red blood cell production. The primary basis for this defect is that the diseased kidneys are unable to secrete adequate amounts of erythropoietin. Plasma erythropoietin levels are lower than those of nonuremic patients with a comparable degree of uremia. Erythropoiesis is further impaired but not abolished in patients who have undergone bilateral nephrectomy. In addition, red blood cell production may be suppressed by the accumulation of substances that are normally cleared by the kidneys. Iron kinetic measurements reveal impaired incorporation of iron into circulating red blood cells. Thus, it is likely that the anemia is due in part to ineffective erythropoiesis (see Chap. 54). Improvement in the rate of utilization of iron by the bone marrow has been noted following hemodialysis.

A small minority of uremic patients, particularly those with advanced disease, have brisk hemolysis. Red blood cell survival studies indicate that the hemolysis is due to extracorpuscular factors. Both metabolic and mechanical factors contribute to the hemolysis. Some patients may acquire a defect in the hexose monophosphate shunt which renders the red blood cell vulnerable to the formation of Heinz bodies (see Chap. 329). The hemolysis can be aggravated by oxidant drugs or oxidant compounds such as chloramine in the dialysis bath. If the renal failure is due to thrombotic thrombocytopenic purpura or hemolytic-uremic syndrome, patients will have a severe form of microangiopathic hemolytic anemia, with characteristic abnormalities of red blood cell morphology (see Chap. 329).

Treatment of the anemia of uremia should focus on an attempt to reverse the renal failure. The anemia may be modestly improved following hemodialysis. A prompt and dramatic correction of the anemia follows successful renal transplantation. Occasionally, polycythemia may be encountered following the renal engraftment, and may be a harbinger of impending rejection. In those patients who are not candidates for renal transplantation the administration of androgens has proved effective in stimulating erythropoiesis, particularly in patients who have not undergone bilateral nephrectomy.

It is important to be aware of other factors that may aggravate the anemia of renal disease. Uremic patients have a propensity to hemorrhage, owing to a qualitative defect in platelet function. Thus, gastrointestinal blood loss is commonly encountered. Furthermore a small but significant amount of blood loss occurs during hemodialysis. For these reasons some uremic patients become iron deficient. Folic acid deficiency may also occur, owing to the poor nutrition of many patients or to the loss of this vitamin during dialysis.

ANEMIA SECONDARY TO ENDOCRINE FAILURE

A number of hormones, including thyroxine, glucocorticoids, testosterone, and growth hormone are known to affect proliferation of human erythroid cells in vitro. Therefore it is not surprising that a mild to moderate normochromic-normocytic anemia generally accompanies a number of endocrine deficiency states, including hypothyroidism, Addison's disease, hypogonadism, and panhypopituitarism. It is possible that the anemias associated with hypothyroidism and hypopituitarism are related to the decreased need for oxygen transport, since oxygen consumption is reduced when thyroid hormone or growth hormone is lacking.

The anemia of *myxedema* is usually normocytic. Red blood cell life span is normal and erythropoiesis is effective. A minority of patients have macrocytic red blood cells which can usually be attributed to either folic acid or B_{12} deficiency. Patients with myxedema have an increased incidence of pernicious anemia. Hypothyroid patients, particularly females with menorrhagia, often develop iron deficiency and a microcytic anemia. Because the plasma volume may be reduced along with the red blood cell mass, the anemia of hypothyroidism may be masked. Since the signs and symptoms of myxedema are sometimes elusive, this diagnosis should be considered in the evaluation of any patient with unexplained anemia.

The anemia of *Addison's disease* is also masked by a decrease in plasma volume. Untreated patients have an average hemoglobin level of about 13 g/dl. Upon hormone replacement, the plasma volume is rapidly reconstituted and the hemoglobin level falls to 80 percent of its pretreatment value. With continued therapy, the red blood cell mass returns to normal.

Testosterone has a physiologic influence on red blood cell mass. During passage through adolescence the mean hemoglobin level of males increases from 13 to 15 g/dl. Eunuchoid males generally have a mild decrease in hemoglobin, averaging 13 g/dl. Pituitary dysfunction or ablation is associated with a mild normochromic normocytic anemia as well as occasional leukopenia.

The anemias secondary to endocrine failure are all readily corrected when adequate hormone replacement is given.

ANEMIA OF LIVER DISEASE

Patients with chronic liver disease, regardless of etiology, usually have a mild to moderate anemia which is normocytic or slightly macrocytic. An increased plasma volume may artificially lower the hematocrit and make the anemia seem worse than it is. Red blood cell morphology is normal, except for the presence of target cells (see Plate 9-3) and occasional stomatocytes, which have increased deposits of cholesterol and phospholipid, resulting in an increase in the surface area of the membrane. The bone marrow is usually normal. Erythropoiesis fails to compensate for a moderate shortening of red blood cell life span. The anemia persists as long as hepatic function is defective, but it may be corrected if normal hepatic function can be restored.

The situation is much more complex in patients with *alcoholic liver disease.* Many factors can contribute to the development of anemia. Alcohol is a direct suppressor of erythropoiesis. In alcoholics who have continued to drink up to the time of clinical evaluation, the bone marrow often reveals vacuoles in the cytoplasm of red and white blood cell precursors. In addition, ringed sideroblasts may be observed, particularly in patients who are malnourished. In alcoholics there is often suboptimal intake of dietary folic acid and impairment of folate utilization. Furthermore, alcoholics commonly develop significant hemorrhage from gastritis, esophageal varices, or duodenal ulcer, which contributes to the anemia. The risk of gastrointestinal blood loss is further increased by the presence of thrombocytopenia or deficiencies in soluble clotting factors. Although alcoholics usually have increased iron stores, they may become iron-deficient after prolonged gastrointestinal bleeding. Rarely patients with alcoholic cirrhosis develop a severe hemolytic anemia accompanied by the appearance of rigid red blood cells with irregular borders called acanthocytes or "spur" cells (see Plate 9-8). This entity is discussed in detail in Chap. 329. In addition, alcoholics may acquire a defect in the erythrocyte hexose monophosphate shunt, similar to that encountered in patients with uremia.

REFERENCES

Budman DR, Steinberg AD: Hematologic aspects of systemic lupus erythematosus. Ann Intern Med 86:220, 1977

Caro J et al: Erythropoietin levels in uremic nephric and anephric patients. J Lab Clin Med 93:449, 1979

Cartwright GE, Lee GR: The anemia of chronic disorders. Br J Haematol 21:147, 1971

Colman D, Herbert V: Hematologic complications of alcoholism: Overview. Semin Hematol 17:164, 1980

Douglas SW, Adamson JW: The anemia of chronic disorders: Studies of marrow regulation and iron metabolism. Blood 45:55, 1975

Fried W: Erythropoietin and the kidney. Nephron 15:327, 1975

Mowat AG: Hematologic abnormalities in rheumatoid arthritis. Semin Arthritis Rheum 1:195, 1972

Naets JP: Hematologic disorders in renal failure. Nephron 14:181, 1975

Neff MS et al: A comparison of androgens for anemia in patients on hemodialysis. N Engl J Med 304:871, 1981

Smith JR et al: Abnormal erythrocyte metabolism in hepatic disease. Blood 46:955, 1975

Yawata Y, Jacob HS: Abnormal red cell metabolism in patients with chronic uremia: Nature of the defect and its persistence despite adequate hemodialysis. Blood 45:231, 1975

Zucker S et al: Bone marrow erythropoiesis in the anemia of infection, inflammation and malignancy. J Clin Invest 53:1132, 1974

329 HEMOLYTIC ANEMIAS

RICHARD A. COOPER
H. FRANKLIN BUNN

PATHOGENESIS OF RED CELL DESTRUCTION

Red blood cells undergo premature destruction by two general mechanisms. First, red blood cells lyse in the circulation and release their contents directly into the peripheral blood. Intravascular hemolysis may be caused by trauma to the red blood cell, by fixation of complement to the red blood cell, or by exogenous toxins. Second, and more commonly, red blood cells are taken up by macrophages in the spleen and liver (mononuclear-phagocyte system), where they are destroyed and digested (extravascular lysis). The mononuclear-phagocyte system clears the cells from the circulation under two general conditions: first, the presence of surface abnormalities such as bound immunoglobulin for which macrophages have specific receptors; second, the presence of physical characteristics that limit the red blood cells' ability to traverse the fine filtering system of the spleen. Deformation of shape is required for red blood cells to pass through orifices with diameters smaller than their own. Their discoid shape favors deformability, providing a surface area that is 60 to 70 percent in excess of the minimum that is necessary to encompass the content of the cell.

The deformability of red blood cells is determined by three independent variables: (1) the viscoelastic properties of the red blood cell membrane, (2) the ratio of surface area to volume, and (3) the intracellular concentration of hemoglobin and aggregation of hemoglobin into polymer or precipitate.

One or more of these factors play a role in the pathogenesis of the various hemolytic anemias that are described in this chapter. A classification of these anemias is shown in Table 329-1. A number of clinical and laboratory features are shared by various types of hemolytic anemia. Patients with congenital hemolysis often have lifelong anemia and may have a positive family history. Patients with significant red blood cell turnover may be icteric, owing to an increase in unconjugated bilirubin. Splenomegaly is seen in a variety of chronic hemolytic anemias, both congenital and acquired.

LABORATORY DOCUMENTATION OF HEMOLYSIS

The reticulocyte count is the single most useful test in the initial evaluation. Patients with hemolytic anemia generally have a brisk reticulocytosis. The bone marrow predictably reveals erythroid hyperplasia. Since it seldom provides useful additional information, a bone marrow examination is generally not indicated in the evaluation of a patient with hemolytic anemia, unless an associated disorder such as lymphoma is suspected.

A variety of serum tests are useful in establishing the presence of hemolysis (see Table 329-2), among them the test for bilirubin, a tetrapyrrole formed from the oxidative catabolism of heme. *Unconjugated* or *"indirect" bilirubin* circulates in the plasma in transit from the mononuclear-phagocyte system to the liver where it is conjugated. When measured accurately, unconjugated bilirubin is a reliable guide to the presence of increased heme catabolism and is usually elevated in patients with hemolysis. The serum level of conjugated or "direct" bilirubin is normal unless the patient has associated hepatic or biliary dysfunction. Unconjugated bilirubin is also increased in patients with ineffective erythropoiesis where there is enhanced destruction of red cell precursors within the bone marrow. Since circulating unconjugated bilirubin is tightly bound to albumin, it does not pass through renal glomeruli. Thus, patients with hemolytic anemia have acholuric jaundice, whereas the hyperbilirubinemia of liver disease is associated with bilirubin in the urine.

Other serum tests are also useful in the assessment of hemolysis. *Haptoglobin* is an alpha globulin which is present in high concentration (~100 mg/dl) in the plasma (and serum). It binds specifically and tightly to the protein (globin) in hemoglobin. The hemoglobin-haptoglobin complex is cleared within minutes by the mononuclear-phagocyte system, while free haptoglobin has a prolonged circulation time ($t_{\frac{1}{2}}$ = 4 days). Thus, patients with significant hemolysis, either intravascular or extravascular, have low or absent levels of serum haptoglobin. Haptoglobin synthesis is decreased in patients with hepatocellular disease. Conversely, synthesis is enhanced in inflammatory states. Haptoglobin, like $alpha_1$ antitrypsin, orosomucoid, and the third component of complement are acute phase reactants. These facts must be considered in the interpretation of serum haptoglobin. *Hemopexin* is a plasma beta globulin which binds specifically to heme. It becomes depleted in patients with moderate and severe hemolysis. In addition to that bound by hemopexin, some of the heme from circulating free hemoglobin is transferred to albumin, resulting in the formation of *methemalbumin.* This complex is encountered only in severe intravascular hemolysis. Plasma hemoglobin is increased in proportion to the degree of hemolysis, but may be falsely elevated owing to lysis of red cells in vitro.

The urine should be tested in patients suspected of having intravascular hemolysis. Once the haptoglobin binding capacity of the plasma is exceeded, free hemoglobin will permeate renal glomeruli, primarily as $\alpha\beta$ dimers with a molecular weight of 32,000. This filtered hemoglobin is reabsorbed by the proximal tubule. The molecule is catabolized in situ, and the heme iron is incorporated into storage proteins, ferritin and hemosiderin. The presence of hemosiderin in the urine, detected by staining the sediment with Prussian blue, indicates that a significant amount of circulating free hemoglobin has been filtered by the kidneys. When the absorptive capacity of the tubular cells is exceeded, hemoglobinuria will ensue. The presence of hemoglobinuria indicates severe intravascular hemolysis. Sometimes the clinician is faced with the dilemma of whether benzidine-positive heme pigment in the urine is hemoglobin or myoglobin. The easiest way to distinguish between these alternatives is to examine an anticoagulated blood specimen after centrifiguration. Patients with myoglobinuria have normal-appearing plasma. Conversely, the plasma of patients with hemoglobinuria always has a reddish-brown color. Because of its higher molecular weight, hemoglobin has a lower glomerular permeability than myoglobin and is less rapidly cleared by the kidneys.

Tagging red cells with an appropriate isotopic label provides the most direct and precise measure of cell survival. The most commonly used labels are sodium [^{51}Cr]chromate and diisopropylfluoro[^{32}P]phosphate. Such studies are not necessary or indicated in the diagnostic workup of the majority of patients with hemolytic anemia. However, scanning with a collumnated detector can be employed to monitor the sequestration of ^{51}Cr-tagged red cells in the liver and spleen. This approach has proved useful in evaluating patients for possible splenectomy.

TABLE 329-1
Hemolytic anemias

Extracorpuscular	*1* Environmental factors *a* Splenomegaly *b* Antibody: immunohemolytic anemias *c* Mechanical trauma: microangiopathic hemolytic anemia *d* Direct toxic effect: malaria, clostridial infection, etc. *2* Membrane abnormalities *a* Spur cell anemia	Acquired
Intracorpuscular	*b* Paroxysmal nocturnal hemoglobinuria	Acquired
Intracorpuscular	*c* Hereditary spherocytosis (rare: elliptocytosis, stomatocytosis) *3* Abnormalities of red blood cell interior *a* Enzyme defects *b* Hemoglobinopathies	Hereditary

TABLE 329-2
Laboratory evaluation of hemolysis

	Moderate hemolysis (RBC life span 20–40 days)	*Severe hemolysis (RBC life span 5–20 days)*
HEMATOLOGIC		
Routine blood film	Polychromatophilia	Polychromatophilia
Reticulocyte index	↑	↑↑
Bone marrow examination	Erythroid hyperplasia	Erythroid hyperplasia
PLASMA OR SERUM		
Bilirubin	↑ Unconjugated	↑ Unconjugated
Haptoglobin	↓, absent	Absent
Hemopexin	Normal, ↓	↓, absent
Plasma hemoglobin	↑	↑↑
Lactate dehydrogenase	↑ (variable)	↑↑ (variable)
Methemalbumin	0	+ *
URINE		
Bilirubin	0	0
Urobilinogen	Variable	Variable
Hemosiderin	0	+
Hemoglobin	0	+ *

* *Intravascular hemolysis.*

RED CELL MORPHOLOGY AS A CLUE TO DIAGNOSIS

Most hemolytic disorders are associated with a change in the morphologic appearance of red blood cells. Some of these are depicted in Plate 9. Spherocytes are the most common morphologic abnormality in hemolytic diseases, and small numbers occur in many disorders. They are most striking in patients with hereditary spherocytosis and in patients with warm antibody-induced immunohemolytic disease (Plates 9-10 and 9-11). Spherocytes are the hallmark of splenic conditioning. Fragmented red blood cells suggest traumatic injury of the red cell including valve hemolysis, or one of the microangiopathic hemolytic anemias such as thrombotic thrombocytopenic purpura (Plate 9-7), hemolytic uremic syndrome, or disseminated intravascular coagulation. Target-shaped red blood cells which are well filled with hemoglobin occur in patients with hemoglobin C. They are prevalent in sickle cell anemia, where they were first described, and they are found in patients with the underhydrated form of hereditary stomatocytosis. The most common cause of target cells is liver disease (Plate 9-3). Target cells which are deficient in hemoglobin (hypochromic) are the hallmark of the thalassemia syndromes (Plate 9-5).

Spiculated red blood cells often cause confusion because of the frequency with which they are induced as an artifact during the preparation of a blood smear. Under these conditions, they are particularly frequent at the edges of the smear. When surrounded by otherwise normal-appearing red blood cells, spiculated red blood cells can be a clue to diagnosis. They occur, usually in small numbers, in conjunction with uremia or following splenectomy even in the absence of an underlying red blood cell disorder. Bizarrely spiculated red blood cells (acanthocytes) occur in the rare condition abetalipoproteinemia (Chap. 103) and in anorexia nervosa; however, in each of these instances minimal hemolysis is present. As discussed below, acanthocytes are a striking feature of spur-cell anemia (Plate 9-8).

Permanently sickled, crescent-shaped red blood cells (Plate 9-6) are the hallmark of sickle cell anemia (see Chap. 330). Boat-shaped red cells are a clue to the double heterozygous state of hemoglobin SC disease (see Chap. 330). The presence of both crescent-shaped cells and hypochromic target cells on the same smear is suggestive of the doubly heterozygous state, sickle cell–β thalassemia (see Chap. 330).

While in no case can the peripheral blood smear be totally diagnostic, in many it is a low-cost, important clue to the diagnosis. In addition to red blood cell morphology, a large battery of specific diagnostic tests are available for determining the etiology of the various hemolytic anemias. These are discussed in broad outline in Chap. 54 (Table 54-1) and in detail in this chapter.

ENVIRONMENTAL CAUSES OF HEMOLYSIS

SPLENOMEGALY The spleen is particularly efficient in trapping and destroying red blood cells which have minimal defects, often so mild as to be undetectable by in vitro techniques. This unique ability of the spleen to filter mildly damaged red blood cells results from its unusual vascular anatomy. Almost all the blood circulating through the spleen flows rapidly from arterioles in the white pulp to sinuses in the spleen's red pulp, and then on into the venous system. In contrast, a small portion of splenic blood flow (normally 1 to 2 percent) leaves the arterioles of the white pulp to enter a nonendothelialized portion of the spleen. In this sense, it is extravascular, although the entire spleen may be considered as a specialized part of the vascular system. This blood passes into the "marginal zone" of the lymphatic white pulp. Although the cells which occupy this zone are not phagocytic, they serve as a mechanical filter hindering the progress of damaged red blood cells. As red blood cells leave this zone and enter the red pulp, they flow into narrow cords which end blindly but which communicate with sinuses through small openings between the lining cells of the sinuses. These openings, averaging 3 μm in diameter, test the ability of red blood cells to undergo a deformation of shape. Red blood cells which do not pass the stringent test imposed upon them by the spleen filter are engulfed by phagocytic cells and destroyed.

The normal spleen poses no threat to normal red blood cells. However, splenomegaly exaggerates the adverse conditions to which red blood cells are exposed. Splenic enlargement may be considered in three broad categories. In the first are infiltrative disease (such as myeloproliferative disorders, Chaps. 128, 129, and 336), lymphomas (Chap. 130), and storage diseases (such as Gaucher's disease, Chap. 104). In the second are systemic inflammatory diseases leading to splenic hypertrophy. In the third are diseases which cause congestive splenomegaly. Hemolysis may occur whenever the spleen is enlarged. Its occurrence is least predictable in infiltrative diseases of the spleen where substantial splenomegaly may exist with no apparent hemolysis. Inflammatory and congestive splenomegaly are commonly associated with mild to moderate shortening of red blood cell survival.

RED CELL ANTIBODIES Immune hemolysis in the adult may be induced by three general types of antibodies:

1 Alloantibodies acquired by blood transfusions or pregnancies and directed against transfused red blood cells (Chap. 335).
2 Antibodies reactive at body temperature and directed against the patient's own red blood cells (Table 329-3).
3 Antibodies reactive in the cold and directed against the patient's own red blood cells (Table 329-3).

Coombs' antiglobulin test is the major tool for diagnosing these disorders. This test relies on the ability of antibodies prepared in animals and directed against specific human serum proteins to agglutinate red blood cells if these human serum proteins are present on the red blood cell surface. The serum proteins of particular interest are IgG and C3. The ability of anti-IgG or anti-C3 antiserums to agglutinate the patient's red blood cells is referred to as the *direct Coombs test.* At times it is advantageous to know whether there is antibody in the serum of patients which is reactive against other human red blood cells. This is important in cross matching prior to blood transfusion (Chap. 335), and it is of prognostic significance in patients with warm-antibody hemolytic anemia. To determine this, an *indirect Coombs test* is performed by incubating ABO- and Rh-compatible red blood cells with the patient's serum and subsequently performing a direct Coombs test on these incubated red cells.

TABLE 329-3
Hemolysis due to antibodies

I Warm-antibody immunohemolytic anemia
- *A* Idiopathic
- *B* Lymphomas: Chronic lymphocytic leukemia, non-Hodgkin's lymphomas, Hodgkin's disease (infrequent)
- *C* Systemic lupus erythematosus
- *D* Tumors (rare)
- *E* Drugs
  - *1* α-Methyldopa type
  - *2* Penicillin type (hapten)
  - *3* Quinidine type (innocent bystander)

II Cold-antibody immunohemolytic anemia
- *A* Cold agglutinin disease
  - *1* Acute: Mycoplasma infection, infectious mononucleosis
  - *2* Chronic: Idiopathic, lymphoma
- *B* Paroxysmal cold hemoglobinuria

"Warm" antibodies Antibodies which react at body temperature are usually of the IgG class, although occasionally they are of the IgA class. They induce a pattern of hemolysis which affects both the patient's own cells and normal transfused cells. This acquired syndrome is frequently designated *autoimmune hemolytic anemia.* In recent years, as a number of drugs which induce this clinical syndrome have become recognized, attention has focused on the exogenous factors which may underlie the formation of these red blood cell antibodies, and the expression *immunohemolytic anemia* is preferred.

CLINICAL MANIFESTATIONS Warm-antibody immunohemolytic anemia occurs at all ages but is most common in adults, particularly women and older individuals. In approximately one-fourth of patients this disorder occurs as a complication of an underlying disease affecting the immune system, especially chronic lymphocytic leukemia, non-Hodgkin's lymphoma, and systemic lupus erythematosus (SLE). Occasionally, immunohemolytic anemia is seen in patients with advanced, active Hodgkin's disease. Case reports link it to a variety of nonlymphoid neoplasms.

The presentation and course of immunohemolytic anemia are quite variable. In its mildest form, the only manifestation is a positive direct Coombs test. In this instance, insufficient antibody is present on the red blood cell surface to permit the reticuloendothelial system to recognize the cell as abnormal. This is particularly common in SLE. A large fraction of patients with immunohemolytic anemia have a chronic mild anemia and splenomegaly. The direct Coombs test is positive for IgG but seldom for C3, and the indirect Coombs test is negative. In other cases this disorder may be more severe, with hemoglobin levels less than 7.0 g/dl and reticulocyte counts of 30 percent and higher. Spherocytosis is usually marked (Plate 9-11). Coombs' test is positive for IgG and frequently for C3 as well. The large quantity of antibody bound to the cell is also reflected by the indirect Coombs test, which demonstrates antibody not only on the patient's red blood cells but also in the patient's serum. Thrombocytopenia may also be present. The coexistence of immune destruction of red blood cells and platelets is referred to as *Evans' syndrome.* Possibly because they indicate the presence of a large amount of antibody, a positive indirect Coombs test and thrombocytopenia are poor prognostic signs. In its most severe form, immunohemolytic anemia presents with fulminant, overwhelming hemolysis associated with hemoglobinemia, hemoglobinuria, and shock, a syndrome which may be fatal.

Associated findings include hyperbilirubinemia, decreased or absent haptoglobin levels, and occasionally hepatomegaly. Fever and abdominal pain occur in some patients. Venous thrombosis occurs commonly, the most frequent site being the deep veins of the legs, but thrombosis of mesenteric and portal veins has also been reported. Arterial thromboses occur as well.

PATHOGENESIS Little is known about the origin of red blood cell antibodies in the immunohemolytic anemias. Much more information exists concerning the mechanism of destruction of red blood cells coated with IgG antibodies. Although spherocytosis is often a prominent feature of hemolysis in vivo, the simple exposure of normal red blood cells to IgG antibodies does not lead to spherocytosis in vitro. However, human red blood cells coated with IgG antibodies are bound to the surface of monocytes or splenic macrophages and undergo a spherical transformation. The ability to cause this red blood cell–leukocyte interaction is greatest with IgG of subclasses 1 and 3 (the most common subclasses). It is not shared by IgM or IgA. However, C3 on the red blood cell surface also promotes this cell-cell interaction, but binding may be more transient because of the ability of the plasma C3 inactivator to release bound cells. Indeed, IgG and C3 behave in a synergistic fashion in this regard, accounting for the more severe hemolytic disease in patients in whom both IgG and C3 are present on the red blood cell surface. The slow flow compartment of the spleen is particularly efficient in trapping red blood cells which are coated with IgG antibodies, and the spleen is the major site of red blood cell destruction in this disorder.

THERAPY AND PROGNOSIS In the initial evaluation of the patient, it is important to rule out drugs which are known to cause immunohemolytic anemia. This topic is discussed below.

Patients having a mild degree of hemolysis usually do not require therapy. In those with clinically significant hemolysis, initial therapy consists of corticosteroids (e.g., prednisone, 1.0 mg/kg per day). A rise in hemoglobin is frequently noted within 3 or 4 days and occurs in most patients within 1 week. Prednisone is continued until the hemoglobin level has risen to normal values, and thereafter it is tapered slowly over the course of several months. More than 75 percent of patients will achieve a significant and sustained reduction in hemolysis; however, in half of these patients the disease will relapse either during the period of steroid tapering or following the cessation of steroid therapy. Steroids appear to have two modes of action: an immediate effect due to inhibition of the clearance of IgG-coated red blood cells by the mononuclear phagocyte system, and a later effect due to steroid-induced inhibition of antibody synthesis.

Patients with severe anemia may require blood transfusions. Because the antibody in this disease is a "panagglutinin," reacting with all normal donor cells, the usual cross matching is impossible. The goal in selecting blood for transfusion is to avoid administering red cells with antigens to which patients have previously been sensitized and which are known to be associated with complement lysis and intravascular hemolysis. In addition to A and B, Kell, Kidd (Jk_a), Duffy (F_y), and Lewis account for almost all examples of this type of hemolysis. A common procedure is to adsorb the panagglutinin present in patient's serum using the patient's own red cells from which antibody has previously been eluted. Serum freed of autoantibody in this way can then be tested for the presence of alloantibody to specific donor blood groups. ABO-compatible red cells matched in this fashion are administered slowly with attention paid to the possibility of an immediate-type transfusion reaction.

Splenectomy is the second line of therapy in this disorder. It is recommended for patients who cannot tolerate steroid therapy, in whom steroid therapy has been insufficient to control the disease process, or in whom a normal hematologic status can be maintained only with excessive doses of steroids. When red blood cells are labeled with chromium, their site of destruction can be determined. In 75 percent of patients, the spleen is the dominant site, whereas the liver predominates in the remaining patients. However, this test is not generally useful for selecting those patients who would respond to splenectomy. Rather, a favorable response to splenectomy is obtained in approximately two-thirds of patients in whom a splenic pattern of localization is found and in approximately one-third of patients in whom it is not found. Therefore, splenectomy must be undertaken on clinical grounds alone. Unlike hereditary spherocytosis, where splenectomy carries a very low morbidity and mortality, it poses a greater risk to patients with immunohemolytic anemia, particularly those with an underlying disease of the lymphoid system.

In recent years, patients who have been refractory to steroid therapy and to splenectomy have been treated with immunosuppressive drugs. The greatest experience is with azathioprine (Imuran) and cyclophosphamide (Cytoxan). A variable success rate has been reported with each.

In the majority of patients, this disease is controlled by steroid therapy alone, by splenectomy, or by a combination. In most of the remaining patients, a partial degree of control is achieved. Fatalities occur among three categories: first, rare patients with overwhelming hemolysis in whom death is directly attributable to anemia; second, those with major thrombotic events coincident with active hemolysis; third, those whose host defenses are impaired by corticosteroids, splenectomy, and/or immunosuppressives. In patients in whom immunohemolysis develops as a complication of an underlying disorder, the prognosis is dominated by that of the primary disease.

Immunohemolytic anemia secondary to drugs Drugs which have been directly related to immunohemolytic anemia are of three kinds, as distinguished by their three mechanisms of actions: (1) Drugs, such as α-methyldopa (Chap. 267), which induce a disorder identical almost in every respect to the warm-antibody immunohemolytic anemia described above. (2) Drugs of the penicillin type which can become associated with the red blood cell surface and induce the formation of an antibody directed against the red blood cell–drug complex. (3) Drugs, such as quinidine, that form a complex with plasma proteins to which an antibody forms; this drug–plasma protein–antibody complex settles out on red blood cells or platelets to involve them in a destructive process on an "innocent bystander" basis.

α-METHYLDOPA-TYPE ANTIBODIES A positive direct Coombs test is observed in up to 10 percent of patients receiving α-methyldopa therapy in a dose of 2.0 g daily. A small minority of these patients develop spherocytosis and hemolysis, often of severe degree. This "autoimmune" disorder may be triggered by a deficiency of suppressor T lymphocytes. Two distinctive features are that the indirect Coombs test is positive in almost all patients with hemolysis and that the red cells are coated with IgG but not C3. The IgG antibody is directed against the Rh complex. Hemolysis decreases over the course of several weeks after cessation of drug therapy, although the direct Coombs test may remain positive for more than 1 year.

PENICILLIN (HAPTEN)-INDUCED IMMUNOHEMOLYSIS An antibody directed against "penicillinized" red blood cells induces spherocytosis and hemolysis in patients receiving large, intravenous doses of penicillin and penicillin-type antibiotics (e.g., 15 to 20 million units of penicillin per day, or 12 to 15 g oxacillin per day). Hemolysis usually begins 7 to 14 days after the start of penicillin therapy and is associated with spherocytosis and hyperbilirubinemia. The patient's red blood cells are Coombs-positive for IgG during the period of penicillin therapy. An indirect Coombs test can be demonstrated with the patient's serum using normal red blood cells "penicillinized" in vitro. Hemolysis ceases abruptly when penicillin therapy is stopped, although the serum antibody can be demonstrated for many weeks.

INNOCENT BYSTANDER IMMUNOHEMOLYSIS Innocent bystander antibodies may be of either the IgG or IgM class, and the antigen-antibody complexes which adhere to the red blood cell surface are capable of fixing complement. The drug-antibody complex dissociates from the red blood cell, leaving only C3 to be detected by Coombs' test. The pattern of hemolysis may be primarily extravascular red blood cell destruction, or it may be intravascular hemolysis due to complement lysis with hemoglobinemia, hemoglobinuria, and acute renal failure. This is an uncommon form of hemolysis despite the fact that the drugs associated with it are in very common usage. They include quinine and quinidine, isoniazid, sulfonamides, phenacetin, stibophen, *p*-aminosalicylic acid, dipyrone, and various insecticides.

Immune hemolysis due to cold-reactive antibodies Antibodies which are reactive in the cold induce hemolysis under two general conditions. First, in cold agglutinin disease IgM antibodies, usually reactive with the I antigen, occur spontaneously, in the course of a lymphoproliferative disease or as a complication of infectious mononucleosis or mycoplasma pneumonia. Second, in paroxysmal cold hemoglobinuria, antibodies of the IgG class (Donath-Landsteiner) occur spontaneously or as a complication of certain viral diseases or of syphilis.

COLD AGGLUTININ DISEASE *Clinical manifestations.* Agglutination of red blood cells by IgM cold agglutinins is most profound at very low temperatures, and disagglutination occurs quickly upon warming. In most patients agglutination ceases at 32°C. The fixation of complement is a warm-reactive process. Therefore, patients may have very high titers of cold agglutinins as measured at low temperatures, but these antibodies may be inefficient in fixing complement to the cell surface and totally unable to induce agglutination at temperatures achieved in the bloodstream. Most cold agglutinins cause little or no shortening of red blood cell survival.

In mycoplasma pneumonia, cold agglutinins are very common, whereas only the occasional patient will have significant hemolysis about 5 to 10 days after recovery from the infection. Spherocytes may be seen occasionally, but the red blood cell morphology is usually normal. The antibody is directed against the I antigen, and the entire process is self-limited.

The cold agglutinin in infectious mononucleosis is most frequently directed against the i antigen, an antigen accessible on the surface of fetal red blood cells but not adult red blood cells. Therefore, this cold agglutinin is of serologic interest, but rarely induces hemolysis in humans. Antibody directed against the I antigen and complex antibodies involving both antigens have also been reported, with hemolysis.

A chronic form of cold-induced hemolysis occurs in patients spontaneously or in association with lymphoid neoplasms, most commonly affecting individuals in their seventh or eighth decades. The clinical manifestations relate to hemolysis and less commonly to agglutination of red blood cells in capillaries in those portions of the body exposed to low temperature, causing acrocyanosis. Gangrene is uncommon. Hemoglobin levels are usually above 10 g/dl and rarely below 7 g. Reticulocytes are fewer in number than might be anticipated, presumably because of the selective destruction of young cells (including reticulocytes) in this disorder.

In most patients with cold agglutinin disease, the antibody titer is very high (e.g., 1:10,000) at 4°C and very low (e.g., 1:16) at 37°C. In some patients the antibody shows a flatter thermal spectrum with a moderately high titer at 4°C (e.g., 1:320) and a readily demonstrable titer at 37°C (e.g., 1:64). Hemolysis tends to be more severe in this latter group. The Coombs' test demonstrates the presence of C3 on the red blood cell surface, but IgM is usually not found, and IgG is not present.

Pathogenesis. The etiology of the antibody is unknown. It appears to exert its hemolytic effect not through agglutination per se but rather by the fixation of C3 to the red blood cell surface. The liver is particularly efficient at detecting red blood cells coated with C3 in the form of C3b and clearing them from the circulation. A plasma enzyme, C3 inactivator, is capable of cleaving C3b into a small fragment (C3c) which leaves the cell surface and reenters the plasma, and C3d, which adheres to the red blood cell surface where it is recognized as C3 in Coombs' test but not as C3 by the mononuclear phagocyte system. The presence of C3d on the red blood cell surface decreases the ability of IgM anti-I to begin anew the complement sequence and thereby reestablish C3b on the red cell surface. Because of this, red blood cells that have survived in the circulation for a period of time have become "protected," while the younger red blood cells are in greater jeopardy.

Therapy. The cutaneous manifestations of this disorder are best treated by maintaining the patient in a warm environment. Because transfusion of normal blood presents to the patient a large number of red blood cells which have not previously been exposed to the cold agglutinin and are therefore not "protected," transfusion may be associated with an acceleration of the hemolytic process. Splenectomy is usually not of value in this disorder. Corticosteroids are of limited value, although patients with the panthermal variety of cold agglutinin disease may respond favorably to this therapy. Chlorambucil and cyclophosphamide are the most commonly employed agents in those patients in whom therapy is indicated. Although some patients have experienced a dramatic improvement, the effectiveness of this therapy is usually marginal.

Cold agglutinin disease tends to be chronic and unremitting. The overall prognosis is dominated by the underlying lymphoproliferative disease, if present. In those patients in whom cold agglutinin disease appears to arise spontaneously, lymphoproliferative disease may become apparent after several years.

PAROXYSMAL COLD HEMOGLOBINURIA (PCH) Now a rare disorder, PCH was more frequent at a time when tertiary syphilis was more prevalent. It results from the formation of the Donath-Landsteiner antibody, an IgG antibody directed against the P antigen of the red blood cell surface. Attacks are precipitated by exposure to cold and are associated with hemoglobinemia and hemoglobinuria, chills and fever, back, leg, and abdominal pain, headache, and malaise. Recovery from the acute episode is prompt, and between episodes patients are asymptomatic. When this syndrome accompanies acute viral infections (e.g., measles and mumps), it is self-limited. When secondary to syphilis, it responds favorably to specific therapy for this disorder. No specific therapy exists for idiopathic cases. Despite the severity of individual episodes, the natural history of this disease extends over many years.

TRAUMA IN THE CIRCULATION Mechanical trauma can cause hemolysis in three ways: (1) when red blood cells flow through small vessels over the surface of bony prominences and are subject to external impact during various physical activities; (2) when they flow across a pressure gradient created by an abnormal heart valve or valve prosthesis and are disrupted by a shear stress; and (3) when the deposition of fibrin in the microvasculature exposes them to a physical impediment that fragments them (Table 329-4).

External impact Hemoglobinemia and hemoglobinuria have been observed in individuals who have undergone a prolonged march or a prolonged jog, most typically on a hard surface and while wearing thin-soled shoes. The role of direct external trauma in this process has been demonstrated by the fact that hemolysis can be prevented by the insertion of a soft inner sole in the runner's shoes. Similar types of hemolysis have been described following karate and the playing of bongo drums. No abnormality of red blood cell morphology has been demonstrated, even during the acute episode, and no underlying red blood cell abnormality has been uncovered. A large percentage of individuals will develop hemoglobinemia and hemoglobinuria when exposed to the conditions described above. As a result of muscle damage that occurs during some of these activities, myoglobinuria commonly occurs, but renal function is preserved. No specific therapy is required.

Cardiac hemolysis Hemolysis associated with fragmented red blood cells (Plate 9-7) occurs in approximately 10 percent of patients with artificial aortic valve prostheses. This incidence is somewhat greater with valves having stellite rather than silastic occluders, greater with small valves as compared with larger valves, and greater when valves are cloth-covered or when there is a paravalvular leak with increased flow across the prosthesis. Traumatic hemolysis is much less common in recipients of porcine valves. Severe hemolysis may occur after repair of ostium primum or endocardial cushion defects with a prosthetic patch. Mitral valve prostheses have also been associated with hemolysis, but since the pressure gradient across these is lower than across aortic prostheses, the incidence is lower. A moderately shortened red blood cell survival (chromium half-survivals of 15 to 20 days) with little or no anemia occurs in some patients with severe calcific aortic stenosis. Indeed, almost any intracardiac lesion which alters hemodynamics may lead to some shortening of red blood cell survival. In addition, traumatic hemolysis has been observed in patients who have undergone aortofemoral bypass.

CLINICAL MANIFESTATIONS In severe cases hemoglobin levels fall to 5.0 to 7.0 g/dl with reticulocytosis, fragmented red blood cells in the peripheral blood, depressed haptoglobin, elevated serum lactic dehydrogenase, and hemoglobinemia and hemoglobinuria. Iron loss (as hemoglobin or hemosiderin) in the urine may lead to iron deficiency. Direct Coombs test may rarely become positive.

PATHOGENESIS A number of factors combine to cause the fragmentation and destruction of red blood cells in this disorder. Direct mechanical trauma of red blood cells at the time of seating of the occluder of the prosthetic valve, the deposition of fibrin across disrupted attachment points, but probably most important, the shear stress resulting from turbulent blood flow may all result in the fragmentation of red blood cells. The last explains the higher incidence of hemolysis in patients who

TABLE 329-4
Disturbances of the formed elements of blood secondary to intravascular trauma

Etiology	*Fragments*	*Hemolysis*	*Thrombocytopenia*
Impact: march hemoglobinuria, karate, playing bongo drums, etc.	0	+	0
Cardiac (turbulence):			
Aortic valve prosthesis	++++	++++	0
Ostium primum repair	++++	++++	0
Mitral valve prosthesis	++	++	0
Calcific aortic stenoses	+	±	0
Vessel disease: Malignant hypertension, Eclampsia, Renal graft rejection, Hemangiomas, Immune disease (scleroderma)	+++	+	+
Thrombotic thrombocytopenic purpura	++++	++++	++++
Hemolytic uremic syndrome	++++	++++	++++
Disseminated intravascular coagulation	++	±	++++

have a paravalvular leak and therefore greater velocity of blood flow across the aortic orifice during systole.

THERAPY AND PROGNOSIS Iron deficiency should be corrected by the administration of oral iron. The elevated hemoglobin which results may permit a decrease in the cardiac output and a slowing of the hemolytic rate. Corticosteroid therapy has been successful in partially alleviating the hemolysis in some patients. A limitation in physical activity usually lessens the hemolytic rate. When these measures fail, any paravalvular leak must be repaired or the prosthetic valve removed and replaced by a tissue valve.

Deposition of fibrin in the microvasculature Fibrin becomes deposited in the microvasculature where it traps platelets and fragments red blood cells, under three general conditions: (1) abnormalities of the vessel wall in recognized disorders, such as malignant hypertension, eclampsia, rejection of a renal allograft, disseminated cancer, and hemangiomas; (2) two potentially fatal syndromes of unknown etiology, thrombotic thrombocytopenic purpura and the hemolytic uremic syndrome; and (3) disseminated intravascular coagulation.

ABNORMALITIES OF THE VESSEL WALL IN RECOGNIZED DISORDERS The degree of hemolysis induced by this family of disorders is usually quite mild, although the number of fragments in the peripheral blood may be striking. In occasional patients, thrombocytopenia may be severe. In each case, therapy is best directed at the primary disease. Thus, reversal of renal graft rejection, treatment of malignant hypertension and eclampsia, control of cancer, etc., lead to a cessation of the hemolytic process. The relative importance of the primary vascular abnormality and of the deposition of fibrin in causing hemolysis is unclear.

Thrombotic thrombocytopenic purpura (TTP) This disease of unknown etiology affects individuals of all ages but primarily young adults, more often women.

CLINICAL MANIFESTATIONS Hemolysis is a striking feature of this disease. Anemia occurs in association with fragmented red blood cells, nucleated red cells in the peripheral blood, an elevated reticulocyte count, and thrombocytopenia of varying degree. Platelet counts range from 5000 to 100,000 per cubic millimeter. Jaundice is common, and petechiae may be present, although usually to a less striking degree than in idiopathic thrombocytopenic purpura (ITP). Tests of coagulation, such as the prothrombin time, partial thromboplastin time, fibrinogen concentration, and the level of fibrinogen split products, are usually entirely normal. If the coagulation tests indicate disseminated intravascular coagulation, the diagnosis of TTP is doubtful. Erythroid hyperplasia and an increased number of megakaryocytes are present in the bone marrow. The life span of platelets is decreased to hours, and no site of organ localization of destroyed platelets is observed. A positive lupus erythematosus cell test or antinuclear antibody is obtained in approximately 20 percent of patients. Some patients experience significant bleeding of uterine, gastrointestinal, or other origin, but severe bleeding is not common. Fever is present in almost all patients, and many experience nonspecific constitutional symptoms such as nausea, abdominal pain, and arthralgias. The spleen and liver may be palpable.

The course of TTP spans days to weeks in most patients, but occasionally continues for months. As the disease progresses, the brain and kidneys become progressively involved, and their dysfunction is the ultimate cause of death in the majority of patients. Proteinuria and a moderate elevation of blood urea nitrogen may be present on initial presentation, and there is a continued rise in blood urea nitrogen and a fall in urine output as the disease progresses. Neurologic symptoms evolve in more than 90 percent of patients whose disease terminates in death. Initially, there may be changes in mental status such as confusion, delirium, or altered states of consciousness. Focal findings include seizures, hemiparesis, aphasia, and visual field defects. These neurologic symptoms may fluctuate and terminate in coma. Involvement of myocardial blood vessels may be a cause of sudden death in some patients.

PATHOGENESIS The etiology of TTP is unknown. Arterioles are filled with hyalin material, presumably fibrin and platelets, and similar material may be seen beneath the endothelium of otherwise uninvolved vessels. Immunofluorescence studies have shown the presence of immunoglobulin and complement in arterioles. Microaneurysms of arterioles are often present. Controversy exists concerning the specificity of these changes, some authorities noting them in the hemolytic uremic syndrome and in disseminated intravascular coagulation. An association with systemic lupus erythematosus (SLE), scleroderma, and Sjögren's syndrome suggests an immunologic etiology.

DIAGNOSIS The combination of hemolytic anemia with fragmented and nucleated red blood cells, thrombocytopenia, fever, neurologic disorders, and renal dysfunction is virtually pathognomonic of TTP. The diagnosis is further supported by the finding of normal coagulation tests, although occasional patients have an isolated abnormality of coagulation. Although they are not usually required for diagnosis, biopsies of skin and muscle, gingiva, lymph node, or bone marrow will frequently reveal the pathologic abnormalities described above. The major differential diagnosis is idiopathic thrombocytopenic purpura. TTP should be considered in every patient in whom the diagnosis of ITP or Evans' syndrome (ITP plus immunohemolytic anemia) is made. Because the clinical course can fluctuate widely, therapy is difficult to evaluate. The finding of fragmented red blood cells in the peripheral blood is particularly helpful in this regard.

THERAPY AND PROGNOSIS Until recently, this disease was almost universally fatal. A large number of therapeutic modalities have been attempted with variable success. These include corticosteroids, exchange transfusion, splenectomy, heparin, and antiplatelet drugs. Patients are initially treated with high doses of corticosteroids (100 to 1000 mg prednisone per day). However, additional therapy is indicated once the diagnosis has been established. The most consistent improvement has been noted with exchange transfusion or plasmapheresis. It is likely that plasmapheresis is as effective as exchange transfusion. In some patients the response may depend upon the infusion of plasma. Splenectomy may also be effective, but this procedure poses additional risk in these critically ill patients. The additional benefit of antiplatelet drugs (dipyridamole, sulfinpyrazone, dextran, aspirin) is unclear, but they are commonly used together with the therapeutic measures described above. Aspirin may increase the risk of bleeding and should be employed with caution. Vincristine may be effective in otherwise refractory patients. In addition, rare responses to heparin infusion have been reported. Because of the ever-present risk of sudden death, therapy should be instituted promptly. Even deep coma is not a contraindication to therapy since full neurologic recovery is the rule in patients responding to therapy. If treatment is instituted early in the disease, remission occurs in approximately two-thirds of patients. Relapses have been noted but are usually responsive to therapeutic intervention.

Hemolytic uremic syndrome The hemolytic uremic syndrome is a disorder usually encountered in young children with laboratory features similar to those of TTP. Often the patient has a prodrome of a viral-like illness. Less commonly, the disorder appears to be familial. Patients present with acute hemolytic anemia, thrombocytopenic purpura, and acute oliguric renal failure. Most patients have either hemoglobinuria or anuria. Unlike TTP, neurologic manifestations are uncommon. The peripheral blood findings, coagulation tests, and pathologic changes on biopsy specimens are usually indistinguishable from those of TTP. Patients are treated with dialysis and transfusions. The efficacy of corticosteroids, dextran, and heparin is uncertain. The mortality in children ranges from 5 to 20 percent, but is considerably higher in adults.

Disseminated intravascular coagulation (DIC) Red blood cell fragmentation in the microvasculature (microangiopathic hemolytic anemia) is seen in about one-third of patients with DIC (Chap. 334). The degree of hemolysis is much less in DIC than in either TTP or the hemolytic uremic syndrome, and anemia with reticulocytosis and nucleated red blood cells is distinctly rare.

DIRECT TOXIC EFFECTS A variety of infections may be associated with severe hemolysis. The microorganisms in bartonellosis and malaria directly parasitize red blood cells. These two disorders are discussed in detail in Chaps. 169 and 218. Babesiosis also may cause a mild to moderate hemolytic anemia by direct parasitization of red blood cells.

Other infectious organisms exert their damaging effect on red blood cells indirectly. The most striking is that resulting from septicemia with *Clostridium welchii* (Chap. 172). The phospholipase produced by this organism is capable of cleaving the phosphoryl bond of lecithin thereby lysing human red blood cells. A mild, transient hemolysis frequently accompanies bacteremia with diverse organisms such as pneumococci, staphylococci, and *Escherichia coli.*

Hemolysis may result from the direct action of snake and spider venoms on the red blood cell. Although cobra venom is directly lytic in vitro, the clinical disease induced by the bite of the cobra is one of moderate hemolysis associated with spherocytosis. Spider bites are known to induce acute intravascular hemolysis associated with spherocytosis. It is thought that the brown recluse spider which inhabits the central and southern portions of the United States and portions of South America is responsible. The hemolytic disease continues for several days up to 1 week.

Copper has a direct hemolytic effect on red blood cells. Hemolysis has been observed following exposure of individuals to copper salts (such as during hemodialysis). In addition, the transient episodes of hemolysis observed in patients with Wilson's disease are probably due to copper toxicity.

The red blood cell membrane is unstable at temperatures above 49°C. When studied in vitro, the red blood cell undergoes a process of budding, cleavage, and resealing above this temperature. The same process is observed in individuals who have suffered extensive burns. Hemoglobinemia and hemoglobinuria may accompany this process, and spherocytosis is prominent.

MEMBRANE ABNORMALITIES

ACQUIRED DISORDERS OF THE MEMBRANE There are two well-defined acquired disorders of the red blood cell membrane: spur-cell anemia and paroxysmal nocturnal hemoglobinuria (PNH).

Spur-cell anemia Hemolytic anemia with bizarre-shaped red blood cells occurs in some patients with severe hepatocellular disease. Most patients with spur-cell anemia have advanced Laennec's cirrhosis. This hemolytic disorder is observed in approximately 5 percent of patients with manifestations of severe cirrhosis, such as ascites, jaundice, and hepatic encephalopathy. Spur-cell anemia has also been reported in neonatal hepatitis.

CLINICAL MANIFESTATIONS Anemia is moderate to severe, with hematocrit levels ranging from 16 to 30 percent. Thus, the anemia is more severe than is observed in otherwise uncomplicated cirrhosis, in which hematocrit levels are rarely below 28 percent, unless there is accompanying folic acid deficiency, blood loss, iron deficiency, etc. (Chap. 328). Splenomegaly is a constant feature, and the spleen is generally more prominent than in patients who have cirrhosis but who do not have spur-cell anemia. Jaundice is also a constant feature, and hepatic encephalopathy is common. Other tests of liver function are similar to values obtained in most patients with severe cirrhosis, although there is a tendency to longer prothrombin times. Chromium half-survival times of red blood cells are decreased to as short as 6 days (normal being 26 to 32 days), and red cell destruction is localized to the spleen. Normal transfused red blood cells have a survival similar to that of the patient's own red blood cells. Red blood cells are irregularly shaped with multiple spicules, and a small number of bizarre-shaped fragments are commonly seen on peripheral blood smears (see Plate 9-8). Reticulocytes range from 5 to 15 percent.

PATHOGENESIS The surface membrane of spur cells contains 50 to 70 percent excess cholesterol, but its total phospholipid content is normal. In this way, spur cells are distinct from the more usual target red blood cells in liver disease, which possess an excess of both cholesterol and phospholipid. Cholesterol out of proportion of phospholipid decreases the fluidity of the spur-cell membrane, and therefore cell deformability. Normal red blood cells acquire the spur abnormality when incubated in serum from affected patients. This results from the presence in serum of an abnormal low-density lipoprotein with an increased mole ratio of free (unesterified) cholesterol to phospholipid. Thus, red blood cells in spur-cell anemia may be considered to be "innocent bystanders." These rigid, cholesterol-laden red blood cells are detected by the filtering system of the spleen, aided by congestive splenomegaly in cirrhosis. In contrast to circulating spur cells, normal red blood cells which have acquired cholesterol in vitro have an increased surface area and a decreased osmotic fragility, and they have a regular pattern of spicule deformity. This is also true in vivo for normal red blood cells during their initial 24 h in the circulation. However, during continued circulation in vivo in the presence of the spleen, cholesterol-rich spur cells lose surface area and transform to the irregular pattern of spiculation associated with acanthocytes (see "Red Blood Cell Morphology" above). This process of membrane "conditioning" by the spleen continues, and the cell is destroyed in the spleen.

DIAGNOSIS Increasing anemia in a patient with chronic cirrhosis most commonly results from blood loss, folic acid deficiency, or iron deficiency. The hemolytic rate may increase transiently during periods of acute fatty liver. The combination of an elevated reticulocyte count and elevated bilirubin in the presence of the characteristic morphologic abnormality on peripheral blood smear is diagnostic. Red blood cells of similar morphologic appearance are seen in patients with abetalipoproteinemia. However, these individuals have a minimal amount of hemolysis.

Spur cells and acanthocytes must be distinguished from regularly scalloped, crenated red blood cells (echinocytes). These are a frequent artifact on blood smears, and they are present in some patients with uremia ("burr cells") (Plate 9-9). Small, dense crenated spheres (spheroechinocytes) are sometimes seen in congenital nonspherocytic hemolytic anemia due to enzyme deficiencies in the Embden-Meyerhof pathway.

TREATMENT Since normal red blood cells acquire the spur abnormality when transfused into patients with this form of anemia, transfusion therapy is of limited benefit. Attempts to influence red blood cell cholesterol by the use of various lipid-lowering agents have thus far been unsuccessful. Splenectomy has been reported to prevent both the conditioning of red blood cells in the spleen and their premature destruction. However, splenectomy carries a high risk in patients with severe liver disease complicated by portal hypertension and coagulation defects, and it must be reserved for selected patients in whom hemolysis is a major clinical problem and who appear to be relatively good surgical risks.

PROGNOSIS In most patients spur-cell anemia occurs during the late stages of cirrhosis, and more than 90 percent of patients succumb to their underlying liver disease within 1 year of the diagnosis of spur-cell anemia.

Paroxysmal nocturnal hemoglobinuria (PNH) This condition is distinctive among hemolytic disorders in humans because it is an acquired, intracorpuscular defect. It occurs primarily in young adults.

CLINICAL MANIFESTATIONS Anemia is of exceedingly variable degree with hematocrit values of 20 percent and lower in occasional patients and normal values in others. Mild granulocytopenia and thrombocytopenia are commonly present. Although regarded as a classic feature of this disease, gross hemoglobinuria is present only intermittently in most patients, and never occurs in some. Hemosiderinuria is usually present. Other features of diagnostic significance are a low leukocyte alkaline phosphatase and a low red blood cell acetylcholinesterase. Red blood cells are normochromic and normocytic unless iron deficiency has occurred from the chronic loss of iron in the urine. The diagnosis is established by a positive acid hemolysis test or sucrose lysis test, both of which demonstrate the enhanced sensitivity of PNH red blood cells to complement (see below). Venous thromboses are a common complication of this disorder, and they have been reported in peripheral veins as well as in mesenteric, hepatic, portal, and cerebral veins. Thromboses are a common cause of death in patients severely affected with PNH. A second complication, possibly related to thromboses in small veins, is the occurrence of back and abdominal pain similar in character to that which occurs in sickle cell anemia. Headache has also been reported. Since the widespread use of the sucrose lysis test, many patients have been discovered with mild, chronic disease.

PATHOGENESIS The underlying abnormality which affects red blood cells, granulocytes, and platelets in PNH is an inordinate sensitivity to complement. This may be demonstrated in vitro using a complement-fixing antibody. PNH red blood cells fix more C1 than normal red cells per unit of antibody present, and this C1 promotes more C3 fixation per molecule of C1 than is seen with normal red cells. However, antibody is not necessary for the lysis of red blood cells in PNH. Rather, C3 is readily fixed to the red blood cell surface by means of the alternate (properdin) pathway. Careful analytic procedures have demonstrated two and in some cases three separate populations of red blood cells with varying sensitivities to complement in patients with PNH. The clinical manifestations relate directly to the proportion of the red blood cells produced that are most sensitive to complement. Although platelets share with red blood cells this sensitivity to complement, platelet survival is normal in PNH. However, a functional modification of platelets induced by complement may underlie the thrombotic complications of this disease.

Since it affects granulocytes, platelets, and red blood cells but not lymphocytes, this defect is thought to occur because of an acquired change in the pluripotent stem cell which generates these cells. In this respect it is similar to both acute myelogenous leukemia and the myeloproliferative syndromes, disorders which appear to affect the stem cells responsible for platelet, granulocyte, and red blood cell production. Both acute myelogenous leukemia and PNH may be secondary manifestations of a primary bone marrow injury that is manifested initially as aplastic anemia. Moreover, a number of patients with PNH have subsequently developed acute myelogenous leukemia. The red blood cell abnormality characteristic of PNH (complement sensitivity) occurs to a mild degree in some patients with aplastic anemia and in some with myelofibrosis, further linking this series of bone marrow disorders. Thus, although the precise mechanism has not been identified, it appears likely that PNH results from a mutation in the marrow stem-cell pool. The exact phenotypic representation of this presumed mutation is not known.

DIAGNOSIS As indicated above, PNH is commonly undiagnosed for a period of months to years. The classic manifestation of gross hemoglobinuria may be present only intermittently, and an awareness of its presence may be obtained only by repeated questioning of the patient. In some patients, a chronic hemolytic process occurs without gross hemoglobinuria. Therefore, diagnoses such as refractory anemia, hemolytic anemia of unknown etiology, and pancytopenia are common in patients subsequently proven to have PNH. A decreased leukocyte alkaline phosphatase is a clue to the diagnosis, and the presence of hemosiderin in the urine sediment is strongly suggestive. Hemosiderinuria may occur with intravascular hemolysis of any etiology. However, only a few disorders in humans result in intravascular hemolysis. These are PNH, paroxysmal cold hemoglobinuria, hemolytic transfusion reaction, traumatic hemolysis, and hemolysis due to lysins (snake venom, *C. welchii* bacteremia) or to extensive acute burns. The acid hemolysis test is also positive in the rare congenital disorder, hereditary erythrocytic multinuclearity with positive acidified-serum test (HEMPAS). In this latter disorder, complement sensitivity results from an inordinate fixation of C4 molecules per molecule of C1. Since this sensitivity exists in the classic (antibody-mediated) pathway but not in the alternate (properdin) pathway, spontaneous fixation of complement with lysis in vivo is not a feature of the HEMPAS disorder.

It should be noted that chromium survival studies often produce information which is confusing in PNH. This results from the bi- or trimodal population of red blood cells. The cells most sensitive to complement have a very short survival, and they account for a minority of circulating red blood cells, whereas the cells less sensitive to complement have a more normal survival and account for the majority of circulating cells. Thus, the chromium survival is longer than might be anticipated from other measures of hemoglobin turnover.

TREATMENT Transfusion therapy is useful in PNH not only for raising the hemoglobin level but also for suppressing the marrow production of red blood cells during episodes of sustained hemoglobinuria or of sustained painful crisis. The transfusion of blood prior to surgery may reduce the incidence of postoperative thrombotic complications. For reasons that are still unclear, whole blood transfusions frequently cause an exacerbation of the hemolytic process. This can be prevented by using washed red blood cells rather than whole blood.

Therapy with androgens frequently results in a rise of hemoglobin level. Adrenocortical steroids may also be effective in reducing the rate of hemolysis.

Because of iron loss in the urine, iron deficiency is common. An exacerbation of hemolysis often follows the administration of iron because of the formation of a large number of young red blood cells, many of which are sensitive to complement. This may be minimized by suppressing the bone marrow with transfusions.

Splenectomy has been undertaken in some patients with the hope of decreasing the hemolytic rate and the transfusion requirement. However, because of the limited therapeutic benefit and the high risk attendant upon surgery in patients with PNH, splenectomy cannot be recommended.

Anticoagulation with coumarin-type drugs may have some benefit in preventing thromboses, particularly in the postsurgical patient. On the other hand, therapy with heparin has been noted to cause an increased amount of hemolysis in some patients with PNH, and caution must be exercised when using this drug.

PROGNOSIS Most patients with classic PNH have a life expectancy of less than 10 years, although some survive for much longer. A recent series of 17 patients surviving more than 20 years was compiled by questioning hematologists nationally. In more than one-third of these patients, there had been an amelioration of disease symptoms, and in two patients PNH was totally quiescent. The major morbidity relates to venous thromboses. Despite the overwhelming degree of iron deposition in the kidney, death from renal failure is rare. The prognosis is uncertain in patients in whom the manifestations of PNH are more subtle and in whom the diagnosis was made because of the widespread use of the sucrose lysis test. Some patients may lead a normal life.

CONGENITAL ABNORMALITIES OF THE RED CELL MEMBRANE There are three types of inherited abnormalities of the red cell membrane: hereditary spherocytosis, hereditary elliptocytosis, and hereditary stomatocytosis. Each syndrome may represent a group of disorders with a differing structural basis. The molecular nature underlying these disorders has not been completely defined.

Hereditary spherocytosis This is a disease of autosomal dominant inheritance in which intrinsically abnormal red blood cells are destroyed in the presence of an otherwise normal spleen. Its incidence is approximately 1:4500. In 20 percent of patients the absence of hematologic abnormalities in family members suggests that a spontaneous mutation has occurred. The disorder is sometimes clinically apparent in early infancy, but often escapes detection until adult life.

CLINICAL MANIFESTATIONS The major clinical features of hereditary spherocytosis are anemia, splenomegaly, and jaundice. The prominence of the latter finding accounts for its prior designation "congenital hemolytic jaundice" and is due to an increased concentration of unconjugated (indirect-reacting) bilirubin in plasma. Jaundice may be intermittent and tends to be less pronounced in early childhood. Because of the increased bile pigment production, gallstones of pigment type are common, even in childhood. Compensatory normoblastic hyperplasia of the bone marrow occurs with the extension of red marrow into the midshafts of long bones and occasionally with extramedullary erythropoiesis, at times leading to the formation of paravertebral masses visible on chest x-ray. Because the bone marrow's capacity to increase erythropoiesis by six- to tenfold exceeds the usual rate of hemolysis in this disease, anemia is usually mild or moderate and may even be absent in an otherwise healthy individual. Compensation may be temporarily interrupted by episodes of erythroid hypoplasia precipitated by infections, often of a minor nature. Splenomegaly is a constant feature of hereditary spherocytosis. The hemolytic rate may increase transiently during systemic infections which induce further splenic enlargement. Chronic leg ulcers, similar to those observed in sickle cell anemia, occasionally occur.

The characteristic erythrocyte abnormality is the spherocyte (Plate 9-10). The mean corpuscular volume (MCV) is usually normal or slightly decreased, and the mean corpuscular hemoglobin concentration (MCHC) is increased to 35 to 38 g/dl. Spheroidicity may be quantitatively assessed in terms of osmotic fragility (Fig. 329-1). Because spherocytes have a decreased surface area per unit volume, they lyse more readily when exposed to solutions of low salt concentration. On microscopic examination spherocytes are usually detected even when present in very small numbers (see Plate 9-10). However, they will ordinarily not influence the osmotic fragility test unless they constitute more than 1 or 2 percent of the total cell population. A prominent increase in the osmotic fragility of red blood cells following sterile incubation of whole blood for 24 h at 37°C is also characteristic of hereditary spherocytosis. The autohemolysis test is an extension of this latter procedure and measures the amount of spontaneous hemolysis occurring after 48 h of sterile incubation. In hereditary spherocytosis about 10 to 50 percent of the red blood cells are lysed (versus less than 4 percent of normal red blood cells). Autohemolysis of these red blood cells is largely prevented by the addition of glucose prior to incubation.

PATHOGENESIS Although the molecular abnormality in hereditary spherocytosis is unknown, it is likely that it involves the proteins of the cytoskeleton. The spheroidal contour and

FIGURE 329-1
Osmotic fragility of red blood cells in hereditary spherocytosis. When the spleen is present, a small subpopulation of cells which are "conditioned" in the spleen form the fragile "tail" of the osmotic fragility curve. After splenectomy a single population exists which is more osmotically fragile than normal.

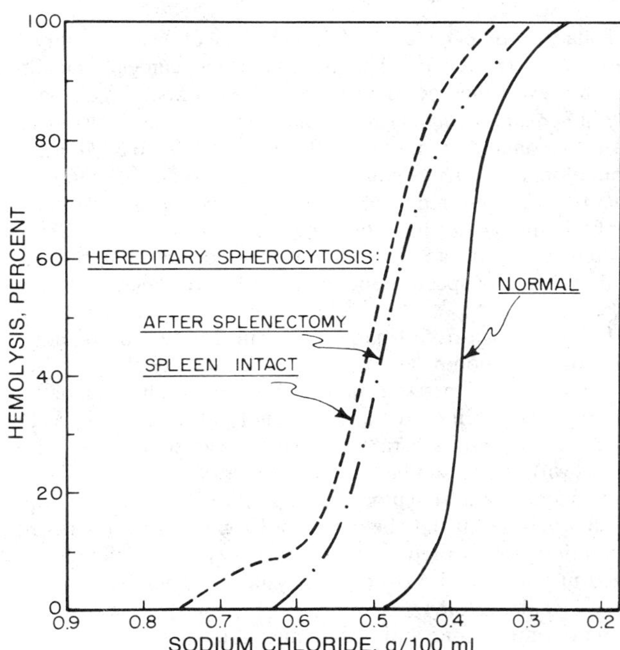

rigid structure of the red blood cells impede their passage through the spleen. There, the red blood cells are exposed to an environment in which their increased metabolic rate cannot be sustained. The first injury imposed upon them by the spleen is a further loss of surface membrane "conditioning," which produces a subpopulation of hyperspheroidal red blood cells in the peripheral blood. These are subsequently destroyed in the spleen. The intracorpuscular nature of the red blood cell defect in hereditary spherocytosis is demonstrated by a diminished life span of the patient's red cells in normal subjects when the spleen is present and a normal survival of normal cells transfused into patients with hereditary spherocytosis.

DIAGNOSIS Hereditary spherocytosis must be distinguished from the spherocytic hemolytic anemias associated with red blood cell antibodies. The family history is helpful, when present. The diagnosis of immune spherocytosis is usually readily established by a positive direct Coombs test. Autohemolysis is increased in immune spherocytosis, but it is not corrected by glucose. Spherocytes, often in considerable numbers, are seen in association with hemolysis induced by splenomegaly in patients with cirrhosis or chronic infections, and a few spherocytes are seen in the course of a wide variety of hemolytic processes, particularly glucose 6-phosphate dehydrogenase deficiency.

TREATMENT AND PROGNOSIS Splenectomy reliably corrects the anemia, although the red blood cell defect persists. The operative risk is low. Red blood cell survival after splenectomy is normal or nearly so. Rare relapses have been reported and are probably attributable to postoperative growth of splenic autotransplants or to hyperplasia of secondary spleens which were overlooked at operation. Because of the potential for gallstones and for episodes of bone marrow hypoplasia or hemolytic crises, splenectomy should be performed in most individuals with hereditary spherocytosis, even those with mild anemia. Splenectomy in children should be postponed until the age of 4 years, if possible, although it may be performed at any age. Beyond age 3, severe infections following splenectomy in hereditary spherocytosis are rare. Because of the increased requirement for folic acid in patients with hemolysis, they sometimes become deficient in this vitamin. Therapy with folic acid may result in an increased hemoglobin level.

Hereditary elliptocytosis Red blood cells of oval or elliptic shape are normally found in birds, reptiles, camels, and llamas; however, they occur in appreciable numbers in humans only in *hereditary elliptocytosis,* a disorder which is transmitted as an autosomal dominant and affects 1 per 4000 to 5000 of the population, a frequency similar to that of hereditary spherocytosis. It is also referred to as *hereditary ovalocytosis.* Less commonly, homozygotes have been encountered with an absence of a red cell membrane protein that is important in stabilizing the interaction of spectrin and actin in the cytoskeleton (Chap. 54).

The great majority of patients manifest only mild hemolysis, with hemoglobin levels above 12 g/dl, reticulocytes less than 4 percent, depressed haptoglobin levels, and red blood cell survivals within or just under the normal range. In 10 to 15 percent of patients the rate of hemolysis is substantially increased with chromium half-survival times of red blood cells as short as 5 days and reticulocytes ranging to 20 percent. Hemoglobin levels rarely fall below 9 to 10 g/dl. Red blood cell destruction occurs predominantly in the spleen, which is enlarged in patients with overt hemolysis, and hemolysis is corrected by splenectomy.

In both the anemic and nonanemic varieties of this disorder the red blood cells are normochromic and normocytic. At least 25 percent and, more commonly, greater than 75 percent of red blood cells are elliptic, with an axial ratio (width/length) of less than 0.78. Patients with hemolysis frequently have microovalocytes, bizarre-shaped red blood cells, and red cell fragments, and these increase in number following splenectomy. The degree of hemolysis does not correlate with the percentage of elliptocytes. Osmotic fragility is usually normal but may be increased in patients with overt hemolysis. The pathogenesis of the red blood cell defect is thought to be similar to that of hereditary spherocytosis.

Hereditary stomatocytosis Stomatocytes are red blood cells having a slit-like central zone of pallor on dried smears. The syndrome of hereditary hemolytic anemia and stomatocytic red blood cells is inherited in an autosomal dominant pattern. It may represent a number of discrete entities. Two major red blood cell defects have been delineated in this syndrome. First, the red blood cells have an increased permeability to sodium and potassium, which is compensated for by an increased active transport of these cations. Second, red cells have an increased surface area associated with an increase in membrane lipid content. In some patients, the red blood cell is swollen with an excess of ions and water and a decreased mean corpuscular hemoglobin concentration (overhydrated stomatocytes, "hydrocytosis"); in other patients the red cell is shrunken with a decreased ion and water content and an increased mean corpuscular hemoglobin concentration (dehydrated stomatocytes, "desiccytosis"). Those patients in whom the red blood cells are overhydrated have true stomatocytes on dried smears. Dehydrated stomatocytes assume the morphology of target cells on dried smears. In both instances, red blood cells are cup- or bowl-shaped when examined in wet preparation. Osmotic fragility is increased in overhydrated stomatocytes and decreased in underhydrated stomatocytes. Autohemolysis is increased and is corrected by glucose.

Most patients have splenomegaly and mild anemia. Splenectomy decreases but does not totally correct the hemolytic process. Its indications are similar to those for hereditary spherocytosis.

DISORDERS OF THE INTERIOR OF THE RED CELL

RED CELL ENZYME DEFECTS During its maturation, the red blood cell loses its nucleus, ribosomes, and mitochondria and thus its capability for protein synthesis and oxidative phosphorylation. The mature circulating red blood cell has a relatively simple pattern of intermediary metabolism (Fig. 329-2) in keeping with its modest metabolic obligations. As discussed in Chap. 54, some ATP must be generated from the Embden-Meyerhof pathway to drive the cation pump which maintains the ionic milieu within the red blood cell. Smaller amounts of energy are needed for the preservation of hemoglobin iron in the ferrous (Fe^{2+}) state, and perhaps for the renewal of the lipids in the red blood cell membrane. About 10 percent of the glucose consumed by the red blood cell is metabolized via the hexose-monophosphate shunt (Fig. 329-2). This pathway protects both hemoglobin and the membrane from exogenous oxidants including certain drugs.

Studies of red blood cell enzyme defects have provided valuable information on the metabolic control of normal erythrocytes. Figure 329-2 shows a large number of recognized specific enzyme deficiency states affecting the glycolytic pathway or the hexose-monophosphate shunt. Many of these enzyme abnormalities appear to be restricted to red blood cells. The long life span of the red blood cell and its inability to synthesize proteins poses a challenge to the stability of its enzymes. Therefore, a mutation resulting in decreased stability will be expressed more readily in the red blood cell compared with other tissues. In other cases, nonerythroid cells may contain isoenzymes that have normal function and stability.

Defects in the Embden-Meyerhof pathway Deficiencies of most of the enzymes of the Embden-Meyerhof (or glycolytic) pathway have been reported. In general, all these enzymopathies have similar pathophysiologic and clinical features. Patients present with a congenital nonspherocytic hemolytic anemia of variable severity. The red blood cells are often relatively deficient in ATP, considering their young age. As a result, there is an increased leak of potassium ion from inside these cells. Abnormalities in red blood cell morphology (see below) also indicate that the red cell membrane is secondarily affected by the enzyme defect. These red blood cells are apt to be rigid and thus more readily sequestered by the mononuclear-phagocyte system.

Some of these glycolytic enzyme deficiencies such as pyruvate kinase (PK) deficiency and hexokinase deficiency are localized to the red blood cell. There is no apparent metabolic abnormality in leukocytes or other cells that have been studied. In other disorders, the enzyme deficiency is more widespread. Glucose phosphate isomerase deficiency and phosphoglycerate kinase deficiency also involve leukocytes, although affected individuals have no apparent abnormalities of white blood cell function. Individuals with deficiency of triose phosphate isomerase have decreased levels of enzyme in leukocytes, muscle cells, and central nervous system fluid. Furthermore, they have a progressive neurologic disorder. Some patients with phosphofructokinase deficiency have a myopathy.

Among the reported defects of glycolytic enzymes, about 95 percent are due to PK deficiency and about 4 percent are due to glucose phosphate isomerase deficiency. The remainder shown in Fig. 329-2 are extremely rare. Most have been encountered in isolated families. There is considerable variability in the clinical manifestation and laboratory findings among reported cases of PK deficiency. This is probably due to the fact that a number of different PK variants have been reported. This heterogeneity probably also applies to the other less common glycolytic enzyme defects. Accordingly, the clinical manifestations of these disorders are quite variable.

GENETICS Most of the glycolytic enzyme defects are inherited in an autosomal recessive pattern. Thus, the parents of affected patients are heterozygotes. Heterozygotes generally possess half-normal levels of enzyme activity which are more than adequate for normal metabolic function. Thus, these individuals are entirely asymptomatic. Since the gene frequency for this group of enzymopathies is low, it is not surprising that true homozygotes are often the offspring of a consanguinous mating. Alternatively, affected individuals may be double heterozygotes, inheriting an abnormal allele from each parent. Phosphoglycerate kinase deficiency is inherited as a sex-linked disorder. Affected males have a severe hemolytic anemia while female carriers may have a mild hemolytic process.

CLINICAL MANIFESTATIONS Patients with severe hemolysis usually present during early childhood with anemia, icterus,

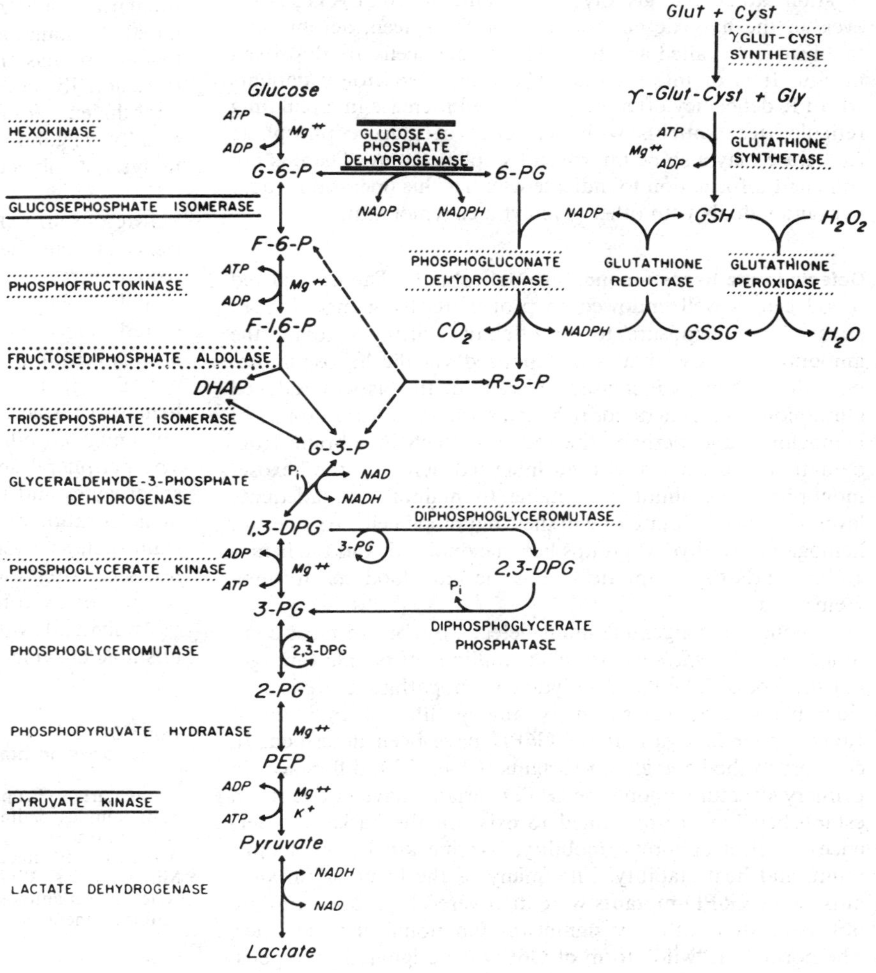

FIGURE 329-2
Metabolic pathways in the red blood cell. The glycolytic pathway is outlined vertically from glucose to lactate. The pentose phosphate pathway is shown on the right. Known enzyme deficiency states are shown. Bold solid lines denote common states, light solid lines less common ones, and dotted lines rare ones. (From WN Valentine, Semin Hematol 8:309, 1971.)

and splenomegaly. Other stigmata of chronic hemolysis are occasionally seen. Occasionally, siblings are similarly affected.

LABORATORY FINDINGS Patients have a normocytic (or slightly macrocytic) normochromic anemia with reticulocytosis. In those with PK deficiency, bizarre erythrocytes are noted on the peripheral smear with large numbers of spiculated red blood cells. Spherocytes are usually infrequent or absent. Hence, the term *congenital nonspherocytic hemolytic anemia* has been applied to these disorders. Unlike hereditary spherocytosis, the osmotic fragility of freshly drawn blood is usually normal. Incubation brings out an osmotically fragile population of red blood cells. When a blood specimen is incubated under sterile conditions for 48 h, an abnormal amount of "autohemolysis" is noted. In contrast to hereditary spherocytosis, the degree of autohemolysis in these disorders is not corrected by the addition of glucose.

The diagnosis of this group of anemias depends upon specific enzymatic assays. An abnormality in enzyme kinetics may be demonstrated. In addition, differences in electrophoretic mobility, pH optimum, or heat stability may be noted. This information is useful in documenting heterogeneity among enzyme variants.

TREATMENT Most patients do not require therapy. Those with severe hemolysis should be given a daily supplement of folic acid (1 mg per day). Blood transfusions may be necessary during a hypoplastic crisis. Patients with PK deficiency may be benefited by splenectomy. Because of their enzymatic defect, the younger cells (reticulocytes) depend on mitochondrial respiration rather than glycolysis for maintenance of ATP. However, in the hypoxic environment of the spleen, aerobic metabolism is curtailed and the ATP-depleted cells are destroyed in situ. It is of interest that following splenectomy patients with PK deficiency often have a marked increase in circulating reticulocytes. Patients with deficiency of glucose phosphate isomerase may also be improved by splenectomy. There is not sufficient information to indicate whether this operation would help individuals with other glycolytic enzymopathies.

Defects in the hexose-monophosphate shunt The normal red blood cell is well endowed to protect itself against oxidant stress. Upon exposure to an offending drug or toxin, the amount of glucose that is metabolized via the hexose-monophosphate shunt is increased severalfold. In this way reduced glutathione is regenerated, protecting the sulfhydryl groups of hemoglobin and perhaps the red blood cell membrane from oxidation. Individuals with an inherited defect in the hexose-monophosphate shunt are unable to maintain an adequate level of reduced glutathione in their red blood cells. As a result, hemoglobin sulfhydryl groups become oxidized, and the hemoglobin tends to precipitate within the red blood cell forming Heinz bodies.

Among the congenital shunt defects, by far the most common is *G6PD deficiency.* It affects millions of people throughout the world. Like the glycolytic enzymopathies, there is considerable genetic heterogeneity among affected individuals. Indeed, over 250 variants of G6PD have been described. In contrast to the hemoglobin variants (Chap. 330) differences in primary structure among the G6PD variants have not yet been established but are presumed to exist on the basis of differences in electrophoretic mobility, enzyme kinetics, pH optimum, and heat stability. Like many of the hemoglobin variants, some G6PD mutants were discovered by chance and are not associated with any significant functional abnormalities. The normal or "wild" form of G6PD is designated by type B. About 20 percent of blacks have a G6PD (designated A+) which differs electrophoretically but is functionally normal. Among the clinically significant G6PD variants, the most common is the so-called A− type encountered primarily in blacks who originated from central Africa. The A− G6PD has the same electrophoretic mobility as the A+ type, but it is unstable and has abnormal kinetic properties. Like the HbS gene, the A− type of G6PD may confer protection against malaria. This variant is found in about 15 percent of black males in the United States. A second relatively common G6PD variant is encountered among peoples of the eastern Mediterranean area, particularly Sephardic Jews.

The G6PD gene is located on the X chromosome. Thus the deficiency state is a sex-linked trait. Affected males (hemizygotes) inherit the abnormal gene from their mothers who are usually carriers (heterozygotes). Because of inactivation of one of the two X chromosomes (Lyon hypothesis, see Chap. 58), the heterozygote has two populations of red blood cells: normal and deficient in G6PD. Most female carriers are asymptomatic. Those who happen to have a high proportion of deficient cells resemble the male hemizygotes.

G6PD activity normally declines about 50 percent during the 120-day life span of the red blood cell. This decay is moderately accelerated in A− red blood cells and markedly so in red blood cells containing the Mediterranean variant. Individuals with the A− variant may have a slightly shortened red blood cell survival, but they are not anemic. Clinical problems arise only when the affected individual is subjected to some type of environmental stress. Most often, hemolytic episodes are triggered by viral and bacterial infections. The mechanism for this is unknown. Drugs or toxins which pose an oxidant threat to the red blood cell also cause hemolysis in individuals deficient in G6PD (see Table 329-5). Of these, sulfa drugs, antimalarials, and nitrofurantoin are most commonly incriminated. Although aspirin is frequently mentioned as a likely offender, it has no deleterious effect in A− individuals. Occasionally, accidental ingestion of toxic compounds such as naphthalene (found in moth balls) can cause severe hemolysis. Finally, metabolic acidosis can precipitate an episode of hemolysis in subjects deficient in G6PD.

CLINICAL AND LABORATORY FEATURES The patient may experience an acute hemolytic crisis within hours of exposure to the oxidant stress. In severe cases, hemoglobinuria and peripheral vascular collapse can develop. Since only the older population of red blood cells is rapidly destroyed, the hemolytic crisis is usually self-limited, even if the exposure to the oxidant continues. During the period of acute hemolysis, a rapid drop in hematocrit is accompanied by a rise in plasma hemoglobin and unconjugated bilirubin and a decrease in plasma haptoglobin. The peripheral smear is often unimpressive, but on occasion spherocytes and fragmented red blood cells may be seen. The demonstration of Heinz bodies requires the use of a supravital stain such as crystal violet. However, Heinz bodies are usually not seen after the first day or so, since these inclusions are readily removed by the spleen.

Individuals with the *Mediterranean type G6PD* have a more unstable enzyme and, therefore, a much lower overall enzyme

TABLE 329-5
Drugs causing hemolysis in subjects deficient in G6PD

Antimalarials: Primaquine, pamaquine, chloroquine, dapsone
Sulfonamides: Sulfanilamide, sulfasoxazole, etc.
Nitrofurantoin
Analgesics: Phenacetin, acetanilid
Miscellaneous: Vitamin K (water-soluble form), probenecid, methylene blue, *p*-aminosalicylic acid, nalidixic acid, quinine,* quinidine,* chloramphenicol*

* *Not known to cause hemolysis in blacks with A− type G6PD.*

activity than blacks with the A− variant. As a result, they have more severe clinical manifestations. Some have a chronic hemolytic anemia, even in the absence of any exposure to oxidants. A minority of patients are exquisitely sensitive to fava beans and will develop a fulminant hemolytic crisis following exposure. Sensitivity to *Vicia fava* is a poorly understood phenomenon that appears to be determined by a separate gene. Favism is not encountered in blacks with the A− variant. Individuals with the Mediterranean variant sometimes have a temporary episode of hemolysis during the newborn period.

The *diagnosis* of G6PD deficiency should be considered in any individual, particularly a black male, who experiences an acute hemolytic episode. The patient should be thoroughly questioned about possible exposure to oxidant agents. A number of screening tests are available to establish the diagnosis. However, since the deficiency occurs primarily in older red blood cells, a false-negative test may be seen during a hemolytic episode when there is a high proportion of young red blood cells. It may be necessary to repeat these diagnostic tests after the patient has recovered. Unusual features in the case should prompt further investigation including a more complete and specific characterization of the enzyme.

TREATMENT Since hemolysis in patients deficient in A− G6PD is usually self-limited, no specific treatment is necessary. Splenectomy does not appear to be of benefit to Mediterranean patients with chronic hemolysis. Blood transfusions are rarely indicated. If a patient develops a severe hemolytic episode with hemoglobinuria, maintaining adequate urine output is important.

Attention should be directed toward the *prevention* of hemolytic episodes. Infections ought to be treated promptly. Subjects deficient in G6PD should be warned about risks posed by oxidant drugs and fava beans. Any black patient about to be given an oxidant drug should be screened for G6PD deficiency.

OTHER DEFECTS OF THE HEXOSE-MONOPHOSPHATE SHUNT A few kindreds have been found to have congenital deficiency in red blood cell glutathione due to a defect in either of the two enzymes responsible for the synthesis of this tripeptide. Affected individuals have a hemolytic anemia with Heinz bodies that is aggravated by oxidant drugs. Deficiency of glutathione reductase has been reported, but its relationship to clinically significant hemolysis is not well established. Sometimes the deficiency state can be corrected by the administration of riboflavin (5 mg per day). There are also isolated reports of deficiencies of glutathione peroxidase and 6-phosphogluconate dehydrogenase, but, again, their association with hemolysis is uncertain.

Other enzyme defects Hemolytic anemia may sometimes be caused by abnormalities in enzymes of nucleotide metabolism. A growing number of individuals with pyrimidine 5′-nucleotidase deficiency have been encountered. Their red cells have marked basophilic stippling. Hemolytic anemia has also been noted in individuals whose red blood cells have supranormal levels of adenosine deaminase and relatively low levels of ATP.

HEMOGLOBINOPATHIES The sickling disorders constitute an important form of congenital hemolytic anemia. Less commonly, hemolysis may be due to the inheritance of an unstable hemoglobin variant. These disorders of hemoglobin are discussed in Chap. 330.

REFERENCES

ANTMAN KH et al: Microangiopathic hemolytic anemia and cancer: A review. Medicine 58:377, 1979

BALLAS SK: Disorders of the red cell membrane: A reclassification of hemolytic anemias. Am J Med Sci 276:4, 1978

BEUTLER E: Red cell enzyme defects as nondiseases and as diseases. Blood 54:1, 1979

BERKOWITZ LR et al: Thrombotic thrombocytopenic purpura: A pathology review. JAMA 241:1709, 1979

BUKOWSKI RM et al: Therapy of thrombotic thrombocytopenic purpura: An overview. Semin Throm Hemo 7:1, 1981

COOPER RA: Abnormalities of cell-membrane fluidity in the pathogenesis of disease. N Engl J Med 297:371, 1977

——— et al: Role of the spleen in membrane conditioning and hemolysis of spur cells in liver disease. N Engl J Med 290:1279, 1974

FORGET BG: Hemolytic anemias, congenital and acquired. Hosp Prac 15:4, 1980

FRANK MM et al: Pathophysiology of immune hemolytic anemias. Ann Intern Med 87:210, 1977

GORDON-SMITH EC: Drug-induced oxidative haemolysis. Clin Haematol 9:557, 1980

LUX SE: Spectrin-actin membrane skeleton of normal and abnormal red blood cells. Semin Hematol 16:21, 1979

MAGALHAES RL et al: Microangiopathic hemolytic anemia in renal allotransplantation. Am J Med 58:862, 1975

PETZ LD, GARRATTY G: *Acquired Immune Hemolytic Anemias.* New York, Churchill Livingstone, 1980

PISCIOTTA AV: Thrombotic thrombocytopenic purpura. Ann Intern Med 92:249, 1980

VALENTINE WN: The Stratton lecture: Hemolytic anemia and inborn errors of metabolism. Blood 54:549, 1979

WILEY JS et al: Characteristics of the membrane defect in the hereditary stomatocytosis syndrome. Blood 46:337, 1975

330 DISORDERS OF HEMOGLOBIN STRUCTURE, FUNCTION, AND SYNTHESIS

H. FRANKLIN BUNN

In 1910, Herrick described a medical student from Jamaica who had a hemolytic anemia in conjunction with elongated "sickled" red blood cells on blood smear. Subsequently, it was shown that all the red blood cells of such patients assume a classic holly leaf or sickle shape following deoxygenation of the blood. In 1949, Itano and Pauling showed that sickle cell anemia was associated with an electrophoretically abnormal hemoglobin. Eight years later, Ingram demonstrated that this hemoglobin (designated HbS) differed from normal HbA by the substitution of valine for glutamic acid at the sixth position of the β chain. Since then, over 350 structurally different human hemoglobin variants have been discovered in widely scattered parts of the world. Generally, a new hemoglobin is named after the place where it is first encountered. No more than a third of these mutant hemoglobins are associated with significant clinical manifestations. The remainder have been discovered by serendipity or as a result of large population surveys. All told, the hemoglobinopathies have taught us many valuable lessons in such diverse areas as the mechanisms underlying red blood cell destruction, the pathophysiology of oxygen transport, the stereochemistry of hemoglobin function, and the genetic bases of protein synthesis.

This chapter focuses on the clinically significant variants. In addition, disorders of the biosynthesis of globin (the thalassemias) and methemoglobinemia are discussed.

GENETIC CONSIDERATIONS The synthesis of each of the subunits of hemoglobin (α, β, γ, δ, ε, ζ) is governed by separate genes. The ε and ζ subunits are found only in embryonic hemoglobin. Normal individuals inherit two β-chain genes (one from each parent), four α-chain genes, and four γ-chain genes. The ε-, γ-, δ-, and β-chain genes occupy adjacent loci on chromosome 11. The ζ and α genes are located on chromosome 16. The structure and function of normal hemoglobin ($\alpha_2\beta_2$) are discussed in Chap. 54. The inheritance of abnormal hemoglobins follows classic mendelian genetics. If two parents are heterozygous for a hemoglobin variant such as HbS, statistically one-quarter of the offspring will be SS homozygotes, another quarter will be normal (AA genotype), and half will have sickle trait (AS) (Fig. 330-1). The commonly encountered hemoglobinopathies such as S, C, and E are β-chain variants. Occasionally, an individual inherits two different β-chain variants, one from each parent. Hemoglobin SC disease is an example of such a double heterozygous state. The gene for β thalassemia is very closely linked to the β-chain structural gene. Therefore, the two genes can be considered allelic. Accordingly, an individual can inherit from one parent (and pass on to a child) either β thalassemia or a β-chain variant, but not both. Among the hemoglobinopathies associated with sickling (described below), only the homozygous state (Hb SS) or double heterozygous state (SThal or SC) has important clinical manifestations. In contrast, the unstable variants and those having abnormal oxygen-binding properties are encountered only in heterozygotes. In many cases, the homozygous state would be incompatible with life.

About 90 percent of these abnormal hemoglobins are single amino acid substitutions, due to a single base substitution in the corresponding triplet codon. The structural information accumulated on human mutant hemoglobins has provided ample verification of the fidelity of the genetic code. Other genetic mechanisms must be invoked to explain the structure of a few interesting hemoglobin variants. The Lepore hemoglobins have arisen because of nonhomologous crossover between the adjacent δ- and β-chain genes, giving rise to a fusion subunit in which the *N*-terminal end has the amino acid sequence of the δ chain and the *C*-terminal end has the sequence of the β chain. Some of the unstable hemoglobins have deletions of one or more residues in sequence within a subunit. Finally there are a few variants which have elongated subunits (e.g., Hb Constant Spring). These have arisen either because of a base substitution in the termination codon or because of a frame shift which puts the termination codon out of phase.

CLINICAL CLASSIFICATION The clinically significant hemoglobin variants are classified in Table 330-1. By far the most important and prevalent type of hemoglobinopathy is due to the presence of sickle hemoglobin, either in the homozygous state or in conjunction with another type of hemoglobin abnormality. The inheritance of an unstable hemoglobin variant may give rise to congenital hemolytic anemia associated with the presence of inclusions of precipitated hemoglobin within the red blood cells (Heinz bodies). Finally, hemoglobin variants may have abnormal functional or spectral properties, resulting in familial erythrocytosis or familial cyanosis.

SICKLE SYNDROMES

SICKLE CELL TRAIT About 8 percent of black Americans are heterozygous for HbS. The gene frequency is highest in central Africa, particularly in regions where malaria is endemic. In some parts of Nigeria, over 30 percent of the population has sickle trait. The gene has persisted because heterozygotes gain a slight protection against falciparum malaria. This is a well-accepted form of balanced polymorphism.

The diagnosis of sickle trait or any of the other sickle syndromes depends upon the demonstration of sickling under reduced oxygen tension. In the widely used sickle preparation, sickled cells can be visualized microscopically after the addition of an oxygen-consuming reagent such as metabisulfite. Many clinical laboratories prefer a solubility test which depends on the fact that deoxyhemoglobin S has a low solubility at high ionic strength. Hemoglobin S also has an increased rate of surface denaturation and will form a precipitate when a dilute solution is shaken vigorously. All these tests are reasonably specific for HbS although some of the unstable variants may give false-positive solubility and mechanical precipitation tests. Therefore, if one of these screening tests is positive, hemoglobin electrophoresis should be performed. Individuals with sickle trait usually have about 35 percent HbS and 60 percent HbA.

Hemoglobin S heterozygotes have minimal clinical prob-

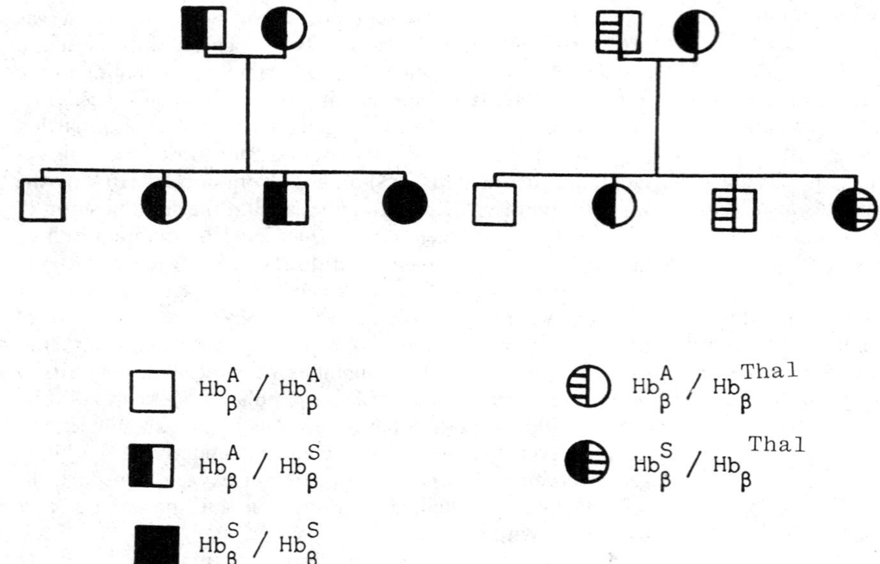

FIGURE 330-1
Diagram of family trees showing inheritance of the homozygous state, sickle cell anemia, SS (left) and the double heterozygous state, sickle β thalassemia (right).

lems. Their overall life expectancy and frequency of hospitalization are no different from those of a comparable group of individuals with hemoglobin A. AS red blood cells require a much lower oxygen tension for sickling than SS red cells. Accordingly, individuals with sickle trait may develop sickle cell crises only if they become severely hypoxic. They may occasionally sustain a splenic infarct. As discussed below, the renal medulla is particularly susceptible to sickling. Many AS individuals have impaired ability to form concentrated urine, and a few have recurrent episodes of painless hematuria as a result of medullary infarction. Infarction due to sickling has been encountered in other organs in sickle trait but is extremely rare. For these reasons, AS individuals should not be placed in any high-risk group for employment or insurance considerations.

SICKLE CELL ANEMIA Sickle cell anemia is a significant cause of morbidity and mortality among black individuals. About 0.15 percent of black children in the United States have the disease. The prevalence is lower among adults because patients with sickle cell anemia have a decreased life expectancy. The protean clinical manifestations of this disorder can all be attributed to a specific molecular lesion: the substitution of valine for glutamic acid at the sixth residue of the β chain.

Molecular pathogenesis Upon deoxygenation, a red blood cell containing HbS changes from a biconcave disk to an elongated crescent-shaped or "sickle"-shaped cell (see Plate 9-6). Electron micrographs, shown in Fig. 330-2, reveal the presence of fibers having a diameter of about 20 nm. It is likely that each sickle fiber consists of a helical polymer with four strands in an inner core and 10 strands in an outer sheath. Both hydrophobic and electrostatic bonds are involved in the stabilization of the helical polymer. In addition, there are probably interactions between neighboring fibers. Sickling, both within the intact red blood cell and in free solution, is greatly affected by the presence of non-S hemoglobin. HbA participates more readily than HbF in copolymerization with HbS.

Cellular pathogenesis As discussed in Chap. 54, the ability of red blood cells to traverse the microcirculation depends in large part on their pliability. As a red blood cell sickles, it becomes rigid, and, as a result, may obstruct capillary blood flow. The deoxygenation of blood from patients with sickle cell disease is associated with a marked increase in viscosity. It is likely that obstruction to flow leads to local tissue hypoxia. As a result, further deoxygenation takes place, leading to further sickling. This vicious cycle may result in the amplification of microscopic obstruction into a larger area of infarction. The oxygen-dependent sickle cycle is ordinarily reversible. However, the membrane of SS red blood cells may become sufficiently damaged so that the cells lose potassium and water, leading to the formation of irreversibly sickled forms. In these cells, the characteristic sickle shape persists even after they are exposed to ambient oxygen tension at room temperature and can readily be seen on examination of Wright-stained blood films (see Plate 9-6). The proportion of irreversibly sickled cells varies considerably among homozygous sicklers and is not correlated with clinical severity. Hemoglobin F is distributed unevenly among red blood cells of SS patients, and composes between 2 and 20 percent of the total hemoglobin (the remainder is almost entirely HbS). Since HbF inhibits the polymerization of HbS, those cells that are relatively rich in HbF are protected from sickling, whereas those cells that have relatively small amounts of HbF are likely to become irreversibly sickled. It is not surprising that these rigid cells are readily culled from the circulation and destroyed. The continuous formation and destruction of irreversibly sickled cells probably contributes significantly to the severe hemolytic anemia shared by all patients with sickle cell anemia. Furthermore, these rigid cells may initiate small-vessel occlusions.

Factors such as acidosis or increased erythrocyte 2,3-DPG, which lower the oxygen affinity of red blood cells, will enhance the formation of deoxyhemoglobin and, therefore, promote intracellular polymerization and eventual sickling. In addition, sickling is highly dependent on hemoglobin concentration. Any pathophysiologic process which tends to pull water out of sickle red blood cells will greatly increase their tendency to sickle. Thus, the hypertonic environment of the renal medulla can cause local sickling and the formation of papillary infarcts, even in individuals with sickle trait.

Clinical manifestations Patients with homozygous sickle cell anemia have a variety of clinical problems broadly outlined in Table 330-2. Signs and symptoms usually do not appear until after the sixth month of life, at which time most of the HbF has been replaced by HbS. Among the *constitutional* manifestations of sickle cell anemia are impairment of growth and devel-

TABLE 330-1
Clinically important hemoglobin variants

I Sickle syndromes
- *A* Sickle cell trait (AS)
- *B* Sickle cell anemia (SS)
- *C* Double heterozygous states: Sickle β thalassemia, sickle C disease (SC), sickle D disease (SD)

II Unstable hemoglobin variants (congenital Heinz body hemolytic anemia)

III Variants with high oxygen affinity: Hb Chesapeake, Hb Yakima, Hb Kempsey, Hb Mälmo, etc.

IV M hemoglobins (see Table 330-3)

FIGURE 330-2
Electron micrograph of deoxygenated SS hemoglobin. A. Transverse section showing bundles of fibers, each about 18 nm in diameter. B. Longitudinal section cut parallel to the long axis of sickling. (From JT Finch et al, Proc Nat Acad Sci USA 70:718, 1973.)

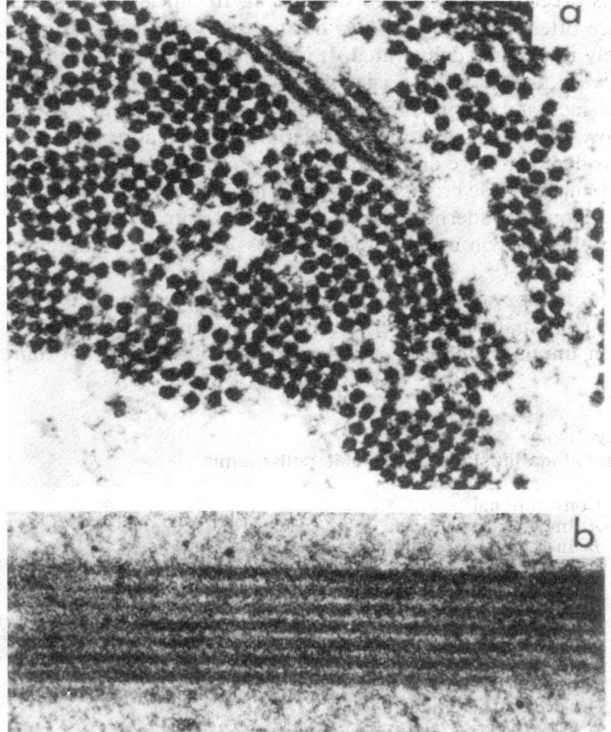

opment and a general failure to thrive. In addition, these patients have an increased tendency to develop serious infections, particularly due to pneumococcus. Sicklers have marked impairment of splenic function, preventing effective clearance of circulating bacteria. With the passage of time, the organ sustains recurrent infarcts and eventually becomes a nubbin of fibrous tissue.

ANEMIA SS homozygotes have a severe hemolytic anemia with hematocrit values between 18 and 30 percent. The destruction of red blood cells is independent of cell age. The mean red blood cell survival is about 10 to 15 days. Those cells having relatively low levels of HbF have a shorter life span, in part due to a greater chance of becoming irreversibly sickled. As a result of accelerated red blood cell breakdown, patients with sickle cell disease have characteristic clinical and laboratory findings discussed in Chap. 54. Even though hemolysis is primarily extravascular, plasma haptoglobin is generally low or absent, and plasma hemoglobin levels are moderately elevated.

The anemia becomes increasingly severe if erythropoiesis is suppressed. There are two main causes of "aplastic crises"—infection and folic acid deficiency. As discussed in Chap. 328, infection brings about a transient reduction in red blood cell production. In SS patients with severe ongoing hemolysis, this usually results in a rapid drop in hematocrit (Table 330-2).

VASOOCCLUSIVE PHENOMENA The morbidity and mortality of sickle cell disease are due primarily to recurrent vasoocclusive phenomena. As shown in Table 330-2, these can be divided into two groups. Throughout their lives, sicklers are plagued by recurrent *painful crises.* These episodes may appear with explosive suddenness and attack various parts of the body, particularly the abdomen, chest, and joints. About a third of painful crises are preceded by a viral or bacterial infection (Table 330-2). The frequency of painful crises is highly variable. A given patient may have months or even years without a crisis and then have a cluster of frequent severe attacks. In some individuals, crises occur more frequently in cold weather, perhaps precipitated by reflex vasospasm. In others, crises come more often in warm weather, during times when patients are likely to become dehydrated. It is often difficult to distinguish between painful sickle crisis and some other type of acute process such as biliary colic, appendicitis, or a perforated viscus. Many patients have undergone exploration because they were considered to have an acute surgical problem. Patients having abdominal sickle crises usually have normal bowel sounds and no rebound tenderness. If the abdominal pain is due to sickling, the surgeon usually finds no gross evidence of infarction or ischemia.

SS homozygotes frequently develop attacks of acute pleuritic chest pain with fever. Although the initial chest x-ray is often unremarkable, an infiltrate may evolve. The important

TABLE 330-2
Clinical manifestations of sickle cell anemia

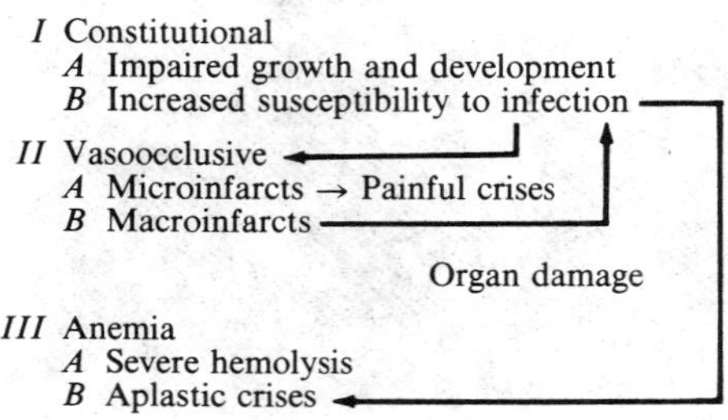
I Constitutional
A Impaired growth and development
B Increased susceptibility to infection
II Vasoocclusive
A Microinfarcts → Painful crises
B Macroinfarcts
Organ damage
III Anemia
A Severe hemolysis
B Aplastic crises

differential is between pneumonitis and pulmonary infarction. Culture and Gram's stain of the sputum will be helpful in establishing the presence of pneumonia. In these patients, pulmonary infarctions are more likely due to thrombosis in situ than to emboli. Occasionally, pulmonary infarcts become secondarily infected.

When a sickle crisis is localized in the extremities, it may mimic osteomyelitis or an acute arthritis such as gout or rheumatoid arthritis. Patients commonly develop acute synovitis with joint effusion. Examination of the joint fluid is helpful in this differential diagnosis. If the effusion is due to sickling, the fluid will be clear and yellow, with a low white blood cell count (100 to 1000 mononuclear cells per cubic millimeter) and an absence of crystals or bacteria. Synovial biopsy may show sickled red blood cells in the lumen of small vessels.

Sickle crises may occasionally involve the central nervous system. Patients can present with a seizure, stroke, or coma. Although such crises are frequently reversible, they may be fatal.

CHRONIC ORGAN DAMAGE By the time that patients reach adulthood, there is often objective evidence of anatomic or functional damage to various tissues, due to the cumulative effect of recurrent vasoocclusive episodes. Almost any organ may be involved, but most commonly the lungs, kidneys, liver, skeleton, and skin.

Cardiopulmonary. Impairment of pulmonary function is a common complication of sickle cell disease. Resting arterial P_{O_2} is usually reduced in part because of intrapulmonary arterial-venous shunting. Since SS red blood cells have decreased oxygen affinity, arterial blood will be significantly undersaturated, leading to an increased tendency for red cells to sickle when they reach the peripheral circulation. SS homozygotes frequently develop congestive heart failure. The chronic severe anemia and hypoxemia impose a sustained burden on the heart. Most patients have a systolic ejection murmur as a result of their hyperdynamic circulation. Even though more oxygen is extracted by the myocardium than any other tissue, SS patients rarely develop myocardial infarction.

Hepatobiliary. Like other patients with congenital hemolytic anemia, those with sickle cell anemia have icterus and an increased tendency to form gallstones. It is often difficult to distinguish between the abdominal pain of acute cholecystitis and that due to a sickle crisis. Jaundice deepens markedly if a patient develops choledocholithiasis, and bilirubin levels as high as 50 mg/dl have been reported. As a rule, cholecystectomy is not recommended unless gallstones cause symptoms. In addition, patients with sickle cell anemia may develop hepatic infarcts which occasionally become infected, resulting in abscess formation. If a significant portion of hepatic parenchyma becomes infarcted, fibrosis and deterioration of liver function may result, with deepening of jaundice.

Genitourinary (see also Chaps. 295 and 298). The hypertonic and acidic environment of the renal medulla promotes sickling, resulting in microinfarcts. Virtually all patients have isosthenuria. The inability of the patient with sickle cell anemia to form concentrated urine means an increased risk of becoming significantly dehydrated. In addition, like those with sickle trait or SC disease, SS homozygotes may develop significant and prolonged painless hematuria as a result of papillary infarcts. Hematuria may be so extensive that iron deficiency develops. ε-Aminocaproic acid has proved to be effective in severe cases but must be used with caution since it may prevent the lysis of clots in the renal pelvis.

A small number of patients develop frank renal failure, sometimes following the nephrotic syndrome. The pathogenesis of the glomerular lesions is not well understood. Mild nitrogen retention is commonly encountered, accompanied by moderate hyperuricemia. However, patients rarely have uric acid nephropathy or gout. Male patients with sickle cell anemia occasionally develop priapism (spontaneous and painful engorgement of the penis). This distressing complication occurs with about equal frequency in prepubertal and postpubertal patients, although the latter are more difficult to treat and may develop impotence following the acute episode. Patients should be treated conservatively with sedation, analgesia, and intravenous fluids. The administration of packed red blood cells may also be effective. Surgical intervention is rarely indicated.

Skeletal. Like other patients with congenital hemolytic anemia, patients with sickle cell anemia demonstrate radiologic abnormalities due to the expansion of red marrow. However, the development of bony infarcts results in more characteristic x-ray abnormalities. The biconcave or "fishmouth" vertebrae are pathognomonic of sickle cell disease. Skeletal infarction generally leads to increased bony trabeculation and sclerosis. Aseptic necrosis of the head of the femur is particularly common in patients with sickle cell disease and can lead to considerable disability. Like infarcts in other organs, bony infarctions are more likely to become infected. In patients who develop osteomyelitis, salmonella is a frequent pathogen.

Ocular. A variety of ocular abnormalities are encountered in patients with SS and SC disease. These include retinal infarcts, peripheral vessel disease, arteriovenous anomalies, vitreous hemorrhage, retinitis proliferans, and retinal detachment. In addition, when viewed with a strong magnifying lens, angulated and "corkscrew" vessels can be seen in the bulbar conjunctiva. The major ocular complications are more commonly encountered in SC patients than in SS patients. The early diagnosis of retinal lesions in SC and SS disease is important since retinal detachment may be prevented by appropriate therapy.

Skin. Chronic skin ulcers often occur in the distal lower extremities. The lesions appear to be commoner in patients with more severe anemia. Ankle ulcers have also been encountered in rare patients with other types of congenital hemolytic anemia. This complication is more commonly seen in tropical areas. Ankle ulcers generally respond to conservative management, such as elevation of the leg, maintenance of strict cleanliness, and application of a mild chemical debriding agent such as Dakin's solution. The weekly application of Unna boots has been effective. In patients with refractory ulcers, a hypertransfusion regimen is probably indicated. Skin grafting should be undertaken only after all other measures have failed.

Neurologic. A variety of central nervous system manifestations may be encountered in sickle cell anemia. Although cerebral thrombosis is the principal neurologic complication, SS patients also have an increased incidence of subarachnoid hemorrhage. A patient has about a 25 percent chance of developing some type of neurologic complication during his lifetime. Hemiplegia is encountered more frequently than coma, convulsions, or visual disturbances. Patients generally make a full recovery, particularly from their first cerebral vascular accident. Preliminary studies in children indicate that a hypertransfusion program is beneficial to those who have sustained a major neurologic complication.

Diagnosis The diagnosis of sickle cell anemia should be considered in any black patient with a hemolytic anemia. The history of painful crises, arthropathy, ankle ulcers, etc., can be very helpful. If a patient has a relatively mild form of the disease, the diagnosis may not have been made during childhood. A number of laboratory tests are useful in distinguishing sickle cell anemia from other hemoglobinopathies. Examination of the peripheral blood smear reveals normochromic normocytic red blood cells, many of which appear as targets. The presence of irreversibly sickled forms is very helpful (see Plate 9-6). In addition, the presence of Howell-Jolly bodies, siderocytes, and occasional normoblasts suggests the absence of effective splenic function. A positive test for sickling, such as the metabisulfite preparation or the solubility test, indicates the presence of HbS but does not distinguish between SS, AS, and double heterozygotes (SThal, SC). Hemoglobin electrophoresis is necessary to establish the diagnosis. Patients with homozygous sickle cell anemia have about 2 to 20 percent HbF and 2 to 4 percent HbA_2. The remainder is HbS. No HbA is detected unless the patient has been transfused within the past 4 months. Patients with sickle thalassemia will have hypochromic microcytic red blood cells, fewer irreversibly sickled forms, and a variable proportion of HbA (0 to 30 percent). SC diseases can be readily diagnosed by hemoglobin electrophoresis. In hemoglobin SD disease, the two hemoglobin variants comigrate during conventional electrophoresis at pH 8.6 but can be separated by agar gel electrophoresis at pH 6.0.

Treatment The understanding of the molecular pathogenesis of sickling has not yet led to an effective form of therapy. A large array of antisickling regimens has been proposed with varying rationale, but thus far none has stood the test of time. Currently accepted management of sickle cell anemia is primarily supportive and conservative. Since patients with sickle cell anemia are at increased risk of developing infections, many of which trigger painful and aplastic crises, it is very important to detect infection early and give appropriate antibiotics promptly. Malaria prophylaxis should be administered in endemic areas. The development of pneumococcal sepsis in children may be prevented by the administration of the polyvalent vaccine.

The anemia of sickle cell disease increases markedly if the patient becomes deficient in folic acid. Since these patients have a continuous increased requirement for folic acid, it is reasonable to maintain them on a daily oral supplement. Testosterone has been demonstrated to increase the red blood cell mass in patients with sickle cell anemia. However, the potential risk of hepatotoxicity, and of priapism in males, limits its utility.

Painful crises should be treated promptly with adequate analgesia and hydration. Some patients feel that their crises can be aborted if treated early. Therefore, it is reasonable to give patients a supply of analgesics such as codeine or meperidine which can be taken at home. However, these patients are at high risk of becoming addicted to opiates. Oxygen should be administered during acute pain crisis if the patient has arterial hypoxemia.

Blood transfusions play a limited role in the management of sickle cell anemia. Between crises, patients tolerate anemia quite well and do not derive much subjective benefit from transfusions. However, partial replacement of the patients' red blood cells by transfused red cells (hypertransfusion) may be an effective way of preventing vasoocclusive crises. In order to lower the viscosity of the patient's blood significantly, it is necessary that over 50 percent of the patient's red blood cells be of donor origin. Hypertransfusion is a reasonable approach to getting a patient through a limited period of risk such as pregnancy or surgery. However, the problems of isoimmunization, iron overload, and hepatitis dictate against its widespread use.

Prevention Genetic counseling can play an important role in the prevention of sickle cell anemia. If both marital partners are AS heterozygotes, they may elect not to have children, knowing that there is a 25 percent chance that their offspring will be homozygous. The antenatal diagnosis of sickle cell anemia can be made in the second trimester of pregnancy by obtaining fetal cells from the amniotic fluid and analyzing the

DNA following digestion with a restriction endonuclease that recognizes the $\beta 6$ valine mutation. If it is established that the fetus is a SS homozygote, the parents may decide to interrupt the pregnancy.

Prognosis The clinical course of patients with sickle cell anemia is highly variable. Many assessments of prognosis that have appeared in the literature have been unduly pessimistic. During the past 30 years there has been considerable improvement in the care of patients with sickle cell anemia. In the United States, an increasing number of patients are surviving into adulthood and even bearing offspring. There has also been a decline in the mortality of SS mothers during pregnancy and childbirth. However, in underdeveloped nations, the mortality in sickle cell anemia remains very high.

No single clinical or laboratory finding is a consistent predictor of prognosis in sickle cell disease. Although those patients who have relatively high amounts of HbF tend to have milder clinical manifestations, this relationship is of no prognostic value in any given patient. Considerable variation in the severity of sickle cell disease has been reported among different ethnic and geographical groups. A group of Shi Arabs from Saudi Arabia has been found to have a very benign form of sickle cell anemia with very high levels of HbF (15 to 30 percent). A mild type of sickle cell anemia has also been seen among the Veddoids of India. SS patients with coexisting α-thalassemia have less severe hemolysis but do not appear to have a significant reduction in vasoocclusive phenomena.

SICKLE β THALASSEMIA This disease is highly variable in its clinical severity and complications. It is commonly encountered in people from the Mediterranean countries as well as those from central Africa. Sickle β thalassemia tends to be milder in blacks, just as homozygous β thalassemia is much less severe in blacks than in the Mediterranean populations. Patients have a congenital hemolytic anemia of variable severity, accompanied by splenomegaly in about 70 percent of cases. They may have all the various types of vasoocclusive phenomena described above for homozygous sickle cell anemia. However, painful crises are generally less frequent and less severe.

Examination of the blood film reveals hypochromic microcytic red blood cells, with polychromatophilia, target cells, stippling, and rare fixed sickle forms. The electrophoretic pattern shows from 60 to 90 percent HbS and 10 to 30 percent HbF. Hemoglobin A will be about 10 to 30 percent if the β-thalassemia gene is capable of producing some β^A chains (β^+ thalassemia, see below). In patients who have sickle β^0 thalassemia, no HbA will be present, and therefore the disorder may be difficult to distinguish from homozygous sickle cell anemia. Hemoglobin A_2 is moderately elevated in sickle β thalassemia, but it is difficult to measure this minor component accurately in the presence of HbS. Most patients with sickle β thalassemia do not require close medical attention or specific therapy. Occasional patients may derive benefit from splenectomy if the spleen is sequestering a significant amount of red blood cells.

SICKLE C DISEASE Although the gene frequency for HbC ($\alpha_2\beta_2{}^{6\mathrm{Glu}\rightarrow\mathrm{Lys}}$) is only one-fourth that for HbS, the prevalence of SC disease among adults is almost as high as SS disease since the former group of patients has a nearly normal life expectancy. These individuals have a mild to moderate hemolytic anemia, usually accompanied by splenomegaly. On peripheral blood smears, target cells and occasional plump sickled forms are seen. Hemoglobin electrophoresis reveals 50 percent HbS, 50 percent HbC. Hemoglobin S copolymerizes with HbC to the same extent as with HbA. The increased tendency of SC red cells to sickle, compared with sickle trait cells, can be explained by two phenomena: increased intracellular hemoglobin concentration and significantly higher-percent HbS. Patients with SC disease may occasionally have painful crises or organ infarcts. They are at particular risk of developing ocular complications described above, including proliferative retinopathy and retinal detachment. In addition, patients with SC disease are at relatively high risk of developing hematuria from renal medullary infarcts and avascular necrosis of the femoral heads. Pregnant women with SC disease have a high rate of complications during pregnancy. Individuals with an electrophoretic pattern suggestive of Hb SC disease but with more severe clinical manifestations are likely to be double heterozygotes for HbS and HbO Arab ($\alpha_2\beta_2{}^{121\mathrm{Glu}\rightarrow\mathrm{Lys}}$).

SICKLE D DISEASE A number of hemoglobins comigrate with HbS on routine electrophoresis. The most commonly encountered variant is HbD Los Angeles ($\alpha_2\beta_2{}^{121\mathrm{Glu}\rightarrow\mathrm{Gln}}$). Hemoglobins S and D can be separated by special electrophoretic methods. The diagnosis of Hb SD disease is suggested by the demonstration of a positive sickle cell preparation in only one of the patient's two parents. SD double heterozygotes have moderately severe anemia.

HOMOZYGOUS HbC DISEASE This disease is a mild congenital hemolytic anemia accompanied by splenomegaly. Red blood cells of CC individuals have markedly increased intracellular hemoglobin concentration. Hemoglobin C has a tendency to form intracellular crystals, particularly if red blood cells are suspended in a hypertonic medium. The blood film reveals striking target cells. Red blood cell osmotic fragility is decreased. Patients rarely develop significant complications. No specific therapy is indicated.

UNSTABLE HEMOGLOBIN VARIANTS

In the early 1950s a group of patients in England were found to have congenital nonspherocytic hemolytic anemia associated with inclusions of precipitated hemoglobin (Heinz bodies) within red blood cells. The presence of an abnormal hemoglobin was suspected by the fact that a precipitate was formed when the patients' hemolysates were gently heated. Currently, over 80 different unstable hemoglobin variants have been identified. The great majority are single amino acid substitutions in the β chain. A few are due to deletion of one or more amino acids within the β chain. Patients present with a hemolytic anemia of variable degree. Severe cases are usually detected in late infancy or early childhood and have jaundice, splenomegaly, and dark-colored urine. An autosomal dominant mode of inheritance can usually be established, although about a fifth of the cases appear to be spontaneous mutants.

Pathogenesis These hemoglobin variants have structural alterations at sites in the molecule that drastically affect its stability and solubility. Many involve an amino acid substitution in the portion of the subunit where heme is inserted. In such instances, the heme may be displaced from the heme pocket. As a result, the abnormal hemoglobin has decreased solubility and forms an intracellular precipitate (Heinz body). Red blood cells which contain this type of inclusion are recognized by the mononuclear-phagocyte system and are either cleansed of their intracellular debris (pitting) or destroyed. The displaced heme moiety is aberrantly catabolized, forming dipyrroles, such as mesobilifuscin, instead of bilirubin. Pigmenturia is probably due to the excretion of these dipyrroles. The degree of instability of these hemoglobin variants and, therefore, the extent of hemolysis vary considerably. In some, such as Hb Zürich, an additional oxidant stress, such as the ingestion of certain drugs, is required for significant hemolysis. In contrast, patients with Hb Hammersmith have continuous and marked red blood cell breakdown. The degree of anemia is influenced not only by the severity of the hemolysis but also by the ability of the blood to unload oxygen. Thus, patients having unstable variants with increased oxygen affinity, such as Hb Köln, may have a near-normal hemoglobin level, i.e., compensated hemolysis. In contrast, the hemoglobin level is apt to be much lower in patients having variants with decreased oxygen affinity such as Hb Hammersmith.

Diagnosis The red blood cell morphology is somewhat variable. Often, patients with a functioning spleen have normal-appearing red blood cells. Slight hypochromia and basophilic stippling are not uncommon. The blood may have to be incubated in order to bring out Heinz bodies. In some cases, red blood cells appear as if a bite had been taken from a margin. It is tempting to speculate that at this site a Heinz body had been pitted. Following splenectomy, red blood cells appear much more abnormal, and Heinz bodies are larger and more numerous. The extent of clinical symptomatology varies markedly with the degree of anemia.

The diagnosis of a congenital Heinz body hemolytic anemia is established by the following laboratory tests and results:

1 *Hemoglobin electrophoresis* will often reveal an abnormal component, usually composing less than 30 percent of the total.
2 *Heinz bodies* can be demonstrated by incubating a freshly drawn sample of blood with a supravital strain.
3 A significant *precipitate* is formed when the hemolysate is incubated at 50°C, or in the presence of 17% isopropanol.
4 The unstable hemoglobins often have an abnormal *oxygen dissociation curve.*

If these tests are negative in a patient with congenital nonspherocytic hemolytic anemia, a defect of one of the red blood cell enzymes is likely.

Treatment The treatment of congenital Heinz body hemolytic anemia is primarily supportive. Anemia is rarely severe enough to warrant blood transfusion. Oxidant drugs should be avoided. Like others with chronic hemolysis, these patients have an increased requirement for folic acid. Those with severe hemolysis should benefit from prophylactic folate therapy. The red blood cell mass may fall during a period of bone marrow suppression, such as that resulting from folate deficiency or acute infection. Although patients with severe hemolysis may benefit from splenectomy, this operation is not curative. Because of the risk of bacterial sepsis in infants and young children who have been splenectomized, this treatment should be postponed until the child is over 4 years old. The diagnostic tests cited above become more abnormal following splenectomy. For this reason, in some cases the diagnosis may not be definitely established until after the operation.

STABLE VARIANTS HAVING ABNORMAL O_2 AFFINITY

In 1966 certain members of a large family were discovered to have erythrocytosis in association with an electrophoretically abnormal hemoglobin, Hb Chesapeake, which had a very high affinity for oxygen. Since then, more than 30 other stable hemoglobin variants have been encountered which also have a significant increase in oxygen affinity. Their structural alterations tend to be at sites which influence hemoglobin's functional behavior. As a result of the hemoglobin's increased oxygen affinity, oxygen unloading to tissues is decreased, and there is an erythropoietin-mediated stimulus to erythropoiesis. Accordingly, these individuals have secondary erythrocytosis. This disorder is manifested in the heterozygous state and fol-

lows an autosomal codominant pattern of inheritance. Hematocrit levels are rarely high enough to cause a significant increase in blood viscosity. Thus, affected individuals are generally asymptomatic and lack any pertinent physical findings other than a ruddy complexion. The diagnosis should be suspected in all patients with unexplained erythrocytosis, particularly when other family members are similarly affected, and can be established by the demonstration of increased oxygen affinity of the whole blood. About two-thirds of the high affinity variants can be readily separated from HbA by electrophoresis. No treatment is indicated. The patient should be reassured that the disorder is benign.

Hemoglobin variants having a marked decrease in oxygen affinity cause one form of familial cyanosis (Table 330-3). Except for this cosmetic problem, affected individuals have no other clinical manifestations. Because of the abnormality of hemoglobin function, arterial blood is partially unsaturated despite normal oxygen tension. Thus, the cyanosis is due to increased levels of deoxyhemoglobin in the blood. Blood values are otherwise normal.

METHEMOGLOBINEMIA

Oxygen transport depends on the maintenance of intracellular hemoglobin in the reduced (Fe^{2+}) state. When hemoglobin is oxidized to methemoglobin, the heme iron becomes Fe^{3+} and is incapable of binding oxygen. Normal red cells contain less than 1 percent methemoglobin. A small amount of hemoglobin autooxidizes as red cells circulate. This process probably occurs by the dissociation of the superoxide anion from oxyhemoglobin:

$$Hb^{2+}O_2 \rightarrow Hb^{3+} + O_2^-$$

Normally, the methemoglobin that is formed is reduced by the following reaction:

$$Hb^{3+} + \text{RedCyt } b_5 \rightarrow Hb^{2+} + \text{OxCyt } b_5$$

Reduced cytochrome b_5 (RedCyt b_5) is regenerated by the enzyme cytochrome b_5 reductase (methemoglobin reductase):

$$\text{OxCyt } b_5 + \text{NADH} \xrightarrow[\text{reductase}]{\text{Cytochrome } b_5} \text{RedCyt } b_5 + \text{NAD}$$

Hereditary methemoglobinemia is due either to the presence of one of the M hemoglobins or to the deficiency of the

TABLE 330-3
Differential diagnosis of cyanosis

I Decreased oxygenation of hemoglobin (↑ deoxyhemoglobin)
- *A* Reduced arterial oxygen tension (common)
  - *1* Pulmonary disease
  - *2* Cardiac right-to-left shunt
- *B* Hemoglobin variant having decreased oxygen affinity (rare): Hb Kansas, Hb Beth Israel

II Methemoglobinemia (rare)
- *A* Hereditary
  - *1* M hemoglobins:
    - *a* HbM Boston ($\alpha_2^{58His \rightarrow Tyr}\beta_2$)
    - *b* HbM Iwate ($\alpha_2^{87His \rightarrow Tyr}\beta_2$)
    - *c* HbM Saskatoon ($\alpha_2\beta_2^{63His \rightarrow Tyr}$)
    - *d* HbM Hyde Park ($\alpha_2\beta_2^{92His \rightarrow Tyr}$)
    - *e* HbM Milwaukee ($\alpha_2\beta_2^{67Val \rightarrow Glu}$)
  - *2* Cytochrome b_5 reductase deficiency
- *B* Acquired
  - *1* Nitrites and nitrates: sodium nitrite, amyl nitrite, nitroglycerin, nitroprusside, silver nitrate
  - *2* Aniline dyes
  - *3* Acetanilid and phenacetin
  - *4* Sulfonamides
  - *5* Other: lidocaine, chlorate, phenazopyridine

enzyme cytochrome b_5 reductase (Table 330-3). These inherited disorders are clinically mild, while the induction of methemoglobinemia by drugs or toxins can be life threatening.

If methemoglobin exceeds 1.5 g/dl (10 percent of the total hemoglobin), affected individuals will have clinically obvious cyanosis. The color of the skin is indistinguishable from the much commoner cyanosis due to impairment of oxygen saturation that may occur in pulmonary and cardiac disorders (Table 330-3). With higher amounts of methemoglobin, patients become symptomatic. At a methemoglobin level of about 35 percent, the affected individual experiences headache, weakness, and breathlessness. Levels in excess of 80 percent are probably incompatible with life.

The toxicity of methemoglobinemia can be readily explained in terms of hemoglobin function. The fact that a certain proportion of the heme moieties is no longer able to bind oxygen is not a serious physiological handicap per se. A proportion of 30 percent methemoglobin is much more deleterious than a 30 percent decrement in red cell mass, because the oxidized hemes have a profound effect on the remaining functional hemes in the hemoglobin tetramer. The conformation of methemoglobin (like that of carboxyhemoglobin) is very similar to that of oxyhemoglobin. Thus, a partially oxidized hemoglobin tetramer has the same tertiary and quaternary structure as a molecule which is comparably oxygenated. In each case, the affinity of the remaining hemes for oxygen is increased. For this reason, methemoglobinemia (as well as carbon monoxide) causes a "shift to the left" of the oxyhemoglobin dissociation curve and, consequently, impaired unloading of oxygen to tissues.

M HEMOGLOBINS Five hemoglobin variants listed in Table 330-3 have abnormal absorbance spectra, owing to the oxidation of the heme iron in the affected subunit. They involve amino acid substitutions of residues responsible for the binding of the heme iron to the globin. These so-called M hemoglobins result in a rare form of congenital and familial cyanosis. Individuals with the α-chain variants HbM Boston and HbM Iwate are cyanotic at birth, while cyanosis does not appear in those with the β-chain variants (HbM Saskatoon, HbM Hyde Park, and HbM Milwaukee) until about 4 to 6 months of age, when fetal hemoglobin has been replaced by adult hemoglobin. As with the unstable and high-affinity variants, an autosomal codominant inheritance pattern is found. Except for cyanosis, patients are asymptomatic.

CYTOCHROME b_5 REDUCTASE (METHEMOGLOBIN REDUCTASE) DEFICIENCY This condition is inherited in an autosomal recessive pattern. The enzyme is a flavoprotein having properties similar to those of liver microsomal cytochrome b_5 reductase. The soluble erythrocyte enzyme is formed by cleavage of a hydrophobic tail from the microsomal enzyme.

Individuals with cytochrome b_5 reductase deficiency have lifelong cyanosis of variable degree, depending on the level of methemoglobin, but usually have no associated symptoms or other physical findings. Some may have mild polycythemia owing to increased oxygen affinity. Others have been noted to be mentally retarded. Untreated individuals usually have 15 to 30 percent methemoglobin. Methemoglobin levels are higher in the older population of red cells because the activity of the abnormal enzyme declines markedly with red cell age. There appears to be considerable heterogeneity in the variant enzymes from different families, as shown by differences in their electrophoretic mobility and kinetic parameters. In these ways, cytochrome b_5 reductase deficiency resembles glucose 6-phosphate dehydrogenase deficiency (Chap. 329).

ACQUIRED METHEMOGLOBINEMIA This disorder is generally due to exposure to certain drugs or toxins. Compounds which can cause clinically significant methemoglobinemia are listed in Table 330-3. Some agents such as nitrite and chlorate oxidize the heme iron directly. Others such as sulfa drugs and aniline must undergo biochemical transformation before they cause methemoglobinemia. Few if any drugs currently in use cause significant methemoglobinemia, unless the individual is unusually susceptible. As might be expected, individuals heterozygous for methemoglobin reductase deficiency are much more likely than normal individuals to develop clinically apparent methemoglobinemia after exposure to an oxidant stress. Thus, the extent of methemoglobinemia depends not only on the dose of the toxic agent but also on the susceptibility of the exposed individual.

DIAGNOSIS Methemoglobinemia should be considered in any cyanotic patient with no evidence of heart or lung disease. If the cyanosis is due to decreased oxygen saturation, a blood specimen will change from a purple to a red color upon mixing with air. In contrast, a blood specimen from a methemoglobinemic individual remains a chocolate brown color irrespective of exposure to air. Methemoglobinemia can be documented by spectroscopic examination of the hemolysate. Individuals with hereditary methemoglobinemia will have lower levels than patients symptomatic from acquired methemoglobinemia. Patients who have ingested an oxidant drug may have an additional hemoglobin derivative called sulfhemoglobin in which the heme group has been modified by covalent attachment of a sulfur atom. Sulfhemoglobinemia tends to cause cyanosis even more readily than methemoglobinemia. Unlike methemoglobin, the absorbance of sulfhemoglobin at 620 to 630 nm is not decreased by the addition of cyanide. The M hemoglobins have characteristic spectral abnormalities which differ from those obtained when normal HbA is partially oxidized. Furthermore, these hemoglobin variants can be detected by hemoglobin electrophoresis.

TREATMENT In individuals with methemoglobin reductase deficiency, the oral administration of methylene blue (100 to 300 mg per day) or ascorbic acid (300 to 500 mg per day) will result in a marked reduction in the level of methemoglobin. The purpose of treatment is primarily cosmetic. Severe toxic methemoglobinemia is treated by the intravenous administration of methylene blue (2 mg/kg, repeat if needed). Within an hour, the methemoglobin level is usually reduced by at least 50 percent. Treatment is neither necessary nor possible in individuals having HbM.

THALASSEMIAS

The thalassemias are a diverse group of congenital disorders in which there is a defect in the synthesis of one (or more) of the subunits of hemoglobin. As a result of decreased production of hemoglobin, the red blood cells are microcytic and hypochromic (Table 54-1). The thalassemias involve a spectrum ranging from subtle morphologic abnormalities to life-threatening disease. In contrast to the qualitative hemoglobin abnormalities listed in Table 330-1, the thalassemias are quantitative abnormalities of subunit synthesis. Thus, the β chains of patients with β thalassemia have normal structure but are produced in reduced and sometimes undetectable amounts. Conversely, patients with α thalassemia have impaired production of α chains. The reduction in globin chain synthesis can be demonstrated in vitro by incubating reticulocytes with labeled amino acids and determining the incorporation of radioactivity into globin subunits (Table 330-4). Most forms of thalassemia can be identified from the information summarized in Table 330-4.

Occasionally, establishing a definitive diagnosis requires measurement of globin chain synthesis or analysis of globin gene structure.

α THALASSEMIA As mentioned at the beginning of this chapter, normal individuals inherit two α-chain genes from each parent. The great majority of cases of α thalassemia can be explained by deletions of α-chain genes, owing to nonhomologous crossover. Specific gene deletions can be identified by analysis of patients' DNA following digestion by restriction endonucleases. The clinical manifestations of α thalassemia depend upon the number of genes deleted (Table 330-4). In the silent carrier state, heterozygous α thalassemia 2 ($\alpha\alpha^0/\alpha\alpha$), one of the four genes is deleted. Affected individuals have no hematologic abnormalities. Individuals with deletion of two of the four α-chain genes (α-thalassemia trait) have either homozygous α thalassemia 2 ($\alpha\alpha^0/\alpha\alpha^0$) or heterozygous α thalassemia 1 ($\alpha^0\alpha^0/\alpha\alpha$). They have microcytic and slightly hypochromic red blood cells but no significant hemolysis or anemia. Hemoglobin electrophoresis is normal except for a decreased amount of HbA_2. Deletion of three α-chain genes ($\alpha^0\alpha^0/\alpha\alpha^0$) produces a well-compensated hemolytic state with microcytic hypochromic red blood cells including many target cells. Intracellular inclusions or Heinz bodies are formed by the precipitation of HbH, a tetramer composed of β chains which accumulates because of the marked impairment of α-chain synthesis. The most severe form of α thalassemia, hydrops fetalis, is usually due to deletion of all four α-chain genes. The affected fetus has red blood cells containing only Hb Barts, a tetramer composed of γ chains. This condition is incompatible with life, since oxygen transport depends upon the presence of heterotetramers such as $\alpha_2\beta_2$ and $\alpha_2\gamma_2$. In orientals both the $\alpha\alpha^0$ and the $\alpha^0\alpha^0$ haplotypes are relatively common; thus both HbH disease and hydrops fetalis are frequently encountered. In contrast, blacks commonly have the $\alpha\alpha^0$ haplotype (gene frequency $\cong 0.15$) but rarely have the $\alpha^0\alpha^0$ haploptype. Therefore HbH disease is very rare in blacks and hydrops fetalis has not been reported. Homozygous α thalassemia 2 is encountered in about 2 percent of blacks and is therefore a relatively common cause of microcytosis in an individual who is otherwise healthy and not iron-deficient.

The elongated α-chain variant Hb Constant Spring, commonly encountered among southeast Asians, also has an α-thalassemia phenotype, and when inherited with the $\alpha^0\alpha^0$ haplotype can cause HbH disease.

β THALASSEMIA Since individuals inherit only one β-chain gene from each parent, affected individuals are either heterozygotes, homozygotes, or double heterozygotes. The gene frequency for β thalassemia approaches 10 percent in southern Italy and certain Mediterranean islands. β Thalassemia is also encountered quite commonly in central Africa, Asia, the south Pacific, and certain parts of India. Statistically, one-quarter of the offspring of two heterozygotes (β-thalassemia trait) will have the homozygous state: β thalassemia major or Cooley's anemia. An individual may inherit a β-thalassemia gene from one parent and a β-chain structural variant from the other (Fig. 330-1). Sickle β thalassemia (discussed above) is a commonly encountered example of such a double heterozygous state.

The molecular pathogenesis of the β thalassemias is more complex and heterogeneous than that of α thalassemia. In contrast to α thalassemia, gene deletion is an uncommon cause of β thalassemia. Among the recognized types of β-gene deletion, an entity known as "pancellular hereditary persistence of fetal hemoglobin" has minimal clinical manifestations owing to efficient synthesis of γ chains on the chromosome in which the β and δ genes are deleted. Hemoglobin Lepore is a variant formed from a nonhomologous crossover between the δ and β genes resulting in the absence of normal β-chain synthesis and therefore a β-thalassemia phenotype. In the great majority of cases of β thalassemia, restriction endonuclease maps reveal no gross abnormalities of the β-globin gene complex. Nevertheless, there are several steps in β-globin synthesis that could go awry and lead to a thalassemic phenotype. A number of cases involve mutations in one of the intervening sequences of the β-globin gene, leading to errors in the processing of mRNA. Others have nonsense mutations in the coding region, causing premature termination of β-globin chains.

Cellular pathogenesis As a result of imbalance in globin chain synthesis, the β thalassemias have varying degrees of ineffective erythropoiesis (Chap. 54) and hemolysis. In β thalassemia major there is a marked relative excess of α-chain production. Free α chains have decreased solubility and will form insoluble aggregates or inclusions within red blood cell precursors in the bone marrow. Like congenital Heinz body hemolytic anemia due to unstable hemoglobin variants, the inclusion bodies in thalassemia bring about abnormalities in membrane permeability as well as entrapment and destruction of red blood cells by the macrophages in the mononuclear-phagoycte system. As a result, β thalassemia is characterized by both intramedullary erythroid destruction and also a shortening of the life span of circulating red blood cells that emerge from the bone marrow. Thus, these patients have the characteristic parameters of both ineffective erythropoiesis (increased plasma iron turnover, decreased incorporation of iron into red blood cells) and peripheral hemolysis. Because these red blood

TABLE 330-4
Classification of the thalassemias

Diagnosis	*Globin chain synthesis in reticulocytes*	*RBC morphology*	*Hb electrophoresis*	*Clinical severity*
α thalassemia:	α/β*			
Silent carrier ($\alpha\alpha^0/\alpha\alpha$)	0.9	Normal	Normal, ↓ A_2	0
α-thalassemia trait [($\alpha\alpha^0/\alpha\alpha^0$) or ($\alpha^0\alpha^0/\alpha\alpha$)]	0.7	↓ MCV†	Normal	0
HbH disease ($\alpha^0\alpha^0/\alpha\alpha^0$)	0.3	↓ MCV Heinz bodies, targets	↑HbH (β_4) (10–15%)	2+
Hydrops fetalis ($\alpha^0\alpha^0/\alpha^0\alpha^0$)	0	↑↑ Nucleated RBC	↑↑ Hb Barts (γ_4)	4+
β thalassemia:	β/α*			
Heterozygous	0.5	↓ MCV, stippling	↑ A_2 (± ↑ HbF)	0 to +
Homozygous (or double heterozygous)	0–0.3	↓ MCV, hypochromic Nucleated RBC, targets bizarre shapes	↑↑ HbF	4+ (major) 2–3+ (intermedia)

* *Normal = 1.*
† *MCV = mean corpuscular volume.*

cells are under double jeopardy, there is an enormous compensatory stimulus to erythropoiesis, resulting both in expansion of the red marrow and in extramedullary hematopoiesis in the liver and spleen. Chain imbalance in β thalassemia is attenuated to a variable degree by the "compensatory" synthesis of γ chains which are able to combine with excess free α chains and form a stable tetramer (HbF). Patients with Cooley's anemia who have a relatively high rate of γ-chain production have a less severe clinical course. Individuals with β thalassemia minor have absent or very mild ineffective erythropoiesis and hemolysis, detectable in some patients by a slight elevation in fecal urobilinogen and a modest shortening of the red blood cell life span.

In the α thalassemias a relative excess production of non-α chains can be detected, leading to the formation of Hb Barts (γ_4) in the newborn and young infant. Children and adults with deletion of 3 α-globin genes usually have HbH β_4. In contrast to the α-chain inclusions found in β thalassemia, the Heinz bodies due to HbH are more stable and develop in mature circulating red blood cells. As a result, HbH disease is primarily a hemolytic disorder without a significant amount of ineffective erythropoiesis.

β thalassemia minor This common entity, also referred to as *β-thalassemia trait,* is rarely associated with significant clinical manifestations. The diagnosis is generally made in patients being evaluated for mild anemia or in follow-up of abnormalities found on routine blood studies. Most individuals with β-thalassemia trait escape diagnosis. About one-fifth of affected individuals have splenomegaly. Icterus is occasionally noted, particularly in those individuals who also have Gilbert's disease, another common and benign congenital disorder (Chap. 317).

In otherwise healthy individuals with β-thalassemia trait, the mean hemoglobin level is about 15 percent lower than in normal persons of the same age and sex; the red blood cell count is usually elevated, and the cells are microcytic. Indeed, at any level of hematocrit, patients with β thalassemia minor will have more marked microcytosis than those with iron deficiency. In contrast, the mean corpuscular hemoglobin concentration is normal. In addition to microcytosis, examination of the blood film reveals occasional target cells, cigar-shaped cells, and a moderate amount of basophilic stippling; the reticulocyte count is normal. Special isotope techniques are required to demonstrate a slightly reduced red blood cell life span. The red blood cells have decreased osmotic fragility. Serum iron is normal unless the patient also happens to be iron-deficient. Hemoglobin electrophoresis is very useful in establishing the diagnosis of β thalassemia minor. Most affected individuals will have a twofold increase in HbA_2 (5 percent versus normal of 2.5 percent). In contrast, HbA_2 is subnormal in iron deficiency and sideroblastic anemias. Patients with β-thalassemia trait who become iron-deficient usually have a "normal" level of HbA_2 which increases to above normal after correction of the deficiency. Almost half of individuals with β thalassemia minor also have moderate elevation of HbF (2 to 5 percent). In the less common state, $\delta\beta$ thalassemia, in which there is a deletion of the adjacent δ and β chain genes, HbA_2 levels will be normal, but HbF is increased (5 to 15 percent).

No treatment is indicated for individuals with β-thalassemia trait. They should be reassured that they do not have a serious hematologic problem. The genetic implications of thalassemia should be explained, particularly to those of childbearing age. Many individuals have been given long-term iron treatment on the mistaken impression that they had iron-deficiency anemia. These patients may gradually develop clinically significant siderosis. Establishing the diagnosis of β thalassemia minor should prevent such inappropriate therapy.

β thalassemia major Also termed Cooley's anemia, this is probably the most severe form of congenital hemolytic anemia. Clinical manifestations generally appear after the first 4 to 6 months of life when the switch from γ-chain to β-chain production usually occurs. Patients develop a severe anemia with a hematocrit of less than 20 unless they are supported by transfusions. Accordingly, patients have all the signs and symptoms associated with severe anemia. In addition, they have findings related to severe intramedullary and peripheral hemolysis and to iron overload. Patients with β thalassemia major often have marked wasting and appear malnourished. Children have slow rates of growth and development. In adolescents, the onset and development of secondary sex characteristics are delayed. Patients have a peculiar skin color due to a combination of icterus, pallor, and increased melanin deposition. They usually have skeletal abnormalities, secondary to expansion of the erythroid marrow. Enlargement of the malar bones may give the characteristic "chipmunk" facies or cause malocclusion of the jaw. Patients invariably have cardiomegaly which may be accompanied by signs of congestive heart failure. Marked hepatomegaly and splenomegaly are always found in these patients.

The *diagnosis* of β thalassemia major should be considered in any patient with a severe hemolytic anemia and hypochromic microcytic red blood cells. Examination of the peripheral blood smear reveals marked variations in the size and shape of red blood cells, including many target cells as well as teardrop and cigar-shaped cells (Plate 9-5). Normoblasts are usually seen, particularly if the patient has undergone splenectomy. Hemoglobin electrophoresis shows the presence of large amounts of HbF and variable amounts of HbA. In patients who are homozygous for β^0 thalassemia, no HbA can be detected. Hemoglobin A_2 is usually increased about twofold, although it can be normal in β thalassemia major.

Patients with β thalassemia major have a short life expectancy. It is unusual for a patient with the most severe form of the disease to survive into adulthood. Most patients have such severe anemia that they are dependent upon transfusions. The chronic administration of large amounts of blood along with an inappropriate increase in iron absorption from the gastrointestinal tract inevitably leads to clinically significant hemosiderosis. As a result of iron overload, these patients develop abnormalities in hepatic, endocrine, and cardiac function. The combination of chronic hypoxia and myocardial siderosis leads to cardiac arrhythmias, congestive failure, and ultimately death.

Homozygotes who survive into adulthood are likely to have a milder form of the disease, designated as *β thalassemia intermedia.* There are several genetic subtypes which are associated with less severe clinical manifestations: (1) β thalassemia with unusually high levels of HbF synthesis, (2) $\beta\delta$ thalassemia in which there is suppression of δ-chain as well as β-chain synthesis, and (3) the presence of heterozygous α thalassemia in combination with homozygous β thalassemia, leading to more balanced subunit synthesis. A milder clinical course is also seen in individuals who are doubly heterozygous for β thalassemia and hereditary persistence of HbF. These patients usually have moderately severe anemia, but do not require transfusions.

Treatment of β thalassemia major is primarily supportive. The obvious benefits of transfusion therapy are partially offset by the risk of iron overload, hepatitis, and isoimmunization. Despite these problems, children with Cooley's anemia fare better if their hemoglobin is maintained at greater than 9 g/dl. In view of the increased demands of the hyperplastic marrow, it is reasonable to maintain these patients on a daily supplement of folic acid. Since splenic sequestration contributes to shortened red blood cell survival, many patients derive some benefit from splenectomy. The prevention and treatment of iron overload is a continuing concern in these patients. Transfusion of young low-density red blood cells, "neocytes," reduces the rate of iron accumulation. Continuous subcutaneous injection of desferrioxamine permits the mobilization and excretion of significant amounts of iron. However, the long-term efficacy of this therapy has not yet been established.

Considerations of genetic counseling and antenatal diagnosis are as relevant in the *prevention* of β thalassemia major as they are for sickle cell anemia (see above). Because of linkages between β thalassemias and restriction enzyme polymorphisms, prenatal diagnosis can sometimes be made by DNA analysis of amniotic fluid cells. However, in most cases it is necessary to take the risk of obtaining fetal red blood cells for globin chain synthesis measurements.

REFERENCES

Alter BP: Prenatal diagnosis of hemoglobinopathies; a status report. Lancet 2:1152, 1981

Benz ES, Forget BG: The thalassemia syndromes: Models for the molecular analysis of human disease. Ann Rev Med 33:363, 1982

Bunn HF, Forget BG: *Human Hemoglobins,* 2d ed. Philadelphia, Saunders, 1983

Castle WB: From man to molecule and back to mankind. Semin Hematol 13:159, 1976

Dean J, Schechter AN: Sickle cell anemia: Molecular and cellular bases of therapeutic approaches. N Engl J Med 299:752, 804, 863, 1978

Jaffe EF: Methemoglobinemia. Clin Hematol 10:99, 1981

Nienhuis AW, Benz EJ: Regulation of hemoglobin synthesis during the development of the red cell. N Engl J Med 197:1318, 1430, 1977

Noguchi CT, Schechter AN: The intracellular polymerization of sickle hemoglobin and its relevance to sickle cell disease. Blood 58:1057, 1981

Powars DR: Natural history of sickle cell disease: The first ten years. Semin Hematol 12:267, 1975

Serjeant GR: *The Clinical Features of Sickle Cell Disease.* New York, American Elsevier, 1974

Weatherall DJ, Clegg JB: *The Thalassemia Syndromes.* Oxford, Blackwell, 1982

Wood WG et al: Developmental biology of human hemoglobins. Prog Hematol 10:43, 1977

331 BONE MARROW FAILURE AND BONE MARROW TRANSPLANTATION

E. DONNALL THOMAS

DEFINITION The bone marrow is a large organ, contained within the marrow cavities of the central bony skeleton. This organ performs a number of functions essential to life, including the production of red blood cells, platelets, and granulocytes. It is also an immunologically competent organ, rich in lymphocytes and in monocyte-macrophages. Bone marrow failure is characterized by hypoplasia of the marrow with a consequent pancytopenia.

APLASTIC ANEMIA

The term *aplastic anemia* should be reserved for patients who have a fatty or "empty" bone marrow due to severe hypoplasia of the erythroid, myeloid, and thrombopoietic cell lines. Life-threatening or severe aplastic anemia is defined as marrow hypoplasia associated with a pancytopenia consisting of at least two of the following: less than 500 granulocytes per cubic millimeter; less than 20,000 platelets per cubic millimeter; or a corrected reticulocyte count of less than 1 percent.

CONGENITAL APLASTIC ANEMIA Constitutional aplastic anemia (Fanconi's anemia) usually appears in childhood and may be associated with multiple congenital anomalies. There is often a positive family history, and chromosomal abnormalities have been observed frequently. If the patient survives the complications of aplasia, there is a high risk of developing leukemia.

ACQUIRED APLASTIC ANEMIA Etiology Acquired aplastic anemia is thought to be due to injury or destruction of a pluripotential hematopoietic stem cell. In more than one-half of the cases no etiologic agent can be incriminated. Despite intensive research, the nature of the injury to the stem cell remains obscure. Some etiologic hypotheses have assumed the continued presence of a "toxin," lack of a necessary humoral factor, or abnormality in the sites (microenvironment) where marrow cells grow. Successful restoration of marrow function by bone marrow transplantation constitutes strong evidence against the persistence of any of these mechanisms. A possible autoimmune mechanism is suggested by the observation that some patients with aplastic anemia have recovered following treatment with the immunosuppressive agent antithymocyte globulin and by the fact that some transplants from normal identical twins have succeeded only after immunosuppressive treatment of the patient with large doses of cyclophosphamide. In vitro studies have shown that a minority of patients have lymphocytes (T cells) that inhibit the development of hematopoietic colonies by marrow cells in agar cultures.

A unifying hypothesis might be as follows: a viral or chemical agent binds to the pluripotent hematopoietic stem cells to produce a haptene which incites an immunologic reaction that injures or destroys the stem cells. By the time that pancytopenia produces symptoms and the patient seeks medical help, the immunologic reaction may have diminished or disappeared. A mechanism of this type would explain some of the puzzling features of aplastic anemia: occasional spontaneous recovery; occasional in vitro evidence of an immune process; occasional response to immunosuppressive therapy; cure by syngeneic marrow infusion without immunosuppressive therapy in some patients but not in others; irreversible marrow failure in the majority of patients.

Drugs and toxins Many drugs and chemical agents have been incriminated as etiologic agents in aplastic anemia. The association has a varying spectrum from predictable dose-related aplasia to idiosyncratic reactions unrelated to dose. Irradiation and cytotoxic drugs produce predictable marrow hypoplasia. Benzene and benzene derivatives may produce either dose-related or idiosyncratic marrow aplasia, and other hematologic abnormalities may either precede or follow the aplasia or occur independently, including hemolytic anemia, refractory pancytopenia with hypercellular marrow, myeloid metaplasia, and leukemia. The mechanisms are unknown.

Chloramphenicol may be associated with two forms of bone marrow toxicity. The more common effect is a reversible, dose-related suppression of erythroid and, on occasion, granulocytic and megakaryocytic precursors. The bone marrow is normocellular with vacuolization of the cytoplasm of erythroid and granulocytic precursors. The marrow morphology usually reverts to normal after cessation of the drug. The second, more serious form of chloramphicol-associated marrow failure is the idiosyncratic reaction which occurs in approximately 1 of

30,000 patients at risk. These patients develop severe pancytopenia and marrow aplasia which is usually irreversible, resulting in death.

Table 331-1 lists some of the other drugs and chemicals thought to be responsible for some cases of aplastic anemia. The establishment of a relationship is often difficult since many patients have had exposure to multiple agents. Furthermore, large numbers of individuals with the same exposure do not develop aplastic anemia. In the case of insecticides, for example, it is usually impossible to determine whether the aplastic anemia was related to the insecticide or represented a chance occurrence of an "idiopathic" aplastic anemia. Of course, "idiopathic" aplastic anemia might be the consequence of a reaction to an unidentifiable agent.

INFECTIOUS HEPATITIS Aplastic anemia is a rare complication of infectious hepatitis. Marrow failure may appear concurrently or some months after the episode of hepatitis. The aplasia tends to be severe with a frequently fatal outcome. Many cases of "idiopathic" aplastic anemia are preceded by apparently benign viral respiratory illness. It is postulated that hepatitis or other viral infections might initiate an autoimmune mechanism, but there is, as yet, no proof of this hypothesis.

Clinical manifestations The clinical manifestations of aplastic anemia are a direct result of the failure of the bone marrow to manufacture red blood cells, platelets, and granulocytes. The symptoms are those of anemia, bleeding, and infection. The development of pancytopenia is not necessarily synchronous, so that some patients may present with anemia, others with bleeding, and others with infection. The development of symptoms is usually insidious, and patients often present to the physician with less than 10 percent of normal bone marrow cellularity.

Physical examination generally reveals pallor. The skin, mucous membranes, and conjunctivae may show petechiae or ecchymoses. There is no lymphadenopathy or hepatosplenomegaly. Fever is often present. The usual signs of localized infection, such as pus formation, may be absent because of granulocytopenia.

The course of the disease is unpredictable in that patients with a mild pancytopenia may recover or may progress to severe pancytopenia. Patients who meet the criteria for severe disease show a mortality of 50 percent within the first 4 months of diagnosis. Thereafter the mortality rate slows, but only about 10 to 20 percent of the patients go on to complete recovery.

TABLE 331-1
Possible etiologic factors in the development of acquired aplastic anemia

- *I* Cause unknown (idiopathic)
- *II* Chemical and physical agents
  - *A* Dose-related
    - *1* Antineoplastic agents
    - *2* Benzene
    - *3* Chloramphenicol
    - *4* Inorganic arsenicals
    - *5* Ionizing irradiation
  - *B* Idiosyncratic
    - *1* Acetazolamide
    - *2* Arsenicals
    - *3* Barbiturates
    - *4* Chloramphenicol
    - *5* Gold
    - *6* Insecticides
    - *7* Phenothiazines
    - *8* Phenylbutazone
    - *9* Pyrimethamine
    - *10* Solvents
    - *11* Sulfa drugs
    - *12* Thiouracils
- *III* Hepatitis and other viral infections
- *IV* Pregnancy
- *V* Paroxysmal nocturnal hemoglobinuria

BONE MARROW FAILURE DUE TO RADIATION INJURY

Radiation injury to the bone marrow is of particular interest because the pluripotential stem cell is extremely limited in its ability to recover from radiation injury. The consequence of such injury is marrow aplasia and severe pancytopenia. Since the bone marrow is widely distributed in the body, most experimental studies of radiation injury to the marrow have involved total-body irradiation, usually accomplished with photons, X-rays, and gamma rays.

Dose units. The roentgen (R) is a measure of radiation exposure in air. The unit which reflects energy transfer to the tissue is the rad. The international unit, the gray (Gy), equals 100 rad. Radiation damage is a function of both the total exposure and of the dose rate. The lower the dose rate, the less will be the biological effect.

CLINICAL PHENOMENA IN RELATION TO DOSE AND TIME AFTER EXPOSURE Diminution in the repair of tissues with a high cellular turnover, such as bone marrow and gut epithelium, results in a spectrum of effects ranging from hypoplasia to total atrophy. The consequences of total-body irradiation exposure are best described by three overlapping syndromes. The cerebral syndrome, characterized by nausea, vomiting, convulsions, and death, occurs after very high exposures, greater than 60 Gy. The gastrointestinal syndrome begins with exposures of approximately 4 Gy and becomes lethal with exposures greater than 20 Gy. It is characterized by vomiting and diarrhea, which is usually greatest 3 to 5 days after exposure.

The hematopoietic syndrome, which occurs following whole-body exposure, may be preceded by anorexia, nausea, and vomiting that is greatest between 6 and 12 h after exposure to doses of irradiation between 2 and 10 Gy. Within 24 h after the exposure the subject is usually asymptomatic and experiences a period of relative well-being until the onset of bleeding or infection. Lymphopenia begins immediately and becomes maximal within 24 to 36 h. Thereafter, the lymphocytes remain at low levels for weeks with recovery occurring over several months. A neutrophilic leukocytosis appears within a few hours after irradiation. Mature granulocytes are not directly damaged, and therefore peripheral blood neutropenia does not begin until the bone marrow reserves are depleted of mature granulocytes. After sublethal and low lethal doses, the minimum granulocyte values occur in 4 to 6 weeks. After high lethal doses, granulocytes diminish more rapidly, and values approach zero within 7 to 10 days. Reticulocyte production is halted immediately, but the long red cell life span results in a slow onset of significant anemia.

Thrombocytopenia develops slowly over a period of approximately 30 days after doses of 2 to 4 Gy. After doses of 6 to 10 Gy, which effectively stop new platelet production, the decline in the platelet count reflects the life span of the platelet, and levels below 20,000 per cubic millimeter develop in approximately 9 days. The bleeding component of the hematopoietic syndrome is due to the lack of platelets and can be corrected by platelet transfusions.

Studies of decreased resistance to infection following total-body exposure have disclosed many contributing factors, including lymphopenia, impaired antibody production, impaired granulocyte function, decreased cellular ability to kill phagocytized bacteria, and damage to skin and bowel which provides portals of entry for infectious agents. However, in the acute hematopoietic syndrome, the most significant factor by far is the quantitative reduction in circulating granulocytes, since there is a high probability of bacterial infection when the granulocyte level falls below 200 cells per cubic millimeter.

BONE MARROW FAILURE DUE TO MARROW REPLACEMENT (MYELOPHTHISIC ANEMIA)

Infiltration of the bone marrow with tumor cells can result in the development of severe pancytopenia. Tumor may be derived from cell lines such as leukemia, lymphoma, or myeloma which are indigenous to the bone marrow, or the marrow may be invaded by metastatic deposits of solid tumor. Among the solid tumors most frequently associated with myelophthisic anemia are carcinoma of the breast, prostate, lung, and thyroid. Other causes of marrow replacement are lipid storage disorders such as Gaucher's disease, osteopetrosis, and the development of fibrosis. Whatever the mechanism of bone marrow replacement, the end result is impaired production of normal formed blood elements with the consequences of anemia, bleeding, and infection. The following findings are not characteristic of aplastic anemia and suggest the presence of a myelophthisic anemia: bone pain, splenomegaly or lymphadenopathy, a "dry tap" marrow aspirate, red cells of abnormal shape, the presence of many nucleated red blood cells, and immature white blood cells in the peripheral blood.

SINGLE CELL LINE DEFICIENCIES

Deficiency of a committed stem cell compartment, whether congenital or acquired, will result in a lack of that particular cell line in the circulating blood. Red cell aplasia can be secondary to a variety of causes, including infection, malnutrition, renal failure, systemic lupus erythematosus, and neoplasms. Patients with pure red cell aplasia are anemic and reticulocytopenic with decreased erythropoietic activity in the bone marrow. Approximately one-half of the cases of pure red cell aplasia are associated with the presence of a thymoma. Many of these patients have an antibody to bone marrow erythroblasts and some respond to immunosuppressive therapy. Neutropenia may occur secondary to bacterial or viral infections. Agranulocytosis induced by drugs is usually reversible if death from infection can be prevented by supportive care. Thrombocytopenia may also be drug-related or idiopathic (see Chap. 332). Hyperplasia of a cell line in the bone marrow with deficiency of that cell line in the peripheral blood usually indicates an immune-mediated destruction of that cell line (hemolytic anemia, idiopathic thrombocytopenia).

MANAGEMENT OF BONE MARROW FAILURE

A presumptive diagnosis of marrow failure, irrespective of cause, poses a life-threatening situation which should be treated as a medical emergency. Appropriate supportive treatment should be started immediately while the cause and course of the illness are being studied.

If marrow aplasia is due to irradiation or a suspected toxin or drug, the patient should be removed from the exposure. History, physical examination, and laboratory studies, including a complete hematologic evaluation, should be completed as quickly as possible. Evaluation of the bone marrow should include a search for malignant cells. Cytogenetic studies of the marrow may be helpful in identifying radiation injury or in the identification of preleukemia presenting as aplastic anemia.

Ultraisolation techniques are effective in preventing infection in neutropenic patients undergoing treatment for leukemia or bone marrow transplantation. Patients with bone marrow failure should be cared for using the most effective available isolation facilities. Particular attention should be paid to oral hygiene and dental care, and intramuscular injections should be avoided or given with sterile precautions using a "Z" needle technique. Meticulous technique should be used for intravenous injections and withdrawals to preserve the patient's veins. A central venous line of the "Hickman" type is used for blood withdrawal, intravenous medications, and hyperalimentation in the supportive care of patients with bone marrow failure.

Platelet transfusions are usually unnecessary at levels above 20,000 per cubic millimeter (see Chap. 335). Below that level, they should be used until values above 20,000 are sustained, especially if there is any evidence of bleeding. If the patient becomes refractory to random donor platelets, the use of platelets from HLA-matched unrelated donors may become necessary. Family member transfusions should not be administered until the possibility of bone marrow transplantation has been excluded because such transfusions might sensitize the patient to the transplantation antigens of the potential marrow donor. Aspirin should be avoided since this agent depresses platelet function.

Granulocyte transfusions (see Chap. 335) may be used to prevent infection in marrow transplant patients who are not in ultraisolation when the granulocyte count falls below 200 per cubic millimeter, but the routine use of prophylactic granulocyte transfusions is controversial and impractical. Granulocyte transfusions are indicated for therapy of any significant infection in a granulocytopenic patient. Packed red blood cells should be given as needed to control the symptoms of anemia, usually to keep the hematocrit above 25 percent.

If the patient is immunosuppressed because of disease or treatment, all blood products should be irradiated with 1.5 Gy before infusion to inactivate lymphocytes that might subsequently proliferate and cause a graft-versus-host reaction.

Since infection is an ever-present danger, bacteriologic cultures should be obtained frequently. The onset of significant fever (38.5°C) should arouse a strong suspicion of infection in the granulocytopenic patient. Fever with clinical signs of bacteremia or fever sustained more than 24 h is an indication for initiating systemic antibacterial therapy even though cultures are negative. Since the most likely bacterial agent is a gram-negative organism from the normal bowel flora, initial therapy usually includes an aminoglycoside active against *Pseudomonas* (gentamicin, tobramycin, amikacin) and carbenicillin or ticarcillin with additional antibiotics added as indicated by culture results (see Chaps. 107 and 111). Subsequently, if cultures are negative but fever persists, therapy with a combination of trimethoprim and sulfamethoxazole or with amphotericin may be considered. Once broad-spectrum antibiotic therapy has been initiated, it should be continued until the granulocyte count rises above 200 per cubic millimeter, even if the clinical signs of infection disappear.

In the treatment of aplastic anemia, corticosteroids have been used in an effort to decrease capillary fragility and reduce the bleeding tendency. Objective benefit from this therapy has not been demonstrated, and it may result in a number of undesirable side effects. Therefore, the use of corticosteroids is not recommended. The use of androgens for the treatment of aplastic anemia is controversial. Several reports describe an apparent benefit from androgen therapy, but none of these involve a controlled clinical trial. Convincing support for androgen therapy is derived from occasional case reports of patients who improve on androgens and relapse when androgens are discontinued. A prospective randomized study reported by the International Aplastic Anemia Study Group failed to show a benefit of androgen therapy in patients with severe aplastic anemia. Androgens have undesirable side effects including virilization, hepatotoxicity, peliosis hepatis, and, after prolonged use, hepatocellular carcinoma.

Whatever the cause of the marrow failure, the physician should keep in mind the possibility of bone marrow transplantation. Accordingly, lymphocytes should be obtained from the patient and all available family members for HLA typing and for mixed leukocyte cultures. Lymphocytes for the mixed leukocyte cultures can be cryopreserved for testing at a later date. Transfusion of blood or its components should be avoided if possible, and family members should not be used as blood donors.

BONE MARROW TRANSPLANTATION

SELECTION OF THE PATIENT Marrow transplantation is a rational therapeutic option only if the patient's disease involves the bone marrow or if hazard to the normal marrow is the limiting factor in the aggressive treatment of a disease. A marrow transplant involves a transplant not only of the donor hematopoietic system but also of the donor lymphoid and macrophage system. The underlying philosophy is illustrated by the three types of diseases for which marrow transplantation has been most widely utilized:

1 *Immunologic deficiency diseases.* Here, the objective is to utilize marrow grafting in order to replace the recipient's genetically defective lymphoid system with the normal lymphoid system of the donor.
2 *Aplastic anemia.* In this instance, the disease process, regardless of etiology, has resulted in loss of the marrow, and the objective is to replace the defective organ with a normal functioning organ.
3 *Acute leukemia.* In this disease the objective is the complete destruction of the leukemic cell population and, unavoidably, normal marrow cells by intensive chemoradiotherapy with restoration of normal marrow function by the transplanted marrow.

SELECTION OF THE DONOR The donor must be in good health, and the donor, or an appropriate advocate, must be capable of giving informed consent for the marrow transplant procedure. The principal risk is from the anesthesia. Beyond these ethical considerations, selection of the donor is largely determined by histocompatibility testing, since the donor must share with the recipient all or part of the major histocompatibility complex, human leukocyte antigens (HLA). Red blood cell incompatibility is not a barrier to marrow transplantation.

Histocompatibility typing (see Chap. 60) An *autologous* marrow graft refers to the removal of a patient's marrow, administration of chemo- and/or radiotherapy, and then return of the patient's own marrow. A *syngeneic* graft describes a graft in which donor and recipient are genetically identical, i.e., identical twins. An *allogeneic* graft describes the situation where donor and recipient are of different genetic origins. A *chimera* is an individual whose body contains living and proliferating cells of different genetic origin.

The HLA region is composed of a series of closely linked genetic loci on chromosome 6 (see Chap. 60). The array of antigens encoded by this region on one chromosome is known as a haplotype. Each individual has two haplotypes, one inherited from each parent. The antigens located at HLA-A, -B, and -C are detected on lymphocytes by serological techniques in a microcytotoxicity assay and that at HLA-D by the mixed leukocyte culture. A locus that is either identical with or closely related to HLA-D, called DR, can now be recognized serologically by typing of B lymphocytes. These closely linked genetic loci, each with a large number of known alleles, make the HLA region by far the most complex genetic polymorphism yet described in human beings.

Despite this complexity, within a family there can be only four haplotypes. Therefore, for a given patient, each sibling has one chance in four of being HLA-identical with the patient. The most widely used transplants are those between HLA-identical siblings, the most compatible form of allogeneic transplant.

An identical twin constitutes a special example of an HLA-identical sibling who is matched not only for HLA but for all genetic loci. Although only a small fraction of patients will have an identical twin, transplants between identical twins have been very effective therapeutically and informative scientifically because the twin provides marrow which is like the patient's own except that it is free of disease. Marrow transplantation from a twin, therefore, is like a perfect "autologous" marrow transplant.

PREPARATION OF THE PATIENT Infants with severe combined immunologic deficiency are conditioned to accept a transplant by the nature of their disease. All other patients are immunologically competent, to a greater or lesser degree, and are therefore able to reject the marrow transplant unless prepared with some form of immunosuppressive therapy. An immunosuppressive regimen commonly used for patients with aplastic anemia consists of large doses of cyclophosphamide. Preparation of the patient with leukemia involves the administration of high-dose chemoradiotherapy designed to kill as many leukemic cells as possible. A commonly used regimen involves the administration of cyclophosphamide followed by total-body irradiation. An irradiation exposure of approximately 10 Gy is necessary for immunosuppression sufficient to permit consistent engraftment of marrow even though only 4 to 5 Gy will cause lethal marrow injury.

Aspiration and infusion of the marrow The pelvic bones are the most readily accessible sites for procurement, although marrow may be obtained from the sternum, the ribs or, from children, the tibia. The marrow donor is taken to the operating room and, under general or spinal anesthesia, multiple marrow aspirations are performed on the anterior and posterior iliac crests. In order to avoid excessive dilution with blood, the point of the aspirating needle must be placed in as many different locations as possible. Usually, some 100 to 150 aspirations are carried out, and the volume of the mixture of blood and marrow cells is from 500 to 800 ml. As each aspiration is performed, the marrow is mixed with heparin and tissue culture medium. When the collection is completed, the marrow is passed through stainless steel screens to break up the marrow particles. It is then transferred to a blood transfusion bag and administered by intravenous infusion. The marrow stem cells pass through the lungs and subsequent growth and reconstitution of the marrow is confined almost exclusively to the medullary cavities.

Support for the patient without marrow function Following marrow transplantation, the stem cells must reach the marrow cavities, proliferate, and undergo the normal maturation process. Two to four weeks are usually required, sometimes longer, before the transplanted marrow starts to be functionally effective in producing the critical formed elements of the peripheral blood. Supportive care is crucial for survival and is the same as that for any kind of complete marrow failure.

In addition, many patients coming to marrow transplantation may have had inadequate nutrition because of their disease or the efforts to treat it. In any event, the preparation for marrow grafting results in nausea and vomiting, and the mucositis associated with therapy and granulocytopenia will result in poor oral intake for at least several weeks. In order to ensure adequate nutrition, a Hickman modification of the Broviac catheter is installed routinely on admission for marrow transplantation. The catheter makes it possible to administer hyperalimentation, medications, and blood products and is also used for drawing blood samples. Although some catheters are removed because of infection or suspected infection, about 90 percent of the patients have the catheter in place for approximately 3 months, the period of time when it is needed.

ENGRAFTMENT AND PROOF OF ENGRAFTMENT After a period of profound granulocytopenia, engraftment is usually signaled by a rise in granulocytes and platelets and the reappearance of reticulocytes. The median time required to reach a granulocyte count of 100 per cubic millimeter is 16 days and to reach 1000 per cubic millimeter, 26 days. The rise in platelet count usually lags a week or two behind the rise in granulocyte count.

Proof of engraftment depends upon the use of cytogenetics and/or blood genetic markers in order to confirm that the regenerating marrow is of donor origin. Cytogenetic evidence of engraftment is most easily demonstrated when donor and recipient are of opposite sex, although banding techniques frequently permit distinction between cells of donor and recipient of the same sex. A variety of red blood cell and isoenzyme differences can be utilized if not obscured by recent blood transfusions. Patients with leukemia prepared for engraftment with cyclophosphamide and total-body irradiation invariably have a regenerating marrow entirely of host type. Patients prepared with cyclophosphamide alone occasionally show persistence of some host cells for a period of a few weeks. A few of these patients have an increasing number of host cells so that the graft is eventually lost and the marrow is repopulated by host cells.

COMPLICATIONS FOLLOWING ENGRAFTMENT The complications that may follow successful marrow engraftment are (1) graft rejection, a problem primarily occurring in patients with aplastic anemia; (2) infection, including early bacterial infections or later opportunistic infections such as cytomegalovirus; (3) acute graft-versus-host disease, the consequence of the immunologic reaction of the engrafted lymphoid elements against the tissues of the recipient; (4) chronic graft-versus-host disease; (5) recurrence of leukemia; and (6) miscellaneous complications such as hemorrhagic cystitis, cardiomyopathy, cataract formation, leukoencephalopathy, and sterility.

CLINICAL RESULTS OF BONE MARROW TRANSPLANTATION

IMMUNODEFICIENCY DISEASES Studies of marrow transplantation for the treatment of infants with the severe combined immunodeficiency syndromes have provided important basic information despite the rarity of these disorders. These patients are unique in that immunosuppressive therapy is not necessary to condition the patient to accept a graft, and because some myeloid function is usually present, rapid marrow engraftment is not essential. One of these patients was the first to be transplanted from an HLA-identical sibling, and some 50 similar patients have been successfully reconstituted in the intervening 10 years. According to the International Bone Marrow Transplant Registry, 63 percent of these patients given identical sibling marrow are alive 6 months after grafting and, presumably, cured.

APLASTIC ANEMIA Because of the poor prognosis on conventional therapy, patients with severe aplastic anemia are logical candidates for marrow transplantation.

Transplantation for severe aplastic anemia using HLA-identical sibling donors Patients with severe aplastic anemia must be prepared for engraftment with immunosuppressive therapy, and the most widely used regimen has been cyclophosphamide, 50 mg/kg on each of 4 days, followed 36 h later by the intravenous infusion of donor bone marrow. The first two successful transplants of this type were reported in 1972, and these recipients are alive and well 9 years after transplantation.

For ethical reasons the initial marrow transplants had to be carried out in patients who had clearly failed to benefit from conventional therapy. As a consequence these end-stage patients had already received multiple transfusions of blood and platelets, and many were severely infected at the time of marrow transplantation. By 1976 the Seattle marrow transplant team had reported a series of 73 patients treated by marrow transplantation. Thirty of these patients are alive and cured 5 or more years after grafting, a long-term survival rate of 41 percent. Several other marrow transplant teams have reported similar results.

A cooperative study was carried out by 28 medical centers in order to compare, prospectively, the results of marrow transplantation from HLA-identical siblings to conventional therapy with steroids and androgens for patients without a marrow donor. The results showed that patients treated by marrow transplantation had a 60 percent survival at 2 years while those treated by conventional methods had a 2-year survival of 25 percent. Most patients in this study were in the first three decades of life. The results showed clearly that if a suitable donor is available, marrow transplantation is superior to conventional management, at least in younger patients.

Although these results were encouraging, there was obviously much room for improvement. Studies of marrow transplantation in dogs had shown that blood transfusions could sensitize an intended marrow transplant recipient, resulting in subsequent rejection of the marrow graft. It seemed likely, therefore, that marrow graft rejection by the human patient might be due to sensitization to minor transplantation antigens by prior transfusions. Accordingly, the Seattle marrow transplant team tried to identify patients with severe aplastic anemia early in the course of the disease and carry out marrow transplantation before blood transfusions were given. In the initial series of 30 such patients, graft failure was observed in only 3, and the actuarial long-term survival rate was 75 percent. Twenty of the twenty-five long-term survivors are entirely well, and five have mild-to-moderate graft-versus-host disease. It is clear, therefore, that patients with severe aplastic anemia and their families should have tissue typing performed immediately upon diagnosis. If a suitable donor can be identified, marrow transplantation should be carried out promptly before transfusions become necessary.

Despite these encouraging results, however, many patients with severe aplastic anemia present to the physician with bleeding and/or infection, and transfusions must be given as a matter of medical necessity. Therefore, marrow transplant teams are investigating other preparative regimens in an effort to improve survival for these patients. These include procarbazine and antithymocyte globulin administered before the standard cyclophosphamide regimen, cyclophosphamide followed by 3-Gy total-body irradiation, a cyclophosphamide regimen followed by 8-Gy total-body irradiation with shielding of the lung to 4 Gy in an attempt to reduce the incidence of interstitial pneumonia, and the use of cyclophosphamide followed by 7.5 Gy of total nodal irradiation. It is too early for a definitive analysis of these regimens.

An analysis of the first 73 patients with severe aplastic anemia disclosed the fact that patients given a small number of marrow cells had an increased probability of graft rejection. Since it was not practical to get more bone marrow cells from the donor, attention was turned to peripheral blood mononuclear cells as an added source of donor cells. The standard cyclophosphamide regimen was administered followed by the marrow transplant. Then, on each of 3 to 5 days following marrow transplantation, buffy coat white blood cells were collected from 4 units of donor blood by a leukapheresis technique and administered intravenously to the recipient without in vitro irradiation. Thirty of forty-three (70 percent) such sensitized patients given marrow plus buffy coat are alive between 10 and 61 months after grafting.

Early transplantation before transfusions are given or, for patients who have been transfused, modified preparative regimens have largely solved the problem of graft rejection. The result has been an overall improvement in long-term survival to approximately 70 to 75 percent.

Transplantation for severe aplastic anemia using identical twin donors Aplastic anemia is not a common disease, and to find that a patient with it has an identical twin is even more uncommon. Nevertheless, at least 13 transplants have been carried out for severe aplastic anemia using an identical twin as the marrow donor. In 10 patients the simple intravenous infusion of marrow without any immunosuppressive treatment resulted in recovery. These results reinforce the concept that aplastic anemia is due to an acquired abnormality of the stem cell which can be corrected by transplantation of normal syngeneic stem cells. However, two patients did not recover following simple intravenous marrow infusion. These two patients were subsequently treated with the cyclophosphamide regimen and given a second infusion of bone marrow from the donor which resulted in complete hematopoietic reconstitution. Although the number of cases is necessarily small, the results suggest that a majority of the cases are likely to be due to a cellular defect correctable by stem cell replacement, but some may be due to immune suppression or abnormal regulators of cell growth. Whatever the mechanism, the rare patient with aplastic anemia who has a genetically identical twin has a 90 percent chance of being cured with marrow transplantation, virtually without risk.

ACUTE LEUKEMIA Acute leukemia (see Chap. 128) served as a prototype malignant disease of the marrow for treatment by intensive chemoradiotherapy and marrow transplantation. In this situation the objectives of the therapeutic approach are, first, to destroy the malignant disease and, second, to replace the destroyed marrow by transplantation of a normal marrow. The problems encountered are those related to transplantation biology, as described for aplastic anemia, and, in addition, the recurrence of leukemia subsequent to marrow transplantation.

Almost all regimens used for preparing the leukemic patient for marrow transplantation have employed supralethal total-body irradiation. This has been done for several reasons: (1) much of the laboratory experience with marrow transplantation in animals has been carried out with supralethal total-body irradiation; (2) irradiation is known to be an effective means of eradicating leukemic cells, but its clinical usefulness is limited because of destruction of normal marrow as well; (3) irradiation penetrates to the so-called privileged sites where leukemic cells may not be readily accessible to chemotherapeutic agents; and (4) irradiation is a powerful immunosuppressive agent.

Transplantation for acute leukemia in relapse using HLA-identical sibling donors For obvious ethical reasons, marrow transplantation was initially attempted only in patients with acute leukemia in relapse after "conventional" chemotherapy had failed. These end-stage patients were poor candidates for any therapeutic procedure because they usually presented with a heavy burden of leukemic cells, were usually granulocytopenic and thrombocytopenic, and often already infected with antibiotic-resistant bacteria and fungi. Nevertheless, the eventual demonstration that some of these patients could be cured was impressive and encouraged renewed efforts to improve the overall results.

In the initial series of 10 patients in Seattle, 10-Gy total-body irradiation was given in preparation for grafting. Four patients died early of infection, and five suffered a relapse of leukemia 2 to 5 months later. One patient is alive in remission with a marrow graft 10 years later.

Because of the high relapse rate, a decision was made to attempt to kill more leukemic cells by giving cyclophosphamide a few days before the administration of total-body irradiation and the marrow transplant. One hundred patients with acute leukemia in relapse were treated on this regimen 5 or more years ago. Many died in the first 3 months of causes related to advanced illness at the time of transplantation, graft-versus-host disease, or opportunistic infections, principally interstitial pneumonia. Recurrence of leukemia was observed in 31 patients, occurring throughout the first 2 years after transplantation. After 2 years, however, no more recurrences of leukemia were observed. Of the 12 survivors, 3 suffer from chronic graft-versus-host disease and 9 are living normal lives in remission now 5 to 9 years after transplantation. An analysis of survival shows that these long-term survivors are very far out on a plateau indicating that these patients, on no maintenance chemotherapy, are probably cured of their disease. These long-term survivors of end-stage acute leukemia are unique and demonstrate the possibility of cure even in the advanced stages of the disease.

Because recurrence of leukemia following marrow transplantation has been a major problem for patients transplanted in relapse, several marrow transplant teams have attempted to achieve a greater antileukemic effect by the administration of other intensive chemotherapy regimens before total-body irradiation and marrow transplantation. These regimens either had no effect on the recurrence of disease or may have reduced the leukemic relapse rate but at a high price in added toxicity and, therefore, without a significant effect on overall survival.

Transplantation for acute lymphoblastic leukemia (ALL) in remission using HLA-identical sibling donors The fact that some patients in the end stages of acute leukemia could apparently be cured by intensive chemoradiotherapy and marrow transplantation led to marrow transplantation earlier in the course of the disease. Some patients with ALL, particularly children in the "good-risk" category, can be cured by combination chemotherapy, but it is widely agreed that once marrow relapse has occurred, long-term survival is rare with therapy in current use. Therefore, the decision was made to transplant patients with this disease in the second or subsequent remission. It was recognized that some of these patients would be lost early to the complications of transplantation, but this risk seemed acceptable if some of the patients could, in fact, be cured.

The initial series involved 22 patients transplanted between April 1976 and December 1977. The median survival in this group of patients was 1 year, which compares favorably to the 6- and 8-month median survival usually achieved with combination chemotherapy. Twelve patients have died of recurrent leukemia. The six survivors are 4 to 5 years post transplantation in continuous remission on no maintenance chemotherapy and are presumed to be cured. One has a moderately severe chronic graft-versus-host disease.

Recurrent leukemia was the major problem in this series of patients. These recurrences, in host-type cells, show that the preparative regimen was often ineffective in eradicating the residual leukemic cell population.

Transplantation for acute nonlymphoblastic leukemia (ANL) in remission using HLA-identical sibling donors In contrast to patients with ALL, patients with ANL in first remission are known to have a poor prognosis. With combination chemotherapy the median duration of the first remission in most reported series is approximately 12 months, and only 15 to 20 percent of the patients are alive at 3 years after initial chemotherapy. Therefore, a study of marrow transplantation in these patients in first remission was considered to be ethically acceptable. The Seattle Marrow Transplant Team reported an initial series of 19 consecutive patients transplanted between March 1976 and March 1978. These patients underwent marrow transplantation a median of 16 weeks following initial treatment or 10 weeks following the achievement of the first complete remission. Eleven (58 percent) of these patients are in continued disease-free remission more than 3 years after grafting. A Kaplan-Meier plot of the probability of survival shows that the long-term survivors are well out on a plateau. Three of the long-term survivors have mild chronic graft-versus-host disease, and eight are entirely well. Only 2 of these 19 patients have suffered a recurrence of leukemia. Evidently, the preparative chemoradiotherapy regimen is capable of eradicating the leukemic cell population in most of these patients. The other six deaths were related to graft-versus-host disease and interstitial pneumonia. Other marrow transplant teams have carried out marrow transplants for patients with ANL in remission with excellent results.

Transplantation for refractory acute leukemia using identical twin donors An occasional patient with acute leukemia will have a normal identical twin. In this situation, a syngeneic transplant offers an opportunity to study the effects of the transplantation regimen on the patient and the disease without the immunologic problems or benefits associated with graft-versus-host disease. The Seattle Marrow Transplant Team has carried out 34 identical-twin transplants in patients whose leukemia had relapsed (18 with ALL and 16 with ANL). Eight are alive in remission on no maintenance chemotherapy 41 to 116 months following transplantation. Analysis of the survival of these patients shows that the long-term survivors are very far out on the plateau and are presumably cured of their disease. Although recurrent leukemia has been a major problem in recipients of syngeneic grafts, the absence of immunologic complications and the apparent cure of approximately one-fourth of the patients indicates clearly that all patients who have a hematologic malignancy and an identical twin should be referred to a transplant center without delay. Transplantation early in the course of the disease, before relapse occurs, should result in an improved number of long-term survivors.

Marrow transplantation for patients with chronic granulocytic leukemia (CGL) The term "chronic" is inappropriate in describing the clinical course of patients with CGL. The conversion to blast crisis and death occurs at a fairly constant rate, and the median survival in most series of patients is approximately 30 to 36 months (see Chap. 129). Although a small fraction of patients may live for a long time in the chronic phase, in general, the outlook for most patients with this disease is quite grim. When the blast crisis of the disease appears, therapy is usually ineffective, and most investigators, despite trials of a wide variety of agents, consider chemotherapy to be ineffective. A subset of those patients whose blasts appear to be more like lymphoblasts (terminal transferase-positive) and with a hypodiploid number of chromosomes may respond for a period of a few months to treatment with vincristine and prednisone.

The Seattle team has attempted marrow transplantation in 27 patients with CGL in blast crisis. These patients were critically ill, and most died soon after transplantation. However, seven are alive and free of disease 3 to 41 months after transplantation. Six patients with CGL in blast crisis were transplanted using an identical twin donor, and one of these patients continues in remission without the Philadelphia chromosome 67 months after transplantation.

In an effort to improve the results, the Seattle team initiated a study of marrow transplantation during the chronic phase of the disease for patients with an identical twin to serve as marrow donor. The objective was to use supralethal chemoradiotherapy and twin marrow transplantation in an effort to eradicate the Philadelphia chromosome-positive clone to prevent the transformation into blast crisis and to cure the disease. An initial group of four patients was treated with dimethylbusulfan, cyclophosphamide, and total-body irradiation followed by twin marrow infusion. The twin donors were examined and found to be clinically and hematologically normal without the presence of the Philadelphia chromosome. A complete hematologic and cytogenetic remission was induced in all four patients. One patient relapsed cytogenetically and hematologically 30 months after transplantation and died of leukemia at 51 months. The other three patients are clinically, hematologically, and cytogenetically normal 54, 57, and 62 months after marrow transplantation. These results of syngeneic marrow transplantation, indicating that the Philadelphia chromosome–positive leukemic clone can be eliminated, suggest that it may be reasonable to carry out marrow transplantation in the chronic phase of the disease utilizing allogeneic donors.

Marrow transplantation for patients with acute leukemia using donors other than HLA-identical siblings The general experience in the United States has been that approximately one-third of the patients with acute leukemia will have an HLA-identical sibling. The majority of patients will not have an HLA-identical sibling, and a cautious exploration of the use of other donors has been initiated by several marrow transplant teams. The Seattle team began to explore marrow transplantation in donor-recipient pairs in which one of the HLA haplotypes was genetically identical and the other haplotype was phenotypically identical for one or more of the HLA loci. For example, the marrow donor might be a parent, in which case the patient's haplotype inherited from that parent would be HLA-identical. The haplotype inherited from the other parent might, by chance, be phenotypically similar to the donor's other haplotype. Similarly, a sibling might be haploidentical with the patient. The results of these transplants carried out to the end of 1980 are as follows: 12 patients with ALL in relapse, no survivors, 4 patients dying of relapsed leukemia; 10 patients with ALL in remission, 4 survivors at 8, 10, 21, and 24 months; 10 patients with ANL in relapse, 2 survivors at 20 and 22 months; and 12 patients with ANL in remission, 7 survivors at 9, 10, 22, 24, 26, 29, and 43 months. It is apparent that for these patients the outcome is largely a function of the stage of the disease in which the transplant was carried out. The incidence of acute graft-versus-host disease and the cause of death were not significantly different from the results described utilizing HLA-identical donor-recipient sibling pairs. There are to date too few patients to permit an analysis according to the family relationship of the donor or according to the HLA locus involved in the mismatch.

Since HLA-A, -B, and -DR typing can now be carried out

serologically, it is technically possible to find a suitably matched unrelated donor, at least for patients with the more common HLA haplotypes, given a large panel of potential donors whose HLA type has been determined.

Two transplants using unrelated donors have been reported for patients with aplastic anemia and two for patients with severe combined immunodeficiency disease. One of the patients with severe combined immunodeficiency disease, transplanted by the Sloan-Kettering team, is the first long-term survivor of an unrelated graft. At last report, 2 years after grafting, the patient suffered moderately severe chronic graft-versus-host disease.

The Seattle team has transplanted a patient with ALL in second remission who received allogeneic marrow from an unrelated but HLA-A, -B, -D, and -DR phenotypically identical unrelated donor. Engraftment occurred promptly and graft-versus-host reaction was not observed. The patient was in good health until the leukemia recurred 1 year later.

These results indicate the feasibility of utilizing unrelated donors for marrow transplantation. For patients with common haplotypes, the search for a marrow donor can now reasonably be extended beyond the immediate family members.

AUTOLOGOUS MARROW TRANSPLANTATION The technique for procuring and cryopreserving marrow has been established for 20 years. It is possible to remove the patient's own marrow, set it aside during intensive chemoradiotherapy, and then return the marrow to the patient in order to avoid subsequent lethal marrow aplasia. The following points are pertinent in considering autologous marrow transplantation: (1) The patient's marrow should not be contaminated with malignant cells. (2) Autologous marrow is of value only in protecting the patient against lethal toxicity to the hematopoietic system. If the regimen of chemoradiotherapy involves lethal toxicity to other organ systems, autologous marrow will not be of benefit. (3) The tumor being treated must show a dose-response curve such that "supralethal" chemoradiotherapy can be expected to result in a significantly enhanced antitumor response. Unfortunately, with currently available agents, only a few tumors appear to fall into this category. (4) The protocol must be designed in such a way that the role of autologous marrow can be demonstrated. In animal systems it is feasible to administer "supralethal" therapy and to demonstrate that animals given syngeneic marrow will survive while those not given marrow will die. For obvious reasons, this kind of controlled experiment cannot be done in humans. Failure to recognize these four principles accounts for much of the current uncertainty about the value of autologous marrow transplantation in the treatment of patients with malignant disease.

Nevertheless, the potential use of autologous marrow is the subject of a new wave of interest and some results are encouraging. The tumors that might be expected to show a significant improvement in response to high-dose chemoradiotherapy inclue the leukemias, Hodgkin's disease, non-Hodgkin's lymphoma, small-cell cancer of the lung, testicular tumors, and ovarian tumors. Several transplant centers are conducting studies of the utility of cryopreserved autologous marrow, and all have reported successful hematopoietic reconstitution in most patients. It is, as yet, too early to evaluate the clinical impact of these studies on the course of the several diseases.

IMMUNOLOGIC ASPECTS OF MARROW TRANSPLANTATION

Marrow graft rejection "Marrow graft rejection" describes a phenomenon in which the transplanted marrow graft functions briefly, but, after a few days or weeks, the peripheral blood counts suddenly drop and marrow biopsy shows the marrow to be devoid of myeloid elements. In some instances, the graft may be rejected so quickly that graft function is never clearly established. Immunologically mediated marrow graft rejection is usually a consequence of sensitization of the recipient by transfusions against antigens present in the donor. In addition, inadequate immunosuppressive therapy before grafting may facilitate marrow graft rejection. Marrow graft rejection is a common problem in patients with aplastic anemia, but is very uncommon in patients with leukemia, which may be due to several factors: (1) Transfusions are usually given to leukemic patients while they are receiving antileukemic chemotherapy which is also immunosuppressive. This chemotherapy may prevent sensitization to transplantation antigens contained in blood products. (2) Leukemia involves the lymphoid system so that the disease process itself may interfere with sensitization. (3) Leukemic patients receive a more intensive immunosuppressive regimen before grafting and are less likely to reject the graft.

Marrow graft rejection is a form of marrow graft failure which may be due to causes other than immunologic mechanisms. With a solid organ, such as the kidney, histologic proof of graft rejection is easily obtained, but such proof cannot usually be obtained with a marrow graft since the myeloid marrow simply disappears. Other possible mechanisms of graft failure include (1) defective or inadequate numbers of "stem cells" in the donor marrow; (2) allogeneic resistance not associated with HLA; and (3) susceptibility of the donor marrow to the same etiologic mechanism(s) responsible for the original disease process.

Acute graft-versus-host disease (GVHD) A "wasting disease" or "runt disease" was described many years ago in newborn mice or in rodents exposed to lethal total-body irradiation and given infusions of allogeneic hematopoietic cells. Over subsequent years these observations were confirmed for other species, including humans, and were recognized to be the consequence of an immunologic reaction of engrafted lymphoid cells, presumably T cells, against the tissues of the host. This graft-versus-host reaction and its consequences are now referred to as "GVHD," which is one of the major complications of marrow transplantation in humans. In Seattle, a series of 262 patients were given a marrow graft from an HLA-identical sibling, and after the graft they received methotrexate designed to prevent GVHD. Nevertheless, 116 (44 percent) developed moderate-to-severe GVHD.

GVHD in humans usually involves the skin, gastrointestinal tract, and/or liver. A skin rash is usually the first sign of GVHD. Intestinal involvement results in diarrhea and may progress to abdominal pain and ileus. Liver disease is characterized by rises of bilirubin, serum glutamic oxaloacetic transaminase, and alkaline phosphatase. Severe immunologic deficiency accompanies GVHD, and death from infection is frequently the terminal event. The distinction between illness due to an active immunologic assault against host tissues, the graft-versus-host reaction, and the consequences of this assault, deranged organ function and infection, is subtle and, therefore, both are considered to be a part of GVHD.

Since GVHD is immunologically mediated, efforts to prevent the development of GVHD have involved the use of immunosuppressive therapy. In animal systems it was found that treatment with immunosuppressive agents must be started before GVHD becomes apparent. Of the many agents studied, methotrexate and cyclophosphamide were found to be useful. The standard Seattle regimen consists of methotrexate, 15 mg/m^2 on day 1 post grafting, and 10 mg/m^2 on days 3, 6, 11, 18, and weekly thereafter through day 102. The Johns Hopkins team has used cyclophosphamide, 7.5 mg/kg for five doses on alternate days, beginning on the first day after marrow grafting followed by additional doses at irregular intervals. Controlled clinical trials of these regimens have not been carried out in humans, and, despite these regimens, GVHD remains a serious problem.

A number of studies have been carried out in animals and in humans in an effort to treat GVHD once it becomes established. Human recipients of HLA-identical marrow have been treated with rabbit or goat antithymocyte globulin, and improvement was observed in some patients. In a clinical trial, without untreated controls because of ethical considerations, prednisone and horse antithymocyte globulin gave equivalent results in the treatment of established human GVHD. Despite these efforts, about one-third of the patients who develop moderate to severe GVHD will die with this complication. It is clear from these studies that the treatment of acute GVHD is unsatisfactory and that new approaches in preventing or treating GVHD must be found.

One such new approach, currently under investigation, involves an agent with unique immunosuppressive properties, cyclosporin A. Other experiments are underway designed to eliminate from the marrow inoculum the immune competent cells believed to be responsible for GVHD while retaining hematopoietic stem cells. These efforts involve treatment of the marrow inoculum with heterologous or xenogeneic antiserums in an effort to destroy the T cells thought to be responsible for the development of GVHD. The recent development of monoclonal antibodies that react with human T cells or subsets of T cells points the way to greatly improved methods of in vitro treatment of marrow. These attractive approaches for the prevention of GVHD require further study for application in human marrow transplantation.

Chronic GVHD Chronic GVHD occurs in approximately one-fourth of those recipients of marrow from an HLA-identical sibling who survive beyond 100 days. It may range from mild to severe and may develop as an extension of acute GVHD or de novo after a period of well-being. The manifestations include skin disease, keratoconjunctivitis, buccal mucositis, esophageal strictures, small- and large-intestinal involvement, pulmonary insufficiency, chronic liver disease, and generalized wasting. Histologically, the disease resembles the systemic collagen vascular diseases, especially morphea and lupus erythematosus profundus. Chronic GVHD may be associated with recurrent and occasionally fatal bacterial infections.

Initial efforts to treat chronic GVHD with short courses of antithymocyte globulin or prolonged treatment with prednisone were ineffective. More recently, the Seattle team treated a series of 21 patients with combinations of prednisone and either procarbazine, cyclophosphamide, or azathioprine. Four of the twenty-one patients died with chronic GVHD. Eleven are alive and leading almost normal lives on treatment, while six have recovered completely and treatment has been discontinued. It appears that combination therapy can modify the course of chronic GVHD, but new approaches must be sought to treat or prevent this disorder.

Recovery of immunologic function Almost all patients given a marrow transplant from an HLA-identical sibling develop a functional graft with adequate levels of circulating granulocytes and platelets. Nevertheless, particularly in the first 3 months after grafting, these patients are susceptible to a wide variety of opportunistic infections. Approximately one-third of patients develop an interstitial pneumonia, and cytomegalovirus can be demonstrated in approximately one-half of these pneumonias. The mortality rate is high. The high incidence of infection is the result of a very slow return of immunologic function, which may be made worse by GVHD and by efforts to prevent or treat GVHD. Fortunately, by the end of the first year after grafting, most patients have recovered immunologically and are able to lead normal lives without an increased incidence of infection.

Tolerance The long-term healthy human recipients of allogeneic marrow transplants are true chimeras. Their myeloid system, lymphoid system, and monocyte-macrophage system are entirely made up of cells of donor origin. Clearly, these donor cells in the recipient are "tolerant" of the hosts' tissues. The studies of this tolerance constitute a fascinating story in immunobiology, but a clear understanding of the state of tolerance has not emerged. At least three mechanisms may be operative, including classical central tolerance, tolerance maintained by "blocking factors," and tolerance related to the presence of "suppressor" cells.

RECURRENT LEUKEMIA AFTER GRAFTING **Frequency of recurrence of leukemia** For patients with leukemia transplanted in relapse or in second remission, an actuarial analysis shows a rather constant rate of recurrence of leukemia in the first year, a decreasing rate in the second year, and few recurrences thereafter. If there were no other causes of death, approximately 35 percent of the patients would be cured while 65 percent will be destined to relapse. Most impressive, and rather unexpected, was the finding that only about 10 percent of patients with ANL transplanted in first remission subsequently relapsed. It is evident that recurrent leukemia after grafting is a major problem for patients transplanted in relapse or in the second or subsequent remission. Recurrent leukemia is only a minor problem for those patients transplanted in the first remission, which may be explained by the presence of only a very small number of residual leukemic cells and/or by the possibility that the leukemic cells of patients in first remission may not yet have acquired resistance to therapeutic agents.

Nature of recurrent leukemia Blood genetic markers and cytogenetic techniques can be used to identify the donor or host origin of the leukemic cells in those patients who relapse following marrow transplantation. In the vast majority of patients the recurrent leukemia is in host-type cells. However, five cases have now been reported in whom the recurrent leukemic cells were shown to be of donor origin.

Graft-versus-leukemia A graft-versus-leukemia effect has been demonstrated in murine systems in several laboratories. In human recipients of allogeneic bone marrow grafts, evidence supporting the existence of a graft-versus-leukemia effect has been difficult to obtain because of the large number of deaths from other causes among patients with severe GVHD. Sophisticated statistical methods have now shown that the relative relapse rate of leukemia was 2.5 times greater in recipients without GVHD than in recipients with GVHD. Recipients of allogeneic marrow who did not develop GVHD had the same relapse rate as recipients of syngeneic marrow, indicating that subclinical GVHD did not reduce the relapse rate.

SOME GENERALIZATIONS ABOUT MARROW TRANSPLANTATION Because of the complexity of the marrow grafting regimens, transplantation should only be undertaken by teams with all of the resources needed to ensure an optimal result. The number of such teams has increased rapidly over the past few years, and in general the clinical results are comparable to those described above.

Two major concerns have delayed a more general application of marrow transplantation. The first is cost. Marrow transplantation is obviously an expensive undertaking, but cost has been reduced appreciably by transplantation earlier in the course of the disease when the patient is in relatively good condition. Three centers (UCLA, Children's Orthopedic Medical Center of Seattle, and the Royal Marsden) have carried out cost analysis studies comparing marrow transplantation with "conventional" therapy and have found marrow transplantation to be less expensive than current chemotherapy regimens.

The second major concern has been that marrow transplantation has been regarded as an experimental procedure. As for all experimental procedures, the ethical problems of exposing a patient and donor to the marrow transplant regimen have limited its use. However, the demonstration of better long-term survival with marrow transplantation compared to conventional therapy for younger patients with severe aplastic anemia or acute leukemia should mitigate the ethical concern. Extension of this form of therapy to other malignant diseases and to other genetic disorders is experimental, but the current rapid rate of progress may soon make a much broader application of marrow grafting a reality.

REFERENCES

Appelbaum FR et al: Treatment of aplastic anemia by bone marrow transplantation in identical twins. Blood 55:1033, 1980

Blume KG et al: Bone marrow ablation and allogeneic marrow transplantation in acute leukemia: Clinical candidacy and outcome. N Engl J Med 302:1041, 1980

Bortin MM, Rimm AA, for the Advisory Committee of the International Bone Marrow Transplant Registry: Severe combined immunodeficiency disease. Characterization of the disease and results of transplantation. JAMA 238:591, 1977

Camitta BM et al: A prospective study of androgens and bone marrow transplantation for treatment of severe aplastic anemia. Blood 53:504, 1979

Clift RA et al: Marrow transplantation from donors other than HLA-identical siblings. Transplantation 28:235, 1979

Fefer A et al: Disappearance of Ph[1]-positive cells in four patients with chronic granulocytic leukemia after chemotherapy, irradiation and marrow transplantation from an identical twin. N Engl J Med 300:333, 1979

Gale RP and the UCLA Bone Marrow Transplant Unit: Current status of bone marrow transplantation in acute leukemia. Transplant Proc 11:1920, 1979

Meyers JD, Thomas ED: Infection complicating bone marrow transplantation, in *Clinical Approach to Infection in the Immunocompromised Host,* LS Young, RH Rubin (eds). New York, Plenum, 1981, p 507

Pahwa R et al: Treatment of the immunodeficiency diseases—Progress toward replacement therapy emphasizing cellular and macromolecular engineering. Springer Semin Immunopathol 1:355, 1978

Powles RL et al: Curability of acute leukemia, in *Topical Reviews in Haematology,* S Roath (ed). London, John Wright & Sons, 1980, p 186

Ramsay NKC et al: Total lymphoid irradiation and cyclophosphamide as preparation for bone marrow transplantation in severe aplastic anemia. Blood 55:344, 1980

Santos GW et al: Bone marrow transplantation—Present status. Transplant Proc 11:182, 1979

Storb R et al: Marrow transplantation in thirty "untransfused" patients with severe aplastic anemia. Ann Intern Med 92:30, 1980

Sullivan KM et al: Chronic graft-versus-host disease in 52 patients: Adverse natural course and successful treatment with combination immunosuppression. Blood 57:267, 1981

Thomas ED: Bone marrow transplantation: Present status and future expectations, in *Update I: Harrison's Principles of Internal Medicine,* KJ Isselbacher et al (eds). New York, McGraw-Hill, 1981, pp 135–152

——— et al: Bone-marrow transplantation. N Engl J Med 292:832, 895, 1975

———: Marrow transplantation for patients with acute lymphoblastic leukemia in remission. Blood 54:468, 1979

———: Marrow transplantation for acute nonlymphoblastic leukemia in first remission. N Engl J Med 301:597, 1979

Tsoi MS et al: Nonspecific suppressor cells in patients with chronic graft-*vs*-host disease after marrow grafting. J Immunol 123:1970, 1979

Weiden PL et al: Antileukemic effect of graft-versus-host disease in human recipients of allogeneic-marrow grafts. N Engl J Med 300:1068, 1979

Clotting disorders

332

PLATELET DISORDERS

HYMIE L. NOSSEL

Platelet disorders may be due to altered number or function of the platelets. Disorders of platelet number include thrombocytopenia and thrombocythemia (thrombocytosis). The most common serious bleeding disorder involving platelets is due to thrombocytopenia.

THROMBOCYTOPENIA

CLINICAL CONSIDERATIONS The normal platelet count ranges from 150,000 to 400,000 per cubic millimeter. A platelet count of less than 100,000 per cubic millimeter is generally considered to constitute thrombocytopenia. Although there is an approximate relationship between the platelet count and severity of bleeding, the hemostatic effects of thrombocytopenia may be aggravated by a sudden drop in the platelet count, infection, or anemia. With platelet counts above 40,000 per cubic millimeter, bleeding may occur after injury or surgery, but spontaneous bleeding is uncommon. Spontaneous bleeding is common with platelet counts between 10,000 and 20,000 per cubic millimeter; with counts below 10,000 per cubic millimeter, it is usual and often severe.

Spontaneous bleeding into the skin manifests as petechiae, purpuric spots, or confluent ecchymoses. In the mouth, blood-filled bullae are almost pathognomonic for thrombocytopenia. Bleeding may occur from any mucosal surface, including the nose and uterus and the gastrointestinal, urinary, or respiratory tracts. The most serious site for spontaneous bleeding is the central nervous system, where it may be fatal. Bleeding due to trauma in a thrombocytopenic patient presents a number of features distinct from bleeding in a patient with a coagulation factor disorder: (1) it occurs immediately after the trauma; (2) in mild cases it may cease in response to local pressure; and (3) it usually stops within 48 h and does not readily recur.

MECHANISMS A low platelet count may result from one or a combination of mechanisms. These include abnormal platelet production, disordered platelet distribution, and increased rate of destruction (Table 332-1).

Defective production of platelets may result from decreased production or from defective maturation. When platelet production is significantly diminished, the number of megakaryocytes visible in a bone marrow aspirate is usually significantly decreased.

Reduced production may result from (1) the administration of drugs such as the cytotoxic agents used in cancer chemotherapy (this is the commonest cause of thrombocytopenia in a large medical center), gold, sulfonamides, ethanol, and irradiation of the bone marrow; (2) generalized decrease in production of all marrow cells (aplastic anemia); (3) marrow replacement or infiltration, including marrow fibrosis, leukemia, and metastatic carcinoma; and (4) congenital deficiency of a thrombopoietic factor.

Defective maturation is associated with vitamin B_{12} or folate deficiency, the myeloproliferative disorders, paroxysmal nocturnal hemoglobinuria, and two hereditary disorders, the Wiskott-Aldrich syndrome and the May-Hegglin anomaly. In these disorders the bone marrow shows a normal or increased number of megakaryocytes, but thrombopoiesis is ineffective in a manner analogous to ineffective erythropoiesis.

Disordered distribution of platelets may be the cause of thrombocytopenia. In normal individuals about 30 percent of the circulating platelets are present in the spleen, whereas with massive splenomegaly up to 80 percent of the total number of circulating platelets may be in the spleen, resulting in thrombocytopenia in the peripheral blood. Thrombocytopenia may occur in any patient with a significantly enlarged spleen. However, the thrombocytopenia is rarely severe enough to produce hemorrhage, and splenectomy will restore the platelet count to normal levels, but is not usually required.

Accelerated destruction of platelets is a frequent cause of thrombocytopenia. The survival time of platelets is markedly decreased from the normal of 10 days to less than 1 day. The commonest causes of accelerated platelet destruction are antibody-mediated platelet injury, increased platelet utilization in disseminated intravascular coagulation, and severe blood loss with multiple transfusions.

Antibody-mediated thrombocytopenia may be due to (1) *autoantibodies* in idiopathic thrombocytopenic purpura, systemic lupus erythematosus, chronic lymphocytic leukemia, and in association with autoimmune hemolytic anemia; (2) alloantibodies associated with pregnancy or transfusion; (3) antibodies associated with the administration of certain drugs such as quinidine, quinine, and sulfonamides.

IDIOPATHIC THROMBOCYTOPENIC PURPURA (ITP) Clinical features This disorder may be considered the prototype thrombocytopenic state. The chief sign is purpura over the limbs, upper chest, and neck. Mucosal bleeding may occur. There is no adenopathy. The spleen is not palpable in 90 percent of patients and when palpable does not usually extend more than 1 cm below the left costal margin. Fever and malaise are uncommon.

The course of the disorder may be acute or chronic. The acute form of the disease occurs most commonly in children between the ages of 2 and 6 years, but is seen in adults as well. In children acute thrombocytopenia often follows an infection. Bleeding starts suddenly, usually being most severe at the onset. The risk of cerebral hemorrhage is greatest at this time. Bleeding usually ceases within a few days, although some patients may display a bleeding tendency for several months. When thrombocytopenia persists for 6 months or more, the disease is considered to be chronic. The chronic recurrent form occurs most often in women between 20 and 40 years of age. Most patients present with easy bruising of insidious onset, and menorrhagia is common. Mucosal bleeding indicates more severe thrombocytopenia. Characteristically, transient remissions occur and may last weeks, months, or years.

Idiopathic thrombocytopenic purpura may present with bleeding localized to one site only, e.g., menorrhagia, hematuria, or epistaxis. In such patients idiopathic thrombocytopenic purpura should be suspected, and the platelet count should be measured.

Laboratory tests Examination of the peripheral blood smear is an important part of the examination and reveals few platelets which are normal morphologically, with an increased percentage of large platelets. The bleeding time is prolonged, usually in proportion to the degree of thrombocytopenia. The whole-blood clotting time test is normal, but clot retraction is poor or absent when the platelet count is below 40,000 per cubic millimeter. Anemia is present only to the extent of blood loss; the erythrocyte sedimentation rate is usually normal. Bone marrow examination reveals megakaryocytes in normal or increased numbers with normal morphology. Increased platelet-associated IgG is the most useful diagnostic finding.

Differential diagnosis In children most acute thrombocytopenia is associated with other disorders. In adults a significant degree of splenomegaly, fever, disproportionate anemia, or a high sedimentation rate suggests another diagnosis. Bone marrow examination is essential in order to exclude other marrow diseases; the histology of the spleen should be examined for the same reason if the spleen is removed for therapeutic reasons. It is important to exclude other diagnoses, in particular drug-induced thrombocytopenia on a sensitization basis because the clinical and hematologic pictures of idiopathic and drug-induced hypersensitivity thrombocytopenic purpura are indistinguishable. A careful history is the only clue to the pos-

TABLE 332-1
Causes of thrombocytopenia

I Production defect
- *A* Reduced thrombopoiesis (reduced megakaryocytes)
  - *1* Marrow injury: drugs, chemicals, radiation, infection
  - *2* Marrow failure: acquired, congenital (Fanconi's syndrome, amegakaryocytic)
  - *3* Marrow invasion: carcinoma, leukemia, lymphoma, fibrosis
  - *4* Lack of marrow stimulus: thrombopoietin deficiency
- *B* Defective maturation (normal or increased megakaryocytes)
  - *1* Vitamin B_{12} deficiency, folic acid deficiency
  - *2* Hereditary: Wiskott-Aldrich syndrome, May-Hegglin anomaly

II Sequestration (disordered distribution)
- *A* Splenomegaly
- *B* Hypothermic anesthesia

III Accelerated destruction
- *A* Antibodies
  - *1* Autoantibodies
    - *a* ITP, systemic lupus erythematosus, hemolytic anemias, lymphoreticular disorders
    - *b* Drugs
  - *2* Alloantibodies
    - *a* Fetal-maternal incompatibility
    - *b* Following transfusions
- *B* Nonimmunologic
  - *1* Injury due to:
    - *a* Infection
    - *b* Prosthetic heart valves
  - *2* Consumption
    - *a* Thrombin in disseminated intravascular coagulation
    - *b* Thrombotic thrombocytopenic purpura
  - *3* Loss by hemorrhage and massive transfusion

sibility of drug-induced thrombocytopenia. Systemic lupus erythematosus and other diseases associated with platelet antibodies should be considered, and appropriate serologic tests for lupus erythematosus should be carried out. When thrombocytopenia results from platelet sequestration in a large spleen, anemia and leukopenia are usually associated. In leukemia, disproportionate anemia is frequent and the marrow is diagnostic. In aplastic anemia, pancytopenia is characteristic, and bone marrow biopsy should reveal hypocellularity. In patients with bone marrow infiltration, large platelets or megakaryocyte fragments may be present, the patient is usually anemic, normoblasts and myelocytes are found in the peripheral blood, and the marrow is diagnostic.

Pathogenesis The thrombocytopenia results from a shortened platelet survival time which is directly proportional to the platelet count. Platelet destruction results from binding of antibody to a platelet-associated antigen which renders the platelets more susceptible to phagocytosis by macrophages. Platelet-bound antibody is best demonstrated by increased platelet-associated IgG. Normal washed platelets have some detectable bound IgG, but the platelets of all patients with ITP have increased platelet-associated IgG; inverse correlations are noted with the platelet count and life span, and corticosteroid-induced responses are accompanied by a decrease in the platelet-associated IgG. The platelet antigens to which the antibodies bind have not been identified, and the term *autoimmune thrombocytopenic purpura* will be appropriate when this is achieved. In some patients with a greater density of IgG binding, C3 fixation occurs. Platelet phagocytosis by macrophages occurs primarily in the spleen, which is the major site of platelet sequestration and also a major site for antibody synthesis, thus explaining the clinically beneficial effect of splenectomy. Corticosteroids are thought to reduce macrophage uptake of antibody-coated platelets and also to interfere with antibody binding to platelets, thus reducing platelet-associated IgG. Without knowledge of the platelet-associated antigen with which the antibodies are reacting, it is not possible to implicate definitely a defect in the immune system as the cause of the production of the antibodies, although this seems likely.

Treatment of acute ITP More than 80 percent of patients with acute ITP will recover in time regardless of therapy; hence conservative management is favored. Treatment should take into account the following possibilities.

1 Corticosteroids do not appear to shorten the duration of thrombocytopenia, but prednisone, 1 mg per kilogram of body weight per day in children or 40 to 60 mg per day in adults, is advisable during the first 2 to 4 weeks because of a possible beneficial effect on capillary integrity.
2 Platelet transfusions should be used in treating life-threatening hemorrhage since they may be of benefit, although they are rapidly destroyed and will not affect the platelet count.
3 About 20 percent of children with ITP fail to recover in 6 months, and their course is similar to that of adults with chronic ITP. Of these 20 percent, about one-third have no or mild symptoms and do not require therapy. Purpura in the remainder can generally be controlled with prednisone. Splenectomy is generally advised if large doses of steroids are required beyond 3 to 6 months, although alternate-day steroid therapy may permit normal growth and minimize other undesirable side effects. In adults with acute ITP, splenectomy is generally advised within 2 to 4 weeks if response to therapy with high-dose prednisone has not occurred.
4 Splenectomy carried out on such patients is beneficial in 85 percent of cases.
5 Immunosuppressive therapy may be considered if splenectomy fails.

Treatment of chronic ITP The most important modes of treatment are the following.

1 Adrenocortical steroids produce a beneficial effect by improving the life span of antibody-coated platelets and by suppressing the phagocytic activity of the macrophages. Antibody synthesis may also be inhibited. A dose of 0.5 mg prednisone per kilogram per day will elevate the platelet count in mild cases; 1 mg/kg may be needed for cases of intermediate severity; 2 mg/kg or more per day may be necessary if the platelet count is less than 10,000 per cubic millimeter. The platelet count usually rises after several days, and by 14 days the majority of patients will show an elevation of platelet level. If improvement does not occur within 2 to 3 weeks or can be maintained only with massive doses of steroids, the spleen should be removed. In the patients who respond to steroids, dosage should be gradually reduced over a several-week period until the platelet count is about 60,000 per cubic millimeter. Splenectomy is favored in patients who fail to recover spontaneously within 3 to 6 months, who require more than 5 to 10 mg prednisone per day, and who are suitable operative risks.
2 Splenectomy removes the major site of platelet destruction and also a significant source of platelet antibody synthesis. Prior to surgery the prednisone dosage should be increased to raise the platelet count. Platelet transfusion may be used in the presence of severe thrombocytopenia but is usually not required in the less severe cases. Eighty percent of patients improve after splenectomy, and the platelet count is restored to normal levels permanently in two-thirds of patients. The count may rise within 24 h or within a week of surgery. There is no certain method of predicting a successful response to splenectomy. Following splenectomy, steroids should be withdrawn gradually over a 3-week period. If steroids are still required to prevent purpura or severe thrombocytopenia, immunosuppression should be considered.
3 Patients in whom splenectomy has failed may show a response to vincristine, cyclophosphamide, or azathioprine. An initial response rate of 50 to 70 percent to each of these drugs has been reported but is often not sustained. The clinical response with each of the three drugs has been approximately the same, but vincristine might be considered as the initial agent because of its marrow sparing effect.
4 Platelet transfusion is often effective in treating life-threatening hemorrhage but should not be used otherwise because of the short platelet life span and because of alloantibody formation.

OTHER AUTOANTIBODY THROMBOCYTOPENIAS Thrombocytopenia occurs in about 10 percent of patients with systemic lupus erythematosus. The thrombocytopenia usually results from platelet autoantibodies, and hemolysis due to red blood cell autoantibodies is often present as well. The treatment and the results of treatment are the same as in ITP. Idiopathic thrombocytopenic purpura may also occur in association with a Coombs-positive hemolytic anemia (Evans syndrome) and in association with chronic lymphocytic leukemia.

Thrombocytopenia due to drugs and chemicals (see Table 332-2) In every adult patient with thrombocytopenia a drug etiology should be considered. Thrombocytopenia may be part of the marrow suppression which occurs with the cytotoxic agents used in the therapy of leukemia, lymphoma, and carcinoma. Generalized marrow depression and consequent pancytopenia may also occur with other drugs such as gold or the sulfonamides. Selective thrombocytopenia may result from a specific effect on the megakaryocytes or as part of a hypersensitivity reaction in the peripheral blood. In the latter case the drug is thought to act as a hapten and bind to a plasma protein to form the primary antigen. Antibodies stimulated by the primary antigen bind the drug, and thrombocytopenia occurs when antigen-antibody complexes form which have a high affinity for the platelet membrane. The drugs most commonly associated with hypersensitivity reactions are quinidine, quinine, and sulfonamides.

The clinical manifestation of drug-induced thrombocytopenia is bleeding. In hypersensitivity reactions bleeding usually occurs within hours or days of initial drug administration, although it may occur after weeks or months of ingestion of the drug. Thrombocytopenia often develops abruptly. Bleeding is often severe and sudden in onset and may be associated with fever and systemic symptoms when toxic suppression of the marrow is involved.

The bone marrow may show increased numbers of megakaryocytes when peripheral blood destruction of platelets is the mechanism of thrombocytopenia (hypersensitivity reactions), or a reduced number of megakaryocytes and other marrow elements in marrow. Evidence of drug hypersensitivity may be demonstrable in vitro. The drug may inhibit clot retraction when added to the patient's blood, but this is an insensitive test. Complement fixation is a far more sensitive test for drug hypersensitivity.

Patients with hypersensitivity thrombocytopenia generally recover briskly in response to withdrawal of the offending drug. Adrenocorticosteroids should be given for control of bleeding, and platelet transfusion is indicated if the bleeding is potentially fatal. Splenectomy is *not* indicated. Patients should be given a card to carry with them, indicating the drug sensitivity. When thrombocytopenia is part of aplastic anemia, the prognosis is that of the cause of the underlying anemia.

Thrombocytopenic purpura due to alloantibodies Alloantibodies may occur following immunization of the mother against fetal platelets with subsequent transplacental transfer of the antibody. The infant may manifest purpura at birth; if it is severe, steroids, exchange transfusion, and transfusion with maternal platelets may be tried.

TABLE 332-2
Drugs implicated in thrombocytopenia

I Suppression of platelet production
- *A* Myelosuppressive drugs
  - *1* Severe: cytosine arabinoside, daunorubicin
  - *2* Moderate: cyclophosphamide, busulfan, methotrexate, 6-mercaptopurine
  - *3* Mild: vinca alkaloids
- *B* Thiazide diuretics
- *C* Ethanol
- *D* Estrogens

II Immunologic platelet destruction
- *A* Clinical suspicion plus convincing experimental evidence
  - *1* Antibiotics: sulfathiazole, novobiocin, *p*-aminosalicylate
  - *2* Cinchona alkaloids: quinidine, quinine
  - *3* Foods: beans
  - *4* Sedatives, hypnotics, anticonvulsants: Sedormid, carbamazepine, Centalun
  - *5* Arsenical drugs used to treat syphilis
  - *6* Digitoxin
  - *7* Methyldopa
  - *8* Stibophen
- *B* Clinical suspicion (major drugs implicated)
  - *1* Aspirin
  - *2* Chlorpropamide
  - *3* Chloroquine
  - *4* Chlorothiazide and hydrochlorothiazide
  - *5* Gold salts
  - *6* Insecticides
  - *7* Sulfadiazine, sulfisoxazole, sulfamerazine, sulfamethazine, sulfamethoxypyridazine, sulfamethoxazole, sulfatolamide

A complement-fixing platelet alloantibody may develop in the blood of a patient following blood transfusion. This disorder results from sensitization of the patient to an antigen in the transfused platelets. The antigen Pl^{A1} occurs in 98 percent of the population and is absent from the platelets of a recipient who develops the disorder. The Pl^{A1} antigen is also absent or decreased in platelets from patients with the congenital disorder thrombasthenia. Thrombocytopenic purpura may develop suddenly about 1 week after the transfusion and may persist for 6 weeks. The mechanism of the thrombocytopenia is not clear. There is some evidence that antibody provoked by Pl^{A1} antigen reacts with the antigen to form soluble immune complexes with a special affinity for the patient's own Pl^{A1}-negative platelets. The mechanism of this special affinity is unclear. If the thrombocytopenia is severe (below 10,000 per cubic millimeter), large doses of steroids and exchange transfusion should be used.

NONIMMUNOLOGIC THROMBOCYTOPENIC PURPURA Nonimmunologic causes of purpura include several forms of platelet injury and consumption.

Platelet injury INFECTION Thrombocytopenia occurring in acute infection may be due to marrow suppression, injury to the platelets caused directly by the organism or by exotoxins released by staphylococci or streptococci or endotoxins from gram-negative organisms. Disseminated intravascular coagulation may occur and contribute to the thrombocytopenia. Recovery from thrombocytopenia may be delayed for days or weeks.

PROSTHETIC HEART VALVES Thrombocytopenia occasionally occurs with or without a hemolytic anemia with fragmented red blood cells in patients with malfunctioning prosthetic heart valves. It has been suggested that extreme turbulence is responsible for the thrombocytopenia.

Platelet consumption DISSEMINATED INTRAVASCULAR COAGULATION In this condition thrombin aggregates platelets and reduces the circulating platelet count. Thrombocytopenia generally persists for longer than the other alterations in coagulation. Patients with diffuse intravascular clotting occasionally have fragmented red blood cells.

THROMBOTIC THROMBOCYTOPENIC PURPURA (TTP) (see also Chap. 329) This is a fulminating, often lethal disorder characterized by a Coombs-negative hemolytic anemia with severely fragmented red blood cells (microangiopathic hemolytic anemia), thrombocytopenic purpura, fever, renal failure, fluctuating levels of consciousness, and specific neurologic defects. Most patients die within a few weeks of the onset of the disease. The anemia is usually severe, the packed cell volume often being below 20 percent with a marked reticulocytosis. An essential diagnostic requirement is the presence of severely fragmented red blood cells in the peripheral blood smear. The diagnosis can be confirmed by the presence of occlusive hyalin accumulations in the lumina of arterioles and capillaries in the absence of vessel wall damage or inflammation. The deposits are inferred to be thrombi composed primarily of platelets and fibrinogen and/or fibrin. Lymph node, marrow, or gingival biopsy specimens may give a positive diagnosis in a significant number of patients. Blood coagulation tests generally show normal values with elevated fibrinogen levels in the early stages of the disease. Hypofibrinogenemia and elevated fibrinogen degradation product levels occur occasionally. Platelet survival is markedly decreased, and fibrinogen survival is only moderately reduced. The cause of TTP is unknown. The evidence does not support disseminated intravascular coagulation as having a primary pathogenic role. Platelet consumption is important, but it is not known whether the platelets or the vessel wall are primarily involved. The red blood cell fragmentation and hemolysis may result from contact with fibrin deposited in vessels.

Acute TTP constitutes a medical emergency. Therapy unfortunately is empiric and quite unpredictable in its effects. The effectiveness of therapy in general or the superiority of one form of therapy over another has not been demonstrated by controlled trial. Hence management is based on the published general experience and the response of the individual patient one is treating. Prior to 1960 most publications reported an acute fulminating course with death within 2 weeks. Since then there have been many reports (varying from 1 to 20 patients) of recovery in quite a high proportion of cases treated intensively with a variety of regimens. Heparin therapy is generally ineffective, whereas drugs inhibiting platelet function (most often either a combination of aspirin and dipyridamole or low-molecular-weight dextran) appear generally to be beneficial. Regimens in which good results have been reported include a combination of antiplatelet agents, corticosteroids, and splenectomy, and more recently antiplatelet agents and plasmapheresis. There are also reports of good results in patients treated with plasma transfusion.

HEMOLYTIC-UREMIC SYNDROME (see also Chap. 298) This syndrome is a disease of infancy (6 to 12 months) or early childhood (until age 6) characterized by the acute onset of fever, renal failure, microangiopathic hemolytic anemia, and thrombocytopenia. Hypertension is often present. A minor febrile illness with diarrhea or respiratory symptoms may precede the illness, and it has been postulated that virus-related immune complexes play a primary role in the pathogenesis of the syndrome. Laboratory studies reveal markedly decreased platelet survival but only moderately decreased fibrinogen survival. An occasional patient may show evidence of disseminated intravascular coagulation. Biopsy reveals hyalin occlusions in the afferent arterioles and glomerular capillaries of the kidneys, but other organs are usually not affected. With regard to therapy, corticosteroids and heparin have equivocal effects. Dialysis and the judicious use of red blood cell transfusions are helpful and with their aid the mortality rate in the acute stage may be as low as 5 percent. The reported incidence of chronic renal disease varies from 10 to 50 percent.

OTHER CAUSES Thrombocytopenia and hemolysis with fragmented red blood cells may also occur with neoplasms, with widespread metastatic tumors, or with acute transplant rejection. They may also occur as a complication of pregnancy or the puerperium when toxemia is present. The pathogenetic mechanism is not established.

PLATELET TRANSFUSIONS (See also Chap. 128)

Platelet transfusions are useful in preventing or stopping bleeding due to thrombocytopenia. Ideally the platelets should be transfused within 6 h of collection since they lose function after that time but are helpful if used within 24 h. Generally, in adults, transfusions involving platelets derived from 8 to 15 units of blood are used. In the absence of antibodies 1 unit of platelets will elevate the count by 5000 to 10,000 per cubic millimeter. The response may be less in the presence of infection or splenomegaly.

Repeated platelet transfusion results in alloimmunization and failure of response to further infusion. Following alloimmunization a satisfactory response to HLA-compatible platelets generally occurs and may persist indefinitely. Platelet transfusions are indicated in the therapy of life-threatening or serious hemorrhage and to tide a patient over an acute period of severe thrombocytopenia of less than 20,000 per cubic millimeter. Conditions in which platelet transfusions may be used, on the basis of these principles, include:

1 Acute leukemia
2 Aplastic anemia with serious hemorrhage
3 Acute thrombocytopenia manifesting serious bleeding
4 Exsanguinating blood loss requiring massive blood transfusion
5 Uremia with bleeding while awaiting dialysis

THROMBOCYTOSIS AND THROMBOCYTHEMIA *Thrombocytosis* is a term used to describe a temporary elevation of platelet count above 400,000 per cubic millimeter which may occur after severe hemorrhage, surgery, or splenectomy and in iron deficiency. Thrombocytosis may also occur in chronic inflammatory disorders and following recovery from acute infection. Malignant diseases such as carcinoma and Hodgkin's disease may also be associated with thrombocytosis.

The term *thrombocythemia* refers to a sustained elevation of platelet count, usually above 800,000 per cubic millimeter. In this condition, which is generally considered to be a myeloproliferative disorder, the spleen is almost always enlarged sufficiently to be detected by abdominal palpation. Thrombocythemia may occur as part of polycythemia vera, chronic myelogenous leukemia, or myelosclerosis, or it may occur alone, in which case it is termed essential (hemorrhagic) thrombocythemia. Patients with essential thrombocythemia frequently manifest spontaneous bleeding as well as venous and arterial thromboses. Platelet function studies such as aggregation and platelet factor 3 activity are often abnormal. The treatment of primary thrombocythemia involves therapy to decrease the autonomous growth of megakaryocytes and thus the excessive platelet production. ^{32}P, busulfan, or another alkylating agent is used for this purpose. Heparin therapy is required if thrombosis develops; aspirin and dipyridamole may prove useful in preventing thrombosis. The prognosis of primary thrombocythemia is that of the basic myeloproliferative disorder.

FUNCTIONAL DISORDERS OF PLATELETS The finding of a prolonged bleeding time in association with a normal platelet count suggests a disorder of platelet function. These disorders can be classified according to mechanism.

Defective adhesion A *defect in adhesion* appears to be the functional disturbance present in von Willebrand's disease, in which the primary defect is in a plasma protein. Platelet aggregation is normal with ADP, epinephrine, thrombin, and collagen, but is usually defective in response to ristocetin. Similar findings due to a primary platelet disorder occur in the Bernard-Soulier (giant-platelet) syndrome in which platelet membrane glycoprotein I is defective.

Defective primary aggregation A defect in the primary aggregation response is characteristic of a congenital disorder termed *thrombasthenia.* This disorder is associated with a severe hemorrhagic diathesis with a markedly prolonged bleeding time, absent clot retraction, and absent platelet aggregation in response to ADP or collagen. A defect in membrane glycoproteins IIb and IIIa and of Pl^{A1} antigen has been identified in the platelets of some patients with this disorder.

Defective platelet release reaction There are two distinct types of functional defect associated with defective ADP release. In one type, termed *storage pool disease,* the storage pool of ADP is defective, and the disorder occurs congenitally with or without albinism. In another type of congenital disorder the storage pool of ADP is normal, but the release reaction is defective. A patient with a congenitally defective release reaction associated with cyclo-oxygenase deficiency has been reported. In other patients the mechanism of defective release has not yet been established. Drugs may impair platelet function by inhibiting the release reaction. Aspirin inhibits release by irreversibly acetylating cyclo-oxygenase, thereby blocking the production of thromboxane A_2, which mediates the release reaction. The aspirin effect persists for the life span of the platelet. Drugs which inhibit platelet release include phenylbutazone, indomethacin, and many others with an anti-inflammatory action. Analgesic drugs without effect on platelets include codeine, acetaminophen (Tylenol), and propoxyphene (Darvon). The plasma expander dextran may also inhibit platelet function and prolong the bleeding time. The drugs which inhibit platelet function do not produce a bleeding diathesis by themselves but may aggravate an underlying disorder of hemostasis. They lengthen the bleeding time of normal individuals, which generally still remains within the normal range. The secondary wave of platelet aggregation in response to ADP and epinephrine is defective, platelet factor 3 activity is reduced, and clot retraction is normal.

Platelets from patients with a myeloproliferative syndrome and from patients with cirrhosis have functional defects which have not been completely characterized. A defect of platelet function occurs in *uremia* and may be associated with generalized bleeding from mucosal surfaces such as the nose, gastrointestinal tract, or renal tract, as well as cutaneous bleeding. This defect in platelet function is reversed by dialysis. It has been reported that infusion of plasma cryoprecipitate will temporarily correct the bleeding tendency in these patients. The mechanism of this effect is unknown. Some patients with *dysproteinemia* may have defective platelet function. In patients with macroglobulinemia or myeloma, the abnormal globulin is thought to coat the platelet and interfere with its proper function.

REFERENCES

ASTER RH: Thrombocytopenia due to enhanced platelet destruction, in *Hematology,* 2d ed, WJ Williams et al (eds). New York, McGraw-Hill, 1977, chap 145

DIXON R et al: Quantitative determination of antibody in idiopathic thrombocytopenic purpura. N Engl J Med 292:230, 1975

MACMILLAN R: Chronic idiopathic thrombocytopenic purpura. N Engl J Med 304:1135, 1981

MONCADA S, VANE JR: Arachidonic acid metabolites and the interactions between platelets and blood vessel walls. N Engl J Med 300:1142, 1979

MUSTARD JF, PACKHAM MA: Clinical pharmacology of platelets. Blood 50:555, 1977

ROSSE WF, LOGUE GL: Immune thrombocytopenia and granulocytopenia, in *Update II: Harrison's Principles of Internal Medicine,* KJ Isselbacher et al (eds). New York, McGraw-Hill, 1982

WEISS HJ: Congenital disorders of platelet function. Semin Hemostasis 17:228, 1980

333 BLEEDING DISORDERS DUE TO VESSEL WALL ABNORMALITIES

HYMIE L. NOSSEL

Vascular defects (nonthrombocytopenic purpuras) are common, but they usually do not cause serious bleeding problems. Bleeding mainly occurs from mucous membranes or into the skin, starts immediately following injury, ceases in less than 24 to 48 h, and rarely recurs. The mechanism of bleeding is thought to be damage to capillary endothelium. The platelet count is usually normal, but tests of platelet function may be normal or abnormal. In those cases where a platelet function defect is demonstrable, the actual role of the vascular defect in the pathogenesis of the bleeding syndrome is uncertain, and there is no current method of diagnosing the vascular defect under such circumstances. In many cases, the diagnosis of a vascular defect underlying the bleeding syndrome is by exclusion. The platelet count and bleeding time are usually normal. A number of disease syndromes may be accompanied by bleeding thought to be due to vascular defects.

INFECTIONS Many severe infections may be associated with bleeding manifestations, especially meningococcemia, septicemia, typhoid fever, subacute bacterial endocarditis, and sometimes childhood viral infections such as measles. Disorders of platelet function, thrombocytopenia, and coagulation (defibrination) may play a role as well as vascular defects.

DRUGS In addition to purpura, urticarial or maculopapular rashes may be present. Drugs which may be associated with purpura include penicillin and the sulfonamides.

SCURVY The pathogenetic mechanism in scurvy is defective intercellular substance of capillary walls. There is a failure in collagen formation associated with defective hydroxyproline synthesis. Ascorbic acid is essential for synthesis of hydroxyproline. In addition, a defect of platelet function has been described in scurvy. Bleeding may occur in the skin, where it is often perifollicular, in the muscles, particularly the calf muscles, in the gastrointestinal tract, or into the urine. Clinical signs which suggest scurvy are swelling of the gums and hyperkeratosis of the skin. If the diagnosis is suspected, it can be confirmed by demonstrating a low ascorbic acid content in the white blood cells. Treatment is administration of vitamin C.

CUSHING'S SYNDROME The basic pathologic defect in this disorder, characterized by excessive cortisol production, is thought to be the protein-wasting effect of the increased blood steroid level with loss of perivascular supporting tissue.

HENOCH-SCHÖNLEIN SYNDROME Also known as anaphylactoid purpura, this disorder is a vasculitis with a characteristic clinicopathologic picture. It occurs most commonly between the ages of 2 and 20. Pathologically, an acute inflammatory reaction of the capillaries and mesangial tissues of the small arterioles is found associated with increased vascular permeability, exudation, and hemorrhage into the tissues. IgA and alternate pathway complement components have been identified in the capillaries of patients with the disease. Food, drugs, and bacteria have been implicated in hypersensitivity angiitis without definitive evidence for any of these. The syndrome is most common in children and is often preceded by streptococcal sore throat 1 to 3 weeks before the onset of hemorrhagic manifestations. The clinical pattern includes:

1 *Purpuric rash,* with either small or large spots. Initially they may be urticarial, and they often have a characteristic distribution on the extensor surfaces of the arms, legs, and buttocks. The character and distribution of the rash may be the only clue to the diagnosis of the disorder. Tests of platelet function and coagulation are normal.
2 *Abdominal manifestations,* including colicky pain due to extravasation of fluid and blood into the intestinal wall.
3 *Polyarthralgia and polyarthritis*—tenderness and swelling are mainly periarticular.
4 *Hematuria,* often with albuminuria and casts, reflecting focal glomerulonephritis which is usually transient. In a minority of cases, the clinical spectrum of acute diffuse glomerulonephritis, with edema and hypertension, may occur and an occasional patient may die in acute renal failure. Five to ten percent develop chronic nephritis. Tests of platelet function and coagulation are normal.

Corticosteroids do not appear to affect the course of the disease but may control edema and joint and abdominal pain.

SENILE PURPURA This condition occurs most commonly in thin, elderly people and usually affects the extensor surfaces of the arms. Irregular dark purple areas with clear-cut margins are present on the arms, and the skin is freely mobile over the deeper tissues. The disorder is thought to be due to atrophy of collagen so that the skin is poorly anchored to deeper tissues and movements easily rupture vessels.

HEREDITARY HEMORRHAGIC TELANGIECTASIA This syndrome is transmitted as a simple dominant trait affecting both sexes equally. The telangiectases are due to multiple dilatations of capillaries and arterioles, which are lined by a thin layer of endothelial cells. The bleeding tendency is thought to be due to mechanical fragility of the dilated vessel. Clinically, the telangiectases may be on any part of the skin as well as the mucosae of the nose and mouth, gastrointestinal tract, or renal tract. Bleeding may occur from any one of these sites in a recurrent fashion. Telangiectases present on the skin blanch on pressure, since the blood is not extravascular but within the capillary dilatation. The diagnosis is made from the clinical triad of telangiectasia, hemorrhage, and familial pattern.

DYSPROTEINEMIA Vascular purpura may occur in macroglobulinemia, multiple myeloma, and cryoglobulinemia. Pathogenic mechanisms may involve damage by the proteins to the vessel walls and capillary anoxia associated with hyperviscosity. Platelet and coagulation function may be disturbed. A malignant type of maculopapular purpura may occur in association with mixed cryoglobulinemia. The vascular lesions are due to immune-complex damage to the vessel walls. Mixed cryoglobulinemia (often a complex of IgG and anti-IgG) may be associated with a variety of disorders including infection and autoimmune disorders. Mixed cryoglobulinemia and purpura may be associated with arthralgia, weakness, and nephritis without an identifiable primary disorder. Plasmapheresis with removal of cryoglobulin will have short-term benefit. Long-term management is that of the underlying disease. In the condition termed *benign hyperglobulinemic purpura,* purpuric spots are found characteristically on the anterior aspects of the lower limbs, in association with an elevated gamma globulin level in the serum.

REFERENCES

CAPRA DJ et al: Hyperglobulinemic purpura. Studies on the unusual anti-globulins characteristic of the sera of these patients. Medicine 50:125, 1971

CREAM JJ et al: Schönlein-Henoch purpura in the adult. Q J Med 39:461, 1970

FAUCI AS: The spectrum of vasculitis. Ann Intern Med 80:660, 1978

GOTTLIEB AJ: in *Hematology,* 2d ed, WJ Williams et al (eds). New York, McGraw-Hill, 1977, chaps 151, 153, 154

WINTROBE MM: *Clinical Hematology,* 8th ed. Philadelphia, Lea & Febiger, 1981

334
DISORDERS OF BLOOD COAGULATION FACTORS

HYMIE L. NOSSEL

CONGENITAL DISORDERS

Congenital disorders of coagulation characteristically involve a single coagulation protein, and transmission of the defect is genetically determined. A severe functional defect may be transmitted either as an autosomal recessive or dominant trait or as an X-linked recessive characteristically manifested in male hemizygotes and in the rare female homozygotes. In many instances a coagulation protein is present in the blood in normal concentrations as measured immunologically but is functionally defective. Since the plasma concentrations of most of the coagulation proteins are very low, evidence for the presence of a normal amount of the protein principally depends on measurement of a normal amount of antigenic activity. The coagulation proteins may then be measured as clot-promoting activity and as antigenic activity. In normal individuals these two activities correlate, whereas in some patients with coagulation factor disorders, clot-promoting activity may be sharply reduced and antigenic activity may be normal, reflecting an abnormal molecule. In other patients both coagulant and antigenic activity may be similarly reduced, due either to fewer molecules or to a defect which reduces both functional and antigenic activity.

HEMOPHILIA Hemophilia is a bleeding disorder due to inherited deficiency in the procoagulant activity of factor VIII, the antihemophilic factor. It is the most common of the congenital coagulation factor disorders, occurring in 1 in 10,000 of the population. The gene is transmitted in a sex-linked recessive pattern. Female heterozygotes (carriers) transmit the disorder to one-half of their sons and the gene to one-half of their daughters. Female carriers rarely manifest any bleeding tendency. The measured level of factor VIII coagulant activity cannot absolutely establish whether the sister of a hemophilic male is a carrier (heterozygote) or is normal. When both factor VIII coagulant activity and antigenic activity are measured, 30 percent of carriers can be detected at the 99 percent level of confidence and 50 percent at the 95 percent confidence level. Males with the disorder (hemizygotes) transmit the gene to all their daughters, who rarely have a bleeding tendency; their sons are all normal. In 30 percent of cases, no family history can be elicited.

Molecular defect Two proteins circulate in plasma, apparently bound to one another, and are referred to as the factor VIII complex. These proteins are the antihemophilic and von Willebrand factors which are under separate genetic control, have distinct biochemical and immunologic properties, and have quite different and essential physiologic functions. The antihemophilic factor, although separated from the von Willebrand and other plasma proteins, has not been purified to homogeneity but appears to have a molecular weight of 285,000 daltons. Treatment with thrombin results in a progressive decrease in molecular size accompanied by an initial increase in activity and subsequent inactivation. Antibodies specific to the molecule may arise in transfused hemophiliacs or in individuals who form autoantibodies, and these antibodies are useful in measuring antihemophilic factor antigen. The function of the antihemophilic factor is to act as a cofactor for factor IX_a in the activation of factor X. Defective activity of this molecule is responsible for hemophilia, but the structural abnormalities responsible for lack of activity have not been determined. Synthesis of the protein is governed by the X chromosome, but the cellular site of synthesis has not been identified. The antihemophilic protein is often referred to as factor VIII coagulant activity, abbreviated VIII:C, and its antigen as factor VIII coagulant antigen, abbreviated VIII:CAg.

The von Willebrand protein constitutes most of the protein in the factor VIII complex. It has been purified and comprises a heterogeneous population of multimers ranging in size from about 850,000 to 12 million daltons. The basic subunit is about 210,000 daltons in size, a disulfide-bonded tetramer of which forms the 850,000-dalton molecule. The molecule contains carbohydrate and is thus a glycoprotein. Antibodies to the protein are readily produced by immunization of rabbits. The von Willebrand protein binds to the surface of platelets and is essential for the normal formation of platelet plugs. Hence deficient activity of the protein produces a prolonged bleeding time test. Von Willebrand protein is synthesized in vascular endothelial cells and in megakaryocytes and is under autosomal control. The von Willebrand protein is often referred to as factor VIII-related protein, abbreviated VIIIR or VIIIvWF, and the antigen as VIIIRAg or VIIIvWFAg.

Clinical features BLEEDING IN GENERAL It will be recalled (Chap. 55) that platelet plug formation is the first line of defense against bleeding, followed by coagulation. Since platelet plug formation is normal in hemophilia, the onset of bleeding is characteristically delayed for several hours or days after injury. Bleeding may, however, persist for several days or weeks since coagulation is important in maintenance of the occlusive plug. The clinical manifestations of hemophilia vary greatly depending on the level of factor VIII coagulant activity (Table 334-1). In milder cases, spontaneous bleeding does not occur, but exsanguinating hemorrhage may follow injury or surgery. In severe cases spontaneous recurrent bleeding episodes are characteristic and may be associated with chronic joint deformity. Large hematomas may be associated with fever, anemia, and hyperbilirubinemia.

BLEEDING IN SPECIFIC LOCATIONS As one would anticipate from the defect in the maintenance stage of hemostasis, bruises, ecchymoses, and deep subcutaneous and intramuscular hematomas occur frequently, whereas petechiae and purpura do not occur. Recurrent hemarthroses are a characteristic feature and often result in permanent joint damage with destruction of the edges of the bones forming the joints, osteophyte formation with limitation of joint movement, and eventual fibrous or bony ankylosis. Bleeding following dental extractions is often a problem. Bleeding also often occurs from mucosal surfaces such as the frenum of the tongue and the urogenital and gastrointestinal tracts. Gastrointestinal hemorrhage is frequently associated with a local lesion. Any organ in the body may be the site of bleeding. Hemorrhage is potentially lethal, owing to local pressure effects when it is intracranial, lingual, laryngeal, retropharyngeal, pericardial, or pleural in location.

Diagnosis Hemophilia should be suspected from the sex of the patient, a familial pattern if present, the age of onset, and the type of bleeding. A family tree should be drawn while taking the history. Laboratory tests establish the diagnosis. Tests of platelet function, bleeding time, and platelet count are normal. Tests of coagulation show a prolonged whole-blood clotting time in severe hemophilia; in mild hemophilia the clotting time may be normal. The prothrombin time is normal, and the partial thromboplastin time is prolonged. Low factor VIII coagulant activity is diagnostic. Factor VIII coagulant antigen activity is generally absent in severe hemophilia but may be reduced or normal in mild or moderate hemophilia. Von Willebrand antigen levels are generally normal.

Treatment Following diagnosis, patients or their parents should be instructed in detail about the care, prognosis, and hereditary nature of the disorder. Children should be reared in as normal a way as is compatible with physical safety since emotional crippling can be as serious as that resulting from hemorrhage. As they grow older, patients should be encouraged to participate in sports such as swimming or golf and to avoid those involving body contact. A vocation should be sought which is not inherently dangerous. The aim should be to encourage patients to become self-supporting adults capable of looking after themselves and living a full life.

The basis for therapy of bleeding episodes is transfusion of material containing factor VIII procoagulant activity which temporarily corrects the specific defect. Whole blood is not used for this purpose, and its use is restricted to restoration of blood volume following severe loss. Plasma with a high factor VIII content may be used, but factor VIII concentrates are the preferred method of treatment since the content of antihemophilic factor is known and the load on the blood volume is less. Following infusion, about 90 percent of the infused activity may be found in the patient's plasma. Hence, if the amount of factor VIII infused and the patient's plasma volume are both known, it is possible to predict the rise in factor VIII level resulting from the infusion. Following transfusion, factor VIII activity disappears rapidly, about half remaining after 12 h, so that repeated infusion is required till the bleeding stops. In the event of major injury or surgery, factor VIII levels should be elevated to above 50 percent of the normal level and maintained above 30 percent at all times until the wound has healed completely. The amount of factor VIII required may be calculated as follows: 1 unit of factor VIII (the average activity in 1 ml normal plasma) per kilogram of body weight elevates the factor VIII level about 1.8 percent of the normal. Following an initial dose of 50 units per kilogram, about 30 units per kilogram should be given every 8 h for the first 2 days. Infusions

TABLE 334-1
Relationship of factor VIII blood levels to severity of bleeding

Factor VIII coagulant activity, % normal	*Type of bleeding*
50–100	None
25–50	Bleeding may be excessive after major trauma
5–25	Severe bleeding after surgical operations and some bleeding after minor trauma; no spontaneous bleeding
1–5	Severe bleeding after minor injury; occasional spontaneous hemorrhages
0	Severe hemophilia with spontaneous bleeding into muscles and joints

every 12 h of a suitably adjusted dose may then be given if clinical progress is satisfactory and factor VIII levels are in the desired range. For dental extraction an initial elevation of the factor VIII level to 50 percent of the normal level should be accompanied by the administration of ε-aminocaproic acid (EACA) (24 g per day in a 70-kg adult, orally for 7 days). The EACA greatly reduces the infusion requirement, probably by inhibiting salivary plasmin which otherwise dissolves clots as they form. A second similar dose of factor VIII should be given on the fourth or fifth day following the procedure. Sockets of extracted teeth should not be sutured since if hemostasis is not effective, blood accumulating under the sutures may track into the soft tissues of the neck or lingual area.

Transfusion of factor VIII is also useful in aborting bleeding into joints if given in the early stages. The factor VIII level in the patient should be elevated to 30 to 50 percent of normal. Acutely swollen joints should be immobilized, and local chilling in the early stages may be beneficial. Aspiration may be helpful but should be performed only after adequate infusion therapy. After bleeding has stopped, active motion without weight bearing is important to prevent chronic limitation of movement. Careful use of physiotherapy and splints may be helpful in preventing and correcting deformities and useful in avoiding later reparative surgery. Development and maintenance of strength of the muscles surrounding the joints should be an important aim of management so that the muscles will be able to assist the joints in weight bearing. Infusion therapy at home permits the early therapy of bleeding episodes which are thereby often aborted with a marked reduction in morbidity, absenteeism from work, time in hospital, and attendance at the outpatient clinic. These factors result in a high degree of patient satisfaction with home infusion therapy. It is important that regular contact between patient and physician be maintained.

For minor bleeding occurring from an accessible site, local measures such as application of thrombin, cold, and gentle pressure may be helpful. Hemophiliacs should not be given intramuscular injections, and following venipuncture, local pressure should be maintained until bleeding has stopped (usually within 5 min). Immunization against tetanus is important because patients with hemophilia may be prone to infection with this organism. Immunizations should be given while the patient is receiving factor VIII replacement therapy. Regular prophylactic care of the teeth should be provided. It is wise to avoid aspirin which increases the hazard of bleeding by impairing platelet function. Acetaminophen and propoxyphene are analgesics which do not impair hemostasis. It has been found that infusion of a synthetic analogue of the antidiuretic hormone [1-deamino-8-D-arginine vasopressin (DDAVP)] will transiently elevate the factor VIII level threefold in normal individuals and in hemophiliacs with measurable activity but not when the factor VIII level is below 1 percent. It has been suggested that DDAVP infusion may be useful to treat or prevent bleeding in hemophiliacs with factor VIII levels of about 10 percent or higher. The place of such therapy remains to be determined.

About 5 percent of hemophiliacs develop antibodies to factor VIII (circulating anticoagulants) which vitiate the beneficial effect of infusion. Such patients should not undergo surgery, and infusion therapy should be avoided as far as possible to avoid unnecessarily raising the antibody titer. (See also circulating anticoagulants below).

Course and prognosis Patients with milder forms of hemophilia usually live a virtually normal life but may have severe hemorrhage after dental extraction, injury, or surgery. Patients with severe disease may require frequent admission to the hospital and may develop crippling joint deformities. Home transfusion therapy permits early treatment of the bleeding and significantly reduces morbidity. The patient or the family can be trained to give infusions at home and thereby avert many visits to the hospital emergency room. Regular contact with an experienced physician should be maintained so that when hospital therapy is required, it is not delayed unnecessarily. Many patients with severe disease may live productive lives, whereas others are chronic invalids. Although life expectancy has been greatly prolonged by replacement therapy, death as a complication of hemorrhage still occurs quite frequently.

VON WILLEBRAND'S DISEASE Von Willebrand's disease is a hereditary hemorrhagic disorder transmitted as an autosomal dominant trait and characterized by a prolonged bleeding time in association with an abnormality in the von Willebrand protein. Reduction in antihemophilic factor activity is often present, apparently as a secondary phenomenon.

The pathogenesis of the prolonged bleeding time appears to involve a defect in platelet adhesion to the subendothelial collagen of the capillary wall. The von Willebrand protein is not required for normal adhesion of platelets to collagen under the flow conditions used for in vitro tests of this function but is required for normal adhesion. Under in vivo flow conditions, the von Willebrand protein is necessary for normal platelet adhesion. Since platelet adherence to the subendothelial tissues is abnormal, hemostatic plug formation is delayed, and the bleeding time is prolonged. Immunofluorescent techniques demonstrate close association of von Willebrand antigen with endothelial cells lining blood vessels throughout the body and also with subendothelial collagen. The von Willebrand factor is required for normal platelet aggregation induced by ristocetin, and in platelet-rich plasma from most patients with von Willebrand's disease ristocetin does not induce platelet aggregation.

Factor VIII complex As discussed in the section on hemophilia, the von Willebrand factor constitutes most of the protein of the factor VIII complex. A number of abnormalities in the behavior of the von Willebrand factor have been described, but the precise structural defects in the molecule have not been identified. The concentration of von Willebrand's protein in plasma can be determined immunologically, the Laurell technique being used most commonly. In most patients with von Willebrand's disease the plasma concentration of antigen is reduced. Normal concentrations of antigen may be associated with an abnormal protein which migrates abnormally on crossed immunoelectrophoresis. In normal plasma the protein occurs in a series of multimeric forms as shown by electrophoresis on agarose, and an abnormal protein may manifest as absent or diminished multimers. The von Willebrand protein binds to the platelet surface, and in the presence of ristocetin platelets are aggregated in a time-dependent reaction varying as a function of the concentration of von Willebrand protein and of ristocetin. This activity of the protein is termed *ristocetin cofactor* activity.

In the most common variety of von Willebrand's disease, with a mild to moderately severe bleeding diathesis, low levels of von Willebrand antigen and of ristocetin cofactor are associated with comparably low levels of antihemophilic factor coagulant activity (generally in the range of 20 to 50 percent of the normal levels). The von Willebrand protein behaves normally on crossed immunoelectrophoresis. In one variant, clinically severe von Willebrand's disease is associated with very low levels (less than 5 percent of the normal levels) of von Willebrand antigen, ristocetin cofactor, and antihemophilic coagulant activity. Too little protein is present to determine behavior on immunoelectrophoresis. In another, usually milder variant, antihemophilic factor and von Willebrand antigen levels are normal and ristocetin cofactor levels may be increased. The abnormal von Willebrand protein is detected by abnormal migration on crossed immunoelectrophoresis. Further analysis of the abnormally migrating von Willebrand protein distinguishes two types of abnormality. In normal plasma large, intermediate, and small multimers occur. In one of the abnormal forms, both the large and intermediate multimers are absent; in the other form only the large multimers are lacking. The mechanism leading to decreased antihemophilic factor activity in von Willebrand's disease is not clear but may reflect an increased clearance rate or decreased synthesis.

Clinical features The true incidence of the disease is not known, but it appears to be one of the most common congenital bleeding disorders. Although transmitted by a dominant autosomal gene, it has been detected more often in women. Symptoms usually appear in childhood and decrease with age. The severity of symptoms may vary among affected members of the same family, some of whom may be asymptomatic. In general the severity of bleeding corresponds to the degree of antihemophilic factor deficiency and of prolongation of the bleeding time. Most commonly the bleeding is mucosal and cutaneous. Epistaxis and easy bruising occur frequently but petechiae are rare. Recurrent gastrointestinal bleeding may be troublesome. Excessive bleeding may accompany surgery and is prevented by transfusion therapy. Hemarthroses occur only in isolated patients with very low levels of antihemophilic factor activity. Menorrhagia and excessive postpartum bleeding are common. During pregnancy the concentrations of all components of the factor VIII complex frequently increase significantly and the bleeding time decreases. These changes are presumably responsible for normal hemostasis observed in many patients after parturition.

Von Willebrand's disease may develop in a previously normal individual, generally in association with a primary disease in which immunoglobulin production is abnormal. The immunoglobulins may be polyclonal (as in systemic lupus erythematosus) or monoclonal.

Diagnosis The extraordinary heterogeneity of the disorder means that no single normal test is sufficient to exclude the diagnosis. In addition, both the antihemophilic factor activity and the bleeding time abnormality may fluctuate widely in an individual on repeated testing. The bleeding time and the antihemophilic factor assay are the most useful tests in the initial evaluation of von Willebrand's disease. The prolonged bleeding time may be regarded as a cardinal feature, while a normal bleeding time excludes a clinically significant abnormality. A low concentration of von Willebrand protein confirms the diagnosis, but a normal level does not exclude it. Crossed immunoelectrophoresis is necessary to detect an abnormal molecule. Ristocetin aggregation of platelets in platelet-rich plasma is a useful in vitro measure of von Willebrand protein function, but testing the patient's plasma mixed with washed normal platelets provides a more sensitive and specific test.

The von Willebrand protein level is increased as an acute phase reactant during pregnancy. High levels have been reported in Kaposi's sarcoma.

Treatment Local measures, as in hemophilia, are used in mild bleeding in von Willebrand's disease. Transfusion of normal plasma has a sustained effect on the factor VIII level in most patients, unlike the brief elevation in hemophilia (see Chap. 55). A cryoprecipitate rich in factor VIII prepared from normal plasma may be used in the therapy of von Willebrand's disease and produces both a prolonged increase in factor VIII activity and improvement in hemostasis. The hemostatic effectiveness of more purified factor VIII preparations is uncertain. Infusion of DDAVP elevates the von Willebrand protein level in plasma transiently. The therapeutic benefit of this phenomenon remains to be determined.

CONGENITAL DEFICIENCY OF OTHER COAGULATION FACTORS Congenital deficiencies of each of the other coagulation factors occur, and may be associated with a hemorrhagic tendency except for a deficiency of factor XII, prekallikrein, and high-molecular-weight kininogen. Laboratory diagnosis is made in a manner similar to that described for hemophilia; the results of different laboratory tests are summarized in Table 55-4. The principles of therapy are similar to those described for hemophilia. Replacement transfusion therapy is modified from that described for hemophilia according to the availability of concentrates and the recovery and in vivo survival times of the deficient factor (Table 55-3).

Factor IX deficiency Factor IX deficiency [also termed plasma thromboplastin component (PTC) or Christmas factor deficiency] occurs about one-sixth as frequently as factor VIII deficiency. The clinical manifestations and inheritance are exactly as in hemophilia, but a different protein is defective and a different concentrate is used in therapy. There is evidence that many patients with factor IX deficiency actually synthesize a factor IX-like protein with antigenic activity but with defective coagulant activity.

Concentrates containing factor IX are used in the treatment of the congenital deficiency. These concentrates (prothrombin complex concentrates) generally contain prothrombin and factors VII, IX, and X. Many of the concentrates contain some activated factors as well; when they are infused very rapidly, intravascular coagulation and thrombosis may result. The indications for use of the concentrates should be severe bleeding in the presence of established deficiency of one or more of the four factors listed above. The infusion should be given slowly.

Factor XI deficiency Clinically, deficiency of factor XI [which is also termed plasma thromboplastin antecedent (PTA)] resembles mild to moderate hemophilia. It is even less common than factor IX deficiency, occurs most often in people of Jewish origin, and is transmitted as an autosomal dominant characteristic. About one-third of affected individuals appear to have no excessive bleeding at all. In individuals who do bleed excessively, the disorder is readily treated with infusions of fresh frozen plasma.

Factor XII deficiency Deficiency of this factor (also known as Hageman factor) is usually asymptomatic, and therapy is not required. The whole-blood clotting time and partial thromboplastin time tests are grossly prolonged. The explanation for the lack of hemorrhagic diathesis is unknown.

Factor XIII deficiency Deficiency of factor XIII appears to be inherited in two patterns—as an autosomal recessive trait in some families, confined to males in others. Clinically, a moderately severe bleeding tendency occurs. Fibrin clots formed in this disorder are not cross-linked and are very susceptible to dissolution by plasmin or by mechanical stress. Excessive bleeding from the umbilicus and production of keloid scar tissue, often on the forehead, following bleeding from injury is suggestive of the disorder. Recurrent abortion in early pregnancy is characteristic. The screening test for factor XIII deficiency is based on solubility of the non-cross-linked clot in 5 *M* urea or 1% monochloroacetic acid. There are other causes of abnormal clot solubility, and the diagnosis should be confirmed by a quantitative assay of factor XIII activity. All other coagulation tests are normal in this disorder. Transfusion with plasma temporarily restores normal hemostasis, the $t_{\frac{1}{2}}$ of the infused activity being 4 to 7 days.

Fibrinogen deficiency Fibrinogen deficiency is generally transmitted as an autosomal recessive trait and may manifest as a complete or partial absence of fibrinogen from the blood plasma. Clinically, the disease resembles moderate or mild hemophilia, but hemarthroses do not occur. When there is complete absence of fibrinogen, the whole-blood clotting time, the one-stage prothrombin time, and thrombin clotting time all are grossly prolonged. Control of bleeding is achieved by transfusion of fibrinogen contained in freshly frozen plasma. With fibrinogen levels above 50 mg/dl, the screening coagulation tests may show only minor abnormality, and a quantitative measure of the fibrinogen level is required to indicate the presence of a deficiency.

Congenital fibrinogen abnormality may also be due to the hereditary synthesis of structurally and functionally abnormal fibrinogen molecules, a situation analogous to some of the hemoglobinopathies. In fibrinogen Detroit the amino acid serine is substituted for arginine at position 19 on the Aα-polypeptide chain; the propositus with this defect presented with a severe bleeding tendency. More than 50 additional patients with molecular abnormalities of fibrinogen have been identified, but amino acid substitutions have been demonstrated in only about half a dozen cases. Some of these patients display a severe hemorrhagic syndrome, some have recurrent thrombosis, whereas others are asymptomatic. The laboratory finding most useful in identifying these abnormalities is a prolonged thrombin clotting time.

ACQUIRED COAGULATION DISORDERS

These disorders occur much more often than do the congenital disorders and constitute the bulk of coagulation disorders encountered.

VITAMIN K DEFICIENCY Vitamin K is a fat-soluble vitamin essential for the synthesis of normal prothrombin and factors VII, IX, and X, which are referred to as the K-dependent coagulation factors. Normal prothrombin has 10 γ-carboxyglutamic acid residues grouped near the NH_2-terminal end of the molecule which bind calcium and via calcium serve to bind phospholipid and factor X_a. Prothrombin synthesized in the absence of vitamin K has glutamic acid in place of the γ-carboxyglutamic acid, since vitamin K is required for postribosomal γ-carboxylation of glutamic acid (see Fig. 334-1). When glutamic acid replaces γ-carboxyglutamic acid, there is defective binding of calcium, phospholipid, and factor X_a to prothrombin. This impaired binding is responsible for the defective biological function of vitamin K–deficient prothrombin. Similar abnormalities are responsible for the defective activity of factors VII, IX, and X.

The natural sources of vitamin K are food and the intestinal bacterial flora. The principal food sources are green leafy vegetables. There are relatively small body stores of vitamin K, and if intake of the vitamin is stopped, deficiency may develop within 1 to 3 weeks. The diagnosis of vitamin K deficiency is confirmed if prolonged prothrombin and partial thromboplastin times are corrected in 12 to 24 h by the parenteral administration of vitamin K.

Etiology In most patients, multiple factors are involved. Vitamin K deficiency may occur from impaired absorption due to lack of bile salts as in obstructive jaundice or biliary fistula. Intestinal malabsorption syndromes can also produce vitamin K deficiency. Oral administration of antibiotics, which leads to decreased gut flora in association with total or partial parenteral alimentation, may lead to vitamin K deficiency.

Clinical features Bleeding associated with deficiency of the vitamin K–dependent factors is similar to that occurring with other coagulation defects. It may be severe or even fatal.

Treatment Proper therapy must involve correction of the underlying cause. Vitamin K administration will immediately correct the defect; it can be administered either as the naturally occurring oil-soluble vitamin K_1 (oral and intravenous forms are available) or as the synthetic vitamin K. Vitamin K_1 is the most potent and rapidly acting form, measurably correcting clotting tests within 6 to 12 h of intravenous administration; it should be used for treatment of hemorrhagic disease in the newborn or for any vitamin K deficiency if bleeding is active. Oral and parenteral preparations of synthetic vitamin K are also available and may be used for treatment in the absence of bleeding and for maintenance vitamin K replacement. Rapid intravenous injection of vitamin K_1 has been associated with anaphylactic reactions and should be avoided. Synthetic preparations should not be used in the neonate since they may cause hemolysis and kernicterus in infants with glucose 6-phosphate dehydrogenase deficiency and in premature infants. Response to therapy should always be confirmed by repeating the prothrombin time 24 h after administration of vitamin K. Failure to correct the prothrombin time signifies failure to absorb the vitamin K or the presence of liver disease. If more urgent correction of the hemostatic defect is required than can be provided by administration of vitamin K, plasma or a concentrate of the vitamin K–dependent factors (prothrombin complex) should be infused.

ANTICOAGULANT DRUGS The commonly used anticoagulant drugs include the coumarin derivatives and heparin. The *coumarins* act by antagonizing the action of vitamin K and lead to the same clotting abnormalities as vitamin K deficiency (Fig. 334-2). Coumarin therapy prolongs the prothrombin and partial thromboplastin time tests and reduces the levels of prothrombin and factors VII, IX, and X. Abnormal bleeding is the chief complication of overdosage, which may be due to error, accident, or attempted suicide. The drugs usually implicated are dicoumarol (half-life 24 h) and warfarin (half-life 40 h). Treatment consists of administration of vitamin K and infusion of plasma or a prothrombin complex concentrate if bleeding is severe.

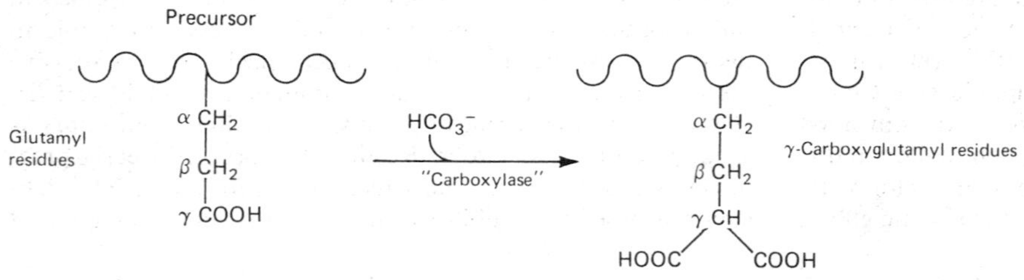

Precursor

Glutamyl residues: α CH_2 — β CH_2 — γ COOH

HCO_3^- "Carboxylase" →

γ-Carboxyglutamyl residues: α CH_2 — β CH_2 — γ CH (HOOC, COOH)

FIGURE 334-1
Vitamin K–dependent carboxylase. Vitamin K is a required cofactor in the reaction that converts glutamyl residues in microsomal precursors of prothrombin to γ-carboxyglutamyl residues in prothrombin.

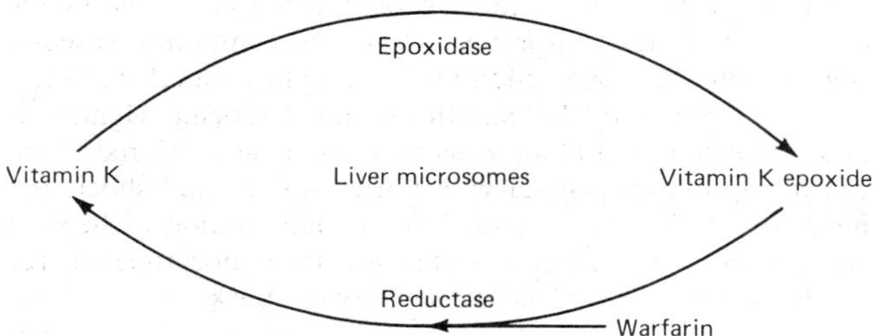

FIGURE 334-2
Vitamin K is converted to vitamin K epoxide by a microsomal epoxidase in the liver, and vitamin K epoxide is converted back to vitamin K by a microsomal reductase. Warfarin blocks the action of the reductase, resulting in accumulation of vitamin K epoxide. The exact way in which this effect of warfarin antagonizes the action of vitamin K in carboxylation of coagulation proteins is not established.

The best known action of *heparin* is the inactivation of thrombin, which prevents it from acting on fibrinogen. Blood contains a naturally occurring inhibitor of thrombin, termed *antithrombin III,* which irreversibly combines with the thrombin molecule on a 1:1 basis and inactivates it. Heparin binds to the lysine residues on the antithrombin III molecule, thereby markedly accelerating the stoichiometric reaction between thrombin and antithrombin III in the inactivation of thrombin. Heparin also acts earlier in the coagulation sequence by accelerating the combination of antithrombin III with factors IX_a, X_a, XI_a, and XII_a. Some of the activated factors, notably factors IX_a and X_a, are inactivated by much lower concentrations of heparin than are required to inactivate thrombin. This may be the reason that low-dose heparin reduces the incidence of postoperative venous thrombosis and pulmonary embolism. All coagulation tests are affected by heparin, including the one-stage prothrombin time. The most sensitive tests usually used to monitor the pharmacologic effect of heparin are the whole-blood clotting time, the partial thromboplastin time, and the thrombin time. An average dose of heparin is cleared from the blood in about 6 h by excretion in the urine and inactivation by a liver heparinase.

The treatment of bleeding associated with an excessive blood level of heparin is relatively simple. Heparin is a strongly negatively charged molecule and is rapidly neutralized, milligram for milligram, by intravenous protamine sulfate which is strongly positively charged. The amount of protamine required to neutralize the circulating heparin can be determined in vitro by a protamine titration test.

LIVER DISEASE Liver disease is one of the commonest causes of impaired coagulation. The principal functional changes appear to be decreased hepatic protein synthesis and increased plasma proteolytic activity, perhaps due to a decrease in the liver's capacity to remove proteases from the circulation. Increased fibrinolytic activity is often found in patients with cirrhosis and liver failure. There is evidence that intravascular coagulation may also occur in liver failure. The net effect of these derangements is to reduce the levels of all coagulation factors except for factor VIII, the level of which is often significantly increased. Hemostasis is frequently further impaired by thrombocytopenia and platelet dysfunction and low antithrombin III levels are often found.

In severe liver disease, a common pattern of hemostatic abnormalities includes a low plasma fibrinogen level, a prolonged prothrombin time, and a normal or prolonged partial thromboplastin time. The normal partial thromboplastin time may be the result of an elevated factor VIII level which can compensate for low levels of the other factors. The reason for the increased factor VIII concentration is not known. A low level of factor VII which does not affect the partial thromboplastin time may also contribute to a disproportionately prolonged prothrombin time. The thrombin clotting time is moderately prolonged in some patients with liver disease. The sialic acid content of the fibrinogen of these patients is increased and may be responsible for the prolonged thrombin clotting time. Heparin infusions may transiently elevate the fibrinogen level, suggesting that hypofibrinogenemia is in part due to catabolism from thrombin-mediated proteolysis, but the low fibrinogen level is often not restored to normal. The effect of heparin on clinical hemostasis is variable; it is apt to be associated with increased bleeding due to the anticoagulant effect of heparin. Fibrinolytic inhibitors appear to have at best a transient beneficial effect. In the management of frank bleeding, infusion of plasma which also contains antithrombin III may be preferable to infusion of coagulation factor concentrates. Some concentrates contain active coagulation enzymes which, being poorly cleared by the failing liver, can aggravate intravascular clotting and compound the problem. If there is an associated vitamin K deficiency it should be treated. In general, bleeding due to liver failure responds poorly to therapy unless improvement in liver-cell function occurs.

ACQUIRED FIBRINOGEN DEFICIENCY

The normal plasma concentration of fibrinogen is 200 to 400 mg/dl. Elevated levels occur during pregnancy, with stress, surgery, or infections, and in many chronic diseases.

Acquired deficiency of fibrinogen may be due to impaired synthesis and/or accelerated destruction of the protein. Impaired synthesis occurs in hepatitis, hepatic necrosis, and following administration of L-asparaginase for the treatment of leukemia. Accelerated destruction usually results from increased blood proteolytic activity. The commonest causes of increased proteolytic activity are discussed in the following section.

DISSEMINATED INTRAVASCULAR COAGULATION

Abbreviated DIC, this condition constitutes a series of syndromes recognized with increasing frequency over the last several years. The pathogenesis, diagnosis, and management of the disorder are complex. The basis of the disorder is generation of thrombin in the circulating blood. The thrombin can be demonstrated in the peripheral blood by its proteolytic activity.

BIOCHEMISTRY AND PHYSIOLOGY The principal target protein for thrombin is fibrinogen. There is evidence that in DIC the actions of thrombin and plasmin on fibrinogen are combined as shown in Fig. 334-3. Following injury the coagulation system is activated and thrombin is formed. Thrombin releases fibrinopeptide A from fibrinogen, which forms fibrin I monomer (reaction 1) and then polymer (reaction 2). Fibrin polymer adsorbs tissue plasminogen activator and accelerates its reaction with plasminogen to form plasmin. Each fibrin molecule in the polymer is then either further proteolysed by thrombin to release fibrinopeptide B and form fibrin II (reaction 3) or by plasmin to release $B\beta1$-42 and form fragment X (reaction 4). High levels of fibrinopeptide A and $B\beta1$-42 have been found in DIC, implying the occurrence of reactions 1 and 4. As noted in Chap. 54, fragment X forms physically weak clots which will not form α-chain cross-links and are readily dissolved by further plasmin action. The rapid conversion of fibrin to fragment X probably explains the relative rarity of thrombi found at autopsy of patients with DIC. Further degradation of fragment X results in the production of nonclottable fibrin degradation products. Tests for increased serum concentrations of the degradation products are important in the diagnosis of disseminated intravascular coagulation. Besides acting on fibrinogen, thrombin also acts on factors V and VIII, initially activating and then inactivating these proteins, resulting in either increased or more often decreased activity of these two factors, depending on the severity of the process and the concentration of thrombin generated. Thrombin also aggregates platelets and causes release of the contents of their granules, resulting in thrombocytopenia and increased plasma concentrations of the platelet-specific proteins. With resolution of the underlying disorder the thrombocytopenia generally persists longer than do the changes in fibrinogen.

The normal concentration of fibrinogen reflects a balance between synthesis and catabolism. Synthesis is in the liver and normally can be increased up to tenfold. The $t_{\frac{1}{2}}$ of fibrinogen in normal individuals is 100 h. The pathways of catabolism are not known nor is the extent to which enzyme action contributes normally. Thrombin action is believed to contribute less than 2 percent to normal fibrinogen catabolism. Coagulated fibrin is removed immediately from the circulating blood, and soluble fibrin and fibrinogen degradation products are removed more rapidly than is fibrinogen. Hence fibrinogen catabolism can be greatly accelerated by excessive enzyme action. If the synthetic reserve capacity is reduced as in liver failure, a lesser increase in catabolic rate would produce hypofibrinogenemia. Excessive proteolysis may reduce the fibrinogen concentration from an elevated level to the normal range or from the normal range to hypofibrinogenemic levels.

EXPERIMENTAL INTRAVASCULAR COAGULATION Intravascular coagulation can be induced experimentally. Rapid injection of thrombin into a large vein causes local thrombosis. Slower infusion of thrombin results in hypofibrinogenemia and usually no thrombi except sometimes in small vessels in the kidneys and adrenals. The reticuloendothelial system, particularly in the liver, removes fibrin and activated coagulation factors from the circulation, and suppression of reticuloendothelial activity enhances susceptibility to disseminated intravascular coagulation. Inhibition of fibrinolysis promotes the occurrence of organ thrombosis. In experimental intravascular coagulation, thrombin action results in reduced levels of fibrinogen, factors V and VIII, and in thrombocytopenia. Hemolysis and fragmented red blood cells may occur owing to red blood cell disruption by contact with fibrin strands, and shock and hemorrhage may be evident. Prior administration of heparin will prevent the coagulation changes, thrombocytopenia, red cell hemolysis, and reduce the severity of shock.

FIGURE 334-3

Postulated scheme of fibrinogen proteolysis in vivo. Half fibrinogen molecules are depicted. Reaction 1, thrombin cleaves the Aα chain of fibrinogen to produce free FPA and fibrin I monomer. Reaction 2, polymerization occurs. In reactions 3 and 4 fibrin is split by thrombin and plasmin into smaller fragments as shown.

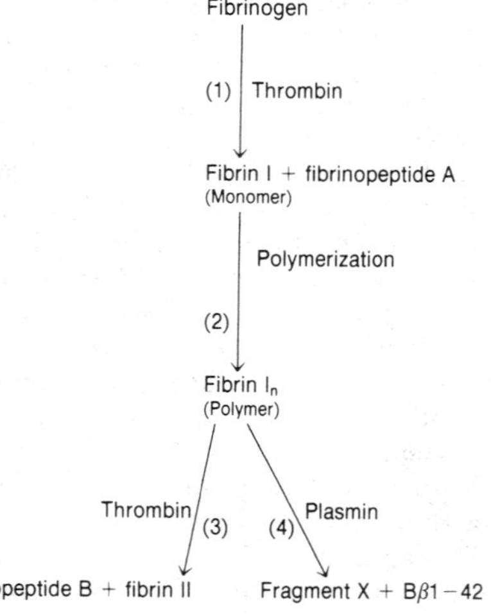

LABORATORY DIAGNOSIS The cardinal laboratory sign of disseminated intravascular coagulation is a quantitative and/or qualitative change in the plasma fibrinogen. The fibrinogen concentration is classically low but may be in the normal range, representing a reduction from a previously elevated level or may actually be elevated if the rate of synthesis exceeds the catabolic rate, even though the latter is elevated. An index of alteration in the fibrinogen molecule is the presence in the blood of increased concentrations of fibrinogen degradation products. These derivatives may be detected by immunologic techniques such as hemagglutination inhibition, immunodiffusion, immunoelectrophoresis, radioimmunoassay, or by their ability to clump certain strains of staphylococci. It is generally inferred that fibrinogen derivatives measured by these tests are derived principally by plasmin proteolysis of fibrin in most clinical circumstances.

Tests which specifically reflect thrombin action in vivo are still at the research stage and include (1) the measurement of free fibrinopeptide A and (2) evidence for the presence of fibrin monomer in solution. Abnormalities in other laboratory tests may be useful as ancillary evidence of disseminated intravascular coagulation. Classically, factor V and VIII activity is reduced and thrombocytopenia is present. The coagulation factor abnormalities often result in a prolonged prothrombin and partial thromboplastin time. However, factor V and VIII levels may be normal or even grossly increased.

CLINICAL SYNDROMES Disorders with hypofibrinogenemia and intravascular coagulation are outlined in Table 334-2.

DIC with hypofibrinogenemia LOCALIZED In certain clinical syndromes, the stimulus to intravascular coagulation appears to be localized, yet the hematologic changes are manifested throughout the circulating blood. Such conditions include the Kasabach-Merritt syndrome, some cases of dissecting aneurysm of the aorta, and occasional cases of massive venous thrombosis or pulmonary embolism. In the Kasabach-Merritt syndrome, a congenital hemangioma is associated with thrombocytopenia, hypofibrinogenemia, and elevated levels of fibrinopeptide A and fibrinogen degradation products. The survival time of radiolabeled fibrinogen in the circulating

TABLE 334-2
Disorders with hypofibrinogenemia and intravascular coagulation

1 Local stimulus to clotting
- *a* Vascular: giant hemangioma, aortic aneurysm, massive thrombosis, or pulmonary embolism
- *b* Tissue damage: burns, retained dead fetus, premature placental separation, amniotic fluid embolism

2 Generalized stimulus to clotting
- *a* Exogenous agents: snake venoms
- *b* Shock: hypovolemic, cardiogenic
- *c* Infections: gram-negative and gram-positive septicemia, viremia, miliary tuberculosis, Rocky Mountain spotted fever, subacute bacterial endocarditis, malaria
- *d* Immunologic: anaphylaxis
- *e* Neoplasms: carcinoma of the prostate, pancreas, lung; leukemia, lymphoma

3 Defective regulation (liver failure): impaired clearance of activated factors and defective fibrinogen synthesis

blood is shortened, and can be prolonged by heparin infusion. The radiolabeled fibrinogen accumulates in the hemangioma. All the hematologic changes revert to normal following extirpation of the hemangioma. This type of case offers a clear demonstration that the stimulus to intravascular coagulation is local, but the increased proteolytic activity may become disseminated through the blood.

Localized tissue damage appears to provide the stimulus for intravascular coagulation in burn injuries, retained dead fetus, premature placental separation, and amniotic fluid embolism.

GENERALIZED In other disease states it seems possible that the stimulus to intravascular coagulation may be generalized. It should be recognized that further work may well result in transfer of diseases from the generalized category to the localized, and vice versa. The disorders in this category with the clearest pathogenesis result from the action of coagulant enzymes present in snake venoms. The proteolytic enzyme may be introduced into the bloodstream by the fangs of the snake or as therapy by the physician. Preparations used therapeutically include Ancrod, derived from the venom of the Malayan pit viper, and reptilase, derived from *Bothrops atrox.* These preparations act specifically on fibrinogen but not on platelets or factors V and VIII, and hence do not alter their levels.

Shock of whatever cause (hypovolemic, cardiogenic) is frequently accompanied by disseminated intravascular coagulation, which rapidly ceases when the shock is reversed. The pathogenesis is unknown but may be related to tissue vascular endothelial cell damage.

Sepsis is one of the commonest of the disorders associated with disseminated intravascular coagulation. Classically, the sepsis is due to gram-negative organisms such as in meningococcemia, but the syndrome may be encountered with infection with gram-positive organisms, viruses, and plasmodia. In animal experimental work, it has been found that endotoxin-induced intravascular coagulation is prevented by prior production of granulocytopenia with nitrogen mustard. Intravascular coagulation can be produced by infusion of extracts of leukocytes from endotoxin-treated animals. On the basis of these findings, it is thought that leukocytes may participate in intravascular coagulation accompanying certain cases with sepsis. Acute hemolysis associated with incompatible blood transfusion reaction or with near-drowning may be associated with disseminated intravascular coagulation, to which procoagulant materials released from the red blood cells contribute. Anaphylactic shock and lesser degrees of acute allergic reactions are frequently accompanied by intravascular coagulation. Disseminated intravascular coagulation may occur in association with malignant neoplasia. Carcinoma of the prostate is the most well recognized of these, but the disorder is also encountered with many other neoplasms, including pancreatic, pulmonary, and gastric neoplasms, acute leukemia, and lymphoma. Thrombosis of large veins and arteries is often recurrent and is particularly associated with neoplastic disease. Some neoplastic cells produce a tissue thromboplastic factor which directly activates factor X without requiring factor VII.

Clinical features present in patients with disseminated intravascular coagulation include the features of the primary condition, which frequently includes shock. Bleeding may be from a single site but is particularly suggestive of disseminated intravascular coagulation when it occurs from multiple bleeding sites, from venipuncture wounds, and from skin suture sites. Purpura and ecchymoses may be present. When the disorder is present chronically, as for example in the Kasabach-Merritt syndrome, the patient experiences no shock or bleeding but will bleed excessively following injury and from venipuncture wounds.

The primary *treatment* of intravascular coagulation is that of the underlying disease. The Kasabach-Merritt syndrome is cured by removal of the hemangioma. Intravascular coagulation associated with placental separation or with fetal death should be treated by removal of the uterine contents. When shock is the precipitating factor, every effort should be made to reverse it as rapidly as possible. Intravascular coagulation associated with metastatic prostatic carcinoma will often diminish very rapidly after the start of estrogen therapy, depending on the responsiveness of the tumor. A second line of therapy involves replacement of blood components. Without question, blood loss should be replaced. If fibrinogen is replaced without effectively controlling clotting, it will merely provide more substrate for the enzymes. Since it is difficult to be certain that clotting is controlled and because of the likelihood of hepatitis virus contamination, fibrinogen is best withheld. If the basic condition has been reversed or if heparin is being given, coagulation factor deficiencies should be replaced with plasma, and significant thrombocytopenia treated with platelet transfusion. When the primary disease cannot be treated effectively, and it is judged that the injury which activates the coagulation system is still active, heparin will inactivate thrombin intravascular clotting and elevate clotting factor levels, but the platelet count almost invariably remains low. Bleeding is frequently enhanced by heparin alone, and platelets and plasma should also be given. Approximately 100 units heparin per kilogram of body weight may be given to initiate therapy followed by 10 to 15 units per kilogram per hour by constant intravenous infusion. The best index of hemostatic effectiveness is cessation or reduction of bleeding. The most rapid and specific indication that coagulation has been interrupted is provided by a drop in fibrinopeptide A concentration to the normal level within 15 min of starting heparin. Of the available laboratory tests, elevation in fibrinogen level and reduction in degradation product level provide evidence that intravascular proteolysis has been interrupted. Larger doses of heparin than usual may be needed in some patients, and smaller than usual doses should be used in the presence of severe thrombocytopenia. When there is a large open wound, as after surgery, the risk of local bleeding limits the usefulness of heparin therapy. Heparin therapy is most useful when gross thrombosis or purpura fulminans is present.

Purpura fulminans is an acute disorder which occurs most often in children following a bacterial or viral infection. Following a latent period after the infection, swollen purple purpuric lesions, possibly with a necrotic center, occur on the limbs, back, buttocks, or face. The laboratory signs of disseminated intravascular coagulation are present; histologically, widespread thrombosis of capillaries and venules with a surrounding perivascular inflammatory reaction is found. Heparin can stop the progress of the disease, and vigorous therapy is recommended for about a week, to be succeeded by warfarin.

Intravascular coagulation with normal or elevated fibrinogen concentrations In a large number of diseases, laboratory changes have been described comprising elevated levels of fibrinogen degradation products, plasma coagulation on addition of protamine or ethanol, and variations in the platelet count, partial thromboplastin time, prothrombin time, and thrombin clotting time. It is contended that these changes reflect increased intravascular coagulation and that although insufficient to produce hypofibrinogenemia, the clotting may be sufficient to produce ischemic tissue damage. A listing of such disorders is given in Table 334-3. It is not clear that the laboratory changes do signify the presence of disseminated intravascular coagulation. It is also not clear to what extent intravascular coagulation, if present, contributes to the pathogenesis of the disorders. With these uncertainties, the role of anticoagulant therapy in these conditions remains to be determined. As in the hypofibrinogenemic syndromes, heparin therapy is most clearly indicated when thrombosis is present.

FIBRINOLYTIC STATES

In certain conditions it is thought that plasmin may be formed in the circulating blood without thrombin and fibrin formation. The only definite condition in this category is produced by the therapeutic infusion of streptokinase or urokinase. In such circumstances, the concentration of fibrinogen and factors V and VIII in the circulating blood may drop, and increased fibrinogen degradation products may be present in the serum, whereas the platelet count may remain in the normal range.

It is uncertain whether a similar state may arise in patients not receiving thrombolytic therapy. Patients have been encountered in which a similar set of laboratory findings has occurred in association with rapid lysis of whole-blood clots formed in vitro and with rapid euglobulin lysis times. These circumstances have been accompanied by generalized oozing of blood. None of these patients has been studied in sufficient detail to know whether intravascular coagulation, i.e., excessive thrombin action, was an accompaniment.

There is evidence that localized plasmin action promotes bleeding following prostatectomy and dental extraction. Systemic administration of an inhibitor of plasmin formation, ε-aminocaproic acid, diminishes postprostatectomy hemorrhage and markedly reduces the requirement for replacement therapy in hemophiliacs undergoing dental extraction. One should be cautious about using EACA in patients diagnosed as having primary fibrinolysis until there is evidence concerning the degree of thrombin action in these patients. There is clinical and pathologic evidence that the drug will promote thrombosis in a potentially disastrous fashion if given alone when intravascular coagulation is present.

CIRCULATING ANTICOAGULANTS

Most naturally occurring circulating anticoagulants are actually antibodies to specific clotting factors. Patients have been described with antibodies to fibrinogen, factors V, VIII, IX, X, XI, and XIII. Antibodies may arise in patients with congenitally deficient factor activity or in patients with a previously normal coagulation system. In the latter case, the antibody may be an isolated finding or may be only part of a complex autoimmune syndrome such as systemic lupus erythematosus.

The clinical findings in patients with *antibody-type circulating anticoagulants* are similar to those in patients with congenital deficiency of the designated factor. The principal difference is that replacement therapy is ineffective in the presence of such anticoagulants. Steroid treatment is generally also ineffective unless the primary disease (e.g., systemic lupus erythematosus) is responsive to steroids. The disorder may persist indefinitely or may remit spontaneously and unpredictably.

Laboratory studies reveal all the features of deficiency of the specific factor. For example, if the antibody is to factor VIII, there is a long partial thromboplastin time, low factor VIII level, and normal prothrombin time. Furthermore, the patient's plasma induces factor VIII deficiency in normal plasma when the two are mixed. The patient's plasma will also inactivate purified factor VIII in a time-dependent reaction. Antibodies to factor VIII are the commonest antibodies encountered; they occur in about 5 to 10 percent of hemophiliacs, transiently and occasionally in postpartum women, in association with penicillin allergy, systemic lupus erythematosus, and rheumatoid arthritis, and at times without apparent cause. Despite lack of laboratory evidence of an increase in specific factor level, infusion of the appropriate concentrate may be lifesaving. There appears to be a difference in the response to immunosuppressive (azathioprine) therapy in patients with antibodies to factor VIII, depending on whether the patient was previously normal or had hemophilia. Antibodies in previously normal individuals have in some instances disappeared as a response to azathioprine therapy, whereas in hemophilia, such therapy has been uniformly ineffective. Because of the likelihood of an anamnestic rise in antibody titer, therapy should be vigorous and prompt. Once hemostasis has been achieved, the rise in inhibitor level will not be deleterious. If hemostasis has not been secured, the high titer of antibody will render further therapy useless. A novel approach to treatment of bleeding in patients with factor VIII inhibitors is the infusion of certain "activated" commercial vitamin K–dependent factor concentrates. Hemostasis is often but not always achieved. The beneficial effect is thought to depend on a poorly defined activated coagulant moiety which bypasses the factor VIII–dependent steps and produces a mild state of intravascular coagulation. A number of reports of thromboembolism, and even of death, in patients receiving these concentrates mandate caution in their use. Patients with impaired liver function may be especially prone to thrombosis following infusion of these concentrates. Nevertheless, their use may be considered when no alternative therapy is feasible.

In addition to the antibody directed against a specific coagulation factor, patients with *systemic lupus erythematosus* may develop antibodies directed against prothrombin activator, or a component of the prothrombin activator complex. The prothrombin activator complex is composed of factor X_a, factor V, and calcium ions bound to the lipoprotein surface of the platelet membrane. In a number of instances, the antibody in systemic lupus appears to be directed against the lipid component. Clinically, there is usually no excessive bleeding other than bruising. Bleeding in these patients depends on the presence of associated thrombocytopenia. Thrombophlebitis has been reported quite frequently. Laboratory features of the disorder include a prolonged whole-blood clotting time, prothrombin time, and partial thromboplastin time. When individual coagulation factors are assayed, the patient's prothrombin level may be low. Other factor assays are normal. A mixture of patient's and normal plasma has a long prothrombin and partial thromboplastin time immediately following mixing. This condition may respond rapidly to steroid therapy, often with return to normal of the coagulation findings within a week, but the coagulation findings themselves are not an indication for steroid therapy, which should be used as indicated for the underlying disease.

TABLE 334-3
Disorders with normal or elevated fibrinogen levels associated with intravascular coagulation

1 Local vascular alterations: glomerulonephritis, nephrotic syndrome with proliferative glomerulonephritis, polyarteritis nodosum, thrombotic thrombocytopenic purpura, hemolytic-uremic syndrome, organ transplant rejection
2 Generalized derangements
  a Hemolysis: paroxysmal nocturnal hemoglobinuria, hemolytic-uremic syndrome
  b Immunologic: systemic lupus erythematosus
  c Infections: bacterial, viral, rickettsial, fungal, malaria, bubonic plague, subacute bacterial endocarditis
  d Neoplasms: gastric, pulmonary, breast, renal

REFERENCES

BIGGS R (ed): *Human Blood Coagulation, Hemostasis and Thrombosis,* 2d ed. Oxford, Blackwell, 1976

——— (ed): *The Treatment of Haemophilia A and B and von Willebrand's Disease.* Oxford, Blackwell, 1978

FEINSTEIN DI, RAPAPORT SI: Acquired inhibitors of blood coagulation, in *Progress in Hemostasis and Thrombosis,* vol 1, TH Spaet (ed). New York, Grune & Stratton, 1972

HOYER CW: The factor VIII complex: Structure and function. Blood 58:1, 1981

LORAND L: Haemorrhagic disorders of fibrin-stabilization, in *Haemostasis,* D Ogston, B Bennett (eds). New York, Wiley, 1977

MINNA JD et al: *Disseminated Intravascular Coagulation in Man.* Springfield, Ill., Charles C Thomas, 1974

ROSENBERG RD, DAMUS PS: Actions and interactions of antithrombin and heparin. N Engl J Med 292:146, 1975

SHARMA GVRK et al: Thrombolytic therapy. N Engl J Med 306:1268, 1982

SUTTIE JW, JACKSON CM: Prothrombin structure, activation and biosynthesis. Physiol Rev 57:1, 1977

WEISS HJ et al: Pseudo-von Willebrand's. N Engl J Med 306:326, 1982

WILLIAMS WJ et al (eds): *Hematology,* 2d ed. New York, McGraw-Hill, 1977, chaps 128–162

Other hematologic disorders

335 BLOOD GROUPS AND BLOOD TRANSFUSION

ELOISE R. GIBLETT

BLOOD GROUP ANTIGENS AND ANTIBODIES

INTRODUCTION Human red blood cell membranes contain over 300 different antigenic determinants, the molecular structure of which is dictated by genes at an unknown number of chromosomal loci. The term *blood group* is applied to any well-defined system of red blood cell antigens controlled by a locus having a variable number of allelic genes, such as *A, B,* and *O* in the ABO system. Twenty-one blood group systems are currently recognized. The term *blood type* refers to the antigen phenotype, which is the serologic expression of the inherited blood group genes.

Alloantibodies specific for the blood group antigens may occur "naturally" (i.e., in the absence of known stimulus by foreign red blood cells) or in response to transfusion or pregnancy. Naturally occurring antibodies tend to be IgM molecules, and many of them (notably excepting anti-A and anti-B) react poorly at body temperature but readily agglutinate red blood cells at 5 to 20°C. Antibodies formed in response to exposure to another person's red blood cells or soluble blood group substances initially belong to the IgM class but usually change to the IgG class within a few weeks or months. In general, these "immune" antibodies react best at body temperature, and special laboratory procedures are required for their detection.

BLOOD GROUP SYSTEMS ABO system: Genes and antigens There are four major allelic genes in this system: A^1, A^2, *B,* and *O.* The locus for these alleles is on the long arm of chromosome 9. The actual products of the first three genes are glycosyltransferases which select specific sugars, *N*-acetyl-D-galactosamine (GalNAc) by the A^1 and A^2 transferases and D-galactose (Gal) by the *B* transferase, attaching them by alpha-linkage to short (oligo) saccharide chains. These chains comprise the carbohydrate moiety of glycolipid and glycoprotein molecules on the red blood cells or in other tissues and fluids. Although the A^1 and A^2 transferases perform the same function, they have different rate constants, so people who inherit an A^1 gene have more A-reactive sites than those with an A^2 gene. The *O* gene product is a protein which cross-reacts immunologically with the *A* and *B* transferase molecules but has no detectable enzyme activity; thus it is functionally "silent."

Nearly all individuals produce "naturally occurring" antibodies against the A or B antigens not present on their own red blood cells, as shown in Table 335-1. This fact is used as the basis for confirming the red blood cell type. Most of the major phenotypes represent more than one genotype. Thus, in the absence of family studies, it is possible to infer the genotype from only three phenotypes: A_1B, A_2B, and O. In routine practice, the ABO type is determined by testing the red blood cells with anti-A and anti-B and by testing the serum against A, B, and O red blood cells. Under special circumstances, a further distinction between A and AB types is made by using anti-A_1, an antiserum prepared by absorbing anti-A typing serum with A_2 red blood cells. The remaining unabsorbed antibodies have A_1 specificity, reacting with A_1 and A_1B, but not with A_2 and A_2B cells. (Alternatively, anti-A_1 is prepared as a lectin from extracts of certain seeds.) The frequencies of the various phenotypes in two American blood donor populations are also given in Table 335-1.

Red blood cells of types O and A_2 have large amounts of another antigen, called H, which is the immediate precursor to A and B. H specificity depends on the presence of a fucose (Fuc) residue attached to the oligosaccharides by a transferase that is the product of a very common gene called *H.* (The H and ABO loci are not genetically linked.) In very rare individuals who fail to inherit an *H* gene from either parent (i.e., they are homozygous for its allele, *h*), the *H* transferase is not made, and the H-determining fucose is not attached. This prevents the addition of specific sugars by the *A* and *B* transferases. As a result, even if an *A* or *B* gene has been inherited, the red blood cells are not agglutinated by anti-A, anti-B, or anti-H, while the serum contains all three antibodies. When a patient requiring transfusion has this so-called O_h (or Bombay) phenotype, special arrangements are necessary to obtain blood of the same rare type from a source such as the Red Cross.

About 80 percent of people are either homozygous or heterozygous for the "secretor," or *Se,* gene, which has no effect on the formation of antigens intrinsic to red blood cells but which activates the *H* gene to produce its fucosyltransferase in secretory tissues. Homozygotes for the apparently inactive allele *se* are called *nonsecretors* because their secretory cells do

TABLE 335-1
Blood types of the ABO system (including Hh)

*Genotype**	*Phenotype*	*Antigens on red blood cells†*	*Antibodies in serum‡*	*Phenotype frequencies in Americans, %*	
				Western European descent	*African descent*
A^1A^1 A^1A^2 A^1O	A_1	A_1, (H)	Anti-B (anti-H)	35	23
A^2A^2 A^2O	A_2	A_2, H	Anti-B (anti-A_1)	10	6
BB BO	B	B, (H)	Anti-A, A_1	8	17
A^1B	A_1B	A, A_1, B	(Anti-H)	3	3
A^2B	A_2B	A, B, H	(Anti-A_1)	1	1
OO	O	H	Anti-A, A_1 Anti-B	43	50
hh	O_h	None	Anti-A, A_1 Anti-B Anti-H	Very rare	Very rare

* *In all types except the last, the* H *allele is present as* HH *or* Hh.
† *(H) indicates occasional presence of weakly reacting H antigen.*
‡ *Antibodies in parentheses are, if present, weak cold agglutinins.*
SOURCE: *Race and Sanger.*

not produce the *H* transferase, so their body fluids lack H, A, and B antigen activities.

Antibodies in ABO system Red blood cells of newborn infants have decreased numbers of H, A, and B reactive sites, and their plasma normally contains very little anti-A or anti-B. The latter finding is due to the fact that fetal immunoglobulin production is minimal, while most of the anti-A and anti-B produced in the mother are IgM molecules which cannot cross the placenta. However, in some type O adults, the anti-A, anti-B, and anti-AB (a cross-reacting antibody sometimes called anti-C) are of the IgG class. Thus, ABO hemolytic disease of the newborn usually occurs in A (or B) infants of O mothers.

It is not acceptable medical practice to transfuse A, B, or AB blood into patients whose red blood cells lack the corresponding antigens, since their plasma contains incompatible antibodies. However, it is acceptable to give A or B blood (preferably as packed red blood cells) to AB recipients, or to give O packed red blood cells (*not* whole blood, except in severe emergencies) to patients of type A, B, or AB when the transfusion requirement exceeds the supply of type-specific blood. Although antibodies with A_1 specificity frequently occur in the plasma of A_2 and A_2B subjects, they are almost always weak cold agglutinins. Thus, if anti-A_1 has been identified in a transfusion patient, it can be ignored unless it reacts in vitro with A_1 red blood cells at 37°C.

Lewis system Antigens in the Lewis system are not produced by red blood cells but rather are taken up as glycosphingolipid molecules from the surrounding plasma. About 80 percent of western Europeans are either homozygous or heterozygous for the *Le* gene. The other 20 percent are homozygous for its presumably inactive allele, *le*. There are two well-defined Lewis antigenic determinants, Le^a and Le^b, both of which are structurally related to the H, A, and B antigens (Table 335-2). The *Le* gene product, like the *H* gene product, is a fucosyltransferase, but it attaches fucose to a different sugar (*N*-acetyl-D-glucosamine instead of D-galactose) in the oligosaccharide chains. The Le^a determinant is a monofucosyl structure which lacks the fucose attached by the *H* transferase. The Le^b determinant has two fucose residues placed there by the *H* and *Le* transferases, in that order.

As shown in Table 335-3, individuals who lack an *Se* gene (i.e., nonsecretors of H, A, and B) cannot produce molecules with the difucosyl structure. If they have an *Le* gene, their secretions and plasma contain a large amount of Le^a, but no Le^b, and their blood cells have the phenotype Le(a+b−). However, secretors of H(A,B) who have an *Le* gene produce only a small amount of Le^a and a much larger amount of Le^b antigen. Their red blood cells are usually Le(a−b+), although they may be Le(a+b+), reacting with both anti-Le^a and anti-Le^b. The red blood cells of *le* homozygotes are Le(a−b−), even if they inherit both *H* and *Se* genes, since they lack the necessary *Le* transferase to form either Le^a or Le^b determinants.

Anti-Le^a and anti-Le^b are fairly common naturally occurring antibodies, produced mainly by subjects of phenotype O, Le(a−b−). Nearly all examples of these antibodies are of the IgM class, so they rarely, if ever, can cross the placenta during pregnancy. Were they to do so, destruction of the infant's red blood cells would be highly unlikely, since the Lewis glycosphingolipids are very poorly developed during fetal life.

Lewis antibodies (particularly anti-Le^a) are complement-binders, and thus anti-Le^a is occasionally the cause of a transfusion reaction with intravascular hemolysis. However, the plasma of Le(a+) donors usually contains enough soluble Le^a

TABLE 335-2
Structure of oligosaccharides with H, A, B, and Lewis specificities

Antigen specificity	*Structure**
H	β-Gal-β-GlcNAc-β-Gal-R† ↑ (on first β-Gal) α-Fuc
A_1 or A_2	α-GalNAc-β-Gal-β-GlcNAc-β-Gal-R ↑ (on first β-Gal) α-Fuc
B	α-Gal-β-Gal-β-GlcNAc-β-Gal-R ↑ (on first β-Gal) α-Fuc
Le^a	β-Gal-β-GlcNAc-β-Gal-R ↑ (on β-GlcNAc) α-Fuc
Le^b	β-Gal-β-GlcNAc-β-Gal-R ↑ ↑ (on β-Gal and β-GlcNAc) α-Fuc α-Fuc

* *See text for explanation of abbreviations. Specific bonds between sugars are omitted.*
† *R is the rest of the molecule, consisting of more monosaccharides, usually attached to peptide or lipid carriers.*
SOURCE: *Watkins.*

TABLE 335-3
Associations of various genes with H, A, B, and Lewis antigen activities

	Antigens on red blood cells		*Antigens in plasma and secretions*			
Genes present	*H, AB*	*Le^a^*	*Le^b^*	*H, AB*	*Le^a^*	*Le^b^*
H, AB, Se, Le	+++		++	+++	+	++
H, AB, sese, Le	+++	+++			+++	
H, AB, Se, lele	+++			+++		
H, Ab, sese, lele	+++					
hh, AB, Se or *sese, Le* / *hh, AB, Se* or *sese, lele*	*	+++			+++	

* *Individuals who lack the H gene belong to the very rare O_h phenotype.*
SOURCE: *Watkins.*

antigen to neutralize the patient's anti-Le^a^ before it can attack the vulnerable red blood cells. Nevertheless, patients whose plasma contains an anti-Le^a^ that strongly hemolyzes Le(a+) red blood cells or agglutinates them at temperatures above 30°C should be given blood from either Le(a−b+) or Le(a−b−) donors. Anti-Le^b^ is virtually never a transfusion hazard.

P system Several structurally related antigens are considered together under the heading of a single system called P. As in the ABO and Lewis systems, the gene products are glycosyltransferases, attaching either D-galactose, *N*-acetyl-D-galactosamine, or *N*-acetyl-D-glucosamine to glycosphingolipids on the red blood cell membrane. P_1 and P, the major antigenic determinants, were previously thought to represent the expression of two allelic genes at the same locus, analogous to A^1 and A^2 in the ABO system. However, these two antigens represent quite different sugar sequences, and the genetic interpretation is complex.

Table 335-4 shows the five interrelated phenotypes in this system, with their corresponding antigens and antibodies. P_1 is the most common phenotype in most populations, while P_1-negative individuals nearly always have the P_2 type. $P_1{}^k$, $P_2{}^k$, and p phenotypes are extremely rare, but they are clinically important, being associated with the presence of naturally occurring antibodies with strong hemolytic activity. On the other hand, anti-P_1, which frequently occurs in people of type P_2, is virtually never capable of causing red blood cell destruction—the exceptions being those rare examples which react strongly with P_1 red blood cells in vitro at 37°C. In patients with paroxysmal cold hemoglobinuria, the so-called Donath-Landsteiner autoantibodies frequently react with globoside, a very common red blood cell glycosphingolipid with P specificity.

I system The I and i antigenic determinants are structurally heterogeneous, biochemically related to the H, A, B, Le, and P antigens. Most people inherit a gene associated with I antigen production, but the red blood cells of newborn infants react very weakly with anti-I and strongly with anti-i. A gradual reversal occurs during the first year or two, representing the development of I antigen in association with branching of carbohydrate chains on the cell membrane. In patients with certain kinds of "marrow stress," particularly thalassemia and hypoplastic anemia, red blood cell i activity increases.

Anti-I is a common antibody, frequently found as a weak cold agglutinin of no clinical concern. In patients with the cold type of autoimmune hemolytic anemia, autoantibodies nearly always have anti-I or anti-I plus i specificity, and most of them belong to the IgM class (see Chap. 329). Anti-i production is associated mainly with lymphoid cell diseases, especially infectious mononucleosis and lymphosarcoma. A patient already having a "marrow-stressing" disorder such as thalassemia may develop an intense autoimmune hemolytic anemia due to anti-i. When transfusions are required, finding compatible blood poses no problem, since the red blood cells of most adults are i-negative. Even patients with strong cold-reacting anti-I antibodies are usually not difficult to transfuse safely if they are kept warm during the infusion. However, since anti-I often fixes complement, washed red cells may be preferable for transfusion to prevent exposure to additional complement components.

MNS system Closely linked genes on chromosome 4 determine the MN and Ss antigens, respectively. Thus, there are four inherited haplotypes: MS, Ms, NS, and Ns. Glycophorin A carries M and N specificity, while S and s are on glycophorin B. Absence of these sialoglycoproteins is associated with rare phenotypes such as En(a-), S^u^, and M^k^, but there are no accompanying hematological abnormalities.

Anti-M and anti-N are usually naturally occurring IgM agglutinins with little capability of destroying red blood cells. Patients on long-term renal dialysis tend to form anti-N as either an auto- or alloantibody. These N-specific autoantibodies have no hemolytic potential, but they are alleged to cause rejection of kidneys kept refrigerated before transplantation.

Formation of anti-S or anti-s usually requires the stimulus of transfusion or pregnancy, and accordingly these antibodies often belong to the IgG class. A third antibody, anti-U, behaves serologically somewhat like anti-S plus anti-s, being formed in sensitized black subjects whose red blood cells have the S^u^ phenotype lacking S and s antigens. All three of these antibodies can hemolyze incompatible red blood cells in vivo, but they are readily detectable by adequate compatibility testing.

Rh system The Rh locus is on chromosome 1. Rh antigenic determinants may be dependent on interaction between red blood cell membrane protein and phospholipid molecules. Many Rh phenotypes have been described serologically, but the underlying biochemical genetics is unknown. It is convenient to envision a stretch of nucleotides at the Rh locus which dictates the structure of a set of three antithetical determinants: C or c, E or e, and D or d (the latter having no corresponding antibody and therefore being simply the absence of D). These sets are thus inherited from each parent as a haplotype, such as CDe, cde, cDE, and so forth. This nomenclature, used by Race and Sanger, is compared with the alternative nomenclature of Wiener in Table 335-5, which also gives the approximate frequencies of the corresponding alleles in Americans of western European, African, and Oriental origins.

The D(Rh_o) antigen is by far the most immunogenic of this or any other blood group system (except for those previously described systems in which the formation of antibodies does

TABLE 335-4
Characteristics of the P phenotypes

Phenotype	*Approximate frequency*	*Antigens on red blood cells*	*Antibodies in plasma*
P_1	75%	P_1, P, P^k	None
P_2	25%	P, P^k	Anti-P_1 (often)
$P_1{}^k$	Very rare	P_1, P^k	Anti-P
$P_2{}^k$	Very rare	P^k	Anti-P
p	Very rare	None	Anti-P_1PP^k

SOURCE: *Race and Sanger.*

not depend on exposure to foreign red blood cells). About 15 percent of Caucasians lack the D(Rh_o) antigen and are Rh-negative. When transfused only once with Rh-positive blood, these Rh-negative persons have about a 50 percent chance of forming anti-D(Rh_o) antibodies, which could cause destruction of any subsequently transfused Rh-positive red blood cells. For this reason, Rh-negative patients are always given Rh-negative blood except when the transfusion requirements of a male or postmenopausal female exceed the available supply. Giving Rh-positive blood to Rh-negative premenopausal females is a very serious matter, because, unless adequate amounts of Rh immunoglobulin are given to prevent immunization, any subsequent pregnancy with an Rh-positive infant will almost always stimulate a secondary immune response, resulting in hemolytic disease of the newborn.

The Rh antigens C, c, E, and e are considerably less immunogenic than D, and it is impractical to match these antigens in donors and recipients. Of course, when previously sensitized patients form the corresponding antibodies, it is necessary to find donor blood lacking the specific antigens. The difficulty of this search varies. For example, about 20 percent of the population lack the c antigen and thus are compatible donors for a patient whose plasma contains anti-c. However, only 2 percent lack the e antigen, so patients with anti-e pose serious problems, especially when large amounts of blood are required. Blood banks often maintain donor calling lists or frozen red blood cells for use in such cases.

A large proportion of patients with acquired hemolytic anemia of the warm type have IgG autoantibodies which react with one or more Rh-associated antigens. In some instances, the specificity is clear-cut (for example, anti-e), but more often the antibodies react with all red blood cells except those of the rare type known as Rh null. These cells lack all known Rh antigens, and the cell membrane is defective, reinforcing the belief that in normal red blood cells, molecules bearing the Rh determinants are an intrinsic part of the membrane protein structure.

Kidd, Kell, Duffy, and Lutheran systems The major antigens of these four clinically important systems and their average phenotype frequencies in Americans of western European and African origins are presented in Table 335-6 along with the frequencies of S and s in the MNS system. Anti-K and anti-Fy^a are frequently encountered antibodies capable of marked alloimmune red blood cell destruction. Even more dangerous are the antibodies in the Kidd system, anti-Jk^a and anti-Jk^b, which are notoriously difficult to detect. Whenever a patient has a hemolytic transfusion reaction after transfusion of blood found to be compatible by the usual laboratory tests, the most likely cause is anti-Jk^a. Antibodies in the Lutheran system have only rarely been reported to cause red blood cell destruction.

Other blood group antigens Many other red blood cell antigens have been described. The Xg^a antigen is of considerable importance to geneticists, since its locus is on the X chromosome. Other antigens are of clinical interest because they occur on the red blood cells of 95 percent or more of most populations, making it difficult to find compatible blood when their antibodies are present in patients requiring transfusion. Many of these antibodies have little ability to destroy red blood cells, even though they consist of IgG molecules and react in vitro at 37°C. Included in this category are most examples of anti-Sd^a (Sid), anti-Yt^a (Cartwright), anti-Yk^a (York), and many others. Nevertheless, both caution and experience are necessary when considering the transfusion of serologically incompatible blood, particularly when the antibodies react in vitro at body temperature. Antibodies with Chido (Ch^a) and Rodgers (Rg^a) specificity are incapable of causing hemolysis. Their respective antigenic determinants are located on the C4d fragment of the fourth component of complement and are thereby taken up from the plasma by red cells.

BIOLOGICAL SIGNIFICANCE OF BLOOD GROUPS Immune reactions The relationship of blood group antigens and antibodies to alloimmune red blood cell destruction has been briefly discussed in the previous sections. Because antigens in the ABO system are present in other tissues, they play a role in determining *histocompatibility,* so that transplantation of ABO-incompatible kidneys and other organs carries a risk of rejection (see Chap. 292). However, successful grafting of ABO-incompatible bone marrow is possible when the patient is immunosuppressed and either given exchange transfusions of plasma compatible with the donor's red blood cells or the patient's own plasma is passed over a column containing oligosaccharides with A and/or B specificity.

Infertility and early fetal loss Both of these effects have been ascribed to ABO incompatibility, although in some instances the data are of marginal significance. Nevertheless, many population geneticists believe that this factor plays a significant role in the processes of natural selection.

Disease-related phenotype changes A and, to a lesser extent, B determinants are subject to certain biochemical changes, such as those caused by bacterial glycosidases and other enzymes. As a result, the red blood cells may develop new specificities, becoming either "polyagglutinable" or having "pseudo-B" characteristics. Another acquired alteration in ABO type occurs in some patients with acute myelocytic leukemia whose original type is A_1 or B. This change in phenotype, with partial or complete loss of agglutinability by anti-A or anti-B, can be a

TABLE 335-5
Rh alleles, their antigenic determinants, and frequencies

	*Associated antigenic determinants**		*Approximate allele frequencies in Americans†*		
Allele	*R-S*	*W*	*Western European descent*	*African descent*	*Oriental descent*
R^1	D, C, e	Rh_o, rh′, hr″	0.45	0.10	0.55
r	c, e	hr′, hr″	0.37	0.15	0.10
R^2	D, c, E	Rh_o, hr′, rh″	0.14	0.10	0.35
R^o	D, c, e	Rh_o, hr′, hr″	0.02	0.60	Low
r''	c, E	hr′, rh″	0.01	Low	Low
r'	C, e	rh′, hr″	0.01	Low	Low
R^z	D, C, E	Rh_o, rh′, rh″	Low	Low	Low
r^y	C, E	rh′, rh″	Low	Low	Low

* *R-S = Race and Sanger; W = Wiener (see references).*
† *Low frequency means less than 0.01. Individuals of African descent have other alleles not listed here, thus accounting for failure of their frequencies to total 1.0.*

diagnostic aid in the early hypoplastic phase of leukemia. The changes in Ii specificity associated with "marrow stress" are described above (see "I System" above).

Other disease relationships The incidence of certain diseases is related to blood type. For example, type O "nonsecretors" have about twice the incidence of duodenal ulcer than do secretors of types A or B. On the other hand, type A carries a higher incidence of tumors of salivary glands, stomach, and pancreas than does type O. Persons with the rare Rh_{null} type, whose red cells lack all the Rh antigens, have some degree of increased hemolysis, as do people with the McLeod phenotype. The latter red blood cells react only weakly with antibodies against antigens of the autosomally controlled Kell system, and they lack Kx, a very common X-linked antigen. Some boys with the X-linked form of chronic granulomatous disease have the McLeod phenotype and others do not. In both instances, the Kx antigen, also a normal granulocyte component, is not detectable on these cells. Individuals (mainly of African origin) who lack both Fy^a and Fy^b—the major antigens in the Duffy system—are protected against infestation by the malarial parasite, *Plasmodium vivax*, presumably because Fy^a and Fy^b act as specific recognition or acceptor sites for the merozoites.

Chromosome mapping Blood genetic markers, including the red and white blood cell allotypes as well as the plasma and blood cell enzyme phenotypes, are very useful for mapping the human chromosomes. Some of these markers are genetically linked to loci for genes causing metabolic diseases, and, as more markers are identified, it will be increasingly possible to predict the development of inherited malfunctions from specimens obtained in utero or from newborn infants. For example, the secretor gene locus is closely linked to the locus of the gene causing myotonic dystrophy. Thus, a determination of the secretor status of a baby at risk can be used to predict the likelihood of its developing this disease, since both characters are inherited as autosomal dominants.

Medicolegal applications When the red blood cell antigens are combined with the other genetic markers in blood, distinguishing one person from another is possible with a probability of about 2 million to 1. This high degree of individuality promotes the usefulness of genetic markers for ruling out paternity, maternity, and monozygosity in nearly all cases where those relationships do not exist.

BLOOD TRANSFUSION

INTRODUCTION Considerable morbidity and, to a lesser extent, mortality are associated with blood transfusion therapy. Responsible medical practice dictates that physicians have sufficient background information to make soundly reasoned judgments concerning the risks as well as the benefits of this procedure. They must decide not only what blood components (if any) are indicated but also what quantities are needed.

WHOLE BLOOD A unit of whole blood consists of approximately 450 ml blood collected into a plastic bag containing 63 ml of either citrate-phosphate-dextrose (CPD) or citrate-phosphate-dextrose-adenine (CPD-A) solution as anticoagulant and preservative. Blood collected in CPD has a refrigerated storage life of only 3 weeks, while CPD-A blood may be kept 5 weeks. At the end of these periods, about 70 to 80 percent of red blood cells are still viable, white blood cells and platelets are nonviable, and clotting factors V and VIII have low levels of activity.

Virtually the only reason to transfuse whole blood is to restore blood volume lost through recent hemorrhage, as with gastrointestinal bleeding, major surgery, or trauma. For assessing blood loss, routine laboratory tests are misleading for several hours after hemorrhage. Both hemoglobin and hematocrit measurements reflect the ratio of red blood cell mass to blood volume, rather than indicating the total circulating red blood cells. Since the compensatory vasoconstriction evoked by hemorrhage initially prevents extravascular fluids from replacing intravascular fluid loss, both laboratory measurements may be falsely high. Clinically, postural hypotension provides a warning that blood transfusion may be required. Pallor, syncope, tachycardia, thirst, and air hunger are useful indicators of massive blood loss (i.e., 1500 ml or more in adults), sometimes requiring immediate transfusion of type O red blood cells that have not been cross matched. In less severe cases, maintaining

TABLE 335-6
The major antigens and phenotypes in five clinically important blood group systems (excepting ABO and Rh)*

			Approximate phenotype frequencies in Americans, %†	
System	*Major antigens*	*Phenotypes*	*Western European descent*	*African descent*
Kidd	Jk^a, Jk^b	Jk(a+b−)	26	55
		Jk(a−b+)	24	7
		Jk(a+b+)	50	38
Kell	K, k, Js^a	K−k+Js(a−)	91	83
		K−k+Js(a+)	Low	15
		K+k−Js(a−)	Low	Low
		K+k+Js(a−)	9	2
		K+k+Js(a+)	Low	Low
Duffy	Fy^a, Fy^b	Fy(a+b−)	18	10
		Fy(a−b+)	33	20
		Fy(a+b+)	49	2
		Fy(a−b−)	Low	68
Lutheran	Lu^a, Lu^b	Lu(a+b−)	Low	Low
		Lu(a−b+)	92	97
		Lu(a+b+)	8	3
(MN) Ss	S, s	S−s+	47	65
		S+s−	10	9
		S+s+	43	24
		S−s−	Low	2

* *See Tables 335-1 and 335-5 for information about ABO and Rh types.*
† *Low means less than 1 percent.*
SOURCE: *ER Giblett, Genetic Markers in Human Blood, Philadelphia, Davis, 1969.*

the blood volume with saline or plasma expanders provides time for accurate blood typing and compatibility testing.

During surgery, blood loss can be measured quite accurately, and there is a tendency to "keep up" or even to "stay ahead" of lost volume by transfusion. Such practices lead to unwarranted use of blood with its attendant hazards. In most adult subjects, blood loss of 500 ml is easily tolerated, being equivalent to the amount given by a blood donor. Judicious use of crystalloid infusions is frequently all that is required to circumvent blood transfusion, even with blood losses up to a liter. In modern medicine, ordering "fresh" blood at any time is not acceptable practice, since proper component therapy is both safer and more scientifically based.

PACKED RED BLOOD CELLS The preparation of packed red blood cells from whole blood involves sedimentation or centrifugation followed by removal of plasma into a satellite bag, all in a closed system. Such packed cells have the same storage periods as whole blood. Removal of the plasma provides protection against circulatory overload as well as against excessive loads of sodium, potassium, citrate, ammonia, and antibodies (particularly anti-A) which might be harmful to the patient. Furthermore, the removed plasma can be used for preparing such products as cryoprecipitate, albumin, and immunoglobulins.

In the absence of recent blood loss, most transfusions are given to patients who need replacement of oxygen-carrying capacity. Packed red blood cells are much preferred to whole blood for this purpose, since the plasma serves no useful purpose and may be detrimental, especially in hypervolemic subjects. Diagnoses most frequently associated with the need for packed red blood cells fall into two major categories of anemia, hypoplastic and hemolytic.

Red blood cell hypoplasia Chronic bone marrow depression may, under favorable circumstances, be treated by bone marrow transplantation from an identical twin or another HLA-compatible sibling (see Chap. 331). However, many patients either have no access to a marrow donor or are unsuitable candidates. The red blood cell mass of these patients can be maintained at functional levels for long periods, provided they do not develop multiple antibodies against red blood cell antigens. These patients are in general more liable to become immunologically refractory to platelets and white blood cells than to red blood cells. Patients whose red blood cell hypoplasia is secondary to marrow invasion by malignancy and/or to various chemo- or radiotherapeutic agents also require red blood cell transfusions. Again, sensitization to transfused platelets and white blood cells creates a greater problem than red blood cell immunization.

Hemolytic anemia In severe cases of inherited nonimmune hemolysis due to intrinsic red blood cell defects (e.g., sickle cell anemia, thalassemia, or severe deficiencies of glucose 6-phosphate dehydrogenase), the only hope of maintaining oxygen-carrying capacity through a crisis is the careful use of red blood cell transfusion. Patients with other forms of nonimmune hemolysis or ineffective erythropoiesis (e.g., vitamin B_{12}, folate, or iron deficiencies) are candidates for transfusion only if they are severely anemic and if the cause cannot be corrected by specific replacement therapy. Whenever any infusion is given to a patient with severe anemia, the possibility of precipitating heart failure must be circumvented by careful monitoring.

Patients with autoimmune hemolytic anemia are very poor candidates for red blood cell transfusion. Not only are they liable to develop new alloantibodies, but they may have already formed such antibodies as the result of earlier transfusion or pregnancy. In the presence of circulating *auto*antibodies, alloantibodies are often difficult to detect, and transfused red blood cells may be rapidly destroyed. Consultation with a blood transfusion expert is desirable in cases where severe anemia with hypoxemia or cardiac failure poses an immediate threat to life.

PLATELETS Platelet concentrates are prepared by centrifugation of platelet-rich plasma to yield about 5×10^{10} platelets from each donor unit. Retention of about 70 ml plasma is necessary to prevent the unfavorable drop in pH which would otherwise occur during storage at room temperature. Prepared in this way and kept under constant agitation, platelets can be stored for up to 3 days and still survive normally with a half-life of about 5 days. Platelets stored in the refrigerator for no more than 24 h may function well immediately after transfusion, but their survival is much shorter. In adult thrombocytopenic patients without consumptive coagulopathy or platelet-specific antibodies, 1 unit of platelet concentrate raises the platelet count by about 10,000 per microliter.

Patients with idiopathic thrombocytopenic purpura produce autoantibodies which react with all human platelets (see Chap. 332), and therefore derive little or no benefit from platelet transfusion. Moreover, the platelets produced by such a hyperactive marrow are highly effective in maintaining hemostasis even at platelet counts as low as 10,000 per microliter. Similarly, in patients with thrombocytopenia due to a consumptive coagulopathy (as in infection or metastatic malignancy) the usefulness of platelet therapy is limited, unless its purpose is to keep the patient from bleeding while the primary cause is being treated.

The most rational use of platelets is to control bleeding in patients either with a temporary loss of platelets not due to immunity (e.g., massive blood replacement, prolonged surgery) or with suppressed platelet production (leukemia, lymphoma, treatment with radio- or chemotherapy). Since platelets are very immunogenic, and typing techniques are not yet practical, this blood component should not be given in the absence of clear indication. Most nonbleeding patients with platelet counts above 10,000 per microliter can maintain adequate hemostasis. Patients in the immediate postoperative period may need to have their platelet counts elevated to as high as 100,000 per microliter. In other bleeding situations, a platelet count of 50,000 per microliter or more suggests other causes for hemorrhage, especially if there is no recent history of ingestion of aspirin or other drugs that interfere with platelet function, which would be reflected by a prolonged bleeding time. The effectiveness of platelet transfusion is assessed by comparing the platelet count before the infusion with counts obtained about 1 and 24 h later.

Choice of blood type Ideally, donors of platelets should have the same ABO and Rh types as the patient, since it is impossible to remove all red blood cells and plasma from the platelet concentrate. When it is necessary to use O donors for A, B, or AB recipients, the plasma may contain sufficient anti-A (or anti-B) to destroy some of the patient's red blood cells. Although this possibility is small, it deserves consideration in children or in adults receiving large numbers of platelet concentrates. When platelets of A, B, or AB donors are given to patients of unlike ABO type, their effectiveness may be somewhat diminished, although this is rarely a major problem. However, it is important that the number of red blood cells in such ABO-incompatible preparations be kept as small as possible.

Since some red blood cells are inevitably present in platelet concentrates, Rh-negative patients should receive platelets from Rh-negative donors whenever feasible, particularly if there is a possibility of subsequent pregnancy. However, lack of platelets from Rh-negative donors should not preclude transfusing Rh-positive donor platelets in a life-threatening situation. Patients who have the potential of becoming mothers can be protected against Rh alloimmunization by an injection of Rh immunoglobulin, about 20 μg for each milliliter of Rh-positive red blood cells present in the infusion. In other Rh-negative patients given platelets from Rh-positive donors, Rh-antibody formation can be expected to occur with a high frequency, but these antibodies do not interfere with the survival of subsequently transfused Rh-positive donor platelets, since they do not themselves contain Rh antigens.

Refractory state Patients who receive random donor platelets on more than one or two occasions frequently develop alloantibodies with either HLA or platelet antigen specificities. Such refractory patients can often be maintained with concentrates prepared by plateletpheresis from siblings compatible for HLA. Platelets from unrelated HLA-compatible donors are less successful than those from relatives, indicating the importance of platelet-specific antigens in alloimmunization. When platelet cross-matching tests become available, this problem should diminish.

WHITE BLOOD CELL TRANSFUSIONS Since it is now possible with platelet transfusions to control bleeding in many patients with hematologic malignancies, hemorrhage is being supplanted by infection as the most frequent cause of death. In general, patients most likely to benefit from neutrophil transfusions are those with severe neutropenia who have documented infections not responsive to appropriate antibiotic therapy. However, the problems of maintaining patients for long periods in this way are even more difficult than those associated with platelets. Neutrophils have a very short life span in the bloodstream, and many questions remain unanswered about the best collection techniques, the feasibility of neutrophil storage, dosage schedules, and long-term effects on donors. Furthermore, alloimmunization to HLA and other antigens is a definite hazard.

PLASMA COMPONENT THERAPY Fresh frozen plasma and cryoprecipitate are major blood component preparations because they are necessary for the care of patients with coagulation disorders, especially hemophilia (see Chap. 334). Pooled plasma is not an acceptable agent for expanding intravascular volume since it has a high hepatitis risk. However, albumin and other salvaged human plasma protein derivatives with high albumin content are commercially prepared for use in special cases, such as nephrosis, certain gastroenteropathies, and severe malnutrition. Immunoglobulin preparations are also commercially made, including specific hyperimmune globulin for preventing the development of certain infectious diseases and for blocking the immune response to Rh antigen.

PLASMAPHERESIS The introduction of cell separators has made plasmapheresis a simple procedure, especially in the treatment of diseases whose course can be modified by removal of autoantibodies or immune complexes. While the number of different diseases that have been managed in this way is considerable, there are only a few where the role of plasmapheresis is uncontested. Even under these circumstances, there is no consensus with regard to frequency or volume of exchange and the nature of replacement fluids.

The most established indication is symptomatic paraproteinemia, especially in association with hyperviscosity or cryoglobulinemia. There is also clinical evidence to show that plasmapheresis can be used successfully as an adjunct in selected patients with myasthenia gravis, Goodpasture's syndrome, thrombotic thrombocytopenic purpura, and rapidly progressive glomerulonephritis. Diseases that do not have an immunological basis have also been treated with plasmapheresis; they include hypertriglyceridemia, hypercholesterolemia, and poisonings due to toxins that are bound to plasma albumin after absorption.

COMPLICATIONS OF BLOOD TRANSFUSION Transfusion reactions are classified as immune or nonimmune. The immunologically mediated reactions may be directed against red or white blood cells, platelets, or at least one of the immunoglobulins, IgA. Other less well defined hypersensitivity reactions also occur. The major nonimmune reactions are due to circulatory overload, massive transfusion, or transmission of an infectious agent.

Immunologically mediated reactions Hemolysis due to red blood cell alloantibodies may occur within the circulation or extravascularly. The very rapid cell destruction associated with *intravascular hemolysis* is usually due to incompatibility within the ABO system, since both anti-A and anti-B fix complement, regardless of whether they are IgM or IgG molecules. Other possibilities to consider are anti-Jk^a, anti-Le^a, and anti-Fy^a. Rh antibodies are only rarely associated with hemoglobinemia. Symptoms include restlessness, anxiety, flushing, chest or lumbar pain, tachypnea, tachycardia, and nausea, followed by the typical findings of shock and renal failure. In comatose or anesthetized patients, the first sign of danger is often oozing of blood from the mucous membranes or operative site, due to intravascular coagulation.

Extravascular hemolysis is most commonly caused by antibodies of the Rh system, but several other antibodies, especially of the Kell, Duffy, and Kidd systems, are among the offenders. The clinical manifestations are usually milder, consisting of malaise and fever. Shock and renal complications rarely, if ever, occur. Some patients have delayed reactions in which the transfused red blood cells have normal survival initially, but about a week later they are rapidly destroyed in the reticuloendothelial system. Such delayed reactions are commonly due to an anamnestic rise in antibodies previously stimulated by transfusion or pregnancy. Rarely, patients are found to have destroyed all the transfused cells in the absence of demonstrable antibodies.

LABORATORY INVESTIGATION Of first importance in the investigation of a hemolytic transfusion reaction is a careful check on the identity of both the donor and the recipient, since clerical errors, especially mistakes in identity, are most frequently involved. Then the necessary steps include demonstrating that red blood cell destruction has occurred, investigating its cause, and determining the status of the patient's renal and coagulation mechanisms.

With recent *intravascular* lysis, the hemoglobin level is elevated in both plasma and urine (blood must be drawn cautiously to avoid red blood cell rupture). Also, depending on the number of red blood cells destroyed, there may be methemalbuminemia accompanied by marked reduction of serum haptoglobin and hemopexin. (Measuring the latter two substances is rarely necessary, and to be meaningful, both tests require knowledge of the pretransfusion levels for comparison.) The best indicator of *extravascular* lysis is a rise in unconjugated bilirubin, accompanied by failure of the hematocrit to reach the expected posttransfusion level.

Having a *pretransfusion* specimen of the patient's blood is very helpful, so that determination of both donor and recipient blood types can be repeated, along with the compatibility test.

If antibodies are detected, this pretransfusion specimen is also valuable for determining specificity, aided by knowledge of the full antigen composition, since alloantibodies are formed only against antigens not present on the patient's own cells. The *posttransfusion* specimen may not contain the offending antibodies, since they could have been completely absorbed by the donor's incompatible red blood cells. However, it is desirable to examine the red blood cells in the posttransfusion sample, both microscopically for agglutinates and by the direct antiglobulin (Coombs) test. A positive result usually means that some of the donor's red blood cells, coated by the patient's antibodies, were still present when the blood was drawn. But it is also possible that the *donor's* plasma contained antibodies, missed during the donor screening procedure, which reacted with the red blood cells of the patient. Thus, if the direct antiglobulin test on the posttransfusion specimen is positive, the plasma of both donor and recipient should be examined for the responsible antibodies. In the absence of ABO incompatibility, significant destruction of a patient's red blood cells by a donor's alloantibodies is distinctly rare. More typically, the antibody-coated red blood cells survive well in vivo, but their presence can lead to a misdiagnosis of acquired hemolytic anemia.

TREATMENT The care of patients with extravascular hemolysis should be conservative, avoiding additional transfusion unless the patient's life is otherwise threatened. Intravascular hemolysis is a far greater hazard, since shock and renal failure can occur. Immediate treatment with an osmotic diuretic is indicated unless acute tubular necrosis has already occurred. Renal blood flow can be increased with appropriate agents, shock controlled symptomatically, and disseminated intravascular coagulation treated with platelet concentrates and fresh frozen plasma, as needed. Management of the coagulopathy is discussed in Chap. 334, and treatment of renal shutdown in Chap. 290.

In the absence of red blood cell destruction, most febrile reactions can be ascribed to immunity against white blood cell, platelet, or plasma antigens. Further laboratory workup is required only when the reaction is unusually severe. For example, patients with antibodies against IgA molecules sometimes undergo severe shock upon exposure to the blood of other human subjects. Such individuals must be transfused only with blood that lacks IgA or with repeatedly washed red blood cells. Patients with antibodies against white blood cells or platelets can usually be given packed red blood cells from which the buffy layer has been removed after centrifugation or by filtration. Some centers use frozen and thawed red blood cells for transfusing patients sensitized to white blood cells, or to retard the occurrence of such sensitization in candidates for bone marrow transplantation.

Nonimmune transfusion reactions Included in this category are circulatory overload, adverse effects of massive transfusion, infections, metabolic shock, air and fat embolisms, thrombophlebitis, and siderosis. The first three are by far the most common.

CIRCULATORY OVERLOAD Patients with renal or cardiac insufficiency are liable to develop circulatory failure and pulmonary edema with even modest amounts of intravenous infusion. Infants are also vulnerable, since their vasculature does not accommodate rapidly to infusions. The onset may be immediate or delayed for up to 24 h after transfusion, with dyspnea and chest pain progressing to the full-blown picture of pulmonary edema. Susceptible patients should be transfused in a sitting position, with the rate of red blood cell flow not exceeding 2 ml/min, depending on body size and degree of impairment. A rise in central venous pressure heralds the danger of administering more red blood cells unless they are exchanged with whole blood removed from the patient.

MASSIVE TRANSFUSION When the amount of stored blood transfused to bleeding patients exceeds the amount of their normal blood volume, complications can include hyperkalemia, ammonia and citrate toxicity, and dilutional coagulopathy. These problems are largely avoided by using blood stored for no more than a week, supplementing with platelet concentrates when indicated. Fresh frozen plasma is rarely indicated. If the factor 8 level or fibrinogen content is low, concentrates such as cryoprecipitate should be considered.

INFECTION Many diseases, such as hepatitis, cytomegalovirus infection, syphilis, malaria, toxoplasmosis, and brucellosis, can be transmitted by transfusion. In addition, blood that becomes infected during handling and storage can cause very severe shock, owing to toxic bacterial metabolites.

Of all the transfusion-transmitted infections, viral hepatitis is by far the most common and most serious in most parts of the world. Presence in donor blood of the hepatitis B virus (HBV) can be inferred by the detection of the hepatitis B surface antigen (HBsAg). All blood banks are required to perform this test. Although this procedure has reduced the incidence of posttransfusion hepatitis by about a third, other non-A, non-B viruses, as yet undetectable on a routine basis, are responsible for a large proportion of this complication. Blood obtained from paid donors carries an especially high risk of hepatitis.

REFERENCES

ANSTEE DJ: The blood group MNSs-active sialoglycoproteins. Semin Hematol 18:13, 1981

GIBLETT ER: Blood group alloantibodies: An assessment of some laboratory practices. Transfusion 17:299, 1977

HAKOMORI S: Blood group ABH and Ii antigens of human erythrocytes: Chemistry, polymorphism and their developmental change. Semin Hematol 18:39, 1981

MARCUS DM: The P blood group system: Recent progress in immunochemistry and genetics. Semin Hematol 18:63, 1981

MARSH WL: Molecular defects associated with the McLeod blood group phenotype, in *Blood Groups and Other Red Cell Surface Markers in Health and Disease,* C Salmon (ed). New York, Masson, 1982

McKUSICK VA, RUDDLE FH: The status of the gene map of the human chromosomes. Science 196:390, 1977

MOHN JF et al (eds): *Human Blood Groups.* New York, Karger, 1977

MOLLISON PL: *Blood Transfusion in Clinical Medicine,* 6th ed. Philadelphia, Lippincott, 1979

MOURANT AE et al: *The Distribution of the Human Blood Groups and Other Biochemical Polymorphisms,* 2d ed. New York, Oxford University Press, 1975

RACE RR, SANGER R: *Blood Groups in Man,* 6th ed. Oxford, Blackwell, 1975

SLICHTER SJ: Controversies in platelet transfusion therapy. Ann Rev Med 31:509, 1980

WATKINS WM: Biochemistry and genetics of the ABO, Lewis, and P blood group systems, in *Advances in Human Genetics,* H Harris, K Hirschhorn (eds). New York, Plenum, 1980, vol 10, pp 1–136, 379–385

WIENER AS: The blood groups: Three fundamental problems—serology, genetics and nomenclature. Blood 27:110, 1966

336 POLYCYTHEMIA VERA

JOHN W. ADAMSON

DEFINITION Polycythemia vera is one of the *myeloproliferative syndromes,* a group which also includes chronic myelogenous leukemia (see Chap. 129), agnogenic myeloid metaplasia (see Chap. 337), and primary hemorrhagic thrombocythemia. Polycythemia vera is characterized by splenomegaly and an increased production of erythrocytes, granulocytes, and platelets; however, the disease is generally dominated by an elevated hemoglobin concentration. Polycythemia vera is gradual in onset and runs a chronic but usually slowly progressive course.

The disease generally begins in late middle life and is slightly more common in males. Only rarely is polycythemia vera found in children or multiple members of a single family. The disease is relatively uncommon in blacks, and occurs with increased frequency in Jews of European extraction.

ETIOLOGY None of the recognized physiologic causes of increased red blood cell production is present in polycythemia vera. The disease must be distinguished from secondary forms of polycythemia, in which an elevated hemoglobin concentration results from increased erythropoietin production. This association may arise through hypoxia, or is occasionally found with certain neoplasms. Polycythemia vera is also distinct from spurious (relative) polycythemia, which results from a decrease in the plasma volume rather than a true increase in red blood cell mass. Also, secondary causes do not explain the splenic enlargement and increased leukocytes and platelets which are typically seen.

Polycythemia vera is a disease of a pluripotent stem cell and appears to arise from a single clone, findings most consistent with the neoplastic origin of the disorder. In polycythemia vera, there is a unique relationship of erythropoietin to red blood cell production. As opposed to the findings in secondary forms of erythrocytosis, urinary erythropoietin excretion and serum levels of erythropoietin in patients with polycythemia vera are substantially reduced or absent. Presumably erythropoietin production is suppressed by the elevated hemoglobin concentration, since phlebotomy results in a rise in both erythropoietin excretion and red blood cell production (provided that there is no deficiency in iron), demonstrating the marrow's ability to respond at least in part to humoral regulation.

In culture, marrow from patients with polycythemia vera forms colonies of hemoglobin-synthesizing cells in the absence of added erythropoietin. This is rarely the case with marrow cells from normal individuals or from patients with secondary erythrocytosis. A reduced production of erythropoietin, the appearance of "endogenous" erythroid colonies in marrow cultures, and the apparently clonal origin from the pluripotent stem cell all suggest that hematopoiesis in polycythemia vera is not regulated by the usual mechanisms.

PATHOPHYSIOLOGY AND SYMPTOMATOLOGY Polycythemia vera produces symptoms associated with increased blood volume and blood viscosity. The hemoglobin concentration, hematocrit, and total blood volume may become markedly elevated, a consequence of the sharply increased red blood cell mass. The plasma volume is usually normal or reduced slightly; occasionally patients with an increased plasma volume are seen. Associated with the expanded blood volume is a consistently elevated increase in cardiac output and a less uniform, but significant, increase in cardiac index. Reduction of the hematocrit and blood volume by phlebotomy leads to a reduction in the stroke volume and cardiac output in these patients and generally to an improvement in exercise tolerance. The increased cardiac output occurs in association with an increase in blood viscosity and, presumably, vascular resistance, associated with the elevated hematocrit.

Complaints related to the disturbed cerebral circulation include headache, dizziness, vertigo, a sense of fullness of the head, rushing in the ears, visual alterations (scotomata, double vision, or blurred vision), tinnitus, syncope, and even chorea. Peripheral vascular symptoms of both arterial and venous insufficiency are common; in one large series, more than 35 percent of patients gave a history of some thrombotic or hemorrhagic event during the course of their disease. The risk of thrombosis may be increased by the accelerated atherosclerosis in this disease. Bleeding is common and comes most often from the nose and from peptic ulcer disease. Intramuscular hemorrhages and increased bruising are also seen. The tendency to increased bleeding may be due to the distended vasculature resulting from the increased blood volume. However, intrinsic platelet dysfunction also may contribute to bleeding, particularly in the gastrointestinal tract. The incidence of peptic ulcer disease is estimated to be four to five times higher in patients with polycythemia vera than in the general population, although the reasons are unclear.

Late in the disease, the spleen may become greatly enlarged, producing symptoms of easy satiety, a sense of intraabdominal fullness and pleuritic chest or left upper quadrant pain secondary to capsular stretching or infarction. Pruritus, occurring particularly after bathing, is reported frequently and may be disabling. Occasionally, urticaria is seen.

The increased cellular proliferation seen with polycythemia vera results in hyperuricemia in 25 to 30 percent of patients and may be associated with secondary gout in 5 to 10 percent. There also may be renal involvement with uric acid nephropathy and formation of urate stones.

LABORATORY FINDINGS The most prominent laboratory feature is an elevated concentration of hemoglobin. Unless altered by iron deficiency, the red blood cells are normochromic and normocytic. Polychromasia is frequently seen, and nucleated red blood cells may be found in the later stages of the disease. These findings represent cells released from extramedullary sites of hematopoiesis or reflect damage to marrow stroma due to fibrosis. The erythrocyte sedimentation rate is frequently very low (0 to 3 mm/h). Ferrokinetic studies in the patient who is not iron-deficient document an increase in red blood cell production, but studies in the presence of iron deficiency cannot be interpreted with certainty.

The white blood cell count is elevated in two-thirds of patients, usually in the range of 15,000 to 25,000 per cubic millimeter, but may be as high as 60,000 per cubic millimeter. An increase in the absolute basophil count (greater than 65 per cubic millimeter) is found in about 70 percent of patients with polycythemia vera. The alkaline phosphatase of circulating neutrophils is increased in more than 80 percent of cases. Serum vitamin B_{12} levels vary and are increased in about one-third of the patients; however, the binding capacity is increased in as many as 75 percent. This is due to an increase in the vitamin B_{12}–binding proteins, transcobalamins I and III.

Thrombocytosis is seen in over half of all patients with polycythemia vera. In vitro studies of platelet function suggest defective platelet adhesiveness and impaired secondary release of adenosine diphosphate in response to epinephrine. However, the contribution of these functional abnormalities to the thrombotic and hemorrhagic events in patients with polycythemia vera is uncertain. Abnormal liver function studies, including an elevated alkaline phosphatase, may occur if there is massive hepatomegaly.

Splenomegaly occurs in 75 percent of patients and may persist even when the elevated hemoglobin concentration has been reduced by repeated phlebotomies. The spleen may become massive late in the disease. Microscopic examination of the spleen reveals multiple foci of extramedullary hematopoiesis and fibrosis. These may become marked, but the follicular pattern of the organ is retained, unlike the loss of normal architectural structure observed in chronic granulocytic leukemia. Occasionally, similar foci may be found in the liver.

The bone marrow generally reflects either erythroid or panhyperplasia without distinctive morphologic features. There is also increased megakaryocyte nuclear ploidy in the face of thrombocytosis. This pattern of platelet regulation is different from that observed in the reactive thrombocytosis associated with inflammation or neoplasia, where megakaryocyte nuclear ploidy is inversely related to the peripheral platelet count. As the disease progresses, fibrosis may appear in central areas of the marrow, and scanning techniques will demonstrate expansion of hematopoietic tissue to more peripheral skeletal sites.

A variety of cytogenetic abnormalities have been reported in polycythemia vera; however, prior treatment with myelosuppressive agents or radioactive phosphorus (^{32}P) has clouded the significance of such observations. Trisomy 1, 8, or 9 has been reported several times in untreated patients, as has 20q−.

DIAGNOSIS The plethoric patient with pancytosis and splenomegaly, and without evidence of chronic cardiac or pulmonary disease, presents few diagnostic problems. However, it is more common to see these patients with less than the full clinical expression of the disease or as individuals in whom an elevated hemoglobin or hematocrit has been discovered at the time of routine laboratory evaluation. Under these circumstances, it is important that the diagnosis of polycythemia vera be made or excluded with certainty in order to direct therapeutic efforts appropriately.

First the question of whether an elevated hemoglobin represents a true increase in red blood cell mass should be answered. Statistically, there is little likelihood that hematocrits consistently near or greater than 60 percent represent simply a decrease in plasma volume. When hematocrit levels are in the range of 50 to 55 percent, however, the likelihood of true erythrocytosis is considerably reduced. The red blood cell mass should be determined directly by isotope dilution using ^{51}Cr-labeled autologous red blood cells. While the plasma volume may be calculated indirectly from the red blood cell mass, it is preferable to measure this compartment independently, using a second label. If the spleen is markedly enlarged, the mixing time in the circulation for the labeled red blood cells may be prolonged, and samples for radioactive counting should be obtained up to 30 to 45 min after injection. The red blood cell mass results are best expressed as a function of the lean body mass, which may be estimated from the patient's height and weight. If the results of such a study are equivocal, the clinical findings must establish whether the patient has a true increase in red blood cell production.

The patient who presents with a hematocrit or hemoglobin in the high normal range, microcytosis, leukocytosis, and iron deficiency should be considered as possibly having polycythemia vera. Evaluation of red and white blood cell morphology, basophil count, and platelet morphology should be carried out to make certain that this is not a patient with polycythemia vera who has bled.

While measurements of red blood cell mass distinguish between spurious and true erythrocytosis, the results do not distinguish between the various forms of polycythemia. If the diagnosis is uncertain, additional indexes which may be helpful include the absolute basophil count, the leukocyte alkaline phosphatase, and radioisotope scanning to quantitate spleen size. This technique is particularly useful in obese individuals or patients in whom the spleen is enlarged but not palpable. Splenomegaly occurs rarely in individuals with secondary erythrocytosis.

If the diagnosis of polycythemia remains obscure, an intravenous pyelogram to exclude hypernephroma, as well as arterial blood gases, should be obtained. Perhaps 20 percent of patients with polycythemia vera may have a hemoglobin oxygen saturation below 92 percent, but almost all will have a saturation equal to or greater than 88 percent. This modest impairment of oxygen loading may be due to decreased diffusing capacity of the lung, possibly triggered by repeated episodes of thromboembolism or thrombosis in situ.

When the diagnosis is not clear following routine investigation, then measurement of serum levels or urinary excretion of erythropoietin may be helpful. Patients with polycythemia vera excrete little or no measurable erythropoietin, while patients with secondary forms of erythrocytosis excrete at least normal and frequently elevated amounts. Measurements of serum erythropoietin may be performed using a bioassay or a radioimmunoassay. Other types of immunologic assays have not been helpful. In vitro growth characteristics of bone marrow cells from patients with polycythemia vera suggest that such determinations may be useful in diagnosis, but experience with these tests is limited.

COURSE AND PROGNOSIS The course of polycythemia vera has been a subject of disagreement, some observers believing that later complications may be hastened by myelosuppressive therapy. About 15 to 20 percent of patients will progress to marrow fibrosis, marked splenomegaly, and anemia; and one view holds that if patients live long enough, all will enter this so-called spent phase of the disease and will require red blood cell transfusions. However, the majority of patients die of vascular complications of their disease, or of unrelated causes. Although the incidence is low, there is a statistically significant association of second hematologic neoplasms in patients with polycythemia vera, including chronic granulocytic leukemia, lymphocytic and histiocytic lymphomas, multiple myeloma, and erythroleukemia (di Guglielmo's syndrome). Some patients with polycythemia vera experience transformation into acute leukemia even in the absence of prior radiation or chemotherapy.

THERAPY Optimal therapy of polycythemia vera remains unsettled. The median survival has been extended to 10 to 12 years with phlebotomy alone, while patients receiving no therapy at all survive only 2 years. However, neither myelosuppressive therapy nor phlebotomy hold any clear advantage for survival. For many years after its introduction in 1940, ^{32}P was the therapy of choice. However, a retrospective analysis of a large number of cases suggested that ^{32}P increased the incidence of acute leukemia to nearly 15 percent while not clearly enhancing survival over other forms of therapy. In order to resolve the major questions regarding the most effective therapy, the incidence of complicating factors and the prognostic implication of certain features such as thrombocytosis or cytogenetic abnormalities, the International Polycythemia Vera Study Group was established. Beginning in 1967, this group prospectively randomized patients who met strict diagnostic criteria into three treatment programs: ^{32}P therapy augmented by phlebotomy, myelosuppressive therapy plus phlebotomy, and phlebotomy alone. Analysis of the survival curves demonstrates similar life expectancies for the various treatment groups. Acute leukemia has occurred predominantly in the group of patients treated with chemotherapy. The long-term results of this study should provide important information concerning the best treatment and the complications of this disease.

Despite the controversy, certain therapeutic tenets meet with agreement. First, phlebotomy is safe, can be done repeatedly, and is preferred in individuals with mild disease, young patients, or those with polycythemia of uncertain etiology. Regardless of eventual decisions involving therapy, phlebotomy should be used initially to reduce the red blood cell mass and blood volume. The end point of phlebotomy therapy should be a hematocrit or hemoglobin value in the low-normal range. This form of treatment may lead to prolonged clinical remission. Iron should not be given if phlebotomy is the primary mode of therapy. Phlebotomy is especially important if a patient with polycythemia vera must undergo emergency surgery, since intra- and postoperative morbidity and mortality are four to five times greater in uncontrolled as opposed to controlled (phlebotomized) patients. Under these circumstances, the red blood cell mass should be reduced acutely by exchange phlebotomies and the blood replaced with a suitable plasma expander. This will prevent the vascular instability associated with too rapid a reduction in total blood volume.

Marrow suppression may be achieved by radiation or chemical agents. Phosphorus 32 is easy to administer, provides long, trouble-free remissions in most cases, and successfully reduces the morbidity associated with the disease. The isotope is incorporated into bone and comes into close proximity to rapidly dividing marrow cells. The regimen recommended by the Polycythemia Vera Study Group consists of the intravenous administration initially of 85.2 MBq ^{32}P per square meter of body surface area. The patient is then followed for a period of 3 months and re-treated at that time, as needed, with a dose 25 percent greater than that given originally. This program may be repeated 3 months later, but is rarely required. Remissions may last 6 to 24 months, during which time the patient is often symptom-free. Radioactive phosphorus therapy may be repeated if relapse occurs. Exposure to ^{32}P probably increases the incidence of leukemia in patients with polycythemia vera, and the risk of leukemic transformation may be related to the cumulative dose of isotope. Thrombocytosis may be troublesome and constitutes an indication for myelosuppressive therapy.

Suppression of marrow function with chemotherapy has been common during the last 15 years. Effective drugs include melphalan, busulfan, and chlorambucil. Busulfan, in doses of 4 to 6 mg per day orally, reduces the white blood cell and platelet counts, but suppression may be unpredictable and prolonged, and the drug is relatively less effective in suppressing erythropoiesis. Moreover, continued use of this drug may lead to pulmonary fibrosis and a syndrome resembling adrenal insufficiency. Chlorambucil, originally employed in the prospective treatment trial by the Polycythemia Vera Study Group, results in a high incidence (greater than 10 percent) of acute leukemia and the study group has recommended against the use of this and other alkylating agents in this disease. Currently, no form of treatment is clearly better than any other in terms of patient survival, but management with ^{32}P may be simpler. Hydroxyurea, a drug active in the DNA synthetic phase of the cell cycle, is currently being evaluated.

Other symptoms associated with polycythemia vera may be managed conservatively. In the case of pruritus, cyproheptadine, 12 to 16 mg per day, may be effective. Allopurinol in doses of 300 mg per day may successfully reduce the number of acute gouty attacks. Symptomatic splenomegaly is usually improved with treatment, although splenectomy or radiation of the spleen followed by splenectomy may be indicated in rare instances. This procedure is associated with a significant degree of morbidity and mortality.

REFERENCES

ADAMSON JW et al: Polycythemia vera: Stem cell and probable clonal origin of the disease. N Engl J Med 295:913, 1976

BERK PD et al: Increased incidence of acute leukemia in polycythemia vera associated with chlorambucil therapy. N Engl J Med 304:441, 1981

FIALKOW PJ: Clonal hematologic disorders, in *Update III: Harrison's Principles of Internal Medicine*, KJ Isselbacher et al (eds). New York, McGraw-Hill, 1982, pp 13–30

KLEIN H: *Polycythemia Vera: Theory and Management*. Springfield, Ill., Charles C Thomas, 1973

MIESCHER PA, JAFFE ER (eds): Polycythemia, parts I and II. Semin Hematol 12:335, 1975; 13:1, 1976

MODAN B, LILIENFELD AM: Polycythemia vera and leukemia: The role of radiation treatment. Medicine 44:305, 1965

SEGEL N, BISHOP JM: Circulatory studies in polycythemia vera at rest and during exercise. Clin Sci 32:527, 1967

337
AGNOGENIC MYELOID METAPLASIA

JOHN W. ADAMSON

DEFINITION Agnogenic myeloid metaplasia is a member of the *myeloproliferative syndromes*. The disease is characterized by progressive splenomegaly, the gradual replacement of marrow elements by fibrosis, varying degrees of anemia, and variable changes in the number of granulocytes and platelets. The disease begins in late middle life and is gradual in onset, chronic, and progressive. Males and females are equally involved, and there is only rare familial occurrence.

ETIOLOGY The disease arises from a pluripotent hematopoietic stem cell. Erythrocytes, granulocytes, and platelets are members of a single clone, while the fibrosis is reactive and not part of the abnormal clone. Nevertheless, marrow fibrosis progresses in the absence of recognizable stimuli. This distinguishes the disease from those conditions such as metastatic neoplasms or infections involving the bone marrow, which also give rise to reactive fibrosis. Extramedullary hematopoiesis is an integral part of the disease and is seen early in its course. There is no evidence supporting the contention that myeloid metaplasia arises in compensation for replacement of the marrow by fibrous tissue.

PATHOPHYSIOLOGY AND SYMPTOMATOLOGY Agnogenic myeloid metaplasia presents most commonly with vague constitutional symptoms associated with anemia, such as fatigue, weakness, and anorexia, or with splenomegaly. An enlarged spleen is seen in virtually all patients; however, the disease progresses slowly and splenomegaly may be present for years prior to diagnosis. The enlargement may become so extensive as to produce symptoms of pain, abdominal fullness, and dyspnea. Hepatomegaly occurs in more than 50 percent of patients and also may become massive, but enlargement of the liver due to myeloid metaplasia does not occur in the absence of splenomegaly. Because of thrombocytopenia or possible platelet dysfunction, petechiae are found in 20 percent of patients, and a history of bleeding is obtained in 10 percent. Less common findings include lymphadenopathy, jaundice, ascites, and bone pain. Weight loss, fever, sweating, and pain in the extremities may occur occasionally and are associated with a hypermetabolic state. The increased cellular turnover results in hyperuricemia in 25 to 30 percent of patients and may be associated with symptomatic gout in 5 percent.

LABORATORY FINDINGS The blood counts of patients with agnogenic myeloid metaplasia are variable. Mild anemia is observed in the majority of patients at the time of diagnosis and progresses during the course of the disease. Eventually, almost all patients become anemic. The recognized mechanisms leading to anemia include ineffective erythropoiesis, increased splenic pooling of red cells, and a variable decrease in red blood cell survival. Low serum folate and megaloblastic maturation may be contributory factors. A membrane defect similar to that found in paroxysmal nocturnal hemoglobinuria with a positive sucrose hemolysis test has been observed in occasional patients; the significance of this finding is unknown. The peripheral blood smear usually shows dramatic changes in red cell and platelet morphology. Basophilic stippling is prominent, and bizarre red cell shapes, including teardrop poikilocytes, fragmented cells, and nucleated red cells are common, as are giant platelet forms.

An elevation in the white blood cell count is found in about 50 percent of patients, and values as high as 50,000 per cubic millimeter may be seen. However, 20 percent of patients are leukopenic, with white blood cell counts less than 4000 per cubic millimeter. Generally, there is a shift to the left in granulocyte maturation, and circulating blast forms may be found. The appearance of these cells does not imply a bad prognosis. An increase in the absolute basophil count may be observed in about 25 percent of patients. The leukocyte alkaline phosphatase activity of circulating neutrophils is elevated in about half the patients, the remainder being equally distributed between normal and low values. Serum vitamin B_{12} levels are normal or slightly elevated, as are vitamin B_{12}–binding proteins. These values usually do not approach those seen with chronic granulocytic leukemia.

A normal or elevated platelet count is frequently found early in the course of the disease, but thrombocytopenia eventually develops in most patients, owing to ineffective production and splenic pooling. The circulating platelets may vary considerably in size and shape, and megakaryocyte nuclei may be found on the peripheral blood smear. In vitro studies of platelet function reflect defective platelet adhesiveness and secondary release of adenosine diphosphate in response to epinephrine. Abnormal liver function tests, including elevated bilirubin and alkaline phosphatase, may be associated with massive hepatomegaly.

Splenomegaly may become massive. There are multiple foci of extramedullary hematopoiesis on pathologic examination, but the normal follicular architecture of the spleen is maintained. Other organs which may be involved include the kidneys, lymph nodes, adrenal glands, and lungs. Bone marrow examination early in the course of the disease may reveal a hypercellular marrow in about 20 percent of patients and may be difficult to distinguish from polycythemia vera. A silver stain of the marrow often reveals increased reticulin deposition. The majority of patients with agnogenic myeloid metaplasia have either obvious patchy collagen fibrosis separating areas of hyperplastic marrow, or diffuse heavy fibrosis with osteosclerosis. Megakaryocytes may be preserved remarkably well in the areas of fibrosis. The degree of fibrosis and osteosclerosis of the marrow generally correlates with one another and also with the degree of splenomegaly. However, there is no clear relationship between the histopathology of the marrow and the peripheral blood counts. In 40 to 50 percent of patients, the appearance of marrow sclerosis is reflected by increased bone density on x-ray examination, involving particularly the axial skeleton and proximal long bones. These x-ray changes result from thickened bone cortex and loss of medullary spaces due to increased and thickened bony trabeculae.

No unique cytogenetic abnormalities have been described in agnogenic myeloid metaplasia; however, certain nonrandom findings, including monosomy 7 and trisomy 9 have been reported in a few patients. Reports of the Philadelphia chromosome in this disorder probably reflect examples of atypical chronic myelocytic leukemia.

DIAGNOSIS A bone marrow biopsy is essential to the evaluation of this disease, and without it, the diagnosis cannot be made with certainty. This disorder may be difficult to distinguish from others of the myeloproliferative syndromes. This is not surprising because there are several reports of apparent transition of one of the myeloproliferative diseases to another.

In chronic myelocytic leukemia, the white blood cell count is usually greater than 20,000 per cubic millimeter, while in agnogenic myeloid metaplasia it is generally 10,000 to 20,000 per cubic millimeter. Leukocyte alkaline phosphatase is usually lower in chronic myelocytic leukemia, and this determination may be useful in distinguishing between the two disorders. Fibrosis of the marrow is found in only 10 to 15 percent of patients with chronic myelocytic leukemia and is usually present only as a preterminal event; osteosclerosis is almost never seen. In the absence of the Philadelphia chromosome, however, the distinction between these diseases is occasionally difficult.

The separation of polycythemia vera and primary hemorrhagic thrombocythemia from agnogenic myeloid metaplasia also may be troublesome because all may present with thrombocytosis, splenomegaly, leukocytosis, and anemia. However, essential thrombocytosis generally is not associated with advanced fibrosis. The most difficult distinction is between agnogenic myeloid metaplasia and the late stages of polycythemia vera, and attempts to separate them may be unwarranted. Approximately 15 to 25 percent of patients with polycythemia vera progress to advanced marrow fibrosis and marked splenomegaly. It is impossible to be certain that a patient with typical agnogenic myeloid metaplasia did not have polycythemia vera initially. Postpolycythemia myeloid metaplasia and myelofibrosis has a relatively poorer prognosis.

Secondary causes of myelofibrosis include metastatic carcinoma, leukemia and lymphomas, tuberculosis, Gaucher's disease, Paget's disease, and exposure to toxins such as benzol or to x-rays. These causes are usually not difficult to distinguish from agnogenic myeloid metaplasia.

COURSE AND PROGNOSIS Agnogenic myeloid metaplasia generally follows a prolonged course, with a median survival of 4 to 5 years from the time of diagnosis; 25 percent of patients may live 15 years. Anemia will occur eventually in most patients, and many will require transfusions. Complicating features of the disease include gout or other problems related to hyperuricemia; portal hypertension due to hepatic fibrosis or hepatic vein thrombosis; and symptoms related to an enlarging spleen. Clinically evident bleeding occurs in about 25 percent. While the degree of splenomegaly appears of no prognostic importance, a low platelet count (less than 100,000 per cubic millimeter), anemia (hemoglobin less than 10 g/dl), and hepatomegaly appear to influence survival adversely.

The major causes of death include infection, congestive heart failure, renal failure, portal hypertension, and hemorrhage. Transformation to acute leukemia occurs in 5 to 10 percent of patients and may be related to radiation or chemotherapy. An unusual and fulminant variant of agnogenic myeloid metaplasia is characterized by rapid progression of fibrosis and pancytopenia without massive splenic enlargement. Death due to marrow failure usually occurs within 1 year of diagnosis.

THERAPY There is no definitive therapy for this disorder, and no treatment has been shown to affect life span favorably. Anemia is treated with transfusions as required. Androgens may be administered to improve the anemia, although they are helpful in less than half the cases. Oxymetholone (2 to 4 mg/kg per day) or fluoxymesterone may be given, particularly if there is marked ineffective erythropoiesis. Corticosteroids may enhance the response to androgens but alone are not helpful. Myelosuppressive therapy is only occasionally indicated, but may be used to control painful splenomegaly or marked thrombocytosis. Chlorambucil or melphalan may be employed, but other blood elements may be depressed and the period of remission is relatively short (4 to 5 months). External radiation to the spleen will reduce its size, but the effects are transient and therapy may lead to severe pancytopenia. Allopurinol (300 mg per day) may be given to reduce the high uric acid level and control its complications.

The role of splenectomy in the treatment of agnogenic myeloid metaplasia is controversial. Late in the course of the disease the hazards of removing a massively enlarged organ are considerable, and intraoperative mortality and postoperative complications, particularly thrombosis and infection, are frequent. Some clinicians have advocated early removal of the spleen, as soon as the diagnosis is made, believing that this will reduce later complications and make management easier. Until this question is resolved, perhaps the only clear indications for splenectomy are hemolysis, severe thrombocytopenia, and intractable symptoms related to the splenomegaly.

REFERENCES

FIALKOW PJ: Clonal hematologic disorders, in *Update III: Harrison's Principles of Internal Medicine,* KJ Isselbacher et al (eds). New York, McGraw-Hill, 1982, pp 13–30

JACOBSON RJ et al: Agnogenic myeloid metaplasia: A clonal proliferation of hematopoietic stem cells with secondary myelofibrosis. Blood 51:189, 1978

LEWIS SM, SZUR L: Malignant myelosclerosis. Br Med J 1:472, 1963

SILVERSTEIN MN: *Agnogenic Myeloid Metaplasia.* Acton, Mass., Publishing Sciences Group, 1975

WARD HP, BLOCK MH: The natural history of agnogenic myeloid metaplasia (AMM) and a critical evaluation of its relationship with the myeloproliferative syndrome. Medicine 50:357, 1971

section 9 | Disorders of bone and bone mineral metabolism

338 SKELETAL REMODELING AND FACTORS INFLUENCING BONE AND BONE MINERAL METABOLISM

STEPHEN M. KRANE
JOHN T. POTTS, JR.

BONE STRUCTURE AND METABOLISM (See also Chap. 341) Bone is a dynamic tissue, constantly remodeling itself throughout life. The skeleton is highly vascular and receives about 10 percent of the cardiac output. The skeleton has extraordinary mechanical functions suited for mobility of vertebrates. The arrangement of compact and cancellous bone provides a combination of strength and density for these mechanical functions. In addition, bone provides a store of calcium, magnesium, phosphorus, sodium, and other ions necessary for the support of a variety of homeostatic functions.

In the following chapters a number of disorders will be discussed in which the metabolism of cartilage, bone, and mineral ions is affected. A brief review of skeletal remodeling, the metabolism of mineral ions, and the major factors which influence mineral metabolism is, therefore, pertinent.

The properties of bone are a function of the organization of its extracellular components. Its structure consists of a solid mineral phase in close association with an organic matrix, consisting of 90 to 95 percent collagen, small amounts of proteoglycans, and noncollagenous proteins including proteins derived from serum (e.g., albumin and an alpha$_2$ glycoprotein) and others synthesized by bone cells, particularly a γ-carboxyglutamic acid–containing (GLA) protein called, by some, osteocalcin. The mineral phase is comprised of calcium and phosphate, best described as a poorly crystalline hydroxyapatite, although the calcium/phosphate molar ratio is less than the 1.67 that hydroxyapatite would require [empiric formula, $Ca_{10}(PO_4)_6(OH)_2$]. In addition, other ions are present, predominantly in the surface layers. The mineral phase of bone is deposited in intimate relation to the collagen fibrils and is found largely in specific locations within the "holes" of the collagen fibrils which result from the manner in which the collagen molecules are packed. This architectural organization of mineral and matrix results in a two-phase material uniquely suited to withstand mechanical stresses. The formation as well as the localization of the inorganic phase is probably determined at least in part by the organic matrix, particularly the collagen.

Bone is formed by cells of mesenchymal origin which synthesize and secrete the organic matrix. Mineralization of the matrix, particularly in *osteons* (haversian systems), begins soon after secretion (primary mineralization) but is not completed until after several weeks (secondary mineralization). As an *osteoblast* secretes matrix which is then mineralized, this cell becomes surrounded by matrix and becomes an *osteocyte,* still connected with its blood supply through a series of canaliculi. Resorption of bone is carried out by cells which include mononuclear cells as well as multinucleated *osteoclasts,* the latter characterized by their elaborately infolded border adjacent to the bone and their location in scalloped resorption spaces (Howship's lacunae) (Fig. 338-1). Some resorption of bone may also take place around the osteocytes. The cells of bone are probably derived from precursor cells in the bone marrow. A hematopoietic stem cell is the likely precursor of the osteoclast, whereas a stromal stem cell is the likely precursor of the osteoblast. It is unlikely that there is transformation between these two cell types or their precursors under physiological or pathological conditions.

In the embryo and in the growing child, bone develops either by remodeling and replacing previously calcified cartilage (endochondral bone formation), or it is formed without a cartilage matrix (intramembranous bone formation). The young new bone, especially in embryos and infants and that newly formed in adults during repair, has a relatively high ratio of cells to matrix and is characterized by coarse fiber bundles of collagen which are interlaced and randomly dispersed (woven bone). In adults, the more mature bone is organized with fiber bundles regularly arranged in parallel or concentric sheets (lamellar bone). In long bones, the lamellar bone is deposited in a highly ordered concentric arrangement around blood vessels along their length and forms the haversian systems. Growth in length of bones is dependent upon proliferation of cartilage cells and the endochondral sequence at the growth plate. Growth in width and thickness is accomplished by formation of bone at the periosteal surface and resorption at the endosteal surface with the rate of formation exceeding that of resorption. In adults, after the epiphyses close, growth in length and endochondral bone formation cease, except for some activity in the cartilage cells beneath the articular surface. However, even in adults, remodeling of bone (remodeling of haversian systems as well as trabecular bone) is a continuous process through life, as can be shown by microradiographic studies utilizing radioisotopes or fluorescence of tetracyclines fixed in bone in regions of new mineralization. Quantitative histomorphometric techniques have been developed utilizing thin, undemineralized sections of standard biopsies from the iliac crest. Newly forming surfaces are characterized by smooth character, uptake of tetracycline, and relatively low mineral density. Actively forming surfaces are covered by active osteoblasts. The osteoid seam which results from the relative lag in mineralization of the newly formed organic matrix is normally no greater than about 12 μm. An index of the rate of bone formation can be obtained by examination of undemineralized sections of bone biopsies obtained from individuals who have received tetracycline for two periods separated by a drug-free interval. The distance between the fluorescent bands on the sections reflects the new bone formed. Resorption areas are characterized by their irregular configurations and the presence of osteoclasts (Fig. 338-1). Resorption precedes formation and is more intense, but it does not persist as long as formation. In adults, approximately 4 percent of the surface of trabecular bone (such as iliac crest) is involved in active resorption, whereas 10 to 15 percent of trabecular surfaces are covered with osteoid. Kinetic studies using isotopes such as radioactive calcium (^{47}Ca) provide estimates that as much as 18 percent of the total skeletal calcium may be deposited and removed each year. Thus bone is an active metabolizing tissue, with its cells dependent upon an intact blood supply. Throughout life bone is constantly being remodeled in a manner somehow related to the continuous mechanical stresses to which it is subjected. Bone also serves as an important reservoir of mineral ions, particularly calcium, which are critical for a variety of processes in other tissues.

FIGURE 338-1

Schematic representation of bone remodeling surfaces in trabecular bone. Most bone surfaces in adults are involved in neither formation nor resorption. Such surfaces are usually smooth, have no osteoid seam, and are covered either by no visible cells or by flattened cells. Active formation surfaces are smooth and covered by osteoblasts which have an osteoid seam (clear), normally no thicker than 12 μm. The calcification front is located at the junction of the osteoid seam and mineralized bone (stippled). Inactive forming surfaces are not covered by osteoblasts but by only a few flattened cells. Active resorbing surfaces are irregular or scalloped and contain multinucleated osteoclasts. The latter are not seen on inactive resorbing surfaces.

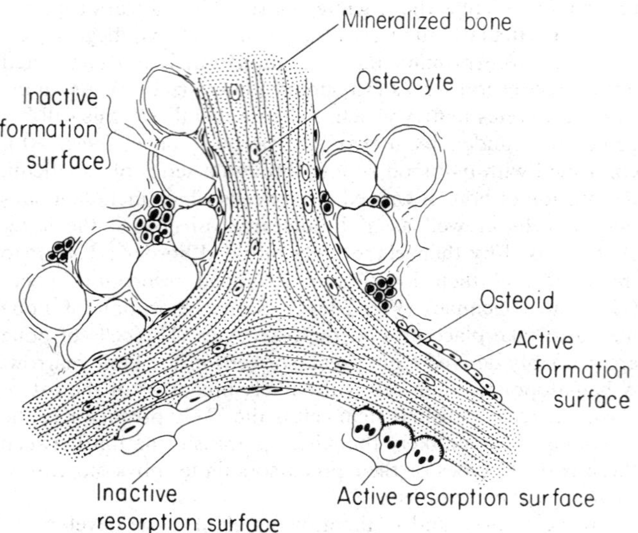

The response of bone to injuries, such as fractures, infection, interruption of blood supply, and the presence of expanding lesions is relatively limited. Dead bone must be resorbed and new bone formed, a process which normally is carried out in association with new blood vessels growing into the involved area. In injuries that severely disrupt the organization of the tissue, such as a fracture in which apposition of fragments is poor and motion exists at the fracture site, the osteoprogenitor stromal cells differentiate into cells with functional capacities other than those of osteoblasts, and repair is accompanied by formation of varying amounts of fibrous tissue and cartilage. In instances in which there is good apposition with fixation and little motion at the fracture site, repair occurs predominantly by bone without other scar tissue. Remodeling of this bone is subsequently accomplished along lines of force determined by mechanical stresses that are somehow translated into biologic response.

Expanding lesions in bone, such as tumors, tend to induce resorption at the surface in contact with the tumor and formation at the outer circumference. A bowing deformity tends to result in increased new bone formation at the concave surface and resorption at the convex surface, all seemingly designed to produce the strongest mechanical structure. Even in a disorder as architecturally disruptive as Paget's disease of bone, remodeling appears to be dictated by mechanical forces. Thus the biologic plasticity of bone is due to the response of cells interacting with each other and the environment.

Mechanisms of bone formation and resorption Bone formation is an orderly process in which inorganic mineral is deposited in relation to an organic matrix. The mineral phase is composed of calcium and phosphorus, and, therefore, the concentration of these ions in the plasma and extracellular fluid influences the rate at which the mineral phase is formed. In vitro, mineralization can proceed, and crystals of hydroxyapatite can grow at concentrations of calcium and phosphorus similar to those in an ultrafiltrate of plasma. However, the concentration of these ions at the sites of mineralization is unknown, and it is possible that the cells involved (osteoblasts, osteocytes) somehow regulate the local concentration of calcium, phosphorus, and other ions. Collagens from a variety of sources can catalyze the nucleation of a mineral phase of calcium and phosphorus from solutions of these ions, and the initial mineral phase is deposited in specific locations in the holes produced by the particular packing arrangement of the collagen molecules. It is likely that the organization of collagen influences the amount and type of mineral phase that is formed in bone. The collagen of bone is similar in its primary structure to that of skin [contains two $\alpha 1(I)$ chains and one $\alpha 2$ chain] but differs in hydroxylation, glycosylation, and the type, number, and distribution of intermolecular cross-links. In addition, the "holes" in the packing structure of the collagen are larger in normally mineralized collagen of bone and dentin than those of a normally unmineralized collagen such as tendon. Other noncollagenous organic components such as GLA proteins and other glycoproteins may also play a role in the formation and localization of the mineral phase of bone. To explain how collagens from tissues that are normally not mineralized can catalyze nucleation of an inorganic phase from solutions similar to normal extracellular fluid, regulation of mineralization by inhibitory substances has been suggested. Inorganic pyrophosphate is a potent inhibitor of mineralization at concentrations several orders of magnitude below those necessary to bind calcium ions. Since alkaline phosphatase, present in osteoblasts and other cells, can catalyze the hydrolysis of inorganic pyrophosphate at neutral pH, this enzyme could play a role in the regulation of mineralization by controlling the concentrations of pyrophosphate. In addition, macromolecular inhibitors such as the proteoglycan aggregates may also influence the rate and extent of mineralization. In cartilage undergoing calcification, membrane-bound vesicles containing mineral have been identified outside the cells, and it has been suggested that this is the initial mineral phase.

In bone, the calcium phosphate solid phase at the inception of mineralization is brushite ($CaHPO_4 \cdot 2H_2O$). As mineralization progresses, the solid phase is a poorly crystalline hydroxyapatite with a relatively low ($\sim$ 1.2) calcium/phosphate molar ratio. With age and maturation, the degree of crystal perfection increases as does the calcium/phosphate ratio. Fluoride ions, when incorporated into the mineral phase, tend to decrease the proportion of amorphous calcium phosphate and increase crystallinity.

There is a limit for the concentration of calcium and phosphorus ions in the extracellular fluid below which the mineral phase will not be formed. A "solubility product" for bone mineral is difficult to calculate since the mineral phase itself is of variable composition and the true nature of species in solution governing this solubility product is not known. Nevertheless when the concentrations of calcium and phosphorus, particularly the latter, in extracellular fluid are excessive, a mineral phase may be formed in areas that are not normally mineralized.

When bone is resorbed, calcium and phosphorus ions from the solid phase are released into solution in the extracellular fluid, and subsequently the organic matrix is also resorbed. It is not entirely clear how these processes occur. A decrease in pH, the presence of a chelating substance, and the operation of a cellular pump mechanism to shift the equilibrium between solids and solution are possibilities to explain mineral release. Resorption occurs at specific sites either adjacent to osteoclasts or surrounding osteocytes and requires normal metabolism of these cells. Osteoclasts are rich in acid phosphatase, a convenient marker for these cells, but the function of this enzyme in mineral resorption is not known. Whereas the activity of alkaline phosphatase, an enzyme found in osteoblasts, may be increased in serum when osteoblast number or function is increased, no such spillover from acid phosphatase is observed. The matrix is resorbed presumably through the action of collagenases and possibly other proteinases released by the resorbing cells; the collagenases attack collagen in a specific manner but are incapable of degrading the protein before the mineral phase is removed. The rate at which resorption occurs is stimulated by parathyroid hormone as well as by other substances such as heparin, prostaglandins of the E series, and protein factor(s) derived from lymphocytes (osteoclast-activating factor). The effect of the hormones is discussed in more detail later.

CALCIUM METABOLISM Before considering the effects of hormones and vitamin D, a brief summary of calcium and phosphorus homeostasis in humans is indicated.

There is about 1 to 2 kg calcium in the average adult human body, of which over 98 percent is in the skeleton. The calcium of the mineral phase at the surface of the crystals is in equilibrium with ions of the extracellular fluid, but only a minor proportion of the total calcium (about 0.5 percent) is exchangeable as determined by isotope dilution techniques. Although the calcium in the extracellular fluid is only a small fraction of the total, its concentration is critical for a variety of functions, and it is kept remarkably constant. In plasma, in normal adults, the range of concentration is 8.8 to 10.4 mg/dl (2.2 to 2.6 m*M*). The calcium in plasma is in three forms: as free ions, bound to plasma proteins, and, to a small extent, as diffusible complexes. The concentration of free calcium ions is of critical importance in regulating the level of neuromuscular irritability as well as a variety of other cellular functions and is subjected to exquisite hormonal control, especially through parathyroid hormone, as described below. The concentration of serum proteins is an important factor in prediction of the concentration of calcium ions; most of the protein binding is to albumin. One formula that approximates the amount of calcium bound to proteins is

$$\%\ \text{protein-bound Ca} = 8 \times \text{albumin (g/dl)} + 2 \times \text{globulin (g/dl)} + 3$$

Another correction is simply to subtract 1 mg/dl from the serum calcium concentration for every 1.0 g/dl serum albumin lower than 4.0 g/dl. Thus the concentration of ultrafiltrable calcium is usually about 50 percent of the total calcium. In most laboratories only total calcium is determined, and therefore knowledge of the concentration of proteins is essential to estimate concentration of calcium ions. Free ions are measured directly as a routine procedure in some laboratories with the use of calcium-specific electrodes.

Decrease in the concentration of free calcium ions in plasma results in increased neuromuscular irritability and the syndrome of tetany. This syndrome is characterized, when fully expressed, by peripheral and perioral paresthesias, carpal spasm, pedal spasm, anxiety, seizures, bronchospasm, laryngospasm, Chvostek's, Trousseau's, and Erb's signs, and lengthening of the QT interval of the electrocardiogram. In infants tetany may be manifested only by irritability and lethargy. The level of calcium ions that determines which features of tetany will be manifested is variable in different individuals. The occurrence of tetany is also influenced by the concentration of other components of the extracellular fluid. For example, hypomagnesemia and alkalosis lower the threshold for tetany, whereas hypokalemia and acidosis raise the threshold.

Increases in total serum calcium are, as a rule, accompanied by increases in calcium ions and may be associated with a variety of symptoms and signs including anorexia, nausea, vomiting, constipation, some degree of hypotonia, depression, and occasionally lethargy and coma. Persistent hypercalcemia, especially when accompanied by normal or elevated levels of serum phosphate, may eventually result in deposition of a solid mineral phase of calcium and phosphate in abnormal sites such as walls of blood vessels, connective tissue about the joints, gastric mucosa, cornea, and renal parenchyma. Hypercalcemia per se alters renal function in addition to the pathological effects of calcium-phosphate deposits in the lumen of renal tubules and in the interstitial areas of the kidney.

The concentration of calcium ions in the extracellular fluid is kept constant by the interaction of a number of processes which constantly feed calcium into and withdraw calcium from the extracellular fluid. Calcium enters the plasma via absorption from the intestinal tract and by resorption of ions from the bone mineral. Calcium leaves the extracellular fluid via secretion into the gastrointestinal tract, urinary excretion, deposition in bone mineral, and, to a minor extent, via losses in sweat. Resorption and formation are usually tightly coupled, approximately 500 mg calcium entering and leaving the skeleton daily (Fig. 338-2).

The average diet in the United States provides about 600 to 1000 mg calcium daily, mostly in the form of dairy products. However, less than half of the calcium in the diet is absorbed in adults. The percentage of calcium absorbed increases during periods of rapid growth in children, in pregnancy, and in lactation, and decreases with advancing age. If adequate vitamin D is available and vitamin D metabolism is normal, a greater percentage of dietary calcium is absorbed (adaptation). Most of the calcium is absorbed in the proximal small intestine, and the efficiency of absorption decreases in the more distal intestinal segments. Both active transport and diffusion-limited absorptive processes are involved; the former is more important in the upper and the latter in the lower intestine. Both are influenced by vitamin D through the action of its metabolites. Adequate calcium absorption requires the availability of a functioning surface. It is possible that all forms of calcium in the diet are not equally absorbed; even with defined salts, calcium as the chloride is probably absorbed more efficiently than that in other preparations.

FIGURE 338-2
Calcium homeostasis. Schematic illustration of calcium content of extracellular fluid (ECF) and bone as well as of diet and feces; magnitude of calcium flux per day as calculated by various methods is shown at sites of transport in intestine, kidney, and bone. Ranges of values shown are approximate and chosen to illustrate certain points discussed in text. In intestine, absorption efficiency varies inversely with dietary calcium (chronic adaptation). This is reflected in typical quantities absorbed and excreted in feces; with 0.5-g intake, 50 percent absorption is depicted to occur (0.25 g), but at 1.5 g only 30 percent (0.5 g). Fecal calcium as a percentage of intake can be as high at low intakes as at high intakes because of the greater significance in the former of the contribution from endogenous fecal calcium, the 0.1 to 0.2 g secreted into the intestinal lumen daily independent of intake. Quantities of calcium depicted as filtered, reabsorbed, and excreted at the kidney are chosen arbitrarily to indicate that at lower rates of filtration of calcium (expected at lower glomerular filtration rates), most is reabsorbed (e.g., 5.85 of 6 g), leading to urinary excretion of 150 mg; at higher rates of filtration (at high dietary calcium intake), slightly less is reabsorbed (e.g., 9.7 of 10 g), leading to a higher urinary excretion, 300 mg. In all situations, renal calcium reabsorption exceeds 95 percent of filtered load. Urinary calcium excretion is seen, therefore, to increase by only 150 mg despite a 1-g increase in dietary intake. In conditions of calcium balance, rates of calcium release from and uptake into bone are equal.

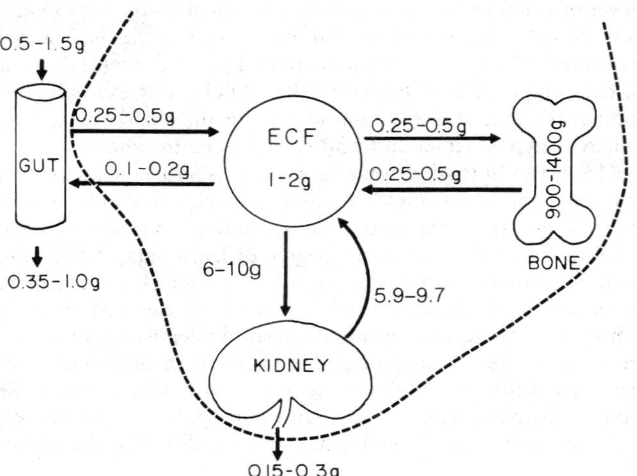

Calcium is also secreted into the lumen of the gastrointestinal tract. When isotopes of radioactive calcium are administered intravenously, radioactivity appears in the feces, leading to calculations of *endogenous fecal calcium* of about 60 to 130 mg per day. Higher estimates of calcium losses in intestinal juices have been made by other approaches. It is generally agreed, however, that no control of calcium balance is exerted by regulation of intestinal calcium secretion. On the other hand, if calcium availability in the diet is low (less than 500 mg per day), positive calcium balance requires an efficiency of absorption greater than 30 to 40 percent if intestinal uptake is to be sufficient to exceed losses via intestinal secretion and to match calcium losses that occur through renal calcium excretion.

The urinary calcium excretion of normal adults on average calcium intakes ranges between a minimum of 100 mg per day to as high as 300 to 400 mg per day. When the dietary calcium is reduced to below 200 mg daily, urinary calcium excretion is usually less than 200 mg per day. However, in most normal individuals the level of dietary intake over a wide range has relatively little effect on the urinary excretion of calcium. Hence in individuals on diets low in calcium, this relative inefficiency of renal calcium conservation leads to negative calcium balance unless calcium absorption is maximally efficient (Fig. 338-2). Calculations of calcium clearance have been reported based on estimation of calcium concentration obtained by ultrafiltration methods. Ratios of calcium to creatinine clearance are thus calculated to be less than 0.05. However, the amount of calcium excreted in the urine is minute compared with that filtered through the glomerulus (about 6 to 10 g per day); it is not certain whether some non-protein-bound, nonionic forms of calcium (e.g., calcium citrate) are cleared at rates considerably greater than others. The excretion of other electrolytes also affects the urinary excretion of calcium. For example, calciuresis is usually proportional to natriuresis; other ions, such as sulfate, also increase calcium excretion.

Maintenance of calcium balance (Fig. 338-2) is dependent upon hormonally supported efficiency of intestinal absorption. Deficiency of parathyroid hormone or vitamin D, intestinal disease, or severe dietary calcium deprivation may provide challenges to calcium homeostasis that cannot be compensated adequately by renal calcium conservation, resulting in negative calcium balance. Increased bone resorption may protect against extracellular fluid calcium depletion and symptomatic hypocalcemia even in states of chronic negative calcium balance but only at the expense of progressive osteopenia.

PHOSPHORUS METABOLISM Phosphorus is not only a major component of the mineral phase of bone but is among the most abundant constituents of all tissues and in some form is involved in almost all metabolic processes. The total amount of phosphorus in the normal adult is about 1000 g, of which about 85 percent is in the skeleton.

In normal plasma most of the phosphorus is present as inorganic orthophosphate in concentrations which range in the fasting state from 2.8 to 4.0 mg (P)/dl. In contrast to calcium, where about 50 percent is bound, only about 12 percent of the phosphorus in plasma is bound to proteins. Free HPO_4^{2-} and $NaHPO_4^-$ normally are about 75 percent of the total plasma phosphorus, and free $H_2PO_4^-$ is 10 percent. Since so many species are present, depending upon pH and other factors, it has been the convention to express concentrations in terms of mass of elemental phosphorus, i.e., milligrams phosphorus per deciliter. Total phosphorus levels are higher in children and tend to rise in women after the menopause. There is a diurnal variation of phosphorus concentration even in conditions of a 24-h fast, mediated in part by the adrenal cortex. Ingestion of carbohydrate depresses serum phosphorus acutely by as much as 1.0 to 1.5 mg/dl, presumably by cellular uptake and formation of phosphate esters. Ingestion of phosphorus per se increases serum levels. Therefore, it is essential for the interpretation of serum levels and urinary clearances that samples be obtained in the fasting state. Decreases in plasma phosphorus also occur during induction of alkalosis.

No definite symptoms result from hyperphosphatemia. However, when high levels are maintained for long periods, the driving force for mineralization is increased, and calcium phosphate deposits may occur in abnormal sites as discussed earlier. Severe acute hypophosphatemia may or may not be accompanied by symptoms. Persistent hypophosphatemia may cause varying degrees of anorexia, dizziness, bone pain, proximal muscular weakness, and waddling gait. In severe hypophosphatemia (which may be aggravated, after hospitalization, by administration of nutrients to alcoholics, or with therapy of diabetic ketoacidosis), sharp elevations in serum creatine phosphokinase (CPK) suggest that rhabdomyolysis may be superimposed on myopathy. This sequence of events also occurs in experimental phosphate depletion in animals. Severe congestive cardiomyopathy has also been noted with chronic hypophosphatemia; restoration of phosphorus deficits leads to prompt reversal of the abnormalities. The bone pain and waddling gait are attributed to the osteomalacia which develops as a result of phosphate depletion. The muscular weakness may be due either to direct effects of hypophosphatemia on nerves and muscle or, in some instances, to the effects of hyperparathyroidism (either primary or secondary) which may have a role in the etiology of the hypophosphatemia. Defective growth in children may also be due to phosphate depletion. Hypophosphatemia results in decreased levels of 2,3-diphosphoglyceric acid and adenosine triphosphate (ATP) in erythrocytes which in turn alter the dissociation of oxyhemoglobin so that less oxygen is delivered in the periphery. Hemolytic anemia may also be produced by the effects of decreased ATP on the ability of erythrocytes to deform in small peripheral vessels.

Whereas only a small proportion of dietary calcium is absorbed from the intestine, phosphorus absorption is remarkably efficient. At low levels of dietary intake (less than 2 mg/kg per day) 80 to 90 percent of ingested phosphorus is absorbed. Even with the higher levels of intake (greater than 10 mg/kg per day) in average diets in the form of dairy products, cereals, eggs, and meat, absorption is about 70 percent. Hypophosphatemia due to deficient intestinal absorption is rarely encountered except in situations where excessive quantities of nonabsorbable antacids are consumed; the antacids bind phosphorus and prevent absorption from the intestinal lumen.

The major control of phosphorus economy is exerted at the level of the kidney. Phosphorus filtered through the glomerulus is largely reabsorbed in the proximal tubule (there is homeostatically important distal reabsorption as well) so that normally only about 10 to 15 percent of the filtered load is excreted. When filtered loads of phosphorus decrease, proximal tubular reabsorption increases. Conversely when phosphorus loads are increased, tubular reabsorption decreases and clearance rises. Thus the urinary excretion of phosphorus normally reflects dietary intake, and conservation or elimination of excessive amounts of the ion depends upon adequate renal handling (Fig. 338-3). There is no good evidence for renal tubular phosphate secretion. Proximal reabsorption of phosphorus is dependent upon parallel sodium reabsorption, but whereas the

sodium rejected by the proximal tubule may be reabsorbed distally, the rejected phosphorus is not. Therefore the effects of volume expansion and decreased sodium reabsorption are to increase phosphorus clearance; similarly diuretics such as acetazolamide, which act proximally, are phosphaturic parallel to the degree to which they are natriuretic.

In contrast to critical features of calcium metabolism as discussed above, negative phosphorus balance (Fig. 338-3) is rarely caused by inadequate phosphorus absorption in the intestine and maintenance of normal phosphorus balance is dependent upon efficiency of renal excretion or conservation of phosphorus. In severe renal failure, hyperphosphatemia results from inadequate renal phosphorus clearance; heritable or acquired renal tubular insufficiency may lead to hypophosphatemia due to inadequate renal conservation of phosphorus.

FIGURE 338-3

Phosphate homeostasis. Schematic illustration of inorganic phosphorus content (termed here phosphate) in extracellular fluid (ECF) and bone as well as diet and feces; magnitude of phosphorus flux per day as estimated by various methods is shown at transport sites in intestine, kidney, and bone. Range of values shown illustrates special features of phosphorus metabolism discussed in text. Intestinal phosphorus absorption is highly efficient, 85 percent at a lower intake (0.5 g of a 0.6-g intake) and 70 percent at a higher intake (1.4 g of a 2.0-g intake). Estimates of magnitude of endogenous fecal phosphate are less well established than for calcium. Contribution of at least 0.15 g is estimated to be added to the nonabsorbed phosphorus to provide a total of 0.2 g fecal phosphorus at the low intake level. At high phosphorus dietary intakes, no correction for endogenous fecal phosphate is calculated. Higher quantities of phosphorus are excreted in urine at all levels of dietary intake than for corresponding intakes of calcium; quantities excreted match closely the quantities absorbed, thereby maintaining phosphorus balance (no correction in this illustration is made for endogenous fecal phosphorus). Note that renal phosphorus reabsorption, in contrast to high and relatively invariant renal calcium reabsorption, varies from a low of 75 percent of filtered load to greater than 85 percent. The compartment labeled ICF refers to intracellular phosphorus, both organic and inorganic; rapid shifts of phosphorus into cells (and corresponding, possibly slower, efflux of phosphorus from cells) contribute to changes in ECF phosphorus. These shifts between ECF and ICF and phosphorus release from and uptake by bone are equal in conditions of phosphorus balance.

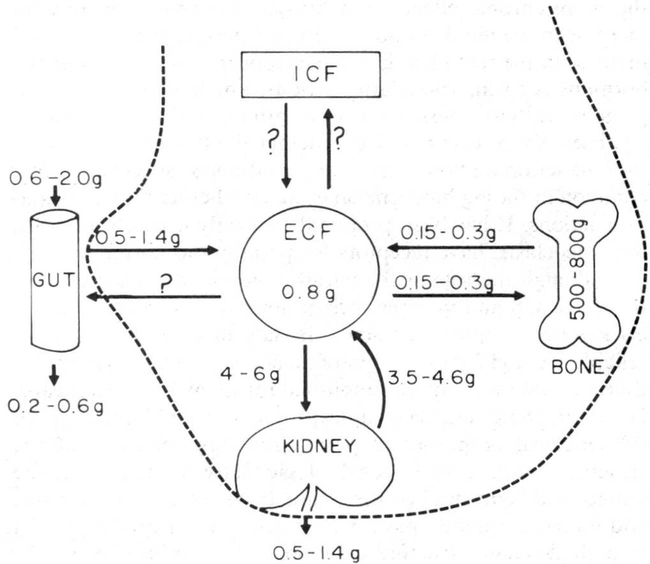

PARATHYROID HORMONE (See also Chap. 339) The physiological function of parathyroid hormone is to maintain extracellular fluid calcium concentration. The hormone acts on bone and kidney directly and indirectly through its effects on synthesis of 1α,25-dihydroxyvitamin D_3 [1α,25-$(OH)_2D_3$] on intestine to increase serum calcium; in turn, parathyroid hormone production is closely regulated by serum ionized calcium concentration. This feedback system involving the parathyroids is one of the most important homeostatic mechanisms for the close regulation of extracellular fluid calcium concentration. Any tendency toward hypocalcemia, as might be induced by calcium-deficient diets, is counteracted by an increased rate of secretion of parathyroid hormone. This in turn (1) acts to increase the rate of dissolution of bone mineral, thereby providing an increased flow of calcium from bone into blood, (2) reduces the renal clearance of calcium, returning more of the calcium filtered at the glomerulus into extracellular fluid, and (3) increases the efficiency of calcium absorption in the intestine. The relative physiological importance of these three actions of parathyroid hormone, stimulation of calcium transport in bone, kidney, and intestine, is not definitely resolved. Most evidence suggests that rapid changes in blood calcium are due to effects of the hormone on bone and, to a lesser extent, on renal calcium clearance; maintenance of calcium balance, on the other hand, is probably due to the effects of the hormone, via control of 1α,25-$(OH)_2D_3$ levels, on efficiency of intestinal calcium absorption (Chap. 340). Evidence from calcium kinetic studies indicates a transfer between extracellular fluid and bone of as much as 500 mg calcium daily (an amount large in relation to the total extracellular fluid calcium pool), and parathyroid hormone is known to influence this movement of calcium from bone into blood. This action of the hormone would tend to preserve calcium concentration in blood acutely at the cost of bone destruction and bone mineral release. However, the action of parathyroid hormone on kidney to preserve calcium by increasing the percentage reabsorption of filtered calcium may also be important in rapid regulation of blood calcium concentration.

There is evidence for a dual action of parathyroid hormone on bone. These two effects have been termed the *calcium replacement* and the *bone remodeling* effects of parathyroid hormone. It can be shown in vitro that there is an increased rate of release of calcium from bone into blood within minutes of the administration of parathyroid hormone; in vivo, a rapid efflux of calcium out of blood, presumably into bone cells, can be shown to precede the release of calcium. On the other hand, the more chronic effects of parathyroid hormone, mainly an increase in the number and activity of osteoclasts and a general increase in the remodeling of bone, appear only hours after the hormone is given. These latter actions, which involve increased protein synthesis, persist for hours after parathyroid hormone has been given. It is not clear whether the two effects of parathyroid action on bone represent a continuous spectrum with a common initiating biochemical event or whether they are separate actions. It has been proposed that only osteoblastic cells, not osteoclasts, have receptors for parathyroid hormone.

Although the role of the parathyroid glands in the prevention of tetany and maintenance of normal plasma calcium levels has been appreciated since the late nineteenth century, a reliable method for extraction of an active principle from parathyroid tissue was not accomplished for many years afterward. However, there has been rapid progress in our knowledge of the chemical properties of parathyroid hormone and of the structural requirements for biologic activity. The complete amino acid sequences of the major forms of bovine, porcine, and human hormones have been defined. The peptides consist of a single-chain structure composed of 84 amino acids. The molecules lack cysteine or cystine; the sequences of the three known forms of the hormone are similar, as is illustrated in Fig. 338-4.

The often discussed possibility that different forms of the hormone are active on bone and kidney is not supported by analyses of the relation between parathyroid hormone structure and physiological actions. The structural requirements for biologic activity of parathyroid hormone have been defined recently by synthesis of peptides based on the structures deduced. Numerous peptides consisting of portions of the amino-terminal 34 residues and various analogues have been synthesized. Synthetic fragments containing the amino-terminal sequence have been shown to exert all the known biologic actions of the hormone on mineral ion transport in kidney and bone. It seems likely that the amino terminal portion of the hormone is also responsible for stimulation of the renal 25-hydroxyvitamin D 1α-hydroxylase and, hence, the action of the hormone to stimulate intestinal calcium absorption.

It can now be concluded on the basis of studies with synthetic peptides that any fragment of parathyroid hormone, in order to be biologically active on bone and kidney, must consist of a continuous peptide sequence beginning with residue 2, valine, and extending as far as residue 26, lysine.

These observations are of particular interest because the biosynthesis and peripheral metabolism of parathyroid hormone have been found to be more complex than initially thought. Furthermore, parathyroid hormone which is extracted from glands differs from both the hormone that is initially synthesized and the hormone found in the peripheral circulation.

FIGURE 338-4

Model illustrating the sequence of human, bovine, and porcine parathyroid hormone. The continuous open circles represent the sequence of human PTH, numbers referring to sequence positions beginning with the amino terminus; sequence positions at which the residues found in the bovine and porcine molecule differ from that found in the human hormone are shown by the circles adjacent to the human sequence. Note relative conservation in the sequence region associated with biologic activity, residues 1 to 34; most sequence differences are found in the middle region of the molecule. (From HT Keutmann et al, Biochemistry 17:5723, 1978.)

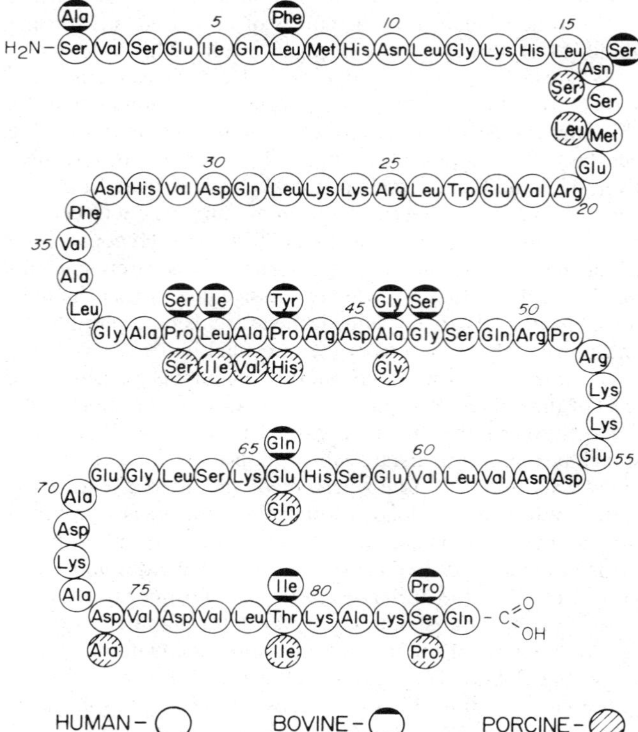

It has also been shown that parathyroid hormone in human plasma is immunologically different from the hormone extracted from human adenomas.

The hormone secreted in vivo from normal bovine and human parathyroid glands and from parathyroid adenomas is indistinguishable by immunologic criteria and by molecular size from the 84-amino acid peptide (molecular weight 9500) extracted from glands. However, much of the immunoreactive material found in the peripheral circulation of humans and animals (cow, dog) is smaller than the extracted or secreted hormone. The principal circulating fragment(s) of immunoreactive hormone (approximate molecular weight 7000) lacks a portion of the critical amino-terminal sequence required for biologic activity and, hence, must constitute a biologically inactive hormonal fragment(s).

Cleavage of the native peptide by an endopeptidase would be expected to result in formation of a second fragment, molecular weight 2000 to 3000, representing the amino-terminal, biologically active, portion of the hormone. There is disagreement in published reports concerning the presence or absence of such a circulating amino-terminal fragment. It is unclear (1) whether peripheral metabolism accounts for most of the circulating fragment(s) of hormone or whether fragments as well as intact hormone are also secreted by the gland and (2) whether peripheral metabolism is a purely catabolic process concerned only with hormone destruction or whether the peripheral cleavage results in formation of a metabolically active amino-terminal fragment of parathyroid hormone with physiologically significant action. Much more work on this issue of hormonal metabolism is required. Present evidence suggests that the liver and kidney are the principal sites at which peripheral metabolism of hormone occurs. Specific cleavages in these organs may serve as points of metabolic control to regulate the concentration of hormonally active polypeptides in the circulation (Fig. 338-5). Peripheral metabolism, in turn, may also be affected by pathological processes, such as renal failure or severe hepatic dysfunction.

The rate of uptake and cleavage of the secreted 84-amino acid peptide is more rapid than the rate of clearance from blood of the smaller, biologically inactive fragment(s) that result from peripheral metabolism and release into the circulation from cleavage sites. Hence, at present it must be concluded that measurements of parathyroid hormone in blood by immunoassay provide only an overall index of parathyroid glandular activity rather than a direct measure of biologically active hormone, since biologically inert fragments rather than intact hormone are the principal circulating form of immunoreactive hormone (Chap. 339). Changes in rate of production or clearance of fragments could change the concentration of immunoreactive hormone without involving corresponding changes in rate of hormone secretion. Such discordance between concentrations of immunoreactive hormone and biologically active peptide seem likely, for example, in renal failure, since the kidney seems to be the principal route of excretion of hormone fragments.

The biosynthesis of parathyroid hormone has been extensively investigated. Several larger molecular forms have been identified in the biosynthetic sequence leading from gene transcription and translation to final packaging of the 84-amino acid peptide in secretory granules prior to secretion. The earliest detected precursor form, termed *preproparathyroid hormone,* consists of 115 amino acids; this molecular form is converted to an intermediate form of 90 amino acids termed *proparathyroid hormone.* The details of intracellular regulation of biosynthesis are still unknown. Parathyroid hormone shares, with other polypeptides and proteins destined for secretion from cells, this complex pattern of initial synthesis as a larger molecule which is then reduced in size by several, apparently highly specific, intracellular cleavages prior to secretion. The hydrophobic regions of the preproparathyroid hormone are similar to, but distinct from, preprotein-specific regions of other cell-secreted proteins and may serve an important role in guiding transport of the polypeptide from sites of synthesis on polyribosomes through the cytoskeleton to secretory granules. Hence, it is possible that hereditary or acquired defects in the cellular control of biosynthesis may lead to deficient secretion of active hormone or to release of incompletely processed precursor forms into the circulation. No direct evidence of such defects has been obtained yet, however. Recently, the coding

FIGURE 338-5
Schematic model of the biosynthesis, secretion, and peripheral metabolism of parathyroid hormone, as well as contributions of these processes to the heterogeneity of circulating, immunoreactive parathyroid hormone (see text for details). Biosynthesis involves initial translation of parathyroid hormone–specific messenger RNA (mRNA) into a polypeptide of 115 amino acids, preproparathyroid hormone (preproPTH) followed by several specific posttranslational cleavages. The first cleavage (1) occurs on or near the endoplasmic reticulum within seconds of synthesis; this cleavage removes the 25-amino acid preproPTH-specific peptide, or leader sequence (represented by a straight line). The product, proPTH, a peptide of 90 amino acids, is converted by a second specific peptidase(s) with removal of the proPTH-specific peptide (represented by a jagged line), forming PTH. (An alternate possibility, not illustrated, is that proPTH is converted to PTH after packing into secretory granules.) PTH, consisting of 84 amino acids (illustrated as a heavy bar with N indicating amino terminus, C, the carboxy terminus), is the principal secretory product of the cell, resulting from exocytosis of secretory granules containing the hormone (indicated by heavy arrow). Some have reported that there is an alternate secretory pathway in which amino-terminal fragments (N) and carboxy-terminal fragments (C) of the molecule are formed by further proteolytic processing within the cell followed by release into the circulation (dotted arrows). Speculations concerning release of precursor forms, or fragments (not yet proved), from the cell into the circulation are indicated by dotted arrows and question marks. Peripheral metabolism involves uptake of the intact hormone by certain organs (liver and kidney being most likely) followed by a third cleavage (3). This last cleavage is presumed to result in formation of an amino-terminal fragment (N) and a carboxy-terminal fragment (C). The carboxy-terminal fragment reenters the circulation, from which it disappears more slowly than the intact hormone, and is taken up and cleaved; hence the concentration of carboxy-terminal fragment is higher than that of intact PTH. The fate of the amino-terminal fragment, presumably derived by peripheral metabolism, is unsettled. The relative contribution of peripheral metabolism and the release of fragments directly from the gland to the heterogeneity of circulating parathyroid hormone is presently disputed and awaits clarification.

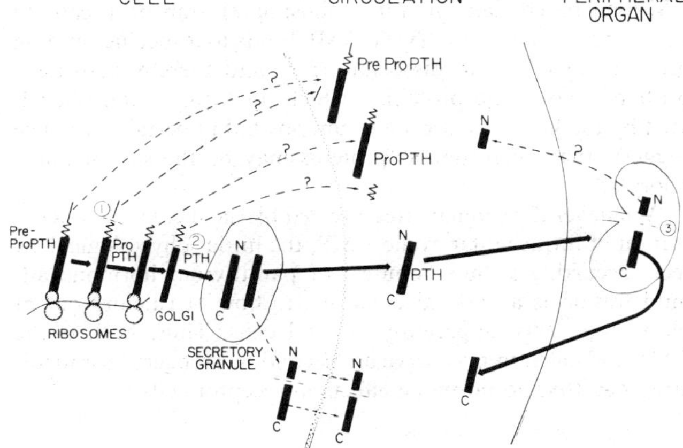

portion of the gene for bovine and human parathyroid hormone has been deduced by structural analysis of DNA prepared biosynthetically from the messenger RNA for parathyroid hormone. There are considerable homologies in the gene structures as well as in the proteins from these two species.

Numerous in vivo and in vitro experiments have shown that blood calcium concentration controls the secretion of parathyroid hormone and that the ionized fraction of blood calcium is the important determinant of hormone secretion. Hormone secretion increases steeply to a maximum value of fivefold above basal rates of secretion whenever calcium concentration falls from normal to the range of 7.5 to 8.0 mg/dl (measured as total calcium). Beta-adrenergic agonists such as epinephrine and histamine II agonists may also increase hormone secretion, but the physiological significance of these secretagogues is not yet established. Furthermore, drugs such as propranolol or cimetidine do not reproducibly decrease circulating parathyroid hormone levels.

Magnesium may influence hormone secretion in the same direction as calcium. It is unlikely that physiological variations in magnesium concentration affect parathyroid secretion, but severe intracellular magnesium deficiency is associated with defective hormone secretion.

The mode of action of parathyroid hormone at the biochemical level involves effects of parathyroid hormone on adenylate cyclase in the cells of the target tissue. Stimulation of enzyme activity during specific hormone–target cell membrane interaction leads to an increase in intracellular cyclic adenosine monophosphate (cyclic AMP). It seems likely that this rapid rise in intracellular cyclic AMP is the initial biochemical step in all the physiological effects of parathyroid hormone. Following the administration of parathyroid hormone there is, within minutes, a rise in urinary cyclic AMP that precedes any observable increase in phosphate excretion. Likewise, the effects on bone adenylate cyclase activity can be detected within 1 min of the addition of parathyroid hormone to a suspension of bone cells. In addition, administration of dibutyryl cyclic AMP, which, as a more soluble analogue of cyclic AMP, penetrates cells more effectively, simulates the actions of parathyroid hormone in parathyroidectomized animals. Dibutyryl cyclic AMP leads to a rise in serum calcium, a lowering of serum phosphate, and an increased excretion of calcium, phosphate, and hydroxyproline in urine.

There are as yet no data concerning the cellular mechanism whereby an increased intracellular concentration of cyclic AMP leads to changes in calcium and phosphate ion translocation. In a number of tissues responsive to hormones through a cyclic AMP mechanism there is evidence for stimulation of protein kinases causing, in turn, phosphorylation of critical proteins that initiate the hormonal effect. The postulated sequence of events in parathyroid hormone–driven, cyclic AMP–mediated calcium (and phosphate) transport can be summarized as follows. Cyclic AMP binds to a specific binding protein, causing it to dissociate from and thereby activate a protein kinase. The protein(s) which, in turn, is phosphorylated by the kinase is at present unknown, but certain evidence suggests that microtubular proteins may be the site of phosphorylation.

Whatever the cellular sites affected by the increased concentration of intracellular cyclic AMP, the initial physiological effect (occurring within minutes) of parathyroid hormone administration is a hypocalcemia due to flow of calcium out of blood into cells, apparently skeletal cells. Thus, both cyclic AMP and calcium may serve as "second messengers" for mediating parathyroid hormone effects in receptor cells.

CALCITONIN (See also Chap. 123) Calcitonin is the potent hypocalcemic, hypophosphatemic peptide hormone which, in many ways, acts as the physiological antagonist to parathyroid hormone. Calcitonin reduces bone resorption and has opposing effects to parathyroid hormone on the kidney in that it increases renal calcium clearance. This hormone has been the subject of intensive physiological studies and has been extensively evaluated as a therapeutic agent of potential value in skeletal disease characterized by excessive resorption. Although calcitonin exerts its hypocalcemic, hypophosphatemic action principally by an inhibition of bone resorption, the initial step in hormone action and the exact sequence of effects on target cells influenced by the hormone are not known.

Present gaps in understanding the physiological role of calcitonin and the effects of the peptide at physiological concentrations on organs other than the bone in turn complicate efforts to understand the biochemical mode of action of the hormone. However, calcitonin may also exert its effects through stimulation of membrane-bound adenylate cyclase in receptor cells in kidney and bone. Calcitonin has been shown to bind to renal cells and to stimulate membrane-bound adenylate cyclase. There is a variable hormonal responsiveness of renal tubular cells to calcitonin, parathyroid hormone, and vasopressin. In some portions of the nephron, cells respond to all three hormones, whereas in others the response is restricted to one or two. In bone, osteoclasts possess calcitonin receptors. Although it is not clear which ion translocation is primary in the overall action of calcitonin, data have pointed to mediation of calcitonin effects on calcium transport and bone metabolism through initial effects on phosphate transport. In this view, calcitonin acts by causing an initial influx of phosphate into cells; this in turn results in effects on calcium transport.

The thyroid gland is the major source of the hormone in mammalian species. Extensive embryologic and histological studies have established that the cells involved in calcitonin synthesis arise originally from neural crest tissue. During embryogenesis these cells migrate into the ultimobranchial body. The latter body or gland arises from the last branchial pouch, hence the name *ultimobranchial body*. In submammalian vertebrates the ultimobranchial body remains as a discrete organ, anatomically separate from the thyroid gland. In mammals the ultimobranchial gland fuses with the thyroid gland, and the calcitonin-secreting cells become part of the thyroid in adult life. Calcitonin is found in all vertebrate classes.

The amino acid sequences of eight calcitonins from six species, including humans, have been determined. The naturally occurring calcitonins consist of a peptide chain of 32 amino acids. There is a considerable amount of variability in sequence. The entire chain of 32 amino acids appears to be required for biologic activity in the whole animal, although fragments function in in vitro systems. The factors that regulate the synthesis of calcitonin in the parafollicular or C cells are not known. Calcitonin from salmon, when tested in various animal species, is 25 to 100 times more potent by weight in lowering serum calcium than are other forms of calcitonin. In fact, the salmon hormone is at least 10 times more potent in humans than human calcitonin. Greater resistance to metabolic destruction may explain in part the greater biologic potency of salmon calcitonin, but the salmon hormone appears to bind more strongly to receptor sites as well. Calcitonin is synthesized as a precursor molecule, the parent molecule being four times larger than calcitonin itself. Analysis of the sequence of the coding portions of the gene for rat calcitonin indicates that at least two peptides flank calcitonin from which they are separated by basic residues. It is likely (in analogy with the common precursor for ACTH and endorphin) that these peptides are released with calcitonin and may have biological actions that, for example, might explain certain pathophysiological features in syndromes associated with excess calcitonin production.

In animals, the concentration of the hormone rises within minutes of induced hypercalcemia. The secretion of the hormone is under the direct control of blood calcium: an increase in calcium causes an increase in calcitonin, and a decrease in calcium causes a decrease in calcitonin. Once secreted, calcitonin disappears rapidly from the circulation with a half-life of 2 to 15 min.

The concentration of calcitonin in the peripheral blood of normal humans is lower than in many other species such as cows, rats, pigs, and sheep. Basal and stimulated immunoreactive calcitonin levels are lower in women than in men and tend to decrease with increasing age to a greater extent in women.

The physiological role of calcitonin is, in many ways, unclear. In many mammals calcitonin acts to lower both blood calcium and blood phosphate; the principal action of calcitonin is inhibition of bone resorption. The importance of calcitonin in increasing urinary calcium and phosphate clearance is synergistic with its effects on bone resorption. The actions of calcitonin on kidney and bone are in turn modulated by the regulation of calcitonin production by serum calcium; hypercalcemia stimulates and hypocalcemia suppresses calcitonin release. The view that calcitonin serves physiologically to protect against hypercalcemia is thus explained by the hypocalcemic effects of calcitonin triggered in response to hypercalcemia.

The role of calcitonin, however, if any, in normal adult humans is unknown. Changes in calcium and phosphate metabolism are not seen in humans despite extremes of variation in hormone production; there are no definite effects attributable to calcitonin deficiency (totally thyroidectomized patients replaced only with thyroxine) or excess (patients with the calcitonin-secreting tumor, medullary carcinoma of the thyroid). Patients with the latter disorder suffer multiple deleterious consequences of their malignancy (see Chap. 123), but no abnormalities in calcium or bone metabolism are detected, perhaps because they become refractory to the skeletal effects of calcitonin.

Medical interest in calcitonin, therefore, at present is centered principally upon its promise as a therapeutic agent and its usefulness, when deployed in radioimmunoassays, for detection of medullary carcinoma (Chap. 123). The effectiveness of calcitonin in the treatment of some patients with Paget's disease of bone is established (Chap. 342).

REFERENCES

Avioli LV, Krane SM (eds): *Metabolic Bone Disease,* New York, Academic, 1977, vol I; ibid, 1978, vol II

Bringhurst FR, Potts JT Jr: Calcium and phosphate distribution, turnover, and metabolic actions, in *Endocrinology,* vol 2, LJ DeGroot (ed). New York, Grune & Stratton, 1979, p 551

Glimcher MJ: Composition, structure, and organization of bone and other mineralized tissues and the mechanism of calcification, in *Handbook of Physiology,* sec 7: *Endocrinology,* vol VII, GD Aurbach (ed). Washington, DC, American Physiological Society, 1976, p 25

Habener JF, Potts JT Jr: Biosynthesis of parathyroid hormone. N Engl J Med 299:580, 635, 1978

———, ———: Chemistry, biosynthesis, secretion, and metabolism of PTH, in *Handbook of Physiology,* sec 7: *Endocrinology,* vol VII, GD Aurbach (ed). Washington, DC, American Physiological Society, 1976, p 313

Hendy GN et al: Nucleotide sequence of cloned cDNAs encoding human preproparathyroid hormone. Proc Natl Acad Sci USA 78:7365, 1981

Jacobs JW et al: Calcitonin messenger RNA encodes multiple polypeptides in a single precursor. Science 213:457, 1981

Jowsey J: *Metabolic Diseases of Bone.* Philadelphia, Saunders, 1977

Krane SM, Schiller AL: Metabolic bone disease: Introduction and classification, in *Endocrinology,* vol 2, LJ DeGroot (ed). New York, Grune & Stratton, 1979, p 839

Munson PL: Physiology and pharmacology of thyrocalcitonin, in *Handbook of Physiology,* sec 7: *Endocrinology,* vol VII, GD Aurbach (ed). Washington, DC, American Physiological Society, 1976, p 443

Potts JT Jr, Aurbach GD: Chemistry of the calcitonins, in *Handbook of Physiology,* sec 7: *Endocrinology,* vol VII, GD Aurbach (ed). Washington, DC, American Physiological Society, 1976, p 423

Sledge CB: Formation and resorption of bone, in *Textbook of Rheumatology,* WN Kelley et al (eds). Philadelphia, Saunders, 1981, p 277

339 DISORDERS OF PARATHYROID GLANDS

JOHN T. POTTS, JR.

PRIMARY HYPERPARATHYROIDISM

NATURAL HISTORY AND INCIDENCE Primary hyperparathyroidism is a generalized disorder of calcium, phosphate, and bone metabolism that results from an increased secretion of parathyroid hormone. The excessive concentration of circulating hormone usually leads to hypercalcemia and hypophosphatemia. There may be multiple associated problems such as recurrent nephrolithiasis, peptic ulcers, mental changes, and bone destruction; however, it has become evident that clinical manifestations may be absent, the disease being detected because an elevated blood calcium level is found during routine blood screening tests.

Prior to the last decade the disease was thought to have a *prevalence* of less than 1 per 10,000 of the population. Recent studies have indicated that the disease is more common than previously suspected. In women over the age of 60, 2 new cases per 1000 of the population per year were found in population screening studies, with half that rate found in men. The *incidence* of the disease in older people is thus at least 10 times greater than believed previously. Lower rates of the disease were found in younger age groups but with an incidence still greater than 1 per 1000 in women over the age of 40.

ETIOLOGY AND PATHOLOGY The pathology in hyperparathyroidism is either disease in a single gland [approximately 85 percent (81 percent adenoma, 4 percent histologically carcinoma)] or hyperplasia of all glands (approximately 15 percent of cases, usually chief-cell hyperplasia). Adenoma of more than one gland with the other glands normal is rare. This view, that either one gland only is abnormal or all glands are abnormal, now accepted by most groups, is helpful to the surgeon in planning exploration of the neck.

An adenoma is most often in the inferior parathyroid glands. However, the tumor is found in an unusual location in 6 to 10 percent of patients; such ectopic parathyroid adenomas may be located in the thymus, the thyroid, the pericardium, or behind the esophagus. Adenomas vary in size from 0.5 to 5 g; in some instances, however, tumors as large as 10 to 20 g are found. The adenoma is usually composed of chief cells; a rim of normal tissue can sometimes be detected encapsulating the adenomatous nodule.

Chief-cell hyperplasia is especially common in those instances of hyperparathyroidism which are familial or which are part of the syndrome of multiple endocrine neoplasia (see Chap. 123). Chief cells are predominant in both hyperplasia and adenoma; cells of a different histological appearance such as oxyphil cells are reported occasionally.

It can be difficult sometimes to distinguish adenoma from hyperplasia. With hyperplasia the enlargement may be so asymmetric that some involved glands appear normal grossly. Even if certain glands are not clearly increased in size, histological examination reveals a uniform pattern of chief cells and *disappearance of fat.* Thus, findings at surgery must be combined with microscopic examination of biopsy specimens of several glands. When an adenoma is present, examination of other glands indicates that they are of normal size, approximately 25 mg average weight, and histologically there is a normal distribution of all cell types (rather than only chief cells) and normal areas of fat.

Parathyroid carcinoma is usually not very malignant in character. Long-term survival without recurrence is common if the entire gland is removed at initial operation without rupture of the capsule. When recurrent, parathyroid carcinoma is usually slow-growing with local spread in the neck; surgical correction of recurrent disease is therefore feasible. Occasionally, parathyroid carcinoma is more aggressive in character with distant metastases (lung, liver, and bone) found at the time of initial operation. It may be difficult initially to decide if the primary tumor is carcinoma; increased numbers of mitotic figures and increased fibrosis of the gland stroma may precede more clear-cut invasive features. Hyperparathyroidism resulting from a parathyroid carcinoma may be clinically indistinguishable from other forms of primary hyperparathyroidism.

The occurrence of hyperparathyroidism in a familial pattern is well documented and may occur without other endocrinologic abnormality. More often, however, hereditary hyperparathyroidism is found as part of a multiglandular endocrinopathy (see Chap. 123). It is now appreciated that there are two or more genetically distinct syndromes with multiple endocrine disorders. The syndrome originally described (Wermer's syndrome) consisted of hyperparathyroidism and tumors of the pituitary and pancreatic islet cells. This multiglandular disorder is often associated with peptic ulcer and gastric hypersecretion (the Zollinger-Ellison syndrome). Another distinct constellation of endocrinologic abnormalities consists of hyperparathyroidism associated with pheochromocytoma and medullary carcinoma of the thyroid. The etiology of these syndromes is not known. The pattern of inheritance is autosomal dominant. Tumors of the thyroid and adrenal medulla are not found in members of kindreds with Wermer's syndrome, and pancreatic and pituitary tumors are not found in the kindreds with medullary carcinoma of the thyroid and pheochromocytoma. Wermer's syndrome is now termed *multiple endocrine neoplasia* (adenomatosis) type I (usually abbreviated MEN I or MEA I), and the syndrome involving thyroid tumors is referred to as MEN II or MEA II. Since the different endocrine tumors can occur at widely separated intervals, hyperparathyroidism and the related endocrine disorders should be carefully and repeatedly searched for in all members of kindreds afflicted with the multiple endocrine neoplasia syndromes (Chap. 123).

Another familial disorder resembles but may be distinct from primary hyperparathyroidism. This entity, termed *familial hypocalciuric hypercalcemia* (FHH) or *familial benign hypercalcemia,* occurs in a pattern compatible with autosomal dominant inheritance. Few, if any, clinical signs or symptoms are found in patients with FHH syndrome; only 3 of 25 patients in one series had kidney stones or any abnormality in renal function. No evidence of any other endocrine abnormalities is seen. Most patients are detected as a result of family screening for hypercalcemia once one member of the kindred is detected; such studies have suggested a higher incidence in FHH of hypercalcemia in the first decade of life in affected family members than in the MEN I families screened as controls. Average values for renal clearance of calcium and magnesium are lower in FHH than in primary hyperparathyroidism (calcium/creatinine clearance ratio of 0.006 ± 0.004 versus 0.024 ± 0.01). Serum magnesium levels are higher in FHH than in primary hyperparathyroidism; PTH levels tend to be lower. Despite these differences in mean values for certain laboratory measurements, no absolute biochemical discriminant segregates FHH from other forms of familial hyperparathyroidism. Clinical distinction seems the most compelling argument that FHH is a distinct entity, especially reports that surgery has not led to a cure of the hypercalcemia unless hypoparathyroidism was induced by total parathyroidectomy. The true nature of this disorder and its proper management remain unclear; surgery should be delayed indefinitely in hypercalcemic patients suspected to be members of an FHH kindred.

SIGNS AND SYMPTOMS Most of the signs and symptoms of hyperparathyroidism reflect known pathophysiological consequences of hypercalcemia. Many organ systems can be affected by hyperparathyroidism. However, characteristically, involvement of the kidneys and skeletal system is most prominent. *Kidney involvement,* due either to deposition of calcium in the renal parenchyma or to recurrent nephrolithiasis, is found in 60 to 70 percent of patients reported in large series prior to 1970. With the increased frequency of detection of asymptomatic individuals in the last decade, the incidence of renal complications appears lower but is still the most common complication of hyperparathyroidism.

Renal stones are usually composed of either calcium oxalate or calcium phosphate. Repeated episodes of nephrolithiasis or the formation of large calculi may lead to urinary tract obstruction and repeated episodes of infection. These complications may also contribute to progressive loss of renal function. Nephrolithiasis and nephrocalcinosis rarely occur in the same patient. Nephrocalcinosis may be accompanied by decreased renal function and phosphate retention.

The classic pattern of bone involvement in hyperparathyroidism is *osteitis fibrosa cystica.* Several decades ago an incidence of osteitis fibrosa cystica of 10 to 25 percent or even higher was reported in patients with hyperparathyroidism. In the United States, at the present time, x-ray evidence of osteitis fibrosa cystica is not commonly found in patients when the diagnosis of hyperparathyroidism is made, even though there may be a long history of renal or other complications of the disease. This reduced frequency of this type of skeletal involvement has not been adequately explained. Bone disease, however, is still a serious issue in hyperparathyroidism. Quantitative bone biopsy studies with histomorphometric analyses reveal microscopic evidence of abnormality in bone turnover in as many as 50 percent of patients, even in the absence of osteitis fibrosa. Thus, although many patients give evidence of excessive effects of parathyroid hormone on bone, only a few develop clinically evident osteitis fibrosa cystica. Present emphasis is focused on a different issue, the frequency of development of osteopenia which is parathyroid hormone–dependent and progressive, indicating the need for surgery, and the diagnostic methods most useful for determining its presence.

Histological examination of bone specimens from patients who do have osteitis fibrosa reveals a number of changes that, when present, define unambiguously the presence of parathyroid overactivity. There is a reduction in the number of trabeculae, an increase in giant multinucleated osteoclasts seen in scalloped areas on the surface of the bone (Howship's lacunae), and a replacement of normal cellular and marrow elements by fibrous tissue. In milder forms of osteitis early changes can sometimes be detected by high-resolution x-rays of the hands. The *phalangeal tufts* may be resorbed, and an irregular outline replaces the normally sharp cortical outline of the bone in the digits. This change is termed *subperiosteal resorption.* Detection of loss of the *lamina dura* of the teeth is less specific but may be helpful diagnostically. Tiny, "punched-out" lesions in the skull, producing the so-called salt-and-pepper appearance, are characteristic.

Severe *osteopenia* without radiological criteria of osteitis fibrosa cystica is associated with long-standing, excessive parathyroid action; there are, however, as yet no criteria to distinguish such a generalized osteopenia from "high-turnover" osteoporosis not related to excess parathyroid hormone action. Bone biopsy followed by quantitative histomorphometry does establish a highly cellular bone with increased numbers of osteoclasts and osteoblasts and increase in the number of active bone-resorbing and forming areas. Criteria useful in establishing that there is progressive bone destruction include (1) serial measurements of bone mass by photon beam densitometry or metacarpal cortical thickness and (2) metabolic studies such as urine calcium excretion on a low calcium intake (less complex than formal balance studies). Patients who exhibit evidence of progressive osteopenia are usually recommended to have surgery on the parathyroids with the rationale that parathyroid hormone–dependent osteopenia may not be reversible and hence must be arrested as early as possible.

In addition, hyperparathyroidism may be associated with symptoms or signs referable to *the central nervous system, neuromuscular function, the gastrointestinal tract, the skin, and the joints.* Sometimes, vague or minor complaints from a patient, particularly neuromuscular or gastrointestinal symptoms, are the only clue to the diagnosis; awareness of the subtle manifestations of the disease may prompt a request for blood calcium determination as part of a diagnostic evaluation.

Central nervous system manifestations of hyperparathyroidism range from mild personality disturbances to severe psychiatric disorders; mental obtundation or coma is seen with severe hypercalcemia. In some instances, the patient experiences multiple vague complaints which can often be mistaken for psychoneurosis. It must be emphasized, however, that mild depression, found frequently in the population without the presence of hyperparathyroidism, cannot be used as the sole clinical criterion for parathyroid surgery.

A distinctive syndrome of *neuromuscular involvement* in hyperparathyroidism has been described by several groups. Proximal muscle weakness, easy fatigability, and atrophy of muscles are clinical features. Abnormal electromyograms and atrophy of muscle fibers without myopathic changes are detected. In some cases, the clinical signs are so striking as to suggest amyotrophic lateral sclerosis or some other incurable primary neuromuscular disorder; in other patients the signs may be minimal. Clinically, the important feature is the complete regression of neuromuscular disease after surgical correction of the hyperparathyroidism.

There may be varied and sometimes subtle manifestations of hyperparathyroidism in the *gastrointestinal tract.* In addition to a variety of vague abdominal complaints, diseases of the stomach and pancreas are frequent. *Duodenal ulcers* have been reported in as many as 25 percent of patients with proven hyperparathyroidism. In patients with hyperparathyroidism resulting from multiple endocrine neoplasia syndrome (MEN I), there is a high incidence of ulcer as a result of the associated pancreatic tumors that secrete excessive quantities of gastrin (the Zollinger-Ellison syndrome). Cases of pancreatitis have been reported in association with hyperparathyroidism, but the absolute incidence is not established. Various mechanisms have been proposed to explain the apparent increased incidence of pancreatitis, but there is no convincing explanation.

It has also been noted that *chondrocalcinosis* and *pseudogout* are seen in sufficiently frequent association with hyperparathyroidism that screening of such patients for hyperparathyroidism is warranted. Occasionally pseudogout is the initial clinical manifestation of the hyperparathyroidism.

DIAGNOSIS The diagnosis of hyperparathyroidism is made primarily on clinical grounds. The immunoassay for parathyroid hormone is of increasing value as a specific diagnostic test for hyperparathyroidism, but there are still numerous problems in interpretation of assay results. The efforts to establish the diagnosis are most exhaustive in patients with clear-cut symptoms, particularly with recurrent kidney stones or symptomatic bone disease. The philosophy of approach is different at the other extreme, a totally asymptomatic patient in whom hypercalcemia is detected coincidentally. However, since hypercalcemia can be the presenting evidence for malignancy or other serious disease, a thorough evaluation of possible etiologies, including hyperparathyroidism, by application of at least standard screening procedures is indicated even in asymptomatic subjects. If the diagnosis of hyperparathyroidism is suspected after such an evaluation, a decision can still be made to follow the patient for a time rather than recommend surgery.

Hypercalcemia is the most common manifestation of hyperparathyroidism. Repeated measurements of plasma calcium should be made in patients with suspected hypercalcemia. One may detect either a sustained hypercalcemia or a pattern of high normal blood calciums alternating with occasional definitely elevated values, an intermittent hypercalcemia. If errors due to altered concentration of blood protein or variation in laboratory range of normal can be eliminated, such findings establish the presence of hypercalcemia. Careful consideration must be given to the justification for surgical exploration in the absence of definite hypercalcemia. There are now numerous reports of so-called normocalcemic hyperparathyroidism, that is, patients with surgically proven hyperparathyroidism with normal calcium but elevated values of immunoreactive PTH (iPTH). Careful scrutiny of the reports reveals that in those with adenomas, the patients were, in fact, hypercalcemic at some time in their course; they could more correctly be described, therefore, as having intermittent hypercalcemia. If there is not even intermittent hypercalcemia but the patients have coexisting conditions that interfere with the calcium-elevating actions of PTH, such as chronic renal failure, severe malabsorption, or vitamin D deficiency, then the lack of calcium elevation need not argue against the presence of true hyperparathyroidism. In confusing, borderline situations where symptoms call for definitive diagnosis, it may be useful to search for postabsorptive hypercalcemia (detectable in certain patients when fasting hypercalcemia is absent) or to use a provocative test with benzothiadiazides (see discussion of thiazide-induced hypercalcemia below).

Hypercalciuria is also commonly seen in hyperparathyroidism. However, it should be kept in mind that parathyroid hormone actually reduces calcium clearance. In fact, the 24-h urine excretion of calcium is lower in patients with hyperparathyroidism than in patients with equivalent degrees of hypercalcemia from nonparathyroid causes.

Serum phosphate is usually low but may be normal, especially if renal failure has developed. Detection of hypophosphatemia is supportive of the diagnosis but is a less stringent criterion than hypercalcemia; phosphate levels are influenced by multiple factors which need to be considered. Samples must be obtained in the morning, under fasting conditions, to be useful; a serum phosphate below normal is not an abnormal finding in the postabsorptive state. Patients with severe hypercalcemia of any cause have been reported to have a low phosphate.

Other electrolyte abnormalities have also been described; however, these abnormalities may not be sufficiently specific to be of diagnostic value. Serum magnesium levels have been reported to be low. Serum chloride and citrate are often elevated, and serum bicarbonate is reduced. The combination of elevated chloride and low phosphate (reflecting the acidosis and renal phosphate wasting, respectively, of hyperparathyroidism) can be used as a diagnostic clue; the chloride/phosphorus ratio in patients with hyperparathyroidism is usually greater than 30, while in those with hypercalcemia of other causes it is less than 30.

Blood alkaline phosphatase (of bone origin) and urinary hydroxyproline concentrations are elevated only when there is significant bone involvement. Renal involvement can be reflected by a decreased concentrating ability, by specific tubular defects such as tubular acidosis, and finally by frank renal failure with the chemical findings of azotemia.

Special tests *Glucocorticoid administration* has been useful in differentiating the hypercalcemia of hyperparathyroidism from that associated with sarcoidosis, multiple myeloma, vitamin D intoxication, and some malignant diseases with osseous metastases. In these diseases doses of hydrocortisone of 100 mg per day (or an equivalent dose of another steroid such as prednisone) given for 10 days often result in a lowering of the serum calcium, whereas ordinarily calcium does not fall in hyperparathyroidism. Occasional false-positive and false-negative results have been reported. The mechanism of the effect is not explained but may reflect the physiological antagonism between glucocorticoids and vitamin D action in vitamin D intoxication and sarcoidosis and the tumor-suppressive action of glucocorticoids in some forms of malignancy.

A variety of tests of parathyroid function are based on the known effects of the hormone on the *renal handling of phosphate.* These tests are designed to take advantage of the decrease in tubular resorption of phosphate caused by parathyroid hormone. The tests are now used less frequently as an aid in the diagnosis of patients with equivocal evidence for hyperparathyroidism due to the difficulty in controlling conditions and to an increased use of cyclic AMP and parathyroid hormone measurements. To perform the test, any of several convenient indices of phosphate handling by the kidneys is determined. Because of the diurnal variation in plasma phosphate concentration and the marked fluctuations in phosphate that occur with eating, long periods of urine collection are not useful in determinations of phosphate clearance.

Phosphate clearance is determined by standard techniques over 1- to 2-h periods. Normal phosphate clearance is 10.8 ± 2.7 ml/min; values 50 percent or more above this figure have been detected in hyperparathyroidism. The ratio of phosphate clearance to creatinine clearance indicates the percentage of filtered phosphate that was reabsorbed. In normal subjects the tubular resorption of phosphate exceeds 85 percent; in hyperparathyroidism tubular resorption of phosphate may be as low as 50 to 60 percent.

Diuretics of the benzothiazide class in the usual doses (chlorothiazide 0.5 g bid) can produce sustained, frank hypercalcemia in patients with hyperparathyroidism and borderline calcium values, the *thiazide provocation* test. Since such a response is not seen in normal subjects (there may be some elevation in blood calcium in normal subjects, but any effect seen is lost in a few days despite continued administration of thiazides), thiazide administration has been suggested as a provocative test for the presence of hyperparathyroidism. In interpreting the results, it should be appreciated that patients with high rates of vitamin D intake and/or underlying bone disease may also develop hypercalcemia with thiazides.

Radioimmunoassay for parathyroid hormone A *radioimmunoassay* for circulating human parathyroid hormone provides a specific test for parathyroid function. Independent assay procedures have been developed in many centers and commercial laboratories. There have been and continue to be, however, numerous problems with the application and interpretation of the assay. Most laboratories still find it necessary to use a nonhomologous assay system (labeled bovine parathyroid hormone and antiserum to bovine parathyroid hormone) to measure human parathyroid hormone; there is variation introduced thereby. There are in plasma several immunologically (and biologically) distinct species of parathyroid hormone. The heterogeneity of plasma immunoreactive parathyroid hormone (iPTH) presents interpretive problems, especially with assays that measure principally the middle and carboxyl regions of the hormone (*C* assays). Assays of sufficient sensitivity to measure the biologically active amino-terminal portion of the hormone (*N* assays) have not been fully evaluated for clinically discriminating value. Despite these problems, when appropriate precautions are observed, presently available immunoassays for parathyroid hormone based on detection of carboxyl fragments can be uniquely useful in the diagnostic evaluation of patients with primary hyperparathyroidism and/or with hypercalcemia.

Many patients with hyperparathyroidism have concentrations of hormone clearly elevated above the normal range. Most workers, however, find that the concentration of hormone in many subjects with proven hyperparathyroidism is no higher than that found in some normal subjects. Patients with hypercalcemia not due to parathyroid disease, however, have undetectable concentrations of parathyroid hormone; in these patients, since parathyroid gland function is normal, secretion is suppressed because of the hypercalcemia. Patients with hypercalcemia due to hyperparathyroidism have detectable, if not elevated, concentrations of hormone despite hypercalcemia. Thus the assay is helpful in the differential diagnosis of hypercalcemia; a clear distinction exists between values found in hypercalcemia of parathyroid and nonparathyroid origin. It has been recently appreciated that in patients with hyperparathyroidism, hormone concentration in blood changes in response to induced changes in blood calcium. This, in part, explains the overlap found between hormone concentrations in patients with hyperparathyroidism and increased blood calcium level when compared with normal subjects with normal calcium concentrations.

These findings emphasize that the disorder of parathyroid function in primary hyperparathyroidism cannot be explained simply on the basis of a fixed rate of hormone secretion; the defect in control of secretion, responsible for excessive hormone production, must be more subtle than simple autonomy. The nature of the cellular defect has not yet been defined.

As illustrated schematically in Fig. 339-1, most useful clinical interpretation of present immunoassays (*C* assays) is best achieved by (1) plotting results of iPTH concentration in each patient against the simultaneously measured calcium concentration and (2) comparing and contrasting the individual test results with the results of such covariant analysis ([iPTH] $\times$ [Ca^{2+}]) with each type of patient group for whom extensive retrospective clinical correlation results have been made. A rectangular domain includes the values found for several hundred normal controls, a domain bounded laterally by the normal upper and lower limits of serum calcium and vertically by the lower limit of assay detection and the highest range of iPTH concentration found in normal subjects. Those patients with surgically documented hyperparathyroidism whose concentration of iPTH overlaps with the upper limit of normal assay values can usually (especially with several repeated assays) be discerned as abnormal because iPTH levels should be undetectable due to hypercalcemia if their parathyroids were normally responsive (see text below and legend to Fig. 339-1 for details of use of the assay in other states such as malignancy and hypoparathyroidism). One disturbing issue in assay interpretation of hypercalcemia not due to parathyroid disease is the possibility that renal failure may falsely elevate iPTH levels when the latter are based on carboxyl fragment detection. Since the kidney is the principal site of excretion of carboxyl fragments of iPTH (Chap. 338), renal failure may lead to a detectable level of the carboxyl fragment (and hence a false-positive result for hyperparathyroidism), despite the fact that sufficient gland suppression has occurred to render iPTH itself undetectable in plasma.

The technique of *percutaneous venous catheter sampling* of the veins of the neck and thorax, and parathyroid hormone radioimmunoassay of the samples so obtained, has been introduced as a method for preoperative localization of parathyroid tissue. In patients in whom a single adenoma is subsequently found at surgery, a marked unilateral gradient in hormone concentration is seen in the small thyroid veins on the side of the neoplasm. In patients who have abnormal parathyroid tissue on both sides of the neck (hyperplasia), on the other hand, gradients in hormone concentration are found on both sides of the thyroid plexus. Because of variations in drainage patterns, however, results of venous catheterization studies often allow a lateralization but not a localization; intramediastinal tumors

FIGURE 339-1
Schematic illustrating results seen when simultaneous measurements of immunoreactive parathyroid hormone (PTH RIA) and serum calcium are made in normal subjects (N), patients with tumor hypercalcemia (TH), hypoparathyroidism (HP), pseudohypoparathyroidism (PHP), chronic renal failure with secondary hyperparathyroidism [CRF (2° HPTH)], and primary hyperparathyroidism (1° HPTH). Enclosed areas indicate the range of values typical for each class of subject measured; note overlap of regions and interrupted scales (see text for details).

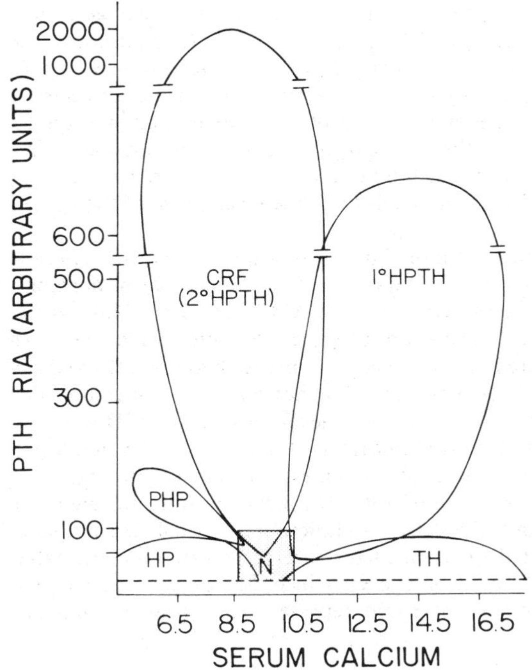

may drain upward into the neck. Hence, it has been found that selective arteriography, guided by the results of venous catheterization, often is helpful in providing a precise anatomic location of the parathyroid tumor. It has been possible to distinguish preoperatively a single adenoma from hyperplasia of all four glands. Since the radiological expertise necessary to perform these angiographic studies is not available in many centers and overall experience is limited, the technique is recommended only for patients who present special diagnostic problems, or in whom previous neck surgery has failed to locate hyperfunctioning parathyroid tissue.

Nephrogenous cyclic AMP Measurements of nephrogenous cyclic AMP may be equivalent in diagnostic value to the parathyroid radioimmunoassay in hyperparathyroidism and other hypercalcemic states. The test requires timed urine collections and measurements of plasma and urinary cyclic AMP. Perhaps because of the requirement for both blood and urine samples, the test has not been extensively applied nor is it available from commercial laboratories, but it is likely to be more widely used in the future because of findings in hypercalcemia associated with tumors not of parathyroid origin (pseudohyperparathyroidism) discussed below.

Total urinary cyclic AMP consists of approximately half derived from plasma (filtered) cyclic AMP and half derived from renal cyclic AMP (the latter synthesized and excreted by renal tubular cells). The test is performed by collecting precisely timed 1- to 3-h morning urine specimens in well-hydrated, resting subjects; midcollection plasma and urine samples are analyzed for creatinine and cyclic AMP (the latter by radioimmunoassay or protein binding assays, prior chromatography being required for plasma cyclic AMP measurements). Nephrogenous cyclic AMP (NcAMP) is given by the formula

$$\text{NcAMP} = \frac{(UcA \cdot V) - (PcA \cdot Ccr)}{Ccr} \times 100$$

and is expressed as nanomoles per minute per deciliter of glomerular filtration rate (GFR) or more correctly as nmol per dl of glomerular filtration (GF) (where $C, P, U,$ and V represent the symbols for clearance, plasma, and urinary concentration and urine flow rate, respectively; cA, cyclic AMP; cr, creatinine). More conveniently, the expression nephrogenous cyclic AMP can be computed by subtracting the plasma cAMP concentration (nanomoles per deciliter, equivalent to nanomoles per deciliter of GFR) from the total urinary cAMP excretion rate, nanomoles per deciliter of GFR. Thus, the expression NcAMP provides a measurement of renal tubular cell synthesis and excretion of cyclic AMP derivable by measuring total urinary cyclic AMP and correcting for the plasma cyclic AMP that is filtered. NcAMP is almost entirely dependent on parathyroid hormone function. Acute challenge or suppression tests of parathyroid function based on oral or intravenous calcium loading lead to prompt falls in NcAMP, attesting to the parathyroid dependence of the parameter. One group has reported mean values of 1.59 ± 0.59 nmol/dl GFR in normal subjects, 4.64 ± 1.95 nmol/dl GFR in more than 100 patients with hyperparathyroidism, and 0.31 ± 0.16 nmol/dl GFR in patients with suppressed parathyroid function (hypoparathyroid). Elevated values found in 90 percent of hyperparathyroid patients compare favorably with results achieved with the most discriminating iPTH measurements. An alternate method that avoids the need to measure plasma cyclic AMP is to measure total urinary cyclic AMP and to relate this to glomerular filtration rate determined by simultaneous estimation of creatinine clearance. This expression, urinary cyclic AMP corrected for GFR (urinary cAMP, nanomoles per deciliter of GFR) was of equivalent value to NcAMP in discriminating normal individuals from patients with primary hyperparathyroidism, but the comparison was not reported in cancer patients (see below) where NcAMP only was evaluated. Total urinary cyclic AMP not corrected for GFR has a much less discriminating value.

DIFFERENTIAL DIAGNOSIS The differential diagnosis of hyperparathyroidism is best considered under three general headings: (1) nephrolithiasis, (2) bone disease, and (3) hypercalcemia. The issues relating to hypercalcemia are medically of greatest concern; recurrent kidney stones or lytic bone disease, however, also lead to differential diagnostic issues.

Nephrolithiasis Nephrolithiasis must be considered in any discussion of the differential diagnosis of hyperparathyroidism. See Chap. 300 for detailed discussion. Recurrent episodes of formation of calcium-containing kidney stones are most often associated with metabolic or renal abnormalities unconnected with hyperparathyroidism. Nonetheless, a detailed search for hyperparathyroidism is indicated in patients who form calcium-containing kidney stones, even if hypercalcemia is not present at the time when nephrolithiasis first occurs.

A difficulty frequently encountered in the differential diagnosis of nephrolithiasis is to distinguish idiopathic hypercalciuria from hyperparathyroidism. In idiopathic hypercalciuria, there is a strong familial incidence, a preponderance in males, an increased urinary excretion of calcium, and a tendency to hypophosphatemia. In most patients the disorder reflects excessive dietary absorption of calcium with high calcium intake leading secondarily to increased urinary calcium (and thereby can be diagnosed). In patients in this category, iPTH should not be elevated; this finding may help in the differential diagnosis.

Hypercalciuria and the formation of calcium-containing stones have been recognized in a number of disorders in addition to hyperparathyroidism and idiopathic hypercalciuria. These include metastatic cancer, multiple myeloma, senile osteoporosis, Cushing's syndrome, phosphate diabetes, milk-alkali syndrome (in the initial phases), vitamin D intoxication, sarcoid, gout, and idiopathic hypercalcemia of infancy. In some instances hypercalcemia is present; in others blood calcium is normal. The differential diagnosis involves a careful examination for the cause of the hypercalcemia when present (as discussed in the preceding section). Hypercalciuria without hypercalcemia is noted with renal tubular disorders such as renal tubular acidosis, in which systemic acidosis may be responsible for increased bone resorption.

Bone disease Discussion of the differential diagnosis of the common types of metabolic bone disease occurs subsequently (see Chap. 341). A few points should be stressed in considering the differentiation of hyperparathyroidism from other skeletal disorders. The only commonly occurring disorder in which hypercalcemia is found together with demineralization and localized areas of bone resorption is malignant disease with osteolytic metastases; patients with severe Paget's disease may develop hypercalcemia during periods of enforced immobilization.

The possibility of underlying hyperparathyroidism should always be considered when solitary bone rarefactions are detected; such a lesion could represent a bone cyst or brown tumor of the bone.

Hypercalcemia: diagnosis and treatment Hyperparathyroidism is a chronic disorder. It is important to obtain historical or clinical evidence of chronicity such as recurrent renal colic, documented hypercalcemia many months earlier, or evidence of occult renal stones. Such evidence of chronicity favors the diagnosis of hyperparathyroidism rather than malignancy. On the other hand, if hypercalcemia has been detected only recently without other historical features of chronicity, the search for other causes of hypercalcemia must be particularly thorough. Moderately elevated calcium with low phosphate suggests hyperparathyroidism in contrast to many other causes of hypercalcemia where phosphate levels are normal or increased. However, severe hypercalcemia per se lowers phosphate. Special assay procedures such as those for iPTH NcAMP and 1,25-dihydroxyvitamin D are proving increasingly helpful, but differential diagnosis is still made largely on clinical grounds.

MALIGNANCY Hypercalcemia due to malignancy is common (as high as 10 to 15 percent in certain types of tumor such as lung carcinoma), often severe and difficult to manage, confusing as to etiology, and sometimes difficult to distinguish from primary hyperparathyroidism. Prior to the recent awareness of the high incidence of hyperparathyroidism, malignancy was listed as the most frequent cause of hypercalcemia (as high as half in series accumulated prior to 1970). Traditionally, hypercalcemia in malignancy was thought to be due either to local invasion and destruction of bone by tumor cells or to the elaboration by the malignancy of systemically active humoral mediators of hypercalcemia. Even when bone metastases are present, locally active mediators that stimulate bone resorptive cells are believed to be responsible for bone destruction and hypercalcemia. One such substance, believed to be a peptide, *osteocyte activation factor (OAF),* has been identified as a product of normal lymphocytes; OAF produced in increased amounts by malignant cells is thought to be the cause of hypercalcemia in hematologic malignancies such as multiple myeloma and lymphoma. The substance has not been purified, and hence no specific assay exists for its detection on blood or tissue fluids; assays have been indirect using malignant cells from bone marrow maintained in tissue culture. *Prostaglandins,* especially of the E series, may be locally active mediators of bone resorption in solid tumors.

Pseudohyperparathyroidism is the term used to define the syndrome of hypercalcemia in patients with malignancies, especially of lung and kidney, in which bone metastases are not detectable, the clinical picture resembles primary hyperparathyroidism (hypophosphatemia accompanies hypercalcemia), and cure or remission of the primary tumor leads to disappearance of the hypercalcemia. Ectopic production by the tumor of parathyroid hormone (PTH) or material closely resembling PTH was long felt to be the mechanism of the hypercalcemia.

Recent investigations using multiple diagnostic studies, tests of serum and urinary mineral ion metabolism, hormone assays, and measurements of NcAMP have led to intriguing, but in several respects confusing, results. Immunoreactive PTH is not elevated in most cases of pseudohyperparathyroidism (Fig. 339-1), although most, but not all, laboratories find detectable rather than suppressed levels of PTH. If PTH were the mediator, produced ectopically by tumor tissue, elevated levels of iPTH would be expected unless chemically and therefore immunologically altered forms of hormone were secreted; on the other hand, if parathyroid function is normal and nonparathyroid-related humoral factors are responsible, undetectable iPTH levels would be expected in hypercalcemic individuals. The low levels of iPTH may represent false-positive signals in the assay or, alternatively, may reflect altered forms of hormone. However, the absence of metabolic acidosis, characteristic of primary hyperparathyroidism, is additional evidence against an exclusive mediation of hypercalcemia by parathyroid hormone in most cases.

Recent evidence has led to further uncertainty. Patients with hypercalcemia and malignancy were found to fall into two groups, independent of the presence of metastases; one group had elevated NcAMP, hypophosphatemia, and increased urinary phosphate clearance—all findings compatible with excessive parathyroid hormone action. On the other hand, these same patients had barely detectable iPTH levels in multiple immunoassays, high rather than low renal calcium clearance, and low-to-normal levels of 1,25-$(OH)_2$-vitamin D, suggesting that the hypercalcemia is mediated by humoral agents distinct from parathyroid hormone, although resembling PTH in certain renal responses. The other group of patients, usually with extensive bone metastases, had low NcAMP, low 1,25-$(OH)_2$-vitamin D, and normal urinary and blood phosphate levels, findings compatible with hypercalcemia due to factors locally active in bone. Further study is required to clarify clinical and biochemical features in patients with hypercalcemia and malignancy. At present absolute discrimination between primary hyperparathyroidism and cancer hypercalcemia cannot be made by any single test. The small numbers of patients studied and the variation in individual as compared to group responses make it difficult to distinguish between hyperparathyroidism and cancer on the basis of iPTH, 1,25-$(OH)_2D_3$, NcAMP, P_i clearance, etc.

In hypercalcemia associated with the presence of malignant cells in bone and bone marrow (solid tumors such as breast carcinoma and hematologic malignancies such as multiple myeloma) radiological examinations utilizing both conventional x-rays and bone scans after administration of radioactive diphosphonate are useful diagnostic aids (some instances of myeloma involvement in bone are not detected by bone scans, however). A tissue diagnosis may be obtained with examination of marrow aspirates. The hypercalcemia of multiple myeloma nearly always falls to normal within a few days of therapy with a glucocorticoid such as prednisone, 40 mg per day.

SARCOIDOSIS In sarcoidosis the hypercalcemia presumably results from increased absorption of calcium from the gastrointestinal tract secondary to exaggerated sensitivity to vitamin D. This enhanced sensitivity may be due to a defect in the production or degradation of 1,25-$(OH)_2D_3$. Administration of vitamin D in doses not affecting 1,25-di$(OH)_3D_3$ levels in normal subjects causes a doubling or tripling of levels of the active metabolite in patients with sarcoidosis, along with increases in urinary calcium. Treatment with prednisone, known to restore elevated serum and urinary calcium to normal, lowered 1,25-$(OH)_2D_3$ levels to normal. Sarcoid patients have suppressed iPTH levels, hence abnormal vitamin D metabolism is not attributable to PTH excess. Clinically, hypercalcemia of sarcoidosis, when present, is usually a manifestation of severe disseminated disease. Hence evidence of pulmonary involvement is usually seen; chest x-ray may reveal a diffuse fibronodular infiltrate and/or prominent hilar adenopathy. An elevated blood gamma globulin may also be detected. In severe cases there may also be direct involvement of bone by the granulomatous process. The most definitive diagnostic procedure is demonstration of noncaseating granulomas by liver or lymph node biopsy, the latter usually of a scalene node. The hypercalcemia of sarcoidosis can present a difficult problem in differential diagnosis, especially since sarcoidosis may have existed for several years with many of the typical features of the disease lacking. In some patients abnormal pulmonary function tests

such as exercise-induced hypoxia or abnormal carbon monoxide diffusion time may be found; such studies, performed in patients whose blood chemical indexes are atypical for primary hyperparathyroidism (low PTH values, normal phosphate), may focus attention on a more detailed search for pulmonary sarcoidosis. Measurement of iPTH in the absence of severe renal failure is helpful; the levels are low or undetectable. Suppression of hypercalcemia with glucocorticoids can be helpful in confusing cases.

VITAMIN D INTOXICATION The chronic ingestion of large doses of vitamin D can produce hypercalcemia. Usually the ingestion of doses in excess of 100,000 units of vitamin D_2 or D_3 for many months is necessary for this complication to occur. (See Chap. 340.)

MILK-ALKALI SYNDROME (BURNETT'S SYNDROME) In this now rare syndrome hypercalcemia and renal failure occur as a complication of long-term ingestion of large amounts of calcium and alkali, usually in the form of milk and absorbable antacids. The syndrome is less prevalent since nonabsorbable antacids have been used in ulcer therapy. Possibly many of these patients have an underlying tendency for excessive gastrointestinal absorption of calcium similar to that predicated to be present in idiopathic hypercalciuria. Alkalosis contributes to deposition of calcium phosphate in abnormal locations including the kidney. Because of the increased incidence of ulcer disease in primary hyperparathyroidism, the possibility that the milk-alkali syndrome may coexist with hyperparathyroidism should always be considered.

THYROTOXICOSIS Significant hypercalcemia is a rare complication of thyrotoxicosis. However, minimal elevations of calcium occur in as many as 25 percent of patients with hyperthyroidism. Hypercalcemia in hyperthyroidism is presumably related to increased bone resorption; iPTH values are not elevated. The diagnosis usually offers no difficulties since, in most cases, it is the thyrotoxicosis rather than the hypercalcemia that brings the patient to the physician. However, particularly in the elderly, the signs of thyrotoxicosis may be minimal. If the serum calcium does not return toward normal as the thyrotoxicosis is brought under control, another cause for the hypercalcemia should be suspected.

ADRENAL INSUFFICIENCY Hypercalcemia occurs in adrenal insufficiency, especially acute adrenal failure. The cause has not been determined. There is evidence that glucocorticoids and vitamin D have opposing actions on blood calcium. High doses of steroids lower blood calcium when given as replacement in adrenal crisis; it is assumed by some that the elevation in calcium in the state of adrenal insufficiency reflects in some way the result of glucocorticoid deficiency. Others, however, have suggested that the hypercalcemia is due merely to hemoconcentration and that the ionized calcium is normal. In any event, in acute adrenal failure hypercalcemia is only a transient phenomenon; blood calcium returns to normal with adrenal replacement therapy.

IDIOPATHIC HYPERCALCEMIA OF INFANCY This is a rare syndrome characterized by hypercalcemia, often in association with multiple congenital cardiovascular lesions. Hypersensitivity to vitamin D has been postulated. The distinctive clinical features and age distribution of the syndrome make it unlikely to be a problem in the differential diagnosis of hypercalcemia in adults.

OTHER CAUSES OF HYPERCALCEMIA Prolonged immobilization of a patient may lead to hypercalcemia, especially in patients with high rates of bone turnover, such as those with Paget's disease. Immobilization may also cause hypercalcemia in young patients who are undergoing rapid growth and, therefore, have higher bone turnover rates. The hypercalcemia and associated hypercalciuria resolve when the patient becomes ambulatory. Hypercalcemia may occur in renal disease as a complication of secondary hyperparathyroidism, particularly in subjects undergoing chronic hemodialysis or renal transplantation.

MEDICAL TREATMENT OF HYPERCALCEMIA The acute treatment of hypercalcemia is usually successful; however, the chronic management of hypercalcemia is unsatisfactory unless the underlying cause can be corrected, because the available therapies are inconvenient or toxic. The serum calcium concentration can be decreased by 3 to 9 mg/dl in 24 to 48 h in most patients, enough to relieve acute symptoms, prevent death from hypercalcemic crisis, and permit diagnostic evaluation.

Hypercalcemia develops because skeletal calcium release is excessive, intestinal calcium absorption is excessive, or renal calcium excretion is inadequate. Understanding the particular pathogenesis helps guide therapy. For example, hypercalcemia in patients with osteolytic metastases or acute immobilization is primarily due to excessive skeletal calcium release and is, therefore, minimally affected by a severe restriction of dietary calcium. On the other hand, patients with vitamin D hypersensitivity or vitamin D intoxication have excessive intestinal calcium absorption, and severe restriction of dietary calcium is extremely beneficial. Decreased renal function or extracellular fluid depletion decreases urinary calcium excretion. If additional abnormalities, such as increased bone breakdown, are present, hypercalcemia will develop. This may happen, for example, when patients with resorptive bone disease become dehydrated. In such situations, increasing the urinary calcium excretion may cure the hypercalcemia, although excessive bone resorption continues.

Hydration, increased salt intake, mild and forced diuresis The first principle of treatment is to increase urinary calcium excretion by maximizing glomerular filtration and urinary sodium excretion. Many hypercalcemic patients are dehydrated because of vomiting, inanition, or hypercalcemia-induced defects in urinary concentrating ability. The resultant drop in glomerular filtration rate is accompanied by an additional drop in renal tubular sodium and calcium clearance. Restoring a normal extracellular fluid volume corrects these abnormalities and increases urine calcium excretion by 100 to 300 mg per day (2.5 to 7.5 mmol per day). Increasing urinary sodium excretion to 400 to 500 meq per day increases urinary calcium excretion even further than simple rehydration. Finally, administering conventional doses of furosemide or ethacrynic acid twice daily depresses the tubular reabsorptive mechanism for calcium and potentiates the above maneuvers (unless the diuretic is allowed to provoke dehydration). The combined use of these three therapies increases urinary calcium excretion to 400 to 800 mg per day (10 to 20 mmol per day) in a hypercalcemic patient. Since this is a substantial percentage of the exchangeable calcium pool, the serum calcium concentration usually falls 1 to 3 mg/dl (0.25 to 0.75 mmol/liter) within 24 h. The combination of fluids, sodium, and furosemide or ethacrynic acid is also adaptable to chronic outpatient treatment, if necessary, using sodium chloride tablets. The usual precautions regarding potassium and magnesium depletion during chronic therapy are necessary; calcium-containing renal calculi are a potential but unlikely complication.

Under life-threatening circumstances, the above therapy can be pursued more aggressively, giving 6 liters of isotonic saline (900 meq sodium) daily plus furosemide in doses up to 100 mg every 1 to 2 h or ethacrynic acid in doses up to 40 mg every 1 to 2 h. Urinary calcium excretions exceeding 1000 mg per day (25 mmol per day) are possible, and the serum calcium may decrease by as much as 4 mg/dl or more within 24 h. Severe potassium and magnesium depletion is inevitable unless replacements are given; pulmonary edema can obviously be precipitated. The potential complications can be averted by careful monitoring of central venous pressure and plasma or urine electrolytes, but the demands on the patient and medical staff are significant. A bladder catheter is usually necessary after the first day to allow the patient to sleep.

Phosphate Patients with primary hyperparathyroidism are frequently hypophosphatemic, and hypercalcemia of other causes may also be complicated by hypophosphatemia. Hypophosphatemia decreases the rate of calcium uptake into bone, increases intestinal calcium absorption, and both directly and indirectly stimulates bone breakdown. All these effects aggravate hypercalcemia, and correcting hypophosphatemia lowers the serum calcium concentration. The usual treatment is 1 to 1.5 g of phosphate phosphorus per day for several days, given in four divided doses to minimize the chances of developing hyperphosphatemia. Such therapy has been administered for prolonged periods in selected patients. It is not known whether toxicity will occur if the phosphate therapy only restores serum inorganic phosphate concentrations to normal.

Raising the serum inorganic phosphate concentration above normal further decreases serum calcium levels. Intravenous phosphate is one of the most dramatically effective treatments available for severe hypercalcemia. A dose of 1500 mg phosphate phosphorus or more intravenously over 6 to 8 h leads to a prompt decrease in serum calcium of 2 to 10 mg/dl in patients with initially normal serum inorganic phosphate concentrations. However, this therapy should be employed only in extreme emergencies for two reasons. First, fatal hypocalcemia can be produced by excessive dosage; frequent serum calcium determinations are necessary if intravenous phosphate is being administered. Second, unlike sodium chloride, sodium phosphate does not remove calcium from the body. In fact, urine calcium generally declines after phosphate administration, and fecal calcium declines or remains the same. The decline in serum calcium reflects a redistribution of calcium within the body. Studies of strontium and calcium kinetics during intravenous phosphate therapy indicate a rapid efflux of calcium from the circulation with no change in calcium entry to the circulation, findings indicative of acute precipitation of calcium phosphate salt. The calcium precipitates not only in bone, but metastatic calcification has also been reported in patients receiving oral or intravenous phosphate therapy for hypercalcemia. Furthermore, hyperphosphatemia can also cause metastatic calcification in normocalcemic animals. Thus, although it is not clear that this metastatic calcification is permanent if therapy is brief, administration of intravenous phosphate just to, but not beyond, the point of hyperphosphatemia is justifiable only as emergency treatment.

Inorganic phosphate is commercially available in liquid, powder, and capsule form for oral use and as a liquid for intravenous use. Preparations differ in their content of phosphorus and associated cation and pH. It is important to calculate doses in terms of phosphate phosphorus (see Table 339-1).

TABLE 339-1
Commercially available phosphate preparations

	1000 mg P	*meq Na*	*meq K*
Oral phosphate preparations:			
Neutraphos (1250-mg capsule)	4 caps	28.5	28.5
Neutraphos-K (1450-mg capsule)	4 caps	—	57
Phos-Tabs (860-mg tablet)	6 tabs	—	51
Fleets Phospho-Soda (liquid)	6.7 ml	40	—
Intravenous phosphate preparations:			
In-Phos	40 ml	65	8
Hyper-Phos-K	15 ml	—	50

SOURCE: *After Neer and Potts, in DeGroot et al.*

Mithramycin For the acute management of hypercalcemia, mithramycin, which inhibits bone reabsorption, is a therapeutic agent of major importance. Mithramycin must be given intravenously, either as a freshly prepared injection or as a 4- to 24-h infusion. The usual dose for the treatment of hypercalcemia is 25 μg per kilogram of body weight; 10 μg/kg can be effective for chronic therapy in some patients. One or two doses per week is usually sufficient; treatment should not be repeated until hypercalcemia recurs because the toxicity of the drug is dependent on the frequency of treatment and the total dosage.

Mithramycin has serious toxic effects; careful monitoring is needed if repeated doses are used. The major side effects are thrombocytopenia, hepatocellular necrosis with increased LDH and SGOT levels, and decreased clotting factors with resultant epistaxis, bruising, hemorrhage, and bleeding gums. Azotemia and proteinuria may occur; renal function should be carefully followed. Hypocalcemia can occur. Hypophosphatemia and hypokalemia may also develop, and nausea, vomiting, stomatitis, and facial swelling can occur. Toxicity is rare when only one or two doses are used and can be minimized by repeating single doses only when hypercalcemia recurs. Toxic effects can usually be reversed by stopping the drug; hemorrhage may be an exception.

Other therapies *Glucocorticoids* increase urinary calcium excretion and decrease intestinal calcium absorption when given in pharmacological doses (e.g., 40 to 100 mg prednisone daily in divided doses), but they also cause negative skeletal calcium balance. In normal subjects and in patients with primary hyperparathyroidism, glucocorticoids neither increase nor decrease the serum calcium concentration. In patients with hypercalcemia due to certain osteolytic malignancies, however, glucocorticoids are strikingly effective as a result of antitumor effects. The malignancies in which hypercalcemia responds to glucocorticoid are, most frequently, hematologic malignancies such as multiple myeloma, leukemias, Hodgkin's disease, and other lymphomas; carcinoma of the breast also responds frequently, at least early in the course of the disease. Other malignancies occasionally produce a glucocorticoid-responsive hypercalcemia, but this is unpredictable and more reliable remedies are available for the hypercalcemia. Glucocorticoids are very effective in treating hypercalcemia due to vitamin D intoxication or vitamin D hypersensitivity of sarcoidosis and tuberculosis. The mechanism of action in the latter circumstances is unclear. In all the above situations, the hypocalcemic effect develops over several days, and the usual glucocorticoid dosage is 40 to 100 mg prednisone (or its equivalent) daily in four divided doses. The side effects of chronic glucocorticoid therapy are well known but may be acceptable in some circumstances.

The hormonal mediator of hypercalcemia secondary to malignancies that cause excessive bone breakdown without actually metastasizing to bone may be a prostaglandin of the E series in some patients but is still undefined in the remainder. Since *prostaglandin synthesis* can be blocked by indomethacin or aspirin, these drugs sometimes correct the hypercalcemia in such patients. The analytical methods necessary to define prostaglandin excess are not widely available, and a therapeutic trial is the accepted diagnostic maneuver. Indomethacin, 25 mg every 6 h, or aspirin in sufficient doses to produce a serum salicylate level of 20 to 30 mg/dl generally lowers the serum calcium concentrations to or toward normal over several days if prostaglandin excess is the cause.

Hypercalcemia complicated by severe renal failure is difficult to manage; dialysis is often the treatment of choice. Peritoneal dialysis can be used to remove 500 to 2000 mg (12.5 to 50 mmol) of calcium in 24 to 48 h and lower the serum calcium concentration by 3 to 12 mg/dl (0.75 to 3.0 mmol/liter), if calcium-free dialysis fluid is used.

Large quantities of phosphate are lost during dialysis, and serum inorganic phosphate concentrations usually fall, thus aggravating hypercalcemia. Therefore, the serum inorganic phosphate concentration should be measured after dialysis, and phosphate supplements added to the diet or to subsequent dialysis fluids if necessary.

Calcitonin decreases the skeletal release of calcium, phosphorus, and hydroxyproline within minutes of its intravenous injection. The subsequent changes in serum calcium and phosphorus depend upon the initial magnitude of skeletal resorption: subjects with the most rapid bone turnover show the greatest reduction in serum calcium concentration. Calcitonin also increases the renal clearance of calcium and phosphorus (and sodium). The most impressive results have been seen in patients with hypercalcemia due to immobilization, thyrotoxicosis, or vitamin D intoxication. These situations are all characterized by a high rate of bone turnover. Surprisingly, calcitonin has been less effective than phosphate or mithramycin in patients with hypercalcemia due to malignancy or hyperparathyroidism, conditions in which bone turnover is also high.

Escape from drug action occurs in patients and animals invariably after 12 to 24 h of high-dose therapy or after several days of continuous therapy with calcitonin. The mechanism of the escape is unknown; until this problem is overcome, the general usefulness of the drug is limited to that of adjuvant therapy. Calcitonin is effective only by intravenous, intramuscular, or subcutaneous injection; doses used are 25 to 50 units every 6 to 8 h, usually in the form of salmon calcitonin (Calcimar).

Summary The various therapies for hypercalcemia are listed in Table 339-2 with their particular indications and principal toxicities. The choice of therapy depends upon the underlying disease, the severity of the hypercalcemia, the serum inorganic phosphate level, and the patient's renal, hepatic, and bone marrow function. Mild hypercalcemia ($<$12 mg/dl or 3 mmol/liter) can usually be managed by hydration, sodium chloride, and small doses of furosemide or ethacrynic acid. Severe hypercalcemia ($>$15 mg/dl or 3.75 mmol/liter) requires rapid correction. Aggressive sodium/calcium diuresis with large doses of furosemide and ethacrynic acid works rapidly but should only be undertaken if appropriate monitoring is available and cardiac function is adequate. Mithramycin is often the drug of choice, since it has the advantages of effectiveness and simplicity of use; the principal contraindication is its potential for toxicity. Renal, hepatic, or bone marrow disease may preclude its use. Hypophosphatemia, if present, should be corrected with oral or, rarely, intravenous phosphate repletion.

Phosphate supplements should never be administered if hyperphosphatemia is present. Intermediate degrees of hypercalcemia can be treated with some combination of these remedies and/or glucocorticoids, with the choice dependent upon the underlying disease. Severe dietary calcium restriction should be employed if intestinal hyperabsorption is present. Glucocorticoids and prostaglandin-synthesis inhibitors, even when effective in a particular disease, work slowly over several days and should not be relied upon as the sole treatment for life-threatening hypercalcemia. Dialysis should be reserved for hypercalcemia complicating acute or chronic renal failure.

The only really satisfactory treatments for chronic use in outpatients are dietary calcium restriction, administration of sodium chloride with or without furosemide and ethacrynic acid, and moderate-dose oral phosphate (the patient is kept normophosphatemic). The more effective remedies (mithramycin, glucocorticoids, high-dose oral phosphate) all have significant toxicity when used chronically.

It is important to stress that the treatment of hypercalcemia must be undertaken in the context of overall patient care. If the underlying disease is unknown or has a reasonable chance of successful definitive therapy, then treatment of the hypercalcemia should be aggressive. If the patient suffers from a disease process, such as malignancy, for which all definitive or effective ameliorative measures have been exhausted, then aggressive therapy of the hypercalcemia is not indicated.

SURGICAL TREATMENT OF HYPERPARATHYROIDISM Once the diagnosis of primary hyperparathyroidism has been made, surgery is the treatment of choice. However, a decision may be made to defer surgery when mild asymptomatic hypercalcemia is discovered in an elderly patient or when other factors such as cardiovascular or pulmonary disease make the patient a poor operative risk. Too little is known about the natural history of hyperparathyroidism to recommend surgery automatically, particularly in older patients, if no signs or symptoms are present that are attributable to hyperparathyroidism. One may elect to follow such a patient if hypercalcemia is not severe, e.g., less than 11.5 to 12.0 mg/dl, and if osteopenia or other signs of bone disease, as well as renal complications, are lacking. If a decision not to operate is made, however, careful serial evaluation of bone and renal function is indicated to guard against silent renal or osseous deterioration. Occasionally, if the relation of vague constitutional symptoms to hypercalcemia is raised, it may be useful to evaluate the symptomatic response following the lowering of blood calcium. Since blood phosphate is low, administering sodium or potassium phosphate in doses of 1 to 2 g phosphate phosphorus daily may be useful. On the other hand, such therapy raises PTH levels, which might be harmful, and may lead to ectopic calcification. Generally, it seems wiser either to follow a patient without treatment or to recommend surgical exploration of the parathyroids.

Parathyroid exploration should be undertaken only by an experienced surgeon with the help of an equally astute pathologist. There are many critical decisions regarding management that can be made only during the operation. The examination of tissue removed at surgery by frozen section should direct the subsequent course of the operation. The usual procedure recommended by the author's colleagues is as follows: if

TABLE 339-2
Summary of useful treatments for hypercalcemia

Therapy	*Therapeutic details*	*Indications*	*Complications*	*Precautions*
MOST GENERALLY USEFUL THERAPIES				
Hydration	2 liters or more	Universal	—	—
High salt intake	Achieve urine Na of 300 meq/day or more	Universal	Edema	—
Furosemide or ethacrynic acid	40–160 mg/day 50–200 mg/day	Universal	↓K and ↓Mg	Measure serum K and Mg
Forced diuresis	4–6 liters fluid IV/day containing 600–900 meq Na plus furosemide every 1–2 h, plus at least 60 meq K/day, plus at least 60 meq Mg/day	Universal	Pulmonary edema; ↓K and ↓Mg	Intensive monitoring, including venous pressure and serum Mg and K
Oral phosphate	250 mg P every 6 h PO	Universal if serum P < 3 mg/dl	Ectopic calcification	Keep serum P below 5–6 mg/dl
Mithramycin	10–25 μg/kg IV, repeat prn	Increased bone resorption	Liver; kidney; marrow toxicity	Monitor platelets CBC, BUN, SCOT
Prednisone or equivalent	5–15 mg every 6 h	Breast cancer, lymphomas, leukemias, multiple myeloma, Vitamin D poisoning, sarcoidosis	Cushing's syndrome if chronic Rx	Alternate-day Rx for chronic use
SPECIAL THERAPIES FOR PARTICULAR USES				
IV phosphate	1500 mg P every 12 h until P 6 mg/dl	Severe hypercalcemia; diuresis or mithramycin contraindicated	Ectopic calcification; severe hypocalcemia	Monitor serum Ca and P closely
Calcitonin	2 units every 4 h subcutaneously	Adjunct when ↑bone reabsorption; paralysis; immobilization	—	—
Indomethacin	25 mg every 6 h PO	Certain types of pseudo-hyperparathyroidism	Na retention; GI bleeding; headache	Careful clinical monitoring
Dialysis	Low-Ca bath	Acute renal failure	Multiple	Monitor serum P after dialysis

an abnormal gland is identified, remove it and search for at least one additional gland. If the second gland is normal in size and normal histologically (frozen section), the hyperparathyroidism was due to a *single adenoma.* For this reason exploration is stopped. Others believe that several glands are involved in all cases and that subtotal parathyroidectomy is the procedure of choice. The risk of the former approach is lack of cure or early recurrence; the risk of the latter is hypoparathyroidism. Further long-term follow-up of patients managed by each procedure seems indicated.

Hyperplasia involves even more difficult questions of surgical management. Once a diagnosis of hyperplasia has been established, it is necessary to identify all the glands. It usually is recommended that three glands be totally removed and that the fourth gland be partially excised; care should be taken to leave a good blood supply for the remaining gland. Some surgeons now advocate transplantation of some of the removed, minced tissue into the muscles of the forearm to avoid delayed vascular failure of residual tissue in the neck. The merits of the two approaches have not yet been compared systematically.

There are documented cases of five or six parathyroid glands, as well as unusual locations for adenomas. If no glandular abnormalities are found in the neck, further exploration must be undertaken. When parathyroid carcinoma is encountered, it is important that the tissue be widely excised; great care should be taken to avoid rupture of the capsule to prevent local seeding of the tumor.

Decline in serum calcium occurs within 24 h after successful surgery; usually blood calcium falls to low normal values for 4 to 5 days until the remaining parathyroid tissue resumes hormone secretion. Severe postoperative hypocalcemia is likely to occur if there has been significant osteitis fibrosa or if there has been injury to the normal parathyroid glands during surgery.

For mild symptomatic hypocalcemia, oral calcium supplementation may suffice; if hypocalcemia is severe, intravenous calcium is necessary. It is usually convenient to prepare a solution of calcium (gluconate or chloride) at a concentration of 1 mg/ml in 5% dextrose in water. The rate and duration of intravenous calcium therapy are determined by severity of symptoms and the response detected by frequently monitoring blood calcium levels. A rate of infusion of 0.5 to 2 (mg/kg)/h or 30 to 100 ml/h of the 1 mg/ml solution usually suffices to relieve symptoms. Generally, parenteral therapy in most instances is required for only a few days. If symptoms and/or need for parenteral calcium continue for more than 4 to 5 days, replacement therapy with vitamin D (or vitamin D metabolites) and/or calcium should be started (see "Hypoparathyroidism," below). A sudden rise in blood calcium after several months on vitamin D replacement therapy may indicate restoration of parathyroid function to normal.

Magnesium deficiency may also complicate the postoperative course of parathyroid surgery and represents an additional cause of tetany. Impaired secretion of parathyroid hormone has been demonstrated in magnesium deficiency. Hypomagnesemia should therefore be corrected whenever detected. $MgCl_2$ is sufficiently soluble to be effective by mouth, but preparations of this compound are not widely available. Accordingly, repletion must usually be parenteral. Only a small fraction of total-body magnesium is present in extracellular fluid, but total-body Mg deficiency is reflected by hypomagnesemia. Since the depressant effect of magnesium on central and peripheral nerve functions is not seen below 4 meq per liter (normal range 1.5 to 2 meq per liter), parenteral replacement can be given at a vigorous rate. A dose as great as 2 meq/kg can be given if severe hypomagnesemia is present. The magnesium is given either as an intravenous infusion over 8 to 12 h or in divided doses intramuscularly (magnesium sulfate, USP, the preparation normally used, is available as a 20% solution, 1 g or 8 meq/ml, or as a more concentrated solution, 50%).

SECONDARY HYPERPARATHYROIDISM

Secondary hyperparathyroidism is also characterized by excessive production of parathyroid hormone. It is encountered in various disease states in which there is resistance to the metabolic actions of parathyroid hormone. Because of the resistance to the action of the hormone, these disease states are usually characterized by a mild degree of hypocalcemia, at least in the ionized fraction of blood calcium, despite the excessive secretion of parathyroid hormone.

Secondary hyperparathyroidism occurs in patients with some forms of osteomalacia, pseudohypoparathyroidism, and chronic renal disease. Correction of the osteomalacia with adequate vitamin D therapy or reversal of renal failure (as with successful renal transplant) should lead to regression of the hyperparathyroidism. This has been documented in patients with a successful renal transplant. In turn, these considerations lead to an important distinction between the character of abnormal growth of parathyroid glands in secondary hyperparathyroidism (reversible) and primary hyperparathyroidism (presumably irreversible). It is not clear, however, that in all patients with long-standing, secondary parathyroid hyperplasia the enlarged glands do revert to normal size and function after removal of the initial stimuli to hyperplasia.

The pathogenesis of the secondary hyperparathyroidism, deficient vitamin D metabolism, intestinal malabsorption, and osteodystrophy in chronic renal failure is difficult to reconstruct (see Chap. 289). A variable picture of bone disease may develop in association with hyperparathyroidism in chronic renal failure. (This is discussed in Chap. 341.) Occasionally, severe bone pain, widespread ectopic calcification, and severe pruritis may develop, and the question of subtotal parathyroidectomy may be raised. While this may be necessary, appreciation of the frequent, although not invariant, reversibility of the parathyroid hyperplasia has led to a more conservative attitude toward surgical intervention. Subtotal parathyroidectomy may lead to severe postoperative hypoparathyroidism. Medical treatment such as reduction of excessive blood phosphate by dietary phosphate restriction and use of nonabsorbable antacids, and better management of renal failure, may reverse ectopic calcification. Selective treatment with vitamin D analogues, especially 1,25-dihydroxyvitamin D_3 [1,25-$(OH)_2D_3$] in doses of 0.25 to 2.0 μg per day (see Chap. 340), has led to improvement in calcium absorption and blood calcium levels. These recent advances in medical therapy may eliminate the need for surgery of the parathyroids in many cases.

The stimulus for hyperplasia of the parathyroids has not been identified. It seems possible that in all conditions in which secondary hyperparathyroidism is found, resistance to hormone action accounts for persistent hypocalcemia in spite of increased hormone secretion. Chronic, even though partly compensated, hypocalcemia may be the stimulus that directly causes parathyroid hyperplasia. Specific aspects of the clinical features and approaches encountered in states of secondary hyperparathyroidism, in pseudohypoparathyroidism, and in osteomalacia (Chap. 341) are reviewed below.

In summary, present knowledge concerning the complex pattern of biosynthesis, secretion, and metabolism of parathyroid hormone, even in normal subjects, must be taken into account in attempting to understand the origins or predict the course of secondary hyperparathyroidism. Attempts to manage hyperparathyroidism by correction of underlying defects is the most reasonable approach (whenever feasible) in view of the potential reversibility of this adaptive disorder of the parathyroids.

HYPOPARATHYROIDISM

Hypoparathyroidism is a metabolic abnormality characterized by hypocalcemia and consequent neuromuscular symptoms; the disease results from a deficiency of parathyroid hormone production or end organ resistance to the action of the hormone.

ETIOLOGY Postoperative hypoparathyroidism The most common cause of hypoparathyroidism is excision of the parathyroids or damage to the glands or their vascular supply during surgery for thyroid disorders, hyperparathyroidism, or radical neck dissections for cancer. Postoperative hypoparathyroidism is now less frequent, not only because of improved awareness of the potential problem during extensive neck surgery, but also because of the increased use of medical therapy for treatment of thyrotoxicosis. Although the symptoms of hypoparathyroidism usually develop several days after the operation, there can be a delay of months to years after neck surgery before the diagnosis is made. Although it has been speculated that in these patients the glands slowly atrophy because of progressive ischemic damage following surgery, it is possible that signs and symptoms of hypocalcemia were overlooked. A different situation can also take place: transient hypoparathyroidism may occur immediately following thyroid surgery. In this situation it seems likely that the glands are initially injured but gradually recover or that a small remnant of remaining parathyroid tissue gradually hypertrophies. In this form of hypoparathyroidism secondary to trauma (analogous to idiopathic forms of the disorder, discussed below), analyses of parathyroid hormone by immunoassay (Fig. 339-1) and by assays, based on cytochemical methods believed to reflect biologically active hormone have substantiated clinical evidence that parathyroid glandular failure may in some cases be partial rather than absolute.

Idiopathic hypoparathyroidism Idiopathic hypoparathyroidism is relatively rare. A total lack of parathyroid function can be detected as (1) an isolated entity (idiopathic hypoparathyroidism), (2) in association with agenesis of the thymus (the Di George syndrome), or (3) in association with a familial disorder in which there may be a deficiency of thyroid, adrenal, and ovarian function, pernicious anemia, and other defects. The Di George syndrome is a rare disorder in which there is congenital absence of the thymus and the parathyroids, organs embryologically derived from the third and fourth branchial pouches. Patients with this syndrome usually die at 1 to 2 years of age of severe hypocalcemia, persistent infection, or both. The immune deficiency is of the cellular type. Delayed hypersensitivity reactions are deficient, and allograft rejections are absent. Humoral and circulating antibody mechanisms are intact. The striking features that result from the absence of the thymus make this syndrome quite distinctive.

The familial syndrome of hypoparathyroidism is unusual in several respects (see Chap. 123). An autoimmune basis for this disease has been suspected. Antibodies to parietal cells, the parathyroids, adrenal cortex, thyroid, and ovary have been detected. However, there are poor correlations between the occurrence of endocrine deficiency and detection of endocrine organ-specific antibodies; some family members have antibodies but no endocrine deficiency. Patients frequently have moniliasis, particularly in the fingernails. Recognition of the associated features is important because of the clinical problems encountered when adrenal failure or anemia develops. Careful periodic evaluation of a given patient or family members with respect to hematopoietic, adrenal, ovarian, and thyroid status is important. The frequency of expression of the disease or of antibodies does not fit any simple pattern of inheritance, although autosomal recessive inheritance has been suggested.

Other causes of true hypoparathyroidism Hypoparathyroidism secondary to radiation therapy is rare. The gland presumably atrophies secondary to radiation damage after radioactive iodine therapy for thyrotoxicosis. An unusual form of hypoparathyroidism occurs in infants born of mothers with hyperparathyroidism. The high level of the circulating calcium in the mother's blood apparently inhibits the activity or development of the parathyroid glands in the infant. This form of hypoparathyroidism is usually transient.

Pseudohypoparathyroidism Pseudohypoparathyroidism is a hereditary disorder characterized by symptoms and signs of hypoparathyroidism in association with distinctive skeletal and developmental defects. The hypoparathyroidism is due to *deficient end organ response* to the endogenous hormone, reflected in deficient to absent increase in urinary cyclic AMP excretion in response to exogenous parathyroid hormone; there is excessive secretion of parathyroid hormone and hyperplasia of the parathyroids, a response to the resistance to hormone action.

Recent studies concerning the biochemical defect in end organ response have clarified the nature of the abnormality in the receptor–adenyl cyclase complex for parathyroid hormone; however, many clinical aspects of pseudohypoparathyroidism remain unclarified, including the relation between the skeletal and developmental defects and the hypoparathyroidism. Relatives of patients with pseudohypoparathyroidism often exhibit skeletal and developmental defects without any symptoms or chemical evidence of hypoparathyroidism, so-called pseudopseudohypoparathyroidism. It has been shown that (1) there is an increased concentration of circulating parathyroid hormone in all subjects with pseudohypoparathyroidism (at least, if studied when they are hypocalcemic prior to the institution of vitamin D therapy) (Fig. 339-1), (2) there is no evidence for circulating antiparathyroid antibodies in any of these patients, and (3) there is evidence that the hormone made by these patients is biologically active.

Since, by definition, all patients with the complete syndrome are hypocalcemic and hyperphosphatemic, it has generally been believed that both bone and kidney are unresponsive, but the pathophysiology is complex. Some patients show an essentially normal phosphaturia following the injection of parathyroid hormone. In one patient with pseudohypoparathyroidism previously treated with vitamin D, the removal of all four parathyroid glands was accompanied by a striking fall in serum calcium, requiring a massive increase in vitamin D to restore serum calcium toward normal. This implied that during long-term vitamin D treatment, there is a significant contribution to extracellular fluid calcium from parathyroid hormone–driven bone resorption when sufficient parathyroid hypersecretion has developed, despite osseous resistance to parathyroid action.

Reports have accumulated concerning patients with hypocalcemia and hyperphosphatemia in whom evidence of osteitis fibrosa has been found by both x-ray and biopsy. This has led to the speculation that the renal end organ defect may be the most severe if not the sole abnormality in some patients. After vitamin D therapy in patients with typical pseudohypoparathyroidism, normal responses in blood and urinary calcium and phosphate levels may occur after administration of parathyroid hormone, although urinary cyclic AMP production remains impaired. Subjects with pseudohypoparathyroidism, unlike those with true hypoparathyroidism, usually excrete less excessive quantities of calcium in urine when their blood calcium is made normal after vitamin D treatment. This suggests that there is some renal end organ response with regard to the action of the increased levels of circulating hormone to reduce renal calcium clearance.

These varied clinical observations suggest that end organ resistance may be less severe in some patients than in others or that vitamin D treatment alters end organ sensitivity. In addition, it may be true that bone is more responsive to hormone than kidney in certain patients with pseudohypoparathyroidism. Several additional clinical reports have appeared proposing an additional clinical subtype, pseudohyperparathyroidism type II, in which it is proposed that the bone and renal receptors for parathyroid-stimulated adenyl cyclase are intact but that there is a failure of normal calcium and phosphate transport systems to respond to the cyclic AMP generated. The difficulty in obtaining clear-cut responses in renal phosphate clearance to injected parathyroid hormone even in normal subjects without carefully standardized conditions and clear indication of partial rather than complete end organ unresponsiveness in pseudohypoparathyroidism suggests the need for considerable caution in defining precise or distinct subtypes of this complex hereditary syndrome. Further work may, however, reveal heterogeneity of the pathophysiology in these peculiar heritable syndromes associated with end organ hyporesponsiveness to PTH.

Earlier suggestions, dating from the observations of Albright that there was an end organ failure in pseudohypoparathyroidism, have been confirmed both by physiological and biochemical studies over the last decade, beginning with the observation of the failure of these patients to respond to PTH injections with an appropriate increase in nephrogenous cyclic AMP. The receptor–adenyl cyclase complex on plasma membranes that responds to parathyroid hormone (and, in addition, with different specificity of binding at the receptor per se for other peptide hormones) consists of at least three distinct components: hormone receptor, enzyme catalytic unit (adenyl cyclase), and a guanyl nucleotide regulatory protein (G unit or N protein). The latter protein mediates the response between receptor occupancy by hormone and stimulation of adenyl cyclase (see Chap. 87). When the G units (N proteins) in red cell membranes were compared in some patients with pseudohypoparathyroidism, normal controls, and subjects with true hypoparathyroidism, G unit extracts from red cells of patients with pseudohypoparathyroidism appeared to contain only about half the normal activity, as assessed by both a bioassay and a direct chemical assay. Although there is variation from patient to patient, a nearly complete discrimination has been found between normal subjects (or hypoparathyroid patients) and those with pseudohypoparathyroidism.

Reports that hormone responsiveness improves in some patients with adjuvant therapy (such as calcium or vitamin D) may also be ultimately understood in light of the partial, rather than total, reduction in G units in this disease. Defective responses to other hormones would be predicted from a generalized reduction in cellular concentration of G units. Although clinically only hypothyroidism has been reported (in association with increased thyrotropin), the blunted responses to prolactin, antidiuretic hormone, and gonadotropin that are reported are compatible with a generalized reduction in G unit cellular concentration.

Many features of the correlations between in vitro findings and physiological defects in vivo are still to be clarified, however, as are hereditary patterns. Studies by one group included findings of completely normal G unit levels in 11 patients from two kindreds with multiple manifestations of defective hormone responsiveness; one kindred exhibited the usual skeletal and developmental defects, while brachydactyly and related abnormalities were absent from the other kindred. One patient studied by another group also had evidence of pseudohypoparathyroidism clinically but normal G units. This clearly indicates genetic heterogeneity even within a single pathophysiological presentation; the predominant group of patients so far tested has a deficit in guanyl nucleotide subunit functions but at least one (or two) other kindred has a type of defect not detected in the present assays, perhaps at a different step in the hormone–receptor–guanyl nucleotide–adenyl cyclase interaction. Also two patients from kindreds with multiple symptomatic patients exhibiting signs and symptoms of hormone unresponsiveness who were devoid of any signs of hypocalcemia but had brachydactyly (hence met the criteria of pseudopseudohypoparathyroidism) had deficient G units by assay but without visible consequence on mineral ion transport.

Even more confusing is a recent report that again raises an older issue concerning the pathophysiology, namely, that the hormone secreted in many of these patients may be biologically defective. Comparisons were made of circulating levels of hormone by immunoassay (employing two different antiserums felt to measure, respectively, only amino-terminal or carboxyl-terminal regions of the hormonal molecule) and by a cytochemical bioassay (felt to reflect biological activity) in six patients with pseudohypoparathyroidism as well as in normal subjects, and patients with hypoparathyroidism or primary and secondary hyperparathyroidism. The study uncovered the surprising finding that the subjects with pseudohypoparathyroidism, unlike all others tested, had high immunoreactive, but low bioactive, hormone levels. Since there is no apparent relation between the defective G unit and defective hormone per se, it is clear that further analysis of both issues in the same patients is needed; a definitive explanation of the syndrome(s) is not yet available.

Little is known about the pathophysiology of the skeletal defects in these patients, although there is a clear hereditary linkage between the biochemical and developmental defects. Pseudohypoparathyroidism is usually found within kindreds in which some other family members have the metabolically normal but developmentally abnormal variant of the disorder, pseudopseudohypoparathyroidism. However, the exact mode of genetic inheritance is still uncertain, and the variable expression of metabolic abnormalities in affected individuals is not understood. Some analyses have suggested that the two linked disorders, pseudopseudohypoparathyroidism and pseudohypoparathyroidism, are transmitted as an X-linked dominant. The sex incidence is 2:1 affected females versus males. However, the disease is extremely rare, and the total number of patients and of involved sibships is small for purposes of suitable statistical analysis. Male-to-male transmission is reported. Furthermore, acceptance of some cases as authentic examples of the syndrome on the basis of literature reports is difficult, particularly with respect to the metabolically normal individuals (those with pseudopseudohypoparathyroidism). Certain of the developmental defects such as short stature, short metacarpal or metatarsal bones, and/or even basal ganglion calcification are found in Turner's syndrome, Gardner's syndrome, basal-cell nevus syndrome, and other hereditary disorders that are believed to be genetically distinct. Detailed studies of quantitative defects in the nucleotide regulatory subunit of the receptor (N protein or G unit) in families in association with careful pedigree analysis, detailed biochemical testing and classification by physical features, and further characterization of hormone activity are needed to permit meaningful genetic classification. Genetic heterogeneity seems likely.

SIGNS AND SYMPTOMS Most of the symptoms of hypoparathyroidism reflect altered neuromuscular irritability due to the decreased concentration of ionized calcium. The age of onset of symptoms is earlier in pseudohypoparathyroidism than in idiopathic hypoparathyroidism.

Tetany and convulsions represent the most serious complications in hypoparathyroidism. Latent tetany can be elicited by tapping the facial nerve and producing a contraction of the facial muscles (Chvostek's sign), or by application of a tourniquet or blood pressure cuff leading to carpopedal spasm (Trousseau's sign). Increased bone density may occasionally be present in hypoparathyroidism; however, there may be no detectable skeletal abnormalities.

A complication perhaps related to the hyperphosphatemia is the frequent occurrence of *soft-tissue calcification*. In pseudohypoparathyroidism the mineral deposits in ectopic sites may include the development of true bone. True bone formation in ectopic sites is never seen in idiopathic hypoparathyroidism. Amorphous deposits of calcium and phosphate are found in the basal ganglia. Calcification of the basal ganglia is noted in as many as half of the patients. Most patients with pseudopseudohypoparathyroidism do not have ectopic calcium deposits.

The skeletal and developmental abnormalities that are found in both pseudohypoparathyroidism and pseudopseudohypoparathyroidism include short stature, round face, short neck, thick, stocky body build, and multiple discrete abnormalities in individual bones of the skeleton. Abnormally short metacarpal and metatarsal bones and sometimes phalanges have been reported. These defects seem to be due to premature closure of the epiphyses. The most classic finding is an *abnormally short fourth and fifth metacarpal and metatarsal.* This defect may be unilateral. Exostoses are frequently reported. Usually only one or two are detected, but occasionally multiple exostoses are found. Radius curvus may be present in some patients.

Multiple abnormalities are detected in tooth formation. The nails may be fragile and skin dry; moniliasis is commonly found in true hypoparathyroidism but not in pseudohypoparathyroidism. Mental deficiency is rather common in patients with pseudohypoparathyroidism. It seems most probable that this is part of the inherited syndrome. In any event, there is little improvement in mental status even with adequate therapy with calcium and vitamin D. Distinctive impairment in olfaction and taste has also been reported in the majority of patients examined. In addition, unusual dermatoglyphic abnormalities have been noted.

In pseudohypoparathyroidism there is an increased incidence of diabetes (or an abnormal glucose tolerance curve) and hypothyroidism. Recent studies have indicated that hypothyroidism, at least in some patients, is due to deficient response to thyrotropin.

DIAGNOSIS AND DIFFERENTIAL DIAGNOSIS Typically, the diagnosis of hypoparathyroidism is considered in a patient who has symptoms of hypocalcemia and is found to have both hypocalcemia and hyperphosphatemia in the presence of normal renal function. Clinically, the patient's history or physical features may be helpful in suggesting the diagnosis. A history of neck surgery with difficulties dating from that time points to postsurgical hypoparathyroidism. Pseudohypoparathyroidism is more likely than true hypoparathyroidism if unusual skeletal and developmental defects are detected or if there is a family history of other sibs with short stature and skeletal abnormalities. However, a definitive diagnosis, particularly for pseudohypoparathyroidism, must be established through application of specific laboratory tests. Three specific tests should be used to establish the diagnosis definitively, namely, the *parathyroid hormone radioimmunoassay, measurement of urinary cyclic AMP excretion* following the administration of parathyroid hormone, and, when available, *measurement of N protein (G unit)* in erythrocyte membranes prepared from blood samples in patients.

Patients with *symptomatic hypocalcemia*, particularly if the history and physical examination suggest chronicity of the hypocalcemia (such as gradual onset of symptoms and evidence of ectopic calcification), would be expected to have secondary hyperparathyroidism if the parathyroid glands are functional. If no parathyroid hormone is detected by radioimmunoassay, notwithstanding the stimulus of marked hypocalcemia, then true hypoparathyroidism is the most likely diagnosis. As noted in Fig. 339-1, not all patients with idiopathic hypoparathyroidism have undetectable levels of iPTH; some patients show values in the lower half of normal. Nonetheless, if not undetectable, the concentrations are lower than expected for the degree of hypocalcemia and thereby confirm the diagnosis. If elevated concentrations of parathyroid hormone are found, pseudohypoparathyroidism due to end organ resistance is more likely. In such cases, renal end organ resistance can be demonstrated by measuring the urinary excretion of cyclic AMP in response to the injection of a standard dose of parathyroid hormone. Synthetic human parathyroid hormone, hPTH 1-34, is now available commercially for investigative use in such tests of hormone responsiveness, an advance over the early use of impure fractions of bovine hormone; potency of the latter was highly variable, complicating interpretation of the tests. Normal subjects, patients with idiopathic or postsurgical hypoparathyroidism, and patients with pseudopseudohypoparathyroidism exhibit a ten- to twentyfold increase in urinary cyclic AMP secretion. In those with pseudohypoparathyroidism, little, if any, response is noted. At least in specialized referral centers, erythrocyte membranes prepared from blood samples of suspected patients can be assayed for concentration of N protein (G unit); patients with pseudohypoparathyroidism have results well below values in normal subjects or those with true hypoparathyroidism.

Hypocalcemia may be encountered not only in hypoparathyroidism but also in malabsorption, osteomalacia secondary to true vitamin D lack or vitamin D resistance, renal failure, hypoproteinemia, pancreatitis, and acute nutritional deficiency with associated hypomagnesemia. In patients with *malabsorption*, true vitamin D lack, vitamin D resistance, or renal failure, the parathyroid hormone concentration by radioimmunoassay is increased. Secondary hyperparathyroidism apparently results from the chronic hypocalcemia that accompanies these diseases. The manifestations of *renal failure*, including phosphate retention, are usually obvious when hypocalcemia is found. Patients with *osteomalacia* usually show a low serum phosphorus, an apparent reflection of the persistence of the action of parathyroid hormone on renal phosphate excretion in spite of the deficiency of vitamin D that interferes with the effective action of the hormone on bone.

Hypoproteinemia causes a reduction in total serum calcium because of reduced binding protein. Subjects with this abnormality have a normal ionized serum calcium concentration and lack symptoms of hypocalcemia. Correction for the total calcium concentration in patients with hypoproteinemia is based on the known binding of calcium by albumin and globulin. Episodes of *acute pancreatitis* are associated with hypocalcemia, but this is present only during the acute phase of the illness. The explanation for the hypocalcemia in pancreatitis, although much discussed, remains unknown.

There is an increasingly frequent recognition of the syndrome of hypocalcemia in patients with *hypomagnesemia.* Severe hypomagnesemia, less than 0.8 meq per liter, reflects serious intracellular magnesium deficits. Recent reports have emphasized that a state of functional hypoparathyroidism is associated with severe hypomagnesemia. Parathyroid hormone secretion is severely blunted or totally blocked in such patients. Earlier reports, especially in animals, suggested that magnesium deficiency may also be associated with reduced peripheral responsiveness to parathyroid hormone, but impaired secretion of the hormone is the more important cause of hypocalcemia. Parenteral correction of the hypomagnesemia over several days restores normal parathyroid responsiveness. For details of therapy with magnesium, see the discussion above under treatment of magnesium deficits following surgery in hyperparathyroidism. Recognition of this syndrome is important to avoid unnecessary and expensive diagnostic evaluation for some unusual cause of parathyroid failure in patients with hypomagnesemia.

TREATMENT The principal aim of treatment is to restore calcium toward normal by use of supplementary dietary calcium and vitamin D and thereby relieve symptoms of increased neuromuscular irritability. However, it is not clear whether the other complications of hypoparathyroidism can be as readily controlled despite therapy which appears to be adequate for regulation of blood calcium. It has been noted that lenticular opacities may progress despite therapy.

There are numerous problems in achieving proper regulation of calcium metabolism in patients with hypoparathyroidism. Continued treatment with adequate doses of vitamin D presents several difficulties. Urinary calcium excretion is often excessive in hypoparathyroidism owing to the lack of the normal parathyroid effect to lower urine calcium clearance. This leads to the anomalous result that patients with hypoparathyroidism may develop nephrolithiasis during therapy which maintains blood calcium only at low normal concentration. Excessive urinary calcium excretion is typically not seen in pseudohypoparathyroidism. Vitamin D intoxication may develop without any apparent change in a dosage of vitamin D and calcium that has been optimal for several years. If hypercalcemia occurs, the long duration of action of vitamin D may result in persistence of hypercalcemia for weeks after the vitamin D has been discontinued. Despite these potential complications, most patients with hypoparathyroidism can be adequately regulated; complications can be avoided if the effects of therapy are continually monitored by frequent determinations of urinary as well as blood calcium concentration.

A practical approach to the chronic treatment of hypoparathyroidism at present involves initial use of less expensive agents with careful attention to complications and the use of newer, more expensive analogues of vitamin D only if more conventional measures prove inadequate. Vitamin D is given, usually as ergocalciferol (vitamin D_2), in a dose of 50,000 to 100,000 units per day; several grams of additional elemental calcium as citrate, lactate, or gluconate are usually provided (calcium lactate contains 13 percent calcium). Appropriate adjustments in dosage are made to achieve a blood calcium of 8.5 to 9.0 mg/dl; it is important to appreciate that often weeks are required before the full effects of an increased dose of vitamin D are manifest. Patients should be seen at frequent intervals, particularly when dose schedules are initially established or readjusted; blood and urine calcium estimations provide the early clues to excessive or inadequate dosage of vitamin D.

Dihydrotachysterol (DHT) or the 1α-hydroxylated active metabolites of vitamin D are theoretically preferable to vitamin D alone because of the defective activity of the renal 1α-hydroxylase in states of hypoparathyroidism or parathyroid hormone resistance (as discussed in Chap. 340 on the metabolism of vitamin D). If a patient is unusually resistant to vitamin D and, therefore, difficult to maintain symptom-free, if the therapeutic margin between hypocalcemia and hypercalciuria in a given patient is excessively narrow, or if one or more episodes of vitamin D intoxication have occurred, dihydrotachysterol in doses of 1.0 to 1.5 mg per day, or 1α,25-$(OH)_2D_3$ in doses of 0.25 to 1.0 μg per day, may be substituted for vitamin D.

In general, it can be concluded that satisfactory maintenance of mineral ion deficits can be achieved in hypoparathyroid subjects with supplemental calcium plus vitamin D or vitamin D analogues. However, vitamin D is not a perfect substitute for parathyroid hormone, particularly in view of different effects on renal calcium conservation and the higher requirement for vitamin D in parathyroid deficiency. Hence all patients with hypoparathyroidism, particularly idiopathic or postsurgical hypoparathyroidism, must be reexamined at appropriate intervals of 6 months to 1 year to ensure adequate treatment schedules and particularly to detect complications, hypercalciuria, or onset of more severe vitamin D intoxication.

REFERENCES

Anast CS et al: Impaired release of parathyroid hormone in magnesium deficiency. J Clin Endocrinol Metab 42:707, 1976

Bell NH et al: Evidence that increased circulating 1α,25-dihydroxyvitamin D is the probable cause for abnormal calcium metabolism in sarcoidosis. J Clin Invest 64:218, 1979

Broadus AE: Nephrogenous cyclic AMP. Recent Progr Horm Res, 37:667, 1981

Drezner M et al: Pseudohypoparathyroidism type II: A possible defect in the reception of the cyclic AMP signal. N Engl J Med 289:1056, 1973

Farfel Z et al: Defect of receptor-cyclase coupling protein in pseudohypoparathyroidism. N Engl J Med 303:237, 1980

Habener JF, Potts JT Jr: Parathyroid physiology and primary hyperparathyroidism, in *Metabolic Bone Disease,* LV Avioli, SM Krane (eds). New York, Academic, 1978, vol II, p 1

Heath H III et al: Primary hyperparathyroidism: Incidence, morbidity, and potential economic impact in a community. N Engl J Med 302:189, 1980

Levine MA et al: Deficient activity of guanine nucleotide regulatory protein in erythrocytes from patients with pseudohypoparathyroidism. Biochem Biophys Res Commun 94:1319, 1980

Nagant De Deuxchaisnes C et al: Dissociation of parathyroid hormone bioactivity and immunoreactivity in pseudohypoparathyroidism type I. J Clin Endocrinol Metab 53:1105, 1981

———, Krane SM: Hypoparathyroidism, in *Metabolic Bone Disease,* LV Avioli, SM Krane (eds). New York, Academic, 1978, vol II, p 218

Neer RM, Potts JT Jr: Medical management of hypercalcemia and hyperparathyroidism, in *Endocrinology,* LJ DeGroot et al (eds). New York, Grune & Stratton, 1979, vol II, p 725

Parfitt AM: Surgical, idiopathic, and other varieties of parathyroid hormone-deficient hypoparathyroidism, in *Endocrinology,* LJ DeGroot et al (eds). New York, Grune & Stratton, 1979, vol II, p 755

Raisz LG et al: Comparison of commercially available parathyroid hormone immunoassays in the differential diagnosis of hypercalcemia due to primary hyperparathyroidism or malignancy. Ann Intern Med 91:739, 1979

Rude RK et al: Parathyroid hormone secretion in magnesium deficiency. J Clin Endocrinol Metab 47:800, 1978

Stewart AF et al: Biochemical evaluation of patients with cancer-associated hypercalcemia. N Engl J Med 303:1377, 1980

340 VITAMIN D

MICHAEL F. HOLICK
JOHN T. POTTS, JR.

Vitamin D is a hormone, not a vitamin. With adequate sunlight, no dietary supplements are needed. The active principle of vitamin D is synthesized under metabolic control via successive hydroxylations in the liver and kidney and is transported through the blood to its target tissues (the small intestine and bone) to help maintain calcium homeostasis. Calcium and phosphate ions, parathyroid hormone (PTH), and possibly other peptide and steroid hormones play major roles directly or indirectly in the regulation of the renal metabolism of vitamin D. Analysis of the physiological control of vitamin D metabolism and studies of hereditary and acquired defects in these metabolic processes have provided new insights into the pathophysiology of several disorders involving calcium, phosphorus, and bone metabolism. These discoveries have made possible several advances, including the chemical synthesis of new vitamin D metabolites and analogues, the clinical use of 1α,25-dihydroxyvitamin D_3 [1α,25-$(OH)_2D_3$] in many vitamin D–resistant disorders, the development and application of assays for measuring vitamin D metabolites in blood to define suspected abnormalities in vitamin D metabolism, and a growing interest in developing more potent analogues for clinical use.

CHEMISTRY AND NOMENCLATURE OF VITAMIN D Vitamin D is a derivative of $\Delta^{5,7}$-diene steroids. [The Δ represents a double bond, the location(s) of which is indicated by the superscript number(s).] Upon exposure to ultraviolet radiation, the cutaneous steroid precursor of vitamin D_3 (7-dehydrocholesterol, *provitamin D_3*) undergoes a photochemical reaction that results in the cleavage of a C—C bond between C_9 and C_{10}, thereby opening ring B to generate a 9,10-secosteroid, *previtamin D_3* (Fig. 340-1). Previtamin D_3, a thermally labile intermediate, undergoes a molecular rearrangement involving its conjugated triene system (three double bonds) to a thermally stable 9,10-secosteroid, vitamin D_3 (Fig. 340-1).

Historically, the subscripts for vitamin D are related to the order in which the compounds were isolated and characterized. What was originally called vitamin D_1 was found to be a mixture of compounds, and the term was consequently dropped. The next two vitamin D compounds, vitamin D_2 (ergocalciferol) and vitamin D_3 (cholecalciferol), were isolated, respectively, from the irradiation products of ergosterol (a $\Delta^{5,7}$-diene steroid found primarily in plants) and 7-dehydrocholesterol (a

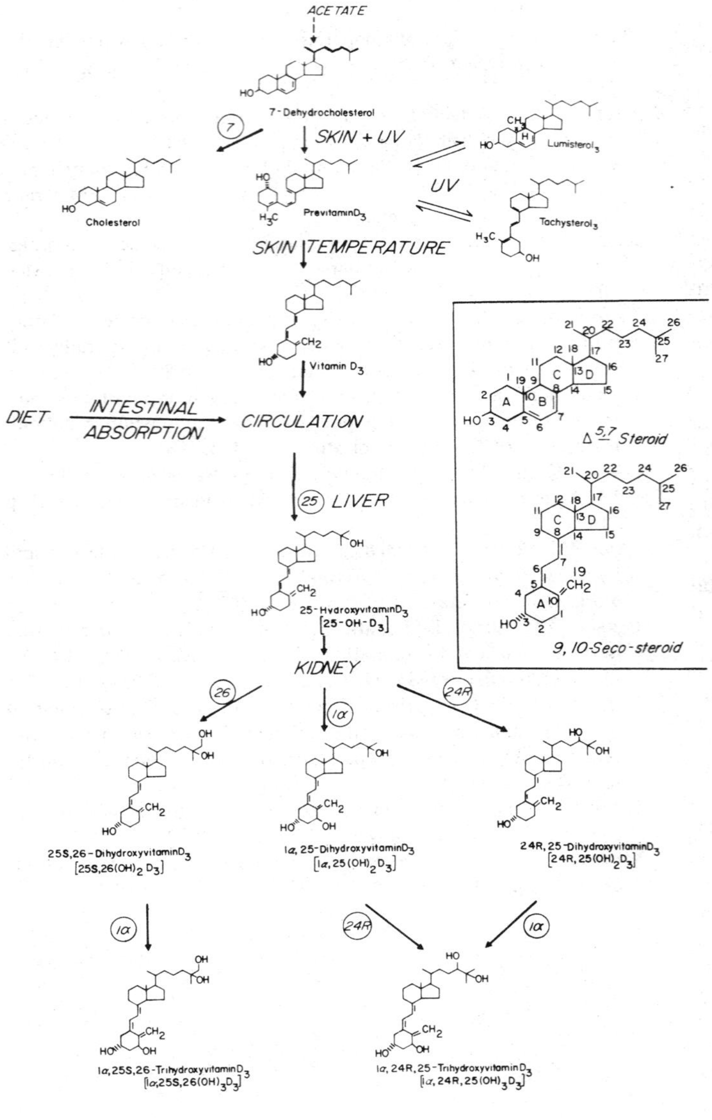

FIGURE 340-1
Photobiogenesis and metabolic pathways for vitamin D production and metabolism. Circled letters and numbers denote specific enzymes: ⑦ = 7-dehydrocholesterol reductase; ㉕ = vitamin D-25-hydroxylase; (1α) = 25-OH-D-1α-hydroxylase; 24R = 25-OH-D-24R-hydroxylase; ㉖ = 25-OH-D-26-hydroxylase. The insert denotes the basic $\Delta^{5,7}$-diene steroid and 9,10-secosteroid structures and nomenclature. In steroid nomenclature, substituents on the steroid ring skeleton that are spatially oriented below the plane of the molecule (drawn as a broken line) are called α *substituents, and those substituents spatially oriented above the plane of the molecule (drawn as a solid line) are called* β *substituents. Because vitamin D is a structural derivative of a $\Delta^{5,7}$-diene steroid, by convention the numbering of the carbon atoms and the stereochemical designation of the functional groups remain the same as for the parent steroid. During the transformation $\Delta^{5,7}$-diene → previtamin D → vitamin D, the geometric position of ring A is altered, thereby changing the stereochemical orientation of its substituents; nonetheless, the original designation(s) of the hydroxyl function(s) on ring A of the steroid precursor are retained. The R,S notation, as in 24R,25-dihydroxyvitamin D_3 specifies the spatial configuration of a substituent at an asymmetric carbon center (see Bell for details).*

$\Delta^{5,7}$-diene steroid precursor of cholesterol present in animal tissues, including human). The only structural difference between vitamins D_2 and D_3 is in their side chains; the side chain for vitamin D_2 differs in that it contains a Δ^{22} and a C_{24}-methyl group. Even though vitamin D_3 is the only endogenous form of vitamin D in human skin, both vitamins D_2 and D_3 are metabolized identically and have equivalent biological potency in most mammals; in the absence of a subscript the term *vitamin D* may refer to either compound.

When vitamin D is chemically manipulated to rotate the A ring through 180°, the C_3-β-OH assumes a geometric position that mimics the C_1-α-OH (Fig. 340-2). These compounds, called *pseudo-1α-hydroxyvitamin D analogues,* include dihydrotachysterol and 5,6-*trans*-vitamin D_3. These analogues are less effective in stimulating intestinal calcium transport on a weight basis than either vitamin D or 1α,25-$(OH)_2D_3$ when vitamin D metabolism is normal. However, because these pseudo-1α-hydroxyvitamin D analogues do not require a renal 1α-hydroxylation to be active on intestinal calcium transport, they are at least 3 to 10 times more potent than vitamin D in disease states that adversely affect the renal 25-hydroxyvitamin D 1α-hydroxylase, such as hypoparathyroidism and chronic renal failure. These pseudo-1α-hydroxy analogues are efficiently metabolized in the liver to their corresponding 25-hydroxy derivatives, which are the biologically active forms. 1α-Hydroxyvitamin D_3 (1α-OH-D_3) is a potent 1α,25-$(OH)_2D_3$ agonist. The structure of this analogue is identical to that of the renal hormone with the exception that it lacks a C_{25}-OH (Fig. 340-2). In humans, this analogue is rapidly metabolized by the liver to 1α,25-$(OH)_2D_3$, the biologically active molecule.

FIGURE 340-2
When vitamin D is treated with I_2 or reduced with H_2, ring A of the vitamin D molecule rotates 180° to reorient spatially the 3β-OH in a pseudo-1α-OH position. These analogues, 5,6-trans-vitamin D_3 and dihydrotachysterol$_3$ (DHT_3), are called pseudo-1α-hydroxy analogues. 1α-OH-D_3 is a synthetic analogue of 1α,25-$(OH)_2D_3$ that lacks a C_{25}-OH. 1α-OH-D_3, 5,6-trans-vitamin D_3, and DHT_3 all undergo a hepatic C_{25}-hydroxylation before they are biologically active.

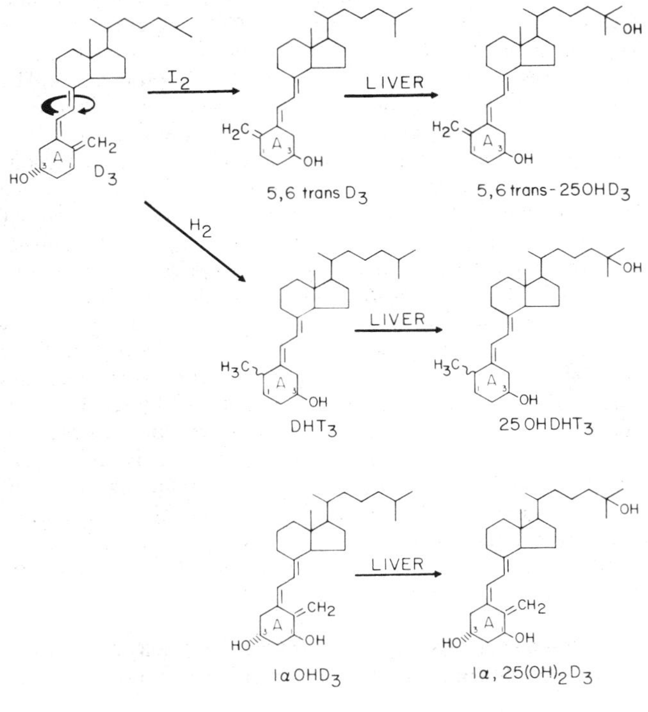

BIOCHEMISTRY, PHYSIOLOGY, AND METABOLISM OF VITAMIN D **Photobiogenesis of vitamin D_3** When skin is exposed to sunlight, the ultraviolet radiation energy that passes through the atmospheric ozone layer (between wavelengths ~ 290 and 320 nm) is responsible for the photochemical conversion of epidermal stores of 7-dehydrocholesterol (provitamin D_3) to previtamin D_3. Previtamin D_3 slowly converts to vitamin D_3 by a temperature-dependent process that takes approximately 48 h; small changes in the skin temperature have little effect on this reaction. This unique process ensures that vitamin D_3 is continuously made in the skin from the previtamin for days after sun exposure (Fig. 340-1). Although melanin in the skin competes with 7-dehydrocholesterol for ultraviolet photons and thus can limit the synthesis of previtamin D_3, the photochemical isomerization of previtamin D_3 to two biologically inert products (lumisterol$_3$ and tachysterol$_3$) appears to be more important for preventing excessive production of previtamin D_3 during prolonged exposure to the sun. Only when skin irradiation is limited and insufficient to produce required quantities of vitamin D_3 is there a need for dietary supplementation to prevent skeletal mineralization defects. Fish-liver oils are a natural source of vitamin D_3 and were used widely for the treatment of rickets early in this century. Now crystalline vitamin D_2 or vitamin D_3 is added to various foodstuffs such as milk, milk products, and cereals. Such supplementations have been effective in preventing rickets in countries that permit them. The daily requirement for vitamin D in adults has not been established; the National Research Council of the United States has recommended an intake of 400 IU per day (1 IU = 0.025 μg). Once vitamin D enters the circulation, either by its absorption in the small intestine from the diet or through the skin, it is transported through the circulation by a specific transport protein, an alpha$_1$ globulin, to the liver for its first hydroxylation.

Metabolism of vitamin D In the liver, vitamin D is metabolized to 25-hydroxyvitamin D (25-OH-D) by hepatic mitochondrial and/or microsomal enzyme(s), vitamin D-25-hydroxylase(s) (Fig. 340-1). 25-OH-D is one of the major circulating metabolites of vitamin D. The concentration of 25-OH-D in the circulation, as with other metabolites of vitamin D, is measured by competitive binding assays in which displacement of radioactive 25-OH-D from binding sites on the plasma transport protein or tissue receptor is used to quantitate 25-OH-D in serum samples. Estimates of the concentration of this metabolite vary somewhat among laboratories; however, there is general agreement that the concentration of 25-OH-D is greater than 5 ng/ml and less than 80 ng/ml. Assays using prior chromatographic separation techniques give lower estimates, perhaps because other vitamin D metabolites may simulate the reaction given by 25-OH-D in this assay. The normal range, apparently independent of method, is lower in Great Britain than in the United States; in Great Britain dietary supplementation with vitamin D is not used, and exposure to sunlight is less than in many regions of the United States. The serum 25-OH-D levels routinely measured reflect both 25-OH-D_2 and 25-OH-D_3. The ratio of these two 25-hydroxylated derivatives depends on the relative amounts of vitamins D_2 or D_3 present in the diet and upon the amount of previtamin D_3 that is produced by exposure to sunlight. It was initially believed that this hepatic hydroxylation was regulated by a product feedback mechanism in such a way that 25-OH-D levels were closely controlled. Now it is clear that this reaction is not tightly regulated; an increase in dietary intake or endogenous production of vitamin D is reflected by elevations in 25-OH-D levels in the serum. The levels can rise to greater than 500 ng/ml when the intake of vitamin D is increased markedly. Serum

25-OH-D levels are reduced in severe chronic parenchymal and cholestatic liver disease.

25-OH-D is not considered biologically active at physiological levels in vivo, but it can be shown to be active in vitro at high concentrations. Normally, after formation in the liver 25-OH-D is bound by the high-affinity vitamin D–binding protein of plasma and is transported to the kidney for an additional stereospecific hydroxylation on either C_1 or C_{24} (Fig. 340-1). The kidney plays a pivotal role in the metabolism of 25-OH-D to biologically active metabolites. The renal mitochondrial 25-OH-D-1α-hydroxylase activity is enhanced by hypocalcemia so that the rate of conversion of 25-OH-D to 1α,25-$(OH)_2$D increases. However, hypocalcemia may not directly control this hydroxylation. Any decrease in the serum calcium level below normal is a stimulus for increased secretion of parathyroid hormone (PTH). In addition to acting on mineral metabolism in the bone and kidney (see Chap. 338), PTH also acts physiologically as a tropic hormone to increase the synthesis of 1α,25-$(OH)_2$D in the renal proximal convoluted tubule. The mechanism by which PTH exerts its influence on the renal metabolism of 25-OH-D is not established; however, the bulk of the available data in humans and animals suggests that the renal production of 1α,25-$(OH)_2$D is closely correlated with the effects of PTH on phosphate metabolism. 1α,25-$(OH)_2$D also influences the renal metabolism of 25-OH-D by diminishing 25-OH-D-1α-hydroxylase activity and enhancing the metabolism of 25-OH-D to 24R,25-dihydroxyvitamin D [24,25-$(OH)_2$D].

24,25-$(OH)_2$D is a circulating metabolite of 25-OH-D that is normally present in serum at concentrations of about 0.5 to 5.0 ng/ml. 24,25-$(OH)_2$D is also a substrate for the renal 25-OH-D-1α-hydroxylase and is converted to 1α,24,25-trihydroxyvitamin D [1α,24,25-$(OH)_3$D]. This trihydroxy metabolite is less potent than 1α,25-$(OH)_2$D in stimulating intestinal calcium transport; whether it has a physiological role in maintaining calcium homeostasis is unclear. The kidney is not the only organ that converts 25-OH-D to 24,25-$(OH)_2$D; cartilage and chondrocyte cultures also metabolize 25-OH-D to 24,25-$(OH)_2$D. 24,25-$(OH)_2$D is equally as potent as 1α,25-$(OH)_2$D in stimulating chondrocyte protein synthesis in vitro, and reports indicate that 24,25-$(OH)_2$D has preferential effects on bone mineralization in a vitamin D–deficient animal model compared with 1α,25-$(OH)_2$D. There are also data to indicate that 24,25-$(OH)_2$D stimulates intestinal calcium absorption in human subjects without increasing renal calcium excretion; these effects, however, are different from those seen with 1α,25-$(OH)_2$D. These observations have led some authors to speculate that 24,25-$(OH)_2$D may play an important role in the expression of vitamin D action, especially on the skeleton; others remain skeptical about the biological importance of 24,25-$(OH)_2$D per se as distinct from actions resulting from its conversion to 1α,24,25-$(OH)_3$D.

The kidney also possesses a third enzyme that metabolizes 25-OH-D to form 25S,26-dihydroxyvitamin D [25,26-$(OH)_2$D]. 25,26-$(OH)_2$D, like 24,25-$(OH)_2$D, is metabolized by the kidney to a metabolite believed to be 1α,25S,26-trihydroxyvitamin D. 25,26-$(OH)_2$D is less active than 1α,25-$(OH)_2$D in inducing intestinal calcium transport, and the physiological function of this dihydroxy metabolite, if any, remains to be defined.

1α,25-$(OH)_2$D is a substrate for the 25-OH-D-24R-hydroxylase and is metabolized to 1α,24,25-$(OH)_3$D, but this conversion is not believed to be important for the expression of biological activity of 1α,25-$(OH)_2$D. Recently, attention has been focused on the metabolic cleavage of the side chain of 1α,25-$(OH)_2$D. These efforts have led to the identification of a 1α,25-$(OH)_2$D metabolite that was formed by an oxidative cleavage of the side chain at C_{23}—C_{24} and is called 1α-hydroxytetranorvitamin D 23-carboxylic acid. The biological function(s), if any, for this metabolite likewise remains to be determined.

Physiology of vitamin D 1α,25-$(OH)_2$D, which is produced by the kidney and also by the placenta during pregnancy, is the only clearly established biologically important form of vitamin D; the potential role of other metabolites remains to be clarified. 1α,25-$(OH)_2$D bound to a vitamin D–binding protein (which may be identical to the transport protein that binds 25-OH-D) is delivered to the intestine, where it is efficiently taken up by specific cytoplasmic receptor proteins to stimulate calcium and phosphate transport from the intestinal lumen into the circulation. Cytoplasmic receptors for 1α,25-$(OH)_2D_3$ have also been discovered in bone cells as well as in tissues that have not classically been recognized as target organs for this hormone, including skin, breast, pituitary glands, parathyroid glands, and beta-islet cells of the pancreas; the physiological importance of these receptors is unknown. Under physiological conditions the action of 1α,25-$(OH)_2$D is believed to be synergistic with that of PTH on bone resorption; effects on bone resorption, of 1α,25-$(OH)_2$D at physiological concentrations independent of PTH are still not clarified. However, like PTH, 1α,25-$(OH)_2$D can independently mobilize bone mineral at supraphysiological levels. Whether 1α,25-$(OH)_2$D has any direct effect on the renal handling of calcium and phosphorus also remains unsettled.

Serum vitamin D and 25-OH-D levels change seasonally and as a function of vitamin D intake. Serum 1α,25-$(OH)_2$D levels, however, appear to be unaltered by seasonal variation, by increases in dietary vitamin D, or by exposure to sunlight; as long as vitamin D supplies and 25-OH-D levels are sufficient, metabolic influences operate on the renal 25-OH-D-1α-hydroxylase to provide a closely regulated circulating concentration of 1α,25-$(OH)_2$D. Estimates of the serum concentration of 1α,25-$(OH)_2$D by several laboratories are in close agreement; values reported range from 25 to 75 pg/ml. The serum half-life of 1α,25-$(OH)_2$D is estimated to be about 3 to 6 h.

Whenever the serum calcium drops below normal, PTH secretion is enhanced; this increased concentration, by mechanisms still unclear, increases the production of 1α,25-$(OH)_2$D. The principal physiological regulation of the production of 1α,25-$(OH)_2$D appears to involve changes in serum calcium levels with reciprocal changes in the PTH secretion rate, the latter controlling, possibly through actions on serum or tissue phosphorus levels, the rate of 1α,25-$(OH)_2$D production. The possible role of hormones and metabolic factors other than PTH on 1α,25-$(OH)_2$D production has been examined, so far, principally in laboratory animals. These studies have demonstrated that estrogen, prolactin, and growth hormone enhance the production of 1α,25-$(OH)_2$D. Humans, as well as other mammals, adapt to increased calcium requirements during growth, pregnancy, and lactation by increasing the efficiency of intestinal calcium absorption; effects on the renal (or placental) 25-OH-D1α-hydroxylase by estrogen, prolactin, and/or growth hormone may prove to be the mediators of these physiological changes in calcium absorption. Most measurements of the circulating concentration of 1α,25-$(OH)_2$D in humans in various physiological or pathophysiological states are based on studies using competitive binding assays in a small number of subjects; data are sometimes conflicting. More information on larger numbers of patients using techniques to measure production and clearance rates of 1α,25-$(OH)_2$D is needed to assess the importance of factors other than PTH on vitamin D metabolism. (See Table 340-1.)

PATHOPHYSIOLOGY OF DISORDERS OF VITAMIN D METABOLISM **Hypovitaminosis D** Inadequate endogenous production of vitamin D_3 in the skin, insufficient dietary supplementation, and/or the inability of the small intestine to absorb adequate amounts of vitamin D from the diet can cause hypovitaminosis D. Disease states equivalent to hypovitaminosis D are caused by (1) drugs that antagonize vitamin D action, (2) alteration in the metabolism of vitamin D, or (3) inadequate response of tissue receptors to vitamin D metabolites.

The pathophysiological consequences of hypovitaminosis D or equivalent disease states are twofold: (1) disturbances in mineral ion metabolism and PTH secretion and (2) mineralization defects in the skeleton (e.g., rickets in children, osteomalacia in adults). Details of these pathophysiological changes, especially on the skeleton, are described in Chap. 341. With regard to calcium metabolism, lack of vitamin D action leads to deficient calcium absorption and eventual hypocalcemia. The latter is accompanied by a compensatory secondary hyperparathyroidism; the increased secretion of PTH and enhanced actions of the hormone (Chap. 339) in causing calcium release via bone resorption and in promoting renal calcium conservation tend to blunt the severity of the hypocalcemia. (Late in the course of otherwise untreated hypovitaminosis D, severe hypocalcemia develops.) Hypophosphatemia is more marked than hypocalcemia, especially in early stages of vitamin D lack. The efficiency of phosphate absorption, like that of calcium absorption, falls with severe vitamin D deficiency or its equivalent state. The increased secretion of parathyroid hormone, although partially effective in minimizing hypocalcemia, leads to severe urinary phosphate wasting. This latter effect may be quantitatively the most significant factor in causing hypophosphatemia. With adequate renal function, the predominant changes in blood chemical values are *severe hypophosphatemia, moderate hypocalcemia* or low-normal blood calcium, and *increased PTH levels.* Blood *25-OH-D levels* are *low.* As discussed in Chap. 341 severe defects in skeletal mineralization accompany these disturbances in mineral ion metabolism.

Although the conversion of vitamin D to 25-OH-D is impaired to varying degrees in chronic, severe cholestatic or parenchymal liver disease, there is no strong correlation between low serum 25-OH-D levels and the development of osteopenia; multiple effects of the primary disease state seem to affect skeletal metabolism as well. A relation between *chronic anticonvulsant therapy* and the development of osteopenia has been well established in Great Britain and the United States; the problem is worse in patients on multiple drug therapy and when vitamin D intake or exposure to sunlight is minimal. It was initially believed that anticonvulsant drugs induced hepatic microsomal enzymes which metabolized vitamin D and 25-OH-D into inactive products. However, these drugs have multiple and complex effects on calcium metabolism. Phenobarbital induces hepatic microsomal enzymes and stimulates bile secretion, both of which have the net effect of decreasing serum vitamin D and 25-OH-D levels. Both phenytoin and phenobarbital influence calcium metabolism by directly inhibiting intestinal calcium transport and bone mineral mobilization.

TABLE 340-1
Serum 1α,25-$(OH)_2$D levels in disorders of calcium and phosphorus metabolism

Disease states	*Serum 1α,25-$(OH)_2D$*
Vitamin D deficiency	↓*
Renal failure:	
GFR > 30 (ml/min)/1.7 m^2	↓ or N
GFR < 30 (ml/min)/1.7 m^2	↓
Hypoparathyroidism	↓ or N
Pseudohypoparathyroidism	↓ or N
Vitamin D–dependent rickets:	
Type I	↓
Type II	N or ↑
X-linked vitamin D–resistant rickets	↓ or N
Tumor-induced osteomalacia	↓ or N
Hyperparathyroidism	↑
Idiopathic hypercalciuria	N or ↑
Sarcoidosis	N or ↑
Tumor hypercalcemia	N or ↓
Vitamin D intoxication	↓ or N

* *It should be noted that serum 1α,25-$(OH)_2D$ concentrations have been found to be normal or even elevated in occasional patients with biopsy-proven osteomalacia and undetectable or low circulating concentrations of 25-OH-D. These patients also have secondary hyperparathyroidism, and it may be that they represent a partially treated state; if a small amount of vitamin D is obtained from the diet or generated in the skin in these patients, the vitamin is efficiently converted to 1α,25-$(OH)_2D$. The net effect is low or undetectable circulating concentrations of 25-OH-D along with normal or elevated concentrations of 1α,25-$(OH)_2D$. However, in extreme vitamin D deficiency, circulating concentrations of 1α,25-$(OH)_2D$ are low or undetectable.*

NOTE: *↓=decreased; N=normal; ↑=increased; GFR=glomerular filtration rate.*

Glucocorticoids used in high doses for suppression of various inflammatory disorders are known to cause disturbances in calcium metabolism and osteopenia, although osteomalacia and rickets per se are not a consequence of glucocorticoid therapy. Like anticonvulsant drugs, actions of glucocorticoids on vitamin D–mediated calcium metabolism are complex and include a direct inhibitory effect on vitamin D–mediated intestinal calcium absorption and bone mineral mobilization and an enhancement of the sensitivity of 1α,25-$(OH)_2D_3$ on bone cells either by stabilizing its receptor or by increasing the affinity or number of receptors for this hormone. Patients receiving chronic glucocorticoid therapy have been reported to have depressed serum 1α,25-$(OH)_2$D levels; the mechanism(s) for this is unknown.

A genetic defect in the hepatic 25-hydroxylation of vitamin D has not been described. However, one heritable disorder of calcium and bone metabolism may involve a defect in renal production of 1α,25-$(OH)_2$D. In the syndrome of *pseudovitamin D–deficient rickets* (also known as *vitamin D–dependent rickets, type I;* see Chap. 341), *low* serum 1α,25-$(OH)_2$D levels and a therapeutic response to physiological doses of 1α,25-$(OH)_2$D (0.25 to 1.0 μg/dl) have been attributed to an inherited deficiency in renal 25-OH-D-1α-hydroxylase activity. In addition, there have been a few reports of patients with a similar phenotype, *pseudovitamin D–resistant rickets* (*vitamin D–dependent rickets, type II*), whose defect appears to be due to *a lack of a (or a defective) 1α,25-$(OH)_2D$ cytoplasmic receptor* rather than defective metabolism of the vitamin. These latter patients have *high serum 1α,25-$(OH)_2D$* levels; therapeutic response to high-dose vitamin D was noted in association with a further increase in the serum 1α,25-$(OH)_2$D levels.

Current reports disagree concerning findings in patients with *X-linked hypophosphatemic rickets;* normal values of serum 1α,25-$(OH)_2$D have been reported in one series, and low values have been reported in another. Since hypophosphatemia is a potent stimulus for the renal 25-OH-D-1α-hydroxylase, in X-linked hypophosphatemic patients with severe hypophosphatemia the serum 1α,25-$(OH)_2$D levels should be high. Thus, even a normal serum 1α,25-$(OH)_2$D level suggests a functional defect in the 25-OH-D-1α-hydroxylase system. It is unclear whether physiological doses of 1α,25-$(OH)_2$D or high doses of vitamin D offer any therapeutic advantage to that seen with phosphate therapy alone (Chap. 341).

In patients with mild to moderate chronic renal failure (glomerular filtration rate > 30 ml/min) with phosphate retention, hyperphosphatemia and acidosis play important roles in suppressing the renal production of 1,25-$(OH)_2$D despite high levels of PTH. As the destruction of the renal cortex progresses, there is a depletion in the renal reserves of the 25-OH-D-1α-hydroxylase to a point at which the kidney is unable to produce sufficient quantities of 1α,25-$(OH)_2$D to maintain calcium homeostasis, even when serum phosphate levels are normal. Under these circumstances replacement therapy with 1α,25-$(OH)_2D$ or one of its analogues is most beneficial (Chap. 341).

Patients with *hypoparathyroidism* and *pseudohypoparathyroidism* have mean serum levels of 1α,25-$(OH)_2D$ that are lower than normal, although there is overlap in individual values with the normal range. In these hypocalcemic patients favorable responses to small replacement doses of 1α,25-$(OH)_2D$ (0.25 to 1.0 μg per day; see Chap. 339), including increases in serum calcium, are seen at a time when the serum 25-OH-D levels are higher than normal. These observations are consistent with the concept that patients with hypoparathyroidism or pseudohypoparathyroidism due to absent or ineffective action of PTH have defective function of renal 25-OH-D-1α-hydroxylase. It is not clear to what extent serum 1α,25-$(OH)_2D$ levels would be restored toward normal if the hyperphosphatemia in these diseases was controlled.

Hypervitaminosis D Vitamin D intoxication occurs after chronic oral ingestion of large doses of vitamin D_2 or D_3 (usually in excess of 50,000 to 100,000 IU daily) for months. In such circumstances, the excessive quantities of ingested vitamin are stored in body fat and released slowly into the bloodstream. Hypervitaminosis D as a result of prolonged sun exposure has not been reported, presumably because of protective mechanisms that include slow release of vitamin D_3 from skin after conversion from previtamin D_3, photoisomerization of previtamin D_3 to lumisterol$_3$ and tachysterol$_3$, skin pigment, and perhaps other still-unrecognized regulatory controls. The consequences of excessive vitamin D action are *hypercalcemia* and *hypercalciuria;* blood phosphate levels are variable but usually normal. In severe, unrecognized, or untreated vitamin D intoxication, the Ca $\times$ P product exceeds the solubility product, and widespread ectopic calcification results, especially in the kidneys, causing renal failure. A marked elevation of serum 25-OH-D levels (usually greater than 100 ng/ml) is found. Because anephric patients who do not synthesize 1α,25-$(OH)_2D$ can be intoxicated with vitamin D, it is believed that high circulating levels of 25-OH-D or other metabolites of vitamin D can directly stimulate intestinal calcium absorption and bone mineral mobilization without undergoing further metabolism. The fact that serum 1α,25-$(OH)_2D$ levels are low to normal rather than elevated in patients with hypervitaminosis D is consistent with this observation.

In some circumstances cessation of the vitamin D ingestion and lowering of oral calcium intake leads to rapid disappearance of the hypercalcemia. On the other hand hypercalcemia may persist for weeks to months after vitamin D ingestion is stopped. Under such circumstances, patients should be treated with a glucocorticoid such as prednisone in doses of 20 to 40 mg per day to control the hypercalcemia and to prevent irreversible renal damage and ectopic calcification. A dramatic lowering of calcium to normal levels can be accomplished within days (see Chap. 339 for diagnostic use of the glucocorticoid suppression test in hypercalcemic disorders). Other measures to treat hypercalcemia (see Chap. 339) can be used acutely in severe cases.

The clinical use of potent vitamin D metabolites and analogues for the treatment of many disorders of calcium metabolism has added a new dimension to the syndrome of vitamin D intoxication. The therapeutic index for 1α,25-$(OH)_2D_3$ is low. This is not surprising when one considers that oral administration of 1α,25-$(OH)_2D_3$ provides relatively high concentrations of the natural hormone in direct contact with its target tissue (the small intestine). More than half of the patients with renal insufficiency treated with 1α,25-$(OH)_2D_3$ in doses of 0.5 to 2 μg per day demonstrate at least transient hypercalcemia. This is quickly alleviated by decreasing the drug dosage (see Chap. 341 for details). It is not known how frequently toxicity develops when lower doses of 1α,25-$(OH)_2D_3$ are used or whether the blood assay for 1α,25-$(OH)_2D_3$ will be a useful indicator of potential toxicity.

Acute vitamin D toxicity due to a single excessive dose of vitamin D_2 or D_3 is not seen; however, one can anticipate that a single overdose of 1α,25-$(OH)_2D_3$ or a potent analogue may cause acute toxicity, including hypercalcemia and hypercalciuria. Treatment of such intoxication should include elimination of calcium from the diet, induction of emesis or gastric lavage if the overdosage is discovered within a relatively short time, and the use of cathartics. Careful monitoring of serum calcium and phosphorus levels should be maintained for at least 24 h after ingestion, and hypercalcemia, if serious, should be treated with measures directed at increasing urinary calcium excretion or blocking bone resorption (see Chap. 339). The usefulness of glucocorticoid therapy in severe toxicity due to an acute overdose of 1α,25-$(OH)_2D_3$ remains to be established.

Other acquired or hereditary disorders of vitamin D metabolism There are several reports, based on the measurement of circulating levels of 1α,25-$(OH)_2D$ in limited numbers of patients, of abnormalities in vitamin D metabolism in disease states such as osteoporosis in elderly women, tumor-induced osteomalacia, sarcoidosis, and idiopathic hypercalciuria. The nature and frequency of disturbances in vitamin D metabolism in these disorders are still uncertain because of both the small number of patients involved and inherent limitations in data provided by present assays for 1α,25-$(OH)_2D$. The assays allow only a static measurement of the serum 1α,25-$(OH)_2D$ concentration. Ultimate definition of significant differences between normal and abnormal states of 1α,25-$(OH)_2D$ production will probably require, in analogy with earlier studies of steroid hormones, formal measurements of production rates of 1α,25-$(OH)_2D$ including metabolic clearance rates. Of particular value, when and if developed, will be tests of the capacity of 1α,25-$(OH)_2D$ production and renal 25-OH-D-1α-hydroxylase reserve.

Calcium absorption is subnormal in the elderly. This may be due to the effect of age on the decreased renal responsiveness to PTH in stimulating 1α,25-$(OH)_2D$ synthesis. Intestinal absorption of calcium from the diet can be improved by treatment with 1α-OH-D_3 or 1α,25-$(OH)_2D_3$, as well as by high doses of vitamin D. Because animal studies showed that estrogen enhances the production of 1α,25-$(OH)_2D$, there has been speculation that the pathogenesis of postmenopausal osteoporosis is, in part, related to estrogen deficiency and/or an imbalance in the circulating levels of estrogens and androgens that in turn adversely influence the renal production of 1α,25-$(OH)_2D$. Serum 1α,25-$(OH)_2D$ levels have been reported to be slightly below normal in some patients with postmenopausal osteoporosis; however, the differences are small, and most values fall within the normal range. Studies are underway to evaluate the potential benefit of long-term therapy with 1α-OH-D_3 or 1α,25-$(OH)_2D_3$ in patients with senile and postmenopausal osteoporosis. Such therapy does increase intestinal calcium absorption, thereby reducing negative calcium balance; however, it remains to be determined whether 1α,25-$(OH)_2D$ deficiency is indeed present in such patients or whether the course of the bone disease is altered by treatment. There have been a few reports that patients with tumor-induced osteomalacia have low serum 1α,25-$(OH)_2D$ levels; after tumor resection, the serum 1α,25-$(OH)_2D$ levels return to normal.

In addition to hyperparathyroidism, disease states that may have enhanced 1α,25-$(OH)_2D$ production include sarcoidosis and idiopathic hypercalciuria. In sarcoidosis, the abnormal calcium metabolism, as manifested by hypercalcemia and hypercalciuria, has been attributed to abnormal sensitivity to vitamin D. During periods of hypercalcemia, 1α,25-$(OH)_2D$ levels are increased in sarcoidosis, which suggests that the apparent hypersensitivity to vitamin D seen in this disease is due to either a defect in the control of the renal production of 1α,25-$(OH)_2D$ or that there is an extrarenal site that can produce this hormone.

In many cases of idiopathic hypercalciuria, which is often familial, there is an inappropriately increased intestinal calcium absorption. Several reports indicate an elevation in 1α,25-$(OH)_2D$ levels in some of these patients, consistent with the speculation that excessive 1α,25-$(OH)_2D$ production could be responsible for the disorder in some patients.

REFERENCES

Barbour GL et al: Hypercalcemia in an anephric patient with sarcoidosis: Evidence for extrarenal generation of 1,25-dihydroxyvitamin D. N Engl J Med 305:440, 1981

Bell PA: The chemistry of the vitamins D, in *Vitamin D*, DEM Lawson (ed). London, Academic, 1978, pp 1–50

Bilezikian JP et al: Response of 1α,25-dihydroxyvitamin D_3 to hypocalcemia in human subjects. N Engl J Med 299:437, 1978

Broadus AE et al: The importance of circulating 1,25-dihydroxyvitamin D in the pathogenesis of hypercalcemia and renal stone-formation in primary hyperparathyroidism. N Engl J Med 302:421, 1981

DeLuca HF: The vitamin D system in the regulation of calcium and phosphorus metabolism. Nutr Rev 37:161, 1979

Eil C et al: A cellular defect in hereditary vitamin D–dependent rickets type II. Defective nuclear uptake of 1,25-dihydroxyvitamin D in culture skin fibroblasts. N Engl J Med 304:1588, 1981

Fieser LD, Fieser M: *Steroids.* New York, Reinhold, 1959, chap 4

Gray TK et al: Vitamin D and pregnancy: The maternal-fetal metabolism of vitamin D. Endocrinol Rev 2:264, 1981

Haussler MR, McCain BS: Basic and clinical concepts related to vitamin D metabolism and action. N Engl J Med 297:974, 1977

Holick MF: The cutaneous photosynthesis of previtamin D_3: A unique photoendocrine system. J Invest Dermatol 76:51, 1981

Scriver CR et al: Serum 1,25-dihydroxyvitamin D levels in normal subjects and in patients with hereditary rickets or bone disease. N Engl J Med 299:976, 1978

Slovik DM et al: Deficient production of 1,25-dihydroxyvitamin D in elderly osteoporotic patients. N Engl J Med 305:372, 1981

341 METABOLIC BONE DISEASE

STEPHEN M. KRANE
MICHAEL F. HOLICK

OSTEOPOROSIS

GENERAL CONSIDERATIONS *Osteoporosis* is the term used for a group of diseases of diverse etiology which are characterized by a reduction in the mass of bone per unit volume to a level below that required for adequate mechanical support function. The reduction in mass is not accompanied by a significant reduction in the ratio of the mineral to the organic phase, nor by any reproducible abnormality in the structure of either the mineral or the organic matrix. Histologically, osteoporosis is characterized by a decrease in cortical thickness and in the number and size of the trabeculae of cancellous bone with normal width of the osteoid seams. Osteoporosis is the commonest of the metabolic bone diseases (disorders in which all the skeleton is involved, presumably as a result of systemic factors acting on the skeleton) and is an important cause of morbidity in elderly subjects.

The remodeling of bone (its formation and resorption) is a continuous process throughout life. Any combination of changes in the rates of formation and resorption which results in bone resorption exceeding bone formation could therefore cause a decrease in bone mass. In osteoporosis the bone mass *is* decreased, indicating that the rate of bone resorption must exceed that of bone formation. Although osteoporosis is a heterogeneous disorder, in most studies formation rate is normal, although low rates are sometimes found. Current evidence suggests that, in normal individuals for many years after closure of the epiphyses and after longitudinal growth has ceased, skeletal mass remains constant and the rates of bone formation and resorption are relatively low and approximately equal. Resorption and formation of bone are normally tightly coupled. However, the rate of remodeling is not uniform throughout the skeleton after epiphyseal closure. Most of the bone surfaces are "inactive" and not involved at any given time either in formation or resorption. It has been proposed that formation and resorption are coupled in space as "remodeling units." Resorption areas are covered by osteoclasts if active; bone formation surfaces are characterized by the presence of osteoid seams and are covered by active osteoblasts. Active surfaces may be randomly distributed, but formation and resorption are locally coupled as units. Resorption precedes formation and is probably more intense, but it does not last as long as formation. As a consequence, there are normally more sites of active formation than of resorption. Bone turnover is high when there are many units active and low when there are few. Unless formation compensates completely for resorption, bone mass would have to decrease. After the age of 40 to 50 skeletal mass begins to decline, at a faster rate in women than in men, and at a different rate in different parts of the skeleton. The loss has been documented quantitatively in selected regions using techniques such as photon densitometry and neutron-activation analysis. For example, the rate of loss is greater in the metacarpals, in the femoral neck, and in the vertebral bodies than in the midshaft of the femur, the tibia, and the skull. Over the next three or four decades the total loss in skeletal mass may be 30 to 50 percent of that present at age 30 or 40. Kinetic studies (using radioactive isotopes of calcium and strontium) and quantitative microradiography (which includes both cortical and cancellous bone) indicate that in most older subjects the resorption rate is high, whereas the bone formation rate remains at a level similar to that of younger adults. At some critical point if the difference between rates of formation and resorption is maintained, loss of bone substance may become so marked that the bone can no longer resist the mechanical forces to which it is subjected, and fracture results. Osteoporosis would then be evident as a clinical problem. The level of reduction in bone mass sufficient to result in fractures after minimal trauma is variable. The strength of the vertebral body may depend upon additional factors such as adequacy of ligamentous support and the age-related changes in the intervertebral disks.

In the process of remodeling of lamellar bone in adults, most of the net resorption occurs at the corticoendosteal surface. The abnormal remodeling in osteoporosis follows the same pattern; the bone loss includes cancellous bone, cortical bone at the endosteal surface, and intracortical bone, resulting in enlargement of the medullary cavity and thinning of the cortex. Since bone formation at the periosteum continues at a very slow rate, the diameter of the bone does not decrease, and the periosteal surface retains its smooth configuration. In addition, the cancellous bone also undergoes progressive resorption, with some trabeculae being resorbed at rates faster than others, particularly those vertebral trabeculae with horizontal orientation.

The cause of this age-associated decrease in bone mass and increase in bone resorption or the accelerated loss in that form of osteoporosis occurring particularly in older women after the menopause is not known. A possible role for calcitonin has been postulated in view of observations that the decrease in mass is similar in a number of different populations throughout the world. Although blacks in the United States have a lower incidence of clinically significant osteoporosis than do whites, they also have a larger initial skeletal mass, such that adequate bone could remain even in the presence of age-associated losses. Estrogens, which are often used to treat osteoporosis, tend to inhibit bone resorption and decrease the hypercalcemia of hyperparathyroidism. A possible role of estrogens in the pathogenesis has been discussed in Chaps. 118 and 340. However, there is no direct evidence of increased parathyroid hormone secretion with increasing age; most determinations of immunoreactive parathyroid hormone levels are normal. Epidemiologic surveys have shown that there is no relation between the degree of bone loss and age of onset or type of menopause. There is also no difference in the calcium intake of osteoporotic compared with control subjects of similar age and sex. Osteoporotic subjects tend to have lower body weight and muscle mass than do controls, but the significance of these findings is uncertain. No consistent changes in adrenocortical function have been documented in osteoporotics, although there are suggestions that subtle alterations in pituitary, adrenal, and gonadal functions may play a role in the production of osteoporosis. The possible role of substances that stimulate bone resorption, such as prostaglandins and osteoclast-activating factors, the latter derived from lymphocytes but modulated by monocytes, has not yet been evaluated. In patients with primary hypogonadism due to gonadal dysgenesis or pituitary failure, osteoporosis is frequently noted radiologically. This has been attributed to the failure to attain full adult skeletal mass rather than to an increased rate of bone loss associated with age.

Another factor implicated in bone loss is the possibility that excessive acid intake, particularly in the form of high-protein diets, results in "dissolution" of bone in an attempt to buffer the extra acid. Prolonged use of heparin as an anticoagulant is also associated with osteoporosis, and heparin potentiates bone resorption in vitro. Patients with osteoporosis have increased numbers of mast cells, presumably capable of producing heparin, in their bone marrow. Circumscribed and diffuse areas of osteoporosis are also seen in patients with systemic mastocytosis.

As mentioned earlier, the remodeling of bone is physiologically responsive to mechanical forces of many types. The early response to immobilization in the normal skeleton is an increase in bone resorption while bone formation remains normal or is decreased; later there is a compensatory increase in bone formation. In osteoporosis, immobilization tends to aggravate the defect by further increasing the gap between formation and resorption. It is, therefore, possible that a sedentary life in an individual with poor musculature would tend to reduce mechanical forces exerted on the skeleton and to increase the tendency to bone loss.

CLASSIFICATION In only a few forms of osteoporosis is the cause certain, such as in that associated with Cushing's syndrome, both endogenous and exogenous. Osteoporosis is also associated with a number of other disorders, but the nature of the relationship is not clear. In the majority of cases of osteoporosis the etiology is not apparent. While most of these occur in older women past the menopause (*senile* or *postmenopausal osteoporosis*), it is not certain how the osteoporosis is related to the postmenopausal state. When osteoporosis occurs in younger individuals, it is usually termed *idiopathic osteoporosis.* In fact, most of these disorders should be considered idiopathic since details of their pathogenesis are not known. A suggested classification is shown in Table 341-1.

GENERAL CLINICAL FEATURES Although osteoporosis is a generalized disorder of the skeleton, its major clinical manifestations involve the axial skeleton. Fractures of long bones are also somewhat more frequent in osteoporotic subjects than in others of similar age without osteoporosis and are most common in the hip, humerus, and wrists. The most frequent symptoms are pain in the back and deformity of the spine. Pain usually results from collapse of the vertebral bodies, especially in the lower dorsal and upper lumbar regions, is typically acute in onset, and often radiates anteriorly around the flank into various portions of the abdomen, depending upon the location of the fracture. Such episodes frequently occur after sudden bending, lifting, or jumping movements which may seem to have been trivial; on some occasions they cannot be related to trauma. The pain may be increased even with slight movements such as turning in bed or by the Valsalva maneuver. Rest in bed in one position may relieve the pain temporarily, but it then may recur in spasms of variable duration. Radiation of pain down one leg is uncommon, and symptoms or signs of spinal cord compression are very rare. The acute episodes of pain may also be accompanied by abdominal distention and ileus, thought to be due to retroperitoneal hemorrhage, but the use of narcotics at this stage also contributes to the ileus. Loss of appetite and apparent muscular weakness, which is probably due to fear of reproducing pain, may also be present. Episodes of pain usually subside after several days to a week, and by 4 to 6 weeks patients may be fully ambulatory and able to resume their normal activities. Although the acute pain may be minimal, many patients continue to have nagging, deep, dull, uncomfortable sensations localized to the area of fracture brought about by straining or sudden changes in position. They may be unable to sit up in bed and have to arise by

TABLE 341-1
Classification of osteoporosis

I Common forms of osteoporosis of unknown cause unassociated with other disease
- *A* Idiopathic osteoporosis (juvenile and adult)
- *B* Postmenopausal osteoporosis
- *C* Senile osteoporosis

II Disorders or conditions in which osteoporosis is a common feature or pathogenesis partially understood
- *A* Hypogonadism
- *B* Hyperadrenocorticism
- *C* Thyrotoxicosis
- *D* Malabsorption
- *E* Scurvy
- *F* Calcium deficiency
- *G* Immobilization
- *H* Chronic heparin administration
- *I* Systemic mastocytosis
- *J* Adult hypophosphatasia
- *K* Associated with other metabolic bone diseases

III Osteoporosis as a feature of heritable disorders of connective tissue
- *A* Osteogenesis imperfecta
- *B* Homocystinuria due to cystathionine synthase deficiency
- *C* Ehlers-Danlos syndrome
- *D* Marfan syndrome

IV Disorders in which osteoporosis is associated but pathogenesis not understood
- *A* Rheumatoid arthritis
- *B* Malnutrition
- *C* Alcoholism
- *D* Epilepsy
- *E* Diabetes
- *F* Chronic obstructive pulmonary disease
- *G* Menkes' syndrome

rolling over on their sides and then propping themselves up. Most patients have disappearance or marked diminution of pain between episodes of vertebral body collapse. Others never have acute episodes but complain of varying degrees of backache often made worse by standing or moving suddenly. Tenderness over involved areas of the spinous processes or rib cage is commonly noted. The collapse fractures of the vertebral bodies are usually anterior, producing a wedge-shaped deformity and contributing to loss in height. This is particularly common in the middorsal region where collapse may be unassociated with pain but result in a dorsal kyphosis and exaggerated cervical lordosis described as a "dowager's" or "widow's" hump. Postural slumping with increase in existing curves also contributes to the loss of height. Generalized skeletal pain is uncommon, and between fractures most patients are free even of pain localized to the spine. Although recurrent episodes of collapse fractures of vertebral bodies, increasing spine deformity, and loss of height are common in osteoporosis, the course of the disorder in any one subject is not predictable, and there may be intervals of several years between fractures.

RADIOLOGICAL FEATURES Prior to fracture and collapse the osteoporotic vertebral body shows a decrease in mineral density, an increase in prominence of vertical striations due to a relatively greater loss of the horizontally oriented trabeculae, and prominence of the end plates. The bodies may become increasingly biconcave because of weakening of the subchondral plates and expansion of the intervertebral disks, resulting in the so-called codfish vertebrae. When collapse occurs, most frequently in lower dorsal and upper lumbar spine, it usually produces a decrease in the anterior height of the vertebral body and irregularity in the anterior cortex (Fig. 341-1). Older compression fractures may show reactive changes and osteophytes about the anterior margins. Although the cortices of long bones may be thin because of excessive endosteal resorption, the outer margins are sharp in contrast to the typical effects of the subperiosteal resorption of hyperparathyroidism. Pseudofractures or Looser's zones are not present in osteoporosis without osteomalacia, but distinguishing osteoporosis from osteomalacia may be impossible on radiological grounds alone.

LABORATORY FINDINGS The concentrations of calcium and inorganic phosphorus in the blood are usually normal in patients with osteoporosis; slight hyperphosphatemia is present in women who are past the menopause. The alkaline phosphatase in uncomplicated instances is normal, although slight increases may be seen after fractures. Only about 20 percent of postmenopausal women with osteoporosis have significant hypercalciuria. Urinary excretion of peptides containing hydroxyproline, an index of bone resorption, is usually normal or slightly increased.

DIFFERENTIAL DIAGNOSIS Since decrease in skeletal mass is an age-associated finding, it is particularly difficult to evaluate asymptomatic decreased bone density in older women, especially when unaccompanied by marked increase in biconcavity of vertebral bodies or fractures. In the presence of bone pain with or without fracture or deformity, it is important to establish the presence or absence of known causes of osteoporosis as listed in Table 341-1 and to be certain that osteoporosis in the broad sense is the correct diagnosis. Malignancies of various types, particularly *multiple myeloma, lymphoma, leukemia,* and *carcinomatosis,* may result in diffuse loss of bone, especially the trabecular bone of the vertebral column, even in the absence of hypercalcemia. The absence of anemia, elevated erythrocyte sedimentation rate, abnormal electrophoretic patterns of serum proteins, and Bence Jones proteinuria is helpful in eliminating the possibility of multiple myeloma. However, needle bone biopsy or marrow aspiration is usually indicated in cases of severe osteoporosis.

Radiological osteoporosis is commonly present in patients with primary *hyperparathyroidism* who may not have specific evidence of osteitis fibrosa (discrete lytic lesions of varying size and subperiosteal resorption) or elevation of serum alkaline phosphatase. Although hyperparathyroidism could accelerate bone loss in the pattern of osteoporosis and contribute to it, it is not clear that excessive secretion of parathyroid hormone is the sole cause of the bone disease, even in these cases, rather than an associated finding. Repeated determinations of serum calcium and phosphorus levels are therefore necessary. An element of secondary hyperparathyroidism may be present in some elderly patients in whom there is impairment of renal function, inadequate oral calcium intake, or decrease of intestinal calcium absorption. Increased numbers of osteoclasts may be found in bone biopsy specimens from such patients.

Osteomalacia may mimic osteoporosis or coexist with it, yet specific radiological signs of osteomalacia may not always be present. Although the presence of abnormalities such as hypophosphatemia would suggest the possibility of osteomalacia, these too may be absent in some cases of osteomalacia, and bone biopsy may be essential for diagnosis, as discussed below. Since osteomalacia of various causes is more responsive to specific therapy than the usual case of osteoporosis, such diagnostic procedures are often warranted and provide, in addition, adequate specimens for examination for the presence of malignant cells.

FIGURE 341-1
Lateral views of the lumbar spine of a 54-year-old man with idiopathic osteoporosis. A typical anterior compression fracture is indicated by the arrow.

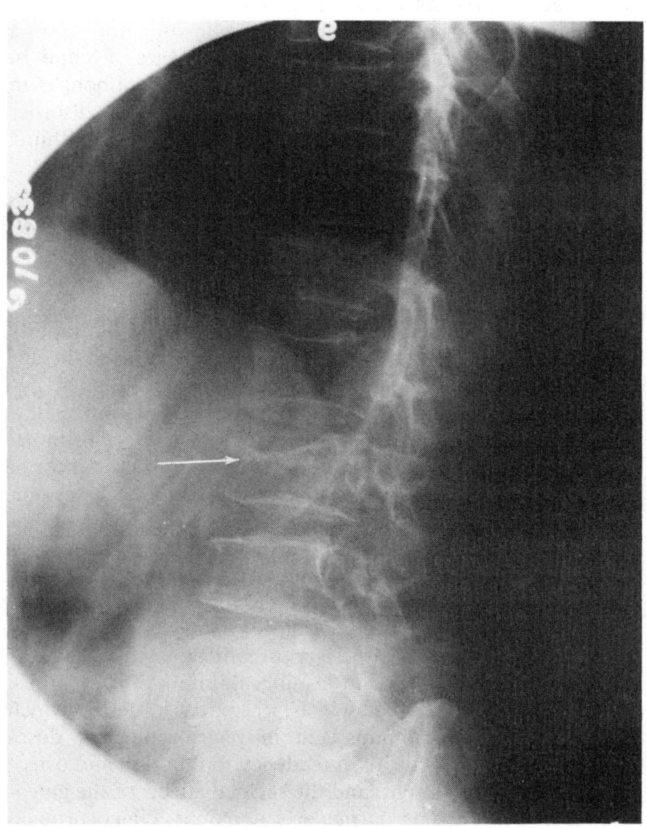

In an occasional patient with *Paget's disease* the radiological features may be almost purely lytic and be confused with osteoporosis. However, high alkaline phosphatase levels and moderately or markedly increased urinary excretion of hydroxyproline-containing peptides are clues to the presence of Paget's disease. Scanning procedures with bone-seeking isotopes are not helpful in differential diagnosis if fractures are present, because in any disease fractures demonstrate preferential uptake of isotope. However, in the absence of fracture, "hot spots" suggest presence of tumor or early Paget's disease, particularly if present in the appendicular skeleton.

IDIOPATHIC OSTEOPOROSIS Most of the comments about osteoporosis in the preceding sections are particularly pertinent to elderly patients, especially women with bone loss sufficient to produce significant symptoms. Although its ultimate cause is unknown, this type of osteoporosis is often termed *senile* or *postmenopausal. Idiopathic osteoporosis* is the term used to describe the disorder in younger men or in premenopausal women in whom no other etiologic factor is detected. It is likely that these patients will eventually be shown to have a number of different disorders with superficial resemblances. In some women the onset of the disease and deterioration of bone appear to be related to pregnancy, whereas in others no adverse effect of pregnancy is observed. Some patients tend to have low levels of serum alkaline phosphatase but not low enough to fit into the group of patients with so-called hypophosphatasia. Estrogens are ineffective in therapy. Losses of calcium and phosphorus are probably excessive, and it is unwise to permit women with osteoporosis to breast-feed their infants since additional calcium losses via lactation are appreciable. It is possible that some patients have a disorder similar to the late-onset forms of osteogenesis imperfecta, although such features as family history, blue scleras, and deafness are lacking. The course of this disorder is variable, and although recurrent episodes of fractures are characteristic, progressive deterioration does not occur in all patients, and in some the clinical problem is rather benign. Juvenile osteoporosis is a rare disorder with onset usually between the ages of 8 and 14 years and characterized by the abrupt appearance of bone pain and fractures after minimal trauma. In many cases the disorder is self-limited, and recovery takes place spontaneously within 4 or 5 years.

GLUCOCORTICOID EXCESS The presence of glucocorticoid excess has not been established in osteoporosis of the idiopathic, senile, or postmenopausal variety. However, osteoporosis commonly accompanies Cushing's syndrome, both endogenous and exogenous, and in some instances is rapidly progressive, especially in children and in women over the age of 50. The rapid progression of bone loss in conditions of glucocorticoid excess is accounted for by a combination of low rates of bone formation (depressed osteoblastic oppositional rate) accompanied by high rates of bone resorption. A part of the latter may be the result of glucocorticoid-induced secondary hyperparathyroidism, although increases in circulating immunoreactive parathyroid hormone have not been found regularly using a variety of immunoassays. Glucocorticoids, however, potentiate the effects of parathyroid hormone and $1,25\text{-(OH)}_2D$ on isolated populations of bone cells. Glucocorticoids depress collagen synthesis in organs other than bone, as evidenced by delayed wound healing, thinning of the dermis, striae, and tendency to blue scleras. In some disorders in which glucocorticoids are administered in pharmacological doses such as rheumatoid arthritis, a tendency to thin skin and osteoporosis is initially present, and the skeletal effects of the glucocorticoids may become particularly apparent. Glucocorticoid excess also results in alteration in the metabolism of vitamin D; blood levels of 25-hydroxyvitamin D_3 ($25\text{-OH-}D_3$) are normal or only slightly decreased, and blood levels of $1\alpha,25$-dihydroxyvitamin D_3 [$1\alpha,25\text{-(OH)}_2D_3$] are low in some patients, particularly in children. Part of the defect in calcium absorption is explainable by the vitamin D abnormalities, but glucocorticoids also inhibit intestinal calcium absorption by a direct, vitamin D–independent action on the intestine. Osteomalacia is not observed histologically, despite the abnormalities in vitamin D metabolism. Once osteoporosis develops in adults with Cushing's syndrome, the abnormal appearance of the vertebrae may persist indefinitely following alleviation of the glucocorticoid excess. In children, however, cure of the Cushing's syndrome may result in striking improvement in the appearance of the spine due to new endochondral bone formation which can surround the less dense, older osteoporotic bone. This does not occur in adults since endochondral bone formation has ceased. Usually withdrawal of glucocorticoids or decrease of the dose by alternate-day schedule may be the only way to halt progression of the osteoporosis. Anabolic steroids are not effective in this regard. The intestinal absorption defect may be helped by administering vitamin D in doses of 50,000 IU three times weekly plus supplemental oral calcium of 1000 to 1500 mg per day. The use of vitamin D metabolites such as $25\text{-OH-}D_3$ or $1\alpha,25\text{-(OH)}_2D_3$ may prove to be more effective. When large doses of vitamin D are used, it is important to monitor serum and urinary calcium and serum 25-OH-D levels at intervals of 2 to 4 months, especially if glucocorticoid dosages are lowered. In Cushing's syndrome, spontaneous, symptomless fractures may occur in bones such as ribs and pubic and ischial rami even in the absence of marked osteoporosis of the spine. These fractures often heal partially with an exuberant calcified callus surrounding a radiolucent zone of nonunion, which superficially resembles the pseudofractures of osteomalacia. If they appear in the thorax superimposed upon the lungs, they may be confused with nodules suggesting primary or metastatic tumor.

GONADAL DEFICIENCY Estrogen lack is present in the postmenopausal woman with osteoporosis, and the administration of estrogen to such an individual reduces the negative calcium balance and decreases urinary hydroxyproline excretion as is consistent with a decrease in bone resorption. However it does not necessarily follow that estrogen deficiency per se is the cause of the osteoporosis. In patients of either sex castrated at an early age, the adult skeleton is smaller to begin with, and therefore age-related losses are more significant.

THYROTOXICOSIS In many patients with hyperthyroidism, there is excessive bone resorption, occasionally marked in degree and far exceeding that in the usual patient with osteoporosis, associated with increased excretion of calcium and phosphorus in urine and feces. The excessive bone resorption is usually accompanied by a compensatory increase in bone formation. Parathyroid hormone secretion is decreased, and levels of $1,25\text{-(OH)}_2D$ are normal or low. If the hyperthyroidism is of short duration, skeletal losses are inconsequential. However, in patients with chronic hyperthyroidism, especially in women after the menopause, this accelerated bone loss becomes clinically significant, and it is important to eliminate hyperthyroidism as a contributing cause of osteoporosis. Although typical osteitis fibrosa (resorption lacunae containing osteoclasts and a fibrous stroma) may be seen on biopsy, even in these cases the skeletal lesions have the appearance of osteoporosis when examined radiologically.

ACROMEGALY Hypercalciuria and overall net negative calcium balance occur in acromegaly, and occasionally osteoporosis is an associated finding. The panhypopituitarism secondary to a pituitary adenoma and gonadal insufficiency may be factors in production of the osteoporosis. In adult animals growth hormone decreases endosteal resorption and stimulates bone formation, and it is therefore unlikely that excessive secretion of growth hormone in itself produces osteoporosis.

DIABETES MELLITUS In several studies individuals with juvenile or adult-onset diabetes mellitus have a decreased bone mass. In some series the incidence of hip fractures has been increased. A more detailed investigation of a large group of diabetic subjects has failed to confirm the presence of abnormal calcium metabolism or bone disease specifically attributable to the diabetes.

CALCIUM DEFICIENCY AND MALABSORPTION Although calcium deficiency may be a factor in some instances of osteoporosis, it cannot be the sole or major cause in idiopathic, senile, or postmenopausal osteoporosis. Osteoporosis is an associated finding in a significant number of cases of steatorrhea, prolonged obstructive jaundice, and lactose intolerance and in patients following gastrectomy. In other patients there are suggestions of a specific defect in calcium absorption or a failure to adapt adequately to a low-calcium diet either by increasing the percentage of dietary calcium absorbed or by decreasing urinary calcium excretion. Presumably adequate vitamin D is available in these instances to prevent osteomalacia.

HERITABLE DISORDERS OF CONNECTIVE TISSUE In the strict sense, the bone disease of osteogenesis imperfecta is osteoporosis. *Osteogenesis imperfecta* is a clinically, genetically, and biochemically heterogeneous disorder. Several different forms have been described. The best known is transmitted as an autosomal dominant trait and is associated with blue scleras and, later, deafness. The bone disease in this form tends to be relatively mild, and the tendency toward fractures may decrease after puberty. Another form, which itself is probably genetically heterogeneous but is likely autosomal recessive, is usually detected shortly after birth and is progressive with recurrent fractures of long bones and kyphoscoliosis. Sclerae are white, and deafness is uncommon. A lethal perinatal type (autosomal recessive) is also seen. Some cases of idiopathic osteoporosis may represent forms of osteogenesis imperfecta. The organization of the collagen in bone and skin is abnormal, and in some instances there likely is a genetic defect in the synthesis of the type I collagen of bone and skin. Osteoporosis is also seen in patients with *homocystinuria* due to cystathionine synthase deficiency, an autosomal recessive trait. Other characteristics of this disorder should suggest its presence, such as ectopia lentis, various deformities of the extremities, mental retardation, decreased pigmentation of hair and skin, and thromboembolism. The diagnosis is established by the finding of homocystine in urine. The defect may be due to the effect of homocysteine or other metabolites in interfering with the cross-linking of collagen.

THERAPY Before considering the various modes of treatment for osteoporosis, it should be emphasized that one is dealing with a group of disorders rather than a single entity. Even in patients considered to fall within the same category, e.g., those with idiopathic osteoporosis, the etiologies may be different. In addition, it is difficult to predict the course and the rate of progression of the disease in any patient, especially when seen initially because of pain and collapse-fracture. Many patients in the idiopathic, senile, and postmenopausal groups have a few episodes of vertebral body collapse with symptom-free intervals of months or years and lose height consistent with the extent of collapse but then go for many years without symptoms or further loss in height. Furthermore, the acute pain associated with vertebral body fracture tends to subside in a matter of weeks, and *any* treatment administered at that time might be considered efficacious. It is evident from the different therapeutic programs available for osteoporosis that therapy is far from ideal, despite claims to the contrary.

General measures Patients who present with acute pain secondary to fracture of vertebral bodies frequently require hospitalization with rest in bed in a position of maximum comfort, local heat, adequate analgesics, and avoidance of constipation. Use of traction or plaster jacket splints is not indicated. As soon as pain permits, it is prudent to have the patient attempt to move out of bed, slowly at first, perhaps with support of a walker or crutches. The patient should not become too fatigued when starting ambulation. Braces of various types are commonly employed, but it has not been proved that they are efficacious in preventing progression of spinal deformity. A well-made corset may provide a sensation of support and comfort. Exercises to correct postural deformity and increase muscle tone are useful. It is also important to instruct patients to avoid sudden painful movements such as jumping and how to lift and carry objects with minimal back strain.

Estrogens and androgens The use of estrogens in postmenopausal women with osteoporosis was first advocated by Fuller Albright and his colleagues. Decrease in urinary calcium and hydroxyproline excretion results from such therapy, especially during the first few months of treatment. Estrogens decrease the rate of bone resorption, but bone formation does not increase and eventually usually decreases. The mean level of circulating $1\alpha,25\text{-(OH)}_2D$ is lower than normal in osteoporotic subjects and is brought to normal by estrogen therapy. Thus, estrogens produce significant, although modest, calcium retention, decrease the difference between formation and resorption, and therefore tend to retard the progress of osteoporosis, but they are not capable of restoring skeletal mass. The magnitude of calcium retention also tends to decrease with continuous therapy. Therefore, it is not surprising that there is no change in radiological features of the osteoporosis with such therapy. It is likely that estrogens have a role in preventing osteoporosis in menopausal women rather than treating clinical disease already developed, although they may be the best therapy in the postmenopausal woman with mild or moderate disease within the first 5 to 6 years following cessation of ovarian function. Testosterone preparations are useful in treatment of men with gonadal deficiency, but there are no convincing reports of their efficacy in men with normal gonadal function. There is also no proved advantage to combinations of estrogens and androgens. The chronic use of estrogens restores menses in some postmenopausal women and induces breast swelling and hyperpigmentation. In women receiving estrogens the risk of mammary carcinoma is not increased, but there is a dose-related increase in the incidence of endometrial carcinoma. Any decision on the use of these hormones must take this risk factor into consideration (see Chap. 118).

Calcium preparations Use of oral calcium preparations in doses of 1.0 to 1.5 g elemental calcium per day increases calcium retention in some osteoporotic subjects and decreases indexes of bone resorption. The elemental calcium content of available preparations varies, depending upon the accompanying anion and the composition, as shown by the examples in Table 341-2. However, as with the use of estrogens, this eventually results in decrease in bone formation and tends to arrest rather than "cure" the osteoporosis. In patients with malabsorption, calcium may be effective in addition to vitamin D given orally in doses of 25,000 to 50,000 IU once or twice weekly. The use of more active metabolites of vitamin D may prove more efficacious. Both serum and urinary calcium should be monitored at intervals of several months to be certain that hypercalcemia and hypercalciuria do not result. Diuretics of the benzothiadiazide class reduce urinary calcium excretion and could be helpful in reducing a negative calcium balance. Calcium preparations might be of greater use in patients with normal gonadal function and relatively mild disease. Intermittent intravenous infusions of calcium have also been advocated, but the efficacy has yet to be established.

Fluoride Fluoride ions are promptly deposited in the skeleton where they become incorporated into the crystal lattice of hydroxyapatite, substituting for hydroxyl ions. This process results in a mineral phase of greater crystallinity. Fluoride ions in chronic high doses also increase new bone formation and in excess produce a form of hyperostosis with dense bones, exostoses, neurological complications due to bony overgrowth, and ligamentous calcification. Fluoride in treating osteoporosis has not resulted in uniformly satisfactory results, possibly because of variations in dosage of fluoride ion, retention of absorbed ion, and calcium intake while on fluoride. The stimulation of new bone formation, a desirable effect not seen with the other agents mentioned previously, is unfortunately associated with the production of bone that is poorly mineralized and also, presumably, structurally unsound. If the dose of fluoride ion is moderate (25 mg per day) and calcium supplements are given in doses of at least 1 g daily plus vitamin D, 50,000 IU twice weekly, considerable new bone may be produced. Significant toxicity is absent, although weight-bearing pain, especially in ankles and knees, is noted by some patients and disappears when fluoride is discontinued. Such therapeutic programs have not been approved for general use.

Other measures Although calcitonin therapy of osteoporosis has been advocated, this therapy probably does not produce benefits greater than attained with supplemental calcium and vitamin D. Oral phosphates (greater than 1 g elemental phosphorus per day in divided doses) may decrease urinary calcium excretion and improve calcium tolerance in patients with marked hypercalciuria. However, phosphate is of no value in the treatment of patients with postmenopausal osteoporosis who have normal levels of serum phosphorus.

RICKETS AND OSTEOMALACIA

The terms *rickets* and *osteomalacia* describe a group of disorders in which there is defective mineralization of the newly formed organic matrix of the skeleton. In *rickets* the growing skeleton is involved; defective mineralization occurs not only in bone but also in the cartilaginous matrix of the growth plate. The term *osteomalacia* is usually reserved for the disorder of mineralization of the adult skeleton in which the epiphyseal growth plates are closed. A number of conditions result in rickets and/or osteomalacia such as inadequate dietary intake of vitamin D, inadequate exposure to ultraviolet radiation to form endogenous vitamin D, intestinal malabsorption of vitamin D, chronic acidosis, renal tubular defects which produce hypophosphatemia or acidosis, and chronic administration of anticonvulsants. In the renal tubular disorders rickets and osteomalacia develop in the presence of normal intestinal function and are not cured by treatment with doses of vitamin D adequate to cure deficiency rickets. Thus the term *vitamin D–resistant* (or *refractory*) has been applied in these instances. Renal insufficiency, especially in children, is also associated with rickets or osteomalacia. A classification of rickets and osteomalacia is given in Table 341-3.

TABLE 341-2
Elemental calcium content in various oral calcium preparations

Calcium preparation	*Elemental calcium content per unit weight or volume*
Calcium citrate	40 mg/300 mg
Calcium carbonate	400 mg/g
Calcium lactate	80 mg/600 mg
Calcium gluconate	40 mg/500 mg
Calcium carbonate + 5 μg vitamin D_2 (os − cal)	250 mg/tablet
Calcium carbonate + glycine (Titralac)	168 mg/tablet
Calcium carbonate + glycine (Titralac)	400 mg/5 ml

PATHOGENESIS AND HISTOPATHOLOGY For mineralization of matrices of skeletal tissues, sufficient calcium and phosphate is required at the mineralization sites. Although it is not known what the optimal concentration is at these sites, mineralization does not proceed normally when the concentrations of calcium and inorganic phosphate in the plasma (and extracellular fluid) are too low. Other conditions required for normal mineralization include intact metabolic and transport functions of osteoblasts and chondrocytes, adequate collagen matrix, possibly phosphorylation or other modifications of matrix components, and low concentrations of inhibitory substances such as proteoglycan aggregates or inorganic pyrophosphate. A specific function of the γ-carboxyglutamic acid–containing proteins synthesized by bone cells in the mineralization process has not been demonstrated, although they appear to bind calcium ions. In cartilage the initial mineral phase is in membrane-bound extracellular vesicles. If the osteoblast continues to produce matrix components which cannot be adequately mineralized, the typical features of rickets and osteomalacia result. If calcification continues to be inadequate, the production of organic matrix (osteoid) must also gradually decrease. In bone there will be an increase in the fraction of the forming surface covered by incompletely mineralized osteoid, an increase in osteoid volume and thickness (the latter normally less than 12 to 14 μm), and a decrease in the calcification or mineralization front. The latter is detected in undemineralized sections by the fluorescence of previously ingested tetracycline or by special stains. There is a marked decrease in the rate of apposition of mineralized bone. A variety of methods are available to measure the thickness of the osteoid seams and the calcification front. In routine histological sections stained with hematoxylin and eosin, if the specimens are not overdecalcified in preparation, the more heavily mineralized areas tend to appear violet or blue, whereas the osteoid seams appear pink. Subtle degrees of osteomalacia may not be appreciated with routine preparations, and undecalcified, thin sections (3 to 5 μm) stained, for example, with Goldner's trichrome method are necessary to establish its presence (Fig. 341-2). Rickets is also characterized by inadequate mineralization of the matrix of cartilage in the growing epiphyseal plate. Calcification in the interstitial regions of the hypertrophic zone is defective, the growth plate increases in thickness, the arrangement of the columns of cartilage cells (usually highly ordered) is disorganized, and there is a variable cupping of the epiphyses. The rachitic bones are often incapable of withstanding usual mechanical stresses and in the process of growth tend to undergo bowing deformities. If rickets is untreated, growth at the epiphyseal plates is slowed, and the eventual length of the long bones is diminished.

It has not been established whether vitamin D, through one of its metabolites, has a major direct effect on mineralization. Its primary role after metabolic conversion to 25-OH-D and $1\alpha,25\text{-(OH)}_2D$ is to regulate and enhance absorption of calcium ions from the intestinal lumen. The pathogenesis of inadequate skeletal mineralization when vitamin D is insufficient, from whatever cause, is probably as follows. Insufficiency of the active metabolites of vitamin D lead to decreased intestinal absorption of calcium and decreased mobilization of calcium from bone, resulting in hypocalcemia. This stimulates increased secretion of parathyroid hormone (PTH) and, later, increased synthesis of PTH and hyperplasia of the parathyroid glands. The increased circulating concentration of PTH tends to raise plasma calcium concentrations but also stimulates increased renal phosphate clearance, which, in turn, produces hypophosphatemia. When the concentration of phosphorus in the extracellular fluid falls below a critical level, mineralization cannot proceed normally. In severe vitamin D lack, normocalcemia cannot be maintained, and the driving force for mineralization is further decreased. The absence of some critical metabolite of vitamin D that acts directly on the skeleton may also play a role in the defective mineralization of rickets and osteomalacia.

TABLE 341-3
Classification of rickets and osteomalacia

I Vitamin D lack
- *A* Dietary deficiency
- *B* Deficient endogenous synthesis

II Gastrointestinal
- *A* Small-intestinal diseases with malabsorption
- *B* Partial or total gastrectomy
- *C* Hepatobiliary disease
- *D* Chronic pancreatic insufficiency

III Disorders of vitamin D metabolism
- *A* Hereditary: pseudovitamin D deficiency or vitamin D dependency, types I and II
- *B* Acquired
  - *1* Anticonvulsants
  - *2* Chronic renal failure

IV Acidosis
- *A* Distal renal tubular acidosis (classic or type I)
- *B* Secondary forms of renal acidosis
- *C* Ureterosigmoidostomy
- *D* Drug-induced disease
  - *1* Chronic acetazolamide ingestion
  - *2* Chronic ammonium chloride ingestion

V Chronic renal failure

VI Phosphate depletion
- *A* Dietary: low phosphate intake plus ingestion of nonabsorbable antacids
- *B* Impaired renal tubular phosphate reabsorption
  - *1* Hereditary
    - *a* X-linked hypophosphatemic rickets (vitamin D–resistant rickets)
    - *b* Adult-onset vitamin D–resistant hypophosphatemic osteomalacia
  - *2* Acquired
    - *a* Sporadic hypophosphatemic osteomalacia (phosphate diabetes)
    - *b* Tumor-associated rickets and osteomalacia
    - *c* Neurofibromatosis
    - *d* Fibrous dysplasia

VII Generalized renal tubular disorders (Fanconi's syndrome)
- *A* Primary renal
- *B* Associated with systemic metabolic abnormality
  - *1* Cystinosis
  - *2* Glycogenosis
  - *3* Lowe's syndrome
- *C* Systemic disorder with associated renal disease
  - *1* Hereditary
    - *a* Inborn errors
      - (*1*) Wilson's disease
      - (*2*) Tyrosinemia
    - *b* Neurofibromatosis
  - *2* Acquired
    - *a* Multiple myeloma
    - *b* Nephrotic syndrome
    - *c* Transplanted kidney
  - *3* Intoxications
    - *a* Cadmium
    - *b* Lead
    - *c* Outdated tetracycline

VIII Primary mineralization defects
- *A* Hereditary: hypophosphatasia
- *B* Acquired
  - *1* Diphosphonate (disodium etidronate) treatment
  - *2* Fluoride treatment

IX States of rapid bone formation with or without a relative defect in bone resorption
- *A* Postoperative hyperparathyroidism with osteitis fibrosa cystica
- *B* Osteopetrosis

X Defective matrix synthesis: fibrogenesis imperfecta ossium

XI Miscellaneous
- *A* Magnesium-dependent conditions
- *B* Axial osteomalacia
- *C* Parenteral alimentation

Phosphate depletion alone can produce osteomalacia as in patients consuming large amounts of nonabsorbable antacids. Excessive renal loss of phosphate due to decreased tubular reabsorption may also result in the hypophosphatemia responsible for the osteomalacia in some of the renal tubular disorders. Secondary hyperparathyroidism is probably not present in many of these patients. It should be emphasized that hypophosphatemia per se produces mineralization defects despite its effect on increasing the activity of the renal 25-OH-D-1α-hydroxylase, but it cannot account for the osteomalacia in all the disorders listed in Table 341-3. In chronic renal failure, for example, plasma phosphate levels are not decreased and usually are increased. Similarly, plasma phosphorus levels are not depressed in infants and children with osteomalacia secondary to hypophosphatasia, a hereditary deficiency in alkaline phosphatase.

CLINICAL FINDINGS The clinical problems of rickets are the result of skeletal deformities, susceptibility to fractures, weakness and hypotonia, and disturbances in growth. In extreme instances of vitamin D–deficiency rickets, hypocalcemia may be sufficient to produce tetany which, when severe, may be

FIGURE 341-2
Photomicrograph of an undemineralized section stained with Goldner method of an iliac crest bone biopsy from a 45-year-old man with chronic renal failure maintained on hemodialysis. Almost the entire surface is covered by osteoid (O) readily distinguished from mineralized bone (MB). The thickness of the osteoid seams exceeds 100 μm in several areas.

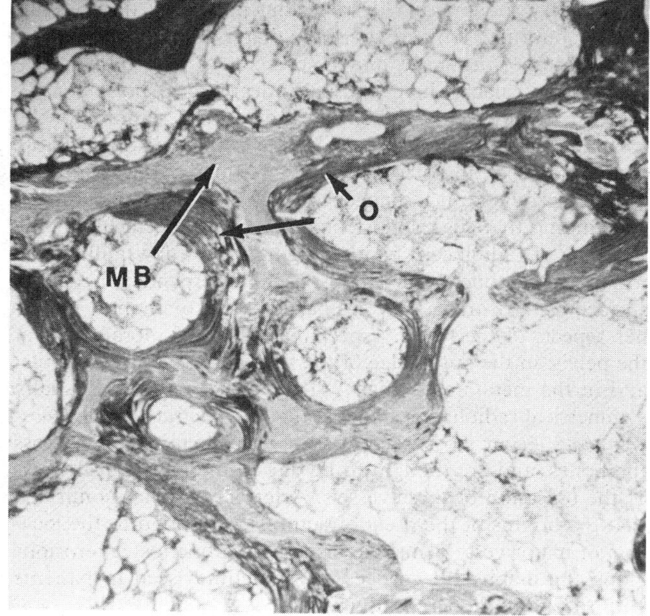

accompanied by laryngeal spasm and convulsive seizures.

In infants and young children features include listlessness, irritability, and often profound hypotonia and muscular weakness. As the disorder progresses, children become unable to walk without support. Abnormal parietal flattening and frontal bossing develop in the skull. The calvaria is softened (craniotabes), and widening of sutures may be evident. Prominence of the costochondral junctions is called the "rachitic rosary," and the indentation of the lower ribs at the site of attachment of the diaphragm is known as *Harrison's groove.* If untreated, progressive deformities of the pelvis and extremities result, with bowing particularly common in the tibia, femur, radius, and ulna. Fractures are frequent, dental eruption is often delayed, and enamel defects are common.

The presentation of osteomalacia in adults usually is not as dramatic as in infants and children. The skeletal deformities may be overlooked, and the features of the underlying disorder may dominate, as, for example, in the vitamin D loss associated with adult celiac disease. Major symptoms, when they occur, include varying degrees of diffuse skeletal pain and bony tenderness. Pain may be especially prominent about the hips and may result in an antalgic gait. Muscular weakness is also common in adult osteomalacia, although it may be difficult to distinguish from hesitancy to move because of skeletal pain. Weakness, usually proximal in distribution, may mimic that of primary muscle disorders and contribute to the waddling gait. In some patients pain and muscular weakness may be sufficient for them to be confined to bed and chair. Many factors, including the secondary hyperparathyroidism, contribute to the myopathy when it is present. Clinical improvement in the myopathy usually results from specific therapy such as vitamin D repletion in nutritional osteomalacia, phosphate replacement in renal hypophosphatemia, or correction of acidosis. Fractures of involved bones may occur with minimal trauma. When the ribs are involved, severe deformities may develop in the thoracic cage, and the collapse of vertebral bodies may produce loss of height.

RADIOLOGICAL FEATURES Radiological changes in the skeleton in rickets and osteomalacia reflect the pathological changes. In rickets the alterations are most evident at the epiphyseal growth plate which is increased in thickness, cupped, and hazy at the metaphyseal border due to decreased calcification of the hypertrophic zone and inadequate mineralization of the primary spongiosa. The trabecular pattern of the metaphyses is abnormal, the cortices of the diaphyses may be thinned, and bowing of the shafts may be present.

In osteomalacia there is usually decrease in bone density associated with loss of trabeculae and variable thinning of the cortices. In some the radiological changes are indistinguishable from those seen in osteoporosis. Trabecular patterns may be blurred, producing a homogeneous ground glass appearance. The finding that suggests osteomalacia more specifically is the presence of radiolucent bands ranging from a few millimeters to several centimeters in length, usually perpendicular to the surface of the bones. They are particularly common at the inner aspects of the femur, especially near the femoral neck, in the pelvis, in the outer edge of the scapula, in the upper fibula, and in the metatarsals (Figs. 341-3 and 341-4). These usually symmetrical radiolucent bands, called *pseudofractures* or *Looser's zones,* occur most often at sites where major arteries cross the bones, and are thought to be due to the mechanical stress of the pulsation of these vessels. Arteriography has confirmed that the origins of the pseudofractures correspond to the location of major vessels in some instances. Subperiosteal erosions along the diaphyseal cortices are sometimes seen in patients with secondary hyperparathyroidism.

In some patients with osteomalacia increased rather than decreased density of bones may be observed. This is seen in patients with renal tubular disorders rather than with vitamin D deficiency and may produce a striking degree of thickening of the cortices and trabeculae of spongy bone. Despite the increase in mass of bone per unit volume, microscopically the trabeculae are covered with abnormally thickened osteoid seams typical of osteomalacia. Similar findings may be noted in patients with chronic renal failure. The reason for the hyperostosis is unknown; the bone is architecturally abnormal and subject to fracture with minimal trauma.

LABORATORY FINDINGS Changes in serum concentrations of calcium, inorganic phosphorus, 25-OH-D, and 1α,25-$(OH)_2D$ vary with the different disorders. In vitamin D deficiency, whether due to dietary lack, inadequate sunlight exposure, or intestinal malabsorption, serum calcium levels are normal or low, whereas phosphorus and 25-OH-D levels are characteristically low, usually < 5 ng/ml depending upon the assay. In contrast, levels of 1,25-$(OH)_2D$ may not be low. In adults phosphorus concentrations less than 2.8 mg/dl are abnormal; in children the lower limit of normal is closer to 4.0 to 4.5 mg/dl. In *severe* states of vitamin D depletion, hypocalcemia may also be seen, occasionally sufficient to produce tetany. Mild acidosis and generalized aminoaciduria may also be found, as a result of secondary hyperparathyroidism. As a rule, patients with renal tubular disorders maintain normal serum calcium levels while hypophosphatemia is characteristic. Other laboratory findings such as glucosuria, aminoaciduria, acidosis,

FIGURE 341-3
Radiographs of the scapula of a 58-year-old woman with phosphate diabetes. The presence of a pseudofracture or Looser's zone is indicated by the arrow.

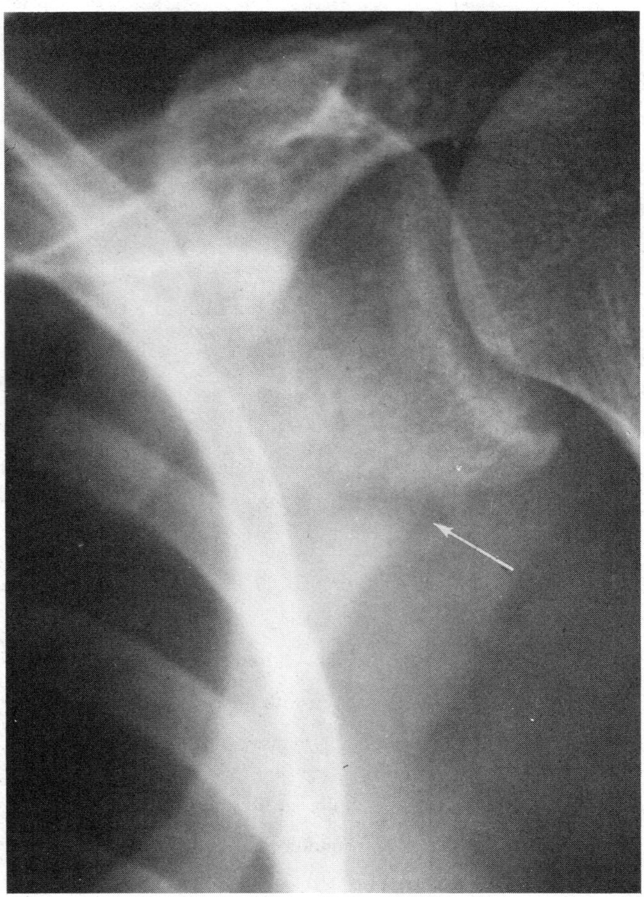

and hypouricemia reflect variable degrees of disturbance of proximal tubular function or features of the underlying disease (e.g., low plasma ceruloplasmin in Wilson's disease or abnormalities of immunoglobulins in multiple myeloma). In chronic renal failure hyperphosphatemia and some degree of hypocalcemia are usually seen accompanied by normal 25-OH-D and low 1α,25-$(OH)_2D$ levels. In nephrotic syndrome serum 25-OH-D levels can be low due primarily to urinary losses of protein-bound 25-OH-D. Serum phosphorus levels are also normal or elevated in hypophosphatasia. Increased excretion of hydroxyproline peptides is a component of those conditions in which secondary hyperparathyroidism and excessive bone resorption are associated with the defect in mineralization. Alkaline phosphatase levels in plasma are usually elevated in rickets or osteomalacia, but typical and even severe osteomalacia, especially that due to renal tubular disorders, may be accompanied by normal or only borderline elevations. Levels may increase during the early phases of therapy.

DIETARY VITAMIN D DEFICIENCY AND INADEQUATE ENDOGENOUS SYNTHESIS Most foods unfortified with vitamin D contain insufficient amounts of the vitamin to prevent rickets in growing children or osteomalacia in adults living in temperate-zone cities. As discussed in Chap. 340, in the absence of supplements, vitamin D must be formed endogenously through the ultraviolet irradiation of precursor 7-dehydrocholesterol in the skin. Many factors decrease the formation of vitamin D_3 from its precursor: increased melanin pigmentation, hyperkeratosis, limited exposure of the body, short days of sunlight, oblique angle of ultraviolet irradiation, and factors in the atmosphere, such as smog, which prevent adequate penetration of ultraviolet radiation. Since fortification of dairy products and routine use of vitamin D supplements for infants have been in effect, deficiency rickets is unusual in the United States. Poor, dark-skinned infants living in crowded northern cities are most susceptible. However, osteomalacia due to vitamin D deficiency still is observed in adults, especially in elderly individuals who tend to remain indoors and whose dietary intake of vitamin D is inadequate (probably less than 70 to 100 IU per day).

VITAMIN D LOSS AND INTESTINAL MALABSORPTION Osteomalacia may be seen in patients with intestinal malabsorption such as in adult celiac disease and regional enteritis. Prior to the discovery of gluten sensitivity in some of these cases, celiac disease was among the more common disorders underlying osteomalacia. Vitamin D absorption, which normally occurs via chylomicrons, is impaired in diseases causing steatorrhea where emulsification of fat is disturbed, such as chronic biliary obstruction. Patients with cholestatic liver disease or extrahepatic biliary obstruction may have low serum levels of 25-OH-D_3 and osteomalacia, due not only to poor vitamin D absorption but also to decreased hepatic production of 25-OH-D_3 and disruption in its enterohepatic circulation. Osteomalacia is less frequent in chronic pancreatic insufficiency. Patients who have had gastric surgery may also develop osteomalacia, possibly due to malfunction of the proximal small bowel. Factors other than failure to absorb vitamin D may contribute to the osteomalacia in patients with small-bowel disease, such as inadequate absorbing surface and failure of intestinal cells to respond to the active metabolites of vitamin D. Secondary hyperparathyroidism is usually present in intestinal malabsorption, as it is in dietary lack of vitamin D. In some studies patients who lack vitamin D, usually associated with intestinal malabsorption, have normal circulating levels of 1α,25-$(OH)_2D$, despite low or undetectable 25-OH-D. In these individuals the normal levels of 1α,25-$(OH)_2D$ may be accounted for by ingestion of sufficient vitamin D in hospital diets to produce substrate 25-OH-D for 1α-hydroxylation by the renal enzyme that is increased in activity due to secondary hyperparathyroidism. In other patients, circulating 1α,25-$(OH)_2D$ levels may not reflect levels at critical target cells.

ABNORMAL METABOLISM OF VITAMIN D Although serum 25-OH-D levels are reduced in some instances of parenchymal and obstructive liver disease, studies have not yet correlated these findings with quantitative histological observations. Patients consuming anticonvulsant drugs such as phenobarbital and/or phenytoin may develop rickets or osteomalacia. For a given intake of vitamin D, patients receiving chronic anticonvulsant drugs have lower serum levels of calcium and 25-OH-D. Consumption of anticonvulsants may be especially important in individuals whose intake of vitamin D is barely optimal, who are nonambulatory and confined indoors, who have chronic recurrent infections, or in whom mild intestinal malfunction exists as in the postgastrectomy state. As dis-

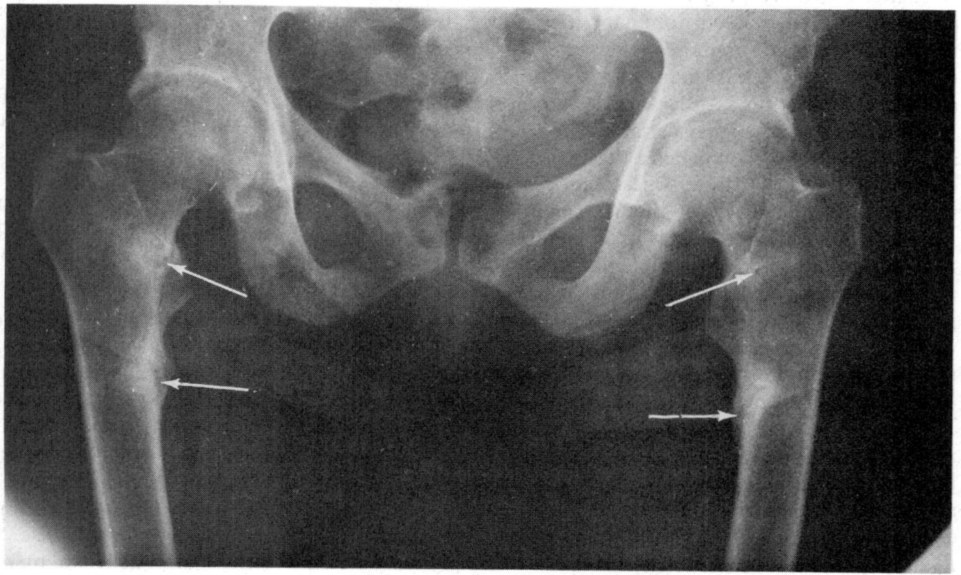

FIGURE 341-4
Radiograph of the femurs of a 47-year-old woman with Fanconi's syndrome of adult onset. The presence of multiple pseudofractures is indicated by the arrows.

cussed in Chap. 340 the anticonvulsant drugs have multiple actions on calcium homeostasis that are dependent and independent of vitamin D metabolism.

A syndrome superficially resembling vitamin D–resistant rickets has been termed *pseudovitamin D deficiency*. Because these patients respond to pharmacological doses of vitamin D, this disease has also been termed *vitamin D–dependent rickets*. These patients have rickets or osteomalacia, a tendency to hypocalcemia but normal or only slightly depressed serum phosphorus levels, a response to a variable but moderate dose of vitamin D which is usually excellent and complete, and an autosomal recessive inheritance. No other renal tubular abnormalities are found. These patients also respond to small doses of $1\alpha,25\text{-(OH)}_2D$ or 1α-OH-D. Most of the cases described have low serum $1\alpha,25\text{-(OH)}_2D$ levels, suggesting a defect in the renal production of $1\alpha,25\text{-(OH)}_2D$; these have been classified as vitamin D–dependent rickets, type I. Vitamin D–dependent rickets, type II, is postulated to result from an impaired responsiveness of target tissues to $1\alpha,25\text{-(OH)}_2D$ since cultured cells from affected subjects have abnormalities in the amount or function of normal $1\alpha,25\text{-(OH)}_2D$ receptors. In these subjects elevated serum $1\alpha,25\text{-(OH)}_2D$ levels are present and increase further when large doses of vitamin D are administered.

Other individuals with rickets unresponsive to 25-OH-D or $1\alpha,25\text{-(OH)}_2D$ treatment have low circulating levels of $24,25\text{-(OH)}_2D$ as currently measured and normalize serum calcium concentrations when synthetic $24,25\text{-(OH)}_2D$ is administered.

Recently, osteomalacia has been reported in patients with bowel diseases who are maintained on chronic total parenteral nutrition. These patients have hypercalcemia, hypercalciuria and negative calcium balance, and normal circulating levels of 25-OH-D. The cause of the bone disease has not been elucidated.

RENAL TUBULAR DISORDERS Rickets and osteomalacia develop in association with a variety of disorders of proximal renal tubular function. These disorders have in common increased renal clearance of inorganic phosphorus and hypophosphatemia with normal or near normal glomerular filtration rate. Most frequently, increased phosphate clearance with resultant hypophosphatemia is an isolated defect with no other abnormalities except for increase in urinary glycine excretion (hyperglycinuria). Primary hypophosphatemia (*phosphate diabetes* and *vitamin D–resistant rickets* are terms applied to these cases especially when the disorder presents in early childhood) is characterized by progressively severe skeletal deformities, dwarfism, and sex-linked dominant inheritance. In some patients there may be spontaneous remissions followed by recurrences in adult life associated, for example, with pregnancy and lactation. Serum 25-OH-D levels are normal while serum $1\alpha,25\text{-(OH)}_2D$ levels have variably been reported as normal and low. There is little evidence that $1\alpha,25\text{-(OH)}_2D_3$ therapy is of specific benefit in a majority of these patients. It is likely that the biochemical defect is not the same in all these kindreds and may not be related to defects in metabolism of vitamin D. Sporadic cases of hypophosphatemia have also been described in adults in whom family histories are negative and where proximal muscle weakness is a prominent feature. Muscle weakness is not characteristic. As mentioned above, in most of the untreated cases of renal tubular disorders with rickets and osteomalacia, secondary hyperparathyroidism is not present.

In other patients the disorder in tubular function may be more widespread, involving (besides phosphorus) glucose, potassium, amino acids, and uric acid; the various combinations are termed the de Toni-Debré-Fanconi syndrome. The more complete renal tubular defects may also occur sporadically or in families. In some instances the lesion is simply part of a more widespread disorder as in Wilson's disease and cystinosis. The acidosis of proximal tubular defects also plays a role in development of osteomalacia, possibly by altering metabolism of vitamin D or altering renal handling of calcium and phosphorus. In this regard osteomalacia has accompanied the hyperchloremic acidosis of ureterocolic anastomosis.

TUMOR-ASSOCIATED (ONCOGENIC) OSTEOMALACIA Osteomalacia and hypophosphatemia with high renal phosphate clearance have been associated with a variety of tumors. The latter have included giant-cell tumors (benign or malignant), reparative granulomas, hemangiomas, fibromas, and other mesenchymal neoplasms. In some instances, removal of the tumor resulted in normalization of renal phosphorus clearance, rise in serum phosphorus levels, and healing of the osteomalacia (or the rickets in children). In several reports serum $1\alpha,25\text{-(OH)}_2D$ levels have been low or undetectable, although chronic administration of sufficient $1\alpha,25\text{-(OH)}_2D$ to raise circulating levels of this metabolite to normal does not alter renal phosphorus clearance or serum phosphorus concentrations. A possible explanation of these events is that some renal toxin is released by the tumor which impairs proximal tubular functions such as 1α-hydroxylation of 25-OH-D *and* phosphate transport.

CHRONIC RENAL FAILURE Histologically osteomalacia is common in patients with chronic renal failure; it often tends to be the predominant phase of renal osteodystrophy in younger patients and is more frequent in those with the lower plasma levels of calcium and phosphorus. There is almost always a component of secondary hyperparathyroidism and osteitis fibrosa accompanying the defect in mineralization. The defect itself probably involves a decreased conversion of 25-OH-D to $1\alpha,25\text{-(OH)}_2D$ because of either insufficient viable renal cortical tissue or the inhibitory effect of hyperphosphatemia on renal 25-OH-D-1α-hydroxylase activity. In addition, there may be a primary defect in intestinal calcium absorption. Part of the secondary hyperparathyroidism may also be due to decreased phosphate clearance and subsequent hyperphosphatemia. In the presence of near-normal plasma concentration of calcium and hyperphosphatemia, it is not clear why mineralization of the organic matrix should be incomplete. Although it has been postulated that inhibitors of mineralization are present to account for this anomaly, the osteomalacic component usually does respond to large doses of vitamin D or dihydrotachysterol or to small doses of $1\alpha,25\text{-(OH)}_2D_3$ or $1\alpha\text{-OH-}D_3$. However, some patients with renal osteodystrophy do not respond to pharmacologic doses of vitamin D_2 nor improve when given small amounts of $1\alpha,25\text{-(OH)}_2D_3$. In some patients with renal osteodystrophy the total bone mass may be increased (osteosclerosis), resulting in increased density of bone seen radiologically. This is particularly evident in the spine where a characteristic appearance is that of dense bone at the superior and inferior margins of the vertebral bodies with more radiolucent central portions ("rugger jersey sign"). Histologically, although there is more bone per unit area, each trabecula is covered by an abnormally wide osteoid seam.

HYPOPHOSPHATASIA Rickets is a feature of this heritable deficiency of alkaline phosphatase in infants and children, although osteomalacia is an inconstant finding in adults with hypophosphatasia. Serum phosphorus levels are not reduced. Phosphorylethanolamine and phosphorylcholine are excreted in excessive amounts in the urine, but it is not clear how this is related to the inadequate skeletal mineralization. There is a direct correlation between plasma alkaline phosphatase and inorganic pyrophosphatase. Since patients with hypophosphatasia are also deficient in pyrophosphatase, it is possible that concentrations in inorganic pyrophosphate, a potent inhibitor of mineralization, are too high to allow normal mineralization at formation sites.

OTHER DISORDERS ASSOCIATED WITH DEFECTIVE MINERALIZATION Disturbances in mineralization may be seen in patients consuming high doses of fluoride ion and in patients with Paget's disease treated with disodium etidronate. Some decrease in mineralization of newly forming matrix, increase in surface covered by osteoid, and increase in the width of the osteoid seams are seen in several conditions that are not usually considered as osteomalacia except by these criteria. Biopsies in some of these conditions show a normal calcification front. Examples include patients with the osteitis fibrosa of hyperparathyroidism in the weeks to months following surgical cure. In these circumstances there is a temporary imbalance between the rate at which mineral is supplied to bone and the rate at which bone matrix is formed. Wide osteoid seams as well as hypophosphatemia are also seen in the bones of children with osteopetrosis in whom there is inadequate resorption of bone and calcified cartilage but active bone formation.

A condition which resembles osteomalacia and is associated with a coarsened, mottled bony trabecular pattern, pseudofractures, and bone pain but normal plasma levels of calcium and phosphorus is *fibrogenesis imperfecta ossium.* Histologically the bone has a distinctive appearance, with wide osteoid seams and a distortion of the birefringent pattern of normal bone suggesting an abnormality in the collagen recently deposited. The nature of the abnormality is not known.

TREATMENT OF RICKETS AND OSTEOMALACIA The therapeutic approach to the various disorders associated with rickets and osteomalacia is somewhat different. In rickets and osteomalacia due to dietary absence of vitamin D or inadequate exposure to sunlight, vitamin D_2 or vitamin D_3 is given orally in doses of 2000 to 4000 IU (0.05 to 0.1 mg) daily for 6 to 12 weeks, followed by daily supplements of 200 to 400 IU, which are adequate to prevent the development of the disorder in otherwise normal subjects. In infants and children such treatment causes improvement in muscle tone and strength, rise in serum calcium and phosphorus, and fall in alkaline phosphatase levels after several weeks. Radiological evidence of healing is first noted within weeks and may be complete by a few months. Calcium supplements and larger initial doses of vitamin D may be necessary in infants and children with tetany. In adults with nutritional osteomalacia healing of pseudofractures may be evident within 3 to 4 weeks after therapy with as little as 2000 IU (0.05 mg) vitamin D daily. Healing is complete usually by 6 months.

Patients with osteomalacia due to intestinal malabsorption do not respond to the relatively small doses of vitamin D that can cure deficiency-nutritional osteomalacia. In the presence of active steatorrhea, oral doses of vitamin D of 40,000 to 100,000 IU (1.0 to 2.5 mg) daily may be required in addition to large doses of calcium (e.g., 15 g calcium lactate or 4 g calcium carbonate orally per day). In some instances oral vitamin D is ineffective, and the parenteral route is required (e.g., 10,000 IU intramuscularly per day). Another approach is the use of ultraviolet irradiation in addition to supplemental calcium. Small doses of 1α-OH-D_3 (2.5 to 5.0 μg daily) or 1α,25-$(OH)_2D_3$ (0.5 to 1.0 μg daily) are also effective in treatment of this form of osteomalacia. Inorganic phosphate therapy is not indicated either in deficiency osteomalacia or in intestinal malabsorption, since hypocalcemia will develop and intestinal calcium absorption will remain inadequate. In all patients in whom large doses of vitamin D are used, monitoring of serum calcium and 25-OH-D levels at intervals is essential. Semiquantitative urinary calcium measurements alone are inadequate.

In patients on anticonvulsants, it is often necessary to continue the drugs while adding supplemental vitamin D and monitoring levels of serum calcium at biweekly intervals and serum 25-OH-D levels bimonthly for the first few months until a therapeutic response (evidence of radiological healing, improvement in symptoms) is obtained. Doses varying from 4000 to 40,000 IU daily have been recommended.

Treatment of rickets and osteomalacia in the presence of renal tubular disorders is more difficult, and there is not uniform agreement as to the exact regimen to be followed. The X-linked form of hypophosphatemic osteomalacia has usually been treated with large doses of vitamin D (from 40,000 IU to several hundred thousand international units or more daily). The use of dihydrotachysterol, a pseudo-1α-OH-D analogue, 0.2 to 0.6 mg, or 1α,25-$(OH)_2D$, 0.5 to 2.0 μg (see below), orally per day, in place of calciferol has the advantage of shorter onset and duration of action. With vitamin D therapy alone, there is radiological evidence of healing in many patients, but this is usually incomplete; some hypophosphatemia persists, linear skeletal growth remains abnormally slow, and bony deformities continue to develop. In addition, the potential hazard of hypercalcemia and its consequences exists. The addition of oral supplements of inorganic phosphate in divided doses of 1.0 to 3.6 g phosphorus daily has improved the clinical and radiological response, allowed the use of smaller doses of vitamin D, and improved the rate of linear growth in many younger subjects. In some adults, therapy with inorganic phosphate alone has been successful in abolishing muscle weakness and bone pain and in producing radiological and histological healing. The addition of vitamin D improves calcium balance and helps decrease secondary hyperparathyroidism and maintain a higher level of serum phosphorus to permit complete healing. In some patients there may be temporary increase in bone pain and rise in serum alkaline phosphatase during the early phases of treatment. In the osteomalacia associated with the chronic acidosis of renal tubular disorders, the use of alkali may be of value in supplementing therapy with phosphate and vitamin D. In patients with ureterosigmoidostomy, oral sodium bicarbonate has reversed acidosis, improved serum phosphate level, and healed the bone disease; with maintenance use of alkali, recurrence of symptoms has been prevented.

Patients with nephrotic syndrome and low serum 25-OH-D levels benefit from modest vitamin D supplementation. In chronic renal failure high doses of vitamin D, similar to those needed to treat osteomalacia of renal tubular disorders, are used. Dihydrotachysterol at doses of 0.2 to 1.0 mg daily is effective in treating hypocalcemia and osteodystrophy resulting from chronic renal failure. 1α,25-$(OH)_2D_3$ and 1α-OH-D_3 in small doses are equally effective in therapy of most cases of renal osteodystrophy. 1α-OH-D_3, which requires hepatic hydroxylation before it is active, is widely used in Europe but is an experimental drug in the United States. 1α,25-$(OH)_2D_3$ is approved for use in the treatment of hypocalcemic patients on chronic hemodialysis. The generic name of this drug is *calcitriol;* it is available in dosages of 0.25 and 0.50 μg. The recommended initial dose is 0.25 μg per day. If after 2 to 4 weeks on this dose the biochemical parameters are unaltered, the dose is increased by 0.25 μg per day every 2 to 4 weeks until a satisfactory clinical biochemical response (including elevation of serum calcium levels and decrease in PTH levels) is obtained. The usual dose is 0.5 to 1.0 μg per day. Because there are no regulatory mechanisms to control the biological responses to 1α-$(OH)D_3$, there is a high incidence of transient hypercalcemia, especially in patients treated initially. Thus, frequent (biweekly) serum calcium determinations are encouraged during the first 1 to 2 months of therapy; they can be made at monthly intervals once a stable dose has been established. Since $1\alpha,25\text{-(OH)}_2D_3$ has a short duration of action and is not stored in fat depots, hypercalcemia is reversed by discontinuing its use or decreasing its dose. Hypercalcemia usually resolves in 2 to 7 days. Phosphate supplements are, of course, contraindicated in the usual patient with chronic renal failure. Occasionally, however, hypophosphatemia may result from the excessive use of nonabsorbable antacids in addition to excessive removal of phosphate through hemodialysis.

In patients who have had rickets in childhood, the abnormal mechanical stress of severe deformities may contribute to the development of degenerative joint disease, particularly in hips and knees. Osteotomies at the proper time after healing has occurred may help to prevent this complication and avoid more extensive arthroplasties later in life.

REFERENCES

Osteoporosis

AVIOLI LV: Osteoporosis: Pathogenesis and therapy, in *Metabolic Bone Disease*, LV Avioli, SM Krane (eds). New York, Academic, 1977, vol 1, p 307

———: What to do with "postmenopausal osteoporosis." Am J Med 65:881, 1978

CHRISTIANSEN C et al: Bone mass in postmenopausal women after withdrawal of oestrogen/gestagen replacement therapy. Lancet 1:459, 1981

DEQUEKER J: Bone and aging. Ann Rheum Dis 34:100, 1975

GALLAGHER JE et al: Intestinal calcium absorption and serum vitamin D metabolites in normal subjects and in osteoporotic patients. J Clin Invest 64:729, 1980

HAHN TJ et al: Altered mineral metabolism in glucocorticoid-induced osteopenia. J Clin Invest 63:750, 1979

Heath H III et al: Calcium homeostasis in diabetes mellitus. J Clin Endocrinol Metab 49:462, 1979

JICK H: Replacement estrogens and endometrial cancer. N Engl J Med 300:218, 1979

JOWSEY J: *Metabolic Diseases of Bone*. Philadelphia, Saunders, 1977

RECKER RR et al: Effect of estrogens and calcium carbonate on bone loss in postmenopausal women. Ann Intern Med 87:649, 1977

SILLENCE DO et al: Clinical variability in osteogenesis imperfecta—Variable expressivity or gene heterogeneity. Birth Defects 15:113, 1979

THOMSON DL, FRAME B: Involutional osteopenia: Current concepts. Ann Intern Med 85:789, 1976

Rickets and osteomalacia

BORDIER P et al: Vitamin D metabolites and bone mineralization in man. J Clin Endocrinol Metab 46:284, 1978

FRAME B, PARFITT AM: Osteomalacia: Current concepts. Ann Intern Med 89:966, 1978

FUKAMOTO Y et al: Tumor-induced vitamin D-resistant hypophosphatemic osteomalacia associated with proximal renal tubular dysfunction and 1,25-dihydroxyvitamin D deficiency. J Clin Endocrinol Metab 49:873, 1979

GOLDRING SR, KRANE SM: Disorders of calcification: Osteomalacia and rickets, in *Endocrinology*, LJ DeGroot (ed). New York, Grune & Stratton, 1979, vol 2, p 853

LIBERMAN UA et al: End-organ resistance to 1,25-dihydroxycholecalciferol. Lancet 1:504, 1980

MANKIN HJ: Rickets, osteomalacia and renal osteodystrophy. J Bone Joint Surg (Am) 56A:101, 352, 1974

PARKER MS et al: Tumor-induced osteomalacia. Evidence of a surgically correctable alteration in vitamin D metabolism. JAMA 245:492, 1981

RASMUSSEN H et al: $1,25(OH)_2D_3$ is not the only metabolite involved in the pathogenesis of osteomalacia. Am J Med 69:360, 1980

SCHOTT GD, WILLS MR: Muscle weakness in osteomalacia. Lancet 1:626, 1976

STEINBACH HL, NOETZLI M: Roentgen appearance of the skeleton in osteomalacia and rickets. Am J Roentgenol 91:955, 1964

342
PAGET'S DISEASE OF BONE

STEPHEN M. KRANE

Paget's disease of bone (osteitis deformans) is among the most common of the chronic skeletal diseases. In the strict sense it is a focal disease, although occasionally it may be widespread. Histologically the initial event is excessive resorption of bone mediated by cells such as osteoclasts, followed by the replacement of normal marrow by vascular, fibrous connective tissue. At some stage and to a variable degree, the resorbed bone is replaced by coarse-fibered, dense trabecular bone organized in haphazard fashion. The irregular and often rapid deposition of this new bone, to a great extent still lamellar, causes an increase in the number of prominent, irregular cement lines which gives the bone its characteristic "mosaic" pattern. Some areas may show evidence of both excessive resorption and the chaotic new bone formation.

INCIDENCE The prevalence of Paget's disease is difficult to determine since it is most often asymptomatic and is detected usually when roentgenograms are obtained for other reasons. On the basis of autopsy examination, the incidence of Paget's disease has been estimated to be about 3 percent in individuals over the age of 40; there is increased likelihood of occurrence with increasing age. Figures based on radiological surveys indicate less than 1 percent in the adult population in the United States, Great Britain, and Australia. However, the incidence varies markedly in different parts of the world; in some areas, including India, Japan, the Middle East, and Scandinavia, the disease is exceedingly rare.

ETIOLOGY Almost a century after the original description of the disorder and despite intensive study and widespread interest, the etiology of Paget's disease is unknown. No convincing evidence of endocrine abnormality has been produced. Although pagetic bone can be exceedingly vascular, out of proportion to any other disorder, it has not been established that the vascular abnormality is primary. The observation that some of the manifestations of the disease can be suppressed with the use of adrenal glucocorticoids, salicylates, and cytotoxic drugs is of interest, although there is not sufficient information to support earlier hypotheses that an inflammatory process is the fundamental lesion. Intranuclear inclusions have been found by electron microscopy in osteoclasts in pagetic bone but not in osteoclasts or any other cells in bone from normal persons or patients with various bone diseases. In some the inclusions are morphologically similar to nucleocapsids of viruses belonging to the measles group. Results obtained using indirect immunofluorescence and immunoperoxidase techniques with several different serums directed against different strains of measles virus support the suggestion that the inclusions are indeed measles virus nucleocapsids. Other evidence suggests that the inclusions are due to respiratory syncytial virus. Despite these observations, a viral etiology has not been proved.

PATHOPHYSIOLOGY The characteristic feature of Paget's disease is increased resorption of bone accompanied by an increase in bone formation, which is usually adequate to compensate. In the early phase bone resorption predominates (for example, in the variant, *osteoporosis circumscripta*), and the bones are exceedingly vascular. This has been termed the *osteoporotic, osteolytic,* or *destructive phase* of disease in which the external calcium balance may be negative. Commonly the excessive resorption is followed closely by formation of new pagetic bone. In this so-called mixed phase of the disease, the rate of bone formation is so geared to that of bone resorption that the magnitude of the increase in bone turnover is not reflected in the overall calcium balance.

As the activity of the disease decreases, a progressive decrease in resorptive rate may occur, eventually leading to the occurrence of hard, dense, less vascular bone (the so-called *osteoplastic* or *sclerotic* phase) and a positive external calcium balance. Techniques measuring disappearance rates of injected radioisotopes of calcium or strontium have shown that the rates of bone turnover may be increased enormously in patients with active Paget's disease, occasionally more than twenty times normal. Quantitative histomorphometry of pagetic bone biopsies confirms the extent of remodeling with findings of marked increase in resorption surfaces with deep scalloped lacunae containing giant osteoclasts with numerous nuclei. Resorption surfaces are also increased with increased numbers of plump osteoblasts lining the edges. The calcification rate is also markedly increased. The normal hematopoietic marrow is replaced by a loose stroma which may be highly vascular. The magnitude of the increase in turnover varies with the extent as well as the activity of the disease. The increase correlates well with the increased levels of plasma alkaline phosphatase, which are higher in Paget's disease than in any other condition with the exception of hereditary hyperphosphatasia. Although increased bone resorption enhances release of calcium and phosphate ions from the inorganic mineral phase of bone, utilization of these ions for new bone formation and, presumably, feedback control of parathyroid hormone secretion usually maintain the concentration of calcium ions in the plasma at normal levels. The concentration of phosphate in the plasma is normal or slightly elevated. When marked imbalance between bone formation and resorption occurs in favor of resorption, as after prolonged immobilization or fractures, urinary calcium excretion may be increased, and rarely hypercalcemia may be encountered. If, on the other hand, bone formation exceeds resorption (relatively uncommon), circulating levels of parathyroid hormone may be increased. Resorption involves the organic phase of bone as well as the mineral phase. Although the inorganic ions of the mineral phase are reutilized for bone formation, amino acids such as hydroxyproline and hydroxylysine released during resorption of the collagen matrix of bone are not reutilized for collagen biosynthesis. The urinary excretion of small peptides containing hydroxyproline is increased, reflecting the increased bone resorption. Peptides of higher molecular weight (about 5000) containing hydroxyproline and other amino acids in proportions characteristic of collagen are also excreted in increased amounts in the urine and are correlated with increased bone formation.

RADIOLOGICAL CHANGES The radiological findings reflect the underlying pathology and the phase of the disease which predominates at the time of the examination. The pelvic bones are most commonly involved, followed by the femur, skull, tibia, lumbosacral spine, dorsal spine, clavicles, and ribs in that order; small bones are not as frequently diseased. The lytic phase of the disease may be overlooked except when it occurs in the skull as *osteoporosis circumscripta,* with areas of sharply demarcated radiolucency in the frontal, parietal, and occipital bones. In the long bones the lytic areas are usually first seen at one end, from which they progress toward the other end with a V-shaped advancing edge. The lesion may produce expansion of the cortex and exhibit other features which suggest malignancy. Usually the lytic area is followed by a zone of increased density, representing the new bone formation of the mixed phase of the disease. In general, the bone shows enlargement with irregularly widened cortex in a coarse, striated pattern and increased density, occasionally focal in distribution. Perpendicular lines of radiolucency (cortical infractions) are frequent and occur on the convex side of bowed long bones, particularly the femur and tibia. Transverse fractures may also occur, some initiated at the sites of these cortical infractions. The remodeling of the pagetic bone usually follows the lines of stress produced by muscle pull or gravity, accounting for the characteristic lateral bowing of the femur or anterior bowing of the tibia and the tendency for most of the dense bone to be deposited on the concave side of the bowed bone. In the skull, in the mixed stage, there is enlargement and thickening, especially of the outer table, with irregular areas of increased density, often spotty (Fig. 342-1). Basilar invagination is common with involvement of the base of the skull. The changes in the pelvis also consist of the combination of bone resorption and new bone formation and are frequently accompanied by a thickening of the pelvic brim, a characteristic of Paget's disease. In the sclerotic phase of the disease, the bone may show uniform increase in density, often in the absence of striations. This is common in the facial bones but is occasionally seen as well in the vertebrae where a homogeneous, dense pattern gives an "ivory" appearance similar to that produced typically by Hodgkin's disease, although the involved vertebrae are not enlarged in Hodgkin's disease.

CLINICAL PICTURE The clinical presentation is variable and is a function of the extent of the disease, the particular bones involved, and the presence of associated complications. Many patients are asymptomatic. In these individuals the disorder is discovered because of radiological findings during the course of examination of the pelvis or spine for an unrelated disease or complaint, or because of the finding of an elevated level of

FIGURE 342-1
Lateral roentgenogram of the skull from a 58-year-old woman with Paget's disease of bone.

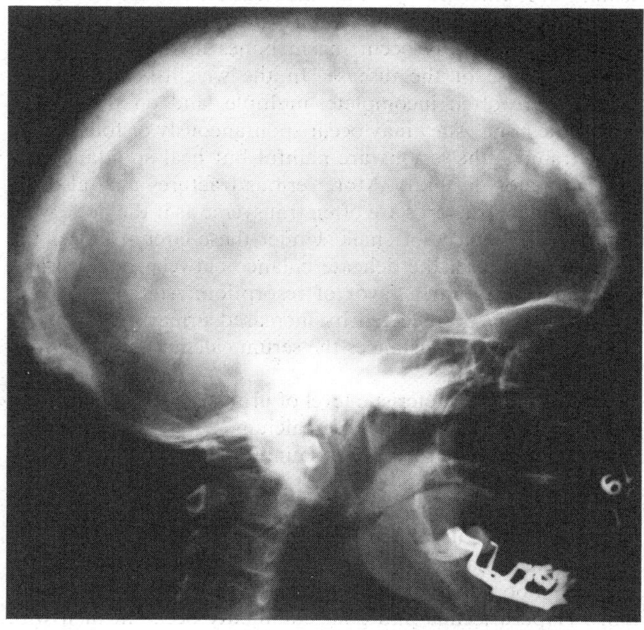

plasma alkaline phosphatase. Other individuals may gradually become aware of a swelling or deformity of a long bone or develop a disturbance in gait due to unequal length of and change in the distribution of mechanical forces in the lower extremities. Enlargement of the skull is often not noticed by the patients, or they may be aware of increasing hat size. Pain in the face and headache are initial complaints in some; backache and pain in the lower extremities are common. The pain is usually dull but may be shooting or knifelike. Back pain is most common in the lumbar region and may radiate into the buttocks or lower extremities. This pain is probably due to the pagetic process itself and to distortion of articular facets and secondary osteoarthritis. Pain in the lower extremities may be associated with the transverse cortical infractions which occur along the convex lateral surface of the femur or the anterior surface of the tibia. Often the new lytic lesions detected on bone scan are the most painful. Pain may also be due to involvement of the hip joint resembling degenerative joint disease and characterized by narrowing of the joint space, bony lipping at the margin of the acetabulum, and deepening of the acetabulum. Angioid streaks of the retina have been observed. Hearing loss is due to direct pagetic involvement of the ossicles of the inner ear or of bone in the region of the cochlea or to impingement on the eighth cranial nerve by pagetic bone narrowing the auditory foramen. More serious neurological complications can result from overgrowth of pagetic bone at the base of the skull (platybasia) due to compression of the brainstem. Compression of the spinal cord with paraplegia has been observed, particularly with involvement of the middorsal spine. Pathological fractures of vertebrae may also produce spinal cord lesions.

COMPLICATIONS Blood flow may be markedly increased in extremities involved with Paget's disease. There is proliferation of blood vessels in pagetic bone, but anatomic and functional studies have not confirmed the presence of arteriovenous fistulas. Although blood flow in the bone itself is increased, there is also cutaneous vasodilatation in the pagetic extremities, which accounts for the increased warmth noted clinically. When the disease is widespread, involving over one-third of the skeleton, the increased blood flow may be associated with *high cardiac output*. In the rare patient so-called high-output heart failure may result. However, heart disease in pagetic individuals is usually accounted for by the same conditions that occur in other patients of similar age. *Pathological fracture* is a frequent complication, usually occurring in bones involved in the destructive phase of the disease. In the weight-bearing bones fractures are often incomplete, multiple, and on the convex side of the bone. They may occur spontaneously or follow only slight trauma; the lesions are painful but heal spontaneously with no major disability. More serious fractures may also occur. Complete fractures are often transverse as if the bone were snapped like a piece of chalk. Under these circumstances the fracture may upset the delicate balance between bone formation and resorption in favor of resorption. At this stage the imbalance may be reflected by increased urinary calcium excretion, and in rare instances the serum calcium level may rise to dangerous levels.

There is no characteristic level of urinary calcium excretion, although there is a tendency for calcium excretion to be higher when the resorptive phase predominates. This may be a factor which accounts for the somewhat higher incidence of *urinary stone* in these patients, although many of the urinary calculi reported may be unrelated to the pagetic process. In addition to secondary changes in the cartilage of the hip joint, similar changes in bones about the knees may result in articular symptoms. Hyperuricemia and gout commonly occur in men with Paget's disease, and calcific periarthritis is also found in high incidence.

Sarcoma is the most dreaded complication. Fortunately, the incidence is probably no greater than 1 percent, although higher incidence has been noted in some series which include many patients with polyostotic involvement. The sarcomas most frequently arise in the femur, humerus, skull, face, and pelvis, and rarely in the vertebrae. In about 20 percent the tumors are multicentric. Histologically, they are usually osteosarcomas, although fibrosarcomas and chondrosarcomas have also been found. Increase in pain and swelling are the most common complaints which lead to recognition of the sarcomas. The level of alkaline phosphatase in the serum of patients with sarcomas reflects the activity and extent of the Paget's disease, although in occasional patients an "explosive rise" of the phosphatase level may accompany the growth of the sarcoma. However, in some patients with limited involvement, phosphatase levels may be only slightly elevated and give no clue to the development of the malignant lesion. The prognosis is extremely poor following the development of sarcomas, and ablative operative therapy is rarely successful. Giant-cell tumors closely resembling reparative granulomas histologically also occur with an increased frequency and are usually benign. Pagetic bone is rarely the site of metastases despite its great vascularity.

THERAPY Most patients require no treatment, since the disease is localized and does not cause symptoms. Indications for therapy include persistent pain in involved bones, neural compression, rapidly progressive deformity resulting in disabling disturbance of posture and/or gait, high-output congestive heart failure, hypercalcemia, severe hypercalciuria with or without formation of renal stones, repeated fractures or nonunion in pagetic bone, and preparation for major orthopedic surgery. *Aspirin* is an effective analgesic, and if it can be tolerated in large enough doses (3.6 to 4.0 g per day) for months or years, disease activity may be suppressed, as shown by decreases in the level of plasma alkaline phosphatase and urinary hydroxyproline excretion. *Indomethacin*, 25 mg three or four times daily, may also relieve pain, especially in the presence of hip involvement. *Glucocorticoids* suppress the disease but only in large doses (greater than 60 mg prednisone per day) which are usually not tolerated and, therefore, are not recommended. It is of interest that the high cardiac output of some patients may be reduced significantly after only a few days of glucocorticoid treatment. Although the use of *sodium fluoride* (80 to 120 mg sodium fluoride per day) for more than a year has produced amelioration of symptoms and decrease in the indexes of activity of the disease, this high dose may lead to poorly mineralized bone. Orthopedic procedures also have a role in the management of selected cases. Total hip replacement may be indicated in the patient with severe hip involvement, and osteotomy is useful to correct marked bowing deformities, particularly of the tibia. In patients with fractures or orthopedic procedures or in patients immobilized for any reason, determinations of urinary and serum calcium levels should be performed at intervals to anticipate the development of hypercalciuria and hypercalcemia. Early ambulation and adequate fluid intake are essential. Preparations of sodium phytate or inorganic phosphate to reduce hypercalciuria may be useful under these circumstances (5 to 6 g neutral sodium phosphate daily in divided doses).

Several agents are effective in reducing the excessive bone resorption of Paget's disease and are of possible therapeutic value. Porcine, salmon, and human *calcitonins* have been administered subcutaneously for prolonged periods to pagetic patients, accompanied by decrease in plasma alkaline phosphatase levels and urinary hydroxyproline excretion. Treatment with calcitonin has produced variable decrease in bone pain, improvement in neurological symptoms, and decrease in elevated cardiac output. Some patients have not continued to respond to porcine and salmon calcitonins because of the development of neutralizing antibodies. These individuals usually continue to exhibit a satisfactory response to human calcitonin. In others in whom diminution in response was not associated with development of antibodies, the development of secondary hyperparathyroidism has been postulated, although this cannot account for resistance in all cases. The calcitonins have a limited usefulness in the treatment of Paget's disease. They are probably most useful in patients with pain corresponding to areas of pagetic involvement, not due to associated joint disease. The dose of salmon calcitonin (the form available in the United States) is 50 to 100 MRC units given subcutaneously daily. In some cases it may be possible to reduce the dose to three times weekly. In severe cases alkaline phosphatase levels, although reduced, do not reach the normal range. The disorder relapses after weeks or months when the calcitonin is discontinued. Some patients develop disturbing nausea, occasionally with vomiting, 30 min to several hours after injection. This may occur after initiating treatment or after months or years of therapy. The etiology is unknown, but the symptoms may be severe enough to discontinue the medication.

Cytotoxic drugs such as mithramycin and actinomycin D are potent agents in pagetic patients. Parenteral administration of mithramycin, 10 to 25 μg/kg for 10 to 14 days, has produced striking decrease in urinary hydroxyproline excretion with subsequent decreases in plasma alkaline phosphatase level and clinical improvement. The indexes of active disease again become abnormal within weeks to months following completion of this course of mithramycin therapy. The drug may continue to be administered as a weekly intravenous bolus. With doses of less than 15 μg/kg, toxicity has been surprisingly low despite potential risks.

Disodium etidronate, a diphosphonate compound, given orally in doses up to 20 mg/kg per day has also been effective in reducing bone resorption in almost all and producing clinical improvement in some. In contrast to the calcitonins, the use of disodium etidronate often brings biochemical abnormalities to normal even in severe cases. Serum alkaline phosphatase and urinary hydroxyproline excretion remain decreased for several months after withdrawal of the drug and only gradually return to pretreatment levels. In doses of 20 mg/kg per day mineralization of new bone may be inhibited and predispose to fracture. Some patients develop disabling pain over pagetic lesions within weeks or months of starting treatment which may be severe enough to warrant discontinuing the drug. Radiographs in some instances show marked increase in bone lysis. This heals when the drug is stopped. It is therefore recommended that doses of 5 mg or occasionally 10 mg/kg per day be used for 6-month periods. Treatment could be reinstituted within 3 to 12 months if biochemical relapse occurs. Other diphosphonate compounds such as the dichloromethylidene or the 3-amino-1-hydroxypropylidine derivatives have been introduced for therapy in Europe. They have a rapid onset of action and apparently do not inhibit mineralization.

REFERENCES

ALTMAN RD, SINGER F (eds): Proceedings of the Kroc Foundation Conference on Paget's Disease of Bone. Arthritis Rheum 23:1073, 1980

AVRAMIDES A: Salmon and porcine calcitonin treatment of Paget's disease of bone. Clin Orthop Relat Res 127:78, 1977

BARRY HC: *Paget's Disease of Bone.* Edinburgh, E and S Livingstone, 1969

FRANCK WA et al: Rheumatic manifestations of Paget's disease of bone. Am J Med 56:592, 1974

KHAIRI MRA, JOHNSTON CC JR: Treatment of Paget's disease of bone (osteitis deformans) with sodium etidronate (EHDP). Clin Orthop Relat Res 127:94, 1977

NAGANT DE DEUXCHAISNES C, KRANE SM: Paget's disease of bone: Clinical and metabolic observations. Medicine 43:233, 1964

RYAN WG: Treatment of Paget's disease of bone with mithramycin. Clin Orthop Relat Res 127:106, 1977

SINGER FR: Human calcitonin treatment of Paget's disease of bone. Clin Orthop Relat Res 127:86, 1977

——— et al: Paget's disease of bone, in *Metabolic Bone Disease,* LV Avioli, SM Krane (eds). New York, Academic, 1978, vol II, p 489

STEINBACH HL: Some roentgen features of Paget's disease. Am J Roentgenol 86:950, 1961

343 HYPEROSTOSIS, NEOPLASMS, AND OTHER DISORDERS OF BONE AND CARTILAGE

STEPHEN M. KRANE
ALAN L. SCHILLER

HYPEROSTOSIS

A number of disease states have in common an increase in the mass of bone per unit volume (hyperostosis). Such increase in bone mass is detected radiologically as increased density of the bone, often associated with a variable degree of disturbance in the architecture of the tissue. In most of these disorders, it is not possible to distinguish between an increase in bone mass due to excessive formation of new bone or decreased resorption of bone already formed. When bone deposition is rapid, the new bone may be of the woven type, but if the process is more chronic, true lamellar bone is formed. The additional bone may be located at the periosteum, within the compact bone of the cortex, or in the trabeculae of the cancellous regions. In the medullary area, the new bone is deposited on and between the trabeculae and encroaches upon the medullary spaces. Typical examples of such responses are seen in areas adjacent to tumors or in association with infection. In some diseases the increase in bone mass may be spotty, as in osteopoikilosis, whereas in others most of the skeleton may be involved, as in the malignant form of osteopetrosis in children. The mechanism of the increase in mass is usually not due to an excessive amount of mineral relative to matrix, except in some disorders such as osteopetrosis where islands of calcified cartilage may persist. (The mineral density of calcified cartilage is greater than that of bone.) In some diseases such as the osteosclerosis of renal insufficiency, the bone mass and radiodensity may be increased, even though the new bone formed is poorly mineralized and contains widened osteoid seams. A classification of the causes of hyperostosis is presented in Table 343-1.

Several of these conditions are discussed in more detail in other chapters, although some general comments are pertinent. Bone that is denser than normal may be seen occasionally in the osteitis fibrosa associated with active hyperparathyroidism. When the hyperparathyroidism is successfully treated, the rate of bone resorption is decreased abruptly out of proportion to the rate of bone formation; this imbalance may lead to the production of areas of bone density greater than in the surrounding skeleton, especially in the healing of brown tumors.

In hypothyroidism, the rates of both bone formation and resorption may be decreased, but the balance may be in favor of formation, resulting in bones that are of increased density but normal architecture. Increased bone density is also observed in some instances of osteomalacia associated with disturbances in renal tubular function. The increased mass of bone occurs together with widened osteoid seams, as in chronic renal glomerular insufficiency. In the vertebral bodies the bone appears denser in transverse bands at the upper and lower margins, with a relatively radiolucent center. This "sandwich" appearance is similar to that seen in some patients with osteopetrosis and has been termed by the British the *rugger jersey sign.*

OSTEOPETROSIS Osteopetrosis (marble bone disease of Albers-Schönberg) is a rare disorder which varies in severity and age of clinical presentation. The most severe form occurs in infants and children and is inherited as an autosomal recessive trait, while a more benign form is transmitted as an autosomal dominant trait. The so-called malignant variant starts in utero and progresses rapidly with marked anemia, hepatosplenomegaly, hydrocephalus, cranial nerve involvement, and death, often due to infection. In the less fulminant form, the anemia is not as severe, neurological abnormalities are not as frequent, and recurrent pathological fractures are the main feature. Although the majority of cases are in infants and children, many are discovered first in adult life when roentgenograms are obtained because of fractures or unrelated diseases. There is no particular predilection for either sex.

The increased bone mass is generally thought to be due to a defect in the normal remodeling of bone. Both bone formation and resorption are depressed, particularly resorption. Islands of unresorbed calcified cartilage encased in bone are frequently seen. The defect in remodeling results in marked disorganization of bone structure with thickened cortices and lack of funnelization of metaphyses. Despite its increased density, the bone is abnormal mechanically and fractures readily. Osteomalacia or rickets is sometimes a component of the osteopetrosis in children (Fig. 343-1).

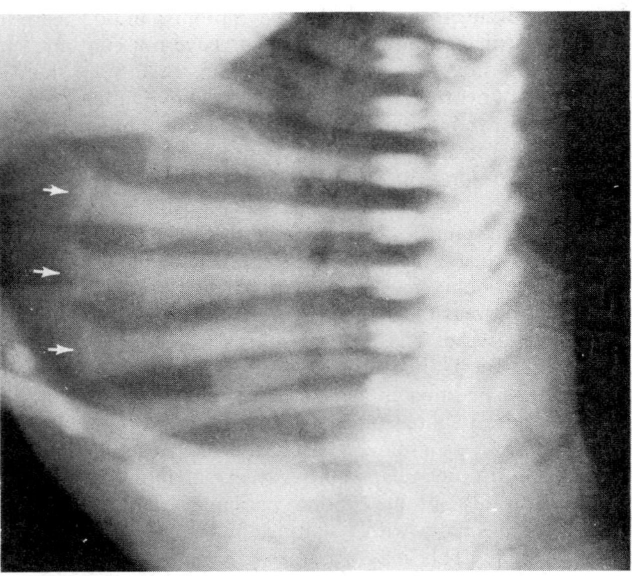

FIGURE 343-1
Lateral roentgenogram of the thorax of a 9-month-old boy with the "malignant" form of osteopetrosis. Note the uniform increase in mineral density of the vertebral bodies and the marked flaring of the ends of the ribs (arrows), indicative of rickets.

TABLE 343-1
Causes of hyperostosis

1 Endocrine disorders
 a Primary hyperparathyroidism
 b Hypothyroidism
 c Acromegaly
2 Radiation osteitis
3 Chemical poisoning
 a Fluoride
 b Elemental phosphorus
 c Beryllium
 d Arsenic
 e Vitamin A intoxication
 f Lead
 g Bismuth
4 Osteomalacic disorders
 a Renal tubular osteomalacia (vitamin D resistance or phosphate diabetes)
 b Chronic renal glomerular failure
5 Osteosclerosis (localized) associated with chronic infection
6 Osteosclerotic phase of Paget's disease
7 Osteosclerosis associated with carcinomatous metastases, malignant lymphoma, and hematologic disorders (myeloproliferative disorders, sickle cell disease, leukemia, multiple myeloma, systemic mastocytosis)
8 Osteosclerosis of erythroblastosis fetalis
9 Unclassified diseases
 a Osteopetrosis (marble bone disease of Albers-Schönberg)
 b Pyknodysostosis
 c Osteomyelosclerosis
 d Hyperostosis corticalis generalisata
 e Hyperostosis generalisata with pachydermia
 f Hereditary hyperphosphatasia
 g Progressive diaphyseal dysplasia (osteopathia hyperostotica multiplex infantilis; Camurati-Engelmann disease)
 h Melorheostosis
 i Osteopoikilosis
 j Hyperostosis frontalis interna

The histological changes are reflected in the roentgenograms (Fig. 343-2), which reveal uniformly dense, sclerotic bone often without distinction between the cortical and cancellous regions. There is persistence of the primary spongiosa with central calcified cartilage cores surrounded by woven bone. Osteoclasts are often increased in number but apparently are not functioning properly. Osteoclasts morphologically may be normal or have loss of thin ruffled borders suggesting a spectrum of changes which may occur in these cells. The variability of the observed changes may reflect heterogeneity in this syndrome, as in the osteopetrosis that occurs spontaneously in rodents. The long bones are usually involved, with increased density along the entire shaft. Foci of increased density may be seen in the epiphyses corresponding to regions of unresorbed calcified cartilage. The metaphyses have a characteristic clubbed or splayed appearance. Horizontal bandings of increased density alternating with zones of decreased density are seen in the long bones and vertebrae and suggest that the defect may be intermittent during periods of growth. The skull, pelvis, ribs, and other bones may also be involved. The phalanges and the distal humerus may appear normal when the disease is not severe.

Encroachment of bone upon the marrow cavity is associated with anemia of the myelophthisic type with foci of extramedullary hematopoiesis in liver, spleen, and lymph nodes and enlargement of these organs. In the malignant form of the disease it is thought that the abundant osteoclasts may crowd out the hematopoietic marrow. Neurological abnormalities are associated with encroachment on cranial nerves, which may result in optic atrophy, nystagmus, papilledema, exophthalmos, and impairment of extraocular motility. Facial paralysis and deafness are frequent; trigeminal lesions and anosmia have also been described. In infants with severe disease, macrocephaly, hydrocephalus, and convulsions may occur. Infections such as osteomyelitis are frequent in these children. Associated renal tubular acidosis has also been described.

In the milder dominant osteopetrosis, about half of the patients have no symptoms, and the disorder is discovered incidentally on roentgenograms. Other such patients present because of fractures, bone pain, osteomyelitis, and cranial nerve palsies.

Fractures are a common complication even with trivial trauma. Healing of such fractures is usually satisfactory, although delayed union may occur. When the disease is manifested first in adult life, fractures may be the only clinical problem. Levels of calcium and alkaline phosphatase in the plasma are usually normal in adults, although in children hypophosphatemia and, occasionally, moderate hypocalcemia have been noted. Serum acid phosphatase levels are usually increased.

The mechanism of the skeletal abnormality in osteopetrosis is not known. However, a disorder resembling osteopetrosis has been described in several strains of mice and rats. In the affected mice bone resorption can be restored by transplanting spleen and bone marrow cells, and the disease can be transferred to normal recipients by spleen cells from affected donors. Transfusion of normal syngeneic bone marrow cells to osteopetrotic rats also reverses the osteopetrosis. Thus the defect in bone resorption may be related to defects in cellular immunity. Several children with severe osteopetrosis have received bone marrow transplants from HLA-identical siblings which resulted in histological and radiological increases in bone resorption, accompanied by improvement in anemia, vision, hearing, and growth and development. In one report, donor (male) nuclei were identified by Y-chromosome analysis in recipient (female) osteoclasts.

Other attempts to affect the altered remodeling of bone in patients with osteopetrosis have been unsuccessful, although there is evidence that administration of parathyroid hormone may increase bone resorption. Despite the extramedullary hematopoiesis in the spleen, splenectomy can occasionally decrease erythrocyte destruction in this organ and increase the life span of the erythrocytes.

FIGURE 343-2
Roentgenogram of the spine and pelvis of a 55-year-old man with the more benign, dominant form of osteopetrosis.

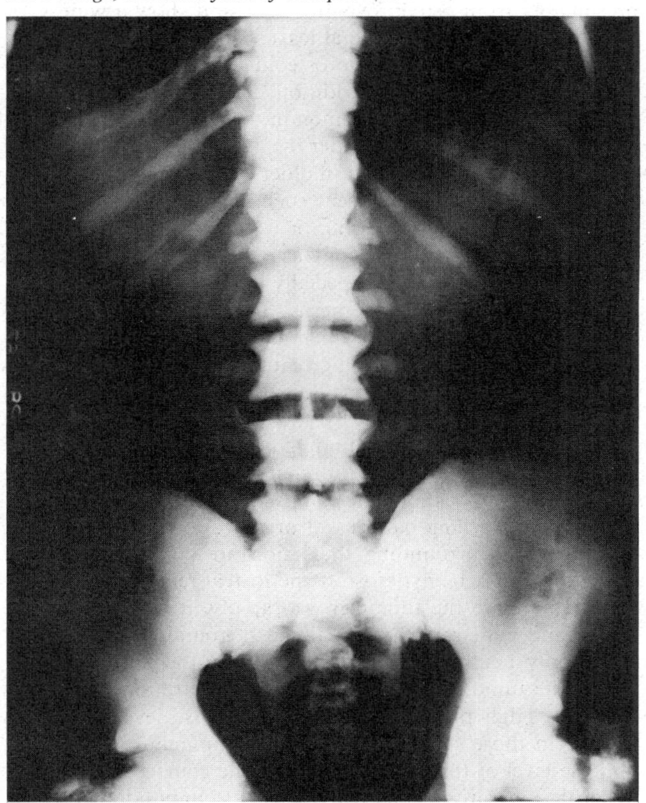

PYKNODYSOSTOSIS *Pyknodysostosis* resembles osteopetrosis but is usually a more benign condition not associated with hepatosplenomegaly, anemia, or cranial nerve involvement. In addition to a generalized increase in bone density, features include short stature, separated cranial sutures, hypoplasia of the mandible, persistence of deciduous teeth, and progressive acroosteolysis of the terminal phalanges. Longevity is usually not decreased, and the patient usually presents to the physician because of frequent fractures. Pyknodysostosis is inherited as a mendelian recessive trait. In one case intermittently elevated levels of plasma calcitonin were found as well as an exaggerated response of the plasma calcitonin to infusions of calcium and glucagon. The gene which determines this disorder may be located on the short arm of a small accrocentric chromosome.

OSTEOMYELOSCLEROSIS *Osteomyelosclerosis* is a disorder in which the marrow cells are replaced by diffuse fibroplasia, occasionally accompanied by osseous metaplasia. When the latter is prominent, increased skeletal density is seen on roentgenograms. Osteomyelosclerosis is probably a phase in the course of the myeloproliferative disorders and is characteristically accompanied by extramedullary hematopoiesis.

A disease distinct from those described above has been termed *hyperostosis corticalis generalisata* (van Buchem's disease). It is characterized by osteosclerosis of the skull (base and calvaria), lower jaw, clavicles, and ribs, and thickening of the diaphyseal cortices of the long and short bones. Alkaline phosphatase levels in the serum are elevated, and histological observations suggest that the disorder is due to increased formation of bone of normal structure. The major clinical manifestations are due to neural compression and consist of optic atrophy, facial paralysis, and perception deafness. In *hyperostosis generalisata with pachydermia* (Uehlinger), the sclerosis is due to increased formation of subperiosteal spongy bone and involves the epiphyses, metaphyses, and diaphyses. Pain, swelling of joints, and thickening of the skin of the lower arms are common.

HEREDITARY HYPERPHOSPHATASIA This disorder is characterized by severe structural deformities of the skeleton with increase in thickness of the calvaria, large homogeneous areas of increased density at the base of the skull, and widening and loss of normal architecture of the shafts and the epiphyses of the long and short bones. There is a failure to deposit normal bone, with haphazard orientation of lamellae suggesting active remodeling. Plasma alkaline phosphatase levels and urinary excretion of hydroxyproline peptides and other collagen degradation products are markedly increased. The disorder is apparently inherited as an autosomal recessive trait. Calcitonin therapy may be of value in some of these patients.

PROGRESSIVE DIAPHYSEAL DYSPLASIA A disorder in which a symmetrical thickening and increased diameter of the diaphyses of long bones occurs, particularly in femurs, tibias, fibulas, radii, and ulnas, has been termed *progressive diaphyseal dysplasia* (Camurati-Engelmann disease). The alkaline phosphatase levels are normal, although the erythrocyte sedimentation rate may be elevated. Pain over affected areas, fatigue, abnormal gait, and muscle wasting are the major manifestations. Clinical and biochemical improvement may result from the use of prednisone or related glucocorticoids.

MELORHEOSTOSIS This rare condition, which usually begins in childhood, is characterized by areas of sclerosis that appear in the bones of one limb. All segments of the bone may be involved, with the dense structures appearing as sclerotic areas which have a "flowing" distribution. The involved limb is often extremely painful.

OSTEOPOIKILOSIS This is a benign disorder usually discovered by chance and is not associated with symptoms. It is characterized by dense spots of trabecular bone less than a centimeter in diameter, usually of uniform density, that are located in the epiphyses and adjacent parts of the metaphyses. All bones may be involved except the skull, ribs, and vertebrae.

HYPEROSTOSIS FRONTALIS INTERNA *Hyperostosis frontalis interna* is an abnormality of the inner table of the frontal bones of the skull first described by Morgagni and consisting of smooth, rounded enostoses covered by dura and projecting into the cranial cavity. These enostoses are usually less than 1 cm at their greatest diameter and usually do not extend posteriorly beyond the coronal suture. The abnormality is found almost exclusively in women, who are frequently obese, hirsute, and who have a variety of neuropsychiatric complaints (Morgagni-Stewart-Morel syndrome). However, hyperostosis frontalis interna has also been seen in women with no obvious illness or particular associated disease. There is no good evidence that the finding in the skull is a manifestation of a generalized metabolic disorder.

NEOPLASMS OF BONE

Primary neoplasms of the skeletal system reflect in their histology the cellular and extracellular components of the skeleton. However, it is not always possible to prove that a tumor arises from the same type of tissue that it produces. The precursor cells of bone tissue are probably derived from histogenetically distinct cell lines in which the osteoclasts arise from hematopoietic cells and the osteoblasts arise from the stromal cell system. The primitive stromal cell could differentiate into chondroblasts and fibroblasts as well as osteoblasts. Neoplasms can arise from all these cell types. Each of these cells can produce its characteristic extracellular matrix, and neoplasms arising from them may thus be recognized. Primary neoplasms of bone can arise also from other hematopoietic, vascular, and neural elements.

PATHOPHYSIOLOGY Tumors in bone induce resorption of normal skeletal tissue by (1) production of factors that directly lyse bone, (2) production of factors that increase the function of osteoclasts in the vicinity of the tumor, (3) modulation of hematopoietic osteoclast precursors into active osteoclasts, and (4) interfering with blood supply. Tumors also produce some reaction in surrounding bone and alter the normal contour. The epiphyseal plate, articular cartilage, cortex, and periosteum of bone often offer a barrier to the spread of neoplastic tissue. Alteration of the contour of the cortex is not due to "expansion" but to remodeling of the bone in the area and formation of new bone with the new contour. Some tumors induce primarily an osteoblastic or sclerotic reaction in surrounding bone, which results in increased radiodensity. Primary neoplasms may appear to be less radiopaque than surrounding bone or more radiopaque, depending upon the degree of calcification or ossification of the matrix and the density of the tissue. Bone tumors may be recognized because of (1) the presence of a mass in the soft tissues, (2) deformity of a bone, (3) pain and tenderness, and (4) pathological fractures. Tumors of bone may also be detected incidentally on roentgenograms obtained for other clinical reasons. Although it is usually possible to classify bone tumors as benign or malignant as described below, prediction of the clinical outcome of these tumors based on histological and radiological criteria may not always be possible.

Bone scans utilizing ^{99m}Tc polyphosphonate may be useful in detecting bone tumors. The extent of the lesions can also be assessed by standard and computerized tomographic techniques. However, proper evaluation and selection of therapy require detailed evaluation of clinical radiographic and histological aspects. There are numerous pitfalls in the clinical diagnosis and interpretation of histological features of tumors of bone. Management of the patient therefore requires cooperation of the orthopedist, oncologist, radiologist, radiotherapist, and pathologist.

BENIGN TUMORS The most common benign tumors, but not necessarily true neoplasms, are *osteochondromas* (exostoses) and *endochondromas* (which may be multiple in Ollier's disease), *benign giant-cell tumors, unicameral bone cysts, osteoid osteomas,* and *nonossifying fibromas* (fibrous cortical defects). As a rule benign tumors are not painful except for osteoid osteomas, benign chondroblastomas, and benign chondromyxoidfibroma. The usual clinical problem is that of slowly progressing mass, pathological fracture, or deformity. Treatment is usually accomplished by resection of the tumor or curettage and bone grafting. In some instances in which wide resection of tissue has been necessary, insertion of metal and plastic prostheses or allograft transplantation has been successful in preserving limb function.

MALIGNANT TUMORS The most common malignant tumor of bone is multiple myeloma (see Chap. 65), which arises from hematopoietic cells. Reticulum-cell sarcoma or primary lymphoma of bone may also arise locally in bone. Malignant tumors of nonhematopoietic origin include osteosarcomas, chondrosarcomas, fibrosarcomas, and Ewing's tumor. Giant-cell tumors may be included here since they may, on occasion, metastasize and are locally destructive. *Osteogenic sarcomas* arise presumably from osteoprogenitor cells and show a wide variation in histopathology, with at least six histologic types. These tumors usually contain some osteoid tissue, at least in small foci, and may contain in addition cartilaginous and fibrous elements. They are most common in the second and third decades and are less common under the age of 10 and over the age of 40 years. When they occur in older individuals, some predisposing cause is usually present such as Paget's disease, prior exposure to ionizing radiation, or a bone infarct. In primary osteogenic sarcomas the lesions usually arise in the metaphyseal region of long bones, especially in the distal femur, proximal tibia, and proximal humerus. The most common symptoms are pain and swelling which may be present for weeks or months. The roentgenographic features of osteosarcomas depend upon the degree of bone destruction, the extent to which mineralized bone is formed by and within the tumor, and the type of reaction in the surrounding bone. Thus the lesions may vary from ones purely lytic in character to those with dense areas containing radiopaque lumps, clouds, or spicules of tumor bone in varying patterns of organization. Discontinuities in the cortex surrounding the lesion are common. In other cases, there may be hyperostotic periosteal reactions of grossly layered bone. If the tumor grows rapidly, it may destroy the cortex and penetrate the soft tissue surrounding the bone; it leaves only a cuff of periosteal new bone at the peripheral margin of the tumor, just at the point of penetration (Codman's triangle). High plasma alkaline phosphatase levels are often present in those sarcomas that are predominantly osteogenic, and the level of this activity parallels the course of the tumor. When lesions are adequately treated by amputation or radiation, the level of alkaline phosphatase falls, and when metastases appear, the level rises again, often reaching values higher than those present initially. When values are initially very high, the course is often rapidly fatal. Metastases occur primarily by the hematogenous route especially to the lung. The prognosis of osteosarcoma is very poor, with radiological evidence of pulmonary metastases usually occurring within a year following a potentially curable surgical amputation. The course varies with the type of tumor; for example, a "telangiectatic" variant has a very poor prognosis, whereas the rare low-grade intramedullary type has a better one. In the typical intramedullary type of osteosarcoma, death occurs within 6 months from the onset of detectable pulmonary metastases, suggesting that the lesions in the lungs were present at the time of amputation or that cells were shed from the tumor during the operation. Use of chemotherapy such as doxorubicin hydrochloride (Adriamycin), dactinomycin, high-dose methotrexate with citrovorum factor rescue, and vincristine has increased survival and seemingly eliminated tumors in some instances. It has even been possible to resect pulmonary metastases in selected patients after chemotherapy and removal of the primary lesion. Reduction of the growth rate of tumor cells by the chemotherapy has made this approach feasible. Nevertheless, these treatment programs have high morbidity and high mortality.

Chondrosarcomas are clinically distinguishable from osteogenic sarcomas. In contrast to the latter, chondrosarcomas usually arise in adulthood and old age, with the peak incidence in the fourth, fifth, and sixth decades. Most are located in the pelvic girdle, ribs, and diaphyseal portions of the femur and humerus; distal portions of the extremities are involved rarely. Chondrosarcomas may also rarely arise by malignant transformation of osteochondromas and enchondromata. As a rule chondrosarcomas are slow growing and slow to recur. Radiographically the lesions appear destructive, with mottled increases in radiodensity which reflect the variable degree of calcification of cartilaginous matrix and ossification. Radical excision is the treatment of choice. Histological grading of the tumor can be valuable for predicting prognosis and determining appropriate surgical therapy.

Ewing's tumor This is a malignant sarcoma composed of small, round cells that occurs most frequently in the first three decades of life. Most are located in some portion of the long bones, although any bone may be involved. Ewing's sarcoma is a highly malignant lesion with a low incidence of cure by ablative surgery with or without radiation. However, aggressive chemotherapy and radiation have proved successful in improving survival of patients with Ewing's sarcoma.

TUMORS METASTATIC TO BONE The skeleton is one of the most common sites of metastases from carcinomas and occasionally even sarcomas. Skeletal metastases may be relatively silent or may produce symptoms by the same mechanisms as primary tumors, i.e., pain, swelling, deformity of a bone, encroachment on hematopoietic tissue in the marrow, compression of spinal cord or nerve roots, and pathological fractures. In addition, rapidly lytic skeletal metastases can result in hypercalcemia and, in some instances, renal insufficiency secondary to the hypercalcemia. The bones involved most commonly are the vertebrae, proximal femur, pelvis, ribs, sternum, and proximal humerus, in that order of frequency. The carcinomas that most frequently metastasize to bone arise in prostate, breast, lung, thyroid, kidney, and bladder.

Malignant cells reach the skeleton via the bloodstream. Those that survive may proliferate and distort the normal architecture, probably by production of substances which cause dissolution of both mineral phase and organic matrix.

Osteolysis most often results from stimulated modulation of osteoprogenitor cells to osteoclasts in the surrounding bone. Tumor cells produce parathyroid hormone-like peptides and other peptides as well as prostaglandins which function to stimulate modulation of osteoclasts from progenitor cells and increase the functional activity of osteoclasts already present. Malignant tumor cells may also secrete osteoclastic activating factor, which normally is lymphocyte-derived. Some carcinoma cells may also act directly to resorb bone. Examples of carcinomatous metastases (which are usually predominantly osteolytic) are those arising from thyroid, kidney and lower bowel. Other tumors induce an *osteoblastic* response in which the new bone arises from skeletal cells and not the tumor itself. The resulting lesion may appear more dense than the surrounding tissue. Occasionally the increase in radiodensity is uniform, simulating osteosclerosis. Carcinoma of the prostate characteristically produces osteoblastic metastases. Carcinoma of the breast produces both osteolytic and osteoblastic metastases. Malignant carcinoid tumors arising from the embryonic foregut and hindgut metastasize to bone with high frequency, producing an osteoblastic reaction. Hodgkin's disease in bone also produces an osteoblastic response both focal and diffuse. More malignant lymphomas in bone produce predominantly destructive lesions. As a rule, osteolytic metastases are the ones associated with hypercalcemia, hypercalciuria, and increased hydroxyprolinuria (reflecting matrix destruction); they are usually associated with normal or slightly increased levels of serum alkaline phosphatase. Osteoblastic metastases, on the other hand, are often accompanied by more marked elevations of serum alkaline phosphatase and may even be associated with hypocalcemia. With some metastases (as in carcinoma of the breast) there may be phases in which osteolysis predominates (with hypercalciuria, hypercalcemia, and normal alkaline phosphatase levels) alternating with phases in which alkaline phosphatase levels rise and the skeletal lesions become more sclerotic.

Treatment of skeletal metastases is usually palliative. In the case of slowly growing localized lesions (as in some instances of carcinoma of the thyroid or occasionally in carcinoma of the kidney) local radiation is useful to relieve pain or reduce compression of surrounding structures. Many patients with carcinomas of breast or prostate survive for years even after extensive skeletal metastases are recognized. Castration and estrogen therapy slow the progress of the lesions in patients with metastatic prostatic carcinoma (see Chap. 127). When patients with mammary cancer are treated with estrogens or androgens, the character of the reaction to the metastases may temporarily shift from a predominantly osteoblastic to a lytic phase with resultant hypercalcemia (see Chap. 126). Mithramycin, which inhibits osteoclast function and is effective in treating hypercalcemia associated with malignant disease, may also be useful in palliation of osteolytic metastases. Dichloromethylene diphosphonate, which has been used to decrease bone resorption in Paget's disease, also decreases the bone resorption secondary to malignant disease. The bone pain in patients with metastatic carcinoma may be relieved by the use of L-dopa. It is also important to recognize that hypercalcemia in patients with malignant tumors is not due solely to skeletal metastases, although this is the most common situation. Production of parathyroid hormone-like polypeptides and other osteolytic substances by extraskeletal neoplasms may also result in elevation of serum calcium levels. Hypercalcemia per se, whether spontaneous or induced by therapy, may produce symptoms such as anorexia, polyuria, polydipsia, depression, and eventually coma. In addition, nephrocalcinosis can result from hypercalcemia, and death may result from renal insufficiency.

OTHER DISORDERS OF BONE AND CARTILAGE

FIBROUS DYSPLASIA (ALBRIGHT'S SYNDROME) Albright and his associates, in 1937, described a syndrome characterized by "osteitis fibrosa disseminata, areas of pigmentation and endocrine dysfunction, with precocious puberty in females." It was subsequently recognized that the bony lesions, called *fibrous dysplasia,* may occur in the absence of the other features of Albright's syndrome. The fundamental nature of the osseous disorder is unknown; the disease does not appear to be heritable, although it has been reported to affect monozygotic twins. The frequency of the disease is approximately the same in both sexes.

Incidence The lesions of fibrous dysplasia may be confined to one bone or be polyostotic in distribution. The disease may be divided into three main categories that are useful for clinical evaluation and therapy: (1) monostotic, (2) polyostotic, and (3) Albright's syndrome and its variants. The monostotic form is the most common. It can be asymptomatic or lead to a pathological fracture. The majority of the lesions are located in the craniofacial bones or ribs; however, any bone can be affected, especially the proximal femur or tibia. Monostotic fibrous dysplasia is most often diagnosed between 20 and 30 years of age. There are usually no associated skin lesions. Approximately a quarter of the individuals with the polyostotic form have more than half the skeleton involved by disease. One side of the body may be affected, and the lesions may be distributed segmentally in a limb, particularly in the lower extremities. Craniofacial lesions are present in approximately half of those with the polyostotic form. Whereas the monostotic form is usually detected in young adults, fractures and skeletal deformities occur in the polyostotic form in childhood; the disease is generally more severe and deforming in patients with early clinical onset. Puberty may lead to quiescence of the lesions, and in some instances lesions worsen during pregnancy. Albright's syndrome is more common in females than males. The occurrence of short stature can be ascribed to premature closure of the epiphyses. The most frequent extraskeletal manifestations are the skin lesions.

Pathology All forms of fibrous dysplasia have an identical histological appearance, although cartilage is more commonly involved in the polyostotic form. Grossly, the marrow cavity is filled by gritty, gray-pink, rubbery tissue that replaces the normal cancellous bone. Often, the endosteal cortical surface is scalloped. Histologically, the lesions contain benign-appearing fibroblastic tissue arranged in a loose whorled pattern (Fig. 343-3). The grittiness is due to numerous irregularly arranged woven bone spicules, most of which lack osteoblastic palisading or rimming, which are embedded in the fibrous tissue. These bone spicules may also have prominent cement lines. In approximately 10 percent of cases, islands of hyaline cartilage are present, and more rarely, particularly in young patients, myxoid tissue may predominate. Examination by polarized light and with the use of special stains indicates a contiguity of collagen fibers of the osseous and marrow tissue. Occasionally, particularly in the polyostotic form, cystic degeneration occurs, characterized by the presence of hemorrhage with hemosiderin-containing macrophages and osteoclast-type giant cells in the periphery of the cyst. Malignant degeneration into a sarcoma (osteosarcoma, chondrosarcoma, fibrosarcoma) occurs rarely, and in most instances these sarcomas arise in previously radiated lesions. Ossifying fibroma of long bones is a peculiar fibrosseous cortical lesion which may be a variant of fibrous dysplasia. It is seen most commonly in the tibial shaft of teenagers. Although clinically benign, it has a tendency to recur if not adequately excised.

FIGURE 343-3
Photomicrograph of the lesion of fibrous dysplasia. Note spicules of dark-staining woven bone (WB) surrounded by loose fibroblastic tissue.

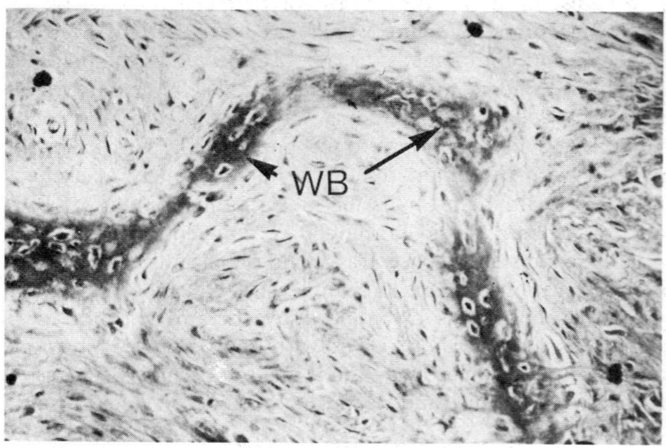

Radiological changes The roentgenographic appearance of the lesions is that of a radiolucent area with a well-delineated, smooth or scalloped border, typically associated with focal thinning of the cortex of the bone (Fig. 343-4). These lesions are not usually cysts in the strict sense, since they are not fluid-filled cavities. They occasionally appear multiloculate. The so-

FIGURE 343-4
Roentgenogram of the upper extremity from a 33-year-old woman with fibrous dysplasia of bone. Typical lesions involve the entire humerus as well as the scapula and proximal ulna.

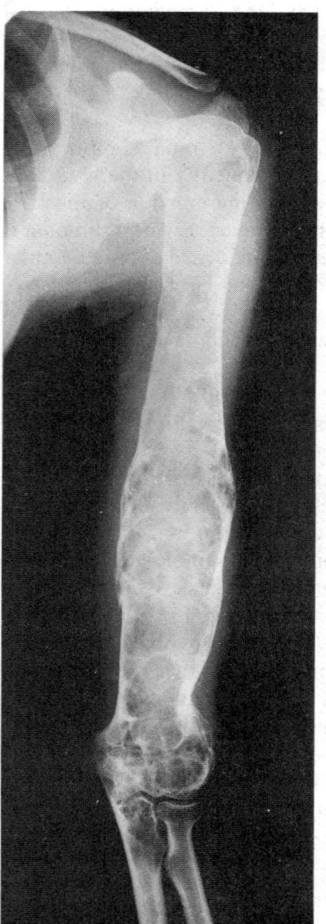

called ground-glass appearance reflects the content of the thin spicules of calcified, woven bone. Frequently, deformities are present such as coxa vara, shepherd's-crook deformity of the femur, bowing of the tibia, Harrison's grooves, and protrusio acetabuli. Involvement of facial bones, usually with lesions of increased radiodensity, may create a leonine appearance (leontiasis ossea) superficially resembling that seen in some patients with leprosy. Advanced skeletal age may be noted, which in females is correlated with sexual precocity but may also be seen in males without sexual precocity. Although the lesions tend to spare the epiphyseal regions before puberty, in older individuals fibrous dysplasia may develop in the epiphyses.

Clinical picture The clinical course is highly variable. Skeletal lesions are usually detected because of deformity or fractures. Symptoms ascribable to bone involvement are headache, seizures, cranial nerve abnormalities, or even spontaneous scalp hemorrhages if there is craniofacial bone disease. In some females and even less commonly in males sexual precocity is the presenting complaint, occasionally present years before the appearance of skeletal symptoms. Serum calcium and phosphorus values are usually normal. In approximately one-third of patients with polyostotic fibrous dysplasia, levels of serum alkaline phosphatase may be elevated to high values, and urinary hydroxyproline excretion is often increased. In some subjects, high cardiac output similar to that seen in extensive Paget's disease may be found. In general, patients with extensive involvement have widespread disease when symptoms first appear, whereas with mild disease at the onset of symptoms extensive disease does not usually develop.

The abnormal cutaneous pigmentation that is seen in most patients with Albright's syndrome consists of isolated dark-brown to light-brown macules which tend to remain on one side of the midline (Fig. 343-5). The border is usually, although not always, irregular or jagged ("coast of Maine") in contrast to the smooth borders of the pigmented macules of neurofibromatosis ("coast of California"). As a rule there are fewer than six of the lesions, which range in size from 1 cm to those covering very large areas, particularly the back, buttocks, or sacral regions. When the lesions are present in the scalp, the overlying hair may be more deeply pigmented than that over the remainder of the scalp. Localized alopecia, associated with osteomas of the skin, has been seen in Albright's syndrome, and such lesions tend to have focal concordance with the skeletal lesions. There is a strong tendency for the pigmentation to be on the same side as the skeletal lesions and actually overlie them.

The sexual precocity of unknown cause is found in females and rarely in males (see also Chap. 118). Premature vaginal bleeding and development of axillary and pubic hair and of breasts are the main features. In the few ovaries that have been examined, no corpora lutea have been seen. The cause of the precocious sexuality is still not clear. In the few cases where measurements have been reported, the females have shown high estrogen levels and low or undetectable gonadotropins. In one studied case gonadotropin levels did not respond to luteinizing hormone–releasing hormone (LHRH). Precocious sexuality is not limited to patients with cranial involvement, and although the characteristic pigmented macules are usually found, this association is not invariable. Another endocrine abnormality present with increased frequency is hyperthyroidism. Rarer associations include Cushing's syndrome, acromegaly, possibly hypogonadotropic hypogonadism, and soft tissue myxomas. Hypophosphatemic osteomalacia may also accompany fibrous dysplasia and resembles the disorder associated with other skeletal and nonskeletal tumors. As mentioned, sarcomatous degeneration may be rarely seen in fibrous dysplasia. Sarcomatous changes are found only in a focus of preexisting fibrous dysplasia, are more common in the polyostotic forms, and have usually been associated with previous radiation of the lesions.

Although the lytic lesions of fibrous dysplasia resemble superficially the brown tumors of hyperparathyroidism, the age of the patient, normocalcemia, increased density of bone in the skull, and areas of cutaneous pigmentation identify the former condition. However, fibrous dysplasia and hyperparathyroidism may coexist. Neurofibromas may involve bone and produce cutaneous pigmentation as well as nodules in the skin. The pigmented macules of neurofibromatosis are more numerous and more widely distributed than in fibrous dysplasia, usually have smooth borders, and tend to involve areas such as the axillary folds. Other lesions which may have a roentgenographic appearance similar to that of isolated fibrous dysplasia are unicameral bone cysts, aneurysmal bone cysts, and nonossifying fibromata. Leontiasis ossea is most often due to fibrous dysplasia, although other disorders may also produce this ap-

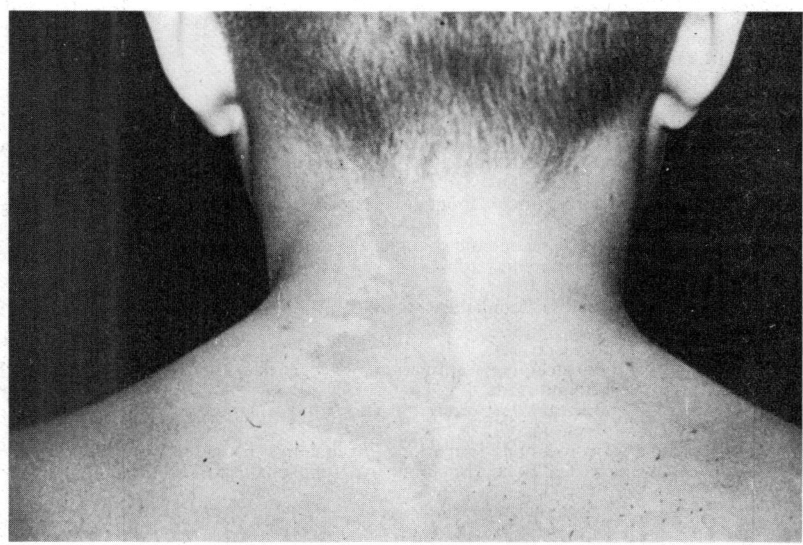

FIGURE 343-5
Typical pigmented café au lait lesion of the skin in an 11-year-old boy with polyostotic fibrous dysplasia. The border has the jagged "coast of Maine" appearance that is characteristic of Albright's syndrome. Note that the lesion is limited to one side (left) of the body.

pearance such as craniometaphyseal dysplasia, hyperphosphatasia, and, in adults, Paget's disease.

Treatment Fibrous dysplasia, when symptomatic, can be managed by a variety of orthopedic operative procedures such as osteotomy, curettage, and bone grafting. Indications for such procedures include progressive deformity, nonunion of fractures, and persistent pain unresponsive to conservative treatment. Calcitonin may be effective in treatment of widespread disease associated with bone pain and high serum alkaline phosphatase levels (see Chap. 342).

DYSPLASIAS AND CHONDRODYSTROPHIES A variety of diseases of bone and cartilage have been called *dystrophies* or *dysplasias*. Classification has been difficult, since the underlying defect is not usually known. It is possible that a biochemical lesion, such as that in the metabolism of the mucopolysaccharides demonstrated in the Hunter and Hurler syndromes, will also be found in a number of these disorders and permit more than a descriptive classification. However, a useful scheme has been proposed by Rubin based on the consideration of errors in modeling of bone and cartilage as departures from normal development (Table 343-2). Other clinical and genetic features form the basis of a classification by Rimoin. Pathological processes in the skeletal dysplasias may be expressed as a deficiency (hypoplasia) or excess (hyperplasia) in relation to normal development. Several of the more common of these will be described.

Spondyloepiphyseal dysplasia The spondyloepiphyseal dysplasias are a heterogeneous group of disorders in which abnormalities of growth occur in various bones including the vertebrae, pelvis, carpal and tarsal bones, and the epiphyses of tubular bones. On the basis of roentgenographic findings, this group can be divided into (1) those with generalized platyspondyly, (2) those with multiple epiphyseal dysplasias, and (3) those with epiphysometaphyseal dysplasias. *Morquio's syndrome,* a mucopolysaccharidosis inherited as an autosomal recessive character and associated with corneal opacities, dental defects, variable disturbances in intellect, and increased urinary excretion of keratosulfate, belongs in the first group. Other forms of spondyloepiphyseal dysplasias show no abnormality in mucopolysaccharide metabolism and are sometimes not recognized until late in childhood. Flat vertebral bodies are associated with other abnormalities in shape and alignment. The disordered development of the capital femoral epiphyses leads to irregularities in shape and flattening of the femoral heads and early onset of osteoarthritis of the hips.

TABLE 343-2
Proposed classification of bone dysplasias

- *I* Epiphyseal dysplasias
  - *A* Epiphyseal hypoplasias
    - *1* Failure of articular cartilage: spondyloepiphyseal dysplasia, congenita and tarda
    - *2* Failure of ossification of center: multiple epiphyseal dysplasia, congenita and tarda
  - *B* Epiphyseal hyperplasia
    - *1* Excess of articular cartilage: dysplasia epiphysalis hemimelica
- *II* Physeal (growth plate) dysplasias
  - *A* Cartilage hypoplasias
    - *1* Failure of proliferating cartilage: achondroplasia, congenita and tarda
    - *2* Failure of hypertrophic cartilage: metaphyseal dysostosis, congenita and tarda
  - *B* Cartilage hyperplasias
    - *1* Excess of proliferating cartilage: hyperchondroplasia
    - *2* Excess of hypertrophic cartilage: enchondromatosis
- *III* Metaphyseal dysplasias
  - *A* Metaphyseal hypoplasias
    - *1* Failure to form primary spongiosa: hypophosphatasia, congenita and tarda
    - *2* Failure to absorb primary spongiosa: osteopetrosis, congenita and tarda
    - *3* Failure to absorb secondary spongiosa: craniometaphyseal dysplasia, congenita and tarda
  - *B* Metaphyseal hyperplasia
    - *1* Excessive spongiosa: familial exostosis
- *IV* Diaphyseal dysplasias
  - *A* Diaphyseal hypoplasias
    - *1* Failure of periosteal bone formation: osteogenesis imperfecta, congenita and tarda
    - *2* Failure of endosteal bone formation: idiopathic osteoporosis
  - *B* Diaphyseal hyperplasias
    - *1* Excessive periosteal bone formation: Engelmann's disease
    - *2* Excessive periosteal bone formation: hyperphosphatasia

Achondroplasia *Achondroplasia* is a physeal dysplasia in which dwarfism results from decrease in the proliferation of cartilage in the growth plate. This disorder of unknown cause is among the more common types of dwarfism and is inherited as an autosomal dominant trait. Histological sections through the growth plate show a thin zone of cartilage cells with absence or abbreviation of the normal columnar arrangement and zone of provisional calcification, although endochondral ossification may not be completely disorganized. Formation of the primary spongiosa is reduced since there is often a transverse bar of bone sealing off the plate from further endochondral ossification. However, formation and maturation of the secondary ossification centers and articular cartilage are not disturbed. Appositional growth at the metaphysis continues, with resulting flare in this region of the bone; intramembranous bone formation at the periosteum is normal. The result of abnormal proliferation at the growth plate, leaving other areas relatively unaffected in the tubular bones, is the production of short bones which are proportionately thick. However, the length of the spine is almost always normal. The appearance of short limbs with a normal trunk is characteristically accompanied by a large head, saddlenose, and an exaggerated lumbar lordosis. The disease is usually recognized at birth. Those who survive the period of infancy usually have normal mental and sexual development, and life span may be normal. However, spinal deformity may lead to cord compression and nerve root encroachment in a significant number of affected individuals, especially those with kyphoscoliosis. Homozygous achondroplasia is a more serious disorder and a cause of neonatal death.

Enchondromatosis (dyschondroplasia, Ollier's disease) This is also a disorder affecting the growth plate in which the hypertrophic cartilage is not resorbed and ossified in a normal fashion. It results in masses of cartilage with disorderly arrangement of the chondrocytes showing variable proliferative and hypertrophic changes. These masses are located in the metaphyses in close association with the growth plate in very young patients but often are diaphyseal in teenagers and young adults. The disorder is usually recognized in childhood by the appearance of deformities or retardation in growth. The most common sites of involvement are the ends of long bones, usually in that region where rate of growth is most marked. The pelvis is often involved, but bone such as ribs, sternum, and skull are seldom affected. There is also a tendency toward unilateral involvement. Chondrosarcoma develops occasionally in the enchondromata. The association of enchondromatosis and cavernous hemangiomata in the soft tissues is known as Maffucci's syndrome.

Multiple exostoses (diaphyseal aclasis or osteochondromatosis) This is a disorder of the metaphysis, inherited as an autosomal dominant character, in which areas of the growth plate become displaced, presumably by growing through a defect in the perichondrium or so-called ring of Ranvier. The spongiosa forms within the mass as vessels invade the cartilage. Therefore, the diagnostic radiographic finding is the direct continuity of the mass to the marrow cavity of the parent bone with absence of underlying cortex. Usually the growth of these exostoses ceases when growth of the adjacent plate ceases. The lesions may be solitary or multiple and are usually located in the metaphyseal areas of long bones with the apex of the exostosis directed toward the diaphysis. Often the lesions produce no symptoms, but occasionally interference with the function of a joint or tendon or compression of nerves may result. Dwarfing is seen occasionally. The metacarpals may be shortened, resembling those seen in Albright's hereditary osteodystrophy. Multiple exostoses are sometimes seen in patients with pseudohypoparathyroidism.

An exostosis may suddenly begin to enlarge long after growth should have ceased, and rarely chondrosarcomas develop from the cartilage cap of an exostosis. Although the exact incidence of this complication is not known, estimates as high as 7 to 11 percent have been made. Pregnancy may stimulate growth of an exostosis which clinically may mimic malignancy. However, the lesion merely undergoes exuberant endochondral ossification and cartilage hyperplasia without malignant changes.

RELAPSING POLYCHONDRITIS See Chap. 353.

TIETZE'S SYNDROME (COSTOCHONDRAL SYNDROME) See Chap. 353.

REFERENCES

Bone and cartilage

ALBRIGHT FA et al: Syndrome characterized by osteitis fibrosa, disseminate areas of pigmentation and endocrine dysfunction, with precocious puberty in females: Report of five cases. N Engl J Med 216:727, 1937

ALTERMAN SL, LIEBER AL: Albright's hereditary osteodystrophy: The effect of treatment during adolescence. Ann Intern Med 63:140, 1965

BAILEY JA: Orthopaedic aspects of achondroplasia. J Bone Joint Surg (Br) 52A:1285, 1970

BENEDICT PH: Endocrine features in Albright's syndrome (fibrous dysplasia of bone). Metabolism 11:30, 1962

——— et al: Melanotic macules in Albright's syndrome and in neurofibromatosis. JAMA 209:72, 1968

DENT CE, GERTNER JM: Hypophosphatemic osteomalacia in fibrous dysplasia. Q J Med 45:411, 1976

GIOVANELLI G et al: McCune-Albright syndrome in a male child: A clinical and endocrinologic enigma. J Ped 92:220, 1978

GRABIAS SL, CAMPBELL, CJ: Fibrous dysplasia. Orthoped Clin N Am 8:771, 1977

GRAF CJ, PERRET GE: Spontaneous recurrent hemorrhage as an unusual complication of fibrous dysplasia of the skull. J Neurosurg 52:570, 1980

HARRIS WH et al: The natural history of fibrous dysplasia: An orthopaedic, pathological and roentgenographic study. J Bone Joint Surg (Br) 44A:207, 1962

RIMOIN DL: The chondrodystrophies. Adv Hum Genet 5:1, 1975

RUBIN P: *Dynamic Classification of Bone Dysplasias.* Chicago, Year Book, 1964

SILLENCE DO et al: Neonatal dwarfism. Pediatr Clin North Am 25:431, 1978

STEENDIJK R: Metabolic bone disease in children, in *Metabolic Bone Disease,* LV Avioli, SM Krane (eds). Academic, New York, 1978, vol II, p 633

Hyperostosis

CANALIS E et al: Dynamic bone morphometry and studies on the effects of serum on bone metabolism in vitro in a case of pycnodysostosis. Metab Bone Dis Rel Res 2:99, 1981

COCCIA PF et al: Successful bone-marrow transplantation for infantile malignant osteopetrosis. N Engl J Med 302:701, 1980

COLLINS DH, DODGE OG: *Pathology of Bone.* London, Butterworth, 1966

DENT CE et al: Studies in osteopetrosis. Arch Dis Child 40:7, 1965

ELMORE SM et al: Pyknodysostosis, with a familial chromosome anomaly. Am J Med 40:273, 1966

GENANT HK: Osteosclerosis in primary hyperparathyroidism. Am J Med 59:104, 1975

GLORIEUX FH et al: Induction of bone resorption by parathyroid hormone in confluent malignant osteopetrosis. Metab Bone Dis Rel Res 3:143, 1981

JAFFE HL: *Metabolic, Degenerative and Inflammatory Disease of Bones and Joints.* Philadelphia, Lea & Febiger, 1972

JOHNSTON CC et al: Osteopetrosis: A clinical, genetic, metabolic and morphologic study of the dominantly inherited benign form. Medicine 47:149, 1968

LORIA-CORTES R et al: Osteopetrosis in children. A report of 26 cases. J Pediatr 91:43, 1977

MILHAUD G et al: Immunologic defect and its correction in the osteopetrotic mutant rat. Proc Natl Acad Sci USA 74:339, 1977

SHELDON J et al: Engelmann's disease (progressive diaphyseal dysplasia). A review and presentation of two cases with abnormal phosphate retention. Metab Bone Dis Rel Res 2:307, 1981

SMITH R et al: Clinical and biochemical studies in Engelmann's disease (progressive disphyseal dysplasia). Q J Med 46:273, 1977

SORELL M et al: Marrow transplantation for juvenile osteopetrosis. Am J Med 70:1280, 1981

THOMPSON RC JR et al: Hereditary hyperphosphatasia. Am J Med 47:209, 1969

VAN BUCHEM FSP et al: Hyperostosis corticalis generalisata. Am J Med 33:387, 1962

WALKER DG: Bone resorption restored in osteopetrotic mice by transplants of normal bone marrow and spleen. Science 190:784, 1975

Neoplasms

CORTES EP et al: Amputation and adriamycin in primary osteosarcoma. N Engl J Med 291:998, 1974

DOUGLAS DL et al: Effect of dichloromethylene diphosphonate in Paget's disease of bone and in hypercalcemia due to primary hyperparathyroidism or malignant disease. Lancet 1:1043, 1980

JAFFE HL: *Tumors and Tumorous Conditions of the Bones and Joints.* Philadelphia, Lea & Febiger, 1958

JAFFE N et al: Adjuvant methotrexate and citrovorum-factor treatment of osteogenic sarcoma. N Engl J Med 291:994, 1974

LICHTENSTEIN L: *Bone Tumors.* St Louis, Mosby, 1972

LODWICK GS: *The Bones and Joints.* Chicago, Year Book, 1971

MANKIN HJ: Current concepts. Advances in diagnosis and treatment of bone tumors. N Engl J Med (in press)

——— et al: Massive resection and allograft replacement in the treatment of malignant bone tumors. N Engl J Med 294:1247, 1976

MINTON JP: The response of breast cancer patients with bone pain to L-dopa. Cancer 33:358, 1974

MOSELEY JE: *Bone Changes in Hematologic Disorders.* New York, Grune & Stratton, 1963

MUNDY GR et al: Osteoclast activating factor: Its role in myeloma and other types of hypercalcemia of malignancy. Metab Bone Dis Rel Res 2:173, 1980

RAISZ LG et al: Hypercalcemia of neoplastic diseases, in *Endocrinology of Calcium Metabolism,* DH Copp, RV Talmage (eds). Amsterdam, Excerpta Medica, 1978, p 64

RODMAN JS, SHERWOOD LM: Disorders of mineral metabolism in malignancy, in *Metabolic Bone Disease,* LV Avioli, SM Krane (eds). New York, Academic, 1978, vol II, p 577

ROSEN G et al: Curability of Ewing's sarcoma and considerations for future therapeutic trials. Cancer 41:888, 1978

SIRIS ES et al: Effects of dichloromethylene diphosphonate on skeletal mobilization of calcium in multiple myeloma. N Engl J Med 302:310, 1980

UNNI KK et al: Conditions that simulate primary neoplasms of bone. S Pathol Ann 15:91, 1981

WEICHSELBAUM RR et al: Preliminary results of aggressive multimodal therapy for metastatic osteosarcoma. Cancer 40:78, 1977

344 OSTEOMYELITIS

JAN V. HIRSCHMANN

DEFINITION *Osteomyelitis* denotes infection of bone. While many types of microorganisms, including viruses and fungi, may cause osteomyelitis, it is usually bacterial in origin.

PATHOGENESIS Organisms reach the bone to cause infection by one of three routes: (1) hematogenous spread, (2) extension from a contiguous site of infection, and (3) direct introduction of organisms into bone by trauma, including surgery.

Acute hematogenous osteomyelitis usually involves bone with rich, red marrow; in children the long bones, especially the femur and tibia, are most frequently affected. The infection begins in the metaphyseal sinusoidal veins, where sluggish blood flow and a paucity of phagocytes favor the growth of organisms. In adults acute hematogenous infection rarely involves the long bones, where adipose tissue has largely replaced the red marrow. Instead, hematogenous osteomyelitis most commonly occurs in the vertebrae, where cellular marrow and an abundant vascular supply exist. The organisms reach the spine directly through the nutrient branches of the posterior spinal artery or, probably less commonly, from retrograde flow through the valveless paravertebral venous plexus of Batson, which drains the vertebral bodies, body wall, and the pelvis. Infection usually begins in the vertebral body near the anterior longitudinal ligament and may spread to adjacent vertebrae by direct extension through the disk space or by a system of freely communicating venous channels. Because the disk in adults possesses no vascular supply, disk space infection in *hematogenous* infections is always secondary to osteomyelitis in an adjacent vertebra.

Osteomyelitis caused by extension from a contiguous site of infection may occur with soft-tissue suppuration resulting from trauma, necrosis of a malignant tumor, radiation therapy, burns, or other causes. In patients with vascular insufficiency from diabetes mellitus or atherosclerosis, organisms commonly enter the soft tissues through a cutaneous ulcer, usually in the foot, causing cellulitis and subsequently osteomyelitis. Osteomyelitis of the skull bones may result from underlying sinus or dental infections.

Direct introduction of organisms into bone may occur with open fractures, the open surgical reduction of closed fractures, or penetrating trauma by bullets or other foreign bodies. Osteomyelitis may also follow insertion of prostheses or other surgical procedures for nontraumatic bone or joint disorders.

PATHOLOGY Pathological findings during the acute phase include neutrophilic inflammation, edema, and vascular congestion. Because of the bone's rigidity, increased intramedullary pressure develops, compromising the blood supply and causing ischemia, cell death, and vascular thrombosis. After several days, the suppurative and ischemic injury may cause the bone to fragment into devitalized segments called *sequestra.* The inflammation spreads via the haversian and Volkmann canals to reach the periosteum, beneath which abscesses may form or through which the purulent material may penetrate to form soft-tissue abscesses or sinus tracts.

With persistent infection, chronic inflammatory cells—lymphocytes, histiocytes, and plasma cells—may join the neutrophils. Fibroblastic proliferation and new bone formation also occur. Osteogenesis from the periosteum may surround the inflammation to form a bony envelope or *involucrum.* Occasionally, a dense fibrous capsule confines the infection to a localized area of suppuration, called *Brodie's abscess.* Rarely, exuberant osteogenesis may result in a sclerotic, nonpurulent osteomyelitis (Garré's sclerosing osteomyelitis).

MANIFESTATIONS Hematogenous osteomyelitis The bacteremia causing hematogenous osteomyelitis may be from a urinary infection, bacterial endocarditis, a distant soft-tissue infection, or another location. Frequently, the original site is not apparent. Intravenous drug abusers, in whom *Pseudomonas aeruginosa* is the most common infecting organism, and patients receiving chronic hemodialysis are especially at risk for hematogenous osteomyelitis, presumably because of frequent bacteremias. Diabetes mellitus also seems to be a predisposing condition, perhaps because of impaired neutrophil function and frequent infections of the skin and urinary tract, sites from which bacteremias frequently originate.

Vertebral osteomyelitis may occasionally begin abruptly with back pain and systemic signs of infection, but usually the onset is insidious and the course gradually progressive. Persistent back pain, exacerbated by movement and commonly unrelieved by heat, analgesics, or bed rest, is the predominant symptom. Fever is usually minimal or absent. Physical examination typically reveals tenderness to percussion and palpation over the affected vertebrae, guarding and splinting on movement, and paravertebral muscle spasm.

Leukocytosis is usually absent, but the erythrocyte sedimentation rate is almost always increased. The earliest roentgenographic changes are erosion of the subchondral bony plate, narrowing of the intervertebral disk space, and involvement of the adjacent vertebra. Bony destruction follows, sometimes with loss of vertebral height, usually anteriorly. Anterior osteogenesis with coarse bony density and sclerosis may occur. Soft-tissue densities, representing paravertebral abscesses, may lie adjacent to the vertebrae. The lumbar vertebrae are most frequently involved, the cervical vertebrae least. While roentgenographic changes may not develop for several weeks following infection, radionuclide scans with technetium pyrophosphate are positive early.

Complications of vertebral osteomyelitis include anterior extension to cause retropharyngeal abscesses, mediastinitis, empyema, pericarditis, subdiaphragmatic abscess, psoas muscle abscess, or peritonitis, depending upon the vertebrae involved. Posterior extension by pus (epidural abscess), bony fragments, or inflammatory tissue can cause spinal cord compression; if infection penetrates the dura to enter the subarachnoid space, meningitis results.

Acute hematogenous osteomyelitis occurring in sites other than the vertebrae is unusual in adults. When it does develop in such locations as the clavicle or the long bones of the extremities, its typical features are pain and evidence of soft-tissue infection over the affected bone.

Hematogenous osteomyelitis acquired in childhood may present in adults as intermittent or persistent drainage from sinus tracts communicating with the involved bone—usually the femur, tibia, or humerus—or as a soft-tissue infection overlying it. Signs of infection may recur after months or years of quiescence. Roentgenographic changes include bony destruction with radiolucent areas, radiopaque sequestra, and formation of an involucrum. A roentgenogram of contrast material injected into a sinus tract (sinogram) may help define the location and extent of involvement.

Posttraumatic osteomyelitis and osteomyelitis from a contiguous infection The clinical features of these forms of osteomyelitis are a varying combination of local pain, draining sinuses, and heat, swelling, tenderness, and erythema over the involved bone. Patients often are afebrile. Persistent pain and loosening of the appliance may be the major manifestations in those with infected orthopedic prostheses. Leukocytosis and an elevated erythrocyte sedimentation rate are present in a minority of patients. Radiographic changes are similar to those in chronic hematogenous osteomyelitis. With plates, nails, screws, pins, or prostheses there is frequently evidence of loosening of the appliance. Radionuclide scans with technetium pyrophosphate are nearly always positive. Since increased uptake in these scans depends in part on bone hyperemia, which may occur with adjacent inflammation alone, there may be difficulty in distinguishing early osteomyelitis from cellulitis or a subcutaneous abscess when the roentgenograms do not show bony destruction.

DIAGNOSIS While radiographic or radionuclide studies may be helpful, definitive diagnosis requires isolation of the responsible organism. If blood cultures are negative (they usually are), patients with suspected vertebral osteomyelitis should undergo needle aspiration of the intervertebral disk space if it appears infected, percutaneous needle biopsy of the infected bone, or open bone biopsy at surgery. Although *Staphylococcus aureus* is the most common cause, aerobic gram-negative bacilli, typically arising from a previous or concurrent urinary infection, are also frequent. Moreover, pyogenic vertebral osteomyelitis is often impossible to differentiate from tuberculous or fungal vertebral osteomyelitis.

In patients with chronic hematogenous osteomyelitis, posttraumatic osteomyelitis, or osteomyelitis from a contiguous infection, the diagnosis is best established by careful cultures, both aerobic and anaerobic, of bone, tissue, or pus from a deep abscess obtained during surgery. These infections are often polymicrobial and sometimes include anaerobic bacteria; precise bacteriologic identification is necessary for appropriate antimicrobial therapy. Cultures of material obtained from draining sinuses are generally unreliable, even if only a single organism grows, because the tracts may become colonized by bacteria present on the skin surface but absent in the infected bone.

TREATMENT Bed rest and appropriate parenteral antimicrobial agents given for 6 to 8 weeks cure most cases of vertebral osteomyelitis.

The antibiotic(s) used in the treatment of osteomyelitis depend on the result of culture and sensitivity tests; the appropriate drugs are detailed in Chap. 141. In general, the first several weeks of therapy should be parenteral in order to achieve adequate levels of antibiotic in bony tissue. If no organisms are culturable, the choice of the antimicrobial necessarily must be based on cultures from other sites or, if these are negative, on the clinician's best estimate of the infecting pathogen. When staphylococcal infection is suspected, a penicillinase-resistant penicillin or a cephalosporin should be used.

External stabilization by traction or brace is indicated for an unstable cervical spine but is unnecessary for most patients with thoracic or lumbar osteomyelitis. Surgery is usually necessary only to drain paravertebral or spinal epidural abscesses. With successful therapy, bony bridging and spontaneous fusion of adjacent vertebral bodies occur, and the erythrocyte sedimentation rate returns to normal.

The main treatment of chronic hematogenous osteomyelitis, posttraumatic osteomyelitis, and osteomyelitis from a contiguous infection is surgery, with antimicrobial therapy an important adjunct. Antibiotics alone rarely cure these infections. The major surgical principles are thorough removal of all necrotic bone and tissue and the elimination of dead space. Rigid bone, unlike soft tissue, does not collapse around a site evacuated of pus; the resultant cavity provides an area for blood, debris, and organisms to collect. This dead space may be obliterated by (1) open packing of the wound, allowing the slow process of granulation to fill the defect, (2) packing the cavity with potentially viable grafts from cancellous bone, (3) transfer of a pedicle of skeletal muscle into the cavity, (4) skin grafting directly onto the granulating bone surface, or (5) constant irrigation to keep the cavity free of debris, followed by one of the methods mentioned above. These surgical measures are accompanied by appropriate parenteral antimicrobial therapy for 3 to 6 weeks. Since there are no controlled studies, the optimal choice and duration of antibiotics are unknown, but antimicrobial therapy is clearly doomed to failure unless the surgical debridement is thorough. Sometimes the location or extent of osteomyelitis makes surgical cure short of amputation impossible. In these patients, if amputation is not performed, treatment is given only for acute exacerbations, such as the formation of overlying soft-tissue abscesses, where surgical drainage and a short course of antibiotics help control the acute manifestations.

Osteomyelitis associated with a prosthesis generally requires removal of the appliance, thorough debridement, and appropriate antimicrobial therapy. With either quiescent or low-grade infection, a new prosthesis may be implanted at the same operation as the removal of its predecessor; otherwise, the therapeutic choices are excision arthroplasty or replacement of the prosthesis later when the infection subsides.

Osteomyelitis associated with plates, screws, rods, or pins used for the open reduction of fractures also requires removal of the appliance, thorough debridement, and antimicrobial therapy if union of the fracture has occurred. In infected fractures with nonunion, the principles of treatment are the establishment of rigid bony stability and debridement of infected material to permit union to occur. Screws, plates, pins, and rods that have not loosened are left in place, and the wound is treated with open irrigation. If the hardware is loose, thus failing to provide rigid stability, it is removed, and stability is attained by other means, such as external fixation with pins above and below the fracture site. When the infection is controlled, bone grafts may be necessary for union to occur, but some fractures will unite without them.

In osteomyelitis associated with vascular insufficiency, especially if it involves multiple bones of the foot in diabetics, cure is seldom possible without amputation.

REFERENCES

BURRI C: *Posttraumatic Osteomyelitis.* Bern, Hans Huber, 1975

JUPITER JB et al: Total hip arthroplasty in the treatment of adult hips with current or quiescent sepsis. J Bone Joint Surg 63A:194, 1981

KELLY PJ, FITZGERALD RH: Symposium on infections in orthopedics. Orthop Clin North Am, October 1975

LEWIS RP et al: Bone infections involving anaerobic bacteria. Medicine 57:279, 1978

MACKOWIAK PA et al: Diagnostic value of sinus tract cultures in chronic osteomyelitis. JAMA 239:2772, 1978

MCHENRY MC et al: Hematogenous osteomyelitis. A changing disease. Cleveland Clin Q 42:125, 1975

MUSHER DM et al: Vertebral osteomyelitis. Still a diagnostic pitfall. Arch Intern Med 136:105, 1976

WALDVOGEL FA et al: Osteomyelitis: A review of clinical features, therapeutic considerations, and unusual aspects. N Engl J Med 282:198, 260, 316, 1970

———, VASEY H: Osteomyelitis: The past decade. N Engl J Med 303:360, 1980

section 10 | Disorders of the joints and connective tissues

345
APPROACH TO DISORDERS OF THE JOINTS

BRUCE C. GILLILAND
MART MANNIK

The causes of joint disorders are numerous and include traumatic, infectious, degenerative, metabolic, immunologic, and neoplastic processes. The purpose of this chapter is to present an approach to the patient with joint disease. Figure 345-1 should serve as a guide to a group of disorders with common manifestations that may be divided further by means of historical, physical, laboratory, or radiological information. Clinical judgment and bedside information become highly important for achieving the correct diagnosis since specific tests are not available for each subgroup. The detailed differential diagnoses are discussed in the appropriate chapters.

Joint symptoms may originate from disease processes involving synovium, cartilage, or structures around the joint (tendons, bursae). Inflammation in joints is characterized by accumulation of inflammatory cells in the synovial tissue and fluid, and may be caused by immunologic events (rheumatoid arthritis), infectious agents (septic arthritis), crystal deposition (gout, pseudogout), or injury. Degenerative joint disease and some metabolic diseases, such as ochronosis, acromegaly, or hyperparathyroidism, are characterized by alterations of cartilage and supporting structures. Pain and stiffness around joints may follow vigorous exercise or trauma. Musculoskeletal complaints of a diffuse nature may be a manifestation of psychological conditions such as depression or anxiety.

The process of arriving at a logical diagnosis, therefore, will depend on the development of the data base consisting initially of historical information followed by the findings of the physical examination. This data base is used to proceed through the diagram in Fig. 345-1. Specific radiographs and laboratory tests, including synovial fluid analysis and in some instances arthroscopy, arthrography, or synovial tissue biopsy, may be required to define the joint disorder.

The history of joint complaints should define the following: duration of joint symptoms; how rapidly the symptoms developed; whether the symptoms were self-limited; the number and location of involved joints (peripheral small joints, proximal large joints, spine); the pattern of involved joints (symmetrical or asymmetrical); the sequence of joint involvement (migrating or additive); swelling or redness of the joints; precipitating causes of joint pain (physical activity); events preceding joint symptoms (trauma, other illnesses); pain at rest; and the presence and duration of morning stiffness. Persistent pain and swelling of more than 6 weeks, involving a few or several joints, suggests a chronic inflammatory arthritis. Involvement of the peripheral joints in a symmetrical distribution points to rheumatoid arthritis, while an asymmetrical pattern of joint involvement raises the possibility of Reiter's syndrome or psoriatic arthritis. Other clues then should be sought, such as a history of urethritis, conjunctivitis, or skin lesions. The sequence of joint involvement also provides useful information. Migratory arthritis is characterized by one joint improving while another is becoming involved. An additive or progressive pattern of arthritis occurs when the initial joint(s) involved remains affected as other joints become inflamed. Migratory arthritis is observed in rheumatic fever and viral illnesses, while an additive pattern occurs in rheumatoid arthritis and other chronic inflammatory arthritides. A history in a young man of persistent low back pain and stiffness often worse in the morning may indicate ankylosing spondylitis. A self-limited episode of polyarthritis lasting a few days to several weeks may have been caused by a viral infection. In a middle-aged person pain and stiffness in weight-bearing joints (hips and knees) following physical activity may be a manifestation of degenerative joint disease. The appearance of pain in a knee after an injury may reflect damage to supporting structures such as menisci or ligaments. A painful shoulder following physical activity may be caused by tendonitis or bursitis. Septic arthritis or crystal deposition disease should be considered in a patient presenting with a history of sudden onset of a very painful, swollen, and erythematous joint. Chills and high fever in this patient would strongly suggest septic arthritis, and further workup and treatment should proceed immediately. Delay in treatment of a bacterial infectious arthritis may result in permanent joint damage. The presence of constitutional symptoms (fever, weight loss, malaise) in a patient with multiple joint symptoms suggests a systemic disease. Constitutional symptoms may accompany rheumatoid arthritis or may be due to an underlying infectious or neoplastic disease with musculoskeletal manifestations. The duration of morning stiffness is a good indicator of the degree of joint inflammation. The question of the duration of morning stiffness is best determined by asking patients at what time they get out of bed and at what time they finally get as loose as they will become. Patients with active rheumatoid arthritis will have several hours of morning stiffness, which will decrease with improvement of the disease. Patients with osteoarthritis will also experience morning stiffness; however, it is short-lived, disappearing after a few minutes of physical activity.

Patients should be questioned about medications since drugs such as procainamide (Pronestyl) can produce a lupus erythematosus syndrome with arthritis. Inquiries should be made about exposure to rubella, mumps, or hepatitis, since these and other viral illnesses may cause arthritis. A history of Raynaud's phenomenon may indicate a connective tissue disorder such as progressive systemic sclerosis. Complaints of bilateral numbness and/or tingling of the thumb and first three fingers are observed in carpal tunnel syndrome due to compression of the median nerve. Chronic inflammatory synovitis is one of the causes of carpal tunnel syndrome. A history of acute iritis in a patient complaining of low back pain suggests ankylosing spondylitis. A history of colitis in a patient with an acutely swollen knee suggests the diagnosis of arthritis associated with inflammatory bowel disease. A promiscuous sexual history raises the possibility of gonococcal arthritis or Reiter's syndrome. The social history should be explored for personal, family, or job-related problems. Fibrositis and musculoskeletal syndromes may reflect underlying depression or anxiety. A positive family history of arthritis may be obtained in patients with rheumatoid arthritis, ankylosing spondylitis, or gout.

A careful and complete physical examination should be performed on all patients with musculoskeletal complaints. This is especially important since musculoskeletal symptoms may be a manifestation of an underlying metabolic, neoplastic, infectious, or rheumatic disease. The skin should be inspected for psoriasis, mucocutaneous lesions of Reiter's syndrome, lesions of vasculitis, and for the presence of subcutaneous nodules. Nodules have a propensity for points of pressure such as the elbow. Nodules are seen in rheumatoid arthritis, rheumatic fever, and gout (gouty tophus). Dryness of the eye and/or mouth may signify Sjögren's syndrome. Painful oral ulcers or a facial butterfly rash may be a manifestation of systemic lupus erythematosus.

The joint examination should include assessment of all joints, even though symptoms are localized to one or a few joints. Joints should be inspected for redness, swelling, and deformity, and muscle atrophy noted. Joints are palpated for tenderness, fluid, synovial proliferation, and bony enlargement. Joint effusions are appreciated best in the knee joint where they can be detected by a fluid wave (bulge sign) or by a patellar click on ballottement of the patella downward on the femur. The bulge sign is more sensitive for detection of small effusions and may permit detection of as little as 5 ml removable synovial fluid. In other joints compression of fluid in the joint may give a palpable transmission of pressure. Synovial hypertrophy is palpable as boggy tissue between and around joint margins. Synovial hypertrophy of the metatarsal joints produces widening of the forefoot and separation of the toes. The structures around the joints (tendons, bursae, soft tissue) are also palpated for tenderness and warmth. Points of insertion of tendons and fascia are examined by applying gentle pressure over these sites. The range of motion of each joint is determined, and crepitus, if any, noted.

The joint examination should distinguish between joint tenderness and tenderness of the surrounding joint structures. Pain elicited on passive motion of a joint usually indicates inflammation of the joint or periarticular structures such as tendons or bursae. Palpable tenderness over a tendon placed on gentle stretch or pain on movement of the tendon indicates

FIGURE 345-1
Approach to joint disorders. (Numbers in parentheses indicate chapters containing detailed discussions.)

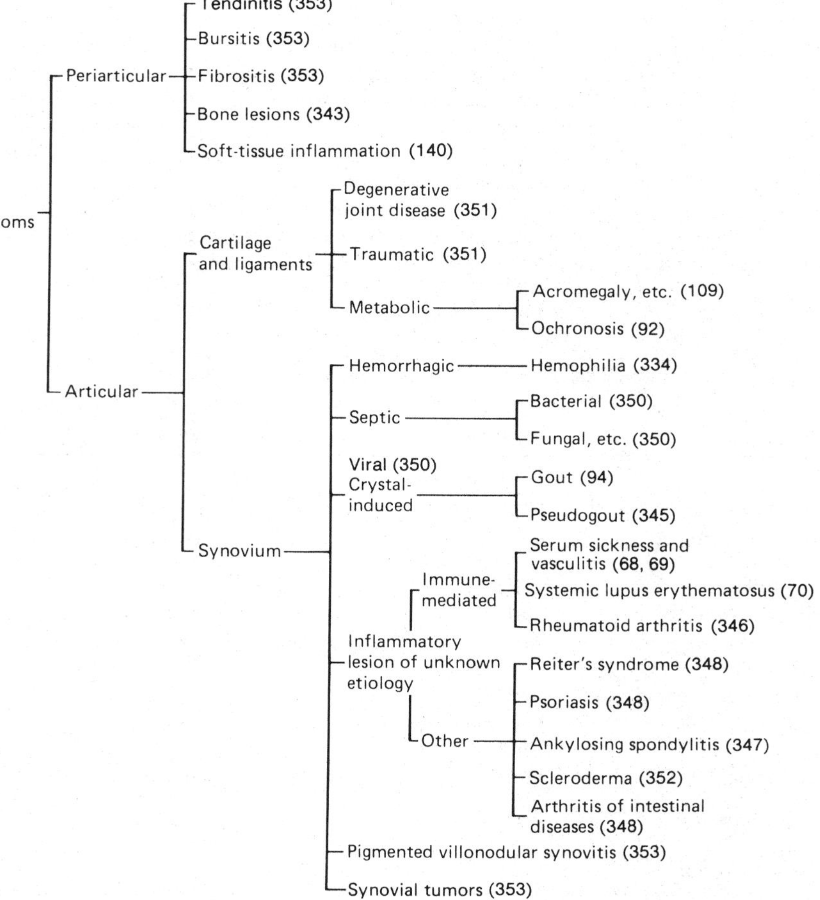

tendonitis. Pressure over an inflamed bursa also usually produces pain. Patients with ankylosing spondylitis or Reiter's syndrome may exhibit tenderness over points of insertion of tendons or fascia, such as at the site of insertion of the Achilles tendon or the plantar fascia with the calcaneus. Evidence for joint involvement is the presence of a joint effusion, warmth over the joint, and tenderness on compression of the joint.

Joint examination should also indicate whether the joint disorder is primarily an inflammatory disease of the synovium or a disease of the cartilage. In acute inflammatory disorders (e.g., septic arthritis and crystal deposition arthritis) the joint is painful, swollen, and warm. The overlying skin is often erythematous. An acute traumatic arthritis also may present as a swollen and warm joint but should be suspected with a history of antecedent trauma. In both of these conditions, further evaluation and treatment should be immediately undertaken. In patients with chronic inflammatory joint disease such as rheumatoid arthritis, the joint is swollen and only mildly warm, and may have a boggy sensation due to underlying synovial hypertrophy. Firm compression, particularly over the involved small joints, will be painful. The overlying skin may show only minimal erythema. In degenerative joint disease, synovial effusion may be found, but the overlying tissues usually do not show inflammation; bony overgrowth at the joint margins may be present. Crepitus may indicate fraying and loss of articular cartilage.

Muscle strength and tenderness should be assessed. Quadriceps atrophy indicates underlying knee disease regardless of cause, and decreased grip strength points to inflammatory disease of the wrists and small joints of the hand. Proximal muscle weakness of the hip and shoulder girdles in a patient with joint complaints suggests polymyositis. Polymyalgia rheumatica should be considered in an elderly patient complaining of muscle aching of the shoulder and hips. Muscle tenderness over specific points, such as the belly of the trapezius, the lateral neck strap muscle, the epicondylar region, the anserine bursa, and the medial aspect of the knee, suggests the diagnosis of fibrositis. Patients with psychogenic rheumatism will complain of pain at most sites of palpation.

The examination of synovial fluid is mandatory to establish the specific diagnosis of infections, crystal-induced arthritides, pigmented villonodular synovitis, and neoplasms involving the joint. Inflammatory joint diseases of unknown cause often can be diagnosed on the basis of the history and physical examination without the examination of synovial fluid. However, the synovial fluid should be examined when possible because it may provide a precise diagnosis or further clues to an accurate diagnosis. Aspiration of a joint should be performed under aseptic conditions.

Table 345-1 lists the characteristics of joint fluid for the major types of arthritis. Normal joint fluid is clear and straw-colored. Turbidity is produced by inflammatory cells and occasionally by a chylous effusion. Fragments of cartilage and fibrin may be present. Normal joint fluid is quite viscous, because of hyaluronic acid. The viscosity is reduced in inflammatory arthritides, especially in chronic rheumatoid arthritis. Viscosity can be grossly evaluated by forcing synovial fluid from the syringe. Fluid of high viscosity forms a string several inches long; fluid of low viscosity drops like water. The mucin clot test correlates with the viscosity. This test is performed by adding acetic acid to joint fluid from which cells and debris have been removed by centrifugation. The formation of a tight, ropy, and persistent clot indicates qualitatively good mucin and the presence of adequate molecules of intact hyaluronic acid. The mucin clot in degenerative joint disease is of good quality and quantity, while in inflammatory joint disease, such as rheumatoid arthritis, the mucin clot is of both poor quality and quantity. Fluid from an inflammatory effusion often forms a fibrin clot which should not be confused with a mucin clot. Normal joint fluid does not contain fibrinogen; therefore, it will not clot spontaneously unless blood enters the joint during the aspiration.

Synovial fluid for cell counts should be collected in an anticoagulant-containing tube. Joint fluid for cell counts should not be diluted in acetic acid, the normal diluent for white blood cell counts, since this will result in the formation of a mucin clot. Normal joint fluid contains less than 200 cells per cubic millimeter, predominantly mononuclear white blood cells. In degenerative joint disease the intraarticular white blood cell count is usually less than 2000 per cubic millimeter and the cells are also predominantly mononuclear. Variable degrees of leukocytosis, consisting mainly of neutrophils, are seen in inflammatory joint diseases; cell counts in septic arthritis are often greater than 50,000 per cubic millimeter. However, septic arthritis should still be considered with lower cell counts. White blood cell counts up to 50,000 per cubic millimeter or even higher may occasionally be found in nonseptic joints. For proper interpretation of the synovial fluid glucose, blood should be drawn simultaneously for glucose analysis; both samples should be obtained 6 h after a meal. The synovial

TABLE 345-1
Synovial fluid characteristics in major joint diseases*

Diagnosis	*Appearance*	*Fibrin clot*	*Mucin† clot*	*WBC/mm³*	*PMN,‡ %*	*Sugar, % of blood level*
Normal	Straw-colored, clear	None	Good	<200	<25	~100
Degenerative joint disease	Slightly turbid	Small	Good	<2,000	<25	~100
Traumatic arthritis	Straw-colored, bloody, or xanthochromic	Small	Good	~2,000	<25	~100
Rheumatoid arthritis	Turbid	Large	Fair to poor	5,000–50,000	>65	~75§
Other types of inflammatory arthritis¶	Turbid	Large	Fair to poor	5,000–50,000	>50	~75
Acute gout or pseudogout	Turbid	Large	Fair to poor	5,000–50,000	>75	~90
Septic arthritis	Very turbid or purulent	Large	Poor	10,000–>100,000	>80	<50
Tuberculous arthritis	Turbid	Large	Poor	~25,000	Variable	<50

* *See text for discussion of synovial fluid complement.*
† *Correlates with viscosity.*
‡ *PMN, polymorphonuclear cells.*
§ *May be less than 50 percent.*
¶ *Includes Reiter's syndrome, psoriatic arthritis, ankylosing spondylitis (peripheral joints), arthritis associated with intestinal diseases.*

fluid glucose level falls with increasing inflammation, and the difference between levels of serum and synovial fluid glucose increases. The level in septic arthritis may be less than 50 percent of the serum glucose. A low synovial glucose level also can be seen in rheumatoid arthritis.

Synovial fluid should be examined under polarized light for the presence of crystals. The crystals of gout and of pseudogout are differentiated by their size, shape, and properties under compensated polarized light. The fluid to be used for examination of crystals should be anticoagulated with heparin, since crystalline anticoagulants may be mistaken for crystals in synovial fluid.

Gram's stain and stains for tubercle bacilli should be performed on the sediment of synovial fluid. Bacterial, fungal, and viral cultures should be obtained when these infections are suspected.

Determination of the joint fluid complement is useful, but specific diagnostic information is not obtained from this measurement. For best interpretation, the joint fluid complement (hemolytic complement, C3 or C4) should be expressed as a function of the total protein concentration in the fluid. Macromolecules of complement or protein do not readily enter the uninflamed synovial cavity, but with inflammation the synovium becomes permeable to these macromolecules. Therefore, synovial fluid complement levels usually correlate with the total protein concentration of the fluid. Normal levels of synovial fluid complement, as related to the total protein of the fluid, are found in joint fluid from normal persons, and from patients with osteoarthritis, gout, and other nonrheumatoid inflammatory arthritides. Patients with rheumatoid arthritis, particularly those with high titers of serum rheumatoid factor, and patients with systemic lupus erythematosus may have low synovial complement levels as related to the total protein in the fluid. The decreased joint fluid complement levels in these patients may be due to the consumption of complement by antigen-antibody complexes in the joint cavity.

Needle biopsy of the synovium can provide precise diagnostic information. With currently available needles, a biopsy can be performed on most large joints with relatively little discomfort. If bedside observations and synovial fluid studies have not yielded a diagnosis, a biopsy should be considered. In a large joint, such as the knee, arthroscopy can facilitate the selection of the site for biopsy. Synovial biopsy may lead to a diagnosis of tuberculosis, coccidioidomycosis, hemochromatosis, sarcoidosis, amyloidosis, pigmented villonodular synovitis, or synovial tumors. A biopsy may support the diagnosis of rheumatoid arthritis, systemic lupus erythematosus, or Reiter's syndrome, but the biopsy alone will not suffice for a diagnosis in these diseases.

REFERENCES

Convery FR, Convery MM: Examination of the joints, in *Textbook of Rheumatology,* WN Kelly et al (eds). Philadelphia, Saunders, 1981, pp 358–383

Fries JF: General approach to the rheumatic disease patient, in *Textbook of Rheumatology,* WN Kelly et al (eds). Philadelphia, Saunders, 1981, pp 353–358

McCarty DJ: Differential diagnosis of arthritis; analysis of signs and symptoms, in *Arthritis and Allied Conditions,* DJ McCarty (ed). Philadelphia, Lea & Febiger, 1979, pp 36–50

———: Synovial fluid, in *Arthritis and Allied Conditions,* DJ McCarty (ed). Philadelphia, Lea & Febiger, 1979, pp 51–69

346 RHEUMATOID ARTHRITIS

BRUCE C. GILLILAND
MART MANNIK

Rheumatoid arthritis (RA) is a chronic systemic disease of unknown etiology, manifested primarily by inflammatory arthritis of the peripheral joints, usually in a symmetrical distribution. Systemic manifestations include hematologic, pulmonary, neurological, and cardiovascular abnormalities.

PATHOGENESIS Joint inflammation in RA is a chronic process usually leading to progressive joint damage. Susceptibility for developing RA may be influenced by the type of immune response which is genetically determined. The histocompatibility antigen HLA-DRw4 is found in 70 percent of patients with RA as compared to 28 percent in controls (for discussion of histocompatibility antigens, see Chap. 60). The etiologic factor(s) that initiates or precipitates the inflammatory process is unknown. An infectious microorganism, viral or bacterial, has not been isolated from joints. In animal models, however, the injection of bacterial cell wall fragments can produce a chronic synovitis. It is conceivable that in genetically susceptible persons exposure to a microorganism may lead to synovitis. The serum and joint fluid of the majority of patients with RA contains antibodies specific for the Fc fragment of IgG (rheumatoid factors). These antibodies are heterogeneous and consist of IgM, IgG, and IgA and are, respectively, termed IgM rheumatoid factors, IgG rheumatoid factors, and IgA rheumatoid factors. The stimulus for synthesis of rheumatoid factors appears to be chronic antigenic challenge. Patients with subacute bacterial endocarditis or with other forms of chronic infection develop rheumatoid factors which disappear from the serum after successful treatment of the infection. These observations suggest that IgG, altered as a result of combining with an antigen, can serve as the immunogenic stimulus for the synthesis of rheumatoid factors (antibodies to IgG). Chronic arthritis does not appear in the above-mentioned patients or in the immunized animals, indicating that the presence of some rheumatoid factors alone does not contribute to the pathogenesis of rheumatoid arthritis. In RA, the reasons for the appearance and continued production of rheumatoid factors remain unknown.

Though the presence of rheumatoid factor in the serum apparently does not lead to the development of rheumatoid arthritis, increasing evidence shows that immunologic mechanisms play an important role in the pathogenesis of synovitis in RA. Lymphocytes and plasma cells in the synovium synthesize immunoglobulins, including some with antibody specificity to IgG. Immunoglobulin deposits, together with complement components, are found in articular cartilage, in synovium, and in phagocytic cells of the synovial membrane. Immunoglobulins, including some with antibody specificity to IgG, and complement can be identified in the phagolysosomes of polymorphonuclear cells in the synovial fluid. Immune complexes composed of IgG and antibodies to IgG exist in synovial fluid. Some of the IgG-containing immune complexes in RA result from self-association of IgG rheumatoid factor. In this reaction the IgG rheumatoid factor molecule serves both as an antibody and as an antigen molecule. The antibody specificity is directed to antigenic determinants on the Fc fragments, present in the same molecule. Thereby two antigen-antibody bonds are formed in the dimerization, leaving the other antibody-binding site free for further concentration-dependent polymerization. Immune complexes generated in this manner do not require an exogenous antigen but are formed by the IgG rheumatoid factors when these IgG molecules possess both the antibody specificity and the antigenic determinant. Immune complexes composed of other antigens and antibodies are present in some patients. The activation of complement by these immune complexes apparently leads to the generation of chemotactic and vasoactive factors, resulting in the influx of neutrophils into the joint. The finding of decreased complement components and total hemolytic complement and the presence of breakdown products of complement in synovial fluid supports this notion. Phagocytosis of immune complexes by polymorphonuclear cells results in the release of lysosomal enzymes capable of producing tissue injury. Superoxide ion (O_2^-) is also liberated during phagocytosis. O_2^- ions damage cell membranes, kill cells, and depolymerize hyaluronic acid. Macrophages that have accumulated in the synovial tissue contribute to release of enzymes that degrade joint structures. Collagenase cleaves collagen to render it susceptible to other proteases, and neutral protease depolymerizes proteoglycans. Prostaglandin production by synovial cells results in stimulation of osteoclasts and bone resorption. Osteoclast-activating factor from mononuclear leukocytes acts similarly on bone.

Large numbers of T cells are present in the synovium. Through release of various lymphokines these cells also contribute to the inflammation of rheumatoid arthritis. The inflammatory process culminates in the destruction of articular cartilage and subchondral bone, especially at the margins of articular cartilage, leading to features that are characteristic of rheumatoid arthritis.

The pathogenic mechanisms of extraarticular manifestations of RA have not been identified with certainty. However, mounting evidence indicates that humoral immune mechanisms involving immune complexes participate in this process. The acute vasculitic lesions of RA contain immunoglobulins and complement components. Patients with such lesions tend to have minimally depressed serum complement level, and these patients frequently have circulating immune complexes containing either IgM rheumatoid factors or IgG rheumatoid factors.

EPIDEMIOLOGY The onset of RA may occur anytime in life. Approximately 70 percent of RA occurs between the third and seventh decades; the peak onset is in the fourth decade. The prevalence in North America ranges from 0.5 to 3.8 percent in women and from 0.15 to 1.3 percent in men, depending on which diagnostic criteria are applied in population studies. Women are affected approximately three times more often than men; however, this difference disappears in older age. RA appears in all races, and climate does not appear to influence the prevalence.

A genetic predisposition for RA is suggested by the previously mentioned association with HLA-DRw4. Severe RA is found at four times the expected rate in first-degree relatives of probands with seropositive disease. Studies of monozygotic twins, however, showed mostly disconcordance for RA. Both genetic predisposition and environmental factors therefore appear to play a role in the development of RA.

PATHOLOGY The synovium develops numerous folds consisting of large villi and spreads to cover the articular cartilage with what is referred to as a *pannus.* The pannus destroys the underlying articular cartilage and subchondral bone. The earliest and most prominent bone erosions occur at the joint margins where the articular cartilage ends and the joint capsule attaches to bone. The bone at these sites in the joint is covered by the synovial membrane as it is reflected from the periosteum to the inner aspect of the joint capsule. Later, fibrous adhesions or even bony ankylosis may unite the opposing joint surfaces. The invasion and destruction of the subchondral bone and the destruction of cartilage are mediated by enzymes emanating from phagocytic cells in the synovial membrane and fluid. The inflammatory process weakens the joint capsule and supporting ligaments. The combination of joint destruction, loss of supporting structures, muscle atrophy, and imbalance of opposing muscle groups results in joint instability and subluxation. Persistent inflammation in the tendon sheaths may cause weakening and even rupture of the tendons.

Hypercellularity of the synovium results from the influx of lymphocytes, plasma cells, and monocytes. The synovial lining cells proliferate and lose their organization. In more chronic disease, lymphocytes form follicles in the synovium.

The so-called rheumatoid nodules are fairly characteristic of RA. The center of the nodule consists of an area of fibrinoid necrosis and cellular debris, surrounded by several layers of palisading large monocytic cells. The periphery is infiltrated with lymphocytes and monocytes. Small-vessel vasculitis is considered to be the initiating event in the formation of the nodule. Nodules are most often found in subcutaneous tissue over pressure points such as the elbows, occiput, and sacrum in bedridden patients. They may be bound to the underlying periosteum. Nodules may appear on the dorsum of the fingers and may be attached to tendons. Solitary or multiple nodules may appear in the lung parenchyma, in the pleura, in heart valves, in myocardium, and rarely in vocal cords.

Vasculitis involving small to medium-sized vessels occurs in RA. The histological picture ranges from focal perivascular accumulation of lymphocytes to necrotizing lesions showing fibrinoid necrosis, disruption of the intima, and infiltration of polymorphonuclear cells. Immunoglobulins and complement deposits can be demonstrated by immunofluorescence in the vessel of acute lesions. Vasculitis of the vasa nervorum may lead to peripheral neuropathy. Nail-fold thrombi, digital gangrene, and leg ulcers may occur. Necrotizing vasculitis involving intestinal wall and coronary and cerebral arteries has also been described.

Atrophy of skeletal muscles with interstitial accumulation of lymphocytes is present. Rarely, myositis occurs that is indistinguishable histologically and clinically from polymyositis.

Enlargement of the lymph nodes draining the affected joints, as well as generalized lymphadenopathy, may be present. Histologically, the nodes show hyperplasia and in some instances may resemble those of giant follicular lymphoma.

CLINICAL MANIFESTATIONS In the majority of patients the onset of RA is insidious. A prodrome of fatigue, weakness, joint stiffness, and vague arthralgias and myalgias may precede the appearance of joint swelling by several weeks. Several joints are usually involved in a symmetrical fashion at the onset, especially those of the hands, wrists, and feet. Disease, in approximately one-third of the patients, however, may initially be confined to one or a few joints, frequently one or both knees, before spreading to other joints in a symmetrical pattern. The pattern of joint involvement may remain asymmetrical in some patients. Unlike the migratory polyarthritis of rheumatic fever, RA usually persists in the initially involved joints as other joints become affected. Some patients may have an acute onset, with fever and multiple swollen, painful joints. Raynaud's phenomenon occurs in some patients.

Examination of the involved joints reveals increased warmth, tenderness, and swelling, which early in the disease may be subtle. The synovium becomes palpable as boggy tissue around the joint margin. The skin over small joints often has a ruddy cyanotic hue; marked erythema is unusual. Muscle weakness and atrophy adjacent to the affected joint often parallel the severity of joint disease. Range of joint motion, especially extension, becomes limited. Flexion contractures and in some instances fibrous or bony ankylosis may develop. Terms such as *swan neck, boutonnière,* and *cock-up toes* are used to describe joint deformities in the hands and feet. Another frequently observed deformity consists of volar subluxation and ulnar deviation of the fingers at the metacarpophalangeal joints (Fig. 346-1). Tenosynovitis and tendon nodules of the flexor tendons adjacent to the metacarpophalangeal joints may restrict flexion of the fingers and cause a trigger finger. Flexion contractures of the knees and hips greatly hinder ambulation.

The duration of morning stiffness may be useful in assessing disease activity. During periods of active joint disease, the patient may complain of morning stiffness lasting an hour or more. With improvement, the duration of morning stiffness decreases. Disease activity in the hands and wrist can be followed by measurement of grip strength, which is performed by having the patient compress a rolled-up, partially inflated sphygmomanometer cuff. Disease activity in the lower extremities is assessed by recording the time required to walk a standard distance (e.g., 50 ft).

Though the disease may occur in any diarthrodial joint, the joints most commonly affected are the metacarpophalangeal, wrist, proximal interphalangeal, knee, ankle, metatarsophalangeal, shoulder, and elbow. Cervical spine disease is common; however, the lower part of the spine is relatively spared. Unilateral sacroiliitis occurs but is of little clinical significance. A serious complication is *subluxation of the atlantoaxial joint,* which may lead to compression of the spinal cord by the odontoid process. Symptoms and signs of cord compression, such as bladder dysfunction, anal sphincter laxity, circumanal hypesthesia, and long-tract signs, should be sought. Sudden death has resulted from laceration of the cord by the odontoid process or from impingement by the odontoid upon the medulla within the foramen magnum. *Temporomandibular disease* may interfere with mastication, and pain from this joint may be referred to the middle ear and throat. *Arthritis in the cricoarytenoid* joints can cause hoarseness or even life-threatening upper-airway obstruction if the joints are fixed in adduction. Tenosynovitis in the wrist may compress the median nerve, causing a carpal tunnel syndrome. Nerve entrapment may also occur at the elbow (ulnar nerve), peroneal region (peroneal nerve), or tarsal region (plantar nerves), producing symptoms of sensory or motor loss.

Popliteal cyst may develop in patients with synovitis of the knee. The cyst forms either from herniation or rupture of the synovium posteriorly through the joint capsule or from communication of the joint with the semimembranosus bursa. The cyst enlarges because synovial fluid is forced into it by motion of the joint and is unable to return. A popliteal cyst may extend down into the calf or rarely up into the posterior thigh. A clinical picture resembling thrombophlebitis is produced by rupture of the popliteal cyst or by rupture of the synovium of the knee even in the absence of a cyst. It is important to remember that a ruptured popliteal cyst and thrombophlebitis can coexist. The diagnosis of a cyst or a ruptured cyst is confirmed by arthrography. Ultrasound can also be employed for demonstration of a cyst. Venogram may be indicated to exclude thrombophlebitis.

Rheumatoid nodules are found in approximately 20 percent of patients and are most commonly located over the extensor surface of the elbows. They may also be present over the extensor surface of the fingers and in other areas exposed to pressure, such as the back of the head and over the sacrum in bedridden patients. The nodules may be freely movable or attached to tendons or the periosteum. They are usually firm and nontender but may be cystic. The overlying skin may break down and lead to chronic drainage. Pressure by eyeglasses at the bridge of the nose may produce an ulcerated rheumatoid nodule which may be mistaken for basal-cell carcinoma. Nodules are usually associated with active disease and a positive test for rheumatoid factor.

The hands of a rheumatoid patient are often cool and damp, reflecting autonomic nervous system dysfunction. Palmer erythema is also seen. In long-standing disease, the skin over the distal extremities often becomes atrophic and bruises easily. These manifestations may be further accentuated in patients on glucocorticosteroids.

Nail-fold thrombi, small infarcts on the volar surface of the hands, digital gangrene, and ulcers of the lower part of the leg and the ankle are manifestations of rheumatoid vasculitis. Both sensory and motor types of neuropathy result from vasculitis of the vasa nervorum. Vasculitis of the cranial, coronary, and mesenteric vessels has been observed.

The most common ocular manifestation is keratoconjunctivitis sicca (Sjögren's syndrome), which occurs in approximately 15 percent of patients. Uveitis is encountered occasionally. Episcleritis may occur; this may evolve into a rheumatoid

FIGURE 346-1

Rheumatoid arthritis. A. Synovial proliferation of the metacarpophalangeal joints and to a lesser degree of the proximal interphalangeal joints. B. Advanced deformities of RA. Subluxation and ulnar deviation of the metacarpophalangeal joints are present. Fingers show swan neck deformity with hyperextension of the proximal interphalangeal joint.

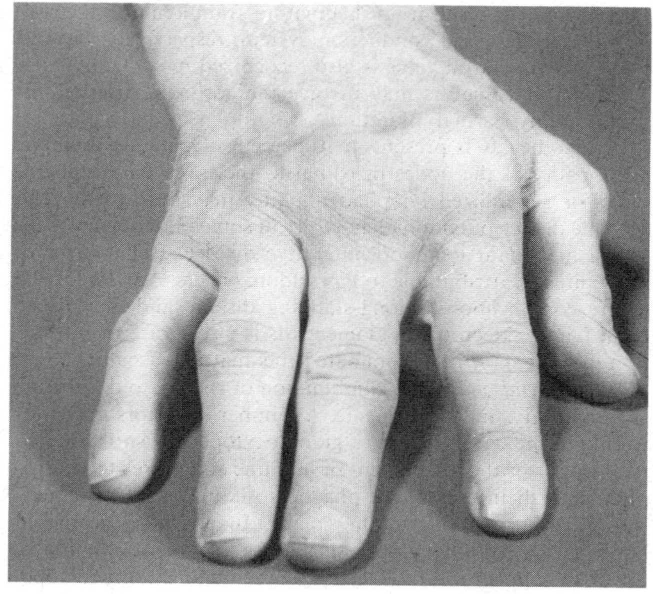

A

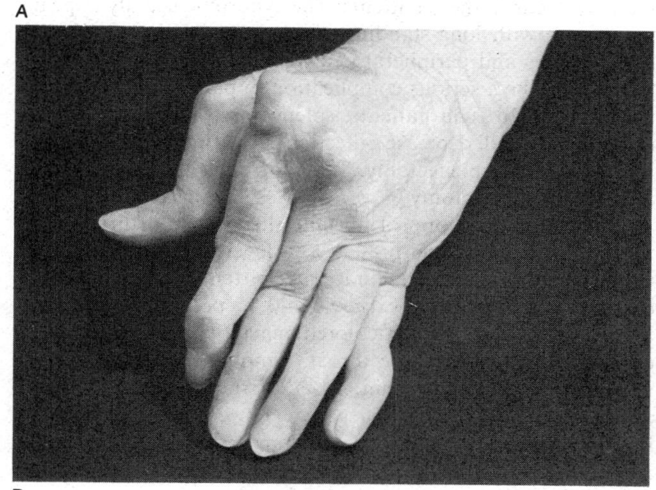

B

nodule that eventually perforates the sclera (scleromalacia perforans).

Pulmonary involvement may take the form of diffuse interstitial fibrosis, single or multiple nodules in the lung parenchyma, or a pleural effusion with or without antecedent symptoms of pleurisy. A distinguishing characteristic of some pleural fluids is their low glucose and high lactic dehydrogenase concentrations. Glucose levels as low as 10 mg/dl may be observed in the absence of infection. Also, the pleural fluid complement level is low compared with the serum level when these values are related to the total protein concentrations of the respective compartments. The pleural fluid may show a distinctive cytological picture, consisting of a background of amorphous necrotic material, large elongated cells, and giant multinucleated cells. Parenchymal rheumatoid nodules may lead to cavitation, which is easily seen on x-ray films. Caplan's syndrome, described originally in Welsh coal miners, is the combination of RA and multiple pulmonary nodules (rheumatoid granulomas) developing in patients with underlying pneumoconiosis. Patients may have impaired pulmonary diffusion in the absence of chest film abnormalities.

Clinical heart disease is unusual, even though evidence of previous pericarditis is often found at necropsy. Rarely, pericarditis with cardiac tamponade occurs. As in the pleural fluid, glucose and complement levels may be reduced. Aortic regurgitation and conduction abnormalities are occasionally seen. These problems result from rheumatoid granulomas in the aortic valve leaflets and conduction system, respectively. Slowed closure of the mitral valve is also recognized in some patients. Rheumatoid vasculitis may involve the coronary arteries, resulting in myocardial infarction.

Splenomegaly is present in 10 percent of patients. Lymphadenopathy of the nodes proximal to the involved peripheral joints or generalized lymphadenopathy may be present. The extreme degree of lymphadenopathy in some patients may suggest a malignant lymphoproliferative disease. Renal involvement directly attributable to RA seldom occurs. Amyloidosis is a rare complication in long-standing disease and may cause renal failure. Necrotizing glomerulitis is also a rare manifestation in patients with disseminated rheumatoid vasculitis.

Felty's syndrome is the combination of rheumatoid arthritis, splenomegaly, and neutropenia. A number of factors may contribute to the development of granulocytopenia. Antibodies to neutrophils or the attachment of immune complexes to neutrophils with their subsequent phagocytosis may lead to sequestration of neutrophils in the spleen. In addition, decreased bone marrow granulocytopoiesis may be due to a serum inhibitor or to suppression by T cells. Anemia and thrombocytopenia may occur in these patients. The syndrome usually appears in patients with long-standing disease. Vasculitis, manifested by leg ulcers and peripheral neuropathy, may be present. Infection may be a serious complication in patients with marked neutropenia. In such patients, splenectomy may improve the neutropenia and decrease infections. Neutropenia, however, may recur after splenectomy. The course of the arthritis is not affected by splenectomy.

Still's disease, a form of juvenile rheumatoid arthritis, may also occur in adults and present as a fever of unknown origin. Clinical manifestations include intermittent episodes of high daily spiking fever often exceeding 40°C, polyarthralgias, myalgias, evanescent salmon-colored maculopapular rash, pericarditis, pneumonitis, sore throat, lymphadenopathy, splenomegaly, and abdominal pain. Tests for rheumatoid factor and antinuclear antibodies are negative. Fewer joints are usually involved and joint destruction seldom occurs. These patients respond well to high doses of salicylates or indomethacin.

CLINICAL COURSE The course of RA is highly variable and unpredictable. Spontaneous remissions and exacerbations are characteristic; remissions are more apt to occur early in the disease. Many patients who early in their disease are diagnosed as having possible RA either turn out to have another disease or completely recover, suggesting that the original diagnosis was in error. Approximately 10 to 20 percent of patients will have either a remission early in their disease or mild intermittent disease which requires little if any medical attention. On the other side, approximately 10 percent of patients will have progressive crippling disease. Most of these patients will have some response to aggressive therapy; however, a few, probably less than 3 percent, will ultimately be confined to bed. The majority of patients fall between these groups. The patients in this middle group experience joint damage to varying degrees over the years, yet most of them are able to continue functioning at work or at home. There are certain features that portend a poor prognosis. These include a high titer of rheumatoid factors, multiple rheumatoid nodules, and vasculitis. A history of mild, intermittent disease over the years will usually continue in this pattern.

LABORATORY FINDINGS Normocytic, normochromic, or hypochromic (hypoproliferative) anemia is often present in active disease. The serum iron level and total iron-binding capacity are low. The ineffective erythropoiesis, also seen with other chronic inflammatory disorders, is due in part to a block in the release of iron from the reticuloendothelial system. Iron therapy is of no value except in those cases where superimposed blood loss has occurred and when no stainable iron can be demonstrated in the bone marrow. Rarely, a Coombs-positive hemolytic anemia is present.

A mild leukocytosis may be present. A few patients may have neutropenia and a mild thrombocytopenia. Eosinophilia of 5 percent or greater has been observed, especially in patients with extraarticular manifestations of vasculitis, pleuropericarditis, pulmonary fibrosis, and subcutaneous nodules.

The erythrocyte sedimentation rate (ESR) is commonly elevated and can be used as an index for following disease activity. However, the ESR may not always reflect the activity of the disease.

Protein electrophoresis often shows a reduced albumin, moderately elevated gamma globulin, and elevated $alpha_2$ globulins. Measurements of immunoglobulins may show increased levels of IgG, IgM, and IgA. These findings, however, are not diagnostic.

Rheumatoid factor as indicated by the latex agglutination test is positive in the majority of patients with RA. Only IgM rheumatoid factor is readily measured by the currently available methods, which include latex agglutination, bentonite flocculation, and sensitized sheep or human red blood cell tests. The basic principle of all these tests is the same because the antigen, human or rabbit IgG, is coated onto a carrier particle (red blood cell, latex, bentonite), allowing agglutination to be visible when rheumatoid factors react with IgG. Methods for detecting IgG and IgA rheumatoid factors remain research tools.

Patients with a variety of nonrheumatoid diseases, usually characterized by chronic inflammation with persistent antigenic challenge, have positive tests for rheumatoid factor. These include other connective tissue diseases (systemic lupus erythematosus, Sjögren's syndrome, polymyositis, scleroderma) and infectious diseases (tuberculosis, leprosy, syphilis, subacute bacterial endocarditis, bacterial bronchitis, parasitic infections, viral hepatitis, infectious mononucleosis, influenza). Positive results are also found in patients with idiopathic pulmonary fibrosis, pneumoconiosis, sarcoidosis, hypergammaglobulinemic purpura, mixed cryoglobulinemia, chronic active hepatitis and cirrhosis, lymphomas, renal allografts, and repeated blood transfusions. An occasional monoclonal IgM (Waldenström's macroglobulin) will show rheumatoid factor activity. Rheumatoid factor has been reported to appear transiently in the serum of army recruits after extensive prophylactic immunizations. Population studies of apparently healthy persons show an increasing prevalence of rheumatoid factor with age. The overall prevalence in persons below the age of 60 is less than 4 percent. However, in persons over the age of 60, positive results have been encountered in 40 percent of subjects in some surveys. The titer of rheumatoid factor in these elderly apparently normal persons is usually low, being less than 1:80.

Rheumatoid factor is usually present either when the patient is first seen or within the first year of disease. The titer of rheumatoid factor correlates poorly with disease activity; therefore, once a definite positive test is found, there is little reason to measure rheumatoid factor repeatedly. However, those patients with high titers tend to have more severe disease and thus a poorer prognosis than seronegative patients. Positive tests are almost always found in patients with nodules or with clinical evidence of vasculitis. A positive test does not make the diagnosis of RA but must be interpreted in the light of other clinical features.

Antinuclear antibodies are found in 20 to 60 percent of patients. Titers of antibodies with specificity for native DNA are usually low; titers of antibodies to single-stranded or denatured DNA may be elevated. Antibodies to an antigen present in Epstein-Barr virus carrying a lymphoblastic cell line can be identified by immunodiffusion or by immunofluorescence in the serum of most patients with RA. These antibodies are referred to as rhematoid arthritis precipitin (RAP) and rheumatoid arthritis nuclear antigen (RANA), respectively. Anti-RAP and anti-RANA may be reacting with the same nuclear antigen. The pathogenic significance of these findings remains to be determined. Serum complement level is usually normal or elevated. Slightly reduced levels have been reported in patients with rheumatoid vasculitis.

Synovial fluid has a turbid appearance because of increased numbers of white blood cells. The cells are predominantly neutrophils and usually range from 10,000 to 50,000 per cubic millimeter. The fluid may clot spontaneously because of the presence of fibrinogen. This fibrin clot should not be confused with the mucin clot formed by adding 1 percent acetic acid to the fluid. In rheumatoid synovial fluid the viscosity is decreased and the mucin clot is poor because of smaller than normal polymers of hyaluronic acid. Cytoplasmic inclusions in polymorphonuclear cells, containing ingested immune complexes, are not specific for RA. Especially in patients with positive tests for rheumatoid factor, the synovial fluid hemolytic complement or complement components, such as C3 and C4, are low when these values are related to the total protein concentration of the synovial fluid. The synovial fluid glucose level, as compared with a simultaneously drawn serum glucose, may be low in some patients, possibly because of decreased transport across the membrane or increased utilization by inflammatory cells.

Radiographs of the joints in early disease show only soft-tissue swelling and mild juxtaarticular osteoporosis. Later, bony erosions, initially quite subtle, appear at the joint margins; these are most readily seen in the small joints of the hands and along the ulnar and radial styloid processes. Joint space narrowing is seen as cartilage is destroyed. In advanced disease, destruction of subchondral bone and diffuse osteoporosis develop. When the cervical part of the spine is involved, flexion and extension films should be obtained to check for atlantoaxial subluxation.

DIAGNOSIS The diagnosis of RA is readily made in the patient with symmetrical inflammatory arthritis of small joints, rheumatoid nodules, characteristic radiographic abnormalities, and a positive test for rheumatoid factor. The patient who presents a history of fatigue and vague arthralgias without definite evidence of arthritis frequently poses a diagnostic problem. Such a patient may be in the prodromal phase of RA; however, these symptoms occur in depressed middle-aged patients, especially women. If the diagnosis is not certain, the patient's course should be followed for objective evidence of rheumatoid arthritis. A premature diagnosis of RA may cause a patient needless anxiety and fear. Other types of inflammatory arthritis deserve consideration, especially in the patient who has only a few joints involved in an asymmetrical distribution. Reiter's syndrome (see Chap. 348), psoriatic arthritis (see Chap. 348), systemic lupus erythematosus (see Chap. 70), and arthritis associated with gastrointestinal diseases (see Chap. 348) should be considered in the differential diagnosis. Some patients with ankylosing spondylitis (see Chap. 347) may have peripheral arthritis. The arthritis of rheumatic fever follows a streptococcal infection and presents as a limited symmetrical polyarthritis and tenosynovitis involving most often the joints of the lower extremities. The arthritis in the prodromal phase of hepatitis B infection may initially mimic RA. Arthritis associated with rubella infection or Lyme disease may also resemble RA, especially in those patients who continue to have recurrent arthritis for several years (see Chap. 350). The arthritis of hemochromatosis (see Chap. 97) may be mistaken for RA especially when there is swelling and bony enlargement of the second and third metacarpophalangeal joints. Chronic sarcoid arthritis with symmetrical joint involvement and evidence of joint destruction may require biopsy of the synovium to distinguish it from RA. Degenerative joint disease is easily distinguished from RA, but erosive osteoarthritis (see Chap. 351) may be confused with RA. In rheumatoid arthritis, the most frequently involved joints of the upper extremity are the metacarpophalangeal, proximal interphalangeal (PIP), and wrists, while in osteoarthritis the distal interphalangeal joints, followed by the PIP, are most often affected. Osteoarthritis also frequently involves the carpometacarpal joint. Calcium pyrophosphate deposition disease may be manifested as a chronic erosive polyarthritis and may mimic rheumatoid arthritis. Distinction from RA will require examination of joint fluid for crystals. The finding of a positive test result for rheumatoid factor in an elderly person with joint pain should not by itself lead to the diagnosis of RA.

The definite diagnosis of RA depends primarily on the presence of characteristic clinical features and the exclusion of other inflammatory arthritides.

TREATMENT General measures Once the diagnosis has been established, the patient and family should be given a clear understanding of the chronic nature of RA. The value of careful and continuous medical supervision should be emphasized. Above all, the patient should be reassured that there is readily available therapy and that severe crippling is usually not the outcome. The patient should be apprised that the majority of patients continue to lead active, productive lives with varying degrees of restricted activity. The patient should be encouraged to continue working within reasonable limits. This in some instances may necessitate retraining in work that is physically less demanding. Depression as a reaction to their disabling illness occurs and requires careful attention. These patients may benefit from antidepressant medications. The question of moving to a warm climate is often raised. The patient may subjectively feel better in a warm climate; however, the course of the disease is not changed.

The goal of therapy is to maintain the patient's ability to function. To accomplish this, every effort should be made to reduce joint inflammation and pain, maintain motion and strength, and prevent and correct joint deformities. The proper utilization of rest, anti-inflammatory drugs, splints, physical therapy, and orthopedic surgery is aimed at preserving function. Adequate rest is important. Patients should be encouraged to take short rest periods during the day and to get a full night's sleep. They should be instructed to maintain a well-balanced diet. There is no evidence that a nutritional deficiency leads to rheumatoid arthritis or that certain foods or vitamins affect the outcome.

Drug therapy The main goals of drug therapy are suppression of inflammation and remission of the disease. Joint pain, which is often the patient's main concern, is usually relieved by achieving these goals. The joint pain of active synovitis is not effectively treated with analgesic drugs alone. When joints are structurally damaged, the pain experienced on weight bearing and motion may require the judicious use of analgesic agents. Drugs used in the treatment of RA can be classified as *anti-inflammatory agents, remission-inducing agents,* and *immunosuppressive (cytotoxic) agents.*

ANTI-INFLAMMATORY AGENTS Anti-inflammatory drugs relieve symptoms and signs of inflammation but do not significantly alter the natural course of rheumatoid arthritis. Salicylates remain valuable and effective drugs and should be given an adequate trial in the initial treatment of RA. They have been shown to be superior to placebo and to be both anti-inflammatory and analgesic. An adequate anti-inflammatory dosage, 3 to 6 g per day, should be administered in divided amounts four times a day, preferably after meals. Determination of the salicylate blood level may be useful when the question of inadequate absorption or compliance is raised. The blood sample should be obtained 2 to 3 h after a regular dose. A level between 15 and 30 mg/dl is in the therapeutic range.

An increase in fecal blood is commonly observed with salicylate usage, regardless of the route of administration. Direct contact of aspirin particles on mucosa may cause superficial gastric erosions and bleeding. Also, salicylates may aggravate peptic ulcer disease. The gastrointestinal upset, a common complaint, can be alleviated by giving the drug with meals and by the use of antacids. Salicylates have been reported to cause urticaria or asthma and nasal polyps. Signs of toxicity such as tinnitus, deafness, hyperventilation, or confusion should be carefully monitored, especially in older patients.

Acetylsalicylic acid (aspirin) is the most effective preparation on weight basis. Choline salicylate, salicylsalicylic acid, or enteric coated preparations may be better tolerated in patients with gastrointestinal upset or with peptic ulcer disease.

Nonsteroidal anti-inflammatory drugs (NSAIDs) provide an alternative to salicylate therapy. The effectiveness of these drugs is comparable to salicylates, and they may be better tolerated in some instances. The NSAIDs, like aspirin, inhibit prostaglandin synthesis and are both anti-inflammatory and analgesic. These drugs can be used in conjunction with salicylates without adverse effects; however, no proven additive therapeutic response has been shown. These drugs include indomethacin (Indocin), ibuprofen (Motrin), fenoprofen (Nalfon), naproxen (Naprosyn), tolmetin (Tolectin), sulindac (Clinoril), and meclofenamate sodium (Meclomen). The usual dose of indomethacin is between 75 and 150 mg per day, in divided doses, and the drug is best tolerated if the dosage is gradually increased to these amounts. Side effects of lightheadedness, headaches, unreal feeling, depression, dyspepsia, or peptic ulcer disease may curb its use. The recommended dose of ibuprofen is between 1200 and 2400 mg per day, in divided doses. Side effects include epigastric pain, diarrhea, peptic ulcer disease, and skin eruptions. The usual dose of naproxen is 250 mg twice a day, and, again, adverse reactions include upper gastrointestinal distress and bleeding. The usual dose for fenoprofen is 600 mg four times per day. Again, gastrointestinal side effects such as dyspepsia, constipation, nausea, and occult blood in the stool may occur. The usual dose of tolmetin is between 600 and 1800 mg in divided doses. The side effects are similar to those of indomethacin. Sulindac is recommended in the dosage of 150 to 200 mg twice daily; the potential side effects are comparable with drugs mentioned above. The usual dose of meclofenamate sodium is between 200 mg and 400 mg per day, administered in three or four equal doses. Side effects include exacerbation of peptic ulcer disease, gastrointestinal bleeding, and diarrhea. All these drugs and acetylsalicylic acid, but not choline salicylate, salicylsalicylic acid, and sodium salicylate, interfere with platelet aggregation and therefore may prolong bleeding time. The NSAIDs as well as aspirin may lead to salt retention and renal insufficiency, especially in older patients with compromised renal function, by interfering with prostaglandin synthesis in the kidney. Rarely these drugs may cause an interstitial nephritis.

Phenylbutazone may be useful for short periods during an acute exacerbation of arthritis but is not recommended for long-term therapy. The dose should not exceed 400 mg per day. Complications include fluid retention, peptic ulcer disease, and bone marrow toxicity, primarily leukopenia.

Glucocorticosteroids are classified as anti-inflammatory drugs since they do not significantly alter the natural course of the disease in spite of their rather dramatic initial suppression of symptoms and signs of inflammation. The use of these agents in a chronic disease such as rheumatoid arthritis is justified in only a few situations. The long-term use of these drugs, even in low doses, leads to significant osteopenia and compression fractures. In patients with severe progressive disease, a dose of 5 to 10 mg of prednisone per day can keep a patient functioning or employed while waiting for remission-inducing drugs to work. An effort should be made to reduce the prednisone to the lowest possible dose required by the patient. The reduction of prednisone in these patients is best achieved by decrements of 1 mg. Patients should be encouraged to take the prednisone in the morning as a single dose. In special circumstances, large doses of prednisone are necessary in patients with rheumatoid vasculitis. Patients who are receiving steroids or have received them in the recent past should be given supplemental steroids when they undergo surgery or develop a severe intercurrent infection.

Intraarticular steroid injections are useful in temporarily suppressing joint inflammation, especially in patients who have monoarticular or oligoarticular disease. In patients with multiple joint involvement, injections of the most symptomatic joints may serve to supplement other forms of therapy. Following injection of small finger joints, inflammation may be suppressed for as long as 1 year. Injections of a single joint should be limited to three or four per year; more frequent injections of glucocorticosteroids into a single joint may damage cartilage. Some patients experience a transient exacerbation of joint inflammation a few hours after injection which is due to a "crystal-induced synovitis" from glucocorticosteroid crystals. Sterile technique is mandatory to prevent infection.

REMISSION-INDUCING AGENTS These agents are given to patients with definite RA who have persistent active synovitis, in the hope of inducing a complete or partial remission. These drugs are often used early in the course of RA before permanent joint damage occurs. They also can be given to patients with long-standing disease experiencing an exacerbation of synovitis. When administering these drugs, aspirin or NSAIDs can be continued. The remission-inducing agents are gold salts, penicillamine, and antimalarials. Gold is most commonly used as the initial remitting agent. If no clinical improvement occurs after a standard course of gold, the patient then can be given a trial of penicillamine. Again, if no clinical improvement occurs, an antimalarial such as hydroxychloroquine or chloroquine might be used. Antimalarials have the advantage of being better tolerated; however, they have the potential risk of eye toxicity.

Gold salts are beneficial in suppressing disease activity in the majority of patients. In a controlled study, patients treated with a total of 1 g gold sodium thiomalate over a 20-week period experienced greater clinical improvement than those given placebo. The clinical improvement was still evident 12 months after stopping gold therapy, but not after 24 months. A later study over a 30-month period showed that patients continued on monthly injections of 50 mg after the initial standard gold course had less joint damage radiographically than a control group. In general, patients with recent onset of RA are more likely to respond than those with long-standing disease. Also, patients who previously failed to respond to an adequate course of gold are not likely to respond to another course.

The two gold salts most commonly used are gold sodium thiomalate (Myochrysine) and gold thioglucose (Solganol); they are administered intramuscularly, usually on a weekly basis. The initial dose is 10 mg, followed by 25 mg the next week. If no adverse effects are noted, 50 mg is given weekly. The beneficial effects of gold therapy usually do not become apparent until at least 400 to 500 mg has been given. If no improvement results after a total dose of 1 g, the drug is discontinued. With a favorable response, the interval between injections is gradually increased until the patient is receiving 50 mg monthly. On maintenance therapy patients may continue to improve or remain in remission. Maintenance therapy may be continued for years and may prevent relapse. Gold therapy should be stopped only after several years of no active disease.

Dermatitis and stomatitis are the most common toxic manifestations of gold therapy. The rash is often pruritic and accompanied by eosinophilia. The appearance of the rash is highly variable and can resemble many types of papulosquamous lesions. The mucocutaneous lesions are reversible when gold therapy is discontinued. Early detection of a rash is important, since continuation of gold may lead to a generalized exfoliative dermatitis. A mild rash may be treated with local steroid preparations; however, systemic steroids may be necessary for severe extensive dermatitis.

Gold toxicity can cause membranous glomerulonephritis, the earliest manifestations being proteinuria and/or hematuria. Renal disease may uncommonly progress to the nephrotic syndrome and renal failure. Histologically the renal lesion consists of typical membranous glomerulonephritis with subepithelial deposits of immune complexes. Bone marrow toxicity may present as an aplastic anemia, agranulocytosis, and/or thrombocytopenia with severe marrow depression. The use of a chelating agent may be necessary for treatment of severe gold toxicity. Toxic reactions to gold have been reported to be more common in patients with the histocompatibility antigens HLA-B8 and HLA-DRw3.

In view of the potential serious toxicity of gold, the decision to use gold carries with it the obligation of careful medical supervision. Each week the patient should be asked about and examined for evidence of skin and/or mouth lesions. White blood cell counts and analysis of the urine for protein should be performed on alternate weeks. Periodic platelet counts are advisable. If rash, proteinuria, or leukopenia appears, administration of gold should be discontinued.

A new oral form of gold, auranofin (gold triethylphosphine), is scheduled for release. The drug is taken daily in divided doses. The efficacy of the oral form is comparable with the intramuscularly injected gold salts. The toxic manifestations are similar to parenteral gold salts. Prescribing this drug still carries the responsibility of closely observing the patient for gold toxicity.

D-Penicillamine was shown in controlled multicenter trials to be effective in RA. Its therapeutic efficacy is comparable to gold salts. It is usually given after a patient has failed to respond to gold salts. To reduce side effects, the drug is given in a graduated dosage schedule, beginning with 250 mg daily for 3 months. The single daily oral dose should be taken on an empty stomach at least 1 h before or at least $1\frac{1}{2}$ h after a meal to permit maximum absorption and to reduce the likelihood of inactivation of the drug by metal binding. If no improvement occurs, the dosage is increased to 500 mg daily for 3 months. A trial of 750 mg daily for 12 more weeks may be indicated in some patients who still have not had a response to penicillamine. Patients are maintained on the dosage at which clinical improvement occurred. Since 125-mg capsules are available, some physicians prefer to adjust the dosage by 125-mg increments. Toxicity includes skin rashes, nausea, loss of taste, nephropathy with proteinuria and nephrotic syndrome, fever, and bone marrow suppression. Various autoimmune syndromes have also occurred with penicillamine administration. These include Goodpasture's syndrome, myasthenia gravis, pemphigus, polymyositis, and lupus erythematosus. Minor skin rashes and pruritus can usually be controlled by the administration of an antihistamine. Decreased taste perception is common and may last for several months, but the perception of taste gradually returns while the therapy is continued. The patient should be encouraged to continue therapy in spite of this unpleasant but transient side effect. Other toxic reactions necessitate discontinuation of therapy. The use of this drug requires following the patient closely; blood counts and tests for proteinuria should be obtained at regular intervals.

In controlled studies both chloroquine and hydroxychloroquine have been shown to be effective. The recommended daily dose of chloroquine is 250 mg, and of hydroxychloroquine, 400 mg. A response is not usually seen until 4 to 6 weeks of therapy, and 4 months of therapy should be given before considering the drug ineffective. Once remission or maximum improvement has occurred, the dosage should be reduced. With a flare, the full dose should again be given. Long-term use of these drugs is curtailed by the risk of blindness from irreversible retinal degeneration. This toxic effect appears to be less common with hydroxychloroquine. The risk can be minimized by following the above dosage schedule and having regular eye examinations. The eyes should be examined by an ophthalmologist prior to initiation of therapy and at 6-month intervals thereafter, or when symptoms indicate. The patient should be advised to wear sunglasses to protect the eyes from bright sunlight. Other complications of antimalarials include neuromyopathy, gastrointestinal distress, band keratopathy, bleaching of hair, and skin tanning on sun exposure.

IMMUNOSUPPRESSIVE (CYTOTOXIC) DRUGS These drugs are reserved for patients who have progressive disease unresponsive to anti-inflammatory and remission-inducing drugs. The rationale for their use is based on evidence that immunologic mechanisms mediate synovitis and other manifestations of RA. These drugs are effective in suppressing the primary humoral and cellular responses, provided that the drug is given in the proper dose and time in relation to the introduction of antigen.

They diminish ongoing cellular immune responses but have little, if any, effect on ongoing humoral immune responses. These drugs are anti-inflammatory, as shown in experimental animals and in human beings. Their action in RA has not been clarified but may be related in large part to their anti-inflammatory properties by decreasing the traffic of monocytes and lymphocytes.

The immunosuppressive drugs that have been used in RA include cyclophosphamide, azathioprine, 6-mercaptopurine, chlorambucil, and methotrexate. Favorable responses have been reported with all these drugs; however, few carefully controlled studies have been performed. A controlled study of cyclophosphamide, over an 8-month period, showed that patients receiving high doses (up to 150 mg per day) had greater improvement than those on a nontherapeutic dose (up to 15 mg per day). Patients treated with the high-dose regimen had improved grip strength, a decrease in the duration of morning stiffness, a decrease in the number of painful swollen joints, and a decrease in the number of new articular erosions. Sedimentation rates did not correlate well with improvement. Controlled studies carried out with azathioprine have also shown favorable results.

The toxicity and side effects of cytotoxic drugs limit their use. These agents can cause bone marrow depression with severe leukopenia, infection (especially with opportunistic microorganisms), sterility, and an increased risk of neoplasia. Because of their mutagenic potential, contraception should be recommended when they are being used. In addition, there are specific adverse manifestations of the individual drugs. Methotrexate is hepatotoxic and causes cirrhosis. Cyclophosphamide causes cystitis, resulting in hemorrhage and bladder wall fibrosis. Alopecia occurs frequently. Immunosuppressive therapy should be considered experimental and, if used at all, should be restricted to patients who have not responded to more conventional forms of therapy. Azathioprine has recently been approved for use in RA; use of the other drugs requires an informed consent from the patient. The care of these patients should be closely supervised, and white blood cell counts should be carefully monitored.

Plasmapheresis may be beneficial in the treatment of RA. Since it is expensive, time-consuming, and potentially risky, only critically ill patients with life-threatening rheumatoid vasculitis or hyperviscosity syndrome should be considered for treatment. The use of long-term plasmapheresis in patients with relentlessly progressive RA, unresponsive to conventional therapy, remains controversial.

Physical therapy This form of treatment plays an important role in the treatment of RA. Heat helps to relieve muscle spasm and reduce stiffness. Paraffin baths and heat lamps can be used at home. Passive range-of-motion exercises can help to prevent or minimize loss of joint motion. Isometric exercises increase muscle strength and thereby help to maintain joint stability. Repetitious forms of exercise should not be performed with joints that have active disease. Splinting of an actively involved joint for short periods of time is useful in reducing pain and possibly inflammation. The use of night splints is helpful in preventing flexion contractures, especially of the knees and wrists. Review and revision of home and work routines, and the use of assistive devices, can enhance the patient's ability to continue functioning at an independent level.

Orthopedic surgery This modality plays an important role in the treatment of RA. Function may be improved by surgical correction of joint deformities and stabilization of certain joints. Resection of the metatarsal heads is often beneficial in relieving forefoot pain. The carpal tunnel syndrome with persistent neurological signs necessitates surgical release and synovectomy. Ruptured tendons should be repaired within a couple of days after their breakage. Removal of rheumatoid synovium involving the extensor hood over the dorsum of the wrist and hands may prevent tendon rupture. Resection of the distal ulna, together with synovectomy of the wrist, helps to relieve pain and improve function. Synovectomy of the knee may be needed when a symptomatic popliteal cyst does not respond to intraarticular corticosteroids.

Atlantoaxial subluxation with symptoms of cord compression may require surgical stabilization. Patients with atlantoaxial subluxation but without evidence of cord compression should protect themselves by wearing a collar, especially when riding in an automobile.

Prophylactic synovectomy may diminish joint pain and temporarily retard progression of the disease in the operated joint. If the disease remains active, the joints treated with synovectomy become reinflamed. Development of total hip prostheses has given new hope to patients with severely damaged hip joints. Results of total knee, ankle, and other large-joint prostheses are encouraging. Rehabilitation of many patients is now possible through orthopedic procedures that improve function and reduce pain.

JUVENILE RHEUMATOID ARTHRITIS

Juvenile rheumatoid arthritis (JRA) consists of several distinct syndromes. Three main subgroups have been identified: systemic-onset disease, polyarticular disease, and pauciarticular disease. In addition, ankylosing spondylitis and rheumatoid arthritis indistinguishable from adult-onset disease may begin in childhood.

Systemic-onset JRA represents 25 percent of juvenile arthritis and is characterized by distinctive extraarticular manifestations in addition to the arthritis. Boys are affected more than girls, and the median age of onset is 5 years. These patients may have high fever (40°C and over). The fever has wide diurnal fluctuations and is highest in the afternoon and evening. Fever may be present for weeks or months before the appearance of arthritis. An evanescent salmon-color nonpruritic macular or maculopapular rash may appear, especially during fever, and is more common on the trunk. Generalized lymphadenopathy, splenomegaly, and hepatomegaly are often present. Cardiac involvement includes pericarditis and, rarely, myocarditis; pneumonitis and pleuritis also occur. Systemic manifestations are self-limited. Approximately one-fourth of this group of patients experience severe, destructive polyarthritis. Laboratory findings include anemia, leukocytosis, and negative tests for rheumatoid factors and antinuclear antibodies. The name *Still's disease* is sometimes used for this form of disease, but this eponym is also used for all forms of JRA.

Pauciarticular arthritis, affecting about 30 percent of patients with JRA, is characterized by female predominance, early age of onset (2 to 4 years), and involvement of one or a few joints, most commonly the knees or ankles. The arthritis is mild, with a good prognosis. Half of the patients experience chronic iridocyclitis, which may lead to band keratopathy, cataracts, and loss of vision. Since eye symptoms may be minimal, patients should have regular slit-lamp examinations, whether or not the arthritis is in remission. Antinuclear antibodies have been found in 50 to 60 percent of these patients; rheumatoid factor is absent.

Polyarticular arthritis occurs in 25 percent of patients, affects predominantly girls at a young age (median age of onset 2 years), and has a relatively good prognosis. The onset is usually insidious; the initial joint involvement is in the small joints of the hands and feet. Twenty-five percent have antinuclear antibodies. The standard tests for rheumatoid factor are negative. With special techniques, IgG and IgA rheumatoid factors have been found in over half the patients that are seronegative by standard methods.

In addition to these three subgroups, 5 to 10 percent of patients have polyarticular disease and a positive rheumatoid factor test. The median age of onset is 12 years, and females predominate. The course and clinical manifestations are those of adult-onset RA. Ankylosing spondylitis may also present in childhood, as pauciarticular disease, and represents 20 percent of patients with juvenile-onset arthritis. The median age of onset is 10 years, and males predominate. Patients experience early hip girdle symptoms; episodes of acute iridocyclitis may occur. Rheumatoid factor and antinuclear antibody tests are negative. The prevalence of HLA-B27 is 75 percent in this group while an increased prevalence of HLA-B27 is not found in the other subgroups of JRA.

The object of therapy in JRA, as in adult-onset RA, is to relieve pain and maintain function. The child should be allowed to lead as normal a life as possible and should be encouraged to participate in the activities of childhood. Only vigorous athletics should be discouraged. Salicylates are the first drug of choice. Patients on salicylates should be followed closely with liver function tests, since these drugs occasionally produce hepatotoxicity. It is recommended that liver function tests plus a prothrombin time be obtained before starting therapy, and then at regular intervals. The abnormal liver function tests return to normal in most patients while they remain on salicylates. Progressive liver dysfunction may necessitate stopping the drug. If salicylates are not effective, gold salts can be given. Antimalarials can also be beneficial in JRA. The use of systemic glucocorticosteroids is seldom indicated in the treatment of JRA. In certain instances, glucocorticosteroids are required for the treatment of uncontrolled systemic JRA or in treating iridocyclitis not controlled by a topical steroid. They are not indicated for the treatment of joint manifestations alone. Immunosuppressive agents are seldom indicated in JRA, since little is known of the long-term effects of these drugs. Physical therapy, the judicious splinting of joints, proper exercise, and adequate rest are all important factors in the treatment of JRA.

SJÖGREN'S SYNDROME

This syndrome consists of dry eyes (keratoconjunctivitis sicca, xerophthalmia), dry mouth (xerostomia), and a connective tissue disease, most commonly rheumatoid arthritis. It can be diagnosed when any two of the three clinical features (dry eyes, dry mouth, arthritis) are present. Patients with only eye and oral involvement are classified as Sjögren's syndrome (SS) and those with an associated connective tissue disease as SS with RA, SS with SLE, etc. The lack of secretions may also involve the entire respiratory tract, vagina, and skin. The syndrome occurs most commonly in middle-aged women; fewer than 10 percent of patients are men. The histological and immunologic findings suggest that abnormalities of both humoral- and cell-mediated immunity are involved in the pathogenesis of Sjögren's syndrome.

The decrease in tears and saliva (sicca syndrome) results from lymphocytic infiltration of the lacrimal and salivary glands. The earliest histological finding is periductal lymphocytic infiltration, which progresses to produce atrophy of the acini. The cells are predominantly small lymphocytes, but large lymphocytes, plasma cells, and reticulum cells may be present. Lymph follicles with germinal centers form in the gland. Hyperplasia of the ductal lining cells narrows and obstructs the duct and leads to its dilatation. Focal hyperplasia of ductal cells produces epimyoepithelial islands surrounded by lymphocytes. Hyalinization of these islands may occur. Later in the course of the disease, the atrophied parenchymal tissue is replaced by adipose tissue. Lip biopsy specimens show infiltrates of plasma cells and lymphocytes in the minor (accessory) salivary glands. Features that are helpful in distinguishing this syndrome from malignant lymphoma are the benign appearance of the small lymphocytes, the preservation of the lobular architecture of the gland, and the presence of epimyoepithelial cells.

The sicca syndrome occurs in approximately 10 to 15 percent of patients with RA; the arthritis usually appears first. In RA, dryness afects the eyes more often than the mouth. Rheumatoid nodules, splenomegaly, leukopenia, and vasculitis may be present in these patients. Sjögren's syndrome is associated less often with systemic lupus erythematosus, polymyositis, scleroderma, and periarteritis nodosa. The syndrome also occurs in some patients with autoimmune liver disease (chronic active hepatitis, primary biliary cirrhosis, and cryptogenic cirrhosis).

Keratoconjunctivitis sicca produces symptoms of burning, itching, and blurring of vision. The patient may complain of a sensation of sand in the eye. Thick secretions accumulate in the conjunctival sac, and the conjunctiva may be reddened. The diagnosis is made by demonstrating decreased lacrimation (Schirmer's test), corneal or conjunctival erosions (rose bengal or fluorescein dye staining), and filamentary keratitis (slit-lamp examination).

Patients with xerostomia may have difficulty in swallowing solid foods, a decrease in taste acuity, and a rapid progression of dental caries. Cracks and fissures may appear at the corners of the mouth. The buccal mucosa has a parchment-like appearance, and the tongue is red and smooth. Bilateral parotid gland enlargement is observed in one-half the patients. Other salivary glands also may enlarge. The glands are usually smooth, firm, and only slightly tender but may be nodular and hard. Fluctuation in size is common. The diagnosis of xerostomia may be confirmed by measurement of salivary flow, by sialography, and by sequential salivary scintigraphy with pertechnetate.

Dryness of the nasal mucosa may cause epistaxis and decreased acuity of smell. Hoarseness may occur with laryngeal dryness. Patients also may have recurrent bronchitis and pneumonitis because of the decrease of protective mucous secretions. Vaginal dryness may cause dyspareunia. Generalized skin dryness may also occur.

Patients with SS may develop a lymphoproliferative disorder referred to as pseudolymphoma. Features of this complication include fever, weight loss, enlarged salivary glands, lymphadenopathy, splenomegaly, and lymphocytic infiltrates in the lung and kidney. Separation of this disorder from a malignant lymphoma is at times difficult. Some patients with pseudolymphoma will go on to develop a malignant lymphoreticular disease involving the salivary glands or extrasalivary sites. These malignant disorders include reticulum-cell sarcoma, lymphosarcoma, giant follicular sarcoma, and Waldenström's macroglobulinemia. Patients with the SS alone are at a greater risk to develop a pseudolymphoma or malignant lymphoma than patients with SS associated with connective tissue disorders.

Other clinical features of SS include vasculitis, Raynaud's phenomenon, hypergammaglobulinemic purpura, hyperviscosity syndrome, and peripheral neuropathy. Single or multiple cranial nerves may be affected; isolated trigeminal nerve neuropathy is most common. Cryoglobulinemia may be associated with glomerulonephritis. Acute pancreatitis may also occur. Lymphocytic infiltrates involving the renal tubules cause renal tubular acidosis. Patients can also develop pulmonary interstitial fibrosis.

A common laboratory feature is normocytic normochromic anemia due to chronic inflammation. Leukopenia and eosinophilia are found in some patients. Hypergammaglobulinemia with elevation of all three major immunoglobulin classes is common. Cryoglobulins may be detected. Rheumatoid factors are found in approximately 50 percent of patients with SS alone and in almost all patients with SS associated with rheumatoid arthritis. Antinuclear antibodies are found in the majority of patients with sicca syndrome alone. Two antinuclear antibodies, anti-SS-A and anti-SS-B in particular, are associated with SS. Anti-SS-A is found in approximately 70 percent of patients with SS alone, 30 percent of patients with SS with SLE, and in less than 10 percent of patients with SS and RA. Anti-SS-B is present in half the patients with SS alone and rarely in patients with SS associated with SLE or RA. Other autoantibodies which may be present in SS include antibodies to thyroglobulin, mitochondria, and salivary and lacrimal ducts.

In the differential diagnosis, parotid gland tumors should be considered when enlargement is unilateral and other features of the syndrome are absent. Features favoring Sjögren's syndrome are the absence of pain, fluctuation in gland size, and the chronicity of the swelling without extension into the adjacent tissues. The differentiation between a benign and malignant lymphoproliferative disease may be difficult and confusing. Enlargement of the lacrimal and salivary glands (Mikulicz's syndrome) may occur in lymphoma, lymphocytic leukemia, and sarcoidosis. The sicca syndrome is usually not present in malignant lymphoproliferative involvement of the salivary and lacrimal glands, but occurs in sarcoidosis. The diagnosis of sarcoidosis is established by the finding of noncaseating granulomas in the involved gland. Dry eyes may also result from senile atrophy of the lacrimal glands.

One of the major goals in the treatment of SS is the alleviation of symptoms caused by lack of secretions. Dry eyes can be temporarily relieved by the use of 0.5% methylcellulose drops or other types of artificial tears. Methylcellulose (1 or 2%) may be used as a mouthwash in patients with dry mouth. Gelatin and glycerine lozenges may be helpful. Vaginal dryness may require lubricants. Systemic steroids are not recommended for treatment of the enlarged glands. Though they may reduce the size of the glands, dryness is not helped. Steroids may be indicated in patients with extrasalivary lymphoid infiltrates and with clinical manifestations of vasculitis. Improvement of the sicca syndrome by treatment with cyclophosphamide has been observed; however, further controlled observations are necessary before immunosuppressive drugs can be recommended for this use. Irradiation of the enlarged parotids is contraindicated because reticulum-cell sarcoma may develop in patients who have received this form of therapy during the early phases of their Sjögren's syndrome.

REFERENCES

Bennett JC: The infectious etiology of rheumatoid arthritis: New considerations. Arthritis Rheum 21:531, 1978

Bujak JS et al: Juvenile rheumatoid arthritis presenting in the adult as fever of unknown origin. Medicine 52:431, 1973

Gottlieb NL: Gold compounds in the rheumatic diseases, in *Textbook of Rheumatology,* WN Kelley et al (eds). Philadelphia, Saunders, 1981, chap 52, pp 796–814

Jaffe IA: D-Penicillamine, in *Textbook of Rheumatology,* WN Kelley et al (eds). Philadelphia, Saunders, 1981, chap 53, pp 815–821

Moutsopoulos HM et al: Sjögren's syndrome (sicca syndrome): Current issues. Ann Intern Med 92:212, 1980

Pope RM et al: The molecular basis of self-association of IgG-rheumatoid factors. J Immunol 115:365, 1975

Schaller JG: The diversity of JRA: A 1976 look at the subgroups of chronic childhood arthritis. Arthritis Rheum 20:6, 1977

Shearn MA: Sjögren's syndrome. Med Clin N Am 61:2, 1977

Simon LS, Mills JA: Nonsteroidal antiinflammatory drugs, parts I and II. N Engl J Med 302:1179, 1237, 1980

Steinberg AD: Immunoregulatory agents, in *Textbook of Rheumatology,* WN Kelley et al (eds). Philadelphia, Saunders, 1981, chap 55, pp 841–861

Ward JR, Samuelson CO Jr: Nonsteroidal anti-inflammatory drugs, in *Update II: Harrison's Principles of Internal Medicine,* KJ Isselbacher et al (eds). New York, McGraw-Hill, 1982, pp 91–110

Williams RC Jr: Rheumatoid arthritis as a systemic disease, in *Major Problems in Internal Medicine,* vol 4, LH Smith Jr (ed). Philadelphia, Saunders, 1974

Winchester RJ: Characterization of IgG complexes in patients with rheumatoid arthritis. Ann NY Acad Sci 256:73, 1975

Zvaifler NJ: Etiology and pathogenesis of rheumatoid arthritis, in *Arthritis and Allied Conditions,* DJ McCarty (ed). Philadelphia, Lea & Febiger, 1979, pp 417–428

347
ANKYLOSING SPONDYLITIS

BRUCE C. GILLILAND
MART MANNIK

Ankylosing spondylitis, a disease that has been called by many names, including rheumatoid spondylitis and Marie-Strümpell disease, is a chronic and usually progressive inflammatory disease involving the articulations of the spine and adjacent soft tissues. The sacroiliac joints are always affected. Involvement of the hip and shoulder joints commonly occurs; peripheral joints are affected less frequently. The disease predominantly affects young men and begins most often in the third decade. A high association has been found between this disorder and the histocompatibility antigen HLA-B27. The clinical features of this disease are distinctly different from those of rheumatoid arthritis. The etiology is not known.

EPIDEMIOLOGY Ankylosing spondylitis is found throughout the world. In the white population, the prevalence in men is 0.5 to 4 per 1000 and in women 0.05 to 0.5 per 1000, depending on the criteria employed.

Hereditary factors play an important role in the development of ankylosing spondylitis. Histocompatibility typing has revealed the presence of HLA-B27 antigen in 88 to 96 percent of spondylitic patients, while in the normal white population 7 percent have this antigen. In blacks, HLA-B27 occurs less frequently, which may account for the lower prevalence of this disease among them.

HLA-B27 is inherited in a mendelian fashion, and HLA-B27 is found in 50 percent of first-degree relatives of those spondylitic patients who are positive for HLA-B27. Within the group of relatives, 20 percent have either symptomatic or asymptomatic spondylitis. Ankylosing spondylitis is seen occasionally in patients who are negative for HLA-B27, indicating that other genetic or environmental factors are necessary for the development of the disease.

Twenty percent of apparently healthy people of both sexes who are positive for HLA-B27 have some clinical features of ankylosing spondylitis or sacroiliitis. Since spondylitis is diagnosed 10 times more frequently in men than women, these studies on apparently healthy people suggest that women have a milder disease. On the basis of these studies the prevalence of ankylosing spondylitis is estimated at 1 percent.

Several diseases that possess clinical features in common with ankylosing spondylitis also occur more frequently in patients with the HLA-B27 antigen. These disorders include Reiter's syndrome, psoriatic spondyloarthritis, *Yersinia* arthritis, spondyloarthritis of inflammatory bowel disease, and acute anterior uveitis. The role of HLA-B27 antigen in the pathogenesis of these disorders is not known. The currently favored hypothesis is that the HLA-B27 antigen, because of a close association with the immune response genes, is only a marker distinguishing a group of individuals whose immune response to an as yet undefined infectious agent leads to one of the HLA-B27 associated forms of the arthritides.

PATHOLOGY The earliest histopathologic changes usually occur in the sacroiliac joints but may start anywhere in the spine. The disease usually progresses up the spine, and occasionally segments will be skipped.

Synovitis of the involved diarthrodial joints of the spine (apophyseal and costovertebral joints) and of the sacroiliac, hip, shoulder, and peripheral joints resembles that of rheumatoid arthritis. Synovial hyperplasia and focal accumulation of lymphoid and plasma cells are seen histologically. Bony erosions and cartilage destruction ensue, followed later by fibrosis and bony ankylosis. In cartilaginous joints (intervertebral disks, manubriosternal, and symphysis pubis), granulation tissue invades the fibrocartilage, and adjacent bone is replaced later by fibrosis and ossification.

Occasionally, fibrous tissue invades the vertebral body to produce a radiolucent cyst which may be confused with an infectious process. Erosions at the anterior corners of the vertebral bodies destroy their normal anterior concavity and give the vertebrae a square appearance on lateral radiographs. Ossification of the outer layers of the annulus fibrosus at its lateral margins produces the syndesmophytes and "bamboo spine" observed radiographically. Ossification also involves the anterior portion of the annulus fibrosus and occasionally the inner aspect of the anterior longitudinal ligament. The radiographic appearance of the ossification at the anterior disk margins has led to the misconception that only the anterior longitudinal ligament is involved. In ankylosing spondylitis, a common site of inflammation is at insertion of ligaments, tendons, and capsules into bone. Bony erosions and new bone formation follow at these sites, most notably at the spinous processes, greater trochanters, pelvic bones, and heels.

Focal medial necrosis at the root of the aorta causes dilatation of the aortic ring. The aortic cusps may be shortened and thickened but are not fused. These processes lead to aortic valve incompetence. Fibrous tissue may enter the membranous septum and invade the atrioventricular bundle, resulting in conduction defects.

MANIFESTATIONS The disease occurs most commonly between the ages of 15 and 40 years and rarely after age 50. The initial symptoms are low back pain and stiffness, often worse in the early morning. Pain in the hips, buttocks, and shoulders is often present. Nocturnal back pain may force the patient to walk around in an attempt to gain relief. In approximately 10 percent of patients, early symptoms resemble sciatica, with pain in the buttocks and in back of the thighs. The pain may alternate from side to side and seldom radiates below the knee. Abnormal findings on neurological examination are unusual. Patients may have the simultaneous onset of peripheral arthritis and back pain; however, peripheral arthritis uncommonly precedes back symptoms in adults. Approximately one-fourth of patients will have peripheral arthritis during the course of their disease, but residual damage of these joints occurs infrequently. Hip disease may be a major cause of disability. Severe involvement early in the disease may result in ankylosis of the hip. Hip involvement, on the other hand, may lead to arthritis indistinguishable from osteoarthritis of the hip. Occasionally, patients may experience anterior chest pain from thoracic skeletal involvement which may mimic angina pectoris. Pleuritic chest pain may occur on deep breathing due to inflammation at the insertion of the costosternal and costovertebral muscles. Other causes of chest pain are involvement of the manubriosternal and sternoclavicular joints. Radicular pain from the lumbar part of the spine may radiate to the abdomen, suggesting visceral disease. Atlantoaxial subluxation and spinal cord compression occur less commonly than in rheumatoid arthritis. Patients with fused cervical spines are especially susceptible to fractures of the neck on falling.

Aortic valve incompetence is present in 3 percent of patients and may result in severe aortic regurgitation, requiring surgical repair. Conduction abnormalities include varying degrees of heart block and left bundle branch block. The conduction defects are more apt to appear in patients with aortic valve incompetence, but they may exist alone. Some patients require implantation of a pacemaker.

Acute anterior uveitis is observed in 20 to 30 percent of patients and may be recurrent. Occasionally, this may be the presenting symptom, calling attention to the diagnosis of ankylosing spondylitis. Amyloidosis is found in a small number of patients at autopsy and is a cause of uremia in this disease. Bilateral upper lobe fibrosis is a recognized late manifestation of ankylosing spondylitis and may mimic tuberculosis. Patients develop chronic productive cough and dyspnea. The disease may progress to dense fibrosis, and death can result from massive hemoptysis.

The constitutional symptoms are usually mild at the onset and throughout the disease, but in a few patients with severe disease, fatigue, anemia, fever, and weight loss may be present.

Symptoms may be persistent or intermittent for months or years. In some patients ankylosis of the spine may progress with little or no pain. The degree of spinal involvement varies among patients, ranging from only sacroiliac joint involvement to complete ankylosis of the spine. Once ankylosis of joints occurs, pain usually disappears.

The *cauda equina syndrome* is a rare complication appearing usually in patients with long-standing and apparently inactive disease. The cause of this syndrome is unclear but may be the result of previous arachnoiditis or ischemia. Symptoms result from the involvement of the lumbosacral nerve roots and include buttock or leg pain, lower extremity weakness, and loss of bladder and rectal sphincter control. Loss of sensation occurs in the saddle area, posterior thighs, and lateral aspects of the feet. The deep tendon reflexes are diminished. Myelography shows posterior diverticula along the lumbar nerve root sheets or throughout the entire dural sac, when the study is done with the patient in the supine position. Neurological manifestations are usually slowly progressive. Adequate treatment is not available.

Physical findings early in the disease may be minimal. Tenderness over the sacroiliac joints can be elicited by direct palpation or percussion, or by maneuvers that stress the joint. The lumbar part of the spine will show loss of the normal lordosis and paraspinal muscle spasm. The anterior flexion of the lumbar spine is judged best by distraction of skin marks made on the back of the patient while standing erect, the upper mark being 10 cm above and the lower mark 5 cm below the lumbosacral junction. Upon full forward flexion these marks should distract more than 5.0 cm in patients below the age of 50 years. Serial measurements in a given patient will reflect the progression of spine involvement. No distraction of such skin marks is seen in a patient with an ankylosed spine. Costovertebral involvement is best measured by chest expansion. The more advanced changes of spondylitis are easily recognized by the rigid spine, often fused in varying degrees of flexion, which may be quite pronounced in the thoracic region of the spine.

LABORATORY FINDINGS The erythrocyte sedimentation rate (ESR) is elevated in the majority of cases, but its level reflects fluctuations of disease activity poorly, and the ESR is normal in 20 percent of patients with mild disease. A mild hypoproliferative anemia may be present during severe active disease. Sheep cell agglutination and latex fixation tests for rheumatoid factor are negative even when peripheral joint disease is present. Mild to moderate elevations of the spinal fluid protein level may be present in active spondylitis. Synovial fluid from peripheral joints usually shows a moderate neutrophilic leukocytosis.

At the onset of symptoms the radiographs of the sacroiliac joints and the spine are often normal and may remain so for variable periods of time, depending on the rate of progression of the disease. Radiographs of the sacroiliac joints in early disease show blurring of the margins, irregular subchondral erosions, and patchy sclerosis. These changes are initially more pronounced in the lower third of the joint. Both sacroiliac joints are characteristically involved, but findings may first appear on one side. With progression, sclerosis becomes more marked, the joint space is lost, and later osteoporosis appears. Similar changes are observed in other articulations of the axial skeleton, including the symphysis pubis and apophyseal joints. At points of tendon insertions (e.g., pelvis, os calcis) the adjacent bone shows erosions, sclerosis, and fluffy new bone formation. Lateral films of the os calcis may show bony spurs at the site of attachment for the Achilles tendon and for the plantar fascia.

Radiographs of the spine in early phases of the disease may show straightening of the lumbar part of the spine and squaring of the lumbar and lower thoracic vertebrae. With progression, syndesmophytes appear along the lateral and anterior surfaces of the intervertebral disks and bridge adjacent vertebrae. They are characteristically present on both lateral sides of the intervertebral disk at any given level and usually arise from the margin of the vertebral body. The widespread distribution of syndesmophytes in advanced disease produces the picture of the "bamboo spine." Syndesmophytes must be differentiated from the osteophytes observed in degenerative joint disease. The syndesmophyte extends vertically from the adjacent vertebral margins along the outer aspect of the intervertebral disk, while the osteophyte projects horizontally before curving to form an intervertebral bridge. The radiographic changes in involved peripheral joints are similar to those of rheumatoid arthritis.

DIAGNOSIS A patient with ankylosing spondylitis in the advanced stage is easily recognized by the characteristic bent-over posture, rigid spine, exaggerated dorsal kyphosis, and waddling gait. When peripheral arthritis is present in the early stages of ankylosing spondylitis, confusion with rheumatoid arthritis may occur. Ankylosing spondylitis is predominantly a disease of young men, but the disease also exists in women in a milder form. HLA-B27 antigen is usually present, rheumatoid factor tests are negative, and rheumatoid nodules are not found. Radiographs of the spine show bilateral sacroiliitis and syndesmophytes, which are features not seen in adult rheumatoid arthritis. Ankylosing spondylitis in children often presents as a peripheral arthritis and, therefore, may be initially diagnosed as juvenile rheumatoid arthritis. Hip, sacroiliac, and spine involvement along with attacks of acute anterior uveitis eventually point to the diagnosis of spondylitis. Older boys are most often affected. HLA-B27 is usually present in these children in contrast to juvenile rheumatoid arthritis in which the prevalence of this antigen does not differ from normal persons.

Differentiation from other diseases with spondylitis early in the course may be difficult. Since the spondylitis is indistinguishable from that associated with ulcerative colitis and regional enteritis and may antedate the bowel disease by months or years, symptoms and signs of intestinal disease should always be sought, especially in female patients. The spondylitis with Reiter's syndrome and psoriatic arthritis have common radiographic features, but differ from ankylosing spondylitis in having a greater tendency for syndesmophytes to appear at only one lateral margin of the intervertebral disk at any given level and to arise beyond the margin of the vertebral body. The distribution of syndesmophytes is more random, and the degree of spinal involvement is usually less than in ankylosing spondylitis. Other clinical features of Reiter's syndrome and psoriatic arthritis allow for easy separation of these diseases from ankylosing spondylitis. Diffuse idiopathic skeletal hyperostosis (DISH, or Forestier's disease with extra spinal involvement) is distinguished from ankylosing spondylitis by the lack of apophyseal and sacroiliac joint involvement and by its more frequent occurrence in men over 50. Laminated new bone formation involves the anterior and lateral spinal ligaments most prominently in the middle to lower thoracic regions, particularly on the right side, and resembles the dripping of candle wax. The radiological findings of sacroiliitis are distinguished from osteitis condensans ilii by the finding of sclerosis on only the ilial side of the joint and the preservation of the joint space in the latter. Sciatica of ankylosing spondylitis can be differentiated from that of disk disease, since it may alternate from side to side, the pain seldom radiates below the knee, and neurological signs are usually absent. Malignancies should be considered in both youngsters and older patients with symptoms of back pain.

TREATMENT The goal of therapy is to prevent or minimize the deformities of the spine inherent in this disease. With minimal deformity, patients may be able to continue working and living in a reasonably normal fashion if hip disease is not severe. Patients should be instructed to maintain an erect posture whether walking, standing, or sitting. They should be encouraged to sleep in a prone position or, if this is not possible, in a supine position on a flat firm mattress using a small pillow or none at all. Breathing exercises should be encouraged.

Drugs will not halt the progression of the disease, but they provide adequate relief to permit maintenance of posture. Phenylbutazone or indomethacin is effective in a maintenance dose of 200 to 300 mg per day for phenylbutazone, and 75 to 150 mg per day for indomethacin. Therapy should be discontinued when symptoms abate. Salicylates or one of the newer nonsteroidal anti-inflammatory drugs (e.g., naproxen) may be effective. Gold and chloroquine have not been beneficial. Any benefit from glucocorticosteroids is outweighed by their side effects. Iritis can usually be treated with intraocular steroids. No effective therapy is available for the lung fibrosis occurring in patients with ankylosing spondylitis.

Surgical correction of extreme flexion deformities of the spine by wedge resection and refusion in an improved position may be helpful in selected patients. The potential danger of spinal cord damage and the long convalescent period should be carefully considered before advising surgery. Patients with crippling hip disease may benefit from total hip replacement.

REFERENCES

CALIN A, FRIES JF: Striking prevalence of ankylosing spondylitis in "healthy" W27 positive males and females. N Engl J Med 293:835, 1975

——— et al: Clinical history as a screening test for ankylosing spondylitis. JAMA 237:2613, 1977

Cohen LM et al: Increased risk for spondylitis stigmata in apparently healthy HLA-W27 men. Ann Intern Med 84:1, 1976

Engleman EG, Engleman EP: Ankylosing spondylitis. Recent advances in diagnosis and treatment. Med Clin N Am 61:347, 1977

Macrae IF, Wright V: Measurements of back movement. Ann Rheum Dis 28:584, 1969

Moll JMH et al: Associations between ankylosing spondylitis, psoriatic arthritis, Reiter's disease, the intestinal arthropathies and Behçet's syndrome. Medicine 53:343, 1974

Resnick D et al: Diffuse idiopathic skeletal hyperostosis (DISH): Forestier's disease with extraspinal manifestations. Radiology 115:513, 1975

———, Niwayama G: Ankylosing spondylitis, in *Diagnosis of Bone and Joint Disorders,* D Resnick, G Niwayama (eds). Philadelphia, Saunders, 1981, pp 1040–1102

348

REITER'S SYNDROME, PSORIATIC ARTHRITIS, ARTHRITIS ASSOCIATED WITH GASTROINTESTINAL DISEASES, AND BEHÇET'S SYNDROME

BRUCE C. GILLILAND
MART MANNIK

REITER'S SYNDROME Reiter's syndrome is characterized by arthritis in association with one or more of the following: urethritis and/or cervicitis, bacillary dysentery, eye inflammation, and mucocutaneous lesions. The HLA-B27 antigen is present in the majority of patients.

Epidemiology, pathogenesis, and pathology Reiter's syndrome occurs most frequently in young men but can develop at any age. It is also recognized in women and represents 15 percent of patients in one reported study. In the United States and Britain, many cases are closely related to sexual exposure. Reiter's syndrome also follows bacillary dysentery. The cause and pathogenesis of Reiter's syndrome are unknown. Several different infectious agents have been associated with Reiter's syndrome, but their role remains uncertain. *Chlamydia* or *Mycoplasma* agents have been recovered from the urethra in some patients with nonspecific urethritis associated with Reiter's syndrome. Arthritis, however, develops in patients whose urethral cultures are negative for these infectious agents, and most patients with nonspecific urethritis do not develop Reiter's syndrome. Arthritis, including urethritis and other features of Reiter's syndrome, may follow *Salmonella, Shigella,* or *Yersinia* infections. Arthritis, however, may be the only feature following these infections.

Histocompatibility typing has shown the presence of HLA-B27 antigen in approximately 80 percent of Caucasian patients with Reiter's syndrome, but this association is lower in blacks. The risk of the HLA-B27 individual with nonspecific urethritis or bacillary dysentery for developing Reiter's syndrome is approximately 20 percent.

Histologically, the cutaneous and mucosal lesions are very similar, even though their gross appearances are different. In the cutaneous lesions the epidermis shows hyperkeratosis, parakeratosis, and acanthosis. Spongiform pustules or microabscesses are present in the epidermis and are formed by focal infiltration of neutrophils, with degeneration of epithelial cells. The dermis shows edema, infiltration of lymphocytes, plasma cells, and neutrophils. The skin lesions are termed *keratodermia blenorrhagica* and are indistinguishable microscopically from those of pustular psoriasis. In the mucosal lesions, the inflammatory changes are similar, but keratinized cells do not accumulate. The synovium in the superficial vascular region shows edema, erythrocyte extravasation, and infiltration of neutrophils and lymphocytes. In synovitis of several months' duration, the synovium resembles that of rheumatoid arthritis, with villous hypertrophy, pannus formation over the articular cartilage, and infiltration of lymphocytes and plasma cells.

Clinical manifestations Reiter's syndrome often begins with urethritis after sexual exposure, followed in a few days to 4 weeks by arthritis which may be accompanied by conjunctivitis and/or mucocutaneous lesions. Urethritis, arthritis, and other features of Reiter's syndrome may also follow bacillary dysentery. Arthritis, however, is often the only manifestation following bacillary dysentery. The onset of the arthritis is usually acute, affecting two or more joints. The joints are usually warm, erythematous, and painful. There is a predilection for joints of the lower extremities; ankles, knees, and metatarsophalangeal and proximal interphalangeal joints of the toes are commonly affected. Arthritis also occurs in the wrist, interphalangeal joints of the hand, costosternal joints, sacroiliac joints, and low part of the back, but is relatively uncommon in the hips and shoulders. Tenderness under the heel may be prominent because of periostitis at the insertion of the plantar fascia. Achilles tendonitis may also be present. The distribution of the arthritis tends to be asymmetrical and is extremely variable; multiple or single joints may be affected. The arthritis usually reaches a maximum within 2 weeks and begins to subside after 2 to 6 weeks. The duration of arthritis is usually from 2 to 4 months, with a spontaneous remission often occurring within the first year. The majority of patients, however, continue to have recurrent attacks of arthritis for several years; these flare-ups may be accompanied by one or more of the other clinical features of the syndrome. Recurrent attacks, similar to the first, may be precipitated by sexual exposure followed by urethritis. Patients with persistent or recurrent arthritis may develop flexion contractures and permanent joint damage.

Urethritis is characterized by a mucopurulent discharge and dysuria, but may be asymptomatic and may be overlooked unless the urethra is milked and the obtained material is cultured. The urethral meatus may be edematous and reddened, and urethral strictures may develop. Prostatitis and seminal vesiculitis occasionally occur, but epididymitis and orchitis are rare. Cystitis, which may be hemorrhagic, can occur and lead to urinary frequency, suprapubic pain, hematuria, and rarely to obstruction of the ureters. In women, urethritis and cervicitis may be asymptomatic. Since gonococcal urethritis may accompany the nonspecific urethritis of Reiter's syndrome, urethral and/or cervical smear and culture should be performed. When gonococcal urethritis is present, the purulent discharge will usually clear when penicillin is given, but will be replaced by the less purulent mucoid discharge of nonspecific urethritis.

Conjunctivitis is usually bilateral, mild, and evanescent, lasting only a few days. It may be present only at the lateral aspect of the tarsal conjunctiva. Conjunctivitis at times may be quite severe and produces burning, itching, and a profuse mucopurulent discharge, which may last several weeks. A nongranulomatous anterior uveitis which appears in some patients may lead to photophobia, glaucoma, cataracts, and even blindness. Subsequent attacks of anterior uveitis may appear in the absence of other clinical features of Reiter's syndrome. Painful superficial keratitis occurs occasionally.

Mucocutaneous lesions occur in over half the patients and appear most commonly on the glans penis, on the palms and soles, and in the mouth. They are typically painless and transient, and may go unnoticed unless the patient is examined carefully. On the glans penis, the lesion begins as a small vesicle, which evolves to a superficial reddened erosion with well-demarcated borders. In the circumcised male, the lesions may be covered with scales. Only a few lesions may be present on the glans penis, usually around the meatus, or lesions may completely circumscribe the glans (circinate balanitis). Lesions are occasionally found on the shaft and prepuce of the penis and on the scrotum. They also have been observed by endoscopy on the mucosa of the urethra and bladder. In the mouth, the lesions begin as small vesicles, papules, or plaques and later become superficial erosions with a surrounding area of erythema. The erosions may be covered by a thin grayish membrane. The mouth lesions are found on the soft palate, buccal mucosa, and the dorsum of the tongue. Keratodermia blenorrhagica describes the cutaneous lesions, which are found most commonly on the soles but are also occasionally observed on the palms, the extremities, and the trunk. These lesions begin as brownish-red macules, which develop into crusted scaling papules. Such lesions may coalesce to cover the sole with a thick layer of crusted scales, which peel off in the ensuing weeks. The nails may become thickened, opaque, and brittle; keratotic debris accumulates under the nail. None of the mucocutaneous lesions leaves residual scarring.

Cardiac conduction abnormalities and aortic regurgitation have been reported. The pathogenesis of the aortic valve incompetence is similar to that of ankylosing spondylitis, resulting from medial necrosis of the aortic root and dilatation of the aortic ring. Neurological abnormalities, including optic neuritis, meningoencephalitis, transient hemiplegia, psychotic reactions, and peripheral neuropathy, are exceedingly rare.

Laboratory findings A mild leukocytosis and an elevated erythrocyte sedimentation rate are often present. Tests for rheumatoid factor are negative. HLA-B27 antigen is found in the majority of patients. Synovial fluid examination shows an increase in white blood cells, predominantly neutrophils, ranging usually from 5000 to 20,000 cells per cubic millimeter. Large mononuclear cells, some containing ingested polymorphonuclear cells, are observed frequently but are not specific for Reiter's syndrome. The viscosity of the fluid may be reduced, and the mucin clot is fair to poor.

Radiographs of the involved joint may show only soft-tissue swelling. With recurrent disease, bony erosions and joint narrowing may appear. A suggestive, but not diagnostic, finding is periosteal new bone formation along the shaft adjacent to the involved joint and on the posterior and inferior aspects of the os calcis. Calcaneal spurs appear later. One or both sacroiliac joints may show irregularity, sclerosis, and fusion. With involvement of the spine, syndesmophytes may be observed and tend to be randomly distributed in the thoracic and lumbar parts of the spine. These syndesmophytes often arise at the upper or lower third of the vertebral body.

Diagnosis The most important immediate differential diagnosis is gonococcal arthritis, because gonococcal urethritis may be present simultaneously. Gonococcal arthritis is confirmed by a positive synovial fluid culture but is not excluded by a negative one. The presence of conjunctivitis or characteristic mucocutaneous lesions is helpful, since these are not associated with gonococcal arthritis. When there is doubt, the arthritis associated with gonococcal urethritis should be treated as gonococcal arthritis, with adequate doses of penicillin (see Chap. 150). If Reiter's syndrome is present, the arthritis will persist, and other features of the syndrome may appear subsequently.

There is usually no problem differentiating Reiter's syndrome from rheumatoid arthritis. The sudden onset preceded by urethritis, the absence of nodules, negative rheumatoid factor, and the asymmetrical joint involvement contrast sharply with the insidious, symmetrical joint disease of rheumatoid arthritis.

Psoriatic arthritis and ankylosing spondylitis share several features of Reiter's syndrome. The pustular form of psoriasis is similar in appearance to keratodermia blenorrhagica but tends not to involve mucous membranes. Psoriatic arthritis presenting as monarticular arthritis or asymmetrical oligoarthritis may be differentiated from Reiter's syndrome by the chronic nature of the skin lesions, the absence of urethritis and conjunctivitis, and the rarity of mucous membrane lesions. At times, however, differentiation of these two diseases may not be possible. Compared with ankylosing spondylitis, the spondylitis associated with Reiter's syndrome is usually less severe and progressive. Dilatation of the aortic ring, conduction abnormalities, calcaneal periostitis and spurs, and iritis occur in both Reiter's syndrome and ankylosing spondylitis. The sudden onset of the peripheral arthritis associated with urethritis and conjunctivitis and typical mucocutaneous lesions help to distinguish Reiter's syndrome. Hip involvement is rare in Reiter's syndrome and common in ankylosing spondylitis.

Treatment The treatment of the nonspecific urethritis with 2 g tetracycline per day for 10 to 14 days may affect the urethritis but probably does not influence the development of arthritis. No treatment is necessary for conjunctivitis and other mucocutaneous lesions; however, iritis may require intraocular glucocorticosteroid therapy. The arthritis is usually responsive to phenylbutazone or indomethacin. With phenylbutazone, a loading dose of 600 to 800 mg is given initially to obtain a rapid therapeutic blood level, followed by a daily maintenance dose of 200 to 300 mg. The dose of indomethacin is 100 to 150 mg per day. Salicylates or one of the newer nonsteroidal anti-inflammatory drugs may be effective in some patients. Local injection of glucocorticosteroids for persistent monarticular disease, plantar fasciitis, or Achilles tendonitis may be helpful. Systemic glucocorticosteroids are rarely indicated. In patients with progressive joint disease unresponsive to conventional therapy, immunosuppressive drugs may be useful. Physical therapy may be required to prevent flexion contractures.

PSORIATIC ARTHRITIS The prevalence of arthritis in patients with psoriasis is higher than that found in the general population, even when degenerative joint disease and rheumatoid arthritis are excluded. Arthritis related to psoriasis occurs in approximately 5 percent of patients with skin disease.

The *etiology* and *pathogenesis* of psoriatic arthritis are not known; however, studies showing aggregation of psoriatic arthritis in first-degree relatives of psoriatic patients suggest that hereditary factors may play a role. Approximately 90 percent of psoriatic patients with sacroiliitis and spondylitis have the HLA-B27 antigen. In patients with only sacroiliitis or spondylitis with normal sacroiliac joints, approximately 40 percent are positive for HLA-B27, while in those with only peripheral arthritis less than 20 percent have this antigen.

The age of onset is similar to that of rheumatoid arthritis, and the sex distribution slightly favors women. Psoriasis usually precedes the onset of arthritis by months or years. In approximately 15 percent of patients, the arthritis precedes the skin lesions. Simultaneous onset of arthritis and skin lesions is uncommon, but arthritis and nail abnormalities often begin together. In general, the prognosis of psoriatic arthritis is more favorable than that of rheumatoid arthritis, except in patients with the severe destructive form of psoriatic arthritis (arthritis mutilans). The course of psoriatic arthritis in most patients is mild, intermittent, and affects only a few joints. Spontaneous remission may occur.

On the basis of the pattern of joint involvement five clinical groups may be distinguished. The first group which includes approximately 70 percent of patients with psoriatic arthritis has monarticular or asymmetrical oligoarticular arthritis involving scattered small joints of the hands and feet. "Sausage" digits are often present and result from inflammation of the interphalangeal joints and of the flexor tendon sheath. A second group composed of about 15 percent of patients has a seronegative symmetrical polyarthritis similar to rheumatoid arthritis. In addition to this group, there are patients with psoriasis, symmetrical polyarthritis, and a positive test for rheumatoid factor. These patients are considered to have coexistent rheumatoid arthritis and psoriasis. A third group has predominantly distal interphalangeal joint involvement. The adjacent nail often has changes of psoriasis. Another very small group has severe destructive polyarthritis with widespread ankylosis which is termed *arthritis mutilans.* Dissolution of bone may occur. Onset of arthritis in this group often occurs before age 20. The last group has sacroiliitis and spondylitis with or without peripheral joint involvement. Men are affected more commonly. Patients with sacroiliitis and peripheral arthritis may have no symptoms or signs of back disease. The clinical features of spine involvement are similar to idiopathic ankylosing spondylitis.

The peripheral joints in psoriatic arthritis are warm, swollen, and tender, and show synovial proliferation. Flexion contractures and ankylosis of joints may occur, with long periods of persistent joint inflammation. No definite correlation exists between the degree of skin involvement and joint disease, but in some patients the activity of both tends to be parallel. A closer temporal relationship has been found between psoriatic nail lesions and arthritis than between the skin lesions and arthritis. Onycholysis is the most characteristic nail lesion. The coexistence of onycholysis, nail pits, and nail ridges is indicative of psoriasis. In addition, the presence of more than 20 nail pits in a patient suggests psoriasis.

Laboratory abnormalities include hypoproliferative anemia and an elevated erythrocyte sedimentation rate, which are nonspecific findings. Tests for rheumatoid factor are negative. Hyperuricemia is observed in 10 to 20 percent of patients, similar to uncomplicated psoriasis and reflects the severity of skin involvement. Synovial fluid and biopsy findings are those of nonspecific inflammation.

Several *radiographic* features are characteristic of psoriatic arthritis. These include severe destruction of isolated joints, osteolysis, bony ankylosis, whittling of the tufts of the terminal phalanges, and the "pencil-in-cup" deformity, which is most commonly observed in the joints of the fingers and toes. Whittling of the distal end of the middle phalanx produces the "pencil" which projects into a widened, cuplike erosion in the joint surface of the terminal phalanx. Bony absorption of phalanges produces the opera-glass deformity of the hands (telescoped fingers). The radiographic findings in spondylitis associated with psoriatic arthritis are similar to those found in spondylitis with Reiter's syndrome.

The *diagnosis* of psoriatic arthritis is suggested by the presence of an inflammatory arthritis in a patient with typical skin or nail lesions of psoriasis. Skin lesions may be quite small and hidden in the scalp, intergluteal fold, or umbilicus. The asymmetry of joint involvement, negative test for rheumatoid factor, and the absence of rheumatoid nodules help to distinguish psoriatic arthritis from rheumatoid arthritis. The differentiation of psoriatic arthritis from Reiter's syndrome and ankylosing spondylitis has been discussed under "Reiter's Syndrome" above. Psoriatic arthritis presenting as an acute arthritis, especially in a toe or finger, may be mistaken for gouty arthritis. In addition, hyperuricemia, which may occur in association with psoriasis, may also be present. The appearance of the joint also may suggest septic arthritis. These diagnostic considerations are easily excluded by examining synovial fluid for sodium urate crystals and for microorganisms with appropriate cultures. Development of acute Heberden's nodes may be confused with psoriatic arthritis, but other features such as Bouchard's nodes at the proximal interphalangeal joints, involvement of the first carpometacarpal joint, and a normal ESR point to the diagnosis of primary osteoarthritis. Fungal disease of the toenails may be mistaken for psoriatic nails; the distinction may require examination of nail scrapings for mycelia.

The *treatment* of the arthritis is similar to that outlined for rheumatoid arthritis. The value of gold has not been established. The use of immunosuppressive agents may be beneficial; methotrexate has been used most extensively. However, in view of their toxicity, these drugs should be restricted to patients with severe psoriasis and destructive polyarthritis. Adequate control of skin disease may lead to improvement of the joint disease in an occasional patient.

ARTHRITIS ASSOCIATED WITH GASTROINTESTINAL DISEASES **Inflammatory bowel disease** The articular manifestations of ulcerative colitis and regional enteritis (Crohn's disease, granulomatous colitis) are similar and will be discussed together. Two patterns of joint involvement may be distinguished: arthritis of peripheral joints and spondylitis. The frequency of peripheral arthritis in regional enteritis is approximately 20 percent and in ulcerative colitis, 10 percent. The frequency of spondylitis in both bowel disorders is 4 percent.

The peripheral arthritis of inflammatory bowel disease (IBD) most commonly begins between the ages of 25 and 45 years and affects both sexes equally. Arthritis usually follows the onset of colitis by 6 months to several years, but uncommonly the onset of both may coincide or the arthritis may precede colitis. Arthritis is more frequent in ulcerative colitis patients who have pseudopolyps or perianal disease and also is more common with extensive colitis than disease limited to the rectum. In regional enteritis, arthritis is more frequent in patients with colon disease and less common with disease limited to the small bowel. Patients with aphthous stomatitis, erythema nodosum, or uveitis are likely also to have arthritis. These extraintestinal manifestations often flare up with exacerbation of colitis.

The typical attack of arthritis presents acutely, reaching a peak within 24 h, and often affects a single joint in the lower extremity. Involvement of other joints, without definite symmetry, may follow over the next few days. Usually fewer than four joints are involved during an episode. The involved joint is usually red, swollen, and painful. The knee and ankle are most frequently affected, followed by the proximal interphalangeal, elbow, shoulder, and wrist joints. The arthritis usually subsides within several weeks, but occasionally lasts for months. Complete resolution without residual damage is the general rule. Some patients may only experience migratory arthralgias as evidence of an attack.

Spondylitis with IBD is indistinguishable from ankylosing spondylitis. However, the usual male preponderance observed in ankylosing spondylitis is not seen in patients with IBD and spondylitis. The onset of spondylitis antedates IBD in approximately one-third of patients. The HLA-B27 antigen is found in 70 percent of these patients. In some patients, spondylitis and bowel disease may have a nearly simultaneous onset, while in others spondylitis follows the onset of colitis. The frequency of

HLA-B27 is lower in these patients compared to those with spondylitis preceding bowel disease. Spondylitis usually progresses regardless of remission of the bowel disease or colectomy. The disease may progress to complete ankylosis of the spine.

Radiographic evidence of sacroiliitis without symptoms is found in patients with IBD, the prevalence ranging from 4 to 15 percent. The majority of these patients will probably not become symptomatic or progress to ankylosing spondylitis. In this group of patients the prevalence of HLA-B27 is not increased.

The peripheral white blood cell count, anemia, and erythrocyte sedimentation rate usually reflect the intestinal disease. Tests for rheumatoid factor are negative. Synovial fluid shows a moderate leukocytosis, in the range of 10,000 cells per cubic millimeter, consisting predominantly of polymorphonuclear leukocytes.

Radiographs of involved peripheral joints usually are normal except for soft-tissue swelling. An occasional patient with recurrent or persistent disease will show small bony erosions and joint space narrowing. Films of the spine show changes indistinguishable from those of ankylosing spondylitis.

Treatment should be directed primarily at the underlying IBD. Joint symptoms can usually be managed with salicylates, phenylbutazone, or other nonsteroidal anti-inflammatory drugs. Glucocorticosteroids used for control of colitis and extraintestinal manifestations, such as erythema nodosum, may lead to suppression of arthritis. Colectomy or systemic glucocorticosteroids are not indicated for treatment of the arthritis alone. Physical therapy is directed toward maintenance of posture in spondylitis and prevention of contractures in the peripheral form of arthritis.

Intestinal bypass arthritis Approximately one-third of patients with jejunocolic and a somewhat smaller percentage of patients with jejunoileal bypass develop arthritic manifestations which occur from several weeks to years following the surgery. These consist of recurrent episodes of migratory polyarthralgia, polyarthritis, and, sometimes, tenosynovitis. Episodes last from a few days to a few weeks. Some patients may experience persistent arthritis for months. The knees, ankles, wrists, and shoulders are most commonly affected. Neck and back symptoms may also occur. Joint damage usually does not occur. However, in some patients with persistent arthritis, erosions of the joint margins have been described. The arthritis may be accompanied by vasculitic skin lesions which can be urticarial, pustular, or nodular. Raynaud's phenomenon also occurs in some of these patients.

Examination of synovial fluid has shown a mild leukocytosis with polymorphonuclear white cells predominating. Circulating immune complexes and cryoglobulins are found in the serum of many bypass patients with arthritis. Immunoglobulins, complement, and antibodies to *Escherichia coli* and other bacteria have been identified in cryoglobulins from these patients.

The pathogenesis of bypass arthritis and vasculitis is postulated to be mediated by immune complexes. Bacterial growth in the blind loop of the intestine leads to absorption of bacterial antigens, and subsequent development of antibodies to these antigens results in formation of immune complexes.

The definitive treatment of bypass arthritis is reconnecting the bowel. When this is not possible, treatment with tetracycline or other appropriate antibiotics to reduce the bacterial flow in the blind loop has produced clinical improvement. Aspirin, phenylbutazone, and other nonsteroidal anti-inflammatory drugs may help to control symptoms. Arthritis and vasculitis are also suppressed with systemic glucocorticosteroids in most patients.

Whipple's disease Whipple's disease (intestinal lipodystrophy) is a rare disorder affecting predominantly middle-aged males and is characterized by arthritis, serositis, diarrhea, malabsorption, weight loss, and lymphadenopathy. The diagnosis is confirmed by the identification of periodic acid Schiff (PAS) staining of bacilliform structures intercellularly or as inclusions in foamy macrophages. Electron microscopy has demonstrated rod-shaped organisms in the lamina propria of the small intestine. The PAS-staining material is thought to consist of partially degraded bacteria. PAS-staining granules can also be seen in abdominal and peripheral lymph nodes and in other tissues.

Arthritis occurs in approximately two-thirds of the patients and usually precedes the appearance of intestinal symptoms by months or years, making the diagnosis of the arthritis difficult. With the onset of intestinal symptoms, the arthritis may subside. The joint disease involves predominantly peripheral joints, affecting knees and ankles most commonly, followed by fingers, hips, shoulders, elbows, and wrists. It is typically acute, migratory, and transient, lasts only a few days, and causes no permanent joint damage. Long, irregular periods of remission are common. Some patients with peripheral joint involvement have radiographic changes in the sacroiliac joints similar to those of ankylosing spondylitis. Synovial fluid usually shows only a mild monocytosis without characteristic foamy macrophages. PAS-positive macrophages have been seen in synovial biopsy tissue. This disease, including the joint manifestations, responds well to therapy with penicillin, 1.2 million units, and streptomycin, 1 g daily for 2 weeks, followed by tetracycline, 1 g daily for 1 year. Relapse while on tetracycline requires administration again of penicillin and streptomycin. Corticosteroids may be necessary in addition to antimicrobials in severely ill patients but are not indicated for the treatment of arthritis alone. Salicylates or phenylbutazone may be helpful in controlling joint symptoms.

BEHÇET'S SYNDROME

Recurrent oral and genital ulcers and eye inflammation characterize Behçet's syndrome. Other manifestations include arthritis, thrombophlebitis, neurological abnormalities, and skin lesions. One or several clinical features may be present at any given time. The peak onset of the disease is in the third decade, but it may occur at any age. Men are affected more often than women. The etiology of this disease is not known.

Epidemiology Behçet's syndrome is found throughout the world with the greatest number of patients being reported from the Middle East and Japan. The prevalence of disease is unknown, but based on a study from Japan, the frequency is in the range of 1 patient per 10,000 persons. Familial aggregation has been observed; however, hereditary factors have not been clearly identified.

Pathology The predominant histopathologic lesion is vasculitis which affects mainly small to medium-size arteries and veins. The blood vessel walls and perivascular tissues are infiltrated predominantly by lymphocytes. Monocytes, plasma cells, and neutrophils may also be present. Swelling and proliferation of endothelial cells are observed. The lumen of the vessel may be narrowed or obliterated. Fibrinoid necrosis and disruption of the vessel wall may be seen.

In patients with active synovitis, the synovium shows hypercellularity consisting of neutrophils and, to a lesser degree, plasma cells. Arterioles have perivascular infiltration of lymphocytes.

Clinical manifestations Oral ulcers are usually the first manifestation and develop in nearly all patients with Behçet's syndrome. These painful ulcers, measuring 2 to 10 mm in diameter, have a central yellowish necrotic base, surrounded by erythema. Their appearance is similar to aphthous ulcers. Herpetiform ulcers also may be present and occur more frequently in women. They may occur as a single lesion or in crops and involve the lips, tongue, gingiva, buccal mucosa, pharynx, and rarely the larynx and nasal mucosa. These ulcers persist for several days to several weeks and heal without scarring.

Genital ulcers are also found in the majority of patients, on the scrotum and rarely on the penis. In females, lesions occur on the labia, vulva, and vaginal wall. Lesions in the vagina may not be painful and may go unnoticed unless a pelvic examination is performed. Perineal lesions are seen in both sexes. The course of genital ulcers is similar to that of the oral ulcers.

Recurrent ocular inflammation is another common feature of this syndrome, manifested by anterior uveitis with hypopyon, conjunctivitis, posterior uveitis, optic neuritis, retinal arteritis, or retinal vein occlusion. Eye lesions may be reversible; however, cataracts, glaucoma, and blindness may ensue.

Arthritis or arthralgias occur in approximately 50 percent of patients and may precede, accompany, or follow other manifestations of Behçet's syndrome. The arthritis is usually asymmetrical and polyarticular, and involves most often large joints such as knees, ankles, and elbows. In a few patients, only a single large joint is involved. Small joints can also be affected. Arthritis tends to occur with other features of Behçet's syndrome, especially with erythema nodosum. The majority of patients experience multiple recurrent episodes of acute inflammatory arthritis, not unlike arthropathy associated with inflammatory bowel disease. In a few patients the arthritis may become chronic. Residual joint damage seldom results even after several years of recurrent arthritis. Sacroiliitis and spondylitis may occasionally be found.

Recurrent and migratory superficial or deep thrombophlebitis is observed in about 25 percent of patients. The lower extremities are most often involved. Pulmonary embolization is an infrequent complication. Thrombosis of the superior or inferior vena cava may develop.

Central nervous system involvement is present in approximately 25 percent of patients, tends to appear later in the course of the disease, and is characterized by exacerbations and remissions. The central nervous system abnormalities include meningoencephalitis, benign intracranial hypertension with papilledema, brainstem lesions, cranial nerve palsies, spinal cord lesions, and psychosis. Peripheral neuropathies are infrequent. Death may result from central nervous system involvement.

Skin lesions are found in the majority of patients and take a variety of forms. These include erythematous papules, vesicles, pustules, pyoderma, and erythema nodosum. Clusters of the erythema nodosum lesions may appear on the lower extremities, as well as on the upper extremities.

A physical finding that is almost a diagnostic feature of Behçet's syndrome is the appearance after 24 h of a pustule surrounded by erythema at the site of a needle puncture. This sign, however, does not develop in all patients.

Colitis, indistinguishable from idiopathic ulcerative colitis, is present in a few patients with Behçet's syndrome. The colonic ulcers in the early inflammatory bowel disease, however, are separated by normal mucosa. Other gastrointestinal manifestations include nausea, diarrhea, abdominal distention, proctitis, and perianal ulcers.

Fever in the range of 38 to 39°C is present during exacerbations and usually reflects the severity of the clinical state. The clinical course of Behçet's syndrome is highly variable, as are the combinations of features that may be present at any given time. Mucocutaneous lesions usually appear with each exacerbation. Disease-free intervals may be measured in weeks, months, or even years. Mortality is especially high in patients with central nervous system involvement.

Laboratory findings Anemia, elevated erythrocyte sedimentation rate, and mild leukocytosis are often present during active disease. A polyclonal elevation of immunoglobulins may occur; complement levels are normal. Antibodies and cellular immunity to mucosal cells have been demonstrated in some patients, but these studies do not have diagnostic value. Coagulation studies may reveal elevated levels of fibrinogen and factor VIII. In addition, a decrease in plasma fibrinolytic activity is found in some patients.

In patients with central nervous system involvement, the cerebrospinal fluid shows a mild pleocytosis consisting of mononuclear cells and an increase in protein.

Synovial fluid from patients with acute arthritis shows white blood cell counts of 20,000 per cubic millimeter or greater, consisting predominantly of neutrophils. In chronic, mild arthritis, the fluid is clear and contains few mononuclear white blood cells.

Cell-mediated immunity to mucosal-cell antigens has been shown by the transformation of patients' lymphocytes when stimulated with mucosal cell extracts. These immunologic studies should be extended to confirm the role of immunity in the pathogenesis of this disorder.

Diagnosis The diagnosis of Behçet's syndrome is readily made when the triad of oral ulcers, genital ulcers, and eye inflammation is present. Since other features such as central nervous system involvement, thrombophlebitis, and arthritis occur frequently in this syndrome, their presence along with oral ulcers, genital ulcers, or eye inflammation should raise the possibility of Behçet's syndrome.

Reiter's and Behçet's syndromes have several clinical features in common. Both have an acute asymmetrical polyarthritis, mucocutaneous lesions, eye inflammation, and neurological abnormalities. In Reiter's syndrome, however, the orogenital lesions are usually not painful, thrombophlebitis is not a common feature, central nervous system manifestations are unusual, and the eye involvement consists mainly of conjunctivitis and less often anterior uveitis. The presence of spondylitis supports the diagnosis of Reiter's syndrome.

Painful oral ulcers also occur in the Stevens-Johnson syndrome. The absence of other features of Behçet's syndrome eventually distinguishes these diseases. Likewise, in patients with recurrent benign aphthous ulcers Behçet's syndrome is excluded by the absence of other manifestations. Patients with ulcerative colitis may have recurrent aphthous ulcers, iritis, arthritis, and erythema nodosum, and this may be confused with Behçet's syndrome with colitis. The colitis of Behçet's syndrome is characterized by the finding of discrete colonic ulcers separated by normal-appearing mucosa. In ulcerative colitis, genital ulcers are not seen, the posterior segment of the eye is not involved, and the aphthous ulcers are usually not as severe.

Treatment No effective form of therapy is available. Any form of treatment is difficult to assess because of the variable natural course of this disease. Prednisone in doses of 40 to 60 mg per day may improve some patients, and local application of steroids to the oral ulcers may be useful. Viscous xylocaine mouthwash helps to reduce pain.

Immunosuppressive drugs including azathioprine, cyclophosphamide, and chlorambucil have been administered to some patients with favorable results. Finally, a few patients have improved after the administration of transfer factor, prepared from normal donors. These forms of treatment remain entirely experimental and must be thoroughly evaluated prior to general acceptance.

REFERENCES

CALIN A: Reiter's syndrome, in *Textbook of Rheumatology,* WN Kelley et al (eds). Philadelphia, Saunders, 1981, chap 65, pp 1033–1046

CHAJEK T, FAINARU M: Behçet's disease. A report of 41 cases and a review of the literature. Medicine 54:179, 1975

GOOD AE: Enteropathic arthritis, in *Textbook of Rheumatology,* WN Kelley et al (eds). Philadelphia, Saunders, 1981, chap 67, pp 1063–1075

GREENSTEIN AJ et al: The extra-intestinal complications of Crohn's disease and ulcerative colitis: A study of 700 patients. Medicine 55:401, 1976

KAMMER GM et al: Psoriatic arthritis: A clinical, immunologic and HLA study of 100 patients. Semin Arthritis Rheum 9:75, 1979

LEVINE ME, DOBBINS WO III: Joint changes in Whipple's disease. Semin Arthritis Rheum 3:79, 1973

SHIMIZU T et al: Behçet disease (Behçet syndrome). Semin Arthritis Rheum 8:223, 1979

STEIN HB et al: The intestinal bypass arthritis-dermatitis syndrome. Arthritis Rheum 24:684, 1981

VERNON-ROBERTS B et al: Synovial pathology in Behçet's syndrome. Ann Rheum Dis 37:139, 1978

WRIGHT V: Psoriatic arthritis, in *Textbook of Rheumatology,* WN Kelley et al (eds). Philadelphia, Saunders, 1981, chap 66, pp 1047–1062

349 CALCIUM PYROPHOSPHATE DEPOSITION DISEASE (PSEUDOGOUT)

BRUCE C. GILLILAND
MART MANNIK

The deposition of calcium pyrophosphate dihydrate crystals in the joint is referred to as calcium pyrophosphate deposition disease (CPDD) and is characterized by acute and chronic inflammatory joint disease, usually affecting older individuals. The acute or subacute form of this arthritis is called *pseudogout,* but this term is also used as a synonym for CPDD. The calcium deposits in articular cartilage (chondrocalcinosis) are detected radiographically in most patients with CPDD. Knee and other large joints are the most frequent sites of involvement.

EPIDEMIOLOGY, PATHOGENESIS, AND PATHOLOGY CPDD occurs in persons of either sex, usually over age 50; its prevalence increases sharply with age. Approximately one symptomatic CPDD patient is observed for every two to three patients with gouty arthritis. An indication of the prevalence of chondrocalcinosis comes from autopsy studies, which have shown that approximately 3 to 5 percent of the adult population have calcium pyrophosphate dihydrate deposits in the knee joints.

CPDD is classified into three groups: a hereditary type, CPDD associated with metabolic disease, and idiopathic CPDD. Reports of hereditary CPDD have come from outside the United States; this disease occurs in individuals in the fourth to sixth decade. Sometimes it is severe, crippling, and involves many joints. Another form of familial disease is oligoarticular and affects older patients.

CPDD appears in association with several metabolic disorders: hyperparathyroidism, hemochromatosis, hypophosphatasia, hypomagnesemia, hypothyroidism, gout, ochronosis, and Wilson's disease. In hypothyroidism, acute arthritis attacks usually occur only after treatment with thyroid hormone. The relationship of these disorders to the pathogenesis of chondrocalcinosis is unknown; furthermore, the association of some of them (e.g., hyperparathyroidism) with chondrocalcinosis may not be greater than with osteoarthritis alone. In general, CPDD has a close association with degenerative joint disease.

Levels of inorganic pyrophosphate are elevated in the synovial fluid of many patients with CPDD but are also elevated in patients with osteoarthritis without evident chondrocalcinosis. Elevated levels of inorganic pyrophosphate most likely reflect increased metabolic activity of cartilage. The concentrations of calcium and pyrophosphate ions in joint fluid do not exceed their solubility product, and therefore it is unlikely that crystals form within synovial fluid. The initial site of crystal formation is believed to be in articular cartilage; however, the mechanism has not been elucidated.

The crystals in synovial fluid are believed to be shed from crystals in the cartilage. Several mechanisms have been postulated for the release of crystals from cartilage into the joint fluid. Lowering of either calcium or pyrophosphate ions in synovial fluid may loosen and shed crystals from cartilage into synovial fluid. This hypothesis is supported by two observations: (1) lowering of the concentration of ionized calcium in joint fluid brings on an acute attack of crystal-induced arthritis; (2) acute attacks of arthritis are associated with illness in which blood calcium concentrations decrease. Crystals may also enter the joint fluid as a consequence of mechanical disruption of cartilage secondary to microfractures of subchondral bone. The occurrence of acute attacks following trauma supports this concept. Another proposed mechanism is the release of crystals resulting from degradation of the cartilage matrix by enzymes. This mechanism may explain the occurrence of pseudogout superimposed on infectious arthritis, gout, or osteoarthritis. The finding of calcium pyrophosphate crystals may sometimes be the result and not the primary cause of joint inflammation.

The presence of calcium pyrophosphate crystals in the synovial fluid leads to an inflammatory response. Acute arthritis can be induced experimentally by the injection of calcium pyrophosphate crystals into a normal joint. Phagocytosis of the crystals by polymorphonuclear leukocytes leads to release of lysosomal enzymes and a chemotactant for leukocytes.

The *pathological changes* in the joint involve deposits of calcium pyrophosphate dihydrate crystals in the joint capsule, synovium, tendons, and ligaments, in the midzonal area of articular hyaline cartilage, and diffusely in fibrocartilage. The menisci of the knee are a common site of crystal deposition. Crystals can be seen at the margin of degenerating cartilage and surrounding the lacunae of chondrocytes; this site is considered the earliest detectable lesion. The deposition of crystals varies from microcrystalline aggregates to large masses intermixed with fibrous tissue. Crystals may also be observed in normal-appearing cartilage.

The synovium in acute arthritis is edematous, with numerous polymorphonuclear leukocytes. In chronic arthritis, mononuclear cell infiltration and fibroblastic proliferation are present; crystals are rarely observed.

CLINICAL MANIFESTATIONS Several patterns of joint involvement are recognized in calcium pyrophosphate deposition disease. Acute attacks occur in approximately 25 percent of patients, and this clinical picture is commonly called *pseudogout.* The onset of the acute attack of pseudogout is rapid and reaches a peak usually in 12 to 36 h. The involved joint is erythematous, swollen, warm, and painful. The acute attack is usually confined to a single joint, but in some patients involvement of other joints may follow in rapid progression. The knee is by far the most frequent site of acute arthritis, but attacks occur in the ankles, wrists, elbows, hips, and cervical and lumbar spine. As in gout, the metatarsal joint of the great toe may be a site of involvement. Furthermore, attacks may be provoked by trauma, surgery, or medical illness. The acute arthritis is usually intermittent, and the same joint is often involved in subsequent attacks. The acute episode usually subsides in 1 to 2 weeks. Between attacks the involved joint appears relatively normal. Most patients have radiographic evidence of chondrocalcinosis.

Approximately 5 percent of patients with calcium pyrophosphate deposition disease have what is termed *pseudorheumatoid disease,* which is characterized by multiple joint involvement with subacute attacks lasting several weeks to several months. The attacks affect one or several joints, then move on to involve other joints. Patients may complain of morning stiffness and fatigue. Synovial proliferation, limitation of joint motion, and flexion deformities can develop.

Another group, predominantly women and representing half the patients with calcium pyrophosphate deposition disease, has a chronic form of the disease. Progressive degenerative joint changes occur in multiple joints. The knees are the most frequently involved, followed by the wrists, metacarpophalangeal joints, hips, shoulders, elbows, and ankles. The joint involvement is usually symmetrical, and flexion contractures may develop. Approximately one-half of the patients with this form of the disease experience intermittent acute attacks. Another group of patients has typical articular chondrocalcinosis without any symptoms. Finally, CPDD may resemble neuropathic arthropathy; in these patients a severe oligo- or polyarticular destructive arthropathy is seen without neurological deficits. Calcium pyrophosphate deposits, however, are also seen in neuropathic arthropathies.

DIAGNOSIS The microscopic examination of *synovial fluid* in an acute attack shows large numbers of polymorphonuclear leukocytes. Calcium pyrophosphate dihydrate crystals are frequently found extracellularly and in polymorphonuclear leukocytes. In chronic arthritis, the crystals are observed less frequently and are most often extracellular. With polarized light, the crystals appear as short blunt rods, rhomboids, and cuboids and polarize light weakly compared to urate crystals. They have weakly positive birefringence under compensated polarized light, in contrast to the strongly negative birefringence of sodium urate crystals. The diagnosis is made by finding typical crystals under compensated polarized light and is supported by radiographic evidence of chondrocalcinosis.

Radiographically, calcifications in articular hyaline cartilage appear as fine linear densities parallel to the subchondral bone surface. In the knee, this line is best observed on a lateral film. Calcifications in fibrocartilage, ligaments, and joint capsule usually appear as more diffuse punctate and linear densities. Common sites of fibrocartilage involvement include the menisci of the knee, articular disk of the distal radioulnar joint, symphysis pubis, and the annulus fibrosis of the intervertebral disk. Evidence for chondrocalcinosis can usually be obtained with radiographs of the knees, wrists, and pelvis. Radiographic findings of osteoarthritis are also present, particularly in patients with chronic CPDD.

Gout and septic arthritis are the main considerations in the *differential diagnosis* of the acute arthritis. Gout and pseudogout are frequently indistinguishable clinically, and the diagnosis depends on the identification of their characteristic crystals under compensated polarized light. Both crystals occasionally have been found together in the synovial fluid of patients with typical radiographic articular calcifications of chondrocalcinosis. Bacterial smears and cultures should be performed on synovial fluid in all patients with an acute monarticular arthritis. The symptoms of osteoarthritis and chronic CPDD are very similar, and radiographic evidence for both is often present. The role played by each is difficult to determine. Pseudogout should be considered when intermittent attacks of acute arthritis occur. The finding of a chronic effusion in patients with symptoms of osteoarthritis also suggests the possibility of pseudogout. The diagnosis should not be made only on the radiographic findings of intraarticular calcific deposits, but depends also on the identification of the characteristic crystals, since other forms of inflammatory arthritis may affect the same joints. Attacks of pseudogout occur in patients without radiographic evidence of chondrocalcinosis, requiring a careful search for calcium pyrophosphate dihydrate crystals in any case of acute arthritis, especially in older patients. On the other hand, radiographic evidence of calcific deposits is found not infrequently in the knees of elderly patients who have no joint symptoms.

TREATMENT Phenylbutazone is usually effective. A loading dose of 600 mg is given, followed by 200 to 300 mg per day until symptoms subside. Indomethacin, 75 to 150 mg per day, or other new nonsteroidal anti-inflammatory agents (NSAIDs) may also be used. Aspiration of the synovial fluid, followed by intraarticular injection of glucocorticosteroids also may be effective. Results of treatment with colchicine are variable but may be useful in those patients who require parenteral therapy. In chronic arthritis, salicylates or the newer NSAIDs may give symptomatic relief. The deposition of calcium pyrophosphate crystals in articular tissues cannot be prevented or reversed.

Hydroxyapatite arthropathy Crystal-induced arthritis is also observed with calcium hydroxyapatite crystals. The frequency of this disease is not known, since the diagnosis is very difficult to establish; because of their small size (0.1 to 1 μm in length), hydroxyapatite crystals cannot be recognized by light microscopy. Electron-microscopic or x-ray diffraction studies are required for the accurate diagnosis of this crystal deposition disease. When the diagnosis can be established, the management of these patients is similar to those with CPDD.

REFERENCES

Howell DS: Diseases due to the deposition of calcium pyrophosphate and hydroxyapatite, in *Textbook of Rheumatology,* WN Kelley et al (eds). Philadelphia, Saunders, 1981, chap 87, pp 1438–1454

McCarthy DJ: Pseudogout and pyrophosphate metabolism, in *Advances in Internal Medicine,* GH Stollerman (ed). Chicago, Year Book, 1980, pp 363–390

Resnick D, Niwayama G: Calcium pyrophosphate dihydrate (CPDD) crystal deposition disease, in *Diagnosis of Bone and Joint Disorders,* D Resnick, G Niwayama (eds). Philadelphia, Saunders, 1981, chap 44, pp 1520–1574

Schumacher HR et al: Arthritis associated with apatite crystals. Ann Intern Med 87:411, 1977

INFECTIOUS ARTHRITIS

BRUCE C. GILLILAND
ROBERT G. PETERSDORF

ACUTE BACTERIAL ARTHRITIS Septic arthritis is a medical emergency requiring prompt recognition and appropriate treatment to avoid permanent joint damage. Microorganisms usually reach the joint by hematogenous spread from a primary infection elsewhere, but occasionally no source can be found. Joint sepsis may also occur by direct extension of infection from adjacent bone or soft tissue. Occasionally no source is evident.

Etiology Acute *bacterial arthritis* is caused by many different types of bacteria; the ones most commonly encountered are *Neisseria gonorrhoeae, Staphylococcus aureus, Streptococcus pneumoniae, Streptococcus pyogenes, Hemophilus influenzae,* and gram-negative bacilli (*Escherichia coli, Salmonella, Pseudomonas* spp., etc.). Septic arthritis due to *H. influenzae* occurs mostly in children under 6 years of age. *S. aureus* is a common infecting agent in septic arthritis observed in intravenous drug addicts. Gram-negative bacillary infections also occur in this group of patients. In addition, joint sepsis with gram-negative bacilli tends to occur in patients with underlying infection of the urinary, biliary, or intestinal tract and in patients with impaired resistance to infection. Osteomyelitis is also a feature of infections with gram-negative bacilli, and joint damage is a common sequel. Patients with *Salmonella* arthritis often have evidence of underlying osteomyelitis. Infectious arthritis of the spine is most often caused by staphylococci. Brucellosis, tuberculosis, and *Salmonella* infections preferentially involve the spine.

An increased susceptibility to joint infection occurs in patients with diabetes, leukemias, or multiple myeloma, and in those receiving corticosteroids or immunosuppressive drugs. Patients with chronic alcoholism are more prone to develop infections, in general, and bacterial arthritis, in particular. In addition, joints previously damaged by trauma or by rheumatoid arthritis are more susceptible to infections.

Manifestations The onset of bacterial arthritis is usually abrupt and accompanied by fever. Shaking chills occur in some patients. One or a few joints may be involved. The affected joint is warm, erythematous, swollen, and painful; however, these signs may be less marked in elderly patients or in those patients receiving corticosteroids or immunosuppressive drugs. Marked guarding of the joint and muscle spasms are common. The knee is involved in approximately one-half of the cases. Other large joints, such as the hips and shoulders, are commonly affected, and the wrists, ankles, elbows, and sternoclavicular and sacroiliac joints less often. However, predilection of the latter two joints for septic arthritis has been observed in intravenous drug abusers. The articulations of the spine or any peripheral joint may be a site of infection. In the spine, infection involves the vertebral body and adjacent intervertebral disk space, and may extend to the adjacent apophyseal joint. Localized tenderness and spasm of the paraspinal or psoas muscles are often present. The diagnosis of septic arthritis of the hip is often delayed, since swelling of this joint is not readily detected. Pain from the hip may be felt in the groin, buttock, or lateral upper thigh, or referred to the anterior knee. The thigh is usually held in adduction, flexion, and internal rotation. In some instances, the thigh becomes edematous and swelling appears in the anterior groin.

Pathology The synovium in the early stages of infection is edematous and infiltrated by neutrophils. An effusion with many neutrophils forms rapidly. Lysosomal proteolytic enzymes released from neutrophils destroy articular cartilage, subchondral bone, and joint capsule. Small abscesses appear in the synovium and subchondral bone, and necrotic debris collects in the joint space. During healing, proliferation of fibroblasts may lead to ankylosis.

Laboratory and x-ray findings Aspiration and examination of joint fluid should be performed immediately in any patient suspected of having a septic joint. Sterile technique should be used in aspirating any joint to avoid inadvertently introducing an infection. Also, the needle should not be inserted into the joint through an overlying area of cellulitis or an infected bursa. The appearance of synovial fluid in infectious arthritis is usually cloudy but may be grossly purulent. The white blood cell count ranges from 10,000 to greater than 100,000 per cubic millimeter, and more than 90 percent of the cells are neutrophils. The peripheral blood often shows a leukocytosis; however, the leukocyte count may be normal in debilitated persons. The concentration of glucose in the joint cavity is often less than 50 percent of a simultaneous blood sugar reading when obtained at least 6 h after a meal, or after cessation of intravenous glucose infusions to allow equilibrium of glucose between blood and synovial fluid. In some patients with gonococcal arthritis, the reduction of synovial fluid glucose may be less marked. Gram's stain frequently reveals microorganisms. Blood and synovial fluid should be cultured for aerobes and anaerobes. Obtaining a positive synovial fluid culture is enhanced by plating the fluid on the appropriate media while still warm. Cultures of the synovial fluid and blood should be performed even if the Gram's stain is negative. Radiographs of the joint early in infection show soft-tissue swelling and distention of the joint capsule, and later show juxtaarticular osteoporosis, periosteal elevation, joint space narrowing due to cartilage destruction, and bony erosions on the articular surface. Radiographic evidence of coexisting osteomyelitis may be present. In the spine, radiographic changes may not be seen for several months. The first changes consist of narrowing of the involved disk space or vertebra and proliferation of bone at the vertebral margins. Subsequently, lytic lesions appear in the vertebra and may extend to the disk space. During healing adjacent vertebrae may become fused. Radioisotope scanning techniques utilizing technetium polyphosphonate or gallium may be useful in distinguishing whether the site of the infection is cellulitis, osteomyelitis, or septic arthritis. Both types of scan are positive in septic arthritis and osteomyelitis, but only the gallium scan is positive in cellulitis. Radioisotope scans may point to infection in such joints as hip, shoulder, spine, and sacroiliac. A positive scan, however, is not specific for infection, since other causes of inflammatory joint disease as well as degenerative joint disease will give a positive scan.

Diagnosis The diagnosis of acute bacterial arthritis can be made by finding microorganisms on Gram's stain of synovial fluid or in synovial tissue, and is confirmed by a positive culture. With involvement of the spine or sacroiliac joint, needle biopsy or open surgical biopsy may be required to obtain tissue for examination and culture. The possibility of infectious arthritis should be entertained in a patient with fever and unilateral sacroiliac or back pain. Other forms of acute arthritis may be mistaken for infectious arthritis. These include gout, pseudogout, Reiter's syndrome, psoriatic arthritis, peripheral arthritis of inflammatory bowel disease, and rheumatic fever. These disorders usually are not associated with chills, high fever, and marked leukocytosis. Crystal deposits of sodium urate or calcium pyrophosphate may be found in joint fluid or a septic joint, and may have played a role in predisposing this joint to infection. On the other hand, the enzymes of the inflammatory process of infectious arthritis may have released into the joint fluid preexisting crystal deposits from synovial tissue or cartilage, a process referred to as "enzymatic strip mining." In patients with rheumatoid arthritis who develop chills and fever and have one or two joints disproportionately more inflamed than others, superimposed infectious arthritis in those joints should be carefully excluded by examination and culture of synovial fluid.

Infection of a bursa or juxtaarticular soft tissue and skin should be distinguished from infectious arthritis. Bursae and tendon sheaths become infected with the same type of microorganisms that invade joints. Care must be taken not to infect a bursa or joint by passing a needle through an overlying area of cellulitis.

Treatment Septic arthritis requires prompt treatment with appropriate antibiotics. The preferred antibiotic regimens for the more common organisms are given in the chapters dealing with these organisms as well as in Chap. 141, which summarizes the properties of each antibiotic. When no organisms are seen on Gram's stain, a penicillinase-resistant penicillin and gentamicin should be given, particularly to those patients with factors known to diminish host resistance. Bactericidal levels of antibiotics are achieved with systemic administration; therefore, direct administration of an antibiotic into the joint is not necessary and may in itself produce a chemical synovitis. During treatment, bactericidal assays of synovial fluid may be performed to assure that therapeutic levels of antibiotic have been achieved. Drainage, recommended when the joint is tightly distended or contains a high neutrophil count, reduces pressure and removes pus that generates proteolytic enzymes. Needle aspiration, during which the joint cavity can be irrigated with sterile saline to enhance removal of inflammatory substances, usually provides adequate drainage. The frequency of aspiration depends on the amount of fluid and the cell count of that which reaccumulates. Aspiration ordinarily is necessary only during the first few days of treatment. Open surgical drainage is usually not indicated except in septic arthritis of the hip or in a joint with chronic suppuration and loculated pus. Splinting of the affected joint may make the patient more comfortable and reduce the degree of flexion deformity. Prolonged splinting, however, should be avoided, since it may lead to a permanent joint stiffness. When the inflammation has subsided, physical therapy will aid the return of joint function. A severely damaged weight-bearing joint may require bony fusion.

GONOCOCCAL ARTHRITIS (See Chap. 150) Gonococcal arthritis is the most common cause of arthritis in young adults, especially women. Pregnancy and menstruation are predisposing factors for bacteremia and arthritis. Patients with homozygous deficiency of a terminal complement component (C5 to C8) are also more susceptible to disseminated *Neisseria* infections, since these organisms are killed by complement-mediated cell lysis requiring the terminal complement components.

Patients with gonococcal arthritis may present with fever, chills, skin lesions, polyarthritis, and a positive blood culture. The polyarthritis usually evolves in a few days to a monoarticular septic arthritis. These two stages have been referred to as the "bacteremic" and "septic joint" phases. The clinical picture, however, is quite variable, and some patients present with monoarticular septic arthritis and few if any systemic manifestations. Diagnosis is confirmed by positive cultures of blood, synovial fluid, or skin lesion. Cultures of synovial fluid, however, are positive in less than half the cases. Arthritis usually responds promptly to antibiotic therapy. The gonococcal organisms associated with disseminated infection are usually very sensitive to penicillin.

TUBERCULOUS ARTHRITIS (See Chap. 174) Tuberculous arthritis is a chronic destructive form of septic arthritis caused by *Mycobacterium tuberculosis.* Approximately 1 percent of patients with tuberculosis have skeletal involvement. Many patients with skeletal tuberculosis do not have evidence for active or even inactive pulmonary disease. Tuberculous arthritis occurs more frequently in nonwhites and men, and tends to involve an older population of patients, in their fifth and sixth decades. Tuberculous arthritis, however, can occur at any age.

The most frequently involved joints are the spine, hips, knees, sacroiliac, wrists, and ankles. In the spine (Pott's disease) the infection begins in the margins of the vertebral bodies and extends into the adjacent disk space. Destruction of bone leads to vertebral collapse and angulation of the spine resulting in kyphosis or gibbus. Extension of the infection into the paraspinal muscles produces a cold abscess which can spread up or down the spine or along the rib and eventually point in the groin, neck, chest wall, or sternum. Cord compression may cause paraplegia, and extension into the meninges results in tuberculous meningitis. A rare complication is the formation of a mycotic aneurysm formed by the erosion of a cold abscess into the aorta. Common clinical manifestations of spinal involvement are back pain, muscle spasm, local tenderness, kyphosis, and referred pain from spinal nerve root compression.

Peripheral or axial joints are infected by direct hematogenous spread or by extension from a tuberculous process in the adjacent bone. A combination of arthritis and osteomyelitis often occurs in skeletal tuberculosis. The tuberculous process produces synovitis with the formation of a pannus of granulation tissue over the articular cartilage. Destruction of articular cartilage initially occurs at the joint margins and gradually progresses. The rate of destruction is slower than in other acute infectious bacterial arthritis. The subchondral bone is involved and areas of necrosis develop. The joint infection can extend to the juxtaarticular soft tissues to produce a cold abscess and eventually a sinus tract.

Tuberculous arthritis has an insidious onset and is usually monarticular, and hips and knees are the most commonly affected peripheral joints. A low-grade fever and night sweats may be present, but most patients do not have prominent constitutional symptoms. The affected peripheral joint is swollen, warm, and tender and has a decreased range of motion. Erythema is minimal, and pain is initially mild. The hypertrophied synovium gives the joint a boggy, doughy feeling. Muscle atrophy, spasm, and contracture of the affected extremity occur. Tenosynovitis of the flexor tendon sheaths of the wrist may compress the median nerve and produce a carpal tunnel syndrome.

The synovial fluid white cell count is usually greater than 10,000 per cubic millimeter, with polymorphonuclear cells predominating. The tubercle bacilli are seen on smears of synovial fluid in approximately 20 percent of patients but are more likely to be found on biopsy of synovial tissue.

Radiographs of peripheral joints in early disease show joint capsule distention and juxtaarticular osteoporosis. Bony erosions at the joint margin, subchondral bone destruction, and joint space narrowing are observed later in the disease. Films of the spine show destruction of the vertebral body, vertebral collapse, and loss of intervertebral disk space.

The diagnosis of tuberculous arthritis is made by demonstrating tubercle bacilli in synovial fluid or tissue by smear, histology, or culture. The tuberculin skin test is almost always positive. Anergy may occur in advanced disease, old age, or severe malnutrition.

Nontuberculous (atypical) mycobacteria (see Chap. 176) (e.g., *M. kansasii, M. marinum, M. intracellulare*) can also cause septic arthritis and infect bursae and tendons. Microorganisms usually reach the joint by hematogenous spread but also can be introduced into the bone or joint by direct inoculation. Involvement of the tendon sheaths in the hand and wrist often occurs and may result in a carpal tunnel syndrome. Peripheral joint involvement is similar to that in tuberculosis. The correct diagnosis depends on a positive culture from synovial or bursal fluid or tissue. Treatment of tuberculosis and nontuberculous mycobacterial infections is described in Chaps. 174 and 176.

MYCOTIC, SYPHILITIC, AND VIRAL ARTHRITIS **Mycotic arthritis** The systemic mycoses (coccidioidomycosis, histoplasmosis, blastomycosis, cryptococcosis, candidiasis, and sporotrichosis) may involve bone and joints. In the primary phase of coccidioidomycosis, a transient polyarthritis, lasting up to 1 month, may occur in association with erythema nodosum (desert arthritis), but no residual joint damage ensues. However, with chronic disseminated disease, arthritis may occur alone or secondary to adjacent bone infection. The arthritis is usually monarticular, affects the knee predominantly, and leads in time to joint destruction. Sporotrichosis arthritis occurs in two distinct clinical forms: in the unifocal form, one or a few joints are chronically affected; while in the multifocal form, multiple joints, skin, and other tissues are involved. Progressive joint damage ensues in the absence of treatment. Young infants receiving parenteral nutrition or patients receiving glucocorticosteroids or immunosuppressive or antibiotic drugs are at risk for *Candida* infections which can involve joints. In other mycotic diseases, joint involvement is infrequent.

Actinomycosis infection due to an anaerobic bacteria-like obligate parasite may involve the spine. The diagnosis of fungal arthritis is established by the identification of the organisms in synovial fluid or in a biopsy specimen. Treatment with amphotericin B is usually successful; however, surgical debridement may be necessary. Penicillin is the drug of choice for actinomycosis.

Syphilitic arthritis This form of arthritis (see Chap. 177) occurs in congenital, secondary, or tertiary syphilis. During the first year of life, congenital syphilis may produce an osteochondritis in the juxtaepiphyseal region which results in the breakdown of bone and articular cartilage (Parrot's pseudoparalysis). At puberty, congenital disease may cause a synovitis which most commonly involves the knees and elbows (Clutton's joints). The joint is often red, swollen, and tender, but pain may be minimal. Synovial fluid shows a leukocytosis, predominantly lymphocytes.

In secondary syphilis, transient polyarthritis and polyarthralgia occur. Gummatous involvement of the synovium may occur in tertiary syphilis and most often involves the larger joints.

In addition to direct involvement of the joint, syphilis also produces a neuropathic joint (Charcot's joint).

The proper diagnosis of the joint disease can be established only after the correct diagnosis of syphilis. A positive serologic test for syphilis is not diagnostic, since biological false-positive tests may occur in rheumatic diseases such as systemic lupus erythematosus.

Viral arthritis A self-limited polyarthritis may be a manifestation of several viral diseases. Three viral infections especially are accompanied by significant arthritis: rubella, type B hepatitis, and arboviruses not found in the western hemisphere (chikungunya and o'nyong-nyong in Africa, and Ross River arthritis in Australia). Other viral infections with arthritis include mumps, infectious mononucleosis, varicella, and adenoviral infections.

Rubella infection may present with a polyarthritis, usually involving the fingers, wrists, and knees symmetrically. The arthritis is seen most often in young adults, especially women. Arthritis is also observed in children and young adults after vaccination with live, attenuated rubella vaccine, and is similar to that observed with natural disease. The onset of arthritis coincides with or shortly follows the appearance of the rash. The arthritis lasts up to 2 weeks or occasionally a month. In a few patients, the arthritis may be recurrent for months to years. Permanent joint damage does not usually occur even with chronic disease. Joint effusions are usually small, and synovial fluid shows mild leukocytosis with either lymphoctyes or neutrophils predominating. Rheumatoid factor tests may be positive.

Arthritis is a relatively common manifestation of type B hepatitis (serum hepatitis). It is often accompanied by a rash, may precede the onset of clinical jaundice by a few days to 2 weeks, or coincide with the appearance of jaundice. Jaundice may not appear in some patients with arthritis; however, liver function tests are abnormal in such patients. The rash is most often urticarial, but can be macular, papular, or petechial. The onset of arthritis is usually abrupt, with symmetrical involvement of both small and large joints. The most commonly involved joints are the fingers, followed by the knee, shoulder, ankle, elbow, and wrist. The arthritis can also be asymmetrical or migratory. Permanent joint damage does not occur. Synovial fluid shows a varying degree of leukocytosis with polymorphonuclear cells. Rheumatoid factor tests usually are negative.

Serum and joint fluid complement levels are usually low during arthritis. Serum complement level returns to normal with the appearance of overt liver disease. Hepatitis B antigen (Australia antigen, hepatitis-associated antigen) can usually be detected in both serum and joint fluid during the prodromal period of hepatitis. The synovitis is thought to be induced by immune complexes consisting of viral antigens and their antibodies.

Lyme arthritis was originally described in patients from the contiguous communities of eastern Connecticut (Old Lyme, Lyme, and East Haddam). Although initially thought to be caused by a virus, a spirochetal etiology seems more likely. Most of the cases have centered in the New England area, but a few cases have appeared on the Pacific coast and in an area in central Wisconsin. Transmission of the causative agent is by the minute tick, *Ixodes damminni.* Most of the cases occur in children and young adults during the summer and fall, probably because they spend more time outdoors in wooded areas. The disease usually begins with a characteristic skin lesion, erythema chronicum migrans, an expanding erythematous annular skin lesion that usually appears on a thigh, buttock, or trunk. The lesion may reach a diameter of 50 cm with central clearing and last a few weeks. Fever, chills, headache, and malaise often accompany the skin lesion. Arthritis occurs in approximately half the patients with erythema chronicum migrans, the onset being several weeks to months after the appearance of the skin lesion. About 25 percent of patients with Lyme arthritis do not have erythema chronicum migrans. Other manifestations of this illness include neurological abnormalities (aseptic meningitis, Bell's palsy) and cardiac conduction abnormalities.

The arthritis is an acute, recurrent, monarticular, or asymmetrical oligoarticular joint disease involving most commonly the knee, followed by other large joints and the temporomandibular joint. The small joints of the feet and hands are occasionally affected. The affected joint is swollen and warm but usually not red. The duration of arthritis in a single joint is approximately 1 week, but it sometimes can persist for several months. The arthritis in some patients may be migratory. Most patients have recurrent attacks, separated by intervals ranging from 1 to several weeks. The number of attacks tends to become less frequent; most of the patients have at least one recurrence in the second and third years of illness. Recurrent attacks of arthritis may be accompanied by fever, fatigue, and malaise. Significant joint damage usually does not occur; however, in a few patients arthritis in the knees has become chronic, with formation of a pannus and damage to cartilage and subchondral bone.

The white blood cell count of the synovial fluid ranges from 2000 to over 50,000 per cubic millimeter and consists mostly of granulocytes. Cryoprecipitate and immune complexes can be demonstrated in the serum of patients early in the disease and may occur with attacks of arthritis. They are nearly always present in the joint fluid.

Treatment consists of salicylates. Aspiration of fluid and injection of glucocorticosteroids may be beneficial in a knee with a tense effusion. Treatment with penicillin usually leads to prompt disappearance of the erythema chronicum migrans, but does not prevent the subsequent arthritis or cardiac or neurological abnormalities. Glucocorticosteroids may be beneficial in the treatment of neurological or cardiac abnormalities.

REFERENCES

BAYER AS et al: Fungal arthritis: III. Sporotrichal arthritis. Semin Arthritis Rheum 9:66, 1979

BURGDORFER W et al: Lyme disease—a tick-borne spirochetosis? Science 216:1317, 1982

CLARK GM: Tuberculosis arthritis, in *Arthritis and Allied Conditions,* 9th ed, JL Hollander, DJ McCarty Jr (eds). Philadelphia, Lea & Febiger, 1979

HOFFMAN GS: Mycobacterial and fungal infections of bones and joints, in *Textbook of Rheumatology,* WN Kelley et al (eds). Philadelphia, Saunders, 1981

LOCKSHIN MD, BRAUSE BD: Infectious arthritis. Disease-a-Month 28(4):1, 1982

MALAWISTA SE, STEERE AC: Viral arthritis, in *Textbook of Rheumatology,* WN Kelley et al (eds). Philadelphia, Saunders, 1981

ROSENTHAL J et al: Acute nongonococcal infectious arthritis: Evaluation of risk factors, therapy and outcome. Arthritis Rheum 23:889, 1980

SCHMID FR: Principles of diagnosis and treatment of infectious arthritis, in *Arthritis and Allied Conditions,* 9th ed, JL Hollander, DJ McCarty Jr (eds). Philadelphia, Lea & Febiger, 1979

SHARP JT: Gonococcal arthritis, in *Arthritis and Allied Conditions,* 9th ed, JL Hollander, DJ McCarty Jr (eds). Philadelphia, Lea & Febiger, 1979

STEERE AC et al: Erythema chronicum migrans and Lyme arthritis: The enlarging clinical spectrum. Ann Intern Med 86:685, 1977

WARD JR, ATCHESON SG: Infectious arthritis. Med Clin North Am 61:313, 1977

351 DEGENERATIVE JOINT DISEASE

MART MANNIK
BRUCE C. GILLILAND

Degenerative joint disease (DJD) is characterized by loss of joint cartilage and by hypertrophy of bone. Synonyms for degenerative joint disease include osteoarthritis and hypertrophic arthritis. Surveys have estimated that over 40 million Americans have radiological evidence of DJD, including 85 percent

of persons over the age of 70. Many persons with radiographic changes, however, have no musculoskeletal complaints. In young persons changes identical to the degenerative changes in advanced age are encountered when cartilage has been damaged by injury, infection, or congenital deformities. The exact mechanisms for cartilage loss in DJD have not been defined, but stress and subchondral bone changes contribute to the damage. Treatment of DJD is directed to amelioration of symptoms, decrease in excessive stress, and corrective procedures in properly selected subjects.

ETIOLOGY AND PATHOGENESIS The joint cartilage, subchondral bone, and joint capsule dissipate the forces of weight bearing and joint function. The joint cartilage has unique properties of compressibility and elasticity due to the combined presence of collagen fibers and proteoglycans. The articular cartilage contains a unique type of collagen, called *type II collagen,* which is composed of three identical α_1(II) polypeptide chains. Collagen fibers provide cartilage with structural integrity. The proteoglycans of cartilage consist of a protein backbone and many glycosaminoglycan side chains with negative charges. These proteoglycan molecules bind a large number of water molecules. Upon compression of cartilage the structural water is released from the proteoglycans and regained upon removal of the compressive force. The loss of compressibility of cartilage secondary to proteoglycan malfunction seems to be a central feature in the development of DJD.

In normal adult cartilage, chondrocytes no longer synthesize DNA or divide. Experimental trauma to cartilage and the pathogenic events of DJD reactivate DNA synthesis and cell division; as a result clusters of chondrocytes form in osteoarthritic cartilage. Chondrocytes are metabolically active and continuously rebuild the matrix of cartilage. The turnover of structural molecules requires the presence of enzymes that can dismantle the "old" structures as new molecules are synthesized and assembled. Such enzymes exist in chondrocytes and are more abundant in osteoarthritic lesions.

In degenerative lesions of joint cartilage the size of the proteoglycan molecules is reduced, owing to either degradation or altered synthesis, and the composition of glycosaminoglycans is altered. In addition, the content of proteases (particularly cathepsin D) and other hydrolases is increased in degenerative lesions. These observations along with the finding of increased metabolic activity and increased cell division in osteoarthritic cartilage indicate that increased degradation and increased synthesis of cartilage matrix occur concurrently. Apparently, as the lesions progress, the synthetic activities cannot keep up with degradative processes, and a progressive net loss of cartilage ensues. During the reparative process the original architecture of collagen fibrils is not achieved, and type I cartilage (normally found in skin, tendons, etc.) is laid down in place of type II collagen. At the same time sclerosis of subchrondral bone continues, and marginal bone overgrowths (spurs) develop.

Epidemiologic studies suggest that wear-and-tear processes play a central role in initiating the degenerative process in cartilage. Work patterns can lead to early involvement of joints that are usually not affected by DJD. For example, foundry workers who exert great leverage on their elbows by lifting metals with long tongs were found to have an increased prevalence of osteoarthritis of these joints. In contrast, the development of DJD is slow in paralyzed limbs. The continued wear-and-tear on joints is thought to cause fatigue fractures of subchondral bone. The repair of these microfractures leads to loss of deformability in subchondral bone and a concomitant decrease in energy dissipation by bone. By this mechanism, the articular cartilage is subjected to increased forces that initiate surface alterations, increase release of enzymes from chondrocytes, and enhance repair processes. In congenital malformations or malalignment of joints normal stresses cause increased wear and tear that leads to early DJD.

PATHOLOGY Early pathological changes of DJD are recognized in the joint cartilage. New bone formation develops in subchondral bone and at the margins of the articular cartilage. Progressive loss of metachromasia (histological evidence of proteoglycan loss) occurs in the cartilage, beginning at the surface. Chondrocytes increase in number and form clusters. With progression of the process the surface of cartilage begins to loosen and flake along superficial collagen fibers that parallel the joint surface; upon reaching the deeper radial layer the damage is reflected in fissuring of cartilage. Abrasion of damaged cartilage may ultimately lead to total loss of the cartilage. This progressive loss of cartilage is apparent radiologically as "joint space" narrowing.

The bone at the joint margins responds to cartilage damage with osteophyte formation. These lesions usually extend from the margin of the joint along the contour of the joint surface. Alternatively, osteophytes may develop within and extend along ligamentous and capsular attachments of the joint margin. The denuded subchondral bone becomes dense, smooth, and glistening, and looks like ivory (eburnation). In addition, cystic areas may develop below the joint surface and become filled with fibrous tissue. These "pseudocysts" are thought to be caused by synovial fluid escaping through cartilaginous defects into underlying cancellous bone. Low-grade inflammatory changes are present in the synovium and joint capsule, but the capsule is subject to thickening with fibrosis.

CLINICAL MANIFESTATIONS Degenerative joint disease is divided into *primary* and *secondary* forms. In primary DJD no predisposing abnormality or cause can be found, and the usual symptoms of the illness begin after the fifth and sixth decades of life. In secondary DJD an underlying abnormality or injury can be found, and the clinical symptoms may begin several decades earlier. The clinical findings in primary and secondary DJD are similar, except that in secondary DJD unusual or single joints are more likely to be involved.

Secondary DJD follows septic arthritis or inflammatory arthritides (e.g., rheumatoid arthritis, psoriatic arthritis) that destroy cartilage. Fractures through the cartilage, lacerations of cartilage, removal of menisci, and aseptic necrosis predispose the affected joints to early development of DJD. Diabetes mellitus and acromegaly also predispose to development of DJD. Local anatomic aberrations are thought to be the most common causes of early development of DJD. Congenitally shallow acetabulums, slipped capital femoral epiphyses, and Legg-Perthes disease are commonly accepted causes of early DJD in the hip. Deviations from the normal matching of the curvatures of the femoral head and the acetabulum are thought to contribute to DJD. The alterations in the congruence of this and other joints, however, need to be evaluated further in relation to the development of what now is termed *primary idiopathic DJD.*

The cardinal complaint in DJD is pain confined to joints, especially on motion and weight bearing. The pain is usually described as aching. Patients complain of definite joint stiffness; this occurs after resting and subsides in a few minutes upon resuming motion. In the morning the stiffness lasts only a short time (usually reported in minutes), whereas the morning stiffness of rheumatoid arthritis lasts an hour or more. With advanced disease pain at night may become prominent in the large joints and spine. On examination the joints may show a restricted range of motion, local tenderness, bony enlargement, small effusions, and crepitus. Erythema and increased heat are unusual in DJD.

DJD of the distal interphalangeal joints of the fingers leads to bony enlargement of the joint. These dorsolaterally located nodules at the base of the terminal phalanx are called *Heberden's nodes.* One-fourth of the patients who have nodes of the distal interphalangeal joints also have similar deformities at the proximal interphalangeal joints, called *Bouchard's nodes.* The primary Heberden's nodes usually evolve insidiously and without pain. However, some patients develop redness, swelling, and tenderness that last a few weeks or months. Subsequently the initial relatively soft and painful swelling is replaced by a hard, bony, painless enlargement. Heberden's nodes are more common in females than in males, and in females heredity seems to play a role. The mother and sisters of a woman with Heberden's nodes are more likely to have the nodes than controls of the same age and sex. The presence of Heberden's and Bouchard's nodes does not imply DJD in weight-bearing joints.

Osteoarthritis may develop in single or multiple joints of the hands as a result of trauma (e.g., "baseball fingers," "karate fingers"). Metacarpophalangeal joints are virtually never involved. The carpometacarpal joint of the thumb is frequently involved (Fig. 351-1).

FIGURE 351-1
Degenerative joint disease. A. Heberden's nodes of the distal interphalangeal joints and Bouchard's nodes of the proximal interphalangeal joints of the fingers. The carpometacarpal joints of both thumbs are swollen. B. X-rays of the middle three fingers of the left hand from the same patient. Note the marked joint space narrowing, osteophyte formation in the distal and proximal interphalangeal joints, cystic changes in subchondral bone, and absence of osteoporosis.

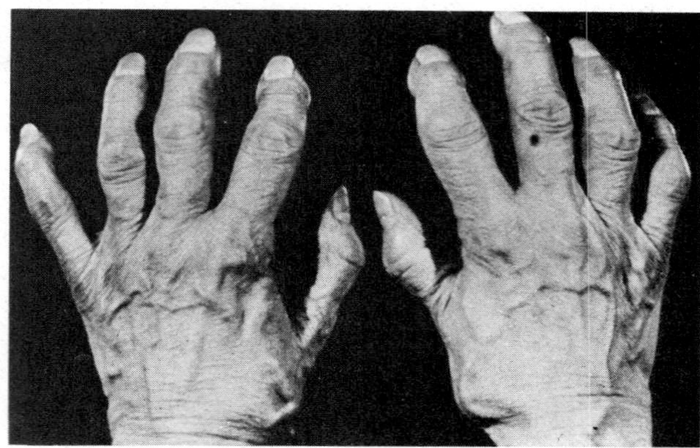

A

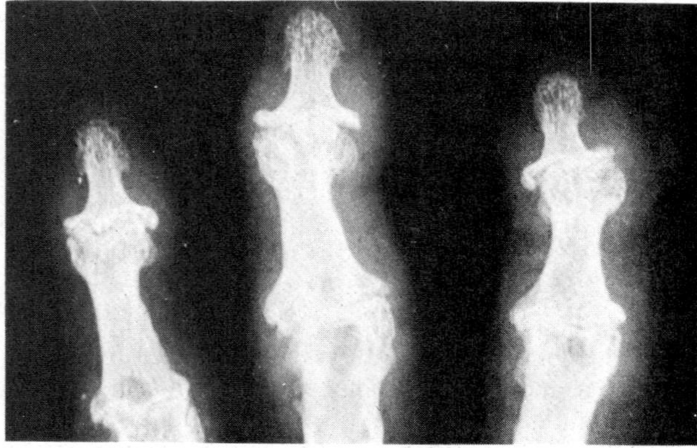

B

DJD of the wrists, elbows, and shoulders is relatively uncommon. However, occupational trauma may enhance DJD in the elbows and shoulders, as in air-hammer workers.

Degenerative joint disease of the spine can involve the apophyseal joints, the intervertebral joints as a consequence of disk disease, or the joints of Luschka in the cervical spine. The latter joints are articulations between the lateral aspects of adjacent vertebral bodies from C2 to C7. The herniation of intervertebral disks is covered in Chap. 366. The involvement of apophyseal joints or joints of Luschka leads to stiffness, pain, decreased motion, and at times to spinal nerve root compression. Radiographs of the spine will show characteristic osteophyte formation, extending from the bodies of vertebrae or extending into the spinal foramina from the apophyseal joints. Most elderly persons have some radiographic changes, but relatively few of the changes become severe enough to cause symptoms and signs.

In the cervical spine the maximum motion occurs between C4 and C5 and between C5 and C6; these articulations are most likely to develop DJD. Development of osteophytes from the margins of the joints of Luschka or the apophyseal joints can cause impingement on nerve roots at the spinal foramens. Radicular pain, muscle spasms or atrophy, paresthesias, and sensory changes will localize the level of root involvement. Cervical traction can provide relief of symptoms and resolution of neurological abnormalities. At times, surgery will be required. Occasionally osteophytes may extend posteriorly from the vertebrae into the spinal canal and result in cord compression. Surgical intervention is required in such situations.

In the lumbar spine, herniated disk disease (see Chap. 366) is more common than impingement of the nerve roots or cauda equina by osteophytes. The syndrome of spinal stenosis supervenes in persons who have anatomic variations with decreased anteroposterior dimensions of the spinal cord or decreased lateral recesses of the canal. In contrast to herniation of an intervertebral disk, the symptoms of spinal stenosis evolve insidiously, back symptoms precede nerve compression symptoms in the legs, and the symptoms are often bilateral. The symptoms of spinal stenosis are increased by exercise, enhanced by the lordotic position, and relieved by flexion of the spine. The onset and relief of symptoms are not as predictable in relation to exercise as in intermittent claudication due to vascular disease of the extremities, and the presence of numbness, tingling, and weakness also serves to distinguish the symptoms from claudication. Myelography is needed to establish the diagnosis with certainty. Laminectomy is indicated when symptoms and signs of spinal stenosis persist.

DJD of the hip is perhaps the most disabling form of the illness, with considerable loss of function in the advanced stages. Early in the course of hip involvement pain occurs on weight bearing and is relieved by rest. Groin pain, at times referred to the knee, is most common. Nocturnal pain evolves later. On examination, the range of motion is decreased and accompanied by pain. Internal rotation of the hip and extension of the hip are the earliest to be limited. Flexion deformities evolve later in the course of the illness. Radiological examination is important to determine the extent of involvement.

Secondary DJD of the hip occurs earlier and may be unilateral. Among the various causes of secondary DJD, avascular necrosis occurs most often in the hips and may be related to underwater diving, alcoholism, corticosteroid therapy, and sickle cell disease. Pain usually antedates radiological changes, but the pain becomes severe when the subchondral bone collapses. Radiographically a characteristic wedge-shaped alteration of bone and discontinuity of the subchondral bone are noted. The destruction of cartilage and loss of subchondral bone lead to rapid development of DJD.

Occupational or sport injuries are frequent causes of degenerative changes in the knees. Torn menisci and ligamentous instability contribute to early changes. Tenderness, limitation of motion by pain, crepitation, and joint effusions may be present. The medial compartment of the knee is more often involved than the lateral compartment. The patellofemoral joint is another site of frequent involvement with DJD. On examination, movement of the knee cap causes crepitus. *Chondromalacia patellae* is typically seen in adolescents and thought to be separate from DJD. The cartilage becomes softened, fibrillated, and eroded. In adolescents lateral subluxation of the patella and trauma may lead to this entity.

Extensive DJD is found late in the course of acromegaly. The early articular changes in acromegaly include thickened synovial tissues and considerable overgrowth of the joint cartilage, presumably in response to the excessive secretion of growth hormone.

Occasionally middle-aged or older women are encountered who have an acute and transient inflammatory joint disease, particularly in the joints of the hands, in association with typical changes of DJD. These patients have tender and red distal and proximal interphalangeal joints. Subsequently Heberden's nodes evolve. Single or several joints may be involved at any one time. On radiographs these patients are seen to have developed osteophytes and subchondral sclerosis but may also have erosions of the joint surface. Periarticular osteoporosis is not present. On histological examination, mild to moderate inflammation is present during the acute phase, with lymphocyte and plasma cell infiltration and even mild pannus formation—quite similar to that in mild rheumatoid arthritis. Some observers refer to this form of DJD as "erosive osteoarthritis." Patients with this disease pattern, however, can be distinguished from patients with rheumatoid arthritis by the characteristic presentation and pattern of joint involvement, the absence of prolonged morning stiffness, absence of typical rheumatoid deformities, lack of palpable synovial hypertrophy, radiological presence of degenerative changes, and negative tests for rheumatoid factor. A weakly positive test for rheumatoid factor does not exclude erosive osteoarthritis, since normal elderly persons may have a positive test.

DIAGNOSIS The usual laboratory tests show no abnormalities in DJD. The erythrocyte sedimentation rate is normal for the age of the patient. The characteristics of joint fluid have been discussed (see Chap. 345). Radiological changes are most helpful for diagnosis. Joint pain in elderly persons without other abnormalities usually means DJD. However, caution should be exercised in ascribing joint complaints to DJD on the basis of radiographic changes alone, because spurs, lipping, and joint space narrowing also occur in rheumatoid arthritis, pseudogout, and gout and as a long-term consequence of joint space infection.

TREATMENT Following evaluation of a patient with DJD, realistic goals for treatment should be established. Reassurance is important, because patients frequently equate any joint disease with total disability. The progression of DJD tends to be slow. The presence of Heberden's nodes does not lead to loss of essential hand functions but may cause cosmetic complaints and loss of fine functions. Involvement of weight-bearing joints with DJD, however, can lead to severe disability. Steps should be taken to eliminate excessive and recurrent trauma. A weight-reduction program should be initiated for overweight individuals. Moderate exercise is recommended, but vigorous activity that produces prolonged pain and discomfort should be avoided.

Aspirin in an adequate dose (2 to 4 g per day) is the drug of choice for relief of pain. Other salicylate preparations may be equally useful (sodium salicylate, choline salicylate, salicyl salicylate). Indomethacin (25 mg tid or qid) provides relief in some patients who do not benefit from salicylates. A number of other nonsteroidal anti-inflammatory drugs such as naproxen, tolmetin, or sulindac may be tried. Phenylbutazone (100 mg bid to qid) should be employed only for short periods, and care must be exercised to detect toxicity (see Chap. 346). All these drugs may lead to gastric irritation, and occasionally to peptic ulcer.

Local heat is useful in many patients with mild DJD. In severe joint involvement, physical therapy with infrared heat, ultrasound, or hot packs may help to relieve pain. Isometric exercises may be useful, especially to strengthen the quadriceps muscle when knees are involved. Cervical traction may be helpful in relieving compression of the nerve roots.

Patients with intractable pain and advanced DJD can benefit significantly from orthopedic procedures, including debridement and removal of loose bodies, osteotomy, partial prosthetic replacement, and total joint replacement. Outstanding results have been achieved with total hip replacement in patients who were disabled by DJD of the hips. Knee and ankle replacement with prosthetics will provide relief of intractable pain and improve mobility. The potential benefits should be carefully weighed against the risks of each patient who is being considered for these procedures.

REFERENCES

Howell DS: Degradative enzymes in osteoarthritic human articular cartilage. Arthritis Rheum 18:167, 1975

——— et al: The pathogenesis of osteoarthritis. Semin Arthritis Rheum 5:365, 1976

Mankin HJ: The reaction of articular cartilage to injury and osteoarthritis. N Engl J Med 291:1285, 1974

Moskowitz RW: Clinical and laboratory findings in osteoarthritis, in *Arthritis and Allied Conditions,* 9th ed, DJ McCarty (ed). Philadelphia, Lea & Febiger, 1979, p 1161

Paine KWT et al: Clinical features of lumbar spinal stenosis. Clin Orthop 115:77, 1976

Peter JB et al: Erosive osteoarthritis of the hands. Arthritis Rheum 9:365, 1966

Ward J, Samuelson CO: Nonsteroidal anti-inflammatory drugs, in *Update II: Harrison's Principles of Internal Medicine,* KJ Isselbacher et al (eds). New York, McGraw-Hill, 1982, pp 91–110

352 PROGRESSIVE SYSTEMIC SCLEROSIS (DIFFUSE SCLERODERMA)

BRUCE C. GILLILAND
MART MANNIK

Progressive systemic sclerosis (PSS) is a multisystem disorder characterized by fibrosis that involves the skin (scleroderma) and a variety of internal organs, most notably the gastrointestinal tract, lungs, heart, and kidney. The clinical hallmark of PSS is the tight, firm skin, which may be present several years before visceral involvement becomes apparent. In some patients, however, visceral disease occurs in the absence of skin involvement. Although the disease is not always progressive, the survival of these patients is determined by the severity of visceral involvement.

ETIOLOGY AND PATHOGENESIS This disease has a worldwide distribution but is apparently rare in Asia, especially among the Chinese, Indians, and Malaysians. The onset of disease is usually in the third to fifth decades, and women are affected four times as often as men. The etiology and pathogenesis of PSS are not known, and the role of heredity has not been clarified. Several examples of familial PSS have been reported. The increased fibrosis in the various organ systems is considered to be due to the overproduction of normal collagen. Tissue culture of skin fibroblasts from patients with scleroderma synthesize increased amounts of collagen compared with appropriate controls. Qualitative abnormalities of collagen have not been documented in PSS.

The primary event in systemic sclerosis is postulated to be endothelial cell injury in blood vessels ranging from small arteries to capillaries. The cause of this endothelial damage is not known, but a serum cytotoxic factor, a nonimmunoglobulin, has been identified in some patients with systemic sclerosis. In small arteries, disruption of endothelial cells leads to platelet aggregation, myointimal cell proliferation, and fibrosis resulting in narrowing, decreased distensibility, and obliteration of the vessels. Increased vascular permeability from endothelial cell damage produces interstitial edema, fibroblast stimulation, and eventually fibrosis in the surrounding tissue. Thus, the early phase of systemic sclerosis is characterized by target organ edema followed later by fibrosis. The number of capillaries in the skin is reduced by this fibrotic process; the remaining capillaries dilate and proliferate to become visible telangiectatic lesions.

The role of immunologic abnormalities in the pathogenesis of PSS has not been established. Autoantibodies occur in this disorder, and PSS is associated with other rheumatic diseases in which immunologic mechanisms are of pathogenetic importance. In particular, patients with combined features of scleroderma, systemic lupus erythematosus, and myositis have been described. PSS is sometimes associated with Sjögren's syndrome. Biopsies of the border of spreading skin lesions contain lymphocytes, suggesting that cell-mediated immunity may participate in the genesis of the lesions. In addition, tissue antigens from the skin of scleroderma patients stimulate release of lymphokines from lymphocytes. Other evidence suggestive of immune mechanisms is the occurrence of scleroderma-like features, Sjögren's syndrome, and antinuclear antibodies in chronic graft-versus-host disease following bone marrow transplantation.

Occupational hazards have been associated with the development of PSS. The occurrence of PSS in coal and gold miners appears to be more common than in nonminers, suggesting that silica dust may be a predisposing factor. Workers exposed to polyvinyl chloride may develop Raynaud's phenomenon, acroosteolysis, and scleroderma-like skin lesions. Nail-fold capillary abnormalities similar to those observed in PSS are also present. In addition, these workers also developed hepatic fibrosis and angiosarcoma. Extensive sclerosis of the dermis and subcutaneous tissue has been noted in patients receiving pentazocine, a nonnarcotic analgesic agent. Absence of Raynaud's phenomenon and sparing of the face and distal extremities distinguish this entity from PSS.

PATHOLOGY In the skin, a thin epidermis overlies compact bundles of collagen which lie parallel to the epidermis. Fingerlike projections of collagen extend from the dermis into the subcutaneous tissue and bind the skin to the underlying tissue. Dermal appendages are atrophied, and rete pegs are lost. Increased numbers of lymphocytes identified as T cells may be present at the border of skin lesions.

In the lower two-thirds of the esophagus, the histological findings consist of a thin mucosa and increased collagen in the lamina propria, submucosa, and serosa. The degree of fibrosis is less than in the skin. Atrophy of the muscularis in the esophagus and throughout the involved portions of the gastrointestinal tract is more prominent than the amount of fibrotic replacement of muscle. Ulceration of the mucosa is often present and may be due to either PSS or superimposed peptic esophagitis. Striated muscles in the upper one-third of the esophagus are relatively spared. Similar changes may be found throughout the gastrointestinal tract, especially in the second and third portions of the duodenum, jejunum, and large intestine. Atrophy of the muscularis of the large intestine may lead to the development of large-mouth diverticula. In the later stages of the disease, the involved portions of the gastrointestinal tract become dilated. Infiltration of lymphocytes and plasma cells in the lamina propria is also present.

With pulmonary involvement, diffuse interstitial fibrosis, thickening of the alveolar membrane, and peribronchial fibrosis are observed. Bronchiolar epithelial proliferation accompanies the pulmonary fibrosis. Rupture of septa produces small cysts and areas of bullous emphysema. Small pulmonary arteries and arterioles show intimal thickening, fragmentation of the elastica, and muscular hypertrophy; this may occur without pulmonary fibrosis and produce pulmonary hypertension.

The synovium in patients with PSS and arthritis is similar to that seen in early rheumatoid arthritis and shows edema with infiltration of lymphocytes and plasma cells. Later in the disease the synovium may become fibrotic. Fibrinous deposits appear on the surfaces of tendon sheaths and in the overlying fascia, and may lead to audible creaking over moving tendons.

Histological features of muscle involvement consist of interstitial and perivascular lymphocytic infiltrations, degeneration of muscle fibers, and interstitial fibrosis. Arterioles may be thickened, and capillaries may be decreased in number.

In the heart, myocardial interstitial fibrosis replaces myocardial fibers. Fibrosis also involves the conduction system, leading to atrioventricular conduction defects and arrhythmias. The wall of smaller coronary arteries may be thickened, and lymphocytic infiltration is seen. Fibrinous pericarditis and pericardial effusions are found in some patients.

Renal involvement is found in over half the patients and consists of intimal hyperplasia of the interlobular arteries, fibrinoid necrosis of the afferent arterioles, including the glomerular tuft, and thickening of the glomerular basement membrane. These lesions result in cortical infarctions and glomerulosclerosis. The renal pathological change is often indistinguishable from that observed in malignant hypertension. Renal vascular lesions, however, may be present in the absence of hypertension. Angiographic renal studies in patients with PSS may show constriction of the intralobular arteries, a finding that simulates the vasospasm of the digital arteries observed in Raynaud's phenomenon. Along with Raynaud's phenomenon, induced by cooling, a decrease in renal blood flow has been observed. These studies are of interest because three-quarters of the deaths from renal involvement in PSS have been shown to occur in the fall and winter.

Primary liver involvement is not common, but diffuse cirrhosis, intrahepatic cholestasis, and chronic passive congestion occur occasionally. Fibrosis of the thyroid may develop. Thickening of the periodontal membrane with replacement of the lamina dura is demonstrated radiographically as widening of the periodontal space and rarely causes loosening of the teeth.

Small arterial and arteriolar lesions are found in many tissues; they consist of concentric acellular thickening of the intima with narrowing or occlusion of the lumen. These lesions are found in the digital arteries and arterioles in patients with PSS and Raynaud's phenomenon. Vascular abnormalities have been described in the lung, skin, kidney, muscle, gastrointestinal tract, pancreas, synovium, vasa vasorum, and the central nervous system. Arteritis with fibrinoid necrosis and infiltration by mononuclear cells of all three layers is occasionally observed.

CLINICAL MANIFESTATIONS PSS usually begins insidiously; the first symptoms often are Raynaud's phenomenon or symmetrical swelling or stiffness of the fingers. Raynaud's phenomenon may precede the skin changes by months or even years. Raynaud's phenomenon occurs in 90 percent of patients with the skin changes of scleroderma. In the early stages, patients may have pitting edema of the face, hands, and feet. The fingers and hands in the early stages are swollen. Subsequently the skin becomes firm, thickened, and leathery in appearance, and tightly bound to the underlying subcutaneous tissue. The skin changes spread to involve the arms, face, upper part of the chest, abdomen, and back. The lower extremities are relatively spared. The taut skin over the fingers gradually limits full extension, and fixed flexion contractures develop. Ulcers may appear on the fingertips and over bony prominences and may become infected. The soft tissue of the fingertips is lost, and in some instances the bone of terminal phalanges is resorbed. The skin may become darkly pigmented even without exposure to the sun; areas of depigmentation and numerous telangiectatic mats often appear on the skin. The skin becomes dry and coarse, and hair is lost. Examination of nail folds with a wide-angle microscope or an ophthalmoscope shows a decrease in the number of capillary loops and dilatation of the remaining loops. Similar changes are also observed in dermatomyositis. In some patients, calcific deposits develop in the subcutaneous and periarticular tissue. The overlying skin may break down, with draining of calcific material. Involvement of the face results in the loss of normal skin wrinkles, loss of facial expression, and inability to open the mouth fully. In disease of many years' duration, the hidebound skin may soften and become pliable, but it will remain atrophic.

The coexistence of *c*alcinosis, *R*aynaud's phenomenon, *e*sophageal hypomotility, *s*clerodactyly, and *t*elangiectasia has been termed the CREST syndrome and initially was considered a benign form of PSS. However, some of these patients have subsequently developed visceral and more extensive cutaneous lesions of PSS.

More than half the patients with PSS complain of pain, swelling, and stiffness of the fingers and knee joints. A symmetrical polyarthritis, resembling rheumatoid arthritis, may be seen. In more advanced stages of the disease, leathery crepitation can be palpated over moving joints, especially the knee. Extensive fibrotic thickening of the tendon sheaths in the wrist can produce a carpal tunnel syndrome. Acute myositis with proximal muscle weakness and enzyme elevation occurs in PSS and is indistinguishable from polymyositis. Patients also develop a distinctive indolent myopathy characterized by mild muscle weakness with few laboratory abnormalities.

Symptoms attributable to esophageal involvement, which are present in more than 50 percent of patients, include epigastric fullness, burning pain in the epigastric or retrosternal regions, and regurgitation of gastric contents. These symptoms, most noticeable when the patient is lying flat or bending over, are due to the reduced tone of the gastroesophageal sphincter and to dilatation of the distal esophagus. Peptic esophagitis frequently occurs and may lead to strictures and narrowing of the lower part of the esophagus. However, it seldom results in bleeding. Dysphagia, particularly of solid foods, may occur independent of other esophageal symptoms and is caused by the loss of esophageal motility due to neuromuscular dysfunction. Gastric involvement, which is not common in PSS, produces symptoms that are difficult to distinguish from esophageal symptoms. Manometry or cineradiography reveals decreased amplitude or disappearance of peristaltic waves in the lower two-thirds of the esophagus. A closer correlation exists between this finding and Raynaud's phenomenon than with cutaneous manifestations of PSS. Later in the course of the illness, dilatation and atony of the lower portion of the esophagus as well as reflux are seen. With gastric involvement, barium studies show dilatation, atony, and delayed gastric emptying.

Symptoms referable to involvement of the small intestine by PSS include bloating and abdominal pain and may suggest intestinal obstruction or paralytic ileus. Malabsorption syndrome with weight loss, steatorrhea, and anemia also occurs secondary to obliteration of the lymphatics by fibrosis or in some patients due to bacterial overgrowth in the atonic intestine. Involvement of the large intestine may cause chronic constipation and fecal impaction with episodes of bowel obstruction. Roentgenographic features of the second and third portions of the duodenum and of the jejunum include dilatation, loss of the usual feathery pattern, and delayed disappearance of barium. Pneumatosis intestinalis, which occasionally occurs in PSS, is seen as radiolucent cysts or linear streaks within the wall of the small intestine. Benign pneumoperitoneum may result from the rupture of these cysts. Barium studies of the large intestine may show dilatation, atony, and large-mouth diverticula. Some patients may have gastrointestinal PSS with little or no cutaneous or other organ involvement.

Patients with pulmonary fibrosis often complain of a dry cough and exertional dyspnea; however, shortness of breath as a presenting complaint is unusual. Bilateral basilar rales may be present. Though pleural involvement is not infrequent at postmortem, pleurisy is unusual. Restriction of chest movement may rarely occur with extensive skin involvement of the thorax. Additional pulmonary problems result from aspiration pneumonia secondary to esophageal malfunction. Superimposed bacterial or viral pneumonia may be a serious complication in patients with pulmonary fibrosis. Malignant alveolar or bronchiolar cell neoplasms have been reported in some patients with PSS and pulmonary fibrosis. However, no other association of PSS with malignancy has been shown. Pulmonary function test results are abnormal even in early disease and show a low diffusion capacity and a low P_{O_2} on exercise. Roentgenograms of the chest may show a pattern of linear densities, mottling, and honeycombing. These changes are more evident in the lower two-thirds of the lungs. Patients may develop pulmonary arterial hypertension without significant interstitial fibrosis, presumably secondary to the proliferative vascular lesion of PSS involving pulmonary arteries and arterioles. These patients complain of shortness of breath, and on physical examination they have an accentuated pulmonic second heart sound, a fixed split second heart sound, and the systolic murmur of pulmonary artery dilation. Electrocardiographic evidence of pulmonary hypertension may also be present.

Cardiac involvement by PSS often goes clinically unrecognized; however, varying degrees of heart block and arrhythmias may be seen. Cardiomyopathy attributable to diffuse myocardial fibrosis may also occur. Other cardiac manifestations may be secondary to pulmonary disease and hypertension. Left ventricular failure develops more frequently than cor pulmonale, even with the presence of pulmonary fibrosis. Acute and chronic pericarditis may develop and occasionally produce tamponade. Cardiac involvement is the cause of death in 15 percent of PSS patients.

Renal failure is the leading cause of death in PSS, accounting for almost half of the deaths. The onset of renal involvement is frequently within 3 years of the diagnosis of PSS. Renal failure, however, can present abruptly at any time in an apparently stable patient and is fatal unless treated. Acute renal failure can develop in association with malignant hypertension or in a setting of mild chronic hypertension. Proteinuria, an abnormal urine sediment, hypertension, azotemia, and microangiopathic hemolytic anemia are clinical features associated with progressive renal disease. It is difficult to predict the patient who will develop renal failure. Microangiopathic anemia may appear several weeks before renal involvement and thereby serve as an indicator of impending renal failure. The presence of chronic pericardial effusion may also be associated with subsequent renal failure.

LABORATORY FINDINGS The erythrocyte sedimentation rate may be elevated. Hypoproliferative anemia related to chronic inflammation is the most common cause of anemia in PSS. Anemia may also be caused by iron deficiency secondary to gastrointestinal bleeding. Bacterial overgrowth due to atony of the small bowel may lead to vitamin B_{12} and/or folic acid deficiency anemia. Microangiopathic hemolytic anemia is most often associated with renal involvement and the presence of fibrin deposition in the renal arterioles. Hypergammaglobulinemia, with elevated levels mainly of IgG, is found in approximately half the patients. Rheumatoid factor, in low titer, is present in 25 percent of patients. Antinuclear antibodies are reported in 40 to 80 percent of patients and include antibodies to nucleolar antigen, deoxyribonucleoprotein, and an extractable nuclear antigen with a molecular weight of 70,000 (called scleroderma-70 antigen). The latter gives a speckled pattern on immunofluorescent tests. Anticentromere antibodies are found mainly in patients with the CREST syndrome.

DIAGNOSIS The diagnosis of PSS presents no difficulty in the presence of Raynaud's phenomenon, with typical skin lesions and visceral involvement. PSS should always be included in the differential diagnosis of patients with Raynaud's phenomenon. Other causes of Raynaud's phenomenon include thoracic outlet (scalenus anticus and cervical rib) syndromes, shoulder-hand syndrome, trauma (jackhammer or vibratory machine operators), previous cold injury, vinyl chloride exposure, and circulating cryoglobulins or cold agglutinins. Linear scleroderma and morphea are localized forms of PSS and may be associated with Raynaud's phenomenon and hypergammaglobulinemia. PSS may be confused with rheumatoid arthritis, systemic lupus erythematosus, or polymyositis when articular or muscle involvement is prominent early in the disease. PSS without cutaneous involvement should be considered in patients with unexplained pulmonary fibrosis, cardiomyopathies, heart block, dysphagia, or malabsorption syndrome. Several conditions have scleroderma-like features but lack the visceral involvement. Scleredema (scleredema adultorum of Buschke) occurs predominantly in children and is characterized by painless edematous induration involving the face, scalp, neck, trunk, and proximal portions of the extremities. Involvement of the hands and feet usually does not occur. Scleredema may be associated with previous streptococcal infection and is usually self-limited, resolving in 6 to 12 months. Histology reveals accumulation of mucopolysaccharides in the dermis and skeletal muscle. A rare entity, scleromyxedema (lichen myxedematosus), is manifested by yellowish papules and may involve the face and hands. Acid mucopolysaccharide deposits are found in the dermis. Monoclonal IgG may be detected in some of these patients. Primary amyloidosis may involve the skin of the extremities and face diffusely to give the appearance of scleroderma. Biopsy will clearly differentiate these entities.

Diffuse fasciitis with eosinophilia A scleroderma-like syndrome consisting of fasciitis, myositis, eosinophilia, and hypergammaglobulinemia has been recognized. Patients usually do not have Raynaud's phenomenon or develop sclerodactyly.

Systemic involvement seldom occurs. Several patients with eosinophilic fasciitis have been reported to have aplastic anemia; however, the significance of the association is not understood. Patients develop tenderness and swelling of the extremities with the onset of symptoms often related to strenuous physical exertion. The skin is firmly bound over areas of nonpitting induration. Biopsy shows perivascular infiltration of histiocytes, eosinophils, lymphocytes, and plasma cells in the dermis, subcutaneous fat and fascia, and underlying muscle. Improvement has been noted with administration of corticosteroids, but spontaneous improvement has also been recorded.

Mixed connective tissue disease This rheumatic syndrome describes patients with clinically overlapping features of scleroderma, systemic lupus erythematosus, and polymyositis. Not all investigators agree that this syndrome is a separate entity but consider it as part of the spectrum of PSS or systemic lupus erythematosus. The serums of all these patients have hemagglutinating antibody specific for an extractable nuclear antigen which is composed largely of ribonucleoprotein and produces a speckled pattern on fluorescent antibody testing. High titers of antibody to nuclear ribonucleoprotein are found in almost all patients with the mixed connective tissue disease, even during clinical remissions. High titers of this antibody, however, are also found in some patients with systemic lupus erythematosus, discoid lupus, rheumatoid arthritis, and progressive systemic sclerosis.

Arthralgias or arthritis is present in most patients with mixed connective tissue disease, but deformities are infrequent. An erythematous rash, similar to that seen in systemic lupus erythematous (SLE), is observed in some patients. In most patients the clinical appearance of the skin over the hands is similar to that seen in scleroderma. Telangiectatic lesions are frequently present. Most patients do not develop severe ulcerations on the digits. Biopsy of skin may show abnormalities comparable with scleroderma; some patients may have immunoglobulin deposits at the dermoepidermal junction similar to patients with SLE. Raynaud's phenomenon and esophageal hypomotility occur frequently. Some patients show heliotropic discoloration of the upper eyelids, and erythematous patches over the dorsum of the fingers similar to those observed in dermatomyositis; myalgias, proximal muscle weakness, elevated levels of muscle enzymes, and electromyographic changes of myositis are found in the majority of patients. Pulmonary abnormalities are common and include decreased diffusing capacity, diffuse interstitial infiltrates, and pleural disease. Occasionally pulmonary involvement is the predominant symptom and is expressed as exertional dyspnea and/or pulmonary hypertension. Other features are pericarditis, trigeminal neuropathy, generalized lymphadenopathy, and splenomegaly. Renal involvement is uncommon and usually mild; however, some patients develop progressive renal failure. Mesangial changes, focal nephritis, or diffuse membranous nephritis are the most frequently observed findings on renal biopsy. Granular deposits consisting of IgG and C3 have been observed in the glomerular basement membrane. Circulating immune complexes are detected in some patients. Anemia, leukopenia, and diffuse hypergammaglobulinemia are often present and respond to glucocorticosteroids. The inflammatory aspects of this disease, such as fever, rash, arthritis, and myositis, all show a favorable response to glucocorticosteroids. The sclerodermal skin manifestations, if treated early, and the pulmonary diffusing capacity may also improve with steroid therapy.

PROGNOSIS In the majority of patients PSS is characterized by a prolonged, relentless course of progressive skin and/or visceral involvement. In some patients remissions occur, including partial improvement of the skin, and the disease progresses slowly; 80 percent of one group of patients were alive 2 years after onset of symptoms, and 20 percent were alive 10 years after onset. Patients with mainly skin involvement have a more gradual and favorable course than those with visceral disease, especially of the heart, kidney, and lung. Among Caucasians the prognosis is worse in males than in females, and it is worse in patients whose onset of disease occurs after 45 years of age. The disease tends to be more severe in blacks, especially in black females. Death stems most often from cardiac, renal, and pulmonary involvement.

TREATMENT Effectiveness of drug therapy in PSS is difficult to evaluate because of the variable course and severity of the disease. Many drugs have been used in the treatment of PSS without any consistent or prolonged benefit. In uncontrolled studies D-penicillamine has been reported to reduce skin thickening and prevent development of significant organ involvement. Reports of beneficial effects of colchicine or chlorambucil have not been documented in controlled studies. Even though no drug or combination of drugs has been proved to stop this disease, management directed at the involved organ systems may prolong life and improve the quality of life.

The management of Raynaud's phenomenon is directed at control of vasospasm. It is important to prevent periods of vasospasm since the resulting ischemia may be a further stimulant for vascular fibrosis and eventual obliteration. Patients should be advised to dress warmly and wear mittens and socks, not to smoke, to remove causes of external stress, and to avoid drugs such as amphetamine and ergotamine. Warmth of the central body induces peripheral vasodilation. Drugs that block sympathetic vasoconstriction, such as reserpine, guanethidine, α-methyldopa, phenoxybenzamine, and prazosin may be useful in the treatment of Raynaud's phenomenon, but their side effects often curtail extended use. Techniques of biofeedback have also been used with variable success for teaching patients to control the temperature of their hands. Surgical sympathectomy usually provides only temporary improvement, and it, along with other forms of therapy, does not prevent progression of the vascular lesion. The response to any therapy for Raynaud's phenomenon is limited by the degree of existing structural narrowing of digital arteries.

Numerous drugs have been claimed to soften the hidebound skin, but documentation in controlled studies is lacking. These drugs include D-penicillamine, colchicine, *p*-aminobenzoic acid, vitamin E, and dimethyl sulfoxide (DMSO). Dryness of the skin may be reduced by avoiding frequent use of detergent soaps and by applying regularly hydrophilic ointments and bath oils. Regular exercise helps to maintain flexibility of extremities and pliability of skin. Massaging the skin several times a day may also be beneficial. Skin ulcers should be kept clean by soaking or by surgical or chemical debridement. Sympatholytic drugs or local nitroglycerine paste may be beneficial in promoting healing. Infected ulcers can usually be treated with topical antibiotics.

Patients with reflux esophagitis are treated with small frequent meals, antacids between meals, and elevation of the head of the bed. Patients should be advised not to lie down for a few hours after a meal, and to avoid coffee, tea, and chocolate, which reduce the pressure of the lower esophageal sphincter. Cimetidine may be beneficial in some patients. Patients with dysphagia should be instructed to chew their food thoroughly and wash it down with fluids. Malabsorption syndrome due to duodenal hypomotility and bacterial overgrowth may improve with intermittent use of appropriate antibiotics. Stool softeners and mild laxatives are usually adequate for the constipation due to involvement of the colon.

Acute myositis is usually responsive to glucocorticosteroids; these drugs should not be used for the indolent form of muscle disease of PSS. Articular symptoms are treated with aspirin or other nonsteroidal anti-inflammatory agents.

The pulmonary fibrosis of PSS is not reversible, and therefore the treatment is directed at symptoms or complications. Pulmonary infection requires prompt treatment with antibiotics. Hypoxia necessitates giving low concentrations of oxygen. The role of glucocorticosteroids in preventing progression of interstitial lung disease is not clear. Pulmonary hypertension in patients with minimal or no interstitial fibrosis may respond to glucocorticosteroids.

Recognition of early renal failure is important in order to preserve remaining function. Renal involvement is usually accompanied by hypertension, but occasional patients may be normotensive. Since most patients have increased renin, drugs that block the renin-angiotensin pathway may be effective in stabilizing or reversing renal failure, as well as lowering the blood pressure. These drugs include propranolol, clonidine, and minoxidil. Another effective drug in treating the renal failure of PSS is captopril, which is an inhibitor of angiotensin converting enzyme. Dialysis may be required in patients with progressive renal failure.

Patients with cardiac failure require careful monitoring of digitalis and diuretic administration. Pericardial effusions may also improve with diuretics. Care should be taken to avoid overdiuresis which may lead to decreased effective plasma volume, decreased cardiac output, and renal failure.

REFERENCES

Battle WM et al: Abnormal colonic motility in progressive systemic sclerosis. Ann Intern Med 94:749, 1981

LeRoy EC: Scleroderma (systemic sclerosis), in *Textbook of Rheumatology,* WN Kelley et al (eds). Philadelphia, Saunders, 1981, chap 76, pp 1211–1230

Maricq HR, LeRoy EC: Progressive systemic sclerosis: Disorders of the microcirculation. Clin Rheum Dis 5:81, 1979

Rodnan GP: Progressive systemic sclerosis (scleroderma), in *Arthritis and Allied Conditions,* 9th ed, DJ McCarty (ed). Philadelphia, Lea & Febiger, 1979, pp 762–809

——— et al: Morphologic changes in the digital arteries of patients with progressive systemic sclerosis (scleroderma) and Raynaud's phenomenon. Medicine 59:393, 1980

Sharp GC: Mixed connective tissue disease and overlap syndromes, in *Textbook of Rheumatology,* WN Kelley et al (eds). Philadelphia, Saunders, 1981, chap 71, pp 1151–1161

Shulman LE: Diffuse fasciitis with eosinophilia: A new syndrome. Arthritis Rheum 20:S205, 1977

353
MISCELLANEOUS ARTHRITIDES AND EXTRAARTICULAR RHEUMATISM

MART MANNIK
BRUCE C. GILLILAND

HYPERTROPHIC OSTEOARTHROPATHY Hypertrophic osteoarthropathy is characterized by the presence of periosteal inflammation and new bone formation, arthritis, and clubbing of the digits. This syndrome frequently results from disorders in the lungs and hence is called *hypertrophic pulmonary osteoarthropathy.* It also occurs in association with disorders of other organs, as well as in familial and idiopathic forms.

In hypertrophic osteoarthropathy the periosteum becomes hyperemic and edematous and is infiltrated with mononuclear cells. The periosteum is lifted, and new bone matrix is put down and calcified. At the same time endosteal bone is resorbed. These changes occur at the distal ends of long bones, at the wrists and ankles, as well as in the metacarpal and metatarsal bones. With progression of the disease, these changes may affect ribs, clavicles, and scapulae. The synovial membrane and joint capsule show edema and mild, chronic inflammation. At the same time soft-tissue edema, fibroblast proliferation, and minimal mononuclear infiltration lead to enlargement of the distal ends of digits, a process termed *clubbing.*

The mechanisms that cause hypertrophic osteoarthropathy are not known, but arteriovenous shunts and humoral and neurogenic factors are suspected because the process may be reversed upon correction of cardiac shunts, removal of pulmonary tumors, and vagotomy.

Hypertrophic osteoarthropathy occurs in 5 to 10 percent of patients with primary intrathoracic malignancies, notably bronchogenic carcinomas and pleural tumors, but is very rare with metastatic tumors of the lung. Chronic suppurative lung lesions, such as lung abscesses, bronchiectasis, and empyema, are frequent causes of hypertrophic osteoarthropathy. However, with decline of these problems, due to antibiotics, tumors are now the most frequent cause. This disorder also may accompany cyanotic cardiac malformations, biliary cirrhosis, ulcerative colitis, and regional enteritis. When no associated disorders have been identified, the disorder is called *idiopathic hypertrophic osteoarthropathy.* Hereditary hypertrophic osteoarthropathy (pachydermoperiostitis) is a disorder characterized by marked thickening of skin of the limbs and face, in addition to the typical features of hypertrophic osteoarthropathy.

Hypertrophic osteoarthropathy frequently occurs with digital clubbing but may precede clubbing or develop without it. Similarly, clubbing of the digits occurs without any evidence of hypertrophic osteoarthropathy. Hypertrophic osteoarthropathy may cause mild arthralgias. Other patients develop severe burning pain in the hands and feet. Erythema and effusions may involve wrists, ankles, and metacarpophalangeal or metatarsophalangeal joints. Tenderness is likely to be present in the joints of these patients as well as over the adjacent bones. Dependency may aggravate these symptoms. At times the periosteal changes evolve without symptoms.

The synovial fluid of these patients usually has a total white blood cell count of less than 500 per cubic millimeter with only a few neutrophils.

Radiographs show increased thickness of the periosteum with new bone formation over the distal ends of bones. However, this may not be evident if the symptoms and signs have been present for only a short time. Lung lesions and other associated diseases must be sought. No specific laboratory tests are available for the diagnosis of hypertrophic osteoarthropathy, and its treatment must be directed toward search for and management of the underlying disorder. The symptoms may be controlled with aspirin or with analgesics. The symptoms and signs of hypertrophic osteoarthropathy may abate completely with treatment of empyema, abscess, or bronchiectasis or upon removal of the tumor.

NEUROPATHIC JOINT DISEASE Neuropathic joint disease, also called *Charcot joints,* develops in a variety of neurological disorders in which proprioception and/or deep pain sensation are disrupted. Increased trauma and stress are thought to occur during joint motion because of relaxation of the supporting structures of the joint. This leads to degeneration of cartilage, recurrent fractures of subchondral bone, and marked proliferation of adjacent bone. Neuropathic joint disease usually involves the knees, hips, ankles, and lumbar spine in tabes dorsalis; the tarsometatarsal, metatarsophalangeal, and tarsal joints in diabetic neuropathy; and the shoulders, elbows, and cervical spine in syringomyelia. Neuropathic joints also occur in meningomyelocele, congenital insensitivity to pain, leprous neuropathy, and peripheral nerve injuries.

On pathologic examination, cartilage degeneration, loose bodies, and marginal osteophytes are seen. The osteophytes are larger and more disorganized than in degenerative joint disease. Fractures occur in the articular facets, osteophytes, epicondyles, or condyles, with callus formation and further osteophyte formation. This process ultimately results in disorganization of the joints, which is characteristic of this disease. These alterations of the bone and joint space are easily recognized radiologically. The synovium shows fibrosis, fragments of calcified cartilage, and hemosiderin deposits.

Neuropathic joint disease, regardless of the underlying disorder, begins insidiously in a single joint and then progresses to involve other joints. The distribution of involved joints is influenced by the underlying neurological disorder. The involved joint enlarges because of effusion and overgrowth of bone; instability develops later. The discomfort is strikingly mild in relation to the structural abnormalities. Intraarticular fractures may cause sudden onset of pain. Examination may show increased mobility and instability. Effusions are common. Crepitus is frequent and marked in the late stages of disease. Many loose bodies may give the joint a feeling of a "bag of bones." The synovial fluid leukocyte count is low, comparable with osteoarthritis, but these fluids tend to be bloody and xanthochromic owing to intraarticular bleeding.

To diagnose a neuropathic joint, the underlying neurological disorder must be identified, but the treatment of the underlying neuropathologic condition seldom influences the progression of the joint disease. Therefore, the treatment should be directed to providing stability and relief of pain. External supports are useful, but the braces have to be carefully adjusted and checked, since patients with neurological disorders are not sensitive to maladjustments. Arthrodesis may provide stability, but these procedures are frequently accompanied by nonunion.

ARTICULAR PROBLEMS IN RENAL HOMOTRANSPLANTATION AND CHRONIC HEMODIALYSIS One to several months after renal homotransplantation, about a third of the recipients develop musculoskeletal complaints. *Avascular necrosis* of bone may occur in these patients. The hips are most frequently involved, but other joints may be affected as well. Corticosteroid therapy is thought to contribute to this problem. Some patients have only transient musculoskeletal pain; in others acute or chronic synovitis and joint effusions may occur. The cause of these abnormalities has not been elucidated. The joint symptoms may last for months and tend to appear first after reduction of steroid dosage. These patients, as well as about 90 percent of all transplant recipients, develop positive tests for rheumatoid factor, but the significance of this remains unknown.

During chronic hemodialysis some patients develop extensive periarticular calcifications. Acute inflammation may evolve at these sites. Phenylbutazone can suppress the attacks, and lowering of serum phosphorus can prevent or dissolve the deposits.

SARCOID ARTHRITIS See Chap. 235.

ARTHROPATHY OF HEMOCHROMATOSIS See Chap. 97.

ARTHRITIS OF FAMILIAL MEDITERRANEAN FEVER See Chap. 236.

HEMOPHILIC ARTHRITIS See Chap. 334.

ARTHRITIS OF LIPID DISORDERS AND LIPID STORAGE DISEASES (See Chap. 103) Patients with familial hyperbetalipoproteinemia may have transient polyarthritis. This synovitis reaches the maximum intensity within 24 h and subsides in 48 h. The joint involvement is migratory, affecting several joints in sequence. The knees and proximal interphalangeal joints are involved most commonly; the ankles, wrists, elbows, shoulders, and hips are less frequently affected. Morning stiffness may be present. The joints may be swollen and erythematous. The synovial fluid has noninflammatory characteristics (less than 400 white blood cells per cubic millimeter) and has good viscosity. The attacks of this migratory arthritis last about a week and occur a few times per year. The cause of this synovitis is not known. Crystals have not been found in synovial fluid. In contrast to podagra, the attacks do not have nocturnal onset but may be brought on by increased activity.

PIGMENTED VILLONODULAR SYNOVITIS Pigmented villonodular synovitis usually affects a single joint, most commonly the knee. However, hip, ankle, tarsus, carpus, and elbow may be involved. The cause of this disorder is unknown. The synovium is brownish in color and covered with elongated and enlarged villi; fusion of villi leads to formation of pedunculated nodules. Histologically the synovial lining cells appear normal, but the stroma of the villi contains large numbers of round and polyhedral cells. Hemosiderin granules and cholesterol crystals are abundant in the cytoplasm of synovial cells and in the interstitial spaces. Multinucleated giant cells may be present. Invasion of other tissues does not occur, but erosion of adjacent bone is seen.

The clinical picture of pigmented villonodular synovitis is characterized by the insidious onset of monarticular swelling in young adults, accompanied by pain. These symptoms tend to be continuous, but exacerbations occur from time to time. Radiological examination may show narrowing of the joint space, bone erosion, and subchondral cysts. The synovial fluid frequently contains blood and is dark brown, indicative of previous episodes of bleeding from the synovium. In some patients, however, the fluid is clear and yellow.

Complete removal of the affected synovium is recommended. With incomplete synovectomy, recurrences are common. Irradiation has been used successfully in some patients.

A localized lesion histologically similar to nodular tenosynovitis occurs in the fingers or as an intraarticular nodule, most often in the knee. The latter will cause symptoms similar to other intraarticular derangements.

TRAUMATIC ARTHRITIS Joints are subjected to many forms of trauma. The immediate damage may include capsular tears, detachment of menisci and joint cartilage, laceration of cartilage, and articular fractures. As a result of such damage hemorrhagic effusions are frequent. The product of such effusions changes to a serous, amber-colored fluid within 2 to 3 weeks. Bleeding may occur from injury of the synovial membrane alone, without damage to bone or cartilage.

The symptoms of joint trauma are obviously confined to the damaged joint. Swelling, ecchymoses, muscular spasms, and tenderness tend to be present. Pain, particularly on motion, is characteristic. Radiological examination is essential to exclude fractures. Obvious rupture of ligaments must be excluded on examination, but internal derangement of the joint may become apparent only later. Air-contrast arthrograms are helpful in defining internal derangements, particularly meniscal tears.

Treatment should include rest and removal of large hemorrhagic effusions. Physical therapy is necessary during convalescence. Orthopedic evaluation should be obtained when repair of tendons, ligaments, or bone or the removal of menisci may be required. Severe damage to a joint hastens the onset of degenerative joint disease.

Patients frequently attribute the onset of a generalized joint disease to trauma. The diagnosis of *traumatic arthritis* should be reserved for patients in whom (1) a specified traumatic insult was severe enough to produce acute pain, swelling, effusion, and dysfunction of the affected joint, (2) the affected joint(s) alone shows the abnormalities mentioned, and (3) these abnormalities did not exist prior to trauma.

RELAPSING POLYCHONDRITIS Relapsing polychondritis is a disease of unknown cause that leads to inflammation and destruction of cartilage. The cartilage loses its characteristic basophilic staining with hematoxylin and eosin. The chondrocytes degenerate, and the cartilage is fragmented and replaced by fibrous connective tissue. Lymphocytes and plasma cells are present at the interface between cartilage and scar tissue. Cell-mediated immunity to cartilage may play an important role in the pathogenesis of this disease.

This disorder occurs predominantly in middle age. Involvement of the ears and nose is most common (in 80 to 90 percent of patients). The disease activity fluctuates and involves different sites. The affected ears or nose become swollen and tender. The destruction of cartilage leads to floppy ears and a collapsed nose. Hearing loss may ensue from collapse of the external auditory meatus. Fever and arthralgias are frequent. Involvement of the larynx, trachea, and bronchi leads to hoarseness, recurrent pulmonary infections, stenosis, and even acute suffocation from collapse of the cartilaginous structures. Episcleritis is seen in about 60 percent of patients. Aortic regurgitation occurs occasionally.

No specific laboratory tests are available, but the erythrocyte sedimentation rate is usually elevated, and mild anemia occurs. Biopsy of cartilage is helpful in establishing the diagnosis. Glucocorticosteroids in moderate doses suppress the disease's activity.

TIETZE'S SYNDROME Tietze's syndrome consists of swelling, pain, and tenderness in the upper costochondral cartilages. The cause of this disorder is unknown. This syndrome tends to evolve gradually but may be acute. Patients often associate the onset with trauma. The involved costochondral joints are swollen and tender but not warm, and the disorder must be differentiated from bacterial infections, rheumatoid arthritis, and other inflammatory arthritides. Single joints are frequently involved, and multiple joint involvement tends to be unilateral. The location and character of the pain may mimic the symptoms of myocardial infarction. Injection with procaine and corticosteroids tends to provide relief. Excision has been tried. Analgesics and physical therapy have been helpful sporadically.

BURSITIS AND TENOSYNOVITIS Bursitis is defined as an inflammation of unknown cause of any of the many bursas between tendons, muscles, and bony prominences. The most common type of bursitis occurs in the shoulder. Other common types of bursitis are *trochanteric bursitis* (bursas around the gluteus medius insertion to the trochanter of the femur), which causes pain on external rotation of the hip and is recognized by tenderness over the trochanteric area; *olecranon bursitis,* recognized by tenderness and inflammation at the point of the elbow; *ischiatic bursitis* (also called "weaver's bottom"), in which tenderness is present over the ischial tuberosities and is caused by prolonged sitting on hard surfaces; *prepatellar bursitis* (also called "housemaid's knee") produced by frequent or prolonged kneeling; *anserine bursitis,* an inflammation of the sartorius bursa, in which tenderness is present at the insertion of the conjoined tendon of the sartorius, semitendinosus, and gracilis muscles on the medial aspect of the tibia, and in which characteristically pain occurs on ascending or descending stairs.

In the shoulder, *subacromial bursitis* and *bicipital tenosynovitis* are the most common problems. In the former the supraspinatus tendon becomes inflamed where it passes under the subacromial bursa. Calcifications are frequently seen adjacent to the tendon, but the presence of calcium does not necessarily relate to the symptoms. With acute subacromial bursitis or supraspinatus tendinitis, the onset of symptoms is sudden and the pain may be severe. Any abduction or external rotation causes agony. Marked tenderness is present over the lateral humeral head below the acromion. In chronic forms, a nagging, intermittent pain may be present, particularly during any motion that includes abduction and rotation of the shoulder.

Bicipital tenosynovitis consists of inflammation of the synovial sheath of the tendon of the long head of the biceps as it passes through the bicipital groove of the humeral head. In the acute form of this illness, pain develops along the biceps area and may radiate to the forearm. Abduction and forceful supination cause an increase in pain. Marked tenderness is present over the bicipital groove. In chronic bicipital tenosynovitis the symptoms are milder but tenderness is present. Muscle atrophy and adhesive capsulitis of the shoulder may develop because of decreased usage. At times chronic inflammation may lead to rupture of the involved tendon.

The treatment of any type of bursitis should include rest, analgesics, and physical therapy upon recovery from the acute phase, to prevent loss of function. Salicylates, phenylbutazone, or other nonsteroidal anti-inflammatory drugs may be helpful. Injection of glucocorticosteroids and local anesthetics hastens recovery and provides marked relief from acute symptoms.

The *frozen shoulder* (termed *adhesive capsulitis* by some) can be the product of intrinsic disease such as bicipital tenosynovitis, immobilization for fractures, or trauma, but in most elderly patients an antecedent cause is not evident. Reflex sympathetic dystrophy is thought to be a significant factor in the development of a frozen shoulder. Disuse and inactivity of the shoulder appear to contribute to the development of this syndrome. The term *adhesive capsulitis* has been used since inflammation of the entire capsule of the glenohumeral joint has been noted, but fibrotic thickening of the capsule without inflammation has also been found. The shoulder pain may progress rapidly or advance gradually to constant pain and inability to use the joint. Tenderness on palpation is found in several areas around the shoulder. Osteoporosis of the shoulder is often present on radiological examination. The symptoms may abate spontaneously in several months or may lead to permanent disuse of the joint. Progressive exercises and nonsteroidal anti-inflammatory drugs provide relief in some patients. Local or even systemic steroids have been helpful in others. Frequent encouragement of patients appears beneficial in this slowly resolving problem.

Tenosynovitis (inflammation of the synovial lining of tendons) occurs with other types of rheumatic disease (rheumatoid arthritis, systemic lupus erythematosus, gout), in bacterial infections (gonococcal, tuberculous), secondary to trauma, and without known causes (idiopathic).

REFLEX SYMPATHETIC DYSTROPHY SYNDROME The reflex sympathetic dystrophy syndrome is a symptom complex characterized by pain, swelling, trophic skin changes, and vasomotor instability in an extremity, usually precipitated by trauma, myocardial infarction, or neurological diseases. Shoulder-hand syndrome and Sudeck's atrophy are the most commonly encountered varieties of reflex sympathetic dystrophy syndrome.

The onset of reflex sympathetic dystrophy syndrome is related to an identifiable event or underlying disease in over two-thirds of patients, including musculoskeletal trauma, myocardial infarction, and central or peripheral nervous system disorders. The pathogenic mechanisms by which these disorders lead to the syndrome remain unknown, but disturbances in the functions of the autonomic nervous system have been evoked.

This syndrome occurs in all age groups and affects males and females equally. In medical practice, however, older persons predominate because of the increased prevalence of underlying disease. In a surgical practice younger persons are more commonly encountered whose disorder is due to trauma.

The affected extremity is distally painful and swollen; the pain may be described as burning in character and involving the entire hand or foot. On examination the entire foot or hand is swollen and extremely tender; these findings, however, may be more pronounced in periarticular areas. The swelling tends to be pitting in character but may become nonpitting. Later, the skin becomes thin and shiny, and superficial desquamation may develop. In some patients increased hair growth may be present, while in others hair loss is found. Thickening of the palmar fascia may be present and develop into Dupuytren's contractures. The vasomotor instability may present as vasoconstriction with cool, pale distal extremities or as vasodilation with warm, red hands or feet with increased perspiration. Frank Raynaud's phenomenon may develop in some patients. With involvement of the upper extremity the shoulder-hand syndrome may develop with shoulder pain and loss of range of motion in this joint. In some patients tenderness and swelling of the contralateral extremity occurs.

The reflex sympathetic dystrophy syndrome can be thought of in three overlapping phases. The initial phase may begin weeks to months after the precipitating event and consists of pain, swelling, and vasomotor disturbances described above. This phase may persist for 3 to 6 months. The above findings subside and the trophic changes in the skin predominate. These findings during the ensuing several months evolve into atrophy of the skin and the development of contractures, leaving the patient with an atrophic, contracted but painless extremity. During the first two phases the abnormalities are potentially reversible, but the last phase is highly refractory to therapy.

The usual laboratory tests are not useful in the diagnosis of the reflex sympathetic dystrophy syndrome and usually reflect only the underlying disease. The x-rays of the affected extremity disclose a rather characteristic patchy or mottled osteopenia. This finding, however, is not pathognomonic and can be seen with disuse osteopenia caused by immobilization or paralysis. In the late phase of the disease the bones give a ground-glass appearance on the radiography. Radionuclide scans with technetium pertechnetate or other similar agents disclose increased uptake in the periarticular areas of the affected extremity and provide objective evidence for involvement of the contralateral side.

The treatment of the reflex sympathetic dystrophy syndrome should begin early. Appropriate mobilization of patients with trauma, myocardial infarcts, and stroke may help to prevent this syndrome. Once the symptoms have started, nonsteroidal anti-inflammatory drugs, analgesics, moderate exercise, and cold or heat applications may prove useful. If these measures provide no relief in 2 to 3 weeks, a course of glucocorticosteroids over a period of 2 to 3 weeks can relieve the symptoms in a high percentage of patients. For example, 60 to 80 mg of prednisone in divided doses is recommended for a period of up to 4 days, followed by tapering the dose at 2- to 4-day intervals. The total period of treatment should last no longer than 3 weeks. In one study, the majority of patients improved on this program, while patients treated with stellate ganglion blockade did not respond.

FIBROSITIS Fibrositis is a nonarticular form of rheumatism characterized by chronic generalized aching and stiffness with persistent tender points in specific areas. The examination of joints is otherwise normal and laboratory tests are normal. Middle-aged females are most commonly affected. The cause of this entity is not known.

The prevalence of fibrositis is not known but it is believed to be among the top five most common rheumatic conditions. The diagnosis of this condition is often not made due to lack of recognition of the symptom complex and the absence of adequate criteria for the diagnosis.

The onset of fibrositis occurs most commonly between the ages of 25 and 40 but is found in younger and older persons as well. The prevalence is about five times higher in females than males. Generalized aches, pains, and stiffness are the most common complaints. These symptoms tend to be more prominent in the morning or evening and are enhanced by changes in the weather. The aching is increased by inactivity and relieved by moderate physical exercise. These patients also complain frequently of generalized fatigue, insomnia, headaches, and anxiety. Patients often describe swelling of joints or of periarticular areas; on examination, however, no evidence of synovitis is found. On physical examination characteristically tender spots are found in the same areas on repeated examinations. These occur (in decreasing frequency) at the upper border of the trapezius muscles, medial aspect of the knees, lateral aspect of the elbows, posterior iliac crests, lumbar spine areas, medial aspect of elbows, and the areas over the sternocleidomastoid muscles. At least five or six tender spots are present, but the number may be much higher. In these tender spots actual nodules may be palpable in some patients. Similar nontender nodules may be found in normal persons.

The diagnosis of fibrositis depends on the recognition of the symptom complex described above. Patients with other rheumatic diseases have similar complaints, but rheumatoid arthritis, systemic lupus erythematosus, polymyositis, and polymyalgia rheumatica can be excluded by physical findings and laboratory tests. Patients with fibrositis have no abnormalities of the joints other than periarticular tenderness, muscle strength is normal, and all laboratory tests and radiological examinations are normal. Fibrositis can be distinguished from psychogenic rheumatic complaints by more bizarre and inconsistent complaints in the latter situation that do not fluctuate during the day, with activity, or with changes in the weather.

In the treatment of fibrositis, physical and mental relaxation with moderate physical activity is important. Stretching exercises are particularly useful. The patients should be provided assurance that they are not suffering from a serious disorder. Salicylates or other nonsteroidal anti-inflammatory drugs provide relief. Furthermore, injections of tender spots with local anesthetics with or without long-acting glucocorticosteroids facilitate the institution of the moderate exercise program.

PSYCHOGENIC RHEUMATISM Psychogenic rheumatism is a term applied to rheumatic symptoms that are manifestations of psychoneurosis. Common complaints are stiffness and limitation of motion and painful joints, tendons, or muscles. These patients are in good general health and have no objective abnormalities of the joints and no tender spots as found in fibrositis. Radiological and laboratory studies are normal. The complaints tend to vacillate and do not fluctuate with activity and alterations in the weather, and the physical findings lack the consistency seen in fibrositis. These patients obtain no relief from nonsteroidal anti-inflammatory drugs.

CARPAL TUNNEL SYNDROME Carpal tunnel syndrome, also called *entrapment neuropathy,* may be due to tenosynovitis, trauma, edema, fibrosis, tuberculosis and other granulomatous diseases, rheumatoid arthritis, acromegaly, amyloidosis, edema of pregnancy, and premenstrual edema. Localized tenosynovitis of unknown cause is the most common basis of the carpal tunnel syndrome, particularly in middle-aged females.

Carpal tunnel syndrome is caused by pressure on the median nerve as it passes through the space formed by the bones of the wrist and the transverse carpal ligament. Any space-occupying process may cause compression and malfunction of the median nerve or other nerves similarly confined, such as the ulnar nerve or the posterior tibial nerve.

Patients with the carpal tunnel syndrome complain of numbness and/or burning pain on the palmar surface of the first three digits of the hand. This pain may be referred proximally up the arm. Characteristically the pain is more severe at night. Abduction of the thumb is weakened, and atrophy of the thenar eminence develops. Dryness of the skin over the thumb and first two fingers is frequent. Pain and tingling may be elicited by sustained flexion of the wrist or by tapping over the median nerve on the flexor surface of the wrist. Nerve conduction studies across the wrist will confirm the diagnosis.

Surgical decompression of the carpal tunnel with release of the transverse ligament and debridement is the definitive treatment when symptoms and signs persist. Analgesics, splinting, and injection of corticosteroids may provide temporary or complete relief.

TUMORS OF THE JOINTS Primary tumors of the joints are relatively uncommon but should be considered a rare cause of monarticular symptoms. In addition, primary bone tumors and metastases to bone may produce articular symptoms when adjacent to joints.

In *synovial chondromatosis* multiple metaplastic growths of cartilage occur in the synovium or tendon sheaths. Later these may calcify and become evident on radiographs. Single joints are involved and include the knee, hip, elbow, and shoulder. The involved joint may enlarge because of effusions. Pain and limitation of motion occur because of loose bodies. Synovectomy is the definitive treatment.

Hemangiomas may occur in the synovial or tenosynovial membranes. Symptoms usually develop in childhood. Bloody effusions occur. The hemangioma should be excised. *Lipomas* may occur in subsynovial fat and extend into the joint space, particularly into the knees.

Synoviomas or synovial sarcomas develop in the immediate periarticular tissues and seldom extend into the synovial cavity. These highly malignant tumors develop in adolescents or young adults. They present as a slowly growing mass adjacent to a joint. Biopsy is required for diagnosis, and radical resection is recommended for treatment.

Synovial chondrosarcoma may occur in joints or tendon sheaths.

Metastatic tumors to bone rarely extend to the synovial cavity. Destruction of adjacent bone and bloody effusions are characteristic.

REFERENCES

Arkin CR, Masi AT: Relapsing polychondritis: Review of current status and case report. Semin Arthritis Rheum 5:41, 1975

Bland JH et al: The painful shoulder. Semin Arthritis Rheum 7:21, 1977

Kozin F et al: The reflex sympathetic dystrophy syndrome (RSDS) III. Scintigraphic studies, further evidence for the therapeutic efficacy of systemic corticosteroids, and proposed diagnostic criteria. Am J Med 70:23, 1981

Massry SG et al: Abnormalities of the musculoskeletal system in hemodialysis patients. Semin Arthritis Rheum 4:321, 1975

Myers BW et al: Pigmented villonodular synovitis and tenosynovitis: A clinical epidemiologic study of 166 cases and literature review. Medicine 59:223, 1980

Rooney PJ et al: Transient polyarthritis associated with familial hyperbetalipoproteinemia. Q J Med 47:249, 1978

Schumacher HR Jr: Articular manifestations of hypertrophic pulmonary osteoarthropathy in bronchogenic carcinoma. A clinical and pathological study. Arthritis Rheum 19:629, 1976

Sinha S et al: Neuroarthropathy (Charcot joints) in diabetes mellitus. Medicine 51:191, 1972

Ward J, Samuelson CO: Nonsteroidal anti-inflammatory drugs, in *Update II: Harrison's Principles of Internal Medicine,* KJ Isselbacher et al (eds). New York, McGraw-Hill, 1982, pp 91–110

Yunus M et al: Primary fibromyalgia (fibrositis): Clinical study of 50 patients with matched normal controls. Semin Arthritis Rheum 11:151, 1981

section 11 Disorders of the central nervous system

354 DIAGNOSTIC METHODS IN NEUROLOGY

RAYMOND D. ADAMS
KEITH H. CHIAPPA
JOSEPH B. MARTIN
ROBERT R. YOUNG

The strict analysis and interpretation of the data elicited by a careful history and examination may prove to be adequate for diagnosis in clinical neurology; special laboratory tests can then do no more than corroborate the initial impression. But it more often happens that the final conclusion as to the nature of the disease is not reached by simple case study. The possibilities may be reduced to two or three, but the correct diagnosis cannot be determined. Under these conditions, one resorts to one or several of the laboratory tests outlined below.

It must be stressed that laboratory procedures should follow rather than precede clinical case study, except in emergencies when the disease threatens life and time does not allow detailed clinical observation. Laboratory procedures are but a part of the clinical method outlined in Chap. 10. They should be undertaken only for the specific purpose of obtaining certain otherwise unavailable data which should shed light on the clinical problem. Some of the procedures are costly, time-consuming, and occasionally dangerous or painful (unless done with skill); many require hospitalization and are misleading if the data are not gathered or interpreted competently. During clinical training every young neurologic physician should gain experience in each of these special procedures and learn to recognize its limitations and to interpret the results correctly. Some of these tests are regularly performed by the general physician or internist.

LUMBAR PUNCTURE AND EXAMINATION OF CEREBROSPINAL FLUID

The information yielded by the examination of the cerebrospinal fluid (CSF) is often of crucial importance.

INDICATIONS FOR LUMBAR PUNCTURE Lumbar puncture is performed for the following reasons:

1 To obtain pressure measurements and to secure a sample of CSF for cellular, chemical, and bacteriologic examination.
2 To aid in therapy by the administration of spinal anesthetics and occasionally antibiotics or antitumor agents.
3 To inject air, as in pneumoencephalography; a radiopaque substance (Pantopaque) or some of the water-soluble contrast media, as in myelography; or a radioactive substance [e.g., indium or radioactive iodinated serum albumin (RISA)] for the study of the dynamics of CSF and the diagnosis of hydrocephalus.

Lumbar puncture carries a risk if the CSF pressure is high (evidenced by headache and papilledema), for it increases the possibility of a fatal cerebellar or tentorial pressure cone. In doubtful cases, it is always wise first to obtain a CT scan to exclude a mass lesion before proceeding to perform a lumbar puncture. However, if it seems important in a given case of suspected increased intracranial pressure to have the information yielded by CSF examination, the lumbar puncture may be performed with a fine-bore (no. 22 or 24) needle as the last part of the clinical study. (Note that if the pressure is over 400 mmHg, one should obtain the necessary sample of fluid and then, according to the suspected clinical disease and patient's condition, administer a unit of urea or mannitol and watch the manometer until the pressure falls.) Dexamethasone (Decadron) should be started in a dose of 4 to 6 mg every 6 h in cases of tumor, cerebral trauma, hemorrhage, and certain types of encephalitis (acute hemorrhagic leukoencephalitis, herpes simplex encephalitis).

Cisternal puncture and lateral cervical puncture (C1–C2), although safe in the hands of the expert, are too hazardous to entrust to those without experience. The lumbar puncture is to be preferred except in obvious instances of spinal block requiring a sample of cisternal fluid or myelography above the lesions, or in rare instances where infection of the skin or subcutaneous tissue render needle penetration dangerous.

Experience teaches the importance of meticulous technique. Lumbar puncture should always be done under sterile conditions. If procaine is injected in and beneath the skin, the procedure should be painless. Failure to enter the lumbar subarachnoid space after two or three trials can usually be corrected by doing the puncture with patients in the sitting position and then assisting them to lie on their side for pressure measurements and fluid removal. The "dry tap" is more often due to an improperly placed needle than to a pathologic obliteration of subarachnoid space by compressive lesion of the spinal cord or chronic adhesive arachnoiditis. A bloody tap due to transfixation of a meningeal vessel may result in hopeless confusion of the diagnosis if it is falsely interpreted as indicating hemorrhage in the subarachnoid spaces and ventricles. Lumbar puncture should be undertaken with particular care in patients with thrombocytopenia or disorders of blood coagulation because serious hemorrhage into the extradural or intradural space may occur.

EXAMINATION PROCEDURES Once the lumbar puncture is successful, some or all of the following aspects of the CSF should be studied: (1) pressure and "dynamics"; (2) gross appearance of CSF including centrifugation, if blood is present, to examine the supernatant for xanthochromia; (3) number and type of cells and presence of microorganisms; (4) protein, sugar, and, in special instances, analysis of pigments; (5) exfoliative cytology using Millipore filters; (6) Wassermann reaction and appropriate serologic precipitation reactions; (7) protein immunoelectrophoresis for determination of gamma globulin levels, and other special biochemical tests (for NH_3, pH, CO_2, enzymes, etc.); and (8) bacteriologic cultures and virus isolation. See the appendix for normal values of CSF.

RADIOLOGIC EXAMINATION OF SKULL AND SPINE

Plain x-rays of the skull or spinal column, according to the nature of the symptoms, constitute an indispensable part of the thorough study of traumatic, spondylitic, and neoplastic diseases but are of relatively little value in others. The procedure is relatively simple, and the findings are interpretable by most general radiologists. Space does not permit an illustration of such common findings as fractures, bone erosion, intracerebral calcifications, premature closure or separation of sutures, or alterations of skull configuration. These have been presented in Taveras and Wood's *Diagnostic Neuroradiology*.

Of more specific value in neurology and neurosurgery are five special radiologic procedures which now permit the visualization of most parts of the brain and spinal cord and their vessels.

COMPUTERIZED TOMOGRAPHY (CT SCAN) This radiologic procedure, which computerizes the absorption offered by brain, CSF, and skull to more than thirty thousand 2- to 4-mm beams of x-ray and permits visualization of the ventricles, subarachnoid space, and the major cisternal fissures and sulci in several horizontal planes (Fig. 354-1*A* to *E*), has become available in most medical centers and has replaced plain x-rays and most of the other contrast procedures such as pneumoencephalography and arteriography. It differentiates epidural, subdural, and intracerebral hemorrhages and deformities of the ventricular system from "mass" lesions, and demonstrates tumors, abscesses, granulomas [when done after an intravenous injection of meglumine diatrizoate (Renografin) or other contrast medium], as well as areas of brain edema and infarction, hydrocephalus, and brain atrophy. The simplicity of this noninvasive procedure, its low risk to patients with expanding lesions, and the low exposure to x-ray have virtually revolutionized diagnostic neurology and neurosurgery.

ANGIOGRAPHY This has been developed over the last 30 years to the point where it is a relatively safe and extremely valuable method in the diagnosis of occluded arteries, aneurysms, and vascular malformations, tumors, abscesses, and intracranial hemorrhages. Its use has diminished greatly since the advent of CT scans. Following local anesthesia, a needle or cannula can be placed percutaneously into the lumen of a bra-

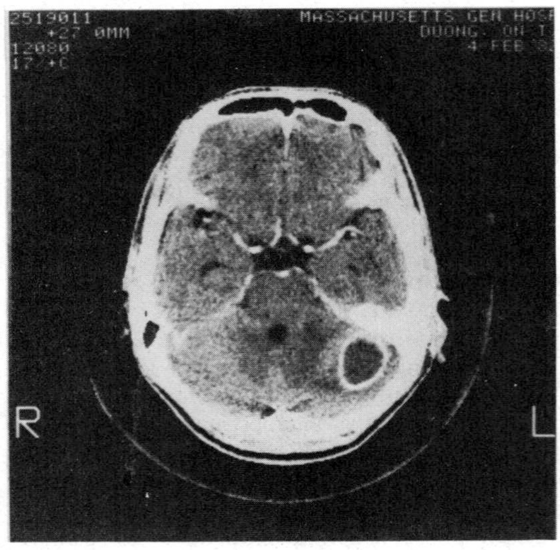

A

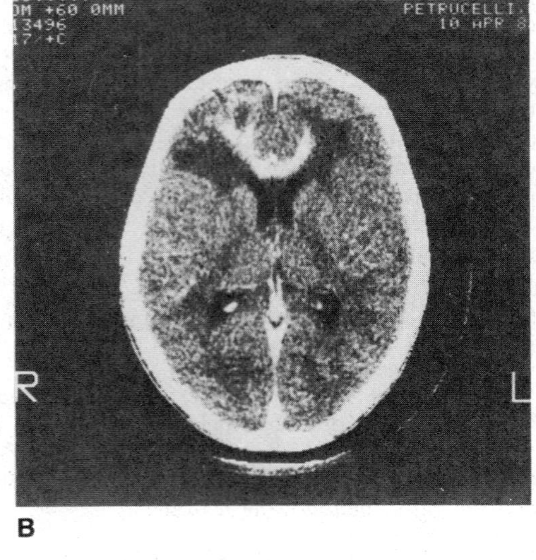

B

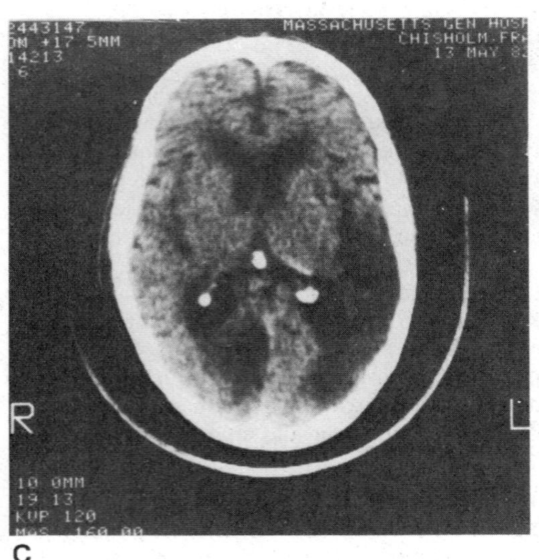

C

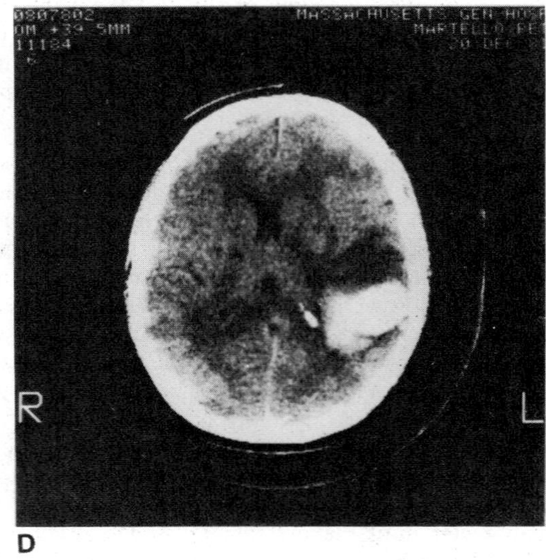

D

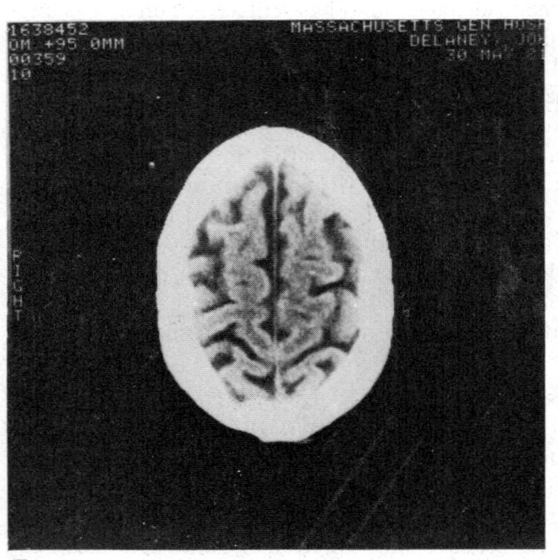

E

FIGURE 354-1
Computerized tomography scans in disease. Frontal lobes above; right hemisphere to viewer's left. A. Left cerebellar abscess arising as a complication of mastoid sinus infection. Typical "ring" enhancement is evident. B. Malignant astrocytoma infiltrating corpus callosum and bifrontal white matter. Edema surrounding tumor in frontal lobes is shown. C. Large cerebral infarcts, bilateral. Infarct on right is in distribution of posterior cerebral artery, that on left in distribution of middle cerebral artery. D. Intracerebral hematoma in left parietal lobe. Blood in hemorrhage is evident without administration of contrast media. E. Cerebral cortical atrophy in Alzheimer's disease.

chial or femoral artery and a catheter can be introduced and threaded along the aorta to cannulate the major arteries in the cervical region. Radiopaque contrast media can be injected to visualize the arch of the aorta, the origins of carotid and vertebral systems and their extent through the neck into the cranial cavity, and occasionally the spinal cord arteries. It is possible to show with clarity cerebral arteries down to about 0.1 mm lumen diameter under optimal conditions, as well as small veins of comparable size, vascular abnormalities (angiomas, aneurysms), occluded arteries, delayed circulation from increased intracranial pressure as with masses or occlusion of dural sinuses and veins, displacement of vessels by mass lesions, or complete failure of intracranial vascular filling with cerebral death. *Digital subtraction venous angiography,* which requires pressure injection of contrast dye into a brachial vein, is currently under investigation as an alternative or adjunct to arterial angiography.

PNEUMOENCEPHALOGRAPHY AND VENTRICULOGRAPHY Injection of air or oxygen into the lumbar subarachnoid space with the patient in the sitting position (pneumoencephalography) permits visualization in considerable detail of the size and position of the ventricles, the subarachnoid space (upper spinal and cerebral), and, indirectly, the structures which lie between the ventricles and the meninges. Hydrocephalus, mass lesions which displace or deform the ventricles, and atrophic states of the cerebrum are revealed by this technique. Ventriculography is accomplished by injection of air or contrast material directly into the lateral ventricles. CT scan has largely replaced both pneumoencephalography and ventriculography.

IOPHENDYLATE (PANTOPAQUE) MYELOGRAPHY AND VENTRICULOGRAPHY By injecting 5 to 15 ml iophendylate through a lumbar puncture needle and then tipping the patient on a tilt table, the entire spinal subarachnoid space may be visualized. The procedure is almost as harmless as the lumbar puncture, provided that the iophendylate is afterward removed through the needle. Ruptured lumbar and cervical disks and spinal cord tumors can be diagnosed accurately. Intraventricular injection of iophendylate is occasionally done to visualize the third and fourth ventricles and the aqueduct of Sylvius in tumors of the posterior fossa when air does not enter from below. In some clinics, air has been used instead of iophendylate to visualize masses within the spinal canal. It is of particular value when combined with polytomography in visualizing the size and position of the spinal cord and its relation to spondylotic bars and spurs. Water-soluble contrast media (e.g., metrizamide) that are self-absorbing have recently become available. Metrizamide injected in the lumbar CSF affords the additional advantage of assessing the subarachnoid space in the body CT scan. The body CT scan allows accurate visualization of the spinal canal at any level and the spinal cord and canal can be seen. It reveals tumors, ruptured disks, etc. that compress or displace the spinal canal and roots and also destructive lesions of the vertebrae. The latter may also be evident in bone scans.

RADIOACTIVE ISOTOPES Radioactive isotopes, such as technetium, are in regular use for the visualization of tumors, inflammatory masses, and some vascular lesions (brain scan) such as "watershed" infarcts that are difficult to demonstrate otherwise. Since this is a simple, noninvasive procedure, the only limitation in its use is the expense. The more the lesion disrupts the blood-brain barrier, the more consistent its demonstration by these methods. Ultrasound can also be used to show displacement of central structures of the brain by a mass lesion.

NUCLEAR MAGNETIC RESONANCE

The recent application of nuclear magnetic resonance (NMR) techniques to brain scanning has permitted visualization of cerebral lesions not evident on CT scans (Fig. 354-2). Although the full usefulness of this technique remains to be determined, the ability of NMR to delineate white matter from gray matter has already indicated its potential importance for localizing lesions in the white matter. The NMR technique, which is noninvasive, does not require exposure to ionizing radiation, and permits delineation of tissues without administration of contrast-enhancing agents, will undoubtedly greatly improve diagnostic ability in the future. Of particular value is the fact that NMR scans do not visualize bone; hence, soft tissue adjacent to bone is easily viewed, making scans through the posterior fossa particularly useful.

POSITRON EMISSION TOMOGRAPHY

Positron emission tomography (PET) is an experimental investigative technique currently available in only a few centers. The procedure involves the systemic administration of positron-emitting radionuclides of oxygen or ^{18}F 2-deoxyglucose (^{18}FDG) combined with computerized tomography. The latter permits three-dimensional localization of the disintegrating positrons with a tissue resolution of about 1 cm. Administration of labeled O_2, CO_2, and ^{18}FDG provide regional quantitation of oxygen uptake, blood flow, and glucose utilization. Studies in patients with cerebrovascular diseases, seizure disorders, and degenerative conditions have been undertaken. In stroke, PET imaging is useful in acute studies to discriminate viable from nonviable tissue. In patients with seizure disorders interictal ^{18}FDG studies may show localized areas of decreased glucose metabolism in and around a seizure focus, with increased glucose metabolism evident during a seizure. Metabolic studies with ^{18}FDG have also shown decreased glucose uptake in the striatum in patients with Huntington's disease who have normal CT scans. Although these studies show great promise in the biochemical analysis of brain functions, the cost of the instrumentation and the technology required to produce isotopes will restrict PET scanning to major medical centers.
promise in the biochemical analysis of brain functions, the cost of the instrumentation and the technology required to produce isotopes will restrict PET scanning to major medical centers.

ELECTROMYOGRAPHY (EMG)

This examination supplements the clinical study of patients with neurologic diseases which affect the neuromuscular apparatus or with primary or secondary diseases of the skeletal musculature. It is described in relation to muscle diseases (see Chap. 369).

ELECTROENCEPHALOGRAPHY (EEG)

The electroencephalographic examination is part of the clinical study of a patient suspected of having a cerebral disease; it is also used in the evaluation of the central nervous system (CNS) effects of many medical diseases.

In addition to the resting record, a number of so-called activating procedures are usually carried out.

1 The patient is requested to breathe deeply 20 times a minute for 3 min. The resulting alkalosis and cerebral vasoconstriction may activate characteristic seizure patterns or other abnormalities.

2 A very powerful light (a stroboscope) is placed over the patient's face and flashed at frequencies from 1 to 20/s with the patient's eyes opened and closed. The EEG may then show abnormal discharges in photosensitive patients.
3 The EEG is recorded after the patient is allowed to fall asleep naturally or following sedative drugs given by mouth or by vein. Procedures 1 and 2 are more commonly employed, but sleep is extremely helpful in bringing out abnormalities, especially where temporal lobe epilepsy and certain other seizures are concerned, and all too often is omitted from study.

Certain preparations are necessary if electroencephalography is to be most useful. The patient should not be sedated and should not have been for a long time without food, for both sedative drugs and relative hypoglycemia modify the normal EEG pattern. The same may be said of mental concentration, extreme nervousness, or drowsiness, all of which tend to suppress the normal alpha rhythm and increase muscle artifacts. When dealing with patients suspected of having epilepsy who are already being treated for it, most physicians prefer to record the first EEG while the patient continues to receive drugs.

TYPES OF NORMAL RECORDINGS The normal EEG in adults is usually easy to recognize. It shows somewhat asymmetric 8- to 12-Hz, 50-μV sinusoidal *alpha* waves in both occipital and parietal regions. These waves wax and wane spontaneously and usually disappear promptly when patients open their eyes or fix their attention on something. Faster waves than 13 Hz of lower amplitude (10 to 20 μV), called *beta* waves, are also seen symmetrically in the frontal regions. Very slow waves (*delta* waves), sharp waves, or other unusual patterns are absent in a normal record. When normal subjects fall asleep, the rhythm slows symmetrically, and characteristic waveforms (vertex sharp waves and sleep spindles) appear; if the sleep is induced by barbiturates or benzodiazepines, an increase in the fast frequencies is seen and is considered to be normal (see Chap. 19).

An occipital response to each flash may be seen in the normal EEG during stroboscopic stimulation and is called the evoked response, or, at faster repetition rates, photic "driving." The clinical utility of this evoked occipital response has increased the scope of electroencephalography in several ways: (1) one can be reasonably sure that a person with such a response can at least perceive light; (2) when this evoked response is absent on one side of the head but present on the other, there is physiologic evidence of a lesion interfering with normal transmission between the thalamus and the occipital lobe on this side; and (3) when the flashing light produces abnormal waves, there is evidence of increased excitability. Actual seizure patterns may be produced in the EEG if the activation procedure is continued; if the sensitivity is still greater, frank myoclonic jerks of face or arms, or, rarely, major convulsions may occur. This finding is to be differentiated from the purely muscular response, also myoclonic, produced normally in contracting scalp muscles and often visible in routine EEGs (photomyoclonus).

TYPES OF ABNORMAL RECORDINGS The most pathologic finding of all is the disappearane of the EEG pattern and its replacement by "electrocerebral silence," which means that the electrical activity of the cortical mantle, measured at the scalp, is below 2 μV and probably absent. Acute intoxication with

FIGURE 354-2
Comparison of images obtained by conventional CT scan (upper three figures) and by inversion recovery nuclear magnetic resonance (NMR) scan (lower three figures) in a patient with biopsy-proven grade II astrocytoma. The CT scan is limited by bone artifacts in lower cuts (upper left). The infiltrating tumor is easily seen in the white matter at all three levels (arrows) in the NMR scans but was not diagnosed with certainty in the conventional CT scan. (Courtesy of F Buonanno and JP Kistler.)

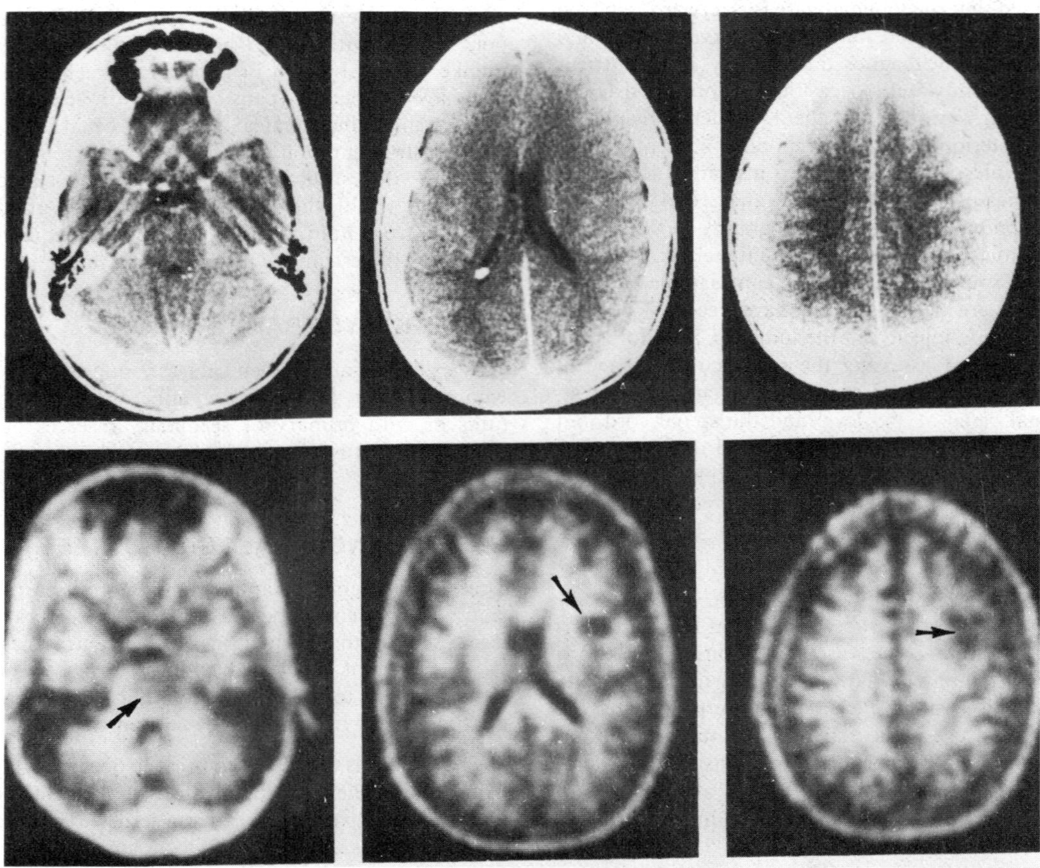

anesthetic levels of drugs, such as barbiturates, can produce this sort of isoelectric EEG. However, in the absence of CNS depressants or extreme hypothermia ($< 70°F$), a record which is "flat" (except for artifacts) all over the head is almost always a result of cerebral hypoxia or ischemia. Such a patient, without EEG activity, reflexes, spontaneous respiration, or muscular activity of any kind for 6 h or more, is said to be in "irreversible coma." The brain of such patients is largely necrotic. There is no chance for neurologic recovery, and the patient may be considered dead, despite the preservation of vegetative (cardiovascular) functions supported by mechanical means, such as respirators. There has been no exception to this statement in more than 750 patients examined at the Massachusetts General Hospital in the past 15 years.

Localized regions with absence of EEG activity may rarely be seen when there is a large area of softening or an extensive surface tumor or clot lying between the cerebral cortex and the electrodes. The localization of this abnormality is precise, but of course the nature of the lesion cannot be ascertained. Most such lesions, however, are too small, relative to the recording arrangement, to be visible, and the EEG may then record abnormal waves arising from functional, though deranged, brain at the borders of the lesion. These abnormal waves are slower and of higher amplitude than normal. Those which are less than 4 Hz with amplitude from 50 to 350 μV are called *delta* waves; those from 4 to 7 Hz are called *theta* waves; and the higher-voltage, faster waves are known as *spikes* or *sharp waves.* These fast and slow waves may be combined, and when a series of them suddenly interrupts relatively normal EEG patterns in a paroxysmal fashion, they are highly suggestive of epilepsy. The ones associated with *petit mal* (absence) spells are 3-Hz spike-and-wave complexes that characteristically appear in all leads of the EEG at the same time and disappear almost as suddenly at the end of the seizure.

NEUROLOGIC CONDITIONS WITH ABNORMAL EEG In the following groups of neurologic disorders, the EEG may be of considerable help in reaching the correct diagnosis.

Epilepsy All types of generalized epileptic seizures (grand mal and petit mal) are associated with some abnormality in the EEG, provided it is being recorded at the time. The EEG is also usually abnormal during the more restricted types of seizure activity (complex partial, myoclonic, focal and Jacksonian) (see Chap. 355). One exception is certain deep temporal lobe foci where the discharge fails to reach the scalp in sufficient amplitude to be seen against the background activity of the normal EEG, particularly if there is a strong alpha rhythm. A nasopharyngeal or sphenoidal lead may localize an epileptic focus in the medial temporal lobe, but rarely does it provide the only EEG evidence of epileptic activity. Other exceptions in which, on occasion, no EEG abnormality may be recorded during a seizure include some of the patients with other focal seizures (sensory, Jacksonian, myoclonic, and epilepsia partialis continua). This fact presumably means that the neuronal discharge is too deep, discrete, fast, or asynchronous to be transmitted by volume conduction through the skull and recorded via the EEG electrode, which is some 2 cm from the cortex. The petit mal, myoclonic jerk, and grand mal patterns correlate closely with the clinical seizure type and may be present in the interictal EEG.

A fact of importance is that between seizures as many as 20 percent of patients with petit mal and 40 percent with grand mal epilepsy show a normal EEG. Anticonvulsant therapy also tends to diminish the EEG abnormalities. The records of another 30 to 40 percent of epileptics, though abnormal between seizures, are nonspecifically so, and therefore the diagnosis of epilepsy can be made only by the correct interpretation of the clinical data in relation to the EEG abnormality.

Brain tumor, abscess, and subdural hematoma Clinically significant intracranial space-occupying lesions are characteristically associated with abnormalities in the EEG, depending on their type and location, in some 90 percent of patients. In addition to diffuse changes, the classic abnormalities are focal or localized slow-wave (usually delta), or, occasionally, seizure activity and decreased amplitude and synchronization of normal rhythms. As a rule, those lesions which expand more rapidly (abscess, some metastases, glioblastoma), especially when situated supratentorially, have the greatest frequency of EEG abnormalities (90 to 95 percent of the latter two and virtually 100 percent of abscesses). Slower growing tumors (astrocytomas) and particularly those outside the cerebral hemispheres (meningiomas, pituitary tumors) often produce no change in the EEG, though they may be very evident clinically. The EEG abnormality has the correct lateralization in as many as 75 to 90 percent of patients with supratentorial tumors or abscesses. A normal EEG and brain scan together almost exclude the presence of a supratentorial brain tumor or abscess. The EEG may be normal, however, in 20 to 25 percent of patients with infratentorial tumors.

Cerebrovascular disease Both the diffuse and localized EEG changes produced by vascular lesions such as cerebral infarcts and intracranial hemorrhages depend on their location and size rather than their type. The EEG has been shown to be useful in the differential diagnosis of vascular hemiplegia. If the lesion responsible is in the internal carotid or a major cerebral artery, an area of decreased normal activity and excessive slowing is practically always seen acutely in the appropriate region. If the hemiplegia is due to small-vessel disease, i.e., a lacunar infarction deep in the cerebrum or brainstem (Chap. 356), the EEG should be normal. Large hemispheral lesions associated with acutely depressed levels of consciousness also produce widespread, diffuse, slow-wave activity of a nonspecific type as is seen with stupor or coma from any cause. Resolution begins after a few days, cerebral edema subsides, and focal activity may then be seen (slow-wave activity or suppression of normal background rhythms). Smaller infarctions are associated with acute focal abnormalities which lateralize the lesion well but do not localize it precisely. In contrast with tumors, further resolution continues, and after 3 to 6 months roughly 50 percent of patients with cerebrovascular accidents have a normal EEG despite the persistence of clinical abnormalities. Under these circumstances the prognosis for further recovery is poor. The EEG may be of lateralizing value in acute subarachnoid hemorrhage, depending upon the extent to which the adjacent cerebrum is affected.

Brain injury Cerebral contusion or laceration produces EEG changes similar to those described for cerebrovascular disease. Diffuse changes often give way to focal ones, especially if the lesions are on the lateral or superior surface of the brain, and these in turn usually disappear over a period of weeks or months unless seizures supervene. Sharp waves or spikes sometimes emerge as the focal slow-wave abnormality resolves. These or failure of the EEG to "normalize" usually precede the occurrence of posttraumatic epilepsy. Following head injury, therefore, serial EEGs may be of prognostic value as regards the prospect of epilepsy.

Diseases which cause coma and states of impaired consciousness The EEG is abnormal in almost all conditions in which there is some impairment of consciousness. With hypothyroidism the rhythms are normal in configuration but are usually slow. In general, the more profound the change in consciousness, the more abnormal the EEG recording. In these latter situations the slow waves (delta) are bilateral, are of high amplitude, and tend to be more conspicuous over the frontal regions. This pertains to such differing conditions as acute meningitis or encephalitis, severe disorders of blood gases, glucose, electrolyte and water balance, uremia, diabetic coma, liver coma, or impairment of consciousness accompanying the large cerebral lesions discussed above. In hepatic coma, the degree of abnormality in the EEG corresponds with the degree of confusion, stupor, or coma. Moreover, paroxysms of bilaterally synchronous large, sharp "triphasic waves" are characteristic, though they may also be seen with other metabolic encephalopathies associated with renal or pulmonary failure. Diffuse degenerative diseases (e.g., Alzheimer's disease and senile dementia) affecting the cerebral cortex are accompanied by relatively slight degrees of diffuse, slow-wave abnormality in the theta (4- to 7-Hz) range. Certain more rapidly progressive ones, such as subacute sclerosing panencephalitis (SSPE), Creutzfeldt-Jakob disease, and to a lesser extent the cerebral lipidoses, have, in addition, very characteristic, almost pathognomonic EEG changes consisting of recurring complex bursts of sharp and slow activity. A normal EEG in a patient who is apathetic, slow, depressed, or forgetful is a point in favor of the diagnosis of an affective disorder or schizophrenia.

An EEG may also assist the physician in caring for a comatose patient when the pertinent history is unavailable. It may point to such otherwise unexpected causes as hepatic encephalopathy (bilaterally synchronous triphasic waves), intoxication with barbiturates or benzodiazepines (excess fast activity), clinically inapparent continuous epileptic discharges, a large space-occupying lesion, or diffuse anoxia-ischemia ("burst-suppression" pattern with repetitive generalized complexes separated by periods with very little EEG).

Other diseases of the cerebrum There are many disorders of nervous function that cause little or no alteration in the EEG. Multiple sclerosis and other demyelinating diseases are examples, though as many as 50 percent of advanced cases will have an abnormal record. Delirium tremens, Wernicke-Korsakoff disease, and withdrawal seizures, despite the dramatic nature of the clinical picture, cause little or no changes in the EEG. Some degree of slowing usually accompanies confusional states which have been designated elsewhere as hypokinetic delirium (see Chap. 21). Interestingly, neuroses and psychoses, such as manic-depressive disorders or schizophrenia, abnormal states due to hallucinogenic drugs such as LSD, and the majority of cases of mental retardation are associated with no important modification of the normal record or with nonspecific abnormalities.

SPECIAL APPLICATIONS OF THE EEG Because the EEG provides information about the status and function of the cerebrum, it is useful as a monitor in the operating room to ensure the presence of a viable brain during the increasingly extensive procedures of modern cardiovascular surgery. EEG apparatus has long been available for indicating the level of anesthesia, and such simple equipment should eventually be used by the anesthetist to monitor both the cardiac and cerebral status of all patients during surgical anesthesia.

It is routine practice now for the EEG to be monitored continuously during carotid endarterectomies, a procedure performed in carefully selected patients suffering from stenotic or ulcerative carotid artery disease. Characteristic EEG changes (particularly voltage attenuation) signal the need for a temporary bypass shunt to maintain sufficient cerebral blood flow to preclude ischemic cerebral damage during surgery.

In the neurosurgical operating room the EEG can be recorded from the exposed brain *(electrocorticogram)*, and seizure patterns can be localized more precisely than from the scalp so that resection of such physiologically abnormal tissue may be undertaken.

The routine EEG can be of value in the diagnosis of hysterical blindness. Similarly, a response evoked by noise during light sleep can be of help in confirming the presence of hearing in a patient who feigns total deafness. These responses may also be helpful in evaluating hearing and vision in infants.

EVOKED RESPONSES

An *evoked response* (sometimes termed an *evoked potential*) is the record of electrical activity produced by groups of neurons within the cord, brainstem, thalamus, or cerebral hemispheres following stimulation of one or another sensory system by means of visual, auditory, or tactile input. The amplitude of these potentials, as recorded from the scalp using ordinary EEG electrodes, ranges from less than 0.5 to 20 μV. Because of their extremely small size, they can rarely be recognized on the ink-written EEG record with the background of ongoing EEG activity, which itself is usually 50 μV or more in amplitude. Therefore, special techniques, requiring simple computers, must be used to extract the evoked response waveform that one is interested in, from the continuous background EEG activity. These techniques are called "averaging" because the process involves repeating 100 to 1000 precisely timed stimuli and recording the electrical activity during a certain brief interval following each stimulus. The random ongoing EEG activity which, at any given point in time following the stimulus, is sometimes negative and at other times positive in polarity, tends to cancel out with sufficient repetition. The evoked response, on the other hand, is time-locked to the stimulus, and at a given time following the stimulus always has the same electrical sign as well as shape. The evoked response thus grows larger with repetition while the background averages out and becomes smaller. It is important to have special amplifiers, to apply the electrodes to the surface of the scalp with great care, and to time stimuli precisely with a minimum of accompanying electrical artifact.

VISUAL EVOKED RESPONSES The evoked response with the longest history of clinical usefulness (since 1971) is the *visual evoked response* produced by a pattern shift (PSVER). During this test, patients are asked to watch an alternating black and white checkerboard pattern which is projected on a screen. When patients watch this pattern shift, it produces a characteristic waveform which can be recorded from the scalp over the posterior portion of the head. Under normal circumstances, this triphasic wave has a distinctive positive peak at 95 to 115 ms latency (usually called P100; see Fig. 354-3) from the time of pattern reversal. This latency, the duration of the response, and the amplitude of the peak are measured; the latency is the most important parameter clinically. Each eye is tested independently.

Many disease processes affecting the optic nerve fibers in their intraocular, orbital, or intracranial portions produce abnormalities of this potential. Glaucoma, compression of the optic nerve, chiasm, or tract by various space-occupying lesions, and degenerative disease of this system often produce a reduction in amplitude and/or prolonged latency of the PSVER. If the visual system is sufficiently affected, no response may be recorded by stimulation of one or both eyes. In a general hospital setting, however, the most common cause of abnormality in this response is optic neuritis, frequently associated with multiple sclerosis. Demyelination of the optic nerve fibers, as a primary demyelinating disease or due to one of the lesions listed above, slows conduction in the nerve fibers so that the latency of the positive peak of the PSVER is prolonged (115 to 200 ms). In fact, almost all patients with optic neuritis, even after the visual acuity has returned to normal, continue to show distinct abnormalities in this PSVER at a time when detailed ophthalmological evaluations reveal no abnormality. In multiple sclerosis, if the PSVER is normal, the neuroophthalmological examination is always normal. We have found no exceptions to this rule in more than 200 patients. When the PSVER is abnormal, the visual fields, visual acuity, pupillary reactions, and optic fundus examination are normal in a considerable number of patients.

Approximately one-half of the patients with multiple sclerosis who have never had visual symptoms also show abnormalities, and this accounts for one of the most useful aspects of the test. If a patient presents with what appears to be the first episode of a neurological illness in which the lesion is in the brainstem or spinal cord, a demonstration by means of an abnormal PSVER of another clinically unsuspected lesion in a different part of the central nervous system (the optic nerves) makes the diagnosis of multiple sclerosis more likely and may spare the patient certain neuroradiological procedures.

Abnormalities in visual acuity have no effect on the PSVER unless the acuity is so poor that the patient cannot see the checkerboard pattern—patients with acuity of 20/200 or better are suitable for testing. The only other requirement is that the patient be cooperative enough to sit still for 20 min and watch the pattern. Infants and children can also be tested by using special techniques.

BRAINSTEM AUDITORY EVOKED RESPONSES *Brainstem auditory evoked responses* (BAERs) are more difficult to obtain than PSVER because BAERs are much smaller, of the order of 0.5 μV. These are produced by clicks transmitted to one of a patient's ears through earphones. The patient may be alert or comatose and need not be particularly cooperative except that an excess of movement or muscle artifact makes the response even more difficult to obtain. BAERs of essentially normal appearance can be recorded from infants and children. BAERs consist of a series of seven waves which appear within the first 10 ms after the click (Fig. 354-3). These (named I to VII) are considered to represent successive activation of the auditory nerve (I) and the brainstem auditory pathways (cochlear nucleus, II; superior olivary complex, III; lateral lemniscus, IV; inferior colliculus, V; and higher auditory centers, VI, VII). A lesion at or between any of these levels either obliterates or delays the appearance of waves from successively higher levels. Multiple sclerosis can, for example, also produce slow conduction between any of the levels in this test. The same is true of other lesions affecting the brainstem, such as small vascular lesions, central pontine myelinolysis, hypoxic damage, and so on. The waves which arise from structures caudal to the lesion are perfectly normal in latency, whereas those arising from structures cranial to the lesion are either obliterated or de-

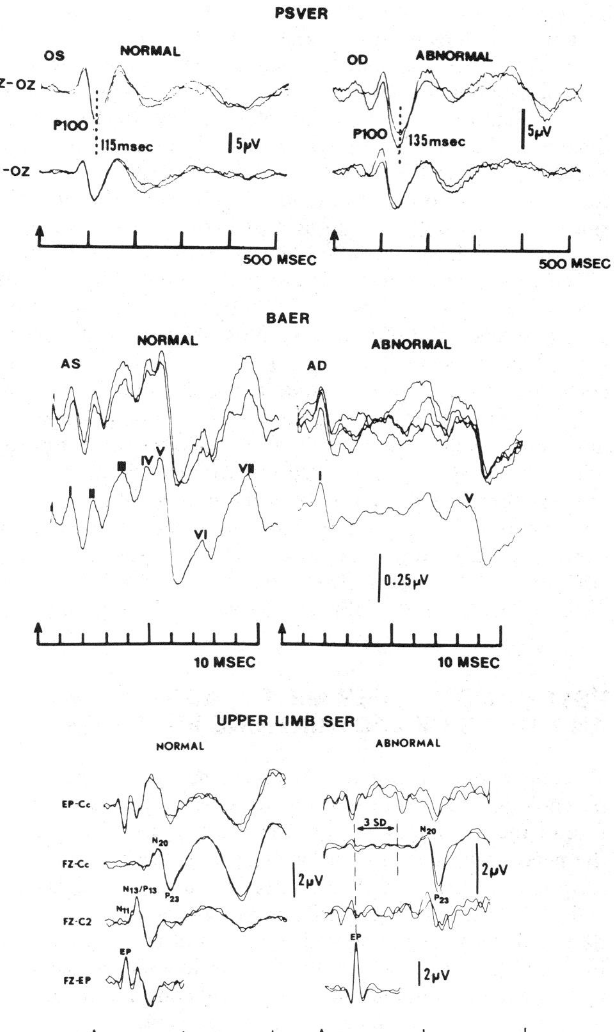

FIGURE 354-3

Evoked responses (ER). PSVER. Pattern-shift visual ER recorded from a patient with multiple sclerosis showing a monocular latency abnormality. Latency of the occipital response (P100) following stimulation of the left eye (OS) was normal at 115 ms; right response (OD) was abnormal because the latency of the P100 peak was delayed at 135 ms. Relative positivity at G2 causes a downward trace deflection. Electrode locations: CZ = vertex, OZ = midline occipital, R = linked ears. [From EB Brooks, KH Chiappa, Clinical applications of evoked potentials, in Neurology, J Courjoun et al (eds), New York, Raven Press, 1982.]

BAER. Brainstem auditory ERs from a patient with multiple sclerosis showing the marked asymmetry which can be present with monaural click stimulation. The responses following left ear (AS) stimulation are normal. The right ear (AD) responses are missing wave III (lower pons) and have a markedly abnormal I–V (cochlear nerve to midbrain) separation of 6.7 ms, evidence of a conduction defect in the pontine auditory tracts on the right. Left ear responses for superimposed trials (above) are produced by N = 1024 clicks each; in the right ear N = 2048 clicks each. The single trace below each is the grand average of the superimposed trials. Recording is from vertex to earlobe of stimulated ear; relative positivity at the vertex produces an upward trace deflection. (Reprinted from KH Chiappa et al, Ann Neurol 7:135, 1980.)

Upper limb SER. Short-latency somatosensory ERs produced by stimulation of the median nerve at the wrist. The left set of responses is from a normal subject; the right set is from a patient with multiple sclerosis who had no sensory symptoms or signs. In the patient, note preservation of the brachial plexus component (EP) and absence of cervical cord (N11) and lower medullary components (N13-P13). The latency of thalamocortical components (N20-P23) was prolonged markedly above the normal mean plus 3 standard deviations for the separation of N20 from the brachial plexus potential. Unilateral stimulation at 5 per second. Each trace is the averaged response to 1024 stimuli, with the superimposed trace a repetition following 1024 stimuli to demonstrate waveform consistency. Recording electrode locations: FZ = midfrontal, EP = Erb's point (supraclavicular), C2 = middle back of neck over C2 cervical vertebra, and Cc = scalp overlying sensoriparietal cortex contralateral to limb stimulated.

layed. This allows one to pinpoint quite accurately the level of the lesion within the brainstem auditory pathways and provides a very neat opportunity for correlation of clinical observations with neurophysiological and occasionally pathological data. This test is useful as a screening test for patients with acoustic neuromas (who always show an abnormality), for patients suspected of having multiple sclerosis, for comatose patients in whom the level of lesion within the central nervous system is not clear, and for other patients in whom documentation of brainstem lesions is important. Hearing loss can often be recognized in this test, since changes in the latency of the first (and, therefore, subsequent) waves are produced, and these must be taken into consideration in the evaluation of the results obtained. Interwave latencies, which are the parameters used to measure central conduction, are not affected by hearing loss or stimulus intensity.

SOMATOSENSORY EVOKED RESPONSES *Somatosensory evoked responses* (SERs) are produced by small painless electrical stimuli administered to large sensory fibers in mixed nerves of the hand or foot. The afferent valley is recorded at many levels as it ascends the somatosensory pathways, and a series of waves can be recorded which reflect activity in peripheral nerve trunks, tracts in the spinal cord, gracile and cuneate nuclei, pontine and/or cerebellar structures, thalamus, thalamocortical radiations, and primary sensory fields of the cortex (see Fig. 354-3). Lesions of the pathways at any level affect the subsequent waves, thus providing localizing and confirmatory data in a similar fashion to the BAER.

Evoked responses can be used for a single evaluation of patients (looking for lesions in the various pathways discussed) or as a quantitative method for following a patient's course to document functional improvement or deterioration as time passes, following therapy, and so on. They also prove useful for on-line monitoring of function in optic nerve, brainstem, or spinal cord during neurosurgical procedures that involve manipulation of those structures. Since BAERs and SERs are unaffected by general anesthesia and high-dose barbiturates, they also can be used to follow CNS function in comatose patients. Longer latency auditory and somatosensory evoked responses have been studied for a number of years. These are largely cortically produced responses, dramatically affected by drowsiness, inattention, and other poorly controllable variables, and have not proved to be clinically useful. Neither have most visual evoked responses produced by stroboscopic flashes. They are very useful in evaluation of visual pathways in infants and young children who are not cooperative enough to watch the checkerboard pattern and in adults during surgery or when comatose. Under other circumstances, pattern-shift PSVERs afford a much more reliable and reproducible response.

PSYCHOMETRY, PERIMETRY, AUDIOMETRY, AND TESTS OF LABYRINTHINE FUNCTION

These methods, drawn largely from the field of physiologic psychology, are of utility in quantitating and defining the nature of the psychic or sensory deficits produced by disease of the nervous system. Limitations of space do not permit a description of them here. The precise indications for doing these tests are (1) to obtain confirmation of a functional disorder in particular parts of the nervous system and to ascertain its nature, and (2) to quantitate the disorder in order to determine, by subsequent examinations, the natural course of the underlying illness (see Chap. 22).

BIOCHEMICAL TESTS

With advances in the biochemistry of metabolic diseases, a number of highly specific tests of serum, CSF, and circulating red and white blood cells have become available. These will be presented in relation to the metabolic diseases of which they are diagnostic.

REFERENCES

Buonanno FS et al: Clinical relevance of two different nuclear magnetic resonance (NMR) approaches to imaging of a low grade astrocytoma. J Comput Assist Tomogr 6:529, 1982

Chiappa KH: *Evoked Potentials in Clinical Neurology.* New York, Raven Press, 1983

———, Ropper AH: Evoked potentials in clinical medicine. N Engl J Med 306:1136, 1982

Klass DW, Daly DD (eds): *Practice of Clinical Electroencephalography.* New York, Raven Press, 1981

Newton TH, Potts DG (eds): *Radiology of the Skull and Brain,* vol 3. St. Louis, Mosby, 1977

Pykett IL: NMR imaging in medicine. Sci Am 246(5):78, 1982

Remond A: *Handbook of Electroencephalography and Clinical Neurophysiology,* vols 1–15. Amsterdam, Elsevier/North-Holland, 1976–1978

Spahlmann R: *EEG Primer.* Amsterdam, Elsevier/North-Holland, 1981

Stalberg E, Young RR (eds): *Clinical Neurophysiology.* London, Butterworths, 1981

Taveras J, Wood EH: *Diagnostic Neuroradiology,* 2d ed, *Golden's Diagnostic Radiology Series,* sec 1. Baltimore, Williams & Wilkins, 1976

Werner SS et al: *Atlas of Neonatal Electroencephalography.* New York, Raven Press, 1977

355 THE EPILEPSIES AND CONVULSIVE DISORDERS

MARC A. DICHTER

The *epilepsies* are a group of disorders characterized by chronic, recurrent, paroxysmal changes in neurological function caused by abnormalities in the electrical activity of the brain. They are common neurological disorders, estimated to affect between 0.5 and 2 percent of the population, and can occur at any age. Each episode of neurological dysfunction is called a *seizure.* Seizures may be *convulsive* when they are accompanied by motor manifestations or may be manifested by other changes in neurological function (i.e., sensory, cognitive, emotional events). Epilepsy can be acquired as a result of neurological injury or a structural brain lesion and can also occur as a part of many systemic medical diseases. Epilepsy also occurs in an *idiopathic* form in an individual with neither a history of neurological insult nor other apparent neurological dysfunction. Isolated, nonrecurrent seizures may occur in otherwise healthy individuals for a variety of reasons, and, under these circumstances, the individual is not said to have epilepsy.

CLASSIFICATION OF SEIZURES

The neurological manifestations of epileptic seizures are varied, ranging from a brief lapse of attention to a prolonged loss of consciousness with abnormal motor activity. The proper classification of the kinds of seizures which an individual is experiencing is important for an appropriate diagnostic workup, prognostic evaluation, and selection of therapy. The classification of epileptic seizures provided in this chapter is based on the International Classification of Epileptic Seizures developed in 1969 and subsequently modified in 1981. It emphasizes the clinical seizure type and ictal (seizure-associated) and interictal (between seizures) electroencephalographic pattern (Table 355-1), whereas etiology, anatomic substrate, and pathways of spread are not major considerations. The older terminology of grand mal, petit mal, and psychomotor or temporal lobe epilepsy has been integrated into the current scheme.

The major underlying premise of this classification is that some seizures (partial or focal seizures) start in a localized area of brain (cortex) and either remain localized or secondarily generalize (that is, spread throughout the brain), whereas other seizures appear to be generalized from their earliest manifestation.

PARTIAL OR FOCAL SEIZURES Partial or focal seizures begin with the activation of neurons in one localized area of cortex. The specific clinical symptoms depend on the area of cortex involved and imply dysfunction in a localized area of cortex. The lesion may be due to birth injury, postnatal trauma, tumor, abscess, infarction, vascular malformation, or some other structural abnormality. The abnormal area of cortex underlying the seizure activity can be identified by the specific neurological phenomena observed during the focal seizure. Partial seizures are classified as *simple* if there is no alteration of consciousness or awareness of the environment and *complex* if there is such a change.

Simple partial seizures Simple partial seizures can occur with motor, sensory, autonomic, or psychic symptoms. A simple partial seizure with motor signs consists of recurrent contractions of the muscles of one part of the body (finger, hand, arm, face, etc.) without loss of consciousness. Each muscular contraction is caused by the discharge of neurons in the corresponding area of the contralateral motor cortex.

The muscle activity of a partial seizure (*ictus*) may remain confined to one area or may spread from the affected area to involve contiguous ipsilateral body parts (i.e., right thumb to right hand to right arm to right side of face). This "Jacksonian march," named after Hughlings Jackson who first described it, is caused by a demonstrable progression of epileptiform discharges in the contralateral motor cortex and may occur over seconds or minutes. The EEG manifestations of this form of seizure are often very striking and consist of regularly occurring spike discharges in the appropriate area of (frontal) motor cortex. Between seizures (interictal period) this region may give rise to irregular spike discharges in the EEG.

Simple partial seizures may have other behavioral manifestations if the seizure discharges occur in other cortical regions. Thus, sensory symptoms (paresthesias, vertiginous feelings, simple auditory or visual hallucinations) occur with epileptiform discharges in the contralateral sensory cortex, and autonomic and psychic symptoms [i.e., the sensation of having experienced something before (déjà vu), unwarranted sense of fear or anger, illusions, and even complex hallucinations] occur with discharges in limbic regions of the temporal and frontal lobes.

TABLE 355-1
Classification of epileptic seizures

1 Partial or focal seizures
- *a* Simple partial seizures (with motor, sensory, autonomic, or psychic signs)
- *b* Complex partial seizures (psychomotor or temporal lobe seizures)
- *c* Secondary generalized partial seizures

2 Primary generalized seizures
- *a* Tonic-clonic (grand mal)
- *b* Tonic
- *c* Absence (petit mal)
- *d* Atypical absence
- *e* Myoclonic
- *f* Atonic
- *g* Infantile spasms

3 Status epilepticus
- *a* Tonic-clonic status
- *b* Absence status
- *c* Epilepsia partialis continua

4 Recurrence patterns
- *a* Sporadic
- *b* Cyclic
- *c* Reflex (photomyoclonic, somatosensory, musicogenic, reading epilepsy)

Complex partial seizures (temporal lobe or psychomotor seizures) Complex partial seizures are episodic changes in behavior in which an individual loses conscious contact with the environment. The onset of these seizures may consist of any of a variety of auras: an unusual smell (as of burning rubber), a feeling that the current experience has happened before (déjà vu), a sudden intense emotional feeling, a sensory illusion such as that of objects growing smaller (*micropsia*) or larger (*macropsia*), or a specifically formed sensory hallucination. Patients may come to recognize these as heralding their seizures, or the memory of the aura may be lost in the postictal amnesia which often occurs if the seizure becomes generalized. During complex partial seizures there may be a cessation of activity with some minor motor activity, such as lip smacking, swallowing, walking aimlessly, or picking at one's clothes (*automatisms*). Complex partial seizures may also be accompanied by the unconscious performance of highly skilled activities such as driving a car or playing complicated musical pieces. When the seizure ends, the individual is amnesic for events which took place during the seizure and may take minutes or hours to recover full consciousness.

Patients with complex partial seizures have EEGs which exhibit unilateral or bilateral spikes or slow wave discharges over temporal or frontotemporal regions both interictally and during seizures. Most of these seizures originate from epileptiform activity in the temporal lobes—especially the hippocampus or amygdala—or other parts of the limbic system, but others have been shown to originate from mesial parasagittal or orbital frontal regions. These seizures are also referred to as *temporal lobe epilepsy* and *psychomotor epilepsy* in older classification schemes.

Although often showing spike discharges or focal slowing during complex partial seizures, exceptionally the surface EEG may be normal. Nasopharyngeal or sphenoidal electrodes may record the abnormal discharges, but in some cases only depth electrodes in the amygdaloid nuclei or other limbic structures will show seizure discharges. The occasional discrepancy between surface and depth electrophysiological events is a particularly difficult problem when trying to use the surface EEG to determine the nature of an abnormal behavior in an individual suspected of having complex partial seizures. (See "Differential Diagnosis of Seizures" below.)

Secondary generalization of partial seizures Simple or complex partial seizures can progress to generalized seizures with loss of consciousness and often with convulsive motor activity. This may occur immediately or after many seconds or a minute or two. In addition, many patients with focal seizures have generalized seizures without an obvious initial focal component which are difficult to distinguish from primary generalized seizures. The presence of an aura or the observation of any focal feature (twitching of one extremity, aphasia, tonic eye deviation) at the onset of the generalized seizure or the presence of a postictal focal neurological deficit (Todd's paralysis) is an important clue to a focal origin to the seizure.

PRIMARY GENERALIZED SEIZURES **Tonic-clonic (grand mal)** One of the most common kinds of epileptic paroxysms is the generalized tonic-clonic seizure. Some of these appear to be primary generalized seizures, and others are the result of secondary generalization from partial seizures. In either case, the seizures follow a common pattern. The primary generalized seizures usually start without warning, although some individuals sense a vague, nonspecific sense of the impending event. The onset is heralded by a sudden loss of consciousness, a *tonic* contraction of the muscles, a loss of postural control, and a cry produced by a forced expiration caused by contraction of the respiratory muscles. The individual falls to the floor in an opisthotonic posture, often sustaining injury, and remains rigid for many seconds. There may be cyanosis as respiration is inhibited. Soon a series of rhythmic contractions of all four limbs occurs. This *clonic* phase can last for a variable period of time and ends when the muscles relax. The individual remains unconscious and unarousable for a period of minutes or longer. There is usually a gradual return to consciousness and often a period of disorientation during recovery. The patient may even be combative if restrained. During the seizure, urinary or fecal incontinence and tongue biting may occur. Postictally there is amnesia for the seizure, and sometimes a retrograde amnesia as well. Headache and drowsiness are common sequelae, and the individual may not return to base-line functioning for days.

The EEG in patients with tonic-clonic seizures shows low-voltage fast (10 Hz or more) activity during the tonic phase, which converts gradually to slower, larger sharp waves throughout both hemispheres. During the clonic phase there are bursts of sharp waves associated with the rhythmical muscular contractions and slow waves coincident with the pauses. Often the excessive muscular activity of the seizure causes artifacts which interfere with ictal EEG recordings. Interictally, the EEG is usually abnormal with polyspike (or spike) and wave or occasionally sharp and slow wave discharges.

Tonic seizures Tonic seizures are a less common form of primary generalized seizure which consist of the sudden occurrence of a rigid posturing of the limbs or torso, often with deviation of the head and eyes toward one side. They are not followed by a clonic phase and are often of shorter duration than tonic-clonic seizures.

Absence seizures (petit mal) Pure absence seizures consist of the sudden cessation of ongoing conscious activity without convulsive muscular activity or loss of postural control. Such seizures may be so brief as to be inapparent. Usually they last for seconds or minutes. The brief lapses of consciousness or awareness may be accompanied by minor motor manifestations such as eyelid fluttering, small chewing movements of the mouth, or mild shaking of the hands. During longer absences, automatisms may occur which may be difficult to distinguish from complex partial seizures. At the end of the absence seizure, the patient regains awareness of the environment very quickly, and there is usually no period of postictal confusion.

Absence seizures almost always begin in young children (6 to 14 years of age) and rarely appear for the first time in adults. These brief seizures may occur hundreds or more times per day and go on for weeks or months before it is recognized that the child is having seizures. In fact, it is not uncommon for these to be first recognized when the child begins having problems with learning.

The EEG is pathognomonic in this form of seizure disorder. During the seizures there are 3-Hz spike-and-wave discharges which appear synchronously throughout all the leads. The EEG is usually normal during the interictal periods. Often the EEG demonstrates that the child is having more seizures than was thought from clinical observation alone.

Absence seizures usually occur in otherwise neurologically normal children. These seizures are usually sensitive to anticonvulsants (see below). Children with this condition often do quite well once it is treated. Approximately one-third outgrow the seizure disorder, one-third continue to have only absence seizures, and one-third have occasional concomitant generalized tonic-clonic seizures.

Absence seizures can be differentiated from absence-like attacks which occasionally occur in complex partial seizures by the lack of aura, immediate recovery from the absence, and typical 3-Hz spike-and-wave EEG pattern.

Atypical absence seizures Atypical absence seizures are similar to absence seizures but coexist with other forms of generalized seizures, such as tonic seizures, myoclonic seizures, or atonic seizures (see below). The EEG is more heterogeneous, containing spike-and-wave discharges at 2 or 4 Hz during the absence attacks and poorly developed background with spike or polyspike activity during interictal periods.

Atypical absence seizures commonly occur in children with some other form of underlying neurological dysfunction and tend to be resistant to medication. In the most severe form of this disorder, the Lennox-Gastaut syndrome, children have several kinds of generalized seizures and often have intellectual impairment.

Myoclonic seizures Myoclonic seizures are sudden, brief, single or repetitive muscle contractions involving one body part or the entire body. In the latter case, the seizure is accompanied by a violent fall, without a loss of consciousness. Myoclonic seizures often coexist with other seizure types but may occur alone. The EEG shows polyspike-and-wave discharges or sharp and slow waves, both ictally and interictally. Although often idiopathic, myoclonic seizures occur as a major neurological symptom in a variety of medical conditions including uremia, hepatic failure, Creutzfeldt-Jakob disease, subacute leukoencephalopathies, and a hereditary degenerative condition, Lafora body disease.

Atonic seizures Atonic seizures are brief losses of consciousness and postural tone not associated with tonic muscular contractions. The individual may simply drop to the floor without apparent cause. Atonic seizures usually occur in children and are often accompanied by other forms of seizures. The EEG contains polyspikes and slow waves. The "drop attacks" of atonic seizures need to be distinguished from cataplexy seen in narcolepsy (where the patient remains conscious), transient brainstem ischemia, or sudden rises in intracranial pressure.

Infantile spasms or hypsarrhythmia This form of primary generalized seizure occurs in infants between birth and approximately 12 months of age and consists of brief synchronous contractions of the neck, torso, and both arms (usually in flexion). Infantile spasms often occur in children with underlying neurological diseases, such as anoxic encephalopathy or tuberous sclerosis, but can rarely occur in an otherwise apparently normal infant. The prognosis for children with this form of seizure disorder is grave, and approximately 90 percent develop mental retardation in addition to their seizures. The EEG is characterized by a very disorganized background, random high-voltage slow waves, spikes and burst suppression (hypsarrhythmia). The spasms and hypsarrhythmia tend to disappear over the first 3 to 5 years of life, only to be replaced by other forms of generalized seizures.

STATUS EPILEPTICUS Prolonged or repetitive seizures without a period of recovery between attacks can occur with all forms of seizures and is defined as *status epilepticus.* When tonic-clonic seizures are involved, this state can be life-threatening (see "Treatment of Seizures"). Absence status, on the other hand, may proceed for some time before it is recognized because the patient does not lose consciousness or have convulsive movements. Status epilepticus of partial seizures is called *epilepsia partialis continua* and may occur with partial motor, sensory, or visceral seizures. Complex partial seizures may also present as status epilepticus.

RECURRENCE PATTERNS All classes of recurrent seizures can occur sporadically or randomly, with no apparent triggering event, or can occur cyclically, i.e., in concert with the sleep-walking cycle or the menstrual cycle (catamenial epilepsy). Epileptic seizures can also occur as evoked reactions to a specific stimulus (reflex epilepsy), although this is relatively infrequent. Examples are seizures triggered by photic stimulation (photomyoclonic or photoconvulsive epilepsy), specific musical compositions (musicogenic epilepsy), tactile stimulation (somatosensory induced epilepsy), or reading (reading or language epilepsy). The latter usually consists of brief myoclonic jerks of the jaw, cheek, and tongue which occur during silent or oral reading and may progress to generalized tonic-clonic seizures.

PATHOPHYSIOLOGY OF EPILEPSY

Epileptic seizures can be induced in any normal human (or vertebrate) brain with a variety of different electrical or chemical stimuli. The ease and rapidity with which these seizures can occur, and the stereotyped nature of the seizures produced suggest that the normal brain, particularly the cerebral cortex, contains within its fine anatomical and physiological structure a mechanism which is inherently unstable and which can be influenced in many different ways to produce a seizure. Thus, many kinds of metabolic abnormalities and anatomical lesions of brain can produce seizures, and conversely, there is no pathognomonic lesion of the epileptic brain.

The hallmark of the altered physiologic state of epilepsy is a rhythmical and repetitive hypersynchronous discharge of many neurons in a localized area of the brain. A reflection of this hypersynchronous discharge can be observed in the electroencephalogram (EEG). The EEG records the integrated electrical activity generated by synaptic potentials in neurons in the superficial layers of a localized area of cortex. Normally, the EEG records unsynchronized activity during periods when the mind is actively working, or mildly synchronized activity when the mind is in a restful state (i.e., alpha waves during relaxation with closed eyes) or during various stages of sleep. In the epileptic focus, neurons in a small area of the cortex are activated in an unusually synchronized manner, and this produces a larger, sharper waveform in the EEG—the *spike discharge.* If the neuronal hypersynchrony is large, a focal, simple seizure follows; if it spreads through the brain and lasts for seconds or minutes, a complex partial or generalized seizure (the *ictus*) will occur and the EEG can have a variety of appearances, depending on which areas of brain are involved and how the primary discharging areas project to the superficial cortex. During the seizure, the EEG may display low-voltage fast activity or high-voltage *spikes* or *spike-and-wave* discharges throughout both hemispheres.

During the interictal spike discharge, the neurons in the epileptic focus undergo a large membrane depolarization (the *depolarizing shift,* or DS) accompanied by action potential generation. After the DS, the neurons hyperpolarize and stop firing for several seconds. In areas around the discharging focus, the neurons are also inhibited, but do not first have the large DS. Thus, it appears as if the epileptic discharge is limited to a localized area of cortex by a ring of inhibition around the focus and slightly delayed inhibition within the focus. When the epileptic focus undergoes a transition from the isolated discharges to a seizure, the post-DS inhibition disappears and is replaced by a depolarizing potential. Neurons in contiguous areas and in synaptically connected distant areas are then recruited into the seizure and become activated. Local cortical circuits, long association pathways (including callosal), and subcortical pathways are all utilized for the spread of the discharges. Thus, a focal seizure can spread locally or generalize throughout the brain. Widely ramifying thalamocortical pathways are likely to be responsible for the rapid generalization of some forms of epilepsy, including absence seizures.

A number of metabolic events occur within the brain during the epileptic discharges which may contribute to the development of the focus, to the transition to seizures, or to postictal dysfunction. During the discharges, extracellular potassium concentration increases and extracellular calcium concentration decreases. Both of these changes have profound effects on neuronal excitability and neurotransmitter release and on neuronal metabolism. Neurotransmitters and neuropeptides are also released in unusually large amounts during seizure discharges. Some of these substances can have prolonged actions on central neurons and may be responsible for prolonged postictal phenomena such as Todd's paralysis. In addition to the ionic effects, seizures produce increases in cerebral blood flow to the primary involved areas, increases in glucose utilization, and alterations in oxidative metabolism and local pH. It is possible that these events are not just consequences of the seizures but actually contribute to the development of the seizure activity and that manipulation of such factors could become an effective means for controlling seizures.

There are many mechanisms by which seizures can develop in either normal or pathological brains. One of the most common methods for producing epilepsy in experimental animals is to block inhibitory mechanisms. For example, agents which antagonize the inhibitory neurotransmitter γ-aminobutyric acid (GABA) are potent convulsants, both in animals and in human beings. A diminution of inhibition may also be involved in some forms of chronic focal epilepsy, as it has been demonstrated that inhibitory terminals on neurons in areas around cortical gliotic lesions are reduced. This reduction of inhibition may allow excess excitation to develop. It has been postulated that some forms of generalized epilepsy could also be due to an abnormality in the GABA-inhibitory system, but this has not yet been firmly established. Several antiepileptic drugs, including phenobarbital, the benzodiazepines, and valproic acid, have been shown to enhance GABA-mediated inhibition in the brain, and this effect is likely to contribute to their antiepileptic actions.

Electrical stimulation is another mechanism by which seizures can easily be produced in a normal brain. At certain current strengths and stimulus frequencies seizure discharges are produced and become self-sustaining beyond the original stimulus. Generalized tonic-clonic seizures result. At lower stimulus parameters, seizure afterdischarges may not occur. However, if a stereotyped subthreshold stimulus is repeated at regular intervals (which may even be as infrequent as one stimulation per day), there is a gradual buildup of response until generalized seizures occur to the same stimulus which was originally subthreshold. Eventually spontaneous seizures may occur without any further electrical stimulation. This phenomenon has been called *kindling*. Its relationship to the pathophysiology of posttraumatic epilepsy or to the issue of whether the occurrence of seizures themselves tends to foster the continued development of a seizure focus in human beings has not been resolved.

THE CAUSES OF EPILEPSY

The likely etiology of a given seizure depends upon the age of the patient and the type of seizure (see Table 355-2). In young infants, anoxia or ischemia before or during birth, intracranial birth injury, metabolic disturbances, such as hypoglycemia, hypocalcemia, and hypomagnesemia, congenital malformations of the brain, and infections are the most common causes of seizures. In the young child, trauma and infections are common causes of epilepsy, although idiopathic seizures account for the majority of patients.

Genetic factors can influence the development of epilepsy and have also been shown to affect EEG patterns in general. Patients with primary generalized seizures, especially absence seizures, have a higher familial incidence of epilepsy than is found in the normal population, and relatives of such patients have higher incidences of dysrhythmic EEGs, even when they do not have seizures. The mode of inheritance of susceptibility to epilepsy appears complicated and probably represents multiple genes with variable penetrance. Even in the highest risk group, however, the chance of a sibling or a child of an individual with generalized seizures also having epilepsy is below 10 percent.

Young children also frequently (approximately 2 to 5 percent of the population) develop seizures with febrile illnesses. These febrile convulsions are short, generalized tonic-clonic convulsions which occur during the early phases of a febrile illness in children between the ages of 3 months and 5 years. Febrile seizures must be distinguished from seizures that are triggered by central nervous system infections which coincidentally produce fever (meningitis or encephalitis). There is minimal likelihood that the child will develop epilepsy or any neurological impairment from the febrile convulsion if the seizure lasts less than 5 minutes, is generalized rather than focal, and is not associated with any interictal EEG abnormalities or abnormalities on neurological exam. There may be a family history of febrile seizure. Febrile seizures are probably best treated with quick and relatively vigorous attempts to keep children from developing excessive fevers during various childhood illnesses but without specific antiepileptic medication. Some pediatricians prefer to maintain children susceptible to febrile convulsions on chronic phenobarbital medication. On the other hand, if the febrile convulsion is prolonged or focal or is associated with an abnormal EEG, or if the child has a neurological abnormality, there is a significant risk of subsequent epilepsy. These children should be treated with chronic antiepileptic therapy. Intermittent antiepileptic medication given at the onset of a febrile illness is ineffective and should be avoided.

In adolescents and young adults, head trauma is a major cause of focal epilepsy. Epilepsy can be caused by any kind of serious head injury, with the likelihood of developing recurrent seizures being proportional to the extent of the damage. Injuries which either cause dural penetration or produce posttraumatic amnesia of more than 24-h duration may result in a 40 to 50 percent incidence of later epilepsy, while the incidence with closed head injuries with cerebral contusion varies from 5 to 25 percent. Brief concussive illnesses or nonpenetrating head injuries without loss of consciousness are not epileptigenic. Seizures which occur immediately or within the first 24 h of injury are not associated with a poor prognosis, whereas seizures occurring after the first day and within the first 2 weeks indicate a high likelihood of posttraumatic epilepsy. Most recurring seizures develop by 2 years after the injury, although longer intervals may occur. Approximately 50 percent of patients with posttraumatic seizures spontaneously recover, 25 percent have medically controllable seizures, and 25 percent have seizures that are much more intractable to antiepileptic medication. The effectiveness of prophylactic anticonvulsant medication after head trauma still requires adequate documentation, although many physicians treat such patients (and other postoperative neurosurgical patients) with phenytoin or phenobarbital to attempt to prevent the development of posttraumatic seizures.

In the adolescent or young adult age group, generalized tonic-clonic seizures tend to be idiopathic or are associated with drug (especially barbiturate) or alcohol withdrawal. Arteriovenous malformations may present as focal seizures in this age group. Between ages 30 and 50, brain tumors become more common causes of seizures and may be present in 30 percent of patients with new focal seizures. In general, the incidence of seizures is higher with slowly growing brain tumors involving the cerebrum, such as meningiomas or low-grade gliomas, than with the more malignant types. However, seizures can occur in individuals with any kind of central nervous system mass lesion, including highly malignant metastatic tumors or completely benign vascular malformations.

Above age 50, cerebrovascular disease is the most common cause of focal or generalized seizures. Seizures can occur acutely in patients with an embolus, hemorrhage, or, more rarely, a thrombosis but more often as a late sequel to these lesions. Seizures can also result from "silent" cerebral infarctions in patients with no known cerebrovascular disease. Brain tumors, either primary or metastatic, also present with seizures in the older age group.

At any age, a variety of medical diseases can produce metabolic disturbances which may present as seizures. Uremia, hepatic failure, hypo- or hypercalcemia, hypo- and hyperglycemia, or hypo- and hypernatremia may be associated with myoclonic seizures or generalized tonic-clonic seizures.

TABLE 355-2
The causes of seizures

Age group	Causes
Infant (0–2 years)	Paranatal hypoxia and ischemia Intracranial birth injury Acute infection Metabolic disturbances (hypoglycemia, hypocalcemia, hypomagnesemia, pyridoxine deficiency) Congenital malformation Genetic disorders
Child (2–12 years)	Idiopathic Acute infection Trauma Febrile convulsion
Adolescent (12–18 years)	Idiopathic Trauma Drug, alcohol withdrawal Arteriovenous malformations
Young adult (18–35 years)	Trauma Alcoholism Brain tumor
Older adult (over 35 years)	Brain tumor Cerebrovascular disease Metabolic disorders (uremia, hepatic failure, electrolyte abnormality, hypoglycemia) Alcoholism

EVALUATION OF THE PATIENT WITH A SEIZURE

Individuals with seizures present to physicians either in an emergency room setting during the acute attack or in an office setting days after the epileptic event. In the former case, the seizure may be the presenting symptom of a serious central nervous system disorder which requires immediate diagnosis and therapy. In the latter case, the seizure may be a symptom of a more chronic neurological dysfunction and a different approach is warranted.

Initial emergency evaluation is directed toward ensuring adequate ventilation and perfusion and stopping the seizure (see "Treatment"). Once the patient is medically stable, the investigation is directed at determining the cause of the seizure. Often a careful history (either from the patient, if recovered, or from a friend or relative), a physical examination, and a few blood studies can provide the diagnosis.

A history suggesting a recent febrile illness accompanied by headaches, change in mental status, or confusion suggests an acute CNS infection (either meningitis or encephalitis) and indicates the need for urgent examination of the CSF. In this context, a complex partial seizure may be the presenting symptom of herpes simplex encephalitis. A history of headache and/or change in mental functioning preceding the seizure, coupled with either signs of increased intracranial pressure or a focal neurological deficit suggests an underlying mass lesion (tumor, abscess, arteriovenous malformation) or a chronic subdural hematoma. Seizures with a clear focal onset or aura are especially worrisome in this regard. A CT scan should be performed for a more definitive diagnosis.

The general physical examination may provide important etiologic information. Gum hyperplasia is usually the result of chronic phenytoin therapy. Exacerbation of a chronic seizure disorder due to intercurrent infection, alcohol, or cessation of therapy is a common cause of patients presenting to an emergency room. Skin examination may reveal the port-wine facial stain of Sturge-Weber disease (with cerebral calcifications being detectable on skull x-ray), or the stigmata of tuberous sclerosis (adenoma sebaceum and shagreen patches) or neurofibromatosis (subcutaneous nodules, café au lait spots). Body or limb asymmetries may indicate hypotrophic somatic development contralateral to a congenital or infantile cerebral lesion.

The history or physical examination may also reveal evidence of chronic alcoholism. Heavy alcohol users commonly have seizures for any of several reasons—alcohol withdrawal *(rum fits),* old cerebral contusion (from falls or fights), chronic subdural hematoma, or metabolic derangements of undernutrition and liver disease. Withdrawal seizures usually occur between 12 and 36 h after cessation of drinking and are brief, generalized tonic-clonic seizures. They occur singly or in a flurry of two or three. After the period of epileptic activity, the seizures do not have to be treated since they are usually self-limiting. Seizures in alcoholics which occur at other times should be treated, but this group of patients presents a particular challenge because of lack of compliance and metabolic problems which complicate drug therapy.

Routine blood studies will indicate if the seizure was caused by hypoglycemia, hypo- or hypernatremia, or hypo- or hypercalcemia. These biochemical abnormalities should be corrected and the cause determined. In addition, other less common causes of seizures which can be sought with the appropriate tests are thyrotoxicosis, acute intermittent porphyria, and lead or arsenic intoxication.

In the older patient, a seizure may indicate an acute cerebrovascular accident or may be a delayed effect of an old cerebral infarct (even a silent one). The manner in which further evaluation proceeds is dictated by the patient's age, cardiovascular status, and accompanying symptoms.

Generalized tonic-clonic seizures can occur in neurologically normal individuals after moderate sleep deprivation. Such seizures can be seen in individuals working double shifts, in college students around examination time, and in soldiers returning from short leaves of absence. After the first seizure, if all investigations are normal, such individuals do not require further treatment.

If the patient's history, physical examination, and blood chemistries are all normal after a seizure, it is likely that the seizure was *idiopathic* and was not caused by a serious underlying CNS lesion. However, tumors or other mass lesions may be entirely asymptomatic, and every adult with an unexplained seizure should have an EEG and a CT scan, both without and with contrast, and should be reexamined at regular intervals (3 to 6 months).

The EEG is important in relation to the differential diagnosis of the seizure, the determination of the cause of the seizure, and the proper classification of the seizure. When the diagnosis of a seizure is in doubt, as, for example, when trying to distinguish seizures from syncope, the presence of a paroxysmal EEG abnormality supports the diagnosis of epilepsy. For this purpose, special activation procedures (sleep recording, photic stimulation, or hyperventilation) or special EEG leads (nasopharyngeal, nasoethmoidal, sphenoidal) for recording from deep structures can be employed. The EEG can also reveal focal abnormalities (spikes, sharp waves, or focal slow waves) which would indicate the possibility of a focal neurological lesion even if the seizure symptomatology appeared generalized from the outset.

The EEG is also used to help classify seizures. It can distinguish focal seizures with secondary generalization from primary generalized seizures and is especially useful in the differential diagnosis of brief lapses of consciousness. Absence seizures are always accompanied by bilateral spike-and-wave discharges, whereas complex partial seizures are accompanied by either focal paroxysmal spikes or slow waves or by a normal surface EEG. In cases of absence seizures, the EEG may reveal that the patient is having many more small seizures than was clinically apparent and may help in monitoring antiepileptic drug therapy.

Skull x-rays were originally an important adjunct to the evaluation of the seizure patient, although the CT scan can now provide more definitive information. X-rays may indicate increased intracranial pressure or a midline pineal shift caused by a mass lesion. Abnormal calcifications may occur with gliomas, meningiomas, or Sturge-Weber disease. Lytic lesions in the skull may indicate unexpected metastatic lesions. Marked skull asymmetries may indicate a long-standing atrophic process, perhaps a result of a congenital malformation or a brain lesion acquired in childhood.

Lumbar puncture is employed in the evaluation of the seizure patient in those situations where acute or chronic CNS infections or subarachnoid hemorrhage are suspected. It is also useful in patients who have a focal seizure, especially a temporal lobe seizure, but a normal CT scan. In this case, an elevated CSF protein would indicate that close follow-up or additional studies may be necesssary to detect an occult brain tumor.

Arteriography and pneumoencephalography were formerly employed to search for tumors or other structural abnormalities in patients with seizures. To a large extent these have been replaced by CT scans. However, the arteriogram is still the procedure of choice when searching for an arteriovenous malformation in a patient with a focal seizure disorder and no other apparent cause, and the pneumoencephalogram would be reserved for those patients in whom a small tumor is suspected (i.e., because of elevated CSF protein or persistent, uncontrolled focal seizures) but who have a normal CT scan.

DIFFERENTIAL DIAGNOSIS OF SEIZURES

SYNCOPE VERSUS SEIZURE Sudden loss of consciousness, usually without convulsive movements, presents a common diagnostic problem in both children and adults (see Chap. 12). Faints are often preceded by a feeling of lightheadedness, of the room spinning, of a flush, and are often, but not always, precipitated by an environmental stimulus such as prolonged standing in a hot, crowded area, the sight of blood, a fright, etc. In older people, pure syncope is most often secondary to cardiovascular problems, such as Stokes-Adams attacks, tachyarrhythmias, or orthostatic hypotension, and these may occur with or without a warning. A clear focal onset of the event (i.e., abnormal smell, head turning, staring, etc.) favors seizure as the cause. In addition, convulsive muscular contractions, tongue biting, or incontinence commonly accompany seizures but are much less common with fainting spells. Occasionally vasovagal or other types of fainting episodes can be accompanied by either clonic movements or brief generalized tonic-clonic seizures. If the original loss of consciousness can be ascribed to a clearly nonepileptic cause (e.g., the patient was having blood drawn or a dental procedure at the time), it is not necessary to regard the episode as a manifestation of epilepsy, and antiepileptic drug therapy is not indicated.

When the origin of a syncopal episode is in doubt, the patient should undergo a complete cardiovascular evaluation and an EEG with sleep recording. If the EEG shows paroxysmal activity (which is often brought out by drowsiness and sleep onset), and the patient has no signs of cardiac arrhythmia with ECG monitoring or of valvular disease on echocardiogram, it is likely that the syncopal episode represented a seizure and the patient should be evaluated and treated accordingly.

TRANSIENT ISCHEMIC ATTACKS AND MIGRAINE Transient ischemic attacks (TIAs) and migraine episodes can present as a transient alteration in neurological function (usually without loss of consciousness) which may be confused diagnostically with focal seizures. Neurological dysfunction due to ischemia (TIA or migraine) is often a negative symptom (i.e., loss of feeling, numbness, visual field deficit, paralysis), whereas deficits due to focal seizure activity are often positive (twitching, paresthesias, visual distortion, or hallucination), although this distinction is not absolute. Brief stereotyped episodes which conform to dysfunction in a single vascular territory in an individual with either known vascular disease, heart disease, or with risk factors for vascular disease (diabetes, hypertension) are more likely TIAs. However, since cerebral infarcts are a common cause of subsequent seizures in older patients, a paroxysmal EEG focus should be sought.

Classic migraine headaches with a visual aura, unilateral headache, and gastrointestinal upset are usually easy to distinguish from seizures. However, some migraine patients have only "migraine equivalents" such as a hemiparesis, numbness, or aphasia and may not have subsequent headache. These episodes, especially when they occur in older individuals, are hard to distinguish from TIAs, but may also represent focal seizures. The presence of loss of consciousness after some forms of vertebrobasilar migraine and the common occurrence of headaches after seizures makes this differential diagnosis more difficult. The slower development of neurological dysfunction in migraine is the most helpful point. Nevertheless, occasionally such patients need to be investigated for all three problems with a CT scan, cerebral angiography, and specialized EEG procedures before a diagnosis can be made. In some cases, a therapeutic trial with antiepileptic drugs (which, interestingly, can prevent migraines as well as seizures in some patients) will be necessary for the final diagnosis.

PSYCHOMOTOR VARIANTS AND "HYSTERICAL" SEIZURES As remarked above, patients with complex partial seizures often have bizarre behavioral manifestations of their seizures. These may consist of abrupt changes in personality, feelings of impending doom, abnormal bodily sensations, episodic forgetfulness, or brief repetitive motor activities such as picking at one's clothes or stamping a foot. Many of these patients also have personality disorders, and a significant proportion have had psychiatric intervention. It is common, especially if these patients do not have tonic-clonic seizures or loss of consciousness and when these patients appear emotionally disturbed, for such episodes of psychomotor seizures to be called psychopathic fugues or hysterical seizures. This incorrect diagnosis is often reinforced by a "normal EEG" interictally, or even during one of the episodes. It must be emphasized that seizures can arise from foci deep in temporal lobe structures with *no* surface EEG manifestations. This has been repeatedly demonstrated with depth electrode recordings. Moreover, deep temporal seizures can be manifested only by the kinds of phenomena described above and may be free of the usual seizure phenomena of motor convulsions and loss of consciousness.

In a small number of cases, individuals present with seizure-like events which upon investigation turn out to be hysterical "pseudoseizures" or frank malingering. Often these individuals have had true seizures in the past or are acquainted with an individual with epilepsy. Such pseudoseizures can be quite difficult to distinguish from true seizures. Hysterical seizures are characterized by nonphysiological events such as a progression of twitching from one hand to the other without spread to subjacent ipsilateral face or leg areas, twitching of all four extremities without loss of consciousness (or with surreptitious loss of consciousness), or careful attention to avoiding injury by moving away from a wall or bed edge while having motor convulsions. In addition, hysterical seizures, especially in adolescent girls, may have frankly sexual overtones, with pelvic thrusting or genital manipulation. While many forms of temporal lobe seizures can occur with normal surface EEGs, generalized tonic-clonic seizures always produce abnormal EEGs both during and after the seizure.

TREATMENT OF SEIZURES

Treatment of the patient with a seizure disorder is directed at eliminating the cause of the seizures, suppressing the expression of the seizures, and dealing with the psychosocial consequences which may occur as a result of the neurological dysfunction underlying the seizure disorder or from the presence of a chronic disability.

If the seizure disorder is a result of a metabolic disturbance, such as hypoglycemia or hypocalcemia, restoration of normal metabolic function is usually accompanied by cessation of the seizures. If the seizures are caused by a structural brain lesion, such as a brain tumor, arteriovenous malformation or cerebral cyst, removal of the offending lesion may eliminate the seizures. However, long-standing lesions, even nonprogressive ones, can result in gliosis and other chronic changes in the cerebral cortex. These changes may lead to chronic epileptic foci which will not be eliminated by the subsequent removal of the original lesion. In such cases, surgical extirpation of the epileptic brain regions may be necessary for control of the epilepsy (see "Neurosurgical Treatment of Epilepsy" below).

PHARMACOLOGIC CONTROL OF EPILEPSY The fundamental modality for the treatment of epilepsy is pharmacologic therapy. The goal is to protect the patient from having seizures without interfering with normal cognitive function (or, in the child, with development of normal intellectual function) and without producing harmful systemic side effects. If possible, the individual should be treated with the lowest possible dose of a single anticonvulsant medication. Precise knowledge of the kind of seizure the patient is having, the spectrum of action of the available anticonvulsant medications, and a few basic pharmacokinetic principles can result in the complete control of approximately 60 to 75 percent of patients with epilepsy. Many patients appear to be resistant to medications or develop unnecessary side effects because the medications chosen are not appropriate for the kind(s) of seizure or are not administered in the optimum doses.

The availability of serum levels of anticonvulsant drugs makes it possible to optimize dosage regimens for individual patients and to monitor drug compliance. Thus, patients can be placed on a medication and after a suitable equilibration period (usually several weeks, but at least five *half-lives*), the amount of medication in the serum can be determined and compared to standard *therapeutic ranges* established for each drug. Utilizing blood levels to adjust doses can compensate for individual patient variability in absorption or metabolism of drugs.

Many anticonvulsant drugs are bound by serum proteins, and it is the unbound, or *free*, drug which is in equilibrium with extracellular spaces within the brain; this level correlates best with seizure control. However, *total* drug is measured in the serum by conventional assays. Under most circumstances, this is adequate for determining if the anticonvulsant is in the therapeutic range. Occasionally, serum anticonvulsant levels will be high, yet the patient continues to have seizures without any pharmacologic side effects of the anticonvulsant. In these cases, it is possible that serum protein binding is higher than expected and that the patient is undermedicated in relation to the free drug available. Increase in dose may produce control without any untoward side effects (despite a blood level above therapeutic range). Similarly, individuals with impaired liver or renal function may have low serum proteins or circulating "toxins" which reduce drug binding. In this case, toxicity may appear at unusually low serum levels because of a relatively higher free level of drug.

Intensive long-term EEG and video monitoring have demonstrated that careful characterization of seizures and selection of anticonvulsant drugs can significantly increase seizure control in many patients whose seizures had previously been considered intractable to conventional antiepileptic drugs. In fact, often these patients can have one or more of their multiple drugs removed while still achieving better control.

INDICATIONS FOR USE OF SPECIFIC DRUGS Generalized tonic-clonic seizures (grand mal) There are three medications which are of proven value in this very common form of seizure—phenytoin [or diphenylhydantoin (Dilantin)], phenobarbital (and other long-acting barbiturates), and carbamazepine (Tegretol) (see Table 355-3). Most patients will be controlled by adequate doses of any one of these, although individual patients may respond better to one or another. The choice among them often relates to minimizing undesirable side effects. Phenytoin is probably the drug of choice producing effective control with no sedation and very little, if any, intellectual impairment. However, phenytoin does produce gum hyperplasia in some individuals and can produce mild hirsutism, which is especially unpleasant for young women. Phenytoin may produce lymphadenopathy and, in very high doses, may be toxic to the cerebellum. Carbamazepine is equally effective and does not have many of the side effects seen with phenytoin. Cognitive function appears as well or even better preserved than with phenytoin. However, carbamazepine causes bone marrow depression with mild to moderate falls in peripheral white count (3.5 to 4 $\times$ 10^3/ml) which can occasionally become severe and which must be watched carefully. In addition, a small number of patients show hepatotoxicity.

Phenobarbital is also effective against tonic-clonic seizures and has none of the side effects mentioned above. It can cause sedation and a dulling of intellect, however, especially early in its use and this may lead to poor compliance. The sedation is dose-dependent and may limit the amount of drug which can be given to achieve complete control. However, if control can be achieved with nonsedative doses of phenobarbital, it may be the safest chronic regimen. In children and in the elderly, phenobarbital can produce a state of hyperactivity and hyperirritability which may limit its usefulness.

In addition to their systemic side effects, all three classes of drugs have neurological toxicities at higher doses. Nystagmus is common at therapeutic blood levels, but ataxia, dizziness, tremor, intellectual dulling, forgetfulness, confusion, and even stupor may occur with increasing blood concentrations. These are reversible when blood levels fall back to therapeutic levels.

Partial seizures, including complex partial seizures (temporal lobe epilepsy) The same drugs which are useful for tonic-clonic seizures are also effective for partial seizures, although carbamazepine appears to be slightly more effective than phenytoin, and the barbiturates less effective. Primidone (Mysoline) is a barbiturate which is metabolized to phenobarbital and phenylethylmalonamide (PEMA) and may be more effective than phenobarbital alone. In general, complex partial seizures are difficult to control, and patients with these seizures often require more than one medication (i.e., carbamazepine and primidone or phenytoin and primidone) and may become candidates for neurosurgical intervention.

Primary generalized absence seizures (petit mal, atypical petit mal) These seizures respond to different classes of medications than either tonic-clonic or focal seizures. For simple absence, ethosuximide (Zarontin) is the drug of choice. These seizures are usually seen in children and the dose is calculated according to body weight (Table 355-3). Side effects include gastrointestinal upset, dizziness, and lethargy, but are not often troublesome. For more difficult to control absence seizures, valproic acid (Depakene) or clonazepam (Clonopin, a benzodiazepine) can be used. Both of these are effective, but valproic acid can cause gastrointestinal irritation, bone marrow suppression, and hepatic dysfunction (including rare instances of fatal progressive hepatic failure which appear to be idiosyncratic rather than dose-related), and clonazepam can cause drowsiness and irritability. Trimethadione (Tridione) was one of the first antiabsence drugs but is now rarely used because of its potential toxicity.

Approximately one-third of children who present with absence seizures also have tonic-clonic seizures at some later time. The question of whether these children should be treated prophylactically with an anti-tonic-clonic seizure medication has not been resolved. Recent evidence indicates that the concurrent use of phenobarbital with antiabsence drugs may interfere with therapy for the absence.

Status epilepticus Generalized tonic-clonic status epilepticus is a life-threatening medical emergency, but overzealous and incautious treatment can produce more harm than good. Patients are in danger from hyperpyrexia and acidosis (from prolonged muscle activity) and less commonly, hypoxia or compromise of respiratory function. Immediate treatment for

TABLE 355-3
Commonly used antiepileptic drugs

Generic name	*Trade name*	*Principal uses*	*Dosage*	*Half-life*
Phenytoin (diphenylhydantoin)	Dilantin	Tonic-clonic (grand mal) Focal Complex partial	300–400 mg/day (3–5 mg/kg—adult; 4–7 mg/kg—child)	24 h (with wide variation)
Carbamazepine	Tegretol	Tonic-clonic Focal Complex partial	600–1200 mg/day (20–30 mg/kg—child)	13–17 h
Phenobarbital	Luminol	Tonic-clonic Focal	60–200 mg/day (1–5 mg/kg—adult; 3–6 mg/kg—child)	90 h (shorter in children)
Primidone	Mysoline	Tonic-clonic Focal Complex partial	750–1000 mg/day (10–25 mg/kg)	Primidone—8 h PEMA—24–48 h Phenobarbital—90 h
Ethosuximide	Zarontin	Absence (petit mal)	750–1250 mg/day (20–40 mg/kg)	60 h (adult) 30 h (child)
Methsuximide	Celontin	Absence	600–1200 mg/day	
Clonazepam	Clonopin	Absence Atypical absence Myoclonic	1–12 mg/day (0.1–0.2 mg/kg)	24–48 h
Sodium valproate	Depakene	Absence Atypical absence (Tonic clonic)	750–1250 mg/day (30–60 mg/kg)	15 h
Trimethadione	Tridione	Absence Atypical absence (Use only with intractable seizures)	900–2100 mg/day (20–60 mg/kg)	6–13 days (for dimethadione)

status is protection of the airway, protection of the tongue (with a soft object, large enough not to be swallowed, between the clenched teeth), protection of the head, and then establishment of a secure parenteral (intravenous) access. A bolus of 50% glucose in water (after blood is drawn for analysis), even if hypoglycemia is not expected, may stop the seizures. All further intravenous medication should be given after preparation for respiratory and circulatory support is available.

Phenytoin (Dilantin), 500 to 1500 mg (13 to 18 mg/kg) in a slow intravenous "push" or in an intravenous drip mixed in normal saline (*not* 5% dextrose in water—phenytoin precipitates in this low pH solution)—in either case no faster than 50 mg/min—is one of the drugs of choice. It does not depress respiration but may produce mild AV block and, if given too rapidly, can cause a fall in blood pressure.

The benzodiazepines, diazepam (Valium) 10 mg or lorazepam (Ativan) 4 mg (followed by another dose if necessary), are also effective in stopping status epilepticus when administered intravenously. However, these drugs may depress respiratory function (or even cause respiratory arrest), and measures for respiratory support should be available before they are administered. The use of a benzodiazepine after phenobarbital administration carries a particular risk. The benzodiazepines are short-acting drugs, and after they are administered, a second, longer-acting anticonvulsant such as phenytoin is usually required to prevent recurrence of seizures.

Phenobarbital, in a dose of 10 to 20 mg/kg (up to 1 g), divided into two to four doses at 30- to 60-minute intervals, can also be administered for status epilepticus. Phenobarbital also causes respiratory depression and should not be used immediately after treatment with intravenous diazepam.

After stopping the seizures it is imperative to determine the cause of the status epilepticus in order to prevent its recurrence. In approximately two-thirds of adults the cause can be determined and is usually tumor, vascular disease, infection, cerebral damage, or precipitous withdrawal from alcohol or antiepileptic medication. In children, the incidence of idiopathic status is higher (approximately 50 percent), and the remaining cases are divided between acute brain illnesses such as purulent meningitis, encephalitis, and dehydration with electrolyte disturbances, and chronic encephalopathies. Status epilepticus is a dangerous condition; the mortality rate may be over 10 percent with another 10 to 30 percent of patients being left with permanent neurological sequelae.

NEUROSURGICAL TREATMENT OF EPILEPSY If a structural lesion (i.e., tumor, cyst, abscess, etc.) is causing recurrent seizures, the removal of that lesion and nearby diseased brain will often eliminate the seizures or make them easier to control. Some patients, however, have uncontrollable seizures without a demonstrable structural lesion. These are often complex partial seizures with ictal and interictal EEG abnormalities emanating from one or both temporal lobes. Many surgical series have shown that if the epileptogenic lesion can be clearly localized to one temporal lobe, neurosurgical removal of that temporal lobe can result in significant improvement in 60 to 80 percent of the patients. Localization often depends on intensive EEG monitoring and even depth electrode recordings from the temporal lobes. In a high percentage of cases the removed temporal lobe can be shown to have microscopic pathology, such as *hippocampal* (or *Ammon's horn*) *sclerosis* (loss of pyramidal cells in the hippocampus), a hamartoma, or cortical ectopia.

Some individuals with complex partial seizures also develop a psychiatric illness characterized most often as a borderline

Therapeutic range	% Protein-bound	Toxic effects: Neurological	Toxic effects: Systemic	Drug interactions
10–20 μg/ml	90	Ataxia Incoordination Confusion	Gum hyperplasia Lymphadenopathy Hirsutism Osteomalacia Skin rash Altered folate metabolism	Level increased by INH, dicumeral, sulfonamides Level decreased by carbamazepine phenobarbital Folate interferes with effects
4–12 μg/ml	80	Ataxia Dizziness Diplopia Vertigo	Bone marrow suppression Gastrointestinal irritation Hepatotoxicity	Level decreased by phenobarbital, phenytoin
10–50 μg/ml	40–60	Sedation Ataxia Confusion Dizziness	Skin rash	Level increased by valproate, phenytoin
2–10 μg/ml	Small for primidone or PEMA	Same as phenobarbital	Same as phenobarbital	
40–100 μg/ml	Small	Ataxia Lethargy	Gastrointestinal irritation Skin rash Bone marrow suppression	
	Small	Ataxia Lethargy	Same as ethosuximide	
5–70 ng/ml	50	Ataxia Sedation Lethargy	Anorexia	May precipitate absence status if given with valproic acid
50–100 μg/ml	80–94	Ataxia Sedation	Hepatotoxicity Bone marrow suppression Gastrointestinal irritation Weight gain Transient alopecia	May precipitate absence status if given with clonazepam
700 μg/ml (for dimethadione)	Small	Sedation Blurred vision	Skin rash Bone marrow suppression Nephrosis Hepatitis	

personality with certain specific behavioral manifestations including hypergraphia, hyperreligiosity, lack of sense of humor, and disordered sexuality. The psychiatric aspects of this illness may result from the epilepsy or may be independently produced by the same underlying brain lesion which produces the epilepsy. The personality disorder may not significantly change after epilepsy surgery, even if the seizures are controlled.

TREATMENT OF A SINGLE SEIZURE Some individuals present with a single, brief generalized tonic-clonic seizure and, after complete evaluation, are found to have a normal EEG and no underlying cause for the seizure. Some of these individuals go on to have recurrent seizures, but an unknown proportion do not. The decision to treat such a patient with several years (at least) of antiepileptic medication must be made on an individual basis, considering the patient's life style, risks from a sudden loss of consciousness, and feelings about medications.

CESSATION OF ANTIEPILEPTIC DRUG THERAPY Many patients with epilepsy require antiepileptic drug therapy for life. However, a large proportion of epileptic patients become seizure-free on appropriate medication, and approximately half of such patients can eventually stop their medications and remain seizure-free. The patient who has had no seizures for 4 years, who has had relatively few seizures before control was attained, who only required a single medication, who has a normal neurological exam and no structural lesion causing the seizures, and who has a normal EEG at the end of the therapeutic period has the best chance of remaining seizure-free if medication is slowly tapered (over 3 to 6 months). An abnormal EEG is not a contraindication to discontinuing medication. When considering the discontinuance of antiepileptic therapy, the consequences of the recurrence of seizures must be carefully considered. One inopportune seizure in a previously well controlled patient who is not used to taking precautions may be a life-threatening event, or lead to loss of a driver's license or loss of employment. Nevertheless, since all medicatons carry some risk of toxicity and since medication compliance in a healthy individual is often variable, it is worth a careful trial of medication tapering in individuals who meet the above criteria and are willing to accept the risk.

EPILEPSY AND PREGNANCY Most women with epilepsy can undergo uneventful pregnancies and deliver healthy babies—even those taking anticonvulsant medications. During the pregnant state, however, body metabolism changes and close attention must be given to antiepileptic drug levels. Sometimes relatively high doses have to be given to ensure therapeutic levels. Most women who are well controlled before pregnancy will remain so during pregnancy and delivery.

One of the most serious complications of pregnancy, toxemia, often presents as a generalized tonic-clonic convulsion in the third trimester. This seizure is a symptom of a severe neurological disturbance and is not a manifestation of epilepsy, nor is it more common in epileptic women. The toxemic state must be treated in order to control the seizures.

There is a two- to threefold higher incidence of fetal malformations in offspring of epileptic women, and this is likely due to a combination of the low incidence of medication-induced malformation and of genetic predisposition in this population. Among those malformations which do occur, a *fetal-hydantoin syndrome* consisting of cleft lip and palate, heart defects, digital hypoplasia, and nail dysplasia has been identified.

Although it would be ideal for women contemplating pregnancy to have their antiepileptic drugs discontinued, it is likely that for a large number of women this would result in recurrence of seizures which would, in the long run, be more harmful for both mother and baby. If patients meet the criteria for discontinuance of medication, this should be done with a suitable interval before pregnancy is to occur. Other patients should be tapered to a minimal effective dosage and followed closely throughout the pregnancy and delivery. Phenobarbital, primidone, or phenytoin can cause transient and reversible deficiency in vitamin K-dependent clotting factors in the neonate, and these should be promptly treated. Some babies are transiently sluggish and hypotonic and may show signs of mild barbiturate withdrawal. These babies should be considered potentially at risk for neonatal problems and should be closely observed in the nursery for the first 2 to 4 days of life.

DRIVING AND EPILEPSY Each state has its own regulations for determining when an individual with epilepsy can obtain a driver's license, and several states have laws about the physician's obligations in either reporting epileptic patients to the registry or informing the patients of their responsibilities to do so. In general, patients can drive after a seizure-free interval (on or off medications) which ranges from 6 months to 2 years. In some states there is no fixed interval, but the individual is required to have a physician's letter attesting to seizure control. It is the physician's responsibility to warn the epileptic patient of the risks of driving when seizures are not under control.

SOCIAL AND EDUCATIONAL REHABILITATION Most people with epilepsy attain adequate control of their seizures and are able to attend school, obtain employment, and live a relatively normal life. Children with epilepsy tend to have more problems in school than their peers, but every effort should be made to keep these children integrated into the mainstream of the educational process while supplying additional help in the form of academic tutoring or psychological counseling.

REFERENCES

COMMISSION ON CLASSIFICATION AND TERMINOLOGY OF THE ILAE: Proposal for revised clinical classification of epileptic seizures. Epilepsia 22:489, 1981

EMERSON R et al: Stopping medication in children with epilepsy. N Engl J Med 304:1125, 1981

LAIDLAW J, RICHENS A (eds): *A Textbook of Epilepsy,* 2d ed. London, Churchill Livingstone, 1982

THURSTON J et al: Prognosis in childhood epilepsy. N Engl J Med 306:831, 1982

WOODBURY D et al (eds): *Antiepileptic Drugs,* 2d ed. New York, Raven Press, 1982

356 CEREBROVASCULAR DISEASES

JAY P. MOHR
CARLOS S. KASE
RAYMOND D. ADAMS

Vascular diseases of the nervous system rank first in frequency among all the neurologic diseases. They remain an excellent approach to the study of neurology since they yield a wide range of disorders of brain function.

The term *cerebrovascular disease* refers to any disease implicating one or more of the blood vessels of the brain in a pathologic process. By *pathologic process* is meant any abnormality of the vessel wall, an occlusion by thrombus or embolus, rupture of a vessel, a failure of cerebral blood flow due to a fall in blood pressure, a change in the caliber of the lumen, altered permeability of the vascular wall, or increased viscosity or other quality of the blood. The pathologic process within the vessel may be described not only according to its grosser aspects—thrombosis, embolism, rupture of a vessel, etc.—but also in terms of the more basic vascular disorder, i.e., atherosclerosis, hypertensive arteriosclerosis, arteritis, trauma, aneurysm, developmental malformation. These processes result in two types of parenchymal changes in the brain, ischemia with or without infarction, and hemorrhage. Other, less common, effects of vascular disease include syndromes of local pressure of an aneurysm, vascular headache (migraine, hypertension, arteritis), and occasionally increased intracranial pressure in hypertensive encephalopathy and venous thrombosis.

Obstruction of the nutrient artery by thrombus or embolus or failure of the systemic circulation and hypotension, if severe and prolonged enough, can deprive brain tissue of blood and oxygen, leading to ischemic disruption of physiologic function and subsequent necrosis (infarction).

Brain infarcts vary greatly in the amount of congestion and hemorrhage found within the softened tissue at autopsy. Some infarcts are pale; others show mild dilatation of vessels and some extravasation of red blood cells; still others are hemorrhagic, with extensive scattering of petechial hemorrhages throughout the damaged gray matter. Thrombotic infarcts are usually pale, while embolic infarcts are sometimes pale, sometimes hemorrhagic. Hemorrhagic infarction is often associated with the fragmentation and migration of embolic material from its original site of arrest, the distal movement of the embolus allowing blood to enter the more proximal part of the infarct.

In hemorrhage an extravasation of blood occurs into the brain tissue, the subarachnoid space, or both. Once the leakage stops, the blood is slowly resorbed over a period of weeks and months. Damage to the brain results from physical disruption of the region directly involved and pressure of the mass of blood on the surrounding tissue.

THE STROKE SYNDROME

The cardinal feature of cerebrovascular disease is the *stroke,* a term that connotes the sudden and dramatic development of a focal neurologic deficit. The deficit may vary from a dense hemiplegia and coma to only a trivial neurologic disorder insufficient to disturb the customary activities of the patient.

Undoubtedly, the most characteristic feature of a stroke is its *temporal profile.* The suddenness of syndrome development stamps the disorder as vascular. The speed of evolution varies from seconds, minutes, or rarely hours, to at most a few days. Sudden onset characterizes strokes from embolism and ruptured aneurysm, the deficit reaching its maximum almost immediately. Thrombotic strokes are also usually sudden in onset, but may develop over a period of several days, usually progressing in a stepwise fashion, i.e., in a series of sudden changes. In parenchymatous hemorrhage the deficit evolves smoothly over minutes or hours. Rapid reversal of the deficit may occur from ischemic cause but never in hemorrhage. Later in the course of a nonfatal stroke, stabilization occurs, and is followed by some degree of improvement, especially in cases with deficits in language function. The improvement is gradual, taking place over weeks and months.

The neurologic deficit in a stroke reflects both the location and the size of the infarct or hemorrhage in the brain. Hemiplegia is the classic sign of vascular disease and occurs with strokes involving the cerebral hemisphere or the brainstem. However, depending on its location, a stroke may also give rise to many other manifestations accompanying or independent of hemiplegia, including numbness, sensory deficit, dysphasia, blindness, diplopia, dizziness, and dysarthria. Familiarity with the neurovascular syndromes outlined in this chapter will aid in locating the lesion in individual cases of stroke and in determining whether the stroke represents ischemia or hemorrhage.

Laboratory assessment of stroke provides further data concerning its site, size, and type of brain lesion, and, if possible, the status of arteries or veins involved in the stroke process. *Computerized tomography* of the brain (CT scan) has proved a most valuable tool for the diagnosis of stroke. Although CT may be normal in the initial days after infarction, a focal area of decreased density rapidly follows, as the infarct liquefies. The intravenous infusion of radiographic contrast material produces a characteristic "enhancement" (high attenuation) of the cortical portions of the infarct, a feature usually seen between 1 and 3 weeks from the onset. Hematomas and hemorrhagic infarcts are detected as areas of high attenuation, the former usually accompanied by prominent mass effect. *Radionuclide brain scanning* successfully images many hematomas and some infarcts in their subacute stage (days to weeks), but hematomas cannot be seen in the late stages (months or years). *Arteriography* with radiopaque dyes demonstrates stenoses and occlusions of the larger vessels and aneurysms and arteriovenous malformations. Embolic occlusions are demonstrable in 75 percent of cases, especially in the initial hours and days after stroke, but in less than 15 percent when arteriography is carried out more than 2 days after the stroke. At that time, the fragmented embolic material may only be found scattered in branches distal to the original site of occlusion, or altogether dissipated. The larger hematomas are seen in arteriograms to cause displacement of vessels (mass effect); and in hemorrhages due to aneurysm, in 85 percent of cases they demonstrate the ruptured aneurysm as well as associated arterial spasm. *Lumbar puncture* regularly yields bloody fluid in ruptured aneurysm or vascular malformation or ventricular extension of a hypertensive hemorrhage. The cerebrospinal fluid (CSF) is clear in bland infarction from either embolus or thrombus.

ISCHEMIC STROKE

The effects of both thrombotic and embolic arterial occlusion relate to the topography of the occluded artery and vary according to the availability of *collateral or anastomotic blood flow.* If the obstruction lies proximal to the circle of Willis, collateral flow via the circle may be adequate to prevent infarction. In occlusion of the internal carotid artery in the neck, anastomotic flow may pass along the external carotid artery and retrograde in the ophthalmic artery or other smaller external-internal connections. In vertebral artery blockage low in the neck, blood may reach the upper part of the vertebral artery via the deep cervical, thyrocervical, occipital artery, or retrograde from the other vertebral artery. If the occlusion is distal to the circle of Willis, i.e., in the stem of one of the cerebral or cerebellar arteries, a series of subarachnoid border zone interarterial anastomoses that join many of the branches of the major cerebral arteries may carry sufficient blood into the compromised tissue to lessen the ischemic damage (Fig. 356-1). The capillary anastomotic system between adjacent brain arteries, although always the source of some collateral supply, is probably inconsequential. Thus in the event of occlusion of a major arterial trunk the extent of infarction ranges from none (rare) to softening throughout the entire territory. Between these two extremes are countless variations in the size, shape, and completeness of an infarct, depending on such ischemic modifying factors as the speed of occlusion (time for compensation), the level of the systemic blood pressure, hypoxia, and altered physical state of the blood.

The *specific neurologic abnormality* depends on the location and size of the infarct or the focus of ischemia. The territory of any vessel, large or small, deep or superficial, may be involved. In involvement of the carotid system, *unilateral* signs predominate: hemiplegia, hemihypesthesia, hemianopia, aphasia, and agnosia. In basilar disease, one more commonly finds *bilateral* signs, motor and/or sensory, in combination with a disturbance of cranial nerves, cerebellum, or other structures localized in or related to the brainstem.

NEUROVASCULAR SYNDROMES

While the clinical picture resulting from the occlusion of any particular artery differs in minor ways from one patient to another, there is sufficient uniformity to permit diagnosis. Partial syndromes are in the majority. The following descriptions apply particularly to infarction and ischemia due to embolism or thrombosis. Although hemorrhage within these vascular territories may give rise to many of the same effects, the total clinical picture is apt to differ because in its deep extension the hemorrhage may involve the territory of more than one vessel and by its mass effect may cause an increase in intracranial pressure.

INTERNAL CAROTID ARTERY Occlusion of the internal carotid artery may be completely asymptomatic. However, most occlusions lead to symptoms, whose severity reflects the highly variable extent of the infarction. Most often the infarct involves some part of the middle cerebral territory, but when the anterior communicating artery is very small, the ipsilateral anterior cerebral territory may be affected too, in which case the anterior part of the hemisphere (the frontal lobe) bears the brunt of the insult, while the region posterior to the rolandic fissure tends to be spared. When both anterior cerebral arteries arise from a common stem on one side, infarction may involve the anterior cerebral territory bilaterally. The posterior cerebral artery is infrequently supplied from the internal carotid rather than from the basilar artery, and its territory, too, may be softened, and thus the entire hemisphere and even part of the other may be involved. The tissue in the territory of the anterior choroidal artery may also be infarcted. When one carotid has been occluded at a previous time, occlusion of the other can contribute to a catastrophic infarction of both the cerebral hemispheres. In such cases, coma with quadriplegia and continuous horizontal conjugate "metronomic" eye movements may be seen.

In symptomatic occlusion of the internal carotid artery the picture resembles that of middle cerebral occlusion with contralateral hemiplegia, hemihypesthesia, and disturbance in behavior with aphasia (in involvement of the dominant hemisphere). When the anterior cerebral territory is also infarcted, the clinical picture will be broadened to include some or all its clinical effects (see below). Such patients are much less responsive than those with lesions in the territory of only one cerebral artery, and often they are in a coma. Headache may also occur with both cerebral thrombosis or embolism in the carotid artery; the pain is situated just above the eyebrow. That associated with occlusion of the middle cerebral artery is usually more lateral, at the temple and, with occlusion of the posterior cerebral artery, in or behind the eye.

When the circulation in one carotid is compromised and collateral flow is restricted, the tissue in the most distal or terminal parts of the territories of the middle and anterior and at

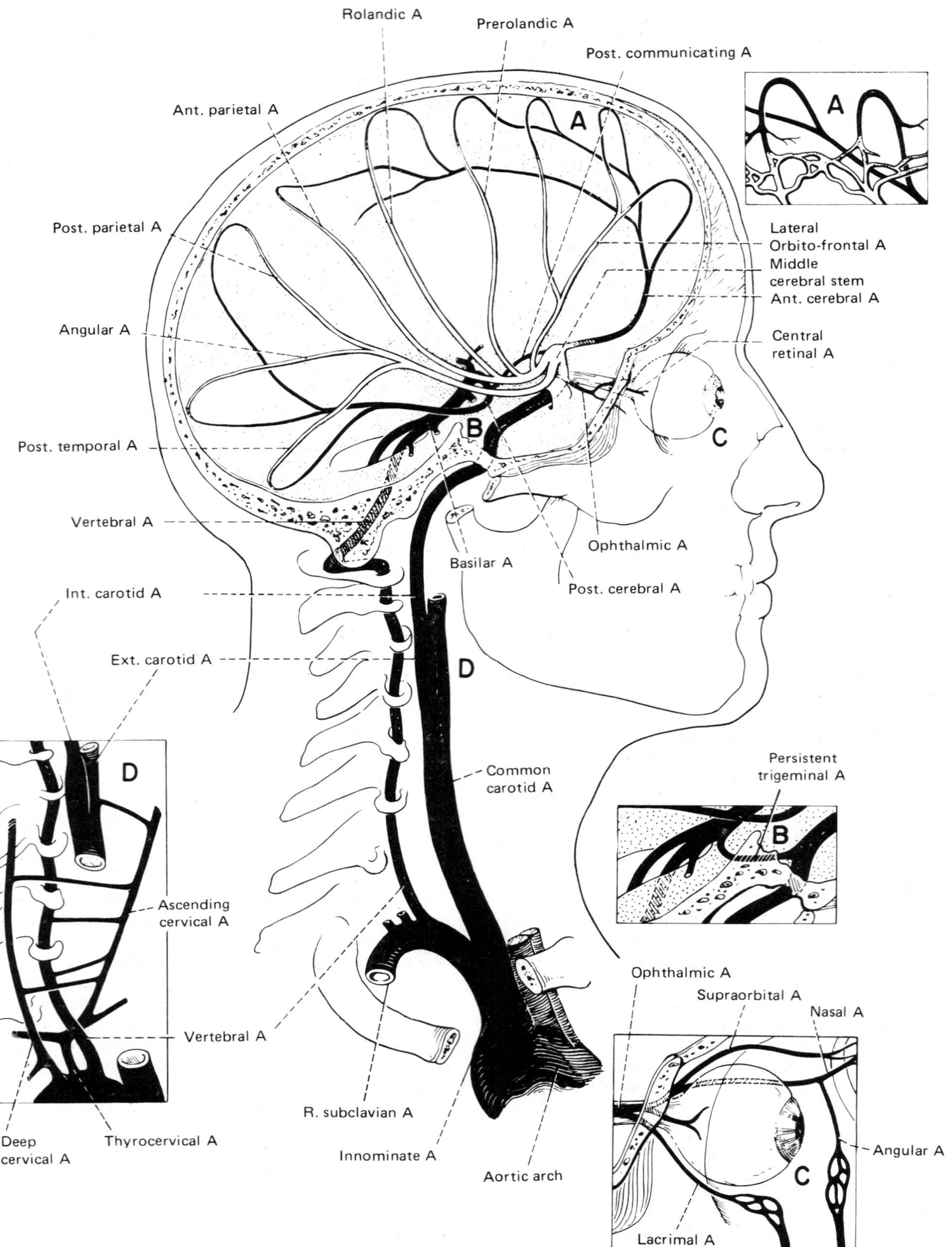

FIGURE 356-1

Arrangement of the major arteries on the right side carrying blood from the heart to the brain. Also shown are vessels of collateral circulation that may modify the effects of cerebral ischemia. For example, the posterior communicating artery connects the internal carotid and the posterior cerebral arteries, and may provide anastomosis between the carotid and basilar systems. Over the convexity, the subarachnoid interarterial anastomoses linking the middle, anterior, and posterior cerebral arteries are shown, with inset A illustrating that these anastomoses are a continuous network of tiny arteries forming a border zone between the major cerebral arterial territories. Occasionally a persistent trigeminal artery connects the internal carotid and basilar arteries proximal to the circle of Willis, as shown in inset B. Anastomoses between the internal and external carotid arteries via the orbit are illustrated in inset C. Wholly extracranial anastomoses from muscular branches of the cervical arteries to vertebral and external carotid arteries are indicated by inset D.

times the posterior cerebral arteries suffers first and most severely. This gives rise to an irregular and asymmetric *border-zone* (watershed) configuration of infarction in which the contiguous distal fields of each vessel are disproportionately affected, the heaviest involvement usually falling on the frontocentral regions of the middle cerebral artery territory. When well developed, the zone of damage forms an elongated strip of variable width extending from the frontal pole to the occipital. Therefore carotid infarcts of less than maximal extent tend to be located distally rather than proximally in the sylvian region. Likewise it is in this most vulnerable region that transient ischemic attack symptoms are liable to arise in carotid stenosis, taking the form of weakness or paresthesias in the upper extremity and, only if more extensive, in the face and tongue. Relative sparing of the posterior part of the hemisphere is reflected in a low incidence of central aphasia and persistent homonymous hemianopia.

In addition to nourishing the brain, the internal carotid artery supplies the optic nerve and retina via the ophthalmic artery (Fig. 356-1). Transient monocular blindness occurs intermittently as a warning symptom prior to the onset of the stroke in approximately 25 percent of cases of symptomatic carotid occlusion. Of interest, and presumably reflecting good collateral blood supply, central retinal artery occlusion rarely appears under such circumstances.

Whereas most cerebral vessels are inaccessible within the skull and topical diagnosis is made only by inference, in carotid disease more direct diagnostic tests are available. Pressure in the central retinal artery is usually reduced on the side of carotid occlusion or severe stenosis and is usually a significant sign when the values for diastole are below 20 mmHg. Dilated collateral channels coursing over the forehead may also suggest carotid occlusion. Supraorbital and supratrochlear arterial pulsations on the rim of the orbit may be prominent but easily suppressed upon simultaneous compression of the preauricular, facial, or superficial temporal branches of the external carotid artery. The usual blood supply from the internal carotid artery via the ophthalmic artery has then been reversed, indicating collateralization of internal carotid from external carotid sources. Retinal embolism, either of shining white or plain type, may point to carotid disease. Severe stenosis within the carotid sinus due to an atherosclerotic plaque—with or without superimposed thrombus—is likely to give rise to a local bruit. Occasionally the murmur results from stenosis at the origin of the external rather than the internal carotid artery. The auscultation of the bruit while the patient performs the Valsalva maneuver is helpful in differentiating external from internal carotid origin: a significant reduction in amplitude characterizes bruits from internal carotid origin, whereas those originating in external carotid stenosis remain unchanged. If the murmur is heard at the angle of the jaw, the stenosis is in the carotid sinus; if lower in the neck, the stenosis is in the common carotid or subclavian artery. (Distal propagation of an aortic valvular murmur must be distinguished from carotid bruits.) An additional sign of carotid occlusion is the presence of an intracranial murmur over the *opposite* carotid artery. This is heard best by placing the bell of the stethoscope over the eyeball. The murmur is presumably due to augmented blood flow through the remaining patent vessel. Pulsation may be reduced or absent in the internal or common carotid arteries in the neck, in the external carotid branch in front of the ear, or in the internal carotid artery when palpated in the pharynx, but minor asymmetries in pulsations are rarely significant when present as an isolated finding. *Because of the possibility* of precipitous onset of unconsciousness, seizures, or an electroencephalographic change, testing the carotid circulation by compressing the artery is not recommended.

Occlusion of the cervical segments of the carotid and subclavian or innominate arteries proximal to the internal carotid is frequently asymptomatic because of the abundant collateral circulation. The following manifestations, for the most part nonneurologic, have been reported when collateral flow proves inadequate: absence of pulsation in carotid and radial arteries, faintness on arising from the horizontal position, recurrent loss of consciousness, headache, neck pain, paresthesias of various parts of the body, transient blindness (unilateral or bilateral), dimness of vision with exercise, premature cataracts, retinal atrophy and pigmentation, atrophy of the iris, leukomas, peripapillary arteriovenous anastomoses, optic atrophy, claudication of the jaw muscles, perforation of the nasal septum, saddle nose deformity, trophic ulceration of the face, facial atrophy (unilateral or bilateral), indolent infections of the face, abnormal facial pigmentation, and loss of hair. Pulseless disease expresses its cerebral effects through occlusion of both carotid arteries. Originally described in Japan, particularly in young women and called Takayasu's disease, it consists essentially of a granulomatous arteritis of unknown cause involving all three major trunks arising from the aortic arch (see Chap. 268). An incomplete aortic arch syndrome consisting of various combinations of carotid, subclavian, or innominate occlusion or stenosis is not uncommon. The majority of the cases of pulseless disease in the United States and Europe, both the partial and the complete syndrome, have been due to severe atherosclerosis. Often this has been mistakenly called *Buerger's disease*.

MIDDLE CEREBRAL ARTERY The cortical branches of this artery supply the lateral surface of the hemisphere. Its territory includes the cortex and white matter of the lateral and inferior aspects of the frontal lobe, the motor cortex, the cortex and white matter of the lateral parietal lobe (sensory cortex, angular and supramarginal convolutions), the lateral and superior parts of the temporal lobe, and the insula. The penetrating branches of the middle cerebral artery arise from the stem of the artery, prior to its cortical surface branches, to supply the putamen, outer globus pallidus, the posterior limb of the internal capsule above the plane of the upper border of the globus pallidus, the adjacent part of the corona radiata, the body of the caudate nucleus, and the superior and lateral portions of the head of the caudate nucleus (Fig. 356-2).

The middle cerebral artery may be occluded in its stem, blocking the mouths of the penetrating vessels as well as the flow to the superficial (cortical) vessels, or its major branches can be blocked individually. Thrombotic occlusion of the stem of the middle cerebral artery is relatively uncommon compared with embolism. The classic picture of infarction of its whole territory is a contralateral hemiplegia, hemianesthesia, homonymous hemianopia, global or total sensorimotor aphasia (left hemisphere), and apractagnosia (right hemisphere). When collateral circulation restricts the ischemia to a part of the territory, the deficit is more limited. Once the major infarction is established, the motor, sensory, and language deficits usually remain static or very little improved after the passage of months or even years. Seldom can the patient ever again communicate effectively. A deceptive sign is the occasional echoic speech that may occur in the early stage, encouraging the family and physician to assume that speech is not severely affected. But these stereotypic greetings, short word utterances, and the repetition of short words generally remain as the only language performance of which the patient is capable.

Occlusion (usually embolic) of the main divisions or individual branches of the middle cerebral artery produces a corresponding partial deficit. The embolus may block the vessel to the anterior or motor part of the hemisphere (superior division) or the posterior or sensory part of the hemisphere (infe-

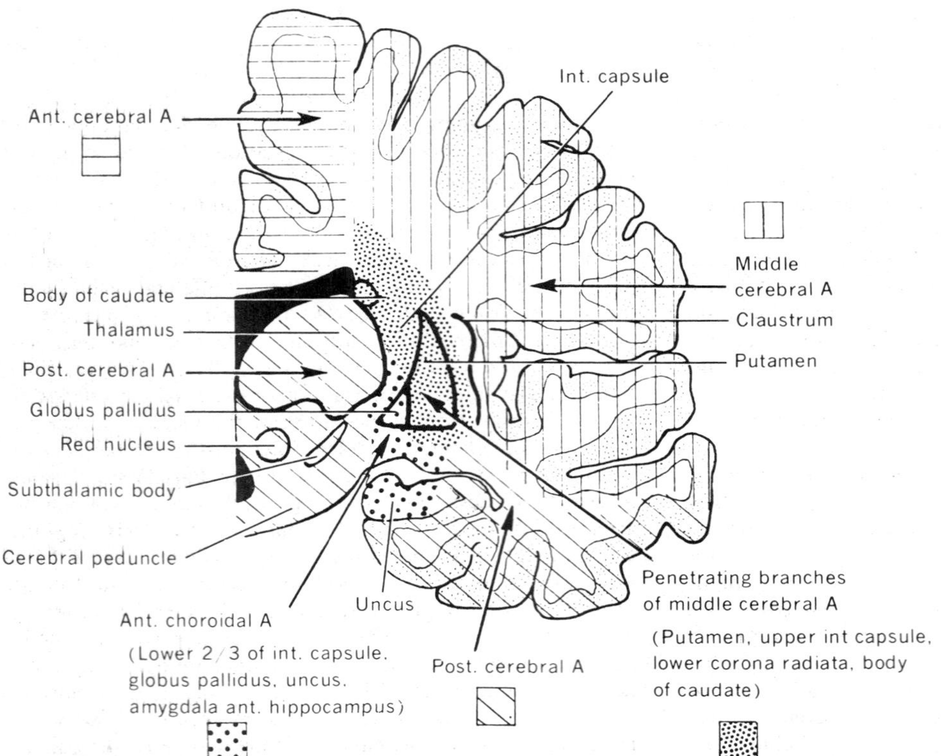

FIGURE 356-2
Diagram of a cerebral hemisphere, coronal section, showing the territories of the major cerebral vessels.

rior division) (Fig. 356-3). Major occlusion of the superior division causes a dense sensorimotor deficit in the face and limbs and total aphasia (left) that mimics the syndrome of occlusion of the stem of the middle cerebral artery or the carotid artery.

Varying degrees of improvement follow occlusions of individual branches of the middle cerebral artery. Within weeks, after branch occlusions affecting the upper division, there is usually sufficient motor improvement that the patient can walk on the spastic leg while motor deficits of arm and face frequently remain severe. The initial total aphasia changes toward predominantly motor aphasia, with improvement in comprehension of spoken and written language and the emergence of a hesitant, grammatically simplified, dysmelodic speech.

Because the upper division gives off its branches in sequence, an occlusion limited to only one of them may elicit a highly circumscribed infarct that fractionates the syndrome even farther. In occlusion of the ascending frontal branch, involving Broca's area and immediate surrounding territory, the sensorimotor deficit is limited to faciobrachial paresis with little weakness of the leg, and the speech disorder consists of an initial mutism with very mild comprehension disorder. Within hours to weeks, the weakness lessens, and a dysmelodic but grammatically appropriate speech appears. Occlusion of rolandic branches produces a sensorimotor paresis with severe dysarthria that may follow a clinical course suggestive of pure motor stroke from a lacunar infarct (see "Lacunar Syndromes" below) but with little sign of dysphasia. When ascending parietal and other posterior branches of the upper division are occluded, the result is a deficit currently described as "conduction" aphasia, and ideomotor dyspraxia affecting both sides of the body, but often no significant sensorimotor deficit. The speech disorder usually improves to a normal or near-normal state within months.

The lower division of the middle cerebral artery is only infrequently occluded alone, but when it is so involved (almost always from an embolus and only with great rarity from thrombosis), the full syndrome of Wernicke's aphasia is the usual result (Chap. 23) when the dominant hemisphere is affected. No hemiparesis occurs, although the larger infarcts may involve the deep white matter, including the visual radiation, and produce hemianopia as well. The deficit remains static for months and even years but tends to improve. In right nondominant lesions a syndrome of apractagnosia results. In less extensive infarcts, the more distal parietal, temporal, and occipital regions are collateralized via the branches of the posterior cerebral artery, and the major involvement is more or less confined to the posterior temporal regions. With lesions in the dominant hemisphere, such patients often show greater deficit on language tests that involve auditory comprehension and perform better, sometimes almost normally, in reading. Within weeks or months, the disorder improves to the point that it is evident only in self-generated efforts at speaking and writing. Especially in the later stages, the deficit resembles the syndrome of conduction aphasia resulting from occlusion of posterior branches of the upper division of the middle cerebral artery. The site and size of the infarct are difficult to predict on clinical grounds alone.

ANTERIOR CEREBRAL ARTERY Through its cortical branches, this artery supplies the anterior four-fifths of the medial surface of the cerebral hemisphere, including the medial part of the orbital surface of the frontal lobe, the frontal lobe, a strip of the lateral surface along the superior border, and the anterior seven-eighths of the corpus callosum. The deep branches, which arise near the circle of Willis, run chiefly to the anterior limb of the internal capsule and inferior part of the head of the caudate nucleus (see Fig. 356-4).

Again the clinical picture will depend on the location and size of the infarct. Occlusion of the stem of the anterior cerebral artery proximal to the anterior communicating artery is usually well tolerated, since collateral flow will come from its mate of the opposite side. The maximal disturbance occurs when both anterior cerebral arteries happen to arise from one anterior cerebral stem, occlusion of which then results in infarction of the anterior cerebral territory of both hemispheres. This may include bilateral pyramidal signs with paraplegia and profound mental symptoms. A complex syndrome of contralateral grasp and sucking reflex, paratonic rigidity (gegenhal-

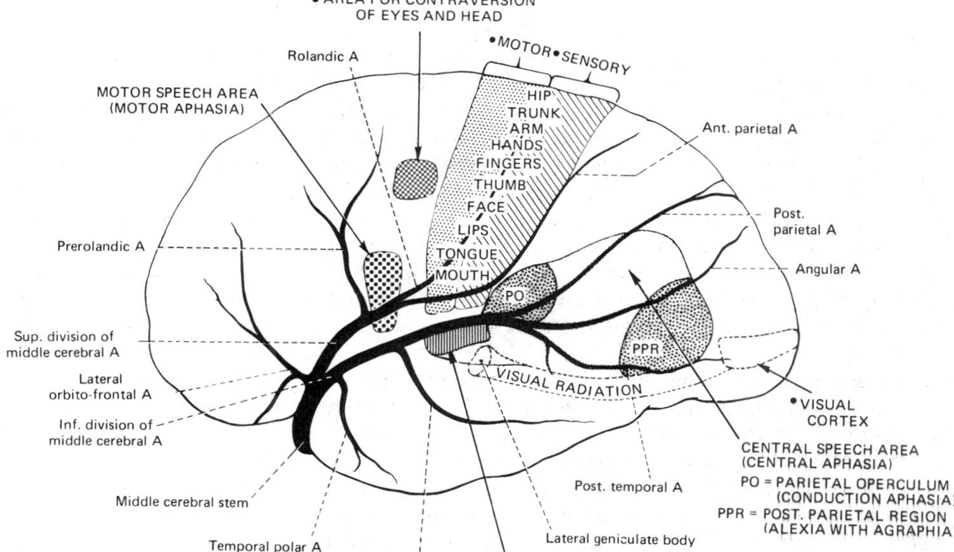

FIGURE 356-3
Diagram of a cerebral hemisphere, lateral aspect, showing the branches and distribution of the middle cerebral artery and the principal regions of cerebral localization.

ten), and unwitting urinary incontinence is often evident. Other disorders in behavior and praxis that may be overlooked in routine clinical evaluations include abulia (a syndrome of slowness, lack of spontaneity, and laconic spoken or motor responses), delay in response, intermittent interruption of behavior, tendency to speak in a whisper, reflexive distraction by sights and sounds, dyspraxia and tactile aphasia of the left limbs (from callosal involvement), and several weeks of mutism with rare echolalia, without disturbed comprehension or hemianopia.

Complete occlusion of one anterior cerebral artery, distal to the anterior communicating, results in infarction in the entire territory and presents clinically as a sensorimotor deficit involving the opposite foot and leg, a lesser degree of paresis of the opposite arm, and sparing of the face and lesser degrees of the mental symptoms.

ANTERIOR CHOROIDAL ARTERY A few incomplete clinicopathologic studies have been the basis of present knowledge of the syndrome of this artery. The syndrome may be so mild as to pass unnoticed and is usually far less than the anticipated contralateral hemiplegia, hemianesthesia (hypesthesia), and homonymous hemianopia. All these symptoms are due to involvement of the posterior limb of the internal capsule and the white matter posterolateral to it, through which the first part of the geniculocalcarine fibers passes.

VERTEBRAL-BASILAR, POSTERIOR CEREBRAL SYSTEM **Posterior cerebral artery** In 70 percent of cases both posterior cerebral arteries arise from the basilar artery; in 22 percent one comes from the basilar and the other one from the internal carotid artery; and in 8 percent both come from the internal carotid. The terminal or cortical branches of this vessel supply the undersurface of the temporal and occipital lobes, as well as the entire medial surface of the occipital lobe including the visual area (areas 17, 18, and 19).

From the more proximal part of the artery between its origin at the bifurcation of the basilar artery and the cortical distribution many important branches arise that supply the midbrain and thalamus. The interpeduncular branches arising near its origin penetrate the brainstem to supply the red nucleus, subthalamic nucleus of Luys, substantia nigra, the most medial part of the cerebral peduncle, the oculomotor nucleus, the reticular substance of the midbrain, the decussation of the superior cerebellar peduncles, rubrothalamic tract, medial longitudinal fasciculus, and the medial lemniscus. The thalamoperforate branches also arise here and pass to the inferior, posterior, medial, and anterior parts of the thalamus. Branches

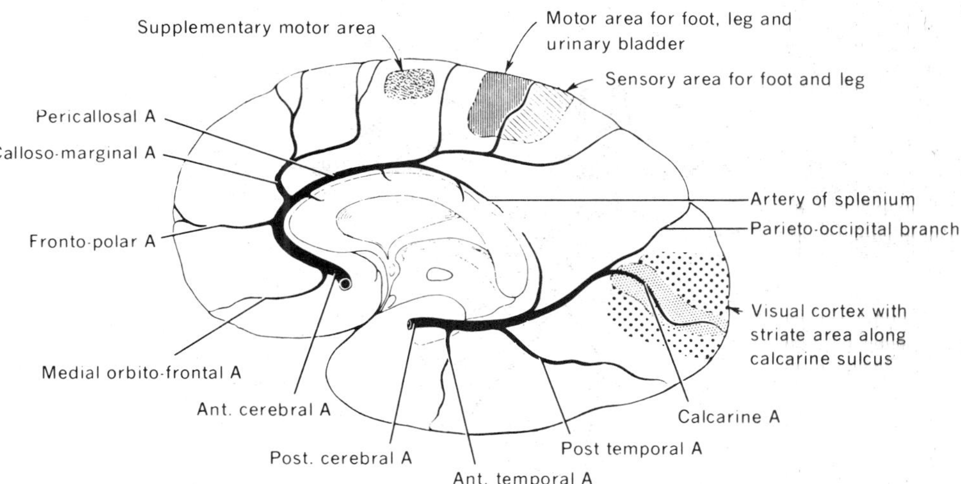

FIGURE 356-4
Diagram of a cerebral hemisphere, medial aspect, showing the branches and distribution of the anterior cerebral artery and the principal regions of cerebral localization.

arising serially along the parent vessel as it encircles the midbrain supply the cerebral peduncle, lateral part of the tegmentum, corpora quadrigemina, pineal gland, lateral geniculate body, choroid plexus, and hippocampus. The thalamogeniculate branches which originate distal to the junction with the posterior communicating artery supply the pulvinar and the posterior lateral nuclei of the thalamus (Fig. 356-5).

For convenience of exposition it is helpful to divide the various syndromes into three groups: (1) anterior and proximal (involving perforating branches), (2) cortical (inferior temporal and medial occipital), and (3) bilateral.

Anterior and proximal The thalamic syndrome of Dejerine and Roussy is due to infarction of the sensory relay nuclei in the thalamus from occlusion of the thalamogeniculate branches. Here a transitory hemiparesis is usually accompanied by a severe sensory loss of the opposite side of the body (deep and cutaneous). In some instances there is a dissociation of sensation, with pain and temperature being more affected than touch, vibration, and position senses, or only one part of the body may be rendered anesthetic. After an interval of time elapses and sensation begins to return, the patient may become chronically afflicted with pain and hyperpathia in the affected parts, or experience distortion of taste, athetotic posturing and ataxia of the hand, and depression of mood.

Central midbrain and subthalamic syndromes, which may be bilateral, are due to occlusion of paramedian branches on one or both sides. The findings include Weber's syndrome (oculomotor palsy with contralateral hemiplegia), paralysis of vertical gaze, stupor or coma, and a movement disorder, most often ataxia. Hemiplegia from infarction of the cerebral peduncle is relatively rare.

Occlusion of the thalamoperforate branches may be manifested by an extrapyramidal movement disorder, including hemiballismus, hemiathetosis with or without deep sensory loss, hemiataxia, or tremor. These syndromes, which Caplan groups under the title "top of the basilar syndrome," are usually temporary.

Cortical syndromes Classically, occlusion of the branches to temporal and occipital lobes gives rise to a homonymous hemianopia because of involvement of the primary visual receptive area or calcarine (striate) cortex. When incomplete, it usually involves the upper quadrants of the visual fields more than the lower. Macular or central vision may be spared because of collateralization of the occipital pole from distal branches of the middle or anterior cerebral artery. Large infarcts of the dominant hemisphere cause alexia, anomia (amnesic aphasia), and impaired memory. The alexia, unaccompanied by agraphia, often is so severe that patients act as if their own written language were foreign. The anomias (dysnomias) are most severe for colors, but may include other visual stimuli such as pictures, musical notes, mathematical symbols, and manipulable objects. Color anomia and amnesic aphasia are more often present in this syndrome than is alexia. Involvement of the hippocampus in the dominant hemisphere alone may produce a profound disturbance in recent memory (Korsakoff's amnesic state), which usually fades within months. Nondominant hemisphere lesions are commonly accompanied by topographic disorientation and dysnomia for faces (so-called prosopagnosia). (See Chap. 24.)

A complete proximal arterial occlusion leads to a syndrome that combines anterior and proximal with cortical syndromes in part or totally. The vascular lesion may be either an embolus or an atherosclerotic thrombus.

Bilateral occipital infarcts These may occur from a single embolism or a succession of emboli in the upper basilar artery. Thrombosis has similar effects, especially if the posterior communicating arteries are unusually small.

Bilateral lesions of the occipital lobes, if extensive, cause total blindness of the cortical type, i.e., a bilateral homonymous hemianopia. The pupillary reflexes are preserved, and fundoscopically the optic disks are normal. Often patients are unaware of their blindness. More frequently the bilateral lesions are incomplete, and a sector of the visual field remains intact. When the remnant is small, vision appears to fluctuate from moment to moment, as patients attempt to capture the image in the island of intact vision. Hysteria may be suspected because of such inconsistencies. In small bilateral calcarine lesions there may be a loss of only central vision (bilateral homonymous central scotomas). In other cases only central vision may remain, leaving the patient with gun-barrel sight.

With bilateral lesions Korsakoff's amnesic state may occur and persist indefinitely. Other common accompaniments are apraxia of ocular movements, inability to enumerate objects, inaccurate visually guided limb movements (optic ataxia), inability to turn the eyes to a precise point in the visual fields (ocular ataxia), to-and-fro movements of eyes, and a tendency to run into obstacles that are seen, as though unable to avoid them. This combination of symptoms is known as Balint's syndrome.

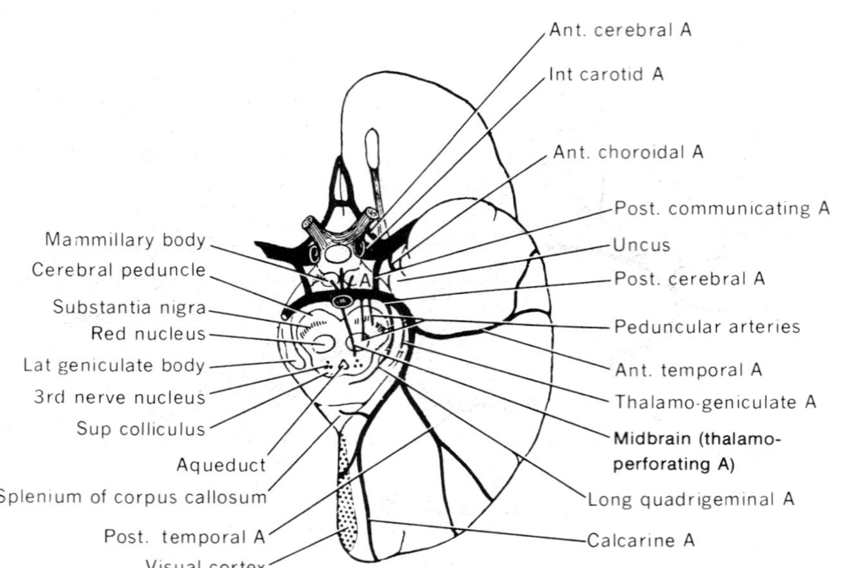

FIGURE 356-5
Inferior aspect of the brain with the branches and distribution of the posterior cerebral artery and the principal anatomic structures.

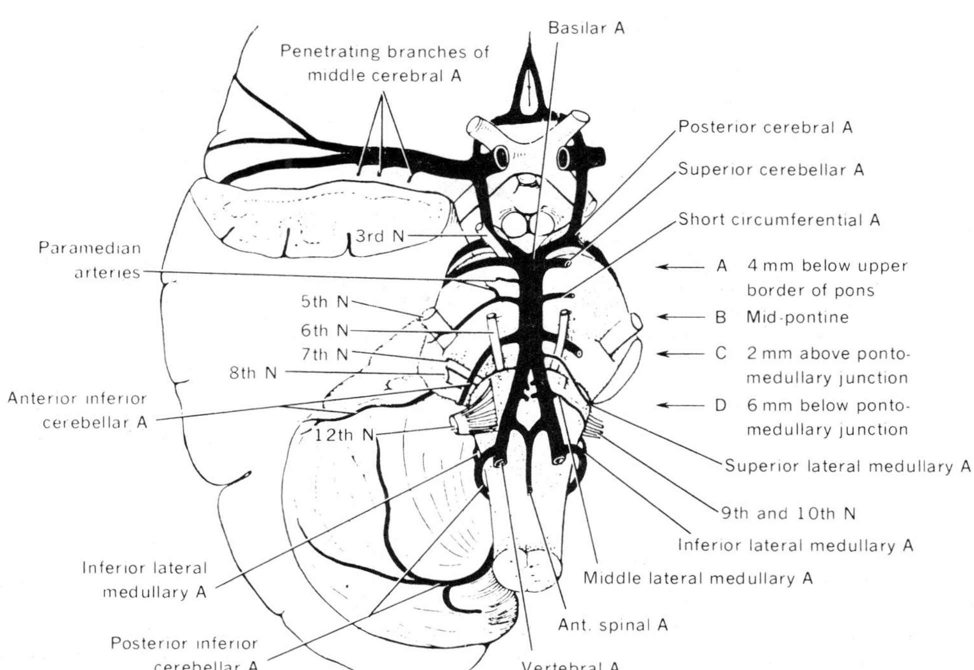

FIGURE 356-6
Diagram of the brainstem at top of figure shows the principal vessels of the vertebral-basilar system. The letters and arrows on the right indicate the levels of the four cross sections A, B, C, and D which follow. Although typical vascular syndromes of the pons and medulla have been designated by sharply outlined shaded areas, the student must appreciate that since satisfactory clinicopathologic studies are far from numerous, the diagrams are not necessarily accurate, nor do they always represent established facts. The great frequency with which infarcts fail to produce a well-recognized syndrome and the special tendency for syndromes to merge with one another must be emphasized.

Vertebral artery The vertebral arteries are the chief arteries of the medulla, and each supplies the lower three-fourths of the pyramid, the medial lemniscus, all or nearly all the retroolivary region (the lateral medullary region), the restiform body, and the posteroinferior part of the cerebellar hemisphere (see Figs. 356-6 to 356-10). The relative sizes of the vertebral arteries vary a good deal, and in approximately 10 percent of cases, one vessel is so small that the other can be considered the only artery of supply to the brainstem. In this case, if collateral inflow from the carotid system via the circle of Willis is unavailable, occlusion would be equivalent to occlusion of the basilar artery or bilateral occlusion of the vertebral arteries. The posterior inferior cerebellar artery is usually a branch of the vertebral artery, but can have a common origin with the anterior inferior cerebellar artery from the basilar artery. It is necessary to keep these anatomic variations in mind when visualizing the effects of vertebral artery occlusion.

The results of vertebral occlusion are quite variable. When there are two good-sized arteries, occlusion on one side occurs not infrequently without any recognizable symptoms and signs or pathologic changes. If the subclavian artery is blocked proximal to the origin of the vertebral artery, exercise of the arm on that side may draw blood from the vertebral-basilar system into the arm, sometimes resulting in the symptoms of basilar insufficiency (the "subclavian steal" syndrome of Fisher). If the occlusion of the vertebral artery is so situated as to block the mouth of one or more arteries supplying the lateral medulla, the most common consequence is the lateral medullary syndrome (see below). When the branch to the anterior spinal artery is blocked, collateral influx from the spinal artery branch of the opposite side is usually sufficient to prevent infarction of the spinal cord and medial aspect of the medulla. If a branch to the pyramid is occluded, that part of the corticospinal tract may be infarcted unless collateral flow is adequate. Rarely, occlusion of the vertebral artery or one of the anterior spinal arteries produces an infarct which involves the medullary pyramid, the medial lemniscus, and the emergent hypoglossal fibers, with resulting contralateral paralysis of arm and leg (face spared), contralateral loss of position and vibration sense, and ipsilateral paralysis and atrophy of the tongue (the medial medullary syndrome; see Fig. 356–10). Vertebral occlusion can also lead to symptoms by blocking the posterior inferior cerebellar artery (see below). Occlusion of the vertebral arteries low in the neck is usually compensated for by anastomotic flow to the upper part of the vertebral arteries via the thyrocervical, deep cervical, and occipital arter-

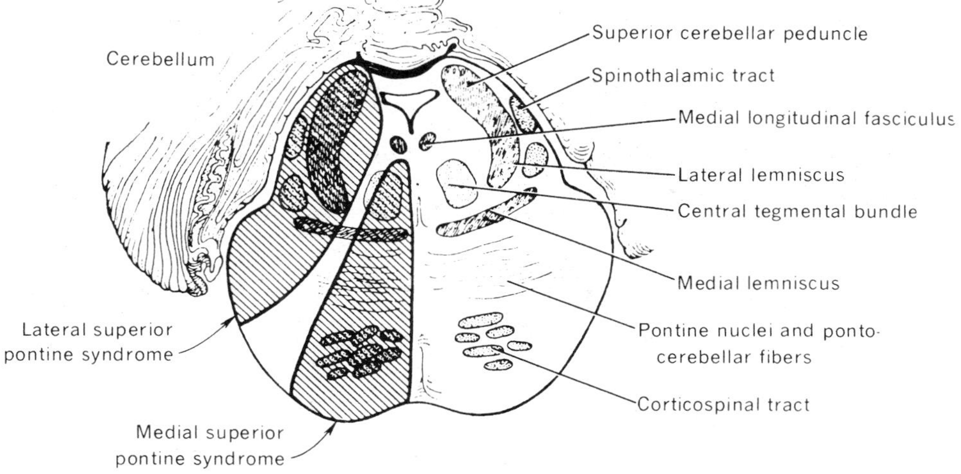

FIGURE 356-7
Medial superior pontine syndrome (paramedian branches of upper basilar artery). Lateral superior pontine syndrome (syndrome of superior cerebellar artery).

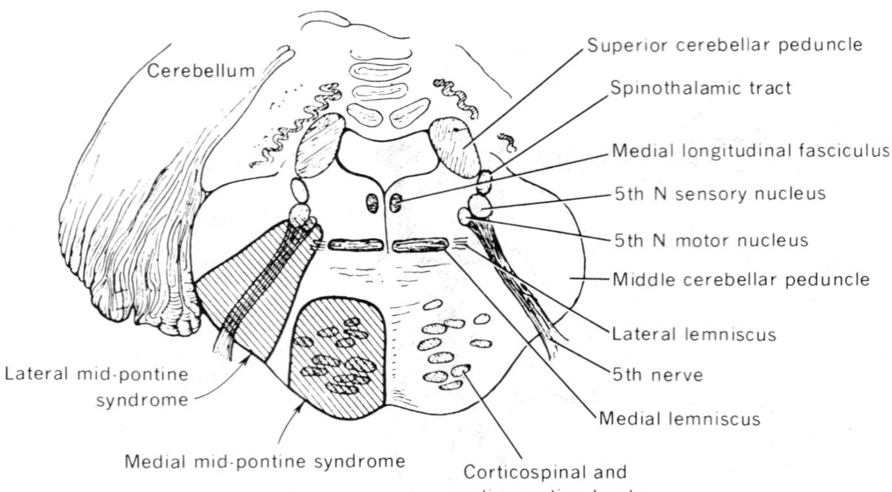

FIGURE 356-8
Medial midpontine syndrome (paramedian branch of midbasilar artery). Lateral midpontine syndrome (short circumferential artery).

ies, or an influx from the anterior part of the circle of Willis may occur.

The *posterior inferior cerebellar artery* supplies the inferior portion of the lateral medullary region, the restiform body, and the inferior surface of the cerebellar hemisphere. It may be occluded at its mouth, i.e., by thrombosis of the vertebral artery, or anywhere along its course. Some patients tolerate obstruction of the vessel with little or no ill effect; in others an extensive infarct results in the cerebellum and/or the posterolateral medulla. In other cases, the symptoms include sudden severe dizziness, nausea, vomiting, ataxia, and nystagmus, a picture that mimics acute labyrinthitis. Occasionally the infarction is of such size that a fatal compression of the brainstem develops within days due to the postinfarction edema of the affected portions of the cerebellum and a pressure-cone at the foramen magnum. Surgical evacuation of the necrotic area may be a lifesaving procedure.

The *lateral medullary syndrome* is produced by infarction of a small wedge of lateral medulla lying posteriorly to the inferior olivary nucleus (see Fig. 356-10). The classic syndrome reflects the involvement of the spinothalamic tract (*contralateral* impairment of pain and thermal sense over half the body, sometimes face); descending sympathetic tract (*ipsilateral* Horner's syndrome of miosis, ptosis, decreased sweating); issuing fibers of the ninth and tenth nerves (hoarseness, dysphagia, *ipsilateral* paralysis of the palate and vocal cord, diminished gag reflex); vestibular disorder (nystagmus, diplopia, oscillopsia, vertigo, nausea, vomiting), involvement of cerebellum, olivo- and/or spinocerebellar fibers, and sometimes restiform body (*ipsilateral* ataxia of limbs, falling or toppling to the ipsilateral side); descending tract and nucleus of the fifth nerve (pain, numbness, impaired sensation over ipsilateral half of the face); nucleus and tractus solitarius (loss of taste); cuneate and gracile nuclei (numbness of *ipsilateral* arm), and hiccup. This syndrome is one of the most striking in neurology. It is almost always due to ischemic necrosis, usually from occlusion of the vertebral artery, not the posterior inferior cerebellar, as shown by the now classic work of Fisher et al.

Occasionally, the occlusion of one vertebral artery involves the site of origin of both the posterior-inferior cerebellar artery and the anterior spinal artery, resulting in a combination of dorsolateral and medial medullary infarctions. Such patients present with the elements of the lateral medullary syndrome, with the addition of contralateral hemiplegia (sparing the

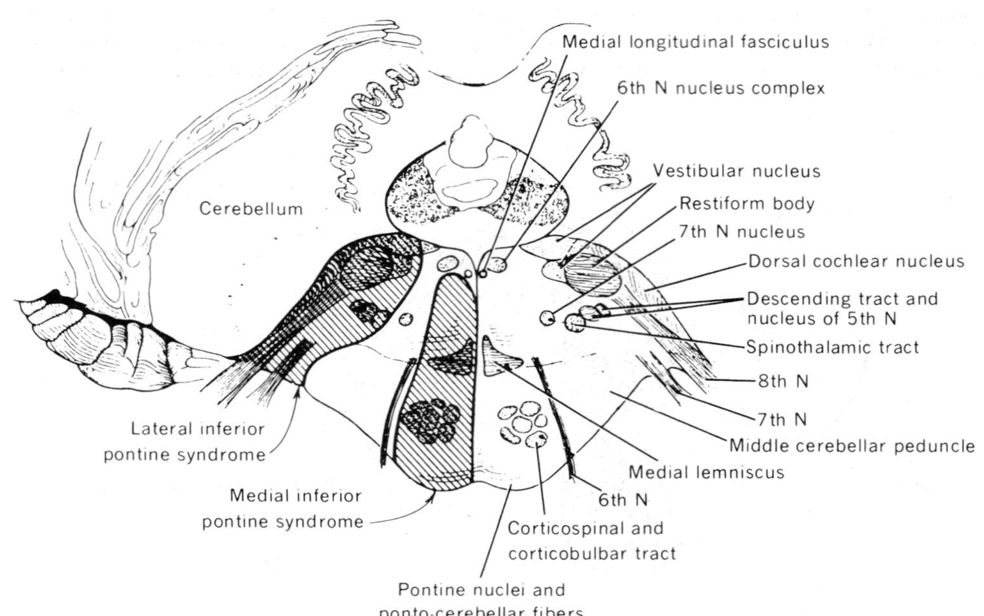

FIGURE 356-9
Medial inferior pontine syndrome (occlusion of paramedian branch of basilar artery). Lateral inferior pontine syndrome (occlusion of anterior inferior cerebellar artery). Total unilateral inferior pontine syndrome (occlusion of anterior inferior cerebellar artery). Lateral and medial syndromes combined.

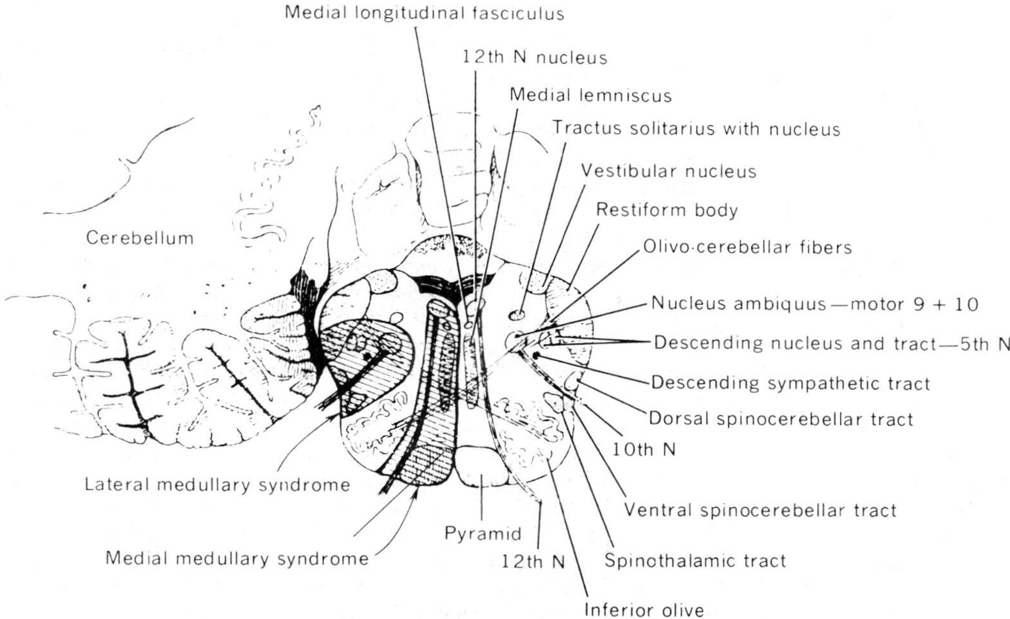

FIGURE 356-10
Medial medullary syndrome (occlusion of vertebral artery or of branch of vertebral or lower basilar artery). Lateral medullary syndrome (occlusion of any five vessels may be responsible—vertebral, posterior inferior cerebellar, or superior, middle, or inferior lateral medullary arteries). Total unilateral medullary syndrome (occlusion of vertebral artery). Combination of medial and lateral syndromes. Lateral pontomedullary syndrome (occlusion of vertebral artery). Combination of lateral medullary and lateral inferior pontine syndromes. Basilar artery syndrome (the syndrome of the lone vertebral artery is equivalent). A combination of the various brainstem syndromes plus those arising in the posterior cerebral artery distribution. The clinical picture combines bilateral long-tract signs (sensory and motor) with cerebellar and peripheral cranial nerve abnormalities.

face), hemisensory deficit for vibration and proprioception, and ipsilateral hypoglossal paralysis. This combination is known as the syndrome of Babinski-Nageotte.

Basilar artery The basilar artery supplies not only the pons and upper part of the cerebellum but also in most cases the inferior temporal and medial occipital lobes and thalamus via the posterior cerebral arteries. Occlusion may occur in the trunk of the basilar artery or in any one of its branches.

The branches of the basilar artery may be conveniently grouped as follows: (1) paramedian, 7 to 10 in number, supplying a wedge of pons on either side of the midline; (2) the short circumferential branches, 5 to 7 in number, supplying the lateral two-thirds of the pons and the middle and superior cerebellar peduncles; and (3) the long circumferential, 2 in number on each side, running laterally around the pons to reach the cerebellar hemispheres (the superior cerebellar artery and the anterior inferior cerebellar artery).

Occlusion of the basilar artery evokes a sizable array of clinical manifestations reflecting involvement of a large number of structures [corticospinal and corticobulbar tracts, cerebellum, middle and superior cerebellar peduncles, medial and lateral lemnisci, spinothalamic tracts, medial longitudinal fasciculi, pontine nuclei, vestibular and cochlear nuclei, descending hypothalamospinal sympathetic fibers, the upper medulla, and the third through the eighth cranial nerves (including the nuclei, their segments within the brainstem, and the peripheral nerves themselves)] (see Figs. 356-6 to 356-10).

The picture of basilar occlusion due to thrombosis may arise in several ways: (1) occlusion in the basilar artery itself, usually in the lower third at the site of an atherosclerotic plaque; (2) occlusion of both vertebral arteries, with closure of the second amounting to basilar obstruction; or (3) occlusion of a single vertebral artery, when there is only one of good size. Thrombosis may also involve only a branch of the basilar artery rather than the trunk (*basilar branch occlusion*). When the obstruction is embolic, the embolus usually lodges at the upper bifurcation of the basilar or in one of the posterior cerebral arteries, since if it is small enough to pass through the vertebral artery, it should easily traverse the length of the basilar artery, which is of greater diameter than either vertebral artery.

The complete basilar syndrome comprises bilateral long-tract signs (sensory and motor) with variable cerebellar and cranial nerve abnormalities and other segmental disorders of brainstem. As a rule the patient is comatose with quadriplegia and cranial nerve abnormalities, and has a clear CSF. The coma is due to lesions in the reticular activating system of midbrain and diencephalon. In the presence of the full syndrome, it is usually not difficult to make the correct diagnosis. In many other instances, the basilar occlusion is well collateralized by anastomoses between the cortical branches of the cerebellar arteries, leaving an infarction confined only to one or more of the branches of the basilar artery at the site of the major basilar occlusion.

Occlusion of individual basilar branches yields highly focal syndromes. The main signs of thrombosis of the *superior cerebellar artery* are severe ipsilateral cerebellar ataxia (middle and/or superior cerebellar peduncles), nausea and vomiting, slurred speech, and loss of pain and temperature sensation over the extremities, body, and face of the opposite side (spinothalamic and trigeminothalamic tracts). Partial deafness, a static tremor of the ipsilateral upper extremity, Horner's syndrome, and bulbar myoclonus have also been reported.

In occlusion of the *anterior inferior cerebellar artery* the extent of the infarct is extremely variable. The size of this artery and the territory it supplies vary inversely with that of the posterior inferior cerebellar artery. The principal findings are ipsilateral deafness, whirling dizziness, nausea and vomiting, nystagmus, tinnitus and cerebellar ataxia (inferior cerebellar peduncle, or restiform body), Horner's syndrome, and paresis of conjugate lateral gaze. Pain and temperature sensation are lost on the opposite side of the body. If the occlusion is close to the origin of the artery, the corticospinal fibers may also be involved, producing a hemiplegia. Occlusion of the *artery to the retroolivary space* will produce the lateral medullary syndrome. Occlusion of a *paramedian branch* will result in infarction of the corticospinal fibers, the adjacent pontine nuclei, and the pontocerebellar fibers on one side of the pons. If the infarct extends deep to reach the tegmentum, as it occasionally does, paralysis of conjugate lateral gaze and a contralateral sensory deficit will result.

In the diagnosis of disease of the brainstem it is impossible from motor signs alone to distinguish a hemiplegia of pontine origin from one of cerebral origin, and one is always dependent on coexisting neurologic phenomena. In a lower brainstem hemiplegia the eyes may move more easily to the side of the paralysis, just the opposite of supratentorial lesions. In brainstem lesions, as in cerebral, a flaccid paralysis gives way to spasticity in the following days, weeks, or months, and there is no satisfactory explanation for the variability in this period of delay. The pattern of sensory disturbance may be helpful in localization. A dissociated sensory deficit over the face or one-half the body usually indicates a lesion within the brainstem, while a sensory loss over one side of the body involving all modalities with no suggestion of dissociation in any region indicates a lesion in the thalamus or deep in the white matter of the parietal lobe. When position sense, two-point discrimination, and tactile localization are affected relatively more than pain, temperature, and tactile sense, a cortical lesion is suggested; the converse suggests a brainstem location. When both motor and sensory manifestations in a given stroke are bilateral, it is almost unequivocal evidence that the lesion lies infratentorially. When hemiplegia or hemiparesis and sensory loss are coextensive, the lesion lies supratentorially. Additional manifestations which point unequivocally to a brainstem site are whirling dizziness, diplopia, cerebellar ataxia, Horner's syndrome, and deafness. The several brainstem syndromes illustrate the important point that the cerebellar system, spinothalamic tract, trigeminal nucleus, and sympathetic fibers can be involved at different levels, and neighborhood phenomena must be used to identify the exact site.

A myriad of eponymic brainstem syndromes, e.g., Weber, Claude, Benedict, Foville, Raymond-Cestan, Millard-Gubler (see Chap. 367), have been described in relation to brainstem lesions. The diagnosis of vascular disorders in this region of the brain is not greatly facilitated by a knowledge of these eponymic syndromes, and it is preferable to memorize the neuroanatomy of the brainstem. The principal syndromes to be recognized are full basilar, vertebral, anterior inferior cerebellar artery, superior cerebellar artery, pontomedullary, and medial medullary branches. Partial syndromes can usually be identified as fragments of the major ones.

MAJOR TYPES OF CEREBROVASCULAR DISEASES AND THEIR FREQUENCY

The six common types of stroke listed in Table 356-1 can be diagnosed with a high degree of accuracy. Since each one requires a special approach, therapy, and management, correct diagnosis is advantageous to the patient. The criteria for diagnosis and the confirmatory laboratory tests are described in the following pages.

The natural frequency of these six types of cerebrovascular lesions has been difficult to ascertain. Obviously clinical diagnosis is not always correct, and clinical services are more heavily weighted with acute strokes and nonfatal cases. An autopsy series inevitably includes many old vascular lesions, particularly infarcts, whose nature cannot be determined, and there is a bias also toward large fatal lesions (usually hemorrhages).

In Table 356-1 we have presented the figures obtained from the NINCDS Stroke Data Book, a recent population study in southern Alabama, and the Harvard Cooperative Stroke Registry. In these studies, a high percentage of appropriate laboratory aids were employed, i.e., four-vessel arteriography, CT scan, CSF examination. For comparison we have included an autopsy series of 179 successive brains examined during the year 1949 by Fisher and Adams.

In all three series the ratio of infarcts to hemorrhages was 4:1, and embolism accounted for approximately one-third of all strokes. Hypertensive hemorrhages, aneurysms, and vascular malformations were conditions diagnosed with the highest degree of reliability. The most frequent sources of error were (1) mistaking a small embolic occlusion for a lacune or vice versa and (2) confusing a thrombotic infarct for an embolus or vice versa. When the most stringent rules for diagnosis are applied, the importance of laboratory testing becomes apparent. In 25 percent of the southern Alabama population study, either the tests were not performed at all because the patient was hospitalized outside a major center or the tests were performed at the wrong time; these cases had to be classified as "ischemia—cause unknown." An earlier problem of mistaking a small hypertensive hemorrhage for an infarct has been virtually eliminated by the CT scan.

ATHEROSCLEROTIC THROMBOSIS

Atherosclerosis in the arteries of the brain is similar to that elsewhere in the body. The atheromatous plaques tend to form at branchings and curves. The severity of the process runs parallel to but is somewhat less severe than that of other arteries—aorta, lower limbs, and heart. Thrombosis is most likely to occur where the plaque narrows the lumen to the greatest degree. The most common sites of thrombosis are the internal carotid artery at the carotid sinus in the neck, the vertebral and basilar arteries in the region of their junction, the main bifurcation of the middle cerebral artery, the posterior cerebral artery as it winds round the cerebral peduncle, and the anterior cerebral artery as it curves upward over the corpus callosum. Hypertension aggravates the atherosclerotic process. Because of abundant collateral arterial pathways, occlusion of the common carotid, brachiocephalic, cervical portion of the vertebral arteries, or subclavian arteries in the upper thorax is not commonly responsible for cerebral ischemia. The vertebral arteries may be narrowed at their origins from the subclavian,

TABLE 356-1
Frequency of common types of stroke

	NINCDS Stroke Data Bank, 925 successive cases (%)*	*Harvard Stroke Series,† 684 successive cases (%)*	*BCH Autopsy Series,‡ 179 successive cases (%)*
Atherosclerotic thrombosis	173 (19)	233 (34)	21 (12)
Lacunae	100 (11)	121 (19)	34 (18.5)
Embolism	198 (21)	215 (31)	57 (32)
Hypertensive hemorrhage	115 (13)	70 (10)	28 (15.5)
Ruptured aneurysms and vascular malformations	104 (11)	45 (6)	8 (4.5)
Indeterminate	235 (25)¶		17 (9.5)
Other§			14 (8.5)

* *NINCDS National Pilot Stroke Data Bank, 1982.*
† *Mohr et al, 1978.*
‡ *Series compiled by Fisher and Adams in an examination of 780 brains during the year 1949 at Mallory Institute of Pathology, Boston City Hospital.*
§ *Hypertensive encephalopathy, cerebral vein thrombosis, meningovascular syphilis, polyarteritis nodosa.*
¶ *These represent clinically or CT-detected infarcts, for which no specific etiologic diagnosis could be made.*

resulting in cerebral infarction. Ordinarily it is rare for the cerebral arteries to be significantly affected beyond their first major branching.

The state of the arterial lumen during the period when the stroke is evolving varies from case to case. Judging from arteriographic and surgical findings in the carotid and vertebral arteries in the neck, it is likely that when prodromal transient ischemic attacks are occurring, atherosclerosis and superimposed thrombus have severely stenosed the affected artery; microembolism may occur, or blood flow is intermittently reduced in the territory distal to the stenosis. In addition, transient ischemic attacks can also occur if the main vessel is totally occluded while a compensating collateral channel is stenotic. Permanent stroke may result from embolism into intracranial arteries arising from the stenotic or occluded main vessel, or it may be due to complete occlusion of a main vessel lacking adequate intracranial collaterals. It is common to find more than one vessel affected by stenosis or occlusion, and then it is especially difficult to decipher the interplay of hemodynamic factors leading to symptoms.

CLINICAL PICTURE In general, the evolution of the clinical picture in cerebral thrombosis is much more variable than in embolism and hemorrhage. In approximately 60 percent of cases, the main part of the stroke (paralysis or other deficit) is preceded by minor signs or by one or more *transient ischemic attacks,* which herald the oncoming vascular catastrophe. Transient ischemic attacks rarely precede embolism and intracerebral hemorrhage. Transient warning attacks in carotid-middle cerebral disease consist of focal symptoms such as mono- or hemiplegia, mono- or hemiparesthesia, blindness in one eye, speech disturbance, etc. These attacks reflect evolving thrombosis of the internal carotid or middle cerebral arteries. In the vertebral-basilar system there may occur dizziness, diplopia, numbness, impaired vision in one or both visual fields, dark vision, dysarthria, etc. The attacks last usually *less than 10 min;* attacks lasting many hours are often documentably associated with embolism. Most frequently only *one or two attacks* precede the final stroke, although as many as hundreds may occur. The stroke comes within the first month in over 25 percent of cases, but may be delayed for months, and in as many as 30 percent of cases, the attacks die away without leading to a stroke. When these minor ischemic attacks are not part of the picture, one must depend on other factors in identifying the cerebrovascular process as one of cerebral thrombosis.

The main part of the thrombotic stroke, whether or not it is preceded by warning attacks, develops in one of several ways. In 60 percent of cases, there is but a single attack, the whole illness developing suddenly, or at most within minutes. A more diagnostic pattern is for the stroke to have a stuttering intermittent progression over several hours or days, but only 14 percent show this stepwise onset. Another type of onset is that in which a partial stroke develops, and after the patient has improved for several hours, there is progression to full paralysis. The affection may involve several parts of the body simultaneously or only one part, such as a limb or one side of the face, and the other parts become involved serially in step-like fashion until the stroke is fully developed. All these various modes of onset bespeak cerebral thrombosis, and when developing over days or weeks, the whole process may be referred to as *thrombosis in evolution.* In 60 percent of cases either the onset or progression of the stroke occurs during sleep or shortly after arising. In fewer than 20 percent of cases, a thrombotic stroke comes on in what appears to be a slow, gradual fashion, but in most of these cases careful inquiry will reveal an uneven or saltatory progression.

Headache, although absent in the majority of cases, is present in approximately 15 percent of cases of cerebral thrombosis. It is not so violent as in cases of intracranial hemorrhage, generally being on one side in the front part of the head in occlusion of the carotid system and at the back of the head or simultaneously in the forehead in basilar disease. Its cause is unknown. It may antedate the other symptoms of the stroke by several days.

Hypertension, an important aggravating factor in atherosclerosis, is present in 60 percent of cases and diabetes mellitus in 25 percent, while evidence of vascular disease elsewhere, e.g., angina pectoris, electrocardiographic abnormality, myocardial infarction, absence of one or several peripheral pulses in the lower limbs, or intermittent claudication occurs in 50 percent. The retinal arteries may show uniform or focal narrowing, but these alterations cannot be correlated with cerebral atherosclerosis. The peak age of atherosclerotic thrombosis of brain arteries is 70 years.

LABORATORY FINDINGS Arteriography is the definitive procedure for the demonstration of arterial occlusion or stenosis and also provides information about collateral flow. Injection into the major cervicocerebral arteries via a catheter introduced from a femoral artery is preferred to direct injection into the carotid artery through a needle. Arteriography carries a risk of neurologic defect in 1 percent of cases studied by experienced arteriographers, but in patients with vessels narrowed by atherosclerosis the risk may be higher. It should be used when the diagnosis of vascular disease is uncertain or when vascular surgery may be possible.

CT scan usually demonstrates a focal area of decreased attenuation values, corresponding to infarcted brain parenchyma. This aspect usually requires 3 to 4 days to develop (CT scans done within the first 24 to 48 h from the onset of infarction are usually normal). Depending on the size of the infarct, mass effect with midline shift may occur if significant brain edema has developed. Between 1 and 3 weeks from onset a "gyral" pattern of cortical enhancement can be seen after intravenous contrast infusion.

Radioactive concentration studies (e.g., technetium, scan) and positron-emission tomography, particularly the latter, often show the infarcts earlier than the CT scan. Scintillation counting over the two sides of the skull after the intravenous injection of radioactive material can provide a comparative index of circulation in the two carotid systems.

Skull x-rays are not remarkable, and the pineal gland will not be shifted unless severe cerebral swelling has occurred, in which case the patient will usually be stuporous or comatose.

The electroencephalogram is still of limited value in indicating infarction or distinguishing it from hemorrhage and from nonvascular conditions. In cerebral infarction the electrical activity may be of a slightly slower frequency and of lower voltage than normal. High-voltage slow waves (3 to 5 per second) are evidence in favor of hemorrhage or tumor.

Lumbar puncture has receded in value as a test for cerebral thrombosis, since the findings are so often normal. The cerebrospinal fluid pressure is normal in patients with cerebral thrombosis, though it may be under increased pressure if the infarct is large and associated with severe swelling of the damaged tissue. Cerebral thrombosis never causes blood in the spinal fluid, which is "crystal clear." A slight increase in the leukocytes of the spinal fluid (three to eight polymorphonuclear leukocytes) is not uncommon in the first few days of the illness. Rarely, and usually only with large infarcts, a brisk, transient pleocytosis (400 to 2000 polymorphonuclear leukocytes per milliliter) occurs on about the third day. A persistent increase in the number of white blood cells of the cerebrospinal fluid suggests the presence of chronic meningitis (syphilis, tuberculosis, torula), granulomatous arteritis, septic embolism, cerebral thrombophlebitis, or a nonvascular process. The total amount of protein may be normal, but frequently it is raised to 50 to 80 mg/dl. Rarely is it over 100, in which case some other diagnosis should be considered.

COURSE AND PROGNOSIS When the patient is seen early in the course of atherosclerotic thrombosis, it is extremely difficult to give an *immediate prognosis.* Where does the patient stand in the stroke process when first examined? Is worsening to be anticipated or not? No rules have yet been laid down which allow one to predict the course. A mild paralysis today may become a disastrous hemiplegia tomorrow, or the patient's condition may only worsen temporarily for a day or two. In basilar artery occlusion, dizziness and dysphagia may progress in a few days to total paralysis and deep coma. The course of the deficit is so often progressive that a cautious attitude on the part of the physician is justified in what appears to be a mild stroke.

Progression of the stroke is probably most often due to increasing narrowing of the involved artery by mural thrombus. In some instances extension of the thrombus along the vessel may block side branches and hinder anastomotic flow. In the basilar artery, thrombus may gradually build up along its entire length. In the carotid system, the thrombus at times propagates distally from the site of origin in the neck to the intracranial supraclinoid portion, and possibly into the anterior cerebral artery, preventing collateral flow from the opposite side. Embolic particles from the site of thrombosis in a cervical vessel may obstruct intracranial vessels to produce a disastrous abrupt change in the clinical picture.

Several other circumstances influence the *immediate prognosis* in cerebral thrombosis. In the case of large infarcts, swelling of the infarcted tissue may occur, tentorial herniation may follow, and the patient dies in 2 to 4 days. Milder degrees of swelling and increased intracranial pressure, though causing an apparent progression for 2 to 3 days, may not prove fatal. In extensive basilar infarction associated with deep coma, the patient seldom lives for more than a few days. If coma or stupor is present from the beginning, survival is largely determined by the success in keeping the airway clear (preventing aspiration pneumonia) and maintaining fluid and electrolyte balance (see Chap. 20). Respiratory and urinary infections are constant dangers, and once they begin, there is usually a rapid decline in the patient's condition as his or her temperature rises.

As for the *eventual, or long-term, prognosis* of the neurologic deficit, there are many possibilities. Improvement is the rule if the patient survives. In small infarcts, improvement may start within hours or a day or two, and restoration may be complete within a week. With severe deficits there may be no significant recovery whatsoever, and after months of assiduous effort at rehabilitation, the patient may remain bereft of speech, with the upper extremity still useless and the lower extremity serving only as an uncertain prop in attempting to walk. Between these two extremes there is every degree of recovery. It is certain that the longer the delay before movement begins, the poorer the prognosis becomes. If recovery does not begin in 1 or 2 weeks, the outlook is gloomy for both motor activity and speech, and it may be said that whatever motor paralysis remains after 5 to 6 months will probably be permanent. Nevertheless aphasia, dysarthria, cerebellar ataxia, and walking may improve for a year or longer. Anosognosia, constructional apraxia, nonsensical logorrhea, and neglect of the paralyzed side all tend to diminish and may disappear within a few weeks. A hemianopia which has not cleared in a few weeks will usually remain permanently, although reading and color discrimination may continue to improve. In lateral medullary infarction difficulty in swallowing may be protracted (4 to 7 weeks), and yet eventually relatively normal function is nearly always restored.

Characteristically, the paralyzed muscles are flaccid in the first days or weeks following a stroke, and the tendon reflexes may be unchanged, slightly increased, or decreased. Gradually spasticity develops, and the tendon reflexes become brisker. This change into spasticity occurs irrespective of the location, superficial or deep, of the lesion interrupting the corticospinal tract. The arm tends to assume a flexed adducted posture, whereas the leg is usually extended and adducted. Function is rarely if ever restored after the slow evolution of spasticity. In some cases with extensive temporoparietal lesions the hemiplegia remains flaccid; the arm dangles and the slack leg must be braced to stand. Bowel and bladder control usually returns. Not infrequently the hemiplegic limbs become tender and ache on manipulation, interfering with the physical therapy program. Nevertheless, physiotherapy should be initiated early in order to prevent contracture of muscles at shoulder, elbow, wrist, knuckles, knee, and ankle, a frequent complication and often the source of pain and added disability, particularly in relation to the shoulder. A typical Sudeck type of pain and bone atrophy of the hand may accompany the shoulder pain (shoulder-hand syndrome) as described in Chap. 7. An annoying, unsteady "dizzy" feeling in the head often persists after damage to the vestibular system in brainstem infarcts.

Recurrent cerebral (epileptic) seizures, while not unknown after thrombotic strokes, are rare. This is in contrast with embolic cortical infarcts where they occur in more than 20 percent of patients. A seizure involving the weakened limbs, followed by transient postictal paralysis may mimic another stroke. Often it takes several days for the paralysis, sensory loss, or aphasia to remit to the preseizure level.

Many patients complain of fatigability and are depressed. These changes appear to occur more commonly after right (nondominant) hemispheric infarcts. The explanation of these symptoms is uncertain; some are expressions of a reactive depression (see Chap. 11). Only a few patients become serious *behavior problems* or are psychotic after a stroke, but paranoid trends, ill temper, stubbornness, and peevishness are recognized sequelae.

Finally, in regard to prognosis, it must be mentioned that having had one thrombotic stroke, the patient is in danger in the ensuing months and years of having a stroke at the same or another site, especially if there is hypertension. Myocardial infarction is also frequent, more so in the few weeks following a cerebral thrombosis. More stroke victims eventually succumb to a heart attack than to another stroke.

TREATMENT The treatment of cerebrovascular disease and strokes may be divided into four parts: (1) general medical management in the acute phase, as outlined in Chap. 20, (2) measures to restore the circulation and arrest the pathologic process, (3) physical therapy and rehabilitation, and (4) preventive measures against strokes and vascular disease.

Measures to restore the circulation and arrest the pathologic process Once a thrombotic stroke has developed fully, no therapy so far devised is of any value in restoring the cerebral tissue or its function. *To be effective, therapy must be preventive.*

MEDICAL MEASURES TO IMPROVE THE BLOOD SUPPLY TO THE BRAIN On the assumption that decrease in the cerebral circulation resulting from the upright position can aggravate cerebral ischemia, some physicians recommend that patients with a stroke as the result of ischemic infarction should remain horizontal in bed for 7 to 10 days. When ambulation starts, special attention should be given to preservation of the systemic circulation and avoidance of orthostatic changes in blood pressure. Treatment of previously unappreciated hypertension is preferably deferred until the later stage of the stroke, when the neurologic deficit has stabilized. The systemic blood pressure must be maintained (correction of blood loss, avoidance of autonomic blocking agents, etc.). Injections of sympathicomimetic drugs have also been recommended as a means of raising the systemic blood pressure above the usual levels. There is no clear evidence that any of these maneuvers influences the course of the cerebral lesion.

ANTICOAGULATION Anticoagulant therapy may prevent transient ischemic attacks, postpone the arrival of an impending stroke, and halt the advance of a progressive thrombotic stroke, or prevent its recurrence. There are few studies to date which satisfy all epidemiologic criteria, and none which conclusively documents the value of anticoagulants nor indicates they are useless in the prevention of thrombotic stroke, or the worsening of an ischemic deficit. All investigators agree, however, that anticoagulants are not of value as treatment for the fully developed, i.e., completed, stroke.

When *anticoagulant therapy* is instituted in an evolving thrombotic stroke, heparin is recommended, intravenously in a dose of approximately 1000 units per hour by continuous drip therapy. In cases with a progressing stroke or with transient ischemic attacks, heparin therapy is maintained for 1 to 2 weeks. The dose is regulated to keep the partial thromboplastin time in the range of 50 to 60 s. While heparin therapy is being given, Coumadin therapy is instituted and continued well-regulated for 6 to 12 months or more. Coumadin therapy can be used alone from the beginning when transient ischemic attacks are fewer than once every few days to a week.

The use of anticoagulant drugs makes an accurate clinical diagnosis imperative. Intracranial hemorrhage must be ruled out by CT scan, or if this procedure is not available, by relying primarily on examination of the cerebrospinal fluid; it is to be remembered, however, that a clear fluid does not necessarily exclude hemorrhage (see "Laboratory Findings" under "Intracranial Hemorrhage" below). A control prothrombin concentration and coagulation time should be measured before therapy is started, but if this is not feasible, the initial doses of anticoagulant drugs can usually be given safely if there is no evidence of active bleeding anywhere in the body. The question whether severe hypertension is a contraindication to anticoagulant therapy has not been accurately answered. There is no reliable evidence that complications are more frequent in the presence of moderate hypertension if the prothrombin activity is maintained between $1\frac{1}{2}$ and 2 times the control value, and therefore the authors have not withheld anticoagulant therapy in these patients; however, when the blood pressure is greater than 220/120, an attempt is made to lower the pressure gradually with hypotensive agents, exercising care not to prejudice further the circulation in the region of the infarct by too great a reduction in the systemic pressure. It is preferable to avoid reduction of the blood pressure in the 2-week period immediately following a thrombotic stroke.

Anticoagulant therapy is relatively safe provided the prothrombin concentration is determined regularly (once a day, for the first 10 days, thence thrice a week, and finally once every 2 weeks) at a laboratory using reliable methods. We prefer to keep the prothrombin time between 16 and 20 s. Therapy can be prolonged for months and years, and only occasionally is it necessary to interrupt treatment because of unexplained disturbances of coagulation. Coumadin overdosage may cause hemorrhage into the brain or subdurally or into the retroperitoneal space, kidney, nose, bowel, skin, or muscle. Most of the extracerebral accidents are not serious, but vitamin K_1 should be administered immediately.

ANTIPLATELET THERAPY Recent data suggest that inhibition of platelet aggregation may be the equivalent of oral anticoagulants in therapy for transient ischemic attacks, reducing the frequency of subsequent attacks, ischemic stroke, death from stroke, and death from nonstroke causes. The effect has been demonstrated only in men, and was most associated with the use of aspirin, in doses of 300 mg four times a day. Disputes as to whether dipyridamole (Persantine) (50 mg three times a day) augments the effect of aspirin are being resolved by an ongoing cooperative study. Opinions are now divided whether this therapeutic approach should precede, supplement, or supplant oral anticoagulants. In many centers, they precede oral anticoagulants, which are then also administered if transient ischemic attacks continue. When anticoagulants are used along with platelet inhibitors, the danger of hemorrhage is increased, necessitating reduced doses of oral anticoagulants and close clinical monitoring.

SURGERY Surgical management of the arterial obstruction in the neck and thorax is achieved by thromboendarterectomy. The region of the carotid sinus is most frequently amenable to such therapy. The carotid sinus may prove tightly stenotic, occluded, or affected with plaque and/or ulcer formation. In experienced hands, these lesions can usually be dealt with safely by endarterectomy. When a thrombus of the internal carotid artery extends higher than the siphon, the surgical approach depends on some form of bypass grafting (transcranial external carotid to middle cerebral), a surgical procedure found technically feasible, and its value is currently under active study. Surgery can also be done at the other sites suitable for surgical management, including the common carotid, innominate, and subclavian arteries. Operation on the vertebral artery at its origin is still of limited value, as proof of its role in preventing transient ischemic attacks and stroke is lacking. Before operation the existence of the occlusive lesion and its extent must be determined by arteriography. Surgery is optimally undertaken at the stage of transient ischemic attacks or early in the course of thrombosis-in-evolution. When total infarction has occurred, surgery will be ineffective even though patency of the vessel is restored. Surgery is not without risk (postoperative strokes still occur in 2 to 3 percent of the cases in the best surgical circumstances), and the less severe the disease process, the less definitive the therapeutic results of surgery. Asymptomatic carotid stenosis need not be routinely treated by endarterectomy, unless progression of the stenosis is documented.

DIETARY MANAGEMENT Recent studies of platelet physiology in the human have isolated a variety of dietary factors that affect platelet aggregation. Due to their high content of the fatty acid eicosapentaenoate, seafood diets, especially mackerel, oysters, and other seafoods, have significantly reduced platelet aggregation throughout the period of their consumption. Other foods producing similar effects include the black tree fungus (extensively used in Chinese cooking), the oils of garlic and onions, and cod liver extracts. It is possible that further discoveries in this area will result in the applicability of dietary manipulations as one of many factors in stroke prevention.

THERAPY FOR CEREBRAL EDEMA In the initial days following major cerebral infarction, cerebral edema may occasionally threaten life. In such instances, dexamethasone in intramuscular doses of 4 to 6 mg every 4 to 6 h may prove helpful. Oral therapy with glycerin in doses of 30 ml every 4 to 6 h or glycerol in doses of 50 g dissolved in 500 ml of 2.5% saline solution given intravenously daily are other forms of therapy available. There are conflicting results from various clinical trials on the value of antiedema agents in acute cerebral infarction. Much of the evidence points to a limited value, in particular of steroids, which in addition are not uncommonly associated with significant complications (severe infection, decompensation of diabetes, upper gastrointestinal bleeding).

CEREBRAL VASODILATORS Despite experimental evidence that these agents increase the cerebral blood flow, as measured by the nitrous oxide method, they have not proved beneficial in careful studies in human stroke cases at the stage of transient ischemic attacks, thrombosis-in-evolution, or in the established stroke. This is true of nicotinic acid, tolazoline (Priscoline), alcohol, papaverine, and inhalation of 5% carbon dioxide. A few clinical trials have suggested that histamine, aminophylline, acetazolamide, and intraarterial papaverine have some merit. In opposition to the use of these methods is the suggestion that vasodilators are harmful rather than beneficial, since by lowering the systemic blood pressure they reduce the intracranial anastomotic flow, or by dilating blood vessels in the normal parts of the brain they divert blood from the area of ischemia.

THROMBOLYTIC AGENTS Fibrinolysin and profibrinolysin activators have not proved helpful in cases of transient ischemia, thrombosis-in-evolution, and the established stroke.

Physical therapy and rehabilitation Beginning within a few days, the joints of the paralyzed limbs should be passively carried through a full range of movement at frequent intervals. Contracture (and periarthritis) must be avoided, especially at the shoulder, elbow, and ankle. Pain, soreness, and aching in the paralyzed limbs may temporarily interfere with exercises. The patient can be placed in a chair after a week or so, or sooner if the lesion is small. Nearly all hemiplegics can learn to walk again to some extent, usually within a 3- to 6-month period, and this should be a primary aim in rehabilitation. A short or long leg brace is often required. Speech therapy is not of proved value, but it may enhance rehabilitation in patients with motor aphasia; in addition, it improves the morale of the patient. Physical therapy seems not to benefit patients with cerebellar ataxia. As the hemiplegic patient improves, and if mentality is preserved, instruction in the activities of daily living, using various special devices, can assist the patient in becoming at least partially independent in the home.

General preventive measures against strokes and vascular disease AVOIDING SITUATIONS IN WHICH STROKES ARE LIKELY TO OCCUR (1) Particular care should be taken to maintain the systemic blood pressure, oxygenation, and intracranial blood flow during surgical procedures, especially in elderly patients. (2) Hypotensive agents, whether given therapeutically or for diagnostic procedures, should be administered with care. (3) In the elderly patient in whom deep sleep might help to precipitate cerebral ischemia, oversedation should be avoided. (4) Systemic hypotension, severe anemia, and polycythemia should be treated promptly. (5) Rapid diuresis may be contraindicated.

FACTORS WHICH DETERMINE ULTIMATE OUTCOME The ultimate solution of the problem of cerebrovascular disease lies in more fundamental fields. Atherosclerosis and hypertension must be prevented or alleviated (see Chap. 267 for prophylaxis of atherosclerosis and Chap. 266 for the treatment of hypertension).

TRANSIENT ISCHEMIC ATTACKS OF CEREBRAL ORIGIN When transient ischemic attacks precede a stroke, they almost always stamp the process as thrombotic. Fully 60 percent of cases of atherothrombic strokes are preceded by transient ischemic attack, the risk of stroke in the population of cases experiencing transient ischemic attack is 6 to 7 percent the first year, and the 5-year cumulative risk reaches an alarming 35 to 50 percent. These attacks belong, therefore, under the heading of cerebral thrombosis, but they are discussed separately here because of their importance clinically and therapeutically.

Attention is directed to these attacks for the reason that their treatment (the administering of anticoagulant drugs or performing surgical endarterectomy at the stage of prodromal symptoms) may prevent a disastrous stroke. There would seem to be little doubt that they are due to transient focal ischemia, and they might be referred to as temporary strokes which fortunately reverse themselves. Corresponding to the higher incidence of atherosclerosis in hypertension and in the male population, about two-thirds of all patients with transient ischemic attacks are hypertensive and/or men.

Clinical picture Thrombosis of virtually any cerebral or cerebellar artery, deep or superficial, can be associated with transient ischemic attacks, e.g., common carotid, internal carotid, middle cerebral, anterior cerebral, ophthalmic, vertebral, basilar, posterior cerebral, the cerebellar arteries, and the penetrating branches to the deep structures of the basal ganglia and brainstem. If the posterior cerebral arteries are included in the vertebral-basilar system, ischemic episodes are slightly more common in that system than in the carotid. Transient ischemic attacks may precede, accompany, or rarely follow the development of a stroke, or they can occur by themselves without leading to a stroke. So far, it has not been possible to distinguish the early cases destined to do well from those in which a full-blown stroke will develop.

Transient ischemic attacks last from a few seconds up to 24 h, the most common duration being a few seconds up to *5 to 10 min*. It is uncommon for recurrent discrete attacks to last more than 30 min. There may be only a few attacks or several hundred. Between attacks, the neurologic examination may disclose no abnormalities. A stroke may ensue after the second episode or may be postponed until hundreds of attacks have occurred over a period of weeks or months. Often, especially when frequent over a long period of time, the attacks gradually cease and no important paralysis occurs, a fact which makes any form of therapy difficult to evaluate.

The neurologic features of the transient episode indicate the territory or artery involved and are fragments borrowed from the stroke which may be approaching. In the *carotid system*, attacks reflect involvement of cerebral hemisphere and eye. The ocular disturbance is ipsilateral; the sensorimotor disturbance is contralateral. Repeated attacks tend to respect their original general site and uncommonly involve only the eye at first, then the hemisphere, when each is affected alone. It is almost unknown for the eye and the brain to be involved simultaneously in a single attack. In the *transient hemisphere attacks*, ischemia occurs foremost in the distal middle cerebral territory and adjacent border zone region, producing weakness or numbness of the opposite hand and arm. However, many different combinations may be seen: face and lips, lips and fingers, fingers alone, hand and foot, etc. Less common manifestations include aphasia, difficulty in calculation (when the dominant hemisphere is involved), and other temporo-parieto-occipital disturbances, such as anosognosia, hemineglect, or visual field defects. In ocular attacks, *transient monocular blindness* is the usual symptom. Many of the latter episodes evolve swiftly and are described as being like a shade falling smoothly over the visual field until the eye is completely but painlessly blind. The attack clears slowly and uniformly. Uncommonly, the visual disorder may take the form of a wedge of missing vision, sudden generalized blurring, or, rarely, a bright light.

The clinical picture in the *vertebral-basilar system* is one of more variation, as many combinations of signs and symptoms may result from simultaneous ischemia of long tracts (motor and sensory) and cranial nerve structures. Occurring in varied combinations, the following manifestations in their approximate order of frequency may be recognized: dizziness; diplopia (vertical or horizontal); dysarthria; perioral numbness; weakness of a part or all of one side, or both sides, or crossed numbness (one side of face and opposite limbs); a feeling of cross-eyedness; dark vision; blurred vision; tunnel vision; partial or complete blindness; pupillary change; ptosis; paralysis of gaze; speechlessness; and dysphagia. Less common symptoms include noise or pounding in the ear or in the head, head or face pain, peculiar head sensations, vomiting, pallor, hiccups, memory lapse, drowsiness, transient unconsciousness (rare), impaired hearing, deafness, a feeling of movement of a part, peduncular hallucinosis, and forced deviation of the eyes.

It is not always easy to identify the territory affected. However, the occurrence of monocular blindness with or without contralateral weakness or numbness always points to the carotid system, as does receptive or sensory aphasia. The hallmarks of vertebral-basilar involvement are dizziness, diplopia, and bilateral weakness and/or numbness, i.e., a disturbance of the long motor or sensory tracts bilaterally.

The attacks may all take approximately the same pattern, or they may vary considerably in detail, although maintaining the same basic pattern. For example, weakness or numbness may involve fingers and face in some episodes and fingers only in others; or dizziness alone may occur in some attacks, while in others diplopia is added to the picture. In basilar artery disease each side of the body may be affected alternately. All the involved parts may be affected simultaneously, or a definite march or spread from one region to another can occur in a period of 10 to 60 s, or even a few minutes; e.g., numbness may spread from the hand to the face, or the reverse. The individual attack may cease abruptly or fade gradually.

Mechanism Ophthalmoscopic observations of the retinal vessels made during episodes of transient monocular blindness may show no abnormalities, or may show arrest of the blood flow in the retinal arteries and breaking up of the venous column to form a "boxcar" pattern, or can even demonstrate white material temporarily blocking the retinal arteries. The abnormalities indicate that in ischemic attacks a temporary, complete, or relatively complete cessation of blood flow occurs locally, possibly with associated microembolism. Hypotension, or postural factors, although long enjoying popularity as the basis of these attacks, do not produce the same type of symptoms. However, altered cerebrovascular reactivity may prove an important mechanism: in Moya-Moya disease (described below), severe bilateral intracranial stenoses are common and are associated with remarkable alterations in cerebrovascular collateral blood supply. In these cases, hyperventilation, which results in vasoconstriction in normal cerebral blood vessels, may precipitate focal symptoms. Similarly, in recent positron-emission studies of cerebral metabolism, cases have been described with severe arterial stenosis and cerebral zones of decreased vascular perfusion which can be corrected by extracranial-intracranial bypass surgery. There is good evidence that the attacks are abolished by anticoagulant drugs, but the mechanism of this is not known. Whatever their exact cause, they are closely related to vascular stenosis due to atherosclerosis and thrombosis.

Cerebral embolism (platelet emboli from sites of atherosclerosis) is frequently suggested as an explanation for recurrent transient ischemic attacks, and indeed this mechanism may underlie the nonstereotyped attacks. The usual source is an ulcerated atheromatous plaque in a stenosed carotid artery. In some cases of documented embolism, the deficit fluctuates from normal to abnormal repeatedly as long as 36 h, giving the appearance of transient ischemic attacks. In others, there is a short-lived deficit of several hours' duration, fulfilling the traditional criteria of transient ischemic attacks, i.e., a deficit of less than 24 h duration. However, if all the attacks are of approximately identical pattern, successive emboli coming from a distance could hardly be expected to enter the same arterial branch. Moreover, one would expect the involved cerebral tissue to be at least partially damaged, leaving some residual signs. The mechanism of single transitory episodes and multiple episodes of different pattern must be clearly distinguished from that of recurrent attacks of the *same pattern.* The former is embolic, the latter is progressing atherostenosis of a proximally located artery.

Arteriography sheds some light on pathogenesis. In the vast majority of series, the dominant finding has been hemodynamically significant stenosis or occlusion of the main artery ipsilateral to the side of the ocular or contralateral to the hemispheral symptoms. Ulceration is often present within the stenosis itself. However, ulceration independent of stenosis does not correlate with transient ischemic attacks as it is present as often in the asymptomatic side.

Differential diagnosis The following conditions must be differentiated from transient ischemic attacks: epileptic seizures, Ménière's syndrome, migraine accompaniments, Stokes-Adams attacks, hypersensitive carotid sinus reflex, transient global amnesia, insulin reactions, attacks of hysteria, anxiety, and depression, akinetic falling spells of the aged, and recurrent cerebral embolism.

Frank motor *convulsions* rarely if ever occur in ischemic attacks. The patient may report a feeling of movement, distortion, drawing, jumping, or jerking, but an isolated frank focal seizure may not have been encountered. Conversely, a cerebral seizure rarely displays as its only manifestation a temporary paralysis of a limb or of one side of the body. Unconsciousness is rare in ischemic attacks, and its occurrence even in only a few attacks indicates another diagnosis (seizure, Stokes-Adams attack, etc.). Incontinence of bowel and bladder, tongue biting, cyanosis, and residual sleepiness or muscle soreness are indicative of a seizure rather than an ischemic episode. In the sensory sphere, the distinction between ischemic episodes and seizures is less clear, for numbness or scintillating visual phenomena are seen in both conditions, and therefore in making a differentiation one must rely on the presence of associated phenomena (dizziness, diplopia, etc.). When numbness appears simultaneously in face, hand, and leg, i.e., when there is no "march," ischemia rather than a seizure is probably responsible.

Dizziness associated with brainstem ischemia is less likely to have a clear rotatory component than that seen in *Ménière's syndrome* or in *labyrinthitis.* In making a diagnosis, however, one depends on the presence of associated symptoms and signs. It is a simple matter to decide that the dizziness is of central origin when there are other evidences of brainstem involvement, by history or by neurologic examination: diplopia, dysarthria, cerebellar ataxia, vertical nystagmus, persistent horizontal nystagmus, numbness, weakness, dysphagia, etc. On the other hand, the isolated presence of the triad—recurrent dizziness, tinnitus, and chronic deafness (i.e., signs of both auditory and vestibular involvement)—is almost certain evidence of Ménière's syndrome. In the early stages the pictures at times resemble each other closely, however, and only an especially thorough search will reveal signs indicating that the disorder is due to ischemia of the brainstem or the cerebellum. Tinnitus of a constant hissing or ringing type is a rare complaint in brainstem vascular disease. When dizziness is the sole symptom in an elderly person, it is often impossible to make an accurate diagnosis, and only after observing the patient for a period of time will the nature of the underlying disease be disclosed. It must be remembered that since both basilar artery disease and Ménière's syndrome are common conditions, the two may coexist.

The visual, sensory, and motor phenomena which precede the headache (or occur in its absence) in some cases of *migraine* bear a close resemblance to ischemic manifestations, but since migraine originates in early life and most characteristically disturbs vision in both eyes, its differentiation from ischemic attacks does not ordinarily pose a problem. An important point is that migrainous accompaniments in 75 percent of cases develop gradually over a period of 5 to 10 min, marching across the affected region, whereas transient ischemic phenomena rarely do this. When vascular disease has its onset in the twenties or thirties, the two may be confused until the history is carefully taken. A migrainous accompaniment may return after a headache-free interval of 10 to 20 years. It is not rare for migrainous accompaniments to appear for the first time in the forties or fifties. Still more important, periodic headaches may not be obvious at this age. Headache, at times of some intensity, can accompany cerebral thrombosis, and in an elderly person the occurrence for the first time of periodic headache associated with numbness or weakness should suggest atherothrombosis rather than migraine.

Stokes-Adams attacks and *hypersensitivity* of the *carotid sinus reflex* cause "collapsing spells" with unconsciousness, confusion, pallor, sweating, and jerking, but almost never do they produce focal neurologic manifestations such as numbness, weakness, or diplopia.

Difficulty in differentiation of these conditions will arise only when the clinical details of the episode are not available, and usually a careful minute-by-minute description of the attack will enable the physician to make the correct diagnosis. Only in an occasional case of basilar artery insufficiency will an ischemic episode result in unconsciousness, usually accompanied by other symptoms such as weakness, numbness, blindness, or dysarthria. In *akinetic falling spells of the aged,* the patient falls either conscious or unconscious without convulsive movements, color change, or alteration in pulse, blood pressure, or respiration. Within a few seconds or a minute or two consciousness is restored.

Treatment The therapy of transient ischemic attacks has already been discussed under "Treatment of Atherosclerotic Thrombosis," where it was pointed out that anticoagulants, antiplatelet agents, or surgical endarterectomy usually stop the attacks and prevent indefinitely the onset of a threatening stroke. Surgery must be seriously considered in carotid and subclavian cases. In many patients the attacks cease spontaneously, and anticoagulant therapy can be withheld if the episodes are few and spaced at long intervals. In nonsurgical cases, however, anticoagulants or drugs that prevent platelet aggregation are indicated if the attacks are of recent onset, and are becoming more frequent, more severe, or of longer duration, or if each attack no longer clears away completely, and a persistent neurologic deficit is accumulating. If anticoagulants are used, they may be replaced by aspirin after 3 to 6 months.

Other measures that have been recommended include administration of phenobarbital, papaverine, or nicotinic acid, inhalation of 5% carbon dioxide, breathing into a paper bag, and stellate block or cervical sympathectomy, but none of these has proved effective under careful clinical testing. On several occasions the authors have been impressed with the salutary effect of having the patient stop smoking cigarettes. For the more general therapeutic measures applicable in these cases, see the section on treatment of atherosclerotic thrombosis, above.

OTHER CAUSES OF THROMBOSIS (INFARCTION) It will be seen from the list at the beginning of this chapter that there are few causes of cerebral arterial occlusion other than thrombosis and embolism. There are fewer still that are important in the stroke picture. In many of those included, the mechanism is ischemia without actual thrombosis.

Venous thrombosis is a rather uncommon condition and rarely mimics a cerebrovascular stroke. Arising in relation to extracranial and intracranial sepsis, surgical operations, parturition, contraceptive pill, polycythemia, sickle cell anemia, and chronic wasting illnesses, particularly in children, it can cause a relatively mild neurologic illness with raised intracranial pressure, headache, visual obscurations, and focal seizures, or on the other hand, it can lead to extensive cerebral infarction and hemorrhage, with grave neurologic manifestations and death.

Systemic hypotension usually results in unconsciousness (syncope) without focal motor and sensory signs. But if the state of vascular collapse persists for a sufficient length of time, ischemia distal to a point of stenosis may result. Infarction will occur in the border zone and adjacent distal regions of major arterial territories of the cerebrum and cerebellum. It has already been mentioned that transient ischemic attacks and persistent strokes often develop under circumstances which suggest that a fall of the systemic blood pressure was the precipitating factor. Hypotension occurs in "simple faint," acute blood loss, myocardial infarction, Stokes-Adams syndrome, traumatic and surgical shock, cardiac arrest or anesthetic accident during surgery, hypersensitivity of the carotid sinus reflex, and in the several types of postural hypotension [idiopathic, postsympathectomy, tabetic, diabetic, with autonomic blocking agents, with reserpine (Serpasil), and on getting up and around after surgery].

Arteriography occasionally causes cerebral infarction. In some cases this is the result of cerebral embolism from a clot forming on the tip of the catheter; in others the embolic material may be fragments of a local atherosclerotic plaque; subintimal contrast injections are no longer a problem since the replacement of direct carotid needle insertion by femoral catheterization.

Carotid occlusion may be the result of direct *trauma* to the neck, or it may be precipitated by a "closed head injury," sometimes of a seemingly trivial nature. Here there is a traumatic dissecting aneurysm in the common or internal carotid arteries manifested arteriographically by an abrupt, elongated narrowing of the vascular lumen ("string sign"). Cases of this type are being recognized with increasing frequency in patients who have had no neck trauma (? medionecrosis) (see further on), and the mechanisms of stroke are either distal low flow from carotid occlusion or embolization into intracranial branches.

Arteritis is no longer a common cause of cerebral thrombosis, at least in North America, owing to the present satisfactory treatment of syphilis. *Necrotizing* or *granulomatous arteritis,* whether limited to the cerebral vessels or occurring as part of a polyarteritis, usually produces a series of small ischemic deficits in brain, optic nerve, or spinal cord; it only rarely mimics a stroke, as it presents as a chronic granulomatous meningitis. *Idiopathic giant-cell arteritis* involving the large arteries arising from the aortic arch is a rare cause of unilateral or bilateral carotid occlusion but must be kept in mind. It appears to be more common in young women in Japan, the aforementioned Takayasu's syndrome or "pulseless disease." *Cranial arteritis* or *temporal arteritis* is usually limited to the extracranial arteries except for the small vessels supplying the optic and oculomotor nerves. Unfortunately, in over 50 percent of cases permanent blindness or a severe impairment of vision results. The process usually involves the internal or common carotid arteries, but rarely causes a stroke (Chap. 69). Occasionally a vertebral-basilar stroke is reported.

Moya-Moya disease is another poorly understood occlusive disease involving large arteries, especially the intracranial portions of the internal carotid and stems of the middle and anterior cerebral arteries, usually bilaterally. Angiographically, a remarkable collateral circulation is developed, involving the deep, i.e., lenticulostriate, arteries (which usually fail to develop such collaterals in other occlusive diseases), as well as transdural anastomoses between external and internal carotid artery branches (the so-called rete mirabile). Most of the patients have been children, and the original vascular lesion is unknown. A typical clinical feature of this condition is the development of cerebral symptoms after hyperventilation, possibly due to constriction of collateral flow channels. Hemorrhage may occur, presumably from later rupture of the anastomotic blood vessels.

Contraceptive therapy is undoubtedly associated with strokes in young women. Major cerebral arteries may be occluded with the usual varieties of syndromes. This is but part of a more generalized affection of the circulatory system; death occurs approximately five times more frequently than in age-matched controls. In those individuals using these agents for 10 years the death rate is 10 times that of controls. An occlusive cerebrovascular lesion is calculated to have an incidence of 13.2 in 100,000 in the treated group and 2.8 in 100,000 in the control group. These statistics, while provocative, are difficult to interpret because there is a small but significant incidence of ischemic strokes in young women, especially during pregnancy. Interestingly, in 25 percent of our patients arteriography of the affected vessel showed it to be normal; or, if at first it was occluded, it later became patent. This means that embolism is the probable basis in at least some of the cases. In postmortem studies the wall of the occluded vessel has shown no inflammatory or other pathological change. Presumably the thrombus formation is due to an abnormality of platelets. Migraine and cigarette smoking appear to be predisposing factors.

Polycythemia is stated to be a cause of cerebral thrombosis, but convincing cases must be rare. *Thrombotic thrombocytopenic purpura* usually leads to multiple microscopic infarcts and fluctuating neurologic symptoms without evidence of stroke.

Idiopathic thrombocytosis with platelet counts of more than 10^6 per milliliter due to megakaryocytosis may result in multiple episodes of focal cerebral ischemia. Antimitotic drugs have suppressed the attacks. *Hyperproteinemia* (greater than 9 to 10 g/dl) may produce impairment of circulation through small cerebral and retinal vessels (Bing-Neal syndrome). The increased viscosity of blood, correctable by bleeding or plasmapheresis, tends to cause more general cerebral symptoms (confusion, coma, blurred vision) rather than strokes. *Sickle cell disease* is associated with obstruction of small vessels, including the cerebral arteries and veins, but has recently been shown to have a high frequency of stenosis or occlusion affecting the extracranial internal carotid artery, with extensive intracranial collateral supply. A *dissecting aortic aneurysm* may involve the large vessels arising from the arch and result in carotid occlusion and hemiplegia, a concomitant fall in systemic blood pressure probably contributing to the picture. "Spontaneous" (nontraumatic) dissection also occurs in the cervical carotid and, less commonly, in intracranial arteries, with resulting occlusion and cerebral infarct.

Fibromuscular dysplasia is also attended at times by stroke. It should be considered in middle-aged individuals, especially women, and in association with vascular diseases of the kidneys. A corrugated appearance of the affected vessels in an arteriogram is the basis of most diagnoses. *Hypoxia* usually produces a diffuse destruction of neurons rather than frank infarction, but bilateral softening of the globus pallidus is a classic feature. *Tentorial and subfalcial herniation* can cause infarction by compression of the posterior and anterior cerebral arteries, respectively. Under the rare types of infarction, it should be mentioned that carotid occlusion has been described following tonsillectomy, in association with *cavernous sinus thrombophlebitis,* and the trigeminal ganglionitis of herpes zoster. Also, a previously transient and harmless migrainous aura can be transformed into a persistent deficit, presumably because of infarction as the result of prolonged arterial spasm. This complication most frequently takes the form of homonymous hemianopia. Finally, a category for *cerebral infarction of undetermined cause* is included, for it must be admitted that in some cases, even after neuropathologic examination, it is impossible to determine the exact cause of an infarct, especially in young adults.

Omitted here is *Binswanger's chronic progressive subcortical encephalopathy,* a rare disease of cerebral white matter tentatively attributed by Binswanger to atherosclerosis. In some instances extensive softening due to atheromatous thrombosis is more or less confined to white matter, which may be border-zone territory between the penetrating cortical arteries and periventricular ones.

LACUNAR SYNDROMES

Infarcts in the deep portions of the cerebral hemispheres and brainstem can result from occlusion of small perforating branches of the circle of Willis and of adjacent anterior, middle, and posterior cerebral and basilar arteries. Occlusion of such individual perforating arteries—the diameters of which are from 100 to 400 μm—produces a small infarct of 2 to 15 mm in diameter. The cavity left after removal of the necrotic tissue has been referred to as a *lacune,* and the clinical pictures that result from such small, deep cerebral infarcts are called *lacunar syndromes.* These are now well-recognized clinicopathologic entities, and they are sufficiently different from infarcts affecting the cerebral surface to warrant separate description.

Lacunar infarcts represent about 10 percent of strokes, and one out of every seven cerebral infarcts corresponds to this type. Their pathogenesis is closely related to arterial hypertension and atherosclerosis of large arteries. The occlusion of the perforating arteries relates to a degenerative process in the media which Fisher has called *lipohyalinosis.* Using serial sections,

Fisher has shown the occlusion to be segmental and to involve relatively circumscribed portions of the artery, generally at some distance from the parent trunk. In other instances, a microatheroma was found in the occluded segment of the perforating artery, usually in close proximity to its point of origin from the main arterial trunk. The location and, at times, the histologic appearance separate this arterial process from the more common atherosclerotic arterial degeneration affecting extracranial and proximal intracranial arteries. These differences account for the distinctive qualities of these two types of strokes in terms of clinical presentation, preceding manifestations, diagnostic findings, therapy, and prognosis.

The clinical presentation in lacunar infarction varies according to the perforating arteries involved, and a number of clinical syndromes have been defined. These correspond to infarcts in the distribution of the perforating branches of the middle cerebral, posterial cerebral, and basilar arteries. In occlusion of a middle cerebral perforator or *lenticulostriate artery,* the lacunar infarct is confined to the basal ganglia (putamen, globus pallidus, and caudate) and the adjacent genu and posterior limb of the internal capsule. The most common lacunar syndrome, *pure motor hemiparesis,* results from an infarct in the posterior limb of the internal capsule. It is characterized by a usually severe hemiparesis or hemiplegia involving arm, leg, face, and trunk, accompanied by mild dysarthria, but without sensory deficit, visual field defect, aphasia, or alteration of consciousness. The unusual combination of a severe or complete flaccid hemiplegia with exquisite preservation of fine tactile sensation, proprioception, vibratory sense, graphesthesia, and stereognosis of the affected limbs is strongly suggestive of a capsular lacune on clinical grounds only. A syndrome of identical characteristics can result from a lacune at the level of the basis pontis (see below), whereas pure motor hemiparesis secondary to medullary pyramidal infarction is characterized by sparing of the face. Although cases of pure motor hemiparesis may show different degrees of severity of weakness in the arm, the leg, and the face, in the majority the degree of weakness of the different segments of the affected side is about the same. This feature points to corticospinal tract involvement at a capsular level and contrasts with the commonly unequal degree of weakness of different parts of the body observed in cortical surface infarctions in the middle or anterior cerebral artery distribution.

Other lacunar syndromes in the lenticulostriate territory are less common and are not as well characterized as pure motor hemiplegia. These include the *dysarthria–clumsy hand syndrome,* in which severe dysarthria, facial palsy, and tongue paresis are associated with clumsiness and mild weakness of the hand due to a lacune involving the genu and anterior limb of the internal capsule; the *hemichorea-hemiballismus syndrome* in association with subthalamic lacunes, with sparing of the internal capsule; and the *mutism* or *anarthria syndrome* from bilateral, nonsimultaneous, capsular lacunes. In the latter situation, a *pseudobulbar syndrome* may develop, in which anarthria or severe dysarthria is accompanied by dysphagia, bilateral spasticity, bilateral Babinski sign, paroxysms of inappropriate crying or laughter, and a short-stepped gait. This combination is usually referred to as a *lacunar state.*

Occlusion of a perforating branch originating from the posterior cerebral artery (one of the *thalamoperforate arteries*) results in a *pure sensory stroke.* This is characterized by a hemisensory syndrome involving face, limbs, and trunk, at times remarkably well defined along the midline of the body. Along with a variety of subjective sensory symptoms (heaviness, heat, burning feeling, changes in size or shape of the limbs), patients present with partial or, less commonly, total loss of superficial and deep sensory modalities on one-half of the body. This contrasts with perfect preservation of motor strength, visual fields, speech function, and level of consciousness. The responsible lacunes have been found in the ventral posterior thalamic nuclei. In very rare instances, this striking sensory syndrome has been accompanied by a mild and transient hemiparesis, and autopsy has documented slight involvement of the posterior limb of the internal capsule adjacent to the expected lacune in the ventral posterior nucleus of the thalamus.

The occlusion of *perforating pontine branches of the basilar artery* has been associated with a variety of lacunar syndromes. The resulting syndromes are most commonly related to the basis pontis, where the descending corticospinal tracts and the exiting cerebellopontine fibers along with the pontine nuclei are the principal structures. Involvement of tegmental structures by pontine lacunes is a rare occurrence. Lacunar syndromes due to lesions in the basis pontis include *pure motor hemiparesis* and the *dysarthria–clumsy hand syndrome,* both clinically indistinguishable from the varieties due to capsular infarcts. A third syndrome, *homolateral ataxia and crural paresis* or *ataxic hemiparesis,* has been correlated with basal pontine lacunar infarcts. It presents with a peculiar combination of hemiparesis that affects the leg more than the arm or face in association with marked cerebellar ataxia of the weak limbs, usually more prominent than the paresis. This is particularly obvious at the level of the upper limb, where the weakness is usually rather slight. The unusual combination of contralateral weakness and cerebellar ataxia affecting the same limbs has been attributed to involvement of corticospinal fibers before decussation and efferent cerebellar fibers after decussation.

A number of other combinations of symptoms and signs have been observed in single cases of brainstem lacunes. These include oculomotor paresis with cerebellar ataxia, dysarthria with cerebellar ataxia, pure motor hemiparesis with internuclear ophthalmoplegia, or abducens palsy, or lateral gaze paresis, all of which indicate tegmental extension of the basis pontis lesion. Most of these cases probably represent lesions larger than the usual lacunes, and their etiology most likely is proximal occlusion of basilar branches by intrinsic atherosclerotic disease or from atheroma of the basilar trunk compromising the ostium of the perforating artery. These latter examples are better classified as *basilar branch occlusions,* a process more related to large-vessel atherostenosis than to intrinsic disease of the primary perforating artery. Finally it should be said that many lacunes are completely asymptomatic, though in combination with others they may cause ill-defined failures of cerebral function.

The clinical presentations of the different lacunar syndromes have a number of features in common. Transient ischemic attacks precede them in about 20 percent of the cases, less often than in large-artery atherosclerosis (50 percent), but more often than in cerebral embolism (5 percent). In about one-third of the cases, the onset is one of progression of the deficit over a period of several hours; not uncommonly it continues for 24 h or more after admission to the hospital. The sudden onset that is commonly associated with stroke in general is manifested by only 50 to 60 percent of the cases of lacunar infarcts. In the remainder one cannot determine the onset because it occurred during sleep without further progression on awakening. The clinical course commonly is one of improvement after a few days of stabilization of the neurologic deficit, and the speed of recovery relates to the completeness of the initial deficit, i.e., those with initially partial syndromes showing the fastest and most complete reversal, not infrequently with return of function to allow independent motor activity within 1 month from the onset. Because of the small size of the infarcts and their tendency toward a rapid recovery of function, lacunes are the stroke type with the lowest mortality (less than 5 percent).

The diagnosis of lacunar infarctions is usually made on

purely clinical grounds. A normal electroencephalogram supports a clinical diagnosis of lacunes, since the same motor or sensory syndrome caused by cortical surface infarction is more likely to be associated with focal slowing. CT scan may provide the positive diagnostic evidence for lacunar infarction. Despite variation in size and location of these infarcts, approximately half of them can be detected if CT scans are performed within 10 days from the onset. Those likely to be missed are smaller than 2 mm or located at the level of the pons, where artifact usually precludes visualization of small, nonhemorrhagic lesions. Angiography is a procedure of little use in the evaluation of lacunar strokes, with the exception of those instances in which an unusually large lacune is detected by CT scan. The latter may indicate that the vessel is occluded proximally, at its origin from the middle cerebral artery stem, where atherosclerosis or embolism may be the causal factor. This rare occurrence needs consideration, as its therapy would be different from that of the usual variety of lacune.

Therapy for lacunes is customarily restricted to initial bed rest, promptly followed by physiotherapy. Control of hypertension is usually not an issue in the acute stage but becomes of theoretical importance following the stroke as a means of preventing recurrence. Anticoagulants or antiplatelet drugs are not currently used, except for those uncommon cases of hemispheral or pontine lacunes secondary to major atherosclerotic disease of the parent vessel (middle cerebral, posterior cerebral, basilar), the latter being thus treated with the aim of preventing its secondary thrombosis.

CEREBRAL EMBOLISM

In most cases of cerebral embolism, the embolic material consists of a fragment which has broken away from a thrombus or a valve vegetation within the heart. Less frequently the source is intraarterial from an atheromatous plaque that has damaged the endothelium and has become ulcerated. Still another mechanism is circulating thrombus that has broken away from the distal (intracranial) end of a thrombus formed in the internal carotid artery. Embolism due to fat, tumor cells, and air is a rare occurrence and seldom enters into the differential diagnosis of strokes. The embolus usually becomes arrested at a bifurcation or other site of narrowing of the lumen. Ischemic pale, hemorrhagic, or mixed infarction usually follows; hemorrhagic infarction, as pointed out earlier, nearly always indicates embolism. Any region of the brain may be affected, but the territory of the middle cerebral artery is most frequently involved, especially the upper division. The two hemispheres are approximately equally affected. Large embolic masses will block larger vessels (sometimes the carotids in the neck), while tiny fragments may reach vessels as small as 0.2 mm, in which case the stroke may clear in a few days and the resultant infarct might be so small as to almost escape detection at autopsy. The fate of embolic material is not fully understood. Often, it remains arrested, plugs the lumen solidly and is organized by fibroblasts from the arterial wall; but in many cases it breaks up into fragments which enter smaller vessels and disappear completely, so that careful pathologic examination fails to reveal their final location. The anatomic diagnosis must then be made by inference, e.g., the absence of a vascular occlusion at the proper site to explain the infarct, the absence of atherosclerosis or other cause for thrombosis in the cerebral vessel, a ready source of embolus, infarcts in other organs such as kidney and spleen (recognized clinically in less than 4 percent of cases), the occurrence of hemorrhagic infarction, and last, but not least, the clinical history.

Because of the rapidity with which occlusion develops in embolism, there is not much time for collateral influx to become established. Thus sparing of territory distal to the site of occlusion is not so common as in thrombosis. However, the ischemia-modifying factors mentioned under thrombosis are still to some extent operative and will influence the size, shape, and severity of the infarct.

Brain embolism is essentially a manifestation of heart disease. Many kinds of heart disease can be associated with embolism. The commonest direct cause is *chronic atrial fibrillation* (approximately 50 percent of all cases of embolism) due to atherosclerotic or rheumatic heart disease, the source of the embolus being mural thrombus deposited within the atrial appendage. In rheumatic heart disease mitral stenosis increases the likelihood of embolism seven times. Atrial fibrillation due to other types of heart disease, usually ischemic, can also lead to embolism. Embolism also occurs during paroxysmal atrial fibrillation or flutter. *Mural thrombus* deposited on the damaged endocardium overlying a myocardial infarct is an important source of cerebral emboli. Emboli can also arise from atrial thrombi associated with severe mitral stenosis without atrial fibrillation. *Cardiac surgery,* especially valvoplasty, may disseminate fragments of thrombus or particles of a calcified valve leaflet. Mitral and aortic valve prostheses are associated with embolism with variable frequencies, depending on the type of prosthesis used and the adequacy of anticoagulation. *Paradoxic embolism* can occur when an abnormal communication exists between the right and left sides of the heart, or when both ventricles communicate with the aorta. Thus embolic material arising in the veins of the lower extremity or, indeed, anywhere in the systemic venous tree may, particularly in conditions of pulmonary hypertension (often from previous pulmonary embolism), bypass the pulmonary circulation and reach the cerebral vessels. Subendocardial fibroelastosis, idiopathic myocardial hypertrophy, cardiac myxomas, and cardiac lesions in trichinosis are rare causes of embolism.

The *vegetations of acute and subacute bacterial endocarditis,* being infected, give rise to septic embolism, which results in several different pathologic pictures in the brain. In some cases the infarcts (they are usually multiple) produce clinical syndromes identical to those due to bland emboli; in others, tiny septic infarcts develop, or as in acute bacterial endocarditis, there may be miliary abscesses into which a small amount of hemorrhage (focal embolic encephalitis) may occur. Meningitis can be a concomitant with septic embolization. Mycotic aneurysm is another complication of septic embolism and may be a source of intracerebral or subarachnoid hemorrhage. *Marantic or nonbacterial endocarditis* occasionally causes cerebral embolism and can produce a most baffling clinical picture, especially when associated, as it often is, with carcinomatosis.

The following sources of embolic material are more difficult to prove or less frequent: (1) *Mural thrombus,* deposited upon ulcerated atheroma in the arch of the aorta or in the carotid arteries, may break loose and find its way into brain arteries. Massage of the carotid sinus, a favorite site for atherosclerosis, may dislodge a mural thrombus and produce a hemiplegia. This is one of the reasons why carotid massage should always be carried out gently. (2) Atheromatous material may be washed out of a large *plaque* in the aorta or carotid arteries and carried distally into the branches of the cerebral tree. (3) The *pulmonary veins* are a source of cerebral emboli, as indicated by the occurrence of cerebral abscesses in association with pulmonary suppurative processes and by the high incidence of cerebral deposits secondary to pulmonary carcinoma. (4) Surgery of the neck and thorax can be complicated by cerebral embolism. A rare type is that which follows thyroidectomy, in which thrombosis in the stump of the superior thyroid artery extends proximally until a section of it, protruding into the lumen of the carotid, is carried away into the cerebral arteries. (5) Foreign bodies (such as shotgun pellets) occasionally are embolized into the intracranial circulation after entering the heart or cervical arteries at the time of the initial injury. (6) As is pointed out in Chap. 258, *prolapsed mitral valve* is a frequently observed abnormality and is a potential but rare source of cerebral embolism.

Cerebral embolism must always have occurred when secondary tumor is deposited in the brain, and cerebral embolism regularly accompanies septicemia. However, the tiny mass of tumor cells or bacteria seldom is large enough to occlude a cerebral artery and produce the picture of a stroke. Nevertheless clinically symptomatic tumor embolism has been reported secondary to *cardiac myxomas* and occasionally with other tumors. It must be distinguished from the *marantic endocarditis* and embolism which occasionally complicate carcinomatosis. Embolism in the course of septicemia usually means that a vegetative endocarditis is present with thrombus formation. *Cerebral fat embolism* is usually related to fractures of large bones. As a rule, the emboli are minute and widely dispersed, giving rise to multiple cerebral petechial hemorrhages; accordingly the clinical picture is usually not focal, as in a stroke. *Cerebral air embolism* is a rare complication of criminal abortion or of cervical and thoracic operations and was formerly encountered as a complication of pneumothorax therapy. This condition is usually difficult to separate on clinical grounds from the deficits following hypotension or hypoxia, which frequently coexist.

Not infrequently at autopsy the diagnosis of cerebral embolism is made with full justification without finding a source. The same is true of embolism elsewhere in the body. Possibly the routine search for a thrombotic nidus is not sufficiently thorough, and small thrombi in the atrial appendage, in the carotid branches, in the endocardium between the papillary muscles of the heart, or in the pulmonary veins may be overlooked. Nevertheless, in some cases studied most carefully, no source of a demonstrable embolus in a cerebral artery can be discovered.

CLINICAL PICTURE Of all strokes, those due to cerebral embolism develop most rapidly. "Like a bolt out of the blue," the full-blown picture evolves within several seconds or a minute, exemplifying most strikingly the temporal profile of a stroke. The neurologic deficit nearly always comes in a single sudden attack, only rarely in stuttering fashion. As a rule, there are no warning episodes whatsoever. This statement is possibly too stringent, for in occasional cases the onset is more gradual or fluctuating, or a transient episode or two may precede the final arrival of the stroke. However, any emphasis on these exceptions is misleading. The embolus strikes at any time of the day or night. Getting up to go to the bathroom is a time of danger.

It is important to realize that an embolus in its passage along an artery may produce a severe neurologic deficit which is only temporary; symptoms disappear as the embolus finally passes into a small branch supplying a relatively silent part of the hemisphere. In other words, embolism is a common cause of a single evanescent stroke. Also it can give rise to multiple transient attacks of differing pattern. Our opinion has already been expressed that recurrent transient ischemic attacks of the same pattern are not likely to be embolic, since successive emboli would hardly be expected to lodge at identical sites.

The neurologic picture will depend on the artery involved and where the obstruction lies. The syndromes related to each cerebrovascular territory are the same as those outlined (under "Neurovascular Syndromes") above. A large embolus may plug the stem of the middle cerebral artery, producing a severe hemiplegia. Eighty percent of Harvard Stroke Registry Series of embolic cases were in middle cerebral artery (11 percent posterior cerebral, 7 percent basilar, and 3 percent carotid arteries). More often the embolus is smaller and passes into one of the branches of the middle cerebral artery, producing a strikingly focal disorder: motor aphasia, a monoplegia (or part thereof), a central type of aphasia with little or no motor paralysis, or a sensorimotor paralysis with little or no involvement of language. Most patients diagnosed as having middle cerebral artery thrombosis prove to have emboli in the middle cerebral artery (or an atherosclerotic thrombosis of the carotid artery). Embolic material entering the vertebral-basilar system occasionally is arrested in the vertebral artery just below its union with the basilar; more often it traverses the vertebral and also the basilar, which is larger, and is not held up until it reaches the upper bifurcation. If arrested here, it abruptly produces deep coma and total paralysis. More often the embolus enters one, or both, of the posterior cerebral arteries and, by infarcting the visual cortex, causes a unilateral or bilateral homonymous hemianopia. Embolic infarction of the undersurface of the cerebellum is common, and the resulting swelling of necrotic brain may cause acute, fatal brainstem compression. Embolic material rarely enters the penetrating branches of the pons.

The general neurologic disturbance associated with embolic strokes is not significantly different from that seen in thrombotic cases, and the reader is referred to the description of the changes in consciousness, respiration, etc., under "Course and Prognosis" above. Again the patient may have a most devastating hemiplegia and yet be alert. Headache is not uncommon. In occlusion of the middle cerebral artery, the headache is usually referred to the ipsilateral temple; in occlusion of the posterior cerebral artery, to the outer half of the eyebrow.

Although the abruptness with which the stroke develops and the lack of prodromal symptoms point strongly to embolism, it is the total clinical picture upon which the diagnosis is based. If hemorrhage is ruled out, particularly by the use of the CT scan, there remains only thrombosis to be excluded. The presence of atrial fibrillation or "sick sinus syndrome," a history of myocardial infarction (recent or in the preceding months), or the occurrence of embolism to other regions of the body all support the diagnosis of embolism. Embolism merits careful consideration in young persons in whom atherosclerosis is rather unlikely. Not infrequently the first sign of myocardial infarction is the occurrence of embolism; therefore, it is advisable to perform an electrocardiogram in all patients with cerebrovascular stroke of uncertain origin and to monitor (Holter monitor) cardiac function for 3 days, even if the initial findings show normal cardiac rhythm.

Acute and *subacute bacterial endocarditis* do not usually present as a stroke due to infarction, although 3 percent of embolic cases are due to this cause, often as the first sign. The signs of endocarditis, anemia, splenomegaly, and often a pleocytosis in the cerebrospinal fluid should point to the correct diagnosis.

Cardiac catheterization and *cardiac surgery,* now being widely used, are a source of significant neurologic disorder, fortunately of decreasing frequency. Formerly as many as 50 percent of patients with open heart surgery suffered a postoperative neurologic complication; now the figure is down to about 25 percent. In 100 successive cases examined pre- and postoperatively by Mohr at the Massachusetts General Hospital there were two types of complications, one being discovered immediately and the other after an interval of days or weeks. The immediate neurologic disorder consisted of a delay in waking up from the anesthesia, a slowness in thinking, a disorientation, agitation, combativeness, visual hallucinations, and poor registration and recall of what was happening. These symptoms, sometimes verging on psychosis, usually cleared within a 5- to 7-day period, although some patients were not completely normal mentally at the time of discharge from the hospital. As the confusion clears, about half of the affected patients will be found to have small visual field defects, dyscalculia, oculomanual ataxia, alexia, and other visual perceptive defects indicative of lesions in the parietooccipital regions of the cerebrum. It is believed that these immediate disorders are related to hypotension and various types of emboli (air, silicon, fat, platelet). In addition, some of the patients have stretch injuries of the lower part of the brachial plaxus (numb, weak hand, and Horner's syndrome) that are manifest as soon as they awaken.

The delayed effects are mainly embolic and are more frequent in cases with prosthetic valve replacements than with arterial homografts. In one series the frequency of embolism was calculated to be 4.6 percent per month in the former group, and 1 percent per month in the latter, if untreated. The Starr-Edwards ball valve has given rise to embolism in 20 to 30 percent of cases over a 4-year period. Warfarin and dipyridamole reduced the rate of embolism from 14.9 percent in the untreated to 1.3 percent in the treated group.

LABORATORY FINDINGS The description under "Atherosclerotic Thrombosis," above, applies for the most part to embolism except insofar as hemorrhagic infarction and septic embolism (focal embolic encephalitis) are concerned. Cerebral embolism in some 30 percent of cases produces a hemorrhagic infarct, which in most instances does not cause the cerebrospinal fluid to be bloody. However, in some excessively hemorrhagic infarcts, the fluid may be grossly bloody and contain as high as 10,000 or more red blood cells per cubic millimeter. The possibility that an embolic infarct is unusually bloody underlines the danger of administering anticoagulants routinely without examination of the cerebrospinal fluid. Also, it is the single exception to the rule that blood in the spinal fluid is unequivocal evidence that the stroke is due primarily to an intracerebral hemorrhage, aneurysm, or vascular malformation. In the milder cases of hemorrhagic infarction, a slight xanthochromia (grade 1 to 3 on the scale of 1 to 10) may appear after a few days.

CT scan is helpful in showing hemorrhagic infarction. The foci of high density consistent with hemorrhagic infarction have been observed within hours from onset. Most commonly, embolic cerebral infarction appears on CT as an area of low attenuation in the parenchyma, often affecting a fraction of the vascular territory of a given artery, as a result of occlusion of a branch or subdivision of that vessel. Multiple independent foci of infarction in the territories of more than one intracranial artery are strong evidence for embolism. The presence of two separate foci of infarction in the middle cerebral artery territory, one deep (in the basal ganglia and internal capsule), the other in the cortical surface, also suggests embolism. Such a combination suggests initial arrest of an embolus at the middle cerebral artery stem (with ischemia in the territory supplied by the lenticulostriate branches), followed by partial fragmentation and migration of embolic material into superficial (cortical) branches of that artery.

In septic embolism resulting from subacute bacterial endocarditis the white blood cells in the cerebrospinal fluid may be increased, usually numbering up to 200 per cubic millimeter and occasionally reaching several hundred; the proportion of lymphocytes and polymorphonuclear leukocytes varies with the acuteness of the septic process. There may also be several hundred or more red blood cells, and a faint xanthochromia is often present. The protein values are elevated, and the sugar content is within normal limits. No bacteria are seen or obtained by culture. In acute bacterial endocarditis there may be either the cerebrospinal fluid formula of subacute endocarditis or a frank purulent meningitis.

Arteriography is often successful (75 percent) in the detection of intracranial branch occlusion in cerebral embolism, if performed within 48 h from the onset. Beyond this period of time, due to the naturally unstable, fragmentary character of the embolic material, the probability of documenting the occlusion falls to as low at 15 percent.

Positive blood cultures will be found in as many as 3 percent of patients presenting with a cerebral embolus in the setting of clinically unobvious bacterial endocarditis. Echocardiography is of limited value in the detection of clinically inapparent cardiac sources of systemic emboli, because particulate matter small enough to produce focal cerebral symptoms is commonly too small to be resolved by this technique. Its main value is in the demonstration of segmental hypokinesis of the ventricular wall or ventricular aneurysms secondary to myocardial infarction, mitral valve prolapse, and the very rare atrial tumors (myxomas). Echocardiography's yield in disclosing mural thrombi in cases of recent myocardial infarction is virtually zero.

COURSE AND PROGNOSIS The remarks made concerning the *immediate prognosis* in atherosclerotic thrombosis apply as well here. As a rule, all but the most aggravated cases survive the initial insult. Massive brainstem infarction as a result of basilar embolism is almost always fatal. The eventual prognosis as to *survival* is determined by the occurrence of further emboli and the gravity of the underlying illness—cardiac failure, rheumatic heart disease, myocardial infarction, bacterial endocarditis, malignant growth, etc. The threat of an early recurrence of embolism is very real, and it is not uncommon to have the second embolus strike within a few days or weeks of the first. Considering these facts and the data of the Framingham series, where atrial fibrillation due presumably to arteriosclerotic heart disease increased the likelihood of a stroke fivefold (compared with age-matched controls) and atrial fibrillation with rheumatic heart disease increased the probability of stroke 17 times (Wolf et al.), the urgency of anticoagulant therapy is thereby emphasized. A cooperative study is currently studying the value of anticoagulation in the acute stage of cerebral embolism. The eventual prognosis regarding the *neurologic deficit* is not different from that given for atherosclerotic thrombosis (see "Course and Prognosis" above). The fact that an embolic episode may last only minutes or hours before clearing up should be stressed, especially in estimating the effect of any therapeutic measure.

TREATMENT The first three phases of therapy—(1) general medical management in the acute phase, (2) measures directed to restoring the circulation, and (3) rehabilitation—are much the same as described under "Treatment of Atherosclerotic Thrombosis" above. Attempted embolectomy at the bifurcation of the common carotid artery has usually failed but should be considered. If pulsation in the temporal artery in front of the ear is present, it means the embolus is not at that bifurcation but has passed up into the internal carotid system, and embolectomy will probably be unsuccessful. Embolectomy of the middle cerebral artery has proved too hazardous, since the penetrating arteries, i.e., lenticulostriates, are frequently occluded by the surgical manipulation. Fibrinolysin therapy has not proved effective.

In the field of prophylaxis there is strong evidence that the use of long-term anticoagulant therapy is effective in the prevention of embolism in cases of atrial fibrillation, myocardial infarction, and valve prosthesis. Prophylactic anticoagulant therapy is recommended for consideration in all cases of permanent and paroxysmal atrial fibrillation without waiting for embolism to occur, and once embolism does occur in 80 percent of cases the first episode will be followed by another embolus to the brain, frequently with severe damage. Although there has been much argument about the value of anticoagulants in thrombosis, they are almost universally recommended in embolism. In at least 14 studies of anticoagulant therapy, there has been a 65 to 90 percent reduction in the number of embolic accidents. Nonetheless, there is no completely randomized series. The treatment is continued for 6 to 12 months to years or for the lifetime of the patient. Platelet inhibition therapy may be of value in those patients whose valvular disease is associated with shortened platelet survival time.

After cerebral embolism has occurred, the question arises as to the necessity of delaying anticoagulant therapy for several days to avoid precipitating bleeding into a hemorrhagic infarct. It is the authors' practice always to perform a lumbar puncture first in order to rule out gross hemorrhage from the infarct and to obtain a CT scan in questionable cases. If the CT scan is normal and/or the cerebrospinal fluid is clear, the authors proceed with intravenous heparin therapy, since there is the constant danger of another embolus breaking away from the heart. One should not do a lumbar puncture in an anticoagulated patient unless absolutely necessary for fear of producing a spinal epidural or subdural hemorrhage and paraplegia. We have not encountered a case in which the use of anticoagulant drugs has increased the degree of hemorrhage within a hemorrhagic infarct, and indications are that such therapy is relatively safe. Rare exceptions to this statement may be expected. The use of anticoagulant therapy in patients with acute myocardial infarction, including those judged to be in the "good risk" category, is advisable. In cerebral embolism associated with subacute bacterial endocarditis, anticoagulant therapy is usually held to be contraindicated because of the danger of intracranial bleeding, and it is preferable to rely on a rapid sterilization of the bloodstream. However, the risks and value of anticoagulation in this setting have never been thoroughly tested.

Valvoplasty and amputation of the atrial appendage have substantially reduced the incidence of embolism in rheumatic heart disease. The need for special care in preventing emboli from entering the carotid arteries during the performance of cardiac valvoplasty is appreciated by all thoracic surgeons.

INTRACRANIAL HEMORRHAGE

This is the third most frequent cause of stroke, accounting for some 25 percent of cases. Although more than a dozen causes of intracranial hemorrhage have been listed (Table 356-2), hypertensive intracerebral hemorrhage, ruptured saccular aneurysm, hemorrhage associated with bleeding disorders, and arteriovenous malformations account for most of the hemorrhages which give rise to the clinical picture of a stroke. Duret hemorrhages, hypertensive encephalopathy, and idiopathic brain purpura will not simulate a stroke and are included only for the sake of completeness.

HYPERTENSIVE INTRACEREBRAL HEMORRHAGE Hypertensive intracerebral hemorrhage is the ordinary, well-recognized brain hemorrhage. Although sometimes the levels of blood pressure are normal (rare) or only in the range of 160/90 to 170/90, usually they are much higher. Hypertensive hemorrhage occurs *within* brain tissue, and rupture of the arteries lying in the subarachnoid space is practically unknown, apart from aneurysm. The extravasation which results from rupture of an artery forms a roughly circular or oval mass, which disrupts the tissue as the bleeding continues and it grows in volume. Adjacent brain tissue is displaced and compressed. If the hemorrhage is large, midline structures are displaced to the opposite side and vital centers are compromised, leading to coma and death. Rupture or seepage into the ventricular system usually occurs, and the spinal fluid becomes bloody in the larger hematomas. A hemorrhage of this type almost never ruptures directly into the subarachnoid space through the cerebral cortex; the blood reaches the subarachnoid spinal fluid via the ventricular system. When the hemorrhage is small and located at a distance from the ventricles, the cerebrospinal fluid may remain clear even on repeated examinations.

Extravasated blood undergoes a series of changes beginning with phagocytosis of the red blood cells at the outer rim, producing a brown-orange zone of hemosiderin-filled macrophages. The mass gradually decreases in size. After a period of some 2 to 6 months, only an orange-stained cleft (color due to presence of hemosiderin and iron in macrophages) is left at the site of the hemorrhage.

Hemorrhages may be classified as massive, small, slit, and petechial. *Massive* refers to huge hemorrhages several centimeters in diameter; *small* to those 1 to 2 cm in diameter; *slit* applies to a special type of small hypertensive hemorrhage which lies subcortically at the junction of white and gray matter and which in the healing stage becomes narrowed to an elongated, thin, orange cavity. *Petechial* hemorrhages are pinpoint in size, usually multiple, and correspond microscopically to round collections of red blood cells in the vicinities of arterioles and capillaries.

In order of frequency, the most common sites for hypertensive hemorrhage are (1) the putamen and adjacent internal capsule (50 percent of cases), (2) various parts of the central white matter (frontal lobe, corona radiata, etc., often extensions from the putamen), (3) thalamus, (4) cerebellar hemisphere, and (5) pons. The vessel involved is usually a penetrating artery. The nature of the vascular lesion which leads to arterial rupture is not fully known, but in the few serially sectioned cases, the hemorrhage appeared to arise from an arterial wall altered by the effects of hypertension, referred to as *segmental lipohyalinosis*. Amyloid has been found in the vessel wall in some cases of multiple cerebral hemorrhages.

Clinical picture The clinical picture has an abrupt onset and evolves gradually and steadily over an appreciable length of time, taking minutes, hours, or occasionally days (average of 1 to 24 h) to reach its peak, depending on the speed of bleeding. Hemorrhages associated with anticoagulant excess may be remarkably leisurely in evolution. Usually there are no recognizable warning or prodromal symptoms. Often the patient has

TABLE 356-2
Causes of intracranial hemorrhage (including intracerebral, subarachnoid, ventricular, and rarely subdural)

1. Hypertensive intracerebral hemorrhage
2. Ruptured saccular aneurysm
3. Ruptured arteriovenous malformation
4. Trauma including posttraumatic delayed apoplexy
5. Hemorrhagic disorders: leukemia, aplastic anemia, thrombopenic purpura, liver disease, complication of anticoagulant therapy, hyperfibrinolysis, hypofibrinogenemia, hemophilia, Christmas disease
6. Undetermined cause (normal blood pressure and no arteriovenous malformation)
7. Hemorrhage into primary and secondary brain tumors
8. Septic embolism and mycotic aneurysm
9. With hemorrhagic infarction, arterial or venous
10. With inflammatory disease of the arteries and veins
11. Miscellaneous rare types: after vasopressor drugs, upon exertion, during arteriography, during painful urologic examination, as a late complication of early-life carotid occlusion, complication of carotid-cavernous arteriovenous fistula, with anoxemia, migraine, teratomatous malformations. (Acute inclusion body encephalitis produces xanthochromia and up to 2000 red blood cells or more per milliliter of cerebrospinal fluid; acute necrotizing hemorrhagic encephalopathy may be associated with up to 100 red blood cells per milliliter of cerebrospinal fluid; tularemia and snake venom poisoning may cause bloody cerebrospinal fluid.)

been well, and headache, dizziness, and epistaxis have not occurred with any consistency as prodromal symptoms. There is no sex or age predilection except that the average age of occurrence is less than in thrombotic infarction. Negroes suffer this type of stroke more frequently than do Caucasians. In the great majority of cases, the hemorrhage comes on while the patient is up and active, and onset during sleep is a rarity. Hypertension is maintained early in the course of the stroke or may even rise higher, so that the existence of hypertension will be easily established when the patient is first examined. Hypertension is usually of the "essential" type, but other causes must always be considered—renal disease, renal artery occlusion, toxemia of pregnancy, pheochromocytoma, aldosteronism, adrenocorticotropic hormone (ACTH) overdosage, injection of excessive amounts of epinephrine, and rarely, violent exertion or an intense emotional experience. Cardiomegaly is usually present. A few of the patients have only slightly elevated or normal blood pressure.

There is ordinarily only one episode of hemorrhage, and recurrence of bleeding from the same site, as occurs in cases of saccular aneurysm, is not encountered. With the use of injection of radioisotope-labeled red blood cells to patients shortly after the onset of intracerebral hemorrhage, it has been shown that no further bleeding occurs beyond 2 to 3 h from the onset. Once bleeding has become arrested, rebleeding in the near future, i.e., after the first few days, is not to be anticipated. The blood spilled into the tissues is removed slowly, over a period of weeks and months, during which time symptoms and signs persist. Hence the neurologic deficit is never transitory in intracerebral hemorrhage, as it so often is in thrombosis and embolism, and, for the same reason, rapid improvement in the neurologic deficit from one examination to another is not to be expected.

The neurologic signs and symptoms vary with the site and size of the extravasation. The most common picture is that associated with a *putaminal hemorrhage,* in which the adjacent internal capsule is implicated. In the large hemorrhages patients lapse almost immediately into a comatose state with hemiplegia, and their condition visibly deteriorates as the hours pass. More often, however, they initially complain of something going awry within the head. In a few minutes the face sags on one side, speech becomes slurred or aphasic, the arm and leg gradually weaken, and the eyes tend to deviate away from the side of the paretic limbs. A carefully taken history often reveals that these events occurred gradually over a period of 5 to 30 min. Gradually the paralysis worsens, the affected limbs become flaccid, pinprick is not appreciated, a Babinski sign appears, speaking becomes impossible, and consciousness gives way to stupor. In the worst cases, signs of upper brainstem compression appear—coma, Babinski sign bilaterally, deep, irregular, or intermittent respiration, dilated fixed pupils, and occasionally decerebrate rigidity.

Thalamic hemorrhage of moderate size also produces a hemiplegia or hemiparesis via pressure on the adjacent internal capsule. The sensory deficit equals or outstrips the motor weakness. Aphasia may be present with lesions of the dominant side and apractagnosia of the nondominant. A homonymous field defect if present usually clears in a few days. Thalamic hemorrhage by virtue of its extension medially and into the subthalamus causes a series of ocular disturbances, including paralysis of vertical gaze, forced deviation of the eyes downward, inequality of pupils, with absence of light reaction, skew deviation with the eye opposite the hemorrhage being displaced downward and medially, ipsilateral ptosis and miosis, absence of convergence, an assortment of lateral gaze abnormalities (paresis or pseudoparesis of the sixth nerve), retraction nystagmus, and tucking in of the eyelids. Neck retraction may be prominent. Hemorrhage into the nondominant thalamus is liable to produce mutism.

Lobar hemorrhages commonly occur in the junction between cortex and white matter of the various cerebral lobes. They can be small and limited to a "slit" in the gray-white matter interphase, or they can enlarge into the underlying white matter and extend into the ventricular cavity, in a manner similar to the putaminal and thalamic varieties. A parieto-occipital location is more common, but any of the other lobes may be involved. In their clinical presentation they share many features with the other types of intracerebral hemorrhage, but lobar hematomas appear to present with seizures more often, and coma is infrequent at the onset. The latter attribute probably reflects their location at a distance from the midline structures that maintain consciousness. Their clinical manifestations vary according to their location: frontal hematomas present with contralateral hemiparesis more severe in the arm; those of dominant temporal location with Wernicke-type aphasia that at times shows a surprising tendency to early improvement; parietal foci produce sensorimotor and visual field deficits, in combination with features of hemi-inattention if nondominant in location; occipital hematomas with isolated homonymous hemianopia. The prognosis in lobar hemorrhage correlates with the size of the hematoma measured by CT scan. Whereas small hematomas are regularly associated with good prognosis, the large ones carry a 60 percent mortality rate. In selected instances, the latter type of lobar hematomas may benefit from surgical evacuation, in particular in those cases that continue to deteriorate clinically after admission.

In *pontine hemorrhage,* deep coma usually ensues in a few minutes, and the clinical picture includes total paralysis, prominent decerebrate rigidity, and small (1 mm) pupils that react to light. Lateral eye movements, evoked by head turning or irrigation of the ears with ice water, are impaired. The cerebrospinal fluid will be bloody. Death usually occurs within a few hours, but there are rare exceptions where consciousness is retained and the clinical manifestations indicate a small lesion in the tegmentum of the pons. These cases of partial hemorrhage of unilateral tegmental location are being diagnosed more often by CT scan. They present with crossed sensory or motor disturbances, gaze palsy, cranial nerve palsies, and Horner's syndrome. Coma is usually not a feature. Although their functional prognosis is poor, they are usually not fatal.

Cerebellar hemorrhage usually develops over a period of several hours, and loss of consciousness at the onset is almost unknown. Repeated vomiting is a hallmark of cerebellar hemorrhage, along with inability to walk or stand, occipital headache, and vertigo. There is a paresis of conjugate lateral gaze of the eyes to the side of the hemorrhage, forced deviation of the eyes to the opposite side, or an ipsilateral sixth nerve weakness. In the most acute phase of the illness there may be little or no evidence of cerebellar disease, and only a minority of cases show nystagmus or cerebellar ataxia of the limbs, although these signs must always be sought. Other ocular signs include "ocular bobbing," blepharospasm, involuntary closure of one eye, skew deviation, maintenance of vertical eye movements, small pupils which continue to react until very late in the illness and exhibit slight inequality. A mild ipsilateral facial weakness and a diminished corneal reflex are common. Dysarthria and dysphagia may be prominent. Contralateral hemiplegia and facial weakness do not occur. The plantar reflexes are flexor early, extensor late. As the hours pass, and occasionally with unanticipated suddenness, the patient becomes stuporous, then comatose as a result of brainstem compression, at which point reversal of the syndrome, even by surgical therapy, is seldom successful.

Ocular signs are important in the localization of intracerebral hemorrhages. In putaminal hemorrhage the eyes are deviated to the side opposite the paralysis; in thalamic hemorrhage the eyes are deviated downward and the pupils may be unreactive; in pontine hemorrhage the eyeballs are fixed and the pupils tiny and reactive; and in cerebellar hemorrhage the eyes are deviated laterally (to the side opposite the lesion) in the absence of limb paralysis.

At each of the above sites the hemorrhage is usually massive and patients survive only a few hours or a few days, succumbing as a result of secondary brainstem insult. Rarely do patients survive once deep stupor supervenes, although in some cases they may linger in an unresponsive state for a week or two. In some 30 percent of cases, however, the hemorrhage is less extensive and survival is possible, hemorrhages into the lobar white matter and the thalamus tending to be somewhat smaller than putaminal or cerebellar hemorrhages.

A *severe headache* occurs in only 50 percent of cases; in many others no headache is noted. *Nuchal rigidity* is frequently found, but again it is so often absent that failure to find it must by no means detract from the diagnosis. If the neck becomes stiff, it will become supple again as coma deepens. *Vomiting* occurs once or twice at the onset of intracerebral hemorrhage, and it is so frequent in cerebral syndromes of hemorrhage compared with infarction that hemorrhage is the leading diagnosis in that setting. But of equal importance is the fact that the patient often is far from comatose and may even be alert and responding accurately when first seen. This is true even with grossly bloody spinal fluid, and thus the adage that hemorrhage into the ventricular system always precipitates coma is quite incorrect. Only if bleeding into the ventricles is massive will coma result. *Seizures,* usually focal, occur in some 10 percent of cases of supratentorial hemorrhage in the first few days, especially in association with subcortical "slit" hemorrhage. The fundi often show hypertensive changes in the arteries. Rarely, fresh preretinal (subhyaloid) hemorrhages occur but are much more common in ruptured aneurysm or arteriovenous malformation.

Many of the less precisely localized neurologic manifestations described under cerebral thrombosis are also encountered in intracerebral hemorrhage, including coma, stupor, drowsiness, confusion, Cheyne-Stokes respiration, bilateral or contralateral grasping and sucking reflexes, incontinence of bowel and bladder, and unilateral and bilateral extensor rigidity.

Although the proper interpretation of this array of clinical data allows the correct diagnosis to be established in most cases, the laboratory examinations described below are helpful, especially in the more difficult small hemorrhages.

Laboratory findings The CT scan has revolutionized the diagnosis of intracerebral hemorrhage and has proved totally reliable in the detection of hemorrhages 1.5 cm or more in diameter situated in the cerebral or cerebellar hemispheres for the first 1 or 2 weeks after the rupture of the vessel. Thereafter, the extravasated blood becomes invisible in the CT scan. Small pontine hemorrhages are visualized less certainly. Hemorrhages are localized with remarkable accuracy, far surpassing that achieved with arteriography. At the same time coexisting hydrocephalus, tumor, cerebral swelling, and displacement of intracranial contents are readily appreciated. The administration of intravenous contrast permits the visualization of dilated vascular channels in cases of hematoma due to a ruptured arteriovenous malformation. The CT scan is particularly helpful in the diagnosis of small brain hemorrhages that do not spill blood into the CSF and were heretofore clinically unrecognizable.

Before the introduction of CT scanning the examination of the cerebrospinal fluid was the most dependable method for the diagnosis of hemorrhage. In cases of massive hemorrhage, the cerebrospinal fluid is often under increased pressure, but in almost half of our cases readings under 200 mm were obtained. The fluid is usually grossly bloody, although not so bloody as in ruptured saccular aneurysm (the count ranging from a few thousand cells up to 1 million). In smaller hemorrhages into central structures the cerebrospinal fluid contains a lesser amount of blood, and in some cases of intracerebral hemorrhage, particularly in those of the "slit" type, between cortex and white matter, it remains free of blood and clear of xanthochromia in repeated taps. In these latter cases, slight xanthochromia may appear after a few days to a week. At times the spinal fluid may be clear grossly but contain some 200 to 400 red blood cells, and it is then difficult to decide if this represents intracranial bleeding or a traumatic tap.

A *traumatic bloody spinal tap* greatly complicates the diagnostic problem. In a bloody tap the pressure tends to be low, the fluid that first flows from the needle is more bloody than that which comes later (third tube less bloody than the first), the fluid often clots in the test tube, and xanthochromia is either absent or at most present only in proportion to the amount of serum bilirubin admixed with the fluid. Bloody fluid due to cerebral hemorrhage is often under increased pressure, there is an even admixture of blood in all samples, the cerebrospinal fluid will not clot, and if more than 8 to 12 h has elapsed since the hemorrhage, a definite xanthochromia will be present in the supernatant fluid after centrifugation, which should always be carried out if there is any question of the reliability of the tap. However, the presence of xanthochromia after centrifugation may be due to the bilirubin contained in the blood spilled by a traumatic tap and therefore is not an infallible index of subarachnoid or brain hemorrhage. The white blood cells of the cerebrospinal fluid are accounted for by the amount of hemorrhage, and their ratio of red blood cells is usually the same as in the circulating blood. After hemolysis of red blood cells, the white blood cell count may be disproportionately increased. In parenchymatous hemorrhage the protein content of the cerebrospinal fluid is proportionately much greater than accounted for by the amount of hemorrhage, presumably due to leakage of high protein fluid from the hemorrhage. Sometimes after a questionably traumatic tap it is worthwhile to perform immediately another puncture at a higher level.

Lumbar puncture is not completely innocuous, since temporal lobe herniation may be precipitated in cases of massive supratentorial hemorrhage or softening. Despite this danger, the procedure is necessary when CT scanning is not available, and if specific therapeutic measures are contemplated, or if any doubt exists as to the diagnosis of cerebrovascular disease. X-ray of the skull early in the stroke sometimes shows a shift of the calcified pineal gland to the side of the cranium opposite the lesion, a change usually not seen in infarction. The electroencephalogram does not show a typical or diagnostic pattern, but high-voltage, slow waves are the most common finding with hemorrhage into the cerebral hemisphere. X-ray of the chest will often show cardiomegaly. Any urinary abnormalities will for the most part reflect coexisting renal disease, although transient glycosuria has been reported to result specifically from intracranial hemorrhage. The white blood cell count often rises to 15,000 to 20,000 per cubic millimeter, a higher figure than in thrombosis. The sedimentation rate is elevated.

Course and prognosis The immediate prognosis is grave, some 60 to 70 percent of patients dying in 1 to 30 days. Either the hemorrhage extends into the ventricular system, or temporal lobe herniation and midbrain compression occur. Sometimes the hemorrhage appears to seep gradually into vital centers. Gastric erosion and gastrointestinal hemorrhage of neurogenic origin may occur at any time within the first week or two. When the hemorrhage is smaller, survival is often the result, and the restitution of motor function, speech, etc., can be excellent, since, in contrast to infarction, the hemorrhage has to some extent pushed brain tissue aside instead of destroying it. Function may be slow to return, because extravasated blood is slow to be resorbed or removed from the tissues. Since rebleeding from the same site is unlikely, the patient may live for many years. In some instances of medium-sized cerebral and cerebellar hemorrhages, the patient survives and his or her condition gradually stabilizes, but definite papilledema appears after several days of increased intracranial pressure. This does not mean that the hemorrhage is increasing in size or swelling, only that papilledema is slow to develop. Healed scars impinging on the cortex are liable to be epileptogenic.

Treatment *The general medical management of the comatose, apoplectic patient is the same as that outlined under "Atherosclerotic Thrombosis"* above, and in Chap. 20. Measures to stem the hemorrhage and restore the integrity of damaged tissue have been relatively ineffective.

Surgical removal of the clot in the acute stage, either by evacuation or aspiration, has seldom proved beneficial except in patients with a hemorrhage lying near the surface and who are not comatose. Acute cerebellar hemorrhage, however, is usually amenable to surgical therapy and is the treatment of choice when the hemorrhage is diagnosed within the first 2 days of onset. In the smaller hemorrhages that reach a subacute stage, when papilledema appears, in many instances it has dictated unnecessary surgical evacuation of the hemorrhage when the patient's condition stabilized. Although the prognosis in hemorrhage into the cerebral hemisphere is probably little altered by surgery, the outlook for cerebellar cases seems to be improved.

Attempts to halt the hemorrhage by lowering the systemic blood pressure through the use of autonomic blocking agents have not been effective, and in many instances the inadvertent occurrence of disastrously low levels of blood pressure has complicated the illness. Artificial hypothermia has been used sporadically, but there are insufficient data to permit appraisal of this procedure. Intermittent compression of the ipsilateral carotid in the neck may be beneficial in acute putaminal cases.

The *only preventive measure* is the use of antihypertensive drugs to lower the blood pressure in cases of essential hypertension. If ACTH or one of the adrenal steroids is being given, toxicity must be watched for. When hypotension threatens during surgical procedures, injections of excessive amounts of vasoconstrictive agents are to be avoided. Toxemia of pregnancy, another cause of cerebral hemorrhage, must be detected early and the hypertension treated.

RUPTURED SACCULAR ANEURYSM This is the fourth most frequent of the cerebrovascular disorders following atherosclerosis, embolism, and hypertensive intracerebral hemorrhage. Saccular aneurysms take the form of small, thin-walled blisters protruding from the arteries of the circle of Willis or the major branches arising therefrom. These saccules or berries, as they have been called, are located for the most part at bifurcations and branchings (Fig. 356-11) and are presumed to be the result of developmental defects in the media and elastica. A small number of aneurysms have been attributed to incomplete involution of embryonic vessels. Owing to the local weakness, the intima bulges outward, covered only by adventitia; the sac gradually enlarges, until finally dissolution of the wall and rupture occur. Saccular aneurysms vary in size from tiny nubbins 2 mm in diameter up to spheric masses 2 or 3 cm in diameter, averaging 8 to 20 mm. Almost all aneurysms have reached a size over 10 mm at the time of their rupture. They vary greatly in form; some are round and connected to the parent artery by a narrower stalk; others are broad-based without a stalk; still others are narrow cylinders. The site of rupture is usually the dome of the aneurysm which may present one or more secondary sacculations but may also occur near the base. Enlargement is the result of dilatation of the lumen and organization of a laminated clot.

In routine autopsies the incidence of ruptured aneurysms is 1.8 percent, of unruptured ones, 2.0 percent. Saccular aneurysms are rare in childhood, even at routine postmortem examination; they increase in frequency to reach their highest plateau of incidence in persons between 35 and 65 years of age. Therefore, they are not congenitally formed anomalies but develop over the years on the basis of the developmental arterial defect. There is an increased incidence of congenital polycystic disease of the kidney and coarctation of the aorta in association with saccular aneurysm. Hypertension is more frequently present than in the average population, but aneurysms occur in persons with normal blood pressure. Atherosclerosis, although present in the walls of some saccular aneurysms, probably plays no part in their formation or enlargement.

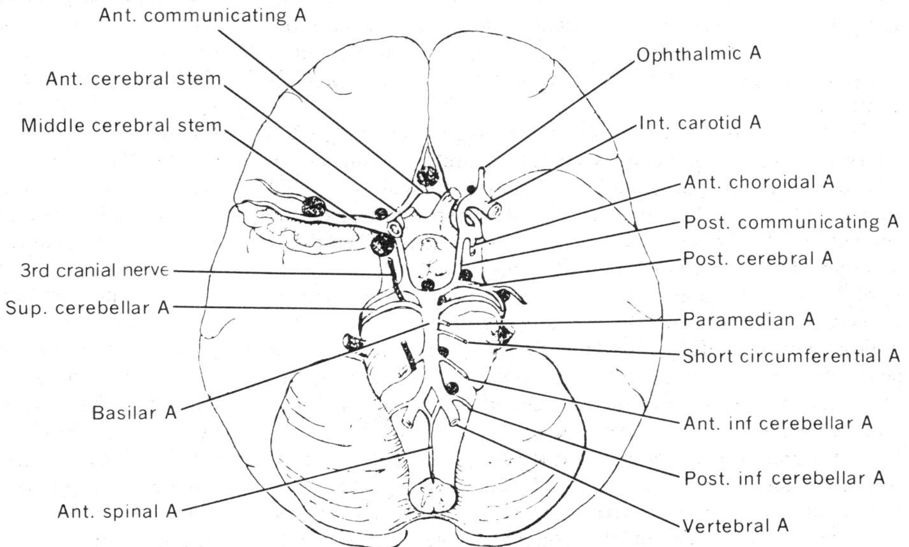

FIGURE 356-11
Diagram of the circle of Willis to show the principal sites of saccular aneurysm. Approximately 90 percent of aneurysms are on the anterior half of the circle.

Approximately 90 to 95 percent of saccular aneurysms lie on the anterior part of the circle of Willis. The four most common sites are (1) in relation to the anterior communicating artery, (2) at the origin of the posterior communicating artery from the stem of the internal carotid, (3) at the first major bifurcation of the middle cerebral artery, and (4) at the bifurcation of the internal carotid into middle and anterior cerebral arteries (see Fig. 356-11). Other sites include the internal carotid in the cavernous sinus (rupture may lead to an arteriovenous fistula without causing subarachnoid hemorrhage), at the origin of the ophthalmic artery, at the junction of the posterior communicating artery with the posterior cerebral, at the bifurcation or at the origin of the basilar artery, and at the origins of the three cerebellar arteries. In 20 percent of cases there is more than one aneurysm, and they may be situated unilaterally or bilaterally.

Several types of aneurysm other than saccular occur, e.g., fusiform, diffuse, globular, and mycotic. The first three are named for their predominant morphologic aspects and consist of enlargement or dilatation of the entire circumference of the involved vessels, usually the internal carotid, vertebral, or basilar arteries. Frequently showing atherosclerotic deposition in their walls, they are often referred to as arteriosclerotic, but most likely they are at least partly developmental in nature. They press on neighboring structures or become occluded by thrombosis and rupture only infrequently. Mycotic aneurysms occur in the setting of infective endocarditis, and they represent acquired pseudoaneurysms resulting from partial destruction of the media of arteries. The arterial injury is due to septic emboli into the arterial wall. These aneurysms are frequently multiple, and they can occur at locations peripheral to the circle of Willis.

Clinical picture Prior to rupture, saccular aneurysms are usually asymptomatic. Occasionally, large aneurysms immediately distal to the cavernous sinus may compress the optic nerves or chiasm, third nerve, hypothalamus, or pituitary gland. In the cavernous sinus they may press on the oculomotor, ophthalmic, or fifth or sixth cranial nerves (Chap. 367). In the posterior fossa, one or more of the cranial nerves may be compressed adjacent to the brainstem. Rarely they cause headache, but by then other signs will usually have appeared.

In most patients there are no warning symptoms; in some, however, minor leakage from the aneurysm sometimes precedes devastating rupture by a few days or weeks. Headache is the chief sign of such an event, but there may be in some instances a transitory unilateral weakness, numbness and tingling, or speech disturbance. Aneurysmal rupture usually occurs while the patient is active rather than during sleep, and in many instances sexual intercourse or other exertion precipitates the ictus.

When rupture occurs, blood under high pressure is discharged into the subarachnoid space (the circle of Willis lies in the subarachnoid space), and the resulting clinical events fall into one of three patterns: (1) in almost 50 percent of cases, the patient may be stricken with an excruciating generalized headache and fall unconscious almost immediately; (2) in the remainder headache may develop as in number 1, but the patient remains relatively lucid; (3) consciousness may be lost quickly without any preceding complaint. If the hemorrhage is massive, a fatal issue may ensue immediately. Decerebrate rigidity may occur at the onset of hemorrhage in association with unconsciousness. Persistent deep coma is accompanied by irregular respiration, attacks of extensor rigidity, and finally respiratory arrest and circulatory collapse. In these rapidly fatal cases, the blood has usually dissected intracerebrally and entered the ventricular system. Death occasionally occurs within 5 min, and ruptured aneurysm must be considered in the differential diagnosis of sudden death.

In mild cases, consciousness, if lost, may be regained within a few minutes as the blood diffuses through the subarachnoid space and the intracranial pressure falls, but a residuum of confusion and amnesia accompanied by severe headache and stiff neck persists for at least several days. It is not uncommon for drowsiness and confusion to last 10 days or longer. If the hemorrhage is confined to the subarachnoid space, there are few or no lateralizing neurologic signs.

Gross lateralizing signs in the form of hemiplegia, hemiparesis, or aphasia are absent in the majority of cases, but can occur and, in the acute stages, are due to an intracerebral clot, or ischemia in the territory of the aneurysm-bearing artery. The aneurysm may rupture partly into the subarachnoid space and partly into brain tissue (subarachnoid-cerebral hemorrhage) and even reach the ventricular system (subarachnoid-ventricular hemorrhage), rendering the patient stuporous or comatose. The initial neurologic deficit may clear in a matter of days, indicating that hemorrhage into tissues was not responsible for the focal signs. The pathogenesis of such manifestations is not fully understood, but a transitory fall in pressure in the circulation distal to the aneurysm is postulated. Transient deficits, still more evanescent, are not uncommon; paresis or aphasia, for example, may be present for only a few minutes or so after the onset of bleeding, constituting a reliable telltale of the site of the ruptured aneurysm. A delayed hemiplegia or other deficit may occur 4 to 9 days after rupture. This is attributable to focal narrowing of a large artery at the base, usually interpreted as vasospasm due to the presence of extravasated blood. Areas of ischemic necrosis of tissue in the territory of the vessel bearing the aneurysm, but sometimes in the territory of other arteries, are frequently found postmortem. These are probably due to vascular spasm because thrombosis is seldom found. A reliable indicator of a high chance of symptomatic delayed vasospasm is the presence of blood clots in the basal cisterns and in the subarachnoid space over the convexity on CT scan at onset. Distribution of the subarachnoid blood in the form of thin sheets rather than thick clots is associated with a very low incidence of delayed vasospasm. A subacute hydrocephalus due to blockage of the CSF pathways by blood may appear after 2 to 4 weeks. Ventriculoatrial shunting provides relief.

Although in most patients the neurologic manifestations do not point to the exact site of the aneurysm, in many instances there are clues to the localization. For example, (1) third nerve palsy (ptosis, diplopia, mydriasis, and oculomotor paralysis) usually indicates an aneurysm at the junction of the posterior communicating artery and the internal carotid stem. The third nerve passes immediately lateral to this point. (2) Transient paresis of one or both of the lower limbs at the onset of hemorrhage is suggestive of an anterior communicating aneurysm which has interfered with the circulation in the anterior cerebral arteries, causing ischemia of the motor areas for the lower extremities. (3) Hemiparesis or aphasia often points to an aneurysm at the bifurcation of the middle cerebral artery which has critically reduced the circulation in the middle cerebral system. (4) Unilateral blindness or amblyopia indicates an aneurysm which lies anteromedially in the circle of Willis (at the origin of the ophthalmic artery, at the bifurcation of the internal carotid artery, or in the anterior communicating region). (5) A stage of retained consciousness with akinetic mutism or abulia favors an aneurysm of the anterior communicating artery which has caused ischemia of or hemorrhage into one or both of the frontal lobes, hypothalamus, or corpus callosum. (6) The side on which the aneurysm lies may be indicated by a unilateral preponderance of headache or preretinal hemorrhages, by the occurrence of monocular pain, or by the lateralization of an intracranial sound heard at the time of rupture of the aneurysm. Sixth nerve palsy, unilateral or bilateral, results from the presence of subarachnoid blood and raised intracranial pressure and is seldom of localizing value. Other neurologic signs which have relatively little localizing value include sucking and grasp reflexes, bilateral Babinski signs, choreoathetosis, and extensor rigidity.

In summary, the clinical sequence of sudden violent headache, collapse, brief unconsciousness and confusion, combined with an absence of prodromal symptoms and a paucity of lateralizing signs, is diagnostic of a ruptured saccular aneurysm.

Other clinical data may be of assistance in reaching a correct diagnosis. Nuchal rigidity is usually present. Examination of the fundi not infrequently reveals smooth-surfaced, sharply outlined collections of blood which cover the retinal vessels—the so-called preretinal or subhyaloid hemorrhages. These are usually a sign of ruptured aneurysm but can occur in hypertensive hemorrhage and cranial trauma. Bilateral Babinski signs are found in the early days following rupture. The patient may appear to be normally alert, while impairment of memory and confabulation are found on more careful testing. A mild fever is commonly observed in the first week. The escaping blood occasionally enters the subdural space and produces a subdural hematoma, evacuation of which may be lifesaving. Aneurysmal rupture may complicate pregnancy, but pregnancy is not associated with an increased incidence of aneurysmal rupture. Spontaneous intracranial bleeding with normal blood pressure should always suggest ruptured aneurysm, ruptured arteriovenous malformation, or hemorrhage into a cerebral tumor.

Laboratory findings Carotid and vertebral angiography is the only certain means of demonstrating an aneurysm and does so effectively in some 85 percent of patients in whom aneurysm appears to be the correct diagnosis on clinical grounds, i.e., in cases of so-called spontaneous subarachnoid hemorrhage. However, in modern times, CT scanning is usually sufficient to arrive at a diagnosis of aneurysm, and immediate angiography can be deferred. By delaying angiography for several days, time will permit any associated arterial narrowing (vasospasm) to develop, and these changes can then be demonstrated. Angiography must include all the intracranial circulation, since multiple aneurysms are present in as many as 20 percent of cases.

A CT scan will detect a localized blood clot within the brain or ventricular system or in the subarachnoid spaces adjacent to the ruptured aneurysm. The use of iodinated intravenous contrast will usually disclose the location of the aneurysm. In addition, any degree of coexistent hydrocephalus will be demonstrated.

X-rays of the skull are usually negative, though in a few patients one or both of the anterior clinoid processes show erosion by the pressure of an adjacent aneurysm, or calcification has occurred in the region of a previous hemorrhage. A calcified pineal gland may be displaced by an intracerebral or subdural clot.

The cerebrospinal fluid is usually extremely bloody, with red blood cell counts reaching to 1 million per cubic millimeter or higher. When the hemorrhage is very slight, there may be only a few thousand cells. It is unlikely that an aneurysm can rupture entirely into brain tissue without some leakage of blood into the subarachnoid fluid, and therefore the diagnosis of ruptured saccular aneurysm must never be made unless blood is present in the spinal fluid. Only unruptured saccular aneurysms which either compress the optic nerves, chiasm, cranial nerves, or brainstem or lie within the cavernous sinus produce symptoms without hemorrhage. Usually deep xanthochromia is found after centrifugation. The cerebrospinal fluid is under greatly increased pressure, as high as 1000 mmH_2O. The subarachnoid bleeding can be distinguished from a bloody tap (see "Laboratory Findings," above, regarding traumatic tap). The white blood cells in the spinal fluid are usually present in the same proportion to red blood cells as in the circulating blood, but in some patients within 48 h a brisk leukocytosis appears, reaching 2000 to 3000 cells per cubic millimeter. After a few days white blood cells contain phagocytized red blood cells and hemosiderin (hemocytoblasts). The glucose level may become subnormal after 2 to 3 days.

A leukocytosis of 15,000 to 18,000 cells per cubic millimeter is common. Any urinary abnormality is usually due to concomitant renal disease. Rarely diabetes insipidus occurs. Transient glycosuria and albuminuria may occur.

Acute subarachnoid hemorrhage may be associated with electrocardiographic abnormalities suggestive of myocardial ischemia. Rarely, life-threatening ventricular arrhythmias occur. The electroencephalogram is of little help in localizing the lesion unless a gross neurologic deficit is present, in which case the lateralization is probably already evident clinically. The abnormality usually consists of slow waves.

Course and prognosis The outstanding characteristic of this condition is the tendency for the hemorrhage to recur. This threat colors all prognostications, and unfortunately there appears to be no way of determining reliably which cases will rebleed. The cause of the intermittency of bleeding is not understood, but may be related to naturally occurring mechanisms of clot lysis.

Patients with the typical clinical picture of spontaneous subarachnoid hemorrhage but in whom the angiogram shows no aneurysm or arteriovenous malformation have a better prognosis than those in whom the lesion is demonstrated.

Treatment General medical management in the acute stage is similar to that described under "Atherosclerotic Thrombosis" above. The earlier the case comes under medical purview and the more severe the impairment of consciousness, the less certain are any known therapeutic measures to be beneficial. Those surviving in good condition for several days have the best outlook, and with the passage of time the risk of recurrent bleeding diminishes. Absolute bed rest is mandatory. Coughing and all forms of exertion are avoided. Straining during bowel movement is forbidden, lest the Valsalva maneuver raise intracranial pressure and prompt a rerupture. Laxatives or general enemas are administered. The patient is fed. Dilantin or phenobarbital may be prescribed to prevent seizures. Sedatives (barbiturates) and analgesics are important in aiding relaxation. Prior recommendations to decrease the arterial blood pressure in order to arrest the hemorrhage and prevent recurrence are now no longer valid since this may aggravate the effects of vasospasm. Hypotensive agents are used to bring blood pressures to normal, but methyldopa (Aldomet) should be avoided as it produces drowsiness, which is easily misdiagnosed as due to hydrocephalus or vasospasm. Promazine intramuscularly is used to control nausea and vomiting. Aspirin should not be given since it may impair clotting and encourage rebleeding.

At present a systemic antifibrinolysin, ε-aminocaproic acid (Amicar), in a dosage of 24 g intravenously per day for 3 weeks is used to impede lysis of the clot at the site of aneurysmal rupture. This measure is effective in reducing the incidence of recurrent subarachnoid hemorrhage. Its use beyond 3 weeks is often associated with thrombophlebitis and pulmonary embolism. Measures to avoid this complication (elastic stockings, frequent assessment of venous flow in the lower limbs by Doppler technique) need to be instituted concomitantly. Because its use may aggravate vasospasm, ε-aminocaproic acid is discontinued if any delayed focal symptoms develop.

The place of repeated drainage of the cerebrospinal fluid by lumbar puncture is still uncertain, although several workers have concluded that it does not affect the outcome of the illness. At present, one lumbar puncture is usually carried out for diagnostic purposes, and thereafter it is performed only for the relief of intractable headache, to detect recurrence of bleeding, or to measure the intracranial pressure prior to surgery.

In maintaining fluid balance, intravenous fluids should be used in adequate doses, since deliberate dehydration may add to the severity of symptoms due to vasospasm. The proper electrolyte combination (a mixture of equal parts of 5% glucose in water and normal saline solution or balanced electrolytes) should be used in order to minimize the danger of aggravating brain swelling. Any abnormality of concentration of electrolytes in the blood must be corrected. If diabetes insipidus has occurred, it should be treated with antidiuretic hormone injection (Pitressin). Disorders of blood coagulation should be corrected. Intravenous hypertonic urea or mannitol may be effective in temporarily reducing the intracranial pressure, but their anticoagulant properties may encourage rebleeding.

Since the attainment of a significant reduction in recurrent hemorrhage by ε-aminocaproic acid, vasospasm has become the most pressing problem. It usually develops between 4 and 10 days after the first rupture and often causes paralytic symptoms. No specific therapy has yet been developed for its prevention. The use of reserpine and kanamycin has now been shown valueless.

After resting in bed for 6 weeks, patients not treated surgically are gradually allowed to resume activity and may return to work in 4 months. It seems logical to advise that heavy labor not be resumed.

Surgical therapy Apart from occasionally evacuating an associated intracerebral clot, surgical treatment is for the most part directed to the prevention of recurrence of the hemorrhage. In recent years, almost all surgical therapy for aneurysms has been *intracranial* (clipping; ligating the neck of the aneurysm under the operating microscope). Other procedures include wrapping the aneurysmal sac by plastic coating; trapping the aneurysm with prior extracranial-intracranial bypass grafting to prevent ischemia in the affected territory; ligation of the main feeding vessel proximal to the aneurysm. Occasionally extracranial and intracranial procedures are combined. Because of the high operative mortality if surgery is undertaken early, the operation has usually been delayed 1 to 2 weeks until the patient's condition has stabilized beyond the period of incidence of vasospasm. However, with a plan to use vigorous hypertensive therapy to counteract vasospasm after the aneurysm is safely ligated, surgery within days has been undertaken in a few centers with mixed success. Before treatment is undertaken, the site, size, and form of the aneurysm must be determined by angiography. At the same time the pattern of the anterior half of the circle of Willis is noted, as it may influence the choice of operative procedure. It has been demonstrated that surgical treatment improves upon the natural outlook for almost all aneurysms. The operative mortality has been reduced to less than 5 percent in experienced hands.

After aneurysmal rupture a chronic obstructive or communicating hydrocephalus may develop, causing persistent stupor. The 20 percent of cases who do not improve spontaneously are relieved by ventriculoatrial shunting.

OTHER CAUSES OF INTRACRANIAL HEMORRHAGE An arteriovenous malformation (AVM) consists of a tangle of abnormal vessels forming an anomalous communication between the arterial and venous systems, really an arteriovenous fistula. It is a developmental abnormality, not a neoplasm, but the constituent vessels enlarge with growth and the passage of time. They vary in size from a small blemish a few millimeters in diameter lying in the cortex or white matter to a huge mass of tortuous channels composing an arteriovenous shunt of sufficient magnitude to raise the cardiac output. Hypertrophic dilated arterial "feeders" approach the main lesion, disappear below the cortex, and break up into a network of thin-walled blood vessels which connect directly with draining veins. The latter often form huge, dilated pulsating channels, carrying away arterial blood. The blood vessels forming the tangle interposed between arteries and veins are usually abnormally thin and do not have the normal structure of arteries or veins. Arteriovenous malformations occur in all parts of the brain, brainstem, and spinal cord, but the larger ones are more frequently found in the posterior half of the hemispheres, commonly forming a wedge-shaped lesion whose base is on the cortex and whose apex reaches the ventricular lining.

Arteriovenous malformations predominate in males over females about 2:1. They may occur in more than one member of a family in the same or successive generations. Although the lesion is present from birth, the onset of complaints is most common in the twenties and thirties, but occasionally it is delayed as late as the fifties. The chief clinical features are cerebral or cerebral-subarachnoid hemorrhage or epileptic seizures occurring in a child or young adult. In 50 percent the first manifestation is a hemorrhage, in 30 percent, a seizure, and in 20 percent, headache, dementia, progressive hemiparesis, hemiatrophy (if onset is early in life), hemisensory syndrome, hemiathetosis, etc. The seizure pattern depends on the site of the lesion; when focal motor in type the seizure may be followed by a temporary postictal paralysis. When hemorrhage occurs, blood may enter the subarachnoid space almost exclusively, producing a picture identical with that of ruptured saccular aneurysm, but since the AVM lies within the cerebral tissue, the bleeding is more likely to be at least partly intracerebral, causing hemiparesis, hemiplegia, or death. In other cases, bleeding may be primarily into the ventricular cavity through the apex of the lesion, producing a temporary severe hydrocephalus with surprisingly modest focal deficits. Before rupture, chronic nondescript headache is a frequent complaint, and sometimes a slowly evolving (over several minutes) and regressing hemiparesis or hemianesthesia are encountered. This may at times simulate migraine. Huge AVMs may produce a slowly progressive neurologic deficit because of local pressure and depletion of blood from adjacent brain tissue, but the array of syndromes produced is only incompletely described. Proptosis has been encountered. When the vein of Galen is involved, hydrocephalus may result. Not infrequently one or both carotid arteries pulsate unusually forcefully in the neck. A loud systolic bruit heard over the carotid in the neck, the mastoid process, or the eyeballs in young adults, although rare, is almost pathognomonic of AVM; faint ones in infancy and early childhood are of little significance. The older patient should be exercised in order to bring out a bruit if none is present at rest. A bruit may also be heard over a spinal angioma of large size. The eye grounds may reveal a retinal vascular abnormality. Preretinal hemorrhages may be found after hemorrhage has occurred. X-ray of the skull occasionally shows crescentic linear calcification in the vicinity of larger AVMs. Most arteriovenous malformations are visible on a CT scan, especially after contrast infusion, as large, tortuous high densities, but are seen more completely in an arteriogram, which will demonstrate those larger than 5 mm in diameter. Small AVMs may be obscured by the resulting hemorrhage, and even at autopsy a careful microscopic search may be necessary to find them.

Most AVMs bleed sooner or later. The bleeding of smaller AVMs is thought to produce a more significant functional deficit than the larger lesions. The first hemorrhage may be fatal, but in more than 90 percent of cases bleeding stops, and the patient survives. Recurrence of hemorrhage with a fatal outcome is a constant danger, but the risk is less than with saccular aneurysm. In patients who have had a hemorrhage the incidence of recurrence is approximately 3 percent per year. The prognosis is better in those patients who have not had a manifest brain hemorrhage than in those who have.

In recent years it has been the practice of neurosurgeons to perform a block dissection of AVMs of suitable size and location. In preparation for surgery, artificial embolization and ligation of feeding arteries has become commonplace. Recently attempts have been made at obliteration by means of intravascular resins, and proton-beam focused irradiation.

Although *intracranial bleeding due to head trauma* does not rightfully fall within the scope of the stroke problem, it must be mentioned here because of the great frequency with which it enters into the differential diagnosis, especially in cases in which the history is inadequate or the patient falls and is injured at the onset of the stroke. *Acute extradural* and *acute subdural hemorrhage* must always be considered in the patient who under unknown circumstances has rather abruptly developed a neurologic deficit such as hemiparesis or confusion, whether the spinal fluid is bloody or not. In *chronic subdural hemorrhage,* which can occur without known trauma, the indefinite picture of drowsiness, confusion, and mild hemiparesis may be erroneously attributed to a stroke, especially in elderly persons. Failure to make the correct diagnosis deprives the patient of lifesaving surgical intervention. There should be no hesitation in subjecting the patient to CT scanning or arteriography whenever subdural hemorrhage cannot be excluded on clinical grounds. *Cerebral contusion and laceration* may be a cause of subarachnoid hemorrhage, and if the patient has fallen, causing a blow to the head at the time of the onset of the stroke, it may be difficult or impossible to decide if the red blood cells in the cerebrospinal fluid are due to a cerebrovascular stroke or to cerebral contusion. Trauma may also cause *acute* or *delayed intracerebral hemorrhage, acute intracerebellar hemorrhage, acute infratentorial subdural hemorrhage, acute brain swelling,* and on rare occasions, extensive *focal infarction* due probably to vasospasm (see Chap. 357).

Several *hemorrhagic hematologic disorders* may be complicated by hemorrhage into the brain. The most frequent of these are leukemia, aplastic anemia, and thrombocytopenic purpura. As a rule this complication signals a fatal issue. Any part of the brain may be involved, and often the lesions are multiple. Usually there is already evidence of abnormal bleeding elsewhere (skin, mucous membranes, kidney) by the time cerebral hemorrhage occurs. Intracranial bleeding is also a complication of anticoagulant therapy; the hemorrhages that develop usually occur in the sites of predilection in hypertensive hemorrhage, but a slight predilection for bleeding into the cerebellum has been observed. They tend to have a leisurely but steady evolution, and attempts to control them by reversal of the anticoagulant effects usually fail. When precipitated by warfarin therapy, treatment by fresh-frozen plasma and vitamin K is recommended; when associated with aspirin therapy or other agents that affect platelet function, fresh platelet infusions, often in massive amounts, are required to control the hemorrhage.

Occasionally *hemorrhages* are of *undetermined origin* both clinically and pathologically. The blood pressure is normal, and neither an aneurysm nor AVM can be demonstrated. In some postmortem cases a careful microscopic search discloses a small angioma in the cerebral tissue at one side of the hemorrhage, and on this basis it is suspected that in other cases, too, an overlooked angioma may have been the cause of the extravasation of blood. Primary intraventricular hemorrhage, a rare event, is at times due to angioma or neoplasm of the choroid plexus, which may not have been seen by the prosector. More often, such intraventricular hemorrhages are the result of a paraventricular bleeding that immediately entered the ventricle without producing a large parenchymal clot. This is often the case for those rare forms of hypertensive hemorrhage arising from the head of the caudate nucleus. Chronic *steroid therapy* may precipitate subarachnoid hemorrhages.

Hemorrhage into primary and secondary brain tumors is not rare, and when it is the first manifestation of the neoplasm, the correct diagnosis may be extremely obscure. Choriocarcinoma, malignant melanoma, renal cell carcinoma, bronchogenic carcinoma, pituitary adenoma, glioblastoma multiforme, and medulloblastoma may present in this way. Careful inquiry may disclose that signs of intracranial tumor growth have preceded the onset of hemorrhage. Examination clinically and by x-ray may reveal evidence of intracranial tumor or of secondary tumor deposits in other organs. A chest film will frequently show metastatic or primary neoplasm and should be performed in all cases of obscure intracerebral hemorrhage. CT scan is of greatest value in this setting, as it may disclose multiple intracranial tumors in addition to the one that bled.

Septic embolism may lead to massive fatal intracranial bleeding via a *mycotic aneurysm.* Any part of the circulatory tree may be involved, but usually the aneurysm (about 0.5 mm in diameter) lies at a branching or forking of a small meningeal branch or a branch of the middle cerebral artery.

On infrequent occasions bleeding within an area of *hemorrhagic infarction* as a result of cerebral embolism or venous thrombosis reaches major proportions, forming an intracerebral hematoma, and the cerebrospinal fluid becomes bloody.

Hypertensive encephalopathy and *toxemia of pregnancy* may result in intracerebral hemorrhages, which can vary in size from petechial to massive.

Idiopathic brain purpura, or hemorrhagic encephalitis, consists of multiple petechial hemorrhages scattered throughout the white matter of the brain. The picture is that of a diffuse cerebral disease. There is never blood in the spinal fluid, and the condition should never be confused with a typical stroke. Exogenous agents (e.g., arsenic) or gram-negative bacteria causing septicemia and shock are the usual cause.

Brainstem hemorrhages secondary to temporal lobe herniation are extremely common but never present as a cerebrovascular stroke.

Inflammatory disease of arteries and veins, especially polyarteritis nodosa and lupus erythematosus, can cause hemorrhage into the nervous system. In polyarteritis, rupture of a vessel may occur on the basis of a concomitant hypertension superimposed on local vascular disease. In lupus erythematosus—if it can be included in the arteritides—hemorrhage is attributable to hypertension or disease of the vascular wall of undetermined nature. Bleeding nearly always occurs into the parenchyma rather than the subarachnoid space.

The rarer types of hemorrhage listed in the classification in Table 356-2 are self-explanatory.

Hemorrhages of *intraspinal* origin may be the result of angiomas, hematomyelia, bleeding into tumors, extradural and subdural extravasation (trauma, anticoagulants, spontaneous), and circulatory changes around benign tumors. Extradural spinal hemorrhage rapidly causes an irreversible paraplegia, and diagnosis must be prompt if function is to be salvaged by surgical drainage.

HYPERTENSIVE ENCEPHALOPATHY

This term refers to an acute syndrome in which severe hypertension is associated with headache, nausea, vomiting, convulsions, confusion, stupor, and coma. Focal or lateralizing neurologic signs, either transitory or lasting, may occur but are infrequent and always suggest some other form of vascular disease (hemorrhage, embolism, or atherosclerotic thrombosis). By the time neurologic manifestations appear, the hypertension has usually reached the malignant stage, with retinal hemorrhages, exudates, papilledema (*hypertensive retinopathy* grade IV, see Chap. 267), and evidence of renal and cardiac disease. In many, but not all cases, the cerebrospinal fluid pressure and the protein values are both elevated, the latter sometimes to over 100 mg/dl. The hypertension may be essential or due to chronic renal disease, acute glomerulonephritis, acute toxemia of pregnancy, pheochromocytoma, Cushing's syndrome, or corticosteroid treatment. Lowering of the blood pressure with hypotensive drugs may reverse the picture in a day or two. If the hypertension cannot be controlled, the outcome is fatal. Neuropathologic examination may reveal a rather normal looking brain, but usually small cerebral infarcts and/or hemorrhages of various sizes from massive to petechial will be found. A cerebellar pressure cone reflects increased volume of tissue secondary to swelling, and in some instances lumbar puncture may have precipitated a fatality. Microscopically there are, in addition to small hemorrhages, clusters of microglial cells, minute cerebral infarcts, and necrosis and thrombosis of arterioles and capillaries.

The term *hypertensive encephalopathy* should be reserved for the above syndrome and not used to refer to chronic recurrent headaches, dizziness, epileptic seizures, recurrent transient ischemic attacks, or small strokes which often occur in association with high blood pressure. For further discussion, see Chap. 267.

INFLAMMATORY DISEASES OF BRAIN ARTERIES

Inflammatory diseases of the vessels of the brain have been mentioned on several occasions in the preceding paragraphs, and here they are discussed briefly.

Meningovascular syphilis, formerly one of the most frequent causes of occlusive vascular disease in patients of all ages, has become a rarity since the introduction of penicillin therapy (see Chap. 177).

Tuberculous meningitis, fungal meningitis, and the subacute forms of bacterial meningitis (influenzal bacillus, staphylococcus, pneumococcus) may also be accompanied by vascular disorders of the occlusive type, in either the cerebral arteries or veins. Occasionally in tuberculous meningitis a stroke may be the first clinical sign of meningitis; more often it develops after the meningeal symptoms are established. It occurs as a result of a form of obliterative endarteritis which produces stenosis and eventual occlusion of the lumen, generally in large proximal intracranial trunks (supraclinoid carotid, middle cerebral stem).

Typhus, schistosomiasis mansoni, mucormycosis, malaria, and *trichinosis* are rare types of infective inflammatory diseases of the arteries and, unlike the above, are not secondary to meningeal inflammation. In typhus and other rickettsial diseases, capillary and arteriolar changes and perivascular inflammatory cells are found in the brain, and presumably they underlie the convulsions, acute psychoses, and coma which reflect the central nervous system involvement. They do not cause strokes, however. The internal carotid artery may be occluded in diabetic patients during orbital and cavernous sinus infections with mucormycosis. In trichinosis the sudden onset of convulsions, aphasia, hemiplegia, and coma may either accompany or, as happens more often, follow the systemic and muscular symptoms. The cause of the cerebral symptoms has not been established. Parasites have been found in the brain; in one of our cases the cerebral lesions were produced by bland emboli arising in the heart and related to a severe myocarditis. Malaria of the malignant or falciparum variety is frequently attended by a clinical state known as *cerebral malaria,* in which convulsions, coma, and sometimes focal symptoms appear to be due to blockage of capillaries and precapillaries by masses of parasitized red blood cells.

The *arteritides of obscure origin* include polyarteritis nodosa, disseminated lupus erythematosus, granulomatous arteritis, giant-cell arteritis, temporal (cranial) arteritis, and rheumatic arteritis (see Chap. 353).

Lupus erythematosus causes cerebral symptoms in over 50 percent of cases. Seizures and psychoses are common. Small cerebral infarcts lead to widespread focal deficits. Accompanying hypertension may precipitate hemorrhage or hypertensive encephalopathy, or endocarditis may cause cerebral embolism.

Temporal arteritis (cranial arteritis) is an uncommon affliction of elderly persons in which the external carotid system, particularly the temporal branches, is the seat of a subacute granulomatous inflammation with an exudate of lymphocytes, monocytes, neutrophilic leukocytes, and giant cells. Usually the most severely affected parts of the artery become thrombosed. Headache or head pain is the chief complaint. Systemic manifestations include anorexia, loss of weight, malaise, and polymyalgia rheumatica. The latter is manifested by pain and stiffness of proximal joints, especially the arms, that occurs on awakening. The inflammatory nature of the illness is indicated by some or several of the following: fever, slight leukocytosis, increased sedimentation rate, and anemia. Occlusion of branches of the ophthalmic artery results in blindness in one or both eyes in over 40 percent of patients, and occasionally an ophthalmoplegia due to involvement of ocular nerves occurs. An arteritis of the aorta and its major branches, including carotid, subclavian, coronary, and femoral arteries, is found at postmortem examination. Significant inflammatory involvement of intracranial arteries is rare, but strokes occur occasionally, on the basis of occlusion of the internal carotid, middle cerebral, or vertebral arteries. The diagnosis depends on the finding of a tender thrombosed or thickened cranial artery and the demonstration of the lesion in a biopsy. Prednisone and ACTH bring striking subjective relief and prevent blindness. See Chap. 357 for further discussion.

Thromboangiitis obliterans of cerebral vessels (Winiwarter-Buerger disease) has not been included in the foregoing list. Despite the large volume of literature on the subject, the pathology remains dubious.

DIFFERENTIATION OF CEREBROVASCULAR DISEASE FROM OTHER NEUROLOGIC ILLNESSES

It has already been stated that the diagnosis of a vascular lesion rests solely on recognition of the stroke syndrome and that without evidence of this the diagnosis must always be in doubt. Three useful criteria in the identification of the stroke have already been emphasized: (1) the tempo of the clinical syndrome, (2) evidence of focal brain disease, and (3) the clinical setting. The temporal profile can usually be defined by means of a clear history of premonitory phenomena, the mode of the onset, and the evolution of the neurologic disturbance taken in relation to the medical status at the time of examination. If these data are lacking, the course may still be determined by extending the period of observation for a few more days or weeks. An inadequate history is probably the most frequent cause of diagnostic errors.

Few other neurologic illnesses mimic cerebrovascular disease. When the details of the history are missing, however, subdural hematoma, brain tumor, brain abscess, and senile dementia may lead to diagnostic difficulties. The reader should refer to Chaps. 354, 358, 359, and 364 for further discussion of differential diagnosis.

A GUIDE TO THE CLINICAL MANAGEMENT OF CEREBROVASCULAR DISEASES

The student, family physician, and internist are not expected to become expert in the diagnosis and treatment of cerebrovascular diseases after having read the jumble of ideas in the preceding pages. But there are certain clinical situations which recur repeatedly and which demand an organized set of responses on the part of the physician if the patient is to receive the benefits of the most advanced medical thought. These reactions devolve upon:

1 A patient who has had a probable stroke and is now comatose
2 A patient who has had an obvious focal neurologic deficit, probably a stroke, and who is responsive
3 A patient who has had an indefinite neurologic disorder which proves to be an inobvious stroke
4 A patient who gives a history of having had a stroke in the past which may or may not relate to the present problem
5 A patient who is believed to have had a mild stroke but actually has some type of nonvascular disease

The authors would suggest the following approach to each of these problems.

THE COMATOSE STROKE PATIENT Here the analysis of the state of coma should proceed in accordance with the scheme outlined in Chap. 20, where it was pointed out that in comas due to cerebrovascular disorders there is nearly always evidence of unilateral hemispheral or segmental brainstem deficits of function, and in some instances changes in CSF. The CT scan, available in most medical centers, has largely replaced lumbar puncture and CSF examination, which carry some degree of risk if there is massive intracranial bleeding.

The usual causes of a comatose stroke are hypertensive hemorrhage, a ruptured saccular aneurysm, or a massive cerebral or brainstem infarct. The diagnostic steps described in preceding sections permit differentiation of these diseases. The clinician's first problem is to make sure the clinical condition is due to a stroke and not to a treatable form of traumatic epidural or subdural hematoma (see Chap. 357), a metabolic disorder, or drug intoxication (Chaps. 243 and 362).

The most that can be done for the cerebrovascular coma patient is to offer supportive measures along the lines indicated in Chap. 20. Measures to control raised intracranial pressure (dexamethasone and glycerol or mannitol) may be beneficial. Surgical intervention is rarely undertaken and is usually unsuccessful; if operation is decided upon (aspiration of the clot and reduction of intracranial pressure), it must be done at once. In ruptured saccular aneurysms, as long as the patient is comatose or stuporous (grade IV in presently used rating scheme), surgery must be deferred and it is wise to postpone arteriography. Even cerebellar hemorrhage, which sometimes yields to surgical intervention, seldom does so once the patient has become comatose. There is no need to undertake arteriography in cases of massive infarction, for it will not lead to any form of definitive therapy. If the patient is in a hospital with limited facilities, there is little point in urgent transfer to a larger medical center while coma persists. Once consciousness is regained, however, and neurologic condition stabilizes, it is important to identify the cases of ruptured aneurysm and arteriovenous malformations and to institute appropriate therapy.

THE NONCOMATOSE STROKE PATIENT The question of diagnosis is seldom in doubt, though a focal convulsion (a rare initial event in stroke) followed by a postictal paralysis must be considered. After the initial events it is the pace of the neurologic deficit and the course toward improvement or worsening that are the best guides in the recognition of the different types of strokes. One must keep foremost in mind the potentially treatable diseases such as carotid stenosis, saccular aneurysm, recurrent transient ischemic attack, and the different types of embolism. ECG, cardiac monitoring, blood cultures, and platelet counts should accompany CT scanning; the latter will exclude a small hemorrhage. The examination of the CSF is also of importance to demonstrate a pleocytosis or signs of intracranial bleeding. Arteriography is one of the most helpful diagnostic aids, but the timing of it should reflect the proximity of the most recent transient ischemic attack or increment of deficit. The more recent the change the more urgently the arteriogram is indicated. An attack the day of admission warrants an arteriogram on the same day, after the CT scan. Carotid occlusion at the sinus level, of a few hours' standing, is amenable to emergency thromboendarterectomy. The diagnosis of embolism should lead to the initiation of anticoagulant therapy at once, to prevent subsequent emboli. However, a massive persistent cerebral deficit discourages all further diagnostic studies and efforts directed toward therapy and prevention.

THE INOBVIOUS STROKE Here the problem is one of a patient who has developed a mild neurologic deficit, the diagnosis of which is obscure. Inexplicable headache, dizziness, mental confusion, or a variety of other minor symptoms have clearly declared their presence. What may be overlooked is the fact that the classic sign of stroke (i.e., hemiplegia) may never appear, yet certain minor signs, if of sudden or acute onset, carry the same diagnostic, prognostic, and therapeutic implications as paralysis.

Five such inobvious stroke syndromes occur regularly. The first of these is a *leaking aneurysm,* presenting as a sudden, generalized headache (unlike any experienced in the past), often having developed during exertion, persisting for hours or days. Examination may disclose no abnormalities, but the neck may be slightly stiff. Casual urinary—less often fecal—incontinence, vague recollection for recent events, and unaccountable delays in answering simple questions may also be present and reflect emerging hydrocephalus in the days after the onset of headache. Ruptured aneurysm occasionally also presents as unexplained severe interscapular back pain. Subdural hematoma, anticoagulant-induced frontal pole hemorrhage, brain tumor, and other entities must be included in the differential diagnosis.

A second type of inobvious stroke is *cerebellar hemorrhage.* Sudden onset of dizziness, repeated uncontrollable vomiting, inability to stand and walk, ipsilateral gaze palsy, ipsilateral facial paresis, and, less often, ipsilateral cerebellar ataxia are often incompletely detected and need to be assembled into the diagnostic syndrome by the examining physician. Considerate of the patient's misery, the physician often defers testing the patient's ability to stand and walk; and finding no obvious hemiparesis, often does not test ocular movements fully; the mild facial asymmetry easily escapes detection in the setting of vomiting and dizziness. Such patients are often assumed to have labyrinthitis, Ménière's disease, alcoholic or drug intoxication, and even viral gastroenteritis, and little thought is given to impending disaster because the patient seems so alert—until brainstem compression suddenly intervenes, with fatal results. CT scan is an essential diagnostic step in the evaluation of all such cases. Hematoma evacuation has proved the only reliable therapeutic step in the acute phase. Cerebellar infarction with progressive edema leading to brainstem compression can produce a similar picture.

The third type of inobvious stroke involves the *posterior cerebral artery territory.* Homonymous hemianopia is often not implicitly appreciated by the patient, whose complaints, if any, center on the need for new eyeglasses, on poor vision in the eye ipsilateral to the visual field loss, or on vague descriptions of blurring of vision. Failure to appreciate the visual environment on that side has often led to embarrassing social experiences or accidents. Accompanying deficits in higher cerebral function, when present, usually require direct testing, including reading, naming of colors or manipulable objects, description of faces, and routes on maps.

The fourth type of inobvious stroke is that of *infarction or subcortical hemorrhage into the nondominant parietal lobe.* If these lesions are of less than massive proportions, the patient will present with minimal or no contralateral motor deficit, but rather with behavioral abnormalities or an acute psychosis. Patients with these lesions are frequently unaware of or unconcerned about their deficits, which tend to occur in the sensory and visual spheres. Inattention for the space on the patient's left side is a prominent finding, but often it needs special testing to be detected; double simultaneous stimulation with visual, tactile, or auditory stimuli consistently results in extinction of the stimulus on the patient's left side; when drawing numbers in a clock, the patient repeatedly mishandles the numbers on the left side of the circle; bisection of lines put in front of him or her is only performed on those located to the patient's right on the field of vision. At times, the mishandling of the left side of the space is apparent in the patient's attitudes and activities, such as lying in bed, eating, shaving, walking, etc. The latter may be the only signs of abnormality detected by family members, and the physician should be alerted to the possibility of these being the manifestations of a strictly focal cerebral lesion that requires investigation, rather than casually misdiagnosing the case as "senility," "cerebral arteriosclerosis," or a psychiatric illness.

The fifth common type of inobvious stroke is an episode of mild paraphasic speech and slightly impaired auditory comprehension that characterizes most examples of *Wernicke's aphasia from embolism.* The patient is often thought to be confused. Most patients perform satisfactorily at a superficial level in making socially appropriate greetings and gestures, and they may approve readily of the examiner's efforts to shorten the interview by posing questions to be answered yes or no. Scrutiny of their remarks and behavior during history-taking will elicit the deficit. Tests involving the naming aloud or spelling of even short words that are the names of objects presented, writing the names of objects, pointing to objects whose names are spelled aloud, and describing the use of objects presented all suffice to bring out errors in word selection, sentence construction, and comprehension. Frequently, a hemianopic or quadrantic visual field defect can be demonstrated by bedside testing.

PATIENT WITH A HISTORY OF PRIOR STROKE This is the time when the identification of the patient "at risk" becomes an important matter, for it offers the best opportunity for medical intercession. Excluding a postconvulsive state, any deficit in neurologic function involving a cerebral or brainstem location that has persisted over a few hours should be taken as evidence of a destructive lesion, even though the deficit appears to have disappeared. The lesion may have been a small embolus, lacunar infarct, transient ischemic attack, or thrombotic occlusion. Electrolyte disturbance, fever, and other "metabolic" states may often cause a transient relapse, and knowledge of such a prior lesion is of immeasurable value in assessing the significance of any focal cerebral disorder that emerges during a general metabolic derangement. A history of the briefer episodic focal deficit compels consideration of transient ischemic attack. In such a setting, migraine, seizure, depression, peripheral neuropathies, and other entities arise in the differential diagnosis. Search for extracranial vascular abnormalities including a carotid bruit is a useful exercise. If the episodes are recurrent, the similarities between episodes, the arterial territory inferred from the symptoms, and their duration are all important features to be studied. Transient ischemic attacks that warn of disaster frequently last only seconds to a few minutes and are often shrugged off by the patient as insignificant. Distal brachial predominance characterizes the attacks in most cases of carotid stenosis. Although many patients experience hundreds of attacks over months before a stroke, most experience few, often only one; the last, sometimes the only, such attack tends to occur within the day(s) before the stroke. The closer in time to the last attack, the more expeditious should be the attempt to find the source (embolic, atherosclerotic, thrombocytosis, lacunar) of the prior deficit.

THE SIMULATED STROKE Since cerebrovascular diseases are by far the most frequent affections of the nervous system in middle and late adult life, there is an understandable tendency to diagnose every disease of the brain in this age period as vascular. If one reviews the hospital records of patients with a brain tumor, encephalitis, chronic subdural hematoma, episodic global amnesia, dementia, normal pressure hydrocephalus, and even depression, it is striking how often the initial diagnosis was one of stroke. This error can be avoided if one insists on having a clear history covering the onset and minute-by-minute and hour-by-hour course of the illness. If an adequate history is not available, one must then resort to a series of examinations to reveal the course of the illness. The data yielded by CT scan, CSF examination, EEG, radionuclide scan, arteriography, etc., are also helpful. If diagnosis is still in doubt, the proper tactic is to keep the patient under observation (possibly at home) until the future course of the illness clarifies the problem. Seldom in such patients is there reason for urgent surgical intervention.

REFERENCES

CAPLAN LR: "Top of the basilar" syndrome. Neurology 30:72, 1980

FISHER CM et al: Lateral medullary infarction—the pattern of vascular occlusion. J Neuropathol Exp Neurol 20:323, 1961

———: Cerebral ischemia—less familiar types. Clin Neurosurg 18:267, 1971

MOHR JP: Valvular disease, cardiac arrest, systemic hypotension, and cardiac surgery, in *Handbook of Clinical Neurology,* GW Bruyn, PJ Vinken (eds). Amsterdam, North-Holland, 1978

——— et al: The Harvard Cooperative Stroke Registry: A prospective registry. Neurology 28:754, 1978

———: Lacunes. Stroke 13:3, 1982

TOOLE JF, YUSON CP: Transient ischemic attacks with normal arteriograms: Serious or benign prognosis. Ann Neurol 1:100, 1977

WOLF PA et al: Epidemiologic assessment of chronic atrial fibrillation and risk of stroke. Neurology 28:973, 1978

357 TRAUMATIC DISEASES OF THE BRAIN

RAYMOND D. ADAMS
ALLAN H. ROPPER
JOSEPH B. MARTIN

Head injury, which is the basis of some of the most frequent and serious neurologic disorders in these times of high-velocity transport, mechanization in industry, and violent street crimes, poses many problems to the practicing physician. To deal effectively with this condition demands a knowledge of the clinical manifestations as well as a sound grasp of fundamental physiologic mechanisms. Physicians must stand prepared at all times, for they may at any moment be summoned to render aid or to assess the clinical status of a person who has suffered an injury of the head or spine. This chapter reviews the salient facts concerning these injuries and outlines an approach to these problems that has been useful to the authors.

PHYSIOLOGIC AND PATHOLOGIC CONSIDERATIONS

The clinical descriptions that are used for various forms of head injury do not always provide insight into the mechanisms of transient or permanent dysfunction that result. The word *concussion,* for example, implies a violent shaking and agitation of an organ or the transient functional impairment that occurs. Yet despite numerous experiments to demonstrate physical evidence of such injury in nerve cells or fiber pathways, we remain largely ignorant of the pathophysiologic process. Concussion is accompanied by slowing and other changes in the electroencephalogram (EEG) and may be best considered as an electrophysiologic disruption of brain function without a morphologic counterpart. On the other hand, the word *contusion* means a bruising or crushing of the brain, and use of the term should be restricted to an injury associated with physical evidence of brain damage. This may be apparent by presence of focal neurologic signs, by focal abnormality on the EEG, by an abnormal CT scan, or by blood in the cerebrospinal fluid (CSF). *Laceration* refers to disruption of brain tissue and usually, but not always, occurs with fracture and dislocation of skull fragments or results from penetrating injuries or missiles.

The mechanism of brain damage in head injury is most often the sudden application of a physical force of considerable magnitude to the head. The size of the area on the skull over which the force is exerted is of importance. High-velocity missiles destroy a small part of the skull and penetrate the cranial cavity without causing significant displacement of the head or brain; heavy, crushing injuries which result from the skull's being compressed between two converging objects may crush the brain. In these two circumstances it is interesting to note that the patient may suffer severe and often fatal injury without immediate loss of consciousness. Hemorrhage, focal destruction of brain tissue, and, if the patient survives for a time, hydrocephalus, meningitis, or abscess are the principal pathologic changes created by injuries of this type. They present little that is difficult to understand.

The common civilian injury is one in which a rapidly moving blunt object strikes the head or the head is flung against a hard surface. Injuries of this type, often termed *blunt head injuries,* are remarkable in two respects: (1) they almost always induce at least a temporary loss of consciousness, and (2) even though the skull is not penetrated and fragments of bone are not driven into its cavity, the brain may suffer gross damage, i.e., contusion, laceration, hemorrhage, swelling, herniation.

The two most frequent circumstances wherein a blunt head injury is sustained are a car accident in which the driver or passenger is flung against the windshield and one in which a pedestrian is struck by a car. In a head-on collision the knees of a passenger strike the lower dashboard and the upper body is catapulted forward and upward so that the cranium strikes the windshield. The driver is protected somewhat by the steering wheel which reduces the momentum. Passengers wearing seat belts receive considerable protection, and in particular the seat belt prevents ejection of the passenger from the car. Lateral collisions cause the head to strike the upper door frame, window, or windshield. Injuries of the cervical spine are often associated, usually occurring at the craniocerebral junction and upper cervical vertebrae.

Pedestrians struck by automobiles are often thrown onto or over the car because the center of gravity of the standing adult is at the level of the umbilicus, which is slightly above the automobile hood. They are flipped upward, and their head tends to rotate toward the car and to strike the hood or windshield. The victims may be flung to the ground, striking their head against the pavement. Motorcycle accidents provide another example of the latter type of deceleration injury and can be reduced in frequency at least 50 percent by protective head gear.

SKULL FRACTURES The skull may be fractured in any type of head injury. With the arrival of the CT scan, it is now customary to search for indications of intracranial lesions in addition to the routine evaluation by x-ray. Fractures assume importance in indicating the site and possible severity of brain damage, in providing an explanation for cranial nerve injuries, and in affording potential pathways for the ingress of bacteria and air or the egress of CSF. Furthermore, the existence of a skull fracture increases the chances of an underlying hematoma (subdural or epidural), up to twentyfold. Significant intracranial lesions accompany two-thirds of skull fractures.

The mechanics of skull fracture have been studied. Blunt injury to the skull results in a deformation of the whole intracranial cavity with a decrease in the diameter occurring in the direction of the impact line. The skull cracks if the elastic tolerance is exceeded. The fracture tends to extend from the center of the impact zone to the base of the skull. Powerful blows produce stellate fractures and fragments of bone may be displaced inward. The direction of the fractures through the base tends to parallel the petrous bones and to extend along the sphenoid bone through the sella and ethmoidal groove. Fractures of the basal skull bones may be accompanied by *hemotympanum* (blood behind the tympanic membrane), ecchymosis over the mastoid process (Battle's sign), periorbital ecchymosis, or *CSF rhinorrhea.* The diagnosis of basilar fracture is often missed on x-ray and should be suspected in the presence of these clinical signs.

Anterior pituitary insufficiency and diabetes insipidus may result from traumatic sellar fractures, hematomas, or pituitary stalk transection.

CRANIAL NERVE INJURY The position of a basal skull fracture may be indicated by signs of cranial nerve damage. Cranial nerves which are particularly liable to injury are the olfactory, optic, oculomotor, trochlear, first and second branches of the trigeminal, facial, and auditory. Anosmia and an apparent loss of taste (actually a loss of perception of aromatic flavors, elementary tastes—salt, sweet, bitter, sour—being retained) occur in approximately 10 percent of severe head injuries, especially of falls on the back of the head, and result from displacement of the brain and shearing of the olfactory nerve filaments. A fracture of the ethmoid plate may also disrupt these filaments. A fracture of the sphenoid bone may lacerate or transect the optic nerve, with partial or complete blindness. The pupil is dilated and unreactive to a direct light stimulus but still takes part in the consensual reflex. The optic disk becomes pale, i.e., atrophic, after an interval of several weeks. Partial injuries may result in a troublesome blurring of vision. Injury to the eighth cranial nerve with petrosal fractures causes loss of hearing and/or postural vertigo and nystagmus immediately after injury. The deafness due to nerve injury must be distinguished from that caused by rupture of the eardrum or the presence of blood in the middle ear, and the vertigo from labyrinthine concussion. In oculomotor nerve injury there is a divergent squint, with loss of internal and vertical movement of the eye and a fixed, dilated pupil. Diplopia only on looking down suggests trochlear nerve affection. Direct injury of the facial nerve by a basal fracture may be present immediately after the injury or may be delayed, coming on after several days. This delayed form is usually transitory, and its mechanism is not known. It may be misinterpreted as an important progression of the traumatic intracranial lesion. Injury to the ophthalamic or maxillary divisions of the trigeminal nerve may be the result either of a basal fracture across the middle cranial fossa or of a direct extracranial injury to the branches of the nerves. Numbness and paresthesias over the area of skin supplied by the nerve or a troublesome neuralgia are the sequelae of these injuries.

If the skin is lacerated over the skull fracture and the underlying meninges are torn, or if the fracture passes through the posterior wall of a nasal sinus, bacteria or air may enter the cranial cavity with resulting meningitis, abscess, and pneumoencephalocele (air in the ventricles). Cerebrospinal fluid may also leak through the cribriform plate or adjacent sinus and present as a watery discharge from the nose (CSF rhinorrhea). Persistence of the rhinorrhea or the occurrence over a period of years of episodes of recurrent meningitis (headache, convulsions, fever, and stiff neck with CSF pleocytosis and sometimes bacteria) is often an indication for a surgical repair of the torn dura mater over the fissure. Depressed fractures are of significance only if the underlying dura is lacerated by spicules of bone or the brain is compressed.

BLUNT HEAD INJURY WITH CONCUSSION Much has been written about the mechanism of coma in closed or blunt head injury. Certain facts concerning this condition stand out clearly: (1) its onset is immediate (not delayed even by seconds); (2) concussive effects on brain function may last for a variable time (seconds, minutes, or hours); (3) the optimal conditions for its production are those in which there is some change in the momentum of the head (i.e., movement is suddenly imparted to it by a blow, or its movement is suddenly arrested). Striking the stationary head of an experimental animal will cause a loss of brainstem reflexes only if the head is free to move, not if it is clamped in one position. This finding alone would stand in refutation of such theories of concussion as a wave of high intracranial pressure due to the indentation of the skull or a subsequent wave of negative pressure, cerebral ischemia, or a general vibration or agitation transmitted via the skull. The speed of acceleration or deceleration of the head necessary for this concussive effect must exceed 7 m/s in the macaque. It is probably less for the heavier human brain. The initial action of the blunt injury of this type is alleged (without proof) to excite the nervous system (the "stars" that one sees with a minor injury, the gasp of the animal), and this is followed by transient paralysis of cerebral function, i.e., abolition of consciousness, suppression of reflexes, arrest of respiration, transitory bradycardia, and fall in blood pressure, etc. The means whereby the latter effects are produced is not established. Equally uncertain is the site of injury, whether diffuse in the cerebral cortex, in the cerebral white matter, or in the diencephalon and midbrain. We favor the idea of diencephalic-mesencephalic injury caused by torsion to this part of the neuraxis by movement of the cerebral hemispheres.

In fatal cases of severe head injury, where this concussive injury must have existed, the brain is almost invariably bruised or lacerated, and often there is hemorrhage, either meningeal or intracerebral. The observation of these gross pathologic findings has led to the widely prevalent view that head injuries are largely matters of bruises and hemorrhages and of urgent operations. That this can hardly be the case is suggested by the fact that some patients survive head injuries almost as severe as the fatal ones and yet make an excellent recovery. At autopsy years later old contusions *(plaques jaune)* and hemorrhages of approximately the same distribution and extent as those observed in some of the immediately fatal cases are found. One can only conclude, therefore, that most of the immediate symptoms of severe head injury, both general and localized, depend on invisible and highly reversible changes in the brain, probably of the same nature as those which underlie concussion. Nevertheless these bruises, lacerations, hemorrhages, localized swellings of tissues, and herniations cannot be disregarded, because they are probably responsible for most of the fatalities that occur 12 to 72 h or more after the injury. Of these lesions the most important are the surface bruising of the brain beneath the point of impact (*coup* injury) and the more extensive lacerations and contusions on the opposite side of the brain (*contrecoup* injuries). The inertia of the malleable brain, which causes it to be flung against the side of the skull that was struck and to be pulled away from the contralateral side, has been invoked to explain these coup-contrecoup contusions. This theory has been further elaborated by Holburn, who points out that the brain is roughly spherical and that all movements of the head describe an arc with its axis centered where skull is attached to spine. Sudden changes in the momentum of the head, therefore, impart a swirling motion to the brain, which may then suffer injury against all rough, bony, and dural prominences (wings of sphenoid bones, petrous parts of temporal bones, rough surfaces of orbital and frontal bones, falx, and tentorium).

PENETRATING INJURIES Bullets and other high-velocity missiles destroy brain tissue in proportion to their size and kinetic energy; high-velocity bullets are the more damaging. The region of brain damage may extend far beyond the missile track. Steel military bullets retain their shape and produce a well-defined brain track with adjacent hemorrhage, while softer lead civilian bullets shatter and fragment, producing smaller, low-velocity fragments. There is a sudden rise in intracranial pressure after bullet injury which stabilizes in several minutes, the ultimate level depending upon the degree of associated hemorrhage. Hemorrhages in the subdural or epidural spaces are frequent.

INTRACRANIAL PRESSURE AND CEREBRAL BLOOD FLOW The physiology of intracranial pressure (ICP) regulation applicable to other pathologic processes such as cerebral hemorrhage, encephalitis, and brain edema is best presented in the context of head trauma. A relationship between clinical outcome and ICP has been established in patients with closed head injury. Approximately 50 percent of patients who die as a result of head injury do so because of uncontrolled rises in ICP; moreover, outcome may be predicted in a graded way on the basis of the level of ICP after acute injury. Modern intensive care units and simplified methods of ICP measurement have made these observations possible.

The components of the intracranial compartment are brain, CSF, and blood. Because the skull limits the total intracranial contents, the volume of these compartments is compromised with expanding lesions within the cranial cavity. The brain is virtually incompressible so that CSF and blood serve as the main buffers of changing intracranial volume. The relationship between increments in intracranial volume and the associated rise in ICP is called *compliance* and approximates an exponential function after the CSF and blood buffers are exceeded. Raised ICP may not be harmful in itself, but secondary damage results either by precipitously decreasing global cerebral perfusion or by herniation of brain tissue. The global damage from increased ICP is therefore ischemic in nature and is related to the balance between blood pressure in the carotid and vertebral arteries and the ICP. The difference between the mean blood pressure and ICP is called the *cerebral perfusion pressure* (CPP). Cerebral perfusion pressure below 40 to 60 torr is considered to be detrimental to nerve cells, and therapy should be directed toward maintaining perfusion levels above this range. Physiologic changes or medications that increase blood pressure do not necessarily increase CPP because increased vascular pressure may exacerbate brain edema in damaged areas, resulting in a further increase in ICP so that perfusion ultimately is lowered.

The relationship of resting ICP, CPP, and compliance are spontaneously interrupted by reflex-induced rises in ICP *(plateau waves).* Periods of raised ICP lasting 2 to 10 min and ranging from 25 to 60 torr occur and are most pronounced in patients with diminished intracranial compliance. Plateau waves are probably due to a temporary loss of cerebrovascular tone with a resultant increase in cerebral blood volume. They are commonly observed on continuous recordings of ICP.

There is, as yet, little consensus about the importance of the complex patterns of blood flow alterations caused by head injury. For several minutes to an hour after acute head injury, cerebral blood flow increases though metabolic demands and O_2 consumption is diminished, a circumstance termed *luxury perfusion.* Autoregulation, the ability of the cerebral vasculature to dilate or constrict in response to decreased or increased perfusion pressure, respectively, is also impaired. Abnormally increased cerebral blood flow contributes to increased ICP by raising blood volume and may also give rise to plateau waves. Occasionally, large-vessel vasospasm, perhaps related to blood in the subarachnoid space, occurs after acute head injury, and it has been suggested that regional ischemia or infarction may occur on this basis.

The blood-brain barrier becomes more permeable after head injury and in badly damaged regions may no longer exist. Barrier abnormalities persist for up to months after injury, accounting for persistent abnormalities on radionuclide brain scans.

CLINICAL MANIFESTATIONS OF HEAD INJURY

Upon being called to see a patient who has had a head injury, the physician will generally find the patient in one of three clinical conditions; each must be dealt with differently. It is usually possible to categorize such patients by assessing their mental and general neurologic status when they are first seen and at intervals of time after the accident. This division of cases depends mainly on an assessment of levels of consciousness, verbal response, and motor response, which for purposes of clinical comparison and estimation of prognosis have been standardized in a rating scale (Table 357-1).

PATIENTS WHO ARE CONSCIOUS OR ARE RAPIDLY REGAINING MENTAL CLARITY WHEN FIRST SEEN (MINOR HEAD INJURY) The typical example is a patient who has been rendered unconscious by a blow to the head and then seems all right. If unconscious, such persons may regain their senses within seconds, minutes, or a few hours. Some are never unconscious at all. They were observed to have been struck on the head and were stunned or "saw stars." By all criteria their head injury was insignificant, at least when judged in terms of life and death and severe brain damage, though in exceptional cases there is always the possibility of skull fracture or the development of an epidural or subdural hematoma. Nevertheless, a troublesome group of symptoms (headaches, giddiness, fatigability, insomnia, and nervousness) may appear at once or within a few days.

Clinically, such patients with minor head injury and brief loss of consciousness are said to have suffered a concussion, which is instantaneous in onset, manifests widespread symptoms of a purely paralytic kind, does not as such comprise any evidence of structural cerebral injury, and is nearly always followed by amnesia for the actual moment of the impact. Patients, if observed immediately after injury, show a complete paralysis of nervous function. In a few instances death has occurred at this time, from respiratory arrest or cardiac arrhythmia, and no lesion is found at postmortem examination. However, the usual sequela is for the pulse and respiration (if they were depressed or arrested) to return at once and for muscle tone, reflexes, voluntary movement, and mental clarity to be regained within a few minutes. Only an amnesia for the accident and the events that immediately preceded (retrograde amnesia) and followed it (anterograde amnesia) will remain.

These relatively trivial head injuries may rarely be followed by a number of other puzzling features, all of which indicate the occurrence of some process in addition to concussion:

1. *Delayed traumatic collapse.* Following an accident a few patients, after walking about and seeming to be mentally normal, will turn pale and fall unconscious for a few minutes. This is a vasomotor syncopal attack and is probably related to injury, pain, and emotional upset. Rarely does the patient exhibit any focal or lateralizing neurologic signs.
2. *Immediate traumatic paraplegia or blindness.* With falls on top of the head, which may injure the motor areas for the lower extremities, both legs may become temporarily weak and numb, sometimes with bilateral Babinski signs and sphincteric incontinence. Temporary blindness may have a similar base in occipital injuries. In several personally observed instances the mechanism was probably the vaso-

TABLE 357-1
Glasgow coma scale for head injury

Eye opening (E):	
Spontaneous	4
To loud voice	3
To pain	2
Nil	1
Best motor response (M):	
Obeys	6
Localizes	5
Withdraws (flexion)	4
Abnormal flexion posturing	3
Extension posturing	2
Nil	1
Verbal response (V):	
Oriented	5
Confused, disoriented	4
Inappropriate words	3
Incomprehensible sounds	2
Nil	1

NOTE: *Coma score = E + M + V. Patients scoring 3 or 4 have an 85 percent chance of dying or remaining vegetative, while scores above 11 indicate 5 to 10 precent likelihood of death or vegetative state and 85 percent chance of moderate disability or good recovery. Intermediate scores correlate with proportional chances of patients recovering.*

spasm of a migraine attack that had been initiated by trauma.

3 *Delayed hemiplegia or monoplegia.* An "interval" paralysis in cases of minor or major injury usually signifies an epidural hemorrhage, a subdural hemorrhage, dissecting aneurysm of the carotid artery, spreading venous thrombosis, or intracerebral hemorrhage.

4 *Acute drowsiness, confusion, and headache,* due presumably to localized and generalized traumatic brain edema. Children who have concussions are especially liable to headache, drowsiness, and vomiting, which may have their onset some hours after the injury. In these children, intravenous infusions and oral intake of water are particularly dangerous; such treatment may prove fatal by inducing severe brain swelling. The contribution of an excessive output of antidiuretic hormone to the water retention is still uncertain but possibly plays a factor. Many patients remain drowsy, confused, or agitated for several hours or even 2 to 3 days after concussion. The majority of these patients have skull fractures; a few may demonstrate a subtle hemiparesis due to a presumed associated contusion. Persistent vomiting is frequent. In such cases a CT scan should be performed to exclude extraparenchymal hematoma and to demonstrate contused regions that may later become edematous. These patients ultimately do well, with rapid recovery of orientation and full ambulation. However, many will describe that they are not "themselves" for up to several weeks, frequently showing a bland affect, decreased spontaneity, and memory difficulties. They should be treated acutely with fluid restriction to avoid exacerbating brain swelling but do not require ICP monitoring. Sedation should be used sparingly.

5 *Posttraumatic syndrome* (see below).

PATIENTS WHO HAVE BEEN UNCONSCIOUS SINCE RECEIVING MAJOR HEAD INJURY **The clinical state** In this group, which includes the patients with the more severe head injuries, the outlook is obviously less favorable and one is concerned at first for the patient's life. However, within this group there is still a wide variation in the severity of the traumatic brain disease. A certain number of patients die at once or within a few minutes, and it may be assumed that the direct injury to the brain or some other organ was of such magnitude as to be incompatible with life. Other patients in this group recover consciousness rapidly after several hours, but a few remain deeply comatose for days or even weeks before doing so. One particular subgroup survives for a matter of hours or days and then the pupils dilate and become fixed and all brainstem reflex mechanisms, including the maintenance of respiration, are paralyzed and the EEG is usually isoelectric (as described in Chap. 354 under "Types of Abnormal Recordings"). In this, the brain-death syndrome, the outlook is hopeless, and the patient's circulation usually fails within a few days. The mortality rate in those who reach a hospital in coma was formerly 50 to 60 percent, but as pointed out by Langfitt, modern methods of critical care have reduced this to 30 percent (see below). Most of the deaths occur in the first 12 to 24 h. Of those alive after 24 h the mortality falls to 10 to 20 percent, and after 48 h to 5 to 10 percent.

Those patients whose illness will end fatally may be moribund from the beginning. The coma is profound. The limbs may be flaccid without reflexes or are rigidly extended (decerebrate rigidity). The corneal and pharyngeal (gag) reflexes are usually present. The pupils are small and unreactive to light, or dilated and fixed, or unequal. The ocular axes are divergent or askew. The jaw sags, the tongue falls back in the throat, saliva drools from the mouth, and swallowing is obviously lost. There may be cardiovascular shock at first for a brief period, with the usual findings of pale and moist skin, weak and rapid pulse, subnormal temperature, and a blood pressure that is difficult to obtain. Within a few hours, however, the temperature usually rises, and this may continue until death, reaching levels of 39 to 40°C. The breathing may be stertorous and later feeble and irregular. The state of consciousness and the temperature chart provide information of great value in appraising the status of the patient. An ascending pulse rate, possibly interspersed by short periods in which there is a bounding, slow pulse, and rising temperature or a combination of fast pulse and subnormal temperature are signs of grave prognostic import.

In those whose prognosis is favorable, the coma is less deep; i.e., there is confusion, stupor, or semicoma (see Chap. 20) and for a time restlessness and combativeness. The reflexes are normal, as are pulse, blood pressure, and respiration. The patient is able to swallow and may or may not speak. There are no obvious neurologic signs.

Once the patient regains consciousness sufficiently to respond to a spoken command, the physician no longer needs to be concerned about survival and may begin to think about the possibility of focal brain damage and prospects for return of neurologic function. There is still a substantial risk in the first 2 or 3 weeks, however, from pneumonia, meningitis, or epidural and subdural hemorrhage, which may intervene and impair the chances of survival. It is often said that death during the first 12 h is the result of the direct injury of the brain usually in association with high ICP and reduced cerebral perfusion. In that which occurs later these factors are still operative, but other complications of cranial trauma, such as intracerebral or subarachnoid hemorrhage, herniation of the temporal lobe, localized or generalized edema, epidural or subdural hemorrhage, meningitis, and pneumonia, assume increasing importance.

There is another group of patients to whom some reference must be made, for they represent difficult problems in diagnosis and therapy. Here a known or evident head injury is not followed by deep or lasting coma, but instead the patients are awake and able to respond to some degree upon arrival at the hospital. Yet as the hours pass, it is apparent that their condition is deteriorating, and within a day or two they lapse into coma. A CT scan may attest to the existence of contusion. The progressive nature of the illness suggests intracerebral, epidural, or subdural hemorrhage; yet at postmortem examination only contusion, localized edema (sometimes generalized), and temporal lobe pressure cone are found to be the basis of the clinical syndrome. The point to remember is that consciousness may return early, i.e., within minutes or hours, after a head injury severe enough to contuse the brain seriously and to lead to death after a few days. Presumably the concussive coma has not been as severe as in most patients who suffer contusive injuries.

Focal and lateralizing neurologic symptoms and signs, as would be anticipated, will be observed with notable frequency in this group of patients. In some the pupillary and ocular abnormalities and decerebrate posturing point unmistakably to upper brainstem lesions, either primary or secondary to temporal lobe–tentorial herniation. These abnormalities are presumably related to hemorrhage and contusion, and inasmuch as they are usually engrafted on a severe concussive injury, they become manifest as consciousness is regained. Local injury to the brain without a disturbance of consciousness occurs exceptionally, and then more often with the penetration of the skull by missiles or a direct glancing blow by a relatively small object (golf ball, stone), and sometimes with depressed fractures. Of the focal symptoms, hemiparesis is probably the most frequent. The weakness in the arm and leg may be evidenced even during coma by the hypotonia, the less frequent movement of the limbs, inequality of tendon reflexes, and a more persistent Babinski sign on one side. Complete hemiplegia is rarely observed. Hemihypesthesia, although occasionally found, is less common, possibly because sensory tests are difficult to interpret until mental clarity is regained. Homonymous hemianopsia is not at all infrequent and may present early as an inattentiveness to visual stimuli on one side. Aphasia, usually of mixed type, may be noted in a number of cases. A series of focal seizures may occur within a few days of the time of injury and is probably due to cortical contusion. Such seizures usually cease after a few days and do not necessarily signify that epilepsy is to be a sequel to the trauma. Diabetes insipidus, disturbances of sleep (reversal of rhythm, somnolence), diplopia, heteronymous visual field defects, and gastrointestinal hemorrhage indicate damage to the hypothalamus and walls of the third ventricle. Midbrain lesions are evidenced by ocular palsies, protracted coma (weeks, months, or years), decerebrate rigidity, crossed ocular-limb paralyses, bilateral Babinski's signs, and later, dysarthria, ataxia of the limbs on one side, and sensory disturbances.

Laboratory findings In this group of patients with severe head injury there is a high incidence of skull fracture. The CSF, which is now seldom examined, is usually sanguineous (red blood cells usually 100,000 per cubic millimeter or less) and under elevated pressure (between 200 and 300 mmH_2O) in the majority of patients. The prognosis is distinctly less good in those with more than 100,000 red blood cells per cubic millimeter and pressures in excess of 300 mmH_2O. Nevertheless death may occur in patients who have no skull fracture, a subnormal intracranial pressure, and relatively clear CSF. The EEG regularly shows focal and diffuse abnormalities. The CT scan is the most definitive diagnostic test and should be obtained at the earliest opportunity in such patients (Fig. 357-1).

Neuropathologic findings In patients who die during the first few hours or days after a severe head injury, hemorrhage and necrosis of tissue will frequently be observed. In 50 consecutive autopsies summarized in Rowbotham's excellent monograph, only 2 showed no macroscopic change. Lacerations of cerebral cortex (28 percent), surface contusions (48 percent), subarachnoid hemorrhage (72 percent), acute subdural hemorrhage (16 percent), and extradural hemorrhage (20 percent) were the usual findings. As a rule, several of these pathologic changes were found in the same case. Skull fractures were discovered in 72 percent.

In another series of 50 cases, 21 percent had associated fractures of limbs, 18 percent chest injuries, and 13 percent abdominal injuries and ruptures of organs.

Recently attention has been called to shearing injuries to tracts in the cerebral white matter; both myelin sheaths and axons are said to be thereby interrupted. This is not surprising for on sectioning the recently traumatized brain one can sometimes actually see macroscopically a series of small hemorrhages and zones of necrosis extending through the hemispheres and corpus callosum along the line of impact. But Strich demonstrated bands of white matter degeneration and disappearance of axis cylinders at long distances from surface contusions in five patients who had remained comatose for long periods after a head injury. And in earlier lesions she found fragmented axons with retraction bulbs. Shearing

FIGURE 357-1
Computerized tomographic (CT) scans from patients with head trauma. A. Acute subdural hematoma with compression of adjacent brain tissue. B. Chronic subdural hematoma, less dense than brain tissue. C. Contusion—traumatic hemorrhage of the frontal and parietal lobes. D. Epidural hematoma in relation to a fracture and tearing of the middle meningeal artery. The lenticular shape of the hemorrhage is typical. E. Skull fractures in the path of a bullet trajectory. By manipulating the windows on the CT scan, fractures and radiodense objects are shown to advantage and appear similar to plain radiographs.

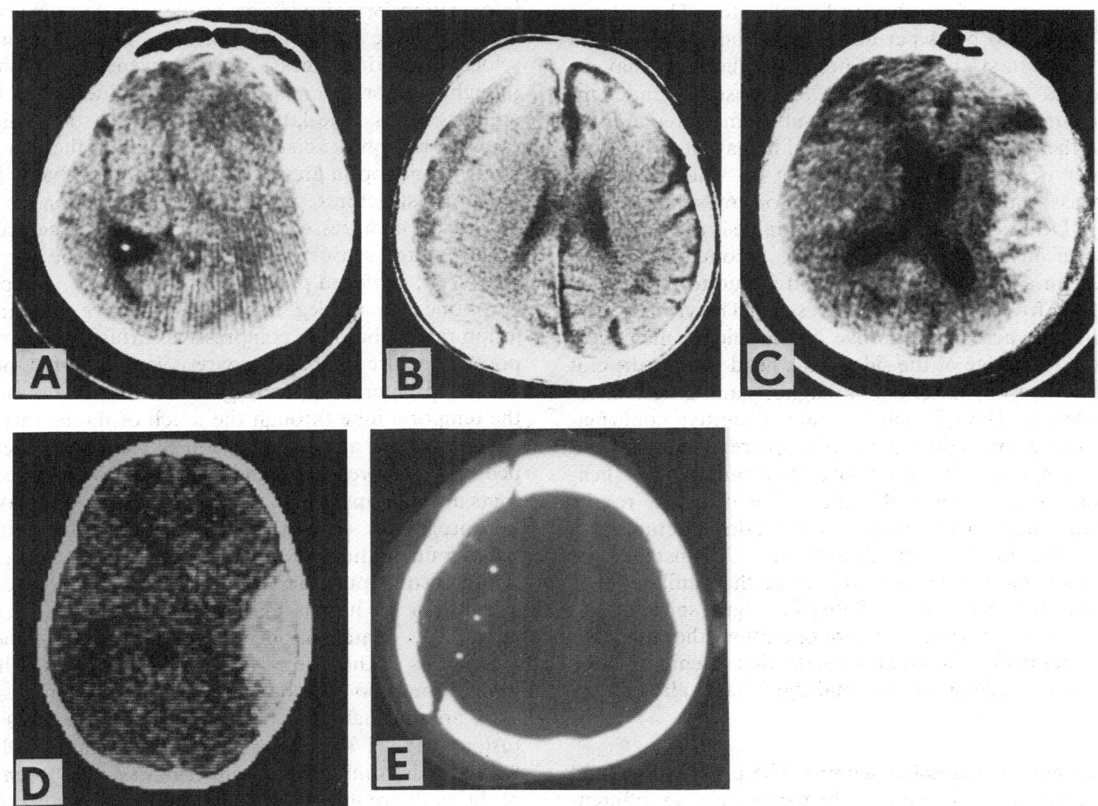

stresses were believed to be the cause. J. H. Adams has confirmed these findings in the brainstem and hemispheral white matter. However, the nature of these changes is still unsettled. Whether they are a primary or secondary wallerian degenerative effect from a destructive cortical and deep white matter lesion is debated. Much has been made of these axonal changes, perhaps more than they deserve. It has even been suggested that they may occur during concussion, but they were not found by Adams in regions related to arousal and coma.

PATIENTS WHO ARE UNCONSCIOUS WHEN FIRST SEEN BUT WHO WERE CONSCIOUS AFTER THE ACCIDENT (PRESENCE OF LUCID INTERVAL) This group of patients is smaller than the other two but is of great importance because it includes many who are in urgent need of surgical treatment. The initial coma may have been brief or there may have been none at all, in which instance one might conclude that there was neither concussion nor contusion. The following conditions must be considered in every case of this type.

Acute epidural hemorrhage This condition is due as a rule to a temporal or parietal fracture with laceration of the middle meningeal artery and vein. Less often there is a tear in a dural venous sinus. The injury, even when it fractures the skull, may not have produced coma. A typical example is seen in a child who has fallen from a bicycle or a swing or has suffered a hard blow to the head in a fight and was only momentarily unconscious. A few hours or a day or two later (exceptionally the interval may be as long as several days or a week, especially with venous bleeding), the child develops headache of increasing severity, vomiting, drowsiness, confusion, seizures (which may be one-sided), and hemiparesis, with slightly increased tendon reflexes and Babinski's sign. As coma develops, the hemiparesis with Babinski's sign may give way to spasticity and Babinski's sign bilaterally. There may be aphasia before consciousness is lost. Respirations become deeper and stertorous, then shallow and irregular, and finally stop. The pulse is often slow (below 60 beats per minute) and bounding, with a concomitant rise in systolic blood pressure. The pupil may dilate on the side of hematoma. The CSF is usually under increased pressure, though normal and subnormal pressures do not exclude the possibility of an epidural hematoma. The fluid may be clear or sanguineous, depending on whether or not there is an associated contusion, laceration, or subarachnoid hemorrhage. Death, which is almost invariable if the clot is not removed surgically, comes at the end of a comatose period, rarely if ever in a conscious patient, and is due to respiratory arrest resulting from brainstem compression. The visualization of a fracture line across the groove of the middle meningeal artery and a knowledge of the side of the head struck (the clot is usually on that side) are of aid in diagnosis and of lateralization of the lesion. The CT scan provides definitive confirmation. The surgical procedure consists of placement of several burr holes (a single one may miss the clot), drainage, identification of the bleeding vessel, and ligation. The operative results are excellent, except in the cases with extended fractures and laceration of the dural venous sinuses, in which instance the epidural hematoma may be bilateral rather than unilateral, as it ordinarily is. If coma, bilateral Babinski's signs, spasticity, or decerebrate rigidity supervene before operation, the prognosis for life becomes poor. This usually means that a temporal lobe herniation and crushing of the midbrain have already occurred.

Acute and chronic subdural hematoma The problems created by the acute and chronic subdural hematoma are so different that they must be discussed separately. In *acute subdural hematomas*, which may be unilateral or bilateral, the latent interval is usually longer than in epidural hemorrhage—many days or 1 to 2 weeks. Headaches, drowsiness, sometimes agitation, slowness in thinking, and confusion, all of which progressively worsen, are the most frequent symptoms. Focal or lateralizing signs (hemiplegia) are late and tend to be less prominent than the disturbance of consciousness. Frequently the acute subdural hematoma is combined with cerebral contusion and laceration, so that the clinical effects of these several lesions are difficult to distinguish; and there are some patients in whom it is impossible before operation to state whether the surface clot is epidural or subdural in location. CT scan provides quick, accurate diagnosis. The x-ray absorptive value of the subdural fluid is about 70 units, the same as blood, and it decreases on the fortieth to seventieth day after subdural clot formation. (The absorptive value of CSF is 8 units, and this rises linearly with high protein content.) If CT scan is not available, the physician must resort to arteriography, which shows inward displacement of cerebral arteries from the skull. The treatment is to place bilateral temporal burr holes and to evacuate the clot. The surgical results are less certain than in chronic subdural hematoma. Once coma has occurred, as many as half the patients die. If the clot that is found is too small to explain the symptoms and the CSF pressure is high, some neurosurgeons proceed to do a right subtemporal decompression. Exceptionally the subdural hematoma forms in the posterior fossa and gives rise to headache, vomiting, pupillary inequality, dysphagia, cranial nerve palsies, ataxia of trunk and gait, and stiff neck, in some combination.

In *chronic subdural hematoma*, the traumatic cause is less clear. The head injury, especially in the elderly person, may be trivial (striking the head against the branch of a tree, or on the mantel of a fireplace during a faint, etc.), and it may have been forgotten completely. A period of weeks then follows when headaches (not invariable), giddiness, slowness in thinking, confusion, exaggeration of certain personality peculiarities, and a seizure or two (rare) are the main symptoms. The initial impression may indicate a vascular lesion, a brain tumor, drug intoxication, or a depressive, senile, or other type of psychosis. As with acute subdural hematoma, the disturbance of consciousness (drowsiness, inattentiveness, incoherence of thought, stupor, or coma) is more prominent than focal or lateralizing signs. The latter usually consist of hemiparesis and rarely of an aphasic disturbance. Hemianesthesia and homonymous hemianopsia are seldom observed, probably because the anatomic structures subserving these functions are deep and not easily compressed (in the case of the geniculocalcarine pathway) and sensory changes are likely to be overlooked in a stuporous, confused patient. Hemiplegia, i.e., complete paralysis of one arm and leg, is usually indicative of an intracerebral lesion rather than of a compressive surface lesion. Another important feature of the hemiparesis is that it may be contralateral or ipsilateral, depending on whether or not herniation of the temporal lobe through the notch of the tentorium into the posterior fossa and compression of the contralateral cerebral peduncle are present; if the latter has occurred, corticospinal signs are then ipsilateral to the clot or bilateral. As the condition progresses, the patient becomes comatose but often with striking fluctuations of awareness. The ipsilateral pupil dilates (Hutchinson's pupillary sign), owing, it is believed, to direct pressure of the herniating temporal lobe upon the oculomotor nerve. The dilated pupil and ptotic eyelid are more reliable indications of the side of the hematoma than the hemiparesis, though they too may be misleading in certain cases. Convulsions are unusual (<15 percent) except in patients with a contusion. The CT scan shows the surface mass of blood clot or fluid and deformity of the ventricular system. Roentgenograms of the skull are usually negative except for a shift of a calcified pineal to one side or an occasional unexpected fracture line. The branches of the middle cerebral artery are separated from the skull and displaced contralaterally in an arteriogram. The CSF may be clear, bloody, or xanthochromic, depending on the presence or absence of recent or old contusion and subarachnoid hemorrhage, and the pressure may be elevated, normal, or subnormal. Of all these diagnostic procedures, CT scan and arteriography are the most reliable.

The acute, rapidly evolving subdural hematomas are due to tearing of bridging veins and direct compression of the brain by an expanding clot of fresh blood. Unlike the epidural arterial hemorrhage, which is progressive, the bleeding is usually arrested by the rising intracranial pressure. The chronic subdural hematoma is believed to gradually expand by becoming encapsulated by fibrous membranes (pseudomembranes) which grow from the dura. In its encysted state, as red corpuscles hemolyze and blood proteins disintegrate, the osmotic pressure rises and fluid enters the hematoma, with the result that the hematoma enlarges and the compressive effects increase. Severe cerebral compression and displacement with temporal lobe–tentorial herniation are the usual causes of death. Treatment consists of placing burr holes and evacuating the clot before deep coma has developed.

Subdural hygromas (collections of blood and CSF in the subdural space) may also form after an injury, as well as after meningitis (in an infant) or rarely following pneumoencephalography (see Chap. 365). In meningitis, it is said that a tear of the arachnoid permits bacteria to enter and excite a serous reaction in the subdural space. Drowsiness, confusion, irritability, and fever are relieved when the subdural fluid is aspirated or drained.

Delayed focal edema from contusion As was mentioned under "Presence of Lucid Interval," the patient with severe blunt injury may be only slightly confused soon after the blow to the head and only later lapse into coma as further bleeding and swelling occur. Although exceptional, this condition must be considered in those patients with a relatively lucid interval.

Cerebral hemorrhage (immediate and delayed) Acute, massive brain hemorrhages are more frequent in elderly than in young patients and are usually fatal within a few hours. The clinical picture is similar to that of hypertensive brain hemorrhage (deepening coma with hemiplegia, a dilating pupil, bilateral Babinski's signs, stertorous and irregular respiration). Indeed the problem that cannot be solved even at postmortem examination is whether the patient had a hemorrhagic type of stroke and then fell or had a fall that caused the head injury and hemorrhage. If the bleeding is slow, there may be an interval of 2 to 3 days between injury and the symptoms of the oncoming hemorrhage. Coma or confusion, if present from the time of the injury, may obscure the signs of the intracerebral hemorrhage. Craniotomy with evacuation of the clot has given a successful result in a few cases.

TRAUMATIC OCCLUSION OF THE CAROTID ARTERY In this relatively rare and most dramatic form of cranial trauma, the patient is usually young and athletic, and the mechanism of the injury is usually unclear. An accident on the playing field is followed after an interval of hours or days by a massive hemiplegia, hemianesthesia, homonymous hemianopsia, and, if left-sided, aphasia. Occlusion is demonstrable by arteriography. Hemorrhage into the wall of the common or internal carotid artery causing a dissecting aneurysm similar to the type which is nontraumatic has been found in a few patients (see Chap. 356). In others injury to the wall of the carotid artery has given rise to embolism of the anterior or middle cerebral artery.

REPEATED CONCUSSION (PUNCH-DRUNK) The cumulative effects of repeated injuries, observed almost exclusively in professional boxers, constitute a type of head injury difficult to classify, for only a few cases have been well studied pathologically. It is a common observation that after a number of years in the ring, pugilists often become forgetful, slow in thinking, and slightly dysarthric. Their movements are stiff and uncertain, especially in the lower extremities; there is an unsteadiness of gait, and occasionally involuntary movements. The plantar reflexes may be extensor on one or both sides. The EEG shows slow waves of theta and sometimes of delta type. The anatomic basis of this disease is not fully known. The postulation of showers of petechial hemorrhages from repeated blows on the jaw should not be given credence until demonstrated pathologically. The brain is atrophied, and the CT scan will reveal dilated lateral ventricles. A low-pressure hydrocephalus from repeated meningeal hemorrhages is another possibility. In at least a half dozen reported cases loss of cortical neurons has been accompanied by senile plaques and fibrillary changes in remaining neurons, as in Alzheimer's disease. The findings of diffuse degeneration of the cerebral white matter have been demonstrated in rabbits and monkeys which have been subjected to repeated concussions and offer another, more acceptable possibility.

PENETRATING AND COMPRESSION INJURIES OF THE BRAIN Penetrations of the brain by high-velocity missiles and shell fragments are occurring with increasing frequency in these times of violent street crimes. But these and the rare compression fractures are more strictly neurosurgical problems and will not be discussed here.

SEQUELAE OF SEVERE HEAD INJURY

The signs of focal brain disease, whether due to open and penetrating or closed head injuries, tend always to ameliorate as the months pass. A hemiplegia is often reduced to a minimal hemiparesis or ineptitude of voluntary motor function with exaggerated reflexes and an equivocal Babinski sign on that side, and aphasia improves to become a stuttering or hesitant paraphasia which is not disabling except in a person whose profession requires much speaking or writing. Many of the signs of brainstem disease improve, often to an astonishing degree.

PROTRACTED TRAUMATIC COMA AND PSEUDOCOMA Of particular interest is the outcome of those rare conditions in which coma persists for weeks or months or even years. Early in the illness these patients, while comatose (i.e., unreceptive to stimuli and unresponsive) or in a state of pseudocoma (receptive and capable of signaling by blinking their eyes but otherwise unresponsive), usually exhibit a variety of neurologic abnormalities: unequal pupils; dilated, fixed pupil and oculomotor palsy on one side and hemiplegia on the other; disturbances of gaze; bilateral corticospinal paralysis with Babinski's sign; extensor postures of arm and leg on one side and flexed arm and extended leg on the other; brainstem attacks (extension of limbs and increased respiration, blood pressure, and sweating on stimulation of any kind); and involuntary movements (tremor, chorea, athetosis). Some remain in this reduced mental state until death (after nearly 10 years in one of the authors' cases, but usually after a few months or a year or two). The majority, however, may regain enough function to leave the hospital; not a few, surprising as it may seem, are restored to full alertness and fairly adequate mental function. Residual weakness of limbs, slurred speech, ocular palsies, ataxia of an arm or leg, or involuntary movements are frequent. During convalescence, language mechanisms may be found disturbed in various ways, i.e., mutism, akinesia or adynamia (lack of volition or impulse to speak or move), dysarthria, and, if there are contusions of the cortex of the dominant hemisphere, an aphasia as well. Any one or a combination of these abnormalities may be present.

The authors have examined the brains in nearly a dozen cases of this type, and nearly all have shown numerous old foci of hemorrhage and ischemic necrosis in the midbrain and subthalamus, especially in the tegmentum and tectum. They were probably due in most instances to temporal lobe herniation and midbrain compression, for one could see where one side of the base and tegmentum had been indented by the free edge of the tentorium. In others there may have been direct injury to the midbrain and pons, with numerous small hemorrhages. Presumably these pathologic changes are not constant, for scattered lesions in the cerebral cortex (contusions of the summits of convolutions, ischemia with necrosis in the depths of sulci) and scattered foci of necrosis and hemorrhage in the cerebral white matter and corpus callosum along the lines of force of the injury have been observed. As stated above several neuropathologists have attributed these white matter lesions to shear strains with axonal injury. We interpret tract degenerations as secondary to focal necrosis of tissue.

EPILEPSY Posttraumatic epilepsy, which occurs in 20 to 40 percent of patients with severe head injury, is one of the most dreaded complications. Its basis is nearly always a contusion or laceration of the cortex. The likelihood of epilepsy is said to be greater in parietal and posterior frontal lesions, but it may arise from lesions in any area of the cerebral cortex. The incidence of epilepsy is much greater in "open" than in "closed" head injuries. Indeed, in cases of pure concussion without contusion or laceration, seizures are not much more frequent than in the general population. The interval between head injury and the first seizure ranges from 3 to 9 months, but it may be much longer, i.e., many years, particularly in children. The longer the interval, the less certain one is of its relation to the traumatic incident. There is a slightly greater tendency for those patients who had seizures at the time of head injury to become subject to recurrent seizures later. The seizures are always of focal character, or grand mal; petit mal is rarely if ever due to trauma. The significance of the different patterns of focal seizures, which vary according to the location of the lesion, has been worked out in detail by Penfield and his associates (see Chap. 355). The frequency of seizures in any given patient varies widely; some patients have only a few, others many, with episodes of status epilepticus. The EEG is of value in diagnosis; a focus of spike or sharp waves is the characteristic finding. Usually the seizures can be controlled by anticonvulsant medications, and only the recalcitrant cases are likely to require excision of the epileptic focus. The surgical results vary according to the methods of selection and technique of operation. Seizures are abolished in approximately 50 percent of cases by excision of the focus. They tend to decrease in frequency as the years pass, and some patients (an estimated 10 to 30 percent) stop having them. A recent suggestion has been made that the routine administration of phenytoin (Dilantin) to all patients with severe head injury will diminish posttraumatic epilepsy.

IMPAIRMENT OF MENTAL FUNCTION Fortunately this is a rare sequela to head trauma. Mental function may be disturbed by focal lesions which produce dysphasia, agnosia, apraxia, etc. Rubens et al. have reported disconnection syndromes from traumatic hemorrhages in the corpus callosum. But usually intellectual functions and memory are relatively well preserved. The exceptions are often elderly persons in whom the injury may have uncovered an early senile dementia or the development at any age of hydrocephalus secondary to subarachnoid hemorrhage. Children and adolescents are more apt to show residual mental and personality disorders.

POSTTRAUMATIC SYNDROME Undoubtedly the most troublesome sequela of head injury is that alluded to above in the discussion of the first group of cases under "Clinical Manifestations of Head Injury"—*headache, giddiness, and nervous instability*. This has been called the "postconcussional syndrome" or the "minor contusion syndrome" (Trotter), or "posttraumatic vasomotor neurosis" (Friedmann). All these terms are objectionable on the grounds that they suggest an explanatory hypothesis, as yet unproved. Headache is the central symptom, at times localized to the part struck. It is variously described as an aching, throbbing, pounding, stabbing, or pressing pain and is remarkable for its variability. The intensification of symptoms by mental and physical effort, straining, stooping, and emotional excitement has already been mentioned. Rest and quiet may relieve them. Thus the headache becomes a major obstacle to convalescence, which demands always a resumption of normal activities. The dizziness is usually not a true vertigo but a giddiness. The patient feels suddenly unsteady, dazed, weak, or faint. However, a certain number of patients report symptoms which suggest a labyrinthine disorder. For example, objects in the environment are said to move momentarily, and looking upward or to the side may cause a sense of unbalance. Or changing one's position in space may evoke momentary vertigo and nystagmus. Labyrinthine tests may show either hypo- or hyperreactivity, or the results may prove to be normal. The data are usually so indefinite that it is impossible to state whether or not the labyrinth and vestibular mechanisms have been injured. Exceptionally, vertigo is accompanied by diminished excitability of both the labyrinth and the cochlea, and one may assume the existence of direct injury to the nerve or end organ. The giddy patient usually is intolerant of noise, emotional excitement, and crowds. Tenseness, restlessness, inability to concentrate, a feeling of nervousness, fatigue, worry, apprehension, and an inability to tolerate the usual amount of alcohol complete the clinical picture. In contrast to the multiple subjective symptoms, detailed tests of intellectual functions and memory show little or no impairment. In a recent study of brainstem auditory evoked potentials, abnormalities have been found in some patients. This syndrome, once established, may persist for months or even years, but usually the symptoms lessen as time passes. Strangely, it is almost unknown in children. Its intensity and duration are augmented by compensation problems and litigation, suggesting a psychopathologic factor.

EXTRAPYRAMIDAL AND CEREBELLAR DISORDERS The question of *posttraumatic Parkinson's syndrome* has been discussed many times, usually with the general conclusion that a true traumatic parkinsonism does not exist. Most patients have merely had paralysis agitans or postencephalitic Parkinson's disease brought to light by head injury, but severe hypoxic damage to basal ganglia is a possibility in patients who had been comatose for a long time. Cerebellar ataxia is a rare consequence of cranial trauma. When present, it is frequently unilateral and due to injury of the superior cerebellar peduncle against the tentorium. If bilateral, it suggests traumatic hemorrhage in the midbrain tegmentum involving the decussation of the brachium conjunctivum. An unsteadiness of gait may also reflect a communicating hydrocephalus.

POSTTRAUMATIC HYDROCEPHALUS The not infrequent examples of posttraumatic hydrocephalus exhibit intermittent headaches, vomiting, confusion, and drowsiness, and autopsy has demonstrated an adhesive basilar meningitis, attributed to subarachnoid or ventricular hemorrhage. Later, mental dullness, apathy, and psychomotor retardation are the principal manifestations. The CSF pressure may then have fallen to a normal level (low-pressure hydrocephalus). Since symptoms like these have been observed occasionally after the rupture of a saccular aneurysm with massive subarachnoid hemorrhage, due presumably to blocking of the aqueduct and fourth ventricle by blood clot, this mechanism has also been suggested as a possible explanation of traumatic hydrocephalus in patients with cerebral contusion. Response to ventriculoatrial shunt may be dramatic.

POSTTRAUMATIC PSYCHIATRIC DISORDERS In contrast to nervousness and nervous instability, which are common sequelae of injuries of all types, posttraumatic psychoses are relatively infrequent. The most distressing psychiatric syndromes have been suspiciousness and paranoid delusions, unaccountable outbursts of violent temper, sometimes with homicidal or suicidal tendencies, progressive hyperactivity, delirium, and mania, and episodes of bizarre behavior with subsequent amnesia, reminiscent of temporal lobe seizures. Alcoholism may provoke some of these behavioral abnormalities. Some of these illnesses are undoubtedly due to residual brain damage in individuals of peculiar personality makeup. However, attempts to account for psychoses of this type by reference to constitutional peculiarities and predisposition, laid bare, so to speak, by head injury, have not been convincing. Approximately 50 percent of patients with combinations of neurologic deficits and disturbances of personality and control of impulses treated at the New York Rehabilitation Center were restored to a level of useful functioning in 1 year.

TREATMENT

The physician who undertakes to treat the "head injury case" must at all times bear in mind that assiduous attention to detail may prove to be lifesaving, and that accurate documentation of all diagnostic findings and therapy is desirable if the medical data are later to be used in the arbitration of insurance claims, worker's unemployment compensation, etc. The suggestions which follow can do no more than serve as guides, for every patient presents a combination of problems that the physician has not encountered before and may not observe again in identical form.

Exact data concerning the patient's medical status before the accident (previous illnesses, work and social record, emotional stability), the nature and precise circumstances of the accident, the duration of retrograde and anterograde amnesia, and all that transpired afterward should be obtained and recorded. Verbatim statements should be written down whenever possible.

The treatment problems presented by each of the three groups of clinical cases discussed above are as follows.

MINOR HEAD INJURY In this group are included patients who (1) were never unconscious at any time, (2) were briefly unconscious at the time of the first examination, or (3) are rapidly regaining consciousness.

Circumstances dictate how each case is managed. If the injury was trivial and the scalp was not lacerated and if patients are entirely clear mentally, little or nothing need be done. When patients are unable to give an accurate account of what has happened and appear still to be somewhat confused or incoherent, they should be compelled to lie down or at least remain in one place. It often happens that the confusion is not detected and patients are permitted to resume activity while still acting in an irrational manner. They may get into their car and attempt to drive, only to have another accident, or if they are athletes they may continue to play a game and make a series of errors.

It is often tempting to discharge the conscious or nearly conscious person who is admitted to a general hospital after only brief observation. However, experience teaches caution. A complete examination, with the patient fully undressed, should be carried out. It is well, if there is any likelihood of litigation, to obtain x-rays of the skull and an EEG. Whether to perform a lumbar puncture will usually depend on how serious the injury was, on the prominence of posttraumatic headache, etc. A simple fracture without involvement of paranasal sinuses requires no special treatment but is believed to contraindicate vigorous athletic activities for several months or a year.

Posttraumatic headache, dizziness, and nervousness are the most difficult symptoms; an optimistic prognosis and the institution of a program of graded mental and physical activities to the point of tolerance stand the best chance of restoring the patient to a useful life. The patient should be told to expect a certain amount of headache and to carry on in spite of it. Meprobamate, 200 mg tid, is useful for anxiety, and a non-habit-forming analgesic medication should be given for the more severe headaches (acetaminophen or aspirin). Insomnia may require a benzodiazepine medication or chloral hydrate at first, but these drugs should be discontinued as soon as possible. If symptoms of anxiety and depression appear, medicines for their suppression should be used as outlined in Chap. 11. Any litigation that may be involved should be settled within 6 to 9 months. To delay settlement usually works against the best interests of patients. The severity of their injury can be ascertained within this period of time, and a longer period of observation only enhances their worries and fears and reduces their motivation to return to work.

PATIENTS WHO ARE UNCONSCIOUS WHEN FIRST SEEN These are the ones that require critical care. Physician and surgeon must collaborate. Operation may be necessary for severe injury that results in contusions, edema, and surface hemorrhages. And these lead to respiratory problems, electrolyte disorders, circulatory changes, and infection, which are essentially medical.

If the physician arrives on the scene of the accident, a hurried examination should be made before the patient is moved in order to determine whether there is dangerous hemorrhage from a laceration of the scalp or other parts of the body and whether there is a likelihood of a fracture-dislocation of the cervical part of the spine, which is occasionally associated with head injury. The patient who is in shock, with cold, clammy skin and feeble pulse, should be covered with warm blankets. In moving an individual with a potential cervical spine injury, the spine should be kept straight at all times and flexion of the neck should be avoided. This can best be done by placing sandbags or firm pillows on either side of the head and warning everyone against neck flexion. An even safer method is to place the patient on a stretcher face down and arrange pillows to assure a clear airway. Bleeding from the scalp can usually be controlled with a firm pad unless an artery is divided, and then a suture becomes necessary.

In the hospital, where all such patients should be taken, the first steps in the emergency ward should be to control shock. This can usually be done by the application of warmth, keeping the head low, and leaving the patient alone for a few minutes. The shock will usually come under control with or without vasopressor drugs or transfusions. Persistent shock is rare in head injury and always raises the suspicion of a ruptured viscera with internal bleeding, extensive fractures, or traumatism of the cervical part of the spinal cord. A quick survey will enable one to estimate the depth of coma, size of pupils, and presence of obvious fractures, and if shock is not present, or after the blood pressure has stabilized, a more detailed examination can be performed. The skull should be carefully inspected and palpated. The hair should be cut off around the scalp wound. A bogginess of the temporal or postauricular region (Battle's sign), bleeding from the nose or ear, extensive conjunctival edema, and hemorrhage are useful signs of underlying skull fracture. However, it should be remembered that rupture of the eardrum or a blow on the nose may also cause bleeding from the ear and nose, respectively. Fractures of the orbital bones may cause displacement of the eye, with resulting diplopia, and fracture of the jaws, disalignment of the teeth, and great discomfort on attempting to open the mouth. Careful notes should be made regarding temperature, pulse, blood pressure, state of consciousness, and responses to vocal and pain stimuli, pupillary size, ocular movements, corneal reflexes, facial movements (spontaneous or during grimace), tone of jaw and limb muscles, swallowing, movements of the limbs, prevailing postures, and reflexes. The Glasgow coma scale (Table 357-1) expresses some of the findings and is now widely used.

As soon as vital functions permit, the patient should be taken to a critical care unit; cervical spine x-rays and a CT scan are obtained. The finding of an epidural or subdural hematoma or large intracerebral hemorrhage would be an indication for surgery and intracranial decompression. If such lesions are not seen and it is evident that the patient is still in coma and critically ill, the following treatment plan should be initiated.

1. An adequate airway must be secured and maintained. In the deeply comatose patient endotracheal intubation is undertaken to protect the airway, assist respiration, should it be required, and also to control respiration for management of increased ICP. In general we have not favored tracheostomy unless respiratory assistance or pulmonary toilet is still needed after 12 to 14 days. Oxygen is given to maintain arterial P_{O_2} levels above 85 torr.
2. Intracranial pressure must be controlled, since it is elevated in the majority of severe head injuries. At first, as the mass of damaged brain increases, the pressure is buffered by displacement of venous blood and CSF. Once exceeded, however, increments of intracranial volume are associated with corresponding rises in ICP. Since the lumbar CSF pressure does not accurately reflect the intracranial pressure and may actually increase the tendency to brain herniation, it has become standard practice in most head injury treatment centers to use a subarachnoid screw device with a hollow bore or ventricular catheter to measure ICP. The pressure can be monitored continuously, disturbances in compliance and falling CPP identified, and appearance of plateau waves noted. The treatment of raised intracranial pressure is best guided by direct measurement but may proceed on a presumptive basis using the clinical state and CT scan as guides. Normal ICP is considered below approximately 15 torr. (In our experience, unilateral pupillary dilatation does not occur below 28 to 34 torr except in middle fossa lesions.) All potentially exacerbating factors must be assiduously eliminated. Hypoxia ($P_{O_2} < 50$ torr), hyperthermia, hypercarbia, awkward head positions, and high mean airway pressures from mechanical ventilation all increase cerebral blood volume and ICP. Many, but not all, patients will have lower ICPs with the head and trunk elevated approximately 60° than when supine.

   Active management of raised ICP in patients with or without surgical lesions then includes induced hypocarbia to an initial P_{CO_2} plateau of 28 to 33 torr; hyperosmolar dehydration with 20% mannitol (0.25 to 1 g/kg every 3 to 6 h), preferably using directly measured ICP as a guide but otherwise aiming for a serum osmolarity of 305 to 315 mosmol per liter, and ventricular or subarachnoid fluid drainage in the few cases where it is possible. Persistently raised ICP after inception of this conservative therapy generally indicates a poor outcome, but some evidence suggests that the addition of high-dose barbiturates may further lower ICP and salvage a small number of patients. The beneficial effects of barbiturates, aside from their sedative and anticonvulsant activities, are unproven. The reader is referred to Chap. 20, "Coma and Other Disorders of Consciousness," for further details of treatment of raised ICP.
3. Stable blood pressure is to be maintained by the use of vasopressor agents, if necessary. Mean blood pressure levels above 110 to 120 torr are thought to be detrimental, particularly if associated with plateau waves, and should be treated with diuretics and beta-adrenergic blockers.
4. Fluid and electrolytes must be administered cautiously, correcting sodium loss, etc. Fluid intake should be kept low—1000–1500 ml per day for hydration worsens edema.
5. There should be prophylactic administration of phenytoin sodium, 100 mg intravenously three times a day, to prevent seizures.
6. Administer cimetidine, 300 mg intravenously every 4 h or hourly, or introduce antacids by nasogastric tube to keep gastric pH above 3.5.
7. The use of large doses of corticosteroids in severe head injury is controversial, but some patients appear to benefit, particularly those less severely injured. Most centers use dexamethasone (Decadron) or its equivalent in a dose of 10 to 20 mg intravenously, followed by 4 to 6 mg every 6 h intravenously or intramuscularly.

As the days pass and the patient remains comatose, it is worthwhile to repeat the CT scan to seek evidence of a surface or intracerebral hemorrhage that may have appeared. Repeated CT scans reduce the need for other invasive procedures and also reduce the number of unnecessary operations by showing the extent of edema, contusion, etc.

In some series of severely head-injured patients mass lesions are treated by surgical decompression in up to 25 percent of patients. In this operated group, 40 percent died as compared to 30 percent for the nonoperated group with diffuse brain injuries. Of the survivors 36 percent made a good recovery, 32 percent were disabled (24 percent moderately and 8 percent severely), 2 percent were left in a vegetative state. Whether more assiduous control of ICP and CPP will produce better results remains to be proven. It has become clear that intensive care salvages some critically ill head-injured patients by concentrating efforts on simple treatments that avoid medical complications and preventable ICP rises. The advisability of any surgical procedure is still much debated, except for the acute epidural hemorrhage.

Once the patient has regained consciousness, the danger of suffocation, aspiration pneumonia, thrombophlebitis, and pulmonary embolism has usually passed, and the therapy can proceed along the lines indicated for the first group.

ASSOCIATED DERANGEMENTS OCCURRING WITH HEAD TRAUMA Injuries outside the cranium should be assiduously searched for at the outset, for they are likely to be forgotten if not initially noted. In particular associated spinal, long-bone, and abdominal injuries may lead to delayed difficulties in management. However, often medical complications dominate the intermediate-term, intensive care of head trauma patients.

Fluid and electrolytes Over one-half of patients who persist in coma for 24 h after head injury develop abnormalities of electrolytes or fluid balance. Frequently these are a consequence of therapy, but the metabolic responses to head trauma are similar to those produced by trauma elsewhere and are important in planning treatment. Daily input-output records and body weights, when possible, are important in management. Restriction of water intake and the use of osmotic agents renders most patients hyperosmolar and hypovolemic, requiring regular monitoring of serum osmolality and sodium concentrations. Diabetes insipidus should be suspected if urine output increases and urine specific gravity is low. Replacement of intravascular volume and water deficit suffices for mild cases, but vasopressin administration is required in persistent cases. Serum osmolality above 320 mosmol per liter should be avoided because of the associated decrease in cardiac output.

Aldosterone and antidiuretic hormone (ADH) secretion in response to stress favor sodium and free water retention, respectively. The latter usually predominates, leading to mild hypervolemic hyponatremia in untreated patients but is submerged by concomitant administration of osmotic agents. Severe hyponatremia (below 122 meq per liter) results from excessive ADH secretion which may occur with raised ICP, basilar skull fractures, and after prolonged mechanical ventilation. Inappropriate ADH secretion is distinguished from iatrogenic water overload by relative urine hyperosmolarity. Adequate correction of hyponatremia can be accomplished by free water restriction in most cases, with care to limit unnoticed intravenous fluids such as antibiotic solutions.

Potassium is lost in large quantities in head injury because of trauma-induced aldosterone hypersecretion and therapeutic osmotic diuresis. Because potassium is predominantly an intracellular ion, hypokalemia is frequently manifested as a hypochloremic alkalosis with normal or minimally depressed serum potassium and requires adequate replacement therapy with KCl.

Respiratory complications A significant number of head-injured patients will have hypoxemia (arterial $P_{O_2} < 70$ torr) acutely after injury without obvious pulmonary pathology. Severe hypoxemia is associated with a poor clinical outcome and should be treated vigorously. Aspiration pneumonia presents a great risk to head-injured patients. Penicillin is appropriate initial therapy for aspiration, which occurs prior to hospitalization, whereas hospital-acquired organisms are usually penicillin-resistant and require therapy based on the results of sputum culture. Aspiration of gastric contents occurs in unresponsive patients with a depressed protective gag reflex and gastric distention. Acid burn injury from aspirated gastric contents, infection, and atelectasis may combine in severe cases to produce the adult respiratory distress syndrome (ARDS) and severe arterial-venous shunting. ARDS also occurs in head injury due to disseminated intravascular coagulopathy, fat embolism, or "neurogenic" pulmonary edema. Treatment is similar to other cases of ARDS with positive end-expiratory pressure (PEEP) to allow lowered, inspired oxygen concentrations and to prevent further atelectasis. The effect of PEEP on ICP is complex but should not be withheld if necessary for oxygenation.

Atelectasis is common to all poorly responsive patients and is treated with chest physical therapy or adequate tidal volumes delivered by mechanical ventilation. Pulmonary embolus is also a major threat to bedridden patients, and intermittent pneumatic calf compression or small doses of subcutaneous heparin may be useful prophylaxis. The latter has not predisposed to intracerebral or gastrointestinal bleeding. Early recognition of deep leg vein thrombosis and aggressive treatment by occlusion of the inferior vena cava may prevent fatal emboli.

Gastrointestinal hemorrhage The majority of severely head-injured patients have endoscopically demonstrable gastric erosions, but only 10 percent have clinically significant hemorrhages. Gastrointestinal bleeding is usually an early complication occurring in the first days to 1 week. Unlike patients in shock or with stress-injured ulceration, head-trauma patients have elevated gastric acidity. The synergistic effect of corticosteroids in causing upper tract hemorrhage has been questioned, but the incidence of viscus perforation, particularly of the cecum, is probably elevated. Prophylactic treatment with frequent antacid administration to keep gastric pH high (above 3.5) or cimetidine has been shown to reduce gastric hemorrhage in other stressful states and is commonly used in head trauma.

Cardiovascular changes Acute head trauma may cause transient apnea and cardiac arrest. In the absence of overwhelming brain damage recovery from arrest is the rule. Subsequently, raised ICP may cause systemic hypertension, either with the classically associated bradycardia or, almost as frequently, with tachycardia. Animal studies suggest that the paramedian medulla is involved in the pressor response. Whether increased peripheral vascular resistance or increased cardiac output is primarily responsible for hypertension is unknown. Cardiac arrhythmias are common, most notably severe sinus bradycardia, nodal rhythm, and Mobitz heart blocks.

Neurogenic pulmonary edema is a form of ARDS in which the alveoli fill with fluid as they would in congestive heart failure but left ventricular end-diastolic pressure (measured by pulmonary capillary wedge pressure) is normal. It seems likely that a pulmonary vascular leak is produced when a sudden shift of intravascular volume occurs from the systemic to pulmonary circulation as occurs transiently with suddenly raised ICP. It is possible that once the pulmonary vasculature has been damaged, an alveolar capillary leak continues despite normalization of intracardiac pressures. The result is pulmonary edema with normal central venous and wedge pressures when measured after the initial injury.

Hematologic complications A large number of head-injured patients demonstrate a mild coagulopathy, and 5 to 10 percent have various degrees of disseminated intravascular coagulation. A correlation may exist between the severity of injury and increased fibrin degradation products. The cause of the coagulopathy is thought to be secondary to highly thromboplastic material released into the systemic circulation by damaged brain.

PROGNOSIS Extensive work by Jennet's group in Glasgow has provided modern data on the outcome in severe head injury using the Glasgow coma scale (Fig. 357-1). They found verbal output, eye opening, and best motor response to be the important predictors of ultimate outcome. Eighty-five percent of patients with aggregate scores of 3 or 4 at 24 h after injury died. Yet a number of patients with poor initial prognosis, including absent pupillary light responses, survived, suggesting that aggressive initial management is justified in virtually all patients. Patients below approximately 20 years of age and particularly children may make remarkable recoveries, even after grave early neurological signs; aggressive treatment efforts are justified, particularly in young patients.

REFERENCES

ADAMS JH et al: Diffuse brain damage of the immediate impact type. Brain 100:489, 1977

AMBROSE J et al: EMI scan in the management of head injuries. Lancet 1:847, 1976

BAKAY L, GLASSAUER FE: *Head Injury*. Boston, Little, Brown, 1980

BECKER DP et al: Outcome from severe head injury with early diagnosis and intensive management. J Neurosurg 47:491, 1977

CAVENESS WF, WALKER AE: *Head Injury*. Philadelphia, Lippincott, 1966

DAVIS KR et al: Computed tomography in head trauma. Semin Roentgenol 12:53, 1977

JENNET B et al: Predicting outcome in individual patients after head injury. Lancet 1:1081, 1976

LANGFITT TW: Measuring the outcome of head injury. J Neurol Neurosurg Psych 48:683, 1978

MARSHALL LF et al: The outcome with aggressive treatment in severe head injury. I: The significance of intracranial pressure monitoring. II: Acute and chronic barbiturate administration in the management of head injury. J Neurosurg 50:20, 1979

ROPPER A et al (eds): *Neurological and Neurosurgical Intensive Care*. Baltimore, University Park Press, 1982

ROWBOTHAM GF: *Acute Injuries of the Head*, 4th ed. Baltimore, Williams & Wilkins, 1964

RUBENS AB et al: Post-traumatic cerebral hemispheric disconnection syndrome. Arch Neurol 34:750, 1975

RUSSELL WR: Cerebral involvement in head injury. Brain 55:549, 1932

WALKER AE: *The Late Effects of Head Injury*. Springfield, Charles C Thomas, 1969

358
NEOPLASTIC DISEASES OF THE BRAIN

RAYMOND D. ADAMS
FRED H. HOCHBERG

Tumors of the central nervous system are of considerable importance in neurologic and oncologic medicine and occupy a distinct field by themselves. It may be said of them generally that they occur in great variety; produce neurologic symptoms because of size, location, and invasive qualities; usually destroy the tissues in which they are situated and displace those around them; are a frequent cause of increased intracranial pressure; and are often lethal. Although patients who harbor such lesions are seen by physicians with neurologic interests, their primary care is often the responsibility of internists, family physicians, pediatricians, and oncologic physicians. Decisions regarding the investigation of a suspected tumor must in the first instance be made as a result of the clinical examination, and the interpretation of neurologic findings requires an understanding of the pathophysiology of tumor growth in the cranial cavity.

For the student of medicine the most important facts to know about CNS tumors are the following: (1) Many types of tumor occur in the cranial cavity and spinal canal, and certain ones are much more frequent than others (see Table 358-1). (2) The largest number of intracranial tumors represent spread of systemic cancers to the brain or its coverings. (3) Certain tumors, such as craniopharyngioma, meningioma, and neurilemmoma, have a disposition to grow in particular parts of the cranial cavity, thereby eliciting certain syndromes and not other ones. (4) Variability in the growth patterns of malignant tumors is another feature; the glioblastoma is usually single and invasive, while tumors of metastatic origin are often multiple and either invasive or compressive. In contrast the more benign tumors, such as meningiomas, are always single and produce symptoms by slow compression of normal structures. These pathologic peculiarities are important, for they have valuable clinical implications, providing the explanation of slowly or rapidly progressive clinical states and the good or poor prognosis after attempted surgical excision.

The one place where pathologic-clinical correlations tend to fail is in the glioma group of tumors, i.e., the astrocytoma-glioblastoma series, and this is all the more regrettable because tumors of this type are so common. Often these gliomas are of mixed type. For example, one part of the tumor is a typical astrocytoma and another an oligodendroglioma. Also the degree of differentiation, or its opposite, the degree of anaplasia, varies from one part of the tumor to another. Therefore, a biopsy sample is often misleading with reference to the prognosis. For example, the clinician may be led to believe that a tumor which on biopsy is composed of astrocytes is benign, whereas actually the main part of it still in the brain is a highly malignant glioblastoma. Another problem is posed by the metastatic tumor which may seed the brain before there is clinical or laboratory evidence of its source, and the CT scan may fail to disclose the number and locale of the brain lesions, particularly in meningeal carcinomatosis.

INCIDENCE OF CENTRAL NERVOUS SYSTEM TUMORS AND THEIR TYPES It was estimated by Posner that in the United States in 1975 there were 365,000 deaths from tumors of all types. Of these, the total number of patients dying of primary tumors of the brain seemed comparatively small (about 8500). However, there were fully 67,000 patients with extracranial tumors who died of metastases to the brain. Thus, approximately 20 percent of all the tumor cases present with neurologic abnormalities at some time in their course. Among neurologic problems, intracranial tumors rank second in frequency (after cerebrovascular diseases).

It is difficult to obtain accurate statistics on the types of intracranial tumors, for most of them have been obtained from the neurosurgical centers in university hospitals, which attract the less easily diagnosable and treatable forms. From the data reported above, intracranial tumors should outnumber primary ones almost 10 to 1. Yet, in almost all reported series (Zulch, Cushing, Olivecrona) less than 15 percent of all tumors of the nervous system are of this type. Autopsy-based studies

TABLE 358-1
Types of intracranial tumor in approximately 15,000 cases in the combined series of Zulch, Cushing, Olivecrona

	Percent
Gliomas:	45
Glioblastoma multiforme	20
Astrocytoma	10
Ependymoma	6
Medulloblastoma	4
Oligodendrocytoma	5
Meningioma	15
Pituitary adenoma	7
Neurilemmoma	7
Metastatic carcinoma	6
Craniopharyngioma and dermoid, epidermoid or teratoma	4
Angiomas and vascular malformations	4
Sarcomas	4
Unclassified (mostly gliomas)	5
Miscellaneous (pinealoma, chordoma, granuloma)	3
	100

reveal metastatic tumors to be more frequent than primary ones, and even the latter figures are not fully reliable for there is a tendency to not examine the brain in cancer patients. With these reservations concerning the natural incidence, the figures in Table 358-1 might be taken as representative.

INTRACRANIAL TUMORS Pathophysiology Since the cranium is filled with three virtually incompressible elements—brain tissue, blood, and cerebrospinal fluid (CSF)—a tumor which adds to brain mass must grow at the expense of the other two elements. As the volume of the tumor and its surrounding brain edema increase, the cerebrospinal fluid is forced out of the ventricles and the cerebral subarachnoid space through the foramen magnum and optic foramens into the spinal and perioptic extensions of the subarachnoid space. The lumbar CSF pressure becomes increased, and the raised perioptic pressure impairs venous return from the optic nerve heads and adjacent retinas, resulting in papilledema ("choked disks"). (See Plate 7-6).

Pressure of the tumor mass on adjacent brain tissue presumably narrows or obliterates venules, particularly in the cerebral white matter. Circulatory slowing and altered permeability of vessels leads to local vasogenic edema of the brain. As the intracranial pressure increases, the cerebral circulation must be maintained. At first this is accomplished by arteriolar dilatation (decreased cerebrovascular resistance). Later, once this compensation proves inadequate, systemic blood pressure increases and the pulse slows (Kohler-Cushing principle).

Inasmuch as the cranial cavity is subdivided by the rigid falx and tentorium, the increase in brain volume occasioned by the tumor and surrounding edema may raise the pressure in one of the cranial compartments to the point that the brain tissue is displaced into an adjacent compartment (where pressure is lower). In this way brain herniations occur—of the inferior part of the cerebellum through the foramen magnum into the cervical canal (cerebellar pressure cone), the medial part of the temporal lobe through the opening in the tentorium into the posterior fossa (temporal lobe–tentorial pressure cone), and the medial, frontal, and parietal lobes beneath the falx into the opposite side (subfalcial pressure cone).

Raised intracranial pressure from the tumor mass or an attendant obstructive hydrocephalus is manifested by generalized headache, slowed mental activity, drowsiness, apathy, and diffuse slowing in the EEG. Regional edema causes a rapidly evolving impairment of the function of the part of the brain involved. Temporal lobe–tentorial pressure cone causes dilatation of the ipsilateral pupil (Hutchinson's pupil) and ptosis of the eyelid; hemiplegia that is either contralateral from the tumor mass or ipsilateral from compression of the opposite cerebral peduncle against the sharp edge of the tentorium; coma (compression, ischemia, and hemorrhages in the upper reticular formation of the brainstem); Cheyne-Stokes and finally arrest of respirations; and high CSF pressure from blockage of the aqueduct of Sylvius and perimesencephalic subarachnoid space (mainly the latter).

A knowledge of these effects of elevated intracranial pressure, regional edema, and herniations is necessary to an understanding of the clinical behavior of intracranial growths.

Clinical and pathologic characteristics Tumors of the brain may exist with hardly any symptoms. Often only a slight deficiency in mental power, a slowness in comprehension, or a loss of capacity in sustaining continuous mental activity suggests any deviation from normal health. Specific signs that would lead to a suspicion of any real cerebral disease may be wholly wanting. In some patients, on the other hand, there is evidence of cerebral disease in the form of a seizure or some other dramatic symptom, but the evidence may not be clear enough to warrant the diagnosis of a cerebral tumor. In a third group, the existence of a new growth in the brain may be determined with much probability by the presence of signs of elevated intracranial pressure, but without symptoms which disclose localization of the growth. Lastly, a particular syndrome may be so clear and definite as to make it probable not only that there is a new growth within the cranium but also that it is located in one particular region and is of a particular histologic type. In other words, these latter tumors create certain unique syndromes seldom evidenced by any other disease.

In the further exposition of this subject, all intracranial tumors are considered in relation to the common clinical circumstances in which they are likely to be encountered, as follows:

1 The patient whose presenting symptom is either a decline in general mental ability or a seizure
2 The patient with unmistakable evidence of headaches and raised intracranial pressure
3 Specific intracranial tumor syndromes

PATIENTS WITH GENERAL SYMPTOMS OF CEREBRAL DISEASE OR A SEIZURE AS THE MAIN COMPLAINT These are the patients who give the most trouble in diagnosis and about whom decisions are often made with a great degree of uncertainty. Their initial symptoms are vague, and not until some time has elapsed will signs of focal brain disease appear; when they do, they are not always of accurate localizing value. Altered psychic function, headache, and seizures are the usual symptoms.

Some *change in mental function* may be found in nearly every patient of this type, but it may be necessary to obtain the observations of a person who knows the patient intimately to learn of it. A lack of persistent application to the tasks of the day, an undue irritability, emotional lability, a "peculiar inertia," faulty insight, forgetfulness, reduced range of mental activity, indifference to common social practices, and lack of initiative and spontaneity, all of which may be falsely attributed to worry, anxiety, or depression, are the usual symptoms. Much of this behavior is accepted by the patient with forbearance, and if he or she has any complaint, it is of being weak, tired, dizzy (nonrotational), or "queer in the head." Inordinate drowsiness, a remarkable equanimity or apathy, and stoicism may be primary findings. Usually within a few weeks or months the drowsiness and mental dullness increase. When questioned, if the psychic inertia is well advanced, a long pause precedes each reply, and at times the patient may not bother to respond at all. Or at the very moment when the examiner has decided that the patient has not heard the question and prepares to repeat it, an appropriate, sensible answer is given, usually in relatively few words. The responses are often much more intelligent than would be expected from the torpid mental state. Headache occurs with increasing frequency in many of the patients. There are, in addition, those who are confused or demented (see Chap. 24). The dullness and somnolence may gradually increase, and finally, as increased intracranial pressure supervenes, they end in stupor or coma.

Mental symptoms of this type cannot be ascribed to disease in any particular part of the brain. Tumors are most likely to be accompanied by intellectual disturbance when they interfere with large association fiber systems of the cerebral white matter; growths limited to the cortex and subcortical white matter are less likely to affect the mind. Much of the drowsiness, torpor, inertia, lack of spontaneity, and general restriction of mental horizon is related to increased intracranial pressure and not to the site and nature of the lesion.

The *headaches* in the "tumor patient" are variable. In some the pain is slight, temporary, and dull in character; in others it may be severe and unendurable, and either dull or sharp, but as a rule it is intermittent. If there are any characteristics of the headache, they would include its nocturnal occurrence, its presence on first awakening, or its deep nonpulsatile quality. However, these are not specific attributes, since migraine, hypertensive vascular headaches, etc., may also begin early in the morning when the patient first awakens. The patient does not always complain of the pain even when it is present and may betray its existence by placing a hand on the forehead and looking distressed.

The mechanism of the headache is not known. In the majority of instances, the intracranial pressure is normal during the first weeks when the headache is present, and one can attribute it only to distortion or alteration of blood vessels in or around the tumor. Later the headache appears to be related to rises in intracranial pressure. Tumors above the tentorium cause headache on the side of and in the vicinity of the tumor, usually in the orbital, frontal, temporal, or parietal regions. Tumors in the posterior fossa usually cause ipsilateral retroauricular or occipital headache. With elevated intracranial pressure, bifrontal and bioccipital headache is the rule, regardless of the location of the tumor.

Vomiting appears in about one-third of the patients with tumor syndromes of this type and usually accompanies the headache. It is more frequent with tumors of the posterior fossa and may precede other signs of intracranial tumor by weeks or months. Some patients may vomit unexpectedly and forcibly, without preceding nausea (projectile vomiting), but others suffer both nausea and great pain. Usually the vomiting is not related to the ingestion of food, often occurring before breakfast.

No less frequent is the complaint of *giddiness* or *dizziness.* As a rule it is not described with accuracy and consists of a more or less confused sensation in the head, coupled with feelings of strangeness and insecurity when the position of the head is altered.

One or more generalized *convulsions* are another major symptom calling attention to the existence of cerebral tumor. Their frequency in various statistical analyses is 20 to 50 percent of all patients with cerebral tumors. The onset of a seizure during adult years and the existence of a localizing aura are always suggestive of tumor. The localizing significance of seizure patterns has already been discussed (see Chaps. 12 and 355). The seizures may occur once or many times and may precede other symptoms for as long as 10 years or more in cases of astrocytoma or meningioma.

The management of patients who present any one of the aforementioned symptoms requires brief discussion. Any clinical problems of these types, especially if accompanied by recurrent headache of a form which the patient recognizes as different from customary headaches; or a seizure, appearing for the first time, justify a careful review of the patient's general behavior. In obtaining further data, one must rely heavily on the observations of other members of the family. A thorough neurologic examination with careful inspection of optic fundi, a test of visual fields, motor, reflex, and sensory functions in the limbs, alertness, memory, facility in language (speaking, reading, writing, and understanding the spoken word), calculation, and tests of visuospatial orientation must follow. Sooner or later other regional or localizing symptoms and signs will be discovered, and it is only by repeated examinations that one will note the earliest stages of a hemiparesis, aphasia, visual field defect, hemianesthesia, etc. Unmistakable signs of increased intracranial pressure eventually become manifest and establish the diagnosis of tumor with reasonable certainty (see "Astrocytoma," below.)

The decision as to the appropriate time for doing confirmatory diagnostic tests requires balanced clinical judgment. Since many of the symptoms described above could be due to any number of metabolic abnormalities or diseases, for a time it is wise to follow the patient by repeated examinations and not proceed too quickly to expensive and difficult diagnostic tests. As more of the clinical picture unfolds, there comes a time when CT scans with single and double doses of contrast, x-rays of the chest (always done to help rule out metastatic carcinoma), radionuclide scans, a localizing EEG, and finally lumbar puncture (for pressure, cells, cytologic examination, protein, and Wassermann reaction) should be done, preferably by admitting the patient to a hospital. The early use of CT scan, even on an emergency basis, allows for the planning of therapy, especially in patients at high risk (those with known systemic malignancy, seizures, or localized clinical deficits). Carotid arteriography is reserved in most medical neurologic clinics for those patients in whom the total clinical syndrome is already strongly suggestive of tumor and further information is needed for the planning of surgery. Most tumor patients with cerebral edema will benefit from the use of corticosteroids during the period of diagnostic studies.

TUMORS WHICH TEND TO PRODUCE GENERAL CEREBRAL SYMPTOMS OR SEIZURES The following tumors are most likely to produce initial convulsions or a vague syndrome of headache, giddiness, vomiting, dull or stuporous state, and psychic changes: metastatic carcinoma, glioblastoma multiforme, astrocytoma, oligodendroglioma, meningioma, and primary reticulum-cell sarcoma (histiocytic lymphoma) of the cerebrum.

Metastatic carcinoma Carcinomas reach the brain by hematogenous spread. Rarely epithelial malignancies, usually of nasopharyngeal origin, may spread to the cranial cavity through cranial and intervertebral foramens or by invading bone. Probably 35 to 40 percent of metastatic tumors originate in the lung, and approximately 15 percent from the breast. Melanomas, carcinomas of the colon, testicular and kidney tumors each account for 10 to 15 percent, while the remainder come from stomach, liver, thyroid, uterus, ovary, and other organs. Carcinoma of the prostate, esophagus, oropharynx, or skin (except for melanocarcinoma) rarely disseminate in the brain. Brain metastases will develop in as many as 80 percent of patients with melanocarcinoma and 25 percent of patients with breast carcinoma. In more than 75 percent of cases the metastases are multiple and are scattered through both the cerebrum and cerebellum with 5 to 10 percent spreading through the meninges. Hemorrhagic metastases are likely to be from the lung, kidney, or uterus (chorioepithelioma). The implanted tumor tissue usually is well vascularized, exciting little tissue reaction but much edema.

The usual clinical picture in metastatic carcinoma of the brain does not differ from that of glioblastoma multiforme. The majority of patients (60 percent) develop neurologic difficulties in a setting of known systemic malignancy, although in as many as 20 percent brain lesions appear before the primary tumor becomes symptomatic. Also in approximately 20 percent of cases secondary tumors invade the brain when the patient is moribund without producing symptoms.

A number of striking clinical neurologic syndromes occur as a result of brain metastases. One such condition, carcinomatous meningoencephalopathy, is particularly difficult to diagnose. Patients may present with headache, nervousness, depressed mood, trembling, mental confusion, and signs of forgetfulness. This syndrome may be the result of diffuse or multiple brain metastases or a number of metabolic and infective and hematologic disorders associated with systemic cancer. Another difficult syndrome is carcinomatosis of the cerebellum resulting in headache and dizziness, but with no signs of ataxia other than those of gait. A third unusual syndrome is meningeal carcinomatosis, with the main symptoms and signs being referable to one or more cranial and spinal nerve roots in combination with diffuse headache, confusion, and hydrocephalus on CT scan. The lumbar CSF usually contains a few white blood cells (lymphocytes) along with elevated protein and diminished glucose, but in some cases is unremarkable. Tumor cells can be identified in stained sections passed through Millipore filters or in centrifuged specimens, even when no malignant cells are seen in routine chamber counts. Cytologic evaluation has thus become a routine method of evaluating CSF in the cancer patient. The highest success rate is with adenocarcinomas of breast or lung, melanoma and lymphoma. Measurement of glucuronidase and carcinoembryonic antigen in the CSF was found by Posner et al. to be of diagnostic help, for the levels of these substances are increased in meningeal carcinomatosis. While elevation of glucuronidase is nonspecific (raised also in chronic infectious meningitis), the carcinoembryonic antigen is a specific marker for CNS metastases. Diagnostic tests will usually reveal the primary tumor and other secondary deposits in the lungs, liver, and lymph nodes.

When the syndromes due to these several varieties of metastatic tumor are fully developed, diagnosis is relatively easy. If only headache and vomiting are present, a common error is to attribute such symptoms to a psychological disorder. One learns by experience with this type of patient to make a psychiatric diagnosis only if the patient presents with all the standard symptoms of one of the psychiatric disorders described in Chaps. 375 and 376. A lumbar puncture, a chest x-ray, sedimentation rate (often increased in metastatic carcinoma but not glioblastoma), and other x-rays (xeromammography, bronchograms and cytology of bronchial washings, gastrointestinal series, barium enema, and pyelograms) are advisable if metastatic cancer is suspected. In most instances the diagnosis of brain metastasis is substantiated by CT scan (over 90 percent of supratentorial and 75 percent of infratentorial lesions) using single or double doses of contrast material administered by vein. Biopsy or resection is often required for diagnosis in the patient with a solitary intracerebral lesion when there is no evidence of systemic malignancy or when definitive therapy is being planned for patients with quiescent cancer.

Virtually all patients benefit from corticosteroids to control brain edema and anticonvulsants to reduce the risk of seizure activity. Localized 40,000- to 50,000-mGy (4000- to 5000-rad) or whole-brain irradiation [40,000 to 50,000 mGy (4000 to 5000 rads)] produces significant diminution of "radiosensitive" metastases such as of small-cell tumors of lung or breast. Cairncross, Kim, and Posner report improvement in cerebral symptoms in 74 percent of 183 cases. In 15 percent there was no change and 11 percent deteriorated. Of those who improved, two-thirds maintained their improvement until death. The median survival period was not significantly prolonged; only 25 percent lived for 6 months and only 8 percent for 1 year, but the relief of cerebral symptoms is often welcomed. Steroids and x-radiation were about as effective for solitary metastases as surgical excision. It may prolong the life of the patient and give palliation in less radiosensitive malignancies. Chemotherapy has proved to be of little value in individuals with metastatic brain lesions, though there are exceptions such as follows intravenous administration of *cis*-platinum and/or methotrexate for metastases from testicular and nasopharyngeal tumors, non-Hodgkin's lymphoma, and chorioepithelioma. The administration of chemotherapeutic agents through the carotid offers a new approach (presently under study) to the treatment of brain metastases. Therapy of meningeal carcinomatosis involves cranial irradiation of the entire neuraxis (cranium and spinal) followed by twice weekly intrathecal or intraventricular methotrexate and/or cytosine arabinoside. A small chamber (Ommaya reservoir) implanted beneath the scalp but in continuity with the subarachnoid space or ventricular system facilitates the administration of the drug.

Radiation necrosis This is the proper place to remark on brain lesions induced by gamma radiation, for such therapy carries a calculable risk. If the total dosage to brain or spinal cord exceeds 60,000 mGy (6000 rads) a neurologic syndrome is likely to result in 9 to 24 or more months. The vessels in the irradiated tissue thicken and become occluded, resulting in a zone of coagulation necrosis where nerve cells and other tissue elements are virtually congealed. Aside from gliosis there is little reaction to the necrosis (if extensive) because of the lack of circulation. The lesion is of gradual onset and progresses until all function of the neural elements is lost. The cerebral lesion, when large, may result in swelling and increased intracranial pressure; the spinal lesion involves both gray and white matter—a transverse myelopathy.

The effects of whole-brain radiation even at the conventional dose of 40,000 to 50,000 mGy (4000 to 5000 rads) in 10 to 15 days also is not without danger. We have observed several patients who became gradually demented after an interval of several months to a year or more. Scattered small lesions all through the cerebrum of monkeys subjected to whole-brain radiation were reported by Caviness et al.

In a fraction of a percent of patients whose brain or nerves have been radiated, a sarcomatous degeneration of connective tissue may occur years later.

Glioblastoma multiforme In all statistical analyses of surgical and postmortem material, glioblastoma multiforme is responsible for more than 25 percent of intracranial gliomas and for more than 90 percent of gliomas of the cerebral hemispheres in adults. Although these tumors frequently occupy more than one lobe of a hemisphere, fewer than 10 percent are multicentric and fewer than 25 percent cross to the opposite hemisphere. Although predominantly cerebral in location similar tumors may be observed in the brainstem, cerebellum, or spinal cord. The peak incidence is in the middle adult life, but no age group is spared.

The glioblastoma is a highly malignant tumor which infiltrates the brain extensively and may attain large size before attracting medical attention. It may extend, especially in young patients, to the meningeal surface or the ventricular wall, which probably accounts for the elevation of protein level (more than 100 mg/dl in many cases), as well as an occasional pleocytosis of 10 to 100 cells or more, mostly lymphocytes. The tumor has a variegated appearance, being a mottled gray, red, orange, or brown, depending on the degree of necrosis, cyst formation, or hemorrhage, whether recent or old. It is highly vascular, and in an arteriogram one can often see a network of abnormal vessels, mistaken at times for a hemangioma, and the displacement of normal vessels which may result from any "mass lesion." The vessels in the tumor are excessively permeable to radioactive phosphorus (^{32}P), radioactive arsenic, mercury, and technetium, which is the basis for radioactive nuclide scanning techniques. Computerized tomography may demonstrate distortion of some part of one lateral ventricle, contralateral displacement of both lateral and third ventricles, as well as contrast enhancement of the tumor mass and a surrounding low-density edema of the brain. The characteristic microscopic pathologic findings are great cellularity with pleomorphism of cells and hyperchromatism of nuclei; identifiable astrocytes with fibrils in combination with astroblasts, tumor giant cells, and cells in mitosis; a curious sarcoma-like neoplastic proliferation of the cells of small vessels (adventitial and endothelial); necrosis, pseudopalisading of viable cells, hemorrhage, thrombosis of vessels, and variable infiltrates of inflammatory cells (lymphocytes and mononuclear leukocytes). Temporal lobe–tentorial herniation, midbrain compression, midbrain and pontine hemorrhages, and increased intracranial pressure are usually the immediate causes of death.

Clinically the diffuse cerebral symptoms and seizures (present in 30 to 40 percent of cases) usually give way to a more definite frontal, temporal, parietooccipital, or callosal syndrome in a few weeks or months. Seldom, however, do the symptoms and signs point to one lobe, and often one is satisfied to be able to specify the region of the hemisphere which is involved.

Astrocytoma The astrocytoma may occur anywhere in the brain or spinal cord. Favored sites are cerebrum, cerebellum, thalamus, optic chiasma, and pons. It is a slowly growing tumor of infiltrative character with a tendency to form large cavities or pseudocysts. Other of these tumors are noncavitating, grayish white, firm, and relatively avascular, almost indistinguishable from normal white matter, with which they may merge imperceptibly. Calcium deposits may occur in parts of the tumor and may be seen in plain x-rays of the skull and even better in CT scans. The CSF is acellular, the only abnormality being increased pressure and elevated protein level, in some cases. In the CT scan the tumor mass shows varying degrees of enhancement and often distorts the lateral and third ventricles. Displaced anterior and middle cerebral arteries are seen on CT scan or carotid arteriogram. At an early stage, however, all radiologic and electrographic tests may be negative. Microscopically, the tumor tissue is composed of well-differentiated astrocytes of fibrillary, protoplasmic, or transitional type.

The majority of cerebral astrocytomas undergo malignant degeneration and present as mixed astrocytomas and glioblastomas.

The astrocytoma may cause trivial symptoms for a long period of time. Seizures, headaches, and bizarre mental symptoms may be present for several years; in a few instances more than 10 years may pass before the diagnosis is made. The average survival period after the first symptoms is 67 months in cerebral growths and 89 months in cerebellar ones. The cystic astrocytoma of the cerebellum (usually in children) is particularly benign, and some patients have lived and remained well as long as 30 years after part of the cyst was excised. In such cases accuracy of the original diagnosis of neoplasm is always open to question. The astrocytoma of the pons, optic nerves, and chiasm are discussed in more detail later on in this chapter (see "Glioma of the Brainstem").

Oligodendrocytoma The oligodendrocytoma is a relatively rare cerebral tumor (5 to 10 percent of gliomas) and is usually slow in its rate of growth (average span of evolution is 66 months). It is generally a soft, solid tumor, rarely cystic, and through its tendency to calcify (spherules and particles of calcium in microscopic sections) often casts a shadow in the roentgenogram of the skull and CT scan. Microscopically it is composed of small round cells with spherical nuclei and cytoplasm that stains poorly, forming a halo around the nucleus. Some of the tumors are mixtures of astrocytomas and oligodendrocytoma. The usual location is some part of the cerebrum. Seizures are uncommon, and generalized or focal symptoms may be present for a long time before the mass of the tumor declares its presence by increased intracranial pressure. Although the CT scan may demonstrate a mass which absorbs contrast material, the histopathologic definition of the tumor awaits biopsy.

Ependymoma and ependymoblastoma Although occasionally this tumor presents as a solitary mass in a cerebral hemisphere in adults, presumably arising from the ependymal wall of the lateral ventricle, its most distinctive form is a papillary growth filling the fourth ventricle of children. It is discussed below.

Therapy of Glioma The use of corticosteroids (dexamethasone, 6 to 8 mg every 6 h) for the control of cerebral edema improves neurologic function during the pre- and postoperative period. The risk of steroid-induced muscle weakness often precludes the more chronic use of these drugs at a high dose. With the exception of patients with deep-seated tumors, a diagnosis of glioma is usually established through operative resection or needle biopsy. The tumor cannot be totally resected; surgical cure is rarely possible. Postoperative treatment of patients with malignant glioma (grade IV) includes irradiation of both the tumor and the surrounding tissue. Radiation therapy may be given on an out-patient basis. Chemotherapy consists mainly of the lipid-soluble nitrosourea, carmustine (BCNU), which is administered by vein or arterial infusion.

The use of postoperative irradiation and chemotherapy improves the median survival time and level of function of most patients, but seldom is there survival beyond 2 years if the glioma is malignant. Patients with less malignant glial tumors (grades II to III) may benefit from irradiation alone.

Meningioma (arachnoidal fibroblastoma or endothelioma) This is a benign tumor composed of specialized arachnoid lining cells, arising usually in places where there are many arachnoid villi. Since these clusters of arachnoid cells penetrate the dura in the vicinity of the venous sinuses, they often appear to originate from the dura itself; hence the old term dural endothelioma. Grossly the tumors are firm, gray-white, lobulated, bulbous, or plaque-like masses and indent or compress but do not invade the brain tissue. Many of them are highly vascular, receiving their blood supply from the branches of the external carotid artery. In size they are variable; those which have produced symptoms usually have attained a size of 3 to 4 cm or more. The cellular composition permits easy identification. The cells are of uniform type and have the peculiar disposition to encircle one another and to form characteristic whorls and psammoma bodies. The common sites of these tumors are the olfactory groove, tuberculum sellae, parasagittal region, sylvian fissure, cerebellopontine angle, and spinal canal. Inasmuch as they lie on the surface of the brain in or next to the dura, changes in the skull are frequent. The skull may be eroded over the tumor, and the meningeal and diploic vessels, which provide part of the blood supply to the tumor, dilate and are usually prominent in CT scans and x-rays. Or the tumor cells may invade the bone and stimulate osteoblastic activity, as a consequence of which a bony bulge may rarely be seen and felt, or an endostosis is visualized on the inner table of the skull x-ray. The meningioma must be listed with bone-metastasizing carcinoma and the cholesteatoma of the base of the skull or posterior fossa as the three tumors most likely to cause a visible erosion of cranial bone in relation to cerebral symptoms (benign exostoses are neurologically asymptomatic).

Offering a broad vascular meningeal surface as they do, meningiomas often elevate the protein level of the CSF. Their striking vascularity accounts for a characteristic "blush" seen in arteriograms and the dense opacification in contrast-enhanced CT scans. The excessive permeability of the vessels, as well as the superficial location of the tumors, makes them ideal subjects for localization with radioactive isotopes. The underlying brain tissue is visibly edematous in CT scans, and this accounts for some of their subacutely evolving symptoms. The displacement without invasion of cerebral tissue probably explains the interruption locally of normal alpha frequencies in the EEG and the sharp waves or theta waves, in contrast to the delta waves so often found with infiltrative gliomas. Multiple meningiomas within the cranium or spinal canal may occur, particularly in cases of neurofibromatosis.

These tumors may be found at any age but are more frequent in advanced years, especially in women. Therapy consists of operative resection with irradiation reserved for nonresectable, recurrent, or malignant varieties.

Histiocytic lymphoma (reticulum-cell sarcoma) These tumors may be primary in the brain (microglioma) or meninges and present a clinical picture nearly identical to that of glioblastoma multiforme. There is a tendency of this tumor to occur in immunosuppressed individuals, in some of whom there is a history of chronic viral parotitis and iridocyclitis, and in children, in association with ataxia-telangiectasia. Sporadic cases are increasingly common. The tumor mass tends to arise in periventricular and subcortical regions of the cerebrum and cerebellum and may be multifocal. Fully three-quarters of patients will benefit from corticosteroid therapy. This clinical improvement is often reflected in CT scans which show diminished or absent contrast enhancement—"a disappearing tumor." The cytologic examination of centrifuged CSF frequently reveals the tumor cells, providing hematologic stains are used. Immunohistologic typing of lymphocyte subtypes in CSF samples may also aid in confirming the diagnosis. The diagnosis can only be made by biopsy in at least 50 percent of patients. Therapy includes the early and often chronic use of corticosteroids followed by irradiation. The tumor is highly radiosensitive.

TUMORS OF INFECTIVE ORIGIN (GRANULOMAS AND PARASITIC CYSTS) Tuberculoma is much less frequent in the United States than it was 30 years ago, and gumma has become almost nonexistent. In fact a patient with serologic syphilis and a positive Wassermann reaction of the CSF has a greater chance of having two diseases, a cerebral tumor and asymptomatic neurosyphilis, than a gumma. The tuberculoma may occur in any part of the brain, but in children it is more likely to develop in the posterior fossa, i.e., in the cerebellum or brainstem, than in the cerebrum. Often there are a small number of cells and an increased protein content in the CSF because the lesion frequently lies contiguous to the meninges; it may at any time give rise to a tuberculous meningitis with typical CSF formula (50 to 300 cells, increased amount of protein, decreased sugar content, and decreased chloride content).

In South America, tuberculoma, cysticercosis, and echinococcus cysts are much more frequent, and one can usually obtain clues as to their nature from similar disease in other parts of the body, especially the lungs, and characteristic changes in the CSF (see Chap. 354). Cysticercus cellulosae and hydatid cysts are common lesions and should always be suspected when seizures, increased intracranial pressure, or diffuse cerebral symptoms develop in the adult. X-rays of the skull and skeletal muscles (e.g., thigh) may reveal characteristic calcific deposits in cysticercosis. Torula and other fungous granulomas and *Schistosoma japonicum* infection may also present as space-occupying cerebral lesions.

PATIENTS WITH SIGNS OF INCREASED INTRACRANIAL PRESSURE WHEN FIRST SEEN A certain number of patients show all the characteristic symptoms and signs of increased intracranial pressure when first seen. These signs are periodic bifrontal and bioccipital headaches which awaken the patient during the night or are present upon awakening, vomiting that may or may not be expected and may or may not be projectile, mental torpor, unsteady gait, sphincteric incontinence, and papilledema. The physician confronted with this clinical problem is forced to take immediate action, for the condition is potentially dangerous. A critical rise in intracranial hypertension may occur at any time and result in coma, respiratory arrest, and death. Admission to a hospital with a neurosurgical service is therefore usually urgent. Nevertheless all the medical aspects of the patient's problem should first be worked out.

Three questions demand immediate answers: (1) Does the patient have a space-occupying intracranial lesion? (2) Where in the cranial cavity is it situated? (3) What is its nature? With respect to the first question it is well to keep in mind that a number of medical conditions may simulate an intracranial growth that causes only the general symptoms of increased intracranial pressure. These are (1) "pseudotumor cerebri," (2) hypertensive encephalopathy, (3) chronic pulmonary disease with hypercapnia and hypoxia, (4) chronic meningitis or adhesive arachnoiditis and/or aqueductal stenosis, (5) thrombosis of cerebral veins and dural sinuses, (6) Addison's disease and hypoparathyroidism, (7) excessive vitamin A and chloramphenicol (Chloromycetin) therapy in children, and (8) withdrawal from corticosteroid therapy in children. Several of these conditions are discussed elsewhere in this book, and it is sufficient to mention them briefly; others have not been considered before and will be discussed in detail.

Pseudotumor syndromes In the condition of *pseudotumor cerebri* (meningeal hydrops) the patient, more often than not a child or obese young woman, complains of headaches of some weeks' standing and when first examined is found to have papilledema, or choked disks, with slightly constricted visual fields and enlarged blind spots. Except for a vague dizziness, diplopia due to a slight abducens weakness, or paresthesias of some part of the body, neurologic signs are conspicuously absent, and the patient appears remarkably "bright" and well. The CSF is under increased pressure and is acellular with normal protein content; a CT scan shows small or normal-sized ventricles. The arteriogram demonstrates patency of venous sinuses and veins. With the use of corticosteroid drugs (dexamethasone, 6 to 12 mg every 6 h) and daily, then biweekly, then weekly lumbar punctures to lower the CSF pressure, most of the patients gradually recover over a period of weeks to months. If the pressure is not controlled, a spinal subarachnoid peritoneal shunt should be installed. Careful attention must be paid to sequential examinations of the blind spot, visual fields, and extent of elevation of the optic disk. Extremely high CSF pressure with episodes of cloudy vision (obscurations) may herald the onset of blindness and require a lumbar-peritoneal shunt as an emergency measure. The cause of the condition is unknown, but not uncommonly it is related to obesity or pregnancy. Radioactive isotope studies reveal slowed absorption of CSF.

Extreme hypertension (diastolic pressures of 120 torr or over), retinal arteriolar changes with hemorrhages and exudates in the periphery of the optic fundi, signs of renal disease, and headache, convulsions, confusion, stupor, or coma (due to multifocal ischemia and brain swelling) are the basis of the diagnosis of *hypertensive encephalopathy* (see Chap. 356). *Chronic emphysema or other lung diseases,* with cyanosis, dyspnea, cough, signs of cor pulmonale with right-sided congestive heart failure, and secondary polycythemia, may be attended by bilateral papilledema, elevated CSF pressure (small ventricles), high venous pressure, severe headache, drowsiness, stupor, or coma, and peculiar lapses in the posture of the outstreched limbs and other contracted skeletal muscles (flapping movements, or asterixis, similar to the flap in impending liver coma). The finding of an elevated P_{CO_2} and diminished arterial oxygen concentration substantiates the diagnosis (see Chap. 362). *Chronic meningitis or adhesive arachnoiditis* due to chronic fibrosing meningeal diseases such as syphilis, postspinal anesthesia arachnoiditis, and cryptogenic meningeal diseases may be attended by headache, papilledema, seizures, blindness, paraplegia, or quadriplegia. Other benign causes of adult hydrocephalus are aqueductal stenosis and the Arnold-Chiari malformation. The CSF protein level may be normal or elevated, with or without a "dynamic block"; the lateral, third, and fourth ventricles are enlarged in the ventriculogram. Syphilis and other chronic meningitides may also cause *aqueductal stenosis* owing to a proliferative gliotic ependymitis, with enlargement of the lateral and third ventricles (see Chap. 364). *Thrombosis of the jugular veins and of the lateral and posterior parts of the superior sagittal sinus* may result in increased intracranial pressure, with otherwise normal CSF and usually small ventricles (see Chap. 359). No explanation can be given for the papilledema with headache, drowsiness, and confusion and elevated CSF pressure observed in conjunction with *Addison's disease,* corticosteroid withdrawal, vitamin A overdosage, and also, in certain rare cases, hypoparathyroidism. In the latter the ventricles are of normal size.

"TRUE" AND "FALSE" LOCALIZING SIGNS If the clinical findings permit the exclusion of the aforementioned conditions, there is reasonable certainty that the patient has an intracranial growth. The problem then is to search for signs that will localize the lesion. In doing this, several pitfalls must be avoided. One common source of error is to place undue reliance on a sign which proves to have no localizing value whatsoever. One should distrust any symptom or sign which develops late, after headache and increased intracranial pressure have been established, for it often turns out to be a false localizing sign. Under these circumstances drowsiness, slowness in response, inattentiveness, and emotional blunting can be found as often with cerebellar as with cerebral growth. Ataxia of gait, urinary incontinence, and psychomotor retardation may occur as part of a communicating hydrocephalus from any cause. Unilateral or bilateral abducens palsy is another common false localizing sign, and reference has already been made to the drooping eyelid, dilated pupil, ipsilateral hemiparesis and bilateral Babinski signs, and coma in temporal lobe herniation. Jacksonian and generalized seizures and ipsilateral or bilateral pyramidal signs may be observed in the advanced stages of a cerebellar tumor. Early and sometimes relatively slight focal signs that may be easily overlooked are sometimes the most reliable guides to the localization of the tumor. Examples are a mild weakness or stiffness and hyperreflexia of an arm and leg in a frontal tumor; ataxia of gait (but not of limbs) and head tilt in cerebellar tumors; paralysis of upward gaze with the Argyll Robertson pupillary phenomenon in pinealomas; pale optic disks and chiasmal field defects in craniopharyngiomas; and homonymous visual inattentiveness and sensory extinction (see Chaps. 17 and 18) in posterior cerebral tumors.

TUMORS WHICH TEND TO PRODUCE ELEVATED INTRACRANIAL PRESSURE WITHOUT CONSPICUOUS LOCALIZING SIGNS The tumors most likely to do this are medulloblastoma, ependymoma of the fourth ventricle, hemangioblastoma, pinealoma, colloid cysts of the third ventricle, gliomas of the tegmentum of the midbrain with blocking of the aqueduct, and craniopharyngioma. In addition, in some of the cerebral gliomas discussed above, particularly those of the corpus callosum and frontal lobes, increased intracranial pressure may precede focal cerebral signs.

Medulloblastoma This is a rapidly growing tumor which arises in the posterior part of the vermis of children and rarely in the cerebellar hemisphere of adults. The tonsils of the cerebellum are forced down into the cervical spinal canal (cerebellar pressure cone) in fatal cases. Seedings of the tumor may be seen on the walls of the third and lateral ventricles, on the meningeal surfaces of the brain, and around the spinal cord. The tumor is solid, reddish-gray, and poorly demarcated from the adjacent brain tissue. It is very cellular, and the cells are small, closely packed with little cytoplasm, many mitoses, and scant stroma; and have a tendency to form clusters or pseudorosettes. Bailey and Cushing introduced the name medulloblastoma in 1925. Although medulloblasts as such have not been described in the fetal or adult human brain and the cell type is not known for certain, the term is retained if for no other reason than its familiarity.

The clinical picture is distinctive. Typically, the patient becomes listless, vomits repeatedly, and has a morning headache. The first diagnosis which suggests itself may be gastrointestinal disease or abdominal migraine. Soon, however, a stumbling gait, frequent falls, unilateral hearing loss, or a squint lead to a neurologic examination and the discovery of papilledema. Ataxia of the limbs may be absent at all times. Decerebrate attacks (tonic cerebellar fits) may occur in the late stages of the disease. CT scan may show a contrast-enhanced cerebellar mass distorting the fourth ventricle. Not uncommonly, obstructive hydrocephalus necessitates the introduction of a ventriculoperitoneal shunt. In such situations, a filter is often interposed to diminish tumor dissemination. The tumor is highly radiosensitive, and surgery with craniospinal x-ray treatment followed by systemic chemotherapy is associated with 5-year survival for the majority of patients. Local recurrence of tumor may be heralded by reemergence of cerebellar signs without contrast enhancement on CT scan. Over 100 examples of systemic dissemination of medulloblastoma have been reported. Most commonly there is involvement of bones of the pelvis, or vertebral bodies, the liver, or lungs.

Ependymoma and papilloma of the fourth ventricle This tumor also arises from the walls of the fourth ventricle, more often in children, and from the lateral ventricles in adults. It is a soft, whitish-gray, lobulated growth composed of small cells arranged in the form of small rosettes around vessels or central clear areas and containing blepharoplasts in their cytoplasm. The clinical syndrome of the fourth ventricle tumor is much like that of the medulloblastoma except for the absence of ataxia of gait. The tumor is not very sensitive to x-ray, and surgical removal offers the only hope of survival. Prolongation of life is sometimes attained through ventriculoatrial shunting of CSF. The papilloma or papillary adenocarcinoma of the choroid plexus of the fourth ventricle gives rise to a similar syndrome but tends to occur later in life.

Hemangioblastoma of the cerebellum The disease of Lindau is described in Chap. 365. Dizziness, ataxia of gait or of the limbs on one side, symptoms and signs of increased intracranial pressure, and in some instances a retinal angioma (von Hippel's disease) and polycythemia constitute the neurologic syndrome. Familial incidence is high; the inheritance pattern is autosomal dominant. Craniotomy with opening of the cerebellar cyst and excision of the mural nodule may be curative.

Some of the retinal lesions can be obliterated by laser beam treatment. Unfortunately the lesions may be multiple (cerebellum and spinal cord) and noncystic.

Pineal tumors Four tumors, histologically different, occur in the pineal area: the pineocytoma and pineoblastoma, the germinoma, the teratoma, and the astrocytoma. The age of the patient at the time of first symptoms varies widely from childhood to early adult life. The germinoma, which resembles the dysgerminoma of the ovary and the seminoma of the testis, is approximately five times more frequent than the tumors of the pineal parenchyma (pineocytomas and pineoblastomas). Teratomas and astrocytomas are relatively infrequent. Germinomas vary histologically. About two-thirds of them are of uniform type, being composed of large epithelial cells separated by a loose reticular network and infiltrated by lymphocytes. The other germinomas take the form of endodermal sinus tumors, embryonal carcinoma, or choriocarcinomas. The pineocytomas and blastomas are poorly differentiated small-cell tumors.

Pineal tumors perch over the dorsum of the upper brainstem, in position to compress the aqueduct of Sylvius (and thereby to cause hydrocephalus), the superior colliculi, and the superior peduncles of the cerebellum. The germinoma may also extend anteriorly into the third ventricle and compress the hypothalamus, but a similar germinoma sometimes arises in the hypothalamic region, having no connection with the pineal gland.

The characteristic clinical picture of the pinealoma is headache, mental obtundation, and unsteadiness of gait in combination with paralysis of upward gaze and slightly dilated, unreactive pupils. Sometimes an ataxia of gait and a spastic weakness of the limbs appear in the late stages of the illness. If the tumor extends to the floor of the third ventricle, diabetes insipidus, delayed sexual development (in adolescents), and visual impairment may occur. The germinoma, which is twice as frequent in males as females, often causes sexual precocity, but only in males.

CT scans reveal the tumor and are helpful in differentiating tumor type. The germinomas, pineocytomas, and astrocytomas appear as homogeneous masses in the pineal region. The teratomas are nonhomogeneous and often contain calcium. Some of the germinomas give rise to a pleocytosis in the CSF, and they may disseminate through the meninges. A radiosensitive x-ray response to 20,000 mGy (2000 rads), which reduces the size of the tumor within a few weeks is also diagnostic. Alpha fetoprotein in blood and CSF correlates with the presence and degree of cellular activity of the endodermal sinus tumor, and elevated chorionic gonadotropins in blood and urine indicate tumors of chorioepithelioma type.

The treatment plan has been undergoing modification in recent years. If hydrocephalus is threatening life, a ventriculoatrial shunt is indicated as an emergency measure. In Japan and Taiwan where pineal tumors make up 4 to 9 percent of all intracranial tumors in both the pediatric and adult brain tumor series (in contrast to 1 percent in the United States), empiric radiation with 20,000 mGy (2000 rads) has been practiced, followed by stereotaxic needle biopsy if the tumor does not shrink. For the germinoma, whole-neuraxis radiation is advised because 10 percent of such tumors spread through the cerebrospinal meninges in the 12 to 36 months following diagnosis. Increasingly in several university centers exploration of the pineal region and total excision is being undertaken.

Colloid (paraphyseal) cyst of the third ventricle This is a papillomatous structure always situated in the anterior extremity of the third ventricle between the interventricular foramens and attached to the roof of the ventricle. Usually it is about a centimeter or two in diameter, is oval or round with a smooth external surface, and is filled with a glairy colloid material. The wall is composed of a layer of epithelial cells surrounded by a capsule of fibrous connective tissue. These benign cysts may exist without causing symptoms for long periods of time; they produce neurologic symptoms by blocking the third ventricle and causing an obstructive hydrocephalus. This tumor should be suspected when the following clinical syndromes are found: confusion or dementia with or without headache, intermittent generalized headaches, gait disturbance, vomiting, blurred vision, dizziness, "frontal lobe" type of incontinence, bilateral paresthesias, and weakness of legs with sudden falls. The larger colloid cysts can be seen in a CT scan, for the colloid has higher absorptive values than CSF and brain tissue. The treatment is surgical excision, but recently, satisfactory results have been obtained by ventriculoatrial shunt of the CSF, leaving the benign growth untouched (see Little and McCarthy). Stereotaxic aspiration of the cyst has been accomplished successfully in a small number of cases.

Craniopharyngioma (suprasellar or Rathke's pouch cyst, hypophyseal duct tumors, adamantinomas, ameloblastomas) This is a benign congenital, or "rest-cell," tumor. By the time it has grown to a diameter of 3 to 4 cm, it is almost always cystic. Usually it lies above the sella turcica, depressing the optic chiasm and extending up into the third ventricle. Less often it is subdiaphragmatic, i.e., within the sella, where it compresses the pituitary body, erodes one part of the wall of the sella or a clinoid process, but seldom balloons the sella like a pituitary adenoma. The tumor is oval, round, or lobulated and has a smooth surface. The wall of the cyst and the solid parts of the tumor consist of cords and whorls of epithelial cells (often with intercellular bridges and keratohyalin), separated by a loose network of stellate cells. The cyst contains dark albuminous fluid and cholesterol crystals. Calcium deposits are found in nearly all of them and can be seen in plain x-rays of the suprasellar region in about 40 percent of cases. The sella beneath the tumor tends to be flattened and enlarged. In children, adiposity, delayed or infantile physical and sexual development (Froehlich's or Lorain syndrome—see Chaps. 109 and 365), headaches, vomiting, dim vision with chiasmal field defects (see Chap. 17), optic atrophy, or papilledema comprise the clinical picture. In adults, waning libido, amenorrhea, slight spastic weakness of the legs, headache without papilledema, and mental dullness and confusion are often found. Later drowsiness, diabetes insipidus, and disturbances of temperature regulation may occur, indicating hypothalamic involvement.

In the differential diagnosis of these several tumor syndromes a careful clinical analysis is often more important than laboratory procedures. Arteriography and electroencephalography are not as helpful as in cerebral tumors. CT scans reveal calcium deposits when these are not seen in plain x-rays, and hydrocephalus and obstruction of the third ventricle are also disclosed. Other tests which, though somewhat hazardous, are likely to give the most useful information are the air ventriculogram, a combined ventriculogram-pneumoencephalogram, a metrizamide cisternogram, or a Pantopaque ventriculogram (injection of radiopaque fluid). Modern neurosurgical techniques reinforced by corticosteroid therapy before and after surgery and careful control of temperature and water balance postoperatively permit complete excision of the tumor in the majority of cases. Large inoperable lesions have been aspirated, and radiotherapy has been beneficial in some of them.

In certain marginal states of hydrocephalus temporary benefit may accrue from the use of acetazolamide (Diamox) in doses of 250 mg three or four times a day, but surgical shunting of CSF has given the best results.

PATIENTS WITH SYMPTOMS AND SIGNS OF A SLOWLY PROGRESSIVE LESION IN A PARTICULAR REGION OF THE CRANIAL CAVITY In this group of conditions general cerebral symptoms and the signs of increased intracranial pressure occur late or not at all. The physician arrives at the correct diagnosis by being able to make an anatomic or regional diagnosis from a set of neurologic findings and by reasoning that the cause must be neoplastic because of the slowly progressive nature of the illness. Special x-rays of the skull, CSF examination, and, depending on the location of the disease, CT scan and either pneumoencephalography or arteriography will usually confirm the clinical impression.

The following tumors produce unique syndromes usually diagnostic of a special type of tumor.

Acoustic neurofibroma or neurinoma This slowly growing benign tumor may occur as a solitary lesion or as a part of the syndrome of neurofibromatosis. By the time of operation the tumor has usually attained a size of 1 to 3 cm in diameter. It arises from the extramedullary part of the eighth cranial nerve, usually within the internal auditory meatus, where the intracranial part of the nerve first acquires the histologic character of a peripheral nerve, i.e., has Schwann cells and fibroblasts. The space it occupies is the cerebellopontine angle, i.e., between the cerebellum, pons, and medulla posteriorly, the petrous pyramid anteriorly, and the tentorium above. The internal auditory meatus is usually enlarged (visible in x-rays), the middle cerebellar peduncle and the anterolateral part of the cerebellum are depressed, and the trigeminal, facial, glossopharyngeal, and vagus nerves are displaced and stretched over the surface of the growth. The fourth ventricle is deformed, displaced, and narrowed (visible in a CT scan or encephalography with water-soluble metrizamide), and there is hydrocephalic enlargement of the aqueduct and of the third and lateral ventricles in the late stages. The tumor is vascular, and the surrounding CSF has a high protein content (CSF protein of 300 mg/dl or over is not infrequent, especially with tumors >3 cm). The microscopic picture is that of a typical neurofibroma (axis cylinders mixed with masses of fibrous connective tissue in interlacing strands, palisaded nuclei, and mononuclear giant cells with mitoses).

The typical clinical syndrome, which usually occurs in adult men or women, consists of tinnitus, deafness, and rotational vertigo (seldom in discrete attacks as in Ménière's syndrome, Chap. 367) of several years' standing, followed by postauricular or suboccipital pain, disturbance in balance, spasms and twitching or slight weakness of the face, paresthesias in the face or facial weakness, dysphonia and dysphagia, and homolateral cerebellar ataxia of the arm and leg. Headache, vomiting, and papilledema (choked disk) are late findings. Variations of this syndrome are numerous. Early in its development only progressive deafness, tinnitus, and vague vertigo may be present, and the abnormal audiogram, impaired vestibular function, abnormal brainstem auditory evoked response (BSAER) test, elevated CSF protein level, widened internal auditory meatus, and obliteration of the lateral recess of the fourth ventricle in a metrizamide encephalogram must be depended upon for diagnosis. Computed tomography using overlapped sections and positive-contrast encephalography improve diagnostic accuracy. Dementia may later be the presenting syndrome, and the deaf ear may be incorrectly attributed to some other disease. Unilateral cerebellar ataxia and dizziness may predominate, and definite signs of involvement of the fifth, seventh, and eighth cranial nerves may not be found. The only treatment is surgical excision using the dissecting microscope. Modern surgical approaches permit total removal in more than two-thirds of all cases. Patients with small (<2 cm) tumors, without facial or brainstem dysfunction, have the best outcome.

The *neurinoma* of the *trigeminal* or *gasserian ganglion* and *meningioma* of the *cerebellopontine angle* may be indistinguishable from an acoustic neurinoma. They should always be considered if the tinnitus, deafness, and the unresponsive labyrinth ("dead labyrinth") are not the initial symptoms of the cerebellopontine angle syndrome. A true *cholesteatoma* of *the temporal bone* may simulate this clinical picture, but usually the facial weakness is early and severe, the ear is deaf, and labyrinthine function is absent, whereas the other cranial nerve signs, cerebellar ataxia, and increased intracranial pressure are absent. The *tumor* of *the glomus jugulare* (a flat ovoid body, found in the adventitia of the jugular bulb, immediately below the floor of the middle ear and near the ramus tympanicus of the ninth cranial nerve) may, like the acoustic neurofibroma, basal meningioma, metastatic cancer, syphilitic meningitis, neurofibroma of other cranial nerves, and vascular malformation, cause unilateral lower cranial nerve palsies (see Chap. 367). It is a purplish-red, highly vascular tumor composed of large epithelioid cells in an alveolar pattern and an abundant capillary network. Partial deafness, facial palsy, dysphagia, and unilateral atrophy of the tongue, combined with a vascular polyp visible in the auditory meatus and a palpable mass below and anterior to the mastoid eminence, often with a bruit, compose the syndrome. The jugular foramen is eroded (visible by x-ray), and the level of CSF protein may be elevated. Arteriography is of value in diagnosis. Women are affected more than men, and the peak incidence is during middle adult life. The tumor grows slowly over a period of many years, sometimes 10 or more. The treatment is x-ray radiation. Surgical excision has been successful, if performed before invasion of the posterior fossa has occurred.

Pituitary adenomas These tumors, which are so common, particularly in late adult life, often are discovered when a patient begins to complain of a visual disturbance. A partial or complete bitemporal hemianopsia progressing to blindness, with optic atrophy, x-ray evidence of an expanded sella turcica and endocrine disorder lead to a diagnosis of pituitary adenoma. Occasionally, if the growth is eccentric, one optic nerve may be compressed with a resulting monocular scotoma. As the growth enlarges, large suprasellar extensions may involve the hypothalamus or temporal lobe, and oculomotor palsy may occur if there is lateral extension. If there are signs of acromegaly, one may assume that an eosinophilic adenoma is present; if not, and signs of pituitary insufficiency are present (amenorrhea without "hot flashes," sexual impotence, etc.—see Chap. 109), the tumor is usually a prolactinoma. Basophilic adenomas, one of the causes of Cushing's syndrome, rarely cause enlargement of the sella or visual symptoms. The diagnosis is made from the endocrine picture (see Chap. 109). The CSF is usually under normal pressure, and protein level is elevated only in exceptional cases. The syndrome of pituitary apoplexy (acute onset of headache, confusion, stupor or coma, blindness, and bilateral ophthalmoplegia) has usually occurred in individuals with a known or occult chromophobe or eosinophilic adenoma of the pituitary gland. The CSF is usually abnormal, i.e., bloody and/or containing white blood cells and an increased level of protein.

Other conditions may rarely expand the sella (craniopharyngioma, carotid aneurysm, cysts of pituitary, and the "empty sella" syndrome), and there are also rather wide normal variations in its size. The empty sella results from a defect in the dural diaphragm of the sella and nontumorous enlargement.

Raised intracranial pressure may occasionally cause the floor of the third ventricle to protrude into the sella. However, in the usual empty sella syndrome, the CSF pressure is normal. Downward herniation of the optic chiasma may cause visual disturbances simulating a pituitary adenoma. This syndrome may also follow surgical excision of a pituitary adenoma or pituitary apoplexy. Most of our patients have been obese women with no endocrine abnormality or at most a slightly reduced release of growth hormone and increased morning prolactin. Hence the diagnosis of pituitary adenoma should not be made because of minor enlargements of the sella in the absence of endocrine and neighborhood neurologic signs. The CT scan or CT with metrizamide injected into the subarachnoid space permits visualization of the suprasellar extension of the tumor or an empty sella. If vision is compromised or endocrine dysfunction is profound (acromegaly or Cushing's disease) transsphenoidal surgical excision is indicated. Proton beam irradiation (or gamma irradiation if proton is not available) is the treatment of choice for non-prolactin-secreting microadenoma. Replacement endocrine therapy is also needed. Bromocriptine is now being used to suppress prolactin production by a microadenoma.

Meningioma of the sphenoid ridge This tumor is situated over the lesser wing of the sphenoid bone. As it increases in size, it may expand medially to encroach on structures in the wall of the cavernous sinus, anteriorly to invade the orbit, or laterally to erode or invade the temporal bone. Most prominent among the symptoms are a slowly developing unilateral exophthalmos, slight bulging of the bone in the temporal region, and roentgenologic evidence of thickening or erosion of the lesser wing of the sphenoid bone. Variants of the clinical syndrome include oculomotor palsy or syndrome of Foix (see Chap. 367), blindness in one eye with optic atrophy but no bony changes (see Susac et al.), anosmia (and sometimes the Kennedy syndrome—see below), mental changes, uncinate fits, and increased intracranial pressure. Sarcomas arising from the skull bones, metastatic carcinoma, orbitoethmoid osteoma, tumors of the optic nerve, and angiomas of the orbit must be considered in the differential diagnosis. Auscultation of the skull, CT scan, x-ray of the skull, ultrasonograms of the orbit, and carotid arteriography are helpful in differentiating these lesions.

Meningioma of the olfactory groove This tumor is a growth derived from arachnoid cells along the cribriform plate. The diagnosis depends on the finding of ipsilateral or bilateral anosmia, ipsilateral or bilateral blindness, often with optic atrophy on one side and papilledema without atrophy on the other (Kennedy syndrome), and mental changes. The tumors may reach enormous size before coming to the attention of the physician. The anosmia, if unilateral, is rarely if ever reported by the patient. The unilateral visual disturbance may consist of a slowly developing unilateral central scotoma. Confusion, forgetfulness, and inappropriate jocularity (witzelsucht) are the usual psychic disturbances. These patients are indifferent to or joke about their blindness. Usually there are x-ray changes along the cribriform plate and an extremely high CSF protein level (200 to 400 mg/dl).

Glioma of the brainstem Astrocytomas of the brainstem (formerly called "bipolar spongioblastomas") are slow-growing, firm, white infiltrating growths which insinuate themselves between tracts and nuclei. They produce a variable clinical picture, depending on their exact location in the medulla, pons, and midbrain (see Chaps. 16 and 17 for syndromes). The characteristic features, in the early stages, are signs of crossed motor or sensory disturbances, which always indicate brainstem disease. Headache, vomiting, and papilledema occur late. The course is slowly progressive over years unless some part of the tumor becomes more malignant (glioblastoma multiforme), in which instance the illness may terminate fatally within months. The main clinical problem is to differentiate among this disease, multiple sclerosis, and vascular malformations of the pons. CT scan, often with intrathecal metrizamide contrast, and pneumoencephalography to visualize the fourth ventricle and aqueduct and occasionally vertebral arteriography are helpful in diagnosis. The treatment is x-ray irradiation and corticosteroids, and if intracranial pressure is increased, a ventriculoatrial shunt.

Glioma of the optic nerves and chiasma This tumor is often found in patients with von Recklinghausen's disease and, like the glioma of the brainstem, arises most frequently during the period of childhood and adolescence. The initial symptoms are dimness of vision with constricted fields, bizarre bilateral field defects of homonymous, heteronymous, and sometimes bitemporal type, blindness, and optic atrophy with or without papilledema. Hypothalamic signs (hypogonadism, adiposity, polyuria, and somnolence) are common. When progressive blindness of one eye is the only symptom, the tumor must be differentiated from a meningioma of the perioptic sheath. X-rays reveal an enlargement of the optic foramen. With this finding and the lack of ballooning of the sella or suprasellar calcification, pituitary adenoma, Hand-Schüller-Christian disease, and craniopharyngioma can be excluded. CT scans and ultrasonograms of the orbit can usually be depended on to establish the diagnosis. The treatment is surgical excision or x-ray, depending on the exact location. Nontumorous gliotic lesions of optic nerves may occur in von Recklinghausen's disease and may be difficult to distinguish from tumors.

Chordoma This is a soft, jelly-like gray-pink growth composed of cords or masses of large cells with granules of glycogen in their cytoplasm and often multiple nuclei and intercellular mucoid material. They are locally invasive but do not metastasize. Any part of the vertebral column or the base of the cranium are the most common sites, especially the base of the skull (from physaliphorous ecchondrosis) or the lumbosacral region (giving rise to a cauda equina syndrome). Those in the base of the skull create a remarkable clinical picture in which all or any combination of cranial nerve palsies from the second to twelfth on one side or both sides are combined with a retropharyngeal mass and erosion of the clivus of the sphenoid bone and the occiput. It is one of the lesions that may present both as an intracranial and as an extracranial mass. The others are the meningioma, neurofibroma, glomus jugulare tumor, carcinoma of sinuses or pharynx, and midline granuloma. The treatment is x-ray therapy.

Nasopharyngeal growths which erode the base of the skull These are rather common in a general hospital and arise from the mucous membrane of the paranasal sinuses or the nasopharynx near the eustachian tube, i.e., the fossa of Rosenmueller (*transitional cell carcinoma, Schmincke tumor*). In addition to symptoms of nasopharyngeal or sinus disease, which may not be prominent, facial pain and numbness (trigeminal), abducens palsy (sixth cranial nerve), and other cranial nerve palsies may occur. Diagnosis depends on inspection and biopsy of a nasopharyngeal mass, biopsy of an involved cervical gland, and x-ray evidence of erosion of the base of the skull (which is not present in all cases). Not uncommonly a "blind" biopsy of the nasopharynx reveals a thin sheet of submucosal neoplasm. The treatment is x-ray therapy. Carcinoma of ethmoid or sphenoid sinuses may produce a similar clinical picture.

PARANEOPLASTIC NEUROLOGIC SYNDROMES Systemic tumors, apart from their tendency to invade the cranial cavity and spinal canal, may engender a number of special diseases of the nervous system, presently designated as *paraneoplastic*. These diseases, which have no direct relation to invading tumor cells, include

1 Limbic encephalitis
2 Cerebellar degeneration
3 Progressive multifocal leukoencephalopathy
4 Myelitides
5 Polyneuropathies (several types)
6 Dermatomyositis and polymyositis (see Chap. 370)
7 Eaton-Lambert type of myasthenia gravis (see Chap. 372)

Each of these diseases can be diagnosed with relative ease from clinical data and certain special laboratory tests. Each is known to occur in the absence of systemic tumor, or it may precede the clinically recognized tumor by 1 to 2 years. The appearance of the neurologic syndrome thus serves to alert the physician to the possibility of an occult tumor, which if found and removed, may permit recovery from the paraneoplastic disease.

These diseases are regularly associated with certain systemic neoplasms and rarely with others. The most frequent connection is with carcinoma of the lung, particularly the oat-cell tumor (which, unfortunately, is also the most frequent lung tumor), carcinoma of the ovary, and gastric carcinoma.

Actually these paraneoplastic diseases are not esoteric rarities that are encountered only in neurologic institutes. Croft and Wilkinson at the London Hospital found one or more of them in 6.6 percent of cancer patients with solid tumors and 2.2 percent of patients with hematologic lymphoid tumors, particularly multiple myeloma and Hodgkin's disease. Table 358-2 is a listing of the several diseases of this category, along with some of their most prominent features.

Limitations of space permit descriptions of only a few of these syndromes. More complete descriptions of the neoplastic polyneuropathies are contained in Chap. 368, the cerebellar degeneration and encephalitides in Chap. 360, and the muscular diseases in Chap. 370.

Limbic encephalitis There have been reports of approximately 50 cases of a subacute encephalopathic process presenting as a confusional state and followed by a defect in retentive memory. This combination of neurological findings is reminiscent of the clinical picture induced by herpes simplex encephalitis, but, as a rule, the onset and clinical course have been more gradual and there has been no rise in neutralizing antibodies to this or other known viruses. The CSF is abnormal (increased protein and pleocytosis) in some cases. Descriptions of the neuropathology are to be found in the articles of Corsellis et al. and of Forno. Neuronal loss occurs mainly in the medial parts of the temporal lobes and is attended by perivascular and mild meningeal infiltrates of lymphocytes and mononuclear cells and microglial and astrocytic reactions. In two of our patients, dying after a long interval of time (years), only neuronal loss and gliosis remained. Similar, but less severe, changes were found in the cerebellum in approximately half of the cases. No effective treatment has been found.

Other less definitive encephalitic diseases arising in conjunction with systemic tumors are oat-cell carcinoma with bulbar encephalitis and adenocarcinoma with optic neuritis.

Cerebellar and spinocerebellar degeneration Subacute or chronic cerebellar degeneration, sometimes associated with intellectual impairment, is a rare effect of tumors. First described in connection with ovarian carcinoma, its linkage has since been established with carcinomas of lung, breast, uterus, gastrointestinal tract, and with lymphoma. The ataxia involves the legs and arms, deranges gait, and may alter speech. The CSF is usually normal except for slightly elevated levels of protein. A diffuse degeneration of Purkinje cells and, to a lesser extent, of granule cells has been reported. Infiltrations of lymphocytes, present in some cases, are completely absent in others.

TABLE 358-2
Remote effects of cancer on the nervous system

Site	*Frequency (no. of cases)*	*Evolution*	*Clinical involvement*	*Cancer*	*Pathology*
BRAIN					
Encephalomyelitis	50	Months to years	Dementia Memory disturbance	Oat cell	Lymphocytic infiltration (all levels of neuraxis)
Dementia Thalamic degeneration Optic neuritis	All anecdotal				?
CEREBELLUM AND BRAINSTEM					
Subacute to chronic cerebellar degeneration	?	Months	Cerebellar ataxia Nystagmus	Lung Ovary Breast Lymphoma	Purkinje cell loss
Cerebellum-brainstem	?	Weeks	Dancing eyes Myoclonic jerks Cerebellar ataxia	Carcinoma Neuroblastoma	?
SPINAL CORD					
Subacute myelitis	25	Months	Extremity weakness with CSF pleocytosis and hyperactive reflexes	Lung (oat cell)	Anterior horn cells Lymphocytic infiltration
Subacute necrotizing myelopathy	10	Hours to days	Transverse cord lesion	Lung Ovary	Cord necrosis
ROOT AND PERIPHERAL NERVE					
Mixed motor-sensory	7% of all cancers	Months	Distal	Lung Ovary Lymphoma	Segmental demyelination
Pure sensory	50	Weeks to months	Pain Sensory loss	Oat cell	Dorsal root ganglionitis

A special syndrome of *opsoclonus* ("dancing eyes"), *myoclonus* of limbs, and *cerebellar ataxia* has also been observed in a number of our own cases, but its pathological basis is not settled. It resembles the myoclonic syndrome associated with some cases of neuroblastoma in children. There is no known therapy; corticosteroids may have helped a few patients.

Progressive multifocal leukoencephalopathy Adult tumor patients are susceptible to acute and subacute encephalitis from herpes simplex and to a more slowly progressive multifocal leukoencephalopathy (PML) related to the oncogenic JC virus and papovaviruses. At least 200 cases of PML have been described. Most of them have occurred in conjunction with Hodgkin's lymphoma or chronic lymphatic leukemia. These patients present with progressive difficulties in intellectual function, motor weakness, hemisensory loss, hemianopsia, and aphasia, i.e., frontal, temporal, or parietal lobe syndromes. The CSF is unremarkable; EEG abnormalities are uniformly present and tend to be focal; and CT scans show hypodense white-matter lesions. Brain biopsy may lead to therapy with antiviral agents, such as cytosine arabinoside or acycloguanosine, but they have been effective only in some of the cases which were proven to have acute herpes simplex encephalitis.

Subacute and chronic myelitis It is still a matter of controversy whether a form of pure degeneration of motor neurons in the brainstem and spinal cord is ever a remote effect of cancer. There is no doubt, however, as to the existence of a rare chronic poliomyelitis that progresses for several months or a year. In one of our cases of Hodgkin's disease it caused a pure, atrophic, areflexic motor paralysis spreading from limb to limb, and in another patient with squamous-cell carcinoma of the bronchus the same signs, plus a syringomyelic analgesia of shoulders and arms, occurred. The anterior horn cell degeneration was accompanied by microglial neuronophagia, gliosis, and lymphocytic infiltrates. A virus could not be seen under the electron microscope.

Mancall and Rosales have described both an acute and subacute transverse necrotizing myelopathy with cancer.

Polyneuropathies Denny-Brown in 1948 described a subacute to chronic sensory polyneuropathy with disabling ataxia in two patients with carcinoma of the lung. Similar cases have since been reported. More frequent, however, has been a subacute or chronic sensorimotor polyneuropathy with increased CSF protein in patients with lung and other tumors (ovary, stomach, breast, colon) and with multiple myeloma. Also, isolated cases of typical acute Landry-Guillain-Barré syndrome have been observed in tumor patients from time to time.

These chronic polyneuropathies may precede or accompany the primary tumor, but their course does not parallel that of the tumor. The polyneuropathy may remit when the tumor is removed, and there may be a response of a polyneuropathy to corticosteroid therapy while the tumor progresses.

The neuropathology is unclear. In some instances axonal degeneration, Wallerian degeneration, and denervation atrophy of muscles are unattended by any sign of inflammatory or vascular reaction. Lymphocytic infiltrates in perivenous regions of the nerve are seen in other cases. The cause(s) of these polyneuropathies is not known.

Neuropathies in cancer patients must not be confused with some of the neuropathies induced by antitumor therapy, e.g., vincristine or isoniazid.

Dermato- and polymyositis are discussed in Chap. 370 and the Eaton-Lambert syndrome in Chap. 372.

PROGNOSIS The prognosis of intracranial tumor is influenced by the nature of the growth, its location, and other factors. As a general rule, unless an operation is performed, almost all intracranial tumors end fatally. Death in most instances is preceded by a critical rise in intracranial pressure and tentorial or foramen magnum herniation. The more malignant tumors, such as the glioblastoma multiforme, medulloblastoma, and metastatic carcinoma, end fatally within a few months to a year, as a rule, whereas the slowly growing meningiomas and astrocytomas often permit survival for many years.

The prospects for recovery after surgery depend largely on the type of tumor. With meningiomas, pinealomas, craniopharyngiomas, and acoustic neurofibromas, if completely excised, there is complete cure. In gliomas the outlook is more bleak. The period of postoperative survival for glioblastoma is only 6 to 12 months; only 20 percent live for a year and 10 percent for 2 years. This dismal statistic has been slightly if at all lengthened by x-ray treatment and chemotherapy (BCNU). Cure is rare, for seldom can complete excision be accomplished. Nevertheless with the slow-growing gliomas, partial excision, the marsupialization of a cyst, irradiation, and chemotherapy, and the relief of increased intracranial pressure by long-term corticosteroid therapy may lead to improvement and resumption of a useful life for many years. With metastatic growth the outlook is dismal, though if there are no metastases in other organs and the cerebral deposit appears to be solitary, as determined by clinical examination and CT scan, operation occasionally results in temporary recovery for a few months or a year or two.

CONCLUSIONS The physician's responsibilities in this field of intracranial tumors are as follows:

1 Diagnosis. It is essential that the physician separate the tumor cases from all the others which pass through his or her hands.
2 Exclusion of the possibility of the intracranial mass as part of a general disease which would contraindicate surgery, e.g., metastatic carcinoma, syphilis, tuberculosis, parasitic infection.
3 Exclusion of the several pseudotumor syndromes.
4 Recognition of the paraneoplastic syndromes and search for the associated tumor.
5 Maintenance of the patient in the best possible condition until surgery can be undertaken (fluids, electrolytes, corticosteroid therapy, etc.).
6 Assisting the surgeon in the postoperative medical management.

(For tumors of spinal cord and nerves, see Chaps. 366 to 368.)

REFERENCES

Bailey P: *Intracranial Tumors,* 2d ed. Springfield, Charles C Thomas, 1948

Cairncross JG et al: Radiation therapy for metastases. Ann Neurol 7:529, 1980

Caviness WF: Experimental observations: Delayed necrosis of the normal monkey brain, in *Radiation Damage to the Nervous System,* HA Gilbert, AR Kagan (eds). New York, Raven Press, 1980

Corsellis JAN et al: Limbic encephalitis and its association with carcinoma. Brain 91:481, 1968

Forno L: Chronic atypical encephalitis. 6th Internat Congress of Neuropathology. Paris, Masson, 1970, p 1156

Hochberg FH, Pruitt A: Assumptions in the radiotherapy of glioblastoma. Neurology 30:907, 1980

———: Neurological aspects of systemic tumors, in *Update I: Principles of Internal Medicine,* KJ Isselbacher et al (eds). New York, McGraw-Hill, 1981

LITTLE JR, MCCARTHY CS: Colloid cysts of the third ventricle. J Neurosurg 40:230, 1974

LUMSDEN CE: Study of tumors by tissue culture, in *Pathology of Tumors of the Nervous System,* 3d ed. DS Russell, LJ Rubenstein (eds). Baltimore, Williams & Wilkins, 1971

MANCALL EL, ROSALES RK: Necrotizing myelopathy associated with visceral carcinoma. Brain 87:639, 1964

MILHORAT TH: *Hydrocephalus and the Cerebrospinal Fluid.* Baltimore, Williams & Wilkins, 1972

OJEMANN RG et al: Evaluation and surgical treatment of acoustic neuroma. N Engl J Med 289:895, 1972

POSNER J, SHAPIRO WR: Brain tumor. Arch Neurol 32:781, 1978

RUSSELL DS, RUBINSTEIN LJ: *Pathology of Tumors of the Nervous System.* Baltimore, Williams & Wilkins, 1977

SCHOLD SC et al: Cerebrospinal fluid biochemical markers of CNS metastases. Ann Neurol 8:597, 1980

SUSAC J et al: The impossible meningioma. Arch Neurol 34:36, 1977

WALKER MD et al: Randomized comparisons of radiotherapy and nitrosoureas for the treatment of malignant glioma after surgery. N Engl J Med 303:1323, 1980

359 PYOGENIC INFECTIONS OF THE CENTRAL NERVOUS SYSTEM

RAYMOND D. ADAMS
ROBERT G. PETERSDORF

Pyogenic infections of the cranial contents originate in one of two ways, by hematogenous spread or by extension from surface structures—the ears—paranasal sinuses, osteomyelitic foci in the skull, penetrating cranial injuries, congenital sinus tracts, or following neurosurgical procedures.

Surprisingly little is known concerning the hematogenous pathway because human autopsy material seldom divulges information on this point and animal experiments involving the injection of virulent bacteria into the bloodstream have yielded somewhat contradictory results. In most instances of bacteremia the nervous system seems not to be infected, yet in certain cases of pneumonia, bacteremia is the only apparent forerunner of meningitis. In chronic suppurative pulmonary disease, septic venous thrombi become sources of emboli to the brain, and in acute and subacute bacterial endocarditis bacterial emboli are found in cerebral and meningeal arteries.

Experimentally, cerebral tissues are resistant to abscess formation. Direct injection of virulent bacteria into the brain of an animal seldom results in abscess formation. In fact, experimental brain abscess has been produced only by injecting the infected culture medium or by first causing necrosis of the tissue and then inoculating it with bacteria. In human beings infarction of brain tissue by arterial occlusion (embolism) or venous occlusion (thrombophlebitis) appears to be the common and perhaps necessary antecedent.

The cranial epidural and subdural spaces are noticeably inaccessible to bloodborne infection in contrast to the spinal epidural space, where infection is frequently hematogenous. Furthermore, the cranial bones and the dura mater, which serves as the inner periosteum of the skull, protect the cranial cavity against the ingress of bacteria. This protective mechanism may fail if suppuration occurs in the middle ear, mastoid cells or frontal ethmoid, and sphenoid sinuses. Two pathways have been demonstrated in postmortem material:

1 Infected thrombi may form in diploic veins and spread along these vessels into the dural sinuses (into which they flow) and from there in retrograde fashion along the meningeal veins in the brain.

2 An osteomyelitic focus may form, with erosion of the inner table of bone and invasion of the dura, subdural space, piarachnoid, and even the brain substance. Each of these pathways may be visualized in some fatal cases of epidural abscess, subdural empyema, leptomeningitis, cranial venous sinusitis, meningeal thrombophlebitis, and brain abscess. However, in many cases coming to autopsy the pathway cannot be determined.

Hematogenous infections following bacteremia usually permit a single strain or species of virulent organism to gain entry to the cranial cavity (meningococcus, pneumococcus, *Hemophilus influenzae,* or more rarely staphylococcus or gram-negative bacillus). In contrast, septic cerebral emboli from lung abscess or bronchiectasis, or in congenital heart disease, and thrombotic or direct extension from ear or sinus infections may be caused by multiple organisms, which are often anaerobes and consist of peptostreptococci, *Bacteroides,* fusobacteria, *Veillonella, Propionibacterium acnes, Actinomyces,* and others (see Chap. 173). These mixed infections present more complex problems in therapy. If the causative organism is an anaerobe, culture even from the pus of an abscess may be unsuccessful, although the organism can often be demonstrated by Gram's stain. Even in so-called neighborhood infections, however, the bloodstream may be the pathway by which bacteria gain access to the meninges. It has been shown in experimental meningeal infections in mice, for example, that following intranasal infection, bacteria circulate through the blood to reach the meninges via the leptomeningeal vessels.

ACUTE BACTERIAL MENINGITIS

DEFINITION Bacterial meningitis may be defined as an inflammation of the piarachnoid and the fluid residing in the space which it encloses and also that in the ventricles of the brain. Since the subarachnoid space is continuous around the brain, spinal cord, and the optic nerves, an infective agent (or tumor cells or blood) gaining entry to any one part of it may extend immediately to all of it, even its most remote recesses; therefore, meningitis is always *cerebrospinal.* It also reaches the ventricles, either directly or by reflux through the basal foramens of Magendie and Luschka.

PATHOLOGY The effect of bacteria or other organisms in the subarachnoid space is to cause an inflammatory reaction in the pia and arachnoid and in the cerebrospinal fluid (CSF); in pyogenic meningitis, pus accumulates in this space. The infective agent or its toxin, if allowed sufficient time to act, injures those structures which lie within the subarachnoid space (cranial and spinal roots) or ventricles (choroid plexuses) and adjacent to it (pial arteries and veins, underlying cerebral and cerebellar cortices, subpial white matter of the spinal cord, peripheral fibers of optic nerves, ependymal and subependymal tissues). In addition, purulent material may interfere with the flow of CSF from the ventricles or along the subarachnoid space over the brainstem, with resulting obstructive hydrocephalus. Although the outer arachnoidal membrane proves to be a remarkably effective barrier to the extension of infection, some reaction in the cranial subdural space and even the inner surface of the dura and spinal epidural space may occur. This happens more often in infants, approximately 15 percent of whom develop subdural effusions in response to meningitis, than in adults.

The most immediate clinical effects of acute subarachnoid suppuration, distinguishing it from infections in other parts of the body, are severe headache, vomiting, drowsiness, stupor, or coma, and, occasionally, convulsions. The one clinical sign of importance is stiffness of the neck (resistance to passive movement) on forward bending. Kernig and Brudzinski's signs are of the same nature but less reliable. Any circumstance which prolongs the meningitis should increase the risk of injury to all the enumerated structures; this accounts for many features of the clinical picture in the subacute and chronic varieties of meningeal infection.

ETIOLOGY The causes of bacterial meningitis vary with age as follows:

1 *Streptococcus pneumoniae* (see Chap. 146) causes 30 to 50 percent of cases in adults, 10 to 20 percent in children, and up to 5 percent of cases in infants.
2 *Neisseria meningitidis* (see Chap. 149) causes from 10 to 30 percent of cases in adults and from 30 to 40 percent in children up to age 15. It is a rare cause in infants.
3 *Hemophilus influenzae,* type B (see Chap. 156) is responsible for 35 to 45 percent of cases in children, but for only 1 to 3 percent in adults and for virtually none in infants.

Also important in the etiology of meningitis are *Staphylococcus aureus* and *Staph. epidermidis,* the latter accounting for 75 percent of infections associated with shunting procedures for hydrocephalus; group B streptococci, particularly in infants; anaerobic or microaerophilic streptococci and gram-negative bacilli, usually in association with brain abscess, epidural abscess, head trauma, neurosurgical procedures, or cranial thrombophlebitis; *Escherichia coli* and other Enterobacteriaceae such as *Klebsiella-Enterobacter, Proteus,* and *Citrobacter;* and *Pseudomonas,* usually as a consequence of lumbar puncture, spinal anesthesia, or shunting procedures to relieve hydrocephalus, also are important causes of meningitis. Heretofore, gram-negative bacilli were associated most often with neonatal meningitis, but the spectrum has shifted to adults with the predisposing causes cited. The outcome in this group has been notoriously poor. Rare meningeal pathogens include *Salmonella, Shigella, Clostridium perfringens,* and *N. gonorrheae.*

The changing etiology of bacterial meningitis is reflected by the appearance of *Listeria monocytogenes* as a major pathogen, particularly in elderly, debilitated patients or in those with immunosuppression secondary to transplantation, therapy for cancer, or with connective tissue diseases. Alcoholism and high-dose steroids also appear to be predisposing factors. The mortality rate in the adult group with severe underlying disease is 70 percent.

EPIDEMIOLOGY AND CLINICAL SETTING Pneumococcal, *H. influenzae,* and meningococcal infections have a worldwide distribution, tending to occur more often in males and during the fall, winter, and spring. *H. influenzae* meningitis is the most frequent meningeal infection in children between 2 months and 3 years of age. Meningococcal infections occur most often in children and adolescents, but they are also encountered throughout most of adult life with a sharp decline after age 50. Pneumococcal meningitis predominates in adults over 40 years of age.

A variety of factors apart from age predispose to the development of certain types of acute bacterial meningitis. Acute otitis media and mastoiditis occur in about 25 percent of patients with pneumococcal meningitis and pneumonia in another 25 percent. Recent head injury is recorded in 10 to 20 percent of patients with pneumococcal meningitis and may give rise to recurrent meningitis because of persistent cerebrospinal fluid rhinorrhea. Pneumococcal meningitis also occurs in patients with sickle cell disease, and in urban general hospitals many adults who develop pneumococcal infections suffer from chronic alcoholism. Immunoglobulin deficiency, whether congenital or acquired, and splenectomy also predispose patients to pneumococcal infection. Adults who develop *H. influenzae* meningitis should be suspected of harboring an anatomical defect (dermal sinus tract, old fracture, empty-sella syndrome) or abnormality of immune defenses. Meningitis caused by *Staph. aureus* usually follows neurosurgical procedures or a penetrating cranial wound. This organism and *Staph. epidermidis* account for the majority of cerebral ventricular shunt infections and occasionally neonatal omphalitis and meningitis. Gram-negative bacillary infections also complicate neurosurgical operations and other nosocomial diseases, and are assuming progressively greater importance in meningitis in adults.

PATHOGENESIS The three common meningeal pathogens are invasive and depend upon antiphagocytic capsular or surface antigens for survival in the tissues of the infected host; all express their pathogenicity largely in the form of extracellular proliferation. All three are inhabitants of the nasopharynx in a significant part of the population. It is evident from the frequency with which the carrier state is detected that nasal colonization is not a sufficient explanation for infection of the meninges. The factors which predispose the colonized patient to bloodstream invasion, which is the usual route by which bacteria reach the meninges, are obscure but include antecedent viral infections of the upper respiratory passages or, as in the case of the pneumococcus, infections in the lung. Once bloodborne, the factors which lead to meningeal localization of bacteria are unknown, but it has been postulated that pneumococci, *H. influenzae,* and meningococci possess a unique predilection for the meninges. Other possibilities are that the entry of bacteria into the subarachnoid space is facilitated by disruption of the blood-CSF barrier by trauma, circulating endotoxin, or an initial viral infection of the meninges.

Avenues other than the bloodstream by which bacteria can gain access to the meninges include congenital neuroectodermal defects, craniotomy sites, diseases of the middle ear and paranasal sinuses, and cranial trauma, notably skull fractures. Occasionally brain abscesses may rupture into the subarachnoid space or ventricles, infecting the meninges. The isolation of anaerobic streptococci, *Bacteroides* spp., or *Actinomyces,* or a mixture of microorganisms in the CSF should suggest the possibility of a brain abscess occurring as an antecedent to meningitis.

SYMPTOMATOLOGY Fever, headache, seizures, vomiting, impairment of consciousness, and stiff neck and back are common to bacterial meningitis irrespective of its etiology. When the initial symptoms are pain in the neck or abdomen, a confusional state or delirium, the diagnosis is much more difficult. Three patterns of onset have been documented. In approximately 25 percent of patients, meningitis has a fulminant onset and patients become seriously ill within 24 h, usually without antecedent respiratory tract infections. In over 50 percent, meningitis develops over 1 to 7 days and is associated with respiratory symptoms. Slightly less than 20 percent have meningeal symptoms after 1 to 3 weeks of respiratory symptoms.

In children, the onset is often nonspecific. Fever and vomiting are more frequent than headache. There is a higher incidence of seizures, and the error of misinterpreting seizures as febrile convulsions is greater.

There are certain special clinical features that correlate with particular types of meningitis. Meningococcal meningitis should always be suspected in epidemics of meningitis, when the evolution is extremely rapid, when the onset is attended by a morbilliform, petechial, or purpuric skin eruption, larger ecchymoses and lividity of skin of lower parts of the body, and if circulatory collapse has occurred. Since a rash accompanies approximately 50 percent of meningococcal infections, its presence should dictate immediate institution of therapy for a neisserial infection, even though similar rashes may be observed with echo 9 meningitis and rarely staphylococcal, *H. influenzae,* and streptococcal meningitis. Pneumococcal meningitis is usually preceded by an infection in the lungs, ears, and sinuses, and the heart valves may be affected. In addition a pneumococcal etiology should be suspected in patients suffering from alcoholism, sickle cell disease, and basal skull fracture, and following splenectomy. *Hemophilus influenzae* meningitis usually follows upper respiratory and ear infections in young children.

The signs of meningeal irritation—stiff neck or positive Kernig and Brudzinski's signs—may be absent in the very young, the very old, or the severely obtunded. Signs of focal cerebral disease, although seldom prominent, are more frequent in pneumococcal and influenzal meningitis and are associated with a comparatively poor prognosis. Seizures are encountered most often in infants with *H. influenzae* meningitis. In some instances they are caused by hypoglycemia or penicillin neurotoxicity, especially the latter if they are preceded by myoclonus of the face and extremities. Some of the more transitory focal cerebral signs may represent postictal phenomena (Todd's paralysis), whereas stable, local, cerebral lesions are probably the result of vasculitis and occlusion of cerebral veins with infarction of cerebral tissue, or they may connote localization of pus as occurs in brain abscess or subdural empyema. Abnormalities involving the third, fourth, and sixth as well as other cranial nerves are particularly frequent with pneumococcal meningitis.

LABORATORY FINDINGS The alterations of the cerebrospinal fluid are diagnostic. The number of leukocytes in the CSF ranges between 1000 and 100,000 per milliliter but averages 5000 to 20,000. Cell counts above 50,000 per milliliter raise suspicion of the possibility of a brain abscess having ruptured into the ventricle (ventricular empyema). Neutrophilic leukocytes generally predominate, but an increasing proportion of mononuclear cells are found in the exudate as the infection continues, especially in partially treated meningitis. In the early stages careful cytological examination may reveal some of the mononuclear cells to be myelocytes or young neutrophils. Later as treatment takes effect, the proportions of lymphocytes, plasma cells, and histiocytes steadily increase.

The pressure of the *cerebrospinal fluid* is so consistently elevated (above 180 mm water) that a normal or low pressure on the initial lumbar puncture in a case of suspected bacterial meningitis should raise the possibility that the needle was partially occluded or that the spinal arachnoid space was blocked.

The *protein levels* of CSF are higher than 45 mg/dl in 90 percent of cases, and most determinations fall in the range of 150 to 500 mg/dl.

The sugar concentration of CSF is depressed, usually to a level lower than 40 mg/dl or less than 40 percent of the blood sugar concentration (measured concomitantly), provided the latter is less than 250 mg/dl. However in atypical or "culture-negative cases," other conditions associated with a depressed CSF glucose should be considered. These include hypoglycemia from any cause, sarcoidosis of the central nervous system, meningeal carcinomatosis or gliomatosis, fungal or tuberculous meningitis, and subarachnoid hemorrhage. In acute cases of pyogenic meningitis, the CSF glucose concentration often approaches zero.

Gram's stain of sedimented CSF permits identification of the causative agent in most cases of bacterial meningitis; pneumococci and *H. influenzae* are identified more readily than meningococci. Small numbers of gram-negative diplococci present within leukocytes may be indistinguishable from nuclear material which may also be gram-negative and of the same shape. In such cases a thin film of uncentrifuged CSF may lend itself more readily to morphological interpretation than a smear of sedimented CSF. The commonest error in reading gram-stained smears of CSF is misinterpretation of precipitated dye or debris as gram-positive cocci, or a confusion of pneumococci with *H. influenzae. Hemophilus* organisms may stain heavily at the poles so that they resemble gram-positive diplococci, and older pneumococci often lose their capacity to take a gram-positive stain.

Cerebrospinal fluid cultures are positive in 70 to 80 percent of cases. When brain abscess is suspected, anaerobic cultures should be made, and meningococci should be cultured under 10% CO_2 (see Chap. 136). Partially treated meningitis poses a most difficult problem in diagnosis because cultures are often negative. The measurement of bacterial antigen in the CSF by countercurrent immune electrophoresis (CIE) to determine the presence of a specific capsular polysaccharide associated with *H. influenzae, S. pneumoniae,* and *N. meningitidis* has been helpful. It has limited value in *E. coli* and streptococcal group B infections. The concentration of bacterial antigen diminishes as treatment progresses. Failure to detect antigen does not rule out bacterial meningitis.

The *Limulus* amebocyte gelation assay for endotoxin has not been of practical value. The level of CSF lactic acid exceeds 35 mg/dl (range 35 to 700) in bacterial meningitis and falls below 35 mg/dl in viral meningitis. The levels of the LDH isoenzymes 4 and 5 are elevated markedly (mean, 113 units; normal, 2 to 7), whereas the level is on an average of 23 units in viral meningitis and the isoenzymes consist mainly of fractions 1 and 2. Isoenzymes 4 and 5 probably come from neutrophilic leukocytes and 1 and 2 from brain tissue.

In addition to CSF cultures, *blood cultures* should always be obtained because they are positive in 40 to 60 percent of patients with *H. influenzae* and with meningococcal and pneumococcal meningitis and may provide the only definitive clue to the causative agent (if CSF cultures are negative). Routine cultures of the pharynx or external ear are as often misleading as helpful because pneumococci, *H. influenzae,* and meningococci are such common inhabitants of these locations. However, culture of pus from the middle ear or sinuses is often helpful.

The *blood leukocyte count* is generally elevated, and usually there is a shift to the left. Most patients with meningitis are sufficiently ill to require determination of blood urea nitrogen and serum electrolytes. These may be abnormal because of severe dehydration and may reveal inappropriate secretion of antidiuretic hormone (ADH) with resultant hyponatremia.

ROENTGENOGRAPHIC STUDIES Patients with bacterial meningitis should have x-rays of the chest, skull, and sinuses as soon as possible after admission. Chest x-rays are particularly important because they may reveal a silent area of pneumonitis or abscess. Sinus and skull films may provide clues to the presence of cranial osteomyelitis, paranasal sinusitis, or skull fracture. Computerized tomography (CT scan) is usually not necessary in bacterial meningitis and is normal early in most infections. In severe cases there may be evidence of cerebritis, vascular occlusions, and encephalomalacia. Later in the course, CT will detect hydrocephalus, brain abscess, and subdural effusions or subdural empyema.

COMPLICATIONS OF BACTERIAL MENINGITIS The longer the duration of meningitis and the less effective the treatment, the greater the chances that complications and neurological residua will develop. The cranial nerve palsies which occur in some 10 to 20 percent of cases usually disappear within a few weeks. Approximately 20 percent of patients over 3 years of age have partial or complete neurosensory deafness. If it is partial, there may be some recovery. The cochlea may be damaged by infection as it passes from the meninges along the cochlear duct. Deafness is especially frequent with meningococcal meningitis. If focal and lateralizing neurological signs last for some days or occur late in the course of meningitis, they are usually indicative of a vasculitis and cerebral infarction. Such lesions are most extensive in children with *H. influenzae* meningitis who are inadequately treated. If these lesions are extensive, they may leave the child retarded and epileptic. Persistent coma is more common in pneumococcal meningitis in adults, and in *H. influenzae* in children should raise the suspicion of obstructive hydrocephalus and subdural effusions.

DIFFERENTIAL DIAGNOSIS The diagnosis of bacterial meningitis is not difficult, providing a high index of suspicion is maintained. All febrile patients with lethargy, headache, or confusion of sudden onset, even if only low-grade fever is present, should be subjected to lumbar puncture. It is particularly important to consider meningitis in febrile, confused alcoholic patients. Too often the symptoms are mistakenly ascribed to inebriation, delirium tremens, or hepatic encephalopathy until the CSF reveals a meningitis.

Bacterial meningitis can be diagnosed definitively only by examination of the CSF. Viral meningoencephalitis and tuberculous, leptospiral, and fungal meningitides often enter into the differential diagnosis. Also to be considered are Behçet's syndrome, a disease characterized by recurrent oral and genital ulcers along with meningitis, and Mollaret's meningitis, which consists of recurrent episodes of fever, headache, and meningeal irritation accompanied by a leukocytosis in the CSF.

The diagnosis of other intracranial suppurative diseases is detailed below.

PROGNOSIS The mortality rate of *H. influenzae* or meningococcal meningitis has remained fixed at 5 to 15 percent for many years. Also in meningococcal infection, because of the fulminating nature of the disease and the often complicating adrenocortical necrosis (Waterhouse-Friderichsen syndrome), the mortality rate remains significant. Old age, infancy, abrupt onset, bacteremia, coma, seizures, and a variety of concomitant diseases including alcoholism, diabetes mellitus, multiple myeloma, and head trauma all worsen the prognosis. The triad of pneumococcal meningitis, pneumonia, and endocarditis has a particularly high fatality rate.

It is often impossible to explain the death of the patient or at least to trace it to a single specific mechanism. Bacteremia with hypotension or brain swelling and bilateral temporal or uncal and cerebellar herniation are clearly implicated in the deaths of some patients during the initial 48 h. These events may occur in bacterial meningitis of any etiology; however, some observations suggest that they are more important in meningococcal infection. There is experimental evidence that acute centrally mediated respiratory failure (rather than circulatory collapse) is the major mechanism of early death. Deaths occurring later during the course of illness may be attributed to cerebral necrosis and respiratory failure, often consequent to aspiration pneumonia.

TREATMENT **Antimicrobials** Bacterial meningitis is a medical emergency; the rapid destruction of bacteria in the meninges and in the CSF is essential to survival. For this reason, bactericidal drugs should be used where possible. The following therapeutic regimens are recommended:

1 For adults with *pneumococcal* or *meningococcal meningitis,* penicillin G, 20 to 24 million units intravenously each day in four to six divided doses, is recommended; for children the dose of penicillin G should be 300,000 units per kilogram of body weight; and for neonates, 150,000 to 200,000 units per kilogram of body weight.
2 For children over 2 months of age with *H. influenzae* or uncomplicated meningitis of unknown etiology, ampicillin, 300 to 400 mg per kilogram of body weight intravenously in divided doses, plus chloramphenicol, 100 to 200 mg/kg per day intravenously, should be given. The reason for the use of two drugs is the progressive increase in the number of ampicillin-resistant *H. influenzae* from patients with meningitis; a few strains of chloramphenicol-resistant *H. influenzae* have also been reported. In order to avoid interference between the two drugs, ampicillin should be given 30 min before chloramphenicol. Once the etiologic organism and its sensitivity have been determined, chloramphenicol can be discontinued if the organism is sensitive to ampicillin. In adults with *H. influenzae* meningitis, the daily doses of ampicillin and chloramphenicol are 12 and 4 to 6 g, respectively (administered intravenously either as a constant infusion or in divided doses).
3 In adult patients with any of these types of bacterial meningitis who may be allergic to the penicillins, chloramphenicol in a dosage of 4 to 6 g per day intravenously may be used. The cephalosporins are questionable alternates for pneumococcal meningitis, and there have been some failures also in *H. influenzae* and meningococcal meningitis; hence, chloramphenicol is preferred in infections due to these organisms.
4 For meningitis due to Enterobacteriaceae (excepting *Pseudomonas*), the drug of choice is gentamicin in dosage of 5 mg/kg per day administered intramuscularly or intravenously in divided doses at 6-h intervals. This drug can be given intravenously, but many prefer the intramuscular route to avoid high blood levels which may lead to respiratory paralysis and permanent damage to inner ears. Chloramphenicol, 4 to 6 g per day in adults and 50 to 100 mg/kg in children, should be given intravenously. Because of gentamicin's poor penetration into the CSF, the drug should also be given intrathecally in doses of 2.0 to 5.0 mg per day as long as CSF cultures remain positive. Some prefer intracisternal to intralumbar administration to assure better mixing of drug. The treatment for *Pseudomonas* meningitis is similar except that carbenicillin in doses of 30 to 40 g per day should be substituted for chloramphenicol.
5 Meningitis due to *S. aureus* should be treated with nafcillin, 12.0 g per day intravenously (200 to 300 mg/kg in children). Because penetration of the penicillins into the CSF is variable, even when the meninges are inflamed, the course of the infection should be monitored carefully, and chloramphenicol should be added if symptoms persist or the CSF remains infected. Intrathecal bacitracin, 5000 to 10,000 units given very slowly in 10 ml of CSF in adults, may be added in refractory cases. Some of the third-generation cephalosporins may have better penetrability into the CSF than earlier drugs of this class, but more experience is needed. Patients allergic to the penicillins should receive vancomycin, 2.0 g intravenously in divided doses.
6 When the etiology of meningitis is unknown, the drugs of choice are as follows: in adults, ampicillin 12 g per day in divided doses; in children, ampicillin 400 mg/kg and chloramphenicol 100 mg/kg; and in neonates, ampicillin 100 to 200 mg/kg and gentamicin 5 mg/kg.
7 Foci of infection in the paranasal sinuses, mastoids, in an infected shunt, or in cranial osteomyelitis should be identified so that appropriate drainage may be carried out when the acute episode of meningitis has subsided.
8 In most patients bacterial meningitis need not be treated for longer than 10 days except when there is a persistent parameningeal focus of infection. Antibiotics should be administered in full doses parenterally (preferably intravenously)

throughout the period of treatment. Treatment failures with several drugs, notably ampicillin, are attributable to oral or intramuscular administration, resulting in inadequate concentration in the CSF.

9 Repeated lumbar punctures are not necessary to follow the course of therapy as long as the patient is doing well. The CSF sugar may remain low for a number of days after cultures become negative and should occasion concern only if bacteria are present. Likewise, persistent but steadily diminishing mononuclear pleocytosis, following pyogenic meningitis, is the rule.

Adrenocortical steroids The few controlled studies available have demonstrated that steroids exert no beneficial effects in pyogenic meningitis. These drugs should not be used except possibly in overwhelming meningococcal sepsis or as an adjunct to intravenous mannitol in severe cerebral edema.

Other forms of therapy Intrathecal administration of enzymes to lyse excessive subarachnoid cellular exudate which may be associated with spinal block or hydrocephalus in the subacute stages of bacterial meningitis is of no value. There is also no evidence to support the therapeutic efficacy of repeated drainage of CSF. In fact, increased CSF pressure in the acute phases of bacterial meningitis is largely a consequence of cerebral edema, and lumbar puncture may predispose to temporal lobe or cerebellar herniation and death. Mannitol and urea have been employed apparently successfully in some cases of severe brain swelling with unusually high initial CSF pressures ($>$ 400 mmH_2O). Either should be accompanied by dexamethasone in relatively high doses. An adequate but not excessive amount of parenteral fluids should be given, and phenylhydantoin should be given to control seizures (see Chap. 355). In children care should be taken to avoid hyponatremia and water intoxication—a cause of brain swelling. Subdural effusions should be drained repeatedly by subdural taps; if they persist after the infection has subsided, surgical removal may become necessary.

RECURRENT MENINGITIS

Recurrent attacks of bacterial meningitis usually follow in the wake of trauma. The interval between the traumatic episode and the initial bout of posttraumatic meningitis may be as long as several years. *S. pneumoniae* is the usual bacterial pathogen. Often it proves to be one of the higher serologic types, reflecting the predominance of such strains in nasal carriers. *Cerebrospinal fluid rhinorrhea* is present in most of these patients but may be transient. The patient with recurrent meningitis of inapparent origin should always be suspected of having a fistulous connection between the nasal sinuses and the subarachnoid space. The fistula is usually traumatic (old basal skull fracture), and the site is the frontal or ethmoid sinuses or the cribriform plate. The rhinorrhea may be difficult to demonstrate except by injection of a dye, such as carmine red, or radioactive albumin into the spinal fluid and watching for its appearance in nasal secretions. Cerebrospinal fluid rhinorrhea may also be detected by measuring the glucose concentration of nasal secretions. The usual mucous secretions contain little glucose, but in CSF rhinorrhea the amount approximates that in CSF. The prognosis in recurrent meningitis is remarkably benign, and the mortality is much lower than in ordinary pneumococcal meningitis. Nevertheless, vaccination of these patients with pneumococcal vaccine is indicated, and long-term prophylactic chemotherapy with penicillin V should be considered. Treatment of recurrent meningitis is similar to that for first bouts. Attempts to demonstrate CSF rhinorrhea should be made only after the acute infection has subsided; if evidence of a fistula is found, surgical repair should be considered. Recurrent meningitis due to *N. meningitidis* has been reported in a patient with C8 and IgA deficiency.

Other causes of recurrent meningitis include congenital dermal sinus tract, empty-sella syndrome, and tumors at the base of the skull.

SUBDURAL EMPYEMA

DEFINITION Subdural empyema is a suppurative process in the cranial subdural space between the inner surface of the dura and the outer of the arachnoid. The proper term for this condition is not *abscess* but *empyema,* indicating suppuration in a preformed space. About three-fourths of cases are unilateral, and the remainder bilateral, usually in the parafalcial region.

ETIOLOGY The infection usually gains entry to the subdural space from the frontal or ethmoid sinuses, or, less often, from the mastoid cells. These cases are termed *primary* subdural empyema. Occasionally the subdural space becomes infected by extension of bacteria from the CSF or from a brain abscess. Rarely has it been observed with bloodstream infections. The flora in subdural empyema is usually polymicrobial and consists of anaerobes (streptococci and *Bacteroides*) and aerobes (*H. influenzae, Staph. aureus, Klebsiella,* and *E. coli*). *Secondary* subdural empyema usually follows neurosurgical drainage of a chronic subdural hematoma.

PATHOLOGY A collection of subdural pus in quantities of a few milliliters to 100 to 200 ml lies over the cerebral hemisphere. It is often mistaken for meningitis. The arachnoid, when cleared of exudate, is cloudy, and thrombosis of meningeal veins may be seen. The underlying cerebral hemisphere is depressed, and in fatal cases there is often an ipsilateral temporal lobe pressure cone. Microscopic studies demonstrate various degrees of organization of the exudate on the inner surface of the dura, and infiltration of the underlying pia with small numbers of neutrophilic leukocytes, lymphocytes, and mononuclear cells. There is superficial thrombophlebitis; the thrombi in cerebral veins appear to begin on the outer side (toward the empyema). The thrombosis extends to other dural sinuses, and the superficial layers of the cerebral cortex undergo ischemic necrosis, which probably accounts for the unilateral seizures and signs of disordered cerebral function.

SYMPTOMATOLOGY AND LABORATORY FINDINGS The usual history includes chronic sinusitis and mastoiditis with a recent flare-up and evidence of local pain and increase in purulent nasal or aural discharge. Generalized headache, fever, and a depressed sensorium are the first indications of intracranial spread. They are followed within a few days by localizing signs including focal motor seizures, hemiplegia, hemianesthesia, and aphasia. Stupor or coma develops rapidly as the cerebral symptoms progress. Fever is usually present, but the neck is not always stiff. When CSF is examined, increased pressure, raised white blood cell count in the range of 50 to 1000 per milliliter including both neutrophils and lymphocytes, elevated protein concentration (75 to 300 mg/dl), and normal sugar values are the usual findings. The CSF is sterile. Lumbar puncture poses a distinct risk because it may precipitate transtentorial herniation. In the type of subdural empyema that follows drainage of a chronic subdural hematoma, the onset is more indolent, fever is lower, and there is usually a local wound infection.

DIAGNOSIS Skull films may show involvement of the sinus or mastoid. The most useful diagnostic procedures are the CT scan and carotid arteriography, which disclose inward displacement of meningeal vessels and contralateral shift of the anterior cerebral arteries. CT scans are not always positive in primary subdural empyemas, and angiography is the procedure of choice. In secondary empyemas, CT scan is invariably positive. Four conditions need to be distinguished clinically from subdural empyema: cerebral thrombophlebitis, brain abscess, acute hemorrhagic leukoencephalitis, and acute hemorrhagic viral (inclusion body) encephalitis (see Chap. 360).

TREATMENT Drainage of pus is the single most important part of treatment. In particular, it is important to institute drainage early because delaying it sharply increases the mortality rate. Appropriate antibiotic therapy consists of 20 million units of penicillin per day plus chloramphenicol, 4 g per day, aimed particularly at *Bacteroides*, administered intravenously. Without such massive antimicrobial therapy and surgery, most patients will die, usually within 7 to 14 days, often while the unsuspecting physician and surgeon are waiting for better localization of an assumed cerebral abscess, the most commonly mistaken diagnosis. On the other hand, successfully treated patients may make a surprisingly good recovery, including full or partial resolution of their focal neurological deficits.

EXTRADURAL ABSCESS

This condition is almost invariably associated with osteomyelitis in a cranial bone which originates from an infection in the ear or paranasal sinuses. Pus and granulation tissue accumulate on the outer surface of the dura, separating it from the cranial bone. Symptomatically, the effects are those of a local inflammatory process: frontal or auricular pain, purulent discharge from the sinuses or ear, and fever and local tenderness. Sometimes the neck is slightly stiff. Localizing neurological signs are usually absent. Rarely a fifth and sixth cranial nerve palsy appears with infections of the petrous part of the temporal bone (petrositis with Gradenigo's syndrome), or a focal seizure may occur. The CSF is usually clear and under normal pressure but may contain a few lymphocytes and neutrophils (20 to 100 per milliliter) and slightly raised protein concentration. Treatment consists of antibiotics aimed at the appropriate pathogen which may be *Staph. aureus,* anaerobic streptococci, *Bacteroides* spp., or Enterobacteriaceae. The primary sinusitis or mastoiditis, from which the extradural infection has arisen, may require surgical drainage.

SPINAL EPIDURAL ABSCESS

This type of abscess possesses unique clinical features and constitutes an important neurological and neurosurgical emergency. It is discussed in Chap. 366.

INTRACRANIAL THROMBOPHLEBITIS

The lateral, cavernous, and superior longitudinal sinuses are relatively uncommon sites of infection. Usually there is evidence that the intracranial process has extended from the middle ear and mastoid cells, the paranasal sinuses, and skin around the upper lip, nose, and eyes.

LATERAL SINUS THROMBOPHLEBITIS In lateral sinus thrombophlebitis, which usually follows chronic mastoiditis, the earache and mastoid tenderness are succeeded, after a period of days to a few weeks, by generalized headache and papilledema. As a rule there are no other neurological signs. As a diagnostic aid, compression of the jugular veins separately, during the Queckenstedt maneuver, will demonstrate failure of the CSF pressure to rise when the ipsilateral one is compressed (Tobey-Ayer test). When the intracranial pressure is greatly elevated, the suspicion of cerebellar abscess is raised, but this process is usually characterized by other neurological signs, especially nystagmus to the side of the lesion and ataxia of the arm and leg.

CAVERNOUS SINUS THROMBOPHLEBITIS In this condition, which is usually secondary to oculonasal infections, the clinical syndrome is one of orbital edema, chemosis, venous congestion, and evidence of palsy of the third, fourth, ophthalmic fifth, and sixth cranial nerves. Later spread through the circular sinus to the opposite cavernous sinus results in bilateral symptoms and signs. The posterior part of the cavernous sinus may be infected via the superior and inferior petrosal veins without the occurrence of orbital edema or ophthalmoplegia. The CSF is usually normal unless there is associated meningitis or subdural empyema. The only effective therapy in the fulminant variety, associated with thrombosis of the anterior portion of the sinus, has been antimicrobial therapy usually aimed at coagulase-positive staphylococci (see Chap. 147), and occasionally gram-negative pathogens as well. Anticoagulants have been used occasionally, but their value has not been proved. Cavernous sinus thrombosis must be differentiated from mucormycosis which may cause a similar clinical picture in uncontrolled diabetics or in immunosuppressed patients (see Chap. 184).

THROMBOPHLEBITIS OF THE SUPERIOR LONGITUDINAL SINUS Although occasionally asymptomatic, the typical clinical syndrome is one of unilateral convulsions and hemiplegia, first on one side of the body, then on the other, because of extension into the superior cerebral veins. The paralysis may be predominantly monoplegic and involve mainly the legs. Headache, papilledema, and increased intracranial pressure may accompany these signs. The diagnosis can be corroborated by demonstrating a sluggish circulation and failure of the superior sagittal sinus to fill during the late stage of the carotid arteriogram. Treatment consists of large doses of antibiotics and temporization until the thrombus recanalizes.

All types of thrombophlebitis, especially those related to ear and paranasal sinus infection, may be complicated by other forms of intracranial suppuration including bacterial meningitis, subdural empyema, or brain abscess. Therapy in these patients must be individualized. The initiating focus should be brought under control by surgery if necessary, once the patient's condition permits such a procedure. To operate on the primary focus before medical treatment is instituted is to court disaster. The better plan is to institute antibiotic therapy; surgery on the ears or sinuses should be decided upon only after the infection is well controlled.

ASEPTIC THROMBOSIS OF INTRACRANIAL VENOUS SINUSES This may develop after sinus and ear infections and may lead to an obscure increase in intracranial pressure because of the occlusion of one lateral or superior sagittal sinus. The more common conditions which may be accompanied by aseptic thrombosis are postpartum and postoperative states, which are often characterized by thrombocytosis and hyperfibrinogenemia; congenital heart disease and marasmus in infants; sickle cell disease; and primary or secondary polycythemia.

BRAIN ABSCESS

PATHOGENESIS Most of the focal suppurative intracranial processes of this type are linked to chronic ear and sinus or pulmonary infections. Nearly half of all brain abscesses are secondary to disease of the middle ear and mastoid cells, and of these about one-third arise in the anterolateral part of the cerebellar hemisphere and the remainder (lying above the tegmen tympani) in the middle and inferior part of the temporal lobe. Frontal sinusitis accounts for roughly 10 percent of the cases, the abscess being almost invariably situated in the anterior and inferior part of the frontal lobe. Of the remaining cases, a small portion are due to penetrating wounds or postoperative infections, and the rest are metastatic. Of the latter, about half are traceable to a primary septic focus in the lung, usually bronchiectasis, empyema, lung abscess, or bronchopleural fistula, and in the rest, the source of infection may be the skin, bone, i.e., a focus of osteomyelitis, or the heart. In 5 to 10 percent of cases, the source cannot be ascertained. Brain abscess is almost never a consequence of bacterial meningitis.

Brain abscesses are particularly frequent with congenital heart disease with right-to-left shunts (e.g., tetralogy of Fallot), and they may also complicate arteriovenous vascular abnormalities of the lung, as in cases of familial telangiectasia. With cranial trauma the location of the abscess will depend on the site of the penetrating wound. Metastatic abscesses are most likely to occur in the distal territory of the middle cerebral arteries. In contrast to the otogenic and rhinogenic abscesses, they may be multiple.

Bacterial endocarditis rarely gives rise to brain abscess. Instead, the picture is one of focal embolic encephalitis with or without signs of embolic vascular disease elsewhere (see Chap. 259). In subacute endocarditis the emboli are sterile and cause only infarction, miliary foci of tissue necrosis, focal meningeal inflammation, and mycotic aneurysms. The CSF may contain a small number of neutrophilic leukocytes, lymphocytes, and red blood cells; the protein level may be elevated, but cultures are sterile and sugar values remain normal. In acute bacterial endocarditis, miliary abscesses and purulent meningitis may develop, or there may be infarcts, and subarachnoid or intracerebral hemorrhages secondary to rupture of a mycotic aneurysm. Rarely do the miliary abscesses progress to large ones. Rapidly evolving cerebral signs in endocarditis are nearly always caused by embolic infarction or hemorrhage.

ETIOLOGY The most common organisms causing brain abscess are streptococci, most of which are anaerobic or microaerophilic. These organisms are often found in combinations with other anaerobes, notably *Bacteroides,* and may also be combined with Enterobacteriaceae, such as *E. coli, Klebsiella-Enterobacter,* and *Proteus.* Staphylococci also may cause brain abscess, but pneumococci, meningococci, and *H. influenzae* rarely do so. In addition to *Bacteroides* and anaerobic streptococci, anaerobic actinomyces, veillonellae, and fusobacteria have been isolated. The bacterial species vary with the site of the abscess; staphylococcal abscesses are usually a consequence of penetrating head trauma or of bacteremia; enteric organisms are almost always associated with otitic infections, while anaerobic streptococci are commonly metastatic from the lung.

PATHOLOGY Localized inflammatory necrosis and edema, septic thrombosis of vessels, and aggregates of degenerating leukocytes (suppurative encephalitis), represent the early reaction to bacterial invasion of the brain. This is followed within a few weeks by encapsulation of the liquefied brain and of accumulated pus. The lesion becomes encapsulated by fibroblasts and newly formed vessels, and the capsule thickens over a period of weeks. The meninges adjacent to the abscess, especially near the point of entry of infection, are infiltrated by neutrophils, lymphocytes, and plasma cells.

CLINICAL MANIFESTATIONS In patients with chronic ear, sinus, or pulmonary infections, a recent reactivation of the infection usually precedes the onset of cerebral symptoms. In a number of patients evidence of central nervous system invasion is acute and fever, headache, vomiting, increasing obtundation, seizures, and a variety of localizing neurological signs appear within a few days. In other patients, bacterial invasion of the brain substance may be asymptomatic or may be attended only by a transitory focal neurological disorder, as may happen with lodgment of a septic embolus. Sometimes stiff neck accompanies generalized headache, suggesting the diagnosis of meningitis (especially a partially treated one). However, the CSF shows only a few cells, normal or slightly increased protein concentration, and normal sugar concentration. These early symptoms may subside or they may appear to respond to antimicrobials, but within a few weeks, recurrent headache, slowness in mentation, focal or generalized convulsions, and obvious signs of increased intracranial pressure provide evidence of an inflammatory mass in the brain. At this stage, the symptoms of infection are not conspicuous. While fever is characteristic of the invasive phase best described as suppurative encephalitis, as the abscess becomes encapsulated, the temperature returns to normal. Indeed, if the invasive stage of cerebral infection is inconspicuous, the entire clinical picture does not differ from that of brain tumor. In the later stages of abscess formation, the CSF pressure is usually elevated and there is nearly always pleocytosis between 25 and 300 cells per milliliter consisting both of neutrophils and lymphocytes and an elevation of protein between 75 and 300 mg per 100 ml with CSF glucose remaining normal.

The focal neurological signs depend on the location of the abscess as follows.

Temporal lobe abscess Headache is usually on the side of the abscess and is localized to the frontotemporal region. If the abscess lies in the dominant hemisphere, there is a dysphasia of the amnestic type (inability to name objects). A homonymous upper quadrantic field defect may also be demonstrable—the inferior portion of the optic radiation is interrupted—and this may be the only sign in abscess of the right temporal lobe. Contralateral motor or sensory defects in the limbs tend to be minimal, though weakness of the lower face is often observed.

Cerebellar abscess Headache in the postauricular or suboccipital region is usually the first symptom and may at first be ascribed to infection in the mastoid cells. Coarse nystagmus and gaze weakness to the side of the lesion and a cerebellar ataxia of the ipsilateral arm and leg are present in most patients, though the ataxia may be difficult to demonstrate if the patient is very ill. As a rule, the signs of increased intracranial pressure are more prominent than those of focal cerebral disease. Mild contralateral or bilateral pyramidal signs are evidence of ipsilateral brainstem compression; in the late stages as consciousness becomes impaired they are ominous signs.

Frontal lobe abscess Headache, drowsiness, inattention, and general impairment of mental function are prominent. Hemiparesis with unilateral motor seizures and motor or expressive dysphasia are the most frequent neurologic signs.

DIAGNOSIS The diagnosis of a brain abscess depends on (1) a demonstrated source of infection in the ears, sinuses, or lungs or the presence of a right-to-left cardiac shunt, (2) evidence of increased intracranial pressure, and (3) focal cerebral or cerebellar signs. Although the CSF shows a characteristic inflammatory reaction, lumbar puncture in brain abscess is potentially dangerous, particularly when intracranial pressure is obviously elevated and the information to be derived is not specific enough to justify the risk.

The CT scan is the most valuable procedure for visualizing an abscess(es). It also shows distortion of the ventricles, surrounding edema of white matter, and the thickness of the capsule, and it enables close follow-up of therapy. The use of iodine will enhance the selectivity of the CT scan. CT scanning permits the visualization of an abscess from the early stage of focal cerebritis to a densely encapsulated mass, or if early treatment is instituted, disappearance of the abscess. If CT scanning is not available, ^{99m}Tc imaging (radionuclide scan) is a reliable method for localizing brain abscess. Generally only a CT scan is required to make the diagnosis. If both tests are negative, there is little likelihood of cerebral abscess. Scanning procedures have supplanted arteriography in most instances.

When the typical clinical picture is present and CT scan corroborates the presence of a mass lesion, the diagnosis is easy. If there is no source of infection and there are only signs and symptoms of a mass lesion, the diagnosis includes differentiation of abscess from tumor, subdural hematoma, and hemorrhage. Sometimes only surgical exploration will settle the issue. Once the inflammatory nature of the intracranial mass has been established, brain abscess must then be distinguished from subdural empyema, intracranial thrombophlebitis with hemorrhage and infarction of brain, necrotizing viral encephalitis, and acute hemorrhagic leukoencephalitis.

TREATMENT During the stage of acute suppurative cerebritis, intracranial operation accomplishes little and probably causes only additional trauma and swelling of brain tissue. There is good evidence that many brain abscesses visible by CT scanning can be cured at this stage by the administration of adequate doses of antimicrobials. Since the bacteriologic diagnosis must be presumptive, the best regimen consists of 20 million units of penicillin G intravenously in divided doses and 4 to 6 g chloramphenicol, both drugs being given intravenously in divided doses. This choice of antimicrobial agents is based on the preponderance of anaerobic streptococci and *Bacteroides* that are usually isolated from the abscess in such patients. If there is evidence of staphylococcal infection, adequate amounts of nafcillin or oxacillin should be given. Treatment should be continued for 6 weeks, and if there is clinical improvement and recovery during the course of therapy, surgical intervention can be withheld. The initial elevation of intracranial pressure and threatening temporal lobe or cerebellar pressure cone should be managed by intravenous injection of urea, mannitol, or dexamethasone. Persistence or progression of high intracranial pressure manifested by deepening coma and threat of herniation often forces operation, regardless of the stage of the abscess. Likewise, clear-cut evidence of a mass lesion which is not improving with antimicrobial therapy is an indication for surgery. The usual methods of treatment are unroofing and drainage by aspiration. If superficial and encapsulated, total excision is sometimes attempted; if deep, aspiration and the injection of antimicrobial agents into the abscess are the only possible treatment methods, and they may have to be repeated. Guidance of the needle with CT scan has improved the technique strikingly. With earlier diagnosis, which is largely due to CT scans, abscesses have been treated earlier and the mortality has fallen to approximately 10 percent. However, patients with multiple metastatic abscesses tend to do less well.

Neurological residua, particularly focal epilepsy, is a troublesome sequel. Following successful treatment of a cerebral abscess in patients with congenital heart disease, correction of the cardiac anomaly is indicated to prevent recurrence.

PROGNOSIS Earlier diagnosis has improved the outlook. However, if brain abscess is not recognized and treated, it terminates either by development of a tentorial or foramen magnum pressure cone or by rupture of the abscess into the ventricles (ventricular empyema). Rarely the abscess becomes thickly encapsulated and chronic; in this form it may be only mildly symptomatic over a period of months or years.

REFERENCES

CHERUBIN CE et al: Listeria and gram-negative bacillary meningitis in New York City, 1972–1979. Am J Med 71:199, 1981

ELLNER JJ, BENNETT, JE: Chronic meningitis. Medicine 55:341, 1976

FEIGIN RD, DODGE PR: Bacterial meningitis: Newer concepts of pathophysiology and neurologic sequelae. Pediatr Clin N Am 23:541, 1976

KAUFMAN DM et al: Subdural empyema: Analysis of 17 cases and review of the literature. Medicine 54:485, 1975

LUKEN MG III, WHELAN MA: Recent diagnostic experience with subdural empyema. J Neurosurg 52:764, 1980

NEW PJ, DAVIS KR: The role of CT scanning in diagnosis of infections of the central nervous system, in *Current Clinical Topics in Infectious Diseases,* JS Remington, MN Swartz (eds). New York, McGraw-Hill, 1980, vol 1, pp 1–33

RAHAL JJ JR: Diagnosis and management of meningitis due to gram-negative bacilli in adults, in *Current Clinical Topics in Infectious Diseases,* JS Remington, MN Swartz (eds). New York, McGraw-Hill, 1980, vol 1, pp 68–84

SCHOENBAUM SC et al: Infections of cerebrospinal fluid shunts: Epidemiology, clinical manifestations and therapy. J Infect Dis 131:543, 1975

STEVENS EA et al: Computed tomographic brain scanning in intraparenchymal pyogenic abscesses. Am J Roentgenol 130:111, 1978

SWARTZ MN: Intracranial infections, in *The Science and Practice of Clinical Medicine,* vol 5: *Neurology,* RN Rosenberg (ed). New York, Grune & Stratton, 1980, pp 1–40

VEEDER MH et al: Recurrent bacterial meningitis associated with C8 and IgA deficiency. J Infect Dis 144:399, 1981

YOSHIKAWA TT et al: Role of anaerobic bacteria in subdural empyema. Am J Med 58:99, 1975

360 VIRAL DISEASES OF THE CENTRAL NERVOUS SYSTEM: ASEPTIC MENINGITIS AND ENCEPHALITIS

DONALD H. HARTER
ROBERT G. PETERSDORF
RAYMOND D. ADAMS

Viruses can affect the central nervous system (CNS) in a variety of ways. Although much is known about the nature and replication of viruses, correlation between viral properties and the type of the neurological disease produced is inadequate or incomplete. Viruses that differ widely in their morphology, chemical composition, and replication can provoke identical clinical and pathologic changes in the CNS. As more becomes known, it may be possible to correlate clinical patterns or pathologic changes with specific viral properties.

It is helpful to consider the time between the patient's first exposure to the viral agent and the appearance of disease, that is, to distinguish between CNS infections of a "fast" or "slow" nature. In fast or acute viral disease, neurological changes occur very shortly after the patient first becomes infected by the virus. The illness follows a course of one to several weeks. In slow viral disease, the neurological changes appear months to years after viral invasion, are insidious in development, and progress slowly.

ACUTE VIRAL CNS DISEASE

Most viral CNS infections are the end result of preceding infection in other tissues and organs. There is usually a phase of extraneural viral replication before the nervous system becomes involved. Acute viral CNS infections are classified according to the clinical findings presented by the patient or, more indirectly, by the part of the nervous system involved by the disease process. In these terms, acute viral CNS disease is defined as meningitis, encephalitis, or myelitis, depending on the patient's symptoms and signs and the location of the infection. It is often difficult, however, to arrive at a single satisfactory localization on the basis of clinical findings alone. This leads to the use of compound terms such as meningoencephalitis or encephalomyelitis to describe the disease. This manner of classification is less than satisfactory because it gives no clear idea about the virus causing the condition.

Viruses vary in size, morphology, chemical composition, and effect on the host. Their common characteristics include a genome, which is either RNA or DNA surrounded by a protective protein shell; the fact that they multiply only inside the cell; and the fact that the initial step in replication involves separation of the genome from its protective shell. They are divided into two broad categories on the basis of their nucleic acid content and then into major families and genera (Table 360-1). Certain common properties of viruses are important determinants of the disease they produce. Herpesviruses have a tendency to remain latent in cells. Togaviruses and bunyaviruses are transmitted by insect vectors. Enteroviruses replicate in the gastrointestinal tract and are transmitted by the oral-fecal route. Myxoviruses contain a segmented genome which is prone to genetic recombination. Selection of the most effective methods of virus isolation depends in great measure on the virus's properties. Knowledge of a virus's biochemical composition is of help in determining whether antiviral therapy can be used. Understanding the biological features of viruses within the major families and genera permits associations which are impossible when the location of the disease process is considered alone (see Chap. 196).

TABLE 360-1
Viruses of vertebrates

RNA-containing	*DNA-containing*
Picornavirus:*	Parvovirus:
Enterovirus*	Parvovirus
Cardiovirus	Adeno-associated virus
Rhinovirus	Papovavirus*
Aphthovirus	Papillomavirus
Calicivirus	Polyomavirus*
Reovirus:	Adenovirus:
Reovirus	Mastadenovirus
Orbivirus	Aviadenovirus
Rotavirus	Iridovirus
Togavirus:*	Herpesvirus*
Alphavirus*	Poxvirus:
Flavivirus*	Orthopoxvirus
Rubivirus*	Parapoxvirus
Pestivirus	Avipoxvirus
Orthomyxovirus:	Capripoxvirus
Influenza virus C	Leporipoxvirus
Paramyxovirus:*	Suipoxvirus
Paramyxovirus*	
Morbillivirus*	
Pneumovirus	
Rhabdovirus:*	
Lyssavirus*	
Vesiculovirus	
Retrovirus:	
Oncovirus	
Spumavirus	
Lentivirus	
Bunyavirus*	
Arenavirus*	
Coronavirus	

* *Virus families and groups of neurologic importance.*

ASEPTIC OR VIRAL MENINGITIS Etiology The term *aseptic meningitis* was first introduced by Wallgren over 50 years ago to designate a disease characterized by an acute onset, meningeal symptoms, fever, cerebrospinal fluid (CSF) pleocytosis, and bacteriologically sterile cultures. The illness had a relatively benign clinical course of short duration, and recovery was the rule. With introduction of more refined methods of viral isolation and the use of new culture techniques to define other microorganisms, it became clear that aseptic meningitis is a syndrome of multiple etiologies. When viral infection produces the syndrome, the condition may be more properly referred to as viral meningitis.

Epidemiology Aseptic meningitis affects between 3500 and 6500 persons in the United States every year. Although all ages are involved, more than 90 percent of the patients are under age 30. The peak incidence of aseptic meningitis is regularly in the late summer. The majority of cases seen in the summer are due to picornaviruses other than polioviruses, such as the coxsackie- and echoviruses. Mumps meningitis occurs more often in the winter and late spring. Both sexes are affected equally by enteroviruses, but there is a 2:1 or 3:1 male predominance in the meningitis produced by mumps.

Clinical picture The symptoms and signs of viral meningitis are similar irrespective of the particular virus involved. The onset of illness is acute. There may be a prodromal "flu-like" illness before the onset of meningitis, as in lymphocytic choriomeningitis (LCM). This biphasic pattern of illness also may be observed in young children with poliomyelitis or in illness due to other insect-borne viruses (see Chaps. 208 and 209). CNS involvement is manifested by an intense frontal or retroorbital headache. Malaise, nausea and vomiting, listlessness, and photophobia may be present. As a rule, there is little impairment of consciousness. The patient may be drowsy and slightly confused but is usually oriented to surroundings and is rational. Stupor and coma occur rarely. The temperature is usually elevated in the range of 38 to 40°C. There is neck stiffness on forward flexion. Kernig's and Brudzinski's signs are present in most cases but may be absent in patients with minimal meningeal irritation. Stiffness of the spine may be such that a child will sit with the head retracted and the arms extended posteriorly in the form of a tripod. Signs of focal damage to the central nervous system are rarely present. Occasionally, strabismus or diplopia, asymmetry of tendon reflexes, and an inconstant extensor plantar response may be found.

Clinical findings outside the nervous system may provide clues to the virus involved in the infection. Parotitis in association with viral meningitis suggests mumps. Skin rash has been a prominent feature of coxsackievirus or echovirus infections (see Chap. 205). Blotchy or punctate maculopapular rashes which involve the extremities and which occur chiefly in the summertime are commonly due to echovirus. Herpangina (large, painful vesicles in the posterior one-third of the oropharynx) are usually caused by coxsackieviruses. Sharp pains in the chest aggravated by deep respiration or coughing suggest the pleurodynia seen with Coxsackie B viruses.

Laboratory findings The lumbar CSF is usually under increased pressure and clear or slightly turbid in appearance. Slight turbidity can be demonstrated by holding a tube containing CSF to the light and agitating the fluid with a gentle finger tap. CSF usually contains 10 to 100 cells per cubic millimeter. At times, the cell count rises to levels of 3000 per cubic millimeter or greater. Elevated cell counts are associated with LCM virus infection. The cells are usually more than three-fourths lymphocytes or mononuclear cells. Polymorphonuclear cells may predominate in the early phases of aseptic meningitis. The CSF protein and sugar concentrations are usually normal. Isolated instances of depressed CSF sugar in patients with infections due to mumps or herpes simplex virus (HSV) have been reported, but these are rare. If the patient presents with a spinal fluid which contains less sugar than expected, meningitis due to bacteria, mycobacteria, or fungi should receive first attention. In viral meningitis, gram stain and india ink preparations fail to identify an organism; bacterial and fungal cultures are negative. Although certain viruses (such as mumps virus) can be recovered from CSF with relative ease, in most cases of viral meningitis, it is usually impossible to recover the responsible viral agent from the patient's CSF. The white cell count in the blood is usually normal, but leukopenia is present in about one-third of patients.

The specific viral diagnosis can usually be made by performing serologic tests on acute and convalescent serums and by attempting to isolate viruses from feces, urine, and throat washings. Attempts to isolate the agent from blood are usually unsuccessful.

Differential diagnosis The syndrome of viral or aseptic meningitis can be caused by a number of different infectious and noninfectious agents. The majority of cases of viral origin are due to picornaviruses, togaviruses, herpesviruses, paramyxoviruses, and arenaviruses. The list of nonviral infectious causes of the aseptic meningitis syndrome is extensive. It includes intracranial infections located near the meninges (otitis, mastoiditis, vertebral osteomyelitis); brain abscess; partially treated bacterial meningitis; and fungal, rickettsial, protozoan, or helminthic infections.

Also, there are a number of infrequently encountered neurological diseases in which the CSF findings resemble viral meningitis. These include (1) Behçet's disease, characterized by uveitis, genital and oral ulcers, and focal neurological abnormalities; (2) Vogt-Koyanagi and Harada's diseases, which combine uveitis, depigmentation of the hair and skin about the eyes, loss of eyelashes, and deafness; and (3) Mollaret's meningitis.

Noninfectious causes of the aseptic meningitis syndrome include the intrathecal introduction of drugs and agents for diagnostic tests and tumors in close proximity to the cerebral ventricles or that invade the subarachnoid space. Cytological examination of cells in the CSF will distinguish neoplastic meningeal infiltration from viral meningitis. Systemic diseases such as sarcoidosis, disseminated lupus erythematosus, and infective endocarditis may be associated with aseptic meningitis.

Treatment The treatment of viral meningitis is symptomatic. Antiviral agents are not indicated in uncomplicated cases. Fever and other symptoms resolve in 3 to 5 days, and patients are usually entirely well within 2 weeks. CSF abnormalities are most pronounced from the fourth to sixth day, but the CSF white blood cell count may remain elevated for several weeks in patients who are otherwise asymptomatic. Initial therapy with antimicrobial agents may be appropriate if the initial elevation is not completely typical for viral infection. In most instances, patients recover from viral meningitis without sequelae. A limited number of patients may develop muscular weakness and other forms of motor disability. A very small number of patients may have recurrent attacks of viral meningitis; the multiple episodes are often due to different viruses.

Prognosis It is important to recognize that viral meningitis is an acute and self-limited illness and to realize that it may mimic life-threatening CNS infections which are potentially treatable. Most important to appreciate is the similarity between viral meningitis and partially treated bacterial meningitis, tuberculous meningitis, or fungal meningitis. If the CSF changes are not completely characteristic of viral meningitis or if the patient's clinical response is atypical, it is important to perform repeated lumbar punctures and to reexamine the CSF within a relatively brief period of time, until the clinical picture becomes clear.

VIRAL ENCEPHALITIS **Definition** The term *encephalitis* is used when there is clinical and/or pathological evidence of involvement of the cerebral hemispheres, brainstem, or cerebellum by the infectious process. It is customary to divide viral encephalitis into primary and postinfectious or parainfectious forms and to consider whether the disease is sporadic or epidemic. The primary form of the disease occurs when the encephalitis is the presenting form of the disease and is due to direct invasion and replication of virus within the CNS. The term *postinfectious* or *parainfectious* is used to describe an encephalitis which follows or occurs in combination with other viral illnesses or administration of certain vaccines. The cause of the encephalitis in such cases is believed to be a hypersensitivity reaction. The pathologic picture is typical of multifocal perivenous demyelination. The virus cannot be recovered from the CNS. If the inflammatory condition extends into the spinal cord, the term encephalomyelitis is used.

Clinical picture When encephalitis is the primary illness, such as with togaviruses and herpesviruses, there may be a minor illness consisting of such systemic symptoms as headache, myalgia, malaise, and upper respiratory symptoms. These nonspecific symptoms may occur several days before neurological complaints and signs are recognized.

The onset of neurological symptoms is abrupt. There is alteration in the patient's state of consciousness with lethargy, drowsiness, or stupor. The patient's behavior may be abnormal as a consequence of confusion, disorientation, and hallucinations. A convulsion or series of convulsions may occur at the start of the illness, and epileptic seizures may be the sole presenting symptom. The patient usually complains of headache, nausea, and vomiting. Fever is usually present, and there may be stiffening of the neck on forward bending. Focal neurological abnormalities are found, depending on the portion of the nervous system involved by the inflammatory process. Involvement of the cerebral hemispheres may result in aphasia, signs of corticospinal and corticobulbar tract lesions, involuntary movements, ataxia, sensory defects, and loss of retentive memory.

Laboratory examinations General laboratory tests are usually of little help in the diagnosis of encephalitis. They may provide evidence of systemic disease, such as abnormal lymphocytes in infectious mononucleosis, cells in the urinary sediment with inclusions characteristic of cytomegalovirus infection, and elevated amylase and transaminase levels in mumps and certain picornavirus infections.

Lumbar puncture, followed by examination of the CSF, is the most important diagnostic test. The CSF is usually under normal or slightly elevated pressure, clear or slightly turbid, and contains an increased number of white cells (in the range of 50 to 500 per cubic millimeter), a slight-to-moderate elevation of protein content, and a normal glucose level. There may be a predominance of polymorphonuclear leukocytes in the early phase of the illness. The protein content will often rise as the total cell count diminishes. In HSV encephalitis, the CSF may be slightly bloody or xanthochromic and contain a significant number of red blood cells. This reflects the sometimes hemorrhagic nature of HSV encephalitis. Occasionally a viral encephalitis may exist without CSF abnormalities, which makes the diagnosis even more difficult.

The electroencephalogram (EEG) may be of diagnostic help in suspected encephalitis. Diffuse or bilateral abnormalities can be defined by the EEG in patients who present with focal or unilateral neurological deficits. A number of EEG changes may be seen, but the most common pattern is a diffuse slow wave activity with disruption of normal rhythms, punctuated at times with periodic high-amplitude bursts and spike-and-wave complexes. Computerized tomography (CT) and radionuclide scans may be helpful in demonstrating intracranial mass lesions or localized foci of infection about or within the brain. The cerebral cortex may be enhanced diffusely.

Diagnosis When presented with a patient with suspected viral encephalitis, it is important to exclude nonviral infections for which potential treatment is available. A number of conditions can mimic viral encephalitis (Table 360-2). It is imperative to consider these alternative causes when the patient is first evaluated. Once the diagnosis of primary viral encephalitis is secure, it is important to determine if the illness is occurring as part of an epidemic or as an isolated sporadic event. Knowledge of the seasonal, geographic, and age group occurrence of the disease can often furnish enough information to make an informed guess about the correct viral etiology. During the summer and early fall, togaviruses, bunyaviruses, and picornaviruses may prevail. Some of these viruses may produce milder disease than others; some, such as western equine and California encephalitis viruses, affect a predominantly young age group. In the winter, epidemic encephalitis is more often associated with paramyxovirus, varicella-zoster (V-Z), Epstein-Barr (EB), or rubella virus infection. HSV is responsible for more cases of nonepidemic sporadic encephalitis cases than any other virus.

The course of viral encephalitis is variable. It may be a short-lived, benign illness or a devastatingly severe one which leaves the patient with pronounced impairment of cerebral functions. Severe sequelae may be associated with certain viruses (HSV, eastern equine encephalitis, Japanese encephalitis, and St. Louis encephalitis). Other viruses cause milder disease (California encephalitis, western equine encephalitis). The acute phase of the disease usually lasts a few days to a week. Resolution can be abrupt or gradual. The disease may be complicated by a salt-wasting syndrome resulting from hypothalamic involvement and/or alterations in temperature or respiratory control centers owing to brainstem involvement. These events may occur rapidly and require prompt recognition and correction. Neurological defects may continue to improve over a period of weeks to months.

In most instances of epidemic encephalitis, the viral diagnosis is made by serologic tests of acute and convalescent phase serums. Three major serologic tests are employed: complement-fixation, hemagglutination-inhibition, and neutralization. Because the serologic test is crucial for viral diagnosis, it is imperative to obtain an acute-phase serum as soon as the diagnosis of viral encephalitis is suspected. In vector-transmitted encephalitis which does not result in fatality, the blood is the most likely tissue source of viral isolation. Isolation of virus from blood is difficult, however, because viremia is usually brief and occurs before the onset of neurological symptoms. In fatal cases, the virus can often be isolated from brain and spinal cord by inoculation of susceptible animals and tissue culture cells.

When HSV encephalitis is suspected, greater urgency is required in arriving at a viral diagnosis because there is a definite advantage in initiating antiviral therapy as quickly as possible (see Chap. 210). A significant number of patients with HSV encephalitis present with fever and neurological findings compatible with a bilateral space-occupying lesion of the medial parts of the temporal and the orbital parts of the frontal lobes. A severe retentive memory defect is a frequent sequela. HSV can be best demonstrated in brain tissue obtained by biopsy. Examination of the tissue by light, electron, and immunofluorescence microscopy and inoculation of a brain homogenate into cell cultures and animals permit a specific diagnosis of HSV early in the course of the patient's illness. However, many neurologists object to biopsy as a diagnostic procedure because the risks and sequelae outweigh the dangers of treatment. Moreover, enhanced CT scans often reveal the bitemporal lesions which, when added to the clinical picture and a CSF pleocytosis, make the diagnosis fairly certain.

Encephalitis may present as an infrequently encountered manifestation of a systemic disease such as measles, varicella, or neoplasia. When this is the case, the encephalitis occurs after the more characteristic features of the disease have become evident. Rarely, the systemic disease may appear after the diagnosis of encephalitis has been established.

TABLE 360-2
Nonviral conditions mistaken for acute viral encephalitis

Infection:	
Bacterial	Early or imperfectly treated meningitis
	Brain abscess
	Parameningeal infections
	Illness due to mycobacteria, spirochetes, mycoplasma
Fungi	Cryptococcus, *Coccidioides immitis,* histoplasma, candida, nocardia, blastomyces
Rickettsia	Rocky Mountain spotted fever
Protozoa	"Fresh water" amebiasis, malaria, toxoplasma
Metazoa	Cysticerosis, trichinella, and others
Intoxication	Salicylates, barbiturates, heavy metals, tick paralysis
Endocrine and metabolic disorders	Acute sodium, calcium, or carbohydrate imbalance; porphyria, pheochromocytoma
Systemic diseases	Sarcoidosis, hyperglobulinemia, collagen disease, neoplasms, endocarditis with embolization
Acute psychotic disorders	

SOURCE: *After Brown.*

UNUSUAL FORMS OF VIRAL ENCEPHALITIS *Reye's syndrome* (acute encephalopathy with fatty degeneration of the viscera) is a form of postinfectious encephalopathy in which the encephalopathy appears to be secondary to the effects of liver disease. It occurs 1 to 6 days after influenza or other viral illness in children 2 months to 15 years in age. There is severe and persistent vomiting, delirium, convulsions, and coma. An extremely elevated blood ammonia level, prolonged prothrombin time, elevated serum aminotransferases, and mild hypoglycemia are the characteristic laboratory abnormalities.

Acute cerebellar ataxia may be associated with a number of different viruses (picornaviruses, V-Z, and EB virus). The illness usually afflicts children between the ages of 1 and 5 years. The majority of patients have had a preceding mild infectious illness a week or so before the onset of neurological signs. The onset of the illness is characteristically abrupt with prominent ataxia of the trunk and limbs. Complete recovery is the rule, but a permanent cerebellar deficit may ensue in patients when ataxia is profound in the early stages of the illness. In some instances of varicella-zoster infection, the cerebellar lesions are of the parainfectious, demyelinating type (see Chap. 361).

Acute hemorrhagic leukoencephalitis is an infrequently encountered inflammatory disease of the brain which is often preceded by some form of systemic viral illness, most often an upper respiratory tract infection. The disease is marked by an acute onset, progressively deepening disturbance of consciousness, fever, seizures, and focal cortical abnormalities. The course is rapid and usually fatal. There is a peripheral leukocytosis, and the CSF frequently contains mononuclear and polymorphonuclear leukocytes. The cause of the disease is unknown. It has not been linked to infection by a specific virus or group of viruses and may well be allergic in nature. A virus has not been recovered from brain tissue. Treatment includes vigorous control of intracranial pressure and seizures and aggressive use of corticosteroids in high dosage (see Chap. 361).

Limbic encephalitis is a form of encephalitis localized to the temporal and frontal lobes—the limbic part of the brain. It is encountered as a remote effect of malignancy—most commonly carcinoma of the lung. A viral etiology such as HSV has been suspected, but never proved. Patients with limbic encephalitis have marked impairment of recent memory manifested by a confabulatory-amnestic state, and generalized seizures. The patient's CSF often contains a limited number of lymphocytes and mononuclear cells. The EEG is characterized by paroxysmal and/or slow waves over one or both temporal lobes. Pathologic changes are most pronounced in the hippocampal formation and amygdaloid nuclei. Encephalitis with predilection for the brainstem has also been reported as a remote effect of tumor.

Encephalitis lethargica (von Economo's disease) first occurred during and for about 10 years after World War I. A causative viral agent was never identified, but the clinical and pathologic features were those of a viral infection of the thalamus and midbrain. The disease was characterized by pronounced somnolence and ophthalmoplegia. A high proportion of survivors developed a parkinsonian syndrome months or years after the encephalitis. Sporadic case reports of patients with the clinical features of encephalitis lethargica appear even to the present time.

MYELITIS Viral infection of the central nervous system may localize in the parenchyma of the spinal cord producing myelitis. Poliovirus infection with damage to spinal motor neurons is the prototype of a viral infection localized chiefly to the spinal cord. Vaccination has markedly reduced but not eliminated poliomyelitis because patients who have not been vaccinated remain susceptible. Spinal paralytic disease has also been described with other enteroviruses (coxsackieviruses and echoviruses). The illness is characterized by an asymmetric flaccid paralysis of the limbs; it is usually less severe and has a higher rate of recovery from muscular weakness than poliomyelitis.

Other viruses have also been reported to affect the spinal cord directly. Herpesvirus infection in the genital and perineal region has been associated with paralysis of sphincter function, probably indicative of direct viral involvement of the sacral spinal cord. Myelitis due to V-Z virus (aside from the ganglionitis and unilateral poliomyelitis) is another very rare cause of a leukomyelitis resulting in bilateral weakness of the legs with occasional ankle clonus or extensor plantar responses. Sphincter disturbances are present in two-thirds of patients and a sensory level in about one-half of patients. The CSF contains from 25 to 125 cells per cubic millimeter; the protein content may be normal or elevated. Recovery of function is the rule.

There may also be delayed involvement of the white matter of the spinal cord following viral infection. This is a parainfectious demyelinative process that interrupts sensory and motor tracts at one level and is termed an acute transverse myelitis. It begins with the abrupt onset of bilateral weakness of the legs and concomitant involvement of ascending sensory pathways. Urinary bladder and bowel functions are usually disturbed early in the course of the illness. An exanthem or respiratory infection not uncommonly precedes neurological symptoms. Acute myelitis in the absence of encephalitis has been described in association with measles, V-Z, echovirus, HSV, and infectious mononucleosis. It has also been observed after rabies and smallpox vaccination. Virus isolation from CSF has been unsuccessful. A small proportion of patients with acute transverse myelitis will later develop multiple sclerosis. Acute spinal epidural abscess should be considered and excluded in patients who present with an acute nontraumatic transverse spinal cord syndrome.

CNS DISEASES DUE TO SLOW VIRUS INFECTION

In slow virus infections, a protracted period, often on the order of months or years, passes between the introduction of the infectious agent and the appearance of clinical illness. Once neurological disease is established, it may progress slowly over many months or years. The reasons why a certain virus will cause acute illness in one patient and slow infection in another are still largely unknown. Viruses causing slow infections do not appear to share any common features. No single virus property can be correlated with the slow virus disease process. The factors invoked to explain slow virus infections include (1) a defect in the composition of the virus; (2) a change in the virus's antigenicity; (3) an altered or defective host immune response; (4) a special property of the virus which permits it to remain latent or to become integrated in the host cell's genome; or (5) a yet incompletely understood and possibly unique method of replication.

Slow virus CNS diseases affect the parenchyma of the cerebral hemispheres and, in some instances, the cerebellum, brainstem, and spinal cord. These infections are not grouped by their topography, i.e., the part of the nervous system that they damage, or by their clinical presentation. Some slow viruses provoke a mild conventional inflammatory response during the time they are clinically silent; others are able to reside within cells for long periods without causing detectable cytopathic changes. The role of immunity in slow virus infection is largely unknown. Some slow virus infections occur in the presence of elevated levels of circulating antibodies; in others, there may be no detectable immune response.

Because infective agents causing some human slow CNS diseases have not been demonstrated to contain nucleic acid, the slow viral CNS infections are divided into those due to conventional viruses and those due to unconventional agents whose viral nature has not been fully established (Table 360-3). There are currently six well-defined neurological diseases due to slow viruses. No consistently effective therapy is now available for any of the six. Conventional viruses have been recovered from the CNS of patients with subacute sclerosing panencephalitis (SSPE), progressive multifocal leukoencephalopathy (PML), progressive rubella encephalitis, and persistent viral infection in immunodeficient patients. Each of these is based on an inflammatory reaction in the CNS. Kuru and Creutzfeldt-Jakob disease (CJD) share common neuropathologic features which are noninflammatory. They produce fine vacuolation of nervous tissue and hence are referred to as the subacute spongiform virus encephalopathies. Although these diseases have been shown to be of infectious etiology by the transmission of neurological illness to higher primates, their causative agents remain incompletely characterized. They are classified as the slow virus infections due to unconventional agents.

SUBACUTE SCLEROSING PANENCEPHALITIS (INCLUSION-BODY ENCEPHALITIS) This progressive and ultimately fatal disease of children and adolescents had been suspected to be of viral origin since its initial description by Dawson in 1932. Measles virus or a virus very closely related to measles virus has been recovered from the brains of patients with the disease. The disorder may be considered to be a slow form of measles encephalitis (see Chap. 200).

SSPE occurs in patients between the ages of 4 and 20; 80 percent are under 11. The disease affects boys 3 to 10 times as frequently as girls. The incidence has fallen recently. Most patients are from rural areas or small towns. Characteristically, they are entirely well until the disease begins. The onset of usually insidious mental deterioration, often expressed by a decline in the patient's schoolwork, is the presenting symptom. Incoordination, ataxia, and myoclonic jerks develop within a few months along with abnormalities of the pyramidal and extrapyramidal motor systems. Cortical blindness, papilledema, and optic atrophy may be present; focal chorioretinitis has been described. A few cases have occurred in association with infectious mononucleosis.

The patient becomes bedridden within 6 to 9 months. Death results from superimposed pulmonary or urinary tract infections or from decubiti. Signs of meningeal irritation are absent.

The CSF gamma-globulin level, as determined by electrophoresis, quantitative immunochemical assay, or colloidal gold curve, is elevated, but the fluid is otherwise normal. The EEG typically shows a "burst suppression" pattern characterized by synchronous and symmetrical spike and high-voltage slow wave activity followed by electrical inactivity. Elevated levels of measles antibody are found in the serum and CSF.

Pathologic findings include lymphocyte and mononuclear infiltrations about small cerebral arteries and veins, intranuclear and intracytoplasmic inclusions in neurons and glial cells, and varying degrees of destruction of medullated nerve fibers. The lesions occur in the cerebral gray and white matter, brainstem and cerebellum.

Measles virus is the etiologic agent. Electron-microscopic studies show that the intranuclear inclusions in brain cells are composed of hollow tubular filaments resembling the internal nucleocapsid component of a paramyxovirus. Staining of brain tissue from patients with the disease demonstrates measles virus antigen in the inclusions. An agent serologically identical with measles virus and having the properties of measles virus has been recovered from brain by cocultivating cell cultures originating from brain tissue with established laboratory cell lines.

Attempts to transmit the disease to animals have met with variable results. Ferrets inoculated with suspensions of brain from patients with the disease develop a nonfatal neurological disorder with EEG changes.

There is evidence that SSPE patients have clinical measles at an unusually early age, but SSPE appears many years after the patient's initial rubeola infection. A few reported cases may have been related to measles vaccination. The risk of SSPE following measles vaccination is far less, however, than the risk of encephalitis or SSPE following natural measles.

SSPE patients lack antibody to one of the measles virus proteins (the M or matrix protein) despite high titers of antibodies to the other viral proteins. The M protein is a nonglycosylated protein localized to the inner surface of the viral membrane; it is important in the assembly of the virus particle at the cell surface. SSPE brain cells do not appear capable of synthesizing the M protein even in normal amounts. The reason for this selective defect in a single viral protein has not been ascertained.

Isoprinosine[1] has been reported by some to affect the course of the disease favorably in an open therapeutic trial, but there is controversy about the drug's effectiveness.

PROGRESSIVE MULTIFOCAL LEUKOENCEPHALOPATHY This rare neurological condition, first described in 1958, usually occurs in patients who have leukemia, malignant lymphoma, carcinomatosis, immunosuppressive therapy, or a variety of other chronic disease processes. The disease is consistently associated with disorders of cell-mediated immunity with which deficits in humoral antibody response may or may not coexist.

The disease affects adults of both sexes, and its duration from onset of symptoms to death is 1 to 6 or more months. The neurological signs and symptoms reflect a diffuse, asymmetric involvement of the cerebral hemispheres. Hemiplegia, hemianopsia, aphasia or dysarthria, and organic mental changes are frequent; visual field abnormalities and complete or incomplete transverse myelitis may develop. Headache and convulsive seizures are rare, but EEG abnormalities consisting of diffuse or focal abnormalities are often present. Lesions in the white matter may be recognized on CT scans. CSF is normal.

The pathologic changes consist of multiple areas of demyelination with little or no perivascular infiltration and abnormal mitotic figures in astrocytes. The presence of distinctive intranuclear inclusions in oligodendrocytes first suggested that the disease was of a viral etiology. Electron-microscopic observations show the intranuclear inclusion bodies to be composed of closely packed spheres, which have the physical dimensions and properties of the polyomavirus genus of the papovaviruses.

By employing tissue cultures derived from human fetal brain it has been possible to recover a new human polyomavirus serotype (JC virus) from the brains of PML patients. Abundant virus particles are present in brain. Rapid identification of the virus in brain is possible using fluorescent antibody staining or electron-microscopic agglutination with monospecific hyperimmune rabbit serum. Serologic diagnosis using the patient's serum is unreliable. The virus has not been demonstrated in tissues other than brain; the disease has not been transmitted to animals.

There are isolated reports of clinical remission with cytosine arabinoside, but no cures. Death usually occurs within 6 months of onset.

PML may result from the activation of a polyomavirus which has been latent in brain or other tissues since childhood infection. Alternatively, there may be certain individuals who fail to acquire immunity in childhood and have their first encounter with the virus when a disease which interferes with cell-mediated immunity develops. The demyelination which

TABLE 360-3
Slow virus diseases of the CNS

Conventional viruses	Subacute sclerosing panencephalitis (SSPE) (inclusion-body encephalitis) Progressive multifocal leukoencephalopathy (PML) Progressive rubella encephalitis Persistent viral disease in immunodeficient patients
Unconventional virus-like agents	Kuru Creutzfeldt-Jakob Disease (CJD) ? Familial Alzheimer's disease

[1] *This drug has not been approved by the Food and Drug Administration at the time of publication.*

occurs may be related to virus-induced damage of oligodendroglia, cells which appear to be required for the normal maintenance of myelin.

PROGRESSIVE RUBELLA ENCEPHALITIS A chronic progressive encephalitis developing in the second decade of life and sharing some of the features of SSPE has been described in patients with congenital rubella (see Chap. 201).

Deterioration of mental and motor functions begins after a stable period of 10 or more years. The CSF has an increased cell count, and the protein and IgG levels are elevated. High titers of antibody to rubella virus can be detected in both the serum and CSF. Rubella virus has been recovered from the brain by use of the cocultivation technique.

Unlike SSPE, patients with rubella panencephalitis have the stigmata of congenital rubella before the onset of progressive disease. Myoclonus is less constant, and the EEG does not show the burst suppression observed in SSPE. Histologic examination of the brain shows mineralization of old lesions and an inflammatory reaction, but not the inclusion bodies characteristically found in SSPE.

The clinical picture of progressive rubella encephalitis also resembles the rare case of juvenile paresis which may occur in patients with congenital syphilis. The immune status of patients with rubella encephalitis has not been fully defined, and the pathogenesis of the disease remains obscure.

PERSISTENT VIRAL DISEASE IN IMMUNODEFICIENT PATIENTS Persistent or chronic neurological infections of the nervous system may occur in immunodeficient patients. Enteroviruses may be recovered from the CSF of agammaglobulinemic patients over a period of many years, during which time there is a persistent CSF pleocytosis. A chronic or subacute encephalitis has also been described in children with congenital hypogammaglobulinemia. A specific virus has not been associated with this disorder. Other nonviral infections such as toxoplasmosis, cryptococcosis, and other fungal infections, and pneumocystis infections may be associated with altered immune states (see Chap. 137).

KURU Kuru, or "trembling with fear," is a progressive and fatal neurological disorder which occurs exclusively among natives of the New Guinea highland. The disease is rare and seems to be disappearing; its elucidation represented a major hallmark in microbiology.

Difficulty in walking is usually the first sign of kuru. This usually progresses from a minor disturbance in gait to marked ataxia with lurching and staggering. Eventually, ambulation becomes so incoordinated that patients are unable to walk independently or to use their limbs because of intention tremor. Patients display an inability to perform rapid alternating movements, hypotonia, and abnormal involuntary movements which take the form of myoclonus, athetosis, or chorea. Slurring of speech and convergent strabismus appear as the disease progresses. There are no abnormalities in the blood or CSF. Dementia develops in the later phases of the disease. The illness terminates fatally in 4 to 24 months, usually from decubitus ulcers or bronchopneumonia. Approximately 80 percent of adults afflicted with the disease are women. The incubation period may be longer than 30 years in older patients.

Pathologic changes are limited to the CNS and include widespread neuronal loss, intense astrocytosis and microglial proliferation, loss of myelinated fibers, and the presence of plaque-like bodies. Perivascular cuffing by lymphocytes and mononuclear cells is rarely present.

It was the close similarity between the neuropathologic and clinical findings found in kuru and in scrapie, a slow infectious disease of sheep, that suggested the possibility that kuru might be caused by a virus or some closely related infectious agent. The infectious origin of kuru was confirmed subsequently by the transfer of a kuru-like syndrome in chimpanzees 10 to 82 months after intracerebral inoculation of suspensions of brain from human cases. Disease has also been produced in chimpanzees by inoculation of tissues other than brain. The clinical illness in chimpanzees appears 3 to 11 months after inoculation. The disease has also been successfully transmitted to a number of new world and old world monkeys as well as to minks and ferrets. The specific agent responsible for the disease has not been fully characterized.

Cannibalism is the probable mode of transmission of kuru. Native custom in New Guinea dictated that bone marrow, viscera, and brain be cooked and eaten. The agent may be introduced by conjunctival, nasal, or skin contamination during the practice of ritual cannibalism. The marked predilection of kuru for the adult female may be explained by the observation that cannibalism appears more prevalent among women and that males who practice cannibalism seldom eat the bodies of women. The recent influx of foreign settlers into the kuru area has led to increasing rejection of cannibalistic practices and this is turn may be responsible for the progressive decline in the number of cases of kuru since 1960. Oral feeding of kuru agent to squirrel monkeys has been reported to produce the disease.

CREUTZFELDT-JAKOB DISEASE CJD is an invariably fatal degenerative disease of the CNS which afflicts persons between 40 and 80 years of age and presents as a rapidly evolving dementia with myoclonic seizures. Unlike kuru, the disease is not geographically limited.

Although CJD may have a diverse clinical presentation, it is usually first manifested by rapidly evolving mental changes similar to those seen in the presenile dementias. Impairment of reasoning and judgment, memory disturbances, and bizarre behavior are usually the first symptoms. The patient may complain of distortions in the shape and appearances of objects. Hallucinations, delusional ideas, and confusion occur as the disease progresses and are nearly always accompanied by cerebellar ataxia and myoclonic movements. As the condition worsens, the patients become mute, stuporous, spastic, and rigid. Only rarely has a second member of a family been affected. The disease progresses rapidly; death usually terminates the illness within 3 to 12 months often from intercurrent infection. There are no abnormalities in the CSF, but the EEG reveals characteristic periodic bursts of slow waves.

The cerebrum and cerebellum are affected predominantly. Widespread status spongiosus nerve cell loss in gray matter and intense gliosis are seen. Vacuoles are located within the neuropil, i.e., within axons, dendrites, and glial fibers. There is no inflammatory reaction. In the spinal cord, anterior horn cells may be damaged or lost and there may be degeneration of the corticospinal tracts.

A neurological disease with the clinical and pathologic features of CJD can be induced in chimpanzees 11 to 71 months after incubation with brain suspensions from patients with CJD. It is also possible to transmit the disease to monkeys, the domestic cat, and guinea pigs. Neutralizing antibodies to the Creutzfeldt-Jakob agent have not been demonstrated in the serums of patients with the disease or of primates with the experimental disease.

There is an unexpectedly high incidence of previous brain or eye operations among patients with CJD. Human-to-human transmission has occurred by corneal transplantation and by implantation of contaminated stereotactic electroencephalographic electrodes after an incubation period of 15 to 20 months.

The Creutzfeldt-Jakob agent has been found in lymph nodes, liver, kidney, spleen, lung, cornea, and CSF of patients afflicted with the disorder. The agent is also present in leukocytes of infected guinea pigs.

Exposure to breath, saliva, nasopharyngeal secretions, urine, or feces of the Creutzfeldt-Jakob patient should not be of special concern, but the patient's CSF and blood should be considered a potential source of infection. Maximum caution should be taken to avoid accidental percutaneous exposure to blood, CSF, or tissue. Guidelines for the handling of materials from patients with these disorders have been developed. These should be rigorously applied to all patients who have evidence of rapid intellectual deterioration, particularly if it is associated with myoclonic activity, when no space-occupying lesion is demonstrated in the brain.

Claims have been made that amantadine hydrochloride (Symmetrel) is therapeutically effective in CJD, but these claims have not been substantiated in most subsequent investigations.

One familial form of Alzheimer's disease (presenile dementia) may also have an infectious etiology. Brain tissues from a restricted number of patients with familial Alzheimer's disease have induced neurological disease and spongiform changes in chimpanzees. However, many other isolation attempts from patients with familial and nonfamilial Alzheimer's disease have been negative. It seems highly improbable that Alzheimer's disease and senile dementia are caused by a slow virus.

REFERENCES

Brown P: Viral encephalitis, in *Current Diagnosis 5,* HF Conn, RB Conn (eds). Philadelphia, Saunders, 1977, p 126

Chonmaitree T et al: The clinical relevance of 'CSF viral culture.' JAMA 247:1843, 1982

Freeman JM: The clinical spectrum and early diagnosis of Dawson's encephalitis. J Pediatr 75:590, 1969

Gajdusek DC: Unconventional viruses and the origin and disappearance of kuru. Science 197:943, 1977

——— et al: Precautions in medical care of, and in handling material from, patients with transmissible virus dementia (Creutzfeldt-Jakob disease). N Engl J Med 297:1253, 1977

Hall WW, Choppin PW: Measles-virus proteins in the brain tissue of patients with subacute sclerosing panencephalitis. Absence of the M protein. N Engl J Med 304:1152, 1981

Ho M: Acute viral encephalitis, in *Handbook of Clinical Neurology,* PJ Vinken, GW Bruyn (eds). Amsterdam, Elsevier/North-Holland 1977, vol 34, p 63

Karandanis D, Shulman JA: Recent survey of infectious meningitis in adults: Review of laboratory findings in bacterial, tuberculous and aseptic meningitis. S Med J 69:449, 1976

Kennard C, Swash M: Acute viral encephalitis. Its diagnosis and outcome. Brain 104:129, 1981

Modlin JF et al: Epidemiology of subacute sclerosing panencephalitis. J Pediatr 94:231, 1979

Padgett BL et al: JC papovavirus in progressive multifocal leukoencephalopathy. J Infect Dis 133:686, 1977

Richardson EP: Progressive multifocal leukoencephalopathy. N Engl J Med 265:815, 1961

Roos R et al: The clinical characteristics of transmissible Creutzfeldt-Jakob disease. Brain 96:1, 1973

Singer JI et al: Management of central nervous system infections during an epidemic of enteroviral aseptic meningitis. J Pediatr 96:559, 1980

Weil ML et al: Chronic progressive panencephalitis due to rubella virus simulating subacute sclerosing panencephalitis. N Engl J Med 292:994, 1975

Whitley RJ et al: Herpes simplex encephalitis: Vidarabine therapy and diagnostic problems. N Engl J Med 304:313, 1981

Wilfert CM et al: Persistent and fatal central-nervous-system echovirus infections in patients with agammaglobulinemia. N Engl J Med 296:1485, 1977

361 MULTIPLE SCLEROSIS AND OTHER DEMYELINATING DISEASES

JACK P. ANTEL
BARRY G. W. ARNASON

The demyelinating diseases comprise an important group of neurological disorders both because of the frequency with which they occur and the disability which they cause. Demyelinating diseases share in common the pathologic feature of focal or patchy destruction of myelin sheaths in the central nervous system accompanied by an inflammatory response. Some degree of axonal damage may occur as well, but demyelination always predominates. No cause has been determined for any of the conditions considered to be demyelinating diseases. Current opinion holds that autoimmunity or viral infection is likely to be implicated in their pathogenesis.

Myelin loss occurs in other entities as well, but in these an inflammatory response is lacking. Included are genetically determined defects in myelin metabolism, exposure to toxins such as carbon monoxide, and opportunistic viral infection of oligodendrocytes (e.g., progressive multifocal leukoencephalopathy) against a background of immune incompetence. These entities, which are usually not classified as demyelinating diseases, are discussed in Chaps. 360 and 364.

Three demyelinating diseases can be distinguished on the basis of clinical history, examination, and pathologic findings:

1 Multiple sclerosis
2 Acute disseminated encephalomyelitis (including postinfectious and postvaccinal encephalomyelitis)
3 Acute necrotizing hemorrhagic encephalomyelitis

MULTIPLE SCLEROSIS

This disease presents in the form of recurrent attacks of a focal neurologic disorder with a predilection for spinal cord, optic nerves, and brain. Attacks occur, remit, and recur, seemingly randomly and capriciously over many years. The disease begins most commonly in early adult life. The frequency of flare-ups is greatest during the first 3 to 4 years of disease, but a first attack, which may have been so mild as to escape medical attention and can barely be recalled, may not be followed by another attack for 10 to 20 years. During typical episodes, symptoms worsen over a period of a few days to 2 to 3 weeks and then remit. Recovery is usually rapid over a period of weeks, although at times it may extend over several months. Remission may be complete, particularly after early attacks; more often remission is incomplete and as one attack follows another, a stepwise downward progression ensues with increasingly permanent deficit.

The extent of recovery varies markedly between patients and from one attack to the next in the same person. In perhaps as many as one-third of cases the disease declares itself as a slowly but inexorably progressive illness. This is particularly likely to be the case if the onset is after age 40. In cases with earlier onset a series of attacks and remissions may occasionally be engrafted on a slower course of incipient worsening, but more frequently after many years of attacks there is a gradual deterioration. Occasional patients die rapidly; most do not, and the average survival is better than 30 years after onset of disease.

Multiple sclerosis is pleomorphic in its presentation. The clinical picture is determined by the location of foci of demyelination; certain parts of the nervous system are preferentially involved. Classic features include impaired vision, nystagmus, dysarthria, decreased perception of vibration and position sense, ataxia and intention tremor, weakness or paralysis of one or more limbs, spasticity, and bladder problems.

Diagnosis requires proof of at least two episodes of clear-cut neurologic deficit and of lesions at more than one site within the central nervous system. While corroborative laboratory tests are available, the diagnosis of multiple sclerosis remains predominantly clinical. When signs pointing to damage of white matter tracts in optic nerves, brainstem, and spinal cord are present together and more than one attack is known to have occurred, the diagnosis can be made with greater than 95 percent certainty. In the early years of the disease, when few relapses have occurred and fixed deficits are mild, the diagnosis may prove difficult and single or multiple focal lesions due to other causes must be excluded.

PATHOLOGY Many scattered, discrete areas of demyelination, termed *plaques,* are the pathologic hallmark of multiple sclerosis. Macroscopically, plaques appear as gray-pink sharply defined areas which stand out against the surrounding white matter of the central nervous system. Lesions may extend into gray matter, although nerve cell bodies are seen to be preserved on microscopic examination. Plaques vary in size from a few millimeters to several centimeters; larger ones form by coalescence of smaller ones and by expansion of their margins. Plaques may be found anywhere in the white matter but typically occur in the paraventricular areas of the cerebrum and subpially, and within the brainstem and spinal cord. Their topography conforms to that of the venous drainage of the brain and spinal cord, and no particular anatomical structures are respected. The peripheral nervous system is not affected. At autopsy the number of plaques found invariably exceeds the number expected on the basis of physical signs. Many plaques, therefore, are clinically silent; this establishes that substantial impulse conduction occurs across regions of demyelination. In fact, autopsy studies indicate that 20 percent of multiple sclerosis cases are totally silent, clinically, during life.

The microscopic features of multiple sclerosis lesions depend on their age. Typically lesions of different ages and evidence of new activity about the margins of old lesions are encountered. Active multiple sclerosis lesions feature lymphocyte and monocyte-macrophage accumulations about venules and at plaque margins where myelin is being destroyed. The invasion of white matter by inflammatory cells is held responsible for the myelin breakdown. Macrophages (microglia) are believed to be the vectors of myelin breakdown. They also function as scavengers of myelin debris; fat-laden macrophages may persist for months, perhaps for years, after the acute inflammatory response has subsided. Plasma cells accumulate within plaques and are usually found at or near their centers.

An astroglial response at or just beyond the margins of acutely demyelinating lesions is characteristic. In established, inactive plaques, a thick mat of fibrillary gliosis throughout the demyelinated regions is usual, and only a few residual perivascular macrophages are found. Oligodendrocyte number is reduced within plaques, indicating that this cell type is lost in multiple sclerosis. Indeed, death of oligodendrocytes may be the primary event.

Only limited regeneration of myelin occurs in multiple sclerosis. The reason for this is unclear but may relate to loss of

oligodendrocytes. At the pial margins of the spinal cord remyelination by peripheral nerve Schwann cells that have invaded the central nervous system may be encountered. Despite assiduous search, viral inclusions have not been detected in multiple sclerosis lesions.

Axons within plaques tend to be spared, although in acute lesions frank necrosis with loss of axons can sometimes occur. At least 10 percent of multiple sclerosis plaques show marked axonal loss, and ultrastructural studies indicate that loss of axons may be more general than can be appreciated by routine histology. All gradations of pathologic change between the extremes described above are encountered.

The pathologic features of multiple sclerosis fail to account for the hour to hour and day to day waxings and wanings in function so characteristic of the disease. Conduction of impulses through demyelinated nerve is compromised and is further altered by transient changes in the internal milieu such as alterations in temperature and in electrolyte balance or by stress. Fever, or even minor increases in body temperature, such as may follow a hot bath or exercise, may cause a failure of conduction through demyelinated regions and lead to evanescent symptoms and signs. The mechanism of this fatigability is unknown, but some type of conduction block is assumed to occur. It is important to distinguish transient fluctuations in symptomatology of the type just described from attacks of disease.

ETIOLOGY The cause or causes of multiple sclerosis remain unknown. A role for immune-mediated or infectious factors has been proposed, but the data to support these postulates are fragmentary and indirect.

Epidemiology Epidemiologic studies have established several facts which will ultimately have to be incorporated into any coherent theory of the disease. Average age at onset of the first clinical episode of multiple sclerosis (MS) falls within the third and fourth decades, onset being somewhat later in males than in females. Females account for 60 percent of cases. For disease to begin in childhood or beyond the sixth decade is uncommon but not unknown.

In general, incidence in temperate climatic zones exceeds that in tropical zones; but variations within regions with similar climates do exist; hence the effect is not simply one of latitude or temperature. The incidence of multiple sclerosis in northern Europe, Canada, and the northern United States is approximately 10 new cases each year per hundred thousand persons between the ages of 20 and 50. The incidence in Australia, New Zealand, and the southern United States is one-third to one-half of that just given; in Japan, elsewhere in the orient, and in Africa, multiple sclerosis is rare. Epidemiologic evidence also suggests that persons migrating from high- to low-risk regions as children are partially protected from MS. The data are consistent with the existence of a geographically restricted environmental factor, possibly a virus, which influences development of multiple sclerosis.

Genetic factors There is some suggestion that multiple sclerosis may be more common in higher socioeconomic groups. The incidence of multiple sclerosis among American Indians and blacks is lower than among caucasians living in the same regions. This suggests that genetic factors also influence disease susceptibility. Blood relatives of multiple sclerosis patients (parents, siblings) have an eightfold increased risk of developing multiple sclerosis. This could reflect an interplay of several genetic factors, shared exposure to an environmental factor, or a combination of the two. A study of multiple sclerosis in identical twins has revealed concordance for multiple sclerosis to be slightly greater than that for fraternal twins, yet even among identical twins, multiple sclerosis in one twin is more common than in both. Family studies have failed to reveal any predictable genetic pattern but do argue for a genetically determined predisposition to disease.

Certain histocompatibility antigens (HLA) occur more often in patients with multiple sclerosis. Among Caucasians with the disease the HLA-B7 and Dw2 region alleles occur with increased frequency. Most illnesses with which an HLA association has been shown are autoimmune or infectious in nature, a finding which is in keeping with current thought about the etiology of multiple sclerosis. Many American blacks with multiple sclerosis express the HLA-B7 allele; this allele is rare in blacks in Africa among whom MS is unknown. It follows that an HLA-linked genetic factor which predisposes to multiple sclerosis exists, but inasmuch as the vast majority of persons bearing B7 or Dw2 do not develop the disease, additional genetic or environmental factors must play a role. The HLA-B12 allele is less frequent in MS than in the population at large. This finding suggests that genetically determined protective factors may operate in MS.

Autoimmune factors The lesions of multiple sclerosis are mimicked by those of experimental allergic encephalomyelitis (EAE), an autoimmune disease induced in animals by immunization with myelin. Lesions of EAE are demyelinating, perivenular, plaque-like, occur in chronic and recrudescent forms, and have an inflammatory infiltrate composed of lymphocytes, macrophages, and plasma cells. In EAE, T lymphocyte sensitivity to a single antigen known as myelin basic protein can be shown to be the cause of the disease; yet in multiple sclerosis, sensitivity to myelin basic protein cannot be demonstrated. This indicates that, if multiple sclerosis should prove to be an autoimmune process, as the clinical and histologic parallels with EAE might suggest, the antigen is something other than myelin basic protein. Attempts to find any antigen to which only multiple sclerosis patients react have failed.

Changes in peripheral blood lymphocytes occur during attacks of multiple sclerosis. Suppressor T-cell levels fall just prior to attacks and rise as attacks end. Whether this change relates to the etiology of multiple sclerosis is not known. Loss of suppressor cell function, for whatever reason, could permit a latent autoimmune response to become an active one. Alternatively the elusive multiple sclerosis antigen could be present both on suppressor T cells and on oligodendrocytes.

Hyperactivity of circulating B cells also occurs in multiple sclerosis; this is particularly the case during the attacks. Excessive IgG production within the CNS is also characteristic; whether this reflects the presence of some stimulator of B cells in the brain in multiple sclerosis or is the result of a defect in immune regulation is not known. Viral infection of brain remains a possible cause of multiple sclerosis, despite the fact that all attempts to isolate, rescue or "passage" a virus from multiple sclerosis brains or to visualize a virus within them have failed.

Precipitating factors Various infections, injury, and even emotional upsets have been claimed to precipitate a first attack of multiple sclerosis. Evidence in support of these claims remains anecdotal and unpersuasive. The probability that an attack of multiple sclerosis will occur during the first 6 months after pregnancy is greater than chance would predict, but this observation is counterbalanced by a decreased risk of an attack during the second and third trimesters of pregnancy. In established cases, trauma, including lumbar puncture, myelography, and surgery, has not been shown to relate to attacks or to progression of disability nor has emotional turmoil been shown to alter the tempo at which the disease evolves. Experience has also shown that vaccinations do not provoke attacks of multiple sclerosis.

CLINICAL MANIFESTATIONS The first attack of MS may declare itself as a single symptom or sign (45 percent) or as more than one (55 percent). Approximately 40 percent of MS patients will have an episode of optic neuritis, either as their first difficulty or at some point along the course of their disease. Optic neuritis presents as loss of vision, partial or total, usually in one eye, rarely in both, and often associated with pain on movement of the eye. Macular vision tends to be most affected (central scotoma), but a wide range of field defects may occur. Disturbances of color perception sometimes provide an early indication of mild disease. Fewer than half of optic neuritis patients will show evidence of an inflamed optic nerve head (papillitis); most show no changes in the optic disc at the outset, indicating that the demyelinating lesion is developing some distance behind the nerve head (retrobulbar neuritis). Both forms of optic neuritis will be followed by optic nerve atrophy, detected as pallor of the optic disc.

It is important to recognize that most cases of optic neuritis occur as an isolated event. At most, 40 percent of individuals with optic neuritis subsequently go on to develop multiple sclerosis; unfortunately it is difficult to predict who will and who will not develop the disease. The optic nerve is an extension of the brain, and lesions of multiple sclerosis are confined to central nervous system white matter. Whether optic neuritis occurring alone constitutes a forme fruste of multiple sclerosis with but a single attack is not known; no other cause for optic neuritis has been determined. Approximately one-third of patients with optic neuritis recover completely, one-third partially, and one-third little or not at all. Visual evoked potential testing reveals prolonged latencies of the evoked potential in the occipital cortex in more than 80 percent of established cases of multiple sclerosis; less than half of these can describe an antecedent optic neuritis. Clearly subclinical involvement of the optic pathways is common.

Symptoms and signs of neurologic dysfunction arising from brainstem, cerebellar, and spinal cord lesions are frequent in multiple sclerosis. Diplopia may occur either because the third, fourth, or sixth cranial nerve pathways are damaged along their course within the central nervous system or because an internuclear ophthalmoplegia (INO) has developed (see Chap. 17). An INO reflects involvement of the medial longitudinal fasciculus. The sign consists of an inability to adduct one eye on attempted lateral gaze together with full abduction of the other eye, which shows horizontal nystagmus. Bilateral INO in a young adult is virtually diagnostic of multiple sclerosis, although a few instances of bilateral INO in systemic lupus erythematosus are on record. Another clinical feature of brainstem involvement is either facial hypesthesia, or tic douloureux (fifth cranial nerve). When tic douloureux occurs in a young adult, the possibility of underlying multiple sclerosis should be seriously entertained. Bell's palsy or hemifacial spasm (seventh cranial nerve), vertigo, vomiting, and nystagmus (vestibular connections of the eighth cranial nerve) are also frequent; less commonly there is complaint of deafness. Involvement of cerebellar connections or of spinocerebellar pathways results in ataxia which can affect speech (scanning), head or trunk (titubation), limbs (intention tremor), and stance and gait. Cerebellar ataxia may be combined with sensory ataxia due to involvement of the spinal cord.

Spinal cord lesions produce a myriad of motor and sensory problems. Corticospinal tract interruption results in the classical features of upper motor neuron dysfunction (weakness, spasticity, hyperreflexia, clonus, Babinski response, loss of abdominal skin reflexes). Posterior column lesions cause loss, or diminution, of joint-position and vibration senses as well as the frequently encountered complaints of tingling or tightness of the extremities and of band-like sensations about the trunk. Less often, pain and temperature sensations are lost or diminished, reflecting spinothalamic tract involvement. Partial lesions of sensory tracts or of the root entry zones of sensory nerves can produce painful dysesthesias. On occasion, spinal cord lesions will result in paroxysmal symptoms including tonic spasms which can be painful.

Symptoms of bladder dysfunction, including hesitancy, urgency, frequency, and incontinence are common features of spinal cord involvement. Equally common is bowel dysfunction, particularly constipation. Males with multiple sclerosis, if questioned, often complain of sexual impotence. Patients with multiple sclerosis may experience an electric shock-like sensation on flexion of the neck, called Lhermitte's sign.

Severe spinal cord lesions can result in loss of function, sometimes total, below the level of the lesion; less complete lesions can result in the hemicord syndrome of Brown-Séquard (see Chap. 366). When either of these events occurs, it is referred to as a transverse myelitis. A single episode of transverse myelitis not followed by subsequent progression of disease may, as with an isolated episode of optic neuritis, represent a forme fruste of multiple sclerosis, and again as with optic neuritis, approximately one-third of patients with transverse myelitis recover completely, one-third partially, and one-third not at all. It must be stressed that spinal cord involvement is the predominating feature in most advanced cases of multiple sclerosis.

Cerebral symptoms may occur in multiple sclerosis due to extensive involvement of subcortical and central white matter. With extensive lesions of brain, intellect may suffer, sometimes disastrously. By far, the most frequent emotional feature of multiple sclerosis is depression. Euphoria, when it occurs, indicates widespread cerebral disease and is often associated with dementia and pseudobulbar palsy. Three to five percent of patients will have one or more epileptic seizures, presumably because of extension of plaques into gray matter. Focal neurologic signs of cerebral origin, such as hemiparesis, homonymous hemianopsia and dysphasia, while seen in multiple sclerosis, are rare.

Neuromyelitis optica and multiple sclerosis An ill-defined symptom complex known as Devic's syndrome, or neuromyelitis optica, is considered by some, for dubious reasons, to be an entity distinguishable from multiple sclerosis. The complex is characterized by acute optic neuritis, usually bilateral, which is followed, or less frequently preceded, within hours to weeks by transverse myelitis. The cerebrospinal fluid may show a pleocytosis with polymorphonuclear cells and a protein content that is higher than is usual for multiple sclerosis. Pathologic examination in fatal cases reveals more tissue destruction and cavitation than is expected in multiple sclerosis, although this may bespeak no more than the intensity of the process. Some cases of neuromyelitis optica evolve over time into typical multiple sclerosis; those that do not may be compared to instances of optic neuritis and transverse myelitis occurring as isolated events. In the orient, multiple sclerosis presents with bilateral optic nerve and spinal cord involvement more frequently than is the case in the occident. Such cases are often classified as Devic's disease, but at autopsy they cannot be distinguished from multiple sclerosis.

COURSE OF ILLNESS AND PROGNOSIS The clinical course is unpredictable. In general, symptoms which appear acutely and those referable to sensory paths and the cranial nerves have a more favorable prognosis than those developing insidiously or involving motor and especially cerebellar function. According to McAlpine, 80 percent of cases that have a purely exacerbating and remitting disease have unrestricted function after 10 years. Of cases in which exacerbations and remissions are superimposed on a progressive tempo of evolution, 50 percent are disabled after 10 years. In cases that have a purely progressive course from the outset (in these the brunt of the disease usually falls on the spinal cord) long-term prognosis for ambulation is poor.

Rarely multiple sclerosis may be fulminant and fatal within weeks to months. Such cases, which are referred to as acute multiple sclerosis, show intense inflammatory responses within their plaques. Onset in such cases may be with headache, vomiting, delirium, convulsions, even coma, plus an array of signs indicating severe compromise of cortical, brainstem, optic nerve, and spinal cord function. The distinction from acute disseminated encephalomyelitis may be difficult in life; at autopsy the lesions are larger and more like those of multiple sclerosis.

DIFFERENTIAL DIAGNOSIS The diagnosis of multiple sclerosis becomes secure when signs referable to multiple lesions of central nervous system white matter have developed and remitted at different times. Particularly in the early phases of disease, the neurologic symptoms may suggest discrete dysfunction of the nervous system, and other causes of focal disease must be excluded. An excellent clinical rule is that multiple sclerosis should not be diagnosed when all the patient's symptoms and signs can be explained by a single lesion. A common aphorism is that multiple sclerosis presents with symptoms in one leg and signs in both.

Conditions to be excluded vary depending on the sites of the lesions. Abrupt monocular loss of vision may result from impaired vascular supply to the optic nerve, including embolic and thrombotic occlusion of the carotid, ophthalmic, or central retinal arteries, or as an accompaniment of migraine. When monocular visual loss is more gradual, compressive lesions affecting the optic nerve or an optic nerve glioma need to be considered. Diseases of the macula and retina can usually be excluded by careful funduscopic examination. When optic neuropathy is bilateral, toxic factors such as drugs, nutritional deficiencies, or compressive perichiasmal lesions must be considered.

In patients presenting with acute or progressive spinal cord disease the presence of focal lesions affecting the cord and of degenerative-nutritional diseases which selectively affect spinal cord tracts should be considered. Patients with progressive spastic paraplegia should be evaluated for the presence of intrathecal or extradural neoplasm and for cervical spondylosis. Such evaluation often requires a CT body scan and myelography. Hereditary ataxias can present as degeneration of multiple central nervous system tracts, with or without involvement of the peripheral nervous system. Degeneration of posterior columns and corticospinal and spinocerebellar tracts is common in these disorders. Hereditary ataxias are slowly progressive and feature stereotyped symmetric involvement as well as a family history consistent with autosomal dominant, or recessive, inheritance. Amyotrophic lateral sclerosis usually presents with prominent lower motor neuron signs (atrophy, weakness, and fasciculations) in addition to pyramidal signs (spasticity, hyperreflexia) and without sensory abnormalities. Subacute combined degeneration of the cord can be excluded by symmetry of spinal symptoms and by a normal serum vitamin B_{12} level, by a normal bone marrow, and a normal Schilling test.

When progressive brainstem dysfunction occurs, posterior fossa tumor as well as brainstem encephalitis should be excluded. Single cranial nerve palsies, particularly Bell's palsy, trigeminal sensory neuropathy, or tic douloureux may occur as part of the multiple sclerosis picture, but evidence of multifocal disease must be present before they can be ascribed to multiple sclerosis. When vertigo is the complaint and nystagmus is detected, inner ear disease should be considered as well as the possibility that barbiturates or phenytoin have been taken.

There are several multifocal and recrudescent diseases of the central nervous system which may mimic multiple sclerosis. Systemic lupus erythematosus and other vasculitides may cause scattered and recurring lesions within brain, brainstem, and spinal cord. Behçet's disease is characterized by recurrent episodes of focal brain disease, spinal fluid pleocytosis, oral and genital ulcers, and uveitis. Other disorders to be excluded include meningovascular syphilis, cryptococcosis, toxoplasmosis, other chronic nervous system infections, and sarcoidosis.

When complaints are vague and findings minimal, a diagnosis of conversion reaction (hysteria) may come to mind. This diagnosis should always be made on the basis of positive criteria for hysteria and never as a "diagnosis by exclusion." Early in its course, multiple sclerosis is mislabeled as hysteria with distressing frequency.

A firm diagnosis of multiple sclerosis should only be made when the evidence is unequivocal. Aside from the distress that such a diagnosis causes, it will serve to explain almost any subsequent neurologic event and may divert attention away from other possibly treatable diseases.

LABORATORY TESTS Although the diagnosis of multiple sclerosis continues to depend on its clinical features, laboratory aids have become increasingly useful as supports for the diagnosis. In the vast majority of patients with multiple sclerosis, one or more tests will be abnormal, although normal results do not rule out this diagnosis.

The cerebrospinal fluid in multiple sclerosis patients typically reveals only a slight or no increase in cell number. Ninety percent of patients show fewer than 10 cells per cubic millimeter in their spinal fluid; cell counts greater than 50 are rare. The cells in the spinal fluid are predominantly T lymphocytes, although rare plasma cells may be found. Some correlation exists between the extent of pleocytosis and disease activity. Evidence that the cells in the spinal fluid are activated not only during exacerbations of disease but also during seeming remission has been presented; this indicates that disease activity smolders at all times, even though neither the physician nor the patient may be able to detect changes. The spinal fluid of 90 percent of patients contains less than 60 mg/dl of total protein; a protein of greater than 100 mg/dl should raise questions about whether the diagnosis is correct.

The most characteristic spinal fluid finding in multiple sclerosis is an increase in immunoglobulin G (IgG) which contrasts with relatively normal total protein and albumin concentrations. IgG levels are increased in 80 percent of multiple sclerosis patients; the increase is greatest in long-standing cases with severe neurological deficits. Early in the disease, when the diagnosis is most in doubt, IgG values are often normal. IgG levels do not change in any meaningful way with relapses and remissions. Most of the IgG in the spinal fluid is synthesized within the central nervous system. The increased IgG fraction in the spinal fluid explains the first-zone abnormality of the colloidal gold curve, a test of historical interest and still of some practical value in multiple sclerosis.

When the spinal fluid IgG from multiple sclerosis patients is subjected to electrophoresis or isoelectric focusing, it fractionates into a restricted number of bands (termed oligoclonal bands). Oligoclonal banding of IgG has also been found in the spinal fluid in a number of acute and chronic central nervous system infections; in these the bands have been shown to be antibodies to the infective agent. In multiple sclerosis, the IgG bands have not been shown to be directed against any single viral or intrinsic brain antigen; more likely they represent a heterogeneous group of antibodies directed against many antigens. The number of bands in the spinal fluid increases as the disease evolves. It has also been suggested that high levels of IgG and many oligoclonal bands are associated with a severe course.

Within spinal fluid, myelin debris as well as myelin basic protein appears during attacks of disease. Myelin basic protein levels can be measured by radioimmunoassay; their level seems to reflect the extent of myelin breakdown since myelin basic protein levels also increase in other disorders associated with white matter breakdown such as stroke.

Conduction of nerve impulses along axons denuded of their myelin is slowed. Evoked potential testing provides a sensitive means to detect slowed conduction of visual, auditory, or somatosensory impulses. Such tests employ repetitive sensory stimuli and utilize computer averaging techniques to record the electric responses evoked during the conduction of these stimuli along visual, auditory, or somatosensory afferent pathways. In normal subjects, the pattern of the evoked potentials and time for conduction are highly predictable. One or more of the evoked potential tests will reveal slowing of conduction in 80 percent of MS patients; in 30 to 40 percent of patients, abnormal evoked responses are detected without any clinical symptoms or signs in the involved pathway being apparent. Evoked potential testing may confirm the presence of additional sites of disease in suspected cases with only a single clinically detectable lesion (see Chap. 354).

Computerized tomography (CT) of the brain may reveal low-density lesions within white matter, usually in a paraventricular or subcortical distribution. The incidence of abnormality discovered by CT scanning is reported to range from 10 to 50 percent. Similar lesions may be noted in optic nerves and brainstem. At times, enhancement may be revealed by iodine infusion; this finding indicates the presence of acute lesions and a disruption of the blood-brain barrier. Enhancement may disappear as the clinical symptoms resolve. Cortical atrophy with enlarged ventricles is also found in some patients.

Elevated spinal fluid IgG, abnormal evoked potentials, and low-density lesions on CT scan provide useful adjuncts in evaluation of the patient with suspected multiple sclerosis; however, the clinical findings remain paramount in establishing the diagnosis.

TREATMENT OF MS No effective treatment for multiple sclerosis is known. Therapeutic efforts are directed toward (1) amelioration of the acute episode, (2) prevention of relapses, and (3) relief of symptoms.

In acute flare-ups of disease, glucocorticoid treatment may lessen the severity of symptoms and speed recovery; however, ultimate recovery is not improved by this drug nor is the extent of permanent disability altered. Glucocorticoids likely act chiefly via mechanisms other than through modulation of the immune response. They may improve the ability of demyelinated nerve to conduct and reduce edema and inflammation within plaques. Usual regimens utilize either ACTH to stimulate endogenous glucocorticoid synthesis or prednisone. ACTH is preferred by many clinicians since the only controlled trials that demonstrated the efficacy of glucocorticoid therapy in flare-ups of multiple sclerosis and in acute optic neuritis were performed with this drug. ACTH is commonly given in a dose of 80 units daily intravenously for 3 to 7 days, followed by intramuscular injections, in periodically decreasing doses over the next 2 to 3 weeks. Prednisone, 15 mg qid., is sometimes given rather than ACTH, again over 3 to 7 days with gradually tapering doses over the next 2 to 3 weeks. Since prednisone is taken by mouth, the treatment is simpler than with ACTH and an admission to the hospital may sometimes be avoided. Use of long-term daily or alternate-day steroids is not advised.

Immunosuppressive agents such as azathioprine (Imuran) have been claimed to reduce the number of relapses in several series, but there is no consensus about the efficacy of this drug. Although the question of efficacy remains unresolved, the abnormal B-cell response seen in the blood in multiple sclerosis returns to normal levels with azathioprine treatment. The efficacy of treatment with cyclophosphamide, antithymocyte serum, plasmapheresis, and interferon are currently under investigation.

Symptomatic treatment should address both the physical and psychological needs of patients. Patients should avoid excess fatigue and extremes of temperature and eat a balanced diet. Diets containing low levels of saturated fats have been advocated; their efficacy is doubtful. The use of belladonna alkaloids and bethanechol chloride can help bladder dysfunction. Periodic checks for urinary tract infection should be performed. Bowel training can alleviate disorders of bowel function. Drugs available for the treatment of spasticity include diazepam, baclofen, and dantrolene sodium. Painful dysesthesias, facial twitching, tic douloureux, and tonic spasms may respond to carbamazepine or phenytoin. Occasionally trigeminal root injection is required to relieve tic douloureux (see Chap. 367).

ACUTE DISSEMINATED ENCEPHALOMYELITIS

Acute disseminated encephalomyelitis may be defined as a monophasic encephalitis or myelitis of abrupt onset characterized by symptoms and signs indicative of damage chiefly of the white matter of the brain or spinal cord. The process may be severe, and even fatal, or mild and evanescent. Pathologic features are those of innumerable minute foci of perivenular lymphocyte and mononuclear cell infiltration with demyelination. The topography of the demyelination corresponds to that of the inflammatory infiltrates. The condition most commonly follows vaccinations against rabies or smallpox or acute infectious illnesses, especially measles, but may occur without any obvious antecedent. The cause is uncertain but is believed by some to represent a hypersensitivity, perhaps to myelin basic protein, and to be the human counterpart of experimentally induced EAE.

ETIOLOGY The entity has been described after two types of vaccination: after rabies vaccination with the Semple vaccine, which contains brain tissue and which is now seldom used, and after vaccination against smallpox, which is now seldom performed.

Shortly after introduction of rabies vaccination by Pasteur it became evident that neuroparalytic accidents could follow this procedure. After a course of injections a sudden encephalitic or myelitic catastrophe might occur coincident with hypersensitivity-type reactions at the sites of vaccine injection. The process clearly involved hypersensitivity to nervous system antigens and came to be looked upon as the human counterpart of EAE. The incidence was variously reported as between 1 in 1000 and 1 in 5000 persons vaccinated. An identical syndrome has followed inoculation with noninfected brain material, indicating that killed rabies virus was not the cause; with the introduction of duck embryo killed rabies virus vaccine (which is free of myelinated nervous tissue), the condition has disappeared. Neuroparalytic accidents were most frequent in young adults, the peak age of occurrence corresponding to that of onset of multiple sclerosis.

Smallpox vaccination was followed by an identical complication, the incidence averaging perhaps 1 case per 5000 persons vaccinated but with marked differences between vaccination programs. The complication almost always occurred in conjunction with a primary take rather than a booster-type response. The encephalitis usually followed the peak of the vaccination response by a few days to a week or more but on occasion preceded it. The complication was unknown in children less than 2 years of age; in infants, smallpox vaccination was sometimes associated with an encephalopathy with brain swelling, i.e., toxic encephalopathy.

One case of measles in 1000 is complicated by significant neurologic complications, which are often severe. The mortality rate averages 20 percent, and half the survivors are left with significant residual damage. The syndrome usually follows the rash by a few days. It bears no relationship to the severity of measles itself. Abnormal spinal fluid and changes in the electroencephalogram are observed in perhaps half the children who contract measles, suggesting that subclinical neurologic involvement may be much more widespread than is usually appreciated. A subtle decline in performance and changes in behavior following measles may reflect this inapparent nervous system involvement. Measles vaccination has drastically reduced the frequency of this complication.

An identical clinical picture formerly was seen as a complication of smallpox and is still encountered during or following chickenpox and extremely rarely as a complication of rubella. Demyelinating encephalomyelitis is very rare in mumps; instead there is often a true viral meningitis. A clinical picture identical to postinfectious encephalomyelitis has been described after mycoplasma infections. Despite its striking association with measles, the occurrence of the same clinical picture after several different infections fits better with the postulate that the basic process involves hypersensitivity rather than a direct viral infection of the brain and spinal cord. Sensitivity to myelin basic protein has, in fact, been demonstrated in several instances. All attempts to isolate a virus have failed.

CLINICAL MANIFESTATIONS The disease usually begins abruptly. Headache and delirium may give way to lethargy and coma. Coma has an ominous prognosis. Seizures at the onset or shortly thereafter are not infrequent. There may be stiffness of the neck, other signs of meningeal irritation, and fever. Focal signs may be engrafted on this picture, and spinal cord involvement with flaccid paralysis of all four limbs is particularly common. Monoparesis and hemiplegia are also seen. Tendon reflexes may be lost initially only to become hyperactive later; extensor plantar responses are the rule, and sphincter control is generally lost. Sensory loss is variable but may be extensive and severe. Brainstem involvement may be reflected by nystagmus, ocular palsies, and pupillary changes. Some cases may present as a purely spinal cord syndrome and in mild instances with minor signs such as a facial palsy. Chorea and athetosis are rare. Cerebellar signs may predominate, particularly in cases associated with chickenpox. The spinal fluid almost always shows an increase in protein (50 to 100 mg/dl) and lymphocytes (10 to several hundred cells); rarely it is normal. The mortality is 20 percent, and perhaps half the survivors have residual deficits.

The diagnosis is not difficult if there is a history of rabies or smallpox vaccination or of measles. In cases without such a history, distinction from viral encephalitis may be difficult and at times not possible. Reye's syndrome (see Chap. 360) may be difficult to distinguish from acute disseminated encephalomyelitis. Vomiting at onset, a normal spinal fluid, hyperammonemia, and raised intracranial pressure should suggest Reye's syndrome; frequent convulsions and focal signs argue against it. A distinction from acute multiple sclerosis may not be possible.

PREVENTION AND TREATMENT Since smallpox has been eradicated, there is no longer reason to vaccinate against it. Use of duck embryo and human diploid vaccine in rabies prophylaxis has eliminated neuroparalytic accidents, and measles vaccination has drastically reduced what used to be the largest group of postinfectious encephalomyelitides.

Administration of high doses of glucocorticoids every 4 to 6 h is the treatment of choice though controlled trials have not been carried out.

ACUTE NECROTIZING HEMORRHAGIC ENCEPHALOMYELITIS

Acute necrotizing hemorrhagic encephalomyelitis is a rare tissue destructive disease of the central nervous system which occurs with explosive suddenness within a few days of an upper respiratory infection. The pathologic findings are distinctive. On sectioning the brain, much of the white matter of one or both hemispheres is seen to be destroyed almost to the point of liquefaction. The involved tissue is pink or yellowish-gray and flecked with multiple small hemorrhages. Sometimes similar changes are localized to the brainstem or spinal cord. On histological examination the core lesion resembles that of acute disseminated encephalomyelitis in showing perivenular foci of demyelination, all of like age. As in acute disseminated encephalomyelitis lymphocytes and macrophages are present in the regions of myelin loss, but superimposed and dominating the picture is an intense polymorphonuclear infiltrate in keeping with the necrotizing nature of the process. The vessels themselves are partially necrotic; they may contain platelet or fibrin thrombi within their lumens and fibrin deposits beyond their walls. Multiple small hemorrhages at sites of vessel damage are an invariable feature, as is a violent inflammatory reaction in the meninges. Large necrotic foci form by coalescence of smaller lesions in the hemispheres, brainstem, or spinal cord.

The clinical course of the illness resembles that of acute disseminated encephalomyelitis save for its apoplectiform onset and rapidity of progress, sometimes leading to death within 48 h. Neurological signs are frequently unilateral, reflecting disease in one cerebral hemisphere, or bilateral. It is probable that certain patients showing an explosive myelitic illness are suffering from a necrotizing myelitis of similar type, but pathologic evidence in support of this view has been difficult to obtain. The cerebrospinal fluid examination discloses a more intense reaction than in other demyelinating diseases. Often a polymorphonuclear pleocytosis of up to 2000 cells and a considerable increase in amount of protein are detected. In cases of slower evolution the cell counts are lower and cells are mainly of the mononuclear type.

The etiology of this disease is not established; however, the entire clinical-pathologic entity bears a close resemblance to a hyperacute form of EAE which can be induced in animals by administration of endotoxin, pertussis vaccine, or its histamine sensitizing factor coincident with or shortly after injection of myelin in adjuvant. The lesions in this experimental disease can perhaps be considered as those of a Sanarelli-Shwartzman reaction within the brain, superimposed on an acutely demyelinating process. Rarely a lesion like acute necrotizing hemorrhagic encephalomyelitis occurs in multiple sclerosis.

The differential diagnosis of this disorder includes acute encephalitis, particularly those types causing tissue necrosis (herpes simplex, arbovirus), acute bacterial cerebritis, septic embolic occlusion of an artery, thrombophlebitis, and suppurative brain abscess. The similarity of acute necrotizing hemorrhagic encephalomyelitis to acute disseminated encephalomyelitis suggests that steroid therapy may be beneficial.

REFERENCES

ADAMS RD, KUBIK CS: The morbid anatomy of the demyelinative disease. Am J Med 12:510, 1952

BAUM HM, ROTHSCHILD BB: The incidence and prevalence of reported multiple sclerosis. Ann Neurol 5:420, 1981

ELLISON GW, MYERS LW: Immunosuppressive drugs in multiple sclerosis: Pro and con. Neurology 30(part2):28, 1980

LAMPERT PW: Autoimmune and virus-induced demyelinating diseases. A review. Am J Pathol 91:176, 1978

MCALPINE D et al: *Multiple Sclerosis—A Reappraisal.* London, Churchill Livingstone, 1972

WHITAKER JN: Current views regarding the etiology and pathogenesis of multiple sclerosis, in *Update IV: Harrison's Principles of Internal Medicine,* KJ Isselbacher et al (eds). New York, McGraw-Hill, 1983, pp 39–48

362
METABOLIC DISEASES OF THE NERVOUS SYSTEM

MAURICE VICTOR
RAYMOND D. ADAMS

Included under this title is a large and varied group of neurologic disorders united by one particular attribute—that of deranging in some way the metabolism of nervous tissue. This derangement must be ascribed in the final analysis to some fundamental and often unique biochemical abnormality of the neurons involved. In a sense this can be said of all disease processes, but it is in the metabolic disorders that the importance of biochemical factors is most evident.

The metabolic diseases of the nervous system can be divided readily into two distinct categories—acquired and inherited. In the acquired type, a disturbance of cerebral function is usually consequent upon disease in some other organ system—heart (and circulation), lungs (and respiration), kidneys, liver, pancreas, and endocrine glands. The inherited type, as the name indicates, is characterized by an inborn abnormality of metabolism, which affects both the brain and other organs; reference is made here to conditions such as the aminoacidurias with mental defect, the mucopolysaccharidoses, the lipidoses, the lipoproteinemias, several of the leukodystrophies, hepatolenticular degeneration (Wilson's disease), porphyria, galactosemia, and the glycogen storage diseases.

In this chapter, emphasis will be on the acquired metabolic diseases listed in Table 362-1, and appropriately so, insofar as they are essentially disorders of adult life and a major source of concern to internist and neurologist alike. In fact no other category of disease so clearly exemplifies the interdependence of these two medical disciplines.

The inherited metabolic diseases, on the other hand, are fundamentally disorders of infancy and early childhood and are more appropriately considered in a textbook of pediatrics. One group of these diseases, the lysosomal storage diseases, is discussed in Chap. 104. Other inherited diseases, which permit survival to adolescence or early adult life or which have their onset during these periods, are discussed in this and in other chapters of this book, to which the reader will be referred.

ACQUIRED (SECONDARY) METABOLIC DISEASES OF THE NERVOUS SYSTEM

METABOLIC DISEASES PRESENTING AS A SYNDROME OF EPISODIC CONFUSION, STUPOR, OR COMA The *syndrome of impaired consciousness* has been described in detail in Chap. 20. There it was pointed out that metabolic disturbances are frequent causes of impaired consciousness and that their presence must always be considered when there are no focal or lateralizing signs of cerebral disease and no cellular changes in the spinal fluid. Intoxication with alcohol and other drugs figures prominently in the differential diagnosis.

Anoxic encephalopathy This is one of the most frequent and disastrous accidents encountered in the emergency and operating rooms of every general hospital. The basic disorder is a lack of oxygen to the brain, resulting from a failure of the heart and circulation or of the lungs and respiration. Often both are responsible, and one cannot say which predominates—hence the ambiguous allusion in clinical records to "cardiorespiratory failure." The conditions which most often lead to anoxic encephalopathy are (1) suffocation (from drowning, strangulation, aspiration of vomitus or blood, compression of the trachea by hemorrhage or a surgical pack, or foreign body in the trachea); (2) carbon monoxide (CO) poisoning, in which respiration fails first and then cardiovascular functions; (3) diseases which paralyze the muscles of respiration (Landry-Guillain-Barré syndrome) or damage the central nervous system diffusely (trauma and vascular diseases of the brain, epilepsy), again with respiratory failure being the initial factor, preceding cardiac failure; and (4) myocardial infarction, hemorrhage, shock, and circulatory collapse, cardiac arrest during inhalation of spinal anesthesia, and infective and traumatic shock, in all of which cardiac action is paralyzed before respiration.

CLINICAL FEATURES Mild degrees of hypoxia induce only inattentiveness, impaired judgment, and motor incoordination and have no lasting effects. With severe hypoxia or anoxia, as occurs with cardiac arrest, consciousness is lost within seconds, but recovery will be complete if breathing, oxygenation of blood, and cardiac action are restored within 3 to 5 min. If anoxia persists beyond this time, serious and permanent injury to the brain results, particularly to those parts with marginal efficiency of their circulation (globus pallidus, cerebellum, hippocampus, and parietooccipital lobes in "border-zone regions"). Clinically, it is difficult to judge the precise degree of hypoxia since slight heart action or an imperceptible blood pressure may serve to maintain the circulation to some extent. Hence some individuals have made an excellent recovery after cerebral anoxia that allegedly lasted 8 to 10 min or longer. *An important clinical rule is that degrees of hypoxia which at no time abolish consciousness rarely if ever cause permanent damage to the nervous system.* Also, generally speaking, subjects who demonstrate intact brainstem function when the acute hypoxic event has terminated (as indicated by normal ciliospinal and pupillary light responses, intact doll's head eye movements, and oculovestibular responses) tend to have a better outlook for recovery of consciousness and perhaps all of their faculties. Conversely, absence of these reflex activities and the presence of pupils that are persistently fixed to light suggest a hopeless outlook.

The most severe degrees of anoxia are manifested by a state of complete unawareness and unresponsiveness with abolition of the brainstem reflexes. Natural respiration cannot be sustained; only *cardiac action and blood pressure are maintained.* No electrical activity is seen in the EEG (it is isoelectric). This is the *brain death syndrome.* When caused by anoxia-hypotension it is always irreversible. At autopsy nearly all the cerebral, cerebellar, and brainstem tissues are found to be destroyed. One must exercise extreme caution in concluding that the patient has "brain death," because anesthesia, drug intoxication, and hypothermia may also cause deep coma and an isoelectric EEG, but permit recovery. Such cases have been brought increasingly to public attention because of ethical and moral issues that surround the question of discontinuing medical therapy. In the authors' experience "brain death" victims usually cannot be sustained for more than several days; in other words, the problem settles itself, and it is not so difficult as the cases in which the patient has suffered severe but somewhat lesser degrees of cerebral damage, as described below.

Patients who have suffered a severe but lesser degree of hypoxia will have stabilized breathing and heart action by the time they are first seen. Yet such patients may be profoundly comatose, with eyes slightly divergent and motionless but with reactive pupils, inert and flaccid or intensely rigid limbs, and diminished tendon reflexes. Within a few minutes after cardiac action and breathing have been restored, generalized convulsions and isolated or grouped twitches of muscles (myoclonus) may supervene. If the damage has been severe, coma persists, decerebrate postures may be present or occur upon pinching the limbs, and bilateral Babinski signs can be evoked. In the first 24 to 48 h death may terminate this state in a setting of rising temperature, deepening coma, and circulatory collapse. Or, with lesser degrees of injury, where the cerebral and cerebellar cortices are partly or completely destroyed but brainstem-spinal structures remain intact, the individual may survive in a state referred to as "irreversible coma" or "persistent vegetative state." Some of these patients remain mute, unresponsive, and unaware of their environment for weeks, months, or years. The medical profession is searching for criteria that will accurately predict this hopeless state early in the comatose period, but the data are as yet insecure. If intoxication can be excluded, the presence of fixed dilated pupils and paralysis of eye movement for 24 to 48 h, along with marked slowing of the EEG, usually signifies irreversible cerebral damage. We have not observed deep coma of this type, lasting more than 5 days, to be attended by recovery.

Patients with still lesser degrees of injury improve after a period of coma. Consciousness is regained, and then various degrees of confusion, visual agnosia, extrapyramidal rigidity, or movement disorder (action or intention myoclonus, choreo-

TABLE 362-1
Classification of the acquired metabolic disorders of the nervous system

1 Presenting as a syndrome of episodic confusion, stupor, or coma
- *a* Hypoxic-hypotensive encephalopathy
- *b* Hypercapnic encephalopathy
- *c* Hypoglycemic and hyperglycemic encephalopathies
- *d* Hepatic and portal-systemic encephalopathy
- *e* Uremic and dialysis encephalopathy
- *f* Encephalopathies due to electrolyte disturbances

2 Presenting as a progressive extrapyramidal syndrome
- *a* Acquired hepatocerebral degeneration
- *b* Kernicterus
- *c* Hypoparathyroidism

3 Presenting as cerebellar ataxia
- *a* Hyperthermia
- *b* Hypothyroidism

4 Causing psychosis or dementia
- *a* Cushing's disease and steroid encephalopathy
- *b* Thyroid psychosis
- *c* Hyperparathyroidism
- *d* Addison's disease (adrenal insufficiency)
- *e* Pancreatic encephalopathy

athetosis) become manifest. Some of these patients quickly pass through this acute hypoxic phase and proceed to make a full recovery; others are left with permanent neurologic sequelae. The *posthypoxic syndromes* that we have observed most frequently are (1) *persistent coma or stupor;* and, with lesser degrees of cerebral injury, (2) *dementia,* with or without extrapyramidal signs; (3) *visual agnosia;* (4) *parkinsonism;* (5) *choreoathetosis;* (6) *cerebellar ataxia;* (7) *intention or action myoclonus;* and (8) *Korsakoff's amnesic state. Seizures* may or may not continue to be a problem.

A relatively uncommon and unexplained phenomenon is *delayed postanoxic encephalopathy.* Initial improvement, which appears to be complete, is followed after a variable period of time (2 to 10 days, occasionally longer) by a relapse, characterized by apathy, confusion, irritability, and occasionally agitation or mania. A few patients have recovered from this second episode, but in most of them there has been progression of the neurologic syndrome, with shuffling gait, diffuse rigidity and spasticity, coma, and death after 1 to 2 weeks. Postmortem examination of these cases has shown the major abnormality to be widespread cerebral demyelination. Exceptionally, yet another delayed syndrome occurs, where a period of hypoxia is followed by a slow, deteriorative state, affecting basal ganglia more than cerebral cortex and white matter, which then progresses for weeks to months until the patient is mute, rigid, and helpless.

The essential *mechanism* in hypoxic encephalopathy is a lack of oxygen and an arrest of all aerobic metabolic processes necessary to sustain the Krebs tricarboxylic cycle and the electron transport system. Lactic acid accumulates in the tissues. Deprived of their source of energy, neurons proceed to catabolize themselves in an attempt to maintain their activity and in so doing damage themselves to such a degree that they cannot survive. The phenomenon of delayed progression is not understood but may be due to the blockage or exhaustion of some enzymatic process during the period when brain metabolism is restored or even increased (as in hyperthermia or with seizures or increased motor activity).

DIAGNOSIS This depends on (1) the history of the hypoxic event and evidence of reduced oxygenation of arterial blood ($P_{O_2} < 40$ mmHg), CO intoxication (the latter is indicated by its spectroscopic band or cherry red color of the skin for a few minutes to hours after the episode), blood pressures below 70 mmHg systolic, or cardiac arrest; and (2) the typical clinical sequences of events outlined above after a possible hypoxic episode has terminated. Renal damage (anuria) and myocardial infarction may also have occurred (see Chap. 20) and provide corroborative evidence of hypoxia.

TREATMENT The treatment of anoxic encephalopathy is directed mainly at the prevention of a critical degree of hypoxic injury. After a clear airway is secured, artificial respiration, external thoracic cardiac massage, open-chest surgery, and the use of a cardiac defibrillator or pacemaker all have their place, and every second counts in their prompt utilization. Once cardiac and pulmonary function are restored, there is some evidence that reducing cerebral metabolic requirements by continuous hypothermia or administration of barbiturates for 48 to 72 h may prevent the delayed worsening referred to above. Oxygen may be of value during the first hours, but is probably of little use after the blood becomes well oxygenated. Dexamethasone administered intravenously in doses of 6 to 12 mg every 6 h helps to combat brain (cellular) swelling. Seizures should be controlled by the methods indicated in Chap. 358. If the seizures are severe, continuous, and unresponsive to drugs, the use of curare and controlled respiration may be required. Often the seizures cease after a few days. If they persist, they are often myoclonic, and mephobarbital (Mebaral), in divided doses up to 500 mg per day, phenobarbital, 300 mg per day, or clonazepam, 8 to 12 mg daily in divided doses, may be useful in their control. Keeping the patient quiet in bed for 10 days, even if consciousness was regained early, may help to prevent the delayed form of postanoxic encephalopathy. Thiopental therapy to reduce brain metabolism has proved to be feasible and safe in a clinical setting, but there are no data regarding its efficacy.

Hypercapnic encephalopathy Chronic emphysema, chronic fibrosing lung disease, and in some instances a seeming inadequacy of the respiratory center lead to chronic respiratory acidosis, with an elevation of P_{CO_2} and a reduction in arterial P_{O_2}. Secondary polycythemia and cor pulmonale often accompany these diseases of the lungs, and pulmonary infection may be superimposed.

The clinical syndrome consequent upon hypercapnia (and hypoxia) comprises generalized or bilateral frontal or occipital headache, often intense and persistent for hours; papilledema; mental dullness, drowsiness, confusion, stupor, and coma; a fast-frequency action tremor and coarse twitching of all muscles that are in a state of sustained contraction; and an inability to maintain a fixed posture or interruption of a voluntary movement because of brief lapses of sustained muscle contraction (asterixis). Intermittent drowsiness, indifference and inattention to the environment, reduction of psychomotor activity, imperception of the sequence of events, and forgetfulness constitute the more subtle manifestations of this syndrome.

In fully developed cases, the cerebrospinal fluid (CSF) is under increased pressure, P_{CO_2} may exceed 75 mmHg, and oxygen saturation of arterial blood ranges from 85 to 40 percent. The EEG reveals slow activity, in the delta and theta range, sometimes bilaterally synchronous. The mechanism of the cerebral disorder is said to be CO_2 narcosis, but the biochemical details are not known. The danger of administering morphine or sedatives, which depress the respiratory center (now insensitive to CO_2), or the inhalation of oxygen, which removes the sole stimulus to the respiratory center, is now widely recognized.

Forced ventilation with an intermittent positive-pressure respirator, treatment of heart failure with digitalis and diuretics, venesection to reduce the viscosity of the blood, and antibiotics to combat pulmonary infection are the most effective therapeutic measures. If stupor or coma persists, the arterial O_2 level should be rechecked; it may be critically reduced. Or the pH of the CSF may be very low, in the range of 7.15 to 7.25. In CO_2 narcosis, correction of the acidosis of blood is easier than that of CSF, which tends to lag.

Unlike pure hypoxic encephalopathy, hypercapnia rarely causes prolonged coma, and in our experience it has not led to irreversible brain damage. The papilledema and the intermittent lapses of sustained postures or asterixis (the latter are also characteristic of liver failure, uremia, and rarely other metabolic disorders) are important diagnostic features. The syndrome of hypercapnia is apt to be mistaken for brain tumor, a confusional psychosis of nondescript type, or a disease causing myoclonus or chorea. In the latter instance it must be distinguished from a chronic extrapyramidal syndrome, as described further on in this chapter.

Hypoglycemic encephalopathy (see also Chaps. 20 and 116) This condition is a relatively infrequent but important cause of episodic confusion, convulsions, and coma. The essential biochemical abnormality is a critical lowering of the blood glucose level to less than 25 to 30 mg/dl (lower in infants), which, if it lasts for about 90 min, leads to exhaustion of the cerebral glucose reserve. Within this brief span of time, as cerebral oxidation proceeds without exogenous glucose, the lipid and protein components of neurons are metabolized, and irreversible damage occurs. Long before the 90 min have elapsed, however, the severely hypoglycemic patient becomes deeply comatose.

The most common causes of hypoglycemic encephalopathy are (1) accidental or deliberate overdose of insulin or of an oral antidiabetic agent, (2) an islet cell, insulin-secreting tumor of the pancreas, (3) rarely an alcoholic debauch, (4) acute nonicteric hepatic encephalopathy of childhood (Reye's syndrome), (5) glycogen storage disease in infancy, and (6) an idiopathic state in the neonatal period. In the past, hypoglycemic encephalopathy was a rather frequent complication of "insulin shock" therapy of schizophrenia. In functional hyperinsulinism the hypoglycemia is rarely of sufficient severity or duration to damage the central nervous system.

As the level of blood glucose descends, to about 30 mg/dl, the initial symptoms appear—nervousness, hunger, flushed facies, headache, palpitation, anxiety, sweating, and trembling—and these gradually give way to confusion, drowsiness, and occasionally excitement or overactivity. In the next stage, forced sucking, grasping, motor restlessness, muscular spasms, and finally decerebrate rigidity occur, in that sequence. Myoclonic twitching and convulsions may develop in some patients but are by no means the rule. Blood levels of approximately 10 mg/dl are associated with deep coma, dilation of pupils, pale skin, shallow respirations, bradycardia, and hypotonicity of limb musculature—the so-called medullary phase of hypoglycemia. If glucose is administered before this medullary phase appears, the patient is restored to normalcy, retracing the aforementioned steps in reverse order. However, once the medullary phase is reached, and particularly if it persists for a time before the hypoglycemia is corrected by intravenous glucose or spontaneously, by the so-called gluconeogenic activities of the adrenal glands and liver, recovery is delayed for a period of days or weeks and may be incomplete.

A huge dose of insulin that produces intense hypoglycemia, even of relatively brief duration (30 to 60 min), is more dangerous than a series of less severe hypoglycemic episodes from smaller doses of insulin, possibly because the former impairs or exhausts essential enzymes. This condition cannot then be overcome by large quantities of glucose given intravenously.

The major *neuropathologic effect* is on the cerebral cortex; nerve cells degenerate and are replaced by microgliacytes and astrocytes. The distribution of lesions is similar though not identical to that in hypoxic encephalopathy (there is a tendency for the cerebellar cortex to be spared in hypoglycemic encephalopathy). The sequelae of the two disorders are also much alike.

In addition to coma, lesser and more chronic forms of hypoglycemia may produce two other syndromes. One of these, termed *subacute hypoglycemia,* is characterized by drowsiness and lethargy, diminution in psychomotor activity, deterioration of social behavior, and confusion. Oral or intravenous glucose will immediately alleviate the symptoms. In the other more *chronic syndrome* there is a gradual deterioration of intellectual function, raising the question of a presenile dementia, and in some reported instances there are tremor, chorea, rigidity, cerebellar ataxia and rarely signs of lower motor neuron involvement ("hypoglycemic amyotrophy"). These subacute and chronic forms of hypoglycemia have been observed with islet-cell hypertrophy or tumor, carcinoma of the stomach, fibrous mesothelioma, carcinoma of the cecum, and hepatoma. Supposedly an insulin-like substance is elaborated by the nonpancreatic tumors.

The major clinical differences between hypoglycemia and hypoxia lie in the clinical setting and the mode of evolution of the neurologic disorder. Hypoglycemia usually disturbs cerebral function more slowly than hypoxia, over a period of 30 to 60 min rather than suddenly, within seconds or a few minutes. The recovery phase and sequelae of the two conditions bear close resemblance. *Recurrent hypoglycemia,* as occurs with an islet-cell tumor, may masquerade for some time as an episodic confusional psychosis or convulsive illness, and diagnosis awaits a period of demonstrably low blood glucose or hyperinsulinism (see Chap. 116).

The correction of the hypoglycemia at the earliest moment is the obvious therapy. It is not known whether hypothermia or other measures will increase the safety period in hypoglycemia or alter the outcome.

Hyperglycemic coma Two hyperglycemic syndromes have been described, mainly in diabetics: (1) hyperglycemia with ketoacidosis, and (2) hyperosmolar nonketotic hyperglycemia. These are described in Chap. 114.

Hepatic and portal-systemic encephalopathy Chronic hepatic insufficiency with portal-caval shunting of blood is often punctuated by episodes of stupor, coma, and other neurologic symptoms, a state referred to as hepatic stupor or coma. Also, there are a number of hereditary hyperammonemic syndromes of infancy which may lead to episodic coma with or without seizures. A special type of nonicteric hepatic encephalopathy, first described by Reye and his associates, occurs in children, presenting as an acute toxic encephalopathy (acute brain swelling) in conjunction with rapid enlargement of the liver, fine droplets of fat in hepatocytes, high SGOT and other liver enzymes, and very high levels of ammonium in the blood (see Chap. 322).

CLINICAL FEATURES The central feature of the syndrome is a derangement of consciousness, presenting first as mental confusion with increased or decreased psychomotor activity, followed by progressive drowsiness, stupor, and coma. The confusional state that occurs before coma intervenes is frequently combined with characteristic lapses of sustained muscle contraction (asterixis) and an EEG abnormality consisting of paroxysms of bilaterally synchronous slow waves, in the delta range, which at first are interspersed with alpha activity and which later, as the coma deepens, displace all normal activity. A variable, fluctuating rigidity of the trunk and limbs, grimacing, suck and grasp reflexes, exaggeration or asymmetry of tendon reflexes, Babinski signs, and focal or generalized seizures round out the clinical picture.

The syndrome of hepatic encephalopathy usually evolves over a period of days to weeks and often terminates fatally. In some patients the syndrome does not advance beyond the stage of mild mental dulling and confusion with asterixis and EEG changes. In this relatively mild form it must be differentiated from other acute confusional psychoses and deliria. If the metabolic disorder persists for months and years, a mild dementia and a disorder of posture and movement may gradually appear (grimacing, tremor, dysarthria, ataxia of gait, choreoathetosis), and the condition must then be distinguished from the other dementing and extrapyramidal syndromes (see further on in this chapter).

The striking neuropathologic finding in patients who die in a state of hepatic coma is a diffuse increase in the number and size of the protoplasmic astrocytes (Alzheimer type II astrocytes) in the deep layers of the cerebral cortex, lenticular nuclei, thalamus, substantia nigra, cerebellar cortex, and red, dentate, and pontine nuclei, with little or no visible alteration in the nerve cells or other parenchymal elements. The pathogenesis of hepatic encephalopathy is not fully understood, but the most plausible hypothesis relates it to an abnormality of nitrogen metabolism, wherein ammonium (NH_4^+) or some other amines, which are formed in the bowel by the action of urease-containing organisms on dietary protein and are carried to the liver in the portal circulation, fail to be converted into urea, either because of hepatocellular disease or portal-systemic shunting of blood, or both. As a result, these substances reach the systemic circulation, where they interfere with cerebral metabolism in some obscure way.

Despite our incomplete understanding of the role of disordered nitrogen metabolism in the genesis of hepatic coma, an awareness of this relationship has provided the few effective means of treating this disorder: restriction of dietary protein; mechanical cleansing of the colon; oral administration of neomycin or kanamycin, which suppresses the urease-producing organisms in the bowel; and the use of lactulose, an inert sugar that acidifies the colonic contents. Should these measures not control the protein intolerance, surgical exclusion of the bowel may be undertaken, but this operation carries a high risk of mortality. More recent methods of treatment, the practicality of which remains to be established, include the use of keto analogues of essential amino acids (which theoretically should supply a nitrogen-free source of essential amino acids), and bromocriptine, a dopamine agonist, which is thought to enhance dopaminergic transmission.

In acute hepatitis, delirious, confusional, and comatose states also occur, but their mechanisms are not understood. Blood ammonium levels are usually elevated, but of unclear significance, because of the large number of associated metabolic abnormalities.

Uremic encephalopathy Episodic confusion and stupor and other neurologic symptoms may accompany any form of severe renal disease, acute or chronic. In addition, a number of neurologic syndromes complicate chronic hemodialysis and kidney transplantation. Chronic polyneuropathy, the most common neurologic complication of renal failure, is discussed in Chap. 291.

The initial cerebral symptoms attributable to uremia consist of apathy, fatigue, inattentiveness, and irritability; later, confusion, disturbances of sensory perception, hallucinations, and stupor supervene. Clouding of the sensorium is practically always associated with twitching of the muscles and myoclonic jerks, and the patient may convulse. We have observed this twitch-convulsive phenomenon in association with a variety of diseases, such as widespread neoplasia, delirium tremens, diabetes with necrotizing pyelonephritis, and lupus erythematosus, all of which were associated with renal failure, only modestly elevated blood urea nitrogen, and normal or subnormal serum calcium and magnesium.

The prognosis of uremic encephalopathy, if associated with irreversible and progressive renal disease, is poor and can only be managed with dialysis or renal transplantation. Convulsions, which occur in about one-third of cases, often preterminally, respond to relatively low plasma concentrations of phenytoin and phenobarbital.

Opinions vary as to the cause of uremic encephalopathy and the twitch-convulsive syndrome. The brain shows hyperplasia of protoplasmic astrocytes in some cases, but never to the degree observed in hepatic encephalopathy. Cerebral edema is notably absent. Restoration of renal function completely corrects the neurologic syndrome attesting to an abnormality at a subcellular level. Whether this is caused by the retention of organic acids, elevation of phosphate in the CSF, or by the action of other toxins has never been settled.

"Disequilibrium syndrome" and dialysis encephalopathy These terms refer to syndromes that commonly complicate hemodialysis or peritoneal dialysis. Under *disequilibrium syndrome* are included headaches, nausea, muscular cramps, nervous irritability, agitation, drowsiness, and convulsions. The headache develops in approximately 70 percent of patients, while the other symptoms are observed in 5 to 10 percent, usually in those undergoing rapid dialysis or in the early stages of a dialysis program. The symptoms tend to occur in the third or fourth hour of dialysis and last for several hours. Sometimes the symptoms appear 8 to 48 h after completing dialysis. Originally these symptoms were attributed to the rapid lowering of serum urea, leaving the brain with a higher concentration of urea than the serum and resulting in a shift of water into the brain to equalize the osmotic gradient ("reverse urea syndrome"). Now the condition is attributed to a shift of water into the brain as in volume expansion due to water intoxication and inappropriate secretion of antidiuretic hormone.

Dialysis encephalopathy or *dialysis dementia* is an unusual complication of chronic hemodialysis. It begins with a stuttering dysarthria and apraxia of speech, to which are added facial and then generalized myoclonus, focal and generalized seizures, personality changes, intellectual decline, and EEG abnormalities, the last of which consist of synchronous or multifocal bursts of slow wave discharges associated with spikes and sharp waves. The CSF is normal except for increased pressure in some cases. At first these symptoms are intermittent, occurring during or immediately after dialysis and lasting for only a few hours, but gradually they become more persistent and eventually permanent. Once established, the syndrome is usually steadily progressive over a 1- to 15-month period (average survival of 6 months in 42 cases analyzed by Lederman and Henry). Some patients have a waxing and waning course and survive for several years. In some patients the myoclonus and seizures subside for several months under the influence of clonazepam.

No consistent neuropathologic changes have been found in the fatal cases, and the pathogenesis of this syndrome is still obscure. Current speculation centers on the role of aluminum. Alfrey and his associates found that the cerebral gray matter of patients who died from dialysis encephalopathy contained a much greater amount of aluminum than tissue from dialysis patients without encephalopathy. The aluminum may be derived from the dialysate or orally administered aluminum gels, or both. These authors suggested that dialysis encephalopathy represents a form of aluminum intoxication, a view that has received support from recent observations that interruption of aluminum intake may reverse the symptoms of encephalopathy.

Kidney transplantation involves an increased risk of developing reticulum-cell sarcoma, Wernicke's encephalopathy, and central pontine myelinolysis. Systemic fungal infections are found at autopsy in about 45 percent of patients who have had renal transplants and long periods of immunosuppressive treatment, and in about one-third of these patients there is central nervous involvement. *Aspergillus, Candida, Nocardia,* and *Histoplasma* are the usual organisms found in that order of frequency. Other central nervous system infections that complicate transplantation are toxoplasmosis and cytomegalic inclusion disease.

Encephalopathies due to electrolyte disturbances Limitation of space permits only brief reference to this important group of metabolic encephalopathies.

Metabolic acidosis (arterial pH < 7.30, $P_{CO_2} < 35$, $HCO_3 <$ 10 meq per liter) due to diabetes mellitus, renal failure, lactic acidosis, or poisoning with an acidic substance produces a syndrome characterized by drowsiness, stupor, and coma with dry skin and Kussmaul breathing, described in Chap. 113. Coma due to acidosis is a particularly prominent feature of many of the metabolic diseases of infancy and childhood, including the various forms of hyperammonemia, isovaleric acidemia, maple syrup urine disease, methylmalonic aciduria, the ketotic form of hyperglycinemia, propionic acidemia, lactic acidemia, and lysosomal acid phosphatase deficiency. Extreme degrees of *hyperosmolality* of the blood may develop in the course of diabetes mellitus (blood glucose greater than 400 mg/dl) and in *hypernatremic dehydration,* resulting in both instances in convulsions, tremulousness, and coma. In some instances the movement disorder resembles chorea or the myoclonic twitching of uremia. *Hyponatremia,* usually with water intoxication, is another cause of episodic coma, especially in infants. *Hypokalemia* may be associated with a stuporous-confusional state, sometimes accompanied by striking changes in personality and behavior.

In children more than adults, cholera being an exception, extremely *severe diarrhea* may be attended by an encephalopathy. Irritability, weakness, headache, seizures, stupor, and coma may develop over a period of 2 to 3 days and carry a grave prognosis unless promptly relieved. Presumably this is a metabolic encephalopathy due to loss of fluids and electrolytes and can be corrected by their replacement. In the more protracted illness of *typhoid fever,* approximately half the patients develop a delirium, and a small number will exhibit meningism and become comatose with twitching and seizures or spasticity and hyperactive reflexes in the legs, all of which are transitory.

Other encephalopathies of this type, associated with adrenal insufficiency and hypo- and hyperparathyroidism, are considered at the end of this chapter in relation to the endocrine psychoses.

METABOLIC DISEASES PRESENTING AS EXTRAPYRAMIDAL SYNDROMES These syndromes are usually of mixed type, i.e., they include a number of basal ganglionic and cerebellar symptoms in various combinations. They may emerge in a variety of clinical settings—as a sequela of kernicterus or of hypoxic or hypoglycemic encephalopathy, or as part of hepatocerebral degeneration of acquired or familial type, or with calcification of the basal ganglia and cerebellum, a disorder which also takes a familial or acquired form.

The extrapyramidal symptoms that result from severe *anoxia* and *hypoglycemia* have been described in the preceding section. Chronic *parathyroid hypofunction,* either idiopathic or following surgery in the area of the thyroid, may rarely give rise to intracranial calcifications and an extrapyramidal motor syndrome. Somewhat more common is the familial form of basal ganglionic-cerebellar calcification in which choreoathetosis and rigidity are prominent (*Fahr's syndrome*). Some of these patients are mentally retarded, others are intellectually intact. The familial form of calcification is inherited as an autosomal recessive trait, and usually has its onset in adolescence and early adult life. The serum calcium levels are usually normal, and there is no explanation of the calcification.

The development of an extrapyramidal syndrome in late childhood and adolescence should always suggest (1) Wilson-Westphal-Strümpell hepatocerebral degeneration (Chap. 98) and (2) Hallervorden-Spatz disease (Chap. 364). Only kernicterus and the acquired form of hepatocerebral degeneration remain to be discussed here.

Kernicterus This is an important cause of generalized choreoathetosis and rigidity in children and adults, the result of excessive hemolysis (Rh incompatibility) or other forms of hyperbilirubinemia in the neonatal period.

The symptoms of kernicterus appear in the jaundiced neonate on the second or third postnatal day. The infant becomes listless, sucks poorly, develops respiratory difficulties, and becomes stuporous as the jaundice intensifies. The serum bilirubin is over 25 mg/dl. The majority of infants with this disease die within the first week or two of life. Many of those who survive are mentally retarded, deaf, and totally unable to sit, stand, or walk. But there are exceptional patients, obviously less damaged, who are mentally normal or at most only slightly backward. These are the ones who develop a variety of persistent neurologic sequelae—choreoathetosis, dystonia, and rigidity of the limbs—a picture not too different from that of cerebral spastic diplegia with involuntary movements. Kernicterus should always be suspected if an extrapyramidal syndrome is accompanied by bilateral deafness and palsy of upward gaze.

Neonates who die in the acute stage of kernicterus show a characteristic yellow staining of nuclear masses in the basal ganglia, brainstem, and cerebellum—a finding from which the disease takes its name. In surviving patients the pathologic change consists of a symmetrically distributed nerve cell loss and gliosis in the subthalamic nucleus, the globus pallidus, thalamus, and oculomotor and cochlear nuclei; these lesions are the result of the hyperbilirubinemia. In the newborn, unconjugated bilirubin can pass through the poorly developed blood-brain barrier into these central and brainstem nuclei, where it has a direct toxic effect. Acidosis and hypoxia exacerbate the effect. Also, in the newborn, the development of hyperbilirubinemia is enhanced by the transient deficiency of the enzyme glucuronyl transferase, essential for the conjugation of bilirubin. Hereditary hyperbilirubinemia, due to lack of this enzyme (*Crigler-Najjar syndrome*), may have the same effect on the nervous system as hyperbilirubinemia due to excessive hemolysis (Rh incompatibility).

Phototherapy and exchange transfusions with female blood designed to prevent high levels of unconjugated serum bilirubin have been shown to protect the nervous system. If the blood bilirubin level can be held to less than 20 mg/dl (16 mg/dl in prematures), the nervous system escapes damage.

Acquired (non-Wilsonian) hepatocerebral degeneration Patients who survive an episode or several episodes of hepatic coma are occasionally left with residual neurologic abnormalities, such as tremor of the head or arms, asterixis, grimacing, choreatic twitching of the limbs, dysarthria, ataxia of gait, or impairment of intellectual function, and these symptoms may worsen with repeated attacks of stupor and coma. In other patients with hepatic failure, these neurologic abnormalities become manifest in the absence of discrete episodes of hepatic coma. In either event, patients thus afflicted deteriorate neurologically over a period of months or years. As the condition evolves, a rather characteristic dysarthria, mild ataxia, wide-based, unsteady gait, and choreoathetosis, mainly of the face, neck, and shoulders, are joined in a common syndrome. Mental function is slowly altered—a simple dementia with lack of concern and indifference to the illness evolves. A coarse rhythmic tremor of the arms, appearing with certain sustained postures, mild corticospinal tract signs, and diffuse EEG abnormalities complete the clinical picture. Other less frequent signs are muscular rigidity, grasp reflexes, tremor in repose, nystagmus, asterixis, and action or intention myoclonus. Many of the neurologic abnormalities that occur as part of acute hepatic encephalopathy may also be observed in patients with chronic hepatocerebral degeneration; the only difference is that the abnormalities are evanescent in the former and irreversible in the latter.

The chronic cerebral symptoms, like the transient ones, may occur with all varieties of chronic liver disease. Portocaval shunts are always present; jaundice, ascites, and esophageal varices are manifest in most of the cases.

Chronic hepatocerebral degeneration, like acute hepatic coma, is characterized by a widespread hyperplasia of protoplasmic astrocytes in the deep layers of the cerebral and cerebellar cortices as well as in thalamic and lenticular nuclei and many other nuclear structures of the brainstem. In addition, in the chronic disease, medullated fibers and nerve cells are destroyed in the affected areas, and polymicrocavitation is prominent at the corticomedullary junction, in the striatum (particularly in the superior pole of the putamen), and in the cerebellar white matter. Protoplasmic astrocytic nuclei contain periodic acid Schiff (PAS) positive glycogen granules. Nerve cells may appear swollen and chromatolyzed, accounting, we believe, for the so-called Opalski cells. The similarity of the neuropathologic lesion in the familial (Wilson's) and acquired forms of liver disease suggests a common hepatogenesis.

METABOLIC DISEASES PRESENTING AS CEREBELLAR ATAXIA, PSYCHOSIS, OR DEMENTIA The association of *myxedema and a cerebellar type of ataxia* has been mentioned sporadically in medical writings since the latter part of the nineteenth century. The neuropathologic basis of this disorder remains unclear, as does the pathogenesis. The damaging effects of *hyperthermia,* like those of anoxia and hypoglycemia, involve the brain diffusely; in the case of hyperthermia, however, the changes are disproportionately severe in the cerebellum. The acute manifestations of profound hyperthermia are coma and convulsions, frequently complicated by shock and renal failure. Patients who survive the initial stage of the illness frequently show signs of widespread cerebral affection, such as confusion, dementia, and pseudobulbar and spastic paralysis. These abnormalities tend to resolve gradually, leaving the patient with a more or less pure disorder of cerebellar function. This disorder has its basis in a degeneration of the Purkinje cells, with gliosis throughout the cerebellar cortex, as well as degeneration of the dentate nuclei.

Already the point has been made that milder degrees of episodic stupor and coma, if persistent, may present as a state of protracted confusion that is impossible to distinguish from dementia. Chronic portal-systemic encephalopathy, the syndromes of chronic hypoglycemia, and dialysis encephalopathy all have a similar clinical effect.

In the *endocrine encephalopathies* the clinical phenomena are even more abstruse. Confusional states may be combined with agitation, hallucinations, delusions, anxiety, and depression. And the time course of the illness may be in terms of weeks and months, rather than days. Such a derangement of higher nervous function may follow the *administration of ACTH or corticosteroid* agents, and the same symptoms have been reported in *Cushing's disease.* The neurology of *thyrotoxicosis* has proved to be peculiarly elusive. Allusions to thyrotoxic psychosis are widely recorded in the medical literature; mental confusion, seizures, manic or depressive attacks, delusions, and chorea occur in various combinations with muscular weakness and atrophy, periodic paralysis, and myasthenia. Treatment of the hyperthyroidism gradually restores the patient to a normal mental state leaving one with no explanation of what had happened to the nervous system. The reactions of *myxedematous patients* are slowed and their psychomotor activity is reduced, but only in a small proportion is there a major change in cerebral function, taking the form of drowsiness or extreme somnolence, inattentiveness, and apathy. These symptoms can be reversed within a few weeks by thyroid medication. In *hyperparathyroidism,* when the serum calcium levels reach 15 mg/dl or higher, the patient sinks into a quiet state of inattentiveness, lethargy, and confusion. Stupor, coma, and death may be caused by extreme degrees of hypercalcemia such as occur occasionally in cases of excessive vitamin D administration and metastatic carcinoma of the bones. *Addison's disease* (adrenal insufficiency) may be attended by episodic confusion, stupor, or coma, without special identifying features. Hypoglycemia and hypotension, with diminished cerebral circulation, are thought to be the underlying mechanisms, and measures which correct them appear to be beneficial.

The term *pancreatic encephalopathy* was introduced by Rothermich and Von Haam in 1941 to describe a syndrome of agitation and confusion, sometimes with hallucinations and clouding of consciousness, dysarthria, and changing rigidity of the limbs, in association with acute pancreatic disease. The status of this entity is uncertain. A uniform neuropathologic change has not been discerned. Pallis and Lewis suggest that before such a clinical diagnosis can be seriously entertained in a patient with acute pancreatitis one should exclude delirium tremens, cerebral circulatory insufficiency from shock, renal failure, hypoglycemia, diabetic acidosis, hyperosmolality syndrome, hypokalemia, and hypo- or hypercalcemia, any one of which may complicate the underlying disease(s).

HEREDITARY METABOLIC DISEASES OF THE NERVOUS SYSTEM

As stated above these will receive only cursory treatment, for most of them effect pathologic change in the nervous system during the pediatric age period and seldom does the affected individual survive to adulthood.

As a group these diseases share certain characteristics. Essentially all of them involve many tissues, e.g., white blood cells, fibroblasts, endothelial cells, and hepatocytes, although the nervous system may be the only organ whose functions are clinically deranged. Thus, the diseases appear primarily neurologic even though they are truly multisystemic. Advantage can be taken of this fact by the knowledgeable clinician who can utilize the more accessible nonnervous cells for cytologic diagnosis. Of the more than 100 hereditary metabolic diseases that possess a known metabolic marker, the majority, particularly those that express themselves in the first days, weeks, months, and years, are of recessive type. The organism is usually normal at birth and does not express its enzymatic defect until later, having been protected in utero by the mother. Once the disease strikes, however, it tends to be global and devastating in its effects, blighting the development of the brain and preventing the attainment of the so-called milestones of psychomotor maturation. The remainder of the genetic metabolic diseases are of dominant or sex-linked recessive inheritance; they can begin at any age and usually are of slower evolution. Their effects may not become apparent until adult life and are then more likely to be restricted to certain systems of neurons, giving rise to the aforementioned neurologic syndromes (seizures, cerebellar ataxia, dystonia and choreoathetosis, dementia, progressive spasticity, polyneuropathy, etc.).

A new neurologic principle emerges in connection with this group of diseases—that in the early epochs of life each disease tends to have its favorite age of onset (neonatal, early or late infantile, childhood, or adolescence) and that each of these epochs of life is marked by a disposition to certain metabolic diseases and not to others. Thus the evolving syndrome depends not only on the nature of the disease but also on the age and state of maturation of the nervous system at the moment it strikes. Pursuant to this principle one can subdivide and group the diseases according to the age of the afflicted organism and according to the clinical syndrome, as shown in Table 362-2. It is evident from this table that the late-onset (mendelian dominant) diseases are more likely to express themselves as recognizable syndromes of diagnostic value than are the early-onset, recessive ones.

Of the many diseases listed in Table 362-2 only the few observed to begin in late adolescent and adult years are of interest to internists and family practitioners. They are the ones that must occasionally figure in the differential diagnosis of acquired diseases of the nervous system. A noteworthy attribute of the entire group is their chronicity and progressive nature. The diseases described below are examples personally observed by the authors.

ADULT METACHROMATIC LEUKODYSTROPHY (MLD) This is one of the more frequent hereditary metabolic diseases of the nervous system. While the majority of cases appear in early childhood, some 25 percent or more manifest their first symptoms beyond the twenty-first year of life. Cases among men have outnumbered those in women two to one. The mode of inheritance is autosomal recessive in almost all instances. The onset is insidious and the course protracted, over 20 or more years.

In our experience mental symptoms tend to dominate the clinical picture. Failing scholastic performance, forgetfulness, and irrationality occur early in the illness but may be obscured by peculiarities of personality, such as suspiciousness, delusional thinking, and bizarre actions. These latter qualities may raise the question of schizophrenia or immature ("borderline") personality development. Sooner or later a mild cerebellar ataxia presenting as awkwardness and falling, mild pyramidal signs, masked facies, and bizarre postures stamp the illness as neurologic. Eventually the patient's mental processes deteriorate to the point where he or she is totally helpless, demented, mute, incontinent of sphincteric control, and bedfast.

Specific diagnostic tests include (1) the demonstration of a diminished aryl-sulfatase A activity in white blood cells, serum, and urine, (2) increased excretion of sulfatides in urine, (3) slowed conduction velocity in nerves, and (4) deposits of metachromatic material in nerve biopsies.

No treatment is presently available.

One must add adult MLD to the growing list of inherited metabolic diseases that cause early mental changes. The others are Wilson's hepatolenticular degeneration, adult lipidoses, mucolipidoses, cerebrotendinous xanthomatosis, the myoclonic epilepsies, and basal ganglia calcinoses. All of these are clinically separable from the major "functional psychoses" of this age period, by virtue of the progressive impairment of cognitive function, other neurologic findings, the EEG, and certain radiologic and biochemical tests.

In *adrenoleukodystrophy* either bronzing of the skin and Addison's disease or cerebral symptoms may be the initial manifestation. The cerebral lesions may present as a homonymous hemianopia, cortical blindness, hemiparesis, aphasia, or dementia. Usually the signs are asymmetrical at first and progress intermittently. A relatively pure polyneuropathic and myelopathic form has also been described. The diagnosis is usually settled by the finding of a low blood cortisol level in a male with cerebrospinal demyelinating disease, although recently a purely spinal type, taking the form of a progressive spastic paraparesis, has been described in the heterozygote (female carrier). Corticosteroid replacement therapy helps the Addison's disease but has no effect on the neurologic disorders. The latter progress intermittently over a few years, and usually the outcome is fatal.

ADULT LIPID STORAGE DISEASES Apart from some of the juvenile forms of cerebral lipidoses that are protracted into adult life, there are several that only become clinically visible in adults. These must be considered as rare variants of the more common ones of earlier life, the delay in onset being due to a less severe deficiency of some of the missing enzymes described in Chap. 104, or to other eccentricities of the biochemical mechanism.

G_{M2} *gangliosidosis* has been observed in young adults. Many are from non-Jewish families, and males and females in the same generation are equally affected. Generalized seizures may mark the beginning of a cerebral disorder that later is evidenced by alterations of behavior and intellectual decline. A progressive ataxia and mild signs of corticospinal disease, the combination of which interferes with independent locomotion, clarifies the diagnosis. The fundi and visual function are normal in most cases, but we have seen typical cherry red macular spots. The liver and spleen are normal or slightly enlarged. The CSF protein is normal. Computerized tomography (CT scan) reveals a modest ventricular enlargement. G_{M2} ganglioside is shown to be increased by thin-layer chromatography of tissue obtained by cerebral biopsy. Membranous cytoplasmic bodies

TABLE 362-2
Classification of the hereditary metabolic diseases

I Diseases which begin in the neonatal period and are often fatal (seizures, respiratory difficulty, unresponsivity)
- *A* Diseases of the urea cycle
- *B* Pyridoxine dependency
- *C* Maple syrup urine disease
- *D* Congenital lactic acidosis

II Diseases of infancy and early childhood
- *A* Phenylketonuria and other abnormalities of amino acid metabolism (mental retardation and seizures, blond hair, fair skin); see Chaps. 91 and 92
- *B* Lysosomal storage diseases
  - *1* Lipidoses: Tay-Sachs disease and Sandhoff variant, Niemann-Pick disease, Gaucher's disease (seizures and myoclonia, blindness, auditory startle, psychomotor regression, and in some diseases enlarged liver and spleen); see Chap. 104
  - *2* Mucopolysaccharidoses (psychomotor regression, corneal clouding, skeletal disorder, infiltrates of liver, spleen, lungs, marrow); see Chap. 106
  - *3* Mucolipidoses (syndromes with elements of the lipidoses and mucopolysaccharidoses)
  - *4* Leukodystrophies: globoid body leukodystrophy, metachromatic leukodystrophy, Pelizaeus-Merzbacher disease, Canavan's disease (psychomotor regression, spasticity of legs, areflexia, blindness); see Chap. 104

III Late childhood–adolescent diseases
- *A* Ataxia-telangiectasia (oculomotor apraxia, cerebellar ataxia, athetosis, later telangiectasia of conjunctivae and ears); see Chap. 365
- *B* Leigh's subacute necrotic encephalomyelopathy (ophthalmoplegia, respiratory disorder, mental regression, paralysis)
- *C* Wilson's hereditary hepatocerebral degeneration (Kaiser-Fleischer corneal rings, extrapyramidal signs, liver dysfunction); see Chap. 98
- *D* Hallervorden-Spatz disease (extrapyramidal syndrome); see Chap. 364
- *E* Lesch-Nyhan hyperuricosemia (choreoathetosis, mental retardation, self-mutilation); see Chap. 94

IV Late adolescent–early adult diseases; see Chap. 104
- *A* G_{M2} gangliosidosis (intellectual regression, seizures, ataxia, pyramidal signs)
- *B* Variant of metachromatic leukodystrophy (personality change, dementia, spastic weakness of limbs, ataxia)
- *C* Late form of neuropathic Gaucher's disease (seizures, polymyoclonus, mental deterioration)
- *D* Juvenile dystonic lipidosis or Niemann-Pick disease types C and D (mental decline, dystonic movements of tongue and limbs, paralysis of upward gaze)
- *E* Ceroid lipofuscinosis (dementia, ataxia, seizures)
- *F* Wilson's hepatocerebral degeneration (as in III C above)
- *G* Mucolipidoses (mental deterioration, gargoyle facial features, hyperplasia of gums)
- *H* Cerebrotendinous xanthomatosis (mental decline and personality changes, cerebellar ataxia, spastic quadriparesis, xanthometous deposits on tendons)
- *I* Mucopolysaccharidoses: Maroteaux-Lamy and Morquio types (dwarfism, spastic quadriparesis, hydrocephalus)

are visualized by electron microscopy of rectal, appendicular, and cortical neurons. A slowly developing dementia, cerebellar ataxia, polymyoclonus, and failing vision may characterize the clinical picture in other cases.

Kuf's ceroid lipofuscinosis is another form of lipid storage disease that only becomes evident in adolescence or early adult life. Usually the disease begins with mental deterioration, followed by seizures, ataxia, increasing rigidity, athetotic posturing, and corticospinal signs. Skin and conjunctival biopsies (electron-microscopic examination) showed lipofuscin storage material in fibroblasts and endothelial cells.

Another of our patients who began to have seizures, severe polymyoclonus, and mild intellectual deterioration was found, after several studies, to have *Gaucher's disease.* His spleen had been ruptured in an accident several years before, and when the surgical specimen was reviewed Gaucher cells were seen. A deficiency of glucose cerebroside splitting enzyme was found in white blood cells and skin fibroblasts. We also have under observation several members of a family with Gaucher's disease, who developed seizures, cerebellar ataxia, and blunting of intellectual function in early adult life. Several adolescent cases of *types C and D of Niemann-Pick disease* have been verified, in which the opening symptoms of the illness were dystonic movements of tongue, jaw, and limbs in association with a gradual decline of intellectual function and paralysis of vertical (upward) gaze. Foam cells were found in the bone marrow and liver.

In sum, one should at least consider some of these rare forms of hereditary metabolic diseases whenever an adolescent or young adult becomes demented, shows a psychiatric syndrome with decline in cognitive functions, has seizures, especially with polymyoclonus, failing vision, and cerebellar ataxia in combination with corticospinal signs or a progressive polyneuropathy. (See Chaps. 104 and 364 for further details.)

REFERENCES

ADAMS RD, FOLEY JM: The neurological disorder associated with liver disease. Metabolic and toxic diseases of the nervous system. Proc Assoc Res Nerv Ment Dis 32:198, 1953

———, VICTOR M: *Principles of Neurology,* 2d ed. New York, McGraw-Hill, 1981

ALFREY AC et al: The dialysis encephalopathy syndrome. Possible aluminum intoxication. N Engl J Med 294:184, 1976

CREMER GM et al: Myxedema and ataxia. Neurology 19:37, 1969

LEDERMAN RS, HENRY CE: Progressive dialysis encephalopathy. Ann Neurol 4:199, 1978

MALAMUD N et al: Heat stroke. A clinicopathologic study of 125 fatal cases. Mil Surg 99:397, 1946

MARKS R, ROSE FC: *Hypoglycemia.* Oxford, Blackwell, 1965

MOSER HW et al: Adrenoleukodystrophy: Studies of the phenotype, genetics and biochemistry. Johns Hopkins Med J 147:217, 1980

NADEL AM, WILSON WP: Dialysis encephalopathy. A possible seizure disorder. Neurology 26:1130, 1976

PALLIS CA, LEWIS PD: *The Neurology of Gastrointestinal Disease.* London, Saunders, 1974

PLUM F (ed): *Brain Dysfunction in Metabolic Disorders.* New York, Raven, 1974

———, POSNER JB: *Diagnosis of Stupor and Coma,* 3d ed. Philadelphia, Davis, 1980

RASKIN NH, FISHMAN RA: Neurologic disorders in renal failure. N Engl J Med 294:143, 204, 1976

ROTHERMICH NO, VON HAAM E: Pancreatic encephalopathy. J Clin Endocrinol 1:872, 1941

STANBURY JB et al (eds): *The Metabolic Basis of Inherited Disease,* 4th ed. New York, McGraw-Hill, 1978

SWAIMAN KF et al: Metabolic disorders of the central nervous system, in *The Practice of Pediatric Neurology,* KF Swaiman, FS Wright (eds). St Louis, Mosby, 1975, pp 359–479

VICTOR M et al: The acquired (non-wilsonian) type of chronic hepatocerebral degeneration. Medicine 44:345, 1965

WILKINSON DS, PROCKOP LD: Hypoglycemia: Effects on the nervous system, in *Handbook of Clinical Neurology,* PJ Vinken, BW Bruyn (eds). Amsterdam, North-Holland, 1976, vol 27, chap 4, pp 53–78

363
DEFICIENCY DISEASES OF THE NERVOUS SYSTEM

MAURICE VICTOR
RAYMOND D. ADAMS

The general aspects of deficiency disease have been presented in Chap. 76, and the reader should review them as an introduction to this discussion of deficiency diseases of the nervous system. The term *deficiency* is used here in its strictest sense, to designate those diseases or syndromes which result from the *lack of an essential nutrient in the diet or from a conditioning factor which increases the need for that nutrient.* The neurological diseases which comprise this category are the following:

1 Wernicke's disease and Korsakoff's psychosis
2 "Alcoholic" cerebellar degeneration
3 Nutritional polyneuropathy (neuropathic beriberi)
4 Pellagra
5 Deficiency amblyopia
6 The syndrome of amblyopia, painful neuropathy, and orogenital dermatitis (Strachan's syndrome)
7 Subacute combined degeneration of the spinal cord (vitamin B_{12} deficiency)
8 Vitamin-responsive, genetically determined diseases

Some general principles are applicable to all of the diseases under consideration. Of the known vitamin deficiencies, only those of the B group are of importance in neurologic disease (vitamin E deficiency is under suspicion but is not a proven cause of human disease). A lack of B vitamins affects the brain, spinal cord, and peripheral nerves of humans. Thiamine chloride, nicotinic acid, pyridoxine, pantothenic acid, and riboflavin all play a role in carbohydrate metabolism, upon which the central nervous system depends for its principal source of energy. These vitamins function as coenzymes in the Krebs tricarboxylic acid cycle, and, in addition, thiamine is involved in the hexose-monophosphate shunt. Vitamin B_{12} is known to be required for the conversion of methylmalonyl- to succinyl coenzyme A and for the conversion of homocystine to methionine.

Except for subacute combined degeneration of the spinal cord (vitamin B_{12} deficiency), it is not possible to relate the deficiency diseases in humans to the lack of one particular vitamin. For example, polyneuropathy may result from any one of several vitamin deficiencies [thiamine chloride, pyridoxine (vitamin B_6), pantothenic acid, and probably vitamin B_{12}]. Moreover, pellagra, beriberi, and Strachan's syndrome are probably related to a deficiency of several vitamins. These generalizations should not obscure the fact that certain manifestations of deficiency disease are related to the lack of a specific nutrient (e.g., the ocular signs of Wernicke's disease to a deficiency of thiamine).

In the western world the nutritional disorders of the nervous system are observed most often in the alcoholic population of large urban centers. Alcohol acts mainly by displacing food in the diet, but it also increases the demand for B vitamins, which are necessary to metabolize the carbohydrate furnished by alcohol itself, and it may impair the gastrointestinal absorption of vitamins. Dietary faddism, impaired absorption of dietary nutrients (as occurs in sprue or following the resection of stomach and small bowel), and the use of certain drugs (e.g., isoniazid and hydralazine, which interfere with the enzymatic function of pyridoxine) account for a relatively small number of cases of deficiency disease.

Each of the deficiency diseases may occur in pure form and will be so described. More often, however, they occur in various combinations. Stated in another way, it is usual for deficiency diseases to involve both the central and peripheral nervous systems, an attribute which this category of disease shares with the hereditary metabolic disorders. Also, the examination of patients with deficiency disease frequently discloses nonneurologic signs of malnutrition such as general wasting, lesions of the skin and mucous membranes, and circulatory abnormalities.

WERNICKE'S DISEASE (WERNICKE'S ENCEPHALOPATHY, POLIOENCEPHALITIS HEMORRHAGICA SUPERIORIS) **History** In 1881, Carl Wernicke described an illness of acute onset characterized by mental disturbance, paralysis of eye movements, and ataxic gait. Swelling of the optic discs and retinal hemorrhages were also said to be present, and in all three of his patients there was a progressive depression of the state of consciousness leading to death, so that a fatal outcome was at one time thought to be a universal feature of this disease. Wernicke described focal vascular lesions, primarily affecting the gray matter around the third and fourth ventricles and aqueduct of Sylvius. He regarded the disease as inflammatory in nature and suggested the name *acute superior hemorrhagic polioencephalitis.* Since Wernicke's time, views regarding this disease have undergone considerable modification.

Symptoms and signs The crux of the clinical picture is the *ocular disturbance* (the clinical diagnosis of Wernicke's disease can hardly be made without it) which consists of weakness or paralysis of the lateral recti, nystagmus that is both horizontal and vertical, and various palsies of conjugate gaze. These signs show a considerable diversity. The disorder of conjugate movement varies from a nystagmus on extreme gaze to a complete loss of ocular movement in that direction. This applies to both horizontal and vertical movements; abnormalities of the former are somewhat more frequent. Paralysis of downward gaze is an unusual finding, but internuclear ophthalmoplegia is common. Ptosis and retinal hemorrhages are observed rarely. The lateral rectus palsy is always bilateral, though not necessarily symmetrical, and is accompanied by diplopia and internal strabismus. With complete ocular paralysis nystagmus is absent, but it becomes evident as the weakness improves. In advanced stages of the disease there may be complete loss of ocular movement, and the pupils, which ordinarily are spared, may become miotic and nonreacting.

The *ataxia* affects stance and gait predominantly. It may be so severe initially that the patient is unable to stand or walk without support. Vestibular responses to caloric stimulation are characteristically absent in these patients. With specific treatment the gross disorder of equilibrium improves and the patient is left with a wide-based, uncertain gait. The mildest degree of ataxia may be brought out only by special tests, such as heel-to-toe walking. In contrast to the gross disorder of locomotion is the relative infrequency of clear-cut intention tremor of the limbs. The latter abnormality, when present, affects the legs more than the arms. Scanning speech is present only in isolated cases.

A *derangement of mental function* is found in all but 10 percent of patients and takes one of several forms: (1) The most common is a *global confusion state,* characterized by profound apathy, listlessness, inattentiveness, indifference to the surroundings, and disorientation. Unconsciousness as part of the initial episode is distinctly rare, but mild drowsiness is common. Spontaneous speech is minimal. Many questions directed to the patient go unanswered, or he or she may suspend the conversation in the middle of a sentence and nod off to sleep. The patient is readily roused from this state, however. Whatever questions the patient answers betray disorientation in time and place, misidentification of those around him or her, and an inability to grasp the meaning of the illness or immediate situation. Many of the patient's remarks are irrational and show no consistency from one moment to another. Under these circumstances a more extensive evaluation of intellectual function is seldom possible. (2) Some patients, at the time they are first seen, already show the disorder of retentive memory and otherwise alert state of mind that characterizes Korsakoff's psychosis (see Chap. 21 and further on in this chapter). (3) A relatively small number of patients, less than 20 percent in our series, show the symptoms of alcohol withdrawal, either delirium tremens or a variant thereof.

The symptoms of Wernicke's disease may all appear simultaneously and rather acutely, but more often the ophthalmoplegia and ataxia precede the mental signs by a few days and sometimes by a week or two.

Wernicke's disease is usually associated with other nutritional diseases, both neurologic and nonneurologic. In more than 80 percent of patients, *nutritional polyneuropathy* of varying degrees of severity is evident. Occasionally, *amblyopia* or *spinal spastic ataxia* may be added to the clinical picture. Many patients in the chronic stage of the disease demonstrate impaired olfactory discrimination, a defect that is most likely related to the diencephalic lesions (see below).

The advanced stages of beriberi heart disease are rarely observed in association with Wernicke's disease, although indications of *disordered cardiovascular function* such as tachycardia, exertional dyspnea, postural hypotension, and minor electrocardiographic abnormalities are common. Occasionally patients may die suddenly, the mode of death suggesting "cardiovascular collapse." It has been shown that Wernicke's disease is characterized by a state of high cardiac output which is out of proportion to the oxygen consumption. This is probably due to an abnormal state of peripheral vasodilatation, which in turn may be related to thiamine deficiency. Postural hypotension and syncope are related to impaired function in the autonomic nervous system, more specifically to a defect in the sympathetic outflow.

Ancillary findings Vestibular function, as measured by the response to standard caloric testing, is always impaired bilaterally and more or less symmetrically in the acute stages of Wernicke's disease (*vestibular paresis*). The cerebrospinal fluid (CSF) is normal or shows only a modest elevation of protein content; protein values above 100 mg/dl or a CSF pleocytosis should always suggest the presence of a complicating illness. In untreated cases of Wernicke's disease, there is invariably an elevation of the *blood pyruvate,* and a marked reduction in the *blood transketolase* (a thiamine-dependent enzyme of the hexose monophosphate shunt). Diffuse slowing of the EEG, mild to moderate in degree, occurs in about one-half of the patients. On the other hand, total cerebral blood flow and cerebral oxygen and glucose consumption may be greatly reduced in the acute stages of the disease and may persist for several weeks after the institution of treatment (Shimojyo et al.).

Course of the illness Death occurs in 15 to 20 percent of hospitalized patients and is usually due to a complicating infection (pneumonia, pulmonary tuberculosis, and septicemia being the most common) or to cirrhosis of the liver.

Patients who recover do so in a characteristic manner. Ocular palsies may begin to improve within hours after the administration of thiamine and practically always within several days. Failure of the patient to respond in this manner should raise doubts about the diagnosis of Wernicke's disease. Sixth nerve palsies, ptosis, and vertical gaze palsies recover completely, within a week or two in most cases, but vertical nystagmus may occasionally persist for several months. Horizontal gaze palsies recover completely as a rule, but in more than half the cases a fine horizontal nystagmus remains as a permanent sequela of the disease.

Ataxia improves somewhat more slowly than the ocular abnormalities. Almost half the patients recover incompletely and are left with a slow, shuffling, wide-based gait and inability to walk tandem. The residual gait disturbance and horizontal nystagmus provide a means of identifying obscure and chronic cases of dementia as alcoholic-nutritional in origin. Vestibular function, as measured by caloric testing, improves at about the same rate as the ataxia of stance and gait, i.e., over a period of weeks or months, and recovery is usually, but not always, complete.

The symptoms of apathy, drowsiness, and profound confusion recede gradually, and as they do, the *defect in retentive memory and learning (Korsakoff's psychosis)* stands out more clearly. The features of Korsakoff's psychosis (amnesic or amnesic-confabulatory syndrome) are described in Chap. 21. Here it is important to emphasize that in the alcoholic, nutritionally deficient patient Wernicke's disease and Korsakoff's psychosis are not separate diseases, but that the changing ocular and ataxic signs and the transformation of the global confusional state into an amnesic syndrome are successive stages in the recovery of a single disease process. Stated in another way, Korsakoff's psychosis is but the psychic component of Wernicke's disease. Hence the symptom complex should be called Wernicke's disease with or without Korsakoff's psychosis or the Wernicke-Korsakoff syndrome when both components of the disease are present.

The outcome of Korsakoff's psychosis varies. Complete or almost complete recovery occurs in only 20 percent of patients. In the remainder recovery is slow and incomplete. Depending on the severity of the residual symptoms, the patient may or may not be able to lead a supervised existence out of a hospital. The residual mental state is characterized by large gaps in memory, without confabulation, and an inability of the patient to sort out events in their proper temporal sequence. If the patient is seen for the first time during this stage, the diagnosis of "alcoholic deteriorated state" or "organic brain syndrome due to alcohol" is commonly made.

Pathologic changes Postmortem examination in patients who die in the acute stages of Wernicke's disease reveals symmetrically located lesions in the paraventricular regions of the thalamus and hypothalamus, the mammillary bodies, the periaqueductal region of the midbrain, the floor of the fourth ventricle, and the anterior lobe of the cerebellum, particularly the vermis. Lesions are invariably found in the mammillary bodies and less consistently in the other areas. Microscopically, the principal change consists of varying degrees of necrosis of parenchymal structures. Many nerve cells and fibers are destroyed; others remain intact and are seen against a background of reactive glial elements, both astrocytes and microgliacytes. The blood vessels are prominent, owing to adventitial and endothelial proliferation. Hemorrhagic lesions are present in a small proportion of cases and usually give the appearance of being of recent origin. The oculomotor and vestibular nuclei are regularly involved to a relatively slight degree.

Clinical-pathologic correlations The ocular muscle and gaze palsies are attributable to lesions of the sixth and third nerve nuclei. The lesions of the vestibular nuclei are probably responsible for the loss of caloric responses and for the gross abnormality of equilibrium that characterizes the initial stage of the disease. The lack of significant destruction of nerve cells in these lesions accounts for the rapid improvement in oculomotor and vestibular function.

The persistent ataxia of stance and gait is attributable to the loss of neurons in the superior vermis of the cerebellum; ataxia of individual movements of the legs is attributable to an extension of the lesion into the anterior parts of the anterior lobes. The cerebellar lesions of Wernicke's disease are indistinguishable from those of *alcoholic cerebellar degeneration* (see below). The latter designation is used when the cerebellar abnormalities occur on a background of alcoholism and malnutrition, without the characteristic ocular and mental disorder.

The amnesic defect is related to lesions in the diencephalon, more specifically to those in the medial dorsal nuclei of the thalamus. Lesions in the mammillary bodies are probably not critical in respect to memory function since they are found in patients with Wernicke's disease who had shown no disorder of memory during life.

Etiology and pathogenesis Nutritional deficiency is now established as the causal factor. Wernicke's disease has been encountered in prisoner-of-war camps and in wasting diseases of varied origin where alcohol played no part. The specific factor that is responsible for most, if not all, of the symptoms of the Wernicke-Korsakoff syndrome is a deficiency of thiamine. The marked sensitivity of the ocular abnormalities to the administration of thiamine accounts for their rapid abatement after the ingestion of one or two meals. The quality of prompt reversibility suggests that the ocular signs are due to a biochemical abnormality and not to irreversible structural changes. On the other hand, the slow and incomplete recovery of the memory defect suggests that this symptom is the result of irreversible structural changes, presumably in the medial dorsal nuclei of the thalamus.

How a deficiency of thiamine produces the paraventricular lesions of the Wernicke-Korsakoff syndrome is not clear. McEntee and Mair have pointed out that the lesions lie in the monoamine-containing pathways and have presented evidence that 3-methoxy-4-hydroxyphenylglycol, the primary brain metabolite of norepinephrine, is decreased in the CNS of patients with Korsakoff's psychosis; the administration of clonidine, a putative alpha-noradrenergic agonist, seemed to improve the memory disorder in these patients. These authors theorized that damage to the ascending norepinephrine-containing neurons in the brainstem and diencephalon may be the basis for the amnesia.

Blass and Gibson have suggested that a genetically determined defect in transketolase may be operative in the pathogenesis of Wernicke's disease. They found that transketolase in fibroblasts cultured from patients with this disease bound thiamine pyrophosphate (TPP) less avidly than did the transketolase from control lines. This defect in transketolase would presumably be insignificant if the diet were adequate, but would be deleterious if the diet were low in thiamine. These findings, if corroborated, would explain why only a small proportion of alcoholics develop Wernicke-Korsakoff disease.

Treatment of the Wernicke-Korsakoff syndrome Wernicke's disease represents a medical emergency, and its recognition demands the immediate administration of thiamine. A delay of a few hours may be crucial in determining whether the patient who presents only ocular and ataxic signs will be prevented from developing mental signs and whether the patient with early Korsakoff changes will be restored to a state of mental competency. Although 2 to 3 mg thiamine is sufficient to modify the ocular signs, much larger doses are usually employed—50 mg intravenously and 50 mg intramuscularly, the latter dose being repeated each day until the patient resumes a normal diet. The other B vitamins may be given by mouth in the dosages outlined in Chap. 76. If the patient cannot or will not eat, parenteral feeding and administration of B vitamins become necessary.

A particular danger attends the treatment of the severely depleted alcoholic patient with intravenous glucose solutions. This may exhaust the patient's reserve of B vitamins and either precipitate Wernicke's disease where it was not present before or cause a rapid worsening of an early form of the disease. For this reason, B vitamins must be administered in all alcoholic patients requiring parenteral glucose. If there are signs of cardiac failure, rapid digitalization should be undertaken. Since these patients are confused and forgetful, they must be supervised continually, preferably on a medical ward.

A special problem in management arises when the patient recovers from the acute phase of the illness and the amnesic psychosis becomes prominent. The disposition of the patient to family, nursing home, or mental institution should be undertaken on the basis of the severity of the mental illness as well as the capacity of the family unit and social circumstances.

"ALCOHOLIC" CEREBELLAR DEGENERATION This term is applied to a nonfamilial type of cerebellar ataxia which occurs in adult life against a background of prolonged ingestion of alcohol. The symptoms may evolve slowly over a long period, but much more frequently they evolve in subacute fashion (over several weeks or months), after which they remain stationary. Often they are present in mild form and worsen after an attack of pneumonia or delirium tremens.

The signs are those of cerebellar dysfunction, affecting stance and gait predominantly. The legs are involved more severely than the arms, and nystagmus and speech disturbances occur relatively infrequently. Once established, the signs change very little, although some improvement of gait (due mainly to recovery from associated polyneuropathy) may follow the cessation of drinking. The essential pathologic changes consist of degeneration of varying severity of all the neurocellular elements of the cerebellar cortex, particularly of the Purkinje cells, with a striking topographic restriction to the anterior and superior aspects of the vermis and adjacent parts of the anterior lobes of the cerebellum. The disorder of stance and gait is related to the lesion in the vermis, and the ataxia of the limbs to the involvement of the anterior lobes. A similar clinical-pathologic syndrome is observed occasionally in nutritionally depleted nonalcoholic patients.

NUTRITIONAL POLYNEUROPATHY (See also Chap. 83) In the United States, nutritional polyneuropathy is essentially a disease of the alcoholic population. As has been mentioned above, it is present in more than 80 percent of patients with the Wernicke-Korsakoff syndrome, but it also occurs frequently as the only manifestation of deficiency disease. The peripheral neuropathy of alcoholics ("alcoholic polyneuropathy") does not differ in any fundamental way from that of beriberi. The clinical features of nutritional polyneuropathy and its identity with beriberi are discussed in Chap. 83, and the nutritional disorder is explained in greater detail in Chap. 368. A deficiency of thiamine chloride, pyridoxine, pantothenic acid, vitamin B_{12}, and perhaps folic acid has been demonstrated in individual cases to cause nutritional polyneuropathy. In the alcoholic patient it is difficult to incriminate any particular one of these vitamins.

PELLAGRA This disease is described in Chap. 83. The comments here are concerned only with the neurologic manifestations, which in themselves are quite diverse. Pellagra is essentially an encephalopathy, although involvement of other parts of the nervous system may occur. The early mental symptoms—insomnia, fatigue, nervousness, irritability, and feelings of depression—may be mistaken for those of a psychoneurosis. However, careful examination as the disease advances will reveal slowing and inefficiency of mental processes and impairment of memory. Pellagra may not only be the cause of insanity but occasionally may result from it, because certain mental illnesses, including alcoholism, are accompanied by anorexia and unbalanced diet.

The manifestations of involvement of the spinal cord have not been clearly delineated, perhaps because the mental state of the patients has precluded accurate testing. In general, there is evidence of both posterior and lateral column involvement, predominantly the former. Neuropathic signs are frequent and difficult to distinguish from other types of nutritional polyneuropathy. Other manifestations such as tremors, extrapyramidal rigidity, sucking and grasping reflexes, and coma (referred to in the past as "nicotinic acid deficiency encephalopathy") have indiscriminately been included in the pellagrous syndrome, as have various disorders of the special senses.

A *spastic paretic syndrome,* apart from the other symptoms and signs of pellagra, may be a rare manifestation of deficiency disease. The chief clinical signs are spastic weakness of the legs with absent abdominal and increased tendon reflexes, clonus, and extensor plantar responses. These signs are usually accompanied by other manifestations of nutritional deficiency, such as Wernicke's disease and retrobulbar and peripheral neuropathies. Spastic weakness of the legs has also been observed in conjunction with chronic liver disease.

Pathologic changes The distinctive neuropathologic changes in pellagra are most readily discerned in the large cells of the motor cortex, the cells of Betz, although the same changes are seen to a lesser extent in the smaller pyramidal cells of the cerebral cortex and cells of the basal ganglia, cranial motor and dentate nuclei, and anterior horns of the spinal cord. The affected cells appear swollen and rounded with eccentric nuclei and loss of the Nissl particles. This central neuritis of pellagra, as it is called, is probably not dependent on injury to the axons of the Betz cells but appears to represent a primary affection of the whole motor cell. The spinal cord lesions take the form of a symmetrical degeneration of the dorsal columns, especially those of Goll, and to a lesser extent of the corticospinal tracts. The posterior column degeneration affects a specific system of fibers and may be secondary to degeneration of the dorsal root ganglion cells. The pathogenesis of the corticospinal tract lesion in pellagra is not known.

DEFICIENCY AMBLYOPIA (NUTRITIONAL OPTIC NEUROPATHY, TOBACCO-ALCOHOL AMBLYOPIA) These terms refer to a characteristic form of visual impairment that complicates nutritional disease and is due to a lesion in the optic nerve, more or less confined to the zone of the papillomacular bundle. The cornea and other parts of the refractive mechanism are uninvolved, hence the term amblyopia.

The main symptom is dimness or blurring of vision for near and distant objects, which worsens progressively for several days or weeks. In addition to a reduction in visual acuity, examination discloses the presence of bilateral, more or less symmetrical central or centrocecal scotomata, which are larger for colored than for white test objects. Pallor of the temporal portion of the optic disc is observed in some cases. Untreated, this condition progresses to irreversible optic atrophy.

Deficiency amblyopia was particularly prevalent during World War II and the Korean war, in prisoner-of-war camps of the far east. Although this form of amblyopia had previously been described in association with beriberi and pellagra, the peak incidence among prisoners did not coincide with either of these syndromes but with the syndrome of orogenital dermatitis and "burning feet" (see below, under "Strachan's Syndrome").

In the United States most, if not all, of the cases of retrobulbar neuropathy attributed to the toxic effects of alcohol or tobacco—so-called tobacco-alcohol amblyopia—are of nutritional origin. Optic neuropathy may occur as the only manifestation of deficiency disease, but more often it is combined with other nutritional syndromes, such as peripheral neuropathy and the Wernicke-Korsakoff syndrome.

Although the nutritional origin of this type of amblyopia seems established, the specific nutrient that is responsible is uncertain. Observations in both humans and experimental animals indicate that a deficiency of thiamine or vitamin B_{12} or perhaps riboflavin may cause degenerative changes in the optic nerves. It has been suggested that the combined effects of vitamin B_{12} deficiency and chronic poisoning with cyanide (generated in tobacco smoke) are responsible for "tobacco amblyopia." Vitamin B_{12} deficiency is a rare but established cause of optic neuropathy, but the notion that cyanide or other substances in tobacco smoke have a damaging effect upon the optic nerves is supported neither by logic nor by experimental data.

Since a specific nutritional deficiency can rarely be determined in this disorder, treatment consists of the administration of a balanced diet, supplemented with B vitamins, and the interdiction of alcohol where this is a factor.

SYNDROME OF AMBLYOPIA, PAINFUL NEUROPATHY, AND OROGENITAL DERMATITIS (STRACHAN'S SYNDROME) Beginning with the observations of Strachan, in 1888, and 1897, there have been many reports from diverse sources concerning a neurologic syndrome which is undoubtedly nutritional in origin but which cannot be forced into the boundaries of the classical deficiency diseases, beriberi and pellagra. Strachan attributed the disorder to malaria. Originally known as "Jamaican neuritis," the syndrome was soon recognized among the undernourished population of many other tropical countries. Large numbers of patients with this syndrome were observed also in the beseiged population of Madrid during the Spanish Civil War and later during World War II, among prisoners of war in the middle and far east. In the United States, patients with this syndrome are found occasionally among the alcoholic population.

Strachan's syndrome is essentially a disorder of the peripheral and optic nerves. The peripheral nerve disorder is characterized mainly by sensory symptoms and signs (paresthesias of the extremities, painful hyperesthesia of the feet, loss of superficial and deep sensation, and ataxia). On the other hand, foot drop and muscle weakness occur very rarely. A frequently associated disorder is failing vision, which may go on to complete blindness and pallor of the optic discs. In general, deafness and vertigo are rare complications, but in some outbreaks among prisoners of war these symptoms were so common as to earn the epithet "camp dizziness." In all these respects the syndrome differs from beriberi. Along with the neurologic signs there may be varying degrees of stomatoglossitis, corneal degeneration, and genital dermatitis. These mucocutaneous lesions are often spoken of together as the *orogenital syndrome* and are quite distinct from those of pellagra.

There have been only a few pathologic studies of this syndrome. Aside from the damage to the papillomacular bundle in the optic nerve, the most consistent abnormality has been a loss of medullated fibers in each column of Goll adjacent to the midline. This indicates a systematized degeneration of the central process of the bipolar sensory neuron of the lumbosacral spinal ganglia. The fact that the primary sensory neuron is the chief site of disease is consistent with the predominant sensory symptomatology. There are no reliable data concerning the specific deficiencies (vitamin or other) that cause this disease.

SUBACUTE COMBINED DEGENERATION (SCD) OF THE SPINAL CORD (See also Chap. 327) This is the term used to designate the spinal cord disease that results from vitamin B_{12} deficiency. The brain, optic nerves, and peripheral nerves may also be involved but far less often than the spinal cord. The neurologic manifestations of vitamin B_{12} deficiency, and the hematologic ones (pernicious anemia), are clearly different from the other deficiency diseases insofar as their usual cause is not a lack of vitamin B_{12} in food but an inability to transfer minute amounts of this nutrient across the intestinal mucosa ("starvation in the midst of plenty," as Castle has aptly phrased it). Such a nutritional disorder is referred to as a *conditioned deficiency,* since it depends upon the lack of an intrinsic factor in the gastric secretion (see Chap. 327).

Clinical manifestations Symptoms of nervous system disease are present in the large majority of patients with pernicious anemia. The patient first notices general weakness and paresthesias consisting of tingling, "pins and needles" feelings, or other vaguely described sensations. The paresthesias tend to be constant, to progress steadily, and to be the source of much distress. They are localized in the distal parts of the limbs in a symmetric distribution; the lower extremities may be involved before the upper ones or vice versa. As the illness progresses the gait becomes unsteady, and movements of the limbs, especially of the legs, become stiff and awkward.

Early in the course of the illness, when only paresthesias are present, there may be no objective signs. Later, the neurologic examination discloses a disorder of the posterior or lateral columns of the spinal cord, predominantly of the former. Loss of vibration sense is by far the most consistent sign; it is more pronounced in the legs than in the arms, and frequently it extends over the trunk. Position sense is involved somewhat less frequently. The motor signs include loss of power, spasticity, changes in the tendon reflexes, clonus, and extensor plantar responses. These signs are usually limited to the legs. At first the patellar and Achilles reflexes are found to be diminished as frequently as they are increased, and they may even be absent. With treatment the reflexes may return to normal or become hyperactive. The gait at first is predominantly ataxic, later ataxic and spastic. If the disease remains untreated, an ataxic paraplegia with variable degrees of spasticity and contracture may develop.

Isolated instances of loss of superficial sensation below a segmental level on the trunk do occur, implicating the spinothalamic tracts, but such a finding should always suggest the possibility of some other disease of the spinal cord. The defect of cutaneous sensation may take the form of a blunting of touch, pain, and temperature sensation over the limbs in a distal distribution, implicating the peripheral nerves, but such findings are also uncommon.

The nervous system involvement in vitamin B_{12} deficiency is characteristically, though not always, symmetric. A definite asymmetry of motor or sensory findings, maintained over a period of weeks or months, should always cast doubt on the diagnosis.

Mental signs are frequent, ranging from irritability, apathy, somnolence, suspiciousness, and emotional instability to a marked confusional or depressive psychosis, or even to intellectual deterioration. Visual impairment is infrequent and presents with roughly symmetrical centrocecal scotomata. If involvement of the optic nerve is severe, optic atrophy may occur. Although dementia and amblyopia are relatively uncommon, they may be the initial manifestations of the disease.

Neuropathologic changes The pathologic process takes the form of diffuse, although uneven, degeneration of the white matter. At first there is swelling of myelin sheaths, characterized by separation of myelin lamellae and formation of intramyelinic vacuoles. This is followed by a coalescence of small foci of tissue destruction into larger ones, imparting a vacuolated appearance to the tissue. The myelin sheaths and the axis cylinders are both affected, the former perhaps earlier and to a greater extent than the latter. There is relatively little fibrous gliosis in the early lesions, but in the more chronic ones gliosis is pronounced. The changes begin in the posterior columns of the lower cervical and upper thoracic cord and spread from this region up and down the cord, as well as forward into the lateral columns. The lesions are not limited to specific systems of fibers within the posterior and lateral funiculi but are scattered irregularly through the white matter.

The pathogenesis of the nervous system lesions in vitamin B_{12} deficiency is not well understood. It has been proposed that impairment of DNA synthesis in vitamin B_{12} deficiency accounts for the hematologic abnormalities and particularly for the production of megaloblasts; however, since neurons do not divide, this factor does not appear to be operative in regard to the central nervous system. One of the better-understood functions of vitamin B_{12} is its role as a coenzyme in the methylmalonyl CoA mutase reaction. In this reaction, which is a key step in propionate metabolism, methylmalonyl CoA is transformed to succinyl CoA, which subsequently enters the Krebs cycle. It has been shown that impairment of this metabolic step may lead to production of abnormal fatty acids (Cardinale et al.). Since fatty acids are important building blocks of cell membranes and of myelin, it is conceivable that this biochemical abnormality may in some way be responsible for the nervous system lesions.

Treatment The treatment of the neurologic manifestations of vitamin B_{12} deficiency differs in no way from the treatment of the other manifestations of pernicious anemia. Theoretically, 1 μg per day of parenterally administered vitamin B_{12} is adequate, but in practice much larger doses are used.

The most important factor influencing *response* to treatment is the duration of the disease. Recovery may be complete if therapy is instituted within a few weeks of the onset of symptoms. For this reason SCD and the other neurologic complications of vitamin B_{12} deficiency represent medical emergencies. If symptoms have been present for longer than a month or two, only partial recovery can be expected, and in long-standing cases the best that can be expected is the arrest of progression of the symptoms.

The chief obstacle to early diagnosis is the lack of parallelism between the hematologic and neurologic signs. This is particularly the case in patients who have received folic acid, which serves to maintain a hematologic remission for an indefinite period while the neurologic signs worsen, often to an irreversible stage. Under these circumstances the most reliable diagnostic procedure is the Schilling test (see Chap. 327).

HEREDITARY VITAMIN-RESPONSIVE DISEASES An important development in the understanding of hereditary disorders of the nervous system is the recognition that some of them are due to a genetically deranged mechanism for the control of vitamin utilization. In some instances the defect is only quantitative and, by loading the organism with a great excess of the vitamin in question, the disability can be diminished or reversed. These disorders are referred to as *vitamin-dependency states* or *vitamin-responsive disorders.* The following disorders (and the responsible vitamin deficiency) fall into this category: lactic acidosis and certain instances of Leigh's disease and maple syrup urine disease (thiamine); certain cases of homocystinuria and infantile convulsions (pyridoxine); methylmalonic aciduria (cobalamin); propionic acidemia (biotin); and Hartnup disease (niacin).

The biochemical mechanisms involved are not yet clear. It is presumed that the vitamin or cofactor stabilizes a genetically deficient enzyme or facilitates its interaction with its substrate. Awareness of these states is of great practical significance, since administration of specific cofactors in appropriate dosage may restore to normal function a person who would otherwise die or be severely disabled. Careful therapeutic trials should be undertaken whenever one of the above disorders is documented by precise enzymatic assays. Even among patients who have apparently similar enzyme defects, there still appears to be considerable heterogeneity. Thus some patients may respond very favorably to the administration of the cofactor, while others may show no improvement.

PROTEIN-CALORIE MALNUTRITION (PCM) AND MENTAL RETARDATION Although not a problem of immediate concern to the internist, any discussion of the nervous disorders associated with malnutrition would be incomplete without some reference to infantile malnutrition and mental retardation.

During the past two decades evidence has accumulated from observations of children and animal experimentation that gross insufficiency of food in early life can interfere with brain development, leaving the child temporarily or permanently mentally enfeebled. And since there are more than 100 million children in the world who are suffering from malnutrition, this stands as one of the most important public health problems.

The evidence appears to indicate that a reduction of all the essential elements of diet but particularly of protein impairs the function and alters the chemistry of the brain in all species studied, including humans. In the latter the most definite effects occur when the deficiency is in early life, whether antenatal or postnatal, viz., in infancy. Once the maturation and development of the brain are complete, general nutritional or protein deficiency harm the nervous system little if at all.

Two overlapping clinical syndromes have been defined in malnourished infants and children—kwashiorkor and marasmus. Kwashiorkor is a syndrome of weanling children consisting of edema (and sometimes ascites), hair changes (sparsity and depigmentation), and stunting of growth due to protein deficiency. The edema is due to hypoalbuminemia, and there is in addition an abnormal pattern of blood amino acids as well as a fatty liver. There are sometimes skin changes suggestive of pellagra or riboflavin deficiency but no signs of polyneuropathy or subacute combined degeneration of the cord. Marasmus consists of an extreme degree of cachexia and growth failure in early infancy. The latter infants usually have been weaned early or were never breast-fed. Common to both groups of children is an apathy and indifference to the environment, combined with irritability when handled or moved. The children are underactive, and even after an adequate diet has been instituted, their tendency is to follow with the eyes rather than to move. At one stage of early convalescence a small number of the kwashiorkor children pass through a phase of rigidity and tremor which has not been explained.

In contrast to the devastating effects of PCM upon body growth, the brain weight of these severely undernourished children is only slightly reduced. Nevertheless, on the basis of experiments in dogs, pigs, and rats, it is evident that early (prenatal and early postnatal) malnutrition retards cellular proliferation in the brain. All cells are affected, including oligodendroglia, with a proportional reduction in myelin. Also, the process of dendritic branching may be retarded by early malnutrition. A limited number of studies in humans suggest that PCM has a similar effect upon the brain during the first 8 months of life. Details of these studies cannot be given here, but an excellent review has been provided by Winick.

In animals, varying degrees of recovery from the effects of early malnutrition are possible if normal nutrition is reestablished during the vulnerable periods. Presumably this is true for humans as well, although it remains to be proved. In every series of severely undernourished infants and young children who have been followed for many years, a variable percentage have been left mentally backward to a modest degree; the majority recover, however (Latham; Birch et al.). As matters presently stand one cannot be certain that protein-caloric undernutrition is the sole cause of either subnormal brain development or of mental retardation. Not only has it proved difficult to assess the mental function of malnourished infants and young children, but it has been virtually impossible to isolate the effects of infection, which is almost always present in these subjects, and of social deprivation, inherited intellectual defects, and other factors. For a cautious analysis of this problem the reader should turn to the monographs of Scrimshaw and Gordon and of Dodge et al.

REFERENCES

Adams RD, Victor M: *Principles of Neurology,* 2d ed. New York, McGraw-Hill, 1981

Birch HG et al: Relation of kwashiorkor in early childhood and intelligence at school age. Pediatr Res 5:579, 1971

Blass JP, Gibson GE: Abnormality of a thiamine-requiring enzyme in patients with Wernicke-Korsakoff syndrome. N Engl J Med 297:1367, 1977

Cardinale GJ et al: Effect of methylmalonyl coenzyme A: A metabolite which accumulates in vitamin B_{12} deficiency on fatty acid synthesis. J Biol Chem 245:3771, 1970

Dodge RR et al: *Nutrition and the Developing Nervous System.* St. Louis, Mosby, 1975

Latham MC: Protein-calorie malnutrition in children and its relation to psychological development and behavior. Physiol Rev 54:541, 1974

McEntee WJ, Mair RG: Memory enhancement in Korsakoff's psychosis by clonidine: Further evidence for a nonadrenergic deficit. Ann Neurol 7:466, 1980

Pallis CA, Lewis PD: *The Neurology of Gastrointestinal Disease.* New York, Saunders, 1974

Potts AM: Tobacco amblyopia. Surv Ophthalmol 17:313, 1973

Rosenberg LE: Vitamin-responsive inherited diseases affecting the nervous system, in *Brain Dysfunction in Metabolic Disorders,* F Plum (ed) Assoc Res Nerv Ment Dis. New York, Raven Press, 1974, vol 53, pp 263–270

Scrimshaw NS, Gordon JE (eds): *Malnutrition, Learning and Behavior.* Cambridge, MIT Press, 1968

Shimojyo S et al: Cerebral blood flow and metabolism in the Wernicke-Korsakoff syndrome. J Clin Invest 46:849, 1967

Victor M: Polyneuropathy due to nutritional deficiency and alcoholism, in *Peripheral Neuropathy,* PJ Dyck et al (eds). Philadelphia, Saunders, 1975, pp 1030–1066

———, Adams RD: On the etiology of the alcoholic neurologic diseases. With special reference to the role of nutrition. Am J Clin Nutr 9:379, 1961

——— et al: A restricted form of cerebellar degeneration occurring in alcoholic patients. Arch Neurol 1:577, 1959

——— et al: Deficiency amblyopia in the alcoholic patient. A clinicopathologic study. Arch Ophthalmol 64:1, 1960

——— et al: *The Wernicke-Korsakoff Syndrome. A Clinical and Pathological Study of 245 Patients, 82 with Postmortem Examinations.* Philadelphia, Davis, 1971

Winick M: *Malnutrition and Brain Development.* New York, Oxford University Press, 1976

364 DEGENERATIVE DISEASES OF THE NERVOUS SYSTEM

Alzheimer's disease and Parkinson's disease

EDWARD P. RICHARDSON, JR.
RAYMOND D. ADAMS

The term *degenerative* as applied to diseases of the nervous system is used to designate a group of disorders in which there is gradual, generally symmetric, relentlessly progressive wasting away of neurons for reasons still unknown. Many of the conditions so designated depend on genetic factors and thus appear in more than one member of the same family; this general group of diseases is, therefore, frequently referred to as *heredodegenerative.* A number of other conditions, not apparently differing in any fundamental way from the hereditary disorders, occur only sporadically, i.e., as isolated instances in a given family. For all diseases of this class Sir William Gowers in 1902 suggested the term *abiotrophy,* by which he meant "defective vital endurance" of the structures affected, leading to their premature death. This term, of course, tells nothing of the true nature of the defects. It is to be assumed that their basis must be some disorder of the metabolism of the neurons themselves.

Within relatively recent times there has been some elucidation of the nature of a number of metabolic nervous disorders which, in their symmetric distribution and gradually progressive course, resemble the degenerative diseases under discussion. It is to be expected that with advances in knowledge others of the latter group will eventually find their place in the metabolic category. It is possible that some of these diseases may turn out to be the result of atypical virus infections, as has been demonstrated in one disease previously classified with the degenerative group, Creutzfeldt-Jakob disease, also called subacute spongiform encephalopathy (see Chap. 360).

The degenerative diseases of the nervous system manifest themselves by a number of common syndromes easily distinguished by their clinical attributes, the recognition of which can assist the clinician in arriving at the diagnosis of a disorder of this class. Some of these syndromes and the particular diseases which give rise to them are summarized in the following paragraphs.

GENERAL CONSIDERATIONS It is a characteristic of the degenerative diseases that they begin insidiously and run a gradually progressive course which may extend over many years. The earliest changes may be so slight that it is frequently impossible to assign any precise time of onset. However, as with other gradually developing conditions, the patient or his family may give a history implying an abrupt appearance of disability. This is particularly likely to occur if there has been an injury, or if some other dramatic event has taken place in the patient's life, to which illness might conceivably be related. In such a case, skillful taking of the history may bring out that the patient or family has suddenly become aware of a condition which had, in fact, already been present for some time but had passed unnoticed. Whether trauma or other stress may bring on or aggravate one of the degenerative diseases is still a question that cannot be answered with certainty. From all that is known it would seem highly improbable that this could happen. In any event, it must be kept in mind that the disease processes under discussion by their very nature develop spontaneously, that is to say, without relation to external factors.

The family history is of great importance, but one cannot always be immediately satisfied with that obtained on first contact with the patient. One reason for this is that patients or their relatives may be ashamed to disclose a neurologic disease that has occurred in the family. Another is that it may not be realized that an illness is hereditary when other members of the family have a much less severe form of the disorder such that the patient and family may have been unaware of the abnormality—as not infrequently occurs in the hereditary ataxias and related conditions. Moreover, in modern western families the small sibships may prevent even well-established hereditary diseases from expressing themselves. It must, of course, be remembered that familial occurrence of a disease does not always mean that it is hereditary; it may indicate instead that more than one member of a family has been exposed to the same infectious or toxic agent.

Another significant feature of the degenerative nervous diseases is that in general their ceaselessly progressive course is uninfluenced by all medical or surgical measures. Dealing with a patient with this type of illness is often, therefore, an anguishing experience for all concerned. Yet symptoms can often be alleviated by wise and skillful management, and the physician's kindly interest may be of great help even when curative measures cannot be offered.

The bilaterally symmetric distribution of the changes brought about by these diseases has already been mentioned. This feature alone may serve to distinguish conditions in this group from many other diseases of the nervous system. At the same time, it should be pointed out that, in the earliest stages, greater involvement on one side or in one limb is not uncommon. Sooner or later, however, despite the asymmetric beginning, the inherently generalized nature of the process asserts itself.

A striking feature of a number of disorders of this class is the almost selective involvement of anatomically or physiologically related systems of neurons. This is clearly exemplified in amyotrophic lateral sclerosis, in which the process is almost entirely limited to cortical and spinal motor neurons, and in certain types of progressive ataxia, in which the Purkinje cells of the cerebellum are alone affected. Many other examples could be cited (e.g., Friedreich's ataxia) in which certain neuronal systems disintegrate, leaving others perfectly intact. An important group of the degenerative diseases has therefore been called "system diseases" ("progressive cerebrospinal system atrophies"), and many of these are strongly hereditary. It must be realized, however, that selective involvement of neuronal systems is not exclusively a property of the degenerative group, since several disease processes of known cause have similarly circumscribed effects on the nervous system. Diphtheria toxin, for instance, selectively attacks the myelin of the peripheral nerves, and triorthocresyl phosphate affects particularly the corticospinal tracts in the spinal cord as well as the peripheral nerves. Another example is the special vulnerability of the Purkinje cells of the cerebellum to hyperthermia. On the other hand, several of the conditions included among the degenerative diseases are characterized by pathologic changes that are diffuse and unselective. These exceptions nevertheless do not detract from the importance of affection of particular neuronal systems as a distinguishing feature of many of the diseases under discussion.

Typically, the pathologic process in the nervous system is one of slow involution of nerve cell bodies or their prolongations as nerve fibers, unaccompanied by any intense tissue reaction or cellular response. The cerebrospinal fluid (CSF), therefore, shows little if any change—at most a slight elevation of protein, without abnormalities in pressure, cell count, or in other constituents. Moreover, since these diseases invariably result in tissue loss, rather than in new tissue formation (as with neoplasms or inflammation), x-ray visualization of the ventricular system or subarachnoid space shows either no change or an enlargement of these compartments. These negative laboratory findings thus help to distinguish the degenerative disorders from the other large classes of progressive diseases of the nervous system—tumors and infections.

CLASSIFICATION Since etiologic classification is impossible, subdivision of the degenerative diseases into individual syndromes rests on descriptive criteria, based largely on pathologic anatomy but to some extent on clinical aspects as well. In the terms used to designate many of these syndromes, the names of a number of distinguished neurologists and neuropathologists are commemorated. A useful way of keeping in mind the various disease states is to group them according to the outstanding clinical features that may be found in an actual case. The classification outlined in Table 364-1 and described below is based on such a plan.

SYNDROMES IN WHICH PROGRESSIVE DEMENTIA PREDOMINATES

In the disease entities about to be discussed, the clinical picture is dominated by gradual loss of intellectual capacities, i.e., by dementia. Other neurologic abnormalities, except in the terminal stages, are absent or relatively insignificant. (For further discussion of dementia, including its clinical evaluation, Chaps. 22, 23, and 24 should be consulted.)

DIFFUSE CEREBRAL ATROPHY: SENILE DEMENTIA, ALZHEIMER'S DISEASE Some degree of shrinkage in size and weight of the brain, i.e., "atrophy," has been shown to be the inevitable accompaniment of advancing age. In many instances, this is of no clinical significance, and there are many very old people who remain alert and perceptive, with keen intellect, to the end. Nevertheless, severe degrees of diffuse cerebral atrophy are as a general rule associated with some evidence of dementia. When these changes occur in old age (and the definition of when old age begins is largely subjective), it is usual to speak of *senile dementia.* That this is a fairly frequent condition is common experience. Much more infrequent is a pathologically identical progressive dementia with diffuse brain atrophy coming on well before the senile period—a presenile dementia. This condition, classically described in 1906 by Alois Alzheimer, has since become generally known as *Alzheimer's disease.* The distinction between the two conditions is purely clinical; pathologically, they differ only in that the characteristic abnormalities tend to be more severe and widespread in cases beginning at an earlier age than at the senile period.

There is a tendency in medical circles to view the pathologic changes in Alzheimer's disease as the inevitable consequences of age. The writers suggest, however, that the disease is age-linked, since similar pathologic changes have been produced in a number of ways in experimental animals.

Pathology The brain presents a generally shrunken appearance, with diffuse atrophy of the convolutions and symmetric enlargement of the lateral and third ventricles. Frequently, these changes are especially pronounced in the frontal and temporal lobes. Microscopically, there is widespread loss of nerve cells, most apparent in the cerebral cortex, but often present likewise in the basal ganglia, with secondary glial proliferation. In addition, two types of lesions give this disease process its distinctive character: (1) microscopic deposits of amorphous material, scattered throughout the cerebral cortex and most easily seen with silver-staining methods—the "neutritic plaques" (so called because of their content of fragmented axons and dendrites, as well as glial fibrils)—and (2) the Alzheimer fibrillary change in nerve cells. The latter abnormality consists of the presence within the cytoplasm of thick fiber-like strands of silver-staining material, often in the form of loops, coils, or tangled masses. Recent investigations have greatly advanced knowledge of the structural aspects of these lesions, in that the neuritic plaques are now known to contain amyloid, and the fibrillary change is characterized by masses of paired helical filaments. Their pathogenesis is still unknown, however. Of interest is the observation of Bowen et al. of a reduction of choline acetyltransferase, the key enzyme in the synthesis of the neurotransmitter acetylcholine, in the cerebral cortex of cases of Alzheimer's disease. This suggests that impairment of cholinergic transmission may play a part in the clinical expression of the disease. Recently the demonstration of aluminum in the neurofilamentous tangles and of amyloid, an IgG, in capillaries and neuritic plaques has excited the interest of biochemists and immunologists.

Clinical aspects Although Alzheimer's disease has been described as occurring during every age period, it is most frequently a disease of the later decades of life. A number of well-documented familial cases have been recorded, but there is not sufficient evidence to indicate that this is truly a hereditary disorder. Most of the cases actually seen in practice are sporadic. The onset is insidious and subtle, with changes most noticeable first in memory for recent happenings and in range of mental activity. Emotional disturbances such as depression, anxiety, or odd, unpredictable quirks of behavior, may be salient features in the early stages. Progression is very slow and gradual, and unless the condition is earlier brought to a close by the effects of advanced age, it may smolder on for some 10 or more years.

In the milder cases, including those of the senile period, the noteworthy features are those of simple dementia, as described in Chap. 24. More unusual disorders of thought and intellect, including aphasia, apraxic disturbances, and abnormalities of space perception, may be seen, especially in the presenile group. Exceptionally, and only in the advanced stages of the disease, extrapyramidal signs appear; the patient walks in a shuffling manner with short steps, and there is a generalized stiffness of the musculature with slowness and awkwardness of all movements. These abnormalities have been attributed to involvement of the basal ganglia. Terminally the patient may become nearly decorticate, losing all ability to perceive, think, speak, or move. Additional investigative procedures, including the usual blood and CSF determinations, do not yield any conclusive or pertinent data. There is a diffuse slowing in the electroencephalogram in the more advanced stages of the disease. The enlargement of the ventricular system and subarachnoid space resulting from the diffuse brain atrophy can be demonstrated by computerized tomography (CT scan) and pneumoencephalography; otherwise, no characteristic roentgenographic findings are seen. During the course of the illness, occasional convulsive seizures may occur, but they are relatively rare and should raise suspicion of other diseases. Terminally, in a state of total helplessness, the patient dies from intercurrent disease. Institutional care is usually necessary long before the end.

Differential diagnosis Several disease states for which effective treatment is available may give rise to progressive intellectual deterioration closely resembling what may be seen with the diffuse cerebral atrophy above described. It is imperative that these be looked for. Specific examples include chronic subdural hematoma, chronic "normal pressure" hydrocephalus, frontal glioma or meningioma, bromide intoxication, myxedema, pernicious anemia (vitamin B_{12} deficiency), and neurosyphilis. Various other forms of intoxication, infection, metabolic disorder, or neoplasm may have to be considered. Of these several conditions that simulate the Alzheimer-senile dementia complex "normal pressure hydrocephalus" is one that has yielded most dramatically to therapy. As originally pointed out by Hakim and Adams, an obstruction to CSF flow in the

TABLE 364-1
Clinical classification of the degenerative diseases of the nervous system

- *I* Syndrome in which progressive dementia is an outstanding feature, in the absence of other prominent neurologic signs
  - *A* Diffuse cerebral atrophy
    - *1* Senile dementia
    - *2* Alzheimer's disease
  - *B* Circumscribed cerebral atrophy (Pick's disease)
- *II* Syndrome in which progressive dementia is combined with other neurologic signs
  - *A* Principally in adults
    - *1* Huntington's chorea
    - *2* Cerebrocerebellar degeneration
  - *B* In children and adults
    - *1* Amaurotic family idiocy (neuronal lipidoses)
    - *2* Leukodystrophy
    - *3* Familial myoclonus epilepsy
    - *4* Hallervorden-Spatz disease
    - *5* Wilson's disease (hepatolenticular degeneration, Westphal-Strumpell pseudosclerosis)
- *III* Syndrome chiefly manifested by gradual development of abnormalities of posture or involuntary movements
  - *A* Paralysis agitans (Parkinson's disease)
  - *B* Supranuclear ophthalmoplegia (Steele-Richardson-Olszewski syndrome)
  - *C* Dystonia musculorum deformans (torsion dystonia)
  - *D* Hallervorden-Spatz disease and other restricted dyskinesias
  - *E* Familial tremor
  - *F* Spasmodic torticollis
- *IV* Syndrome chiefly manifested by slowly developing ataxia
  - *A* Cerebellar degenerations
  - *B* Spinocerebellar degenerations (Friedreich's ataxia, Marie's hereditary ataxia)
- *V* Syndrome with slowly developing muscular weakness and wasting
  - *A* Without sensory changes; motor system disease
    - *1* In adults
      - *a* Amyotrophic lateral sclerosis
      - *b* Progressive muscular atrophy
      - *c* Progressive bulbar palsy
      - *d* Primary lateral sclerosis
    - *2* In children or young adults
      - *a* Infantile muscular atrophy (Werdnig-Hoffmann disease)
      - *b* Other forms of familial progressive muscular atrophy (including Wohlfart-Kugelberg-Welander syndrome)
      - *c* Hereditary spastic paraplegia
  - *B* With sensory changes
    - *1* Progressive neural muscular atrophy
      - *a* Peroneal muscular atrophy (Charcot-Marie-Tooth)
      - *b* Hypertrophic interstitial neuropathy (Déjerine-Sottas)
    - *2* Miscellaneous forms of chronic progressive neuropathy
- *VI* Syndrome chiefly manifested by progressive visual loss
  - *A* Hereditary optic atrophy (Leber's disease)
  - *B* Pigmentary degeneration of the retina (retinitis pigmentosa)

ventricles or basal meninges will greatly enlarge the ventricles, and, after this has happened, the CSF pressure may gradually return to normal levels. Forgetfulness and reduced mental activity (without agnosia, apraxia, or aphasia) are accompanied by an awkward, unsteady, short-stepped gait and in some instances by sphincteric incontinence. Worsening of the condition results in a marked impairment of intellectual activity and finally an inability to walk or even to stand up. The plantar reflexes become extensor and grasp and sucking reflexes appear. The ventricles are greatly enlarged (span of lateral ventricles greater than 55 mm), radionuclides placed in subarachnoid space reflux into the ventricles, and air during pneumoencephalography will not enter the cerebral subarachnoid spaces. Previous subarachnoid hemorrhage (trauma, aneurysmal rupture), chronic meningitis (syphilitic, idiopathic), Paget's disease of base of skull, and tumors of benign type (cysts of third ventricle) are some of the causes. Other cases are idiopathic. A ventriculoatrial or ventriculoperitoneal shunt relieves the symptoms in a few weeks.

Marked underactivity (mental and physical), extreme drowsiness, increased ratio of sleep to wakefulness, and hypothermia, when combined with ataxia, slow speech, and prolonged tendon reflexes should always raise suspicion of hypothyroidism. Episodic stupor or coma (with or without seizures), cerebellar ataxia, and choreoathetosis suggest hepatic failure. Other metabolic disorders, chronic intoxications, and chronic infections, e.g., syphilitic meningomyelitis, must be excluded by clinical signs and laboratory tests described in Chaps. 177, 240, and 360. In addition to careful clinical assessment special radiologic procedures such as CT scan and pneumoencephalography or carotid angiography may be necessary. Vascular disease of the brain is often included in the differential diagnosis, but dementia on the basis of cerebrovascular disorders characteristically progresses in a halting or stepwise fashion with conspicuous focal cerebral signs, whereas the progression in senile dementia or Alzheimer's disease is gradual and steady and focal signs are absent. A depressive psychosis may also resemble a degenerative disease and must be differentiated along the lines suggested in Chap. 24. No specific therapy is known for Alzheimer's disease. Recent evidence of impaired central cholinergic transmission has led to the use of acetylcholine precursors such as lecithin and choline or an anticholinesterase drug such as physostigmine, but there are no convincing data in support of their beneficial effects. The management should be along the lines of that described in Chaps. 21 and 24 for the delirious and demented patient.

PICK'S DISEASE (CIRCUMSCRIBED CEREBRAL ATROPHY) This remarkable form of cerebral disease, which is characterized by the circumscription of the atrophy (lobar sclerosis), was first described in a series of publications by Arnold Pick in Prague, around the turn of the century. In the differential diagnosis of dementia in the presenile period, it is often mentioned in the same breath with Alzheimer's disease. It is, however, an extremely rare condition as compared with diffuse cerebral atrophy of the Alzheimer type.

Pathology So striking are the gross pathologic changes in the brain that in typical cases the diagnosis can be made at a glance. One sees severe atrophy of the anterior portions of the frontal and temporal lobes, and there is a curiously sharp line of demarcation between the atrophied portions and the remainder of the brain, which appears normal or nearly so. In some cases, the frontal atrophy is more prominent; in others, the temporal lobes are more severely involved; in general, both regions are affected. Rarely, the disorder has a predominantly unilateral localization—as in cases described originally by Pick. Characteristically, there likewise are atrophic changes in a number of subcortical structures: caudate nucleus, putamen, thalamus, and substantia nigra, and in the descending frontopontine fiber system. In the diseased regions, the local destruction of central and convolutional white matter may be out of proportion to the degree of loss of nerve cell bodies in corresponding areas of the cortex. A noteworthy histologic feature of this condition is the occurrence of numerous swollen "ballooned" nerve cells in the atrophic regions, a finding which has been interpreted as an axonal reaction or retrograde cell change secondary to the degenerative process in the periphery. Another frequent nerve cell change is the presence of spheric intracytoplasmic inclusions that stain deeply with silver impregnation methods; the significance of these is unknown. Under the electron microscope they are seen to be composed of masses of straight filaments clearly differing from the aggregates of helical filaments in Alzheimer's disease. These histologic changes, it must be added, are not found in every case of lobar atrophy. In a few, the atrophic regions show innumerable neuritic plaques and neurofibrillary changes of Alzheimer type.

Clinical aspects If Pick's disease has any distinguishing clinical features, they are unusually severe signs of frontal lobe or temporal lobe involvement (see Chap. 24). The clinical differentiation of Alzheimer's and Pick's diseases during life is difficult and probably of no practical importance. As a general rule, rigidity and pronounced grasping and sucking release phenomena are early and pronounced changes in Pick's disease. In CT scans the shrinkage of the cortex and the low density of white matter may be diagnostic. Familial occurrence is on record in a number of instances. Progression is slow and relentless, the average duration of Pick's disease being about 7 years.

Differential diagnosis The considerations noted above with respect to Alzheimer's disease apply to Pick's disease as well.

SYNDROME COMBINING DEMENTIA WITH OTHER NEUROLOGIC SIGNS

HUNTINGTON'S DISEASE (CHRONIC PROGRESSIVE HEREDITARY CHOREA) This condition, which genetically follows the pattern of a mendelian dominant trait, was classically described in 1872 by George Huntington, who, with his father and grandfather, both physicians, observed cases in members of a family living near their home on Long Island, New York. Unmistakable in its typical form, the affliction combines progressive dementia with bizarre involuntary movements (chorea) and odd postures. Atypical cases have also been recognized (see below), but in general the disorder runs true to form. The estimated frequency of the disease is 5 cases per 100,000 population.

Pathology The brain has a generally atrophic appearance, especially noticeable in the frontal lobes. Particularly characteristic is severe bilateral atrophy of the caudate nucleus, which becomes flattened and concave instead of projecting as a convex rounded eminence into the anterior horn of the lateral ventricle. The putamen, likewise, is shrunken, although not to the same extent as the caudate nucleus. The globus pallidus is generally involved to some degree, but less severely than the caudate nucleus and putamen. Microscopically, the affected regions show severe nerve cell loss with reactive glial changes.

Of considerable interest with regard to pathogenesis has been the discovery that the caudate and putamen in the brains of patients with Huntington's chorea are deficient in glutamic acid decarboxylase as well as the inhibitory transmitter γ-aminobutyric acid (GABA). There is also a deficiency of choline acetyltransferase, the enzyme required for acetylcholine synthesis and of several neuropeptides, including substance P, enkephalins, and cholecystokinin.

Clinical aspects This distressing condition generally makes its appearance in early to middle adult years. Its typical hereditary nature (mendelian dominant) has been emphasized, but what appear to be sporadic cases do occur (an impression that may be the result of incomplete family histories). The involuntary movements (bizarre grimacing, respiratory irregularity, faulty articulation of speech, and irregular, arrhythmic, unpatterned movements of the limbs, imparting to the gait a peculiar dancing quality) tend to be less quick and more athetoid than in Sydenham's chorea (see Chap. 15). A few reported cases which on genealogic and pathologic grounds must be classified with Huntington's chorea have shown progressive rigidity, rather than choreiform movements. This is most characteristic of cases in which the onset occurs at a younger age (juvenile form). As a general rule, dementia runs parallel with the motor disorder. Occasionally it may appear before or after chorea; very rarely it may be slight or lacking altogether. The advance of the disease is slow. There is increasing disability because of both involuntary movements and mental changes, terminated after many years by death from intercurrent infection or, not rarely, by suicide.

Differential diagnosis There is no difficulty in the recognition of typical cases. The relatively late onset, the slowly progressive course, the prominent dementia, and lack of association with rheumatic fever help to exclude Sydenham's chorea. Treated cases of Parkinson's disease, when overdosed with L-dopa, may develop a widespread chorea, and the early dementia that occurs in some patients will reproduce the picture of Huntington's chorea. Phenothiazine drugs may induce generalized chorea, unassociated with dementia. Finally, there is a form of self-limited chorea that may appear in older persons without identifiable cause. Hepatolenticular degeneration (Wilson's disease) and nonfamilial forms of hepatocerebral degeneration may display clinical abnormalities resembling those of Huntington's chorea, but the specific changes characteristic of these disorders, including liver disease, corneal Kayser-Fleischer rings (in Wilson's disease), and the typical biochemical abnormalities, are absent in Huntington's chorea. Choreoathetosis appearing during the second postnatal year and lasting throughout life is due to hypoxic birth injury or kernicterus. Sporadic cases of choreiform movements beginning in middle or late life may present a difficult problem in exact diagnosis. The occasional cases of violent choreiform movements produced by vascular lesions, classically in the subthalamic region, are characterized by sudden onset, unilateral distribution (hemiballismus), and a tendency to improve after a period of initial severity. A few cases of acute choreoathetosis have accompanied hyperthyroidism. Virus encephalitis may occasionally be associated with choreiform movements; acute development, fever, and pleocytosis in the cerebrospinal fluid help in recognition of such cases.

Treatment It is impossible to halt the progress of this disease by any of the suggested forms of treatment. Chlorpromazine in doses of 25 to 50 mg three times daily and haloperidol, 2 to 4 mg three times daily, help to control the chorea. Three phenothiazines—perphenazine (Trilafon), fluphenazine (Prolixin), and trifluoperazine (Stelazine)—also reduce to some extent the chorea but result in an undesirable sedation. L-Dopa usually makes the chorea worse and if given in a dosage of 3.0 g per day is said to evoke chorea in an asymptomatic descendant of choreic patients, but both false-negative and false-positive effects have been observed. The finding of low levels of excitatory and inhibitory transmitter substances would suggest that agents which raise their levels might be of value therapeutically.

DEMENTIA WITH ATAXIA The progressive cerebellar degenerations of late life, and some cases of spinocerebellar degeneration, may be accompanied by significant dementia, the pathologic basis for which is not always easily demonstrated. These disorders are dealt with more fully below in the section devoted to conditions manifested by ataxia.

LIPIDOSES OF THE NERVOUS SYSTEM The conditions to be considered here differ from other degenerative disorders in that the underlying pathologic change is more suggestive of a biochemical abnormality, and indeed a defect in hexose aminidase A or B or both has been demonstrated in some of them. They are characterized by a more or less widespread derangement of lipid metabolism, which results in abnormal accumulations of lipids in the cytoplasm of cells of the nervous system and often of other organs as well. (For information relating to the problem of the lipidoses in general, Chaps. 104 and 365 should be consulted.) This process leads to abnormal function and, eventually, to death of the affected nerve cells. There is ample evidence for hereditary transmission of these disorders, the basis for which must consist of genetically determined abnormalities of enzyme systems concerned with intracellular lipid metabolism. This group of diseases is currently the subject of much intensive biochemical and ultrastructural investigation, such that for several of them it has been possible to identify the enzymes that are deficient.

Special clinical types The forms of lipidoses which affect the nervous system exclusively have often been classified together in the earlier literature as *amaurotic family idiocy.* This term emphasizes the important hereditary aspect, but it is not satisfactory, since it can be correctly applied only to cases occurring in infancy. Of interest to the internist is a group of diseases that cause dementia and various other neurological abnormalities during late childhood, adolescence, and early adult life. In the older child and adult, blindness (amaurosis) may never develop, and "idiocy," strictly speaking, implies defective intelligence existing from earliest infancy. Another name that has been given to this group of lipidoses is *cerebromacular degeneration,* but it is accurate only for patients with the combination of cerebral lesions and degeneration of the macular part of the retina.

Within the group of diseases that have been designated as amaurotic family idiocy, the following varieties are generally distinguished.

TAY-SACHS DISEASE This is the classic form of neuronal lipidosis occurring in infants, almost exclusively in Jewish families. It is characterized by extremely widespread involvement (see Chap. 104 for further details).

LATE INFANTILE FORM (JANSKÝ-BIELSCHOWSKY) This variety, which is rare, begins at a somewhat later age than Tay-Sachs disease (age 3 to 4 years) and has a more chronic course. It is biochemically and pathologically (by electron microscopy) distinguishable from both Tay-Sachs disease and juvenile ceroid lipofuscinosis, but has features in common with both. However, vision and the appearance of the retina may be normal.

JUVENILE FORM (BATTEN-SPIELMEYER-VOGT) This form of lipidosis is not confined to patients of Jewish parentage. Clinically, the onset is between the ages of 5 to 10 years, and the course is relatively prolonged, with death at the time of adolescence or early adulthood. Visual impairment is usually the first symptom, followed by cerebellar ataxia, polymyoclonus, and dementia. The retinal lesions take the form of pigmentary degeneration (atypical retinitis pigmentosa). The intraneuronal accumulations differ considerably from those encountered in lipidoses of the Tay-Sachs and Janský-Bielschowsky types, both under light and electron microscopy, although, in common with these disorders, they have the histochemical properties of a glycolipid. Their chemical composition has not as yet been fully determined, but can be classed with the lipofuscins.

ADULT FORM This is an extremely rare disorder, with mental regression often preceding ataxia, athetosis, or other extrapyramidal signs and pursuing a very prolonged course. In all essential respects, it is identical with the juvenile form, except that retinal lesions may be completely absent. The storage material in neurons is in the form of curvilinear bodies and shares certain staining reactions with ceroid and lipofuscin. Recently an adult form with prominent proximal muscular atrophy (due to degeneration of anterior horn cells) and mild dementia has been observed (Kolodny)

Generalized lipidoses with central nervous system involvement In addition to the group of lipidoses exclusively affecting the nervous system, there are a number of more generalized disorders of lipid metabolism in which the nervous system participates.

GENERALIZED GANGLIOSIDOSIS Two rare forms of generalized lipidosis in infants have lately been recognized, both of them characterized by abnormal accumulations of gangliosides in many organs in addition to the nervous system. One of them closely resembles Tay-Sachs disease in that the substance that accumulates abnormally is the same monoganglioside (G_{M2} in the Svennerholm classification) that is present in excess in the neurons in Tay-Sachs disease. This is generally referred to as *Tay-Sachs disease with visceral involvement.* The other, termed *generalized gangliosidosis,* is characterized by excessive amounts of G_{M1} ganglioside.

NIEMANN-PICK DISEASE This disease is discussed in Chap. 104. The typical accumulation of large amounts of lipid in macrophages (reticuloendothelial cells) in many organs, including particularly the liver and spleen, is accompanied by lipidosis of the nervous system, similar to that occurring in the various forms of amaurotic family idiocy. The lipid involved here is mainly sphingomyelin and the disease is caused by a deficiency of sphingomyelinase. The clinical picture may combine a defect in vertical gaze with dystonia or choreoathetosis. Often elements of cerebellar ataxia are added to the dystonic gait disorder.

MUCOPOLYSACCHARIDOSES These disorders belong to a group in which there are abnormalities of connective tissue in many organs. In the Hurler variety, mental retardation is a prominent clinical feature, along with clouding of corneas and certain skeletal abnormalities. In the brain there are striking intraneuronal accumulations of lipid (ganglioside) resembling those found in Tay-Sachs disease. The peculiar facial appearance of patients affected with the disease has led to its being referred to in the older literature as gargoylism. Further studies have revealed six different subtypes. The Morquio and Maroteaux-Lamy forms cause neurological symptoms of hydrocephalus and cervical cord compression in adolescents and adults.

GAUCHER'S DISEASE This generalized metabolic disorder of childhood, described in Chap. 104, resembles Niemann-Pick disease in many respects, inasmuch as it likewise is characterized by extensive lipid accumulations in various organs, especially the spleen, liver, and bone marrow. The nervous system, however, is much less regularly affected; it may be entirely normal in cases occurring in late childhood or adult life, although it usually is involved in infants. The accumulating lipid is glucocerebroside.

Clinical aspects The majority of cases of lipidosis occur in infancy and childhood, after a period of normal development. Motor regression, disinterest, and loss of visual capacity are the leading features and are well covered by the term *amaurotic family idiocy.* At later stages the limbs become enfeebled and the reflexes exaggerated. The fundamental change—"cherry red spots" at maculae, surrounded by a gray halo—gives the diagnosis. Its absence suggests the possibility of another infantile cerebral disease, i.e., spongy degeneration of the white matter, in which progressive blindness is combined with psychomotor regression (see below). Excessive startle to sound (auditory myoclonus) is another characteristic finding of infantile cerebral lipidosis of Tay-Sachs type. Later the child becomes decerebrate and dies in 2 to 3 years. In patients with onset later in life cerebellar ataxia, epilepsy, and myoclonic dementia suggest the diagnosis, especially when associated with atypical retinitis pigmentosa. In the adult form polymyoclonia, choreoathetosis, and dementia may be conjoined and retinas are normal. (See Chap. 365 for differential diagnosis.)

LEUKODYSTROPHIES The disorders to be considered here, which typically show an autosomal recessive pattern of inheritance, are characterized by a widespread disintegration of white matter in association with a remarkable sparing of the nerve cell bodies in the gray matter. The leukodystrophies may be considered to represent disorders of metabolism involving components of the myelin sheath. Some of them are related to the neuronal lipidoses previously discussed.

Pathology The distinguishing feature is diffuse disintegration of myelin at all levels of the central nervous system and often of the peripheral nerves as well. As a rule, axons suffer damage to approximately the same degree as the myelin sheaths. Three of the major varieties of leukodystrophy (see below) are characterized by the presence, within the devastated regions, of lipid breakdown products of myelin which show distinct histochemical differences from the familiar lipid products encountered in all the other disease processes destroying myelin, such as infarction, traumatic necrosis, secondary fiber tract degeneration, demyelinative lesions in multiple sclerosis, and so on. The relative intactness of the nerve cell bodies forms a striking contrast to the extensive white matter lesions.

Varieties of leukodystrophy METACHROMATIC LEUKODYSTROPHY This is now known to be a genetically determined metabolic disorder of sphingolipid metabolism in which cerebroside sulfate (sulfatide) accumulates excessively in many organs, especially brain and kidneys, because of deficient activity of the enzyme cerebroside sulfatase. Since neutral cerebrosides and sulfatides are among the chief lipid components of myelin, all myelin-containing parts of the nervous system, both central and peripheral, are affected in this disease. The metabolic abnormality is well tolerated by other organs, as far as their functional integrity is concerned, but in the nervous system the excessive accumulation of sulfatides leads to breakdown of myelin at all levels. Sulfatides have the property of altering the absorption spectrum of dyes such as toluidine blue and cresyl violet, so that in their presence the color obtained is purple or red or even brown instead of the expected blue or violet—a phenomenon known as *metachromasia*. The name *metachromatic leukodystrophy* comes from the fact that the diseased cerebral white matter stains intensely metachromatically because of the large amounts of phagocytosed sulfatide that accompany the breakdown of the myelin. Metachromatic material indicative of sulfatide can also be readily demonstrated postmortem in kidney tubule cells, Kupffer cells of the liver, and in other organs, unaccompanied by any evidence of tissue damage. In the gallbladder the sulfatide deposits apparently do lead to destructive tissue changes, with the result that nonfunctioning of the gallbladder on radiographic examination is one of the manifestations of the disease.

The disease is mostly seen in infants and children, but it occurs not infrequently in adults, including a few of fairly advanced age. In these personality changes, impairment of intellectual function and a mixture of pyramidal and peripheral nerve signs will finally lead to the appropriate diagnostic tests (peripheral nerve conduction velocities, nerve biopsy, and measurement of arylsulfatase A).

KRABBE'S GLOBOID BODY LEUKODYSTROPHY In this variety, first described by Krabbe in 1916 as a familial disorder of infants, the lipid breakdown products also are atypical as compared with those occurring in most pathologic processes which destroy myelin. They differ histochemically from the metachromatic material just described in several ways, including absence of metachromasia. Typical of this disorder is the presence of unusual multinucleated phagocytic cells (globoid cells) which contain galactocerebrosides. In this disease, the biochemical abnormality is apparently the result of a deficiency of galactocerebroside β-galactosidase. As with metachromatic leukodystrophy, this disorder affects the peripheral as well as the central nervous system. Globoid cells are not seen in the peripheral nerves, but electron microscopy shows characteristic inclusions in microphages.

SPONGY DEGENERATION OF THE NERVOUS SYSTEM (VAN BOGAERT, BERTRAND, CANAVAN) This rare inherited disease of infants is generally classified with the leukodystrophies because the cerebral white matter is the chief site of pathologic changes. Characteristic of the disease is a fine-meshed spongy degeneration of the tissue associated with breakdown of myelin in some regions and, probably, failure of myelination in others. This spongy state is apparently the result of a large increase of water, some of which is within the myelin sheaths, resulting in their disruption. The pathologic findings suggest failure of regulation of intracellular fluid balance, perhaps mainly affecting glial cells, but the biochemical and enzymatic defects that underlie this disease have not yet been identified.

PELIZAEUS-MERZBACHER DISEASE In this condition, characterized clinically by a pronounced male sex-linked familial tendency and a very chronic course, the white matter lesions are patchy and irregular, rather than evenly distributed as in the other forms of leukodystrophy. Furthermore, there is relative sparing of axons. Another distinguishing feature of this disorder is that the breakdown products of the myelin, although very sparse (as would be expected from the prolonged course), are of the usual sort regularly seen with myelin destruction, rather than being atypical as in metachromatic leukodystrophy. What has been called *sudanophilic leukodystrophy* may well be identical with Pelizaeus-Merzbacher disease. The underlying basis for the lesions is still wholly unknown.

ADRENOLEUKODYSTROPHY This disease, which is transmitted as a sex-linked trait, is characterized by a combination of degeneration of the cells of the adrenal cortex and a widespread sudanophilic degeneration of myelinated fibers in large foci in the brain. Distinctive membrane-bound crystal-like inclusions have been identified in adrenal cortical cells, in macrophages in the demyelinated zones in the brain, in Schwann cells, and in the Leydig cells of the testis. The presence of these cytologic changes in various tissues suggests a generalized metabolic disorder, but the destructive lesions occur only in the adrenal cortex and the brain. A distinctive biochemical abnormality has lately been identified in this disorder—the presence of disproportionate quantities of long-chain (e.g., C-26) fatty acids in some lipids. These can now be demonstrated in cultured fibroblasts and possibly in plasma. Moreover, it is now realized that the disorder may occur in a chronic, less severe form in adults, with a clinical picture of slowly progressive spastic paraparesis, peripheral neuropathy, and minimal encephalopathic changes. This variant is called *adrenomyeloneuropathy*.

Clinical aspects The symptoms and signs in all the forms of leukodystrophy are mainly those indicative of involvement of tracts of sensory and motor fibers (corticospinal, thalamocortical, geniculocalcarine, pontocerebellar, and cerebellomesencephalic) in combination with a progressive dementia. In the early stages there is weakness and unsteadiness of gait. Likewise prominent are spasticity and exaggeration of tendon reflexes, referable to the destructive lesions in the corticospinal motor system. In contrast to the neuronal lipidoses and other gray matter diseases, seizures are rare. In metachromatic leukodystrophy there is at first hypotonia, then spastic weakness of limbs, but because of later involvement of the peripheral nervous system, muscle-stretch reflexes are lost. The clinical features of adrenoleukodystrophy are described in Chap. 362.

On the whole, though, clinical differentiation of leukodystrophy from other forms of diffuse progressive cerebral disease is difficult. The metachromatic and globoid cell varieties can now be accurately identified by demonstrating the enzymatic deficiency in tissue cultures of leukocytes or fibroblasts, and metachromatic leukodystrophy can be recognized by the presence of sulfatides in the urine. In the other varieties of leukodystrophy, except for adrenoleukodystrophy and its variant forms in which low serum cortisol levels and unresponsiveness to ACTH are demonstrable, there are as yet no reliable biochemical tests whereby the diagnosis can be made during life. The disease can generally be identified in a brain biopsy, but this is a procedure which is justifiable only under very rare circumstances—such as direction of therapy, genetic counseling, or a carefully thought-out research project in which a specimen of fresh tissue might lead to some new insight into an otherwise hopeless disease. (See Chap. 362 for further account of the adult leukodystrophies.)

Differential diagnosis Familial occurrence, signs referable to a disorder of long projection and associative fiber systems, and relative lack of convulsive manifestations may suggest the diagnosis during life. Final verification, however, requires either the demonstration of a specific biochemical abnormality or the characteristic morphologic changes postmortem.

PROGRESSIVE FAMILIAL MYOCLONIC EPILEPSY (UNVERRICHT-LUNDBORG-LAFORA DISEASE) This rare disorder forms a distinct clinicopathologic syndrome characterized by recessive heredity. Typically, it appears in adolescence or early adult life, beginning with generalized convulsive seizures, which are followed after an interval of years by myoclonic jerks of increasing frequency and severity and progressive dementia. Death follows, usually within 5 to 10 years. The pathologic features suggest a disorder of nerve cell metabolism, the nature of which is under current investigation.

Pathology In many of the cases on record, distinctive intracytoplasmic inclusion bodies within nerve cells may be found at all levels in the central nervous system, although they are most frequent in the cerebral cortex, dentate nucleus of the cerebellum, substantia nigra, and thalamus. These bodies were initially described by Gonzalo Lafora (1911) and are generally known as Lafora bodies. Material with similar staining properties has also been found in heart-muscle fibers and in liver cells in several cases. They have been found to be composed of polymers of glucose (polyglucosans), but the reasons for the accumulation of these polysaccharides are still unknown.

Clinical aspects The onset in most cases is at about the time of puberty. The convulsive seizures, with which the disorder usually begins, are in no way distinctive. The myoclonic jerks are sudden, asymmetric or symmetric brief contractions of muscle groups of the limbs, face, and trunk, occurring arrhythmically and unpredictably, usually with sufficient force to displace the parts affected. They characteristically are provoked by all sorts of stimuli, but occur spontaneously as well. The sudden contractions may interfere seriously with willed movements, or may cause the patient to fall abruptly. The disorder progresses gradually, running a course over several years, with the terminal stage being characterized by profound dementia and total helplessness. Treatment with anticonvulsant medication may relieve the generalized convulsive seizures and reduce the frequency of the myoclonic jerks, but has no effect on the dementia.

Differential diagnosis Other forms of progressive familial dementia with myoclonus may have to be considered. These are discussed elsewhere in the descriptions of Creutzfeldt-Jakob disease (Chap. 360) and the lipidoses. There is in addition a more benign form of myoclonic epilepsy which begins in childhood or adolescence and permits survival to middle age or longer. In cases of this kind, some degree of ataxia is frequently observed; and, although there are no distinctive pathologic changes, degeneration of fiber systems related to the cerebellum have been found. In Unverricht-Lafora myoclonic epilepsy, convulsive seizures are more prominent than in the other disorders mentioned. The diagnosis of these different forms of myoclonus is based on clinical picture and course of illness. All forms of treatment have hitherto been ineffective.

HALLERVORDEN-SPATZ DISEASE This unusual disorder, often familial, is associated with a rather variable clinical picture in which abnormalities of posture and muscle tone, involuntary movements, and progressive dementia predominate. Pathologically, there are characteristic abnormalities in the basal ganglia, suggesting a localized disorder of metabolism. The features of the condition were classically described in an affected family by Hallervorden and Spatz (1922).

Pathology Distinctive for this condition is the accumulation of large amounts of pigmented material in the globus pallidus and zona reticulata of the substantia nigra, resulting in grossly visible brownish discoloration of these regions. Microscopically, there are irregular pigmented, ferruginous concretions and granules of varying brownish or greenish hues, depending on the stains used. Although much of this pigment contains iron, serum iron and ferritin are normal, and there is no systemic disorder of iron metabolism. There also is loss of nerve cells and fibers. Another feature of the disease is the presence of focal swelling of axons, most probably in their terminal portions; this is especially pronounced in the regions affected by the pigmentary disorder, but typically can be found at all levels of the central nervous system, including the cerebral cortex.

Clinical aspects The disorder typically makes its appearance in childhood or adolescence, with abnormalities in muscle tone and movements such as rigidity and choreoathetosis. Abnormal postures of the trunk characteristic of torsion spasm (dystonia) may be seen. Cerebellar ataxia and myoclonus are also present in some instances, or the clinical picture may be reminiscent of parkinsonism. Speech becomes indistinct, and there is progressive intellectual impairment. Eventually, the involuntary movements give way to increasing generalized rigidity, and death comes as a rule about 10 years after onset.

Differential diagnosis No feature of the clinical picture serves to distinguish this particular disorder from other conditions showing dementia with extrapyramidal motor abnormalities. Wilson's disease must be excluded by appropriate laboratory tests. The clearly progressive course sets this condition apart from clinically similar abnormalities resulting from accidents or illnesses at birth or in the neonatal period. It has recently been demonstrated that there is a selective uptake of radioactive iron by the basal ganglia which may be helpful in diagnosis. At present no effective treatment is known. A recent (unpublished) attempt at using a chelating agent (deferoxamine mesylate) in one case led to no definite benefit, and L-dopa and other antiparkinsonian medications, tryptophan, and megavitamin therapy have been of only temporary and questionable help.

FAMILIAL HEPATOLENTICULAR DEGENERATION (WILSON'S DISEASE) This condition is discussed in Chap. 98.

ACQUIRED HEPATOCEREBRAL DEGENERATION This condition is discussed in Chap. 362.

EXTRAPYRAMIDAL SYNDROMES OF ABNORMAL POSTURE OR INVOLUNTARY MOVEMENT

PARALYSIS AGITANS (PARKINSON'S DISEASE) This by no means rare condition was named and classically described by James Parkinson in 1817. His remarkably complete account gives this definition:

Involuntary tremulous motion, with lessened muscular power, in parts not in action and even when supported; with a propensity to bend the trunk forward, and to pass from a walking to a running pace, the senses and intellects being uninjured.

Typically, paralysis agitans is a disorder of middle or late life, with very gradual progression and a prolonged course. Although it has been seen to occur in families (the estimated familial incidence is 1 to 2 percent), it usually is sporadic. It is well recognized, however, that the epidemic encephalitis of von Economo, which occurred in a worldwide distribution in the years following World War I, was followed by a syndrome clinically indistinguishable from paralysis agitans. It is usual in such instances to speak of postencephalitic parkinsonism, whereas the term *Parkinson's disease* should be reserved for true paralysis agitans of unknown cause. Paralysis agitans bears no consistent relation to any known disease process such as arteriosclerosis, trauma, or intoxication, although such conditions have often been invoked as etiologically significant and may at times produce somewhat similar clinical manifestations.

Pathology Despite the general medical familiarity with the condition and an extensive literature on the subject, it cannot be said that the pathologic changes of paralysis agitans are yet fully understood. The only regularly observed changes have been in the aggregates of melanin-containing nerve cells in the brainstem (substantia nigra, locus coeruleus), where there are varying degrees of nerve cell loss with reactive gliosis (most pronounced in the substantia nigra) along with distinctive eosinophilic intracytoplasmic inclusions (Lewy bodies, after their description by F. H. Lewy in 1913). Changes have also been described in other structures of the basal ganglia, but they are not clearly different in nature or degree from what may be encountered in other patients of similar age without extrapyramidal motor disorders. The histopathologic evidence therefore suggests that paralysis agitans can be considered as belonging with the system diseases, the affected system being that of the pigmented nuclei of the brainstem. Significantly, extensive lesions in these same pigmented nuclei characterize the pathologic findings in postencephalitic parkinsonism, in which Lewy bodies typically are absent, and in the Shy-Drager syndrome (Chap. 12). Recent biochemical studies, which show a decrease of dopamine in the caudate nucleus and putamen—an alteration consistently found on experimental ablation of the substantia nigra—lend further support to the idea that Parkinson's disease is indeed a disorder of a particular neuronal system (see Chap. 15).

Clinical aspects In its fully developed form, this disorder cannot be mistaken for any other. The stooped posture, the stiffness and slowness of movement, the fixity of facial expression, and the rhythmic tremor of the limbs which subsides on active willed movement or complete relaxation are familiar to every clinician. Although symmetric in the later stages, the disorder typically begins asymmetrically, e.g., as a slight tremor of the fingers of one hand or in one leg. Also typical are more or less general hypokinesia and stiffness of the musculature so that even where tremor is inapparent, the disease may betray itself by a somewhat staring and immobile facial expression, a monotonous voice, a general slowness and diminution of all motor activity, and a curious lack of the little spontaneous movements of postural change that are so characteristic of the normal individual. When tremor is minimal, patients often are able to alleviate it by resting their hands on a table or the arms of a chair or by keeping them in their pockets. The tremor, although fluctuating from moment to moment in amplitude, characterizes the later course. The tremor is generally most pronounced in the hands but may involve the legs (and thus secondarily the trunk), lips, tongue, and neck muscles, and is easily seen in the eyelids when they are lightly closed. Its frequency is 4 to 5 per second, but another faster tremor (7 to 8 per second) predominates in some patients. There is no total paralysis, although general enfeeblement of voluntary movement is characteristic of the fully developed disorder. Together with the stooped attitude, there is the typical festinating gait, whereby the patient, prevented by the abnormality of postural tone from making the appropriate reflex adjustments required for effective walking, progresses with quick shuffling steps at an accelerating pace as if to catch up with the body's center of gravity. Clinical examination of the tendon and plantar reflexes discloses no abnormalities. There are no sensory changes, although deep aching in joints and muscles is common. Eventually, patients may become so incapacitated by rigidity and tremor as to be helpless in caring for themselves. It has often been observed, however, that even severely disabled patients may, under great emotional stress, perform complex motor acts quickly and efficiently. Although the temporary alleviation under extreme provocation can never be long maintained, it is nevertheless true that the severity of the symptoms is considerably influenced by emotional factors, being aggravated by anxiety, tension, and unhappiness, and minimal when the patient is in a contented frame of mind. Despite the inherently progressive nature of the condition, much can be achieved with good medical management, and patients may continue for years to live effective, happy lives in spite of this affliction. Intellectual deterioration is not a consistent feature of paralysis agitans, but it must be conceded that in very advanced stages of the condition dementia may be encountered.

Differential diagnosis In typical cases, this is not difficult. The extrapyramidal syndromes associated with most diseases of known cause or established nature such as cerebral vascular disease, cerebral hypoxia (including carbon monoxide asphyxia), or metallic poisoning differ from paralysis agitans in a number of respects, such as atypical behavior or tremor, presence of signs of pyramidal tract deficit, or early onset of dementia. The differentiation from postencephalitic parkinsonism may be impossible; a clear history of an attack of epidemic encephalitis (prolonged somnolence, disturbance of consciousness, diplopia) and relatively early age of onset of the disorder and the presence of tics, localized spasms, and oculogyric crises may be the only clues to this diagnosis. In recent years, a neurologic disorder strikingly similar to Parkinson's disease has been seen following the prolonged administration of large amounts of reserpine and phenothiazine drugs, which subsides on withdrawal of the offending drug—a matter of considerable theoretic and practical importance. Parkinsonism is rarely, if ever, produced by cerebral neoplasms.

Treatment Although there is no treatment that is known to halt or reverse the neuronal degeneration that presumably underlies Parkinson's disease, methods are now available which can bring about a considerable degree of relief from symptoms in many patients. An important part of any therapeutic program is the maintenance of optimum general health and neuromuscular efficiency by planned programs of exercise, activity, and rest; expert physical therapy may be of great help in achieving these ends. In addition, the patient often needs much emotional support in meeting the stress of the illness, in comprehending its nature, and in carrying on courageously in spite of it. Along with these general supportive measures, which are applicable to many chronic illnesses, patients generally require a carefully thought-out program of treatment specifically aimed at counteracting the pathophysiologic disorder that produces their disabilities. This treatment is nearly always medical (with drugs), but a stereotoxic surgical procedure is a possibility in selected cases.

The medical treatment has been discussed fully by Growdon. He enunciates several principles, as follows.

The drug therapy should be adapted to the patient's needs, which vary with the stage of the disease and the predominant manifestation(s). Usually anticholinergic drugs are most effective in suppressing tremor at rest and propranolol is best for action tremor. L-Dopa improves akinesia and postural imbalance; anticholinergic drugs have little effect on these two abnormalities.

The decision about whether to treat with a drug(s) and the choice of drug(s) is influenced by the stage of the disease. The scale of Hoehn and Yahr is recommended:

Stage I—Unilateral involvement
Stage II—Bilateral involvement but no postural abnormalities
Stage III—Bilateral involvement with mild postural imbalance; patient leads independent life
Stage IV—Bilateral involvement with postural instability; patient requires substantial help
Stage V—Severe, fully developed disease; patient restricted to bed and chair

For patients with mild disease (stages I and II) no medication may be required, or only an anticholinergic drug. Levodopa is required for stages III, IV, and V; and in each instance one uses the lowest dose that gives satisfactory benefit. This reduces chances of short-term side effects, dyskinesias, on-off phenomenon, mental confusion, and loss of efficacy.

The anticholinergic drugs in use share the capacity to block muscarinic receptors and thereby to reduce cholinergic transmission. They are effective not only in relieving the rest tremor of mild Parkinson's disease but also may be combined with levodopa in the treatment of the severe forms of the disease. The anticholinergic drugs also reverse the dystonia and parkinsonian symptoms of neuroleptic drugs.

Currently available anticholinergic drugs are trihexyphenidyl (Artane), benztropine (Cogentin), biperiden (Akineton), and procyclidine (Kemadrin). The usual dose of trihexyphenidyl is 1 to 2 mg qid. Benztropine has both anticholinergic and antihistaminic properties; the usual dose is 0.5 to 1.0 mg tid. The optimal dose of all these medications varies for each patient and often needs adjusting. Low doses of these drugs cause dry mouth but few if any other side effects. Larger doses should be given with caution for in the elderly they may cause confusion, visual and tactile hallucinations, narrow-angle glaucoma, and urinary retention.

Amantadine (Symmetrel), a drug found by accident to be effective in Parkinson's disease (because of its capacity to release stored dopamine from presynaptic terminals), may be used in the early stages in doses of 100 mg bid. Larger doses may have side effects such as skin changes (livido reticularis), ankle edema, and mental confusion. Amantadine has an additive effect when given with levodopa.

Propranolol (Inderal), a beta-adrenergic antagonist, is helpful in suppressing the fast-frequency action tremor in Parkinson's disease and in the hereditary tremor syndrome. The usual dose is 40 to 80 mg tid. In large doses it may slow the heart rate and lower blood pressure, which are disadvantages in Parkinson patients with a tendency to orthostatic hypotension. Metoprolol (Lopressor), a specific beta_1-adrenergic antagonist, is also effective and is safer in patients with suspected asthma.

Levodopa, which increases the dopamine levels in the striatum and restores neurotransmitter balance between dopamine and acetylcholine, improves akinesia and postural disorders (and sometimes rest tremor) in 75 percent of patients. Levodopa is available in 100-, 250-, and 500-mg tablets. The therapeutic range is 2.0 to 8.0 g per day. It is advisable to begin with a low dose, 100 mg tid, and to increase it gradually over several weeks in order to avoid side effects such as nausea, vomiting, and orthostatic hypotension. A combination of levodopa with a DOPA decarboxylase inhibitor (Sinemet) is most popular; the latter component prevents destruction of levodopa in the bloodstream and permits a lower dose to be effective. There are two commercially available preparations: carbidopa in the United States (Sinemet) and benserazide in Canada and Europe (Madopar). The ratio of decarboxylase inhibitor to levodopa is 1:10. The required dosage ranges from 300 to 2000 mg per day, and the timing of the doses should be individualized. This is the cornerstone of therapy; it may be combined with an anticholinergic drug and amantadine.

Bromocryptine, a dopamine agonist, has also been found to have a therapeutic effect. Unlike levodopa, which is converted to dopamine, bromocryptine has a direct action. The dose is 2.5 mg tid, but commonly doses of 50 to 100 mg per day are required for maximum benefit. Goodwin et al., who compare it with L-dopa, observed some patients to respond better to the bromocryptine and some to L-dopa. The quality of the response is much the same, as are the side effects. The on-off phenomenon was observed in only 1 percent, whose daily dose was 40 mg.

One of the most difficult problems in treating patients with Parkinson's disease is the management of side effects, particu-

larly to levodopa. For the acute gastrointestinal symptoms, beginning with a low dose and taking it with meals and snacks is the best means of control. Usually the nausea ceases after a few weeks. The use of phenothiazine drugs is not advised, for they block dopamine receptors and counteract the effect of levodopa. To minimize the orthostatic effects, the measures discussed in Chap. 12 should be employed.

The dyskinesias which may begin after prolonged treatment are more difficult to manage. After 3 to 5 years of treatment the therapeutic index for levodopa narrows, and there may be a brief period of dyskinesia (usually athetosis of the neck) after each effective dose. The on-off phenomenon, which consists of an abrupt onset of weakness and akinesia lasting for a few minutes to an hour, is another problem, and it may alternate with dyskinesia. In some patients the therapeutic index becomes so narrow that a dose variation of 50 to 100 mg may change the status of the patient from a paralyzing akinesia to a severe choreoathetosis. Loss of efficacy of therapy also occurs; instead of a single dose giving a therapeutic effect for 5 to 6 h, it may last only an hour or more.

For all these complications, a cautious withdrawal of the drug, leaving the patient on antiacetylcholine medication, for 1 to 2 weeks and then restarting it at the lowest possible dose is advised. Interruption of treatment carries a high risk and should be carried out in a hospital, for the patient may become completely immobile, mute, and rigid and develop aspiration pneumonia, thrombophlebitis, or a cardiac arrhythmia.

Progressive dementia, which eventually overtakes one-third to one-half the patients in later years, may render them less tolerant to medication. Visual and tactile hallucinations are especially prominent in this group of patients.

As many as a quarter of patients with Parkinson's disease have depressive symptoms. They should be treated along the lines suggested in Chap. 376.

Another important advance in the attempt to relieve the symptoms of Parkinson's disease has been the development of stereotaxic surgery. This involves the placement of precisely localized focal lesions in the central nuclei of the brain, either in the globus pallidus or ventrolateral thalamus, contralateral to the side of the body chiefly affected. The best results occur in patients who are relatively young and in good general health with sound mentality, in whom unilateral tremor or rigidity, rather than akinesia, is the predominant symptom. Opinions among neurosurgeons still differ as to the best way of making the lesion, and studies are still in progress as to what its ideal location should be. Success with L-dopa has greatly diminished the call for surgical therapy.

PROGRESSIVE SUPRANUCLEAR PALSY (STEELE-RICHARDSON-OLSZEWSKI SYNDROME) This clinicopathologic entity, described in 1963 by Richardson, Steele and Olszewski, affects elderly individuals in approximately the same age period as paralysis agitans. And it is among the group of parkinsonian patients that most of the examples of this disease are to be found. The authors encounter several cases each year.

The clinical features are quite distinctive. Disturbances of balance and gait with unexpected falls; rigidity of the neck and other trunk muscles, resembling Parkinson's disease; "masking" of the face; reduction in the volume of the voice; extreme flexion or extension dystonia of the neck; and difficulty in looking down are all early symptoms. Any one of them may first bring patients to a physician. They progress over months and years, until patients are virtually anarthric with total loss of voluntary control of eye movements, and severe cervical and truncal rigidity. Patients eventually become bedfast. Tremor is rarely seen. In contrast there are no impairments of mentation (in most instances), or of vision, hearing, somatic sensation, or voluntary power; and signs of corticospinal involvement are minimal or absent.

A loss of neurons and gliosis are found on postmortem examination all through the tectum and tegmentum of the midbrain, subthalamic nuclei of Luys, vestibular nuclei, and to some extent ocular nuclei. Remarkable, indeed, and setting the disease apart from most other degenerative diseases, is the presence in surviving neurons of neurofibrillary accumulations of distinctive type, which resemble those of Alzheimer's disease in light-microscopic examination but are shown to differ from them on electron microscopy in that they are composed of straight rather than paired helical filaments.

The cause of the disease is unknown. A slow virus is suspected, but attempts to transfer it to monkeys by the intracerebral inoculation of brain tissue have failed.

Treatment has been unsuccessful. Relatively little benefit comes from the administration of the antiparkinsonian series of drugs, although they should be tried; occasionally L-dopa has helped to diminish some of the symptoms.

The diagnosis should be considered whenever an elderly patient begins to fall repeatedly and inexplicably and has extrapyramidal symptoms with a rigid neck and paralysis of conjugate gaze.

DYSTONIA MUSCULORUM DEFORMANS (TORSION SPASM) This is a clinical term denoting a state characterized by slow, nonrhythmic, involuntary movements which produce abnormal, at times bizarre, postures of the trunk and limbs. With passage of time, these postures tend to become more or less fixed. Underlying the clinical disorder may be any of several pathologic conditions, such as the residual lesions of epidemic encephalitis, the pigmented deposits of Hallervorden-Spatz disease (described above), hepatolenticular degeneration (Wilson's disease), or the scars of cerebral birth injury in the broad sense, or kernicterus. More frequent and puzzling, however, is the hereditary form known as *dystonia musculorum deformans* (torsion dystonia), which has a relatively early onset and progressive course without a definitive lesion.

Pathology Until lately, very few cases of dystonia musculorum deformans not due to one of the definable disease processes indicated above had been adequately studied neuropathologically. Reported results from the few that had been examined led to uncertainty as to what the pathologic-anatomic basis of the clinical state might be, although it was generally assumed that the basal ganglia were diseased. A careful study by Zeman and Dyken in 1967, which included comparison of the findings in patients with the disease with control material, demonstrated that there is, in fact, no definable neuronal or other histologically demonstrable disease process to which the clinical abnormalities can reasonably be attributed. These negative findings, which are perhaps surprising, must not be interpreted as indicating that there is "no disease" in the brain, but rather that the pathologic state is not one that can be disclosed by the usual histopathologic techniques. It may well be that current studies of the pathophysiology of neurotransmitters will result in the elucidation of this disease. So far, this has not occurred however.

Clinical aspects The motor abnormalities are described in Chap. 15. In the early stages, the involuntary muscular contractions are intermittent and variable in location and severity, but typically interfere with motor performance by superimposing an unwanted posture upon parts in use. One leg may briefly be pulled into a flexed or extended position or one shoulder elevated. Later the lingual, pharyngeal, neck, and thoracic muscles participate, and grimacing may occur. These latter may also be the first and only signs of disease for several years. Progression may be relatively rapid in cases with onset during early childhood, but is slow in those beginning in late childhood or adult life. The end result is extreme disability, with grossly distorted postures of the trunk and contractures of the limbs. Affection of face and tongue muscles results in faulty articulation of speech, which eventually becomes incomprehensible. The tendon and plantar reflexes, which can be assessed only during moments of relaxation of the affected parts, are characteristically normal.

Mental function is usually of normal or superior quality, especially in the patients with recessive forms of the disease. However, with severe derangement of all available methods of communication, an adequate evaluation of mental capacity may be impossible.

According to Eldridge, who has made the most careful epidemiologic study of torsion dystonia, two types are distinguishable. The most severe type of early onset occurs almost exclusively in Ashkenazi Jews. The patients are always normal the first few years of life. The dystonic movements and postures are appendicular (either peripheral or proximal) and there is no evidence of other neurological abnormality. The milder form is autosomal dominant of later onset (often in midadult life), less rapidly progressive, more often restricted to one part of the body, and with varied ethnic predominance. Sporadic cases are not infrequent and may be restricted to the trunk musculature. All laboratory data in both types are negative.

Spasmodic torticollis (writer's cramp, buccolingual dystonia; see below) is a restricted form of dystonia, but it typically does not progress to involve the musculature generally. However, torticollis may be an early symptom in cases which later show the typical generalized motor abnormalities.

Differential diagnosis Hepatolenticular degeneration should be seriously considered in any case presenting these motor symptoms, and appropriate measures should be undertaken for its investigation (see Chap. 362). The progressive course, and possibly the family history, differentiate the degenerative group from the "symptomatic" dystonias resulting from infections or metabolic disorders occurring at birth or later. Hallervorden-Spatz disease, however, cannot be distinguished on clinical grounds alone. Rare instances of Niemann-Pick or other lipid storage diseases may begin in adult life with a dystonic syndrome, and phenothiazine-induced (tardive) dyskinesia must be considered in all cases of restricted or generalized dystonia in adults, especially if they have or have had a psychiatric illness.

Treatment This is most unsatisfactory. Dystonia is notoriously unresponsive to drug therapy, although antispasmodic drugs such as those used for parkinsonism should be tried. Trihexyphenidyl (Artane) in high doses (12 to 16 mg per day) is beneficial in some cases. Neurosurgical treatment of the sort used for Parkinson's disease has been sufficiently promising to be worth serious consideration in every case, especially if the patient is young.

SPASMODIC TORTICOLLIS AND OTHER RESTRICTED DYSKINESIAS With advancing age a large variety of degenerative "movement disorders" come to light. Supposedly there is loss of neurons in certain parts of the motor system. Groups of muscles begin to manifest arrhythmic involuntary spasms. The patient's lack of success in suppressing them and recognition that they are beyond voluntary control distinguish them from the common tics, habit spasms, and mannerisms described in Chap. 15. If the muscle contraction is frequent and prolonged, an aching pain accompanies it and may be mistakenly blamed for the spasm. Worsening under stress and improvement during quiet and relaxation are typical of this group of disorders.

Surely the most frequent and familiar type is torticollis, wherein an adult, more often a woman, becomes aware of turning of the head to one side as she walks. It gradually worsens to a point where it may be more or less continuous, not even relieved when lying down. Rarely, more than one member of a family is afflicted. On the assumption of a psychogenic factor in the illness many patients receive psychotherapy, but always without benefit. When followed over the years, the condition is observed to remain limited to the same muscles (scalene, sternocleidomastoid, and upper trapezius). There is little if any response to various drugs. Section of upper cervical roots bilaterally (anterior and posterior roots) is the only form of treatment that has given satisfactory results. It is beneficial in approximately 80 percent of cases.

Other restricted dyskinesias involve the neck in combination with facial muscles, the orbicularis oculi (blepharospasm and blepharoclonus), the throat, and respiratory muscles ("spastic dysarthria," respiratory, and phonatory spasms). All these conditions, once started, are persistent, unpleasant, and relatively unresponsive to all modes of therapy other than denervative surgical procedures. Presumably, the abnormality lies in the basal ganglia, but its pathologic substratum has never been divulged. The facial-cervical dyskinesias caused by phenothiazine drugs resemble these idiopathic disorders and may continue after the withdrawal of medication (tardive dyskinesias). Antiparkinson drugs are sometimes helpful in all these restricted dyskinesias.

FAMILIAL TREMOR One of the commonest hereditary disorders of the human nervous system is that which gives rise to a fast-frequency (6 to 7 or 7 to 8 per second) action tremor. This may appear at any age but more often during adolescence and adult years; once started, it lasts throughout life. Alcohol suppresses it. The heredity is dominant. Probably all cases are not the same, for some have tremors of slower frequency, looking more like those of Parkinson's disease but lacking the slowness of movement, rigidity, and flexed postures. In patients of advanced age it is called *senile tremor.* Imbibition of alcohol suppresses the fast-frequency forms, as does a beta-adrenergic blocking agent (propranolol) in doses of 20 to 40 mg three times daily. The slightly slower rhythmic action tremors of frequencies (approximately 6 per second) and alternate-beat type do not consistantly respond to propranolol or alcohol. Usually the tremor is the only abnormality, but in a few patients a cerebellar ataxia or an extrapyramidal syndrome may appear years later. The pathologic basis is unknown.

SYNDROMES OF SLOWLY DEVELOPING ATAXIA

The conditions about to be considered are distinguished clinically by progressive unsteadiness in standing and walking, along with more or less impaired coordination of other motor acts. Pathologically, they are characterized by degeneration of the cerebellum and/or its related fiber systems, and thus constitute classic examples of the system diseases. Although sporadic instances occur, hereditary transmission is an outstanding feature in many cases; thus, this group of disorders is often referred to as the *hereditary ataxias.* Their subdivision into more or less separate entities is largely arbitrary, with pathologic changes of varying distribution underlying clinically indistinguishable symptom complexes. Furthermore, there is considerable overlapping with other forms of hereditary nervous disease, so that in a given case a remarkable combination of defects may be encountered. These facts have led to the idea that in the ataxias there is a group of closely related genetically determined abnormalities which may occur together in an almost infinite series of combinations with other neurologic disorders so that it is not possible to separate well-defined disease pictures. Nevertheless, certain constellations of symptoms and pathologic findings occur with sufficient regularity to warrant their separation for purposes of discussion. The classification about to be given is not entirely satisfactory but is designed to be of practical help to the physician confronted with a case.

CEREBELLAR DEGENERATIONS To be discussed here are the forms of progressive ataxia which are associated with pathologic changes predominantly in the cerebellum. The more strictly spinocerebellar diseases of which Friedreich's ataxia is the classic variety will be discussed in Chap. 365. Friedreich's ataxia is a disease of late childhood and adolescence.

The adult-onset types of cerebellar degeneration include both hereditary and sporadic diseases and, in addition, the rather rare subacute spinocerebellar degeneration associated with the presence of carcinoma of various types elsewhere in the body. The hereditary and sporadic forms of cerebellar degeneration resemble one another so closely that, for the purposes of the present discussion, they will all be referred to as *hereditary cerebellar degeneration.* Most cases are seen in adults, with the onset occurring in early or middle periods.

Pathology In hereditary cerebellar degeneration the cerebellum is obviously atrophied. In one group of cases, cortical cerebellar atrophies, these changes are chiefly localized to the superior vermis and adjacent parts of the cerebellar cortex, whereas in an even larger group, the entire cerebellar cortex is affected. Microscopically there is loss of nerve cells principally affecting the Purkinje cells, although the granule cells are often involved as well. In most cases, there is an associated atrophy of nerve cells in the inferior olivary nuclei in a distribution dependent on the location and extent of the changes in the cerebellar cortex. It no longer seems justifiable to separate the cases with associated olivary degeneration from the rest and to designate them as "cerebello-olivary degeneration," as has been done in the past. In a second group, *olivopontocerebellar degeneration,* there are extensive degenerative changes in the pontine nuclei, middle cerebellar peduncles, and olivary nuclei.

In all varieties of cerebellar degeneration, affection of other neuronal systems—as, for instance, the cerebral cortex and basal ganglia or the optic or cochlear neurons—may be encountered. In some cases, there are changes in the dentate and roof nuclei of the cerebellum and their projections in the superior cerebellar peduncles (*dentatorubral atrophy*), but these are often found in association with more diffuse cerebellar or spinocerebellar degeneration.

Carcinomatous cerebellar (*spinocerebellar*) degeneration is characterized by extensive cell loss in all parts of the cerebellar cortex, occasionally associated with inflammatory (lymphocytic) infiltrations in the perivascular and subarachnoid spaces. In addition there are degenerative changes in the long-fiber tracts of the spinal cord. These lesions do not depend on the presence of tumor implants anywhere in the nervous system or its coverings, but rather are thought to be due to an obscure infectious (? metabolic) process, somehow resulting from the presence of carcinoma.

Clinical aspects In the hereditary form of pure cerebellar degeneration the abnormality appears first in the legs, resulting in abnormal stance and an unsteadiness of gait of the peculiar wavering, lurching character so typical of cerebellar ataxia (see Chap. 15). This has been correlated with the localization of changes in the superior vermis of the cerebellum and adjacent parts of the cerebellar cortex. With more extensive cerebellar involvement, a disturbance in articulation and rhythm of speech occurs that reduces its comprehensibility, and the arms likewise become ataxic. There may be nystagmus, but it is often absent. Affection of other neuronal systems causes additional neurologic abnormalities, such as exaggerated tendon reflexes, extensor plantar responses, rigidity, tremor, and dementia (*cerebrocerebellar degeneration*). Progression is gradual and slow, being measured in years and sometimes decades, and appears not to shorten life.

No specific treatment is available for any of the progressive ataxias, although encouragement to remain active is beneficial to health in general. Gait training is of relatively little value in enabling the patient to compensate for his disability.

We have not been able to clinically differentiate a cortical parenchymatous from the olivopontocerebellar degeneration with any degree of consistency, though the latter tends to be sporadic, speech is affected early, and extrapyramidal signs of other type appear late. In dentatonigral degeneration, gaze palsy and spasticity are combined with cerebellar ataxia.

In the cases associated with carcinoma, the tempo of evolution of the process is relatively rapid, with severe disability coming on within a period of months. Vertigo, diplopia, and nausea may be prominent. In an occasional patient, the neurologic symptoms have appeared before there was any obvious evidence of carcinoma. Opsoclonus (rapid side-to-side jerking of the eyes) and oscillopsia (movement back and forth of objects seen) may be conjoined. In contrast to the consistently normal cerebrospinal fluid findings in the forms of cerebellar degeneration noted above, the cerebrospinal fluid may show increased lymphocytes and protein.

Differential diagnosis The slow but relentless progression in the absence of abnormalities in the other parts of the nervous system and of the cerebrospinal fluid distinguishes the hereditary group from other diseases and other forms of cerebellar ataxia such as may occur with hereditary metabolic diseases, neoplastic, infectious, or demyelinative disease; with drug intoxications (e.g., barbiturates); or with hyperpyrexia. The degenerative disorders under discussion tend to occur slowly over many years in a setting of otherwise good general health, and in the absence of other neurologic symptoms and signs; this, together with the other clinical differences, distinguishes them from such hereditary metabolic diseases as juvenile Gaucher disease, juvenile Niemann-Pick disease, and juvenile hexoseaminidase deficiency and from alcoholic cerebellar ataxia or deficiency disease, with or without Wernicke-Korsakoff syndrome. Alcoholic cerebellar degeneration usually develops rapidly, and then may remain more or less unchanged for the remainder of the patient's life (Chap. 372). The form of spinocerebellar degeneration associated with carcinoma may be distinguished from direct carcinomatous involvement of the nervous system by the symmetry of the findings and the absence of increased intracranial pressure.

SYNDROME OF MUSCULAR WEAKNESS AND WASTING, WITHOUT SENSORY CHANGES

MOTOR SYSTEM DISEASE This general term is used to designate a progressive disorder of motor neurons in the cerebral cortex, brainstem, and spinal cord, manifested clinically by muscular weakness, atrophy, and spasticity, with exaggeration of tendon reflexes in varying combinations. In its typical form this is a disease of middle life, generally appearing in the fifth or sixth decade. Customarily a subdivision is made on the basis of the particular grouping of symptoms and signs observed. Thus, the most frequent form, in which muscular atrophy and hyperreflexia are combined, is called *amyotrophic lateral sclerosis.* Rather more rare are the cases in which weakness and atrophy exist alone without clinical evidence of corticospinal tract dysfunction; for these, the term *progressive muscular atrophy* is used. Where the disorder affects predominantly the musculature innervated by the cranial nerves, it is usual to speak of *progressive bulbar palsy*. Very rarely, the clinical state is dominated by spasticity and hyperreflexia without obvious muscular wasting; such cases are classed as *primary lateral sclerosis.* It seems very likely that these subgroupings are anything other than clinical variants of the same disease process, which is another classic example of a system disease. Most cases are sporadic, but occasionally this disorder occurs in families in a manner suggesting genetic transmission. Familial motor system disease is discussed further on.

Pathology Widespread selective atrophy and loss of motor nerve cells exist at all levels of the central nervous system, including the Betz cells in the motor areas of the cerebral cortex. Some evidence of disease in the corticospinal motor system is usually found pathologically, even when physical signs referable to such changes were not observed during life. The atrophy of fibers in skeletal muscles is typically that due to loss of motor innervation.

Clinical aspects The disease begins insidiously and may be well advanced before the patient is aware of it. Although often asymmetric initially, the weakness and muscular wasting gradually become bilateral and widespread. Classically, the disorder is first evident in the small muscles of the hands, but it may begin in one or both of the legs, or in muscles supplied by cranial nerves. Vague feelings of discomfort in the muscles, tightness, coldness, numbness (without objective sensory changes), and recurrent cramps may be early symptoms. The progressive enfeeblement and atrophy of the musculature are accompanied by widespread visible fascicular twitchings of groups of muscle fibers, a classic feature that can be related to degeneration of the motor nerve cells supplying the involved muscles. Despite extensive involvement of skeletal muscles generally, sphincter control remains intact. Sooner or later the disease affects muscles supplied by the brainstem, resulting in weakness, atrophy, and fasciculations in the tongue and facial musculature associated with dysarthria and impairment of chewing or swallowing. The ocular nuclei, oddly enough, are invariably spared. In most cases, the weakness and muscular wasting are accompanied by exaggeration of tendon reflexes, extensor plantar reflexes and spasticity, to a degree dependent on the severity of degeneration in the corticospinal (pyramidal) motor system. Affection of corticobulbar fibers results in manifestations of pseudobulbar palsy such as involuntary crying or laughter, exaggerated reflex movements of the muscles of facial expression, and sucking reflexes. These latter may be the first manifestations of the disease. Progression is unhalting and relatively rapid, leading to extensive paralysis, with death from respiratory weakness or aspiration pneumonia, generally within about 2 to 5 years or more from onset. Intelligence and awareness are typically preserved to the end.

Differential diagnosis Spinal cord compression from tumors in the cervical region or from cervical spondylosis with osteophytes projecting into the vertebral canal can at times give rise to weakness, wasting, and fasciculations in the upper limbs and spasticity in the legs, thus closely resembling amyotrophic lateral sclerosis. The absence of cranial nerve involvement may be helpful in differentiation, although some compressive lesions at the foramen magnum may implicate the twelfth cranial (hypoglossal) nerve, with resulting affection of the tongue. Absence of pain or of sensory changes, normal function of bowels and bladder, normal roentgenographic studies of the spine, and absence of changes in the composition or dynamics of the cerebrospinal fluid are all points in favor of motor system disease and against spinal cord compression. Where doubt exists, CT scans and contrast myelography should be performed in order to visualize the cervical spinal canal.

A small number of patients who have motor system disease will have had poliomyelitis years before and another special variety is that in which an immunologically incompetent person (affected by carcinoma, lymphoma, and corticosteroids) develops a pure amyotrophy that progresses over several months to a year and at autopsy is found to be a chronic poliomyelitis.

Chronic inflammatory disorders of the meninges and spinal cord, exemplified by syphilitic meningomyelitis or some cases of adhesive arachnoiditis, may have to be considered. These conditions can readily be recognized by cerebrospinal fluid changes and, if necessary, by abnormal myelographic findings. Nutritional myelopathy can be excluded by history and on other clinical grounds.

Although fasciculations are a prominent feature of motor system disease, they are not, in the absence of weakness, muscle atrophy, or loss of tendon reflexes, valid signs of it, for they may occur in a variety of metabolic or toxic disorders (e.g., thyrotoxicosis, salt depletion) as well as in otherwise healthy individuals. Careful clinical evaluation suffices in such instances to exclude serious neurologic disease (cf. page 2199).

Progressive weakness from intrinsic disease of muscle (myopathy, polymyositis) may occasionally be difficult to distinguish from progressive muscular atrophy of the type under discussion; yet the differentiation is important from the standpoint of prognosis or treatment. Under such circumstances, the diagnosis can be made by muscle biopsy and electromyography.

There is no known treatment for any form of motor system disease.

INFANTILE MUSCULAR ATROPHY (WERDNIG AND HOFFMANN), AMYOTONIA CONGENITA (OPPENHEIM) The form of progressive muscular atrophy described by Werdnig and Hoffmann is a disease of infants and young children, typically afflicting several members of a family. Pathologically, it closely resembles the adult disease described above. Amyotonia congenita is a purely clinical term, used to designate abnormal laxness of somatic musculature observed at birth or in early infancy; it may occur in a number of different pathologic processes, including Werdnig-Hoffmann disease. For further details of these conditions, Chap. 365 should be consulted.

Other forms of familial progressive muscular atrophy In addition to the infantile form there are several other familial syndromes of progressive muscular atrophy. They begin later in childhood, adolescence, and adult life and, though progressive, are extremely chronic. One form affects predominantly the proximal limb muscles (Wohlfart-Kugelberg-Welander syndrome) and must be distinguished from limb girdle dystrophy. In any given family the disease tends to have the same pattern and time course in all affected members.

HEREDITARY SPASTIC PARAPLEGIA This very rare disorder is characterized by weakness and spasticity of the legs, with early onset (childhood or adolescence) and slow progression. Later the arms may be affected, but usually to a lesser degree. The pathologic changes closely resemble those of Friedreich's ataxia, and in some instances this condition is in fact an incomplete form of Friedreich's disease in which spastic weakness overshadows minimal or absent ataxia and sensory changes. The relation to Friedreich's ataxia and other neurologic diseases is further confirmed by the occurrence of pes cavus, scoliosis, and optic atrophy in some cases of this kind. In addition there are pure forms of progressive spastic paraplegia presenting in both childhood and late adult life which have no other neurologic or somatic abnormalities. In the light of present knowledge, some of these may be identified as adrenomyeloneuropathy, a variant of adrenoleukodystrophy (see above), and a very small number may be found to have a rare adult form of G_{M2} gangliosidosis (hexoseaminidase deficiency)—which in young children results in Tay-Sachs disease. The diagnosis is made by the family history, by excluding other possible causes of bilateral spastic weakness of the limbs, and by appropriate biochemical studies. A combination of optic atrophy and spastic paraparesis beginning in childhood is called Behr's syndrome.

SYNDROMES COMBINING WEAKNESS AND WASTING WITH SENSORY CHANGES

PROGRESSIVE NEURAL MUSCULAR ATROPHY The degenerative disorders characterized by progressive weakness and wasting of skeletal muscles combined with sensory changes are chronic diseases of peripheral nerves, often occurring as hereditary conditions. Although clinical and pathologic subvarieties exist, there is no sharp dividing line between them, and they are best considered together under the designation given above, in which the term *neural* emphasizes the peripheral nerve affection. Chronic peripheral neuropathy is an associated disorder in some of the hereditary ataxias and is regularly encountered in the classic form of Friedreich's ataxia. It is also a component of adrenomyeloneuropathy. An additional connecting link with other genetically determined nervous diseases is the occurrence of progressive optic atrophy or pigmentary degeneration of the retina in some cases. Common to all is for the peripheral neuropathy to begin distally and to progress in a centripetal fashion and for the feet and legs to become first affected, with involvement of the hands and more proximal parts only after a considerable interval.

The two most frequent forms of hereditary polyneuropathy, peroneal muscular atrophy and hypertrophic interstitial polyneuropathy, are described in Chap. 368. Brief reference is also made there to a rare form known as Refsum's disease.

Treatment Although no specific treatment is available (except possibly in Refsum's disease, as indicated in Chap. 368), patients whose disease is of slow progression and in whom conditions are otherwise favorable may be greatly helped by measures to ensure a stable walking surface, such as corrective shoes, braces to prevent foot drop, and even orthopedic procedures to stabilize the joints.

SYNDROME OF PROGRESSIVE VISUAL LOSS

As already stated in previous sections, progressive impairment or loss of vision, due to degenerative changes in the visual system (retinas and optic nerves), may be an accompaniment of morbid processes affecting the nervous system diffusely—in particular, the nervous system lipidoses and the hereditary ataxias. Occasionally, however, the peripheral visual system is the major, or only, site of disease. In such cases, the disorders are strongly hereditary. For detailed discussion of these conditions, standard reference works on ophthalmology should be consulted. Nevertheless, two entities, because of their close relationship with other degenerative diseases of the nervous system, warrant some discussion here.

HEREDITARY OPTIC ATROPHY (LEBER) This rare condition is characterized by the relatively rapid development of bilateral blindness with optic atrophy, coming on in early adult life. It was first thoroughly described by Leber in 1871. Typically, it occurs as a sex-linked recessive trait, chiefly affecting men, but it may be seen in women. The manner of genetic expression is not fully understood.

Pathology Common to all cases examined pathologically is loss of retinal ganglion cells with secondary degeneration of optic nerve fibers. In addition involvement of other neural systems (corticospinal and spinocerebellar) has been seen in several instances.

Clinical aspects The onset generally is in the second or third decade. The condition often begins asymmetrically, with blurring of vision in one eye followed in days or weeks by similar affection of the other eye. Vision then deteriorates rapidly over ensuing weeks or months, generally with eventual total blindness as a result, although arrest before this stage has been seen, or even a little improvement after initial steady progression. In the early stages, examination of the visual fields shows large central scotomas. The optic disks may be normal at first, or may be swollen (optic neuritis); later the appearance is typically that of optic atrophy, with pale, clearly outlined disks.

Differential diagnosis Multiple sclerosis may at times act in a manner identical with that just described, but without a definite hereditary background and with a much better outlook for improvement of vision. Toxic or nutritional amblyopia can generally be excluded by history and associated clinical findings. In some cases it may be necessary to eliminate the possibility of a tumor compressing the chiasmal region and optic nerves, although some evidence of bitemporal defects would be then expected, rather than bilateral central scotomas alone. In addition to careful roentgenograms of the skull and cerebrospinal fluid examination, pneumoencephalographic visualization of the chiasmal region may be indicated in cases of serious doubt. Early onset of optic atrophy with spastic weakness of legs and ataxia (Behr's syndrome) should also be distinguishable on clinical grounds.

PIGMENTARY DEGENERATION OF THE RETINA (RETINITIS PIGMENTOSA) This may at times occur as a relatively independent disorder, although it is often associated with other abnormalities, of which cataracts, deaf-mutism, and mental deficiency are outstanding. It is strongly hereditary, chiefly as a recessive trait, although dominant inheritance has been seen. Pigmentary degeneration of the retina is one of the features of the Laurence-Moon-Biedl syndrome. It likewise occurs in a considerable variety of neurologic diseases, including the hereditary ataxias, familial neuropathies, and some of the neuronal lipidoses (ceroid lipofuscinosis).

Pathology The principal lesion is a degeneration of the rods and cones, associated with displacement of melanin-containing cells from the pigment epithelium into more superficial parts of the retina. Other retinal structures are relatively intact. There is no inflammation so that the term *retinitis* is inappropriate.

Clinical aspects The disorder typically begins in childhood, first as night blindness. The visual fields become concentrically narrowed from the periphery to the center, until eventually (by adolescence, or perhaps not until middle age) very little useful vision remains. Ophthalmoscopic examination may be normal at first, but generally discloses irregular patches of dark pigment in the periphery of the retina. When cataracts are likewise present, as sometimes is the case, visual acuity may be significantly improved by their removal. The frequent association of the retinal lesions with other neurologic abnormalities has been mentioned in previous paragraphs.

Differential diagnosis Chorioretinitis from other causes (e.g, syphilis) may present a similar ophthalmoscopic appearance and should be excluded. The hereditary background and the progressive course, with night blindness and peripheral constriction of the visual fields, may lead to the diagnosis even in the rare cases where pigmentary deposits in the retina are absent. The slowly progressive or relatively stationary tapetoretinal degenerations of childhood can be distinguished clinically and by electroretinogram. In most instances, the opinion of a qualified ophthalmologist must be obtained.

REFERENCES

Advances in Neurology, vol 23: *Huntington's Disease.* New York, Raven Press, 1979

BRADY RO: Sphingolipidoses and other lipid metabolic disorders, in *Basic Neuro-Chemistry,* 2d ed. Boston, Little, Brown, 1976, pp 556–568

ELDRIDGE F: The torsion dystonias literature review. Genetic and clinical studies. Neurology, vol 2, no 11, suppl, 1970

GAMBETTI P et al: Myoclonic epilepsy with Lafora bodies: Some ultrastructural, histochemical and biochemical aspects. Arch Neurol 25:483, 1971

GOODWIN RB et al: Comparison of the effects of Bromocriptine and levo-dopa in Parkinson's disease. J Neurol Neurosurg Psychiatry 40:474, 1977

GROWDON JH: Medical treatment of extrapyramidal diseases. *Update III: Harrison's Principles of Internal Medicine,* KJ Isselbacher et al (eds). New York, McGraw-Hill, 1982

HAKIM S, ADAMS RD: The special neurological problem of hydrocephalus with normal CSF pressure. J Neurol Sci 17:527, 1971

KATZMAN R et al: *Alzheimer's Disease: Senile Dementia and Related Disorders.* New York, Raven Press, 1978

KLAWANS KL: Pharmacology of tardive dyskinesia. Am J Psychiatry 28:463, 1973

MORELL P et al: Diseases involving myelin, in *Basic Neurochemistry,* 2d ed, pp 581-604

MOSER H et al: Adrenoleukodystrophy: Increased plasma content of saturated very long chain fatty acids. Neurology 31:1241, 1981

SMITH CM, SWASH M: Possible biochemical basis of memory disorder in Alzheimer disease. Ann Neurol 3:471, 1978

STEELE JC: Progressive supranuclear palsy. Brain 95:693, 1972

TERRY RD, DAVIES P: Dementia of the Alzheimer type. Ann Rev Neurosci 3:77, 1980

VINKEN PJ, BRUYN GW (eds): *Handbook of Clinical Neurology,* vol 13: *Neuroretinal Degenerations.* Amsterdam, North-Holland, 1972

———, ——— (eds): *Handbook of Clinical Neurology,* vol 21: *System Disorders and Atrophies.* Amsterdam, North-Holland, 1975, part I

———, ——— (eds): *Handbook of Clinical Neurology,* vol 22: *System Disorders and Atrophies.* Amsterdam, North-Holland, 1975, part II

YAHR MD (ed): *Basal Ganglia,* vol. 55: Assoc. for Res. Nerv. and Mental Dis. New York, Raven Press

365 DEVELOPMENTAL AND OTHER CONGENITAL ABNORMALITIES OF THE NERVOUS SYSTEM

RAYMOND D. ADAMS
G. ROBERT DeLONG

The human nervous system is subject to a variety of developmental abnormalities which may be traced to genetic faults or diseases acquired in utero, at birth, or during the early years of life. These conditions may be manifest at birth or may be recognized only in late infancy and childhood, after some degree of maturation of the nervous system has occurred. Together they comprise the principal problems of pediatric neurology, and to discuss them fully would be pointless in a textbook of medicine. But many individuals so afflicted reach adolescent and adult age and come under the care of internists and general physicians; hence some understanding of the basic problems in this field is requisite.

Adult disorders of the nervous system that originate in early life may be classified under the following headings:

1 Congenital malformations of head, spine, and other structures, including dwarfism
2 Diseases which retard motor, speech, and intellectual development
3 Hereditary diseases which begin during childhood and persist throughout lifetime, some progressing
4 Epilepsy

Unlike many of the common neurologic problems that begin in adult years, those of infancy and childhood bring to light a number of pathogenic mechanisms unique to the early period of life. A genetic fault or exogenous agent may destroy the embryonal germ plasm in the first three postconceptional months, thereby blighting the formation and subsequent development of the nervous system as well as other somatic structures. Again, more subtle hereditary factors may alter the complex program of cerebral maturation so that it will not unfold in an even and harmonious way, leaving the person at certain times deficient in certain skills such as dexterity, speaking, reading, mathematics, music appreciation, etc. Or a disease may strike the rapidly maturing nervous system at birth (a unique event with its own possibilities of pathogenesis) or in the first years of life, leaving the victim with fixed and persistent deficits, such as retarded intellect, cerebral palsy, and epilepsy, for the entire span of life. For example, the myelination of the brain, which is one of the main developmental processes in infancy, is thought by some investigators to be permanently impaired by protein malnutrition. Finally, an unusually large proportion of special hereditary diseases declare themselves during childhood and continue into adult years, such as von Recklinghausen's neurofibromatosis and tuberous sclerosis.

MALFORMATIONS OF CRANIUM, SPINE, AND LIMBS Certain alterations in the size and shape of the head observed in the adult can nearly always be assumed to have their origin during the intrauterine period or early childhood. Beyond the first 4 to 5 years the brain (to which the skull always accommodates) has approximated adult size, and the sutures are so firmly closed that disease acquired later will have relatively little effect on the skull. Enlargement of the head is due either to macrocephaly with enlargement of brain (macroencephaly) (ventricles not enlarged significantly) or to hydrocephalus. Macroencephaly may be an incidental finding, often familial, in persons entirely normal neurologically or may be associated with neurological disorders as in the syndrome of cerebral gigantism (macroencephaly, tall stature, mental dullness, and seizures). Smallness of the head (microcephaly) is related to lack of brain growth or to a destructive lesion of brain early in life. Unusual shape of head is usually caused by craniostenosis. If the sagittal suture fuses too early, the head is long and narrow (dolichocephaly) with prominent brow and occiput; if the coronal suture closes prematurely, the head is wider than long (brachycephaly). Closure of all sutures produces a characteristic tower skull (turricephaly), shallow orbits, and bulging eyes. The latter condition, if not recognized early and suture lines excised, may prevent brain growth and raise intracranial pressure. Apert's syndrome (craniostenosis with "mitten hands" or syndactyly) is associated often with enlarged ventricles and mental retardation. Achondroplasia results in a normal-sized skull which looks disproportionately large compared with the short limbs.

Hydrocephalus of infancy and early childhood causes frontal bossing and variable degrees of cranial enlargement (usually over 60.0 cm, which is above the 97th percentile). In more than 60 percent of cases the underlying condition is an Arnold-Chiari malformation, followed in frequency by meningeal fibrosis around the brainstem from subarachnoid hemorrhage or meningitis, aqueductal stenosis and Dandy-Walker syndrome (failure of foramens of Magendie and Luschka to open), posterior fossa cysts, etc.

Of course there are wide variations in head size and shape, some familial, as every haberdasher knows, but the importance of all these abnormal deviations is that they continue throughout life, and the hydrocephalic states may arrest only to give trouble at a later age period. The main point to be remembered is that the cranial circumference is a valuable index of cerebral volume, and reflects disease originating in the early period of life.

ABNORMALITIES OF THE SPINE A remarkable variety of lifelong neurologic syndromes is associated with abnormality of the vertebral column. Some of these, such as hemivertebra, platybasia, fusion of the atlas and occiput or of vertebrae (Klippel-Feil syndrome), or congenital dislocation of the atlas, are the consequence of a malformation of the spine itself, and the enclosed spinal cord may or may not be involved. Others, such as spina bifida occulta, spinal meningocele or myelomeningocele, or dysraphism, involve the whole neural tube, including spinal cord, investing meninges, vertebral bodies, and even the overlying skin and subcutaneous tissues. Finally there is a group of hereditary metabolic diseases that alter the spine progressively during childhood and adolescence (e.g., the mucopolysaccharidoses).

Primary malformations of vertebrae These are most frequent in the upper cervical region. The *Klippel-Feil deformity* consists of maldevelopment and fusion of two or more cervical vertebrae, resulting in a short neck of limited mobility. The hairline is low, often at the level of the first thoracic vertebra. There may or may not be associated neurologic symptoms or signs. The importance of the spinal deformity lies in its frequent association with other abnormalities, especially those of platybasia and syringomyelia, the symptoms of which may not become manifest until adolescence or adult life. Also maldevelopment of the cervical or lumbar spine is commonly associated with genitourinary anomalies.

Platybasia and basilar impression This is a rare maldevelopment in which either the base of the skull is flattened or the occiput and upper cervical spine are invaginated in the posterior fossa. Often the foramen magnum itself is imperfectly developed, or the atlas and occiput are fused. The exact teratogenesis of these anomalies is uncertain. The conditions may be asymptomatic, but often there is "crowding," distortion, or compression of the spinal cord, medulla, and lower cranial and cervical spinal nerves.

The resulting clinical picture is variable. Symptoms may be present from early life or may begin in late childhood, adolescence, or even adult years. Early symptoms consist of "dizzy" or "weak" spells and downward nystagmus on tilting the head; evidences of increased intracranial pressure such as headache; occipital neuralgia; vomiting; transient paresthesias in the occipital region, neck, or arm; facial paresthesias, deafness, nasal voice, and dysphagia; cerebellar ataxia; and spastic weakness of the legs. The symptoms may first be intermittent and at any time in the course of the illness may be aggravated by straining, moving the head, or placing the head and neck in certain positions. Inspection alone provides a clue to diagnosis. The whole configuration of the head and neck is abnormal. The neck is short; the ears and hairline are low; the neck movements are obviously restricted; and the normal cervical lordosis is lost or greatly exaggerated, sometimes to the extent that the occiput lies almost on the upper dorsal spine and shoulders.

Instability of the junction of axis on atlas (atlantoaxial dislocation) may cause compression of the spinal cord. This may also occur as a consequence of rheumatoid arthritis, Morquio's disease (probably a type of mucopolysaccharidosis), other debilitating diseases, and trauma (tearing of ligaments which bind the odontoid process to the body of the first cervical vertebra). The odontoideum is a condition in which the odontoid is detached from the body of the axis; it may be either congenital or acquired. Patients with this condition may have transient symptoms of ataxia, neck discomfort, and long-tract signs including quadriparesis and may become quadriplegic after forced flexion of the neck. The treatment is surgical.

Platybasia and these related anomalies of the spine should be suspected in all cases presenting progressive cerebellar, brainstem, and cervical cord syndromes. Many of these cases have been misdiagnosed as multiple sclerosis. Others present a typical syringomyelic syndrome and have been so labeled. The clinical suspicion of platybasia and other spine anomalies can be confirmed by a true lateral roentgenogram of the skull. In such a projection the extension of a line drawn from the hard palate to the posterior border of the foramen magnum (Chamberlain's line) and another through the spine and body of the first cervical vertebra (Bull's line) when extended, instead of being more or less parallel as they normally are, intersect. The relation of cervical vertebrae is also seen. An acquired form of *basilar impression* occurs with rickets and Paget's disease. It is usually asymptomatic but sometimes involves the lower cranial nerves and may cause normal-pressure hydrocephalus.

Arnold-Chiari malformation This condition, in which medulla and inferior-posterior portions of the cerebellar hemispheres project caudally through the foramen magnum, often to the level of the second cervical vertebra, is a common cause of hydrocephalus. It is usually associated with a spinal meningocele or myelomeningocele, and often there are deformities of the cervical spine and cervicooccipital junction. The symptoms of hydrocephalus dominate the clinical picture in infants. But, in milder cases, there may develop during adolescence or adult years any one of the several syndromes described above under "Platybasia and Basilar Impression." There is, in addition, a second type of Arnold-Chiari malformation in patients who have no meningomyelocele. Often it is associated with syringomyelia. When platybasia and the Arnold-Chiari malformation coexist, it is generally impossible to decide which of the two is responsible for the clinical findings.

The treatment of platybasia and the Arnold-Chiari malformation has not been entirely satisfactory. If clinical progression is slight or uncertain, it is probably advisable to do nothing. If progression is certain and disability is increasing, upper cervical laminectomy and enlargement of the foramen magnum are indicated. Often this procedure halts the course of the illness or results in improvement. The surgical procedure must be done cautiously, however, for extensive manipulation of these structures may aggravate the symptoms or even cause death (see review by Salam and Adams).

Malformations associated with a defect in closure of the neural arch These take the forms of craniorachischisis totalis, craniocele, spinal meningocele, meningomyelocele, spina bifida occulta, and sinus tracts. Since these conditions seldom figure in adult neurology, only some of the late complications are mentioned here.

Sinus tracts in lumbosacral or occipital regions are of importance, for they may be sources at any age of bacterial meningitis. They are often indicated by a small dimple in the skin or by a tuft of hair along the posterior surface of the body in the midline. (The pilonidal sinus, in the opinion of the authors, should not be included in this group.) They may be associated with dermoid cysts at the central part of the tract. Evidence of such tracts should be sought in every instance of meningitis, especially when infection has recurred.

There are, in addition, other *congenital cysts* and benign *tumors* which may produce progressive symptoms and signs by compressing the spinal cord or by implicating nerve roots. So-called tethering of the spinal cord is caused by a stout filum terminale exerting downward traction on the cord; the traction may injure the conus medullaris and lower spinal segments.

Several clinical syndromes of delayed progressive disease (in the adolescent or adult) have been delineated:

1 Progressive spastic weakness of some of the already weakened muscles of the legs in a patient known to have had a meningocele or myelomeningocele. Presumably the spinal cord, which is securely attached to the lumbar vertebrae, is stretched during the period of rapid lengthening of the vertebral column.
2 An acute cauda equina syndrome following some unusual activity or incident, e.g., rowing or a fall in a sitting position, in patients who have had an asymptomatic or symptomatic spina bifida or meningocele. The implicated sensory and motor roots are believed to be injured by sudden or repeated stretching. Weakness of bladder control, impotence (in the male), and numbness of feet and legs or footdrop compose the clinical syndrome.
3 Progressive cauda equina syndrome in the lumbosacral region.
4 Syringomyelia (see Chap. 366).

MALFORMATIONS OF THE EXTREMITIES These malformations include syndactylism, clinodactyly along with broad hands and transverse palmar (simian) line (common with mongolism), club feet, and arthrogryposis multiplex, but rarely are they of concern to internists.

DWARFISM IN RELATION TO NEUROLOGIC DISEASE Dwarfs (in contrast to midgets, who are more or less normally proportioned) suffer usually from a disorder of cartilaginous growth. Their head and trunk are large and out of proportion to their limbs. Achondroplasia would be an example. But it is noteworthy that the majority of mentally retarded individuals fall below average in statural growth, and in a few dwarfism is part of any one of many special syndromes. Persons with Down's syndrome and with most of the other chromosomal abnormalities are examples, and there are others in which an inherited or acquired metabolic defect of definable type blights brain and skeletal growth (e.g., cretinism and mucopolysaccharidoses). Microcephaly characterizes many of the dwarfs with cerebral diseases.

The 30 or 40 neurologic syndromes with statural underdevelopment and neurologic diseases are described and illustrated in the atlas of mental retardation by Holmes et al.

THE PHAKOMATOSES

This is a unique group in which neurologic abnormalities are combined with congenital defects of skin, retina, and other organs. The terms *congenital ectodermal dysplasias, congenital neurocutaneous syndromes,* or *phakomatoses* (Greek *phakos,* "lentil," "mole," or "freckle") are used frequently to designate this general class of disorders. The major syndromes include *neurofibromatosis, tuberous sclerosis, encephalotrigeminal syndrome,* and rarely the *cerebelloretinal hemangioblastomatosis.* A variant of the encephalotrigeminal syndrome is the *myelocutaneous* (Klippel-Trénaunay) *syndrome,* in which a vascular malformation of spinal cord and meninges is associated with a vascular nevus within the area of skin innervated by the involved spinal segments and gigantism of an affected arm. Recently it has been suggested that *ataxia telangiectasia* be included with this group of conditions (see review of neurocutaneous diseases by Adams).

NEUROFIBROMATOSIS (VON RECKLINGHAUSEN'S DISEASE) This is an inherited disease (mendelian dominant), in which spots of increased skin pigmentation are combined with multiple neurofibromas. Its incidence is 1 per 3000; about 50 percent of cases arise as mutations. It has been characterized as a maldevelopment of cells of neural crest origin. The pigmented spots are irregular in shape with relatively even borders, vary in size from a few millimeters to several centimeters, and are of brownish coffee color (café au lait). They are most prominent over the trunk, in the axilla (axillary freckles), and about the pelvis. Similar lesions occur in individuals without neurofibromatosis, but in such instances are generally smaller than 1.5 cm in diameter and fewer than five in number. The tumors arise from the neurilemmal sheath (Schwann cells) and fibroblasts of the peripheral nerve. They are usually multiple and vary in size from minute lesions to large tumors several centimeters in diameter. The majority are smoothly rounded or lobulated, soft or firm, and can sometimes be seen or felt along the course of a peripheral nerve. Often they sink into the subcutaneous fat on gentle pressure. Like the pigmented lesions, the tumors are more frequent over the trunk than on the extremities. The pigmented areas, because of giant melanosomes in pigment epithelial cells, become increasingly apparent with age; also the tumors of nerve sheaths are often not demonstrable early in life. Most of the tumors are asymptomatic; but occasionally, if they attain a large size or occupy an unusual position, they may produce pressure upon contiguous structures. Tumors of the spinal nerve roots may compress the spinal cord and at the same time extend through the intervertebral foramens to form a large mass in the posterior mediastinum (dumbbell tumors). Acoustic neurinomas, usually bilateral in patients with neurofibromatosis, may produce deafness and other symptoms and signs of a cerebellopontine angle lesion (Chap. 358). Other histopathologic types of tumor (meningioma, glioma) are encountered more often in neurofibromatosis than in the general population. Diffuse overgrowth of Schwann cells and fibroblasts may also occur, giving rise to plexiform neuromas. They may cause hideous deformities, often with overgrowth of underlying bone. Bone cysts may also form. Most of these associated tumors are rare in infancy and childhood, though pontine glioma and glioma of the optic nerve and chiasm are exceptions to the clinical rule. The latter condition should always be considered in the differential diagnosis of unilateral (rarely bilateral) blindness, proptosis, and extraocular muscle paralysis in childhood, especially if there are signs of von Recklinghausen's disease. Enlargement of the optic foramens, demonstrable by roentgenogram and CT scan of the orbit, is a valuable aid in diagnosis. *Pulsating exophthalmos* (usually due to an orbital hemangioma) may result from congenital absence of part of the sphenoid bone. *Pheochromocytoma* is an infrequent accompaniment of the disease. In about 5 to 10 percent of cases of neurofibromatosis one of the tumors will become sarcomatous.

Fibrous dysplasia, congenital vertebral anomalies, local gigantism of an extremity, subperiosteal bone cysts, and pseudoarthrosis of the tibia may be associated with neurofibromatosis. Scoliosis is a common skeletal deformity in children with this disease, so that neurofibromatosis must be added to the list of neurogenic kyphoscolioses (the others are syringomyelia, Friedreich's ataxia, and poliomyelitis). Stenosis of the aqueduct of Sylvius with obstructive hydrocephalus is at times observed in neurofibromatosis. Also there may be a mild degree of mental retardation, related presumably to developmental abnormalities of the cerebral cortex. Spina bifida, hypospadias, glaucoma, and elephantiasis are occasionally seen. An association of vascular stenoses (renal, cerebral, or pulmonic) and neurofibromatosis has been recognized.

About one-third of cases of neurofibromatosis are discovered accidentally on routine examination, there being no complaints. Another third of these patients come seeking advice about the cosmetic aspects of the disease, and the remainder have neurologic syndromes. Those with prominent neurologic signs tend to have few cutaneous lesions. There is no treatment for the disease other than excision of symptomatic tumors.

TUBEROUS SCLEROSIS (BOURNEVILLE'S DISEASE) This curious disease, of dominant inheritance, is manifested by the clinical triad of convulsive seizures, mental deficiency, and adenoma sebaceum. The latter are fine, wart-like lesions distributed predominantly in a butterfly distribution over the cheeks and forehead. The individual adenomas vary in size from 0.1 to 1.0 cm and are elevated and pinkish or pinkish yellow in color. In addition, the skin over the lower part of the back may be thick, rough, and of yellowish color like sharkskin or pigskin (shagreen patch). Actually the earliest lesions are foliate hypopigmented spots ("white spots") over the trunk and limbs, which are seen most clearly under ultraviolet light (Wood's lamp). They are distinguishable on the basis of size, shape, and character from avascular nevi and vitiligo, and are highly diagnostic, often providing the earliest clue to mental retardation or infantile epilepsy. The mental deficiency may be relatively stationary or progressive. The seizures are usually generalized but may be focal. Retinal tumors and other visible malformations may be conjoined.

The most advanced examples of tuberous sclerosis usually are to be found in institutions for the mentally retarded, but it would be a mistake to assume that all are so severely disabled. In general hospital clinics it is not at all unusual to see patients with average intelligence and only seizures and a few skin lesions. Occasionally a focal cerebral syndrome will prove at biopsy to have a typical "tuber" or an associated glioma as its basis in a patient not known to have this disease. Family history is frequently unhelpful; approximately one-half of cases are sporadic (? mutation).

The lesions of the skin are pathologically fibromas and not true adenomas. Some are rather vascular and suggest telangiectasia. The brain lesions consist of areas of malformed cortex with extensive astrogliosis and a peculiar mixture of glioblasts and monster nerve cells. Calcification may or may not be present. Masses of subependymal glial tissue account for nodules which project into and form "candle gutterings" on the walls of the ventricles that are often seen in computerized tomography and pneumograms. In Bourneville's original case, death was due to rhabdomyoma of the heart, and most cases of this benign tumor of heart muscle are associated with tuberous sclerosis. This disease is also combined with tumorous malformations of kidney, liver, adrenal glands, and pancreas.

The diagnosis is aided by CT scans and roentgenograms of the skull. Calcified nodules occur particularly in the temporal lobes and adjacent to the ventricles. If large, they may obstruct the foramen of Monro, causing a unilateral or bilateral hydrocephalus. The center of the nodule tends to be more densely radiopaque than the periphery. The electroencephalogram is usually abnormal but without specific pattern. The cerebrospinal fluid may be normal; rarely, the total protein level is elevated.

The only treatment is symptomatic. The prognosis for life beyond the third decade is poor. Death is usually due to seizures, associated tumors, or intercurrent diseases. Genetic counseling is an obligation of the physician.

CEREBELLORETINAL HEMANGIOBLASTOMATOSIS (HIPPEL-LINDAU SYNDROME) As the name implies, the syndrome consists of a vascular malformation of the retina and cerebellum. The retinal lesions are capillary angiomas, usually multiple, causing progressive loss of vision; the cerebellar lesion consists of a slowly growing hemangioblastoma, frequently multiple, with a large cystic component, lending itself to surgical removal; spinal and medullary hemangioblastomas also occur. The clinical symptoms and signs consist of progressive cerebellar ataxia, headache, and papilledema. Seldom is a vascular bruit audible over the head. Polycythemia, possibly related to the production of erythropoietin, has been observed in many cases and has in a few instances disappeared after excision of the tumor. The disease is transmitted as an autosomal dominant, but many cases are sporadic. Rarely do these tumors appear before adolescence. The cerebellar lesions may be multiple and associated with one or more spinal hemangioblastomas. One should consider this diagnosis in all patients with a cerebellar tumor syndrome (see Chap. 358). Not all have a retinal lesion—the von Hippel part of the disease. The hemangioblastoma of the cerebellum is usually but one part of a constellation of abnormalities including angiomas and cysts of the liver, pancreas, and kidneys, and tumors of the epididymis and kidney, the latter being the cause of death in some cases. Pheochromocytomas have been described in this and in other of the phakomatoses. Syringomyelia has been observed in a few cases, and if a careful search is made, a hemangioblastoma can often be found in relation to the syrinx at some level.

The cerebellar hemangioblastoma demands surgical treatment, and if the nodule of the tumor is found in the wall of the cyst and is excised, the results can be excellent; if the tumor cannot be operated on because of size or multiplicity, radiation may be tried. The retinal lesions, when small, can be arrested by photocoagulation.

ENCEPHALOTRIGEMINAL SYNDROME (STURGE-WEBER DISEASE) This disease consists of capillary or cavernous hemangiomas, within but not always limited to the cutaneous distribution of the trigeminal nerve and of a predominantly venous hemangioma of the leptomeninges. If the skin lesion is within the area of supply of the ophthalmic division of the trigeminal nerve, the occipital lobes are more commonly involved, whereas a facial nevus is more often associated with involvement of the parietal and frontal lobes. The intracranial and cutaneous lesions may occur separately. The disease is usually sporadic; familial occurrence is exceptional.

Pathologically, in addition to the large number of abnormal blood vessels in the meninges, the subjacent cortex is progressively destroyed, due probably to stagnation of blood flow and consequent hypoxia, and in some cases a band of calcium develops within the lesion. This band, following the convolutional pattern as it does, is responsible for the characteristic "railroad track" roentgenographic picture. Deeply situated arteriovenous malformations rarely coexist.

The first neurologic symptom is usually a focal seizure on the side opposite the skin lesion. Transient postictal (Todd's) paralysis or permanent paralysis may follow the seizure. Sensorimotor paralysis or permanent visual field defect, the most frequent findings, may be either of insidious onset with slow progression or apoplectic. Hemorrhage into the meninges has been reported, but this must be a rare event. Possibly occlusion of cortical vessels is, in certain instances, responsible for neurologic deficits. Blindness in the eye on the side of the nevus is frequent and is nearly always due to glaucoma. Most patients with this malformation survive for many years, often with residual mental defects and hemiparesis.

The lesions are usually too extensive to be treated surgically, though hemispherectomy has been advised by some surgeons for intractable epilepsy. Anticonvulsant medication is indicated, but the seizures may be difficult to control.

Hemangioma of the trunk or upper or lower extremity may be associated with a spinal cord vascular malformation (Klippel-Trénaunay syndrome). The extremity may be hypertrophied. The cord lesion may bleed into or cause infarction in the nervous tissue, producing a spinal sensorimotor paralysis. Surgical exploration and decompression are seldom beneficial to the patient.

ATAXIA TELANGIECTASIA This condition has attracted considerable interest because of theoretical implications of its apparent cause and pathogenesis. Inherited as a recessive trait, the disease is characterized neurologically by a progressive cerebellar ataxia, apraxia of ocular movement, and choreoathetosis beginning during the early years of life. Telangiectases of bulbar conjunctivas and skin, especially about the ears, neck, and in flexor creases at the elbows and knees, appear somewhat later in childhood or adolescence. Recurring pulmonary and sinus infections have been prominent in many cases, and a deficiency in the IgA globulins and a defect of delayed cellular hypersensitivity are found. The diagnosis can be supported by the finding of abnormal humoral and cell-mediated immunity and of raised levels of alpha fetoprotein and cytogenetic abnormalities. Fibroblasts and lymphocytes from patients with this disease have enhanced in vitro radiosensitivity, attributed to deficiencies in enzyme systems that repair DNA. The associated pathologic changes consist of an extensive loss of Purkinje cells of the cerebellum and possibly degeneration of the neurons in other parts of the basal ganglia. Dysplasia of the thymus has been well documented, and death usually occurs by the second or third decade of life from infection or a reticuloendothelial tumor.

FAMILIAL DYSAUTONOMIA (RILEY-DAY SYNDROME)

This disease is characterized by autonomic instability (abnormal sweating, loss of vasomotor control, labile hypertension), impaired taste with absence of fungiform papillae, diminished pain and temperature sensation, hyporeflexia, episodic fever, vomiting attacks, and lack of lacrimation (alacrima), with corneal ulceration. Studies by Sedgewick and Boder show the disease to be inherited in a pattern consistent with an autosomal recessive trait and to be limited to Ashkenazi Jews.

The clinical manifestations become apparent soon after birth with difficulty in feeding (dysphagia) and moving and are increasingly evident in childhood. A few patients reach adult years, but the mortality rate is high because of recurrent pulmonary infections with inappropriate autonomic responses. Emotional instability presents a problem in most patients. Although intelligence has been within normal limits in some patients, in others it has been slightly subnormal. Growth seems to be delayed for unclear reasons, and the natural tendency is to undernutrition and scoliosis. Neuropathic (Charcot) joints due to lack of pain and related injury have been reported.

Proof of the disturbance of the autonomic nervous system comes from special tests such as absence of skin flare after histamine and skin stroking (loss of axonal reflex), and hypersensitivity to both cholinergic and adrenergic agents. Nerve conduction velocities are decreased. Quantitative pathologic studies of peripheral and autonomic nervous systems have shown marked depletion of small-caliber axons in peripheral nerves (which could account for the deficit in pain and temperature appreciation), and decreased numbers of small neurons in the dorsal root ganglia, in sympathetic ganglia, and in the ciliary ganglia (which could account for some of the dysautonomic features). Intermediolateral cell columns of the spinal cord are normal, as is the rest of the central nervous system.

By inference it is suggested that the disease is due to a unitary biochemical defect, probably a deficiency of a single enzyme and perhaps related to the "nerve growth factor."

In the differential diagnosis one must consider other forms of small-fiber polyneuropathy with analgesia and dysautonomia (including congenital indifference to pain and amyloidosis) (see Chap. 368), as well as the Shy-Drager syndrome (a degenerative disease of lateral horn cells and basal ganglia) (see Chap. 364).

Picrotoxin is said to increase tearing of eyes. Chlorpromazine in conjunction with phenobarbital may control vomiting attacks. The Heller-type myotomy has been successful in some few instances in improving esophageal function. Orthopedic measures are needed to stabilize neuropathic joints. Injury must be avoided and wounds treated carefully.

ABNORMALITIES OF MOTOR FUNCTION (CEREBRAL PALSY)

In this category of neurologic defect a major disturbance of motor function, usually nonprogressive, has been present since infancy or childhood. The popular term for these conditions is *cerebral palsy.* The name is not altogether appropriate, nor is such a crude classification of nervous disorders particularly useful from the viewpoint of the physician, because it results in a collocation of diseases of widely differing etiologic and anatomic types. The hereditary and acquired and the intrauterine, natal, and postnatal diseases lose their identity. Nevertheless, the term has been adopted as a slogan for fund-raising societies and for a major rehabilitation movement throughout the United States, and it will not soon disappear from medical terminology.

CLINICAL ASPECTS OF MOTOR DISTURBANCES WHICH HAVE BEEN PRESENT SINCE INFANCY OR CHILDHOOD Motor abnormalities which have had their onset early in life are so numerous and diverse in their manifestations that it is necessary to refer to the discussion of the motor system (Chaps. 14 and 15) in order to interpret them. To ascertain etiologic factors, it is helpful to attempt to categorize a given case according to the extent and nature of the abnormality. A careful history of possible prenatal, perinatal, or postnatal insults to the developing nervous system must always be sought; certain correlations of these factors with the resulting pattern of neurologic deficit are outlined below. Many patients with these motor abnormalities of infancy and childhood, which are relatively frequent, reach adult years.

SPECIAL TYPES **Infantile spastic and rigid paralyses** The pattern of paralysis or rigidity is important, for it provides information as to the etiology and possible pathogenic mechanism.

Cerebral spastic diplegia (Little's disease) In 1862 Little called attention to the concurrence of "Abnormal parturition, difficult labours, premature birth, and asphyxia neonatorum" and of a spastic weakness that affected legs more than arms. He emphasized the prenatal or natal origin, the diplegic distribution of the paralysis (legs more than arms), and the nonprogressive course. Little was of the opinion that asphyxia caused the cerebral damage. According to present thinking, two groups can be identified. One is associated with prematurity and consists predominantly of a mild spastic paraplegia; head size and intelligence are less diminished than in other forms of the disease. The incidence of this form of cerebral palsy has declined significantly since the introduction of neonatal intensive care, and some results indicate that it can be virtually eliminated by expert management of premature infants.

The second group is more varied and is regularly associated with term birth and difficult parturition, in which instance the main insult is intrapartum hypoxia and asphyxia. Here the medical profession is confronted with one of the gravest of pediatric neuroligic problems, where in a few minutes (5 to 10) of compromise of cardiac and/or respiratory function result in death or, even worse, the tragedy of life-long mental retardation and paralysis. The factors that determine hypoxic-ischemic injury to the brain have been investigated by Windle and by Myers. Cardiac standstill with severe hypoxia and relatively normal CO_2 results in restricted destruction of the inferior colliculi and the cranial nerve nuclei; the cerebral and cerebellar cortices are relatively unaffected. If hypoxia and hypotension are less severe and more prolonged, and particularly if CO_2 and tissue lactic acid increase, there is an entirely different pattern of cerebral injury. The border-zone areas between the main cerebral and cerebellar arteries (i.e., the frontal, parietal, lateral occipital and hippocampal cortices, the globus pallidi, certain of the thalamic nuclei, the deep periventricular white matter, and the deep folia of the cerebellum) become edematous and necrotic. Myers points out that the high tissue lactic acid is the main factor and that elevated blood glucose and the higher content of glycogen in brainstem nuclei result in great increases in the lactic acid in the tissue.

This second type of hypoxic-hypotensive damage is the one most frequently observed in humans and accounts for such pathologic entities as cerebral ulegyria, atrophic lobar sclerosis, and état marbré of basal ganglia. The important point that obstetricians and pediatricians must keep in mind is that every additional minute of insufficient brain perfusion and oxygenation may be disastrous.

Infants who suffer these insults have low Apgar scores (reflections of poor circulation and breathing), do not respond, and will need respiratory and circulatory support. These are the infants who, if they survive, are likely to later minifest spastic quadriplegia, severe spastic diplegia, and athetosis.

Three types of cerebral palsy may be distinguished: the

paraplegic, the diplegic, and the generalized and pseudobulbar. These differ from one another only with respect to the severity of affection of the arms and bulbar musculature. Pure paraplegias and pure pseudobulbar cases are relatively rare. Usually all four extremities are involved, but the legs much more than the arms, which is the real meaning of diplegia. As a rule the damage to the nervous system is recognized at birth or soon thereafter by some abnormality of breathing, sucking and swallowing, color of mucous membranes, or responsiveness. These latter signs may indicate either a congenital defect of the nervous system or birth injury of the brainstem. However, the stiff, awkward movements of the legs, maintained in an extended, adducted posture, do not usually attract attention until several weeks or months have passed. Seizures occur in some cases, and it is not uncommon to observe a delay in all normal developmental sequences, especially those which depend on the motor system. Once walking is attempted, usually much later than in the normal child, the characteristic stance and gait become manifest. The legs are advanced stiffly in short steps, each describing part of the arc of a circle; adduction is often so strong as to lead to actual crossing (scissors gait), with lower legs slightly splayed out and the feet flexed and turned in, the heels not touching the ground. In the adolescent and adult, the legs tend to be short and small, but the muscles are not markedly atrophic, as in infantile muscular atrophy and dystrophy. Passive manipulation of the limbs reveals marked spasticity in the extensors and adductors and also slight shortening of the calf muscles. The hands and arms may be affected only slightly, if at all; there may be awkwardness and stiffness of the fingers; in a few, pronounced weakness and spasticity are noted. Speech may be well articulated or noticeably slurred, and in some instances the face is set in a spastic smile. The deep-tendon reflexes are exaggerated, those in the legs more than in the arms, and the plantar reflexes are extensor. Usually there is no disturbance of sphincteric function, though delay in acquiring voluntary control is usual. Athetotic postures and movements of the face, tongue, and hands are present in some patients and may actually conceal the pyramidal weakness. Ataxic and hypotonic forms also exist. In sum, birth injury usually means hypoxic-ischemic encephalopathy, a condition which is potentially preventable.

The condition must be distinguished from familial types of spastic paraparesis, which are well-recognized clinical entities (Chap. 364).

Infantile hemiplegia, double hemiplegia, and quadriplegia Hemiplegia is a not uncommon condition of infancy and childhood, and the functional difference between the two sides may be noticed soon after birth or during the first 6 to 12 months of life. The condition develops usually as a consequence of a predominantly unilateral infection or thrombosis of cerebral arteries that may have happened before or after birth or during childhood. The parents may be the first to notice that movements of prehension and exploration are carried out with only one arm. The affection of the leg is usually recognized later, i.e., during the first attempt to stand and walk.

Mental defect may be associated with infantile hemiplegia but is even less common than with cerebral diplegia and much less than in bilateral hemiplegia. Convulsions occur in 35 to 50 percent of children with congenital hemiplegia, and these may persist throughout life. If the hemiplegia was acquired during childhood, seizures often accompany the onset. They may be generalized but are frequently unilateral and limited to the hemiplegic side. Often, after a series of seizures, the affected side will be weak for several hours or longer (Todd's paralysis).

In double hemiplegia, a much less frequent condition, the bilateral weakness of face, arms, and legs arises under conditions of more severe acquired cerebral disease and at any age. The arms are severely affected, in contrast to their minimal involvement in cerebral diplegia.

The quadriplegic state differs from bilateral hemiplegias in that the bulbar musculature is not involved. The condition is relatively rare but may result from a bilateral cerebral lesion. However, one should also be alerted to the possibility of a high cervical cord lesion. Although this may occasionally result from cysts, tumors, and other malformations, it is usually produced in the infant by a fracture-dislocation of the cervical spine, induced during a difficult breech delivery. Similarly, in *paraplegia,* with weakness or paralysis limited to the legs, the lesion may be either a cerebral form of diplegia or a spinal one. Sphincteric disturbances and a definite loss of somatic sensation below a certain level on the trunk always favor a spinal localization. Congenital cysts, tumors, and diastematomyelia are more frequently the cause of paraplegia than of quadriplegia. An additional cause of infantile paraplegia is spinal infarction from thrombotic complications of umbilical artery catheterization.

Encephaloclastic disorders underlie all these conditions. The pathologic change is essentially that of ischemic necrosis. In many cases, the lesions must have been incurred in utero and thus are not dependent on perinatal events. For the most part, the lesions reflect not pure asphyxia (anoxia) but circulatory insufficiency (ischemia) resulting from hypotension or circulatory collapse. The ischemia of circulatory failure tends to affect the tissues lying in arterial border zones. In the premature infant, ischemia followed by hyperperfusion may result in hemorrhage in the deep central structures and periventricular matrix zones.

CONGENITAL EXTRAPYRAMIDAL SYNDROMES IN INFANCY AND CHILDHOOD

The spastic and rigid cerebral diplegias discussed above shade almost imperceptibly into the congenital extrapyramidal syndromes. Many such patients are found in every cerebral palsy clinic, and they ultimately may reach adult medical clinics. Pyramidal tract signs may be completely absent, and the inexperienced student, familiar only with the pure cerebral spastic diplegia syndrome, is always puzzled as to their classification. Some extrapyramidal cases of this type undoubtedly are attributable to severe perinatal hypoxia; others represent separate diseases such as erythroblastosis fetalis with kernicterus. In the interest of being able to state accurately the probable pathologic basis and future course of these illnesses, it is desirable to separate the extrapyramidal syndromes due to prenatal and natal diseases, which usually become manifest during the first year of life, from the acquired or hereditary postnatal syndromes such as familial athetosis, dystonia musculorum deformans, and cerebellar ataxia. The latter are discussed in Chap. 364.

CONGENITAL CHOREOATHETOSIS (DOUBLE ATHETOSIS) Probably the most frequent representative of this group, this condition is like the spastic states in that it may not be recognized at birth but only after several months or a year have elapsed. The nature of the chorea and athetosis has been discussed in Chap. 15. Syndromes may be mixed, however. All combinations of chorea, athetosis, ballismus, myoclonus, and even dystonia may be found in a single case, or one or another type of movement disorder may predominate. However, in all instances there is in addition a primary defect in voluntary movement.

Choreoathetosis in infants and children varies in severity. In some the disorder is so mild that the abnormal movements are misinterpreted as restlessness or "the fidgets"; in others, every voluntary act is marred by intense involuntary movements, leaving the patient nearly helpless. The severely handicapped patients, even with the help of rehabilitation clinics and corrective orthopedic operations, rarely achieve a degree of motor control that will permit them to lead an independent life, and they continually need supportive treatment and help as adults. Intelligence may be well preserved.

Kernicterus is of importance in this context for it may also be a cause of generalized athetosis in children and adults. It is true that the majority of infants who suffer this disease die within the first week or two of life, and those who survive are often mentally retarded, deaf, and totally unable to sit, stand, or walk, so that the tendency is always to put them in homes for the feebleminded. But there are exceptional patients, obviously less damaged, who are mentally normal or at most only slightly backward. These are the ones who develop a variety of other neurologic sequelae that persist throughout life. Either athetosis or ataxia may be present, and a few have also shown rigid limbs and a picture not too different from that of cerebral spastic diplegia with involuntary movements. Kernicterus should always be suspected if an extrapyramidal syndrome is accompanied by bilateral deafness and palsy of upward gaze. The neuropathologic changes in these surviving patients with milder cases consist of symmetrically distributed nerve-cell loss and gliosis in the subthalamic nucleus of Luys, the globus pallidus, thalamus, and oculomotor and cochlear nuclei. These lesions are the result of the hyperbilirubinemia. In the newborn, unconjugated bilirubin can pass through the poorly developed blood-brain barrier into these central and brainstem nuclei, where it is directly toxic. Acidosis and hypoxia exacerbate the effect.

CONGENITAL AND ACQUIRED ATAXIAS The combination of cerebral diplegia with cerebellar ataxia has already been mentioned. In these patients difficulty in standing and walking cannot be attributed to spasticity or paralysis. Incoordination, similar to that seen in cerebellar disease, and hypotonia are the principal findings. The motor defect may be so great that the individual is never able to sit or stand; the muscles are of normal size, and voluntary movements, though weak, are possible in all the limbs. In less severe cases sitting, standing, and walking are merely delayed, and with advancing years cerebellar ataxia and tremor become manifest. Relative improvement may occur in later years. The tendon reflexes are present, and the plantar reflexes are either flexor or extensor. Many of these patients suffer a degree of amentia and retardation of speech development that results in their placement in homes for the feebleminded. In relatively few of the recorded cases have the pathologic changes of this condition been studied, though they are increasingly recognized in CT scans. Aplasia or hypoplasia of the cerebellum has been reported only a few times. Sclerotic lesions of the cerebellum are more common.

The hereditary ataxias are likely to begin at a later age and are progressive. They are discussed in Chap. 364.

MENTAL RETARDATION

Mentally retarded (feebleminded) individuals pose special problems not only in childhood but also as adults. They become the concern of the internist for several reasons. Firstly, failure to recognize the mentally subnormal patient means that one depends on a history that is inadequate, instead of turning to the guardian; also one must rely more on objective signs of disease than on subjective complaint. Then, too, the reactions of such patients to drugs and fever may be unexpectedly devastating and less predictable. Recognition of the type of disease underlying impaired mentality also becomes important in genetic counseling for the prevention of similar disease in other members of the family.

The more severely retarded individuals nearly always are forced to reside in institutions, and the brain is so extensively damaged that many do not survive beyond childhood. There are special severe types of mental retardation, such as Down's syndrome, that are less lethal, and many persons with such conditions live with their families until adulthood. Their condition raises a number of interesting problems for the internist (i.e., the tendency to develop leukemia and premature senile dementia). Other milder forms of mental subnormality are much more numerous, however, amounting to 3 percent of the general population, and they are more often familial and occur more frequently in the lower economic stratum of society. Their anatomic basis is uncertain. In many instances they probably represent examples of persons who fall within the lower distribution of normal human intelligence.

The clinical manifestations of mental retardation are relatively easy to perceive. Silly behavior and inability to give a sensible account of the medical problem constitute one useful datum. Slowness in motor development, inability to learn and poor school progress (individuals unable to pass the sixth grade usually have an IQ of 60 to 70), lack of a concept of time or space, and inability to secure and hold a job or to perform more than the menial tasks of society are other useful indexes. The differentiation of the various classes of mental backwardness by clinical criteria is facilitated if the framework of reference in Table 365-1 is used.

In spite of the wide spectrum of specific disease entities causing mental retardation, perhaps half of all mentally retarded persons cannot presently be classified in terms of specific etiology by clinical criteria. Many of these cases are familial, the patients coming from families in which other members are retarded or have important mental disorders, and the heritable factors may be polygenic. There also appears to be another group of disorders, due to single gene defects affecting only the brain, which have been poorly defined clinically and pathologically; included are several types of maldevelopment of the cerebral cortex. An important and varied group of X-linked recessive disorders causing mental retardation in males has recently come to medical attention. In some of these affected males there are physical stigmata including macro-orchidism, prognathism, large ears, and dolichocephaly; an identifiable abnormality of the X chromosome, called the *fragile X,* appears when the cells are grown in folate-deficient media. Finally, infantile malnutrition as a cause of impaired brain growth and consequent poor mental development has received much attention. Malnutrition during the first two years of life, when coupled with other socioeconomic deprivations, may result in retarded brain growth and mental development that persist into adult life. If, however, such children are "rescued" by refeeding and placement in a stimulating and supportive environment, the effects of early malnutrition are largely reversible, and normal mental development can result.

CLINICAL CHARACTERISTICS As an aid to the general physician who must undertake the diagnosis and management of backward children, the following comments may be of some value. Mental retardation manifests itself most obviously in the spheres of motor, language, social, and intellectual development. Severely retarded children at idiot level with IQs of less than 20 and unable to look after themselves often do not sit up, walk, or stand, and if any one of these motor activities is acquired, it appears late and is imperfectly performed. Language is not mastered, or at most a few words are understood and uttered. Patients are continuously idle and can only vocalize in a meaningless way. They do not interact with people and objects around them, nor do they make known their needs for water, food, excretion, etc. They do nothing for themselves and exhibit only primitive emotional reactions. Physical growth is usually retarded, nutrition may be poor, and susceptibility to respiratory infections is common. Sphincteric control may never be secured. A variety of physical deformities, particularly microcephaly, is common in this group. Such persons are to be found among the adult populations of state hospitals. Affections of the nervous system which have their onset later in life are usually not attended by bodily disfigurement.

If the mental defect is less pronounced, with an IQ of 20 to 50 (i.e., imbecile), or 50 to 70 (i.e., moron), and if specific motor defects do not coexist, then sitting, walking, and speech are acquired, but after a delay in many cases. The existence of a cerebral defect may be noted for the first time when the child fails to speak normally during the second and third years of life and seems not to be able to learn the usual household tasks and play activities as well as other children. However, delay in speech development must not by itself be taken as a mark of mental retardation, for some children who are obviously intelligent and who show remarkable talent in communicating by gesture are slow in talking. Also the deaf child may be singled out by indifference to noise and reduced vocalization but otherwise normal development. Toilet training also may be difficult to accomplish in the retarded child, but again it may be delayed in an otherwise normal child.

Within the spectrum of types of mental retardation, even within a group of persons of similar IQs, there are vast differences and contrasts in overall behavioral functioning. Some mentally retarded persons are pleasant and amiable, and achieve a rather satisfactory social adjustment; this is especially true of simple mental retardates. At the opposite extreme is the ill-understood syndrome of autism, associated with varying degrees of retardation, in which the child or older person fails to manifest any kind of interpersonal, social contact—including communicative language—and demonstrates a limited and bizarre interest primarily in inanimate objects (see "Autism" below). It is impossible to list all variations of mental retardation here, but the point should be made that all aspects of intellectual life and personality are touched in differing degrees. Many retarded individuals are dull, apathetic, and underactive. Others display an incessant hyperactivity, characterized by a very short attention span, a restless inquisitive searching of the environment, and low frustration tolerance; they may be destructive or recklessly fearless, and may seem strangely impervious to injury. Some display a peculiar anhedonia and are indifferent to either punishment or reward. Strangely, as with the mentally normal but hyperactive, inattentive child, improvement in these children can often be achieved by using amphetamines. Other aberrant types of behavior, such as violent aggressiveness and even self-mutilation, are not uncommon. Rhythmic rocking, rolling, head banging, and bouncing movements feature the motor activities of retarded persons, and may be performed hour after hour without fatigue, often to the accompaniment of bleating sounds, squeals, and other ejaculations. Here the abnormality is not the appearance of rhythmic movements of the body, which are to be observed at one period in the development of many normal children, but their persistence. Music may encourage rhythmic movement and gives pleasure to many retarded children and adults.

It is apparent that the clinical and behavioral characteristics of individuals with retarded development cannot be adequately described by a single parameter, the IQ. There are many other factors which determine the social success of retarded children and should give direction to their education and training. These include recognition of specific sensory or motor handicaps, such as blindness and deafness as well as athetosis or hemiplegia; specific language or speech deficits; behavioral disturbances, such as autism or hyperactivity; and the presence of seizures. Measures can be taken which help the handicapped person to compensate for these deficiencies. This becomes a primary consideration in functional diagnosis and in guiding the parents or guardians.

The least severely retarded individual (IQ of 50 to 70) grows and develops in many ways not different from normal ones, and he or she can be taught useful occupational skills. A few of these persons can work under careful supervision. All scholastic pursuits are relatively unsuccessful, and vocational training is of more value than other types of education.

TABLE 365-1
Types of mental retardation

- *I* Mental defect with associated developmental abnormalities in nonnervous structures
  - *A* Those affecting cranioskeletal structures
    - *1* Microcephaly
    - *2* Macrocephaly
    - *3* Hydrocephalus (including myelomeningocele with Arnold-Chiari malformation and associated cerebral anomalies)
    - *4* Down's syndrome (mongolism)
    - *5* Cretinism (congenital hypothyroidism)
    - *6* Mucopolysaccharidoses (Hurler, Hunter, Morquio, and Sanfilippo types)
    - *7* Acrocephalosyndactyly (craniostenosis)
    - *8* Arthrogryposis multiplex congenita (some cases)
    - *9* Rare specific syndromes: e.g., Rubinstein-Taybi
    - *10* Dwarfism, short stature: Russell-Silver dwarf, Seckel's bird-headed dwarf, Cockayne-Neel dwarf, etc.
    - *11* Hypertelorism, median-cleft-face syndromes, agenesis of corpus callosum
  - *B* Those affecting nonskeletal structures
    - *1* Neurocutaneous syndromes: tuberous sclerosis, Sturge-Weber, neurofibromatosis (uncommonly)
    - *2* Congenital rubella syndrome (deafness, blindness, congenital heart disease, small stature)
    - *3* Chromosomal disorders: Down's syndrome, some cases of Klinefelter's syndrome (XXY), XYY, Turner's (XO) syndrome (occasionally), others
    - *4* Laurence-Moon-Biedl syndrome (retinitis pigmentosa, obesity, polydactyly)
    - *5* Eye disorders: toxoplasmosis (chorioretinitis), galactosemia (cataract), congenital rubella
    - *6* Prader-Willi syndrome (obesity, hypogenitalism)
- *II* Mental defect without developmental anomalies in nonnervous structures, but with focal cerebral and other neurologic abnormalities
  - *A* Cerebral spastic diplegia and quadriplegia
  - *B* Cerebral hemiplegia, unilateral or bilateral
  - *C* Congenital choreoathetosis or ataxia
    - *1* Kernicterus
    - *2* Status marmoratus
  - *D* Congenital atonic diplegia
  - *E* Posthypoglycemic, posttraumatic, postmeningitic, and postencephalitic states
  - *F* Those associated with other neuromuscular abnormalities (muscular dystrophy, Friedreich's ataxia, etc.)
  - *G* Cerebral degenerative diseases (lipidoses)
  - *H* Lesch-Nyhan syndrome
- *III* Mental defect without signs of other developmental abnormality or neurologic disorder (epilepsy may or may not be present)
  - *A* Simple mental retardation, familial mental retardation [including X-linked (fragile X)]
  - *B* Some cases of encephaloclastic disease (hypoxia, hypoglycemia)
  - *C* Infantile autism
  - *D* Associated with inborn errors of metabolism (phenylketonuria, other aminoacidurias, organic acidurias)
  - *E* Congenital infections (some cases of congenital syphilis, cytomegalic inclusion disease)

SPECIAL VARIETIES OF MENTAL RETARDATION Several of the special types of mental retardation are discussed in other chapters (see "Lipidoses and Cerebral Sclerosis," in Chap. 364). In the following pages are presented only those with special features likely to be seen in adults.

Down's syndrome (mongolism) This is a unique condition, and, although accounting for only about 1 percent of all mental defectives, it is the reason for nearly one-third of the admissions to state schools for the mentally retarded. The degree of mental retardation varies from mild to severe and is associated with a curious facial configuration and a dwarfed physical stature. Many stigmata of Down's syndrome can be recognized in the neonatal period. The head tends to be small and round, with sloping forehead. The ears are set low and are oval, with small lobules. The eyes slant slightly upward and outward owing to the presence of a medial epicanthal fold, which partly covers the angle of the palpebral fissure. The bridge of the nose is generally absent or poorly developed. The mouth tends to hang open, and the tongue is usually enlarged, heavily fissured, and protruding. Gray-white specks of depigmentation are seen in the iris (Brushfield's spots). The little fingers are often short and curved inward (clinodactyly), owing to a hypoplastic middle phalanx. The hands are broad and simian-like, with a single transverse palmar crease. A number of other characteristic dermal markings are noted in fingers and toes. Lenticular opacities and congenital heart lesions (septal defects) are found in some cases. At birth these children are of average size, but at later periods of life they are characteristically small. The average adult person with Down's syndrome never exceeds the stature of a 10-year-old child.

Aside from having a rather rounded shape, which conforms to that of the skull, a subnormal weight, and a relatively simple convolutional pattern, with particular smallness of the frontal lobes and superior temporal convolutions, the brain shows no specific abnormalities.

The mortality rate is high in the first years of life, death usually being due to respiratory infections, interventricular cardiac lesion with failure, or leukemia. Of the patients who survive to puberty, many live to middle adult life and many then suffer a premature form of Alzheimer's cerebral degeneration (onset in the majority by the age of 40).

Older mothers are more apt to have Down's syndrome babies than are young mothers. The mean age of the mother at the time of birth of these children is 37. Trisomy of chromosome 21 or translocation of parts of this chromosome has been found (also by amniocentesis) with Down's syndrome and is responsible for the disorder.

Cretinism and childhood hypothroidism True endemic cretinism occurs in parts of the world where there is iodine deficiency and in infants who suffer a dysgenetic disorder of thyroid function. The frequency is greater than that of phenylketonuria. For iodine deficiency to produce cretinism the mother must be lacking in iodine during the pregnancy, especially in the first trimester. Diagnosis rests on the clinical picture, for in the iodine deficiency state measures of thyroid function may be normal. Jaundice, umbilical hernia, noisy respirations, hypotonia, depression of reflexes, and lethargy are present at birth. The coarse features, large tongue, and constipation become manifest later. One of the authors (DeLong), who has examined 76 cretins born of iodine-deficient mothers, observed the emergence of a pattern of neurologic abnormality consisting of mental deficiency, deaf-mutism (or lesser degrees of hearing loss), and a combination of flexed posture with spasticity-rigidity of proximal limb musculature. This persists throughout adult life. In the dysgenetic cretin the diagnosis can be confirmed by measurement of T_3T_4.

Childhood hypothyroidism and myxedema resemble the adult forms of diseases described in Chap. 111.

Gargoylism (Hunter-Hurler disease) This condition is discussed in Chap. 92.

Phenylketonuria (phenylpyruvic oligophrenia) This condition is discussed in Chap. 92.

Galactosemia Another congenital metabolic disease, galactosemia is transmitted by a single, autosomal recessive gene. It is characterized clinically by mental defect, cataract, nausea, vomiting, hepatomegaly, jaundice, and the excretion of large quantities of galactose in the urine (Chap. 101).

Autism Autism is a mysterious and provocative condition identified in young children. Long considered primarily psychiatric, it is now generally thought to represent an organic defect in brain development. It is characterized by failure of children to develop communicative language or any form of social communication. By contrast, they often show motor and other skills far beyond what is to be expected of a mentally retarded person. Often they are obsessively preoccupied with inanimate objects, such as lights, running water, or spinning objects. Most of the youngsters prove later to be retarded, and the ultimate prognosis depends largely on the child's IQ. Some few gradually acquire language and may then exhibit certain exceptional talents, such as in mathematics. Upon reaching adult life they are found to retain all the above characteristics. Not more than 1 in 20 will seem to have made any progress. Imprecision of diagnosis allows the inclusion of other brain diseases under the rubric of autism. The patients at a later age do not resemble schizophrenics, despite claims that autism is an unusually precocious form of schizophrenia. No biochemical abnormality has been discovered. Brain volume appears to be normal by contrast studies and gross examination, but few detailed histopathologic studies have been made. CT studies and pneumoencephalograms show that some children with features of autism have left-sided medial temporal lobe atrophic lesions. This finding is consistent with our understanding of the role of the medial temporal lobes in mediating language, affective, motivational, and social behavioral functions in human beings. It is also consistent with the finding that up to 30 percent of autistic children eventually manifest temporal lobe epilepsy. There is no therapy for this condition.

Simple mental retardation Although presented last, this category includes the great number of cases of defective mentality of indeterminate etiology in which neither somatic nor neurologic abnormality is exhibited. The degree of mental impairment tends to be mild (moron, educable) or moderate (imbecile, trainable). Penrose found that this group of retardates constituted 25 percent of 1280 institutionalized individuals, and of course those who are in institutions represent only the more severely damaged individuals in our society. Their physical appearance is usually not strikingly abnormal; yet many of the aforementioned characteristics of the mentally retarded individual are to be observed. Seizures occur in a significant number, being several times more frequent than in a normal population. Within the limits of their intelligence, the success of these individuals in learning to look after themselves is often determined by how effectively their parents and teachers have inculcated or reinforced good work habits and stable personality traits. The brighter ones can profit to some extent from formal education. Those less well endowed may be trained to care for their personal wants and needs and may profit from a limited amount of manual training. Special schools and classes are of great help. Later in life supervised work situations are possible solutions to their occupational needs.

Society, in the final analysis, determines the eventual disposition of these unfortunates. Many of them, being not unattractive and giving less trouble than many other defective persons, are able to adjust to foster families and live in a community. They need protection, for they are easily led astray and may commit infractions of the law, usually of a minor sort. Institutionalization is required when family and society cannot or do not wish to look after them. Reproductivity is frequently impaired in those with severe mental defects but may be distressingly undisturbed in many of the less defective individuals.

The problem of eugenics assumes great importance. This type of mental defect is often seen in families in which one or both of the parents are dull or retarded. The term *familial* may be applied to this group. However, the majority of cases are sporadic. Probably multiple etiologic factors may lead to simple mental retardation. The pathologic change is variable, ranging from "no demonstrable lesion" to several different gross and microscopic abnormalities.

EPILEPSY

The majority of adult patients with recurrent seizures acquire the tendency toward seizures during childhood. They represent the sequelae of disease processes which may have begun and ended in the distant past. In early life the pattern of the seizures varies widely, depending in part on the level of maturation of the nervous system. Certain types such as fragmented neonatal seizures, infantile spasms, photic epilepsy, febrile seizures, etc., are peculiar to the earlier periods of life. Others, such as petit mal, grand mal, and psychomotor, are identical in child and adult. The latter types are discussed in Chap. 12.

REFERENCES

ADAMS RD: Neurocutaneous disease, in *Dermatology in General Medicine,* 2d ed, TB Fitzpatrick et al (eds). New York, McGraw-Hill, 1979

COOPER IS: *Involuntary Movement Disorders.* New York, Hoeber-Harper, 1969

HOLMES LB et al: Mental retardation, in *An Atlas of Diseases with Associated Physical Abnormalities.* New York, Macmillan, 1972

MYERS RE: A unitary theory of causation of anoxic and hypoxic brain pathology, in *Advances in Neurology,* S Fahn et al (eds). New York, Raven Press, 1979, vol 26

SALAM M, ADAMS RD: Arnold-Chiari malformation, in *Handbook of Clinical Neurology.* Amsterdam, North-Holland, 1978

SEDGEWICK RP, BODER E: Ataxia telangiectasia, in *Handbook of Clinical Neurology.* Amsterdam, North-Holland, 1972, vol 14, pp 267–334

WINDLE WF Selective vulnerability of the CNS of rhesus monkeys to asphyxia, in *Symposium on Selective Vulnerability of CNS to Hypoxaemia,* JP Schade et al (eds). Oxford, Blackwell Scientific, 1963

366
DISEASES OF THE SPINAL CORD

RAYMOND D. ADAMS
JOSEPH B. MARTIN

Diseases of the nervous system may at times limit themselves to the spinal cord and also produce a number of distinctive syndromes. This relates to special anatomic features such as great length in proportion to width, peripheral location of medullated fibers next to the pia, tight envelopment by meninges, arrangement of blood vessels, and relationship to vertebrae. Because of the frequency and gravity of these diseases, and the special difficulties attendant upon diagnosis, we have grouped them in a special chapter under a series of relatively common syndromes, the basis of which will be better understood after reading Chaps. 14 and 18.

GLOBAL PARALYSIS OF LEGS OR ALL EXTREMITIES DUE TO MASSIVE TRANSVERSE LESION OF THE SPINAL CORD

This condition may best be considered in relation to trauma, one of the most frequent causes of it, but it also occurs with certain types of myelitis, infarction, and hemorrhage in the spinal cord, and rapidly advancing compressive myelopathy.

INJURIES TO THE SPINE AND SPINAL CORD Although injuries to the spinal cord may be the sole manifestation of a traumatic disease, it is seldom that the vertebral column is not harmed at the same time. Often there is an associated head injury, as is pointed out in Chap. 357.

A useful classification of spinal injuries is one which divides them into fracture-dislocations, pure fractures, and pure dislocations. The relative frequency of these types is about 3:1:1. Direct violence to the spine is an uncommon cause of vertebral disruption; except for stab and bullet wounds, most spine injuries are the result of force *applied at a distance.* All three types of injury are produced by a similar mechanism, usually a vertical compression of the spinal column to which flexion is almost immediately added. Or, in the neck the mechanism may be one of extension. The two important variables in the mechanics of vertebral injury are the nature of the bones and joints and the strength, direction, and point of impact of the force.

Strength, direction, and point of impact of the force If the injuring body striking the cranium is hard and the velocity is high, a skull fracture occurs, the elastic quality of the skull absorbing the force of the injury. If the injuring body is soft yet heavy, the spine and particularly its cervical portion will be the part injured. If the neck happens to be rigid and straight and the force is quickly applied to the head, the atlas and the odontoid process of the axis may break. If the force is less quickly applied and removed, an element of flexion occurs. Flexion movements plus a vertical force constitute the essential factors in the majority of fracture-dislocation or pure dislocation injuries.

The other common mechanism of cord injury is sudden extension of the neck. It is especially frequent in civilian motor accidents and in forward falls, and more often it affects supporting structures of the head than spinal nerves or cord. Cervical spondylosis adds to the hazards of spinal injury. Lesser degrees of extension injuries of the neck, which have no direct impact on the spinal cord, nerve roots, or peripheral nerves, are the common whiplash injuries. They are a source of pain, emotional upset, and litigation.

A special type of spine injury, occurring most often in military life, is that in which missiles of high velocity pass through the vertebral canal and destroy the spinal cord. In some cases they may strike the vertebral column without entering the spinal canal and agitate it so violently that the cord suffers injury. The term given to temporary spinal paralysis is *spinal concussion.* This condition may also be produced by violent falls flat on the back.

A study of 2006 cases collected from the literature by Jefferson shows that most vertebral injuries occur at the first to second cervical, fourth to seventh cervical, and eleventh thoracic to second lumbar vertebrae. Industrial accidents most often involve the dorsolumbar vertebrae. Accidents caused by falling with head down, as in diving accidents, affect the cervical region. In the authors' neuropathologic material, the usual circumstances of spinal injury were a state of alcoholic intoxication and a fall down a flight of stairs, automobile accidents, crushing industrial accidents, gunshot or stab wounds, and birth injury, in that order of frequency. The majority of these fatal cases had fracture-dislocations or dislocations of the cervical spine.

Mechanism of spinal cord injury The spinal cord may escape injury even though there is vertebral dislocation, especially in regions where the spinal canal is large, i.e., in the cervical and lumbar regions. Rarely the spinal cord may be damaged without radiologic evidence of fracture or dislocation. One cannot easily determine the full extent of spinal injury by radiology or even at autopsy because of the difficulty in examining the vertebrae. By far the most satisfactory technique for demonstrating the degree of spine injury and the presence of a tearing of ligaments with dislocation is the x-ray, taken laterally, but one must be careful to avoid flexion or extension of the neck, for it may inflict further injury to the spinal cord. The most frequently established mechanism is a vertebral dislocation with or without fracture. The upper vertebrae are displaced anteriorly, and there is a break in the posterior longitudinal ligament and the capsule of the intervertebral disk. The spinal cord is most often subjected to a shearing force between the pedicles of the vertebra above and the body and laminae of the vertebra below the dislocation.

When the cervical spine is sharply extended, especially in the presence of cervical spondylosis, the damage to the spinal cord is due to the sudden narrowing of the spinal canal. The spinal cord is caught between the lamina of the lower vertebra and body of the higher one. Also, the ligamentum flavum may buckle and compress the cord. There may be no x-ray evidence of the spinal lesion. A congenital stenosis or a spondylytic narrowing of the spinal canal predisposes to this type of injury.

In direct trauma of the spine, as when it is struck in some part by a bullet, the means of spinal concussion is said to be *agitation.* Little is known of the underlying pathology. This term has led to much confusion because it is not employed here in the usual sense of cerebral concussion, i.e., a transient interruption of neural function by trauma without proved structural change.

Pathology of spinal cord injury As a result of squeezing or shearing of the cord, there is destruction of gray matter and a variable amount of hemorrhage, chiefly in the more vascular parts. These changes are maximal at the level of injury and one or two segments above and below it. Rarely is the cord cut in two, and seldom is the pia-arachnoid lacerated. The condition is best designated as *traumatic necrosis of the spinal cord.* As the lesion heals, cavitation or a gliotic focus results. Months or years later a diverticulation of the central canal into the cavity may result in a traumatic syringomyelia. Attempts to distinguish such pathologic entities as hematomyelia, concussion, contusion, and hematorrhachis are of little value either clinically or pathologically.

As with most lesions, the total disease picture includes an irreversible structural lesion and a disorder of function, each of which may vary in degree. The extent and permanence of the clinical manifestations are determined by the relative proportions of these two. An exception to this statement might be made for gunshot wounds of the vertebrae. Here the explosive force of the missile may shatter myelinated fibers with maximal functional disturbance.

CLINICAL EFFECTS OF SPINAL CORD INJURY The "classic" description of traumatic paraplegia by Riddock cannot be excelled. He divided the clinical picture into two stages: spinal shock and reflex activity.

Spinal shock or muscular flaccidity The loss of function which is inflicted at the time of injury (fourth to fifth cervical vertebrae—quadriplegia, thoracic vertebrae—paraplegia, both with paralysis of bladder and bowel sphincters and loss of sensibility below the level corresponding to the spinal lesion) is accompanied by a complete or almost complete suppression of reflex activity of all spinal segments below the lesion. This is the condition known as *spinal shock.* The plantar reflexes are at first variable and may be absent, flexor, or extensor. The lower extremities lose heat if left uncovered and swell if dependent. Sweating is abolished. Cutaneous ulcerations may develop over bony prominences. Urine and feces are retained to the point where overflow and involuntary leakage results. Occasionally there is priapism because of venous congestion. A paralytic ileus may occur.

Reflex activity If the lumbosacral segments are undamaged, spinal shock wears off in 2 to 3 weeks. The first sign of this is contraction of the hamstrings and flexion or extension of the toes on plantar stimulation. Then gentle and later strong involuntary flexor spasms make their appearance. Ankle jerks and then knee jerks return. Retention of urine and feces becomes less complete, and at irregular intervals urine is expelled by active contraction of the detrusor muscle. Reflex defecation and sweating also appear. At times flexor spasms and later extensor spasms, often accompanied by profuse sweating and micturition, all occur after stimulation of the skin, viz., the *mass reflex.* This stage of reflex activity may last for years, unless sepsis intervenes, in which case the state of spinal shock may return.

Less complete lesions of the spinal cord may result in little or no spinal shock or extensor spasm. Incomplete voluntary motor paralysis, a flaccid atrophic paralysis, variable sensory impairment in the arms, a spastic weakness of the legs, and a partial or complete Brown-Séquard syndrome are some of the resulting clinical pictures.

The end stage may be permanent and complete disability, rarely consistent with survival for more than a few months or years; or a gradual improvement and complete or almost complete recovery may occur. Any residual symptoms after 6 months are likely to be permanent.

The level of the cord lesion can be determined by the clinical picture. A complete paralysis of arms and legs usually indicates a dislocation at the fourth to fifth cervical vertebrae. If the legs are paralyzed and the arms can still be abducted and flexed, the dislocation is likely to be at the fifth to sixth cervical. Paralysis only of hands and of legs indicates the level of vertebral disorder to be the sixth to seventh cervical. When the motor paralysis involves muscles above the knees and sensory loss includes the twelfth thoracic dermatone, the site is the eleventh to twelfth thoracic. If the paralysis is below the knees and the first lumbar escapes, the lesion is at the twelfth thoracic, first lumbar vertebrae. Prognosis for the latter group of patients, with preponderantly cauda equina lesions, is better than for those with injury to the eleventh to twelfth thoracic vertebrae. In all cases of spinal cord injury any elicitable movement or preserved sensation during the first 48 to 72 h gives a favorable prognosis for recovery.

Treatment In general, the treatment for spinal cord injuries is conservative and symptomatic. The degree of injury can be lessened by ensuring that no movement of cervical spine (especially flexion) is made from the moment of the accident. Mannitol and corticosteroid therapy, as for brain swelling (Chap. 358), may reduce the swelling of spinal cord tissue. Hypothermia is beneficial in spinal cord trauma in experimental animals but has few advocates as a treatment for humans. If the spinal cord injury is associated with dislocation of the vertebrae, traction on the neck is necessary to secure proper alignment. This is accomplished by a head halter attached through the head of the bed over a pulley to a weight of 10 to 15 lb or, even better, the use of tongs which fasten onto the skull (Crutchfield). In thoracic crush injuries, hyperextension can be maintained by placing a narrow pillow under the affected area. Traction should be continued for 4 to 6 weeks, and then a brace may be substituted. In some centers for the treatment of spinal cord injury early fixation and traction of spine have almost completely replaced decompression by laminectomy. The latter are reserved for x-ray-visible intraspinal bone fragments and dislocations that are irreducible by traction. Comparison of conservative and operative results shows little difference, according to Gillingham et al.

The aftercare of patients with paraplegia and disturbance of vesical or rectal functions is similar to that of patients with like symptoms from other causes. Decubitus ulceration can be prevented by special skin care. Intermittent drainage of the bladder by catheter is of value in preventing infection, stone formation, and contracture and in securing return of function. Daily enemas are usually the most effective means of controlling fecal incontinence. Physiotherapy, muscle reeducation, and the application of proper braces are all important in the rehabilitation of the patient. All this is best carried out in centers for rehabilitation of spine injuries. Although one hopes that the paraplegic patient will eventually walk, using caliper braces, a more realistic objective is ambulation in a wheelchair.

MYELITIS The spinal cord appears to be vulnerable to three types of inflammatory processes, all of which have been called *myelitic.* First there are the specific viral infections which tend to involve principally the gray matter (hence called *poliomyelitic*). Zoster and the three viruses of poliomyelitis are the most frequent causes of this type. Secondly, all the subacute and chronic primary meningeal infections may induce damage of the spinal roots and outer surfaces of the spinal cord, i.e., to the white matter of posterior, lateral, and anterior funiculi (meningoradiculitis and meningomyelitis), or there may be occlusion of meningeal vessels. Syphilis offers the best known and formerly the most numerous examples of this category of inflammatory disease, viz., tabes dorsalis (which is essentially a treponemal lumbosacral meningoradiculitis), syphilitic meningomyelitis, and arteritis with myelomalacia. Tuberculous meningitis and fungous meningitis provide other examples. Thirdly, there is a group of primary inflammations of white matter, the leukomyelitides. Most of the leukomyelitides are of unknown cause. Three varieties of the latter have been delineated: (1) postinfectious and postvaccinial myelitis, (2) demyelinative myelitis (acute or chronic relapsing multiple sclerosis), and (3) acute or subacute necrotizing myelitis. Although the white (and gray) matter may be the site of an infective inflammatory process as in abscess, tuberculoma, gumma and parasitic inflammations, and particularly schistosomiasis (in thoracolumbar segments), such conditions are rare.

Whereas any one of the above forms of chronic meningitis or leukomyelitis may induce the clinical picture of a transverse cord lesion, this lesion is usually due to one of the demyelinative or necrotizing forms of myelitis. A painless (rarely painful) paraplegia, beginning simultaneously in both legs, or more often first in one leg and then the other, or in sacral segments, ascends to the abdomen and thorax. Either sensory or motor symptoms may initiate the disease, but both are present as it progresses. Like all cord lesions with involvement of tracts, the loss of sensory and motor function affects all parts of the body below a certain level, sphincters as well, and, if acute, overflow incontinence and obstipation are included. In only a few patients will vaccination against smallpox, rabies inoculation, or a frank chickenpox or measles be found to have preceded the neurologic symptoms by days to 1 to 2 weeks; in all the rest, the illness develops without explanation. The conjunction of retrobulbar neuritis with the cord lesion is called *neuromyelitis optica* or *Devic's disease.* This is not a disease but a syndrome occurring in necrotizing myelitis (usual cause), multiple sclerosis, and postinfectious myelitis. If the spinal cord lesion is severe and paralysis is complete, spinal shock supervenes, with the same flaccidity and areflexia of legs described under spinal cord trauma (above). The cerebrospinal fluid (CSF) may be normal or may contain lymphocytes and mononuclear leukocytes (numbering from 20 to 1000 or more per milliliter), and the protein is sometimes raised. If the cord lesion swells, as it rarely does, there may be a dynamic block (positive Queckenstedt test). When the latter is found, it always suggests the possibility of a *spinal epidural abscess,* another important and treatable cause of a rapidly developing transverse cord lesion with spine ache and fever. Subacute necrotizing myelitis is a less well-defined condition in which a succession of obscure inflammatory (?) vascular lesions convert a state of spastic paraplegia with sensory loss to a flaccid one (as the lower parts of the spinal cord are involved). Of passing interest is the observation in some forms of myelitis (postzoster, idiopathic) of a spinal, focal segmental myoclonus resembling restricted myoclonus of cerebral origin (see Hoehn and Cherington). It may indicate the level of a motor or sensory tract lesion.

Treatment of the demyelinative and necrotizing myelitides consists of ACTH (40 units twice a day for a week, then once a day for 2 to 3 weeks) or prednisone (60 mg per day for 3 weeks). Improvement usually occurs, but the relation to therapy is uncertain. Administration of other immunosuppressants (cyclophosphamide) or plasmapheresis is advocated by some. Except for patients with the postinfectious form of myelitis there is always danger of later progression or relapse. Prevention of decubitus ulceration, early catheterization and bladder care, and rehabilitation measures, the usual procedures in the management of the paraplegia patients, must also be employed.

SPINAL EPIDURAL ABSCESS Children or adults may be affected. An injury to the back, often trivial, at the time of a furunculosis or other skin infection or a bacteremia may permit seeding of the spinal epidural space or of vertebral body. The latter gives rise to osteomyelitis with extension to the epidural space. The suppurative process is accompanied at first only by fever and aching in the region of the spine and later by radicular pain. After several days or a few weeks there is a rapid onset and progression of paraplegia, sensory loss in the lower parts of the body, urinary and fecal retention, and sphincteric incontinence. Percussion of the spine elicits tenderness over the site of the infection. Examination reveals all the signs of transverse cord lesion with spinal shock. The CSF contains small numbers of cells (neutrophilic leukocytes and lymphocytes), and the protein is relatively high (100 to 400 mg/ml). More importantly there is a dynamic block (positive Queckenstedt test). If not treated surgically by laminectomy and drainage at the earliest possible moment, the spinal cord lesion, which is due in part to ischemia (compression mainly of veins), becomes irreversible. Emergency myelography must be used to determine the level of block and the operative site. At an early stage bone scan is more revealing of an early osteomyelitis of the spine than plain x-rays. Antibiotic therapy must also be given.

Another circumstance in which an acute spinal epidural abscess may develop is in a patient with some combination of chronic medical diseases in whom a septicemia occurs. Here the symptoms of spine disease may be minimal until the onset of the spinal cord lesion some weeks later. Staphylococci or some other organism may reach the epidural or subdural spinal space via a lumbar puncture needle during epidural anesthesia or a laminectomy. The localization is then over lumbar and sacral roots. Pain may be severe and neurologic symptomatology minimal.

Subacute pyogenic infections and granulomatous infections (tubercular, fungal) may also arise in the spinal epidural space causing symptoms and signs of disorder of spinal tracts at the level of the lesion. The clinical picture is less dramatic, and the diagnosis depends on the demonstration, in a patient with weakness and/or sensory loss or ataxia of the legs, of a partial or complete block by contrast myelography. Bone scans are helpful when there is concomitant vertebral infection. Somatosensory evoked potentials will reveal a block between the cauda equina and the brainstem. The treatment depends on the nature of the underlying disease and the general condition of the patient (see Chap. 359).

INFARCTION OF SPINAL CORD (MYELOMALACIA) AND HEMORRHAGE (HEMATOMYELIA) Unlike the brain, the spinal cord is rarely the site of vascular disease. The spinal arteries are not susceptible to atherosclerosis, and emboli rarely lodge here. As was stated in relation to chronic meningeal infections, an endarteritis of surface arteries may lead to thrombosis with devastating ischemic necrosis of the spinal cord. Polyarteritis nodosa may have a similar effect though the localization in the nervous system in this disease is usually peripheral. Atherosclerotic thrombosis of the aorta or dissecting aortic aneurysms may cause myelomalacia by occluding nutrient arteries at cervical, thoracic, or lumbar levels. Paralysis during cardiac surgery requiring clamping of the aorta for more than 30 min and vertebrobasilar (thyrocervical branch) and aortic arteriography may result in the syndrome. Infarction of the gray matter of the upper cervical cord segments and medulla oblongata may follow vertebral angiography. Sudden development of symptoms referable to lesions of spinal tracts (sensory or motor or both) always bespeaks an infarctive or hemorrhagic vascular lesion of the spinal cord. The onset of symptoms in such cases is more rapid than in the myelitides.

Hemorrhage into the spinal cord is rare. Aside from the aforementioned traumatic variety of hematomyelia, it is usually traceable to a vascular malformation, hereditary telangiectasia (Osler-Rendu-Weber disease), or a hematologic disease including anticoagulant therapy. Epidural hemorrhages with spinal cord compression may occur with hematologic disorders and anticoagulant therapy. The latter requires vitamin K therapy and immediate surgical decompression.

SUBACUTE OR CHRONIC SPINAL SYNDROMES

These take several forms for the reason that the responsible diseases have a variety of different localizations in the tracts and gray matter. Most of the remaining diseases of the spinal cord may be grouped around the following syndromes.

SPASTIC ATAXIC PARAPARESIS The gradual development of ataxia and weakness of the legs is the common manifestation of several diseases. In late childhood or adolescence a syndrome of this type which begins insidiously and progresses steadily over a period of years usually indicates the existence of Friedreich's ataxia or some other type of hereditary spinocerebellar degeneration. In early adult life multiple sclerosis, benign tumors (neurofibroma or meningioma), and chronic adhesive spinal arachnoiditis are the more frequent causes of it. And in middle and late years of life late deteriorative forms of spinal multiple sclerosis and cervical spondylosis are the most frequent causes, followed by syringomyelia, and subacute combined degeneration (B_{12} vitamin deficiency).

CERVICAL SPONDYLOSIS The cervical intervertebral disks degenerate to some degree in the majority of individuals by the sixth and seventh decades of life. This results in narrowing of the disks, especially in the most mobile parts of the cervical spine (fourth to fifth cervical, fifth to sixth cervical, sixth to seventh cervical, and seventh cervical to first thoracic segments) and spur formation on the margins of the adjacent vertebrae. There are anterior beaking and posterior osteophytes which protrude centrally with narrowing of the spinal canal or laterally so as to impinge on spinal roots in the intervertebral canals. This condition is incorrectly called *hypertrophic arthritis,* for there is no consistent association with arthritis of this type in other joints. The more appropriate term *cervical spondylosis* refers to a wear and tear (traumatic?) phenomenon.

The clinical symptomatology is variable. When a group of asymptomatic patients beyond 50 years is surveyed, a few will be found to have slight limitation in neck motions, mild pain in shoulders or an arm, a history of questionable cervical-disk disease in the past, and sometimes a diminution of an arm reflex or a numb finger or two. A few even have had an unexpected Babinski sign on one side.

Abrupt onset of an arm pain, numbness of one side of a hand or two or three fingers, and a diminished reflex, a not-infrequent clinical state in middle and late adult life, are attributed to osteophytic impingement on a root. But the pathology of such nerve lesions is uncertain. Rest with traction often relieves the symptoms while the osteophyte obviously remains. No ruptured disk is seen in the cervical myelogram. Such conditions must be distinguished from brachial neuritis (plexitis), ruptured cervical disk, and costoclavicular and carpal tunnel syndromes.

Central posterior spurring with or without congenital narrowing of the spinal canal and hypertrophy of the ligamentum flavum can compress the spinal cord. In lateral x-rays one can see that the canal in its anteroposterior dimension is reduced to 10 to 11 mm. The column of contrast medium in the myelogram is obstructed, and in an air myelogram with laminography the compression of spinal cord is visualized. The clinical syndrome consists of a spastic weakness of legs (often one more than the other) and posterior column signs (impaired vibratory and position senses and ataxia). Other long-tract sensory changes are less frequent. Slight sensory, motor, and reflex changes are usually found in one or both hands and arms. A lesion at the fourth to fifth cervical segments may result in an increase in all tendon reflexes, particularly finger jerks; a lesion at the fifth to sixth cervical segments may diminish biceps reflexes leaving triceps and finger jerks hyperactive; a lesion at the sixth to seventh cervical segments diminishes the triceps reflexes on one or both sides. The onset of symptoms is insidious and the course slowly or intermittently progressive over several years.

Immobilization of the head with a cervical collar has stopped the progression of symptoms in some cases. Posterior laminectomy, if several interspaces are involved, or anterior fusion of the vertebral bodies, if only one or two, has resulted in improvement in the majority of patients and has halted the progression in others.

In the elderly the differential diagnosis of cervical spondylosis, cervical disk herniation, diabetic neuropathy, pernicious anemia with myelopathy, and amyotrophic lateral sclerosis, in combination with age changes in lumbosacral nerves, represents one of the most vexing of all neurologic problems. Since several of these conditions may be conjoined, the physician can separate their effects only by meticulous clinical examination and appropriate laboratory tests.

RHEUMATOID ARTHRITIS WITH VERTEBRAL SUBLUXATION In this form of arthritis of the spine destruction of ligamentous structures adjacent to affected joints may permit a subluxation with spinal cord compression. Spastic weakness of the legs and sphincteric incontinence are combined with sensory loss and areflexia in arms and variable ataxia and other signs of posterior column disease in lower parts of the body. Lateral x-rays of the cervical spine show the subluxation. Traction and fusion of the cervical spine are necessary to correct the condition (see Hughes).

MULTIPLE SCLEROSIS Probably an ataxic paraparesis ranks as the most common manifestation of an established form of multiple sclerosis. Asymmetric involvement of limbs and signs of cerebral, optic nerve, brainstem, and cerebellar manifestations provide important information for the diagnosis of this disease, but unfortunately these structures are not always involved. Often the patient presents with late onset of symptoms (age 50 to 65) of slow progression. In the study of such cases diagnosis depends on (1) evidence of earlier attacks of disease (not always remembered); (2) evidence of delayed retinocortical conduction of patterned visual stimuli, showing that optic nerves have been damaged; and (3) increased gamma globulin in the CSF. Often a cervical myelogram is necessary to rule out spondylosis or tumor. Purely spinal involvement may occur, no lesions being found outside the spinal cord even at autopsy. See Chap. 361 for further details.

FRIEDREICH'S ATAXIA This classic form of hereditary ataxia, first clearly depicted by Nikolaus Friedreich of Heidelberg in 1863, constitutes a relatively distinct symptom complex which generally runs true to form, although it overlaps other heredodegenerative syndromes, particularly the spinocerebellar atrophies, chronic familial polyneuropathies, and progressive optic atrophy (discussed in Chaps. 364 and 367). In some families, the disorder occurs with dominant inheritance; usually it is a recessive trait.

Clinical aspects As with other progressive ataxias, the disorder first appears in the legs, affecting the individual during late childhood. The patient, previously healthy, begins to stagger and lurch in walking and is unsteady on standing, often in a tremulous fashion. Clumsiness and intention tremor of the hands and arms appear later along with faulty articulation and abnormal rhythm (scanning) of speech. These symptoms usually result from changes in the dorsal root ganglia, the spinocerebellar tracts, and cerebellum; it is not easy to ascertain the relative contribution of lesions in each structure to the ataxia. The limbs, in addition to being ataxic, generally show considerable weakness. Examination usually discloses nystagmus and skeletal deformities: kyphoscoliosis, the basis of which is not certain, and a peculiar foreshortening and high arching of the feet (pes cavus) with cocking of the toes (sometimes called the "Friedreich foot" and best ascribed to atrophy and contractures of the musculature of the feet at a time when the bones of the feet are malleable). Typically, there is the unusual combination of total absence of tendon reflexes with extensor plantar reflexes (Babinski sign). This results from the presence of degeneration of pyramidal tracts together with a mild affection of peripheral sensory neurons and degeneration of the posterior columns. The presence of the latter is further indicated by impairment of position and vibration sense in the extremities and, in some patients, of the sensations of pain, temperature, and light touch in a distal and roughly symmetric distribution. Mentation is usually preserved, though a few of the patients have been of low intelligence or have become demented late in the course of the disease. Survival beyond early adult life is rare, with death frequently the result of associated cardiomyopathy.

Occasionally very mild or fragmentary forms of the disorder (such as pes cavus and absent or hyperactive tendon reflexes) may be encountered with little if any disability or progression. Such abnormalities are most likely to be seen in other members of the family of a patient afflicted with the fully developed form of the disease.

Pathology The principal changes in the spinal cord and dorsal root ganglia are typical of a chronic degenerative process. The cerebellum is variably affected. In addition to the neuropathologic changes there is in some cases a peculiar form of myocardial degeneration resulting in fiber loss and fibrosis. There are no other associated visceral lesions.

Differential diagnosis The classic form of Friedreich's ataxia is readily recognizable and cannot easily be confused with other conditions. It is to be expected, however, that variations in the clinical manifestations may occur because of the variable pathologic changes. Chronic familial polyneuropathies are particularly difficult to distinguish since they also give rise to sensory ataxia, but signs of pyramidal tract disease are absent (see Chap. 368). Hereditary forms of cerebellar ataxia with pyramidal signs (hyperactive tendon reflexes) and sensory disturbances are also known to occur in the adolescent or adult. Familial spastic paraplegia with or without optic atrophy (Behr's syndrome) is another closely related disease. In the absence of a family history, and with atypical clinical findings, further diagnostic studies to exclude tumor, chronic basal meningitis, chronic barbiturate intoxication, or congenital malformation will be necessary.

No treatment is of proven value. The recent reports of disturbed pyruvate metabolism have not been confirmed. Physical medicine and rehabilitation measures are of little value in ataxia.

SYPHILITIC MENINGOMYELITIS Here as in multiple sclerosis the degree of alteration of vibratory and position sense and ataxia is variable. Some patients with primary lateral sclerosis, such as Erb described, have almost pure pyramidal spasticity and weakness of the legs requiring differentiation from motor system disease and familial spastic paraplegia. In others sensory ataxia and posterior column signs predominate. The confirmation of diagnosis depends on the finding of a positive Wassermann reaction in the CSF, but a late and advancing form of the disease may appear with a negative CSF in a known syphilitic patient. See Chap. 177 for a discussion of pathology and treatment.

SUBACUTE COMBINED DEGENERATION OF SPINAL CORD AND BRAIN DUE TO VITAMIN B_{12} DEFICIENCY AND SYNDROME OF NUTRITIONAL COMBINED SYSTEM DISEASE (STRACHAN SYNDROME) These two forms of the more treatable diseases of the spinal cord are fully described in Chap. 363.

Progressive spastic or spastic-ataxic paraparesis may also develop in conjunction with hepatic decompensation.

SPASTIC PARAPARESIS WITH OR WITHOUT CERVICOBRACHIAL AMYOTROPHY Although a few such cases are traced to multiple sclerosis, syringomyelia, cervical pachymeningitis, or cervical meningomyelitis, the purely motor syndrome is nearly always traceable to primary lateral sclerosis, possibly a variant of amyotrophic lateral sclerosis. Paralysis, atrophy, and fascicular twitching of hands and arms are joined with spastic weakness and hyperreflexia in legs with Babinski signs (see Chap. 364). Some of these spastic parapareses or quadripareses with pure corticospinal degeneration evolve over a year or two and are nonfamilial. Cervical spondylosis and high cervical tumors must also be considered in the differential diagnosis. Pure spastic paraparesis may occur in multiple sclerosis, spondylosis, liver failure, hereditary spastic paraplegia with or without dementia, and one form of hereditary adrenoleukodystrophy.

SEGMENTAL SENSORY DISSOCIATION WITH BRACHIAL MUSCULAR ATROPHY (SYRINGOMYELIC SYNDROME)

This syndrome is most often ascribable to a syringomyelia, but examples have been found in patients with intramedullary cord tumors, delayed traumatic myelopathy, postradiation myelopathy, syphilitic cervical pachymeningitis, cervical spondylosis, extramedullary tumors of the high cervical canal and foramen magnum, and necrotizing myelitis.

SYRINGOMYELIA This is a term that refers to a cavity (from the Greek *syrinx*, meaning "pipe" or "tube"). The cavity occupies the central parts of the spinal cord in the cervical region but may extend upward into the medulla oblongata (syringobulbia) or downward into the thoracic or even lumbar segments. In approximately 5 percent of cases studied postmortem, an intramedullary tumor (hemangioblastoma or glioma) has been found in or near some part of the syrinx. The syrinx is independent of, but connected with, the central canal, replaces the gray matter of the posterior or anterior horns of the spinal cord, and interrupts the crossing pain and temperature fibers in the anterior commissure in several successive cord segments. The cavity is lined with astrocytic glia and a few thick-walled blood vessels. It may enlarge the spinal cord and the central canal is dilated. The CSF in the cavity always has a relatively low protein level unless a tumor is present.

The cause of the disease is unknown, but in about half of the cases is clearly linked to malformations such as the type I Chiari malformation (see Chap. 365) at the craniocervical junction. Familial incidence is rare. A blastomatous formation akin to tuberous sclerosis or central von Recklinghausen's disease but with a tendency for the abnormal tissue to cavitate is one explanation. A hydromyelia, sometimes associated with hydrocephalus in early life, may through continuous movement and injury of the cervical segments of the spinal cord, result in diverticulation of the central canal. However, hydromyelia is absent in another group of cases of syringomyelia. It has been postulated that a Chiari formation or some other anomaly at the craniospinal junction that prevents opening of the foramen of Magendie and directs the ventricular pressure into the central canal of the spinal cord may contribute to the development of syringomyelia. But this could not apply to all cases, for in many autopsied cases the upper spinal canal is atretic or occluded.

The clinical triad upon which the diagnosis is based consists of (1) segmental sensory loss or dissociation (loss of pain and temperature sense and preservation of sense of touch) over neck, shoulders, and arms, (2) amyotrophy, and (3) thoracic scoliosis. Symptoms may begin in late childhood and adolescence, but more often in adult life, and progress irregularly, often being arrested for long periods of time. The segmental sensory loss or dissociation and amyotrophy are caused by cavitation, destruction, and stretching of the ventral commissural fibers and by extension of the cavity into the anterior and posterior horns. Analgesia and thermoanesthesia account for painless ulcers, injuries, and burns; Charcot joints, also seen rarely in this disease, result from repeated injury of the denervated joint tissue. Areflexia without atrophy may be due to involvement of the afferent as well as efferent limbs of the reflex arc, but destruction of anterior horn cells is the more frequent cause, particularly if accompanied by muscle atrophy. A useful clinical rule is that a neurologic disease which leaves all deep tendon reflexes in the arms intact is usually not syringomyelia. Horner's syndrome on the affected side may result from involvement of cells of the intermediolateral cell column of the first and second thoracic segments of the spinal cord. Occipitocervical pain intensified by cough and aching or burning pains in the neck or arms is a troublesome complaint in a third of the patients. Pyramidal tract signs in the legs tend to appear late in the disease course and are attributable to extension of the syrinx into the lateral columns of the cord to interrupt the corticospinal tracts. They are also related to the Chiari malformation, which may compress the upper cervical cord segments. If the cavity enlarges the spinal cord, a spinal subarachnoid block may result, and prolonged pressure may cause widening of the spinal canal and erosion of pedicles. The kyphoscoliosis, which may antedate other evidence of disease by several years, is thought to result from asymmetric weakness of paravertebral muscles. Short neck and dysplastic features, atlantoaxial fusion, basilar invagination, and bifid or fused vertebrae are congenital abnormalities of the spine and base of skull that are found in about one-third of the patients.

A syrinx in the brainstem (syringobulbia) usually extends into the lateral tegmentum of the medulla, being so placed as to result in nystagmus and sensory impairment over one or both sides of the face. Unilateral palatal and vocal cord paralysis, as well as weakness and atrophy of one side of the tongue, are other clinical signs which call attention to lesions at this level of the neuraxis. Syringobulbia never occurs without syringomyelia.

The association of cavitation of the spinal cord with myelomeningocele (so-called myelodysplasia), Arnold-Chiari malformation, platybasia, and other congenital defects about the cervicocranial junction are commented on in Chap. 365. The diagnosis is confirmed in the majority of patients by the radiologic demonstration of spinal abnormalities, an abnormal myelogram showing obstruction below the foramen magnum (patient must be supine), and in a few instances by a body CT scan showing an enlarged cervical cord with central cavitation.

The treatment of syringomyelia is far from satisfactory. The fact that the disease process may remain stationary for some months or years before progressing makes evaluation of any mode of therapy difficult. Decompression of a distended syrinx and Chiari malformation up to the foramen magnum alleviates or prevents progression of the symptoms and signs resulting from local compression of ascending and descending spinal tracts, but relief is not always lasting. The spinal cord symptoms due to the syringomyelia have responded the least, according to Logue and Edwards. Reducing the pressure within the cavity by occluding the upper end of the central canal, opening it, or making a ventriculosubarachnoid shunt has given unpredictable results. X-ray treatment, based on the belief that symptoms result from gliomatous malformation of the cord which subsequently cavitates, is probably worthless, unless there is an underlying tumor. As matters now stand all patients should have a myelogram, and if a Chiari malformation is present, the cervical cord and medulla should be decompressed.

OTHER SYNDROMES CAUSING ASYMMETRIC WEAKNESS OF LEGS, SENSORY LOSS (ATAXIA), AND SPHINCTERIC DISTURBANCES

Here a miscellany of diseases (vascular malformations, chronic adhesive arachnoiditis following spinal anesthesia, and infections and metabolic and nutritional diseases, etc.) would have to be considered, but only spinal cord tumors will be discussed.

SPINAL CORD TUMORS Space-occupying lesions within the spinal canal can be conveniently divided into two groups: (1) those which arise within the substance of the spinal cord and invade and destroy tracts and central gray structures (intramedullary) and (2) those outside the spinal cord (extramedullary), either in the vertebral bodies and epidural tissues (extradural), or in the meninges, or roots (intradural). The relative frequency of spinal tumors in these different locations in a general hospital is about 5 percent intramedullary, 40 percent intradural-extramedullary, and 55 percent extradural. The percentage of extradural lesions in a general hospital population is usually higher than in most neurosurgical services, which often do not include many of the lymphomas, metastatic carcinomas, etc., most of which are extradural.

The cellular origin of the intramedullary gliomas has been mentioned in the section on intracerebral tumors. The proportions of the different cell types differ, however. Ependymoma makes up 40 percent of the cases, and the remainder are more or less evenly distributed among astrocytomas, glioblastomas, hemangiomas, and hemangioblastomas. The hemangioma is the common source of spontaneous hematomyelia, and the hemangioblastoma may give rise to a syringomyelia. Of the intradural-extramedullary tumors, neurofibromas and meningiomas are the most common.

Symptomatology Patients with spinal cord tumor are likely to manifest one of two clinical pictures: either a purely sensorimotor spinal tract and rarely a syringomyelic syndrome or a radicular-spinal syndrome, nearly always painful.

Compression of sensorimotor spinal tracts The predominant clinical syndrome relates to spinal cord compression. With intraspinal tumors, the onset of the compressive symptoms is usually gradual over a period of weeks and months, and the course is progressive. The initial disturbance is likely to be motor, and often the distribution is asymmetric. With cervical lesions the order of motor impairment is first the arm, then the ipsilateral and contralateral leg, and finally the opposite arm. With thoracic lesions one leg usually becomes weak and stiff before the other one. Subjective sensory symptoms (tingling paresthesias) of spinal tract involvement take the same pattern. Pain and temperature are more likely to be affected than touch, vibration and position senses and are contralateral to the maximum motor weakness (Brown-Séquard syndrome). Nevertheless the posterior columns are also frequently involved. Voluntary control over bladder and bowel usually becomes diminished coincident with motor paralysis of the legs. If the compression is relieved, there is recovery from these sensorimotor symptoms often in the reverse order of their affection. The first part affected is the last to recover, and sensory symptoms disappear before motor.

Compressive-irritative radicular symptoms This syndrome of spinal cord compression is often combined with radicular pain, i.e., pain in the distribution of a spinal root. It is described as knifelike or as merely a dull ache with superimposed sharp pains which are intensified by cough, sneeze, or strain and with radiation in a distal direction, i.e., away from the spine. Segmental sensory changes (paresthesias, hyperalgesia, impairment of pain and touch) or motor disturbances (spasm, cramp, twitching, atrophy, fascicular twitching, and loss of tendon reflex) and an ache in the spine are the usual manifestations of a compressive-irritative lesion of roots. Tenderness of spinous processes over the growth is found in half the patients. These segmental changes, particularly the sensory ones, often precede the signs of spinal cord compression by months or years if the lesion is benign. Sphincter disturbances usually appear late.

The clinical findings are (1) spastic weakness of the legs, in one leg more than in the other, with thoracolumbar lesions, and of the arms and legs with cervical lesions, (2) a sensory level for pain on the trunk below which pain sense is reduced or lost, (3) posterior column signs, and (4) a spastic bladder under weak voluntary control.

The diagnosis is established by x-rays of the spine (erosion of vertebrae, widened spinal canal), lumbar puncture, and electromyography to demonstrate the fasciculations and denervation resulting from involvement of motor roots. The most important diagnostic test of all is contrast myelography for the direct visualization of the compressive lesion. A CT body scan obtained with metrizamide injection into the subarachnoid space provides accurate localization of the lesion. Occasionally lumbar puncture may exacerbate the symptoms and signs.

Special spinal syndromes Unusual clinical syndromes may be found in patients with tumors near the foramen magnum. They may produce a quadriparesis with pains in the back of the head and stiff neck, a weakness and atrophy of the hands and dorsal neck muscles, and either bizarre sensory changes or no sensory loss whatsoever. Lesions of the tenth, eleventh, and twelfth thoracic and the first lumbar vertebrae may result in a curious syndrome of mixed cauda equina and spinal cord symptoms. *Lesions of the cauda equina* alone, always difficult to separate from those of the plexus and multiple nerves, are usually attended in the early stages with pain (present in 80 percent of cases, especially at night, and worsened by jolting) which is variously combined with an asymmetric, atrophic, areflexic paralysis, radicular sensory loss, and later sphincteric disorder (see Fearnsides and Adams). This must be distinguished from *tumors of the conus medullaris* (lower sacral segments of spinal cord) in which there are early disturbances of sphincters of the bladder and bowel, back pain, hypesthesia, and anesthesia over the sacral dermatomes, a lax anal sphincter with loss of anal and bulbocavernosus reflexes, and sometimes weakness of gluteal and hamstring muscles. A Babinski sign means that the spinal cord is involved above the third lumbar segment. Pain and stiffness of the back may precede signs of spinal cord disease or dominate the clinical picture in some extramedullary tumors. Extravertebral (presacral or pelvic) tumors such as neuroblastomas, rhabdomyosarcomas, carcinomas of cervix or body of uterus, or prostatic carcinomas may simulate the conus medullaris syndrome.

Pathology, anatomy, and physiology Peculiarities of anatomic structure are decisive factors in determining the symptomatology of tumor growths. The structure of the spine is described in Chap. 6, "Pain in the Back and Neck." Epidural growths arise from hematogenous deposits or tumors which extend from the vertebral bodies or from extraspinal spaces through intervertebral foramens.

Intramedullary growths not only invade but also compress and distort fasciculi in the adjacent white matter. As the cord enlarges from the tumor growing within it or is compressed from a tumor growing without, the free space around the cord is consumed and the CSF below the lesion becomes isolated or loculated from the rest of the CSF above. This can be demonstrated by a positive Queckenstedt test, Froin's syndrome of xanthochromia and clotting of CSF, and interruption of the flow of a contrast medium in the subarachnoid space (myelogram).

Differential diagnosis Several problems may arise in the diagnosis of patients with spinal cord tumors. In the early stages spinal tumor must be distinguished from other diseases which cause pain over certain segments of the body, i.e., those affecting the gallbladder, kidney, stomach and intestinal tract, pleura, etc. Here the localization of the pain to a dermatome, its intensification by effort, segmental sensory changes, and minor alterations of motor, reflex, or sensory function in the legs will usually provide the clues to the compressive-irritative radicular lesion. Examination of the CSF, x-ray of the spine, bone scan, and myelography will settle the diagnosis in most instances.

If symptoms and signs of disorder of sensory and motor tracts of the spinal cord are present, there is still the problem of locating the segmental level of the lesion. At first the sensory and motor deficiencies may be more pronounced in those parts of the body farthest removed from the lesion, i.e., in feet or lumbosacral segments. Later these sensory and motor levels may ascend, but at any time they may continue to be far below the lesion. Of greatest help in determining the level of the lesion are the locality of the root pains and atrophic paralysis and lastly the upper level of hypalgesia.

Once vertebral and segmental levels are settled, there is still the necessity of determining whether the lesion is neoplastic and extradural, intradural-extramedullary, or intramedullary. This is important from the standpoint of etiologic diagnosis. If there is a visible or palpable spinal deformity, positive bone scan, or x-ray evidence of vertebral destruction, one may confidently assume an extradural localization. Without x-ray changes one still suspects extradural lesion if root pain developed early and is bilateral, spine ache is prominent, and percussion tenderness is marked, if motor symptoms below the lesions precede sensory changes, and sphincter disturbances are late. To distinguish clinically between intradural-extramedullary and intramedullary lesions is almost impossible. Radicular pain, asymmetry of signs of motor and sensory tract involvement, and early CSF blockage (positive Queckenstedt test and high protein) favor the extramedullary localization. With extradural lesions one must differentiate between ruptures of disk, spondylosis (hypertrophic spurring and osteophyte formation in cervical spinal canal), tuberculous caries, other pyogenic, fungous, and syphilitic granulomatous lesions, metastatic carcinoma, and lymphoma. With intradural-extramedullary lesions, meningioma, neurofibroma, meningeal carcinomatosis, cholesteatoma, teratomatous cyst, or meningomyelitic process is most likely. Intramedullary lesions are usually gliomas or vascular malformations. A normal or relatively low protein in the CSF, and a negative myelogram will serve to rule out intraspinal tumors or granulomatous lesions in most instances.

Treatment This varies with the nature of the lesion and the clinical condition of the patient. Intradural-extramedullary tumors should be removed. Laminectomy, decompression, sometimes surgical enucleation of tumor, marsupialization of cysts, and x-ray therapy are the treatment of intramedullary gliomas. Intramedullary ependymomas may in some instances be removed (Fisher and Mansuy). Extradural malignant growths are best managed by the use of opiates for pain, *x-ray therapy,* endocrine therapy (for carcinoma of breast and prostate), or chemotherapy. Sometimes laminectomy and decompression are necessary for diagnosis and prevention of irreversible compressive effects and infarction of the spinal cord. However, Posner and his associate (Greenberg et al.) have shown that the outcome from medical therapy differs little from that of surgical therapy. This statement is said to apply to both lymphoma and metastatic carcinoma, but in the authors' experience there are exceptions. With tuberculous caries, immobilization of the spine in hyperextension and antituberculous therapy are indicated, and laminectomy should be reserved for exceptional cases with complete and irreversible spinal block. For spondylosis, surgery (extradural decompression) is advised if there are serious neurologic deficits. Syndromes of lesser severity or elderly patients with other important diseases may best be treated with a Thomas collar to immobilize the spine.

In conclusion it is always well to remind oneself that of the more than 30 diseases of the spinal cord, there are available effective means of treating only a few—spondylosis, extramedullary spinal cord tumors, syphilis (meningomyelitis and tabes), epidural granulomas (pyogenic, tuberculous, fungous), subacute combined degeneration, and nutritional myelopathy. The physician's major responsibility is to determine whether the patient has one of the treatable diseases.

INJURIES TO SPINAL ROOTS, PLEXUSES, AND PERIPHERAL NERVES See Chaps. 6 and 368.

REFERENCES

Baker AS et al: Spinal epidural abscess. N Engl J Med 293:463, 1975
Enberg RN, Kaplan JR: Spinal epidural abscess in children. Clin Pediatr 13:247, 1974
Fearnsides MR, Adams CBT: Tumors of cauda equina. J Neurol Neurosurg Psychiatry 41:24, 1978
Fisher G, Mansuy L Total removal of intramedullary ependymomas. Surg Neurol 14:243, 1980
Gillingham FJ et al: Acute cervical spinal cord injury. Early management and long term results. Acta Neurochir 41:73, 1978
Greenberg HS et al: Epidural spinal cord compression from metastatic tumor: Results with new treatment proposal. Ann Neurol 8:361, 1980
Hoehn MM, Cherington M: Spinal myoclonus. Neurology 27:942, 1977
Hughes JT: Spinal cord involvement by C4–5 vertebral subluxation in rheumatoid arthritis. Ann Neurol 1:575, 1977
Kuhn WG Jr: Care and rehabilitation of patients with injuries to the spinal cord and cauda equina: Preliminary report on 113 cases. J Neurosurg 4:40, 1947
Logue V, Edwards MR: Syringomyelia and its surgical treatment. J Neurol Neurosurg Psychiatry 44:273, 1981
Prather GC, Mayfield FH: *Injuries of the Spinal Cord.* Springfield, Ill., Charles C Thomas, 1953
Schlick H, Stille D: Clinical symptomatology of intraspinal tumors, in *Handbook of Clinical Neurology,* vol 19: *Tumors of the Spine and Spinal Cord,* PJ Vinken, GW Bruyn (eds). Amsterdam, North-Holland, 1975
Wyburn-Mason R: *Vascular Abnormalities and Tumors of the Spinal Cord.* London, Kimpton, 1943

367 DISEASES OF THE CRANIAL NERVES

MAURICE VICTOR
RAYMOND D. ADAMS

The cranial nerves are susceptible to many diseases that rarely if ever affect the spinal peripheral nerves, and for that reason alone they deserve to be considered separately. Reference has already been made to some of these diseases in Chaps. 17 and 18. But there the emphasis was on the cardinal manifestations of disordered cranial nerve function and the ways of demonstrating them. Here we are concerned with the principal syndromes by which the cranial nerve disorders express themselves and the diseases which cause them.

SYNDROME OF ANOSMIA AND AGEUSIA AND RELATED DISORDERS OF OLFACTION The delicate filaments of the olfactory nerve pass from the nasal mucous membrane through the cribriform plate of the ethmoid bone to the olfactory bulbs and thence to central structures concerned with olfactory perception. Disturbances in olfaction, which are not numerous, may be subdivided into three groups, as follows:

1 Quantitative abnormalities: reduction (hyposmia, anosmia) and increase (hyperosmia).
2 Qualitative abnormalities: distorted smell (dysosmia or parosmia)
3 Illusions and hallucinations caused by local diseases in the nose, central neurologic diseases, or psychiatric conditions

Unlike vision and hearing there is no easy way of quantitating the sense of smell. The Elsberg olfactomotor used years ago proved to be too capricious and clumsy a method. The usual way of demonstrating the olfactory defect is to ask the patient to sniff a nonirritating scent first with one nostril occluded, then the other. Vanilla, lemon, scented soap, tobacco, and coffee can be distinguished by most people, though not always named correctly. Biopsies of the nasal mucosa reveal the state of the receptor elements and the presence of nasal diseases. Douek has discussed these methods and the differing olfactory capacities of males and females (in smelling the lactone, exaltolide) in the various periods of the life cycle.

Unilateral anosmia is rarely a complaint. Only by the separate testing of smell in each nostril can it be recognized. Bilateral anosmia, on the other hand, does bring patients to medical attention. Interestingly, the usual complaint is of a loss of taste (ageusia), for the reason that taste to a large extent depends on the volatile substances in food, and the sensation of flavor is a combination of smell and taste. Such patients retain the capacity to differentiate perfectly the elementary taste sensations of sweet, sour, bitter, and salty.

Regarding the nasal diseases responsible for bilateral hyposmia or anosmia the most frequent are those in which hypertrophy and hyperemia of the nasal mucosa block access of olfactory stimuli to the receptor cells. Heavy cigarette smoking, it is said, is the most frequent cause of anosmia. Chronic rhinitis of allergic, vasomotor, or infective types are common causes, and it is known that metabolic disorders and hormones may also induce congestion and swelling of the nasal mucosa. In cases of allergic rhinitis, biopsies of the nasal mucosa have shown that the sensory epithelial cells are still present, but their cilia are shortened and deformed, and are buried under surrounding mucosal cells. The occurrence of a permanent hyposmia or anosmia may follow influenza, viz., *postinfluenzal anosmia.* In this instance the sensory epithelium of the olfactory zone is destroyed by the virus and replaced by respiratory epithelial and goblet cells and scar tissue. There is also a group, quite rare, of congenital anosmias, one type of which is associated with an hypothalamic defect (Kallman's syndrome of congenital anosmia with hypogonadotropic hypogonadism). Another type of congenital anosmia occurs in albinos. The receptor cells are present but are hypoplastic, lack cilia, and do not project above the surrounding supporting cells.

Aberrations of smell may follow basal skull fractures and accompany intracranial lesions such as ethmoid tumors and nasal meningoceles. *Cranial trauma* is followed by uni- or bilateral impairment of smell in 5 to 10 percent of cases. Frontal injuries and fractures disrupt the ethmoid plate and the olfactory axons which perforate it. Sometimes there is an associated cerebrospinal fluid (CSF) rhinorrhea resulting from a tearing of the dura overlying the paranasal sinuses. If the anosmia is unilateral, it is usually on the side of the CSF leak, and this fact aids in localization of the fistula. Anosmia may also follow blows to the occiput or operations in the posterior fossa, performed in the semireclining position which allow the frontal lobes and olfactory bulbs to pull away from the orbital surface of the skull. Once traumatic anosmia develops it is usually permanent; only about 10 percent ever improve or recover. Perversion of the sense of smell may occur as a phase in the recovery process. *Meningioma* of the inferior frontal region is the most frequent neoplastic cause of anosmia (one-half of Cushing's series), and another cause is glioma of the frontal lobe. Occasionally pituitary adenomas, craniopharyngiomas, suprasellar meningiomas, and aneurysms of the anterior part of the circle of Willis extend forward and damage olfactory structures. These tumors and hamartomas may also induce seizures in some of which there may be olfactory hallucinations, indicating involvement of the uncus.

Parosmia and *dysosmia* are terms used to designate subjective distortions of olfactory perception. Strictly speaking, dysosmia is an olfactory illusion. As already stated this may be a feature of an intranasal disease that partially impairs smell, or it may represent a phase in the recovery from a neurogenic anosmia. Most parosmic disturbances consist of disagreeable or foul odors, and they may be accompanied by distortions of taste. Such distortions, according to Zilstaff, have been observed in schizophrenic and neurosyphilitic patients and in middle-aged individuals, mostly women, without known nasal or other disease or parageusia. Dysosmia may also be a symptom in elderly patients with depression. Every article of food has an extemely unpleasant odor *(cacosmia).* Sensations of disagreeable taste are often added *(cacogeusia).* Little is known of the physiologic basis of the perversions of smell sensation. In idiopathic cases small doses of $ZnSO_4$, given orally, are claimed to be beneficial. Minor degrees of parosmia are not necessarily abnormal, for unpleasant odors have a way of lingering for several hours and of being reawakened by other olfactory stimuli, as every pathologist knows (phantosmia).

A patient who claims to be smelling an odor that no one else can smell (no objective stimulus) and who is convinced of its presence and personal reference has an *olfactory hallucination.* Aside from alcohol withdrawal, in which olfactory hallucinations are occasionally associated with other types of hallucinations, and uncal seizures, in which they are brief and clearly related to a derangement of consciousness and other epileptic components, olfactory hallucinations usually signify a psychiatric disease. A huge range of odors may be reported, most of them foul. Some patients perceive the smell as emanating from themselves (intrinsic hallucinations). Others perceive the source to be external (extrinsic). Both types vary in intensity and are remarkable with respect to their indefatigability. According to Pryse-Phillips, who catalogued the psychiatric illnesses in 137 patients with olfactory hallucinations, most were associated with schizophrenia and depressive illnesses. In schizophrenia, where the hallucinations are seldom dominant, the stimulus was usually interpreted as arising externally and intending to harm the patient. In patients with depressions and olfactory delusions of reference, the hallucinations most often come from their own body and dominate the patient's thought processes. All manner of ways may be used to get rid of the stench, the usual ones being excessive washing, deodorants, and social withdrawal. In all these psychiatric states the senses of smell and taste are notably intact.

SYNDROME OF RETROBULBAR NEUROPATHY The acute development of impaired vision in one eye or both eyes (in the latter case the eyes may be affected either simultaneously or successively) gives rise to a number of interesting and troublesome problems. The most frequent clinical setting is one in which a child, adolescent, or young adult notes a rapid diminution of vision in one eye (as though a veil or haze covered every object seen). The condition may progress to complete blindness within a few days. The optic disc and retina may appear normal, but in some cases the optic disc is elevated or "choked" and the disc margins are obscure and surrounded by hemorrhages (papilledema). This latter condition, called papillitis, is distinguished from the papilledema of increased intracranial pressure by the effect on visual acuity. In retrobulbar neuropathy there is often pain on movement of or pressure on the eye. After some few days or weeks the other eye may become similarly involved, the blindness then being complete except for slight peripheral vision. The pupillary light reflex is impaired. In a high percentage of patients, no cause can be found, and after several more weeks there is spontaneous recovery. Vision returns to normal in the majority of instances; sometimes a scotoma is left, or even blindness. The optic disc later becomes slightly pale in many of the patients. The CSF may be normal or may contain from 10 to 200 lymphocytes, and the protein content, particularly the gamma globulin portion, may be increased.

A considerable number of such patients (15 to 35 percent) will develop other symptoms and signs consistent with multiple sclerosis within 10 to 15 years, and even more will do so if the patients are observed for longer periods. Less is known about children with retrobulbar neuropathy, but the prognosis for them is considerably better than that for adults. Formerly the syndrome was blamed on sinusitis and treated as such, but Cushing long ago proved the error of the assumption. Sinus disease only rarely affects vision except for an occasional mucocele which presses on an ocular or optic nerve. Demyelinative disease is the only common cause of a unilateral retrobulbar neuritis; regression of symptoms may be hastened by the administration of ACTH or corticosteroids (see Chap. 361).

Other causes of *unilateral optic neuropathy* include postinfectious encephalomyelitis, posterior uveitis (sometimes with reticulum-cell sarcoma), vascular lesions of the optic nerve, and tumors (glioma of optic nerve, von Recklinghausen's neurofibromatosis, meningioma, metastatic carcinoma, and fungus infections).

Simultaneous impairment of vision in the two eyes, with central or centrocecal scotomas, usually is due not to a demyelinative process but to a toxic or nutritional disorder. The former condition (so-called tobacco-alcohol amblyopia) is observed most commonly in the chronic alcoholic patient (see Chap. 363). Impairment of visual acuity evolves over several days or weeks, and examination discloses bilateral, roughly symmetric central or centrocecal scotomas, the peripheral fields being intact. With appropriate therapy (nutritious diet and B vitamins), partial or complete recovery is possible, although some patients are left with a permanent defect in central vision and pallor of the temporal portions of the optic discs. The same disorder may be seen in nonalcoholic patients, under conditions of severe nutritional deprivation and in pernicious anemia. Impairment of vision due to *methyl alcohol intoxication* is more abrupt in onset and is characterized by large symmetric central scotomas, as well as by symptoms of systemic disease and acidosis (see Chap. 242). Treatment is directed mainly to correction of the acidosis. A list of other drugs having a toxic effect on the optic nerve has been compiled by Leibold; included are chloramphenicol, ethambutol, isoniazid, streptomycin, sulfonamides, digitalis, ergot, disulfiram (Antabuse), and heavy metals.

Isolated optic atrophies have been described in degenerative diseases. There are several types, the most frequent being Leber's disease, dominant congenital or early infantile optic atrophy, and optic atrophy with diabetes mellitus and deafness (see Glaser). Rarely amblyopia is due to cranial arteritis, some other vascular disease, or diabetes. In the adult syphilitic meningitis may lead to optic neuritis and atrophy (see Chaps. 177 and 364).

Migraine may cause transient blindness, sometimes without headache.

SYNDROME OF BITEMPORAL HEMIANOPSIA This type of visual disorder is usually related to a pituitary adenoma (ballooned sella shown in skull films) but may also be due to a craniopharyngioma, saccular aneurysms of the circle of Willis, meningioma of the tuberculum sellae (normal sella or thickened tuberculum by radiography), and rarely sarcoidosis, metastatic carcinoma, and Hand-Schüller-Christian disease. The lesion is always in the chiasm, involving the decussating nasal fibers from each retina.

SYNDROMES OF HOMONYMOUS HEMIANOPSIA See Chap. 17.

SYNDROME OF VISUAL AGNOSIA See Chap. 24.

SYNDROME OF OPHTHALMOPLEGIA Rarely, children or adults may have one or more attacks of ocular palsy in conjunction with an otherwise typical migraine (*migrainous ophthalmoplegia*). The muscles innervated by the oculomotor or, less often, the abducens nerve are affected. Presumably, intense vascular spasm in branches of the ophthalmic artery causes a transitory ischemia of nerve. Arteriograms, done after the onset of the palsy, usually reveal no abnormality. Recovery is the rule.

The acute development of a sixth or third nerve palsy on one side is a relatively common occurrence in the adult. An isolated sixth nerve palsy frequently proves to be due to neoplasm—pontine glioma in children and metastatic tumor from the nasopharynx in adults. In third nerve lesions due to compression by aneurysm, tumor, or temporal lobe herniation, enlargement of the pupil is an early sign, because of the peripheral location of the pupilloconstrictor fibers. Infarction of the third nerve, as occurs in diabetes mellitus or, rarely, in cranial arteritis, spares the pupil. In more than half the patients with isolated sixth or third nerve palsies no cause can be assigned; fortunately, most of them recover in a few weeks to months. Acute palsy of the fourth nerve is relatively uncommon; usually it is due to trauma. Exophthalmic ophthalmoplegia and myasthenia gravis must always be ruled out. Combined unilateral ocular palsies of painful type (Tolosa-Hunt syndrome) is indicative of parasellar granuloma. An acute onset of bilateral opthalmoplegia, visual loss, and drowsiness occurs in pituitary apoplexy.

The slow development of a complete ophthalmoplegia on one side is most often due to an aneurysm (may also be of acute onset), tumor, or inflammatory process in the cavernous sinus or at the superior orbital foramen (syndrome of Foix) (see Table 367-1).

Gaze palsies or mixed ophthalmoplegia and gaze palsies, due usually to vascular, demyelinative, or neoplastic processes in the brainstem, are discussed in Chap. 17.

SYNDROME OF FACIAL PAIN (TRIGEMINAL NEURALGIA, TIC DOULOUREUX) The most striking disorder of the trigeminal nerve is tic douloureux. This occurs in middle-aged and elderly persons and consists of excruciating paroxysms of pain in the lips, gums, cheek, or chin, and, very rarely, in the distribution of the ophthalmic division of the fifth nerve. The pain seldom lasts more than a few seconds or a minute or two but may be so intense that the patient winces; hence the term *tic*. The paroxysm recurs frequently, both day and night, for several weeks at a time. Another characteristic feature is the initiation of pain by obvious stimuli applied to certain areas on the face, lips, or tongue, or by movement of these parts, the so-called trigger zones. Sensory loss cannot be demonstrated. In studying the relation between stimuli applied to the trigger zone and the pain paroxysm, it is found that the adequate stimulus for precipitating an attack is touch and possibly tickle, rather than pain or temperature. Usually a spatial and temporal summation of impulses is necessary to trigger an attack, which is followed by a refractory period of up to 2 or 3 min. This suggests that the mechanism for the paroxysmal pain involves the nucleus of the spinal root of the fifth nerve.

The diagnosis of this disorder rests upon these strict clinical criteria, and the condition must be distinguished from other forms of facial and cephalic neuralgia and pain arising from diseases of the jaw, teeth, or sinuses. Tic douloureux is usually without assignable cause, although occasionally it is a manifestation of multiple sclerosis (may be bilateral) or of herpes zoster. Very rarely a tumor, and to a degree that cannot be estimated, a redundant artery in the posterior fossa, causes an early irritative lesion in the nerve or its root and produces pain clinically indistinguishable from that of tic douloureux. Usually, however, space-occupying lesions, such as aneurysms, neurofibromas, or meningiomas, produce a loss of sensation.

The conventional treatment for tic douloureux is alcohol or phenol injection of the affected nerve at the foramen ovale and rotundum or section of the root of the trigeminal nerve between the ganglion and the brainstem. Stereotaxic electrolytic lesions have also been made. Antiepileptic drugs such as phenytoin (Dilantin) and dibenzazepine (Tegretol) have been found to suppress or shorten the duration of the attacks. Temporizing and using these drugs may permit a spontaneous remission to occur. Most of the patients with severe pain come to surgery.

Anesthesia and analgesia of the face may be induced by stilbamidine (formerly used in the treatment of kala azar and multiple myeloma) and by trichloracetic acid. Pain and itching may occur during recovery. An idiopathic form of benign trigeminal neuropathy has also been observed, and leprosy may involve these nerves.

Tonic spasm of the masticatory muscles, known as *trismus*, is symptomatic of tetanus, although it may occur in patients treated with phenothiazine drugs; lesser degrees may be associated with disease of the pharynx and temporomaxillary joint, the teeth, and gums.

SYNDROME OF FACIAL PALSY (BELL'S PALSY) AND FACIAL SPASM The seventh cranial nerve is mainly a motor nerve supplying all the muscles concerned with facial expression on one side. The sensory component is small (the nervus intermedius of Wrisberg); it conveys taste impulses from the anterior two-thirds of the tongue and probably cutaneous impulses from the anterior wall of the external auditory canal. The taste fibers traverse the lingual nerve (a branch of the mandibular) but then leave this nerve to join the chorda tympani. Secretomotor fibers innervate the lacrimal gland through the greater superficial petrosal nerve, and others travel to the sublingual and submaxillary glands via the chorda tympani.

Several other anatomic facts are worth remembering. The motor nucleus of the seventh nerve is anterior and lateral to the abducens nucleus, and in their intrapontine course the facial nerve fibers hook around the abducens nucleus before they emerge from the pons at a point just lateral to the corticospinal tract. After leaving the pons they enter the internal auditory meatus with the acoustic nerve. The facial nerve then bends sharply forward and downward around the anterior boundary of the vestibule of the inner ear. At this angle lies the sensory (geniculate) ganglion. The nerve continues its course in its own bony channel, the facial canal, and makes its exit from the skull at the stylomastoid foramen. It then passes through the parotid gland and subdivides to supply the facial muscles, the stylomastoid muscle, and the posterior belly of the digastric muscle. Within the facial canal, just distal to the geniculate ganglion, it gives off the branch to the sphenopalatine ganglion, i.e., the greater superficial petrosal nerve, and somewhat more distally it gives off a small branch to the stapedius muscle and is joined by the chorda tympani.

A complete interruption of the facial nerve at the stylomastoid foramen paralyzes all muscles of facial expression. The

TABLE 367-1
Cranial nerve syndromes

Site	*Cranial nerves involved*	*Eponymic syndrome*	*Usual cause*
Sphenoid fissure	III, IV, ophthalmic V, VI	Foix	Invasive tumors of sphenoid bone, aneurysms
Lateral wall of cavernous sinus	III, IV, ophthalmic V, VI, often with proptosis	Foix Tolosa-Hunt	Aneurysms or thrombosis of cavernous sinus, invasive tumors from sinuses and sella turcica, sometimes benign granuloma responsive to steroids
Retrosphenoid space	II, III, IV, V, VI	Jacod	Large tumors of middle cranial fossa
Apex of petrous bone	V, VI	Gradenigo	Petrositis, tumors of petrous bone
Internal auditory meatus	VII, VIII		Tumors of petrous bone (dermoids, etc.), infectious processes, acoustic neuroma
Pontocerebellar angle	V, VII, VIII, and sometimes IX		Acoustic neuromas, meningiomas
Jugular foramen	IX, X, XI	Vernet	Tumors and aneurysms
Posterior laterocondylar space	IX, X, XI, XII	Collet-Sicard	Tumors of parotid gland, carotid body, and secondary tumor
Posterior retroparotid space	IX, X, XI, XII, and Bernard-Horner syndrome	Villaret Mackenzie Tapia	Tumors of parotid gland, carotid body, secondary tumor, lymph node tumors, tuberculous adenitis

corner of the mouth droops, the creases and skin folds are effaced, the forehead is unfurrowed, and the palpebral fissure is conspicuous because the eyelids will not close. Upon attempted closure of the lids, the eye on the paralyzed side is seen to roll upward (Bell's phenomenon). The lower lid sags also, and the punctum falls away from the conjunctiva, permitting tears to spill over the cheek. Food collects between the teeth and lips, and saliva may dribble from the corner of the mouth. The patient complains of a heaviness or numbness in the face, but no sensory loss is demonstrable and taste is intact.

If the lesion is in the facial canal above the junction of the facial nerve with the chorda tympani but below the geniculate ganglion, all the above symptoms occur and, in addition, taste is lost over the anterior two-thirds of the tongue on the same side. If the nerve to the stapedius is paralyzed, there is hyperacusis (painful sensitivity to loud sounds), and the sound produced by moving the jaw and facial muscles is no longer present in the ear on the affected side. If the geniculate ganglion or the motor root proximal to it is involved, lacrimation may be reduced. Lesions at this point may also affect the adjacent auditory nerve, causing deafness, tinnitus, or dizziness. Intrapontine lesions that paralyze the face usually affect the abducens nucleus and often the corticospinal and sensory tracts.

If the peripheral facial paralysis has existed for some time and return of motor function has begun but is incomplete, a kind of contracture (actually a continuous diffuse contraction) of facial muscles may appear. The palpebral fissure becomes narrowed and the nasolabial fold deepens. Attempts to move one group of facial muscles result in contraction of all of them (associated movements, or synkinesis). Facial spasms develop and persist indefinitely, being initiated by every facial movement (see below). Anomalous regeneration of the seventh nerve fibers may result in other curious disorders. If fibers originally connected with the orbicularis oculi become connected with the orbicularis oris, closure of the lids may cause a retraction of the mouth; or if fibers originally connected with muscles of the face later come to innervate the lacrimal gland, anomalous tearing (crocodile tears) may occur with any activity of the facial muscles, such as eating (Bogorad's syndrome). With the passage of time, the face and even the tip of the nose become pulled to the unaffected side.

The most common disease affecting the facial nerve is *Bell's palsy,* presumably due to an inflammatory reaction of undetermined type in or around the nerve near the stylomastoid foramen. The onset is acute, and maximum paralysis is usually attained by 48 h; pain behind the ear may have preceded the paralysis for a day or two. Occasionally taste sensation is lost, and more rarely hyperacusis is present. In some cases there is mild pleocytosis in the cerebrospinal fluid. Fully 80 percent of patients recover within a few weeks or months. Electromyographic evidence of denervation after 10 days indicates a long delay until regeneration occurs, and sometimes it is incomplete. Thus electromyography may be of value in distinguishing temporary conduction defects from a pathologic interruption in continuity of nerve fibers. Incomplete paralysis in the first week is the most favorable prognostic sign. Protection of the eye during sleep, massage of the weakened muscles, and a splint to prevent drooping of the lower part of the face are the measures generally employed in the management of such cases. The use of prednisone during the first week may be beneficial. Unroofing of the facial nerve in the facial canal has been suggested, but there is no evidence that this measure is helpful, and it may be harmful.

Tumors which invade the temporal bone (carotid body, cholesteatoma, dermoid) may produce a facial palsy, but the onset is insidious and the course progressive. The Ramsay Hunt syndrome, presumably due to herpes zoster of the geniculate ganglion, consists of a severe facial palsy associated with a vesicular eruption in the pharynx, external auditory canal, and other parts of the cranial integument; often the eighth cranial nerve is affected as well. Acoustic neuromas frequently involve the facial nerve. Vascular lesions or tumors are the common forms of pontine disease which may cause facial palsy. Bilateral facial paralysis (facial diplegia) occurs in acute idiopathic polyneuritis and in a variety of sarcoidosis known as *uveoparotid fever* (*Heerfordt's syndrome*). *Melkersson's syndrome* consists of a rarely encountered triad of recurrent facial paralysis, recurrent—and eventually permanent—facial (particularly labial) edema, and, less constantly, plication of the tongue. The cause is unknown. In the far east, leprosy frequently involves the facial nerve.

A curious disorder is the *facial hemiatrophy of Romberg.* It occurs mainly in females and is characterized by a disappearance of fat in the dermal and subcutaneous tissues on one side of the face. It usually begins in adolescence or early adult years and is slowly progressive. In its advanced form the face is gaunt and the skin is thin, wrinkled, and rather brown. The hair may turn white and fall out, and the sebaceous glands become atrophic. The muscles and bones are as a rule not involved. Sometimes it becomes bilateral. The condition is a form of lipodystrophy, and the localization within a dermatome suggests the operation of some neural factor of unknown nature. The treatment is transplantation of skin and subcutaneous fat by a plastic surgeon.

The facial muscles on one side may be affected by irregular clonic contractions of varying degree (*hemifacial spasm*). This condition may represent a transient or permanent sequela to a Bell's palsy but may also appear as a benign phenomenon in adults who have never had a Bell's palsy. Hemifacial spasm may also be due to an irritative lesion of the facial nerve (e.g., an acoustic neuroma, an aberrant artery which compresses the nerve and is relieved by surgery, or a basilar artery aneurysm). A fine fibrillary activity of the facial muscles (*facial myokemia*) may be caused by a plaque of multiple sclerosis. In the most common form, however, the cause and pathology are unknown. An involuntary recurrent spasm of both eyelids (*blepharospasm*) may occur in elderly persons as an isolated phenomenon or with varying degrees of spasm of the facial muscles. Relaxant and tranquilizing drugs are of little help, although in many cases this disorder may subside spontaneously. In very severe and persistent instances, the only effective treatment has been crushing of the branches of the facial nerve or nerve decompression (from vessels) intracranially.

Complete loss of taste, *ageusia,* may result from bilateral affection of the seventh cranial nerves but is more often due to damage of the lingual epithelium and taste buds (glossitis from fungal infections, drying, and atrophy). Dysgeusia, already mentioned above in connection with parosmia, is most often due to drug ingestion, the drug or some product thereof being excreted in the saliva.

All these forms of nuclear or peripheral facial palsy must be distinguished from the supranuclear type. In the latter the frontalis and orbicularis oculi muscles are involved less than those of the lower part of the face, since the upper facial muscles are innervated by corticobulbar pathways from both motor cortices, whereas the lower facial muscles are innervated only by the opposite hemisphere. In supranuclear lesions there may be a dissociation of emotional and voluntary facial movements, and often some degree of paralysis of the arm and leg or an aphasia (in dominant hemisphere lesions) is conjoined.

SYNDROME OF BENIGN RECURRENT VERTIGO AND MÉNIÈRE'S DISEASE *Ménière's disease,* or *Ménière's syndrome,* is the name applied to recurrent aural vertigo, accompanied by tinnitus and deafness. The latter symptoms may be absent during the initial attacks of vertigo, but they invariably appear as the disease progresses and are increased in severity during an acute attack. With milder forms of the syndrome the patient may complain more of head discomfort and of difficulty in concentration than of vertigo and may be considered neurotic. Provided that deafness is not complete, the recruitment phenomenon can be demonstrated (see Chap. 13).

Ménière's disease has its onset most frequently in the fifth decade of life, though younger adults and the elderly are not spared. The pathological changes in Ménière's disease are said to consist of a dilatation of the endolymphatic system which leads to a degeneration of the delicate vestibular and cochlear hair cells. The relation of these changes to paroxysmal disorder of labyrinthine function is unknown. During an acute attack, rest in bed is the most effective treatment, since the patient can usually find a position in which vertigo is minimal. Dimenhydrinate (Dramamine) or cyclizine (Marezine) in doses of 25 to 50 mg tid is useful in the more protracted cases. A low-salt diet is still used in treatment, but its value is difficult to judge. Mild sedative and hypnotic drugs may help the anxious patient between attacks. Usually the deafness is unilateral and progressive, and when it is complete, the vertiginous attacks cease. However, the course is variable, and if the attacks persist in a severe manner, permanent relief can be obtained by surgical destruction of the labyrinth or section of the vestibular portion of the eighth nerve intracranially.

Another disorder of labyrinthine function is characterized by the occurrence of paroxysmal vertigo and nystagmus with the assumption of certain critical positions of the head. This is the *positional vertigo of Bárany,* of the so-called benign paroxysmal type (see Chap. 13).

There are many other causes of aural vertigo, such as purulent labyrinthitis complicating meningitis, serous labyrinthitis due to infection of the middle ear, "toxic labyrinthitis" due to drug intoxication (e.g., from alcohol, quinine, streptomycin, gentamycin, and other antibiotics), motion sickness, trauma, and hemorrhage into the internal ear. In these instances the attacks of vertigo tend to last longer than in the recurrent form, but in other respects the symptoms are similar. Streptomycin or gentamycin may damage the fine hair cells of the vestibular end organs and cause a permanent disorder of equilibrium especially in older patients.

There has been described a dramatic clinical syndrome, characterized by the abrupt onset of severe vertigo, nausea, and vomiting, without tinnitus or hearing loss. The vertigo persists for several days or weeks, and labyrinthine function is permanently ablated on one side. Occlusion of the labyrinthine division of the internal auditory artery would logically explain this syndrome, but so far postmortem confirmation of this hypothesis has not been obtained.

Vertigo of vestibular nerve origin may occur with diseases that involve the nerve in the petrous bone or the cerebellopontine angle. Except that it is less severe and is less frequently paroxysmal, it has many of the characteristics of labyrinthine vertigo. The adjacent auditory division of the eighth cranial nerve may also be affected, which explains the frequent association of vertigo with tinnitus and deafness. The function of the eighth cranial nerve may be disturbed by tumors of the lateral recess (especially acoustic neuroma), as well as by meningeal inflammation in this region or, very rarely, by compression from an abnormal vessel.

Vestibular neuronitis and *benign recurrent vertigo* are the names that have been applied to a clinical syndrome which occurs mainly in middle aged and sometimes young adults or children and is characterized by the abrupt onset of vertigo, nausea, and vomiting, without impairment of hearing. The attacks are brief and leave the patient for some days with a mild positional vertigo. They may occur once or recur and vary in severity. The cause is unknown. The medical treatment is the same as for Ménière's disease.

A particular variety of paroxysmal vertigo of childhood affects children. The attacks occur in a setting of good health and are of sudden onset and brief duration. Pallor, sweating, and immobility are prominent manifestations, and occasionally vomiting and nystagmus occur. No relation to head posture or movement has been observed. The attacks are recurrent but tend to cease spontaneously after a period of several months or years. The outstanding abnormal finding is demonstrated by caloric testing, which shows impairment or loss of vestibular function, bilateral or unilateral, frequently persisting after the attacks have ceased. Cochlear function is unimpaired. The pathologic basis of this disorder has not been determined.

Cogan has described a peculiar syndrome in young adults, in which a nonsyphilitic interstitial keratitis is associated with vertigo, tinnitus, nystagmus, and rapidly progressive deafness. The prognosis for life and vision is good, but the deafness is usually permanent. The causation of Cogan's disease is not understood, although several patients later developed aortitis and a vasculitis that resembles periarteritis nodosa.

The question of *viral infections of cranial nerves* is always raised by these acute palsies of the facial, trigeminal, and auditory nerves, especially when the affection is bilateral, involves several nerves in combination, or is associated with pleocytosis of CSF. Actually, the only proven viral cause in this group of cases is that of herpes zoster, and search for this virus from cases of Bell's palsy or of vestibular neuronitis has not been rewarding. Since perceptive deafness, vertigo, and other disorders of cranial nerve function have been observed in conjunction with the parainfectious encephalomyelitis of varicella, measles, rubella, mumps, and scarlet fever and also with Landry-Guillain-Barré syndrome, an allergic cause must be considered. Nothing is known of the pathology of the peripheral lesion or of the localization of a virus in the nervous system in these diseases. We have studied a number of cases of acute bilateral facial palsy, and of unilateral facial palsy, numbness, and deafness or vertigo with pleocytosis of CSF, and have had no success in isolating the causative agent. There is no treatment other than symptomatic; fortunately the prognosis for complete recovery is excellent.

SYNDROME OF DEAFNESS See Chap. 17.

SYNDROME OF GLOSSOPHARYNGEAL NEURALGIA Glossopharyngeal neuralgia resembles trigeminal neuralgia in many respects. The pain is intense and paroxysmal; it originates in the throat, approximately in the tonsillar fossa. In some cases the pain is localized in the ear or may radiate from the throat to the ear, because of implication of the tympanic branch (Jacobson's nerve). Spasms of pain may be initiated by swallowing. There is no demonstrable sensory or motor deficit. A trial of phenytoin or dibenzazepine is the recommended therapy, but if this is unsuccessful, division of the nerve near the medulla is the treatment of choice.

Very rarely, herpes zoster may involve the glossopharyngeal nerve. One may occasionally observe a glossopharyngeal palsy in conjunction with vagus and accessory nerve palsies due to a tumor or aneurysm in the posterior fossa. Hoarseness due to vocal cord paralysis, some difficulty in swallowing, deviation of the soft palate to the sound side, anesthesia of the posterior wall of the pharynx, and weakness of the upper part of the trapezius and sternocleidomastoid muscles compose the syndrome (see Table 367-1, jugular foramen syndrome).

SYNDROME OF DYSPHAGIA AND DYSPHONIA Complete interruption of the intracranial portion of one vagus nerve results in a characteristic paralysis. The soft palate droops ipsilaterally and does not rise in phonation. There is loss of the gag reflex on the affected side, as well as of the "curtain movement" of the lateral wall of the pharynx, whereby the faucial pillars move medially as the palate rises in saying "ah." The voice is hoarse, slightly nasal, and the vocal cord lies immobile in the cadaveric position, i.e., midway between abduction and adduction. There may also be loss of sensibility at the external auditory meatus and back of the pinna. Usually no change in visceral function can be demonstrated.

Complete bilateral paralysis is said to be incompatible with life, and this is probably true if the nuclei are involved in the medulla by poliomyelitis or some other disease. However, in the cervical region, both vagi have been blocked with procaine (Novocain) for the treatment of intractable asthma, without mishap. The pharyngeal branches of both vagi may be affected in diphtheria; the voice has a nasal quality, and regurgitation of liquids through the nose occurs during the act of swallowing.

The vagus nerve may be implicated at the meningeal level by tumors and infectious processes and within the medulla by tumors and vascular lesions, e.g., the lateral medullary syndrome of Wallenberg, and by motor system disease. Herpes zoster may attack this nerve. Polymyositis and dermatomyositis, which cause hoarseness and dysphagia by direct involvement of laryngeal and pharyngeal muscles, may be confused with diseases of the vagus nerves. Also dysphagia is a symptom in some patients with myotonic dystrophy (see Chap. 32 for discussion of nonneurologic dysphagia).

The recurrent laryngeal nerves, especially the left, are most often damaged as a result of thoracic disease. Aneurysm of the aortic arch, an enlarged left atrium, and tumors of the mediastinum and bronchi are much more frequent causes of an isolated vocal cord palsy than are intracranial disorders.

When confronted with a case of laryngeal palsy, the physician must attempt to determine the site of the lesion. If it is intramedullary, there are usually other signs, such as ipsilateral cerebellar dysfunction, loss of pain and temperature sensation over the ipsilateral face and contralateral arm and leg, and ipsilateral Bernard-Horner syndrome. If the lesion is extramedullary, the glossopharyngeal and spinal accessory nerves are frequently involved (jugular foramen syndrome, see above). If it is extracranial in the posterior laterocondylar or retroparotid space, there may be a combination of ninth, tenth, eleventh, and twelfth cranial nerve palsies and Bernard-Horner syndrome. Combinations of these lower cranial nerve palsies have a variety of eponymic designations, listed in Table 367-1. If there is no sensory loss in the palate and pharynx, or no palatal weakness or dysphagia, the lesion is below the origin of the pharyngeal branches, which leave the vagus nerve high in

TABLE 367-2
Brainstem syndromes which involve cranial nerves

Eponym	*Site*	*Cranial nerve(s) involved*	*Tracts and nuclei involved*	*Signs*	*Usual cause*
Weber's syndrome	Base of midbrain	III	Corticospinal tract	Oculomotor palsy with crossed hemiplegia	Vascular occlusion, tumor, aneurysm
Claude's syndrome	Tegmentum of midbrain	III	Red nucleus and brachium conjunctivum	Oculomotor palsy with contralateral cerebellar ataxia and tremor	Vascular occlusion, tumor, aneurysm
Benedikt's syndrome	Tegmentum of midbrain	III	Red nucleus, corticospinal tract, and brachium conjunctivium	Oculomotor palsy with contralateral cerebellar ataxia, tremor, and corticospinal signs	Softening, hemorrhage, tuberculoma, tumor
Nothnagel's syndrome	Tectum of midbrain	Unilateral or bilateral III	Superior cerebellar peduncles	Ocular palsies, paralysis of gaze, and cerebellar ataxia	Tumor
Parinaud's syndrome	Tectum of midbrain	Supranuclear mechanism for upward gaze	High midbrain tegmentum, in region of posterior commissure	Paralysis of upward and sometimes downward gaze; fixed pupils, divergence of eyes	Pinealoma
Millard-Gubler syndrome and Raymond-Foville syndrome	Base of pons	VII and often VI	Corticospinal tract	Facial and abducens palsy and contralateral hemiplegia; sometimes palsy of gaze to side of lesion	Softening or tumor
Avellis's syndrome	Tegmentum of medulla	X	Corticospinal tract Sometimes descending pupillary fibers, with Bernard-Horner syndrome	Paralysis of soft palate and vocal cord and contralateral hemiplegia	Softening or tumor
Jackson's syndrome	Tegmentum of medulla	X, XIII	Corticospinal tract	Avellis' syndrome plus ipsilateral tongue paralysis	Softening or tumor
Wallenberg's syndrome	Tegmentum of medulla	Spinal V, IX, X, XI	Lateral spinothalamic tract Descending pupillodilator fibers Spinocerebellar and olivocerebellar tracts	Ipsilateral V, IX, X, XI palsy, Bernard-Horner syndrome, and cerebellar ataxia Contralateral loss of pain and temperature sense	Occlusion of vertebral or posterior inferior cerebellar

the cervical region. The usual site of disease is then the mediastinum.

SYNDROME OF BULBAR PALSY This syndrome is the result of weakness or paralysis of those muscles which are supplied by the motor nuclei of the lower brainstem, i.e., the motor nuclei of the fifth, seventh, and ninth to twelfth cranial nerves. Strictly speaking, the motor nuclei of the fifth and seventh nerves lie outside the bulb, which is the old name for the medulla oblongata. Involved are the muscles of the jaw and face, the tongue, pharynx, larynx, sternocleidomastoid, and upper trapezius. If development is rapid, as may happen in diphtheria or poliomyelitis, there is no time for muscle atrophy. The more chronic disease, progressive bulbar palsy (a form of motor system disease), or tumors or aneurysms of the posterior fossa result in marked wasting and fasciculation of the tongue, sternocleidomastoid, and trapezius muscles. The condition must be distinguished from progressive muscular dystrophy and a restricted form of polymyositis which may be limited to neck muscles; however, these latter disorders seldom affect the tongue. It must also be differentiated from pseudobulbar palsy (see Chap. 14).

MULTIPLE CRANIAL NERVE PALSIES As will be readily understood, several cranial nerves may be affected by the same disease process. One of the clinical problems is to determine whether the lesion lies within or outside the brainstem. Lesions lying on the surface of the brainstem are featured by involvement of adjacent cranial nerves (often occurring in succession) and late and rather slight involvement of the long sensory and motor pathways and segmental structures lying within the brainstem. The opposite is true of intramedullary, intrapontine, and intramesencephalic lesions. The extramedullary lesion is more likely to cause bone erosion or enlargement of the foramens of exit of cranial nerves (seen radiographically). The intramedullary lesion involving cranial nerves often produces a crossed sensory or motor paralysis (cranial nerve signs on one side of the body and tract signs on the opposite side). In this way a number of distinctive syndromes, to which eponyms have been attached, are produced. These are listed in Table 367-2.

Involvement of multiple cranial nerves outside the brainstem is frequently the result of trauma (sudden onset), localized infections such as herpes zoster (acute onset), granulomatous disease including Wegener's granuloma (subacute onset), or tumors and saccular aneurysms (chronic development). Of the tumors, neurofibromas, meningiomas, cholesteatomas, carcinomas, and sarcomas have all been reported. The chordoma (see Chap. 358) may implicate a succession of lower cranial nerves. Owing to their anatomic relationships, the multiple cranial nerve palsies form a number of distinctive syndromes, listed in Table 367-1.

From time to time one observes a benign form of multiple cranial nerve involvement on one or both sides of the face. The disease may recur over a period of years with variable degrees of recovery between attacks. Sarcoidosis is found to be the cause of some, and chronic glandular tuberculosis (scrofula), the cause of others. The condition is called *polyneuritis cranialis multiplex.* The malignant granuloma of the nasopharynx may also affect multiple cranial nerves, as do also nasopharyngeal tumors, platybasia, and adult Arnold-Chiari malformation. A purely motor disorder without atrophy raises the question always of myasthenia gravis (see Chap. 372).

REFERENCES

ADAMS RD, VICTOR M: *Principles of Neurology,* 2d ed. New York, McGraw-Hill, 1981

BRODAL A: *Neurological anatomy,* in *The Cranial Nerves,* 3d ed. New York, Oxford University Press, 1980, pp 448–577

COGAN DG: *Neurology of the Ocular Muscles,* 2d ed. Springfield, Ill., Charles C Thomas, 1956

———: *Neurology of the Visual System.* Springfield, Ill., Charles C Thomas, 1966

DOUEK E et al: Olfaction and its disorders. Proc R Soc Med 68:467, 1975

GLASER JS: Heredofamilial disorders of the optic nerve, in *Genetic and Metabolic Eye Disease,* MF Goldberg (ed). Boston, Little, Brown, 1974

———: *Neuro-ophthalmology.* Hagerstown, Md., Harper & Row, 1978

LEIBOLD JE: Drugs having a toxic effect on the optic nerve. Intern Ophthalmol Clin 11:137, 1971

MAYO CLINIC STAFF: *Clinical Examinations in Neurology,* 5th ed. Philadelphia, Saunders, 1981

PRYSE-PHILIPS W: Disturbances in the sense of smell in psychiatric patients. Proc R Soc Med 68:472, 1975

WOLFSON RJ (ed): *The Vestibular System and Its Diseases.* Philadelphia, University of Pennsylvania Press, 1966

368
DISEASES OF THE PERIPHERAL NERVOUS SYSTEM

RAYMOND D. ADAMS
ARTHUR K. ASBURY

Disease of the peripheral nervous system stands as one of the most difficult subjects in neurology. Since the structure and function of this system are relatively simple, one might suppose that knowledge of its diseases would be complete. Such is not the case. At present a suitable explanation cannot be offered in more than a third of patients who enter a general hospital with a disease of the peripheral nervous system, nor have the pathologic changes been fully determined in many of them. Moreover, the physiologic basis of many of the symptoms of peripheral nerve disease continues to elude experts in the field.

With these rather discouraging remarks behind us, we shall attempt to present a distillate of our personal experience that may be of value to the reader.

GENERAL CONSIDERATIONS It is well to have clearly in mind the extent of the peripheral nervous system and the scope of the possible pathogenetic mechanisms whereby it can be affected.

The peripheral nervous system (PNS) includes all nervous structures lying outside the pia-arachnoid membrane of the spinal cord and brainstem, with the exception of the optic nerves and olfactory bulbs, which are special extensions of the brain. The parts of it within the spinal canal and cranial cavity and attached to the ventral and dorsal surfaces of the cord and ventrolateral surface of the brainstem are the *spinal* and *cranial nerve roots,* respectively. The dorsal roots (sensory) containing afferent fibers (the central axonal processes of the dorsal root ganglion cells) extend for a variable distance into the posterior columns (funiculi) of the spinal cord. The efferent ventral roots, composed of the emerging axons of anterior and lateral horn cells, finally terminate on muscle fibers or in sympathetic or parasympathetic ganglia. Traversing, as they do, the subarachnoid space, and lacking an epineural and in part a perineural sheath, the cranial and spinal roots are bathed by cerebrospinal fluid (CSF), the lumbosacral roots presenting the longest exposure. The vast extent of the peripheral ramification of cranial and spinal nerves is noteworthy, as are their thick protective sheaths of perineurium and epineurium and their unique vascular supply through longitudinal arrays of richly anastomosing nutrient arterial branches. Sensory endings, freely branching or corpuscular, are the site of termination of the peripheral axons of dorsal root ganglion cells. Sympathetic afferent fibers, arising on blood vessels and in viscera, and the sympathetic and parasympathetic ganglia, with their rami communicantes and peripheral extent, complete this system. Segments of myelin, special extensions of Schwann cell plasma membrane, cover all the axons of the extraneuraxial parts of the PNS, but always maintain a morphologically independent though symbiotic relation to it. Indeed the PNS has been defined as the Schwann cell part of the nervous system.

These many anatomic features inform us of the possible pathways and mechanisms of peripheral nerve disease. Pathologic processes (e.g., viral infections) directed at the anterior or lateral horn cells of the spinal cord, the nerve cells of dorsal root ganglia, or the nerve cells of sympathetic or parasympathetic ganglia may reflect themselves secondarily in degeneration of axons and myelin sheaths of the peripheral nerve fibers of these cells. Disease processes involving the oligodendrocytes or astrocytes in the ventral or dorsal columns (funiculi) of the spinal cord, wherein lie the axons of anterior horn cells or dorsal root ganglia cells, may also affect the function and structure of the peripheral nervous system. A pathologic process in the leptomeninges and CSF may damage the anterior and posterior roots in proportion to their length in transit through the subarachnoid space; and the posterior roots may be more affected because of their intimate relation to groups of specialized arachnoidal cells (villi), where CSF is absorbed. Pathogenic processes confined to various components of connective tissue may affect the peripheral nerves which lie enveloped within their sheaths. Special biochemical disorders may involve the most metabolically active and richly vascularized parts of the PNS, the dorsal root and autonomic ganglia. Diffuse or localized arterial diseases injure nerves by narrowing or obliterating the intrinsic vessels (vasa nervorum), thus curtailing their blood supply. Noxious agents which selectively damage the Schwann cells or their membranes composing the myelin sheaths cause demyelination of peripheral nerves but leave axons intact. Finally one might suppose that axoplasm of either motor or sensory nerve fibers or their peripheral endings and end organs might each have their particular affinities to pathogenic agents.

All this is theoretical and somewhat speculative. At present we can cite examples of diseases which are based on only a few of these potential disease pathways, e.g., diphtheria toxin, which acts directly on the membranes of the Schwann cells near the dorsal root ganglia and adjacent nerves; polyarteritis nodosa, which causes widespread occlusion of vasa nervorum; tabes dorsalis, in which there is a treponemal meningoradiculitis of lumbosacral segments; and arsenic, which damages the axoplasm of sensory and motor fibers because of its combination with the rich store of axoplasmic mercaptans, SH radicles. But analogous anatomic possibilities doubtless are implicated in other diseases whose mechanisms remain to be divulged (see Table 368-1).

Pathologically several distinct processes are recognized, although they are not disease-specific and may be present in varying combinations in any given patient. The major processes are Wallerian degeneration, segmental demyelination (focal myelin sheath degeneration), and axonal degeneration. The myelin sheaths themselves are the most susceptible element of nerve, for they may break down as part of a primary process involving the Schwann cells (or some component thereof) or secondarily to axonal or nerve cell destruction. When the myelin sheath itself degenerates, the highly structured lipoprotein disintegrates into fine particles, which are then converted into cholesterol esters and removed by macrophages via the bloodstream. Breakdown of axons causes fragmentation of myelin into blocks or ovoids in which lie fragments of axons. This is a feature typical of Wallerian degeneration. Degeneration of both axon and myelin sheath may occur either distal to axonal interruption (Wallerian degeneration) or as a "dying back" phenomenon in more generalized, metabolically and nutritionally determined polyneuropathies (axonopathies). In segmental demyelination, recovery may be rapid, because the intact axon need only become remyelinated over denuded segments to become functional once more. In contrast, with Wallerian degeneration and axonopathies, recovery is slower, often requiring months to a year or more, because the axon must regenerate and reconnect its peripheral ending before function returns. The rate of axonal regrowth is about 1 to 2 mm per day.

Aside from differences in pathologic pathway and the effects of disease on parenchymal elements of nerve, the various forms of polyneuropathy are distinguished by other characteristics of the lesions and by the topography of the nerve fiber changes. In fact these are the only available criteria for "differential diagnosis." In acute idiopathic polyneuritis and infectious mononucleosis, infiltrations of lymphocytes, plasma cells, and other mononuclear cells in the spinal roots, sensory and sympathetic ganglia, and nerves and a frequent perivenous location of myelin destruction characterize the disease. In polyarteritis nodosa with polyneuropathy, "necrotizing panarteritis" with occlusion and focal infarction of nerve and, less often, rupture and hemorrhage are the dominant findings. In amyloid polyneuropathy, the deposits of this foreign material in endoneurial connective tissue and the walls of vessels secondarily affecting the nerve fibers either by compression or ischemia are the basis of diagnosis. In diphtheritic polyneuropathy, the aforementioned location in and around the roots and sensory ganglia, the purely demyelinative character of the nerve fiber change, and the lack of inflammatory reaction permit its identification under the microscope. Certain toxic polyneuropathies (glue-sniffers' neuropathy) are associated with a special type of axonal swelling and proliferation of neurofilaments. Other polyneuropathies (carcinomatous, nutritional, porphyric, arsenical, uremic) are topographically symmetric but

TABLE 368-1
Principal causes of peripheral neuropathy

1 Exogenous neurotoxic
- *a* Metals: arsenic, lead, mercury, axonopathies thallium
- *b* Drugs: nitrofurantoin and related nitrofurazones, isoniazid, thalidomide, vincristine, diphenylhydantoin, stilbamidine, tetraethylthiuram disulfide, hydralazine, perhexilene, cis-platinum, sodium cyanate, misonidazole, aurothioglucose
- *c* Organic substances: carbon disulfide, acrylamide, solvents including *n*-hexane and methyl-*n*-butyl ketone, and trichloroethylene, immune serums, tetrachlorobiphenyl, dimethylaminopropionitrile, buckthorn toxin, and organophosphorus compounds including triorthocresyl phosphate

2 Deficiency states and metabolic axonopathies
- *a* Chronic alcoholism, beriberi, pellagra, subacute combined degeneration, pregnancy, chronic gastrointestinal disease
- *b* Carcinoma of lung, diabetes mellitus, porphyria, amyloidosis, multiple myeloma, macroglobulinemia, uremia, hypoglycemia, lupus erythematosus, hypothyroidism

3 Specific inflammatory states and infections (mostly demyelinative)
- *a* Acute idiopathic polyneuritis (Landry-Guillain-Barré syndrome)
- *b* Polyneuropathy, complicating acute or chronic infection: diphtheria, Boeck's sarcoid, infectious mononucleosis
- *c* Local infection of nerves: leprosy, herpes zoster

4 Vascular disease (mostly Wallerian degenerations): polyarteritis nodosa, arteriosclerosis, diabetes mellitus, rheumatoid arthritis

5 Genetically determined disorders: progressive hypertrophic polyneuropathy, peroneal muscular atrophy, and others

6 Polyneuropathy of obscure origin: chronic progressive or recurrent polyneuropathy are not presently distinguishable from one another by histopathologic means. They await more definitive study. The least is known about the familial types of polyneuropathy. Although patterns of inheritance can be recognized, the underlying biochemical link has been discovered in only a few genetically determined neuropathies, and the mechanism by which a particular biochemical abnormality leads to nerve dysfunction is not known in any. Indeed, in many types of disease it is not even known whether the primary process is affecting a sensory, motor, or sympathetic neuron in its entirety (neuronopathy) or only its axon or Schwann cell sheath.

Concerning mononeuropathies, these are usually due to local events. Compression, violent stretch, laceration from penetrating injuries, and ischemia are understandable, and the pathologic sequence of events is readily reproduced in animals. Of localized infections of single nerves only leprosy, sarcoid, and zoster represent identifiable disease states. For the larger number of acute lesions the pathology has yet to be defined, since they are usually benign, reversible states, which allow no opportunity for pathological examination.

The clinician is usually faced with two problems: (1) to establish the existence of disease of the peripheral nervous system and (2) to ascertain its nature and the possibilities of treatment. When muscular weakness, areflexia, atrophy, and sensory loss are demonstrable and conform to the region of distribution of one or many nerves, this is not difficult. The tendency for these diseases to affect the feet and lower legs more than the proximal parts, and the legs more than the arms, the frequent sparing of the trunk, the escape of vesical and anal sphincters, phenomena which probably reflect involvement of the largest and longest nerves, already commented upon in Chaps. 14 and 18, are relatively certain clues to diagnosis. But at times pain or dysesthesias may be the major symptoms, and the other subjective and objective neurologic findings are more difficult to put in evidence. Or the disorder may be purely motor, raising a question of myopathy, of motor end plate disorder, or of anterior horn cell disease; again, only paresthesias, ataxia, and sensory loss may be found, suggesting as alternative possibilities a disease of the posterior roots or the posterior columns of the spinal cord, such as tabes dorsalis. Under these circumstances one must resort to a number of laboratory procedures, such as (1) biochemical tests to rule in or out those metabolic or toxic states which will produce neuropathy, (2) measurement of nerve conduction velocity (lowered in chronic nerve disease but not in spinal cord or muscle diseases), (3) electromyography, which distinguishes disorders of muscle due to primary disease (myopathy), denervation, and neuromuscular blockade, (4) CSF examination (increase in protein and sometimes in cells with radicular and meningeal diseases), and (5) nerve (usually sural) and muscle biopsy.

Taking advantage of all available clinical and laboratory techniques and knowledge of the natural course of illnesses, the physician will find it helpful to be familiar with the peripheral nerve syndromes listed in Table 368-2. Stated another way, whenever one of the syndromes in this table can be identified, one is justified in considering any one of the several diseases of the peripheral nervous system listed in that subdivision.

SYNDROME OF ACUTE ASCENDING MOTOR PARALYSIS WITH VARIABLE DISTURBANCE OF SENSORY FUNCTION

Only minor semeiologic differences separate (1) acute idiopathic polyneuritis of Landry-Guillain-Barré, (2) acute infectious mononucleosis, (3) porphyria, (4) diphtheritic polyneuropathy, (5) acute idiopathic hepatitis with polyneuritis, and (6) other acute toxic polyneuropathies. These are the diseases which induce this syndrome.

ACUTE IDIOPATHIC POLYNEURITIS Landry-Guillain-Barré syndrome This disease seems to occur at all seasons, as if it is an endemic process, and it affects children and adults of all ages and both sexes. Its cause is unknown; all attempts to isolate a virus or microbial agent have failed. A mild respiratory or gastrointestinal infection has preceded the neuritic symptoms by 1 to 3 weeks in approximately half the patients. Other preceding events include surgical procedures, viral exanthems, antirabies inoculations and influenza vaccinations, and a similar state may occur during the course of Hodgkin's disease, other malignant diseases, and lupus erythematosus.

The principal symptoms of peripheral nerve involvement have certain unique qualities. The weakness, which advances over a period of days, involves proximal as well as distal limb and also trunk muscles. There may be pain, but it is exceptional; paresthesias (tingling and numbness) are frequent but are occasionally absent throughout the illness, and sensory im-

TABLE 368-2
Principal neuropathic syndromes

I Syndrome of acute ascending motor paralysis with variable disturbance of sensory function
- *A* Acute idiopathic polyneuritis (Landry-Guillain-Barré syndrome)
- *B* Infectious mononucleosis and polyneuritis
- *C* Hepatitis and polyneuritis
- *D* Diphtheritic polyneuropathy
- *E* Porphyric polyneuropathy
- *F* Toxic polyneuropathies (triorthocresyl phosphate poisoning, solvent neuropathy)

II Syndrome of subacute sensorimotor paralysis
- *A* Symmetric polyneuropathies
  - *1* Alcoholic polyneuropathy and beriberi
  - *2* Arsenic polyneuropathy
  - *3* Lead polyneuropathy
  - *4* Nitrofurantoin and other intoxications
- *B* Asymmetric polyneuropathies
  - *1* Diabetic
  - *2* Polyarteritis nodosa
  - *3* Subacute idiopathic polyneuritis
  - *4* Sarcoidosis

III Syndrome of chronic sensorimotor polyneuropathy
- *A* Acquired
  - *1* Carcinoma, myeloma, and other malignancy
  - *2* Chronic polyneuritis
  - *3* Paraproteinemias
  - *4* Uremia
  - *5* Beriberi
  - *6* Diabetes
  - *7* Connective tissue diseases
  - *8* Amyloidosis
  - *9* Leprosy
- *B* Genetically determined disorders
  - *1* Peroneal muscular atrophy (Charcot-Marie-Tooth disease)
  - *2* Hypertrophic polyneuropathy (Dejerine-Sottas disease)
  - *3* Hereditary sensory neuropathy
  - *4* Portuguese amyloidosis (Andrade's disease) and other types
  - *5* Heredopathia atactia polyneuritiformis (Refsum's disease)
  - *6* Abetalipoproteinemia
  - *7* Tangier disease
  - *8* Giant axonal neuropathy
  - *9* Metachromatic leukodystrophy

IV Syndrome of chronic relapsing polyneuropathy
- *A* Idiopathic polyneuritis
- *B* Porphyria
- *C* Beriberi or intoxications

V Syndrome of mononeuropathy
- *A* Pressure palsies
- *B* Traumatic neuropathies
- *C* Idiopathic brachial and sciatic neuritis
- *D* Serum neuritis
- *E* Zoster
- *F* Tumor invasion with neuropathy
- *G* Leprosy
- *H* Paratubercular (polyneuritis cranialis multiplex)

pairment is usually minimal (polyneuropathy is predominantly motor). The enfeeblement of muscle is so acute that it is not attended by atrophy, though hypotonia and areflexia are obvious. There is usually tenderness on deep pressure or squeezing of muscles. At an early stage the arms may be spared or their muscles may be less weakened than the leg muscles. Facial diplegia, occurring in half of all cases, usually comes later, after the arms are affected. However, other cranial nerves (ocular, bulbar) are often implicated. When retention of urine occurs, catheterization is seldom required for more than a few days.

Variants of the clinical syndrome take several forms: a predominantly descending motor paralysis; ophthalmoplegic polyneuritis with ataxia and little if any weakness of the limbs; a painful, mainly sensory polyneuritis. Subacute or chronic asymmetrical polyneuritis is a different disease.

The temperature is usually normal, and lymphadenopathy and splenomegaly do not occur. Electrocardiographic alterations of minor degree have often been reported. The CSF is under normal pressure and is acellular; elevations of protein level are found in most cases, but the values on the first lumbar puncture in the first few days of the disease are usually normal or only slightly raised. In about 10 percent of patients a pleocytosis of 10 to 50 cells per milliliter (rarely to 200 cells per milliliter, predominantly lymphocytes and mononuclear cells) is found. The white blood cell count and differential count tend soon to fall within normal limits.

The pathological changes in fatal cases have had a consistent pattern and form. When the disease is fatal within a few days, perivascular, lymphocytic infiltrates are found. These are generally associated with foci of demyelination, the predominant pathologic effect on nerve. In some instances, not only is myelin sheath attacked, but also Wallerian degeneration occurs, implying that axons have been interrupted more proximally. Inflammation of roots accounts, evidently, for the CSF changes. Infiltrates in liver, spleen, lymph nodes, heart, and other organs are usually found and reflect the systemic nature of the disease. From a pathogenetic standpoint, most of the evidence suggests that the clinical manifestations of this disorder are the result of an intense immunologic reaction directed at peripheral nerve, specifically myelin sheath.

The differential diagnosis includes poliomyelitis (distinguished usually by epidemic occurrence, meningeal symptoms, fever, and pure areflexic paralysis) and acute myelitis (marked by sensorimotor paralysis below a given spinal level and sphincteric paralysis). The forms of acute polyneuropathy described below must also be differentiated from this syndrome.

Corticosteroids (prednisone) are not currently favored for treatment of acute idiopathic polyneuritis, but we have occasionally observed dramatic improvement within hours after the administration of prednisone. This experience may only reflect the natural history of the disorder and not a therapeutic effect of prednisone, because recent large controlled studies of the use of corticosteroid medications in acute idiopathic polyneuritis have not shown beneficial effects. Prednisone is often effective in the management of more chronic or relapsing type of demyelinative polyneuritis (see below). Plasmapheresis has resulted in dramatic improvement in some cases, but its role in therapy remains uncertain. Respiratory assistance is given when the vital capacity falls below 800 to 1000 ml, and tracheostomy or placement of an endotracheal tube is usually performed at this time, especially if the patient has difficulty in removing secretions from the pharynx and tracheobronchial tree. Careful tracheal toilet, treatment of bronchial and pulmonary infections by the use of an appropriate antibiotic, and support of the blood pressure by vasopressor agents in the face of hypotension complete the therapeutic regimen. The best results are obtained by an efficient respiratory unit skilled in maintaining adequacy of ventilation and of cerebral circulation. Under the most ideal conditions the mortality is reduced to less than 5 percent.

Physiotherapy (passive-movement positioning of limbs and later mild resistance exercises) should be given as soon as movement returns to avoid joint contractures. Decisions to discontinue respiratory aid and to close the tracheostomy are based on the degree of recovery of the patient's respiratory mechanism.

Prognosis for complete recovery is good. More than 75 percent of patients are restored to normal function; the remaining usually have only a mild residual deficit, but a few are severely disabled. Speed of recovery varies. Usually it takes place within a few weeks or months, but if nerves have degenerated, their regeneration may require 6 to 18 months.

Infectious mononucleosis with polyneuritis This is a disease of young individuals. Three neurologic syndromes have been described with this disease: (1) ascending sensorimotor paralysis, identical with that of the Landry-Guillain-Barré syndrome, (2) aseptic meningitis, and (3) meningoencephalitis. All three appear during the midphase of the infection. The polyneuritis varies in severity and has rarely been fatal. The few autopsied cases have shown heavy infiltrations of lymphocytes, monocytes, and plasma cells in the nerves, roots, and meninges. The CSF contains a few or as many as several hundred mononuclear cells, and the protein level is raised. The diagnosis is suggested by the other typical physical and laboratory findings in this disease (see Chap. 212).

Infectious hepatitis with polyneuritis Rapidly evolving polyneuritis of the Landry-Guillain-Barré type may be associated with acute hepatitis. In our experience with this syndrome, the polyneuritis has followed the jaundice after several days or a few weeks and has the same relation to it as to respiratory or intestinal infections. Recovery from both the hepatitis and the polyneuritis has been the rule. The pathological changes in roots and nerves are identical with those described above for acute idiopathic polyneuritis.

Diphtheritic polyneuropathy Typical diphtheria (see Chap. 165) follows pharyngeal and laryngeal infections. Local action of the exotoxin may paralyze pharyngeal and laryngeal muscles within a few days and may also cause blurring of vision due to loss of accommodation. But these and other cranial nerve symptoms may be overlooked. The first signs of the neuropathy, coming 4 to 8 weeks later, are then an acute to subacute weakness of limbs with paresthesias and distal loss of vibratory and position sense. The weakness characteristically involves all four extremities at the same time or may descend from arms to legs. After a few days to a week or more the patient may be unable to stand or walk, and occasionally the paralysis is so severe and extensive as to impair respiration. The CSF protein level is usually elevated (50 to 200 mg/dl). After the pharyngeal infection is controlled, death in diphtheria is due usually to myocardiopathy or to polyneuropathy with respiratory paralysis.

Postmortem examination discloses a demyelination without inflammatory reaction of spinal roots, sensory ganglia, and adjacent spinal nerves. Axons, anterior horn cells, peripheral nerves distally, and muscle fibers remain normal.

The disease should be considered in all cases of acute polyneuropathy. Throat culture may demonstrate the *Corynebacterium* many weeks after the throat infection has subsided. Usually the history of nasal voice, dysphagia, blurred vision, and numb lips with a throat infection several weeks before provides the clue to the diagnosis. The ECG may be abnormal at the time of polyneuritis. Occasionally the polyneuropathy has followed a local wound infection with *Corynebacterium.* Titers of antitoxin in the blood and a positive Schick test reaction have usually not been helpful (for treatment see Chap. 165).

The prognosis for full recovery is excellent, once respiratory paralysis and cardiac disorders are circumvented.

Porphyric polyneuropathy As was stated in Chap. 99, a severe, rapidly advancing, more or less symmetric polyneuropathy with or without psychosis (delirium, confusion) and convulsions may occur in the course of acute intermittent porphyria. The neuropathy may affect principally the motor or both the sensory and motor nerves; it may begin in the feet and legs and ascend, or it may begin in the arms and later spread to the trunk and legs. Often it is predominantly proximal in distribution, and in some instances the motor paralysis is more severe than the sensory loss. The CSF protein level is usually normal.

The course of polyneuropathy is variable. If the disease is mild, it may be quite transitory, with regression of symptoms in a few weeks. If severe, it may rapidly progress to a fatal issue in a few days, the advance occurring without warning, or it may progress in a saltatory fashion over a period of weeks, finally resulting in a severe sensorimotor paralysis that may regress only over a period of months. Disorder of the central nervous system is more likely to precede the acute severe forms of neuropathy, but it may not appear at all.

The pathologic changes in the peripheral nervous system vary according to the stage of the illness at which death occurs. If the patient dies in the first few days, the myelinated fibers may appear entirely normal, despite an almost complete paralysis. If symptoms were present for weeks, a severe degeneration of both the axons and myelin sheaths often is found in most of the peripheral nerves. No inflammatory reaction, vascular lesion, or other change distinguishes this form of neuropathy. The relation between the metabolic abnormality centering about porphyrin biosynthetic pathway in the liver and nervous dysfunction has never been satisfactorily explained.

See Chap. 99 for a discussion of treatment.

The prognosis for ultimate recovery is excellent, though relapse of the porphyria may result in further involvement of the peripheral nervous system (see "Relapsing Polyneuropathy" below).

Polyarteritis nodosa with polyneuropathy Occasionally this form of neuropathy develops as rapidly as acute idiopathic polyneuritis. Most of the cases evolve more slowly, however, and the syndrome has been either symmetric or asymmetric in its distribution. For this reason the description will be given in the next section. At times a cutaneous nerve biopsy may be needed to distinguish this acute form from acute idiopathic polyneuritis. The presence of constitutional symptoms, fever, or eosinophilia should provide clues to diagnosis.

Other toxic polyneuropathies that may cause paralysis in a few days An example is triorthocresyl phosphate intoxication, in which the purely motor paralysis ultimately proves to be due to involvement of upper and lower motor neurons, and thallium, which may cause an acute sensorimotor polyneuropathy (see Chap. 239 for discussion of other chemical agents). The acute stages are accompanied by an encephalopathy with delirium and coma. Abusive inhalation of hexacarbon solvents may induce a fulminant polyneuropathy. Stilbamidine, used in the treatment of kala azar, produces a purely sensory neuropathy restricted in many instances to the trigeminal nerves.

SUBACUTE SENSORIMOTOR PARALYSIS

SYMMETRIC DISTRIBUTION Reference is made here to a neurologic disorder that develops over a period of a few weeks and pursues a variable course. The distribution is distal and graded in severity, and usually affects feet first, later spreading to the legs, thighs, and hands. Pain, hypersensitivity of skin, tenderness of muscles, and a mixture of dysesthesias and paresthesias are often prominent features of this clinical state. A purely symmetric syndrome of this type should direct attention to nutritional disorders (alcoholic beriberi), possible exogenous toxins (arsenic, nitrofurantoin), or metabolic abnormalities (myeloma, uremia).

Alcoholic polyneuropathy and beriberi All data point to a common nutritional factor for both these diseases, though it remains unclear whether the deficiency is one of thiamine, pyridoxine, pantothenic acid, or several of the B vitamins. We have not been able to define a form of polyneuropathy due solely to the direct effect of alcohol.

In North America and western Europe this form of polyneuropathy is rarely observed in the nonalcoholic person. Pure starvation does not produce it, the ideal conditions being a vitamin B deficiency in the face of a relatively high carbohydrate consumption. Of course, eccentricity of diet, gastrointestinal disorders, sprue, rice diet for hypertension with neglect of vitamin supplements all may create the necessary circumstances for such a neuropathy.

After several months (approximately two to three) of dietary inadequacy, numbness, tingling, and tenderness of the feet appear and are accompanied by weakness of the more distal muscles of the lower extremities, spreading within a few days to the calves and later the thighs. The leg muscles are always affected before the thighs, and foot drop, accompanied by weakness of the plantar flexors, is the first stage of the motor paresis. Involvement of the thighs is indicated by difficulty in arising from a squatting position. The tendon reflexes (ankle and knee jerks) are abolished, the skin and muscles are tender and vibratory, and position and touch senses are diminished to a variable degree, increasing as the disease progresses. Numbness and sensitivity of the fingers, hands, and forearms, weakness of hand grip, and wrist drop are next to appear. Cranial structures are usually spared unless Wernicke's disease is conjoined, in which instance there will be bilateral abducens and lateral gaze palsy and nystagmus, as well as cerebellar ataxia of gait, confusion, and memory defect (Korsakoff's psychosis). Involvement of vagus nerves with dysphonia and dysphagia has been reported and also involvement of other autonomic fibers in exceptional cases. If pellagra or nutritional myelopathy also occur, signs of retrobulbar neuropathy, deafness, and pyramidal tract signs may be found, resembling subacute combined degeneration.

This form of neuropathy produces a manifest sensorimotor disorder, which demands medical attention in only about half the patients in whom the diagnosis can be made. Once started, the syndrome often progresses over a period of days and weeks until the patient is confined to bed. But many alcoholics come to the physician with only a subclinical neuropathy (thin leg muscles, questionable sensory disorder over the shins and feet, and reduced or absent tendon reflexes). They give no history of having had a subacute symptomatic polyneuropathy. If untreated, the symptomatic form may progress over weeks and months to a severe atrophy of leg muscles, the polyneuropathy then becoming chronic. Edema is not infrequent (wet beriberi) and is due to dependency of limbs and stasis, more than to coincidental myocardial involvement or nutritional hypoproteinemia.

Alcoholic Laennec's cirrhosis and a nutritional anemia as well as autonomic dysfunction, weight loss, myocardiopathy, hypoglycemia, and electrolyte disturbance may coexist. The CSF is normal in nearly all the cases (rarely is the protein level elevated).

The pathologic changes in this neuropathy consist mainly of axonal degeneration with destruction of both axon and myelin sheath, but variable amounts of segmental demyelination may also occur. Cursory studies show the most pronounced lesions to be in the distal parts of the longest and largest myelinated fibers in the crural and, to a lesser extent, the brachial nerves. Vagi, phrenic, and trunk nerves are implicated only in the more advanced and fatal cases. Anterior horn cells and sensory ganglion cells undergo chromatolysis indicating axonal damage. Exceptionally, spinal roots and posterior columns of the spinal cord have shown degenerative changes. Recovery awaits remyelination and regeneration.

The disease process is invariably arrested by adequate diet, and the amount of B vitamins in the average food ration of the American public will be curative, though there is no harm in supplementing the diet with B vitamins (see Chap. 76). Positioning and splinting paralyzed limbs to prevent contracture are important. Occasionally pain and tenderness are so severe as to require analgesic medication. The pain may be of a burning type (causalgic) with excessive perspiration and only slight weakness and reflex changes. Called the *burning foot syndrome,* this has been ascribed to pantothenic acid deficiency, but we have not been able to prove its relation to this vitamin or to separate it clearly from the usual alcoholic neuropathy. Cooling lotions, propoxyphene, aspirin, and codeine are needed. Sometimes sympathetic blocking agents are helpful. The pain subsides after some few weeks.

The prognosis for full functional recovery is good, but if the paralysis is complete, one may anticipate a period of invalidism for 6 months or more. Vitamins do not hasten recovery. The tendon reflexes may remain absent or diminished. Fatalities have usually been the result of coincidental beriberi heart disease or cirrhosis rather than of the polyneuropathy. Vitamin supplements will prevent the polyneuropathy.

Arsenic polyneuropathy Nerve involvement from chronic arsenic poisoning is relatively infrequent. The symptoms develop rather slowly over a period of weeks and have the same sensory and motor distribution as was described in beriberi. A single acute ingestion of arsenic may be followed in 14 to 21 days by a more rapidly advancing polyneuropathy. The condition may be preceded by mental disturbances, convulsions, confusion, and coma, i.e., arsenic encephalopathy. Diagnosis is based on the subacute course of the polyneuropathy coupled with symptoms of gastrointestinal disorder, anemia, jaundice, brownish cutaneous pigmentation, hyperkeratosis of palms and soles, and white transverse banding of nails (Mees's lines). Although arsenic intoxication may be accidental, its occurrence should always arouse suspicion of homicidal or suicidal intent.

See Chap. 239 for diagnostic tests and treatment.

Poisoning due to mercury, thallium, antimony, and nitrofurantoin may produce a similar picture; the first three of these intoxications respond to British antilewisite (BAL).

Lead neuropathy Lead neuropathy occurs following chronic exposure to lead, and its most characteristic feature is the predominantly motor affection involving mainly the upper extremities. The radial nerves are most frequently involved, producing wrist and finger drop with few or no sensory manifestations. Less commonly, weakness of the proximal shoulder-girdle muscle occurs, and in the lower extremities foot drop may appear. Lead neuropathy is seldom combined with encephalopathy. Important associated findings are anemia, basophilic stippling of red blood cells, lead line along the gingival margins, colicky abdominal pain, and constipation. Neuropathy usually affects adults and is infrequent in children. In contrast, lead encephalopathy, manifested by increased intracranial pressure, convulsions, blindness, and coma, occurs almost exclusively in children. The diagnosis of lead neuropathy is established by the history of lead exposure, the characteristic motor involvement, the associated medical findings, and increased urinary excretion of lead and coproporphyrins. Treatment consists of withdrawal from exposure to lead and measures to eliminate body stores of lead (see Chap. 239). Recovery may be slow.

Nitrofurantoin neuropathy The earliest symptoms of nitrofurantoin neurotoxicity are tingling or dysesthesias of the toes and feet, followed shortly by similar sensations in the fingers. If the offending agent is not discontinued, this may progress to a severe sensorimotor, distal, symmetric polyneuropathy. Usually neuropathic symptoms appear only after the drug has been administered in high dosage for several weeks or months; exceptionally rare patients have experienced dysesthesias after brief exposures. Patients with chronic renal failure and azotemia are particularly prone to neurotoxicity with nitrofurantoin, presumably because of diminished excretion in the urine and consequent high tissue levels of the drug. To make matters more difficult to interpret, the uremic state itself may be responsible for a polyneuropathy that is clinically similar, so that the distinction between uremic polyneuropathy and nitrofurantoin neuropathy in the presence of chronic renal failure may be impossible.

Other toxic polyneuropathies Vincristine causes a subacute, mainly sensory polyneuropathy with impairment of tendon reflexes in the legs. A host of other compounds with therapeutic uses can produce polyneuropathy, generally subacute in evolution. These are listed in Table 368-1 and are reviewed extensively by Spencer and Schaumburg.

SUBACUTE ASYMMETRIC POLYNEUROPATHIES The most notable examples of this syndrome are diabetes mellitus, polyarteritis nodosa and other vasculitides, and a more or less obscure form of idiopathic polyneuritis. Rarely, sarcoidosis presents in this fashion.

Diabetic neuropathy Only about 15 percent of patients with diabetes mellitus have both symptoms and signs of neuropathy, but more than 50 percent either complain of neuropathic symptoms or exhibit slowing of nerve conduction velocity. Neuropathy is most common in diabetics over 50 years of age, is uncommon under 30 years of age, and is rare in childhood diabetes.

A number of clinical syndromes have been delineated, as follows: (1) diabetic ophthalmoplegia (described in Chaps. 17 and 367); (2) acute mononeuropathy; (3) painful, asymmetric mononeuropathy multiplex, which may pursue an acute, subacute, or chronic course and from which the patient usually recovers; (4) symmetric proximal motor neuropathy, which is often attended by burning pain, thigh wasting, and weight loss and from which recovery is the rule; (5) distal, symmetric, primarily sensory polyneuropathy, affecting feet and legs more than hands in a chronic, slowly progressive manner; and (6) an autonomic neuropathy involving bowel, bladder, and circulatory reflexes. Combinations of these neuropathies often coexist, particularly the autonomic disturbance in conjunction with other types.

The acute mononeuropathy involves most commonly the femoral or sciatic nerves and is presumably due to occlusion of vessels within or supplying the nerve. The outlook for recovery is good.

Painful, asymmetric mononeuropathy multiplex tends to occur in older patients with mild or unrecognized diabetes. Pain often begins in the low back or hip and spreads to thigh and knee on one side. It usually has a deep, burning character with superimposed, tearing, lancinating jabs and a propensity for becoming most severe at night. Muscle weakness and atrophy are usually most evident in pelvic girdle and thigh, although the distal muscles may not be spared. The upper extremities are usually unaffected. Sensory loss for position, vibration, touch, and pain is not generally severe and may conform to either a multiple nerve or root distribution, or to both. The vesical and anal sphincters may be involved, and the knee jerk is often lost on the affected side. Recovery from this type of neuropathy is the rule, although months and even years are often required. There is a tendency for the same syndrome to recur after a lapse of months or years in the opposite lower extremity.

A somewhat similar syndrome is encountered in elderly diabetics, in which one finds bilateral proximal and pelvic girdle weakness, wasting, weight loss, absent knee jerks, and often sphincteric symptoms and sexual impotence. Improvement tends to occur after some months, perhaps coincidentally with better control of the diabetes. It is unclear whether this diabetic neuropathy has the same basis as the painful asymmetric mononeuropathy multiplex. Both have been included under the general rubric of *diabetic amyotrophy.*

When the clinical picture is dominated by lancinating pain and sensory ataxia, with only slight weakness and bowel and bladder derangements, it resembles that of tabes dorsalis so closely that the condition goes by the name of *diabetic tabes.*

The distal, symmetric, primarily sensory form is the most common type of diabetic neuropathy. Numbness and tingling with relatively little pain are the main symptoms and are usually confined to the feet and lower legs. The ankle jerks are rarely preserved. Trophic changes in the form of deep ulcerations and neuropathic joints are occasionally encountered, presumably caused by injury to severely denervated skin and joints. Muscle weakness is usually mild, but in some cases a crural weakness with only minor sensory disturbance may predominate.

Pathologically, severe nerve fiber loss is a prominent finding in this form of neuropathy. In addition, evidence of segmental demyelination and remyelination of remaining axons is apparent in teased nerve fiber preparations. Since myelin is formed from the cell membranes of Schwann cells, one may infer that the Schwann cell is at least one target of the pathologic process in the distal, symmetric type of diabetic neuropathy. Whether the nerve fiber loss is explained by this same process remains uncertain. The basement membranes of blood vessels in these nerves do not appear abnormal under the light microscope but are altered in electron micrographs.

Symptoms of autonomic involvement include impairment of sweating and vascular reflexes, nocturnal diarrhea, atonic bladder, sexual impotence, and occasionally postural hypotension. The basis for this type of nerve damage is unknown.

In all forms of diabetic neuropathy, the CSF protein level may be elevated (50 to 200 mg/dl), and similar increases may be seen in diabetics with no clinical evidence of neuropathy. An explanation for this phenomenon has not been discovered.

Many uncertainties persist about the pathogenesis of the diabetic neuropathies. Both the cranial mononeuropathies (diabetic ophthalmoplegia) and the proximal asymmetric mononeuropathy multiplex are thought to be ischemic in origin secondary to disease of the vasa nervorum. The other forms are rather vaguely ascribed to an undefined metabolic defect perhaps involving polyol pathways.

The only known treatment is meticulous regulation of the diabetes mellitus along the lines described in Chap. 114. Maintenance of the blood sugar level in a relatively normal range is desirable, for there is some evidence that uncontrolled hyperglycemia is harmful. Vitamin supplements may have some merits, but no clear results have been obtained. Improvement and eventual recovery may be expected over a period of months, but during that time the management of the painful forms of neuropathy may be trying, because analgesic medication is required and one is faced with the possibility of drug addiction.

Polyarteritis nodosa with polyneuropathy Involvement of the intraneural vessels happens in perhaps as many as 90 percent of cases (autopsy figures), and a symptomatic form of neuropathy develops in more than one-half. Such involvement may be the principal clue to the diagnosis of the underlying disease when, up to that time, the main components of the clinical picture—abdominal pain, hematuria, fever, eosinophilia, hypertension, vague limb pains, and possibly asthma—have not fully declared themselves.

As was stated above, the polyneuropathy may develop acutely and be diffuse and more or less symmetric in distribution, but more often it is subacute, multiple, and asymmetric, i.e., a mononeuropathy multiplex. Both spinal and cranial nerves may be affected. No two cases are identical. The CSF protein level is usually normal. Muscle biopsy, taken near the motor point so as to include nerve, is useful in corroborating the clinical impression in the majority of cases. Central nervous system is involved less frequently, somewhat less than one-half of all cases; the lesion may occur concomitantly with those of the peripheral nerves.

Fatal issue is the rule. Corticosteroid therapy has not been successful in most cases. Spontaneous remission and therapeutic arrest are known, however, and a healed or healing form has been observed at autopsy, death having been due to other causes (see Chap. 69).

Subacute asymmetric idiopathic polyneuritis A few patients who consult the physician with an illness which at first glance has all the appearance of acute idiopathic polyneuritis will have an asymmetric pattern and continue to become worse over a period of weeks or months. Nerve conduction slowing and prolonged distal latencies signify a demyelinative neuropathy. Some have an extremely high CSF protein level (600 to 1500 mg/dl), with a virtual Froin CSF syndrome (xanthochromia and spontaneous clotting). The higher concentration of protein fluids may be accompanied by headache, papilledema, and high CSF pressure, possibly because of the osmotic effect of the protein in increasing CSF volume. As the months pass, some symptoms improve as others appear. Ultimately most patients recover, though late fatality is known to occur; corticosteroids in full doses (30 to 45 mg of prednisone daily or twice this amount on alternate days) have proved to be beneficial in the majority of cases but may have to be continued over a period of months.

These subacute forms of idiopathic polyneuritis are different from the acute type. This type of polyneuritis merges with the chronic and relapsing type described below.

Sarcoidosis Another cause of subacute or chronic polyneuropathy, sarcoidosis, is discussed in Chap. 151. It may be associated with signs of central nervous system involvement (stalk of the pituitary with diabetes insipidus and the cerebellum with ataxia) or with lesions in muscles (polymyositis). Facial nerve weakness is the single most common manifestation of peripheral nerve involvement as in Heerfordt's syndrome of chronic parotitis with facial nerve involvement (see Chap. 151).

CHRONIC SENSORIMOTOR PARALYSIS AND OTHER POLYNEUROPATHIC SYNDROMES

Here slowly progressive weakness, muscular atrophy, and reflex loss are associated with paresthesias, pain, sensory loss and ataxia, and autonomic disturbances in various combinations. The onset may be easily dated or insidious and the advance of the disease steady or intermittent. According to whether sensory or motor symptoms appear first, ataxia or muscular weakness may introduce the disease. Because of the chronicity paralysis is accompanied by atrophy of muscles of such degree as to simulate the spinal forms of muscular atrophy or muscular dystrophy, especially in small children in whom sensory functions are nearly impossible to test. In some cases the distribution of sensory and motor abnormalities is quite asymmetric, suggesting a mononeuropathy multiplex. This is true of leprous neuritis, for example, where only one or a few of the nerves of arms and legs may be affected. More often, however, and this applies to most of the familial and the acquired polyneuropathies (chronic polyneuritis), the distribution is relatively symmetrical and the nerves in the distal parts of the lower extremities appear to bear the brunt of the disease.

In the chronic forms of polyneuropathy, presumably because of the time factor, and other more obscure reasons, one witnesses the emergence of a number of unusual neuropathic syndromes. It is as though the pathogenic agent has been able to selectively injure sensory or motor fibers or one size of sensory and autonomic fibers. As a consequence any one of the following syndromes may appear:

1 A sensory syndrome with ulcers of the feet and Charcot arthropathy. This is observed in the chronic familial type of neuropathy described by Denny-Brown.
2 A relatively pure sensory ataxia with paresthesias and areflexia, as in the Levy-Roussy familial polyneuropathy.
3 Pseudosyringomyelic syndrome in which there is mainly a loss of pain and temperature (but usually paresthesias and slight loss of touch, vibratory, and position sense as well), motor power is relatively good and tendon reflexes are absent, and autonomic disturbances are variably prominent. The familial amyloid polyneuropathy of Andrade tends to present in this way.
4 Autonomic polyneuropathy with mydriasis and loss of pupillary reflexes, diminished lacrimation and salivation, achlorhydria of stomach, loss of sweating, orthostatic hypotension, impotence, and diminished contractibility of bowel and bladder, all together or in various combinations, especially in partial syndromes. A pure dysautonomia has been described by the authors and, as was stated above, in one form of diabetic neuropathy autonomic function may be disturbed.
5 Myokymia and the continuous muscular activity syndrome with mild weakness and continuous rippling and wave-like contractions of the muscles. Electrophysiological studies indicate an involvement of distal parts of motor nerve fibers (see Chap. 374).

These syndromes are fully described in the monographs on peripheral nerve diseases by Bradley and by Dyck et al.

ACQUIRED FORMS Carcinomatous and myelomatous polyneuropathy Here several syndromes have been observed. The most frequent is a slowly developing symmetric sensory or sensorimotor polyneuropathy that may accompany the development of a carcinoma or multiple myeloma. Severe weakness, atrophy, ataxia, and sensory loss of the limbs may advance to the point where the patient is confined to a wheelchair or bed. In some instances this may happen months or even a year or more before a small malignant tumor is found. The CSF protein level is often moderately elevated. This form of polyneuropathy has occurred most frequently with carcinoma of the lung but actually has been joined to every tumor. It may accompany either a solitary plasmacytoma of bone or multiple myeloma and in a few instances has been seen in macroglobulinemia without tumor formation. Another predominantly sensory polyneuropathy with good strength but severe ataxia is a relatively rare syndrome with lung tumor. Rarely in the immunologically suppressed patient with certain tumors such as Hodgkin's disease there may develop an acute polyneuritis of Landry-Guillain-Barré type rather than a chronic type. Thus polyneuropathy must be added to polymyositis or dermatomyositis, with which it is frequently conjoined as a neurologic complication of malignant tumor growths. A peculiar type of myasthenia (Eaton-Lambert syndrome), spinocerebellar degeneration (particularly with carcinoma of the ovary), and multifocal leukoencephalopathy, the other neurologic complications of neoplasia, may coexist. The pathology of the neuropathy has been incompletely defined. The only known therapy consists of removing or controlling the tumor growth, which has resulted at times in improvement. Corticosteroid therapy has helped some patients.

Paraproteinemia (see Chap. 63) More than a dozen patients with mild chronic sensorimotor neuropathies have been seen on our wards in recent years in whom no associated metabolic disturbance other than an abnormality of the immunoglobulins was found. In general, three protein abnormalities have occurred: (1) isolated macroglobulinemia (IgM), (2) diffuse increase in all three immunoglobulins (IgM, IgG, and IgA), and (3) other monoclonal gammopathies, most frequently involving κ and λ light chains. In macroglobulinemia, light chain disorders, and diffuse immunoglobulinemia (not to be confused with multiple myeloma), the neuropathies have been chronic, some exquisitely so, relatively mild, and occasionally sensory disorder exceeds motor and is distributed in a multiple nerve trunk pattern. Electrophysiologic studies indicate that the process is usually demyelinating in nature. An excess of plasma cells may be found in the bone marrow. Either prednisone or chlorambucil has at times led to reversal of neuropathy, although recovery has usually been incomplete. A specific disorder of IgA immunoglobulin is found in ataxia-telangiectasia (see Chap. 374), in which peripheral nerve dysfunction is evidenced by hyporeflexia, lowered nerve conduction velocities, and severe axonal loss in a sural nerve biopsy.

Cryoglobulinemia, either the essential idiopathic form or that which is associated with myeloma, lymphoma, connective tissue disease, or chronic infection, occasionally results in a peripheral neuropathy. Pain and paresthesias are prominent symptoms, often precipitated by exposure to cold. Weakness and muscle atrophy may appear, usually in the legs more than arms and sometimes in asymmetric pattern. The pathogenic mechanism is thought to be vascular, but pathologic changes are unsettled. The use of prednisone or the alkylating agent chlorambucil has induced remission, often incomplete.

Uremic polyneuropathy Uremic patients whose renal impairment is chronic may develop a slowly progressive sensorimotor paralysis of the legs and then of the arms. Almost as frequently, the polyneuropathy has developed subacutely. Muscle atrophy, areflexia, and distal distribution in the limbs of neurologic defect leave little doubt of the peripheral nerve character of the disorder. Improvement has been observed after treatment with chronic hemodialysis, and recovery is the rule after successful renal transplantation. The CSF protein level may be moderately elevated (50 to 150 mg/dl).

The pathology is that of a nonspecific degeneration of large myelinated fibers in nerves and spinal roots. Axons degenerate with the expected chromatolysis of their cell bodies. Amyloid deposit in the nerve has not been found; there is no evidence of vitamin deficiency or of diabetes during life and no sign of polyarteritis nodosa at autopsy. The neuropathy has been observed with all types of chronic kidney disease.

Beriberi In all the regions of the world where nutrition is borderline and treatment for an evolving beriberi may of necessity be delayed or even impossible to obtain, the motor paralysis and atrophy of the legs and, to a lesser extent, thighs and arms may reach an extreme degree. Thus this disease, though subacute in its evolution, becomes a frequent cause of chronic polyneuropathy. Uncontrolled diabetes may behave similarly.

Chronic polyneuropathy with connective tissue diseases In a clinic where many patients with connective tissue disease are being studied, occasional examples of either subacute or chronic polyneuropathy or a mononeuropathy have appeared. The latter are usually related to rheumatoid arthritis and are difficult to distinguish from pressure palsies clinically. The polyneuropathy is diffuse, often symmetric, and variably painful. Little is known of its cause, mechanism, or pathology. Some of the most extremely painful polyneuropathies we have seen, extending over long periods of time, have had only minimal sensory loss, weakness, or reflex change in some part of the body, and the diagnosis has been difficult. An unexpected rise in CSF protein level or electromyographic evidence of denervation may sometimes prove to be important leads. Occasionally a chronic symmetric polyneuropathy may accompany lupus erythematosus. It may be due to a small-vessel arteritis. Perhaps more of the obscure polyneuropathies fall into this group of connective tissue diseases than is presently realized.

Chronic relapsing polyneuritis Prineas and McLeod have reviewed large series of cases of subacute to chronic relapsing polyneuritis, which appear to bear no clear relationship to Landry-Guillain-Barré (LGB) syndrome. "Heaviness" and weakness of the legs and difficulty in walking were the initial symptoms in half of the cases, but in one-fourth of them the first sensory and motor symptoms were localized to the arms, and in one to cranial structures. The interval from first symptom to maximal level of weakness ranged from 3 weeks to 16 months. Half of the patients were unable to walk at the peak of the illness. Proximal limb muscles were usually more affected than distal. The tendon reflexes were abolished. Sensory impairment tended always to be less than motor and in several was undetectable by the standard clinical tests. Pain may be a prominent feature of some cases.

Most patients of this kind (the authors have been seeing two or three per year) have attacks or relapses lasting several weeks. In the relapses, unlike the acute LGB syndrome, respiratory difficulties and life-threatening paralysis rarely occur.

The CSF protein is almost invariably elevated, and in some there are few lymphocytes. Sensory nerve conduction is absent and motor nerve conduction is slowed in a pattern characteristic of primary demyelination. There is focal inflammation and demyelination of axons in nerve biopsies, a combination of changes believed to be characteristic of LGB syndrome. "Onion bulb" formations of Schwann cells are seen in some biopsies. No antibodies to any of the common viruses have been found. Prednisone in doses of 40 to 60 mg per day for weeks to months has been followed by a remission in the majority of cases; and in the few that did not respond, cyclophosphamide in a dose of 50 to 150 mg per day for 2 to 4 months has been effective. Most of the patients will improve but will be left with some deficits, and one of five will recover completely. Odd variants of this syndrome have included hypertrophied nerves, an elevated sedimentation rate, an enlarged spleen, or coarse tremor of the hands (worse when receiving corticosteroids).

Hypothyroid neuropathy Although nerve involvement is infrequent, a number of myxedematous patients will complain of numbness and weakness of feet and legs and to a lesser extent, the hands. Weakness of distal muscles; areflexia; and diminution of vibratory, joint-position, and touch-pressure sensations are the usual findings. The nerve conduction velocities are diminished and CSF protein is increased. Subjective improvement and at times a definite disappearance of the abnormalities follow thyroid replacement therapy. Dyck and Lambert observed excessive deposition of glycogen in nerve tissues.

Amyloidosis with chronic polyneuropathy As was pointed out in Chap. 106, primary amyloidosis may occur as a sporadic or a familial disease, the latter being particularly common in Portugal and Brazil. The polyneuropathy usually begins in middle adult life, is often severe, and is usually preceded by gastrointestinal symptoms (anorexia, indigestion, diarrhea). Sensory and motor nerve fibers are affected; in the familial varieties autonomic disturbance may predominate. Symmetry of involvement is the rule. The tongue may be enlarged and weak, and ocular muscles may be paretic. A carpal tunnel syndrome may be observed as the only neurologic abnormality in some cases. Cerebrospinal fluid protein level is elevated. The diagnosis is suggested by the clinical picture, the polyneuropathy being combined with hepatomegaly (often jaundice), anemia, cardiac enlargement, and EEG change. The nerves are probably enlarged in some patients. Restricted syndromes (eye muscles, tongue, etc.) are known. Presently there is no treatment for primary amyloidosis.

Leprous neuritis This is the classic example of an infectious neuritis, for the inflammatory reaction in the nerve is evoked by the leprous bacillus. Two major forms are recognized, tuberculoid and lepromatous, but intermediate forms are frequent. Tuberculoid (high-resistance) leprosy is restricted to a single patch of hypesthetic skin in any location. If a superficially placed nerve trunk, typically a cutaneous nerve, courses just beneath the area of affected skin, it may be engulfed in the inflammatory reaction, resulting in an associated mononeuropathy. Such a nerve may be palpably enlarged and beaded. Lepromatous (low-resistance) leprosy is marked by immunologic tolerance and widespread cutaneous anesthesia and anhidrosis, sparing only the warmest parts of the body, notably the axilla, groin, and beneath the scalp hair. Motor signs (focal weakness and atrophy) result from damage to mixed nerves lying close to the skin, particularly median, ulnar, peroneal, and facial nerves.

Diagnosis depends on the character of the clinical picture, skin and nerve changes often being associated.

See Chap. 175 for diagnostic tests and therapy.

GENETICALLY DETERMINED NEUROPATHIES Three chronic familial polyneuropathies (peroneal muscular atrophy, hereditary sensory neuropathy, and progressive hypertrophic polyneuropathy) have been recognized for many years, but in none has an associated metabolic disturbance been discovered. Several other genetically determined neuropathies have been described (Refsum's disease, abetalipoproteinemia, metachromatic leukodystrophy, and Tangier disease) with which a known metabolic disorder is associated. Familial amyloidosis with neuropathy also belongs to the group and is discussed above.

Peroneal muscular atrophy (Charcot-Marie-Tooth disease) This is a dominant hereditary disease with onset during adolescence or adult years. There is chronic degeneration of peripheral nerves and roots, resulting in distal muscle atrophy, beginning in the feet and legs and later involving the hands. Early symptoms are muscular wasting and weakness, affecting the extensor and everter muscles of the feet and producing an equinovarus deformity. Later, all muscles below the middle third of the thigh may atrophy, resulting in a "stork leg" appearance of the legs. After a period of years, atrophy of hand and forearm muscles develops. The wasting seldom extends above the elbows or above the middle third of the thighs. The feet are short and arched, sometimes with perforating ulcers. Pain, paresthesias, and cramps are common. The objective sensory disorder is usually rather slight but conspicuous enough to enable one to distinguish this polyneuropathy from progressive (spinal) muscular atrophy. There is impairment of position and vibratory sensation in the feet, and touch and pain sensation are lost in the feet. Reflexes are absent in the involved limbs. The progression of the illness is very slow, and it may arrest at any stage (see Chap. 364 for more complete descriptions). Generally speaking, in those families with onset during adolescence, nerve conduction velocities are very slow (10 to 30 m/s) and pathologically one sees hypertrophic neuropathy with "onion bulb" formation (see next section). In families with adult onset in the fourth or fifth decade, nerve conduction velocities are normal or minimally reduced and the pathology is that of axonal loss.

Progressive hypertrophic polyneuropathy (Déjerine-Sottas disease) This type of neuropathy is infrequent and is familial, usually with a recessive type of inheritance pattern. It begins in childhood and is slowly progressive. Pain and paresthesias in the feet are early symptoms, followed by development of symmetric weakness and wasting of the distal portion of the limbs. Sensation is impaired in a distal distribution, and the tendon reflexes are absent. Miotic pupils, nystagmus, and kyphoscoliosis have been observed in some cases. Patients are usually confined to a wheelchair at an early age. Morphologically the nerves are thickened and enlarged because of excessive endoneurial collagen deposition and a prominent myxoid interstitium. Nerve fibers are reduced in number; those remaining have thinned or absent myelin sheaths, and each is surrounded by a lamellated collar of Schwann cells and connective tissue referred to as an "onion bulb" formation. Such hypertrophic changes in nerve are not specific for this condition, but may also occur diffusely in Refsum's disease (see below), certain forms of peroneal muscular atrophy, acquired forms of relapsing polyneuropathy, or a single nerve in multifocal distribution, and possibly diabetes mellitus. Palpable thickening of the ulnar and peroneal nerves may be conspicuous. In the absence of palpable enlargement of nerves, the diagnosis can be established by biopsy of a cutaneous nerve. The treatment is symptomatic.

Hereditary sensory neuropathy Both a dominant and a recessive inheritance pattern are recognized in this disorder. Exquisitely slow progression of distal cutaneous sensory loss of extreme degree is the clinical expression. Recurrent injury to the insensitive hands and feet leads often to mutilation and loss of digits.

Chronic polyneuropathy with ichthyosis, deafness, and retinitis pigmentosa (Refsum's disease) This rare, genetically determined disorder begins in childhood or early adolescence, and the polyneuropathy is sensorimotor, distal, and symmetric in distribution, affecting legs more than arms. Sometimes an attack of polyneuropathy may develop subacutely and later regress. Although the nerves may not be enlarged clinically, hypertrophic changes with "onion bulb" formation are an unfailing pathologic feature. The metabolic defect results in a tissue accumulation of phytanic acid, a tetramethylated 16-carbon fatty acid. The relation between this biochemical lesion and the polyneuropathy remains uncertain. Diets low in phytanic acid may be beneficial.

Abetalipoproteinemia (Bassen-Kornzweig syndrome, acanthocytosis) (see also Chap. 103) The clinical manifestations of this unusual syndrome include (1) near absence of β-lipoprotein in the serum, (2) retinitis pigmentosa, (3) acanthocytosis of the red blood cells, and (4) a chronic, progressive neurologic deficit, usually beginning in childhood. Extreme proprioceptive sensory loss, ataxia, and areflexia are the most constant features, although muscular weakness and atrophy, kyphoscoliosis, and corticospinal signs may also be encountered. The main burden of the neurologic disorder falls upon the peripheral nervous system, but the relation between the neuropathy and the deficiency of β-lipoprotein remains unknown.

Tangier disease (see also Chap. 103) In this rare recessively inherited disorder, marked by near absence of plasma high-density lipoprotein and low serum cholesterol, approximately one-half of patients will exhibit neuropathy. A distinctive clinical picture has been described in three such patients, which consisted of severe progressive asymmetric cutaneous anesthesia to pain and temperature over scalp, face, and limbs with sparing of distal parts.

Giant axonal neuropathy The clinical features of this autosomal recessive disorder form a readily recognizable constellation. These include onset before age 5, insidious progression of distal weakness, tightly coiled "kinky" hair, and minor central nervous system involvement with EEG changes. Cutaneous nerve biopsy discloses segmental giant axonal ballooning by masses of neurofilaments, a finding which is diagnostic. Current evidence indicates that this is a generalized disorder affecting intermediate-sized filaments in many cell types.

Metachromatic leukodystrophy (see also Chap. 364) Massive sulfatide accumulation throughout the central and peripheral nervous systems, and to a lesser extent in other organs, occurs in this disorder, apparently because of congenital absence of the degradative enzyme sulfatase. The abnormality is transmitted as an autosomal recessive trait. Progressive cerebral deterioration is the most obvious clinical aspect, but hyporeflexia, muscular atrophy, and diminished nerve conduction velocity indicate a neuropathic element. Metachromatically staining granules accumulate in the cytoplasm of Schwann cells in all peripheral nerves, as well as in central white matter. Sural biopsy may be used to establish the diagnosis, even early in the course of the illness.

RELAPSING POLYNEUROPATHY

Two diseases most regularly take this form: porphyria, in which the attacks recur because of the administration of barbiturates or spontaneous relapses, and idiopathic polyneuritis. The latter has no proven cause. Enlargement of nerves may occur in the latter disorder so that it is probable that some patients with hypertrophic polyneuropathy may fall into this category. Amyloidosis or leprosy may also cause palpable enlargement of nerves, but by an obviously different mechanism.

MONONEUROPATHY OR MULTIPLE NEUROPATHY

This group of diseases differs in that one or a few of the nerves are involved in the disease process. The finding of a mononeuropathy implies a local cause, usually trauma or compression. Diagnosis rests on the finding of motor, reflex, or sensory changes confined to the territory of a particular nerve. A part of a plexus may also be involved. One variety, mononeuropathy multiplex, which has already been discussed, is due to leprosy, sarcoid, diabetes, and polyarteritis nodosa.

COMMON BRACHIAL AND CRURAL MONONEUROPATHIES

Brachial palsies The fifth to eighth cervical and first thoracic spinal nerves innervate the muscles of the shoulder girdles and upper extremities. The brachial plexus is formed by components of these nerves, and lesions of the nerves or their branches result in characteristic palsies. The following are the brachial palsies most likely to be observed on the medical wards of a hospital.

LONG THORACIC NERVE This nerve is derived from the fifth, sixth, and seventh cervical nerves and supplies the serratus magnus muscle. Paralysis of the serratus magnus muscle results in inability to raise the arm over the head from a forward position, and there is winging of the medial border of the scapula on pushing forward against resistance. It is injured most commonly by pressure on the shoulder, from either a sudden blow or prolonged pressure from carrying heavy weights. It is also involved at times in diabetic patients and as a manifestation of brachial and serum neuritides and in other idiopathic forms of neuritis (pleurodynia, Coxsackie disease).

SUPRASCAPULAR NERVE This nerve is derived from the fifth and sixth cervical nerves and supplies the supra- and infraspinatus muscles. Lesions may be diagnosed by the presence of weakness of abduction and external rotation of the arm and atrophy of the supra- and infraspinatus muscles. The nerve may be injured by blows on the top of the shoulder and fracture dislocations of the shoulder joint.

UPPER BRACHIAL PLEXUS PARALYSIS This is due to injury to the fifth and sixth cervical nerves and roots caused most commonly by forceful separation of the head and shoulder during difficult parturition or by pressure in the supraclavicular region during anesthesia. Headlong falls may also produce this injury. The muscles affected are the biceps, deltoid, brachialis anticus, supinator longus, supra- and infraspinatus, and rhomboids. The arm hangs at the side, internally rotated, with the elbow extended. The forearm is pronated. Hand motion is unaffected. The prognosis for spontaneous recovery is generally good, especially in cases of birth injury. This condition as a result of birth injury (Erb-Duchenne brachial plexus palsy), which may persist throughout life, is discussed in Chaps. 14 and 365.

LOWER BRACHIAL PLEXUS PARALYSIS This is due to injury to the eighth cervical and first thoracic roots as a result of traction on the abducted arm in falls, during operation, and with tumors of the apex of the lung (superior sulcus or Pancoast's syndrome). Injury may occur during birth (Déjerine-Klumpke brachial plexus injury). There is paralysis and wasting of the small muscles of the hand and a characteristic claw-hand deformity. Sensory loss is limited to the ulnar border of the hand and inner side of forearm, and there may be an associated paralysis of the cervical sympathetic nerve with Horner's syndrome if the first thoracic motor root is involved.

LESIONS OF THE CORDS OF THE BRACHIAL PLEXUS The lateral and medial cords are most commonly affected. Dislocation of the head of the humerus, pressure of the cervical ribs, and stab wounds are the most frequent causes. Injury to the lateral cord results in paralysis of the biceps and coracobrachialis muscles and all muscles supplied by the median nerve except the intrinsic hand muscles. There is some loss of sensation over the radial aspects of the forearm. Involvement of the medial cord, as may occur in compression by the cervical rib, results in paralysis of the muscles supplied by the ulnar nerve together with the median-innervated intrinsic muscles of the hand and sensory loss over the ulnar aspect of the hand and forearm. Sternum splitting operations may compress the lower brachial plexus by displacement of the clavicle. Usually it is the medial cord of the brachial plexus that is affected.

AXILLARY NERVE This nerve arises from the posterior cord of the brachial plexus and supplies the teres minor and deltoid muscles. It may be involved in injuries resulting from fractures of the neck of the humerus, serum neuritis, brachial neuritis, or as a part of a disease of unknown cause. The anatomic localization depends on the recognition of a paralysis of abduction of the arm, wasting of the deltoid muscle, and a patch of impaired sensation over the outer aspect of the shoulder.

MUSCULOCUTANEOUS NERVE This nerve is derived from the fifth and sixth cervical roots and is a branch of the lateral cord of the brachial plexus. It innervates the biceps and brachialis anticus muscles. Lesions of the nerve result in weakness of elbow flexion. Rarely is it injured alone.

RADIAL NERVE This nerve is derived from the fifth to eighth cervical roots and is the termination of the posterior cord of the brachial plexus. It innervates the triceps muscle and the supinator and extensor muscles of the forearm and hand. Complete radial paralysis results in inability to extend the elbow, paralysis of supination of the forearm, and complete wrist and finger drop. Sensation is impaired over the posterior aspect of the forearm and a small area over the radial aspect of the dorsum of the hand. The nerve may be injured in the axilla, for example in "crutch" palsy, but most commonly traumatism occurs in the mid-arm where the nerve winds around the humerus. Common types of injury at this site are fractures and pressure palsies incurred during sleep.

MEDIAN NERVE This nerve is derived from the sixth cervical to the first thoracic root and is formed by the union of two heads from the medial and lateral cords of the brachial plexus. It innervates the pronators of the forearm, long finger flexors, and abductor and opponens muscles of the thumb and is a sensory nerve to the palmar aspect of the hand. Complete median nerve paralysis results in wasting of the affected muscles and inability to pronate the forearm, weakness of wrist flexion, paralysis of flexion of the index finger and terminal phalanx of the thumb, weakness of flexion of the remaining fingers, weakness of abduction and opposition of the thumb, and sensory impairment over the radial two-thirds of the palmar aspect of the hand and over the distal phalanges of the dorsum of the index and third fingers. The nerve may be injured in the axilla by shoulder dislocation and in any part of its course by laceration, stab, or gunshot wounds. The wrist is the most common site of external injury. Compression of the nerve at the wrist (carpal tunnel syndrome) may be secondary to prolonged occupational pressure, tenosynovitis with arthritis, or local infiltration, for example, by a thickening of connective tissue and deposit of amyloid with multiple myeloma or of mucopolysaccharides. Other systemic diseases associated with carpal tunnel syndrome are acromegaly, hypothyroidism, and rheumatoid arthritis. Incomplete lesions of the median nerve between the axilla and wrist may result in *causalgia* (see Chap. 2). The treatment of carpal tunnel syndrome is surgical section of the carpal ligament.

ULNAR NERVE This nerve is derived from the eighth cervical and first thoracic roots. It innervates the ulnar flexor of the wrist, the inner half of the deep finger flexors, the adductors and abductors of the fingers, the adductor of the thumb, the two medial lumbricals, and muscles of the hypothenar eminence. It is the sensory nerve to the fifth and ulnar half of the fourth fingers and the ulnar border of the hand. Complete ulnar paralysis results in a characteristic claw-hand deformity owing to wasting of the small hand muscles and hyperextension of the fingers at the metacarpophalangeal joints and flexion at the interphalangeal joints. The flexion deformity is most pronounced in the fourth and fifth fingers. Sensory loss occurs over the fifth finger, the ulnar aspect of the fourth finger, and the ulnar border of the palm. The ulnar nerve is most commonly injured at the elbow because of fracture or dislocation involving the joint. *Delayed ulnar palsy* may occur many years after an injury to the elbow joint which has resulted in a cubitus valgus deformity of the joint. Because of the deformity, the nerve is stretched in its course over the ulnar condyle. The superficial location of the nerve at the elbow makes it a common site of pressure palsy. Prolonged pressure on the base of the palm may result in damage to the deep palmar branch of the ulnar nerve, causing weakness of small hand muscles but no sensory loss.

Crural palsies The twelfth thoracic, first to fifth lumbar, and first, second, and third sacral nerve roots compose the lumbosacral plexuses and innervate the muscles of the lower extremities and "saddle" region. The following are the common crural palsies.

LUMBOSACRAL PLEXUS LESIONS The lumbosacral plexus is subject to a number of disease processes, mostly secondary. Diseases of the upper plexus produce unilateral weakness in flexion and adduction of hip, extension of knee, and sensory loss over anterior thigh and leg; those of lower plexus cause weakness of posterior thigh, leg, and foot muscles with loss of sensation over the fifth lumbar and first and second sacral roots.

The diseases that affect the plexus are carcinoma of cervix and prostate, retroperitoneal tumors, iliopsoas hemorrhages from ruptured aneurysms and hemophilia, neuralgic amyotrophy, abdominal and thoracolumbar operations, and diabetes mellitus. These are discussed more fully by Adams and Victor.

LATERAL FEMORAL CUTANEOUS NERVE This nerve is derived from the second and third lumbar roots. It is a sensory nerve supplying the lateral aspect of the thigh. The nerve enters the thigh beneath the lateral end of the inguinal ligament and then enters the fascia lata, where it may become constricted. Compression of the nerve results in uncomfortable paresthesias along its cutaneous distribution and in sensory impairment. The condition is called *meralgia paresthetica* (mentioned below). The definitive treatment is surgical sectioning of the nerve at the inguinal ligament but this is seldom necessary.

OBTURATOR NERVE This nerve is derived from the second, third, and fourth lumbar roots. It supplies the adductor muscles of the thigh, and injury to the nerve results in almost complete paralysis of adduction of the thigh. The nerve is most frequently injured during the course of a difficult labor and also as a result of dislocation of the hip or an obturator hernia. It may be affected in diabetes, polyarteritis nodosa, osteitis pubis, and retroperitoneal and pelvic malignant tumors.

FEMORAL NERVE This nerve is derived from the second, third, and fourth lumbar roots. It supplies the iliacus, pectineus, sartorius, and quadriceps muscles and carries sensory impulses from the anteromedial aspect of the thigh and medial side of the lower leg. Following injury to the nerve, there is paralysis of extension of the knee, with wasting of the quadriceps muscle and also some weakness of hip flexion. The knee jerk is abolished. The nerve may be involved in fractures and dislocation of the hip and in fractured pelvis. It may be affected in diabetes, polyarteritis nodosa, and in retroperitoneal, pelvic, or abdominal lesions such as tumor, psoas abscess, or retroperitoneal hemorrhage. Because the femoral artery may also be severed, wounds in the femoral triangle may be fatal.

SCIATIC NERVE This nerve is derived from the fourth and fifth lumbar and first and second sacral roots. It provides the motor innervation of the hamstring muscles and all those below the knee; it carries sensory impulses from the posterior aspect of the thigh and posterior and lateral aspects of the leg and entire sole. In complete sciatic paralysis, the knee cannot be flexed and all muscles below the knee are paralyzed. The sciatic nerve is commonly injured in fractures of the pelvis or femur, in gunshot wounds of the buttock and thigh, by lying or sitting insensate and compressing the nerve in the lower buttock area, and by the inadvertent injection of toxic substances such as paraldehyde. It may also be involved by pelvic tumors and in both diabetes mellitus and polyarteritis nodosa. Cryptogenic forms also occur and are actually more frequent than those with an identifiable cause. A ruptured lumbar disk often simulates sciatic neuropathy. Incomplete lesions of the sciatic nerve occasionally result in causalgia.

COMMON PERONEAL NERVE This nerve is one of the terminal divisions of the sciatic nerve in the popliteal fossa. It supplies the dorsiflexors of the foot and toes and everters of the foot and sensation to the dorsum of the foot and lateral aspect of the lower half of the leg. These functions are lost with lesions which completely interrupt the nerve. Pressure or sleep palsy is one of the most frequent types of injury, the compression being of that part of the nerve which passes over the head of the fibula. It is also commonly involved by fractures involving the upper end of the fibula and in diabetic neuropathy, polyarteritis nodosa, and operations on the knee. Some are idiopathic, as pointed out by Berry and Richardson, who analyzed 70 personally observed cases.

TIBIAL NERVE This nerve is the other of the two terminal divisions of the sciatic nerve in the popliteal fossa. It supplies all the calf muscles and the flexors of the foot. Complete paralysis of the nerve results in a calcaneovalgus deformity of the foot, which no longer can be plantar-flexed. There is loss of sensation over the plantar aspect of the foot.

SOME DISEASES WHICH INVOLVE SINGLE NERVES OR PLEXUSES

INFECTIONS In faucial diphtheria, selective involvement of the vagi and nerves to the ciliary muscles of the eye results in palatal paralysis and paralysis of accommodation. The palatal palsy occurs in the first 2 weeks of infection and the loss of accommodation about a week later. Both tend to improve rapidly. In cutaneous diphtheria, involvement of nerves locally results in paralysis of the muscles supplied by the spinal segment from which the infected region is innervated. In leprosy, granulomatous involvement of skin and cutaneous nerves, particularly in the cooler parts of the body, dominates the clinical picture. Several nerves become involved at sites where they lie superficially, for instance, the median nerve at the wrist, the ulnar nerve at the elbow, and the peroneal nerve on the dorsum of the foot. Herpes zoster is a sensory neuritis of viral cause, characterized by acute inflammation of one or more posterior root ganglia, spinal nerves, and roots and gray matter of the spinal cord. Lancinating pain and hyperalgesia over the skin surface supplied by affected roots occur for 3 or 4 days, followed by the appearance of a segmental herpetic eruption. If the inflammatory process spreads to involve adjacent motor roots of anterior horns of the cord, segmental motor weakness and wasting appear. Paralysis of the oculomotor nerves may occur in conjunction with involvement of the gasserian ganglion (ophthalmoplegic zoster). Facial paralysis may occur with involvement of the geniculate ganglion (Ramsay Hunt syndrome). Sarcoidosis may involve single or multiple peripheral nerves, producing asymmetric mononeuritis or polyneuritis. Unilateral or bilateral facial paralysis is common in association with parotitis and uveitis in sarcoidosis.

TRAUMA External trauma may result in complete transection of a peripheral nerve or may block conduction without interrupting the anatomic continuity of the involved nerve, a state called *neuropraxia.* Complete division of a mixed peripheral nerve results in paralysis and sensory loss corresponding to the region supplied by the damaged nerve. Recovery of function after complete division can take place only when the divided ends lie in apposition or have been sutured. Growth of nerve fibers proceeds at a rate of 1 to 2 mm a day, and the recovery time can be estimated by the distance between the site of injury and the destination of the nerve. An early indication of regeneration is the presence of tingling sensation below the lesion (Tinel's sign which is due to sensitivity of thinly myelinated regenerating fibers) on tapping along the nerve. Sensory recovery precedes the return of motor power. All forms of cutaneous sensation begin to return together. Appreciation of pain and temperature improves, but the stimuli are poorly localized for some time. Eventually there is recovery of the discriminative aspects of sensation, including localization of sensory stimuli, postural sense, recognition of slight differences in temperature, and appreciation of very light touch.

PRESSURE PALSIES AND ENTRAPMENT NEUROPATHIES A period of prolonged compression of a nerve against an underlying bone results in temporary paralysis owing to myelin sheath damage. Mild degrees of compression (neuropraxia) are followed by fairly rapid recovery, in 2 to 12 weeks. Severe compression, such as may occur during a bout of alcoholic intoxication, deep sleep, or anesthesia, may result in focal disintegration of myelin, damage to axons, and Wallerian degeneration of distal segments. In this situation, recovery will be slow as regeneration takes place. Common varieties of pressure palsy are radial nerve paralysis with wrist drop due to prolonged pressure against the back of the arm (Saturday night palsy), ulnar palsy due to repeated trauma to the nerve at the elbow, especially after an old fracture that changes the relation of the nerve to the bicipital groove, and peroneal nerve palsy with foot drop caused by compression of the nerve against the fibula, as in sitting with legs crossed or during obstetric procedures with legs in stirrups.

The entrapment neuropathies result from chronic compression of a nerve against bone at a point where it passes through a narrow space. Slowly the perineurium and epineurium thicken and strangulate the nerve with injury to some of its larger, more peripheral, fibers. Several unique syndromes are known: (1) median nerve entrapment in carpal tunnel (see above); (2) *meralgia paresthetica,* a sensory neuropathy characterized by pain and paresthesia over the lateral aspect of the thigh because of compression of the lateral femoral cutaneous nerve at the level of Poupart's ligament or in the fascia lata; (3) Morton's toe from pressure of plantar nerves against metatarsal bone, giving rise to pain and paresthesia of third and fourth toes on walking; and (4) tarsal tunnel syndrome, entrapment of the distal posterior tibial nerve at the ankle with pain and numbness of the sole of the foot and weakness of plantar flexion of the toes. Pressure on nerve roots in the cervical and lumbar regions by *herniated intervertebral disks* results in pain, sensory impairment, and variable motor weakness corresponding to the area supplied by the involved root (see Chap. 137). Compression of the medial cord of the brachial plexus by a *cervical rib or by some other malformation of the thoracic outlet* (thoracic outlet syndrome) results in atrophy of small hand muscles and sensory loss in the ulnar nerve distribution. Usually the subclavian artery is also compressed. When the median nerve is compressed at the wrist beneath the transverse carpal ligament (carpal tunnel syndrome), there are pain and paresthesias in the palmar surface of the hand and first three fingers, then atrophy, weakness in flexor of thumb and opponens muscle, and sensory impairment over the median nerve distribution.

TUMOR Peripheral nerves may be compressed or invaded by primary or metastatic tumors arising in other tissues. Solitary tumors of nerve sheaths, or neuromas, commonly occur along the roots of spinal nerves, chiefly in the thoracic and lumbar regions. Compression of the nerve root and adjacent spinal cord may occur. Root compression causes pain referred to the distribution of the involved nerve, and there may be associated sensory impairment and motor weakness. Lymphomatosis and carcinomatosis of the cranial and spinal meninges may implicate single or multiple nerve roots. Tumor cells may be found in the cerebrospinal fluid. Solitary neuromas may involve any of the peripheral nerves, producing local pain and tenderness to palpation. Multiple neuromas occur in von Recklinghausen's disease and are associated with multiple congenital anomalies, as well as kyphoscoliosis, cutaneous pigmentation, and cutaneous fibromas. The treatment of solitary expanding nerve tumors of the limbs is surgical, the nature and extent of the procedure depending upon the character of the individual tumor.

IDIOPATHIC NEUROPATHY *Bell's palsy* is due to inflammation of the facial nerve in the facial canal as a result of an obscure, possibly infective process. Edema may play a part leading to compression of nerve fibers, with resulting acute unilateral paralysis of facial muscles (see Chap. 367).

Brachial neuritis is an acute affection of the brachial plexus, characterized by the acute or subacute onset of severe pain in the neck, arm, and hand, followed by moderate muscle weakness, slight numbness or hyperesthesia, and depressed reflexes in the involved arm. The pain is usually severe and constant and is aggravated by moving the arm or stretching the brachial plexus. Muscle wasting is rarely severe, but some cases of brachial neuritis, especially those described by the term *neuralgic amyotrophy,* may be followed by localized paralysis and atrophy of the shoulder girdle and arm muscles. Some of these have a familial incidence. Recovery slowly occurs over a period of months. Symptomatic treatment, including complete rest of the involved arm and analgesics in the acute phase, followed by mild massage and exercise, usually suffices.

Sciatic neuritis causes pain in the lumbar region and behind the leg from buttock to ankle. The pain is aching or burning in quality and is aggravated by movement or straining. The sciatic nerve is tender to palpation or stretching. There may be slight weakness of the hamstrings and muscles below the knee. The ankle jerk is absent. Sensory impairment is usually slight. It is necessary to distinguish the symptoms of sciatic neuritis from those of sciatic compression. In compression (e.g., by tumor) the onset is more gradual, symptoms are progressive, muscle wasting is more conspicuous, the nerve is less tender to palpation, and sensory loss is greater. The course of sciatic neuritis is stationary at first, followed by slow improvement.

Serum neuritis develops several days after the onset of serum sickness. The fifth cervical nerve root is most commonly involved, with pain, paralysis, and atrophy corresponding to the distribution of the nerve. Occasionally the entire brachial plexus may be involved, and there is sometimes, but rarely, a generalized polyneuritis. The cause is not known, but the condition is attributed to endoneurial edema, comparable to the urticaria of serum sickness, with compression of affected roots or nerves. Recovery is usually complete but may take weeks or months.

Polyneuritis cranialis is a relapsing and remitting mononeuropathy multiplex restricted to the cranial nerves. It is usually associated with indolent tuberculous cervical adenitis (scrofula) or sarcoidosis. Treatment of the underlying condition will halt the cranial nerve palsies.

REFERENCES

ADAMS RD, VICTOR M: *Principles of Neurology*. New York, McGraw-Hill, 1977

ASBURY AK: The neuroaspects of disease of the peripheral nervous system, in *Update IV: Harrison's Principals of Internal Medicine*, KJ Isselbacher et al (eds). New York, McGraw-Hill, 1983

———, JOHNSON PC: *Pathology of Peripheral Nerve*. Philadelphia, Saunders, 1978

BERRY H, RICHARDSON PM: Common peroneal palsy: A clinical and electrophysiological review. J Neurol Neurosurg Psychiatry 39:1162, 1976

BRADLEY WG: *Disorders of Peripheral Nerve*. Oxford, Blackwell Scientific Publications, 1974

DYCK PJ, LAMBERT EH: Polyneuropathy associated with hypothyroidism. J Neuropathol Exp Neurol 29:631, 1970

——— et al: *Peripheral Neuropathy*, 2d ed. Philadelphia, Saunders, 1982

HAYMAKER W, WOODHALL B: *Peripheral Nerve Injuries*. Philadelphia, Saunders, 1953

PRINEAS JW, MCLEOD JG: Chronic relapsing polyneuritis. J Neurol Sci 27:427, 1976

SPENCER PS, SCHAUMBURG HH: *Experimental and Clinical Neurotoxicology*. Baltimore, Williams & Wilkins, 1980

VINKEN PJ, BRUYN GW: Diseases of nerves, in *Handbook of Clinical Neurology*. Amsterdam, North-Holland, 1970, vols 7, 8

section 12 | Diseases of striated muscle

369 APPROACH TO CLINICAL MYOLOGY

ROBERT R. YOUNG
WALTER G. BRADLEY
RAYMOND D. ADAMS

GENERAL CONSIDERATIONS

Striated muscle tissue constitutes the principal organ of locomotion as well as a vast metabolic reservoir. Disposed in more than 600 separate muscles, this tissue comprises as much as 40 percent of the weight of an adult man. Intricacy of structure undoubtedly accounts for its diverse susceptibilities to disease.

A single muscle is composed of thousands of fibers which course for variable distances along its longitudinal axis. In some muscles the fibers extend the entire length of the muscle, but more often insert laterally into tendons (bipennate); in others they are joined end to end by connective tissue. Each fiber is a relatively large and complex multinucleated cell varying in length from a few millimeters to several centimeters (34 cm in the human sartorius muscle) and in diameter from 10 to 100 μm. Although the fiber normally represents an indivisible anatomic and physiologic unit, disease may affect only one part of it, leaving the remainder to atrophy, degenerate, or regenerate, depending on the nature and severity of the disease. Cell nuclei, which are oriented parallel to the longitudinal axis of the fiber and number into the thousands, lie beneath the plasmalemmal membrane (the sarcolemma) and hence are called *sarcolemmal*. The cytoplasm (sarcoplasm) of the cell is abundant and contains myofibrils and various other organelles such as mitochondria, Golgi apparatus, and endoplasmic reticulum. The myofibrils in turn are composed of longitudinally oriented interdigitating filaments (myofilaments) of contractile proteins (actin and myosin). The transverse regular arrangement of actin (I, isotropic) and myosin (A, anisotropic) myofilaments produces the characteristic striations of skeletal muscle. There are two tubular systems of endoplasmic reticulum, one oriented longitudinally between myofibrils and one transversely (T tubules) at the A-I band junction. The latter is a specialized structure and, with the two lateral cisternae of the longitudinal sarcoplasmic reticulum, forms a triad. Physiologically the T tubules are deep invaginations of the sarcolemma; hence they enclose an extracellular space. Droplets of stored fat, glycogen, various proteins, many enzymes, and myoglobin, the latter imparting the red color to muscle, can also be identified within the sarcoplasm or its organelles.

Histochemistry has been widely used to study diseased muscle and the results have been summarized in a monograph by Dubowitz and Brooke. Histochemical stains of normal muscle show two classes of fibers, one staining darkly and the other lightly. The former is rich in oxidative enzymes and the latter in glycolytic enzymes. Oxidative-rich fibers (type I) are supplied by neurons that are normally designated "slow twitch" and are engaged predominantly in tonic postural muscular reactions; glycolytic-rich fibers (type II) are termed "fast twitch" and are involved mainly in phasic reactions. But in such stains (ATPase at pH 9.4 is most commonly used) there are other intermediate types, subclasses referred to as IIA, IIB, and IIC. Fiber types are found to react differently in certain diseases and in disuse and denervation atrophy, as will be elaborated further on in this chapter.

The individual muscle fibers are enveloped by delicate strands of connective tissue (endomysium) which provide for their support and permit unity of action. The blood vessels, of which there may be several for each fiber, and nerve filaments lie within the endomysium. Similar sheets of collagen (perimysium) bind together groups or fascicles of fibers and surround the entire muscle (epimysium). The muscle fibers are attached at their ends to tendon fibers, which in turn connect with the skeleton. By this means contraction maintains posture and effects movement.

Specialized endings of sensory nerves wrap themselves around small striated muscle fibers described as *intrafusal* because they are grouped into fusiform bundles of 4 to 12 within a connective tissue capsule, termed the *muscle spindle.* These are scattered within each muscle and lie in parallel to the great mass of extrafusal fibers described above. By means of a complex feedback arrangement, the spindle afferent nerve impulses permit the central nervous system to monitor changes in muscle length. Another specialized intramuscular sensory organ is found at the ends of extrafusal muscle fibers where they attach to a tendon. The latter, called *Golgi tendon organs,* are in series between muscle and tendon fibers; afferent nerve impulses from them reflect the tension produced by contraction.

Other notable characteristics of muscle are its natural mode of activation, i.e., innervation, and the necessity of intact nerve supply for the maintenance of its nutrition. Each muscle fiber (intra- or extrafusal) receives a nerve twig from a motor nerve cell in the anterior horn of the spinal cord or nucleus of a cranial nerve, which joins it at a point called the *neuromuscular junction* (also called the *motor end plate*). Acetylcholine is liberated from presynaptic vesicles in the nerve terminals and transmits the nerve impulse to the muscle fiber. There is a gap (synaptic gap) of 200 to 500 Å between the nerve terminal and the postsynaptic membrane of the muscle fiber. The nerve terminal lies in a groove in the muscle (the primary synaptic cleft from which radiate secondary synaptic clefts). Acetylcholine receptors and cholinesterase, which play a special role in neuromuscular transmission, are concentrated postsynaptically at this junction zone. Groups of noncontiguous muscle fibers with a common innervation from one anterior horn cell constitute the "motor unit" which is the basic physiologic unit in all reflex, postural, and voluntary activity. In addition to motor nerve fibers within the muscle nerve, there are the two types of large sensory fibers (proprioceptive), one from the muscle spindles and the other from the Golgi tendon organs, which participate in reflex control of muscle activity. There are also small fibers from free nerve endings which subserve pain sensation, and postganglionic sympathetic fibers to blood vessels.

It would be a mistake to predicate that apparent similarity of structure renders all muscles equally susceptible to disease. In point of fact, no disease affects all muscles in the body, and each neuromuscular disease has as one of its features a unique distribution of muscle involvement. These topographic differences between diseases provide incontrovertible evidence of unique structural qualities, not presently disclosed by the light or electron microscope. One factor may relate simply to fiber size. Consider, for example, the large diameter and length of the fibers of the gluteus and paravertebral muscles in comparison with the ocular muscles. Again, the number of fibers composing a motor unit may be of significance in explaining selective vulnerability; e.g., in the ocular muscles the motor units contain only 6 to 10 muscle fibers, whereas in the gastrocnemius, each motor unit contains as many as 2000 fibers. There are also individual differences in vascular patterns of supply, permitting some muscles to withstand the effects of hypoxia or vascular occlusion (as occurs transiently during forceful contraction) better than others. Metabolic differences among fibers within any one muscle have been revealed by histochemical studies, certain fibers being richer in glycolytic and poorer in oxidative enzymes than others. But there must surely exist other metabolic differences, as yet unknown.

Regarding the pathogenesis of myopathic disease, one may envisage causative agents which affect each of the different components of sarcoplasm, namely, an enzyme, an essential substrate, the filamentous proteins, the endoplasmic reticulum, or the sarcolemma itself. The endomysial connective tissue also could be the primary pathway in disease, since it so closely invests the muscle. Inadequacy of blood supply in relation to the metabolic requirements of active muscle, or frank ischemia from vascular occlusion, could be postulated as another mechanism of disease. Finally, the nerve or its cell of origin in the spinal cord is known to bear the brunt of certain pathologic processes paralyzing all the muscle fibers of that motor unit and removing its unique trophic influence on muscle.

Normal muscle possesses a limited capacity to regenerate, a point often forgotten. Acute destructive processes of the muscle fiber, e.g., inflammatory, metabolic, and certain other diseases, are usually followed by fairly complete restoration of the muscle cells, providing some part of each fiber has survived and the endomysial sheaths of connective tissue have not been disturbed. Unfortunately many pathologic processes of muscle are chronic and unrelenting and completely destroy the muscle fibers. Under such conditions any regenerative activity fails to keep pace with the disease, and the loss of muscle fibers is permanent.

MYOPATHOLOGY

Several basic disorders may be distinguished by means of muscle biopsy and postmortem examination:

1. *Denervation atrophy.* This consists of reduction in size of fibers within denervated motor units due to removal of the trophic influence nerve normally exerts on muscle. Denervated muscle fibers maintain their sarcolemmal integrity but lose myofibrils in excess of other constituents. They become shrunken, angulated, and excessively stained by histochemical reactions for oxidative enzymes. The intact motor units enlarge by collateral sprouting from intact nerves. This is best revealed by grouping of fibers of one histochemical type.
2. *Segmental necrosis of muscle fibers* with myophagia and regeneration (by forking or branching). This is the typical change in idiopathic polymyositis (in combination with infiltrates of inflammatory cells), in infective polymyositis (in the presence of trichina, toxoplasma, etc.), in Zenker's degeneration, in Duchenne's and other dystrophies, in alcoholic polymyopathy, and in Meyer-Betz paroxysmal myoglobinuria.
3. *Structural faults in muscle fibers.* These include sarcoplasmic masses and ringbinden in myotonic dystrophy, glycogen masses in glycogen storage diseases, lipid aggregates in lipid storage diseases, rod (nemeline) and other cytoplasmic bodies in the congenital myopathies, hyperplasia, aggregation, and other abnormalities of mitochondria, and nuclei in the center of fibers in centronuclear myopathy.
4. *Disturbances in number and size of fibers* as a reflection of abnormalities of growth, maturation, and aging. Many states of dwarfism and congenital myopathies of a myotubular type present principally as numerical or volumetric changes, which must be distinguished from denervation atrophy, disuse effects, cachexia, and work hypertrophy. Certain dis-

eases may affect only one fiber type; for example, all forms of disease leading to disuse of the muscle produce atrophy of type II fibers.

5 *Disorders of conduction apparatus* (neuromuscular junctions, sarcolemma, and sarcoplasmic reticulum), in which nerve fibers and muscle fibers appear to be intact and the abnormality can be revealed only by special physiologic, morphologic, pharmacologic, or biochemical techniques. Myasthenia gravis, botulism, and the periodic paralyses fall into this category.

NERVE PATHOLOGY

Two basic processes can be distinguished in nerve by biopsy and postmortem examination:

1 *Segmental demyelination,* where Schwann cells and/or myelin sheaths are damaged, leaving axons intact.
2 *Axonal degeneration,* where axons are disrupted, leading to secondary degeneration of the myelin sheath.

Whenever the axon is destroyed at any point along nerve, the rest of the nerve fiber (both axon and myelin sheath) that is disconnected from the nerve cell degenerates within a few days, a process called *Wallerian degeneration.*

Each of the above processes can be caused by a number of diseases and may occur separately or together, as in diabetic neuropathy. Moreover, mild forms of focal damage such as ischemia or compression may cause segmental demyelination whereas more severe forms, axonal degeneration. Both processes paralyze muscle and both will undergo natural repair, namely, remyelination after segmental degeneration and axonal regeneration after axonal degeneration. Repair of segmental demyelination can be relatively rapid; for example, return of muscle power after paralysis from diphtheritic or Landry-Guillain-Barré disease may take only a few weeks. Regeneration after axonal lesions which must begin from the intact end of the fiber is extremely slow; it proceeds at a rate of 1 to 2 mm per day.

Repeated attacks of nerve disease may result in fiber loss and permanent paralysis. If the basal lamina and endoneurium of individual nerve fibers are disrupted, the regenerating axons are misdirected and may form a neuroma.

Infiltration of inflammatory cells, angiitis, and deposits of amyloid are important diagnostic findings in a nerve biopsy.

BIOPSY OF MUSCLE AND NERVE If muscle or nerve biopsy is to be of maximal diagnostic value, both the surgical and microscopic techniques must be exacting. The muscle chosen for study should show evidence that it has been affected but not totally destroyed by the disease in question, and it should not recently have been studied electromyographically since the trauma of the needle electrodes produces focal destructive lesions. Muscle biopsy is indicated (1) to aid in the differentiation among neuropathic atrophy, dystrophy, metabolic myopathy, and polymyositis; (2) to corroborate the diagnosis of diffuse diseases of connective tissue and blood vessels (e.g., polyarteritis nodosa, lupus), or special infections (e.g., trichinosis, toxoplasmosis); (3) for diagnosis of metabolic diseases involving muscle (e.g., glycogen and lipid storage diseases) and the special myopathies (nemaline and central core myopathies); and (4) in the scientific study of disorders of neuromuscular transmission apparatus (e.g., myasthenia gravis, periodic paralysis), usually by a combination of electrophysiologic, pharmacologic, histochemical, and electron microscopic techniques. In most instances, it is possible to distinguish histologically the effects of denervation, the dystrophies and other necrotizing myopathies, special disfigurative myopathies, and polymyositis.

The muscle biopsy is performed under local or general anesthesia. The local anesthetic must be confined to the skin and superficial fascia. Three cylinders of muscle about 2 cm long and 0.5 cm in diameter are taken. One specimen for histology is kept at its original length in a biopsy clamp, and fixed in 10% neutral formalin, embedded in paraffin, sectioned in a cross and longitudinal fashion, and stained by hematoxylin and eosin, phosphotungstic acid hematoxylin, and Gomori trichrome methods. The second specimen for histochemistry is rapidly frozen in liquid nitrogen, sectioned transversely in a cryostat, and stained by various histochemical reactions (e.g., myosin ATPase, mitochondrial oxidative enzymes, phosphorylase). The third piece in a biopsy clamp is fixed in glutaraldehyde for electron microscopy. Special techniques may be applied, if it is desirable to visualize the intramuscular nerves and myoneural junctions, such as the methylene blue–cholinesterase method of Cöers and Woolf.

Biopsies of nerves for which there must be more rigorous indications (special problems, research) may be taken under local or general anesthesia. The sural nerve is a commonly biopsied sensory nerve, and the whole nerve or a fraction (fascicular biopsy) may be taken. The nerve is fixed under tension to stretch the fibers and is processed by the fixation, staining, and embedding techniques of routine microscopy, phase optics, and electron microscopy. When studied by ordinary microscopy, nerve biopsies provide less useful histopathologic data than muscle biopsy. Before fixation, these biopsies can also be studied physiologically in vitro where fibers of all sizes can be stimulated and their activity recorded. In contrast to routine nerve conduction studies where only the largest fibers can be sampled, this in vitro technique affords a rapid, semiquantitative assessment of the effects of the disease process on fibers of each of the different sizes contained within the nerve.

BIOPHYSICS AND BIOCHEMISTRY OF NEUROMUSCULAR DISEASE

The biochemical tests presently in use fall into two categories: measurement of serum electrolytes, enzymes, and other chemicals and detection of myoglobin and abnormal amounts of creatine and creatinine in the urine. In certain diseases biochemical studies performed on muscle removed at biopsy may be diagnostic.

ELECTROLYTES AND THEIR EFFECTS ON NEUROMUSCULAR EXCITABILITY In the resting state all nerve and muscle fibers are *polarized* with the interior of the cell negative to the outside surface by a potential difference of 70 to 90 mV. This *resting membrane potential* is closely related to the electrochemical equilibrium for potassium ions, the interior of the cell being some 30 times richer in this ion than the extracellular fluid on the outside of the nerve or muscle membrane. At equilibrium, the chemical forces tending to promote diffusion of K ions outward (down their concentration gradient) are counterbalanced by electrical forces, since the relative external positivity opposes the movement of further K ions to the outside. At the resting potential, the situation for Na ions is quite the opposite. Since their external concentration is 10 to 12 times that within the cell, they tend to be driven inward because of both their concentration gradient and the electrical attraction of the relative negativity inside the cell. Under resting conditions, however, these forces are ineffective by virtue of the very low permeability of the sarcolemma to Na ions. Any leakage of Na into the cell is overcome, initially by the diffusion of an equal amount of K outward, and subsequently by the metabolically active expulsion of Na ions (*sodium pump*).

The membrane permeability to Na is controlled by the membrane potential—depolarization producing increased permeability to Na due to activation of sodium carriers in the nerve cell. With slight electrically or chemically mediated depolarization there is a brief influx of Na, but the subsequent diffusion of K outward repolarizes the membrane and, therefore, reduces its permeability to Na. This is the "passive decay" of change in resting potential. If, when the depolarization is greater and a *threshold* is reached at which the outward K current is unable to stabilize the situation, the membrane is further depolarized, it then becomes progressively more permeable to Na, and an explosive *regenerative Na current* develops. Na rushes down its chemical and electrical gradients into the cell which eventually approaches the equilibrium potential for Na with the interior of the cell now 20 to 40 mV positive. This *action potential* lasts a millisecond or less because the membrane now becomes almost impermeable to Na and much more permeable to K. The resulting efflux of K repolarizes it to the resting level.

The regenerative Na current cannot be activated by another depolarizing stimulus during the *refractory period* until the membrane has been repolarized. If this process of recovery is delayed, *depolarization inactivation* of the Na current prevents the development of further action potentials until the resting membrane potential has been restored. These various membrane phenomena responsible for the resting and action potentials do not themselves depend directly upon energy-rich substrates, though such metabolically active processes are essential for the sodium pump and the long-term maintenance of resting ionic concentrations.

Because the region of membrane at the site of the action potential becomes polarized oppositely to the remainder, *action currents* flow into the former from the surrounding regions and depolarize them. The depolarization may reach the threshold for development of an action potential there, and new zones of increased Na permeability then spread in this way in an all-or-none fashion down the length of the nerve or in both directions from the center of the muscle membrane as a *conducted action potential.*

Clearly, these events, the hallmarks of all excitable tissues, are modified by the concentration of K ions in extracellular fluids. Other ions, particularly Ca, Mg, and Cl, are also influential.

The *neuromuscular junction* (motor end plate) has properties of special importance. Here a motor nerve twig indents the surface of the muscle fiber which it innervates. The membranes of the two cells, the neurilemma and the sarcolemma, remain separated by a narrow space, the *synaptic cleft.* Across this space acetylcholine diffuses, liberated from presynaptic vesicles by the arrival of *nerve action potentials.* It is estimated that the arrival of a single nerve impulse at the terminal will liberate the acetylcholine of 60 to 100 vesicles, each containing about 10,000 molecules. Ca ions facilitate the release of packets (*quanta*) of acetylcholine from the vesicles, and botulinus toxin, aminoglycoside antibiotics, or a very high concentration of Mg ions interfere with this release. Acetylcholine receptors on the specialized, chemically excitable area of muscle membrane which forms the postsynaptic portion of the end plate react to the presence of acetylcholine with a local increase in the conductance of Na, K, and other small cations, producing a depolarization which can be recorded as the *end plate potential.* Thus, the spontaneous release of quanta of acetylcholine produces miniature end plate potentials in the postsynaptic membrane. If the depolarization of the membrane is large enough, current flow into it from the neighboring electrically excitable areas of muscle membrane depolarizes it toward the threshold potential. Once the threshold is reached, an independent, all-or-nothing *muscle action potential* arises and, in the same manner as the nerve action potential is conducted, propagates over the surface of the sarcolemma toward both ends of the fiber.

The electrical change appears to be distributed from the surface of the muscle fiber inward to all the myofibrils via the transverse tubular system (T system) to activate the longitudinal sarcoplasmic reticulum, and thus the contractile mechanism. Calcium is released from the depolarized membrane of the sarcoplasmic reticulum into the sarcoplasm, activates myosin adenosine triphosphatase (ATPase), energy is released by the dephosphorylation of adenosine triphosphate (ATP), crossbridges form between the actin and myosin filaments, and they slide past one another shortening each sarcomere and producing tension. The resultant shortening constitutes the ultrastructural equivalent of contraction.

This mechanical change or *twitch* lasts a great deal longer than the action potential. A second electrical wave can, therefore, arrive before the muscle fiber has relaxed, prolonging the contraction, and if the anterior horn cell fires (or the motor axon is stimulated) at frequencies of 10 to 20 per second, the twitches fuse into a prolonged contraction (tetanus). The mechanical event can thus be smoothed into a continuous process, but the electrical potentials remain a series of peaks of external negativity, separated by plateaus during part of which the membrane is in its resting polarized state.

This *repolarization* after passage of an action potential is necessary if the membrane is to be capable of transmitting a second impulse. At the end plate, repolarization is possible only if acetylcholine is removed, a process of hydrolysis achieved by the enzyme cholinesterase. If this fails, the end plate remains depolarized and cannot respond to further nerve impulses. *Anticholinesterases* such as neostigmine (Prostigmin), pyridostigmine (Mestinon), edrophonium (Tensilon), physostigmine (Eserine), diisopropyl fluorophosphate (DFP), tetraethylpyrophosphate (TEPP), and several of the "nerve gases" and pyrophosphate insecticides act in this way to paralyze muscle. These substances and the so-called depolarizing blocking agents (succinylcholine and decamethonium) paralyze by maintaining the end plate region in a depolarized state (depolarization inactivation), refractory to the arrival of further nerve impulses. Curare-like substances and possibly antibodies to receptor substance, the so-called competitive blocking agents, paralyze muscle in a different way by occupying receptor sites for acetylcholine on the postjunctional membrane, thereby preventing the neurotransmitter from depolarizing the muscle fiber. The toxin of puffer fish (tetrodotoxin) and the toxin of paralytic shellfish (saxotoxin) produce paralysis by blocking the Na channels of the excitable nerve and muscle membranes.

Biochemical disturbances may account not only for impairment of neuromuscular activity, resulting in weakness or paralysis, but also for its enhancement, reflected in excessive irritability to mechanical or other stimuli. "Spontaneous" discharges may occur, or a single nerve impulse may set off a train of action potentials in nerve or muscle. Hypocalcemic and hypomagnesemic *tetany* ensues in this way when the membrane of the nerve fiber becomes unstable. Ca and Mg both tend to stabilize the membrane, and changes in their concentrations within the range seen clinically affect conduction in peripheral nerve rather than function at the neuromuscular junction where their actions, opposite or competitive, require changes in concentrations usually incompatible with life. Ischemic paresthesias also arise on the basis of irritability and instability of polarization of axons. Some types of axonal myokymia (Isaac's syndrome) and certain benign fasciculations as well as the common cramps of calf and foot muscles (painful, sustained, involuntary contractions with motor units discharging at frequencies above 25 per second) may be due to increased excitability of the peripheral parts of the motor nerve. Hyponatremia or Na loss predisposes to cramps, as does the unaccustomed use of a muscle. Quinine, procainamide, diphenhydramine (Benadryl), and warmth tend to prevent them. At least one form of myotonia, a noncalcium-related irritability of the sarcolemmal membrane, is related to abnormally low chloride permeability of the sarcolemma. A high chloride conductance normally buffers the sarcolemma against the depolarizing action of extracellular K ions released during the preceding impulse.

The mechanism by which the muscle action potential initiates the contractile process is termed *excitation-contraction coupling;* the energy for this process is derived from the interaction of ATP with the special muscle proteins. The pyrophosphate bonds of ATP supply the energy and must be replenished constantly, a reaction which involves interchanges with the muscle phosphogen, creatine diphosphate, where high-energy phosphate bonds are stored. These interchanges in both directions require the action of creatine phosphokinase (CPK). The intracellular calcium which, as noted above, is released by the muscle action potential must be reaccumulated within the sarcoplasmic reticulum before actin and myosin filaments can slide back past one another with relaxation. This reuptake of calcium (*relaxing factor*) requires the expenditure of considerable energy. When ATP is lacking, the muscle remains contracted as in *rigor mortis* or the electrically silent *contracture* of phosphorylase deficiency (McArdle's syndrome). The same sort of contracture occurs under normal conditions in the "catch muscles" of certain mollusks.

Reconstitution of ATP requires oxidative or glycolytic metabolism. Muscle fibers differ in their content of oxidative versus glycolytic enzymes; the latter determine their ability to sustain anaerobic metabolism during periods of tonic contraction when intramuscular blood flow is compromised. Muscle cells with primarily aerobic metabolism have high concentrations of oxidative enzymes, are rich in mitochondria, contain greater concentrations of myoglobin (appear red), have slower rates of contraction and relaxation, fire more tonically, and are less fatigable than muscle cells poor in oxidative enzymes and myoglobin ("pale") but rich in glycolytic enzymes, which fire phasically in short bursts. The speed of contraction, a function of the exact type of the myosin ATPase, is low in the former and high in the latter type of muscle cell. The activity of calcium-activated myosin ATPase at pH 9.4 has been used to classify muscle fibers into two major types: type I ("red") possesses low and type II ("pale") high activity. Type II fibers may be subdivided into type IIA (fast oxidative, fatigue-resistant) and type IIB (fast glycolytic, easily fatigued) fibers. All the muscle fibers within one motor unit are of the same metabolic type.

To summarize, the muscle fiber, which is totally dependent on nerve for its stimulus to normal contraction, may be paralyzed in a number of ways. There may be failure of nerve to conduct an impulse, insufficient release of acetylcholine to depolarize the muscle cell, damage or inaccessibility of the postjunctional membrane to normally released acetylcholine, or the presence of a pharmacologic agent preventing repolarization of the end plate. Finally, the sarcolemmal membrane itself may fail to distribute the muscle impulse throughout the fiber, or the metabolic or contractile elements of the muscle may be temporarily or permanently deficient. Similarly, fascicular twitching, cramps, and muscle spasms may be due to excessive activity at a number of points in the neuromuscular apparatus. There may be instability of the nerve fiber, as in tetany, or unexplained hyperirritability of the motor neuron, as in amyotrophic lateral sclerosis. The threshold level for mechanical activation or electrical reactivation of the sarcolemmal membrane may be reduced, as with myotonia, or a change may occur within the muscle fiber itself, which, once shortened, may have insufficient energy for restoration to a relaxed state (contracture).

When the musculature is acutely and diffusely weakened, or when twitchings, spasms, and cramps occur, serum electrolytes should be studied. They reflect extracellular levels, and the ECG (see Chap. 249) may reveal alterations in intracellular content in cardiac muscle, which tends to parallel that of skeletal muscle. If the *plasma level of potassium falls below 2.5 meq or rises above 7 meq per liter,* weakness of extremity and trunk muscles results. When the concentration reaches 2 or 9 meq per liter, there is almost invariably flaccid paralysis of these muscles and later of the respiratory ones as well, only those of cranium, e.g., extraocular, tending to be spared. In addition, the tendon reflexes are diminished or absent. The reaction of muscle to percussion is also reduced or abolished, suggesting impairment of transmission along the sarcolemmal membranes themselves. Hypocalcemia of 7 mg/dl or less (as in rickets or hypoparathyroidism) or relative reduction in the proportion of ionized calcium (as in hyperventilation) causes increased irritability of the neurilemma (and to a lesser extent sarcolemma) and spontaneous discharge of sensory and motor nerve fibers, i.e., tetany (see Chap. 370) and sometimes convulsions. Frequent repetitive and finally prolonged spontaneous discharges appear in the electromyogram (EMG). Hypercalcemia above 12 mg/dl (as in vitamin D intoxication, hyperparathyroidism, and carcinomatosis) causes lethargy and weakness, perhaps on a central basis. *Magnesium deficiency* (from decreased intestinal absorption or increased renal losses due to diuretics, gentamycin, or primary renal diseases) with serum levels less than 1.0 meq per liter results in tetanic muscle spasms and convulsions: a considerable *increase in magnesium levels* leads to muscle weakness and depression of central nervous function (confusion). The weakness of muscle may be due, in part at least, to reduced release of acetylcholine at the motor end plate.

CHANGES IN SERUM LEVELS OF ENZYMES ORIGINATING IN MUSCLE CELLS In all diseases which cause extensive damage to striated muscle fibers, intracellular enzymes leak out of the fiber and enter the blood. Those which are now being measured in most hospital laboratories are the transaminases, lactic acid dehydrogenase, aldolase, and creatine phosphokinase. But high concentrations of these enzymes are found in heart muscle and/or liver cells; hence raised serum values may be due to myocardial infarction or hepatitis, as well as to the necrobiotic diseases of striated muscle (polymyositis, muscle trauma, muscle infarction, Meyer-Betz paroxysmal myoglobinuria, and the more rapidly advancing muscular dystrophies). For the serum levels to be interpretable, one must have evidence of the integrity of heart and liver. Isoenzyme patterns are of some value in separating the enzyme derived from skeletal muscle from that of other organs. Creatine phosphokinase (CPK), though present in heart and brain, is found in highest concentration in striated muscle. The normal level is 0 to 65 IU per liter of serum and it may exceed 20,000 IU in patients with destructive lesions of striated muscle. Even more interesting is its rise in some patients with progressive muscular dystrophy before there is enough destruction of fibers for the disease to be clinically manifest. Moreover, about 75 percent of the unaffected female carriers of Duchenne's pseudohypertrophic muscular dystrophy may now be identified because they often show slight elevations of serum CPK level. All workers are agreed that alterations of serum enzyme levels are nonspecific for dystrophy since they occur in all types of disease which injure or destroy the muscle fiber. Moreover, in the more slowly evolving types of dystrophy, such as that of Landouzy-Déjerine, the serum levels of CPK may be normal. It was hoped that the values would always be normal in denervation paralysis and muscular atrophy, but unfortunately they may be slightly elevated in patients with progressive muscular atrophy and amyotrophic lateral sclerosis. Sometimes one sees a patient with elevated CPK levels in the blood for which no explanation can be found and elevated levels in hypothyroidism are also not understood.

ENDOCRINOPATHIES In a number of disorders of endocrine glands, muscle weakness may be a prominent feature, and occasionally it becomes even a chief complaint. While these diseases are discussed in detail elsewhere (Chaps. 372 and 374), it should be noted that such weakness, local or generalized, acute or chronic, may occur in the absence of changes in serum electrolytes or enzymes. Specific hormone assays are then necessary for diagnosis. This is particularly true of thyrotoxicosis, where severe muscle paresis may appear without the classic signs of Graves' disease and of Cushing's disease.

MYOGLOBINURIA The red pigment, myoglobin, responsible for much of the color of muscle, is an iron protein compound present in the sarcoplasm of striated skeletal and cardiac fibers. Of the total body hematin compounds, about 25 percent is in muscle, the remainder in red blood corpuscles and other cells. Destruction of striated muscle, regardless of the process, liberates myoglobin, and because of its relatively small size, the molecule filters through the glomerulus and appears in the urine, imparting to it a burgundy red color. The serum is effectively cleared and retains its normal color. In contrast, hemolysis of red blood corpuscles, which frees hemoglobin, colors both serum and urine because of the high renal threshold. Myoglobinuria should thus be suspected when the urine is deep red and the serum normal in color. As in hemoglobinuria, the guaiac and benzidine tests are positive, and the final demonstration depends on spectroscopic analysis, which shows an absorption band at 581 nm, or immunologic methods which are infinitely more sensitive than spectroscopic ones. The urine does not fluoresce, as it does in porphyria. Myoglobin appears in the urine in the following conditions: spontaneous myoglobinuria of unknown cause, e.g., Meyer-Betz paroxysmal myoglobinuria; as a result of crushing or infarction of muscles; in rare cases of polymyositis and alcoholic and other myopathies such as McArdle's disease, carnitine palmityl transferase deficiency, following extreme muscular activity, and after the ingestion of certain toxic substances (from fish poisoned by waste products, as in Haff disease).

CREATINURIA Creatine, an amino acid, is a prominent constituent of striated muscle tissue. It may be ingested (exogenous creatine) but is also synthesized in the liver from glycine, arginine, and methionine and then delivered to the skeletal muscles, which contain the largest amount of this compound of any organ (150 mg per 100 g fresh weight muscle tissue). Creatinine, the anhydride of creatine, is a degradation product which is excreted in the urine. The creatinine content of muscles is low (about 5 mg/dl), since it diffuses readily through the sarcolemma. Normal male serum contains 0.2 to 0.6 mg/dl creatine; female serum, 0.4 to 0.9 mg. Creatinine serum levels range from 0.8 to 1.4 mg and are increased only in serious renal disease. Adult 24-h urine excretion of creatine averages from 60 to 150 mg in normal men and 100 to 300 mg in women. Creatinine excretion is remarkably constant at 1.0 to 1.6 g per day. In diseases such as progressive muscular dystrophy, the creatine content of the muscle fiber is diminished, and there is a decrease in creatinine excretion, increase in creatine excretion, and hypercreatinemia. The same alterations occur in neurogenic atrophy and with reduction in muscle mass in polymyositis, hyperthyroidism, Addison's disease, and male eunuchoidism. Ingestion of 1 to 3 g creatine will not significantly raise its level in blood or urine in a normal person, for the muscles are not saturated, but in an individual with a reduced muscle mass, creatinemia and creatinuria result. This type of creatine tolerance test thus merely indicates reduction in functional muscle mass. Studies of creatine and creatinine are now seldom used in the investigation of neuromuscular disease.

PHYSIOLOGY OF NEUROMUSCULAR ACTIVITY

ELECTROMYOGRAPHY Normally, a muscle twitch can be produced by a brief electrical pulse, less than 1 ms long (Faradic), because it stimulates motor nerve fibers within the muscle. After denervation, contraction can be produced only by much longer pulses (galvanic), which are necessary to stimulate the muscle fibers directly. This difference (Erb's reaction of degeneration) led to the plotting of strength-duration curves, a technique which is rarely necessary now.

The *motor unit* is defined as a motor neuron, its axon, and all the muscle fibers which it innervates. All movement, posture, and reflex activity are interpreted in terms of the integrated discharge of large numbers of these motor units by spinal and supraspinal mechanisms. Strength of muscle contraction can be reduced to the number of motor units enlisted at a given time, the frequency of their discharge, and the speed of contraction to the phasic versus tonic recruitment of units. A tendon or muscle stretch reflex is caused by a volley of sensory impulses from receptors within muscle spindles which briefly activate a group of the large (alpha) spinal motor neurons. Effectiveness of movement is related to the manner in which motor units of different muscles are activated and inhibited in reciprocal relations. Coordination of movements, posture, and automatic movements such as walking and running are understandable in terms of more complex spinal integrations of muscles. Paralysis represents the reverse, an inactivation of motor units or whole muscles, complete only upon severance of the peripheral motor innervation and followed then by extreme atrophy of muscle fibers with fibrillation and unusual generalized hypersensitivity to acetylcholine.

The striated muscles are numerous, scattered, and, in some instances, of large size. As a result, no small series of leads (cf. ECG) will give an average picture of their electrical activity. They must be tested laboriously, one at a time, because disease may be spread irregularly through many of them, so that normal findings in one area do not exclude the possibility of pathologic phenomena close by. External plate or surface electrodes, such as those used in ECG and EEG, will pick up potentials representing the chance summation of many motor units, giving only an average picture. A more detailed physiologic analysis requires fine concentric needle electrodes to be placed carefully within a muscle so as to register the activity of only a small number of motor units or muscle fibers.

As an impulse travels from the center toward either end of an active muscle fiber, current begins to flow outward through the normally polarized region under the recording electrode toward the depolarized zone. Therefore, as in Fig. 369-1, the recording electrode becomes slightly positive relative to the reference electrode, and the beam of the cathode ray oscilloscope (CRO) is deflected, by convention, downward (at A). When the depolarized region moves under the recording electrode, the latter rapidly becomes quite negative (upward deflection at B). As the active region moves further down the sarcolemma, away from the electrode, the membrane under the latter slowly becomes repolarized. Current again begins to flow outward through the membrane toward the distant depolarized region, and the electrode, therefore, becomes relatively positive once again, as at C, before becoming isopotential to the reference electrode at rest. The net result is a triphasic action potential recorded on the CRO as in Fig. 369-1, with a very rapid negative-going phase, a configuration typical of fibrillations recorded from denervated and spontaneously active single muscle fibers. Because these potential changes are completed in less than 5 ms, the inertia-free CRO must be used to record them (ink writers do not have the necessary frequency response).

RECORDING OF MOTOR UNIT ACTIVITY The simple triphasic potentials discussed above result from the activity of single muscle fibers, but in healthy muscle, single fibers are not independently active. Normally, excitation arrives via the motor nerves so that all the fibers of one motor unit are activated by any one impulse from the motor neuron (as indicated in Chap. 14). The size of the normal motor units varies from several muscle fibers per motor axon in extraocular or laryngeal muscles to several thousand muscle fibers per axon in some of the large limb-girdle muscles. In each motor unit, the fibers are not of uniform diameter, length, or shape, and their spatial orientation with regard to the electrode will vary. In normal muscle, the fibers of one motor unit are not packed tightly together in groups but are spread out in one general region of the muscle interspersed with the fibers of adjacent motor units. Such muscle activated by its nerve, therefore, produces rather complex motor unit potentials, presumably the result of summation of potentials of varying characteristics from each fiber of the motor unit within recording range of the electrode.

THE NORMAL ELECTROMYOGRAM Normal muscle is electrically silent when it is at rest. Once *insertion activity*, produced by the trauma of placing the needle, has died down, the electrodes record no propagated action potentials. When a muscle is voluntarily contracted, action potentials appear on the CRO screen. As a slowly progressive contraction begins, potentials of one motor unit appear at rates of 4 to 5 per second and increase to 8 to 10 per second; with increasing power of contraction, a second, or even third, unit will be *recruited*, slightly larger in size than the first. As the contraction becomes even stronger, more and larger motor units enter the picture, and their potentials begin to overlie each other until there results a disorderly crowd of action potentials of many sizes and shapes, firing at rates of about 20 per second. Since individual motor unit potentials can no longer be distinguished, this is referred to as a complete *interference pattern*. Obviously, a muscle contracting weakly because of less than full effort or disease of central or peripheral nervous or muscular systems will have fewer than normal active fibers and will produce a smaller total potential than normal. However, unless reduction in output is sufficient either to break up the interference pattern just described so that individual motor unit potentials become identifiable or to reduce its amplitude strikingly, one obtains no certain electrical evidence of abnormality. As long as a normal muscle is held actively contracted, the interference pattern continues. Gradual relaxation will result in a progressive dropping out of motor units until a few are left firing, then one, then none.

Skeletal muscle may also be artificially stimulated by the application of brief electric pulses through the skin overlying its motor nerve. With proper stimulating conditions, there will be one maximal muscle response for each shock, the form of which will depend upon the number of motor units activated and the number sampled by the recording electrodes. If repeated shocks are given, each response will have the same form and amplitude, until fatigue supervenes. Normal muscle will follow rates of stimulation greater than 25 per second for periods of at least 60 s before decrement of the action potential indicates the failure of some fibers to respond, probably because of failure of nerve impulse transmission at branching points of the terminal axon. This ability of muscle to follow repetitive stimulation is altered in certain diseases.

FIGURE 369-1

The shaded area represents the zone of the action potential which is negative to all other points on the fiber surface. It is shown at three points in its course (from left to right) along the fiber. At each point, the correspondingly lettered portion of the triphasic muscle action potential displayed on the cathode ray oscilloscope (CRO) reflects the potential difference between the active (vertical arrow) and reference (Ref.) electrodes. Polarity in this and subsequent figures is negative upward as depicted. The time calibration is on the CRO screen; for further details see test.

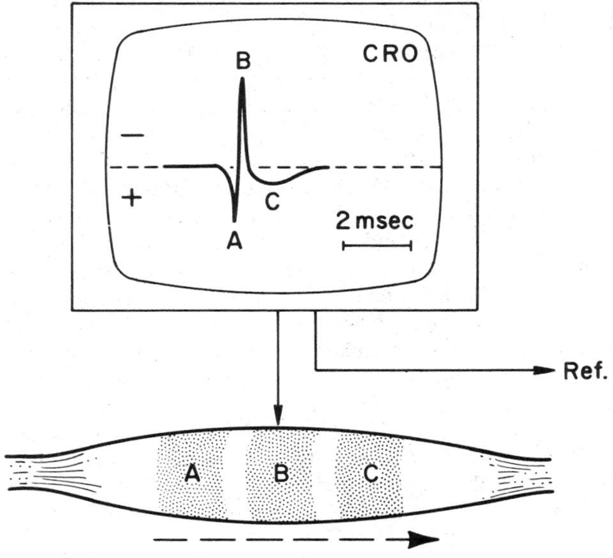

THE ABNORMAL ELECTROMYOGRAM Deviations from normal are detected in (1) the occurrence of "spontaneous" activity during relaxation (fibrillations, positive sharp waves, and fasciculations); (2) abnormalities in the amplitude, duration, and shape of single-motor-unit potentials; (3) a decrease in the number of motor units which can be recruited; (4) alteration in size, duration, or interpotential interval of action potentials recorded during graded single or successive voluntary or electrically induced muscular contractions; (5) the demonstration of special phenomena, such as myotonia, coupling (tetany), bizarre high-frequency potentials, or electrical silence during obvious shortening of the muscle (contracture); and (6) the documentation of various movement disorders.

Spontaneous activity during complete relaxation At the moment the needle is placed in the muscle, there is usually a brief burst of action potentials which cease once the needle is stable, providing it is not in a position to irritate an intramuscular nerve fiber. Myotonic muscle is extremely irritable; long runs of high-frequency discharges, waxing and waning in frequency with a "dive-bomber" sound, may be produced and recur at the slightest movement of the needle. Irritability is also found with conditions which dispose to muscle cramp, in polymyositis and in certain denervated muscles. Spontaneous activity of motor units and of single muscle fibers, known respectively as *fasciculation* and *fibrillation*, are abnormal.

Fibrillation The two phenomena of fibrillation and fasciculation are often confused. Fasciculation, discussed below, consists of synchronous contraction of *groups of muscle fibers* integrated by a single axon into a motor unit. Fibrillation is the contraction of *single muscle fibers* and appears only when destruction of a motor axon has disintegrated its motor unit.

When a motor neuron is destroyed by disease, or when its axon is severed, the distal part of the axon degenerates, a process which takes several days. The muscle fibers formerly innervated by the branches of the dead axon, viz., the muscle unit, are disconnected from the nervous system. For reasons which are still obscure, the chemosensitive region of the sarcolemma at the motor end plate "spreads" after denervation to involve the entire surface of the muscle fiber. Then, 10 to 25 days after death of the axon, the denervated fibers develop spontaneous activity, similar perhaps to that found in the sinoatrial (SA) node of the heart; i.e., each fiber contracts at its own rate and without relation to the activity of its fellows. There results a totally random conglomeration of brief, triphasic fibrillation potentials and diphasic positive sharp waves. The latter are usually the more easily recognized signs that muscle fibers have been denervated. Fibrillation and positive sharp-wave activity continue until the muscle fiber is reinnervated by the outgrowth of new axons, either from the proximal (central) end of the damaged nerve or from nearby healthy nerve fibers, or until the fiber is replaced by connective tissue, a process which may not take place for many years.

Fibrillation and positive sharp-wave activity are prominent in patients with neuropathies or other lesions affecting the peripheral nervous system but are also seen with primary diseases of muscle, such as polymyositis or muscular dystrophy, where necrosis of one segment of a muscle fiber disconnects the distal portion of that fiber from the centrally placed portion containing the neuromuscular junction. The distal segment of muscle, which is functionally isolated ("denervated"), develops fibrillation and positive sharp-wave activity. Though these spontaneous potentials signify that muscle fibers or portions of fibers are denervated, their presence does not guarantee that the underlying disease process primarily affects nerve fibers. An alternative explanation of fibrillation potentials postulates a lowered resting membrane potential (−65 mV) in denervated and damaged fibers, which makes the muscle fiber more easy to discharge.

Fasciculation An involuntary single contraction of a motor unit in isolation is termed fasciculation. Since a large number of muscle fibers contract together, visible dimpling or twitching of the skin occurs, though ordinarily not enough power is exerted to move a joint. The form of the accompanying EMG potential, like that of an ordinary motor unit, is relatively constant for any one fasciculating unit. Commonly, it will have three to five phases, a duration of 5 to 15 ms (somewhat less in the facial muscles), and an amplitude of several millivolts. With "benign fasciculations" seen in normal subjects, the same unit tends to repeat at a fairly regular rate of 1 per second, or even faster, indicating a rhythmic activation of the fibers by the responsible axons. With the "malignant fasciculations" described below, the rate is considerably slower at 1 per 3 or 4 s and slightly less regular.

Traditionally, fasciculation is believed to be a sign of chronic, slowly advancing, destructive disease of the anterior horn cells, such as amyotrophic lateral sclerosis and progressive spinal muscular atrophy. In these diseases, fasciculation potentials are numerous and may exceed 15 ms in duration. They are often seen in the early stages of acute poliomyelitis but are recorded less commonly than in the chronic diseases mentioned, perhaps because the affected cells die too rapidly. They are also seen with compressive root lesions, certain exceptional motor neuropathies, and early in the disease course of some patients with acute idiopathic polyneuritis. With peripheral lesions such as those caused by herniated nucleus pulposis (ruptured disk), large numbers of axons may be affected with the result that the fasciculations (or even cramps) may be more obvious to the patient than the twitching with disease of anterior horn cells. In all these cases, the damaged neuron seems to be "irritated" by the disease process, fires repetitively, and, in so doing, produces activity in all the muscle fibers that it innervates. It has been shown that fasciculation may also follow peripheral nerve lesions, giving way to fibrillation upon death of the axon. More important is the fact that fasciculation, particularly in the calves and hands, occurs occasionally in many normal persons and constantly in some, and so it need not be evidence of disease at all. Shivering induced by low temperature and the twitchings associated with depressed serum calcium levels are sometimes confused with fasciculation.

Abnormalities in motor unit potentials The following abnormalities in amplitude, duration, and shape of motor unit potentials can be noted.

ENLARGED POTENTIALS IN PARTIALLY DENERVATED AND REINNERVATED MUSCLE Early in the course of denervation, any motor units with functional connections to the spinal cord are unaffected, and though the number of motor unit potentials appearing during contraction is reduced, the configurations of the remaining ones are quite normal. In time, those remaining often increase in amplitude, perhaps to two to three times normal, and become longer in duration and *polyphasic* (more than four phases). Such large and, sometimes, *giant potentials* arise from motor units, as in Fig. 369-2*C*, containing more than the usual number of muscle fibers spread out over a greatly enlarged territory within the muscle. Presumably, new nerve twigs have *sprouted* from undamaged axons, reinnervated previously denervated fibers, and added them to their own motor units. Some of these reinnervated units may become extremely polyphasic and prolonged, a finding pathognomonic of reinnervation. These units are to be differentiated from (1) those with lesser degrees of "polyphasicity" which are of normal duration and account for as much as 25 percent of the activity recorded from normal muscles, particularly at the end plate zone, and (2) the polyphasic but brief units seen with primary muscle disease. The histochemical counterpart of the motor unit enlargement is *fiber* type grouping. Subsequent denervation of such a large motor unit produces *grouped atrophic fibers.*

REDUCED AMPLITUDE AND DURATION OF ACTION POTENTIALS Diseases such as polymyositis, the muscular dystrophies, and other myopathies which destroy scattered fibers within a motor unit or render them nonfunctional, as in Fig. 369-2*B*, obviously reduce the population of fibers per motor unit. When such a unit is activated, its potential is, therefore, of lower voltage and shorter duration than normal, and it may also appear polyphasic as the compound motor unit potential is fragmented into its constituent single-fiber potentials. When most of the muscle fibers are affected, the motor unit potentials from these very small units may be difficult to differentiate from fibrillation potentials, and when destruction of all fibers is completed, electrical activity ceases. These small, brief voluntary motor unit potentials, with their characteristic high-pitched crackling sound from the audio monitor, occur in all forms of progressive muscular dystrophy but, unfortunately, are indistinguishable from those of polymyositis, dermatomyositis, and other chronic myopathies. In the myositides, however, fibrillation potentials, as noted above, may often be seen as well. In myasthenia gravis, where transmission of impulse fails progressively at one neuromuscular junction after another in any one motor unit, the EMG potential of that unit may be normal at first and become more *myopathic* as fatigue progresses. Potentials from muscles which are chronically weak in myasthenics are then proportionately myopathic. It can be seen, therefore, from Fig. 369-2*B* that the motor unit potentials will appear equally myopathic whether the disease process directly affects single muscle fibers within the unit as in dystrophy, disturbs neuromuscular transmission at single junctions as in myasthenia gravis, or blocks transmission of the nerve impulse in single axon terminals as probably occurs in thyrotoxic and certain carcinomatous "myopathies."

DECREASE IN NUMBER OF MOTOR UNITS AVAILABLE Diseases which reduce the population of functional lower motor neurons or motor axons within the peripheral nerve obviously decrease the number of motor units which can be recruited in the affected muscles. The number of motor units available for activation varies then in proportion to the strength of a maximal voluntary contraction, appearing no longer as an interference pattern but only as a *single-unit pattern* or a *mixed pattern.*

FIGURE 369-2
The shaded muscle fibers are functional members of one motor unit; the axon, which enters from the upper left, branches terminally to innervate the appropriate muscle fibers. The motor unit action potential produced by each motor unit is seen in the upper right; its duration is measured between the two vertical lines. The normal-appearing but unshaded fibers belong to other motor units. A. The normal situation is schematized with five muscle fibers in the active unit. B. In this myopathic unit, only two fibers remain active; the other three (shrunken) have been affected by one of the primary muscle diseases. C. Four fibers which belonged to other motor units and had been denervated have now been reinnervated by the terminal axon sprouting from the healthy active motor unit. Both the motor unit and its action potential are now larger than normal. Note that only under these abnormal circumstances do fibers in the same unit lie next to one another.

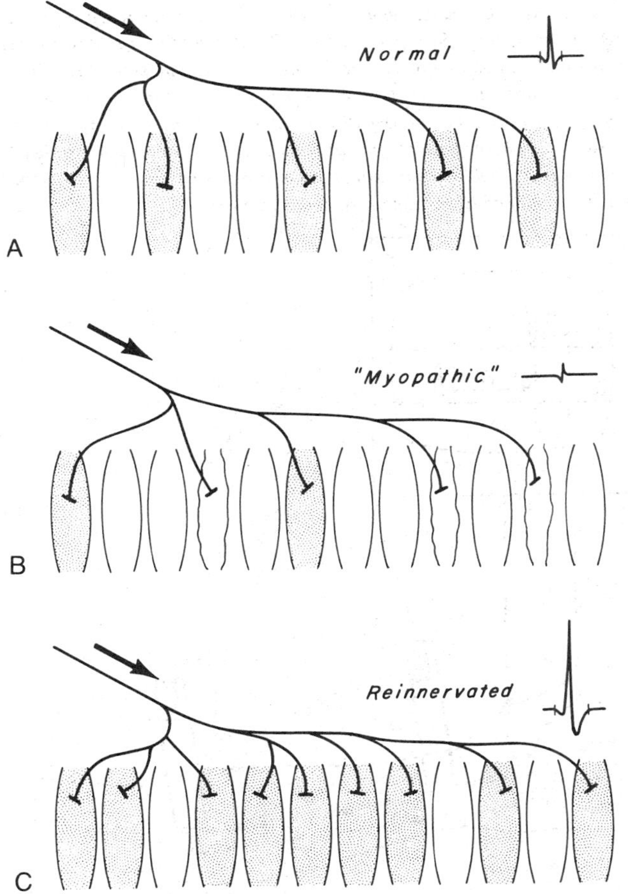

DECREASE IN NUMBER OF MUSCLE FIBERS If muscle power is reduced in diseases such as dystrophies or other myopathies, where individual muscle fibers are affected, there will be little or no reduction in the number of motor units available for recruitment, though each unit will consist of fewer muscle fibers than normal. A maximal voluntary effort will then be associated with a normally complete interference pattern despite marked weakness. Because fewer muscle fibers are active, the amplitude of the pattern will be reduced from normal. A highly complex interference pattern of less than usual amplitude, in the face of dramatic weakness, is the hallmark of a so-called myopathic process.

PROGRESSIVE REDUCTION OR INCREMENT WITH SUCCESSIVE CONTRACTIONS In certain disorders, the size of the initial motor unit potential is normal with voluntary contraction, as is the size of the compound muscle action potential produced by an electric stimulus applied to the nerve. However, during a minimal contraction or after two or three stimuli, at rates as low as 1 to 15 per second, the amplitude of the potentials falls off, though not to zero, and then increases again after the fourth or fifth stimulus. This pattern of "decrement," maximal with the fourth or fifth stimulus, is characteristic of *myasthenia gravis.* Like the partial block at the neuromuscular junction produced by curare, it may be relieved by neostigmine—the pathophysiology is largely postjunctional in both cases. Progressive decline of action potentials with repetitive stimulation may occur in poliomyelitis, in myotonia, or in certain other diseases of the motor unit, but the pattern described for myasthenia gravis is not then present.

In some cases of oat-cell carcinoma of the lung and rarely sarcoidosis with muscular weakness, the Eaton-Lambert syndrome, a condition with somewhat opposite findings, may be observed. If electrical stimulation through nerve is rapid (20 to 30 per second) or follows a brief voluntary contraction, muscle action potentials which were small or practically absent with the first stimulus now increase in voltage with each successive one until a more nearly normal amplitude is attained. This phenomenon is unaffected by neostigmine, but it may be reversible with guanidine (20 to 35 mg/kg per day in divided doses). The pathophysiology of this "reversed" myasthenic syndrome is prejunctional and compromises release of acetylcholine, as does botulinus toxin or the aminoglycoside antibiotics (see Chap. 339).

By the use of single-fiber EMG techniques, it is possible to record what is termed "jitter" and thereby measure accurately (within tens of microseconds) the performance of single pairs of neuromuscular junctions. Characteristic quantitative abnormalities are found in patients with myasthenia gravis or other disorders of neuromuscular transmission. This technique also provides insights, hitherto unavailable, into the pathophysiology of other diseases of peripheral nerve and muscle.

SPECIAL ABNORMALITIES IN THE EMG In *myotonia,* the sarcolemmal membrane is irritable, and muscle contraction persists despite voluntary attempts at relaxation. The symptom is prominent in several hereditary diseases, myotonia congenita (Thomsen's disease), dystrophia myotonica (Steinert's disease), and hyperkalemic periodic paralysis (adynamia episodica hereditaria); minor forms occur sporadically under other circumstances, and it can be produced by drugs interfering with chloride conductance in humans and animals. Myotonia consists of high-frequency repetitive discharges which wax and wane in amplitude and frequency, producing a "dive-bomber" sound on the audio monitor. It is produced mechanically by percussion or movement of the needle electrode. The characteristic electrical picture is also seen following voluntary contraction or electrical stimulation of the muscle via its motor nerve. The voluntary motor unit potentials appear normal, but they are not followed by the silence which normally occurs on relaxation. Instead there is a burst of rapid activity which may take as long as several minutes to subside. Some of the potentials of this prolonged discharge have the duration, amplitude, and form of single-fiber activity, while others appear to have the characteristics of motor unit potentials. If the muscle is activated repeatedly at short intervals, the late discharge becomes briefer and briefer and eventually disappears as the myotonia diminishes temporarily.

Bizarre high-frequency discharges without waxing and waning (*pseudomyotonia*) are seen in hypothyroidism or with certain types of denervation. High-frequency coupling of action potentials into doublets, triplets, or higher multiples of single units, indicating instability in repolarization of the nerve fiber, occurs in tetany and facial spasm.

Contracture, as with cramping in McArdle's disease, percussion and contraction myoedema, and percussion fasciculation, has no electrical counterpart (the EMG is silent). This aspect of these phenomena is important in their definition.

EMG IN DIFFERENTIAL DIAGNOSIS OF MOVEMENT DISORDERS

EMG techniques, often employing surface rather than needle recordings, are very helpful in differentiating among parkinsonian, essential-familial, anxiety, thyrotoxic, and cerebellar tremors; in separating minor degrees of asterixis from tremor; in the recognition of myoclonus; and in differentiating "spasticity" from rigidity. EMG recordings of blink reflexes can document clinically undetectable lesions of the brainstem (as with multiple sclerosis).

ELECTRONEUROGRAPHY

Conduction velocity of nerve Painless and harmless techniques are widely used for both percutaneous stimulation of the larger peripheral motor and sensory nerve fibers and recording of their conducted action potentials. These routine techniques provide numerical data which are of considerable clinical interest. The results of these *motor and sensory nerve conduction studies*, expressed simply as latency in milliseconds or conduction velocity in meters per second, are more objective than the results of electromyography and afford certain information unavailable from EMG studies.

An accessible nerve is stimulated through the skin by surface electrodes, and the resulting compound action potential is recorded by electrodes on the skin (1) over the nerve more proximally in the case of orthodromic activity in large sensory fibers stimulated in the digital nerves, or (2) over the muscle more distally in the case of motor fibers in a mixed nerve (Fig. 369-3). The conduction time from the most distal stimulating electrode, measured in milliseconds from the stimulus artifact to the onset of the response, is also termed the *distal* or *peripheral latency*. If a second stimulus can be applied to a mixed nerve more proximally (or if recording electrodes can be placed more proximally in the case of sensory fibers), a new and longer conduction time can be measured. When the distance (in millimeters) between the two sites of stimulation of motor fibers or recording of sensory fibers is divided by the difference in conduction times (in milliseconds), a *maximal conduction velocity* (in meters per second) is obtained which describes the velocity of propagation of the action potentials in the largest and fastest nerve fibers. These velocities in normal subjects vary roughly from a minimum of 40 or 45 m/s, depending upon which nerve is studied, to a maximum of 75 or 80 m/s. Values are lower in infants, reaching the adult range by the age of 2 to 4 years. Normal values also exist for peripheral latencies from the distalmost site on various mixed nerves to the appropriate muscles; when one stimulates the median nerve at the wrist, for example, the latency (Fig. 369-3*A*) for conduction through the carpal tunnel to the abductor pollicis brevis muscle in the thenar eminence is always less than 4.5 ms in normal adults. Similar tables of normal values have been compiled for orthodromic sensory conduction velocities and distal latencies. Nerve conduction velocity is affected by fiber diameter and degree of demyelination. Unmyelinated or segmentally demyelinated fibers conduct impulses much more slowly, as do fibers with smaller diameters.

When motor fibers in a mixed nerve are stimulated and every one is in functional continuity with its many muscle fibers, the compound action potential of many hundreds of microvolts derived from the many firing muscle fibers can easily be recorded from electrodes on the skin over the muscle. However, when one is dealing with sensory potentials, activity is recorded from nerve fibers themselves; one lacks the "amplification" provided by all the muscle fibers in one motor unit, and much greater electronic amplification is required. In the clinic, therefore, sensory potentials may, under abnormal circumstances, be very small or absent even when powerful computer-averaging techniques are used, and sensory conduction measurements are often impossible to record, though at other times they may be abnormally slow. In contrast, a reliable mo-

FIGURE 369-3

The median nerve may be stimulated through the skin at the wrist (1) or in the antecubital fossa (2), and the resultant compound muscle action potential may be recorded as the potential difference between a surface electrode over the thenar eminence (arrow) and a reference electrode (Ref.) more distally. Sweep 1′ on the CRO depicts the stimulus artifact (moment of stimulation at 1) followed by the muscle potential. The distal latency is the time A′ on the CRO sweep (3.0 ms, for example) which corresponds to conduction over distance A in the hand. The same is true for sweep 2′ where stimulation is at point 2, and the time from artifact to response is A′ + B′. The maximal motor conduction velocity from points 2 to 1 is obtained by dividing distance B by time B′.

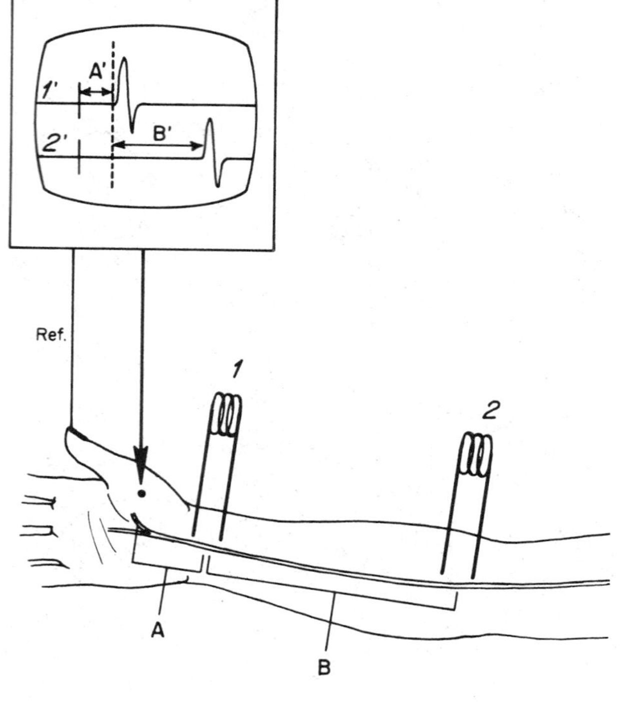

tor conduction velocity is possible if one functional nerve fiber remains.

These conduction velocities reflect the status of surviving nerve fibers and, if the latter are unaffected by the disease process, may be normal despite widespread denervation; e.g., following incomplete transection of a nerve by a sharp object, the maximal motor conduction velocity may be normal in the few remaining fibers, although the muscle involved is almost paralyzed. In most neuropathies, the axon itself is primarily affected either because of disease of the cell body with "dying-back" changes peripherally or because of damage to the axon with distal Wallerian degeneration. This is true for typical alcoholic, nutritional, paracarcinomatous, uremic, other metabolic, and most diabetic neuropathies. The axons which remain intact may conduct impulses normally so that, when the larger fibers have been affected, the remaining fibers with smaller diameters, that naturally conduct more slowly, account for a slightly slower maximal conduction velocity. Also, segmental demyelination may be present even in these primarily axonal neuropathies. Though it is of lesser importance, it may further decrease the conduction velocity to a slight degree.

The total reduction in velocity is often not great enough to place any single value outside the range of normal, although at other times velocity may be slightly below normal to 35 or 40 m/s at worst. Ordinary nerve conduction studies can usually, therefore, be used to document the presence of neuropathy in the disease under question only by comparison of values recorded from a population of patients with those from a control group of the same age and sex. Techniques have recently been devised to study conduction in longer and more proximal segments of nerve than is possible routinely. These involve accurate measurements of latencies for F waves and H reflexes—both of which require conduction in nerves going from the periphery of a limb to the spinal cord and back again. The F wave passes antidromically from the point stimulated up the axon of an alpha motor neuron that lies in the anterior horn of the spinal cord and then returns orthodromically down the same axon. The H wave passes up the nerve along IA fibers through the spinal monosynaptic connection with the alpha motor neuron and then orthodromically down the motor axon. Thus conduction along proximal sensory and motor nerves and spinal roots can be measured. By use of these methods, the diagnostic yield of nerve conduction studies is increased so that the chance of a patient with one of these axonal neuropathies having a diagnostically abnormal test rises to 80 or 90 percent.

Though most diseases of peripheral nerves do not necessarily produce a clear-cut reduction of nerve conduction velocity as it is routinely measured, other, relatively uncommon disorders, such as acute idiopathic polyneuritis (Landry-Guillain-Barré syndrome), diphtheria, metachromatic leukodystrophy, Krabbe's disease, and the hypertrophic neuropathies including Déjerine-Sottas disease and many cases of Charcot-Marie-Tooth disease, that affect Schwann cells primarily, produce segmental demyelination with marked reduction in conduction velocities which are usually in the range of 10 m/s.

Focal compression of nerve, as in the various entrapment syndromes, also produces localized slowing of conduction, because of narrowing of axons and demyelination at the site of compression. The demonstration of such localized slowing of conduction affords ready confirmation of nerve entrapment; for example, if the peripheral latency in the median nerve (Fig. 369-2*A*) exceeds 5.0 ms while that in the ulnar nerve remains normal, compression of the median nerve in the carpal tunnel is extremely likely. Similar focal slowing of conduction may be recorded from the ulnar nerve at the elbow or peroneal nerve at the fibular head when either is compressed (see Chap. 368). A normal conduction time, however, cannot rule out an entrapment syndrome.

Microneurography Disease of peripheral nerve may produce the electromyographic evidences of denervation discussed above, but more quantitative observations of neural function can be made by studies of the electrical activity of nerves themselves. Hagbarth, Struppler, and colleagues have, by means of very fine needle electrodes placed within human peripheral nerves in situ, pioneered the recording of single-fiber activity from muscle afferent and autonomic and cutaneous fibers within peripheral nerves. This *microneurography* promises to be of critical importance in the understanding of many aspects of human physiology and disease but will likely remain a research technique.

CLINICAL MANIFESTATIONS OF MUSCLE DISEASE

The large number and diversity of diseases of striated muscle exceed the number of symptoms and signs by which they express themselves clinically. Different diseases thus must share certain common symptoms and even syndromes. To avoid excessive repetition in the description of individual diseases, there is some advantage to discussing in one place the clinical manifestations seen in *clinical myology*. (See Table 369-1 for a syndromic classification of muscle disease.)

Weakness and paralysis Assuming there are no signs of disease of the corticospinal tracts of the spinal cord and nerve fiber disease, reduced strength of contraction, reflected in diminished power of single contractions [peak or power factor (PF) in performance] or of repeated contractions [endurance factor (EF)], stands as an indubitable sign of muscle disease. Fatigability per se less reliably denotes muscle affection, since it is most often due to some psychic aberration linked to anxiety and depression or to systemic illness (see Chap. 11). It is noteworthy that slight weakness of muscle may be present, even though tests of PF, because of the crudeness of clinical measurement, lack of quantitation, and the uncertainty of gaining the patient's full cooperation, may seem to reveal no definite diminution in power. Theoretically, with milder degrees of weakness, a diminution of EF elicited in a series of timed contractions against a fixed resistance (ergogram) may more reliably demonstrate the disorder than does PF. Furthermore, sustained or repeated maximal muscle contraction over a given period of time evinces optimally the myasthenic reaction, i.e., a rapid failure of contraction, and the restoration of power within minutes by rest. This, in fact, in combination with a restoration of power, i.e., disappearance of the myasthenic state, by neostigmine and edrophonium (Tensilon) stands as the most valid clinical criterion of the various forms of myasthenia gravis.

Qualitative changes in the contractile process In addition, other qualities of muscular contraction and relaxation may be discovered by observing, during one or a series of maximal actions of a group of muscles, the speed and efficiency of contraction and relaxation. Slow waves of contraction in a muscle such as the quadriceps may be seen on change in posture (contraction myoedema) in hypothyroidism. Here it is often associated with percussion myoedema and slowness of tendon reflex. Slowness in relaxation is another indication of a thyroid deficiency state, accounting for the complaints of uncomfortable tightness and firmness of proximal limb muscles.

A prolonged failure of relaxation with afterdischarge is a characteristic of myotonia, as in congenital myotonia (Thomsen's disease), dystrophia myotonica (Steinert's disease), and paramyotonia congenita (von Eulenburg's disease). But a true myotonia, with its long electrical discharges of action poten-

TABLE 369-1
Syndromic classification of muscle diseases

I Acute (days) or subacute (weeks) paralytic disorders of muscle (may cause weakness *or* paralysis)
- *A* Rarely fulminant myasthenia gravis
- *B* Polymyositis and dermatomyositis
- *C* Alcoholic myopathy
- *D* Acute paroxysmal myoglobinuria (*Note:* First attack of episodic weakness may enter into differential diagnosis; see below)
- *E* Botulism
- *F* Organophosphate poisoning
- *G* Acute spinal or peripheral nerve diseases (denervation paralysis where paralysis is often severe and widespread and atrophy may or may not be present)
  - *1* Poliomyelitis
  - *2* Acute idiopathic polyneuritis or other forms of polyneuropathy (porphyria, beriberi, etc.)
  - *3* Rarely polyarteritis nodosa with polyneuropathy

II Chronic (i.e., months to years) paralytic disorders of muscle (weakness usually with severe atrophy)
- *A* Progressive muscular dystrophy
  - *1* Duchenne type
  - *2* Facioscapulohumeral type (Landouzy-Déjerine)
  - *3* Limb girdle type (Erb's and Leyden-Moebius)
  - *4* Distal type (Welander's)
  - *5* Myotonic dystrophy (Steinert's disease)
  - *6* Progressive ophthalmoplegic and oculopharyngeal types
- *B* Chronic polymyositis
- *C* Chronic thyrotoxic and other metabolic myopathies
- *D* Chronic slowly progressive or relatively stationary polymyopathies
  - *1* Central core disease
  - *2* Rod body (nemaline) and related polymyopathies
  - *3* Pleoconial, megaconial, and myotubular polymyopathies
  - *4* Glycogen storage disease
  - *5* Congenital benign hypotonia and congenital universal hypoplasia of muscle
- *E* Progressive muscular atrophies and other forms of motor system disease (amyotrophic lateral sclerosis, progressive bulbar palsy) and infantile muscular atrophy (Werdnig-Hoffmann disease)
- *F* Chronic neural muscular atrophies such as peroneal muscular atrophy (Charcot-Marie-Tooth), hypertrophic polyneuritis (Déjerine-Sottas), amyloid polyneuropathy, chronic nutritional, arsenical, leprous, and other polyneuropathies

III Episodic weakness of muscle
- *A* Myasthenia gravis
- *B* Symptomatic myasthenia of other types
  - *1* With lupus erythematosus disseminatus
  - *2* With polymyositis
  - *3* With rheumatoid arthritis
  - *4* With nonthymic carcinoma
- *C* Familial periodic paralysis (hypokalemic)
- *D* Hereditary adynamia (hyperkalemic periodic paralysis, or Gamstorp's disease)
- *E* Paramyotonia congenita (von Eulenburg's disease)
- *F* Hyper- and hypokalemia (including primary hyperaldosteronism)
- *G* Acute thyrotoxic myopathy (also thyrotoxic periodic paralysis)

IV Stiffness, soreness, involuntary spasm, and cramp
- *A* Congenital myotonia (Thomsen's disease), paramyotonia congenita, and myotonic dystrophy
- *B* Tetanus
- *C* Tetany
- *D* Black widow spider bite
- *E* Hypothyroidism with pseudomyotonia (Debré-Semelaigne and Hoffmann's syndromes)
- *F* Myopathy resulting from myophosphorylase deficiency (McArdle's syndrome) and other forms of contracture
- *G* Contracture with Addison's disease
- *H* Idiopathic cramp syndrome

V Myalgic states
- *A* Connective tissue diseases (rheumatoid arthritis, menopausal arthritis, lupus erythematosus, polyarteritis nodosa, scleroderma, polymyalgia rheumatica, polymyositis)
- *B* Localized fibrositis or fibromyositis
- *C* Many forms of polyneuritis
- *D* Trichinosis
- *E* Myopathy of myoglobinuria and McArdle's syndrome
- *F* Myopathy with hypoglycemia
- *G* Bornholm's disease
- *H* Anterior tibial syndrome

VI Localized muscle mass(es)
- *A* Rupture of a muscle
- *B* Muscle hemorrhage
- *C* Muscle tumor
  - *1* Rhabdomyosarcoma
  - *2* Desmoid
  - *3* Angioma
  - *4* Metastatic nodules
- *D* Localized idiopathic myopathy
- *E* Localized and generalized myositis ossificans
- *F* Fibrositis (myogelosis)
- *G* Granulomatous infections
  - *1* Sarcoidosis
  - *2* Tuberculosis
- *H* Pyogenic abscess (pyomyositis)

tials, unlike the electrically silent myoedema and contracture (see below), requires strong contraction for its elicitation, is more evident after a period of relaxation, and tends to disappear with repeated contractions. This persistence of contraction is demonstrable upon tapping a muscle (percussion myotonia), a phenomenon easily distinguished from the local bulge (myoedema) induced by a sharp tap of a muscle in the myxedematous or cachetic patient.

Increase in power in a series of voluntary contractions in the absence of myotonia is a feature of the Eaton-Lambert syndrome often associated with carcinoma of the lung.

The effect of cold on muscle contraction may also prove informative; either paresis or myotonia, lasting for a few minutes, may be evoked or enhanced by cold as in the paramyotonia of von Eulenberg.

Myotonia and myoedema must be distinguished from the recruitment and spread of involuntary spasm induced by strong and repeated contractions of limb muscles in patients with mild or *localized tetanus,* which is not a phenomenon of muscle but is due to an abolition of inhibitory spinal mechanisms.

The repeated contraction of forearm and leg muscles after the application of a tourniquet (above arterial pressure) to the proximal part of the limb will often elicit latent tetany. The latter state must be separated from ordinary cramp by its special mode of development and duration, its enhancement by hyperventilation, and the presence of accompanying tingling and prickling paresthesias. Tetany also differs from true contracture.

In *true contractures* a group of muscles, after a series of strong contractions, may remain shortened for many minutes, unable to relax because of failure of the metabolic mechanism necessary for relaxation; the muscle in this shortened state remains electrically silent in the electromyogram, in contrast to the tremendous high-voltage, rapid discharges observed with cramp, tetanus, and tetany. Such contracture occurs in McArdle's phosphorylase deficiency, where it is aggravated by arterial occlusion, but it has been seen in deficiencies of phosphofructokinase (Tarui's disease) and in other glycolytic enzymes (Chap. 100).

Pseudocontracture (fibrous contracture) which inevitably follows all conditions which occasion prolonged fixation and complete inactivity of the normally innervated muscle, is another common disorder. The muscle fibers are shortened with loss of sarcomeres; fibrosis may also occur. The condition is distinguished from ankylosis by the springy nature of the resistance coincident with increased tautness of muscle and tendon during passive motion, and from *Volkmann's contracture,* where there is evident fibrosis of muscle and the surrounding tissues due to ischemic injury, usually after a fracture of the forearm.

Topography of paralysis: Patterns of paralysis In the majority of the diseases under consideration, some of the muscles are affected and others are spared. Each disease exhibits its own pattern. Moreover, the topography or distribution of involvement tends to follow the same pattern in all patients with the same disease. Thus, determination of the topography of muscular involvement provides one of the most valid diagnostic attributes of a disease, ranking next in importance after altered quantity and quality of contraction.

To ascertain the extent and severity of muscle weakness, one undertakes a systematic examination of all the main groups of muscles from forehead to feet. The patient is asked to contract each group quickly with as much force as can be mustered, while the examiner opposes the movement and offers a graded resistance in accordance with the degree of residual power. If the weakness is unilateral, one has the advantage of being able to compare it with the action of muscles on the normal side. If it is bilateral, the physician must refer to an idea of what constitutes normalcy, based on experience in muscle testing. Ocular, facial, lingual, pharyngeal, laryngeal, cervical, shoulder, upper arm, lower arm and hand, truncal, pelvic, thigh, and lower leg-foot muscles are examined quickly in this order. To facilitate description and comparison, a rating scale must be used. A widely accepted one is that devised by the Medical Research Council of Great Britain, containing six graded steps, from normal power to paralysis, which are readily distinguishable: 5 represents normal power; 4, weakness with ability to overcome resistance by the examiner; 3, weakness with ability only to overcome gravity; 2, severe weakness, movement only possible with gravity eliminated; 1, trace of movement; 0, no movement. Another scale is that of DeMyer, which rates muscle contractions as *normal* (100 percent), *mildly weak* (75 percent), *moderately weak* (50 percent), *severely weak* (25 percent), and *paralyzed* (0 percent). With practice one can distinguish pseudoparalysis from pain, unwillingness to cooperate, and feigned weakness (see Chap. 14).

The following topographic patterns are so well known that they constitute a core of essential clinical knowledge in this field.

1 Ocular palsies presenting more or less exclusively as diplopia, ptosis, or strabismus, sometimes in association with exophthalmos, enophthalmos, and pupillary change.

As a rule muscle diseases do not affect the pupil, and in most instances their effects are bilateral. In single-nerve lesions the neural origin is revealed by the combination of paralyses of eye muscles or sympathetic and parasympathetic paralysis of the pupil. When weakness of the orbicularis oculi muscle (muscle of eye closure) is added to ocular palsies and ptosis, it nearly always signifies myopathic disease.

Myasthenia gravis, progressive ocular dystrophy of Kiloh and Nevin, exophthalmic ophthalmoplegia of thyroid disease, curare-sensitive nonmyasthenic ophthalmoplegias, myotonic dystrophy of Steinert, ocular dystrophy with retinitis pigmentosa [and heart block, dwarfism, ovarian dysgenesis, (Kearns-Sayre syndrome)], centronuclear myopathy, and botulism are the principal conditions to be considered. When ptosis or weakness of eye closure occurs alone or in combination with weakness of other skeletal muscles, one should think of Landouzy-Déjerine facioscapulohumeral dystrophy, oculopharyngeal dystrophy, and the nemaline form of congenital myopathy.

2 Bilateral facial palsy presenting as an inability to smile and expose teeth and to close eyes. Mild bilateral facial weakness is observed in myasthenia gravis, and ptosis and ocular palsies are usually conjoined (90 percent of cases) in this disease. The same is true of myotonic dystrophy. More severe or complete facial palsy occurs in facioscapulohumeral dystrophy, in Landry-Guillain-Barré syndrome (nearly always with other weaknesses), in sarcoidosis, in Melkersson's syndrome (associated with multiply furrowed tongue, called lingua plicata), and in combination with abducens palsies in the Moebius syndrome. Sometimes polyneuritis cranialis multiplex causes bilateral facial paralysis.

3 Bulbar palsy presenting as dysphonia, dysarthria, and dysphagia with or without a hanging jaw or facial weakness. Myasthenia gravis is the most frequent cause of this syndrome and must also be considered whenever there is the solitary finding of a hanging jaw or fatigue of jaws while eating or talking; but usually ptosis and ocular palsies are conjoined. The same is true of myotonic dystrophy and botulism. Progressive bulbar palsy may be the basis of this syndrome, and the diagnosis is most obvious when the tongue is withered and twitching. The neurologic condition known as pseudobulbar palsy is readily distinguished by the lack of atrophy of muscle, the mode of onset (often sudden), and the associated clinical findings. Platybasia and the Arnold-Chiari malformation may also reproduce some of these findings by involving the lower cranial nerves and their nuclei. Diphtheria and bulbar poliomyelitis may present in this way. Pure dysphagia may be an early manifestation of polymyositis.

4 Cervical palsy presenting often as the hanging-head syndrome, or inability to lift the head from the pillow. The patient may be unable to hold up the head owing to weakness of the posterior neck muscles, or to lift it from a pillow because of weakness of the anterior neck muscles. If this condition is severe, the head may loll unless it is held up by the patient's hands.

This condition occurs most often in idiopathic polymyositis, dermatomyositis, and myasthenia gravis. It tends to be combined with dysphagia. The major types of progressive muscular dystrophy, when advanced, usually weaken neck flexors and extensors, but seldom to the point where the head must be held in the hands. Rarely syringomyelia, syphilitic meningoradiculitis, subacute poliomyelitis (in conjunction with carcinomatosis), motor system disease, or Kugelberg-Welander syndrome may differentially paralyze the neck muscles.

5 Bilateral brachial palsy presenting sometimes as the dangling-arm syndrome. Weakness, atrophy, and fasciculations of hands and arms and sometimes of the shoulders characterize the commonest syndrome of motor system disease, namely, amyotrophic lateral sclerosis. Primary muscle disease hardly ever selects these parts or weakens them disproportionately to other muscles. A diffuse arm weakness may also occur early in acute idiopathic polyneuritis and porphyric polyneuropathy, but it soon becomes part of a more generalized paralysis. A painful unilateral paralysis of shoulder muscles can be due to acute brachial plexopathy (Parsonage-Turner syndrome) or the neuropathy of serum sickness.

6 Bilateral crural palsy presenting as lower-leg weakness with floppy feet and inability to walk on the heels and toes, or as paralysis of all leg and thigh muscles. In lower-leg weakness, polyneuropathy is the usual explanation, although peroneal and anterior tibial muscles are often weakened in dystrophy. Diabetic polyneuropathy may weaken thigh and pelvic muscles asymmetrically with little sensory change but often with pain. In total leg and thigh weakness, one first thinks of a disease of the spinal cord, in which case there is often loss of control of the bladder and bowel sphincters, as well as loss of sensory function below a certain level. Motor system disease may also begin in these parts and affect them out of proportion to others. Thus the differential diagnosis of patterns of leg weakness involves more diseases than do the restricted paralyses of other parts of the body.

7 Limb-girdle palsies presenting as inability to raise the arms or to arise from a squatting, kneeling, or sitting position. Three groups of diseases most often manifest themselves in this fashion—poly- and dermatomyositis, the progressive muscular dystrophies, and the acute proximal polyneuropathies, the Landry-Guillain-Barré syndrome, and acute porphyric neuropathy. The Duchenne, Becker, and Leyden-Moebius type tend first to affect the muscles of the pelvic girdle and lumbar region, resulting in a waddling gait, difficulty in arising from the floor or in climbing stairs without the assistance of the arms, lumbar lordosis, and protuberant abdomen. The Landouzy-Déjerine type affects muscles of face and shoulder girdles foremost, and is manifested by incomplete eye closure, pouting lips, inability to raise the arms above the head, winging of the scapulae, and thinness of the upper arms (Popeye appearance). The lower parts of the deltoid muscle may be relatively spared. In polymyositis, weakness may be limited to either neck muscles or those of the shoulder or pelvic girdles, but sometimes it involves all muscles, including distal ones as well, though the muscles of the face and eyes are almost always spared. Most of the relatively nonprogressive congenital myopathies (central core, nemaline, mitochondrial, centronuclear, multicore, reducing body) cause greater weakness of proximal than of distal muscles. The characteristic feature of the muscular dystrophies is the *selective* muscle involvement, for instance, affecting biceps and brachioradialis while sparing until later triceps, deltoids, and gastrocnemii. Polymyositis tends to produce a more nonselective weakness. A metabolic myopathy, such as the adult form of acid-maltase deficiency or prolonged hypokalemia, may affect only the pelvic and thigh muscles. Proximal muscles are occasionally implicated in progressive spinal muscular atrophy, as in the syndrome first described by Kugelberg and Welander. Full investigations including EMG, measurement of serum creatine phosphokinase, and muscle biopsy are required to establish the diagnosis.

8 Distal limb palsies presenting usually as foot drop, with steppage gait (and pes cavus), weakness of all lower leg muscles, and later wrist drop and weakness of hand grips (claw hand). The principal cause of this neuromuscular syndrome is familial polyneuropathy, such as the peroneal muscular atrophy of Charcot-Marie-Tooth, hypertrophic polyneuropathy of Déjerine and Sottas, and the hereditary polyneuropathy of Refsum. Chronic nonfamilial polyneuropathies may also present in this fashion. Rarely this syndrome is due to the distal progressive muscular dystrophy of Welander. Steinert's myotonic dystrophy also weakens peroneal and posterior tibial muscles as well as those of the forearm, sternomastoid, face, and eyes.

Despite exceptions, a first approximation is that girdle weakness means myopathy and distal weakness neuropathy.

9 Generalized or universal paralyses: limb and cranial muscles—involved either in attacks or in persistent, progressive deterioration. When acute in onset and episodic, this syndrome is usually traceable to an inherent disorder which may be associated with an electrolyte imbalance, as in familial hypokalemic, normokalemic, or hyperkalemic periodic paralysis. One variety of the former type is associated with hyperthyroidism, especially in Orientals. A paresis, rather than paralysis of acute onset that lasts many weeks, is a feature of a peculiar disease called paroxysmal myoglobinuria of Meyer-Betz, and at times of a severe form of idiopathic or parasitic polymyositis (trichinosis) as well. Polymyositis of the idiopathic type may involve all limb and trunk muscles but usually spares the facial and ocular muscles, and trichinosis causes only mild ocular and lingual weakness. In infants a chronic and persistent generalized weakness of all muscles except those of the eyes always raises the question of the Werdnig-Hoffmann infantile muscular atrophy or, if it is in lesser degree, of one of the relatively nonprogressive congenital myopathies or polyneuropathy. In all these diseases, paucity of movement, hypotonia, and retardation of motor development may be more obvious in the infant than weakness.

Universal ascending paralysis, developing over a few days, with involvement of cranial (including ocular) muscles, is usually due to the idiopathic polyneuritis of Landry-Guillain-Barré. Acute porphyric neuropathy must also be considered. Slow onset and progression of paralysis, atrophy, and fasciculation of limb and trunk muscles, without sensory loss, over months to years characterize motor system disease. Mild degrees of generalized weakness are features of a number of metabolic myopathies, such as thyrotoxic myopathy, glycogen storage disease, vitamin D deficiency, and rickets.

10 Paralysis of single muscles or a group of muscles. This is almost always neuropathic, or rarely spinal. Muscle disease does not need to be considered except in its earliest stages when the weakness is mild.

Age of onset and rate of development of paralysis In most neuromuscular diseases the mode of onset and the progression of the weakness are slow. This statement applies to the muscular dystrophies, the congenital and metabolic myopathies, the spinal muscular atrophies, and the chronic familial polyneuropathies. A subacute development of muscular weakness (weeks to months) characterizes dermatomyositis-polymyositis and certain ones of the polyneuritides and nutritional-metabolic polyneuropathies. An acute weakness, i.e., developing over a period of days, is usually not due to a disease of muscles, the only exceptions being acute intoxications with neuromuscular blocking agents or acute electrolyte changes, such as hypo- or hyperkalemia (periodic paralyses). The usual causes of acute neuromuscular paralyses are polymyelitis, acute polyneuritis of the Landry-Guillain-Barré type, porphyric or toxic polyneuropathy (thallium, triorthocresyl phosphate) due to Pb.

Muscle weakness may begin at birth or shortly thereafter, presenting as the "floppy baby syndrome." This may have a central origin, as in hypotonic or other forms of cerebral palsy, or a peripheral one, as in the several congenital polymyopathies or polyneuropathies. Benign congenital hypotonia is the most frequent disorder and can be separated from the common Werdnig-Hoffmann spinal muscular atrophy which is marked by its progressivity and signs of denervation.

Volumetric changes in muscle Altered volume of muscular mass stands as another feature of disease which may be evidenced in all except the most obese patient. There are, of course, innate differences in muscle development, a greater salience of muscle in men than in women, and differences due to use and disuse. Greatly increased size and strength of muscles occur in pure form (hypertrophia musculorum vera) and may also be observed in *congenital myotonia* (circus freaks with phenomenal muscular development often have this disease), in rare instances of a pathologic cramp syndrome, in some patients destined to develop muscular dystrophy, and in de Lange's syndrome of congenital athetosis with feeblemindedness. Muscle enlargement in progressive muscular dystrophy more often takes the form of pseudohypertrophy, where increased size is accompanied by weakness. Here large and small fibers are mixed with fat cells which have replaced many of the degenerated muscle fibers. Other muscles are atrophied in the same patient. If a mass develops rapidly in a muscle, hemorrhage, either spontaneous or associated with a bleeding diathesis or trauma, is the usual cause. A slowly developing mass in a muscle always raises question of a tumor (rhabdomyosarcoma, angioma, metastatic carcinoma) or granuloma. Cachexia, malnutrition, and lipodystrophy tend to reduce muscle bulk without significantly reducing power of contraction (pseudoatrophy). Denervation due to lesions of the peripheral nerve or spinal cord, which if complete leads to a loss of bulk up to 75 percent of the original volume within 3 months, is invariably attended by paralysis. The most severe degrees of atrophy usually signify denervation or dystrophy. Plain soft tissue radiographs and CT scans aid in diagnosis.

Twitches, spasms, cramps, and contracture Fascicular twitches during rest, if pronounced and combined with muscular weakness and atrophy, are typical of motor neuron disease (amyotrophic lateral sclerosis, progressive muscular atrophy, or progressive bulbar palsy); but they may be seen in lesser degree in other diseases of gray matter of the spinal cord (e.g., syringomyelia or tumor), in lesions of anterior roots (e.g., ruptured intervertebral disk), and in peripheral neuropathies. Widespread fascicular twitches spreading in a wavelike pattern along the entire length of a muscle with associated weakness progressing to complete flaccid paralysis within minutes forms the striking clinical picture of organic phosphate insecticide poisoning. The same sequence evolving at a slightly slower pace may occur in poliomyelitis. Fasciculations during contraction indicate, instead, a state in which the muscle is excessively irritable, often for reasons that are not known, or a condition which has previously denervated many motor units, so that during contraction the few remaining enlarged units cannot be recruited smoothly. One may observe this latter phenomenon years after poliomyelitis has left a muscle weakened. *Benign fasciculations,* a common finding in otherwise normal individuals, can usually be distinguished by the lack of muscular weakness and atrophy; *myokymia* and the syndrome of "continuous muscle fiber activity" are rare forms of spasm in which innumerable twitchings impart a rippling appearance to the muscle.

Cramps at rest or with movement (action cramps) are frequently reported in motor system disease, tetany, and dehydration after excessive sweating and salt loss and in other metabolic diseases (uremia, hypocalcemia, and hypomagnesemia), but there is a benign form (idiopathic cramp syndrome), in which no other neuromuscular disturbance can be found. One form of it is known as the *stiff-man syndrome;* this appears to be an obscure disease of the central nervous system for which diazepam is the specific therapy. Continuous spasm, with no demonstrable disorder at a neuromuscular level, intensified by the action of muscles, is a common manifestation of tetanus and also follows the bite of the black widow spider (Chap. 374).

Palpable abnormalities of muscle Altered structure and function of muscle are not accurately revealed by palpation. Of course, the difference between the firm hypertrophied muscle of a well-conditioned athlete and the slack muscle of a sedentary person is as apparent to the palpating finger as to the eye. And the persistent contraction in myxedema, contracture, tetanus, cramp, etc., is easily felt. In muscular dystrophy the muscles are said to have a "doughy" or "elastic" feel, but this is difficult to judge. In the Pompé type of glycogen storage disease attention may be attracted to the musculature by an unnatural firmness and increase in bulk. The swollen, edematous weak muscles in acute paroxysmal myoglobinuria or severe polymyositis may feel taut and firm but are usually not tender. Areas of tenseness in muscles which otherwise function normally, a state called *myogelosis,* may be found in patients with fibrositis or fibromyositis, and their nature has not been divulged by biopsy.

A mass developing in one part of a muscle, or throughout a muscle, poses a special clinical problem. It may, if chronic, be a tumor (rhabdomyosarcoma, angioma, metastatic carcinoma, or desmoid) or a granulomatous inflammation (sarcoid, tuberculoma, or mycosis). Hard masses are usually calcium (myocalcinosis) or bone deposit (myositis ossificans). If a muscle mass develops rapidly, hemorrhage, either spontaneous or traumatic, must be considered. A ruptured tendon may take this form but always causes a bulge which, for obvious reasons, becomes manifest on contraction, and the muscle exhibits a diminished power of contraction.

Tendon (phasic stretch) reflexes Muscle stretch or tendon reflexes should be graded. At the Massachusetts General Hospital, ++ indicates the average response, + obtainable by reinforcement or summation, +++ lively, and ++++ pathological with clonus. The tendon reflexes are altered by the majority of causes of muscle weakness, particularly those which involve peripheral nerves. In muscular dystrophy and polymyositis they tend to be reduced in proportion to the reduction in muscular power. In the myopathy of hypothyroidism, in which the contractile process is slowed, there is a characteristic prolongation of the tendon reflex, and the opposite condition of quickening and brevity of the tendon reflex is less reliably demonstrated in hyperthyroidism. In peripheral neuropathies the tendon reflexes are usually lost at an early stage before much weakness appears. Increased tendon reflexes in atrophic, weak muscles are characteristic of amyotrophic lateral sclerosis due to the unique combination of upper and lower motor neuron lesions.

Muscle pain Pain localized to a group of muscles is extremely severe in wry neck, fibrositis and fibromyositis, acute brachial neuritis, radiculitis, Bornholm's disease, or pleurodynia, but little is known of its cause in any of these diseases. In contrast, the established forms of muscle disease are usually painless. In polymyositis pain is present in about half the patients, and may sometimes indicate coincident involvement of connective tissues and joint structures. Tenderness of muscle is a variable state normally, and it tends to be more definite in polyneuritis, poliomyelitis, and polyarteritis nodosa than in polymyositis and in the various forms of dystrophy and other myopathies in which there is usually no increase in the sensitivity of muscle tissue.

REFERENCES

ADAMS RD: *Diseases of Muscle: A Study in Pathology,* 3d ed. Hagerstown, Md. Harper & Row, 1975

BRADLEY WG: *Disorders of Peripheral Nerves.* Oxford, Blackwell, 1974

BUCHTHAL F, SIMPSON JA (eds): *Handbook of Electroencephalography and Clinical Neurophysiology,* vol 16: *Electromyography,* part A: *Nervous and Muscular Evoked Potentials.* Amsterdam, Elsevier, 1976

———, ——— (eds): *Handbook of Electroencephalography and Clinical Neurophysiology,* vol 16: *Electromyography,* part B: *Neuromuscular Disease.* Amsterdam, Elsevier, 1973

DUBOWITZ V, BROOKE M: *Muscle Biopsy: A Modern Approach.* Philadelphia, Saunders, 1973

DYCK PJ ET AL: *Peripheral Neuropathies,* 2d ed. Philadelphia, Saunders, 1982

GOODGOLD J, EBERSTEIN A: *Electrodiagnosis of Neuromuscular Diseases,* 2d ed. Baltimore, Williams & Wilkins, 1977

KATZ B: *Nerve, Muscle and Synapse.* New York, McGraw-Hill, 1966

STÅLBERG E, TRONTELJ J: *Single Fibre Electromyography.* London, Unwins, 1978

WALTON JN (ed): *Disorders of Voluntary Muscle,* 4th ed. London, Churchill-Livingstone, 1981

370
ACUTE AND SUBACUTE MYOPATHIC PARALYSIS

WALTER G. BRADLEY
MARIA SALAM-ADAMS

It is a fairly safe clinical rule that an abrupt onset of widespread paralysis (one that develops within minutes to hours) is usually due to a lesion of motor tracts in the central or peripheral nervous systems. The most frequent diseases of this type are a cerebrovascular accident, poliomyelitis, or a polyneuropathy. However, disorders of the neuromuscular junction and some myopathic states may occasionally cause paralysis which develops in an acute or subacute manner. Botulism manifests itself as a fulminant paralysis, beginning in ocular and other cranial muscles, and extending to trunk and limb muscles with terminal respiratory failure (see Chap. 171). Myasthenia gravis (Chap. 372) produces paralysis of a similar distribution but which usually develops more slowly. Neuromuscular blockade with paralysis may be induced acutely during the administration of the aminoglycoside antibiotics.

By contrast, most of the myopathies are chronic in course. The relatively small number of diseases of the skeletal muscle which cause acute or subacute paralysis are considered in this chapter. They include the polymyositis-dermatomyositis complex, conditions causing rhabdomyolysis and myoglobinuria, muscle paralysis from hyper- and hypokalemia (including the periodic paralyses) and certain endocrine (hyperthyroid, hypo- or hyperadrenal) myopathies, and drug-induced myopathies. Disorders of muscle energy metabolism (Chap. 374) may cause exercise-induced weakness. It must be emphasized that the same disease entity (e.g., polymyositis) may cause an acute, subacute, or chronic syndrome in different patients and that their description here or in Chap. 371 (chronic myopathy) is arbitrary.

DERMATOMYOSITIS AND POLYMYOSITIS

DEFINITION Polymyositis is an inflammatory disease of skeletal muscles, with lymphocytic infiltration producing muscle fiber damage and degeneration. Dermatomyositis is a condition where polymyositis is associated with inflammation of the skin, which produces the characteristic rash. These relatively common diseases are often associated with other connective tissue disorders, such as rheumatoid arthritis, rheumatic fever, lupus erythematosus, and scleroderma, or with a malignancy.

HISTORY Polymyositis has been known since the original description by Wagner in 1863 and 1887, and the dermatomyositic form was first recorded by Unverricht in 1887. Recent knowledge will be found in the reviews by Adams and Victor (1981), and Bradley (1980).

ETIOLOGY The cause of the disease is unknown. The two main theories are that the disease is due to a viral infection or to an autoimmune disturbance. Almost all attempts to isolate an infective agent have been unsuccessful. Several electron-microscopic observations of virus-like particles in muscle fibers have not been confirmed by positive culture of a virus. Rising titers of antiviral antibodies have not been demonstrated, nor has a polymyositic illness been induced in animals by injection of extracts of affected muscles. A disease resembling polymyositis may be provoked in laboratory animals by injection of sterile muscle extracts with Freund's adjuvant, or by viruses such as the Coxsackie group. The close association of polymyositis and diseases of connective tissue favors the notion of a common etiology or pathogenesis. Dermatomyositis and polymyositis are frequently associated in older patients with a malignancy. In a small number of cases the influenza virus and *Toxoplasma* infection have been demonstrated. Thus dermatomyositis-polymyositis is a syndrome which probably has a number of different causes.

CLASSIFICATION Bohan and Peter (1975) recommended separation of the dermatomyositis-polymyositis group into the following categories: adult polymyositis; adult dermatomyositis; childhood dermatomyositis, which is often accompanied by a vasculitis; dermatomyositis-polymyositis with malignancy; the overlap group with dermatomyositis-polymyositis and one of the other established collagen-vascular disorders such as rheumatoid arthritis. Additional categories which have been described are polymyositis with sarcoidosis, giant-cell myositis with thymoma, and inclusion body myositis (with intranuclear and cytoplasmic filamentous virus-like inclusion). It is not certain that all of these conditions have different etiologies, but current evidence indicates sufficient clinical and pathological differences that their separation appears justified.

CLINICAL MANIFESTATIONS The inflammatory myopathies have a number of different clinical manifestations.

Polymyositis Though this may cause an acute, subacute, or chronic syndrome, the onset is usually insidious, progressing over weeks, months, or even years. The disease may develop at any age and in either sex. Females outnumber males 2:1. A respiratory or obscure systemic illness may precede the muscle weakness, but in many patients the first symptoms develop during excellent health.

The patients first become aware of weakness of the proximal limb muscles, especially the hips and thighs, and find difficulty in arising from the squatting or kneeling position, climbing or descending stairs. With shoulder girdle affection they cannot put an object on a high shelf or comb their hair. In restricted forms of the disease only the neck muscles, the shoulder muscles, or the quadriceps may be involved. Pain of an aching type in the buttocks, thighs, and calves is experienced in a variable percentage of cases (15 to 50 percent) and often indicates a combination of polymyositis and arthritis or other connective tissue disease. The muscles however may be tender to palpation. Early symptoms of dysphagia and weakness of extensor muscles of the neck in a patient with a chronic myopathy suggest the diagnosis of polymyositis.

When the patient is first seen, there may be weakness of the muscles of the posterior and anterior neck, the pharynx and larynx, the trunk and upper and lower girdles, the upper arms and thighs. Ocular muscles are almost never affected except in a rare association with myasthenia gravis. The distal muscles are spared in about 75 percent of cases. Atrophy and reduction in tendon reflexes, though present, are not as pronounced as in denervating conditions; and when the reflexes are disproportionately reduced, one must think of carcinoma with polymyositis and polyneuropathy. Occasionally, the reflexes may appear paradoxically brisk in dermatomyositis-polymyositis.

In reviews of polymyositis and dermatomyositis a surprising number of cardiac abnormalities have been observed. ECG changes, arrhythmias, and heart failure have been reported. Among fatal cases about half show clinical evidence of severe cardiac disease and have necrosis of myocardial fibers at autopsy, usually with only a modest inflammatory reaction. In a few cases there are symptoms such as cough and dyspnea due to interstitial pneumonitis and fibrosis. Arthralgia, Raynaud's phenomenon, and a low-grade fever may also be present.

Dermatomyositis The skin changes may precede or follow the muscle syndrome and may be of various types including a localized or diffuse erythema, maculopapular eruption, scaling eczematoid dermatitis, or even an exfoliative dermatitis. Of particular importance is the distribution of the skin changes, with the occurrence of a lilac-colored (heliotrope) change in the skin over the eyelids, the bridge of the nose, the cheeks, forehead, chest, elbows, knees, knuckles, and around the fingernails. Itching may be troublesome in some cases. The skin lesions may be subtle and thus easily overlooked. Periorbital and perioral edema is frequent, particularly in more fulminating episodes. The skin lesions may occasionally ulcerate. Periarticular and subcutaneous calcification may occur. Signs of other connective tissue diseases are more frequent (in one-third to one-half of all patients) than in pure polymyositis. In those patients with an overlap syndrome with scleroderma, involvement of the distal muscles, the esophagus, and small bowel is more frequent. A considerable number of patients over the age of 50 have an underlying malignancy.

Childhood dermatomyositis Inflammatory myopathy in childhood is frequently associated with skin involvement, and clinical or pathological evidence of vascular damage. There is degeneration and loss of capillaries in the skeletal muscles. Ischemic infarction of other organs in the body, including the kidneys, intestines, and rarely brain, may complicate the disease. Consequently, authors of some series of cases have reported mortality rates of up to one-third in childhood dermatomyositis, though others have found that the prognosis is better than in adult dermatomyositis-polymyositis.

Connective tissue diseases with polymyositis or dermatomyositis (the overlap group) This combination includes rheumatic fever, rheumatoid arthritis, scleroderma, lupus erythematosus, or other established collagen-vascular disorders. The diagnosis rests on the demonstration of the appropriate clinical and laboratory abnormalities, together with myositis. The diagnosis is often difficult in the overlap group since arthritis may appear to produce muscle weakness. Sometimes reliance must be placed on measurement of muscle enzymes in the serum, electromyography, and even muscle biopsy. Though patients in this overlap group respond to corticosteroid therapy, the prognosis for recovery of function is poorer than in pure dermatomyositis-polymyositis.

Carcinoma with polymyositis or dermatomyositis This syndrome is placed in a separate category, although the muscle and skin changes are indistinguishable from those in the above forms of the disease. Approximately 8 percent of all adults who have polymyositis or dermatomyositis are found to have some type of malignancy. The incidence of this neoplastic syndrome is much higher in patients with dermatomyositis over the age of 50, and in this age group the search for an underlying malignancy is obligatory. The malignancy frequently involves the lung but may derive from any organ of the body. The polymyositis may antedate the clinical manifestations of the malignancy by one to two years. The myositis is a paraneoplastic syndrome, the cause of which may lie in an altered immune status or an occult viral infection of the muscle.

LABORATORY FINDINGS In all forms of polymyositis the serum levels of several of the muscle enzymes such as creatine kinase, aldolase, SGOT, SGPT, and LDH are usually elevated. Serum $alpha_2$ and gamma globulin values may be raised. Tests for circulating rheumatoid factor and antinuclear antibodies are positive in less than half of the cases. Myoglobin is occasionally found in the urine when the muscle destruction is acute and extensive. The sedimentation rate is raised in about two-thirds of cases. The electromyogram reveals an increased insertional activity, fibrillation potentials, and "typical myopathic pattern" in about half of the patients. The ECG is abnormal in a few of the cases. The muscle biopsy, if taken from an affected muscle, will demonstrate the typical pathological changes of myositis. Since the lesions have a patchy distribution, it is recommended to biopsy at least two muscles and to select muscles which show active clinical involvement.

PATHOLOGY The principal changes in muscle tissue consist of infiltrates of inflammatory cells (lymphocytes, mononuclear leukocytes, plasma cells, and rare neutrophilic leukocytes), and widespread destruction of muscle fibers with phagocytic reaction. Perivascular (usually perivenular) inflammatory cell infiltration is the hallmark of polymyositis; interstitial inflammatory cell infiltration is also a prominent feature of the disease, but degrees of it may be seen in other conditions as a secondary reaction (e.g., facioscapulohumeral muscular dystrophy). Evidence of muscle fiber regeneration is almost invariable. Many of the residual muscle fibers are small, with increased numbers of sarcolemmal nuclei. Either the degeneration of muscle fibers or the infiltration of inflammatory cells may predominate in any given biopsy specimen. Perifascicular atrophy of muscle fibers, type 2 muscle fiber atrophy, and muscle infarcts may also be found. At autopsy there may be inflammatory and vascular changes in the skin and other organs.

DIAGNOSIS Patients with pure polymyositis are often suspected of having progressive muscular dystrophy because of the similar distribution of weakness in the proximal and trunk muscles. Polymyositis is unlike muscular dystrophy, however, in that the development is much more rapid, individuals may be affected at all ages (few of the muscular dystrophies begin after 30 years of age), and the pharyngeal, posterior neck, and esophageal muscles are often affected. Also in polymyositis-dermatomyositis, the limb-girdle musculature tends to be more diffusely involved than in the muscular dystrophies where there is selective involvement. Nevertheless, in rare patients, it may be difficult, even with biopsy, to distinguish chronic polymyositis from a rapidly advancing muscular dystrophy. This is particularly true of facioscapulohumeral muscular dystrophy where interstitial inflammatory cell infiltration is commonly found early in the disease. Such doubtful cases should always be given an adequate trial of corticosteroid therapy.

A few patients with polymyositis-dermatomyositis and malignancy will exhibit signs of one of the other paraneoplastic syndromes such as polyneuropathy, subacute cerebellar degeneration, multifocal leukoencephalopathy, or the Eaton-Lambert type of myasthenic syndrome; the latter is most often associated with a small-cell carcinoma of the lung.

The diagnosis of polymyositis is not always easy. Patients with pain, but little weakness, may be thought to be hysterical or neurotic. Polymyositis may not be recognized if it occurs in the presence of other collagen-vascular disorders. It is important to determine the serum creatine kinase in such patients. Polymyalgia rheumatica presents with muscle pain and high sedimentation rate; the muscle biopsy discloses only type 2 fiber atrophy, but the temporal artery biopsy may show giant-cell arteritis (Chap. 353). Toxoplasmosis, coxsackie and influenza virus, and other specific infections may occasionally produce a syndrome indistinguishable from polymyositis; antibody screening will reveal the diagnosis. Paroxysmal myoglobinuria, corticosteroid myopathy, thyrotoxic myopathy, and diabetic amyotrophy are other conditions that may enter into the differential diagnosis.

Trichinosis may be confused with idiopathic polymyositis, particularly if the history of pork ingestion is not obtained. The high eosinophil count in the blood, the relatively slight weakness, the conjunctival edema, the ocular and lingual weakness, the symptoms of cerebral involvement (hemiplegia, aphasia, coma, epilepsy, etc.), the positive skin reaction to trichina antigen, and the muscle biopsy establish the diagnosis in most cases (see Chap. 226).

In the final analysis, the diagnosis of idiopathic polymyositis-dermatomyositis must be based on four criteria: clinical picture, EMG, elevation of creatine kinase in the serum, and a positive muscle biopsy. However, in only 25 percent of cases are *all* these criteria satisfied.

TREATMENT Corticosteroids in high dosage are the accepted treatment for severe dermatomyositis-polymyositis, though there is no controlled trial to prove their effectiveness. We have obtained the best results from the use of prednisone, starting at a dose of 1 to 4 mg per kilogram of body weight per day (60 to 80 mg per day for adults). This may need to be continued for 3 months before improvement occurs. When there is significant remission of the weakness, the dose may be reduced every 4 weeks by 5 mg per day. At about 40 mg per day, the schedule is changed to 80 mg every other day in order to reduce the incidence of corticosteroid side effects. Children and patients with acute-subacute dermatomyositis-polymyositis tend to improve more rapidly than those with chronic polymyositis. If the dosage is reduced too rapidly, or to too low a level, relapse will occur, necessitating return to higher dosage. Prednisone therapy may have to be continued for several years, but an attempt should be made to withdraw the therapy every year to determine if the disease is still active. Immunosuppressant drugs should be tried when the disease is severe and when the response to corticosteroids is inadequate or when relapses are frequent. Azathioprine (2.5 to 3.5 mg/kg per day in divided doses) is the most easily used immunosuppressant. Cyclophosphamide and methotrexate have been used with benefit. The aim of cytotoxic therapy is to lower the total lymphocyte count to about 800 per cubic millimeter, while maintaining the hemoglobin level above 12 g/dl, the total white cell count above 3000 per cubic millimeter, and the platelet count above 125,000 per cubic millimeter. Weekly blood counts are required to control immunosuppressant therapy. The combined use of prednisone and a cytotoxic drug usually allows a lower dose of prednisone to be used. Physiotherapy and rehabilitative devices are important in the long-term treatment of patients with dermatomyositis-polymyositis.

Elderly patients, particularly those with dermatomyositis, should be reexamined regularly for a malignancy. If a malignant lesion is found, it should be treated, since the muscle weakness may disappear if the tumor is eradicated. However, a response to corticosteroids can usually be obtained in patients with polymyositis associated with a malignancy.

Serum creatine kinase activity cannot be used to determine disease activity in patients being treated with prednisone for dermatomyositis-polymyositis. This drug lowers the serum creatine kinase activity in a way which is not fully understood, but which is not related to the suppression of muscle inflammation.

PROGNOSIS The overall mortality rate of individuals with dermatomyositis-polymyositis is about four times that of the general population; death is due usually to pulmonary, renal, and cardiac complications. The majority of patients improve with therapy. Many patients make a full functional recovery, though some weakness of the shoulders and hips, usually not disabling, remains at the conclusion of treatment. Relapse may occur at any time. Corticosteroids should not be discontinued too soon, for the relapse which may follow is often more difficult to treat than the original presentation. About one-half of the patients with this disease recover within 5 years after the onset of the symptoms, but about 20 percent still have active disease requiring continued therapy.

SARCOIDOSIS AND POLYMYOSITIS Polymyositis may develop in patients with sarcoidosis, and the muscle will contain noncaseating tubercles with Langhans-type multinucleate giant cells. Regenerating multinucleate myoblasts can however resemble Langhans' giant cells, which has led to misdiagnosis in many of the cases reported to have "sarcoid myositis" in the literature. A giant-cell or granulomatous polymyositis, sometimes associated with myasthenia gravis, has been recorded in patients with thymomas.

A syndrome of acutely developing painful focal inflammatory nodules, sometimes occurring sequentially in different muscles, has been termed "focal nodular myositis." The pathological appearance and response to therapy is indistinguishable from polymyositis. The differential diagnosis includes muscle infarcts such as can occur in polyarteritis nodosa.

RHABDOMYOLYSIS AND MYOGLOBINURIA

In any disease that results in rapid destruction of a large mass of striated muscle, myoglobin and other muscle proteins enter the bloodstream and may appear in the urine, which becomes dark red or burgundy colored. Myoglobin may be separated from hemoglobin by spectroscopy or radioimmunoassay. When myoglobinuria is severe, renal damage may ensue and lead to anuria. The mechanism of renal damage is not clear; probably it is not simply a mechanical obstruction of the tubules by precipitated myoglobin. However, alkalinization of the urine by ingestion of sodium bicarbonate is said to protect the kidney by preventing the formation of myoglobin casts, but in severe cases it is of doubtful value and the sodium may actually be harmful in the presence of anuria. Therapy is the same as in anuria following surgical shock (see Chap. 30).

A number of conditions may cause myoglobinuria, usually with the acute onset of weakness or paralysis:

1 *Crush injury* or infarction of a large mass of muscle.
2 *Excessive muscular contraction* as in forced marches, uncontrolled convulsions, or severe hyperthermia.
3 *Acute idiopathic polymyositis* and *viral myositis* (e.g., due to influenza virus).
4 *Drugs* and *toxins.* A number of agents are toxic to muscle, and under appropriate conditions may cause rhabdomyolysis. Some snake venoms contain potent myotoxins. Haff disease was acute rhabdomyolysis reported from the Bay (Haff) of Konigsberg, Germany, which resulted from the eating of fish contaminated by industrial toxins. A number of myotoxic drugs may cause myoglobinuria, including the intake of large amounts of alcohol. *Alcoholic myopathy* usually occurs in chronic alcoholics during a severe drinking bout. All the limb and trunk muscles may be affected, though the ocular and cranial muscles are spared. Signs of cardiac failure may occur. Most patients recover within a few weeks but may relapse in another bout of drinking. Muscle fiber regeneration restores power but may be impaired by the presence of polyneuropathy or other neurological syndromes associated with chronic alcoholism. The condition is probably due to a transient suppression of the conversion of inactive to active myophosphorylase during bouts of alcoholism, perhaps exacerbated by hypokalemia.

Coma from barbiturates, narcotics, and alcohol may precipitate myoglobinuria, perhaps due to prolonged compression and ischemic necrosis of muscles.

Malignant hyperthermia is a syndrome of acute rise in

body temperature usually associated with severe muscle rigidity, precipitated in susceptible individuals by exposure to succinylcholine and the gaseous anesthetics, especially halothane. The anesthetic agents cause uncontrolled contraction of muscle, and stimulation of anaerobic respiration, perhaps by blocking the reuptake of sarcoplasmic calcium by the sarcoplasmic reticulum. Body temperature may rise 10° in 10 min, and there is severe lactic acidosis. The condition therefore has a high mortality rate. Treatment consists of withdrawal of all anesthetic agents, rapid central cooling, and administering dantrolene sodium, which blocks release of calcium by the sarcoplasmic reticulum. If the patient survives, there may be extensive muscle fiber destruction with myoglobinuria. The condition is often inherited in an autosomal dominant fashion and is sometimes associated with a variety of musculoskeletal abnormalities including congenital ptosis, strabismus, high arched palate, pectus carinatum, dislocation of the patellae, kyphoscoliosis, congenital myopathies, and muscular hypertrophy. Susceptible family members may be detected by the elevation of serum creatine kinase and by the vitro contracture of the muscle fibers in a biopsy when exposed to halothane and succinylcholine.

5 *Metabolic myopathies.* Severe exertion in a patient with a deficiency of an enzyme for energy metabolism, such as myophosphorylase (McArdle's disease), phosphofructokinase, carnitine palmityltransferase, or myoadenylate deaminase, may cause muscle cramps and myoglobinuria.

6 *Idiopathic myoglobinuria.* Recurrent episodes of muscle weakness and myoglobinuria, often precipitated by exertion, may occur in patients where none of the above biochemical causes has been found. This may occasionally be familial (Meyer-Betz disease).

The recent introduction of an extremely sensitive radioimmunoassay has allowed the detection of myoglobinuria and myoglobinemia in many chronic myopathies, including the muscular dystrophies.

POTASSIUM DISTURBANCES AND ACUTE PARALYSIS

Severe hypokalemia ($<$2.5 meq per liter) or hyperkalemia ($>$7.0 meq per liter) of any cause may produce acute or subacute paresis or paralysis. Hyperkalemia causes hyperpolarization of the sarcolemma, raising the threshold for depolarization by the end-plate potential. Hypokalemia produces depolarization of the sarcolemma, which chronically activates the voltage-dependent "off-gate" of the sarcolemmal sodium channels (see Chap. 369).

Familial periodic paralysis of the hypo- or hyperkalemic type (see Chap. 43) causes recurrent attacks of acute paralysis. In these conditions the changes in serum potassium are much less than in the above conditions (about 3.0 and 5.5 meq per liter, respectively) and are probably secondary to primary abnormalities of sarcolemmal electrolyte metabolism.

ENDOCRINE MYOPATHIES

Thyroid dysfunction may be associated with neuromuscular disorders, most of which are chronic (see Chap. 111). Occasionally proximal, mainly upper limb girdle weakness may develop subacutely in thyrotoxic myopathy. Acute or subacute bulbar paralysis has been described in hyperthyroidism, but most such cases are due to an associated myasthenia gravis. Exophthalmic ophthalmoplegia (endocrine exophthalmos) may occasionally develop in a subacute manner with exophthalmos, chemosis, and external ophthalmoplegia (i.e., sparing pupillary and ciliary muscles). In this condition there is acute edema of the muscles and connective tissues of the orbits, often with some infiltration by inflammatory cells. Patients usually have increased T_3 and T_4 levels. An abnormal antibody having thyroid-stimulating activity (long-acting thyroid stimulating factor, or LATS) is present in many patients. Rarely, no clear abnormality of thyroid function can be demonstrated.

Thyrotoxic periodic paralysis is largely restricted to the oriental races, with recurrent hypokalemic attacks and paralysis similar to familial hypokalemic periodic paralysis, but without a family history. This syndrome is cured by correction of the hyperthyroidism. The cause of this syndrome is unknown.

Hypoadrenalism (acute adrenal failure and Addison's disease) causes weakness and lassitude. Hypercorticism, whether spontaneous or iatrogenic, causes increased skeletal muscle protein catabolism, often with the development of proximal myopathy which may occasionally be subacute (Chap. 112). Muscle weakness can occur with primary and secondary hyperparathyroidism and osteomalacia (Chap. 339). Approximately half of all patients with acromegaly will develop muscle weakness with evidence of segmental muscle fiber necrosis and elevated serum creatine kinate levels.

TOXIC MYOPATHIES

Certain chemical agents can cause a myopathy which may be subacute or chronic depending on dosage. This may sometimes be associated with myoglobinuria (see above) if there is rapid muscle fiber necrosis. In addition to the drugs mentioned above, chloroquine, emetine, vincristine, and ε-aminocaproic acid have significant myotoxicity. Several of the hypocholesterolemic drugs, such as 20,25-diazocholesterol and clofibrate, cause myotonia with muscle stiffness and weakness due to replacement of the sarcolemmal cholesterol with desmosterol.

REFERENCES

Bradley WG: Inflammatory diseases of muscle, in *Textbook of Rheumatology*, WN Kelley et al (eds). Philadelphia, Saunders, 1981, vol 2, chap 79, pp 1255–1276

Curie S: Inflammatory myopathies, in *Disorders of Voluntary Muscles*, 5th ed, JN Walton (ed). London, Churchill Livingstone, 1981, chap 15

DiMauro S: Metabolic myopathies, in *Handbook of Clinical Neurology*, PJ Vinken, GW Bruyn (eds). Amsterdam, North Holland, 1980, vol 41, chap 6, pp 175–234

Engel A: Metabolic and endocrine myopathies, in *Disorders of Voluntary Muscles*, 5th ed, JN Walton (ed). London, Churchill Livingstone, 1981, chap 18

Spiegel TM, Pearson CM: Polymyositis, in *Update III: Harrison's Principles of Internal Medicine*, KJ Isselbacher et al (eds). New York, McGraw-Hill, 1982.

Walton JN, Adams RD: *Polymyositis*. Edinburgh, Churchill Livingstone, 1955

371
PROGRESSIVE MUSCULAR DYSTROPHY AND CHRONIC MYOPATHIES

WALTER G. BRADLEY
JEAN J. REBEIZ

There are chronic diseases affecting the neuromuscular system, some spinal, others neural or muscular, and thus the differential diagnosis of chronically progressive muscle weakness is extensive (see Table 369–1). It includes diseases of the lower motor neuron, such as amyotrophic lateral sclerosis and the hereditary spinal muscular atrophies (see Chap. 364); diseases of the peripheral nerves, such as the chronic motor and sensorimotor polyneuropathies (see Chap. 368); diseases of neuromuscular junction transmission, such as myasthenia gravis and the myasthenic syndrome (see Chap. 372); and diseases of the skeletal muscle fiber itself, which are described in this chapter. There are many different chronic myopathies (see Table 369–1), including inherited, inflammatory, metabolic, endocrine, toxic, and paraneoplastic myopathies. The separation of these disorders is based upon the distribution of muscle involvement, the course and associations of the myopathy, and the results of such investigations as the serum enzyme levels, electrophysiology, muscle biopsy pathology, and biochemistry. Many of these conditions are inherited, including the muscular dystrophies, the myotonic disorders, and many of the congenital and metabolic myopathies.

THE MUSCULAR DYSTROPHIES

HISTORY AND TERMINOLOGY The term *progressive muscular dystrophy (dystrophia musculorum progressiva)* has been applied to a group of chronic inherited myopathies since the middle of the nineteenth century. The name of the author of the original description of each disease is often applied eponymously to that condition. The muscular dystrophies include the pseudohypertrophic muscular dystrophy of young males (Duchenne) and of older males (Becker), limb-girdle muscular dystrophy (first so termed by Walton and Nattrass, combining the crural form of Leyden and Möbius and the juvenile dystrophy of Erb), facioscapulohumeral muscular dystrophy (Landouzy and Déjerine), and the distal, ocular, and oculopharyngeal muscular dystrophies. The basis of the separation of the muscular dystrophies from other inherited myopathies is purely historical; the dystrophies were the first recognized familial degenerations of muscle, and later-discovered inherited primary myopathies have not been included in this group.

CAUSE AND PATHOGENESIS The cause of the muscular dystrophies is genetic. Although in many instances a family history cannot be obtained by direct questioning, in approximately 40 to 50 percent of cases there are other affected individuals among the members of the pedigree upon careful examination. Various forms of inheritance are found in the muscular dystrophies, including autosomal dominant and recessive and sex-linked recessive patterns. In Duchenne muscular dystrophy in particular about one-third of the cases are due to new spontaneous mutation.

Several hypotheses of the etiology of the muscular dystrophies have been advanced in recent years. The *neural hypothesis* proposes that the primary defect lies in the lower motor neuron. The *vascular hypothesis* proposes a circulatory insufficiency as the cause of the muscle degeneration. More likely is the *hypothesis that the genetic defect causes a structural or enzymatic metabolic defect in the muscle fiber itself.* Current evidence suggests that a sarcolemmal defect may underlie Duchenne dystrophy. Such a defect may produce focal disruption of the sarcolemma, allowing large concentrations of calcium to enter the muscle fiber, thereby poisoning the mitochondria and activating calcium-dependent proteolytic enzymes. These changes would lead to muscle fiber necrosis and to many of the biochemical changes seen in necrotizing myopathies such as increased lysosomal enzymes and protein catabolism, as well as release of enzymes such as creatine kinase (CK) and lactic dehydrogenase (LDH) into the serum.

THE CHILDHOOD TYPE OF PSEUDOHYPERTROPHIC DYSTROPHY OF DUCHENNE Although several of the different types of muscular dystrophy may begin in infancy and childhood (e.g., myotonic dystrophy, facioscapulohumeral muscular dystrophy), the most frequent and dreaded form in this age period is that first described by Duchenne.

The severe sex-linked recessive pseudohypertrophic type is the most thoroughly studied of the muscular dystrophies. Though the muscle fiber degeneration probably begins in fetal life, most cases are clinically normal at birth. Gait disturbances usually bring the child to the physician between the ages of 3 and 7 years. Onset of symptoms after the age of 10 is more likely to be associated with the mild Becker type of x-linked muscular dystrophy.

Females transmit the disease, but generally only males suffer from it. The carrier female may be identified with about 70 percent accuracy by the presence of an abnormally high serum CK level. Additional aid in carrier detection may be obtained by finding ECG abnormalities and myopathic changes in the muscle biopsy and EMG.

The most frequent initial complaints relate to the early involvement of the pelvifemoral muscles, the extensors of the hips and knees, and the dorsiflexors of the ankles. This lower limb weakness results in a waddling gait, the tendency for toe walking, and difficulty in running, climbing stairs, and rising from the floor. The onset is insidious and the course is slowly progressive over years. Later, shoulder girdle, neck flexor, and trunk muscles become affected, and usually the child is confined to a wheelchair by the age of 12 years. Death generally occurs during the second decade of life due to respiratory muscle failure or pneumonia. Obesity and scoliosis may additionally impair respiratory function. Sudden cardiac failure can occasionally occur.

In the early stages of the disease, the calves and sometimes the quadriceps and deltoid muscles are unusually large and firm, though weak (pseudohypertrophy). The pelvic girdle muscle weakness causes a waddling (Trendelenburg) gait, and a curious manner of arising from the floor by "climbing up the legs" (Gowers' sign). An exaggerated lumbar lordosis develops to maintain balance, producing a protuberant abdomen. Though virtually every skeletal muscle in the body eventually becomes pathologically affected, early in the disease the weakness has a selective distribution affecting the iliopsoas, quadriceps, glutei, and anterior tibial muscles in the lower extremities, and the serrati, pectorals, latissimi, biceps, and brachioradialis muscles in the upper extremities. The forearm and hand muscles, and the gastrocnemius and foot muscles retain good power until late in the illness. Facial muscles are entirely spared, or are minimally affected later in the course of the illness. Early in the disease the tendon reflexes in the arms are preserved, and even at the late stage it is usually possible to obtain ankle reflexes.

The intelligence is reduced in boys with Duchenne dystrophy, with IQs of below 75 in about one-third and below 50 in about 5 percent. The distribution of IQ in Duchenne dystrophy follows a Gaussian curve shifted to the left by about 15 points compared with the normal. When present, mental retardation is evident from the earliest age and is not progressive.

Cardiac involvement is commonly observed in the late

stages of the disease, manifesting as tachycardia and also by signs of decompensation. Prolongation of the PR interval, slowing of QRS complex, high R waves in the right precordial leads, deep Q waves in the left precordial leads, bundle branch block, and elevation or depression of the ST segment are seen in the ECG. These changes are frequently present early in the course of the disease.

The serum CK activity is usually raised several hundredfold in the first few months of life, falling slowly until the time of death. The muscle biopsy in the early months of life shows necrosis, regeneration, and "supercontracted" or "hyaline" muscle fibers. Fibrosis and replacement of lost muscle fibers by lipocytes develop early. Late in the disease, few muscle fibers remain, and active muscle fiber degeneration becomes uncommon.

A clinically and pathologically similar disease occurs rarely in females. Some of these have Turner's syndrome (XO chromosome pattern), so that the abnormal gene on the X chromosome is allowed to manifest. Other female cases have a chromosomal translocation producing the same result. Lyonization (inactivation of one X chromosome early in embryonic development) may account for a small number of female cases resembling Duchenne muscular dystrophy; a similar explanation is given for carrier females manifesting weakness in later life. Autosomal recessive limb-girdle muscular dystrophy may be responsible for a small number of female children with a Duchenne-like picture.

BECKER PSEUDOHYPERTROPHIC MUSCULAR DYSTROPHY This is a sex-linked recessive disease similar to Duchenne dystrophy, but pursuing a milder course with a better prognosis. Walking is possible in most patients beyond age 16 years, and many patients live to the fifth and sixth decades. The distribution of muscle involvement and pseudohypertrophy is similar to that of the Duchenne form. Cardiological changes are less frequent than in the Duchenne form, and CK levels in the serum, though raised, are not as high. The muscle pathology is generally similar to, but less severe than, that in Duchenne muscular dystrophy. Tests similar to those used to detect female carriers of Duchenne muscular dystrophy reveal changes in about 50 percent of carriers of Becker muscular dystrophy.

FACIOSCAPULOHUMERAL (LANDOUZY-DÉJERINE) MUSCULAR DYSTROPHY This disease is inherited as an autosomal dominant disorder, usually with complete penetrance. Males and females are equally affected. Facioscapulohumeral muscular dystrophy often begins in the second and third decades, though facial weakness from an early age with difficulty in whistling and blowing up balloons is common. The degree of involvement is variable; some patients have few symptoms by age 50 years, while others are significantly incapacitated before the age of 20 years.

The pattern of muscular involvement differs from that of the other dystrophies, as indicated by the name. Weakness of facial muscles is nearly always present. The orbicularis oris is particularly affected, together with weakness of the orbicularis oculi muscles, diffuse flattening of the face, and pouting of the lips. Usually it is weakness of the pectoral girdle muscles (pectorals, periscapular, triceps, biceps, and brachioradialis) with winging of the scapulae, which brings the patient to the physician. The tibial and peroneal groups may become weak, with footdrop, relatively early in the disease. In contrast, the pelvifemoral, forearm, and intrinsic hand muscles are maintained until an advanced stage. Pseudohypertrophy and cardiac and intellectual involvement are virtually unknown. The average patient lives out a normal life span but may become incapacitated late in life.

This disease, like limb-girdle muscular dystrophy, must be distinguished from the proximal forms of hereditary spinal muscular atrophy (see Chaps. 364 and 365), based upon the results of laboratory investigations. The serum CK activity is two to five times normal, and the EMG is myopathic. Muscle biopsy shows a moderately necrotizing myopathy, often with slight interstitial inflammatory cell infiltration in the early stage of the disease. This may simulate polymyositis, but perivascular inflammation is rare. Treatment of patients having facioscapulohumeral muscular dystrophy and inflammatory cell infiltration has unfortunately not resulted in clinical improvement, though the serum CK activity may be lowered.

LIMB-GIRDLE MUSCULAR DYSTROPHY This form of muscular dystrophy was first clearly recognized by Walton and Nattrass in 1954. It may affect either sex, the onset usually being in the second and third decades. An autosomal recessive pattern is seen in about one-third of the cases, though rarely there is a dominant pattern. In some cases, muscle weakness begins in the shoulder girdle muscles (Erb type), while in others it begins in the pelvic girdle (Leyden-Möbius type). Weakness spreads to the other limb girdle within 1 to 20 years. The distribution of muscle involvement is selective and rather similar to that in Duchenne muscular dystrophy. Pseudohypertrophy of the calves and other muscles is seen in a small proportion of cases. Cardiac and intellectual changes are rare. The course of the illness is variable, but usually the rate of progression is slow. Severe disability does not occur until middle life when the disease has been present for 20 years or more. Facial muscles are generally spared. Several limited forms have been recognized, including one remaining restricted to the quadriceps muscles for many years. The serum CK level, the muscle pathology, and the EMG changes are similar to those seen in Becker muscular dystrophy.

The purity of this entity has been much debated. A review of patients with this pattern of muscle involvement shows many cases with hereditary spinal muscular atrophy. Other diseases such as polymyositis and certain of the metabolic and endocrine myopathies may also cause a similar picture (see below).

MYOTONIC DYSTROPHY Myotonic dystrophy (dystrophia myotonica, myotonia dystrophica, Steinert's disease) is a dominantly inherited disease characterized by myotonia, muscle wasting of a characteristic pattern, cataracts, testicular atrophy, frontal baldness, and cardiac abnormalities.

The myotonia may be more prominent in the early years than the other manifestations. Although the disease usually begins in early adult life, it may be observed in infancy and childhood. Indeed a particularly severe neonatal form occurs in infants born of mothers with myotonic dystrophy. In the neonatal type, the muscles are thin and weak, without myotonia, and death may occur in the early weeks of life from respiratory muscle weakness. Myotonia (Chap. 369) consists of an inability to relax a muscle normally after strong contraction and is the result of repetitive discharges of muscle fibers. Most characteristically, it is demonstrated in the thenar eminences and forearm muscles. The patient's inability to let go after shaking hands may give the clue to the diagnosis. This difficulty tends to be worse in the cold, to disappear after repeated contractions, and to return after inactivity. Idiomuscular contraction elicited by direct percussion of the muscle (percussion myotonia) is also prolonged in myotonic dystrophy.

The distribution of muscle weakness and atrophy is characteristic of this disease. There is ptosis without ophthalmoplegia. A mild facial myopathy often causes a dull expressionless facies, particularly when associated with a characteristically long facial structure. The voice is often nasal and monotonous. Atrophy of the temporalis and sternocleidomastoid muscles is disproportionately marked. Thus flexion of the neck is weak, while extension is moderately strong. Usually all the limb muscles are weak, particularly proximally but sometimes distal weakness and wasting of the upper and lower limbs is prominent and can occasionally mimick peroneal muscular atrophy. Rarely mild distal sensory impairment can also occur. The tendon reflexes are reduced, and contractures may occur late in the illness. Mental retardation is a common finding, and in some cases appears to be progressive. The brain weight in such cases may be reduced by more than 200 g, and there may be abnormalities of the cortical lamination of neurons.

These patients, whether male or female, also develop progressive alopecia, usually frontal, at an early age. Testicular atrophy with androgen deficiency usually appears in males, associated with sterility and sometimes impotence. Ovarian insufficiency may develop late in females. There is an increased secretion of insulin in response to a glucose load in a small proportion of patients. Reduced levels of IgG, due to an increase in catabolism, have been reported in many patients. Abnormalities in the membranes of certain cells, including red blood cells, have been observed by several investigators.

The lens opacities in myotonic dystrophy are two types. The first consists of fine dust-like subcapsular deposits which often appear colored and scintillate under the slit lamp. This appearance is so characteristic as to be virtually diagnostic. The second type is the usual senile cataract, which may occur at an unusually early age. Myotonic dystrophy affects the gastrointestinal tract, causing weakness and dilatation of the esophagus and colon.

Heart disease frequently appears in patients with well-developed dystrophia myotonica. Cardiac conduction defects, with prolonged PR intervals and heart block, may cause sudden death. More benign arrhythmias may also occur.

The EMG shows both electrical myotonia and myopathic changes. The muscle biopsy shows a nonspecific degeneration and atrophy, sometimes with particular atrophy type 1 fibers and ringed fibers (ringbinden) with sarcoplasmic masses and rows of central nuclei. The serum CK activity may be moderately elevated.

Myotonic dystrophy is inherited as a mendelian autosomal dominant trait, but with incomplete penetrance. The pattern in families is very variable. Some individuals bearing the gene may be severely disabled from childhood, while others may have only cataracts in old age or never manifest signs of the disease. Clinical examination, electromyography, and slit-lamp examination aid in the early recognition of individuals bearing the gene. Linkage exists between the gene for myotonic dystrophy and the secretor gene which allows blood group substances to be secreted into the saliva. In about 5 percent of families, favorable genetic features allows the use of the secretor status of the fetus, detected at amniocentesis, to be used for antenatal genetic counseling in myotonic dystrophy.

Quinine, phenytoin, or procainamide in routine dosages often relieve the myotonia but have no effect upon the myopathic symptoms. Few patients gain great benefit from these drugs.

OTHER FORMS OF MYOTONIA Three forms of nondystrophic congenital myotonia are recognized. *Myotonia congenita of Thomsen* is dominantly inherited and manifests with myotonia and mild muscle hypertrophy from early life. The recessively inherited *myotonia congenita of Becker* frequently has an onset at the end of the first or beginning of the second decade and may be associated with mild muscle weakness later in life. Neither disease has extramuscular manifestations, in contradistinction to myotonic dystrophy. *Paramyotonia congenita of von Eulenberg* is a rare dominantly inherited disorder with myotonia and periodic attacks of muscle weakness precipitated by cold. This condition has some similarities to the periodic paralyses (Chap. 373).

CHRONIC PROGRESSIVE EXTERNAL OPHTHALMOPLEGIA AND OCULOPHARYNGEAL MUSCULAR DYSTROPHY Isolated dystrophic involvement of the extraocular muscles is another relatively rare form of chronic myopathy. These disorders must be differentiated from other causes of ophthalmoplegia, and Drachman has emphasized the heterogeneity of the chronic progressive external ophthalmoplegia syndrome ("ophthalmoplegia plus"). Two separate syndromes have been identified. *Ocular myopathy* consists of a progressive external ophthalmoplegia (sparing the pupils and muscles of accommodation), ptosis, and sometimes later developing weakness of the orbicularis oculi and proximal upper limb girdle muscles. The inheritance pattern is variable. It may begin in childhood, adolescence, or early adult life, and slowly progresses for many years. The electromyogram and muscle biopsy are myopathic, and frequently the latter shows abnormal accumulations of structurally altered mitochondria. Some of these patients, whose symptoms begin in childhood, have the Kearns-Sayre syndrome (chronic progressive external ophthalmoplegia, atypical retinitis pigmentosa, cardiac conduction defects, short stature, and ovarian dysgenesis).

The second form, *oculopharyngeal muscular dystrophy,* was demonstrated to be a myopathy by Hayes, Adams, and Victor. There is a progressive ptosis and dysphagia developing in later life (often beyond 50 years of age), sometimes with limb-girdle muscular involvement late in the course. The disease is inherited as a mendelian dominant trait, and there is often French-Canadian ancestry. The patient complains of increasing difficulty in swallowing and eventually suffers inanition.

DISTAL MUSCULAR DYSTROPHY Familial progressive distal muscle weakness is usually due to the neuropathic type of peroneal muscular atrophy. However, rare cases have electromyographic and muscle pathological changes of myopathies. The disorder usually begins in middle adult life and is slowly progressive, but produces only moderate disability. Welander found an autosomal dominant transmission in some of her families. The disorder is rare and appears concentrated mainly in Scandinavia.

TREATMENT OF THE MUSCULAR DYSTROPHIES There is no specific treatment for any of the muscular dystrophies, and therefore the role of the physician is to provide physical aids which attempt to circumvent the weakness, and to support the patient and relatives. A wide variety of drugs have been used without success, though this continues to be an area of active research. Two factors are important in the management of these patients: avoidance of prolonged bedrest and inactivity, and encouragement of the patients to maintain as full a life as possible. Obesity should be prevented. Pseudocontractures and skeletal deformities can often be prevented by passive and active stretching exercises, splinting, and surgical correction. The techniques of rehabilitation medicine, with physiotherapy, splints and braces, wheelchairs, hoists, and other aids, can greatly benefit the patient and make the lives of the relatives more bearable.

It is a frequent error to assume that patients with slowly progressive proximal muscular weakness have muscular dystrophy, when in fact some treatable disorder such as polymyositis, or endocrine or metabolic myopathy, is the cause. Thus full investigation including muscle biopsy is indicated in every patient.

OTHER CHRONIC, SLOWLY PROGRESSIVE, OR RELATIVELY STATIONARY MYOPATHIES

POLYMYOSITIS AND DERMATOMYOSITIS Polymyositis and dermatomyositis may present as chronic progressive myopathies with symptoms extending over months or years. The course may at times however be acute or subacute and the features of this disease are described in Chap. 370.

METABOLIC MYOPATHIES This term is precise, covering myopathies in which the metabolic defect is known, such as an enzyme defect as in McArdle's disease, a deficiency of a biochemical substrate as in carnitine deficiency, or abnormal electrolyte metabolism as in calcium or potassium disturbances. The separation of these conditions from myopathies due to other biochemical causes (endocrine, toxic, etc.) or to as yet unknown biochemical causes (muscular dystrophies, congenital myopathies) is arbitrary. Metabolic myopathies often cause chronic progressive weakness and thus are considered here, though several may be characterized by acute, subacute, or periodic weakness.

Glycogen storage diseases Deficiency of several of the enzymes of the glycolytic pathway may cause myopathies, in most of which there is glycogen accumulation within the muscle fibers. These are considered more fully in Chap. 100. *Type II glycogenosis* (α-1,4-glucosidase or acid maltase deficiency) may be of three types. In the infantile type (Pompe's disease) a progressive impairment of cardiac and skeletal muscle function is due to excessive deposition of glycogen. Symptoms start in the first weeks or months of life. Death from congestive cardiac failure and respiratory muscle weakness occurs usually within the first year. *Childhood* and *adult* forms of acid maltase deficiency usually present as a slowly progressive limb-girdle muscle weakness. Cardiac involvement is rare. In all types, the serum enzymes (creatine kinase etc.) may be raised 2 to 12 times above normal. The EMG is myopathic, and it frequently shows electrical myotonia in the adult form. Muscle biopsy shows a marked amount of glycogen in muscle fibers in the infantile form, and lesser degrees of accumulation in the childhood and adult types. The glycogen is contained both in membrane-bound lysosomes and free in the sarcoplasm. As to pathogenesis there is an absence of the lysosomal enzyme α-1,4-glucosidase, with inability to digest excessive accumulations of glycogen. The three forms of the disease are probably separate genetic entities, though at present the exact biochemical basis for their differences is not clear. All are autosomal recessive traits. Diagnosis can be made by measuring α-1,4-glucosidase in muscle, leukocytes, or urine.

Type V glycogenosis (myophosphorylase deficiency, McArdle's disease) is a condition in which muscle glycogen cannot be rapidly broken down to glucose l-phosphate during severe or ischemic work. This results in a fall in ATP concentration within the muscle fibers, and consequent painful muscle contractures which are electrically silent on EMG. Symptoms do not usually begin until the second or third decade for reasons which are not clear. Rhabdomyolysis may be precipitated by severe exertion. A few patients develop a mild chronic myopathy in later life. This condition is genetically heterogeneous, some patients having an intramuscular protein which is enzymatically inactive but reacts with antibodies against myophosphorylase, while others have no such identifiable protein. Most cases are inherited in an autosomal recessive fashion, though rare cases have a dominant pattern.

A number of other deficiencies of glycolytic enzymes can affect skeletal muscle, including phosphofructokinase deficiency which is clinically similar to McArdle's disease, and brancher and debrancher enzyme deficiencies (Chap. 100).

Myopathies associated with disorders of lipid metabolism Carnitine is required for the entry of long-chain fatty acids into mitochondria where they undergo beta oxidation. Long-chain fatty acylcoenzyme A is converted to long-chain fatty acylcarnitine by the enzyme carnitine acyltransferase (or carnitine palmityltransferase), which is located on the inner mitochondrial membrane. Fatty acid oxidation provides a major part of the energy source of skeletal muscle during sustained exercise. Deficiency of carnitine impairs long-chain fatty acid oxidation, leading to the accumulation of neutral triglycerides in muscle fibers. Two forms of this disorder are recognized. The *myopathic type of carnitine deficiency* presents with chronic progressive or occasionally fluctuating diffuse proximal muscle weakness in adult life. Carnitine deficiency and triglyceride accumulation is restricted to the skeletal muscle, and probably results from inability of the muscle to accumulate carnitine from the plasma. The disorder may improve with high-dose carnitine therapy (6+ g per day of L-carnitine), with a replacement of the normal diet by one rich in medium-chain fatty acids, and for an unknown reason, with corticosteroids (prednisone, 30 to 60 mg per day). *Systemic carnitine deficiency* presents in infancy or childhood with progressive muscle weakness and liver and kidney dysfunction. Carnitine levels are low in the serum, muscle, and other tissues of the body, probably as a result of impaired synthesis of carnitine in the liver and kidney. The disease is frequently lethal but may respond to oral carnitine therapy. Both forms of carnitine deficiency are probably inherited in an autosomal recessive manner.

Carnitine palmityltransferase deficiency might be expected to cause a similar clinical syndrome to carnitine deficiency. However, for reasons not yet clear, deficiency of this enzyme produces cramps on exercise, frequently complicated by attacks of myoglobinuria. The condition usually presents in early adult life and is not associated with significant triglyceride accumulation in muscle fibers. Attacks of rhabdomyolysis are particularly frequent with exertion in the fasting state, and patients with this deficiency are generally unable to produce ketoacids during fasting. This is presumably due to the enzyme deficiency also involving the liver. Treatment with diets high in either medium-chain fatty acids or carbohydrates may help prevent attacks.

Mirochondrial myopathies This term is usually restricted to myopathies in which skeletal muscle mitochondria are structurally abnormal and/or are present in excessive numbers. The latter causes mitochondrial accumulation in subsarcolemmal areas where they are easily seen with oxidative enzyme histochemical stains. Such mitochondrial-rich fibers stain red in trichrome stains ("ragged red fibers"). An increasing number of different mitochondrial myopathy syndromes are being recognized, though in few is the exact biochemical defect yet known. *Chronic progressive external ophthalmoplegia* and the *Kearns-Sayre syndrome* referred to above are mitochondrial myopathies affecting the extraocular and proximal limb-girdle muscles. *Nonthyrotoxic hypermetabolic myopathy* (Luft's disease) is a rare disease where oxidative posphorylation in skeletal muscle mitochondria is loosely coupled, i.e., oxidative phosphorylation is preserved, but oxidation is not regulated by the ADP concentration. This causes uncontrolled and rapid oxidation of substrate by mitochondria. Excessive heat production and diffuse skeletal muscle weakness are hallmarks of the condition. A deficiency of the ability of mitochondria to retain calcium ions may be responsible.

Rare cases of *specific cytochrome deficiencies* have been

found either in infants with severe myopathies or in young adults with exertional fatigue. Hyperlacticacidemia is a feature of many of these mitochondrial myopathies, and a mitochondrial defect may well underlie subacute necrotizing encephalomyelopathy (Leigh's disease). Little effective therapy is available for any of these disorders, though reduction of the gross acidemia is important.

Vitamin D deficiency myopathy Calcium and vitamin D are important for skeletal muscle function (see Chaps. 340 and 341). Patients with vitamin D deficiency, whether due to dietary causes, chronic renal disease, or chronic anticonvulsant therapy (especially phenytoin), may suffer from a chronic painful proximal myopathy. Muscle weakness is often difficult to assess due to the degree of pain, and wasting is relatively mild. Electromyography is frequently normal, and the muscle biopsy usually shows only nonspecific type 2 fiber atrophy. Diagnosis rests on finding a low serum calcium level, osteomalacia in the bones, and a low serum vitamin D level. Therapy with vitamin D results in improvement within weeks.

Myopathies associated with alterations in serum potassium These usually are acute, subacute, or periodic syndromes and are considered in Chaps. 370 and 374.

ENDOCRINE MYOPATHIES

Chronic progressive muscle weakness of predominantly limb-girdle distribution is seen in a number of different endocrine diseases. Therefore, endocrinological investigations are important in any patient with a limb-girdle syndrome.

THYROID DISORDERS (See Chap. 111) *Hyperthyroidism* causes clinical symptoms of weakness of mainly upper limb girdle muscles in about 25 percent of cases, though up to 50 percent of cases have weakness on examination and 85 percent have electromyographic evidence of a myopathy. The serum CK and muscle biopsy are usually normal. The myopathy responds quickly to correction of the hyperthyroidism. *Exophthalmic ophthalmoplegia* occurs in Graves' disease, though its cause may be independent of the metabolic state. The paralysis of extraocular muscles is due to edema and inflammatory cell infiltration of the orbital contents, including these muscles. The pathogenesis of the disease is still far from clear. Treatment with guanethidine eyedrops, prednisone, or orbital decompression may be required in severe cases. *Hypothyroidism* may cause a number of different neurological syndromes, including a cerebellar degeneration, encephalopathy, peripheral neuropathy, or myopathy. The latter usually presents with mild chronic proximal weakness, often with cramps and aching muscles. There may be hypertrophy of the muscles in the Debré-Semelaigne syndrome of cretinous children, and associated with painful cramps in adults (Hoffman's syndrome). Slowly relaxing reflexes are indicative of hypothyroidism. The serum CK is usually normal but may be quite elevated in some cases, and the EMG is normal or myopathic, occasionally with electrical myotonia. Mild nonspecific abnormalities are found in the skeletal muscle biopsy. The condition responds within a few weeks to thyroid replacement.

ADRENAL DISORDERS (See Chap. 112) The *hypercorticoid state,* whether from Cushing's disease or more commonly from iatrogenic corticosteroid therapy, causes a proximal myopathy with weakness and some wasting. Symptoms usually progress insidiously and are dependent on both dose and duration of therapy. Prednisone, 60 mg per day, will cause some degree of myopathy in almost every patient within 2 months. The fluorinated corticosteroids appear particularly prone to cause a myopathy. Corticosteroids increase skeletal muscle protein catabolism with consequent atrophy, particularly of type 2 muscle fibers. The serum CK activity is almost invariably normal, the EMG is normal or mildly myopathic, and the muscle biopsy shows no abnormality. Corticosteroid myopathy can be mistaken for an exacerbation of inflammatory myopathy in patients with polymyositis. A rise of serum CK activity may help indicate that the inflammation is responsible, but at times the diagnosis rests on reducing the dose of corticosteroids and then determining whether the symptoms worsen or improve. *Hypoadrenalism* may cause mild nonspecific weakness and fatigue.

PITUITARY DISORDERS (See Chap. 109) Pituitary disorders are rarely associated with significant neuromuscular problems. In the early stages of acromegaly, there may be increased muscle strength, though later this is replaced by the mild nonspecific weakness of hypopituitarism.

DRUG-INDUCED MYOPATHIES

Drugs may affect all parts of the neuromuscular apparatus causing weakness. Thus a neuropathy may be caused by toxins like the hexacarbons and organophosphorus compounds, while the neuromuscular junction may be blocked by curare and the aminoglycoside antibiotics. The skeletal muscles are also susceptible to drugs and toxins, some of which may cause a subacute myopathy with rhabdomyolysis and myoglobinuria (see Chap. 370), while others cause a more chronic syndrome. The acuteness of the presentation often depends on dosage.

Chronic alcoholism may cause a variety of neurological disorders, including the Wernicke-Korsakoff syndrome, cerebellar degeneration, peripheral neuropathy, and myopathy. Acute alcoholic myopathy is considered in Chap. 370. The chronic progressive proximal "myopathy" seen in debilitated alcoholics usually has the EMG and muscle histochemical findings of chronic denervation and reinnervation. Thus the condition is likely to be due to a proximal alcoholic polyneuropathy.

Corticosteroid myopathy has been described above. Penicillamine may cause an inflammatory myositis indistinguishable from polymyopsitis, which gradually remits on withdrawal of the drug. The mechanism of induction of the autoimmune myositis is not clear. ε-Aminocaproic acid, chloroquine, emetine, and vincristine can produce chronic myopathies, though emetine has greater toxic effects on the heart, and vincristine on the peripheral nerves.

VITAMIN DEFICIENCY

The peripheral nervous system is more susceptible to deficiencies of vitamins (especially vitamins B_1, B_6, and B_{12}) than is the skeletal muscle. However, in animals, α-tocopherol deficiency causes a profound necrotizing myopathy, and such a condition may rarely occur in humans. Vitamin D deficiency myopathy is described above.

CHRONIC MUSCLE WASTING IN MALIGNANCY

Cachexia in patients with a malignancy has several causes. Investigation often shows severe muscle fiber atrophy, particularly affecting type 2 fibers, together with evidence of a necrotizing myopathy and a polyneuropathy. Occasionally, inflammatory cell infiltrates can also be seen (neuromyositis). The association of dermatomyositis and polymyositis with malignancy is well documented (see Chap. 370). Neuromuscular junction dysfunction may occasionally develop in patients with a malignancy, particularly of the lung, producing the myasthenic syndrome of Eaton and Lambert (see Chap. 372). These latter conditions may result from vitamin-nutritional deficiencies induced by the hypermetabolic neoplasm, though it is possible that toxic factors released into the circulation and autoimmune processes may play a part in the pathogenesis.

CONGENITAL MYOPATHIES

Central core disease, nemaline myopathy, and mitochondrial and centronuclear ("myotubular") myopathies are well-established clinicopathological entities, though each may comprise several different genetic disorders. Congenital fiber type disproportion, multicore disease, minicore disease, reducing body myopathy, fingerprint myopathy, and zebra body myopathy are less clearly established disorders. Common to this entire group are the appearance of weakness and hypotonia in infancy (the floppy baby syndrome) and delayed motor milestones. When these children begin to walk, they are unsteady, fall easily, and cannot run or jump. The congenital myopathies may occasionally be static, or the progression is so slow that during childhood the growth of muscles may outstrip the advance of the disease. Underdevelopment of the muscles is a prominent feature. Weakness is greater in proximal than in distal muscles. Ocular muscles are particularly involved in centronuclear and mitochondrial myopathies. Congenital skeletal muscle abnormalities (high palate, hip dislocation, pes cavus) are frequent, and a marfanoid appearance may be present in nemaline myopathy. The serum CK activity is usually normal, and the EMG is myopathic. The diagnosis rests on the demonstration of the specific muscle biopsy changes, and usually requires histochemical and ultrastructural techniques. In none of the congenital myopathies is the biochemical cause known. Many clinically similar cases have no specific pathological alterations in the muscle and therefore still remain to be characterized. "Central hypotonia" (the clinical syndrome of hypotonia with evidence of central nervous system damage) or neonatal myotonic dystrophy (see above) must be considered in cases with no clearly established muscle pathology. There is no known treatment for any of these congenital myopathies. The prognosis is favorable (compared to the dystrophies), and in many instances muscle function improves as the child grows.

REFERENCES

ADAMS RD: *Diseases of Muscle,* 3d ed. New York, Harper & Row, 1975

BETHLEM J: *Myopathies.* Philadelphia, Lippincott, 1977

BRADLEY WG: Inherited diseases of skeletal muscle, in *Recent Advances in Clinical Neurology,* WG Mathews (ed). Edinburgh, Churchill Livingstone, 1975

DIMAURO S: *Metabolic myopathies,* in *Handbook of Clinical Neurology,* PG Vinken, GW Bruyn (eds). Amsterdam, North Holland, 1979, vol 41

MARKESBERY WR et al: Distal myopathy: Electron microscopic and histochemical findings. *Neurology,* 27:727, 1977

MOKRI B, ENGEL HG: Duchenne dystrophy: Electron microscopic findings pointing to a basic or early abnormality in the plasma membrane of the muscle fiber. *Neurology* 25:1111, 1975

WALTON JN: *Disorders of Voluntary Muscle,* 4th ed. London, Churchill Livingstone, 1981

372

MYASTHENIA GRAVIS, NEUROMUSCULAR JUNCTION DISORDERS, AND EPISODIC MUSCULAR WEAKNESS

WALTER G. BRADLEY
RAYMOND D. ADAMS

The characteristic feature of most of the disorders of the neuromuscular junction is the marked variation in the strength of a muscle induced by repeated contractions. However, such disorders may also cause sustained muscle weakness which may follow an acute, subacute, or chronic course. Even with sustained weakness, variation with exertion is frequently seen, and dramatic fluctuations may be induced by pharmacological agents affecting neuromuscular transmission (Chap. 370). Recurrent attacks of transient muscle weakness which are unrelated to exercise are more suggestive of the periodic paralysis syndrome (Chap. 374). It should be emphasized that diseases of the neuromuscular junction, particularly myasthenia gravis, are often difficult to diagnose. It is therefore important to have a high index of suspicion for these conditions and to undertake appropriate diagnostic investigations in any patient with remotely suggestive symptoms.

MYASTHENIA GRAVIS

DEFINITION This disease, first described in 1672 by Thomas Willis, is characterized by weakness and undue fatigability on exercise. It most frequently affects the oculomotor, facial, laryngeal, pharyngeal, proximal limb, and respiratory muscles. Partial recovery with rest and after administration of an anticholinesterase drug is an important characteristic.

Recent advances in knowledge of myasthenia gravis were reviewed by Juguilon and Bradley.

CLINICAL PATTERN Myasthenia gravis occurs at all ages and in both sexes, but females are affected twice as often as males. The peak incidence for females is in the third decade, while in males the incidence is highest in the sixth and seventh decades. Twenty percent of cases have their onset before the twenty-first year of life. No significant familial occurrence has been noted, except for neonatal myasthenia gravis (see below). However, there is a higher than expected frequency of other autoimmune disorders within the families of people with myasthenia as well as in the individual patient. The prevalence is variously estimated to be between 2 and 10 per 100,000.

The onset is often insidious but may be subacute and rarely acute. Weakness of ocular muscles with drooping of the eyelids, which may be unilateral at first, and diplopia occur in 90 percent of cases. This is often transient and intermittent but may progress to complete paralysis of ocular movement. The pupils are never affected. Facial and pharyngeal muscles are weak in 70 percent of the cases. The facial muscle involvement gives rise to a characteristic smile (the "myasthenic snarl") where the lips elevate but do no retract. The tongue may be weak and is sometimes bilaterally furrowed.

Weakness of the laryngeal and pharyngeal muscles may cause choking, aspiration of food, and nasal regurgitation. The voice is nasal, weak, and may fatigue to the point of unintelligibility with prolonged talking. Involvement of masseter muscles may impair chewing and even prevent closure of the mouth ("hanging-jaw sign"). These patients habitually hold a hand under the jaw both to close the mouth and to hold up the head because of the frequently associated weakness of the extensor muscles of the neck.

Weakness of limb muscles is also present in advanced cases of myasthenia gravis, but seldom occurs in the absence of involvement of muscles innervated by cranial nerves. The proximal muscles, especially those of the neck and shoulder girdle, are most severely affected. In the most severe stage, weakness may be universal.

Easy fatigability (i.e., rapid increase in weakness with repeated muscle contraction) and relatively prompt partial recovery after rest can be elicited by history or clinical examination in most cases. The disease may be aggravated by a number of factors, including infections, fever, general debilitation, loss of sleep, and menstruation. A number of drugs may precipitate or exacerbate myasthenia gravis (see below).

Muscular atrophy is not seen in the majority of patients, but it may be present due to partial denervation if the process has been of long duration. The tendon reflexes are generally preserved and usually there is no evidence of impairment of sphincter or sensory functions.

Approximately 10 percent of myasthenic patients, particularly older males, have a thymoma. A few such cases also have aplastic anemia or a giant-cell myositis.

The course of the disease is very variable. In about 20 percent of patients it remains restricted to the ocular muscles. In others, the disease may become severe enough to cause respiratory and bulbar paralysis. Relapses and partial or complete remissions occur in up to half of the patients, particularly in the first few years. Severe myasthenia gravis is a life-threatening disease with a mortality rate of 5 to 10 percent in the first few years.

PATHOGENESIS A series of discoveries has led to the currently accepted theory that myasthenia gravis is the result of specific immunological damage and loss of acetylcholine receptors from the postsynaptic membrane of the neuromuscular junction. These observations include: (1) the reduced amplitude of miniature end-plate potentials; (2) the demonstration by I-labeled α-bungarotoxin applied to excised intercostal muscle biopsies of a 70 to 90 percent reduction in the number of acetylcholine receptors at each neuromuscular junction; (3) the electron-microscopic findings of postsynaptic membrane damage with accumulation of immunoglobulin and complement; and (4) the demonstration that immunization of experimental animals with purified acetylcholine receptor protein produces a disorder of neuromuscular transmission which is virtually identical with human myasthenia gravis.

It has now been demonstrated that 85 percent of patients with active generalized myasthenia gravis have circulating antibodies against human acetylcholine receptors. These antibodies bind to the receptor on the postsynaptic membrane of the neuromuscular junction, but only rarely do they appear to have a curare-like action that blocks the physiological activation of the receptors by acetylcholine. This receptor-antibody interaction binds complement, thereby increasing the degradation of the postsynaptic membrane and its acetylcholine receptor. If this process is active, the skeletal muscle is unable to synthesize acetylcholine receptors at a sufficient rate to maintain the normal number of receptors at the neuromuscular junction, with consequent lowering of the amplitude of the end-plate potential produced by each motor nerve depolarization. As a result, the amplitude of many of the end-plate potentials is at or below the critical depolarization potential required to fire the muscle fiber action potential. Such muscle fibers will either not respond, or respond to only a few motor nerve action potentials before becoming fatigued and weak.

The thymus gland plays an as yet unidentified pathogenetic role in myasthenia gravis. About 65 percent of patients with this disease have thymic hyperplasia, while 10 percent have thymomas. Myasthenia gravis improves in 50 to 80 percent of patients after thymectomy. Myoid (muscle-like) cells are present in normal thymus, and the close association of skeletal muscle antigens and immunologically responsive cells may allow the development of autoantibodies to the muscle acetylcholine receptor protein. Alternatively, there may be a circulating thymus-derived factor responsible for enhancing the effect of acetylcholine receptor antibodies on receptor turnover.

DIAGNOSIS The diagnosis of myasthenia gravis is often delayed because the complaints such as tiredness and blurring of vision are relatively nonspecific and because the strength is normal unless sustained muscle contraction is tested. Many patients are thought to have psychogenic disorders in the early stages of their disease. The characteristic pattern of myasthenic fatigability is easily demonstrated by having the patient make a repetitive or sustained movement of symptomatic muscles. Thus if the patient looks upward for 2 to 3 min, the eyelids progressively droop until they cover the pupils. Strength returns to fatigued muscles after a few minutes' rest.

Anticholinesterase tests Intravenous injection of edrophonium (Tensilon), a short-acting anticholinesterase, will briefly improve the weakness and fatigability. The test should be fractioned by injecting 1 mg and observing the effect for 2 min, then injecting 3 mg and observing the effect for a further 2 min, before administering the final 6 mg if no dramatic improvement has been observed. Fractionation is required since in some patients, weakness will improve with small doses, but larger doses will block the response by producing excessive cholinergic effects. Side effects include bradycardia, nausea, abdominal cramps, dizziness, and blurred vision due to the cholinergic effects on muscarinic sites. Though these are rarely severe, the edrophonium test must be done cautiously with a syringe of atropine and immediate respiratory assistance available. Intramuscular injection of neostigmine, 0.5 to 2.0 mg, may be used as a diagnostic test if the edrophonium test is equivocal. The effect is slower, peaking 10 to 30 min after injection and lasting about 2 h. However, cholinergic side effects are common, and the test should be preceded by an intravenous injection of atropine, 0.4 to 0.6 mg, given 10 min previously.

Acetylcholine receptor antibodies About 85 percent of patients with active generalized myasthenia gravis can be demonstrated to have abnormally high serum titers of antibodies to human acetylcholine receptor. The frequency of antibodies is lower in patients with inactive ("burnt out") myasthenia gravis and in those with pure ocular myasthenia. The titer of antibodies does not bear a direct relation to the severity of the disease since the activity of the antibody in inducing increased acetylcholine receptor turnover is also important. The best diagnostic test for myasthenia gravis would be the direct determination of the average acetylcholine receptor number per neuromuscular junction, but this requires biopsy of a motor point in muscle and electron microscopy, and is currently purely a research procedure.

Electrophysiological tests The characteristic decremental response of greater than 10 percent from the first to the fifth response on maximum stimulation of a nerve to an involved muscle at a frequency of two to five per second is seen in 60 to 95 percent of the patients with myasthenia gravis. This response is due to the loss of acetylcholine receptors at the neuromuscular junction which lowers the safety factor for transmission. In the normal state, repeated nerve stimulation results in a lowering of the amount of acetylcholine released per impulse, though even this reduced amount is more than adequate to ensure neuromuscular transmission (i.e., there is usually a safety factor of 3 or 4). When the number of receptors is severely decreased, the normal physiological fall of acetylcholine released with repeated stimulation causes failure of activation of some end plates. On the other hand, in the normal state immediately after maximum voluntary contraction, there is an augmentation of the amount of acetylcholine released per impulse. Similarly patients with myasthenia gravis demonstrate posttetanic facilitation electrophysiologically. Single fiber EMG may demonstrate the variable dropout ("blocking") of individual muscle fibers from a motor unit, and the variable time of activation of individual muscle fibers ("increased jitter") results from the end-plate potential being close to threshold. Acetylcholinesterase inhibitors increase the action of acetylcholine at the end plates and thus improve all the electrophysiological parameters.

Curare sensitivity The curare test is now only of historical interest since the discovery of more direct diagnostic tests. The reduction of the number of acetylcholine receptor molecules at each neuromuscular junction, and the consequent reduction of the safety factor for transmission, makes patients with myasthenia gravis extremely sensitive to factors causing additional neuromuscular blockade such as curare. One-tenth of the normal paralyzing dose of *d*-tubocurarine (16 mg/kg intravenously) is sufficient to paralyze a patient with myasthenia gravis. The risks of this test are major. A safer regional curare test has been introduced. In this, an injection of 0.3 mg of *d*-tubocurarine in 20 ml saline is given into a hand vein after occlusion of the arterial supply to the arm by inflating a sphygmometer cuff around the arm to above arterial pressure. Repetitive stimulation of distal median or ulnar nerves brings out the myasthenic decrement in more than 95 percent of patients with generalized myasthenia gravis. Despite its relative safety, respiratory support should be available when one is undertaking this test.

CT scan of the mediastinum Though the CT scan of the mediastinum is not a diagnostic test for myasthenia gravis, the risk of a thymoma in patients with this disease necessitates this investigation. A thymoma can usually be demonstrated, but false-positive results can occasionally occur from thymic hyperplasia. If there is any question of a tumor of the thymus, exploration is indicated since many thymomas are malignant because of their local invasiveness. Antistriational antibody titers are increased in about two-thirds of patients with myasthenia gravis and thymomas and are present in only 10 percent of patients with myasthenia gravis without a thymoma.

TREATMENT In view of the significant mortality of myasthenia gravis, it is important to examine patients as an emergency whenever symptoms of respiratory or bulbar weakness appear. Respiratory infections are a threat and should be treated vigorously with appropriate antibiotics. It is important to exclude the presence of a number of conditions which may add to the weakness of myasthenia gravis, such as hyperthyroidism or rarely hypothyroidism. The possibility that drugs such as the aminoglycoside antibiotics, curare-type drugs, and magnesium may play a part in the symptoms needs to be considered.

The currently available therapeutic modalities are anticholinesterases, corticosteroids, thymectomy, plasmapheresis, and immunosuppressants. However there is still no complete agreement as to the optimal way of using these therapeutic modalities.

The most widely accepted plan is to try first the effect of the anticholinesterase drugs. Neostigmine (Progstigmin) in oral tablet form (15 mg) or pyridostigmine bromide (Mestinon) in oral tablet form (60 mg) improves neuromuscular transmission within 15 to 30 min; the maximal effect is obtained in approximately 2 h, lasting for about 4 h. This dose, or multiples thereof, is administered every 4 h during the waking day, and if there is a nocturnal respiratory problem, a delayed-release form is given at bedtime. A syrup is available for small children and for tube feeding. To prevent the muscarinic effects of the anticholinesterase, atropine sulfate tablets, 0.4 to 0.6 mg, may be administered twice daily orally. Excessive doses of anticholinesterases may worsen neuromuscular transmission ("cholinergic block"). If a patient is not responding well to anticholinesterases, it is possible to distinguish overdosage from underdosage by injecting 10 mg of edrophonium. Strength will improve if there is underdosage but will remain the same or decrease with overdosage.

Most mild myasthenic patients can be maintained at a virtually normal functional level by the strategic use of anticholinesterase drugs. Some 15 to 20 percent of patients will eventually have a spontaneous remission. However, the symptoms in many cases with more severe disease are not suppressed by anticholinesterases, and for them other therapeutic modalities must be tried.

Thymectomy must be considered for every patient with severe generalized or rapidly progressive myasthenia gravis. In a series of patients subjected to thymectomy compared with nonsurgical patients matched for age and severity of the disease, the remission rate and degree of improvement is nearly twice as high in the surgical group as in the control group. Approximately 25 to 35 percent of patients will remit within a few months after thymectomy, and 60 to 80 percent will improve. Thymectomy, usually with x-irradiation, is unquestionably indicated in patients with a thymic tumor demonstrated by CT scan. The sternum-splitting operation is to be preferred because of the more complete removal compared with the simpler transcervical approach. Thymectomy is best done in centers where physicians and surgeons are familiar with the special problems of postoperative care of myasthenic patients. If the myasthenia gravis is severe, preoperative plasmapheresis or corticosteroid therapy should be used to improve the condition.

High-dose corticosteroid treatment increases muscle strength in the majority of patients with myasthenia gravis. However, prolonged relatively high dose therapy is required, with the consequent risks of side effects. Corticosteroids are usually only used with severe generalized myasthenia gravis where response to anticholinesterase drugs is inadequate. Their use in pure ocular myasthenia gravis does not seem justified. The administration of high-dose corticosteroids (prednisone, 60 mg per day) may worsen the myasthenia gravis during the first 7 to 10 days of treatment, and consequently patients should be admitted to a hospital during this period. This may be circumvented by starting treatment with 15 to 20 mg prednisone per day and gradually increasing the dosage over 2 to 4 weeks to 60 mg per day. The usual precautions for patients taking high-dose corticosteroid therapy should be instituted, including an antiulcer regimen, administration of potassium supplements, and monitoring for hypertension and diabetes mellitus. Anticholinesterases should be continued. After maximal improvement, the corticosteroid dose may be slowly reduced to the level where the optimal improvement is just maintained. A change to alternate-day dosage will reduce the incidence of corticosteroid side effects. Later it may be possible to reduce the dose of anticholinesterase medication.

Plasmapheresis is a recent addition to the therapeutic armamentarium. A complete exchange of the plasma can be achieved by 5 to 6 large-volume (2.5-liter) plasma exchanges over 2 weeks, with reinfusion of the patients blood cells suspended in artificial plasma. Synthesis of acetylcholine receptor antibody is relatively slow, with half-life of synthesis of about 6 weeks.

Following plasmapheresis there is a gradual rise in the acetylcholine receptor levels at the end plates, with clinical improvement. As the antibody level rises and the receptor level begins to fall, symptoms return. At this time, single or multiple plasma exchanges are undertaken. Evidence indicates that optimal suppression of antibody synthesis is best achieved by immunosuppression with drugs like azathioprine (about 2 mg/kg per day) and corticosteroids. The use of cytotoxic drugs necessitates weekly blood counts to ensure that the cellular elements in the blood are not excessively suppressed.

By the proper use of these methods, the mortality and morbidity rates in myasthenia gravis have been significantly reduced, and the majority of patients are able to return to a productive life.

NEONATAL MYASTHENIA GRAVIS Myasthenia gravis affects about 16 percent of babies born to mothers with myasthenia gravis as a result of maternal acetylcholine receptor antibodies reaching the baby via the placenta. There is typically involvement of ocular, bulbar, and respiratory muscles, and it may be necessary to provide respiratory support. The disease is self-limiting within 3 to 6 weeks, simultaneous with the spontaneous clearing of maternal antibodies from the baby's circulation. Anticholinesterase may be needed during this period.

CONGENITAL MYASTHENIA GRAVIS

Rare patients are encountered with a lifelong muscle fatigue demonstrated to be due to deficiency of neuromuscular transmission by electrophysiological tests. The clinical syndromes are variable and may in some cases spare extraocular and bulbar muscles. Detailed investigation of these patients shows that they do not have circulating acetylcholine receptor antibodies, though they often respond to anticholinesterase drugs. Several different defects may be responsible for this syndrome, including a specific deficiency of acetylcholine receptors, functionally abnormal acetylcholine receptors, the deficient release of acetylcholine from the presynaptic terminals, and the absence of acetylcholinesterase from the neuromuscular junction.

TRANSIENT PARALYSIS WITH DRUGS

The aminoglycosides and certain other antibiotics may cause severe neuromuscular weakness lasting hours to days and simulate myasthenia gravis. Neomycin, streptomycin, kanamycin, gentamicin, cholistin, and polymyxin B are the most clearly incriminated of these drugs. They appear to have both pre- and postsynaptic neuromuscular blocking effects. Magnesium and lithium salts, quinine, procainamide, and beta-adrenergic blocking drugs may also exacerbate or precipitate myasthenia gravis. Penicillamine occasionally induces a syndrome which is indistinguishable from myasthenia gravis and gradually remits on withdrawal of the drug.

THE MYASTHENIC SYNDROME OF EATON AND LAMBERT

The myasthenic syndrome is associated with a small-cell carcinoma of the lung in more than 90 percent of cases. Weakness in these patients is usually in the upper and lower proximal limb-girdle muscles and is often accompanied by aching and stiffness. Contrary to the situation in myasthenia gravis, ocular and bulbar muscles are usually spared and tendon reflexes are depressed or absent. Patients will often show marked weakness on the first attempt at muscle contraction, but repeated efforts *increase* muscle strength. On electromyography with rapid frequencies of neuromuscular stimulation (20 to 30 per second), this is seen as an initial low-voltage muscle action potential, which increases in amplitude; it diminishes in amplitude with low frequencies (1 to 2 per second). The syndrome appears to be due to a defect of calcium-mediated release of acetylcholine from nerve terminals of the neuromuscular junction. Anticholinesterases usually have little effect on the weakness. Tubocurarine and decamethonium make it worse, even in very small doses. Guanidine hydrochloride in oral doses of 250 mg three or four times a day dramatically improves strength in many patients. The condition may precede the appearance of the malignant tumor by as long as 2 years. In a few patients, no other disease has developed after a period of many years.

BOTULINUS POISONING

This toxin, discussed in Chap. 171, affects neuromuscular transmission by blocking the release of acetylcholine from the presynaptic terminal of the neuromuscular junction. The electrophysiological changes are similar to those seen in the myasthenic syndrome and differ from those of myasthenia gravis. The ocular and other cranial muscles are most sensitive, but severe intoxication can cause a generalized paralysis. The smooth muscles innervated by the parasympathetic nervous system are also affected by the toxin. The paralysis will improve with gradual elimination of the toxin, and with guanidine. Respiratory support may be needed.

REFERENCES

Drachman DB: Myasthenia gravis. N Engl J Med 298:136, 186, 1975

Fenichel GM: Clinical syndromes of myasthenia in infancy and childhood. Arch Neurol 35:97, 1978

Juguilon AC, Bradley WG: New insights into myasthenia gravis, in *Update III: Harrison's Principles of Internal Medicine,* KJ Isselbacher et al (eds). New York, McGraw-Hill, 1982, pp 223–234

Osserman KE (ed): *Symposium on Myasthenia Gravis.* New York, Grune & Stratton, 1975

Simpson JA: Myasthenia gravis and myasthenic syndromes, in *Disorders of Voluntary Muscle,* 4th ed, JN Walton (ed). London, Churchill Livingstone, 1981

Viets HR, Schwab RS: In *Symposium on Myasthenia Gravis,* KE Osserman (ed). New York, Grune & Stratton, 1975

373 TRANSIENT AND PERIODIC MUSCLE PARALYSIS

WALTER G. BRADLEY
RAYMOND D. ADAMS

This group of neuromuscular disorders is characterized by attacks of acutely developing diffuse paralysis, which spontaneously recover to complete normality, usually within a few hours. These conditions, the periodic paralyses, cause recurrent attacks which are usually associated with alterations of serum potassium concentration. The clinical features differ from the acute and subacute monophasic conditions described in Chap. 370, where recovery is much slower. They also differ from the disorders of neuromuscular transmission (Chap. 372), where there is sustained weakness with superadded exercise-induced fatigue. They differ from the numerous central nervous system causes of transient loss of muscle power, which include syncope, seizures, transient ischemic attacks of the brain, cataplexy, hydrocephalic attacks, and idiopathic drop attacks. It is most important to realize that any cause of excessively high ($>$ 8 meq per liter) or low ($<$ 2.5 meq per liter) serum potassium will produce diffuse muscle paresis by an effect on the resting sarcolemmal membrane potential (Chap. 369). Hyperkalemia causes hyperpolarization, preventing the end-plate potential from reaching the critical depolarization potential required to fire the muscle fiber. Hypokalemia produces depolarization, which produces depolarization inactivation (closure of the off-gate) of sodium channels in the sarcolemma. Conditions such as excessive potassium administration and renal failure cause hyperkalemia; and primary hyperaldosteronism (Conn's syndrome) and diuretic (kaluretic) and corticosteroid therapy may cause hypokalemia.

In contrast the familial periodic paralyses cause attacks of considerably greater muscle weakness than expected from the change in serum potassium. In fact, some patients have paralytic attacks without change in the serum potassium concentration. These observations suggest that the serum potassium changes may be secondary to some basic abnormality in the sarcolemma.

At least five different syndromes of transient muscle weakness have now been identified: (1) familial hypokalemic periodic paralysis, (2) hyperthyroidism with hypokalemic periodic paralysis, (3) familial hyperkalemic periodic paralysis (adynamia episodica hereditaria of Gamstorp), (4) paramyotonia congenita of von Eulenberg, and (5) normokalemic periodic paralysis. In each of these conditions, over a period of a few minutes or hours the patient develops a disorder of skeletal muscle which may vary from mild weakness of limb muscles to total paralysis and which subsides and disappears completely after a few hours or days. There are a few clinical features which suggest the exact type of periodic paralysis that is present, but generally the diagnosis rests on determining the serum potassium level in an attack and on tests which attempt to precipitate paralytic attacks either by increasing or decreasing the serum potassium concentration.

FAMILIAL HYPOKALEMIC PERIODIC PARALYSIS **Clinical pattern** Familial hypokalemic periodic paralysis is probably the commonest of the periodic paralyses, though it is still a rare disorder. It is usually inherited as a mendelian dominant trait. The patients have a normal strength except during well-demarcated episodes in which intense weakness or complete paralysis of limb and trunk muscles develops. The attacks begin in the second decade and are more frequent in adolescence or early adult years.

A single attack may last from a few minutes to several days, the average duration being 12 to 48 h. The attacks seldom occur more frequently than every 4 to 6 weeks. During the episode, marked hypotonia of the affected muscles and hyporeflexia are found. The paralyzed muscles are refractory to electrical stimulation. The facial, pharyngeal, thoracic, and diaphragmatic muscles are rarely affected, but respiratory embarrassment and death have been reported. Cardiac muscle is not involved, though there may be ECG changes related to the hypokalemia.

The attacks are precipitated by several factors, such as rest after exercise, ingestion of NaCl, or a large high-carbohydrate meal. Attacks often begin during sleep and are present upon awakening. Profuse diaphoresis may precede the attack. Often no precipitating cause can be discovered. Patients can often abort an attack by gentle exercise as soon as the first symptoms are perceived.

In the average patient, there is no evidence of progressive muscular disease, and physical examination between attacks frequently demonstrates no abnormality. Rarely, there may be eyelid myotonia exacerbated by cold. Exceptionally, some degree of weakness, usually mild, persists after the termination of the attack and is cumulative in successive attacks. This sometimes causes a slowly progressive vacuolar myopathy of pelvifemoral muscles during middle and late adult life (Goldflam).

Pathology Despite the striking paralysis, muscle biopsies often are normal, even in an acute paralytic attack. At other times, there is a significant vacuolization of muscle fibers. The vacuoles are filled with clear fluid, but in glycogen stains a few positive-reacting granules may be seen. Under the electron microscope the vacuoles appear to originate from dilatation of the longitudinal endoplasmic reticulum. In the chronic state the vacuoles probably communicate with the extracellular space.

Pathogenesis During the attack, the serum potassium level drops sharply, though rarely below 2.9 meq per liter. This apparently results from the sudden passage of potassium into the cells of the body since the urinary excretion of potassium diminishes at the same time. The intracellular potassium level of muscle has been demonstrated to rise during the attack. The resting membrane potential of the sarcolemma is decreased both in the interictal period and to a greater extent during the attack. The primary abnormality in familial hypokalemic periodic paralysis is not known but may be of one or more of the ion channels and ion pumps in the sarcolemma (Layzer). As was stated above, the entry of potassium into the muscle may be a secondary process. The relation to excess carbohydrate intake is probably connected with the fall in serum potassium level and rise in intracellular levels of potassium in muscle and liver which occur during rapid glycogen storage. However, the timing of these two events differs. The initial potassium changes occur during the first few hours after carbohydrate ingestion, while the attack of periodic paralysis is frequently delayed for 8 to 12 h.

Diagnosis This rests on the finding of a low serum potassium concentration in a spontaneous attack. The diagnosis can be confirmed by the precipitation of a paralytic attack by the intravenous infusion of glucose, 2 g per kilogram of body weight, followed 10 min later by the intravenous injection of 10 to 20 units of soluble insulin. The serum potassium concentration, ECG, and muscle strength should be followed at 15-min intervals; the attack usually begins within $1\frac{1}{2}$ hours and may be aborted by oral or if necessary intravenous potassium. Patients do not develop a paralytic attack when given 30 to 150 meq of potassium orally, unlike the reaction seen in the hyperkalemic form of periodic paralysis.

Treatment Episodes of familial hypokalemic periodic paralysis are treated by the oral administration of potassium salts in doses of 30 to 120 meq until the attack is relieved. In the rare instances where acute respiratory or pharyngeal paralysis appears, it may be necessary to give potassium intravenously, though great care should be taken with this route of administration. In patients with frequent attacks of familial hypokalemic periodic paralysis, 60 to 120 meq of potassium per day by mouth in divided doses and avoidance of meals high in carbohydrate are helpful in preventing attacks.

Acetazolamide (Diamox), up to 2 g per day in divided doses, may also prevent paralytic attacks. This effect is paradoxical, since this carbonic anhydrase inhibitory diuretic is mildly kaluretic, and the presumptive action appears to rest on the alkalosis which it induces.

HYPERTHYROIDISM WITH HYPOKALEMIC PERIODIC PARALYSIS Attacks of hypokalemic periodic paralysis are frequently due to thyrotoxicosis, particularly in Orientals. These attacks are identical to those in the familial condition, but patients generally do not have a positive family history. The pathogenesis of this condition is not clearly understood, but the attacks disappear with correction of the hyperthyroidism.

FAMILIAL HYPERKALEMIC PERIODIC PARALYSIS (ADYNAMIA EPISODICA HEREDITARIA OF GAMSTORP) This is also a mendelian dominant condition and is characterized by periods of weakness or paralysis of skeletal muscle not unlike those of familial hypokalemic periodic paralysis. The onset is between the ages of 5 and 10 years. The attacks are frequent and may last for one to many hours, and they tend to occur during rest after physical exertion, particularly if the patient is wet, cold, or hungry. Tingling of lips, fingers, or toes may occur at the onset of the attack. Weakness varies in degree. Respiratory embarrassment is virtually never seen. Between attacks, the patient is symptom-free, though in some cases mild weakness persists for days or weeks at a time. Some patients have clinical and electromyographic myotonia.

The diagnosis rests on the finding of a serum potassium concentration that rises transiently in the attack. Paralysis may be present with a serum potassium concentration of 5.5 meq per liter. The diagnosis can be confirmed by the precipitation of an attack by the oral administration of 30 to 150 meq of potassium. The ECG, muscle strength, and serum potassium should be monitored every 15 min. This test should be avoided if there is renal or cardiac impairment, and the patient should have an intravenous route for the administration of glucose and insulin if reversal of the hyperkalemia or paralysis is necessary. Muscle biopsy is usually normal, and electromyography shows electrical silence in the paralyzed muscles.

The pathogenesis of familial hyperkalemic periodic paralysis is uncertain but is probably due to some abnormality of sarcolemmal ion channels or ion pumps. An increased sodium permeability has been suggested as an explanation of the observed partial depolarization of the sarcolemmal membrane during the interictal period and the greater depolarization during the attack. If correct, the release of potassium from muscle into the serum is a compensatory flux tending to repolarize the sarcolemma.

The acute attack should be treated by oral glucose; a kaluretic diuretic such as the thiazides prevents attacks in some patients. However, the latter agents may exacerbate the myotonia in patients where this is prominent. Acetazolamide, up to 2 g per day in divided doses, is often effective in preventing attacks.

PARAMYOTONIA CONGENITA OF VON EULENBERG The principal feature of this disease is stiffness (myotonia) and weakness or paralysis following exposure to cold. It is inherited as a mendelian dominant trait. The myotonic features of this disease are usually the most prominent, though in some cases there are rare attacks of weakness similar to those of periodic paralysis which may or may not be related to cold. The serum potassium concentration may rise in attacks, and the administration of potassium may induce an attack. The resting membrane potential of muscle fibers during the attack is reduced. The myotonia in this syndrome may be limited to the eyelids or tongue. Muscle biopsy reveals no abnormality; vacuolization is seldom seen.

NORMOKALEMIC PERIODIC PARALYSIS A few reports of patients having attacks of periodic paralysis without changes in the serum potassium concentration have appeared. Some of these attacks respond to the intravenous infusion of sodium chloride; attacks may be precipitated by oral potassium administration, and not by intravenous glucose and insulin. Thus, there are features linking this condition to familial hyperkalemic periodic paralysis, but its nosological position remains to be clarified.

REFERENCE

LAYZER RB: Periodic paralysis. Ann Neurol 11:547, 1982

374 OTHER MAJOR MUSCLE SYNDROMES

WALTER G. BRADLEY
RAYMOND D. ADAMS

THE SPASM AND STIFFNESS SYNDROMES Quite apart from spasticity and rigidity, which are forms of excessive motility due to a disinhibition of spinal motor mechanisms (see Chaps. 14 and 15), there are forms of muscular spasm that can be traced to abnormalities of motor neurons themselves or of their terminal axons, or to the sarcolemma of muscle fibers and their intrinsic conducting apparatus. Examples of each type of abnormality have been discovered. Thus, muscles may go into spasm because of unstable depolarization of terminal axons in myokymia, hypokalemic tetany, pseudohypoparathyroidism, and motor system disease. The contraction of muscle may be normal but persists despite attempts at relaxation in myotonia (usually it subsides after repeated contractions except in the state known as myotonia paradoxica where it increases); after one or a series of contractions the muscle may be slow in relaxing, in hypothyroidism, or may lack the energy to relax in the contracture of McArdle's phosphorylase deficiency and phosphofructokinase deficiency. Soreness and tenderness without spasm follow overworking of unconditioned muscle and rhabdomyolysis in Meyer-Betz myoglobinuria, McArdle's phosphorylase deficiency, and carnitine palmityltransferase deficiency.

Each of these conditions evokes complaint, termed by the patient as cramp or spasm, which is variably painful and interferes with free and effective voluntary activity. Each condition has its own identifying clinical characteristics, registered also in the electromyogram, and a gratifying response to therapy may be obtained. Premium attaches, therefore, to the clinical differentiation of cramp, spasm, tetany, tetanus, and contracture, of which the following descriptions are presented.

Fasciculations As described in Chap. 369, fasciculations are spontaneous contractions of groups of muscle fibers which on electromyography are seen to be the result of the discharge of one motor unit. Isolated fasciculations are usually not associated with an underlying disease, but diffuse fasciculations are seen in denervating conditions of muscle, particularly amyotrophic lateral sclerosis, wherein they are combined with weakness, atrophy of muscle, and reflex changes. Fasciculations may also be profuse in overdose or intoxication with anticholinesterases.

Muscle cramps These are isolated painful involuntary contractions of all or part of one or more muscles, and most commonly they affect the calf or foot. The muscle is usually felt to be "in a knot." Because they cause a limp, the term "charley horse" is often applied. Most normal people have experienced a cramp at some time, though some individuals appear particularly prone to develop them. They often occur at night and are seen more frequently in older persons. Vigorous exercise predisposes to the development of cramps. Frequent but otherwise indistinguishable cramps occur in diseases of the anterior horn cells and motor nerves such as amyotrophic lateral sclerosis and the spinal muscular atrophies; in disorders of muscles, particularly the later-onset muscular dystrophies; and in certain other conditions such as pregnancy, dehydration, and sodium loss.

The mechanism of production of cramps is unclear but appears to involve overactivity of the membranes of nerve and muscle. Electromyography shows numerous high-frequency muscle action potentials, and in the pre- and postcramp phases there continues to be excessive discharge of muscle action potentials. The pain of the cramp appears in excess of what would be expected from the degree of muscle contraction and probably is the result of focal ischemia or accumulation of metabolites in the contracting group of muscle fibers.

Massage of the knotted muscle fibers and vigorous stretching will "break the cramp," though there remains hyperexcitability with a tendency to recurrence for several minutes afterward. If the cramp is severe, a soreness of the muscle may persist for a day or two. Quinine sulfate, 300 mg at night or up to 300 mg tid, with procainamide (250 mg tid) or diphenhydramine hydrochloride (Benadryl) 50 mg at bedtime, may help to prevent frequent cramps.

Tetanus and the stiff-man syndrome In *tetanus*, the skeletal muscles are persistently contracted, owing to the inhibitory effect of the tetanus toxin on the activity of Renshaw spinal interneurons, whose function is to inhibit the alpha motoneurons. This disinhibition of the spinal reflex arc causes localized and generalized muscle spasms, often precipitated by voluntary contraction, startle, visual or auditory stimulation. Sleep tends to suppress the spasms, as does spinal anesthesia and curare. Eventually, there is sustained contraction of the muscle from continuous reflex discharge. The electromyogram shows a sustained pattern of motor unit action potentials. The spasms of rabies are probably similar, but arise from higher central nervous system centers. There is experimental evidence that tetanus toxin has a neuromuscular blocking effect like botulinum toxin, though there is no evidence that the effect is significant in human cases (see Chap. 170).

The *stiff-man syndrome* bears many resemblances to tetanus, and though there is no known infective cause, the autopsy examination of one such case showed chronic encephalomyelitis. In others no pathologic change was observed. The usual picture is that of an adult man or woman who begins to complain of intermittent, then more or less continuous, spasms of limb and trunk muscles. The spasms are variably painful. The condition may become generalized, causing overall muscle stiffness. Electromyography shows continuous motor unit activity, which must arise from the central nervous system sources since it is abolished by general and spinal anesthesia, as well as by nerve block and curare. In its mild form, the stiff-man syndrome is difficult to distinguish from a psychogenic disorder, but the overall similarity of individual cases and the lack of psychological predisposition in most of them emphasizes the organic nature of the syndrome. The condition probably arises from excessive activation of alpha and gamma motoneurons in the spinal cord, perhaps as a result of a deficiency of GABA, the inhibitory transmitter of spinal neurons. The condition often responds well to diazepam (5 to 15 mg tid) or baclofen (20 mg tid).

Tetany As pointed out in Chap. 369, hypocalcemia and hypomagnesemia of any cause may induce cramp-like involuntary spasms which in their milder form tend to be distal (carpopedal spasm) but may spread to involve virtually all muscles of the body. Stimulation of the nerve leading to a muscle at fast frequencies (15 to 20 per second) characteristically reproduces the spasm, and hyperventilation and ischemia increase the tetanic activity. The Trousseau's sign takes advantage of this latter phenomenon, carpal spasms being induced by occlusion of the blood supply to the arm. That hypocalcemic tetany is due to increased excitability of the distal segments to the motor nerves is shown by the following facts: (1) the nerve is excessively sensitive to percussion [tapping over the facial nerve anterior to the tragus of the ear induces facial twitching (Chvostek's sign)]; (2) electromyography shows fast frequencies of doublets and triplets of motor unit action potentials; (3) ischemia of the nerve induces the cramp; and (4) there are usually associated sensory symptoms including paresthesias from hyperexcitability of the sensory nerve fibers. Hypocalcemia also causes an increased excitability of the muscle fibers themselves, and hence nerve block does not completely eradicate the tetany.

Hyperventilation from psychogenic causes may produce tetany as a result of lowering of the blood P_{CO_2} with consequent alkalosis and reduced concentration of ionized calcium.

Myokymia As indicated in Chap. 369, myokymia is a slow, writhing, continuous movement of small parts of one or more muscles, which in its most florid form produces a "bag of worms" appearance. It is sometimes difficult to separate profuse fasciculations from myokymia, but only the latter may produce stiffness of muscles on passive movements and postural change. The movements continue at rest and in sleep, hence the term *continuous muscle fiber activity*. They are unrelated to exercise. Any part of the body may be affected, and the condition may become generalized; it is then associated with hyperhydrosis and an increased metabolic rate from the muscular contractions. Electromyography shows that the contractions are produced by triplets or multiplets of motor unit action potentials firing at intervals of about 20 ms. Some patients have clinical and electrophysiological evidence of a mild peripheral neuropathy, hence the misnomer "neuromyotonia." A somewhat similar condition occurs in chondrodystrophic myopathy (Schwartz-Jampel syndrome). The motor unit action potentials are abolished by curare, but not by nerve block or spinal anesthesia. This indicates that the disorder originates from spontaneous discharges of the terminal parts of the motor axons, though the exact pathogenesis is uncertain. Carbamazepine (Tegretol), 200 mg tid or qid, or phenytoin (Dilantin), 100 mg tid or qid, will usually produce a considerable suppression of the continuous muscle fiber activity.

Myotonia As defined in Chap. 369, myotonia is the delayed relaxation of a muscle after contraction, where this is associated with a primary continuous sustained firing of the muscle fiber action potentials. It is seen in its archetypal form in myotonia congenita and myotonic dystrophy (Chap. 371) and is a primary disorder of the sarcolemma. However, the term myotonia is often misused to describe delayed muscular relaxation of a variety of causes where the defect does not lie in the sarcolemma, such as the delayed relaxation in hypothyroidism, where delayed spinal reflex time and delayed relaxation of myofibrils may be responsible.

Contracture As defined in Chap. 369, true contracture is a primary condition of the muscle contractile machinery where contracted myofibrils are unable to relax or relaxation is delayed. This is to be distinguished from pseudocontracture (e.g., "contracture of the tendo Achillis") where tonus of the shortened muscle is unbalanced by paralysis of its antagonist or where damage to a muscle has resulted in fibrosis with shortening. Such damage may be the result of trauma or ischemia (Volkmann's contracture) or of a necrotizing myopathy like Duchenne's muscular dystrophy.

True contracture occurs also in rigor mortis and in nonlethal conditions where the skeletal muscle is deprived of ATP, since the latter is required to allow breakage and sliding apart of the actin-myosin cross bridges of the myofibrils. Deficiency of at least two enzymes of the glycolytic pathway, myophosphorylase deficiency (McArdle's disease) and phosphofructokinase deficiency (Tarui's disease), causes contracture during ischemic or strenuous exercise because the production of ATP is impaired by anaerobic glycolysis. These true contractures are variably painful, and characteristically the electromyogram of the shortened muscle is silent since the sarcoplasm is not being activated. The cause of pain is, however, not clear but may relate to swelling of the contracted muscle. A similar contraction may occur in a rare syndrome where calcium reuptake from the sarcoplasm into the longitudinal endoplasmic reticulum of the muscle fibers is deficient.

Myalgic syndromes Diffuse muscle pain is a frequent expression of a large variety of systemic infections, e.g., influenza, coxsackievirus and other viral illnesses, brucellosis, dengue, Colorado tick fever, glanders, measles, malaria, relapsing fever, rheumatic fever (cf., growing pains), salmonellosis, toxoplasmosis, trichinosis, tularemia, and leptospirosis. When this pain is remarkably intense and especially if it is localized to one group of muscles, the most likely diagnosis is epidemic myalgia (also termed pleurodynia, devil's grip, painful neck, Bornholm disease) due to a coxsackievirus of group B type. Poliomyelitis might also be accompanied by intense pain at the onset of the neurologic involvement. In the Guillain-Barré syndrome, pains in the back and limbs may precede the onset of paralysis in about one-third of the cases. Herpes zoster is another well-known cause of segmental pain. Inflammation in the spinal nerves and dorsal root ganglia, which may precede the vesicular skin eruption by as long as 72 to 96 h, is the cause of the segmental pain in herpes zoster. Inflammation in spinal ganglia may be responsible for the pain in poliomyelitis and the Guillain-Barré syndrome.

Fibrositis and fibromyositis (see Chap. 353) would appear by definition to represent an inflammation of the fibrous tissues of the muscles, fascia, aponeuroses, and probably nerves. However there is little pathological data to clarify what is a rather poorly characterized syndrome. In patients with these conditions, a muscle or a group of muscles becomes painful and tender, frequently related to minor trauma or change in the weather, particularly with cold or dampness. The neck and shoulders are the common sites. Firm, tender zones several centimeters in diameter are found within the muscles, and active pressure or contraction increases the pain. Usually the condition clears up in a few days, but often recurs. Local heat and massage, and aspirin or nonsteroidal anti-inflammatory drugs, such as indomethacin or ibuprofen, help relieve the pain.

Diffuse muscular soreness and aching may at times be the initial symptom in rheumatoid arthritis, preceding the signs of joint involvement by a period of weeks or months. These symptoms may occasionally be seen in polymyositis-dermatomyositis and more frequently in patients with a low-grade nonspecific collagen-vascular disorder ("rheumatism"). Patients are aware that symptoms are worse in cold or damp weather and that aching and stiffness are especially worse in the morning, after rest, and hours or even a day after moderate exertion. An increased sedimentation rate, a positive rheumatoid factor test, or other laboratory abnormalities are occasionally found. The muscle biopsy appearance is almost invariably normal, except for type 2 fiber atrophy. This condition usually responds to nonsteroidal inflammatory drugs. The risks of corticosteroid therapy are not justified in this benign condition, though such drugs usually relieve the symptoms.

In *polymyalgia rheumatica*, a condition of the elderly, diffuse myalgia and malaise are associated with a high sedimentation rate. The condition may overlap with cranial arteritis, and temporal artery biopsy may reveal giant-cell arteritis in both conditions. High-dose corticosteroid therapy (prednisone, 60 to 100 mg daily or alternate daily) is frequently required in these conditions.

Exertional myalgia is a syndrome, the causes of which are gradually being elucidated. A limited number of enzyme deficiencies in the pathways of energy metabolism of skeletal muscle have been identified in a minority of patients with this syndrome. Myophosphorylase deficiency (McArdle's disease) and phosphofructokinase deficiency, which are described in Chaps. 100 and 371, cause painful muscle contracture during sustained severe exertion or ischemic exercise. The pointer to these deficiencies is demonstration of a lack of the normal rise of venous blood lactate during and following ischemic exercise (the ischemic lactate test). The exact diagnosis rests upon the histochemical and biochemical demonstration of the enzyme deficiency in a muscle biopsy specimen. Carnitine palmityltransferase deficiency (Chap. 371) causes muscle pains after sustained exercise, particularly in the fasting state. The diagnosis here rests upon the biochemical demonstration of the enzyme deficiency in a muscle biopsy specimen. Myoadenylate deaminase deficiency may be associated with a syndrome similar to that of carnitine palmityltransferase deficiency. Myoadenylate deaminase catalyzes the deamination of adenosine monophosphate to inosine monophosphate; this prevents the accumulation of adenosine monophosphate derived from high-energy phosphate-saving enzymic reaction in skeletal muscle (2 ADP $\rightarrow$ ATP + AMP). Myoadenylate deaminase apparently is important in skeletal muscle since accumulation of adenosine monophosphate causes inhibition of the vital step of phosphorylation of ADP to ATP. Thus deficiency of the enzyme causes deficiency of ATP production, and thus exertional myalgia. Diminished exercise tolerance and exertional myalgia may be seen in patients with deficiency of the mitochondrial cytochromes (especially cytochrome b).

All of these deficiencies of enzymes of the energy metabolic pathways may cause myoglobinuria (Chap. 370).

LOCALIZED MUSCLE MASSES A mass in one or more muscles may have a variety of different causes and significances.

Muscle or tendon rupture giving rise to a large bulge upon contraction is usually caused by a violent strain attended by an audible snap and then a bulge when the muscle is contracted. A weakening in contractile power and mild discomfort are usually noted by the patient. The biceps brachii is the muscle most often affected. Treatment is by immediate surgical repair, and if this is delayed, little can be done for the condition. *A muscle hernia* results from a deficiency in the deep fascia overlying the muscle (either spontaneous or secondary to surgery or trauma) which allows the muscle to bulge through on contraction.

Hemorrhage into the muscle may occur as a consequence of trauma, as a complication of the use of anticoagulants, and in hematologic diseases such as hemophilia and leukemia.

Tumors include desmoid tumor (a benign massive growth of fibrous tissue in parturient women and after surgery), fibrosarcoma (a highly malignant tumor), rhabdomyoma, rhabdomyosarcoma (a highly malignant tumor of skeletal muscle fibers with a strong liability to local recurrence and metastasis), and a metastatic tumor.

Thrombosis of arteries, or more often *veins*, may cause congestion and infarction of muscles.

Focal inflammation of muscle where a bacterial infection (pyomyositis), or a noninfective condition such as a focal nodular myositis which is actually a form of localized polymyositis, may cause acutely developing painful swellings in muscles. Rarely, parasitic infections (e.g., trichinosis) cause muscle swelling and tenderness.

Myositis ossificans refers to the deposition of bone within the substance of a muscle. Two types are recognized. Localized *myositis ossificans circumscripta* occurs in a single muscle or group of muscles after one or more episodes of trauma. The muscle is gradually replaced by masses of cartilage, and within 4 to 7 weeks, a solid mass of bone develops. This is most frequently seen in the pectoralis, biceps, brachii, and thigh muscles of young adults. Symptoms tend to subside with rest.

Generalized myositis ossificans is a progressive widespread ossifying process in many muscles of unknown cause. It is unrelated to trauma and tends to occur in young persons. A familial incidence is noted in some cases. The first stage appears to be an interstitial myositis or fibrositis with proliferation of connective tissue. The latter undergoes cartilaginous and osteoid transformation, the mass displacing and replacing muscle fibers. Nearly 75 percent of all reported cases have a variety of congenital abnormalities, the most frequent of which is a failure of development of the great toes or thumbs, and less often other digits. The first symptom is often a firm swelling in a paravertebral or cervical muscle with mild tenderness or discomfort. The overlying skin may be reddened and slightly edematous. Within 6 to 12 months, bony masses are palpable within the muscle and are visible upon x-ray. As the disease advances limitation of movement, contractures, and deformity become increasingly evident, and occasionally the patient is converted into a virtual "stone man." Scoliosis, rigidity of the spine, abnormal postures, and a limited expansion of the thorax may ultimately occur. The disease may undergo spontaneous remissions and exacerbations, and may halt at a point where the patient is still capable of adequate functioning. However, major disability and death from pneumonia may occur. No medical treatment is of proven value. Agents which remove calcium from the body (such as oral phytate and ethylenediaminetetraacetic acid) and prednisone have been tried without significant benefit.

This condition should be distinguished from calcinosis universalis, which usually occurs in relation to scleroderma or dermatomyositis. In calcinosis universalis there is deposition of calcium salts in the skin, subcutaneous tissue, and occasionally epimysium, while in myositis ossificans there is actual bone formation within the muscles themselves. Vitamin D calcinosis, resulting from prolonged ingestion of large doses of vitamin D, may also produce widespread deposition of masses of calcium salts around muscles, joints, and subcutaneous tissues.

REFERENCES

Adams RD: *Diseases of Muscle*, 3d ed. New York, Harper & Row, 1975

Layzer RB, Rowland LP: Cramps. *N Engl J Med* 285:31, 1971

Walton JN: *Disorders of Voluntary Muscle*, 4th ed. London, Churchill Livingstone, 1981

section 13 | Major psychiatric disorders

375 NEUROSES

THOMAS P. HACKETT
ELEANOR M. HACKETT

Freud was the first to speak of "psychoneuroses." He described four specific subtypes which have been termed *anxiety neurosis, phobia, obsessive-compulsive neurosis,* and *hysteria.* Freud believed that psychoneuroses were caused by unconscious conflicts. In psychoanalytic terms these conflicts produce anxiety, which is in turn defended against by pathological mechanisms which compose the symptoms of the neuroses (e.g., phobia, compulsion, hysterical paralysis). The term *psychoneurotic* has been shortened over the years to *neurotic* and has been used more generally to describe a group of abnormal but nonpsychotic behaviors. Some theorists feel that the neuroses lie on a quantitative continuum between normalcy and psychosis. Others believe that the differences between normal, neurotic, and psychotic behavior are qualitatively distinct.

Neurotic patients find their abnormal and uncomfortable behavior and symptoms unacceptable. They realize that there is something wrong; their ability to test reality is intact, and they have insight into their condition. Psychotics, on the other hand, generally lack these insights. The term *neurosis,* however, remains unspecific; for this reason some feel it should be deleted from the psychiatric nomenclature. In fact, the *Diagnostic and Statistical Manual of Mental Disorders* of the American Psychiatric Association (DSM III) no longer lists neuroses. Instead, the text refers to anxiety disorders (phobic disorders, anxiety states, panic disorder, and obsessive-compulsive disorder) and somatoform disorders (hysteria and conversion hysteria). Because many dispute this new nosology and because the term *neurosis* has become part of our medical vocabulary, it will be retained in this section.

It should be kept in mind that many of the symptoms described in this chapter occur in mild form in nonneurotic individuals. There are many people who tend to respond with anxiety to any new situation, others who go to great lengths to avoid fearful objects and situations, and still others who are excessively careful and painstaking in their meticulous approach to their work. Such behavior can be quite compatible with normal life. Only when these individual symptoms or symptom clusters interfere seriously with life and livelihood should they be diagnosed as neurotic.

ANXIETY NEUROSIS Definition Anxiety neurosis, known also as panic disorder, is a condition characterized by sudden attacks of extreme apprehension, accompanied by either a sense of impending doom or the fear of becoming insane and/ or losing control. The diagnosis of anxiety neurosis may be made only in the absence of other diagnosed mental disorders, recent physical exertion, or life-threatening situations.

Epidemiology Anxiety neurosis is common. It affects 2 to 5 percent of the general population. Two-thirds of those affected are women. It is said that approximately 10 to 14 percent of patients seen by cardiologists have anxiety neurosis. Lost time at work and the cost of treatment combine to make this an expensive problem.

Clinical picture The principal symptom of anxiety neurosis is sudden panic. The anxiety neurotic is sure that the symptoms are those of serious illness. The anxiety is an intense fear described as unlike anything previously experienced. There is a sense of depersonalization, as though the surrounding world has changed. The symptoms are dyspnea, palpitations, chest pain, choking or smothering sensations, feelings of unreality, sweating, faintness, and trembling. Because the symptoms so frequently focus on the cardiovascular system, this disorder has been called neurocirculatory asthenia or irritable heart. Other organ systems, such as the gastrointestinal tract, can also be the targets (e.g., irritable colon).

Course of illness and prognosis The first anxiety attack is apt to begin suddenly between adolescence and the early thirties. Attacks may be as infrequent as once or twice a year or as often as once a day. Even when infrequent, these spells are memorable. They are described with the same type of anguish as is severe pain. Between spells the individual may complain of chronic anxiety, frequently connected with the anticipation of forthcoming spells. Generally the patient will view the condition as physical in nature and will therefore consult a physician. In one series 100 percent of the patients studied had consulted at least one doctor, while 70 percent had consulted more than 10.

Although such anxiety can be crippling, most sufferers manage to adapt to it with minimal life change. Only about 15 percent of the patients in one series described their symptoms as moderate or severely disabling. With the assistance of pharmacotherapy and psychotherapy, substantial improvement can be made. Drug abuse and alcoholism are the main complications and usually are the result of the use of these substances to control panic.

Etiology The causes of anxiety neurosis are elusive. Stressful life experiences seem to play their part, as do genetic factors. Panic attack patients are known to have a lower exercise tolerance than normal individuals, and they develop high blood levels of lactic acid following exercise. An intravenous infusion of sodium lactate can bring on all of the symptoms of anxiety neurosis in those predisposed to this disorder; abnormal lactate levels may therefore be linked to its cause.

Clinical management There are a variety of physical illnesses that present with the symptoms of anxiety neurosis and which should be ruled out before the diagnosis of anxiety neurosis is established. Cardiac arrhythmias; myocardial infarction; mitral valve prolapse; sedative or hypnotic withdrawal syndromes; metabolic abnormalities, especially of the thyroid gland; encephalopathies; pulmonary edema; carcinoid tumor; and pheochromocytoma are but a few of a large list with which the physician should be familiar.

Once the diagnosis of anxiety neurosis has been made, it is important to explain the link between anxiety and symptom to the patient. It is bad practice to belittle symptoms by saying that there is nothing physically wrong. By dismissing the symptom, the doctor dismisses the patient.

The treatment of anxiety consists primarily of reassurance and the use of anxiolytic drugs such as the benzodiazepines. Diazepam, 5 mg orally tid, or oxazepam, 15 to 30 mg orally tid, are the most commonly used antianxiety agents. Beta-adrenergic blockers, such as propranolol, either alone or in conjunction with anxiolytics, have also offered symptomatic relief. The dosage is not standard but varies from 10 to 20 mg of propranolol tid. These agents do not, however, offer much help in the control of panic attacks.

The treatment of panic attacks has been greatly enhanced by the use of monoamine oxidase (MAO) inhibitors or tricyclic antidepressants (TCAs). There is considerable evidence that phenelzine in a dosage of 45 mg per day or imipramine, 150 mg a day, can reduce or abolish panic attacks. The latency of response from initiation of therapy to disappearance of symptoms is 3 to 14 days. Discontinuation of these drugs often results in the reappearance of panic. Maintenance by these agents for the control of panic attacks may be required for an indefinite period.

PHOBIA **Definition** Phobias, also referred to as phobic disorders, are irrational fears specifically linked with objects (e.g., snakes), activities (e.g., public speaking), or situations (e.g., going over bridges). Moments of phobic confrontation are fraught with immense anxiety and often with uncontrolled panic as described in the previous section. The phobic patient rearranges life as much as possible to avoid the problem. Although phobics realize that their fears are unreasonable and are additionally disturbed by their irrational reactions, they are powerless to correct their phobias by force of reason or desire. While many individuals are made uncomfortable by similar objects and situations, even to the point of avoidance, the diagnosis of phobia or phobic disorder is only made when the fear and avoidance interfere with the individual's life. Agoraphobia, the most common type of phobia, is the dread of open or public places. The individual panics at the thought of visiting public places and consequently remains at home, usually in the company of a helpful, caring person.

Epidemiology Phobias are thought to occur in 0.5 percent to 1 percent of the general population. However, many of them are so circumscribed that they never come to the attention of a physician. Phobias represent less than 5 percent of the neurotic disorders in patients over 18 who seek help.

Clinical picture The phobic individual typically becomes panicky in the presence of the precipitating object or situation. The panic reaction differs from that described under anxiety neurosis in that it is not free-floating, but specifically linked to the situation at hand. The occasion may be public speaking, being caught in a traffic jam, or being threatened by a barking dog. Massive fear, depersonalization, tremulousness, and sweating descend upon the victim along with the compelling urge to escape. The result is an avoidance of any circumstance that might allow a recurrence. At its most extreme, the individual shuns all contact with the environment outside the home. Others lead a reasonably normal life as long as the phobic association can be avoided.

Course of illness and prognosis In general, phobic disorders first afflict individuals in late childhood or early adulthood. While periods of remission are possible, the more likely course is an unremitting persistence of the phobia unless there is therapeutic intervention. Even with optimum management, the problem may persist. Complications are the same as those in panic disorder.

Etiology There is some reason to believe that sudden separation from parents or important people in childhood may predispose to this disorder. Animal phobias and social phobias seem to run in families; whether this is environmental or inherited is undetermined.

It is unclear whether the initial panic reaction stimulates the phobia along the lines of classical conditioning theory (i.e., the panic happens to occur while the patient is in an open square and therefore the square subsequently triggers another attack) or whether the phobia stimulates the panic.

The fact that MAO inhibitors and TCAs often improve phobic disorders indicates that they may have a specific rather than a general biochemical substrate.

Clinical management Phobias do not usually yield to traditional psychotherapy, whether it be insight-oriented or supportive. Behavior therapy has had some success, but it is most useful when combined with drug treatment. While the use of antianxiety agents or beta blockers alone is of limited value, the most promising advance in treating phobias has been in the use of MAO inhibitors and TCAs. (See section on clinical management of anxiety and panic reactions on page 2202.)

OBSESSIVE-COMPULSIVE NEUROSIS Definition Obsessive-compulsive neurosis is an illness characterized by obsessions and compulsions which occur in the absence of other psychiatric disorders. Obsessions are recurrent ideas (e.g., the idea of becoming infected by shaking hands) that insistently and undesirably intrude upon consciousness. Compulsions are repetitive, stereotyped acts or rituals (e.g., washing one's hands incessantly to prevent infection) which follow on the heels of obsessions. They are performed to prevent some future undesirable happening. Failure to perform the compulsion elicits anxiety; completion of the ritual activity provides temporary relief of tension. Obsessive thoughts and compulsions are part of our normal array of everyday experiences. Obsessive-compulsive behavior becomes a psychiatric disorder when it interferes with everyday living.

Epidemiology Obsessive-compulsive neurosis is an uncommon psychiatric condition. The incidence is from 0.5 percent to 2.5 percent of psychiatric patients. It occurs equally in both sexes. Most obsessive-compulsive individuals seem to be first-born or only children. Numerous studies document the above-average intelligence and the higher social class of these patients when compared with other psychiatric patients.

Clinical picture About one-fourth of the obsessive-compulsive patients who come to a physician complain of anxiety or depression accompanying the presenting symptoms. These patients may seek help because they are afraid of hurting somebody or of injuring themselves. They fear the loss of control. Obsessive thoughts of homicide (e.g., poisoning offspring) may result in the development of avoidance patterns and multiple rituals (e.g., counting all roach poison containers). Ideas of contamination (e.g., becoming infected by patting a dog) or doubt about whether one has left a light burning in a room may result in the more common compulsions such as hand-washing or checking. Obsessional symptoms almost invariably produce a depressed, unpleasant state of mind. Even when the compulsion is performed, the dysphoric mood seldom clears; the respite is momentary and the obsession returns.

Course of illness and prognosis The onset usually occurs in adolescence or early adulthood. Only 15 percent begin after the age of 35. Generally a period of seven or more years passes between the onset of the condition and the search for professional help. The problem may present in an acute fashion or more slowly over time. Total remissions are rare, although partial remissions do occur.

The course can be complicated by abuse of alcohol and drugs when these are used to control symptoms. These patients do not usually require hospitalization. When hospitalization is lengthy, the prognosis is markedly worse. In some individuals obsessive-compulsive neurosis may dominate the entire life pattern and so impair the sufferer that invalidism will result. In one follow-up study it was found that 20 percent of the 88 patients treated were symptom-free and socially adapted after 4 years. Another 50 percent were improved in their symptoms and socially adapted. The remaining 30 percent were still plagued by their problem and poorly adapted socially. There are a few factors that correlate with a good prognosis: mild symptoms, prompt search for help, good premorbid personality, and no abnormal patterns of character.

Suicide is not common among obsessive-compulsives, even when depressed. The fear that obsessive people have about injuring others or acting impulsively is almost never realized. Correlation between obsessive-compulsive disorder and homicide or impulse disorders is nonexistent.

Etiology While many obsessive individuals have close relatives with some form of psychiatric illness, the role of genetics is unclear. Between 50 and 60 percent of obsessive-compulsive patients date the onset of their disorder to a stressful life event, such as a pregnancy or the death of a friend.

Clinical management Although psychotherapy has been found to be of limited value in this condition, it can provide reassurance that the impulses are seldom acted upon, that embarrassing acts are not apt to be performed, and that the individual is not apt to become insane.

Some dramatic responses have been reported with the use of the TCAs, but these are not uniform. Clomipramine, a drug not available in the United States, is said to be antiobsessional. MAO inhibitors and anxiolytics, beta-adrenergic blockers, tryptophan, and lithium carbonate have all been tried, but with no outstanding success.

Electroconvulsive therapy (ECT) is of value for those patients with marked depressive affect and no satisfactory response to pharmacotherapy. Psychosurgery, particularly cingulotomy, has been said to be successful, but has not been widely enough applied to be recommended without reservation.

HYSTERIA Definition Hysteria, known also as somatization disorder, has a written history as old as that of schizophrenia. From the ancient Egyptians through Sigmund Freud, many theories have been devised to explain its manifestations. Despite the causes assigned to it, hysteria has preserved a basic identity over the centuries. It has always been associated with physical symptoms ranging from multiple mundane complaints such as headache and constipation to bizarre paralyses and paresthesias. These occur without known pathophysiological cause. The presentation of the illness is often dramatic.

Despite the consistency of the basic clinical picture, there are enough exceptions and variations to provide a complicated and confusing nosology. The problem manifests itself in two basic forms. Some consider these two different illnesses; others believe they are part of the same disease. (1) Hysteria (also known as Briquet's syndrome or somatization disorder) is a polysymptomatic, recurrent condition usually of several years' duration presenting before the age of 30 as a complicated medical illness without apparent organic cause. (2) Conversion hysteria (conversion disorder) is characterized by the presence of one symptom, called a conversion symptom, usually involving a single body system, typically the nervous system. Common conversions are blindness, aphonia, amnesia, and paralysis. The symptom can occur at any age, is usually sudden in onset, and is related in time to an external stress or to an inner psychological problem. The term *conversion* is used to designate the presence of an underlying psychic conflict which has been converted into a motor or sensory symptom (e.g., trigger-finger paralysis). Conversion symptoms are found in many psychiatric conditions, such as schizophrenia and affective disorders. Conversion hysteria is only diagnosed when the single symptom itself is the major problem. The following discussion will deal with hysteria in general terms and will include both forms.

Epidemiology It is estimated that between 1 to 2 percent of the female population suffers from hysteria. It is rarely found in men. Hysteria and conversion symptoms are generally found in backward societies and among the poorly educated. A history of conversion symptoms is most commonly associated with hysteria in women and with sociopathy in men. Conversion disorder in the absence of other forms of psychiatric disturbance is rarely seen today.

Clinical picture The hysterical patient presents a complicated history generally involving multiple organ systems and a variety of complaints. The account is usually colorful and exaggeration plays a role. The review of systems typically produces an abundance of symptoms: dizziness, dyspnea, anxiety, fatigue, headache, weakness, weight loss, constipation, back pain, abdominal pain, joint pain, and indigestion. A hallmark of this disorder is the presence of sexual and menstrual problems. A history of mental difficulty, especially depression, is frequent. Suicide attempts are made, most of which do not succeed. Contact with multiple physicians is the rule. Some of the doctors are deified, others condemned. Multiple surgery is often part of the past history. Frequent hospitalizations, x-ray procedures, and tests are also part of the picture.

Etiology The St. Louis group has turned up two important findings: (1) hysteria runs in families, and (2) a significant relationship exists between hysteria and sociopathy. Men who are first-degree relatives of hysterics are apt to show sociopathy and alcoholism. Women related in the first degree to male felons are apt to be hysterics.

Course of illness and prognosis The disease usually begins in childhood, adolescence, or early adulthood. Typically the illness waxes and wanes, but rarely is the patient free of symptoms. Most of these patients do not improve. They are as crippled by hysteria as they would be by an organic process. In fact, it is not uncommon for a patient to develop a systemic disease in an organ system hit by conversion symptoms in the past. Some believe that the early symptoms of a neurologic disorder may predispose the patient to the development of conversion symptoms. Single conversion symptoms, although they are very often a part of hysteria, can occur in isolation. When this happens, the disease may have a shorter course. The main complications of hysteria are depression, drug dependence, multiple surgery, suicide, divorce, and missed diagnoses. The patient labeled as a hysteric may be quickly written off by a doctor who may subsequently miss an organic disease.

Clinical management Hysterics are by no means the easiest patients to treat. They frequently anger the physician by failing to improve or by developing alternate symptoms as soon as one group has cleared. Also they switch doctors and are attention seekers. Although many hysterical patients are referred for psychotherapy, most of them drop out. It is of value to have a psychiatric consultant verify the diagnosis and help in management, especially when depression is part of the picture. A good doctor-patient relationship is essential for long-term management. The principal goal should be to prevent doctor shopping, unnecessary surgery, divorce, and suicide.

REFERENCES

AMERICAN PSYCHIATRIC ASSOCIATION: *Diagnostic and Statistical Manual of Mental Disorders,* 3d ed, 1980

HACKETT TP, CASSEM, NH (eds): *Massachusetts General Hospital Handbook of General Hospital Psychiatry.* St. Louis, Mosby, 1978, chaps 7, 8, 26

NEMIAH JC: Anxiety state, phobic disorder, obsessive-compulsive disorder, somatoform disorders, and dissociative disorders, in *Comprehensive Textbook of Psychiatry/III,* 3d ed, HI Kaplan et al (eds). Baltimore, Williams & Wilkins, 1980, vol 2, pp 1483–1516, 1525–1561

SHEEHAN DV et al: The treatment of endogenous anxiety with phobic, hysterical and hypochondriacal symptoms. Arch Gen Psych 37:51, 1980

WOODRUFF RA et al: *Psychiatric Diagnosis.* New York, Oxford, 1974, pp 45–100

376
AFFECTIVE DISORDERS

THOMAS P. HACKETT
ELEANOR M. HACKETT

Affective disorders are a group of clinical conditions having as their common denominator a disturbance of mood. Used in this context, *mood* is a prolonged emotional tone dominating an individual's outlook. Depression and elation, either alone or in alternation, are the moods most common to affective disorders. Depression alone is by far the more common. Cognitive, physical, psychological, and interpersonal disturbances accompany the prevailing mood. Thus, slowed thinking, lassitude, impotence, and the distancing of friends often attend depression, just as racing thoughts, hyperactivity, hypersexuality, and false bonhomie accompany mania.

There has been much dispute since the beginning of this century about the terminology for and the classification of depressive illness. The terms *affective disorder* and *mood disorder* are currently preferred because they include states of elation as well as depression. In order to separate states of depression which alternate with mania from the more common types of depression which are uncomplicated by mania, the terms *unipolar* and *bipolar* have been introduced. The person with a unipolar disorder suffers from depression alone, while the individual with bipolar disorder suffers from either mania alone or mania alternating in cyclic fashion with depression.

A useful method of classifying affective disorders is to separate them into those that are primary and those that are secondary to other illnesses. Primary affective disorders originate out of context with other illness (either psychiatric or nonpsychiatric). Manic depressive illness is an example of a primary affective disorder. Secondary affective disorders occur in response to psychiatric or medical illness such as alcoholism, schizophrenia, heart disease, or cancer. (See Fig. 376-1.)

Whether the disorder is primary or secondary, its recognition by the clinician is important for at least three reasons: (1) While depressive illness is the most common of the psychiatric disorders, it is estimated that nonpsychiatric physicians overlook or misdiagnose half of the depressions they encounter in practice. (2) Most affective disorders can be successfully treated or at least controlled. (3) The risk of suicide among patients with mood disorders is considerable; suicide remains the tenth most common cause of death in this country.

EPIDEMIOLOGY

Primary and secondary affective disorders are said to be among the most common conditions found in the practice of medicine. The chance of developing a depression during the course of a lifetime ranges from 8 to 20 percent. However, only 20 to 25 percent of depressed people receive treatment for their depression. Twice as many females as males suffer from mood disorders. While it was once thought that primary affective disorders were more common in the middle and upper classes, this has not been consistently demonstrated.

CLINICAL PICTURE

DEPRESSION Because sadness is a normal part of the human condition, any discussion of mood disorders involves the confusing search for the demarcation between normal and pathological mood. When does sorrow become depression? While this point can rarely be located exactly, there are diagnostic guidelines. In depression the sense of sadness is all-pervasive. The individual is plagued with the constant presence of hopelessness. Feelings of worthlessness, inadequacy, and incompetence hound him or her. Activities and interests once pleasurable and stimulating become stale. Depressed persons isolate themselves by withdrawing from friends and family. Not infrequently, work habits deteriorate. Blue collar workers become easily fatigued. Office workers and professionals experience indecisiveness, slowed thinking, difficulty concentrating, and poor memory. The cognitive component of depression can be so severe that it presents as pseudodementia.

There are eight criteria which form the diagnostic core of depression as defined by the American Psychiatric Association in their *Diagnostic and Statistical Manual of Mental Disorders* (DSM III). These are (1) poor appetite with weight loss or increased appetite with weight gain; (2) insomnia or hypersomnia; (3) psychomotor agitation or retardation; (4) loss of interest or pleasure in usual activities or decrease in sexual drive; (5) loss of energy, and feelings of fatigue; (6) feelings of worthlessness, self-reproach, or inappropriate guilt; (7) diminished ability to think or concentrate; and (8) recurrent thoughts of death or suicide. The patient with five of these eight symptoms is definitely depressed; the patient with four is probably depressed. According to DSM III the depressed state must be present for 1 month to be called depression.

MASKED DEPRESSION Masked depression is a common variant of either primary or secondary depression. A patient with a masked depression will complain of a physical symptom, typically chronic pain, which fails to respond to analgesics. Physical and laboratory findings are usually negative or inconclusive, and the patient's description of the distress is apt to be vague. Depression will be denied, should the patient be questioned, but not infrequently the physician can learn of a loss or disappointment that might explain the onset of the symptom. Even if no precipitating event can be unearthed, the physician should consider the presence of an underlying depression when a symptom such as pain, easy fatigue, irritability, or malaise persists without explanation. The first step in the management of such a patient is to determine the presence of any of the eight DSM III criteria used for depression. Once the diagnosis of masked or underlying depression is made or strongly suspected, a program of therapy can be started.

There are a variety of medical illnesses which present with symptoms suggesting depression. Various anemias; vitamin B_{12} deficiency; infectious diseases; thyroid, parathyroid, and adrenal conditions; multiple sclerosis; organic brain syndrome; subdural hematoma; cancer of the pancreas; and carcinoid tumor are a few of the conditions noted to begin with a depression. Consequently, a thorough examination of all organic sources of depression should be made before specific antidepressant therapy is started.

As the number of medications used by physicians increases, we become aware that many can produce some of the symptoms of depression. Reserpine was one of the first such agents to be implicated. It and methyldopa produce severe depression with a large representation of DSM III criteria. Propranolol, oral contraceptives, corticosteroids, barbiturates, and diazepam also have the capacity to produce a depression. Often the severity of depressive symptoms is dose-related and can be remedied by decreasing drug consumption.

MANIA The clinical picture in mania is, in most ways, the reverse of that seen in depression. A list of criteria adapted from DSM III and used to diagnose a manic episode follows.

The manic patient experiences one (or more) distinct period(s) with a predominantly elevated, expansive, or irritable mood. The elevated or irritable mood must be a prominent part of the illness and relatively persistent, although it may alternate or intermingle with depressive moods.

The manic episode must require hospitalization or last at

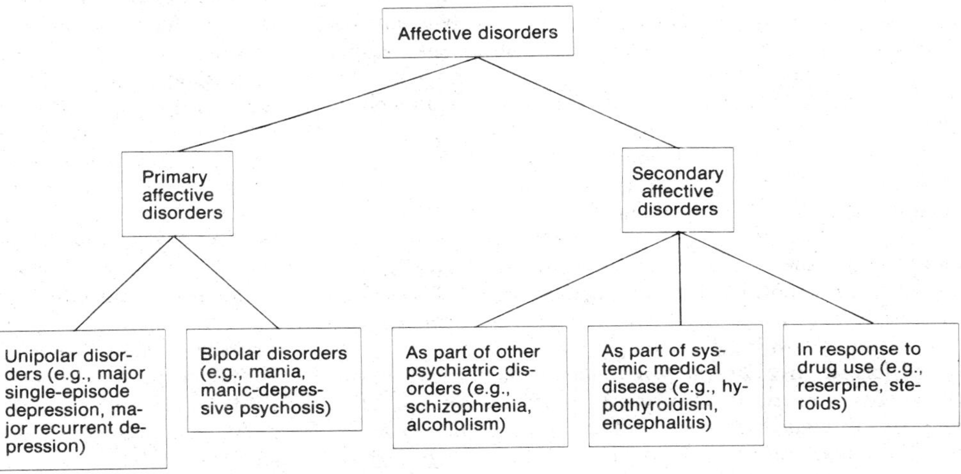

FIGURE 376-1
Suggested nosology of affective disorders. (Adapted from GL Klerman, in Comprehensive Textbook of Psychiatry/III, HI Kaplan et al.)

least 1 week. During most of the episode at least three of the following symptoms must persist in significant degree (four symptoms if the mood is only irritable): (1) increased activity (socially, at work, or sexually) or physical restlessness; (2) unusual verbosity or pressure to keep talking; (3) flight of ideas or subjective experience that thoughts are racing; (4) inflated self-esteem (grandiosity, which may be delusional); (5) decreased need for sleep; (6) distractability, i.e., attention is too easily drawn to unimportant or irrelevant external stimuli; and (7) excessive involvement in activities that have a high potential for unrecognized painful consequences, e.g., buying sprees, sexual indiscretions, foolish business investments, and reckless driving.

Hypomania represents a milder degree of a manic episode, but this term has also been used to depict unusually animated or colorful normal behavior. In such form it need not arouse concern unless it is totally out of character for the individual. Hypomania is a personality trait found in many talented people.

COURSE OF ILLNESS AND PROGNOSIS

In general, mood disorders tend to become manifest a bit later in life than do schizophrenia or the neuroses. Depressions most frequently begin in the fourth decade of life. For mania the mean age of onset is in the early thirties. When the first manic episode takes place in an individual over 50, an organic cause should be sought (e.g., alcohol, CNS illness, tumor).

It is well known that most affective disorders are self-limited with good prognoses even in the absence of therapeutic intervention. It is safe to state that, with treatment, 70 to 85 percent of patients with acute affective disorders, both primary and secondary, have marked to complete remission. Before 1950 the approximate duration of acute depressive episodes was 6 to 8 months. With current somatic treatments, including drug therapy, the length of the acute illness has been reduced to a matter of weeks.

About 15 percent of patients with depression become chronically depressed. This tends to occur as the patient advances in age and as social supports decline. There is a high risk for recurrence in major affective disorders, both primary and secondary. Approximately half of these individuals have more than one episode of illness. Manic episodes tend to recur in about 75 percent of the cases. Before the advent of the phenothiazines and electroconvulsive therapy (ECT), episodes of mania used to average 3 months in length; this has been decreased with chemotherapy.

Suicide is the major complication in this disorder. In the course of a life of primary or secondary depression, there is a 15 percent chance of suicide. Suicide is more likely among depressed patients above 40, among males, and among patients who have suicidal thinking. It is a mistake to think that because a person talks about suicide, he or she is unlikely to attempt it.

ETIOLOGY

GENETIC STUDIES Good evidence exists for the presence of a genetic predisposition toward mood disorders. There is an increased frequency of the illness in families of depressed patients compared with the general population. A greater concordance for affective disorders is found in monozygotic twins than in dyzygotic twins. There is a 12 to 25 percent chance that first-degree relatives of those with bipolar affective disorders will be similarly affected. Relatives of patients with affective disorders have more psychiatric abnormalities than are found in the general population. Also, the characteristics of the affective disorder, such as the age of onset, are similar within families. The nature of the genetic link, however, remains unknown. There is a suggestion that bipolar disorders may be transmitted by an X-linked dominant gene associated with Xg^a blood type and color blindness. It is important to bear in mind that 25 percent of monozygotic twins are discordant for affective disorder, so there are clearly nongenetic influences at work here as well.

Recent work suggests that HLA-linked genes on chromosome 6 influence susceptibility to depressive disorders. There is need for replication of this research before firm conclusions can be drawn. Since the immune system is also involved with the HLA site, this linkage, should it prove true, might help to explain the clinically observed relationship between depression and disease onset.

BIOLOGICAL STUDIES The biology of the affective disorders is more richly documented than any other category of mental illness. There have been three major avenues of investigation: (1) neurochemical, (2) neurophysiological, and (3) neuroendocrine.

Neurochemical studies The biogenic amine hypothesis is often cited to explain affective disorders. A study of the depression associated with the use of reserpine in the treatment of the hypertensive patient gave origin to this theory. It was found that reserpine depleted the intraneuronal concentrations of norepinephrine, dopamine, and serotonin. Based on this observation, a theory logically followed that naturally occurring depressions may be associated with a deficiency of these central neurotransmitters, particularly norepinephrine and serotonin. This supposition was bolstered when it was learned that monoamine oxidase inhibitors increase the concentration of these neurotransmitters by interfering with their destruction within the presynaptic neuron; their antidepressant effect was attributed to this action. The biogenic amine hypothesis is supported by the observation that tricyclic antidepressants block the presynaptic uptake of norepinephrine and/or serotonin, thereby reducing depression by increasing the amount of neurotransmitter available. It is worthy of note that all antidepressants, as well as drugs such as reserpine which produce depression as a side effect, influence amine metabolism at the pre- or postsynaptic receptor.

Work with a metabolite of norepinephrine, 3-methoxy-4-hydroxyphenylglycol (MHPG), has helped to identify subtypes of unipolar depression and to aid in the selection of the correct antidepressant medication. For example, unipolar depressions characterized by low urinary levels of MHPG, indicating inadequate norepinephrine metabolism, usually respond to certain noradrenergically active tricyclic antidepressants such as imipramine. Other subgroups of unipolar depression will undoubtedly be identified with clues to aid in the choice of treatment.

Despite the attractiveness of the amine hypothesis, it has flaws. It does not explain why therapeutic results with antidepressants are so inconsistent. Furthermore, repeated efforts in clinical studies to demonstrate a disorder of the neurotransmitter in the body fluids of the depressed patient have failed.

Less work has been done on the neurochemical basis of mania, but it is believed to be due to an excess of norepinephrine, just as depressions are thought to be caused by a dearth of this neurotransmitter.

Neurophysiological studies There are characteristic changes in the sleeping EEG of the depressed patient. These have been used to separate primary from secondary depressions. The rapid eye movement (REM) latency (time between sleep onset and first REM period) is shortened in primary depression.

Similarly, there is increased REM density (ratio of sum of eye movements to the length of REM sleep) in primary depressions. In patients who have a good response to antidepressant treatment, sleep abnormalities may return to normal within a few days.

Neuroendocrine studies Most of the endocrine findings have been made in the study of primary depressions and do not apply to the manic phase of bipolar illness. About half of the patients with primary depression have increased blood levels of cortisol and show further evidence of a disturbance in steroid metabolism; they fail to suppress cortisol levels when given the glucocorticoid dexamethasone. Control subjects given a low dose of dexamethasone (1 mg at bedtime, followed by measurement of plasma cortisol at 8:00 A.M. and 4:00 P.M. the following day), show feedback suppression of pituitary ACTH output which, in turn, produces a decrease in blood cortisol levels. In patients with primary depression, only 50 percent show suppression to a low dose of dexamethasone. Dexamethasone suppression returns to normal when the depression responds to treatment. It also normalizes in bipolar patients during the manic phase. The dexamethasone suppression test is currently under investigation with the hope that it will serve as a diagnostic aid in separating primary from secondary depressions.

STRESSFUL LIFE EVENTS AND LOSS While an obvious relationship should exist between the onset of depression and disappointment, setbacks, or loss, the relationship is not as direct as one might suppose. Only 20 percent of a population exposed to loss becomes clinically depressed. It is therefore thought that some other factor, either genetic, biological, or emotional, must be present to produce depression.

It is, nonetheless, important to investigate the occurrence of recent stress or loss in the depressed patient's life. The term *reactive depression* has been used to describe the secondary affective disorder that comes in the wake of psychological or physical stress. The symptomatology is the same as that described earlier and the clinical picture is in no way different, although such depressions are apt to be hidden by the patient. Reactive (or secondary) depressions that occur in response to serious medical conditions (e.g., cancer, heart disease) represent the most common type of affective disorder found in the practice of medicine and are the depressions most frequently overlooked by the practicing physician. It is important to bear in mind that reactive depression can develop (see "Clinical Picture") in a patient who never complains of being depressed.

CLINICAL MANAGEMENT

SUICIDE PRECAUTIONS Management of the depressed patient should include the option of psychiatric consultation or referral. Suicide terminates at least 25,000 lives each year in this country. This official tally is probably half the actual figure. Primary and secondary depressions are the conditions that take the highest toll. There are few guidelines to identify the potential suicide victim. Most suicides are not impulsive, but planned. Furthermore, the intention of suicide is more often than not communicated by depressed patients to friends or family. With a depressed patient, the physician should always ask about thoughts of suicide. Thinking of suicide is not, in itself, the principal danger. The presence of a plan for suicide is far more grave. Hopelessness seems to be the bridge between depression and suicide. Suicide is three times more common in men than in women and more common among older people, especially those who have lost a mate through death, separation, or divorce. A family history of suicide or a previous attempt at suicide increases the risk for self-destruction. There is no single trait that stands out as highly predictive of suicide. As a consequence, clinical judgment and index of suspicion must serve as guides to the potentially suicidal patient. The only rule of thumb is that all suicidal threats need to be taken seriously and all patients who threaten to kill themselves should be evaluated by a psychiatrist.

TREATMENT OF MANIA Mania is much less often encountered in the practice of medicine than depression, but it requires a swift response by the physician. Hospitalization is usually required to prevent the patient from impulsive and aggressive behavior which might jeopardize a career or result in injury to self or others. Judgment is so poor in this disorder that patients may gamble away fortunes or make reckless promises. Almost invariably the patient will resist hospitalization, so the doctor must be firm and sure in the insistence that in-patient care is required. Medication is necessary to reduce manic behavior. Oral or parenteral haloperidol, 2 to 10 mg, may reduce the patient's exuberance to a more manageable level. Once the problem is brought under control by hospitalization, lithium carbonate can be started.

ANTIDEPRESSANT MEDICATION Once the diagnosis of depression is made according to DSM III criteria, one should consider using an antidepressant (Table 376-1). Tricyclic antidepressants (TCAs) are the most commonly employed antidepressants and generally are the first to be used. The choice of TCA is largely governed in terms of possible sedative or anticholinergic side effects. Amitriptyline (Elavil) and doxepin (Sinequan) are highly sedating and highly anticholinergic. One would tend to use them in depressions in which nervousness, tension, insomnia, and motor restlessness predominate. When the patient's activity is retarded and agitation is not a problem, imipramine or desipramine are the proper choices since neither is sedating. The therapeutic dose for all of the above medications ranges from 75 to 300 mg qd. The initial dose should be 25 mg qd; this can be increased by increments of 25 mg qd to 150 mg, which is the target dose in most cases. When a sedating TCA is given, the entire dose can be taken at bedtime. Otherwise, it is given in divided doses.

Troublesome anticholinergic side effects are tachycardia, blurred vision, urinary retention, constipation, and dry mouth. Postural hypotension may also occur. Desipramine is low in anticholinergic properties and should be used for patients with medical conditions intolerant of such side effects (e.g., benign prostatic hypertrophy, glaucoma, or congestive heart failure). Because a number of the TCAs prolong cardiac conduction, caution must be used in prescribing these for patients with arrhythmias.

There are important drug interactions to be remembered. When TCAs are used in conjunction with alcohol, the antidepressant effect is decreased and sedation is marked. When used with guanethidine, the latter's antihypertensive effect is reduced. Epinephrine administration in patients receiving a TCA can result in a hypertensive crisis, because of inhibition of catecholamine uptake.

TCAs are metabolized slowly and tend to have a long mean plasma half-life. They do not begin to produce symptomatic improvement until about 3 weeks have passed. Insomnia, anorexia, and low libido begin to improve first; but the patient does not usually achieve a sense of well-being and psychological normalcy before 4 weeks have passed. Once most symptoms of depression have disappeared, the dose can be reduced by half and continued for 6 months to a year. There is some evidence that longer periods of pharmacotherapy produce longer remissions once the medication is stopped.

If one TCA fails to produce improvement, another TCA can be tried. If TCAs fail, one can then use a monoamine oxidase (MAO) inhibitor. When changing from a TCA to a MAO inhibitor, a drug-free period of 1 week should be observed in order to remove the risk of a hypertensive crisis. There has been a general reluctance to use MAO inhibitors because of the danger of inducing a hypertensive crisis if foods containing tyramine are consumed. Tyramine stimulates the release of noradrenalin, which, in turn, cannot be metabolized because the MAO enzymes are inhibited. This brings about hypertensive crisis. Because of this, patients taking an MAO inhibitor should be carefully instructed to avoid foods with a high tyramine content, such as sardines, chicken liver, fermented cheese, red wine, and beer. There are a number of other cautions regarding drugs to be avoided because of deleterious MAO inhibitor interactions. Meperidine, ganglionic blockers, and sympathomimetic amines are examples of agents the MAO inhibitor patient should avoid. The student is advised to consult a psychopharmacological text for full disclosure. The MAO inhibitors have two great advantages over the TCAs: (1) they have few anticholinergic side effects, and (2) they do not sedate. Phenelzine and tranylcypromine are two commonly used MAO inhibitors. The former is given in a dose of 15 mg tid; the latter 20 mg bid. The symptomatic response is the same as for the TCAs. Three to six weeks are required for symptom relief. Once relief is obtained, the maintenance dose should be reduced to one-half or two-thirds of the induction dose. Treatment is continued for 6 months to a year and then gradually reduced to 0 level if the patient remains asymptomatic. Patients who fail to respond to either agent should be referred to a psychiatrist.

ELECTROCONVULSIVE THERAPY Electroconvulsive therapy (ECT) is thought by many to be the most effective treatment for depression, especially for unipolar depression. Temporary memory impairment is the major drawback. Use of unilateral ECT produces less memory disturbance than does bilateral. Patients with drug-resistant depressions, or those acutely suicidal, are usually considered for ECT.

LITHIUM SALTS Lithium salts have been used since 1949. Lithium is the drug of choice in the treatment of hypomania and acute mania as well as in the control of recurrent mania, bipolar illness, and, in some instances, unipolar depression. It is usually administered in 300-mg tablets or capsules in the form of lithium carbonate. Generally, a dose of 600 to 1200 mg per day produces an acceptable blood level of 1.0 to 1.5 meq per liter. Because it takes 1 to 2 weeks to act effectively against mania, the patient should be hospitalized and sedated with an antipsychotic drug until the lithium has taken effect. Since lithium is not specifically an antidepressant, the depression should be controlled by an antidepressant or by ECT before lithium treatment is initiated. When using lithium, it is most important to monitor the blood concentration closely. Once the necessary dose of lithium carbonate has been attained to control mania, the dose can be reduced to maintain a plasma level of 0.6 to 1.0 meq per liter. The dose necessary for proper maintenance varies considerably and must be determined on an individual basis by following blood levels.

TABLE 376-1
Clinical characteristics of some common antidepressants

Drug	*Chemical structure*	*Clinical indications*	*Advantages over other antidepressants*	*Anticholinergic effects*	*Other toxicity*	*Usual daily dosage ranges—adults**	*Therapeutic blood levels (including all active metabolites)†*
Amitriptyline (Elavil, others)	Tricyclic	Major depressions; depression with agitation	Slightly better results than Imipramine	+++	Cardiotoxicity	150–300 mg/day	50–150 ng/ml‡
Imipramine (Tofranil, others)	Tricyclic	Major depression; retarded depression	Less sedation	++	Cardiotoxicity	150–300 mg/day	225–240 ng/ml
Amoxepine (Asendin)	Tricyclic	Major depression; retarded depression	More rapid onset of action is claimed	++	Cardiotoxicity	200–400 mg/day	300–800 ng/ml
Maprotiline (Ludiomil)	Tetracyclic	Major depression; dysthymic disorder; anxious depression	Less cardiotoxicity, more rapid onset of action claimed	+	Reduced cardiotoxicity	150–225 mg/day	200–600 ng/ml
Phenelzine (Nardil)	Hydrazine derivative	Mild/moderate anxious depression	Effective in some patients who do not respond to tricyclics	—	Risk of hypertensive crises	30–60 mg/day	Platelet MAO inhibition 80%
Carbamazepine (Tegretol)	Similar to tricyclic	Bipolar major depression unresponsive to tricyclic	May block switch from depression to mania	—	Early history of aplastic anemia complications; requires hematologic monitoring	600–1200 mg/day	6–8 μg/ml
Lithium	Monovalent cation	Prophylaxis of bipolar depression	Prevents major mood swings in either direction	—	Possible renal toxicity	900–1500 mg/day	0.6–1.5 meq/liter

* *Children, elderly patients, and patients with focal or generalized CNS pathology will ordinarily have lower tolerance and require reduced dosages.*
† *Levels vary from laboratory to laboratory; the values given are only approximate.*
‡ *Level of the metabolite nortriptyline.*

Although most patients experience no side effects, nausea and diarrhea are the most common. A fine resting hand tremor frequently makes its appearance but is unimportant unless it leads to difficulty writing; at this point one can predict impending intoxication. The central nervous system signs of lithium intoxication are weakness, slurred speech, ataxia, increasing tremor, and drowsiness. These reactions can be expected when the blood levels reach 2 to 4 meq per liter.

Other toxic side effects are nephrogenic diabetes insipidus, which is thought to be due to an interference with the activity of antidiuretic hormone on the renal tubules; a possible interstitial nephritic reaction, the pathophysiology of which is still debated; a diffuse, benign, nontoxic goiter, which not infrequently develops following long use of lithium salts (generally the patient remains euthyroid and the condition is not serious.). It is well to record serum creatinine levels on a monthly basis during the first year of treatment.

Few patients complain of mental side effects from the use of lithium, although some hypomanic patients yearn for a return of their hypomanic energy. This type of individual is often noncompliant.

Lithium continues to be used for a variety of conditions with varying success. It has altered the lives and improved the prospect of many patients with bipolar depression whose futures were bleak and whose activity was severely limited by the inroads of their disease. Lithium as a prophylactic agent is indisputably effective in reducing the severity, duration, and frequency of mood swings in bipolar affective disorders.

PSYCHOTHERAPY The value of psychotherapy in the treatment of major affective disease remains to be demonstrated. It is clear that a supportive relationship is helpful in carrying the patient over the course of illness, but the theory that insight has specific curative value remains unproven. The use of a psychotherapeutic relationship together with chemotherapy seems by far the most valuable application of good medical care.

HOSPITALIZATION Manic patients, suicidal patients, and patients whose depression may have a correctable organic cause frequently require hospitalization. With the advent of somatic therapies, the need for hospitalization has been dramatically reduced over the last decade. The average hospital stay is now generally less than a month.

REFERENCES

American Psychiatric Association: *Diagnostic and Statistical Manual of Mental Disorders,* 3d ed, 1980

Cassem NH: Psychiatry, in *Scientific American Medicine,* E Rubenstein, DD Federman (eds). New York, Scientific American, sec 13, 1978

Hackett TP, Cassem NH (eds): *Massachusetts General Hospital Handbook of General Hospital Psychiatry.* St. Louis, Mosby, 1978, chaps 10, 11, 13, 26

Kaplan HI et al (eds): *Comprehensive Textbook of Psychiatry/III,* 3d ed. Baltimore, Williams & Wilkins, 1980, vol 2, pp 1305–1358

Klerman GL: Affective disorders, in *The Harvard Guide to Modern Psychiatry,* AM Nicholi (ed). Cambridge, Belknap, 1978, pp 253–282

Schildkraut JJ: The biochemistry of affective disorders: A brief summary, in *The Harvard Guide to Modern Psychiatry,* AM Nicholi (ed). Cambridge, Belknap, 1978, pp 81–92

Woods BT: Medical and neurological aspects of depression, in *Update III: Harrison's Principles of Internal Medicine,* KJ Isselbacher et al (eds). New York, McGraw-Hill, 1982, pp 167–184

377 SCHIZOPHRENIA

THOMAS P. HACKETT
ELEANOR M. HACKETT

Insanity was mentioned in writing as early as 1400 B.C., and since then references to mental illness have been commonplace in the chronicles of medicine. Emil Kraepelin was among the first to focus on separating insanity into *manic-depressive psychosis* and *dementia praecox,* the former a disorder of mood and the latter a disorder of thought. The term *schizophrenia* replaced the term *dementia praecox* early in this century. There are as yet no basic objective criteria for confirming the diagnosis, no laboratory tests, no single known cause, no consistent premorbid history, and no definite outcome for this disease. However, all experienced clinicians are agreed that a disease exists. They agree that schizophrenia is a thought disorder existing in a relatively clear sensorium and characterized chiefly by lack of logic, confused associations, detachment from reality, auditory hallucinations, and delusions, often of a persecutory nature. Characteristically in the company of this disordered thinking is found diminished or inappropriate affect. Schizophrenia is always accompanied by deterioration in the everyday activities of work, personal hygiene, and interpersonal affairs. According to present convention this diagnosis is not made in the presence of determined organic mental disorder or mental retardation. There is some debate as to whether the diagnosis should be made before the passage of 6 months of illness. If the disease lasts for less than 6 months, it is referred to as *acute schizophrenia* or *schizophreniform disorder* (see below).

EPIDEMIOLOGY Schizophrenia afflicts 1 percent of the population in cultures around the world. Its incidence has remained remarkably constant in our country during the past century, despite extraordinary changes in life-style, social mobility, scientific advancement, and medical achievement. In this country alone it is estimated that the cost of this disease in treatment and lost wages is at least $20 billion each year. One of every two mental health beds in the United States is now occupied by a schizophrenic. The world's schizophrenic population is estimated at more than 10 million.

Schizophrenia is a disease of youth and occurs most frequently between the ages of 15 and 45. The incidence is about equal for males and females. In this country it affects nonwhites in greater numbers than whites and large-city dwellers more often than rural people. Geographic mobility seems to correlate with an increased incidence.

CLINICAL PICTURE Schizophrenia means "splitting." In his choice of this term Eugen Bleuler did not mean splitting into multiple personalities, but rather splitting from reality. Thoughts and associations become fragmented. Affect becomes inappropriate.

Most perceptual peculiarities in schizophrenia are found at one time or another in normal people. Fantasies, daydreams, sleeping dreams, and nightmares all present a phantasmagoria of perceptions which the normal individual is able to separate into real and unreal. The schizophrenic is unable to make this distinction.

Traditionally schizophrenia was divided into four subtypes: catatonic, hebephrenic, paranoid, and simple. The boundaries of these four subtypes have become less clear with increased study and with the development of antipsychotic medication, which has alleviated many of the more florid symptoms of this disease. Since the terms are still in use, however, it is important to become familiar with their meanings.

Catatonia is characterized by stupor, posturing, mutism, negativism, rigidity, or excitement. Whether in the stuporous or excited phase, care must be taken to see that the patients do not injure themselves or others.

Hebephrenia is characterized by disturbances in affect and a marked regression to disorganized behavior. In this primitive form of schizophrenia, inappropriate giggling, posturing, and gesturing abound. Laughter and grimacing occur for no apparent reason.

Paranoid schizophrenia is characterized by delusions of persecution and/or grandeur. This form of schizophrenia tends to occur in individuals who show less deterioration and less regression than in the catatonic and hebephrenic subtypes. Hallucinations, if present, are persecutory. It usually occurs later than the other schizophrenic forms, sometimes beginning in mid-life. The individual may successfully cover symptoms.

Simple schizophrenia is characterized by social inadequacy and withdrawal and is generally not hallucinatory or delusional. These individuals experience an insidious loss of interest, drive, ambition, and initiative. Shallow in response, the simple schizophrenic is often a tramp, a drifter, an itinerant laborer.

It has been found that patients can experience different forms of schizophrenia at different times in their lives; therefore these categories are not mutually exclusive.

According to current convention, what has been known as *acute schizophrenia* has been renamed *schizophreniform disorder.* This differs from the more chronic schizophrenia as described above in that its duration is less than 6 months. Otherwise the clinical picture is identical. For these specific cases, onset and recovery are more swift, recurrence is uncommon, and a family history of schizophrenia is no more frequently found than occurs in a normal population. It does seem to be a separate entity from an epidemiological and etiological point of view.

Since the advent of neuroleptic drugs, schizophrenia in many cases does not progress to its final flowering as described in the categories above. It is important therefore to consider the full range of perceptual, cognitive, verbal, behavioral, affective, and somatic symptoms which can afflict the schizophrenic in varying combinations.

Perceptual disorders Perceptual symptoms include feelings of depersonalization, derealization, and déjà vu. Hallucinations are common, especially auditory hallucinations. Sometimes voices will seem to talk about, talk to, or threaten the patient. Thought broadcasting is another perceptual aberration. Patients think they hear their own thoughts aloud. Visual hallucinations are less common and often occur in combination with tactile, proprioceptive, or auditory hallucinations. Schizophrenic hallucinations of all kinds occur by day as well as by night in contrast to hallucinatory experiences in conjunction with organic conditions, which occur mainly in the evening and at night.

The schizophrenic patient seems more sensitive to sensory stimuli than the ordinary person. Some observers think that this hypersensitivity is genetic. Some believe that these individuals actually perceive more visual stimuli in a given period of time than do normal people. Therefore withdrawal may be a defensive maneuver to escape excessive stimulation. The major function of the neuroleptics in the treatment of schizophrenia may well be to facilitate inhibitory processes.

Cognitive disorders A hallmark of schizophrenia is disordered thinking within the context of an unclouded sensorium. Foremost among the cognitive signs of schizophrenia are delusions, i.e., false ideas that cannot be corrected by reasoning or even by the evidence presented by the patient's own senses. Delusions symptomatic of schizophrenia and helpful for diagnosis are thought insertion (the delusion that thoughts of others are being inserted into the patient's mind), thought broadcasting (the delusion that the patient's thoughts are being broadcast aloud for others to hear), thought withdrawal (the delusion that thoughts are being pulled out of the patient's head), and delusions of control by others. Most frequently schizophrenic delusions are of persecution, but sometimes there are delusions of grandeur as well. The patient may feel controlled by alien powers or followed by enemies. There is a tendency for some schizophrenics to incorporate science fiction and scientific terms into delusional content.

"Concrete thinking" is another form of schizophrenic thought disorder. The ability to abstract or to make valid generalizations is lost. When asked to describe similarities between a leaf, a flower petal, and a palm frond, the schizophrenic often fails to find the similarities or comes up with an idiosyncratic response. When asked the meaning of "rolling stones gather no moss," the schizophrenic is apt to reply "stones that move don't get green."

Psychoanalytic theory describes a "loss of ego boundaries" for the schizophrenic patient, who finds it difficult to see self as separate from others. Identity may be sensed as fused with objects or with other people. This lack of sense of self sets the stage for the schizophrenic delusion that the minds of others can be read or that others can control the mind or behavior of the schizophrenic.

Disorders of verbal behavior Schizophrenic verbal disorders take several forms: excessive concreteness, symbolism (the use of symbols in idiosyncratic ways that make speech difficult to understand), incoherence, the making of neologisms (new words), mutism, echolalia (repetition of the words of others), and verbigeration (excessive and often senseless speech).

Behavioral disorders Behavioral disorders include stereotyped behavior and mannerisms (e.g., lacing and unlacing shoes repetitively), echopraxia (i.e., repeating the motions of others), automatic obedience, negativism, deteriorated appearance and manners, stupor, waxy flexibility (i.e., limbs stay in whatever position they are placed, even when uncomfortable or awkward), lack of enthusiasm, withdrawal, suicide, and homicide.

Dysfunctions of affect Affective disturbances include reduced emotional responses, anhedonia (i.e., emotional emptiness, hopelessness, lack of ability to experience or even imagine pleasant emotion), inappropriate responses (e.g., smiling when hearing of the death of a pet), generally abnormal emotions (e.g., feeling of exhaltation, feelings of oceanic oneness with the universe, religious ecstasies), and lack of empathy and sympathy (resulting from social withdrawal).

Somatic disorders Oddly enough, schizophrenic patients seem less apt to suffer from somatic disease than other people. They also suffer less frequently from allergies. They do often, however, present with hypochondriacal complaints. A common disorder among hospitalized schizophrenics is chronic constipation, which sometimes develops into megacolon.

COURSE OF ILLNESS AND PROGNOSIS The clinical onset of schizophrenia is generally preceded by certain peculiarities of behavior such as shyness, reclusiveness, and social withdrawal. These concern the patient's family for years before the disease becomes evident. By the mid-twenties, delusions, hallucinations, and other signs of marked psychopathology make their appearance and lead to hospitalization. Starting college, marriage, divorce, or loss of a parent are often coincident with onset. Before the use of antipsychotic agents, the schizophrenic's life was largely spent in and out of hospitals. A combination of pharmacotherapy, the deinstitutionalization movement, and policies of early discharge have substantially reduced the amount of hospitalized time for schizophrenics. Current observation indicates that only 30 percent remain permanently and severely handicapped.

The prognosis for a given episode is difficult to assess. In the case of acute schizophrenia or schizophreniform disorder the prognosis is good by definition. Complete recovery for the chronic schizophrenic, while always possible, is unusual. Far more frequent is a course of acute exacerbations with interims characterized by increasing impairment. There are a few factors said to influence the prognosis for schizophrenics favorably: a negative family history or a family history of affective disorder, an acute onset with a show of affect, the presence of precipitating events, an adequate premorbid social adjustment, and an absence of personality disturbance before the onset of schizophrenia. The outlook is less positive if there is a family history of schizophrenia, an insidious onset without precipitating events, affective blunting, or a poor premorbid personal and social adjustment. There is, however, no single factor that relates specifically to outcome other than duration. If there is no remission in 1 or 2 years, the outcome is gloomy.

ETIOLOGY **Genetic studies** There is no specific genotype for schizophrenia. However, it does occur more frequently in close relatives of schizophrenics (10 to 15 percent) than it does in the general population (1 percent). The number of relatives suffering from schizophrenia affects the likelihood of an individual's developing the disease. Children with two schizophrenic parents have a 40 percent chance of becoming schizophrenic; those with one parent affected have a 12 percent chance.

Studies of monozygotic and dizygotic twins have shown that concordance rates of schizoprenia in monozygotic twins may be two to six times as high as concordance rates for dizygotic twins. Adoption studies provide a method for separating environmental from genetic influences. Normal children adopted by individuals who develop schizophrenia do not show increased rates of schizophrenia. Identical twins raised in separate environments have the same concordance rate for schizophrenia as do those raised together. Children of schizophrenics raised in nonschizophrenic families have a higher incidence of schizophrenia than found in the normal population. Work has also been done with children of monozygotic twins discordant for schizophrenia. It was found that children of the nonpsychotic twin were equally at risk for schizophrenia as the children of the schizophrenic twin. These findings leave little question that genetic factors are important in the transmission of schizophrenia. It is equally important, however, to remember that 50 percent of monozygotic twins studied have been discordant for schizophrenia. There clearly are other factors at work.

Biological studies The dopamine hypothesis currently offers the most popular explanation for a biochemical mechanism in schizophrenia. There is thought to be an overactivity at the dopamine synapses in the limbic forebrain of schizophrenics which results in a functional excess of dopamine. Although no direct evidence of an excess of dopamine exists in schizophrenics, there is much supporting evidence for this assumption. In keeping with this theory is the demonstration by microelectrode recording that antipsychotic drugs such as the phenothiazines act by blockading dopamine receptors. The clinical potency of antipsychotic medications has been correlated with their ability to compete with dopamine at stereospecific dopamine binding sites. Furthermore, there is evidence that the schizophrenic-like psychosis produced by amphetamines is evoked either by a release of dopamine or by a heightened sensitivity in the dopamine receptors in the brain. Recently, postmortem study of schizophrenic brains has found that they contain an unusual number of neuroleptic binding sites when compared with controls. This may, however, be the result of chronic antipsychotic drug consumption. To date there is no evidence of increased turnover of dopamine in schizophrenics, and the specific nature of defect in the dopamine system has not been identified.

Platelet monoamine oxidase (MAO) activity has been reported as abnormal in some schizophrenics. Since MAO is important in the breakdown of dopamine and other catecholamine neurotransmitters, this is not unexpected. Reduced platelet MAO activity is said to occur in long-standing schizophrenia.

Recent work with the computerized tomographic (CT) scan has demonstrated increased cerebral ventricular size in some chronic schizophrenic patients. This finding correlates with poor response to antipsychotic drugs as well as to poor performance on neuropsychological tests.

Psychological and social theories During this century several theories have emerged which have helped in the understanding of the clinical features of schizophrenia but which have been less definitive in etiological terms. Adolf Meyer postulated that schizophrenia was a reaction to life stress. Harry Stack Sullivan and his followers have emphasized the importance of interpersonal relationships. Sullivan felt that the schizophrenic had been deprived from early in development of the chance to learn important interpersonal skills. Possessive, hostile, and ambivalent mothers and inadequate, absent, or assaultive fathers have been implicated by some as schizophrenogenic. Being trapped in the "double bind" (i.e., receiving conflicting signals, usually from parents) has also been singled out as an especially detrimental interpersonal problem for schizophrenics. Examples of such a double bind would be (1) being asked to express an opinion and then being condemned for holding such an opinion, and (2) being encouraged to go out and buy new clothes and then being criticized for the purchases brought home.

It seems clear, however, that no single psychological or social cause can be guaranteed to cause schizophrenia, just as no single biological mechanism can be causally implicated. The etiology of this disease is most likely polygenous.

CLINICAL MANAGEMENT While there is no specific cure for schizophrenia, there are several therapeutic approaches which consist of various combinations of hospitalization, psychotherapy, pharmacotherapy, and electroconvulsive therapy.

Hospitalization Until the advent of antipsychotic medication, the schizophrenic was almost invariably hospitalized. More than half of hospitalized patients remained as inpatients for an average of 3 years. Today that situation has changed dramatically. Most acute patients are now hospitalized for a period of only 7 to 21 days. Chemotherapy, in combination with a sturdy program of aftercare in an outpatient setting, has made this policy of early discharge a reasonable and effective plan in many cases. While hospitalization (short or long) is still the rule for patients with acute schizophrenia or acute exacerbations of a chronic process, there has been much interest in attempting to control these acute symptoms with rapid tranquilization in an outpatient setting.

Psychotherapy It is generally agreed that insight-oriented psychotherapy is ineffective in schizophrenia. However, supportive and goal-directed psychotherapy which focuses on giving specific advice about everyday matters such as job seeking, interpersonal relations, and altering behavior has been most helpful. A combination of drug therapy and task-oriented psychotherapy is thought to be the best treatment approach.

Drug therapy The usefulness of antipsychotic drug therapy in the prevention of relapse in schizophrenia has been amply proved. There are three common classes of drugs used in the treatment of schizophrenia in this country: the phenothiazines, the thioxanthenes, and the butyrophenones. All classes of antipsychotic medication have demonstrated effectiveness in alleviating the principal symptoms of schizophrenia such as hallucinations, delusions, combativeness, anxiety, hostility, hyperactivity, negativism, insomnia, and poor general self-care.

To manage the patient with acute schizophrenia, 300 to 500 mg daily of chlorpromazine or its equivalent will be required, either orally or parenterally. Some antipsychotics have greater sedating properties than others. Chlorpromazine should be used with patients who are agitated and truculent. Patients who are quietly psychotic can be given oral haloperidol, 6 to 10 mg daily.

The treatment of the schizophrenic, whether psychopharmaceutical or otherwise, is best handled by a psychiatrist. The question of hospitalization is often difficult to decide even for the most experienced clinician, especially if the patient must be committed. While antipsychotic drugs often remedy target symptoms such as belligerence, agitation, insomnia, and anorexia with dramatic speed, overall improvement requires a few weeks of treatment and demands close monitoring. Drug maintenance over a lifetime is often needed in the treatment of chronic schizophrenia.

Side effects can be expected in the course of antipsychotic drug treatment. All effective antipsychotic agents carry some risk of producing extrapyramidal effects. Acute dystonia including oculogyric crisis can occur, although drug-induced parkinsonism is more common. Benztropine, 1 to 2 mg daily, or trihexyphenidyl, 5 to 15 mg daily, usually brings relief when given parenterally and can be given orally with antipsychotic medication to prevent emergence of extrapyramidal symptoms.

Of all the complications of antipsychotic medication, tardive dyskinesia is the most dreaded. It occurs late in the course of treatment usually in older patients and consists of buccolingual facial dyskinesia. More severe cases show choreoathetoid movements of the tongue, mouth, face, and neck. As yet there is no effective treatment for tardive dyskinesia.

Cardiovascular effects tend to be mild, although orthostatic hypotension is commonly found. Agranulocytosis is a rare, but potentially fatal, side effect. It occurs early in treatment, is not dose-related, and is identified by fever and sore throat early in the course of treatment.

It is important to keep in mind that antipsychotic drugs have a wide margin of safety and are, in fact, regarded by some as the safest drugs in clinical medicine. Furthermore, they are neither addicting nor is there any evidence that tolerance to the antipsychotic effect occurs.

Electroconvulsive therapy (ECT) ECT is of questionable value when compared with antipsychotic medication in the treatment of most schizophrenics. It is occasionally used to treat catatonic states, to treat the acutely suicidal schizophrenic patient, or to treat the patient who is intolerant of neuroleptic medication.

REFERENCES

American Psychiatric Association: *Diagnostic and Statistical Manual of Mental Disorders,* 3d ed, 1980

Kaplan HI et al (eds): *Comprehensive Textbook of Psychiatry/III,* 3d ed. Baltimore, Williams & Wilkins, 1980, vol 2, pp 1093–1304

Kety SM: Genetic and biochemical aspects of schizophrenia, in *The Harvard Guide to Modern Psychiatry,* AM Nicholi (ed). Cambridge, Belknap, 1978, pp 93–102

Lazare A (ed): *Outpatient Psychiatry: Diagnosis and Treatment.* Baltimore, Williams & Wilkins, 1979, chaps 19, 20, 21, 29

Manschrek TC: Schizophrenic disorders. *N Engl J Med* 305:1628, 1981

Woodruff RA et al: *Psychiatric Diagnosis.* New York, Oxford, 1974, pp 25–44

APPENDIX

APPENDIX | LABORATORY VALUES OF CLINICAL IMPORTANCE

INTRODUCTORY COMMENTS

Since *Principles of Internal Medicine* is a textbook used internationally, in preparing the Appendix we have taken into account the fact that the system of international units (SI, Système international d'unités) is being adopted by many laboratories. To this end, where possible and appropriate, we have expressed common laboratory values in terms of both traditional units and SI units. *Values in SI units appear in brackets* after values in traditional units. The use of SI units in medicine was endorsed by the Thirtieth World Health Assembly (May 1977) with the purpose of implementing an international language of measurement.[1] The SI *base* units, SI *derived* units, and other units of measurement referred to in this Appendix are listed in the table to the left.

Quantity	*Name of unit*	*Symbol for unit*	*Derivation of units*
SI BASE UNITS			
Length	meter	m	
Mass	kilogram	kg	
Time	second	s	
Thermodynamic temperature	Kelvin	K	
Amount of substance	mole	mol	
SI DERIVED UNITS			
Force	newton	N	$(m \cdot kg)/s^2$
Pressure	pascal	Pa	$N \cdot m^2$
Work, energy	joule	J	$N \cdot m$
Celsius temperature	degree Celsius	°C	K
OTHER UNITS RETAINED FOR USE			
Time	minute	min	
	hour	h	
	day	d	
Volume	liter	L	

RADIATION DERIVED UNITS

Quantity	*Old unit*	*SI unit*	*Name for SI unit (and abbreviation)*	*Conversion*
Activity	Curie (Ci)	Disintegrations per second (dps)	becquerel (Bq)	1 Ci = 3.7 $\times 10^{10}$ Bq; 1 mCi = 37 mBq; 1 μCi = 0.037 MBq or 37 GBq; 1 Bq = 2.703 $\times 10^{-11}$ Ci
Absorbed dose	rad	Joule per kilogram (J/kg)	gray (Gy)	1 Gy = 100 rad; 1 rad = 0.01 Gy; 1 mrad = 10^{-3} cGy
Exposure	roentgen (R)	Coulomb per kilogram (C/kg)	—	1 C/kg = 3876 R; 1 R = 2.58 $\times 10^{-4}$ C/kg; 1 mR = 258 pC/kg
Dose equivalent	rem	Joule per kilogram (J/kg)	sievert (Sv)	1 Sv = 100 rem; 1 rem = 0.01 Sv; 1 mrem = 10 μSv

TABLE A-1
SI prefixes and their symbols

Factor	*Prefix*	*Symbol for prefix*
10^9	giga	G
10^6	mega	M
10^3	kilo	k
10^2	hecto	h
10^1	deka	da
10^{-1}	deci	d
10^{-2}	centi	c
10^{-3}	milli	m
10^{-6}	micro	μ
10^{-9}	nano	n
10^{-12}	pico	p
10^{-15}	femto	f
10^{-18}	alto	a

ASCITIC FLUID

See Table 39-1, page 210.

BODY FLUIDS AND OTHER MASS DATA

Body fluid, total volume: 50 percent (in obese) to 70 percent (lean) of body weight
- Intracellular: 30 to 40 percent of body weight
- Extracellular: 20 to 30 percent of body weight

Blood:
- Total volume:
  - Males: 69 ml per kilogram of body weight
  - Females: 65 ml per kilogram of body weight
- Plasma volume:
  - Males: 39 ml per kilogram of body weight
  - Females: 40 ml per kilogram of body weight
- Red blood cell volume:
  - Males: 30 ml per kilogram of body weight (1.15 to 1.21 liters per square meter of body surface area)
  - Females: 25 ml per kilogram of body weight (0.95 to 1.00 liters per square meter of body surface area)

[1] The SI for the Health Professions, *Geneva, World Health Organization, 1977.*

$$\text{meq/liter} = \frac{\text{mg/dl} \times 10 \times \text{valence}}{\text{atomic weight}}$$

$$\text{mg/dl} = \frac{\text{meq/liter} \times \text{atomic weight}}{10 \times \text{valence}}$$

CEREBROSPINAL FLUID

Cells: < 5 per cubic millimeter, all lymphocytes
Pressure, initial (horizontal position): 7 to 20 cmH_2O [0.7 to 2.0 kPa]
Creatinine: 0.4 to 1.5 mg/dl [35 to 133 μmol per liter]
Glucose:[2] 44 to 100 mg/dl [2.8 to 4.2 mmol per liter] or 50 to 70 percent of plasma level
pH:[2] 7.34 to 7.43
Protein:
  Lumbar: 14 to 45 mg/dl; gamma globulin <12 percent of total protein [0.14 to 0.45 g per liter]
  Cisternal: 10 to 20 mg/dl [0.10 to 0.20 g per liter]
  Ventricular: 1 to 15 mg/dl [0.01 to 0.15 g per liter]
  $Gamma_1$ globulin (IgG): 2.0 to 5.0 mg/dl (lumbar) [0.02 to 0.05 g per liter]

CHEMICAL CONSTITUENTS OF BLOOD[3]

See also "Function Tests," especially "Metabolic and Endocrine."

Acetoacetate, plasma: <0.3 mmol per liter
Albumin, serum: 3.5 to 5.5 g per 100 ml [35 to 55 g per liter]
Aldolase: 0 to 8 units per liter [0 to 130 nmol/s per liter]
α-Amino nitrogen, plasma: 3.0 to 5.5 mg/dl [2.1 to 3.9 mmol per liter]
Aminotransferases, serum:
  Aspartate (AST, SGOT): 10 to 40 Karmen units; 6 to 18/dl units per liter [100 to 300 μmol/s per liter]
  Alanine (ALT, SGPT): 10 to 40 Karmen units; 3 to 26 units per liter [50 to 430 μmol/s per liter]
Ammonia, whole blood, venous: 80 to 110 μg/dl [47 to 65 μmol per liter]
Amylase, serum: 60 to 180 Somogyi units per deciliters; 0.8 to 3.2 units per liter [13 to 53 nmol/s per liter]
Arterial blood gases:
  $[HCO_3^-]$: 21 to 28 meq per liter [21 to 28 mmol per liter]
  P_{CO_2}: 35 to 45 mmHg [4.7 to 6.0 kPa]
  pH: 7.38 to 7.44
  P_{O_2}: 80 to 100 mmHg [11 to 13 kPa]
Ascorbic acid, serum: 0.4 to 1.0 mg/dl [23 to 57 μmol per liter]
  Leukocytes: 25 to 40 mg/dl [1420 to 2270 μmol per liter]
Barbiturates, serum: nondetectable
  Phenobarbital, "potentially fatal" level (Schreiner): approximately 9 mg/dl [390 μmol per liter]
  Most short-acting barbiturates: 3.5 mg/dl [150 μmol per liter]
Base, total, serum: 145 to 155 meq per liter [145 to 155 mmol per liter]
β-Hydroxybutyrate, plasma: <0.5 mmol per liter
Bilirubin, total, serum (Malloy-Evelyn): 0.3 to 1.0 mg/dl [5.1 to 17 μmol per liter]
  Direct, serum: 0.1 to 0.3 mg/dl [1.7 to 5.1 μmol per liter]
  Indirect, serum: 0.2 to 0.7 mg/dl [3.4 to 12 μmol per liter]
Bromides, serum: nondetectable
  Toxic levels: >17 meq per liter; 150 mg/dl [17 mmol per liter]
Bromsulphalein, BSP (5 mg per kilogram of body weight, intravenously): 5 percent or less retention after 45 min
Calcium, ionized: 2.3 to 2.8 meq per liter; 4.5 to 5.6 mg/dl [1.1 to 1.4 mmol per liter]
Calcium, serum: 4.5 to 5.5 meq per liter; 9 to 11 mg/dl [2.2 to 2.7 mmol per liter]
Carbon dioxide–combining power, serum (sea level): 21 to 28 meq per liter; 50 to 65 volume percent [21 to 28 mmol per liter]
Carbon dioxide content, plasma (sea level): 21 to 30 meq per liter; 50 to 70 volume percent [21 to 30 mmol per liter]
Carbon dioxide tension, arterial blood (sea level): 35 to 45 mmHg [4.7 to 6.0 kPa]
Carbon monoxide content, blood: nondetectable symptoms with over 20 percent saturation of hemoglobin
Carcinoembryonic antigen (CEA): 0 to 2.5 ng/ml (in healthy nonsmokers) [0 to 2.5 μg per liter]
Carotenoids, serum: 50 to 300 μg/dl [0.9 to 5.6 μmol per liter]
Ceruloplasmin, serum: 27 to 37 mg/dl [1.8 to 2.5 μmol per liter]
Chlorides, serum (as Cl^-): 98 to 106 meq per liter [98 to 106 mmol per liter]
Cholecalciferol:
  1,25-dihydroxycholecalciferol: 20 to 60 pg/ml [48 to 144 nmol per liter]
  25-hydroxycholecalciferol: 8 to 42 ng/ml [20 to 100 μmol per liter]
  Cholesterol: see Table A-3
Complement, serum:
  Total hemolytic (CH_{50}): 150 to 250 units per milliliter
  C3: 55 to 120 mg/dl [0.55 to 1.20 g per liter]
  C4: 20 to 50 mg/dl [0.20 to 0.50 g per liter]
Copper, serum (mean ± 1 SD): 114 ± 14 μg/dl [17.9 μmol per liter]
Cortisol (competitive protein binding): 5 to 20 μg/dl at 8:00 A.M. [0.14 to 0.55 μmol per liter]
Creatine phosphokinase, serum (total):
  Females: 10 to 70 units per milliliter [0.17 to 1.18 mmol/s per liter]
  Males: 25 to 90 units per milliliter [0.42 to 1.51 mmol/s per liter]
  Isoenzymes, serum: fraction 2 (MB) < 5 percent of total
Creatinine, serum: < 1.5 mg/dl [< 133 μmol per liter]
Digoxin serum:
  Therapeutic level: 1.2 ± 4 ng/ml [1.54 ± 0.5 nmol per liter]

TABLE A-2
Pressures: Intracardiac and intraarterial

Site	*Representative, mmHg*	*Range*
Aorta:		
Systolic	120	100–140 mmHg [13.3–18.7 kPa]
Diastolic	70	60–90 mmHg [8.0–12.0 kPa]
Atrium:		
Left (mean)	8	2–12 mmHg [0.3–1.6 kPa]
Right (mean)	3	0–5 mmHg [0–0.07 kPa]
Pulmonary artery:		
Systolic	25	15–30 mmHg [2.0–4.0 kPa]
Diastolic	10	3–13 mmHg [0.4–1.7 kPa]
Wedge (mean)	9	5–13 mmHg [0.7–1.7 kPa]
Ventricle, left:		
Systolic	120	100–140 mmHg [13.3–18.7 kPa]
Diastolic	8	4–12 mmHg [0.5–1.6 kPa]
Ventricle, right:		
Systolic	25	15–30 mmHg [2.0–4.0 kPa]
Diastolic	3	0–5 mmHg [0–0.7 kPa]
Venous, antecubital	100	5–14 cmH_2O [0.5–1.4 kPa]

SOURCE: *Based on data in Altman, Dittmer (eds), Respiration and Circulation, Bethesda, Federation of American Societies for Experimental Biology, 1971.*

[2] *Since cerebrospinal fluid concentrations are equilibrium values, measurement of blood plasma obtained at the same time is recommended.*
[3] *Values in parentheses are those found in children.*

Toxic level: > 2.4 ng/ml [>3.2 nmol per liter]
Dilantin, plasma:
Therapeutic level: 10 to 20 μg/ml [40 to 79 μmol per liter]
Toxic level: >30 μg/ml [>119 μmol per liter]
Ethanol, blood:
Mild to moderate intoxication: 80 to 200 mg/dl [17 to 43 mmol per liter]
Marked intoxication: 250 to 400 mg/dl [54 to 87 mmol per liter]
Severe intoxication: >400 mg/dl [>87 mmol per liter]
Fatty acids, free (nonesterified), plasma: <0.7 mmol per liter
Ferritin, serum: 15 to 200 ng/ml [15 to 200 μg per liter]
Fibrinogen, plasma: 160 to 415 mg/dl [0.5 to 1.4 μmol per liter]
Fibrinogen split products: titer 1:4 or less
Folic acid, serum: 6 to 15 ng/ml [14 to 34 nmol per liter]
Folic acid, red cell: 150 to 450 ng/per milliliter of cells, [340 to 1020 nmol per liter cells]
γ-Glutamyl transferase (transpeptidase), serum: 4 to 60 units per liter [0.07 to 1.00 μmol/s per liter]
Gastrin, serum: 40 to 200 pg/ml [40 to 150 ng per liter]
Globulins, serum: 2.0 to 3.0 g/dl [20 to 30 g per liter]
Glucose (fasting), plasma:
Normal: 75 to 105 mg/dl [4.2 to 5.8 mmol per liter]
Diabetes mellitus: >140 mg/dl (on more than one occasion) [>7.8 mmol per liter]
Glucose, 2 h postprandial, plasma:
Normal: <140 mg/dl [<7.8 mmol per liter]
Impaired glucose tolerance: 140 to 200 mg/dl [7.8 to 11.1 mmol per liter]
Diabetes mellitus: >200 mg/dl [>11.1 mmol per liter] (on more than one occasion)
Hemoglobin, blood (sea level):
Males: 14 to 18 g/dl [8.7 to 11.2 mmol per liter]
Females: 12 to 16 g/dl [7.4 to 9.9 mmol per liter]
Hemoglobin A_{1c}: up to 6 percent of total hemoglobin
Immunoglobulins, serum:
IgA: 90 to 325 mg/dl [0.9 to 3.2 g per liter]
IgE: <0.025 mg/dl [<0.00025 g per liter]
IgG: 800 to 1500 mg/dl [8.0 to 15 g per liter]
IgM: 45 to 150 mg/dl [0.45 to 1.5 g per liter]
Iron, serum:
Males and females (mean ± 1 SD): 105 ± 35 μg/dl [19 ± 6 μmol per liter]
Iron-binding capacity, serum (mean ± 1 SD): 305 ± 32 μg/dl [55 ± 6 μmol per liter]
Saturation: 20 to 45 percent
Ketones, total: 0.5 to 1.5 mg/dl [5 to 15.0 mg per liter]
Lactate dehydrogenase, serum:
200 to 450 units per milliliter (Wrobleski)
60 to 100 units per milliliter (Wacker)
25 to 100 units per liter [0.4 to 1.7 μmol/s per liter]
Lactic acid, blood: <1.2 mmol per liter
Lead, serum: <20 μg/dl [<1.0 μmol per liter]
Lipase, serum: 1.5 units (Cherry-Crandall)
Lipids: see Table A-3
Lipids, triglyceride, serum: see Table A–3
Lithium, serum:
Therapeutic concentration: 0.6 to 1.2 mmol/L
Toxic concentration: > 2 mmol/L [> 2 mmol per liter]
Magnesium, serum: 1.5 to 2.5 meq per liter; 2 to 3 mg/dl [0.8 to 1.3 mmol per liter]
Nitrogen, nonprotein, serum: 15 to 35 mg/dl [0.15 to 0.35 g per liter]
5′-Nucleotidase, serum: 0.3 to 2.6 Bodansky units per deciliter [27 to 233 nmol/s per liter]
Osmolality, serum: 280 to 300 mosmol per kilogram of serum water
Oxygen content:
Arterial blood (sea level): 17 to 21 volume percent
Venous blood, arm (sea level): 10 to 16 volume percent
Oxygen percent saturation (sea level):
Arterial blood: 97 percent [0.97 mol/mol]
Venous blood, arm: 60 to 85 percent [0.60 to 0.85 mol/mol]
Oxygen tension, blood: 80 to 100 mmHg [11 to 13 kPa]
pH, blood: 7.38 to 7.44
Phosphatase, acid, serum:
Bessey-Lowry method: 0.10 to 0.63 unit [28 to 175 nmol/s per liter]
Bodansky method: 0.5 to 2.0 units
Fishman-Lerner (tartrate sensitive): <0.6 unit per deciliter (up to 0.15 unit per deciliter)
Gutman method: 0.5 to 2.0 units
International units: 0.2 to 1.8 [3 to 30 nmol/s per liter]
King-Armstrong method: 1.0 to 5.0 units
Shinowara method: 0.0 to 1.1 units
Phosphatase, alkaline, serum:
Bessey-Lowry method: 0.8 to 2.3 units (3.4 to 9 units[3])
Bodansky method: 2.0 to 4.5 units (3.0 to 13.0 units[3]) [0.18 to 0.40 nmol/s per liter]
Gutman method: 2.0 to 4.5 units (3.0 to 13.0 units[3])
International units: 21 to 91 per liter at 37°C [0.4 to 1.5 μmol/s per liter]
King-Armstrong method: 4.0 to 13.0 units (10.0 to 20.0 units[3])
Shinowara method: 2.2 to 8.6 units
Phospholipids, serum: 150 to 250 mg/dl (as lecithin) [48 to 81 mmol per liter]
Phosphorus, inorganic, serum: 1 to 1.5 meq per liter; 3 to 4.5 mg/dl [1.0 to 1.4 mmol per liter]
Potassium, serum: 3.5 to 5.0 meq per liter [3.5 to 5.0 mmol per liter]
Proteins, total, serum: 5.5 to 8.0 g/dl [55 to 80 g per liter]
Protein fractions, serum:
Albumin: 3.5 to 5.5 g/dl (50 to 60 percent) [35 to 55 g per liter]
Globulin: 2.0 to 3.5 g/dl (40 to 50 percent) [20 to 35 g per liter]
$alpha_1$: 0.2 to 0.4 g/dl (4.2 to 7.2 percent) [2 to 4 g per liter]
$alpha_2$: 0.5 to 0.9 g/dl (6.8 to 12 percent) [5 to 9 g per liter]
beta: 0.6 to 1.1 g/dl (9.3 to 15 percent) [6 to 11 g per liter]
gamma: 0.7 to 1.7 g/dl (13 to 23 percent) [7 to 17 g per liter]
Pyruvic acid, blood: <0.15 mmol per liter [<150 μmol per liter]
Quinidine, serum:
Therapeutic range: 1.5 to 3 μg/ml [4.6 to 9.2 μmol per liter]
Toxic range: 5 to 6 μg/ml [15.4 to 18.5 μmol per liter]
Salicylate, plasma: 0 mmol per liter
Therapeutic range: 20 to 25 mg/dl [1.4 to 1.8 mmol per liter]
Toxic range: >30 mg/dl [2.2 mmol per liter]
Sodium, serum: 136 to 145 meq per liter [136 to 145 mmol per liter]
Steroids: see "Metabolic and Endocrine" under "Function Tests"
Transaminase, serum glutamic oxaloacetic (SGOT, AST): 10 to 40 Karmen units per milliliter; 6 to 18 units per liter [0.10 to 0.30 μmol/s per liter]
Transaminase, serum glutamic pyruvic (SGPT, ALT): 10 to 40 Karmen units per milliliter; 3 to 26 units per liter [0.05 to 0.43 μmol/s per liter]
Transferase, γ-glutamyl, serum: 4 to 60 units per liter [0.07 to 1.00 μmol/s per liter]
Triglycerides: see Table A-3

Urea nitrogen, whole blood: 10 to 20 mg/dl [3.6 to 7.1 mmol per liter]
Uric acid, serum:
  Males: 2.5 to 8.0 mg/dl [0.15 to 0.48 mmol per liter]
  Females: 1.5 to 6.0 mg/dl [0.09 to 0.36 mmol per liter]
Vitamin A, serum: 20 to 100 μg/dl [0.7 to 3.5 μmol per liter]
Vitamin B_{12}, serum: 200 to 600 pg/ml [148 to 443 pmol per liter]
Zinc, serum (mean ± 1 SD): 120 ± 20 μg/dl [18 ± 3 μmol per liter]

FUNCTION TESTS

Circulation

Arteriovenous oxygen difference: 30 to 50 ml per liter
Cardiac output (Fick): 2.5 to 3.6 liters per square meter of body surface area per minute
Circulation time:
  Arm to lung, ether: 2 to 12 s
  Arm to tongue:
    Calcium gluconate: 12 to 18 s
    Decholin: 10 to 16 s
    Saccharin: 9 to 16 s
Ejection fraction, stroke volume/end-diastolic volume (SV/EDV):
  Normal range: 0.55 to 0.78
  A_1: 0.67
Left ventricular work:
  Stroke work index: 30 to 110 (g·m)/m^2
  Left ventricular minute work index: 1.8 to 6.6 [(kg·m)/m^2]/min
  Oxygen consumption index: 110 to 150 ml per liter
Pressures, intracardiac and intraarterial: see Table A-2
Pulmonary vascular resistance: 20 to 120 (dyn·s)/cm^5 [2 to 12 kPa·s per liter]
Systemic vascular resistance: 770 to 1500 (dyn·s)/cm^5 [77 to 150 kPa·s per liter]
Systolic time intervals: see Table A-4

Gastrointestinal See also "Stool."

Absorption tests:
  D-Xylose absorption test: After an overnight fast, 25 g xylose is given in aqueous solution by mouth. Urine collected for the following 5 h should contain 5 to 8 g [33 to 53 mmol] (or >20 percent of ingested dose). Serum xylose should be 25 to 40 mg per 100 ml 1 h after the oral dose [1.7 to 2.7 mmol per liter].
  Vitamin A absorption test: A fasting blood specimen is obtained and 200,000 units of vitamin A in oil is given by mouth. Serum vitamin A levels should rise to twice fasting level in 3 to 5 h.
Gastric juice:
  Volume:
    24 h: 2 to 3 liters
    Nocturnal: 600 to 700 ml
    Basal, fasting: 30 to 70 ml/h
  Reaction:
    As pH: 1.6 to 1.8
    Titratable acidity of fasting juice: 15 to 35 meq/h [4 to 10 μmol/s]
  Acid output:
    Basal:
      Females (mean ± 1 SD): 2.0 ± 1.8 meq/h [0.6 ± 0.5 μmol/s]
      Males (mean ± 1 SD): 3.0 ± 2.0 meq/h [0.8 ± 0.6 μmol/s]
    Maximal [after subcutaneous histamine acid phosphate 0.004 mg/kg and preceded by 50 mg promethazine (Phenergan); or after betazole (Histalog) 1.7 mg/kg or pentagastrin 6 μg/mg]:
      Females (mean ± 1 SD): 16 ± 5 meq/h [4.4 ± 1.4 μmol/s]
      Males (mean ± 1 SD): 23 ± 5 meq/h [6.4 ± 1.4 μmol/s]
    Basal acid output/maximal acid output ratio: 0.6 or less
Gastrin, serum: 60 to 200 pg/ml [60 to 200 ng per liter]
Secretin test (pancreatic exocrine function): 1 unit per kilogram of body weight, intravenously
  Volume (pancreatic juice): >2.0 ml/kg in 80 min
  Bicarbonate concentration: >80 meq per liter [>80 mmol per liter]
  Bicarbonate output: >10 meq in 30 min [>10 mmol in 30 min]

Metabolic and Endocrine

ACTH, 8 A.M.: < 80 pg/ml [<3.8 pmol per liter]
Adrenal cortex function tests: see Chap. 112
Adrenal medulla function tests: see Chap. 113
Adrenal steroids, plasma:
  Aldosterone, 8 A.M.: 1 to 5 ng/dl [0.03 to 0.15 nmol per liter] (patient supine, 100 meq Na and 60 to 100 meq K intake)
  Cortisol:
    8 A.M.: 9 to 24 μg/dl [248 to 662 nmol per liter]
    4 P.M.: 3 to 12 μg/dl [82 to 331 nmol per liter]
  Dehydroepiandrosterone (DHEA): 0.2 to 0.9 μg/dl [0.7 to 3.1 nmol per liter]
  Dehydroepiandrosterone sulfate (DHEA sulfate): 50 to 250 μg/dl [130–650 nmol per liter]
  11-Deoxycortisol (compound S): < 1 μg/dl [<30 nmol per liter]

TABLE A-3
Plasma lipid concentration in normal subjects*

	Total plasma cholesterol, ng/dl		*Plasma LDL-cholesterol, ng/dl*		*Plasma HDL-cholesterol, ng/dl*		*Plasma triglyceride, ng/dl*	
Age	*Men*	*Women*	*Men*	*Women*	*Men*	*Women*	*Men*	*Women*
19	113–197	120–203	62–130	59–137	30–63	35–74	37–148	39–132
29	133–244	130–229	70–165	71–164	31–63	37–83	46–249	40–172
39	146–270	141–245	81–189	75–172	29–62	34–82	54–321	41–194
49	158–276	152–268	98–202	79–186	30–64	34–87	58–327	47–228
59	156–276	169–294	88–203	89–210	28–71	37–91	58–286	56–257
69	158–274	171–297	98–210	92–221	30–78	35–98	57–267	60–241
70+	151–270	167–288	80–186	96–206	31–75	33–92	58–258	60–235

* *5th and 95th percentiles not ideal ranges for white men and women; data are too fragmentary to ascertain whether these values apply to other groups.*
SOURCE: *The Lipid Research Clinics Population Studies Data Book, Vol 1, The Prevalence Study, NIH Publication No 80–1529, Bethesda, National Institutes of Health, July 1980.*

TABLE A-4
Systolic time intervals in normal individuals (in milliseconds)

Regression equation	*SD of index*
QS_2 (M) = −2.1 HR + 546	14
QS_2 (F) = −2.0 HR + 549	14
PEP (M) = −0.4 HR + 131	13
PEP (F) = −0.4 HR + 133	11
LVET (M) = −1.7 HR + 413	10
LVET (F) = −1.6 HR + 418	10

NOTE: *QS_2 = total electromechanical systole, PEP = preejection phase, LVET = left ventricular ejection time, HR = heart rate, M = male, F = female, SD = standard deviation of the systolic time interval index.*
SOURCE: *AM Weissler, CL Garrard, Mod Concepts Cardiovasc Dis 40:1, 1971.*

17-Hydroxyprogesterone:
  Women: follicular phase, 6 to 110 ng/dl [18 to 330 nmol per liter]; luteal phase, 50 to 350 ng/dl [150 to 1050 nmol per liter]
  Men: 6 to 300 ng/dl [18 to 900 nmol per liter]
Adrenal steroids, secretion rates:
  Aldosterone: 50 to 250 μg per day [138 to 690 nmol per day]
  Cortisol: 5 to 25 mg per day [14 to 69 μmol per day]
Adrenal steroids, urinary excretion:
  Aldosterone: 2 to 10 μg per day [5.6 to 28 nmol per day]
  Cortisol, free: 20 to 100 μg per day [54 to 276 nmol per day]
  17-Hydroxycorticosteroids: 2 to 10 mg per day [5.4 to 27.6 nmol per day]
  17-Ketosteroids:
    Men: 7 to 25 mg per day [24.5 to 87.5 μmol per day]
    Women: 4 to 15 mg per day [14 to 52.5 μmol per day]
Angiotensin II, plasma, 8 A.M.: 10 to 30 pg/ml [10 to 30 nmol per liter]
Antidiuretic hormone, plasma:
  Random fluid intake: 1 to 3 μU/ml [1 to 3 ng per liter]
  Fluid deprivation, 18 to 24 h: 6 to 10 μU/ml [6 to 10 ng per liter]
Calcitonin, plasma: < 50 pg/ml [< 50 pmol per liter]
Catecholamines, urinary excretion:
  Free catecholamines: <100 μg per day [<590 nmol per day]
  Epinephrine: <50 μg per day [<295 nmol per day]
  Metanephrines: <1.3 mg per day [<6.2 μmol per day]
  Vanillylmandelic acid (VMA): <8 mg per day [<40 μmol per day]
Glucagon, plasma: 50 to 200 pg/ml [14 to 56 pmol per liter]
Gonadal function tests: see Chaps. 117 and 118
Gonadal steroids, plasma:
  Estradiol:
    Women: 20 to 60 pg/ml [0.07 to 0.22 nmol per liter], higher at ovulation
    Men: <50 pg/ml [<0.18 nmol per liter]
  Progesterone:
    Men, prepubertal girls, and postmenopausal women: <2 ng/ml [6 nmol per liter]
    Women, luteal: peak >5 ng/ml [>16 nmol per liter]
  Testosterone:
    Women: <100 ng/dl [<3.5 nmol per liter]
    Men: 300 to 1000 ng/dl [105 to 350 nmol per liter]
    Prepubertal boys and girls: 5 to 20 ng/dl [0.175 to 0.702 nmol per liter]
Gonadotropins, plasma:
  Women, mature, premenopausal, except at ovulation:
    FSH: 5 to 30 mU/ml [5 to 30 units per liter]
    LH: 5 to 25 mU/ml [5 to 25 units per liter]
  Ovulatory surge:
    FSH: 5 to 20 mU/ml [5 to 20 units per liter]
    LH: 15 to 40 mU/ml [15 to 40 units per liter]
  Postmenopausal:
    FSH: >40 mU/ml [>40 units per liter]
    LH: >40 mU/ml [>40 units per liter]
  Men, mature:
    FSH: 5 to 20 mU/ml [5 to 20 units per liter]
    LH: 5 to 20 mU/ml [5 to 20 units per liter]
  Children of both sexes, prepubertal:
    FSH: <5 mU/ml [<5 units per liter]
    LH: <5 mU/ml [<5 units per liter]
Growth hormone, after 100 g glucose by mouth: <5 ng/dl [<230 pmol per liter]
Insulin, serum or plasma, fasting: 6 to 26 μU/ml [43 to 186 pmol per liter]
Oxytocin, plasma:
  Men and preovulatory women: 0.5 to 2 μU/ml [0.5 to 2 mU per liter]
  Ovulating women: 2 to 4 μU/ml [2 to 4 mU per liter]
  Lactating women: 5 to 10 μU/ml [5 to 10 mU per liter]
Pancreatic islet function tests: see Chap. 114
Parathyroid function tests: see Chap. 339
Pituitary function tests: see Chaps. 109 and 110
Pregnancy tests: see Chap. 118
Prolactin, serum: 2 to 15 ng/ml [2 to 15 μg per liter]
Renin-angiotensin function tests: see Chap. 112
Thyroid function tests:
  Dynamic tests of thyroid function: see Chap. 111
  Radioactive iodine uptake, 24 h: 5 to 30 percent (range varies in different areas due to variations in iodine intake)
  Resin T_3 uptake: 25 to 35 percent (varies among laboratories; for calculation of indices of resin T_3 uptake, see Chap. 111)

TABLE A-5
Normal values of echocardiographic measurements in adults

	Range, cm	*Mean, cm*	*Number of subjects*
Age (years)	13 to 54	26	134
Body surface area (m^2)	1.45 to 2.22	1.8	130
RVD—flat	0.7 to 2.3	1.5	84
RVD—left lateral	0.9 to 2.6	1.7	83
LVID—flat	3.7 to 5.6	4.7	82
LVID—left lateral	3.5 to 5.7	4.7	81
Posterior LV wall thickness	0.6 to 1.1	0.9	137
Posterior LV wall amplitude	0.9 to 1.4	1.2	48
IVS wall thickness	0.6 to 1.1	0.9	137
Mid IVS amplitude	0.3 to 0.8	0.5	10
Apical IVS amplitude	0.5 to 1.2	0.7	38
Left atrial dimension	1.9 to 4.0	2.9	133
Aortic root dimension	2.0 to 3.7	2.7	121
Aortic cusps' separation	1.5 to 2.6	1.9	93
Percentage of fractional shortening*	34% to 44%	36%	20%
Mean rate of circumferential shortening (Vcf),† or mean normalized shortening velocity	1.02 to 1.94 circ/s	1.3 circ/s	38

* $\frac{\text{LVIDd} - \text{LVIDs}}{\text{LVIDd}}$

† $\frac{\text{LVIDd} - \text{LVIDs}}{\text{LVIDd} \times \text{Ejection time}}$

RVD = Right ventricular dimension
LVID = Left ventricular internal dimension; d = end diastole; s = end systole
LV = Left ventricle
IVS = Interventricular septum
SOURCE: *From H Feigenbaum, Echocardiography, in Heart Disease—A Textbook of Cardiovascular Medicine, E. Braunwald (ed). Philadelphia, Saunders, 1980.*

TABLE A-6
Amplitude of Q, R, S, and T waves in scalar electrocardiogram of 100 normal adults*

	I	*II*	*III*	aV_R	aV_L	aV_F	V_1	V_5	V_6
Patients with Q wave	38%	41%	50%	—	38%	40%	0%	60%	75%
Q amplitude:									
Mean	0.4	0.6	0.9	—	0.4	0.7	0	0.3	0.3
Range	0 to 1.0	0 to 1.6	0 to 2.3	—	0 to 1.1	0 to 1.7	0	0 to 1.8	0 to 1.8
R amplitude:									
Mean	5.6	8.9	4.5	1.3	3.4	6.0	1.9	12.6	10.2
Range	1.0 to 10.0	2.0 to 16.9	1.0 to 12.1	0 to 2.9	0 to 8.2	0 to 13.8	1.0 to 6.0	7.0 to 21.0	5.0 to 18.0
S amplitude:									
Mean	2.0	2.1	2.4	7.0	2.6	—	8.0	2.5	1.3
Range	0 to 5.0	0 to 3.7	0 to 6.4	2.2 to 11.8	0 to 5.8	—	3.0 to 13.0	0 to 5.0	0 to 2.0
T amplitude:									
Mean	1.9	2.3	1.0	—	0.3	1.7	1.0	3.3	1.0
Range	1.0 to 3.0	1.0 to 4.0	−2.0 to 2.0	—	−1.0 to 2.0	0 to 4.0	−2.0 to 2.0	2.0 to 7.0	1.0 to 4.0

* *Values of Q, R, S, and T amplitudes are in millimeters (1 mm = 0.1 mv).*
SOURCE: *From J D Cooksey, et al, Clinical Vectorcardiography and Electrocardiography, 2d ed. Chicago, Year Book Medical Publishers, 1977. Used by permission.*

Reverse triiodothyronine (rT_3), serum: 10 to 40 ng/dl [0.128 to 0.512 nmol per liter]
Thyroxine (T_4), serum radioimmunoassay: 4 to 12 μg/dl [50 to 154 nmol per liter]
Triiodothyronine (T_3), serum by radioimmunoassay: 80 to 100 ng/dl [1.2 to 1.5 nmol per liter]
Thyroid stimulating hormone (TSH): <5 μU/ml [<5 mU per liter]

Pulmonary See Tables A-7 and A-8.
Arterial blood gas measurements in normal subjects (sea level):

TABLE A-7
Summary of values useful in pulmonary physiology

	Symbol	Typical values: Men	Typical values: Women
PULMONARY MECHANICS			
Spirometry—volume-time curves:			
Forced vital capacity	FVC	≥4.0 L	≥3.0 L
Forced expiratory volume in 1 s	FEV_1	>3.0 L	>2.0 L
FEV_1/FVC	FEV_1%	>60%	>70%
Maximal midexpiratory flow	MMF (FEF 25–27)	>2.0 L/s	>1.6 L/s
Maximal expiratory flow rate	MEFR (FEF 200–1200)	>3.5 L/s	>3.0 L/s
Spirometry—flow-volume curves:			
Maximal expiratory flow at 50% of expired vital capacity:	$\dot{V}$max 50 (FEF 50%)	>2.5 L/s	>2.0 L/s
Maximal expiratory flow at 75% of expired vital capacity	$\dot{V}$max 75 (FEF 75%)	>1.5 L/s	>1.0 L/s
Resistance to airflow:			
Pulmonary resistance	RL (R_L)	<3.0 cmH_2O/s/L	
Airway resistance	Raw	<2.5 cmH_2O/s/L	
Specific conductance	SGaw	>0.13 cmH_2O/s	
Pulmonary compliance:			
Static recoil pressure at total lung capacity	Pst TLC	25 ± 5 cmH_2O	
Compliance of lungs (Static)	CL	0.2 L/cmH_2O	
Compliance of lungs and thorax	C(L+T)	0.1 L/cmH_2O	
Dynamic compliance of 20 breaths per minute	C dyn 20	0.25 ± 0.05 L/cmH_2O	
Maximal static respiratory pressures:			
Maximal inspiratory pressure	MIP	>90 cmH_2O	> 50 cmH_2O
Maximal expiratory pressure	MEP	>150 cmH_2O	> 120 cmH_2O
LUNG VOLUMES			
Total lung capacity	TLC	6–7 L	5–6 L
Functional residual capacity	FRC	2–3 L	2–3 L
Residual volume	RV	1–2 L	1–2 L
Inspiratory capacity	IC	2–4 L	2–4 L
Expiratory reserve volume	ERV	1–2 L	1–2 L
Vital capacity	VC	4–5 L	3–4 L
GAS EXCHANGE (SEA LEVEL)			
Arterial O_2 tension	Pa_{O_2}	95 ± 5 mmHg	
Arterial CO_2 tension	Pa_{CO_2}	40 ± 2 mmHg	
Arterial O_2 saturation	Sa_{O_2}	97 ± 2%	
Arterial blood pH	pH	7.40 ± 0.02	
Arterial bicarbonate	HCO_3^-	24 + 2 meq/L	
Base excess	BE	0 ± 2 meq/L	
Diffusing capacity for carbon monoxide (single breath)	DL_{CO}	25 ml CO/min/mmHg	
Dead space volume	V_D	50 ± 25 ml	
Physiologic dead space: dead space–tidal volume ratio (rest)	V_D/V_T	≤35% V_T	
(exercise)		≤20% V_T	
Alveolar-arterial difference for O_2	A-a D_{O_2}	≤20 mmHg	

P_{CO_2}, seated (mean ± 1 SD): 38.0 ± 2.9 mmHg (no change with age) [5.0 kPa]

P_{O_2}:

Seated (mean ± 1 SD): (104.2 ± 0.27 mmHg) × age in years [13.8 kPa]

Supine (mean ± 1 SD): (103.5 ± 0.42 mmHg) × age in years [13.8 kPa]

Renal

Clearances (corrected to 1.72 m^2 body surface area):

Measures of glomerular filtration rate:

Inulin clearance (Cl):

Males (mean ± 1 SD): 124 ± 25.8 ml/min [2.1 ± 0.4 ml/s]

Females (mean ± 1 SD): 119 ± 12.8 ml/min [2.0 ± 0.2 ml/s]

Endogenous creatinine clearance: 91 to 130 ml/min [1.5 to 2.2 ml/s]

Urea: 60 to 100 ml/min [1.0 to 1.7 ml/s]

Measures of effective renal plasma flow and tubular function:

p-Aminohippuric acid clearance (Cl_{PAH}):

Males (mean ± 1 SD): 654 ± 163 ml/min [10.9 ± 2.7 ml/s]

Females (mean ± 1 SD): 594 ± 102 ml/min [9.9 ± 1.7 ml/s]

Concentration and dilution test:

Specific gravity of urine:

After 12 h fluid restriction: 1.025 or more

After 12 h deliberate water intake: 1.003 or less

Phenolsulfonphthalein:

After intravenous injection:

Excretion in urine in 15 min: 25 percent or more

Excretion in urine in 2 h: 55 to 75 percent

Protein excretion, urine: <150 mg in 24 h [<0.15 g per day]

Males: 0 to 60 mg in 24 h [0 to 0.06 g per day]

Females: 0 to 90 mg in 24 h [0 to 0.09 g per day]

Specific gravity, maximal range: 1.002 to 1.028

Tubular reabsorption, phosphorus: 79 to 94 percent of filtered load

HEMATOLOGIC EXAMINATIONS

See also "Chemical Constituents of Blood."

Bone marrow See Table A-9.

Erythrocytes and hemoglobin See also Table A-10.

Carboxyhemoglobin:

Nonsmoker: 0 to 2.3 percent

Smoker: 2.1 to 4.2 percent

Fragility, osmotic:

Slight hemolysis: 0.45 to 0.39 percent

Complete hemolysis: 0.33 to 0.30 percent

Haptoglobin, serum (mean ± 1 SD): 128 ± 25 mg/dl [1.3 ± 0.2 g per liter]

TABLE A-8
Prediction equations for spirometric tests, lung volumes, and gas exchange in adults

Variable	*Sex*	*Age (A)*	*Height (H)*	*Weight (W)*	*Constant (C)*	*Standard deviation (SD)*
PULMONARY MECHANICS						
Spirometry—volume-time curves* (H in inches):						
FVC	M	−0.025	+0.148	—	−4.241	0.74
	F	−0.024	+0.115	—	−2.852	0.52
FEV_1	M	−0.032	+0.092	—	−1.260	0.55
	F	−0.025	+0.089	—	−1.932	0.47
MEFR	M	−0.047	+0.109	—	+2.010	1.66
(FEF 200-1200)	F	−0.036	+0.145	—	−2.532	1.19
MMF	M	−0.045	+0.047	—	+2.513	1.12
(FEF 25-75)	F	−0.030	+0.060	—	+0.551	0.80
Spirometry—flow-volume curves† (H in centimeters):						
Vmax 50	M	−0.015	+0.069	—	−5.400	1.422
(FEF 50%)	F	−0.013	+0.035	—	−0.444	1.22
Vmax 75	M	−0.012	+0.044	—	−4.143	1.026
(FEF 75%)	F	−0.014	—	—	+3.042	0.936
Lung volumes‡ (H in meters; W in kilograms):						
TLC	M	—	+6.92	−0.017	−4.30	0.67
	F	−0.015	+6.71	—	−5.77	0.48
FRC	M	+0.015	+5.30	−0.037	−3.89	0.56
	F	—	+5.13	−0.028	−4.50	0.41
RV	M	+0.022	+1.98	−0.015	−1.54	0.38
	F	+0.007	+2.68	—	−3.42	0.32
VC	M	−0.020	+4.81	—	−2.81	0.50
	F	−0.022	+4.04	—	−2.35	0.40
Gas exchange§ (H in meters; W in kilograms)						
DLCO	M	−0.20	+32.5	—	−17.6	5.1
	F	−0.16	+21.2	—	−2.66	3.6

NOTE: *Answer = (A × age) + (H × height) + (W × weight) + C ± 2 SD. Example: The normal value and lower limit for the FEV_1 are sought in a man, age 40 years, height 183 cm, and weight 91 kg. The following equation gives the normal value:*
FEV_1 = (−0.032 × 40) + (0.092 × 72) + (−1.260) = 4.08 liters
The lower limit of normal:
4.08 − (2 × SD) = 4.08 − (2 × 0.55) = 2.98 liters
Only 2.5% of a normal population will fall below this value (2 SD below the mean).

* *Morris et al, Am Rev Respir Dis 103:57, 1971.*
† *Knudson et al, Am Rev Respir Dis 113:587, 1976.*
‡ *Grimby G, Söderholm B, Acta Med Scand 173:199, 1963.*
§ *Coates, JE, Lung Function and Application in Medicine, Davis, 1965.*

TABLE A-9
Differential nucleated cell counts of bone marrow

	Normal, mean %*	*Range†*	*AGL*	*CGL*	*CLL*	*Multiple myeloma*	*Hemolytic anemia*
Myeloid:	56.7						
Neutrophilic series:	53.6						
Myeloblast	0.9	0.2–1.5	↑↑↑	↑			
Promyelocyte	3.3	2.1–4.1		↑			
Myelocyte	12.7	8.2–15.7		↑			
Metamyelocyte	15.9	9.6–24.6		↑			
Band	12.4	9.5–15.3		↑			
Segmented							
Eosinophilic series	3.1	1.2–5.3		↑			
Basophilic series	<0.1	0–0.2		↑			
Erythroid:	25.6						
Pronormoblasts	0.6	0.2–1.3					↑↑
Basophilic normoblasts	1.4	0.5–2.4					↑↑
Polychromatophilic normoblasts	21.6	17.9–29.2					↑↑
Orthochromatic normoblasts	2.0	0.4–4.6					↑↑
Megakaryocytes	<0.1						
Lymphoreticular:	17.8						
Lymphocytes	16.2	11.1–23.2			↑↑↑		
Plasma cells	1.3	0.4–3.9				↑↑↑	
Reticulum cells	0.3	0–0.9					

* *From MM Wintrobe et al, Clinical Hematology, 8th ed, Philadelphia, Lea & Febiger, 1981.*
†*Range observed in 12 healthy men.*
NOTE: *AGL = acute granulocytic leukemia, CGL = chronic granulocytic leukemia, CLL = chronic lymphocytic leukemia.*

Hemochromogens, plasma: 3 to 5 mg/dl [0.03 to 0.05 g per liter]
Hemoglobin, fetal: <2 percent of total
Hemoglobin, A_2 (HbA_2): 1.5 to 3.5 percent
"Life span":
  Normal survival: 120 days
  Chromium, half-life ($t_{\frac{1}{2}}$): 28 days
Methemoglobin: up to 1.7 percent of total
Plasma iron turnover rate: 20 to 42 mg in 24 h (0.47 mg/kg)
Protoporphyrin, free erythrocyte (EP): 16 to 36 μg/dl red blood cells [0.28 to 0.64 μmol per liter]
Reticulocytes: 0.5 to 2.0 percent of red blood cells
Sedimentation rate:
  Westergren: <15 mm in 1 h
  Wintrobe:
    Males: 0 to 9 mm in 1 h
    Females: 0 to 20 mm in 1 h

Leukocytes See Table A-11.

Platelets and coagulation

Bleeding time:
  Ivy method, 5-mm wound: 1 to 9 min
  Duke method: 1 to 4 min
Clot retraction, qualitative: apparent in 60 min, complete in <24 h, usually <6 h
Coagulation time (Lee-White):
  Majority and range (glass tubes): 9 to 15 min, 2 to 19 min
  Majority and range (siliconized tubes): both 20 to 60 min
Prothrombin time (Quick's one stage): comparable to normal control (with most thromboplastins, 11 to 15 s)
Partial thromboplastin time [PTT (Nye-Brinkhouse method)]: comparable to normal control (with standard technique, 68 to 82 s; activated, 32 to 46 s)
Plasma thrombin time: 13 to 17 s
Platelets (Brecher-Cronkite method): 290,000 (150,000 to 440,000) per cubic millimeter [2.9×10^{11} per liter]
Whole-clot lysis: >24 h

Schilling test

Excretion in urine of orally administered radioactive vitamin B_{12} following "flushing" parenteral injection of vitamin B_{12}: 7 to 40 percent

STOOL

Bulk:
  Wet weight: <197.5 (115 ± 41) g per day
  Dry weight: <66.4 (34 ± 16) g per day
Coproporphyrin: 400 to 1000 μg in 24 h [610 to 1500 nmol per day]

TABLE A-10
Erythrocytes and hemoglobin: Normal values at various ages

Age	*Red blood cell count,* millions/mm³*	*Hemoglobin,* g/dl*	*Vol. packed RBCs,* ml/dl*	*Corpuscular values: MCV, fl*	*MCH, pg*	*MCHC, g/dl*	*MCD, μm*
Days 1–13	5.1 ± 1.0†	19.5 ± 5.0†	54.0 ± 10.0†	106–98	38–33	36–34	8.6
Days 14–60	4.7 ± 0.9	14.0 ± 3.3	42.0 ± 7.0	90	30	33	8.1
3 months to 10 years	4.5 ± 0.7	12.2 ± 2.3	36.0 ± 5.0	80	27	34	7.7
11–15 years	4.8	13.4	39.0	82	28	34	
Adults:							
Females	4.8 ± 0.6	14.0 ± 2.0	42.0 ± 5.0	90 ± 7	29 ± 2	34 ± 2	7.5 ± 0.3
Males	5.4 ± 0.9	16.0 ± 2.0	47.0 ± 5.0	90 ± 7	29 ± 2	34 ± 2	7.5 ± 0.3

* *The range of values represents almost the extremes of observed variations (93 percent or more) at sea level. The blood values of healthy persons should fall well within these mean ± SD figures.*
NOTE: *MCV = mean corpuscular volume, MCH = mean corpuscular hemoglobin, MCHC = mean corpuscular hemoglobin concentration, MCD = mean corpuscular diameter.*
SOURCE: *MM Wintrobe et al, Clinical Hematology, 8th ed, Philadelphia, Lea & Febiger, 1981.*

TABLE A-11
Leukocytes: Normal values

	Percent	Average	Minimum	Maximum
Total number, per mm^3		7,000	4,300	10,000
Neutrophils:				
Juvenile and band	1–21	520	100	2,100
Segmented	25–62	3,000	1,100	6,050
Eosinophils	0.3–5	150	0	700
Basophils	0.6–1.8	30	0	150
Lymphocytes	20–53	2,500	1,500	4,000
Monocytes	2.4–11.8	430	200	950

Fat (on diet containing at least 50 g fat): <7.0 (4.0 ± 1.5) g per day when measured on a 3-day (or longer) collection
  Percent of dry weight: <30.4 (13.3 ± 8.07)
  Coefficient of fat absorption: >93 percent
Fatty acid:
  Free: 1 to 10 percent of dry matter
  Combined as soap: 0.5 to 12 percent of dry matter
Nitrogen: <1.7 (1.4 ± 0.2) g per day
Protein content: minimal
Urobilinogen: 40 to 280 mg in 24 h [67 to 470 μmol per day]
Water: approximately 65 percent

URINE

See also "Metabolic and Endocrine" under "Function Tests."

Acidity, titratable: 20 to 40 meq in 24 h [20 to 40 mmol per day]
α-Amino nitrogen: 0.4 to 1.0 g in 24 h [28 to 71 mmol per day]
Ammonia: 30 to 50 meq in 24 h [30 to 50 mmol per day]
Amylase: 35 to 260 Somogyi units per hour
Amylase/creatinine clearance ratio [(Cl_{am}/Cl_{cr}) × 100]: 1 to 5
Calcium (10 meq or 200 mg calcium diet): <7.5 meq in 24 h; <150 mg in 24 h [<3.8 mmol per day]
Catecholamines: <100 μg in 24 h
Copper: 0 to 25 μg in 24 h [0 to 0.4 μmol per day]
Coproporphyrins (types I and III): 100 to 300 μg in 24 h [150 to 460 nmol per day]
Creatine, as creatinine:
  Adult males: <50 mg in 24 h [<0.38 mmol per day]
  Adult females: <100 mg in 24 h [<0.76 mmol per day]
Creatinine: 1.0 to 1.6 g in 24 h [8.8 to 14 mmol per day]
Glucose, true (oxidase method): 50 to 300 mg in 24 h [0.3 to 1.7 mmol per day]
5-Hydroxyindoleacetic acid (5-HIAA): 2 to 9 mg in 24 h [10 to 47 μmol per day]
Ketones, total (mean ± 1 SD): 50.5 ± 30.7 mg in 24 h
Lactic dehydrogenase: 560 to 2050 units in 8 h urine
Lead: <0.08 μg/ml; <120 μg in 24 h [0.39 μmol per liter]
Protein: <150 mg in 24 h [<0.05 g per day]
Porphobilinogen: none
Potassium: 25 to 100 meq in 24 h (varies with intake) [25 to 100 mmol per day]
Sodium: 100 to 260 meq in 24 h (varies with intake) [100 to 260 mmol per day]
Urobilinogen: 1 to 3.5 mg in 24 h [1.7 to 5.9 μmol per day]
Vanillylmandelic acid (VMA): <8 mg per day [<40 μmol per day]
D-Xylose excretion: 5 to 8 g within 5 h after oral dose of 25 g [33 to 53 mmol in 5 h]

INDEX

(Page numbers in **boldface** indicate major discussions.)